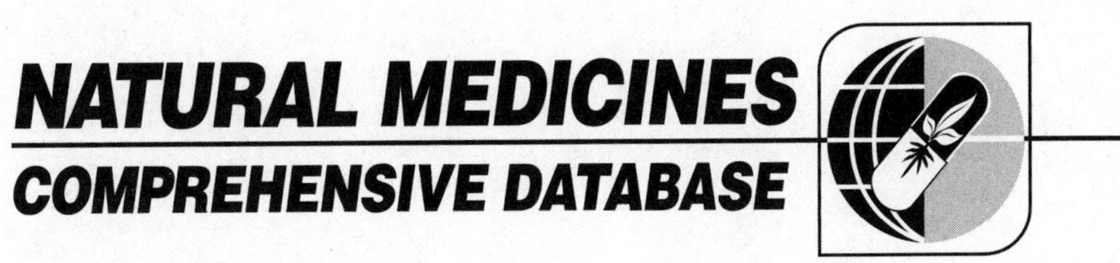

Eighth Edition

Published by Therapeutic Research Faculty

3120 W. March Lane • PO Box 8190 • Stockton CA 95208
phone (209) 472-2244 • fax (209) 472-2249
mail@naturaldatabase.com • www.naturaldatabase.com

Compiled by the Editors of:

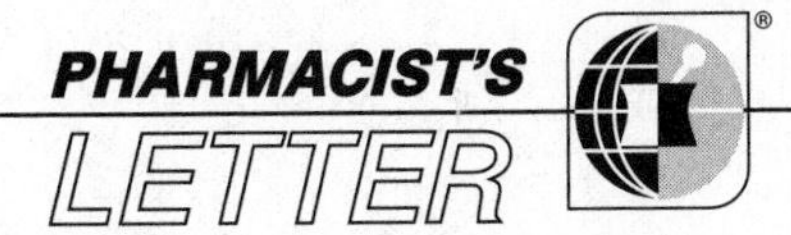

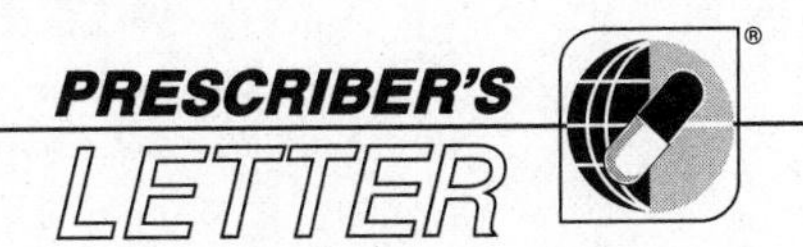

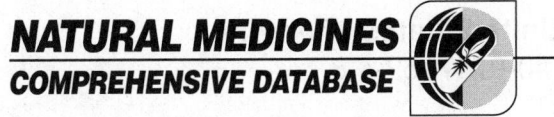

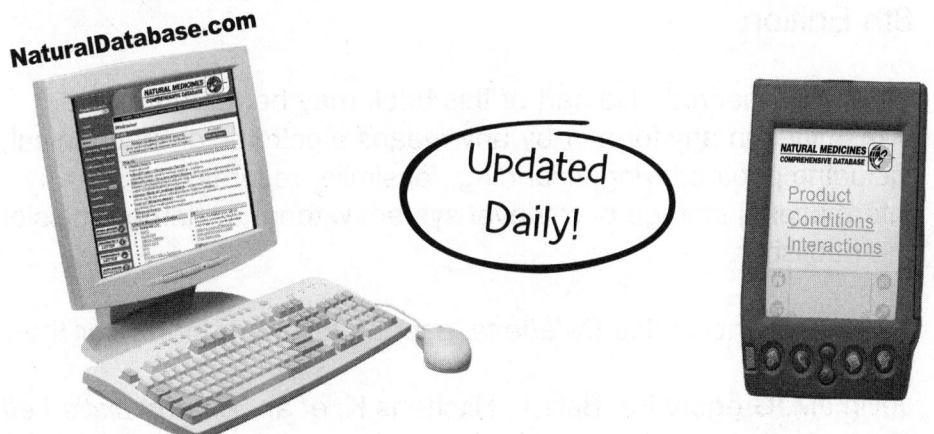

When referencing this *Database*, use the following format for the citation:

Jellin JM, Gregory PJ, Batz F, Hitchens K, et al. *Pharmacist's Letter/ Prescriber's Letter Natural Medicines Comprehensive Database*. 8th ed. Stockton, CA: Therapeutic Research Faculty; 2006:pg xx-xx.

The authors have compiled a comprehensive database of clinically important data on natural medicines. Errors, inaccuracies, or omissions are always possible in a work of this sort. The publisher assumes no responsibility for any patient care based on the application of the data contained in this database. Health professionals who use this database must rely on their own judgment before applying this data to any specific medical situation. People who are not health professionals should seek appropriate professional guidance on the use of any medicinal agent before using it.

For information on obtaining additional copies of this edition, or access to the Web version or the PDA version of *Natural Medicines Comprehensive Database*, or to make use of *Natural Medicines Comprehensive Database CONSUMER Version*, or for a subscription to *Prescriber's Letter* or *Pharmacist's Letter*, see the last pages of this book, or contact:

Therapeutic Research Faculty, 3120 W. March Lane,
PO Box 8190, Stockton, CA 95208
TEL: 209-472-2244 • FAX: 209-472-2249
E-MAIL: mail@NaturalDatabase.com • WEBSITE: www.NaturalDatabase.com

---

Printed in the United States of America
ISBN #0-9747062-4-8

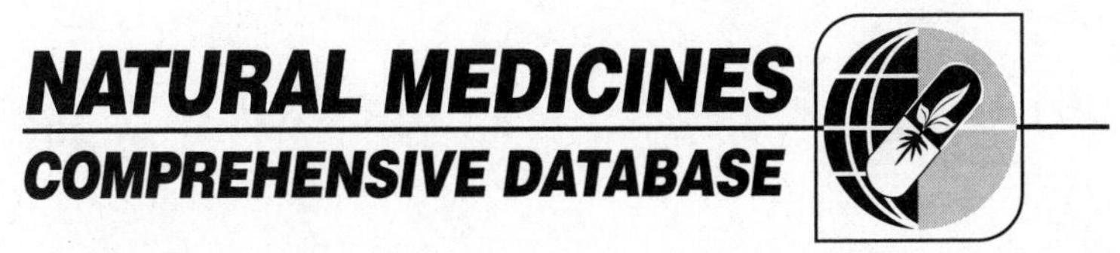

Table of Contents

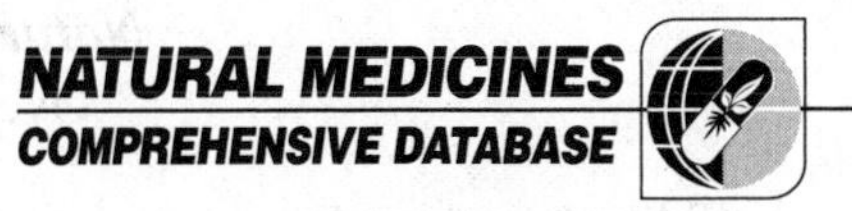

Dear User:

What makes this 8th edition different from other references on this subject?

Natural Medicines Comprehensive Database provides users scientifically reliable evidence-based data presented in an easy-to-use, practical manner. This *Database* neither advocates for or against the use of natural medicines. This *Database* is intended to provide objective, scientific data in a format that facilitates access and use of the data. No other resource makes such a comprehensive collection of data as scientifically reliable and as easy to use.

This *Database* was created by the editors of *Pharmacist's Letter* and *Prescriber's Letter*. These seasoned drug information professionals have been analyzing drug information and publishing drug advisory *Letters* for over 20 years. Hundreds of thousands of pharmacists, physicians, and others subscribe to these *Letters* for trustworthy advice about drug therapy.

The first edition of this *Database* was released in September 1999. Seven new editions have been released in the span of seven years. *Natural Medicines Comprehensive Database* has grown not only in volume, but also in recognition. It is now recognized as the scientific gold standard for evidence-based information on this topic. Leaders in conventional medicine as well as complementary, alternative, and integrative medicine recognize the *Database* as the unbiased, clinically relevant resource. This *Database* is in wide use throughout the English speaking world.

In the most recent year, many new references are cited…new drug interactions have been added…and the safety and effectiveness ratings have been altered for several products based on important new findings. We also continue to add many new brand name products in the brand name listings each day. In some sections readers are referred to the website. This is due to the simple fact that we cannot fit any more pages into this volume.

As good as this book is, it cannot compare to the website version of *Natural Medicines Comprehensive Database* (www.naturaldatabase.com). Thousands of users are transitioning to the Web or PDA versions. By using the *Database* on the Web, users are able to do fast, easy, and highly sophisticated searches, and get information that is updated DAILY by our researchers. Users of the Web-based *Database* also get the complete patient education series providing a Patient Education Handout for each product in the *Database*. There is far more data on the website than can be fit into this printed volume.

The website now also has a *"Natural Product Effectiveness Checker"* to see the effectiveness of each product... *"Natural Product / Drug Interaction Checker"* that checks each ingredient of each natural product... *"Disease/ Medical Conditions Checker"* to find products that might be effective for a condition...*Brand Product Finder*, and more. The entire website has been named one of the 12 most trusted medical websites.

Subscribers to the website also get emailed updates and continuing education that is fully accredited for physicians, pharmacists, nurse practitioners, physician assistants, and dietitians.

This year we released an entirely new PDA version that has many of these same features and is updated daily.

There is now a new consumer website, *Natural Medicines Comprehensive Database - CONSUMER VERSION* that is licensed by health care organizations who wish to provide their members with trustworthy information on natural medicines.

We hope you enjoy this new edition. If you have suggestions, comments, or inquiries, please don't hesitate to contact us: email: mail@NaturalDatabase.com; phone: (209) 472-2244.

Sincerely,

Jeff M. Jellin

Jeff M. Jellin, Pharm.D.
Editor-in-Chief

Natural Medicines Comprehensive Database

Overview of Editorial Principles and Process

Editorial principles

Evidence-Based Foundation:

Natural Medicines Comprehensive Database is built strictly on the evidence. Many aspects of medicine are influenced by tradition and beliefs passed from one person to another. This is especially true in the area of natural medicines. Some natural medicines are used due to traditional or folkloric beliefs, and some are the subject of excessive marketing claims or excessive extrapolations from test tube or animal studies.

Natural Medicines Comprehensive Database is a welcome addition to the world's literature on natural medicines because it curtails perpetuation of myths and age-old beliefs and replaces these with findings from reliable science. *Natural Medicines Comprehensive Database* gives users reliable information that answers their practical questions about the use of any product in this *Database*.

To do this, each product monograph in the *Database* is supported by the best available scientific evidence. This evidence is analyzed and evaluated using the same high standards used to evaluate evidence related to pharmaceuticals. We do not believe that there should be different standards of evidence for pharmaceuticals and natural products. When evidence does not exist or is severely deficient for a particular product (which is often the case), this deficiency is clearly acknowledged with a statement indicating a lack of data.

To gather the scientific data, editors, researchers, and contributors systematically review medical journals from around the world. From these journals, hundreds of articles are reviewed and analyzed. Once filtered and analyzed, the reliable data providing clinically relevant information is then added to product monographs. This does not mean that only flawless studies are analyzed. But it does mean that the data that make it into the *Database* are scientifically reliable. The higher quality research data carry much more weight for addition to the *Database*.

This approach is highlighted by our Effectiveness ratings. Each natural product is assigned an Effectiveness rating based on the quality of the evidence for a given indication. See the table below.

Levels of Evidence for Assessing Effectiveness

Effectiveness Rating	Level of Evidence
Effective	The product has passed a rigorous scientific review equivalent to a review by the FDA, Health Canada, or other governmental authority and has been found to be effective for a specific indication as an OTC drug, orphan drug, or prescription drug product.
Likely Effective	Reputable references generally agree that the product is effective for the given indication, based on two or more randomized, controlled, clinical trials involving several hundred to several thousand patients, giving positive results for clinically relevant end-points and published in established, refereed journals.
Possibly Effective	Reputable references suggest that the product might work for the given indication based on one or more clinical trials giving positive results for clinically relevant end-points.
Possibly Ineffective	Reputable references suggest that the product might not work for the given indication based on one human study giving negative results for clinically relevant end-points.
Likely Ineffective	Reputable references generally agree that the product is not effective for the given indication, based on two or more randomized, controlled, clinical trials giving negative results for clinically relevant end-points and published in established, refereed journals.
Ineffective	Most reputable references agree that the product is not effective for the given indication, or multiple high-quality studies resulted in negative results; there are no equally reliable human studies offering convincing contradictory data.

Because a high level of evidence is required for a product to be rated Likely Effective or above, relatively few products achieve this rating.

Our system for assigning a level of evidence is different from some other systems. Some systems use a scale of letters and numbers (e.g., A-I, A-II, B-I, etc). We've chosen to use terminology that is more colloquial and accessible. It's not always easy to remember what "B-II" means. It's more intuitive to use terms such as "Likely Effective" or "Possibly Effective." The end result is the same. Data are added to the *Database* based on an evidence-based rating scale.

Evidenced-Based:

Natural Medicines Comprehensive Database is more evidence-based than any other major resource on this topic. Evidence-based medicine is a relatively new concept that imposes strict standards on the collection and interpretation of study results. The topic of natural medicines has traditionally not been held to the highest standards of research and interpretation of study results. Many studies and reports on natural medicines do not meet high standards of evidence-based medicine.

Often, clinicians are faced with questions that cannot be answered from an evidenced-based perspective. Some publications simply pass off answers as evidence-based when they are not. *Natural Medicines Comprehensive Database* takes a different approach. We adhere to high standards of evidence-based medicine and when such data do not exist, we give clinicians information that will help as best as is possible. And we clearly indicate by the use of our rating scales, and the text of our entries in the *Database* the strength of the evidence for any particular entry.

We are not hesitant to tell users that the data on a particular topic are not strong enough to give a rating. When we have enough evidence to make a rating we do. When we do not have strong enough evidence, we tell users what we do have. We take into account safety issues as well as factors such as government approvals or recalls. We take seriously our responsibility to give clinicians the most reliable and most helpful information that we have available, and to characterize strong evidence-based data as such.

We realize that there are some publications that are not evidence-based, but proclaim to be. These are often written by proponents of natural medicines. There are also a few publications that are highly evidence-based, like *Natural Medicines Comprehensive Database*, but lack the comprehensiveness of this *Database*. Published reviews of natural medicine resources confirm that *Natural Medicines Comprehensive Database* provides more evidence-based data, and more practical data than other resources.

Unbiased & Reliable Information:

The information contained in the *Database* is unbiased and reliable. It is unbiased because our team of editors, researchers, and contributors evaluate the data for these products without a predetermined notion about the value of the products. Our Effectiveness and Safety ratings are based upon what the evidence says, not based on traditional uses, personal opinions of the editors, or marketing claims. Our team does not have a bias for or against natural products.

The information is reliable because it is drawn from scientific evidence that is analyzed, evaluated, and peer reviewed. Every study is thoroughly evaluated and critiqued to assess its value before adding to the *Database*. Material contained in the *Database* is peer reviewed by physicians, pharmacists, and dietitians. Practitioners who subscribe to the *Database* are also routinely offered the opportunity to comment and critique on information contained in the *Database*. This not only helps ensure that the information is reliable, but also that it is practical and meets the needs of practitioners on the front lines of health care.

Practical & Current Information:

In addition to providing evidence-based information that is unbiased and reliable, a top priority of the *Database* is to provide the most current and practical information. To be practical, the *Database* must be current. To stay current, literature from journals around the world are reviewed on a daily basis. New literature is prioritized based on its potential practical impact. We believe in patient safety first, therefore, safety concerns get top priority. A newly discovered drug-natural product interaction or serious adverse event would be added to the *Database* within

24 hours. New clinical trials that document either positive or negative outcome are also given a high priority and are typically added to the *Database* within one week. Other information regarding mechanisms of action and pharmacologically active constituents are typically added within 1-4 weeks, depending on significance.

In addition to review for quality and reliability, all information added to the *Database* is reviewed for relevance. New data that don't have practical clinical relevance are generally given the lowest priority or are not added to the *Database*.

Editorial Process for Updating *Natural Medicines Comprehensive Database*

Natural Medicines Comprehensive Database is different than many other publications on the subject. It's different because it's updated literally on a daily basis. New information is being researched and added to the *Database* every work day.

For many publications on this topic, the process works as follows: A systematic review of the literature is conducted. Data are gathered and evaluated, and a monograph is written or updated. This process is repeated periodically.

We do it differently. We start similarly for new monographs. We systematically review the literature, analyze the data and write or update a monograph. After that we don't stop. On a daily basis, we continue to look for new data. As new information is discovered, it is critically assessed and if relevant, added to the *Database*. At this time, the new data must be integrated with all the previous findings. In many cases, new data don't agree with old data. In this event, a thorough analysis and review of all data is conducted to assess the reason for different findings and to determine the practical bottom-line for practitioners.

In summary:
We do…

- Use an evidence-based approach
- Systematically review the literature
- Critically assess the literature
- Utilize reliable, relevant data
- Weigh the quality of the data; more weight is given to higher quality data and less weight to lesser quality data
- Peer review
- Focus on practical, clinically relevant data
- Monitor and review new literature on a daily basis
- Update the *Database* daily
- Invite users to communicate with our editors about the content of the *Database*

We do NOT…

- Use traditional or folklore as "evidence"
- Rely on product manufacturer promotional material for our scientific data
- Base ratings on unpublished manufacturer-sponsored studies
- Base our scientific data on non-scientific material from Internet sites
- Have a bias for or against natural products
- Take any advertising or sponsorship...ever.

Natural Medicines Comprehensive Database Team

EDITOR-IN-CHIEF
Jeff M. Jellin, Pharm.D.
Editor, *Pharmacist's Letter* and *Prescriber's Letter*

EDITOR
Philip J. Gregory, Pharm.D.

ASSISTANT EDITOR
Gayle Nicholas Scott, Pharm.D., BCPS, ELS

PROJECT MANAGEMENT
Timothy Swaim, Editorial Project Manager

CONTRIBUTING EDITORS
Forrest Batz, Pharm.D.
Robert Bonakdar, M.D.

RESEARCHERS & WRITERS
Mary Birchfield, Pharm.D.
Judith Marshall, R.Ph.
Jennifer Obenrader, Pharm.D.
Kathy Hitchens, Pharm.D., MSBA
John Benz, R.Ph., MBA, BCPS
Jacintha Cauffield, Pharm.D., BCPS
Camene Wilson, Pharm.D.
Nicole Howard, Pharm.D.
Marie Mulligan, M.D.
Ben Mills, M.D., M.P.H.
James Ables, Pharm.D.
John Cathey, M.S., Pharm.
Gary Holt, R.Ph., Ph.D.
Paul Roberts, R.Ph.
Lynn Limon, Pharm.D.
John Morozumi, Pharm.D.
Loan Cat, Pharm.D.
Gary Choy, Pharm.D.
Tina Madej, R.Ph.
Sandra Downing, Pharm.D.
Lori Kolczak, R.Ph.

EDITORIAL REVIEW
Dan Perri, B.Sc.Pharm., M.D.
University of Toronto, Ontario, Canada
Barbara Miller, Pharm.D.
Kaiser Permanente
Vivian Dickerson, M.D.
Past President, American College of Obstetricians & Gynecologists
Samueli Center for Complementary & Alternative Medicine
University of California, Irvine
Cyndey McQueen, Pharm.D.
Clinical Assistant Professor
University of Missouri, Kansas City
Wadie Najm, M.D.
Samueli Center for Complementary & Alternative Medicine
University of California, Irvine
Shiraz Mishra, M.D., Ph.D.
Samueli Center for Complementary & Alternative Medicine
University of California, Irvine
Kevin Clausen, Pharm.D.
Assistant Professor
Nova Southeastern University
Kelly Shields, Pharm.D.
Assistant Clinical Professor
Ohio Northern University
Stephen McKernan, B.Sc. Pharm., N.D., D.O.
Conroe Family Practice Residency Program, Conroe, Texas
Ben Mills, M.D., M.P.H.
Robin O'Brien, BSc, B.Sc. Pharm, PharmD, BCOP
Drug Information Pharmacist, Vancouver, British Columbia, Canada
Mary Wilson, Ph.D., R.D.
Eastern Kentucky University
Vincent Ferrari, B.Sc. Pharm.
Richard Filice, R.Ph.
John Weeks, M.D.
Private Practice
Joe Pepping, Pharm.D.
Kaiser Permanente

EDITORIAL ADVISORY BOARD
Jim Beattie, MLIS, AHIP
Bio-Medical Library
University of Minnesota
Robert T. Browne, M.D., FAAFP
Narinder Duggal, M.D., B.Sc.Pharm.
Liberty Bay Internal Medicine, Poulsbo, WA
Rex Force, Pharm.D., BCPS
Associate Professor of Pharmacy Practice and Family Medicine
Idaho State University
Harley Goldberg, D.O.
Director of Integrative Medicine, Kaiser Permanente
Mark Graber, M.D.
Research Director, Div of Emergency Medicine
Associate Professor of Clinical Surgery and Family Medicine
University of Iowa Hospitals and Clinics
Charlie Green, R.Ph.
Green Bros Pharmacy
Past President, American Pharmacists Association
Brian Harrington, M.D., MPH, FAAFP
Past Program Director, Darnall Family Medicine Residency Program
Current Teaching Faculty, So. Colorado Family Medicine Residency Program
Assistant Clinical Professor, University of Colorado Health Sciences Center
Mark Hess, M.D., FACP
Wright State University
Terry Ann Jankowski, MLS, AHIP
Information Management Librarian
Health Sciences Libraries, University of Washington
Alan T. Marty, M.D.
Deaconess Hospital Resource Center for Healthy Living
Sarah McCord, MLIS
Health Sciences Library
Washington State University
Adam Perlman, M.D., M.P.H.
The Institute for Complementary & Alternative Medicine
David E. Rosenthal, M.D., FACP
Abington Memorial Hospital
Joseph E. Scherger, M.D., M.P.H.
Clinical Professor
University of California, San Diego
Cynthia Thomson, Ph.D., R.D.
Assistant Professor, Department of Nutritional Sciences
University of Arizona
Raul Zimmerman, M.D.
Family Practice Residency Program
Halifax Medical Center

Natural Medicines Comprehensive Database Team

SPECIAL CONSULTANTS

Karen Davidson, Pharm.D.
Senior Associate Editor,
Pharmacist's Letter and *Prescriber's Letter*

Crystal Amos, B.Sc.Pharm., ACPR
Assistant Editor,
Pharmacist's Letter and *Prescriber's Letter*

Melissa Blair, Pharm.D., BCPS, CDE
Assistant Editor,
Pharmacist's Letter and *Prescriber's Letter*

Kayla Dotson, Pharm.D.
Assistant Editor,
Pharmacist's Letter and *Prescriber's Letter*

Tanveer Khan, Pharm.D.
Assistant Editor,
Pharmacist's Letter and *Prescriber's Letter*

Tony Martin, Pharm.D., MBA
Assistant Editor,
Pharmacist's Letter and *Prescriber's Letter*
Continuing Education Director

Melissa Murfin, PA-C, Pharm.D.
Assistant Editor,
Pharmacist's Letter and *Prescriber's Letter*

Kimberly Palacioz, Pharm.D.
Assistant Editor,
Pharmacist's Letter and *Prescriber's Letter*

Joseph A. Woelfel, Ph.D., FASCP, R.Ph.
Assistant Editor,
Pharmacist's Letter and *Prescriber's Letter*

Neeta O'Mara, Pharm.D., BCPS
Drug Information Consultant,
Pharmacist's Letter and *Prescriber's Letter*

Wan-Chi Tom, Pharm.D.
Drug Information Consultant,
Pharmacist's Letter and *Prescriber's Letter*

Karen Wilson
Editorial Liaison,
Pharmacist's Letter and *Prescriber's Letter*

DATABASE COORDINATORS

Linda Hneitina
Erin Lawler
Julie McCloud

EDITORIAL SUPPORT STAFF

Jocosa Bottemiller
Stephanie Feilzer-Pate
Tyler Nagata
Minda Paglinawan
Ryan Thomas

WEBSITE MANAGEMENT

Mike Acosta
Charles Callistro
Wes Johnson
David Prothero
Jon Rombough
Harold Sohrweide

STAFF

Georgene Albertini
Myleen Arcangel
Rhonda Bigelow
Annie Burt
Janna Foster
Jan Garr
Tillie Giovannetti
Haydee Gobert
Sharon Gunishaw
Danae Harris
Russ Johnson
Jessalyn Ka
Kasey Kaufman
Sheryl Kaufman
Cheryl Laughlin
Keith Marston
Linda McDonald
Rachel McGehee
Ygraine Montgomery
Kristen Moorman
Marji Mullins
Gemma Perez
Gloria Rios
Cessy Rios
Lisa Shawhan
Donna Stewart
Becky Thornburg
Neng Vang
Kathy Webb

How to Get Data From
Natural Medicines Comprehensive Database

Monograph Name
Every one of the 1,000 plus monographs in the *Natural Medicines Comprehensive Database* is given a name based on the most widely used or most recognized name. These appear in ALL CAPS at the top of every monograph.

Also Known As
Many natural medicines go by a variety of names. The most common name is chosen as the name of the monograph. Other colloquial, non-scientific names are included in this section. These names are all indexed at the end of the book for easy reference. This makes finding a natural medicine by any of its names quick and easy.

In many cases, different natural medicines may have similar sounding names. For example, there are numerous varieties of ginseng: Siberian ginseng, American ginseng, Panax ginseng, and others. The *Database* has a separate monograph for each of these. This section will alert you when there are other monographs that have similar names.

Scientific Names
This section contains all botanical, chemical, or other scientific names. Often there is not just one botanical or scientific name for a natural medicine. In these cases, we have provided as many scientific names as are known. We have also included any synonyms. For plants, a family name is also listed.

People Use This For
There are a wide variety of uses for most natural medicines. Not all uses have been validated through scientific study. In this field, ALL known uses are listed without regard for scientific evidence of effectiveness. A use listed in this section does NOT mean the product is effective for that use. Efficacy is discussed in the Effectiveness section (see below).

Safety
For each natural medicine in the *Database* you get an evidence-based safety rating.

These are PRACTICAL ratings that are STANDARDIZED throughout the *Natural Medicines Comprehensive Database*.

You will see that different routes of administration of a product often get different safety ratings. For example, camphor is rated "LIKELY SAFE" when used topically, but it is rated "UNSAFE" when used orally.

Questions often come up about using products during pregnancy or lactation, or in children. If there are safety considerations that apply specifically to children, a special mention in the safety field will address the concern. Every listing includes a rating for safety in PREGNANCY and LACTATION.

Our team has been very meticulous in analyzing the medical literature and applying principles of evidence-based medicine to assign the safety ratings. Each rating is assigned according to specific criteria:

LIKELY SAFE = The product has undergone a rigorous scientific evaluation equivalent to a review by the FDA, Health Canada, or other governmental authority and has been found to be safe when used appropriately. Or reputable references generally agree that the product is safe when used appropriately based on two or more randomized, controlled, clinical trials involving several hundred to several thousand patients and published in refereed journals; or based on large-scale post-marketing surveillance showing a low incidence of significant adverse effects.

POSSIBLY SAFE = Reputable references agree that the product might be safe when used appropriately, and there are sufficiently rigorous human studies reporting no serious adverse effects.

POSSIBLY UNSAFE = There is some evidence suggesting that use of the product might be unsafe.

LIKELY UNSAFE = Reputable references or reliable literature report that the product can be harmful, based on human studies or reliable case reports of significant adverse effects.

UNSAFE = The product has undergone a rigorous scientific evaluation or a review by a reliable regulatory agency and found to often cause clinically significant harm to humans. Or large-scale post-marketing surveillance shows a high incidence of significant adverse effects.

Effectiveness

For each natural medicine in the *Database* you get an evidence-based effectiveness rating.

These are PRACTICAL ratings that are STANDARDIZED throughout the *Natural Medicines Comprehensive Database.*

The "effectiveness" rating differs depending on the use, so you will often see more than one rating for a product.

Our team has been very meticulous in analyzing the medical literature, and applying principles of evidence-based medicine to assign the efficacy ratings. Each product is rated by the following scale:

EFFECTIVE = The product has passed a rigorous scientific review equivalent to a review by the FDA, Health Canada, or other governmental authority and has been found to be effective for a specific indication as an OTC drug, orphan drug, or prescription drug product.

LIKELY EFFECTIVE = Reputable references generally agree that the product is effective for the given indication, based on two or more randomized, controlled, clinical trials involving several hundred to several thousand patients, giving positive results for clinically relevant end-points and published in established, refereed journals.

POSSIBLY EFFECTIVE = Reputable references suggest that the product might work for the given indication based on one or more clinical trials giving positive results for clinically relevant end-points.

POSSIBLY INEFFECTIVE = Reputable references suggest that the product might not work for the given indication based on one human study giving negative results for clinically relevant end-points.

LIKELY INEFFECTIVE = Reputable references generally agree that the product is not effective for the given indication, based on two or more randomized, controlled, clinical trials giving negative results for clinically relevant end-points and published in established, refereed journals.

INEFFECTIVE = Most reputable references agree that the product is not effective for the given indication, or multiple high-quality studies resulted in negative results; there are no equally reliable human studies offering convincing contradictory data.

When possible, we have included one very useful bit of information in the Effectiveness section. This section includes the SPECIFIC FORMULA OR EXTRACT that was used in studies that found the product to be effective or ineffective. This information is not easily found elsewhere, but it is very important. For example, a significant study was published in the *Journal of the American Medical Association* providing evidence that ginkgo has a positive role in delaying the progression of Alzheimer's disease. Its effects have been likened to *Aricept*. Many published works, and many ginkgo manufacturers have since stated ginkgo's effectiveness in this area. But this information is not useful without knowing what formulation of ginkgo was shown to have a positive effect. The *Natural Medicines Comprehensive Database* states that the formulations of ginkgo that contain Egb 761 (Tanakan) or LI 1370 (Lichtwer Pharma), consisting of 24-25% flavone glycosides and 6% terpene lactones, are the formulations in the prominent studies that were shown to have beneficial effect. It cannot be inferred from this that other formulations of ginkgo will also have the same effect.

Mechanism of Action and Active Ingredients

In this field you will find a description of the known constituents and pharmacological actions that might be attributable to these constituents. Keep in mind that most natural medicines are used because people have observed, or think they observed, some benefit to using the product. In many cases there has been relatively little scientific inquiry into the active ingredients and the exact mechanism of action. Also recognize that most herbal medicines are combinations of many constituents. It is quite possible that herbal medicines work by the combined effects of multiple constituents, and the concept of identifying a single specific active ingredient is flawed. Even when a single, specific active ingredient is identified, it is possible that other active ingredients may be discovered later. For example, authorities used to think that St. John's wort exerted its effect due to hypericin content. More recent findings suggest that hyperforin exerts significant activity.

Adverse Reactions
In this field you get information about all the known adverse reactions and side effects associated with the product. These are typically derived from the side effects reported in clinical trials and from reliable case reports regarding adverse effects. In some cases, certain adverse reactions are suspected based on pharmacological properties of the product. Information about suspected adverse reactions and documented adverse reactions is clearly distinguished.

Known allergies are also listed. This can help you anticipate potential problems. For example, people who are allergic to one herb coming from the asteraceae family might also be allergic to other herbs in the same family.

Interactions
There are five separate fields listing different categories of possible interactions. For each product, this *Database* lists Possible Interactions with...

Herbs and Other Dietary Supplements
Drugs
Foods
Lab Tests
Diseases and Conditions

This is a very important part of the *Database*. There are hundreds of potential interactions...and many practitioners are not on the look-out for them. The usual computerized checking systems do not have all this info...and patients do not recognize the potential problems like they do with regular drugs. To use the information in these interaction fields, it is important to understand the origin of the data. In some cases, it comes from documented reports. In other cases, the data are theoretical, based on the pharmacological profile of the natural medicine. For example, horse chestnut seed contains coumarin derivatives and theoretically increases bleeding time. At this point in time, there are very few well-documented interactions. Much of the information regarding potential interactions is theoretical. A synopsis of documented reports and theoretical predictions appears in this field. We have also prepared a separate pair of charts in the back of the book to give you a listing of the potential interactions between drugs and natural medicines.

Drug Influences on Nutrient Levels and Depletion
Some nutrients are thought to be depleted from the body by certain drugs. Data about nutrient depletion appear in this field. This is the only field in the *Database* that appears ONLY for those natural medicines that are involved in nutrient depletion interactions. Most of these include vitamins and minerals. The natural medicines listed in this *Database* are typically the substances that are being depleted, and are not the entities causing the depletion. For this reason, the editors have chosen to only list this field when there are important data to present.

Dosage and Administration
The dosages in this field are not necessarily recommended doses, safe doses, or efficacious doses. If clinical trials have been conducted, then the doses used in the studies are listed. Other doses listed are the common or traditional doses or those typically used in supplements. Many products included in this *Database* may not be safe or effective. This needs to be considered even when a typical dose is listed.

Comments
This field presents a potpourri of info. For example, the comments on Siberian ginseng point out that it is a completely different herb than American or Panax ginseng. American or Panax ginseng is considerably more expensive. It is said that the Soviet Union wanted to provide its athletes with any advantage offered by ginseng but wanted a less expensive version. Therefore, Siberian ginseng became popular, and this is why most studies on Siberian ginseng are written in Russian.

Scattered throughout the *Database* you will see statements like, "None known." This means that data do not exist, or the literature is too contradictory, or the studies are not of high enough quality. This information is valuable because it is important for practitioners to know what is NOT known. Many references state that certain products are effective, or safe, etc. when data do not exist to support this conclusion. This *Database* states when there is insufficient information to meet the reliability standards of this *Database*.

References

This *Database* is thoroughly referenced with thousands of reference citations. In each monograph you will see numbers in parentheses appearing at the end of statements. These refer to reference citations that are listed in the back of the book in numerical order. The fact that so many references were used to create this *Database* allows this *Database* to be both a scientific consensus of clinical information and a comprehensive collection of data on natural medicines.

Brand Names Listing

There are really two separate databases of natural products within the *Natural Medicines Comprehensive Database*. There is a compilation of over 1000 monographs on natural medicines or ingredients. There is another database consisting of several thousand brand name products and their ingredients. Each brand name listing provides the name of the manufacturer and all of the ingredients. This information is towards the back of the book following the reference citations.

Within the Brand Name listing, you will sometimes find the term **"Editor's Comment."** In these instances there will be some important commentary from the editors related to the particular brand name product. For example, the listing of all the ingredients in a brand name product may serve to answer some questions about the product, but the use of all these ingredients in COMBINATION form may require additional commentary. Or, there may be some data related to this particular brand that the editors wish for you to know about. For example, some brand name products contain substances derived from animal organs. Since there is some theoretical risk of contamination with diseased animal tissue (e.g., mad cow disease), our editors have included an "Editor's Comment" about this risk.

Keep in mind that manufacturers can change the ingredients of their brand name products at any time. This has been creating problems for years. Remember when *Ex-Lax* contained phenolphthalein? Some people did not realize that it was changed to contain sennosides and docusate sodium. The same thing happens frequently with natural medicines.

"Tell The Editors" Form

It is unrealistic to believe that all clinicians, researchers, and other experts will always agree with every statement in this *Database*. The Editors recognize that new information is surfacing all the time and new interpretations develop all the time. A team of researchers and editors work full-time to constantly update this *Database*. These editors respect intelligent differences of opinion, and in fact, invite and encourage any professional user of this *Database* to share new knowledge or new interpretations with us. If you recommend a change to any statement in this *Database*, please use the form at the back of the book and send it to us. Please include the reference citation. The Editors review all suggestions. We thank you for helping to make this the best resource possible.

General Index

There are a couple of different ways you can find data on a particular product in this *Database*. One way is to just flip to the listing…it's all in alphabetical order based on the most common name. If you don't see a listing for the product you want, you can use the index in the back of the book. The index is very complete. It allows you to search by scientific name, common names, and botanical name of every product in the *Database*. Keep in mind that the index does NOT include brand names. These are listed in the brand name section in alphabetical order.

Comparison of *Natural Medicines Comprehensive Database* Book, Web, and PDA Versions:

Everything in the Book version of the *Database* is also on the website (NaturalDatabase.com) and PDA version. Whether you get the Book, Web, or PDA version (or a combination of the versions) depends on your specific needs.

The Book version allows you to quickly flip through a few pages to find the answers you need. Some practitioners like to keep a copy handy so they can go over the info face-to-face with their patients.

The Web version offers the same great content with some additional capabilities that can only be made available in the dynamic online format.

The new PDA version gives you the *Natural Database* on your Palm or Pocket PC. The PDA version gives you new functions - unlike anything before.

Updated Daily

The Web and PDA versions of the *Database* are updated daily. Log onto the website or synch your PDA to get the most updated information. Our team of editors and researchers work full-time to continuously add the latest data.

Searchability

The Web and PDA versions feature easy, fast searching. You can find any data very quickly and easily.
For example you can use:

Natural Product Effectiveness Checker to find the effectiveness rating of any product for any condition.
Disease/Medical Condition Checker to find which products are effective for any given condition.
Natural Product/Drug Interaction Checker to find any potential interactions between any natural products (including all ingredients of the natural brand name products) and any conventional drug.
Brand Product Finder to find the ingredients, manufacturer, comments, etc of brand name natural products.

Patient Education

The web version provides a full set of Patient Education Handouts covering all of the monographs in the book. This allows you to provide patient-friendly information to your patients interested in these products. The patient information is updated right along with the professional monographs, so your patients get the most up-to-date information. And the Web version can pull in the health organization's name and logo to add to the Patient Handouts.

Research Abstracts

The *Natural Medicines Comprehensive Database* is a great clinical tool. It's also an efficient research tool. The *Database* is completely referenced with several thousand reference citations from the primary peer-reviewed literature. New citations are added all the time. Citations are typically linked directly to the original abstract so you can see the original research publication.

Colleagues Interact

Colleagues Interact is an online discussion group that allows users to post questions and discuss interesting cases.

Emailed Updates

Web users can also elect to receive emailed updates about the latest additions to the *Database*.

Continuing Education

The Web version provides complete continuing education courses that compare conventional and natural treatments for various conditions. This is fully accredited for physicians, pharmacists, nurse practitioners, nurses, physician assistants, and dietitians.

Tell the Editors

Users of the *Natural Medicines Comprehensive Database* website can instantly click and send comments to the Editors. This is useful to suggest changes to the *Database* or to point out interesting findings to the Editors.

5-HTP

Also Known As
5-hydroxytryptophan, L-5 HTP, Oxitriptan.
CAUTION: See separate listing for L-tryptophan.

Scientific Names
5-hydroxytryptophan; L-5 hydroxytryptophan.

People Use This For
Orally, 5-HTP is used for sleep disorders, depression, anxiety, migraine and tension-type headaches, fibromyalgia, binge eating associated with obesity, premenstrual syndrome (PMS), premenstrual dysphoric disorder (PMDD), attention deficit-hyperactive disorder (ADHD), cerebellar ataxia, Ramsey-Hunt syndrome, Down syndrome, and as adjunctive therapy in seizure disorder and Parkinson's disease.
In combination with carbidopa, 5-HTP is used for treating intention myoclonus and as an orphan drug for treating post-anoxia myoclonus.

Safety
POSSIBLY UNSAFE ...when used orally. There is a lot of controversy about the safety of 5-HTP. There is some concern that 5-HTP might cause eosinophilia myalgia syndrome (EMS) (902,919,7067,10084). However, there is speculation that only certain contaminated 5-HTP products may cause this serious adverse effect. So far, there is not enough evidence to know if EMS is caused by 5-HTP, contaminants, or other unknown factors (919,7067,10084). Until more is known, advise patients against using 5-HTP.
PREGNANCY AND LACTATION: POSSIBLY UNSAFE ...when used orally (919); avoid using.

Effectiveness
POSSIBLY EFFECTIVE

Depression. Taking 5-HTP orally seems to significantly improve symptoms of depression (903,10853), including in patients with treatment-resistant depression (904). There is evidence that 5-HTP might be comparable to the conventional antidepressants fluvoxamine (Luvox) and imipramine (Tofranil) (904,2203).

Fibromyalgia. Taking 5-HTP orally appears to improve symptoms of primary fibromyalgia syndrome (PFS), including pain severity, morning stiffness, and sleeplessness (913,10285,10286).

POSSIBLY INEFFECTIVE

Tension headache. Taking 5-HTP orally doesn't seem to reduce pain intensity or the number of days with headache in patients with chronic tension-type headaches (2204).

INSUFFICIENT RELIABLE EVIDENCE to RATE

Alzheimer's disease. Preliminary evidence suggests that taking 5-HTP orally does not improve symptoms of Alzheimer's disease (918).

Anxiety. There's preliminary evidence that taking 5-HTP orally might help reduce symptoms of anxiety disorders (915).

Cerebellar ataxia. There is preliminary evidence that taking 5-HTP orally might help decrease cerebellar ataxia (916).

Obesity. Preliminary evidence suggests that taking 5-HTP orally might help reduce appetite, caloric intake, and weight in obese patients (914).

Palatal myoclonus. There is preliminary evidence that taking 5-HTP orally might help reduce contractions in patients with palatal myoclonus (917).

More evidence is needed to rate 5-HTP for these uses.

Mechanism of Action
5-HTP (5-Hydroxytryptophan) is related to both L-tryptophan and serotonin. In the body L-tryptophan is converted to 5-HTP, which can then be converted to serotonin. 5-HTP readily crosses the blood-brain barrier and increases central nervous system (CNS) synthesis of serotonin (10853). Serotonin can affect sleep, appetite, temperature, sexual behavior, and pain sensation. Serotonin also has a significant role in depression, anxiety, and aggression (901). Since 5-HTP can increase synthesis of serotonin, 5-HTP is used for several disease states where serotonin is believed to play a significant role including depression, insomnia, obesity, and numerous other conditions.

Adverse Reactions
Orally, 5-HTP can cause gastrointestinal (GI) side effects such as heartburn, stomach pain, belching and flatulence, nausea, vomiting, diarrhea, and anorexia (2203,10858). There is also concern that 5-HTP, like L-tryptophan, can cause asymptomatic eosinophilia and eosinophilia myalgia syndrome (EMS) (902,919,7067). There is speculation that many commercial 5-HTP products may contain contaminants from the peak X family, a group of impurities that might cause EMS (919,10084). However, the presence of the peak X family or other contaminants has not been verified in all cases of EMS. So far there is not enough evidence to determine if 5-HTP, a contaminant, or some other factor is responsible for EMS (902,919,7067,10084). Until more is known, tell patients to avoid taking 5-HTP supplements.

Interactions with Herbs & Other Dietary Supplements

HERBS AND SUPPLEMENTS WITH SEROTONERGIC PROPERTIES: Theoretically, 5-HTP might increase the therapeutic and adverse effects of products that increase serotonin levels, including Hawaiian baby woodrose, L-tryptophan, S-adenosylmethionine (SAMe), and St. John's wort (901).

Interactions with Drugs

ANTIDEPRESSANT DRUGS: Combining serotonergic antidepressants with 5-HTP might increase the risk of serotonergic side effects including serotonin syndrome and cerebral vasoconstrictive disorders such as Call-Fleming syndrome (8056). These drugs include the selective serotonin reuptake inhibitors (SSRIs) such as fluoxetine (Prozac), paroxetine (Paxil), sertraline (Zoloft), and others; and tricyclic and atypical antidepressants such as amitriptyline (Elavil), clomipramine (Anafranil), imipramine (Tofranil), and others.
CARBIDOPA (Lodosyn): Combining 5-HTP and carbidopa can increase the risk of serotonergic side effects. Carbidopa is sometimes used with 5-HTP to minimize peripheral 5-HTP metabolism and boost the amount that reaches the brain. But this combination might also increase the risk of some side effects including hypomania, restlessness, rapid speech, anxiety, insomnia, and aggressiveness. Combining carbidopa and 5-HTP might also cause an eosinophilia myalgia syndrome (EMS)-like reaction including scleroderma-like skin changes. It is suspected that a decrease in 5-HTP metabolism and an increase in either serotonin or a metabolite, kynurenine, are responsible for this adverse effect (1403,1404).
DEXTROMETHORPHAN (Robitussin DM, others): Combining serotonergic drugs such as dextromethorphan with 5-HTP might increase the risk of serotonergic side effects including serotonin syndrome and cerebral vasoconstrictive disorders such as Call-Fleming syndrome (8056).
MEPERIDINE (Demerol): Combining serotonergic drugs such as meperidine with 5-HTP might increase the risk of serotonergic side effects including serotonin syndrome and cerebral vasoconstrictive disorders such as Call-Fleming syndrome (8056).
MONOAMINE OXIDASE INHIBITORS (MAOIs): Combining serotonergic drugs such as one of the MAOIs with 5-HTP might increase the risk of serotonergic side effects including serotonin syndrome and cerebral vasoconstrictive disorders such as Call-Fleming syndrome (8056).
PENTAZOCINE (Talwin): Combining serotonergic drugs such as pentazocine with 5-HTP might increase the risk of serotonergic side effects including serotonin syndrome and cerebral vasoconstrictive disorders such as Call-Fleming syndrome (8056).
TRAMADOL (Ultram): Combining serotonergic drugs such as tramadol with 5-HTP might increase the risk of serotonergic side effects including serotonin syndrome and cerebral vasoconstrictive disorders such as Call-Fleming syndrome (8056).

Interactions with Foods

None known.

Interactions with Lab Tests

None known.

Interactions with Diseases or Conditions

DOWN SYNDROME: 5-HTP is reported to cause seizures in some patients with Down syndrome. In one case series, 15% of patients receiving long-term 5-HTP treatment experienced seizures (5050).

Dosage and Administration

ORAL: For depression, the typical dose of 5-HTP is 150-300 mg daily (903,2203). For the treatment of primary fibromyalgia syndrome (PFS), 5-HTP 100 mg 3 times daily has been used for up to 1 month (10286). For post-anoxic myoclonus, 5-HTP has an orphan drug status. The sponsor of the orphan drug is Circa Pharmaceuticals (phone: 516-842-8383).

Comments

5-HTP is often produced commercially from the seeds of the African plant Griffonia simplicifolia.

7-KETO-DHEA

Also Known As

3-acetoxyandrost-5-ene-7,17-dione, 3Beta-Acetoxyandrost-5-ene-7, 17-dione , 5-androsten-3-beta-17-one-DHEA, 7-ODA, 7-oxo-dehydroepiandrosterone-3-acetate, 7-oxo-DHEA, 7-oxo-DHEA-acetate.
CAUTION: See separate listing for DHEA.

Scientific Names

3-acetyl-7-oxo-dehydroepiandrosterone; 3beta-acetoxy-androst-5-ene-7,17-dione.

People Use This For

Orally, 7-keto-DHEA is used to increase metabolism and thermogenesis to promote weight loss, to improve lean body mass and build muscle, to increase activity of the thyroid gland and immune system, to boost memory, and to reduce aging.

Safety

There is insufficient reliable information available about the safety of 7-keto-DHEA.
Pregnancy and Lactation: Insufficient reliable information available; avoid using.

Effectiveness

INSUFFICIENT RELIABLE EVIDENCE to RATE

Obesity. There is preliminary evidence that 7-keto-DHEA might significantly decrease body weight and fat composition in obese females (5842). More evidence is needed to rate 7-keto-DHEA for this use.

Mechanism of Action

7-keto-DHEA is a metabolite of dehydroepiandrosterone (DHEA) which is formed in the body (5837). Unlike DHEA, 7-keto-DHEA is not converted to androgens and estrogens (5837,5840,5842). Oral or topical administration of 7-keto-DHEA does not affect plasma levels of steroid hormones (10404,10405). Similarly to DHEA, 7-keto-DHEA is rapidly converted to the sulfated form, known as 7-keto-DHEAS (10404).

7-keto-DHEA is thought to be beneficial in weight loss by increasing metabolism and thermogenesis. Early evidence in animals suggests 7-keto-DHEA can increase thermogenesis, possibly by stimulation of thermogenic enzymes in the liver (5837); however this effect has not yet been reported in humans. Clinical evidence suggests 7-keto-DHEA might increase basal metabolism.

In obese patients, 7-keto-DHEA can significantly increase the thyroid hormone triiodothyronine (T3) when used over 4 weeks (5842). Other preliminary evidence suggests that 7-keto-DHEA improves chemically-induced and age-related memory impairment (5839). 7-keto-DHEA may have immunomodulatory effects by stimulating interleukin-2 production by human lymphocytes in vitro (5841).

After oral administration, 7-keto-DHEA is not found in blood. It is rapidly converted to 7-keto-DHEAS, the primary form in which it is found. The half-life of 7-keto-DHEAS is about 2.17 hours, the time to peak plasma levels is about 2.2 hours, and the apparent volume of distribution is about 540 L (10404).

Adverse Reactions

None reported.

Interactions with Herbs & Other Dietary Supplements

None known.

Interactions with Drugs

None known.

Interactions with Foods

None known.

Interactions with Lab Tests

TRIIODOTHYROXINE (T3): In obese patients, 7-keto-DHEA may increase T3 levels (5842).

Interactions with Diseases or Conditions

None known.

Dosage and Administration

ORAL: For weight loss, 100 mg twice daily has been used (5842).

ABSCESS ROOT

Also Known As

American Greek Valerian, Blue Bells, False Jacob's Ladder, Sweatroot.
CAUTION: See separate listing for Jacob's Ladder.

Scientific Names

Polemonium reptans.
Family: Polemoniaceae.

Comments

At the date of publication, this product was not a common ingredient used in brand name supplements marketed to consumers. Details about this product are available in the online version of *Natural Medicines Comprehensive Database.* See www.naturaldatabase.com.

ABUTA

Also Known As

Bejunco de Cerca, Butua, False Pareira, Pareira, Patacon, Velvetleaf.
CAUTION: See separate listing for Pareira.

Scientific Names

Cissampelos pareira.
Family: Menispermaceae.

Comments

At the date of publication, there was very little scientific information available about this product. Our staff is continually analyzing the available information on natural medicines and will add data to the online version of *Natural Medicines Comprehensive Database* as it becomes available. See www.naturaldatabase.com.

ACACIA

Also Known As

Arabic Gum, Gomme Arabique, Gomme de Senegal, Gum Acacia, Gum Arabic, Gum Senegal, Gummae Mimosae, Kher.
CAUTION: See separate listings for Acai and Cassie Absolute.

Scientific Names

Acacia senegal, synonyms Acacia verek, Mimosa senegal, Senegalia senegal.
Family: Fabaceae/Leguminosae.

People Use This For

Orally, acacia is used to reduce cholesterol levels.
In manufacturing, acacia is used as a pharmaceutical ingredient in making emulsions and troches, a demulcent for throat or stomach inflammation, a masking agent for acrid substances (e.g., capsicum), and as a film-forming agent in peel-off skin masks.

Safety

LIKELY SAFE ...when used orally and appropriately in amounts commonly found in foods. Acacia has Generally Recognized As Safe status (GRAS) for use in foods in the US (4912).
POSSIBLY SAFE ...when used orally and appropriately in medicinal amounts (8072).
PREGNANCY AND LACTATION: Insufficient reliable information available; avoid using.

Effectiveness

POSSIBLY INEFFECTIVE

Hypercholesterolemia. Taking acacia orally doesn't seem to reduce cholesterol levels. Five grams twice daily for 4 weeks doesn't seem to affect any plasma lipid levels (8072).

There is insufficient reliable information available about the effectiveness of acacia for its other uses.

Mechanism of Action
Acacia is the gum that is exuded from the acacia tree. Acacia gum is a water-soluble dietary fiber. It consists mostly of arabic acid which becomes arabinose, galactose, and arabinosic acid when hydrolyzed. It is almost completely soluble in twice its weight of water (16,8072).

Adverse Reactions
Orally, acacia can cause minor gastrointestinal disturbances such as gas, bloating, and loose stools. These effects may subside with continued use (8072).

Interactions with Herbs & Other Dietary Supplements
None known.

Interactions with Drugs
AMOXICILLIN (Amoxil, Trimox): Acacia can reduce the absorption of amoxicillin. Separate dose times by at least 4 hours (12654).

Interactions with Foods
None known.

Interactions with Lab Tests
None known.

Interactions with Diseases or Conditions
None known.

Dosage and Administration
ORAL: Acacia is usually dissolved in water to make a mucilage. The usual dose is 1 to 4 teaspoons (5263).

Comments
Avoid confusion with sweet acacia (Acacia farnesiana).

ACAI

Also Known As
Acai Palm, Amazon Acai, Assai Palm, Cabbage Palm.
CAUTION: See separate listing for Acacia.

Scientific Names
Euterpe oleracea, synonym Euterpe badiocarpa.
Family: Arecaceae/Palmae.

People Use This For
Orally, acai is used for osteoarthritis, hypercholesterolemia, and for improving general health.
As a food, the acai berry is consumed raw and as a juice. The juice is also used commercially as a beverage and in ice cream, jelly, and liquors.
In manufacturing, acai berry is used as a natural food colorant.

Safety
There is insufficient reliable information available about the safety of acai.
Pregnancy and Lactation: Insufficient reliable information available; avoid using.

Effectiveness
There is insufficient reliable information available about the effectiveness of acai.

Mechanism of Action
The applicable part of acai is the fruit or berry. Acai juice is often prepared by macerating the fruit. The juice is viscous and contains about 2.4% protein and 5.9% lipids (13087). The fruit pulp contains about 4% protein and 12% lipids. Other constituents include calcium, phosphorus, iron, and thiamine (13088).
Acai berry contains numerous polyphenols and anthocyanins. The most abundant are cyanidin-3-glucoside, ferulic acid, epicatechin, p-hydroxy benzoic acid, and pelargonidin-3-glucoside. Others include gallic acid and several derivatives, catechin, and ellagic acid (13087).
The anthocyanins are pigments that give the ripe fruit its purple color. Anthocyanins are also potent antioxidants.

Acai fruit pulp has a very high antioxidant capacity. It has more antioxidant content than cranberry, raspberry, blackberry, strawberry, or blueberry (13087).

Adverse Reactions
None reported.

Interactions with Herbs & Other Dietary Supplements
None known.

Interactions with Drugs
None known.

Interactions with Foods
None known.

Interactions with Lab Tests
MAGNETIC RESONANCE IMAGING (MRI): Consumption of acai fruit might increase T1-weighted MRI signal and decrease T2-weighted MRI signal in imaging studies of the gastrointestinal tract (13088).

Interactions with Diseases or Conditions
None known.

Dosage and Administration
No typical dosage.

Comments
Acai is pronounced AH-sigh-EE. Acai is a palm tree widely distributed in the northern area of South America. Acai gained popularity in North America after being promoted by Dr. Nicholas Perricone as a "Superfood for Age-Defying Beauty" on the Oprah Winfrey show.

ACEROLA

Also Known As
Barbados Cherry, Puerto Rican Cherry, West Indian Cherry.
CAUTION: See separate listings for Cherokee Rosehip, Rose Hip, and Vitamin C.

Scientific Names
Malpighia glabra; Malpighia punicifolia.
Family: Malpighiaceae.

People Use This For
Orally, acerola is used to treat or prevent scurvy, colds, heart disease, cancer, pressure sores, retinal hemorrhages, tooth decay, gum infections, atherosclerosis, depression, hay fever, for preventing blood clots, collagen disorders, and to enhance physical endurance.

Safety
POSSIBLY SAFE ...when used orally (6,15).
PREGNANCY AND LACTATION: Insufficient reliable information available; avoid using.

Effectiveness
POSSIBLY EFFECTIVE

Scurvy. Taking acerola orally might prevent scurvy due to its vitamin C content (6,15).

There is insufficient reliable information available about the effectiveness of acerola for its other uses.

Mechanism of Action
The applicable part of acerola is the fruit. Acerola contains 1000-2330 mg of vitamin C per 100 grams (6). Vitamin C is an essential coenzyme required for normal metabolic function. It is important for collagen formation and tissue repair. Vitamin C is involved in tyrosine metabolism, folic acid conversion, carbohydrate metabolism, synthesis of lipids and proteins, iron metabolism, resistance to infections, and cellular respiration. Vitamin C also acts as an antioxidant (6,15). It regenerates and restores oxidized vitamin E (127,128). Acerola fruit also contains vitamin A, thiamine, riboflavin, and niacin (6).

Adverse Reactions
Orally, the vitamin C in acerola can cause nausea, abdominal cramps, fatigue, insomnia, and sleepiness. Doses greater than 1 gram might cause diarrhea (15).

Interactions with Herbs & Other Dietary Supplements
VITAMIN C SUPPLEMENTS: Due to vitamin C content in acerola, concomitant use of acerola with vitamin C supplements might increase the risk of adverse effects associated with vitamin C.

Interactions with Drugs
ESTROGENS: Concomitant use of estrogens with acerola might increase absorption and therapeutic effects due to vitamin C content (129,130).
FLUPHENAZINE (Prolixin): Concomitant use with acerola decreases blood levels due to vitamin C content (15).
WARFARIN (Coumadin): Concomitant use with acerola can reduce anticoagulant activity of warfarin due to its vitamin C content (506).

Interactions with Foods
IRON: Concomitant use of iron with acerola increases GI absorption of iron from foods (ferric) but not from supplements (ferrous) due to vitamin C content (15).

Interactions with Lab Tests
STOOL OCCULT BLOOD TESTS: The vitamin C in acerola can cause false-negative results if it is ingested 48-72 hours before amine-dependent tests (506).
URINE GLUCOSE TESTS: Doses of vitamin C greater than 500 mg can cause false-decreases with glucose oxidase tests (e.g., Clinistix). The vitamin C in acerola might also cause false increases with cupric sulfate tests (e.g., Clinitest) (15).

Interactions with Diseases or Conditions
GOUT: The vitamin C in acerola might increase uric acid levels (15).
KIDNEY STONES (Nephrolithiasis): The vitamin C in acerola in large doses might cause precipitation of urate, cystine, or oxalate stones (15).

Dosage and Administration
No typical dosage.

ACETYL-L-CARNITINE

Also Known As
Acetyl-Levocarnitine, Acetyl Carnitine, ALC, ALCAR, Carnitine Acetyl Ester, Gamma-Trimethyl-Beta-Acetylbutyrobetaine, L-Acetylcarnitine, Levacecarnine, N-Acetyl-Carnitine, N-Acetyl-L-Carnitine, ST-200, Vitamin B(t) Acetate.
CAUTION: See separate listings for L-Carnitine and Propionyl-L-Carnitine.

Scientific Names
2-(acetyloxy)-3-carboxy-N,N,N-trimethyl-1-propanaminium inner salt; (3-carboxy-2-hydroxy-propyl)trimethylammonium hydroxide inner salt acetate.

People Use This For
Orally, acetyl-L-carnitine is used for Alzheimer's disease, age-related memory deficits, senile depression, Down syndrome, alcoholism-related cognitive deficits, and cerebrovascular insufficiency after stroke. It is also used for peripheral neuropathies, diabetic neuropathy, neuropathy due to anti-viral drugs used in the treatment of AIDS, facial paralysis, male infertility, symptoms of age-related testosterone deficiency, and Peyronie's disease.
Intravenously, acetyl-L-carnitine is used for dementia and cerebral ischemia.
Intramuscularly, acetyl-L-carnitine is used for peripheral neuropathy with pain.

Safety
LIKELY SAFE ...when used orally and appropriately. Acetyl-L-carnitine has been used safely in clinical trials lasting up to 33 months (42,1589,1594,1595,1596,1597,1598,1599,3600,3601,9105,9791,10076,12743,12745).
POSSIBLY SAFE ...when used parenterally and appropriately under medical supervision (1591,1592,12743).
PREGNANCY AND LACTATION: Insufficient reliable information available; avoid using.

Effectiveness

POSSIBLY EFFECTIVE

Age-related cognitive impairment. Taking acetyl-L-carnitine orally seems to improve some measures of cognitive function and memory in elderly people with age-related mental impairment (42,3600,3601).

Age-related testosterone deficiency. Taking acetyl-L-carnitine orally, in combination with propionyl-L-carnitine, seems to help symptoms of androgen decline in older men. The combination taken for 6 months seems to be similar to testosterone for improving sexual dysfunction, depression, and fatigue (12353).

Alzheimer's disease. Acetyl-L-carnitine might slow the rate of disease progression, improve memory, and improve some measures of cognitive function and behavioral performance in some patients with Alzheimer's disease. It is more likely to show some effect in those with early-onset Alzheimer's disease who are less than 66 years of age and have a faster rate of disease progression and mental decline (1594,1595,1596,1597,1598,1599,9105,10391). Acetyl-L-carnitine has not been compared with cholinesterase inhibitors such as donepezil (Aricept).

Chronic cerebral ischemia. Administering a single dose of acetyl-L-carnitine intravenously seems to produce short-term improvements in cerebral blood flow in people with chronic cerebral ischemia (1591,1592).

Cognitive impairment. Taking acetyl-L-carnitine orally seems to improve memory and visuospatial capacity in 30-60 year-old chronic alcoholics with cognitive impairment (1589).

Diabetic neuropathy. Patients with neuropathy related to type 1 or type 2 diabetes seem to have improved symptoms after taking acetyl-L-carnitine 1500-3000 mg daily in divided doses for a year. Acetyl-L-carnitine seems to increase nerve fibers, regenerate nerve fiber clusters, and improve vibratory sensations. However, research is conflicting on whether it can modestly improve nerve conduction velocity. In patients who have neuropathic pain as the most significant symptoms, taking acetyl-L-carnitine 1000 mg two to three times daily also decreases neuropathy-related pain within six months of beginning treatment. Doses of 500 mg three times daily do not seem to reduce pain. Acetyl-L-carnitine also seems more likely to be effective for reducing pain in patients with a shorter duration of diabetes and patients with poorly-controlled type 2 diabetes (1593,12743,12753,13007).

Infertility. Taking acetyl-L-carnitine orally, in combination with L-carnitine for 6 months, seems to increase sperm motility in men with infertility (12352). Some pregnancies occurred after taking these carnitines, but not enough to be statistically significant (12352). Taking acetyl-L-carnitine orally, in combination with L-carnitine and nonsteroidal anti-inflammatory drugs (NSAIDs), seems to improve male infertility caused by abacterial prostatovesiculoepididymitis, an inflammation of the prostate gland, seminal vesicles, and epididymis. The carnitines increase sperm count and motility. The carnitines are used following 2 months of treatment with NSAIDs (9791).

Peyronie's disease. Taking acetyl-L-carnitine orally seems to help treat acute and early chronic Peyronie's disease (10076). Acetyl-L-carnitine appears to be more effective than tamoxifen for reducing pain and inhibiting disease progression.

INSUFFICIENT RELIABLE EVIDENCE to RATE

Antiretroviral toxic neuropathy. Acetyl-L-carnitine taken orally might relive symptoms of distal symmetrical polyneuropathy caused by antiretroviral treatment in patients with HIV disease, according to preliminary clinical research (12745,12747).

Depression. Some clinical research suggests acetyl-L-carnitine might decrease symptoms of dysthymia and depression in elderly people (3602,3603,3604).

More evidence is needed to rate acetyl-L-carnitine for these uses.

Mechanism of Action

Acetyl-L-carnitine occurs naturally in the body. Endogenous carnitines exist as a "carnitine pool" consisting of L-carnitine and several acetyl-carnitine esters. Intracellular enzymes and cell membrane transporters can rapidly interconvert the carnitines to the needed form and transport them between the tissues and extracellular space. Acetyl-L-carnitine, the most important carnitine ester, is converted to L-carnitine in the body by carnitine acetyltransferase (10395,12744). The body obtains some carnitine from the diet, primarily from red meats and dairy products. The body can also synthesize carnitines from the amino acids, lysine and methionine. The kidney aids in keeping carnitine levels stable. Normally, greater than 90% of filtered carnitine is reabsorbed. If dietary intake of carnitines decreases, carnitine reabsorption becomes even more efficient (12744). Carnitines play an important role in lipid metabolism and energy production. They are essential for normal mitochondrial function, acting as a transporter of long-chain fatty acids into the mitochondria for beta-oxidation (12745,12748,12756,13007).

Carnitine deficiency from inborn disorders of carnitine metabolism most often presents with symptoms of progressive cardiomyopathy and skeletal muscle weakness, and less frequently with fasting hypoglycemic coma (12748).

Acetyl-L-carnitine is structurally related to acetylcholine. It also serves as a precursor to acetyl coenzyme A, and contributes acetyl groups to acetylcholine (10395). It also seems to promote acetylcholine release and increases choline acetyltransferase activity (44). These effects have lead to the study of acetyl-L-carnitine in Alzheimer's disease, in which there is substantial cholinergic neuronal loss and acetylcholine depletion (1594). It may also lessen oxidative stress and prevent oxidative damage in the brain better than L-carnitine (12688).

Carnitine levels are lower in people with complications of diabetes (12746). In diabetic neuropathy, there is damage to sensory neuronal membranes. This causes an increase in sodium channels and therefore an increase in spontaneous neuronal firing. Acetyl-L-carnitine is thought to slow neuronal degeneration or help in the regeneration and repair of neurons and therefore decrease excessive excitability and firing. Acetyl-L-carnitine might improve peripheral as well as autonomic neuropathy (12749,12750,12751,12752,13007). Additionally, preliminary clinical research suggests that acetyl-L-carnitine might also improve glucose utilization, possibly by increasing expression of glycolytic and gluconeogenic enzymes (12754).

In HIV patients, acetyl-L-carnitine might slow the loss of CD4 lymphocytes by reducing apoptosis and increasing the serum level of insulin-like growth factor 1 which protects against apoptosis (3605). Lower plasma levels of acetyl-L-carnitine are also associated with neuropathy in people who take HIV drugs (3606). Preliminary research suggests it might increase the activity of nerve growth factor and promote peripheral nerve regeneration. It might also have analgesic properties. However, it doesn't seem to affect viral load or CD4 or CD8 cell counts (12745). Preliminary research suggests acetyl-L-carnitine might also prevent cisplatin (Platinol-AQ) and paclitaxel (Taxol)-induced neuropathy (12755).

Acetyl-L-carnitine and L-carnitine are present in human sperm and seminal fluid (3607). Their levels increase in sperm during the maturation process in the epididymis and coincide with the acquisition of progressive motility (3608,3609). Levels of acetyl-L-carnitine, and the ratio of acetyl-L-carnitine to L-carnitine, have been reported to be lower in infertile semen and sperm samples with low motility (3610,3611), and an increase in sperm motility is seen in vitro when acetyl-L-carnitine or L-carnitine is added to the sample (3612). Preliminary research also suggests acetyl-L-carnitine may increase testosterone production and improve testicular function (12686,12687).

In patients with alcohol-induced cirrhosis, serum levels of L-carnitine and its esters are sometimes increased, possibly due to increased L-carnitine biosynthesis (1931,1948).

Adverse Reactions

Orally, acetyl-L-carnitine is generally well tolerated (10391,12756). It may cause nausea, vomiting, gastrointestinal upset, and agitation (restlessness and motor overactivity) (1596,1599,12743,13007). One of its metabolites can cause the urine, breath, and sweat to have a fishy odor (12756).

Side effects reported in people with Alzheimer's disease include psychiatric disturbances such as depression, mania, confusion and aggression, but it is not clear whether these are due to acetyl-L-carnitine or the disease itself (1594,1595,1596,1597,1598,1599,9105,10391).

Acetyl-L-carnitine is used for age-related testosterone deficiency. Unlike testosterone, it doesn't cause prostate enlargement or increase prostate-specific antigen when taken orally for 6 months (12353).

Interactions with Herbs & Other Dietary Supplements

D-CARNITINE: D-carnitine might compete with L-carnitine in active transport systems. Taking D-carnitine might cause symptoms of L-carnitine deficiency, and theoretically acetyl-L-carnitine deficiency (1946,12760); avoid using.

Interactions with Drugs

ACENOCOUMAROL (Sintrom): Taking L-carnitine 1 gram/day seems to significantly increase the anticoagulant effects of acenocoumarol. Acenocoumarol is an oral anticoagulant similar to warfarin, but shorter-acting (9878,12165). In one case, INR was stable in the normal range of 1.99-2.94 and then increased to 4.65 after L-carnitine was started and continued for 10 weeks. INR normalized after discontinuation of L-carnitine (12165). This interaction has only been reported with L-carnitine, but theoretically could occur with acetyl-L-carnitine.

WARFARIN (Coumadin): Use acetyl-L-carnitine cautiously in patients taking warfarin. L-carnitine can significantly increase the anticoagulant effects acenocoumarol, a shorter-acting oral anticoagulant similar to warfarin (9878,12165).

ZIDOVUDINE (AZT, Retrovir): Zidovudine inhibits the transport of L-carnitine into muscle. This might cause the muscle weakness seen in patients treated with zidovudine. Whether acetyl-L-carnitine can reverse or prevent this effect is unknown. Low serum carnitine levels are found in some people with HIV infection (3617).

Drug Influences on Nutrient Levels and Depletion

SOME DRUGS CAN AFFECT ACETYL-L-CARNITINE LEVELS:

CARBAMAZEPINE (Tegretol): Carbamazepine can reduce carnitine levels. Whether this reduction is clinically important is unknown. The reduction in carnitine levels might be more significant when other factors are present that also lower carnitine levels such as other drugs that deplete carnitine, vegetarianism, or diabetes (1911,12758).

CEFDITOREN PIVOXIL (Spectracef): Taking cefditoren chronically can induce carnitine deficiency because of its pivalate content. Using cefditoren short-term is unlikely to have any clinically significant effect on carnitine (12759).

PHENOBARBITAL (Luminal): Phenobarbital can reduce carnitine levels. Whether this reduction is clinically important is unknown. The reduction in carnitine levels might be more significant when other factors are present that also lower carnitine levels such as other drugs that deplete carnitine, vegetarianism, or diabetes (1911,12758).

PHENYTOIN (Dilantin): Phenytoin can reduce carnitine levels. Whether this reduction is clinically important is unknown. The reduction in carnitine levels might be more significant when other factors are present that also lower carnitine levels such as other drugs that deplete carnitine, vegetarianism, or diabetes (1911,12758).

PIVAMPICILLIN (Pondocillin): Taking pivampicillin chronically can induce carnitine deficiency because of its pivalate content. Using pivampicillin short-term is unlikely to have any clinically significant effect on carnitine (12759).
VALPROIC ACID (Depakote): Valproic acid can reduce carnitine levels. Whether this reduction is clinically important is unknown. The reduction in carnitine levels might be more significant when other factors are present that also lower carnitine levels such as other drugs that deplete carnitine, vegetarianism, or diabetes (1911,12758).

Interactions with Foods
None known.

Interactions with Lab Tests
None known.

Interactions with Diseases or Conditions
HYPOTHYROIDISM: Avoid using acetyl-L-carnitine in patients with hypothyroidism. L-carnitine seems to inhibit the activity of thyroid hormone in target tissues (12761). Theoretically this might occur with acetyl-L-carnitine.
SEIZURES: An increase in seizure frequency or severity has been reported in people with a history of seizures who have used L-carnitine orally or intravenously (3616). Theoretically, this might occur with acetyl-L-carnitine.

Dosage and Administration
ORAL: In Alzheimer's disease, 1500-4000 mg daily has been used, usually divided into two or three doses during the day (1594,1595,1599).
In age-related memory impairment, 1500-2000 mg daily has been used (3601).
For depression in the elderly, 1500-3000 mg daily in divided doses has been used (3602,3603).
In some infertile men, 4000 mg daily has been used to improve sperm function (3607).
For Peyronie's disease, 1 gram twice daily for 3 months has been used (10076).
For male infertility, 1 gram of acetyl-L-carnitine plus 2 grams of L-carnitine daily has been used (12352).
For male infertility secondary to abacterial prostatovesiculoepididymitis, acetyl-L-carnitine 500 mg plus carnitine 1 gram every 12 hours has been used following 2 months of treatment with nonsteroidal anti-inflammatory drugs (9791).
For symptoms of age-related testosterone deficiency, 2 grams of acetyl-L-carnitine plus 2 grams of propionyl-L-carnitine daily has been used (12353).
For diabetic neuropathy, 1500 to 3000 mg per day in divided doses has been used. A higher dose of 1000 mg two to three times daily seems to be more effective for improving vibratory sensations and reducing neuropathy-related pain (12743,13007).
INTRAVENOUS: Single doses of 1500 mg have been used in people with chronic cerebral ischemia (1591,1592).
INTRAMUSCULAR: In people with peripheral neuropathy, 500-1000 mg daily has been used (1593).

Comments
The body can convert L-carnitine to acetyl-L-carnitine and vice versa. But, no one knows whether the benefits of acetyl-L-carnitine are from the intact molecule, from its acetate metabolite or some other activated form, or from its conversion to L-carnitine. For now, tell patients not to substitute one form of carnitine for another (12744).

ACKEE

Also Known As
Akee, Aki, Anjye, Arbre Fricasse, Ishin, Seso Vegetal.

Scientific Names
Blighia sapida, synonym Cupania sapida.
Family: Sapindaceae.

People Use This For
Orally, ackee is used as a treatment for colds, fever, edema, and epilepsy.
For food uses, the ripe fruit is eaten.

Safety

LIKELY SAFE ...when the ripe fruit is eaten as a food (12415).
UNSAFE ...when the unripe fruit is ingested. It can cause severe hypoglycemia, convulsions, and death (12415). Unripe ackee is unsafe even when cooked (12416). The US has recently begun to allow the import of canned ripe ackee on a limited basis. However, all other forms of ackee are illegal in the US because of safety concerns (12422).
CHILDREN: UNSAFE ...when the unripe fruit is ingested. Children are more sensitive to the toxic effects of ackee than adults (12415). There is insufficient reliable information available about the safety of the ripe fruit for children.
PREGNANCY AND LACTATION: UNSAFE ...when the unripe fruit is ingested (12415). There is insufficient reliable information available about the safety of the ripe fruit during pregnancy and breast-feeding; avoid using.

Effectiveness

There is insufficient reliable information available about the effectiveness of ackee.

Mechanism of Action

The applicable part of ackee is the fruit. It contains fatty acids including linoleic, palmitic, and stearic acids, as well as a significant amount of arginine (12417). The unripe fruit contains the toxin hypoglycin A, which is present in 100 times higher concentrations than in the ripe fruit. Hypoglycin A and its metabolite methlenecyclopropylacetic acid are potent hypoglycemic agents. They also cause liver toxicity (12415). By inactivating flavoprotein acyl-CoA dehydrogenases and inhibiting the oxidation of long-chain fatty acids, the toxins inhibit gluconeogenesis and induce hypoglycemia (5609,5610). Animal research suggests that early administration of sugar or glucose might lessen toxicity and mortality (12418).
Renal excretion of dicarboxylic acids in urine is highly suggestive of hypoglycin A poisoning (12416,12417).

Adverse Reactions

Orally, ackee can cause Jamaican vomiting sickness. Symptoms of Jamaican vomiting sickness include acute onset of severe vomiting after ackee ingestion, which subsides. This is usually followed by another bout of vomiting, seizures, coma, and death within 12 hours. The severity of poisoning appears to be dose dependent with more severe toxicity seen in children (12416). It causes severe hypoglycemia known as toxic hypoglycemic syndrome (THS) and liver damage (5602,12416). Early administration of sugar or glucose might lessen toxicity and mortality (12418).
Chronic ingestion of canned ackee fruit has been associated with cholestatic liver disease (12418).
Urticaria and anaphylaxis has been reported after ingestion of ackee (5610).

Interactions with Herbs & Other Dietary Supplements

None known.

Interactions with Drugs

None known.

Interactions with Foods

None known.

Interactions with Lab Tests

None known.

Interactions with Diseases or Conditions

None known.

Dosage and Administration

No typical dosage.

Comments

Ripe ackee is eaten as food in West Africa and in the Caribbean (12415). Ackee is also found in southern Florida and Central America (5602,5609). It is a dietary staple in Jamaica (12415,12417). But most ackee products have been banned from import into the US for the past 3 decades because of concerns about poisoning from unripe fruit (12422). Unripe ackee is a frequent cause of poisoning in Africa and the Caribbean. Poisonings may occur as epidemics when the unripe fruit is eaten during times of food shortage, particularly in children (12415).
Avoid use of unripe fruit and seeds or water in which unripe ackee has been cooked due to toxicity (5602).

ACONITE

Also Known As
Aconiti Tuber, Autumn Monkshood, Blue Monkshood Root, Chuan-wu, Monkshood, Monkshood Tuber, Wolfsbane.

Scientific Names
Aconitum napellus; Aconitum species.
Family: Ranunculaceae.

People Use This For
Orally, aconite is used for pain, facial paralysis, joint pain, arthritis, gout, rheumatic complaints, inflammation, pleurisy, pericarditis sicca, fever, skin and mucosal diseases, disinfection, and wound treatment. Aconite is also used orally as a cardiac depressant and an agent to induce mild sweating.

Topically, aconite is used as a counterirritant in liniment. Aconite is also used topically for facial neuralgia, rheumatism, and sciatica.

Safety
UNSAFE ...when used orally. Aconite root is a strong, fast-acting poison that affects the heart and CNS (11). All species of this herb are dangerous. Severe poisoning has been reported after ingestion of 0.2 mg of aconitine or 6 grams of processed and cured aconite (3490). Even when used in the therapeutic dose range, aconite can cause toxicity including nausea, vomiting, dizziness, muscle spasms, hypothermia, paralysis of respiratory system, and heart rhythm disorders (2,11). ...when used topically. Aconite can be absorbed through the skin and cause significant toxicity (12).

PREGNANCY AND LACTATION: UNSAFE ...when used orally or topically (11,12); avoid using.

Effectiveness
There is insufficient reliable information available about the effectiveness of aconite.

Mechanism of Action
The applicable part of aconite is the root. Aconite contains alkaloids including aconitine, mesoconitine, and hypaconitine, which have widespread effects on cardiac, neural, and muscle tissue by activating sodium channels (559,3490). In the heart muscle, this activation enhances inward currents during the plateau phase of the cardiac action potential, prolonging repolarization, and inducing after depolarization, leading to tachyarrhythmias (2634).

Adverse Reactions
Orally, aconite causes symptoms of intoxication including nausea, vomiting, weakness, sweating, restlessness, dizziness, numbness, paresthesias (beginning in the mouth and then spreading to the limbs), hypotension, palpitations, hypokalemia, metabolic and/or respiratory acidosis, cardiac toxicity (sustained ventricular tachycardia, ventricular fibrillation), reduced consciousness, and death (558,559,561,562,563,3490). Symptoms of intoxication usually begin 30 minutes after ingestion of aconite (559). Life-threatening symptoms and fatalities have been reported after aconite ingestion (3490,3491). No specific antidote is available. Cardioversion has been reported to be ineffective, but the use of antiarrhythmic agents such as amiodarone has been successful in some cases (2634,3490). Some Chinese medicine practitioners still commonly use aconite rootstocks in their preparations. They cure the rootstocks of aconite by soaking in water (with frequent changes to fresh water) and then boiling or steaming for prolonged periods of time. The process hydrolyzes the aconite alkaloids into less toxic derivatives, but toxicities and fatalities can also occur after ingestion of these cured and processed aconite roots (2634,3490). Aconite is also a common ingredient in numerous homeopathic products. Since most homeopathic products are so diluted that they contain virtually no active molecules, these products are not likely to have any pharmacological or toxic effects.

Interactions with Herbs & Other Dietary Supplements
None known.

Interactions with Drugs
None known.

Interactions with Foods
None known.

Interactions with Lab Tests
None known.

Interactions with Diseases or Conditions
None known.

Dosage and Administration

ORAL: No typical dosage. But people have used homeopathic preparations of aconite of 6c to 30c potency strength. A 6c potency is made by diluting one part of aconite tincture to 99 parts of water or alcohol. One part of the resulting solution is taken and diluted again with 99 parts of water or alcohol. The process done six times resulting in a 6c potency (5011).
TOPICAL: No typical dosage.

ACTIVATED CHARCOAL

Also Known As

Animal Charcoal, Charcoal, Gas Black, Lamp Black, Medicinal Charcoal, Vegetable Carbon.
CAUTION: See separate listing for Coffee Charcoal.

Scientific Names

Carbon.

People Use This For

Orally, activated charcoal is used as an antiflatulent, for reducing blood lipid levels, acute management of poisonings, preventing hangover, and cholestasis of pregnancy.

Safety

LIKELY SAFE ...when used orally short-term (12392,12393).
PREGNANCY AND LACTATION: POSSIBLY SAFE ...when used orally short-term (126).

Effectiveness

LIKELY EFFECTIVE

Poisoning. Taking activated charcoal orally is effective when used as part of a standard treatment for some acute poisonings (12392,12393).

INSUFFICIENT RELIABLE EVIDENCE to RATE

Cholestasis. Taking activated charcoal orally seems to help treat cholestasis of pregnancy, according to preliminary clinical research (12400).
Flatulence. Research is conflicting about the effectiveness of taking activated charcoal orally to reduce flatus and gas (12395,12396).
Hypercholesterolemia. Research is conflicting about the effectiveness of taking activated charcoal orally to reduce serum cholesterol levels (12397,12398,12399).
More evidence is needed to rate activated charcoal for these uses.

Mechanism of Action

Charcoal is made from peat, coal, wood coconut shell, or petroleum. It is activated by increasing the surface area. Heating charcoal to a high temperature in the presence of oxidizing gas such as steam, carbon dioxide, and gas or with an activating agent such as phosphoric acid or zinc chloride causes a highly developed internal pore structure in charcoal. To meet USP standards, the surface area must be at least 900 meters squared per gram (12392).
Activated charcoal adsorbs many drugs, increasing clearance and decreasing elimination half-life. It binds unabsorbed drugs in the gastrointestinal tract. It also binds drugs that diffuse from the circulation into the intestine and interrupts enterohepatic and enterogastric circulation of drugs (12392).
Activated charcoal is included in some hangover remedies. However, ethanol adsorbs poorly to charcoal (12400). There is no reliable evidence that activated charcoal prevents hangover.

Adverse Reactions

Orally, activated charcoal can cause constipation and black stools. More serious, but rare adverse effects include GI obstruction and pulmonary aspiration. When given with cathartics, activated charcoal can cause electrolyte abnormalities and metabolic acidosis, particularly in infants (12392).

Interactions with Herbs & Other Dietary Supplements

MICRONUTRIENTS: Activated charcoal may cause reduced absorption of micronutrients (15).

Interactions with Drugs

ALCOHOL (Ethanol): Alcohol may lower the adsorptive capacity of activated charcoal (12400).
ORAL DRUGS: Activated charcoal may reduce or prevent absorption of drugs including acetaminophen, carbamazepine, dapsone, digoxin, disopyramide, nadolol phenylbutazone, phenytoin, phenobarbital, piroxicam, quinine, propoxyphene, sotalol, theophylline, and tricyclic antidepressants (12392,12400); avoid co-administration, except in overdose.
SYRUP OF IPECAC: Activated charcoal adsorbs and inactivates syrup of ipecac; avoid co-administration (12394).

Interactions with Foods

ALCOHOL (Ethanol): Alcohol may lower the adsorptive capacity of activated charcoal (12400).
MICRONUTRIENTS: Activated charcoal can reduce absorption of micronutrients (15).

Interactions with Lab Tests

SERUM CHOLESTEROL: Some research suggests activated charcoal might reduce serum total cholesterol and LDL cholesterol concentrations and test results (12397,12398).

Interactions with Diseases or Conditions

GI OBSTRUCTION: Use of activated charcoal is contraindicated in intestinal obstruction. It should be administered cautiously in decreased peristalsis (12393).

Dosage and Administration

ORAL: For lowering drug levels in overdose or poisoning, 50 to 100 grams is given initially, followed by charcoal every 2 to 4 hours at a dose equivalent to 12.5 grams per hour. For children, lower doses 10-25 grams are used (12392).

ADENOSINE

Also Known As

A5MP, Adenine Nucleoside, Adenine Riboside, Adenosine Phosphate, ADP, AMP, ATP.

Scientific Names

Adenosine; Adenosine Monophosphate (AMP); Adenosine-5-monophosphate (A5MP); Adenosine Diphosphate (ADP); Adenosine Triphosphate (ATP).

People Use This For

Orally, adenosine monophosphate (AMP) is used for treating herpes zoster and porphyria cutanea tarda.
Sublingually, adenosine triphosphate (ATP) is used to increase physical energy.
Intravenously, adenosine is used for treating surgical and neuropathic pain, pulmonary hypertension, supraventricular tachycardia, and controlling blood pressure during anesthesia and surgery. It is also used for pharmacological cardiac stress tests.
Intrathecally, adenosine is used to treat neuropathic pain.
Intramuscularly, adenosine phosphate is used for treating varicose veins, bursitis, tendonitis, tenosynovitis, pruritus, multiple sclerosis, neuropathy, herpes zoster and herpes simplex infections, and improving coronary and peripheral blood flow.
Intravenously, adenosine triphosphate is used for treating acute renal failure, multiple organ failure, pulmonary hypertension, cystic fibrosis, lung cancer, cachexia associated with cancer, and controlling blood pressure during anesthesia and surgery. It is also used for pharmacological cardiac stress tests.

Safety

LIKELY SAFE ...when adenosine is used intravenously and appropriately. Adenosine (Adenocard, Adenoscan) is an FDA-approved prescription drug (15). ...when adenosine monophosphate (adenosine phosphate, AMP) is used intramuscularly and appropriately. Adenosine monophosphate is an FDA-approved prescription drug (15).
POSSIBLY SAFE ...when adenosine triphosphate (ATP) is used intravenously and appropriately. ATP appears to be safe when up to 75 mcg/kg per minute is given intravenously for 30 hours every 2 weeks for 28 weeks, although doses higher than 50 mcg/kg per minute cause a higher incidence of adverse effects (9149,9154).
PREGNANCY AND LACTATION: Insufficient reliable information available; avoid using.

Effectiveness

EFFECTIVE

Paroxysmal supraventricular tachycardia. Administering adenosine intravenously improves paroxysmal supraventricular tachycardia (15).

POSSIBLY EFFECTIVE

Cachexia. Administering adenosine triphosphate (ATP) given intravenously every 2 to 4 weeks at a dose of up to 75 mcg/kg per minute over 30 hours seems to stabilize body composition, appetite, and dietary intake, and to improve quality of life in people with advanced non-small-cell lung cancer and other tumors (9149,9151,9152).

Venous stasis ulcers. Administering adenosine monophosphate intramuscularly might relieve edema, pruritus, dermatitis, and erythema of varicose ulcers (15).

INSUFFICIENT RELIABLE EVIDENCE to RATE

Herpes zoster (shingles). There is preliminary clinical research that suggests adenosine monophosphate given intramuscularly might be useful for herpes zoster (shingles) infection and to treat and prevent post-herpetic neuralgia (9155,10067). Intramuscular adenosine monophosphate might also be useful for treating other kinds of herpes infections, according to limited clinical research (9590).

Lung cancer. Preliminary clinical studies suggest that adenosine triphosphate (ATP) is not effective for treating non-small-cell lung cancer (9151,9154).

Neuropathic pain. Some clinical research suggests that adenosine given intrathecally might relieve neuropathic pain (9157).

More evidence is needed to rate adenosine for these uses.

Mechanism of Action

Adenosine is a purine nucleotide that is present in all human cells. It contains a purine base, adenine; plus a ribose sugar; and can have one to three phosphate groups (9148). Adenosine is used pharmacologically as an adenosine base, and as the mono- and triphosphate salts. Adenosine is involved in many physiological processes including cellular metabolism, nucleic acid synthesis, neurotransmission, muscle contraction, cardiac function, platelet function, vasodilation, and liver glycogen metabolism (9148,9150). Adenosine triphosphate (ATP) is broken down to adenosine diphosphate (ADP), then to adenosine monophosphate (AMP), and then to adenosine. The ultimate metabolite of adenosine is uric acid. This conversion occurs rapidly. The half-life of adenosine and ATP given by rapid intravenous injection is 0.6 to 1.5 seconds (9148).

Adenosine and ATP both have negative inotropic, dromotropic, and chronotropic effects on the heart.

Adenosine and ATP, after degradation to adenosine, stimulate the release of potassium in the sinoatrial (SA) and atrioventricular (AV) nodal cells, which depresses cardiac conduction (9148). Adenosine and ATP given intravenously works for paroxysmal supraventricular tachycardia by causing a transient AV block, and therefore preventing re-entrant atrial tachyarrhythmias (15).

ATP and its degradation products, ADP and adenosine, may help attenuate ischemic tissue trauma.

These compounds seem to slow the progression of ischemia involved in alterations of cellular energy and depletion of ATP stores (10066). ATP might also prevent cachexia in people with cancer by crossing the cell membrane and changing metabolic activity. Weight loss seems to occur due to conversion of glucose to lactate in peripheral tissues followed by gluconeogenesis from lactate in the liver. ATP seems to inhibit gluconeogenesis, which might contribute to maintenance of body fat and cell mass in people with cancer (9149,9151,9153,9159).

During intravenous infusion of 25 to 75 mcg/kg per minute, ATP is taken up by the erythrocytes and reaches dose-dependent plateau levels that are 1.5 to 1.7 times higher than baseline within 24 hours. After the infusion is stopped, the half-life of ATP in erythrocytes is 6 hours (9158). Preclinical research suggests that ATP might be active orally (9160).

Adverse Reactions

Intravenously, adenosine can cause general discomfort, breathing more deeply or frequently, headache, flushing, chest pressure or pain, and nausea. Sinus bradycardia and atrial fibrillation can also occur. Adenosine given by rapid intravenous injection can cause small but significant decreases in blood pressure and mean arterial pressure (9148). Intravenously, adenosine triphosphate (ATP) commonly causes dyspnea (sometimes severe) and chest pain, particularly at doses greater than 50 mcg/kg per minute (9154). Headache, palpitations, hypotension, nausea, sweating, flushing, lightheadedness, insomnia, coughing, and anxiety can also occur (9148,9151,9152,9154,9158). When given by rapid intravenous injection, adenosine and ATP adverse effects are likely to be mild and transient because of their extremely short half-lives (9148). Following intramuscular injection, adenosine monophosphate (AMP) can cause local erythema, rash, slight flushing, dizziness, diuresis, and palpitations. Hypotension, dyspnea, epigastric discomfort, and nausea may also occur. Anaphylactic reactions have also been reported (15).

Interactions with Herbs & Other Dietary Supplements

CAFFEINE-CONTAINING HERBS/SUPPLEMENTS: Concomitant use can decrease therapeutic effects of adenosine. Methylxanthines, such as caffeine, are competitive antagonists of adenosine on cell surface receptors (9157). It is recommended that caffeine-containing herbs be stopped 24 hours prior to pharmacological stress tests (11770). However, caffeine appears more likely to interfere with dipyridamole (Persantine) than adenosine-induced stress testing (11771). Herbs that contain caffeine include coffee, black tea, green tea, guarana, mate, and cola.

Interactions with Drugs

ANTIGOUT DRUGS: Adenosine triphosphate (ATP) can cause hyperuricemia and uricosuria, and might reduce the effectiveness of drugs used to prevent and treat gout (9152,9158). Some of these drugs are allopurinol (Zyloprim), colchicine, and probenecid (Benemid).

CARBAMAZEPINE (Tegretol): Carbamazepine given concurrently with adenosine might have an additive effect on heart block (15).

DIPYRIDAMOLE (Persantine): Dipyridamole decreases the metabolism of adenosine and can increase its pharmacologic and toxic effects. Intravenous infusion of adenosine in patients who are taking dipyridamole can cause dizziness, bradycardia, and syncope. Dipyridamole should be discontinued for several days prior to an adenosine heart scan (12209).

METHYLXANTHINES: Aminophylline, caffeine, and theophylline might block the effects of adenosine since methylxanthines are competitive antagonists of adenosine on cell surface receptors (9157). It is recommended that methylxanthines and methylxanthine-containing products be stopped 24 hours prior to pharmacological stress tests (11770). However, methylxanthines appear more likely to interfere with dipyridamole (Persantine) than adenosine-induced stress testing (11771).

Interactions with Foods

CAFFEINE: Caffeine might decrease the effectiveness of adenosine since caffeine and other methylxanthines are competitive antagonists for adenosine receptors (9157). It is recommended that caffeine-containing foods and beverages be stopped 24 hours prior to pharmacological stress tests (11770). However, caffeine appears more likely to interfere with dipyridamole (Persantine) than adenosine-induced stress testing (11771).

Interactions with Lab Tests

ELECTROCARDIOGRAM (ECG,EKG): Adenosine triphosphate (ATP) can cause EKG changes such as ST and T wave changes, which can indicate cardiac ischemia (9152).

URIC ACID: Adenosine triphosphate (ATP) can cause hyperuricemia and uricosuria (9152,9158).

Interactions with Diseases or Conditions

GOUT: Adenosine triphosphate (ATP) can cause hyperuricemia and uricosuria, and might precipitate gout (9152,9158).

HEART DISEASE: Adenosine triphosphate (ATP) can cause cardiac ischemia and chest pain. It might worsen symptoms in patients with heart diseases such as angina and myocardial infarction (9152).

Dosage and Administration

INTRAMUSCULAR: For symptomatic relief of varicose vein complications, adenosine monophosphate 25 mg once or twice weekly followed by 25 mg two to three times weekly has been used (15). For bursitis and tendonitis, adenosine monophosphate 20 mg one to three times daily or every hour for five doses on each of the first three days, followed by 20 mg daily as needed thereafter has been used. Alternatively, 100 mg daily for the first three days, followed by alternate day injections has been used (15).

INTRAVENOUS: For paroxysmal supraventricular tachycardia, adenosine 6 mg given rapidly over 1 to 2 minutes is used. If not effective within 1 to 2 minutes, 12 mg can be given and repeated if necessary. For use with thallium in pharmacologic cardiac stress testing, adenosine is given at a dose of 140 mcg/kg per minute over 6 minutes (total dose of 0.84 mg/kg) (15). For preventing cachexia in patients with advanced cancer, adenosine triphosphate (ATP) has been given every 2 to 4 weeks at a dose of up to 75mcg/kg per minute over 30 hours (9149,9151,9152).

Comments

Adenosine is used pharmacologically as adenosine base, and as the mono- and triphosphate salts. Do not confuse adenosine (Adenocard) with adenosine phosphate. They cannot be used interchangeably (15).

ADRENAL EXTRACT

Also Known As
ACE, Adrenal Complex, Adrenal Cortex Extract, Adrenal Factors, Adrenal Substance, Glandular, Whole Adrenal Extract.

Scientific Names
None.

People Use This For
Orally, adrenal extract is used for low adrenal function; fatigue; stress; impaired resistance to illness; and for treating severe allergies, asthma, eczema, psoriasis, rheumatoid arthritis, and other inflammatory conditions.
Sublingually, adrenal extract is used for stress induced fatigue or exhaustion, poor stress tolerance, general fatigue, allergies, auto-immune disorders, depression, physical or emotional stress, inflammation, low blood pressure, hypoglycemia, drug and alcohol withdrawal, and discontinuing cortisone drugs.
Intravenously, adrenal extract has been used for treating adrenal cortical insufficiency, hyperkalemia, ulcerative colitis, status thymicolymphaticus, and preventing spontaneous abortion.

Safety
LIKELY UNSAFE ...when used parenterally. Use of injectable adrenal extract has been associated with at least 50 cases of serious bacterial infections at injection sites (6620). Adrenal extracts are derived from animals so there is concern about contamination with diseased animal parts. So far, there are no reports of disease transmission to humans due to use of contaminated adrenal extracts.
There is insufficient reliable information available about the safety of adrenal extract for its other uses.
PREGNANCY AND LACTATION: Insufficient reliable information available; avoid using.

Effectiveness
There is insufficient reliable information available about the effectiveness of adrenal extract.

Mechanism of Action
Adrenal extracts are derived from raw cow, pig, or sheep adrenal glands gathered from slaughterhouses (6620).
No human studies are reported regarding the absorption or efficacy of adrenal extracts.

Adverse Reactions
Orally, no adverse reactions have been reported; however, adrenal extracts are derived from raw cow, pig, or sheep adrenal glands gathered from slaughterhouses and possibly from sick or diseased animals (6620). Products made from contaminated or diseased organs might present a human health hazard. There is also some concern that adrenal extracts produced from cows in countries where bovine spongiform encephalitis (BSE) has been reported might be contaminated with diseased tissue. Countries where BSE has been reported include Great Britain, France, The Netherlands, Portugal, Luxembourg, Ireland, Switzerland, Oman, Belgium, and others (1825); however, there have been no reports of BSE transfer to humans from contaminated adrenal extract products. Until more is known, tell patients to avoid these products unless country of origin can be determined. Patients should avoid products that are produced in countries where BSE has been found.
Intravenously, adrenal extract can cause infection and abscess at the site of injection (6620). In 1996, the FDA issued a nationwide alert regarding an injectable adrenal cortex extract after more than 50 cases of serious bacterial infections at injection sites were reported (6620).

Interactions with Herbs & Other Dietary Supplements
None known.

Interactions with Drugs
None known.

Interactions with Foods
None known.

Interactions with Lab Tests
None known.

Interactions with Diseases or Conditions
IMMUNODEFICIENCY: Theoretically, adrenal extracts might increase the risk of infection. Adrenal extracts might harbor pathogens. Injectable adrenal extract reportedly caused more than 50 serious infections at injection sites (6620); avoid using.

Dosage and Administration
No typical dosage.

ADRUE

Also Known As
Chintul, Guinea Rush, Jointed Flat Sedge, Piripiri.

Scientific Names
Cyperus articulatus, synonym Cyperus corymbosus.
Family: Cyperaceae.

Comments
At the date of publication, this product was not a common ingredient used in brand name supplements marketed to consumers. Details about this product are available in the online version of *Natural Medicines Comprehensive Database.* See www.naturaldatabase.com.

AFRICAN WILD POTATO

Also Known As
Bantu Tulip, Hypoxis Plant, South African Star Grass, Sterretjie.
CAUTION: See separate listing for Potato.

Scientific Names
Hypoxis hemerocallidea, synonym Hypoxis rooperi.
Family: Hypoxidaceae or Liliaceae

People Use This For
Orally, the African wild potato is used for bladder and urinary disorders including cystitis, prostate problems including prostatic hyperplasia and prostate cancer, lung disease, and cancer. It is also used in maintaining health in individuals who are HIV positive, for TB, "yuppie flu," arthritis, and psoriasis.
Topically, the African wild potato is used for wound healing.

Safety
POSSIBLY SAFE ...when used orally and appropriately. African wild potato has been taken with apparent safety for up to 18 months (5327,5328,7198).
PREGNANCY AND LACTATION: Insufficient reliable information available; avoid using.

Effectiveness
POSSIBLY EFFECTIVE

Benign prostatic hyperplasia (BPH). African wild potato taken orally, alone or in combination with other beta-sitosterol sources, seems to reduce urinary symptoms and improve quality of life (5327,5328,7198).

There is insufficient reliable information available about the effectiveness of African wild potato for its other uses.

Mechanism of Action
The African wild potato tuber contains 3.5%-4.5% lignans, particularly norlignan glucoside (5944). Preliminary human trials indicate the African wild potato glucoside constituent is non-toxic (4284). It also contains beta-sitosterol and beta-sitosterolin, and is sometimes used as a source of beta-sitosterol (5327,5328,7198). The activity of the African wild potato is attributed to the phytosterols that inhibit the production of prostaglandin synthase (5944). Animal research suggests that African wild potato might lower blood glucose levels, but this hasn't been seen in humans (11236).

Adverse Reactions
Orally, the African wild potato is usually well tolerated. In some patients it can cause nausea, indigestion, gas, diarrhea, or constipation (5327,5328). The beta-sitosterol constituent has been associated with erectile dysfunction and loss of libido (5942).

Interactions with Herbs & Other Dietary Supplements

CAROTENE, VITAMIN E: The beta-sitosterol may reduce absorption and blood levels of alpha- and beta-carotene and vitamin E (5814).
CHOLESTEROL LOWERING HERBS/SUPPLEMENTS: The beta-sitosterol constituent of African wild potato might have additive effects with herbs and supplements that also lower cholesterol levels (5331,5336). Some of these herbs and supplements include chromium, flaxseed, garlic, guar gum, niacin, oat bran, psyllium, red yeast, and others.

Interactions with Drugs

None known.

Interactions with Foods

CAROTENE, VITAMIN E: The beta-sitosterol constituent of African wild potato may reduce absorption and blood levels of alpha- and beta-carotene and vitamin E (5814).

Interactions with Lab Tests

CHOLESTEROL: The beta-sitosterol constituent of African wild potato may decrease total serum cholesterol and low-density lipoprotein (LDL) levels (5331,5336).

Interactions with Diseases or Conditions

SITOSTEROLEMIA (PHYTOSTEROLEMIA): The beta-sitosterol constituent of African wild potato can exacerbate sitosterolemia, a rare inherited lipid storage disease (5326,10305). People with this disorder have increased absorption of cholesterol and beta-sitosterol from the diet, and decreased clearance of beta-sitosterol. Total body stores of beta-sitosterol are increased up to 17-fold. Elevated hepatic beta-sitosterol levels competitively inhibit cholesterol catabolism, contributing to hypercholesterolemia (3663). Patients with sitosterolemia are prone to premature coronary artery disease and xanthomas (3661,3662). Beta-sitosterol and its glycoside sitosterolin are contraindicated in patients with sitosterolemia. However, beta-sitosterol appears to be safe for heterozygous carriers of sitosterolemia (10457).

Dosage and Administration

ORAL: For benign prostatic hyperplasia (BPH), African wild potato containing 60 to 130 mg of beta-sitosterol divided into 2-3 doses daily has been used (5327,5328).

Comments

The African wild potato is native to South Africa (5944).

AGA

Also Known As

Fly Agaric, Soma.

Scientific Names

Amanita muscaria.
Family: Amanitaceae.

People Use This For

Orally, aga is used as a hallucinogen. It is also used orally in homeopathic dilutions for nerve pain, fever, anxiety, alcohol poisoning, and joint pains.

Safety

UNSAFE ...when used orally (18).
PREGNANCY AND LACTATION: UNSAFE ...when used orally due to its toxicity (18); avoid using.

Effectiveness

There is insufficient reliable information available about the effectiveness of aga.

Mechanism of Action

The applicable part of aga is the fruiting body. Aga is not a true hallucinogen. The illusions that occur with aga ingestion are a misinterpretation of sensory stimuli. These mind altering effects are due to the isoxazoles ibotenic acid, muscimol, muscazone, and traces of muscarine (18).

Adverse Reactions
Orally, people develop symptoms within 30-90 minutes of using aga. The effects peak at 2-3 hours. Toxicity can occur after ingesting a single aga mushroom. Mind-altering effects have occurred with ingestion of 2-4 mushrooms, and 20 large mushrooms have been ingested with survival. Death due to aga ingestion is rare, less than 1%. The mushrooms can cause drowsiness, confusion, illusions, and mania (18).

Interactions with Herbs & Other Dietary Supplements
None known.

Interactions with Drugs
None known.

Interactions with Foods
None known.

Interactions with Lab Tests
None known.

Interactions with Diseases or Conditions
None known.

Dosage and Administration
No typical dosage.

Comments
Aga is a mushroom with a red cap that is spotted with white. It grows in sandy, acidic soils in the US. It is known as "fly agaric" because ibotenic acid and muscimol are toxic to the common housefly.

AGAR

Also Known As
Agar-Agar, Agarweed, Chinese Gelatin, Colle du Japon, Gelosa, Japanese Isinglas, Layor Carang, Vegetable Gelatin.

Scientific Names
Gelidiella acerosa; Gelidium amanasii; Gelidium cartilagineum; Gelidium crinale; Gelidium divaricatum; Gelidium pacificum; Gelidium vagum; Garacilaria confervoides.
Family: Sphaerococcaceae. Species of the genera Pterocladia; Ahnfeltia; Acanthopeltis; Suhria.

People Use This For
Orally, agar is used as a bulk laxative for chronic constipation.
In dentistry, agar is used to make dental impressions.
In manufacturing processes, agar is used as an ingredient in emulsions, suspensions, gels, and hydrophilic suppositories.

Safety
LIKELY SAFE ...when used orally with at least 250 mL of water (12).
PREGNANCY AND LACTATION: Insufficient reliable information available.

Effectiveness
EFFECTIVE

Constipation. Taking agar orally seems to help decrease constipation by producing a bulk laxative effect (11).

Mechanism of Action
Agar consists of two major polysaccharides, neutral agarose and charged agaropectin. Agarose is the gelling fraction (11).

Adverse Reactions
Potential to cause esophageal or bowel obstruction if taken with insufficient volume of water (12).
Possibly can increase cholesterol levels (11).

Interactions with Herbs & Other Dietary Supplements
None known.

Interactions with Drugs
ORAL DRUGS: The fiber in agar can impair absorption of oral drugs (19).

Interactions with Foods
None known.

Interactions with Lab Tests
None known.

Interactions with Diseases or Conditions
BOWEL OBSTRUCTION OR DIFFICULTY SWALLOWING: Contraindicated (12).

Dosage and Administration
ORAL: A typical dose is 4-16 grams, one to two times daily (12). Take each dose with at least 250 mL of water (11).

AGRIMONY

Also Known As
Ackerkraut, Agrimoniae herba, Agromonia, Cocklebur, Fragrant Agrimony, Funffing, Funffingerkraut, Herba Agrimoniae, Herba Eupatoriae, Herbe d'Aigremoine, Herbe de Saint-Guillaume, Liverwort, Stickwort.
CAUTION: See separate listings for Hemp Agrimony, Liverwort, and Potentilla.

Scientific Names
Agrimonia eupatoria; Agrimonia procera, synonym Agrimonia odorata.
Family: Rosaceae.

People Use This For
Orally, agrimony is used for sore throat, upset stomach, mild diarrhea, gallbladder disorders, tuberculosis, bleeding, corns, warts, as a gargle, antitumor agent, cardiotonic, diuretic, sedative, and antihistamine.
Topically, agrimony is used as a mild astringent and for mild skin inflammation. The ethanolic extracts of agrimony are used for their antiviral properties.

Safety
LIKELY SAFE ...when the dried above ground parts are used orally and appropriately short-term (2,12). ...when used topically (2).
POSSIBLY UNSAFE ...when used orally or topically in excessive doses due to its high tannin content (12).
PREGNANCY AND LACTATION: POSSIBLY UNSAFE ...when used orally because of the possible effects on the menstrual cycle (4,12).

Effectiveness
There is insufficient reliable information available about the effectiveness of agrimony.

Mechanism of Action
The applicable parts of agrimony are the dried, above ground parts. The aerial plant parts contain 4% to 10% condensed tannins which can account for its astringent properties (6). Because of the tannin content and astringent properties of agrimony, it is thought to be helpful for gastrointestinal conditions such as diarrhea.

Adverse Reactions
The use of agrimony can cause photodermatitis and can affect blood pressure (6).

Interactions with Herbs & Other Dietary Supplements
None known.

Interactions with Drugs
ANTIDIABETES DRUGS: Monitor blood glucose levels closely due to claims that agrimony has hypoglycemic effects (19).

Interactions with Foods
None known.

Interactions with Lab Tests
None known.

Interactions with Diseases or Conditions
None known.

Dosage and Administration
ORAL: The typical dosage of agrimony is 3 grams per day (2).
TOPICAL: A poultice is commonly applied several times daily using approximately 10% water extract, which is prepared by boiling the herb at low heat for 10-20 minutes (8).

AHCC

Also Known As
Basidiomycetes Extract, Fungi Extract.

Scientific Names
Active hexose correlated compound.

People Use This For
Orally, AHCC is used for cancer and liver damage.

Safety
There is insufficient reliable information available about the safety of AHCC.

Effectiveness
There is insufficient reliable information available about the effectiveness of AHCC.

Mechanism of Action
AHCC is an extract derived from fungi in the Basidiomycetes family. AHCC is a mixture of polysaccharides, amino acids, lipids, and minerals. Oligosaccharides make up about 74% of AHCC (13093).
AHCC is thought to act as a biological response modifier. AHCC seems to have antioxidant effects. It also seems to increase activity of natural killer (NK) cells in patients with cancer. In animal models, it also seems to protect against carbon tetrachloride-induced liver damage, prevent diabetes, and decrease thymic apoptosis induced by dexamethasone (13093).
The precise mechanism of action of AHCC is not known.

Adverse Reactions
None reported.

Interactions with Herbs & Other Dietary Supplements
None known.

Interactions with Drugs
None known.

Interactions with Foods
None known.

Interactions with Lab Tests
None known.

Interactions with Diseases or Conditions
None known.

Dosage and Administration
No typical dose.

Comments
AHCC is commonly used in Traditionally Chinese medicine (TCM).

ALCHEMILLA

Also Known As
Feuilles d'Alchemille, Frauenmantelkraut, Lady's Mantle, Leontopodium, Lion's Foot, Marienmantel, Nine Hooks, Silerkraut, Stellaria.
CAUTION: See separate listing for Alpine Lady's Mantle.

Scientific Names
Alchemilla xanthochlora; Alchemilla vulgaris.
Family: Rosaceae.

People Use This For
Orally, alchemilla is used for mild diarrhea, heavy menstrual flow, diabetes, menopausal complaints, painful menses, gastrointestinal disorders, as a relaxant for muscle spasms, an anti-inflammatory, a diuretic, and as a gargle for mouth and throat inflammation.
Topically, alchemilla is used as an astringent for bleeding, to improve wound healing, for ulcers, eczema, skin rashes, and as a bath additive for treating lower-abdominal ailments.

Safety
POSSIBLY SAFE ...when used orally and appropriately. Alchemilla has been used for many years without reports of significant toxicity (6,8,12).
There is insufficient reliable information available about the safety of the topical use of alchemilla.
PREGNANCY AND LACTATION: Insufficient reliable information available; avoid using.

Effectiveness
There is insufficient reliable information available about the effectiveness of alchemilla.

Mechanism of Action
The applicable parts of alchemilla are the above ground parts. Alchemilla contains 6-8% tannins (8), which might account for its perceived astringent activity (6). An aqueous extract of Alchemilla xanthochlora demonstrates lipid peroxidation and superoxide anion scavenging activity (6). Flavonoid extracts inhibit proteolytic enzymes, including elastase, trypsin, and alpha-chymotrypsin. This property suggests alchemilla might have a role in protecting conjunctive and elastic tissues (6).

Adverse Reactions
Rarely, alchemilla can cause liver damage (8).

Interactions with Herbs & Other Dietary Supplements
None known.

Interactions with Drugs
None known.

Interactions with Foods
None known.

Interactions with Lab Tests
None known.

Interactions with Diseases or Conditions
None known.

Dosage and Administration
ORAL: For diarrhea, a typical dose is one cup tea, prepared by steeping 1-4 grams above ground parts in boiling water for 10 minutes and then straining (8), used up to three times per day between meals. The average amount used per day is 5-10 grams. Equivalent preparations can also be used (2). Diarrhea persisting for more than 3-4 days should be medically evaluated (8).
TOPICAL: No typical dosage.

Comments
Although the German Standard License warns about possible liver damage, some experts consider the concern to be exaggerated (8).

ALDER BUCKTHORN

Also Known As

Alder Dogwood, Arrow Wood, Black Dogwood, Buckthorn, Dog Wood, Frangula, Frangulae Cortex, Glossy Buckthorn.
CAUTION: See separate listings for European Buckthorn, Sea Buckthorn, and Cascara.

Scientific Names

Frangula alnus, synonym Rhamnus frangula.
Family: Rhamnaceae.

People Use This For

Orally, alder buckthorn is used as a laxative, as a tonic, and as a component in the Hoxsey cancer formula.

Safety

LIKELY SAFE ...when used orally and appropriately for no more than 8 to 10 days (12). Only properly aged bark should be used, and the recommended dose should not be exceeded (12).
POSSIBLY UNSAFE ...when used orally for more than 8 to 10 days (12).
CHILDREN: LIKELY UNSAFE ...when used orally in children younger than 12 years of age (12); avoid using.
PREGNANCY AND LACTATION: LIKELY UNSAFE ...when used orally (12); avoid using.

Effectiveness

POSSIBLY EFFECTIVE

Constipation. Taking alder buckthorn orally seems to relieve constipation (3,4,7,12). Alder buckthorn has laxative effects comparable to cascara (3).

There is insufficient reliable information available about the effectiveness of alder buckthorn for its other uses.

Mechanism of Action

The applicable part of alder buckthorn is the bark. The anthraglycosides and particularly the diglycosides are cathartic in the large intestine (1,8,11). They can increase intestinal motility by inhibiting stationary contractions, stimulating propulsive contractions, stimulating active chloride secretion, and increasing water and electrolytes in the intestinal contents (2). The fresh bark contains free anthrone, which can cause severe vomiting and is destroyed by aging the bark naturally for one year or artificially with heat and aeration (2). Anthroid laxative use is not associated with an increased risk of developing colorectal adenoma or carcinoma (6138).

Adverse Reactions

Orally, alder buckthorn can cause cramp-like discomfort (2). Chronic use can cause pseudomelanosis coli (pigment spots in intestinal mucosa) which is harmless, usually reverses with discontinuation (2), and is not associated with an increased risk of developing colorectal ademoma or carcinoma (6138). Chronic use or abuse of the bark can lead to potassium depletion, albuminuria, and hematuria. Potassium depletion can lead to disturbed heart function and muscle weakness (2). The fresh or improperly aged bark can cause severe vomiting due to the presence of the free anthrone, an emetic constituent.

Interactions with Herbs & Other Dietary Supplements

LICORICE: Concomitant use of alder buckthorn with licorice can increase the risk of potassium depletion (2).
POTASSIUM DEPLETING HERBS: Theoretically, concomitant use of alder buckthorn with horsetail plant or licorice rhizome increases the risk of potassium depletion.
STIMULANT LAXATIVE HERBS: Theoretically, concomitant use of alder buckthorn with other stimulant laxative herbs can increase the risk of potassium depletion. Stimulant laxative herbs include aloe dried leaf sap, wild cucumber fruit (Ecballium elaterium), blue flag rhizome, butternut bark, cascara bark, castor oil, colocynth fruit pulp, gamboge bark exudate, jalap root, black root, manna bark exudate, podophyllum root, rhubarb root, senna leaves and pods, and yellow dock root (19).

Interactions with Drugs

CORTICOSTEROIDS: Concomitant use of corticosteroids with alder buckthorn can increase the risk of potassium depletion (2).
DIGOXIN (Lanoxin): Theoretically, overuse or abuse of alder buckthorn can increase the risk of adverse effects from cardiac glycoside drugs (19).
DIURETIC DRUGS: Overuse of alder buckthorn might compound diuretic-induced potassium loss (19).
There is some concern that people taking alder buckthorn along with potassium depleting diuretics might have an increased risk for hypokalemia. Initiation of potassium supplementation or an increase in potassium supplement dose may be necessary for some patients. Some diuretics that can deplete potassium include chlorothiazide (Diuril), chlorthalidone (Thalitone), furosemide (Lasix), and hydrochlorothiazide (HCTZ, HydroDIURIL, Microzide), and others.

ORAL DRUGS: Theoretically, alder buckthorn can reduce absorption of some drugs due to reduced gastrointestinal transit time (19).
STIMULANT LAXATIVES: Concomitant use might compound fluid and electrolyte loss (19).

Interactions with Foods
None known.

Interactions with Lab Tests
COLORIMETRIC TESTS: Alder buckthorn can discolor urine (pink, red, purple, orange, rust), interfering with diagnostic tests that depend on a color change, due to its anthraquinone content (1,12,275).
POTASSIUM: Excessive use of alder buckthorn can cause potassium depletion, reducing serum potassium concentrations and test results (1,2,4,12,19).

Interactions with Diseases or Conditions
GI CONDITIONS: Alder buckthorn is contraindicated in individuals with intestinal obstruction; abdominal pain of unknown origin; and intestinal inflammation, including appendicitis, Crohn's disease, irritable bowel syndrome (IBS), and ulcerative colitis (12).

Dosage and Administration
ORAL: The typical dose of alder buckthorn is 0.5-2.5 grams of the dried bark (4) or as a tea, which is prepared by steeping 2 grams of the herb in 150 mL boiling water for 5-10 minutes and then straining (12). The average dose per day of the bark is 1 gram (3) or 20-30 mg of the hydoxyanthracene derivatives calculated as glycofrangulin A (2). The common dose of the liquid extract: (1:1 in 25% alcohol) is 2-5 mL three times daily (2). The individual dose of the bark is the minimum amount required to produce a soft stool (2). Limit its use to a maximum of seven to ten days. This preparation should be used only if no effect can be obtained through change of diet or the use of bulk-forming laxative products (2).

Comments
Avoid confusion with European buckthorn. The American Herbal Products Association (AHPA) recommends the following label statement: "Do not use this product if you have abdominal pain or diarrhea. Consult a healthcare provider prior to use if you are pregnant or nursing. Discontinue use in the event of diarrhea or watery stools. Do not exceed dose. Not for long-term use." (12). Today, alder buckthorn is primarily used as a dye.

ALETRIS

Also Known As
Ague, Aloerot, Blazing Star, Colic Root, Crow Corn, Devil's-bit, Stargrass, Starwort, True Unicorn Root, Whitetube Stargrass.

Scientific Names
Aletris farinosa.
Family: Liliaceae or Nartheciaceae.

People Use This For
Orally, aletris is used for rheumatism, as a general tonic, a sedative, to relieve menstrual disorders, as a laxative, an antiflatulent, an antispasmodic, for colic, as an antidiarrheal, and a diuretic. It is also used orally for infertility, dyspepsia, and to prevent miscarriage.

Safety
POSSIBLY SAFE ...when used orally and appropriately (6,12).
PREGNANCY AND LACTATION: POSSIBLY UNSAFE ...when used orally due to the possibility that aletris contains components that cause estrogenic activity (11) and oxytocin (Pitocin) antagonism (12); avoid using.

Effectiveness
There is insufficient reliable information available about the effectiveness of aletris.

Mechanism of Action
The applicable part of aletris is the root. Some aletris constituents may have estrogenic activity (6).

Adverse Reactions
Orally, small doses of aletris may induce colic, stupefaction, and vertigo (6).

Interactions with Herbs & Other Dietary Supplements
None known.

Interactions with Drugs

ANTACIDS: Theoretically, due to reports that aletris increases stomach acid, aletris might decrease the effectiveness of antacids (19).
H2-BLOCKERS: Theoretically, due to reports that aletris increases stomach acid, aletris might decrease the effectiveness of H2-blockers (19). The H2 blockers include cimetidine (Tagamet), ranitidine (Zantac), nizatidine (Axid), and famotidine (Pepcid).
PROTON PUMP INHIBITORS (PPIs): Theoretically, due to reports that aletris increases stomach acid, aletris might decrease the effectiveness of PPIs (19). PPIs include omeprazole (Prilosec), lansoprazole (Prevacid), rabeprazole (Aciphex), pantoprazole (Protonix), and esomeprazole (Nexium).

Interactions with Foods

None known.

Interactions with Lab Tests

None known.

Interactions with Diseases or Conditions

GASTROINTESTINAL (GI) DISEASES: Aletris can irritate the GI tract. It is contraindicated in individuals with infectious or inflammatory GI conditions (19).
HORMONE SENSITIVE CANCERS/CONDITIONS: Aletris might have estrogenic effects (6). Women with hormone sensitive conditions should avoid aletris. Some of these conditions include breast cancer, uterine cancer, ovarian cancer, endometriosis, and uterine fibroids.

Dosage and Administration

ORAL: Aletris is typically used as the powdered root, a liquid extract, and an infusion (18). One common dosage recommendation is 0.3 to 0.6 grams three times daily (18). The infusion is prepared by adding 1.5 grams of aletris to 100 mL of water, and the fluid extract (1:1) is commonly produced with 45% ethanol water (18).

ALFALFA

Also Known As

Feuille De Luzerne, Lucerne, Medicago, Phytoestrogen, Purple Medick.

Scientific Names

Medicago sativa.
Family: Fabaceae/Leguminosae.

People Use This For

Orally, alfalfa is used as a diuretic, for kidney conditions, bladder and prostate conditions, asthma, arthritis, rheumatoid arthritis, diabetes, indigestion, and thrombocytopenic purpura. It is also used orally as a source of vitamins A, C, E, and K4; and minerals calcium, potassium, phosphorous, and iron.

Safety

LIKELY SAFE ...when the above ground parts are used orally and appropriately (4,6,12).
LIKELY UNSAFE ...when excessive amounts of seeds are used. The seed have been associated with pancytopenia (5,6).
PREGNANCY AND LACTATION: POSSIBLY UNSAFE ...when used orally in medicinal amounts. Alfalfa contains constituents with possible estrogenic activity (4,11).

Effectiveness

POSSIBLY EFFECTIVE

Hypercholesterolemia. Taking alfalfa seeds orally seems to lower total cholesterol and low-density lipoprotein (LDL) cholesterol in patients with high cholesterol levels (5816).

There is insufficient reliable information available about the effectiveness of alfalfa for its other uses.

Mechanism of Action

The applicable parts of alfalfa are the above ground parts. The alfalfa leaf contains saponins which appear to decrease plasma cholesterol without creating a change in HDL levels (4). Constituents of alfalfa seem to decrease cholesterol absorption, and increase excretion of neutral steroids and bile acids (4,6). Alfalfa contains manganese which might be responsible for hypoglycemic effects (4). Alfalfa contains medicagol which appears to have antifungal properties. Alfalfa also contains isoflavonoids including coumetrol, genistein, biochanin A, and daidzein which all seem to have estrogenic properties (11).

Adverse Reactions
Alfalfa might cause photosensitivity (605). Ingestion of ground alfalfa seeds is associated with a case of pancytopenia (381). Stems and leaves are reportedly free of systemic lupus erythematosus (SLE) triggering substance(s) found in seeds (4). There is one case report of listeriosis traced to the consumption of contaminated alfalfa tablets from which Listeria monocytogenes was isolated (5600).

Interactions with Herbs & Other Dietary Supplements
HERBS WITH CLOTTING POTENTIAL: Excessive use of herbs that contain vitamin K, an essential coagulation factor, can increase the risk of clotting in people using anticoagulants. These herbs include alfalfa, parsley, nettle, plantain, and others.
VITAMIN E: Alfalfa contains saponins which interfere with the absorption or activity of vitamin E (11).

Interactions with Drugs
CONTRACEPTIVE DRUGS: Excessive doses of alfalfa may interfere with contraceptive drugs. Alfalfa contains isoflavonoids with estrogenic effects (4).
ESTROGENS: Excessive doses of alfalfa may interfere with hormone therapy due to estrogenic effects of isoflavonoids alfalfa (4).
PHOTOSENSITIZING DRUGS: Excessive doses of alfalfa may potentiate drug-induced photosensitivity (605).
WARFARIN (Coumadin): Alfalfa contains large amount of vitamin K (4,6). Concomitant use can reduce the anticoagulant activity of warfarin.

Interactions with Foods
None known.

Interactions with Lab Tests
CHOLESTEROL: Alfalfa seed might lower serum cholesterol concentrations and test results in individuals with type II hyperlipoproteinemia (4).

Interactions with Diseases or Conditions
DIABETES: Alfalfa might reduce blood sugar levels; monitor closely (4).
HORMONE SENSITIVE CANCERS/CONDITIONS: Because alfalfa seems to have estrogenic effects (11), women with hormone sensitive conditions should avoid alfalfa. Some of these conditions include breast, uterine, and ovarian cancer, and endometriosis and uterine fibroids.
KIDNEY TRANSPLANT: There is one report of acute kidney transplant rejection in a patient who took black cohosh and an alfalfa supplement together. The mechanism for this disease interaction is not known, but it is more likely due to alfalfa than black cohosh. Alfalfa is thought to have immune stimulating effects that might counteract the immunosuppressant effects of cyclosporine (12174).
SYSTEMIC LUPUS ERYTHEMATOSUS (SLE): Consumption of seeds (not stems/leaves) might reactivate latent disease (6,605).

Dosage and Administration
ORAL: A typical dosage is 5-10 grams, or as steeped strained tea, three times a day (4).
Liquid extract (1:1 in 25% alcohol) 5-10 mL three times a day has also been used (4).

ALGIN

Also Known As
Alginates, Sodium Alginate.
CAUTION: See separate listings for Laminaria and Bladderwrack.

Scientific Names
Ascophyllum nodosum; Laminaria digitata; Macrocystis pyrifera.
Family: Lessoniaceae.

People Use This For
Orally, algin is used to lower serum cholesterol levels and to reduce absorption of strontium, barium, tin, cadmium, manganese, zinc, and mercury. Algin is also orally for the prevention and treatment of hypertension.
In foods, algin is used in candy, gelatins, puddings, condiments, relishes, processed vegetables, fish products, and imitation dairy products.
In manufacturing, algin is used as a binding and disintegrating agent in tablets, as binding and demulcent in lozenges, and as film in peel-off facial masks.

Safety
LIKELY SAFE ...when used orally in amounts typically found in foods (11).
PREGNANCY AND LACTATION: Insufficient reliable information available.

Effectiveness
There is insufficient reliable information available about the effectiveness of algin.

Mechanism of Action
Algin is the purified carbohydrate product extracted from brown seaweed by use of dilute alkali. Algin is comprised of the sodium salt of alginic acid, a linear polymer of L-guluronic and D-mannuronic acid. Although mannuronic acid is the major component, there is variation depending on the algal source (13). Cholesterol lowering effects may be related to viscosity of gel and inhibiting cholesterol absorption (11). Hypotensive effects may be due to laminine dioxalate (11). Algin is believed, but not confirmed, to be indigestible (11).

Adverse Reactions
None reported.

Interactions with Herbs & Other Dietary Supplements
None known.

Interactions with Drugs
ORAL DRUGS: The fiber in algin can impair absorption of oral drugs (19).

Interactions with Foods
None known.

Interactions with Lab Tests
BLOOD PRESSURE: Theoretically, algin might lower blood pressure and blood pressure readings (11).
CHOLESTEROL: Theoretically, algin might reduce serum cholesterol concentrations and test results (11).

Interactions with Diseases or Conditions
None known.

Dosage and Administration
No typical dosage.

Comments
Algin is isolated from a variety of brown algae (seaweeds, Class: Phaeophyceae), particularly from the genera Ascophyllum, Macrocystis, and Laminaria (11).

ALKANNA

Also Known As
Alkanet, Alkanna Radix, Anchusa, Dyer's Bugloss, Henna, Orchanet, Radix Anchusae.
CAUTION: See separate listing for Henna.

Scientific Names
Alkanna tinctoria, synonyms Alkanna lehmanii, Alkanna tuberculata, Anchusa bracteolata, Anchusa tuberculata, Lithospermum lehmanii.
Family: Boraginaceae.

People Use This For
Orally, alkanna is used for diarrhea and gastric ulcers.
Topically, alkanna is used to heal skin wounds, as an astringent, and for skin diseases.

Safety

LIKELY UNSAFE ...when products containing hepatotoxic pyrrolizidine alkaloid (PA) constituents are used orally. Repeated exposure to low concentrations of hepatotoxic PAs can cause severe veno-occlusive disease. Hepatotoxic PAs might also be carcinogenic and mutagenic (12841,12842). Tell patients not to use alkanna preparations that are not certified and labeled as hepatotoxic PA-free. ...when products containing hepatotoxic PAs are used topically on abraded or broken skin. Absorption of hepatotoxic PAs through broken skin can lead to systemic toxicities (12841). Tell patients not to use topical alkanna preparations that are not certified and labeled as hepatotoxic PA-free. There is insufficient reliable information available about the safety of topical UPA-free alkanna on unbroken skin.

PREGNANCY: LIKELY UNSAFE ...when used orally. Alkanna preparations containing hepatotoxic pyrrolizidine alkaloid (PA) constituents might be teratogenic and hepatotoxic (12841,12842). There is insufficient reliable information available about the safety of alkanna products that do not contain hepatotoxic PAs when used during pregnancy.

LACTATION: LIKELY UNSAFE ...when used orally. Hepatotoxic pyrrolizidine alkaloid (PA) constituents in alkanna are excreted in breast-milk (12841,12842). There is insufficient reliable information available about the safety of alkanna products that are PA-free during lactation; avoid using.

Effectiveness

There is insufficient reliable information available about the effectiveness of alkanna.

Mechanism of Action

The applicable part of alkanna is the root. Alkanna contains alkannin and shikonin, which might have antioxidant activity and anti-inflammatory activity (12853).

Alkanna contains various pyrrolizidine alkaloids (PAs), some of which are toxic. PAs are most concentrated in the plant roots, but may be found in all plant parts. PAs, particularly unsaturated PAs, can cause hepatotoxicity. Cyclic diesters such as retrorsine and senecionine are the most hepatotoxic. Liver toxicity may result from PA-enhanced oxidative stress, but the exact mechanism of toxicity is unknown. Single doses of 10 to 20 mg PAs or chronic ingestion of amounts less than 10 mcg can cause veno-occlusive disease. PAs are metabolized by cytochrome P450 3A4 (CYP3A4) to toxic dehydroalkaloids and pyrroles. Enzyme inducers such as phenobarbital seem to enhance toxicity (12841,12860). Pyrroles are excreted as N-acetyl cysteine conjugates. Some researchers speculate that early administration of N-acetyl cysteine might reduce toxicity (11988). Metabolism is also affected by pregnane X receptor induction of CYP3A4. Genetic or drug induced variation in CYP3A4 or pregnane X receptor activity can affect the degree of PA toxicity by increasing or decreasing its metabolism (12841,12842). Hepatotoxic PAs are also toxic to the lungs. Pneumotoxicity occurs as pulmonary hypertension and right ventricular hypertrophy. Hepatotoxic PAs are carcinogenic and mutagenic. There are sufficient amounts of hepatotoxic PAs in herbal products to cause toxicity (12841,12842).

Adverse Reactions

Orally, alkanna might cause toxicity. The major concern about alkanna preparations is the hepatotoxic pyrrolizidine alkaloid (PA) content. These constituents are hepatotoxic, pneumotoxic, carcinogenic, and mutagenic (12841,12842). Chronic exposure to other plants containing hepatotoxic PA constituents is associated with veno-occlusive disease (4021). Subacute veno-occlusive disease causes vague symptoms with persistent liver enlargement (4021). Symptoms of acute veno-occlusive disease include colicky pains in epigastrium, vomiting and diarrhea, and ascites formation within several days. Enlargement and induration of the liver occurs within a few weeks (12842).

Interactions with Herbs & Other Dietary Supplements

HEPATOTOXIC PYRROLIZIDINE ALKALOID (PA)-CONTAINING HERBS: Concomitant use is contraindicated due to the risk of additive toxicity. Herbs containing hepatotoxic PAs include borage, butterbur, coltsfoot, comfrey, gravel root, hemp agrimony, hound's tongue, and the Senecio species plants dusty miller, alpine ragwort, groundsel, golden ragwort, and tansy ragwort (12841).

HERBS THAT INDUCE CYTOCHROME P450 3A4 (CYP3A4): Theoretically, herbs that induce CYP3A4 might increase the conversion of hepatotoxic PAs to toxic metabolites, enhancing toxicity (12841,12860). Herbs that induce CYP3A4 include St. John's wort and garlic.

Interactions with Drugs

CYTOCHROME P450 3A4 (CYP3A4) INDUCERS: Hepatotoxic pyrrolizidine alkaloids (PAs) are substrates of cytochrome P450 3A4 (CYP3A4) (12841,12860). Theoretically, drugs that induce CYP3A4 might increase the conversion of PAs to toxic metabolites. Some drugs that induce CYP3A4 include carbamazepine (Tegretol), phenobarbital, phenytoin (Dilantin), rifampin, rifabutin (Mycobutin), and others.

Interactions with Foods

None known.

Interactions with Lab Tests
None known.

Interactions with Diseases or Conditions
LIVER DISEASE: Theoretically, hepatotoxic pyrrolizidine alkaloids (PAs) might exacerbate liver disease (12841,12842).

Dosage and Administration
No typical dosage.

ALLSPICE

Also Known As
Aqua Pimentae, Clove Pepper, Jamaica Pepper, Kiln-Dried Allspice, Pimenta, Pimento, Spanish Pimienta, Water of Pimento.

Scientific Names
Pimenta dioica, synonyms Pimenta officinalis, Eugenia pimenta.
Family: Myrtaceae.

People Use This For
Orally, allspice is used for dyspepsia, flatulence, menorrhagia, vomiting, diarrhea, fever, colds, and as a purgative. It is also used orally for hypertension, diabetes, abdominal pain, and obesity.
Topically, allspice is used for muscle pain, toothache, and as an antiseptic.
In dentistry, some dentists use eugenol, a constituent of allspice, as a local antiseptic for teeth and gums.
In foods, allspice is used as an aromatic spice.
In manufacturing, it is used in toothpaste as a flavoring.

Safety
LIKELY SAFE ...when used orally in amounts commonly found in foods. Allspice has Generally Recognized As Safe status (GRAS) the US (4912).
There is insufficient reliable information available about the safety of allspice used medicinally.
PREGNANCY AND LACTATION: There is insufficient reliable information available about the safety of allspice used medicinally during pregnancy and lactation.

Effectiveness
There is insufficient reliable information available about the effectiveness of allspice.

Mechanism of Action
The applicable parts of allspice are the unripe fruit (berries) and leaf. Allspice contains eugenol, which might explain some of its traditional uses for toothache, muscle pain, and as an antiseptic (12889,12890).
Eugenol might also contribute to the antioxidant and antimutagenic properties of allspice that are suggested by preliminary research (12890).
Preliminary research suggests that allspice leaf has hypotensive properties (12891).

Adverse Reactions
Topically, allspice can cause allergic dermatitis in sensitive people (12635).

Interactions with Herbs & Other Dietary Supplements
None known.

Interactions with Drugs
ANTICOAGULANT/ANTIPLATELET DRUGS: Theoretically, combining allspice with an antiplatelet or anticoagulant drug might increase the risk of bleeding. Eugenol, a constituent of allspice, is reported to have antiplatelet activity; however, this interaction has not been reported in humans (12889). Antiplatelet agents include aspirin, clopidogrel (Plavix), dipyridamole (Persantine), ticlopidine (Ticlid), and others. Anticoagulant agents include heparin and warfarin (Coumadin).

Interactions with Foods
None known.

Interactions with Lab Tests
None known.

Interactions with Diseases or Conditions

None known.

Dosage and Administration

No typical dosage.

ALOE

Also Known As

Aloe Capensis, Aloe Perfoliata, Burn Plant, Cape Aloe, Elephant's Gall, Ghrita-Kumari, Hsiang-Dan, Kanya, Kumari, Lily of the Desert, Lu-Hui, Miracle Plant, Plant of Immortality.

Scientific Names

Aloe vera, synonyms Aloe barbadensis, Aloe indica; Aloe africana; Aloe arborescens, synonyms Aloe natalenis, Aloe frutescens, Aloe ucriae; Aloe ferox, synonym Aloe supralaevis; Aloe perryi; Aloe spicata.
Family: Aloaceae or Asphodelaceae.

People Use This For

Orally, aloe is used for osteoarthritis, inflammatory bowel diseases including ulcerative colitis, fever, itching and inflammation, and as a general tonic. Aloe is also used orally for gastroduodenal ulcers, diabetes, asthma, and radiation-related mucositis. Aloe latex is used orally as a laxative for constipation, epilepsy, asthma, colds, bleeding, amenorrhea, colitis, depression, diabetes, glaucoma, multiple sclerosis, hemorrhoids, varicose veins, bursitis, osteoarthritis, and vision problems.
Topically, aloe is used for burns, wound healing, psoriasis, sunburn, frostbite, inflammation, osteoarthritis, and cold sores. It is also applied topically as an antiseptic and as a moisturizer.

Safety

POSSIBLY SAFE ...when used orally or topically, and appropriately (11982,11984).
LIKELY UNSAFE ...when used orally in high doses. Ingesting aloe latex 1 gram/day for several days can cause nephritis, acute renal failure, and death (8,8961).
CHILDREN: POSSIBLY UNSAFE ...when used orally in children. Children younger than 12 years may experience abdominal pain, cramps, and diarrhea (4).
PREGNANCY: POSSIBLY UNSAFE ...when used orally. There is some concern based in anecdotal reports that aloe latex might induce abortion and stimulate menstruation (8,19).
LACTATION: POSSIBLY UNSAFE ...when used orally. Genotoxic aloe-emodin might pass into breast-milk; avoid using (4,19).

Effectiveness

POSSIBLY EFFECTIVE

Constipation. Taking aloe latex orally as a stimulant laxative seems to relieve constipation due to the cathartic effects of the anthraquinones in the aloe (4,5,8).

Psoriasis. Applying aloe extract 0.5% cream topically 3 times daily for 4 weeks significantly improves and increases the resolution of psoriatic plaques compared to placebo (101,12096). Aloe extract cream seems to reduce desquamation, erythema, and infiltration (12096).

INSUFFICIENT RELIABLE EVIDENCE to RATE

Burns. Applying aloe gel topically seems to improve healing of partial thickness burns (101).

Diabetes. Preliminary evidence suggests that taking one tablespoon (15 mL) of aloe gel daily for 42 days can significantly decrease blood glucose levels in women with type 2 diabetes (12164).

Frostbite. Applying aloe gel topically seems to enhance tissue survival following frostbite injury (101).

Genital herpes. There is some evidence that applying aloe extract 0.5% cream 3 times daily increases healing rates compared to aloe gel or placebo. Some patients heal within 5 days of use compared to 12 days with placebo (12164).

Hyperlipidemia. Preliminary evidence suggests that taking 10 mL or 20 mL of aloe orally daily for 12 weeks can reduce total cholesterol by about 15%, low-density lipoprotein (LDL) cholesterol by about 18%, and triglycerides by about 25% to 30% in patients with hyperlipidemia (12164).

Pressure ulcers. Preliminary evidence suggests that applying aloe gel does not improve the healing rate of pressure ulcers compared to management with moist saline gauze (12160).

Radiation-induced skin toxicity. Radiation therapy for cancer often causes erythema, skin desquamation, and itching. Applying 98% aloe gel three times daily throughout radiation treatment and after treatment does not seem to reduce these radiation-related side effects in patients being treated for breast cancer (12098,12163). Applying 100% aloe gel 6-8 times per day also does not seem to reduce these radiation related side effects in people treated for other cancers. Some evidence suggests that aloe gel might prolong the time before radiation-related side effects occur (12159).

Ulcerative colitis. Preliminary evidence suggests that some patients with mild to moderate ulcerative colitis who take aloe gel 25-50 mL twice daily have significantly reduced symptoms (11984).
Wound healing. Applying an aloe gel extract (Carrington Dermal Wound Gel) to surgical wounds might actually delay wound healing (11982).
More evidence is needed to rate aloe for these uses.

Mechanism of Action

The applicable parts of aloe are the gel and latex.
Aloe gel is the clear, jelly-like substance obtained from the thin-walled mucilaginous cells in the center of the leaf. The active constituents include emodin anthrone, dithranol, chrysarobin, and allantoin (10377,11982).
Aloe latex is obtained from the cells just beneath the leaf skin. Aloe latex belongs to the anthraquinone family of laxatives and contains a tricyclic anthracene nucleus (16). It is likely that the anthracene derivatives are cleaved into aloe-emodin anthrone in the colon. Anthrones irritate mucous membranes, causing increased mucous secretion and peristalsis. Aloe latex increases motility of the colon and therefore, increases propulsion and reduces transit time. It also causes fluids and electrolytes to be secreted in the lumen causing a feeling of distention. The cathartic effects occur within 10 hours. Water and electrolyte reabsorption are inhibited (8).
Aloe latex causes a loss of potassium from cells paralyzing the intestinal muscles. With continued use, increasing doses are needed for a laxative effect (8). Anthranoid laxatives have not been associated with an increased risk of developing colorectal adenoma or carcinoma (6138).
The carboxypeptidase and salicylate components of aloe gel can inhibit bradykinin, a pain-producing agent. The magnesium lactate component can inhibit histamine, which may reduce itching (101). The C-glucosyl chromone component appears to reduce topical inflammation (8223).
Aloe gel might inhibit the synthesis of thromboxane A2, a potent vasoconstrictor. By inhibiting thromboxane A2, aloe gel is thought to increase microcirculation and prevent ischemia in wounds, which may speed the healing of burns and frostbite (101,8224,12161,12162).
Aloe gel also seems to have antibacterial and antifungal properties (101).
In vitro, aloe gel seems to have an antioxidant effect and decreased levels of colorectal prostaglandin E2 and interleukin-8. These effects may explain why aloe gel seems to help some patients with inflammatory bowel disease (12158).
Preliminary research suggests that aloe gel might also have hypoglycemic effects (11983).
In animal models, aloe seems to prevent the inhibition of wound contraction caused by silver sulfadiazine (SSD). SSD is often applied to wounds, especially burn wounds, to prevent infection. But SSD seems to slow wound healing by inhibiting contraction and epithelialization. Applying aloe in conjunction with SSD seems to improve the speed of wound healing compared to SSD alone (12097). However, there is also evidence SSD improves the rate of wound healing better than aloe when each product is used alone (12161). This suggests that there might be a synergistic effect when SSD and aloe are used together.
In animal models of frostbite, aloe gel seems to be more effective for improving tissue survival than pentoxifylline. The combination of pentoxifylline plus aloe gel seems to be better than either agent alone (12162).
When applied to psoriatic plaques, aloe extract cream seems to reduce cellular desquamation, erythema, and infiltration. This results in reduction or resolution of the plaques (12096).

Adverse Reactions

Orally, aloe gel is well tolerated (11984). Aloe latex occasionally causes abdominal pain and cramps (4). Long-term use or abuse of aloe can cause diarrhea, sometimes with blood; potassium depletion; albuminuria; hematuria; muscle weakness; weight loss; heart disturbance; and pseudomelanosis coli (pigment spots in intestinal mucosa) (4). Pseudomelanosis coli is believed to be harmless, and usually reverses with discontinuation of aloe. It is not directly associated with an increased risk of developing colorectal adenoma or carcinoma (6138). There is also concern that aloe latex might adversely affect the kidneys. Nephritis and acute renal failure are primarily associated with prolonged use of high doses, 1 gram/day or more (8961).
Topically, aloe gel appears to be well tolerated (11982). Topical use has not been linked to significant side effects.

Interactions with Herbs & Other Dietary Supplements

CARDIAC GLYCOSIDE-CONTAINING HERBS: Theoretically, overuse of aloe can increase the risk of cardiac glycoside toxicity due to potassium depletion. Watch for possible interactions with herbs that contain cardiac glycosides such as black hellebore, Canadian hemp roots, digitalis leaf, hedge mustard, figwort, lily of the valley roots, motherwort, oleander leaf, pheasant's eye plant, pleurisy root, squill bulb leaf scales, and strophanthus seeds (19).
HERBS & SUPPLEMENTS WITH HYPOGLYCEMIC POTENTIAL: Preliminary research suggests aloe gel might lower blood glucose levels (11983) and have additive effects when used with other herbs and supplements that also lower glucose levels. This might increase the risk of hypoglycemia in some patients. Some herbs and supplements with hypoglycemic effects include alpha-lipoic acid, bitter melon, chromium, devil's claw, fenugreek, garlic, guar gum, horse chestnut, Panax ginseng, psyllium, Siberian ginseng, and others.
LICORICE/HORSETAIL: Theoretically, concomitant use of aloe with horsetail or licorice rhizome increases the risk of potassium depletion and hypokalemia (19).

STIMULANT LAXATIVE HERBS: Theoretically, concomitant use of aloe with other stimulant laxative herbs may increase the risk of potassium depletion and hypokalemia. Stimulant laxative herbs include wild cucumber fruit (Ecballium elaterium), blue flag rhizome, alder buckthorn, European buckthorn, butternut bark, cascara bark, castor oil, colocynth fruit pulp, gamboge bark exudate, jalap root, black root, manna bark exudate, podophyllum root, rhubarb root, senna leaves and pods, and yellow dock root (19).

Interactions with Drugs

ANTIDIABETES DRUGS: Preliminary research suggests aloe gel might lower blood glucose levels (11983) and have additive effects when used with antidiabetes drugs. This might increase the risk of hypoglycemia in some patients. Monitor blood glucose levels closely. Some antidiabetes drugs include glimepiride (Amaryl), glyburide (DiaBeta, Glynase PresTab, Micronase), insulin, metformin (Glucophage), pioglitazone (Actos), rosiglitazone (Avandia), and others.

DIGOXIN (Lanoxin): Theoretically, overuse of aloe increases the risk of adverse effects from the cardiac glycoside drugs due to potassium depletion. Overuse of aloe, along with cardiac glycoside drugs, can increase the risk of toxicity (19).

DIURETIC DRUGS: Overuse of aloe might compound diuretic-induced potassium loss, increasing the risk of hypokalemia (19). Initiation of potassium supplementation or an increase in potassium supplement dose may be necessary for some patients. Some diuretics that can deplete potassium include chlorothiazide (Diuril), chlorthalidone (Thalitone), furosemide (Lasix), hydrochlorothiazide (HCTZ, HydroDIURIL, Microzide), and others.

SEVOFLURANE (Ultane): There is a case of excessive intraoperative blood loss in a patient who took aloe 4 tablets/day for 2 weeks prior to surgery for hemangioma. The specific dose of aloe is unknown. Sevoflurane inhibits thromboxane A2 and therefore might decrease platelet aggregation and prolong bleeding time. Aloe vera also seems to inhibit thromboxane A2, prostaglandins, and therefore might also decrease platelet aggregation. Taking Aloe vera preoperatively might have contributed to excessive intraoperative bleeding (12181). Advise patients to avoid taking Aloe vera tablets at least 2 weeks prior to elective surgery.

STIMULANT LAXATIVES: Due to cathartic laxative effects of aloe, concomitant use with other stimulant laxatives might compound fluid and electrolyte loss (19).

ORAL DRUGS: Aloe can reduce drug absorption of some drugs due to decreased GI transit time (19).

Interactions with Foods

None known.

Interactions with Lab Tests

BLOOD GLUCOSE: Preliminary research suggests aloe gel might lower blood glucose levels (11983).

COLORIMETRIC DIAGNOSTIC TESTS: Aloe latex discolors alkaline urine (red) and can interfere with diagnostic tests that depend on a color change (4).

Interactions with Diseases or Conditions

DIABETES: Preliminary research suggests aloe gel might lower blood glucose levels (11983). Monitor blood glucose levels closely.

GASTROINTESTINAL (GI) CONDITIONS: Aloe latex is contraindicated in individuals with intestinal obstruction, acute intestinal inflammation (Crohn's disease, ulcerative colitis, appendicitis), ulcers, abdominal pain of unknown origin, nausea, and vomiting due to the irritating effect of anthranoid aloins (19).

HEMORRHOIDS: Aloe latex is contraindicated in hemorrhoids due to the possibility of stenosis, thrombosis or prolapse (19).

KIDNEY DISORDERS: High doses of aloe latex have been linked to nephritis and renal failure (8961). Theoretically, taking aloe latex orally might exacerbate kidney disorders.

Dosage and Administration

ORAL: For ulcerative colitis, 100 mL of a 50% solution has been used twice daily (11984).
For constipation, the typical dose is 100-200 mg aloe or 50 mg aloe extract taken in the evening (8).

TOPICAL: For psoriasis, aloe extract 0.5% cream applied 3 times daily has been used (12096).

Comments

Aloe of the Bible is an unrelated fragrant wood used as incense (5).

The FDA required manufacturers to remove or reformulate all over-the-counter (OTC) laxative products containing aloe from the US market by November 5th, 2002. The FDA previously requested safety data, but the manufacturers decided it was not worth the expense of conducting studies (8229, 8443).

ALPHA HYDROXY ACIDS

Also Known As

AHA, Alpha-hydroxyethanoic Acid, Apple Acid, Citric Acid, Dihydroxysuccinic Acid, Glycolic Acid, Hydroxyacetic Acid, Hydroxycaprylic Acid, Hydroxypropionic Acid, Hydroxysuccinic Acid, Lactic Acid, Malic Acid, Mixed Fruit Acid, Monohydroxysuccinic Acid, Tartaric Acid.

Scientific Names

Hydroxysuccinic acid; Monohydroxysuccinic acid (Malic acid); 2-hydroxypropionic acid (Lactic acid); Hydroxyacetic acid (Glycolic acid); Dihydroxysuccinic acid (Tartaric acid); Gluconolactone.

People Use This For

Orally, malic acid (an alpha hydroxy acid) is used with magnesium for treating pain and tenderness associated with fibromyalgia.

Topically, alpha hydroxy acids are used for moisturizing and removing dead skin cells, for treating acne and improving the appearance of atrophic acne scars, improving the appearance of photo-aged skin, and firming and smoothing skin. Alpha hydroxy acids are also used to treat xerosis (pathologic dry skin), ichthyosis (disorder with hyperkeratinization and scaling of skin), and decreasing hyperpigmentation associated with melasma.

Safety

LIKELY SAFE ...when used topically and appropriately (947,949,952,10101). Preparations containing concentrations of 10% or less can be safely used for self-treatment if used appropriately (6079,10102). However, higher concentrations should only be used under the supervision of a dermatologist (6079,10101,10103).

POSSIBLY SAFE ...when malic acid (an alpha hydroxy acid) is used orally and appropriately. Malic acid has been safely used for up to 6 months (3262).

POSSIBLY UNSAFE ...when used topically and inappropriately. Inappropriate use of high concentrations of alpha hydroxy acids can cause skin burns (10103).

PREGNANCY AND LACTATION: LIKELY SAFE ...when used topically and appropriately (947,949,952). There is insufficient reliable information available about the safety of the oral use of malic acid during pregnancy and lactation; avoid using.

Effectiveness

LIKELY EFFECTIVE

Dry skin. Applying alpha hydroxy acids in a lotion or cream daily can improve dry skin (949,955).

Wrinkled skin. Applying alpha hydroxy acids in a lotion, cream, or solution daily can decrease wrinkles and other signs of photo-damaged skin (952,953,954,8011). However, applying alpha hydroxy acids in short-contact skin peels is not effective (953).

POSSIBLY EFFECTIVE

Acne. Applying alpha hydroxy acids seems to help reduce acne (947).

Atrophic acne scars. Applying glycolic acid, an alpha hydroxy acid, as a facial peel or lotion seems to improve the appearance of atrophic acne scars. Serial applications of 70% glycolic acid can significantly improve the appearance of atrophic acne scars when compared to daily usage of 15% glycolic acid lotion. However, 15% glycolic acid lotion seems to be moderately effective in persons who can not tolerate facial peeling (10101).

Melasma. Applying 10% glycolic acid, an alpha hydroxy acid, as a lotion for 2 weeks followed by a facial peeling program using 50% glycolic acid every month for 3 consecutive months seems to reduce pigmentation in patients with epidermal-type and mixed-type melasma. However, dermal-type melasma does not appear to respond to glycolic acid facial peels (10102).

INSUFFICIENT RELIABLE EVIDENCE to RATE

Fibromyalgia. Malic acid, an alpha hydroxy acid, used orally with magnesium hydroxide (Super Malic tablets) might help reduce pain and tenderness associated with fibromyalgia (3262).

Ichthyosis. There is some preliminary evidence that alpha hydroxy acid preparations, such as lactic acid at 8% to 12% concentration or glycolic acid, mandelic acid and others at 5-10% concentration, might be useful for treating ichthyosis. These alpha hydroxy acids used daily for 1 to 3 weeks might improve the appearance of skin (10104).

More evidence is needed to rate alpha hydroxy acids for these uses.

Mechanism of Action

Alpha hydroxy acids are a group of natural acids found in foods including citric acid (citrus fruits), glycolic acid (sugarcane), lactic acid (sour milk), malic acid (apples), tartaric acid (grapes), gluconolactone, and others (6064,10104). Hyperkeratinization is thought to contribute to acne, dry skin, and photo-aging. Alpha hydroxy acids work by exfoliating the top layers of dead skin cells (948,950,6064,6079). Alpha hydroxy acids seem to improve the appearance of aging skin by increasing smoothness and reducing dark spots (6064). The degree of exfoliation is determined by the type, concentration, and pH of the alpha hydroxy acid; and other ingredients in the product. The lower the pH of the alpha hydroxy acid, the more rapidly it is absorbed into the skin (6079). Alpha hydroxy acids that are small in molecular size per volume are more active and penetrate the skin more deeply than larger-size alpha hydroxy acids. Glycolic acid is smallest in molecular size followed by lactic, pyruvic, malic, tartaric, and citric acid (10102). Glycolic acid reverses photo-damage to the skin by increasing glycosaminoglycans, including hyaluronic acid, collagen and its precursors, and factor 13A. This contributes to epidermal and dermal growth factors and mast cell degranulation, resulting in the production of thicker and less fragmented elastic fibers and an increase in epidermal volume and tightening of superficial skin layers. There is also preliminary evidence that glycolic acid stimulates fibroblasts and increases cell proliferation in a dose-dependent manner to produce a new zone of collagen (10101). Lactic acid solutions increase skin firmness by increasing the thickness of the epidermal and dermal layers. This effect is concentration dependent; a 5% solution acts at the epidermal layer, while a 12% solution increases the thickness of both layers (8011).

The exfoliating action of alpha hydroxy acids reduces the thickness of the stratum corneum by diminishing corneocyte cohesion at the lower, newly forming levels, but not the mature upper levels, of the stratum corneum. This improves the flexibility of the stratum corneum and the skin surface. The exact mechanism of this effect is unknown. However, some researchers think alpha hydroxy acids interfere with the function of the enzymes involved in the formation of ionic sulfate and phosphate bonds in the stratum corneum (10104). There is concern, however, that the barrier function of the stratum corneum may be reduced, but current evidence suggests alpha hydroxy acids either have no effect or slightly increase the barrier function of the stratum corneum (951,7842).

A combination of the alpha hydroxy acid, malic acid, plus magnesium hydroxide seem to decrease pain and tenderness in patients with fibromyalgia, but the mechanism is not known (3262).

Adverse Reactions

Orally, the alpha hydroxy acid, malic acid, seems to be well tolerated. Some patients can experience gastrointestinal upset including diarrhea and nausea (3262).

Topically, alpha hydroxy acids are generally well tolerated when used in concentrations at or below 10% (947,949,952,10101,10102). However, these products can increase sensitivity to the sun and ultraviolet (UV) light. This can increase damage to the skin, and after long-term use might increase the risk of skin cancer. Advise patients to protect themselves from the sun by using sunscreen and/or protective clothing.

Also, tell patients to test the product on a small area of skin before applying it to a larger area. Adverse reactions can range from mild irritation, a tingling sensation, and stinging to severe redness, swelling, itching, blistering, bleeding, rash, burns, and skin discoloration (6079,6080,10101). Higher concentrations can cause severe skin irritation, burning, sloughing, and limited frosting and whitening to scar areas which sometimes results in transient hyperpigmentation (10101,10102).

There is a report of first and second degree burns with airway compromise resulting after an application of a 10% citric acid facial peel that was left on the face for four hours. After treatment, the patient had permanent facial and neck scars (10103).

Interactions with Herbs & Other Dietary Supplements

MAGNESIUM: Malic acid (an alpha hydroxy acid) is used with magnesium hydroxide for reducing pain and tenderness associated with fibromyalgia (3262).

Interactions with Drugs

None known.

Interactions with Foods

None known.

Interactions with Lab Tests

None known.

Interactions with Diseases or Conditions

INDIVIDUALS WITH SENSITIVE SKIN: Alpha hydroxy acids can worsen skin conditions by causing skin irritation and sloughing (6079,6080,10101).

Dosage and Administration

ORAL: For fibromyalgia, malic acid (an alpha hydroxy acid) 600-1200 mg twice daily with magnesium hydroxide 150-300 mg twice daily (Super Malic) has been used. This is equivalent to 3-6 Super Malic tablets twice daily (3262).
TOPICAL: For treating photo-aged skin, alpha hydroxy acid products are typically used in a concentration of 8% as lactic acid, tartaric acid, gluconolactone, or glycolic acid. They are usually applied to facial or other photo-aged skin twice daily (950,952). The alpha hydroxy acid glucolactone has also been used in a 14% solution. For increasing skin firmness and smoothness, solutions and lotions containing 5 to 12% lactic acid have been used on the face two times daily for up to 16 weeks (955,8011). For improving the appearance of atrophic acne scars, serial glycolic acid (GA) facial peels of 20%, 35%, 50%, and 70% are applied biweekly. Peels are applied first for 2 minutes and then the exposure time is gradually increased up to 4-5 minutes as tolerated with each application before applying the next stronger solution. Repetitive use of 70% GA at least 6 times is usually needed before improvement is seen. For patients unable to tolerate facial peels, long-term daily use of 15% GA lotion has been used (10101).
For decreasing pigmentation associated with melasma, a 10% lotion of the glycolic acid (GA) is applied with a sunscreen to facial skin nightly for 2 weeks followed by a facial peeling program. A 50% GA peel is applied three times to the face and left on for a period of 2-5 minutes each time (first peel 2 minutes, second peel 4 minutes, and third peel 5 minutes). The peeling program is done monthly for 3 consecutive months (10102).

Comments

Alpha hydroxy acid-containing cosmetic products may lack concentration information on labeling. Try to use products that identify the concentration of active ingredients.

ALPHA-GPC

Also Known As

Alpha-glycerylphosphorylcholine, Choline Alphoscerate, Glycerophosphorylcholine, GPC, GroPCho.
CAUTION: See separate listings for Choline, Lecithin, Phosphatidylcholine, and Soy.

Scientific Names

L-alpha-glycerylphosphorylcholine.

People Use This For

Orally and intramuscularly, alpha-GPC is used for Alzheimer's disease, vascular dementia, ischemic dementia, multi-infarct dementia, stroke, transient ischemic attack (TIA), improving memory and cognitive function, and learning.

Safety

POSSIBLY SAFE ...when used orally and appropriately. There is some evidence that taking alpha-GPC 400 mg three times daily (1200 mg/day) seems to be safe when used for up to 6 months (12102,12176). ...when used intramuscularly and appropriately. There is some evidence that administering alpha-GPC from 1000-1200 mg/day intramuscularly seems to be safe when used for 28 to 90 days (12100,12102).
PREGNANCY AND LACTATION: Insufficient reliable information available; avoid using.

Effectiveness

INSUFFICIENT RELIABLE EVIDENCE to RATE

Alzheimer's disease. Preliminary evidence suggests that taking alpha-GPC 1200 mg/day significantly improves cognitive function in Alzheimer's patients after 3 and 6 months of treatment (12176).
Dementia. Giving alpha-GPC intramuscularly might improve symptoms of vascular (multi-infarct) dementia. These patients who get a prescription only formulation of alpha-GPC (Delecit; not available in the US) 1000 mg/day intramuscularly seem to have improved cognitive function, behavior, mood, and functionality (12101).
Stroke. Stroke and transient ischemic attack (TIA) patients who receive alpha-GPC within 10 days post-stroke might have improved outcomes. Preliminary evidence suggests that these patients who get alpha-GPC 1200 mg/day intramuscularly for 28 days, followed by 400 mg three times daily (1200 mg/day) orally for 6 months, have improved recovery including improved cognitive and behavioral function (12102).
More evidence is needed to rate alpha-GPC for these uses.

Mechanism of Action

Alpha-GPC is a breakdown product of phosphatidylcholine derived from plant sources such as soy. Following administration, alpha-GPC is rapidly metabolized by glycerolphosphorylcholine diesterase to form glycerophosphate and choline (12100).
Alpha-GPC is thought to work for dementia and improving memory and learning because it increases plasma levels of choline and therefore also increase production of acetylcholine and phosphatidylcholine (12100).
Alpha-GPC is also a precursor to membrane phospholipids. Therefore, alpha-GPC might improve neuronal functioning by improving neuronal membrane fluidity (12101).
After intramuscular injection of alpha-GPC 1000 mg (405 mg of choline), plasma choline levels significantly increase by about 27% within 30 minutes. Choline levels quickly fall after this peak, following a first order pharmacokinetic process. After 6 hours, choline plasma levels return to normal endogenous amounts, which is about 9.7 micromoles/L (12100).
Levels of alpha-GPC-derived choline in the brain are thought to increase much more slowly, but also remain elevate for longer period of time (12100).
The cholinergic effects of alpha-GPC seem to counteract the attention and memory impairment effects of cause by the anticholinergic drug scopolamine (12103).

Adverse Reactions

Orally, alpha-GPC seems to be well tolerated. Some patients can experience heartburn or upset stomach, nausea, diarrhea, dizziness, skin rash, and headache (12102).
Intramuscularly, alpha-GPC can cause headache, heartburn, diarrhea, insomnia or excitation, flushing, confusion, and erythema at the injection site (12101).

Interactions with Herbs & Other Dietary Supplements

None known.

Interactions with Drugs

SCOPOLAMINE: Alpha-GPC seems to partially counteract the attention and memory impairment effects caused by scopolamine given intramuscularly (12103). It is not known if alpha-GPC is capable of decreasing the beneficial anti-motion sickness effects of the scopolamine patch (Transderm Scop).

Interactions with Foods

None known.

Interactions with Lab Tests

None known.

Interactions with Diseases or Conditions

None known.

Dosage and Administration

ORAL: For Alzheimer's disease, a prescription only formulation of alpha-GPC (Gliatilin; not available in the US) 1200 mg/day has been used (12176).
For stroke and transient ischemic attacks (TIA), alpha-GPC 1200 mg/day intramuscularly starting within 10 days post-stroke, followed by 400 mg three times daily orally has been used (12103).
INTRAMUSCULAR: For vascular dementia, a prescription only formulation of alpha-GPC (Delecit; not available in the US) 1000 mg/day given intramuscularly has been used (12101).
For stroke and transient ischemic attacks (TIA), alpha-GPC 1200 mg/day intramuscularly starting within 10 days post-stroke, followed by 400 mg three times daily orally has been used (12103).

Comments

Alpha-GPC is regulated as a prescription drug used for Alzheimer's disease in European countries. It is known as brand names Gliatilin and Delecit and generic name choline alphoscerate. In the US, alpha-GPC is only available as a dietary supplement, mostly in products promoted to improve memory.

ALPHA-KETOGLUTARATE

Also Known As

A-Ketoglutaric Acid, AKG, Alpha-Ketoglutaric Acid, Alpha KG.

Scientific Names

2-Oxopentanedoicic acid, 2-Oxoglutaric acid.

People Use This For

Orally, alpha-ketoglutarate is used for treating chronic kidney and gastrointestinal dysfunction, bacterial overgrowth, intestinal toxemia, liver dysfunction, and chronic candidiasis. It is also used as an adjunct to diet and training for improving peak athletic performance, and improving amino acid metabolism in hemodialysis patients.

Intravenously, alpha-ketoglutarate is used for preventing ischemic injury during heart surgery, improving renal blood flow after heart surgery, and preventing muscle protein depletion after surgery or trauma.

Safety

POSSIBLY SAFE ...when used orally and appropriately (5311). ...when used intravenously and appropriately (5308,5309,5310,5311,5312,5313).

PREGNANCY AND LACTATION: Insufficient reliable information available; avoid using.

Effectiveness

POSSIBLY EFFECTIVE

Ischemic reperfusion injury. Intravenous use of alpha-ketoglutarate seems to help decrease ischemic injury during heart surgery (5312,5313).

Muscle catabolism. Alpha-ketoglutarate seems to help reduce muscle protein depletion after surgery or trauma (5309,5310).

There is insufficient reliable information available about the effectiveness of alpha-ketoglutarate for its other uses.

Mechanism of Action

Alpha-ketoglutarate, the carbon skeleton of glutamate and glutamine, is an intermediate compound in the Krebs cycle (5308). As a precursor of glutamate, alpha-ketoglutarate is taken up by fibroblasts involved in wound healing (5314). The availability of alpha-ketoglutarate determines the recovery of muscle protein synthesis after surgical trauma (5309). Some evidence suggests that rapidly growing cells use alpha-ketoglutarate when cellular glutamine uptake is limited (5314). Hemodialysis patients who take alpha-ketoglutarate with calcium carbonate have improved amino acid metabolism and reduced hyperphosphatemia (5311).

Adverse Reactions

None reported.

Interactions with Herbs & Other Dietary Supplements

None known.

Interactions with Drugs

None known.

Interactions with Foods

None known.

Interactions with Lab Tests

None known.

Interactions with Diseases or Conditions

None known.

Dosage and Administration

ORAL: To improve amino acid metabolism in hemodialysis patients, 1.187 grams are typically used three times daily (5311).

INTRAVENOUS: For cardiac surgery, a dose of 28 grams of alpha-ketoglutarate has been added to blood cardioplegia (5312,5313). For preventing muscle protein depletion after surgery or trauma, 280 mg/kg of body weight is added to parenteral nutrition (5310).

Comments

Suppliers of athletic nutritional supplements claim alpha-ketoglutaric acid may be an important adjunct to proper diet and training for the athlete desiring peak performance. They base this claim on studies that show excessive ammonia in the body can combine with alpha-ketoglutarate to reduce ammonia toxicity. So far, the only studies that show alpha-ketoglutarate can reduce ammonia toxicity have been performed in hemodialysis patients (5311).

ALPHA-LINOLENIC ACID

Also Known As

ALA, Essential Fatty Acid, LNA, n-3 Fatty Acid, n-3 Polyunsaturated Fatty Acid, Omega-3 Fatty Acids, Omega-3 Polyunsaturated Fatty Acid.
CAUTION: See separate listings for Blue-Green Algae, Chasteberry, DHA, Emu Oil, English Walnut, EPA, Fish Oil, Flaxseed Oil, Gamma-Linolenic Acid, Lecithin, Safflower, Sea Buckthorn, and Sour Cherry.

Scientific Names

Alpha-Linolenic Acid.

People Use This For

Orally, alpha-linolenic acid is used to treat hypertension, rheumatoid arthritis (RA), multiple sclerosis (MS), lupus, diabetes, hypercholesterolemia, renal disease, ulcerative colitis, and Crohn's disease. It is also used to treat chronic obstructive pulmonary disease (COPD), migraine headache, skin cancer, depression, and allergic and inflammatory conditions such as psoriasis and eczema. Alpha-linolenic acid is also used to prevent cardiovascular disease, cancer, the common cold, and upper respiratory tract infections.

Safety

LIKELY SAFE ...when used orally in amounts typically found in foods (7141,7142,7144).
There is insufficient reliable information available about the safety of alpha-linolenic acid when used in amounts exceeding those typically found in foods.
PREGNANCY AND LACTATION: LIKELY SAFE ...when used orally in amounts typically found in foods (7141,7142,7145). There is insufficient reliable information available about the safety of alpha-linolenic acid during pregnancy and lactation when used in amounts exceeding those typically found in foods; avoid using.

Effectiveness

POSSIBLY EFFECTIVE

Atherosclerosis. Epidemiological research suggests high dietary intake of linolenic acid reduces calcified atherosclerotic plaque in the coronary arteries. Most dietary linolenic acid is alpha-linolenic acid (only a small fraction is gamma-linolenic acid). For every gram of linolenic acid consumed, risk of coronary artery calcification drops by 62% (12990).

Cardiovascular disease. High dietary intake of alpha-linolenic acid over a period of 6 years seems to reduce the risk of a first myocardial infarction (MI) by as much as 59% in both men and women (7152). In women, a high dietary intake of alpha-linolenic acid over 10 years seems to reduce the risk of fatal ischemic heart disease by 65% (7153). For prevention of secondary MI, starting a Mediterranean diet rich in alpha-linolenic acid and low in saturated fat and cholesterol after an initial MI appears to reduce the rate of occurrence of a second MI and death rate. Over a 27 month period, patients using this diet seem to be 73% less likely to have a second MI and 70% less likely to die from any cause, compared to the standard postinfarction diet (7150). However, it is difficult to separate effects of alpha-linolenic acid from those of other dietary, lifestyle, or drug interventions (12917). Overall, increasing dietary intake of alpha-linolenic acid by 1.2 grams per day appears to decrease the risk of fatal coronary heart disease, in people with existing heart disease, by at least 20% (12978). It is not known if alpha-linolenic acid supplements have these same benefits. Some research suggests alpha-linolenic acid has a greater effect on coronary heart disease when intake of fish oils is low (12989).

Hypertension. Epidemiological research associates high dietary intake of linolenic acid with reduced risk of hypertension. Most dietary linolenic acid is alpha-linolenic acid (only a small fraction is gamma-linolenic acid). Eating a diet high in linolenic acid seems to reduce risk of hypertension by about a third (12991).

INSUFFICIENT RELIABLE EVIDENCE to RATE

Respiratory infections. Preliminary clinical research suggests alpha-linolenic in combination with linoleic acid might reduce the number of recurrent respiratory infections in children (10785). More evidence is needed to rate alpha-linolenic acid for this use.

Mechanism of Action

Alpha-linolenic acid is an essential omega-3 fatty acid. Dietary alpha-linolenic acid is found primarily in vegetable oils such as flaxseed (linseed) oil, canola (rapeseed) oil, and soybean oil; and also in red meat and dairy products (1337). It is also found in margarines and salad dressings that contain vegetable oils (7141,7142). Walnuts and other edible nuts also contain significant amounts of alpha-linolenic acid. Alpha-linolenic acid is found in smaller amounts in green leafy vegetables and chocolate (7141). Alpha-linolenic acid is also a component of human breast milk, infant formulas, and intravenous fat emulsions (7143). The body converts small amounts of alpha-linolenic acid into longer and more unsaturated omega-3 fatty acids, such as eicosapentaenoic (EPA) and docosahexaenoic acids (DHA). In some disease states, such as type 1 diabetes, chronic alcoholism, and schizophrenia, the amount of alpha-linolenic acid converted to longer chain fatty acids is reduced (7165); however, the reason for this is not known. Alpha-linolenic acid does not seem to have the same physiological effects as EPA and DHA. The amount of EPA made from alpha-linolenic acid is not likely to be clinically significant. Conversion of alpha-linolenic acid to DHA is even less. High dose or long-term consumption of modest amounts of dietary alpha-linolenic acid does not duplicate the effects of preformed EPA+DHA on triglyceride concentrations, on tissue DHA concentrations, or on in vitro susceptibility to oxidation of low-density lipoprotein (LDL) cholesterol (7141,7165,12918).

Omega-6 fatty acids, such as linoleic acid, that are found in corn, safflower, sunflower, and peanut oils compete for enzyme systems that elongate alpha-linolenic acid into EPA and DHA (7142). The Western diet, including vegetarian diets, usually provides a disproportionate amount of omega-6 fatty acids. For example, the typical Western diet often includes an omega-6 to omega-3 fatty acid ratio of 20-30:1 (7148,7149). There is some concern that a diet high in omega-6 fatty acids can lead to long-chain omega-3 fatty acid deficiency and produce a physiologic state that is favorable for platelet aggregation and clot formation and an increased risk of heart disease (7141,7142). The ideal omega-6 to omega-3 fatty acid ratio in the diet should probably be no more than 4:1 (7141,7148). Some researchers theorize that adding omega-3 fatty acids, such as alpha-linolenic acid, can normalize this ratio and therefore decrease the risk of heart disease. Dietary alpha-linolenic acid significantly increases the concentrations of omega-3 fatty acids such as EPA and DHA in platelet phospholipids and plasma lipids (7149,7166).

Although alpha-linolenic acid seems to have beneficial effects on the cardiovascular system and might reduce risk of heart disease, it does not appear to have a significant effect on cholesterol levels (7146,7165). Alpha-linolenic acid may slightly increase triglyceride levels (12918). Alpha-linolenic acid seems to increase arterial compliance and decrease cardiac workload (7165). There is also some evidence that alpha-linolenic acid has antiarrhythmic effects, but researchers are not sure if this is due to alpha-linolenic acid itself, or due to the longer-chain fatty acids EPA and DHA, to which some alpha-linolenic acid is converted (7153,7156). A reduced risk of abnormally prolonged myocardial repolarization is associated with a diet higher in alpha-linolenic acid (12988). Alpha-linolenic acid does not affect measures of coagulation or serum activity of factors associated with coagulation (10323).

Some researchers are interested in alpha-linolenic acid for prevention of breast cancer. There is some evidence that women with higher levels of alpha-linolenic acid in breast adipose tissue have a lower risk of breast cancer. Fatty acid composition of adipose tissue is thought to reflect past dietary intake, so researchers think high intake of alpha-linolenic acid might have a cancer protective effect (7168). However, there is some concern that high dietary intake of alpha-linolenic acid might actually increase the risk for prostate cancer (1334,1336,2558,2559,7147,7823,7824). Typical figures reported are that men with the highest intakes of alpha-linolenic acid have 2-4 times the risk of prostate cancer than men with the lowest intake (1336,2558,7147,7824). It's been suggested that alpha-linolenic acid could increase sex hormone levels or formation of free radicals in prostate cell membranes (2558,7823), but these mechanisms haven't been confirmed. Also, it's been found that alpha-linolenic acid levels in biopsy samples are actually lower in more aggressive tumors (7167). Of the food sources of alpha-linolenic acid, prostate cancer risk is most strongly associated with red meat intake (1336,1337,2558). However, some research shows an increase in prostate cancer risk after adjustment for meat intake or animal fat (7823,7147). Both alpha-linolenic acid from animal sources and alpha-linolenic acid (ALA) from vegetable sources have been associated with an increased risk of prostate cancer (2558). There aren't any studies which have investigated whether alpha-linolenic acid supplements affect prostate cancer risk.

There is some evidence that alpha-linolenic acid might have a beneficial effect on immune function (10785). However, in adults, dietary fatty acids don't seem to affect immune response (10786).

Adverse Reactions

Orally, alpha-linolenic acid from dietary sources is very well tolerated; however, alpha-linolenic acid is high in calories and may result in weight gain if consumed in excess. Patients should be advised that it's best to substitute alpha-linolenic acid in the diet for other sources of fat, such as saturated fats. Very high intake of alpha-linolenic acid from some dietary sources, such as margarine, which also contain high concentrations of linoleic and trans-fatty acids, can increase the risk of heart disease and myocardial infarction. This effect is probably attributable to trans-fatty acid content, and not alpha-linolenic acid (7155).

Epidemiologic research suggests that high dietary intake of alpha-linolenic acid might increase risk for prostate cancer (1337,2558,7823,7147,12978). Other research suggests alpha-linolenic acid doesn't increase the overall risk of prostate cancer, but it might increase the risk of advanced prostate cancer. In contrast, the longer-chain omega-3 fatty acids in fish oils are associated with a decreased risk of total and advanced prostate cancer (12961).

Tell men not to be concerned about moderate dietary intake of alpha-linolenic acid (e.g., canola, soybean, and flaxseed oils), especially if this replaces intake of oils rich in omega-6 fatty acids.

Interactions with Herbs & Other Dietary Supplements
None known.

Interactions with Drugs
None known.

Interactions with Foods
None known.

Interactions with Lab Tests
BLOOD PRESSURE: Alpha-linolenic acid might decrease diastolic blood pressure in patients with hypertension when consumed in place of dietary linoleic acid (7151).
TRIGLYCERIDES: Alpha-linolenic acid might increase triglyceride levels (12918).

Interactions with Diseases or Conditions
HYPERTRIGLYCERIDEMIA: Alpha-linolenic acid might increase triglyceride levels and potentially worsen hypertriglyceridemia. (12918).
PROSTATE CANCER: Some research suggests high dietary intake of alpha-linolenic acid might increase the risk for advanced prostate cancer. Theoretically, taking alpha-linolenic acid supplements might adversely affect prostate cancer. Advise men with prostate cancer or with a high risk for prostate cancer to avoid taking alpha-linolenic acid supplements (12978).

Dosage and Administration
ORAL: For primary prevention of coronary heart disease, approximately 1.2-2 grams per day from dietary sources seems to be associated with the greatest benefit (7152,7153,7156). For secondary prevention of coronary heart disease, approximately 1.6 grams per day as part of a Mediterranean diet appears to be beneficial (7150). Fatty acid dosing is often done based on percentage of daily calories it provides. Some researchers suggest that alpha-linolenic acid should make up roughly 1% of daily calories. This comes to approximately 2 grams based on a 2000 kilocalorie diet (149,7165).

Comments
Use caution in extrapolating information about other omega-3 fatty acids, including EPA and DHA, to alpha-linolenic acid. Although very small amounts of alpha-linolenic acid are converted to long-chain fatty acids, clinical effects may be different (12918).

ALPHA-LIPOIC ACID

Also Known As
a-Lipoic Acid, Acetate Replacing Factor, ALA, Alpha-Lipoic Acid Extract, Biletan, Lipoic Acid, Lipoicin, R-alpha-lipoic acid, RS-alpha-lipoic acid, S-alpha-lipoic acid Thioctacid, Thioctan, Thioctic Acid.

Scientific Names
Alpha Lipoic Acid; 1,2-dithiolane-3-pentanoic acid; 1,2-dithiolane-3-valeric acid; 6,8-thioctic acid; 5-(1,2-dithiolan-3-yl) valeric acid; 6,8-dithiooctanoic acid.

People Use This For
Orally, alpha-lipoic acid is for diabetes, peripheral neuropathy, cardiac autonomic neuropathy, retinopathy, cataracts, and glaucoma. Alpha-lipoic acid is also used orally for dementia, HIV/AIDS, cancer, liver disease, Wilson's disease, cardiovascular disease, and lactic acidosis caused by inborn errors of metabolism. Intravenously, alpha-lipoic acid is used for improving insulin-resistance and glucose disposal in type 2 diabetes, diabetic neuropathy, and Amanita mushroom poisoning.

Safety
POSSIBLY SAFE ...when used orally and appropriately. Oral alpha-lipoic acid has been used safely in clinical trials lasting from 4 months to 2 years (3540,3541,3542,10148). ...when used intravenously and appropriately. Intravenous alpha-lipoic acid has been used safely in clinical trials lasting up to 3 weeks (3540,3557,10148,12106).
PREGNANCY AND LACTATION: Insufficient reliable information available; avoid using.

Effectiveness

POSSIBLY EFFECTIVE

Diabetes. Alpha-lipoic acid used orally or intravenously seems to improve insulin sensitivity and glucose disposal in patients with type 2 diabetes (3545,3874,3875,3876). Patients who took alpha-lipoic acid 600 to 1800 mg orally or 500 to 1000 mg intravenously daily had significant improvement in insulin resistance and glucose effectiveness after four weeks of oral treatment or after 1 to 10 days of intravenous administration (3545,3874,3875,3876). However, alpha-lipoic acid doesn't seem to lower glycosylated hemoglobin (HgbA1c) levels in patients with type 2 diabetes.

Peripheral neuropathy. Giving alpha-lipoic acid orally or intravenously 600 mg to 1200 mg/day seems to reduce symptoms of peripheral neuropathy in diabetes patients. Alpha-lipoic acid seems to improve neuropathic sensory symptoms such as burning, pain, numbness, and prickling of the feet and legs. It also seems to improve objective measures such as ratings of neurological deficit and disability. Onset of symptom improvement occurs within 3 to 5 weeks with oral and intravenous dosing (3540,3541,3557,3868,10148,12106). However, lower doses have not been shown to be effective (3869).

POSSIBLY INEFFECTIVE

Alcohol-related liver disease. People with alcohol-related liver disease taking alpha-lipoic acid orally 300 mg per day for six months did not demonstrate significant improvement compared to placebo (3880).

Cardiac autonomic neuropathy. Taking alpha-lipoic acid orally appears to improve autonomic nerve function indices, measured by ECG, in patients with cardiac autonomic neuropathy, but symptoms don't seem to significantly improve (3542).

HIV-related dementia. Taking alpha-lipoic acid orally had no effect on HIV-associated cognitive impairment in a small trial comparing alpha-lipoic acid alone or in combination with selegiline (Deprenyl) and placebo (1556).

INSUFFICIENT RELIABLE EVIDENCE to RATE

Amanita mushroom poisoning. Alpha-lipoic acid has been used orally in combination with other treatments for Amanita mushroom poisoning. Its use is controversial. Reports are anecdotal, and experimental evidence does not support its effectiveness. Some researchers recommend against its use (105,1548,1549,3871,3879).

Dementia. Preliminary evidence suggests that taking alpha-lipoic acid might decrease the decline in cognitive function in patients with various subtypes of dementia when used over a period of about 337 days (12152).

More evidence is needed to rate alpha-lipoic acid for these uses.

Mechanism of Action

Alpha-lipoic acid was identified as a vitamin when it was isolated 50 years ago, but was reclassified upon the finding that it is synthesized in humans and animals (3871). Endogenous alpha-lipoic acid is a coenzyme that, together with pyrophosphatase, is involved in carbohydrate metabolism and production of adenosine triphosphate (ATP). Exogenous alpha-lipoic acid and the metabolite, dihydrolipoic acid (DHLA), have antioxidant activity and can scavenge free radicals both intra- and extra-cellularly (3871). Alpha-lipoic acid is both water and fat soluble and can regenerate endogenous antioxidants, such as vitamin E, vitamin C, and glutathione, and prevent oxidative damage (1547,1550,3546,3871). Alpha-lipoic acid is about 30% absorbed from dietary or supplemental sources, and is reduced to DHLA in many tissues (1561,3871,3872). Preliminary data suggests that these antioxidant effects might provide protection in cerebral ischemia, excitotoxic amino acid brain injury, mitochondrial dysfunction, diabetes, diabetic neuropathy, and other causes of damage to brain or neural tissue (1561,3546,3871,10148). In experimental diabetic models, alpha-lipoic acid increases neuronal blood flow, improves neuronal glucose uptake, increases amounts of reduced glutathione in neurons, and improves neuronal conduction velocity (3873,3878). Preliminary evidence suggests that DHLA in combination with vitamin E might prevent oxidative stress in cardiac ischemia-reperfusion injury (3871,3877). The antioxidant effects of alpha-lipoic acid might be beneficial in liver diseases in which oxidative stress is a factor (3879). Alpha-lipoic acid has shown promise in experimental models to prevent aminoglycoside-induced cochlear damage, and metal (lead, arsenic, cadmium, mercury) and chemical (hexachlorobenzene, n-hexane) poisoning (3871,3879,3881,3882,3883,3884). Children treated with alpha-lipoic acid, alone or in combination with vitamin E, showed normalized organ function and lessened indices of oxidative damage following radiation exposure in the Chernobyl accident (3871). Case reports indicate that it may be helpful in various inborn errors of metabolism which result in lactic acidosis (1554,1555,1557). Preliminary data suggests that alpha-lipoic acid can inhibit replication of the human immunodeficiency virus (HIV) by inhibiting reverse transcriptase (1280,3871). Reactive oxygen species may act as intracellular messengers for HIV gene expression and transcription, and the antioxidant effects of alpha-lipoic acid could inhibit this process (1562,1563). Alpha-lipoic acid supplementation might improve blood antioxidant status and blood peroxidation products, and increase T-helper lymphocytes and T-helper to T-helper suppressor cell ratio, based on a small open trial in HIV positive patients (3885).

Adverse Reactions

Orally, skin rash has been reported after use of alpha-lipoic acid.
Intravenously, local allergic reactions have occurred at the injection site (1547). Paresthesias have been reported to worsen temporarily at the beginning of therapy. Alpha-lipoic acid can cause gastrointestinal upset, including nausea and vomiting, and headache. Adverse effects are more common in patients receiving higher intravenous doses (3557).
Laboratory studies suggest that very large doses of alpha-lipoic acid can cause fatal toxicity in thiamine deficient animals. For people who are taking high doses of alpha-lipoic acid and are at risk for thiamine deficiency (e.g. alcoholics), thiamine supplementation may be warranted (3871).

Interactions with Herbs & Other Dietary Supplements

HERBS WITH HYPERGLYCEMIC POTENTIAL: Theoretically, herbs that increase blood glucose levels might antagonize the antidiabetic effects of alpha-lipoic acid (3545). Herbs with hyperglycemic potential include ephedra, ginger, gotu kola, and the above ground parts of the stinging nettle.
HERBS WITH HYPOGLYCEMIC POTENTIAL: Theoretically, alpha-lipoic acid might have additive effects with herbs that decrease blood glucose levels (3545). Herbs with hypoglycemic potential include devil's claw, fenugreek, garlic, guar gum, horse chestnut, Panax ginseng, psyllium, and Siberian ginseng.

Interactions with Drugs

ANTIDIABETES DRUGS: Theoretically, concomitant use might cause additive hypoglycemic effects (3545). Dosing adjustments for insulin or oral hypoglycemic agents may be necessary; however, in one study, co-administration of single doses of alpha-lipoic acid and glyburide or acarbose (Precose, Prandase) did not cause detectable drug interactions in healthy volunteers (3870).
CHEMOTHERAPY: Theoretically, concomitant use might decrease the effectiveness of chemotherapy. Preliminary evidence from an unpublished study suggests antioxidants may decrease the effectiveness of chemotherapy (391).

Interactions with Foods

None known.

Interactions with Lab Tests

BLOOD GLUCOSE: Alpha-lipoic acid might decrease blood glucose levels and test results in patients with type 2 diabetes. Alpha-lipoic acid reduces insulin resistance and improves blood glucose disposal in patients with type 2 diabetes (3545); however, alpha-lipoic acid has no effect on glycosylated hemoglobin (HgbA1c) levels (3540,3557).
T HELPER/SUPPRESSOR LYMPHOCYTE RATIO: Alpha-lipoic acid might increase the T helper/suppressor ratio in patients infected with the human immunodeficiency virus (HIV) (3885).
TRIIODOTHYROXINE (T3): Preliminary evidence suggests alpha-lipoic acid might lower T3 levels (8946), but effects on thyroid function have not been reported in clinical trials (3540,3541,3542).

Interactions with Diseases or Conditions

DIABETES: Alpha-lipoic acid can decrease blood glucose levels (3545). Dosing adjustments for insulin or oral hypoglycemic agents may be necessary.
THIAMINE DEFICIENCY: Laboratory studies suggest that very large doses of alpha-lipoic acid can cause fatal toxicity in thiamine deficient animals. Supplementation might be needed for people taking high-dose alpha-lipoic acid who have thiamine-depleting conditions such as alcoholism (3871).
THYROID DISORDERS: Theoretically, concomitant use might interfere with therapy for hyperthyroid or hypothyroid conditions; monitor use (8946).

Dosage and Administration

ORAL: For treatment of diabetes and peripheral neuropathy, doses of 600 and 1200 mg daily has been used (3540,3541,3868). For cardiac autonomic neuropathy in patients with type 2 diabetes, 800 mg daily has been used (3542).
INTRAVENOUS: For peripheral neuropathy in patients with type 2 diabetes, doses 600 mg and 1200 mg daily has been used (3540,3541,3557,10148).

Comments

High doses of alpha-lipoic acid are approved in Germany for the treatment of diabetic neuropathy (3871).

ALPINE CRANBERRY

Also Known As

Cowberry, Dry Ground Cranberry, Foxberry, Lingen, Lingenberry, Lingon, Lingonberry, Lowbush Cranberry, Moss Cranberry, Partridgeberry, Red Bilberry, Redberries, Red Whortleberry, Rock Cranberry, Shore Cranberry, Vine of Mount Ida.
CAUTION: See separate listings for Cranberry, Cramp Bark, and Uva Ursi.

Scientific Names

Vaccinium vitis-idaea.
Family: Ericaceae.

People Use This For

Orally, alpine cranberry is used for urinary tract irritation, gout, arthritis and kidney stones. It is also used orally as a urinary tract disinfectant, diuretic, and antiviral.

Safety

LIKELY UNSAFE ...when the preparations of the leaves are used orally long-term because the arbutin constituent could be toxic (18).
There is insufficient reliable information available about the safety of of alpine cranberry leaf used orally, short-term.
CHILDREN: LIKELY UNSAFE ...when used orally in children under 12 years of age because alpine cranberry might be hepatotoxic (18).
PREGNANCY AND LACTATION: LIKELY UNSAFE ...when used orally because constituents have mutagenic effects (18); avoid using.

Effectiveness

There is insufficient reliable information available about the effectiveness of alpine cranberry.

Mechanism of Action

The applicable part of alpine cranberry is the leaf or berry. When ingested, alpine cranberry releases hydroquinones. In alkaline urine, the hydroquinones act as a disinfectant. Because hydroquinones can cause liver damage, long-term use is not recommended. There is also concern about long-term use because the constituents, arbutin and hydrochinon, are mutagenic and carcinogenic (18).

Adverse Reactions

Orally, alpine cranberry may cause nausea and vomiting due to its high tannin content (18).

Interactions with Herbs & Other Dietary Supplements

None known.

Interactions with Drugs

None known.

Interactions with Foods

None known.

Interactions with Lab Tests

None known.

Interactions with Diseases or Conditions

LIVER DISEASE: Theoretically, the hydroquinones in alpine cranberry may worsen liver disease (18).

Dosage and Administration

ORAL: The typical daily dose is 2 grams of dried leaf or one cup of tea taken orally. The tea is prepared by steeping 2 grams dried leaf in 150 mL of boiling water for 10-15 minutes and straining (18).

Comments

Alpine cranberry leaves are sometimes used as a substitute for bearberry (uva ursi) leaves (18).

ALPINE LADY'S MANTLE

Also Known As

Alchemillae alpinae herba.
CAUTION: See separate listing for Alchemilla (Lady's Mantle).

Scientific Names

Alchemilla alpina.
Family: Rosaceae.

Comments

At the date of publication, this product was not a common ingredient used in brand name supplements marketed to consumers. Details about this product are available in the online version of *Natural Medicines Comprehensive Database.* See www.naturaldatabase.com.

ALPINE RAGWORT

Also Known As

Ragwort, Senecio Herb.
CAUTION: See separate listing for Golden Ragwort and Tansy Ragwort.

Scientific Names

Senecio nemorensis.
Family: Asteraceae/Compositae.

People Use This For

Orally, alpine ragwort is used for diabetes mellitus, hemorrhage, high blood pressure, spasms, and as a uterine stimulant. It is also used orally to control bleeding after tooth extraction.

Safety

LIKELY UNSAFE ...when products containing hepatotoxic pyrrolizidine alkaloid (PA) constituents are used orally. Repeated exposure to low concentrations of hepatotoxic PAs can cause severe veno-occlusive disease. Hepatotoxic PAs might also be carcinogenic and mutagenic (12841,12842). Tell patients not to use alpine ragwort preparations that are not certified and labeled as hepatotoxic PA-free. ...when products containing hepatotoxic PAs are used topically on abraded or broken skin. Absorption of hepatotoxic PAs through broken skin can lead to systemic toxicities (12841). Tell patients not to use topical alpine ragwort preparations that are not certified and labeled as hepatotoxic PA-free.
There is insufficient reliable information available about the safety of topical PA-free alpine ragwort on unbroken skin.
PREGNANCY: LIKELY UNSAFE ...when used orally. Alpine ragwort preparations containing hepatotoxic pyrrolizidine alkaloid (PA) constituents might be teratogenic and hepatotoxic (12841,12842). There is insufficient reliable information available about the safety of alpine ragwort products that do not contain hepatotoxic PAs when used during pregnancy.
LACTATION: LIKELY UNSAFE ...when used orally. Hepatotoxic pyrrolizidine alkaloid (PA) constituents in alpine ragwort are excreted in milk (12841,12842). There is insufficient reliable information available about the safety of alpine ragwort products that do not contain hepatotoxic PAs when used during lactation.

Effectiveness

There is insufficient reliable information available about the effectiveness of alpine ragwort.

Mechanism of Action

The applicable parts of alpine ragwort are the above ground parts. Alpine ragwort contains various pyrrolizidine alkaloids (PA), some of which are toxic. PAs are most concentrated in the plant roots, but may be found in all plant parts. PAs, particularly unsaturated PAs, can cause hepatotoxicity. Cyclic diesters such as retrorsine and senecionine are the most hepatotoxic. Liver toxicity may result from PA-enhanced oxidative stress, but the exact mechanism of toxicity is unknown. Single doses of 10-20 mg PAs or chronic ingestion of amounts less than 10 mcg can cause veno-occlusive disease. PAs are metabolized by cytochrome P450 3A4 (CYP3A4) to toxic dehydroalkaloids and pyrroles. Enzyme inducers such as phenobarbital seem to enhance toxicity (12841,12860). Pyrroles are excreted as N-acetyl cysteine conjugates. Some researchers speculate that early administration of N-acetylcysteine might reduce toxicity (11988).
Metabolism is also affected by pregnane X receptor induction of CYP3A4. Genetic or drug-induced variation in CYP3A4 or pregnane X receptor activity can affect the degree of PA toxicity by increasing or decreasing its

metabolism (12841,12842). Hepatotoxic PAs are also toxic to the lungs. In animals, pneumotoxicity occurs as pulmonary hypertension and right ventricular hypertrophy. Hepatotoxic PAs are carcinogenic and mutagenic. There are sufficient amounts of hepatotoxic PAs in herbal products to cause toxicity (12841,12842).

Adverse Reactions

Orally, alpine ragwort might cause toxicity. The major concern about alpine ragwort preparations is the hepatotoxic pyrrolizidine alkaloid (PA) content. These constituents are hepatotoxic, pneumotoxic, carcinogenic and mutagenic (12841,12842). Chronic exposure to other plants containing hepatotoxic PA constituents is associated with veno-occlusive disease (4021). Subacute veno-occlusive disease causes vague symptoms with persistent liver enlargement (4021). Symptoms of acute veno-occlusive disease include colicky pains in epigastrium, vomiting and diarrhea, and ascites formation within several days. Enlargement and induration of the liver occurs within a few weeks (12842).

Alpine ragwort can cause an allergic reaction in individuals sensitive to the Asteraceae/Compositae family. Members of this family include ragweed, chrysanthemums, marigolds, daisies, and many other herbs.

Interactions with Herbs & Other Dietary Supplements

HEPATOTOXIC PYRROLIZIDINE ALKALOID (PA)-CONTAINING HERBS: Concomitant use is contraindicated due to the risk of additive toxicity. Herbs containing hepatotoxic PAs include alkanna, boneset, borage, butterbur, coltsfoot, comfrey, European buckthorn, forget-me-not, gravel root, groundsel, hemp agrimony, and hound's tongue; and the Senecio species plants dusty miller, groundsel, golden ragwort, and tansy ragwort (12841).

HERBS THAT INDUCE CYTOCHROME P450 3A4 (CYP3A4): Theoretically herbs that induce CYP3A4 might increase the conversion of hepatotoxic PAs to toxic metabolites, enhancing toxicity (12841,12860). Herbs that induce CYP3A4 include St. John's wort and garlic.

Interactions with Drugs

CYTOCHROME P450 3A4 (CYP3A4) INDUCERS: Hepatotoxic pyrrolizidine alkaloids (PA) are substrates of cytochrome P450 3A4 (CYP3A4) (12841,12860). Theoretically, drugs that induce CYP3A4 might increase the conversion of PAs to toxic metabolites. Some drugs that induce CYP3A4 include carbamazepine (Tegretol), phenobarbital, phenytoin (Dilantin), rifampin, rifabutin (Mycobutin), and others.

Interactions with Foods

None known.

Interactions with Lab Tests

None known.

Interactions with Diseases or Conditions

CROSS-ALLERGENICITY: Alpine ragwort may cause an allergic reaction in individuals sensitive to the Asteraceae/Compositae family. Members of this family include ragweed, chrysanthemums, marigolds, daisies, and many other herbs.

LIVER DISEASE: Theoretically, hepatotoxic pyrrolizidine alkaloids (PA) might exacerbate liver disease (12841,12842).

Dosage and Administration

No typical dosage.

Comments

Avoid confusion with golden ragwort (Senecio aureus) also referred to as squaw weed.

ALPINIA

Also Known As

Catarrh Root, China Root, Chinese Ginger, Colic Root, East India Catarrh Root, East India Root, Galanga, Galangal, Galangal Officinal, Galangal Root, Galgant, Gargaut, Gao Liang, India Root, Lesser Galangal, Rasna, Rhizome Galangae.

CAUTION: See separate listing for Ginger.

Scientific Names

Alpinia officinarum, synonym Languas officinarum.

Family: Zingiberaceae.

People Use This For
Orally, alpinia is used as a stimulant, antiflatulent, antibacterial, antispasmodic, anti-inflammatory agent, and for fever.

Safety
LIKELY SAFE ...when used orally in amounts commonly found in foods. Alpinia has Generally Recognized As Safe (GRAS) status in the US (4912).
POSSIBLY SAFE ...when used orally and appropriately in medicinal amounts (12).
PREGNANCY AND LACTATION: There is insufficient reliable information available about the safety of alpinia when used in medicinal amounts during pregnancy and lactation; avoid using.

Effectiveness
There is insufficient reliable information available about the effectiveness of alpinia.

Mechanism of Action
The applicable part of alpinia is the rhizome. Alpinia is related to ginger in its botanical and pharmacological properties. The gingerols and diaryheptanoids constituents are potent inhibitors of PG synthetase (prostaglandin biosynthesizing enzyme). Their structures indicate they can also be active against 5-lipoxygenase, an enzyme involved in leukotriene biosynthesis (6). Some constituents possess antifungal activity while others inhibit prostaglandin biosynthesis and can inhibit leukotriene biosynthesis. The other Alpinia genus plants are also pharmacologically active (6).

Adverse Reactions
None reported.

Interactions with Herbs & Other Dietary Supplements
None known.

Interactions with Drugs
ANTACIDS: Theoretically, due to reports that alpinia increases stomach acid, alpinia might decrease the effectiveness of antacids (19).
H2-BLOCKERS: Theoretically, due to reports that alpinia increases stomach acid, alpinia might decrease the effectiveness of H2-blockers (19). The H2 blockers include cimetidine (Tagamet), ranitidine (Zantac), nizatidine (Axid), and famotidine (Pepcid).
PROTON PUMP INHIBITORS (PPIs): Theoretically, due to reports that alpinia increases stomach acid, alpinia might decrease the effectiveness of PPIs (19). PPIs include omeprazole (Prilosec), lansoprazole (Prevacid), rabeprazole (Aciphex), pantoprazole (Protonix), and esomeprazole (Nexium).

Interactions with Foods
None known.

Interactions with Lab Tests
None known.

Interactions with Diseases or Conditions
None known.

Dosage and Administration
ORAL: The typical dose of alpinia is 2-4 grams of the herb per day or one cup of the tea 30 minutes before meals (18). The tea is prepared by steeping 0.5-1 grams in 150 mL hot water for 10 minutes and then straining.

AMARANTH

Also Known As
Chua, Huantli, Lady Bleeding, Love-Lies-Bleeding, Lovely Bleeding, Ramdana, Pilewort, Prince's Feather, Red Cockscomb, Ramdana, Velvet Flower.
CAUTION: See separate listings for Bulbous Buttercup, Lesser Celandine, and Potentilla.

Scientific Names
Amaranthus hypochondriacus, synonyms Amaranthus frumentaceus, Amaranthus leucocarpus.
Family: Amaranthaceae or Chenopodiaceae.

People Use This For
Orally, amaranth is used for ulcers, diarrhea, and inflammation of the mouth and throat. It is also used orally to treat hypercholesterolemia.
In foods, amaranth is used similarly to wheat as a cereal grain.

Safety
There is insufficient reliable information available about the safety of amaranth.
Pregnancy and Lactation: Insufficient reliable information available; avoid using.

Effectiveness
POSSIBLY INEFFECTIVE

Hypercholesterolemia. Amaranth muffins added to a National Cholesterol Education Program (NCEP) step-one low-fat diet failed to reduce cholesterol levels in a group of hypercholesterolemic adults beyond the reduction achieved by a group who ate only the low-fat diet (6188).

There is insufficient reliable information available about the effectiveness of amaranth for its other uses.

Mechanism of Action
The applicable part of amaranth is the whole plant. Amaranth is considered an astringent (18). The leaf contains a small amount of vitamin C (3833). There is preliminary evidence that suggests that amaranth seed can reduce serum cholesterol. It seems to reduce total cholesterol and low density lipoprotein (LDL) cholesterol, while increasing high density lipoprotein (HDL) cholesterol. Additionally, it seems to have a minimal effect on very low density lipoprotein (VLDL) cholesterol (5063).

Adverse Reactions
None reported.

Interactions with Herbs & Other Dietary Supplements
None known.

Interactions with Drugs
None known.

Interactions with Foods
None known.

Interactions with Lab Tests
None known.

Interactions with Diseases or Conditions
None known.

Dosage and Administration
ORAL: People typically prepare amaranth as a tea, adding 1 teaspoon of leaves to 1 cup of cold water. The tea is taken cold, 1 to 2 cups a day. As a tincture amaranth is dosed up to 1 teaspoon (5263).

Comments
Avoid confusion with bulbous buttercup (Ranunculus bulbosus) or lesser celandine (Ranunculus ficaria), also known as pilewort.

AMBRETTE

Also Known As
Abelmosk, Ambretta, Egyptian Alcee, Gandapura, Kasturidana, Kasturilatika, Latakasthuri, Latakasturi, Lathakasthuri, Muskadana, Muskmallow, Musk Seed, Okra, Target-Leaved Hibiscus.

Scientific Names
Abelmoschus moschatus, synonym Hibiscus abelmoschus.
Family: Malvaceae.

Comments
At the date of publication, there was very little scientific information available about this product. Our staff is continually analyzing the available information on natural medicines and will add data to the online version of *Natural Medicines Comprehensive Database* as it becomes available. See www.naturaldatabase.com.

AMERICAN ADDER'S TONGUE

Also Known As

Dog's Tooth Violet, Erythronium, Lamb's Tongue, Rattlesnake Violet, Serpent's Tongue, Snake Leaf, Yellow Snakeleaf, Yellow Snowdrop.
CAUTION: See separate listing for English Adder's Tongue.

Scientific Names

Erythronium americanum.
Family: Liliaceae.

Comments

At the date of publication, this product was not a common ingredient used in brand name supplements marketed to consumers. Details about this product are available in the online version of *Natural Medicines Comprehensive Database.* See www.naturaldatabase.com.

AMERICAN BITTERSWEET

Also Known As

False Bittersweet, Waxwork.

Scientific Names

Celastrus scandens.
Family: Celastraceae.

Comments

At the date of publication, this product was not a common ingredient used in brand name supplements marketed to consumers. Details about this product are available in the online version of *Natural Medicines Comprehensive Database.* See www.naturaldatabase.com.

AMERICAN CHESTNUT

Also Known As

None.
CAUTION: See separate listing for European Chestnut.

Scientific Names

Castanea dentata, synonym Castanea americana.
Family: Fagaceae.

People Use This For

Orally, American chestnut is used for cough, pertussis, respiratory ailments, as an antirheumatic, sedative, tonic, and astringent agent.
Topically, American chestnut is used for pharyngitis.
In foods, an extract of American chestnut is used in beverages.

Safety

LIKELY SAFE ...when used orally in amounts commonly found in foods. American chestnut has Generally Recognized As Safe status (GRAS) for use in foods in the US (4912).
There is insufficient reliable information available about the safety of the oral or topical use of American chestnut for medicinal purposes.
PREGNANCY AND LACTATION: Insufficient reliable information available; avoid using.

Effectiveness

There is insufficient reliable information available about the effectiveness of American chestnut.

Mechanism of Action

American chestnut contains 8-9% tannins (11), which exerts an astringent effect on the mucosal tissue. This effect dehydrates the tissue, reducing internal secretions and forming external cells into a protective layer (12).

Adverse Reactions
Orally, though no cases have been reported, adverse effects from the use of American chestnut are theoretically possible. Plants with at least 10% tannins may cause gastrointestinal disturbances, kidney damage, and necrotic conditions of the liver (12). Some animal experiments show that tannins may cause cancer; others show they may prevent it (12). Regular consumption of herbs with high tannin concentrations correlates with increased incidence of esophageal or nasal cancer (12).

Interactions with Herbs & Other Dietary Supplements
TANNIN-CONTAINING HERBS: Herbs that contain high percentages of tannins (such as American chestnut) may cause precipitation alkaloid constituents of other herbs (19).

Interactions with Drugs
ORAL DRUGS: Theoretically, concomitant oral administration may cause precipitation of some drugs due to the high tannin content of American chestnut. Separate administration of oral drugs and tannin-containing herbs by the longest period of time practical (19).

Interactions with Foods
None known.

Interactions with Lab Tests
None known.

Interactions with Diseases or Conditions
None known.

Dosage and Administration
ORAL: People typically prepare American chestnut as a tea with 1 teaspoon of leaves and bark boiled in a covered container with 2 cups of water for 30 minutes. The liquid is cooled slowly in the closed container and taken cold, 1 to 2 cups per day (5254).

Comments
American chestnut (Castanea dentata) has been devastated by fungal disease. Chestnut leaves used in commerce usually come from European chestnut (Castanea sativa) or other Castanea species (11).

AMERICAN DOGWOOD

Also Known As
Bitter Redberry, Box Tree, Boxwood, Budwood, Cornel, Cornelian Tree, Dog-Tree, Dogwood, False Box, Green Ozier, Osier, Rose Willow, Silky Cornel, Swamp Dogwood.
CAUTION: See separate listing for Jamaican Dogwood.

Scientific Names
Cornus florida.
Family: Cornaceae.

Comments
At the date of publication, this product was not a common ingredient used in brand name supplements marketed to consumers. Details about this product are available in the online version of *Natural Medicines Comprehensive Database*. See www.naturaldatabase.com.

AMERICAN ELDER

Also Known As
American Elderberry, Common Elderberry, Elder Flower, Elderberry, Sweet Elder.
CAUTION: See separate listings for Dwarf Elder, Elderberry, and Elderflower.

Scientific Names
Sambucus canadensis.
Family: Adoxaceae/Sambucaceae or Caprifoliaceae.

People Use This For

Orally, American elder is used for asthma, bronchitis, bruises, cancer, flatulence, colds, edema associated with weak heart function, epilepsy, fever, gout, headache, neuralgia, psoriasis, rheumatism, to stimulate healing, for sore throat, sores, swelling, syphilis, toothache, as a cathartic laxative, as a diaphoretic, as a diuretic, emetic, eye wash, mouthwash, poultice, "purifier", and stimulant.

In foods, American elder is cooked and eaten and used to make elderberry wine. American elder is also used as a flavor component in foods and beverages.

In manufacturing, extracts of American elder are used in perfumes.

Safety

LIKELY SAFE ...when the flower is used in amounts found in foods. The flowers have Generally Recognized as Safe (GRAS) status in the US (4912). Cooked, ripe fruit has few if any adverse effects (6).

POSSIBLY SAFE ...when flowers are used orally for medicinal purposes (12).

POSSIBLY UNSAFE ...when leaves, stems, or unripe fruit are used. All these parts contain cyanogenic glycosides (12). Limit juice consumption to avoid toxicity (6).

PREGNANCY AND LACTATION: LIKELY UNSAFE ...when the leaves, stems, or unripe fruit are used (6). There is insufficient reliable information available about the safety of the flower or cooked fruit; avoid using.

Effectiveness

There is insufficient reliable information available about the effectiveness of American elder.

Mechanism of Action

The applicable parts of American elder are the flower and ripe fruit. Elder flowers are believed to have diuretic and laxative effects (6). They are a rich source of vitamin C (19). Elder leaves (6) and unripe berries (12) contain cyanogenic glycosides. If ingested, the leaves or unripe berries can cause cyanide poisoning (6). Sambucus species contain plant lectins with hemagglutinin characteristics that might be useful in blood typing and other blood testing (11).

Adverse Reactions

Orally, ingesting several glasses of American elderberry juice can cause nausea, vomiting, weakness, dizziness, numbness, and stupor (6).

Interactions with Herbs & Other Dietary Supplements

None known.

Interactions with Drugs

CYTOCHROME P450 3A4 (CYP3A4) SUBSTRATES: There is preliminary evidence that American elder can inhibit the cytochrome P450 3A4 (CYP3A4) enzymes (6450). Theoretically, American elder might increase levels of drugs metabolized by CYP3A4; however, this interaction has not been reported in humans. Some drugs metabolized by CYP3A4 include lovastatin (Mevacor), ketoconazole (Nizoral), itraconazole (Sporanox), fexofenadine (Allegra), triazolam (Halcion), and numerous others. Use American elder cautiously or avoid in patients taking these drugs.

Interactions with Foods

None known.

Interactions with Lab Tests

None known.

Interactions with Diseases or Conditions

None known.

Dosage and Administration

No typical dosage.

Comments

Though making a pea shooter from an American elder stem seems innocuous, it is not a good idea. The stem contains cyanogenic glycosides and has been reported to cause toxicity in children (6).

AMERICAN HELLEBORE

Also Known As

American Veratrum, American White Hellebore, Bugbane, Devil's Bite, Earth Gall, False Hellebore, Green Hellebore, Green Veratrum, Indian Poke, Itchweed, Tickleweed, Veratro Verde.
CAUTION: See separate listings for Black Hellebore, Pheasant's Eye, and White Hellebore.

Scientific Names

Veratrum viride, synonym Veratrum eschscholtzii.
Family: Liliaceae or Melanthiaceae.

People Use This For

Orally, American hellebore has been used as an antispasmodic, diuretic, sedative, antipyretic, and for hypertension. In manufacturing, American hellebore has been used as an insecticide.

Safety

LIKELY UNSAFE ...when used orally (18,1502) or topically. The alkaloids can be absorbed through unbroken skin and should be avoided (18).
UNSAFE ...when used orally in large amounts. American hellebore can cause death (18).
PREGNANCY AND LACTATION: LIKELY UNSAFE ...when used orally or topically; avoid using.

Effectiveness

There is insufficient reliable information available about the effectiveness of American hellebore.

Mechanism of Action

The applicable part of American hellebore is the rhizome and root. The principal active constituents are steroid ester alkaloids (13,18), which reduce blood pressure even in small doses (13,18,1502). At therapeutic dosages, they have cardiac depressant, bradycardic, and sedative effects (13,18). The alkaloids inhibit inactivation of sodium-ion channels in excitable cells, especially those regulating cardiac activity (18).

Adverse Reactions

Orally, American hellebore in therapeutic amounts can cause numerous adverse effects, including irritation of mucous membranes and cardiac depression (18). Large doses can cause sneezing, lacrimation, salivation, vomiting, diarrhea, burning sensations in the mouth and pharynx, dysphagia, paresthesias, vertigo, possible blindness, paralysis, mild convulsions, bradycardia, arrhythmias, hypotension, and death due to cardiac arrest or asphyxiation (17,18).

Interactions with Herbs & Other Dietary Supplements

None known.

Interactions with Drugs

None known.

Interactions with Foods

None known.

Interactions with Lab Tests

None known.

Interactions with Diseases or Conditions

CARDIAC DISEASE: Theoretically, American hellebore can worsen cardiac disease by depressing cardiac activity or causing bradycardia (13,18).
GI IRRITATION: American hellebore can irritate the gastrointestinal tract and is contraindicated in individuals with infectious or inflammatory gastrointestinal conditions (19).

Dosage and Administration

No typical dosage.

Comments

Avoid confusion with European hellebore and pheasant's eye.

AMERICAN IVY

Also Known As

American Woodbine, Creeper, False Grapes, Five Leaves, Ivy, Virginia Creeper, Wild Woodbine, Wild Woodvine, Woody Climber.
CAUTION: See separate listings for Gelsemium, Honeysuckle, and Woodbine.

Scientific Names

Parthenocissus quinquefolia.
Family: Vitaceae.

People Use This For

Orally, American ivy is used for digestive disorders. It is also used orally to stimulate sweating, as an astringent, and a tonic.

Safety

There is insufficient reliable information available about the safety of American ivy.
Pregnancy and Lactation: Insufficient reliable information available; avoid using.

Effectiveness

There is insufficient reliable information available about the effectiveness of American ivy.

Mechanism of Action

The applicable part of American ivy is the bark. There is insufficient reliable information available about the possible mechanism of action and active ingredients.

Adverse Reactions

Orally, ingestion of the berries, containing 2% oxalic acid, is considered poisonous. There is one case of a child's death following ingestion of the berries (18).

Interactions with Herbs & Other Dietary Supplements

None known.

Interactions with Drugs

None known.

Interactions with Foods

None known.

Interactions with Lab Tests

None known.

Interactions with Diseases or Conditions

None known.

Dosage and Administration

ORAL: People typically drink a tea made from the ground bark (18).

Comments

Avoid confusion with woodbine (Clematis virginiana). Also, avoid confusing American ivy with gelsemium or honeysuckle, which are also known as woodbine.

AMERICAN MISTLETOE

Also Known As

Eastern Mistletoe, Mistletoe.
CAUTION: See separate listing for European Mistletoe.

Scientific Names

Phoradendron leucarpum, synonyms Phoradendron flavescens, Phoradendron serontium, Viscum leucarpum, Viscum flavescens; Phoradendron macrophyllum; Phoradendron tomentosum.
Family: Viscaceae.

People Use This For
Orally, American mistletoe is used as a smooth muscle stimulant to increase blood pressure, and to increase uterine and intestinal contractions. It is also used as an abortifacient.

Safety
LIKELY UNSAFE ...when the flower, fruit, leaf, or stem are used orally (6,515). All American mistletoe plant parts are considered toxic (6).
PREGNANCY: LIKELY UNSAFE ...when used orally. American mistletoe is considered an abortifacient (19).
LACTATION: LIKELY UNSAFE ...when used orally (6,515); avoid using.

Effectiveness
There is insufficient reliable information available about the effectiveness of American mistletoe.

Mechanism of Action
The applicable parts of American mistletoe are the flower, fruit, leaf, and stem. The constituent phoratoxins produce dose-dependent hypertension or hypotension, bradycardia, and increased uterine and intestinal motility. Phoratoxins can cause contraction of smooth muscle, vasoconstriction, and cardiac arrest, similar to the cardiotoxins from cobra venom (6).

Adverse Reactions
Some people who have ingested American mistletoe have reported nausea, bradycardia, hypertension, delirium, hallucinations, vasoconstriction, and cardiac arrest. Diarrhea and vomiting from ingestion of this product can lead to dehydration, hypovolemic shock, and cardiovascular collapse. Acute gastroenteritis has occurred following ingestion of a few berries. Deaths have been reported after ingestion of teas used as an abortifacient (mistletoe species not identified) (6). However, no fatalities were reported in a review of 1754 accidental American mistletoe exposures extracted from the American Association of Poison Control Centers national data collection system from 1985-1992. Ingestion of one to three berries or one or two leaves of American mistletoe is unlikely to result in any significant toxicity (3706).

Interactions with Herbs & Other Dietary Supplements
None known.

Interactions with Drugs
None known.

Interactions with Foods
None known.

Interactions with Lab Tests
None known.

Interactions with Diseases or Conditions
HEART DISEASE: Avoid in individuals with heart disease; theoretically, may exacerbate.

Dosage and Administration
No typical dosage.

Comments
American mistletoe is considered likely unsafe; avoid using. Avoid confusion with European mistletoe, as well as mistletoe from Australia, Korea, New Zealand, and other areas. Mistletoe is a parasite. Some Australian mistletoe species are reported to extract toxic constituents from the host plant on which they grow (515), suggesting the importance of identifying the host plant before use of mistletoe is considered.

AMERICAN PAWPAW

Also Known As
Custard Apple, Dog-Banana, Pawpaw.
CAUTION: See separate listings for Papaya and Papain.

Scientific Names
Asimina triloba, synonym Annona triloba.
Family: Annonaceae.

People Use This For

Orally, in Homeopathy, American pawpaw is used for treating fever, vomiting, and inflammation of the mouth and throat.

Safety

There is insufficient reliable information available about the safety of American pawpaw.
Pregnancy and Lactation: Insufficient reliable information available; avoid using.

Effectiveness

There is insufficient reliable information available about the effectiveness of American pawpaw.

Mechanism of Action

The applicable parts of American pawpaw are the bark, leaf, and seed. American pawpaw contains multiple acetogenin constituents; of these asimin, asiminacin and asininecin are reported to be highly cytotoxic (258). Based on preliminary animal studies and in vitro studies of human cancer lines, scientists report some acetogenins show activity against certain lung and breast cancers (256). An acetogenin mixture also demonstrates pesticide activity (257).

Adverse Reactions

Topically, American pawpaw extract can cause contact dermatitis (1525).

Interactions with Herbs & Other Dietary Supplements

None known.

Interactions with Drugs

None known.

Interactions with Foods

None known.

Interactions with Lab Tests

None known.

Interactions with Diseases or Conditions

None known.

Dosage and Administration

No typical dosage.

AMERICAN SPIKENARD

Also Known As

Indian Root, Life of Man, Life-of-Man, Old Man's Root, Pettymorell, Small Spikenard, Spignet, Spikenard.

Scientific Names

Aralia racemosa.
Family: Araliaceae.

Comments

At the date of publication, there was very little scientific information available about this product. Our staff is continually analyzing the available information on natural medicines and will add data to the online version of *Natural Medicines Comprehensive Database* as it becomes available. See www.naturaldatabase.com.

AMERICAN WHITE POND LILY

Also Known As
Cow Cabbage, Pond Lily, Water Cabbage, Water Lily, Water Nymph.

Scientific Names
Nymphaea odorata, synonyms Nymphaea maximilianii, Nymphaea rosea.
Family: Nymphaeaceae.

Comments
At the date of publication, this product was not a common ingredient used in brand name supplements marketed to consumers. Details about this product are available in the online version of *Natural Medicines Comprehensive Database.* See www.naturaldatabase.com.

ANDIROBA

Also Known As
Andiroba-Saruba, Bastard Mahogany, Brazilian Mahogany, Carapa, Cedro, Crabwood, Iandirova, Mahogany, Requia.

Scientific Names
Carapa guianensis.
Family: Meliaceae.

Comments
At the date of publication, there was very little scientific information available about this product. Our staff is continually analyzing the available information on natural medicines and will add data to the online version of *Natural Medicines Comprehensive Database* as it becomes available. See www.naturaldatabase.com.

ANDRACHNE

Also Known As
None.

Scientific Names
Andrachne aspera; Andrachne cordifolia; Andrachne phyllanthoides
Family: Euphorbiaceae.

Comments
At the date of publication, this product was not a common ingredient used in brand name supplements marketed to consumers. Details about this product are available in the online version of *Natural Medicines Comprehensive Database.* See www.naturaldatabase.com.

ANDROGRAPHIS

Also Known As
Andrographolide, Bhunimba, Bidara, Carmantina, Chiretta, Chuan Xin Lian, Chuan Xin Lin, Creat, Fa-Tha-Lai-Jone, Gubak, Indian Echinacea, Kalamegha, Kariyat, King of Bitters, Kirta, Nabin Chanvandi, Poogiphalam, Sadilata, Sambilata, Shivaphala, Supari, Takila, Vizra Ufar, Yavatikta.

Scientific Names
Andrographis paniculata, synonym Justicia paniculata.
Family: Acanthaceae.

People Use This For

Orally, andrographis is used for preventing and treating the common cold, influenza, pharyngotonsillitis, allergies, sinusitis, and to treat HIV/AIDS. Andrographis is also used orally for anorexia, atherosclerosis, snake and insect bites, bronchitis, cachexia, prevention of cardiovascular disease, cholera, colic, diabetes, diarrhea, flatulence, gastritis, gonorrhea, hemorrhoids, hepatomegaly, drug-induced hepatotoxicity, and other hepatic disorders. Other uses include myocardial ischemia, jaundice, leprosy, leptospirosis, malaria, familial Mediterranean fever, pharyngitis, pneumonia, pruritus, pyelonephritis, rabies, skin wounds, skin diseases, syphilis, tuberculosis, tonsillitis, and ulcers. Andrographis is also used as an astringent, antiseptic, antidote, analgesic, antipyretic, anti-inflammatory, antithrombotic, expectorant, anthelmintic, laxative, and tonic.

Safety

LIKELY SAFE ...when used orally and appropriately, short-term. A specific andrographis extract (Kan Jang) has been safely used in short-term clinical trials lasting 4-7 days (2744,2748,2773,2774,10441,10795,13016).
POSSIBLY SAFE ...when used orally and appropriately long-term. A specific andrographis extract (Kan Jang) has been safely used in one clinical trial using low doses lasting 3 months (2772).
CHILDREN: POSSIBLY SAFE ...when used orally and appropriately, short-term. Andrographis, in combination with other herbs, has been given to children with apparent safety for up to one month (12381,12382).
PREGNANCY: LIKELY UNSAFE ...when used orally due to abortifacient effects; avoid using (12).
LACTATION: Insufficient reliable information available; avoid using.

Effectiveness

POSSIBLY EFFECTIVE

Common cold. Taking andrographis orally seems to significantly improve symptoms of the common cold when started within 72 hours of symptom onset. Some symptoms can improve after 2 days of treatment (2744,2773), but it typically takes 4-5 days of treatment before there is maximal symptom relief (2744,2773,2774,5784,10795,12380). Andrographis is often given in combination with Siberian ginseng for treating colds (12380). Some research suggests this combination relieves cold symptoms better than Echinacea or placebo in children (12381). There is some preliminary evidence that taking andrographis prophylactically might decrease the risk of developing a cold by about 50% after 2 months of continuous treatment (2772), but more evidence is needed.

Pharyngotonsillitis. There is some evidence that high doses of andrographis are comparable to acetaminophen after 3 and 7 days of treatment for fever and sore throat associated with pharyngotonsillitis (2748).

Most clinical trials used Andrographis paniculata dried extract (Kan Jang, Swedish Herbal Institute), standardized to contain 4-5.6 mg of the constituent andrographolide per tablet (2744,2772,2773,2774,5784).

INSUFFICIENT RELIABLE EVIDENCE to RATE

Familial Mediterranean fever. Preliminary clinical research suggests a combination of andrographis, Siberian ginseng, schisandra, and licorice reduces the duration, frequency, and severity of attacks of familial Mediterranean fever in children (12382).

Influenza. Preliminary evidence suggests that patients with influenza who take a specific Andrographis extract in combination with Siberian ginseng have symptom relief more quickly compared to patients taking amantidine. Patients who take this combination also seem to have a reduced risk of post-influenza complication such as sinusitis or bronchitis (10441).

More evidence is needed to rate andrographis for these uses.

Mechanism of Action

The applicable parts of andrographis are the leaf and rhizome (12,2758,2767). Several active constituents have been identified, including andrographolide; deoxyandrographolide, and other diterpenes (2750,2760,2768,2771).
Although andrographis is used for a wide variety of indications in Ayurvedic and herbal medicine, clinical evidence of effectiveness in humans is limited to the common cold. People use andrographis for the common cold because it is thought to have immunostimulant properties. There is some preliminary evidence that it might increase antibody activity and phagocytosis by macrophages (2766).
Preliminary evidence also suggests that andrographis might have mast cell-stabilizing and antiallergy activity (2750,2751).
Andrographis has traditionally been used for infectious diseases. Antibacterial activity was not detected by one group of investigators, but preliminary evidence suggests potential use against bacteria in raw water, human roundworm (Ascaris lumbricoides), Toxoplasma gondii, malaria, and E. coli enterotoxin secretion (2752,2753,2764,2767,2777,2779,2780,2781).
People use andrographis for HIV/AIDS because some of its constituents have been found to have anti-HIV in vitro (2765). High doses of the purified andrographolide constituent can also increase CD4+ cell counts in HIV patients. Andrographolide is thought to work through correction of T-lymphocyte function rather than by direct inhibition of viral replication (6767).
There is interest in using andrographis as an anticancer agent. Extracts of andrographis inhibit proliferation of HT-29 colon cancer cells in vitro. This activity has been attributed to the diterpine constituents andrographolide;

deoxyandrographolide; and 14-deoxy-11,12-didehydroandrographolide. The andrographolide constituent also inhibits proliferation of breast, brain, lung, skin, ovarian, prostate, and renal cancer cells in vitro (10302).
Andrographis might also have leukemia cell differentiation-inducing activity (2766,2768).
Possible analgesic, antipyretic, and anti-ulcerogenic effects of andrographis have been described (2753,2754).
Andrographis might protect the liver against hepatotoxic drugs (e.g., acetaminophen) and chemicals possibly by increasing bile flow, bile salt, and bile acids (2761,2762,2763,2778). The andrographis constituent, andrographolide, is a more potent hepatoprotectant than silymarin, an active constituent of milk thistle (Silybum marianum) (2762,2778).
Andrographis may be beneficial in cardiovascular disease. Early evidence suggests that andrographis might lower blood pressure, prevent arteriosclerosis, inhibit platelet aggregation, and reduce myocardial ischemia and reperfusion injury (2755,2756,2757,2758,2759,2760,2782,2783).
Andrographis is reported to have abortifacient activity. The mechanism of abortifacient action is unknown (2771).
Preliminary evidence suggests that andrographis might also have detrimental effects on male and female fertility. In animals, andrographis decreased fertility of both males and females (2769,2770,2776); however, this has not been demonstrated in humans.

Adverse Reactions

Orally, andrographis is generally well tolerated (12380,12381,12382). Side effects reported in clinical trials include allergic reactions, urticaria, fatigue, headache, diarrhea, nausea, vomiting, drowsiness, dry mouth, metallic taste, dizziness, heartburn, decreased short-term memory, and runny nose (2743,2773,13016).
Large doses of andrographis are reported to cause gastrointestinal (GI) distress, anorexia, and emesis (2743). High doses of the purified andrographolide constituent, 5 mg/kg three times daily, have caused headache, fatigue, rash, abnormal taste, diarrhea, itching, lymphadenopathy, and anaphylactic reactions. The andrographolide constituent may also cause dose-related increases in liver enzymes such as ALT, which return to normal when andrographolide is discontinued (6767); however, these effects have not yet been reported in humans.
Preliminary evidence suggests that andrographis might impair male and female fertility (2769,2770,2776), but this has not been demonstrated in humans.

Interactions with Herbs & Other Dietary Supplements

HERBS & SUPPLEMENTS WITH HYPOTENSIVE ACTIVITY: Theoretically, concomitant use with andrographis might enhance therapeutic effects and increase the risk of hypotension (2755,2760).
HERBS WITH ANTICOAGULANT/ANTIPLATELET POTENTIAL: Theoretically, concomitant use of andrographis with herbs that have anticoagulant or antiplatelet activity might enhance therapeutic effects and increase the risk of bleeding (2758,2759). These include angelica, clove, danshen, garlic, ginger, ginkgo, Panax ginseng, horse chestnut, red clover, turmeric, and others.

Interactions with Drugs

ANTICOAGULANT/ANTIPLATELET DRUGS: Theoretically, concomitant use with andrographis might enhance therapeutic effects and increase the risk of bleeding (2758,2759).
ANTIHYPERTENSIVE DRUGS: Theoretically, concomitant use with andrographis might enhance therapeutic effects and increase the risk of hypotension (2755,2760).
IMMUNOSUPPRESSANTS: Theoretically, andrographis might interfere with immunosuppressive drugs because of its immunostimulant activity (2766). Immunosuppressant drugs include azathioprine (Imuran), basiliximab (Simulect), cyclosporine (Neoral, Sandimmune), daclizumab (Zenapax), muromonab-CD3 (OKT3, Orthoclone OKT3), mycophenolate (CellCept), tacrolimus (FK506, Prograf), sirolimus (Rapamune), prednisone (Deltasone, Orasone), and other corticosteroids (glucocorticoids).

Interactions with Foods

None known.

Interactions with Lab Tests

None known.

Interactions with Diseases or Conditions

BLEEDING DISORDERS: Theoretically, andrographis might have antiplatelet activity and increase the risk of bleeding in patients with bleeding disorders (2758,2759).
HYPOTENSION: Theoretically, andrographis might lower blood pressure and exacerbate hypotension (2755,2760).
INFERTILITY: Theoretically, andrographis might have detrimental effects on male and female fertility (2769,2770,2776). Avoid in couples with infertility.

Dosage and Administration

ORAL: For treating the common cold, 400 mg three times daily has been used (2744,2773,2774,5784). For preventing the common cold, a dose of 200 mg daily for 5 days each week has been used (2772). For relieving fever and sore throat in pharyngotonsillitis, doses of 3 grams and 6 grams daily has been used (2748). For influenza, a combination of a specific Andrographis extract 178-266 mg plus Siberian ginseng 20-30 mg (Kan Jang) three times daily for 3-5 days has been used (10441).

Most of the clinical trials have used andrographis dried extract (Kan Jang, Swedish Herbal Institute), standardized to contain 4-5.6 mg andrographolide.

Comments

Andrographis is native to Asian countries such as India and Sri Lanka, and is cultivated and naturalized in other areas of the world. Andrographis products have reportedly been used in Scandinavia for more than a decade (2772). One writer credits Andrographis with arresting the 1919 flu epidemic in India, although this has not been verified (2774).

Some Internet vendors offer andrographis augmented to contain up to 30% andrographolide (2746). The safety and effectiveness of andrographis preparations with augmented andrographolide content is unknown.

ANDROSTENEDIOL

Also Known As

4-AD, 4-Androstenediol, 5-AD, 5-Androstenediol, Androdiol.

CAUTION: See separate listing for Androstenedione.

Scientific Names

4-androstene-3beta,17beta-diol; 5-androstene-3beta,17beta-diol.

People Use This For

Orally, androstenediol is used to increase endogenous testosterone production to increase energy, enhance recovery and growth from exercise, heighten sexual arousal and function, and to promote a greater sense of well being.

Safety

POSSIBLY UNSAFE ...when used orally; the potency and purity of androstenediol products can differ significantly from the product label (10641).

PREGNANCY AND LACTATION: Insufficient reliable information available; avoid using.

Effectiveness

POSSIBLY INEFFECTIVE

Athletic conditioning. Androstenediol taken orally, 100 mg twice per day, does not seem to add any significant increase in muscle strength or size when used for 12 weeks in conjunction with high-intensity resistance training (1905).

There is insufficient reliable information available about the effectiveness of androstenediol for its other uses.

Mechanism of Action

Androstenediol, a prohormone, is a weak steroid hormone and is a direct precursor of testosterone (1905).

Androstenediol can be converted to estradiol, estrone, dehydroepiandrosterone (DHEA), and testosterone; and may increase levels of these hormones (1905,10162).

Androstenediol also decreases high-density lipoprotein cholesterol (HDL-C) levels. It also increases low-density lipoprotein cholesterol LDL-C/HDL-C and apolipoprotein A/apolipoprotein B lipid ratio, which are considered to be indicators of coronary heart disease risk (1905).

Adverse Reactions

Orally, androstenediol can increase endogenous testosterone production and increase levels of estrone and estradiol (1905,10162).

Theoretically, androstenediol may cause masculinization and increased growth of facial hair in women.

Interactions with Herbs & Other Dietary Supplements

None known.

Interactions with Drugs

ESTROGENS: Intake of androstenediol can increase levels of the estrogens, estradiol, and estrone (1905). Theoretically, concomitant use with androstenediol might increase therapeutic and adverse effects of estrogens. Some of these drugs include CombiPatch, Estraderm Transdermal, Kestrone, Vivelle Transdermal, and others.
TESTOSTERONE: Androstenediol is a precursor to testosterone and can increase levels of testosterone (1905). Theoretically, concomitant use with androstenediol might increase therapeutic and adverse effects of testosterone. Some of these drugs include Androderm Transdermal, AndroGel, Depo-Testosterone, Testex, Testoderm, and others.

Interactions with Foods

None known.

Interactions with Lab Tests

ESTRADIOL AND ESTRONE ASSAYS: Androstenediol can increase levels of estrone and estradiol (1905).
HIGH DENSITY LIPOPROTEIN (HDL) CHOLESTEROL: Androstenediol can lower HDL levels (1905).
TESTOSTERONE: Androstenediol is a precursor to testosterone and can increase levels of testosterone (1905).

Interactions with Diseases or Conditions

BREAST CANCER: Androstenediol can increase levels of estrone and estradiol (1905). Theoretically, use of androstenediol might increase the risk of hormone-sensitive cancers such as breast cancer.
HEART DISEASE: There is some concern that androstenediol might increase the risk of coronary heart disease (1905).
HORMONE SENSITIVE CANCERS/CONDITIONS: Androstenediol can increase levels of estrone, estradiol, and testosterone (1905). Theoretically, androstenediol might increase the risk of or aggravate hormone sensitive conditions. Some of these conditions include endometriosis, uterine fibroids, uterine cancer, and ovarian cancer.
PROSTATE CANCER/CONDITIONS: Androstenediol can increase levels of testosterone (1905). There is also preliminary evidence that androstenediol might stimulate prostate cancer cell growth (10161). There is concern androstenediol might aggravate prostate conditions such as benign prostate hypertrophy (BPH) or prostate cancer (10161,10162).

Dosage and Administration

For improving muscle strength and size of weight trainers, 100 mg twice daily has been used (1905).

Comments

In January 2005 legislation went into affect in the Unites States called the Anabolic Steroid Control Act of 2004. This reclassifies androstenediol from a dietary supplement to an anabolic steroid, which is a schedule III controlled substance (8639).

ANDROSTENEDIONE

Also Known As

Andro, Androstene.
CAUTION: See separate listings for Androstenediol and Androstenetrione.

Scientific Names

4-androstene-3,17-dione; Androst-4-ene-3,17-dione.

People Use This For

Orally, androstenedione is used to increase endogenous testosterone production to enhance athletic performance, increase energy, keep red blood cells healthy, enhance recovery and growth from exercise, and to heighten sexual arousal and function.

Safety

POSSIBLY UNSAFE ...when used orally. Androstenedione has been associated with significant side effects, including increased risk of breast, pancreatic, and prostate cancer (672,3861,6000). In addition, there are safety concerns that the potency and purity of androstenedione products can differ significantly from the product labeling (10641).
CHILDREN: LIKELY UNSAFE ...when used orally. Androstenedione could potentially cause premature closure of the bone growth plates (674).
PREGNANCY: LIKELY UNSAFE ...when used orally. Androstenedione might induce labor (673).
LACTATION: Insufficient reliable information available; avoid using.

Effectiveness

LIKELY INEFFECTIVE

Athletic conditioning. Taking androstenedione orally in doses of 100-300 mg per day does not significantly increase muscle strength, muscle size, or lean body mass when used for 2-3 months in conjunction with weight training (1365,1905,6000,7514).

There is insufficient reliable information available about the effectiveness of androstenedione for its other uses.

Mechanism of Action

Androstenedione is a steroid hormone produced by the adrenal glands, testes, and ovaries (3861). It is a direct precursor of testosterone and estrone in both men and women (674). Androstenedione production peaks in the mid-twenties and declines steadily after age 30 (1365). A lot of people use it as an alternative to anabolic steroids to increase testosterone levels, improve athletic performance, and build muscle. Short-term use (less than one month) can sometimes increase testosterone levels (1905,3861,10696); however, with continued use, testosterone levels return to normal (1365,1905,6000,7236,7514,10696). The acute pharmacokinetic response seems to diminish after 28 days of supplementation (10696). When used for longer than one month, luteinizing hormone secretion seems to decline by about a third, and dehydroepiandrosterone (DHEA) concentrations rise (1905,8138,10696). This suggests androstenedione might actually down-regulate testosterone synthesis (1905,10696). Androstenedione also does not seem to have anabolic effects and does not significantly affect markers of muscle anabolism or growth; increase lean body mass or physical strength; or produce any perceived changes in mood, health, or libido (1365,1905,3862,7236). Furthermore, androstenedione consistently increases estrogen levels (1905,3861,3862,6000,7236,8138). This might increase the risk of estrogenic side effects in both men and women using androstenedione (674,6000). Androstenedione also lowers high-density lipoprotein (HDL) cholesterol (1905,8138). Some androstenedione products are combined with herbal aromatase and 5-alpha-reductase inhibitors to prevent these adverse effects on hormones and lipids. However, these combinations don't seem to help (8138).

Adverse Reactions

Orally, side effects can be different for men and women. In men, androstenedione might decrease endogenous testosterone production and increase estrogen. Theoretically, androstenedione might cause decreased spermatogenesis, acne, testicular atrophy, gynecomastia, behavioral changes, and potentially increase the risk of pancreatic and prostate cancer (672,674,6000). There is preliminary evidence that androstenedione might stimulate prostate cancer cell growth (672). There is also some concern that androstenedione might increase risk of heart disease in men. Androstenedione decreases high-density lipoprotein (HDL) cholesterol (1905,6000). Some androstenedione products are combined with other supplements such as dehydroepiandrosterone, puncture vine, saw palmetto, indole-3-carbinol, and chrysin (DION) to lessen the adverse effects of androstenedione, lipids, and on hormones such as increased estradiol and dihydrotestosterone (DHT), which is associated with increased prostate cancer risk. However, this combination does not seem to help (8138). Some male patients might also be at risk for developing priapism. There is one case report of two episodes of priapism associated with androstenedione use in a 30-year-old man (5089).

In women, androstenedione theoretically might cause masculinization with the deepening of voice, hirsutism, acne, clitoral hypertrophy, menorrhea, male-pattern baldness, and coarsening of the skin (674). There is also some concern that androstenedione might cause or worsen depression in women. Some women with severe major depression seem to have increased endogenous androstenedione concentrations; however, it is not known if supplements can actually cause this adverse effect (6796).

In children, androstenedione might cause premature bone growth plate closure and decrease adult height (674). Androstenedione might cause early development of secondary sex characteristics in boys; and acne, oligomenorrhea or amenorrhea, hirsutism, and virilization in girls. Testosterone derivatives similar to androstenedione have also been associated with hepatic toxicity (3861). Consider monitoring liver function tests (LFTs) in patients using androstenedione.

Interactions with Herbs & Other Dietary Supplements

None known.

Interactions with Drugs

ESTROGENS: There is some concern that taking androstenedione with estrogens might increase estrogenic effects and potential side effects. Androstenedione is a precursor to estrogen and seems to increase estrogen levels (674).

Interactions with Foods

None known.

Interactions with Lab Tests

ESTRONE ASSAYS: Androstenedione is a precursor to estrone and might increase results of estrone assays (674,1905).
HIGH DENSITY LIPOPROTEIN (HDL) CHOLESTEROL: Androstenedione can lower HDL levels (7236).
NANDROLONE: Trace contamination of androstenedione with 19-norandrostenedione can result in positive urine test results for nandrolone use (1906).
TESTOSTERONE: Androstenedione is a precursor to testosterone and can increase results of total and free testosterone assays during the first month of androstenedione use. However, testosterone levels tend to normalize when androstenedione is used for longer than 1 month (674,1905).

Interactions with Diseases or Conditions

DEPRESSION: Theoretically, androstenedione supplementation might cause or worsen depression in women. There is evidence that some women with severe major depression have elevated endogenous androstenedione levels (6796). However, it is not known if taking androstenedione supplements causes this adverse effect.
HORMONE SENSITIVE CANCERS/CONDITIONS: Androstenedione is a precursor to testosterone and estrogen and seems to increase estrogen levels (674). Men and women with hormone sensitive conditions should avoid androstenedione. Some of these conditions include breast, uterine, ovarian and prostate cancer; endometriosis; and uterine fibroids.
LIVER DISEASE: There is some concern that androstenedione might adversely affect the liver. So far there are no cases of this adverse effect, but steroids similar to androstenedione have been associated with liver abnormalities. Androstenedione should be avoided by people with hepatic disease (3861). Consider checking liver function tests (LFTs) in patients taking androstenedione.
PROSTATE CANCER: There is some concern that androstenedione might increase the risk of developing prostate cancer. There is preliminary evidence that androstenedione can stimulate human prostate tumor cell growth (672). Avoid using in patients with prostate cancer.

Dosage and Administration

ORAL: For improving muscle strength and size in weight trainers, 50-150 mg twice daily has been used in studies. However, androstenedione does not seem to be effective for this use (1365,1905,3861,6000,7514).

Comments

Androstenedione gained popularity as the supplement used by the baseball homerun hitter Mark McGwire and other professional sports players. In January 2005 legislation went into affect in the Unites States called the Anabolic Steroid Control Act of 2004. This reclassifies androstenedione from a dietary supplement to an anabolic steroid, which is a schedule III controlled substance (8639).

ANDROSTENETRIONE

Also Known As

6-Oxo, ADT.
CAUTION: See separate listing for Androstenedione and Androstenediol.

Scientific Names

4-androstene-3,6,17-trione, synonym androst-4-ene-3,6,17-trione.

People Use This For

Orally, androstenetrione is used to increase testosterone levels and improve athletic performance.

Safety

POSSIBLY UNSAFE ...when used orally. There is no scientifically reliable information about androstenetrione. However, promoters indicate that it can increase testosterone levels. If this is true, this product may not be safe due to the adverse effects associated with elevated testosterone levels.
PREGNANCY AND LACTATION: POSSIBLY UNSAFE ...when used orally. There is no scientifically reliable information about using androstenetrione during pregnancy or lactation. Promoters indicate that it can increase testosterone levels. If this is true, this product may not be safe due to the adverse effects associated with elevated testosterone levels; avoid using.

Effectiveness

There is insufficient reliable information available about the effectiveness of androstenetrione.

Mechanism of Action

Androstenetrione is an aromatase inhibitor. It blocks conversion of testosterone to estrogen (12167,12168). Theoretically, as a result of falling estrogen levels, the body is thought to compensate by further increasing testosterone levels.

Promoters of androstenetrione say that it increases total testosterone by 188% and free testosterone by 226% over 3 weeks of use. Despite this claim by marketers of androstenetrione, there is no scientifically reliable research in humans that validates this information.

Adverse Reactions

There is no data regarding oral use of androstenetrione in humans. However, androstenetrione might increase testosterone levels. Theoretically, androstenetrione might cause testosterone-like side effects including spermatogenesis and infertility, acne, testicular atrophy, gynecomastia, behavioral changes, cardiovascular disease, and potentially increase the risk of pancreatic and prostate cancer.

Interactions with Herbs & Other Dietary Supplements

None known.

Interactions with Drugs

None known.

Interactions with Foods

None known.

Interactions with Lab Tests

ESTRONE ASSAYS: Androstenetrione is thought to have aromatase inhibitor activity. Theoretically, this could cause decreased estrogen levels.

TESTOSTERONE: Androstenetrione is thought to have aromatase inhibitor activity. Theoretically, this could cause increased testosterone levels.

Interactions with Diseases or Conditions

HORMONE SENSITIVE CANCERS/CONDITIONS: Androstenetrione is thought to have aromatase inhibitor activity. This might decrease estrogen levels and increase testosterone levels. Men with hormone sensitive conditions such as prostate cancer should avoid androstenetrione.

LIVER DISEASE: Androstenetrione is thought to have aromatase inhibitor activity. This might decrease estrogen levels and increase testosterone levels. Increased testosterone is associated with liver abnormalities. Androstenetrione should be avoided by people with hepatic disease. Consider checking liver function tests (LFTs) in patients who take androstenetrione.

PROSTATE CANCER: Androstenetrione is thought to have aromatase inhibitor activity. This might decrease estrogen levels and increase testosterone levels. Men with hormone sensitive conditions such as prostate cancer should avoid androstenetrione.

Dosage and Administration

No typical dosage.

Comments

Androstenetrione is promoted as an alternative to "prohormones" such as androstenedione. Marketers claim that androstenetrione increases the body's natural testosterone levels and therefore is free from the negative side effects of prohormones. There is no reliable evidence to substantiate these claims.

ANGEL'S TRUMPET

Also Known As

Devil's Trumpet.

CAUTION: See separate listing for Jimson Weed (Datura stramonium).

Scientific Names

Brugmansia suaveolens, synonym Datura suaveolens.

Family: Solanaceae.

People Use This For

Orally, Angel's trumpet is used to induce hallucinations and euphoria; and to treat asthma.

Safety

UNSAFE ...when used orally (5624,5625,5626,5627). All parts of the plant contain tropane alkaloids and are considered poisonous (5624,5625,5627); the foliage and seeds contain the highest concentration of toxic alkaloids (5627).
CHILDREN: UNSAFE ...when used orally (5624,5625,5626,5627). Severe toxicity has occurred in cases of accidental ingestion and in teenagers experimenting with Angel's trumpet for recreational use (5626).
PREGNANCY AND LACTATION: UNSAFE ...when used orally. The entire plant is considered poisonous (5624,5627); avoid using.

Effectiveness

There is insufficient reliable information available about the effectiveness of Angel's trumpet.

Mechanism of Action

The applicable parts of Angel's trumpet are the leaf and flower. Angel's trumpet contains tropane alkaloids, particularly atropine, hyoscyamine, and hyoscine (scopolamine), which are responsible for the anticholinergic effects and toxicity (5625,5627).

Adverse Reactions

Orally, Angel's trumpet can cause severe toxicity. Ingestion of Angel's trumpet can cause acute anticholinergic poisoning, which often requires medical attention (5624,5625,5626,5627). Oral use has been associated with delirium, dilated pupils, hyperactivity, disorientation, intense thirst, dry skin and mucous membranes, flushing, fever, widened pulse pressure, systolic hypertension, tachycardia (5624,5625), audio-visual disassociation (5627), hyperexcitability, visual hallucinations, anxiety, amnesia, combativeness, ataxia, clonus, muscular weakness, expressive aphasia, muscular paralysis, seizure, urinary retention (5624,5625), decreased GI motility (5627), alternating levels of consciousness, convulsions, and coma (5624,5625). Death may result from respiratory arrest (5624). Each flower contains approximately 0.20 mg of atropine and 0.65 mg of scopolamine. Reports suggest ingestion of tea made from 3-6 flowers can produce hallucinations, and 9 flowers can produce total paralysis (5624).

Interactions with Herbs & Other Dietary Supplements

None known.

Interactions with Drugs

ANTICHOLINERGIC DRUGS: Concomitant use may increase anticholinergic effects and adverse effects. Drugs include amantadine, atropine, belladonna alkaloids, phenothiazines, scopolamine, and tricyclic antidepressants (506).

Interactions with Foods

None known.

Interactions with Lab Tests

None known.

Interactions with Diseases or Conditions

CONGESTIVE HEART FAILURE (CHF): Angel's trumpet might cause tachycardia and exacerbate CHF due to its hyoscyamine (atropine) and scopolamine content (5625).
CONSTIPATION: Angel's trumpet might cause constipation due to its hyoscyamine (atropine) and scopolamine content (5625,5627).
DOWN SYNDROME: Caution, patients with Down syndrome might be hypersensitive to the antimuscarinic effects (mydriasis, positive chronotropic heart effects, etc.) of hyoscyamine (atropine) and scopolamine contained in Angel's trumpet (15).
ESOPHAGEAL REFLUX: Angel's trumpet might delay gastric emptying due to anticholinergic effects, exacerbating reflux (5626).
FEVER: Angel's trumpet might increase the risk of hyperthermia in patients with fever due to its hyoscyamine (atropine) and scopolamine content (5624).
GASTRIC ULCER: Angel's trumpet might delay gastric emptying and exacerbate gastric ulcers due to anticholinergic effects of hyoscyamine (atropine) and scopolamine content (5626,5627).
NARROW-ANGLE GLAUCOMA: Angel's trumpet might increase ocular tension in patients with narrow-angle (angle-closure) glaucoma due to anticholinergic effects of hyoscyamine (atropine) and scopolamine (5627).
OBSTRUCTIVE GI TRACT DISEASE: Angel's trumpet might exacerbate obstructive GI tract diseases (including atony, paralytic ileus, and stenosis) due to its hyoscyamine (atropine) and scopolamine content (15).
TACHYARRHYTHMIAS: Angel's trumpet might cause tachycardia due to its hyoscyamine (atropine) and scopolamine content (5625).
ULCERATIVE COLITIS: Angel's trumpet might suppress intestinal motility, which might produce paralytic ileus and precipitate toxic megacolon, due to its hyoscyamine (atropine) and scopolamine content (5626).
URINARY RETENTION: Angel's trumpet might increase urinary retention due to its hyoscyamine (atropine) and scopolamine content (5625,5627).

Dosage and Administration
No typical dosage.

Comments
Angel's trumpet is usually cultivated as an ornamental plant in the southeastern US (5625,5626) and may be confused with jimson weed which grows wild throughout the US (5621,5622).

ANGELICA

Also Known As
Angelicae Fructus, Angelicae Herba, Dang Gui (Angelica root), European Angelica, Garden Angelica, Root of the Holy Ghost, Wild Angelica.
CAUTION: See separate listing for Dong Quai.

Scientific Names
Angelica archangelica, synonyms Angelica officinalis, Archangelica officinalis; Angelica atropurpurea; Angelica sylvestris; Angelica curtisi.
Family: Apiaceae/Umbelliferae.

People Use This For
Orally, angelica is used for dyspepsia, flatulence, and loss of appetite (anorexia). It is also used as a diuretic, as a diaphoretic, for inducing menstrual flow, as an abortifacient, antiseptic, expectorant, and for the plague. Topically, angelica is used for neuralgia and rheumatism, and skin disorders. It is also used as part of a multi-ingredient preparation for treating premature ejaculation.

Safety
POSSIBLY SAFE ...when used orally in amounts commonly found in foods. Angelica has Generally Recognized as Safe (GRAS) status in the US, however, Canada does not allow Archangelica as a food ingredient (12,4912). ...when used topically, short-term as part of a multi-ingredient preparation (SS Cream). This preparation was used safely for premature ejaculation in a clinical trial where the cream was applied and left on the glans penis for one hour (2537). More evidence is needed to determine its safety after prolonged, repetitive use. There is insufficient reliable information available about the safety of angelica when used orally for medicinal purposes.
PREGNANCY AND LACTATION: LIKELY UNSAFE ...when used orally. Angelica is reported to be a menstrual and uterine stimulant (4,12); avoid using.

Effectiveness
POSSIBLY EFFECTIVE

Dyspepsia. A specific combination product containing angelica (Iberogast, Enzymatic Therapy) seems to improve symptoms of dyspepsia. The combination includes angelica plus peppermint leaf, clown's mustard plant, German chamomile, caraway, licorice, milk thistle, celandine, and lemon balm (7049,12724).
A meta-analysis of studies using this combination product suggests that taking 1 mL orally three times daily over a period of four weeks significantly reduces severity of acid reflux, epigastric pain, cramping, nausea and vomiting compared to placebo (13089).
Premature ejaculation. In one controlled clinical trial, a multi-ingredient cream preparation containing Panax ginseng root, Angelica root, Cistanches deserticola, Zanthoxyl species, Torlidis seed, clove flower, Asiasari root, cinnamon bark, and toad venom (SS Cream) was applied to the glans penis one-hour prior to intercourse and washed off immediately before intercourse. Men suffering from premature ejaculation who were treated with the cream had significantly improved ejaculatory latency compared to placebo (2537).

There is insufficient reliable information available about the effectiveness of angelica for its other uses.

Mechanism of Action
The applicable parts of angelica are the root, tops, and seed. Angelica contains furanocoumain constituents including angelicin, bergapten, imperatorin, and xanthotoxin, which can be photosensitizing (5,8,12). The coumarin constituents of related Angelica species can inhibit human platelet aggregation in vitro (736). The related species, Angelica sinensis (Dong Quai), can lower prothrombin time in rabbits when coadministered with warfarin (737). It is not known if angelica also has this effect.
The constituent alpha-angelica lactone may have calcium antagonist effects (11). Angelica contains volatile oils. Volatile emissions from the angelica root might have fungistatic activity (6).
A multi-ingredient preparation containing angelica root is thought to work in premature ejaculation by increasing the penile vibratory threshold and reducing the amplitude of penile somatosensory evoked potentials (2537).

Adverse Reactions

Orally, angelica herb and seed might cause photosensitivity reactions (2,6,12). Patients who take angelica orally or apply it topically should be advised to avoid prolonged exposure to the sun.
Large doses of angelica can cause severe poisoning (5).
Topically, when the multi-ingredient cream preparation (SS Cream) is applied to the glans penis, sporadic erectile dysfunction, excessively delayed ejaculation, mild pain, local irritation, and burning has occurred (2537).

Interactions with Herbs & Other Dietary Supplements

HERBS WITH ANTICOAGULANT/ANTIPLATELET POTENTIAL: Theoretically, concomitant use with herbs that have antiplatelet/anticoagulant activity might increase the risk of bleeding in some people. These herbs include clove, danshen, garlic, ginger, ginkgo, Panax ginseng, red clover, turmeric, and others.

Interactions with Drugs

ANTACIDS: Theoretically, due to reports that angelica increases stomach acid, angelica might decrease the effectiveness of antacids (19).
ANTICOAGULANT/ANTIPLATELET DRUGS: Excessive doses of angelica herb and seed might potentiate therapeutic effects and adverse effects of anticoagulants (736).
H2-BLOCKERS: Theoretically, due to reports that angelica increases stomach acid, angelica might decrease the effectiveness of H2-blockers (19). The H2 blockers include cimetidine (Tagamet), ranitidine (Zantac), nizatidine (Axid), and famotidine (Pepcid).
PHOTOSENSITIZING DRUGS: Angelica might increase photosensitization and side effects; concomitant use with these drugs should be avoided (6,12).
PROTON PUMP INHIBITORS (PPIs): Theoretically, due to reports that angelica increases stomach acid, angelica might decrease the effectiveness of PPIs (19). PPIs include omeprazole (Prilosec), lansoprazole (Prevacid), rabeprazole (Aciphex), pantoprazole (Protonix), and esomeprazole (Nexium).

Interactions with Foods

None known.

Interactions with Lab Tests

None known.

Interactions with Diseases or Conditions

None known.

Dosage and Administration

ORAL: For dyspepsia, A specific combination product containing angelica (Iberogast, Enzymatic Therapy) and several other herbs has been used in a dose of 1 mL three times daily (7049,12724,13089). Traditionally 4.5 grams per day of the root have been used. The 1:5 tincture has been dosed at 1.5 grams per day (2). Do not store angelica root preparations in plastic, because plastic can react with the essential oil (8).

Comments

There has been confusion in the past between angelica and water hemlock. Water hemlock is highly toxic (6). According to legend, humans began to use the angelica root after an angel explained to them that the plant was a cure for the plague (6). Angelica is often planted in herb gardens as a decorative border and to protect other herbs from the wind (6).

ANGOSTURA

Also Known As

Angustura, Carony Bark, Cusparia, Cusparia Bark, True Angostura.

Scientific Names

Angostura trifoliata, synonyms Galipea officinalis, Bonplandia trifoliata, Cusparia febrifuga, Cusparia trifoliata.
Family: Rutaceae.

Comments

At the date of publication, there was very little scientific information available about this product. Our staff is continually analyzing the available information on natural medicines and will add data to the online version of *Natural Medicines Comprehensive Database* as it becomes available. See www.naturaldatabase.com.

ANISE

Also Known As
Aniseed, Anisi Fructus, Phytoestrogen, Semen Anisi, Sweet Cumin.

Scientific Names
Pimpinella anisum.
Family: Apiaceae/Umbelliferae.

People Use This For
Orally, anise is used for dyspepsia and as a pediatric antiflatulent and expectorant. Anise is also used orally to increase lactation, induce menstruation, facilitate birth, increase libido; and to alleviate the symptoms of male climacteric, which is the period of life after reproduction functions stop.
Topically, anise is used for lice, scabies, and psoriasis treatment.
In foods, anise is used as a flavoring agent, and has a sweet, aromatic taste characteristic of black licorice. It is commonly used in alcohols and liqueurs, such as Ouzo, Benedictine, Boonekamp, and Danziger Goldwasser. It is also used in dairy products, gelatins, meats, candies, breath fresheners.
In manufacturing, anise is often used as a fragrance in soap, creams, perfumes, and sachets.

Safety
LIKELY SAFE ...when used orally in amounts commonly found in food. Anise and anise oil have Generally Recognized As Safe (GRAS) status in the US (4912).
POSSIBLY UNSAFE ...when used topically. Anise contains furanocoumarin constituents that may cause photosensitivity reactions when skin is exposed to UV light. The constituent bergapten is also believed to be carcinogenic (4).
LIKELY UNSAFE ...when the undiluted oil is used orally. Ingestion of 1-5 mL can cause nausea, vomiting, seizures, and pulmonary edema (4).
PREGNANCY: POSSIBLY UNSAFE ...when used orally in medicinal amounts due to possible abortifacient activity (4,12).
LACTATION: POSSIBLY UNSAFE ...when used orally in medicinal amounts (4). Anise has traditionally been used to promote lactation, however the safety has not been established.

Effectiveness
There is insufficient reliable information available about the effectiveness of anise.

Mechanism of Action
The applicable parts of anise are the dried fruit, seed, and oil. Anise seed is rich in calcium and iron (19). Trans-anethole is a major component of the anise oil, and is responsible for its characteristic taste, smell, and medicinal properties. Anethole has a structure that is similar to catecholamines including adrenaline, noradrenaline, and dopamine; and to the hallucinogenic compound myristicin as well (4). Anethole and the anethole polymers, dianethole and photoanethole might be responsible for the estrogenic activity (4,11). The constituent bergapten can cause photosensitivity and may be carcinogenic (6). Anise also includes the furanocoumarins umbelliferone, umbelliprenine, bergapten, and scopoletin (6).

Adverse Reactions
Allergic reactions to anise may include reactions of the skin, respiratory, and GI tract, and photosensitivity. Anise is not considered a primary irritant, but its use has been associated with skin and mouth irritation and sensitization. Excessive doses of anise can cause adverse neurological effects. The ingestion of 1-5 mL of the oil can cause nausea, vomiting, seizures, and pulmonary edema (4).

Interactions with Herbs & Other Dietary Supplements
None known.

Interactions with Drugs
CONTRACEPTIVE DRUGS: Theoretically, concomitant use of large amounts of anise might interfere with contraceptive drugs through competition for estrogen receptors (4).
ESTROGENS: Theoretically, concomitant use of large amounts of anise might interfere with hormone replacement therapy through competition for estrogen receptors (4).
MONOAMINE OXIDASE INHIBITORS (MAOIs): Theoretically, large doses of anise might interfere with MAOI therapy (4).
TAMOXIFEN (Nolvadex): Theoretically, large doses of anise might interfere with tamoxifen because of its potential estrogenic effects (4).

Interactions with Foods
None known.

Interactions with Lab Tests
BLOOD PRESSURE: Theoretically, anise might increase blood pressure and blood pressure readings, due to the catecholamine activity of the constituent anethole (4,11).
HEART RATE: Theoretically, anise might increase heart rate and pulse rate due to the catecholamine activity of the constituent anethole (4,11).

Interactions with Diseases or Conditions
HORMONE SENSITIVE CANCERS/CONDITIONS: Because anise might have estrogenic effects (4,11), women with hormone sensitive conditions should avoid using it. Some of these conditions include breast cancer, uterine cancer, ovarian cancer, endometriosis, and uterine fibroids.
SKIN CONDITIONS: Anise oil can be potentially irritating and photosensitizing. Avoid anise in cases of dermatitis and inflammatory or allergic skin reactions (4).

Dosage and Administration
ORAL: The typical dose of anise is 0.5-1 grams of the dried fruit or .05-.2 mL of the essential oil, three times per day (4). The tea is prepared by steeping 1-2 teaspoons of the crushed seed for 10-15 minutes and then straining (4). As an expectorant, one cup of tea is commonly taken in the morning and/or at night. As an antiflatulent, one tablespoon of the tea is usually taken several times a day. For nursing babies and infants, the typical dose is one teaspoon of the tea (8).

ANNATTO

Also Known As
Achiote, Achiotillo, Annotta, Arnotta, Bija, Lipstick Tree, Roucou.

Scientific Names
Bixa orellana.
Family: Bixaceae.

People Use This For
Orally, annatto is used to treat diabetes, diarrhea, fevers, heartburn, malaria, hepatitis; and as an antioxidant, diuretic, and purgative.
Topically, annatto is used for burns, vaginitis, and as an insect repellent.
In foods, annatto is used as a coloring agent.

Safety
LIKELY SAFE ...when used orally in amounts commonly found in foods. Annatto has Generally Recognized As Safe status (GRAS) for use in foods in the US (4912).
PREGNANCY AND LACTATION: There is insufficient reliable information available about the safety of annatto during pregnancy and breast-feeding.

Effectiveness
There is insufficient reliable information available about the effectiveness of annatto.

Mechanism of Action
The applicable part of annatto is the seed. Researchers think the coloring principles are carotenoids, mostly bixin and norbixin (11), which do not have vitamin A activity (11).

Adverse Reactions
None reported.

Interactions with Herbs & Other Dietary Supplements
None known.

Interactions with Drugs
ANTIDIABETES DRUGS: Monitor blood glucose levels closely due to claims that annatto has hyperglycemic effects (19).

Interactions with Foods
None known.

Interactions with Lab Tests
None known.

Interactions with Diseases or Conditions
None known.

Dosage and Administration
ORAL: People typically use 1 to 2 grams of powdered leaf in tablets or capsules twice daily. Annatto is also used as a 4:1 tincture in a dose of 2 to 4 mL twice daily (5255).

Comments
This product is used commercially as a food coloring agent (11).

APPLE

Also Known As
Apples.

Scientific Names
Malus sylvestris
Family: Rosaceae.

People Use This For
Orally, apples are used to control diarrhea or constipation; and for the softening, passage, and collection of gallstones. Apples are also used for treating cancer, diabetes, dysentery, fever, heart ailments, scurvy, warts, and cleaning teeth.

Safety
LIKELY SAFE ...when used orally in food amounts. Tell patients to avoid eating apple seeds, which can be toxic (6).
PREGNANCY AND LACTATION: There is insufficient reliable information about the safety of apple in medicinal amounts during pregnancy and lactation; avoid using.

Effectiveness
INSUFFICIENT RELIABLE EVIDENCE to RATE

Gallbladder disease. There is some preliminary evidence apple juice used orally for seven days, with olive oil used on the seventh day before going to bed, might be effective for the softening, passage, and collection of gallstones in the stool (3472).

Lung cancer. There is some preliminary evidence that increasing apple consumption might decrease the risk of developing lung cancer (3470).

More evidence is needed to rate apple for these uses.

Mechanism of Action
The applicable part of apple is the fruit. The pectin in apples probably accounts for their effect on diarrhea and constipation. Pectin absorbs water in the gastrointestinal (GI) tract and swells to a gummy mass. The mass provides bulk which tends to normalize bowel function (6). Apples also contain phloretin, which has antibacterial activity (6). There is some interest in using apples for improving lung function. There is some evidence that consuming five or more apples per week can improve lung function as measured by maximum forced expiration in one second (FEV1) (3469). The constituent quercetin is an antioxidant flavonoid found in high concentrations in apples. Quercetin is thought to be responsible for apples potential benefit in preventing lung cancer (3469,3470).

Adverse Reactions
No adverse reactions are generally known or predicted to occur with apple fruit. However, one death is attributed to ingestion of a large amount (a cupful) of apple seeds, which contain hydrogen cyanide (HCN) (6). Ingestion of large amounts of seeds may cause cyanide poisoning, leading to death. To release cyanide, seeds must be hydrolyzed in the stomach, and several hours may elapse before poisoning symptoms occur (6). Patients allergic to other fruits in the Rosaceae family can also be allergic to apples. Cross-reactivity among the apple fruit and other members of the Rosaceae family, including apricot, almond, plum, peach, pear, and strawberry, has been demonstrated (7129).

Interactions with Herbs & Other Dietary Supplements
None known.

Interactions with Drugs

FEXOFENADINE (Allegra): Apple juice can significantly decrease oral absorption and blood levels of fexofenadine when used together. Apple juice decreases bioavailability of fexofenadine by about 78%. Apple juice seems to inhibit organic anion transporting polypeptide (OATP), which is involved in drug uptake in the gut, liver, and kidney (7046). It's not yet known how long apple juice inhibits OATP. Separating administration times might not prevent this interaction. Tell patients it's best to take their medications with a plain glass of water.

Interactions with Foods

CROSS-ALLERGENICITY: Patients allergic to other fruits in the Rosaceae family can also be allergic to apples. Cross-reactivity among the apple fruit and other members of the Rosaceae family, including apricot, almond, plum, peach, pear, and strawberry, has been demonstrated (7129).

Interactions with Lab Tests

None known.

Interactions with Diseases or Conditions

CROSS-ALLERGENICITY: Patients allergic to other fruits in the Rosaceae family can also be allergic to apples. Cross-reactivity among the apple fruit and other members of the Rosaceae family, including apricot, almond, plum, peach, pear, and strawberry, has been demonstrated (7129).

Dosage and Administration

ORAL: People typically use 500 mg apple pectin capsules daily as a supplement. Dried apple peels are used to make a tea: 1 to 2 teaspoons with 1 cup simmering water. The usual dose is from 1 to 3 cups per day (5250,5263,6006). For the softening of gallstones, one liter of apple juice used daily for seven days with 1 cup of olive oil used on the seventh day before going to bed has been used (3472).

APPLE CIDER VINEGAR

Also Known As

Cider Vinegar.
CAUTION: See separate listing for Apple.

Scientific Names

Malus sylvestris.
Family: Rosaceae.

People Use This For

Orally, apple cider vinegar is used alone or with honey for weight loss, leg cramps and pain, upset stomach, sore throats, sinus problems, high blood pressure, arthritis, to help rid the body of toxins, stimulate thinking, slow the aging process, regulate blood pressure, reduce cholesterol, fight infection, and osteoporosis.
Topically, apple cider vinegar is used for acne, as a skin toner, as an ingredient in hair rinse, to soothe sunburn, for shingles, insect bites, and to prevent dandruff. It is also used in the bath for vaginitis.
In foods, apple cider vinegar is used as a flavoring agent.

Safety

LIKELY SAFE ...when used orally as a food flavoring. ...when used topically, diluted.
POSSIBLY UNSAFE ...when used orally in amounts of 250 mL per day long-term. There is one report of an individual who developed hypokalemia, elevated renin levels, and osteoporosis after 6 years of ingesting 250 mL apple cider vinegar per day (5911).
There is insufficient reliable information available about the safety of apple cider vinegar for its other uses.
PREGNANCY AND LACTATION: There is insufficient reliable information available about the safety of annatto in medicinal amounts during pregnancy and lactation.

Effectiveness

There is insufficient reliable information available about the effectiveness of apple cider vinegar.

Mechanism of Action

Cider vinegar is fermented juice from crushed apples. Like apple juice, it probably contains some pectin; vitamins B1, B2, and B6; biotin; folic acid; niacin; pantothenic acid; and vitamin C. It also contains small amounts of the minerals sodium, phosphorous, potassium, calcium, iron, and magnesium (5912).

Adverse Reactions
Orally, there has been one published report of an individual who developed hypokalemia, high renin levels, and osteoporosis after ingesting 250 mL apple cider vinegar daily for 6 years.

Interactions with Herbs & Other Dietary Supplements
HERBS WITH CARDIAC ACTIVITY: Theoretically, the overuse of apple cider vinegar can increase the risk of cardiotoxicity due to potassium depletion. Cardioactive herbs include digitalis, lily-of-the-valley, pheasant's eye, and squill.
HORSETAIL, LICORICE: Theoretically, overuse of apple cider vinegar can increase the risk of potassium depletion from overuse of horsetail or licorice.
STIMULANT LAXATIVE HERBS: Theoretically, overuse of apple cider vinegar and stimulant laxative herbs can increase the risk of potassium depletion. Stimulant laxative herbs include aloe vera, alder buckthorn, European buckthorn, cascara sagrada, castor oil, rhubarb, and senna.

Interactions with Drugs
DIGOXIN (Lanoxin): Theoretically, overuse of apple cider vinegar could decrease potassium levels, increasing the risk of toxicity for cardiovascular drugs such as digoxin (Lanoxin) (5911).
DIURETIC DRUGS: Overuse of apple cider vinegar might compound diuretic-induced potassium loss (5911). There is some concern that people taking apple cider vinegar along with potassium depleting diuretics might have an increased risk for hypokalemia. Initiation of potassium supplementation or an increase in potassium supplement dose may be necessary for some patients. Some diuretics that can deplete potassium include chlorothiazide (Diuril), chlorthalidone (Thalitone), furosemide (Lasix), hydrochlorothiazide (HCTZ, Hydrodiuril, Microzide), and others.
INSULIN: Theoretically, overuse of apple cider vinegar concomitantly with insulin might cause hypokalemia (5911).

Interactions with Foods
None known.

Interactions with Lab Tests
POTASSIUM LEVEL: Theoretically, long-term use or high doses can reduce serum potassium level and increase urine potassium level (5911).
URINARY ANION GAP: In one case report, long-term use of 250 mL apple cider vinegar per day was associated with high positive urinary anion gap (5911).

Interactions with Diseases or Conditions
DIABETES: Theoretically, long-term use or high doses of apple cider vinegar might increase potassium loss of individuals using insulin.
OSTEOPOROSIS: Theoretically, long-term use or high doses might cause osteoporosis (5911).

Dosage and Administration
TOPICAL: For vaginitis add 3 cups of apple cider vinegar to hot bath and soak, spreading legs to allow water into vagina (5910).

APRICOT

Also Known As
Amygdaloside, Armeniaca, Chinese Almond, Laetrile, Madelonitrile, Vitamin B17.

Scientific Names
Prunus armeniaca, synonyms Amygdalus armeniaca, Armeniaca vulgaris.
Family: Rosaceae.

People Use This For
Orally, apricot is used for asthma, cough, constipation, hemorrhage, infertility, eye inflammation, spasm, and vaginal infections. Laetrile, the semi-synthetic derivative of amygdalin constituent, has been fraudulently acclaimed as a cancer treatment.
In manufacturing, apricot oil is used in cosmetics or as a vehicle for pharmaceutical preparations.

Safety

POSSIBLY SAFE ...when apricot oil is used topically (6).
LIKELY UNSAFE ...when apricot kernels are taken orally because they are a source of cyanide. Acute poisonings may progress to respiratory failure, coma and death within 15 minutes (4). The lethal dose is 50-60 kernels (12) but amount may vary (4). Chronic poisoning can also occur (4).
CHILDREN: POSSIBLY SAFE ...when apricot oil is used topically (6). LIKELY UNSAFE ...when apricot kernels are ingested. The lethal dose is 7-10 kernels (12) but amount may vary (4).
PREGNANCY AND LACTATION: POSSIBLY SAFE ...when apricot oil is used topically (6). LIKELY UNSAFE ...when apricot kernels are ingested (4,12).

Effectiveness

INEFFECTIVE

Cancer. Taking apricot orally is not effective for treating cancer (4,5).

There is insufficient reliable information available about the effectiveness of apricot for its other uses.

Mechanism of Action

The applicable parts of apricot are the kernel (seed) and oil. Apricot contains fruit acids, a variety of sugars, vitamins C and K, beta-carotene, thiamine, niacin, and iron. The seed contains the glycoside amygdalin which yields laetrile and hydrocyanic acid (6). Related glucosides include prunasin, sambunigrin and prulaurasin (6673). Several popular theories that have now been disproved claimed preferential uptake and conversion of amygdalin to hydrogen cyanide in tumor cells. Actually, research shows that amygdalin is slowly hydrolyzed to HCN in the stomach, rapidly absorbed via the GI tract, and then diffused through the body (4).

Adverse Reactions

Apricot may cause acute poisoning, with symptoms including dizziness, headache, nausea, vomiting, drowsiness, dyspnea, palpitations, marked hypotension, convulsions, paralysis, coma, and death (4). Apricot may also cause chronic poisoning, with symptoms of increased blood thiocyanate, goiter, thyroid cancer, optic nerve lesions, blindness, ataxia, hypertonia, cretinism and mental retardation. Demyelinating lesions and neuromyopathies reportedly occur secondary to chronic exposure, including long-term therapy (4).

Interactions with Herbs & Other Dietary Supplements

None known.

Interactions with Drugs

None known.

Interactions with Foods

None known.

Interactions with Lab Tests

None known.

Interactions with Diseases or Conditions

None known.

Dosage and Administration

No typical dosage.

Comments

The apricot seed constituent, amygdalin, is the generic name for laetrile, which is also referred to as amygdaloside, madelonitrile, or vitamin B17 (6673). In 1984, amygdalin, was classified prescription-only to protect the general public (4). In 1987, laetrile was ruled to be an unapproved drug and its importation into the USA under an affidavit system created in 1977 ended (6672).
The FDA is seeking a permanent injunction against three corporations for unlawfully promoting and marketing laetrile (injectable and oral) and apricot seeds for treating cancer on their Internet websites (6669). The companies named in the action are Without Cancer, Inc. and The Health World International, Inc. both located in Florida, and Health Genesis Corporation located in Arizona.

ARECA

Also Known As
Areca Nut, Betel Nut, Betel Quid, Gubak, Pinag, Pinlag, Poogiphalam, Puga, Supari, Tantusara.

Scientific Names
Areca catechu.
Family: Arecaceae/Palmae.

People Use This For
Orally, areca is used as a recreational drug because of its central nervous system (CNS) stimulating properties.
It is also used orally for treatment of schizophrenia, glaucoma, as a mild stimulant, and digestive aid.
In veterinary medicine, an extract of areca is used for expelling tapeworms in cattle, dogs, and horses; as a cathartic; and for treating intestinal colic in horses.

Safety
LIKELY UNSAFE ...when used orally, long-term or in high doses. Constituents of areca have documented carcinogenic potential and have been commonly associated with precancerous lesions and squamous cell carcinoma in long-term users (6,17). Other constituents are poisonous. Ingesting 8-30 grams of areca nut can cause death (6). There is insufficient reliable information available about the safety of short-term use of areca.
PREGNANCY AND LACTATION: LIKELY UNSAFE ...when used orally. Areca has carcinogenic potential as well as central nervous system (CNS) stimulant and cholinergic properties and might adversely affect pregnancy and nursing infants (6,17); avoid using.

Effectiveness
INSUFFICIENT RELIABLE EVIDENCE to RATE

Schizophrenia. There is preliminary evidence that areca might be helpful for schizophrenia. Some patients with schizophrenia who chew areca nut seem to have less severe symptoms (6081). More evidence is needed to rate areca for this use.

Mechanism of Action
The applicable part of areca is the nut. Researchers think alkaloid components have cholinergic action similar to pilocarpine, but with greater central nervous system (CNS) action (6). The most abundant alkaloid is arecoline (6081). Arecoline's cholinergic effects are thought to be the reason for improvement in psychotic symptoms in patients with schizophrenia who chew areca nut (6081). Arecoline also has anthelmintic activity (6). The constituents arecaidine, and arecoline have carcinogenic potential (6); and chewing areca nut has been associated with oral cancer (329). Areca was also historically tried for glaucoma due to its cholinergic effects.

Adverse Reactions
Orally, areca may cause pupil dilation, increased salivation, vomiting, diarrhea, gingivitis, and periodontitis (6). High doses can cause convulsions and death (6). Chewing areca nut results in red-stained mouth, lips, and feces (18). Chewing areca quids is likely to produce central nervous system (CNS) stimulation similar to caffeine and tobacco (6). Areca quid chewing can cause oral submucous fibrosis in susceptible individuals (327,328,329). Chronic use of areca has also been associated with cardiovascular disease, diabetes, asthma (326), and oral cancer (329).

Interactions with Herbs & Other Dietary Supplements
None known.

Interactions with Drugs
ANTICHOLINERGIC DRUGS: Theoretically, due to cholinergic effects areca nut can interfere with anti-cholinergic drug therapy (6). Avoid concomitant use.
CHOLINERGIC DRUGS: Theoretically, due to cholinergic effects areca nut can increase the effects and risk of side effects of cholinergic drugs (6). Avoid concomitant use.
PROCYCLIDINE: Concomitant use can reduce anticholinergic effects of procyclidine (Kemadrin) given to treat the extrapyramidal effects of fluphenazine (19).

Interactions with Foods
None known.

Interactions with Lab Tests
FECAL LAB TESTS: Chewing areca nuts stains feces red (18). This coloration may interfere with fecal lab tests.

Interactions with Diseases or Conditions
ASTHMA: Areca may aggravate asthma (6).

Dosage and Administration

ORAL: An average of approximately 11 whole nuts per day is commonly used (6081).

Comments

Areca nut is chewed alone or in the form of quids, a mixture of tobacco, powdered or sliced areca nut, and slaked lime wrapped in the leaf of "betel" vine (Piper betel) (6).

ARENARIA RUBRA

Also Known As

Common Sandspurry, Sabline Rouge, Sandwort.

Scientific Names

Spergularia rubra.
Family: Caryophyllaceae.

Comments

At the date of publication, this product was not a common ingredient used in brand name supplements marketed to consumers. Details about this product are available in the online version of *Natural Medicines Comprehensive Database.* See www.naturaldatabase.com.

ARISTOLOCHIA

Also Known As

Birthwort, Guang Fang Ji, Long Birthwort, Pelican Flower, Red River Snakeroot, Sangree Root, Sangrel, Serpentaria, Snakeroot, Snakeweed, Texas Snakeroot, Virginia Serpentary, Virginia Snakeroot.

Scientific Names

Aristolochia auricularia; Aristolochia clematitis; Aristolochia fangchi; Aristolochia heterophylla; Aristolochia kwangsiensis; Aristolochia manshuriensis; Aristolochia moupinensis; Aristolochia reticulata; Aristolochia serpentaria; other Aristolochia species.
Family: Aristolochiaceae.

People Use This For

Orally, aristolochia is used as an aphrodisiac, anticonvulsant, immune stimulant, to promote menstruation, and to treat snakebite. It is also used to treat allergic gastrointestinal colic and gallbladder colic. Other uses include arthritis, gout, rheumatism, eczema, and wound treatment.

Safety

UNSAFE ...when used orally. Aristolochia contains aristolochic acid, which is nephrotoxic and carcinogenic (6073,6118). The FDA considers all products containing aristolochic acid to be unsafe and adulterated (6118).

PREGNANCY AND LACTATION: UNSAFE ...when used orally; avoid using (6118).

Effectiveness

There is insufficient reliable information available about the effectiveness of aristolochia.

Mechanism of Action

The applicable parts of aristolochia are the above ground parts and root. Aristolochia contains aristolochic acid which is nephrotoxic and carcinogenic. Aristolochic acid and possibly other aristolochia constituents damage DNA, which causes fibrotic destruction of the kidney and development of tumors (12782). Aristolochic acid has been associated with cancers of the kidney, bladder, stomach, and lung, and lymphoma in rodents and cancers of the bladder, ureter, and/or renal pelvis in people with aristolochic acid-associated nephropathy (6118).

Adverse Reactions
Orally, use of aristolochia can cause end-stage renal failure and urothelial carcinoma of the bladder (12782). There have been more than 100 cases of nephropathy, referred to as "Chinese herb nephropathy", characterized by interstitial fibrosis and associated with tea believed adulterated with aristolochia. This was originally reported in Belgium with accidental substitution of aristolochia for another herb. Of these cases, 43 progressed to end stage renal failure requiring dialysis or transplantation (564,6073) and 18 developed urothelial carcinomas of the bladder, ureter, and/or renal pelvis (6073). Many cases of nephropathy associated with aristolochia use have been reported worldwide (12783,12784,12785,12786,12787). The risk of developing urothelial carcinoma seems to be related to cumulative intake of the herb (6073).

Interactions with Herbs & Other Dietary Supplements
None known.

Interactions with Drugs
None known.

Interactions with Foods
None known.

Interactions with Lab Tests
KIDNEY FUNCTION TESTS: Aristolochia can cause nephropathy and abnormal kidney function results (564).

Interactions with Diseases or Conditions
RENAL DISEASE: Aristolochia causes interstitial fibrosis and might accelerate renal failure in people with pre-existing renal disease (12782).

Dosage and Administration
No typical dosage.

Comments
The FDA considers all products containing aristolochic acid to be unsafe and adulterated (6118). The FDA intends to automatically detain, without physical examination, any product which contains plants known or suspected to contain aristolochic acid, or which might be adulterated with plants known to contain aristolochic acid. Each detained product will be released only after the responsible party provides direct analytical evidence that it is free of aristolochic acid (6118). Aristolochia is also banned in Germany, Austria, France, Great Britain, Belgium, and Japan (367).
Health Canada, the Canadian health authority, removed five aristolochia-containing Chinese herbal medicine products from sale. The products include, Touku Natural Herbal Rheumatic Pills, two brands of Tri-Snakegall & Fritillary Powder, Tracheitis Pills, and Gastropathy Capsules (367).

ARNICA

Also Known As
Arnica Flos, Arnica Flower, Arnikablüten, Bergwohlverleih, Fleurs d'Arnica, Kraftwurz, Leopard's Bane, Mountain Tobacco, Wolf's Bane, Wundkraut.

Scientific Names
Arnica montana; Arnica fulgens; Arnica sororia; Arnica latifolia; Arnica cordifolia.
Family: Asteraceae/Compositae.

People Use This For
Topically, arnica is used for the inflammation and immune system stimulation associated with bruises, aches, and sprains. It is also used orally for mouth and throat inflammation, insect bites, superficial phlebitis, and as an abortifacient.
In foods, arnica is a flavor ingredient in alcoholic beverages, nonalcoholic beverages, frozen dairy desserts, candy, baked goods, gelatins, and puddings.
In manufacturing, arnica is used in hair tonics and anti-dandruff preparations. The oil is used in perfumes and other cosmetic preparations.

Safety

POSSIBLY SAFE ...when used in amounts commonly found in foods. Arnica has Generally Recognized As Safe status (GRAS) for use in foods in the US (4912). Canadian regulations do not allow its use as a food ingredient (12). ...when used topically for short-term use on unbroken skin (12).
LIKELY UNSAFE ...when taken orally. Arnica is considered poisonous and has caused severe or fatal poisonings (5). It can be cardiotoxic and cause large increases in blood pressure (5,17). Arnica is irritating to mucous membranes and can cause gastroenteritis, muscle paralysis (voluntary and cardiac), an increase or decrease in pulse rate, heart palpitations, shortness of breath, and death (4,17).
PREGNANCY AND LACTATION: LIKELY UNSAFE ...when used orally or topically; avoid using (12).

Effectiveness

POSSIBLY INEFFECTIVE

Wisdom tooth extraction. Taking arnica orally doesn't seem to reduce the postsurgical complications of third molar extraction. Arnica does not appear to improve pain, swelling, or wound infection associated with wisdom tooth removal (10630).

There is insufficient reliable information available about the effectiveness of arnica for its other uses.

Mechanism of Action

The applicable part of arnica is the flowerhead. The sesquiterpene lactones of arnica are the active constituents and produce anti-inflammatory and analgesic effects (102). They also can have some antibiotic activity (5). Two constituents of arnica, helenalin and 11 alpha,13-dihyrohelenalin, have been shown to inhibit human platelet function (104).

Adverse Reactions

Arnica taken orally can cause irritation of mucous membranes, drowsiness, stomach pain, vomiting, diarrhea, tachycardia, shortness of breath, coma, and death (4,6,11). Arnica can cause an allergic reaction in individuals sensitive to the Asteraceae/Compositae family. Members of this family include ragweed, chrysanthemums, marigolds, daisies, and many other herbs. Topically, arnica can cause contact dermatitis and mucous membrane irritation (6,11).

Interactions with Herbs & Other Dietary Supplements

None known.

Interactions with Drugs

ANTICOAGULANT/ANTIPLATELET DRUGS: There is some concern that arnica might potentiate the effects of anticoagulant and antiplatelet drugs and possibly increase the risk of bleeding. Constituents of arnica can decrease platelet aggregation in vitro (104). However, this effect has not yet been demonstrated in humans. Until more is known, use cautiously in patients taking anticoagulant or antiplatelet drugs. Some of these drugs include aspirin, clopidogrel (Plavix), dalteparin (Fragmin), enoxaparin (Lovenox), heparin, ticlopidine (Ticlid), warfarin (Coumadin), and others.

Interactions with Foods

None known.

Interactions with Lab Tests

PLATELET FUNCTION: Theoretically, arnica might inhibit platelet function and test results (104).

Interactions with Diseases or Conditions

BROKEN SKIN: Avoid the use of arnica on broken or damaged skin (2,4).
CROSS-ALLERGENICITY: Arnica can cause reactions in individuals allergic to plants in the Asteraceae/Compositae family. Members of this family include ragweed, chrysanthemums, marigolds, daisies, and many other herbs (12,17).
GASTROINTESTINAL (GI) IRRITATION: Arnica can irritate the gastrointestinal (GI) tract. Arnica is contraindicated in individuals with infectious or inflammatory GI conditions (19).

Dosage and Administration

TOPICAL: The typical dose of arnica is 2 grams of the flowerheads in 100 mL of water (8). As a poultice, the tincture of arnica is diluted three to ten times with water (8). As a mouthwash, the tincture is diluted ten times (8); the mouthwash should not be swallowed. Ointments commonly contain a maximum of 20-25% of the tincture or 15% of the oil (8). The tincture is usually 1:10 (2), and the oil is usually 1:5 in vegetable fixed oil (2,8).

ARRACH

Also Known As
Dog's Arrach, Goat's Arrach, Goosefoot, Netchweed, Oraches, Stinking Arrach, Stinking Goosefoot, Stinking Motherwort.

Scientific Names
Chenopodium vulvaria.
Family: Chenopodiaceae or Amaranthaceae.

Comments
At the date of publication, this product was not a common ingredient used in brand name supplements marketed to consumers. Details about this product are available in the online version of *Natural Medicines Comprehensive Database.* See www.naturaldatabase.com.

ARROWROOT

Also Known As
Maranta.

Scientific Names
Maranta arundinacea.
Family: Marantaceae.

People Use This For
Orally, arrowroot is used as a nutritional food for infants and convalescents. Babies cut teeth on arrowroot cookies. It is also used as a dietary aid in gastrointestinal disorders and acute diarrhea.
Topically, arrowroot is used as a soothing agent for painful, irritated or inflamed mucous membranes.
In foods, arrowroot is used as an ingredient in cooking.

Safety
LIKELY SAFE ...when the starch from the root or rhizome are used orally in amounts found in foods (12).
POSSIBLY SAFE ...when used orally or topically in medicinal amounts (12).
PREGNANCY AND LACTATION: POSSIBLY SAFE ...when used in amounts found in foods. There is insufficient reliable information available about the safety of larger amounts used during pregnancy and lactation; avoid using.

Effectiveness
There is insufficient reliable information available about the effectiveness of arrowroot.

Mechanism of Action
The applicable part of arrowroot is the starch from the root and rhizome. Animal data suggests that arrowroot may reduce deposited cholesterol in the aorta and heart muscle. This may be due to an increase in the elimination of cholesterol in the form of bile acids (18).

Adverse Reactions
None reported.

Interactions with Herbs & Other Dietary Supplements
None known.

Interactions with Drugs
None known.

Interactions with Foods
None known.

Interactions with Lab Tests
None known.

Interactions with Diseases or Conditions
None known.

Dosage and Administration

ORAL: Arrowroot starch is extracted from the chopped root and rhizome by a specific process using water. The powdered starch is usually boiled with water and used orally (18).

Comments

Arrowroot is often replaced with cheaper starches, including potato, corn, wheat, or rice starch (18).

ARTICHOKE

Also Known As

Alcachofa, Alcaucil, Artichaut Commun, Artichoke Extract, Artichoke Leaf, Artichoke Leaf Extract, Artischocke, Cardo, Cardo de Comer, Cardon d'Espagne, Cardoon, Garden Artichoke, Gemuseartischocke, Globe Artichoke, Kardone, Tyosen-Azami.

Scientific Names

Cynara cardunculus, synonym Cynara scolymus.
Family: Asteraceae/Compositae.

People Use This For

Orally, artichoke is used for dyspepsia, hyperlipidemia, nausea, alcohol-induced hangover, and irritable bowel syndrome (IBS). It is also used orally as a diuretic and choleretic. Artichoke is also used orally for treating snakebites, renal insufficiency, anemia, edema, arthritis, cystitis, liver dysfunction, preventing gallstones, lowering blood pressure, as a hypoglycemic, stimulant, and a tonic.

In foods, artichoke leaves and extracts are used as flavoring agents in beverages. The constituents, cynarin and chlorogenic acid, are sometimes used as sweeteners.

Safety

LIKELY SAFE ...when used orally in amounts commonly found in foods. Artichoke has Generally Recognized As Safe status (GRAS) for use in foods in the US (4912).

POSSIBLY SAFE ...when used orally and appropriately in therapeutic amounts (2056,11773). Artichoke extract appears to be safe for up to 23 months (11773).

PREGNANCY AND LACTATION: There is insufficient reliable information about the safety of therapeutic amounts of artichoke used during pregnancy or lactation; avoid using.

Effectiveness

POSSIBLY EFFECTIVE

Dyspepsia. Artichoke leaf extract seems to significantly reduce symptoms such as nausea, vomiting, flatulence, and abdominal pain in functional dyspepsia and dyspepsia associated with biliary disease. Improvement can take up to 2 to 8 weeks of treatment (2056,11429,12208). Artichoke leaf extract needs to be given to 11.5 patients for 6 weeks in order for one patient to have markedly or completely improved symptoms (12208).
Some studies have used a specific extract called ALE LI 220 (HeparSL forte, Berlin, Germany).

Hyperlipidemia. Artichoke extract seems to modestly reduce total and low-density lipoprotein (LDL) cholesterol, and the LDL/high density lipoprotein (HDL) ratio over 6 to 12 weeks of treatment. Artichoke extract may work better in people with higher cholesterol levels (6282,11773).

POSSIBLY INEFFECTIVE

Hangover. Artichoke extract doesn't seem to prevent alcohol-induced hangover (11774).

INSUFFICIENT RELIABLE EVIDENCE to RATE

Irritable bowel syndrome (IBS). There is preliminary evidence that artichoke extract might reduce abdominal pain and cramping, bloating, flatulence, and constipation associated with IBS after 6 weeks of treatment (2562). More evidence is needed to rate artichoke for this use.

Mechanism of Action

The applicable parts of artichoke are the leaf, stem, and root. The primary constituents include up to 2% phenolic acids, primarily chlorogenic acid, cynarin, and caffeic acid. Artichoke also contains up to 4% sesquiterpene lactones, and 1% flavonoids including scolymoside, cynaroside, and luteolin (2056). Artichoke's therapeutic benefit in dyspepsia has centered around its choleretic effects, or ability to stimulate bile flow, which has been demonstrated in several studies (2056). This might explain its use as a hangover remedy (11774). Constituents responsible for this effect are thought to be cynarin, chlorogenic acid, and scolymoside (2056).

Antiemetic, spasmolytic, and carminative effects of artichoke have also been described. These effects may be responsible for the potential beneficial effects in patients with irritable bowel syndrome (IBS) (2562). Cynarin and chlorogenic acid may also have cholesterol-lowering effects, although studies with cynarin for hyperlipidemia have produced mixed results (1423,1424).

Artichoke might reduce cholesterol synthesis (11773). Cynaroside and its derivative, luteolin, might also indirectly inhibit HMG-CoA reductase (1425,1426,2056). Several constituents are reported to have antioxidant activity (1422). Preliminary research suggests that artichoke leaf extract might also protect liver cells from damage (1421,1422,2056,3269). A mixture of polyphenols and flavonoids including caffeic acid, chlorogenic acid, cynarin, luteolin-7-O-glycoside (cynaroside), and luteolin might contribute to hepatoprotective activity (3269,2056).

Adverse Reactions

Orally, artichoke extract might increase flatulence in some patients (2562). Artichoke can also cause an allergic reaction in some patients. Patients sensitive to the Asteraceae/Compositae family may be at the greatest risk. Members of this family include ragweed, chrysanthemums, marigolds, daisies, and many other herbs.
Topically, allergic contact dermatitis can occur with the use of artichoke. This has been attributed to the constituent cynaropicrin (11).

Interactions with Herbs & Other Dietary Supplements

None known.

Interactions with Drugs

None known.

Interactions with Foods

None known.

Interactions with Lab Tests

None known.

Interactions with Diseases or Conditions

BILE DUCT OBSTRUCTION: Theoretically, artichoke might worsen bile duct obstruction by increasing bile flow (2056); avoid using.
CROSS-ALLERGENICITY: Artichoke might cause an allergic reaction in individuals sensitive to Asteraceae/Compositae family plants. Members of this family include ragweed, chrysanthemums, marigolds, daisies, and many other herbs (2056).
GALLSTONES: Theoretically, artichoke might worsen gallstones by increasing bile flow (2056); use with caution.

Dosage and Administration

ORAL: For dyspepsia, 320 mg to 640 mg artichoke leaf extract three times daily has been used (11429,12208). Some studies have used a specific extract called ALE LI 220 (HeparSL forte, Berlin, Germany).
For irritable bowel syndrome (IBS), 640 mg leaf extract three times daily has been used (2562).
For lowering serum cholesterol, an artichoke extract 1800 to 1920 mg per day in 2 to 3 divided doses has been used. The isolated constituent cynarin 60-1500 mg per day has also been used to lower cholesterol (1423,1424,2056,11773).

Comments

Avoid confusion with Jerusalem artichoke (Helianthus tuberosus).

ARUM

Also Known As

Adder's Root, Bobbins, Cocky Baby, Cuckoo Pint, Cypress Powder, Dragon Root, Friar's Cowl, Gaglee, Kings and Queens, Ladysmock, Lords and Ladies, Parson and Clerk, Portland Arrowroot, Quaker, Ramp, Starchwort, Wake Robin.
CAUTION: See separate listing for Beth Root.

Scientific Names

Arum maculatum.
Family: Araceae.

People Use This For

Orally, arum is used for colds and inflammation of the throat. It is also used orally to stimulate sweating and as an expectorant.

Safety

UNSAFE ...when used orally (18).
PREGNANCY AND LACTATION: UNSAFE ...when used orally because of its toxicity (18); avoid using.

Effectiveness

There is insufficient reliable information available about the effectiveness of arum.

Mechanism of Action
The applicable part of arum is the root. Arum can cause severe mucous membrane irritation and bleeding. This is probably due to sharp oxalate crystals present in the root. These injure the mucous membranes, and may also introduce impurities into the wounds. Arum also contains cyanogenic glycosides, but the levels are probably too low to cause poisoning (18).

Adverse Reactions
Orally, arum can cause swelling of the tongue, bloody vomiting, and bloody diarrhea (18).

Interactions with Herbs & Other Dietary Supplements
CALCIUM, IRON, ZINC: Concurrent use might decrease mineral absorption. Arum contains oxalate (18), which can bind multivalent metal ions in the gastrointestinal tract and decrease mineral absorption.

Interactions with Drugs
None known.

Interactions with Foods
CALCIUM, IRON, ZINC: Concurrent use might decrease mineral absorption from foods. Arum contains oxalate (18), which can bind multivalent metal ions in the gastrointestinal tract and decrease mineral absorption.

Interactions with Lab Tests
None known.

Interactions with Diseases or Conditions
None known.

Dosage and Administration
No typical dosage.

ASAFOETIDA

Also Known As
Assant, Devil's Dung, Food of the Gods, Fum, Giant Fennel, Heeng.

Scientific Names
Ferula assa-foetida; Ferula foetida; Ferula pseudalliacea, synonym Ferula rubricaulis.
Family: Apiaceae/Umbelliferae.

People Use This For
Orally, asafoetida is used for chronic bronchitis, asthma, pertussis, hoarseness, hysteria, flatulent colic, chronic gastritis, dyspepsia, irritable colon, convulsions, as a nerve stimulant in treating neurasthenia. It is also used orally for amenorrhea, croup, insanity, and sarcomas.
Topically, asafoetida is used for corns and calluses.
In manufacturing, asafoetida is used as a fragrance or fixative in cosmetics, and it is used as a flavoring ingredient in foods and beverages.
Other uses for asafoetida include its use as a cat, dog, and wildlife repellent.

Safety
LIKELY SAFE ...when used orally in amounts commonly found in foods. Asafoetida has Generally Recognized As Safe status (GRAS) for use in foods in the US (4912).
POSSIBLY SAFE ...when used orally and appropriately (12).
CHILDREN: UNSAFE ...when used orally in infants due to the possible risk of methemoglobinemia (4).
PREGNANCY: UNSAFE ...when used orally in medicinal amounts; asafoetida might cause abortion (4).
LACTATION: UNSAFE ...when used orally due to possible risk of methemoglobinemia in infants (4).

Effectiveness
There is insufficient reliable information available about the effectiveness of asafoetida.

Mechanism of Action
The applicable part of asafoetida is the root resin. Asafoetida may contain sulfur compounds in its volatile oil which may protect against fat-induced hyperlipidemia. Asafoetida may contain coumarin constituents with anticoagulant activity (4). There is some evidence to suggest that its constituents treat irritable bowel syndrome (IBS) (4).

Adverse Reactions

Orally, 50-100 mg of asafoetida may cause convulsions in people with nervousness (12). There is one report of methemoglobinemia in an infant (4). Large amounts are reported to cause swelling of the lips, belching, flatulence, diarrhea, headache, or convulsions (18).
Topically, genital organ swelling was reported after external use of asafoetida on the abdomen (18).

Interactions with Herbs & Other Dietary Supplements

None known.

Interactions with Drugs

ANTICOAGULANT/ANTIPLATELET DRUGS: Theoretically, asafoetida might increase the risk of bleeding (4).
ANTIHYPERTENSIVE DRUGS: Theoretically, concomitant use may increase therapeutic effects of antihypertensive therapy due to hypotensive activity of asafoetida (4).

Interactions with Foods

None known.

Interactions with Lab Tests

None known.

Interactions with Diseases or Conditions

BLEEDING DISORDERS: Theoretically, asafoetida might increase the risk of bleeding (4).
CENTRAL NERVOUS SYSTEM (CNS) CONDITIONS: Asafoetida is contraindicated in people with CNS conditions that could result in convulsions (12).
GASTROINTESTINAL (GI) IRRITATION: Asafoetida can irritate GI tract. It is contraindicated in individuals with infectious or inflammatory gastrointestinal conditions (19).
HYPERTENSION: Theoretically, asafoetida might interfere with blood pressure control (4).
HYPOTENSION: Theoretically, asafoetida might interfere with blood pressure control (4).

Dosage and Administration

ORAL: A typical dose is 300-1000 mg powdered resin three times daily (4). Tincture of asafoetida (concentration unspecified), 2-4 mL (4), or 20 drops as a single dose (18) have also been used.
TOPICAL: No typical dosage.

Comments

Asafoetida resin is produced by solidifying juice exuded from incisions in living roots of Ferula foetida and other Ferula species. Asafoetida is known to have putrid odor and tastes bitter. The acrid taste is the basis for its name, devil's dung (6). Various species of this plant have somewhat different constituents. The related species Ferula communis, contains toxic coumarin constituents. Other related species are Ferula galbaniflua and Ferula rubricaulis. These seem to cause contact dermatitis (4).

ASARABACCA

Also Known As

Asaroun, Asarum, Azarum, False Coltsfoot, Hazelwort, Public House Plant, Snakeroot, Wild Ginger, Wild Nard.
CAUTION: See separate listings for Bitter Milkwort, Coltsfoot, Ginger, and Senega.

Scientific Names

Asarum europaeum.
Family: Aristolochiaceae.

People Use This For

Orally, asarabacca is used for acute and chronic bronchitis, bronchial spasms, and bronchial asthma. It is also used orally as an emetic; antitussive; menstrual stimulant; abortifacient; and to treat pneumonia, angina pectoris, migraines, liver disease, jaundice, and dehydration.

Safety

POSSIBLY SAFE ...when used orally and appropriately short-term (12).
POSSIBLY UNSAFE ...when used orally in large amounts or long-term (12). Large doses have been associated with significant side effects, including burning tongue, gastroenteritis, diarrhea, skin rashes, and partial paralysis (18). ...when the essential oil is taken orally. The essential oil contains a potential hepatocarcinogenic constituent, beta-asarone (12).
UNSAFE ...when aristolochic acid-contaminated asarabacca is used orally. Asarabacca is commonly contaminated with aristolochic acid, which is nephrotoxic and carcinogenic. The FDA considers all products containing aristolochic acid to be unsafe and adulterated. Only products analytically verified to be aristolochic acid-free should be used (6118).
PREGNANCY: LIKELY UNSAFE ...when used orally. Asarabacca might act as a menstrual or uterine stimulant (12); contraindicated.
LACTATION: Insufficient reliable information available; avoid using.

Effectiveness

There is insufficient reliable information available about the effectiveness of asarabacca.

Mechanism of Action

The applicable part of asarabacca is the rhizome. The constituent phenylpropanol may be responsible for the effects of asarabacca on bronchitis/bronchial asthma. Some products are standardized for content of this constituent (18). The emetic and spasmolytic effects may be due to the constituent trans-isoasarone (18). Local anesthetic effect demonstrated in humans may be due to constituents, trans-isoasarone and trans-isomethyleugenol (18).

Adverse Reactions

Orally, asarabacca may cause nausea and vomiting (12). Severe poisoning has also been reported (553). Symptoms of poisoning include burning of tongue, gastroenteritis, diarrhea, skin rashes, and partial paralysis (18). Asarabacca is commonly contaminated with aristolochic acid, which is nephrotoxic and carcinogenic (6118).

Interactions with Herbs & Other Dietary Supplements

None known.

Interactions with Drugs

None known.

Interactions with Foods

None known.

Interactions with Lab Tests

None known.

Interactions with Diseases or Conditions

GASTROINTESTINAL (GI) IRRITATION: Asarabacca can irritate the GI tract; contraindicated in individuals with infectious or inflammatory GI conditions (19).

Dosage and Administration

ORAL: Typically, 30 mg of the extract made from dried asarabacca is used in adults and children over 13 years old (18).

Comments

Asarabacca has been reported as obsolete for medicinal use (18); safer alternatives are available. Avoid confusion with bitter milkwort (Polygala amara), or senega (Polygala senega) also known as snakeroot. Asarabacca is frequently contaminated with aristolochic acid, which is nephrotoxic and carcinogenic. The FDA considers all products containing aristolochic acid to be unsafe and adulterated (6118). The FDA intends to automatically detain, without physical examination, any product which contains plants known or suspected to contain aristolochic acid, or which might be adulterated with plants known to contain aristolochic acid. Each detained product will be released only after the responsible party provides direct analytical evidence that it is free of aristolochic acid (6118).

ASH

Also Known As

Bird's Tongue, Common Ash, European Ash, Weeping Ash, White Ash.
CAUTION: See separate listings for Northern Prickly Ash and Southern Prickly Ash.

Scientific Names

Fraxinus americana; Fraxinus excelsior.
Family: Oleaceae.

Comments

At the date of publication, there was very little scientific information available about this product. Our staff is continually analyzing the available information on natural medicines and will add data to the online version of *Natural Medicines Comprehensive Database* as it becomes available. See www.naturaldatabase.com.

ASHWAGANDHA

Also Known As

Ajagandha, Amangura, Amukkirag, Asan, Asgand, Asgandh, Asgandha, Ashagandha, Ashvagandha, Ashwaganda, Ashwanga, Asoda, Asundha, Asvagandha, Aswagandha, Avarada, Ayurvedic Ginseng, Clustered Wintercherry, Ghoda Asoda, Indian Ginseng, Kanaje Hindi, Kuthmithi, Samm Al Ferakh, Turangi-Ghanda, Winter Cherry, Withania.
CAUTION: See separate listings for Blue Cohosh, Canaigre, Codonopsis, Ginseng American, Ginseng Panax, Ginseng Siberian, and Winter Cherry.

Scientific Names

Withania somnifera, synonym Physalis somnifera.
Family: Solanaceae.

People Use This For

Orally, ashwagandha is used for arthritis, anxiety, insomnia, tumors, tuberculosis, and chronic liver disease. Ashwagandha is also used as an "adaptogen" to increase resistance to environmental stress, and as a general tonic. It is also used orally for immunomodulatory effects, improving cognitive function, decreasing inflammation, preventing the effects of aging, for emaciation, infertility in men and women, menstrual disorders, and hiccups. It is also used orally as an aphrodisiac, and emmenagogue; and for treating asthma, leukoderma, bronchitis, backache, and arthritis.
Topically, ashwagandha is used for treating ulcerations, backache, and hemiplegia.

Safety

POSSIBLY SAFE ...when used orally and appropriately, short-term (3710,11301).
There is insufficient reliable information available about the safety of ashwagandha when used long-term or topically.
PREGNANCY: LIKELY UNSAFE ...when used orally. Ashwagandha has abortifacient effects (12).
LACTATION: Insufficient reliable information available; avoid using.

Effectiveness

There is insufficient reliable information available about the effectiveness of ashwagandha.

Mechanism of Action

The applicable parts of ashwagandha are the root and berry. Ashwagandha contains several active constituents including alkaloids (isopelletierine, anaferine), steroidal lactones (withanolides, withaferins), and saponins (4116,11301). Ashwagandha does not contain nicotine as some researchers have reported (3710). Preliminary animal evidence suggests ashwagandha may have a variety of pharmacological effects including analgesic, antipyretic, anxiolytic, immunomodulatory, sedative, hypotensive, anti-inflammatory, and antioxidant effects (3710,3711,4113,4116,11301). It might also stimulate respiratory function, cause smooth muscle relaxation, and stimulate thyroid synthesis and/or secretion (3710).
Some researchers think ashwagandha has a so-called "anti-stressor" effect. Preliminary evidence suggests ashwagandha might suppress stress-induced increases of dopamine receptors in the corpus striatum of the brain (3710). It also appears to reduce stress-induced increases of plasma corticosterone, blood urea nitrogen, and blood lactic acid (11301). Ashwagandha might also have anxiolytic effects, possibly by acting as a gamma-aminobutyric acid (GABA) mimetic agent. It might also have anticonvulsant activity, by binding to the GABA receptor (3710).

Ashwagandha and its constituents also seem to have immunomodulatory effects. The withanolides and sitoindosides seem to cause a mobilization of macrophages, phagocytosis, and lysosomal enzymes (11301). Preliminary evidence suggests ashwagandha might reduce cyclophosphamide-induced immunosuppression and leukopenia (3711,4114). Ashwagandha also seems to increase bone marrow cell and white blood cell count in radiation-treated animals (3711). It remains unclear, however, what net effect whole ashwagandha preparations have on the immune system (3710,3711).

Adverse Reactions

Orally, ashwagandha seems to be well tolerated at typical doses. Large doses may cause gastrointestinal (GI) upset, diarrhea, and vomiting secondary to irritation of the mucous and serous membranes (3710).

Interactions with Herbs & Other Dietary Supplements

HERBS/SUPPLEMENTS WITH SEDATIVE PROPERTIES: Theoretically, concomitant use with herbs that have sedative properties might enhance therapeutic and adverse effects (11301). Some of these include 5-HTP, calamus, California poppy, catnip, hops, Jamaican dogwood, kava, St. John's wort, scullcap, valerian, yerba mansa, and others.

Interactions with Drugs

BENZODIAZEPINES: Theoretically, ashwagandha might increase the effects of benzodiazepines (3710). There is preliminary evidence that ashwagandha might have an additive effect with diazepam (Valium) and clonazepam (Klonopin) (3710). This may also occur with other benzodiazepines such as alprazolam (Xanax), flurazepam (Dalmane), lorazepam (Ativan), and midazolam (Versed).

CNS DEPRESSANTS: Theoretically, ashwagandha's sedative effect may potentiate the effects of barbiturates, other sedatives, and anxiolytics (3710).

IMMUNOSUPPRESSANTS: Theoretically, ashwagandha might decrease the effectiveness of immunosuppressant therapy because of its potential immunostimulating effects. There is preliminary evidence that ashwagandha might decrease immunosuppression caused by cyclophosphamide (3711,4114). It might also decrease the effectiveness of other immunosuppressant drugs such as azathioprine (Imuran), basiliximab (Simulect), cyclosporine (Neoral, Sandimmune), daclizumab (Zenapax), muromonab-CD3 (OKT3, Orthoclone OKT3), mycophenolate (CellCept), tacrolimus (FK506, Prograf), sirolimus (Rapamune), prednisone (Deltasone, Orasone), and other corticosteroids (glucocorticoids).

THYROID HORMONE: Theoretically, ashwagandha might have additive effects when used with thyroid supplements. There is preliminary evidence that ashwagandha might boost thyroid hormone synthesis and/or secretion (3710).

Interactions with Foods

None known.

Interactions with Lab Tests

THYROID FUNCTION TESTS: Theoretically, ashwagandha might suppress thyroid stimulating hormone (TSH) or increase triiodothyronine (T3) or thyroxine (T4) values. There is some evidence that ashwagandha might stimulate thyroid hormone synthesis or secretion (3710).

Interactions with Diseases or Conditions

PEPTIC ULCER DISEASE: Theoretically, ashwagandha should be avoided by people with peptic ulcer disease because of its irritant effect on the gastrointestinal (GI) tract (3710).

Dosage and Administration

ORAL: People typically use 1 to 6 grams daily of the whole herb in capsule or tea form (3710). The tea is prepared by boiling ashwagandha roots in water for 15 minutes and cooled. The usual dose is 3 cups daily. Tincture or fluid extracts are dosed 2 to 4 mL 3 times per day.

TOPICAL: No typical dosage.

Comments

The name Ashwagandha is from the Sanskrit language and is a combination of the word ashva, meaning horse, and gandha, meaning smell. The root has a strong aroma that is described as "horse-like" (3710). In Ayurvedic, Indian, and Unani medicine, ashwagandha is described as "Indian ginseng". Ashwagandha is sometimes substituted or adulterated with a similar plant, Withania coagulans (3710). Avoid confusing ashwagandha with Physalis alkekengi, also known as winter cherry.

ASPARAGUS

Also Known As

Asparagi Rhizoma Root, Asperge, Garden Asparagus, Sativari, Shatavari, Spargelkraut, Spargelwurzelstock, Sparrow Grass.

Scientific Names

Asparagus officinalis, synonym Asparagus longifolius.
Family: Asparagaceae or Liliaceae.

People Use This For

Orally, asparagus is used along with copious fluid consumption as "irrigation therapy" to increase urine output. It is also used orally for treating urinary tract infections and other inflammatory conditions of the urinary tract, preventing kidney and bladder stones, rheumatic joint pain and swelling, female hormone imbalances, dryness in the lungs and throat, AIDS, to prevent anemia due to folic acid deficiency, as a laxative, for neuritis, and for treating parasitic diseases and cancer.
Topically, asparagus is used for cleaning the face, drying sores, and acne.
In foods, the newly-formed shoots, or spears, are eaten as a vegetable. The seed and root extracts of asparagus are used in alcoholic beverages.

Safety

LIKELY SAFE ...when used in amounts commonly found in foods. Asparagus seed and root extract have Generally Recognized As Safe status (GRAS) for use in foods in the US (4912).
POSSIBLY SAFE ...when used orally and appropriately for medicinal purposes (2,12).
There is insufficient reliable information available about the safety of the topical uses of asparagus.
PREGNANCY: POSSIBLY UNSAFE ...when used for medicinal purposes; asparagus extracts have been used as a contraceptive (6); avoid using.
LACTATION: There is insufficient reliable information available about the safety of asparagus in medicinal amounts during breast-feeding.

Effectiveness

There is insufficient reliable information available about the effectiveness of asparagus.

Mechanism of Action

The applicable parts of asparagus are the rhizome and root. Asparagus is a vitamin E rich plant source (19). The asparagus root has diuretic effects in animal experiments (2). Asparagus also has hypotensive, antibacterial, and antiviral effects in vitro (11). Fibers from the plant can have mutagen-adsorbing (cancer-preventing) activity (11). The saponin constituents can irritate mucous membranes and can be cytotoxic (6,3901). Asparagus can also cause urinary tract irritation (19).

Adverse Reactions

Orally, asparagus can cause mucous membrane irritation (3901).
Topically, asparagus can cause allergic skin reactions (2).

Interactions with Herbs & Other Dietary Supplements

None known.

Interactions with Drugs

None known.

Interactions with Foods

None known.

Interactions with Lab Tests

None known.

Interactions with Diseases or Conditions

EDEMA: Irrigation therapy with asparagus is contraindicated in individuals with edema caused by heart or kidney disorders (2).
KIDNEY DISEASE: Asparagus is contraindicated in individuals with inflammatory kidney disease because the mucosal irritant effect of asparagus can exacerbate this condition (2,6,12).

Dosage and Administration
ORAL: Typically, asparagus is used daily as a tea prepared by steeping 40-60 grams of the cut rhizome or root in 150 mL of boiling water for 5-10 minutes and then straining (2). Ensure ample fluid intake when used as "irrigation therapy" (2,18).
TOPICAL: No typical dosage.

Comments
Asparagus seeds are used medicinally in a few cultures. The consumption of asparagus spears produces a pungent odor in the urine of some people.

ASPARTATES

Also Known As
Aspartate Chelated Minerals, Aspartate Mineral Chelates, Aspartic Acid, L-Aspartic Acid, Mineral Aspartates. CAUTION: See separate listing for Chelated Minerals.

Scientific Names
None.

People Use This For
Orally, aspartates are used to increase absorption of mineral supplements and enhance athletic performance.

Safety
There is insufficient reliable information available about the safety of aspartates.
Pregnancy and Lactation: Insufficient reliable information available; avoid using.

Effectiveness
INSUFFICIENT RELIABLE EVIDENCE to RATE

Hepatic encephalopathy. Preliminary clinical research suggests an L-ornithine-L-aspartate infusion might reduce hepatic encephalopathy in some patients with hepatic cirrhosis (10655). More evidence is needed to rate aspartates for this use.

Mechanism of Action
Aspartate is an amino acid that is metabolized in resting muscles (5141). People theorize that aspartate mineral salts of copper, iron, magnesium, manganese, potassium, or zinc have better absorption or improve athletic ability. There is no evidence to suggest that this is true (5133). Except in cases of mineral deficiency, such as iron-deficiency anemia, a well-balanced diet typically provides the RDA of minerals (5133).

Adverse Reactions
None reported.

Interactions with Herbs & Other Dietary Supplements
None known.

Interactions with Drugs
None known.

Interactions with Foods
None known.

Interactions with Lab Tests
None known.

Interactions with Diseases or Conditions
None known.

Dosage and Administration
No typical dosage.

ASPEN

Also Known As
American Aspen, European Aspen, Populi Cortex, Populi Folium, Trembling Aspen, Quaking Aspen, Zitter-Pappel.

Scientific Names
Populus tremuloides; Populus tremula.
Family: Salicaceae.

People Use This For
Orally, aspen is used as a component in various medicinal herbal combinations for treating rheumatic disorders, prostate discomforts, sciatica, neuralgia, and bladder problems.

Safety
There is insufficient reliable information available about the safety of aspen.
Pregnancy and Lactation: Insufficient reliable information available; avoid using.

Effectiveness
There is insufficient reliable information available about the effectiveness of aspen.

Mechanism of Action
The applicable parts of aspen are the bark and leaf. Aspen contains salicin, a precursor to salicylate (3700), and therefore aspen may have anti-inflammatory activity (2,7).

Adverse Reactions
Topically, salicin is associated with skin rashes (4). Pollen sensitization and allergic contact dermatitis may occur following contact with the bud resin (2).

Interactions with Herbs & Other Dietary Supplements
SALICYLATE-CONTAINING HERBS: Theoretically, concomitant use with aspen may potentiate effects of other herbs that contain salicylates (19).

Interactions with Drugs
None known.

Interactions with Foods
ALCOHOL: Theoretically, concomitant use with aspen increases the incidence, severity, and risk of salicylate-induced gastrointestinal bleeding (15).

Interactions with Lab Tests
Theoretically, salicylate-containing herbs may interfere with lab tests affected by salicylates, such as serum uric acid, urine glucose, vanillylmandelic acid (VMA), and 5-HIAA tests.

Interactions with Diseases or Conditions
SALICYLATE HYPERSENSITIVITY: Theoretically contraindicated, due to salicylate (salicin) content. Avoid or use aspen with caution in people with active peptic ulcer disease, diabetes, gout, hemophilia, hypoprothrombinemia, kidney, or liver disease (15).

Dosage and Administration
ORAL: People typically use 1 to 5 grams of powdered aspen bark. A liquid is prepared using 1 to 2 teaspoons of the bark simmered in a cup of water for 10 to 15 minutes. This is taken three times daily. The liquid extract is commonly dosed 1 to 5 mL (223,5253).

ASTAXANTHIN

Also Known As
Microalgae, Ovoester.
CAUTION: See separate listing for Beta-Carotene.

Scientific Names
3,3'-dihydroxy-4,4'-diketo-beta-carotene; 3S,3'S-astaxanthin; 3R,3'R-astaxanthin; 3R,3'S-astaxanthin.

People Use This For

Orally, astaxanthin is used for macular degeneration, Alzheimer's and Parkinson's diseases, stroke, cancer, and hypercholesterolemia.
Topically, astaxanthin is used for sunburn.

Safety

LIKELY SAFE ...when used in amounts found in foods. Astaxanthin has Generally Recognized As Safe (GRAS) status in the US (4912). There is insufficient reliable information available about the safety of oral use of astaxanthin supplements or the topical use of astaxanthin.
PREGNANCY AND LACTATION: Insufficient reliable information available; avoid using.

Effectiveness

There is insufficient reliable information available about the effectiveness of astaxanthin.

Mechanism of Action

Astaxanthin is a reddish carotenoid pigment found in the microalgae Haematococcus pluvialis. Salmon, trout, red sea bream, shrimp, lobster, fish eggs, and many bird species also contain substantial amounts of astaxanthin (4326,4332). It is a powerful antioxidant that is structurally similar to beta-carotene (8467). Astaxanthin contains the highest relative antioxidant activity when compared with alpha-tocopherol, alpha-carotene, beta-carotene, lutein, and lycopene (10634). The concentration of astaxanthin is 1% to 3% in microalgae. A 4-ounce portion of farmed Atlantic salmon contains about 0.5 to 1.1 mg of astaxanthin; 4 ounces of sockeye salmon contains about 4.5 mg (8467).
Preliminary data suggests astaxanthin may decrease the oxidative liver damage caused by carbon tetrachloride. It seems to decrease oxidative consumption of glutathione (GSH) and increase hepatoprotective antioxidant activity (8454). There is also preliminary data that suggests that astaxanthin might have gastroprotective effects against Helicobacter pylori, possibly by inhibiting inflammation and acting as an antioxidant (4341).
Evidence also suggests that astaxanthin might stimulate immunity (4335,4336). Additional animal research suggests astaxanthin might protect against mammary cancer, liver cancer, bladder cancer, and oral cancer (4337,4338,4339,4340). It seems to suppress the growth of tumor cells by increasing concentrations of gamma-interferon and increasing the activity of cytotoxic T lymphocytes. It appears that astaxanthin needs to be part of the diet prior to tumor development to inhibit tumor growth (8453).
Preliminary research also suggests that astaxanthin may be able to prevent the oxidative damage caused by ultraviolet (UVA) light (8490).

Adverse Reactions

None reported. However, another carotenoid substance that is chemically related to astaxanthin, canthaxanthin, caused crystals in the retina and loss of visual acuity in one patient (8455). This effect has not been observed with astaxanthin, but patients who have visual changes while taking astaxanthin should stop taking it immediately.

Interactions with Herbs & Other Dietary Supplements

CAROTENOIDS: Other carotenoids may decrease the absorption of astaxanthin, by competing for absorption in the gastrointestinal tract. Carotenoids include beta-carotene, lutein, canthaxanthin, and lycopene (8456).

Interactions with Drugs

None known.

Interactions with Foods

CAROTENOID-CONTAINING FOODS: Carotenoids present in food may decrease the absorption of astaxanthin (8456). Carotenoids are found in a wide variety of vegetables and have high concentrations in carrots and tomatoes.

Interactions with Lab Tests

None known.

Interactions with Diseases or Conditions

None known.

Dosage and Administration

No typical dosage.

ASTRAGALUS

Also Known As

Astragali, Beg Kei, Bei Qi, Buck Qi, Huang Qi, Hwanggi, Membranous Milk Vetch, Milk Vetch, Mongolian Milk, Ogi.
CAUTION: See separate listing for Tragacanth.

Scientific Names

Astragalus membranaceus, synonym Phaca membranacea; Astragalus mongholicus.
Family: Fabaceae/Leguminosae or Papilionaceae.

People Use This For

Orally, astragalus is used for treating the common cold and upper respiratory infections; to strengthen and regulate the immune system; and to increase the production of blood cells particularly in individuals with chronic degenerative disease or in individuals with cancer undergoing chemotherapy or radiation therapy. It is also used orally for chronic nephritis, diabetes, as an antibacterial, antiviral, tonic, liver protectant, anti-inflammatory, antioxidant, as a diuretic, vasodilator, and as a hypotensive agent.
Topically, astragalus is used as a vasodilator and to speed healing.
In combination with Ligustrum lucidum (glossy privet), astragalus is used orally for treating breast cancer, cervical cancer, and lung cancer.

Safety

POSSIBLY SAFE ...when used orally and appropriately (12). Significant toxic reactions have not been reported (11,303); however, specific safety evaluations have not been performed. ...when used topically (12).
PREGNANCY AND LACTATION: Insufficient reliable information available.

Effectiveness

INSUFFICIENT RELIABLE EVIDENCE to RATE

Breast cancer and lung cancer. There is preliminary evidence that adjunctive use of astragalus in combination with glossy privet (Ligustrum lucidum) might increase survival rates in patients being treated conventionally for breast or lung cancer (303).
Common cold. There is preliminary evidence that long-term ingestion of astragalus might reduce the risk of catching the common cold (303).
Hepatitis. There is preliminary evidence that intravenous use of astragalus might be beneficial for patients with chronic hepatitis (303).
More evidence is needed to rate astragalus for these uses.

Mechanism of Action

The applicable part of astragalus is the root. Astragalus contains a variety of active constituents including more than 40 saponins such as astragaloside, several flavonoids, polysaccharides, multiple trace minerals, amino acids, and coumarins (11,303). Astragalus is an antioxidant. It inhibits free radical production, increases superoxide dismutase, and decreases lipid peroxidation (303). Astragalus is often promoted for its effects on the immune system, liver, and cardiovascular system. Astragalus seems to improve the immune response by potentiating the effects of interferon, and increasing antibody levels of IgA and IgG in nasal secretions (303). It also seems to improve the response of mononuclear cells and stimulate lymphocyte production (10777). Additionally, there is preliminary evidence that astragalus extracts can restore or improve immune function in cases of immune deficiency (423,3713). For example, astragalus seems to restore suppressed T-cell function in cancer patients (423). In animal models, an astragalus extract can reverse cyclophosphamide-induced immune deficiency (3713). Lower doses of astragalus appear to stimulate the immune system, but doses in excess of 28 grams might suppress immunity (303). When administered intravenously, some evidence suggests astragalus extract might increase proliferation and differentiation of bone marrow stem cells and progenitor cells (303). Astragalus also shows evidence of broad-spectrum antibiotic activity (303). In individuals with chronic hepatitis, astragalus seems to improve liver function as demonstrated by improvement in serum glutamate pyruvate transaminase (SGPT) levels (303). Astragalus is also thought to cause vasodilation and increase cardiac output which might be beneficial in angina, congestive heart failure, and post-myocardial infarction (303).

Adverse Reactions

The toxicity of astragalus root is reportedly "very low" (11). Although side effects have not been reported, doses greater than 28 grams might cause immunosuppression (303).

Interactions with Herbs & Other Dietary Supplements

None known.

Interactions with Drugs

CYCLOPHOSPHAMIDE: Some evidence suggests astragalus might reduce immunosuppression caused by cyclophosphamide (Cytoxan, Neosar) (303,3713).
IMMUNOSUPPRESSANTS: Theoretically, concurrent use might interfere with immunosuppressive therapy (303); avoid concurrent use. Immunosuppressant drugs include azathioprine (Imuran), basiliximab (Simulect), cyclosporine (Neoral, Sandimmune), daclizumab (Zenapax), muromonab-CD3 (OKT3, Orthoclone OKT3), mycophenolate (CellCept), tacrolimus (FK506, Prograf), sirolimus (Rapamune), prednisone (Deltasone, Orasone), and other corticosteroids (glucocorticoids).

Interactions with Foods

None known.

Interactions with Lab Tests

None known.

Interactions with Diseases or Conditions

AUTO-IMMUNE DISORDERS: Astragalus might increase immune system activity and may not be appropriate for individuals with auto-immune disorders (303).
ORGAN TRANSPLANT RECIPIENTS: Astragalus might interfere with immunosuppressive therapy; avoid concurrent use (303).

Dosage and Administration

ORAL: Astragalus powder 1-30 grams per day is typically used (11,303). For enhancing immune function for prevention of the common cold, 4-7 grams per day is commonly used (303). In some cases, people have used astragalus powder 30-60 grams per day (303). However, this should be avoided because some research suggests that doses greater than 28 grams per day offers no additional benefit and might even cause immune suppression (303). Astragalus decoction 0.5-1 L per day (maximum of 120 grams of whole root per liter of water) has been used (303). As a soup, mix 30 grams in 3.5 L of soup and simmer with other food ingredients (303).
TOPICAL: No typical dosage.

Comments

Astragalus is most commonly used in combination with other herbs (303).

ATRACTYLODES

Also Known As

Bai Zhu, Byaki-jutsu, Cang Zhu, Cangzhu, Chang Zhe, Jutsu, Red Atractylodes, So-jutsu.

Scientific Names

Atractylodes lancea, synonyms Atractylodes chinensis, Atractylodes ovata, Atractylis lancea, Atractylis ovata; Atractylodes japonica; Atractylodes macrocephala.
Family: Asteraceae/Compositae.

People Use This For

Orally, atractylodes is used for indigestion, stomach ache, abdominal distension, edema, diarrhea, anorexia, and rheumatism.

Safety

There is insufficient reliable information available about the safety of atractylodes.
Pregnancy and Lactation: Insufficient reliable information available; avoid using.

Effectiveness

There is insufficient reliable information available about the effectiveness of atractylodes.

Mechanism of Action
The applicable part of atractylodes is the rhizome. The rhizomes of several closely related atractylodes species contain a variety of constituents including sesquiterpenoids such as atractylenolides and atractylon, essential oils that contain beta-eudesmol and hinesol, and L-phenylalanine (12445,12446,12447,12457).
Atractylodes is used in Japanese (Kampo) and Traditional Chinese Medicine (TCM) for gastrointestinal complaints. Preliminary research suggests that extracts of atractylodes might delay gastric emptying and inhibit gastric secretion (12448). The beta-eudesmol constituent seems to have an H2-antagonist effect (12449).
Beta-eudesmol and hinesol seem to enhance intestinal motility (12450). Some atractylodes species may also modulate the intestinal immune system (12452,12453).
Extracts of Atractylodes macrocephala, japonica, and lancea seem to have cyclooxygenase (COX)-1 and COX-2 inhibitory activity, suggesting these species might have analgesic and anti-inflammatory effects (12451,12452,12454).
Atractylodes might have antifungal activity and activity against HIV protease (12455,12456). The constituents, atractylenolides and atractylin, seem to inhibit the growth of leukemia cells (12457).

Adverse Reactions
Atractylodes can cause an allergic reaction in people sensitive to the Asteraceae/Compositae family (12450). Members of this family include ragweed, chrysanthemums, marigolds, daisies, and many other herbs.

Interactions with Herbs & Other Dietary Supplements
None known.

Interactions with Drugs
None known.

Interactions with Foods
None known.

Interactions with Lab Tests
None known.

Interactions with Diseases or Conditions
CROSS-ALLERGENICITY: Atractylodes may cause an allergic reaction in individuals sensitive to the Asteraceae/Compositae family (12450). Members of this family include ragweed, chrysanthemums, marigolds, daisies, and many other herbs.

Dosage and Administration
No typical dosage.

Comments
Atractylodes is used in Traditional Chinese Medicine (TCM) formulations with other herbs for treating lung cancer (ninjin-yoei-to) and complications of peritoneal dialysis in chronic renal failure (shenling baizhu san) (12458,12459).

AUTUMN CROCUS

Also Known As
Colchicum, Crocus, Fall Crocus, Meadow Saffran, Meadow Saffron, Mysteria, Naked Ladies, Upstart, Vellorita, Wonder Bulb.
CAUTION: See separate listing for Saffron.

Scientific Names
Colchicum autumnale; Colchicum speciosum; Colchicum vernum.
Family: Colchicaceae or Liliaceae.

People Use This For
Orally, autumn crocus is used for arthritis, gout, and familial Mediterranean fever.

Safety
UNSAFE ...when used orally for self-medication because it is a potential poison (6,500). Human intoxication can occur when corms, which are the underground bulb-like stems, are mistaken for onions and ingested (6).
PREGNANCY AND LACTATION: UNSAFE ...when used orally because autumn crocus is a potential mutagen and toxin (500); avoid using.

Effectiveness
There is insufficient reliable information available about the effectiveness of autumn crocus.

Mechanism of Action
The applicable parts of autumn crocus are the seed, tuber, and flower. The seeds of this plant contain at least 0.4% colchicine, which is the constituent responsible for its therapeutic benefit (2).

Adverse Reactions
Orally, autumn crocus can cause burning of the mouth and throat, thirst, nausea, vomiting, diarrhea, liver necrosis, hypovolemic shock, kidney impairment, multiorgan failure, and death (6,553). Long-term use of colchicine is associated with agranulocytosis, aplastic anemia, and peripheral neuritis (6). Human intoxication can occur when corms, which are the underground bulb-like stems, are mistaken for onions or when contaminated milk is ingested (6).
Topically, handling fresh corm slices can cause finger numbness (6).

Interactions with Herbs & Other Dietary Supplements
None known.

Interactions with Drugs
COLCHICINE: Avoid concomitant use of autumn crocus with colchicine because it can increase therapeutic and adverse effects (2).

Interactions with Foods
None known.

Interactions with Lab Tests
URIC ACID: Autumn crocus can lower serum uric acid concentrations and test results due to its colchicine content (8).

Interactions with Diseases or Conditions
None known.

Dosage and Administration
ORAL: Dosing is related to the colchicine content (2). Due to its toxic potential, use the standardized, FDA-approved colchicine. Gout and familial Mediterranean fever require diagnosis, treatment, and monitoring by a medical professional.

Comments
Colchicine is available by prescription and used to treat acute gout attacks and familial Mediterranean fever (506).

AVENS

Also Known As
Benedict's Herb, Bennet's Root, Colewort, Geum, Herb Bennet.

Scientific Names
Geum urbanum.
Family: Rosaceae.

People Use This For
Orally, avens is used to treat diarrhea, catarrhal colitis, uterine bleeding, intermittent fevers, and ulcerative colitis.
In foods, avens is used as a source of food flavoring.

Safety
LIKELY SAFE ...when used in amounts typically found in foods. The Council of Europe allows avens as a natural source of food flavoring (4).
There is insufficient reliable information available about the safety of avens for its other uses.
PREGNANCY AND LACTATION: POSSIBLY UNSAFE ...when used orally because avens seems to have an affect on the menstrual cycle (4); avoid using.

Effectiveness
There is insufficient reliable information available about the effectiveness of avens.

Mechanism of Action
The applicable parts of avens are the above ground parts. The tannin-type constituents of avens have an astringent action; this supports the traditional use of avens for treating diarrhea (4).

Adverse Reactions
None reported.

Interactions with Herbs & Other Dietary Supplements
None known.

Interactions with Drugs
None known.

Interactions with Foods
None known.

Interactions with Lab Tests
None known.

Interactions with Diseases or Conditions
None known.

Dosage and Administration
ORAL: People typically use 1-4 grams steeped in boiling water, strained, three times a day (4). Liquid extract (1:1 in 25% alcohol) 1-4 mL three times a day has also been used (4).

Comments
Avens is very rarely used medicinally today (18).

AVOCADO

Also Known As
Abokado, Ahuacate, Alligator Pear, Avocato.

Scientific Names
Persea americana; Persea americana var. americana, synonyms Laurus persea, Persea gratissima, Persea leiogyna, Persea persea.
Family: Lauraceae.

People Use This For
Orally, avocado fruit is used to reduce serum cholesterol levels, as an aphrodisiac and to stimulate menstrual flow. Unsaponifiable fractions of the oil are used to treat osteoarthritis. The seeds, leaves, and bark are used for dysentery and diarrhea.
Topically, avocado oil is applied to soothe and heal skin, treat sclerosis of the skin, pyorrhea, and arthritis. The fruit pulp is used topically to promote hair growth and hasten wound healing. The seeds, leaves, and bark are used to relieve toothache.
In foods, avocado fruit is edible.

Safety
LIKELY SAFE ...when the fruit is consumed in amounts commonly found in foods (668,669,670,671).
POSSIBLY SAFE ...when unsaponifiable fractions of avocado oil are used orally and appropriately in medicinal amounts. Unsaponifiable fractions of avocado oil appear to be safe for up to 6 months (10693).
There is insufficient reliable information available about the safety of avocado for its other uses.
PREGNANCY AND LACTATION: There is insufficient reliable information available about the safety of avocado used in medicinal amounts during pregnancy and lactation.

Effectiveness

POSSIBLY EFFECTIVE

Hypercholesterolemia. An avocado-enriched diet high in monounsaturated fatty acids seems to lower total serum cholesterol, low-density lipoprotein (LDL) cholesterol, and apolipoprotein B. It may also increase high-density lipoprotein (HDL) serum cholesterol levels (668,669,670,671).

Osteoarthritis. Taking unsaponifiable fractions of avocado and soybean oils orally appears to significantly improve pain and overall disability. It seems to be more effective for hip than knee osteoarthritis (10693).

There is insufficient reliable information available about the effectiveness of avocado for its other uses.

Mechanism of Action

The applicable parts of avocado are the fruit, leaves, and seed. Among fruits, avocado contains more protein and fiber than most. It also contains manganese, phosphorous, iron, potassium, vitamin E, vitamin C, Beta-carotene, thiamin, riboflavin, nicotinic acid, and folate. It is relatively low in sodium and simple sugars. Avocado is rich in oil (15-30 g/100 g fresh fruit) that is mainly monounsaturated. It is a good source of linoleic acid. Its high fiber content might be responsible for its cholesterol-lowering effects (11010).

Unsaponifiable fractions of avocado and soybean oils may reduce the progression of joint space loss in patients with osteoarthritis who have advanced joint space narrowing of the hip (10694). Preliminary evidence suggests this combination can inhibit cartilage degradation and promote cartilage repair in osteoarthritic chondrocytes (10695).

Adverse Reactions

Allergic cross-sensitivity may be seen in latex-sensitive individuals (6197,7853).

Interactions with Herbs & Other Dietary Supplements

None known.

Interactions with Drugs

WARFARIN (Coumadin): Avocado may antagonize the anticoagulant effects of warfarin, but there has been only one case report of this interaction (667).

Interactions with Foods

None known.

Interactions with Lab Tests

CHOLESTEROL: Avocado can lower serum total cholesterol, LDL cholesterol, and apolipoprotein B concentrations and test results. Avocado can increase serum HDL cholesterol concentrations and test results (668,669,670,671).

Interactions with Diseases or Conditions

LATEX ALLERGY: People who are allergic to latex should avoid eating avocado because of the possibility of cross hypersensitivity between latex and avocado (6197,7853).

Dosage and Administration

ORAL: For lowering cholesterol, avocado is dosed in relation to dietary calorie content or fat intake (668,669,670,671,675). For osteoarthritis, 300 mg daily (a combination of one-third avocado and two-thirds soybean unsaponifiables) has been used (10693).

BA JI TIAN

Also Known As

Indian Mulberry, Morinda, Morindae radix, Noni.

CAUTION: See separate listing for Morinda.

Scientific Names

Morinda officinalis.

Family: Rubiaceae.

People Use This For

Orally, ba ji tian is used for cancer, cholecystitis, debility, enuresis, polyuria, hernia, impotence, premature ejaculation, back pain, depression, increasing white blood cell count, stimulating the endocrine system, improving kidney function, strengthening the skeletal and nervous systems, and as a kidney tonic to strengthen the yang.

Safety
LIKELY SAFE ...when used orally and appropriately (12).
PREGNANCY AND LACTATION: Insufficient reliable information available; avoid using.

Effectiveness
There is insufficient reliable information available about the effectiveness of ba ji tian.

Mechanism of Action
The applicable part of ba ji tian is the root. The root contains several active constituents, including an iridoid lactone called morindolide, iridoid glucosides including morofficinaloside, anthraquinones, a monoterpene glycoside, sterols including beta-sitosterol, an ursane-type triterpene, a lactone compound, and 24-ethylcholesterol (448,451,452). However, the roles of specific constituents have not been described. Constituents reported to have antidepressant activity have been isolated (succinic acid, nystose, 1F-fructofuranosylnystose, inulin-type hexasaccharide, and heptasaccharide) (449). Ba ji tian is thought to work in depression by increasing serotonergic effects (3558). A study in mice reported that ba ji tian had anti-fatigue properties, reversed radiation-induced leukopenia, and reduced excitability of the parasympathetic nervous system associated with hypothyroidism (453).

Adverse Reactions
None reported.

Interactions with Herbs & Other Dietary Supplements
None known.

Interactions with Drugs
None known.

Interactions with Foods
None known.

Interactions with Lab Tests
None known.

Interactions with Diseases or Conditions
DYSURIA: Theoretically, ba ji tian may exacerbate urinary difficulties. Ba ji tian is reported to stimulate the kidneys. Use with caution (12).

Dosage and Administration
No typical dosage.

Comments
In some commercial preparations, Morinda officinalis is combined with Morinda citrifolia.

BAEL

Also Known As
Bel, Bengal Quince, Bilva, Bilwa, Indian Bael, Shivaphala.

Scientific Names
Aegle marmelos.
Family: Rutaceae.

Comments
At the date of publication, there was very little scientific information available about this product. Our staff is continually analyzing the available information on natural medicines and will add data to the online version of *Natural Medicines Comprehensive Database* as it becomes available. See www.naturaldatabase.com.

BAIKAL SKULLCAP

Also Known As

Chinese Skullcap, Huang Qin, Huangquin, Hwanggum, Ogon, Ou-gon, Scullcap, Scute, Skullcap, Wogon.
CAUTION: See separate listing for Skullcap.

Scientific Names

Scutellaria baicalensis, synonym Scutellaria macrantha.
Family: Lamiaceae/Labiatae.

People Use This For

Orally, Baikal skullcap is used to treat respiratory and gastrointestinal infections, allergic rhinitis, jaundice, viral hepatitis, nephritis, pelvic inflammation, sores or swelling, and fever. It is also used orally for scarlet fever, headache, irritability, red eyes, flushed face, seizures, epilepsy, hysteria, nervous tension, and a bitter taste in the mouth.

In combination with shung hua, the Baikal skullcap constituent baicalin is used to treat upper respiratory tract infections. In combination with other herbs, Baikal skullcap is used to treat attention-deficit hyperactivity disorder (ADHD), prostate cancer, bronchiolitis, osteoarthritis, and hemorrhoids.

Safety

POSSIBLY SAFE ...when used orally and appropriately (5549,5550,5551). ...when used by injection, short-term. An intravenous preparation that includes Baikal skullcap, forsythia, and honeysuckle has been used with apparent safety in children for up to 7 days (12613). There is insufficient reliable information about the safety of Baikal skullcap when used long-term.

PREGNANCY AND LACTATION: Insufficient reliable information available; avoid using.

Effectiveness

INSUFFICIENT RELIABLE EVIDENCE to RATE

Bronchiolitis. Preliminary clinical research suggests a combination of Baikal skullcap, forsythia, and honeysuckle given intravenously might decrease the duration of symptoms of bronchiolitis in children with respiratory syncytial virus (RSV) infection (12613). More evidence is needed to rate forsythia for this use.

Mechanism of Action

The applicable parts of Baikal skullcap are the root and, to a lesser extent, the above ground parts. Most pharmacological activity has been attributed to flavonoid constituents, including baicalin, baicalein, wogonin, and scutellarein. These flavonoids all appear to bind to GABA-A receptors with possibly benzodiazepine-like effects (6290,6291). The constituent baicalein has weak antipyretic properties (5541) and might also have antimutagenic (6294) and alpha-glucosidase activity (6292), according to preliminary evidence.

Baicalin has potent anti-inflammatory properties (5541). Preliminary research suggests baicalin might decrease inflammation and relieve pain, possibly by inhibiting proinflammatory cytokines, nitric oxide, and prostaglandin E2 (12847,12848). Some evidence suggests it can inhibit tumor growth and suppress carcinoma cell proliferation (5541). Baicalin might inhibit HIV-1 infection and replication by inhibiting HIV reverse transcriptase (5541). Baicalein and baicalin are reported to be more active free-radical scavengers than alpha-tocopherol (vitamin E) (5541,6293). Baikal skullcap also appears to have antibacterial and antiviral properties, as well as antifungal activity, particularly against Candida albicans (5541,6295). It also might have diuretic and antihypertensive properties (5541).

Adverse Reactions

Orally, Baikal skullcap is generally well tolerated. However, several case reports implicate Baikal skullcap products in hepatotoxicity (4284). Baikal skullcap can cause pneumonitis (9185). Use of Baikal skullcap as an intramuscular injection can cause fever and a sudden drop in the leukocyte count (5541). Theoretically, Baikal skullcap could cause sedation (6290,6291).

Interactions with Herbs & Other Dietary Supplements

HERBS WITH SEDATIVE PROPERTIES: Theoretically, concomitant use with herbs that have sedative properties might enhance therapeutic and adverse effects (6290,6291). Some of these include 5-HTP, calamus, California poppy, catnip, hops, Jamaican dogwood, kava, St. John's wort, skullcap, valerian, yerba mansa, and others.

Interactions with Drugs

ALCOHOL (Ethanol): Theoretically, Baikal skullcap can potentiate the sedative effects of alcohol (6290,6291); use with caution.
ANTIDIABETES DRUGS: Theoretically, concomitant use might enhance blood glucose lowering effects due to alpha-glucosidase inhibitor activity of the constituent baicalein (6292). Monitor blood glucose levels closely.
BENZODIAZEPINES: Theoretically, concomitant use with benzodiazepines can cause additive therapeutic and adverse effects (6290,6291); use with caution.
CNS DEPRESSANTS: Theoretically, concomitant use of Baikal skullcap and drugs with sedative properties can cause additive therapeutic and adverse effects (6290,6291); use with caution.

Interactions with Foods

None known.

Interactions with Lab Tests

BLOOD GLUCOSE: Theoretically, Baikal skullcap might reduce postprandial blood glucose concentrations and test results due to alpha-glucosidase activity (6292).

Interactions with Diseases or Conditions

DIABETES: Theoretically, Baikal skullcap could have hypoglycemic activity (6292). Use in diabetics might increase the risk of hypoglycemic episodes; use with caution.
STOMACH DYSFUNCTION: Baikal skullcap should not be used by individuals with stomach or spleen dysfunction (5544).

Dosage and Administration

ORAL: A typical dose is 6-15 grams of Baikal skullcap, toasted to moderate the effect (5544). A typical dose of the Baikal skullcap constituent baicalin to treat viral hepatitis is 500 mg three times daily (5541). A typical dose to treat an upper respiratory tract infection is a tablet containing 50 mg of the Baikal skullcap constituent baicalin in combination with 100 mg of shung hua. Two to three tablets are taken four to six times per day (5541).

Comments

Common substitutions for Scutellaria baicalensis (Baikal skullcap) in Chinese medicine include Scutellaria viscidula, Scutellaria amonea, and Scutellaria ikoninikovii (5541).

BAMBOO

Also Known As

Arrow Bamboo, Yadake.

Scientific Names

Pseudosasa japonica, synonyms Arundinaria japonica, Sasa japonica.
Family: Poaceae/Gramineae.

Comments

At the date of publication, there was very little scientific information available about this product. Our staff is continually analyzing the available information on natural medicines and will add data to the online version of *Natural Medicines Comprehensive Database* as it becomes available. See www.naturaldatabase.com.

BANABA

Also Known As

Banaba Extract, Corosolic Acid, Crape Myrtle, Crepe Myrtle, Pride-of-India, Pyinma, Queen's Crape Myrtle.

Scientific Names

Lagerstroemia speciosa; synonyms Lagerstroemia flos-reginae, Munchausia speciosa.
Family: Lythraceae.

People Use This For

Orally, banaba is used for diabetes and weight loss.

Safety

POSSIBLY SAFE ...when banaba extract is used orally for 15 days (11954). The safety of long-term use is unknown.
PREGNANCY AND LACTATION: Insufficient reliable information available; avoid using.

Effectiveness

INSUFFICIENT RELIABLE EVIDENCE to RATE

Diabetes. Preliminary clinical research suggests that orally administered banaba extract, standarized to 1% corosolic acid, might lower blood sugar in people with type 2 diabetes (11954). More evidence is needed to rate banaba for this use.

Mechanism of Action

The applicable part of the banaba tree is the leaf. Active constituents include corosolic acid and the ellagitannins lagerstroemin, flosin B, and reginin A (11954,11955,11956). In diabetic animals and in humans with type 2 diabetes, banaba extract lowers blood glucose (11954,11955). In vitro research suggests that the ellagitannins have an insulin-like effect (11956). Research on lagerstroemin suggests that it might activate insulin receptors (11957).

The banaba constituent valoneic acid seems to have xanthine oxidase activity similar to or better than allopurinol, according to in vitro research (11958).

In genetically diabetic obese mice, banaba seems to suppress weight gain (11959). However, this antiobesity effect has not been tested in nondiabetic animals or humans.

Adverse Reactions

None reported.

Interactions with Herbs & Other Dietary Supplements

HERBS WITH HYPOGLYCEMIC POTENTIAL: Theoretically, banaba might have additive effects with herbs that decrease blood glucose levels (11954). Herbs with hypoglycemic potential include alpha-lipoic acid, devil's claw, fenugreek, garlic, guar gum, horse chestnut, Panax ginseng, psyllium, and Siberian ginseng.

Interactions with Drugs

ANTIDIABETES DRUGS: Theoretically, banaba might enhance the blood glucose-lowering effects of hypoglycemic drugs (11954). Monitor blood glucose levels closely. Some antidiabetes drugs include glimepiride (Amaryl), glyburide (Diabeta, Glynase PresTabs, Micronase), insulin, metformin (Glucophage), pioglitazone (Actos), rosiglitazone (Avandia), and others.

Interactions with Foods

None known.

Interactions with Lab Tests

BLOOD GLUCOSE: Banaba can lower blood sugar resulting in lower blood glucose test results (11954).

Interactions with Diseases or Conditions

DIABETES: Banaba can affect blood sugar control, and blood glucose levels should be monitored closely (11954).

Dosage and Administration

ORAL: For lowering blood sugar in people with type 2 diabetes, 16 to 48 mg per day has been used (11954).

Comments

Banaba is the Tagalog name for a species of crepe myrtle that is native to the Philippines and Southeast Asia (11954).

BARLEY

Also Known As

Cereal Fiber, Dietary Fiber, Hordeum, Mai Ya, Pearl Barley, Pot Barley, Scotch Barley.

Scientific Names

Hordeum vulgare; Hordeum distychum.
Family: Poaceae/Gramineae.

People Use This For

Orally, barley is used for bronchitis, diarrhea, gastritis, inflammatory bowel conditions, and cancer prevention. It is also used for lowering blood sugar, blood pressure, and cholesterol, and for promoting weight loss. It is also used for increasing strength and stamina.

Topically, barley is used for treating boils.

In foods, barley is utilized as a source of vitamins, carbohydrates, proteins, and fatty oils.

In manufacturing, barley is used as a food grain, natural sweetener, and as an ingredient for brewing beer and making alcoholic beverages.

Safety

LIKELY SAFE ...when used orally and appropriately (4819,4820,4821,5104,10166,10435,11134,11463,11986).
PREGNANCY: LIKELY SAFE ...when used orally in amounts commonly found in foods (19).
POSSIBLY UNSAFE ...when barley sprouts are consumed in relatively high doses. Excessive amounts of barley sprouts should not be consumed during pregnancy (19).
LACTATION: Insufficient reliable information available; avoid using.

Effectiveness

POSSIBLY EFFECTIVE

Gastric cancer. Epidemiologic evidence suggests that dietary fiber consumed in the diet might reduce the incidence of stomach cancer (10435).

Hypercholesterolemia. Taking barley orally seems to reduce total cholesterol and low-density lipoprotein (LDL) cholesterol when added to the National Cholesterol Education Program's Step I diet (11134,11986). The effect of barley on cholesterol appears to be dose dependent. Taking 0.4, 3, or 6 grams of soluble fiber from barley daily reduces total cholesterol by 14%, 17%, and 20% respectively. LDL is lowered by 17% to 24%. Barley also seems to lower triglycerides by 6% to 16% and increase high density lipoprotein (HDL) cholesterol by 9% to 18% (11986). However, barley that is highly enriched with beta-glucan doesn't seem to affect cholesterol. This lack of effect seems to be the result of processing the barley into a highly enriched beta-glucan product (10166). Taking barley orally also seems to produce modest, but significant reductions in systolic, diastolic, and mean arterial blood pressures in non-hypertensive patients with moderate hypercholesterolemia (11463).

POSSIBLY INEFFECTIVE

Colorectal cancer. Dietary cereal fiber, including barley fiber, doesn't seem to the reduce the risk of colorectal cancer (160,4819,4820,4821,5104).

There is insufficient reliable information available about the effectiveness of barley for its other uses.

Mechanism of Action

The applicable part of barley is the grain. Barley contains 5% to 10% beta-glucan, a soluble fiber (10166). The fiber content of barley is likely responsible for the observed reduction of cholesterol levels in healthy and hypercholesterolemic people (11134). Researchers think soluble fiber such as barley might increase the excretion of bile acids or neutral sterols (cholesterol precursors), increase catabolism of low-density lipoprotein (LDL) cholesterol, and reduce fat absorption (11986).
Researchers also think that the beta-glucan contained in barley helps control appetite by slowing stomach emptying, prolonging the feeling of fullness, and stabilizing blood sugar (11135). Several mechanisms have been proposed for reducing blood pressure, including an increase in electrolyte and water excretion, alteration of gastric emptying time, and an increase in fecal mineral loss (11463).
Barley contains hordenine, a sympathomimetic. There have been no reports of stimulant effects in humans (11136).
The enzyme, diastase, is responsible for barley's ability to ferment (216).

Adverse Reactions

Orally, beer made with barley can cause anaphylaxis in sensitive individuals (317). Occupational exposure to barley flour can cause asthma (1300).

Interactions with Herbs & Other Dietary Supplements

HERBS AND SUPPLEMENTS WITH HYPOGLYCEMIC EFFECTS: There is some evidence that barley might lower blood glucose (11135). Theoretically, concomitant use with other herbs and supplements that decrease blood glucose levels might increase the risk of hypoglycemia. Some of these products include bitter melon, ginger, goat's rue, fenugreek, kudzu, willow bark, and others.

Interactions with Drugs

ANTIDIABETES DRUGS: Theoretically, concomitant use might enhance blood glucose lowering effects (11135). Monitor blood glucose levels closely. Some antidiabetes drugs include glimepiride (Amaryl), glyburide (DiaBeta, Glynase PresTab, Micronase), insulin, pioglitazone (Actos), rosiglitazone (Avandia), and others.
ORAL DRUGS: Theoretically, fiber can reduce the absorption of some drugs by reducing the gastrointestinal transit time (11135)

Interactions with Foods

None known.

Interactions with Lab Tests

CHOLESTEROL: Barley might reduce serum total cholesterol and LDL cholesterol concentrations and test results (11134).
GLUCOSE: Barley might reduce blood glucose concentrations and test results (11135).
URINE DRUG SCREENS: The barley constituent, hordenine, can yield false-positive test results with ELISA, RIA and TLC urine assays for a number of opiate drugs. Positive urine test results should be confirmed with the more sensitive GC/MS or HPLC assay (1302).

Interactions with Diseases or Conditions

CELIAC DISEASE: The gluten content in barley can exacerbate celiac disease (11137); avoid using.

Dosage and Administration

ORAL: For lowering cholesterol, 3 grams of barley oil extract or 30 grams of barley bran flour or 0.4 to 6 grams of soluble fiber from barley added to a National Cholesterol Education Program (NCEP) Step I diet has been used (11134,11986). For reducing blood pressure, 3-6 grams barley flakes, barley flour, or pearled barley daily, combined with a National Cholesterol Education Program (NCEP) Step I diet has been used in non-hypertensive patients with moderate hypercholesterolemia (11463).

Comments

Barley is a common grain that is used world-wide as a food and in the brewing processes of alcoholic beverages. Avoid confusion with malt extract products that do not contain the enzyme diastase and are intended for use as bulk laxatives (13).

BASIL

Also Known As

Basilici Herba, Common Basil, Garden Basil, Munjariki, St. Josephwort, Surasa, Sweet Basil, Vanatulasi, Varvara.
CAUTION: See separate listing for Holy Basil.

Scientific Names

Ocimum basilicum.
Family: Lamiaceae/Labiatae.

People Use This For

Orally, basil is used for stomach spasms, kidney conditions, before and after childbirth to promote blood circulation, and to treat snakebites and insect bites. It is also used orally as an appetite stimulant, antiflatulent, diuretic, lactation stimulant, gargle and mouth astringent, and in maggot-infested nasal disease. Basil is also used to treat head colds, worms and warts.
In foods, basil is used as an oil or oleoresin at levels usually below 0.005%.

Safety

LIKELY SAFE ...when used orally in amounts commonly found in foods. Basil has Generally Recognized As Safe (GRAS) status in the US (4912).
POSSIBLY SAFE ...when the above ground parts are used orally and appropriately short-term (2,8,12).
POSSIBLY UNSAFE ...when the above ground parts of basil are used orally long-term. ...when the oil of basil is used orally (12). Both the above ground parts and the oil contain estragole which shows evidence that it might be hepatocarcinogenic (8) and mutagenic (2).
CHILDREN: LIKELY SAFE ...when the above ground parts are used as a spice. POSSIBLY UNSAFE ...when used orally in larger amounts due to the estragole constituents (2,8).
PREGNANCY AND LACTATION: LIKELY SAFE ...when the above ground parts are used as a spice. POSSIBLY UNSAFE ...when used in larger amounts due to the estragole constituent of the essential oil. Estragole might have mutagenic effects (2,12).

Effectiveness

There is insufficient reliable information available about the effectiveness of basil.

Mechanism of Action

The applicable parts of basil are the above ground plant parts. The basil plant is a rich source of vitamin C, calcium, magnesium, potassium, and iron (19). The basil constituents methyl cinnamate, methyl chavicol, ocimene, cineole, and linalool have insecticidal activities (11). The volatile oil of basil can have antagonistic activity on worms (11). The essential oil contains up to 85% estragole (2) (methyl chavicol), which can produce liver tumors in mice (11). The constituent, xanthomicrol, can have cytotoxic and antineoplastic activities (11).

Adverse Reactions
Orally, basil is known to cause hypoglycemia (6002). Due to the adverse effects of the constituents of basil, CAUTION should be used in long-term treatment, which may be unsafe (12).

Interactions with Herbs & Other Dietary Supplements
None known.

Interactions with Drugs
None known.

Interactions with Foods
None known.

Interactions with Lab Tests
None known.

Interactions with Diseases or Conditions
None known.

Dosage and Administration
ORAL: The typical dose of basil leaf for distention or flatulence is 1 cup of the fresh brewed tea 2-3 times a day between meals. The tea is prepared by steeping 2-4 grams in 150 mL boiling water for 10-15 minutes and straining (8). For chronic flatulence the usual oral dose is 1 cup 2-3 times daily between meals for 8 days, then stopped for 14 days, and resumed for another 8 days (8).

BAYBERRY

Also Known As
Candleberry, Myrica, Southern Bayberry, Southern Wax Myrtle, Tallow Shrub, Vegetable Tallow, Wax Myrtle, Waxberry.
CAUTION: See separate listings for Sweet Gale and Tung Seed.

Scientific Names
Morella cerifera, synonyms Myrica cerifera, Myrica pumila; Morella caroliniensis, synonyms Myrica pensylvanica, Morella pensylvanica, Myrica caroliniensis, Myrica heterophylla.
Family: Myricaceae.

People Use This For
Orally, bayberry is used for head colds, mucous colitis, diarrhea, as an antipyretic, a circulatory stimulant, and an emetic in large doses.
Topically, bayberry is used as a gargle for sore throat, as a douche for leukorrhea (vaginal discharge), for indolent ulcers, and wound healing.

Safety
POSSIBLY UNSAFE ...when used orally. The root bark and berries contain high amounts of tannins (6). Large doses may have mineralocorticoid activity (4). Root bark can also contain a carcinogen (5).
There is insufficient reliable information available about the safety of bayberry for its other uses.
PREGNANCY AND LACTATION: POSSIBLY UNSAFE ...when used orally or topically because of possible carcinogenic, or mineralocorticoid activities; avoid using (4,5).

Effectiveness
There is insufficient reliable information available about the effectiveness of bayberry.

Mechanism of Action
The applicable parts of bayberry are the root bark and berry. The tannin constituents of bayberry are responsible for its astringent action (4).

Adverse Reactions
Orally, bayberry can cause gastrointestinal irritation, vomiting, liver damage (possibly due to tannin content), and can act as an irritant and sensitizer (6).

Interactions with Herbs & Other Dietary Supplements
None known.

Interactions with Drugs
None known.

Interactions with Foods
None known.

Interactions with Lab Tests
None known.

Interactions with Diseases or Conditions
HYPERTENSION: Consuming large amounts of tannin-containing herbs such as bayberry can cause sodium and water retention and possibly increase blood pressure (4).

Dosage and Administration
ORAL: The typical dose of bayberry is 0.6-2 grams powdered bark, steeped in boiling water and strained, used 3 times a day (4). The liquid extract of bayberry (1:1 in 45% alcohol) is typically used 0.6-2 mL three times a day (4).
TOPICAL: No typical dosage.

Comments
Bayberry is a shrub that is commonly found in Texas and the eastern US. The wax extract taken from the berries is used in fragrances and candles.

BEAN POD

Also Known As
Cannelli Beans, Common Bean, Green Bean, Kidney Bean, Legume, Navy Bean, Phaseoli fructus, Pinto Bean, Seed-Free Bean Pods, Sine Semine, Snap Bean, Starch Blocker, String Bean, Wax Bean, White Kidney Bean.

Scientific Names
Phaseolus vulgaris; Phaseolus vulgaris varieties.
Family: Fabaceae/Leguminosae.

People Use This For
Orally, bean pod is used for hypercholesterolemia, weight loss and obesity, urinary tract infections, kidney or bladder stones, and for the promotion of urine flow. It is also used orally as a diuretic and for diabetes.

Safety
POSSIBLY SAFE ...when used orally and appropriately. Bean pod extracts seem to be safe when used for 2-3 months (10633,12186).
POSSIBLY UNSAFE ...when large amounts of fresh bean husks are ingested. Raw bean husks contain lectins that can cause gastrointestinal upset. Cooking destroys lectins (18).
PREGNANCY AND LACTATION: Insufficient reliable information available; avoid using.

Effectiveness
INSUFFICIENT RELIABLE EVIDENCE to RATE

Hypercholesterolemia. There is preliminary evidence that a bean pod and carob extract might modestly decrease cholesterol levels and increase excretion of fat in the feces of overweight and obese patients (10633).
Obesity. Preliminary evidence suggests that taking a specific bean pod extract (Phase 2, Pharmachem Labs) does not significantly decrease weight or triglycerides in obese patients (12186).
More evidence is needed to rate bean pod for these uses.

Mechanism of Action
The applicable part of bean pod is the pod without the seeds. Bean pod is a source of dietary fiber, which suggests it might modestly reduce lipids. It might also bind cholic acids and fat, thereby reducing fat absorption (10633). Extracts of bean pod are often referred to as carbohydrate absorption blockers and are promoted for weight loss. Bean pod extracts seem to inhibit alpha-amylase in vitro. Blocking alpha-amylase might decrease carbohydrate breakdown and absorption in the GI tract and theoretically result in fewer calories ingested (12186).

Adverse Reactions
Orally, bean pod extracts might cause nausea, vomiting, diarrhea, and stomach pains (11265). Consuming large amounts of green bean husks, or raw green beans, can cause vomiting, diarrhea, and gastroenteritis due to the content of the plant protein lectin. Cooking usually destroys lectins (18).

Interactions with Herbs & Other Dietary Supplements
None known.

Interactions with Drugs
ANTIDIABETES DRUGS: Monitor blood glucose levels closely due to claims that bean pod has hypoglycemic effects (19).

Interactions with Foods
None known.

Interactions with Lab Tests
None known.

Interactions with Diseases or Conditions
DIABETES: Monitor blood glucose level closely due to claims that bean pod has hypoglycemic effects (19).

Dosage and Administration
ORAL: For hypercholesterolemia, bean pod extract 300-600 mg three times daily, combined with carob gum 50-100 mg three times daily, has been used (10633).
For obesity, a specific bean pod extract (Phase 2, Pharmachem Labs) 1500 mg twice daily taken with lunch and dinner has been used (12186).

BEAR'S GARLIC

Also Known As
Broad-leaved Garlic, Ramsons, Wild Garlic.

Scientific Names
Allium ursinum.
Family: Liliaceae or Alliaceae.

Comments
At the date of publication, this product was not a common ingredient used in brand name supplements marketed to consumers. Details about this product are available in the online version of *Natural Medicines Comprehensive Database.* See www.naturaldatabase.com.

BEE POLLEN

Also Known As
Bee Pollen Extract, Buckwheat Pollen, Honeybee Pollen, Honey Bee Pollen, Maize Pollen, Pine Pollen, Pollen, Pollen D'Abeille.
CAUTION: See separate listings for Bee Venom, Honey, and Royal Jelly.

Scientific Names
None.

People Use This For
Orally, bee pollen is used for nutrition, as an appetite stimulant, to improve stamina and athletic performance, for premature aging, premenstrual syndrome (PMS), hay fever or allergic rhinitis, mouth sores, rheumatism, painful urination, prostate conditions, and radiation sickness. It is also used orally for bleeding problems including coughing or vomiting blood, bloody diarrhea, nosebleed, cerebral hemorrhage, and menstrual problems. Bee pollen is also used for gastrointestinal (GI) problems including constipation, diarrhea, enteritis, colitis, as a general tonic, diuretic, and for alcohol intoxication.
Topically, bee pollen is used for skin care in skin softening products, and for treating eczema, pustular eruptions, and diaper rash.

Safety
POSSIBLY SAFE ...when used orally and appropriately, short-term (7062,7063,12008). There is some evidence that taking bee pollen extracts for up to approximately 30 days is safe (7063). There is also preliminary evidence that taking 2 tablets twice daily of a specific combination product containing royal jelly 6 mg, bee pollen extract 36 mg, and bee pollen plus pistil extract 120 mg (Femal, Natumin Pharma) per tablet for up to 2 months seems to be safe (12008).

PREGNANCY: POSSIBLY UNSAFE ...when used orally. There is some concern that bee pollen might have uterine stimulant effects (5,6,11); avoid using.
LACTATION: Insufficient reliable information available; avoid using.

Effectiveness

POSSIBLY INEFFECTIVE

Athletic performance. Taking bee pollen orally doesn't seem to increase athletic performance or stamina (7062,7063).

INSUFFICIENT RELIABLE EVIDENCE to RATE

Premenstrual syndrome (PMS). Preliminary evidence suggests that a specific combination product (Femal, Natumin Pharma) seems to decrease some symptoms of PMS including irritability, weight increases, and edema when given over a period of 2 menstrual cycles. This product contains royal jelly 6 mg, bee pollen extract 36 mg, and bee pollen plus pistil extract 120 mg per tablet. It is given as 2 tablets twice daily (12008). More evidence is needed to rate bee pollen for this use.

Mechanism of Action

Bee pollen refers to the pollen from flowers that collects on the legs and bodies of worker bees. It can also include amounts of nectar and bee saliva. Bee pollen composition varies depending on plant source and geographic region. Up to 50% of bee pollen may be polysaccharides. The other constituents include lipids, protein, simple sugars, vitamin C, and carotenoids (5). Proponents often claim that enzymes in bee pollen provide a variety of therapeutic benefits. However, any enzymes in bee pollen are likely to be digested in the gastrointestinal (GI) tract. There is no reliable evidence indicating that bee pollen enzymes or other constituents in bee pollen offer any therapeutic benefit.

Adverse Reactions

Orally, bee pollen seems to be well tolerated in most patients. There is one report of dizziness in a patient who took a combination product containing royal jelly, bee pollen extract, and a bee pollen plus pistil extract (12008). Patients with pollen allergies are at risk for serious allergic reactions. Allergic reactions can include itching, swelling, shortness of breath, light headedness, and anaphylaxis. Chronic allergy symptoms due to bee pollen include gastrointestinal (GI) and neurologic symptoms and eosinophilia (5,6,11). There have also been two cases of acute hepatitis associated with bee pollen use. One case involved ingestion of two tablespoons of pure bee pollen daily for several months. Another case involved ingestion of 14 tablets per day of a combination herbal product containing bee pollen, chaparral, and 19 other herbs for 6 weeks (1351). In this case it is not known if bee pollen or another herb might have caused the adverse event.

Interactions with Herbs & Other Dietary Supplements

None known.

Interactions with Drugs

None known.

Interactions with Foods

None known.

Interactions with Lab Tests

LIVER FUNCTION TESTS: Bee pollen might increase alkaline phosphatase (Alk Phos), alanine aminotransferase (ALT), aspartate aminotransferase (AST), lactate dehydrogenase (LDH), total bilirubin, prothrombin time (PT), and test results. Bee pollen has been associated with two cases of acute hepatitis and abnormally high results for these tests (1351).

Interactions with Diseases or Conditions

LIVER DISEASE: Use of bee pollen has been associated with two cases of acute hepatitis (1351). Avoid using in patients with existing liver disease.
POLLEN ALLERGY: Patients with pollen allergies are at risk for serious allergic reactions. Allergic reactions can include itching, swelling, shortness of breath, light headedness, and anaphylaxis (5,6).

Dosage and Administration

ORAL: For premenstrual syndrome (PMS), two tablets twice daily of a specific combination containing royal jelly 6 mg, bee pollen extract 36 mg, and bee pollen plus pistil extract 120 mg (Femal, Natumin Pharma) per tablet for two menstrual cycles has been used (12008).

Comments

Pollens come from various plants, including buckwheat, maize, pine (songhuafen), rape, and typha (puhuang) (11). Avoid confusion with bee venom, honey, and royal jelly.

BEE VENOM

Also Known As

Apis Venenum Purum, Apitoxin, Bald-Faced Hornet, Bee Sting Venom, Bumblebee Venom, Honeybee Venom, Mixed Vespids, Pure Bee Venom, Wasp Venom, White-Faced Hornet, Yellow Hornet, Yellow-Jacket Venom.
CAUTION: See separate listings for Bee Pollen, Honey, and Royal Jelly.

Scientific Names

Apis mellifera (Honeybee); Bombus terrestis (Bumblebee); Vespula maculata (Hornet, Wasp).
Family: Apidae; Vespidae.

People Use This For

Parenterally, bee venom is used for rheumatoid arthritis, neuralgias, multiple sclerosis, desensitization to bee stings (venom immunotherapy), tendonitis and tendosynovitis, and muscle conditions such as fibromyositis and enthesitis.

Safety

LIKELY SAFE ...when used by subcutaneous injection by a trained medical professional (2619,6070). Purified bee venom for subcutaneous injection is an FDA approved product (2619).
PREGNANCY AND LACTATION: POSSIBLY SAFE ...when used by subcutaneous injection by a trained medical professional. Significant adverse effects to fetus or mother have not been reported. However, some clinicians decrease maintenance dose by half during pregnancy (2619). POSSIBLY UNSAFE ...when used by subcutaneous injection in high doses. High doses of bee venom can increase release of histamine, which can cause uterine contraction (2619); avoid using in high doses.

Effectiveness

LIKELY EFFECTIVE

Bee sting allergy. Subcutaneous use of bee venom seems to be effective for bee sting desensitization in patients with severe allergy to bee stings. Bee venom immunotherapy provides 98-99% protection from systemic reactions to bee stings. Once immunotherapy is stopped, the risk of a systemic reaction over the next 5 to 10 years is about 5-15% (6043,6075,6076). Bee venom is an FDA-approved subcutaneous injectable product for the treatment of severe allergies to bee stings (2619).

POSSIBLY INEFFECTIVE

Osteoarthritis. Some early reports seemed to indicate a possible benefit of injected bee venom in the treatment of arthritis; however, results are conflicting and most clinical studies do not show a benefit (6045).

There is insufficient reliable information available about the effectiveness of bee venom for its other uses.

Mechanism of Action

Bee venom contains several physiologically active components. Two of the most toxic compounds are melittin and phospholipase A2 (PLA2). Melittin constitutes 30-50% of dry bee venom (6041,6045,6046), and PLA2 makes up about 10-12% of bee venom (6041). Melitin is a potent hemolytic (6042,6045) that causes mast cell degranulation and activates PLA2 (6045). Other constituents in bee venom include hyaluronidase, apamin, mast cell degranulating peptide (MCD peptide), procamine, secapin, tertiapin, and other small peptides including adolapin (6). Some other components are histamine, dopamine, and noradrenaline (6041). In desensitization to bee stings, hymenoptera venom stimulates an allergenic response, decreases leukocyte sensitivity to the allergen, and increases the number of T-suppressor cells (2619). There were early suggestions that bee venom could be a useful treatment in patients with arthritis. This theory was largely due to purported anti-inflammatory effects of bee venom, and the observation that many beekeepers don't develop arthritis (6). While some components in bee venom have been shown to have anti-inflammatory effects, studies have also shown that some components of bee venom are pro-inflammatory. For example, activators of PLA2 such as melittin, are thought to cause an increase in the synthesis of cytokines (tumor necrosis factor and interleukin 1) and stimulate arachidonic acid release resulting in an immune or inflammatory response (6044,6071).

PLA2 is an enzyme which catalyzes the hydrolysis of phospholipid bonds, destroying the major component of cell membranes and leading to cell death (6041,6046). PLA2 causes smooth muscle contraction, blood pressure reduction, increased capillary permeability, and mast cell destruction. PLA2 also reduces blood coagulation, possibly by reducing the activity of coagulation factors II, V, and VIII (6046). Melittin might also be partially responsible for bee venom's anticoagulant effects (6046). Some components in bee venom seem to cause neutrophil degranulation and superoxide production (6,6044), but other actions of bee venom components seem to decrease superoxide production (6,6041,6045,6072). The formation of superoxide anions can be destructive to tissues. The melittin component of bee venom possesses antimicrobial activity, but due to its hemolytic effects, melittin is unsuitable as a treatment for infections (6042). Hyaluronidase is an enzyme which hydrolyzes hyaluronic acid. The adhesive properties of hyaluronic acid hold cells together, so once hydrolyzed, other venom components can penetrate into the cell. For this reason, hyaluronidase is termed a spreading factor (6041). Apamin is a neurotoxin (6045). It blocks many inhibitory effects, including alpha-adrenergic, cholinergic, and neurotensin-induced relaxation, by blocking calcium-dependent potassium channels (6041). MCD peptide is chemically similar to apamin. It causes mast cell degranulation and release of histamine at extremely low concentrations. Histamine causes dilation and increased permeability of capillaries (6041). The constituent adolapin inhibits inflammation and the prostaglandin-synthase system (6). In animals, whole bee venom, melittin, and apamin have also been shown to cause increases in cortisol levels (6039,6040). The mechanism of other peptides is not yet understood (6041).

Adverse Reactions

Parenterally, local erythema and swelling at the injection site are the most common reactions to bee venom treatment (1343). Less common adverse effects ranging from itching, urticaria, edema, malaise, and anxiety to anaphylaxis occur in about 20% of patients (1343). Adverse reactions most often occur during the dose increase phase of immunotherapy, particularly with rapid dose increases (1343,6077). Risk of adverse effects seems to be increased in people treated with honeybee venom (1343,6077). Women seem to have more severe and more frequent adverse effects (1343). Anaphylaxis is most likely to occur in extremely sensitive individuals or in the case of an overdose (2169,6074,6077). Other adverse reactions include chest tightness, palpitations, dizziness, nausea, vomiting, diarrhea, somnolence, respiratory distress, hypotension, confusion, fainting, and laryngeal edema or asthma (1343,2619,6070,6078). Uncommon reactions are abdominal pain, incontinence, chest pain, or visual disturbances (6078). Rarely, coagulation abnormalities can occur, and are usually associated with severe reactions to bee stings (6046).

Interactions with Herbs & Other Dietary Supplements

None known.

Interactions with Drugs

None known.

Interactions with Foods

None known.

Interactions with Lab Tests

PROTHROMBIN TIME (PT): Bee venom might increase the prothrombin time (PT) and partial thromboplastin time (PTT) (6046). The PLA2 component of bee venom seems to reduce the activity of clotting factors II, V, and VIII (6046).

Interactions with Diseases or Conditions

None known.

Dosage and Administration

PARENTERAL: Bee venom is used subcutaneously, intradermally, and intra-arterially for these uses. For arthritis, purified, sterile bee toxin (apitoxin 2 mg/mL) has been used starting with 0.05-0.1 mL. The dose is gradually increased to 0.25 mL, 0.5 mL, and 1 mL, with dose intervals usually from 5 to 7 days. For bee venom immunotherapy in people hypersensitive to bee stings, increased doses of venom are given at selected intervals, usually weekly (6078). There are many possible protocols for immunotherapy. Some start with 0.0001 or 0.001 mcg of venom extract (6077). This is continued until a maintenance dose is achieved, usually 100 micrograms per venom. Once the maintenance dose is achieved, therapy can continue for years. Patients have varying sensitivities to venom and tolerability to immunotherapy, so it is not possible to provide a general dosing schedule for all patients. Venom immunotherapy should only be done by physicians thoroughly familiar with the use of these products, including the treatment of anaphylactic and other adverse reactions. It is also advised to have injectable epinephrine and emergency facilities nearby in case an anaphylactic reaction occurs (2619,6074,6078). Alcohol and tincture of iodine rapidly destroy the activity of bee venom and should not be applied at the site of injection. In China, bee venom is also commonly administered by electrophoresis, ultrasonophoresis, and acupuncture.

Comments

Avoid confusion with bee pollen, honey, and royal jelly. Other venoms are derived from related members of the insect order, Hymenoptera (6).

BEER

Also Known As

Alcohol, Ethanol.
CAUTION: See separate listings for Barley, Hops, Wine, and Yeast.

Scientific Names

None.

People Use This For

Orally, beer is used for reducing the risk of cardiovascular disease, including coronary heart disease, atherosclerosis, heart failure, and myocardial infarction (MI), and for reducing the risk of ischemic stroke and type 2 diabetes. It is also used to reduce the risk of mortality after an acute MI and in people with ischemic left ventricular (LV) dysfunction. Additionally, beer is used orally for preventing cognitive decline in later life, Alzheimer's disease, loss of bone mineral density, cancer, gallstones, kidney stones, and Helicobacter pylori (H. pylori) infection. Beer is also used orally as an appetite and digestive stimulant, and to promote lactation.

Safety

LIKELY SAFE ...when used orally in moderation. Beer seems to be safe when 24 oz or less is consumed daily (2060).
POSSIBLY UNSAFE ...when consumed in large amounts. More than 24 oz per day can cause significant adverse effects (2060,6840).
PREGNANCY: LIKELY UNSAFE ...when used orally. Alcohol is a teratogen. Use during pregnancy, especially during the first two months after conception, is associated with significant risk of spontaneous abortion, fetal alcohol syndrome, and developmental and behavioral dysfunction in infants and children exposed to alcohol in utero (8100); avoid using.
LACTATION: LIKELY UNSAFE ...when used orally. Alcohol is secreted in breast milk. Chronic use can cause abnormal psychomotor development, and disrupt the infant's sleep wake pattern. Alcohol also seems to reduce milk production (11878); avoid using.

Effectiveness

LIKELY EFFECTIVE

Cardiovascular disease. Consumption of alcoholic drinks, including beer, by otherwise healthy people seems to reduce the risk of developing cardiovascular disease. Moderate alcohol use (one to two drinks per day) reduces the risk of coronary heart disease, atherosclerosis, and myocardial infarction (MI), by approximately 30% to 50% when compared with nondrinkers (2267,2268,2271,6888,6892,8648,8649,10128,11879). Alcohol reduces the risk of ischemic stroke, but increase the risk of hemorrhagic stroke. Light to moderate alcohol consumption reduces ischemic stroke risk (2271,2279,6834,6842,6893). However, there is evidence that consuming any amount of alcohol can increase the risk of hemorrhagic stroke (841,2271,6842). There is some evidence that light to moderate consumption of alcoholic drinks can reduce the risk of all-cause mortality in people who are middle-aged or older (2058,6823,6837,6843). Light to moderate consumption of alcohol might also reduce the risk of cardiovascular mortality in otherwise healthy people (2058,2270,6835,6837). Light to moderate alcohol consumption in the year prior to first acute MI is associated with a reduced cardiovascular and all-cause mortality risk compared with non-drinkers (8650). Consumption of one alcoholic beverage per day or consuming alcohol on at least 3 to 4 days per week is a good rule of thumb for people who drink alcohol. Tell patients not to exceed two drinks per day. More than two drinks daily can increase the risk of cardiovascular and overall mortality (841,2060,2261,6173,6890,8648,11879). In men with established coronary heart disease (CHD), consumption of 1-14 alcoholic drinks per week, including beer, doesn't seem to have any effect on cardiovascular disease or all-cause mortality compared with men who drink less than one drink per week. Consuming three or more drinks per day is associated with increased mortality in men with a history of heart attacks (6173).

POSSIBLY EFFECTIVE

Cognitive function. Elderly men who have a history of consuming one alcoholic drink per day seem to maintain better general cognitive function during their late 70s and 80s compared to non-drinkers (6824,6829). However, consumption of more than four drinks per day during middle age seems to be associated with significantly poorer cognitive function later in life (6824).

Diabetes. People who consume alcohol in moderate amounts seem to have a lower risk of developing type 2 diabetes (6172,6891). Diabetes patients who consume alcohol in moderate amounts seem to have a reduced risk of coronary heart disease compared with non-drinkers with type 2 diabetes. The risk reduction is similar to that found in healthy people who consume light to moderate amounts of alcohol (8653,8654).

Heart failure. There is some evidence that consuming one to four alcoholic drinks per day reduces the risk of heart failure in persons aged 65 years or older (8104).

Helicobacter pylori (H pylori). There is evidence that suggests that moderate to high consumption of alcohol, more than 75 grams, per week from beverages such as beer and wine can reduce the risk of H. pylori infection (8034).

POSSIBLY INEFFECTIVE

Cancer. Although wine consumption has been associated with some reductions in cancer mortality, beer consumption does not seem to have this effect (2058). In fact, there is some evidence that beer consumption might slightly increase cancer-related mortality (6823,6843). There is some evidence that consumption of one or more alcoholic drinks might increase mortality from breast cancer (6843).

INSUFFICIENT RELIABLE EVIDENCE to RATE

Alzheimer's disease. There is preliminary evidence that suggests one to two alcoholic drinks per day can reduce the risk of Alzheimer's disease in both men and women compared to non-drinkers (6603).

Anxiety. The effect of alcohol on anxiety is complex and may be affected by the psychological state of the user. It sometimes reduces anxiety, sometimes increases it, and sometimes has no effect (2266).

Bone mineral density. There is also preliminary evidence that suggests moderate alcohol consumption in postmenopausal women is associated with increased bone mineral density in the trochanter, femoral neck, midradius, and lumbar spine (6825,6836,8655). Alcohol intake of one-half to one drink per day seems to have the greatest effect on bone mineral density compared with non-drinkers and heavy drinkers of alcohol (8655).

More evidence is needed to rate beer for these uses.

Mechanism of Action

Beers vary in ethanol content between 2-6%, with typical American beers averaging 4-5% ethanol by volume (17). Ethanol is a central nervous system (CNS) depressant (2263).

Several mechanisms have been proposed for the protective effects of alcohol against coronary heart disease. One to two alcoholic drinks per day increases HDL cholesterol by about 12% (6892) and apolipoprotein A-I by about 2.2% (8649). The increase in HDL cholesterol levels might account for approximately 50% of the cardioprotective effect of moderate alcohol consumption (2261,6838,6841). Moderate alcohol consumption also decreases LDL cholesterol by 5-17%, triglycerides by 5-10%, and apolipoprotein B levels by 3.7% (6841,8649). There is concern that moderate alcohol consumption can increase systolic blood pressure (6841). However, there is evidence light to moderate alcohol consumption does not increase the risk of hypertension and may actually decrease the risk (8102). Effects of alcohol on blood clotting include a reduction in clotting potential and enhancement of clot breakdown (2261). Alcohol consumption decreases platelet aggregation, possibly via inhibition of prostaglandin synthesis (6892). Moderate alcohol consumption is also associated with an increase in plasma levels of tissue-type plasminogen activator, an indicator of fibrinolytic capacity (6894). Light to moderate alcohol consumption produces a reduction in coronary narrowing due to atherosclerosis (2261,6840,8652).

High levels of homocysteine are a risk factor for cardiovascular disease. Homocysteine breakdown and removal requires folate and vitamin B6, and alcohol is an antagonist of folate metabolism (8101). However, there is evidence that an increased intake of dietary folate or the use if supplemental folate, 400 mcg/day, in moderate alcohol users can lower homocysteine levels compared to nonusers of alcohol (8101). However, beer contains folate and vitamin B6 (pyridoxine), and its presence may explain why the increase in plasma homocysteine levels seen with other alcoholic beverages is not seen with beer (6832).

Dark beers contain flavonoids (6892). These polyphenolic compounds, which are found in higher concentrations in red wine, have antioxidant properties and may contribute to protection against CHD by reducing oxidation of LDL cholesterol (2268).

Possible mechanisms by which alcohol could have a protective effect against ischemic stroke include increasing HDL and prostacyclin, decreasing fibrinogen, and inhibiting platelet aggregation (6842). There is evidence that suggests that moderate intake of alcohol increases cerebral blood flow (8651). Moderate alcohol consumption is associated with a lower prevalence of white matter changes and brain infarcts on magnetic resonance imaging in adults 65 years of age or older compared to non-drinkers and heavy drinkers (8651).

The protective effect of alcohol against cardiovascular disease is lost at higher intakes of alcohol (greater than 1-2 drinks per day). High alcohol consumption can cause increased homocysteine levels, hypertension, hemorrhagic stroke, fatal arrhythmias, and direct damage to heart muscle (alcoholic cardiomyopathy) (2060,2261,2267,2270,8101,8102,8103). Certain alcoholic beverages, in particular red wine, may be more protective than other alcoholic beverages such as beer. However, a difference in lifestyle among wine, beer, and other alcohol beverage drinkers, including diet and social class, might also explain why some alcoholic beverages appear to offer more protection than others against coronary heart disease (10129).

Moderate alcohol intake may be protective against the development of type 2 diabetes due to an increase in insulin sensitivity (6891).

Moderate alcohol consumption may be protective against postmenopausal bone loss due to an increase in estrogen levels, increased calcitonin secretion, and reduced parathyroid hormone secretion (6825,6836,8655). However, heavy and chronic alcohol consumption reduces bone mineral density, possibly due to increased calcium and magnesium excretion, increased cortisol secretion, and reduced osteoblast activity (6836,8656). Chronic alcoholics also often have other risk factors for osteoporosis, including poor nutrition, smoking, sedentary lifestyle, and lower body weight (6825,6836).

Preliminary studies suggest that substances in beer may have inhibitory effects on heterocyclic amines, which are carcinogenic substances formed during cooking of some foods (6833).

Beer stimulates gastric acid secretions and gastrin release. This may explain why moderate to high alcohol consumption from beverages such as beer seems to prevent Helicobacter pylori infection (8034).

Adverse Reactions

Orally, beer can cause a variety of side effects due to the alcohol content. The side effects depend on the amount ingested and can vary among individuals. Some common side effects include flushing, confusion, emotional lability, perceptual and sensational disturbances, blackouts, lack of coordination and trouble walking, central nervous system (CNS) depression, drowsiness, respiratory depression, hypothermia, hypoglycemia, nausea, vomiting, diarrhea, abdominal pain, and others. Chronic heavy ethanol ingestion (three or more alcoholic drinks per day) can lead to physical dependence, malnutrition, amnesia, dementia, somnolence, cardiac myopathy, hepatotoxicity, and cirrhosis. Other effects of chronic abuse are pancreatitis, hypomagnesemia, skeletal myopathies, Wernicke's encephalopathy, Korsakoff's psychosis, chronic cerebellar syndrome, mouth cancer, esophageal cancer, pharyngeal cancer, laryngeal cancer, and liver cancer (6843,9004). There is evidence heavy alcohol consumption is associated with the mutation of the p53 gene in individuals with esophageal carcinoma (9005). There is also some evidence that heavy consumption of wine is associated with the highest risk of esophageal cancer compared with heavy consumption of beer and spirits (9004). Chronic intake of three or more drinks per day is associated with an increased risk of all-cause mortality, ischemic stroke, and hypertension (2261,6892,8102). Heavy alcohol consumption (fifteen or more drinks per week) is also associated with a higher percentage of white matter changes and larger ventricular and sulcal size on magnetic resonance imaging of the brain, suggesting heavy alcohol consumption decreases cerebral blood flow and may contribute to brain atrophy (8651).

Consumption of any amount of alcohol can increase the risk of hemorrhagic stroke (841,2271). Daily consumption of one or more alcoholic drinks in women might increase the risk of breast cancer by 2-15% and increase mortality from breast cancer by as much as 30% (6843,8100,9006). There is also evidence suggesting that women who consume alcohol daily have an increased risk of developing breast cancer increases when the daily intake of folate is 300 mcg or less (9006).

Beer made with barley can cause anaphylaxis in sensitive individuals (317). There have been occasional reports of asthma triggered by beer consumption (6174).

Some research suggests an association between alcohol consumption and an increased risk for pancreatic cancer, but other studies do not support this association (8038).

Study results of a possible association between beer consumption and increased waist-to-hip ratio are inconsistent. There is evidence that suggests that consumption of more than six beers per week is associated with a larger waist-to-hip ratio than those consuming an equivalent amount of hard liquor or wine. However, an association between moderate alcohol intake equivalent to approximately 3 beers per week or less and waist-to-hip ratio does not seem to exist (10164,10165). It also is unclear whether waist-to-hip ratios associated with the intake of wine, beer, or other alcoholic beverages have any clinical significance (9007).

Interactions with Herbs & Other Dietary Supplements

HERBS/SUPPLEMENTS WITH SEDATIVE PROPERTIES: Theoretically, concomitant use of beer with herbs that have sedative properties might enhance adverse effects (2262). Some of these include 5-HTP, calamus, California poppy, catnip, hops, Jamaican dogwood, kava, St. John's wort, scullcap, valerian, yerba mansa, and others.

Interactions with Drugs

ASPIRIN: Concomitant use of aspirin with alcohol can increase the risk of gastrointestinal (GI) bleeding (2262).

BARBITURATES: Concomitant consumption of large amounts of alcohol may decrease metabolism of barbiturates (2262). Some of these sedative medications include pentobarbital (Nembutal), phenobarbital (Luminal), secobarbital (Seconal), and others.

BENZODIAZEPINES: Concomitant consumption of large amounts of alcohol may decrease metabolism of benzodiazepines (2262).

CEFAMANDOLE (Mandol): Cefamandole antibiotics can cause a disulfiram-like reaction when taken with alcohol (2262).

CEFOPERAZONE (Cefobid): Cefoperazone can cause a disulfiram-like reaction when taken with alcohol (2262).

CHLORPROPAMIDE (Diabinese): Chlorpropamide can cause a disulfiram-like reaction when taken with alcohol (506).

CISAPRIDE (Propulsid): Concomitant use of beer with cisapride (Propulsid) might increase blood alcohol levels and effects (2262).

CNS DEPRESSANTS: Concomitant use of beer with antihistamines, barbiturates, benzodiazepines, and tricyclic antidepressants may increase sedative and other adverse effects (2262).

DISULFIRAM (Antabuse): The alcohol content of beer can cause a disulfiram reaction when taken within 12 hours of disulfiram (2262). Patients taking disulfiram should not drink any alcoholic beverages including beer.

ERYTHROMYCIN: Concomitant use of erythromycin with alcohol can increase blood alcohol levels and effects (2262).

GRISEOFULVIN (Fulvicin): Griseofulvin can cause a disulfiram-like reaction when taken with alcohol (2262).

H2-BLOCKERS: Concomitant use of cimetidine (Tagamet) and ranitidine (Zantac) with alcohol may increase blood alcohol levels and adverse effects (2262).

HEPATOTOXIC DRUGS: Concomitant use of beer with acetaminophen, isoniazid, or phenylbutazone can increase the risk of hepatotoxicity (2262).

METFORMIN (Glucophage): Concomitant consumption of large amounts of alcohol may increase the risk of

lactic acidosis with metformin (Glucophage) (2262).
METRONIDAZOLE (Flagyl): Metronidazole can cause a disulfiram-like reaction when taken with alcohol (2262).
NARCOTIC DRUGS: Concomitant consumption of large amounts of alcohol may decrease metabolism of narcotics (2262).
NONSTEROIDAL ANTI-INFLAMMATORY DRUGS (NSAIDs): Concomitant use of nonsteroidal anti-inflammatory drugs with alcohol can increase the risk of gastrointestinal (GI) bleeding (2262).
PHENYTOIN (Dilantin): Concomitant consumption of large amounts of alcohol may induce metabolism, reducing therapeutic effectiveness of phenytoin (Dilantin) (2262).
SULFONAMIDE ANTIBIOTICS: Sulfonamide antibiotics can cause a disulfiram-like reaction when taken with alcohol (2262).
TOLBUTAMIDE (Orinase): Tolbutamide can cause a disulfiram-like reaction when taken with alcohol (2262).
WARFARIN (Coumadin): Acute alcohol intoxication can decrease metabolism and increase effects of warfarin (Coumadin) (2262). In contrast, chronic intoxication can induce metabolism of warfarin, reducing therapeutic effectiveness (2262).

Interactions with Foods
FOOD: Chronic use of alcohol might interfere with absorption of B vitamins and other nutrients (2263).

Interactions with Lab Tests
FOLATE: Chronic alcohol ingestion may decrease folate levels and test results (2263).
LIVER FUNCTION TESTS: Chronic alcohol ingestion can increase alkaline phosphatase (Alk phos), alanine aminotransferase (ALT), aspartate aminotransferase (AST), gamma-glutamyltransferase (GGT), and bilirubin test results (2263).
MEAN CORPUSCULAR VOLUME (MCV): Chronic alcohol ingestion can increase MCV (2263).
TRIGLYCERIDES: Chronic alcohol ingestion can increase triglycerides (2263).

Interactions with Diseases or Conditions
ASTHMA: There have been occasional reports of asthma triggered by beer consumption (6174).
GOUT: Alcohol use can exacerbate gout (2263).
HEART CONDITIONS: Alcohol use can exacerbate variant angina, congestive heart failure (2261,2263,6889), and idiopathic cardiomyopathy (6889).
HIGH BLOOD PRESSURE: Consuming three or more alcoholic drinks a day can increase blood pressure and exacerbate hypertension (2261).
HYPERTRIGLYCERIDEMIA: Alcohol ingestion can exacerbate hypertriglyceridemia (2261,2263,6892).
INSOMNIA: Alcohol use may exacerbate insomnia (2263).
LIVER DISEASE: Alcohol use can exacerbate liver disease (2261).
NEUROLOGICAL CONDITIONS: Alcohol use can exacerbate degenerative neurological conditions (6889).
PANCREATITIS: Alcohol use can exacerbate pancreatitis (2261).
PEPTIC ULCER DISEASE (PUD)/GASTROESOPHAGEAL REFLUX DISEASE (GERD): Alcohol use can exacerbate PUD and GERD (2261,2263).
PORPHYRIA: Alcohol use can exacerbate porphyria (2261).
PSYCHIATRIC DISORDERS: Consuming three or more drinks of alcohol a day can also exacerbate psychiatric disorders and increase cognitive impairment (2261).

Dosage and Administration
ORAL: For reducing the risk of cardiovascular disease and ischemic stroke one or two drinks, 12 oz, per day has been used (2261,2271,6835,6837,6840,6841,6842,6888,6892,6893,8648,8649,8650,10128). Up to four glasses per day has been associated with reducing the risk for heart failure (8104). Up to one drink per day has been associated with less cognitive decline in older men (6824,6829). Three drinks per day to two drinks per week and have been associated with reduced risk of type 2 diabetes in healthy men (6172,6891). Up to seven drinks per week has been associated with reducing the risk of coronary heart disease in people with type 2 diabetes (8653,8654). Consumption of more than 75 grams of alcohol from beverages such as beer has been associated with reducing the risk of Helicobacter pylori infection (8034). Alcohol intake is often measured in number of "drinks." One drink is equivalent to a 4 oz or a 120 mL glass of wine, 12 oz of beer, or 1 oz of spirits.

BEESWAX

Also Known As
Bleached Beeswax, White Beeswax, White Wax, Yellow Beeswax, Yellow Wax.

Scientific Names
Apis cerana; Apis mellifera.
Family: Apidae.

People Use This For

Orally, beeswax is used for lowering lipids, as an anti-inflammatory, anti-ulcer, for diarrhea, hiccups, and pain relief.

In foods and beverages, white beeswax and beeswax absolute are utilized as stiffening agents.

In manufacturing, yellow and white beeswax are used as thickeners, emulsifiers, and as stiffening agents in cosmetics. Beeswax absolute is used as a fragrance ingredient in soaps and perfumes. White beeswax and beeswax absolute are also used as tablet polishing components in pharmaceutical products.

Safety

LIKELY SAFE ...when used orally in amounts commonly found in foods. Beeswax has Generally Recognized As Safe (GRAS) status in the US (4912). ...when used orally as a medicinal agent (11). ...when used topically (11).

PREGNANCY AND LACTATION: There is insufficient reliable information available about the safety of medicinal amounts of beeswax during pregnancy and lactation.

Effectiveness

There is insufficient reliable information available about the effectiveness of beeswax.

Mechanism of Action

A natural mixture of high molecular weight alcohols isolated and purified from beeswax, termed D-002, had mild anti-inflammatory effects in experimental animals (4052). In rats, injected D-002 partially inhibited experimentally-induced gastric damage (4053,4054). Concomitant use of beeswax and nonsteroidal anti-inflammatory drugs (NSAIDs) may protect against NSAID-induced ulcers (4053,4054).

Adverse Reactions

Orally, beeswax may cause allergic reactions (11).

Interactions with Herbs & Other Dietary Supplements

None known.

Interactions with Drugs

None known.

Interactions with Foods

None known.

Interactions with Lab Tests

None known.

Interactions with Diseases or Conditions

None known.

Dosage and Administration

No typical dosage.

Comments

The three major beeswax products are yellow beeswax, white beeswax, and beeswax absolute. Yellow beeswax is the crude product obtained from the honeycomb. White beeswax is derived from yellow beeswax by bleaching, and beeswax absolute is derived from yellow beeswax by extraction with alcohol. Beeswax is obtained from the honeycomb of the honeybee (Apis mellifera) and other Apis species.

BEET

Also Known As

Fodder Beet, Garden Beet, Mangel, Mangold, Red Beet, Sugarbeet, Yellow Beet.

Scientific Names

Beta vulgaris.

Family: Chenopodiaceae.

People Use This For

Orally, beets are used as a supportive therapy in the treatment of liver diseases and fatty liver.

Safety
LIKELY SAFE ...when used in amounts commonly found in foods.
There is insufficient reliable information available about the safety of beets used medicinally.
PREGNANCY AND LACTATION: There is insufficient reliable information available about the safety of beets used medicinally during pregnancy and breast-feeding.

Effectiveness
There is insufficient reliable information available about the effectiveness of beets.

Mechanism of Action
The applicable part of beet is the root. Animal data suggests that beets may be effective against fat deposition in the liver. A component called betaine may play a role (18).

Adverse Reactions
Orally, ingestion of large quantities of beets could lead to hypocalcemia and kidney damage because of the oxaluric acid content (18).

Interactions with Herbs & Other Dietary Supplements
None known.

Interactions with Drugs
None known.

Interactions with Foods
None known.

Interactions with Lab Tests
None known.

Interactions with Diseases or Conditions
KIDNEY DISEASE: Ingestion of large quantities of beets could worsen kidney disease (18).

Dosage and Administration
ORAL: Beet is used as a standardized granular powder (18).

BELLADONNA

Also Known As
Belladone, Deadly Nightshade, Devil's Cherries, Devil's Herb, Divale, Dwale, Dwayberry, Great Morel, Indian Belladonna, Naughty Man's Cherries, Poison Black Cherries.
CAUTION: See separate listings for Bittersweet Nightshade, Henbane, and Scopolia.

Scientific Names
Atropa belladonna; Atropa acuminata.
Family: Solanaceae.

People Use This For
Orally, belladonna is used as a sedative, as an antispasmodic in bronchial asthma and whooping cough, and as a cold and hay fever remedy, for Parkinson's disease, intestinal and biliary colic, motion sickness, and as anesthetic.
Topically, belladonna is used in liniments for rheumatism, sciatica, and neuralgia; and in medicinal plasters for treating psychiatric disorders, hyperkinesis, hyperhidrosis, and bronchial asthma.
Rectally, belladonna is used in hemorrhoid suppositories.

Safety
POSSIBLY SAFE ...when the standardized extract is used orally and appropriately under the supervision of a medical professional trained in the use of belladonna (2). Belladonna is available as a prescription drug in the US and has a narrow therapeutic index.
LIKELY UNSAFE ...when the standardized extract is used orally without professional medical supervision (12). ...when the unstandardized leaf, root, or other preparation is used orally (12).
There is insufficient reliable information available about the safety of belladonna for its other uses.
CHILDREN: POSSIBLY SAFE ...when used orally in children older than 6 years old only under professional medical supervision. LIKELY UNSAFE ...when the leaf, root, or extract is used orally in children under six years old (12). There is insufficient reliable information available about the safety of the topical or rectal use

of belladonna in children.
PREGNANCY: LIKELY UNSAFE ...when the leaf or root are used orally without medical supervision. There is insufficient reliable information about the safety of belladonna for its other uses during pregnancy.
LACTATION: LIKELY UNSAFE ...when the leaf, root, standardized extract, or other preparation are used orally. Use should be avoided because it can reduce milk production and is secreted into breast milk (15). There is insufficient reliable information available about the safety of belladonna for its other uses during lactation.

Effectiveness

There is insufficient reliable information available about the effectiveness of belladonna.

Mechanism of Action

The applicable parts of belladonna are the leaf and root. Its anticholinergic activity is due to the 0.3% to 0.5% tropane alkaloid constituents; mainly l-hyoscyamine, but it also contains traces of l-scopolamine and atropine (dl-hyoscyamine) (11). On extraction, most of the l-hyoscyamine is racemized to atropine (11).

Adverse Reactions

Orally, belladonna can cause dry mouth, decreased perspiration, dilation of pupils, blurred vision, red dry skin, hyperthermia, tachycardia, difficulty urinating, hallucinations, spasms, acute psychosis, convulsions, and coma (2,11,553).

Interactions with Herbs & Other Dietary Supplements

None known.

Interactions with Drugs

ANTICHOLINERGIC DRUGS: Belladonna can increase the anticholinergic effects and adverse effects of amantadine, antihistamines, phenothiazines, procainamide, quinidine, tricyclic antidepressants, and others (2).

Interactions with Foods

None known.

Interactions with Lab Tests

None known.

Interactions with Diseases or Conditions

CONGESTIVE HEART FAILURE (CHF): Belladonna might cause tachycardia and exacerbate CHF due to its hyoscyamine (atropine) and scopolamine content (15).
CONSTIPATION: Belladonna might cause constipation due to its hyoscyamine (atropine) and scopolamine content (15).
DOWN SYNDROME: Caution, patients with Down syndrome might be hypersensitive to the antimuscarinic effects (mydriasis, positive chronotropic heart effects, etc.) of hyoscyamine (atropine) and scopolamine contained in belladonna (15).
ESOPHAGEAL REFLUX: Belladonna might delay gastric emptying and decrease lower esophageal pressure, promoting gastric retention and exacerbating reflux due to its hyoscyamine (atropine) and scopolamine content (15).
FEVER: Belladonna might increase the risk of hyperthermia in patients with fever due to its hyoscyamine (atropine) and scopolamine content (15).
GASTRIC ULCER: Belladonna might delay gastric emptying and exacerbate gastric ulcers due to its hyoscyamine (atropine) and scopolamine content (15).
GASTROINTESTINAL (GI) INFECTIONS: Belladonna might suppress GI motility causing retention of infecting organisms or toxins due to its hyoscyamine (atropine) and scopolamine content (15).
HIATAL HERNIA: Belladonna might delay gastric emptying and decrease lower esophageal pressure, promoting gastric retention and exacerbating reflux due to its hyoscyamine (atropine) and scopolamine content (15).
NARROW-ANGLE GLAUCOMA: Belladonna might increase ocular tension in patients with narrow-angle (angle-closure) glaucoma due to its hyoscyamine (atropine) and scopolamine content (2,15).
OBSTRUCTIVE GASTROINTESTINAL (GI) TRACT DISEASE: Belladonna might exacerbate obstructive GI tract diseases (including atony, paralytic ileus, and stenosis) due to its hyoscyamine (atropine) and scopolamine content (15).
TACHYARRHYTHMIAS: Belladonna might cause tachycardia due to its hyoscyamine (atropine) and scopolamine content (2,15).
TOXIC MEGACOLON: Belladonna might suppress intestinal motility, which might produce paralytic ileus and exacerbate toxic megacolon, due to its hyoscyamine (atropine) and scopolamine content (2,15).
ULCERATIVE COLITIS: Belladonna might suppress intestinal motility, which might produce paralytic ileus and precipitate toxic megacolon, due to its hyoscyamine (atropine) and scopolamine content (15).
URINARY RETENTION: Belladonna might increase urinary retention due to its hyoscyamine (atropine) and scopolamine content (2,15).

Dosage and Administration

ORAL: The belladonna leaf powder is typically an average single dose of 50-100 mg. The maximum single dose is 200 mg, which is equivalent to 0.6 mg total alkaloids, calculated as hyoscyamine. The maximum daily dose is 600 mg, which is equivalent to 1.8 mg total alkaloids, calculated as hyoscyamine. The root powder is commonly used in an average single dose of 50 mg. The maximum single dose is 100 mg, which is equivalent to 0.5 mg total alkaloids, calculated as hyoscyamine. The maximum daily dose of the root powder is 300 mg, equivalent to 1.5 mg total alkaloids calculated as hyoscyamine. The belladonna extract has an average single dose of 10 mg. The maximum single dose is 50 mg, equivalent to 0.73 mg total alkaloids calculated as hyoscyamine, and the maximum daily dosage is 150 mg, equivalent to 2.2 mg total alkaloids calculated as hyoscyamine (2).
TOPICAL: No typical dosage.
RECTAL: No typical dosage.

Comments

The name, belladonna, means beautiful lady. The belladonna berry juice has been used historically in Italy to dilate the pupils of women giving them a striking appearance (11). Avoid confusion with bittersweet nightshade (Solanum dulcamara) and henbane (nightshade).

BENZOIN

Also Known As

Benzoe, Gum Benjamin, Gum Benzoin, Sumatra Benzoin.

Scientific Names

Styrax benzoin; Styrax paralleloneurum.
Family: Styracaceae.

People Use This For

Orally, benzoin is used for throat and bronchial inflammation.
Topically, benzoin is used as an antiseptic, astringent, skin protectant, and styptic on small cuts. Benzoin is also used topically for skin ulcers, bedsores, cracked nipples, and fissures of the lips and anus.
By inhalation, benzoin is used to treat laryngitis, croup, and other respiratory conditions.
In combination with other herbs, benzoin tincture (benzoin, aloe, storax, and tolu balsam) is used as a skin protectant.
In dentistry, benzoin is used for gum inflammation and oral herpes lesions.
In manufacturing, benzoin is used in making pharmaceutical preparations.

Safety

POSSIBLY SAFE ...when preparations of the gum resin are used orally for medicinal purposes (12). ...when used topically (11). Tincture of benzoin can cause contact dermatitis.
There is insufficient reliable information available about the safety of benzoin for its other uses.
PREGNANCY AND LACTATION: Insufficient reliable information available; avoid using.

Effectiveness

There is insufficient reliable information available about the effectiveness of benzoin.

Mechanism of Action

The applicable part of benzoin is the gum resin. Benzoin has antiseptic, stimulant, expectorant, astringent, diuretic, and skin protectant effects (11,13).

Adverse Reactions

Topically, the compound benzoin tincture (benzoin, aloe, storax, and tolu balsam) can cause contact dermatitis (11) and should be avoided in sensitive individuals.

Interactions with Herbs & Other Dietary Supplements

None known.

Interactions with Drugs

None known.

Interactions with Foods

None known.

Interactions with Lab Tests
None known.

Interactions with Diseases or Conditions
SENSITIVE INDIVIDUALS: Avoid contact with benzoin and the compound benzoin tincture due to contact dermatitis (11).

Dosage and Administration
ORAL: No typical dosage.
TOPICAL: A typical dosage is a few drops of compound benzoin tincture (USP) every two hours (6002). Compound benzoin tincture contains 100 grams of benzoin powder, 20 grams of aloe powder, 80 grams of storax, and 40 grams of tolu balsam per 1000 mL of tincture (16).
INHALATION: People typically add 5 mL of a compound benzoin tincture (USP) to 473 mL of hot water or place the tincture directly on a handkerchief (6002).

Comments
Benzoin is the gum resin of Styrax species trees. Avoid confusion with Siam benzoin (Styrax tonikensis), which is used only in manufacturing and has no medicinal uses (11,13).

BERGAMOT OIL

Also Known As
Bergamot, Bergamot Orange, Bergamota, Bergamotier, Bergamoto, Bergamotte, Bergamotto Bigarade Orange, Oleum Bergamotte.
CAUTION: See separate listings for Bitter Orange and Sweet Orange.

Scientific Names
Citrus bergamia, synonym Citrus aurantium var. bergamia.
Family: Rutaceae.

People Use This For
Topically, bergamot oil is used to treat psoriasis in conjunction with long-wave ultraviolet light. Bergamot oil is also used topically for vitiligo, mycosis fungoides, and as an insecticide to protect the body against lice and other vermin.
By inhalation, bergamot oil is used as aromatherapy for anxiety.
In foods, bergamot oil is widely used as a citrus flavoring agent, up to 0.02% in gelatins and puddings.
In manufacturing of cosmetics, bergamot oil is used (up to 3% in perfumes and 0.25% in creams and lotions), in soaps, and suntan oils.

Safety
LIKELY SAFE ...when bergamot oil is used orally in amounts commonly found in foods. Bergamot oil has Generally Recognized As Safe status (GRAS) for use in foods in the US (4912).
POSSIBLY UNSAFE ...when used topically. Bergamot oil can act as a photosensitizer and can induce malignant changes (6).
CHILDREN: POSSIBLY UNSAFE ...when large amounts are ingested. Bergamot oil can cause intestinal colic, convulsions, and death (12).
PREGNANCY AND LACTATION: POSSIBLY UNSAFE ...when used topically (6).

Effectiveness
INSUFFICIENT RELIABLE EVIDENCE to RATE

Anxiety. There's preliminary evidence that suggests using bergamot oil as aromatherapy does not help reduce anxiety in patients receiving concurrent radiotherapy (11452). More evidence is needed to rate bergamot oil for this use.

Mechanism of Action
Bergamot oil is obtained from the peel of Citrus bergamia. The photosensitivity of bergamot oil is linked to the furocoumarin constituents, bergapten (5-methoxypsoralen) (11019), and xanthotoxin (8-methoxypsoralen) (6).

Adverse Reactions
Frequent contact with the peel or oil of bergamot can cause erythema, blisters, pustules, dermatoses leading to scab formation, and pigment spots (18).
Topically, photosensitivity can also occur, especially in fair-skinned people (11909).

Interactions with Herbs & Other Dietary Supplements
None known.

Interactions with Drugs
PHOTOSENSITIZING DRUGS: Topically due to bergapten content use of bergamot oil can compound photosensitizing effects and increase the risk of side effects (11909). Concomitant use should be avoided.

Interactions with Foods
None known.

Interactions with Lab Tests
None known.

Interactions with Diseases or Conditions
None known.

Dosage and Administration
No typical dosage.

BETA GLUCANS

Also Known As
Beta Glucan, Beta 1,3 Glucans, Beta-Glucan, Beta-Glucans, Beta Glycans, Beta-Glycans, Grifolan (GRN), Lentinan, PGG Glucan, PGG-Glucan, Poly-[1-6]-Beta-D-Glucopyranosyl-[1-3]-Beta-D-Glucopyranose, Schizophyllan (SPG), SSG, Yeast-Derived Beta Glucan.
CAUTION: See separate listings for Barley, Brewer's Yeast, Maitake Mushroom, Oats, Saccharomyces Boulardii, Salep, and Shiitake Mushroom.

Scientific Names
1-3,1-6-beta-glucan; beta-1,3-D-glucan; beta-1-6,1,3-beta-glucan.

People Use This For
Orally, beta glucans are used for hypercholesterolemia, diabetes, cancer, and HIV/AIDS. Beta glucans are also used orally as an immunostimulant in people with conditions that may compromise their immune system such as chronic fatigue syndrome, physical and emotional stress, and patients receiving chemotherapy or radiation treatment. It is also used orally for colds (common cold), flu (influenza), allergies, hepatitis, Lyme disease, asthma, ear infections, aging, ulcerative colitis and Crohn's disease, fibromyalgia, rheumatoid arthritis, and multiple sclerosis.
Topically, beta glucans are used for dermatitis, eczema, wrinkles, bedsores, wounds, burns, diabetic ulcers, and radiation burns.
Intravenously and intramuscularly, beta glucans are used for treating cancer and as an immunostimulant in patients with HIV/AIDS and AIDS-related disorders. It is also used intravenously for preventing sepsis in trauma patients after undergoing exploratory laparotomy or thoracotomy and for preventing infection in surgical patients.
Subcutaneously, beta glucans are used for treating and reducing the size of subcutaneous tumors resulting from malignant metastatic disease.
In manufacturing, beta glucans are used as a food additive in products such as salad dressings, frozen desserts, sour cream, and cheese spreads.

Safety
LIKELY SAFE ...when used orally in amounts commonly found in foods. Beta glucans derived from baker's yeast or brewer's yeast (Saccharomyces cerevisiae) have Generally Recognized As Safe (GRAS) status in the US (4912).
POSSIBLY SAFE ...when used orally and appropriately, short-term in medicinal amounts. There is some evidence that yeast-derived beta-glucans 15 grams per day can be used safely for up to 8 weeks (7272). ...when used intravenously or intramuscularly and appropriately. Both yeast and fungal beta-glucans seem to be safe when soluble forms are used (7261,7263,7264,7266,7267,7269,7270,7271). Particulate beta glucans may not be safe. There is preliminary evidence that intravenous beta glucans in the microparticulate form might cause serious side effects such as hepatosplenomegaly, granuloma formation, and microembolization (7241). Most studies evaluating parenteral use of beta glucans have used specific forms including PGG-glucan (Betafectin) from a proprietary strain of Saccharomyces cerevisiae (7269,7270,7271) and specific fungal-derived beta glucans lentinan and schizophyllan (SPG) (7261,7263,7264,7266,7267). Lentinan and SPG have been safely used in studies lasting for up to 12 months (7263,7264,7267). PGG-glucan has been safely used in studies when given 24 hours prior to surgery

and lasting up to 96 hours after surgery (7269,7270,7271).
There is insufficient reliable information available about the safety of beta glucans when used subcutaneously or topically.
PREGNANCY AND LACTATION: Insufficient reliable information available; avoid using.

Effectiveness

POSSIBLY EFFECTIVE

Cancer. Giving the specific fungal beta glucans lentinan and schizophyllan intravenously or intramuscularly seems to prolong survival time of cancer patients when used in addition to conventional cancer treatment regimens. Lentinan 1-2 mg once or twice weekly for at least 1 year increases survival time by 6-9 months in people with advanced (stage III or IV) unresectable cancers (7266). Schizophyllan 20-40 mg once or twice weekly for at least 1 year significantly improves 4-5 year survival rates in people with cervical cancer and head and neck cancer (7261,7263,7264).

HIV/AIDS. There is preliminary evidence that giving the specific fungal beta glucans lentinan 2-10 mg once or twice weekly intravenously can increase levels of CD4 cells by 5.5-18% and decrease p24 antigen levels (a marker of viral replication) by 11.5% after 12-20 weeks of treatment in asymptomatic patients with HIV (7267).

Hypercholesterolemia. Taking yeast-derived beta glucans 7.5 grams twice daily appears to reduce serum total cholesterol concentrations by 6-8% in patients with hypercholesterolemia after 7-8 weeks of treatment (7272). However, barley that is highly enriched (75% by weight) with beta glucan doesn't seem to affect cholesterol. This lack of effect seems to be the result of processing the barley into a highly enriched beta glucan product (10166). More research is needed to determine if improved processing methods can produce beta-glucan enriched products that can lower cholesterol.

Postoperative infection. A proprietary beta glucans preparation from Saccharomyces cerevisiae called PGG-glucan given intravenously 12-24 hours before and 4-96 hours after surgery at 0.5-1 mg/kg per dose reduces the occurrence of postoperative infection by 10-16%, decreases the number of days of intravenous antibiotic use by 10 days, and shortens the length of stay in the intensive care unit (ICU) by 3 days in surgical patients at high risk for infection (7269,7271). Administering beta glucans intravenously also seems to help prevent sepsis in trauma patients following exploratory laparotomy or thoracotomy. There is some evidence that intravenous soluble yeast-derived beta glucans 50 mg/M2 daily for 7 days decreases the rate of septic morbidity by 39.5% in trauma patients following exploratory surgical procedures (7268).

There is insufficient reliable information available about the effectiveness of beta glucans for their other uses.

Mechanism of Action

Beta glucans are polysaccharides that consist of (1-3)-beta-D-linked polymers of glucose that are either non-branched or with 1-6-beta-branches (3394,7242). Beta glucans are primary components in cell walls of bacteria, fungi, yeasts, algae, lichens, plants such as oats and barley, and are excreted extracellularly by various fungi (3394,7242,7250). The beta glucans most extensively studied to date are yeast-derived beta glucans from Saccharomyces cerevisiae; the fungal-derived beta glucans such as lentinan from Lentinus edodes, gifolan (GRN) from Grifola frondosa, schizophyllan (SPG) from Schizophyllum commune, SSG from Sclerotinia sclerotiorum; and beta glucans from oats (7241,7248,7273). Mammals cannot digest and absorb beta glucans because they lack the enzyme beta-1-3-glucanase needed to break down large beta glucan molecules. Since beta glucans cannot be absorbed orally, clinical studies have usually administered beta glucans by the parenteral route (3393). Beta glucans seem to have antibacterial, antiviral, antifungal, antiparasitic, and antitumor activity; and might promote recovery from sepsis and immunosuppression associated with various disease states or conditions such as HIV infection or whole body radiation (7238,7243,7250). Laboratory findings suggest beta glucans specifically bind to monocyte and macrophage cell lines, increase the proliferation and activation of macrophages, and increase the production of cytokine interleukin-1 (IL-1) by macrophages which in turn promotes the release of IL-2 by T-cells (7243,7248,7249,7250,7252,7268). Beta glucans also seem to have anticancer effects. Beta glucans don't seem to have direct antitumor or antibacterial activity, but are thought to act as biological response modifiers (BRMs) that restore or enhance humoral and cell-mediated immune responses (3394,7237,7251). Beta glucans increase macrophage phagocytosis of tumor cells, increase the cytotoxicity of natural killer cells (NK), and stimulate the release of interleukin-1 (IL-1) and tumor necrosis factor (TNF) (7237,7238,7240,7265). Beta glucans bind to a beta glucan receptor on macrophages, neutrophils, and NK cells and seem to activate a complement receptor on the cells which bind to tumor or bacterial cells that are opsonized with complement and antibodies (7237,7239,7248,7269,7270,7271). Many cells, including cancer cells and bacteria, can acquire mechanisms to resist the action of complement, but there is some evidence that beta glucans can override this mechanism and allow the phagocytosis to occur (7237).
For wound healing after surgery, there is some evidence beta glucans can decrease inflammation, and accelerate the repair of surgical wounds by stimulating macrophages and increasing macrophage infiltration, causing increased tissue granulation and enhanced re-epithelization of tissue (7246).
For hypercholesterolemia, beta glucans are thought to lower cholesterol by forming a layer adjacent to the intestinal mucosa that delays or prevents cholesterol absorption (7273,10166). Beta glucans might also bind bile acids in the intestinal lumen (7272,10166).

Adverse Reactions

Orally, yeast-derived beta glucans seem to be well-tolerated. No adverse effects have been reported (7272). Intravenously, beta glucans can cause chills and fever (7267,7271), redness, pain and swelling at the injection site, lymph node swelling (7261,7263), joint pain, lower back pain, headache, diarrhea, dizziness, flushing (7267), hypotension, hypertension, vasodilation, nausea, vomiting, leukocytosis (7270,7271), hives (7267), maculopapular rash (7270,7271), and excessive urination (7267).

Interactions with Herbs & Other Dietary Supplements

None known.

Interactions with Drugs

IMMUNOSUPPRESSANTS: Theoretically, beta glucans might decrease the effects of immunosuppressants because of its immunostimulant effects (7243,7248,7249,7250,7252,7268). Immunosuppressant drugs include azathioprine (Imuran), basiliximab (Simulect), cyclosporine (Neoral, Sandimmune), daclizumab (Zenapax), muromonab-CD3 (OKT3, Orthoclone OKT3), mycophenolate (CellCept), tacrolimus (FK506, Prograf), sirolimus (Rapamune), prednisone (Deltasone, Orasone), and other corticosteroids (glucocorticoids).

Interactions with Foods

None known.

Interactions with Lab Tests

WHITE BLOOD CELL COUNT: Beta glucans can cause a transient increase in the number of white cells (leukocytosis) (7270).

Interactions with Diseases or Conditions

ACQUIRED IMMUNODEFICIENCY SYNDROME (AIDS) or AIDS-RELATED COMPLEX (ARC): Keratoderma of the palms and soles can develop in patients with AIDS/HIV or ARC who are receiving yeast beta glucans. The condition can begin during the first two weeks of therapy and resolves two to four weeks after discontinuation of beta glucans (7252).

Dosage and Administration

ORAL: For hypercholesterolemia, 7.5 grams twice daily of yeast-derived beta glucans fiber added to juice has been used (7272).

INTRAVENOUS: For HIV infection, 1-10 mg of the fungal beta glucan lentinan, administered over 10-30 minutes and given once to twice weekly has been used (7267). To prolong survival time in patients with cancer, 1-2 mg of the fungal beta glucan lentinan or 20-40 mg of the fungal beta glucan schizophyllan (SPG) administered once or twice weekly for at least one year has been used (3393,7261,7263,7264,7266). To prevent infection in trauma patients undergoing exploratory surgical procedures, 50 mg/M2 of soluble yeast-derived beta-glucan per day for 7 days has been used (7268). In surgical patients at high-risk for infection, 0.5-2 mg/kg of PGG-glucan given 1-6 hours before surgery and then repeated 4 hours, 48 hours, and 96 hours after surgery has been used (7270,7271).

Comments

There are several beta glucan supplement products that claim beta glucan taken orally can only be absorbed if the product is prepared by a special patented process that micronizes beta glucan particles to a size of 1 micron or less. However, there is no reliable evidence to support such a claim.

BETA-CAROTENE

Also Known As

A-Beta-Carotene, Carotenes, Carotenoids, Provitamin A.
CAUTION: See separate listings for Astaxanthin and Vitamin A.

Scientific Names

Beta-carotene.

People Use This For

Orally, beta-carotene is taken as a dietary source of vitamin A; and to reduce photosensitivities, including erythropoietic protoporphyria (EPP) and polymorphous light eruption. Beta-carotene is also used orally for decreasing exercise-induced asthma; and to reduce the risk of some cancers, cardiovascular disease, cataracts, and age related macular degeneration. Additionally, beta-carotene is used to treat AIDS, alcoholism, Alzheimer's disease, depression, epilepsy, headache, heartburn, hypertension, infertility, Parkinson's disease, psoriasis, rheumatoid arthritis, schizophrenia, and vitiligo.

Safety

LIKELY SAFE ...when used orally and appropriately in amounts commonly found in foods (139,4844,6393).
POSSIBLY SAFE ...when used orally as a dietary supplement. Doses up to 300 mg per day have been used with apparent safety for conditions such as erythropoietic protoporphyria (11793). However, doses as low as 20 mg per day have been associated with increased risk of lung and prostate cancer in people who smoke. Although there is no evidence of significant adverse effects of beta-carotene in nonsmokers, the mechanism for cancer promotion is unknown. If beta-carotene supplements are used, it may be prudent to limit daily consumption to 7 mg per day until more is known about its long-term toxicity (11786).
POSSIBLY UNSAFE ...when used orally in people who smoke or have a history of asbestos exposure. Supplemental beta-carotene 20 mg daily for 5-8 years seems to increase the risk of lung cancer, prostate cancer, intracerebral hemorrhage, and cardiovascular and total mortality in people who smoke cigarettes or have a history of high-level exposure to asbestos (1371,3359,3937,3959,6393,11786). Beta-carotene from foods does not seem to have this effect.
CHILDREN: LIKELY SAFE ...when used orally in amounts commonly found in foods (4844).
POSSIBLY SAFE ...when used orally as a dietary supplement. High doses (greater than 60 mg per day) have been used with apparent safety for conditions such as erythropoietic protoporphyria (11793). However, doses as low as 20 mg per day have been associated with increased risk of lung and prostate cancer in adults who smoke. Although there is no evidence of significant adverse effects of beta-carotene in nonsmokers, the mechanism for cancer promotion is unknown. Supplemental beta-carotene in children should be limited to specific medical indications.
PREGNANCY AND LACTATION: LIKELY SAFE ...when used orally and appropriately in amounts commonly found in foods (139,6393,4844). POSSIBLY SAFE ...when used orally as a dietary supplement. Although there is no evidence of significant adverse effects of beta-carotene in nonsmokers, the mechanism for promotion of some cancers is unknown. If used, it may be prudent to limit daily consumption of supplemental beta-carotene to 7 mg per day until more is known about its long-term toxicity (11786). There is insufficient reliable information available about the safety of large doses of beta-carotene in pregnancy and lactation.

Effectiveness

EFFECTIVE

Erythropoietic protoporphyria (EPP). Taking beta-carotene orally can reduce photosensitivity in patients with EPP, a genetic disorder resulting in defective porphyrin metabolism (11793).

POSSIBLY EFFECTIVE

Age-related macular degeneration (AMD). Taking beta-carotene orally 15 mg, combined with vitamin C 500 mg, vitamin E 400 IU, and elemental zinc 80 mg daily seems to provide a risk reduction of 27% for visual acuity loss and a risk reduction of 25% for progression of AMD in patients with advanced AMD (7303,11326). Patients with monocular or binocular intermediate AMD or monocular advanced AMD are at high risk for advanced AMD. Theoretically, these patients may also benefit from beta-carotene and antioxidant-zinc supplementation (11326). There isn't enough evidence to know if this combination is beneficial for people with less advanced macular disease. Supplemental beta-carotene with antioxidants, but without zinc, doesn't seem to have any significant effect on AMD (7303,7304). Additionally, there is preliminary evidence that a high dietary intake of beta-carotene might decrease the risk of AMD (5922). Other dietary carotenoids such as lycopene, lutein, and zeaxanthin may provide greater protection from radiation and oxidative damage in the retina than beta-carotene (6110,8446).

Breast cancer. There is some evidence that a diet rich in beta-carotene may reduce the risk of breast cancer in premenopausal women, especially those at high risk due to family history or high alcohol intake (1444,10132).

Chronic obstructive pulmonary disease (COPD). The prevalence of bronchitis and dyspnea in male smokers with chronic obstructive pulmonary disorder (COPD) seems to be lower in those patients who consume a diet containing high amounts of beta-carotene (2580). But taking beta-carotene supplements doesn't seem to help (2580).

Exercise-induced asthma. Taking a mixture of beta-carotene isomers orally seems to prevent exercise-induced asthma (1474).

Oral leukoplakia. Taking beta-carotene orally seems to induce remission in patients with oral leukoplakia. There's an increased risk of disease progression over 12 months if beta-carotene is stopped (1472).

Osteoarthritis. Taking beta-carotene orally doesn't seem to prevent osteoarthritis, but it might slow progression of the disease (5881).

Ovarian cancer. There is some evidence a diet rich in carotenoids, including beta-carotene and especially alpha-carotene, can decrease the risk of ovarian cancer in postmenopausal women (10133).

Post-partum complications. Taking beta carotene orally seems to reduce the occurrence of post-partum diarrhea and fever in malnourished women. All-trans beta-carotene (synthetic beta-carotene) taken weekly before, during, and after pregnancy reduces, but does not eliminate, the occurrence of post partum diarrhea and fever (2581).

Pregnancy-related complications. Taking beta-carotene orally seems to reduce pregnancy-related maternal mortality and night blindness in malnourished women. All-trans beta-carotene (synthetic beta-carotene) taken weekly before, during, and after pregnancy seems to reduce pregnancy-related mortality and night blindness (6153,6154). But synthetic beta-carotene does not reduce fetal and early infant mortality (6152).

Sunburn. Taking beta-carotene orally seems to modestly reduce the risk of sunburn in individuals who are sensitive to sun exposure. There is some evidence that 25 mg of mixed beta-carotene daily for 12 weeks reduces skin redness after exposure to UV light in sun-sensitive individuals (6134). However, beta-carotene is unlikely to have much effect on sunburn risk in most people (11792). Also, it doesn't seem to reduce the incidence of solar keratoses or skin cancers associated with sun exposure (1297,2599,11302).

POSSIBLY INEFFECTIVE

Alzheimer's disease. Intake of dietary or supplemental beta-carotene doesn't seem to have any effect on Alzheimer's disease risk (10131).

Cataracts. Taking elemental beta-carotene orally 15 mg, in combination with vitamin C 500 mg, vitamin E 400 IU, and zinc 80 mg daily for 6.3 years does not seem to have any effect on the development or progression of age-related lens opacities (cataracts) or the need for cataract surgery in well-nourished people 55-80 years of age. However, it is unknown whether earlier intervention and/or a longer period of treatment with supplements would have any effect on cataracts (7304).

Prostate cancer. Beta-carotene doesn't seem to decrease prostate cancer risk in most men (148,1473,2406,7895,12877). In the Physicians' Health Study, 22,071 US male physicians took 50 mg of beta-carotene every other day for nearly 13 years. Beta-carotene provided no overall protective effect. Some subgroups of men such as those with low beta-carotene levels (less than 153.25 ng/mL) or high body mass index might benefit (1473,12877).

Stroke. Taking all-trans beta-carotene (synthetic beta-carotene) orally, 20 mg/day for a median of six years may have no effect on the overall incidence of stroke in male smokers (1371). Additionally, there is some evidence that beta-carotene actually increases the risk of intracerebral hemorrhage by 62% in patients who also drink alcohol (1371,3359).

LIKELY INEFFECTIVE

Cancer. Beta-carotene 20-50 mg daily, or 50 mg on alternate days, does not affect the incidence of a variety of cancers in adults, including uterine cancer, cervical cancer, thyroid cancer, bladder cancer, skin cancers (melanoma, basal cell carcinoma, squamous cell carcinoma) brain cancer, and blood cancer (140,1297,1448,2599,2642,2646,2657,3949).

Cardiovascular disease. Taking beta-carotene orally doesn't reduce the risk of heart disease and cardiovascular mortality. Large population studies of dietary or supplemental beta-carotene show mixed results (3933,7386,7387), but large-scale controlled clinical trials are more definitive. In male and female patients with no history of cardiovascular disease, dietary beta-carotene and beta-carotene 20-50 mg daily or every other day has no effect on death rates from cardiovascular causes (1448,2646,2657,3935,10130). In people with coronary heart disease, beta-carotene 25 mg daily in combination with selenium and vitamin C and vitamin E doesn't seem to protect from cardiovascular disease progression and related events such as myocardial infarction (MI) (7388). In people who smoke, beta-carotene 20-30 mg daily actually increases cardiovascular mortality by 12% to 26% (2642,3949). In men who smoke and have had a prior MI, the risk of fatal coronary heart disease increases by as much as 43% with beta-carotene 20 mg daily (3937). These adverse effects do not seem to occur in people who eat foods high in beta-carotene content (1440,2657,7714,7715,7716). A Science Advisory from the American Heart Association states that the evidence does not justify use of antioxidants such as beta-carotene for reducing the risk of cardiovascular disease (12142).

Lung cancer. Taking beta-carotene 20 to 30 mg daily actually seems to increase the risk of lung cancer by 18% to 28%, in people who smoke (especially those smoking more than 20 cigarettes per day), former smokers, people exposed to asbestos, and those who ingest significant amounts of alcohol (one or more drinks per day) in addition to smoking (139,1471,2582,2642,3949,11303,11786). However, beta-carotene from food does not seem to have this adverse effect.

INSUFFICIENT RELIABLE EVIDENCE to RATE

Chemotherapy toxicity. Observational research suggests that greater dietary intake of beta-carotene appears to lower the incidence of adverse effects in children undergoing chemotherapy for lymphoblastic leukemia (11997).

Colorectal cancer. There is some evidence that increasing dietary content of beta-carotene can decrease the incidence of colorectal cancer (10244). But other evidence shows no benefit (3962). Prospective randomized trials show that taking beta-carotene supplements alone or in combination with other antioxidants such as vitamin C or vitamin E probably does not reduce the risk of colorectal cancer (12185).

Esophageal cancer. Taking beta-carotene supplements alone or in combination with other antioxidants such as vitamin A or vitamin E plus vitamin C doesn't seem to reduce the risk of esophageal cancer (12185).

Gastric cancer. Some evidence suggests that taking beta-carotene orally 30 mg daily might increase the rate of regression of premalignant gastric lesions in patients at risk for gastric cancer (2579). But pooling the results from other studies suggests that beta-carotene doesn't significantly decrease risk of gastric cancer (12185). Preliminary evidence suggests that beta-carotene 15 mg daily plus vitamin E and selenium might decrease gastric cancer incidence in the high-risk, malnourished Chinese population (2658). But this combination does not seem to affect mortality (2658,12185). Taking beta-carotene in combination with vitamin A, vitamin C, or vitamin E does not seem to reduce the risk of gastric cancer. Taking beta-carotene in combination with both vitamin C and vitamin E also does not seem to reduce the risk of gastric cancer (12185).

Pancreatic cancer. Taking beta-carotene supplements alone or in combination with other antioxidants such as vitamin A or vitamin E doesn't seem to reduce the risk of pancreatic cancer (12185). More evidence is needed to rate beta-carotene for these uses.

Mechanism of Action

Beta-carotene belongs to a class of red, orange, and yellow pigments called carotenoids. There are hundreds of varieties of provitamin A carotenoids, which are present in many fruits, grains, oils, and vegetables (2628,8044). Commercially available beta-carotene is produced synthetically or from palm oil, algae, or fungi (11786).

Beta carotene is converted to retinal, which is essential for vision and is subsequently converted to retinoic acid, which is used for processes involving growth and cell differentiation (7135,8044). The typical dietary intake of beta-carotene in American adults varies from 0.5 to 6.5 mg per day (2628). Beta-carotene is closely related to alpha-carotene; both are precursors for vitamin A (2628). Beta-carotene and other carotenoids provide approximately 50% of the vitamin A needed in the American diet (8044).

Absorption of beta-carotene is variable. The intestine has a limited capacity to absorb intact beta-carotene (8044). The amount of beta-carotene absorbed from food is only about 5% to 30% of that from synthetic supplements due to complexes it forms with proteins and fiber. Heating food may break down these complexes (2628). Carotenoid absorption is improved by dietary fat. Carotenoids are mainly carried in the blood on low-density lipoproteins (LDLs) (2628). The amount of beta-carotene absorbed and converted to vitamin A also depends upon the individual's vitamin A status, beta-carotene body stores, and the amount of beta-carotene ingested (2628,8044). Some of the ingested beta-carotene is converted to vitamin A in the intestinal mucosa (2628). Although beta-carotene is partly metabolized to vitamin A, high intake of beta-carotene does not result in vitamin A toxicity because the proportion converted to vitamin A decreases as beta-carotene intake increases (8044). Beta-carotene also has activity independent of its conversion to vitamin A (139,1470).

Beta-carotene consists of a number of isomers. Synthetic beta-carotene, the form used in most of the clinical studies, is composed of the all-trans form. Natural beta-carotene sources contain 9-cis-, 13-cis-, and 15-cis-beta-carotene (1474). The 9-cis-beta-carotene isomer is poorly absorbed, and most of it is converted to all-trans-beta-carotene in the intestine (2628). The cis isomers account for less than 5% of carotenoids in plasma, but 10% to 25% of carotenoids in the tissues are beta-carotene cis isomers (2628). Little is known about the pharmacology of beta-carotene and the differences that may exist between the various isomers and the natural and synthetic forms (2628).

Beta-carotene seems to have antioxidant activities and prevent lipid peroxidation (139). Serum beta-carotene levels seem to be inversely related to C-reactive protein levels and the white blood count. These markers are markers of inflammation and are associated with tumor recurrence and arteriosclerotic cardiovascular disease events (10135).

It has been proposed that the antioxidant effects may help prevent cancer by reducing free radical-induced DNA damage (2592,2599). There seems to be an inverse relationship between dietary carotenoid intake, or serum beta-carotene levels, and the incidence of various cancers. In-vitro studies show that beta-carotene inhibits tumor cell growth (2592,2628). There is preliminary evidence that carotenoids, including beta-carotene, can inhibit breast cancer cell growth regardless of estrogen receptor status (8045). However, dietary beta-carotene is not substantially concentrated in breast adipose tissue. Breast adipose tissue concentrations are only slightly higher than serum concentrations (10243). There is also evidence that the inhibitory effect on cancer cell growth by certain statin drugs with a closed ring structure, such as mevastatin and lovastatin (Mevacor), may be enhanced when used with carotenoids (8046). However, anticancer effects of beta-carotene supplementation have not been effectively demonstrated in humans.

There is some concern that beta-carotene metabolites with pharmacological activity can accumulate and have carcinogenic effects (6377,6393). Components of cigarette smoke can degrade beta-carotene, and lower concentrations of beta-carotene have been reported in both active and passive smokers (2592,2593). Smoking might enhance production of carcinogenic beta-carotene oxidation metabolites which, if not neutralized by other antioxidants (such as tocopherol and ascorbate, which are also often depleted in smokers), could lead to increased risk of lung cancer (2628,6377). In addition, beta-carotene metabolites might increase the binding of carcinogenic metabolites to DNA and inhibit gap-junction communication between normal cells and tumor cells. Beta-carotene itself might also increase the levels of certain cytochrome P450 (CYP450) dependent enzymes that can hydroxylate and activate certain compounds into their highly carcinogenic forms (6393), as well as increase catabolism of retinoic acid, which controls lung epithelial cell proliferation and differentiation (2592).

Adverse Reactions

Orally, beta-carotene is typically well tolerated and safe when used in appropriate amounts. High doses can cause yellow or orange skin pigmentation called carotenoderma (11786). Although beta-carotene is partly metabolized to vitamin A, high intake of beta-carotene does not result in vitamin A toxicity because the proportion converted to vitamin A decreases as beta-carotene intake increases (8044).

Advise smokers and people with a history of asbestos exposure not to use beta-carotene supplements. Beta-carotene in doses of 20 mg per day for 5-8 years has been associated with an increased risk of lung and prostate cancer and increased total mortality in people who smoke cigarettes, and in people with a history of high-level asbestos exposure (3959,6393,11303,11786). In people who smoke, beta-carotene 20 to 30 mg daily also seems to increase cardiovascular mortality by 12% to 26% (2642,3949). In men who smoke and have had a prior myocardial infarction (MI), the risk of fatal coronary heart disease increases by as much as 43% with beta-carotene 20 mg daily (3937). These adverse effects do not seem to occur in people who eat foods high in beta-carotene content (1440,2657).

There is some evidence that beta-carotene in combination with selenium and vitamin C and vitamin E might lower high-density lipoprotein 2 (HDL2) by 15%, which is considered to be the most cardioprotective component of HDL (7388). Beta-carotene 20 mg daily increases serum concentrations of beta-carotene and alpha-carotene, beta-cryptoxanthin, and retinal. Additionally, beta-carotene supplementation lowers serum lutein concentrations. Increased or decreased levels of carotenoids may be responsible for the untoward effects of beta-carotene supplementation (10134). More research is needed to determine the mechanism of the adverse effects of beta-carotene supplements.

Interactions with Herbs & Other Dietary Supplements

None known.

Interactions with Drugs

HMG-CoA REDUCTASE INHIBITORS ("Statins"): Concomitant use of beta-carotene in combination with selenium, vitamin C, and vitamin E appears to decrease the effectiveness of the combination of simvastatin (Zocor) and niacin (7388). This combination of antioxidants can lower high-density lipoprotein 2 (HDL-2) levels by 15% and reduce the HDL-2-raising effects of HMG-CoA reductase inhibitors and niacin by more than 50% in people with heart disease (7388). Theoretically, beta-carotene could reduce the effectiveness of other HMG-CoA reductase inhibitors such as atorvastatin (Lipitor), fluvastatin (Lescol), lovastatin (Mevacor), and pravastatin (Pravachol).

NIACIN: Concomitant use of beta-carotene in combination with selenium, vitamin C, and vitamin E appears to decrease the effectiveness of the combination of niacin and simvastatin (Zocor) (7388). This combination of antioxidants can lower high-density lipoprotein 2 (HDL-2) levels by 15% and reduce the HDL-2-raising effects of HMG-CoA reductase inhibitors and niacin by more than 50% in people with heart disease (7388).

Drug Influences on Nutrient Levels and Depletion

SOME DRUGS CAN AFFECT BETA-CAROTENE LEVELS:

BILE ACID SEQUESTRANTS: Cholestyramine (Questran) and colestipol (Colestid) can reduce absorption of fat-soluble vitamins, including beta-carotene (4454,4457,4458,4461,5919). Serum levels of beta-carotene can be reduced (4457,4461), but this is probably only in proportion to the lowering of cholesterol (on which beta-carotene is transported). Supplements aren't usually needed (4461).

COLCHICINE: Colchicine can cause disruption of intestinal mucosal function, resulting in malabsorption (4543). Limited evidence suggests that short-term treatment with colchicine 1.9 to 3.9 mg/day can reduce absorption and serum levels of beta-carotene (4543). Long-term use of 1 to 2 mg/day does not affect beta-carotene levels (5921). Advise patients that this is unlikely to be clinically significant.

MINERAL OIL: Mineral oil reduces absorption of fat-soluble vitamins, including beta-carotene (4454,4495,4496). This isn't likely to be clinically significant when mineral oil is used for four months or less (4496).

NEOMYCIN: Oral neomycin sulfate in doses of 4 to 12 grams per day can reduce beta-carotene absorption, but this isn't likely to be clinically significant with short-term use (5916).

ORLISTAT (Xenical): Orlistat can decrease absorption of beta-carotene and other fat soluble vitamins (6001). Recommend that patients take a multivitamin supplement, and separate the dosing time by at least two hours from orlistat (6001).

PROTON PUMP INHIBITORS: Loss of stomach acid can reduce absorption of a single dose of beta-carotene (31), but it isn't known if this is clinically significant, or if it occurs with dietary beta-carotene. Some of these drugs include Lansoprazole (Prevacid), Omeprazole (Prilosec, Losec), Rabeprazole (Aciphex), and Pantoprazole (Protonix, Pantoloc).

Interactions with Foods

ALCOHOL (Ethanol): High consumption of alcohol can decrease serum concentrations of beta-carotene and other carotenoids such as alpha-carotene and beta-cryptoxanthin, and increase serum concentrations of retinol. Researchers are concerned increased retinol concentrations might promote carcinogenesis (10134). Further study is needed to determine whether this effect actually occurs.

OLESTRA (fat substitute): Olestra may interfere with supplemental beta-carotene activity. Olestra lowers serum beta-carotene concentrations in healthy people by 27% (2392).

Interactions with Lab Tests

HIGH-DENSITY LIPOPROTEIN 2 (HDL-2): Beta-carotene in combination with selenium, vitamins C, and vitamin E seems to lower HDL-2 levels (7388). This combination can lower HDL-2 levels by 15% in people with heart disease (7388).

Interactions with Diseases or Conditions

ANGIOPLASTY: There is some concern that when antioxidant vitamins, including beta-carotene, are used together they might have harmful effects in patients after angioplasty. A combination of beta-carotene 30,000 IU, vitamin C 500 mg, and vitamin E 700 IU daily started 30 days before angioplasty, and continued for 6 months thereafter, seems to prevent beneficial vascular remodeling in patients after angioplasty by promoting fibrosis at the site of angioplastic intervention (11000). Tell patients to avoid taking supplements of these vitamins immediately before and following angioplasty without the supervision of a healthcare professional.
SMOKERS: Cigarette smoking decreases serum concentrations of beta-carotene and other carotenoids, and depletes body stores of beta-carotene (7722,10134). However, beta-carotene supplementation should not be recommended because supplemental beta-carotene in doses greater than 20 mg per day is associated with a significantly higher risk of lung and prostate cancer in smokers (139,3949,3959,6382,6393). Tell smokers to avoid taking beta-carotene supplements.

Dosage and Administration

ORAL: For erythropoietic protoporphyria (EPP), dosage is based on age. For age 1 to 4, the daily dose is 60-90 mg; age 5 to 8 years, 90-120 mg; age 9 to 12 years, 120-150 mg; age 13 to 16 years, 150-180 mg; and age 16 and older, 180 mg. If adequate photoprotection is not provided by theses doses, beta-carotene can be increased by 30-60 mg per day for children under 16 years old, and up to a total of 300 mg per day for people older than age 16 (11793).
For decreasing the risk of prostate cancer in men with plasma beta-carotene concentrations less than 153.25 ng/mL, 50 mg every other day has been used (1473). For oral leukoplakia, 30 mg orally twice daily for a total of 6 months has been used (1472). For preventing sunburn in sun-sensitive people, beta-carotene 25 mg orally daily has been used (6134). For preventing gastric cancer in people at high risk, 15-30 mg daily has been used (2579,2658). For treating age-related macular degeneration (AMD), beta-carotene 15 mg plus vitamin C 500 mg, zinc oxide 80 mg, and vitamin E 400 IU has been given daily (7303).
The Institute of Medicine has reviewed beta-carotene, but did not make recommendations for daily intake, citing lack of sufficient evidence. Consuming 5 servings of fruit and vegetables daily provides 6-8 mg of beta-carotene. Routine use of beta-carotene supplements is not necessary in the general population (4844). Beta-carotene requires some dietary fat for absorption, but supplemental beta-carotene is similarly absorbed when taken with high-fat (36 grams fat) or low-fat (3 grams fat) meals (2628,6133).
Beta-carotene supplements are available in both oil matrix gelatin capsules and water-miscible forms. Some clinical trials have used water-miscible beta-carotene (10%) beadlets. The water miscible form seems to produce a significantly higher response in plasma beta-carotene (approximately 47% to 50%) than oil matrix gelatin capsules (10136).

Comments

The American Heart Association recommends obtaining antioxidants, including beta-carotene, from a diet high in fruits, vegetables and whole grains rather than through supplements until more information is known from randomized clinical trials (1440). Similar statements have been released by the American Cancer Society, the World Cancer Research Institute in association with the American Institute for Cancer Research, and the World Health Organization's International Agency for Research on Cancer (1470).

BETA-SITOSTEROL

Also Known As

24-ethyl-cholesterol, Angelicin, B-sitosterol 3-B-D-glucoside, B-sitosterolin, Beta sitosterin, Beta Sitosterol, Beta-sitosterol glucoside, Beta-sitosterol glycoside, Betasitosterol, Cinchol, Cupreol, Phytosterols, Plant Sterols, Quebrachol, Rhamnol, Sitosterin, Sitosterol, Sitosterolins, Sitosterols, Sterinol, Sterolins.
CAUTION: See separate listing for Sitostanol.

Scientific Names

22,23-dihydrostigmasterol; 24-beta-ethyl-delta-5-cholesten-3beta-ol; 24-ethyl-cholesterol; 3-beta-stigmast-5-en-3-ol.

People Use This For

Orally, beta-sitosterol is used for coronary heart disease and hypercholesterolemia, benign prostatic hyperplasia (BPH) and prostatitis, and gallstones. It is also used orally for enhancing sexual activity and for preventing colon cancer. Beta-sitosterol is also used orally for boosting the immune system, preventing immune suppression and inflammation following participation in a marathon, common cold and flu (influenza), HIV/AIDS, rheumatoid arthritis, tuberculosis, psoriasis, allergies, cervical cancer, fibromyalgia, systemic lupus erythematosus, asthma, alopecia, bronchitis, idiopathic thrombocytopenia purpura (ITP), migraine headache, chronic fatigue syndrome, and symptoms of menopause.
In foods, beta-sitosterol is added to some margarines designed for use as part of a cholesterol-lowering diet and for preventing heart disease.

Safety

LIKELY SAFE ...when used orally and appropriately. Beta-sitosterol has been safely used in studies lasting up to 18 months (5327,5328,5329,5330,5331,5332,5333,5334,5336,5337,5338,5339,7198,10638).

PREGNANCY AND LACTATION: Insufficient reliable information available; avoid using.

Effectiveness

LIKELY EFFECTIVE

Benign prostatic hyperplasia (BPH). Taking beta-sitosterol orally significantly improves urinary symptoms, increases maximum urinary flow, and decreases postvoid residual urine volume; however, it does not affect prostate size (5327,5328,5329,7195,7198).

Hypercholesterolemia. Taking beta-sitosterol orally significantly reduces total and low-density lipoprotein (LDL) cholesterol levels, but has little or no effect on high-density lipoprotein (HDL) cholesterol levels (5330,5331,5332,5333,5334,5336,6668,7195,8528,10638).

POSSIBLY INEFFECTIVE

Tuberculosis. There is some evidence that taking beta-sitosterol orally as an adjunct to conventional treatment for tuberculosis can increase lymphocyte counts; however, beta-sitosterol does not seem to decrease the time to cure based on negative sputum culture (5337).

LIKELY INEFFECTIVE

Gallbladder disease. Taking beta-sitosterol orally isn't effective for treating gallstones (5338,5339).

There is insufficient reliable information available about the effectiveness of beta-sitosterol for its other uses.

Mechanism of Action

Beta-sitosterol is a plant sterol. It has a chemical structure similar to cholesterol with an ethyl group added at position 24. The average diet provides about 175-200 mg of beta-sitosterol, but less than 5% is actually absorbed when consumed orally. Therefore these plant sterols do not cause some of the atherogenic adverse effects associated with cholesterol from animal products. Beta-sitosterol is commonly added to margarines as a cholesterol reducing aid. Fats are needed to solubilize plant sterols so margarines are an ideal vehicle.

Soybean phytosterols containing 48% beta-sitosterol, 26% campesterol, and 21% stigmasterol have been added to ground beef (8528). Capsules containing beta-sitosterol may not disperse properly in the gut, limiting their ability to reduce cholesterol absorption (5814). Beta-sitosterol actually inhibits intestinal absorption of cholesterol by competing for the limited space in mixed micelles, which decreases cholesterol absorption by about 50% (5814). Because there is less cholesterol available in the body, compensatory mechanisms kick in and increase cholesterol synthesis in the liver (5814).

For prostatic hyperplasia, animal research suggests that beta-sitosterol might inhibit 5-alpha-reductase activity, although finasteride (Proscar) appears to be more potent (11739). Laboratory research suggests beta-sitosterol might have antiproliferative effects on the prostate, possibly by inhibiting growth factors (11234). In animals, beta-sitosterol shrinks the prostate, but this has not been shown in humans (11759).

There is some preliminary evidence that beta-sitosterol might also have anticancer and immunostimulant effects. Beta-sitosterol can inhibit the growth of human colon cancer cells in vitro (3667,3668). Mixtures of beta-sitosterol and its glycoside sitosterolin seem to also enhance proliferative responses of T-cells in vitro (3669,5342). Beta-sitosterol might also reduce the mild immune suppression and inflammation seen in marathon runners after a race (5335).

Adverse Reactions

Orally, beta-sitosterol is usually well tolerated. In some patients it can cause nausea, indigestion, gas, diarrhea, or constipation (5327,5328).

Interactions with Herbs & Other Dietary Supplements

CAROTENE, VITAMIN E: Beta-sitosterol may reduce absorption and blood levels of alpha- and beta-carotene and vitamin E (5814).

CHOLESTEROL LOWERING HERBS/SUPPLEMENTS: Beta-sitosterol might have additive effects with herbs and supplements that also lower cholesterol levels. Some of these herbs and supplements include chromium, flaxseed, garlic, guar gum, niacin, oat bran, psyllium, red yeast, and others.

Interactions with Drugs

EZETIMIBE (Zetia): Ezetimibe inhibits intestinal absorption of beta-sitosterol and reduces plasma concentrations in people with and without sitosterolemia. In people with mild to moderate hypercholesterolemia, ezetimibe reduces beta-sitosterol levels by 41% (11985,11989).

PRAVASTATIN (Pravachol): There is some evidence that pravastatin can lower blood levels of beta-sitosterol (3672). Theoretically, this might occur with other HMG-CoA reductase inhibitors ("statins"); however, simvastatin (Zocor) does not seem to affect beta-sitosterol levels (3673). Other statin drugs include atorvastatin (Lipitor), cerivastatin (Baycol), fluvastatin (Lescol), and lovastatin (Mevacor).

Interactions with Foods

CAROTENE, VITAMIN E: Beta-sitosterol may reduce absorption and blood levels of alpha- and beta-carotene and vitamin E (5814).

Interactions with Lab Tests

CHOLESTEROL: Beta-sitosterol decreases total serum cholesterol and low-density lipoprotein (LDL) levels (5331,5336).

Interactions with Diseases or Conditions

SITOSTEROLEMIA (Phytosterolaemia): Taking beta-sitosterol can exacerbate sitosterolemia, a rare inherited lipid storage disease (5326,10305). People with this disorder have increased absorption of cholesterol and beta-sitosterol from the diet, and decreased clearance of beta-sitosterol. Total body stores of beta-sitosterol are increased up to 17-fold. Elevated hepatic beta-sitosterol levels competitively inhibit cholesterol catabolism, contributing to hypercholesterolemia (3663). Patients with sitosterolemia are prone to premature coronary artery disease and xanthomas (3661,3662). Beta-sitosterol and its glycoside sitosterolin are contraindicated in patients with sitosterolemia. However, beta-sitosterol appears to be safe for heterozygous carriers of sitosterolemia (10457).

Dosage and Administration

ORAL: For benign prostatic hyperplasia (BPH) and prostatitis, a typical dose is 60 to 130 mg of beta-sitosterol divided into 2-3 doses daily (5327,5328,5329). For hypercholesterolemia, the usual dose is 800 mg to 6 grams per day divided and given before meals. Beta-sitosterol is typically given in conjunction with a low-fat diet (5327,5328,5329,5330,5331,5332,5333,5334,5336,5337,5338,5339,10638). One supplier suggests that doses should be taken at least 30 minutes, but not more than 90 minutes, before meals for maximum effect on cholesterol absorption (3658).

Comments

Beta-sitosterol is a supplement that is also found in the functional food product Take Control. The FDA authorized the use of labeling health claims for foods containing plant sterol esters, including beta-sitosterol, for reducing the risk of coronary heart disease (CHD) (6668). This rule is based on the FDA's conclusion that plant sterol esters may reduce the risk of CHD by lowering blood cholesterol levels. Although there is plenty of evidence that beta-sitosterol does lower cholesterol levels, there is no proof that long-term use actually lowers the risk of developing CHD. Avoid confusing beta-sitosterol with sitostanol, the saturated beta-sitosterol derivative contained in Benecol (5340). Both sitostanol and beta-sitosterol are used for lowering cholesterol levels in people with hypercholesterolemia and appear to be equally effective (7196).

BETAINE ANHYDROUS

Also Known As

Betaine, Cystadane, Trimethyl Glycine, Trimethylglycine, TMG.
CAUTION: See separate listing for Betaine Hydrochloride.

Scientific Names

Trimethylglycine anhydrous.

People Use This For

Orally, betaine anhydrous is used for homocystinuria caused by cystathionine beta-synthase deficiency, 5,10-methylenetetrahydrofolate reductase deficiency, or cobalamin cofactor metabolism defect. It is also used orally for hyperhomocysteinemia, homocystinuria not responsive to pyridoxine, and nonalcoholic steatohepatitis.

Topically, betaine anhydrous is used as an ingredient in toothpastes to reduce the subjective symptoms of dry mouth.

Safety

LIKELY SAFE ...when used orally and appropriately (698,10631). Betaine anhydrous is an FDA-approved prescription product.

PREGNANCY AND LACTATION: Insufficient reliable information available; avoid using.

Effectiveness

EFFECTIVE

Homocystinuria. Betaine anhydrous reduces plasma homocysteine levels by 20-30% (15). Betaine anhydrous is FDA-approved for this indication.

POSSIBLY EFFECTIVE

Dry mouth. Applying betaine anhydrous topically as an ingredient of toothpastes seems to reduce the subjective symptoms of dry mouth (6812).

INSUFFICIENT RELIABLE EVIDENCE to RATE

Cardiovascular disease. There is some evidence that betaine supplementation for 3 weeks can produce a small, 5.5% to 8%, decrease in plasma homocysteine levels in people with normal homocysteine levels, <15 micromol/L. It is not clear whether this reduction results in a decreased risk for cardiovascular disease (6810).

Steatohepatitis. Preliminary evidence suggests that betaine supplementation might be useful for nonalcoholic steatohepatitis. Use for 12 months seems to normalize liver enzymes and improve the degree of steatosis, necroinflammatory grade, and stage of fibrosis (10631).

More evidence is needed to rate betaine anhydrous for these uses.

Mechanism of Action

Betaine anhydrous occurs naturally in the body. It is the major metabolite of choline. It is present in small amounts in foods such as beets, spinach, cereals, seafood, and wine. Betaine is a methyl group donor. It reduces homocysteine levels by remethylating homocysteine to methionine (15). Elevated homocysteine levels can be reduced by two mechanisms: trans-sulfuration to cysteine using pyridoxine as a cofactor, or remethylation to methionine. This latter reaction uses either 5-methyltetrahydrofolate derived from folic acid as a methyl donor, and either vitamin B12 or betaine anhydrous as a cofactor (6810). In patients with homocystinuria, total plasma homocysteine concentrations are very high, >50 micromol/L, compared to normal levels in the population of 5 to 15 micromol/L (3047,6810). Levels greater than 15 micromol/L are referred to as hyperhomocysteinemia and have been identified as a risk factor for cardiovascular disease (3047). The potential role of betaine anhydrous in lowering normal or slightly elevated homocysteine levels in order to reduce the risk of cardiovascular disease is not known. It has been suggested that the betaine content of wine may contribute to the lower incidence of cardiovascular disease in countries with a high wine consumption such as France, but it is not known whether the levels present, approximately 3 mg per glass, have any significant effect (6811). Preliminary studies suggest that betaine supplementation may increase methionine and S-adenosyl-L-methionine (SAMe) synthesis from homocysteine in the liver when these compounds have been inhibited by ethanol; betaine may also reduce ethanol-induced liver damage (6813). Topically, betaine anhydrous has been reported to reduce the irritant effects of sodium lauryl sulfate on the skin and oral mucosa, and may reduce subjective symptoms of dry mouth (6812).

Adverse Reactions

Orally, betaine anhydrous can cause nausea, GI distress, diarrhea, and body odor (698,10631).

Interactions with Herbs & Other Dietary Supplements

None known.

Interactions with Drugs

None known.

Interactions with Foods

None known.

Interactions with Lab Tests

None known.

Interactions with Diseases or Conditions

None known.

Dosage and Administration

ORAL: For homocystinuria, a maintenance dose of 3 grams is typically taken twice daily in both adults and children. Dose titration is preferable in children. For children under three years old, the starting dose is 100 mg/kg per day, increased in weekly intervals in increments of 100 mg/kg daily. All patients can receive dose increases until plasma homocysteine concentrations are undetectable or very low, which can require doses up to 20 grams per day. Dissolve the powder in water immediately before administration (15). For reducing plasma homocysteine levels, 3 grams betaine anhydrous twice daily orally has been used (6810). For nonalcoholic steatohepatitis, 20 grams daily, in two divided doses has been used (10631).

TOPICAL: Betaine anhydrous has been added to toothpastes in a concentration of 4% for treatment of symptoms of dry mouth (6812).

Comments
Betaine anhydrous has Orphan Drug status in the US. Avoid confusion with betaine hydrochloride, a dietary supplement with variable purity and potency that has not been demonstrated safe or effective for treating homocystinuria.

BETAINE HYDROCHLORIDE

Also Known As
Betaine, Betaine HCl, Trimethyl Glycine, Trimethylglycine, TMG.
CAUTION: See separate listing for Betaine Anhydrous.

Scientific Names
Trimethylglycine hydrochloride.

People Use This For
Orally, betaine hydrochloride is used as a supplemental source of hydrochloric acid, to treat hypokalemia, and as a liver protectant. It is also used for allergic rhinitis, anemia, asthma, atherosclerosis, candidiasis, diarrhea, food allergies, gallstones, inner ear infection, rheumatoid arthritis, and thyroid disorders.

Safety
There is insufficient reliable information available about the safety of betaine hydrochloride.
Pregnancy and Lactation: Insufficient reliable information available; avoid using.

Effectiveness
There is insufficient reliable information available about the effectiveness of betaine hydrochloride.

Mechanism of Action
Betaine hydrochloride is a source of hydrochloric acid (9). Some people use it due to inaccurate claims that many conditions are due to inadequate gastric acid.

Adverse Reactions
Orally, betaine hydrochloride can theoretically irritate gastric or duodenal ulcers or impede ulcer healing by increasing gastric acid. Theoretically, it might also cause heartburn (9).

Interactions with Herbs & Other Dietary Supplements
None known.

Interactions with Drugs
None known.

Interactions with Foods
None known.

Interactions with Lab Tests
None known.

Interactions with Diseases or Conditions
GASTRIC AND DUODENAL ULCERS: Theoretically, betaine hydrochloride can irritate ulcers or impede healing by increasing gastric acid; avoid using in patients with gastric or duodenal ulcers (9).

Dosage and Administration
No typical dosage.

Comments
Avoid confusion with betaine anhydrous. Betaine is manufactured in various salt forms around the world, including betaine hydrochloride. The purity and potency of these dietary supplement products can vary. There are no data to support the effectiveness of betaine hydrochloride in any condition, including homocystinuria. Use only the FDA-approved betaine anhydrous for the treatment of homocystinuria (see separate listing for betaine anhydrous).

BETH ROOT

Also Known As
Birthroot, Coughroot, Ground Lily, Jew's Harp Plant, Indian Balm, Indian Shamrock, Lamb's Quarters, Milk Ipecac, Pariswort, Rattlesnake Root, Snakebite, Stinking Benjamin, Three-Leafed Nightshade, Wake Robin.
CAUTION: See separate listing for Arum.

Scientific Names
Trillium erectum.
Family: Liliaceae or Trilliaceae.

People Use This For
Orally, beth root is used for long, heavy menstruation and pain relief. It is also used orally as an astringent and expectorant.
Topically, beth root is used for varicose veins and ulcers, hematomas, and hemorrhoid bleeding.

Safety
POSSIBLY UNSAFE ...when used orally. Beth root is a gastrointestinal irritant (12).
There is insufficient reliable information available about the safety of beth root for its other uses.
PREGNANCY AND LACTATION: LIKELY UNSAFE ...when used orally; avoid using. Beth root might have menstrual or uterine stimulant activity (12,18).

Effectiveness
There is insufficient reliable information available about the effectiveness of beth root.

Mechanism of Action
The applicable parts of beth root are the rhizome, and dried root and leaf. There is insufficient reliable information about the possible mechanism of action or active ingredients.

Adverse Reactions
Orally, ingestion of large amounts of the plant or volatile oil might produce GI irritation severe enough to cause vomiting (12,18). In pregnant women, the drastic purgative effects can cause reflex uterine contractions.
Topically, beth root causes extreme irritation (18).

Interactions with Herbs & Other Dietary Supplements
None known.

Interactions with Drugs
None known.

Interactions with Foods
None known.

Interactions with Lab Tests
None known.

Interactions with Diseases or Conditions
CARDIAC CONDITIONS: Due to potential cardiotoxicity from the convallamarin-like glycoside, patients with a cardiac condition should be cautioned against the use of this herb (6002).

Dosage and Administration
ORAL: No typical dosage.
TOPICAL: The ground plant parts are used as a poultice (18).

BETONY

Also Known As
Bishopswort, Bishop Wort, Hedge Nettles, Wood Betony.

Scientific Names
Stachys officinalis, synonyms Betonica officinalis, Stachys betonica.
Family: Lamiaceae/Labiatae.

People Use This For
Orally, betony is used to treat diarrhea, irritation of mucous membranes, stress and tension, headache, facial pain, coughs as an expectorant, bronchitis, asthma, as an antiflatulent, and as a sedative. It is also used orally to treat heartburn, gout, nervousness, bladder and kidney stones, and for bladder inflammation.
In combination with other herbs, betony is used to treat of neuralgia and anxiety.

Safety
POSSIBLY SAFE ...when the dried above ground parts are used orally in medicinal amounts (5,6,12).
POSSIBLY UNSAFE ...when used in large amounts because it contains 15% tannins and these can cause gastrointestinal irritation (5,12).
PREGNANCY: POSSIBLY UNSAFE ...when used orally; avoid using (6).
LACTATION: Insufficient reliable information available; avoid using.

Effectiveness
There is insufficient reliable information available about the effectiveness of betony.

Mechanism of Action
The applicable parts of betony are the dried above ground parts. The high tannin content (15%) is responsible for its astringent properties (5). The glycoside mixture can have a hypotensive effect, possibly explaining its effectiveness in mild anxiety states and headache (5,6). One constituent, stachydrine, is a systolic depressant that is also active against rheumatism (6).

Adverse Reactions
Large doses can cause significant GI irritation due to the tannin component (5,6).

Interactions with Herbs & Other Dietary Supplements
None known.

Interactions with Drugs
ANTIHYPERTENSIVE DRUGS: Theoretically, betony might have additive effects with blood pressure lowering drugs due to hypotensive activity of the glycosides found in betony. It might also interfere with the activity of pressor drugs (5,6).

Interactions with Foods
None known.

Interactions with Lab Tests
None known.

Interactions with Diseases or Conditions
None known.

Dosage and Administration
ORAL: Betony is typically taken as a tea or an infusion (6002). Use small doses to avoid gastrointestinal (GI) irritation.

BHT (BUTYLATED HYDROXYTOLUENE)

Also Known As
Butylated Hydroxytoluene, Butylhydroxytoluene, Dibutylated Hydroxytoluene.

Scientific Names
2,6-di-tert-butyl-p-creosol.

People Use This For
Orally, BHT is used for genital herpes and acquired immunodeficiency syndrome (AIDS).
Topically, BHT is used for herpes simplex labialis.
In foods, BHT is used as an antioxidant.

Safety

LIKELY SAFE ...when used orally as a food additive (10292,10293). BHT has Generally Recognized As Safe (GRAS) status for food use in the US (4912).
There is insufficient reliable information available about the safety of BHT for its other uses.
CHILDREN: LIKELY SAFE ...when used orally as a food additive (10292).
PREGNANCY AND LACTATION: LIKELY SAFE ...when used orally as a food additive (10292).

Effectiveness

INSUFFICIENT RELIABLE EVIDENCE to RATE

Herpes labialis (cold sores). There is preliminary evidence that suggests that topical application of BHT might be helpful for herpes simplex labialis. Topical application of BHT may decrease the time from lesion formation to dry crust formation by about 0.4 days; and it may decrease the duration of the vesicle-ulcer stage by about 0.8 days (10294). More evidence is needed to rate BHT for this use.

Mechanism of Action

BHT is a synthetic phenolic, hydrophobic chemical that is used extensively as an antioxidant in foods, pharmaceutical preparations, and other manufacturing processes (10293,10697). BHT may exert antiviral effects by interfering with membrane function in viruses that have a lipid envelope. BHT is lipid soluble and remains in highly lipid soluble regions, such as membranes (10295,10697). However, BHT does not appear to affect plaque diameter in cells infected with herpes simplex virus (HSV) (10295).

Adverse Reactions

Orally, BHT can cause severe gastritis characterized by severe epigastric pain, nausea, and vomiting. Symptoms may progress to weakness, dizziness, confusion, slurred speech, unsteady gait, and loss of consciousness (10303,10698,10699). BHT is highly lipid soluble. It may cross the blood brain barrier, causing psychotropicsymptoms (10303). BHT has been associated with development of cancer; however, BHT does not appear to increase the incidence of cancer in the amounts consumed in the diet. Some evidence suggests that BHT may actually decrease the formation of cancer (10292,10293).

Interactions with Herbs & Other Dietary Supplements

None known.

Interactions with Drugs

None known.

Interactions with Foods

None known.

Interactions with Lab Tests

None known.

Interactions with Diseases or Conditions

None known.

Dosage and Administration

ORAL: No typical dosage. However, the typical dietary consumption of BHT is less than 0.1 mg/kg/day (10292).
TOPICAL: For treating herpes simplex labialis, BHT 15% in mineral oil applied 4 times daily for 5 days has been used (10294).

BIFIDOBACTERIA

Also Known As

B. bifidum, Bifido, Bifidobacteria bifidus, Bifidobacterium, Bifidum, Probiotics.
CAUTION: See separate listings for Lactobacillus, Saccharomyces boulardii, and Yogurt.

Scientific Names

Bifidobacterium adolescentis; Bifidobacterium bifidum; Bifidobacterium breve; Bifidobacterium infantis; Bifidobacterium lactis; Bifidobacterium longum.
Family: Actinomycetaceae.

People Use This For

Orally, bifidobacteria are used for preventing acute diarrhea in infants and children; preventing necrotizing enterocolitis in neonates; treating atopic eczema in infants; preventing traveler's diarrhea; improving immune function; and replenishing intestinal normal flora depleted by diarrhea, radiation, chemotherapy, antibiotics, or other causes. Bifidobacteria are also used orally for candidiasis, the common cold and flu (influenza), hepatitis, hypercholesterolemia, lactose intolerance, mastitis, mumps, and cancer. They are also used orally to treat ulcerative colitis and pouchitis following surgery for ulcerative colitis.

Safety

LIKELY SAFE ...when used orally and appropriately. Bifidobacteria has been safely used in clinical trials lasting up to one year (162,1233,1731,3261,6087,11379,12769,12775,13054).

CHILDREN: POSSIBLY SAFE ...when used orally and appropriately. Bifidobacteria seem to be safe in children including those under two years of age and critically ill neonates when used for up to 8 months (161,3162,3169,3458).

PREGNANCY AND LACTATION: Insufficient reliable information available; avoid using.

Effectiveness

POSSIBLY EFFECTIVE

Antibiotic-induced gastrointestinal adverse effects. Ingestion of Bifidobacterium longum can reduce stool frequency, abdominal discomfort, and stool clostridial spore count when used in patients concurrently taking erythromycin (1233).

Atopic dermatitis (eczema). Giving infants Bifidobacterium lactis orally seems to help reduce the severity of atopic eczema and the markers for allergic responses including soluble CD4 in serum and eosinophilic protein X in urine (3458).

Chronic pouchitis. Taking bifidobacteria orally seems to help treat chronic pouchitis, a complication of surgery for ulcerative colitis. Continuous oral treatment for one year with a specific concentrated formulation of Lactobacillus, Bifidobacterium, and Streptococcus (VSL#3) seems to maintain remission in 85% of patients (6087,12769). Daily consumption of bifidobacteria is usually required to maintain effectiveness, although effects may persist a week after discontinuation (1731).

Helicobacter pylori (H pylori). Bifidobacteria, in combination with Lactobacillus species and the probiotic yeast Saccharomyces boulardii seems reduce the adverse effects of Helicobacter therapy, but doesn't seem to improve compliance (12763).

Irritable bowel syndrome (IBS). Consuming Bifidobacterium infantis 1 billion cells daily in a malted milk drink for 8 weeks seems to significantly reduce symptoms of IBS such as abdominal pain and bloating, and bowel movement difficulty. Improvement is seen within 1 week of treatment. It does not seem to reduce bowel movement frequency or quality of stool (13054). A specific bifidobacteria combination probiotic containing strains of viable lyophilized bacteria species including Bifidobacterium, Lactobacillus, and Streptococcus (VSL#3), also appears to improve IBS symptoms (11379).

Necrotizing enterocolitis (NEC). Bifidobacterium infantis in combination with Lactobacillus acidophilus seems to reduce the incidence of NEC and NEC-associated mortality in critically ill neonates (3162).

Rotaviral diarrhea. Bifidobacterium bifidum combined with Streptococcus thermophilus or the Bifidobacterium Bb12 strain appears to reduce the incidence of diarrhea and rotavirus shedding in infants (153,161,3169).

Traveler's diarrhea. Bifidobacterium in combination with Lactobacillus acidophilus, Lactobacillus bulgaricus, or Streptococcus thermophilus seems to decrease the chance of developing traveler's diarrhea (155).

INSUFFICIENT RELIABLE EVIDENCE to RATE

Radiation sickness. There is preliminary evidence that antibiotic-resistant Bifidobacterium longum can help improve short-term survival in the treatment of radiation sickness. In combination with prophylactic antibiotics, bifidobacteria appear to inhibit colonization and overgrowth of intestinal opportunistic pathogens, preventing post-irradiation sepsis (3457).

Ulcerative colitis. Bifidobacterium breve and Bifidobacterium bifidum plus Lactobacillus acidophilus seem to prevent relapse in patients with ulcerative colitis when used as an adjunct to treatment with sulfasalazine (Azulfidine), mesalamine (Asacol, Pentasa, others) and steroids (12775). In patients intolerant to 5-aminosalicylic acid, bifidobacteria plus lactobacilli and Streptococcus thermophilus seems to prevent increases in pathogenic bacteria and relapse in some patients with ulcerative colitis (3261).

More evidence is needed to rate bifidobacteria for these uses.

Mechanism of Action

Bifidobacteria are anaerobic, rod-shaped, Gram-positive bacteria that normally colonize in the human colon (1060,1137). Bifidobacteria appear to be the most important organisms in the intestine for providing a microbial barrier to infection. Bifidobacteria produce antimicrobial substances that have activity against many gram-positive and gram-negative organisms (1060,12774). Bifidobacteria belong to a group of bacteria called lactic acid bacteria. Lactic acid bacteria, which also include the lactobacilli species, are also found in fermented foods like yogurt and cheese (1055,3589). Bifidobacteria are used therapeutically as so-called probiotics, the opposite of antibiotics.

They are considered "friendly" bacteria and are used with the purpose of re-colonizing areas of the body where they normally would occur. The human body relies on the normal flora for several functions, including metabolizing foods, absorbing nutrients, and preventing colonization by pathogenic bacteria. Probiotics such as bifidobacteria are typically used in cases when a disease occurs or might occur due to depleted normal flora. For example, treatment with antibiotics can kill off pathogenic bacteria and also the normal flora of the gastrointestinal and genitourinary tracts. The theory is that taking Bifidobacterium probiotics during antibiotic treatment can prevent or minimize normal flora depletion and pathogenic bacteria colonization. Bifidobacteria given in combination with lactobacillus concurrently with clindamycin seem to prevent increases in the number of Bacteroides fragilis bacteria (1055,3589,11382).

Bifidobacteria, especially Bifidobacterium bifidum, are the predominant intestinal flora of breast-fed infants (161). The antimicrobial substances that bifidobacteria produce might contribute to the protection that breast-feeding provides against gastrointestinal infections in infants (1060).

Bifidobacteria are also in the adult colon, but are less predominant (1060). When used orally, some species of bifidobacteria, such as Bifidobacterium infantis, and some strains of Bifidobacterium breve and Bifidobacterium longum, pass through the gut and bind to the intestinal mucosa, preventing attachment of pathogenic coliform bacteria (1137,1731). Bifidobacteria disappear from the feces within 2 weeks of discontinuation of bifidobacteria, suggesting that there is no long-term colonization (1117,4363). For continued effect, bifidobacteria must be used regularly.

In addition to acting as a barrier to pathogenic bacterial adhesion, some researchers think bifidobacteria and other probiotics might have immunomodulating effects (1137). Quantitative differences in the composition of intestinal microflora appear to affect immunological homeostasis (3458). Bifidobacteria seem to modulate non-specific cellular and humoral immunity possibly by stimulating lymphocyte and macrophage activity and cytokine production by mononuclear cells (6099). Due to these immunomodulating effects, some researchers think bifidobacteria and other probiotics might not only fight intestinal pathogens, but might also be helpful for conditions such as inflammatory bowel disease and pouchitis (6087). The addition of Bifidobacterium lactis to milk enhances cellular immunity in healthy middle-aged and elderly people, improving phagocyte function and natural killer cell activity, and increasing production of interferon-alpha (1055,1117). In infants, bacterial colonization appears to be essential in the development of oral tolerance instead of sensitization to dietary antigens (3458).

There is also some preliminary evidence that bifidobacteria and other probiotics might help protect against cancer. Bifidobacteria decrease fecal enzymes such as beta-glucuronidase, beta-glucosidase, nitroreductase, and urease, which are involved in the metabolic activation of some mutagens and carcinogens (6099). Bifidobacteria might also fight cancer by alteration of colonic physiochemical conditions and production of antitumorigenic or antimutagenic compounds in the colon (1154). Most researchers agree that the effectiveness of bifidobacteria and other probiotics for all indications depends on their ability to colonize an area of tissue. To do this, bifidobacteria preparations must contain live and viable organisms. Products stored for long periods of time or stored improperly may contain few live and active organisms to start with. For oral preparations, bacteria must also remain viable after passing through the gut (3589). Bifidobacterium longum is particularly resistant to gastric acid (3589). They must also be able to latch on to the intestinal epithelium. Bifidobacteria strains might vary in their effectiveness due to differences in their ability to adhere to epithelial cells (1137). Complex sugars, such as fructo-oligosaccharides, inulin, and oligofructose, are selectively fermented by bifidobacteria in the colon, and increase indigenous bifidobacteria quantities (4363). The addition of oligosaccharides to bifidobacteria also seems to enhance the activity of bifidobacteria (1117). However, there are no trials confirming the clinical benefit of combining bifidobacteria with complex sugars.

Adverse Reactions

Orally, bifidobacteria seem to be well tolerated by most people. In children, bifidobacteria can cause diarrhea (3169). Adverse effects from ingestion of bifidobacteria have not been reported; however, with other probiotics, patients can sometimes experience gastrointestinal upset including bloating and flatulence. This effect is usually mild and typically subsides with continued use. Most bifidobacteria species are considered nonpathogenic and nontoxigenic; however, the Bifidobacterium dentium species, has been associated with dental caries (1137,1236). Sepsis with the Bifidobacterium longum species has occurred in one patient following acupuncture. This was likely due to needle contamination. This effect would not be expected to occur from taking oral bifidobacteria supplements in most healthy patients (1236).

Interactions with Herbs & Other Dietary Supplements

None known.

Interactions with Drugs

ANTIBIOTIC DRUGS: There is some concern that concomitant administration of antibiotics might decrease the effectiveness of bifidobacteria. Since bifidobacteria preparations usually contain live and active organisms, simultaneously taking antibiotics might kill a significant number of the organisms (1740). Tell patients to separate administration of antibiotics and bifidobacteria preparations by at least 2 hours.

Interactions with Foods

None known.

Interactions with Lab Tests
None known.

Interactions with Diseases or Conditions
IMMUNODEFICIENCY: There is some concern that bifidobacteria preparations might cause pathogenic colonization in patients who are immunocompromised. Although this has not occurred specifically with bifidobacteria, there have been rare cases involving other probiotic species such as lactobacillus. Pathogenic colonization seems to be more likely to occur in severely immunocompromised patients (4380,4391,4393,4398). Use with caution in these patients.

Dosage and Administration
ORAL: The strength of bifidobacteria preparations is usually quantified by the number of living organisms per dose.
For irritable bowel syndrome, Bifidobacterium infantis 1 billion cells daily in a malted milk drink has been used (13054).
For chronic pouchitis, a dose of 600 billion bacteria consisting of species of Lactobacillus, Bifidobacterium, and Streptococcus (VSL#3) given once daily has been used (12769).
As an adjunct in Helicobacter pylori treatment, a dose of 5 billion bacteria consisting of Bifidobacterium lactis and lactobacillus acidophilus has been given once daily (12763).

BILBERRY

Also Known As
Airelle, Black Whortles, Bleaberry, Blueberry, Burren Myrtle, Dwarf Bilberry, Dyeberry, Huckleberry, Hurtleberry, Myrtilli Fructus, Trackleberry, Whortleberry, Wineberry.
CAUTION: See separate listings for Blueberry and Bog Bilberry.

Scientific Names
Vaccinium myrtillus.
Family: Ericaceae.

People Use This For
Orally, bilberry is used to improve visual acuity including night vision, and to treat degenerative retinal conditions, varicose veins, atherosclerosis, venous insufficiency, and hemorrhoids. It is also used orally for angina; diabetes; arthritis; gout; dermatitis; and prevention and treatment of gastrointestinal (GI), kidney, and urinary tract symptoms and diseases.
Topically, it is used for mild inflammation of the mouth and throat mucous membranes.

Safety
LIKELY SAFE ...when the fruit is used in amounts commonly found in foods. Bilberry has Generally Recognized As Safe status (GRAS) for use in foods in the US (4912).
POSSIBLY UNSAFE ...when the leaves are used orally in high doses or for prolonged use. Death can occur with chronic use of 1.5 g/kg/day (2).
PREGNANCY AND LACTATION: There is insufficient reliable information available about the safety of bilberry fruit used in medicinal amounts during pregnancy and lactation.

Effectiveness
POSSIBLY EFFECTIVE

Retinopathy. Taking bilberry fruit orally seems to improve retinal lesions from diabetic or hypertensive retinopathy (39,40). Clinical studies of bilberry's effectiveness have used formulations containing 25% of the bioflavonoid complex anthocyanoside.

POSSIBLY INEFFECTIVE

Night vision. Bilberry fruit extract 160 mg taken three times daily for 21 days does not seem to improve night visual acuity and contrast sensitivity in men with good vision and normal night vision (8139). A single dose of anthocyanosides, the active constituents of bilberry, does not significantly improve night vision (9738,9739).

There is insufficient reliable information available about the effectiveness of bilberry for its other uses.

Mechanism of Action
The applicable parts of bilberry are the fruit and leaf. Astringent tannin components of bilberry dried, ripe fruit are responsible for the potential benefits in diarrhea and irritation of the mouth and throat mucosa. Anthocyanadin (anthocyanoside) constituents increase the synthesis of glycosaminoglycans, decrease vascular permeability, reduce basement membrane thickness, and aid in the redistribution of microvascular blood flow and the formation of interstitial fluid. An anthocyanadin pigment found in bilberry fruit might have anti-ulcer and gastroprotective

effects (6). Preliminary evidence indicates these constituents are widely distributed in the body after oral administration and are eliminated by the kidneys (8140). Laboratory research also suggests that anthocyanadins have anti-inflammatory and anti-edema effects (8141). Bilberry leaves contain polyphenols, tannins, flavonoids (1265) and a relatively high concentration of chromium (9.0 ppm) (8). Preliminary evidence suggests that a bilberry leaf extract might have blood glucose, triglyceride, and cholesterol lowering effects (1264). The chromium in bilberry leaf is theorized to play a role in potential blood glucose lowering activity (8). Bilberry leaf also contains a glucokinin, neomirtilline, that seems to lower blood glucose (1264). Some researchers think that flavonoids in bilberry leaf might also be useful for diabetic circulatory disorders (8).

Adverse Reactions

None reported.

Interactions with Herbs & Other Dietary Supplements

HERBS WITH HYPOGLYCEMIC POTENTIAL: Theoretically, bilberry leaf might have additive effects with herbs that decrease blood glucose levels (1264). Herbs with hypoglycemic potential include devil's claw, fenugreek, garlic, guar gum, horse chestnut, Panax ginseng, psyllium, Siberian ginseng, and others.

Interactions with Drugs

ANTIDIABETES DRUGS: Theoretically, concomitant use of bilberry leaf might require dosing adjustment of anti-diabetes drugs. Preliminary evidence suggests that bilberry leaf extract might have blood glucose lowering activity (1264); monitor closely.

Interactions with Foods

None known.

Interactions with Lab Tests

BLOOD GLUCOSE: Theoretically, bilberry leaf might lower blood glucose and test results. Preliminary evidence suggests that a bilberry leaf extract might have blood glucose lowering activity (1264).
TRIGLYCERIDES: Theoretically, bilberry leaf might lower serum triglycerides and test results. Preliminary evidence suggests that a bilberry leaf extract might have triglyceride lowering activity (1264).

Interactions with Diseases or Conditions

DIABETES: Theoretically, bilberry leaf might lower blood glucose. Preliminary evidence suggests that a bilberry leaf extract might have blood glucose lowering activity (1264); monitor closely.

Dosage and Administration

ORAL: The typical dose of the dried, ripe berries is 20-60 grams daily. People also drink a decoction of the berries, which is prepared by adding 5-10 grams, 1-2 teaspoons, of mashed berries in cold water, bringing the water to a simmer for 10 minutes, and then straining. A dose of 160 mg of bilberry extract taken twice daily has been used in patients with retinopathy (39). Clinical studies of bilberry's effectiveness have used formulations containing 25% of the bioflavonoid complex anthocyanoside. Bilberry leaf is commonly used as a tea. The tea is prepared by steeping 1 gram, 1-2 teaspoons, finely chopped dried leaf in 150 mL boiling water for 5-10 minutes, then straining; avoid prolonged use (8). For improving night vision, anthocyanosides have been used as a single dose of 12, 24, or 36 mg or as 12 or 24 mg 2 times daily for 4 days (9738,9739).
TOPICAL: The berries are usually applied as a 10% decoction, made by boiling the dried berries in water for 10 minutes and straining (2).

Comments

During World War II, British pilots in the Royal Air Force ate bilberry jam to improve their night vision; however, subsequent clinical studies indicate that bilberry probably doesn't help night vision (8139).

BIOTIN

Also Known As

Coenzyme R, D-Biotin, Vitamin H, W Factor.

Scientific Names

Cis-hexahydro-2-oxo-1H-thieno[3,4-d]-imidazole-4-valeric acid.

People Use This For

Orally, biotin is used for preventing and treating biotin deficiency associated with pregnancy, long-term parenteral nutrition, malnutrition, rapid weight loss, and multiple carboxylase deficiency. It is also used orally for hair loss, brittle nails, seborrheic dermatitis of infancy, diabetes, and mild depression.

Safety

LIKELY SAFE ...when used orally and appropriately (1900,8468).
CHILDREN: POSSIBLY SAFE ...when used orally and appropriately (173).
PREGNANCY AND LACTATION: POSSIBLY SAFE ...when used orally and appropriately (1901).

Effectiveness

LIKELY EFFECTIVE

Biotin deficiency. Taking biotin orally is effective for preventing or treating biotin deficiency (1901).

POSSIBLY EFFECTIVE

Brittle nails. Taking biotin orally seems to increase the thickness of fingernails and toenails in people with brittle nails (171).

POSSIBLY INEFFECTIVE

Seborrheic dermatitis. Taking biotin orally doesn't seem to improve seborrheic dermatitis of infancy (8469).

INSUFFICIENT RELIABLE EVIDENCE to RATE

Alopecia areata. There is some preliminary evidence that biotin given orally in combination with zinc and topical clobetasol propionate (Olux, Temovate) might be helpful for alopecia areata (6932).

Diabetes. Very preliminary clinical research suggests that a combination of biotin and chromium (Diachrome) might lower hemoglobin A1c levels in patients with type 2 diabetes (12385,12390). But biotin alone doesn't seem to affect glucose or insulin levels in people with type 2 diabetes (11579).

Peripheral neuropathy. There is preliminary evidence that intramuscular or oral biotin might help decrease symptoms of peripheral neuropathy in diabetic patients (8468).

More evidence is needed to rate biotin for these uses.

Mechanism of Action

Biotin is a vitamin that is found in small amounts in numerous foods. In food, biotin is protein bound and is cleaved by the enzyme biotinidase. Biotin is also synthesized in animals by intestinal microflora. Researchers think biotin is stored in the mitochondria, and that it acts as a coenzyme in bicarbonate-dependent carboxylation reactions (6243).
Biotin-containing enzymes are involved in gluconeogenesis, fatty acid synthesis, propionate metabolism, and the catabolism of leucine in mammals (173). Pyruvate decarboxylase is a biotin-dependent enzyme. Decreased activity of this enzyme during biotin deficiency may result in accumulation of pyruvate or decreased aspartate concentration (8468).
Biotin deficiency is difficult to detect because of the lack of assay techniques to determine biotin concentrations in blood (8501). Symptoms of deficiency include thinning of the hair, frequently with loss of hair color, and red scaly rash around the eyes, nose, and mouth. Neurological symptoms, including depression, lethargy, hallucinations, and paresthesias of the extremities, are also common in biotin deficiency (6243). Biotin deficiency is most likely to occur in people with congenital biotinidase deficiency, malabsorption syndromes, such as short-gut syndrome, during pregnancy, and in people receiving long-term parenteral nutrition (6243,7878,8501). There is some evidence that diabetes may produce a biotin-deficient state (8468).
Biotin supplementation can reduce the activity of interleukins and interferons and reduce the number of lymphocytes (7879). Blood glucose concentrations decrease as plasma and tissue concentrations of biotin increase in people with and without diabetes, but this effect is far more dramatic in people with diabetes (7880).
After oral administration, biotin is completely absorbed. About half of the dose of biotin is excreted within 24 hours (8758). Biotin is recycled endogenously. This may be the reason why deficiency symptoms take a long time to develop and are rarely seen in humans (173).

Adverse Reactions

Orally, there is one case of eosinophilic pleuropericardial effusion with high-dose biotin 10 mg per day in combination with pantothenic acid 300 mg for 2 months (3914). Whether eosinophila in this case is related to high-dose biotin use is unknown. However, biotin is well tolerated when used at recommended dosages (6243). Biotin in doses of 10 mg per day have been taken without adverse effects (6243).

Interactions with Herbs & Other Dietary Supplements

None known.

Interactions with Drugs

None known.

Drug Influences on Nutrient Levels and Depletion

SOME DRUGS CAN AFFECT BIOTIN LEVELS:
CARBAMAZEPINE: Taking carbamazepine can reduce biotin absorption (172,176).
PHENOBARBITAL: Taking phenobarbital can reduce biotin levels (175,176).
PHENYTOIN: Taking phenytoin can reduce biotin levels (175,176).
PRIMIDONE: Taking primidone can reduce biotin absorption (172,176).

Interactions with Foods

EGG WHITES: Consumption of large amounts of egg whites can cause biotin deficiency (173,6243).

Interactions with Lab Tests

FREE THYROXINE (FT4): There is one report of a false-high FT4 on the assay by the Boehringer Mannheim ES 700 analyzer due to high serum biotin levels in a neonate (170).
THYROID STIMULATING HORMONE (TSH): There is one report of a false-low TSH on the assay by the Boehringer Mannheim ES 700 analyzer due to high serum biotin levels in a neonate (170).

Interactions with Diseases or Conditions

BIOTINIDASE DEFICIENCY: Biotin requirements may be higher in people with genetic biotinidase deficiency (6243).
RENAL DIALYSIS: Biotin requirements may be higher in people receiving hemodialysis or peritoneal dialysis (6243).

Dosage and Administration

ORAL: There is no recommended dietary allowance (RDA) established for biotin. The adequate intakes (AI) for biotin are 7 mcg for infants 0-12 months, 8 mcg for children 1-3 years, 12 mcg for children 4-8 years, 20 mcg for children 9-13 years, 25 mcg for adolescents 14-18 years, 30 mcg for adults over 18 years and pregnant women, and 35 mcg for lactating women (6243). In the treatment of diabetic peripheral neuropathy, oral biotin 5 mg daily has been used for up to 130 weeks. This was preceded by 12 weeks of intramuscular treatment (8468).
INTRAMUSCULAR: In the treatment of diabetic peripheral neuropathy, intramuscular biotin 10 mg daily for six weeks, then three times weekly for six weeks, followed by an oral dose has been used (8468).

BIRCH

Also Known As

Betula, Betulae folium, Downy Birch, Silver Birch, White Birch.

Scientific Names

Betula pendula, synonym Betula verrucosa; Betula pubescens, synonym Betula alba.
Family: Betulaceae.

People Use This For

Orally, birch is used as a diuretic, for rheumatic ailments, "irrigation therapy" (use of a mild diuretic along with copious fluid intake to increase urine flow), to treat pyelonephritis, ureteritis, cystitis, urethritis, for arthritis, rheumatism, loss of hair, skin rashes, and in "spring cures" for "purifying the blood."

Safety

POSSIBLY SAFE ...when used orally and appropriately (12).
PREGNANCY AND LACTATION: Insufficient reliable information available; avoid using.

Effectiveness

There is insufficient reliable information available about the effectiveness of birch.

Mechanism of Action

The applicable part of birch is the leaf. The aquaretic and possibly saluretic effects are due to the flavonoid constituents of the birch leaf. Aquaretics increase urine volume (water loss) but not electrolyte excretion (512). The high vitamin C content of the leaf can enhance the effect (8).
Birch pollen contains the allergens Bet v 1 and Bet v 2 (birch pollen profilin), which are responsible for allergic reactions in sensitive people (12192).

Adverse Reactions

Birch pollen can cause allergic reactions. People who are sensitive to wild carrot, celery, or mugwort spices are more likely to also be sensitive to birch. This has been called the "celery-carrot-mugwort-spice syndrome" (12192).

Interactions with Herbs & Other Dietary Supplements

None known.

Interactions with Drugs

DIURETIC DRUGS: Theoretically, birch might interfere with diuretic therapy (512).

Interactions with Foods
None known.

Interactions with Lab Tests
None known.

Interactions with Diseases or Conditions
CROSS-ALLERGENICITY: Birch pollen can cause allergic reactions in patients who are sensitive to other plants and spices including wild carrot, mugwort, and celery (12192). This has been called the "celery-carrot-mugwort-spice syndrome" (12192).
HYPERTENSION: Theoretically, birch leaf might increase sodium retention and worsen hypertension (512).

Dosage and Administration
ORAL: The typical dose of birch leaf is several times daily as a tea, which is prepared by steeping 2-3 grams of finely cut dried leaf in 150 mL boiling water for 10-15 minutes and straining (2,8). The tea should be taken with plenty of water (8).

BISHOP'S WEED

Also Known As
Ajava Seeds, Ajowan, Ajowan Caraway, Ajowan Seed, Ajowanj, Bishop's Flower, Bishops Weed, Bullwort, Carum, Flowering Ammi, Omum, Yavani.
CAUTION: See separate listings for Goutweed and Khella.

Scientific Names
Ammi majus, synonym Ammi glaucifolium.
Family: Apiaceae/Umbelliferae.

People Use This For
Orally, bishop's weed is used for digestive disorders, asthma, angina, kidney stones, and as a diuretic. Topically, bishop's weed is used for psoriasis and vitiligo.

Safety
There is insufficient reliable information available about the safety of bishop's weed.
PREGNANCY: LIKELY UNSAFE ...when used orally. The active constituent, khellin, has uterine stimulant activity (19); avoid using.
LACTATION: Insufficient reliable information available; avoid using.

Effectiveness
There is insufficient reliable information available about the effectiveness of bishop's weed.

Mechanism of Action
The applicable parts of bishop's weed are the seeds (7161). Bishop's weed contains several active ingredients including khellin, 8-methoxsalen, xanthotoxin, bergapten, and umbelliferone (1332,7162). The constituent, khellin, seems to have calcium channel blocking effects. There is some evidence it might also increase high-density lipoprotein (HDL) levels without affecting total cholesterol or triglyceride concentrations (2522,7162). The 8-methoxsalen (8-MOP, methoxypsoralen) constituent is one of the first agents used along with ultraviolet-A (UVA) radiation to treat psoriasis. It binds pyrimidine bases in DNA and suppresses cell division. This constituent also seems to contribute to the phototoxicity caused by bishop's weed (15,2528). Another constituent, xanthotoxin, also seems to have antipsoriatic activity (7162). The bergapten (5-methoxypsoralen) has antipsoriatic activity and antiplatelet activity (7162). Bergapten also appears to inhibit the cytochrome P450 3A4 (CYP3A4) system, which might lead to numerous interactions with drugs metabolized by this system (7029). The umbelliferone constituent is a hydroxycoumarin. Some researchers are interested in coumarins such as umbelliferone from bishop's weed because of in vitro evidence that they can inhibit reverse transcriptase in human immunodeficiency virus (HIV) replication (1332,1333). Further research is being done to see if these constituents have this effect in humans. Although people use bishop's weed for kidney stones, animal models show that it does not seem to decrease calcium oxalate deposition in the kidneys (2526).

Adverse Reactions

Orally, bishop's weed can cause nausea, vomiting, and headache (7161). Bishop's weed can also cause allergic reactions including rhinitis and urticaria in sensitive patients (2520). There is some concern that bishop's weed might increase liver enzymes. The isolated constituent khellin can increase transaminase levels (2522); however, so far this effect has not been reported for bishop's weed. Bishop's weed might also cause photosensitivity due to the 8-MOP constituent. In some patients bishop's weed can also cause contact dermatitis (2520,2521). There is also concern based on preliminary evidence that bishop's weed might cause ophthalmic changes, such as pigmentary retinopathy (2527).
Topically, bishop's weed might cause skin malignancies in patients predisposed to cancer (6002).

Interactions with Herbs & Other Dietary Supplements

HEPATOTOXIC HERBS: Theoretically, bishop's weed might have additive effects with herbs that cause hepatotoxicity. The khellin constituent can cause elevated transaminase levels in some patients (2522). Other products that might affect the liver include borage, chaparral, uva ursi, and others (2,2522).
HERBS WITH ANTICOAGULANT/ANTIPLATELET POTENTIAL: Concomitant use of herbs that affect platelet aggregation might increase the risk of bleeding. These herbs include angelica, anise, arnica, asafoetida, bogbean, boldo, capsicum, celery, chamomile, clove, fenugreek, feverfew, garlic, ginger, ginkgo, Panax ginseng, horse chestnut, horseradish, licorice, meadowsweet, onion, prickly ash, papain, passionflower, poplar, quassia, red clover, turmeric, wild carrot, wild lettuce, willow, and others (7162).
PHOTOSENSITIZING HERBS: Theoretically, bishop's weed might have an additive effect with products that increase sun sensitivity, such as St. John's wort (2521,7162).

Interactions with Drugs

ANTICOAGULANT/ANTIPLATELET DRUGS: There is some concern that bishop's weed might have additive effects with anticoagulant or antiplatelet drugs and possibly increase the risk of bleeding. The bergapten constituent of bishop's weed has antiplatelet effects. Some anticoagulant or antiplatelet drugs include aspirin, clopidogrel (Plavix), dalteparin (Fragmin), enoxaparin (Lovenox), heparin, ticlopidine (Ticlid), warfarin (Coumadin), and others (7162).
CYTOCHROME P450 3A4 (CYP3A4) SUBSTRATES: Theoretically, bishop's weed might inhibit elimination and increase blood levels of drugs metabolized by cytochrome P450 3A4 (CYP3A4) isoenzymes (7029). The bergapten constituent of bishop's weed is the same constituent as in bitter orange, which inhibits CYP3A4. Some drugs metabolized by CYP3A4 include alprazolam (Xanax), amitriptyline (Elavil), amiodarone (Cordarone), buspirone (Buspar), cerivastatin (Baycol), citalopram (Celexa), felodipine (Plendil), fexofenadine (Allegra), itraconazole (Sporanox), ketoconazole (Nizoral), lansoprazole (Prevacid), losartan (Cozaar), lovastatin (Mevacor), ondansetron (Zofran), prednisone (Deltasone, Orasone), sertraline (Zoloft), sibutramine (Meridia), sildenafil (Viagra), simvastatin (Zocor), verapamil (Calan, Covera-HS, Isoptin), and many others.
HEPATOTOXIC DRUGS: Theoretically, bishop's weed might have additive adverse effects on the liver when used with hepatotoxic drugs. The khellin constituent of bishop's weed can increase liver transaminases (2,2522). Some drugs that can adversely affect the liver include acetaminophen (Tylenol), amiodarone (Cordarone), carbamazepine (Tegretol), isoniazid (INH), methotrexate (Rheumatrex), methyldopa (Aldomet), and many others.
PHOTOSENSITIZING DRUGS: Theoretically, concomitant use might result in increased photosensitivity. Bishop's weed constituents seem to cause photosensitivity (2521,7162). Some drugs that cause photosensitivity include amitriptyline (Elavil), quinolones (Ciprofloxacin, others), sulfa drugs (Septra, Bactrim, others), and tetracycline.

Interactions with Foods

None known.

Interactions with Lab Tests

HIGH-DENSITY LIPOPROTEIN (HDL): Theoretically, bishop's weed might increase HDL levels. The isolated bishop's weed constituent, khellin, seems to increase in HDL levels without affecting total cholesterol or triglycerides (2522).
LIVER FUNCTION TESTS: There is some concern that bishop's weed might increase liver function tests in some patients. It is known that the isolated constituent khellin can increase aspartic acid transaminase (AST) and alanine aminotransferase (ALT, SGPT) (2522). However, this effect has not yet been reported specifically for bishop's weed.

Interactions with Diseases or Conditions

LIVER DISEASE: Theoretically, bishop's weed might exacerbate liver dysfunction in patients with liver disease. The isolated khellin constituent of bishop's weed is known to increase liver enzymes in some patients (2522).

Dosage and Administration

No typical dosage.

Comments
The prescription drug methoxsalen (Oxasoralen, Methoxypsoralen) was originally prepared from bishop's weed, but is now made synthetically (9,15). Bishop's weed is sometimes confused with its more used relative, khella (Ammi visnaga). The two species do have some common chemical constituents and pharmacological effects. Bishop's weed is more commonly used for dermatological conditions, and khella is usually used for cardiac and pulmonary conditions (7161). The isolated active constituent, khellin, is also used medicinally for angina pectoris, asthma, in conjunction with phototherapy for vitiligo, psoriasis, and alopecia areata (9,560,849,868).

BISTORT

Also Known As
Adderwort, Dragonwort, Easter Giant, Easter Mangiant, Oderwort, Osterick, Patience Dock, Red Legs, Snakeweed, Sweet Dock.

Scientific Names
Polygonum bistorta.
Family: Polygonaceae.

People Use This For
Orally, bistort is used for digestive disorders, particularly diarrhea.
Topically, bistort is used for mouth and throat infections, and for wounds.

Safety
There is insufficient reliable information available about the safety of bistort.
Pregnancy and Lactation: Insufficient reliable information available; avoid using.

Effectiveness
There is insufficient reliable information available about the effectiveness of bistort.

Mechanism of Action
The applicable parts of bistort are the rhizome and root. Bistort contains 15-21% tannins, which have astringent effects. Tannins work internally by dehydrating mucosal tissue, which reduces secretions. Externally, tannin astringent effects result in a protective layer of constricted, harder cells. Plants with at least 10% tannins can cause gastrointestinal upset, kidney damage, and liver damage. Animal data conflicts with respect to the carcinogenicity of tannins. They may be carcinogenic or may have anti-carcinogenic effects. An increased risk of esophageal or nasal cancer may be linked to people who regularly ingest herbs with high tannin concentrations (12).

Adverse Reactions
None reported.

Interactions with Herbs & Other Dietary Supplements
TANNIN-CONTAINING HERBS: Theoretically, herbs that contain high percentages of tannins, such as bistort, may cause precipitation of constituents of other herbs (19).

Interactions with Drugs
ORAL DRUGS: Theoretically, concomitant use may cause precipitation of some drugs due to the high tannin content of bistort (19). Separate administration of oral drugs and tannin-containing herbs by the longest period of time practical (19).

Interactions with Foods
None known.

Interactions with Lab Tests
None known.

Interactions with Diseases or Conditions
None known.

Dosage and Administration
ORAL: The rhizome and root are powdered and used to make an infusion (18).
TOPICAL: The powdered root is used as an extract or ointment (18).

BITTER ALMOND

Also Known As

Amygdala Amara, Badama, Bitter Almond Oil, Vatadha, Vathada, Volatile Almond Oil.
CAUTION: See separate listing for Sweet Almond Oil.

Scientific Names

Prunus dulcis, synonyms Prunus amygdalus, Amygdalus communis, Amygdalus dulcis, Prunus communis, Prunus dulcis var. amara.
Family: Rosaceae.

People Use This For

Orally, bitter almond is used as an antispasmodic, local anesthetic, for its narcotic properties, as a cough suppressant, and as an antipruritic.

Safety

POSSIBLY SAFE ...when the HCN (hydrocyanic acid)-free oil is used orally in amounts commonly found in foods. HCN free oil is also known as FFPA (free form prussic acid). FFPA bitter almond oil has Generally Recognized As Safe (GRAS) status in the US (4912).
LIKELY UNSAFE ...when the volatile oil containing HCN is used orally (11,12). ...when large amounts of HCN-free volatile oil are used orally. Ingesting 50-60 mL benzaldehyde can cause fatal CNS depression and respiratory failure (11).
PREGNANCY AND LACTATION: LIKELY UNSAFE ...when the volatile oil containing HCN is used orally (11). There is insufficient reliable information available about the safety of the oral of the HCN-free oil during pregnancy and breast-feeding; avoid using.

Effectiveness

There is insufficient reliable information available about the effectiveness of bitter almond.

Mechanism of Action

The applicable part of bitter almond is the volatile oil. The bitter almond kernel contains 3-4% amygdalin, which is hydrolyzed to poisonous hydrocyanic acid (HCN, prussic acid). The volatile oil contains 95% benzaldehyde and 2% to 4% HCN. For food and flavor use, HCN is removed. High doses of benzaldehyde can have narcotic properties and the potential for adverse reactions (11).

Adverse Reactions

Orally, 50-60 mL of benzaldehyde (sole constituent of HCN-free oil) can have high toxicity and be fatal due to CNS depression with respiratory failure (11). There is a report of one death of an adult after ingestion of 7.5 mL of the volatile oil (11).

Interactions with Herbs & Other Dietary Supplements

None known.

Interactions with Drugs

CNS DEPRESSANTS: Theoretically, bitter almond oil use with CNS depressants increases the risk of severe or fatal CNS and respiratory depression.

Interactions with Foods

None known.

Interactions with Lab Tests

None known.

Interactions with Diseases or Conditions

None known.

Dosage and Administration

No typical dosage.

Comments

The volatile oil of bitter almond contains 95% benzaldehyde and 2-4% poisonous HCN. It is made by water maceration and steam distillation of partially defatted bitter almond (Prunus amygdalus amara), apricot (Prunus armeniaca), peach (Prunus persica), and plum (Prunus domestica) kernels. The fixed almond oil (sweet almond oil) is prepared by pressing the kernels of both sweet almond and bitter almond and contains no benzaldehyde or hydrocyanic acid (HCN). Sweet almond does not yield a volatile oil (11). Bitter almond volatile oil consists of distilled, partially defatted oil of the kernels of bitter almond (Prunus amygdalus amara) and kernels of other Prunus species.

BITTER MELON

Also Known As

African Cucumber, Balsam Pear, Balsam-Apple, Balsambirne, Balsamo, Bitter Apple, Bitter Cucumber, Bitter Gourd, Bittergurke, Carilla Gourd, Cerasee, Chinli-Chih, Cundeamor, Karavella, Karela, Kathilla, Kerala, Kuguazi, K'u-Kua, Lai Margose, Momordique, Pepino Montero, P'u-T'ao, Sorosi, Sushavi, Wild Cucumber.
CAUTION: See separate listing for Ivy Gourd.

Scientific Names

Momordica charantia, synonym Momordica murcata.
Family: Cucurbitaceae.

People Use This For

Orally, bitter melon is used to treat diabetes, psoriasis, gastrointestinal upset, ulcers, colitis, constipation, intestinal worms, urinary tract stones (kidney stones), fever, and hepatic disease. It is also used orally to induce menstruation and as supportive therapy for patients with AIDS/HIV.
Topically, bitter melon is used for skin abscesses and wounds, and anorectal herpes lesions.

Safety

POSSIBLY SAFE ...when used orally and appropriately, short-term. Extract of bitter melon fruit appears to be safe for up to 7 weeks (36).
There is insufficient reliable information available about the safety of bitter melon when used topically.
PREGNANCY: LIKELY UNSAFE ...when used orally. Bitter melon juice can stimulate menstruation and cause abortion (19).
LACTATION: Insufficient reliable information available; avoid using.

Effectiveness

INSUFFICIENT RELIABLE EVIDENCE to RATE

Diabetes. Bitter melon fruit, fruit juice, and extract seem to improve glucose tolerance, reduce blood glucose levels, and lower glycosylated hemoglobin (HbA1c) in patients with type 2 diabetes (34,35,36,38,12530). But all studies have been small, short-term, or uncontrolled. More evidence is needed to rate bitter melon for this use.

Mechanism of Action

The applicable parts of bitter melon are the fruit and seeds, and less commonly the leaves and roots.
The bitter melon fruit and fruit extracts seem to have hypoglycemic activity in humans and animal models of diabetes (34,35,36,3762,3763,3764,3765,7700,8179). Bitter melon fruit extract might also protect against hyperinsulinemia (7700). Bitter melon contains an insulin-like polypeptide called polypeptide P, plant insulin, or p-insulin. P-insulin has pharmacologic effects similar to bovine insulin with an onset of action between 30 and 60 minutes, and a peak effect at about four hours (37,38). Preliminary evidence suggests that an aqueous extract of bitter melon fruit can slow the progression of microalbuminuria and diabetic nephropathy (8179).
Bitter melon contains several other constituents with a variety of pharmacological effects. Flavonoids in bitter melon seem to have a cholesterol lowering effect. There's also some preliminary evidence that they might raise hemoglobin, and increase white and red blood cell counts (8180). Constituents called alpha- and beta-momorcharin seem to have immunosuppressive activity in vitro and in animal models (3724). However, other constituents have antitumor, antileukemia, and antiviral activity (3722,3723). A bitter melon protein from the seed and fruit called momordica anti-human immunodeficiency virus (HIV) protein (MAP30) has antiviral and antitumor activity in vitro (3720,3721,7540). It inhibits HIV and herpes simplex viruses, including acyclovir-resistant strains (7539,7540). It appears to inhibit HIV by inhibiting reverse transcriptase. MAP30 is also a N-glucosidase, which inhibits HIV ribosomal protein synthesis and might make viral and plasmid DNA inactive (7542,7543). MAP30 also seems to inhibit HIV integrase, which prevents integration of viral DNA into the genetic material of healthy cells (7542). Another protein, MRK29, found in the seed and fruit of a smaller variety of bitter melon found in Thailand, appears to inhibit HIV reverse transcriptase and to increase tumor necrosis factor (TNF) activity (7541). There's some preliminary evidence that an ethanolic extract of bitter melon seed might also have antispermogenic and androgenic properties, suggesting potential use as a male contraceptive (7538).

Adverse Reactions
None reported.

Interactions with Herbs & Other Dietary Supplements
HERBS & SUPPLEMENTS WITH HYPOGLYCEMIC POTENTIAL: Bitter melon can lower blood glucose levels (34,35,36) and might have additive effects when used with other herbs and supplements that also lower glucose levels. This might increase the risk of hypoglycemia in some patients. Some herbs and supplements with hypoglycemic effects include alpha-lipoic acid, chromium, devil's claw, fenugreek, garlic, guar gum, horse chestnut, Panax ginseng, psyllium, Siberian ginseng, and others.

Interactions with Drugs
ANTIDIABETES DRUGS: Bitter melon can lower blood glucose levels (34,35,36) and might have additive effects when used with antidiabetes drugs. This might increase the risk of hypoglycemia in some patients. Monitor blood glucose levels closely. An additive effect of chlorpropamide (Diabinese) and bitter melon has been reported (8181). Some antidiabetes drugs include glimepiride (Amaryl), glyburide (Diabeta, Glynase PresTabs, Micronase), insulin, metformin (Glucophage), pioglitazone (Actos), rosiglitazone (Avandia), and others.

Interactions with Foods
None known.

Interactions with Lab Tests
BLOOD GLUCOSE: Bitter melon extracts, fruits, and fruit juice can lower blood glucose and test results in patients with type 2 diabetes (34,35,36).
GLYCOSYLATED HEMOGLOBIN (HbA1c): Bitter melon extract can lower HbA1c in type 2 diabetes patients after 7 weeks of treatment (36).

Interactions with Diseases or Conditions
DIABETES: Bitter melon can lower blood glucose levels (34,35,36) and might have additive effects when used with antidiabetes drugs. This might increase the risk of hypoglycemia in some patients. Monitor blood glucose levels closely.

Dosage and Administration
No typical dosage.

Comments
Bitter melon is used as a vegetable in India and other Asian countries (7538,7541). Bitter melon is used as an ingredient in some kinds of curries. A reduction in blood sugar after eating foods spiced with curry has been described in a patient taking chlorpropamide (Diabinese) (8181).

BITTER MILKWORT

Also Known As
European Bitter Polygala, European Senega, Evergreen Snakeroot, Flowering Wintergreen, Little Pollom, Snakeroot.
CAUTION: See separate listings for Asarabacca and Senega.

Scientific Names
Polygala amara.
Family: Polygalaceae.

Comments
At the date of publication, this product was not a common ingredient used in brand name supplements marketed to consumers. Details about this product are available in the online version of *Natural Medicines Comprehensive Database.* See www.naturaldatabase.com.

BITTER ORANGE

Also Known As

Aurantii Pericarpium, Chisil, Fructus Aurantii, Green Orange, Kijitsu, Neroli Oil, Seville Orange, Shangzhou Zhiqiao, Sour Orange, Synephrine, Zhi Qiao, Zhi Shi.
CAUTION: See separate listings for Bergamot Oil, Oswego Tea, and Sweet Orange.

Scientific Names

Citrus aurantium, synonyms Citrus amara, Citrus bigarradia, Citrus vulgaris.
Family: Rutaceae.

People Use This For

Orally, bitter orange peel is used as an appetite stimulant and for dyspepsia. Bitter orange fruit and peel are also used orally for weight loss and nasal congestion. The bitter orange flower and its oil are used orally for gastrointestinal (GI) disturbances, duodenal ulcers, constipation, regulating blood lipid levels, lowering blood sugar in diabetes, blood purification, functional disorders of liver and gallbladder, stimulation of the heart and circulation, frostbite, as a sedative for sleep disorders, for kidney and bladder diseases, general feebleness, anemia, imbalances of mineral metabolism, impurities of the skin, hair loss, as a tonic, antiflatulent, and for cancer. Other uses include prolapsed uterus, prolapsed anus or rectum, diarrhea, and blood in the stools.
Topically, bitter orange peel is used for inflammation of the eyelid, conjunctiva, and retina. It is also used for retinal hemorrhage, exhaustion accompanying colds, headaches, neuralgia, muscular pain, rheumatic discomfort, bruises, phlebitis, and bed sores.
In aromatherapy, the essential oil of bitter orange is used topically and by inhalation as an analgesic.
In foods, bitter orange oil is used as a flavoring agent.
In manufacturing, bitter orange oil is used in pharmaceuticals, cosmetics, and soaps.

Safety

LIKELY SAFE ...when used orally in the amounts found in foods. Bitter orange has Generally Recognized As Safe (GRAS) status in the US (4912).
POSSIBLY SAFE ...when the essential oil is used topically or by inhalation as aromatherapy (6972,7107).
POSSIBLY UNSAFE ...when used orally for medicinal purposes. Bitter orange juice and extract have been safely used, short-term in healthy adults in small controlled trials (2040,11269). But there is concern that bitter orange might be associated with severe adverse effects in some patients due to its stimulant effects. There are case reports of ischemic stroke, and cardiotoxicity including tachyarrhythmia, syncope, and myocardial infarction in otherwise healthy patients who have taken bitter orange extract alone or in combination with other stimulants such as caffeine (2040,6979,12030,13039,13067).
There is insufficient reliable information available about the safety of other forms of bitter orange.
CHILDREN: LIKELY SAFE ...when used orally in the amounts found in foods. Bitter orange has Generally Recognized As Safe (GRAS) status in the US (4912). POSSIBLY UNSAFE ...when used orally for medicinal purposes. There are case reports of cardiotoxicity including tachyarrhythmia, syncope, and myocardial infarction in otherwise healthy adults who have taken bitter orange extract in combination with other stimulants such as caffeine (2040,6979,12030,13039).
PREGNANCY AND LACTATION: LIKELY SAFE ...when used orally in the amounts found in foods. Bitter orange has Generally Recognized As Safe (GRAS) status in the US (4912). POSSIBLY UNSAFE ...when used orally for medicinal purposes. There are case reports of cardiotoxicity including tachyarrhythmia, syncope, and myocardial infarction in otherwise healthy adults who have taken bitter orange extract in combination with other stimulants such as caffeine (2040,6979,12030,13039). The effects of bitter orange on a fetus or in a breast-feeding infant are not known; avoid using.

Effectiveness

POSSIBLY EFFECTIVE

Tinea corporis, tinea cruris, and tinea pedis. Applying bitter orange oil seems to help treat tinea corporis, cruris, or pedis (6972).

INSUFFICIENT RELIABLE EVIDENCE to RATE

Obesity. Preliminary clinical research suggests that a combination of bitter orange, caffeine, and St. John's wort may be helpful for weight reduction when used with caloric restriction and exercise (11268). More evidence is needed to rate bitter orange for this use.

Mechanism of Action

The applicable parts of bitter orange are the peel, flower, leaf, and fruit. Bitter orange has numerous active constituents and pharmacological effects; however, the amount of each constituent can vary depending on the part of the plant used.

The flavonoid content is higher in the flowers than the leaves (6971). The flavonoids are also present in the peel. These flavonoids include limonene, hesperidin, neohesperidin, naringin, and tangaretin (12193).

The fruit and peel of bitter orange contain the adrenergic agonists synephrine and octopamine (2080,4800,11267). Synephrine is structurally similar to epinephrine. Octopamine is similar to norepinephrine (11995,12193,12378).

There are at least 6 isomers of synephrine. Different isomers of synephrine can have somewhat different pharmacological effects. It is unclear which isomer or isomers are contained in bitter orange. Some references suggest that bitter orange contains only p-synephrine. Other references suggest that it contains only m-synephrine, which is also known as phenylephrine. Phenylephrine (m-synephrine) is the alpha-adrenergic agent used as an over-the-counter nasal decongestant (Neosynephrine). Some bitter orange product labels indicate that the product contains both p-synephrine and m-synephrine. In laboratory analysis, both of these isomers have been detected in at least one commercial bitter orange product (13136). But it is unknown if these commercial bitter orange product may be spiked with one or more synthetic synephrine isomers. More research is needed to determine which isomer(s) of synephrine occur naturally in bitter orange extracts in order to better understand the pharmacological effects of bitter orange products.

Synephrine and octopamine naturally occur in the human body. Trace amounts are part of the pool of circulating amines in humans (12379).

In the body tyramine is converted to octopamine, which then gets converted to synephrine (12193). Like tyramine, octopamine and synephrine are substrates of monoamine oxidase (11995,12378).

The exact physiological function of octopamine and synephrine is unclear. They were once referred to as "false neurotransmitters," but it is now thought that they might act as true neurotransmitters (12193).

Octopamine and synephrine might have a role in fat cell lipolysis. Octopamine seems to have an insulin-like effect on glucose uptake by fat cells (11995). Preliminary research suggests that migraine and cluster headaches might be related to excess levels of synephrine and octopamine (11996).

Both synephrine and octopamine are selective beta-3 adrenoreceptor agonists. Synephrine also appears to be an alpha-1 agonist. Octopamine appears to also affect alpha-2 receptors (12193).

Fresh bitter orange fruit contains approximately 0.02% synephrine (11267). The concentration tends to be smaller in larger fruits, and higher in smaller fruits. In freshly squeezed bitter orange juice, the synephrine concentration is 57 mcg/mL (12193). Drying the fruit seems to increase synephrine concentrations to approximately 0.35%. Dried extracts contain approximately 3% synephrine. Octopamine levels are much lower, usually <0.03% (11267). Since octopamine concentration is so low, it's not known if its effects in humans is significant.

Commercially available bitter orange extracts usually contain 1% to 6% synephrine. But some manufacturers boost synephrine content to as much as 30%. These preparations are often promoted for weight loss due to purported thermogenic effects (4800). In animal models, synephrine causes weight loss, but also increases cardiovascular toxicity (6969).

Animal models suggest that bitter orange can cause vasoconstriction and increase mean arterial pressure (MAP), but reduce portal pressure (6975). Synephrine given intravenously in men increases systolic blood pressure, but doesn't seem to increase diastolic blood pressure or heart rate (12193). Bitter orange plus a synthetic preparation of the active components synephrine and N-methyltyramine have been used successfully to treat infectious shock in preliminary research. N-methyltyramine seems to increase blood pressure by increasing norepinephrine release (6978).

Preliminary research suggests that synephrine might have antidepressant effects, possibly by promoting norepinephrine release (12376,12377).

Bitter orange peel is also commonly used for dyspepsia due to its spasmolytic effects. Bitter orange peel might also have anti-inflammatory activity, which might be due to the flavonoids naringin and nobiletin (1281).

Bitter orange preparations have a variety of antimicrobial properties. The oil of the bitter orange peel seems to have insecticidal activity (6973). Two flavonoids of the bitter orange fruit, neohesperidin and hesperidin, also seem to have antiviral activity against rotavirus infection (6976). Preliminary research indicates that bitter orange constituents auraptene, marmin, tangeretin, nobiretin, and a psoralen compound, might have antitumor effects (6974).

Bitter orange also contains furocoumarins. The furocoumarins bergapten and oxypeucedanin in bitter orange oil are photosensitizing (11019). The furocoumarins bergamottin, dihydroxybergamottin, and bergapten in the fruit and juice can inhibit the cytochrome P450 3A4 (CYP3A4) isoenzyme (7029). Bitter orange appears to selectively inhibit intestinal CYP3A4, but not hepatic CYP3A4 (7029,11269). These are the same constituents found in grapefruit that are responsible for numerous drug interactions. However, grapefruit juice contains a significantly higher concentration of these constituents than bitter orange juice (7029). Research on the effects of bitter orange on P-glycoprotein is conflicting (7029,11269,11270,11362). Dihydroxybergamottin appears to inhibit CYP3A4, but not P-glycoprotein (11270).

Adverse Reactions

Orally, bitter orange, which contains the adrenergic agents synephrine and octopamine, might theoretically cause hypertension and cardiovascular toxicity (2040,6969,6979).
Synephrine is similar to phenylephrine and the ephedrine contained in the herb ephedra. Theoretically, synephrine might cause similar side effects such as myocardial infarction, stroke, seizure, and other serious side effects; however, in one clinical trial of bitter orange extract there were no significant changes in blood pressure, heart rate, or electrocardiogram measurements in normotensive patients (11268).
There is one case report of myocardial infarction in a patient without a history of cardiovascular disease who took a supplement containing 300 mg of bitter orange for a year. The supplement also contained guarana and green tea, both of which are sources of caffeine (12030).
In another case, a woman experienced unremitting tachycardia after taking a bitter orange extract 500 mg containing 6% synephrine (30 mg). The patient discontinued bitter orange extract for one month and then took it again. Upon this rechallenge, the patient experienced another episode of unremitting tachycardia. Tachycardia resolved when the bitter orange was discontinued (13067).
There is also a case report of syncope, tachyarrhythmia, and QT prolongation in a young, healthy woman who took a specific combination product containing bitter orange (Xenadrine EFX) just prior to exercising. This product also contained other stimulants including caffeine, theobromine, phenylethylamine, tyamine, and others. The tachyarrhythmia and QT interval normalized within 24 hours of discontinuing the product (13039).
In another case, an otherwise healthy man experienced ischemic stroke after taking a specific combination product containing bitter orange (Stacker 2 Ephedra Free) for 1 week. The patient initially took 1 capsule daily and then increased to 2 capsules daily 4 days before presentation and diagnosis. According to the product label at the time of this case, each capsule provided approximately 6 mg synephrine and 200 mg caffeine (13091).
Photosensitivity can also occur, especially in fair-skinned people (11909).

Interactions with Herbs & Other Dietary Supplements

PANAX GINSENG: Theoretically, Panax ginseng might prolong the QT interval on electrocardiogram (ECG). Other stimulant products such as bitter orange also increase the QT interval. Theoretically, combining Panax ginseng and bitter orange might have an additive effect on the QT interval and increase the risk for arrhythmias (4322,11355).
STIMULANTS: Theoretically, herbs and supplements with stimulant properties, such as caffeine, coffee, cola nut, ephedra, guarana, and mate, might increase the risk of hypertension and adverse cardiovascular effects with bitter orange due to synephrine content (6979).

Interactions with Drugs

CYTOCHROME P450 3A4 (CYP3A4) SUBSTRATES: Bitter orange juice can inhibit cytochrome P450 3A4 (CYP3A4) metabolism of drugs (7029), causing increased drug levels and potentially increasing the risk of adverse effects. But the extent of the effect of bitter orange on drug interactions is unknown. Bitter orange selectively inhibits intestinal CYP3A4, but not hepatic CYP3A4. Its effect on P-glycoprotein, which strongly overlaps with CYP3A4 interactions, is unclear (7029,11269,11270,11362). It has no effect on cyclosporine which seems to be more dependent on hepatic CYP3A4 and P-glycoprotein than intestinal CYP3A4 (11270). Some possible drug interactions with bitter orange include calcium channel blockers (diltiazem, nicardipine, verapamil), chemotherapeutic agents (etoposide, paclitaxel, vinblastine, vincristine, vindesine), antifungals (ketoconazole, itraconazole), glucocorticoids, cisapride (Propulsid), losartan (Cozaar), fexofenadine (Allegra), and numerous others.
DEXTROMETHORPHAN (Robitussin DM, others): Bitter orange juice can inhibit cytochrome P450 3A4 (CYP3A4) metabolism (11362), causing increased dextromethorphan levels and potentially increasing the risk of adverse effects.
FELODIPINE (Plendil): Consumption of bitter orange juice 240 mL can significantly increase felodipine levels. Bitter orange juice inhibits cytochrome P450 3A4 (CYP3A4) metabolism of felodipine (7029).
INDINAVIR (Crixivan): Bitter orange juice slightly increases indinavir levels, but this effect is likely to be clinically insignificant. Bitter orange selectively inhibits intestinal cytochrome P450 3A4 (CYP3A4). The metabolism of indinavir seems to be more dependent on hepatic CYP3A4 (11269). The effect of bitter orange on other protease inhibitors has not been studied.
MIDAZOLAM (Versed): Bitter orange juice can significantly inhibit cytochrome P450 3A4 (CYP3A4) metabolism of the midazolam, and potentially increase drug levels and adverse effects (7029).
MONOAMINE OXIDASE INHIBITORS (MAOIs): Theoretically, concurrent use of MAOIs with synephrine-containing bitter orange preparations might increase the blood pressure raising effects of synephrine and potentially cause hypertensive crisis. Bitter orange contains tyramine, octopamine, and synephrine, which are MAO substrates (11267,11995,12378). Tell patients taking MAOIs to avoid using bitter orange. Some MAOIs include phenelzine (Nardil), tranylcypromine (Parnate), and others (2040).
QT INTERVAL-PROLONGING DRUGS: Bitter orange in combination with other stimulants such as caffeine might prolong the QT interval in some patients (13039). Theoretically, bitter orange could have an additive effect when combined with drugs that prolong the QT interval and potentially increase the risk of ventricular arrhythmias. Drugs that prolong the QT interval include amiodarone (Cordarone), disopyramide (Norpace), dofetilide (Tikosyn), ibutilide (Corvert), procainamide (Pronestyl), quinidine, sotalol (Betapace), thioridazine (Mellaril), and many others.
STIMULANT DRUGS: Theoretically, drugs with CNS stimulant properties, such as phenylpropanolamine,

pseudoephedrine, and caffeine, might increase the risk of hypertension and adverse cardiovascular effects of bitter orange due to synephrine content (2040,6979).

Interactions with Foods

CAFFEINE: Theoretically, large amounts of caffeine-containing beverages might increase the risk of hypertension and adverse cardiovascular effects with bitter orange due to synephrine content (6979).

Interactions with Lab Tests

None known.

Interactions with Diseases or Conditions

HEADACHE: Theoretically, bitter orange might trigger migraine or cluster headache due to its synephrine and octopamine content (11996).
HYPERTENSION: Theoretically, bitter orange fruit, peel, or juice might worsen hypertension due to synephrine content (2040,6979).
NARROW-ANGLE GLAUCOMA: Theoretically, bitter orange fruit, peel, or juice might worsen narrow-angle glaucoma due to synephrine content (2040,6979).
LONG QT INTERVAL SYNDROME: Bitter orange in combination with other stimulants such as caffeine might prolong the QT interval in some patients (13039). Theoretically, taking bitter orange might increase the risk of ventricular arrhythmias in patients with long QT interval syndrome.
TACHYARRHYTHMIAS: Theoretically, bitter orange might worsen tachyarrhythmias due to synephrine content (2040,6979).

Dosage and Administration

ORAL: For weight loss, bitter orange extract 975 mg in combination with St. John's wort 900 mg and caffeine 528 mg per day has been used (11268). Bitter orange extracts commonly contain from 1.5% to 6% synephrine (6969).
TOPICAL: For treatment of fungal skin infections, pure oil of bitter orange has been applied once daily for one to three weeks (6972).

Comments

Bitter orange is a small tree that produces an extremely sour and bitter citrus fruit. It's generally not considered an edible fruit, but it is eaten in Iran and Mexico (12193). Due to the fruit's acidity it is popular for making marmalades and liquors such as triple sec, grand marnier, cointreau, and curacao. The dried peel of the fruit is also used as a seasoning.

In Asian medicine, the entire dried unripe fruit is used primarily for digestive disorders (12193). In Western countries the dried peel of the fruit has historically been used to stimulate appetite. This is in surprising contrast to bitter orange's primary use today, as a component of weight loss products.

BITTERSWEET NIGHTSHADE

Also Known As

Bitter Nightshade, Bittersweet, Blue Nightshade, Common Nightshade, Deadly Nightshade, Dulcamara, Fellen, Fellonwood, Felonwort, Fever Twig, Mortal, Scarlet Berry, Snake Berry, Staff Vine, Violet Bloom, Woody, Woody Nightshade.
CAUTION: See separate listings for Belladonna and Henbane.

Scientific Names

Solanum dulcamara.
Family: Solanaceae.

People Use This For

Orally, bittersweet nightshade is used for chronic eczema, itchy skin conditions, acne, furuncles, skin abrasions, warts, as an antirheumatic, diuretic, narcotic, sedative, and for inflammation.
Topically, bittersweet nightshade is used for chronic eczema.

Safety

POSSIBLY SAFE ...when used orally or topically and appropriately (2,18).
LIKELY UNSAFE ...when the leaves or berries are used orally. The plant contains the toxic compounds solanine, solanidine, and dulcamarin (6).
CHILDREN: LIKELY UNSAFE ...when used orally; unripe berries have caused poisonings. A lethal dose is estimated to be 200 berries (18). There is insufficient reliable information available about the safety of bittersweet nightshade when used topically in children; avoid using.
PREGNANCY: LIKELY UNSAFE ...when used orally. The alkaloids of the plant, solasodine, soladulcine, and related compounds have been linked to malformations in animals (6); avoid using. There is insufficient reliable information available about the safety of bittersweet nightshade when used topically during pregnancy; avoid using.
LACTATION: LIKELY UNSAFE ...when orally; avoid using. There is insufficient reliable information available about the safety of bittersweet nightshade when used topically; avoid using.

Effectiveness

There is insufficient reliable information available about the effectiveness of bittersweet nightshade.

Mechanism of Action

The applicable part of bittersweet nightshade is the stem. It has astringent, antimicrobial, and mucous membrane-irritating actions (2). The steroidal alkaloid constituents of the stem can have anticholinergic effects (2). The component, solasodin, can prevent inflammation (2).

Adverse Reactions

Orally, the bittersweet nightshade plant can cause the symptoms of solanine poisoning, commonly associated with old potatoes. Symptoms include scratchy throat, headache, vertigo, dilated pupils, speech difficulties, subnormal temperature, vomiting, diarrhea, GI bleeding, cyanosis, convulsions, circulatory and respiratory depression, and even death (6). The ingestion of unripe berries can cause poisoning in children (18).

Interactions with Herbs & Other Dietary Supplements

None known.

Interactions with Drugs

None known.

Interactions with Foods

None known.

Interactions with Lab Tests

None known.

Interactions with Diseases or Conditions

GI IRRITATION: Bittersweet nightshade can irritate the gastrointestinal tract. It is contraindicated in individuals with infectious or inflammatory gastrointestinal conditions (19).

Dosage and Administration

ORAL: The typical dose of the bittersweet nightshade stem is 1-3 grams of the dried herb per day, and can be taken as a tea, which is prepared by steeping the herb in 150 mL boiling water for 5-10 minutes and straining (2).
TOPICAL: The stem is used as a compress prepared by steeping 1-2 grams of the dried herb in 250 mL boiling water for 5-10 minutes and straining (2).

Comments

Bittersweet nightshade is a perennial vine-like plant that is found throughout the United States, Canada, and Eurasia and is a member of the same family that includes tomatoes and potatoes.

BLACK ALDER

Also Known As
Betula Alnus, Common Alder, English Alder, European Alder, European Black Alder, Owler.

Scientific Names
Alnus glutinosa, synonyms Betula glutinosa, Alnus barbata.
Family: Betulaceae.

Comments
At the date of publication, there was very little scientific information available about this product. Our staff is continually analyzing the available information on natural medicines and will add data to the online version of *Natural Medicines Comprehensive Database* as it becomes available. See www.naturaldatabase.com.

BLACK BRYONY

Also Known As
Black Bindweed, Blackeye Root, Lady's-Seal.

Scientific Names
Dioscorea communis, synonyms Tamus communis, Tamus edulis.
Family: Dioscoreaceae.

People Use This For
Orally, black bryony is used as an emetic.
Topically, black bryony is used as a counterirritant, to treat bruises, strains, torn muscles, gout, rheumatic disorders, hair loss, and for improving blood circulation to the scalp.

Safety
POSSIBLY UNSAFE ...when the fresh root is used topically. Skin contact can cause severe skin irritation (3829).
UNSAFE ...when used orally. Black bryony can cause seizures, respiratory and kidney failure (18).
PREGNANCY AND LACTATION: Insufficient reliable information; avoid using.

Effectiveness
There is insufficient reliable information available about the effectiveness of black bryony.

Mechanism of Action
The applicable part of black bryony is the root. It can stimulate external nerve endings. Applied topically, it acts as a mechanical irritant, penetrating the skin with tiny, needle-like crystals of calcium oxalate (3829). The rhizome contains histamine (3829), which can have a role in producing skin irritation (3829). In rats, an ethanolic extract of the root exhibited local anti-inflammatory activity (3828).

Adverse Reactions
Orally, black bryony can cause severe mouth, pharyngeal and GI irritation, as well as vomiting, diarrhea, spasms, colic, decreased kidney function, and respiratory depression (18).
Topically, the fresh root can cause reddening of skin (18). The fresh plant used topically can cause skin irritation, rash, swelling, pustules, wheals, and mucous membrane irritation (18).

Interactions with Herbs & Other Dietary Supplements
None known.

Interactions with Drugs
None known.

Interactions with Foods
None known.

Interactions with Lab Tests
None known.

Interactions with Diseases or Conditions
None known.

Dosage and Administration

ORAL: No typical dosage.
TOPICAL: The fresh root is scraped and the pulp rubbed into affected areas (223).

BLACK COHOSH

Also Known As

Baneberry, Black Snakeroot, Bugbane, Bugwort, Macrotys, Phytoestrogen, Rattle Root, Rattle Top, Rattlesnake Root, Rattleweed, Snakeroot, Squaw Root.
CAUTION: See separate listings for Blue Cohosh and White Cohosh.

Scientific Names

Actaea racemosa, synonym Cimicifuga racemosa; Actaea macrotys.
Family: Ranunculaceae.

People Use This For

Orally, black cohosh is used for symptoms of menopause, inducing labor in pregnant women, premenstrual syndrome (PMS), dysmenorrhea, nervous tension, dyspepsia, rheumatism, fever, sore throat, cough, as an insect repellent, and as a mild sedative.
Topically, black cohosh is used for acne, mole and wort removal, improving appearance of the skin, and rattlesnake bites.

Safety

POSSIBLY SAFE ...when used orally and appropriately. Black cohosh has been safely used in studies lasting up to 6 months (141,4614,4620,7054,9437,9494,13143). But there is concern that black cohosh might cause liver damage in some patients. There are a few case reports that link black cohosh to liver failure and autoimmune hepatitis (4383,10692,12006,11906,13144). There is no conclusive evidence that black cohosh is the cause of liver damage in these patients. Until more is known, monitor liver function in patients who take black cohosh.
PREGNANCY: LIKELY UNSAFE ...when used orally in pregnant women who are not at term. Black cohosh has menstrual and uterine stimulant effects, which can increase the risk of miscarriage (3382); avoid using. There is insufficient reliable information about the safety of black cohosh for labor induction. Some midwives use black cohosh to induce labor in pregnant women at term. Observational reports suggest that this practice does not appear to adversely affect the mother or fetus, but there are no clinical trials to support the safety of this practice (1122).
LACTATION: POSSIBLY UNSAFE ...when used orally. There is some concern that black cohosh, particularly in large doses, may adversely affect a nursing child (3382). Until more is known, tell nursing mothers to avoid taking black cohosh.

Effectiveness

POSSIBLY EFFECTIVE

Menopausal symptoms. Taking black cohosh orally seems to modestly reduce symptoms of menopause, such as hot flashes, in perimenopausal women. (4620,9437,10987,11913,13143). Some research suggests that black cohosh might be as effective as estrogen replacement for some patients (4620,10987). Treatment for 4 weeks is often required before there is significant improvement in symptoms.

POSSIBLY INEFFECTIVE

Breast cancer-related hot flashes. Black cohosh does not seem to reduce hot flashes in breast cancer survivors (7054).

Most clinical studies on the effectiveness of black cohosh have used a specific black cohosh formulation standardized to contain 1 mg triterpene glycosides, calculated as 27-deoxyacetin (Remifemin, GlaxoSmithKline).

There is insufficient reliable information available about the effectiveness of black cohosh for its other uses.

Mechanism of Action

The applicable parts of black cohosh are the rhizome and root. The active constituents of black cohosh include phytosterin; isoferulic acid; fukinolic acid; caffeic acid; salicylic acid; sugars; tannins; long-chain fatty acids; and triterpene glycosides, including acetein, cimicifugoside, and 27-deoxyacetin (4618,9432).
Fukinolic acid is a potent inhibitor of neutrophil elastase, which is important in inflammatory responses. Inhibition of neutrophil elastase is a possible mechanism by which black cohosh exerts anti-inflammatory action (9432).
The presence of an isoflavone, formononetin, is doubtful (1122,4616,9431). Earlier reports of isoflavone content may have been a result of contamination with other similar plant species (4615).
Black cohosh has estrogen-like effects that are exerted by an unknown mechanism (4618,4619). Clinically, it doesn't appear to affect endometrial tissue or hormone levels such as estradiol, luteinizing hormone (LH), follicle-stimulating hormone (FSH), and prolactin (9437,10987). Laboratory research suggests that extracts of black cohosh don't bind to estrogen receptors, up-regulate estrogen-dependent genes, or stimulate the growth of estrogen-dependent tumors in experimental animals (4619,7860,9996,9998). But there is some evidence from animal studies that

black cohosh can suppress pituitary secretion of luteinizing hormone (LH) (12064). Preliminary clinical evidence also suggests that black cohosh might increase osteoblast activity (10987).

It's thought that black cohosh might have selective estrogen receptor modulating (SERM) effects and therefore have estrogenic effects in some tissues and antiestrogenic effects in other tissues. For example, in animal models, there is preliminary evidence that black cohosh might have a modest estrogenic effect on bone and suppress LH, but it doesn't seem to stimulate an increase in uterine weight (12064).

Research on breast cancer cells suggests that black cohosh doesn't promote tumor growth (9435,9436,11911). Some constituents of black cohosh seem to inhibit breast cancer cell growth (11912). Animal research suggests that black cohosh doesn't increase or decrease risk of breast cancer (9999). But black cohosh does seem to increase metastatic cancer in animals with existing cancer (9999). Therefore, black cohosh shouldn't be used by women with existing breast cancer or women with a high risk of developing breast cancer.

Preliminary research also suggests that an black cohosh extract can inhibit proliferation of prostate cancer cells in vitro (13145).

In vitro research suggests black cohosh might increase the toxicity of the chemotherapy drugs doxorubicin (Adriamycin) and docetaxel (Taxotere) (10000,13101); however, black cohosh seemed to decrease the cytotoxicity of cisplatin on breast cancer cells in an animal model (13101).

The acetein constituent seems to have activity against the human immunodeficiency virus (HIV). In vitro it seems to decrease replication of HIV in lymphocytes (13004).

Adverse Reactions

Orally, black cohosh can commonly cause gastrointestinal upset (3382,4383,4615,4616). Other potential adverse effects include rash, headache, dizziness, weight gain, feeling of heaviness in the legs, and cramping (3382,7054,10987).

There is concern that black cohosh might cause liver disease. Several cases of liver toxicity have been described in women taking black cohosh products alone or in combination with other herbs. In many cases, women developed liver failure and required immediate liver transplantation (4383,10692,12006,11909,13144). In one case, a woman developed autoimmune hepatitis after 3 weeks of taking black cohosh. Symptoms resolved 2 weeks after discontinuing black cohosh (11906).

Hepatitis can occur with no identifiable cause, raising the possibility that black cohosh and hepatitis might have been coincidental. Also, plant misidentification can occur, resulting in accidental substitution of a hepatotoxic plant (11910). These cases do not provide conclusive evidence that black cohosh is responsible for liver disease. Until more is known, monitor liver function in patients who take black cohosh.

Some patients taking tamoxifen plus black cohosh have experienced endometrial hyperplasia and vaginal bleeding. However, these effects are more likely due to tamoxifen than black cohosh (7054).

There is one case report of seizures in a woman who used black cohosh, evening primrose oil, and chasteberry (10988).

There has been a case report of severe complications, including seizures, renal failure, and respiratory distress, in an infant whose mother was given an unknown dose of black and blue cohosh at 42 weeks gestation to induce labor (1122,9492,9493). However, this adverse effect may have been attributable to blue cohosh.

Studies on black cohosh mutagenicity, teratogenicity, and carcinogenicity have been negative (4615).

Interactions with Herbs & Other Dietary Supplements

HEPATOTOXIC HERBS AND SUPPLEMENTS: There is some concern that black cohosh can adversely affect the liver (4383,10692,12006,11906,11909,13144). Theoretically, concomitant use with other potentially hepatotoxic products might increase the risk of developing liver damage. Some of these products include androstenedione, chaparral, comfrey, DHEA, germander, kava, niacin, pennyroyal oil, red yeast, and others.

Interactions with Drugs

CISPLATIN (Platinol-AQ): Preliminary evidence suggests that black cohosh might decrease the cytotoxic effect of cisplatin on breast cancer cells in an animal model (13101). Advise patients receiving cisplatin chemotherapy to avoid black cohosh.

HEPATOTOXIC DRUGS: There is concern that black cohosh might be linked to cases of liver failure and autoimmune hepatitis (4383,10692,12006,11906,11909,13144). Theoretically, taking black cohosh with hepatotoxic drugs might increase the risk of liver damage. Advise patients against combining black cohosh with potentially hepatotoxic drugs. Some drugs that can adversely affect the liver include acetaminophen (Tylenol), amiodarone (Cordarone), carbamazepine (Tegretol), isoniazid (INH), methotrexate (Rheumatrex), methyldopa (Aldomet), and many others.

Interactions with Foods

None known.

Interactions with Lab Tests

None known.

Interactions with Diseases or Conditions

BREAST CANCER: Preliminary evidence suggests that black cohosh might increase the risk of metastasis in existing breast cancer. Women with a history of breast cancer or women at risk for breast cancer should avoid black cohosh (9999).

HORMONE-SENSITIVE CANCERS/CONDITIONS: Black cohosh doesn't seem to affect estrogen receptors, but it hasn't been studied for longer than 2 months in women with hormone-sensitive conditions (7054). Until more is known, women with hormone-sensitive conditions should avoid black cohosh. Some of these conditions include uterine cancer, ovarian cancer, endometriosis, and uterine fibroids.

KIDNEY TRANSPLANT: There is one report of acute kidney transplant rejection in a patient who took black cohosh and an alfalfa supplement together. The mechanism for this disease interaction is not known, but it is more likely due to alfalfa than black cohosh. Alfalfa is thought to have immune stimulating effects that might counteract the immunosuppressant effects of cyclosporine (12174).

LIVER DISEASE: There is concern that black cohosh might be linked to cases of liver failure and autoimmune hepatitis (4383,10692,12006,11906,11909,13144). Theoretically, black cohosh might exacerbate liver problems in patients with existing liver disease such as hepatitis. Advise these patients to avoid taking black cohosh.

Dosage and Administration

ORAL: For menopause and premenstrual syndrome (PMS), most clinical studies have used a specific black cohosh extract (Remifemin, Enzymatic Therapy, and Phytopharmica) standardized to contain 1 mg triterpene glycosides, calculated as 27-deoxyacetin, per 20 mg tablet. Most studies used doses of 40-80 mg twice daily, providing 4-8 mg triterpene glycosides for up to 6 months (141,4614,4620,7054,9494). The manufacturer now claims that improvement in the extraction process permits using their currently recommended lower dose of 20 mg twice daily, providing 2 mg triterpene glycosides (4615). This formulation and lower dose has also been used in two clinical trials (9437,13143).

Comments

Black cohosh was first used medicinally by Native Americans who introduced it to European colonists (9997).
It was introduced into Germany in the late 19th century. Remifemin, a branded black cohosh product, has been used in Germany since the mid-1950s to manage menopause (141). Black cohosh was also used as the main ingredient in Lydia Pinkham's Vegetable Compound (3382).
One clinical study used the product Menofem (Pharmaton) which contains 20 mg black cohosh extract per dose (10987). This product is not available in the US or Canada. Another product called Menofem (Vitamin Plus Company) contains unspecified quantities of black cohosh and a variety of other ingredients. These products are not interchangeable.
The genus name of black cohosh, cimicifuga, comes from the Latin words for "bedbug" and "repel." Although less fragrant than other species of the genus, black cohosh was used as an insect repellent, hence the common name "bugbane." Do not confuse black cohosh with two unrelated plants, blue cohosh and white cohosh.

BLACK CURRANT

Also Known As

Cassis, European Black Currant, Ribes Nigri Folium (black currant leaf), Ribes Nero.
CAUTION: See separate listings for Borage, Evening Primrose Oil, Gamma Linolenic Acid (GLA), and Omega-6 Fatty Acids.

Scientific Names

Ribes nigrum.
Family: Grossulariaceae.

People Use This For

Orally, black currant seed oil is used for menopausal symptoms, premenstrual syndrome, dysmenorrhea, mastodynia, and for boosting immunity. Black currant berry is used orally for coughs. Black currant dried leaf is used orally for arthritis, gout, rheumatism, diarrhea, colic, hepatitis, liver ailments, convulsions, and inflammatory disorders of the mouth and throat. Black currant dried leaf is also used for coughs and colds, whooping cough, disinfecting the urine, promoting diuresis, treating bladder stones, and as a cleansing tea.
Topically, black currant leaf is used for the treatment of wounds and insect bites.
In foods, black currant berry is utilized as a flavor component in liqueurs, for flavorings, and as a food.

Safety

LIKELY SAFE ...when used in amounts commonly found in foods. Black currant juice, leaves, and flower have Generally Recognized As Safe (GRAS) status in the US (4912).
POSSIBLY SAFE ...when black currant berry or seed oil is used orally and appropriately in medicinal amounts (4016).
There is insufficient reliable information available about the safety of black currant dried leaf.
PREGNANCY AND LACTATION: Insufficient reliable information available; avoid using.

Effectiveness

There is insufficient reliable information available about the effectiveness of black currant.

Mechanism of Action

The applicable parts of black currant are the seed oil, berry, flower, and leaf.
Black currant seed oil is obtained by pressing the seeds found in the fruit of black currant. Black currant seed oil contains 6-19% gamma-linolenic acid (GLA), an omega-6 fatty acid, and approximately 13% alpha-linolenic acid (ALA), an omega-3 fatty acid (512,515,4016). GLA may be beneficial for people who are unable to metabolize cis-linolenic acid to GLA, and produce adequate prostaglandin E1 (PGE-1). People with this condition have an imbalance in the ratio of inflammatory to non-inflammatory prostaglandins. GLA is thought to improve this ratio (512,4016). GLA also reduces production of interleukin 1 (IL-1)-beta, which may be involved in inflammation in diseases such as rheumatoid arthritis (12470). Preliminary research suggests that a hydroalcoholic extract of black currant leaves has anti-inflammatory action (9238).
Black currant seed oil may increase immune response in healthy elderly people by reducing prostaglandin E2 (PGE-2) production, which contributes to the decline in T cell-mediated function associated with aging. Black currant seed oil supplementation improves delayed-type hypersensitivity skin testing response and improves immune response in peripheral blood mononuclear cells (4016). However, whether black currant seed oil supplementation results in better health in elderly people is unknown.
There is also evidence that GLA may be a good source of nutrition in critical care patients and neonates who might have low stores of essential fatty acids (9238).
Preliminary evidence suggests GLA might have an antiestrogenic effect and might hasten the response to tamoxifen (Nolvadex) in women with estrogen-sensitive breast cancer (5902). GLA also seems to modulate the sensitivity of breast cancer cells to paclitaxel (Taxol) and fulvestrant (Faslodex), enhancing malignant cell killing without adverse effects on normal cells (8133,11791). However, other research suggests that taking GLA alone might stimulate the growth of breast cancer cells at low concentrations and inhibit growth at higher concentrations (11339).

Adverse Reactions

None reported.

Interactions with Herbs & Other Dietary Supplements

None known.

Interactions with Drugs

None known.

Interactions with Foods

None known.

Interactions with Lab Tests

None known.

Interactions with Diseases or Conditions

None known.

Dosage and Administration

No typical dosage.

BLACK HAW

Also Known As

Blackhaw, Nanny Bush, Southern Black Haw, Stag Bush, Viburnum.

Scientific Names

Viburnum prunifolium; Viburnum lentago; Viburnum rufidulum.
Family: Adoxaceae/Viburnaceae or Caprifoliaceae.

People Use This For

Orally, black haw is used as a tonic, uterine sedative, antidiarrheal, diuretic, antispasmodic, to treat painful menses, preventing miscarriage, asthma, and as a postpartum antispasmodic.

Safety

LIKELY SAFE ...when the stem bark is used orally in amounts commonly found in foods. Black haw has Generally Recognized As Safe status (GRAS) for use in foods in the US (4912).
POSSIBLY SAFE ...when the root bark is used orally and appropriately in medicinal amounts (12).
PREGNANCY: POSSIBLY UNSAFE ...when used orally. Some evidence suggests black haw has uterine relaxant effects (11); avoid using.
LACTATION: Insufficient reliable information available.

Effectiveness

There is insufficient reliable information available about the effectiveness of black haw.

Mechanism of Action

The applicable parts of black haw are the root bark and stem bark. The root bark has several active constituents, including scopoletin, tannins, oxalic acid, salicin, salicylic acid biflavone, iridoid glycosiders, coumarins, urolic acid, and oleanolic acid (11,296,9241). Scopoletin is thought to be a uterine relaxant (11).
Black haw has spasmolytic activity in the uterus and other smooth muscle. It has been reported to cause vasoconstriction (9241).

Adverse Reactions

None reported.

Interactions with Herbs & Other Dietary Supplements

CALCIUM, IRON, ZINC: Concurrent use might decrease mineral absorption. Black haw contains oxalic acid (oxalate) (11,296), which can bind multivalent metal ions in the gastrointestinal (GI) tract and decrease mineral absorption.

Interactions with Drugs

None known.

Interactions with Foods

CALCIUM, IRON, ZINC: Concurrent use might decrease mineral absorption from foods. Black haw contains oxalic acid (oxalate) (11,296), which can bind multivalent metal ions in the gastrointestinal (GI) tract and decrease mineral absorption.

Interactions with Lab Tests

None known.

Interactions with Diseases or Conditions

ASPIRIN ALLERGY: Theoretically, the salicylate constituents in black haw could trigger allergic reaction in individuals with aspirin allergy or asthma.
KIDNEY STONES (Nephrolithiasis): Avoid the use of black haw because it contains oxalic acid and might increase stone formation in individuals with a history of kidney stones (11,12).

Dosage and Administration

ORAL: People typically use 2 teaspoons of the dried bark in 1 cup of water, boiled and simmered for 10 minutes. This is taken three times daily. In tincture form, black haw is taken 5 to 10 mL three times daily (5253).

Comments

Black haw is a shrub that has serrated oval leaves, clusters of white flowers, and blue-black berries. It is native to the woodlands of central and southern North America (4201).

BLACK HELLEBORE

Also Known As

Christe Herbe, Christmas Rose, Christmas Rose Plant, Melampode.
CAUTION: See separate listings for American Hellebore, Pheasant's Eye, and White Hellebore.

Scientific Names

Helleborus niger.
Family: Ranunculaceae.

People Use This For

Orally, black hellebore is used for nausea, worm infestations, regulating menstruation, acute nephritis, head colds, as a laxative, and as an abortifacient.

Safety

LIKELY UNSAFE ...when used orally. Black hellebore contains cardiac glycosides with structure, activity, and adverse effects similar to digitalis (3).
PREGNANCY: LIKELY UNSAFE ...when used orally because it can have menstrual stimulant (19) or abortifacient effects (18); avoid using.
LACTATION: LIKELY UNSAFE ...when used orally (3); avoid using.

Effectiveness

There is insufficient reliable information available about the effectiveness of black hellebore.

Mechanism of Action

Black hellebore root contains cardioactive glycosides with digitalis-like effects (18). It also contains saponins that irritate mucous membranes and can cause toxicity (18). Black hellebore is a GI irritant (19), and the fresh plant has local irritant properties (19).

Adverse Reactions

Orally, black hellebore can cause GI irritation (19). The symptoms of poisoning from black hellebore include scratchy throat or mouth, salivation, nausea, vomiting, diarrhea, dizziness, shortness of breath, spasm, and asphyxiation (18).
Topically, the fresh plant may cause irritation or inflammation when handled (19).

Interactions with Herbs & Other Dietary Supplements

CARDIAC GLYCOSIDE-CONTAINING HERBS: Contraindicated; concomitant use can increase the risk of cardiac glycoside toxicity. Cardiac glycoside-containing herbs, including black hellebore, Canadian hemp roots, digitalis leaf, hedge mustard, figwort, lily-of-the-valley roots, motherwort, oleander leaf, pheasant's eye plant, pleurisy root, squill bulb leaf scales, and strophanthus seeds (19).
LICORICE/HORSETAIL: Theoretically, overuse/misuse of licorice rhizome or horsetail plant with cardiac glycoside-containing herbs increases the risk of toxicity due to potassium depletion (19).
OTHER CARDIOACTIVE HERBS: Avoid concomitant use with other cardioactive herbs due to unpredictability of effects and adverse effects. Other cardioactive herbs include calamus, cereus, cola, coltsfoot, devil's claw, European mistletoe, fenugreek, fumitory, ginger, Panax ginseng, hawthorn, white horehound, mate, parsley, quassia, scotch broom flower, shepherd's purse, and wild carrot (4).
STIMULANT LAXATIVE HERBS: Theoretically, overuse or misuse of stimulant laxatives with cardiac glycoside-containing herbs increases the risk of cardiac toxicity due to potassium depletion. Stimulant laxative herbs include aloe dried leaf sap, blue flag rhizome, alder buckthorn, European buckthorn, butternut bark, cascara bark, castor oil, colocynth fruit pulp, gamboge bark exudate, jalap root, black root, manna bark exudate, podophyllum root, rhubarb root, senna leaves and pods, wild cucumber fruit (Ecballium elaterium), and yellow dock root (19).

Interactions with Drugs

DIGOXIN (Lanoxin): Black hellebore contains cardiac glycosides. Using black hellebore in combination with digoxin might have additive effects and increase the risk of toxicity (18,19).
DIURETIC DRUGS: Theoretically, concomitant use of potassium depleting diuretics and black hellebore can increase the risk of cardiac glycoside toxicity due to potassium depletion (506). Some diuretics that can deplete potassium include chlorothiazide (Diuril), chlorthalidone (Thalitone), furosemide (Lasix), hydrochlorothiazide (HCTZ, Hydrodiuril, Microzide), and others.
MACROLIDE ANTIBIOTICS: Theoretically, concomitant use might increase risk of cardiac glycoside toxicity (17). Some of these drugs include erythromycin, azithromycin, and clarithromycin.
QUININE: Theoretically, concomitant use of quinine and black hellebore can increase the risk of cardiac glycoside toxicity (506).

STIMULANT LAXATIVES: Theoretically, overuse or misuse of stimulant laxatives can increase the risk of cardiac glycoside toxicity due to potassium depletion (19,506).
TETRACYCLINE ANTIBIOTICS: Theoretically, concomitant use might increase risk of cardiac glycoside toxicity (17).

Interactions with Foods
None known.

Interactions with Lab Tests
None known.

Interactions with Diseases or Conditions
GASTROINTESTINAL (GI) INFLAMMATION: Black hellebore can aggravate gastrointestinal inflammation, contraindicated (19).
HEART DISEASE: Self-medication is contraindicated; requires diagnosis, treatment, and monitoring (515).

Dosage and Administration
No typical dosage.

Comments
Avoid confusion with white hellebore (Veratrum album). Black hellebore is an obsolete and dangerous natural product (18).

BLACK HOREHOUND

Also Known As
Ballota, Black Stinking Horehound.
CAUTION: See separate listing for White Horehound.

Scientific Names
Ballota nigra.
Family: Lamiaceae/Labiatae.

People Use This For
Orally, black horehound is used for nausea, vomiting, sedation in hysteria and hypochondria, nervous dyspepsia increasing bile flow, whooping cough, and as an antispasmodic. It is also used orally for symptomatic relief of nervous disorders in adults and children, especially mild sleep disorders, and for cough.
Topically, black horehound is used as a mild astringent and for gout.
Rectally, black horehound is used as an enema against ascaridae, or intestinal worms.

Safety
POSSIBLY SAFE ...when the above ground parts are used orally and appropriately in medicinal amounts (12). There is insufficient reliable information available about the safety of topical or rectal use of black horehound.
PREGNANCY: LIKELY UNSAFE ...when used orally; black horehound may affect the menstrual cycle (4). There is insufficient reliable information available about the safety of black horehound used topically or rectally during pregnancy.
LACTATION: Insufficient reliable information available; avoid using.

Effectiveness
There is insufficient reliable information available about the effectiveness of black horehound.

Mechanism of Action
The applicable parts of black horehound are the above ground parts. Chemicals isolated from black horehound include flavonoids (apigenin-7-glucoside, vicenin-2, tangeretin), diterpenoids (ballotinone, ballonigrine, 7-alpha-acetoxymarrubiin, ballotenol, preleosibirin, 13-hydroxyballonigrinolide), and phenylpropanoids (caffeoyl-L-malic acid, verbascoside, forsythoside B, arenarioside, ballotetroside, alyssonoside, lavandulifolioside, angoroside A). In vitro studies indicate that caffeoyl-L-malic acid, verbascoside, forsythoside B, and arenarioside are able to bind to dopaminergic D2, benzodiazepine and morphine (mu) receptors. Verbascoside, forsythoside B, caffeoyl-L-malic acid, arenarioside, and ballotetroside (in order of decreasing potency) also have antioxidant properties, as demonstrated by scavenging of reactive oxygen species and reducing their release from polymorphonuclear neutrophils in vitro (5880). Black horehound also has antiemetic (4,18), sedative, mild astringent (4), antispasmodic, and stimulant effects (18). Preliminary evidence suggests that the aqueous extracts of black horehound may reduce arterial blood pressure and heart rate and increase gallbladder secretions (18).

Adverse Reactions
None reported.

Interactions with Herbs & Other Dietary Supplements
None known.

Interactions with Drugs
DOPAMINE AGONISTS: Theoretically, black horehound might have additive effects when used with dopamine agonists. Some constituents of black horehound bind to dopamine D2 receptors in vitro (5880); however, this has not yet been reported in humans. Some dopamine agonists include bromocriptine (Parlodel), levodopa (Dopar, component of Sinemet), pramipexole (Mirapex), ropinirole (Requip), and others.

Interactions with Foods
None known.

Interactions with Lab Tests
None known.

Interactions with Diseases or Conditions
PARKINSON'S DISEASE: Theoretically, black horehound might affect therapy for Parkinson's disease. Some constituents of black horehound bind to dopamine D2 receptors in vitro (5880); however, this has not yet been reported in humans.
SCHIZOPHRENIA, PSYCHOTIC DISORDERS: Theoretically, black horehound might adversely affect people with schizophrenia and psychotic disorders. Some constituents of black horehound bind to dopamine D2 receptors in vitro (5880); however, this has not yet been reported in humans.

Dosage and Administration
ORAL: The typical dose of black horehound is 2-4 grams of the above ground parts or one cup of tea three times daily (4). The tea is prepared by steeping 2-4 grams of the above ground parts in 150 mL boiling water for 10-15 minutes and then straining. The usual dose of the liquid extract, 1:1 in 25% alcohol, is 1-3 mL three times daily (4). The common dose of the tincture, 1:10 in 45% alcohol, is 1-2 mL three times daily (4).
TOPICAL: No typical dosage.

Comments
Avoid confusion with white horehound.

BLACK MULBERRY

Also Known As
Mulberry, Purple Mulberry.

Scientific Names
Morus nigra.
Family: Moraceae.

Comments
At the date of publication, there was very little scientific information available about this product. Our staff is continually analyzing the available information on natural medicines and will add data to the online version of *Natural Medicines Comprehensive Database* as it becomes available. See www.naturaldatabase.com.

BLACK MUSTARD

Also Known As
Mustard.
CAUTION: See separate listings for Clown's Mustard Plant, Hedge Mustard, and White Mustard.

Scientific Names
Brassica nigra, synonym Sinapis nigra.
Family: Brassicaceae/Cruciferae.

People Use This For

Orally, black mustard oil is used for the common cold, rheumatism, and osteoarthritis. Black mustard seed is used for inducing vomiting, as a diuretic, and as an appetite stimulant.

Topically, black mustard seed is used as a poultice for pneumonia, pleurisy, osteoarthritis, lumbago, aching feet, and as a counterirritant.

In foods, black mustard is a flavoring agent in mustard condiments, foods, and beverages; and is a culinary spice.

Safety

LIKELY SAFE ...when used orally in the amounts commonly found in foods. Black mustard has Generally Recognized As Safe (GRAS) status in the US (4912).

POSSIBLY SAFE ...when used topically and appropriately, short-term (3,272).

LIKELY UNSAFE ...when the seed is used orally as an emetic. Black mustard seed is an irritant and exposes the esophageal tissue to corrosive effects (19). Ingesting a large amount of the seed can cause irritant poisoning (12). ...when pure mustard powder is applied topically for more than 15-30 minutes. Pure mustard powder can cause severe burns when applied to the skin for an extended period (12). ...when the undiluted oil used orally. Black mustard oil is an extremely powerful topical irritant. Ingesting large amounts can cause irritant poisoning (12). ...when inhaled (11).

CHILDREN: LIKELY UNSAFE ...when used orally (12,19). There is insufficient reliable information available about the safety of black mustard for its other uses in children.

PREGNANCY: LIKELY UNSAFE ...when used orally. Black mustard might have abortifacient and menstrual stimulant effects (19). There is insufficient reliable information available about the safety of black mustard for its other uses during pregnancy; avoid using.

LACTATION: Insufficient reliable information available; avoid using.

Effectiveness

There is insufficient reliable information available about the effectiveness of black mustard.

Mechanism of Action

The applicable parts of black mustard are the seed, oil, and powder. Black mustard powder contains the glucosinolate sinigrin, which produces allyl isothiocyanate when mixed with warm water (3,6,11). Allyl isothiocyanate has strong antimicrobial (bacterial and fungi) properties (11), lacrimatory effects, and can act as a counterirritant when diluted (1:50) (6,11). The glucosinolate products can have protective effects against carcinogens (11).

Allyl isothiocyanate also forms the basis for toxic agents such as the "mustard gases" and antineoplastic agents (11). Mustard oil is absorbed through the skin and eliminated through the lungs. This could explain its inclusion in liniment preparations to treat lung congestion (11).

Black mustard has powerful irritant properties that can cause pain and increase inflammation of the skin (6,11,18).

Adverse Reactions

Orally, large amounts of black mustard seed can lead to vomiting, stomach pain, diarrhea, somnolence, cardiac failure, breathing difficulties, coma, and possibly death (18). The isothiocyanate constituents can cause endemic goiters (6,11). In rare cases, black mustard oil exacerbates stomach and intestinal ulcers (18,19) and causes kidney irritation (19).

Topically, allyl isothiocyanate in black mustard can cause skin blistering and necroses (6,11,18), but contact allergies are rare (18).

Interactions with Herbs & Other Dietary Supplements

None known.

Interactions with Drugs

ANTACIDS: Theoretically, due to reports that black mustard increases stomach acid it might decrease the effectiveness of antacids (19).

H2-BLOCKERS: Theoretically, due to reports that black mustard increases stomach acid it might decrease the effectiveness of H2-blockers (19). The H2 blockers include cimetidine (Tagamet), ranitidine (Zantac), nizatidine (Axid), and famotidine (Pepcid).

PROTON PUMP INHIBITORS (PPIs): Theoretically, due to reports that black mustard increases stomach acid it decrease the effectiveness of PPIs (19). PPIs include omeprazole (Prilosec), lansoprazole (Prevacid), rabeprazole (Aciphex), pantoprazole (Protonix), and esomeprazole (Nexium).

Interactions with Foods

None known.

Interactions with Lab Tests

None known.

Interactions with Diseases or Conditions

ASTHMA: Coughing, sneezing, and possible asthma attacks can result from handling mustard flour (18).
GI IRRITATION: Black mustard can irritate the gastrointestinal tract. Contraindicated in individuals with infectious or inflammatory gastrointestinal conditions (19).

Dosage and Administration

TOPICAL: No typical dosage. However, traditionally a mustard plaster is prepared by using 100 grams of ground mustard seed with warm water to make a paste. The paste is packed in linen and applied to the affected area for 10 minutes (3-5 minutes for children over 6 years old) (18). Mustard plaster applied for longer than 15-30 minutes is associated with severe burns and skin necroses (12). Treatment should not exceed two weeks (19). As a counterirritant, black mustard oil is typically used in concentrations from 0.5% to 5% and as frequently as 3-4 times daily (3,272).

Comments

There are approximately 40 different species of mustard plant. Three different types are typically used to make the mustard condiment. Black mustard (Brassica nigra) is the most pungent. White mustard (Brassica alba) is the most mild and is used to make traditional American yellow mustard. Brown mustard (Brassica juncea) is dark yellow, has a pungent taste, and is used to make Dijon mustard.

BLACK NIGHTSHADE

Also Known As

Garden Nightshade, Houndsberry, Kakamachi, Petty Morel, Poisonberry.

Scientific Names

Solanum nigrum.
Family: Solanaceae.

People Use This For

Orally, black nightshade is used for gastric irritation, cramps, as an antispasmodic, pain reliever, sedative, and narcotic.
Topically, black nightshade is used for psoriasis, hemorrhoids, and abscesses. The bruised, fresh leaves are used topically to treat inflammation, burns and ulcers.

Safety

LIKELY UNSAFE ...when used orally (4009).
There is insufficient reliable information available about the safety of black nightshade for its other uses.
PREGNANCY AND LACTATION: LIKELY UNSAFE ...when used orally because of concerns it could be teratogenic (4009); avoid using.

Effectiveness

There is insufficient reliable information available about the effectiveness of black nightshade.

Mechanism of Action

Most of the toxic effects of black nightshade can be attributed to the solanine constituent. The green fruits have higher solanine concentrations and are therefore more toxic than the other plant parts. However, among plant strains, toxicity varies widely (4009).

Adverse Reactions

Orally, ingestion of large quantities of the green berries or fresh foliage with high alkaloid content can result in overdose. Symptoms include nausea, vomiting, headache, and in rare cases, dilation of the pupils (18). At doses of 200-400 mg, solanine can cause gastroenteritis, tachycardia, dyspnea, vertigo, drowsiness, lethargy, twitches of the arms and legs, and cramping. Other symptoms of poisoning include diarrhea, panic, excitation, coma, hyperthermia. This is followed later by a dazed state, paralysis, and rarely, death due to respiratory arrest and hypothermia (4009).

Interactions with Herbs & Other Dietary Supplements

None known.

Interactions with Drugs

None known.

Interactions with Foods

None known.

Interactions with Lab Tests
None known.

Interactions with Diseases or Conditions
None known.

Dosage and Administration
ORAL: No typical dosage.
TOPICAL: A handful of herb is placed in boiling water for 10 minutes, and used as a compress or a rinse (18).

Comments
Black nightshade is sometimes referred to as petty morel. This name is a corruption of the original, petit morel. Originally, black nightshade was called petit morel to differentiate it from the more poisonous species, deadly nightshade that is known as great morel. Black nightshade has a musk-like fragrance when wilting (18).

BLACK PEPPER AND WHITE PEPPER

Also Known As
Black Pepper, Blanc Poivre, Kosho, Krishna, Maricha, Pepe, Pepper, Pepper Extract, Pepper Plant, Peppercorn, Pfeffer, Pimenta, Pimienta, Piper, Piperine, Poivre, Poivre Noir, Vellaja, White Pepper.

Scientific Names
Piper nigrum.
Family: Piperaceae.

People Use This For
Orally, black pepper is used for stomach upset, bronchitis, and cancer. White pepper is used orally for stomach upset, malaria, cholera, and cancer.
Topically, black pepper is used for treating neuralgia and scabies. Black and white pepper are also used topically as a counterirritant for pain.
In foods and beverages, black pepper, white pepper, and pepper oil are used as flavoring agents.

Safety
LIKELY SAFE ...when used orally in amounts commonly found in foods. Black and white pepper have Generally Recognized As Safe (GRAS) status in the US (4912).
POSSIBLY SAFE ...when used orally and appropriately in medicinal amounts (12). ...when black pepper oil is used topically. Black pepper oil is nonirritating and is typically well tolerated (11).
CHILDREN: LIKELY SAFE ...when used orally in amounts commonly found in foods (11).
POSSIBLY UNSAFE ...when used orally in large amounts. Fatal cases of pepper aspiration have been reported in some patients (5619,5620). There is insufficient reliable information available about the safety of topical pepper oil when used in children.
PREGNANCY: LIKELY SAFE ...when used orally in amounts commonly found in foods (11).
LIKELY UNSAFE ...when used orally in large amounts. Black pepper might have abortifacient effects (11,19); contraindicated. There is insufficient reliable information available about the safety of topical pepper when used during pregnancy.
LACTATION: LIKELY SAFE ...when used orally in amounts commonly found in foods (11). There is insufficient reliable information available about the safety of black and white pepper when used in medicinal amounts during breast-feeding.

Effectiveness
There is insufficient reliable information available about the effectiveness of black pepper and white pepper.

Mechanism of Action
The applicable part of black pepper and white pepper is the fruit. Piper nigrum is said to have antiflatulent and diuretic properties (11), antimicrobial and insecticidal effects (18). It is thought to influence liver and metabolic functions (11), stimulate thermal receptors, induce sweating, and stimulate taste buds causing a reflex increase in gastric secretions (18). It might also have lipolytic activity related to the outer layer of the fruit (11). Piper nigrum contains piperine which increases oral absorption of drugs and other substances, possibly by modulating intestinal membrane dynamics (3757). Some evidence suggests piper nigrum might protect against colon cancer (3761); however, other evidence suggests black pepper might induce hepatic enzymes (3760) or cause liver tumors (3759).

Adverse Reactions

Orally, pepper can cause a burning aftertaste.
Topically, eye contact with ground pepper can cause redness of eyes and swelling of eyelids (5619). Deaths due to aspiration of large amounts of pepper have been reported (5619,5620).

Interactions with Herbs & Other Dietary Supplements

SPARTEINE: Piperine increases the bioavailability of sparteine, a constituent of scotch broom (19).

Interactions with Drugs

PHENYTOIN (Dilantin): Concomitant administration speeds absorption and slows elimination of phenytoin (Dilantin) (537).
PROPRANOLOL (Inderal): Concomitant administration speeds and increases absorption, and increases serum concentrations of propranolol (Inderal) (538).
THEOPHYLLINE: Concomitant administration increases absorption and serum concentrations of theophylline (Theo-Dur) (538).

Interactions with Foods

None known.

Interactions with Lab Tests

SERUM DRUG ASSAYS: Black pepper and white pepper can increase phenytoin, propranolol, and theophylline serum concentrations and test results (537,538).

Interactions with Diseases or Conditions

None known.

Dosage and Administration

ORAL: A typical dose of black pepper and white pepper ranges from 300-600 mg (18); up to 1.5 grams per day have been used (18).
TOPICAL: No typical dosage.

Comments

Black pepper is the dried, full grown but unripe fruit of Piper nigrum (11). White pepper is the dried ripe fruit of Piper nigrum with the outer covering that is known as a pericarp removed (11). Pepper oil is distilled from black pepper (11). Indian long pepper contains higher concentrations of piperine. Red pepper and cayenne contain no piperine.

BLACK PSYLLIUM

Also Known As

Brown Psyllium, Dietary Fiber, Fleaseed, Fleawort, French Psyllium, Plantain, Psyllion, Psyllios, Psyllium Seed, Spanish Psyllium.
CAUTION: See separate listings for Blond Psyllium, Buckhorn Plantain, Great Plantain, and Water Plantain.

Scientific Names

Plantago psyllium, synonym Psyllium afra; Psyllium indica, synonym Psyllium arenaria.
Family: Plantaginaceae.

People Use This For

Orally, black psyllium is used for chronic constipation and for softening stools in conditions such as hemorrhoids, anal fissures, anorectal surgery, and pregnancy. It is also used orally for diarrhea, irritable bowel syndrome (IBS), reducing elevated cholesterol, dysentery, and treating cancer.

Safety

LIKELY SAFE ...when used orally with appropriate fluid intake (4,12,272).
LIKELY UNSAFE ...when used orally without adequate fluid intake because it can cause esophageal obstruction (2,4,18). ...when the seeds of non-commercial preparations of black psyllium are chewed, crushed, or ground because they release a pigment that deposits in renal tubules (11) and can be nephrotoxic (6). This pigment has been removed from most commercial products (6).
PREGNANCY AND LACTATION: LIKELY SAFE ...when used orally with appropriate fluid intake (272).

Effectiveness

EFFECTIVE

Constipation. Taking black psyllium orally works as a bulk laxative and reduces constipation (272).

POSSIBLY EFFECTIVE

Hypercholesterolemia. Taking black psyllium orally seems to reduce total and LDL cholesterol, and the LDL:HDL ratio (6,11).

There is insufficient reliable information available about the effectiveness of black psyllium for its other uses.

Mechanism of Action

The applicable part of black psyllium is the seed. Its constituents are not absorbed and have no systemic effects (1). Black psyllium seed forms a mucilaginous mass when mixed with water and has a bulk laxative effect (1,4,6). In people with diarrhea, the mucilage absorbs water, provides mass, and prolongs gastrointestinal transit (1,6). In individuals with constipation, the mucilage absorbs water, swells, and stimulates peristalsis, reducing gastrointestinal transit time (1,4,6). Black psyllium can decrease abdominal pain in people with irritable bowel syndrome (IBS) by reducing rectosigmoidal pressure (405). Psyllium reduces peak blood glucose levels by slowing carbohydrate absorption (1,6) and can decrease cholesterol by absorbing dietary fats in the gastrointestinal tract, thereby preventing systemic absorption. It can also increase cholesterol elimination in the fecal bile acids (1,6,11,12). Chewing or crushing the seeds can release a pigment that deposits in renal tubules (11) and can be nephrotoxic (6). This pigment is removed from most commercial products (6).

Adverse Reactions

Orally, black psyllium can cause transient flatulence and abdominal distention (4). When consumed without water, it can cause esophageal (4) and bowel obstruction (4,604). Chewing or crushing the seeds can release a pigment that deposits in the renal tubules (11) and can be nephrotoxic (6). This pigment is removed from most commercial products (6). Allergic reactions to black psyllium include allergic rhinitis, conjunctivitis, urticaria, and asthma (18). Occupational exposure to black psyllium can cause sensitization, of which symptoms include sneezing, watery eyes, chest congestion, and anaphylactoid reaction (6).

Interactions with Herbs & Other Dietary Supplements

VITAMIN/MINERAL SUPPLEMENTS: The long-term use of black psyllium with vitamin or mineral supplements can reduce the absorption of calcium, iron, zinc, and vitamin B12 (1,12). Supplements should be taken one hour before or four hours after black psyllium to avoid this interaction (4,12).

Interactions with Drugs

ANTIDIABETES DRUGS: Black psyllium can reduce blood glucose levels in patients with type 2 diabetes (10091) and might have additive effects on glucose levels when used with antidiabetes drugs. Monitor blood glucose levels closely. Medication dose adjustments may be necessary. Some antidiabetes drugs include glimepiride (Amaryl), glyburide (Diabeta, Glynase PresTab, Micronase), insulin, pioglitazone (Actos), rosiglitazone (Avandia), and others.
CARBAMAZEPINE (Tegretol): Black psyllium can reduce carbamazepine absorption (539).
DIGOXIN (Lanoxin): Concomitant use might reduce digoxin absorption (1), requiring dose adjustment (12).
LITHIUM: Black psyllium use can reduce serum lithium levels (540). The fiber in lithium might decrease the absorption of lithium.

Interactions with Foods

NUTRIENT ABSORPTION: The long-term use of black psyllium with meals can reduce nutrient absorption requiring vitamin or mineral supplementation (12).

Interactions with Lab Tests

BLOOD GLUCOSE: Theoretically, black psyllium might lower postprandial blood glucose levels and test results (1,6,1405).
SERUM CHOLESTEROL: Black psyllium can lower total cholesterol and LDL cholesterol levels, LDL:HDL ratio, and test results (1,6,1405).

Interactions with Diseases or Conditions

DIABETES: Black psyllium can lower blood glucose levels in people with type 2 diabetes by retarding carbohydrate absorption (1405,8064). Monitor blood glucose levels closely. Doses of conventional antidiabetes medications may require adjustment. Also, warn patients with diabetes that some commercial blond psyllium products can contain added sugars and other absorbable carbohydrates which might increase blood glucose levels.
GI CONDITIONS: Black psyllium is contraindicated in people with fecal impaction, GI atony (1), GI tract narrowing, and obstruction or conditions that can lead to obstruction, such as spastic bowel (1,2,4,12,18).
HYPERSENSITIVITY: Some patients can have severe hypersensitivity reactions to black psyllium. This is more likely to occur in patients with previous occupation exposure to black psyllium (2328,2329,2330,8079,9246). Blond psyllium is contraindicated in these patients.
PHENYLKETONURIA: Avoid products containing aspartame (Nutrasweet) (272).

SWALLOWING DISORDERS: Patients with swallowing disorders might be at greater risk for esophageal obstruction when using blond psyllium. Blond psyllium is contraindicated in these patients (8080,8081).

Dosage and Administration

The amount of black psyllium seed required for an individual can vary. For best results, start with small amounts and increase to the desired response. Follow the package labeling when available.
ORAL: As a laxative, the typical dose of black psyllium seed is 10-30 grams per day (2,18), in divided amounts. Mix 10 grams seed in 100 mL water, to be followed by at least 200 mL water (18). Avoid chewing or crushing the seeds which can release a pigment that deposits in renal tubules (11). Adequate fluid intake is necessary and should be at least 150 mL water for each 5 grams of drug. The FDA labeling recommends at least 8 ounces (a full glass) of water or other fluid with each dose. Taking this product without enough liquid can cause choking (12). Black psyllium should be taken 30-60 minutes after a meal or the administration of other drugs (272).

Comments

Black psyllium is an aggressive-growing, perennial weed found throughout the world. The plant was spread with the colonization of the New World and was nicknamed "Englishman's foot" by the North American Indians. The FDA requires that psyllium be labeled: "WARNING: Taking this product without adequate fluid may cause it to swell and block your throat or esophagus and may cause choking. Do not take this product if you have difficulty in swallowing. If you experience chest pain, vomiting, or difficulty in swallowing or breathing after taking this product, seek immediate medical attention" (12).

BLACK ROOT

Also Known As

Beaumont Root, Bowman's Root, Culvers, Culveris Root, Hini, Oxadoddy, Physic Root, Purple Leptandra, Tall Speedwell, Tall Veronica, Veronica Virginica Root, Whorlywort.
CAUTION: See separate listings for Brooklime (Veronica beccabungo), Veronica (Veronica officinalis), Indian Physic, and Comfrey.

Scientific Names

Veronicastrum virginicum, synonyms Leptandra virginica, Veronica virginica.
Family: Scrophulariaceae.

People Use This For

Orally, black root is used for chronic constipation and disorders of the liver and gallbladder. It is also used as an emetic and to treat bilious fever.

Safety

POSSIBLY SAFE ...when the dried root is used orally (12). The dried root has a milder action than the fresh root (18).
POSSIBLY UNSAFE ...when the fresh root is used orally (12).
PREGNANCY: LIKELY UNSAFE ...when the fresh root is used orally because it has abortifacient and teratogenic effects (19). There is insufficient reliable information available about the safety of using the dried root; avoid using.
LACTATION: Insufficient reliable information available; avoid using.

Effectiveness

There is insufficient reliable information available about the effectiveness of black root.

Mechanism of Action

The applicable parts of black root are the rhizome and root. Black root is stated to have antiflatulent, laxative, and bowel evacuant properties (18). It can stimulate bile flow into the duodenum and induce sweating. It contains tannic acid, which has astringent properties that act on the GI mucosa. Tannic acid can also form insoluble complexes with alkaloids, glycosides, and certain heavy metals (6002).

Adverse Reactions

Orally, black root can cause abdominal pain or cramps, changes in stool color or odor, drowsiness, headache, nausea, and vomiting. Hepatotoxicity has been reported after ingestion of large amounts (6002).

Interactions with Herbs & Other Dietary Supplements
POTASSIUM DEPLETING HERBS: Theoretically, concomitant use with horsetail plant or the licorice rhizome can increase the risk of potassium depletion (19).
STIMULANT LAXATIVE HERBS: Theoretically, concomitant use with other stimulant laxative herbs can increase the risk of potassium depletion. Stimulant laxative herbs include aloe dried leaf sap, wild cucumber fruit (Ecballium elaterium), blue flag rhizome, alder buckthorn, European buckthorn, butternut bark, cascara bark, castor oil, colocynth fruit pulp, gamboge bark exudate, jalap root, manna bark exudate, podophyllum root, rhubarb root, senna leaves and pods, and yellow dock root (19).

Interactions with Drugs
DIGOXIN (Lanoxin): Theoretically, the overuse or abuse of black root can increase the risk of adverse effects of cardiac glycoside drugs. Black root chemically binds with the glycosides while in the gastrointestinal (GI) tract, which may reduce their effectiveness if used concomitantly (6002).
DIURETIC DRUGS: Overuse of black root might compound diuretic-induced potassium loss (19).There is some concern that people taking black root along with potassium depleting diuretics might have an increased risk for hypokalemia. Initiation of potassium supplementation or an increase in potassium supplement dose may be necessary for some patients. Some diuretics that can deplete potassium include chlorothiazide (Diuril), chlorthalidone (Thalitone), furosemide (Lasix), hydrochlorothiazide (HCTZ, Hydrodiuril, Microzide), and others.

Interactions with Foods
None known.

Interactions with Lab Tests
None known.

Interactions with Diseases or Conditions
GALLSTONES/BILE DUCT OBSTRUCTION: Black root is contraindicated, because it theoretically has bile stimulatory effects and could aggravate these conditions (19).
GASTROINTESTINAL (GI) INFLAMMATION: Black root is contraindicated in individuals with inflammation of the GI tract due to the irritant, emetic, and stimulant laxative effects (19).
HEMORRHOIDS: Theoretically, black root is contraindicated due to its cathartic properties (19).
MENSTRUATION: Theoretically, black root is contraindicated due to its cathartic properties (19).

Dosage and Administration
ORAL: People typically use one teaspoon of dried black root in one cup boiling water, which is allowed to steep for 30 minutes, to make a tea. The suggested dose is 1/3 cup before each meal. A black root tincture is taken as 2-4 drops in water. The powdered root bark is taken in a dose of 1-4 grams (223,5263).

Comments
Black root grows in the US and Canada and has a bitter and nauseous taste.

BLACK SEED

Also Known As
Ajenuz, Arañuel, Baraka, Black Cumin, Black Caraway, Charnuska, Cominho Negro, Cominho-Negro, Fennel Flower, Fennel-Flower, Fitch, Kalajaji, Kalajira, Kalonji, Love in a Mist, Mugrela, Nigelle de Crète, Nutmeg Flower, Nutmeg-Flower, Roman-Coriander, Schwarzkümmel, Toute Épice.
CAUTION: See separate listings for Caraway, Coriander, Cumin, Fennel, and Nutmeg.

Scientific Names
Nigella sativa.
Family: Ranunculaceae.

People Use This For
Orally, black seed is used for treating gastrointestinal conditions including gas, colic, diarrhea, dysentery, constipation and hemorrhoids. It is also used orally for respiratory conditions, including asthma, allergies, cough, bronchitis, emphysema, flu and congestion. Additionally, it is used orally as an antihypertensive, immunoprotectant, anticancer agent, and vermifuge. It is used orally for women's health: including as a contraceptive, for stimulation of menstruation, and increasing milk flow.
Topically, black seed is used for inflammatory conditions including rheumatism, headache and skin conditions. Traditionally, black seed has been used for headache, toothache, nasal congestion, and intestinal worms. It has also been used for conjunctivitis, abscesses, and parasites.

In combination with cysteine, vitamin E, and saffron, black seed is used to decrease cisplatin-induced side effects. In foods, black seed is used as a flavoring or spice.

Safety

LIKELY SAFE ...when used orally in amounts found in foods (6).
There is insufficient reliable information available about the safety of black seed for its other uses.
PREGNANCY: LIKELY UNSAFE ...when used orally in amounts exceeding those found in food.
Black seed may decrease or inhibit uterine contractions (241) and may have contraceptive activity (242).
LACTATION: Insufficient reliable information available; avoid using.

Effectiveness

There is insufficient reliable information available about the effectiveness of black seed.

Mechanism of Action

In allergic conditions, black seed might have antihistamine effects. Although not yet demonstrated in humans, low concentration of the constituent nigellone has been shown to inhibit the release of histamine from mast cells in animals (233). Black seed is thought to have immunoprotectant effects. Preliminary evidence suggests it may help minimize chemotherapy-induced decreases in hemoglobin and leukocyte counts. It may also enhance the production of certain human interleukins and alter macrophages (234). Black seed is also used as an anticancer agent. According to preliminary studies, black seed may inhibit stomach tumors, carcinoma, and Ehrlich ascites carcinoma (236,239). The black seed constituents thymoquinone and dithymoquinone are actually cytotoxic toward human cells (238). Although some evidence suggests thymoquinone may offer protection against chemically induced hepatotoxicity (237,240), a study in rats indicates that black seed may actually be hepatotoxic. A fixed oil from black seed is reported to have anti-eicosanoid and antioxidant effects, which may support anti-inflammatory activity (235), but this effect has not been studied in humans. The essential oil may have antimicrobial and anthelmintic activity, particularly against staphylococcus as well as other gram-positive and gram-negative bacteria (243,1516). Black seed may have anti-oxytocic potential, and may inhibit spontaneous contractions (241). It may also have contraceptive activity (242).

Adverse Reactions

Topically, black seed oil can cause allergic contact dermatitis (6). Black seed may be associated with hepatotoxicity based on preliminary animal research (245).

Interactions with Herbs & Other Dietary Supplements

None known.

Interactions with Drugs

None known.

Interactions with Foods

None known.

Interactions with Lab Tests

None known.

Interactions with Diseases or Conditions

None known.

Dosage and Administration

No typical dosage.

Comments

Black seed is reported to have been used for over 2000 years. Recordings mention it as far back as 1400 years. Black seed was found in the tomb of King Tutankhamen (6).
An issued patent covers the use of black seed to stimulate immune-competent cells in humans; however, this should not be taken as evidence for the safety and efficacy of black seed as an immunostimulant (246).

BLACK TEA

Also Known As

Black Leaf Tea, English Tea, Tea.

CAUTION: See separate listings for Caffeine, Cola nut, Coffee, Green Tea, Guarana, Mate, and Oolong Tea.

Scientific Names

Camellia sinensis, synonyms Camellia thea, Camellia theifera, Thea bohea, Thea sinensis, Thea viridis.

Family: Theaceae.

People Use This For

Orally, black tea is used for improving mental alertness, and cognitive performance. It is also used for headache, hypotension, atherosclerosis, and myocardial infarction; preventing Parkinson's disease; and reducing the risk of gastrointestinal cancer, ovarian cancer, and breast cancer. It is also used for stomach disorders, vomiting, diarrhea, preventing dental caries and kidney stones, and as a diuretic. In combination with various other products, black tea is used orally for weight loss.

In foods, black tea is consumed as a hot or cold beverage.

Safety

LIKELY SAFE ...when used orally in moderate amounts (9222,9223,9224,9228,9233,9234,9235,9236).

POSSIBLY UNSAFE ...when used orally long-term or in high doses. Black tea contains a significant amount of caffeine. Chronic use, especially in large amounts, can produce tolerance, habituation, psychological dependence, and other significant adverse effects. Doses greater than 250-300 mg per day have been associated with significant adverse effects such as tachyarrhythmias and sleep disturbances (11832). These effects would not be expected to occur with the consumption of decaffeinated black tea.

LIKELY UNSAFE ...when used orally in very high doses. The fatal acute oral dose of caffeine is estimated to be 10-14 grams (150-200 mg per kilogram). Serious toxicity can occur at lower doses depending on variables in caffeine sensitivity such as smoking, age, prior caffeine use, etc (11832).

CHILDREN: POSSIBLY SAFE ...when used in food and beverage amounts (4912,11833).

PREGNANCY: POSSIBLY SAFE ...when used orally in moderate amounts. Due to the caffeine content of black tea, mothers should closely monitor their intake to ensure moderate consumption. Fetal blood concentrations of caffeine approximate maternal concentrations (4260). Use of caffeine in pregnancy is controversial; however, moderate consumption has not been associated with clinically important adverse fetal effects (2708,2709,2710,2711,9606). Caffeine crosses the human placenta, but is not considered a teratogen. Mothers should keep caffeine consumption below 300 mg per day. This is similar to the amount of caffeine found in about 3 cups of coffee or tea (2708).

POSSIBLY UNSAFE ...when used orally in large amounts. Caffeine crosses the placenta, producing fetal blood concentrations similar to maternal levels (4260). Mothers should avoid consuming more than 300 mg of caffeine daily or more than 3 cups of tea or black tea per day (2708). High maternal doses of caffeine throughout pregnancy have resulted in symptoms of caffeine withdrawal in newborn infants (9891). High doses of caffeine have been associated with spontaneous abortion, premature delivery, and low birth weight (2709,2711). Fetal birth weight is reduced by 28 grams for every 100 mg-per-day of caffeine consumed during pregnancy. But this is unlikely to be clinically important except for women consuming more than 600 mg of caffeine daily (9606).

LACTATION: POSSIBLY SAFE ...when used orally in moderate amounts. Due to the caffeine content of black tea, nursing mothers should closely monitor caffeine intake. Breast milk concentrations of caffeine are thought to be approximately 50% of maternal serum concentrations. Minimal consumption would likely result in limited exposure to a nursing infant (9892). POSSIBLY UNSAFE ...when used orally in large amounts. Consumption of black tea might cause irritability and increased bowel activity in nursing infants (6026). Large doses or excessive intake of black tea should be avoided during lactation.

Effectiveness

LIKELY EFFECTIVE

Mental alertness. Consumption of black tea and other caffeinated beverages seems to prevent a decline in alertness and cognitive capacity when consumed throughout the day (4221,4224).Caffeine can improve mental performance and alertness following prolonged sleep deprivation (10205). Combining caffeine with taurine seems to provide a small improvement in mental performance (9899).

POSSIBLY EFFECTIVE

Atherosclerosis. Epidemiological evidence shows that black tea consumption seems to reduce the risk of severe aortic atherosclerosis, especially in women (3450).

Hypotension. Consuming caffeinated beverages seems to increase blood pressure in elderly people with postprandial hypotension (11834,11835).

Kidney stones (nephrolithiasis). Women consuming black tea seem to have an 8% decreased risk of developing kidney stones (4216).

Myocardial infarction (MI). There is some evidence that people who consume black tea have a lower risk of MI (4222,8119,8121). Consuming black tea for at least one year before a heart attack also seems to reduce the risk of subsequent death (8120).

Parkinson's disease. There is some evidence from large-scale epidemiological studies that people who consume caffeinated beverages such as coffee, tea, and cola have a decreased risk of Parkinson's disease. For men, the effects seem to be dose related. For example, men consuming a total of 421-2716 mg of caffeine from any source daily seem to have the greatest reduction in risk. However, there seems to be a significant reduction in risk even with consumption of as little as 124-208 mg caffeine per day (6022). In women, the effects do not seem to be dose related. Moderate consumption of caffeine (equivalent to one to four cups black tea daily) seems to provide the most reduction in risk (1238). Drinking black tea appears to reduce the incidence of Parkinson's disease among people who smoke (9236).

POSSIBLY INEFFECTIVE

Breast cancer. People who drink black tea do not seem to have a lower risk of breast cancer (9235).

Gastrointestinal cancer. People who drink black tea do not seem to have a lower risk of colon cancer, stomach cancer, or rectal cancer (9222,9223,9224,9233,9234).

Ovarian cancer. People who drink black tea do not seem to have a lower risk of ovarian cancer (9228).

INSUFFICIENT RELIABLE EVIDENCE to RATE

Osteoporosis. There is some preliminary evidence that black tea might be beneficial for preventing osteoporosis by improving bone mineral density (6404). More evidence is needed to rate black tea for this use

Mechanism of Action

The applicable parts of black tea are the leaf and stem. Black tea is different than green and oolong teas. Black tea is fully fermented tea. Oolong tea is partially fermented. Green tea is not fermented.

Polyphenols such as flavonoids including catechins, thearubigins, and theaflavins are abundant in black tea, and are thought to be responsible for many of its proposed benefits as an antioxidant (6032,6033,9232). Black tea contains 2% to 4% caffeine (519). Black tea also contains significant amounts of gallic acid, an antioxidant with antimutagenic and anticarcinogenic activities (8123). Polyphenols, such as thearubigin, in tea also appear to have antimutagenic effects and may protect DNA (12523).

It's often thought that green tea has more polyphenols, and therefore greater potential health benefits, than black tea. But there is some evidence that suggests there is no difference in quantity and quality of polyphenols between green and black teas (12087).

Theaflavins are effective antioxidants, which may be beneficial for preventing atherosclerosis and cardiovascular disease (9232). Consumption of a theaflavin-enriched green tea extract has been shown to produce mild reductions in low-density lipoprotein (LDL) levels (11308). In addition, a single dose of black tea can increase the concentration of antioxidants in serum (6032,6033). However, drinking black tea on a regular basis does not appear to significantly reduce lipoprotein oxidation (9230,9231). Preliminary evidence suggests that consumption of four cups of black tea might restore blood vessel dilation to near-normal in people with heart disease. Constituents other than caffeine are thought to be responsible for this effect. Acute or chronic consumption of black tea does not seem to inhibit platelet aggregation in people with coronary heart disease and is unlikely to be responsible for the reported beneficial effect of black tea on heart disease (8905). Earlier conflicting evidence had suggested that an inhibitory effect on platelets resulted from a higher concentration of flavonoids than is attainable with oral intake (8028,8029).

Black tea might also have a negative effect on a cardiac risk factor. There is evidence suggesting that black tea increases homocysteine levels, possibly due to the high concentration of polyphenols in tea (8035). It is unknown whether this effect decreases any of the benefits black tea may have in reducing cardiovascular disease.

Caffeine, a constituent of black tea, has been reported to cause increases and decreases in blood glucose. In people with type 2 diabetes, acute administration of caffeine impairs postprandial glucose metabolism, while acute abstention from caffeine reduces postprandial glucose levels by 21%. Whether these effects also occur with caffeinated beverages and herbs is unknown (12374). Other research in obese people suggests that caffeine ingestion may contribute to insulin resistance (12375). However, one study found that type 1 diabetics taking 200 mg of caffeine twice daily had increased frequency and intensity of warning signs of hypoglycemia. This may be due to a reduction in blood flow to the brain and an increase in glucose utilization by the brain (6024).

For osteoporosis, the mechanism is not known, but it is thought that isoflavonoids in black tea have weak estrogenic effects that might be beneficial for postmenopausal women with low endogenous estrogen levels (6404). Tea consumption seems to raise prolactin levels in women (an indicator of estrogen activity) in a dose-dependent manner (8122).

The caffeine in black tea stimulates the central nervous system (CNS), heart, muscles, and possibly the pressor centers that control blood pressure (2722). Possible mechanisms include adenosine receptor blockade and phosphodiesterase inhibition (2722). By blocking adenosine receptors, caffeine is thought to increase the release of neurotransmitters such as dopamine (6370). Caffeine also decreases airway resistance and stimulates respiration, via adenosine receptor blockade and phosphodiesterase inhibition (11836). It has also been proposed that caffeine may decrease GABA and serotonin signaling (6370). Caffeine stimulates gastric acid secretion, and increases plasma catecholamine levels (11837). Caffeine can have positive inotropic and chronotropic effects on the heart (11836). Caffeine can also acutely elevate both diastolic and systolic blood pressure, but might not have this effect in habitual users (2722).

Caffeine exerts a diuretic effect, with water losses estimated at 1.17 mL per milligram of caffeine (2712). Tachyphylaxis to the diuretic effect develops rapidly, diminishing fluid losses associated with caffeine intake (10206).

Caffeine-containing beverages consumed during moderate endurance exercise do not appear to compromise bodily hydration status (2713). Caffeine does not substantially affect the fluid status of people who drink caffeinated beverages on a regular basis (10206). The caffeine content is also thought to be responsible for black tea's effects on cognitive performance (4221,4224).

For prevention of Parkinson's disease, caffeine in black tea may prevent adenosine's inhibition of dopaminergic transmission. This may result in a reduction in the clinical expression of Parkinsonism (6022).

Adverse Reactions

Orally, black tea, due to its caffeine content, can cause insomnia, nervousness, restlessness, gastric irritation, nausea, vomiting, tachycardia, quickened respiration, tremors, delirium, convulsions, and diuresis. Large doses can produce headache, anxiety, agitation, ringing in the ears, premature heartbeat, and arrhythmia (11832,11838). In fatal overdose, the cause of death is usually ventricular fibrillation (11838). In infants, black tea can cause microcytic anemia (631). The caffeine in black tea may exacerbate sleep disturbances in patients with acquired immunodeficiency syndrome (AIDS) (10204).

Although acute administration of black tea can cause increased blood pressure, regular consumption does not seem to increase either blood pressure or pulse, even in mildly hypertensive patients (1451,1452,2722).

Tolerance to caffeine is a widely held belief, but there is little supportive clinical evidence. If it exists, it appears to be of little clinical significance (11839). Withdrawal symptoms such as irritability, sleepiness, delirium, nausea, vomiting, rhinorrhea, nervousness, restlessness, anxiety, muscle tension, muscle pains, and flushed face have been described. However, these symptoms may be from nonpharmacological factors related to knowledge and expectation of effects. Clinically significant symptoms caused by caffeine withdrawal may be uncommon (2723,11839).

Some evidence shows caffeine is associated with fibrocystic breast disease, breast cancer, and endometriosis in women; however, this is controversial since findings are conflicting (8043). Restricting caffeine in women with fibrocystic breast conditions doesn't seem to affect breast nodularity, swelling, or pain (8996).

There is evidence that daily consumption of strong black tea (2 liters) or black tea solids (4 grams) can raise plasma homocysteine levels, however it is unclear if lower doses have this effect (8035). There is also some evidence consumption of black tea (greater than 1 cup per day) may increase the risk of colon cancer (8041).

Epidemiological evidence regarding the relationship between use of caffeine, a constituent of black tea, and the risk for osteoporosis is contradictory. Caffeine can increase urinary excretion of calcium (2669,10202,11317). Women identified with a genetic variant of the vitamin D receptor appear to be at an increased risk for the detrimental effect of caffeine on bone mass (2669). However, moderate caffeine intake, less than 300 mg per day, does not seem to significantly increase osteoporosis risk in most postmenopausal women with normal calcium intake (2669,6025,10202,11317).

Combining ephedra with caffeine or caffeinated beverages can increase the risk of adverse effects. Jitteriness, hypertension, seizures, temporary loss of consciousness, and hospitalization requiring life support have been associated with the combined use of ephedra and caffeine (2729). There is also a report of ischemic stroke in an athlete who consumed ephedra 40-60 mg, creatine monohydrate 6 grams, caffeine 400-600 mg, and a variety of other supplements daily for six weeks (1275).

The caffeine in black tea can cause anaphylaxis in sensitive individuals, although true IgE-mediated caffeine allergy seems to be relatively rare (11315).

Interactions with Herbs & Other Dietary Supplements

CAFFEINE-CONTAINING HERBS/SUPPLEMENTS: Concomitant use can increase caffeine therapeutic and adverse effects. Natural products that contain caffeine include coffee, tea (black or green), guarana, mate, and cola.

CALCIUM: High caffeine intake from foods and beverages including black tea increases urinary calcium excretion (2570).

CREATINE: There is some concern that combining caffeine, a constituent of black tea, with ephedra, and creatine might increase the risk of serious adverse effects. There is a report of ischemic stroke in an athlete who consumed creatine monohydrate 6 grams, caffeine 400-600 mg, ephedra 40-60 mg, and a variety of other supplements daily for 6 weeks (1275). Caffeine might also decrease creatine's possible beneficial effects on athletic performance. Some researchers think caffeine can inhibit phosphocreatine resynthesis (2117,4575).

EPHEDRA (ma huang): Use of ephedra with black tea can increase the risk of stimulatory adverse effects due to its caffeine content. There is evidence that using ephedra with caffeine might increase the risk of serious life-threatening or debilitating adverse effects such as hypertension, myocardial infarction, stroke, seizures, and death (6486,10307). Tell patients to avoid taking black tea with ephedra and other stimulants.

IRON: Black tea appears to reduce absorption of non-heme iron from foods (8904). Infants given tea to drink have an increased risk of microcytic anemia (631). Theoretically, black tea might reduce the absorption of iron supplements. For most patients, this effect will not be clinically significant. Advise patients with iron deficiency to consume tea between meals rather than with meals to lessen this interaction (8904).

MAGNESIUM: Consuming large amounts of black tea can increase excretion of magnesium (11939).

Interactions with Drugs

ADENOSINE (Adenocard): The caffeine in black tea is a competitive inhibitor of adenosine at the cellular level. However, caffeine doesn't seem to affect supplemental adenosine because high interstitial levels of adenosine overcome the antagonistic effects of caffeine (11771). It is recommended that methylxanthines and methylxanthine-containing products be stopped 24 hours prior to pharmacological stress tests (11770). However, methylxanthines appear more likely to interfere with dipyridamole (Persantine) than adenosine-induced stress testing (11771).
ALCOHOL (Ethanol): Concomitant use of alcohol can increase caffeine serum concentrations and the risk of caffeine adverse effects. Alcohol reduces caffeine metabolism (6370).
ANTICOAGULANT/ANTIPLATELET DRUGS: Theoretically, the caffeine in black tea might increase the risk of bleeding when used concomitantly with these agents. Caffeine is reported to have antiplatelet activity (8028,8029); however, this interaction has not been reported in humans. Antiplatelet agents include aspirin, clopidogrel (Plavix), dipyridamole (Persantine), ticlopidine (Ticlid), and others. Anticoagulant agents include heparin and warfarin (Coumadin).
ANTIDIABETES DRUGS: Theoretically, concomitant use of caffeine, because of its caffeine content, and diabetes drugs might interfere with blood glucose control. Data are conflicting. Reports claim that caffeine might increase or decrease blood sugar (6024,8646).
CIMETIDINE (Tagamet): Cimetidine interacts with the caffeine in black tea and decreases caffeine clearance by 31% to 42% (11736).
CLOZAPINE (Clozaril): The caffeine in black tea might interact with clozapine and cause acute exacerbation of psychotic symptoms. Caffeine can increase effects and toxicity of clozapine. Caffeine doses of 400-1000 mg per day inhibit clozapine metabolism (5051).
CONTRACEPTIVE DRUGS: Theoretically, concomitant use might increase caffeine concentrations and the risk adverse effects, due to the caffeine contained in black tea. Contraceptive drugs decrease the rate of caffeine clearance by 40% to 65% (2714,11737).
DIPYRIDAMOLE (Persantine): The caffeine in black tea might inhibit dipyridamole-induced vasodilation (11770,11772). It is recommended that methylxanthines and methylxanthine-containing products be stopped 24 hours prior to pharmacological stress tests (11770). Methylxanthines appear more likely to interfere with dipyridamole (Persantine) than adenosine-induced stress testing (11771).
DISULFIRAM (Antabuse): Concomitant use can decrease clearance and increase the half-life of caffeine, increasing effects and risk of adverse effects (11840).
EPHEDRINE: Use of ephedrine with caffeine-containing products can increase the risk of stimulatory adverse effects. There is evidence that using ephedrine with caffeine might increase the risk of serious life-threatening or debilitating adverse effects such as hypertension, myocardial infarction, stroke, seizures, and death (6486,10307). Tell patients to avoid taking caffeine with ephedrine and other stimulants.
ESTROGENS: Concomitant use can increase serum concentrations of caffeine, a constituent of black tea, and the risk of caffeine adverse effects. Estrogen inhibits caffeine metabolism (2714).
FLUCONAZOLE (Diflucan): Concomitant use might increase the effects of caffeine in black tea. Fluconazole decreases caffeine clearance by approximately 25% (11022).
FLUVOXAMINE (Luvox): Concomitant use can increase serum concentrations of caffeine, a constituent of black tea, and the risk of caffeine adverse effects. Fluvoxamine reduces caffeine metabolism (6370).
LITHIUM: Abrupt withdrawal of the caffeine in black tea can increase serum lithium levels (609), worsening lithium tremor (610).
MEXILETINE (Mexitil): Concomitant use might increase the effects and adverse effects of caffeine in black tea. Mexiletine can decrease caffeine elimination by 50% (1260,11741).
MONOAMINE OXIDASE INHIBITORS (MAOIs): Theoretically, concomitant intake of large amounts of black tea with MAOIs might precipitate a hypertensive crisis, due to the caffeine contained in black tea. This is based on the claim that intake of large amounts of caffeine with MAOIs might precipitate a hypertensive crisis (15).
PHENOTHIAZINES: The tannins in black tea might cause precipitation of solutions of fluphenazine (Permitil, Prolixin), chlorpromazine (Thorazine), haloperidol (Haldol), prochlorperazine (Compazine), thioridazine (Mellaril), and trifluoperazine (Stelazine) (626,627).
PHENYLPROPANOLAMINE: Concomitant use of phenylpropanolamine and black tea might cause an additive increase in blood pressure due to the caffeine in black tea (11738).
QUINOLONE ANTIBIOTICS: Concomitant use can decrease caffeine clearance and increase effects and risk of adverse effects (606,607,608). Quinolones include ciprofloxacin (Cipro), enoxacin (Penetrex), norfloxacin (Chibroxin, Noroxin), sparfloxacin (Zagam), trovafloxacin (Trovan), and grepafloxacin (Raxar).
RILUZOLE (Rilutek): Theoretically, concomitant use of riluzole and caffeinated beverages such as black tea might increase serum caffeine and riluzole concentrations and the risk of adverse effects of both caffeine and riluzole. Caffeine and riluzole are both metabolized by cytochrome P450 1A2, and concomitant use might reduce metabolism of one or both agents (11739).
STIMULANT DRUGS: Due to the CNS stimulant effects of the caffeine constituent of black tea, concomitant use can increase the risk of adverse effects (11832). Some stimulant drugs include diethylpropion (Tenuate), epinephrine, phentermine (Ionamin), pseudoephedrine (Sudafed), and many others.
TERBINAFINE (Lamisil): Theoretically, concomitant use of terbinafine and caffeinated beverages such as black tea might increase serum caffeine concentrations and the risk of adverse effects. Terbinafine decreases

the rate of caffeine clearance (11740).
THEOPHYLLINE: The caffeine in black tea can increase theophylline levels (11862).
TRICYCLIC ANTIDEPRESSANTS (TCAs): The tannins in black tea might cause precipitation of solutions of amitriptyline (Elavil) or imipramine (Tofranil, Janimine) (626,627).
VERAPAMIL (Calan, Covera, Isoptin, Verelan): Theoretically, concomitant use of verapamil and caffeinated beverages such as black tea might increase plasma caffeine concentrations and the risk of adverse effects. Verapamil increases plasma caffeine concentrations by 25% (11741).

Interactions with Foods

IRON: Black tea may interfere with the absorption of iron in the diet. People who are iron-deficient should not drink black tea. Black tea doesn't seem to affect iron status in people with normal iron stores (631,9237).
MILK: When taken together, milk might bind the antioxidants in black tea and reduce their beneficial effects (220); however, in one study this interaction did not occur (6032).

Interactions with Lab Tests

5-HYDROXYINDOLEACETIC ACID: Black tea might increase urine 5-hydroxyindoleacetic acid concentrations and test results, due to its caffeine content. Caffeine can increase urine catecholamine concentrations (15).
BLEEDING TIME: Theoretically, black tea might increase bleeding time. Caffeine is reported to have antiplatelet activity (8028,8029). However, the significance of these effects in humans is not known.
CATECHOLAMINE: Caffeine can increase plasma catecholamine levels (8646).
CREATINE: The caffeine in black tea can increase urine creatine levels (1701).
DIPYRIDAMOLE THALLIUM IMAGING: Black tea might interfere with dipyridamole thallium imaging studies, due to its caffeine content. Caffeine attenuates the characteristic cardiovascular responses to dipyridamole and has altered test results (11742).
FERRITIN: Drinking black tea may cause a reduction in serum ferritin in iron-deficient people (631,9237).
GLUCOSE: Caffeine, a constituent of black tea, has been reported to cause increases and decreases in blood glucose (8646).
HEMOGLOBIN: Drinking black tea may cause a reduction in hemoglobin in iron-deficient people (631,9237).
IRON: In people with iron deficiency, black tea may further reduce the concentration of serum iron (631,9237).
LACTATE: The combination of ephedrine, a constituent of ephedra, and caffeine, a constituent of black tea, can increase blood lactate levels (8646).
NEUROBLASTOMA TESTS: Black tea (due to its caffeine content) might cause false-positive diagnosis of neuroblastoma, when diagnosis is based on tests of urine vanillylmandelic acid (VMA) or catecholamine concentrations. Caffeine can increase urine catecholamine and VMA concentrations (15).
PHARMACOLOGICAL STRESS TESTS: The caffeine in black tea is a competitive antagonist for adenosine receptors (11771). It is recommended that caffeine and caffeine-containing products be stopped 24 hours prior to pharmacological stress tests (11770). However, caffeine appears more likely to interfere with dipyridamole (Persantine) than adenosine (Adenocard) stress testing (11771). The interaction between caffeine and dipyridamole is unlikely to be significant in stress testing if the heart rate increase is greater than 5% after dipyridamole infusion (11772).
PHEOCHROMOCYTOMA TESTS: Black tea (due to its caffeine content) might cause false-positive diagnosis of pheochromocytoma, when diagnosis is based on tests of urine vanillylmandelic acid (VMA) or catecholamine concentrations. Caffeine can increase urine catecholamine and VMA concentrations (15).
PULMONARY FUNCTION TESTS: People may need to avoid caffeine and caffeinated beverages such as black tea for at least four hours prior to lung function testing. Forced expiratory volume in one minute (FEV1) seems to show a small improvement up to two hours after caffeine use. Mid-expiratory flow rates may also improve with caffeine for up to four hours (9607).
URATE: Black tea might falsely increase serum urate test results determined by the Bittner method, due to its caffeine content. Caffeine causes false elevations in serum urate test results determined by the Bittner method (11844).
URINARY CALCIUM: Caffeine, a constituent of black tea, can increase urinary calcium levels (11317).
VANILLYLMANDELIC ACID (VMA): Black tea might increase urine VMA concentrations and test results, due to its caffeine content. Caffeine can increase urine VMA concentrations (15).

Interactions with Diseases or Conditions

ANEMIA: Drinking black tea may worsen anemia in people with iron deficiency (631,9237).
ANXIETY DISORDERS: The caffeine in black tea might aggravate anxiety disorders (11743).
BLEEDING DISORDERS: Theoretically, caffeine in black tea might aggravate these conditions. Caffeine is reported to have antiplatelet activity (8028,8029); however, this interaction has not been reported in humans. Caffeine can prolong bleeding time and increase the results of a bleeding time test (1701).
CARDIAC CONDITIONS: Caffeine in black tea can induce cardiac arrhythmias in sensitive individuals (11845); use with caution.
DIABETES: Some research suggests that caffeine (a constituent of black tea) may impair postprandial glucose metabolism in people with diabetes and contribute to insulin resistance. The effect of caffeinated beverages such as black tea and herbs has not been studied (12374,12375). Caffeine in black tea may enhance the frequency and intensity

of hypoglycemic warning symptoms in type 1 diabetics. This may increase the ability of diabetics to detect and treat hypoglycemia early. However, it might also increase the frequency of hypoglycemic events (6024); use with caution. Caffeine has been reported to cause increases and decreases in blood glucose (8646); use with caution.
GLAUCOMA: Drinking caffeinated black tea increases intraocular pressure. The increase occurs within 30 minutes and persists for at least 90 minutes (8540).
HORMONE-SENSITIVE CANCERS/CONDITIONS: Because black tea might have weak estrogenic effects (6404), women with hormone-sensitive conditions should avoid high doses of black tea. Some of these conditions include breast, uterine, and ovarian cancer, and endometriosis and uterine fibroids.
HYPERTENSION: The caffeine in black tea might increase blood pressure in people with high blood pressure. However, this doesn't seem to occur in people who consume black tea or other caffeinated products regularly (1451,1452,2722).
OSTEOPOROSIS: Consuming caffeinated black tea can increase urinary excretion of calcium. Caffeine consumption should be limited to less than 300 mg per day (approximately 2-3 cups of black tea). Adequate calcium supplementation may partially compensate for calcium losses (2669,10202,11317). Postmenopausal women identified with a genetic variant of the vitamin D receptor should use caffeine with caution (2669).

Dosage and Administration

ORAL: A typical dose as a stimulant is several cups per day. The typical dose of caffeine for headache or restoring mental alertness is up to 250 mg per day (2718,11743). For reducing the risk of heart attack and kidney stones, a dose of at least one cup per day has been used (4216,4222,4224). For preventing atherosclerosis, consumption of 125-500 mL (1-4 cups) of brewed black tea daily has been used (3450). For preventing Parkinson's disease, men consuming 421-2716 mg total caffeine (approximately 5-33 cups of black tea) daily have the lowest risk of developing Parkinson's disease. However, a significantly lower risk is also associated with consumption of as little as 124-208 mg of caffeine (approximately 1-3 cups of black tea) daily (6022). In women, more moderate caffeine consumption seems to be best; equivalent to approximately 1-4 cups of black tea per day (1238).

Comments

Camellia sinensis leaves and stems are used to manufacture green tea (non-fermented), oolong tea (partially fermented), and black tea (fermented) (4218). Black tea is the more frequently ingested variety. Leaves used for green tea are prepared immediately after harvest, which limits enzymatic changes. Leaves used for black tea are fermented before preparation, promoting enzymatic changes. Consequently, black tea and green tea have different chemical constituents (8115).

BLACK WALNUT

Also Known As

Nogal Americano, Nogueira-preta, Noyer Noir, Schwarze Walnuss, Walnut.
CAUTION: See separate listing for English Walnut.

Scientific Names

Juglans nigra.
Family: Juglandaceae.

People Use This For

Orally, black walnut is used for diphtheria, leukemia, syphilis, and as an anthelmintic.
Topically, black walnut is used as a gargle, hair dye, insecticide, and for wounds.

Safety

POSSIBLY SAFE ...when used orally and appropriately, short-term (12).
POSSIBLY UNSAFE ...when used topically because it contains the constituent juglone (2). Daily use of the juglone-containing bark of a related species (English walnut) is associated with increased risk of tongue cancer and lip leukoplakia (2,12).
PREGNANCY AND LACTATION: POSSIBLY UNSAFE ...when used topically (12); avoid using. There is insufficient reliable information about the safety of black walnut used orally during pregnancy or lactation; avoid using.

Effectiveness

There is insufficient reliable information available about the effectiveness of black walnut.

Mechanism of Action
The applicable part of black walnut is the hull. Black walnut hulls contain approximately 45% tannins (19) which exert an astringent effect on the mucosal tissue. Tannins work internally by dehydrating mucosal tissue, which reduces secretions. Externally, tannin astringent effects result in a protective layer of constricted, harder cells. Plants with at least 10% tannins can cause gastrointestinal upset, kidney damage, and liver damage. Animal data conflicts with respect to the carcinogenicity of tannins. They may be carcinogenic or may even have anti-carcinogenic effects. An increased risk of esophageal or nasal cancer may be linked with people who regularly ingest herbs with high tannin concentrations (12).

Adverse Reactions
None reported.

Interactions with Herbs & Other Dietary Supplements
TANNIN-CONTAINING HERBS: Theoretically, herbs such as black walnut contain high percentages of tannins, which might cause precipitation of constituents of other herbs (19).

Interactions with Drugs
ORAL DRUGS: Theoretically, concomitant oral administration might cause precipitation of some drugs due to the high tannin content of black walnut hulls (19). Separate administration of oral drugs and tannin-containing herbs by the longest period of time practical (19).

Interactions with Foods
None known.

Interactions with Lab Tests
None known.

Interactions with Diseases or Conditions
None known.

Dosage and Administration
No typical dosage.

BLACKBERRY

Also Known As
Bramble, Dewberry, Goutberry, Rubi Fruticosi Folium, Rubi Fruticosi Radix, Thimbleberry.
CAUTION: See separate listing for Raspberry.

Scientific Names
Rubus plicatus, synonyms Rubus fruticosus, Rubus affinis.
Family: Rosaceae.

People Use This For
Orally, blackberry is used for diarrhea and edema.
Topically, blackberry is used as a mouth rinse for mild inflammation of the mucosa of the oral cavity and throat.

Safety
POSSIBLY SAFE ...when used orally, short-term (12).
There is insufficient reliable information available about the safety blackberry for its other uses.
PREGNANCY AND LACTATION: Insufficient reliable information available; avoid using.

Effectiveness
There is insufficient reliable information available about the effectiveness of blackberry.

Mechanism of Action
The applicable part s of blackberry are the leaf and root. Tannin constituents in the leaf have an astringent effect and are thought to help relieve mucosal inflammation and diarrhea (12).

Adverse Reactions
None reported.

Interactions with Herbs & Other Dietary Supplements
None known.

Interactions with Drugs
None known.

Interactions with Foods
None known.

Interactions with Lab Tests
None known

Interactions with Diseases or Conditions
None known.

Dosage and Administration
No typical dosage.

BLACKTHORN

Also Known As
Pruni Spinosae Flos, Pruni Spinosae Fructus, Sloe Berry, Sloe Flower, Wild Plum Flower.

Scientific Names
Prunus spinosa.
Family: Rosaceae.

People Use This For
Orally, blackthorn flower is used for common colds, ailments of the respiratory tract, bloating, general exhaustion, dyspepsia, kidney and bladder ailments, and to treat and prevent gastric spasms. Blackthorn flower is also used orally as a laxative, diuretic, diaphoretic, expectorant, and as a component in "blood cleansing" teas.
Blackthorn berry is used as a mouth rinse (gargle) for mild inflammation of the oral and pharyngeal mucosa. The syrup and wine of the blackthorn berry are used for purging the bowels and as a diuretic. The berry marmalade is used for dyspepsia.
Topically, blackthorn flower is used for rashes, skin impurities, and "blood purification."
In foods, blackthorn flower is utilized in herbal teas as a coloring agent.

Safety
POSSIBLY UNSAFE ...when used orally. Fresh blackthorn berries and seeds contain cyanogenic glycosides, which can cause toxicity (12).
PREGNANCY AND LACTATION: POSSIBLY UNSAFE ...when used orally; avoid using. Fresh blackthorn flowers and seeds contain cyanogenic glycosides that can be teratogenic (12).

Effectiveness
There is insufficient reliable information available about the effectiveness of blackthorn.

Mechanism of Action
The applicable parts of blackthorn are the berries and dried flowers. Blackthorn berries contain tannins. The astringent properties of the tannin constituents can contribute to the reduction of mucous membrane inflammation (7). Fresh blackthorn berries and seeds contain cyanogenic glycosides, which can cause toxicity (12).

Adverse Reactions
None reported; however, blackthorn berries and seeds contain cyanogenic glycosides, which can be toxic (12).

Interactions with Herbs & Other Dietary Supplements
None known.

Interactions with Drugs
None known.

Interactions with Foods
None known.

Interactions with Lab Tests
None known.

Interactions with Diseases or Conditions
None known.

Dosage and Administration
ORAL: No typical dosage. However, traditionally blackthorn berry tea is used as a mouth rinse up to two times per day. The tea is made from 1-2 grams of berries in 150 mL of boiling water (12). Blackthorn flower is also used as a tea, 1-2 cups during the day or 2 cups in the evening. The tea is prepared by steeping 1-2 heaping teaspoons of dried flower (1-2 grams) in 150 mL boiling water for 5-10 minutes and then straining (18). Blackthorn is for short-term use only (12).

BLADDERWORT

Also Known As
None.
CAUTION: See separate listing for Bladderwrack.

Scientific Names
Utricularia vulgaris.
Family: Lentibulariaceae.

Comments
At the date of publication, this product was not a common ingredient used in brand name supplements marketed to consumers. Details about this product are available in the online version of *Natural Medicines Comprehensive Database.* See www.naturaldatabase.com.

BLADDERWRACK

Also Known As
Black Tang, Bladder Fucus, Blasentang, Cutweed, Fucus, Kelp, Kelp-Ware, Knotted Wrack, Marine Oak, Meereiche, Quercus Marina, Rockweed, Rockwrack, Schweintang, Seawrack, Tang, Varech.
CAUTION: See separate listings for Algin, Bladderwort, and Laminaria.

Scientific Names
Fucus vesiculosus; Ascophyllum nodosum; other Fucus species.
Family: Fucaceae.

People Use This For
Orally, bladderwrack is used for thyroid disorders, iodine deficiency, lymphadenoid goiter, myxedema, obesity, arthritis, and rheumatism. Bladderwrack is also used orally for arteriosclerosis, digestive disorders, heartburn, "blood cleansing", to increase energy, constipation, bronchitis, emphysema, genitourinary disorders, decreased resistance to disease, and anxiety.
Topically, bladderwrack is used for skin diseases, burns, aging skin, and insect bites.

Safety
POSSIBLY UNSAFE ...when used orally. Bladderwrack can contain high concentrations of iodine and heavy metals (12788,12789). Ingesting more than 150 mcg iodine per day can cause hyperthyroidism or exacerbate existing hyperthyroidism (12788). Heavy metal poisoning has also been reported (645).
PREGNANCY AND LACTATION: LIKELY UNSAFE ...when used orally (12788,12789); avoid using.

Effectiveness
There is insufficient reliable information available about the effectiveness of bladderwrack.

Mechanism of Action
The applicable part of bladderwrack is the entire plant. Bladderwrack is a brown algae (seaweed).
Bladderwrack contains high concentrations of iodine, which is present in varying amounts. It can also contain heavy metals such as arsenic and cadmium. Bladderwrack is also a source of fiber, minerals such as iron, and vitamin B12 (12789).
Preliminary clinical research suggests bladderwrack might extend the menstrual cycle and have anti-estrogenic effects in premenopausal women. It may also increase progesterone levels (12790).
Preliminary research suggests that extracts of bladderwrack also might have antibacterial, anti-HIV, and antioxidant activity (12791,12792,12793).

Fucoidan, a sulfated polysaccharide derivative of bladderwrack, seems to be active against a variety of viruses including the herpes virus, HIV, and cytomegalovirus (12794). Other preliminary research suggests that fucoidan might have antifertility effects by preventing the binding of sperm to egg (12795). Fucoidan also seems to stimulate the activity of transforming growth actor (TGF)-beta to increase fibroblast proliferation, which suggests it might be useful for treatment of wound healing (12796). Preliminary research also suggests that fucoidan also has anticoagulant, fibrinolytic, and antiplatelet adhesion effects (12797). Other preliminary research suggests that it might have antiangiogenic and antitumor activity (12798).

Preliminary clinical research suggests topical administration of bladderwrack extract might reduce skin thickness and other signs of aging (12799).

Adverse Reactions

Orally, bladderwrack can induce or exacerbate hyperthyroidism (12788,12789). The iodine in bladderwrack can cause idiosyncratic reactions. Prolonged, high intake of dietary iodine is associated with goiter and increased risk of thyroid cancer (7135). There is one case report of heavy metal poisoning where arsenic poisoning occurred with ingestions of a contaminated kelp product (645). Another case of arsenic-related poisoning with bladderwrack ingestion 400 mg three times a day for 3 months resulted in renal tubular necrosis and interstitial fibrosis (12800).

Interactions with Herbs & Other Dietary Supplements

HERBS WITH ANTICOAGULANT/ANTIPLATELET POTENTIAL: Theoretically, concomitant use of bladderwrack with herbs that might affect platelet aggregation might increase the risk of bleeding in some people (12797). These herbs include angelica, clove, danshen, fenugreek, feverfew, garlic, ginger, ginkgo, Panax ginseng, poplar, red clover, turmeric, and others.

Interactions with Drugs

ANTICOAGULANT/ANTIPLATELET DRUGS: Bladderwrack seems to have anticoagulant effects (12797). Theoretically, taking bladderwrack with antiplatelet or anticoagulant drugs might increase the risk of bruising and bleeding. Some of these drugs include aspirin; clopidogrel (Plavix); nonsteroidal anti-inflammatory drugs (NSAIDs) such as diclofenac (Voltaren, Cataflam, others), ibuprofen (Advil, Motrin, others), naproxen (Anaprox, Naprosyn, others); dalteparin (Fragmin); enoxaparin (Lovenox); heparin; warfarin (Coumadin); and others.

ANTITHYROID DRUGS: Theoretically, concomitant use may result in additive hypothyroid activity, and may cause hypothyroidism (7135). Some of these medications include methenamine mandelate (Methimazole), methimazole (Tapazole), potassium iodide (Thyro-Block), and others.

Interactions with Foods

None known.

Interactions with Lab Tests

ACTIVATED PARTIAL THROMBOPLASTIN TIME (aPTT): Theoretically, bladderwrack might increase aPTT test results due to the heparin-like activity of one of its constituents (12797).

ESTRADIOL: In premenopausal women, bladderwrack seems to lower 17-beta-estradiol levels in a dose-dependent manner (12790).

PROGESTERONE: In premenopausal women, bladderwrack seems to increase progesterone levels in a dose-dependent manner (12790).

RADIOACTIVE IODINE UPTAKE: Theoretically, bladderwrack might interfere with the results of thyroid function tests using radioactive iodine uptake (12789).

THYROID STIMULATING HORMONE (TSH): Theoretically, bladderwrack might increase serum TSH levels and test results (7135).

THYROXINE (T4): Theoretically, bladderwrack might increase serum T4 levels and test results (7135).

Interactions with Diseases or Conditions

INFERTILITY: Preliminary research suggests bladderwrack might impair fertility (12795). Avoid use in women trying to conceive.

IODINE ALLERGY: Avoid bladderwrack use in people sensitive to iodine (7135).

THYROID DYSFUNCTION: Prolonged use or excessive amounts of iodides may cause or exacerbate thyroid gland hyperplasia, thyroid adenoma, goiter, and hypothyroidism. Bladderwrack contains significant amounts of iodine, which might exacerbate hyper- or hypothyroidism (7135).

Dosage and Administration

No typical dosage.

Comments

Avoid confusion with bladderwort.

BLESSED THISTLE

Also Known As

Carbenia Benedicta, Cardo Santo, Carduus, Carduus Benedictus, Cnici Benedicti Herba, Cnicus, Holy Thistle, St. Benedict Thistle, Spotted Thistle.
CAUTION: See separate listing for Milk Thistle.

Scientific Names

Cnicus benedictus.
Family: Asteraceae/Compositae.

People Use This For

Orally, blessed thistle is used for loss of appetite and indigestion; and as an antidiarrheal, expectorant, antibiotic, and diuretic. It is also used orally for promoting lactation, and for treating colds and fever.
Topically, blessed thistle is used as a poultice for boils, wounds, and ulcers.
In manufacturing, blessed thistle is used as a flavoring in alcoholic beverages.

Safety

LIKELY SAFE ...when used orally in amounts commonly found in foods. Blessed thistle has Generally Recognized As Safe status (GRAS) for use in foods in the US (4912).
POSSIBLY SAFE ...when used orally and appropriately (12).
PREGNANCY: LIKELY UNSAFE ...when used orally (4,12); avoid using.
LACTATION: Insufficient reliable information available; avoid using.

Effectiveness

There is insufficient reliable information available about the effectiveness of blessed thistle.

Mechanism of Action

The applicable parts of blessed thistle are the flowering tops, leaves, and upper stems. Blessed thistle may have bacteriostatic properties due to the volatile oil content. The sesquiterpene lactone constituent, cnicin, may have antibacterial and antitumor activity (11). Metabolism of the constituents, arctiin and tracheoloside, following oral ingestion results in compounds that inhibit cyclic-AMP phosphodiesterase and histamine release from mast cells (11). Blessed thistle contains 8% tannins (4).

Adverse Reactions

Orally, when blessed thistle is used in high doses (greater than five grams per cup of tea), it can cause stomach irritation and vomiting (12). Blessed thistle may cause an allergic reaction in individuals sensitive to the Asteraceae/Compositae family. Members of this family include ragweed, chrysanthemums, marigolds, daisies, and many other herbs.

Interactions with Herbs & Other Dietary Supplements

None known.

Interactions with Drugs

ANTACIDS: Theoretically, due to reports that blessed thistle increases stomach acid, blessed thistle might decrease the effectiveness of antacids (19).
H2-BLOCKERS: Theoretically, due to reports that blessed thistle increases stomach acid, blessed thistle might decrease the effectiveness of H2-blockers (19). The H2 blockers include cimetidine (Tagamet), ranitidine (Zantac), nizatidine (Axid), and famotidine (Pepcid).
PROTON PUMP INHIBITORS (PPIs): Theoretically, due to reports that blessed thistle increases stomach acid, blessed thistle might decrease the effectiveness of PPIs (19). PPIs include omeprazole (Prilosec), lansoprazole (Prevacid), rabeprazole (Aciphex), pantoprazole (Protonix), and esomeprazole (Nexium).

Interactions with Foods

None known.

Interactions with Lab Tests

None known.

Interactions with Diseases or Conditions

CROSS-ALLERGENICITY: Blessed thistle may cause an allergic reaction in individuals sensitive to the Asteraceae/Compositae family. Members of this family include ragweed, chrysanthemums, marigolds, daisies, and many other herbs.

GASTROINTESTINAL (GI) IRRITATION: Blessed thistle may irritate the GI tract. It is contraindicated in individuals with infectious or inflammatory GI conditions (19).

Dosage and Administration

ORAL: The typical dose of the dried, flowering tops is 1.5-3 grams as a tea three times daily. The tea is prepared by steeping the dried, flowering tops in boiling water and then straining. 1.5-3 mL of the liquid extract, 1:1 in 25% alcohol, is commonly taken three times daily (4).

TOPICAL: No typical dosage.

Comments

Blessed thistle was commonly used during the Middle Ages to treat the bubonic plague and as a tonic for monks. Avoid confusion with milk thistle (Silybum marianum).

BLOND PSYLLIUM

Also Known As

Blond Plantago, Dietary Fiber, Englishman's Foot, Indian Plantago, Ispaghula, Ispagol, Pale Psyllium, Plantaginis ovatae semen, Plantaginis ovatae testa, Sand Plantain, Spogel.

CAUTION: See separate listings for Black Psyllium, Buckhorn Plantain, Great Plantain, and Water Plantain.

Scientific Names

Plantago ovata, synonyms Plantago fastigiata, Plantago insularis, Plantago ispaghula, Plantago decumbens.

Family: Plantaginaceae.

People Use This For

Orally, blond psyllium is used for constipation, softening stools in patients with hemorrhoids and during pregnancy, anal fissures, post-anorectal surgery. It is also used for diarrhea, irritable bowel syndrome (IBS), hyperlipidemia, hypertension, diabetes, dysentery, cancer, ulcerative colitis, weight control, and end-stage renal disease.

Topically, blond psyllium is used as a poultice for furunculosis (boils).

In food manufacturing, blond psyllium is used as a thickener or stabilizer in some frozen dairy desserts.

Safety

LIKELY SAFE ...when used orally and appropriately. Blond psyllium preparations have been safely used in doses up to 20 grams per day for up to 6 months (1376,2324,2327,6261,6262,8060,8061,8066,8423,9422,10095,13102).

PREGNANCY AND LACTATION: LIKELY SAFE ...when used orally and appropriately (272).

Effectiveness

EFFECTIVE

Constipation. Taking blond psyllium orally is effective as a bulk laxative for reducing constipation or softening stools (8424,9423,10092). Some evidence suggests that blond psyllium alone can relieve constipation and improve stool consistency as effectively as preparations containing blond psyllium plus senna (8424) or docusate sodium (10088).

LIKELY EFFECTIVE

Hyperlipidemia. Taking blond psyllium orally reduces cholesterol levels in patients with mild to moderate hypercholesterolemia. Blond psyllium seed husk or seed added to food or as a separate supplement in a dose of approximately 10-12 grams daily, in combination with a low-fat or a high-fat diet, can reduce levels of total cholesterol by 3% to 14%, low density lipoprotein (LDL) cholesterol by 5% to 10%, and apolipoprotein B by 8.8% after 7 weeks or more of treatment. It also significantly reduces the LDL to high-density lipoprotein (HDL) ratio after 6 months of treatment (1376,2324,2327,6261,6262,8060,8061,8066,10095).

There is evidence the LDL:HDL ratio can be reduced further when psyllium is consumed with a diet containing approximately 12% of energy as monounsaturated fatty acids and 29% of total fat (8067).

Some evidence suggests that psyllium seed might be more effective than the seed husk for lowering cholesterol (8069).

Psyllium seems to be less effective in older patients. There is some evidence that it lowers LDL cholesterol levels to a lesser degree in patients 60 years or older compared to patients under 60 (2326). Blond psyllium does not significantly increase HDL levels and may actually lower HDL cholesterol levels in some patients. However, the magnitude of change in the HDL level is much less than changes in total and LDL cholesterol levels (1376,8433,10095). Blond psyllium also does not seem to lower triglycerides (13102).

Blond psyllium seems to be most effective when consumed with foods at mealtime (8062). Breakfast cereal containing blond psyllium can modestly decrease total cholesterol and LDL cholesterol, by 5% and 9% respectively (1584,6263,8060,8061).

Blond psyllium in combination with pectin, guar gum, and locust bean gum in a dose of 15 grams daily with a low-fat diet, reduces total cholesterol by 6.4% and LDL cholesterol by 10.5% after six months of treatment (8431).

Patients taking a combination of simvastatin (Zocor) 10 mg and blond psyllium (Metamucil) 15 grams daily seem to have cholesterol lower in comparable amounts as those patient taking just simvastatin 20 mg/day (13102).

A combination of blond psyllium with colestipol, at half their usual doses seems to be as effective as colestipol alone (8432). Blond psyllium also seems to reduce colestipol and cholestyramine side effects such as constipation and abdominal pain (8432,9424).

In children with hypercholesterolemia, psyllium supplementation can further decrease LDL cholesterol levels by 7% to 15% when added to a low fat, low cholesterol diet, National Cholesterol Education Program (NCEP) Step 1 diet. However, psyllium supplementation added to a more stringent low fat, low cholesterol diet, NCEP Step 2 diet, may have less of an additional effect in lowering LDL cholesterol (8073,8074,8075,8076).

POSSIBLY EFFECTIVE

Diabetes. Taking blond psyllium seed husk orally seems to significantly reduce postprandial serum glucose, insulin levels, serum total cholesterol, and low-density lipoprotein (LDL) cholesterol levels in patients with type 2 diabetes and hypercholesterolemia (1405,8058,8064,10091,10099,12552). Blond psyllium seems to reduce postprandial blood glucose levels by about 14% to 20%, total cholesterol by about 9%, and LDL cholesterol by 13% (1405,8058). Blonde psyllium also seems to lower postprandial glucose levels in patients with type 1 diabetes (12553,12554). Blond psyllium's maximum effect on the glucose levels occurs when psyllium is mixed and consumed with foods (8064,10091). Blond psyllium does not lower postprandial glucose in people who do not have diabetes (9249).

Diarrhea. Taking blond psyllium orally seems to delay gastric emptying, slow colonic transit, increase fecal viscosity, and improve fecal consistency in patients with diarrhea (5246,8419,8420,8421). Psyllium is also used in combination with calcium carbonate and calcium phosphate, weight ratio 4:1:1, and seems to be as effective as loperamide in reducing the frequency and urgency associated with diarrhea (8422). In patients receiving enteral tube feedings, psyllium does not decrease the frequency of stools, but it may decrease the number of liquid stools (8423,9422). Preliminary clinical evidence suggests blond psyllium might also be useful in treating postcholecystectomy diarrhea (10097). Taking blond psyllium orally seems to reduce diarrhea associated with the use of misoprostol (Cytotec). There is preliminary evidence that blond psyllium relieves diarrhea associated with misoprostol use and prevents its reoccurrence when used throughout misoprostol therapy (8429).

Hemorrhoids. Taking blond psyllium orally, with micronized purified flavonidic fraction (MPFF, Daflon), seems to help to relieve bleeding from nonprolapsed hemorrhoids. Psyllium husk used with micronized purified flavonidic fraction relieves bleeding more rapidly than psyllium husk used alone or psyllium husk used with rubber band ligation (8077).

Hypertension. Taking psyllium fiber (husks) orally, with soy protein, seems to help reduce systolic blood pressure by about 8 mmHg and diastolic blood pressure by about 2 mmHg in adult men and women (10458).

Irritable bowel syndrome (IBS). Taking blond psyllium orally seems to improve some symptoms of IBS. There is some controversy about the clinical benefits of blond psyllium seed husk for IBS. There is evidence that shows no benefit (8425), but the majority of evidence shows that blond psyllium seed husk can relieve constipation and improve abdominal pain, diarrhea, and overall well-being (2316,8426,8427,8428). There is also some evidence that a combination of blond psyllium and propantheline (Pro-Banthine) relieves constipation, incomplete bowel evacuation, abdominal pain, constipation, and straining associated with IBS. Patients typically experience relief after four weeks of treatment (8428).

Orlistat (Xenical) side effects. Taking blond psyllium orally with each dose of orlistat seems to relieve orlistat side effects such as flatulence, borborygmi, abdominal cramps, oily spotting, and fecal incontinence without decreasing the weight-reducing effect of orlistat (5245).

Ulcerative colitis. There is some evidence 10 grams of blond psyllium seeds taken orally twice daily might be as effective as 500 mg of mesalamine (Asacol) taken three times daily in preventing the relapse of ulcerative colitis (2385). Blond psyllium also appears to relieve gastrointestinal symptoms in adult patients with ulcerative colitis in remission, including abdominal pain, diarrhea, loose stools, urgency, bloating, incomplete evacuation, mucus discharge, and constipation (10086). However, in patients with juvenile ulcerative colitis in remission, blond psyllium does not appear to have an effect on fecal bile acid excretion, an indicator of disease progression (10090).

POSSIBLY INEFFECTIVE

Colorectal adenoma. Taking blond psyllium orally 3.5 grams per day does not seem to reduce the risk of colorectal adenoma recurrence. There is some evidence that it might actually increase the risk of adenoma recurrence, particularly in people with high dietary calcium intake.

However, more evidence is needed to determine the relationship of psyllium and calcium to colorectal adenoma (7585).

End-stage renal disease (ESRD). Taking blond psyllium orally does not seem to reduce potassium, phosphate, or ammonia concentrations in patients with ESRD (9248).

INSUFFICIENT RELIABLE EVIDENCE to RATE

Fat redistribution syndrome. Consumption of a high fiber diet with adequate energy and protein might prevent fat deposition in patients with HIV. A one-gram increase in total dietary fiber may decrease the risk of fat deposition by 7% (12517). More evidence is needed to rate blonde psyllium for this use.

Mechanism of Action

The applicable parts of blond psyllium are the seed and seed husk. The blond psyllium husk and intact seed contain water-soluble fibers that form a viscous gel in the intestine (2387). Most commercial preparations contain purified seed husk. The inner seed components, the endosperm and the plant embryo, are responsible for the majority of the allergic reactions to blond psyllium. The inner seed parts, which sometimes contaminate commercially produced psyllium seed husks, seem to be responsible for allergenicity, rather than the husk itself (9245). There is some evidence that the soluble fibers undergo partial fermentation by bacteria in the colon (2393,5246,8071), but the bulking effect of psyllium is primarily a result of intact material (10096). When psyllium seed husk is mixed with water, the mucilage has a bulk laxative effect and stimulates peristalsis, which decreases gastrointestinal transit time (8421). In patients with diarrhea, the mucilage increases the water-holding capacity and viscosity of stools, which delays gastric emptying and improves stool consistency (5246,8420,8421). It also prolongs gastrointestinal transit time, possibly by delaying the production of gaseous fermentation products (5246). The polysaccharides in psyllium that form into a gel in the intestine also lubricate stool contents and provide greater ease during defecation (8421). In patients with irritable bowel syndrome (IBS), blond psyllium is thought to normalize bowel function and relieve symptoms of abdominal pain by reducing rectosigmoidal pressure (405). Blond psyllium is also thought to maintain remission in adult patients with ulcerative colitis since fermentation of blond psyllium in the colon yields butyrate, a short-chain fatty acid known to inhibit cytokine production and have an anti-inflammatory effect (2385).

Blond psyllium seems to decrease serum cholesterol levels by adsorbing dietary fats in the gastrointestinal tract and decreasing systemic absorption of the fat. Cholesterol elimination in fecal bile acids also seems to be increased by blond psyllium (1376,8065,8070,8072). Increasing elimination of bile acids increases their production and turnover in the liver, which lowers serum cholesterol. Blond psyllium does not bind to cholesterol or bile acids, but they probably become trapped in the mucilloid matrix and are then expelled. This mechanism also seems to inhibit cholesterol stone formation. Because bile acid sequestrants work by different mechanisms than blond psyllium, together their effects on cholesterol is additive (2387,9425,9426).

There seems to be an inverse relationship between cholesterol and blood urea nitrogen (BUN) levels (8068). This may explain why psyllium is not useful for lowering BUN in end-stage renal disease (ESRD).

Psyllium, by itself, does not affect the absorption of carcinogens in the gastrointestinal tract. The soluble fiber formed by psyllium does not bind to carcinogens. However, wheat bran, which provides insoluble fiber does bind carcinogens. Some evidence suggests that psyllium might improve the chemoprotective effect of wheat bran (9250). A diet that includes an equal combination of psyllium and wheat bran might decrease the risk of breast and colon cancer. In addition, psyllium might help maintain normal cell proliferation in the colon (8082,8083).

In patients with diabetes, blond psyllium reduces postprandial blood glucose levels, probably by delaying the rate of digestion and absorption of carbohydrates (1405,8064). However, psyllium does not seem to reduce postprandial blood glucose when it is given to people without diabetes (9249).

Adverse Reactions

Orally, blond psyllium can cause transient flatulence, abdominal pain, diarrhea, constipation, dyspepsia, and nausea (1376). Starting with a low dose and slowly titrating to the desired dose can often minimize gastrointestinal side effects. There is some concern that blond psyllium can cause esophageal or bowel obstruction when consumed without water or in patients with swallowing disorders (604,8080,8081). Tell patients to consume plenty of water when taking blond psyllium. Suggest at least 240 mL of fluid for every 3.5-5 grams of seed husk or 7 grams of seed (1376,8080,8081). Occasionally, headache, backache, rhinitis, increased cough, and sinusitis have also been reported in patients taking psyllium (1376). Some patients can have an allergic response to blond psyllium. Allergy symptoms include allergic rhinitis, sneezing, conjunctivitis, urticarial rash, itching, flushing, and dyspnea. More serious symptoms include wheezing, facial and body swelling, chest congestion, chest and throat tightness, cough, diarrhea, hypotension, loss of consciousness, and anaphylactic shock. Occupational exposure or repeated ingestion of psyllium can cause sensitization, which can lead to serious allergic reactions (2328,2329,2330,8079,9246). Severe allergic reactions may occur after eating a small quantity of cereal that contains blond psyllium. At least one cereal (Heartwise, Kellogg Co.) has increased the purity of the psyllium it contains, which has decreased the incidence of allergic reactions (9244). A warning of the potential for allergic reactions is on the label of all cereals that contain psyllium (9247). Patients hypersensitive to psyllium usually have marked eosinophilia and an elevated psyllium-specific IgE antibody serum level (2328,2329). There is concern that individuals allergic to English plantain weed, Plantain lanceolata, pollen might also react to psyllium husk dust; however, it appears that there is little cross-allergenicity between these plants and is probably of no clinical significance (8057,9244).

Blond psyllium has a tendency to plug feeding tubes. This can be avoided if blond psyllium is mixed with water and pushed through the feeding tube in less than 5 minutes (8423).

Interactions with Herbs & Other Dietary Supplements

IRON SUPPLEMENTS: Use of blond psyllium with iron supplements can reduce iron absorption (2340,2367,10089). There is some evidence that blond psyllium decreases the absorption of iron by forming a highly stable complex in the intestine (2340,2367). Take supplements one hour before or four hours after psyllium to avoid this interaction.
RIBOFLAVIN SUPPLEMENTS: Psyllium seems to slightly reduce the absorption of riboflavin by about 5%, but this is unlikely to be clinically significant (10094).

Interactions with Drugs

ANTIDIABETES DRUGS: Blond psyllium can reduce blood glucose levels in patients with type 2 diabetes (1405) and might have additive effects on glucose levels when used with antidiabetes drugs. Monitor blood glucose levels closely. Medication dose adjustments may be necessary. Some antidiabetes drugs include glimepiride (Amaryl), glyburide (Diabeta, Glynase PresTab, Micronase), insulin, pioglitazone (Actos), rosiglitazone (Avandia), and others.
CARBAMAZEPINE (Tegretol): Blond psyllium can reduce carbamazepine absorption and serum levels (539).
DIGOXIN (Lanoxin): Theoretically, psyllium might reduce digoxin absorption. However, some evidence suggests that the effect of psyllium on digoxin absorption is not clinically significant (10098).
ETHINYL ESTRADIOL: Concurrent use of blond psyllium with ethinyl estradiol results in a slight increase in the extent of ethinyl estradiol absorption and a slower rate of absorption. This is unlikely to be clinically significant (12421).
LITHIUM: There is one case report of reduced serum lithium levels associated with psyllium use. This was reversed when psyllium was stopped (540). The fiber in lithium might decrease the absorption of lithium.
WARFARIN (Coumadin): There used to be concern that blond psyllium might decrease absorption of warfarin and other oral drugs due to its fibrous content. But blond psyllium does not seem to affect warfarin absorption or warfarin levels (12420).

Interactions with Foods

NUTRIENT ABSORPTION: Despite concern that long-term use of psyllium with meals can reduce nutrient absorption, possibly requiring vitamin or mineral supplementation, use of blond psyllium husk for up to six months did not clinically alter vitamin or mineral status in a review of eight human trials (1376). Blond psyllium does not reduce the absorption of calcium (9243).

Interactions with Lab Tests

CHOLESTEROL: Blond psyllium reduces serum total cholesterol and LDL cholesterol levels, LDL:HDL ratio, and test results (1405,1376).
GLUCOSE: Blond psyllium can reduce postprandial blood glucose levels and test results (1405).

Interactions with Diseases or Conditions

DIABETES: Blond psyllium can lower blood glucose levels in people with type 2 diabetes by retarding carbohydrate absorption (1405,8064). Monitor blood glucose levels closely. Doses of conventional antidiabetes medications may require adjustment. Also, warn patients with diabetes that some commercial blond psyllium products can contain added sugars and other absorbable carbohydrates which might increase blood glucose levels.
GASTROINTESTINAL CONDITIONS: Blond psyllium is contraindicated in people with fecal impaction, GI tract narrowing, obstruction, or conditions that can lead to obstruction, such as spastic bowel (604).
HYPERSENSITIVITY: Some patients can have severe hypersensitivity reactions to blond psyllium. This is more likely to occur in patients with previous occupation exposure to blond psyllium (2328,2329,2330,8079,9246). Blond psyllium is contraindicated in these patients.
PHENYLKETONURIA: Some blond psyllium preparations are sweetened with aspartame (Nutrasweet) and should be avoided in patients with phenylketonuria (272).
SWALLOWING DISORDERS: Patients with swallowing disorders might be at greater risk for esophageal obstruction when using blond psyllium. Blond psyllium is contraindicated in these patients (8080,8081).

Dosage and Administration

ORAL: As a bulk laxative for constipation, blond psyllium seed 7-40 grams per day, in 2-4 divided doses is commonly used (6248,9423,10088).
For diarrhea, 7-18 grams of blond psyllium, in 2-3 divided doses, has been used (8419,8420) or 5 grams of a combination of blond psyllium, calcium carbonate, and calcium phosphate, weight ratio 4:1:1, has been used twice daily (8422).
For decreasing diarrhea in patients receiving tube feedings, up to 30 grams of blond psyllium has been used daily in divided doses of 2.5-7.5 grams per dose. It may be given through the feeding tube, mixed with the enteral feeding, or by bolus followed by a flush with water. However, psyllium may cause clogging of the feeding tube when either of these techniques is used (8423,9422).
For chronic diarrhea associated with postcholecystectomy diarrhea, blond psyllium 6.5 grams three times daily has been used (10097).
For diarrhea associated with the use of misoprostol, blond psyllium 3.4 grams twice daily has been used (8429).
For irritable bowel syndrome (IBS), blond psyllium seed husk, 10-30 grams in two to three divided doses, has

been used daily (2316,8426,8427,8428). Blond psyllium seed husk 10 grams twice daily with propantheline 15 mg three times daily has also been used (8428).
For reducing the gastrointestinal (GI) side effects of orlistat, 6 grams three times daily with each orlistat dose has been used (5245).
For maintaining remission in patients with ulcerative colitis, 10 grams of blond psyllium seeds, taken twice daily, has been used (2385).
For relieving bleeding from non-prolapsed hemorrhoids, 3.5 grams of psyllium seed husk, twice daily for three months, has been used in addition to treatment with micronized purified flavonidic fraction (MPFF, Daflon) 1500 mg twice daily for five days, followed by 1000 mg twice daily for three weeks (8077).
For hyperlipidemia, blond psyllium seed husk 3.4 grams three times daily or 5.1 grams twice daily has been used (2324,8433,6261,6262,6264,8066,10095). However, doses up to 20.4 grams per day have been tried (1376). Psyllium-enriched cereal containing 12 grams of soluble fiber per day has been also used (1584,6263,8060,8061). A mixture of 2.1 grams of psyllium, 1.3 grams of pectin, 1.1 grams of guar gum and 0.5 grams of locust bean gum has been used three times daily (8431). A combination of 2.5 grams of blond psyllium powder (Metamucil) with 2.5 grams of colestipol, taken three times daily, has also been used (8432). A combination of simvastatin (Zocor) 10 mg and blond psyllium (Metamucil) 15 grams daily has also been used (13102).
In children with hypercholesterolemia, psyllium-enriched cereal containing 5-10 grams of psyllium has been used daily (8073,8075,8076).
For type 2 diabetes and hypercholesterolemia, blond psyllium 15 grams in three divided doses has been used (10099).
For reducing the glycemic index of food in patients with type 2 diabetes, blond psyllium 15 grams in three divided doses with a carbohydrate meal has been used (10091).
For treating end-stage renal disease (ESRD), 8.7 grams daily of blond psyllium has been used (9248).
For hypertension, blond psyllium husks 15 grams daily has been used for 8 weeks (10458).
Tell patients to ensure adequate fluid intake. Inadequate fluid intake can lead to choking and esophageal or bowel obstruction. Suggest a minimum of 240 mL per 5 grams or less of blond psyllium husk or 7 grams of blond psyllium seed (1376,8080,8081). To minimize some of the common gastrointestinal side effects, suggest that patients start with a low dose and titrate slowly to the desired dose.

Comments

There are some blond psyllium-containing foods with labeling that claim these foods, when consumed as part of a low-fat diet, may reduce the risk of coronary heart disease (CHD) (6264). It is true that blond psyllium can help lower cholesterol levels; however, there is not yet proof that taking blond psyllium reduces the risk of developing heart disease. Despite its effectiveness in lowering cholesterol levels, blond psyllium has not yet been included in the stepwise approaches to dietary therapy such as the American Heart Association Step I or Step II diets for hypercholesterolemia (2321,8430). Most clinical studies have used a specific blond psyllium powder preparation (Metamucil) (1376,6261) or psyllium seed husk-containing foods such as cereals, breads, or snack bars (8433,6262). The FDA allows foods containing at least 1.7 grams of psyllium per serving to be labeled with the claim that it may reduce the risk of heart disease when it is consumed as part of a diet low in fat and cholesterol (11018).

BLOODROOT

Also Known As

Bloodwort, Blood Root, Coon Root, Indian Plant, Indian Red Paint, Pauson, Red Indian Paint, Red Puccoon, Red Root, Sanguinaria, Snakebite, Sweet Slumber, Tetterwort.
CAUTION: See Separate listing for Yarrow.

Scientific Names

Sanguinaria canadensis.
Family: Papaveraceae.

People Use This For

Orally, bloodroot is used as an emetic, cathartic, antispasmodic, and expectorant. Bloodroot is also used orally for bronchitis, asthma, croup, laryngitis, pharyngitis, deficient capillary circulation, nasal polyps, rheumatism, warts, cancer (Fell technique), dental analgesic, fever, and as a general tonic.
Topically, bloodroot is used as an irritant and debriding agent.
In dentistry, bloodroot is used topically to reduce plaque.

Safety

POSSIBLY SAFE ...when used orally and appropriately short-term (4).
POSSIBLY UNSAFE ...when excessive doses are used orally; sanguinarine, although thought to be poorly absorbed, is a toxic alkaloid (6,12).
There is insufficient reliable information available about the safety of bloodroot for its other uses.
PREGNANCY: LIKELY UNSAFE ...when used orally (12); avoid using.
LACTATION: POSSIBLY UNSAFE ...when used orally (4); avoid using.

Effectiveness

There is insufficient reliable information available about the effectiveness of bloodroot.

Mechanism of Action

The applicable part of bloodroot is the rhizome. The isoquinolone alkaloid constituents, primarily sanguinarine, appear to have antimicrobial, antifungal, anti-inflammatory, and antihistamine activity (11446,11448). The negative ion of sanguinarine can bind to dental plaque and exert antiplaque activity (11446). Bloodroot also seems to exhibit cardiotonic (exerts a favorable effect on the heart) actions, possibly by inhibiting Na/K-ATPase activity and producing a positive inotropic effect (11447).

Adverse Reactions

Orally, bloodroot may cause nausea, vomiting (12), slight central nervous system (CNS) depression, and narcosis (6). High doses may cause hypotension, shock, coma, and glaucoma (6).
Topically, skin contact with fresh bloodroot can cause irritation or contact dermatitis (19). Avoid contact with the eyes and mucous membranes because of its irritant properties.

Interactions with Herbs & Other Dietary Supplements

None known.

Interactions with Drugs

None known.

Interactions with Foods

None known.

Interactions with Lab Tests

None known.

Interactions with Diseases or Conditions

GASTROINTESTINAL (GI) IRRITATION: Bloodroot can irritate the GI tract and is contraindicated in individuals with infectious or inflammatory gastrointestinal conditions (19).
GLAUCOMA: Bloodroot might affect glaucoma treatment. Do not exceed the recommended dose (12).

Dosage and Administration

ORAL: The typical dose of the bloodroot rhizome is 60-500 mg three times a day (4). The usual dose of the liquid extract, 1:1 in 60% alcohol, is 0.06-0.3 mL three times a day (4). The tincture, 1:5 in 60% alcohol, is dosed at 0.3-2 mL three times a day (4).
TOPICAL: No typical dosage.
EMETIC DOSE: As an emetic, 1-2 g of the rhizome; 1-2 mL of the liquid extract, 1:1 in 60% alcohol; or 2-8 mL of the tincture, 1:5 in 60% alcohol have been used (4).

Comments

During the mid-1800s, topical preparations of the bloodroot extracts were used in the Fell Technique for treatment of breast tumors (6).

BLUE COHOSH

Also Known As

Blue Ginseng, Caulophyllum, Papoose Root, Squaw Root, Yellow Ginseng.
CAUTION: See separate listings for Black Cohosh, White Cohosh, Ginseng American, Canaigre, Codonopsis, Ginseng Siberian, Ginseng Panax, and Ashwaganda.

Scientific Names

Caulophyllum thalictroides.
Family: Berberidaceae or Leonticaceae.

People Use This For

Orally, blue cohosh is used for stimulating the uterus and inducing labor, inducing menstruation, as an antispasmodic, as a laxative, and for colic, sore throat, cramps, hiccups, epilepsy, hysterics, inflammation of the uterus, and rheumatic conditions.

In foods, the roasted seeds of blue cohosh are used as a coffee substitute.

Safety

LIKELY UNSAFE ...when used orally (4,12). Poisonings have occurred after ingestion of blue cohosh eaf or seeds (4).

PREGNANCY AND LACTATION: LIKELY UNSAFE ...when used orally. Blue cohosh is a uterine stimulant and can induce labor (12047). Several blue cohosh constituents are potentially teratogenic and might cause congenital malformations in newborns (1122,7110). Use of blue cohosh near term can cause life-threatening toxicity in the infant (1207,9492,9493,12047). Many midwives still use blue cohosh to facilitate delivery. This dangerous practice should be avoided (1122,1207).

Effectiveness

There is insufficient reliable information available about the effectiveness of blue cohosh.

Mechanism of Action

The applicable parts of blue cohosh are the rhizome and root. Blue cohosh has several pharmacological effects. However, most of these effects are undesirable. Blue cohosh constricts coronary arteries and seems to decrease the flow of oxygen to the heart (3383). Blue cohosh also contains several alkaloid constituents that are suspected teratogens. There is some evidence that the constituent anagyrine might cause birth defects in humans (7110). Another constituent, N-methylcytosine also seems to be teratogenic (7110). N-methylcytosine seems to act similarly to nicotine, which can increase blood pressure, stimulate the small intestine, and produce hyperglycemia the developing fetus (7110). Blue cohosh also contains taspine, which is chemically related to morphine and its congeners (7110). Taspine seems to be cytotoxic and lethal to embryos even at very low concentrations (7110). There is preliminary evidence that blue cohosh might have estrogenic effects. A blue cohosh extract seems to enhance estradiol binding to estrogen receptors and increase estradiol-induced transcription activity in estrogen-responsive cells (6180). In animal models, it also decreases luteinizing hormone (LH) levels and increases serum ceruloplasmin oxidase activity, which is a measure of estrogenic activity in the liver (6180).

Adverse Reactions

Orally, blue cohosh can cause significant adverse effects including mucous membrane irritation, stomach upset including diarrhea and cramping, chest pain (angina), hypertension, and hyperglycemia (6002).

Neonatal acute myocardial infarction (MI), congestive heart failure (CHF), and shock has occurred following maternal use of a blue cohosh combination product one month before delivery (566,3383). There is also a case report of severe complications, including seizures, renal failure, and respiratory distress, in an infant whose mother was given an unknown dose of black and blue cohosh at 42-weeks gestation to induce labor (1122,9492,9493). In another case, a mother was advised to drink a blue cohosh tea to induce labor. The infant experienced a seizure during delivery and 2 days later it was discovered that the infant was experiencing an evolving ischemic stroke (12047). Due to these life-threatening side effects pregnant women should be advised not to ingest any blue cohosh product during pregnancy.

Interactions with Herbs & Other Dietary Supplements

None known.

Interactions with Drugs

ANTIDIABETES DRUGS: There is some concern that blue cohosh might increase blood glucose levels (6002). Theoretically, it might decrease the effectiveness of medicines used for diabetes.

ANTIHYPERTENSIVE DRUGS: Constituents in blue cohosh might increase blood pressure by causing coronary vasoconstriction (6002). Theoretically, this might decrease the effectiveness of drugs used for angina and high blood pressure.

NICOTINE: Blue cohosh can increase the effects of nicotine (6002).

Interactions with Foods

None known.

Interactions with Lab Tests

None known.

Interactions with Diseases or Conditions

CARDIOVASCULAR CONDITIONS: There is some concern that blue cohosh might worsen cardiovascular conditions such as angina and hypertension. There is evidence that blue cohosh can cause coronary vasoconstriction and decrease oxygen flow to the heart. It might also increase blood pressure (6002). Avoid using in these patients.
DIABETES: There is some concern that blue cohosh might worsen diabetes. It can increase blood glucose levels in some patients (6002).
DIARRHEA: Blue cohosh might worsen symptoms in patients with diarrhea (4). Blue cohosh seems to increase gastrointestinal motility (5).
HORMONE SENSITIVE CANCERS/CONDITIONS: Because blue cohosh might have estrogenic effects (6180), women with hormone sensitive conditions should avoid blue cohosh. Some of these conditions include breast cancer, uterine cancer, ovarian cancer, endometriosis, and uterine fibroids.

Dosage and Administration

ORAL: The typical dose of the dried rhizome or root is 0.3-1 grams or as a tea three times daily. The tea is prepared by steeping the herb in 150 mL boiling water and then straining. The usual dose of the liquid extract (1:1 in 70% alcohol) is 0.5-1.0 mL three times daily (4).

Comments

Cohosh is from the Algonquin word "rough", referring to the appearance of the roots (7110). Blue cohosh was listed in the US Pharmacopoeia from 1882 to 1905 for inducing labor (7110).

BLUE FLAG

Also Known As

Iris, Sweet Flag, Water Flag.
CAUTION: See separate listing for Orris.

Scientific Names

Iris versicolor; Iris caroliniana; Iris virginica.
Family: Iridaceae.

People Use This For

Orally, blue flag is used as a laxative and diuretic and for dermatological, anti-inflammatory, and antiemetic uses. It is also used as a bile stimulant, for liver dysfunction, and specifically for skin eruptions.

Safety

LIKELY UNSAFE ...when used orally; contraindicated in all but small doses (4). The fresh root can cause nausea, vomiting, and mucosal irritation (4,12). The blue flag oil is a mucous membrane irritant (4).
PREGNANCY AND LACTATION: LIKELY UNSAFE ...when used orally (4,12); avoid using.

Effectiveness

There is insufficient reliable information available about the effectiveness of blue flag.

Mechanism of Action

The applicable part of blue flag is the rhizome. There is insufficient reliable information available about the possible mechanism of action and active ingredients. Some related species can be toxic (4).

Adverse Reactions

Orally, blue flag can cause nausea and vomiting, and the fresh root can irritate mucosa or skin (4,19). The volatile oil constituent irritates mucous membranes and can cause lacrimation, eye inflammation, irritation of the throat, and headache (4).

Interactions with Herbs & Other Dietary Supplements

POTASSIUM DEPLETING HERBS: Theoretically, concomitant use with horsetail plant or the licorice rhizome increases the risk of potassium depletion.
STIMULANT LAXATIVE HERBS: Theoretically, concomitant use of blue flag with other stimulant laxative herbs can increase the risk of potassium depletion. Stimulant laxative herbs include aloe dried leaf sap, wild cucumber fruit (Ecballium elaterium), alder buckthorn, European buckthorn, butternut bark, cascara bark, castor oil, colocynth fruit pulp, gamboge bark exudate, jalap root, black root, manna bark exudate, podophyllum root, rhubarb root, senna leaves and pods, and yellow dock root (19).

Interactions with Drugs

DIGOXIN (Lanoxin): Theoretically, overuse or abuse of this product increases the risk of adverse effects from cardiac glycoside drugs.
DIURETIC DRUGS: Overuse of blue flag might compound diuretic-induced potassium loss (19). There is some concern that people taking blue flag along with potassium depleting diuretics might have an increased risk for hypokalemia. Initiation of potassium supplementation or an increase in potassium supplement dose may be necessary for some patients. Some diuretics that can deplete potassium include chlorothiazide (Diuril), chlorthalidone (Thalitone), furosemide (Lasix), hydrochlorothiazide (HCTZ, Hydrodiuril, Microzide), and others.

Interactions with Foods

None known.

Interactions with Lab Tests

None known.

Interactions with Diseases or Conditions

GASTROINTESTINAL IRRITATION: Blue flag can irritate the GI tract and is contraindicated in individuals with infectious or inflammatory gastrointestinal conditions (19).

Dosage and Administration

No typical dosage.

Comments

Little is known about blue flag's phytochemical, pharmacological, or toxicological properties, or those of its constituents. Some related species can be toxic (4). Though orris root is sometimes used as a common name for blue flag, it is also used to describe the Iris species.

BLUE-GREEN ALGAE

Also Known As

AFA, BGA, Blue-Green Micro-Algae, Cyanobacteria, Dihe, Klamath Blue/Green Algae, Spirulina, Tecuitlatl.

Scientific Names

Microcystis aeruginosa; Microcystis wesenbergii; other Microcystis species; Spirulina maxima; Spirulina platensis; Spirulina pacifica; other Spirulina species; Anabaena species; Lyngbya wollei; Aphanizomenon flos-aquae.

People Use This For

Orally, blue-green algae is used as a source of dietary protein, B-vitamins, and iron. It is also used orally for weight loss, oral leukoplakia, and obstetric and gynecological disorders. Blue-green algae is also used orally for attention deficit-hyperactivity disorder (ADHD), premenstrual syndrome, allergic rhinitis, diabetes, stimulating the immune system, stress, fatigue, anxiety, depression, improving memory, increasing energy and metabolism, lowering cholesterol, decreasing cardiovascular disease, wound healing, and for promoting digestion and bowel health.

Safety

POSSIBLY SAFE ...when non-contaminated, non-microcystin containing species of blue-green algae are used orally (9171).
POSSIBLY UNSAFE ...when contaminated blue-green algae are used orally. Blue-green algae can be contaminated with microbes, heavy metals (including mercury, cadmium, lead, or arsenic), and radioactive divalent and trivalent metal ions (6).
LIKELY UNSAFE ...when any microcystin-containing blue-green algae products are used orally (3535,3536,9171); avoid using all untested blue-green algae products.
CHILDREN: LIKELY UNSAFE ...when any microcystin-containing blue-green algae products are used orally. Children are more sensitive to poisoning by microcystins produced by blue-green algae (3536).
PREGNANCY AND LACTATION: Insufficient reliable information available; avoid using.

Effectiveness

POSSIBLY EFFECTIVE

Oral leukoplakia. Taking spirulina blue-green algae orally seems to reduce oral leukoplakia in people who chew tobacco (6).

POSSIBLY INEFFECTIVE

Weight loss. Taking spirulina blue-green algae doesn't seem to help reduce weight (6).

There is insufficient reliable information available about the effectiveness of blue-green algae for its other uses.

Mechanism of Action

Blue-green algae are a mixture of single celled organisms that have biochemical and cellular similarities to both plant and animal species. While these organisms have the ability to perform photosynthesis like plants, they lack a cell wall. Like animal species, they form many complex glycoproteins. Spirulina and aphanizomenon are the species that have been studied most intensively. Spirulina blue-green algae consists of approximately 65% crude protein, high concentrations of B vitamins, phenylalanine, and iron and other minerals (6). The B vitamins are thought to be analogs of vitamin B12 and nutritionally insignificant (6). The phenylalanine content is promoted as being responsible for reducing appetite and causing weight loss (6). The FDA reviewed this claim and found no evidence to support using blue-green algae for weight loss (6). The iron in spirulina blue-green algae has been found to be highly bioavailable in humans (6). As much as 1.5-2 mg of iron can be absorbed from a dose of 10 grams of blue-green algae (6).

Spirulina blue-green algae has a high concentration of vitamin B12. However, consumption of spirulina does not appear to decrease mean corpuscular volume (MCV) when added to a vegetarian diet (9467). For reasons that are not clear, the vitamin B12 in spirulina is not bioactive (9477).

A constituent called C- phycocyanin that is found in some species of blue-green algae may have anti-inflammatory actions. In addition, it may bind to reactive oxygen species (ROS), such as hydroxyl free radicals, resulting in antioxidant effects (9468,9469). Preliminary evidence suggests that the antioxidant effect may decrease the toxicity of lead (9470). Evidence suggests that spirulina blue-green algae might reduce serum lipids, liver triglycerides, and gastric secretions (6). It might also protect against the effects of gamma radiation, enhance the regression of oral carcinoma, and have antiviral effects (6).

Blue-green algae seems to have immunomodulatory effects. The blue-green algae species Spirulina platensis may increase the concentration of immune globulin A (IgA) in the gastrointestinal tract, without increasing concentrations of IgG or IgE. This effect may decrease the risk of food allergies (9434,10267). Preliminary research suggests that Spirulina species can inhibit mast cell-mediated allergic reactions (9173). Spirulina platensis also appears to increase immune function by increasing the activity of macrophages, increase phagocytosis, and increase the concentration of interleukin-1 (IL1) (10267). The species of blue-green algae Aphanizomenon flos-aquae (AFA) may stimulate the immune system by stimulating the activity and motility of T lymphocytes, B lymphocytes and natural killer cells. AFA slightly increases the phagocytic activity of polymorphonuclear (PMN) leucocytes (2534). AFA contains 1.9-2.9 times less of the polyunsaturated fatty acids (PUFA), alpha-linolenic acid, and 32-44 times less linoleic acid than soybean oil. Preliminary evidence suggests that an AFA-supplemented diet may be more effective than the soybean oil-supplemented diet at lowering triglycerides and total cholesterol (2535). Preliminary research suggests that AFA might improve utilization of proteins and increase synthesis of enzymes involved with digestion and nutrient utilization (9242).

Researchers at the National Cancer Institute have isolated an antiviral protein, cyanovirin-N (CV-N), which might prove useful in treating human immunodeficiency virus (HIV) infection. Isolated from the blue-green algae Nostoc ellipsosporum, CV-N binds irreversibly to sites on the viral envelope, inactivating HIV and inhibiting its entry into cells. CV-N has unique temperature (heat and cold) stability which might allow for its use in applications not typical for proteins. The researchers hypothesize that, attached to a solid matrix, CV-N might be used to adsorb and remove HIV from infected blood products. This unpublished research was presented at the Microbicides 2000 International Conference (1375).

Adverse Reactions

Orally, blue-green algae appear to cause few adverse effects when non-contaminated products are used. Blue-green algae can be contaminated with the toxic blue-green algae species Microcystis aeruginosa, which produces potent hepatotoxins called microcystins (9171). Microcystin-containing blue-green algae products can cause hepatotoxicity, jaundice, abdominal pain and distention, nausea, vomiting, weakness, excessive thirst, rapid and weak pulse, shock, and death (3535,9172). Symptoms of poisoning usually occur 30 minutes to 24 hours after ingestion (3535). Children are more sensitive to microcystin poisoning than adults (3536).

There is concern that blue-green algae might cause or worsen autoimmune disorders due to its immune-stimulating effects. In one case a patient with pemphigus vulgaris had a disease flare after taking a supplement containing spirulina blue-green algae. In another case, a woman developed dermatomyositis within 1-2 days after taking a supplement containing blue-green algae (12171). More evidence is needed to determine if blue-green algae is responsible for these effects.

Interactions with Herbs & Other Dietary Supplements

None known.

Interactions with Drugs

None known.

Interactions with Foods

None known.

Interactions with Lab Tests

LIVER FUNCTION TESTS: Increases in liver function tests, ALT (alanine aminotransferase, formerly SGPT), and AST (aspartate aminotransferase, formerly SGOT), suggest possible consumption of microcystin-contaminated blue-green algae (9172).

Interactions with Diseases or Conditions

PEMPHIGUS VULGARIS: In one case, a patient with well-controlled pemphigus vulgaris took a supplement containing spirulina blue-green algae and within 7-10 days developed a disease flare. The immunostimulatory effects of spirulina blue-green algae are thought to exacerbate this and other autoimmune disorders (12171).
PHENYLKETONURIA: Theoretically, the phenylalanine content of Spirulina species blue-green algae products might exacerbate phenylketonuria (6); avoid Spirulina species blue-green algae products (6).

Dosage and Administration

ORAL: The typical dose of spirulina blue-green algae is 3-5 grams daily before meals (6002).

Comments

Blue-green algae are commonly found in tropical or subtropical alkaline waters that have a high-salt content, but some species such as Aphanizomenon grow in large fresh water lakes (6002,9171). The natural color of these algae can give bodies of water a dark-green appearance (6). Blue-green algae (cyanophyta) comprises thousands of species, including Spirulina species of blue-green algae and non-Spirulina species of blue-green algae (3536). Most commercial products contain Aphanizomenon flos-aquae, Spirulina maxima, or Spirulina platensis. The altitude, temperature, and sun exposure where the blue-green algae are grown dramatically influence the constituents and the species mixture (9242). Commercial Spirulina species of blue-green algae are usually grown under controlled conditions while some non-spirulina blue-green algae (Klamath blue-green algae and others) are grown in natural setting (lakes, etc.) where contamination and microcystin production may be more likely (3536). Hepatotoxic microcystins have been found in both Spirulina and non-Spirulina products (3536,9171). Select blue-green algae products that have been tested for contamination with heavy metals, microbes, or microcystins (3536). While blue-green algae products are promoted as an excellent source of dietary protein, they are no better than meat or milk and are estimated to cost more than 30 times as much as beef on a per gram basis (6).

BLUEBERRY

Also Known As

Blueberries, Highbush Blueberry, Hillside Blueberry, Lowbush Blueberry, Rabbiteye Blueberry.
Caution: See separate listing for Bilberry (Vaccinium myrtillus).

Scientific Names

Vaccinium angustifolium, synonyms Vaccinium brittonii, Vaccinium lamarckii, Vaccinium pensylvanicum; Vaccinium virgatum, synonyms Vaccinium ashei, Vaccinium amoenum; Vaccinium corymbosum, synonym Vaccinium constablaei; Vaccinium pallidum, synonyms Vaccinium altomontanum, Vaccinium vacillans.
Family: Ericaceae.

People Use This For

Orally, blueberry is used for preventing cataracts and glaucoma, ulcers, urinary tract infections (UTIs), multiple sclerosis, fever, varicose veins, hemorrhoids, improving circulation, and as a laxative. It is also used for colic, labor pain, and as a tonic after miscarriage. The dried fruit and leaves are used for diarrhea. Tea made from the dried leaves is used for sore throat and other inflammations of the mouth or mucous membranes of the throat. Blueberry juice is used as a contrast agent in magnetic resonance imaging (MRI).
By inhalation, fumes of burning dried blueberry flowers are inhaled for treatment of insanity.

Safety

LIKELY SAFE ...when used orally and appropriately (12).
PREGNANCY AND LACTATION: Insufficient reliable information available; avoid using.

Effectiveness

There is insufficient reliable information available about the effectiveness of blueberry.

Mechanism of Action

The applicable parts of the blueberry are the fruit and leaves. Blueberry fruit is high in fiber and vitamin C. Blueberries also contain anthocyanins and proanthocyanidins, which appear to have antioxidant activity (900,907,908). Ethyl acetate extracts of blueberry fruit inhibit ornithine decarboxylase, which is a key enzyme in tumor progression (888). Preliminary research from animal models suggests that the antioxidant effects of blueberry extracts might have anticancer activity and potentially reduce normal oxidative cellular damage that occurs with aging (888,908,1419,9429). Blueberry, like its relative, the cranberry, also appears to prevent bacterial adhesion to the bladder and bacterial colonization (2813,6757); however, clinical studies have not yet been performed.

Adverse Reactions

None reported.

Interactions with Herbs & Other Dietary Supplements

None known.

Interactions with Drugs

ANTIDIABETES DRUGS: Theoretically, blueberry leaf might lower blood glucose (909); however, this effect has not yet been reported in humans. Until more is known, monitor blood glucose levels more closely in patients with diabetes who are taking blueberry. Dose adjustments may be necessary in patients taking diabetes medications.

Interactions with Foods

None known.

Interactions with Lab Tests

BLOOD GLUCOSE: Theoretically, blueberry leaf might lower blood glucose and test results (909); however, this effect has not yet been reported in humans.
MAGNETIC RESONANCE IMAGING (MRI): Because of the high concentration of manganese in blueberry juice, it may act as a negative contrast agent in MRI of the gastrointestinal tract (9427).
TRIGLYCERIDES: Theoretically, blueberry leaf, which is related to the bilberry, might lower serum triglycerides and test results (909); however, this effect has not yet been reported in humans.

Interactions with Diseases or Conditions

DIABETES: Theoretically, blueberry leaf might lower blood glucose (909); however, this effect has not yet been reported in humans. Until more is known, monitor blood glucose levels more closely in patients with diabetes who are taking blueberry. Dose adjustments may be necessary in patients taking diabetes medications.

Dosage and Administration

No typical dosage.

Comments

Don't confuse blueberry with bilberry. Blueberry in the US refers to the species of Vaccinium listed in this monograph. However, elsewhere in the world, blueberry may refer to the European plant, Vaccinium myrtillus, which is called bilberry in the US.

BOG BILBERRY

Also Known As

Moosbeere, Western-Huckleberry.
CAUTION: See separate listing for Bilberry.

Scientific Names

Vaccinium uliginosum, synonyms Vaccinium gaultherioides, Vaccinium occidentale.
Family: Ericaceae.

People Use This For

Orally, bog bilberry is used for mucous membrane inflammation of the gastric and intestinal tract, diarrhea, and bladder complaints.

Safety

POSSIBLY UNSAFE ...when used orally in large amounts. Poisoning has been reported when individuals ingest fruit from fungus-infested plants (18).
There is insufficient reliable information available about the safety of dried bog bilberry fruit used in medicinal amounts.
PREGNANCY AND LACTATION: POSSIBLY UNSAFE ...when used orally in large amounts; avoid using (18).

Effectiveness

There is insufficient reliable information available about the effectiveness of bog bilberry.

Mechanism of Action

The applicable part of bog bilberry is the dried, ripe fruit. The active constituents of bog bilberry are tannins, anthocyanoside, and flavonoids (18).

Adverse Reactions

Orally, poisonings from the ingestion of large quantities of the bog bilberry fruit are rare and could have been due to contamination with a fungus, Sclerroyina megalospora (18). The symptoms of poisoning include queasiness, vomiting, states of intoxication, feelings of weakness, and visual disorders (18).

Interactions with Herbs & Other Dietary Supplements

None known.

Interactions with Drugs

None known.

Interactions with Foods

None known.

Interactions with Lab Tests

None known.

Interactions with Diseases or Conditions

None known.

Dosage and Administration

ORAL: The usual dose of bog bilberry is one cup of the unsweetened tea once or twice daily (18). The tea is prepared by steeping 2 heaping teaspoons of the dried, ripe fruit in 250 mL cold water for 10-12 hours and then straining.

Comments

Avoid confusion with bilberry fruit or bilberry leaf.

BOGBEAN

Also Known As

Buckbean, Marsh Trefoil, Menyanthes, Water Shamrock.

Scientific Names

Menyanthes trifoliata.
Family: Menyanthaceae.

People Use This For

Orally, bogbean is used for rheumatism, rheumatoid arthritis, loss of appetite, and dyspepsia.
In food manufacturing, bogbean is used as a flavoring agent.

Safety

LIKELY SAFE ...when used orally in amounts commonly found in foods. The Council of Europe lists bogbean as a natural food flavoring (4).
POSSIBLY SAFE ...when used orally in medicinal amounts (12).
POSSIBLY UNSAFE ...when used orally in excessive amounts. Bogbean leaf preparations can irritate the GI tract (4).
PREGNANCY AND LACTATION: POSSIBLY UNSAFE ...when used orally due to the lack of toxicity information and its possible purgative action (4); avoid using.

Effectiveness

There is insufficient reliable information available about the effectiveness of bogbean.

Mechanism of Action

The applicable part of bogbean is the leaf. The bitter principles, or iridoids, can stimulate saliva and gastric juices (2,4). Bogbean can have purgative actions (4). An unidentified constituent has hemolytic activity (4).

Adverse Reactions

Orally, excessive doses of bogbean can irritate the GI tract, and cause diarrhea, pain, nausea, and vomiting. Theoretically, it can cause bleeding (4).

Interactions with Herbs & Other Dietary Supplements

None known.

Interactions with Drugs

ANTICOAGULANT/ANTIPLATELET DRUGS: Theoretically, bogbean can increase the risk of bleeding.

Interactions with Foods

None known.

Interactions with Lab Tests

None known.

Interactions with Diseases or Conditions

DIARRHEA, DYSENTERY, COLITIS: Contraindicated (12).
PEOPLE AT RISK FOR BLEEDING: Theoretically, bogbean can increase bleeding risk.

Dosage and Administration

ORAL: The typical dose of bogbean is 1-3 grams of the dried leaf three times daily or as a tea three times daily. The tea is prepared by steeping 1-3 grams of the dried leaf in 150 mL boiling water for 5-10 minutes and then straining (2,4). The common dose of the liquid extract (1:1 in 25% alcohol) is 1-2 mL three times daily (4). The tincture (1:5 in 45% alcohol) is usually given as 1-3 mL three times daily (4).

Comments

The bogbean fruit resembles a small bean and is commonly found in swamps or bogs, which is the reason for its name (6002).

BOIS DE ROSE OIL

Also Known As

Cayenne Rosewood Oil, Distilled Oil from Aniba Rosaeodora Wood, Rosewood Oil.

Scientific Names

Aniba rosaeodora, synonym Aniba duckei.
Family: Lauraceae.

Comments

At the date of publication, there was very little scientific information available about this product. Our staff is continually analyzing the available information on natural medicines and will add data to the online version of *Natural Medicines Comprehensive Database* as it becomes available. See www.naturaldatabase.com.

BOLDO

Also Known As

Boldine, Boldo Folium, Boldoak Boldea, Boldus, Boldus Boldus.

Scientific Names

Peumus boldus, synonyms Boldea fragrans, Peumus fragrans.
Family: Monimiaceae.

People Use This For

Orally, boldo is used for mild gastrointestinal (GI) spasms, gallstones, rheumatism, cystitis, hepatic disease, and gonorrhea. It is also used as a diuretic, sedative, bile stimulant, and antiseptic.

Safety

LIKELY SAFE ...when used in amounts commonly found in foods. Boldo has Generally Recognized As Safe status (GRAS) for use in foods in the US (4912).
LIKELY UNSAFE ...when used excessively for oral medicinal purposes; the volatile oil (2.5% in leaf) contains ascaridole (4). If taken by mouth, ascaridole-free preparations should be used (2).
PREGNANCY AND LACTATION: UNSAFE ...when the volatile oil is used orally, due to ascaridole (4).

Effectiveness

There is insufficient reliable information available about the effectiveness of boldo.

Mechanism of Action

The applicable part of boldo is the leaf. The alkaloidal constituents are responsible for actions that include stimulating bile and bile flow, stimulating stomach function, and diuresis (4). The diuretic and mild urinary antiseptic properties probably result from the irritant volatile oil (4). There's some evidence that the boldine constituent may inhibit thromboxane A2 production, resulting in antiplatelet activity (5191).

Adverse Reactions

Orally, boldo can cause convulsions.
Topically, boldo can irritate the skin (4).

Interactions with Herbs & Other Dietary Supplements

None known.

Interactions with Drugs

ANTICOAGULANT/ANTIPLATELET DRUGS: There is some concern that boldo might have additive effects when used with anticoagulant or antiplatelet drugs and increase the risk of bruising and bleeding. Boldo constituents may have antiplatelet effects (5191). Some of these drugs include aspirin, clopidogrel (Plavix), nonsteroidal anti-inflammatory drugs (NSAIDs) such as diclofenac (Voltaren, Cataflam, others), ibuprofen (Advil, Motrin, others), naproxen (Anaprox, Naprosyn, others), dalteparin (Fragmin), enoxaparin (Lovenox), heparin, and others.
WARFARIN (Coumadin): Boldo may have additive effects with warfarin and increase the international normalized ratio (INR). Boldo constituents may have antiplatelet activity (5191).

Interactions with Foods

None known.

Interactions with Lab Tests

None known.

Interactions with Diseases or Conditions

BILE DUCT OBSTRUCTION: Contraindicated (12).
GALLSTONES: Boldo should not be used for self-medication of gallstones, which requires monitoring (12).
KIDNEY DISORDERS: Avoid boldo products which are not certified as ascaridole-free (4).
LIVER DISEASE: Contraindicated (8,12).

Dosage and Administration

ORAL: The typical dose of boldo is 60-200 mg of the dried leaf three times daily or as a tea three times a day. The tea is prepared by steeping 1 gram of the dried leaf in 150 mL boiling water for 5-10 minutes and then straining (2,4). The common dose of the liquid extract, 1:1 in 45% alcohol, is 0.1-0.3 mL three times daily (4). The tincture, 1:10 in 60% alcohol, is usually given as 0.5-2 mL three times daily (4). The average daily dose of the boldo leaf by infusion is 3 grams (2).

Comments

Fossilized boldo leaves that are over thirteen thousand years old have been found in Chile with the imprints of human teeth on them (6002).

BONESET

Also Known As

Agueweed, Crosswort, Feverwort, Indian Sage, Sweating Plant, Teasel, Thoroughwort, Vegetable Antimony.
CAUTION: See separate listings for Gravel Root and Sage.

Scientific Names

Eupatorium perfoliatum.
Family: Asteraceae/Compositae.

People Use This For

Orally, boneset is used as an antipyretic, diuretic, laxative, emesis, and cathartic.
Boneset is also used to treat influenza (especially with aching muscles), acute bronchitis, nasal inflammation, rheumatism, edema, dengue fever, and pneumonia; and as a stimulant and a diaphoretic.

Safety

POSSIBLY UNSAFE ...when used orally in excessive amounts. Large doses are both cathartic and emetic. Though the alkaloids have not been characterized, hepatotoxic pyrrolizidine alkaloids (PAs) are common in this genus (12842).
PREGNANCY AND LACTATION: POSSIBLY UNSAFE ...when used orally, due to possible hepatotoxic pyrrolizidine alkaloid content (12842); avoid using.

Effectiveness

There is insufficient reliable information available about the effectiveness of boneset.

Mechanism of Action

The applicable parts of boneset are the dried leaf and flowering parts. Preliminary research suggests boneset might have cytotoxic and mild antibacterial activity (12854).

Adverse Reactions

Orally, boneset can cause an allergic reaction in individuals sensitive to the Asteraceae/Compositae family. Members of this family include ragweed, chrysanthemums, marigolds, daisies, and many other herbs.

Interactions with Herbs & Other Dietary Supplements

None known.

Interactions with Drugs

None known.

Interactions with Foods

None known.

Interactions with Lab Tests

None known.

Interactions with Diseases or Conditions

CROSS-ALLERGENICITY: Boneset can cause an allergic reaction in individuals sensitive to the Asteraceae/Compositae family. Members of this family include ragweed, chrysanthemums, marigolds, daisies, and many other herbs.

Dosage and Administration

ORAL: Traditionally one cup of tea, prepared by steeping 1-2 grams herb in 150 mL boiling water, has been used three times daily. The liquid extract, 1:1 in 25% alcohol, has been used 1-2 mL three times daily. 1-4 mL of the tincture, 1:5 in 45% alcohol, has also been used three times daily (4).

Comments

Avoid confusion with gravel root (Eupatorium purpureum), also known as boneset.

BORAGE

Also Known As

Bee Plant, Beebread, Borage Oil, Borago, Burage, Burrage, Common Borage, Common Bugloss, Cool Tankard, Huile De Bourrache, Ox's Tongue, Talewort, Starflower.
CAUTION: See separate listings for Black Currant, Evening Primrose Oil, Gamma Linolenic Acid, and Omega-6 Fatty Acids.

Scientific Names

Borago officinalis.
Family: Boraginaceae.

People Use This For

Orally, borage seed oil is used for rheumatoid arthritis (RA), atopic eczema, infantile seborrheic dermatitis, neurodermatitis, and stress. It is also used for premenstrual syndrome (PMS), diabetes, attention deficit-hyperactivity disorder (ADHD), acute respiratory distress syndrome (ARDS), alcoholism, inflammation, and for preventing heart disease and stroke. Borage flower and leaves are used for fever, cough, depression. Borage is also used for adrenal insufficiency, for "blood purification", as a diuretic, to prevent inflammation of lungs and peritoneum, as a cardiac tonic, as a sedative, to induce sweating, and to increase circulatory capacity. Borage is also used to increase breast milk production and to treat bronchitis and colds.
Topically, borage is used for infantile seborrheic dermatitis, and as an emollient poultice.
In foods, borage is eaten in salads and soups.
In manufacturing, borage is used in skin care products.

Safety

POSSIBLY SAFE ...when used orally and appropriately. Only products that are certified and labeled as hepatotoxic pyrrolizidine alkaloid (PA)-free should be used (8458). Products containing hepatotoxic PAs are considered unsafe. ...when used topically and appropriately (7630). Advise patients not to apply products that contain hepatotoxic PAs on abraded or broken skin. Absorption of hepatotoxic PAs through broken skin can lead to systemic toxicities (12841). Suggest that patients use preparations that are certified and labeled as hepatotoxic PA-free.
LIKELY UNSAFE ...when products containing hepatotoxic pyrrolizidine alkaloid (PA) constituents are used orally. Repeated exposure to low concentrations of hepatotoxic PAs can cause severe veno-occlusive disease. Hepatotoxic PAs might also be carcinogenic and mutagenic (12841,12842). Tell patients not to use borage preparations that are not certified and labeled as hepatotoxic PA-free. There is insufficient reliable information available about the safety of using topical PA-free borage products on unbroken skin.
CHILDREN: POSSIBLY SAFE ...when used orally and appropriately. Only products that are certified and labeled as hepatotoxic pyrrolizidine alkaloid (PA)-free should be used (11341). ...when used topically and appropriately (7630,13305). Advise patients not to apply products that contain hepatotoxic PAs on abraded or broken skin. Absorption of hepatotoxic PAs through broken skin can lead to systemic toxicities (12841). Suggest that patients use preparations that are certified and labeled as hepatotoxic PA-free. LIKELY UNSAFE ...when products containing hepatotoxic pyrrolizidine alkaloid (PA) constituents are used orally. Repeated exposure to low concentrations of hepatotoxic PAs can cause severe veno-occlusive disease. Hepatotoxic PAs might also be carcinogenic and mutagenic (7631,11882,11883,12841,12842). Tell patients not to use borage seed oil preparations that are not certified and labeled as hepatotoxic PA-free.
PREGNANCY: LIKELY UNSAFE ...when used orally. Borage preparations containing pyrrolizidine alkaloid (PA) constituents might be teratogenic and hepatotoxic (12841,12842). There is insufficient reliable information available about the safety of using borage seed oil products that do not contain hepatotoxic PAs during pregnancy.
LACTATION: LIKELY UNSAFE ...when used orally. Hepatotoxic pyrrolizidine alkaloid (PA) constituents in borage are excreted in milk (12841,12842). There is insufficient reliable information available about the safety of using borage products that do not contain hepatotoxic PAs during lactation.

Effectiveness

POSSIBLY EFFECTIVE

Acute respiratory distress syndrome (ARDS). There is some evidence that borage seed oil might reduce the number of days in the intensive care unit (ICU) and the duration of ventilator requirement in patients with ARDS when used orally in combination with eicosapentaenoic acid (EPA) (7629).

Rheumatoid arthritis (RA). There is some evidence that taking borage seed oil in combination with conventional analgesics or anti-inflammatory agents might help decrease symptoms of RA after six weeks of treatment. The improvement appears to be sustained for up to 24 weeks. Borage seed oil can decrease the number of tender joints by 36%, the tender joint score by 45%, the number of swollen joints by 28%, and the swollen joint score by 41% (1985,8458).

POSSIBLY INEFFECTIVE

Atopic dermatitis (eczema). Taking borage seed oil orally 500-2000 mg daily for up to 24 weeks does not seem to improve symptoms of atopic dermatitis in adults or children (7632,7633,11341).

INSUFFICIENT RELIABLE EVIDENCE to RATE

Dermatitis. There is some preliminary evidence that topical application of borage seed oil might be helpful for infantile seborrheic dermatitis. It seems to heal infantile seborrheic dermatitis within 1 to 3 weeks (7630,13305). More evidence is needed to rate borage for this use.

Mechanism of Action

The applicable parts of borage are the seed oil, flowers, and leaves.

Borage oil contains 18% to 26% gamma-linolenic acid (GLA), an omega-6 fatty acid (8013). The leaves and flowers of borage do not contain GLA (7162).

GLA reduces production of interleukin 1 (IL-1)-beta, which may be involved in inflammation in diseases such as rheumatoid arthritis (RA) (12470). GLA is rapidly metabolized to dihomogammalinolenic acid (DGLA). DGLA is a precursor to prostaglandin E1 (PGE1), which has potent anti-inflammatory properties (8013,12088,12089).

Borage seed oil, in combination with fish oil, modulates the immune system by decreasing the serum activity of interleukin 10 (IL-10) and interleukin 4 (IL-4) and changing the activity of other cytokines (7635). Borage seed oil can decrease the activity of tumor necrosis factor (8459).

GLA contained in borage seed oil might also reduce the growth of tumors (8013).

GLA is also thought to lower triglycerides, increase high-density lipoprotein (HDL) levels, decrease blood pressure, have antiplatelet effects, and prolong bleeding time (1979,7634,8470).

GLA might also have an antiestrogenic effect. It seems to modulate the sensitivity of breast cancer cells to paclitaxel (Taxol) and fulvestrant (Faslodex), enhancing malignant cell-killing without adverse effects on normal cells (8133,11791). However, other research suggests that GLA alone can stimulate the growth of breast cancer cells at low concentrations and inhibit growth at higher concentrations (11339).

It has been theorized that low arachidonic acid levels in breast milk of atopic mothers might increase the risk of atopy in infants; however, maternal oral supplementation with borage seed oil does not increase concentrations of arachidonic acid in breast milk (6106).

Borage flower and dried leaves contain rosmarinic acid, which might have antioxidant effects (12855).

Borage contains various pyrrolizidine alkaloids (PAs), some of which are toxic. PAs are most concentrated in the plant roots, but may be found in all plant parts. Borage products contain variable amounts of hepatotoxic PAs. The total amount is usually less than 0.001% relative to the dry weight.

PAs, particularly unsaturated PAs, can cause hepatotoxicity. Cyclic diesters such as retrorsine and senecionine are the most hepatotoxic. Liver toxicity may result from PA-enhanced oxidative stress, but the exact mechanism of toxicity is unknown. Single doses of 10-20 mg PAs or chronic ingestion of amounts less than 10 mcg can cause veno-occlusive disease. PAs are metabolized by cytochrome P450 3A4 (CYP3A4). Hepatotoxicity may result from biotransformation of PAs by CYP3A4 into toxic dehydroalkaloids and pyrroles, which may then serve as alkylating agents (11882). Enzyme inducers such as phenobarbital seem to enhance toxicity (12841,12860). Pyrroles are excreted as N-acetyl cysteine conjugates. Some researchers speculate that early administration of N-acetyl cysteine might reduce toxicity (11988).

Metabolism is also affected by pregnane X receptor induction of CYP3A4. Genetic or drug induced variation in CYP3A4 or pregnane X receptor activity can affect the degree of PA toxicity by increasing or decreasing its metabolism (12841,12842). Hepatotoxic PAs are also toxic to the lungs. In animals, pneumotoxicity occurs as pulmonary hypertension and right ventricular hypertrophy. Hepatotoxic PAs are carcinogenic and mutagenic. There are sufficient amounts of hepatotoxic PAs in herbal products to cause toxicity (12841,12842).

Adverse Reactions

Orally, borage seed oil can cause soft stools, diarrhea, belching, and bloating (8013,11341).

Borage can also cause significant toxicity. The major concern about borage preparations is the hepatotoxic pyrrolizidine alkaloid (PA) content. These constituents are also potentially pneumotoxic, carcinogenic, and mutagenic (12841,12842). Chronic exposure to other plants containing hepatotoxic PA constituents has been associated with veno-occlusive disease (4021). Subacute veno-occlusive disease causes vague symptoms with persistent liver enlargement (4021). Symptoms of acute veno-occlusive disease include colicky pains in epigastrium, vomiting and diarrhea, and ascites within several days.

Enlargement and induration of the liver occurs within a few weeks (12842).

Interactions with Herbs & Other Dietary Supplements

HEPATOTOXIC PYRROLIZIDINE ALKALOID (PA)-CONTAINING HERBS: Concomitant use is contraindicated due to the risk of additive toxicity. Herbs containing hepatotoxic PAs include alkanna, butterbur, coltsfoot, comfrey, European buckthorn, gravel root, hemp agrimony, hound's tongue; and the Senecio species plants dusty miller, alpine ragwort, groundsel, golden ragwort, and tansy ragwort (12841).

HERBS THAT INDUCE CYTOCHROME P450 3A4 (CYP3A4): Theoretically, herbs that induce CYP3A4 might increase the conversion of hepatotoxic PAs to toxic metabolites, enhancing toxicity (12841,12860).

Herbs that induce CYP3A4 include St. John's wort and garlic.

HERBS WITH ANTICOAGULANT/ANTIPLATELET POTENTIAL: Theoretically, concomitant use of borage seed oil with herbs that also have constituents that might affect platelet aggregation could increase the risk of bleeding in some people (1979). These herbs include angelica, clove, danshen, garlic, ginger, ginkgo, Panax ginseng, red clover, turmeric, and others.

Interactions with Drugs

ANESTHESIA: Theoretically, concomitant use can increase the risk of seizures, based on one case report of evening primrose oil (another source of gamma linolenic acid) and possibly other drugs (613).
ANTICOAGULANT/ANTIPLATELET DRUGS: Borage seed oil contains gamma linolenic acid (GLA) that might have anticoagulant effects (1979). Theoretically, taking borage seed oil along with anticoagulant or antiplatelet drugs might increase the risk of bruising and bleeding. Some of these drugs include aspirin; clopidogrel (Plavix); nonsteroidal anti-inflammatory drugs (NSAIDs) such as diclofenac (Voltaren, Cataflam, others), ibuprofen (Advil, Motrin, others), and naproxen (Anaprox, Naprosyn, others); dalteparin (Fragmin); enoxaparin (Lovenox); heparin; warfarin (Coumadin); and others.
CYTOCHROME P450 3A4 (CYP3A4) INDUCERS: Hepatotoxic pyrrolizidine alkaloids (PAs) are substrates of cytochrome P450 3A4 (CYP3A4) (12841,12860). Theoretically, drugs that induce CYP3A4 might increase the conversion of PAs to toxic metabolites. Some drugs that induce CYP3A4 include carbamazepine (Tegretol), phenobarbital, phenytoin (Dilantin), rifampin, rifabutin (Mycobutin), and others.
NONSTEROIDAL ANTI-INFLAMMATORY DRUGS (NSAIDs): Theoretically, concomitant use of nonsteroidal anti-inflammatory drugs (NSAIDs) with borage seed oil might decrease the anti-inflammatory effect of borage seed oil (8459). However, borage seed oil is used commonly with NSAIDs in rheumatoid arthritis (RA), so the clinical significance of this potential interaction is uncertain (1985,8458).

Interactions with Foods

None known.

Interactions with Lab Tests

BLEEDING TIME: Borage seed oil might prolong bleeding time. Borage seed oil contains gamma linolenic acid (GLA), which can inhibit platelet aggregation (1979).
LIPID PROFILE: Borage seed oil might affect lipid levels. Borage seed oil contains GLA, which can lower plasma triglycerides and increase high-density lipoprotein (HDL) cholesterol (1979).

Interactions with Diseases or Conditions

BLEEDING DISORDERS: There is some concern that borage seed oil might prolong bleeding time and increase the risk of bruising and bleeding. Borage seed oil contains gamma linolenic acid (GLA), which can inhibit platelet aggregation (1979).
LIVER DISEASE: Theoretically, borage products containing hepatotoxic pyrrolizidine alkaloids (PA) might exacerbate liver disease (12841,12842).

Dosage and Administration

ORAL: For rheumatoid arthritis, 1.1 or 1.4 grams of borage seed oil daily for up to 24 weeks has been used (8458). For atopic dermatitis, 500-2000 mg borage seed oil daily has been used for up to 24 weeks (7632,11341).
TOPICAL: For infantile seborrheic dermatitis, 0.5 mL of borage seed oil applied two times daily for 10-12 days has been used. After the lesions resolve, borage seed oil has been applied 2-3 times each week until the infants reach six to seven months of age (7630).

BORON

Also Known As

Borate, Borates, Boric Acid, Boric Anhydride, Boric Tartrate, Sodium Borate.

Scientific Names

Boron; B; atomic number 5.

People Use This For

Orally, boron is used for promoting bone health, treating osteoarthritis, as an aid for building muscles and increasing testosterone levels, and for enhancing cognitive function and fine motor skills.
Topically, boric acid, the most common form of boron, is used as an astringent, to prevent skin infection, and as an ophthalmological irrigant.

Safety

LIKELY SAFE ...when used orally and appropriately. Boron is safe in amounts that do not exceed 20 mg per day, the Tolerable Upper Intake Level (UL) (7135). ...when used topically and appropriately. Boric acid, the most common form of boron, can be safely applied to non-broken skin (6).
POSSIBLY UNSAFE ...when used orally in high doses. Tell patients to avoid exceeding the UL of 20 mg per day.

Higher doses might theoretically cause adverse effects on the testes and male fertility (7135). Poisoning has occurred after ingestion of equivalent of 2.12 grams boron per day for 3-4 weeks (17).
CHILDREN: LIKELY SAFE ...when used orally and appropriately. Boron is safe in children in amounts that do not exceed the UL of 3 mg per day in children 1 to 3 years; 6 mg per day in children 4 to 8 years; 11 mg per day in children 9 to 13 years; 17 mg per day in adolescents 14 years or older (7135). The UL for infants has not been determined (7135). POSSIBLY UNSAFE ...when used orally in high doses. Tell patients to avoid exceeding the UL of 3 mg per day in children 1 to 3 years; 6 mg per day in children 4 to 8 years; 11 mg per day in children 9 to 13 years; and 17 mg per day in adolescents 14 years or older (7135). Higher doses might theoretically cause adverse effects on the testes and male fertility (7135).
PREGNANCY AND LACTATION: LIKELY SAFE ...when used orally and appropriately. Boron is safe in amounts that do not exceed the UL of 20 mg per day for pregnant or lactating women 19-50 years, or 17 mg per day for pregnant or lactating women ages 14 to 18 (7135). POSSIBLY UNSAFE ...when used orally in high doses. Tell patients to avoid exceeding the UL of 20 mg per day for pregnant or lactating women 19-50 years, or 17 mg per day for pregnant or lactating women ages 14 to 18 (7135). Higher doses might theoretically cause adverse effects in the developing fetus (7135).

Effectiveness

POSSIBLY INEFFECTIVE

Athletic conditioning. Taking boron orally doesn't seem to help increase lean body mass, muscle mass, or testosterone levels (944).

INSUFFICIENT RELIABLE EVIDENCE to RATE

Cognitive function. There is preliminary evidence that taking boron orally might improve cognitive function and fine motor skills in older people (943).

Osteoarthritis. Preliminary evidence suggests that boron might be useful for decreasing symptoms of osteoarthritis (941).

More evidence is needed to rate boron for these uses.

Mechanism of Action

Boron is a trace mineral for which a clear biological function in humans has not been established. There is some evidence, though, that boron might have a role in reproduction and development (945,7135). Boron is well absorbed from dietary beverages including prune and grape juice; wine; coffee; milk; and in some geographical locations, water (7135). Avocados, peanuts, pecans, apples, dried beans, and potatoes also contain boron (7135). Boron is excreted unchanged in the urine, with a half-life of 21 hours (7135).

Boron seems to be important in mineral metabolism and membrane function (943). Diets higher in boron seem to increase serum 17-beta-estradiol levels in postmenopausal women using estrogen replacement therapy (945). Supplemental boron may increase serum estradiol levels in postmenopausal women (945) and healthy men (937). Boron together with exercise seems to result in lower serum magnesium levels and modestly lower serum phosphorus concentrations (942). The lower serum phosphorus concentrations are diminished by exercise (940). Preliminary evidence suggests that boron may have a role in hand-eye coordination, attention span, and short-term memory (7135).

Adverse Reactions

Orally, boron appears to have a low toxicity (7135). Adverse reactions in doses below 10 mg per day (937) are unlikely. Chronic use of 1 gram daily of boric acid or 25 grams daily of boric tartrate can cause dermatitis, alopecia, anorexia, and indigestion (7135). Boric acid/borate can be fatal when taken orally in doses of 300 mg/kg (6). Large doses can result in acute poisoning. Children who have ingested 5 grams or more of borates can have persistent nausea, vomiting, and diarrhea leading to acute dehydration, shock, and coma. Adults who have ingested 15-20 grams of borate can exhibit nausea, vomiting, diarrhea, epigastric pain, hematemesis, and a blue-green discoloration of feces and vomit (17). Poisoning symptoms in adults and children may also include skin erythema, desquamation, exfoliation, hyperexcitability, irritability, tremors, convulsions, weakness, lethargy, headaches, and depression (17).

Interactions with Herbs & Other Dietary Supplements

MAGNESIUM: Boron supplements can reduce urinary excretion of magnesium and increase serum levels in women (940,9529,9623). In young women, age 18 to 25 years, the effect appears to be greater in sedentary than athletic women (940). In postmenopausal women, the effect is more marked in women with low dietary magnesium intake (9623). The clinical significance of these effects, and whether they occur in men, isn't known.
PHOSPHORUS: Supplemental boron might reduce serum phosphorus concentrations in some individuals (942).

Interactions with Drugs

ESTROGENS: Concomitant administration may increase serum estrogen levels (945).

Interactions with Foods

None known.

Interactions with Lab Tests

BONE MINERAL DENSITY (BMD): Supplemental boron may increase BMD and BMD measurements in young athletic females (942).
MAGNESIUM: Supplemental boron may reduce magnesium excretion and increase magnesium levels in women (940,9529,9623). Whether this occurs in men is unknown.
PHOSPHORUS: Supplemental boron might reduce serum phosphorus concentrations and test results in some individuals (942).

Interactions with Diseases or Conditions

HORMONE SENSITIVE CANCERS/CONDITIONS: Because boron might have estrogenic effects (945), women with hormone sensitive conditions should avoid supplemental boron or high amounts of boron from foods. Some of these conditions include breast cancer, uterine cancer, ovarian cancer, endometriosis, and uterine fibroids.
KIDNEY DISEASE/IMPAIRED KIDNEY FUNCTION: Theoretically, avoid supplements; boron appears to be largely excreted by kidneys (939).

Dosage and Administration

ORAL: There is no RDA for boron since an essential biological role for it has not been identified (7135).
Dietary intake of boron varies. Diets considered to be high in boron provide approximately 3.25 mg boron per 2000 kcal/day. Diets considered to be low in boron provide 0.25 mg boron per 2000 kcal/day (943).
The Tolerable Upper Intake Level (UL), the maximum dose at which no adverse effects would be expected, is 20 mg per day for adults and pregnant or lactating women over 19 years (7135). For adolescents 14 to 18 years and pregnant or lactating women 14 to 18 years, the UL is 17 mg per day (7135). For children 9 to 13 years, the UL is 11 mg per day; children 4 to 8 years, 6 mg per day; and children 1 to 3 years, 3 mg per day. A UL has not been established for infants (7135).

Comments

Boron was used as a food preservative between 1870 and 1920, and during World Wars I and II (945).

BOVINE CARTILAGE

Also Known As

Antitumor Angiogenesis Factor (anti-TAF), Bovine Tracheal Cartilage (BTC), Catrix, Catrix-S, Glycosaminoglycan Polysulphuric Acid Complex, Processed Bovine Cartilage, Psoriacin, Psoriacin-T, Rumalon.
CAUTION: See separate listings for Shark Cartilage and Chondroitin Sulfate.

Scientific Names

None.

People Use This For

Orally, bovine cartilage is used for rheumatoid arthritis, osteoarthritis, ulcerative colitis, scleroderma, psoriasis, allergic reactions caused by chemical toxins, herpes infection, glioblastoma multiforme, and cancer.
Topically, bovine cartilage is used for non-healing ulcerated wounds, moist lesions including pruritus ani, external hemorrhoids, acne, poison oak or poison ivy dermatitis, mandibular alveolitis (dry socket), and psoriasis.
Rectally, bovine cartilage is used for internal hemorrhoids and anal fissures.
Subcutaneously, bovine cartilage is used for osteoarthritis; rheumatoid arthritis; psoriasis; ulcerative colitis; regional enteritis; progressive systemic sclerosis; glioblastoma multiforme; inoperable squamous cancer of the nose; and cancers of the pancreas, lung, ovary, rectum, prostate, cervix, and thyroid.
Intramuscularly, bovine cartilage is used for osteoarthritis.

Safety

POSSIBLY SAFE ...when used orally, topically, subcutaneously, or intramuscularly and appropriately. Bovine cartilage has been used orally, topically, subcutaneously, and intramuscularly for up to five years without significant adverse effects (2009,2010,8242). Orally, up to 20 kg total have been used without evidence of toxicity. Subcutaneously, up to 40 grams per week and 300 grams total have been injected without evidence of toxicity. Intramuscularly, a complex including bovine cartilage and bone marrow (Rumalon) has been used safely when given in a total of ten treatment courses over five years. However, since these preparations are derived from animals, there is concern about contamination with diseased animal parts (see Adverse Reactions) (1825). So far, there are no reports of disease transmission to humans due to use of contaminated bovine cartilage.
PREGNANCY AND LACTATION: Insufficient reliable information available; avoid using.

Effectiveness

POSSIBLY EFFECTIVE

Acne. Applying bovine cartilage topically seems to help reduce acne (2009).

Anal fissures. Rectal use of bovine cartilage seems to help treat anal fissures (2009).

Anal pruritus. Applying a 5% bovine cartilage cream topically at least twice daily seems to help relieve itching within three days (2009).

Hemorrhoids. Rectal use of bovine cartilage seems to be help reduce hemorrhoids (2009).

Mandibular alveolitis. Applying bovine cartilage topically seems to be help treat mandibular alveolitis (2009).

Osteoarthritis. Administering bovine cartilage subcutaneously seems to help reduce symptoms of osteoarthritis (2009). However, intramuscular administration does not seem to be beneficial (8242).

Poison oak and poison ivy dermatitis. Applying a 5% bovine cartilage cream topically seems to help resolve dermatitis within one to two weeks (2009).

Psoriasis. There is some evidence that bovine cartilage can help patients with psoriasis when used topically or subcutaneously. However, churning symptoms, the appearance of new papules as the original lesions fade, may occur for three to six weeks during treatment. These are thought to result from release of psoriagens from present lesions. Eventually, these psoriagens seem to be excreted or metabolized, and then symptoms improve (2009).

Rheumatoid arthritis (RA). Administering bovine cartilage subcutaneously seems to help reduce symptoms of RA (2009).

There is insufficient reliable information available about the effectiveness of bovine cartilage for its other uses.

Mechanism of Action

Bovine cartilage is typically derived from bovine trachea rings. Some researchers think that bovine cartilage provides the needed biochemical components to support resynthesis of cartilage in individuals with osteoarthritis. It might also have anti-inflammatory effects (2009). Bovine cartilage is also thought to have immunoregulatory, hygroscopic-drying, and wound-healing activity (2009).

Adverse Reactions

Orally, bovine cartilage can cause osmotic diarrhea, nausea, and scrotal edema (2009). Subcutaneously, bovine cartilage might initially cause local redness, swelling, and itching (2010). To minimize initial local allergic reaction after subcutaneous administration, the first treatment dose should be limited to 2.5 grams, and administered in combination with oral diphenhydramine 25 mg for the first four treatments (2010). The appearance of new psoriatic papules (2009) and nephrotic syndrome (2011) has also occurred with use of bovine cartilage. Intramuscularly, bovine cartilage might initially cause local redness, rash, swelling, and itching (8242). Bovine cartilage can also cause local allergic reaction (2010). Since these products are derived from bovine tissues, there is some concern about the transmission of bovine spongiform encephalopathy to humans (1825). However, transmission of bovine disease to humans has not been reported with these products.

Interactions with Herbs & Other Dietary Supplements

None known.

Interactions with Drugs

None known.

Interactions with Foods

None known.

Interactions with Lab Tests

None known.

Interactions with Diseases or Conditions

None known.

Dosage and Administration

ORAL: For ulcerative colitis, a dose of 3 grams four times daily has been used (2009).

TOPICAL: For anal pruritus, a 5% cream applied two or more times daily has been used (2009). For poison ivy/oak dermatitis, a 5% cream has been applied every two hours initially and less frequently as itching is controlled (2009). For acne, a 5% cream has been applied at least twice daily after washing (2009). For mandibular alveolitis, powdered bovine cartilage mixed with saline to form a paste, packed into the dry socket following tooth extraction has been used (2009). For psoriasis, parenteral therapy followed by 5% ointment applied two to three times daily after bathing has been used (2009).

RECTAL: As a stool softener for hemorrhoids and anal fissures, bovine cartilage 2.2 grams in the form of a 2% suppository administered at least three times daily with oral dioctyl sodium sulfosuccinate (DSS) 100 mg twice daily has been used (2009).

SUBCUTANEOUS (SC): In general, 5-25 grams is usually given weekly or biweekly for most indications. An

exception is osteoarthritis, where doses up to 40 grams have been used. For psoriasis, doses of up to 75 grams have been used. For cancer, doses of 100-300 grams have been used, followed by an oral maintenance dose of 3 grams every eight hours for a maximum dose for the course of treatment of 20 kilograms. Bovine cartilage solutions for subcutaneous injection are usually prepared in a concentration of 50 mg/mL (diluted 1:10 with 1% lidocaine to alleviate discomfort). Doses of 25-50 mL (1.25-2.5 grams) are slowly injected in different sites with an 18-gauge needle until the total dose (e.g., 5-300 grams) is reached. Common sites of administration include the flanks, anterior thorax, abdomen, or anterior thighs, where subcutaneous space is readily distensible (2009,2010). To minimize initial local allergic reaction, the first treatment dose should be limited to 2.5 grams, and administered with oral diphenhydramine 25 mg for the first four treatments (2010).
INTRAMUSCULAR (IM): For osteoarthritis, a complex including bovine cartilage and bone marrow (Rumalon) has been used. It has been given in a total of ten treatment courses over five years. Each course consists of 15 total injections of 2 mL of the complex, administered twice weekly. Two courses are given each year (8242).

Comments
Catrix is a name which refers to activated acid-pepsin-digested bovine tracheal cartilage of calf origin (2009).

BOXWOOD

Also Known As
Boxwood Extract, Bush Tree, Buxaceae, Buxus, Dudgeon, SPV 30, SPV-30, SPV30.

Scientific Names
Buxus sempervirens, synonyms Buxus colchica, Buxus hyrcana.
Family: Buxaceae.

People Use This For
Orally, boxwood is used to treat HIV/AIDS and to boost immunity. Boxwood is also used for arthritis and as a "blood detoxifying agent."

Safety
POSSIBLY SAFE ...when the leaf extract is used orally and appropriately. There is some evidence that the boxwood leaf extract can be used safely for up to 16 months (5643).
LIKELY UNSAFE ...when the whole leaf is used orally (12,18). The whole boxwood leaf can cause life-threatening side effects including seizures, paralysis, and death by asphyxiation (18).
PREGNANCY AND LACTATION: LIKELY UNSAFE ...when the whole leaf is used orally (12,18); avoid using. There is insufficient reliable information available about the safety of the boxwood leaf extract when used during pregnancy and lactation; avoid using.

Effectiveness
INSUFFICIENT RELIABLE EVIDENCE to RATE

HIV/AIDS. There is preliminary evidence that a specific boxwood leaf extract (SPV30) 990 mg per day might delay disease progression in HIV-infected patients. It seems to delay decreases in CD4 cell counts, increases in viral load, and/or progression to AIDS in asymptomatic patients with CD4 counts greater than 350 cells per microliter and a relatively low viral load. A higher dose of 1980 mg per day does not seem to be effective possibly due to oxidative stress induced by flavonoids in the extract (5643). More evidence is needed to rate boxwood for this use.

Mechanism of Action
The applicable part of boxwood is the leaf. More than 20 steroidal alkaloids and four steroidal alkamines have been isolated from the boxwood extract. The extract containing cyclobuxine D and buxamine appears to be active against HIV; however, the mechanism is not known (4447). There is some speculation that flavonoids in the boxwood extract inhibit viral replication; however, there is not yet scientific evidence to support this.

Adverse Reactions
Orally, boxwood leaf extract can cause diarrhea and abdominal cramps. Ingestion of whole-leaf boxwood can cause serious side effects including vomiting, diarrhea, severe clonic spasms, paralysis and death secondary to asphyxiation (18). The extract, however, does not seem to have these effects (5643).
Topically, the fresh plant can also cause contact dermatitis (18).

Interactions with Herbs & Other Dietary Supplements
None known.

Interactions with Drugs
None known.

Interactions with Foods
None known.

Interactions with Lab Tests
None known.

Interactions with Diseases or Conditions
None known.

Dosage and Administration
ORAL: For HIV, a specific boxwood leaf extract (SPV30) 330 mg every 8 hours has been used (5643). Higher doses do not appear to be effective (5643).

Comments
Boxwood extract (SPV 30) is not usually found on store shelves. Most users get it through Internet sources or AIDS buyers' clubs.

BRAHMI

Also Known As
Bacopa, Jalanimba, Jalnaveri, Nira-Brahmi, Sambrani Chettu, Thyme-Leave Gratiola.
CAUTION: See separate listing for Gotu Kola.

Scientific Names
Bacopa monnieri, synonym Bacopa monniera; Herpestis monniera; Moniera cuneifolia.
Family: Scrophulariaceae.

People Use This For
Orally, brahmi is used to aid learning, and for anxiety, memory problems, attention deficit-hyperactivity disorder (ADHD), allergic conditions, and irritable bowel syndrome.
Brahmi has also been used orally for treating backache, hoarseness, mental illness, epilepsy, rheumatism, sexual dysfunction in both men and women, as a nerve tonic, cardiotonic, and as a diuretic.

Safety
POSSIBLY SAFE ...when used orally and appropriately for up to 12 weeks (10058).
PREGNANCY AND LACTATION: Insufficient reliable information available; avoid using.

Effectiveness
POSSIBLY EFFECTIVE

Cognitive function. Taking 300 mg brahmi extract per day for 12 weeks seems to improve verbal learning, memory, and information processing in healthy men and women (10058).

POSSIBLY INEFFECTIVE

Irritable bowel syndrome (IBS). Brahmi appears to be no more effective than placebo in preventing relapse of IBS (10059).

There is insufficient reliable information available about the effectiveness of brahmi for its other uses.

Mechanism of Action
The applicable part of brahmi is the leaf. Pharmacological activity of brahmi is attributed to the saponin bacoside and bacopasaponin constituents (10060,10061). Some evidence suggests purified bacosides A and B may facilitate learning ability and cognitive performance. Possible mechanisms for cognitive improvement include modulation of acetylcholine release, choline acetylase activity, and muscarinic cholinergic receptor binding (10058). Brahmi may also act as a mast cell stabilizer for allergic conditions (10060).

Adverse Reactions
Orally, brahmi can cause nausea, dry mouth, and fatigue (10058).

Interactions with Herbs & Other Dietary Supplements
None known.

Interactions with Drugs
None known.

Interactions with Foods
None known.

Interactions with Lab Tests
None known.

Interactions with Diseases or Conditions
None known.

Dosage and Administration
ORAL: For cognitive function improvement, a dosage of 300 mg brahmi extract per day has been used (10058).

Comments
Brahmi is a well-known herb in India and is frequently used in Ayurvedic herbal preparations. The name "brahmi" is derived from Brahma, a mystical creator of the Hindu pantheon. Centella asiatica (gotu kola) and Merremia gangetica have also been referred to by the name "brahmi," but most authorities associate brahmi with Bacopa monnieri (10061).

BRANCHED-CHAIN AMINO ACIDS

Also Known As
BCAA, Isoleucine, Leucine, L-Isoleucine, L-Leucine, L-Valine, Valine.
CAUTION: See separate listing for Whey Protein.

Scientific Names
2-amino-3-methylvaleric acid; 2-amino-4-methylvaleric acid; 2-amino-3-methylbutanoic acid.

People Use This For
Orally, branched-chain amino acids are used to enhance exercise performance, prevent fatigue, improve concentration, and reduce protein and muscle breakdown during intense exercise. They are also used for amyotrophic lateral sclerosis (ALS, Lou Gehrig's disease), latent portosystemic encephalopathy, and chronic hepatic encephalopathy. Branched-chain amino acids have also been used orally to treat anorexia in cancer patients, tardive dyskinesia, McArdle's disease (a genetic glycogen metabolic disorder), spinocerebellar degeneration, and to attenuate muscle-wasting during bed rest.
Intravenously, branched-chain amino acids are used for acute hepatic encephalopathy and in conditions of high metabolic stress due to severe trauma or sepsis.

Safety
LIKELY SAFE ...when used intravenously and appropriately. Branched-chain amino acids are an FDA-approved injectable product (13309).
POSSIBLY SAFE ...when used orally and appropriately, short-term. Branched-chain amino acids have not been associated with significant adverse effects in studies lasting from 1-2 weeks up to 6 months (68,72,73,74,10117,10146,10147).
CHILDREN: POSSIBLY SAFE ...when used orally and appropriately, short-term. Branched-chain amino acids have been safely used in children in studies lasting 2 weeks (13307,13308).
PREGNANCY AND LACTATION: Insufficient reliable information available; avoid using.

Effectiveness
POSSIBLY EFFECTIVE

Anorexia. Taking branched-chain amino acids orally seems to reduce anorexia and improve the overall nutritional status in elderly malnourished hemodialysis patients. A combination of branched-chain amino acids consisting of valine, leucine, and isoleucine may rapidly improve appetite and caloric intake, increasing plasma albumin levels and anthropometric measurements (10147). There is also some preliminary evidence that oral branched-chain amino acids might be helpful for anorexia in cancer patients (71).

Hepatic encephalopathy. Taking branched-chain amino acids orally can improve liver function tests and nitrogen balance in patients with chronic hepatic encephalopathy (68,69,82,690). Oral branched-chain amino acids are recommended for malnourished chronic hepatic encephalopathy patients who cannot tolerate protein supplementation (69,4274). When the enteral route is unavailable and in patients who cannot tolerate general purpose amino acid solutions, intravenous solutions with branched-chain amino acids can be used for nutritional support; however, most patients can tolerate standard amino acid mixtures (4274). In patients with latent hepatic encephalopathy taking branched-chain amino acids orally long-term seems to help improve psychomotor function and driving ability (684,685). There is also some preliminary evidence that intravenous branched-chain amino acids might be helpful for reversing coma in acute hepatic encephalopathy. So far, findings are conflicting (66,81,686,687,688,689,4274).

Mania. A tyrosine-free amino acid drink containing leucine, isoleucine, and valine, seems to diminish acute manic symptoms within 6 hours. When taken daily for 7 days, it seems to continue to improve symptoms over a 2-week period (10117).

Muscle breakdown. Taking branched-chain amino acids orally seems to reduce muscle breakdown during exercise (694).

Tardive dyskinesia. Taking branched-chain amino acids orally seems to reduce symptoms of tardive dyskinesia (72,10146,13307). A branched-chain amino acid drink containing valine, isoleucine, and leucine seems to reduce tardive dyskinesia movements by 30-60% in adult and pediatric patients who are taking antipsychotic drugs (10146,13307).

POSSIBLY INEFFECTIVE

Athletic performance. Taking branched-chain amino acids orally doesn't seem to enhance exercise or athletic performance (692).

LIKELY INEFFECTIVE

Amyotrophic lateral sclerosis (ALS, Lou Gehrig's disease). Early studies indicated that taking branched-chain amino acids orally are effective for ALS; however, more recent studies show no benefit and possibly excess loss of pulmonary function and mortality among patients using branched-chain amino acids (678,679,680,681).

INSUFFICIENT RELIABLE EVIDENCE to RATE

Diabetes. There is some preliminary evidence that ingestion of carbohydrates with an amino acid/protein mixture consisting of leucine 25%, phenylalanine 25%, and a wheat protein hydrolysate 50%, may increase the insulin response in patients with type 2 diabetes. Whether dietary supplementation of such a mixture can increase the efficacy of glucose-lowering medications or reduce dependency on insulin is unknown (10118).

Spinocerebellar degeneration (SCD). There is some preliminary clinical evidence that oral branched-chain amino acids might have a beneficial effect on symptoms of SCD (73).

More evidence is needed to rate branched-chain amino acids for these uses.

Mechanism of Action

Branched-chain amino acids are essential amino acids, including leucine, isoleucine, and valine (66,10116). Branched-chain amino acids are found in dietary protein, such as meat, dairy products, and legumes, and account for 15% to 25% of the total daily intake of protein (10116). Branched-chain amino acids act in numerous metabolic processes as modulators of protein synthesis, as substrates for protein synthesis, and as precursors in the synthesis of alanine and glutamine (10110,10116).

Branched-chain amino acids, in particular leucine, act as signaling molecules to stimulate protein synthesis (10110). Branched-chain amino acids seem to simulate pancreatic islet cells to release insulin, which is required for maximal stimulation of protein synthesis (10105,10108,10109,10110,10112,10113,10114). Skeletal muscle is the major site where branched-chain amino acids stimulate protein synthesis and are metabolized (78,10110). Branched-chain amino acids also stimulate protein synthesis in the adipose tissue and liver but not in the kidney (10111). In the heart, branched-chain amino acids seem to have a specific anabolic effect on heart protein metabolism (13306). Evidence indicates most, if not all, of the effects of protein synthesis in skeletal muscle is attributable to leucine alone (10108). The brain and kidney are involved in branched-chain amino acid metabolism but to a lesser degree than skeletal muscle (78). The sensitivity of branched-chain amino acids to stimulate protein synthesis appears to decline with age (10110).

The metabolism and degradation of branched-chain amino acids is linked to the production of alanine and glutamine and the maintenance of glucose homeostasis. The relationship between branched-chain amino acids and glucose metabolism is that they are associated with the glucose-alanine cycle. Branched-chain amino acids are continuously released from the liver and transported to skeletal muscle. Uptake of branched-chain amino acids by the muscle stimulates the transamination of branched-chain amino acids, which results in the production of glutamine and also the transfer of nitrogen from BCAA to pyruvate to produce alanine. Alanine circulates to the liver to support hepatic gluconeogenesis. The glucose-alanine cycle might account for greater than 40% of the glucose produced during prolonged exercise (10116). The oral administration of branched-chain amino acids before exercise increases serum ammonia levels during exercise (693,694); and appears to decrease muscle breakdown (694) and inhibit muscle glycogen degradation during exercise (77).

In the ischemic heart, infusion of branched-chain amino acids solution might contribute to energy production by reducing formation of myocardial lactate (13306).

Branched-chain amino acids also cross the blood brain barrier rapidly. Branched-chain amino acids play a role in the oxidation and synthesis of the excitatory neurotransmitter glutamate. Researchers think that dietary intake of branched-chain amino acids may be necessary to maintain pools of glutamate in the central nervous system (10107). Increased intake of branched-chain amino acids seems to decrease the synthesis of amine neurotransmitters such as dopamine, noradrenaline, and serotonin. Branched-chain amino acids decrease peripheral levels of aromatic amino acids, which are precursors of amine neurotransmitters, and reduce the amount of aromatic amino acids that is available for transport to the brain. An excess of neurotransmitters is associated with disorders such as tardive dyskinesia (10146). Branched-chain amino acids also compete with aromatic amino acids such as tryptophan, tyrosine, phenylalanine, and methionine for access to the neural amino acid transport system that allows amino acid entry into the brain (66,79,80,2719,10146). This competitive inhibition is used therapeutically for amino acid imbalances that produce false neurotransmitters in pathologic conditions such as hepatic encephalopathy (66,2719). Branched-chain amino acids are also used in hepatic encephalopathy as an energy source to prevent endogenous catabolism of proteins and reduce ammonia detoxification in the brain by increasing ammonia metabolism in skeletal muscle (69).

There is preliminary evidence diets deficient in branched-chain amino acids, including leucine, might be associated with decreased appetite and the development of anorexia. Continued consumption of such a diet is thought to cause a conditioned taste aversion and involve several neurotransmitters in the brain, including norepinephrine, GABA, serotonin, dopamine, and nitric oxide. However, the exact mechanism for this is unknown (10115). Supplementation of malnourished elderly patients with branched-chain amino acids seems to reduce anorexia and improve nutritional indices. Branched-chain amino acids might compete with tryptophan, a precursor for serotonin, for uptake across the blood brain barrier. By decreasing the synthesis of serotonin, branched-chain amino acids might increase appetite (10147).

There is some evidence daily administration of branched-chain amino acids containing leucine, isoleucine, and valine can decrease acute symptoms of mania, possibly by attenuating central dopaminergic overactivity and neurotransmission (10117).

Branched-chain amino acids might also reduce symptoms of tardive dyskinesia related to increased phenylalanine due to decreased clearance. Phenylalanine is a precursor of tyrosine, which is a precursor of dopamine. Increased phenylalanine can increase dopaminergic activity. Excessive dopaminergic activity is associated with tardive dyskinesia. Branched-chain amino acids might reduce plasma phenylalanine by increasing protein synthesis and insulin release, resulting in lower levels of phenylalanine in cerebrospinal fluid (13307).

There is evidence that ingestion of carbohydrates with an amino acid/protein mixture consisting of leucine, phenylalanine, and a wheat protein hydrolysate can increase the insulin response in type 2 diabetic patients. This suggests that amino acids might stimulate pancreatic beta cells to secrete insulin, independent of glucose stimulation (10118). Branched-chain amino acids might also promote protein synthesis and energy production in heart and skeletal muscle in people with type 2 diabetes (13006).

Adverse Reactions

Orally and intravenously, branched-chain amino acids can increase plasma ammonia levels (693,694), which can lead to fatigue and loss of motor coordination. Branched-chain amino acids can also cause nausea (10117). Short-term use of 60 grams of branched-chain amino acids containing leucine, isoleucine, and valine for 7 days in patients with normal metabolic function seems to increase levels of ammonia, but not to toxic plasma levels (10117). Liver function should be monitored if high doses or long-term use of branched-chain amino acids is used (10117).

Branched-chain amino acids should be used cautiously before or during activities where performance depends on motor coordination (75).

Orally, there has been one case report of hepatic encephalopathy in a chronic alcoholic. This resolved when dietary branched-chain amino acids were discontinued and recurred with rechallenge (691).

Increased mortality was reported in one study using branched-chain amino acids in the treatment of amyotrophic lateral sclerosis (ALS) (679).

Interactions with Herbs & Other Dietary Supplements

None known.

Interactions with Drugs

ANTIDIABETES DRUGS: Some evidence suggests that branched-chain amino acids might stimulate insulin release (10105,10110,10113,10114,10118). Theoretically, branched-chain amino acids might have an additive hypoglycemic effect with antidiabetic medications such as chlorpropamide (Diabinese), glipizide (Glucotrol), glyburide (DiaBeta), insulin, tolbutamide (Orinase), and others.

DIAZOXIDE (Hyperstat, Proglycem): Theoretically, the use of diazoxide might decrease the stimulation of protein synthesis by branched-chain amino acids (10110,10114). The significance of this and how muscle mass might be affected requires further study.

GLUCOCORTICOIDS (Decadron, Solu-Medrol, Deltasone): Theoretically, the use of glucocorticoids, such as dexamethasone, methylprednisolone, and prednisone, might decrease the stimulation of protein synthesis by branched-chain amino acids and increase the metabolism of branched-chain amino acids (10106). The significance of this and how muscle mass might be affected requires further study.

LEVODOPA: Theoretically, branched-chain amino acids may compete with levodopa for transport systems in the intestine and brain and decrease the effectiveness of levodopa (66,2719).

THYROID HORMONE (Cytomel, Triostat): There is evidence the use of some thyroid hormones (T3, L-triiodothyronine, liothyronine) can decrease metabolism of branched-chain amino acids. The significance of this and how muscle mass might be affected requires further study (10106).

Interactions with Foods

None known.

Interactions with Lab Tests
None known.

Interactions with Diseases or Conditions
AMYOTROPHIC LATERAL SCLEROSIS (ALS, Lou Gehrig's disease): The use of branched-chain amino acids has been associated with accelerated pulmonary failure and increased mortality when used in patients with ALS (679,681).
BRANCHED-CHAIN KETO ACIDURIA: Patients with branched-chain keto-aciduria are unable to effectively oxidize branched-chain amino acids, resulting in increased blood concentrations of branched-chain amino acids and branched-chain alpha-keto acids. Seizures and severe mental and physical retardation can result without proper dietary modification or if intake of branched-chain amino acids is increased (10107).
CHRONIC ALCOHOLISM: Dietary use of branched-chain amino acids in alcoholics has been associated with hepatic encephalopathy (691).
IDIOPATHIC HYPOGLYCEMIA: Intake of leucine has been reported to precipitate hypoglycemia in infants with idiopathic hypoglycemia. Some research suggests leucine stimulates the release of insulin (10105).

Dosage and Administration
ORAL: For latent or chronic hepatic encephalopathy, 240 mg/kg/day up to 25 grams of branched-chain amino acids have been used (68,685,690).
For mania, a 60 gram branched-chain amino acid drink containing valine, isoleucine, and leucine in a ratio of 3:3:4 has been used every morning for 7 days (10117).
For tardive dyskinesia, a branched-chain amino acid drink containing valine, isoleucine, and leucine at a dose of 222 mg/kg taken three times daily for 3 weeks has been used (10146).
For anorexia and improving the overall nutritional status in elderly malnourished hemodialysis patients, granules of branched-chain amino acids consisting of valine, leucine, and isoleucine at a dose of 4 grams taken three times daily has been used (10147).
The estimated average requirement (EAR) of branched-chain amino acids is 68 mg/kg/day (leucine 34 mg, isoleucine 15 mg, valine 19 mg) for adults (11120). However, some researchers think earlier testing methods may have underestimated this requirement and that the requirement is about 144 mg/kd/day (13310).
Other researchers think the EARs for children are also low (13308). EARs for branched-chain amino acids for children are: ages 7-12 months, 134 mg/kg/day; 1-3 years, 98 mg/kg/day; 4-8 years, 81 mg/kg/day; boys 9-13 years, 81 mg/kg/day; girls 9-13 years, 77 mg/kg/day; boys 14-18 years, 77 mg/kg/day; girls 14-18 years, 71 mg/kg/day (11120).
INTRAVENOUS (IV): For all types of hepatic encephalopathy in patients who are intolerant to standard amino acid solutions and cannot take oral therapy, a typical dose of commercially available branched-chain amino acid solution (e.g., HepatAmine) is 80-120 grams per day, which provides 28-43 grams of branched-chain amino acids per day (68,266,687,689).

BREWER'S YEAST

Also Known As
Baker's Yeast, Brewers Yeast, Faex Medicinalis, Levure De Biere, Medicinal Yeast.
CAUTION: See separate listing for Saccharomyces boulardii.

Scientific Names
Saccharomyces cerevisiae.
Family: Saccharomycetaceae.
Candida utilis.
Family: Candidaceae.

People Use This For
Orally, brewer's yeast is used for diarrhea, loss of appetite, chronic acne, premenstrual syndrome, furunculosis, and high chromium type diabetes. It has also been used as a source of B vitamins and protein.

Safety
POSSIBLY SAFE ...when used orally and appropriately, short-term.
There is insufficient reliable information available about the safety of the long-term use of brewer's yeast.
CHILDREN: POSSIBLY SAFE ...when used orally and appropriately; however, diarrhea should be evaluated by a medical professional before using brewer's yeast (2).
PREGNANCY AND LACTATION: Insufficient reliable information available; avoid using.

Effectiveness

POSSIBLY EFFECTIVE

Premenstrual syndrome (PMS). There is some evidence that taking a specific brewer's yeast preparation orally in combination with vitamins and minerals (Sillix Donna, Giuliani) might help reduce symptoms of PMS (7845).

INSUFFICIENT RELIABLE EVIDENCE to RATE

Clostridium difficile colitis. There is a case report of resolution of recurrent Clostridium difficile colitis after use of brewer's yeast for four months in combination with a 30-day course of vancomycin. Before this treatment, the patient experienced four relapses; after this treatment, there were no further relapses (6432). It is not clear what benefit, if any, the yeast product provided in the treatment. More evidence is needed to rate brewer's yeast for this use.

Mechanism of Action

Brewer's yeast can have some action against C. difficile and enterotoxic E. coli. It reduces water and electrolyte influx into the intestines stimulated by the C. vibrio toxin. Brewer's yeast can increase the activity of intestinal disaccharidases, saccharidases, maltase, and lactase to alleviate diarrhea symptoms (2). Preliminary evidence suggests that brewer's yeast can reduce infection caused by Brucella species, by increasing activity of phagocytic cells (7846). It can also increase insulin release (6004).

Adverse Reactions

Orally, brewer's yeast can cause migraine-like headaches in sensitive individuals, intestinal discomfort, and flatulence (2). Allergic reactions to brewer's yeast can occur in hypersensitive individuals. Symptoms include itching, urticaria, local or general exanthemas, and Quincke's edema (2). Crohn's disease can be exacerbated by brewer's yeast with dietary or occupational exposure (7645).

Interactions with Herbs & Other Dietary Supplements

None known.

Interactions with Drugs

ANTIFUNGALS: These drugs can reduce yeast activity (2).

MONOAMINE OXIDASE INHIBITORS (MAOIs): Brewer's yeast is contraindicated, because concomitant use can increase blood pressure (2).

Interactions with Foods

None known.

Interactions with Lab Tests

ANTIMICROBIAL TESTS: Brewer's yeast can confound results. Report the use of brewer's yeast to the lab (2).

Interactions with Diseases or Conditions

CROHN'S DISEASE: Dietary intake of Brewer's yeast can increase the severity of Crohn's disease (7645).

Dosage and Administration

ORAL: The typical dose is 6 grams of brewer's yeast per day (2).

Comments

Brewer's yeast is obtained as a by-product from the brewing of beer made from an extract of grains and hops.

BROMELAIN

Also Known As

Bromelains, Bromelainum, Bromelin, Pineapple Enzyme, Plant Protease Concentrate.
CAUTION: See separate listing for Papain.

Scientific Names

Ananas comosus (Pineapple), synonyms Ananas ananas, Ananas duckei, Ananas sativus, Bromelia ananas, Bromelia comosa.
Family: Bromeliaceae.

People Use This For

Orally, bromelain is used for acute postoperative and post-traumatic conditions of swelling, especially of the nasal and paranasal sinuses. It is also used orally for burn debridement, anti-inflammatory action, allergic rhinitis, prevention of epinephrine-induced pulmonary edema, smooth muscle relaxation, stimulation of muscle contractions, inhibition of blood platelet aggregation, enhanced antibiotic absorption, cancer prevention, shortening of labor, and enhanced excretion of fat. Bromelain is also used orally for mild ulcerative colitis.

In combination with trypsin and rutin, bromelain is used orally for osteoarthritis.

Safety

POSSIBLY SAFE ...when used orally and appropriately (960,6252).

PREGNANCY AND LACTATION: Insufficient reliable information available; avoid using.

Effectiveness

POSSIBLY EFFECTIVE

Osteoarthritis. Taking bromelain orally as a specific combination with trypsin and rutin (Phlogenzym) seems to reduce pain and improve knee function in patients with osteoarthritis. This bromelain combination product seems to be comparable to diclofenac (Voltaren) 50 mg three times daily for one week, then twice daily for two weeks (6252).

POSSIBLY INEFFECTIVE

Myalgia. Bromelain 300 mg three times daily, immediately following an intense exercise regimen, does not seem to delay onset of muscle soreness and has no effect on pain, flexibility, or skeletal weakness (10622).

INSUFFICIENT RELIABLE EVIDENCE to RATE

Knee pain. There's some evidence that taking bromelain orally can reduce mild acute (duration of less than 3 months) knee pain in otherwise healthy patients. Doses of 400 mg bromelain daily seem to be more effective than 200 mg daily in relieving pain, stiffness, and physical function of the knee (11457).

Trauma. Preliminary clinical research suggests bromelain might reduce swelling and pain after surgery or trauma (960); but it doesn't seem to reduce swelling after oral surgery (957).

Ulcerative colitis. Anecdotal evidence suggests that bromelain might improve some symptoms of ulcerative colitis in people with persistent disease despite standard therapy (6253).

More evidence is needed to rate bromelain for these uses.

Mechanism of Action

Bromelain is a general name for proteolytic enzymes obtained from the stem and fruit of the pineapple (9183). Bromelain contains constituents that interfere with the growth of malignant cells and inhibit platelet aggregation. It also possesses fibrinolytic activity and skin debridement properties (10639). The platelet aggregation inhibition action may be related to proteolytic activity. Fibrinolytic activity and an increase in adenosine monophosphate (AMP) may be key in the anti-cancer properties (10639). Bromelain might also exert an anti-inflammatory effect by altering leukocyte migration and activation. However, there is some question whether bromelain reaches concentrations required for anti-inflammatory activity outside of the gastrointestinal tract. Plasma contains proteinase inhibitors that may inactivate bromelain (9183). A polyenzyme preparation containing bromelain can increase the release of reactive oxygen species by polymorphonuclear neutrophils in healthy people (962).

Adverse Reactions

Orally, bromelain may cause gastrointestinal (GI) disturbances or diarrhea. Immunoglobulin E (IgE)-mediated allergic reactions to bromelain may occur and include a cross-allergenicity between bromelain and wheat flour, celery, papain, carrot, fennel, cypress pollen, and grass pollen. Cross-allergenicity may also occur with members of the Asteraceae/Compositae plant family. Some of these herbs include ragweed, chrysanthemums, marigolds, daisies, echinacea, and many other herbs (959,9184).

Interactions with Herbs & Other Dietary Supplements

HERBS WITH ANTICOAGULANT/ANTIPLATELET POTENTIAL: Theoretically, bromelain can increase the risk of bleeding when used concomitantly with herbs that have anticoagulant or antiplatelet potential (10639). Some of these herbs include alfalfa, angelica, aniseed, arnica, asafoetida, celery, chamomile, clove, fenugreek, feverfew, fucus, garlic, ginger, horse chestnut, licorice, meadowsweet, poplar, northern and southern prickly ash, quassia, red clover, and willow.

MAGNESIUM: Acts as a reducing agent and activates bromelain (11).

ZINC (an oxidizing agent): Concomitant use inhibits bromelain activity (11).

Interactions with Drugs

ANTICOAGULANT/ANTIPLATELET DRUGS: Theoretically, concomitant use might cause additive anticoagulant/antiplatelet effects and increase the risk of bleeding (10639).

TETRACYCLINE ANTIBIOTICS: Concomitant therapy increases plasma and urine tetracycline levels (2).

Interactions with Foods
POTATO PROTEIN and SOYBEAN: These foods can inhibit bromelain activity (958,961).

Interactions with Lab Tests
None known.

Interactions with Diseases or Conditions
PINEAPPLE ALLERGY: People allergic to pineapple might also have allergic reactions to bromelain (959).

Dosage and Administration
ORAL: For osteoarthritis, a combination enzyme product (Phlogenzym), which contains rutin 100 mg, trypsin 48 mg, and bromelain 90 mg, given 2 tablets 3 times daily has been used (6252). For delayed onset muscle soreness, bromelain 300 mg three times daily immediately following an intense exercise regimen has been used (10622).
For acute knee pain, bromelain 200 mg to 400 mg daily for 30 days has been used (11457).

BROOKLIME

Also Known As
Beccabunga, Mouth-Smart, Neckweed, Speedwell, Water Pimpernel, Water Purslane.
CAUTION: See separate listings for Black Root and Veronica.

Scientific Names
Veronica beccabunga.
Family: Scrophulariaceae.

Comments
At the date of publication, there was very little scientific information available about this product. Our staff is continually analyzing the available information on natural medicines and will add data to the online version of *Natural Medicines Comprehensive Database* as it becomes available. See www.naturaldatabase.com.

BROOM CORN

Also Known As
Darri, Durri, Guinea Corn, Sorghum.

Scientific Names
Sorghum bicolor, synonyms Sorghum vulgare, Andropogon sorghum, Holcus bicolor, Milium nigricans, Panicum caffrorum.
Family: Poaceae/Gramineae.

People Use This For
Orally, broom corn is used for digestive disorders.
In foods, broom corn is used as a cereal grain.

Safety
LIKELY SAFE ...when consumed in food amounts (18). Although the fruit contains cyanogenic glycosides, the concentrations are very low (18).
There is insufficient reliable information available about the safety of broom corn used in amounts larger than those found in foods.
PREGNANCY AND LACTATION: Insufficient reliable information available.

Effectiveness
There is insufficient reliable information available about the effectiveness of broom corn.

Mechanism of Action
The applicable part of broom corn is the seed. Broom corn contains a high percentage of starch and a small amount of protein and fatty oil. It also contains thiamine and riboflavin. Dhurrin, a cyanogenic glycoside, is present in a very low amount in the fruit, 0.005-5 mg per 100 grams. In contrast, the foliage contains a much higher level, 250-700 mg per 100 grams. Broom corn is thought to have a soothing effect on the alimentary tract (18).

Adverse Reactions
None reported.

Interactions with Herbs & Other Dietary Supplements
None known.

Interactions with Drugs
None known.

Interactions with Foods
None known.

Interactions with Lab Tests
None known.

Interactions with Diseases or Conditions
None known.

Dosage and Administration
No typical dosage.

BRYONIA

Also Known As
Bryoniae Radix, Devil's Turnip, English Mandrake, Ladies' Seal, Tamus, Tetterberry, White Bryony, Wild Hops, Wild Nep, Wild Vine, Wood Vine.
CAUTION: See separate listings for European Mandrake and Podophyllum (American Mandrake).

Scientific Names
Bryonia cretica; Bryonia alba.
Family: Cucurbitaceae.

People Use This For
Orally, bryonia is used as a laxative, emetic, diuretic, for gastrointestinal diseases, respiratory tract diseases, arthritis, liver disease, metabolic disorders, and for prophylaxis against infections.

Safety
LIKELY UNSAFE ...when the root is used orally (2). ...when the berries are ingested; 40 berries might be fatal (18).
CHILDREN: LIKELY UNSAFE ...when the berries are ingested; 15 berries can be fatal (18). ...when the root is used orally (2).
PREGNANCY: UNSAFE ...when the root is used orally because it can cause abortion (2). ...when the berries are ingested (2).
LACTATION: LIKELY UNSAFE ...when the root is used orally (2). ...when the berries are ingested (2).

Effectiveness
There is insufficient reliable information available about the effectiveness of bryonia.

Mechanism of Action
The applicable part of bryonia is the root. The resin from bryonia has strong purgative effects (18). Some evidence suggests the aqueous extract might be effective against tumors (18). Other evidence suggests the methanol extract could have hypoglycemic effects (18).

Adverse Reactions
Orally, bryonia can cause dizziness, vomiting, convulsions, colic, bloody diarrhea, abortion, nervous excitement, and kidney damage (2). Large doses can cause anuria, collapse, spasms, paralysis, and death (2).
Topically, skin contact with fresh bryonia may cause irritation (19). Ingestion of 15 berries is likely to be fatal to a child. Ingestion of 40 berries is likely to be fatal for adults (18).

Interactions with Herbs & Other Dietary Supplements
None known.

Interactions with Drugs
None known.

Interactions with Foods
None known.

Interactions with Lab Tests
None known.

Interactions with Diseases or Conditions
GASTROINTESTINAL (GI) IRRITATION: Bryonia may irritate the GI tract. It is contraindicated in individuals with infectious or inflammatory GI conditions (19).

Dosage and Administration
No typical dosage.

Comments
Bryonia is no longer used as an emetic or laxative due to safety concerns (2).

BUCHU

Also Known As
Barosmae Folium, Bookoo, Bucco, Bucku, Diosma, Round Buchu, Short Buchu.

Scientific Names
Agathosma betulina, synonyms Barosma betulina, Hartogia betulin, Parapetalifera betulina; Agathosma crenulata, synonyms Barosma crenulata, Diosma crenulata, Parapetalifera crenulata, Parapetalifera odorata; Agathosma serratifolia, synonyms Barosma serratifolia, Diosma serratifolia, Parapetalifera serrata, Parapetalifera serratifolia.
Family: Rutaceae.

People Use This For
Orally, buchu is used as a urinary tract disinfectant in cystitis, urethritis, prostatitis, acute cystitis, kidney infections, and venereal disease.
In manufacturing, the oil from buchu is used to give a fruit flavor (often black currant) to foods.

Safety
LIKELY SAFE ...when the leaf is used in amounts commonly found in foods. Buchu has Generally Recognized As Safe status (GRAS) for use in foods in the US (4912).
POSSIBLY SAFE ...when the leaf is used orally and appropriately in medicinal amounts (2,12).
POSSIBLY UNSAFE ...when excessive amounts of buchu leaf are taken orally or when the oil is ingested. Buchu contains pulegone, a known hepatotoxin (4). Pulegone is a major component of the oil.
PREGNANCY: LIKELY UNSAFE ...when used in medicinal amounts; buchu is reported to be an abortifacient (4).
LACTATION: POSSIBLY SAFE ...when used in food amounts. There is insufficient reliable information available about the safety of using larger amounts; avoid using.

Effectiveness
There is insufficient reliable information available about the effectiveness of buchu.

Mechanism of Action
The applicable part of buchu is the leaf. Buchu camphor (also known as diosphenol) is the principal constituent of the oil. Researchers believe this constituent may be responsible for buchu's reported diuretic and antiseptic effects (5).

Adverse Reactions
Orally, buchu leaf can cause GI and kidney irritation (4,6) and increase menstrual flow (6). Buchu is also a reported abortifacient (4).

Interactions with Herbs & Other Dietary Supplements
None known.

Interactions with Drugs
ANTICOAGULANT/ANTIPLATELET DRUGS: May possibly enhance the effects of anticoagulants (6002).

Interactions with Foods
None known.

Interactions with Lab Tests
None known.

Interactions with Diseases or Conditions
KIDNEY INFECTION: Contraindicated (4,12).
URINARY TRACT INFLAMMATION: Contraindicated (4,12).

Dosage and Administration
ORAL: The typical dose is 1 cup of tea (steep 1 gram dry leaf in 150 mL boiling water 5-10 minutes, strain) several times per day (8).

Comments
Liver function should be monitored in people who use buchu because of its potential hepatotoxicity.

BUCKHORN PLANTAIN

Also Known As
Buckhorn, Chimney-Sweeps, English Plantain, Headsman, Hoary Plantain, Plantaginis lanceolatae herba, Plantain, Ribgrass, Ribwort, Ribwort Plantain, Ripplegrass, Soldier's Herb, Spitzwegerichkraut.
CAUTION: See separate listings for Great Plantain, Blond Psyllium, Black Psyllium, and Water Plantain.

Scientific Names
Plantago lanceolata.
Family: Plantaginaceae.

People Use This For
Orally, buckhorn plantain is used to treat inflammation of mucous membranes in the respiratory tract, for the common cold, cough, bronchitis, and fevers.
Topically, buckhorn plantain is used for pharyngeal mucous membrane inflammation, inflammation of the skin, wound healing, and to arrest hemorrhages.

Safety
POSSIBLY SAFE ...when used orally and appropriately (2). ...when used topically (2).
PREGNANCY AND LACTATION: LIKELY UNSAFE ...when used orally or topically.
Some evidence suggests buckhorn plantain affects muscle tone of the uterus (4275).

Effectiveness
There is insufficient reliable information available about the effectiveness of buckhorn plantain.

Mechanism of Action
The applicable parts of buckhorn plantain are the above ground parts. The tannin constituents have an astringent and antibacterial effect (18). Mucilage constituents are believed to be responsible for reducing local irritation and protecting mucous membranes from irritants (7).

Adverse Reactions
Buckhorn plantain is an allergen and a common problem in the early spring (3901).

Interactions with Herbs & Other Dietary Supplements
None known.

Interactions with Drugs
None known.

Interactions with Foods
None known.

Interactions with Lab Tests
None known.

Interactions with Diseases or Conditions
None known.

Dosage and Administration
ORAL: People typically use one cup tea (steep 2-3 grams chopped plant parts in 150 mL boiling water for 10 minutes, strain) several times daily (8,18); average amount is 3-6 grams per day (2).
TOPICAL: No typical dosage.

Comments

Avoid confusion with common plantain (Plantago major). CAUTION: Digitalis leaves resemble plantain leaves; adulteration of plantain with digitalis has been reported (3905). Be careful not to confuse buckhorn plantain with digitalis, which is an unsafe product (2,12).

BUCKWHEAT

Also Known As

Buchweizen, Grano Turco, Sarrasin, Silverhull Buckwheat.

Scientific Names

Fagopyrum esculentum, synonyms Fagopyrum sagittatum, Fagopyrum vulgare; Fagopyrum tataricum, synonym Polygonum tataricum.
Family: Polygonaceae.

People Use This For

Orally, buckwheat is used to improve venous and capillary tone, to prevent hardening of the arteries, and for diabetes. It is also used orally to alleviate venous stasis and varicose veins.

Safety

POSSIBLY SAFE ...when used orally and appropriately (11438,11442).
PREGNANCY AND LACTATION: Insufficient reliable information available; avoid using.

Effectiveness

INSUFFICIENT RELIABLE EVIDENCE to RATE

Diabetes. Preliminary evidence suggests that consuming dietary buckwheat may improve long-term glucose tolerance in patients with diabetes (11438,11442). More evidence is needed to rate buckwheat for this use.

Mechanism of Action

The applicable parts of buckwheat are the leaves and flowers (18). The active constituents of buckwheat include the tocopherols, phenolic acids, and flavonoids. Many flavonoids including rutin, orientin, quercetin, quercitrin, isoorientin, isovitexin, and vitexin have been isolated in buckwheat grain (11431,11439). Buckwheat contains naphthadianthrones, which have photosensitizing effects. Phototoxicity has occurred in animals that ingest large quantities of buckwheat (18).

Dietary buckwheat is largely consumed as flour, used as an ingredient in foods such as bread, pancakes, and noodles. Buckwheat flour contains up to 12% protein, 69% carbohydrates, 3% lipids, and 14% water; as well as a well-balanced composition of amino acids. A buckwheat protein product, extracted from buckwheat flour, contains up to 66% protein, 6% carbohydrates, 22% lipids, and 3% water; as well as an unchanged well-balanced composition of amino acids (11434).

Buckwheat may improve overall glucose tolerance in diabetes by increasing the sensitivity of beta cells to glucose (11438,11442). Buckwheat is reported to have antioxidant activity, possibly through free radical scavenger and anti-lipid peroxidation activities (11432,11444). Preliminary animal research suggests this antioxidant activity might reduce the progression of renal failure (11433). Animal evidence also suggests buckwheat may possess anti-allergenic properties. Although the mechanism is not completely understood, the anti-allergenic action may be associated with histamine release inhibition and cytokine expression in mast cells (11441).

Adverse Reactions

Orally, allergic reactions to buckwheat in adults and children can include skin sensitization, allergic rhinitis, asthma, and anaphylaxis (11435,11436,11437). Occupational exposure to buckwheat, or household exposure through sleeping on a buckwheat husk stuffed-pillow can cause sensitization, of which symptoms include allergic rhinitis and asthma (11437,11443).

Interactions with Herbs & Other Dietary Supplements

None known.

Interactions with Drugs

None known.

Interactions with Foods

None known.

Interactions with Lab Tests

None known.

Interactions with Diseases or Conditions

BUCKWHEAT ALLERGY: Patients with buckwheat allergies are at risk for serious allergic reactions. Allergic reactions can include skin sensitization, allergic rhinitis, asthma, and anaphylaxis (11435,11437).
CELIAC DISEASE: Although some debate exists over the safety of buckwheat in a gluten-free diet, both the Celiac Disease Foundation and the Gluten Intolerance Group consider buckwheat an acceptable food item (11440,11445).

Dosage and Administration

ORAL: For diabetes, 70-100 g buckwheat flour or grain daily has been used (11438,11442).

BUGLE

Also Known As

Ajuga, Bugula, Carpenter's Herb, Middle Comfrey, Middle Confound, Sicklewort.
CAUTION: See separate listing for Comfrey.

Scientific Names

Ajuga reptans.
Family: Lamiaceae/Labiatae.

Comments

At the date of publication, this product was not a common ingredient used in brand name supplements marketed to consumers. Details about this product are available in the online version of *Natural Medicines Comprehensive Database.* See www.naturaldatabase.com.

BUGLEWEED

Also Known As

Archangle, Ashangee, Bugle Weed, Green Wolf's Foot, Gypsy Weed, Gypsywort, Hoarhound, Lycopi Herba, Paul's Betony, Sweet Bugle, Virginia Water Horehound, Water Bugle, Water Hoarhound, Water Horehound, Wolfstrapp.
CAUTION: See separate listings for Horehound, Black Horehound, and Veronica.

Scientific Names

Lycopus americanus; Lycopus europaeus; Lycopus virginicus.
Family: Lamiaceae/Labiatae.

People Use This For

Orally, bugleweed is used for mild hyperthyroidism, premenstrual syndrome, breast pain, nervousness, insomnia; and bleeding, especially nosebleeds and heavy bleeding during menses.

Safety

POSSIBLY SAFE ...when used orally and appropriately (12).
PREGNANCY: LIKELY UNSAFE ...when used orally (12,19) because it has anti-gonadotropic and anti-thyrotropic activity (7,19); avoid using.
LACTATION: LIKELY UNSAFE ...when used orally (12,19) because it might have anti-prolactin activity (7,19); avoid using.

Effectiveness

There is insufficient reliable information available about the effectiveness of bugleweed.

Mechanism of Action

The applicable parts of bugleweed are the above ground parts. Bugleweed demonstrates anti-gonadotropic and anti-thyrotropic activity. It also seems to lower serum prolactin levels (7) and inhibit peripheral deiodination of T4 (2). Bugleweed can also have hypoglycemic activity (19).

Adverse Reactions

Orally, bugleweed rarely can cause thyroid enlargement during extended therapy or with large amounts (7). The sudden discontinuation of bugleweed can result in a sudden increase in thyroid function (2) and prolactin secretion (7).

Interactions with Herbs & Other Dietary Supplements

THYROID-SUPPRESSING HERBS: Theoretically, concomitant use of bugleweed with other thyroid suppressing herbs can have additive therapeutic and adverse effects (19). Herbs with thyroid-suppressing effects include balm leaf and the wild thyme plant (19).

Interactions with Drugs

ANTIDIABETES DRUGS: Theoretically, concomitant use of bugleweed can increase the risk of hypoglycemia (19). Blood glucose levels should be monitored closely.
THYROID HORMONE: Concomitant use of bugleweed is contraindicated because bugleweed may reduce the effects of thyroid hormones by blocking peripheral conversion of thyroxin to T3 (19).

Interactions with Foods

None known.

Interactions with Lab Tests

RADIOACTIVE ISOTOPES: Bugleweed can interfere with diagnostic procedures using radioactive isotopes (2).
THYROID FUNCTION TESTS: Bugleweed might improve thyroid function and test results in mildly hyperthyroid patients (2).

Interactions with Diseases or Conditions

DIABETES: Theoretically, bugleweed can interfere with blood glucose control and increase the risk of hypoglycemia (19). Blood glucose levels should be monitored closely while using bugleweed in diabetic patients.
THYROID DISEASE: Bugleweed is contraindicated in thyroid enlargement, thyroid hypofunction (2,12,19), and during administration of other thyroid treatments (12).

Dosage and Administration

ORAL: The typical dose of bugleweed is 0.2-2 grams per day of the above ground parts or equivalent preparations (7). The dose must be carefully individualized, taking age and weight into consideration (2).

BULBOUS BUTTERCUP

Also Known As

Crowfoot, Cuckoo Buds, Frogsfoot, Frogwort, Goldcup, King's Cup, Meadowbloom, Pilewort, St. Anthony's Turnip.
CAUTION: See separate listings for Buttercup and Poisonous Buttercup.

Scientific Names

Ranunculus bulbosus.
Family: Ranunculaceae.

People Use This For

Orally, bulbous buttercup is used for skin diseases, arthritis, gout, neuralgia, influenza, and meningitis.

Safety

LIKELY UNSAFE ...when used orally or topically because it can cause severe local irritation (18).
PREGNANCY AND LACTATION: LIKELY UNSAFE ...when used orally or topically (18); avoid using.

Effectiveness

There is insufficient reliable information available about the effectiveness of bulbous buttercup.

Mechanism of Action

The applicable parts of bulbous buttercup are the latex and the whole fresh flowering plant. When the fresh plant is crushed or cut into small pieces, the glycoside ranunculin is enzymatically changed into a severely irritating protoanemonin, which, in turn, rapidly degrades into the less toxic anemonin (18). Both protoanemonin and ranunculin are destroyed to an unknown extent during the drying process (2). The constituents ranunculin, protoanemonin, anemonin, and labenzym can cause drowsiness, fatigue and depressive moods. Protoanemonin present in the freshly harvested, bruised plant is severely irritating to skin and mucous membranes (18).

Adverse Reactions

Orally, ingestion of bulbous buttercup can cause severe irritation of the gastrointestinal tract, with colic and diarrhea (18).
Topically, irritation of the urinary tract can also occur. Skin contact can cause blisters and burns which are difficult to heal (18).

Interactions with Herbs & Other Dietary Supplements

None known.

Interactions with Drugs

None known.

Interactions with Foods
None known.

Interactions with Lab Tests
None known.

Interactions with Diseases or Conditions
None known.

Dosage and Administration
No typical dosage.

Comments
This product is rarely used. Avoid confusing bulbous buttercup with lesser celandine and amaranth; these plants are also referred to as pilewort (18).

BUPLEURUM

Also Known As
Bei Chai Hu, Chi Hu, Chinese Thoroughwax, Hare's Ear Root, Sho-saiko-to, Shrubby Hare's-ear, Sickle-leaf Hare's-ear, Thoroughwax.

Scientific Names
Bupleurum chinense; Bupleurum exaltatum; Bupleurum falcatum; Bupleurum fruticosum; Bupleurum longifolium; Bupleurum multinerve; Bupleurum octoradiatum; Bupleurum rotundifolium; Bupleurum scorzonerifolium.
Family: Apiaceae/Umbelliferae.

People Use This For
Orally, bupleurum is used for fevers, flu, the common cold, cough, fatigue, headache, tinnitus, liver disorders, premenstrual syndrome (PMS), dysmenorrhea, depression, anorexia, cancer, inflammation, lung congestion, malaria, angina, epilepsy, pain, muscle cramps, rheumatism, asthma, bronchitis, indigestion, ulcers, hemorrhoids, diarrhea, constipation, as a sedative, antioxidant, antiseptic, antifungal, antiviral, as an immune stimulant, and for reducing cholesterol and triglyceride levels. It is also used orally for increasing sweating, as a protectant against kidney problems, a liver tonic, and a spleen and stomach toner.
In combination, bupleurum is used in many herbal formulas. It is included in a Chinese herbal formula used for treating thrombocytopenic purpura and in a Japanese herbal formula (Sho-saiko-to, TJ-9, Xiao-chai-hu-tang) used for various chronic liver diseases. Bupleurum is used orally in combination with Panax ginseng and licorice to help stimulate adrenal gland function, particularly in patients with a history of long-term corticosteroid use.

Safety
There is insufficient reliable information available about the safety of bupleurum.
Pregnancy and Lactation: Insufficient reliable information available; avoid using.

Effectiveness
There is insufficient reliable information available about the effectiveness of bupleurum.

Mechanism of Action
The applicable part of bupleurum is the root (12). Compounds isolated from Bupleurum species used in traditional Chinese medicine include saikosaponins, polysaccharides, and polyacetylenes. Saikosaponins are triterpenoid saponins, known as saikosides (6). While the saikosaponin content of some species is very similar (3151), that of other species varies considerably, as well as pharmacologic activity (3152). The saikosaponin content is highest in Bupleurum falcatum (2-8%) and Bupleurum chinense (1.7%). For infections, including the flu and the common cold, bupleurum is theorized to work by improving immune function. Bupleurum falcatum is reported to cause proliferation of B-lymphocytes and stimulate them to produce immunoglobulins in vitro. It is also reported to stimulate in vitro macrophage activity, possibly by increasing the number of antibody-binding sites on the cell surface (2598). The constituent saikosaponin-d has immunoregulatory actions on T-lymphocytes, including promotion of interleukin-2 (IL-2) production and IL-2 receptor expression (3160). It also increases macrophage activity, IL-1 production and antibody response (3161). Bupleurum also is reported to have antitussive properties (6). For peptic ulcers, bupleurum is thought to decrease gastric acid and pepsin secretion and have mucosal protecting effects (3154,3155). Bupleurum is also reported to have antitumor (3157), antibacterial (3170), anti-inflammatory (2597,3166,3167,3168), antispasmodic (3167), antioxidant (3154,3155,3156), antiplatelet (3159), and hepatoprotectant effects (3163,3164,3165); however these effects have not been demonstrated in humans.

Adverse Reactions
Orally, bupleurum can cause increased bowel movements, flatulence, and sedation (3148). The Japanese herbal formula, Sho-saiko-to, which contains bupleurum, has been associated with eosinophilic pneumonia (354), pulmonary edema (361), and multiple cases of pneumonitis (355,356,357). Sho-saiko-to, used in combination with interferon-alpha in people with chronic active hepatitis, has been associated with multiple cases of pneumonitis (358,359,360).

Interactions with Herbs & Other Dietary Supplements
None known.

Interactions with Drugs
None known.

Interactions with Foods
None known.

Interactions with Lab Tests
None known.

Interactions with Diseases or Conditions
None known.

Dosage and Administration
ORAL: A dose of 1.5 to 6 grams per day of bupleurum root has been used (3148). As a fluid extract (1:2), 1.5-3 mL daily, up to 25-60 mL per week has been used (3148).

Comments
The Japanese herbal formula, Sho-saiko-to, which contains bupleurum, enhances the anti-HIV-1 activity of lamivudine (Epivir, 3TC) in vitro (362).

BURDOCK

Also Known As
Arctium, Bardana, Bardana-minor, Bardanae Radix, Bardane, Beggar's Buttons, Burr Seed, Clotbur, Cocklebur, Cockle Buttons, Edible Burdock, Fox's Clote, Gobo, Great Bur, Great Burdocks, Happy Major, Hardock, Harebur, Lappa, Love Leaves, Orelha-de-gigante, Personata, Philanthropium, Thorny Burr.

Scientific Names
Arctium lappa; Arctium minus; Arctium tomentosum.
Family: Asteraceae/Compositae.

People Use This For
Orally, burdock is used as a diuretic, "blood purifier", antimicrobial, and an antipyretic. It is also used to treat anorexia nervosa, gastrointestinal (GI) complaints, rheumatism, gout, cystitis, syphilitic disorders, and chronic skin conditions including acne and psoriasis. It is also used for hypertension, arteriosclerosis, hepatitis, and other inflammatory conditions. Burdock is also used for treating colds, catarrh, cancers, and as an aphrodisiac.
Topically, burdock is used for dry skin (ichthyosis), acne, psoriasis, and eczema.
The root of burdock is consumed as a food.

Safety
LIKELY SAFE ...when used in amounts commonly found in foods (12659,12660). There is insufficient reliable information available about the safety of burdock in medicinal doses.
Pregnancy and Lactation: Insufficient reliable information available; avoid using.

Effectiveness
There is insufficient reliable information available about the effectiveness of burdock.

Mechanism of Action
The applicable parts of burdock are the root, seed, and leaf. Extracts of burdock root appear to have antitussive activity and may increase immunological activity (12661). Other preliminary research suggests it might have anti-inflammatory and free radical scavenging activity (12663). Burdock root extract might also protect the liver from toxicity caused by ethanol and carbon tetrachloride, possibly due to its antioxidant activity (12659).
Preliminary research suggests that constituents in burdock seed might inhibit platelet activating factor (12619).
Burdock seeds contain arctiin, which may have a protective effect against cancer (12664). Preliminary research also suggests arctiin might be converted into estrogenic and antiestrogenic compounds by intestinal bacteria (12665).
It's too early to know if arctiin or burdock has hormonal activity in vivo.
Burdock leaf may have antibacterial and anticandidal effects (12666).

Adverse Reactions
Orally, burdock can cause an allergic reaction in individuals sensitive to the Asteraceae/Compositae family. Rarely, it has caused anaphylaxis (12660). Members of the Asteraceae/Compositae family include ragweed, chrysanthemums, marigolds, daisies, and many other herbs. Burdock tea has also been associated with anticholinergic symptoms including dry mouth, dizziness, blurred vision, weakness, inability to urinate, and dilated pupils. It is unclear whether burdock or a contaminant in the tea caused these symptoms (12662).
Topically, burdock can cause contact dermatitis (12667).

Interactions with Herbs & Other Dietary Supplements
None known.

Interactions with Drugs
ANTICOAGULANT/ANTIPLATELET DRUGS: Theoretically, taking burdock with anticoagulant or antiplatelet drugs might increase the risk of bleeding due to decreased platelet aggregation. Burdock might reduce platelet aggregation by inhibiting platelet activating factor (12619). Some of these drugs include aspirin, clopidogrel (Plavix), dalteparin (Fragmin), enoxaparin (Lovenox), heparin, ticlopidine (Ticlid), warfarin (Coumadin), and others.

Interactions with Foods
None known.

Interactions with Lab Tests
None known.

Interactions with Diseases or Conditions
CROSS-ALLERGENICITY: Burdock may cause an allergic reaction in individuals sensitive to the Asteraceae/Compositae family (12660). Members of this family include ragweed, chrysanthemums, marigolds, daisies, and many other herbs.

Dosage and Administration
No typical dosage.

Comments
Burdock has been associated with atropine poisoning as a result of being adulterated with root of belladonna or deadly nightshade (12662).

BURNING BUSH

Also Known As
Adiptam, Burnet Saxifrage, Dictamo Blanco, Dittany, Fraxinella, Gas Plant, Herba Dictamni Herba.
CAUTION: See separate listing for Wahoo.

Scientific Names
Dictamnus albus, synonyms Dictamnus caucasicus, Dictamnus fraxinellus.
Family: Rutaceae.

People Use This For
Orally, burning bush is used for digestive and urogenital disorders, cramps, stomach disorders, epilepsy, to treat worm infestations, and to promote hair growth. It is also used as a spasmolytic, as a stimulant, tonic, diuretic, to promote menstruation, as birth control, and to aid in the expulsion of the afterbirth.
Topically, burning bush is used for treating wounds, eczema, impetigo, scabies, arthritis, rheumatism, fever, hepatitis, skin inflammation, thread fungus, uterine hemorrhages, as a sedative for adults and children, and as a tonic.

Safety
There is insufficient reliable information available about the safety of burning bush.
Pregnancy and Lactation: Insufficient information available; avoid using.

Effectiveness
There is insufficient reliable information available about the effectiveness of burning bush.

Mechanism of Action
The applicable parts of burning bush are the leaf and root. There is some evidence that burning bush decreases the ability of a tropical liver fluke called Clonorchis sinesis to lay eggs. This same liver fluke can occur in sushi if the fish has been imported from Asia. Burning bush leaf contains psoralen, xanthotoxin, auraptene, and bergapten. These furocoumarins can cause phototoxic reactions when they are applied topically (18).

Adverse Reactions
Topically, skin contact with burning bush can cause phototoxicity (18).

Interactions with Herbs & Other Dietary Supplements
None known.

Interactions with Drugs
None known.

Interactions with Foods
None known.

Interactions with Lab Tests
None known.

Interactions with Diseases or Conditions
None known.

Dosage and Administration
No typical dosage.

Comments
Avoid confusion with Wahoo, also referred to as burning bush. Burning bush has a distinctive lemon or cinnamon scent. Its oil is easily flammable (18).

BURR MARIGOLD

Also Known As
Water Agrimony.

Scientific Names
Bidens tripartita.
Family: Asteraceae/Compositae.

Comments
At the date of publication, this product was not a common ingredient used in brand name supplements marketed to consumers. Details about this product are available in the online version of *Natural Medicines Comprehensive Database.* See www.naturaldatabase.com.

BUTANEDIOL (BD)

Also Known As
1,4-BD, 1,4-butylene glycol, 1,4-dihydroxybutane, 1,4-tetramethylene glycol, 2(3H)-Furanone di-dihydro, BD, BDO, Butane-1,4-diol, Butylene glycol, Tetramethylene glycol, Tetramethylene-1,4-diol.
CAUTION: See separate listings for Gamma Hydroxybutyrate (GHB) and Gamma Butyrolactone (GBL).

Scientific Names
1,4-butanediol.

People Use This For

Orally, butanediol has been used to stimulate growth hormone production and muscle growth, for bodybuilding, weight loss, and insomnia.

Safety

UNSAFE ...when used orally. Butanediol, and the closely related products gamma hydroxybutyrate (GHB) and gamma butyrolactone (GBL) have been linked to at least 131 serious illnesses, including 5 deaths (1318,3678,10640).
PREGNANCY AND LACTATION: UNSAFE ...when used orally (1318,3678).

Effectiveness

There is insufficient reliable information available about the effectiveness of butanediol.

Mechanism of Action

Butanediol is converted to gamma hydroxybutyrate (GHB, see separate listing) in the body (3678,5813). It is a powerful hypnotic, producing potentially dangerous sedative effects (3679). GHB can be converted in the brain to the neurotransmitter gamma aminobutyric acid (GABA) (3699), and specific GHB uptake systems, transport systems, and receptors have also been identified (713,3699,5800,5801). Stimulation of GHB receptors reduces dopamine release in the brain (713,3699,5801), and GHB has also been reported to affect the endogenous opioid system, raising dynorphin levels (3682,5803). GHB induces REM and non-REM sleep, hypothermia, abnormalities on the EEG similar to those seen in petit mal epilepsy (5800,5803); and it stimulates growth hormone secretion (5804).

Adverse Reactions

Orally, butanediol, like gamma butyrolactone (GBL), is metabolized to gamma hydroxybutyrate (GHB), and therefore causes similar toxic effects, including breathing problems, respiratory depression requiring intubation, coma, amnesia, combativeness, confusion, agitation, vomiting, urinary and fecal incontinence, seizures, bradycardia, and death (1318,3678,3679,10640). Butanediol, GHB, and GBL have been linked to at least 131 serious illnesses, including 5 deaths (1318,3678,10640). Non-fatal toxicity has been reported with doses of 1 to 14 grams. Death has occurred with doses of 5 to 20 grams (1318). Withdrawal symptoms, including insomnia, tremor, anxiety, hallucinations, and delirium can occur in chronic users of butanediol and GBL, as well as GHB (1430,10375). GHB-like withdrawal has also occurred in a patient who presented with butanediol toxicity (1318).

Interactions with Herbs & Other Dietary Supplements

None known.

Interactions with Drugs

ALCOHOL (Ethanol): Concomitant use with butanediol and its metabolite GHB may increase the risk of serious CNS and respiratory depression (1430,3678).
AMPHETAMINES: Concomitant use with GHB (a metabolite of butanediol) has been associated with severe side effects. Theoretically, concomitant use may also antagonize the effects of GHB (3682).
ANTICONVULSANTS: Theoretically, GHB (a metabolite of butanediol) may antagonize the effects of GHB (3682).
ANTIPSYCHOTIC DRUGS: Concomitant use with GHB (a metabolite of butanediol) has been associated with severe side effects. Antipsychotics can potentiate the effects of GHB (3682).
BENZODIAZEPINES: Concomitant use with GHB (a metabolite of butanediol) has been associated with severe side effects Benzodiazepines can potentiate the effects of GHB (3682).
CNS DEPRESSANTS: Concomitant use with GHB (a metabolite of butanediol) has been associated with severe side effects. Additive sedative effects with butanediol may occur (3682,3679).
HALOPERIDOL (Haldol): Theoretically, Haloperidol may antagonize the effects of GHB (a metabolite of butanediol) (3682).
NALOXONE (Narcan): Theoretically, concomitant use with GHB (a metabolite of butanediol) may antagonize the effects of GHB (3682).
NARCOTIC DRUGS: Concomitant use with GHB (a metabolite of butanediol) has been associated with severe side effects. Concomitant use of GHB with narcotic drugs can potentiate the therapeutic and adverse effects of narcotic analgesics (3682,3679).
RITONAVIR (Norvir): Concomitant use of the protease inhibitor-type antiretroviral drugs ritonavir and saquinavir with GHB (a metabolite of butanediol) reportedly caused a near-fatal reaction, probably due to inhibition of GHB metabolism (1431).
SAQUINAVIR (Fortovase, Invirase): Concomitant use of the protease inhibitor-type antiretroviral drugs ritonavir and saquinavir with GHB (a metabolite of butanediol) reportedly caused a near-fatal reaction, probably due to inhibition of GHB metabolism (1431).
SKELETAL MUSCLE RELAXANTS: Concomitant use with GHB (a metabolite of butanediol) has been associated with severe side effects. Concomitant use with GHB can potentiate the therapeutic and adverse effects of skeletal muscle relaxants (3682).

Interactions with Foods

ALCOHOL: Concomitant use with butanediol and its metabolite GHB may increase the risk of serious CNS and respiratory depression (1430,3678).

Interactions with Lab Tests

None known.

Interactions with Diseases or Conditions

BRADYCARDIA: GHB (a metabolite of butanediol) should be avoided since it can cause bradycardia conditions (4259).
EPILEPSY: GHB (a metabolite of butanediol) should be avoided due to its possible capacity to induce seizures (10658).
HYPERTENSION: GHB (a metabolite of butanediol) should be avoided since it may increase blood pressure (10658).

Dosage and Administration

ORAL: Doses of 0.25 to 1 gram butanediol have been used for stimulating growth hormone release and muscle growth and treating insomnia, but are considered unsafe (3678).

Comments

Butanediol is used industrially to make floor stripper, paint thinner, and other solvent products (3678). It is illegal to sell any product for human consumption containing butanediol (3678). Some manufacturers have substituted butanediol in products previously containing GHB or GBL, but the effects of butanediol are just as dangerous (3679). GBL, GHB, and BD are associated with at least 122 reports of serious adverse effects including dangerously low respiratory rates (intubation might be required), unconsciousness, coma, vomiting, seizures, slowed heart rate, and death (4259).

BUTCHER'S BROOM

Also Known As

Box Holly, Jew's Myrtle, Knee Holly, Kneeholm, Pettigree, Sweet Broom, Rusci Aculeati, Rusci Aculeati Rhizoma.
CAUTION: See separate listings for Scotch Broom and Spanish Broom.

Scientific Names

Ruscus aculeatus.
Family: Ruscaceae.

People Use This For

Orally, butcher's broom is used for hemorrhoids, gallstones, atherosclerosis, and for symptoms of chronic venous insufficiency such as pain, heaviness, leg cramps, leg edema, varicose veins, peripheral vascular disease, itching, and swelling. Butcher's broom is also used as a laxative, diuretic, an anti-inflammatory, and to facilitate the healing of fractures.
As food, the rhizome shoots are eaten in some cultures in a manner similar to asparagus.

Safety

POSSIBLY SAFE ...when used orally and appropriately short-term (9932,10068,10069,10070). The use of butcher's broom is not associated with any significant toxicity for up to 3 months of use.
PREGNANCY AND LACTATION: Insufficient reliable information available; avoid using.

Effectiveness

POSSIBLY EFFECTIVE

Chronic venous insufficiency. Taking butcher's broom orally alone, or in combination with vitamin C and hesperidin, seems to relieve chronic venous insufficiency symptoms including pain, heaviness, leg cramps, itching, and swelling (9932,10068,10070).

INSUFFICIENT RELIABLE EVIDENCE to RATE

Orthostatic hypotension. Some clinical research suggests that butcher's broom taken orally might relieve orthostatic hypotension (10069). More evidence is needed to rate butcher's broom for this use.

Mechanism of Action

The applicable parts of butcher's broom are the rhizomes and roots. The steroidal saponin constituents, ruscogenin and neoruscogenin, produce vasoconstrictive effects by direct activation of alpha-adrenergic receptors. This activation, in turn, stimulates the release of noradrenaline at the vascular wall (10069). Butcher's broom appears to have venotonic properties that reduce venous capacity and pooling of blood in the legs. It also seems to have a protective effect on capillaries, vascular endothelium, and smooth muscle (10068,10070). The flavonoid content might help strengthen blood vessels, lessen capillary fragility, and sustain healthy circulation (10069).

Adverse Reactions

Orally, butcher's broom can cause nausea, gastritis, and diarrhea (10068).

Interactions with Herbs & Other Dietary Supplements

HERBS WITH ALPHA-ADRENERGIC AGONIST ACTIVITY: Theoretically, butcher's broom might have an additive effect on herbs and supplements with alpha-agonist properties (10069). Some of these include bitter orange and ephedra.

HERBS WITH ALPHA-ADRENERGIC ANTAGONIST ACTIVITY: Theoretically, butcher's broom might reduce the effects of herbs and supplements with alpha-antagonist properties (10069). Some of these include yohimbe and saw palmetto.

Interactions with Drugs

ALPHA-ADRENERGIC AGONISTS: Theoretically, butcher's broom might have an additive effect on drugs with alpha-agonist properties (10069). Some of these include pseudoephedrine (Sudafed), phenylpropanolamine (Afrin, Drixoral Non-Drowsy), and others.

ALPHA-ADRENERGIC ANTAGONISTS: Theoretically, butcher's broom might reduce the effects of drugs with alpha-antagonist properties (10069). Some of these include doxazosin (Cardura), terazosin (Hytrin), yohimbine (Aphrodyne), and others.

Interactions with Foods

None known.

Interactions with Lab Tests

None known.

Interactions with Diseases or Conditions

None known.

Dosage and Administration

ORAL: For relieving symptoms of chronic venous insufficiency, butcher's broom 150 mg root extract, combined with 150 mg hesperidin and 100 mg ascorbic acid, has been used twice daily (10068).

BUTTERBUR

Also Known As

Blatterdock, Bog Rhubarb, Bogshorns, Butter-Dock, Butterfly Dock, Capdockin, Exwort, Flapperdock, Langwort, Petasites, Petasitidis folium, Petasitidis rhizoma, Petasitidis hybridus, Plague Root, Umbrella Leaves.

Scientific Names

Petasites hybridus, synonyms Petasites officinalis, Tussilago hybrida.
Family: Asteraceae/Compositae.

People Use This For

Orally, butterbur is used for pain, stomach upset, gastric ulcers, headaches including migraine headaches, chronic cough, chills, anxiety, plague, fever, insomnia whooping cough, asthma, allergic rhinitis (hay fever), and for irritable bladder and urinary tract spasms. Butterbur is also used orally as an antispasmodic and appetite stimulant. Topically, butterbur is used to improve wound healing.

Safety

POSSIBLY SAFE ...when used orally and appropriately. Rhizome extracts that are free of hepatotoxic pyrrolizidine alkaloid (PA) constituents seem to be safe when used for up to 16 weeks (7230,12840,13003). Tell patients not to use butterbur products that are not certified and labeled as hepatotoxic PA-free. Preparations containing hepatotoxic PAs are likely unsafe.
LIKELY UNSAFE ...when products containing hepatotoxic pyrrolizidine alkaloid (PA) constituents are used orally. Repeated exposure to low concentrations of hepatotoxic PAs can cause severe veno-occlusive disease. Hepatotoxic PAs might also be carcinogenic and mutagenic (12841,12842). Tell patients not to use butterbur preparations that are not certified and labeled as hepatotoxic PA-free. ...when products containing hepatotoxic PAs are used topically on abraded or broken skin. Absorption of hepatotoxic PAs through broken skin can lead to systemic toxicities (12841). Tell patients not to use topical butterbur preparations that are not certified and labeled as hepatotoxic PA-free. There is insufficient reliable information available about the safety of topical PA-free butterbur on unbroken skin.
CHILDREN: POSSIBLY SAFE ...when used orally and appropriately. There is some evidence that a specific pyrrolizidine alkaloid (PA)-free butterbur extract (Petadolex, Weber&Weber, GmbH & Co, Germany) can be safely used in children aged 6-17 years for up to 4 months (13121).
PREGNANCY: LIKELY UNSAFE ...when used orally. Butterbur preparations containing hepatotoxic pyrrolizidine alkaloid (PA) constituents might be teratogenic and hepatotoxic (12841,12842). There is insufficient reliable information available about the safety of using butterbur products that do not contain hepatotoxic PAs during pregnancy.
LACTATION: LIKELY UNSAFE ...when used orally. Hepatotoxic pyrrolizidine alkaloid (PA) constituents in butterbur are excreted in milk (12841,12842). There is insufficient reliable information available about the safety of using butterbur products that do not contain hepatotoxic PAs during lactation.

Effectiveness

POSSIBLY EFFECTIVE

Allergic rhinitis (hayfever). Taking petasins, isolated from butterbur, may decrease symptoms of allergic rhinitis. In addition, petasins can decrease concentrations of inflammatory mediators (7595,10336,10337). Some research suggests that butterbur petasins may be as effective as cetirizine (Zyrtec) (7595). Whole butterbur root extract that is not standardized for petasin content (Petaforce) seems to reduce response to adenosine monophosphate challenge in patients with allergic rhinitis (11941). But this extract doesn't seem to improve peak nasal inspiratory flow, nasal and eye symptoms, or quality of life any better than placebo when taken for 2 weeks (11942).

Migraine headache. Taking butterbur orally seems to prevent migraine headache. A specific butterbur rhizome extract standardized to 15% petasin and isopetasin (Petadolex, Weber&Weber, GmbH & Co, Germany), and hepatotoxic pyrrolizidine alkaloids (PA)-free, can reduce the frequency, intensity, and duration of migraine headache when used over a period of 16 weeks (7230,12840,13003). This butterbur extract seems to reduce the frequency of migraine by about 48% (13003). Doses of at least 75 mg twice daily seem to be necessary for significant benefit. Lower doses of 50 mg twice daily may not be effective in adults (13003). There is also preliminary evidence that this butterbur extract can decrease the frequency of migraine headaches in children aged 6-17 years (13121).

INSUFFICIENT RELIABLE EVIDENCE to RATE

Respiratory conditions. There is some preliminary evidence that butterbur might be helpful for treating asthma and chronic bronchitis (7596). More evidence is needed to rate butterbur for this use.

Mechanism of Action

The applicable parts of butterbur are the leaf, rhizome, and root. The active constituents of butterbur are the sesquiterpene compounds, petasin, and isopetasin. Butterbur extracts also contain volatile oils, flavonoids, tannins, and pyrrolizidine alkaloids. Some butterbur extracts are standardized to contain a minimum of 7.5 mg petasin and isopetasin (7229).
Butterbur is thought to have antispasmodic effects on smooth muscle and vascular walls. It might also exert anti-inflammatory effects by inhibiting leukotriene synthesis (7229,7597).
In allergic rhinitis (hayfever), butterbur and purified petasin decrease blood concentrations of histamine and leukotrienes (10336). They also appear to decrease priming of mast cells in response to contact with allergens (10337).
Butterbur contains various pyrrolizidine alkaloids (PA), some of which are toxic. PAs are most concentrated in the plant roots, but may be found in all plant parts. PAs, particularly unsaturated PAs, can cause hepatotoxicity. Cyclic diesters such as retrorsine and senecionine are the most hepatotoxic. Liver toxicity may result from PA-enhanced oxidative stress, but the exact mechanism of toxicity is unknown. Single doses of 10-20 mg PAs or chronic ingestion of amounts less than 10 mcg can cause veno-occlusive disease. PAs are metabolized by cytochrome P450 3A4 (CYP3A4) to toxic dehydroalkaloids and pyrroles. Enzyme inducers such as phenobarbital seem to enhance toxicity (12841,12860). Pyrroles are excreted as N-acetyl cysteine conjugates. Some researchers speculate that early administration of N-acetylcysteine might reduce toxicity (11988).
Metabolism is also affected by pregnane X receptor induction of CYP3A4. Genetic or drug induced variation in CYP3A4 or pregnane X receptor activity can affect the degree of PA toxicity by increasing or decreasing its metabolism (12841,12842). Hepatotoxic PAs are also toxic to the lungs. In animals, pneumotoxicity occurs as

pulmonary hypertension and right ventricular hypertrophy. Hepatotoxic PAs are carcinogenic and mutagenic. There are sufficient amounts of hepatotoxic PAs in herbal products to cause toxicity (12841,12842). Methods to remove hepatotoxic PAs from butterbur extracts are available (7231).

Adverse Reactions

Orally, butterbur is generally well tolerated (12386). It can cause belching, headache, itchy eyes, diarrhea, asthma, pruritus, stomach upset, fatigue, and drowsiness. However, it seems to cause less drowsiness and fatigue than cetirizine (Zyrtec) (7595,12386).

The major concern about butterbur preparations is the hepatotoxic pyrrolizidine alkaloid (PA) content. These constituents are hepatotoxic, pneumotoxic, carcinogenic and mutagenic (12386,12841,12842). Chronic exposure to other plants containing hepatotoxic PA constituents is associated with veno-occlusive disease (4021). Subacute veno-occlusive disease causes vague symptoms with persistent liver enlargement (4021). Symptoms of acute veno-occlusive disease include colicky pains in epigastrium, vomiting and diarrhea, and ascites formation within several days. Enlargement and induration of the liver occurs within a few weeks (12842). Butterbur theoretically might cause an allergic reaction in individuals sensitive to the Asteraceae/Compositae family. Members of this family include ragweed, chrysanthemums, marigolds, daisies, and many other herbs (12841).

Interactions with Herbs & Other Dietary Supplements

HEPATOTOXIC PYRROLIZIDINE ALKALOID (PA)-CONTAINING HERBS: Concomitant use is contraindicated due to the risk of additive toxicity. Herbs containing hepatotoxic PAs include alkanna, borage, coltsfoot, comfrey, gravel root, hemp agrimony, and hound's tongue; and the Senecio species plants dusty miller, alpine ragwort, groundsel, golden ragwort, and tansy ragwort (12841).

HERBS THAT INDUCE CYTOCHROME P450 3A4 (CYP3A4): Theoretically, herbs that induce CYP3A4 might increase the conversion of hepatotoxic PAs to toxic metabolites, enhancing toxicity (12841,12860). Herbs that induce CYP3A4 include St. John's wort and garlic.

Interactions with Drugs

CYTOCHROME P450 3A4 (CYP3A4) INDUCERS: Hepatotoxic pyrrolizidine alkaloids (PA) are substrates of cytochrome P450 3A4 (CYP3A4) (12841,12860). Theoretically, drugs that induce CYP3A4 might increase the conversion of PAs to toxic metabolites. Some drugs that induce CYP3A4 include carbamazepine (Tegretol), phenobarbital, phenytoin (Dilantin), rifampin, rifabutin (Mycobutin), and others.

Interactions with Foods

None.

Interactions with Lab Tests

LIVER FUNCTION TESTS (LFTs): Butterbur can cause increases in liver enzyme activity (7595).

Interactions with Diseases or Conditions

CROSS-ALLERGENICITY: Theoretically, butterbur might cause an allergic reaction in individuals sensitive to the Asteraceae/Compositae family. Members of this family include ragweed, chrysanthemums, marigolds, daisies, and many other herbs (12841).

LIVER DISEASE: Theoretically, pyrrolizidine alkaloids (PA) might exacerbate liver disease (12841,12842).

Dosage and Administration

ORAL: For migraine headache prophylaxis, a pyrrolizidine alkaloid free butterbur rhizome extract standardized to 15% petasin and isopetasin (Petadolex, Weber&Weber, GmbH & Co, Germany) has been used in doses of 50 to 100 mg twice daily with meals (7230,13003). Higher doses seem to be more effective. Lower doses of 50 mg twice daily may not be effective in adults (13003). Some researchers suggest taking the extract for 4-6 months, then tapering the dose until migraine incidence begins to increase (7229). In children with migraine, a dose of 25 mg twice daily has been used in children aged 6-9 years and 50 mg twice daily in older children. Three times daily dosing has been used in children who don't respond to the twice daily dose (13121).

For seasonal allergic rhinitis, an extract of butterbur (ZE 339, Zeller AG) standardized to 8-16 mg of petasin has been used 3-4 times daily (7595,10336). Whole butterbur root extract (Petaforce) 50 mg twice daily has also been used for allergic rhinitis (11941).

BUTTERCUP

Also Known As
Acrid Crowfoot, Bachelor's Buttons, Blisterweed, Burrwort, Globe Amaranth, Gold Cup, Meadow Buttercup, Meadowbloom, Tall Buttercup, Yellows, Yellowweed.
CAUTION: See separate listings for Poisonous Buttercup, Bulbous Buttercup, Cornflower, and Feverfew.

Scientific Names
Ranunculus acris; Ranunculus acris subsp. friesianus, synonym Ranunculus friesianus.
Family: Ranunculaceae.

People Use This For
Orally, buttercup is used for arthritis, blisters, bronchitis, chronic skin complaints, and nerve pain.

Safety
LIKELY UNSAFE ...when the fresh plant is used orally or topically because it can cause severe local irritation (18).
There is insufficient reliable information about the safety of the medicinal use of the dried, cut above ground parts of buttercup.
PREGNANCY AND LACTATION: LIKELY UNSAFE ...when the fresh plant is used orally or topically (18). Buttercup might also stimulate uterine contractions (19). There is insufficient reliable information about the safety of the dried, cut above ground parts of buttercup used during pregnancy and lactation.

Effectiveness
There is insufficient reliable information available about the effectiveness of buttercup.

Mechanism of Action
The applicable parts of buttercup are the fresh above ground parts. When the fresh plant is crushed or cut into small pieces, the glycoside ranunculin is enzymatically changed into a severely irritating protoanemonin, which, in turn, rapidly degrades into the less toxic anemonin (18). Both protoanemonin and ranunculin are destroyed to an unknown extent during the drying process (2).

Adverse Reactions
Orally, ingestion of buttercup may cause severe irritation of the gastrointestinal tract, with colic and diarrhea. Irritation of the urinary tract can also occur.
Topically, skin contact may cause blisters and burns which are difficult to heal (18). Buttercup can also cause phototoxic skin reactions (19).

Interactions with Herbs & Other Dietary Supplements
None known.

Interactions with Drugs
None known.

Interactions with Foods
None known.

Interactions with Lab Tests
None known.

Interactions with Diseases or Conditions
None known.

Dosage and Administration
No typical dosage.

BUTTERNUT

Also Known As

Butternussbaum, Lemon Walnut, Nogal Ceniciento, Noyer Cerdré, Oil Nut, White Walnut.

Scientific Names

Juglans cinerea.
Family: Juglandaceae.

People Use This For

Orally, butternut is used for gallbladder disorders, hemorrhoids, and skin diseases. It is also used orally as a stimulant laxative, antimicrobial, antineoplastic, antiparasitic, and tonic.

Safety

POSSIBLY SAFE ...when used orally and appropriately (12).
PREGNANCY AND LACTATION: LIKELY UNSAFE ...when used orally in large amounts, it can be cathartic (12); avoid using.

Effectiveness

There is insufficient reliable information available about the effectiveness of butternut.

Mechanism of Action

The applicable part of butternut is the bark. It is reported to have cathartic properties (12,19).

Adverse Reactions

Orally, butternut can cause diarrhea and gastrointestinal irritation (19).

Interactions with Herbs & Other Dietary Supplements

CARDIAC GLYCOSIDE-CONTAINING HERBS: Stimulant laxative herbs such as butternut can cause potassium depletion increasing the risk of cardiac toxicity. Cardiac glycoside-containing herbs include black hellebore, Canadian hemp roots, digitalis leaf, hedge mustard, figwort, lily-of-the-valley roots, motherwort, oleander leaf, pheasant's eye plant, pleurisy root, squill bulb leaf scales, and strophanthus seeds (18,19).
LICORICE/HORSETAIL: Theoretically, concomitant use with horsetail plant or licorice rhizome increases the risk of potassium depletion (19).
STIMULANT LAXATIVE HERBS: Theoretically, concomitant use with other stimulant laxative herbs may increase the risk of potassium depletion. Stimulant laxative herbs include aloe dried leaf sap, blue flag rhizome, alder buckthorn, European buckthorn, cascara bark, castor oil, colocynth fruit pulp, gamboge bark exudate, jalap root, black root, manna bark exudate, podophyllum root, rhubarb root, senna leaves and pods, wild cucumber fruit (Ecballium elaterium), and yellow dock root (19).

Interactions with Drugs

CORTICOSTEROIDS: Overuse of butternut might compound corticosteroid-induced potassium loss (2).
DIGOXIN (Lanoxin): Theoretically, overuse of butternut bark increases the risk of adverse effects of cardiac glycoside drugs, including digoxin (Lanoxin).
DIURETIC DRUGS: Overuse of butternut might compound diuretic-induced potassium loss (19). There is some concern that people receiving butternut along with potassium-depleting diuretics might be at an increased risk for hypokalemia. Initiation of potassium supplementation or an increase in potassium supplement dose may be necessary for some patients. Some diuretics that can deplete potassium include chlorothiazide (Diuril), chlorthalidone (Thalitone), furosemide (Lasix), hydrochlorothiazide (HCTZ, Hydrodiuril, Microzide), and others.
ORAL DRUGS: Concomitant use with butternut bark might reduce absorption of drugs due to reduced gastrointestinal transit time (19).
STIMULANT LAXATIVES: Concomitant use might compound fluid and electrolyte loss (19).

Interactions with Foods

None known.

Interactions with Lab Tests

None known.

Interactions with Diseases or Conditions

None known.

Dosage and Administration
No typical dosage.

CABBAGE

Also Known As
Colewort, Kale, Red Cabbage, White Cabbage.

Scientific Names
Brassica oleracea; Brassica oleracea var. capitata.
Family: Brassicaceae/Cruciferae.

People Use This For
Orally, cabbage is used for gastritis, gastric and duodenal ulcers, gastric pain, gastric hyperacidity, and Roemheld syndrome. Cabbage is also used orally to treat asthma, morning sickness, and prevent osteoporosis. It is also used orally to prevent lung cancer, stomach cancer, colorectal cancer, breast cancer, and other cancers.
Topically, cabbage leaves and cabbage leaf extracts are used to relieve swelling and to reduce breast engorgement.

Safety
LIKELY SAFE ...when used orally in amounts commonly found in foods. ...when used topically and appropriately, short-term. Significant side effects have not been reported in short-term studies (6781,6782,6783,6784).
POSSIBLY SAFE ...when used orally and appropriately in medicinal amounts (18).
PREGNANCY: There is insufficient reliable information available about using cabbage in medicinal amounts during pregnancy; avoid using.
LACTATION: LIKELY SAFE ...when used topically and appropriately, short-term. Significant adverse effects have not been reported in short-term studies (6781,6782,6783,6784). POSSIBLY UNSAFE ...when used orally in amounts commonly found in foods. There is some evidence that exclusively breast-fed infants develop colic if mothers consume cabbage as little as once per week (6789).

Effectiveness
POSSIBLY EFFECTIVE

Breast engorgement. Whole cabbage leaves seem to produce subjective relief similar to the standard practice of applying chilled gel-packs to the engorged breast of lactating women (6781,6784). Both chilled and room temperature cabbage leaves seem to provide the same relief (6782). A cabbage leaf extract applied as a cream has also been tried. The cabbage leaf extract cream seems to provide subjective relief, but not significantly better than a placebo cream (6783).

INSUFFICIENT RELIABLE EVIDENCE to RATE

Cancer. There is some evidence that people who consume large amounts of cabbage and other Brassica vegetables such as kale, broccoli, and cauliflower have a lower risk of developing some cancers, such as lung cancer, stomach cancer, and rectal cancer (6790,6792,6793). More evidence is needed to rate cabbage for this use.

Mechanism of Action
The applicable part of cabbage is the leaf. Cabbage, like other dark leafy vegetables, contains high amounts of vitamin K1 (11285). Cabbage contains modest amounts of calcium, vitamin C, vitamin A, vitamin E, and several B vitamins. Cabbage also contains other active constituents including chlorogenic acid, caffeic acid, and goitrin. These constituents seem to have antithyroid effects, possibly by inhibiting iodine uptake (7162). There is some interest in cabbage for breast cancer prevention because it contains constituents called glucosinolates such as indole-3-carbinol. Indole-3-carbinol is released from cabbage when it is chewed and is thought to change how estrogen is metabolized. Estrogen can be converted to either 16-alpha-hydroxyestrone or 2-alpha-hydroxyestrone. The 16-alpha-hydroxyestrone metabolite is thought to have a role in developing cancer. The 2-alpha-hydroxyestrone seems to protect against breast cancer. Indole-3-carbinol induces cytochrome P450 1A1 (CYP1A1) and 1A2 (CYP1A2), which shifts metabolism away from 16-alpha-hydroxyestrone in favor of 2-alpha-hydroxyestrone (7175,7176,7177,7179,7180,7181,7182,7187). This means that indole-3-carbinol might boost levels of a protective estrogen metabolites and decrease levels of a harmful ones. Indole-3-carbinol and other glucosinolates, including S-methyl cysteine sulfoxide, might also have anticarcinogenic properties.
These constituents seem to inhibit the enzymatic transformation of pro-mutagens (6790). Cabbage also has antioxidant effects (5234,6791).

Adverse Reactions
None reported.

Interactions with Herbs & Other Dietary Supplements
None known.

Interactions with Drugs

ACETAMINOPHEN (Tylenol, others): Cabbage can increase metabolism and decrease levels of acetaminophen. A diet that includes daily consumption of cabbage and Brussels sprouts decreases acetaminophen levels by as much as 16%. Cabbage seems to boost elimination through glucuronide conjugation (3952).

CYTOCHROME P450 1A2 (CYP1A2) SUBSTRATES: There is some concern that cabbage might decrease the effectiveness of numerous drugs. Cabbage might increase drug metabolism and elimination by stimulating cytochrome P450 1A2 (CYP1A2) activity (7176,7187). Some drugs metabolized by CYP1A2 include clozapine (Clozaril), cyclobenzaprine (Flexeril), fluvoxamine (Luvox), haloperidol (Haldol), imipramine (Tofranil), mexiletine (Mexitil), olanzapine (Zyprexa), pentazocine (Talwin), propranolol (Inderal), tacrine (Cognex), theophylline, zileuton (Zyflo), zolmitriptan (Zomig), and others.

GLUCURONIDATED DRUGS: Cabbage seems to boost elimination through glucuronide conjugation (3952). Theoretically, cabbage might also lower levels of other drugs that are metabolized through glucuronide conjugation including acetaminophen (Tylenol, others) and oxazepam (Serax), haloperidol (Haldol), lamotrigine (Lamictal), morphine (MS Contin, Roxanol), zidovudine (AZT, Retrovir), and others.

OXAZEPAM (Serax): Cabbage can increase metabolism and decrease levels of oxazepam. A diet that includes daily consumption of cabbage and brussels sprouts decreases oxazepam levels by as much as 17%. Cabbage seems to boost elimination through glucuronide conjugation (3952). Theoretically, cabbage might also lower levels of other drugs that are metabolized through glucuronide conjugation including acetaminophen (Tylenol, others) and oxazepam (Serax), haloperidol (Haldol), lamotrigine (Lamictal), morphine (MS Contin, Roxanol), zidovudine (AZT, Retrovir), and others.

WARFARIN (Coumadin): Cabbage might decrease the anticoagulant effects of warfarin due to its high vitamin K content (19).

Interactions with Foods

None known.

Interactions with Lab Tests

INTERNATIONAL NORMALIZED RATIO (INR)/PROTHROMBIN TIME (PT): Theoretically, cabbage might decrease coagulation test results due to high vitamin K content (11285).

THYROID STIMULATING HORMONE (TSH): Ingesting large quantities of cabbage juice might elevate TSH test results (7162).

Interactions with Diseases or Conditions

HYPOTHYROIDISM: There is some concern that cabbage might worsen hypothyroidism. Cabbage constituents have antithyroid properties and there is some evidence that cabbage can boost TSH levels (7162); avoid using.

Dosage and Administration

ORAL: Cabbage is typically chopped and pressed for its juice. For augmenting the diet, 1 liter of juice has been consumed daily. For gastric pain and hyperacidity, people typically use 1 teaspoon of the juice 3 times daily before meals (18).

TOPICAL: For breast engorgement, cabbage leaves were prepared in clinical studies by stripping out the large vein of the cabbage leaf, cutting a hole for the nipple, and then rinsing and chilling the leaf. The chilled cabbage leaf is worn inside the bra or as a compress under a cool towel until the cabbage leaf reaches body temperature (approximately 20 minutes). This procedure is repeated 1-4 times daily for 1-2 days (6781,6784).

CADE OIL

Also Known As

Alquitran de Enebro, Goudron de Cade, Juniper Tar, Juniper Tar Oil, Kadeol, Oil of Cade, Oil of Juniper Tar, Oleum Cadinum, Oleum Juniperi Empyreumaticum, Pix Cadi, Pix Juniper, Pix Oxycedri, Pyroleum Juniperi, Pyroleum Oxycedri, Wacholderteer.

CAUTION: See separate listing for Juniper.

Scientific Names

Juniperus oxycedrus.

Family: Cupressaceae or Pinaceae.

People Use This For

Topically, cade oil is used for itching, psoriasis, eczema and seborrhea, parasitic skin conditions, hair loss, scalp conditions, cancers, as an antiseptic in wound dressings, and in analgesic and antipruritic preparations. In manufacturing, cade oil is an ingredient in dermatologic creams and ointments, and in anti-dandruff shampoos.

Safety
There is insufficient reliable information available about the safety of cade oil.
Pregnancy and Lactation: Insufficient reliable information available; avoid using.

Effectiveness
There is insufficient reliable information available about the effectiveness of cade oil.

Mechanism of Action
Cade oil contains volatile oils with several constituents. Cade oil is thought to have antipruritic and keratolytic activity, and antimicrobial activity in vitro (11).

Adverse Reactions
None reported.

Interactions with Herbs & Other Dietary Supplements
None known.

Interactions with Drugs
None known.

Interactions with Foods
None known.

Interactions with Lab Tests
None known.

Interactions with Diseases or Conditions
None known.

Dosage and Administration
No typical dosage.

Comments
Avoid confusion with juniper berry (Juniperus communis). Cade oil is obtained by distilling the wood of the juniper tree (Juniperus oxycedrus).

CAFFEINE

Also Known As
Anhydrous Caffeine, Caffeine and Sodium Benzoate, Caffeine Anhydrous, Caffeine Citrate, Citrated Caffeine, Methylxanthine, Methylxanthines.
CAUTION: See separate listings for Black Tea, Green Tea, Oolong Tea, Coffee, Cola Nut, Guarana, and Mate.

Scientific Names
1,3,7-trimethylxanthine.

People Use This For
Orally, caffeine is used in combination with analgesics and ergotamine for treating migraine headaches. It is used orally with analgesics for simple headaches and preventing and treating postoperative and postdural puncture headaches. It is also used orally for asthma, gallbladder disease, attention-deficit hyperactivity disorder (ADHD), neonatal apnea, increasing blood pressure in hypotension, increasing mental alertness, and enhancing athletic performance. In combination, caffeine is used with ephedrine or other stimulants and diuretics for weight loss. Very high doses are used as euphoriants, often in combination with ephedrine as an alternative to illicit stimulants.
Topically, caffeine cream preparations have been used for reducing erythema and itching in dermatitis.
Rectally, caffeine is used in combination with ergotamine for migraine headaches.
Parenterally, caffeine is used for postoperative and postdural puncture headache, neonatal apnea, acute respiratory depression, and as a diuretic. It is also used for extending the length of seizure with electroconvulsive therapy.
In foods, caffeine is used as an ingredient in soft drinks, energy drinks, and other beverages.

Safety

LIKELY SAFE ...when used orally, parenterally, or rectally and appropriately. Caffeine has Generally Recognized As Safe (GRAS) status in the US (4912). Caffeine is an FDA-approved product and a component of several over-the-counter and prescription products (4912,11832).

POSSIBLY UNSAFE ...when used orally, long-term or in high doses. Chronic use, especially in large amounts, can produce tolerance, habituation, psychological dependence, and other significant adverse effects. Doses greater than 250-300 mg per day have been associated with significant adverse effects such as tachyarrhythmias and sleep disturbances (11832).

LIKELY UNSAFE ...when used orally in very high doses. The fatal acute oral dose of caffeine is estimated to be 10-14 grams (150-200 mg per kilogram). Serious toxicity can occur at lower doses depending on variables in caffeine sensitivity such as smoking, age, prior caffeine use, etc (11832).

CHILDREN: POSSIBLY SAFE ...when used orally or intravenously and appropriately in neonates (6371). ...when used in amounts commonly found in foods and beverages (4912,11833).

PREGNANCY: POSSIBLY SAFE ...when used orally in amounts commonly found in foods. Mothers should closely monitor their intake of caffeine. Use of caffeine in pregnancy is controversial; however, moderate consumption has not been associated with clinically important adverse fetal effects (2708,2709,2710,2711,9606). Caffeine crosses the human placenta, but is not considered a teratogen. Fetal blood and tissue levels are similar to maternal concentrations (4260). Mothers should keep caffeine consumption below 300 mg per day. This is similar to the amount of caffeine found in about 3 cups of coffee or tea (2708). POSSIBLY UNSAFE ...when used orally in large amounts. Caffeine crosses the placenta, producing fetal blood concentrations similar to maternal levels (4260). Mothers should avoid consuming more than 300 mg of caffeine daily or more than 3 cups of tea or coffee per day (2708). High maternal doses of caffeine throughout pregnancy have resulted in symptoms of caffeine withdrawal in newborn infants (9891). High doses of caffeine have been associated with spontaneous abortion, premature delivery, and low birth weight (2709,2711). Fetal birth weight is reduced by 28 grams for every 100 mg per day of caffeine consumed during pregnancy. But this is unlikely to be clinically significant except for women consuming more than 600 mg of caffeine daily (9606).

LACTATION: POSSIBLY SAFE ...when used orally in amounts commonly found in foods. Nursing mothers should closely monitor caffeine intake. Breast milk concentrations of caffeine are thought to be approximately 50% of maternal serum concentrations. Minimal consumption would likely result in limited exposure to a nursing infant (9892). POSSIBLY UNSAFE ...when used orally in large amounts. Caffeine is excreted slowly in infants and may accumulate. Caffeine can cause sleep disturbances, irritability, and increased bowel activity in breast-fed infants exposed to caffeine (2708,6026).

Effectiveness

EFFECTIVE

Headache. Taking caffeine orally in combination with analgesics is effective for treating simple headache. Caffeine is an FDA-approved product for use with analgesics for improving pain relief (2718,11832).

Migraine headache. Taking caffeine orally in combination with acetaminophen and aspirin is effective for treating migraine headache. Caffeine is an FDA-approved product for use with analgesics for the treatment of migraine (2715,2716,2717).

Postoperative headache. Using caffeine orally or intravenously is effective for preventing postoperative headache (2725,2726). Caffeine is an FDA-approved product for preventing headache in postoperative patients who regularly consume caffeinated products.

LIKELY EFFECTIVE

Mental alertness. Consumption of caffeinated beverages seems to prevent a decline in alertness and cognitive capacity when consumed throughout the day (4221,4224). Caffeine can improve mental performance and alertness following prolonged sleep deprivation (10205). Combining caffeine with taurine seems to provide a small improvement in mental performance (9899).

POSSIBLY EFFECTIVE

Asthma. Taking caffeine orally appears to improve airway function modestly in people with asthma for up to four hours (9607).

Athletic performance. Caffeine seems to increase physical endurance (11832) and may increase the time to exhaustion during physical exertion (10203). Caffeine doesn't seem to affect activity requiring high exertion over a short period of time such as sprinting and lifting (11832).

Gallbladder disease. Consumption of caffeinated beverages that provide 400 mg or greater of caffeine per day is associated with significantly reducing the risk of developing symptomatic gallstone disease (3345,8032). The effect seems to be dose-dependent. Consumption of 800 mg caffeine per day has the greatest reduction in risk (3345).

Hypotension. Consuming caffeinated beverages seems to increase blood pressure in elderly people with postprandial hypotension (11834,11835).

Neonatal apnea. Using caffeine orally or intravenously seems to improve neonatal apnea of prematurity in infants 28-32 weeks postconception (6023,6371). Caffeine citrate seems to reduce the number of apnea episodes by at least 50% over 7-10 days of treatment (6371).

Parkinson's disease. There is some evidence from large-scale epidemiological studies that suggests people who consume caffeinated beverages such as coffee, tea, and cola have a decreased risk of Parkinson's disease. Men consuming 3-4 cups (28 oz) of caffeinated coffee per day, or 421-2716 mg total caffeine, had the lowest risk of developing Parkinson's disease. However, a significantly lower risk was also associated with consumption of as little as 124-208 mg of caffeine (6022). In women, more moderate caffeinated coffee consumption seems to be best; 1-3 cups per day (1238). Caffeine does not appear to provide additional protection from Parkinson's disease in cigarette smokers (9236).

Postdural puncture headache. Using caffeine orally or intravenously seems to help prevent postdural puncture headache (2727,2728).

Weight loss. Taking caffeine orally in combination with ephedrine seems to help reduce weight, short-term (695,696,1704,8647). Caffeine 192 mg in combination with ephedra 90 mg per day for 6 months seems to cause a modest weight reduction (5.3 kg) in people with a body mass index (BMI) between 25-40 kg per meter squared. This combination, along with limiting fat intake to 30 percent of calories and moderate exercise, also seems to reduce body fat, decrease low-density lipoprotein (LDL) cholesterol, and increase high-density lipoprotein (HDL) cholesterol. Even in carefully screened and monitored otherwise healthy adults, caffeine/ephedra combinations can cause small changes in blood pressure and heart rate (8647).

POSSIBLY INEFFECTIVE

Attention deficit-hyperactivity disorder (ADHD). Most research suggests caffeine doesn't significantly reduce ADHD symptoms in children when used at tolerable doses (10755,10756,10757,10758,10759,10760). The use of caffeine in adolescents and adults with ADHD hasn't been studied.

Mechanism of Action

Caffeine is a methylxanthine compound and is structurally related to theophylline, theobromine, and uric acid (6372). It is 100% bioavailable after oral administration and is metabolized principally in the liver to paraxanthine, theophylline, and theobromine (6370). The half-life of caffeine is about six hours (8644).

Caffeine stimulates the central nervous system (CNS), heart, muscles, and possibly the pressor centers that control blood pressure (2722). Possible mechanisms include adenosine receptor blockade and phosphodiesterase inhibition (2722). By blocking adenosine receptors, caffeine is thought to increase the release of neurotransmitters such as dopamine (6370). Caffeine also decreases airway resistance and stimulates respiration, via adenosine receptor blockade and phosphodiesterase inhibition (11836). It has also been proposed that caffeine may decrease GABA and serotonin signaling (6370). Caffeine stimulates gastric acid secretion, and increases plasma catecholamine levels (11837). Caffeine can have positive inotropic and chronotropic effects on the heart (11836). Caffeine can also acutely elevate both diastolic and systolic blood pressure, but might not have this effect in habitual users (2722).

Caffeine is often combined with analgesics. Caffeine seems to increase the efficacy and onset of analgesic activity by about 40% (11834). Caffeine itself might also have a mild analgesic effect (11835,11836). The mechanism of analgesic effect is unclear. Caffeine might block mediators of pain such as adenosine receptors or inhibit cyclooxygenase (COX)-2 synthesis. It might also cause mood changes that modify the perception of pain (11837).

Caffeine exerts a diuretic effect, with water losses estimated at 1.17 mL per milligram of caffeine (2712). Tachyphylaxis to the diuretic effect develops rapidly, diminishing fluid losses associated with caffeine intake (10206). Caffeine-containing beverages consumed during moderate endurance exercise do not appear to compromise bodily hydration status (2713). Caffeine does not substantially affect the fluid status of people who drink caffeinated beverages on a regular basis (10206). Caffeine's CNS stimulant effects are thought to improve vigilance and psychomotor performance (2720,10205). For improving athletic performance, caffeine has been shown to decrease perceived levels of exertion, which enables the athlete to feel less tired and increase their performance (6370). Caffeine alone or in combination with ephedrine can improve anaerobic exercise performance. Caffeine seems to enhance muscle metabolism and increases time to exhaustion and oxygen deficit, which may lead to better performance (8646). Studies have also suggested caffeine possibly influences cardiovascular stress reactivity, either by potentiating the stress response itself or adding to the level reached during stress (6372). Caffeine may cause a slight decrease in heart rate after consumption and appears to raise blood pressure during psychological stress (6372). Large amounts of caffeine, >10 mg/kg/day, can also produce tachycardia and premature ventricular contractions (6372).

Caffeine has been reported to cause increases and decreases in blood glucose. In people with type 2 diabetes, acute administration of caffeine impairs postprandial glucose metabolism, while acute abstention from caffeine reduces postprandial glucose levels by 21%. Whether these effects also occur with caffeinated beverages and herbs is unknown (12374). Other research in obese people suggests that caffeine ingestion may contribute to insulin resistance (12375). However, one study found that type 1 diabetics taking 200 mg of caffeine twice daily had increased frequency and intensity of warning signs of hypoglycemia. This may be due to a reduction in blood flow to the brain and an increase in glucose utilization by the brain (6024). For preventing Parkinson's disease, caffeine may protect dopaminergic neurons in the brain. This effect appears to be related to modulation of adenosine receptors (10201). This may result in a reduction in the clinical expression of Parkinsonism (6022).

Evidence suggests that tolerance to caffeine's neuroendocrine and cardiovascular effects may develop during consumption throughout the day, but tolerance appears to be lost during overnight abstinence of caffeine (6372).

Preliminary evidence also suggests caffeine may increase plasma levels of cortisol and adrenocorticotrophic hormone (ACTH), decrease levels of extracellular potassium, and increase levels of intracellular calcium in skeletal muscle; but the mechanisms are poorly understood (6370). Caffeine may be beneficial in the prevention of cardiovascular disease. There is evidence caffeine inhibits platelet aggregation and suppresses thromboxane formation during blood clotting (8028,8029). There is also evidence caffeine might be associated with decreased levels of testosterone and increased levels of estrone and sex-hormone binding globulin. These findings might explain why some studies have reported associations between caffeine and hormone-dependent conditions such as fibrocystic disease, osteoporosis, breast cancer, and endometriosis (8043).

Caffeine in green tea seems to work synergistically with other constituents such as catechins and theanine to produce weight loss in animals (11960). Caffeine is often used in combination with ephedra for weight loss and seems to have additive pharmacodynamic effects. A single dose of ephedra in combination with caffeine can increase heart rate from 67 beats per minute to 82 beats per minute in young, healthy people. The combination also increases systolic blood pressure and to a lesser extent, diastolic pressure (8644). Caffeine in combination with ephedra also increases oxygen consumption. Whether the increased oxygen consumption is an indication of a significant increase in metabolism and contributes to weight loss is unknown (8645).

Adverse Reactions

Orally, caffeine can cause insomnia, nervousness, restlessness, gastric irritation, nausea, vomiting, tachycardia, quickened respiration, tremors, delirium, convulsions, and diuresis. Large doses can produce headache, anxiety, agitation, ringing in the ears, premature heartbeat, and arrhythmia (11832,11838). In fatal caffeine overdose, the cause of death is usually ventricular fibrillation (11838). Insomnia is a frequent adverse effect in children (10755). Caffeine may cause feeding intolerance and gastrointestinal irritation in infants (6023). Caffeine may exacerbate sleep disturbances in patients with acquired immunodeficiency syndrome (AIDS) (10204).

Some evidence shows caffeine is associated with fibrocystic breast disease, breast cancer, and endometriosis in women; however, this is controversial since findings are conflicting (8043). Restricting caffeine in women with fibrocystic breast conditions doesn't seem to affect breast nodularity, swelling, or pain (8996).

Although acute administration of caffeine can cause increased blood pressure, regular consumption does not seem to increase either blood pressure or pulse, even in mildly hypertensive patients (1451,1452,2722).

Tolerance to caffeine is a widely held belief, but there is little supportive clinical evidence. If it exists, it appears to be of little clinical significance (11839). Withdrawal symptoms such as irritability, sleepiness, delirium, nausea, vomiting, rhinorrhea, nervousness, restlessness, anxiety, muscle tension, muscle pains, and flushed face have been described. However, these symptoms may be from nonpharmacological factors related to knowledge and expectation of effects. Clinically significant symptoms caused by caffeine withdrawal may be uncommon (2723,11839).

Epidemiological evidence regarding the relationship between caffeine use and the risk for osteoporosis is contradictory. Caffeine can increase urinary excretion of calcium (2669,10202,11317). Women identified with a genetic variant of the vitamin D receptor appear to be at an increased risk for the detrimental effect of caffeine on bone mass (2669). However, moderate caffeine intake, less than 300 mg per day, does not seem to significantly increase osteoporosis risk in most postmenopausal women with normal calcium intake (2669,6025,10202,11317).

Combining ephedra with caffeine can increase the risk of adverse effects. Jitteriness, hypertension, seizures, temporary loss of consciousness, and hospitalization requiring life support has been associated with the combined use of ephedra and caffeine (2729). There is also a report of ischemic stroke in an athlete who consumed ephedra 40-60 mg, creatine monohydrate 6 grams, caffeine 400-600 mg, and a variety of other supplements daily for six weeks (1275).

Caffeine can cause anaphylaxis in sensitive individuals, although true IgE-mediated caffeine allergy seems to be relatively rare (11315).

Interactions with Herbs & Other Dietary Supplements

CAFFEINE-CONTAINING HERBS/SUPPLEMENTS: Concomitant use can increase therapeutic and adverse effects. Natural products that contain caffeine include coffee, black or green tea, guarana, mate, and cola nut.

CALCIUM: High caffeine intake from foods and beverages increases urinary calcium excretion (2570).

CREATINE: There is some concern that combining caffeine, ephedra, and creatine might increase the risk of serious adverse effects. There is a report of ischemic stroke in an athlete who consumed creatine monohydrate 6 grams, caffeine 400-600 mg, ephedra 40-60 mg, and a variety of other supplements daily for 6 weeks (1275). Caffeine might also decrease creatine's possible beneficial effects on athletic performance. Some researchers think caffeine can inhibit phosphocreatine resynthesis (2117,4575).

EPHEDRA (Ma Huang): Use of ephedra with caffeine can increase the risk of stimulatory adverse effects. There is evidence that using ephedra with caffeine might increase the risk of serious life-threatening or debilitating adverse effects such as hypertension, myocardial infarction, stroke, seizures, and death (1275,6486,10307). Tell patients to avoid taking caffeine with ephedra and other stimulants.

Interactions with Drugs

ADENOSINE (Adenocard): Caffeine is a competitive inhibitor of adenosine at the cellular level. However, caffeine doesn't seem to affect supplemental adenosine because high interstitial levels of adenosine overcome the antagonistic effects of caffeine (11771). It is recommended that methylxanthines and methylxanthine-containing products be stopped 24 hours prior to pharmacological stress tests (11770). However, methylxanthines appear more likely to interfere with dipyridamole (Persantine) than adenosine-induced stress testing (11771).

ALCOHOL (Ethanol): Concomitant use of alcohol can increase caffeine serum concentrations and the risk of caffeine adverse effects. Alcohol reduces caffeine metabolism (6370).

ANTICOAGULANT/ANTIPLATELET DRUGS: Theoretically, caffeine might increase the risk of bleeding when used concomitantly with these agents. Caffeine is reported to have antiplatelet activity (8028,8029); however, this interaction has not been reported in humans. Antiplatelet agents include aspirin, clopidogrel (Plavix), dipyridamole (Persantine), ticlopidine (Ticlid), and others. Anticoagulant agents include heparin and warfarin (Coumadin).

ANTIDIABETES DRUGS: Theoretically, concomitant use of caffeine and diabetes drugs might interfere with blood glucose control. Data are conflicting. Reports claim that caffeine might increase or decrease blood sugar (6024,8646).

CIMETIDINE (Tagamet): Concomitant use can increase serum caffeine concentrations, and the risk of caffeine adverse effects. Cimetidine decreases the rate of caffeine clearance by 31-42% (11736).

CLOZAPINE (Clozaril): Co-administration can acutely exacerbate psychotic symptoms. Caffeine can also increase the effects and toxicity of clozapine. Caffeine doses of 400-1000 mg per day inhibit clozapine metabolism (5051).

CONTRACEPTIVE DRUGS: Theoretically, concomitant use might increase caffeine concentrations and the risk adverse effects. Oral contraceptives decrease the rate of caffeine clearance by 40-65% (2714,11737).

DIPYRIDAMOLE (Persantine): Caffeine inhibits dipyridamole-induced vasodilation (11770,11772). It is recommended that methylxanthines and methylxanthine-containing products be stopped 24 hours prior to pharmacological stress tests (11770). Methylxanthines appear more likely to interfere with dipyridamole (Persantine) than adenosine-induced stress testing (11771).

DISULFIRAM (Antabuse): Concomitant use can increase caffeine serum concentrations, and the risk of adverse effects. Disulfiram decreases the rate of caffeine clearance (11840).

EPHEDRINE: Use of ephedrine with caffeine can increase the risk of stimulatory adverse effects. There is evidence that using ephedrine with caffeine might increase the risk of serious life-threatening or debilitating adverse effects such as hypertension, myocardial infarction, stroke, seizures, and death (1275,6486,10307). Tell patients to avoid taking caffeine with ephedrine and other stimulants.

ESTROGENS: Concomitant use can increase serum caffeine concentrations and the risk of caffeine adverse effects. Estrogen inhibits caffeine metabolism (2714).

FLUCONAZOLE (Diflucan): Concomitant use might increase the effects of caffeine. Fluconazole decreases caffeine clearance by approximately 25% (11022).

FLUVOXAMINE (Luvox): Concomitant use can increase caffeine serum concentrations, and the risk of caffeine adverse effects. Fluvoxamine reduces caffeine metabolism (6370).

LITHIUM: Abrupt caffeine withdrawal might increase serum lithium levels (609). There are two case reports of lithium tremor that worsened upon abrupt coffee withdrawal (610).

MEXILETINE (Mexitil): Concomitant use can increase serum caffeine concentrations and the risk of caffeine adverse effects. Mexiletine reduces caffeine metabolism (1260,11741).

MONOAMINE OXIDASE INHIBITORS (MAOIs): Theoretically, concomitant intake of large amounts of caffeine with MAOIs might precipitate a hypertensive crisis (15).

PHENYLPROPANOLAMINE: Concomitant use of phenylpropanolamine and caffeine might cause an additive increase in blood pressure (11738).

QUINOLONE ANTIBIOTICS: Concomitant use can increase serum caffeine concentrations and the risk of caffeine adverse effects. Quinolones decrease caffeine clearance (606,607,608). Quinolones (fluoroquinolones) include ciprofloxacin (Cipro), enoxacin (Penetrex), gatifloxacin (Tequin), levofloxacin (Levaquin), lomefloxacin (Maxaquin), moxifloxacin (Avelox), norfloxacin (Noroxin), ofloxacin (Floxin), sparfloxacin (Zagam), and trovafloxacin (Trovan).

RILUZOLE (Rilutek): Theoretically, concomitant use might increase serum caffeine and riluzole concentrations and the risk of adverse effects of both caffeine and riluzole. Caffeine and riluzole are both metabolized by cytochrome P450 1A2, and concomitant use might reduce metabolism of one or both agents (11739).

STIMULANT DRUGS: Due to the CNS stimulant effects of caffeine concomitant use can increase the risk of adverse effects (11832). Some stimulant drugs include diethylpropion (Tenuate), epinephrine, phentermine (Ionamin), pseudoephedrine (Sudafed), and many others.

TERBINAFINE (Lamisil): Concomitant use can increase serum caffeine concentrations and the risk of caffeine adverse effects. Terbinafine decreases the clearance of intravenous caffeine by 19% (11740).

THEOPHYLLINE: Theoretically, concomitant use might increase serum theophylline concentrations and the risk of adverse effects. Large amounts of caffeine might inhibit theophylline metabolism (11741).

VERAPAMIL (Calan, Covera, Isoptin, Verelan): Theoretically, concomitant use might increase plasma caffeine concentrations and the risk of adverse effects. Verapamil increases plasma caffeine concentrations by 25% (11741).

Interactions with Foods

None known.

Interactions with Lab Tests

5-HYDROXYINDOLEACETIC ACID: Caffeine might increase urine 5-hydroxyindoleacetic acid concentrations and test results. Caffeine can increase urine catecholamine concentrations (15).
BLEEDING TIME: Caffeine is reported to have antiplatelet activity and theoretically affect bleeding time (8028,8029). However, the significance of these effects in humans is not known.
CATECHOLAMINE: Caffeine can increase plasma catecholamine levels (8646).
CREATINE: Caffeine can increase urine creatine levels (1701).
DIPYRIDAMOLE THALLIUM IMAGING: Caffeine might interfere with dipyridamole thallium imaging studies. Caffeine attenuates the characteristic cardiovascular responses to dipyridamole and has altered test results (11742).
GLUCOSE: Caffeine has been reported to cause increases and decreases in blood glucose (8646).
LACTATE: The combination of ephedrine, a constituent of ephedra, and caffeine can increase blood lactate levels (8646).
NEUROBLASTOMA TESTS: Caffeine might cause false-positive diagnosis of neuroblastoma, when diagnosis is based on tests of urine vanillylmandelic acid (VMA) or catecholamine concentrations. Caffeine can increase urine catecholamine and VMA concentrations (15).
PHARMACOLOGICAL STRESS TESTS: Caffeine is a competitive antagonist for adenosine receptors (11771). It is recommended that caffeine and caffeine-containing products be stopped 24 hours prior to pharmacological stress tests (11770). However, caffeine appears more likely to interfere with dipyridamole (Persantine) than adenosine (Adenocard) stress testing (11771). The interaction between caffeine and dipyridamole is unlikely to be significant in stress testing if the heart rate increase is greater than 5% after dipyridamole infusion (11772).
PHEOCHROMOCYTOMA TESTS: Caffeine might cause false-positive diagnosis of pheochromocytoma, when diagnosis is based on tests of urine vanillylmandelic acid (VMA) or catecholamine concentrations. Caffeine can increase urine catecholamine and VMA concentrations (15).
PULMONARY FUNCTION TESTS: People may need to avoid caffeine for at least four hours prior to lung function testing. Forced expiratory volume in one minute (FEV1) seems to show a small improvement up to two hours after caffeine use. Mid-expiratory flow rates may also improve with caffeine for up to four hours (9607).
URATE: Caffeine might falsely increase serum urate test results determined by the Bittner method. Caffeine causes false elevations in serum urate test results determined by the Bittner method (11844).
URINARY CALCIUM: Caffeine can increase urinary calcium levels (11317).
VANILLYLMANDELIC ACID (VMA): Caffeine might increase urine VMA concentrations and test results. Caffeine can increase urine VMA concentrations (15).

Interactions with Diseases or Conditions

ANXIETY DISORDERS: Caffeine might aggravate anxiety disorders (11743).
BLEEDING DISORDERS: Theoretically, caffeine might aggravate bleeding disorders. Caffeine is reported to have antiplatelet activity (8028,8029); however, this interaction has not been reported in humans. Caffeine can prolong bleeding time and increase the results of a bleeding time test (1701).
CARDIAC CONDITIONS: Caffeine can induce cardiac arrhythmias in sensitive individuals (11845); use with caution.
DIABETES: Some research suggests that caffeine may impair postprandial glucose metabolism in people with diabetes and contribute to insulin resistance. The effect of caffeinated beverages and herbs has not been studied (12374,12375). Caffeine may enhance the frequency and intensity of hypoglycemic warning symptoms in type 1 diabetics. This may increase the ability of diabetics to detect and treat hypoglycemia early. However, it might also increase the frequency of hypoglycemic events (6024); use with caution. Caffeine has been reported to cause increases and decreases in blood glucose (8646); use with caution.
GLAUCOMA: Caffeine increases intraocular pressure. The increase occurs within 30 minutes and persists for at least 90 minutes after drinking caffeinated beverages (8540).
HYPERTENSION: Consuming caffeine might increase blood pressure in people with high blood pressure. However, this effect might be less in habitual caffeine users (2722).
OSTEOPOROSIS: Caffeine can increase urinary excretion of calcium. Caffeine consumption should be limited to less than 300 mg per day (approximately 2-3 cups of coffee). Adequate calcium supplementation may partially compensate for calcium losses (2669,10202,11317). Postmenopausal women identified with a genetic variant of the vitamin D receptor should use caffeine with caution (2669).

Dosage and Administration

ORAL: The typical dose of caffeine for headache or restoring mental alertness is up to 250 mg per day (2718,11743). For fatigue, the common dose is 150-600 mg (11832). For increasing exercise performance, 2-10 mg/kg or more has been used. However, doses in excess of 10 mg/kg can result in urine levels greater than the 12 mcg/mL allowed by the International Olympic Committee and the National Collegiate Athletic Association (6370). For weight loss, the ephedrine and caffeine combination products are commonly dosed 20 mg/200 mg three times per day (695,696,1704).

For postdural puncture headache, 300 mg orally has been used (2727,2728). For preventing symptomatic gallstone disease, consumption of 400 mg or greater of caffeine per day has been used for risk reduction (3345,8032). For preventing Parkinson's disease, men consuming 3-4 cups (28 oz) of caffeinated coffee per day or 421-2716 mg total caffeine had the lowest risk of developing Parkinson's disease. However, a significantly lower risk was also associated with consumption of as little as 124-208 mg of caffeine (6022). In women, more moderate caffeinated coffee consumption seems to be best; 1-3 cups per day (1238).
INTRAVENOUS: For apnea in infants, one study used an initial intravenous dose of caffeine benzoate of 10 mg/kg. Some infants required a second dose of 5 mg/kg 18-24 hours later (6023). Another study used a 20 mg/kg loading dose of caffeine citrate intravenously followed by a daily dose of 2.5 mg/kg intravenously or orally for 10 days for maintenance (6371). For postdural puncture headache, 500 mg caffeine sodium benzoate in 1000 mL normal saline infused over 90 minutes following anesthesia has been used (2727,2728).

Comments
People with voice disorders, singers, and other voice professionals are often advised against the use of caffeine; however, this recommendation has been based on anecdotal evidence. Now preliminary research seems to indicate that caffeine ingestion may actually adversely affect subjective voice quality. Further study is necessary to confirm these preliminary findings (2724). The use of caffeine in combination with ephedra for weight loss is controversial. Some authorities think the combination of caffeine and ephedra should only be used with physician supervision (8640). Others call for FDA licensing as a prescription drug (8641). One cup of coffee, tea, and cocoa contain approximately 75-200 mg, 50 mg, and 5 mg of caffeine respectively (6372). A 12 oz bottle of cola drink contains approximately 30-50 mg caffeine (6372).

CAJEPUT OIL

Also Known As
Cajeputi Aetheroleum, Cajuput, Paperbark Tree Oil, Punk Tree.
CAUTION: See separate listings for Niauli Oil and Tea Tree Oil.

Scientific Names
Melaleuca leucadendra, synonym Kajuputi leucadendra, Myrtus leucadendra; Melaleuca quinquenervia.
Family: Myrtaceae.

People Use This For
Orally, cajeput oil is used as an expectorant, tonic, to treat colds, headaches, toothache, and indolent tumors.
Topically, cajeput is used for its anti-parasitic effect in scabies and tinea versicolor. Cajeput oil is also used either alone or in combination with other ingredients in commercially available antiseptic liniments to treat rheumatic and neuralgic discomforts.
As an inhalant, it is used as an expectorant and tonic.
In dentistry, cajeput oil is used to relieve dry socket discomfort.
In food and beverages, it is used as a flavoring in very small amounts.

Safety
LIKELY SAFE ...when cajeput oil is used orally in amounts commonly found in foods. Cajeput oil has Generally Recognized As Safe status (GRAS) for use in foods in the US (4912).
POSSIBLY SAFE ...when used topically on unbroken skin (2,7).
POSSIBLY UNSAFE ...when inhaled. Inhalation can cause bronchospasm (7).
There is insufficient reliable information available about the safety of cajeput oil for its other uses or in amounts exceeding those found in food.
CHILDREN: LIKELY UNSAFE ...when used topically on facial areas, especially the nose (2,7) because it might cause bronchospasm.
PREGNANCY AND LACTATION: Insufficient reliable information available; avoid using.

Effectiveness
There is insufficient reliable information available about the effectiveness of cajeput oil.

Mechanism of Action
Cajeput oil contains 14-65% cineole (7,11), which is reported to have antispasmodic, antimicrobial and fungicidal properties (7). Cineole may act as a counterirritant (7). Cineole is identical to eucalyptol (215).

Adverse Reactions
Orally, use of cajeput oil can lead to dyspepsia (7).
Topically, use can produce hypersensitivity, allergic reactions, and irritation of mucous membranes (7).
Inhalation can cause bronchospasm (7).

Interactions with Herbs & Other Dietary Supplements
None known.

Interactions with Drugs
None known.

Interactions with Foods
None known.

Interactions with Lab Tests
None known.

Interactions with Diseases or Conditions
ASTHMA: Inhalation of cajeput oil may provoke bronchospasm (7).

Dosage and Administration
No typical dosage.

Comments
Avoid confusion with tea tree oil (Maleleuca alternifolia) and niauli oil (Malaleuca viridiflora). Cajeput oil is produced by steam distillation of fresh leaves and twigs of Melaleuca leucadendra and Melaleuca quinquenervia.

CALABAR BEAN

Also Known As
Chop Nut, Esere Nut, Faba Calabarica, Legume, Ordeal Bean, Physotigma.

Scientific Names
Physostigma venenosum.
Family: Fabaceae/Leguminosae.

People Use This For
Orally, calabar bean is used for visual disorders, constipation, epilepsy, cholera, and tetanus. Calabar bean is a source of the prescription drug physostigmine (Isopto Eserine, Antilirium).

Safety
UNSAFE ...when used orally. The calabar bean is extremely toxic. Its active constituent, physostigmine, can cause death by impairing heart contractility and causing respiratory paralysis (6).
PREGNANCY AND LACTATION: UNSAFE ...when used orally (6); avoid using.

Effectiveness
There is insufficient reliable information available about the effectiveness of calabar bean.

Mechanism of Action
The applicable part of calabar bean is the dried, ripe seed. The major constituent, physostigmine, prolongs activity of neurotransmitter acetylcholine (6). It increases parasympathetic nervous system and striated muscle tone, stimulates glandular secretions, increases GI peristalsis, reduces heart rate, and causes pupil contraction leading to a reduction in intraocular pressure (18).

Adverse Reactions
Orally, overdose of physostigmine, the constituent of calabar bean, causes cholinergic crisis characterized by excessive salivation and sweating, constricted pupils of eye, nausea, vomiting, diarrhea, bradycardia or tachycardia, hypotension or hypertension, confusion, seizures, coma, severe muscle weakness, paralysis, and death (15).

Interactions with Herbs & Other Dietary Supplements
None known.

Interactions with Drugs
ANTICHOLINERGIC DRUGS: Physostigmine, a constituent of calabar bean, reverses the effect of belladonna and other drugs with anticholinergic action. These drugs include antihistamines, some emetics, some anti-Parkinson agents, and phenothiazines (15).

Interactions with Foods
None known.

Interactions with Lab Tests
None known.

Interactions with Diseases or Conditions
Avoid in patients with Parkinson's disease, bradycardia, asthma, gangrene, diabetes, cardiovascular disease, and mechanical obstruction of intestinal or urogenital tract.

Dosage and Administration
No typical dosage.

Comments
Historically, African tribes used calabar bean, the "ordeal bean," to identify witches and people possessed by evil spirits. They believed that people who regurgitated the bean and lived were innocent. Ritual uses continue in Africa despite being outlawed (6). Subjects of the "ordeal" can increase their chance of survival by not chewing the bean and swallowing it whole. Chewing releases the toxic constituents.

CALAMINT

Also Known As
Basil Thyme, Lesser Calamint, Mill Mint, Mountain Balm, Mountain Mint.

Scientific Names
Calamintha nepeta, synonyms Clinopodium nepeta, Melissa nepeta, Satureja calamintha, Satureja nepeta.
Family: Lamiaceae/Labiatae.

Comments
At the date of publication, this product was not a common ingredient used in brand name supplements marketed to consumers. Details about this product are available in the online version of *Natural Medicines Comprehensive Database.* See www.naturaldatabase.com.

CALAMUS

Also Known As
Bach, Cinnamon Sedge, Flagroot, Gladdon, Grass Myrtle, Kalmus, Myrtle Flag, Myrtle Sedge, Sadgrantha, Sweet Cinnamon, Sweet Calamus, Sweet Cane, Sweet Flag, Sweet Grass, Sweet Myrtle, Sweet Root, Sweet Rush, Sweet Sedge, Ugragandha, Vacha, Vayambur.

Scientific Names
Acorus calamus; Acorus americanus; Acorus gramineus; Acorus sp.
Family: Acoraceae.

People Use This For
Orally, calamus is used for digestive disorders including ulcers, gastritis, and flatulence, acute and chronic dyspepsia, anorexia; and to stimulate appetite and digestion. Calamus is also used orally as a sedative, to induce sweating, and for rheumatoid arthritis, and stroke.
Calamus is also chewed to remove the smell of tobacco, as a stimulant, as a euphoric, and as a hallucinogen.
Topically calamus is used for skin disease.
In foods, calamus is utilized in cooking as a spice.

Safety
LIKELY UNSAFE ...when used orally. The FDA prohibits calamus use in food products (4912) due to the presence of the carcinogenic constituent, beta-isoasarone in three of the four distinct species. However, the beta-isoasarone content can vary widely among species from 0% to 96% (6); some products may be safer than others.
PREGNANCY AND LACTATION: LIKELY UNSAFE ...when used orally; avoid using (4,500).

Effectiveness
There is insufficient reliable information available about the effectiveness of calamus.

Mechanism of Action

The applicable part of calamus is the rhizome. The constituent asarone, which is chemically related to reserpine, may explain calamus' sedative effects (6). It is not known exactly which constituent is responsible for calamus' ability to relieve smooth muscle spasms, though it is probably not isoasarone, because preparations without isoasarone have a measurable spasmolytic effect (6).

Adverse Reactions

Calamus oil may contain beta-isoasarone, a known carcinogen associated with kidney damage, tremors, and convulsions.

Interactions with Herbs & Other Dietary Supplements

HERBS WITH SEDATIVE PROPERTIES: Theoretically, concomitant use with supplements that have sedative properties might enhance therapeutic and adverse effects or calamus. Some of these include 5-HTP, calamus, California poppy, catnip, hops, Jamaican dogwood, kava, St. John's wort, scullcap, valerian, yerba mansa, and others.

Interactions with Drugs

ANTACIDS: Theoretically, due to reports that calamus increases stomach acid, calamus might decrease the effectiveness of antacids (19).
CNS DEPRESSANTS: Theoretically, concomitant use with drugs with sedative properties can cause additive effects and side effects (4).
H2-BLOCKERS: Theoretically, due to reports that calamus increases stomach acid, calamus might decrease the effectiveness of H2-blockers (19). The H2 blockers include cimetidine (Tagamet), ranitidine (Zantac), nizatidine (Axid), and famotidine (Pepcid).
MONOAMINE OXIDASE INHIBITORS (MAOIs): Theoretically, calamus might potentiate the effects and adverse effects of monoamine oxidase inhibitor drugs (4).
PROTON PUMP INHIBITORS (PPIs): Theoretically, due to reports that calamus increases stomach acid, calamus might decrease the effectiveness of PPIs (19). PPIs include omeprazole (Prilosec), lansoprazole (Prevacid), rabeprazole (Aciphex), pantoprazole (Protonix), and esomeprazole (Nexium).

Interactions with Foods

None known.

Interactions with Lab Tests

None known.

Interactions with Diseases or Conditions

None known.

Dosage and Administration

ORAL: 1-3 grams of the rhizome has been used three times daily (4). As a tea one cup tea, prepared by steeping 1-3 grams of the rhizome in 150 mL of boiling water for 5-10 minutes, has been used three times daily (4). 1-3 mL of the liquid extract, 1:1 in 60% alcohol, has been used three times daily (4). 2-4 mL of the tincture, 1:5 in 60% alcohol, has been used three times daily (4).

Comments

Four different species of Calamus exist, each in a different geographic region of the world. The North American variety is isoasarone free and the European form contains less than 10% isoasarone in the volatile oil. Others contain up to 96% carcinogenic beta-isoasarone in the volatile oil (5).

CALCIUM

Also Known As

Bone Meal, Calcium Acetate, Calcium Aspartate, Calcium Carbonate, Calcium Chelate, Calcium Chloride, Calcium Citrate, Calcium Gluconate, Calcium Lactate, Calcium Lactogluconate, Calcium Orotate, Calcium Phosphate, Di-calcium Phosphate, Heated Oyster Shell-Seaweed Calcium, Hydroxyapatite, Oyster Shell Calcium, Tricalcium Phosphate.
CAUTION: See separate listing for Dolomite.

Scientific Names

Calcium; Ca; atomic number 20.

People Use This For

Orally, calcium is used for treatment and prevention of hypocalcemia, osteoporosis, rickets, and latent tetany. It is also used orally for hypoparathyroidism, osteomalacia, premenstrual syndrome (PMS), leg cramps associated with pregnancy, and reducing the risk of colorectal cancer. Calcium is also used orally for diarrhea and rectal epithelial hyperproliferation following intestinal bypass, hypertension, elevated levels of low-density lipoprotein (LDL), elevated fluoride levels in children, and elevated lead levels. Calcium carbonate is used orally as an antacid. Calcium carbonate and calcium acetate are also used orally as phosphate binders in renal failure. Calcium is also used for metformin-related vitamin B12 deficiency.

Intravenously, calcium gluconate, acetate, gluceptate and chloride are used for severe hypocalcemia and hypocalcemic tetany, and during cardiopulmonary resuscitation. Calcium gluconate and gluceptate are also given intramuscularly when intravenous administration is not possible.

Safety

LIKELY SAFE ...when used orally and appropriately. Calcium is safe when used in doses that do not exceed the tolerable upper intake level (UL) of 2.5 grams (7555). Although higher doses have been used safely, taking doses that exceed the UL are more likely to cause side effects. ...when used intravenously and appropriately (12928,12946).

POSSIBLY UNSAFE ...when used orally in high doses. Doses that exceed 2.5 grams of elemental calcium are more likely to cause side effects such as hypercalcemia, milk-alkali syndrome, nephrocalcinosis, and renal insufficiency (7555).

PREGNANCY AND LACTATION: LIKELY SAFE ...when used orally and appropriately (945,1586,3263,3264). There is insufficient reliable information available about the safety of the intravenous use of calcium during pregnancy and lactation.

Effectiveness

EFFECTIVE

Dyspepsia. Taking calcium carbonate orally as an antacid is effective for treating dyspepsia (1843). Calcium carbonate has FDA approval as an antacid.

Hyperkalemia. Administering calcium gluconate intravenously can reverse hyperkalemia (12946). Intravenous calcium gluconate is FDA-approved for hyperkalemia.

Hypocalcemia. Taking calcium orally is effective for treating and preventing hypocalcemia. Intravenous calcium gluconate, acetate, gluceptate, or chloride is effective for severe hypocalcemia or hypocalcemic tetany (12928).

Renal failure. Taking calcium carbonate or calcium acetate orally is effective as a phosphate binder in renal failure. Calcium acetate (PhosLo) appears to control hyperphosphatemia better than sevelamer (Renagel). Calcium citrate is not recommended for this purpose because it increases aluminum absorption and does not bind phosphate as efficiently as calcium acetate or calcium carbonate (12943,12944).

LIKELY EFFECTIVE

Corticosteroid-induced osteoporosis. Taking calcium in combination with vitamin D as adjunctive therapy seems to be effective for reducing bone mineral density loss in people using corticosteroids long-term (982,1046,1830,1831,1832,4462,4463,4464,4465,4466,4467,12945).

Fetal bone mineralization. Calcium supplementation in pregnant women who have low dietary calcium intake (less than 562 mg elemental calcium per day), increases fetal bone mineralization and density. However, in women with adequate dietary intake, calcium supplementation doesn't offer any additional benefit (3263,3264).

Hyperparathyroidism. Taking calcium orally reduces parathyroid hormone levels in patients with chronic renal failure and secondary hyperparathyroidism (1827,1828,1829). In elderly women, the combination of calcium and vitamin D reverses secondary hyperparathyroidism and reduces hip fracture risk (8818).

Osteoporosis. Taking calcium orally is effective for preventing and treating bone loss and osteoporosis. Maximal bone growth occurs in the teenage years, and then bone density in women remains relatively constant until age 30-40. After age 40, bone loss typically occurs at rates of 0.5% to 1% per year. In men, this occurs several decades later. Bone loss is more pronounced if dietary calcium intake is below the RDA, which is the case for many Americans (2571,2578).

Bone loss in premenopausal women over 40 can be reduced significantly by supplementing with 1000 mg calcium/day (2578). But in the 5 years immediately after menopause, calcium supplementation has very little effect on bone loss (2569,2570,2575,2576). The rapid loss of estrogen causes a high bone resorption rate, which increases serum calcium levels and therefore decreases intestinal absorption of calcium (2570). After this period, calcium supplementation has a significant benefit on bone loss. The typical rate of bone loss in postmenopausal women who are not taking calcium supplements is 2% per year (2572,2576). Calcium 1000-1600 mg/day (as carbonate, citrate, lactate gluconate, or citrate malate) decreases this rate by 0.25% to 1% annually (977,979,981,2569,2571,2572,2575,2576,2578,6850). The greatest reductions (1% or more) are seen in the first 1-2 years of supplementation when bone remodeling foci can be filled in (2569,2576). After this period, the differences in rate of loss between supplemented and unsupplemented women are closer to 0.25% per year (2569,2577).

Despite the "first year effect" it is estimated that 30 years of continuous calcium supplementation after menopause might result in a 10% improvement in bone mineral density, and a 50% overall reduction in fracture rates, compared with women who do not take calcium supplements (2570).

Most studies show that long-term calcium supplementation decreases primary fracture rates for specific bones by 30% to 35% for vertebral bone and 25% for hip bone (2576). Supplements must be continued indefinitely since the effects of 2 years of calcium supplements on bone mineral density are largely lost within 2 years after discontinuing the supplements (981,2576,6853,12932). Multiple clinical studies and meta-analyses suggest efficacy for calcium plus vitamin D for primary prevention (980,1836,8818,10932,12926,12930,12933,12934,12952). Calcium supplementation also seems to reduce bone turnover during weight reduction in postmenopausal women (987).

The usefulness of calcium in preventing osteoporosis in men is not as well-studied as in women. Some evidence suggests calcium 1000 mg/day taken for 2 years might improve trabecular or cortical bone mass by 2% to 4% (980,8827,8873). Dietary supplementation with calcium and vitamin D seems to moderately reduce bone loss measured in the femoral neck, spine, and total body, and seems to reduce the incidence of nonvertebral fractures (980).

Calcium has additive effects on bone density with other agents such as vitamin D, estrogens, or calcitonin. Whereas calcium alone generally reduces or prevents loss of bone density, combination with other agents can produce small increases in bone density ranging from 0.3% to 3.3% depending on the combination and dosages used (978,980,1836,2570,2571,2572,2576). The full potential of osteoporosis treatments cannot be realized without adequate calcium intake (2569,2570,2571,2572). Advise patients taking agents such as estrogens, calcitonin, bisphosphonates, or raloxifene (Evista) to ensure that their daily calcium intake meets the RDA. Use supplements if necessary.

In some cases, calcium supplements might not be beneficial. Calcium supplements don't seem to be effective for preventing bone mineral density loss in lactating women (988), after bone marrow transplantation (1817), or for preventing bone loss associated with renal transplantation (4823).

There is also concern that calcium might not be effective for secondary prevention of fractures in elderly patients. Calcium 1000 mg/day with or without vitamin D 800 IU/day for 2-5 years does not significantly reduce fracture risk in elderly women or men who have had a previous fracture compared to placebo (13073). Another study also suggests that calcium 1000 mg/day plus vitamin D 800 IU/day might not prevent a second fracture in elderly patients, or prevent a first fracture in elderly patients with other risk factors such as low body weight (<58 kg, 127.6 pounds), smoking, family history of hip fracture, or fair or poor self-reported health (12929). However, these studies have been criticized for failing to measure vitamin D levels and low adherence to study protocol (12931). One of these studies did not use a placebo control (12929).

Premenstrual syndrome (PMS). There seems to be a link between low dietary calcium intake and symptoms of PMS (6847). Taking calcium 1-1.2 grams daily seems to significantly reduce depressed mood, water retention, and pain associated with PMS (1822,1823,1824). Calcium seems to decrease symptom scores by about 18% compared to placebo (1822). Increasing dietary calcium intake is also associated with a decreased risk of developing PMS. Women consuming an average of 1283 mg/day of calcium from foods seem to have about a 30% lower risk of developing PMS compared to women consuming an average of 529 mg/day of calcium (13094); however, taking calcium supplements does not appear to be associated with the risk of developing PMS.

POSSIBLY EFFECTIVE

Colorectal cancer. High intake of dietary or supplemental calcium seems to reduce the risk of adenoma recurrence and colorectal cancer (970,994,1047,8820,12118,12120,12950). Vitamin D might be an important factor. People with lower than average vitamin D levels don't seem to get any benefit from calcium supplements (12118).

Fluorosis. Taking calcium orally in combination with ascorbic acid (vitamin C) and vitamin D supplements seems to be effective for reducing excessive fluoride levels in children and improving symptoms of fluorosis (990).

Hypercholesterolemia. Taking calcium orally in conjunction with a low-fat diet seems to be effective for treating mild to moderate hypercholesterolemia. Calcium carbonate 400 mg three times daily produced a 4.4% reduction in low-density lipoprotein (LDL) cholesterol and a 4.1% increase in high-density lipoprotein (HDL) after six weeks of treatment when used in combination with a low-fat diet (American Heart Association step 1) starting eight weeks prior to calcium carbonate (2557).

Hypertension. Calcium supplementation produces a very modest reduction in blood pressure, usually around 1-2 mmHg. Calcium might be more effective for certain subpopulations of patients, such as salt-sensitive people and patients with low baseline dietary calcium intake (945,972,974,976,984,1818,1819,1820,1821,6852,13138). Taking calcium orally also seems to be help for reducing blood pressure in patients with end-stage renal disease (ESRD) (975).

Ischemic stroke. There is some evidence that increasing dietary calcium intake might decrease the relative risk of ischemic stroke in women (4822).

Pregnancy-related complications. Taking calcium orally seems to be effective for reducing pregnancy-related hypertension and pre-eclampsia in women with insufficient dietary calcium intake (971,973,1833,1834,8828). Calcium 2 grams daily appears to reduce pre-eclampsia occurrences up to sevenfold among women at high risk. Supplementation in women with adequate dietary intake does not seem to affect pre-eclampsia. There is also some evidence that calcium 1 gram twice daily (as a mixture of salts) can reduce pregnancy-related leg cramps during the second half of pregnancy (2567).

Tooth retention. Taking calcium and vitamin D orally appear to beneficially affect tooth retention in the elderly population (8816).

Weight loss. Adults and children with low calcium intake are more likely to gain weight, have a higher body mass index (BMI), and be overweight or obese compared to people with high calcium intake (8824,12124,12125,12126,12127). Increasing calcium consumption from dairy products seems to increase weight reduction in people on a calorie restricted diet (8824,8830,12128). Increasing calcium from dairy products such as yogurt to a total calcium intake from 800-1100 mg seems to result in more weight and body fat loss than consuming less calcium. An increase in calcium consumption of 900-1000 mg/day seems to be associated with an 8-9 kilogram reduction in body weight (8824,12050,12051,12127). But increasing calcium intake by taking supplements does not seem to be beneficial for helping weight loss (12051,12052,13138).

POSSIBLY INEFFECTIVE

Elevated lead concentrations. Taking calcium orally doesn't seem to reduce lead concentrations in lactating women. Lead is mobilized along with calcium from bone during pregnancy and lactation, resulting in increased serum concentrations of lead. Calcium supplementation does not significantly decrease these elevated lead concentrations (1586).

INSUFFICIENT RELIABLE EVIDENCE to RATE

Metformin-related vitamin B12 deficiency. Calcium supplementation might reduce a metformin-induced decrease in vitamin B12 levels (8834).

Seizures. Preliminary clinical evidence suggests calcium might help control seizures resulting from sudden declines in serum ionized calcium (8835).

More evidence is needed to rate calcium for these uses.

Mechanism of Action

The bones and teeth contain greater than 99% of the calcium in the human body. Calcium in bone is present mainly as hydroxyapatite (1834).

Calcium is also present in blood, extracellular fluid, muscle, and other tissues. It is essential for nerve transmission, muscle contraction, vascular contraction, vasodilation, glandular secretion, cell membrane and capillary permeability, enzyme reactions, respiration, renal function, and blood coagulation. It also plays a role in neurotransmitter and hormone release and storage, uptake and binding of amino acids, cyanocobalamin (vitamin B12) absorption, and gastrin secretion (15).

Calcium in bone is a reserve source of calcium that can be mobilized to maintain extracellular calcium concentrations. About half of serum calcium is bound to plasma proteins. The free or ionized calcium is tightly regulated and is a useful clinical indicator of calcium status (1834).

Calcium balance is generally positive during growth, neutral in the mature adult, and negative in older adults. Calcium is lost in varying amounts through the feces, urine, sweat, and sloughed skin cells. Reduced estrogen levels in women result in reduced calcium absorption and retention, increased bone turnover, and lower bone mass (1834,8833,8838,8839).

Calcium absorption varies with age, environmental and dietary conditions, and race (1837,8870). People of Asian and African descent absorb calcium more efficiently than Caucasians (1837). Elderly women, in general, have an impaired intestinal response to vitamin D. This impairment can further contribute to negative calcium balance and bone loss (8833,8838). In healthy premenopausal women, the proportion of dietary calcium absorbed varies from 10% to 60%, and is positively correlated with body mass index, dietary fat, and serum vitamin D level (6851). It is inversely correlated with total dietary calcium, dietary fiber, alcohol intake, and physical activity (6851). There is a link between a low fat, high fiber diet and poor calcium absorption, possibly due to a faster rate of intestinal transit (6851).

There is also a link between weight loss and calcium absorption. Weight loss of 5% or greater is associated with decreased bone mass and increased risk of fracture. Weigh loss seems to decrease calcium absorption and increase parathyroid hormone. Taking calcium supplements during weight loss seems to suppress the increased bone resorption (12117).

Calcium exhibits threshold absorption. Below the threshold, an increase in calcium intake results in improved response; above the threshold, increased calcium intake has no effect. The many variables of calcium absorption complicate interpretation of calcium absorption studies (1834,8823). Some evidence suggests that calcium citrate and heated oyster shell-seaweed calcium are absorbed better than calcium carbonate, while other research indicates similar bioavailability (1838,1839,1840,1841,1842,1847,8832).

Calcium carbonate absorption is decreased by estrogen or vitamin D deficiency (8823).

Preliminary evidence suggests that calcium-rich mineral waters appear to have similar bioavailability when compared to oral calcium supplements (8836).

Calcium absorption is not impaired due to lactose intolerance. However, lactose intolerance could limit dairy calcium intake (8837). Contrary to laboratory evidence, lactose does not enhance calcium bioavailability in lactose tolerant people (4824).

As an antacid, calcium carbonate reacts with gastric hydrochloric acid. Calcium carbonate is the most potent antacid on a weight basis, followed by sodium bicarbonate (1843).

Calcium is sometimes used for renal patients because it can bind with phosphate in the gut, preventing its absorption and reducing the hyperphosphatemia associated with renal failure. Calcium carbonate and calcium acetate are used for this purpose. Calcium citrate is not recommended because it increases aluminum absorption. Conversely, hypophosphatemia causes an increase in intestinal calcium absorption and increased calcium in the

blood, which can inhibit formation of new bone (3372,8821), and potentially lead to a greater risk of renal calcium stone formation (3372).
Calcium may help to lower serum cholesterol levels by forming insoluble complexes with saturated fatty acids in the gut, causing them to be excreted in the feces without being absorbed (2557).
For weight loss, calcium seems to modulate diet-related adiposity by inhibiting lipogenesis, increasing lipolysis, and promoting fat loss. Increasing dietary calcium intake may result in reduced body weight, primarily by reducing fat mass (8824,8825,8870). Calcium seems to repartition dietary energy from adipose tissue to lean body mass (12119). Dairy products containing calcium seem to be more effective at regulating adiposity than elemental calcium supplements (12121).
Evidence also suggests that inadequate dietary intake of calcium can play a role in the development of hypertension, stroke, and cardiovascular disease (8817). Calcium might lower blood pressure by increasing renal sodium excretion (12122).
In women, calcium levels may be lower in the premenstrual period (due to effects of variations in estrogen levels on calcium absorption and metabolism), which may contribute to the mood changes and other symptoms associated with premenstrual syndrome (PMS) (2639,6847).
There is also interest in using calcium for cancer prevention. Preliminary evidence suggests calcium may have an antiproliferative effect on colorectal cancer cells (8820,8870,10019). Calcium taken orally also seems to reverse rectal epithelial hyperproliferation caused by excessive output of fecal bile acids and lipids after intestinal bypass (1826).

Adverse Reactions

Orally, calcium can cause belching and flatulence (1843). Although constipation is frequently cited as an adverse effect of calcium, there is no scientific substantiation of this side effect (1843,1844,1845).
Calcium carbonate has been reported to cause acid rebound, but this is controversial (12935,12936).
Prolonged ingestion of large amounts of calcium carbonate (usually greater than 20 grams per day) can cause hypercalcemia, milk-alkali syndrome (1843), nephrocalcinosis, and renal insufficiency (6122). In patients with impaired renal function, doses as low as 4 grams per day might cause hypercalcemia and milk-alkali syndrome (1843,6849).
There is concern that calcium supplements, both oyster shell and refined calcium products, can be contaminated with lead (997,6459,6460). In one report, 8 of 23 nationally available calcium carbonate products contained small amounts of lead (6459). However, these findings are likely clinically insignificant. The amount of lead in these calcium supplements is substantially less than that found in common foods, such as green salads, grapes, and wine. Also, calcium significantly decreases lead absorption. Small amounts of lead in a calcium supplement would not likely be significantly absorbed or achieve clinically relevant levels in the body (6460). So far, there have not been reports of significant lead toxicity from appropriate use of calcium supplements (996). Epidemiological evidence suggests that a high intake of dietary calcium might increase the risk for prostate cancer (4825,12949).

Interactions with Herbs & Other Dietary Supplements

MAGNESIUM: Calcium supplements can decrease the absorption of dietary magnesium, but only at very high, supra-therapeutic doses (2600 mg per day). However, in people with adequate magnesium stores, calcium doesn't have any clinically significant effect on long-term magnesium balance. Advise patients at high risk for magnesium deficiency to take calcium supplements at bedtime, instead of with meals, to avoid inhibiting dietary magnesium absorption (4623,7555,11159).
VITAMIN D: Concomitant administration with vitamin D increases active absorption of calcium in the small intestine (7555).

Interactions with Drugs

BISPHOSPHONATES: Calcium supplements decrease absorption of bisphosphonates. Advise patients to take bisphosphonates at least 30 minutes before calcium, but preferably at a different time of day (12937). The bisphosphonates include alendronate (Fosamax), etidronate (Didronel), ibandronate (Boniva), risedronate (Actonel), and tiludronate (Skelid).
CALCIPOTRIENE (Dovonex): Calcipotriene is a vitamin D analog used topically for psoriasis. It can be absorbed in sufficient amounts to cause systemic effects, including hypercalcemia (12938). Theoretically, combining calcipotriene with calcium supplements might increase the risk of hypercalcemia. Tell patients not to take calcium supplements if they are taking calcipotriene.
CALCIUM CHANNEL BLOCKERS: Calcium when given intravenously may decrease the effects of calcium channel blockers. It is used in the management of calcium channel blocker overdose. But there's no evidence that dietary or supplemental calcium when taken orally interacts with calcium channel blockers (12939,12947). The calcium channel blockers include nifedipine (Adalat, Procardia), verapamil (Calan, Isoptin, Verelan), diltiazem (Cardizem), isradipine (DynaCirc), felodipine (Plendil), amlodipine (Norvasc), and others. Intravenous calcium gluconate has been used before intravenous verapamil (Isoptin) to prevent or reduce the hypotensive effects without affecting the antiarrhythmic effects (6124).
DIGOXIN (Lanoxin): Hypercalcemia increases the risk of fatal cardiac arrhythmias with digoxin (12940).
DILTIAZEM (Cardizem, Dilacor, Tiazac): Hypercalcemia can reduce the effectiveness of verapamil in atrial fibrillation (10574).
ESTROGENS: Estrogen increases supplemental calcium absorption in postmenopausal women (995).

LEVOTHYROXINE (Synthroid, Levothroid, Levoxyl, and others): Calcium reduces levothyroxine absorption, probably by forming insoluble complexes (5082). Calcium carbonate supplements reduce effectiveness of levothyroxine in patients with hypothyroid (5081,5082,6137). Advise patients to take levothyroxine and calcium supplements at least four hours apart.
QUINOLONE ANTIBIOTICS: Taking calcium at the same time as quinolones reduces quinolone absorption. Calcium forms insoluble complexes with quinolones (4412,10339). Advise patients to take these drugs at least 2 hours before, or four to six hours after calcium supplements (10339). Quinolones include ciprofloxacin (Cipro), levofloxacin (Levaquin), ofloxacin (Floxin), moxifloxacin (Avelox), gatifloxacin (Tequin), gemifloxacin (Factive), and others.
SOTALOL (Betapace): Calcium appears to reduce the absorption of sotalol, probably by forming insoluble complexes (10018). Advise patients to separate doses by at least two hours before or four to six hours after calcium.
TETRACYCLINE ANTIBIOTICS: Calcium decreases the absorption of tetracyclines by forming insoluble complexes (1843). Advise patients to take these drugs at least two hours before, or four to six hours after calcium supplements. Tetracyclines include demeclocycline (Declomycin), doxycycline (Vibramycin), and minocycline (Minocin).
THIAZIDE DIURETICS: Thiazides reduce calcium excretion by the kidneys (1902). Using thiazides along with moderately large amounts of calcium carbonate increases the risk of milk-alkali syndrome (hypercalcemia, metabolic alkalosis, renal failure). Advise patients to consult their physician about appropriate calcium doses, and to have their serum calcium levels and/or parathyroid function monitored regularly. These diuretics include chlorothiazide (Diuril), hydrochlorothiazide (HydroDIURIL, Esidrix), indapamide (Lozol), metolazone (Zaroxolyn), chlorthalidone (Hygroton), etc.
VERAPAMIL (Calan, Covera, Isoptin, Verelan): Hypercalcemia can reduce the effectiveness of verapamil in atrial fibrillation (10574).

Drug Influences on Nutrient Levels and Depletion

SOME DRUGS CAN AFFECT CALCIUM LEVELS:
ALUMINUM SALTS: Large doses of aluminum salts (aluminum hydroxide 1-3 grams four times daily, e.g., 90-260 mL Maalox daily) bind dietary phosphate, causing hypophosphatemia. This induces movement of calcium from bone into the blood, increasing urinary calcium excretion (4400). There are reports of negative calcium balance after short-term use of large doses of aluminum-containing antacids, and of osteomalacia after prolonged use of large doses, especially in people with a low dietary phosphate intake, or a low dietary calcium intake (less than 250 mg per day) (4400,5979). Advise patients to avoid taking large doses of aluminum-containing antacids for prolonged periods, unless they are taking them for hyperphosphatemia associated with chronic renal failure.
ANTICONVULSANTS: Phenytoin (Dilantin), fosphenytoin (Cerebyx), phenobarbital, and carbamazepine (Tegretol) decrease calcium absorption by increasing metabolism of vitamin D, which is needed for calcium absorption (2675). Hypocalcemia and osteomalacia have occurred, especially with prolonged therapy and use of more than one of these drugs concurrently (2675). Advise patients taking these medications for six months or more that they may also need vitamin D and calcium supplements. Other anticonvulsants such as gabapentin (Neurontin), felbamate (Felbatol), lamotrigine (Lamictal), levetiracetam (Keppra), tiagabine (Gabitril), and topiramate (Topamax) do not have these effects.
CHOLESTYRAMINE (Questran): Cholestyramine can reduce absorption of vitamin D, which in turn reduces absorption of calcium. Occasionally this can lead to osteomalacia, usually in patients receiving large doses of cholestyramine (more than 32 grams per day), or prolonged therapy (more than two years). It can also occur in the presence of additional risk factors such as ileal resection or primary biliary cirrhosis (which deplete the bile acids needed for vitamin D absorption) (4458,5655,5809,5838). However, cholestyramine (24 grams/day) for treatment of hyperlipidemia in otherwise healthy men doesn't seem to affect vitamin D or calcium levels (2672).
CORTICOSTEROIDS: Corticosteroids, in daily doses equivalent to 7.5 mg prednisone or more, cause significant bone loss, osteoporosis, and increased risk of fractures. The severity increases with duration of therapy. Mechanisms include decreased absorption and increased excretion of calcium, reduction in sex hormones, and inhibition of bone formation. Advise adults taking prednisone 7.5 mg/day (or equivalent doses of other corticosteroids) for six months or longer to maintain a daily calcium intake of 1500 mg/day. They may also need a vitamin D supplement (e.g., 800 IU/day). Monitor serum calcium (1832,4462,4463,4464,4465,4466,4467).
DIURETICS: Loop diuretics increase urinary calcium excretion and may reduce serum calcium levels, especially at higher doses (1902,4412). Loop diuretics include furosemide (Lasix), bumetanide (Bumex), ethacrynic acid (Edecrin), and torsemide (Demadex).
FLUOROQUINOLONES: Fluoroquinolones form complexes with calcium in the gastrointestinal tract, which could reduce absorption of both the fluoroquinolone and calcium if taken at the same time (4412). Significant effects on calcium levels are unlikely when fluoroquinolones are taken at least two hours before, or four to six hours after calcium supplements or calcium-containing foods. Fluoroquinolones include ciprofloxacin (Cipro), levofloxacin (Levaquin), ofloxacin (Floxin), moxifloxacin (Avelox), gatifloxacin (Tequin), and others.
H2 BLOCKERS and PROTON PUMP INHIBITORS (PPIs): Absorption of some calcium supplements, especially calcium carbonate, is reduced when gastric acid is reduced. However, there isn't any evidence that acid suppressive drugs reduce serum calcium levels. There also isn't any evidence that cimetidine affects parathyroid

hormone (PTH) or calcium levels in healthy people, but there are conflicting reports about cimetidine's effect on PTH and calcium levels in people with primary hyperparathyroidism (2738,4330,4331,5060). H2 blockers include cimetidine (Tagamet), ranitidine (Zantac), nizatidine (Axid), and famotidine (Pepcid). PPIs include omeprazole (Prilosec), lansoprazole (Prevacid), rabeprazole (Aciphex), pantoprazole (Protonix), and esomeprazole (Nexium).
LEVOTHYROXINE: Levothyroxine (Synthroid, Levothroid, Levoxyl) may accelerate bone remodeling and turnover, increase the rate of bone loss at several sites including the spine and hips, and cause a negative calcium balance (27,2685,2695,2697,2721). This is most likely when high doses are used for suppressive therapy in thyroid cancer, nodules, or goiter, rather than replacement doses for hypothyroidism. Clinically significant bone loss is most likely in postmenopausal women, but negative effects have also been reported in premenopausal women and men (28,29,2685,2695). Advise patients to have regular thyroid function tests to monitor for appropriate levothyroxine dose (2684,2695,2698,2721). Also check to see patients daily intakes of calcium and vitamin D meet the recommendations for their age and gender (2684).
MAGNESIUM SALTS: Large doses of magnesium salts may cause hypocalcemia. This is most likely with intravenous doses sufficient to produce hypermagnesemia, such as in the treatment of acute myocardial infarction or premature labor (2730,2731). High magnesium levels increase urinary calcium excretion, possibly due to changes in the renal threshold for calcium absorption, or reduced parathyroid hormone secretion (2730,2731). Calcium supplementation is unlikely to be needed with short-term, intravenous magnesium therapy. Oral magnesium supplements (e.g., magnesium oxide 576 mg/day) do not affect calcium absorption (4623).
MINERAL OIL: Mineral oil can interfere with calcium utilization and retention by reducing absorption of both calcium and vitamin D (4495). Advise patients against regular or long-term use of mineral oil.
STIMULANT LAXATIVES: Prolonged use of high doses of stimulant laxatives can reduce dietary calcium and vitamin D absorption, and possibly lead to osteomalacia (11530). Advise patients to limit stimulant laxatives to short-term use of recommended doses. Some stimulant laxatives include cascara (CitraMax Plus), senna (Senokot), bisacodyl (Dulcolax), and others.
TETRACYCLINES: Tetracyclines form complexes with calcium in the gastrointestinal tract, which could reduce absorption of both the tetracycline and calcium if taken at the same time (4412). Significant effects on calcium levels are unlikely when tetracyclines are taken at least two hours before, or four to six hours after calcium supplements or calcium-containing foods. Tetracyclines include demeclocycline (Declomycin), doxycycline (Vibramycin), and minocycline (Minocin).

Interactions with Foods

CAFFEINE: High caffeine intake from foods and beverages increases urinary calcium excretion (2570). Intake of more than 300 mg/day (three to four cups of coffee, or six 12 oz cola drinks) is linked to increased bone loss and increased fracture rates in elderly women, especially when calcium intake is low (2669,2670). Advise patients to ensure that their calcium intake from food and supplements is at the recommended level for their age and sex.
FIBER: Certain constituents of dietary fiber inhibit calcium absorption. These include phytic acid (found in wheat bran), oxalic acid (found in spinach and rhubarb), and uronic acid (a common plant fiber constituent) (7555,12942). Separate administration of calcium supplements from these foods by two hours.
IRON, ZINC, MAGNESIUM: Calcium supplements may decrease the absorption of dietary iron, zinc, and magnesium. However, in people with adequate stores of these minerals, this doesn't have any clinically significant effect on the long-term status of iron, zinc, or magnesium in the body (1848,1849,1850,7135,7308,8822,8831). Advise people at high risk for deficiency of these minerals to take calcium supplements at bedtime, instead of with meals, to avoid inhibiting dietary mineral absorption (7308).
SODIUM: High sodium intake from foods increases urinary calcium excretion (1834,2570). A calcium intake of 1000 mg/day is needed to prevent bone loss in postmenopausal women ingesting 2000 mg sodium chloride daily. About 1500 mg/day calcium is needed if sodium chloride intake is 3000 mg/day (2570).

Interactions with Lab Tests

11-HYDROXYCORTICOSTEROIDS: Calcium gluconate given intravenously may increase plasma 11-hydroxycorticosteroid concentrations and test results (275).
17-HYDROXYCORTICOSTEROIDS: Calcium gluconate may reduce urinary 17-hydroxycorticosteroid concentrations and test results. One case of this interaction is reported (275).
BONE MINERAL DENSITY (BMD): Supplemental calcium taken orally may prevent or reduce the rate of bone mineral loss as reflected in BMD measures (977,978,981).
GASTRIN: Calcium carbonate may increase serum gastrin concentrations and test results within 30-75 minutes after calcium carbonate ingestion (275).
GLUCOSE: Calcium gluconate may decrease serum glucose concentrations and test results. This interaction was reported in newborns (275).
I-131 UPTAKE: Calcium gluconate may decrease serum uptake of I-131 (275).
INSULIN: Calcium gluconate may increase plasma insulin concentrations and test results. This interaction was reported in newborns (275).
LIPASE: Calcium ions may falsely decrease test results when measuring serum lipase concentrations greater than 5 mmol/L using the method of Teitz (275). Calcium ions do not affect test results when measuring serum lipase concentrations up to 5 mmol/L using the method of Teitz (275).

MAGNESIUM: Calcium gluconate can falsely decrease test results for serum magnesium measured by titan-yellow, but will not affect test results measured by the dihydroxyazobenzene method (275). Calcium gluconate can falsely decrease test results for urine magnesium measured by titan-yellow (275).

Interactions with Diseases or Conditions

HYPERCALCIURIA (CALCIUM OXALATE STONES): Restricting intake of animal protein and salt, combined with a normal dietary calcium intake, appears to provide greater protection from recurrent kidney stones than a low-calcium diet (8826).
HYPERPARATHYROIDISM: Hyperparathyroid activity predisposes individuals to increased calcium absorption (12948).
HYPERPHOSPHATEMIA: Use cautiously in patients with high serum phosphate levels. The product of serum phosphate and calcium levels should not exceed 60 to prevent precipitation of calcium phosphate and oft tissue calcification (6479).
HYPOPHOSPHATEMIA: Use cautiously in patients with low serum phosphate levels. If calcium intake increases without a concurrent increase in phosphorus intake, phosphorus absorption can decrease, worsening phosphorus deficiency (8821).
HYPOTHYROIDISM: Patients taking levothyroxine (L-thyroxine, Levothroid, Synthroid) replacement therapy should separate administration of levothyroxine and calcium carbonate by four hours. Calcium carbonate reduces levothyroxine absorption and effectiveness in hypothyroid patients on levothyroxine replacement therapy (5081,5082,6137).
RENAL INSUFFICIENCY: Calcium carbonate supplementation increases the risk of hypercalcemia and alkalosis (7555).
SARCOIDOSIS: This condition results in increased risk of excessive calcium absorption and hypercalcemia (12951).
SMOKING: Cigarette smoking decreases intestinal calcium absorption (1846).

Dosage and Administration

ORAL: For preventing hypocalcemia, 1 gram elemental calcium daily is typically used. Calcium replacement requirements in people with hypocalcemia can be estimated by clinical condition or serum calcium determinations, but a typical starting dose is 1-2 grams daily (12928).
For heartburn, calcium carbonate as an antacid is usually 0.5-1.5 grams as needed (1843).
For hyperphosphatemia in adults with chronic renal failure, the initial dose of calcium acetate is 1.334 grams (338 mg elemental calcium) with each meal, increasing to 2-2.67 grams (500-680 mg elemental calcium) with each meal if necessary (12943,12944).
For prevention of osteoporosis in postmenopausal women, doses of 1-1.6 grams elemental calcium daily in divided doses (as carbonate, citrate, lactate gluconate, or citrate malate) have been used (977,979,981,2569,2571,2575,2576,2578,8838,8871), and should be chosen to bring the total daily calcium intake from diet and supplements up to the relevant dietary reference intake (see below) (981,2569,2571,2575,2578,8838,8870).
For prevention of bone loss in premenopausal women over 40, a dose of 1 gram daily has been used (2578).
For pregnant women with low dietary calcium intake, the dose for increasing fetal bone density ranges from 300-1300 mg/day beginning at gestation week 20-22 (3263,3264). A dose of 1-1.2 grams calcium per day as calcium carbonate has reduced symptoms of premenstrual syndrome (PMS) (1822,1824).
For treatment of secondary hyperparathyroidism in people with chronic renal failure, doses of 2-21 grams calcium carbonate daily have been used (1827,1828,1829).
For treatment of secondary hyperparathyroidism in elderly women, elemental calcium 1200 mg daily, combined with 800 IU vitamin D daily, has been used (8818).
To prevent bone loss associated with chronic corticosteroid therapy, divided daily doses of 1 gram of elemental calcium daily is used (12945).
For reducing the risk of recurrence of colorectal adenomas, calcium carbonate 3 to 4 grams (1.2-1.6 grams calcium) daily has been used (970,994,1047,8820,12118).
As an adjunct to other treatments for hypertension, 1-1.5 grams calcium daily has been used (945,972,974,976,984,1818,1819,1820,1821,6852). Typical doses used to reduce the risk of pre-eclampsia are 1-2 grams elemental calcium daily as calcium carbonate (971,973,1833,1834,8828).
For treating diarrhea and rectal epithelial hyperproliferation due to intestinal bypass, a dose of 2.4-3.6 grams daily calcium as calcium carbonate has been used (1826).
For hypercholesterolemia, 400 mg calcium (as calcium carbonate) three times daily has been used in conjunction with a low-fat diet (2557).
High serum fluoride levels and symptoms of fluorosis in children have been reduced with calcium 125 mg twice daily, in combination with ascorbic acid and vitamin D (990).
For weight loss, increasing calcium consumption from dairy products to a total consumption of 800-1000 mg/day in combination with a calorie-restricted diet seems to increase weight loss (12050,12051,12052).
Calcium carbonate and calcium citrate are the two most commonly used forms of calcium (945,8832). Calcium carbonate contains 400 mg calcium/gram and calcium citrate contains 211 mg calcium/gram (1000 mg elemental calcium = 2500 mg calcium carbonate = 4700 mg calcium citrate). Absorption of calcium from supplements is

greatest when taken with food in doses of 500 mg or less since the active transport system for calcium in the small bowel is easily saturated (6122,8832). Calcium supplements are usually divided into two doses daily (8871).
Calcium citrate may be preferable in people with achlorhydria or taking drugs that reduce gastric acidity (e.g., H2 antagonists, proton pump inhibitors) (1816,8832).
The daily Dietary Reference Intakes (DRI) for elemental calcium are: Age 1-3 years, 500 mg; 4-8 years, 800 mg; 9-18 years, 1300 mg; 19-50 years, 1000 mg; 51+ years, 1200 mg; Pregnant or Lactating (under 19 years), 1300 mg; Pregnant or Lactating (19-50 years), 1000 mg (7555,8839). The daily upper intake level (UL) for calcium is 2.5 grams for everyone over one year of age (3094).
INTRAVENOUS: For emergency management of hypocalcemia, 100-200 mg of elemental calcium can be given intravenously as a bolus, and a central vein should be used whenever possible. One milliliter of calcium chloride provides 27 mg of elemental calcium, and 1 mL of calcium gluconate provides 9 mg (12928). For management of hyperkalemia, 20 mL of 10% calcium gluconate administered over 5-10 minutes in adults (0.5mL/kg in children), and as a slow infusion over 20-30 minutes for patients taking digoxin (12946).

Comments

Calcium-rich foods include milk and dairy products, kale and broccoli, as well as the calcium-enriched citrus juices, mineral water (6356), canned fish with bones, and soy products processed with calcium.
In the US and Canada, foods containing at least 200 mg calcium with less phosphorus content than calcium are allowed to be labeled with a health claim for osteoporosis. In the US, the health claim may read "Regular exercise and a healthy diet with enough calcium helps teen and young adult white and Asian women maintain good bone health and may reduce their high risk of osteoporosis later in life." Canada recently updated its health claim wording to emphasize the importance of vitamin D and to broaden the claim to beyond women: "A healthy diet with adequate calcium and vitamin D, and regular physical activity, help to achieve strong bones and may reduce the risk of osteoporosis" (11940).

CALCIUM D-GLUCARATE

Also Known As

Calcium Glucarate, Calcium-D Glucarate, Calcium-D-Glucarate, D-Glucarate (GA).
CAUTION: See separate listing for Calcium.

Scientific Names

D-glucaro-1,4-lactone (1,4 GL).

People Use This For

Orally, calcium D-glucarate is used for preventing breast, prostate, and colon cancer; and for removing carcinogens, toxins, and steroid hormones from the body.

Safety

There is insufficient reliable information available about the safety of calcium D-glucarate.
Pregnancy and Lactation: Insufficient reliable information available; avoid using.

Effectiveness

There is insufficient reliable information available about the effectiveness of calcium D-glucarate.

Mechanism of Action

Glucaric acid is combined with calcium to form calcium D-glucarate. Glucaric acid is found in tissues and body fluids. Glucaric acid is also found in foods such as fruits and vegetables including oranges, apples, Brussels sprouts, broccoli, and cabbage (772,3952). Dietary sources provide from 1.12-1.73 mg/100 grams (broccoli and potatoes) to a high of 4.53 mg/100 grams (oranges) (772).
There is a lot of interest in using calcium D-glucarate for preventing estrogen-related cancer such as breast cancer and other hormone-related cancers. Calcium D-glucarate is thought to decrease estrogen levels by affecting estrogen's elimination. Estrogen is normally metabolized hepatically in phase II metabolism by combining with glucuronic acid. It's then excreted in the bile, but a bacterial enzyme in the intestine called beta-glucuronidase normally breaks the estrogen-glucuronide bond, allowing estrogen to be reabsorbed. Calcium D-glucarate works at this step by inhibiting beta-glucuronidase. Blocking this enzyme is thought to decrease the amount of estrogen that is reabsorbed and lower circulating estrogen levels. There is some evidence that beta-glucuronidase activity might be increased in patients with hormone-dependent cancers like breast and prostate cancer (773,774). Dietary glucarate can inhibit beta-glucuronidase activity and inhibits animal models of mammary tumor development (775). In vitro, D-glucarate decreases tumor cell proliferation (776).
Urinary excretion of D-glucaric acid may be an indicator of drug metabolizing enzyme activity in people with impaired renal function (778).

Adverse Reactions
None reported.

Interactions with Herbs & Other Dietary Supplements
None known.

Interactions with Drugs
ALCOHOL (Ethanol): Theoretically, concomitant use with alcohol might decrease calcium D-glucarate activity. There is some evidence that urinary excretion of D-glucarate is increased in people consuming alcohol (779).
GLUCURONIDATED DRUGS: Theoretically, calcium D-glucarate might increase the clearance of drugs that undergo glucuronidation. Some of these drugs include acetaminophen, atorvastatin (Lipitor), diazepam (Valium), digoxin, entacapone (Comtan), estrogen, irinotecan (Camptosar), lamotrigine (Lamictal), lorazepam (Ativan), lovastatin (Mevacor), meprobamate, morphine, oxazepam (Serax), and others (772,3952).
KANAMYCIN: Theoretically, D-glucarate may increase the rate of kanamycin elimination and possibly reduce the risk of drug-induced renal impairment (777).

Interactions with Foods
ALCOHOL (Ethanol): Theoretically, concomitant use with alcohol might decrease calcium D-glucarate activity. There is some evidence that urinary excretion of D-glucarate is increased in people consuming alcohol (779).

Interactions with Lab Tests
None known.

Interactions with Diseases or Conditions
None known.

Dosage and Administration
No typical dosage.

CALENDULA

Also Known As
Garden Marigold, Gold-Bloom, Holligold, Marigold, Marybud, Pot Marigold, Zergul.
CAUTION: See separate listing for Tagetes.

Scientific Names
Calendula officinalis.
Family: Asteraceae/Compositae.

People Use This For
Orally, calendula flower is used as an antispasmodic, to initiate menstrual periods, to reduce fever, for treating cancer, and for inflammation of oral and pharyngeal mucosa. Calendula has also been used orally for gastric and duodenal ulcers and dysmenorrhea.
Topically, calendula is used as an anti-inflammatory and for poorly healing wounds and leg ulcers. It is also used topically for nosebleeds, varicose veins, hemorrhoids, proctitis, and conjunctivitis.

Safety
LIKELY SAFE ...when the flower preparations are used orally or topically and appropriately (4).
PREGNANCY: LIKELY UNSAFE ...when used orally; contraindicated due to spermatocide, antiblastocyst, and abortifacient effects. There is insufficient reliable information available about the safety of the topical use of calendula during pregnancy (4).
LACTATION: Insufficient reliable information available; avoid using.

Effectiveness
There is insufficient reliable information available about the effectiveness of calendula.

Mechanism of Action
The applicable part of calendula is the flower. Calendula is used for wound healing due to potential anti-inflammatory effects. The faradiol monoester is believed to play an important role in the anti-inflammatory activity. Some evidence suggests the water-soluble flavonoids might be responsible for the wound-healing effects (515). Preliminary data suggests that calendula may inhibit human immunodeficiency virus (HIV) replication (11455). Calendula also shows some evidence of antibacterial and antitumor activity (4).

Adverse Reactions

Orally, calendula can cause allergic reactions.
Topically, calendula can cause eczematous allergic reactions. Calendula-specific patch testing is recommended prior to usage to determine allergenic potential. Testing is particularly necessary in individuals sensitive to the Asteraceae/Compositae family (10691,11458). Members of this family include ragweed, chrysanthemums, marigolds, daisies, and many other herbs. Despite the widespread use of calendula and the occurrence of allergies to other family members, there has been only one report of anaphylaxis (11152).

Interactions with Herbs & Other Dietary Supplements

None known.

Interactions with Drugs

CNS DEPRESSANTS: Theoretically, concomitant use of calendula with drugs having sedative properties might cause additive therapeutic and adverse effects. A saponoside constituent in Calendula has been reported to increase hexobarbital sleep time in animals (19).

Interactions with Foods

None known.

Interactions with Lab Tests

None known.

Interactions with Diseases or Conditions

CROSS-ALLERGENICITY: Calendula may cause an eczematous allergic reaction in individuals sensitive to the Asteraceae/Compositae family (10691,11458). Members of this family include ragweed, chrysanthemums, marigolds, daisies, and many other herbs.

Dosage and Administration

ORAL: One cup of the tea is commonly taken three times daily; the tea is prepared by steeping 1-2 grams of the dried flowers in 150 mL boiling water for 5-10 minutes and then straining (2,4). The typical dose of the liquid extract, 1:1 in 40% alcohol, is 0.5-1 mL three times daily (4). The tincture, 1:5 in 90% alcohol, is usually given as 0.3-1.2 mL three times daily (4).
TOPICAL: The tea is commonly used as a gargle, mouthwash, or poured over an absorbent cloth and applied as a poultice to skin ailments (3). For topical use, 2-4 mL of the tincture is usually diluted into 0.25-0.5 L water. Ointments typically contain 2-5 grams of the herb in 100 grams ointment (2).

Comments

Avoid confusion with ornamental marigolds of the Tagets genus, which are commonly grown in vegetable gardens (11).

CALIFORNIA POPPY

Also Known As

Poppy California, Yellow Poppy.
CAUTION: See separate listing for Corn Poppy.

Scientific Names

Eschscholzia californica.
Family: Papaveraceae.

People Use This For

Orally, California poppy is used for insomnia, sedation, aches, nervous agitation, enuresis in children, and diseases of the bladder and liver.
In combination with other herbs, California poppy is used orally for depression, neurasthenia, neuropathy, various psychiatric conditions, foehn illness (sleep and mood disturbance associated with strong, warm wind in the Alps), vasomotor dysfunction, sensitivity to weather changes, and sedation.

Safety

POSSIBLY SAFE ...when used orally and appropriately. The dried aqueous extract of California poppy appears to be safe for up to 3 months (12583). Long-term safety is unknown.
PREGNANCY AND LACTATION: Insufficient reliable information available; avoid using.

Effectiveness

INSUFFICIENT RELIABLE EVIDENCE to RATE

Anxiety. Preliminary clinical research suggests California poppy, in combination with magnesium and hawthorn (Sympathyl, not available in the US), might be useful in treating mild to moderate anxiety disorders (12583). More evidence is needed to rate California poppy for this use.

Mechanism of Action

The applicable parts of California poppy are the dried, above ground parts. California poppy contains the alkaloids californine and protopine. Preliminary research suggests that California poppy can prolong sleep time and has spasmolytic, sedative, and anxiolytic activity. Protopine seems to have benzodiazepine-like activity (12596,12597,12691).

The effects of California poppy extract are reversed by flumazenil (Romazicon). However, California poppy does not seem to have anticonvulsant or muscle relaxant effects. California poppy extract might have peripheral analgesic effects (12692).

Preliminary research suggests the California poppy constituents californine and protopine may be metabolized by cytochrome P450 (CYP450) enzymes. There is no research using human CYP450 isoenzymes to know if these constituents are CYP450 substrates that may be involved in drug interactions (12597).

California poppy is sometimes ingested or smoked as a substitute for marijuana. It reportedly causes mild euphoria lasting for about 20 to 30 minutes, but does not appear to be habit forming (12596,12597). California poppy use is detectable in urine (12597).

Adverse Reactions

Orally, California poppy can cause muscular stiffness, "morning sluggishness," and nausea, when used in combination with magnesium and hawthorn (12583).

Interactions with Herbs & Other Dietary Supplements

HERBS WITH SEDATIVE PROPERTIES: Theoretically, concomitant use with supplements that have sedative properties might enhance therapeutic and adverse effects of California poppy (12596,12597). Some of these supplements include 5-HTP, calamus, catnip, hops, Jamaican dogwood, kava, St. John's wort, skullcap, valerian, yerba mansa, and others.

Interactions with Drugs

BENZODIAZEPINES: Theoretically, concomitant use of California poppy with benzodiazepines may cause additive effects and side effects (12596,12597). Some benzodiazepines include clonazepam (Klonopin), diazepam (Valium), lorazepam (Ativan), and others.

CNS DEPRESSANTS: Theoretically, concomitant use of California poppy with drugs with sedative properties may cause additive effects and side effects (12596,12597).

Interactions with Foods

ALCOHOL: Theoretically, California poppy may increase the risk of drowsiness and impair motor skills; avoid concomitant use (12596,12597).

Interactions with Lab Tests

None known.

Interactions with Diseases or Conditions

None known.

Dosage and Administration

ORAL: No typical dosage. However, traditionally a tea (made by steeping 2 grams herb in 150 mL boiling water 10-15 minutes, strain) has been up to four times daily (12).

Comments

California poppy is the state flower of California. Avoid confusion with corn poppy (Papaver rhoeas). The California poppy (Eschscholzia californica) is sometimes confused with the opium poppy (Papaver somniferum). Both are members of the Papaveraceae family, but they are members of different genera (12596,12597).

CALOTROPIS

Also Known As

Ak, Akada, Alarka, Arka, Mudar Bark, Muder Yercum, Sodom-Apple.

Scientific Names

Calotropis procera, synonym Asclepias procera.
Family: Apocynaceae or Asclepiadaceae.

People Use This For

Orally, calotropis is used for toothache, syphilis, digestive disorders, diarrhea, boils, ulcers, swellings, rheumatism, epilepsy, hysteria, cramps, fever, joint pain, muscular spasm, and constipation, cancer, warts, leprosy, elephantiasis, worms, fever, gout, and snake bites.
In inhalation therapy, smoke from the bark is inhaled for coughs, asthma, and to induce sweating.

Safety

LIKELY UNSAFE ...when used orally, especially in high doses. Calotropis contains cardiac glycosides. High doses can cause vomiting, diarrhea, bradycardia, convulsions, and death (18).
There is insufficient reliable information available about the safety of calotropis for its other uses.
PREGNANCY AND LACTATION: LIKELY UNSAFE ...when used orally (18); avoid using.

Effectiveness

There is insufficient reliable information available about the effectiveness of calotropis.

Mechanism of Action

Calotropis contains cardioactive glycosides (cardenolides) (13,18) that show some antitumor effects on human cells in vitro (18). Calotropis also has expectorant and diuretic properties (18). Animal studies of calotropis extract have shown anti-inflammatory (3823), antibacterial (3824), antipyretic, analgesic, and neuromuscular blocking activity (3822). In one animal study, the extract produced contractions that were blocked by atropine; this supports a use in constipation (3822). In another animal study, an extract of the root showed significant anti-ulcer activity against aspirin, indomethacin, ethanol, indomethacin + ethanol, or stress-induced ulcerations. his anti-ulcer activity may be attributable to the inhibition of 5-lipoxygenase (3825).

Adverse Reactions

Orally, high doses can cause vomiting, diarrhea, bradycardia, convulsions, and death (18).

Interactions with Herbs & Other Dietary Supplements

CARDIAC GLYCOSIDE-CONTAINING HERBS: Concomitant use can increase the risk of cardiac glycoside toxicity. Cardiac glycoside-containing herbs include black hellebore, Canadian hemp roots, digitalis leaf, hedge mustard, figwort, lily-of-the-valley roots, motherwort, oleander leaf, pleurisy root, squill bulb leaf scales, strophanthus seeds, and uzara (19).
CARDIOACTIVE HERBS: Avoid concomitant use with cardioactive herbs due to unpredictability of effects and adverse effects. These include calamus, cereus, cola, coltsfoot, devil's claw, European mistletoe, fenugreek, fumitory, ginger, Panax ginseng, hawthorn, white horehound, maté, parsley, quassia, scotch broom flower, shepherd's purse, and wild carrot (4).
LICORICE/HORSETAIL: Theoretically, the overuse or misuse of licorice rhizome or horsetail plant increases the risk of toxicity due to potassium depletion (19).
STIMULANT LAXATIVE HERBS: Theoretically, the overuse or misuse of stimulant laxatives increases the risk of cardiac toxicity due to potassium depletion. Stimulant laxative herbs include aloe dried leaf sap, blue flag rhizome, alder buckthorn, European buckthorn, butternut bark, cascara bark, castor oil, colocynth fruit pulp, gamboge bark exudate, jalap root, black root, manna bark exudate, podophyllum root, rhubarb root, senna leaves and pods, wild cucumber fruit (Ecballium elaterium), and yellow dock root (19).

Interactions with Drugs

DIGOXIN (Lanoxin): Theoretically, concomitant use with calotropis increases the risk of cardiac glycoside toxicity.
DIURETIC DRUGS: Theoretically, concomitant use of caltropis and potassium depleting diuretics can increase the risk of cardiac glycoside toxicity due to potassium depletion (13,18). Some diuretics that can deplete potassium include chlorothiazide (Diuril), chlorthalidone (Thalitone), furosemide (Lasix), hydrochlorothiazide (HCTZ, Hydrodiuril, Microzide), and others.
STIMULANT LAXATIVES: Theoretically, concomitant use with calotropis may increase risk of cardiac glycoside toxicity due to potassium loss.

Interactions with Foods
None known.

Interactions with Lab Tests
None known.

Interactions with Diseases or Conditions
None known.

Dosage and Administration
ORAL: As an expectorant or diuretic, 200 to 600 mg daily; as an emetic, 2-4 grams daily has been used (18).
TOPICAL: Calotropis is applied as a powder (18).

Comments
In India, calotropis has been used as a suicidal and infanticidal poison (215).

CAMPHOR

Also Known As
Camphora, Camphor Tree, Cemphire, Gum Camphor, Karpoora, Laurel Camphor.

Scientific Names
Cinnamomum camphora, synonym Laurus camphora.
Family: Lauraceae.

People Use This For
Topically, camphor is used to relieve pain. It has been used to treat warts, cold sores, hemorrhoids, and osteoarthritis. It has also been applied topically as an analgesic and an antipruritic. It has been used as a counterirritant, and to increase local blood flow. Camphor has frequently been used topically to treat respiratory tract diseases involving mucous membrane inflammation. It is sometimes used topically to treat cardiac symptoms. Camphor is also used topically as an eardrop, and for treating minor burns.
In inhalation therapy, camphor is used as an antitussive.
Orally, camphor is used as an expectorant, antiflatulent, and for treating respiratory tract diseases.

Safety
LIKELY SAFE ...when used topically in low concentrations, short-term. Concentrations ranging from 0.1% to 11% seem to be safe for short-term topical use on intact skin (272,10327). ...when used by inhalation, appropriately (272).
POSSIBLY SAFE ...when used topically and appropriately short-term. Camphor in combination with glucosamine, shark cartilage, and chondroitin appears to be safe when applied topically on an as-needed basis for up to eight weeks (10327).
LIKELY UNSAFE ...when used topically on broken or injured skin. Application of camphor to broken skin can result in systemic absorption and toxicity (272).
UNSAFE ...when used orally. Ingestion of camphor can cause significant toxicity including death (12). Oral preparations of camphor are no longer available in the US (159).
CHILDREN: POSSIBLY UNSAFE ...when used topically (4814). Young children might be more susceptible to the adverse effects associated with even minor systemic absorption of camphor. UNSAFE ...when used orally. Ingestion of camphor can cause significant toxicity including death (4814).
PREGNANCY AND LACTATION: UNSAFE ...when used orally. Ingestion of camphor can cause serious toxicity including death (17). There is insufficient reliable information available about the safety of camphor when used topically during pregnancy and lactation.

Effectiveness
EFFECTIVE

Cough. Camphor is FDA-approved as a topical antitussive (chest rub) in concentrations less than 11% (4814).
Pain. Camphor is FDA-approved for topical use as an analgesic and anesthetic in concentrations of 3% to 11% (272,4814). It is in many topical products for cold sores, insect stings and bites, minor burns, and hemorrhoids (272).
Pruritus (itching). Camphor is FDA-approved for topical use as an antipruritic agent in concentrations of 3% to 11% (272,4814).

POSSIBLY EFFECTIVE

Osteoarthritis. A topical cream containing camphor, glucosamine sulfate, and chondroitin sulfate seems to reduce the severity of symptoms of osteoarthritis by about half. Symptom relief is most likely due to the counterirritant effect of camphor and not the other ingredients (10327).

There is insufficient reliable information available about the effectiveness of camphor for its other uses.

Mechanism of Action

The applicable part of camphor is the wood distillate. Camphor seems to exert its effect as a nasal decongestant by inducing local vasoconstriction (16). Camphor's counterirritant action is also due to vasoconstriction, which often improves local circulation, and therefore provides analgesic and antipruritic effects (16). Camphor also has weak expectorant effects.

Adverse Reactions

Orally, camphor can cause significant toxicity. Symptoms of camphor toxicity occur rapidly and start with nausea and vomiting, oral and intestinal burning, feeling of warmth, and headache. This can progress to confusion, vertigo, excitement, restlessness, delirium, hallucinations, muscular excitability, tremors, jerky movements, epileptiform convulsions, and depression. This is sometimes followed by central nervous system depression and coma. Death can occur from respiratory failure or status epilepticus (17). Other adverse effects that can occur after oral ingestion include tachycardia, mydriasis, visual disturbances, urinary retention, albuminuria, mild transient elevations of aspartate dehydrogenase and lactic dehydrogenase (LDH), and rarely, hepatic failure (17). While adults have recovered after ingesting as much as 42 grams of camphor, as little as 2 grams is usually enough to produce significant toxic effects. Much less is required to cause toxicity in children. In children, ingestion of as little as 700-1000 mg of camphor has been fatal. For example, 20 mL of a 5% camphor product can be lethal in a child (4814). In patients who survive camphor ingestion, recovery from toxicity is usually slow.

Although topical application of camphor is not as likely to cause adverse effects, some camphor can be absorbed through intact skin. A considerable amount of camphor can also be absorbed when used by inhalation. Excessive use of camphor either topically or by inhalation can result in the development of symptoms of toxicity (17). Topical use of camphor has also been associated with contact eczema (12). There is also a report of increased liver enzymes in an infant who received a camphor-containing topical cold remedy. The liver enzymes normalized after stopping treatment (4608). Camphor products can contain safrole, which has been found to be a mild carcinogen in vitro (12); however, carcinogenic effects due to use of safrole-containing camphor preparations have not yet been reported in humans (12).

Due to the potential risk, camphor products should only be used short-term.

Interactions with Herbs & Other Dietary Supplements

None known.

Interactions with Drugs

None known.

Interactions with Foods

None known.

Interactions with Lab Tests

LIVER FUNCTION TESTS: Oral use of camphor can cause transient elevations of liver enzymes in both adults and children. There is also a report of increased liver enzymes in an infant who received a camphor-containing topical cold remedy. The enzymes affected included aspartate aminotransferase (AST), alanine aminotransferase (ALT), alkaline phosphatase, and lactate dehydrogenase (LDH). The liver enzymes normalized after stopping the topical cold formula (4608).

Interactions with Diseases or Conditions

GASTROINTESTINAL (GI) IRRITATION: Camphor might irritate the GI tract, and is contraindicated in individuals with infectious or inflammatory GI conditions (19).

Dosage and Administration

TOPICAL: For itching, cold sores, and hemorrhoids, a 0.1%-3% ointment is typically used three to four times daily (272). As an counterirritant, a 3%-11% ointment is typically used three to four times daily (272). As an antitussive, a thick layer of 4.7%-5.3% camphor ointment is applied to the throat and chest as a thick layer.

The area may be covered with a warm, dry cloth or left uncovered (272). For osteoarthritis, a topical cream containing camphor (32 mg/g), glucosamine sulfate (30 mg/g), and chondroitin sulfate (50 mg/g), has been used as needed on sore joints for up to 8 weeks (10327).

INHALATION: 1 tablespoon of solution per quart of water is placed directly into a hot steam vaporizer, bowl, or washbasin. Sometimes 1.5 teaspoons of solution are added to a pint of water and boiled. The medicated vapors are breathed. This inhalation may be repeated up to three times a day (272).

ORAL: Camphor is unsafe for oral use (12).

Comments
Camphor is a well-established folk remedy and is commonly used. The American Academy of Pediatrics recommends non-prescription camphor products should not exceed 11% strength. They also recommend that camphor not be used in treating children (4814). Camphorated oil (20% camphor in cottonseed oil) was removed from the US market due to toxicity in the 1980s.

CANADA BALSAM

Also Known As
Balm of Gilead, Balsam, Balsam Canada, Balsam Fir, Balsam Fir Canada, Balsam of Fir, Canada Turpentine, Canadian Balsam, Eastern Fir.
CAUTION: See separate listing for Oregon Fir Balsam.

Scientific Names
Abies balsamea, synonym Pinus balsamea.
Family: Pinaceae.

People Use This For
Topically, Canada balsam is used for hemorrhoids and as an antiseptic.
In dentistry, Canada balsam is used in root canal sealers and dentifrices.
Historically, Canada balsam has been used for burns, sores, cuts, tumors, heart and chest pains, cancer, mucous membrane inflammation, colds, coughs, warts, wounds, urogenital complaints, and as a pain-reliever.
In foods, Canada balsam is an ingredient in foods and beverages.
In manufacturing, Canada balsam is used in cosmetics as a fixative and fragrance and in ointments and creams. It is also used as a cement for lenses and prepared microscope slides.

Safety
LIKELY SAFE ...when used orally in amounts commonly found in foods. Canada balsam has Generally Recognized As Safe status (GRAS) for use in foods in the US (4912).
POSSIBLY SAFE ...when used topically (11).
There is insufficient reliable information available about the safety of Canada balsam used orally in medicinal amounts.
PREGNANCY AND LACTATION: Insufficient reliable information available; avoid using.

Effectiveness
There is insufficient reliable information available about the effectiveness of Canada balsam.

Mechanism of Action
There is insufficient reliable information available about the possible mechanism of action and active ingredients.

Adverse Reactions
None reported.

Interactions with Herbs & Other Dietary Supplements
None known.

Interactions with Drugs
None known.

Interactions with Foods
None known.

Interactions with Lab Tests
None known.

Interactions with Diseases or Conditions
None known.

Dosage and Administration
ORAL: People typically take 2 to 6 tablespoons of weak tea of Canada balsam. As a tincture (1:5 with 50% ethanol), Canada balsam is usually dosed 5 to 20 drops.
TOPICAL: A weak liquid is usually applied to affected areas (5276).

Comments

Avoid confusion with poplar (Populus tacamahacca, P. balsamifera, P. candicans) or spruce (Picea excelsa) also known as balm of Gilead. Oregon fir balsam (Pseudotsuga menziesii) has been detected as an adulterant in Canada balsam (Abies balsamea) (11). Canada balsam is an oleoresin (rather than a true balsam) collected from punctures in the bark of the Canadian balsam tree (Abies balsamea).

CANADIAN FLEABANE

Also Known As

Butterweed, Canadian Horseweed, Canadian-Fleabane, Canadian Trailing Arbutus, Coltstail, Flea Wort, Hogweed, Horsewood, Prideweed.

Scientific Names

Conyza canadensis, synonym Erigeron canadensis.
Family: Asteraceae/Compositae.

Comments

At the date of publication, there was very little scientific information available about this product. Our staff is continually analyzing the available information on natural medicines and will add data to the online version of *Natural Medicines Comprehensive Database* as it becomes available. See www.naturaldatabase.com.

CANADIAN HEMP

Also Known As

Bitter Root, Catchfly, Dogbane, Fly-Trap, Honeybloom, Indian Physic, Indian-Hemp, Milk Ipecac, Milkweed, Wallflower, Wild Cotton.
CAUTION: See separate listings for Gentian and Indian Physic.

Scientific Names

Apocynum cannabinum.
Family: Apocynaceae.

People Use This For

Orally, Canadian hemp is used for arthritis, asthma, coughs, edema, and syphilis. It is also used orally for valvular insufficiency, senile heart, and to strengthen weak heart muscles following pneumonia. Canadian hemp is also used orally as a diuretic.
Topically, the fresh juice of Canadian hemp is used for warts.

Safety

LIKELY UNSAFE ...when used orally. Contains digitalis-like cardiac glycosides that can cause toxicity (18).
There is insufficient reliable information available about the safety of Canadian hemp for its other uses.
PREGNANCY AND LACTATION: LIKELY UNSAFE ...when used orally due to toxic potential of digitalis-like cardiac glycosides (18); avoid using.

Effectiveness

There is insufficient reliable information available about the effectiveness of Canadian hemp.

Mechanism of Action

The applicable part of Canadian hemp is the root. Canadian hemp contains cardenolide or digitalis-type glycosides, including cymine. These may cause bradycardia with low blood pressure, increased heart contractions, and reflex hypertension. It also may increase diuresis. It is more irritating to the intestinal mucosa than digitalis and strophanthus preparations. It has a lower therapeutic effect on atrial fibrillation than digitalis (18).

Adverse Reactions

Canadian hemp causes topical irritation of the gastrointestinal mucous membranes. This can cause nausea and vomiting more commonly than in other cardenolide glycoside containing plants (such as digitalis). It can also cause bradycardia with low blood pressure, increased heart contractions, and reflex hypertension (18).

Interactions with Herbs & Other Dietary Supplements

CARDIAC GLYCOSIDE-CONTAINING HERBS: Canadian hemp is contraindicated with these herbs, and concomitant use can increase the risk of cardiac glycoside toxicity. Cardiac glycoside containing herbs include black hellebore, digitalis leaf, hedge mustard, figwort, lily-of-the-valley roots, motherwort, oleander leaf, pheasant's eye plant, pleurisy root, squill bulb leaf scales, strophanthus seeds, and uzara (19).

Interactions with Drugs

DIGOXIN (Lanoxin): Theoretically, concomitant use of Canadian hemp with digoxin (Lanoxin) might increase therapeutic effects and adverse effects (19).

DIURETIC DRUGS: Theoretically, concomitant use of potassium depleting diuretics and Canadian hemp can increase the risk of cardiac glycoside toxicity due to potassium depletion (19). Some diuretics that can deplete potassium include chlorothiazide (Diuril), chlorthalidone (Thalitone), furosemide (Lasix), hydrochlorothiazide (HCTZ, Hydrodiuril, Microzide), and others.

Interactions with Foods

None known.

Interactions with Lab Tests

None known.

Interactions with Diseases or Conditions

None known.

Dosage and Administration

ORAL: Some people take 10 to 30 drops of the liquid extract three times daily or 0.3 to 0.6 mL of the tincture (1:10) (18).

TOPICAL: No typical dosage.

Comments

The tough, fibrous barks of both Canadian hemp and Indian hemp have been used as a substitute for hemp; hence, both are known as hemp (18).

CANAIGRE

Also Known As

Red American Ginseng, Wild Red American Ginseng, Wild Red Desert Ginseng.

CAUTION: See separate listings for Ashwaganda, Blue Cohosh, Codonopsis, Ginseng American, Ginseng Panax, and Ginseng Siberian.

Scientific Names

Rumex hymenosepalus.
Family: Polygonaceae.

People Use This For

Orally, canaigre is used for improving physical and athletic stamina, cognitive function and concentration, and work efficiency or athletic stamina; and as a general tonic to improve well-being. It is also used orally for soothing irritated or inflamed tissues, as a diuretic, as an antidepressant, as an astringent, and to treat leprosy. In manufacturing, it is used for tanning leather and dying wool.

Safety

LIKELY SAFE ...when used orally (12). The petioles, or stems, are edible like rhubarb (6). There is some speculation that the high tannin content may be carcinogenic (5,6); avoid excessive amounts.

PREGNANCY AND LACTATION: Insufficient reliable information available; avoid using.

Effectiveness

There is insufficient reliable information available about the effectiveness of canaigre.

Mechanism of Action

The applicable part of canaigre is the root. The high tannin content, 25%, has astringent effects when applied topically. The leucoanthocyanin fraction may have antitumor activity (6).

Adverse Reactions

None reported.

Interactions with Herbs & Other Dietary Supplements
None known.

Interactions with Drugs
None known.

Interactions with Foods
None known.

Interactions with Lab Tests
None known.

Interactions with Diseases or Conditions
None known.

Dosage and Administration
No typical dosage.

Comments
Avoid confusion with Panax ginseng, Siberian ginseng, and American ginseng. Canaigre root is botanically unrelated to the ginsengs. A 1976 Herb Trade Association policy states that "any herb products consisting of whole or part of Rumex hymenosepalus should not be labeled as containing 'ginseng' " (5).

CANANGA OIL

Also Known As
None.
CAUTION: See separate listing for Ylang Ylang Oil.

Scientific Names
Cananga odorata forma. macrophylla, synonym Canangium odoratum forma. macrophylla.
Family: Annonaceae.

People Use This For
In foods, cananga oil is used as a flavoring agent in gelatins, puddings, and beverages.
In manufacturing, cananga oil is used to make fragrances in cosmetics and soaps.

Safety
LIKELY SAFE ...when used orally in amounts commonly found in foods. Cananga oil has Generally Recognized As Safe (GRAS) status in the US (4912).
POSSIBLY SAFE ...when used topically (11).
PREGNANCY AND LACTATION: Insufficient reliable information available; avoid using.

Effectiveness
There is insufficient reliable information available about the effectiveness of cananga oil.

Mechanism of Action
There insufficient reliable information available about the possible mechanism of action and active ingredients.

Adverse Reactions
Cananga oil can cause allergic skin reactions in sensitive people (5244).

Interactions with Herbs & Other Dietary Supplements
None known.

Interactions with Drugs
None known.

Interactions with Foods
None known.

Interactions with Lab Tests
None known.

Interactions with Diseases or Conditions
None known.

Dosage and Administration
No typical dosage.

Comments
Cananga oil is used predominately as a food and cosmetic ingredient. Avoid confusion with ylang ylang oil (oil from Canangium odorata genuina).

CANELLA

Also Known As
Barbasco, Curbana, Macambo, White Cinnamon, White Wood, Wild Cinnamon.

Scientific Names
Canella winteriana, synonyms Canella alba, Laurus winteriana, Winterana canella.
Family: Canellaceae.

Comments
At the date of publication, there was very little scientific information available about this product. Our staff is continually analyzing the available information on natural medicines and will add data to the online version of *Natural Medicines Comprehensive Database* as it becomes available. See www.naturaldatabase.com.

CANTHAXANTHIN

Also Known As
Canthaxanthine, Carophyll Red, CI Food Orange 8, Colour Index No. 40850, E161, Roxanthin Red 10.
CAUTION: See separate listing for Beta-carotene.

Scientific Names
4,4-diketo-beta-carotene; Beta,beta-carotene-4,4-dione; Canthaxanthin.

People Use This For
Orally, canthaxanthin is used to reduce photosensitivity associated with erythropoietic protoporphyria (EPP); and light-sensitive skin diseases including polymorphous light eruptions, drug-induced photosensitivity and solar urticaria. It is also used orally to color the skin and produce an artificial suntan.
In foods, canthaxanthin is used as a food coloring additive and added to animal feed to enhance the color of chicken skins, egg yolks, salmon, and trout.
In manufacturing, canthaxanthin has been used in cosmetics and as a tablet excipient.

Safety
LIKELY SAFE ...when used orally in amounts commonly found in foods. Canthaxanthin has Generally Recognized As Safe (GRAS) status in the US (4912), but is not to exceed 30 mg per pint of liquid food or per pound of solid or semisolid food (5630).
POSSIBLY UNSAFE ...when used orally in doses to treat and reduce photosensitivities. Development of retinal changes has been reported in patients with erythropoietic protoporphyria (EPP) being treated with canthaxanthin to prevent photosensitization, including deposition of crystals around the macula of the retina (5644), slowing of dark-adaptation curves, and decreased amplitudes in electroretinograms (1326,5632,5638). Deposition of retinal crystals appears dose related (5638). Evidence suggests individuals taking a cumulative dose of 37 grams will have retinal changes 50% of the time, while those taking a total cumulative dose of 60 grams of canthaxanthin will demonstrate definite retinal changes upon examination (5636,5641).
LIKELY UNSAFE ...when used orally in large amounts to color and produce an artificial tan (5628,5629). Retinal changes have been reported in individuals ingesting large amounts of canthaxanthin chronically for tanning purposes (5636,5639,5641). Altered eye function, decreased visual acuity (5639), and aplastic anemia (5635) have also been reported.
PREGNANCY AND LACTATION: POSSIBLY UNSAFE ...when consumed in doses to treat and reduce photosensitivities due to reported retinal changes with use (5632); avoid using. LIKELY UNSAFE ...when used orally in large amounts for artificial tanning purposes due to reported retinal changes with use (5639); avoid using.

Effectiveness

POSSIBLY EFFECTIVE

Erythropoietic protoporphyria (EPP). Taking canthaxanthin orally seems to reduce photosensitivity reactions in EPP (rash, itching, or eczema) due to sunlight exposure (1326,5644).

There is insufficient reliable information available about the effectiveness of canthaxanthin for its other uses.

Mechanism of Action

Canthaxanthin is a carotenoid that is found naturally and produced synthetically (5637). It is not a precursor of vitamin A, has no vitamin A activity, is highly lipid soluble (5635), and accumulates in fatty tissue (5632). Oral canthaxanthin is thought to color the skin by accumulating in the epidermis and subcutaneous fat tissue (5635). Evidence suggests canthaxanthin and other carotenoids protect against photosensitization due to their antioxidant activity against reactive oxygen species by deactivating electronically excited molecules or acting as chain-breaking agents (1326,5649). In vitro and in vivo animal studies suggest canthaxanthin may inhibit the growth and transformation of tumor cells (5642,5647,5648) by inducing the gap junctional communication between cells (5649).

Adverse Reactions

Orally, large amounts of canthaxanthin can cause orange-brown coloration of the skin (5632), brick-red coloration of stools (5631), orange discoloration of plasma (5632), discolored body secretions (5634), diarrhea, nausea, stomach cramps, dry and itchy skin (5634), urticaria (5637), welts, gold and yellow crystalline deposits around the macula of the retina (5632,5635,5636,5638,5639,5640,5641), and hepatitis (5635). Decreased visual acuity (5639), diminished retinal sensitivity (5641), and aplastic anemia (5635) have been associated with large doses of canthaxanthin ingestion. A fatal case of aplastic anemia (5635) associated with the ingestion of canthaxanthin for tanning purposes has been reported. The patient refused treatment with human blood products due to religious beliefs and died (5635).

Interactions with Herbs & Other Dietary Supplements

None known.

Interactions with Drugs

None known.

Interactions with Foods

None known.

Interactions with Lab Tests

VITAMIN A ASSAYS: Canthaxanthin can interfere with carotene and vitamin A laboratory assays (5634).

Interactions with Diseases or Conditions

VITAMIN A HYPERSENSITIVITY: Individuals with known hypersensitivities to vitamin A and carotenoids might also be hypersensitive to canthaxanthin.

Dosage and Administration

ORAL: The typical dose for reducing and treating photosensitivities associated with erythropoietic protoporphyria (EPP) is 60 to 90 mg daily on average for three to five months per year (5640). The typical dose for artificial tanning is 120 mg per day for several days (5633).

Comments

Orobronze (canthaxanthin) is sold in Canada as a nonprescription drug for artificial tanning purposes as 30 mg oral capsules (5631,5633). Oral tanning preparations containing canthaxanthin have been found to be readily available to consumers in the United States through mail order and tanning salons despite the FDA warning (5635,5638). A combination product containing beta-carotene and canthaxanthin (Phenoro: 10 mg beta-carotene and 15 mg canthaxanthin) is used in Europe for treatment of photosensitivities associated with EPP (5637). Other combination products containing beta-carotene and canthaxanthin are manufactured (Carotinoid-N, Apotrin), but are not available in the US (1326,5628).

CAPERS

Also Known As
Cabra, Cappero, Himsra.

Scientific Names
Capparis spinosa, synonym Capparis rupestris.
Family: Capparaceae.

People Use This For
Orally capers are used for diabetes, fungal infections, and leishmaniasis.
Topically, capers are used for skin disorders, improving the function of enlarged capillaries, and dry skin.
Capers are also consumed as a food, and used as a flavoring.

Safety
LIKELY SAFE ...when used orally in amounts commonly found in foods (4912). The pickled flower buds are commonly used without reports of adverse effects.
There is insufficient reliable information available about the safety of the medicinal use of capers.
PREGNANCY AND LACTATION: LIKELY SAFE ...when used orally in amounts typically found in foods; avoid large amounts (4912). There is insufficient reliable information available about the safety of medicinal use of capers during pregnancy and lactation.

Effectiveness
There is insufficient reliable information available about the effectiveness of capers.

Mechanism of Action
The applicable parts of capers are the unopened flower bud and aerial parts. Capers contain alkaloids, lipids, flavonoids such as quercetin and rutin, and glucosinolates (12738,12739). A constituent of the aqueous extract of capers, p-methoxy benzoic acid, seems to have hepatoprotective effects (12740). Other preliminary research suggests that capers might have antioxidant, antibacterial, and antifungal effects (12738,12741).
Preliminary research suggests that capers might have antihyperglycemic activity. This effect appears to be independent of insulin secretion. It might inhibit production of glucose by the liver or increase uptake of glucose by peripheral tissues (12736).

Adverse Reactions
Topically, capers can cause contact dermatitis (12742).

Interactions with Herbs & Other Dietary Supplements
HERBS WITH HYPOGLYCEMIC POTENTIAL: Theoretically, capers might have additive effects with herbs that decrease blood glucose levels (12736). Herbs with hypoglycemic potential include devil's claw, fenugreek, guar gum, Panax ginseng, Siberian ginseng, and others.

Interactions with Drugs
ANTIDIABETES DRUGS: Theoretically, capers might reduce blood glucose levels (12736) and might have additive effects on glucose levels when used with antidiabetes drugs. Monitor blood glucose levels closely. Medication dose adjustments may be necessary. Some antidiabetes drugs include glimepiride (Amaryl), glyburide (DiaBeta, Glynase PresTab, Micronase), insulin, pioglitazone (Actos), rosiglitazone (Avandia), and others.

Interactions with Foods
None known.

Interactions with Lab Tests
BLOOD GLUCOSE: Theoretically, capers might lower blood glucose and test results (12736).

Interactions with Diseases or Conditions
DIABETES: Theoretically, capers might alter blood sugar control in people with diabetes (12736).
Blood glucose levels should be monitored closely.

Dosage and Administration
No typical dosage.

CAPSICUM

Also Known As

African Chillies, African Pepper, Bird Pepper, Capsaicin, Cayenne, Chili Pepper, Garden Pepper, Goat's Pod, Grains Of Paradise, Green Chili Pepper, Green Pepper, Hot Pepper, Hungarian Pepper, Ici Fructus, Katuvira, Louisiana Long Pepper, Louisiana Sport Pepper, Mexican Chilies, Mirchi, Oleoresin capsicum, Paprika, Pimento, Red Pepper, Sweet Pepper, Tabasco Pepper, Zanzibar Pepper.
CAUTION: See separate listings for Grains of Paradise and Indian Long Pepper.

Scientific Names

Capsicum frutescens; Capsicum annuum; Capsicum chinense; Capsicum baccatum; Capsicum pubscens; and other Capsicum species.
Family: Solanaceae.

People Use This For

Orally, capsicum is used for dyspepsia, flatulence, colic, diarrhea, cramps, toothache, to improve peripheral circulation, for reducing blood clotting tendencies, seasickness, swallowing dysfunction, alcoholism, malaria, fever, hyperlipidemia, and preventing arteriosclerosis and heart disease.
Topically, capsicum is used for the pain of shingles; and for post-herpetic, trigeminal, diabetic, post-mastectomy, and post-surgical neuralgias; prurigo nodularis; HIV-associated peripheral neuropathy; and fibromyalgia. It is also used as a counterirritant to desensitize nerves and to create a feeling of warmth. Capsicum is also used to relieve muscle spasms, as a gargle for laryngitis, and as a deterrent to thumb-sucking or nail biting.
As an inhalational provocation test, capsicum is used to distinguish sensory hyperreactivity of the airways from asthma.
In foods, capsicum is used as a condiment.
In manufacturing, capsicum is the main ingredient used in many self-defense sprays, also referred to as pepper spray.

Safety

LIKELY SAFE ...when used orally in amounts typically found in food. Capsicum has Generally Recognized As Safe (GRAS) status in the US (4912). ...when used topically and appropriately. The active capsicum constituent capsaicin used in topical preparations is an FDA-approved over-the-counter product (272).
POSSIBLY SAFE ...when used orally and appropriately, short-term in medicinal amounts (12403,12404). ...when used topically and appropriately (7038,10650).
POSSIBLY UNSAFE ...when used orally, long-term or in high doses. Long-term use or use of excessive doses can sometimes cause hepatic or renal damage (12404).
CHILDREN: POSSIBLY UNSAFE ...when used topically in children under 2 years old (272).
There is insufficient reliable information available about the safety of oral use in children.
PREGNANCY: LIKELY SAFE ...when used topically and appropriately (272). There is insufficient reliable information available about the safety of capsicum during pregnancy when used orally in medicinal amounts.
LACTATION: LIKELY SAFE ...when used topically and appropriately (272). POSSIBLY UNSAFE ...when used orally. Dermatitis can sometimes occur in breast-fed infants when mothers ingest foods heavily spiced with capsicum peppers (739).

Effectiveness

LIKELY EFFECTIVE

Pain. Applying capsicum topically temporarily relieves pain from rheumatoid arthritis (RA), osteoarthritis, psoriasis, and neuralgias including shingles and diabetic neuropathy. The active capsicum constituent capsaicin used in topical preparations is FDA-approved for these uses. For musculoskeletal pain, for every 8.1 patients treated with 0.025% capsaicin, one would achieve at least a 50% reduction in pain.
For neuropathic pain, the number needed to treat using capsaicin 0.075% for eight weeks is 5.7 (272,12401).

POSSIBLY EFFECTIVE

Fibromyalgia. Applying cream containing 0.025% of the active capsicum constituent capsaicin 4 times daily to tender points for 4 weeks seems to reduce tenderness in patients with fibromyalgia (7038).

Prurigo nodularis. Applying a cream containing 0.025% to 0.3% of the active capsicum constituent capsaicin 4-6 times daily seems to relieve burning sensations, erythema, pruritus, and healing of skin lesions over a period of 2 weeks to 33 months. Symptoms, however, may return after discontinuation of therapy (10650).

POSSIBLY INEFFECTIVE

HIV-associated peripheral neuropathy. Applying capsaicin topically does not seem to relieve symptoms of HIV-associated peripheral neuropathy (3891).

INSUFFICIENT RELIABLE EVIDENCE to RATE

Dyspepsia. Preliminary evidence suggests that red pepper powder in capsules taken before meals 3 times daily reduces symptoms of functional dyspepsia. In some patients, there seems to be a worsening of symptoms before improvement (12410).

Irritable bowel syndrome (IBS). Preliminary evidence suggests that capsicum fruit taken orally doesn't help symptoms of IBS (12403).

Peptic ulcers. There is preliminary evidence that suggests people who eat capsicum fruit (chili) an average of 24 times per month appear to be less likely to have an ulcer than people who eat chili an average of 8 times per month. This applies to chili in the form of chili powder, chili sauce, curry powder, and other chili-containing foods (12053).

Swallowing dysfunction. Preliminary evidence suggests that elderly patients at risk for aspiration pneumonia due to swallowing dysfunction have improved swallowing reflexes after dissolving a capsaicin-containing lozenge in their mouth before each meal (13100).

More evidence is needed to rate capsicum for these uses.

Mechanism of Action

The applicable part of capsicum is the fruit. Capsicum contains the constituent capsaicin, which makes it taste hot. When used topically, capsaicin binds to nociceptors in the skin, initially causing neuronal excitation and heightened sensitivity. This is felt as itching, pricking, or burning. Capsaicin also causes cutaneous vasodilation. The mechanism for these effects is thought to be the result of selective stimulation of afferent C fibers, which act as thermoreceptors and nociceptors, and release of substance P, a sensory neurotransmitter that mediates pain. This is followed by a refractory period with reduced sensitivity. After repeated applications, persistent desensitization occurs, possibly the result of substance P depletion. Pain relief may also be caused by degeneration of epidermal nerve fibers (12401,12404,12410).

Capsaicin also stimulates the unmyelinated slow C-fibers of the sensory nervous system, which can induce cough, dyspnea, nasal congestion, and eye irritation after inhalation (5885). Some research with inhaled capsaicin suggests that severity of ACE inhibitor cough correlates with sensitivity to inhaled capsaicin (12411,12412,12413,12414).

In people with swallowing dysfunction, capsaicin is thought to provide sensory stimulation that increases the swallowing reflex (13100).

Capsaicin seems to have antiplatelet effects (12406,12407).

Some evidence shows capsicum extract has antibacterial properties (12402).

Some researchers theorize that the capsaicin constituent might also have gastroprotective effects.

Preliminary evidence suggests that capsicum protects against alcohol and non-steroidal anti-inflammatory drug (NSAID) damage to the GI mucosa. This has also led to the hypothesis that capsaicin might decrease the risk of peptic ulcer disease (12053). However, with heavy ingestion, capsaicin has been associated with necrosis, ulceration, and carcinogenesis (12404).

Capsaicin is thought to be metabolized by the cytochrome P450 (CYP450) system to active metabolites. Whether these substances can cause cancer or protect against cancer by altering carcinogen metabolism is an area of active research (12404).

Adverse Reactions

Orally, capsicum can cause upper abdominal discomfort including fullness, gas, bloating, nausea, epigastric pain and burning, diarrhea, and belching (12403,12410). Sweating and flushing of the head and neck, lacrimation, headache, faintness, and rhinorrhea have also been reported (7005,12410). Excessive amounts of capsaicin can lead to gastroenteritis and hepatic necrosis (12404). There are also reports of dermatitis in breast-fed infants whose mothers' food is heavily spiced with capsicum (739). Capsicum can also decrease blood coagulation (7006).

Topically, capsicum can cause burning, stinging, and erythema. About one in 10 patients who use capsaicin topically discontinue treatment because of adverse effects. Side effects tend to diminish with continued use (12401).

Exacerbation of ACE-inhibitor cough has been reported in patients using topical capsaicin and taking ACE-inhibitors (12414).

Skin contact with fresh capsicum fruit can cause irritation or contact dermatitis (12408). Inhalation of capsicum can cause cough, dyspnea, nasal congestion, eye irritation, and allergic alveolitis (5885).

Capsicum can be extremely irritating to the eyes and mucous membranes. Capsicum oleoresin, an oily extract in pepper self-defense sprays, causes intense eye pain. It can also cause erythema, blepharospasm, tearing, shortness of breath, and blurred vision. In rare cases, corneal abrasions have occurred (12408,12409).

Interactions with Herbs & Other Dietary Supplements

COCA: Theoretically, concomitant use of capsicum (including exposure to the capsicum in pepper spray) and coca might increase the effects and risk of adverse effects of the cocaine in coca (1394).

Interactions with Drugs

ACE INHIBITORS (ACEIs): There is one case report of a topically applied cream containing capsaicin contributing to the cough reflex in a patient using an ACE-inhibitor (12414). But it is unclear if this interaction is clinically significant.
ANTICOAGULANT/ANTIPLATELET DRUGS: Theoretically, capsicum might increase the effects and adverse effects of antiplatelet drugs (12406,12407).
COCAINE: Theoretically, concomitant use of capsicum (including exposure to the capsicum in pepper spray) and cocaine might increase cocaine effects and the risk of adverse effects, including death (1394).
THEOPHYLLINE: Theoretically, oral administration of capsicum before or at the same time as theophylline might enhance theophylline absorption (12405).

Interactions with Foods

None known.

Interactions with Lab Tests

BLEEDING TIME: Capsicum has led to increased fibrinolytic activity and may lead to prolonged times in coagulation studies (7006).

Interactions with Diseases or Conditions

DAMAGED SKIN: Capsicum is contraindicated in situations involving injured skin. Do not apply capsicum if the skin is open.

Dosage and Administration

ORAL: For swallowing dysfunction in the elderly, 1 lozenge containing 1.5 mcg of capsaicin is dissolved in the mouth before each meal (13100).
TOPICAL: For pain syndromes, including rheumatoid and osteoarthritis, neuropathy, and fibromyalgia, creams contain the active capsicum constituent capsaicin and are typically applied 3-4 times daily. It can take up to 14 days for the full analgesic effect. Most creams contain 0.025% to 0.075% capsaicin concentrations. Higher potency preparations may be used for diabetic neuropathy (272,12401). For prurigo nodularis, 0.025% to 0.3% of the active capsicum constituent capsaicin 4-6 times daily has been used (10650). Tell patients to make sure they wash their hands after applying capsaicin cream. Tell patients they can use a diluted vinegar solution to remove capsicum cream. The active constituent, capsaicin is not water washable. Warn against using capsicum preparations near the eyes or on sensitive skin (12409).

Comments

In nature, capsaicin occurs only as a trans stereoisomer. However, civamide, the cis isomer also has activity. Products labeled capsaicin sometimes include nonivamide which is an adulterant or pelargonic acid vanillylamide, referred to as "synthetic capsaicin" (7007). Capsaicin is being studied for use in treating urinary urgency as an intravesical injection (6002). Capsicum powder has been reported to prevent radiation-induced damage to bacterial DNA and thereby protect certain bacteria (Escherichia coli, Bacillus megaterium, and Bacillus pumilus spores) from gamma irradiation used to preserve some foods (5886).

CARAWAY

Also Known As

Anis des Vosges, Apium Carvi, Carvi Fructus, Cumin des Pres, Haravi, Karwiya, Krishan Jeeraka, Krishnajiraka, Kummel, Kummich, Roman Cumin, Semen Cumini Pratensis, Semences de Carvi, Wiesen-Feldkummel, Wild Cumin.

Scientific Names

Carum carvi, synonym Carum velenovskyi.
Family: Apiaceae/Umbelliferae.

People Use This For

Orally, caraway is used for digestive problems including dyspepsia, distention, flatulence, and mild spastic conditions of the gastrointestinal tract. Caraway oil is also used as an expectorant, to promote lactation and menstruation, to relieve menstrual cramps, for incontinence, and as an antibacterial and laxative.
Topically, caraway is used as a component of mouthwashes and in skin rubs to improve local blood flow.
In foods, caraway is used as a cooking spice.
In manufacturing, caraway oil is used as a flavoring agent in pharmaceutical compounding. Caraway oil is commonly utilized as a fragrance in the manufacturing of toothpaste, soap, and cosmetics.

Safety

LIKELY SAFE ...when used orally in amounts commonly found in foods. Caraway has Generally Recognized As Safe (GRAS) status in the US (4912).
POSSIBLY SAFE ...when caraway oil is used orally in medicinal amounts (6740,6741,6742,10075). ...when used orally, short-term. There is some evidence that caraway seed can be used safely for up to 8 weeks (12724).
PREGNANCY AND LACTATION: POSSIBLY UNSAFE ...when used in medicinal amounts (4912,6746). Caraway oil has been used to stimulate menstruation (6746); avoid using.

Effectiveness

POSSIBLY EFFECTIVE

Dyspepsia. Taking caraway oil orally as a specific combination with peppermint oil (Enteroplant) seems to relieve non-ulcerative dyspepsia, including symptoms of fullness and mild gastrointestinal (GI) spasms (6740,6741,10075). The combination of enteric-coated peppermint oil 90 mg and caraway oil 50 mg, which is not available in the US, appears to be comparable to cisapride for relieving dyspepsia (6740,6741,10075). A specific combination product containing caraway (Iberogast, Enzymatic Therapy) also seems to improve symptoms of dyspepsia. The combination includes caraway plus clown's mustard plant, peppermint leaf, German chamomile, licorice, milk thistle, angelica, celandine, and lemon balm (7049,12724). A meta-analysis of studies using this combination product suggests that taking 1 mL orally three times daily over a period of four weeks significantly reduces severity of acid reflux, epigastric pain, cramping, nausea and vomiting compared to placebo (13089).

There is insufficient reliable information available about caraway for its other uses.

Mechanism of Action

The applicable parts of caraway are the seed, fruits, and oils. The caraway fruits contain 2% to 7% volatile oil, consisting mainly of carvone and limonene (7). Caraway seed also contain carveol, dihydrocarveol, thymol, and flavonoids (12736). There's preliminary evidence that peppermint oil in combination with caraway oil can reduce gastroduodenal motility when administered orally in enteric-coated capsules (6742). Preliminary evidence also indicates that the volatile oil constituent carvone induces glutathione S-transferase (GST), which might inhibit carcinogenesis (11,911). Caraway might also have antihistamine activity (12735). Caraway might also have antibacterial and antiulcer effects (12736).

Preliminary research suggests that caraway might have anti hyperglycemic activity. This effect appears to be independent of insulin secretion. It might inhibit production of glucose by the liver or increase uptake of glucose by peripheral tissues (12736).

Adverse Reactions

Orally, caraway oil when used in combination with peppermint oil may cause a substernal burning sensation, belching, nausea, and vomiting (6741,6742,10075).

Interactions with Herbs & Other Dietary Supplements

HERBS WITH HYPOGLYCEMIC POTENTIAL: Theoretically, caraway might have additive effects with herbs that decrease blood glucose levels (12736). Herbs with hypoglycemic potential include devil's claw, fenugreek, guar gum, Panax ginseng, and Siberian ginseng.

Interactions with Drugs

ANTIDIABETES DRUGS: Theoretically, caraway might reduce blood glucose levels (12736) and might have additive effects on glucose levels when used with antidiabetes drugs. Monitor blood glucose levels closely. Medication dose adjustments may be necessary. Some antidiabetes drugs include glimepiride (Amaryl), glyburide (DiaBeta), Glynase PresTab, Micronase), insulin, pioglitazone (Actos), insulin, pioglitazone (Actos), rosiglitazone (Avandia), and others.

Interactions with Foods

None known.

Interactions with Lab Tests

BLOOD GLUCOSE: Theoretically, caraway might lower blood glucose and test results (12736).

Interactions with Diseases or Conditions

DIABETES: Theoretically, caraway might alter blood sugar control in people with diabetes (12736). Blood glucose should be monitored closely.

Dosage and Administration

ORAL: For non-ulcerative dyspepsia, caraway oil 50-100 mg per day has been used in combination with peppermint oil (6740,6741,10075). A specific combination product containing caraway (Iberogast, Enzymatic Therapy) and several other herbs has been used in a dose of 1 mL three times daily (7049,12724,13089).

Comments
Superstitions held that caraway had the power to prevent the theft of any object that contained the seed and to keep lovers from losing interest with one another (6002).

CARDAMOM

Also Known As
Bai Dou Kou, Cardamon, Cardomomi Fructus, Ela.

Scientific Names
Elettaria cardamomum, synonym Amomum cardamomum.
Family: Zingiberaceae.

People Use This For
Orally, cardamom is used for dyspepsia, intestinal spasm, irritable bowel syndrome (IBS), common cold, cough, bronchitis, inflammation of the mouth and pharynx, liver and gallbladder complaints, loss of appetite, and tendency toward infection. It is also used as an antiflatulent, laxative, and as a stimulant and for urinary problems.
In foods, cardamom is consumed as a spice in many parts of the world.

Safety
LIKELY SAFE ...when used orally and appropriately (2).
PREGNANCY AND LACTATION: Insufficient reliable information available; avoid using amounts greater than those used in food.

Effectiveness
There is insufficient reliable information available about the effectiveness of cardamom.

Mechanism of Action
The applicable part of cardamom is the seed. The active principals of cardamom are thought to be volatile oils, including cineole (2,11). Volatile oils are believed to have antispasmodic (11), antiflatulent, virustatic (2,18), and motility-enhancing effects (18).

Adverse Reactions
None reported.

Interactions with Herbs & Other Dietary Supplements
None known.

Interactions with Drugs
None known.

Interactions with Foods
None known.

Interactions with Lab Tests
None known.

Interactions with Diseases or Conditions
GALLSTONES: The cardamom seed can trigger gallstone colic (spasmodic pain) (18) and is not recommended for self-medication in patients with gallstones (2).

Dosage and Administration
ORAL: The typical dose of cardamom is 1.5 grams of the ground seeds per day. The usual dose of the tincture is 1-2 grams per day (2).

CARLINA

Also Known As

Carlinae Radix, Dwarf Carline, Eberwurz, Ground Thistle, Racine de Carline Acaule, Radix Cardopatiae, Radix Chamaeleontis Albae, Silberdistelwurz, Southernwood Root, Stemless Carlina Root.

Scientific Names

Carlina acaulis.
Family: Asteraceae/Compositae.

Comments

At the date of publication, there was very little scientific information available about this product. Our staff is continually analyzing the available information on natural medicines and will add data to the online version of *Natural Medicines Comprehensive Database* as it becomes available. See www.naturaldatabase.com.

CARNOSINE

Also Known As

B-alanyl-L-histidine, B-alanyl histidine, L-carnosine.
CAUTION: See separate listing for L-Carnitine.

Scientific Names

Beta-alanyl-L-histidine.

People Use This For

Orally, carnosine is used to prevent aging and for preventing or treating complications of diabetes such as neuropathy, cataracts, and renal dysfunction.

Safety

There is insufficient reliable information available about the safety of carnosine.
Pregnancy and Lactation: Insufficient reliable information available; avoid using.

Effectiveness

There is insufficient reliable information available about the effectiveness of carnosine.

Mechanism of Action

Carnosine is a naturally occurring di-peptide found in skeletal muscle, heart, brain, and other innervated tissues. Carnosine is formed by a process involving the enzyme carnosine synthetase, which bonds the amino acids beta-alanine and L-histidine. The enzyme carnisinase maintains the carnosine equilibrium by inactivating carnosine located in tissues or blood (3381,3391). Carnosine seems to be concentrated in actively contracting muscles. In patients with muscular dystrophies carnosine levels may be lower. The concentration of carnosine in muscles also appears to correlate with age. Older patients have lower muscle carnosine levels (3391). Preliminary information also suggests that carnosine may play a role in the regulation of intracellular calcium and contractility in cardiac tissue (3390).

Carnosine is of interest as an anti-aging product because of its effects on advance glycosylation end-products (AGEs). AGEs are abnormal, cross-linked, and oxidized proteins that might play a role in the aging process. Animal studies show carnosine may diminish the glycosylation of these proteins, preventing them from inducing cellular damage (3364,10210,10645). Because carnosine appears to diminish the effects of protein glycosylation, there is some interest in using carnosine for complications of diabetes such as cataracts, neuropathy, and kidney failure, which arise from glycosylation (3364).

There is some animal evidence that carnosine can help prevent lipid peroxidation within the cell membranes. Carnosine may block malondialdehyde (MDA) production, which is a toxic lipid peroxidation end-product. Animal studies show carnosine can inhibit MDA-induced protein changes and MDA-induced toxicity (3364,3381,10644). Blocking MDA might decrease oxidative damage to lipids, as well as to enzymes and DNA. This raises the question of whether carnosine might play a role in preventing atherosclerosis, joint inflammation, and cataract formation (3364,3381).

Carnosine may also play a role in the prevention of Alzheimer's disease. The anti-glycating and antioxidant activities of carnosine are both implicated in the neuronal and endothelial cell damage of Alzheimer's disease (10645). Carnosine binds heavy metals and may provide some protection from zinc and copper mediated neurotoxicity (7219). The ability of carnosine to bind heavy metals may also be important in its ability to act as an antioxidant (10211).

Adverse Reactions
None reported.

Interactions with Herbs & Other Dietary Supplements
None known.

Interactions with Drugs
None known.

Interactions with Foods
None known.

Interactions with Lab Tests
None known.

Interactions with Diseases or Conditions
None known.

Dosage and Administration
No typical dosage.

Comments
There is very little scientific information about this product. Our staff is continually analyzing the available information on natural medicines and will add data here as it becomes available.

CAROB

Also Known As
Locust Bean, Locust Pods, St. John's Bread, Sugar Pods.

Scientific Names
Ceratonia siliqua.
Family: Fabaceae/Leguminosae.

People Use This For
Orally, carob is used for acute nutritional disorders, celiac disease, obesity, diarrhea, dyspepsia, entero-colitis, vomiting during pregnancy, and sprue. It is also used for improvement of lipid profiles and excretion of fat in feces. In infants, it is used for vomiting, retching cough, and diarrhea.
In foods and beverages, carob is used as a flavoring agent and as a chocolate substitute. Carob flour and extracts are also used as ingredients in food products.

Safety
LIKELY SAFE ...when used orally in amounts commonly found in foods. Carob has Generally Recognized As Safe (GRAS) status (4912). ...when used orally in medicinal amounts (12).
PREGNANCY AND LACTATION: Insufficient reliable information available; avoid using.

Effectiveness
INSUFFICIENT RELIABLE EVIDENCE to RATE

Obesity. There is preliminary clinical evidence that a carob and bean pod extract might modestly improve lipid profiles and excretion of fat in feces of overweight and obese patients (10633). More evidence is needed to rate carob for this use.

Mechanism of Action
The applicable part of carob is the fruit. Tannins contained in carob strongly inhibit digestive enzymes. Animal data suggest that a 15% carob gum diet fed for 2-6 weeks may result in weight loss. Decreases in blood glucose levels, decreases in cholesterol plasma levels, decreases in insulin levels, and an increases in glucose tolerance are also suggested (11).

Adverse Reactions
None reported.

Interactions with Herbs & Other Dietary Supplements
None known.

Interactions with Drugs
None known.

Interactions with Foods
None known.

Interactions with Lab Tests
None known.

Interactions with Diseases or Conditions
None known.

Dosage and Administration
ORAL: For improvement of lipid profiles and excretion of fat in feces, carob gum 50-100 mg three times daily, combined with bean pod (Phaseolus vulgaris, kidney bean) 300-600 mg three times daily, has been used (10633).

Comments
Avoid confusing carob with carob tree, Jacaranda procera and Jacaranda caroba. The term "carat" evolved from the use of carob seeds as weight units for measuring gold (6).

CARRAGEENAN

Also Known As
Carrageenin, Carragheenan, Chondrus Extract, Irish Moss, Irish Moss Extract, Mousse D'Irlande.

Scientific Names
Chondrus crispus; Euchema species; Gigartina mamillosa and other Gigartina species; related red algae.
Family: Gigartinaceae.

People Use This For
Orally, carrageenan is used to soothe mucous membranes irritated by coughs, bronchitis, tuberculosis, and intestinal problems. The French use a form that has been degraded by low pH and high temperatures to treat peptic ulcers, and as a bulk laxative; this degraded form has lost the gelling properties of the original product.
Topically, carrageenan is used for anorectal symptoms.
In manufacturing, carrageenan is used as a binder, emulsifier, thickening agent, and as a stabilizer in pharmaceuticals, foods, and toothpaste. Carrageenan is also an ingredient in weight loss products.

Safety
LIKELY SAFE ...when used orally in food amounts (11).
POSSIBLY UNSAFE ...when the degraded form is used orally. The degraded form is broken down into a lower molecular weight product that is partially absorbed. There is concern about the safety of this form because it has been linked to lesions in the colons of animals (11).
PREGNANCY AND LACTATION: LIKELY SAFE ...when used in food amounts (11). There is insufficient reliable information available about the safety of using larger amounts; avoid using.

Effectiveness
There is insufficient reliable information available about the effectiveness of carrageenan.

Mechanism of Action
Carrageenan has been reported to lower blood cholesterol, reduce gastrointestinal (GI) secretions and food absorption, and increase water content of the gut when large amounts are given. Parenterally it has shown anticoagulant, hypotensive, and immunosuppressive activities; it may also have anti-inflammatory properties (11).

Adverse Reactions
None reported.

Interactions with Herbs & Other Dietary Supplements
None known.

Interactions with Drugs

ANTICOAGULANT/ANTIPLATELET DRUGS: Carrageenan may increase the risk of bleeding in patients taking anticoagulants (6002).
ANTIHYPERTENSIVE DRUGS: Carrageenan may enhance hypotensive effects of antihypertensive agents (6002).
ORAL DRUGS: Carrageenan can impair gastrointestinal (GI) absorption of oral drugs (6002).

Interactions with Foods

None known.

Interactions with Lab Tests

None known.

Interactions with Diseases or Conditions

None known.

Dosage and Administration

ORAL: A one cup decoction of carrageenan is sometimes used two to three times daily. The decoction is prepared by adding 1 ounce of the dried plant in 1-1.5 pints boiling water, simmer and strain. The decoction can be sweetened with lemon, honey, or cinnamon (6002).

Comments

Carrageenan consists of hydrocolloids from various red algae or seaweeds.

CASCARA

Also Known As

Bitter Bark, Buckthorn, California Buckthorn, Cascara Sagrada, Chittem Bark, Dogwood Bark, Purshiana Bark, Rhamni Purshianae Cortex, Sacred Bark, Sagrada Bark, Yellow Bark.

Scientific Names

Frangula purshiana, synonym Rhamnus purshiana.
Family: Rhamnaceae.

People Use This For

Orally, cascara is used for constipation, as a laxative, for gallstones, liver ailments, cancer, as a bitter tonic.
In foods and beverages, a bitterless extract of cascara is sometimes used as a flavoring agent.
In manufacturing, cascara is used in the processing of some sunscreens.

Safety

POSSIBLY SAFE ...when used orally and appropriately, short-term. Cascara seems to be safe when used for less than one week (272). Cascara was formerly FDA-approved as safe and effective, but this designation was removed in 2002 because of lack of supporting evidence (8229).
POSSIBLY UNSAFE ...when used orally, long-term. Using cascara for more than one to two weeks can lead to dependence and electrolyte loss, specifically low levels of potassium (272).
CHILDREN: POSSIBLY UNSAFE ...when used orally in children. Cascara should be used cautiously in children due to the risk of electrolyte loss, specifically low levels of potassium (272).
PREGNANCY: Insufficient reliable information available; avoid using.
LACTATION: POSSIBLY UNSAFE ...when used orally. Cascara is excreted into breast milk and might cause diarrhea (272).

Effectiveness

LIKELY EFFECTIVE

Constipation. Taking cascara orally has laxative effects and helps for treating constipation (272). Cascara was formerly FDA-approved as safe and effective, but this designation was removed in 2002 because of lack of supporting evidence (8229).

There is insufficient reliable information available about the effectiveness of cascara for its other uses.

Mechanism of Action

The applicable part of cascara is the dried bark. The anthraglycoside constituents in cascara are cascarosides A and B. These stimulate peristalsis and evacuation leading to its stimulant laxative effect (6). Cascara exerts its effect on the large intestine and does not have much effect on the small intestine. Bacteria in the intestine are required to transform the anthraglycosides into stimulant laxatives. The fresh bark contains free anthrone which is an emetic compound that can cause severe vomiting. But the free anthrone is destroyed by aging the bark for at least one year, or by artificial aging with heat and aeration (2). Anthroid laxative use is not associated with an increased risk of developing colorectal ademoma or carcinoma (6138).

Adverse Reactions

Orally, cascara can commonly cause mild abdominal discomfort, colic, and cramps. Long-term use can lead to potassium depletion, albuminuria, hematuria, disturbed heart function, muscle weakness, finger clubbing, and cachexia (4). In some cases, chronic use can also cause pseudomelanosis coli. Pseudomelanosis coli (pigment spots in intestinal mucosa) is believed to be harmless, usually reverses with discontinuation, and is not directly associated with an increased risk of developing colorectal ademoma or carcinoma (6138). Fresh or improperly aged cascara bark can cause severe vomiting due to the presence of free anthrone constituents. There is also some concern about potential liver problems. In one case, cascara aged bark 425 mg (containing approximately 21 mg cascaroside) three times daily for three days resulted in cholestatic hepatitis, ascites, and portal hypertension. Symptoms resolved over about three months following discontinuation of cascara (6895). This adverse effect is suspected to be the result of a hypersensitivity reaction.

Interactions with Herbs & Other Dietary Supplements

DIGITALIS, LILY OF THE VALLEY, SQUILL: Overuse of cascara can increase the risk of cardiac toxicity; these herbs are also cardiac glycoside-containing herbs (19), and because of potassium loss (4).
LICORICE: Using cascara concomitantly with licorice can increase the risk of potassium depletion (2).
POTASSIUM DEPLETING HERBS: Theoretically, concomitant use of cascara along with horsetail plant or licorice rhizome can increase the risk of potassium depletion.
STIMULANT LAXATIVE HERBS: Theoretically, cascara used concomitantly with other herbs that are stimulant laxatives can increase the risk of potassium depletion. Stimulant laxative herbs include aloe, wild cucumber fruit (Ecballium elaterium), blue flag rhizome, alder buckthorn, European buckthorn, butternut bark, castor oil, colocynth fruit pulp, gamboge bark exudate, jalap root, black root, manna bark exudate, podophyllum root, rhubarb root, senna leaves and pods, and yellow dock root (19).

Interactions with Drugs

CORTICOSTEROIDS: Concomitant use of corticosteroids along with cascara can increase the risk of potassium depletion (2).
DIGOXIN (Lanoxin): Theoretically, overuse of cascara increases the risk of adverse effects of cardiac glycoside drugs.
DIURETIC DRUGS: Overuse of cascara might compound diuretic-induced potassium loss (19). There is some concern that people taking cascara along with potassium depleting diuretics might have an increased risk for hypokalemia. Initiation of potassium supplementation or an increase in potassium supplement dose may be necessary for some patients. Some diuretics that can deplete potassium include chlorothiazide (Diuril), chlorthalidone (Thalitone), furosemide (Lasix), hydrochlorothiazide (HCTZ, Hydrodiuril, Microzide), and others.
ORAL DRUGS: Theoretically, cascara can reduce the absorption of some drugs due to the reduced transit time through the GI tract (19).
STIMULANT LAXATIVES: Concomitant use of cascara along with other laxatives can cause electrolyte and fluid depletion.

Interactions with Foods

None known.

Interactions with Lab Tests

COLORIMETRIC TESTS: Cascara can discolor urine (pink, red, purple, orange, rust), interfering with diagnostic tests that depend on a color change, due to its anthraquinone content (275).
POTASSIUM: Excessive use of cascara can cause potassium depletion, reducing serum potassium concentrations and test results (19).

Interactions with Diseases or Conditions

GASTROINTESTINAL (GI) CONDITIONS: Cascara is contraindicated in people with intestinal obstruction, or acute intestinal inflammation. This includes people with Crohn's disease, ulcerative colitis, and appendicitis. It is also contraindicated for people who have ulcers, and abdominal pain of unknown origin (2,4,8).

Dosage and Administration

ORAL: 20-30 mg per day of the active ingredient, hyroxyanthracene derivatives, has been used. This is calculated as cascaroside A, from the cut bark, powder, or extracts (2). A typical dose includes 1 cup of tea which is made by steeping 2 grams of finely chopped bark in 150 mL of boiling water for 5-10 minutes, and then straining (18). The cascara liquid extract is given in a dose of 2-5 mL three times daily (4). The appropriate amount of cascara is the smallest dose that is necessary to maintain soft stools (2).

Comments

Cascara is no longer an FDA-approved drug. It may be sold as a dietary supplement, but not as a drug. The FDA notified manufacturers to remove or reformulate all over-the-counter (OTC) laxative products containing cascara from the US market by November 5, 2002, citing lack of safety and efficacy studies. The FDA gave manufacturers the chance to submit safety and efficacy data; however, the companies decided the expense of conducting safety and efficacy studies exceeded potential profits (8229,8442,8443).

CASCARILLA

Also Known As

Bahama Cascarilla, Sweet Bark, Sweet Wood Bark.

Scientific Names

Croton eluteria, synonym Clutia eluteria.
Family: Euphorbiaceae.

Comments

At the date of publication, this product was not a common ingredient used in brand name supplements marketed to consumers. Details about this product are available in the online version of *Natural Medicines Comprehensive Database*. See www.naturaldatabase.com.

CASEIN PEPTIDES

Also Known As

Bovine Casein Hydrosylate, C12 Peptide, Casein Decapeptide, Casein-derived Peptide, Casein Hydrosylate, Casein Peptide, Casein Protein Hydrosylate, Casein Tripeptide, Hydrolyzed Casein, Hypotensive Peptides, Milk Protein Hydrosylate, Sour Milk Peptides.

Scientific Names

Casein protein hydrosylate.

People Use This For

Orally, casein peptides are used for hypertension, hyperlipidemia, anxiety, fatigue, epilepsy, intestinal disorders, cancer prevention, and to reduce stress.

Safety

There is insufficient reliable information available about the safety of casein peptides.
Pregnancy and Lactation: Insufficient reliable information available; avoid using.

Effectiveness

INSUFFICIENT RELIABLE EVIDENCE to RATE

Hypertension. Preliminary evidence suggests that taking a specific casein peptide, C12 peptide, 100-200 mg twice daily for one day does not significantly reduce systolic or diastolic blood pressure 6 hours after administration (13044). More evidence is needed to rate casein peptide for this use.

Mechanism of Action

Casein peptides are break-down products of casein protein. Casein protein is the primary protein of milk. It makes up 76% to 86% of all milk proteins (13045). Casein is the component of milk that solidifies in the curdling process. When casein protein is consumed, proteolytic digestive enzymes hydrolyze casein into several peptides called casein peptides (13046). Many of these peptides are thought to have a variety of biological activities.
Some casein peptides affect immune functions, including increasing or decreasing proliferation of lymphocytes, increasing antibody formation, increasing phagocytosis, and increasing natural killer cell activity (13046).
Some casein peptides seem to have blood pressure lowering effects in animal models. In 1965 it was discovered that hypertensive patients who drank sour milk had reduced blood pressure. Later it was found that sour milk

contained two tri-peptides, Val-Pro-Pro and Ile-Pro-Pro, which had a blood pressure lowering effect (13044). These peptides are thought to inhibit angiotensin-converting enzyme (ACE) similarly to the ACE inhibitor antihypertensive drugs (13044,13046,13048). When taken orally these ACE inhibiting casein peptides seem to be absorbed intact, without digestive degradation, according to animal models (13052).
Some casein peptides have opioid receptor stimulating properties (13052).
Casein peptides stimulate various intestinal secretions. In isolated rat jejunum, casein peptides stimulate mucin and mucus production (13049). Casein peptides also seem to stimulate cholecystokinin secretion from rat intestinal cells (13050).

Adverse Reactions

None reported.

Interactions with Herbs & Other Dietary Supplements

None known.

Interactions with Drugs

ANTIHYPERTENSIVE DRUGS: Some casein proteins, such as C12 peptide, have ACE inhibitor properties and might reduce blood pressure (13044,13046,13048). Theoretically, combining these casein proteins with antihypertensive drugs might increase the risk of hypotension.

Interactions with Foods

None known.

Interactions with Lab Tests

None known.

Interactions with Diseases or Conditions

MILK ALLERGY: Patients with milk allergy are allergic to the proteins contained in milk. Fragments of milk proteins, such as casein peptides, might also be allergenic in these patients (13047,13051). Advise these patients not to use products containing casein peptides.

Dosage and Administration

ORAL: For hypertension, a specific casein peptide, C12 peptide, 100-200 mg twice daily has been used (13044).

CASHEW

Also Known As

East Indian Almond.

Scientific Names

Anacardium occidentale.
Family: Anarcardiaceae.

People Use This For

Orally, cashew is used for gastrointestinal ailments.
Topically, cashew is used as a skin stimulant and cauterizing agent for ulcers, warts, and corns.
Cashew is also consumed as a food.

Safety

LIKELY SAFE ...when used in amounts commonly found in foods. Cashew has Generally Recognized As Safe status (GRAS) for use in foods in the US (4912).
There is insufficient reliable information available about the safety of cashew when used in medicinal amounts.
PREGNANCY AND LACTATION: There is insufficient reliable information available about the safety of medicinal amounts of cashew during pregnancy and lacation.

Effectiveness

There is insufficient reliable information available about the effectiveness of cashew.

Mechanism of Action
The applicable part of cashew is the nut. A dried ethanolic extract is effective in vitro against gram-positive bacteria Bacillus subtilis and Staphylococcus aureus. Alkyl phenols contained in the cashew nut shell are strong skin irritants. Cashew contains alkyl phenols that are chemically related to constituents in poison ivy, poison oak, mango, and ginkgo. The adverse reactions resulting from cashew are related to the adverse reactions that sometimes occur with these other irritants. Roasted cashew nuts are free of the alkyl phenols (18).

Adverse Reactions
Topically, contact can lead to redness and nodule and blister formation.

Interactions with Herbs & Other Dietary Supplements
None known.

Interactions with Drugs
None known.

Interactions with Foods
None known.

Interactions with Lab Tests
None known.

Interactions with Diseases or Conditions
None known.

Dosage and Administration
No typical dosage.

Comments
Acajou oil, oleum anacardiae, and fatty oil are extracted from cashew nuts (18).

CASSIA AURICULATA

Also Known As
Avaram, Avari Panchaga Choornam, Kalpa Herbal Tea, Ranawara, Tanner's Cassia.
CAUTION: See separate listing for Cassia Cinnamon.

Scientific Names
Cassia auriculata, synonym Senna auriculata.
Family: Cesalpiniaceae.

People Use This For
Orally, Cassia auriculata is used for diabetes, conjunctivitis, rheumatism, constipation, jaundice, liver disease, and urinary tract disorders.

Safety
There is insufficient reliable information available about the safety of Cassia auriculata.
Pregnancy and Lactation: Insufficient reliable information available; avoid using.

Effectiveness
There is insufficient reliable information available about the effectiveness of Cassia auriculata.

Mechanism of Action
The applicable parts of Cassia auriculata are the flower, seed, leaves, root, bark, and unripe fruit. The flower is most commonly used. Animal research suggests that Cassia auriculata flower alone or in combination with other herbs has antihyperglycemic activity, reducing blood glucose and glycosylated hemoglobin, and increasing insulin levels. It may act by stimulating beta-cells to release more insulin (12366,12370). It seems to be similar to acarbose (Precose) in alpha-glucosidase inhibitory activity (12369). Cassia auriculata flower also seems to have antihyperlipidemic and antioxidant effects in diabetic animals (12367,12371). Cassia auriculata leaf extract also reduces blood sugar in normal and diabetic animals (12368).

Cassia auriculata leaf extract shows potential use for liver disease. In animal models of alcoholism, it protects against free radical damage. It restores hepatic levels of glutathione, which is involved in protective antioxidant activity, and serum vitamin E and C levels. It also lowers hepatic enzymes, suggesting that it prevents damage

to hepatic parenchymal cells (12372).
There is no reliable published research in humans.

Adverse Reactions
None reported.

Interactions with Herbs & Other Dietary Supplements
HERBS WITH HYPOGLYCEMIC POTENTIAL: Theoretically, Cassia auriculata might have additive effects with herbs that decrease blood glucose levels (12366,12370). Herbs with hypoglycemic potential include devil's claw, fenugreek, guar gum, Panax ginseng, and Siberian ginseng.

Interactions with Drugs
ANTIDIABETES DRUGS: Theoretically, Cassia auriculata may reduce blood glucose levels (12366,12370) and might have additive effects on glucose levels when used with antidiabetes drugs. Monitor blood glucose levels closely. Medication dose adjustments may be necessary. Some antidiabetes drugs include glimepiride (Amaryl), glyburide (DiaBeta, Glynase PresTab, Micronase), insulin, pioglitazone (Actos), rosiglitazone (Avandia), and others.
CARBAMAZEPINE (Tegretol): Theoretically, Cassia auriculata flower may increase carbamazepine levels. Research in animals suggests that concurrent administration may cause a significant rise in carbamazepine blood levels. The mechanism of this interaction is unknown (12373).

Interactions with Foods
None known.

Interactions with Lab Tests
None known.

Interactions with Diseases or Conditions
None known.

Dosage and Administration
No typical dosage.

Comments
Cassia auriculata is an evergreen shrub that grows widely in India and other parts of Asia.
It is used in Ayurvedic medicine (12366).

CASSIA CINNAMON

Also Known As
Bastard Cinnamon, Canton Cassia, Cassia, Cassia Aromaticum, Cassia Bark, Cassia Lignea, Chinese Cinnamon, Cinnamomum, Cinnamomi Cassiae Cortex, Cinnamon, Cinnamon Flos, Cortex Cinnamomi, False Cinnamon, Nees, Rou Gui, Sthula Tvak, Taja, Zimbluten.
CAUTION: See separate listings for Cassia Auriculata and Cinnamon bark.

Scientific Names
Cinnamomum aromaticum, synonym Cinnamomum cassia.
Family: Lauraceae.

People Use This For
Orally, cassia cinnamon is used for type 2 diabetes, gas (flatulence), muscle and gastrointestinal spasms, preventing nausea and vomiting, diarrhea, infections, the common cold, and loss of appetite. It is also used for impotence, enuresis, rheumatic conditions, testicle hernia, menopausal symptoms, amenorrhea, and as an abortifacient. Cassia cinnamon is also used orally for angina, kidney disorders, hypertension, cramps, cancer, and as a blood purifier.
Topically, cassia cinnamon is used in suntan lotions, nasal sprays, mouthwashes, gargles, toothpaste, and as a counterirritant in liniments.
In food and beverages, cassia cinnamon is used as a flavoring agent.

Safety

LIKELY SAFE ...when used orally in amounts commonly found in foods. Cassia cinnamon has Generally Recognized As Safe (GRAS) status in the US (4912).
POSSIBLY SAFE ...when used orally and appropriately in medicinal doses (11347).
PREGNANCY AND LACTATION: There is insufficient reliable information available about the safety of cassia cinnamon when used in medicinal amounts during pregnancy and breast-feeding; avoid using.

Effectiveness

POSSIBLY EFFECTIVE

Diabetes. Taking cassia cinnamon orally seems to improve type 2 diabetes. Some research suggests that taking cassia cinnamon 1 to 6 grams for 40 days can lower fasting serum glucose by 18-29%, triglycerides by 23% to 30%, low-density lipoprotein (LDL) cholesterol by 7-27%, and total cholesterol by 12-26% (11347).

There is insufficient reliable information available about the effectiveness of cassia cinnamon for its other uses.

Mechanism of Action

The applicable parts of cassia cinnamon are the bark and flower. Cinnamaldehyde is found in the volatile oil fraction of cassia cinnamon. The cassia cinnamon bark contains about 1400 to 1900 ppm cinnamaldehyde (3919). Cinnamaldehyde seems to have antibacterial activity (11244). It may also have immunomodulating, anti-tumor, and antioxidant activity (11245,11246,11247).

Polyphenolic polymers such as hydroxychalcone found in cassia cinnamon seem to potentiate insulin action. These compounds seem to increase phosphorylation of the insulin receptor, which increases insulin sensitivity. Increased insulin sensitivity may improve blood glucose control and lipid levels. Cinnamon extracts also seem to activate glycogen synthetase and increase glucose uptake (11247,11248,11249,11973).

Adverse Reactions

Topically, allergic skin reactions and stomatitis from toothpaste flavored with cassia cinnamon have been reported (11915,11920).

Interactions with Herbs & Other Dietary Supplements

HERBS & SUPPLEMENTS WITH HYPOGLYCEMIC POTENTIAL: Cassia cinnamon can lower blood glucose levels (11347) and might have additive effects when used with other herbs and supplements that also lower glucose levels. This might increase the risk of hypoglycemia in some patients. Some herbs and supplements with hypoglycemic effects include alpha-lipoic acid, bitter melon, chromium, devil's claw, fenugreek, garlic, guar gum, horse chestnut, Panax ginseng, psyllium, Siberian ginseng, and others.

Interactions with Drugs

ANTIDIABETES DRUGS: Cassia cinnamon may lower blood glucose levels, and have additive effects in patients treated with antidiabetic agents; use with caution (11347). Dose adjustments to diabetes medications might be necessary. Some antidiabetes drugs include glimepiride (Amaryl), glyburide (DiaBeta, Glynase PresTab, Micronase), insulin, metformin (Glucophage), pioglitazone (Actos), rosiglitazone (Avandia), and others.

Interactions with Foods

None known.

Interactions with Lab Tests

BLOOD GLUCOSE: Cassia cinnamon might lower blood glucose levels in some patients (11347).

Interactions with Diseases or Conditions

DIABETES: Cassia cinnamon might lower blood glucose in patients with type 2 diabetes (11347). Tell patients with diabetes to use cassia cinnamon products cautiously and monitor blood glucose levels very closely. Dose adjustments to diabetes medications might be necessary.

Dosage and Administration

ORAL: For type 2 diabetes, 1 to 6 grams (1 teaspoon = 4.75 grams) of cassia cinnamon daily for 40 days has been used (11347).

Comments

There are a lot of different types of cinnamon. Cinnamomum verum (Ceylon cinnamon) is the type used most commonly in the Western world. Cinnamomum aromaticum (Cassia cinnamon or Chinese cinnamon) is also commonly used. In many cases, the cinnamon spice purchased in food stores contains a combination of these different types of cinnamon. So far, only cassia cinnamon has been shown to have any effect on blood glucose in humans. However, Cinnamomum verum also contains the hydroxychalcone polymer thought to be responsible for lowering blood sugar (11247).

CASSIE ABSOLUTE

Also Known As
Huisache, Popinac Absolute, Sweet Acacia.

Scientific Names
Acacia farnesiana, synonyms Acacia smallii, Mimosa farnesiana.
Family: Fabaceae/Leguminosae.

People Use This For
Orally, cassie absolute is used as an antispasmodic, antidiarrheal, stimulant, aphrodisiac, to treat fever, rheumatoid arthritis (RA), pulmonary tuberculosis, and stomach cancer.
Topically, cassie absolute is used for dry skin and as an insecticide.
In India, tea made from cassie absolute leaves is used for gonorrhea, and the root is chewed for sore throat.
In foods, cassie absolute is a flavor ingredient in foods and beverages.
In manufacturing, cassie absolute is used as a fragrance in perfumes.

Safety
LIKELY SAFE ...when used orally in amounts commonly found in foods. Cassie absolute has Generally Recognized As Safe status (GRAS) for use in foods in the US (4912).
There is insufficient reliable information available about the safety of cassie absolute used in medicinal amounts.
PREGNANCY AND LACTATION: Insufficient reliable information available; avoid using.

Effectiveness
There is insufficient reliable information available about the effectiveness of cassie absolute.

Mechanism of Action
Cassie absolute is reported to have antispasmodic, aphrodisiac, astringent, demulcent, antidiarrheal, antipyretic, antirheumatic and stimulant properties (11). It contains glycosides which reportedly have anti-inflammatory and bronchodilator effects (1505).

Adverse Reactions
None reported.

Interactions with Herbs & Other Dietary Supplements
None known.

Interactions with Drugs
None known.

Interactions with Foods
None known.

Interactions with Lab Tests
None known.

Interactions with Diseases or Conditions
None known.

Dosage and Administration
No typical dosage.

Comments
Cassie absolute is an extract of Acacia farnesiana flowers. Limited pharmacologic and toxicologic information is available (11).

CASTOR

Also Known As

African Coffee Tree, Bofareira, Castor Oil Plant, Eranda, Gandharva Hasta, Mexico Weed, Palma Christi, Ricin, Tangantangan Oil Plant, Wonder Tree.

Scientific Names

Ricinus communis; Ricinus sanguines.
Family: Euphorbiaceae.

People Use This For

Orally, castor seeds are used for birth control, constipation, leprosy, and syphilis. Castor oil is used orally as a stimulant laxative for constipation, to stimulate labor, and to promote the flow of breast milk.
Topically, castor seed paste is used as a poultice for inflammatory skin disorders, boils, carbuncles, abscesses, inflammation of the middle ear, and migraine headaches. Castor oil is used topically as an emollient and to dissolve cysts, growths, or warts, and to soften bunions and corns.
Intravaginally, castor oil is applied as a cervical abortifacient and vaginal contraceptive.
Ophthalmically, castor oil is used in the eyes to soothe the irritated conjunctiva after the presence of foreign bodies.

Safety

LIKELY SAFE ...when castor oil is used orally and appropriately, short-term (16).
POSSIBLY SAFE ...when the hulled castor seed is used orally and appropriately, short-term. There is some evidence that a single dose of castor seed with the outer coat removed (hulled) can be used safely (7127,7128).
POSSIBLY UNSAFE ...when castor oil is used orally in high doses or for extended periods. Taking castor oil for greater than one week or exceeding the typical dose of 15-60 mL per day can increase the risk of fluid and electrolyte disturbances (272).
UNSAFE ...when the whole seed is used orally. Safety depends on whether or not the seed is chewed or if the outer coat is ruptured. Chewing as few as 1-6 whole seeds can be lethal in an adult. If the seed is swallowed intact, poisoning is less likely; however, prompt medical attention should be sought after ingestion of any whole castor seed (5611).
There is insufficient reliable information available about the safety of castor when applied topically.
CHILDREN: POSSIBLY SAFE ...when castor oil is used orally and appropriately, short-term (16).
POSSIBLY UNSAFE ...when castor oil is used orally in high doses or for extended periods. Taking castor oil for greater than one week or exceeding the typical children's dose of 1-15 mL per day, depending on age, can increase the risk of fluid and electrolyte disturbances (272). UNSAFE ...when the whole seed is used orally. The chewed or uncoated seeds can cause severe toxic effects (5611,5612) and death (5611). There is insufficient reliable information available about the safety of the hulled seed or topical use of castor in children.
PREGNANCY: POSSIBLY SAFE ...when castor oil is used orally in pregnant women at term. Midwives routinely use castor oil for labor induction in pregnant women at term. This practice does not appear to adversely affect the mother or fetus (1122,7191). However, castor oil should not be used without the supervision of a clinician. LIKELY UNSAFE ...when castor oil is used orally in pregnant women who are not at term. Castor oil might induce premature labor and induce miscarriage (12); avoid using. UNSAFE ...when the whole seed is used orally. The chewed or uncoated seeds can cause severe toxic effects, including death (6,5611); avoid using. There is insufficient reliable information available about the safety of using the hulled seed or topical use of castor during pregnancy.
LACTATION: Insufficient reliable information available; avoid using.

Effectiveness

POSSIBLY EFFECTIVE

Constipation. Taking castor oil orally is effective as a stimulant laxative for reducing constipation (272).
Contraception. Taking the hulled castor seed orally seems to be effective as a contraceptive. There is some evidence that a single dose of seeds with the outer coat removed (hulled) can work as a contraceptive for up to 8-12 months (7127,7128).
Parturition. A single 60 mL dose of castor oil appears to stimulate labor within 24 hours in at least 50% of women at term pregnancy with no prior signs of labor (7191). There is also some evidence that women at term pregnancy with premature membrane rupture who take castor oil have a higher incidence of labor onset and a lower incidence of cesarean section than women who take no medication (1122).

There is insufficient reliable information available about the effectiveness of castor for its other uses.

Mechanism of Action

The applicable parts of castor are the seeds and oil. Castor oil is produced by cold pressing ripe seeds. Unlike the seeds, castor oil does not contain the deadly poison ricin (16,17). Castor oil is a glyceride that can be absorbed from the intestine and metabolized as a fatty acid (272). Castor oil is hydrolyzed in the duodenum by pancreatic lipase to release ricinoleic acid, which might have stimulant laxative effects (6,272). Although the exact mechanism of ricinoleic acid is unknown, the laxative effect appears to result from fluid secretion induced by cyclic adenosine monophosphate, rather than the increased peristalsis due to an irritant effect (272). Onset of bowel evacuant action is usually within 2 hours, but sometimes can take up to 6 hours (16).

In pregnancy, castor oil is thought to induce labor by producing hyperemia in the intestinal tract, which causes reflex stimulation of the uterus (16). Castor oil might also increase prostaglandin production, which stimulates uterine activity (7191).

Castor seeds are best known for their toxic effects. They contain the toxic glycoprotein ricin. Ricin can be fatal when ingested, inhaled, or given intravenously. Ricin is an N-glycosidase that affects an RNA subunit and interferes with protein synthesis, causing cell death (6,5611). Toxic effects typically occur 2-5 days after ingestion (5611).

There is some preliminary evidence that ricin might also have analgesic effects and activity against leukemia (6).

It is unclear how castor seeds work as a contraceptive; however, its effects do not seem to be hormonally mediated (7127,7128).

Adverse Reactions

Orally, castor oil, like all stimulant laxatives, can cause abdominal discomfort, cramping, nausea, and faintness (15,272). Nausea can also occur because of the unpleasant taste of castor oil (7191). Using flavored products might reduce this effect. Castor oil can also cause fluid and electrolyte loss, particularly potassium, which can result in hypokalemia. It can also cause malabsorption from intestinal hypermotility (15,272). Chronic ingestion over long periods of time can lead to cathartic colon (15). There is some concern that castor oil might cause amniotic fluid embolism. There is one case of amniotic fluid embolism and cardiopulmonary arrest within one hour of ingestion of 30 mL of castor oil at full-term pregnancy (1219).

Orally, castor seed can cause severe toxicity. Chewing whole seeds can cause nausea, vomiting, diarrhea, abdominal pain, dehydration, shock, hemolysis, severe fluid and electrolyte disturbances, peripheral vascular collapse, renal failure secondary to hypovolemia, and death. Cellular damage to liver, kidneys, and pancreas typically occurs 2-5 days after ingestion (5611,5612). As few as 1-6 seeds can be lethal in humans (6,5611). Rupture of the seed hull seems to be necessary to cause toxicity. Swallowing seeds whole, without chewing, is less likely to cause toxic effects; however, prompt medical attention should be received after ingestion of any whole seed. Serum chemistries should be monitored for at least 5 days after ingestion in symptomatic patients (5611).

Hulled castor seeds, with the outer coat carefully removed, seem to be well-tolerated, and without toxic side effects (7127,7128); however, some patients taking hulled seeds can have transient anorexia and weight loss (1727).

Topically, the castor plant, crushed seeds, or seed dust can cause dermatitis in some patients (5611). Castor seed is also an inhalant allergen in workers in the coffee industry (6). Anaphylaxis can occur in these patients after exposure to castor beans, plants, or dust (5611).

Interactions with Herbs & Other Dietary Supplements

CARDIAC GLYCOSIDE-CONTAINING HERBS: Theoretically, castor oil can increase the risk of cardiac glycoside toxicity due to stimulant laxative effects, which can lead to fluid and electrolyte imbalances (19).

LICORICE/HORSETAIL: Theoretically, concomitant use with horsetail or licorice rhizome increases the risk of potassium depletion (18).

MALE FERN: Concomitant use with oil-soluble anthelmintic herbs, such as the male fern, should be avoided due to enhanced absorption of castor oil (19).

STIMULANT LAXATIVE HERBS: Theoretically, concomitant use with other stimulant laxative herbs might increase the risk of potassium depletion (19).

WORMSEED: Concomitant use with wormseed oil might reduce both toxicity and efficacy of wormseed oil (19).

Interactions with Drugs

CORTICOSTEROIDS: Concomitant use of corticosteroids and castor oil may increase the risk of potassium depletion (18).

DIGOXIN (Lanoxin): Theoretically, concomitant use can increase the risk of adverse effects of cardiac glycoside drugs due to fluid and electrolyte loss.

DIURETIC DRUGS: Overuse of castor oil might compound diuretic-induced potassium loss (19). There is some concern that people taking castor oil along with potassium depleting diuretics might have an increased risk for hypokalemia. Initiation of potassium supplementation or an increase in potassium supplement dose may be necessary for some patients. Some diuretics that can deplete potassium include chlorothiazide (Diuril), chlorthalidone (Thalitone), furosemide (Lasix), hydrochlorothiazide (HCTZ, HydroDIURIL, Microzide), and others.

ORAL DRUGS: Theoretically, castor oil may reduce absorption of drugs due to reduced transit time (19).

Advise patients to separate administration of castor oil and oral drugs.
STIMULANT LAXATIVES: Concomitant use of castor oil and laxatives may lead to electrolyte and fluid depletion (19).

Interactions with Foods
None known.

Interactions with Lab Tests
None known.

Interactions with Diseases or Conditions
INTESTINAL DISORDERS: Avoid using in patients with intestinal obstruction abdominal pain of unknown origin, biliary tract obstruction and other biliary disorders (7).

Dosage and Administration
ORAL: For constipation, 15 mL is commonly used (15).
For total colonic evacuation, such as before surgery, or radiologic or colonoscopic procedures, the dose for adults and children over 12 is 15-60 mL given 16 hours prior to surgery or colonic examination (15).
For children age 2-11 years, 5-15 mL is typically used. In children younger than 2 years, 1-5 mL is commonly used.
For induction of labor, a variety of dosage regimens have been used (1122). Single doses vary from 5-120 mL (1122).
A one-time dose of 60 mL in fruit juice is a commonly used regimen (7191). Other regimens that have been used include 5 mL in peppermint tea every 2 hours, 15 mL three times daily, 30 mL every 2 hours, 30 mL every 6 hours, 30 mL every 3 hours for 3 doses, 60 ml daily, and 60 mL daily for 2 days (1122).
Castor oil is most effective when taken on an empty stomach (7).
TOPICAL: No typical dosage. A paste made with ground seeds applied to affected skin twice daily has been used; treatment takes up to 15 days (18). For use on intact skin; avoid use on broken or damaged skin.

Comments
Castor oil has been used medicinally for centuries and was mentioned in the Ebers Papyrus (16). The taste of castor oil is bland, followed by a slightly bitter and usually nauseating taste (16). Castor oil is sometimes flavored with cinnamon, peppermint, or other flavorings to mask the unpleasant taste (16).

CASTOREUM

Also Known As
Canadian Beaver, European Beaver, Siberian Beaver.

Scientific Names
Castor canadensis; Castor fiber.
Family: Castoridae.

People Use This For
Orally, castoreum is used for absence of menstrual periods, painful menses, hysteria, restless sleep, and as a calming and restorative agent.
In foods and beverages, castoreum extract is used as a flavoring agent.
In manufacturing, castoreum tincture is used as a fragrance or fixative in cosmetics and soaps.

Safety
LIKELY SAFE ...when used in amounts commonly found in foods. Castoreum has Generally Recognized As Safe (GRAS) status in the US (4912). ...when used topically. Castoreum tincture is reported to be nontoxic in dermatological tests (11).
There is insufficient reliable information available about the safety of castoreum for its other uses.
PREGNANCY AND LACTATION: Insufficient reliable information available; avoid using.

Effectiveness
There is insufficient reliable information available about the effectiveness of castoreum.

Mechanism of Action
Castoreum is reported to have calming and sedating effects (11).

Adverse Reactions
None reported.

Interactions with Herbs & Other Dietary Supplements
None known.

Interactions with Drugs
None known.

Interactions with Foods
None known.

Interactions with Lab Tests
None known.

Interactions with Diseases or Conditions
None known.

Dosage and Administration
No typical dosage.

Comments
Castoreum is a secretion collected from scent glands of Canadian, European, and Siberian beavers. Castoreum from the Canadian beaver is considered superior in quality to that of the Siberian beaver (11).

CAT'S CLAW

Also Known As
Cats Claw, Griffe Du Chat, Life-Giving Vine of Peru, Samento, Uña De Gato, Una De Gato.
CAUTION: See separate listing for Cat's Foot.

Scientific Names
Uncaria guianensis; Uncaria tomentosa.
Family: Rubiaceae.

People Use This For
Orally, cat's claw is used for diverticulitis, peptic ulcers, colitis, gastritis, hemorrhoids, parasites, Alzheimer's disease, and leaky bowel syndrome. Cat's claw is also used orally viral infections including herpes zoster, herpes simplex, and human immunodeficiency virus (HIV). It is also used orally for wound healing, arthritis, asthma, allergic rhinitis, cancer (especially urinary tract cancer), gonorrhea, dysentery, birth control, bone pains, and "cleansing" the kidneys.

Safety
POSSIBLY SAFE ...when used orally, short-term. A specific freeze-dried aqueous extract seems to be safe when used for up to four weeks (7317). Another extract of cat's claw, free of tetracyclic oxindole alkaloids, seems to be safe when used for up to 24 weeks (8661).
PREGNANCY: POSSIBLY UNSAFE ...when used orally. There is concern that cat's claw might be unsafe based on its use as a contraceptive (12); avoid using.
LACTATION: Insufficient reliable information available; avoid using.

Effectiveness
POSSIBLY EFFECTIVE

Osteoarthritis. Taking a specific freeze-dried cat's claw extract (Uncaria guianensis) orally appears to relieve knee pain related to physical activity within one week of treatment, but it does not decrease pain at rest or decrease knee swelling (7317).

Rheumatoid arthritis (RA). Taking a specific cat's claw extract (Uncaria tomentosa) orally, containing pentacyclic oxindole alkaloids but free of tetracyclic oxindole alkaloids, appears to modestly improve symptoms of RA. Taken orally in combination with sulfasalazine or hydroxychloroquine for 24 weeks, cat's claw seems to reduce the number of painful and swollen joints (8661).

There is insufficient reliable information available about the effectiveness of cat's claw for its other uses.

Mechanism of Action

The applicable part of cat's claw is the root and bark. The major alkaloid of cat's claw is rhynchophylline. There is some evidence that it might have cardiovascular effects including dilating peripheral blood vessels, lowering heart rate, and possibly lowering blood cholesterol. Rhynchophylline might also inhibit sympathetic nervous system activity (6).

Cat's claw is thought to work for osteoarthritis due to anti-inflammatory effects. It seems to inhibit the production of prostaglandin E2 and tumor necrosis factor-alpha (TNF-alpha) (7317). There is interest in using cat's claw for rheumatoid arthritis. The pentacyclic oxindole alkaloids found in cat's claw seem to exhibit immunomodulatory effects, enhancing phagocytosis and altering lymphocyte activity. However, these effects appear to be antagonized by the tetracyclic oxindole alkaloids also found in cat's claw, suggesting greater effectiveness of extracts without this alkaloid (8661).

There is also interest in cat's claw for cancer and viral infections because some of its constituents seem to have antioxidant, immunostimulant, and antiviral effects (7225,7317). These constituents include quinovic acid alkaloids and the alkaloids pteropodine and isopteropodine (7225). Extracts of cat's claw also might have antimutagenic activity. There is preliminary evidence that cat's claw extracts can induce tumor cell death (apoptosis) (7224,8969), and inhibit proliferation of leukemia and lymphoma cells (7225). However, cat's claw does not appear to be cytotoxic to normal cells (7227,8969). Cat's claw may also exert antiestrogenic effects, although the mechanism is not yet completely understood (8660).

Some cat's claw alkaloids may have a beneficial effect on memory loss caused by cholinergic dysfunction. These alkaloids seem to enhance central cholinergic transmission by increasing acetylcholine levels or by affecting dopaminergic systems that can enhance cholinergic function (7226). Another constituent, uncarine E, might also affect the glutamateric system, which might also play a critical role in memory and cognition (7226).

Adverse Reactions

Orally, cat's claw can cause headache, dizziness, and vomiting (7317).

Interactions with Herbs & Other Dietary Supplements

None known.

Interactions with Drugs

ANTIHYPERTENSIVE DRUGS: Since cat's claw may lower blood pressure, exercise caution when using cat's claw with antihypertensive drugs.

CYTOCHROME P450 3A4 (CYP3A4) SUBSTRATES: There's preliminary evidence that cat's claw can inhibit cytochrome P450 3A4 (CYP3A4) enzymes (6450). Theoretically, cat's claw might increase levels of drugs metabolized by CYP3A4; however, so far, this interaction has not been reported in humans. Some drugs metabolized by CYP3A4 include lovastatin (Mevacor), ketoconazole (Nizoral), itraconazole (Sporanox), fexofenadine (Allegra), triazolam (Halcion), and numerous others. Use cat's claw cautiously or avoid in patients taking these drugs.

IMMUNOSUPPRESSANTS: Theoretically, cat's claw may interfere with immunosuppressant therapy (7225) due to immunostimulating activity. It stimulates phagocytosis and increases respiratory cellular activity and the mobility of leukocytes. Immunosuppressant drugs include azathioprine (Imuran), basiliximab (Simulect), cyclosporine (Neoral, Sandimmune), daclizumab (Zenapax), muromonab-CD3 (OKT3, Orthoclone OKT3), mycophenolate (CellCept), tacrolimus (FK506, Prograf), sirolimus (Rapamune), prednisone (Deltasone, Orasone), and other corticosteroids (glucocorticoids).

Interactions with Foods

None known.

Interactions with Lab Tests

None known.

Interactions with Diseases or Conditions

AUTOIMMUNE DISEASES: There is some concern that cat's claw might adversely affect patients with autoimmune disorders because of its immune stimulating effects (7225). Avoid using in patients with multiple sclerosis, systemic lupus erythematosus (SLE), or other autoimmune disorders without the advice of a healthcare professional.

HYPOTENSION: Cat's claw might reduce blood pressure and exacerbate hypotension (6).

Dosage and Administration

ORAL: For osteoarthritis of the knee, 100 mg daily of a specific freeze-dried aqueous cat's claw extract has been used (7317). For rheumatoid arthritis, 60 mg daily in three divided doses of a specific cat's claw extract (free of tetracyclic oxindole alkaloids) has been used (8661).

Comments
Cat's claw was ranked as the seventh most popular herb in US sales in 1997 (2). Two species of cat's claw are of primary interest for medicinal use: Uncaria tomentosa and Uncaria guianensis. Uncaria tomentosa is most commonly used in the US, and Uncaria guianensis is typically used in Europe (6).

CAT'S FOOT

Also Known As
Antennariase Dioicae Flos, Cat's Ear Flower, Cudweed, Katsenpfotchenbluten, Life Everlasting, Mountain Everlasting.
CAUTION: See separate listings for Cudweed, Cat's Claw, and Ground Ivy.

Scientific Names
Antennaria dioica, synonym Gnaphalium dioicum.
Family: Asteraceae/Compositae.

Comments
At the date of publication, this product was not a common ingredient used in brand name supplements marketed to consumers. Details about this product are available in the online version of *Natural Medicines Comprehensive Database.* See www.naturaldatabase.com.

CATECHU

Also Known As
Black Catechu: Acacia Catechu, Acacia Catechu Heartwood Extract, Black Catechu, Black Cutch, Cachou, Cashou, Catechu nigrum, Cutch, Dark Catechu, Khair, Khadira, Pegu Catechu.
Pale Catechu: Cube Gambir, Gambier, Gambir, Gambir Catechu, Terra Japonica, Uncaria Gambier Leaf/Twig Extract.

Scientific Names
Black catechu: Acacia catechu, synonym Mimosa catechu.
Family: Fabaceae/Leguminosae.
Pale catechu: Uncaria gambir, synonyms Nauclea gambir, Ourouparia gambir.
Family: Rubiaceae.

People Use This For
Orally, catechu is used for diarrhea, chronic mucous membrane inflammation, dysentery, colitis, bleeding, indigestion, osteoarthritis, and cancer. Catechu is used orally in some parts of the world as an antifertility drug. Topically, catechu is used for skin diseases, hemorrhoids, traumatic injuries, to stop bleeding, and for dressing wounds. Catechu is included in mouthwashes and gargles for gingivitis, stomatitis, pharyngitis, and oral ulcers. In foods and beverages, catechu is used as a flavoring agent.

Safety
LIKELY SAFE ...when used orally in amounts commonly found in foods. Catechu has Generally Recognized As Safe status (GRAS) for use in foods in the US (4912). There is insufficient reliable information available about the safety of catechu when used orally in medicinal amounts. There is also insufficient reliable information available about the safety of topical use of catechu.
PREGNANCY AND LACTATION: LIKELY SAFE ...when used orally in amounts commonly found in foods. Catechu has Generally Recognized As Safe status (GRAS) for use in foods in the US (4912). There is also insufficient reliable information available about the safety of catechu when used orally in medicinal amounts. There is insufficient reliable information available about the safety of topical use of catechu.

Effectiveness
There is insufficient reliable information available about the effectiveness of catechu.

Mechanism of Action

The applicable parts of catechu are the leaf and stem (12851). Researchers think the astringent and antibacterial properties of catechu result from its high tannin content (11). Gambrine (in pale catechu) has hypotensive effects (11). D-catechin (in black and pale catechu) causes blood vessel constriction (11). Fisetin (in black catechu) and (+)-catechin (in black and pale catechu) and may protect against liver damage; (+)-catechin (cianidanol) is also thought to protect against experimentally-induced ulcers in animals (11); (+)-catechin (cianidanol) is associated with fatal hemolytic anemia (9).

Preliminary research suggests black catechu modestly inhibits cyclooxygenase (COX)-1 (12851).

Methylcatechin, which is one of the major metabolites of (+)-catechin, inhibits the binding of monocytes to vascular endothelial cells. This suggests that the catechins found in catechu may reduce atherosclerosis (9444).

Adverse Reactions

None reported.

Interactions with Herbs & Other Dietary Supplements

None known.

Interactions with Drugs

None known.

Interactions with Foods

None known.

Interactions with Lab Tests

None known.

Interactions with Diseases or Conditions

None known.

Dosage and Administration

No typical dosage.

Comments

Though black catechu and pale catechu differ somewhat chemically, they are used for the same purposes at the same dose (11). Unstandardized products may contain high amounts of aflatoxin, a metabolite of Aspergillus, which is toxic and may lead to certain cancers.

CATNIP

Also Known As

Catmint, Catswort, Field Balm, Menta De Gato.

CAUTION: See separate listing for Schizonepeta.

Scientific Names

Nepeta cataria.

Family: Lamiaceae/Labiatae.

People Use This For

Orally, catnip is used for insomnia; migraine headaches; cold; flu; fever; hives; and gastrointestinal (GI) upset, including indigestion, colic, cramping, and flatulence. It is also used orally for conditions associated with anxiety, diuresis, as a tonic, for upper respiratory tract infections, and headaches. Additionally, catnip is also used orally for lung and uterine congestion, eradicating worms, and for initiating menses in girls with delayed onset of menstruation.

Topically, catnip has been used for arthritis, hemorrhoids, and as a poultice to relieve swelling.

As an inhalant, catnip is smoked for respiratory conditions and recreationally for inducing a euphoric high.

In manufacturing, catnip is used as a pesticide and insecticide.

Safety

POSSIBLY SAFE ...when used orally and appropriately (6,12). Significant adverse effects have not been reported when catnip tea is used in cupful amounts (6).

POSSIBLY UNSAFE ...when used orally in excessive doses. Higher doses may be associated with significant adverse effects (6). ...when inhaled by smoking dried leaves. Smoking the dried leaves of catnip has been associated with a euphoric high (6), which might impair judgment; however, whether catnip can truly produce this effect in humans remains controversial (6).

There is insufficient reliable information available about the safety of topically applied catnip.

CHILDREN: POSSIBLY UNSAFE ...when used orally. One child developed stomach pain and irritability followed by lethargy and hypnotic state after ingesting catnip leaves and tea (5,2596).

PREGNANCY: LIKELY UNSAFE ...when used orally. Catnip tea has been reported to have uterine stimulant properties (12); avoid using.

LACTATION: Insufficient reliable information available; avoid using.

Effectiveness

There is insufficient reliable information available about the effectiveness of catnip.

Mechanism of Action

The applicable part of catnip is the flowering tops. The pharmacological effect that catnip is famous for is the euphoric state it induces in cats. It is thought that the constituent cis-trans-nepetalcatone produces the characteristic stimulation in cats only when they smell it (5). Although humans have used catnip to induce a euphoric high, whether or not this effect actually occurs in humans is controversial. In humans, the constituent nepetalactone is thought to be responsible for catnip's calming effects in insomnia, anxiety, gastrointestinal (GI) conditions, and migraine headache. Nepetalactone is the major component (80% to 95%) of the volatile oil of catnip and is structurally related to the valepotriates found in valerian. Catnip provides approximately 0.2% to 1% volatile oil. Catnip reportedly also has antipyretic and diaphoretic effects, which have been attributed to its use for colds, flu, and fever. Other reported pharmacological effects, include diuretic and stimulation of gallbladder activity (6).

Adverse Reactions

Catnip abuse may result in headache and malaise. Large amounts of tea may cause vomiting (6). One case report exists of a nineteen-month-old child who developed a stomachache and irritability, followed by lethargy and a hypnotic state after ingesting raisins soaked in catnip tea and chewing on the tea bag (5,2596).

Interactions with Herbs & Other Dietary Supplements

HERBS WITH SEDATIVE PROPERTIES: Theoretically, concomitant use of catnip with herbs that have sedative properties might enhance therapeutic and adverse effects. Some of these supplements include 5-HTP, calamus, California poppy, catnip, hops, Jamaican dogwood, kava, St. John's wort, scullcap, valerian, yerba mansa, and others.

Interactions with Drugs

CNS DEPRESSANTS: Theoretically, concomitant use with drugs with sedative properties may cause additive effects and side effects (19).

Interactions with Foods

None known.

Interactions with Lab Tests

None known.

Interactions with Diseases or Conditions

PELVIC INFLAMMATORY DISEASE (PID) and MENORRHAGIA: Because catnip is also used to stimulate menstruation, theoretically it is contraindicated in pelvic inflammatory disease (PID) and excessive menstrual bleeding (12).

Dosage and Administration

ORAL: People typically use two 380 mg capsules three times daily at meals or prepared as a tea using 1-2 teaspoons in 6 ounces of boiling water (6006).

CATUABA

Also Known As
Caramuru, Catuaba Casca, Chuchuhuasha, Golden Trumpet, Pau De Reposta, Piratancara, Tatuaba.

Scientific Names
Erythroxylum catuaba.
Family: Erythroxylaceae.

Comments
At the date of publication, there was very little scientific information available about this product. Our staff is continually analyzing the available information on natural medicines and will add data to the online version of *Natural Medicines Comprehensive Database* as it becomes available. See www.naturaldatabase.com.

CEDAR leaf

Also Known As
American Arborvitae, Arborvitae, Eastern Arborvitae, Eastern White Cedar, Hackmatack, Northern White Cedar, Swamp Cedar, Thuga, Thuja, Tree of Life, White Cedar.
CAUTION: See separate listings for Cedar Leaf Oil, Cedarwood Oil, and Cedarwood.

Scientific Names
Thuja occidentalis.
Family: Cupressaceae.

People Use This For
Orally, cedar leaf is used to treat respiratory tract infections, in conjunction with antibiotics for bacterial skin infections and herpes simplex, for bronchitis, rheumatism, trigeminal neuralgia, and strep throat. It is also used as an abortifacient.
Topically, cedar leaf is used to manage joint pain, arthritis, and muscle rheumatism.

Safety
LIKELY SAFE ...when used orally in amounts commonly found in foods if thujone-free (12).
POSSIBLY SAFE ...when used orally as a medicinal for occasional use in recommended amounts (12); not for long-term use.
There is insufficient reliable information available about the safety of cedar leaf for its other uses.
PREGNANCY: UNSAFE ...when used orally due to abortifacient activity (12); avoid using.
LACTATION: Insufficient reliable information available; avoid using.

Effectiveness
There is insufficient reliable information available about the effectiveness of cedar leaf.

Mechanism of Action
Cedar leaf is reported to be a urinary irritant (19), a uterine stimulant, and affect menstrual cycle (12). Thujone, a constituent, is a neurotoxin that can cause convulsions (1304). The glycoprotein and polysaccharide fractions have been used therapeutically (18). Some evidence suggests the polysaccharides might have antiviral and immunostimulating (1305) properties, and might inhibit HIV-1-specific antigens and reverse transcriptase activity (1306).

Adverse Reactions
Orally, symptoms of overdose include queasiness, vomiting, painful diarrhea, and mucous membrane hemorrhage. Deaths have been reported (18). Other side effects include asthma, CNS stimulation, and seizures (6002).

Interactions with Herbs & Other Dietary Supplements
THUJONE CONTAINING HERBS: Avoid; concomitant use may increase the risk of thujone toxicity.
Thujone-containing herbs include oak moss, oriental arborvitae, sage, tansy, tree moss, and wormwood (2,4,12).

Interactions with Drugs
ANTICONVULSANTS: Cedar leaf may lower the seizure threshold in those individuals taking anti-convulsants (6002).

Interactions with Foods
None known.

Interactions with Lab Tests
None known.

Interactions with Diseases or Conditions
GI CONDITIONS: Cedar leaf can irritate gastrointestinal tract. Contraindicated in individuals with infectious or inflammatory gastrointestinal conditions (19).

Dosage and Administration
ORAL: The typical dose of liquid extract (unspecified concentration) is 2-4 mL only for occasional use (12).
TOPICAL: No typical dosage.

Comments
Avoid confusion with other Thuja species.

CEDAR LEAF OIL

Also Known As
American Arborvitae, Arborvitae, Eastern Arborvitae, Eastern White Cedar, Hackmatack, Northern White Cedar, Swamp Cedar, Thuja Oil, Tree of Life, White Cedar.
CAUTION: See separate listings for Cedar leaf, Cedarwood Oil, and Cedarwood.

Scientific Names
Thuja occidentalis.
Family: Cupressaceae.

People Use This For
Orally, cedar leaf oil is used as an immune stimulant, expectorant, and diuretic.
Topically, cedar leaf oil is used to treat skin diseases, condyloma, cancers, as an insect repellent, nd as a counterirritant to treat warts.
In foods and beverages, cedar leaf oil is used as a flavoring.
In manufacturing, cedar leaf oil is used as a fragrance in cosmetics and soaps.

Safety
LIKELY SAFE ...when used orally in amounts commonly found in foods. Cedar leaf oil that is thujone-free has Generally Recognized As Safe status (GRAS) for use in foods in the US (4912).
POSSIBLY SAFE ...when used topically (11).
UNSAFE ...when used orally for medicinal use (11). A constituent, thujone, is a neurotoxin (1304).
PREGNANCY: UNSAFE ...when used orally or topically due to toxicity and uterine stimulant activity (11); avoid using.
LACTATION: UNSAFE ...when used orally or topically due to toxicity (11); avoid using.

Effectiveness
There is insufficient reliable information available about the effectiveness of cedar leaf oil.

Mechanism of Action
Thujone, a constituent of cedar leaf oil, is a neurotoxin that can cause convulsions (1304). Polysaccharides have demonstrated in vitro antiviral, immunostimulating (1305), inhibition of HIV-1-specific antigens and reverse transcriptase activity (1306).

Adverse Reactions
Orally, use of cedar leaf oil can result in poisoning. Symptoms of thujone poisoning include hypotension, convulsion, and death (11). Other side effects include asthma, CNS stimulation, and seizures (6002).

Interactions with Herbs & Other Dietary Supplements
THUJONE CONTAINING HERBS: Avoid; concomitant use may increase the risk of thujone toxicity. Thujone-containing herbs include oak moss, oriental arborvitae, sage, tansy, tree moss, and wormwood (2,4,12).

Interactions with Drugs
ANTICONVULSANTS: Cedar leaf oil may lower the threshold in those individuals taking anti-convulsants (6002).

Interactions with Foods
None known.

Interactions with Lab Tests
None known.

Interactions with Diseases or Conditions
None known.

Dosage and Administration
ORAL: People typically use 2 to 4 mL of the liquid extract (5263).
TOPICAL: No typical dosage.

Comments
Avoid confusion with other Thuja species. Cedar leaf oil is produced by steam distillation of Thuja occidentalis leaves and twigs (11).

CEDARWOOD

Also Known As
Ashe Juniper, Cedar, Eastern Red Cedar, Red Cedarwood, Red Juniper, Texas Cedarwood, Virginia Cedarwood.
CAUTION: See separate listings for Cedar Leaf Oil, Cedar leaf, and Cedarwood Oil.

Scientific Names
Juniperus virginiana.
Family: Cupressaceae.

People Use This For
Orally, cedarwood is used for cough, bronchitis, rheumatism, venereal warts, and skin rash.

Safety
POSSIBLY SAFE ...when the berry or leaf is used orally (12).
There is insufficient reliable information available about the safety of the oral or topical use of the bark, seed or twig.
PREGNANCY AND LACTATION: LIKELY UNSAFE ...when the berry or leaf are used orally. Virginia cedarwood berry or leaf is contraindicated in pregnancy (12). There is insufficient reliable information available about the safety of the oral or topical use of cedarwood bark, seed, or twig; avoid using.

Effectiveness
There is insufficient reliable information available about the effectiveness of cedarwood.

Mechanism of Action
Steam distillation of Virginia cedarwood produces an oil that contains alpha- and beta-cedrene, cedrol, and cedreol. It also contains the toxic constituent thujone (11).

Adverse Reactions
None reported.

Interactions with Herbs & Other Dietary Supplements
THUJONE CONTAINING HERBS: Avoid; concomitant use may increase the risk of thujone toxicity. Thujone-containing herbs include oak moss (12), oriental arborvitae (12), sage (2,4,12), tansy (2,4,12), tree moss (12), and wormwood (2,12).

Interactions with Drugs
BARBITURATES: Theoretically, inhaling red cedar chip fragrance might reduce efficacy of hexobarbital or pentobarbital (19). Some of these sedative medications include pentobarbital (Nembutal), phenobarbital (Luminal), secobarbital (Seconal), and others.

Interactions with Foods
None known.

Interactions with Lab Tests
None known.

Interactions with Diseases or Conditions
None known.

Dosage and Administration
No typical dosage.

Comments
Avoid confusion with cedarwood oil.

CEDARWOOD OIL

Also Known As
None.
CAUTION: See separate listings for Cedar leaf, Cedar Leaf Oil, and Cedarwood.

Scientific Names
Juniperus ashei, synonym Juniperus mexicana (Cedarwood Oil Texas); Juniperus virginiana (Cedarwood Oil Virginia).
Family: Cupressaceae.
Cedrus atlantica (Cedarwood Oil Atlas).
Family: Pinaceae.

People Use This For
Topically, cedarwood oil is used for alopecia areata. It is also used topically as an insect repellent.
In manufacturing, cedarwood oils are used as fragrance or fixatives in cosmetics, soaps, and perfumes.

Safety
POSSIBLY SAFE ...when used topically and appropriately. Cedarwood oil (Cedrus atlantica) has been used safely for up to 7 months (5177). The maximum use level in perfumes is 0.8%.
PREGNANCY AND LACTATION: Insufficient reliable information available; avoid using.

Effectiveness
POSSIBLY EFFECTIVE

Alopecia areata. Applying cedarwood oil topically in combination with other essential oils seems to be effective for treating alopecia areata. Cedarwood oil (Cedrus atlantica) in combination with the essential oils from thyme, lavender, and rosemary seem to improve hair growth by 44% after 7 months of treatment (5177).

There is insufficient reliable information available about the effectiveness of cedarwood oil for its other uses.

Mechanism of Action
Steam distillation of Virginia cedarwood produces an oil that contains alpha- and beta-cedrene, cedrol, and cedreol. It also contains the constituent thujone (11). It's not clear how cedarwood oil (Cedrus atlantica) works in alopecia areata, but it may have a stimulatory effect on hair growth (5177). Dermatological studies have shown that all three cedarwood oils (Virginia, Texas, Atlas) are generally non-toxic (11); however, there is other evidence that cedarwood oil (probably Virginia) can produce tumors on mouse skin (11).

Adverse Reactions
There is some evidence that cedarwood oil (Virginia and/or Texas) is an allergenic and is a local irritant (11).

Interactions with Herbs & Other Dietary Supplements
THUJONE CONTAINING HERBS: Avoid; concomitant use may increase the risk of thujone toxicity.
Thujone-containing herbs include oak moss (12), oriental arborvitae (12), sage (2,4,12), tansy (2,4,12), tree moss (12), and wormwood (2,12).

Interactions with Drugs
None known.

Interactions with Foods
None known.

Interactions with Lab Tests
None known.

Interactions with Diseases or Conditions
None known.

Dosage and Administration

TOPICAL: For the treatment of alopecia areata, a combination of the essential oils including cedarwood (Cedrus atlantica) 2 drops or 94 mg, rosemary 3 drops or 114 mg, thyme 2 drops or 88 mg, and lavender 3 drops or 108 mg, all mixed with 3 mL jojoba oil and 20 mL grapeseed oil has been used. Each night, the mixture is massaged into the scalp for 2 minutes with a warm towel placed around the head to increase absorption (5177).

Comments

There are several cedarwood oils with different physical and chemical properties, each produced by steam distillation of wood from various trees. The most common are: cedarwood oil Virginia (synonym cedar oil, red cedarwood oil), cedarwood oil Atlas (synonym cedarwood oil Moroccan), and cedarwood oil Texas (cedarwood oil mountain, Mexican).

CELERY

Also Known As

Ache des Marais, Ajamoda, Apii Fructus, Celeriac, Celery Fruit, Celery Seed, Celery tuber, Fruit de Celeri, Smallage, Selleriefruchte, Selleriesamen.

Scientific Names

Apium graveolens.
Family: Apiaceae/Umbelliferae.

People Use This For

Orally, celery is used to treat rheumatism, gout, hysteria, nervousness, headache, weight loss due to malnutrition, loss of appetite, and exhaustion. Celery is also used as a sedative, mild diuretic, urinary antiseptic, digestive aid, menstrual stimulant, antiflatulent, aphrodisiac, to reduce lactation, for regulating bowel movements, stimulating glands, and for blood purification.

Safety

LIKELY SAFE ...when the oil or seeds are consumed in amounts commonly found in foods. Celery seed has Generally Recognized As Safe (GRAS) status in the US (4912).
POSSIBLY SAFE ...when used orally and appropriately in medicinal amounts (12).
PREGNANCY: LIKELY UNSAFE ...when the oil or seeds are used orally in larger amounts; celery might have uterine stimulant or abortifacient effects (4,19).
LACTATION: There is insufficient reliable information available about the safety of medicinal amounts of celery during lactation; avoid using.

Effectiveness

There is insufficient reliable information available about the effectiveness of celery.

Mechanism of Action

The applicable parts of celery are the fruit and seed. Sedative, diuretic, and antispasmodic effects of celery seed may be due to phthalide constituents (d-limonene, selinene, and related phthalides) (4,6). Celery plant extracts have hypotensive and hypoglycemic effects (4). In preliminary research, 5 of 23 celery-based preparations displayed antiarthritis effects; none of the extracts displayed anti-inflammatory or antipyretic effects. The activity of celery seed is thought to be dependent on processing at low temperatures (6131). Another constituent, apiogenin, has shown evidence of antiplatelet activity. The essential oil can increase kidney inflammation by irritating epithelial tissue (8). Celery juice has been reported to have bile stimulating activity (4). Celery seed oil has shown bacteriostatic effects (4). Celery also contains the furocoumarins bergapten and celereodise, a dihydrofurocoumarin glycoside (isoquercitrin), and the coumarin glycoside apiumoside (6). Celery is a rich plant source of calcium, magnesium, and iron (19).

Adverse Reactions

Celery can cause contact dermatitis (19). Mild allergic reactions to anaphylactic reactions have also been documented (12192). Allergic reactions to celery are more likely in patients who are also sensitive to mugwort, birch, dandelion, or wild carrot (12192). This has been called the "celery-carrot-mugwort-spice syndrome" (12192). Consuming large amounts of celery seed oil can induce CNS depression (6). Contact with celery stems could lead to photosensitivity (4).

Interactions with Herbs & Other Dietary Supplements

None known.

Interactions with Drugs

CNS DEPRESSANTS: Theoretically, concomitant use with these drugs may cause additive effects (4).
PHOTOSENSITIZING DRUGS: Theoretically, concomitant use might result in increased photosensitivity (6178). Some drugs that cause photosensitivity include amitriptyline (Elavil), quinolones (Ciprofloxacin, others), sulfa drugs (Septra, Bactrim, others), and tetracycline.
LEVOTHYROXINE (Synthroid, Levothroid, Levoxyl, and others): Celery seed might decrease the effects of levothyroxine replacement therapy (10646). The mechanism for this interaction is unknown.

Interactions with Foods

None known.

Interactions with Lab Tests

THYROXINE (T-4): Celery seed might decrease thyroxine (T-4) serum levels and test results (10646). The mechanism for this interaction is unknown.

Interactions with Diseases or Conditions

CROSS-ALLERGENICITY: Celery can cause allergic reactions in patients who are sensitive to other plants and spices including wild carrot, mugwort, birch, and dandelion (12192). This has been called the "celery-carrot-mugwort-spice syndrome" (12192).
KIDNEY CONDITIONS: Contraindicated in kidney disorders; celery might increase inflammation (8).

Dosage and Administration

ORAL: 0.5-2 grams of dried fruit three times daily has been used. One cup of tea, prepared by simmering 1 gram of fresh crushed dried fruit in 150 mL boiling water 5-10 minutes, has been used three times daily (4,8). 0.3-1.2 mL of the liquid extract, 1:1 in 60% alcohol, has been used three times daily (4).

Comments

Furanocoumarin content increases 100-fold in injured or diseased celery (6). Celery is available in capsule form, containing 450 or 505 mg of the oil. The ancient Greeks used celery to make wine, which was served as an award at athletic games (6002).

CENTAURY

Also Known As

Bitter Herb, Common Centaury, Drug Centaurium, Lesser Centauru, Minor Centaury.

Scientific Names

Centaurium erythraea, synonyms Erythraea centaurium, Centaurium minus, Centaurium umbellatum.
Family: Gentianaceae.

People Use This For

Orally, centaury is used orally for anorexia and dyspepsia.
In beverages, centaury is used as a flavoring.

Safety

LIKELY SAFE ...when used orally in amounts commonly found in foods. Centaury has Generally Recognized As Safe status (GRAS) for use in foods in the US (4912).
POSSIBLY SAFE ...when used orally in medicinal amounts (12). There is no documented toxicity (4).
PREGNANCY AND LACTATION: Insufficient reliable information available; avoid the use of centaury in amounts greater than those commonly found in foods.

Effectiveness

There is insufficient reliable information available about the effectiveness of centaury.

Mechanism of Action

The applicable parts of centaury are the dried, above ground parts. The bitter constituents amarogentin, gentiopicroside, swertiamarin, and the related bitters (3,7) can act as an appetite stimulant, although with less activity than comparable bitter herbs (4). Its antipyretic activity can result from the phenolic acid constituents. The constituent, gentiopicrin, can have antimalarial properties. Animal evidence suggests that centaury has anti-inflammatory activity (4).

Adverse Reactions

None reported.

Interactions with Herbs & Other Dietary Supplements
None known.

Interactions with Drugs
None known.

Interactions with Foods
None known.

Interactions with Lab Tests
None known.

Interactions with Diseases or Conditions
None known.

Dosage and Administration
ORAL: The typical dose of centaury is 2-4 grams or as a tea three times daily. The tea is prepared by steeping 2-4 grams in 150 mL boiling water (4). The average daily dose of centaury is 6 grams (2). The usual dose of the liquid extract (1:1 in 25% alcohol) is 2-4 mL three times daily (4).

CEREUS

Also Known As
Night Blooming Cereus, Sweet Scented Cactus.

Scientific Names
Selenicereus grandiflorus, synonyms Cereus grandiflorus, Cactus grandiflorus.
Family: Cactaceae.

People Use This For
Orally, cereus is used for angina pectoris, edema associated with weak heart function, and as a cardiac stimulant (sometimes instead of digitalis). Cereus is also used orally for urinary ailments, hemoptysis, menorrhagia, dysmenorrhea, hemorrhage, cystitis, and shortness of breath.
Topically, cereus is used as a skin stimulant for rheumatism.

Safety
POSSIBLY SAFE ...when the flower or stem is used orally for non-cardiac conditions (12). Although it contains cactine, which may have a digitalis-like effect, there are no reports of human toxicity (12).
POSSIBLY UNSAFE ...when used orally to self-medicate for cardiac conditions.
There is insufficient reliable information available about the safety of cereus for its other uses.
PREGNANCY AND LACTATION: Insufficient reliable information available; avoid using.

Effectiveness
There is insufficient reliable information available about the effectiveness of cereus.

Mechanism of Action
The applicable parts of cereus are the flower, stem, and young shoots. There is some evidence that cereus can stimulate the heart and dilate peripheral vessels (18), as well as stimulate spinal cord motor neurons (18). Researchers think tyramine, a cardiotonic amine, can strengthen heart muscle action (4). The reputed digitalis effect of cereus is claimed to be non-cumulative (12).

Adverse Reactions
Orally, fresh cereus juice may cause burning of the mouth, queasiness, nausea, vomiting, and diarrhea (4,18).
Topically, it may cause itching and skin pustules (18).

Interactions with Herbs & Other Dietary Supplements
None known.

Interactions with Drugs
DIGOXIN (Lanoxin): Cereus may potentiate the actions of cardiac glycosides and may enhance the effect of other cardiac drugs (6002).
MONOAMINE OXIDASE INHIBITORS (MAOIs): Theoretically, excessive doses of cereus may interact with MAOIs, because of the tyramine content (4).

Interactions with Foods
None known.

Interactions with Lab Tests
None known.

Interactions with Diseases or Conditions
HEART CONDITIONS: Theoretically, cereus may affect individuals with existing heart conditions or interfere with therapy (4).

Dosage and Administration
ORAL: Typical doses are fluid extract (1:1) 0.6 mL one to ten times daily (4,18), tincture of cereus (1:10) 0.12-2 mL two to three times daily (4,18), or tincture in sweetened water (1:10) 10 drops three to five times daily (18). Should not be used as self-medication for cardiac conditions.

CESIUM

Also Known As
Caesium, Cesium-137, Cesium Chloride, CsCl, High pH Therapy.

Scientific Names
Cesium; Cs; atomic number 55.

People Use This For
Orally, cesium is used for treating cancer and depression.
Radioactive cesium (cesium-137) is used as radiation therapy in cancer patients.
In industry, radioactive cesium is also used in instruments that measure thickness, moisture, and liquid flow.

Safety
POSSIBLY UNSAFE ...when used orally in large doses. There is no reliable evidence about the safety of cesium from clinical trials. There is a case report of life-threatening hypokalemia, hypotensive syncope, and prolonged QT interval on electrocardiogram (ECG) in a patient who took cesium 3 grams/day for several weeks (12178). The safety of lower doses is not known.
PREGNANCY AND LACTATION: Insufficient reliable information available; avoid using.

Effectiveness
INSUFFICIENT RELIABLE EVIDENCE to RATE

Cancer. Preliminary evidence suggests that cesium in combination with other vitamins and minerals might reduce mortality rate in some patients with various types of cancer (7613). More evidence is needed to rate cesium for this use.

Mechanism of Action
Cesium is an alkali metal element, structurally similar to lithium, sodium, and potassium (Group 1A on the periodic table). It is stable in its naturally occurring state. Unstable or radioactive cesium is formed by nuclear fission of uranium and plutonium (3894).
Preliminary research on breast and skin cancer cells suggests that cesium might have an anti-tumor effect. It might also stimulate the release of catecholamines (7612).

Adverse Reactions
Orally, cesium can cause nausea, diarrhea, and anorexia. Tingling of the lips, hands, and feet may also occur (7671). In one case, a female patient who took cesium 3 grams/day for several weeks experienced repeated episodes of diarrhea and then numbness or tingling of the lips. The patient was later admitted to the emergency room after having an episode of hypotensive syncope. She was found to be hypokalemic, disoriented, and had a prolonged cardiac QT interval on electrocardiogram ECG). Symptoms reemerged on rechallenge and resolved gradually over several days when cesium was discontinued (12178). Symptoms reemerged on rechallenge and resolved gradually over several days when cesium was discontinued (12178). It is not known if these symptoms developed due to potassium loss related to diarrhea or due to a direct effect of cesium on potassium channels.
Cesium-137 in high exposures can cause serious burns and death (3894).

Interactions with Herbs & Other Dietary Supplements
None known.

Interactions with Drugs

CORTICOSTEROIDS: Theoretically, drugs that deplete potassium, such as corticosteroids, in combination with cesium might lower serum potassium levels and test results (7670,7671).

DIURETIC DRUGS: Theoretically, people taking cesium along with potassium depleting diuretics might have lower serum potassium levels and test results (7670,7671). Initiation of potassium supplementation or an increase in potassium supplement dose may be necessary for some patients. Some diuretics that can deplete potassium include chlorothiazide (Diuril), chlorthalidone (Thalitone), furosemide (Lasix), hydrochlorothiazide (HCTZ, Hydrodiuril, Microzide), and others.

Interactions with Foods

None known.

Interactions with Lab Tests

POTASSIUM: Theoretically, cesium might lower potassium levels (7670,7671).

Interactions with Diseases or Conditions

None known.

Dosage and Administration

ORAL: A typical dosage is 6 to 9 grams in 3 divided doses (7613).

Comments

Cesium therapy is sometimes called "high pH therapy." According to proponents, oral administration of cesium chloride increases the pH of tumor cells, which are described as very acidic. There is no scientific research that indicates tumor cells differ in pH from normal cells or that cesium affects the pH of tumor or normal cells. Tell patients these are claims without supporting research.

CETYLATED FATTY ACIDS

Also Known As

Cerasomal-cis-9-cetylmyristoleate, Cetyl Laureate, Cetyl Myristate, Cetyl Myristoleate, Cetyl Oleate, Cetyl Palmitate, Cetyl Palmitoleate, Cetylated Monounsaturated Fatty Acids, Cetylmyristoleate, CM, CMO.

Scientific Names

Cis-9-cetylmyristoleate.

People Use This For

Orally, cetylated fatty acids are used for rheumatoid arthritis (RA), osteoarthritis, systemic lupus erythematosus (SLE), multiple sclerosis (MS), ankylosing spondylitis, Reiter's syndrome, Behcet's syndrome, Sjogren's syndrome, psoriasis, fibromyalgia, emphysema, benign prostate hyperplasia (BPH), silicone breast disease, leukemia and other cancers, and relief of various types of back pain.

Topically, cetylated fatty acids are used for osteoarthritis.

Safety

POSSIBLY SAFE ...when used orally or topically and appropriately. A blend of cetylated fatty acids (Celadrin, Proprietary Nutritionals, Inc.) has been used safely when taken orally for 68 days (8924). A topical cream containing a cetylated fatty acid blend (Celadrin, Proprietary Nutritionals, Inc.) has also been safely used when applied twice daily for up to 30 days (12076,13104).

PREGNANCY AND LACTATION: Insufficient reliable information available; avoid using.

Effectiveness

POSSIBLY EFFECTIVE

Osteoarthritis. Taking a specific blend of cetylated fatty acids (Celadrin, Proprietary Nutritionals, Inc.) 350 mg combined with 50 mg soy lecithin, and 75 mg fish oil seems to decrease pain and improve knee range of motion and function in patients with knee osteoarthritis; however, it does not appear to improve morning stiffness (8924). Applying the same specific blend of cetylated fatty acids topically either alone or in combination with menthol also seems to decrease pain and improve functionality in patients with knee osteoarthritis (12076,13104,13105).

There is insufficient reliable information available about the effectiveness of cetylated fatty acids for their other uses.

Mechanism of Action

Cetylated fatty acids include cetyl myristoleate, cetyl myristate, cetyl palmitoleate, cetyl laureate, cetyl palmitate, and cetyl oleate. Many products that contain cetyl myristoleate also contain a mixture of these other cetylated fatty acids.

There is interest in cetyl myristoleate for osteoarthritis because it is a substance isolated from mice that are immune to chemically-induced arthritis (677). Researchers also hypothesize that cetyl myristoleate and other cetylated fatty acids might have surfactant effects. These fatty acids might cause lubrication of joints and muscles, softening of tissues, and increased pliability. It is thought that they might also be a modulator of the immune system and a mediator of inflammatory process. Another proposed mechanism of action is possible inhibition of 5-lipoxygenase, a mediator of inflammation (8924,12076). But the evidence to back these theories is very preliminary.

Adverse Reactions

None reported.

Interactions with Herbs & Other Dietary Supplements

None known.

Interactions with Drugs

None known.

Interactions with Foods

None known.

Interactions with Lab Tests

None known.

Interactions with Diseases or Conditions

None known.

Dosage and Administration

ORAL: For osteoarthritis, a specific blend of cetylated fatty acids (Celadrin, Proprietary Nutritionals, Inc.) 350 mg plus 50 mg of soy lecithin, and 75 mg of fish oil taken 6 times daily has been used (8924).

TOPICAL: For osteoarthritis, a specific blend of cetylated fatty acids (Celadrin, Proprietary Nutritionals, Inc.) applied twice daily to the affected joint has been used (12076,13104).

CHANCA PIEDRA

Also Known As

Chanca-Piedra Blanca, Child Pick-a-Back, Derrière-Dos, Des Dos, Dukong Anak, Feuilles la Fievre, Memeniran, Meniran, Niruri, Pitirishi, Quebra Pedra, Quinina Criolla, Quinine Créole, Rami Buah, Sacha Foster, Sasha Foster, Seed on the Leaf, Shatter Stone, Stone Breaker, Tamalaka, Turi Hutan.

Scientific Names

Phyllanthus niruri.

Family: Euphorbiaceae.

People Use This For

Orally, chanca piedra is used for urinary tract infections and inflammation, kidney stones, urethral or vaginal mucous discharge, as a diuretic, an antiflatulent, aperitif, appetite stimulant, liver tonic, and blood purifier. It is also used orally for diabetes, gallstones, colic, stomachache, dyspepsia, intestinal infections, constipation, dysentery, flu, tenesmus, jaundice, hepatitis B, abdominal tumors, fever, pain, venereal problems, syphilis, gonorrhea, malaria, tumors, caterpillar stings, cough, edema, itching, miscarriage, rectitis, tremors, typhoid, vaginitis, anemia, asthma, bronchitis, thirst, tuberculosis, and vertigo.

Safety

There is insufficient reliable information available about the safety of chanca piedra.

Pregnancy and Lactation: Insufficient reliable information available; avoid using.

Effectiveness

POSSIBLY INEFFECTIVE

Hepatitis B. Taking chanca piedra orally doesn't seem to be effective for treating hepatitis B (3924,3925).

There is insufficient reliable information available about the effectiveness of chanca piedra for its other uses.

Mechanism of Action

Chanca piedra is thought to have multiple properties; antispasmodic, antiviral, bactericidal, antipyretic, and diuretic. It is also thought that chanca piedra reduces blood sugar and protects the liver (517); however, not all of these properties are supported by scientific evidence. In vitro, the constituent niuriside, inhibits specific HIV-protein binding activity, but does not protect cells from acute HIV infection (3927). In isolated animal tissue, an extract from the related plant, Phyllanthus sellowianus, has antispasmodic activity (3921). Preliminary studies in humans show the related species, Phyllanthus amarus, has diuretic, hypotensive and hypoglycemic effects (3928).

Adverse Reactions

None reported.

Interactions with Herbs & Other Dietary Supplements

None known.

Interactions with Drugs

ANTIDIABETES DRUGS: Monitor blood glucose levels closely due to claims that chanca piedra has hypoglycemic effects (19).

Interactions with Foods

None known.

Interactions with Lab Tests

None known.

Interactions with Diseases or Conditions

None known.

Dosage and Administration

ORAL: People typically use 1 to 2 grams of powdered herb in tablets or capsules twice daily. Chanca piedra is also taken as a 4:1 tincture in a dose of 1 to 3 mL twice daily (5255).

Comments

Older studies published in India were reportedly conducted with Phyllanthus niruri, which is thought to be indigenous to the West Indies (271). A report from India mentions Phyllanthus niruri is a synonym for Phyllanthus amarus (3928); however, these appear to be different species (513,816).

CHAPARRAL

Also Known As

Creosote Bush, Greasewood, Hediondilla, Jarilla, Larreastat.

Scientific Names

Larrea divaricata; Larrea tridentata, synonyms Larrea mexicana, Zygophyllum tridentatum.
Family: Zygophyllaceae.

People Use This For

Orally, chaparral is used for cancer, arthritis, venereal disease, tuberculosis, bowel cramps, colds, and chronic cutaneous disorders. It is also used orally for weight loss, as a tonic, antiparasitic, antiflatulent, "blood purifier" for genitourinary and respiratory tract infections, and a treatment for musculoskeletal inflammation, skin diseases, GI conditions, CNS conditions, chickenpox and snakebite pain.

Safety

LIKELY UNSAFE ...when used orally; avoid using. There are reports of serious poisoning, acute hepatitis, kidney and liver damage, and irreversible renohepatic failure (568,569,570,571,3497,11121,11122,11129).
PREGNANCY AND LACTATION: LIKELY UNSAFE ...when used orally; avoid using.
There are reports of serious poisoning, acute hepatitis, kidney and liver damage, and irreversible renohepatic failure (568,569,570,571,3497,11121,11122,11129).

Effectiveness

There is insufficient reliable information available about the effectiveness of chaparral.

Mechanism of Action

The applicable part of chaparral is the leaf. Nordihydroguaiaretic acid (NDGA), a constituent of chaparral, may have antioxidant properties and also selectively inhibits lipoxygenases. It is also involved with platelet -derived growth factor receptors and the protein kinase C intracellular signally family, which suggests it might have anticancer activity. It may also induce apoptosis (cellular death) in tumor cells (11123,11124). NGDA might also be responsible for the nephropathy and hepatotoxicity associated with chaparral. The exact mechanism of toxicity is unknown (11125). NDGA might also have antifungal and antiviral activity (11126,11127).
Preliminary research suggests NGDA undergoes glucuronidation in the liver (11125).

Adverse Reactions

Orally, chaparral can cause symptoms of hepatotoxicity including jaundice, fatigue, abdominal pain (right upper quadrant), dark urine, light stools, nausea, diarrhea, weight loss, fever, and anorexia. It can cause cirrhosis, cholestasis, cholangitis, acute hepatitis, kidney and liver failure (3497) There are multiple reports of hepatotoxicity, including at least two requiring liver transplant (568,569,570,571,3497,11121,11122). Consumption of chaparral tea has been associated with cystic renal disease and cystic adenocarcinoma of the kidney (11129). Preliminary information suggests low doses of chaparral can be used safely (10417). Tell patients until further information is available, chaparral should be considered unsafe.
Topically, chaparral can cause contact dermatitis (11128).

Interactions with Herbs & Other Dietary Supplements

HEPATOTOXIC HERBS: Theoretically, chaparral might have additive effects with herbs that cause hepatotoxicity (568,569,570,571,3497,11121,11122). Other products that might affect the liver include bishop's weed, borage, uva ursi, and others.

Interactions with Drugs

HEPATOTOXIC DRUGS: Theoretically, chaparral might have additive adverse effects on the liver when used with hepatotoxic drugs (568,569,570,571,3497,11121,11122). Some drugs that can adversely affect the liver include acetaminophen (Tylenol), amiodarone (Cordarone), carbamazepine (Tegretol), isoniazid (INH), methotrexate (Rheumatrex), methyldopa (Aldomet), and many others.

Interactions with Foods

None known.

Interactions with Lab Tests

LIVER FUNCTION TESTS: As a hepatotoxin, chaparral might increase liver function tests including alkaline phosphatase, aspartic acid transaminase (AST,SGOT) alanine aminotransferase (ALT, SGPT), total bilirubin, gamma-glutamyltransferase, and lactate dehydrogenase (568,569,570,571,3497,11121,11122).

Interactions with Diseases or Conditions

LIVER DISEASE: Theoretically, chaparral might exacerbate liver dysfunction in patients with liver disease (568,569,570,571,3497,11121,11122).

Dosage and Administration

No typical dosage.

Comments

Herp-Eeze is a dietary supplement promoted for preventing and treating herpes infections. The manufacturer states that a patented manufacturing process renders the product nontoxic. However, toxicity information about this product is limited to the manufacturer's claims (267).

CHASTEBERRY

Also Known As

Agnolyt, Agnus-Castus, Chaste Tree Berry, Chinese Vitex, Gattilier, Hemp Tree, Mang Jing Zi, Monk's Pepper, Vitex, Viticis Fructus.

Scientific Names

Vitex agnus-castus; Vitex trifolia; Vitex rotundifolia.
Family: Verbenaceae.

People Use This For

Orally, chasteberry is used for menstrual irregularities including dysmenorrhea, secondary amenorrhea, metrorrhagia, oligomenorrhea, and polymenorrhea. Chasteberry is also used for symptoms of menopause, for symptoms of premenstrual syndrome (PMS) including cyclical mastalgia, luteal-phase dysfunction (corpus luteum insufficiency), and other symptoms. It is also used orally for treating female infertility, preventing miscarriage in patients with progesterone insufficiency, controlling postpartum bleeding, aiding in expulsion of the placenta, increasing lactation, and treating fibrocystic breasts. It is used for promoting urination, treating benign prostatic hyperplasia (BPH), and reducing sexual desire. Chasteberry is also used for acne, nervousness, dementia, rheumatic conditions, colds, dyspepsia, spleen disorders, headaches, migraine, eye pain, body inflammation and swelling, and insect bites and stings.

Safety

LIKELY SAFE ...when used orally and appropriately. Chasteberry has been used safely in studies, lasting from 3 months up to 1.5 years (7055,7076,7077,7078,7079).

PREGNANCY AND LACTATION: POSSIBLY UNSAFE ...when used orally. Theoretically, the hormonal effects of chasteberry might adversely affect pregnancy or lactation (10979,11456). Avoid use.

Effectiveness

POSSIBLY EFFECTIVE

Premenstrual syndrome (PMS). Taking chasteberry orally seems to decrease some symptoms of PMS, especially breast pain or tenderness (mastalgia), edema, constipation, irritability, depressed mood or mood alterations, anger, and headache (7055,7076,7078,7079). In some patients these symptoms can be decreased by as much as 50% (7055). Chasteberry may not be as effective for symptoms of bloating (7055).

Premenstrual dysphoric disorder (PMDD). Taking chasteberry 20-40 mg/day for 8 weeks seems comparable to fluoxetine 20-40 mg/day for relieving symptoms of PMDD. However, chasteberry seems to be somewhat more effective for physical symptoms such as breast tenderness, swelling, cramps, and food cravings. Fluoxetine seems to be somewhat more effective for psychological symptoms such as depression, irritability, insomnia, nervous tension, and feeling out of control (12207).

Some clinical studies have used a specific extract of chasteberry (Agnolyt) standardized to contain 6% of the constituent agnoside. In the US, this formulation is found in the brand product Femaprin (Nature's Way).

INSUFFICIENT RELIABLE EVIDENCE to RATE

Infertility. There is some preliminary clinical evidence that taking chasteberry orally can increase the chance of getting pregnant in women who are infertile due to relative progesterone deficiency. However, chasteberry does not seem to work quickly. It can take from 3-7 months of treatment to achieve pregnancy (7077).

Mechanism of Action

The applicable part of the chasteberry tree is the fruit. The active constituents of chasteberries are the essential oils, iridoid glycosides, flavonoids, and diterpenes (7012,7013,10121). The primary essential oils consist of limonene, cineol, pinene, and sabinene (7013). The primary flavonoids include casticin, kaempferol, quercetagetin, orientin, and isovitexin (7013). The primary diterpenes include vitexilactone, rotundifuran, and 6-beta,7 beta-diacetoxy-13-hydroxy-labda-8,14-dien (10122). The relevant iridoid glycosides are aucubin and agnoside. Many chasteberry extracts are standardized to contain 6% agnoside (7012). Although not generally considered key constituents, chasteberries also contain several essential fatty acids, including oleic acid, linolenic acid, palmitic acid, and stearic acid (7012).

The therapeutic effects of chasteberry have primarily been attributed to its indirect effects on various neurotransmitters and hormones. Chasteberry seems to affect dopamine, and possibly acetylcholine and opioid receptors (7014,7015,10122). Chasteberry extracts contain multiple active constituents that seem to have agonistic effects at pituitary dopamine (D2) receptors when used in higher doses. This dopaminergic activity inhibits basal and thyrotropin-releasing hormone (TRH)-stimulated prolactin release (7014,7015,11456). In women with hyperprolactinemia, chasteberry seems to suppress prolactin release. This may normalize luteal phase defects in the menstrual cycle (9988). In healthy men, chasteberry's hormonal effects seem to be dose dependent. Lower doses of chasteberry extract of approximately 120 mg per day seem to increase prolactin release. Higher doses seem to suppress prolactin release (7016). Chasteberry doesn't appear to affect testosterone (7016).

Preliminary research suggests chasteberry also might have estrogen and progestin activity (10979,11456). Chasteberry appears to be selective for beta estrogen receptors. The beta estrogen receptor predominates in the heart, vasculature, bone, and bladder (11456). Other preliminary research suggests that chasteberry might inhibit the growth of breast cancer cells and other cancer cells such as ovarian, cervical, gastric, colon, and lung (9990,9991,12648). However, due to the possible estrogenic effect of chasteberry, the safety of chasteberry in estrogen-sensitive conditions is unknown.

In addition to hormonal effects, essential oils of chasteberry also seem to have antibacterial and antifungal effects. Extracts of chasteberry have moderate in vitro activity against a variety of gram-negative and gram-positive bacteria (12838).

Other preliminary research suggests chasteberry might have analgesic and antihistaminic activity (12649,12650).

Adverse Reactions

Orally, chasteberry is usually well tolerated. However, some patients can experience gastrointestinal upset, headache, nausea, itching and urticaria, rash, acne, and intramenstrual bleeding (7055,7076).

Interactions with Herbs & Other Dietary Supplements

None known.

Interactions with Drugs

ANTIPSYCHOTIC DRUGS: Theoretically, chasteberry might interfere with the action of dopamine antagonists such as antipsychotic drugs due to dopaminergic effects of chasteberry (7014,7015). Some of these antipsychotic drugs include chlorpromazine (Thorazine), clozapine (Clozaril), fluphenazine (Prolixin), haloperidol (Haldol), olanzapine (Zyprexa), perphenazine (Trilafon), prochlorperazine (Compazine), quetiapine (Seroquel), risperidone (Risperdal), thioridazine (Mellaril), and thiothixene (Navane).

CONTRACEPTIVE DRUGS: Theoretically, chasteberry can interfere with the efficacy of oral contraceptives because chasteberry seems to have hormone modulating activity (10979,11456).

DOPAMINE AGONISTS: Theoretically, chasteberry might potentiate the actions of dopaminergic agonists due to dopaminergic effects of chasteberry (10122). Some of these drugs include bromocriptine (Parlodel), levodopa (Dopar, component of Sinemet), pramipexole (Mirapex) ropinirole (Requip), and others.

ESTROGENS: Theoretically, chasteberry can interfere with the efficacy of hormone replacement therapy because chasteberry seems to have hormone modulating activity (10979,11456).

METOCLOPRAMIDE (Reglan): Theoretically, chasteberry might interfere with the action of dopamine antagonists such as metoclopramide due to dopaminergic effects of chasteberry (7014,7015).

Interactions with Foods

None known.

Interactions with Lab Tests

None known.

Interactions with Diseases or Conditions

HORMONE SENSITIVE CANCERS/CONDITIONS: Because chasteberry seems to have hormonal effects and might affect estrogen levels (6180), women with hormone sensitive conditions should avoid chasteberry. Some of these conditions include breast, uterine, and ovarian cancer, and endometriosis and uterine fibroids.

IN VITRO FERTILIZATION: There is some evidence that using chasteberry during in vitro fertilization procedures might prevent an ensuing pregnancy despite having a viable embryo. In one case, a woman undergoing in vitro fertilization began taking chasteberry. During her fourth in vitro fertilization treatment cycle she was found to have signs of ovarian hyperstimulation syndrome and a viable embryo did not result in pregnancy (6556).

Dosage and Administration

ORAL: For premenstrual syndrome (PMS) and other conditions doses vary considerably. The dosing regimen used depends on the formulation of chasteberry. In one study a specific chasteberry extract (Ze440) 20 mg per day has been used (7055). In a study using a different specific chasteberry extract (Agnolyt), 4 mg daily has been used (7076). One capsule (Femicur) containing 1.6-3.0 mg of dried fruit extract (6.7-12.5:1) has been used twice daily (7079). For premenstrual dysphoric disorder, 20-40 mg/day has been used (12207).
Crude herb extracts are typically used in doses of 20-240 mg per day up to 1800 mg per day in 2-3 divided doses (7055).

Comments

Historians say that monks chewed chaste tree parts to make it easier to maintain their celibacy.

CHAULMOOGRA

Also Known As

Gynocardia Oil, Hydnocarp, Hydnocarpus, Oleum Chaulmoograe.

Scientific Names

Hydnocarpus kurzii, synonym Taraktogenos kurzii; Hydnocarpus anthelminthicus; Hydnocarpus species.
Family: Flacourtiaceae.

People Use This For

Topically, chaulmoogra is used for skin disorders, psoriasis, and eczema.
Parenterally, chaulmoogra is used for leprosy.

Safety

LIKELY UNSAFE ...when used orally. The seeds are considered very toxic due to their cyanogenic glycoside content (18).

There is insufficient reliable information available about the safety of chaulmoogra for its other uses.

PREGNANCY AND LACTATION: Insufficient reliable information available; avoid using.

Effectiveness

There is insufficient reliable information available to rate the effectiveness of chaulmoogra.

Mechanism of Action

The applicable part of chaulmoogra is the seed. Chaulmoogra is thought to have sedative, antipyretic, and skin effects (18). In mice, intraperitoneal and subcutaneous administration of chaulmoogra fatty acids demonstrated antimicrobial activity against Mycobacterium leprae (3826). The cyanogenic glycoside content of the seeds renders them extremely poisonous (18).

Adverse Reactions

Orally, ingestion of the seed can cause cough, dyspnea, laryngospasms, nephrotoxicity, visual disorders, head and muscle pain, and central paralysis (18).

Topically, use can cause skin irritation (18).

Interactions with Herbs & Other Dietary Supplements

None known.

Interactions with Drugs

None known.

Interactions with Foods

None known.

Interactions with Lab Tests

None known.

Interactions with Diseases or Conditions

None known.

Dosage and Administration

ORAL: No typical dosage.

TOPICAL: People typically use chaulmoogra as a powder, oil, emulsion, or in ointments (18).

PARENTERAL: No typical dosage.

Comments

Chaulmoogra seeds provided the elemental materials for synthesizing the first antileprostatic agents (6002).

CHEKEN

Also Known As

Arryan, Chekan, Myrtus.

Scientific Names

Luma chequen, synonyms Eugenia chequen, Myrtus chequen.

Family: Myrtaceae.

Comments

At the date of publication, this product was not a common ingredient used in brand name supplements marketed to consumers. Details about this product are available in the online version of *Natural Medicines Comprehensive Database.* See www.naturaldatabase.com.

CHELATED MINERALS

Also Known As

Chelated Boron, Chelated Calcium, Chelated Chromium, Chelated Cobalt, Chelated Copper, Chelated Iron, Chelated Magnesium, Chelated Manganese, Chelated Molybdenum, Chelated Potassium, Chelated Selenium, Chelated Trace Minerals, Chelated Vanadium, Chelated Zinc.
CAUTION: See separate listings for Aspartates and individual minerals.

Scientific Names

Mineral-amino acid complex.

People Use This For

Orally, chelated minerals are used as dietary mineral supplements (marketed to be more bioavailable than non-chelated minerals), for supporting normal growth, stabilizing bipolar disorder, building strong muscles and bones, and improving immune function and overall health.

Safety

There is insufficient reliable information available about the safety of chelated minerals.
Pregnancy and Lactation: Insufficient reliable information available; avoid using.

Effectiveness

INSUFFICIENT RELIABLE EVIDENCE to RATE

Bipolar disorder. There is preliminary evidence that suggests that some cases of bipolar disorder may be stabilized with a chelated mineral supplement. A randomized, placebo-controlled trial in adults with bipolar disorder is presently underway (10651,10660). More evidence is needed to rate chelated minerals for this use.

Mechanism of Action

The term, chelated mineral, refers to the formation of a complex between a mineral and an amino acid. Evidence supports the importance of chelated minerals in the central nervous system (CNS), citing a beneficial psychotropic effect, although the exact mechanism is not fully understood (10651,10660).

Adverse Reactions

Orally, chelated minerals can cause nausea (10660). Fatty liver-hemorrhagic syndrome is reported in commercial chickens that are fed diets containing chelated minerals (1162).

Interactions with Herbs & Other Dietary Supplements

None known.

Interactions with Drugs

None known.

Interactions with Foods

None known.

Interactions with Lab Tests

None known.

Interactions with Diseases or Conditions

None known.

Dosage and Administration

See separate listings for specific minerals.

Comments

There is very little scientific information about this product. Our staff is continually analyzing the available information on natural medicines and will add data here as it becomes available.

CHENOPODIUM OIL

Also Known As

Epazote, Jesuit Tea, Mexican Tea.
CAUTION: See separate listings for Wormseed, Wormwood Oil, and Wormwood.

Scientific Names

Chenopodium ambrosioides; Chenopodium anthelminticum.
Family: Chenopodiaceae.

People Use This For

Orally, chenopodium oil has been used as an oral antiparasitic against roundworms and hookworms.

Safety

UNSAFE ...when used orally due to toxicity (11).
PREGNANCY AND LACTATION: UNSAFE ...when used orally due to toxicity (11).

Effectiveness

There is insufficient reliable information available about the effectiveness of chenopodium oil.

Mechanism of Action

The constituent ascaridole is thought to paralyze roundworms, hookworms, and dwarf tapeworms but not large tapeworms within the intestines (11). However, toxicity precludes its clinical use for these helminth infections. Chenopodium oil may explode when heated or treated with acids due to high ascaridole content (11). Handle with caution.

Adverse Reactions

Orally, chenopodium oil can cause skin and mucous membrane irritation, vomiting, headache, vertigo/dizziness, kidney and liver damage, temporary deafness, convulsions, circulatory collapse, paralysis, and death (11).

Interactions with Herbs & Other Dietary Supplements

None known.

Interactions with Drugs

PHOTOSENSITIZING DRUGS: Theoretically, concomitant use of chenopodium oil can increase risk of adverse effects. Chenopodium species are associated with photosensitivity (19).

Interactions with Foods

None known.

Interactions with Lab Tests

None known.

Interactions with Diseases or Conditions

None known.

Dosage and Administration

No typical dosage.

Comments

Authorities disagree on whether chenopodium oil is the distilled oil of fresh above ground flowering and fruiting parts (11) or seed oil (18) of Chenopodium ambrosioides.

CHEROKEE ROSEHIP

Also Known As

Chinese Rosehip, Fructus Rosae Laevigatae, Jinyingzi.
CAUTION: See separate listings for Acerola, Vitamin C, and Rose Hip.

Scientific Names

Rosa laevigata, synonym Rosa cherokeensi; Rosa chinensis, synonyms Rosa sinica, Rosa indica, Rosa roulettii; Rosa ternata; Rosa nivea; Rosa camellia.
Family: Rosaceae.

People Use This For
Orally, Cherokee rosehip is used for male sexual dysfunction (nocturnal emission, spermatorrhea, neurasthenia), gynecologic problems (leukorrhea, uterine bleeding), night sweats, polyuria, enuresis, chronic diarrhea, chronic cough, hypertension, and enteritis.

Safety
POSSIBLY SAFE ...when used orally and appropriately. It contains vitamin C as a major constituent (11).
POSSIBLY UNSAFE ...when used orally in large amounts. Hyperoxaluria, hyperuricosuria, hematuria, and crystalluria can occur in some people taking 1 gram of vitamin C (67 grams of Cherokee rosehip) or more per day (3042). Prolonged use of large amounts of vitamin C can increase its metabolism, and scurvy might occur when intake is reduced (15).
PREGNANCY: POSSIBLY UNSAFE ...when used orally in large doses because it is associated with newborn scurvy (15). There is insufficient reliable information available about the safety of smaller amounts.
LACTATION: Insufficient reliable information available.

Effectiveness
There is insufficient reliable information available about the effectiveness of Cherokee rosehip.

Mechanism of Action
Cherokee rosehip contains vitamin C (approximately 1.5%) (11). An antidiarrheal effect occurs in humans (11).

Adverse Reactions
Orally, the vitamin C in Cherokee rosehip may cause nausea, abdominal cramps, fatigue, insomnia, and sleepiness. Doses greater than 1 gram may cause diarrhea (15).

Interactions with Herbs & Other Dietary Supplements
VITAMIN CONTAINING HERBS: Due to the vitamin C content, concomitant use of Cherokee rosehip with other products containing vitamin C increases total dose of vitamin C and may increase risk of adverse effects.

Interactions with Drugs
ALUMINUM: Concomitant use interacts with the vitamin C in Cherokee rosehip and can increase aluminum absorption, but the clinical significance of this is unknown (3046). Administer Cherokee rosehip with vitamin C two hours before or four hours after antacids (3046).
ASPIRIN: Theoretically, the vitamin C in large amounts of Cherokee rosehip might decrease excretion of aspirin (15).
CHOLINE MAGNESIUM TRISALICYLATE (Trilisate): The vitamin C in Cherokee rosehip can increase urinary excretion of ascorbic acid and decrease excretion of salicylates such as choline magnesium trisalicylate. But this may not have a clinically significant effect on salicylate plasma levels (3046).
ESTROGENS: Theoretically, the vitamin C in large amounts of Cherokee rosehip might increase absorption and effects of estrogen (129,130).
FLUPHENAZINE (Prolixin): Concomitant use with Cherokee rosehip decreases blood levels due to vitamin C content (15).
WARFARIN (Coumadin): Theoretically, the vitamin C in large amounts of Cherokee rosehip might reduce anticoagulant activity (506).

Interactions with Foods
IRON: Theoretically, the vitamin C in Cherokee rosehip might increase GI absorption of food iron (ferric) but not supplement iron (ferrous) (15).

Interactions with Lab Tests
STOOL OCCULT BLOOD TESTS: Theoretically, large amounts of Cherokee rosehip may cause a false-negative result if ingested 48-72 hours before amine-dependent tests due to vitamin C content (506).
URINE GLUCOSE TESTS: Theoretically, large amounts of Cherokee rosehip (containing greater than 500 mg vitamin C) may cause false decreases with glucose oxidase tests (e.g. Clinistix) and may cause false increases with cupric sulfate tests (e.g. Clinitest) (15).

Interactions with Diseases or Conditions
DIABETES: Large amounts may affect blood sugar control because of the vitamin C content (15).
GOUT: Theoretically, the vitamin C in large amounts of Cherokee rosehip might increase uric acid levels (15).
KIDNEY STONES (Nephrolithiasis): Theoretically, the vitamin C in large amounts of Cherokee rosehip might cause precipitation of urate, cystine, or oxalate stones (15).

Dosage and Administration
No typical dosage.

Comments

Cherokee rosehip contains vitamin C (approximately 1.5%) (11).

CHERRY LAUREL WATER

Also Known As

Common Cherry Laurel, Laurocerasus Leaves.
CAUTION: See separate listing for Wild Cherry.

Scientific Names

Prunus laurocerasus, synonyms Laurocerasus officinalis, Cerasus laurocerasus, Laurocerasus ottinii, Laurocerasus vulgaris, Prunus grandifolia.
Family: Rosaceae.

People Use This For

Orally, cherry laurel water is used as a sedative, pain reliever, antispasmodic, for treating cough, colds, insomnia, stomach and intestinal spasms, vomiting, and cancer.
Topically, cherry laurel water is used in eye lotions.
As an inhalant, cherry laurel water is used as an aromatic, and breathing stimulant.

Safety

POSSIBLY SAFE ...when used orally and appropriately (18).
LIKELY UNSAFE ...when use orally in high doses. Cherry laurel water contains 0.1% hydrocyanic acid (11). Overdose can be fatal (18).
PREGNANCY AND LACTATION: Insufficient reliable information available; avoid using.

Effectiveness

There is insufficient reliable information available about the effectiveness of cherry laurel water.

Mechanism of Action

Contains prunasin, a cyanogenic glycoside (11,18).

Adverse Reactions

Orally, adverse effects have not been reported with typical doses. However, cherry laurel water contains 0.1% hydrocyanic acid (11), and overdoses can cause significant toxicity and death (18).

Interactions with Herbs & Other Dietary Supplements

None known.

Interactions with Drugs

None known.

Interactions with Foods

None known.

Interactions with Lab Tests

None known.

Interactions with Diseases or Conditions

None known.

Dosage and Administration

ORAL: People typically use a dose of 2 to 8 mL cherry laurel water (223,5267).

Comments

Cherry laurel water is produced by water distillation of cherry laurel (Prunus laurocerasus) leaves.
Avoid confusion with wild cherry bark, sweet bay leaf (laurel).

CHERVIL

Also Known As
Garden Chervil, Salad Chervil.

Scientific Names
Anthriscus cerefolium, synonyms Anthriscus longirostris, Scandix cerefolium.
Family: Apiaceae/Umbelliferae.

People Use This For
Orally, chervil is used as a diuretic, expectorant, digestive aid, and an antihypertensive. Juice from fresh chervil is used for eczema, gout, and abscesses.
In foods and beverages, chervil is used as a flavoring agent.

Safety
LIKELY SAFE ...when used orally in amounts commonly found in foods. Chervil and chervil extract have Generally Recognized As Safe (GRAS) status in the US (4912).
There is insufficient reliable information available about the safety of the oral use of chervil in medicinal amounts.
PREGNANCY AND LACTATION: LIKELY UNSAFE ...when used orally in medicinal amounts. Chervil contains estragole which might be mutagenic (12).

Effectiveness
There is insufficient reliable information available about the effectiveness of chervil.

Mechanism of Action
The applicable parts of chervil are the dried flowering parts and leaf. Chervil is a plant source rich in calcium and potassium (19). Estragole, the major constituent of the volatile oil, is reported to produce tumors in mice (11).

Adverse Reactions
None reported.

Interactions with Herbs & Other Dietary Supplements
None known.

Interactions with Drugs
None known.

Interactions with Foods
None known.

Interactions with Lab Tests
None known.

Interactions with Diseases or Conditions
None known.

Dosage and Administration
ORAL: Chervil is typically prepared by adding 1 teaspoon of fresh or dried herb to water. The dose is up to 1 cup a day, unsweetened, consumed a mouthful at a time (5263).

CHICKEN COLLAGEN

Also Known As
Chicken Type II Collagen, Type II Collagen.

Scientific Names
Chicken collagen type II.

People Use This For
Orally, chicken collagen is used to treat pain syndromes associated with rheumatoid arthritis, osteoarthritis, gouty arthritis, juvenile rheumatoid arthritis, post-surgical joint pain, post-traumatic pain, fibrositis, back pain, and neck pain.

Safety
There is insufficient reliable information available about the safety of chicken collagen.
Pregnancy and Lactation: Insufficient reliable information available; avoid using.

Effectiveness
There is insufficient reliable information available about the effectiveness of chicken collagen.

Mechanism of Action
The rationale of using chicken collagen for pain syndromes is based on the theory of oral tolerance. This theory hypothesizes that oral administration of small quantities of antigens causes biological processes that suppress inflammation at the cellular level, suppress response to delayed-hypersensitivity antigens, and eliminate the cells that respond to antigens. Although evidence suggests this theory might be true in animals, it is unproven in humans (3126). Based on the theory of oral tolerance, when individuals with rheumatoid arthritis take oral collagen, the collagen should cause certain areas of the gut to generate T-cells that are absorbed by the body. Then, in the body, these T-cells are activated by joint collagen and they secrete cytokines that suppress inflammation. Cytokines thought to be involved include interleukin 4, 10, and transforming growth factor beta (3111,3112,3125). Oral administration of collagen is also believed to decrease the expression of pro-inflammatory cytokines including interleukins 1, 2, 6, and 8; tumor necrosis factor alpha; and interferon gamma (3111). So far, the studies determining the efficacy of chicken collagen demonstrate conflicting results (3125,3112), but these studies have used microgram doses.

Adverse Reactions
Although no significant adverse effects have been reported in the small trials of chicken collagen (3111,3112), allergic reactions to other collagen products have occurred, e.g., bovine collagen used in corneal shields, catgut suture for eye surgery, and dietary collagen in the form of gelatin (3127). If large doses are used, side effects associated with glucosamine sulfate or chondroitin might occur. These include nausea, heartburn, diarrhea and constipation, drowsiness, skin reactions, and headache (2608).

Interactions with Herbs & Other Dietary Supplements
None known.

Interactions with Drugs
None known.

Interactions with Foods
None known.

Interactions with Lab Tests
None known.

Interactions with Diseases or Conditions
ALLERIGES: Theoretically, individuals who are allergic to chicken or eggs should not use chicken collagen. Collagen products have been associated with allergic reactions (e.g., bovine collagen used in corneal shields, catgut suture for eye surgery, and dietary collagen in the form of gelatin) (3127).

Dosage and Administration
ORAL: For rheumatoid arthritis, doses of 20 to 2500 mcg per day of chicken collagen have been used. For juvenile arthritis, doses of 100 mcg per day for the first month then 500 mcg per day thereafter have been used (3111,3112).

Comments
The manufacturer of Colloral, an oral chicken collagen product, stopped product development because it failed to demonstrate efficacy in humans (3128). Bovine collagen products have also been used in the treatment of rheumatoid arthritis.

CHICKWEED

Also Known As
Star Chickweed, Starweed.

Scientific Names
Stellaria media, synonym Alsine media.
Family: Caryophyllaceae.

People Use This For
Orally, chickweed is used for constipation, bronchial asthma, stomach and bowel problems, blood disorders, lung disease, obesity, scurvy, psoriasis, rabies, itching, and muscle and joint pain.
Topically, chickweed is used for skin problems including boils, abscesses, and ulcers.
In foods, chickweed is eaten in salads or served as cooked greens.

Safety
LIKELY SAFE ...when used orally (12).
There is insufficient reliable information available about the safety of the topical use of chickweed.
PREGNANCY AND LACTATION: Insufficient reliable information available; avoid using in amounts greater than those found in food.

Effectiveness
There is insufficient reliable information available about the effectiveness of chickweed.

Mechanism of Action
The applicable part of chickweed is the leaf. While chickweed does contain some vitamin C, the concentrations are too small to be effective (6).

Adverse Reactions
Orally, chickweed is generally well-tolerated (6). There are, however, some poorly documented human cases of paralysis from consumptions of large amounts of chickweed tea (6). There is one case of alleged nitrate toxicity leading to paralysis, but the chickweed implicated in this case may have been contaminated (12).

Interactions with Herbs & Other Dietary Supplements
None known.

Interactions with Drugs
None known.

Interactions with Foods
None known.

Interactions with Lab Tests
None known.

Interactions with Diseases or Conditions
None known.

Dosage and Administration
ORAL: People typically use 1155 to 3450 mg per day in 2 to 3 divided doses. One chickweed supplier suggests three daily doses based on body weight: under 100 pounds, 385 mg per dose; 100 to 175 pounds, 770 mg; and over 175 pounds, 1155 mg. Chickweed is also prepared as a tea with 1 to 2 teaspoons in 6 ounces of boiling water. Chickweed is available as a tincture of unspecified concentration with a typical dose of 1 to 5 mL per day (6006).
TOPICAL: No typical dosage.

CHICORY

Also Known As
Blue Sailors, Cichorii Herba, Cichorii Radix, Common Chicory Root, Hendibeh, Kasani, Succory, Wild Chicory.
CAUTION: See separate listing for Inulin.

Scientific Names
Cichorium intybus.
Family: Asteraceae/Compositae.

People Use This For

Orally, chicory is used as a tonic, diuretic, laxative, liver protectant, to balance the stimulant effect of coffee, for loss of appetite, dyspepsia, liver and gallbladder disorders, cancer, and tachycardia.
Topically, chicory leaves are used as a poultice for swelling and inflammation.
In foods, chicory leaves are often eaten like celery, and the roots are boiled and eaten. Chicory is used as a culinary spice, and the leaf buds and roots are eaten as vegetables.
In food manufacturing, chicory is used as a flavoring component in foods and beverages. The roasted root is also ground and used in coffee mixes to enhance richness and as a coffee substitute.

Safety

LIKELY SAFE ...when consumed in amounts commonly found in food. Chicory and chicory extract have Generally Recognized As Safe (GRAS) status in the US (4912).
POSSIBLY SAFE ...when used orally in medicinal amounts (2,12).
There is insufficient reliable information available about the safety of chicory for its other uses.
PREGNANCY: LIKELY UNSAFE ...when used orally due to concerns that chicory can induce menstruation or miscarriage (19).
LACTATION: Insufficient reliable information available; avoid using.

Effectiveness

There is insufficient reliable information available about the effectiveness of chicory.

Mechanism of Action

The applicable parts of chicory are the root and dried above ground parts. Chicory root has a mild laxative effect and stimulates bile production. It is also believed to slow the heart rate (2,11), perhaps due to the presence of a digitalis-like compound (5). Chicory has a sedative effect that has been attributed to the constituent lactucopicrin (5) and other water-soluble components (6). The sedative effect antagonizes the stimulant effects of coffee and tea (6). The sesquiterpene alkaloid constituents show evidence of bacteriostatic properties (11).
The extracts seem to have anti-inflammatory activity (11). Chicory is a rich source of beta-carotene (19).

Adverse Reactions

Topically, chicory can cause contact dermatitis (6,11). It can cause an allergic reaction in individuals sensitive to the Asterceae/Compositae family. Members of this family include ragweed, chrysanthemums, marigolds, daisies, and many other herbs.

Interactions with Herbs & Other Dietary Supplements

None known.

Interactions with Drugs

None known.

Interactions with Foods

None known.

Interactions with Lab Tests

None known.

Interactions with Diseases or Conditions

CHICORY ALLERGY: Contraindicated (11).
CROSS-ALLERGENICITY: Chicory may cause an allergic reaction in individuals sensitive to the Asteraceae/Compositae family. Members of this family include ragweed, chrysanthemums, marigolds, daisies, and many other herbs.
GALLSTONES: Chicory should be used with medical supervision due to chicory's bile stimulating effects (2,6,11).

Dosage and Administration

ORAL: The typical dose of chicory is one cup of the tea, which is prepared by steeping 2-4 grams of the root in 150 mL boiling water for 10 minutes and then straining (18). The average dose of chicory is 3-5 grams of root per day (18).
TOPICAL: No typical dosage.

Comments

Chicory can be contaminated with bacteria (6,3807) or foreign substances, including fungicides (6).

CHINESE CLUB MOSS

Also Known As
Huperazon, Qian Ceng Ta.
CAUTION: See separate listing for Huperzine A.

Scientific Names
Huperzia serrata.
Family: Lycopodiaceae.

People Use This For
Orally, Chinese club moss is used for Alzheimer's disease, general memory disorders, fever, inflammation, blood loss, irregular menstruation, and as a diuretic.

Safety
There is insufficient reliable information available about the safety of Chinese club moss.
Pregnancy and Lactation: Insufficient reliable information available; avoid using.

Effectiveness
There is insufficient reliable information available about the effectiveness of Chinese club moss.

Mechanism of Action
Chinese club moss contains the alkaloid huperzine A, a reversible acetylcholinesterase (AChE) inhibitor which crosses the blood-brain barrier (3082).

Adverse Reactions
None reported with Chinese club moss.
Orally, huperzine A which is found in Chinese club moss can cause dizziness, nausea, and sweating (3140).

Interactions with Herbs & Other Dietary Supplements
None known.

Interactions with Drugs
ACETYLCHOLINESTERASE (AChE) INHIBITORS: Theoretically, concurrent use with Chinese club moss might have additive effects with drugs that promote acetylcholine activity because huperzine A has AChE inhibitor properties (3082). AChE inhibitors and cholinergic drugs include bethanechol (Urecholine), donepezil (Aricept), echothiophate (Phospholine Iodide), edrophonium (Enoln, Reversol, Tensilon), neostigmine (Prostigmin), physostigmine (Antilirium), pyridostigmine (Mestinon, Regonol), succinylcholine (Anectine, Quelicin), and tacrine (Cognex).
ANTICHOLINERGIC DRUGS: Theoretically, concurrent use of anticholinergic drugs and Chinese club moss might decrease the effectiveness of Chinese club moss or the anticholinergic drug. In an animal model, huperzine A, an active constituent of Chinese club moss, reversed cognitive deficits induced by scopolamine (3135). Anticholinergic drugs include atropine, benztropine (Cogentin), biperiden (Akineton), procyclidine (Kemadrin), and trihexyphenidyl (Artane).
CHOLINERGIC DRUGS: Theoretically, concurrent use with Chinese club moss might have additive effects with drugs that promote acetylcholine activity because huperzine A has AChE inhibitor properties (3082). AChE inhibitors and cholinergic drugs include bethanechol (Urecholine), donepezil (Aricept), echothiophate (Phospholine Iodide), edrophonium (Enoln, Reversol, Tensilon), neostigmine (Prostigmin), physostigmine (Antilirium), pyridostigmine (Mestinon, Regonol), succinylcholine (Anectine, Quelicin), and tacrine (Cognex).

Interactions with Foods
None known.

Interactions with Lab Tests
None known.

Interactions with Diseases or Conditions
VARIOUS DISEASES: Acetylcholinesterase (AchE) inhibitors are used with caution or are contraindicated in people with asthma, chronic obstructive pulmonary disease, cardiovascular disease, obstruction of the intestinal or urogenital tracts, gastrointestinal ulcer disease, or seizures (15). Avoid using Chinese club moss in people with these conditions until more is known about its effects in humans.

Dosage and Administration
No typical dosage.

Comments
Be careful not to confuse club moss and Chinese club moss. Only Chinese club moss contains huperzine A.

CHINESE CUCUMBER

Also Known As
Chinese Snake Gourd, Compound Q, Gua Lou, Gua Luo Ren, Tian Hua Fen, Trichosanthes.

Scientific Names
Trichosanthes kirilowii, synonym Trichosanthes japonica.
Family: Curcurbitaceae.

People Use This For
Orally, Chinese cucumber root is used for HIV/AIDS, cough, fever, swelling, tumors, and diabetes.
A starch extract of the root is used for treating abscesses, amenorrhea, jaundice and hepatitis, frequent urination, and tumors. Chinese cucumber fruit and seed are also used orally for coughing, reducing fever, swelling, tumors, and diabetes.
Intramuscularly, Chinese cucumber root is used to induce abortions.
Intravaginally, Chinese cucumber fruit is used as an abortifacient.

Safety
POSSIBLY SAFE ...when the fruit and seed are used orally and appropriately (12).
LIKELY UNSAFE ...when the root is used orally or by injection. Extracts of Chinese cucumber root can be toxic (6).
There is insufficient reliable information available about the safety of Chinese cucumber for its other uses.
PREGNANCY: LIKELY UNSAFE ...when the root, fruit, or seed are used orally or by injection.
Chinese cucumber root can be toxic. Chinese cucumber fruit and seeds are thought to have abortifacient effects and possible teratogenicity (6).
LACTATION: Insufficient reliable information available; avoid using.

Effectiveness
There is insufficient reliable information available about the effectiveness of Chinese cucumber.

Mechanism of Action
The applicable parts of Chinese cucumber are the fruit, seed, and root.
Chinese cucumber root contains several constituents that have activity against the human immunodeficiency virus (HIV). The constituents trichosanthin and protein "TAP 29" can block HIV replication and some evidence suggests they might selectively kill HIV infected cells (6).
Other constituents of the root, trichosanthin and momorcharin, can have abortifacient effects. Trichosanthin injected intramuscularly or extra-amniotically can induce first-trimester abortions. It has also been used to terminate ectopic pregnancies (6). A sponge containing Chinese cucumber juice might induce abortions when inserted intravaginally (6).
Trichosanthin and momorcharin might cause birth defects (12).
Trichosanthin also has antitumor activity. It has been used to treat invasive moles and certain types of liver tumors. A water extract of the root might have hypoglycemic activity in individuals with normal blood glucose. Subsequent fractionation of the extract yielded five compounds. The activity of one of these suggests it might be useful in reducing blood sugars in individuals with diabetes (4045).
Some evidence suggests a 50% ethanolic extract of the fruit might have protective effects against ulcers (4044).
Preliminary evidence suggests three triterpene compounds isolated from the seed might have anti-inflammatory effects (4042). A 50% ethanolic seed extract might have anti-inflammatory and analgesic effects (4043).

Adverse Reactions
Orally, Chinese cucumber fruit can cause mild diarrhea and gastric discomfort (12).
Chinese cucumber root extracts are extremely toxic, particularly when they are injected. Trichosanthin injections can be fatal. They can also cause severe reactions including seizures, fever, lung and cerebral edema, cerebral hemorrhage, and heart damage. People receiving trichosanthin injections to cause abortion can develop a severe allergy. After a single exposure, the risk of anaphylaxis from a second exposure can persist for more than a decade (6).

Interactions with Herbs & Other Dietary Supplements

HERBS WITH HYPOGLYCEMIC POTENTIAL: Theoretically, due to reported hypoglycemic activity concomitant use may potentiate effects of other herbs with hypoglycemic effects (4045). Herbs with hypoglycemic potential include devil's claw, fenugreek, garlic, guar gum, horse chestnut, Panax ginseng, psyllium, and Siberian ginseng.

Interactions with Drugs

ANTIDIABETES DRUGS: Theoretically, concomitant use with Chinese cucumber may have additive effects and adverse effects (4045). Monitor blood glucose levels closely, dose adjustment may be needed.

Interactions with Foods

None known.

Interactions with Lab Tests

BLOOD GLUCOSE: Theoretically, use of Chinese cucumber root may decrease blood glucose levels and test results (4045).

Interactions with Diseases or Conditions

DIABETES: Theoretically, use of Chinese cucumber root may alter blood glucose control (4045).

Dosage and Administration

No typical dosage.

CHIRATA

Also Known As

Bitter Stick, Bitterstick, Chirayta, Chiretta, East Indian Balmony, Indian Bolonong, Indian Gentian, Kairata, Kirata, Yin Du Zhang Ya Cai.

Scientific Names

Swertia chirayita, synonyms Swertia chirata, Gentiana chirata, Gentiana chirayita.
Family: Gentianaceae.

People Use This For

Orally, chirata is used as a bitter tonic, antipyretic, laxative, anthelmintic, for dyspepsia, loss of appetite, skin diseases, and cancer.
In India, it has been used as an anti-malarial, combined with the seeds of Guilandina Bonducella.
In manufacturing, chirata is used for alcoholic and non-alcoholic beverages.

Safety

LIKELY SAFE ...when used orally in amlunts commonly found in foods.
Chirata has Generally Recognized As Safe status (GRAS) for use in foods in the US (4912).
There is insufficient reliable information available about the safety of chirata in medicinal amounts.
PREGNANCY AND LACTATION: Insufficient reliable information available; avoid using.

Effectiveness

There is insufficient reliable information available about the effectiveness of chirata.

Mechanism of Action

The applicable parts of chirata are the above ground parts. The extract is reported to have anti-inflammatory activity in animals (11). Chirata seems to stimulate gastric juice secretion (18). The swerchirin constituent seems to have antimalarial activity, amarogentin is reported to have hepatoprotective activity, and xanthones might have antituberculous activity (11).

Adverse Reactions

None reported.

Interactions with Herbs & Other Dietary Supplements

None known.

Interactions with Drugs

None known.

Interactions with Foods
None known.

Interactions with Lab Tests
None known.

Interactions with Diseases or Conditions
DUODENAL ULCERS: May exacerbate (18); avoid using.

Dosage and Administration
ORAL: People typically use 0.5 to 2 grams of the powdered herb or 2 to 4 mL of the liquid extract (223).

Comments
Adulteration reported with Andrographis paniculata, roots of Rubia cordifolia, and Swertia species, including Swertia angustifolia (11).

CHITOSAN

Also Known As
Chitosan Ascorbate, Deacetylated chitosan, Enzymatic polychitosamine hydrolisat, HEP-30, Mono-carboxymethylated chitosan, N-Carboxybutyl Chitosan, N,O-Sulfated Chitosan, O-Sulfated N-Acetylchitosan, Sulfated N-Carboxymethylchitosan, Sulfated O-Carboxymethylchitosan, Trimethyl chitosan chloride.

Scientific Names
Chitosan.

People Use This For
Orally, chitosan is used for weight loss. It is also used orally by some people with renal failure on chronic hemodialysis for reducing high cholesterol, improving anemia, enhancing physical strength, appetite, and sleep. Chitosan is also used for Crohn's disease.
Topically, chitosan is used for treating periodontitis and promoting donor site tissue regeneration in plastic surgery.
In pharmaceutical manufacturing, chitosan is used as an excipient in tablets, as a disintegrant to improve drug dissolution, as a vehicle for parenteral drug delivery devices, and as a carrier in controlled release drug systems.

Safety
POSSIBLY SAFE...when used orally for up to 4 weeks (1942,9609,9610,10022,10023,10024,10025,11307).
...when used topically (1944,1945,4269,4270).
PREGNANCY AND LACTATION: Insufficient reliable information available; avoid using.

Effectiveness
POSSIBLY EFFECTIVE

Periodontitis. Applying chitosan ascorbate topically seems to help in the treatment of periodontitis (1945).

Plastic surgery. Applying N-carboxybutyl chitosan topically seems to help promote donor site tissue regeneration in plastic surgery (1944).

Renal failure. Taking chitosan orally, by patients with renal failure on chronic hemodialysis, seems to be effective for reducing high cholesterol; improving anemia; and enhancing physical strength, appetite, and sleep (1942).

POSSIBLY INEFFECTIVE

Weight loss. Taking chitosan orally, without a reduction in food intake, doesn't seem to cause weight loss in healthy people (3243,3244,9986). It doesn't seem to have any effect on fecal fat excretion (9987,10020). Some studies suggest that chitosan can help reduce weight when used in combination with a 1000 to 1200 calorie per day diet; but these studies have methodological flaws and are unreliable (9610,10022,10023,10024,10025).

INSUFFICIENT RELIABLE EVIDENCE to RATE

Crohn's disease. Preliminary clinical research suggests a combination of chitosan and ascorbic acid taken orally might help Crohn's disease. This combination seems to increase fecal excretion of fat, which might decrease intestinal inflammation (9609).

Hypercholesterolemia. The effect of chitosan on cholesterol is controversial. Some studies show a modest decrease in cholesterol, while others show no effect (1942,3243,3244,9986,11307).

More evidence is needed to rate chitosan for these uses.

Mechanism of Action

Chitosan is the N-deacetylated form of chitin that is extracted from the shells of crustaceans such as shrimp, lobster, and crab (9987). Chitosan is a polysaccharide containing copolymers of glucosamine and N-acetylglucosamine (10021). There are high molecular weight and low molecular weight forms of chitosan. Low molecular weight forms are created by cleaving a typical chitosan polymer into a smaller molecule. One such low molecular weight chitosan is called enzymatic polychitosamine hydrolisat or HEP-30 (Libracol).

For reduction of cholesterol, some evidence suggests that positively charged chitosan polymers bind to negatively charged bile acids, thus lowering cholesterol levels (10743). However, the effect of chitosan on cholesterol in humans is questionable (1942,3243,3244,9986). It is theorized that the lower molecular weight chitosan polymers such as HEP-30 might be more effective for lowering cholesterol. The thinking is that because it is smaller and more soluble it might be better able to adhere to fats in the gut and increase fat elimination. But so far there is no published evidence to support this.

For weight loss chitosan is promoted as a fat blocker, similar to orlistat (Xenical). Like for lowering cholesterol, it is thought to work by binding to negatively charged dietary fat and bile acids in the intestine, decreasing absorption. However, studies in healthy humans suggest chitosan doesn't affect fat excretion (9987,10020).

In patients with Crohn's disease, chitosan seems to increase fat excretion when combined with ascorbic acid (9609).

Reported hemostatic and wound-healing activity is believed to be due to an enhancement of macrophages, fibroblasts, and polymorphonuclear leukocytes; this appears to be independent of the classical coagulation cascade (1943,9608). Chitosan ascorbate acts as a surgical cement in treatment of periodontitis, protecting periodontal pockets from oxygen and allowing for proliferation of periodontal tissues (1945).

Scientists are interested in the potential for chitosan to enhance absorption of drugs, such as peptides, that normally can't cross the intestinal mucosa. In laboratory research, chitosan appears to increase permeation and intestinal absorption of hydrophilic macromolecules, such as low molecular weight heparin (10021).

Adverse Reactions

People with shellfish allergies should use chitosan with caution (9987).

Interactions with Herbs & Other Dietary Supplements

None known.

Interactions with Drugs

None known.

Interactions with Foods

None known.

Interactions with Lab Tests

CHOLESTEROL: Chitosan may reduce serum cholesterol levels, and test results in patients with renal failure on chronic hemodialysis (1942).

HEMOGLOBIN: Chitosan may increase serum hemoglobin levels, and test results in patients with renal failure on chronic hemodialysis (1942).

UREA/CREATININE: Chitosan may reduce blood urea and creatinine levels, and test results in patients with renal failure on chronic hemodialysis (1942).

Interactions with Diseases or Conditions

RENAL FAILURE: Chitosan may reduce serum cholesterol, urea, and creatinine levels; and increase hemoglobin levels in patients on chronic hemodialysis (1942).

Dosage and Administration

ORAL: For treating renal failure with chronic hemodialysis, 1.35 grams has been used three times daily (1942).

TOPICAL: No typical dosage.

Comments

Chitosan is a mucopolysaccharide component of crab, lobster, shrimp, and other marine organism exoskeletons.

CHIVE

Also Known As

Chives, Cives.

Scientific Names

Allium schoenoprasum, synonym Allium sibiricum.
Family: Liliaceae or Alliaceae.

People Use This For

Orally, chives are used to expel parasitic worms.
In foods, chives are used commonly as a food flavoring agent.

Safety

LIKELY SAFE ...when used orally in amounts commonly found in food amounts. Chives have Generally Recognized As Safe status (GRAS) for use in foods in the US (4912).
POSSIBLY SAFE ...when used orally in medicinal amounts (12).
PREGNANCY AND LACTATION: There is insufficient reliable information about the safety of medicinal amounts of chives during pregnancy and breast-feeding; avoid using.

Effectiveness

There is insufficient reliable information available about the effectiveness of chives.

Mechanism of Action

The applicable parts of chives are the above ground parts. There is insufficient reliable information available about the possible mechanism of action and active ingredients.

Adverse Reactions

Orally, intake of large quantities of chives can lead to dyspepsia (18).

Interactions with Herbs & Other Dietary Supplements

None known.

Interactions with Drugs

None known.

Interactions with Foods

None known.

Interactions with Lab Tests

None known.

Interactions with Diseases or Conditions

None known.

Dosage and Administration

No typical dosage.

CHLORELLA

Also Known As

Bulgarian Chlorella, Bulgarian Green Algae, Freshwater Green Algae, Freshwater Seaweed, Green Alga, Green Algae, Seaweed.

Scientific Names

Chlorella pyrenoidosa; Chlorella vulgaris; other Chlorella species.

People Use This For

Orally, chlorella is used as a food supplement and source of nutrients, including protein, nucleic acids, fiber, vitamins, and minerals. Chlorella is also used orally for cancer prevention, stimulating the immune system, improving response to flu vaccine, increasing white blood cell counts (e.g., in people with HIV infection or cancer), preventing colds, to protect the body from the effects of radiation (e.g., during cancer therapy), to protect the body from toxic metals such as lead and mercury, and to slow aging. It is also used orally to increase beneficial flora in the gastrointestinal tract in order to improve digestion, and to help treat ulcers, colitis, Crohn's disease, and diverticulosis. Chlorella is also promoted for the prevention of stress-induced ulcers; treatment of constipation, bad breath, and hypertension; as an antioxidant; to reduce serum cholesterol; to increase energy; to detoxify the body; and as a source of magnesium to promote mental health, relieve premenstrual syndrome (PMS), and reduce asthma attacks. It is also used orally for fibromyalgia.
Topically, chlorella is used for treating ulcers, postirradiation dermatitis, vulval leukoplakias, and trichomoniasis.

Safety

POSSIBLY SAFE ...when used orally and appropriately short-term. Chlorella appears to be safe for up to 2 months (5890,10388).

There is insufficient reliable information about the safety of chlorella for its other uses.

PREGNANCY AND LACTATION: Insufficient reliable information available; avoid using.

Effectiveness

INSUFFICIENT RELIABLE EVIDENCE to RATE

Fibromyalgia. Preliminary clinical research shows subjective improvements in general symptom and pain scores in people with fibromyalgia taking chlorella tablets plus a liquid extract containing malic acid daily for two months (5890).

Glioma. Early research suggests chlorella tablets plus chlorella liquid extract might help people with glioma better tolerate chemotherapy and radiotherapy, possibly by improving immune system function; however, there appears to be no effect on tumor progression or survival (6804).

More evidence is needed to rate chlorella for these uses.

Mechanism of Action

Chlorella is a single-celled, freshwater green alga, also referred to as seaweed (5850). The whole plant is processed for medicinal use and is a rich source of chlorophyll. The cell wall must be broken down before it can be digested by humans (5890). Chlorella contains significant amounts of protein, lipid, carbohydrates, fiber, nucleic acids, vitamins, and minerals (5890). There is some evidence that consuming chlorella can increase serum vitamin B12 levels (5848). However, it has been suggested that the vitamin B12 found in chlorella might be in an inactive form which can raise serum levels without contributing biological activity (5849).

In vitro and animal research indicates that substances in chlorella might have antitumor, antibacterial, antifungal, and antiviral activities (5850,5891,5892,10388).

Chlorella might stimulate the immune system by increasing the number and activity of macrophages and polymorphonuclear leukocytes. It might also stimulate interleukin production (10388). A polysaccharide from the cell wall of chlorella might also induce production of interferon (6804). However, chlorella doesn't seem to affect antibody response to influenza vaccine in humans (10388). The photosensitizing components in chlorella have been identified as pheophorbides (5847).

Adverse Reactions

Orally, chlorella can cause diarrhea, abdominal cramping, flatus, and nausea, especially during the first week of treatment (5890,6804). It can also cause fatigue (10388). Green discoloration of the feces has also been reported, presumably due to the chlorophyll content of chlorella (6804). Allergic reactions, including asthma and anaphylaxis, have been reported in people taking chlorella, and in those preparing chlorella tablets (3900,5847). Photosensitivity reactions have also occurred following ingestion of chlorella (3900,5852). Rarely, chlorella and other algae causes infections in humans (11011).

Interactions with Herbs & Other Dietary Supplements

None known.

Interactions with Drugs

WARFARIN (Coumadin): Chlorella contains significant amounts of vitamin K, which may inhibit the anticoagulant activity of warfarin (Coumadin) and related drugs (3900).

Interactions with Foods

None known.

Interactions with Lab Tests

None known.

Interactions with Diseases or Conditions

ALLERGIES, INCLUDING IODINE SENSITIVITY: Chlorella has been associated with significant allergic reactions (5847), and is also reported to contain iodine (10275).

IMMUNODEFICIENCY: Chlorella preparations might cause pathogenic colonization, particularly in patients who are immunocompromised (11011). Use with caution in these patients.

Dosage and Administration

ORAL: For fibromyalgia, doses of 10 gram tablets plus 100 mL liquid extract (Wakasa Gold) daily have been used (5890). For improving tolerability of chemotherapy and radiotherapy in people with brain tumors, chlorella tablets, up to 20 grams daily, plus 150 mL liquid extract daily have been used (6804).

TOPICAL: No typical dosage.

Comments
Since chlorella is a naturally occurring organism, its content can vary with growing, harvesting, and processing conditions. By varying the cultivation conditions, it has been reported that a dried preparation of chlorella can contain from 7-88% protein, 6-38% carbohydrate, and 7-75% fat (5851). Most chlorella sold in the United States is cultivated in Japan or Taiwan (3900). Processing of the chlorella cultures includes destroying the cell walls, dehydration and sterilization (5851). Commercially available products include tablets and liquid extracts. The latter contains "chlorella growth factor", which is described as a water soluble extract of chlorella containing amino acids, peptides, proteins, vitamins, sugars, and nucleic acids (5890).

CHLOROPHYLL

Also Known As
None.
CAUTION: See separate listing for Chlorophyllin.

Scientific Names
Chlorophyll a; Chlorophyll b; Chlorophyll c; Chlorophyll d.

People Use This For
Orally, chlorophyll is used for reducing colostomy odor, bad breath, constipation, detoxification, and wound healing.
Intravenously, chlorophyll is used for treating chronic relapsing pancreatitis.

Safety
LIKELY SAFE ...when used orally (1324).
POSSIBLY SAFE ...when used intravenously (1324).
PREGNANCY AND LACTATION: Insufficient reliable information available.

Effectiveness
POSSIBLY EFFECTIVE

Pancreatitis. Administering chlorophyll intravenously seems to help reduce pain and other symptoms in patients with chronic relapsing pancreatitis (1324).

POSSIBLY INEFFECTIVE

Colostomy odor. Taking chlorophyll orally doesn't seem to reduce colostomy odor (1322).

There is insufficient reliable information available about the effectiveness of chlorophyll for its other uses.

Mechanism of Action
Chlorophyll contains components that are activated by light. It appears that chlorophyll can cause a photosensitization when it is taken internally (1326). Derivatives of chlorophyll which have been extracted from silkworm droppings seem to have a cytotoxic effect on certain cancer cells (1314,1315). Certain carotenoids such as beta-carotene and canthaxanthin seem to prevent or lessen the photosensitivity that results from taking chlorophyll (1326).

Adverse Reactions
None reported.

Interactions with Herbs & Other Dietary Supplements
CAROTENOIDS (Beta-carotene, Canthaxanthin): Theoretically, carotenoids may prevent or lessen chlorophyll-induced photosensitivity (1326).

Interactions with Drugs
PHOTOSENSITIZING DRUGS: Theoretically, concomitant use may exacerbate effects (1326).

Interactions with Foods
None known.

Interactions with Lab Tests
None known.

Interactions with Diseases or Conditions
None known.

Dosage and Administration

ORAL: No typical dosage.
INTRAVENOUS: For pancreatitis an infusion of 5-20 mg water soluble chlorophyll-a per day for 1-2 weeks, followed by intermittent administration has been used (1324).

Comments

Avoid confusion with chlorophyllin, a semisynthetic derivative of chlorophyll. Commercial sources of chlorophyll include alfalfa (Medicago sativa) and silk worm droppings (11). Chlorophyll is a group of related green pigments found in photosynthetic organisms including Chlorophyll a (found in higher plants, red and green algae), Chlorophyll b (found in higher plants), Chlorophyll c (found in brown algae, diatoms, flagellates), and Chlorophyll d (found in red algae).

CHLOROPHYLLIN

Also Known As

None.
CAUTION: See separate listing for Chlorophyll.

Scientific Names

Chlorophyllin.

People Use This For

Orally, chlorophyllin is used for controlling body, fecal, and urine odors, and for treating constipation and flatulence.

Safety

POSSIBLY SAFE ...when used orally (1321,1323).
PREGNANCY AND LACTATION: Insufficient reliable information available; avoid using.

Effectiveness

POSSIBLY INEFFECTIVE

Urinary odor. Taking chlorophyllin orally doesn't seem to be effective for controlling urinary odor in incontinent geriatric patients with indwelling catheters (1323).

INSUFFICIENT RELIABLE EVIDENCE to RATE

Body and fecal odor. Preliminary evidence suggests that taking chlorophyllin orally might help reduce body and fecal odors in geriatric patients (1321).
Constipation. Preliminary evidence suggests that taking chlorophyllin orally might reduce constipation in geriatric patients (1321).
Flatulence. Preliminary evidence suggests that taking chlorophyllin orally might reduce flatulence in geriatric patients (1321).
More evidence is needed to rate chlorophyllin for these uses.

Mechanism of Action

Chlorophyllin has antimutagenic activity in human lymphocytes (in vitro) (1312). Mechanisms may include reduced carcinogen DNA-binding (in fish) (1309), reduced chromosome damage (in vitro) (1311), and reduced carcinogen-induced cell transformation (in vitro) (1307). Bacteriologic studies failed to confirm reports of antibacterial properties for chlorophyllin (1321).

Adverse Reactions

None reported.

Interactions with Herbs & Other Dietary Supplements

None known.

Interactions with Drugs

None known.

Interactions with Foods

None known.

Interactions with Lab Tests

None known.

Interactions with Diseases or Conditions

None known.

Dosage and Administration

ORAL: Typically, 100 mg per day is used for controlling urinary odor in incontinent geriatric patients with indwelling catheters (1323).

Comments

Avoid confusion with Chlorophyll.

CHOLINE

Also Known As

Choline Bitartrate, Choline Chloride, Intrachol, Lipotropic Factor, Methylated Phosphatidylethanolamine.
CAUTION: See separate listings for Alpha-GPC, Lecithin, and Phosphatidylcholine.

Scientific Names

Trimethylethanolamine; (beta-hydroxyethyl) trimethylammonium hydroxide.

People Use This For

Orally, choline is used for liver disease including chronic hepatitis and cirrhosis, hypercholesterolemia, depression, memory loss, Alzheimer's disease and dementia, and schizophrenia. It is also used orally for body building, delaying fatigue in endurance sports, preventing neural tube defects, Huntington's chorea, Tourette's disease, cerebellar ataxia, complex partial seizures, asthma, and as a supplement in infant formulas.
Intravenously, choline has orphan drug status for TPN-associated hepatic steatosis.

Safety

LIKELY SAFE ...when used orally and appropriately (3094). ...when used intravenously and appropriately (5173,5174).
POSSIBLY UNSAFE ...when used orally in excessive doses. High doses can increase the risk of adverse effects. Tell patients not to exceed 3.5 grams per day for adults over age 18 (3094).
CHILDREN: LIKELY SAFE ...when used orally and appropriately (3094). POSSIBLY UNSAFE ...when used orally in excessive doses. High doses can increase the risk of adverse effects. Tell patients not to exceed 1 gram daily for children 1-8 years of age, 2 grams daily for children 9-13 years of age, and 3 grams daily for children 14-18 years of age (3094).
PREGNANCY AND LACTATION: LIKELY SAFE ...when used orally and appropriately. Doses up to 3 grams daily for pregnant and lactating women up to 18 years of age, and 3.5 grams daily for women 19 years and older are not likely to cause adverse effects (3094). There is insufficient reliable information about the safety of choline used in higher doses in pregnant or lactating women.

Effectiveness

LIKELY EFFECTIVE

Hepatic steatosis. Administering choline intravenously is effective for treating total parenteral nutrition-associated hepatic steatosis in patients with choline deficiency (5163,5174).

POSSIBLY EFFECTIVE

Asthma. Taking choline orally seems to decrease the severity of symptoms, number of symptomatic days (5165), and the need to use bronchodilators (5166) in patients with asthma. There is some evidence that higher doses of 3 grams daily might be more effective than lower doses of 1.5 grams daily (5165).

Neural tube birth defects. Epidemiological evidence suggests that women who have a high dietary choline intake around the time of conception have a lower risk of having offspring with a neural tube defect, compared to women with lower intake (13134).

POSSIBLY INEFFECTIVE

Alzheimer's disease. Taking choline orally does not reduce symptoms of Alzheimer's disease (5170).

Athletic performance. Taking choline orally doesn't seem to be effective for delaying fatigue in endurance sports (5164).

Cerebellar ataxia. Taking choline orally doesn't seem to reduce cerebellar ataxia (5161,5173).

LIKELY INEFFECTIVE

Age-related memory impairment. Taking choline orally does not improve memory in elderly people with memory loss (5170).

Schizophrenia. Taking choline orally does not reduce symptoms of schizophrenia (5171,5172).

INSUFFICIENT RELIABLE EVIDENCE to RATE

Complex partial seizures. There is anecdotal evidence that high doses of choline, 12-16 grams daily, might be helpful for some patients with complex partial seizures (5162).
More evidence is needed to rate choline for this use.

Mechanism of Action

Choline has traditionally been considered a B vitamin. However, this is controversial because choline can be synthesized by the human body (5139). Choline is produced in the liver via the methylation of phosphatidylethanolamine. S-adenosylmethionine is the methyl donor for this reaction (1949).

Choline is also readily available in the typical diet (5139). Foods that supply large amounts of choline are liver, muscle meats, fish, nuts, beans, peas, eggs, and others. A typical diet provides 200-600 mg daily.

Deficiency of choline is uncommon except in people receiving long-term total parenteral nutrition (TPN) (5139,5174). Choline deficiency related to long-term TPN use can result in fatty liver and liver damage. Adding choline to the TPN solution usually resolves liver abnormalities (1949). This indicates that dietary choline is required in addition to the choline normally synthesized by the body (5139,5174).

Human breast milk contains choline. Choline is added to infant formulas from cow milk and soy (3094).

Choline, or its metabolites, are needed for the synthesis of cell membrane phospholipids and as methyl donors for the synthesis of other compounds (1949). For example, the choline metabolite betaine is a methyl donor during the methylation of homocysteine to form methionine (1949). Choline concentrates in nervous tissue (272). There is preliminary evidence that supplemental choline during pregnancy and lactation probably affects the birth, death, and migration of cells in the hippocampus during fetal brain development and possibly changes the distribution and morphology of neurons responsible for memory function in the brain (1949). Choline also seems to play a role in the development of neural tube defects (13134).

Some researchers are interested in choline for Alzheimer's disease because it is a precursor to acetylcholine. However, there is evidence that oral choline does not affect concentrations of choline metabolites such as acetylcholine in the brain. This might be the reason oral choline does not seem to be effective for neurodegenerative disorders of cholinergic transmission (5175). In asthma, choline is thought to have anti-inflammatory effects by lowering lipophosphatidylcholine levels (5165). Some researchers speculate that choline might also have a role in cancer prevention (5178,5179,5180). In animal models, long-term withdrawal of choline from the diet can cause hepatocarcinoma (5178,5180).

Adverse Reactions

Orally, adverse reactions can include sweating, a fishy body odor, gastrointestinal distress, and vomiting (5160,5163). Large doses can cause diarrhea (272).

Interactions with Herbs & Other Dietary Supplements

None known.

Interactions with Drugs

None known.

Interactions with Foods

None known.

Interactions with Lab Tests

None known.

Interactions with Diseases or Conditions

None known.

Dosage and Administration

ORAL: For asthma, 500-1000 mg three times daily has been used (5165,5166). An average diet supplies 200-600 mg of choline daily (272). Adequate Intake (AI), as established by the Food and Nutrition Board of the National Institute of Medicine, for adults is 550 mg per day for males and lactating women; females, 425 mg per day; pregnant females, 450 mg per day (3094). For children 1-3 years the AI is 200 mg per day; 4-8 years, 250 mg per day; 9-13 years, 375 mg per day (3094); for infants less than 6 months, 125 mg per day; infants 7-12 months, 150 mg per day (3094).

Daily Upper Intake Levels (UL, the highest level of intake that is likely to pose no risk of adverse effects) for choline are 1 gram daily for children 1-8 years, 2 grams for children 9-13 years, 3 grams for children 14-18 years, and 3.5 grams for adults over 18 years of age (3094).

Comments

Many people think choline, phosphatidylcholine, and lecithin are synonymous. Choline is a component of phosphatidylcholine, which is a component of lecithin. Although closely related, these terms are not synonymous. See separate listings for Phosphatidylcholine and Lecithin.

CHONDROITIN SULFATE

Also Known As

CDS, Chondroitin Polysulfate, CPS, CS, CSA, CSC, GAG, Galactosaminoglucuronoglycan Sulfate.

Scientific Names

Chondroitin 4-sulfate; chondroitin 4- and 6-sulfate.

People Use This For

Orally, chondroitin sulfate is used for osteoarthritis. Chondroitin sulfate is frequently used in combination with other products, including manganese ascorbate, glucosamine sulfate, glucosamine hydrochloride, or N-acetyl glucosamine for osteoarthritis. Chondroitin sulfate is also used orally for ischemic heart disease, osteoporosis, and hyperlipidemia. Chondroitin is also used in a complex with iron for treating iron-deficiency anemia.

Intramuscularly, chondroitin sulfate is used for osteoarthritis.

Topically, chondroitin sulfate is used for keratoconjunctivitis sicca (dry eyes), as a viscoelastic agent in cataract surgery, and as a medium for preservation of corneas used for transplantation. Chondroitin sulfate is also used topically in combination with other products for osteoarthritis.

Safety

LIKELY SAFE ...when used orally and appropriately. Chondroitin sulfate has been used safely in studies lasting from 2 months to 6 years (1342,1955,1970,1971,1972,2533). However, since chondroitin is often derived from bovine cartilage there is some concern about contamination with diseased animal parts (1825). So far, there are no reports of disease transmission to humans due to use of contaminated chondroitin preparations.

...when used topically and appropriately as an ophthalmic product, which is an FDA-approved, prescription-only product that also contains sodium hyaluronate (Viscoat).

POSSIBLY SAFE ...when used intramuscularly (10149). ...when used topically and appropriately short-term. Chondroitin in combination with glucosamine, shark cartilage, and camphor appears to be safe when applied topically on an as-needed basis for up to eight weeks (10327).

PREGNANCY AND LACTATION: Insufficient reliable information available; avoid using.

Effectiveness

LIKELY EFFECTIVE

Eye surgery. Applying chondroitin sulfate topically, in combination with sodium hyaluronate, to the eye is effective as a surgical aid in cataract extraction or lens implantation. A combination product containing chondroitin sulfate and sodium hyaluronate (Viscoat) is an FDA-approved, prescription ophthalmic product (266).

Osteoarthritis. Taking chondroitin sulfate orally seems to relieve symptoms of osteoarthritis. Treatment with chondroitin sulfate for 2-4 months is usually required before significant improvement is experienced (1342). Chondroitin doesn't seem to prevent osteoarthritis, but might help slow progression of established disease. Adding chondroitin sulfate to conventional analgesics or nonsteroidal anti-inflammatory drugs (NSAIDs) is significantly more effective than analgesics or NSAIDs alone for reducing pain and improving functionality indices in patients with osteoarthritis of the hip and knee. Some evidence suggests that chondroitin may allow dosage lowering or discontinuation of NSAIDs after 6 to 8 weeks (322,323,324,1342,1970,1971,1972,2533,4237,7256,10149,10150,10310).

Intermittent treatment with chondroitin might also be effective. Patients who take chondroitin sulfate 800 mg/day for 3 months followed by 3 months of no treatment and then again for 3 months seem to have significantly reduced symptoms. Chondroitin dosed intermittently also seems to prevent joint space narrowing compared to placebo. This suggests that intermittent dosing can also slow disease progression (12148).

Chondroitin sulfate combined with glucosamine HCl and manganese ascorbate (Cosamin-DS) is also effective, but it is not known if this combination is more effective than the individual components alone (4237).

A topical preparation of chondroitin sulfate in combination with glucosamine sulfate, shark cartilage, and camphor also seems to reduce arthritis symptoms. But any symptom relief is most likely due to the counterirritant effect of camphor and not the other ingredients (10327). There's no research showing that chondroitin is absorbed topically. Don't recommend topical chondroitin products.

POSSIBLY EFFECTIVE

Dry eyes. Administering chondroitin sulfate as an ophthalmic preparation seems to lessen dry eyes (1974).

INSUFFICIENT RELIABLE EVIDENCE to RATE

Myocardial infarction (MI). There is some preliminary evidence that oral chondroitin sulfate might lower the risk of MI; or reduce the recurrence of MI in people who have previously had a MI or who have unstable angina (1955,8126). More evidence is needed to rate chondroitin sulfate for this use.

Mechanism of Action

Chondroitin sulfate belongs to a class of very large molecules called glucosaminoglycans (GAGs), which are made up of glucuronic acid and galactosamine. Chondroitin is manufactured from natural sources, such as shark and bovine cartilage. Pure chondroitin is a relatively large molecule, weighing about 16,900 daltons. The species or tissue of origin, and the extraction method used, can affect the size of the molecule (8128). People use chondroitin for osteoarthritis because it is endogenously found in cartilaginous tissues of most mammals and serves as a substrate for the formation of the joint matrix structure (1972,1973,6738). There is some evidence that chondroitin sulfate protects cartilage against degradation by inhibiting the action of the enzyme leukocyte elastase, by decreasing the migration of polymorphonuclear leukocytes, and by increasing the synthesis of proteoglycans and hyaluronic acid (6738,7256). Some researchers think chondroitin might have cardiovascular applications due to potential antiatherogenic properties; laboratory studies suggest that chondroitin might protect against atherosclerosis (1955,8125).

Chondroitin might be useful in cancer monitoring. There is evidence that measurements of endogenous chondroitin sulfate in the peritumoral stromal tissue of the prostate can be a useful biomarker in the disease progression of prostate cancer. The concentration of chondroitin sulfate is increased in the prostate tissue of men with prostate cancer when compared to tissue samples of cancer-free men. When used with the Gleason score and the prostate-specific antigen (PSA) level, the peritumoral chondroitin sulfate measurement can allow practitioners to more accurately assess the progression of prostate cancer (8962).

Preliminary evidence suggests that chondroitin or other GAGs might prevent calcium oxalate crystallization in the urinary tract (8127). Since chondroitin is a minor component, approximately 4%, of the low molecular weight heparinoid mixture, danaparoid (Orgaran), some concern has been expressed about possible anticoagulant activity of chondroitin sulfate. However, significant hematological changes have not been found in studies (760).

Early evidence suggesting that chondroitin is not absorbed orally (4202,10315) has been refuted by more recent studies. Studies show that people absorb 8-18% of orally administered chondroitin (3242,4203,4205,4237). Lower molecular weight derivatives of chondroitin formed in the gastrointestinal tract are more readily absorbed and might also contribute to the pharmacological activity of orally administered chondroitin (3242).

Early evidence suggesting chondroitin might show promise as an HIV therapy adjunct has been refuted. More recent laboratory information suggests that chondroitin does not have anti-HIV activity (1263,1335,8662). However, preliminary research suggests that the chemically oversulfated form of chondroitin has activity against HIV, herpes simplex virus, and human cytomegalovirus (10616).

Adverse Reactions

Orally, chondroitin sulfate is usually well-tolerated. Some patients can have epigastric pain and nausea. Diarrhea, constipation, eyelid edema, lower limb edema, alopecia, and extrasystoles have also been reported in clinical trials (322,323,324,1342,1970,1971,1972,2533,4237,7256,10149,10150,10310), but it's not known if chondroitin sulfate is the cause of these adverse events.

Concern has been expressed about possible anticoagulant activity of chondroitin sulfate. However, hematological changes have not occurred in patients taking chondroitin sulfate in clinical trials (760).

Since chondroitin is usually produced from bovine cartilage, typically the trachea, there is some concern about the potential risk of contamination with diseased animals and transmission of bovine spongiform encephalopathy (BSE, mad cow disease) and other diseases. Although bovine trachea tissue does not seem to carry a high risk of BSE disease infectivity, in some cases manufacturing methods might lead to contamination with other diseased animal tissues. So far there are no reports of BSE or other disease transmission to humans from dietary supplements containing animal materials and the risk of potential disease transmission is thought to be low.

Interactions with Herbs & Other Dietary Supplements

None known.

Interactions with Drugs

WARFARIN (Coumadin): There is concern that high-dose chondroitin sulfate (2400 mg per day) combined with high-dose glucosamine (3000 mg per day) may enhance the effects of warfarin (Coumadin) as measured by the INR (11389). Chondroitin is a small component of a heparinoid and might have weak anticoagulant activity. Glucosamine is also a small component of heparin, but it does not seem to have anticoagulant activity. Interactions with warfarin have not been reported at recommended dosages of chondroitin or glucosamine.

Interactions with Foods

None known.

Interactions with Lab Tests

ANTI-FACTOR Xa: Theoretically, because chondroitin is a component of danaparoid, chondroitin sulfate administered by injection might increase the anti-factor Xa level and test results. No significant hematological changes were noted in a group of patients during six months of oral chondroitin therapy (760).

INTERNATIONAL NORMALIZED RATIO (INR), PROTHROMBIN TIME (PT): High dose chondroitin sulfate (2400 mg per day), combined with high dose glucosamine (3000 mg per day), may increase the INR in patients anticoagulated with warfarin (Coumadin). There is one case report of an increased INR associated with concomitant use of warfarin a glucosamine-chondroitin supplement that was taken above recommended dosages (11389).

Interactions with Diseases or Conditions

ASTHMA: Chondroitin might exacerbate asthma possibly by an unidentified allergic mechanism. Use chondroitin cautiously in patients with asthma (10002).

COAGULATION DISORDERS: Theoretically, parenterally administered chondroitin sulfate might affect coagulation and increase the risk of bleeding when used in patients with clotting disorders; avoid use.

PROSTATE CANCER: Preliminary clinical research suggests that chondroitin may cause the spread or recurrence of prostate cancer (8962). The chondroitin sulfate proteoglycan, versican, seems to facilitate invasion of cancer cells into the prostate stroma (11761). This effect has not been shown with supplemental chondroitin sulfate. But until more is known, advise men with prostate cancer or those at increased risk for prostate cancer to avoid chondroitin.

Dosage and Administration

ORAL: For osteoarthritis, the typical dose of chondroitin sulfate is 200-400 mg two to three times daily (1970,1971,1972,4237,10149) or 1000-1200 mg as a single daily dose (1971,7256). Intermittent dosing also seems to be effective. One study has used 800 mg/day for 3 months followed by 3 months of no treatment, and then 3 months of treatment again (12148).

For prevention of recurrent myocardial infarction (MI), 10 grams daily in 3 divided doses for 3 months, followed by 1.5 grams in 3 divided doses as maintenance therapy has been used (1955).

TOPICAL: For osteoarthritis, topical administration of a cream containing 50 mg/g of chondroitin sulfate, 30 mg/g of glucosamine sulfate, 140 mg/g of shark cartilage, and 32 mg/g of camphor has been used as needed for sore joints for up to 8 weeks (10327).

INTRAMUSCULAR: For osteoarthritis, chondroitin polysulfate 50 mg twice weekly for 8 weeks every 4 months has been used (10149). Parenteral chondroitin sulfate products are not available in the US.

Comments

Although chondroitin sulfate and glucosamine sulfate are frequently marketed together in combination products (760), there is no evidence that the combination has greater benefit than either product alone. There is great variability among chondroitin and chondroitin plus glucosamine products. Actual content versus label claim varies from 0 to 115%. Low-cost chondroitin products (less than $1 per 1200 mg chondroitin) seem to contain little chondroitin, but some higher-priced products may also contain less chondroitin than claimed (8128).

The National Institutes of Health (NIH) is sponsoring a clinical trial of chondroitin sulfate and glucosamine sulfate. The 24-week, parallel group, double-blind RCT includes five separate treatment arms, in which patients will ingest: placebo, glucosamine sulfate 500 mg three times per day, chondroitin 400 mg three times per day, a combination of glucosamine sulfate and chondroitin, or celecoxib (Celebrex) (11012).

Tell patients to look out for chondroitin plus glucosamine combination products that also contain manganese (e.g., Cosamin-DS). Remind patients to adhere to product directions. When taken at doses slightly higher than the recommended dose, these products can sometimes supply greater than the tolerable upper limit (UL) for manganese of 11 mg per day. Ingestion of more than 11 mg per day of manganese might cause significant central nervous system toxicity (7135).

CHROMIUM

Also Known As

Chromic Chloride, Chromium Acetate, Chromium Chloride, Chromium Nicotinate, Chromium Picolinate, Chromium Polynicotinate, Chromium Trichloride, Chromium Tripicolinate, Chromium III, Chromium III Picolinate, Chromium 3+, Cr III, Cr3+, Glucose Tolerance Factor-Cr, GTF, GTF-Cr, Trivalent Chromium.

Scientific Names

Chromium; Cr; atomic number 24.

People Use This For

Orally, chromium is used for improving glycemic control in type 1 and 2 diabetes, impaired glucose tolerance (prediabetes), corticosteroid-induced hyperglycemia and reactive hypoglycemia, for hypercholesterolemia, and for increasing high-density lipoprotein (HDL) cholesterol levels in patients taking beta-blockers.
It is also used orally for weight loss, to increase muscle mass and fat-free mass, and decrease body fat.
Chromium is also used orally to enhance athletic performance, to increase energy and vigor, and to treat dysthymic disorder (a mild form of depression) and atypical depression.
Intravenously, chromium is used as a supplement in total parenteral nutrition (TPN).

Safety

LIKELY SAFE ...when used orally and appropriately. Chromium is safe in amounts found in foods or supplemental amounts not exceeding adequate intake (AI) levels. The AI for chromium is different based on gender and age. For men aged 14 to 50, the AI is 35 mcg per day. For men aged 51 and older, the AI is 30 mcg. For women aged 19 to 50 years, the AI is 25 mcg per day. For women aged 51 and older, the AI is 20 mcg (7135).
POSSIBLY SAFE ...when used orally and appropriately, short-term in amounts greater than adequate intake (AI) levels. Short-term, chromium picolinate has been safely used in doses up to 1000 mcg per day (1934,6867,7135,7137); however, there is insufficient information to establish safe and tolerable upper intake levels (7135). There is also some concern that long-term supplemental use may not be safe due to potential mutagenic effects (6863,6869).
Until more is known, tell patients not to take chromium supplements long-term.
CHILDREN: LIKELY SAFE ...when used orally and appropriately. Chromium is safe in amounts not exceeding the adequate intake (AI) levels (7135). For infants 0 to 6 months, the AI is 0.2 mcg per day; 7 to 12 months, 5.5 mcg. For children 1 to 3 years, the AI is 11 mcg; 4 to 8 years, 15 mcg. For boys 9 to 13 years, the AI is 25 mcg. For girls 9 to 13 years, the AI is 21 mcg; 14 to 18 years, 24 mcg. There is insufficient reliable information available about the safety of chromium in higher amounts when used in children.
PREGNANCY: LIKELY SAFE ...when used orally and appropriately. Chromium is safe in amounts not exceeding adequate intake (AI) levels. The AI for pregnant women aged 14 to 18 years is 29 mcg per day.
For pregnant women aged 19 to 50 years, it is 30 mcg per day (7135). POSSIBLY SAFE ...when used orally in amounts exceeding the adequate intake (AI) levels. There is some evidence that pregnant patients with gestational diabetes can safely use chromium in doses of 4-8 mcg per kilogram (1953); however, patients should not take chromium supplements during pregnancy without medical supervision.
LACTATION: LIKELY SAFE ...when used orally and appropriately. Chromium is safe in amounts not exceeding adequate intake (AI) levels. The AI for lactating women aged 14 to 18 years is 44 mcg per day.
For lactating women aged 19 to 50 years it is 45 mcg per day (7135). Chromium supplements do not seem to increase normal chromium concentration in human breast milk (1937). There is insufficient reliable information available about the safety of chromium in higher amounts when used in breast-feeding women.

Effectiveness

POSSIBLY EFFECTIVE

Beta blocker-induced dyslipidemia. Taking chromium 600 mcg daily for 2 months seems to increase high-density lipoprotein (HDL) levels by 16% in men who take beta-blockers (5040).
Diabetes. There is some evidence that taking chromium picolinate orally can decrease fasting blood glucose and insulin levels, and decrease glycosylated hemoglobin (HbA1c) in people with type 2 diabetes (6862,6867,7137). Higher doses might be more effective and work more quickly. Taking 500 mcg twice daily significantly decreases HbA1c after 2 months of treatment. Taking 100 mcg twice daily can take up to 4 months to decrease HbA1c levels. Higher doses of 200 mcg three times daily or 500 mcg twice daily also seem to reduce triglyceride and total serum cholesterol levels after 2 to 4 months of treatment. This suggests that chromium might also be beneficial for patients with metabolic syndrome (syndrome X) (1934,6867). But there is speculation that chromium supplements might only help patients with low chromium levels. It doesn't seem to help all patients with type 2 diabetes (8927). It only seems to have a blood glucose-lowering effect in 40% to 80% of people with elevated blood glucose (6858). Chromium levels are sometimes below normal in patients with diabetes (7058).
Epidemiological research links lower toenail chromium levels to diabetes and cardiovascular disease, but there is no clinical evidence to suggest that chromium supplements can lower disease risk (11908). There is preliminary evidence that chromium picolinate might also have the same benefits in patients with type 1 diabetes (1935) and in patients who have diabetes secondary to corticosteroid use (5039). Very preliminary clinical research suggests that a combination of biotin and chromium (Diachrome) might lower hemoglobin A1c levels in patients with type 2 diabetes (12385,12390). However, there's no reliable research to suggest that biotin plus chromium is any more effective that chromium alone.
There isn't enough evidence to recommend chromium for all diabetes patients. Consider trial use in interested patients to see if it helps. Use chromium picolinate preparations; chromium chloride may not be as effective (7060). Remind patients that chromium is not an alternative to conventional medicines and should not be used in place of conventional treatments.
Hypoglycemia. Taking chromium orally seems to help prevent reactive hypoglycemia. Treatment for 3 months with chromium chloride 200 mg daily seems to improve symptoms and increase blood glucose levels in patients with reactive hypoglycemia following an oral glucose load (6859).

POSSIBLY INEFFECTIVE

Athletic conditioning. Taking chromium orally doesn't seem to enhance body building, strength, or lean body mass. There is some evidence that suggests taking chromium can increase weight loss, body fat loss, and lean body mass in people taking chromium picolinate 200-400 mcg per day in conjunction with resistance training (6860,6861,6868). But the results of these studies are unreliable due to questionable methods (6861). More reliable studies show that adding chromium picolinate or chloride 177-200 mcg daily to a weight-training program has no additional beneficial effect on body composition (6861,6862).

Imparied glucose tolerance (Prediabetes). Some evidence suggests that prediabetes patients with impaired glucose tolerance do not have improved glucose tolerance after taking chromium picolinate 400 mcg twice daily for 3 months (13053).

INSUFFICIENT RELIABLE EVIDENCE to RATE

Atypical depression. Preliminary clinical research suggests chromium picolinate might help atypical depression (10309).

Dysthymia. There is some preliminary evidence that chromium might improve the response to antidepressants in people with dysthymic disorder (a mild form of depression). Chromium picolinate or chromium polynicotinate 200 mcg once or twice daily appears to improve mood in patients who have only a partial response to antidepressants such as sertraline or nortriptyline (2659).

Obesity. Taking chromium picolinate orally might produce modest weight loss of about 1.1 kg compared to placebo over 72-90 days (11962). But not all studies have found this benefit (6860).

More evidence is needed to rate chromium for these uses.

Mechanism of Action

Chromium is an essential trace element. The activity of chromium depends on its valance state. Metallic chromium, or chromium 0, has no activity. The other two common forms, chromium III (Cr III) and chromium VI (Cr VI), have different activities. Cr VI is typically used in chemical and welding industries and is carcinogenic to humans. Cr III is the form found in foods and supplements.

Chromium is sometimes referred to as glucose tolerance factor (GTF), but GTF is actually a complex of molecules found in the body that includes chromium bound to single molecules of glycine, cysteine, glutamic acid, and two molecules of nicotinic acid. Chromium is thought to be the active component of the complex. Some dietary sources of chromium include canned foods (due to chromium leaching from the can), meats and animal fats, fish, brown sugar, coffee, tea, some spices, calf liver, whole wheat bread, rye bread, and brewer's yeast (7061).

Symptomatic chromium deficiency is rare. When it does occur, it is most often due to malnutrition, pregnancy, stress, or long-term use of chromium deficient total parenteral nutrition (TPN) (6863). Although not yet confirmed, some researchers suspect that tissue levels of chromium might decline with age (6863). People with diabetes may also have lower chromium levels (7058,11907,11908). Low chromium levels are associated with impaired glucose, insulin, and lipid metabolism, and resultant increased cardiovascular risk (11907).

Some athletes might also be at risk for low chromium levels since strenuous aerobic exercise seems to increase urinary excretion of chromium (6860,6861). However, exercise-induced losses seem to be less in those who regularly exercise (6862). People who strength train seem to have increased absorption of chromium (7136). It is difficult to measure chromium status to determine who might require supplementation. Blood chromium levels are not in equilibrium with chromium stores and, therefore, do not provide a good indicator of chromium status (6859). However, elevated blood chromium levels may indicate excessive chromium exposure (11786). Levels in the urine and hair do not reflect overall chromium status (6867). There is no reliable method available to diagnose chromium deficiency, other than observing the outcome following supplementation in patients suspected of being deficient (3859,6869). Symptoms of chromium deficiency can include impaired insulin function and glucose tolerance, increased serum cholesterol and triglycerides, neuropathy, weight loss, decreased respiratory function, and nitrogen metabolism abnormalities (6863,6869,11786).

Discovery of the role of chromium in insulin function occurred when patients on long-term TPN developed symptoms of diabetes that did not respond to insulin, but were reversed by chromium (6869). Because of the symptoms associated with chromium deficiency, researchers have speculated that chromium supplementation might be an effective treatment for diabetes and hypercholesterolemia. There is some evidence that patients with diabetes might have lower than normal levels of chromium due to increased chromium excretion (6858). However, patients with diabetes also seem to have increased gastrointestinal absorption of chromium. It's also theorized that patients with diabetes may not be able to adequately convert chromium from the diet to a usable form in the body (6867).

Chromium seems to be transported to insulin-sensitive cells by transferrin, in response to increases in plasma insulin levels (6869). It is suspected to potentiate insulin by increasing receptor numbers and affinity, and increasing insulin binding to cells (6859,6867). In animal models, a chromium-containing peptide called chromodulin has been identified, which potentiates the actions of insulin at its receptors, including activation of receptor tyrosine kinase activity (6869). In patients with diabetes, these actions seem to translate into decreased insulin resistance, improved glucose tolerance, and lower blood glucose levels (6862). Researchers are interested in chromium for treatment of obesity and metabolic syndrome (syndrome X) due to its potential effects on lipids and body composition.

Some research suggests that chromium might also sensitize insulin-sensitive glucoreceptors in the brain, resulting in appetite suppression, activation of the sympathetic nervous system, stimulation of thermogenesis, and down-regulation of insulin secretion (6170,6860).

It is also theorized that chromium might enhance glucose utilization in the brain and stimulate norepinephrine release (2659). Preliminary clinical research suggests that chromium decreases endocrine responses to serotonin receptor stimulation, which could produce antidepressant activity (8929). Chromium is also hypothesized to increase muscle mass by increasing amino acid uptake into muscle cells via potentiation of insulin activity (6862).

Chromium supplements come in several salt forms. The most common are chromium picolinate, chromium nicotinate, chromium polynicotinate, and chromium chloride.

Chromium picolinate is a complex of chromium and picolinic acid, which is a naturally occurring metabolic derivative of tryptophan.

Chromium polynicotinate is often referred to as niacin bound chromium because it includes chromium bound to molecules of niacin.

Adding the picolinate or nicotinate salt increases absorption, retention, and accumulation of chromium compared to inorganic salts such as chromium chloride (6861,6864,9141). Some manufacturers suggest that chromium polynicotinate is better absorbed that chromium picolinate. But there is not scientific support for this.

When ingested, most chromium is excreted unabsorbed in the feces. The small percentage that is absorbed, typically 0.4% to 2.5%, is rapidly excreted in the urine (7135). Once absorbed, chromium concentrates in the kidney, heart, liver, brain, muscle, spleen, testes, epididymis, and lungs (6863).

Chromium picolinate seems to be handled differently in the body than dietary chromium (6869). There is some evidence that chromium picolinate can enter cells unchanged and then produce hydroxyl radicals when the chromium is released, which might cause DNA damage (1299,6869). This may be due to its higher solubility and lipophilicity compared with other chromium compounds (11786). The clinical significance of this potential harmful effect is not known.

Adverse Reactions

Orally, chromium in the trivalent form (Cr III) is generally well tolerated. However, some patients can experience cognitive, perceptual, and motor dysfunction at doses as low as 200-400 mcg per day of chromium picolinate (1935). Chromium picolinate has also been associated with weight gain in young women who do not exercise and in those on a weight-lifting program (1938). Some patients can also experience headaches, insomnia, sleep disturbances, irritability, and mood changes (6860). Acute chromium toxicity can cause vomiting, diarrhea, hemorrhage, and blood loss into the gastrointestinal tract resulting in cardiogenic shock (11786).

Chronic use of chromium picolinate in higher doses might cause significant adverse effects. In some cases, doses of 600-2400 mcg per day can cause anemia, thrombocytopenia, hemolysis, hepatic dysfunction, and renal failure in some patients (554); however, it is not clear if chromium is responsible for these effects. For example, chromium picolinate has been associated with chronic interstitial nephritis and acute tubular necrosis in two case reports, but contradictory laboratory evidence shows that chromium does not seem to cause kidney tissue damage even after long-term, high dose exposure (554,1951,7135).

Acute hepatitis has been reported in a patient taking chromium polynicotinate 200 mcg daily for 5 months (9141). Symptoms resolved when the product was discontinued. Two other cases of hepatotoxicity have been reported in patients who took a specific combination product (Hydroxycut) which contained chromium polynicotinate in addition to several herbs (13037).

A specific combination product (Hydroxycut) containing chromium, caffeine, and ephedra has been associated with seizures (10307). But the most likely causative agent in this case is ephedra.

Hexavalent chromium (CR VI) is 100 times more toxic than trivalent chromium. It can cause hepatic, renal, and cardiac failure (9141). Occupational inhalation of hexavalent chromium can cause ulceration of the nasal mucosa and perforation of the nasal septum, and has been associated with pneumoconiosis, allergic asthma, and increased susceptibility to respiratory tract carcinomas. Industrial hexavalent chromium is considered cytotoxic and genotoxic (6863). It penetrates the cells easily (unlike trivalent chromium) and appears to induce oxidative damage to DNA (7326).

Intravenously, chromium is associated with decreased glomerular filtration rate (GFR) in children who receive long-term chromium-containing total parenteral nutrition (TPN) (11787).

Interactions with Herbs & Other Dietary Supplements

CHROMIUM-CONTAINING HERBS: Herbs that contain chromium, such as horsetail (Equisetum arvense) and cascara (Rhamus purshiana), can increase the risk of chromium toxicity when taken chronically, or when taken with chromium supplements (9141).

IRON: Chromium competes with iron for binding to the transport protein, transferrin, and could predispose people to iron deficiency. This effect is unlikely to be clinically significant at usual supplemental doses of chromium (6861,6865,6866).

VITAMIN C: Concomitant vitamin C use might increase chromium absorption (7135).

ZINC: Theoretically, co-administration might decrease absorption of both chromium and zinc (1950).

Interactions with Drugs

INSULIN: Theoretically, concomitant use might increase the risk of hypoglycemia (1952).
NONSTEROIDAL ANTI-INFLAMMATORY DRUGS (NSAIDs): There is some evidence that NSAIDs might increase chromium levels by increasing chromium absorption and retention. Drugs that are prostaglandin inhibitors seem to increase chromium absorption and retention (7135).
Some of these drugs include ibuprofen (Advil, Motrin, Nuprin, others), indomethacin (Indocin), naproxen (Aleve, Anaprox, Naprelan, Naprosyn), piroxicam (Feldene), aspirin, and others.

Drug Influences on Nutrient Levels and Depletion

SOME DRUGS CAN AFFECT CHROMIUM LEVELS:
ANTACIDS: There is some evidence that antacids might decrease chromium levels by inhibiting absorption of chromium, but the clinical significance of this isn't clear. Increasing gastric pH seems to decrease chromium absorption due to formation of less soluble chromium salts (7135).
CORTICOSTEROIDS: Use of corticosteroids can increase urinary chromium excretion, which might lead to chromium deficiency and/or corticosteroid-induced hyperglycemia (5039).
H2-BLOCKERS: There is some evidence that H2-blockers might decrease chromium levels by inhibiting absorption of chromium, but the clinical significance of this isn't clear. Increasing gastric pH seems to decrease chromium absorption due to formation of less soluble chromium salts (7135).
The H2 blockers include cimetidine (Tagamet), ranitidine (Zantac), nizatidine (Axid), and famotidine (Pepcid).
PROTON PUMP INHIBITORS (PPIs): There is some evidence that PPIs might decrease chromium levels by inhibiting chromium absorption, but the clinical significance of this isn't clear. Increasing gastric pH might decrease chromium absorption due to formation of less soluble chromium salts (7135). PPIs include omeprazole (Prilosec), lansoprazole (Prevacid), rabeprazole (Aciphex), pantoprazole (Protonix, Pantoloc), and esomeprazole (Nexium).

Interactions with Foods

None known.

Interactions with Lab Tests

None known.

Interactions with Diseases or Conditions

BEHAVIORAL AND PSYCHIATRIC DISORDERS: Theoretically, chromium picolinate preparations might affect behavioral and psychiatric conditions. Picolinic acid in chromium picolinate preparations can alter serotonin, dopamine, and norepinephrine metabolism in the central nervous system (1935).
CHROMATE/LEATHER CONTACT ALLERGY: Oral chromium supplements can cause allergic reactions in people with chromate or leather contact allergy, including dermatitis, erythema, and scaling on the extremities (6624).
DIABETES: Chromium might lower blood glucose levels (1939); monitor closely.
LIVER DISEASE: The chromium polynicotinate form of chromium has been linked to hepatotoxicity in three cases (9141,13037). Theoretically, taking chromium polynicotinate might exacerbate symptoms in patients with existing liver disease. Advise these patients to avoid chromium polynicotinate supplements.
RENAL INSUFFICIENCY: Theoretically, chromium supplements might exacerbate renal insufficiency. There are 2 case reports of people taking chromium picolinate who developed interstitial nephritis (554,1951). Advise patients with renal dysfunction to avoid chromium supplements.

Dosage and Administration

ORAL: For lowering blood glucose and lipid levels in patients with type 2 diabetes, 200-1000 mcg daily in divided dose has been used (1934,6867). For increasing serum HDL cholesterol in men taking beta-blockers, 200 mcg three times daily has been used (5040). For corticosteroid-induced hyperglycemia or exacerbation of pre-existing diabetes, 400 mcg per day or 200 mcg three times daily has been used (5039). Chromium picolinate has been used in most studies. For preventing reactive hypoglycemia, 200 mcg daily of chromium chloride has been used (6859). For treating dysthymic disorder (mild depression), 200 mcg once or twice daily of chromium picolinate or polynicotinate has been used (2659).
Daily adequate intake (AI) levels for chromium have been established: Infants 0 to 6 months, 0.2 mcg; 7 to 12 months, 5.5 mcg; children 1 to 3 years, 11 mcg; 4 to 8 years, 15 mcg; boys 9 to 13 years, 25 mcg; men 14 to 50 years, 35 mcg; men 51 and older, 30 mcg; girls 9 to 13 years, 21 mcg; 14 to 18 years, 24 mcg; women 19 to 50 years, 25 mcg; women 51 and older, 20 mcg; pregnant women 14 to 18 years, 29 mcg; 19 to 50 years, 30 mcg; lactating women 14 to 18 years, 44 mcg; 19 to 50 years, 45 mcg. Sometimes chromium amounts are listed in micromols. The conversion factor to micrograms is: 1.92 micromol Cr = 100 mcg (6867).
INTRAVENOUS: No typical dosage.

Comments

Chromium was discovered in France in the late 1790s, but it took until the 1960s before it was recognized as being an important trace element and important for insulin function (7058).

CHRYSANTHEMUM

Also Known As
Florist's Chrysanthemum, Ju Hua, Mum.

Scientific Names
Chrysanthemum morifolium, synonyms Anthemis grandiflorum, Anthemis stipulacea, Chrysanthemum sinense, Chrysanthemum stipulaceum, Dendranthema grandiflorum, Dendranthema morifolium, Matricaria morifolia.
Family: Asteraceae/Compositae.

People Use This For
Orally, chrysanthemum is used to treat angina, hypertension, type 2 diabetes, fever, cold, headache, dizziness, and swelling.
In combination with other herbs, chrysanthemum is used orally to treat prostate cancer. In combination with licorice (Glycyrrhiza uralensis) and Panax notoginseng, it is used to treat precancerous lesions.
As a beverage, chrysanthemum is very popular as a summertime tea in southern China.

Safety
There is insufficient reliable information available about the safety of chrysanthemum.
Pregnancy and Lactation: Insufficient reliable information available; avoid using.

Effectiveness
There is insufficient reliable information available about the effectiveness of chrysanthemum.

Mechanism of Action
The dried chrysanthemum flower contains the essential oil bornol, chrysantheonon, camphor, the alkaloid stachydrine, and several glycosides. It also contains adenine, choline, B vitamins, and substances similar to vitamin A. Some evidence suggests that chrysanthemum might increase coronary vasodilatation and blood flow without increasing coronary contractility or oxygen consumption. Chrysanthemum may also have antibacterial and antipyretic effects. It may also reduce the capillary permeability induced by histamine (5545).
Preliminary information suggests the chrysanthemum product jiangtangkang used by individuals with non-insulin dependent diabetes might improve insulin sensitivity and decrease blood viscosity (5546). A preliminary trial suggests Hua-sheng-ping, a combination of chrysanthemum, licorice (Glycyrrhiza uralensis), and Panax notoginseng can reverse precancerous gastrointestinal lesions (5555). The chrysanthemum constituents chrysin and acetin-7-O-beta-D-galactopyranoside inhibit HIV replication in vitro (5545,5547).

Adverse Reactions
Chrysanthemum flowers may cause photosensitivity and contact dermatitis (5552,5553,5554,5556,5557).
Chrysanthemum flowers may cause an allergic reaction in individuals sensitive to the Asteraceae/Compositae family. Members of this family include ragweed, chrysanthemums, marigolds, daisies and many other herbs.

Interactions with Herbs & Other Dietary Supplements
None known.

Interactions with Drugs
None known.

Interactions with Foods
None known.

Interactions with Lab Tests
None known.

Interactions with Diseases or Conditions
None known.

Dosage and Administration
ORAL: To make the concentrated water extract, 300 mg of the dried chrysanthemum flower are condensed into 500 mL water. A typical dose is 25 mL three times daily or as a tea (5545).

Comments
The name chrysanthemum is from the Greek words for "gold" and "flower."

CHRYSIN

Also Known As
5,7-Chrysin, 5,7-Dihydroxyflavone, Flavone X, Flavonoid, Galangin Flavanone.
CAUTION: See separate listings for Diosmin, Hesperidin, Methoxylated Flavones, Passionflower, Quercetin, and Rutin.

Scientific Names
Chrysin.

People Use This For
Orally, chrysin is used for bodybuilding, anxiety, inflammation, gout, HIV/AIDS, impotence, baldness, and preventing cancer.

Safety
POSSIBLY SAFE ...when used orally and appropriately, short-term. Chrysin 300 mg daily seems to be safe when taken for up to 8 weeks (7514).
PREGNANCY AND LACTATION: Insufficient reliable information available; avoid using.

Effectiveness
POSSIBLY INEFFECTIVE

Athletic conditioning. Taking chrysin orally, in combination with androgen precursors, doesn't seem to be effective for enhancing resistance training in athletes. The combination of chrysin 300 mg with androstenedione, dehydroepiandrosterone (DHEA), puncture vine, indole-3-carbinole, and saw palmetto taken daily for eight weeks does not appear to increase testosterone concentrations, reduce the estrogenic effects of androstenedione, change body composition, or increase strength in response to resistance training (7514).

There is insufficient reliable information available about the effectiveness of chrysin for its other uses.

Mechanism of Action
Chrysin is a flavonoid that occurs naturally in plants such as the passionflower, silver linden, some geranium species, and in honey and bee propolis (4001,7501,7502). Athletes are interested in chrysin for bodybuilding due to its potential effect on testosterone levels. In vitro research shows that chrysin might inhibit aromatase and decrease aromatization of androstenedione and testosterone to estrogen and dihydrotestosterone (7506), but research in humans shows that chrysin does not increase testosterone levels when used in combination with androgen precursors such as androstenedione and dehydroepiandrosterone (DHEA) (7514).

Researchers are also interested in chrysin due to several potential anticancer properties. Chrysin seems to increase glucuronidation by inducing UDP-glucuronosyltransferase 1A1 (UGT1A1), which might reduce the bioavailability of dietary carcinogens (7504,8170). Chrysin might also might inhibit cytochrome P450 1A1 (CYP1A1) and 1A2 (CYP1A2), which could prevent activation of potentially carcinogenic food-derived heterocyclic aromatic amines (7503,8172).

There is also preliminary evidence that chrysin might decrease estrogen synthesis by acting as an aromatase (estrogen synthetase) inhibitor, similar to the breast cancer drugs anastrozole (Arimidex) and letrozole (Femara) (7507,7508).

Chrysin might also have antioxidant properties (7509). Chrysin appears to inhibit xanthine oxidase, suggesting potential use for preventing oxidative injury in ischemia-reperfusion and treating gout (7510).

Chrysin might have activity against the human immunodeficiency virus (HIV). It appears to block HIV transcriptional activation, possibly by blocking casein kinase II (CKII), an enzyme that seems to regulate HIV transcription (7512,8171).

There's also some evidence that chrysin might act as a sunscreen. Chrysin-fed experimental animals are protected from contact hypersensitivity induced by ultraviolet (UV) radiation (7511).

There is some preliminary evidence that chrysin can bind benzodiazepine receptors and might have some anxiolytic effects. Some researchers call it a partial benzodiazepine agonist because it does not seem to affect memory and does not have anticonvulsant, muscle relaxant, or sedative activity (4001,8165,8166,8167).

Some chrysin derivatives appear to have hypoglycemic activity, unlike chrysin, which seems to inhibit insulin release (8169).

The oral bioavailability of chrysin is low. Since it induces the enzyme UGT, specifically UGT1A1, chrysin appears to induce its own elimination (7513). Most chrysin is deactivated by presystemic intestinal as well as hepatic glucuronidation and sulfonation (8168). There is some speculation that the therapeutic usefulness of chrysin might be negligible due to limited systemic bioavailability (7502,7504,7505).

Adverse Reactions
None reported.

Interactions with Herbs & Other Dietary Supplements

ANDROSTENEDIONE: Preliminary research showed that chrysin might increase androstenedione levels and its conversion to testosterone by inhibiting aromatization of androstenedione to estrogen and dihydrotestosterone (7506). However, research in humans shows that chrysin has no effect on androstenedione metabolism and does not increase testosterone levels (7514).

Interactions with Drugs

AROMATASE INHIBITORS: Theoretically, chrysin may have an additive effect on other aromatase inhibitors such as aminoglutethimide (Cytadren), anastrozole (Arimidex), exemestane (Aromasin), and letrozole (Femara) (7507,7508).

CYTOCHROME P450 1A2 (CYP1A2) SUBSTRATES: There is some preliminary evidence that chrysin inhibits CYP1A2 isozymes (7503,8172). Theoretically, chrysin might decrease the metabolism of CYP1A2 substrates and increase serum concentrations. Some substrates of CYP1A2 include clozapine (Clozaril), cyclobenzaprine (Flexeril), fluvoxamine (Luvox), haloperidol (Haldol), imipramine (Tofranil), mexiletine (Mexitil), olanzapine (Zyprexa), pentazocine (Talwin), propranolol (Inderal), tacrine (Cognex), theophylline, zileuton (Zyflo), zolmitriptan (Zomig), and others.

GLUCURONIDATED DRUGS: There is some preliminary evidence that chrysin might induce UDP-glucuronosyltransferase 1A1 (UGT1A1) (7504,7513,8170). Theoretically, chrysin might increase the clearance of drugs that are UGT1A1 substrates, such as acetaminophen (Tylenol), estrogens (Estrace, Premarin, others) and oral contraceptives, entacapone (Comtan), irinotecan (Camptosar), and others.

Interactions with Foods

None known.

Interactions with Lab Tests

None known.

Interactions with Diseases or Conditions

None known.

Dosage and Administration

ORAL: For bodybuilding, chrysin 300 mg daily has been taken as a component of a combination product (Andro-6) that also includes androstenedione, DHEA, puncture vine (Tribulus terrestris), indole-3-carbinole, and saw palmetto (7514).

CHYMOTRYPSIN

Also Known As

A-Chymotrypsin, Chymotrypsin A, Chymotrypsin B, Quimotripsina.

Scientific Names

Alpha-chymotrypsin; chymotrypsinum.

People Use This For

Orally, chymotrypsin is used for reducing inflammation and edema associated with abscesses, ulcers, surgery or traumatic injuries; as an expectorant in asthma, bronchitis, pulmonary diseases, and sinusitis. It is used in minimizing initial rise in serum liver enzymes in burn patients, reducing liver stress, and associated degradative changes during wound repair.

Topically, chymotrypsin is used for inflammatory and infectious disorders.

As an inhalant, chymotrypsin is used for inflammatory and infectious disorders.

Intramuscularly, chymotrypsin is used to reduce inflammation and edema associated with abscesses, ulcers, surgery or traumatic injuries, and as an expectorant in asthma, bronchitis, pulmonary diseases, and sinusitis, and for inflammatory and infectious disorders.

Ophthalmically, chymotrypsin is used as an adjunct in cataract surgery to reduce trauma to the eye.

Safety

LIKELY SAFE ...when used ophthalmically, as approved by the FDA.

POSSIBLY SAFE ...when used orally for inflammation due to surgery or trauma injuries (717,718).

...when used topically for treating burns (716).

There is insufficient reliable information available about the safety of chymotrypsin for its other uses.

PREGNANCY AND LACTATION: Insufficient reliable information available; avoid using.

Effectiveness

EFFECTIVE

Cataracts. Chymotrypsin is effective when used as an adjunct in cataract surgery according to FDA-approved prescription product labeling (9,509).

POSSIBLY EFFECTIVE

Burns. There is some evidence that chymotrypsin might decrease tissue destruction in burn patients (716).

Fractures. Taking chymotrypsin orally seems to be effective for reducing inflammation and edema associated with hand fractures (717,718).

There is insufficient reliable information available about the effectiveness of chymotrypsin for its other uses.

Mechanism of Action

Chymotrypsin has ingredients that have proteolytic, anti-inflammatory, and antioxidant activities that reduce tissue destruction (715).

Adverse Reactions

Orally, anaphylactic reaction (rare) is characterized by dyspnea, urticaria, edema of the glottis or lip, shock and vascular collapse, loss of consciousness, and death (9,509). If hypersensitivity is suspected, a sensitivity test should be performed before administration (9).

Opthamalmically, chymotrypsin leads to increased intraocular pressure (9,509), corneal edema, striation, moderate uveitis (9), iridoplegia, and filamentary keratitis (509).

Interactions with Herbs & Other Dietary Supplements

None known.

Interactions with Drugs

None known.

Interactions with Foods

None known.

Interactions with Lab Tests

None known.

Interactions with Diseases or Conditions

None known.

Dosage and Administration

ORAL: For inflammation, edema and respiratory secretions, 6:1 ratio (trypsin: chymotrypsin) in a combined amount of 100,000 units USP four times daily has been used (717,718). For burns, as 6:1 ratio (trypsin:chymotrypsin) in a combined amount of 200,000 units USP four times daily for 10 days has been used (716).

INTRAMUSCULAR: For inflammation, edema and respiratory secretions: 5000 USP units one to three times daily has been used (9).

OPHTHALMIC: As an adjunct in cataract surgery, 1:5000 or 1:10,000 solution of chymotrypsin in sterile sodium chloride injection (0.9%) injected to irrigate the posterior chamber has been used (9).

TOPICAL: No typical dosage.

CIGUATERA

Also Known As

Ciguatera Poisoning.

Scientific Names

Gambierdiscus toxicus (dinoflagellate).

People Use This For

There are no medicinal uses for this product, but it may be encountered inadvertently by eating tainted fish.

Safety

UNSAFE ...when ingested. Up to 20% mortality has been reported (6).
A single bite of fish contaminated with this toxin will produce symptoms (6).
PREGNANCY: UNSAFE ...when ingested. There has been one report of a fetus being aborted during acute phase of maternal poisoning. However, no lasting adverse effects have been reported in liveborn infants (6).
LACTATION: UNSAFE ...when ingested. Ciguatera is excreted in breast milk; GI symptoms and itching reported in infants breast-fed by symptomatic mothers; infant symptoms resolved with discontinuation of breast-feeding (6).

Effectiveness

There is insufficient reliable information available about the effectiveness of ciguatera.

Mechanism of Action

The applicable part of ciguatera is the toxin. Ciguatoxin increases cell permeability to sodium, causing sustained depolarization (6). Action in humans is dependent on anti-cholinesterase activity and also to a transmitter-like cholinomimetic activity (6).

Adverse Reactions

Poisoning has many different manifestations. But in general, poisoning is characterized by abdominal cramps, nausea, vomiting, diarrhea within 1-6 hours of ingestion; itching, numbness of lips, tongue, throat, paresthesias, blurred vision, hypotension, bradycardia; reversal of hot and cold sensations, and coma (rarely). In severe cases, shock, muscular paralysis, and death are possible (6). GI symptoms usually resolve within 24 hours. Muscle weakness/numbness may last weeks to months (6). Tumultuous fetal movements and intermittent fetal shivering have been reported with maternal poisoning. There has been one case of a fetus aborted during the acute phase of maternal poisoning (6).

Interactions with Herbs & Other Dietary Supplements

None known.

Interactions with Drugs

None known.

Interactions with Foods

None known.

Interactions with Lab Tests

None known.

Interactions with Diseases or Conditions

None known.

Dosage and Administration

No typical dosage.

Comments

Ciguatera poisoning is caused by eating normally safe, bottom-feeding, coral-reef fish that have accumulated ciguatoxin via the marine food chain (6). The red snapper, barracuda, and grouper are most often involved. Florida and Hawaii have the greatest incidence of ciguatera poisoning. Avoid consumption of fish in areas of recently disturbed coral reefs (includes waterfront construction). Ciguatoxic fish appear normal, including smell and taste. Local "rules of thumb" for detection are unsubstantiated. Testing for ciguatoxin is available in some areas (6).
Over 400 (normally safe) fish species may contain toxin, including red snapper, barracuda, parrotfish, jacks, and grouper (6).

CINCHONA

Also Known As

Chinarinde, Ecorce de Quina, Fieberrinde, Jesuit's Bark, Peruvian Bark, Quinine, Red Cinchona Bark.

Scientific Names

Cinchona calisaya, synonyms Cinchona ledgeriana, Cinchona carabayensis, Cinchona officinalis;
Cinchona pubescens, synonym Cinchona succirubra.
Family: Rubiaceae.

People Use This For

Orally, cinchona is used for stimulating appetite, promoting GI secretions, bloating and fullness, hemorrhoids, varicose veins, colds, and leg cramps. It is also used orally for mild attacks of influenza, malaria, fever, cancer, mouth and throat diseases, enlarged spleen, muscle cramps, and gastric disorders.
Topically, cinchona is used in eye lotions for astringent, bactericidal, and anesthetic effects. Cinchona extract is also used topically for hemorrhoids, stimulating hair growth, and managing varicose veins.

Safety

POSSIBLY SAFE ...when used orally and appropriately (12).
LIKELY UNSAFE ...when excessive amounts are used orally. 2 to 8 grams of the quinine constituent (505), or 2.5-8 grams quinidine constituent (17) can cause serious toxicity including death (505); however, the amount of these constituents varies according to the cinchona species (13).
PREGNANCY: LIKELY UNSAFE ...when used orally; avoid using (12).
LACTATION: Insufficient reliable information available; avoid using.

Effectiveness

There is insufficient reliable information available about the effectiveness of cinchona.

Mechanism of Action

The applicable part of cinchona is the bark. The cinchona bark can stimulate saliva and gastric juice secretion (2). The antimalarial effects can be attributed to quinine, an alkaloid constituent. The constituents, quinidine and quinine, have cardiac depressant properties (11).

Adverse Reactions

Orally, cinchona can cause thrombocytopenia, bleeding, and hypersensitivity reactions, including hives and fever (2). Overdose or hypersensitivity to cinchona can cause cinchonism; symptoms include headache (505), nausea, diarrhea, vomiting, ringing in the ears (6), and vision disturbance (8,505).
Topically, the cinchona bark can cause contact dermatitis (11).

Interactions with Herbs & Other Dietary Supplements

HERBS WITH ANTICOAGULANT/ANTIPLATELET POTENTIAL: Theoretically, concomitant use of cinchona bark with herbs that might have anticoagulant or antiplatelet properties might increase the risk of bleeding in some people. These herbs include alfalfa, angelica, clove, garlic, ginger, Panax ginseng, horse chestnut, red clover, and others.

Interactions with Drugs

ANTACIDS: Theoretically, due to reports that cinchona increases stomach acid, cinchona might decrease the effectiveness of antacids (19).
ANTICOAGULANT/ANTIPLATELET DRUGS: Cinchona can increase the drug effects and risk of bleeding due to its quinine content (2).
CARBAMAZEPINE (Tegretol): Cinchona can increase serum drug levels of carbamazepine due to its quinine content (11016).
H2-BLOCKERS: Theoretically, due to reports that cinchona increases stomach acid, cinchona might decrease the effectiveness of H2-blockers (19). The H2 blockers include cimetidine (Tagamet), ranitidine (Zantac), nizatidine (Axid), and famotidine (Pepcid).
PHENOBARBITAL (Luminal): Cinchona can increase serum drug levels of phenobarbital due to its quinine content (504).
PROTON PUMP INHIBITORS (PPIs): Theoretically, due to reports that cinchona increases stomach acid, cinchona might decrease the effectiveness of PPIs (19). PPIs include omeprazole (Prilosec), lansoprazole (Prevacid), rabeprazole (Aciphex), pantoprazole (Protonix), and esomeprazole (Nexium).
QUINIDINE: Cinchona contains quinidine; concomitant use with cinchona can increase the therapeutic and adverse effects of quinidine (505).
QUININE: Cinchona contains quinine; concomitant use with cinchona can increase the therapeutic and adverse effects of quinine (505).

Interactions with Foods

None known.

Interactions with Lab Tests

None known.

Interactions with Diseases or Conditions

GASTRIC OR INTESTINAL ULCERS: Cinchona is contraindicated (8,12) in conditions with an increased risk of bleeding.

Dosage and Administration

ORAL: The typical dose of cinchona is one cup of the tea up to three times daily (18). The tea is prepared by steeping 500 mg of the dried bark in 150 mL boiling water for 5-10 minutes and then straining. The maximum amount of cinchona is 1-3 grams of the bark per day (18) or 0.05-0.2 grams of the essential oil per day (12).
The usual dose of the cinchona liquid extract (4-5% total alkaloids) is 0.6-3 grams per day (18).
The cinchona extract (15-20% total alkaloids) is commonly given as 0.15-0.6 grams per day (18).

Comments

Cinchona bark contains quinine and related alkaloids, including quinidine (a cardiac depressant) and cinchotannic acid (can cause constipation). While quinine is effective for preventing or suppressing malaria caused by susceptible organisms (15), people treated with cinchona bark are exposed to the risks of quinidine, cinchotannic acid, and other alkaloid constituents. It is recommended that only purified quinine, or other appropriate antimalarial agents, be used to prevent or suppress malaria (15). US drug regulations require products containing cinchona derivatives to contain the labeling, "Discontinue use if ringing in the ears, deafness, skin rash or visual disturbances occur" (12).

CINNAMON bark

Also Known As

Batavia Cassia, Batavia Cinnamon, Cannelier de Ceylan, Ceylon Cinnamon, Ceylonzimt, Ceylonzimtbaum, Cinnamomum, Madagascar Cinnamon, Padang-Cassia, Panang Cinnamon, Sri Lanka Cinnamon, Thwak, Tvak.
CAUTION: See separate listings for Cassia Cinnamon.

Scientific Names

Cinnamomum verum, synonyms Cinnamomum zeylanicum, Laurus cinnamomum.
Family: Lauraceae.

People Use This For

Orally, cinnamon bark is used as an antispasmodic, antiflatulent, appetite stimulant, antidiarrheal, antimicrobial, anthelmintic; and for treating the common cold and influenza, gastrointestinal (GI) upset, diabetes, and dysmenorrhea.
Topically, cinnamon bark is used as part of a multi-ingredient preparation for treating premature ejaculation.
In foods, cinnamon is commonly consumed as a spice and as a flavoring agent in beverages.
In manufacturing, the volatile oil is commonly used in small amounts in toothpaste, mouthwashes, gargles, lotions, liniments, soaps, detergents, and other pharmaceutical products and cosmetics.

Safety

LIKELY SAFE ...when consumed in amounts commonly found in foods. Cinnamon bark has Generally Recognized As Safe (GRAS) status in the US (4912).
POSSIBLY SAFE ...when used orally and appropriately in medicinal amounts (4,12). ...when used topically, short-term as part of a multi-ingredient preparation (SS Cream). This preparation was used safely in a clinical trial where the cream was applied and left on the glans penis for 1-hour (2537). Further evaluation is needed to determine its safety after prolonged, repetitive use.
POSSIBLY UNSAFE ...when used orally in excessive amounts or long-term (4,12). Consumption of up to 700 mcg per kilogram of the constituent, cinnamaldehyde, is considered the highest acceptable level (4).
PREGNANCY: LIKELY SAFE ...when consumed in amounts commonly found in foods (4912).
LIKELY UNSAFE ...when used orally in amounts greater than those found in foods (4,12).
LACTATION: LIKELY SAFE ...when consumed in amounts commonly found in foods (4912). There is insufficient reliable information available about using cinnamon bark in amounts greater than those found in foods; avoid using amounts greater than those found in foods.

Effectiveness

POSSIBLY EFFECTIVE

Premature ejaculation. Applying cinnamon bark topically, as part of a multi-ingredient preparation, seems to be helpful for treating premature ejaculation. In one controlled clinical trial, a multi-ingredient cream preparation (SS Cream) containing Panax ginseng root, Angelica root, Cistanches deserticola, Zanthoxyl species, Torlidis seed, clove flower, Asiasari root, cinnamon bark, and toad venom was applied to the glans penis one hour prior to intercourse and washed off immediately before intercourse. Men suffering from premature ejaculation who were treated with the cream had significantly improved ejaculatory latency compared to placebo (2537).

There is insufficient reliable information available about the effectiveness of cinnamon bark for its other uses.

Mechanism of Action

The volatile oils of cinnamon bark are thought to be the active constituents of cinnamon. They seem to be responsible for the proposed antispasmodic, antiflatulent, and appetite stimulating effects (4).

There are approximately 6000 to 30,000 ppm of cinnamaldehyde in cinnamon bark (3919). Cinnamaldehyde makes up 60% to 80% of the volatile oil from the bark (4800). Cinnamaldehyde is thought to have central nervous system (CNS) stimulant effects at low doses and sedative effects at high doses. It is also thought to have hypothermic, antipyretic, antibacterial, and antifungal activity. Cinnamaldehyde might also increase peripheral blood flow, slow heart rate, reduce blood pressure, and possibly affect blood sugar levels (4). However, these pharmacological effects are thought to be fairly weak. Furthermore, much of the active volatile oil in cinnamon is thought to evaporate away when the cinnamon is prepared as a tea (4).

The tannin constituents in cinnamon bark have astringent properties and are thought to be responsible for an antidiarrheal effect (4). A multi-ingredient topical preparation containing cinnamon bark and several other herbs (SS Cream) is thought to work in premature ejaculation by increasing the penile vibratory threshold and reducing the amplitude of penile somatosensory-evoked potentials (2537). There is some preliminary research that suggests the cinnamon bark constituent, methylhydroxychalcone polymer (MHCP), might improve insulin sensitivity. It seems to mimic the activity of insulin, stimulating glucose metabolism. It also appears to work synergistically with insulin, possibly by improving insulin signaling pathways and alternative pathways that cause increased cellular glucose uptake. It may also have antioxidant effects (11247,11248,11973). An extract from Cinnamon cassia, a cinnamon species that also contains MHCP, lowers blood glucose, triglycerides, and total and low-density lipoprotein (LDL) cholesterol in people with type II diabetes (11347).

Adverse Reactions

Orally, no adverse reactions tend to occur with the use of the cinnamon bark; however, the oil can irritate mucous membranes and is a skin irritant and sensitizer.

Topically, cinnamon bark may cause allergic dermatitis in sensitive individuals (12635). When the multi-ingredient cream preparation (SS Cream) has been applied topically to the glans penis, sporadic erectile dysfunction, excessively delayed ejaculation, mild pain, and local irritation and burning has occurred (2537).

Interactions with Herbs & Other Dietary Supplements

HERBS & SUPPLEMENTS WITH HYPOGLYCEMIC POTENTIAL: Cinnamon bark might lower blood glucose levels (11247,11248,11973) and might have additive effects when used with other herbs and supplements that also lower glucose levels. This might increase the risk of hypoglycemia in some patients. Some herbs and supplements with hypoglycemic effects include alpha-lipoic acid, bitter melon, chromium, devil's claw, fenugreek, garlic, guar gum, horse chestnut, Panax ginseng, psyllium, Siberian ginseng, and others.

Interactions with Drugs

ANTIDIABETES DRUGS: Theoretically, cinnamon bark may lower blood glucose levels, and have additive effects in patients treated with antidiabetic agents; use with caution (11247,11248,11973).

Dose adjustments to diabetes medications might be necessary. Some antidiabetes drugs include glimepiride (Amaryl), glyburide (DiaBeta, Glynase PresTab, Micronase), insulin, metformin (Glucophage), pioglitazone (Actos), rosiglitazone (Avandia), and others.

Interactions with Foods

None known.

Interactions with Lab Tests

BLOOD GLUCOSE: Theoretically, cinnamon bark may lower blood glucose levels in some patients (11247,11248,11973).

Interactions with Diseases or Conditions

CARDIOVASCULAR CONDITIONS: There is concern that cinnamon bark might adversely affect patients with cardiovascular conditions such as high or low blood pressure or congestive heart failure. Some constituents in cinnamon bark seem to slow heart rate and might lower blood pressure (4). However, the clinical significance of these effects in patients is not known. Until more is known, advise patients with cardiovascular conditions to avoid or use cinnamon bark preparations cautiously.

DIABETES: Theoretically, cinnamon bark might lower blood glucose in patients with type 2 diabetes (11247,11248,11973). Tell patients with diabetes to use cinnamon bark products cautiously and monitor blood glucose levels very closely. Dose adjustments to diabetes medications might be necessary.

Dosage and Administration

No typical dosage.

Comments

Cinnamon is getting a lot of attention as a treatment for diabetes. There is preliminary evidence that it can lower blood glucose and cholesterol levels in people with type 2 diabetes. So far this benefit has only been found with Cassia Cinnamon (Chinese Cinnamon) in humans (11347). See separate listing for Cassia Cinnamon.
There are lots of different types of cinnamon. Cinnamomum verum (Ceylon cinnamon) is the type used most commonly in the Western world. Cinnamomum aromaticum (Cassia cinnamon or Chinese cinnamon) is also commonly used. In many cases, the cinnamon spice purchased in food stores contains a combination of these different types of cinnamon.

CITICOLINE

Also Known As

CDP-Choline, Cytidine 5-diphosphocholine, Cytidine diphosphate choline.
CAUTION: See separate listings for Choline and Phosphatidylcholine.

Scientific Names

Cytidine 5'-diphosphocholine, synonyms 5'-Cytidine diphosphate choline, Cytidine (5') diphosphocholine.

People Use This For

Orally or parenterally, citicoline is used for Alzheimer's disease and other types of dementia, head trauma, cerebrovascular disease such as stroke, age-related memory loss, Parkinson's disease, and glaucoma.

Safety

POSSIBLY SAFE ...when used orally and appropriately, short-term. Taking citicoline in doses of 1000-2000 mg/day seems to be safe when used for 60 to 90 days (12130).
PREGNANCY AND LACTATION: Insufficient reliable information available; avoid using.

Effectiveness

POSSIBLY EFFECTIVE

Age-related cognitive impairment. People aged 50 to 85 years with poor memory, taking citicoline 1000-2000 mg daily, seem to have improved verbal memory (12130).
Cerebrovascular disease. There is some evidence that citicoline taken orally or given intramuscularly or by intravenous infusion might improve memory and behavior in patients with chronic cerebrovascular diseases, such as stroke (12131).
Ischemic stroke. Stroke patients who receive citicoline 500-2000 mg/day orally within 24 hours of acute ischemic stroke are more likely to have a complete recovery within 3 months compared to placebo (12139).

INSUFFICIENT RELIABLE EVIDENCE to RATE

Alzheimer's disease. Preliminary evidence suggests that taking citicoline 1000 mg/day orally might improve cognitive function in patients with mild to moderate Alzheimer's disease (12131).
Glaucoma. Preliminary evidence suggests that citicoline 1000 mg/day intramuscularly might improve vision in patients with open-angle glaucoma (12132). Taking 1000 mg/day orally also seems to improve visual evoked potentials in patients with glaucoma (12173).
Parkinson's disease. Preliminary evidence suggests that patients who receive citicoline 500 mg/day intramuscularly in conjunction with conventional treatment might have improved rigidity and bradykinesia. But citicoline does not seem to improve tremor (12132).
Vascular dementia. Preliminary evidence indicates that citicoline 500 mg twice daily (1000 mg/day) does not seem to improve symptoms in patients with vascular dementia (12135).
More evidence is needed to rate citicoline for these uses.

Mechanism of Action

Citicoline is an intermediate compound that is formed endogenously in the process of synthesizing phosphatidylcholine from choline (12129,12140).
When taken orally, citicoline is metabolized in the gut to cytidine and choline. Both compounds are absorbed independently and taken up by brain cells. Within the brain cell cytidine is converted to cytidine monophosphate, cytidine diphosphate, and cytidine triphosphate. Choline is phosphorylated to form phosphocholine. Phosphocholine combines with cytidine triphosphate to reform citicoline. Citicoline then rapidly combines with diacylglycerol to from phosphatidylcholine (12129,12140,12195).
In animal models, orally administered citicoline increases brain phosphatidylcholine levels by 23% after 42 days and 30% after 90 days. In humans, a single dose of citicoline increases brain choline levels by about 18% in younger adults. But in older adults, brain choline levels don't seem to increase significantly. It's thought that choline uptake in the brain decreases with age, but cytidine uptake does not decrease (12129).
Age-related cognitive dysfunction, dementia, and other brain disorders have been linked to decreases in cholinergic neurons, decreases in acetylcholine, and alterations in cell membrane composition, including

decreases in choline-containing phospholipids (12129). During episodes of cerebral ischemia and brain trauma, phosphatidylcholine is degraded to free radicals and free fatty acids (12131,12194).
Citicoline is thought to be beneficial for cerebral ischemia by decreasing generation of reactive oxygen species and stabilizing cell membranes (12134,12194,12195).
Citicoline's potential benefits for central nervous system disorders such as dementia, brain trauma, and other conditions is thought to be related to citicoline's effects on brain acetylcholine and phosphatidylcholine levels (12129,12130,12195).
In animal models, citicoline seems to protect against age-related decline in spatial memory (12196).
Citicoline might also affect dopamine levels. In animal models, citicoline increases retinal dopamine levels. Therefore, there is interest in using citicoline for glaucoma and Parkinson's disease (12132).
Citicoline might also help for Parkinson's disease by improving dopaminergic cell survival. Patients with Parkinson's disease tend to have a degeneration of dopaminergic cells over time. Citicoline also seems to increase levels of reduced glutathione, a potent antioxidant. Glutathione levels are found to be decreased in the substantia nigra of Parkinson's patients (12133,12140).
In animal models of brain trauma, citicoline reduces neuronal death, cortical contusion volume, and improves neurological recovery (12137).
In animal models of ischemic stroke, citicoline seems to help reduce neuronal damage, possibly by decreasing neuronal apoptosis (12138).
Citicoline seems to have a pressor effect. In animal models of hemorrhagic shock, intravenous administration of citicoline reverses hypotension. In normotensive rats, intravenous administration of citicoline increases blood pressure (12136). It's not known if therapeutic doses of citicoline affect blood pressure in humans.
Citicoline is readily absorbed when taken orally. Less than 1% is excreted unchanged in the feces. Citicoline has a biphasic peak. The first peak occurs at 1 hour after administration, followed by a higher peak 24-hours post-dose. Citicoline is primarily eliminated through the kidneys. It's half-life is 71 hours (12132).

Adverse Reactions

Orally, citicoline seems to be well-tolerated (12131). The most common side effects appear to be nausea and diarrhea. Some people who take citicoline also experience insomnia, constipation, headache, blurred vision, chest pain, palpitations, hypotension, bradycardia, tachycardia, and skin rash (12130,12132). But these adverse reactions do not appear to occur more often than in people taking placebo (12131).

Interactions with Herbs & Other Dietary Supplements

None known.

Interactions with Drugs

None known.

Interactions with Foods

None known.

Interactions with Lab Tests

None known.

Interactions with Diseases or Conditions

None known.

Dosage and Administration

ORAL: For age-related cognitive impairment, citicoline 1000-2000 mg/day has been used (12130).
For Alzheimer's disease, citicoline 1000 mg/day has been used (12131).
For chronic cerebrovascular diseases, 600 mg/day has been used (12131).
For acute ischemic stroke, citicoline 500-2000 mg/day starting within 24 hours of stroke has been used (12139).
For glaucoma, 1000 mg/day has been used (12173).
PARENTERAL: For age-related cognitive impairment, citicoline 1000 mg/day intravenous infusion has been used (12131).
For Alzheimer's disease, citicoline 200-1000 mg/day intramuscularly has been used (12131).
For chronic cerebrovascular diseases, 200-1000 mg/day intramuscularly or by intravenous infusion has been used (12131).
For glaucoma, 1000 mg/day intramuscularly has been used (12132).

Comments

Citicoline was originally developed in Japan for acute cerebrovascular events. Citicoline was eventually introduced as a prescription drug in many European countries. In these countries it is now frequently prescribed for cognitive impairment related to chronic cerebrovascular disease (12131). In the US citicoline is marketed as a dietary supplement and is often promoted for age-related cognitive impairment.

CITRONELLA OIL

Also Known As
Ceylon Citronella, Java Citronella.
CAUTION: See separate listings for Lemongrass and Stone Root.

Scientific Names
Cymbopogon nardus, synonyms Andropogon nardus, Cymbopogon afronardus, Cymbopogon validus; Cymbopogon winterianus.
Family: Poaceae/Graminaea.

People Use This For
Orally, citronella oil is used as a vermifuge, diuretic, antispasmodic, and digestive stimulant.
Topically, citronella oil is used as a mosquito repellent and insect repellent.
In foods and beverages, citronella oil is used as a flavoring agent.
In manufacturing, citronella oil is used as a fragrance in cosmetics and soaps.

Safety
LIKELY SAFE ...when used orally in amounts commonly found in foods. Citronella oil has Generally Recognized As Safe (GRAS) status in the US (4912).
POSSIBLY SAFE ...when used to topically and appropriately. Citronella oil seems to be safe for most people when applied topically as an insect repellent, but it might be a skin sensitizer in some patients and cause allergic reactions (13084).
LIKELY UNSAFE ...when used orally in large amounts (6,11). ...when inhaled. There have been reports of toxic alveolitis (2).
CHILDREN: LIKELY UNSAFE ...when used orally. There are reports of poisoning in children and one toddler died after ingesting insect repellent that contained citronella oil (2,6,17).
PREGNANCY AND LACTATION: Insufficient reliable information available; avoid using.

Effectiveness
POSSIBLY EFFECTIVE

Mosquito repellent. Citronella oil in concentrations of 0.05% to 10% seems to be effective when applied topically for short-term prevention of mosquito bites. Higher concentrations of citronella oil seem to have a longer duration of action; however, citronella oil 10% provides less than 20 minutes of protection (13077). Since this duration of action is considerable shorter than many other mosquito repellents, such as DEET, citronella oil is generally not recommended (13083).

Mechanism of Action
There is insufficient reliable information available about the possible mechanism of action or active ingredients.

Adverse Reactions
Orally, there has been at least one report of death following ingestion of insect repellent containing citronella oil (2).
Topically, citronella oil is thought to be a skin sensitizer and can potentially cause contact dermatitis (13084).
By inhalation, citronella oil has caused toxic alveolitis (2).

Interactions with Herbs & Other Dietary Supplements
None known.

Interactions with Drugs
None known.

Interactions with Foods
None known.

Interactions with Lab Tests
None known.

Interactions with Diseases or Conditions
None known.

Dosage and Administration
TOPICAL: For preventing mosquito bites, citronella 0.5% to 10% has been used (13077).

Comments

Avoid confusion with lemongrass (Cymbopogon citratus). Citronella oil is the essential oil produced by steam distillation of other Cymbopogon species. Ceylon or Lenabatu citronella oil is produced from Cymbopogon nardus, and Java or Maha Pengiri citronella oil is produced from Cymbopogon winterianus.

CIVET

Also Known As

African Civet, Large Indian Civet, Zibeth.

Scientific Names

Viverra civetta (African Civet), synonym Civettictis civetta.
Viverra zibetha (Indian Civet).
Family: Viverridae.

Comments

At the date of publication, this product was not a common ingredient used in brand name supplements marketed to consumers. Details about this product are available in the online version of *Natural Medicines Comprehensive Database.* See www.naturaldatabase.com.

CLARY SAGE

Also Known As

Clary, Clary Wort, Clear Eye, Eyebright, Muscatel Sage, See Bright.
CAUTION: See separate listings for Sage and Eyebright.

Scientific Names

Salvia sclarea.
Family: Lamiaceae/Labiatae.

People Use This For

Orally, clary sage is used for upset stomach, digestive disorders, and kidney diseases.
Topically, clary sage mucilage is used to remove foreign objects from the eye, to remove thorns and splinters from the skin, and for treating tumors.
In foods and beverages, the oil from clary sage is used as a flavoring agent.
In manufacturing, the oil from clary sage is used as a fragrance in soaps and cosmetics.

Safety

LIKELY SAFE ...when used orally in amounts commonly found in foods. Clary sage has Generally Recognized As Safe status (GRAS) for use in foods in the US (4912).
There is insufficient reliable information available about the safety of medicinal uses of clary sage.
PREGNANCY AND LACTATION: Insufficient reliable information available; avoid using.

Effectiveness

There is insufficient reliable information available about the effectiveness of clary sage.

Mechanism of Action

The applicable parts of clary sage are the flowering top and leaf. The oil has some anticonvulsant activity in animals (11), and it seems to potentiate the effects of hexobarbitone and chloral hydrate (11).

Adverse Reactions

None reported.

Interactions with Herbs & Other Dietary Supplements

None known.

Interactions with Drugs

CHLORAL HYDRATE: Reportedly potentiates narcotic effects (9,11).
HEXOBARBITONE: Reportedly potentiates narcotic effects (9,11).

Interactions with Foods

None known.

Interactions with Lab Tests
None known.

Interactions with Diseases or Conditions
None known.

Dosage and Administration
No typical dosage.

Comments
Avoid confusion with sage leaf (Salvia officinalis).

CLEMATIS

Also Known As
Upright Virgin's Bower.
CAUTION: See separate listings for Traveler's Joy and Woodbine.

Scientific Names
Clematis recta.
Family: Ranunculaceae.

People Use This For
Orally, clematis is used for treatment of rheumatic pains, headaches, varicose veins, syphilis, gout, rheumatism, bone disorders, chronic skin conditions, and as a diuretic.
Topically, clematis is used for blisters and as a poultice to treat purulent wounds and ulcers.

Safety
POSSIBLY UNSAFE ...when the fresh plant is used topically (18).
LIKELY UNSAFE ...when the fresh plant is used orally because it is severely irritating to mucous membranes and the gastrointestinal tract (18).
There is insufficient reliable information available about the safety of the oral or topical use of dried clematis.
PREGNANCY AND LACTATION: LIKELY UNSAFE ...when the fresh plant is used orally.
There is insufficient reliable information available for the safety of the dried plant; avoid using.

Effectiveness
There is insufficient reliable information available about the effectiveness of clematis.

Mechanism of Action
When the fresh plant is crushed or cut into small pieces, the glycoside ranunculin is enzymatically changed into a severely irritating protoanemonin, which, in turn, rapidly degrades into the non-toxic anemonin (18). Both protoanemonin and ranunculin are destroyed to an unknown extent during the drying process (2), and both have fungicidal activity (4). Since Clematis recta contains low levels of protoanemonin-forming agents, the adverse effects and toxicity may not be as severe as compared to other species of Ranunculaceae.
Clematis also contains saponins (18).

Adverse Reactions
Orally, freshly harvested clematis can cause colic, diarrhea, and severe irritation to the gastrointestinal and urinary tracts (18).
Topically, prolonged skin contact can cause slow-healing blisters and burns (18).

Interactions with Herbs & Other Dietary Supplements
None known.

Interactions with Drugs
None known.

Interactions with Foods
None known.

Interactions with Lab Tests
None known.

Interactions with Diseases or Conditions
None known.

Dosage and Administration
ORAL: Clematis recta is available as drops, extracts, and tea (18).
TOPICAL: The tea is used for poultices (18).

Comments
Avoid confusion with other Clematis species (6). Clematis recta is considered a poisonous plant and is rarely used today (18). Plants that are grown in the sun have a higher ranunculin content than those grown in the shade, and therefore have stronger effects (18).

CLIVERS

Also Known As
Barweed, Bedstraw, Catchweed, Cleavers, Cleaverwort, Coachweed, Eriffe, Everlasting Friendship, Gallium, Goose Grass, Goosebill, Gosling Weed, Grip Grass, Hayriffe, Hayruff, Hedge-Burs, Hedgeheriff, Love-Man, Mutton Chops, Robin-Run-in-the-Grass, Scratchweed, Stick-a-Back, Sweethearts.
CAUTION: See separate listing for Potentilla.

Scientific Names
Galium aparine.
Family: Rubiaceae.

People Use This For
Orally, clivers is used as a diuretic, a mild astringent, for dysuria, lymphadenitis, psoriasis, and specifically for enlarged lymph nodes.
Topically, clivers is used for ulcers, festering glands, breast lumps, and skin rashes.

Safety
POSSIBLY SAFE ...when used orally and appropriately (12). There is no documented toxicity (4).
There is insufficient reliable information available about the safety of the topical use of clivers.
PREGNANCY AND LACTATION: Insufficient reliable information available; avoid using.

Effectiveness
There is insufficient reliable information available about the effectiveness of clivers.

Mechanism of Action
The applicable parts of clivers are the dried or fresh above ground parts. Clivers contain tannins, which are reported to have astringent properties (4).

Adverse Reactions
None reported.

Interactions with Herbs & Other Dietary Supplements
None known.

Interactions with Drugs
None known.

Interactions with Foods
None known.

Interactions with Lab Tests
None known.

Interactions with Diseases or Conditions
DIABETES: Use expressed juice with caution (4).

Dosage and Administration
ORAL: Typical doses are 2-4 grams dried above ground parts three times daily, or one cup tea (steep 2-4 grams herb in 150 mL boiling water 5-10 minutes, strain) three times daily (4).
Liquid extract (1:1 in 25% alcohol) 2-4 mL three times daily (4). Expressed juice, 3-15 mL three times daily (4).
TOPICAL: No typical dosage.

CLOVE

Also Known As
Caryophylli Flos, Clous de Girolfe, Flores Caryophylli, Gewurznelken Nagelein, Kreteks, Lavanga, Oil of Clove.

Scientific Names
Syzygium aromaticum, synonyms Caryophyllus aromaticus, Eugenia aromatica, Eugenia caryophyllata, Eugenia caryophyllus.
Family: Myrtaceae.

People Use This For
Orally, clove is used for dyspepsia and as an expectorant. It is also used as an expectorant. Clove oil is used orally for diarrhea, hernia, and halitosis. Clove and clove oil are used orally for flatulence, nausea, and vomiting.
Topically, clove is used for toothache, postextraction alveolitis (dry socket), as a counterirritant for pain, as a dental anesthetic, and for mouth and throat inflammation. In combination with other ingredients, clove is also used topically as part of a multi-ingredient preparation for treating premature ejaculation.
In foods and beverages, clove is used as a flavoring.
In manufacturing, clove is used in toothpaste, soaps, cosmetics, and perfumes.

Safety
LIKELY SAFE ...when used orally in amounts commonly found in foods.
Clove has Generally Recognized As Safe (GRAS) status in the US (4912).
POSSIBLY SAFE ...when clover flower is used topically, short-term, as part of a multi-ingredient preparation (SS Cream). This preparation was used safely for premature ejaculation in a clinical trial where the cream was applied and left on the glans penis for one hour (2537). Further evaluation is needed to determine its safety after prolonged, repetitive use.
LIKELY UNSAFE ...when clove oil is taken orally. Ingesting 5-15 mL of undiluted clove oil can induce high anion gap acidosis, seizures, coagulopathy, acute liver damage, behavioral changes, and coma (17). ...when clove smoke is inhaled. Smoking clove cigarettes can cause respiratory injury (17).
There is insufficient reliable information available about the safety of using clove leaf or flower orally in medicinal amounts.
PREGNANCY AND LACTATION: LIKELY SAFE ...when used orally in amounts found in foods (4912).
There is insufficient reliable information available about the safety of using clove in medicinal amounts during pregnancy and lactation; avoid using.

Effectiveness
POSSIBLY EFFECTIVE

Premature ejaculation. In one controlled clinical trial, a multi-ingredient cream preparation containing clove flower plus Panax ginseng root, Angelica root, Cistanches deserticola, Zanthoxyl species, Torlidis seed, Asiasari root, Cinnamon bark, and Toad venom (SS Cream) was applied to the glans penis one hour prior to intercourse and washed off immediately before intercourse. Men suffering from premature ejaculation who were treated with the cream had significantly improved ejaculatory latency compared to placebo (2537).

INSUFFICIENT RELIABLE EVIDENCE to RATE

Toothache. Clove oil and its constituent eugenol have long been used topically for toothache, but the FDA reclassified eugenol from Category I, meaning that it was safe and effective as it was labeled, to category III, meaning there is insufficient data to support efficacy (272). More evidence is needed to rate clove for this use.

Mechanism of Action
The applicable parts of clove are the oils, flowers, leaves, and stems. Clove oil contains up to 95% eugenol (11). Clove bud oil contains 60% to 90% eugenol, clove leaf oil contains 82% to 88% eugenol, and clove stem oil contains 90% to 95% eugenol (11).
Eugenol contributes to the mild anesthetic and analgesic properties of clove (12892). Applied topically, eugenol depresses sensory receptors involved in pain perception by inhibiting prostaglandin biosynthesis (3,512). Eugenol also has antiplatelet activity (12892).
Some evidence suggests the sesquiterpene constituents might have anticancer activity (838). Other evidence suggests whole cloves might have chemoprotective activity against liver and bone marrow toxicity (6).
Clove oil has antihistaminic and antispasmodic properties, most likely due to eugenyl acetate (6).
Clove oil inhibits gram-positive and gram-negative bacteria. It also has fungistatic action, and anthelmintic and larvicidal properties.
Preliminary research also suggests that clove extracts mimic the activity of insulin (12894).
The multi-ingredient preparation containing clove flower is thought to work in premature ejaculation by increasing the penile vibratory threshold and reducing the amplitude of penile somatosensory evoked potentials (2537).

Adverse Reactions

Orally, clove oil can cause nervous system depression, seizures, lactic acidosis, disseminated intravascular coagulation, hepatic dysfunction (17), and irritation to mucosal tissues (4,6,512). There is one report of disseminated intravascular coagulation and liver failure following clove ingestion by a two-year-old (6). There is one report of depression and electrolyte imbalance following accidental ingestion by a seven-month-old (6).
Topically, clove can cause tissue irritation. Some people can experience allergic dermatitis from clove (12635). Repeated oral application can cause gingival damage and skin and mucous membrane irritation (4,272,512). There is one report of permanent local facial anesthesia and absence of sweating after clove spilled on an individual's face (6). When the multi-ingredient cream preparation containing clove flower (SS Cream) has been applied topically to the glans penis, sporadic erectile dysfunction, excessively delayed ejaculation, mild pain, and local irritation and burning has occurred (2537).
By inhalation, clove cigarettes can cause serious acute respiratory distress, leading to hospitalization. Smoking clove cigarettes increases heart rate, systolic blood pressure, plasma levels of nicotine, and exhaled carbon monoxide. Clove cigarettes also contain significant amounts of nicotine, tar, and carbon monoxide that might cause long-term health effects similar to tobacco smoking (12892).

Interactions with Herbs & Other Dietary Supplements

HERBS WITH ANTICOAGULANT/ANTIPLATELET POTENTIAL: Concomitant use of herbs that have constituents that might affect platelet aggregation could theoretically increase the risk of bleeding in some people. These herbs include angelica, danshen, garlic, ginger, ginkgo, red clover, turmeric, willow, and others (12889).

Interactions with Drugs

ANTICOAGULANT/ANTIPLATELET DRUGS: Eugenol, a constituent of clove, is reported to have antiplatelet activity; however, this interaction has not been reported in humans (12889). Antiplatelet agents include aspirin, clopidogrel (Plavix), dipyridamole (Persantine), ticlopidine (Ticlid), and others. Anticoagulant agents include heparin and warfarin (Coumadin).

Interactions with Foods

None known.

Interactions with Lab Tests

None known.

Interactions with Diseases or Conditions

BLEEDING DISORDERS: Clove oil contains eugenol which has antiplatelet effects (17). Theoretically, taking clove oil might exacerbate bleeding in patients with bleeding disorders.

Dosage and Administration

ORAL: No typical dosage. However, clove products have been used as a fluid extract, 5-30 drops, an oil extract, 1-5 drops (6002).
TOPICAL: As mouthwash, products equivalent to 1% to 5% clove oil have been used (8). A 15% clove tincture can be effective in treating athletes foot (4).

Comments

Clove cigarettes, also called kreteks, generally contain 60% to 80% tobacco and 20% to 40% ground clove. The clove constituent eugenol, like menthol, reduces the harshness of tobacco smoke and can facilitate learning of smoking techniques (12892).

CLOWN'S MUSTARD PLANT

Also Known As

Bitter Candy Tuft, Candytuft.
CAUTION: See separate listings for Black Mustard, Hedge Mustard, and White Mustard.

Scientific Names

Iberis amara, synonym Iberis coronaria.
Family: Brassicaceae/Cruciferae.

People Use This For

Orally, clown's mustard plant is used for gastrointestinal conditions such as dyspepsia, irritable bowel syndrome (IBS), gastritis, and bloating. It is also used for gout, musculoskeletal aches and pains (rheumatism), tachycardia, asthma, bronchitis, and edema (dropsy).

Safety

POSSIBLY SAFE ...when used orally, short-term. There is some evidence that clown's mustard plant extract can be used safely for up to 8 weeks (7049,12724).

PREGNANCY AND LACTATION: Insufficient reliable information available; avoid using.

Effectiveness

POSSIBLY EFFECTIVE

Dyspepsia. A specific combination product containing clown's mustard plant (Iberogast, Enzymatic Therapy) seems to improve symptoms of dyspepsia. The combination includes clown's mustard plant plus peppermint leaf, German chamomile, caraway, licorice, milk thistle, celandine, angelica, and lemon balm (7049,12724). A meta-analysis of studies using this combination product suggests that taking 1 mL orally three times daily over a period of 4-weeks significantly reduces severity of acid reflux, epigastric pain, cramping, nausea, and vomiting compared to placebo (13089).

Mechanism of Action

The applicable parts of clown's mustard plant are the leaves, stem, root, and seeds. The active ingredients and how it might work for gastrointestinal conditions are not known. Some people think it may contain glycosides or flavonoids that could be responsible for any pharmacological effect. However, this has not been verified by scientific studies. Clown's mustard plant does contain the constituent sinapic acid, which has antioxidant properties (7050).

Adverse Reactions

Orally, clown's mustard plant can cause nausea and diarrhea in some patients. Some patients might be hypersensitive to clown's mustard plant. There is one case of a facial rash following oral use (7051).

Interactions with Herbs & Other Dietary Supplements

None known.

Interactions with Drugs

None known.

Interactions with Foods

None known.

Interactions with Lab Tests

None known.

Interactions with Diseases or Conditions

None known.

Dosage and Administration

ORAL: For dyspepsia, a specific combination product containing clown's mustard plant (Iberogast, Enzymatic Therapy) and several other herbs has been used in a dose of 1 mL three times daily (7049,12724,13089).

CLUB MOSS

Also Known As

Lycopodium, Stags Horn, Vegetable Sulfur, Witch Meal, Wolfs Claw.

CAUTION: See separate listings for Chinese Club Moss and Huperzine A.

Scientific Names

Lycopodium clavatum.

Family: Lycopodiaceae.

People Use This For

Orally, club moss is used for bladder and kidney disorders, and as a diuretic.

Safety

POSSIBLY UNSAFE ...when used orally. Club moss contains toxic alkaloids but no poisonings have been reported (18).

PREGNANCY AND LACTATION: POSSIBLY UNSAFE ...when used orally; avoid using.

Effectiveness

There is insufficient reliable information available about the effectiveness of club moss.

Mechanism of Action
The applicable parts of club moss are the plant and spores. Club moss contains potentially toxic alkaloids, including lycopodine, dihydrolycopodine, and traces of nicotine (18).

Adverse Reactions
None reported.

Interactions with Herbs & Other Dietary Supplements
None known.

Interactions with Drugs
None known.

Interactions with Foods
None known.

Interactions with Lab Tests
None known.

Interactions with Diseases or Conditions
None known.

Dosage and Administration
No typical dosage.

Comments
Avoid confusion with Chinese club moss. Only Chinese club moss contains huperzine A.

CNIDIUM

Also Known As
Cnidii monnieri fructus, Cnidium Extract, Cnidium Fruit, Cnidium Fruit Extract, Cnidium monnier, Cnidium monnieri fructus, Cnidium Seeds, Monnier's Snowparsley, She Chuang Zi.

Scientific Names
Cnidium monnieri, synonym Selinum monnieri.
Family: Apiaceae/Umbelliferae.

People Use This For
Orally, cnidium is used for increasing sexual performance and libido, erectile dysfunction, infertility, body building, increasing energy, cancer, osteoporosis, and fungal and bacterial infections.
Topically, cnidium is used for pruritus, rashes, eczema, and ringworm.

Safety
There is insufficient reliable information available about the safety of cnidium.
Pregnancy and Lactation: Insufficient reliable information; avoid using.

Effectiveness
There is insufficient reliable information available about the effectiveness of cnidium.

Mechanism of Action
The applicable parts of cnidium are the fruit, seed, and whole plant. Active constituents of cnidium are thought to be the coumarin derivatives including osthol, imperatorin, isopimpinellin, xanthotoxin, and bergapten (12218).
Additional coumarins have also been identified including cnidimonal, cnidimarin, and others (13020).
Other constituents include hemiterpenoids, monoterpenoids, and aromatic glucosides (13018).
Cnidium is used to improve sexual performance. There is some evidence from an animal model that the coumarin constituents of cnidium fruit have a relaxing effect on the corpus cavernosum. This suggests that cnidium constituents might facilitate penile erection (13019).
An extract of cnidium fruit and the purified osthol and isopimpinellin constituents seem to have an antipuritic effect in animal models. But this effect does not seem to be as potent as the antihistamine diphenydramine (Benadryl) (12218). Other preliminary research suggests cnidium fruit extract inhibits itching induced by substance P without causing sedation. Substance P is increased in patients with skin disorders such as atopic dermatitis and psoriasis (12623).

Cnidium fruit extracts and the osthol constituent also seem to have an antiallergy effect in animal models (12217). Cnidium fruit extracts also seem to have anticancer effects. Extracts have cytotoxic activity against cervical and colorectal cancer cells, and against leukemia cells in vitro. The coumarin constituent osthol seems to have the strongest cytotoxic activity against tumor cells. Both osthol and imperatorin induce apoptosis of HL-60 human leukemia cells (12529).

There is interest in using cnidium to prevent liver damage. Sesquiterpene constituents, torilolone and 1-hydroxytorilin, seem to protect against tacrine-induced liver cytotoxicity in vitro (12572).

There is interest in using cnidium for osteoporosis. Coumarin constituents of the fruit extract seem to stimulate osteoblast proliferation in vitro. Osthol is more active on osteoblast proliferation than imperatorin and bergapten (13017).

Adverse Reactions

None reported.

Interactions with Herbs & Other Dietary Supplements

None known.

Interactions with Drugs

None known.

Interactions with Foods

None known.

Interactions with Lab Tests

None known.

Interactions with Diseases or Conditions

None known.

Dosage and Administration

No typical dosage.

Comments

Cnidium is a native Chinese plant. It has also been identified in the US in Oregon. Cnidium is a Traditional Chinese Medicine (TCM) that has been used for thousands of years, particularly topically for dermatological conditions. It is a common ingredient in Chinese lotions, creams, and ointments.

COCA

Also Known As

Bolivian Coca, Cocaine Plant, Health Inca Tea, Huanuco Coca, Inca Health Tea, Inca Tea, Java Coca, Mate-de-Coca, Mate de Coca, Peruvian Coca, Spadic, Truxillo Coca.

CAUTION: See separate listing for Cocoa.

Scientific Names

Erythroxylum coca; Erythroxylum novogranatense.

Family: Erythroxylaceae.

People Use This For

Orally, coca is chewed for relief of hunger and fatigue, and enhancing physical performance. Coca extracts are used for stimulating stomach function, causing sedation, and treating asthma, colds, and other ailments. Coca is the source of cocaine, which is used nasally, injected, or smoked, for mind-altering effects.

Topically, people use the prescription drug cocaine for corneal, nasal, and throat mucosa anesthesia; severe ophthalmologic pain; and local vasoconstriction.

In manufacturing, decocainized coca extract is used to flavor cola drinks and food products.

Safety

LIKELY SAFE ...when decocainized coca leaf extract is used in amounts commonly found in foods. It has Generally Recognized As Safe (GRAS) status in the US (4912). ...when the constituent, cocaine, is used as an FDA-approved product for topical use.

UNSAFE ...when the constituent, cocaine, is ingested or inhaled as a recreational when the constituent, cocaine, is used orally for medicinal purposes (17). 20 mg of cocaine can cause severe side effects and 1.2 grams can be fatal. Cocaine is a Schedule II controlled substance in the US due to extremely high potential for addiction (17).

PREGNANCY: UNSAFE ...when inhaled or used orally. Coca, and the constituent cocaine, are contraindicated

due to abortifacient and teratogenic effects (17,6187). Coca use is also associated with a high incidence of Sudden Infant Death Syndrome (SIDS) (17).
LACTATION: UNSAFE ...when inhaled. Coca and the constituent, cocaine, are contraindicated. Cocaine is excreted into breast milk and intoxication can occur in infants breast-fed by mothers recently exposed to cocaine (17,18).

Effectiveness

LIKELY INEFFECTIVE

Athletic performance. Chewing coca leaves doesn't seem to improve physical performance. Coca increases heart rate, but does not appear to improve cardiac output or other physiologic responses to physical exercise (9455,9456).

There is insufficient reliable information available about the effectiveness of coca for its other uses.

Mechanism of Action

The applicable part of coca is the leaf. The major active constituent of coca leaves is the alkaloid cocaine. The leaves also contain essential oils that have not been well identified. The concentration of cocaine is higher in coca grown at lower altitudes and in coca grown under drought conditions (9457). Cocaine has local anesthetic, beta-1, beta-2, and alpha-adrenergic stimulating properties (17). Preliminary evidence suggests that other active constituents in coca leaves, besides cocaine, contribute to the stimulatory effects (9461,9462).

When coca leaves are chewed to improve physical performance, heart rate increases, but cardiac output is not increased. Coca leaves appear to cause a decrease in plasma volume, which blunts cardiac output resulting from increased heart rate. Coca leaves do not improve glucose or fat utilization or other physiologic responses to exercise (9455,9456).

Coca paste is made by mashing coca leaves with alkali, kerosene, and sulfuric acid. The concentration of cocaine in coca paste is over 75%. Coca paste is sometimes used by smoking after it is added to tobacco, but only about 6% of the cocaine survives the heat of smoking (9460).

Adverse Reactions

Adverse effects of coca generally pertain to the cocaine constituent. Initially, these effects can include euphoria, hyperactivity, and restlessness. Later tremors, hyperreflexia, and seizures can develop. Finally, coma, hyporeflexia, respiratory depression, cardiovascular depression, and death may occur. In the central nervous system (CNS), cocaine can also cause migraine headaches, stroke, and intracranial and intracerebral hemorrhage (17,5092).

Chewing coca leaves commonly causes anorexia, which often leads to malnutrition. Poor eating habits may contribute to anemia in people that chew coca leaves (9458). Cocaine use is associated with a high incidence of coronary artery disease or other myocardial disease. Up to 38% of cocaine users may have a defect in left ventricular filling (9459). Other cardiovascular adverse effects include extreme elevations of heart rate and blood pressure, vasoconstriction, myocardial ischemia, myocardial infarction, cardiac arrhythmias, cardiomyopathies, myocarditis, endocarditis, aortic rupture, and diffuse micro-aneurysms (17). There is also some evidence that cocaine use can cause platelet activation, platelet microaggregate formation and platelet alpha granule release, which might increase the risk of thrombosis and accelerate the development of atherosclerosis (6374). Cocaine use may cause mesenteric ischemia and rhabdomyolysis-induced renal failure (17). Liver adverse effects include hepatic necrosis, and elevation of serum transaminase and serum creatinine phosphokinase (17). Metabolic adverse effects include lactic acidosis, hyperthermia, hypoglycemia, and hypoxia (17). Use during pregnancy might cause spontaneous abortion, abruptio placentae, and fetal malformation (17). Fetal exposure to cocaine, a constituent of coca, is associated with impaired auditory information processing in newborns (6187). Psychiatric adverse effects include paranoia, depression, and violence (17). Respiratory adverse effects include exacerbation of asthma, thermal airway injury, adult respiratory distress syndrome, pneumothorax, pneumomediastinum, pulmonary thrombosis, bronchiolitis obliterans, pulmonary edema, pulmonary infiltrates, pulmonary vascular disease, and pulmonary hemorrhage (17).

Chronic intranasal cocaine abuse is associated with orbital wall (bone) destruction, acquired nasolacrimal duct obstruction, and orbital cellulitis (1258).

Interactions with Herbs & Other Dietary Supplements

CAPSICUM: Theoretically, concomitant use of coca and capsicum (including exposure to pepper spray which contains capsicum) might increase the effects and risk of adverse effects of the cocaine in coca (1394).
MARIJUANA: Concomitant use can have additive effects, including increased heart rate (17).

Interactions with Drugs

ALCOHOL (Ethanol): Concomitant use of alcohol and coca or the cocaine constituent may have additive negative effects on neurocognitive functioning in the brain (6373).
NIFEDIPINE: Nifedipine (Adalat, Procardia) use just prior to cocaine use increases the likelihood of seizures and death (17).

Interactions with Foods

None known.

Interactions with Lab Tests

URINE DRUG TEST: Using coca preparations can cause a positive urine drug test for cocaine. Even some "decocainized" tea preparations can contain 5 mg of cocaine per bag.

Interactions with Diseases or Conditions

ASTHMA: Cocaine use is associated with more severe exacerbations in people with asthma. One study found exacerbations were more severe among cocaine users, compared to non-users, who presented to an emergency room during an asthma attack (6186).
CARDIOVASCULAR DISORDERS: People with cardiovascular disorders might be at increased risk for cocaine-induced cardiovascular side effects (17).
INTRACEREBRAL HEMORRHAGE: Cocaine use is associated with increased morbidity and mortality in patients who sustain intracerebral hemorrhage (5092).
PLASMA PSEUDOCHOLINESTERASE DEFICIENCY (PPD): People with PPD are at increased risk for cocaine-induced cardiovascular side effects, including seizures and death (17).

Dosage and Administration

No typical dosage.

Comments

Coca is considered unsafe and illegal for self-use. Cocaine, a constituent of coca, is an FDA-approved Schedule C-II drug.
Avoid confusion with cocoa seed (Theobroma cacao). A type of tea, known as Inca tea, health Inca tea, or mate de coca, is made from the leaves of Erythroxylum novogranatense. After preparation in boiling water, the tea contains 0.04% cocaine (9460,9484). This tea is illegal in the US.

COCILLANA

Also Known As

Grape Bark, Guapi, Trompillo, Upas.

Scientific Names

Guarea guidonia, synonym Guarea rusbyi, Sycocarpus rusbyi, Guarea guara, Guarea trichilioides; Guarea spiciflora; and related Guarea species.
Family: Meliaceae.

Comments

At the date of publication, there was very little scientific information available about this product. Our staff is continually analyzing the available information on natural medicines and will add data to the online version of *Natural Medicines Comprehensive Database* as it becomes available. See www.naturaldatabase.com.

COCOA

Also Known As

Cacao, Chocola, Cocoa Bean, Cocoa Butter, Cocoa Oleum, Cocoa Seed, Cocoa Semen, Cocoa Testae, Theobroma, Theobromine.
CAUTION: See separate listings for Coca, Black Tea, Caffeine, Coffee, Cola Nut, Green Tea, Guarana, Oolong Tea, and Mate.

Scientific Names

Theobroma cacao, synonyms Theobroma sativum.
Family: Malvaceae or Sterculiaceae.

People Use This For

Orally, cocoa seed is used for infectious intestinal diseases and diarrhea, asthma, bronchitis, and as an expectorant for lung congestion. The seed coat is used for liver, bladder and kidney ailments, diabetes, as a tonic, and as a general remedy. Cocoa powder, enriched with flavonoid constituents, is used for prevention of cardiovascular disease.
Topically, cocoa butter has been used to treat wrinkles on the skin and to prevent stretch marks during pregnancy.
In foods, cocoa seed is used as a flavoring agent. Chocolate is produced from cocoa powder.
In manufacturing, cocoa butter is used as a compounding base for various pharmaceutical preparations.

Safety

LIKELY SAFE ...when used orally in amounts commonly found in foods (6). ...when used orally in moderate amounts for medicinal purposes (6). ...when used topically. Cocoa butter is used extensively as a base for ointments and suppositories and is generally considered safe (11).
POSSIBLY UNSAFE ...when used in large amounts. Due to the caffeine content, when used in excessive doses, significant adverse effects may occur, including tachyarrhythmias and sleep disturbances (18).
PREGNANCY: POSSIBLY SAFE ...when used in moderate amounts or in amounts commonly found in foods. Due to the caffeine content of cocoa preparations, mothers should closely monitor their intake to ensure moderate consumption. Fetal blood concentrations of caffeine approximate maternal concentrations (4260). Use of caffeine in pregnancy is controversial; however, moderate consumption has not been associated with clinically important adverse fetal effects (2708,2709,2710,2711,9606). Some sources suggest keeping caffeine consumption below 200 mg per day (2078). Chocolate products provide 2-35 mg caffeine per serving (2078) and a cup of hot chocolate provides approximately 10 mg (3900). POSSIBLY UNSAFE ...when used orally in large amounts. Caffeine found in cocoa crosses the placenta producing fetal blood concentrations similar to maternal levels (4260). Although controversial, some evidence suggests that high doses of caffeine might be associated with premature delivery, low birth weight, and loss of the fetus (6). Some sources suggest keeping caffeine consumption below 200 mg per day (2078).
Excessive use of cocoa in pregnancy should be avoided.
LACTATION: POSSIBLY SAFE ...when used in moderate amounts or in amounts commonly found in foods. Due to the caffeine content of cocoa preparations, mothers should closely monitor their intake to ensure moderate consumption. Breast milk concentrations of caffeine are thought to be approximately 50% of maternal serum concentrations. Moderate consumption of cocoa would likely result in very small amounts of caffeine exposure to a nursing infant (6). POSSIBLY UNSAFE ...when used orally in large amounts. Consumption of excess chocolate (16 oz per day) may cause irritability and increased bowel activity in the infant (6026).
Large doses or excessive intake of cocoa should be avoided during lactation.

Effectiveness

There is insufficient reliable information available about the effectiveness of cocoa.

Mechanism of Action

The applicable parts of cocoa are the seed, seed coat, cocoa powder, and butter. Cocoa seed contains oils, tannins, and alkaloids, including theobromine 1-4%, caffeine 0.07-0.36%, trigonelline, and others. Cocoa butter, also referred to as theobroma oil, is the fat obtained from roasted cocoa seeds. It contains oleic acid 37%, stearic acid 34%, palmitic acid 26%, and linoleic acid 2% (13). Cocoa also contains flavonoids, tyramine, phenylethylamine (PEA), magnesium, and possibly N-acylethanolamines (6018,6019). Cocoa has CNS stimulant, cardiac stimulant, coronary dilatory, and diuretic actions (6). Theobromine is the major methylxanthine found in cocoa and has only one-tenth of the cardiac activity of caffeine. In one study, consumption of 1.5 g/kg body weight of chocolate had no acute hemodynamic or physiologic effects on the hearts of healthy, young adults (1373). There has been recent analyses of the health effects of stearic acid, which is found in substantial amounts in cocoa. Unlike other saturated fatty acids, stearic acid does not increase total and low-density lipoprotein (LDL) cholesterol. However, it has been shown that stearic acid can lower high-density lipoprotein (HDL) levels and increase lipoprotein(a). Because of this, the stearic acid content in cocoa products is not thought to provide a reduction in the risk for coronary heart disease as was once proposed (6017,6027). However, preliminary research indicates that flavonoid constituents found in cocoa might be beneficial in cardiovascular disease, much like aspirin. In vitro data has shown that cocoa can stimulate the formation of nitric oxide and inhibit cyclooxygenase formation. In a human trial, patients receiving cocoa powder enriched with flavonoids had decreased epinephrine- or ADP-stimulated expression of fibrinogen-binding glycoprotein IIb-IIIa, indicating that it might inhibit platelet aggregation (6085). Dark chocolate contains higher amounts of flavonoids than milk chocolate (6018). Preliminary evidence suggests a defatted-cocoa extract might also prevent arteries from constricting in the presence of cholesterol. It has been suggested that stearic acid might activate coagulation factor VII and impair fibrinolysis (6027). In contrast, one study concluded that diets high in stearic acid do not increase the tendency toward thrombosis (6020). PEA found in cocoa is structurally and pharmacologically similar to catecholamines and amphetamine. PEA may be a modulator of mood. N-acylethanolamines are pharmacologically related to anandamide, which activates cannabinoid receptors in the brain (6019).

Adverse Reactions

Orally, cocoa can cause allergic skin reactions, shakiness, increased urination, rapid pulse, constipation, and might trigger migraine headaches (6,18). The cocoa in chocolate can cause nausea, gastrointestinal discomfort, borborygmi, and flatus (1373).
Topically, cocoa butter has occasionally caused a rash. In animals, it has been shown to be comedogenic; however, this has not been found in humans (11).

Interactions with Herbs & Other Dietary Supplements

CAFFEINE CONTAINING HERBS/SUPPLEMENTS: The caffeine in cocoa may have an additive effect with other caffeine-containing products, and increase the risk of adverse effects. Natural products that contain caffeine include coffee, tea (black or green), guarana, mate, and cola.

EPHEDRA (Ma Huang): The caffeine in cocoa may potentiate stimulant effects of ephedra and increase risk of adverse effects (1275,1380,6486,10307).

Interactions with Drugs

ADENOSINE (Adenocard): The caffeine in cocoa is a competitive inhibitor of adenosine at the cellular level. However, caffeine doesn't seem to affect supplemental adenosine because high interstitial levels of adenosine overcome the antagonistic effects of caffeine (11771).

ANTIDIABETES DRUGS: Concomitant use might interfere with blood glucose control. Cocoa is reported to have hyperglycemic effects (19).

BETA-ADRENERGIC AGONISTS: Theoretically, concomitant use of large amounts of cocoa might increase cardiac inotropic effects of beta-agonists, due to cocoa's caffeine content (15).
Beta-adrenergic agonists include albuterol (Ventolin, Proventil), metaproterenol (Alupent), terbutaline (Brethine, Bricanyl), and isoproterenol (Isuprel).

CIMETIDINE (Tagamet): Theoretically, concomitant use might increase the effects of caffeine found in cocoa. Cimetidine decreases caffeine clearance by 30-50% (15,506).

CLOZAPINE (Clozaril): Theoretically, co-administration of clozapine and large amounts of cocoa might acutely exacerbate psychotic symptoms, due to cocoa's caffeine content. Caffeine increases the effects and toxicity of clozapine (151). Caffeine doses of 400-1000 mg per day inhibit clozapine metabolism (5051).

CONTRACEPTIVE DRUGS: Theoretically, concomitant use might increase the effects of caffeine found in cocoa. Oral contraceptives reduce caffeine clearance by 40-65% (2714,11737).

DIPYRIDAMOLE (Persantine): Theoretically the caffeine in cocoa might inhibit dipyridamole-induced vasodilation (11770,11772).

DISULFIRAM (Antabuse): Theoretically, concomitant use of disulfiram and large amounts of cocoa might increase the effects of caffeine found in cocoa. Disulfiram reduces caffeine clearance (15).

ERGOTAMINE (Ergomar): Theoretically, concomitant use of ergotamine and large amounts of cocoa might increase the GI absorption of ergotamine, due to cocoa's caffeine content (15).

ESTROGENS: Concomitant use can increase serum caffeine concentrations and the risk of caffeine adverse effects. Estrogen inhibits caffeine metabolism (2714).

FLUCONAZOLE (Diflucan): Concomitant use might increase the effects of caffeine in cocoa. Fluconazole decreases caffeine clearance by approximately 25% (11022).

LITHIUM: Theoretically, abrupt withdrawal of large amounts of cocoa might cause lithium toxicity, due to cocoa's caffeine content. Abrupt caffeine withdrawal reportedly increases serum lithium levels (609).

MEXILETINE (Mexitil): Concomitant use might increase the effects and adverse effects of caffeine in cocoa. Mexiletine can decrease caffeine elimination by 50% (1260,11741).

MONOAMINE OXIDASE INHIBITORS (MAOIs): Theoretically, concomitant use of MAOIs with large amounts of cocoa might precipitate a hypertensive crisis due to cocoa's tyramine content (19).

PHENYLPROPANOLAMINE: Concomitant use of phenylpropanolamine and cocoa might cause an additive increase in blood pressure due to the caffeine in cocoa (11738).

QUINOLONE ANTIBIOTICS: Theoretically, concomitant use might increase the effects of caffeine found in cocoa. Quinolones decrease caffeine clearance (606,607,608).
Quinolones (fluoroquinolones) include ciprofloxacin (Cipro), enoxacin (Penetrex), norfloxacin (Chibroxin, Noroxin), sparfloxacin (Zagam), trovafloxacin (Trovan), and grepafloxacin (Raxar).

THEOPHYLLINE: Theoretically, concomitant use of theophylline and large amounts of cocoa might increase the risk of theophylline toxicity, due to cocoa's caffeine content. Caffeine decreases theophylline clearance 23-29% (506).

VERAPAMIL (Calan, Covera, Isoptin, Verelan): Theoretically, concomitant use might increase the effects of caffeine found in cocoa. Verapamil can increase plasma caffeine levels by 25% (15,506).

Interactions with Foods

GRAPEFRUIT JUICE: Theoretically, concomitant use might increase the caffeine effects of cocoa. Grapefruit might decrease caffeine clearance (4300).

Interactions with Lab Tests

5-HYDROXYINDOLEACETIC ACID: Theoretically, large amounts of cocoa might increase urine 5-hydroxyindoleacetic acid concentrations and test results, due to its caffeine content. Caffeine can increase urine catecholamine concentrations (15).

BLEEDING TIME: Theoretically, large amounts of cocoa might prolong bleeding time and increase test results, due to its caffeine content (1701).

BLOOD PRESSURE: Theoretically, large amounts of cocoa might increase blood pressure, due to its caffeine content (4).

CATECHOLAMINES: Theoretically, large amounts of cocoa might increase urine catecholamine concentrations

and test results, due to its caffeine content (15).
CREATINE: Theoretically, large amounts of cocoa might increase urine creatine concentrations and test results, due to its caffeine content (1701).
PHARMACOLOGICAL STRESS TESTS: The caffeine in cocoa is a competitive antagonist for adenosine receptors (11771). It is recommended that caffeine and caffeine-containing products be stopped 24 hours prior to pharmacological stress tests (11770). However, caffeine appears more likely to interfere with dipyridamole (Persantine) than adenosine (Adenocard) stress testing (11771). The interaction between caffeine and dipyridamole is unlikely to be significant in stress testing if the heart rate increase is greater than 5% after dipyridamole infusion (11772).
URATE: Theoretically, large amounts of cocoa might falsely increase serum urate test results determined by the Bittner method, due to its caffeine content (15).
VANILLYLMANDELIC ACID (VMA): Theoretically, large amounts of cocoa might increase urine VMA concentrations and test results, due to its caffeine content (15).

Interactions with Diseases or Conditions

ANXIETY: Theoretically, large amounts of cocoa might aggravate anxiety disorders, due to the caffeine content (506).
DIABETES: Cocoa might interfere with blood glucose control. Cocoa is reported to have hyperglycemic effects (19).
DEPRESSION: Theoretically, large amounts of cocoa might aggravate depression disorders, due to its caffeine content (506).
GASTRIC ULCERS, DUODENAL ULCERS: Theoretically, large amounts of cocoa might aggravate ulcers, due to its caffeine content (506).
GASTROESOPHAGEAL REFLUX DISEASE (GERD): Cocoa reduces lower esophageal sphincter pressure, and may aggravate GERD (1374).
HEART CONDITIONS: Theoretically, large amounts of cocoa might induce cardiac arrhythmias in sensitive individuals, due to its caffeine content (506).
IRRITABLE BOWEL SYNDROME (IBS): Avoid cocoa-containing products including chocolate which might aggravate IBS (6).
MIGRAINE HEADACHES: Theoretically, cocoa might trigger migraines in sensitive individuals (18).

Dosage and Administration

No typical dosage.

Comments

Avoid confusion with coca leaf (Erythroxylon coca). Bitter chocolate is produced by pressing roasted cocoa kernels between hot rollers. Cocoa powder is produced by expressing the cocoa butter from bitter chocolate and powdering the remaining residue. Sweet chocolate is produced by adding sugar and vanilla to bitter chocolate (13).
The candy company, Mars, Inc., plans to seek a health claim for chocolate from the Food and Drug Administration in the next few years based on preliminary research they sponsored regarding the potential role of cocoa flavonoids in cardiovascular health (1329).

COCONUT OIL

Also Known As

Cocot Palm, Coconut Palm.

Scientific Names

Cocos nucifera.
Family: Arecaceae/Palmae.

People Use This For

Orally, coconut oil is used for weight loss, heart disease, hypercholesterolemia, diabetes, chronic fatigue, Crohn's disease, irritable bowel syndrome (IBS), disease prevention, thyroid conditions, energy, and boosting the immune system.
Topically, coconut oil is used for psoriasis, as a skin emollient.

Safety

LIKELY SAFE ...when used orally and appropriately in amounts commonly found in foods (4912).
POSSIBLY SAFE ...when used topically and appropriately (12356).
There is insufficient reliable information about the safety of coconut oil when used orally in medicinal amounts.
PREGNANCY AND LACTATION: LIKELY SAFE ...when used orally and appropriately in amounts commonly found in foods (4912). There is insufficient reliable information about the safety of coconut oil when used orally or topically in medicinal amounts.

Effectiveness

INSUFFICIENT RELIABLE EVIDENCE to RATE

Psoriasis. Applying coconut oil to the skin before treatment of psoriasis with ultraviolet B (UVB) or psoralen and ultraviolet A (PUVA) phototherapy doesn't seem to improve efficacy (12356). More evidence is needed to rate coconut oil for this use.

Mechanism of Action

Coconut oil is obtained from the dried nut (fruit) of the coconut palm. About half of coconut oil is made up of medium-chain fatty acids. Lauric acid is the major constituent, followed by myristic and palmitic acids. Coconut oil is the most saturated oil compared with palm, soybean, and corn oils; and animal fats such as butter and lard. It contains 76 grams of saturated fatty acids per 100 grams of fat (12357,12358).

Although medium-chain fatty acids undergo rapid metabolism, oils such as coconut oil can raise total and low-density lipoprotein (LDL) levels (12358,12361). Animal research suggests that coconut oil has an atherogenic effect, possibly by increasing pro-inflammatory cytokines such as interleukin (IL)-1beta and tumor necrosis factor (TNF)-alpha (12362). However, other preliminary clinical research suggests that coconut oil lowers postprandial tissue plasminogen activator (tPA) antigen and lipoprotein (a) levels, which might have a beneficial effect on cardiovascular disease (12363).

Topically, coconut oil doesn't block ultraviolet A (UVA) or ultraviolet B (UVB) radiation (12356).

Adverse Reactions

Orally, coconut oil can rarely cause allergic reactions (12359,12360). Coconut oil is high in fat, which can cause weight gain. It also can increase cholesterol (12358).

Interactions with Herbs & Other Dietary Supplements

None known.

Interactions with Drugs

None known.

Interactions with Foods

None known.

Interactions with Lab Tests

CHOLESTEROL: Coconut oil can increase total and low-density lipoprotein (LDL) cholesterol levels and test results (12358).

Interactions with Diseases or Conditions

HYPERCHOLESTEROLEMIA: Coconut oil can increase total and low-density lipoprotein (LDL) cholesterol levels and may adversely affect treatment (12358).

Dosage and Administration

No typical dosage.

COD LIVER OIL

Also Known As

Cod Oil, Fish Oil, Liver Oil, N-3 Fatty Acids, Omega-3 Fatty Acids, Polyunsaturated Fatty Acids.

CAUTION: See separate listings for DHA (docosahexaenoic acid), EPA (eicosapentaenoic acid), Fish Oil, and Shark Liver Oil.

Scientific Names

None.

People Use This For

Orally, cod liver oil is used for hyperlipidemia, hypertriglyceridemia, albuminuria associated with diabetic nephropathy, hypertension, coronary heart disease, osteoarthritis, systemic lupus erythematosus (SLE), and otitis media.

Topically, cod liver oil is used to accelerate wound healing.

Safety

LIKELY SAFE ...when used orally and appropriately (3398,3399,4026).

POSSIBLY UNSAFE ...when used orally in excessive doses. Doses greater than 25 mL daily might decrease blood coagulation and increase the risk of bleeding (4025,4026). There is also some concern about vitamin A and vitamin D toxicity. On average 20 mL of cod liver oil provides 15,000 IU vitamin A and 1500 IU vitamin D (4003,4004).

There is insufficient reliable information available about the safety of cod liver oil when used topically.

PREGNANCY AND LACTATION: Insufficient reliable information available; avoid using.

Effectiveness

LIKELY EFFECTIVE

Hypertriglyceridemia. Taking cod liver oil orally can reduce triglyceride levels by 20% to 50% in patients with hypertriglyceridemia (3399,4026,5705,5706).

POSSIBLY EFFECTIVE

Diabetic nephropathy. There is some evidence that taking cod liver oil orally can reduce albuminuria in type 2 diabetes patients with nephropathy (1025).

Hypertension. Taking cod liver oil orally seems to produce modest, but significant, reductions in systolic and diastolic blood pressure in patients with mild hypertension (1001,1020,3399).

POSSIBLY INEFFECTIVE

Hypercholesterolemia. Taking cod liver oil doesn't seem to decrease serum total or high-density lipoprotein (HDL) cholesterol or triglycerides in patients with familial hypercholesterolemia (10083).

Osteoarthritis. Taking cod liver oil orally, in combination with nonsteroidal anti-inflammatory drugs (NSAIDs), does not seem to decrease pain or inflammation when compared to NSAID treatment alone (3398).

INSUFFICIENT RELIABLE EVIDENCE to RATE

Arrhythmia. Preliminary clinical research suggests cod liver oil might reduce ventricular premature complexes in people with ventricular arrhythmias (7360).

Otitis media. Preliminary clinical evidence suggests that oral cod liver oil, in combination with a children's multivitamin-mineral preparation containing selenium, might prevent or decrease the frequency of otitis media in young children (10151).

More evidence is needed to rate cod liver oil for these uses.

Mechanism of Action

Cod liver oil contains high amounts of long-chain, polyunsaturated fats called omega-3 fatty acids.

Cod liver oil is especially high in the omega-3 fatty acids docosahexaenoic acid (DHA) and eicosapentaenoic acid (EPA). Cod liver oil also contains a significant amount of vitamins A and D. On average, 20 mL of cod liver oil contains 1.8 grams EPA, 2.2 grams DHA, 15,000 IU vitamin A, and 1500 IU vitamin D (4003,4004,4026). Cod liver oil fatty acids compete with arachidonic acid for the cyclooxygenase and lipoxygenase pathways (4026,10080). Cod liver oil's anti-inflammatory effects are likely due to inhibition of leukotriene synthesis (3392,4026,10080).

Because of this effect, there is interest in cod liver oil for heart disease prevention. Cod liver oil also has antithrombotic effects. It decreases blood viscosity and increases red blood cell deformability, increases prostacyclin synthesis and related vasodilation, reduces thrombogenicity of platelets and monocytes, reduces platelet adhesiveness, and reduces platelet count (3399,4005,4022,4025,10077,10080). Preliminary research suggests cod liver oil may be useful in improving long-term graft patency following arterial bypass reconstruction (10082).

In hypertriglyceridemia, cod liver oil is thought to lower triglycerides by decreasing secretion of very low-density lipoproteins (VLDLs), increasing VLDL apolipoprotein B secretion, possibly by increasing VLDL clearance, decreasing VLDL size, and reducing triglyceride transport (3397,3399,4026).

The DHA and EPA fatty acids found in cod liver oil make up a third of all lipids in the brain's grey matter (425). DHA and EPA play a key role in the structural development of retinal, neural, and synaptic membranes and are thought to be important for normal neural function (424,425). Animals who are deficient in omega-3 fatty acids develop learning and vision disturbances (424). In patients with non-insulin dependent diabetic neuropathy, cod liver oil is thought to improve albuminuria by reducing microvascular albumin leakage (1025).

Preliminary research suggests concurrent use of cod liver oil with nonsteroidal anti-inflammatory drug (NSAID) administration may play a role in the prevention of NSAID-induced gastropathy (10081).

Some researchers think low levels of EPA, selenium, and vitamin A might predispose some children to acute otitis media (10151).

Adverse Reactions

Orally, cod liver oil can have a fishy taste and might cause belching, nosebleeds, halitosis, and heartburn. High doses can cause nausea and loose stools. Some gastrointestinal side effects can be minimized if cod liver oil is taken with meals and if doses are started low and gradually increased. Doses greater than 25 mL might also decrease blood coagulation and potentially increase the risk of bleeding (1313,4025,4026). Long-term cod liver oil supplementation is associated with an increased risk of cutaneous malignant melanoma in women (3395). There is one case of lipoid pneumonia as a result of long-term cod liver oil use (3396). There is also some concern about vitamin A and vitamin D toxicity in people using cod liver oil long-term. On average, 20 mL of cod liver oil provides 15,000 IU vitamin A and 1500 IU vitamin D (4003,4004).

Interactions with Herbs & Other Dietary Supplements

HERBS & SUPPLEMENTS WITH ANTICOAGULANT/ANTIPLATELET POTENTIAL: Concomitant use of herbs that constituents that might affect platelet aggregation could theoretically increase the risk of bleeding in some people. These herbs include angelica, borage seed oil, clove, danshen, garlic, ginger, ginkgo, red clover, turmeric, willow, and others.

Interactions with Drugs

ANTICOAGULANT/ANTIPLATELET DRUGS: Concomitant use with anticoagulant or antiplatelet drugs can increase the risk of bleeding (3399,4005,4022,4025,10077,10080). Some of these drugs include aspirin, clopidogrel (Plavix), dalteparin (Fragmin), dipyridamole (Persantine), enoxaparin (Lovenox), heparin, ticlopidine (Ticlid), warfarin (Coumadin), and others.
ANTIHYPERTENSIVE DRUGS: Cod liver oil can lower blood pressure and might have additive effects in patients treated with antihypertensives (1001,1020,3399); use with caution.

Interactions with Foods

None known.

Interactions with Lab Tests

BLOOD PRESSURE: Cod liver oil might moderately lower blood pressure readings (1001,1020,3399,4026).
INTERNATIONAL NORMALIZED RATIO (INR), PROTHROMBIN TIME (PT): High doses of greater than 25 mL per day might decrease blood coagulation, increase INR and PT, and increase the risk of bleeding (1313,4025,4026).
TRIGLYCERIDES: Cod liver oil can reduce serum triglyceride concentrations and test results in patients with hypercholesterolemia (3399,4026,5705,5706).

Interactions with Diseases or Conditions

DIABETES: There has been concern that fish oil and cod liver oil might increase blood glucose levels in patients with diabetes (3397). However there is no reliable scientific support for this concern. Doses from 2-18 grams/day do not seem to affect blood glucose or hemoglobin A1c (HbA1c) (13011).
HYPERTENSION: Cod liver oil can lower blood pressure and might have additive effects in patients treated with antihypertensives (1001,1020,3399,4026); use with caution.

Dosage and Administration

ORAL: For lowering triglycerides, 20 mL of cod liver oil per day has been used (3399,4026). For familial hypercholesterolemia, 30 ml of cod liver oil per day has been used (10083). For lowering blood pressure, 20 mL of cod liver oil per day has been used (3399,4026).

CODONOPSIS

Also Known As

Bastard Ginseng, Bellflower, Bonnet Bellflower, Chuan Dang, Codonopsis Pilosula Modesta, Dangshen, Radix Codonopsis.
CAUTION: See separate listings for Ashwaganda, Blue Cohosh, Canaigre, Ginseng American, Ginseng Panax, and Ginseng Siberian.

Scientific Names

Codonopsis pilosula; Codonopsis tangshen; Codonopsis tubulosa; other Codonopsis species.
Family: Campanulaceae.

People Use This For

Orally, codonopsis is used to treat HIV infection and as a protective adjuvant to radiotherapy in cancer treatment. It is also used orally as a substitute for ginseng in general tonic formulas, as an immune tonic, for weakness, anorexia, chronic diarrhea, dyspnea, palpitations, asthma, cough, thirst, and diabetes.

Safety

POSSIBLY SAFE ...when used orally and appropriately (12).
PREGNANCY AND LACTATION: Insufficient reliable information available; avoid using.

Effectiveness

There is insufficient reliable information available about the effectiveness of codonopsis.

Mechanism of Action
Codonopsis seems to be able to stimulate the central nervous system (CNS). It seems to promote weight gain, increase endurance, increase tolerance to anoxia, elevate temperature, increase macrophage activity, increase red and white blood cell counts, and promote peripheral vasodilation (11). Codonopsis also has hypotensive, adrenergic blocking, radioprotective and ulcer-protective effects (11).

Adverse Reactions
None reported.

Interactions with Herbs & Other Dietary Supplements
None known.

Interactions with Drugs
None known.

Interactions with Foods
None known.

Interactions with Lab Tests
None known.

Interactions with Diseases or Conditions
None known.

Dosage and Administration
ORAL: People typically use 12 to 15 grams codonopsis added to 3 to 4 cups water and boiled until the volume is reduced by one-half. The cooled liquid is taken in 2 doses on an empty stomach (5251).

Comments
No ginseng saponins have been found in codonopsis (11).

COENZYME Q-10

Also Known As
Co Q10, Coenzyme Q10.

Scientific Names
Ubiquinol; Ubiquinone; Ubidecarenone; Mitoquinone.

People Use This For
Orally, coenzyme Q-10 is used for congestive heart failure (CHF), angina, dilated cardiomyopathy, diabetes, hypertension, periodontal disease, cardiotoxicity associated with doxorubicin (Adriamycin) chemotherapy, and breast cancer. It is also used orally for Huntington's disease, Parkinson's disease, muscular dystrophy, increasing exercise tolerance, chronic fatigue syndrome (CFS), and warfarin-induced alopecia. Coenzyme Q-10 is also used orally for stimulating the immune systems of people with HIV/AIDS, life extension, male infertility, idiopathic asthenozoospermia, migraine headache, quinone-responsive mitochondrial encephalomyelopathy, and for preventing "statin"-induced myopathy.
Topically, coenzyme Q-10 is used for treating periodontal disease.

Safety
LIKELY SAFE ...when used orally and appropriately. There have been no reports of significant toxicity associated with coenzyme Q-10 in studies lasting up to 30 months (2134,6037,6038,6407,8163,8938,8939,8940).
...when used topically on the gums (2107).
PREGNANCY AND LACTATION: Insufficient reliable information available; avoid using.

Effectiveness
LIKELY EFFECTIVE

Coenzyme Q-10 deficiency. Taking coenzyme Q-10 orally seems to improve symptoms of coenzyme Q-10 deficiency (8160,8161). Rare cases of documented coenzyme Q-10 deficiency with symptoms of weakness, fatigue, and seizures have been reported.

Mitochondrial encephalomyopathies. Taking coenzyme Q-10 orally seems to reduce symptoms in some patients with genetic and acquired disorders of mitochondrial dysfunction (8159,8162,8163,8912). The onset of effect is slow, with maximal effect at six months (8163). A specific coenzyme Q-10 formulation (UbiQGel) has

FDA Orphan Drug status for mitochondrial encephalomyopathies, including MELAS (myoclonic epilepsy with lactic acidosis and stroke-like episodes) syndrome, Kearns-Sayre syndrome, and MERRF (myoclonus epilepsy with ragged red fibers).

POSSIBLY EFFECTIVE

Congestive heart failure (CHF). Adding oral coenzyme Q-10 to conventional treatments seems to improve quality of life, improve New York Heart Association classification, decrease hospitalization rates, and decrease symptoms of heart failure such as dyspnea, peripheral edema, enlarged liver, and insomnia in patients with mild to severe (New York Heart Association Class II-IV) CHF (6407,6408,6409,8909,12170). However, the effectiveness of coenzyme Q-10 for heart failure is controversial (8910). Some research suggests that coenzyme Q-10 does not improve objective measures of CHF including ejection fraction or exercise tolerance (5090,6037,6038). Tell patients there's no evidence that coenzyme Q-10 can help heart failure when taken alone, but it might be helpful when taken with other heart failure drugs.

HIV/AIDS. Taking coenzyme Q-10 orally seems to improve immune function in people with HIV/AIDS (2123,2124).

Huntington's disease. Ubiquinol, a reduced form of coenzyme Q-10, has FDA Orphan Drug status for Huntington's disease (11873). However, taking coenzyme Q-10 orally in doses of 600 mg per day or less doesn't seem to be effective for slowing the progression or functional decline in patients with Huntington's disease (1357,8940).

Hypertension. Taking coenzyme Q-10 orally with other antihypertensives seems to provide an additional blood pressure lowering effect and might allow dosage reduction or discontinuation of some antihypertensive medications (2122,3365,9890).

Ischemic reperfusion injury. Taking coenzyme Q-10 orally for a week before cardiac bypass or vascular surgery might lessen hypoxic damage during surgery (11902,11903). But other research suggests no effect (11904).

Isolated systolic hypertension. Taking coenzyme Q-10 orally appears to lower systolic blood pressure by about 26% in some people with isolated systolic hypertension after 12 weeks of therapy (8907).

Migraine headache. Taking coenzyme Q-10 orally might be helpful for preventing migraine headaches. Coenzyme Q-10 seems to decrease the frequency of headaches by about 30% and reduce the number of days with headache-related nausea by about 45% (8135,11872). For reducing migraine frequency, the number needed to treat (NNT) using coenzyme Q-10 100 mg TID for 3 months is 3 (11872). Explain to patients that it can take up to 3 months for significant benefit. Taking coenzyme Q-10 prophylactically does not seem to reduce the duration or severity of migraine headaches when they develop (11872).

Muscular dystrophy. Taking coenzyme Q-10 orally seems to improve physical performance in some patients with muscular dystrophies (2127).

Myocardial infarction (MI). Taking coenzyme Q-10 orally seems to decrease the risk of cardiac events in patients with recent MI who are at risk of atherothrombosis. When started in patients within 72 hours of MI and administered for 1 year, coenzyme Q-10 appears to significantly lower the risk of cardiac events including non-fatal MI and cardiac death (10152).

Parkinson's disease. Taking high doses of coenzyme Q-10, 300-1200 mg orally per day, seems to slow functional decline in people with early Parkinson's disease. The effect appears to be dose dependent (8938).

LIKELY INEFFECTIVE

Athletic performance. Taking coenzyme Q-10 orally doesn't improve aerobic power in athletes (2109,2110,8911). Some evidence suggests coenzyme Q-10 might slightly improve tolerance to higher workloads, but more research is needed to tell if coenzyme Q-10 is effective for this purpose (8911).

Periodontal disease. Coenzyme Q-10 applied topically isn't effective for treating periodontal disease (2107,2108). However, preliminary research suggests that taking coenzyme Q-10 orally might be helpful for periodontal disease (8916,8917,8918); more evidence is needed.

INSUFFICIENT RELIABLE EVIDENCE to RATE

Angina. Some preliminary clinical research suggests that taking coenzyme Q-10 orally might improve exercise tolerance in patients with angina (2121).

Breast cancer. There is preliminary evidence that taking coenzyme Q-10 orally might be helpful in advanced breast cancer along with surgery and conventional therapy plus other antioxidants and omega-3 and omega-6 fatty acids (3993,3995).

Diabetes. There is conflicting evidence about the effectiveness of coenzyme Q-10 for diabetes. Some research suggests that taking 200 mg coenzyme Q-10 per day reduces hemoglobin A1c in people with type 2 diabetes (9890,11877). However, other research in type 2 diabetes using the same dose shows no effect on hemoglobin A1c (492). Some research in people with type 1 diabetes also shows no effect (456,2126). In patients with hypertension and coronary artery disease, there is evidence that coenzyme Q-10 might reduce insulin resistance (3365).

Dilated cardiomyopathy. Preliminary evidence suggests that taking coenzyme Q-10 10 mg/kg/day divided into 2-3 doses significantly improves ejection fraction and New York Heart Association (NYHA) classification in children with dilated cardiomyopathy (12199).

Infertility. Preliminary evidence suggests that infertile men with idiopathic asthenozoospermia who take coenzyme Q-10 200 mg/day have increased sperm motility after 6 months of treatment (12169).

Maternally inherited diabetes mellitus and deafness (MIDD). There is some preliminary evidence that taking

coenzyme Q-10 orally might prevent progressive insulin secretory defect, exercise intolerance, and hearing loss in people with a rare form of diabetes called maternally inherited diabetes mellitus and deafness (MIDD) (2125).
Pediatric congestive heart failure. Ubiquinol, a reduced form of coenzyme Q-10, has FDA Orphan Drug status for pediatric congestive heart failure (11873).
Statin-induced myopathy. There is some preliminary evidence that coenzyme Q-10 might lessen muscular adverse effects caused by high-dose HMG-CoA reductase inhibitors ("statins"). In people taking high-dose lovastatin investigationally for cancer treatment, coenzyme Q-10 seems to lessen the effect of statins on muscles (11899,11900). But there are no clinical trials of the effect of coenzyme Q-10 in hypercholesterolemic people taking statins at usual doses.
Warfarin-induced hair loss. There is some preliminary evidence that coenzyme Q-10 might be helpful for preventing warfarin-induced hair loss (455).
More evidence is needed to rate coenzyme Q-10 for these uses.

Mechanism of Action

Coenzyme Q-10 is a vitamin-like compound present in virtually all cells and in especially high concentrations in the heart, liver, kidney, and pancreas. Within the cell, 25-30% of total coenzyme Q-10 is found in the nucleus, 40% to 50% in the mitochondria, 15-20% in the microsomes, and 5-10% in the cytosol. Coenzyme Q-10 is fat soluble and acts similar to a vitamin (2134,11892). Its primary functions include activity as an antioxidant, a membrane stabilizer, and as a cofactor in many metabolic pathways, particularly in the production of adenosine triphosphate (ATP) in oxidative respiration (2134,6037,6048,6410,11892).
The body produces adequate amounts of coenzyme Q-10, so it's not considered a vitamin (11893). It's also ingested in small amounts from dietary sources, including meats and seafood. However, the amounts ingested in foods do not approach therapeutic doses. Coenzyme Q-10 formulated in soy bean oil appears to have superior bioavailability compared to other formulations (457). Peak levels of coenzyme Q-10 after oral administration occur in 5-10 hours, and the half-life is approximately 34 hours (2134,8907).
Many of the therapeutic benefits of coenzyme Q-10 are primarily attributed to its antioxidant effects and its role in the generation of ATP. Genetic or acquired disorders of mitochondrial function cause increases in serum lactate and the lactate/pyruvate ratio, due to impaired oxidative metabolism. Supplementation with coenzyme Q-10 seems to reduce these levels and improve exercise tolerance and function in people with these disorders (8159,8162,8163).
In addition, coenzyme Q-10 may be helpful for people with diseases for which coenzyme Q-10 levels are often lower, including congestive heart failure (CHF), hypertension, periodontal disease, certain muscular diseases, and AIDS (2134,6410).
In the treatment of CHF, the mechanism is thought to involve prevention of oxidative damage. The greatest benefit seems to occur in people with the largest deficiency of coenzyme Q-10 (2134). The effect in the treatment of angina may be due to increased ATP synthesis, reduction of free radicals, or membrane protection (2134). Preliminary evidence suggests that coenzyme Q-10 might enhance endothelium-independent arterial relaxation and improve endothelium-dependent vasodilation, which can lower total peripheral resistance and systolic blood pressure. This effect seems to be caused by increased endothelial production of prostacyclin (PGI2) or increased sensitivity of arterial smooth muscle to PGI2, or both (8908).
Coenzyme Q-10 increases plasma levels of high density lipoprotein (HDL) cholesterol, vitamin E, and vitamin C; and decreases levels of total cholesterol, low density lipoprotein (LDL) cholesterol, and products of lipid peroxidation such as thiobarbituric acid reactive substances (TBARS), malondialdehyde, and diene conjugates.
In patients at risk for future coronary events, coenzyme Q-10 may prevent thrombosis and have protective effects on vascular and myocardial remodeling and endothelial function (10152).
Coenzyme Q-10 levels are highest during the first 20 years of life and decline with age. At age 80, coenzyme Q-10 levels may be lower than at birth. In some kinds of bacteria, coenzyme Q-10 supplements seem to prolong life (11895). However, life-long administration of coenzyme Q-10 to rodents doesn't affect lifespan (11896).
Coenzyme Q-10 can undergo oxidation/reduction reactions in various cell membranes such as lysosomes, Golgi, or plasma membranes. The proton gradient caused by the redox ability of coenzyme Q-10 provides a basis for antioxidant action either directly or by regeneration of vitamin E (tocopherol) and ascorbate (8913). Preliminary research suggests that decreased redox status of coenzyme Q-10 might indicate a higher risk for coronary heart disease in people with familial hyperlipidemia (8914). Fenofibrate (Tricor) and coenzyme Q-10 seem to improve endothelial and non-endothelial forearm vasodilator function in dyslipidemic type 2 diabetic patients (11877).
Coenzyme Q-10 appears to be a factor in Parkinson's disease. Parkinson's disease might be caused by impaired function of the mitochondrial electron transport chain, and particularly the mitochondrial enzymes, complex I and complex II. Coenzyme Q-10 is the electron acceptor for these complexes. People with Parkinson's disease seem to have lower levels of coenzyme Q-10 in platelet mitochondria. Preclinical research suggests that supplementation increases cerebral concentrations of coenzyme Q-10 and reduces the loss of dopamine and dopaminergic axons in experimental models of Parkinson's disease (8938,8939).
There is also interest in using coenzyme Q-10 for Huntington's disease, which is also thought to be a mitochondrial disorder. In animal models of Huntington's disease, orally administered coenzyme Q-10 extends survival and delays development of motor deficits, weight loss, cerebral atrophy, and neuronal changes (8941). Usefulness in humans hasn't been demonstrated at doses of 600 mg per day or less (8940). Some researchers suggest that L-carnitine and coenzyme Q-10 might have an additive or synergistic effect. Both coenzyme Q-10 and L-carnitine are involved with

maintaining mitochondrial energy production in cells and may help protect against oxidative and toxin-induced damage (3653,9603), but it isn't known whether this has any clinical significance.
As a potential prophylactic treatment for migraine headaches, coenzyme Q-10 might work by improving mitochondrial oxidative phosphorylation, which appears to be impaired in some patients with migraines (8135,11897).
HMG-CoA reductase inhibitors ("statins") may reduce serum coenzyme Q-10 levels. Intramuscular levels don't appear to be affected. Some researchers think statin-induced myopathy may be related to mitochondrial dysfunction. Coenzyme Q-10 and cholesterol share common synthetic pathways. Some evidence suggests that statins may block the synthesis of both. But coenzyme Q-10 does not affect the cholesterol lowering effect of statins (11898).
Some drugs inhibit coenzyme Q-10 activity. Preliminary evidence suggests that the negative inotropic effect of some beta-blockers, particularly propranolol (Inderal), and to a lesser extent metoprolol (Lopressor, Toprol), is caused by inhibition of coenzyme Q-10 dependent enzymes in the myocardium (3368,3369,8958). Preliminary in-vitro evidence suggests coenzyme Q-10 might prevent cardiotoxicity caused by phenothiazines and tricyclic antidepressants. It seems to block mitochondrial dysfunction induced by these drugs (8959). Coenzyme Q-10 also seems to protect against doxorubicin (Adriamycin) cardiotoxicity, possibly through correction of coenzyme Q-10 deficiencies and scavenging of free radicals (2134). Researchers are also interested in coenzyme Q-10's possible anticancer effects related to its antioxidant properties. Coenzyme Q-10 might also have immunostimulatory activity (3993). There is also some evidence that coenzyme Q-10 concentrations are lower in cancerous breast tissue than healthy tissue (4846,5158). Some researchers speculate that very low levels of coenzyme Q-10 might be an indicator of a poor prognosis (4846).

Adverse Reactions

Orally, coenzyme Q-10 is generally well tolerated. In clinical studies, there have been no reports of significant adverse effects (2134,6037,6038,6047,8135,8938,8939,8940). Coenzyme Q-10 can cause gastrointestinal side effects such as nausea, vomiting, diarrhea, appetite suppression, heartburn, and epigastric discomfort in less than 1% of patients (2134,3370,8135,8938,8939,8940,10152). Some of these adverse effects can be minimized if total daily doses exceeding 100 mg are divided and administered two to three times per day (3370).
Allergic rash has been reported (11872).

Interactions with Herbs & Other Dietary Supplements

L-CARNITINE: Some researchers suggest that L-carnitine and coenzyme Q-10 might have an additive or synergistic effect. Both coenzyme Q-10 and L-carnitine are involved with maintaining mitochondrial energy production cells and may help protect against oxidative and toxin-induced damage (3653,9603).
RED YEAST: Theoretically, since red yeast has HMG-CoA reductase inhibitor ("statin") constituents (512), it might reduce coenzyme Q-10 levels.

Interactions with Drugs

ANTIHYPERTENSIVE DRUGS: Coenzyme Q-10 can decrease blood pressure and might have additive blood pressure lowering effects when used with antihypertensive drugs (2122,9890); use with caution.
CHEMOTHERAPY: Preliminary evidence suggests that inhibition of coenzyme Q-10 dependent enzymes contributes to the cardiotoxicity associated with doxorubicin (Adriamycin). Theoretically CoQ-10 supplements might prevent this toxicity, but might also lower effectiveness (3368). There is some concern that taking antioxidants such as coenzyme Q-10 might protect tumor cells from chemotherapeutic agents that work by inducing oxidative stress, such as the alkylating agents (e.g., cyclophosphamide, Cytoxan) and radiation therapy (5158,5159). Consider potential risk versus potential benefit before using coenzyme Q-10.
WARFARIN (Coumadin): Concomitant use might reduce the anticoagulation effects of warfarin (2128,6048,6199). Coenzyme Q-10 is chemically similar to menaquinone and may have vitamin K-like procoagulant effects. Four cases of decreased warfarin efficacy thought to be due to coenzyme Q-10 have been reported (2128,6048). However, there is some preliminary clinical research that suggests coenzyme Q-10 might not significantly decrease the effects of warfarin in patients that have a stable INR (11905). Closely monitor patients taking warfarin and coenzyme Q-10. Dose adjustment may be necessary.

Drug Influences on Nutrient Levels and Depletion

SOME DRUGS CAN AFFECT COENZYME Q-10 LEVELS:
HMG CoA REDUCTASE INHIBITORS (statins): HMG CoA reductase inhibitors can reduce serum coenzyme Q-10 levels (4404,4405,4406,4407,4408,4409,4410). They block the synthesis of mevalonic acid, which is a precursor of coenzyme Q-10 (3370).
Statins' effect on coenzyme Q-10 appears to be dose-related. Taking atorvastatin (Lipitor) 10 mg/day or pravastatin (Pravachol) 20 mg/day doesn't seem to decrease levels of circulating coenzyme Q-10 in healthy people (8915). But taking atorvastatin 80 mg/day for 30 days reduces coenzyme Q-10 levels by 52% (12099).
The clinical significance of statins' effect on coenzyme Q-10 levels is unclear. For example, taking simvastatin 20 mg/day for 4 weeks reduces serum coenzyme Q-10 levels about 32%, but levels in muscle may actually increase, up to 47% according to one study (3367).
Some researchers suspect that depletion of coenzyme Q-10 levels might result in statin-related side effects such as myopathy. But so far there is no reliable evidence that coenzyme Q-10 depletion is the cause of statin side effects. There is also no proof that taking coenzyme Q-10 supplements reduces statin side effects.
Other "statin" drugs include lovastatin (Mevacor), simvastatin (Zocor), and fluvastatin (Lescol).

Interactions with Foods

None known.

Interactions with Lab Tests

GLYCOSYLATED HEMOGLOBIN (Hemoglobin A1C, Hg A1C): Some clinical research suggests that coenzyme Q-10 can reduce glycosylated hemoglobin in people with type 2 diabetes (9890,11877). However, other research suggests no effect (456,492). Coenzyme Q-10 doesn't seem to affect fasting blood glucose (9890,11877).
LIVER ENZYMES: Coenzyme Q-10 does not seem to adversely affect liver function. Despite earlier concern that doses greater than 300 mg per day might cause increases in SGOT (Serum Glutamic-Oxaloacetic Transaminase) and LDH (Lactic Dehydrogenase) (2134), doses greater than 600 mg per day given for 30 months have not caused changes in liver function (8938,8939,8940).
T4/T8 RATIO: Coenzyme Q-10 can increase the T4/T8 ratio in normal patients and some HIV-positive patients (2123).

Interactions with Diseases or Conditions

HYPOTENSION, HYPERTENSION: Coenzyme Q-10 might lower blood pressure. It can have additive effects with medications used for hypertension (2122,3365,9890); use with caution.
SMOKING: Cigarette smoking depletes body stores of coenzyme Q-10 (7722).

Dosage and Administration

ORAL: For documented coenzyme Q-10 deficiency, 150 mg daily has been used (8160).
For mitochondrial encephalomyopathies, 150 to 160 mg, or 2 mg/kg/day has been used (8159,8162,8163).
In some cases, doses have been gradually increased to 3000 mg per day (8912).
For heart failure, most studies have used 100 mg per day divided into 2 or 3 doses (6037,6038,6047,8909). Benefits have also been found with 60 mg/day (12170). For reducing the risk of future cardiac events in patients with recent myocardial infarction, 120 mg daily in 2 divided doses has been used (10152).
For angina, 50 mg three times per day has been used (2121).
For hypertension, 120 to 200 mg per day divided into two doses has been used (3365,9890).
For isolated systolic hypertension, 60 mg twice daily has been used (8907).
For HIV/AIDS, 200 mg per day has been used (2123,2124).
For diabetes, 100 mg once or twice daily has been used (456,492,9890).
For Parkinson's disease, 300 mg, 600 mg, and 1200 mg per day in 4 divided doses has been used (8938).
For preventing migraine headache, 100 mg three times daily has been used (11872).
For muscular dystrophy, 100 mg per day has been used (2127).
For quinone-responsive mitochondrial encephalomyopathy, 5 mg/kg/day has been used (3366).
For dilated cardiomyopathy in children, 10 mg/kg/day in divided doses has been used (12199).
For male infertility, coenzyme Q-10 200 mg/day has been used (12169).
To minimize adverse effects, divided daily doses of coenzyme Q-10 are generally recommended when doses exceed 100 mg/day (3370).
TOPICAL: No typical dosage.

Comments

Coenzyme Q-10 was first identified in 1957. The "Q-10" refers to the five-carbon isoprenoid units that are attached to the quinone ring. In humans, coenzyme Q-10 is most prevalent; in other species, coenzymes Q-6, Q-7, Q-8, and Q-9 dominate (11892,11894).
Coenzyme Q-10 is widely used in Japan. Millions of Japanese patients receive coenzyme Q-10 as part of their treatment for cardiovascular disease. The Japanese government approved coenzyme Q-10 for the treatment of congestive heart failure in 1974. Coenzyme Q-10 is also used extensively in Europe and Russia. Most of the coenzyme Q-10 used in the US and Canada is supplied by Japanese companies. Coenzyme Q-10 is manufactured by fermenting beets and sugar cane with special strains of yeast.

COFFEE

Also Known As

Cafe, Espresso, Java, Mocha.
CAUTION: See separate listings for Caffeine, Black Tea, Green Tea, Oolong Tea, Cola Nut, Guarana, Cocoa, and Coffee Charcoal.

Scientific Names

Coffea arabica; Coffea canephora, synonyms Coffea robusta, Coffea bukobensis; Coffea liberica, synonym Coffea arnoldiana; other Coffea species.
Family: Rubiaceae.

People Use This For

Orally, coffee is used for short-term relief of mental and physical fatigue, and to increase performance capabilities and mental alertness. Coffee is also used orally to prevent Parkinson's disease, symptomatic gallstone disease, type 2 diabetes, gastrointestinal cancer, and breast cancer. Other uses include headache, hypotension, weight loss, and attention deficit-hyperactivity disorder (ADHD).
Rectally, coffee is used as an enema to treat cancer.

Safety

LIKELY SAFE ...when used orally and appropriately. Drinking decaffeinated coffee or coffee containing caffeine in low to moderate amounts is safe (15).
POSSIBLY UNSAFE ...when used orally in excessive amounts. Drinking caffeinated coffee in amounts greater than 6 cups per day (about 600 mg caffeine) short-term or long-term can cause caffeinism with symptoms of anxiety possibly progressing to delirium and agitation. Chronic use of caffeine, especially in large amounts, can sometimes produce tolerance, habituation, and psychological dependence. Abrupt discontinuance of caffeine can cause physical withdrawal symptoms (11733).
LIKELY UNSAFE ...when used rectally as an enema. Coffee enemas can cause severe electrolyte abnormalities and sometimes septicemia leading to severe side effects including death (3026,3349).
CHILDREN: POSSIBLY UNSAFE ...when coffee containing caffeine is used orally.
The adverse effects are usually more severe in children than adults (11733).
PREGNANCY: POSSIBLY SAFE ...when used orally in small amounts. Three cups of coffee (approx. 300 mg caffeine) consumed throughout the day seems to be safe (11733). Caffeine crosses the human placenta but is not considered a teratogen. Fetal blood and tissue levels are similar to maternal concentrations (4260).
POSSIBLY UNSAFE ...when used orally in large amounts. More than 3 cups of coffee (300 mg caffeine) consumed daily may be harmful to the fetus (4260). Drinking more than 6 cups of coffee per day increases the risk of spontaneous abortion (2709). Drinking 8 or more cups of coffee per day doubles the risk of stillbirth, when compared to women who do not drink coffee during pregnancy (10621).
LACTATION: POSSIBLY SAFE ...when used orally. Drinking one or two caffeine-containing beverages per day during lactation is not associated with unacceptable levels of caffeine in human milk (11734).
POSSIBLY UNSAFE ...when used orally in large amounts. Caffeine from coffee can cause wakefulness or irritability in breast-fed infants.

Effectiveness

LIKELY EFFECTIVE

Mental alertness. Consumption of coffee and other caffeinated beverages seems to prevent a decline in alertness and cognitive capacity when consumed throughout the day (4221,4224).
Caffeine can improve mental performance and alertness following prolonged sleep deprivation (10205).

POSSIBLY EFFECTIVE

Colorectal cancer. Epidemiological evidence suggests that drinking more than 3 cups of coffee daily may significantly reduce the risk of rectal cancer (9222).
Diabetes. Long-term consumption of caffeinated coffee seems to significantly reduce the risk of developing type 2 diabetes. This effect seems to be dose-dependent (11353,11731). Population research suggests drinking 5 to 6 cups of coffee per day reduces diabetes risk by 61% in women and 30% in men. Drinking 10 or more cups of coffee per day reduces diabetes risk by 79% in women and 55% in men.
This relationship persists regardless of age, weight, and tobacco or alcohol use (11731).
Gallbladder disease. Consumption of caffeinated beverages including coffee, that provide 400 mg or greater of caffeine per day, is associated with significantly reducing the risk of developing symptomatic gallstone disease (3345,8032). The effect seems to be dose-dependent. Consumption of 800 mg caffeine per day (four or more cups of coffee) has the greatest reduction in risk (3345).
Hypotension. Consuming caffeinated beverages like coffee seems to increase blood pressure in elderly people with postprandial hypotension (11834,11835).
Parkinson's disease. There is evidence that people who consume caffeinated beverages such as coffee, tea, and cola have a decreased risk of Parkinson's disease. For men, the effects seem to be dose related. Men consuming the greatest amount of caffeinated coffee, 28 ounces (three to four cups) per day, or a total of 421 to 2716 mg of caffeine from any source daily, seem to have the greatest reduction in risk.
However, a significant reduction in risk exists even with consumption of as little as 124 to 208 mg caffeine per day, approximately 1-2 cups of coffee (6022).
In women, the effects do not seem to be dose related. Moderate consumption of caffeinated coffee, one to three cups daily, provides the most reduction in risk (1238).
Coffee does not appear to provide additional protection from Parkinson's disease in cigarette smokers (9236).

POSSIBLY INEFFECTIVE

Breast cancer. Consumption of coffee doesn't seem to affect breast cancer incidence (9235).
Digestive tract cancers. Drinking coffee doesn't seem to help prevent esophageal cancer, stomach cancer, or colon cancer. Epidemiological research suggests that coffee intake doesn't affect the risk for developing these digestive tract cancers (9222,9223).

INSUFFICIENT RELIABLE EVIDENCE to RATE

Cognitive function. There is preliminary evidence that suggests that higher lifetime coffee consumption might positively affect cognitive function among elderly women aged 80 or more years (10620). More evidence is needed to rate coffee for this use.

Mechanism of Action

Coffee contains 1% to 2.6% caffeine (7,12,13), which is the primary active ingredient. One cup (six ounces) of coffee contains approximately 60-120 mg of caffeine (8042). Other active constituents include chlorogenic acid, caffeol, and diterpenes. Caffeine acts as a central nervous system (CNS) stimulant, increases heart rate and contractility, increases blood pressure, stimulates gastric acid secretion, causes diuresis, relaxes extracerebral vascular and bronchial smooth muscle, and stimulates the release of catecholamines (8033).

Coffee has properties that might be beneficial in preventing cardiovascular disease and others that might increase risk. There is evidence that caffeine prevents platelet aggregation and that coffee containing caffeine increases the fibrinolytic activity in blood (8029,8030). However, diterpene constituents in unfiltered coffee such as cafestol and kahweol are believed to increase serum cholesterol, which may increase cardiovascular disease risk (1353). Cafestol is also thought to increase triglyceride levels by increasing the production of very-low-density lipoprotein (VLDL) particles which subsequently can cause a rise in low-density lipoprotein (LDL) cholesterol levels (8037). There is also evidence the constituent chlorogenic acid in coffee raises homocysteine levels (8035).

Green coffee beans contain high levels of antioxidant polyphenols, which are thought to be antitumorigenic. Most of these polyphenols are destroyed during the roasting process. Some researchers have reported that a new roasting process maintains higher levels of polyphenols without affecting the flavor. They theorize that such coffee might be healthier to drink (6601); however, this has not been demonstrated.

Epidemiological research suggests that drinking coffee might reduce the risk of type 2 diabetes. The mechanism for this observed effect is unknown, but several constituents of coffee might have an effect on glucose regulation. Chlorogenic acid in coffee might inhibit glucose-6-phosphatase, which might lower hepatic glucose production. Antioxidants in coffee might improve insulin sensitivity. Caffeine seems to stimulate pancreatic beta cells to secrete insulin. Coffee also contains magnesium and phytoestrogens, both of which have been associated with a beneficial effect on diabetes risk (11731,11732). However, some research suggests that the caffeine in coffee might have an adverse effect on diabetes. In people with type 2 diabetes, acute administration of caffeine impairs postprandial glucose metabolism, while acute abstention from caffeine reduces postprandial glucose levels by 21%. Whether these effects also occur with caffeinated beverages and herbs is unknown (12374). Other research in obese people suggests that caffeine ingestion may contribute to insulin resistance (12375).

For prevention of Parkinson's disease, caffeine may prevent the inhibition of dopaminergic transmission by adenosine. This may result in a reduction in the clinical expression of Parkinsonism (6022).

Coffee might also have a protective effect on the gallbladder. It seems to enhance gallbladder contractility, stimulate cholecystokinin (CCK) release, and increase colonic motility, which might lower the risk of gallstone disease (3345).

Proponents of caffeinated coffee enemas believe that caffeine is absorbed into the portal circulation, causing dilation of the bile ducts and stimulation of hepatocellular function to detoxify tumor cell metabolism products. However, these claims have not been substantiated (3026,3346,3347,6653).

Adverse Reactions

Orally, coffee containing caffeine can cause headache, diuresis, gastric distress, nervousness, vomiting, insomnia, anxiety, agitation, ringing in the ears, and heart arrhythmias. Coffee containing caffeine increases intraocular pressure, starting about 30 minutes after consumption and persisting for at least 90 minutes. Decaffeinated coffee does not appear to affect intraocular pressure (8540). Insomnia is a frequent adverse effect in children (10755).

Caffeine may cause feeding intolerance and gastrointestinal irritation in infants (6026). Caffeine may exacerbate sleep disturbances in patients with acquired immunodeficiency syndrome (AIDS) (10204).

Although acute administration of caffeine can cause increased blood pressure, regular consumption does not seem to increase either blood pressure or pulse, even in mildly hypertensive patients (1451,1452,2722). Caffeinated coffee consumption consisting of one or more cups per day doesn't seem to increase the risk of developing hypertension in habitual coffee drinkers (8033).

Tolerance to caffeine is a widely held belief, but there is little supportive clinical evidence. If it exists, it appears to be of little clinical significance (11839). Withdrawal symptoms such as irritability, sleepiness, delirium, nausea, vomiting, rhinorrhea, nervousness, restlessness, anxiety, muscle tension, muscle pains, and flushed face have been described. However, these symptoms may be from nonpharmacological factors related to knowledge and expectation of effects. Clinically significant symptoms caused by caffeine withdrawal may be uncommon (2723,11839).

Boiled coffee that is prepared without a filter appears to increase serum cholesterol and triglyceride levels and increase liver aminotransferase enzymes (1353,4200,8036,8539). Drinking one liter of strong, unfiltered coffee daily for two weeks can raise serum cholesterol by 10% and serum triglyceride by 36% (1353). Tell patients to use coffee filters since these effects do not seem to occur with filtered coffee (4200,8036,8539).

Coffee can adversely affect homocysteine levels. Higher homocysteine levels have been associated with cardiovascular disease. One liter of unfiltered strong coffee daily for two weeks can increase plasma homocysteine levels by 10% (1353). The same amount of filtered strong coffee appears to raise plasma homocysteine levels by 20%, although there have been no head-to-head comparisons of filtered versus unfiltered coffee (3344).

A J-shaped association between regular coffee consumption and the risk of developing acute coronary syndromes has been suggested. Moderate consumption of less than 300 mL per day has been associated with a lower risk of developing acute coronary syndromes. However, regular coffee consumption of 300 mL per day or more is associated with an increase in the risk of developing acute coronary syndromes (11318). More than five cups of coffee daily is also associated with myocardial infarction (MI) and unstable angina in patients with existing coronary heart disease (8533).
The association between consumption of coffee and pancreatic cancer is controversial. Coffee may increase the incidence of some types of pancreatic cancers, but it may decrease other types (8535,8536,8537). Some studies do not support this association at all (8038,8040). Patients who are at risk for pancreatic cancer (pancreatitis) should limit their consumption of coffee.
Coffee consumption has also been associated at various times with an increased risk for breast cancer, bladder cancer, colon cancer, and other types of cancers, but there's no good evidence that coffee consumption increases cancer risk (8039,8040,8041).
Some evidence shows caffeine is associated with fibrocystic breast conditions in women, but caffeine restriction doesn't seem to affect breast nodularity, swelling, or pain (8996). Caffeine is associated with endometriosis in women; however, this is controversial since findings are conflicting (8043).
There is preliminary evidence that use of greater than four cups of coffee per day can increase the risk of rheumatoid factor positive rheumatoid arthritis, but this association has not been confirmed (6482).
Combining ephedra with coffee can increase the risk of adverse effects, due to the caffeine contained in coffee. Jitteriness, hypertension, seizures, temporary loss of consciousness, and hospitalization requiring life support has been associated with the combined use of ephedra and caffeine (2729). There is also a report of ischemic stroke in an athlete who consumed ephedra 40-60 mg, creatine monohydrate 6 grams, caffeine 400-600 mg, and a variety of other supplements daily for six weeks (1275).
Rectally, coffee enemas have been associated with three deaths. Two of these deaths are related to severe electrolyte imbalance, and a third is associated with polymicrobial septicemia following use of coffee enema (3026,3347,3349,6652).
There is evidence coffee containing caffeine shortens whole blood fibrinolysis time (8030). There is also some evidence that consumption of three or more cups of caffeinated coffee might increase the risk of Helicobacter pylori infection (8034).
Epidemiological evidence regarding the relationship between caffeine use and the risk for osteoporosis is contradictory. Caffeine can increase urinary excretion of calcium (2669,10202,11317). Women identified with a genetic variant of the vitamin D receptor appear to be at an increased risk for the detrimental effect of caffeine on bone mass (2669). However, moderate caffeine intake, less than 300 mg per day, does not seem to significantly increase osteoporosis risk in most postmenopausal women with normal calcium intake (2669,6025,10202,11317).
Caffeine can cause anaphylaxis in sensitive individuals, although true IgE-mediated caffeine allergy seems to be relatively rare (11315).

Interactions with Herbs & Other Dietary Supplements

CAFFEINE CONTAINING HERBS/SUPPLEMENTS: Concomitant use of coffee and caffeine-containing herbs/supplements constitutes therapeutic duplication (due to the caffeine contained in coffee) which increases the risk of caffeine-related adverse effects. Other natural products which contain caffeine include black tea, cocoa, cola nut, green tea, guarana, and mate.
CALCIUM: High caffeine intake from foods and beverages including coffee increases urinary calcium excretion (2570).
CREATINE: There is some concern that combining caffeine or caffeine-containing beverages and herbs with ephedra, and creatine might increase the risk of serious adverse effects. There is a report of ischemic stroke in an athlete who consumed creatine monohydrate 6 grams, caffeine 400-600 mg, ephedra 40-60 mg, and a variety of other supplements daily for 6 weeks (1275). Caffeine might also decrease creatine's possible beneficial effects on athletic performance. Some researchers think caffeine can inhibit phosphocreatine resynthesis (2117,4575).
EPHEDRA (Ma Huang): Use of ephedra with coffee can increase the risk of caffeine stimulatory adverse effects. There is evidence that using ephedra with caffeine might increase the risk of serious life-threatening or debilitating adverse effects such as hypertension, myocardial infarction, stroke, seizures, and death (1275,6486,10307).
Tell patients to avoid taking coffee with ephedra and other stimulants.
MAGNESIUM: Consuming large amounts of coffee can increase excretion of magnesium (11939).

Interactions with Drugs

ADENOSINE (Adenocard): The caffeine in coffee is a competitive inhibitor of adenosine at the cellular level. However, caffeine doesn't seem to affect supplemental adenosine because high interstitial levels of adenosine overcome the antagonistic effects of caffeine (11771). It is recommended that methylxanthines and methylxanthine-containing products be stopped 24 hours prior to pharmacological stress tests (11770). However, methylxanthines appear more likely to interfere with dipyridamole (Persantine) than adenosine-induced stress testing (11771).
ALCOHOL (Ethanol): Concomitant use of alcohol can increase caffeine serum concentrations and the risk of caffeine adverse effects. Alcohol reduces caffeine metabolism (6370).
ALENDRONATE (Fosamax): Separate coffee ingestion and alendronate administration by two hours. Coffee reduces alendronate bioavailability by 60% (11735).

ANTICOAGULANT/ANTIPLATELET DRUGS: Theoretically, caffeine in coffee might increase the risk of bleeding when used concomitantly with these agents. Caffeine is reported to have antiplatelet activity (8028,8029); however, this interaction has not been reported in humans. There is some evidence that caffeinated coffee might increase the fibrinolytic activity in blood (8030).
Antiplatelet agents include aspirin, clopidogrel (Plavix), dipyridamole (Persantine), ticlopidine (Ticlid), and others. Anticoagulant agents include ardeparin (Normiflo), dalteparin (Fragmin), enoxaparin (Lovenox), heparin, and warfarin (Coumadin).
ANTIDIABETES DRUGS: Theoretically, concomitant use of coffee and diabetes drugs might interfere with blood glucose control due to the caffeine in coffee. However, data are conflicting. Reports claim that caffeine might increase or decrease blood sugar (6024,8646).
CIMETIDINE (Tagamet): Theoretically, concomitant use might increase serum caffeine concentrations and the risk of adverse effects, due to the caffeine contained in coffee. Cimetidine decreases the rate of caffeine clearance by 30% (11736).
CLOZAPINE (Clozaril): Theoretically, co-administration might acutely exacerbate psychotic symptoms, due to the caffeine contained in coffee. Caffeine can increase the effects and toxicity of clozapine. Caffeine doses of 400-1000 mg per day inhibit clozapine metabolism (5051).
CONTRACEPTIVE DRUGS: Theoretically, concomitant use might increase caffeine concentrations and the risk adverse effects, due to the caffeine contained in coffee. Oral contraceptives decrease the rate of caffeine clearance by 40% to 65% (2714,11737).
DIPYRIDAMOLE (Persantine): The caffeine in coffee inhibits dipyridamole-induced vasodilation (11770,11772). It is recommended that methylxanthines and methylxanthine-containing products be stopped 24 hours prior to pharmacological stress tests (11770). Methylxanthines appear more likely to interfere with dipyridamole (Persantine) than adenosine-induced stress testing (11771).
DISULFIRAM (Antabuse): Coffee contains caffeine. Concomitant use can increase caffeine serum concentrations, and the risk of adverse effects. Disulfiram decreases the rate of caffeine clearance (11840).
EPHEDRINE: Use of ephedrine with coffee can increase the risk of stimulatory adverse effects of caffeine. There is evidence that using ephedrine with caffeine might increase the risk of serious life-threatening or debilitating adverse effects such as hypertension, myocardial infarction, stroke, seizures, and death (1275,6486,10307). Tell patients to avoid taking coffee with ephedrine and other stimulants.
ESTROGENS: Theoretically, concomitant use might increase serum caffeine concentrations and the risk of adverse effects, due to the caffeine contained in coffee. Estrogen inhibits caffeine metabolism (2714).
FLUCONAZOLE (Diflucan): Concomitant use might increase the effects of caffeine. Fluconazole decreases caffeine clearance by approximately 25% (11022).
FLUVOXAMINE (Luvox): Coffee contains caffeine. Concomitant use of fluvoxamine can increase caffeine serum concentrations, and the risk of caffeine adverse effects. Fluvoxamine reduces caffeine metabolism (6370).
LITHIUM: Theoretically, abrupt coffee withdrawal might increase serum lithium levels, due to the caffeine contained in coffee. There are two case reports of lithium tremor that worsened upon abrupt coffee withdrawal (609,610).
MEXILETINE (Mexitil): Concomitant use might increase the effects and adverse effects of caffeine in coffee. Mexiletine can decrease caffeine elimination by 50% (1260,11741).
MONOAMINE OXIDASE INHIBITORS (MAOIs): Theoretically, concomitant intake of large amounts of coffee with MAOIs might precipitate a hypertensive crisis, due to the caffeine contained in coffee. This is based on the claim that intake of large amounts of caffeine with MAOIs might precipitate a hypertensive crisis (15).
PHENOTHIAZINES: The tannins in coffee might cause precipitation of solutions of fluphenazine (Permitil, Prolixin), chlorpromazine (Thorazine), haloperidol (Haldol), prochlorperazine (Compazine), thioridazine (Mellaril), and trifluoperazine (Stelazine) (626,627).
PHENYLPROPANOLAMINE: Concomitant use of phenylpropanolamine and coffee might cause an additive increase in blood pressure due to the caffeine in coffee (11738).
QUINOLONE ANTIBIOTICS: Theoretically, concomitant use might increase serum caffeine concentrations and the risk of adverse effects, due to the caffeine contained in coffee. Quinolones decrease caffeine clearance (606,607,608). Quinolones (also referred to as fluoroquinolones) include ciprofloxacin (Cipro), enoxacin (Penetrex), gatifloxacin (Tequin), levofloxacin (Levaquin), lomefloxacin (Maxaquin), moxifloxacin (Avelox), norfloxacin (Noroxin), ofloxacin (Floxin), sparfloxacin (Zagam), and trovafloxacin (Trovan).
RILUZOLE (Rilutek): Theoretically, concomitant use might increase serum caffeine and riluzole concentrations and the risk of adverse effects of both caffeine and riluzole, due to the caffeine contained in coffee. Caffeine and riluzole are both metabolized by cytochrome P450 1A2, and concomitant use might reduce metabolism of one or both agents (11739).
STIMULANT DRUGS: Concomitant use might increase the risk of stimulant adverse effects, due to the caffeine contained in coffee (11832). CNS stimulants include nicotine, cocaine, sympathomimetic amines, and amphetamines.
TERBINAFINE (Lamisil): Theoretically, concomitant use might increase serum caffeine concentrations and the risk of adverse effects, due to the caffeine contained in coffee.
Terbinafine decreases the rate of caffeine clearance (11740).
THEOPHYLLINE: Theoretically, concomitant use might increase serum theophylline concentrations and the risk

of adverse effects, due to the caffeine contained in coffee. Large amounts of caffeine might inhibit theophylline metabolism (11741).
TRICYCLIC ANTIDEPRESSANTS (TCAs): The tannins in coffee might cause precipitation of solutions of amitriptyline (Elavil) or imipramine (Tofranil, Janimine) (626,627).
VERAPAMIL (Calan, Covera, Isoptin, Verelan): Theoretically, concomitant use might increase plasma caffeine concentrations and the risk of adverse effects, due to the caffeine contained in coffee. Verapamil increases plasma caffeine concentrations by 25% (11741).

Interactions with Foods

None known.

Interactions with Lab Tests

5-HYDROXYINDOLEACETIC ACID: Coffee might increase urine 5-hydroxyindoleacetic acid concentrations and test results, due to its caffeine content. Caffeine can increase urine catecholamine concentrations (15).
BLEEDING TIME: Theoretically, coffee might increase bleeding time. Caffeine can prolong bleeding time and increase the results of a bleeding time test (1701). Caffeine is reported to have antiplatelet activity (8028,8029). There is some evidence that caffeinated coffee increases fibrinolytic activity in blood (8030). However, the significance of these effects in humans is not known.
CATECHOLAMINES: Coffee might increase urine catecholamine concentrations and test results, due to its caffeine content. Caffeine can increase urine catecholamine concentrations (8646).
CREATINE: Coffee might increase urine creatine concentrations and test results, due to its caffeine content (1701).
DIPYRIDAMOLE THALLIUM IMAGING: Coffee might interfere with dipyridamole thallium imaging studies, due to its caffeine content. Caffeine attenuates the characteristic cardiovascular responses to dipyridamole and has altered test results (11742).
GLUCOSE: Caffeine, a constituent of coffee, has been reported to cause increases and decreases in blood glucose (8646).
LACTATE: The combination of ephedrine, a constituent of ephedra, and the caffeine in coffee can increase blood lactate levels (8646).
NEUROBLASTOMA TESTS: Coffee (due to its caffeine content) might cause false-positive diagnosis of neuroblastoma, when diagnosis is based on tests of urine vanillylmandelic acid (VMA) or catecholamine concentrations. Caffeine can increase urine catecholamine and VMA concentrations (15).
PHARMACOLOGICAL STRESS TESTS: The caffeine in coffee is a competitive antagonist for adenosine receptors (11771). Caffeine attenuates the characteristic cardiovascular responses to dipyridamole and has altered test results (11742). It is recommended that caffeine and caffeine-containing products be stopped 24 hours prior to pharmacological stress tests (11770). However, caffeine appears more likely to interfere with dipyridamole (Persantine) than adenosine (Adenocard) stress testing (11771). The interaction between caffeine and dipyridamole is unlikely to be significant in stress testing if the heart rate increase is greater than 5% after dipyridamole infusion (11772).
PHEOCHROMOCYTOMA TESTS: Coffee (due to its caffeine content) might cause false-positive diagnosis of pheochromocytoma, when diagnosis is based on tests of urine vanillylmandelic acid (VMA) or catecholamine concentrations. Caffeine can increase urine catecholamine and VMA concentrations (15).
PULMONARY FUNCTION TESTS: People may need to avoid caffeine and caffeinated beverages for at least four hours prior to lung function testing. Forced expiratory volume in one minute (FEV1) seems to show a small improvement up to two hours after caffeine use. Mid-expiratory flow rates may also improve with caffeine for up to four hours (9607).
URATE: Coffee might falsely increase serum urate test results determined by the Bittner method, due to its caffeine content. Caffeine causes false elevations in serum urate test results determined by the Bittner method (11844).
URINARY CALCIUM: Caffeine, a constituent of coffee, can increase urinary calcium levels (11317).
VANILLYLMANDELIC ACID (VMA): Coffee might increase urine VMA concentrations and test results, due to its caffeine content. Caffeine can increase urine VMA concentrations (15).
WHOLE BLOOD FIBRINOLYSIS TIME (Fearnley method): There is evidence caffeinated coffee may increase the whole blood fibrinolysis time (8030).

Interactions with Diseases or Conditions

ANXIETY DISORDERS: The caffeine in coffee might aggravate anxiety disorders (11743).
BLEEDING DISORDERS: Theoretically, caffeine in coffee might aggravate bleeding conditions. Caffeine is reported to have antiplatelet activity (8028,8029); however, this interaction has not been reported in humans. There is some evidence caffeinated coffee may increase fibrinolytic activity in blood (8030). Caffeine can prolong bleeding time and increase the results of a bleeding time test (1701).
CARDIAC CONDITIONS: The caffeine in coffee can induce cardiac arrhythmias in sensitive individuals (16); use with caution.
DIABETES: Some research suggests that caffeine, a constituent of coffee, may impair postprandial glucose metabolism in people with diabetes and contribute to insulin resistance. The effect of caffeinated beverages and herbs has not been studied (12374,12375). The caffeine in coffee may enhance the frequency and intensity of

hypoglycemic warning symptoms in type 1 diabetics. This may increase the ability of diabetics to detect and treat hypoglycemia early. However, it might also increase the frequency of hypoglycemic events (6024); use with caution. Caffeine has been reported to cause increases and decreases in blood glucose (8646); use with caution.
GLAUCOMA: Drinking caffeinated coffee increases intraocular pressure. The increase occurs within 30 minutes and persists for at least 90 minutes (8540).
HEART DISEASE: Consumption of unfiltered (boiled) coffee increases plasma homocysteine levels, serum cholesterol, and triglycerides, which are associated with an increased risk of cardiovascular disease (1353,4200,8036,8539). Some research suggests an association between heart attacks and coffee consumption.
Regular coffee consumption of 300 ml per day or more is associated with an increase in the risk of developing acute coronary syndromes (11318). Heavy coffee consumption also seems to increase risk in people with existing coronary heart disease (8042,8533,8538). More than 5 cups of coffee on a regular basis is associated with myocardial infarction and unstable angina in patients with coronary heart disease (CHD) (8533).
HYPERTENSION: Consuming caffeinated coffee might increase blood pressure in people with high blood pressure. However, this effect might be less in habitual caffeine users (2722).
OSTEOPOROSIS: Consuming caffeinated coffee can increase urinary excretion of calcium. Caffeine consumption should be limited to less than 300 mg per day (approximately 2-3 cups of coffee). Adequate calcium supplementation may partially compensate for calcium losses (2669,10202,11317). Postmenopausal women identified with a genetic variant of the vitamin D receptor should use caffeine with caution (2669).

Dosage and Administration

ORAL: The typical dose of caffeine for headache or restoring mental alertness is up to 250 mg per day, about 2 cups of coffee (2718,11743). For preventing Parkinson's disease, consumption of three to four cups (28 oz) of caffeinated coffee per day or 421 mg to 2716 mg total caffeine has been used to reduce the risk of developing Parkinson's disease. However, a significantly lower risk has also been associated with consumption of as little as 124 mg to 208 mg of caffeine (approximately one to two cups of coffee) (6022). In women, more moderate caffeinated coffee consumption seems to be best; one to three cups per day (1238). For preventing symptomatic gallstone disease, consumption of 400 mg or greater of caffeine per day (two or more cups of coffee) has been used for risk reduction (3345,8032). However, consumption of at least 800 mg caffeine per day (four or more cups of coffee) seems to be associated with the greatest reduction in risk (3345). For preventing type 2 diabetes, long-term consumption of about 900 mg caffeine per day (6 or more cups of coffee per day) has been used (11353).
Use filtered coffee to avoid some adverse effects. Choice of coffee, grind, ratio of coffee to water, and other factors determine flavor and strength of the beverage.
Caffeine content of coffee (per average cup): percolated, 100-150 mg caffeine; instant, 85-100 mg caffeine; and decaffeinated, approximately 8 mg caffeine (13). Darker roasts contain less caffeine due to sublimation during roasting (13).

Comments

Coffee enemas are used as a part of the "Gerson Therapy." Cancer patients are treated with caffeinated coffee, in the form of four-hourly enemas on a daily basis. The enemas are combined with a diet of liver, vegetables, and a variety of oral medications, including potassium, pepsin, Lugol's solution, niacin, pancreatin, and thyroid extracts (3348,6653). The Gerson Therapy is considered an unacceptable medical practice in the US, but continues to be used at The Hospital of the Baja California in Tijuana, Mexico, one mile from the US (3346,3347,3348,6652,6653).

COFFEE CHARCOAL

Also Known As

None.
CAUTION: See separate listings for Activated Charcoal and Coffee.

Scientific Names

Coffea arabica; Coffea canephora; Coffea liberica.
Family: Rubiaceae.

People Use This For

Orally, coffee charcoal is used for nonspecific, acute diarrhea.
Topically, coffee charcoal is used for inflammation of the oral and pharyngeal mucosa, and for festering wounds.

Safety

POSSIBLY SAFE ...when used orally or topically (2).
PREGNANCY AND LACTATION: Insufficient reliable information available; avoid using.

Effectiveness
There is insufficient reliable information available about the effectiveness of coffee charcoal.

Mechanism of Action
Coffee charcoal can have adsorbent and astringent properties (2).

Adverse Reactions
None reported.

Interactions with Herbs & Other Dietary Supplements
None known.

Interactions with Drugs
ORAL DRUGS: Coffee charcoal can reduce the absorption of orally administered drugs (2) and should be separated from oral drug administration by at least two hours.

Interactions with Foods
None known.

Interactions with Lab Tests
None known.

Interactions with Diseases or Conditions
None known.

Dosage and Administration
ORAL: The average single dose of coffee charcoal is 3 grams (18), and the total daily dose is 9 grams per day (2). Store coffee charcoal in a well-sealed container (18). Diarrhea persisting beyond 3 to 4 days should be evaluated by a health care professional (2).
TOPICAL: No typical dosage.

Comments
Coffee charcoal is produced by roasting the outer portion of the coffee beans until blackened or charred.

COLA NUT

Also Known As
Bissy Nut, Guru Nut, Gworo, Kola Nut, Soudan Coffee.
CAUTION: See separate listings for Caffeine, Gotu Kola, Green Tea, Black Tea, Oolong Tea, Coffee, Cocoa, Guarana, Mate.

Scientific Names
Cola acuminata, synonym Sterculia acuminata; Cola nitida, synonym Sterculia nitida; and related species.
Family: Sterculiaceae or Malvaceae.

People Use This For
Orally, cola nut is used for short-term relief of mental and physical fatigue and depressive states, especially those associated with general muscle weakness. It is also used orally for melancholy, atony, exhaustion, dysentery, atonic diarrhea, weight loss, and migraines.
In foods and beverages, cola nut is used as a flavoring ingredient.

Safety
LIKELY SAFE ...when used in amounts commonly found in foods.
Cola nut extract has Generally Recognized As Safe (GRAS) status in the US (4912).
POSSIBLY SAFE ...when used orally and appropriately, short-term. Cola nut has been used safely for up to 12 weeks (12811).
POSSIBLY UNSAFE ...when cola nut is used orally in large amounts or for prolonged periods of time. Chewing cola nut is associated with an increased risk of mouth cancer and gastrointestinal cancer (11963).
LIKELY UNSAFE ...when used orally in very high doses. Cola nut contains caffeine.
The fatal acute oral dose of caffeine is estimated to be 10-14 grams (150-200 mg per kilogram).
Serious toxicity can occur at lower doses depending on variables in caffeine sensitivity such as smoking, age, prior caffeine use, etc (11832).
CHILDREN: LIKELY SAFE ...when used orally in amounts found in foods (4912,11833).

PREGNANCY: POSSIBLY SAFE ...when used orally in amounts found in foods. Due to the caffeine content of cola nut, mothers should closely monitor their intake to ensure moderate consumption. Fetal blood concentrations of caffeine approximate maternal concentrations (4260). Use of caffeine in pregnancy is controversial; however, moderate consumption has not been associated with clinically important adverse fetal effects (2708,2709,2710,2711,9606). Caffeine crosses the human placenta, but is not considered a teratogen. Mothers should keep caffeine consumption below 300 mg per day. This is similar to the amount of caffeine found in about 3 cups of coffee or tea (2708). POSSIBLY UNSAFE ...when used orally in large amounts. Caffeine crosses the placenta, producing fetal blood concentrations similar to maternal levels (4260). Mothers should avoid consuming more than 300 mg of caffeine daily (2708). High maternal doses of caffeine throughout pregnancy have resulted in symptoms of caffeine withdrawal in newborn infants (9891). High doses of caffeine have been associated with spontaneous abortion, premature delivery, and low birth weight (2709,2711). Fetal birth weight is reduced by 28 grams for every 100 mg per day of caffeine consumed during pregnancy. But this is unlikely to be clinically important except for women consuming more than 600 mg of caffeine daily (9606). Teratogenicity studies have not been performed.

LACTATION: POSSIBLY SAFE ...when used orally in amounts found in foods. Due to the caffeine content of cola nut, nursing mothers should closely monitor caffeine intake. Breast milk concentrations of caffeine are thought to be approximately 50% of maternal serum concentrations. Minimal consumption would likely result in limited exposure to a nursing infant (9892). POSSIBLY UNSAFE ...when used orally in large amounts. Consumption of cola nut might cause irritability and increased bowel activity in nursing infants (6026). Large doses or excessive intake of cola nut should be avoided during lactation. Whether potentially carcinogenic constituents of cola nut are transferred via breast milk is unknown.

Effectiveness

INSUFFICIENT RELIABLE EVIDENCE to RATE

Obesity. Preliminary, manufacturer-sponsored clinical research suggests that cola nut in combination with ephedra and willow bark might cause modest weight loss in overweight and obese people. Cola nut 1500 mg per day given in divided doses for 3 months in combination with ephedra and willow bark might cause a 2 kg reduction in weight (12811). This combination might not be appropriate for weight loss due to safety concerns related to ephedra. Ephedra is banned in the US due to severe adverse effects (10055). More evidence is needed to rate cola nut for this use.

Mechanism of Action

The applicable part of cola nut is the seed (nut). Cola nut contains 1% to 2.5% caffeine (12). Cola nut also contains high concentrations of tannins and N-nitroso compounds that are potential carcinogens (11963).

Caffeine is responsible for most of the pharmacologic effects of cola nut. Caffeine is a methylxanthine compound and is structurally related to theophylline, theobromine, and uric acid (6372). It is 100% bioavailable after oral administration and is metabolized principally in the liver to paraxanthine, theophylline, and theobromine (6370). The half-life of caffeine is about six hours (8644).

Caffeine stimulates the central nervous system (CNS), heart, muscles, and possibly the pressor centers that control blood pressure (2722). Possible mechanisms include adenosine receptor blockade and phosphodiesterase inhibition (2722). By blocking adenosine receptors, caffeine is thought to increase the release of neurotransmitters such as dopamine (6370). Caffeine also decreases airway resistance and stimulates respiration, via adenosine receptor blockade and phosphodiesterase inhibition (11836). It has also been proposed that caffeine may decrease GABA and serotonin signaling (6370). Caffeine stimulates gastric acid secretion, and increases plasma catecholamine levels (11837). Caffeine can have positive inotropic and chronotropic effects on the heart (11836). Caffeine can also acutely elevate both diastolic and systolic blood pressure, but might not have this effect in habitual users (2722). Caffeine exerts a diuretic effect, with water losses estimated at 1.17 mL per milligram of caffeine (2712). Tachyphylaxis to the diuretic effect develops rapidly, diminishing fluid losses associated with caffeine intake (10206). Caffeine-containing beverages consumed during moderate endurance exercise do not appear to compromise bodily hydration status (2713). Caffeine does not substantially affect the fluid status of people who drink caffeinated beverages on a regular basis (10206). Caffeine's CNS stimulant effects are thought to improve vigilance and psychomotor performance (2720,10205). For improving athletic performance, caffeine has been shown to decrease perceived levels of exertion, which enables the athlete to feel less tired and increase their performance (6370). Caffeine alone or in combination with ephedrine can improve anaerobic exercise performance. Caffeine seems to enhance muscle metabolism and increases time to exhaustion and oxygen deficit, which may lead to better performance (8646). Studies have also suggested caffeine possibly influences cardiovascular stress reactivity, either by potentiating the stress response itself or adding to the level reached during stress (6372). Caffeine may cause a slight decrease in heart rate after consumption and appears to raise blood pressure during psychological stress (6372). Large amounts of caffeine, >10 mg/kg/day, can also produce tachycardia and premature ventricular contractions (6372). Caffeine, a constituent of cola nut, has been reported to cause increases and decreases in blood glucose. In people with type 2 diabetes, acute administration of caffeine impairs postprandial glucose metabolism, while acute abstention from caffeine reduces postprandial glucose levels by 21%. Whether these effects also occur with caffeinated beverages and herbs is unknown (12374). Other research in obese people suggests that caffeine ingestion may contribute to insulin resistance (12375). However, one study found that type 1 diabetics taking 200 mg of caffeine twice daily had increased frequency and intensity of warning signs of hypoglycemia. This may be due to a reduction in blood flow to the brain and an increase in glucose utilization by the brain (6024). For preventing Parkinson's disease, caffeine may protect dopaminergic neurons in the brain. This effect appears to be related to modulation of adenosine receptors (10201). This may result in a reduction in the clinical expression of Parkinsonism (6022). Evidence suggests that tolerance to caffeine's neuroendocrine and cardiovascular effects may develop during consumption throughout the day, but tolerance appears to be lost during overnight abstinence of caffeine (6372). Preliminary evidence also suggests caffeine may increase plasma levels of cortisol and adrenocorticotrophic hormone (ACTH), decrease levels of extracellular potassium, and increase levels of intracellular calcium in skeletal muscle; but the mechanisms are poorly understood (6370).

Caffeine may be beneficial in the prevention of cardiovascular disease. There is evidence caffeine inhibits platelet aggregation and suppresses thromboxane formation during blood clotting (8028,8029). There is also evidence caffeine might be associated with decreased levels of testosterone and increased levels of estrone and sex-hormone binding globulin. These findings might explain why some studies have reported associations between caffeine and hormone-dependent conditions such as fibrocystic disease, osteoporosis, breast cancer, and endometriosis (8043).

Caffeine is often used in combination with ephedra for weight loss and seems to have additive pharmacodynamic effects. A single dose of ephedra in combination with caffeine can increase heart rate from 67 beats per minute to 82 beats per minute in young, healthy people. The combination also increases systolic blood pressure and to a lesser extent, diastolic pressure (8644). Caffeine in combination with ephedra also increases oxygen consumption. Whether the increased oxygen consumption is an indication of a significant increase in metabolism and contributes to weight loss is unknown (8645).

Adverse Reactions

Orally, cola nut can cause symptoms of caffeine toxicity. Caffeine can cause insomnia, nervousness, restlessness, gastric irritation, nausea, vomiting, tachycardia, quickened respiration, tremors, delirium, convulsions, and diuresis. Large doses can produce headache, anxiety, agitation, ringing in the ears, premature heartbeat, and arrhythmia (11832,11838). In fatal caffeine overdose, the cause of death is usually ventricular fibrillation (11838,11845). Insomnia is a frequent adverse effect in children (10755). Caffeine may cause feeding intolerance and gastrointestinal irritation in infants (6023). Caffeine may exacerbate sleep disturbances in patients with acquired immunodeficiency syndrome (AIDS) (10204).

Some evidence shows caffeine is associated with fibrocystic breast disease, breast cancer, and endometriosis in women; however, this is controversial since findings are conflicting (8043). Restricting caffeine in women with fibrocystic breast conditions doesn't seem to affect breast nodularity, swelling, or pain (8996).

Although acute administration of caffeine can cause increased blood pressure, regular consumption does not seem to increase either blood pressure or pulse, even in mildly hypertensive patients (1451,1452,2722).

Tolerance to caffeine is a widely held belief, but there is little supportive clinical evidence. If it exists, it appears to be of little clinical significance (11839).

Withdrawal symptoms such as irritability, sleepiness, delirium, nausea, vomiting, rhinorrhea, nervousness, restlessness, anxiety, muscle tension, muscle pains, and flushed face have been described.

However, these symptoms may be from nonpharmacological factors related to knowledge and expectation of effects. Clinically significant symptoms caused by caffeine withdrawal may be uncommon (2723,11839).

Epidemiological evidence regarding the relationship between caffeine use and the risk for osteoporosis is contradictory. Caffeine can increase urinary excretion of calcium (2669,10202,11317). Women identified with a genetic variant of the vitamin D receptor appear to be at an increased risk for the detrimental effect of caffeine on bone mass (2669). However, moderate caffeine intake, less than 300 mg per day, does not seem to significantly increase osteoporosis risk in most postmenopausal women with normal calcium intake (2669,6025,10202,11317).

Combining ephedra with caffeine can increase the risk of adverse effects. Jitteriness, hypertension, seizures, temporary loss of consciousness, and hospitalization requiring life support has been associated with the combined use of ephedra and caffeine (2729). There is also a report of ischemic stroke in an athlete who consumed ephedra 40-60 mg, creatine monohydrate 6 grams, caffeine 400-600 mg, and a variety of other supplements daily for six weeks (1275).

Caffeine can cause anaphylaxis in sensitive individuals, although true IgE-mediated caffeine allergy seems to be relatively rare (11315).

Preliminary research suggests that chewing cola nut could increase the risk of oral and gastrointestinal cancer. Cola nut contains high amounts of tannins and N-nitroso compounds, which are carcinogenic. Chewing cola nuts is practiced widely in Nigeria, which has a high incidence of oral and gastrointestinal cancer. The risk may be even higher in smokers (11963).

Interactions with Herbs & Other Dietary Supplements

CAFFEINE CONTAINING HERBS/SUPPLEMENTS: Concomitant use of cola nut and caffeine-containing herbs/supplements constitutes therapeutic duplication (due to the caffeine contained in cola nut) which increases the risk of caffeine-related adverse effects. Other natural products which contain caffeine include black tea, cocoa, coffee, green tea, guarana, and mate.

CALCIUM: High caffeine intake from foods, beverages, and herbs including cola nut increases urinary calcium excretion (2570).

CREATINE: There is some concern that combining caffeine, ephedra, and creatine might increase the risk of serious adverse effects. There is a report of ischemic stroke in an athlete who consumed creatine monohydrate 6 grams, caffeine 400-600 mg, ephedra 40-60 mg, and a variety of other supplements daily for six weeks (1275). Caffeine might also decrease creatine's possible beneficial effects on athletic performance. Some researchers think caffeine can inhibit phosphocreatine resynthesis (2117,4575).

EPHEDRA (ma huang): Use of ephedra with cola nut can increase the risk of stimulatory adverse effects due to its caffeine content. There is evidence that using ephedra with caffeine might increase the risk of serious life-threatening or debilitating adverse effects such as hypertension, myocardial infarction, stroke, seizures, and death (6486,10307). Tell patients to avoid taking cola nut with ephedra and other stimulants.

Interactions with Drugs

ADENOSINE (Adenocard): The caffeine in cola nut is a competitive inhibitor of adenosine at the cellular level. However, caffeine doesn't seem to affect supplemental adenosine because high interstitial levels of adenosine overcome the antagonistic effects of caffeine (11771).

ALCOHOL (Ethanol): Concomitant use of alcohol can increase caffeine serum concentrations and the risk of caffeine adverse effects. Alcohol reduces caffeine metabolism (6370).

AMPHETAMINES: Theoretically, the caffeine in cola nut might increase the risk of additive CNS effects (2719).

ANTIDIABETES DRUGS: Theoretically, concomitant use of caffeine and diabetes drugs might interfere with blood glucose control. Data are conflicting. Reports claim that caffeine might increase or decrease blood sugar (6024,8646).

CIMETIDINE (Tagamet): Theoretically, concomitant use might increase serum caffeine concentrations and the risk of adverse effects, due to the caffeine contained in cola nut. Cimetidine decreases the rate of caffeine clearance by 30% to 50% (11736).

CLOZAPINE (Clozaril): Theoretically, co-administration might acutely exacerbate psychotic symptoms, due to the caffeine contained in cola nut. Caffeine can increase the effects and toxicity of clozapine (151). Caffeine doses of 400-1000 mg per day inhibit clozapine metabolism (5051).

COCAINE: Theoretically, the caffeine in cola nut might increase the risk of additive CNS effects (2719).

CONTRACEPTIVE DRUGS: Theoretically, concomitant use might increase caffeine concentrations and the risk adverse effects, due to the caffeine contained in cola nut. Oral contraceptives decrease the rate of caffeine clearance by 40% to 65% (2714,11737).

DIPYRIDAMOLE (Persantine): The caffeine in cola nut might inhibit dipyridamole-induced vasodilation (11770,11772).

DISULFIRAM (Antabuse): Theoretically, concomitant use might increase serum caffeine concentrations and the risk of adverse effects, due to the caffeine contained in cola nut. Disulfiram decreases the rate of caffeine clearance (15).

EPHEDRINE: Use of ephedrine with caffeine can increase the risk of stimulatory adverse effects. There is evidence that using ephedrine with caffeine might increase the risk of serious life-threatening or debilitating adverse effects such as hypertension, myocardial infarction, stroke, seizures, and death (1275,6486,10307). Tell patients to avoid taking caffeine with ephedrine and other stimulants.

ESTROGENS: Theoretically, concomitant use might increase serum caffeine concentrations and the risk of adverse effects, due to the caffeine contained in cola nut. Estrogen inhibits caffeine metabolism (2714).

FLUCONAZOLE (Diflucan): Concomitant use might increase the effects of caffeine in cola nut. Fluconazole decreases caffeine clearance by approximately 25% (11022).

FLUVOXAMINE (Luvox): Concomitant use can increase caffeine serum concentrations, and the risk of caffeine adverse effects. Fluvoxamine reduces caffeine metabolism (6370).

LITHIUM: Theoretically, abrupt cola nut withdrawal might increase serum lithium levels, due to the caffeine contained in cola nut. There are two case reports of lithium tremor that worsened upon abrupt coffee withdrawal (609,610).

MEXILETINE (Mexitil): Theoretically, concomitant use might increase serum caffeine concentrations and the risk of adverse effects, due to the caffeine contained in cola nut. Mexiletine reduces caffeine metabolism (11741).

MONOAMINE OXIDASE INHIBITORS (MAOIs): Theoretically, concomitant intake of large amounts of cola nut with MAOIs might precipitate a hypertensive crisis, due to the caffeine contained in cola nut. This is based on the claim that intake of large amounts of caffeine with MAOIs might precipitate a hypertensive crisis (15).

NICOTINE: Theoretically, the caffeine in cola nut might increase the risk of additive CNS effects (2719).

PHENYLPROPANOLAMINE: Concomitant use of phenylpropanolamine and cola nut might cause an additive increase in blood pressure due to the caffeine in cola nut (11738).

QUINOLONE ANTIBIOTICS: Theoretically, concomitant use might increase serum caffeine concentrations

and the risk of adverse effects, due to the caffeine contained in cola nut. Quinolones decrease caffeine clearance (606,607,608). Quinolones (also referred to as fluoroquinolones) include ciprofloxacin (Cipro), enoxacin (Penetrex), gatifloxacin (Tequin), levofloxacin (Levaquin), lomefloxacin (Maxaquin), moxifloxacin (Avelox), norfloxacin (Noroxin), ofloxacin (Floxin), sparfloxacin (Zagam), and trovafloxacin (Trovan).
RILUZOLE (Rilutek): Theoretically, concomitant use of riluzole and caffeinated products such as cola nut might increase serum caffeine and riluzole concentrations and the risk of adverse effects of both caffeine and riluzole, due to the caffeine contained in cola nut. Caffeine and riluzole are both metabolized by cytochrome P450 1A2, and concomitant use might reduce metabolism of one or both agents (11739).
TERBINAFINE (Lamisil): Theoretically, concomitant use might increase serum caffeine concentrations and the risk of adverse effects, due to the caffeine contained in cola nut. Terbinafine decreases the rate of caffeine clearance (11740).
THEOPHYLLINE: Theoretically, concomitant use of theophylline and large amounts of cola nut might increase the risk of theophylline toxicity, due to cola nut's caffeine content. Caffeine decreases theophylline clearance 23% to 29% (11741).
VERAPAMIL (Calan, Covera, Isoptin, Verelan): Theoretically, concomitant use might increase plasma caffeine concentrations and the risk of adverse effects, due to the caffeine contained in cola nut. Verapamil increases plasma caffeine concentrations by 25% (11741). Some of these drugs include Calan, Isoptin, and Verelan.

Interactions with Foods

CAFFEINE-CONTAINING BEVERAGES: Concomitant use can have additive therapeutic and adverse effects due to the caffeine content.
GRAPEFRUIT JUICE: Grapefruit juice interacts with the caffeine in cola nut and can increase caffeine levels, its activity, and the risk of adverse effects (504).

Interactions with Lab Tests

5-HYDROXYINDOLEACETIC ACID: Cola nut might increase urine 5-hydroxyindoleacetic acid concentrations and test results, due to its caffeine content. Caffeine can increase urine catecholamine concentrations (15).
BLEEDING TIME: Cola nut might prolong bleeding time and increase test results, due to its caffeine content (1701).
CATECHOLAMINES: Cola nut might increase urine catecholamine concentrations and test results, due to its caffeine content (15).
CREATINE: Cola nut might increase urine creatine concentrations and test results, due to its caffeine content (1701).
DIPYRIDAMOLE THALLIUM IMAGING: Cola nut might interfere with dipyridamole thallium imaging studies, due to its caffeine content. Caffeine attenuates the characteristic cardiovascular responses to dipyridamole and has altered test results (11742).
GLUCOSE: Caffeine has been reported to cause increases and decreases in blood glucose (8646).
LACTATE: The combination of ephedrine, a constituent of ephedra, and caffeine, a constituent of cola nut, can increase blood lactate levels (8646).
NEUROBLASTOMA TESTS: Cola nut (due to its caffeine content) might cause false-positive diagnosis of neuroblastoma, when diagnosis is based on tests of urine vanillylmandelic acid (VMA) or catecholamine concentrations. Caffeine can increase urine catecholamine and VMA concentrations (15).
PHARMACOLOGICAL STRESS TESTS: The caffeine in cola nut is a competitive antagonist for adenosine receptors (11771). It is recommended that caffeine and caffeine-containing products be stopped 24 hours prior to pharmacological stress tests (11770). However, caffeine appears more likely to interfere with dipyridamole (Persantine) than adenosine (Adenocard) stress testing (11771). The interaction between caffeine and dipyridamole is unlikely to be significant in stress testing if the heart rate increase is greater than 5% after dipyridamole infusion (11772).
PHEOCHROMOCYTOMA TESTS: Cola nut (due to its caffeine content) might cause false-positive diagnosis of pheochromocytoma, when diagnosis is based on tests of urine vanillylmandelic acid (VMA) or catecholamine concentrations. Caffeine can increase urine catecholamine and VMA concentrations (15).
PULMONARY FUNCTION TESTS: People may need to avoid caffeine and caffeine-containing beverages and products such as cola nut for at least four hours prior to lung function testing. Forced expiratory volume in one minute (FEV1) seems to show a small improvement up to two hours after caffeine use. Mid-expiratory flow rates may also improve with caffeine for up to four hours (9607).
URATE: Cola nut might falsely increase serum urate test results determined by the Bittner method, due to its caffeine content. Caffeine causes false elevations in serum urate test results determined by the Bittner method (15).
URINARY CALCIUM: Caffeine, a constituent of cola nut, can increase urinary calcium levels (11317).
VANILLYLMANDELIC ACID (VMA): Cola nut might increase urine VMA concentrations and test results, due to its caffeine content (15).

Interactions with Diseases or Conditions

ANXIETY DISORDERS: The caffeine in cola nut might aggravate anxiety disorders (11743).
BLEEDING DISORDERS: Theoretically, caffeine in cola nut might aggravate these conditions. Caffeine is reported to have antiplatelet activity (8028,8029); however, this interaction has not been reported in humans (1701). Caffeine can prolong bleeding time and increase the results of a bleeding time test (1701).
CARDIAC CONDITIONS: Caffeine in cola nut can induce cardiac arrhythmias in sensitive individuals (11845); use with caution.
DIABETES: Caffeine in cola nut may enhance the frequency and intensity of hypoglycemic warning symptoms in type 1 diabetics. This may increase the ability of diabetics to detect and treat hypoglycemia early. However, it might also increase the frequency of hypoglycemic events (6024); use with caution. Caffeine has been reported to cause increases and decreases in blood glucose (8646); use with caution.
GLAUCOMA: Consuming cola nut increases intraocular pressure due to its caffeine content. The increase occurs within 30 minutes and persists for at least 90 minutes (8540).
HYPERTENSION: The caffeine in cola nut might increase blood pressure in people with high blood pressure. However, this doesn't seem to occur in people who regularly consume cola nut or other caffeinated products (1451,1452,2722).
OSTEOPOROSIS: Consuming cola nut can increase urinary excretion of calcium due to its caffeine content. Caffeine consumption should be limited to less than 300 mg per day. Adequate calcium supplementation may partially compensate for calcium losses (2669,10202,11317). Postmenopausal women identified with a genetic variant of the vitamin D receptor should use caffeine with caution (2669).

Dosage and Administration

No typical dosage.

Comments

Cola nut is used widely in Nigeria and many West African countries as part of traditional hospitality and cultural and social ceremonies (11963).

COLLOIDAL MINERALS

Also Known As

Bioelectrical Minerals, Clay Suspension Products, Colloidal Trace Minerals, Humic Shale, Plant-Derived Liquid Minerals.

Scientific Names

Anhydrous aluminum silicates.

People Use This For

Orally, colloidal minerals are used as a supplemental source of trace minerals, a dietary supplement to increase energy, for improving blood sugar levels in diabetes, arthritis symptoms, reducing blood cell clumping, reversing early cataracts, turning gray hair dark again, flushing poisonous heavy metals from the body, improving general well being, reducing aches and pains.

Safety

POSSIBLY UNSAFE ...when used orally. These products contain varying amounts of aluminum, arsenic, lead, barium, nickel and titanium. Some products contain as much as 1800-4400 ppm aluminum and 20 ppm arsenic (1159); generally, foods do not contain more than 10 ppm of aluminum (1159). While no cases of toxicity have been reported, there are concerns about colloidal mineral supplements containing unsafe levels of radioactive metals (1161).
PREGNANCY AND LACTATION: POSSIBLY UNSAFE ...when used orally (1159); avoid using.

Effectiveness

There is insufficient reliable information available about the effectiveness of colloidal minerals.

Mechanism of Action

Commercial colloidal mineral products are derived from clay or humic shale deposits (1159). Clay minerals are layer type aluminosilicates that figure in terrestrial biogeochemical cycles, in the buffering capacity of the oceans, and in the containment of toxic waste materials (1160). Humic shale is a common source of plant-derived colloidal minerals (1157). When mixed with water, the surfaces of clay particles become negatively charged. This allows the particles to bind with ionic minerals, such as magnesium, sodium, calcium, and potassium (1159). The content of trace minerals in individual products depends upon the rock source used (1159). Proponents claim that, due to mineral depletion of soil, many people do not take in the dietary trace minerals once plentiful in the human diet (1158). However, there is no evidence that there is increased bioavailability of ingested minerals in this form (1159).

Adverse Reactions
None reported.

Interactions with Herbs & Other Dietary Supplements
None known.

Interactions with Drugs
None known.

Interactions with Foods
None known.

Interactions with Lab Tests
None known.

Interactions with Diseases or Conditions
HEMOCHROMATOSIS, WILSON'S DISEASE: Theoretically, colloidal minerals could exacerbate conditions in which metal accumulation is a problem.

Dosage and Administration
No typical dosage.

Comments
The medicinal use of clay-based products in modern days was first encouraged by a southern Utah rancher. Historically, some Native American tribes used clay medicinally (1157). There is a tremendous amount of promotional claims for colloidal mineral products. There is no reliable medical evidence to support using these products. Commercial colloidal mineral products are derived from clay or humic shale deposits (1159).

COLLOIDAL SILVER

Also Known As
Colloidal Silver Protein, Silver Protein.

Scientific Names
Silver in suspending agent.

People Use This For
Orally, colloidal silver is used to treat ear infections, emphysema, bronchitis, fungal infections, Lyme disease, Rosacea, sinus infections, stomach ulcers, yeast infections, chronic fatigue syndrome, AIDS, and tuberculosis. It is used orally for antibacterial properties, for food poisoning, to promote rapid healing and subdue inflammation, and to treat gum disease. It is used to improve digestion, and to prevent flu and colds. Colloidal silver is also used for allergies, appendicitis, arthritis, blood parasites, bubonic plague, cancer, cholera, colitis, cystitis, conjunctivitis, atopic dermatitis (cradle cap), diabetes, dysentery, eczema, gastritis, and gonorrhea. Other uses include impetigo; hay fever; herpes; leprosy; leukemia; lupus; lymphangitis; malaria; meningitis; parasitic infections; pneumonia; pneumococci; psoriasis; prostatitis; rhinitis; ringworm; scarlet fever; and septic conditions of the eyes, ears, mouth, and throat. It is also used for Salmonella, septicemia, shingles, skin cancer, syphilis, tonsillitis, toxemia, trench foot, viruses, warts, and yeast infections. Colloidal silver is used during pregnancy to aid the baby's growth and health as well as the mother's delivery and recovery.
Topically, colloidal silver is used for acne, burns, eye infections, fungal infections, throat infections, skin infections, and Staphylococcus infections.

Safety
POSSIBLY SAFE ...when used orally in amounts found in foods. Two liters of water meeting Environmental Protection Agency (EPA) standards can contain up to 200 mcg, plus a regular diet can contain 90 mcg more silver (5525) for a total of 290 mcg. Total daily silver intake should not exceed 14 mcg/kg/day of (980 mcg/day for a 70 kg person). It is likely that taking colloidal silver supplements on top of regular dietary consumption would increase silver intake to an unsafe level.
LIKELY UNSAFE ...when used orally or topically for medicinal purposes. Total daily silver intake should not exceed 14 mcg/kg/day (980 mcg/day for a 70 kg person). Combining colloidal silver supplements with regular dietary intake of silver would likely result in exceeding this amount of silver. Silver accumulates in the body and can lead to an irreversible bluish skin discoloration known as argyria. Neurological deficits, diffuse silver deposition in visceral organs, renal damage, and metal flume fever can occur (5525,5526,8148,8149,10647,10648,12092).

PREGNANCY AND LACTATION: POSSIBLY UNSAFE ...when used orally. Epidemiological evidence links increased silver levels to babies born with developmental anomalies of the ear, face, and neck (5525).

Effectiveness
There is insufficient reliable information available about the effectiveness of colloidal silver.

Mechanism of Action
Compounds that contain inorganic silver are germicidal. Silver binds to the reactive groups of proteins, causing denaturation and precipitation. Silver can also inactivate enzymes by binding to sulfhydryl, amino, carboxyl, phosphate, and imidazole groups. When absorbed, silver is most concentrated in the skin, liver, spleen, and adrenals with lesser amounts in the muscle and brain. The half-life depends on the silver salt used. Half-life can range from days to months. Silver deposited in the skin has a much longer half-life. Silver primarily leaves the body via fecal elimination with active biliary excretion (5525).

Adverse Reactions
Orally or topically, colloidal silver can lead to an irreversible bluish deposition of silver in the mucous and skin membranes known as argyria (5525,8148,8149,10647,10648,12092). Argyria typically first appears in the gingiva with a slate-blue silver line (5525). Toxicity may also present as blueish-gray discoloration of the fingernails (8149,10648). Colloidal silver can also stimulate melanin production in skin. Areas exposed to the sun will become increasingly discolored. Colloidal silver can also cause neurological deficits, diffuse silver deposition in visceral organs, renal damage, and metal flume fever (5525,8148,10647).

Interactions with Herbs & Other Dietary Supplements
None known.

Interactions with Drugs
LEVOTHYROXINE (Synthroid, Levothroid, Levoxyl, and others): Theoretically, levothyroxine might have reduced absorption if given with colloidal silver.
PENICILLAMINE: Theoretically, drugs such as penicillamine (Cuprimine) might have reduced absorption if given with colloidal silver.
QUINOLONE ANTIBIOTICS: Theoretically, quinolones such as ciprofloxacin (Cipro), norfloxacin (Noroxin), ofloxacin and others might have reduced absorption if given with colloidal silver.
TETRACYCLINE ANTIBIOTICS: Theoretically, drugs such as tetracycline might have reduced absorption if given with colloidal silver.

Interactions with Foods
None known.

Interactions with Lab Tests
None known.

Interactions with Diseases or Conditions
None known.

Dosage and Administration
No typical dosage.

Comments
There are many Internet ads for the components of a generator to produce colloidal silver at home. Those who produce colloidal silver at home will likely have no means to assay the product to assure any standard potency. There are many products that are far safer and more effective than colloidal silver. Silver has no known physiological function and is not an essential mineral supplement, contrary to promoters' claims.

COLOCYNTH

Also Known As
Alhandal, Bitter Apple, Bitter Cucumber, Colocynth Pulp, Colocynthidis Fructus, Koloquinthen, Tumba, Vine-of-Sodom, Wild Gourd.

Scientific Names
Citrullus colocynthis, synonyms Colocynthis vulgaris, Cucumis colocynthis.
Family: Cucurbitaceae.

People Use This For
Orally, colocynth is used in combination products for acute and chronic constipation, and for liver and gallbladder ailments.

Safety
UNSAFE ...when used orally. Colocynth was banned by the FDA in 1991, due to toxicity (17).
PREGNANCY AND LACTATION: UNSAFE ...when used orally (17); avoid using.

Effectiveness
There is insufficient reliable information available about the effectiveness of colocynth.

Mechanism of Action
The applicable part of colocynth is the ripe fruit. It contains up to 3% cucurbitacin, a poisonous constituent that irritates mucous membranes, including GI mucosa (2) .

Adverse Reactions
Orally, ingestion of 0.6-1 grams of colocynth can cause severe irritation of the gastric mucosa, bloody diarrhea, kidney damage, hemorrhagic cystitis, and diuresis leading to anuria (2,18). Colocynth ingestion can also cause acute toxic colitis (10653). Doses of 2 grams or more can cause convulsions; paralysis; and if untreated, death from circulatory collapse (18).

Interactions with Herbs & Other Dietary Supplements
POTASSIUM DEPLETING HERBS: Theoretically, concomitant use with horsetail plant or licorice rhizome increases the risk of potassium depletion.
STIMULANT LAXATIVE HERBS: Theoretically, concomitant use with other stimulant laxative herbs may increase the risk of potassium depletion. Stimulant laxative herbs include aloe dried leaf sap, wild cucumber fruit (Ecballium elaterium), blue flag rhizome, alder buckthorn, European buckthorn, butternut bark, cascara bark, castor oil, gamboge bark exudate, jalap root, black root, manna bark exudate, podophyllum root, rhubarb root, senna leaves and pods, and yellow dock root (19).

Interactions with Drugs
DIGOXIN (Lanoxin): Theoretically, overuse/abuse of this product increases the risk of adverse effects of cardiac glycoside drugs.
DIURETIC DRUGS: Colocynth might compound diuretic-induced potassium loss (19). People taking colocynth along with potassium depleting diuretics might have an increased risk for hypokalemia. Some diuretics that can deplete potassium include chlorothiazide (Diuril), chlorthalidone (Thalitone), furosemide (Lasix), hydrochlorothiazide (HCTZ, Hydrodiuril, Microzide), and others.

Interactions with Foods
None known.

Interactions with Lab Tests
POTASSIUM: Excessive use of colocynth might cause potassium depletion, reducing serum potassium concentrations and test results (19).
URINE OUTPUT: Excessive use of colocynth might lead to cessation of urine output (anuria) (18).

Interactions with Diseases or Conditions
GASTROINTESTINAL (GI) CONDITIONS: Colocynth can irritate gastrointestinal tract. It is contraindicated in individuals with infectious or inflammatory gastrointestinal conditions (19).

Dosage and Administration
No typical dosage.

Comments
Colocynth is considered unsafe; avoid using. The use of colocynth is not justified due to significant risks (2). Death has resulted from the consumption of as little as 1 1/2 teaspoons of the powder. In the management of poisoning, a dilute tannic acid solution should be taken, followed by large quantities of albuminous drinks (215).

COLOMBO

Also Known As
Calomba Root, Calumba, Calumbo Root.

Scientific Names
Jateorhiza palmata, synonyms Wateorhiza palmata, Cocculus palmatus, Jateorhiza columba, Jateorhiza miersii, Menispermum columba, Menispermum palmatum.
Family: Menispermaceae.

People Use This For
Orally, colombo is used to treat gastritis, dyspepsia, chronic enterocolitis, and diarrhea.

Safety
There is insufficient reliable information available about the safety of colombo.
Pregnancy and Lactation: Insufficient reliable information; avoid using.

Effectiveness
There is insufficient reliable information available about the effectiveness of colombo.

Mechanism of Action
The applicable part of colombo is the root. Colombo contains alkaloids that have narcotic properties and side effects similar to morphine (7,18). Colombo might increase the resting tone of smooth muscle in the intestinal tract (7,18). In frogs, the alkaloids appear to act as a central nervous system (CNS) paralyzing agent (18). Palmatine, the main alkaloid component, has a similar effect in mammals (18). Colombo's use as a digestive aid is empirically based upon the bitter content, which is believed to increase stomach acid secretion via vagal nerve stimulation (19).

Adverse Reactions
Orally, large doses of colombo may cause vomiting and epigastric pain (18). Overdose can lead to paralysis and unconsciousness (18).

Interactions with Herbs & Other Dietary Supplements
None known.

Interactions with Drugs
ANTACIDS: Theoretically, due to reports that colombo increases stomach acid, colombo might decrease the effectiveness of antacids (19).
H2-BLOCKERS: Theoretically, due to reports that colombo increases stomach acid, colombo might decrease the effectiveness of H2-blockers (19). The H2 blockers include cimetidine (Tagamet), ranitidine (Zantac), nizatidine (Axid), and famotidine (Pepcid).
PROTON PUMP INHIBITORS (PPIs): Theoretically, due to reports that colombo increases stomach acid, colombo might decrease the effectiveness of PPIs (19). PPIs include omeprazole (Prilosec), lansoprazole (Prevacid), rabeprazole (Aciphex), pantoprazole (Protonix), and esomeprazole (Nexium).

Interactions with Foods
None known.

Interactions with Lab Tests
None known.

Interactions with Diseases or Conditions
None known.

Dosage and Administration
ORAL: A typical dose is 2 teaspoons of the boiled root as tea taken every hour (18). For single use, 20 drops of the extract or 2.5 grams of the tincture has been used (18). The root should be stored in a dry area (18).

Comments
Colombo is no longer used as a digestive aid and is rarely used as an antidiarrheal agent because of its morphine-like effects (18).

COLOSTRUM

Also Known As

Bovine Colostrum, Bovine Immunoglobulin, Cow Milk Colostrum, Goat Colostrum, Hyperimmune Bovine Colostrum.

Scientific Names

None.

People Use This For

Orally, bovine colostrum is used for stimulating the immune system, healing injuries, repairing nervous system damage, burning fat, building lean muscle, increasing stamina and vitality, elevating mood and sense of well being, slowing and reversing aging, and as an antibacterial and antifungal agent. Orally, hyperimmune bovine colostrum is also used in treating AIDS-related diarrhea (FDA Orphan Drug Status), diarrhea associated with graft versus host disease following bone marrow transplant, and rotavirus diarrhea in children.

Rectally, bovine colostrum is used for treating colitis.

Safety

LIKELY SAFE ...when used orally and appropriately. There are no reports of significant toxicity in multiple human trials (4901,4903,4904,4905,4906,4907,4908,4909). Bovine colostrum seems to be safe, however, it is derived from animals, and there is some concern about contamination with diseased animal parts (1825). So far, there are no reports of disease transmission to humans due to use of contaminated bovine colostrum.

POSSIBLY SAFE ...when used rectally and appropriately as a 10% enema (9730).

PREGNANCY AND LACTATION: Insufficient reliable information available; avoid using.

Effectiveness

POSSIBLY EFFECTIVE

Infectious diarrhea. Taking bovine colostrum orally seems to reduce infectious diarrhea in children and immunocompromised patients including patients with HIV/AIDS and bone marrow transplant recipients. It seems to be effective against rotaviral diarrhea in children (4903,4904,4909), cryptosporidium-related diarrhea in immunocompromised patients (4905,4906,4907,4908,10659), and diarrhea caused enterotoxigenic Escherichia coli (2067,2068,2069) or Shigella flexneri (2070). Hyperimmune bovine colostrum has FDA orphan status for AIDS-related diarrhea (9840).

Most clinical trials have used colostrum from pregnant cows which have been immunized against specific pathogens. The hyperimmune colostrum provides high antibody titers against organisms for which the cow has been immunized (4905).

INSUFFICIENT RELIABLE EVIDENCE to RATE

Athletic performance. Preliminary evidence suggests oral bovine colostrum may increase athletic performance in events that rely on peak anaerobic power, such as vertical jumping and bicycle sprints, after 8 weeks of supplementation (11453).

Distal colitis. There is some preliminary evidence that a 10% rectal enema of bovine colostrum might be helpful for treating distal colitis (9730).

More evidence is needed to rate bovine colostrum for these uses.

Mechanism of Action

Colostrum is the milky fluid produced by mammals within the first few days after giving birth. Most nutritional colostrum preparations come from cows (3567). Bovine colostrum contains proteins, carbohydrates, fat, vitamins, minerals, and immunoglobulin A (IgA) and immunoglobulin G (IgG) in concentrations approximately 100 times higher than dairy milk (4901). Because of the antibody content, bovine colostrum was thought to offer passive immunotherapy to people with enteric infections; however, bovine colostrum contains only low concentrations of antibodies against enteric pathogens and does not provide high enough titers to prevent disease. Hyperimmune bovine colostrum can be produced by immunizing pregnant cows against specific pathogens (e.g., cryptosporidium or rotavirus) resulting in increased specific colostrum antibody titers (4903). Hyperimmune bovine colostrum has been primarily used in clinical trials; however, the small amounts of antibodies that have been recovered from people who ingested hyperimmune colostrum were nonreactive (2072).

Taking bovine colostrum might increase peak anaerobic power and improve exercise performance; however, the mechanism of action is not yet understood. Animals fed bovine colostrum have shown an increase in skeletal muscle protein synthesis, creating an interest in the use of bovine colostrum for improvement in exercise performance (11453). Oral bovine colostrum supplementation does not appear to affect insulin response or the plasma nutrient absorptive capacity of alanine or glucose, once suggested as possible mechanisms (11454). Some evidence suggests bovine colostrum contains insulin-like growth factors (IGF), and appears to increase serum insulin-like growth factor I (IGF-I) and insulin in athletes (4901). However, separate evidence suggests bovine colostrum does not alter plasma IGF-I (11453).

Bovine colostrum contains growth factors, cytokines, hormones, and other factors biologically active components that might improve growth and repair of the gastrointestinal system (9731). Preliminary data indicate that bovine colostrum reduces indomethacin-induced gastrointestinal injury and addition of colostrum to drinking water prevents experimental small intestinal injury (4911). Some evidence suggests that bovine colostrum promotes small intestinal growth (4901). The phosphatidylethanolamine in hyperimmune bovine colostrum may prevent Helicobacter pylori from binding to the gastric mucosa (2065). The effectiveness of hyperimmune bovine colostrum may decrease when it is taken with a meal (2070), possibly due to stomach acid and digestive enzymes (2071).

Adverse Reactions

Orally, bovine colostrum has caused nausea and vomiting in an individual with HIV-related cryptosporidiosis. Elevated liver function tests and decreased serum hematocrit have also been reported in HIV patients treated for infectious diarrhea (4905). It may cause allergic reaction in individuals allergic to bovine milk products. There is also some concern that bovine colostrum that is obtained from cows in countries where bovine spongiform encephalitis (BSE) has been reported might be unsafe, however, there is no research indicating that colostrum can be contaminated with the BSE-causing prion. Countries where BSE has been reported include Great Britain, France, The Netherlands, Portugal, Luxembourg, Ireland, Switzerland, Oman, and Belgium (1825). Until more is known, tell patients to avoid these products unless country of origin can be determined. Patients should avoid products that are produced in countries where BSE has been found.

Interactions with Herbs & Other Dietary Supplements

None known.

Interactions with Drugs

None known.

Interactions with Foods

MEALS: Taking hyperimmune bovine colostrum with food may decrease antibody activity due to the increase in stomach acid and digestive enzyme secretion (2070,2071,2072).

Interactions with Lab Tests

None known.

Interactions with Diseases or Conditions

BOVINE MILK ALLERGY: Avoid using.

Dosage and Administration

ORAL: For enhanced athletic performance, 125 mL colostrum whey product twice daily or 60 grams bovine colostrum protein powder daily has been used; however, these products are not available in the US (11453,11454,4901). For AIDS-related Cryptosporidium parvum diarrhea, 10 grams powder four times daily for 21 days has been used (4905). For AIDS-related cryptosporidial and other infectious diarrhea, 10-20 grams daily for 10 days has been used (4906). For graft versus host disease following bone marrow transplant, 10 grams per day for 10 days has been used (4907). For rotavirus diarrhea in children 10 grams, equivalent to 3.6 grams antirotavirus antibodies, per day for 4 days has been used (4903). 100 mL four times per day for 4 days has also been used (4904).
RECTAL: For treating distal colitis, 100 mL of a 10% enema of bovine colostrum two times daily has been used for 4 weeks (9730).

Comments

Bovine colostrum is the milk secreted by cows during the first few days after calving (4901). Hyperimmune bovine colostrum is produced by cows immunized against specific pathogens. Bovine colostrum is not on the banned drug list of the International Olympic Committee (4901).

COLTSFOOT

Also Known As

Ass's Foot, Brandlattich, British Tobacco, Bullsfoot, Coughwort, Farfarae Folium Leaf, Fieldhove, Filuis Ante Patrem, Flower Velure, Foal's Foot, Foalswort, Guflatich, Hallfoot, Horsefoot, Horsehoof, Kuandong Hua, Kwandong Hwa, Pas d'Ane, Pas Diane, Pferdefut, Tussilage.

Scientific Names

Tussilago farfara.
Family: Asteraceae/Compositae.

People Use This For

Orally, coltsfoot is used for bronchitis, asthma, laryngitis, pertussis, acute respiratory tract mucous membrane inflammation with cough and hoarseness, acute or mild inflammation of the oral and pharyngeal mucosa, and sore throat.

As an inhalant, coltsfoot is used for coughs and wheezing.

Safety

LIKELY UNSAFE ...when products containing hepatotoxic pyrrolizidine alkaloid (PA) constituents are used orally. Repeated exposure to low concentrations of hepatotoxic PAs can cause severe veno-occlusive disease. Hepatotoxic PAs might also be carcinogenic and mutagenic (12841,12842). Dietary supplement products sold in the US are not required to include the amount of PAs they may contain; therefore, all preparations used orally containing coltsfoot should be considered potentially unsafe (3484). Tell patients not to use coltsfoot preparations that are not certified and labeled as hepatotoxic PA-free.

PREGNANCY: LIKELY UNSAFE ...when used orally. Coltsfoot preparations containing hepatotoxic pyrrolizidine alkaloid (PA) constituents might be teratogenic and hepatotoxic (12841,12842). There is insufficient reliable information available about the safety of using coltsfoot products that do not contain hepatotoxic PAs during pregnancy.

LACTATION: LIKELY UNSAFE ...when used orally. Hepatotoxic pyrrolizidine alkaloid (PA) constituents in coltsfoot are excreted in milk (12841,12842). There is insufficient reliable information available about the safety of using coltsfoot products that do not contain hepatotoxic PAs during lactation.

Effectiveness

There is insufficient reliable information available about the effectiveness of coltsfoot.

Mechanism of Action

The applicable part of coltsfoot is the leaf. Preliminary research suggests that coltsfoot might inhibit platelet aggregation by blocking the binding of platelet activating factor (PAF) to platelet membranes (12859). Coltsfoot might also exert anti-inflammatory activity by blocking arachidonic acid metabolism. Preliminary research on an ethyl acetate extract of coltsfoot suggests antioxidant and neuroprotective activity (12856). The coltsfoot constituent tussilagone has respiratory stimulant and cardiovascular (including pressor) activities, which might explain its use for asthma (12858). Coltsfoot also seems to have antibacterial properties (12857).

Coltsfoot contains various pyrrolizidine alkaloids (PA), some of which are toxic. PAs are most concentrated in the plant roots, but may be found in all plant parts. PAs, particularly unsaturated PAs, can cause hepatotoxicity. Cyclic diesters such as retrorsine and senecionine are the most hepatotoxic. Liver toxicity may result from PA-enhanced oxidative stress, but the exact mechanism of toxicity is unknown. Single doses of 10-20 mg PAs or chronic ingestion of amounts less than 10 mcg can cause veno-occlusive disease. PAs are metabolized by cytochrome P450 3A4 (CYP3A4) to toxic dehydroalkaloids and pyrroles. Enzyme inducers such as phenobarbital seem to enhance toxicity (12841,12860). Pyrroles are excreted as N-acetyl cysteine conjugates. Some researchers speculate that early administration of N-acetylcysteine might reduce toxicity (11988).

Metabolism is also affected by pregnane X receptor induction of CYP3A4. Genetic or drug induced variation in CYP3A4 or pregnane X receptor activity can affect the degree of PA toxicity by increasing or decreasing its metabolism (12841,12842). Hepatotoxic PAs are also toxic to the lungs. In animals, pneumotoxicity occurs as pulmonary hypertension and right ventricular hypertrophy. Hepatotoxic PAs are carcinogenic and mutagenic. There are sufficient amounts of hepatotoxic PAs in herbal products to cause toxicity (12841,12842).

Adverse Reactions

Orally, coltsfoot might cause toxicity. The major concern about coltsfoot preparations is the hepatotoxic pyrrolizidine alkaloid (PA) content. These constituents are hepatotoxic, pneumotoxic, carcinogenic, and mutagenic (12841,12842). Chronic exposure to other plants containing hepatotoxic PA constituents is associated with veno-occlusive disease (4021). Subacute veno-occlusive disease causes vague symptoms with persistent liver enlargement (4021). Symptoms of acute veno-occlusive disease include colicky pains in epigastrium, vomiting and diarrhea, and ascites formation within several days. Enlargement and induration of the liver occurs within a few weeks (12842). There is one case report of fatal hepatic veno-occlusive disease in a neonate associated with regular maternal consumption during pregnancy of an herb tea containing several pyrrolizidine alkaloid herbs, including coltsfoot (575).

Coltsfoot may cause an allergic reaction in individuals sensitive to the Asteraceae/Compositae family (12856). Members of this family include ragweed, chrysanthemums, marigolds, daisies, and many other herbs.

Interactions with Herbs & Other Dietary Supplements

HEPATOTOXIC PYRROLIZIDINE ALKALOID (PA)-CONTAINING HERBS: Concomitant use is contraindicated due to the risk of additive toxicity. Herbs containing hepatotoxic PAs include alkanna, borage, butterbur, comfrey, European buckthorn, gravel root, groundsel, hemp agrimony, and hound's tongue; and the Senecio species plants dusty miller, alpine ragwort, groundsel, golden ragwort, and tansy ragwort (12841).
HERBS THAT INDUCE CYTOCHROME P450 3A4 (CYP3A4): Theoretically, herbs that induce CYP3A4 might increase the conversion of hepatotoxic PAs to toxic metabolites, enhancing toxicity (12841,12860). Herbs that induce CYP3A4 include St. John's wort and garlic.

Interactions with Drugs

ANTICOAGULANT/ANTIPLATELET DRUGS: Concomitant use might increase the risk of bleeding due to decreased platelet aggregation. Coltsfoot has been reported to inhibit platelet aggregation (12859); avoid concomitant use. Some of these drugs include aspirin, clopidogrel (Plavix), dalteparin (Fragmin), enoxaparin (Lovenox), heparin, ticlopidine (Ticlid), warfarin (Coumadin), and others.
ANTIHYPERTENSIVE DRUGS: Theoretically, excessive doses of coltsfoot may interfere with antihypertensive or cardiovascular therapy (12858).
CYTOCHROME P450 3A4 (CYP3A4) INDUCERS: Hepatotoxic pyrrolizidine alkaloids (PA) are substrates of cytochrome P450 3A4 (CYP3A4) (12841,12860). Theoretically, drugs that induce CYP3A4 might increase the conversion of PAs to toxic metabolites. Some drugs that induce CYP3A4 include carbamazepine (Tegretol), phenobarbital, phenytoin (Dilantin), rifampin, rifabutin (Mycobutin), and others.

Interactions with Foods

None known.

Interactions with Lab Tests

None known.

Interactions with Diseases or Conditions

CROSS-ALLERGENICITY: Theoretically, coltsfoot might cause an allergic reaction in individuals sensitive to the Asteraceae/Compositae family (12856). Members of this family include ragweed, chrysanthemums, marigolds, daisies, and many other herbs.
HYPERTENSION, CARDIOVASCULAR DISEASE: Theoretically, excessive amounts of coltsfoot may interfere with therapy for hypertension or cardiovascular disease (12858).
LIVER DISEASE: Theoretically, hepatotoxic pyrrolizidine alkaloids (PA) might exacerbate liver disease (12841,12842).

Dosage and Administration

No typical dosage.

COLUMBINE

Also Known As

Culverwort.

Scientific Names

Aquilegia vulgaris.
Family: Ranunculaceae.

Comments

At the date of publication, there was very little scientific information available about this product. Our staff is continually analyzing the available information on natural medicines and will add data to the online version of *Natural Medicines Comprehensive Database* as it becomes available. See www.naturaldatabase.com.

COMFREY

Also Known As

Ass Ear, Black Root, Blackwort, Bruisewort, Common Comfrey, Consolidae Radix, Consound, Gum Plant, Healing Herb, Knitback, Knitbone, Salsify, Slippery Root, Wallwort.
CAUTION: See separate listings for Black Root and Bugle.

Scientific Names

Symphytum officinale.
Family: Boraginaceae.

People Use This For

Orally, comfrey is used as a tea for gastritis, ulcers, excessive menstrual flow, diarrhea, bloody urine, persistent cough, pleuritis, bronchitis, cancer, angina, as a gargle for gum disease, and pharyngitis.
Topically, comfrey is used for ulcers, wounds, joint inflammation, bruises, rheumatoid arthritis, phlebitis, gout, and fractures.

Safety

POSSIBLY SAFE ...when used topically short-term on unbroken skin at or below a daily dosage of 100 mcg of the hepatotoxic pyrrolizidine alkaloids (PA). Externally-applied pyrrolizidine alkaloids are absorbed through the skin (11990,11992).
UNSAFE ...when used orally because of its potential for acute or chronic liver toxicity. Comfrey contains hepatotoxic PAs. Chronic ingestion of more than 1 mg per day for 2 weeks or more than 0.1 mg per day for longer periods can cause liver disease. PAs may also be carcinogenic (11987). The FDA has recommended removal of oral comfrey products from the market (11988).
PREGNANCY AND LACTATION: UNSAFE ...when used orally or topically. In addition to hepatotoxicity and possible carcinogenicity, the PAs in comfrey might be teratogenic. PAs are absorbed through the skin (11987,11988,11990).

Effectiveness

INSUFFICIENT RELIABLE EVIDENCE to RATE

Bruises and sprains. Preliminary clinical research suggests that applying comfrey topically might improve pain and tenderness of bruises, sprains, and painful conditions of the muscles and joints (11991). More evidence is needed to rate comfrey for this use.

Mechanism of Action

The applicable parts of comfrey are the leaf, rhizome, and root. Comfrey contains symphytine, lasiocarpine, and other pyrrolizidine alkaloids (PA) that are hepatotoxic and carcinogenic, mutagenic, and teratogenic.
Hepatotoxic PAs cause veno-occlusive liver disease. They destroy and damage centrilobular hepatocytes of the liver and also destroy small branches of the hepatic vein. PAs can also damage the lungs, resulting in pulmonary hypertension (11987,11988,11990). The PA content of comfrey varies with time of harvesting and plant age. The roots have 10 times higher concentrations of PAs than the leaves (11990,11991).
PAs are metabolized in the liver by the cytochrome P450 (CYP) enzyme system, specifically by CYP 3A4, to toxic dehydroalkaloids and pyrroles. Enzyme inducers such as phenobarbital seem to enhance toxicity (11990,12841,12860).
Pyrroles are excreted as N-acetyl cysteine conjugates. Some researchers speculate that early administration of N-acetylcysteine might reduce toxicity (11988).
Metabolism is also affected by pregnane X receptor induction of CYP3A4. Genetic or drug-induced variation in CYP3A4 or pregnane X receptor activity can affect the degree of PA toxicity by increasing or decreasing its metabolism (12841,12842).
There are sufficient amounts of hepatotoxic PAs in herbal products to cause toxicity (12841,12842).

Adverse Reactions

Orally, the major concern about comfrey is the hepatotoxic pyrrolizidine alkaloid (PA) content. These constituents are hepatotoxic, pneumotoxic, carcinogenic, and mutagenic (12841,12842). Comfrey can cause acute veno-occlusive disease characterized by sudden abdominal pain, vomiting, ascites, and hepatomegaly. In subacute disease, comfrey can cause ascites, hepatomegaly, abdominal pain, diarrhea, vomiting, and abdominal swelling. Chronic toxicity appears as asthenia and progressive ascites. Hepatic fibrosis and inflammation may resolve, but hepatic failure is common with more severe disease. This may occur as late as 2 years after the initial ingestion. Other signs and symptoms of pyrrolizidine toxicity include bile duct proliferation, fatty changes of the liver, fibrosis, cirrhosis, and vascular lesions (11988). The mortality of comfrey toxicity is 50%. However, toxicity seems to vary among individuals (11990).
Topically, PAs can be absorbed in quantities sufficient to cause toxicity with extended use or in high concentrations (11990).

Interactions with Herbs & Other Dietary Supplements

HEPATOTOXIC HERBS: Theoretically, comfrey might have additive effects with herbs that cause hepatotoxicity (11988,11990). Other products that might affect the liver include chaparral, bishop's weed, borage, kava, uva ursi, and others.
HERBS THAT INDUCE CYTOCHROME P450 3A4 (CYP3A4): Theoretically herbs that induce CYP3A4 might increase the conversion of comfrey to toxic metabolites, enhancing toxicity (11990). Herbs that induce CYP3A4 include St. John's wort and garlic.
HEPATOTOXIC PYRROLIZIDINE ALKALOID (PA)-CONTAINING HERBS: Concomitant use is contraindicated due to the risk of additive toxicity. Herbs containing hepatotoxic PAs include alkanna, borage, butterbur, coltsfoot, forget-me-not, gravel root, hemp agrimony, hound's tongue, lungwort, and the Senecio species dusty miller, alpine ragwort, groundsel, golden ragwort, and tansy ragwort (11988,11990).

Interactions with Drugs

CYTOCHROME P450 3A4 (CYP3A4) INDUCERS: Theoretically, drugs that induce CYP3A4 might increase the conversion of comfrey to toxic metabolites, enhancing toxicity (11990). Some drugs that induce CYP3A4 include carbamazepine (Tegretol), phenobarbital, phenytoin (Dilantin), rifampin, rifabutin (Mycobutin), and others.
HEPATOTOXIC DRUGS: Theoretically, comfrey might have additive adverse effects on the liver when used with hepatotoxic drugs (11988,11990). Some drugs that can adversely affect the liver include acetaminophen (Tylenol), amiodarone (Cordarone), carbamazepine (Tegretol), isoniazid (INH), methotrexate (Rheumatrex), methyldopa (Aldomet), and many others.

Interactions with Foods

None known.

Interactions with Lab Tests

LIVER FUNCTION TESTS: The hepatotoxic pyrrolizidine alkaloids (PA) in comfrey might increase liver function tests including alkaline phosphatase, aspartic acid transaminase (AST, SGOT), alanine aminotransferase (ALT, SGPT), total bilirubin, gamma-glutamyltransferase, and lactate dehydrogenase (11988).

Interactions with Diseases or Conditions

BROKEN, DAMAGED SKIN: Contraindicated. Apply only to unbroken skin. Broken skin might result in exposure to high concentrations of hepatotoxic pyrrolizidine alkaloids (PA) (11990).
LIVER DISEASE: Theoretically, comfrey might exacerbate liver dysfunction in patients with liver disease (11988,11990).

Dosage and Administration

No typical dosage.

Comments

Some products labeled common comfrey or Symphytum officinale actually contain the more toxic prickly comfrey (Symphytum asperum) or Russian comfrey (Symphytum x uplandicum) species (11991).

COMMON STONECROP

Also Known As

Bird Bread, Creeping Tom, Gold Chain, Golden Moss, Jack-of-the-Buttery, Mousetail, Prick Madam, Wall Ginger, Wallpepper.
CAUTION: See separate listing for Ginger.

Scientific Names

Sedum acre.
Family: Crassulaceae

Comments

At the date of publication, this product was not a common ingredient used in brand name supplements marketed to consumers. Details about this product are available in the online version of *Natural Medicines Comprehensive Database.* See www.naturaldatabase.com.

CONDURANGO

Also Known As

Common Condorvine, Condurango Cortex, Eagle-Vine Bark.

Scientific Names

Marsdenia cundurango, synonym Marsdenia reichenbachii; Gonolobus condurango.
Family: Apocynaceae or Asclepiadaceae.

People Use This For

Orally, condurango is used as an appetite stimulant and for dyspeptic complaints, and for stomach cancer.

Safety

LIKELY SAFE ...when used orally and appropriately (2).
PREGNANCY AND LACTATION: Insufficient reliable information available; avoid using.

Effectiveness

There is insufficient reliable information available about the effectiveness of condurango.

Mechanism of Action

The applicable part of condurango is the bark. The condurango alkaloid constituents, which as a group are referred to as condurangin, stimulate salivation and the secretion of gastric juices (8).

Adverse Reactions

Orally, anaphylaxis can occur with the use of condurango bark (1501).

Interactions with Herbs & Other Dietary Supplements

None known.

Interactions with Drugs

None known.

Interactions with Foods

None known.

Interactions with Lab Tests

None known.

Interactions with Diseases or Conditions

LATEX ALLERGY: Cross-sensitivity to condurango can occur in individuals allergic to natural rubber latex (1500), including anaphylaxis (1501). Avoid the use of condurango in these individuals.

Dosage and Administration

ORAL: The typical dose of the bark is 2-4 grams per day (2). The usual dose of the water extract is 200-500 mg per day (2). The common dose of the liquid extract is 2-4 grams per day (2), and the tincture is usually given as 2-5 grams per day (2).

CONJUGATED LINOLEIC ACID

Also Known As

CLA, CLA-FFA, CLA-Free Fatty Acid, CLA-Triacylglycerol, Linoleic Acid.

Scientific Names

cis-9,trans-11 conjugated linoleic acid; Trans-10,cis-12 conjugated linoleic acid.

People Use This For

Orally, conjugated linoleic acid (CLA) is used for cancer, obesity, cachexia, bodybuilding, for limiting food allergy reactions, and for atherosclerosis.

Safety

LIKELY SAFE ...when used orally in amounts found in foods. Conjugated linoleic acid occurs naturally in milk fat, beef, and meat of other ruminant animals (5924,5925,5932,5933).

POSSIBLY SAFE ...when used orally and appropriately in medicinal amounts (2819,2821,3153,4947,10410,11327).

PREGNANCY AND LACTATION: LIKELY SAFE ...when used orally in amounts found in foods (5924,5932,5933). There is insufficient reliable information available about the safety of conjugated linoleic acid when used in medicinal amounts during pregnancy or lactation; avoid using.

Effectiveness

POSSIBLY EFFECTIVE

Obesity. Taking conjugated linoleic acid (CLA) orally seems to improve body composition in patients who are overweight or obese. Taking 0.7 to 4.5 grams/day seems to significantly decrease body fat mass (BFM) and might increase lean body mass (LBM) in some patients. But CLA does not seem to reduce total body weight or body mass index (BMI) (2819,2821,3153,4947,10410,13137). CLA also seems to reduce hunger and improve satiety and feeling of fullness, but this appetite suppression does not necessarily result in a lower energy intake or improved body weight maintenance (11327). There is evidence that the isolated trans-10, cis-12 isomer of CLA can increase hyperproinsulinemia and insulin resistance in patients with abdominal obesity (2821,13026,13137). Hyperproinsulinemia is an independent risk factor for type 2 diabetes and cardiovascular disease. Therefore, CLA might not be a good choice for obese patients; however, most commercial CLA products contain a mixture of CLA isomers. It is not known if these mixed CLA isomer products have this same risk.

INSUFFICIENT RELIABLE EVIDENCE to RATE

Breast cancer. There is preliminary evidence that CLA might help reduce the risk of breast cancer. Postmenopausal women who have a higher intake of CLA in foods, particularly cheese, seem to have a lower risk of developing breast cancer (5058). More evidence is needed to rate CLA for this use.

Mechanism of Action

Conjugated linoleic acid (CLA) refers to a group of conjugated dienoic isomers of linoleic acid, including cis-9, trans-11 linoleic acid and trans-10, cis-12 linoleic acid. Different isomers seem to have different physiological effects (3158,13069). Dairy products and beef are the major dietary sources. Food sources provide both isomers, but typically contain more of the cis-9, trans-11 isomer in a ratio of 30-70:1. Supplements containing CLA usually provide the two isomers in a 50:50 ratio (13069).

Plant oils contain only small amounts of CLA. Plant oils are good sources of linoleic acid, but in humans linoleic acid does not seem to be converted to CLA in significant amounts (5933,13069).

Conjugated linoleic acid can also be produced synthetically by exposing oils rich in linoleic acid, such as safflower and soybean, to a base and heat. This CLA product is high in both the cis-9, trans-11 and the trans-10, cis-12 isomers (3001).

There is a lot of interest in using CLA for weight loss in obesity. Researchers think that CLA might reduce body fat deposits by promoting apoptosis in adipose tissue (3070,5928).

There is some evidence that only the trans-10, cis-12 isomer has an effect on body fat mass (3001). Additional evidence, however, shows the isolated trans-10, cis-12 isomer might also cause hyperproinsulinemia, increase insulin resistance and glycemia, reduce HDL cholesterol in men with abdominal obesity, increase lipid peroxidation, and C-reactive protein (CRP) levels (2821,13026,13137).

There is also interest in using CLA for cancer prevention. Preliminary evidence suggests CLA may be cytotoxic to human breast cancer cells. It may also inhibit the proliferation of human malignant melanoma and colorectal cancer cells (8997).

CLA appears to enhance immune function (5926,5934), increase peripheral blood mononuclear cell production (2810), and inhibit cyclooxygenase and lipoxygenase pathways in tumor cells (5926,5934). CLA might also modulate cellular response to tumor necrosis factor-alpha (TNF-alpha) (5924).

Adverse Reactions

Orally, the most common adverse effect of conjugated linoleic acid is gastrointestinal upset including diarrhea, nausea, loose stools, and dyspepsia (3153,4947). In some cases patients can experience fatigue (3153).

Interactions with Herbs & Other Dietary Supplements

VITAMIN A: Some evidence suggests conjugated linoleic acid might increase vitamin A (retinol) storage in liver and breast tissues (5931).

Interactions with Drugs

None known.

Interactions with Foods

None known.

Interactions with Lab Tests

CHOLESTEROL: Conjugated linoleic acid appears to reduce total, low-density lipoprotein (LDL), and high-density lipoprotein (HDL) cholesterol levels (3153).

Interactions with Diseases or Conditions

DIABETES: Taking the isolated trans-10, cis-12 isomer of conjugated linoleic acid (CLA) seems to increase insulin resistance and glycemia in patients with diabetes. Monitor blood glucose level closely (2821). Most commercial CLA products contain a mixture of CLA isomers. It is not known if these mixed CLA isomer products have this same risk.

METABOLIC SYNDROME: Men with abdominal obesity and metabolic syndrome who take the isolated trans-10, cis-12 isomer of conjugated linoleic acid (CLA) 3.4 grams/day for 12 weeks can develop hyperproinsulinemia and insulin resistance (2821,13026,13137). Hyperproinsulinemia is an independent risk factor for type 2 diabetes and cardiovascular disease. Most commercial CLA products contain a mixture of CLA isomers. It is not known if these mixed CLA isomer products have this same risk.

Dosage and Administration

ORAL: For weight loss in obese patients, a dose of 2 to 7 grams per day has been used. However, doses greater than 3.4 grams per day do not seem to offer any additional benefit (3153,11327).

Comments

An average diet supplies 15-174 mg of conjugated linoleic acid (CLA) daily (2820).

CONTRAYERVA

Also Known As

Contrayerba, Herbe-Chapeau.

Scientific Names

Dorstenia contrayerva; Dorstenia contrajerva.
Family: Moraceae.

Comments

At the date of publication, this product was not a common ingredient used in brand name supplements marketed to consumers. Details about this product are available in the online version of *Natural Medicines Comprehensive Database.* See www.naturaldatabase.com.

COOLWORT

Also Known As

Foam Flower, Mitrewort.

Scientific Names

Tiarella cordifolia.
Family: Saxifragaceae.

Comments

At the date of publication, this product was not a common ingredient used in brand name supplements marketed to consumers. Details about this product are available in the online version of *Natural Medicines Comprehensive Database.* See www.naturaldatabase.com.

COPAIBA BALSAM

Also Known As

Balsam, Copaiba, Copaiba Oleoresin, Copaiva, Jesuit's Balsam.

Scientific Names

Copaifera officinalis; Copaifera langsdorffii; Copaifera reticulata; and other Copaifera species.
Family: Fabaceae/Leguminosae.

People Use This For

Orally, copaiba balsam is used for chronic bronchitis, hemorrhoids, chronic diarrhea, chronic cystitis, urinary tract infections, as a stimulant, and a laxative.
In foods and beverages, copaiba balsam oleoresin is used as an ingredient.
In manufacturing, copaiba balsam oleoresin and oil are used in soaps, cosmetics, and perfumes.
In pharmaceutical preparations, both the oleoresin and oil are used in cough medicines and diuretics.

Safety

LIKELY SAFE ...when used orally in amounts commonly found in foods. Copaiba has Generally Recognized As Safe status (GRAS) for use in foods in the US (4912). ...when used topically (11).
POSSIBLY UNSAFE ...when used orally for medicinal purposes. Copaiba balsam can irritate mucous membranes. Ingesting 5 grams can cause stomach pains (18).
PREGNANCY AND LACTATION: POSSIBLY UNSAFE ...when used orally for medicinal purposes; avoid using.

Effectiveness

There is insufficient reliable information available about the effectiveness of copaiba balsam.

Mechanism of Action

Copaiba balsam contains a volatile oil consisting of alpha and beta-caryophyllene, L-cadinenes, and copene. It also has resins, including diterpenoid oleoresins. Some evidence suggests copaiba balsam might have bacteriostatic (18), diuretic, expectorant, disinfectant, and stimulant activity (11). In addition to these properties, the oil exhibits antibacterial activity (11). Some evidence suggests the oleoresin of the Brazilian Copaifera species might have anti-inflammatory effects (11).

Adverse Reactions

Orally, ingesting 5 grams of copaiba balsam orally can cause stomach pains (18); repeated doses can cause shivers, tremor, groin pain, and insomnia (18). Large amounts may cause vomiting, diarrhea, and measles-like rash (11).
Topically, copaiba balsam can cause contact dermatitis with erythema, papular or vesicular rash, urticaria, petechiae, and the rash may leave brown spots after healing (18).

Interactions with Herbs & Other Dietary Supplements

None known.

Interactions with Drugs

None known.

Interactions with Foods

None known.

Interactions with Lab Tests

None known.

Interactions with Diseases or Conditions

None known.

Dosage and Administration

No typical dosage.

Comments

Copaiba balsam is an oleoresin rather than a true balsam collected from the trunk of Copaifera species trees (11). Copaiba oil is distilled from the oleoresin (11). Copaiba balsam is considered obsolete for medicinal purposes (18).

COPPER

Also Known As

Cuivre, Cupric Oxide, Elemental Copper.

Scientific Names

Copper; Cu; atomic number 29.

People Use This For
Orally, copper is used for treating copper deficiency, anemia due to copper deficiency, zinc-induced copper deficiency, improving wound healing, osteoarthritis, and osteoporosis.

Safety
LIKELY SAFE ...when used orally and appropriately. Copper is safe in amounts that do not exceed 10 mg per day, the Tolerable Upper Intake Level (UL) (7135).
POSSIBLY UNSAFE ...when used orally in high doses. Tell patients to avoid exceeding the UL of 10 mg per day. Higher intake can cause liver damage (7135). Renal failure and death can occur with ingestion of as little as 1 gram of copper sulfate (17).
CHILDREN: LIKELY SAFE ...when used orally and appropriately. Copper is safe in amounts that do not exceed the UL of 1 mg per day for children 1 to 3 years, 3 mg per day for children 4 to 8 years, 5 mg per day for children 9 to 13 years, and 8 mg per day for adolescents (7135). POSSIBLY UNSAFE ...when used orally in high doses. Tell patients to avoid exceeding the UL of 1 mg per day for children 1 to 3 years, 3 mg per day for children 4 to 8 years, 5 mg per day for children 9 to 13 years, and 8 mg per day for adolescents (7135). Higher intake can cause liver damage (7135).
PREGNANCY: LIKELY SAFE ...when used orally and appropriately. Copper is safe in amounts that do not exceed the UL of 8 mg per day for women 14 to 18 years, or 10 mg per day for women 19 and older (7135). POSSIBLY UNSAFE ...when used orally in high doses. Tell patients to avoid exceeding the UL of 8 mg per day for women 14 to 18 years, or 10 mg per day for women 19 and older. Higher intake can cause liver damage (7135).
LACTATION: LIKELY SAFE ...when used orally and appropriately. Copper is safe in amounts that do not exceed the UL of 10 mg per day for breast-feeding women 19 or older, or 8 mg per day for breast-feeding women ages 14 to 18 years (7135). POSSIBLY UNSAFE ...when used orally in high doses. Tell patients to avoid exceeding the UL of 10 mg per day for breast-feeding women 19 or older, or 8 mg per day for breast-feeding women ages 14 to 18 years. Higher intake can cause liver damage (7135).

Effectiveness
LIKELY EFFECTIVE

Copper deficiency. Taking copper orally or intravenously is effective for treating copper deficiency and anemia due to copper deficiency. Copper deficiency is rare. It is seen most commonly in people receiving prolonged parenteral nutrition (7135).

There is insufficient reliable information available about the effectiveness of copper for its other uses.

Mechanism of Action
Copper is an essential trace mineral. It is widely distributed in foods particularly in organ meats, seafood, nuts, seeds, wheat bran cereals, grain products, and cocoa products (7135). Absorption occurs primarily in the small intestine with lesser absorption in the stomach (7135). The majority of copper in the body is in the skeleton and muscles; the liver maintains plasma copper concentrations. Excretion of copper into the gastrointestinal tract regulates copper homeostasis; greater excretion is the result of increased absorption (7135). Biochemically, copper acts as a catalytic agent via the many copper metalloenzymes which act as oxidases (7135). Amine oxidases are important in a variety of processes including allergic reactions, serotonin and catecholamine degradation, and connective tissue development. Ferroxidases, copper enzymes in the plasma, are required for ferrous iron oxidation and binding of iron to transferrin. The main copper protein in plasma Ferroxidase I, also called ceruloplasmin, might have antioxidant functions. Another copper enzyme, cytochrome-c oxidase, is a mitochondrial enzyme that catalyzes the reduction of oxygen to water to fuel ATP synthesis. Cytochrome-c oxidase is most abundant in highly metabolic tissues, including the heart, brain, and liver. Other copper enzymes are responsible for precursors of dopa and melatonin formation, conversion of dopamine to norepinephrine, production of amides, and protection from free radical damage (7135). The activity of copper enzymes decreases with copper depletion (7135). Copper deficiency in humans is rare, but has been associated with excessive zinc intake, intestinal bypass surgery, parenteral nutrition, and malnourished infants (706,707,708). Copper deficiency is manifested by normocytic hypochromic anemia, leukopenia, and neutropenia (7135). In infants and children, osteoporosis may be seen (7135). No single lab test is available to determine copper deficiency. Diagnosis of copper deficiency is made by several indicators, including serum or plasma copper concentration, ceruloplasmin concentration, and erythrocyte superoxide dismutase activity (7135).

Adverse Reactions
Orally, copper is most commonly associated with gastrointestinal side effects including abdominal pain, cramps, nausea, diarrhea, and vomiting. Copper toxicity is rare in humans, except in those people with a hereditary defect in copper homeostasis. Acute hepatic failure has been reported in a patient taking 30 to 60 mg of copper daily for more than 4 years (7135). Renal failure and death can occur with ingestion of as little as 1 gram of copper sulfate (17). Symptoms of acute copper poisoning include nausea, vomiting, bloody diarrhea, hypotension, hemolytic anemia, uremia, and cardiovascular collapse (159). Chronic exposure symptoms include sporadic fever, vomiting, epigastric pain, diarrhea, and jaundice (159).

Interactions with Herbs & Other Dietary Supplements

IRON: In infants, high iron concentrations in formula can reduce absorption of copper and reduce copper status (7135). It isn't known if this is clinically significant, or if it occurs in adults who take iron supplements.
VITAMIN C (ascorbic acid): 1500 mg of vitamin C taken daily decreases serum levels of copper and the copper transport protein, ceruloplasmin, in young men (710). The acidity of vitamin C may convert copper in the gut to a less absorbable form. It's unlikely that this is clinically significant unless dietary copper intake is low (710).
ZINC: Large amounts of zinc can inhibit copper absorption, due to competition for absorption from the gut (706,707,708). Toxic levels of zinc intake can cause significant copper deficiency and associated anemia (706). It's unlikely that normal supplemental doses of zinc would affect copper levels.

Interactions with Drugs

PENICILLAMINE: Copper chelates penicillamine, decreasing its absorption. Separate dose times by at least 2 hours (4412,4453,4531,4535,9630).

Drug Influences on Nutrient Levels and Depletion

SOME DRUGS CAN AFFECT COPPER LEVELS:
ETHAMBUTOL (Myambutol): Ethambutol, and to a greater extent its metabolite, chelates copper (8971). Tissue depletion of copper can occur (8971). It's suggested that copper chelation in the retina might contribute to ethambutol-induced optic neuropathy (4453,4535). Chelation of copper ions in cytochrome-c oxidase may inhibit mitochondrial activity in optic nerve axons (4535). Whether supplemental copper can prevent this side effect isn't known. Preliminary evidence suggests that copper supplements do not inhibit the antimicrobial action of ethambutol (4535).
PENICILLAMINE (Cuprimine, Depen): Penicillamine chelates copper in the gastrointestinal tract and decreases absorption. The need for copper supplementation in diseases such as rheumatoid arthritis (RA) has not been adequately studied. If used, copper supplements should be separated from penicillamine by at least 2 hours (4453,4531,4535,9630).
ZIDOVUDINE (Retrovir, AZT): Decreased plasma copper levels are found in some people with HIV infection treated with zidovudine (4986). However, preliminary evidence suggests this is beneficial; AIDS patients with lower copper levels appear to have a slight survival advantage (8970). Advise patients on zidovudine not to take copper supplements unless recommended by their physician.

Interactions with Foods

None known.

Interactions with Lab Tests

None known.

Interactions with Diseases or Conditions

IDIOPATHIC COPPER TOXICOSIS: Copper supplementation can worsen this genetic condition (7135).
INDIAN CHILDHOOD CIRRHOSIS: Copper supplementation can worsen this genetic condition (7135).
WILSON'S DISEASE: Copper supplementation can worsen this condition or interfere with penicillamine therapy (7135).

Dosage and Administration

ORAL: For copper deficiency, doses up to 0.1 mg/kg cupric sulfate per day have been used. The National Institute of Medicine has determined Adequate Intake (AI) of copper for infants: 0 to 6 months, 200 mcg (30 mcg/kg/day); 7 to 12 months, 220 mcg (24 mcg/kg/day) (7135).
For children, a Recommended Dietary Allowance (RDA) has been set: 1 to 3 years, 340 mcg/day; 4 to 8 years, 440 mcg/day; 9 to 13, 700 mcg/day; 14 to 18 years, 890 mcg/day.
For men and women age 19 years and older, the RDA is 900 mcg/day.
For pregnancy, the RDA is 1000 mcg/day, and lactation 1300 mcg/day for women of all ages (7135).
The average dietary intake of copper by US women is 1.0 to 1.1 mg/day, men consume 1.2 to 1.6 mg/day (7135).
Tolerable Upper Intake Levels (UL) have been established for children and adults. All copper intake by infants should be from food or formula, unless under medical supervision (7135).
The ULs for copper are: children 1 to 3 years, 1 mg/day; 4 to 8 years, 3 mg/day; 9 to 13 years, 5 mg/day; 14 to 18 years (including pregnancy and lactation) 8 mg/day; adults age 19 and older (including lactation), 10 mg/day; pregnancy age 19 and older, 8 mg/day (7135).
INTRAVENOUS: For copper deficiency, 1 to 2 mg per day is added to the parenteral nutrition solution (505).

Comments

There is no evidence that copper supplementation is needed or beneficial for people eating a normal diet, including athletes (703,704,705,709).

CORAL

Also Known As
Calcium Carbonate Matrix, Coral Calcium, Coralline Hydroxyapatite, Sea Coral.
CAUTION: See separate listing for Calcium, Coral Root.

Scientific Names
Goniopora species; Madrepora species; Porites species.

People Use This For
Orally, coral is used as a calcium supplement; to treat multiple sclerosis; and to treat and prevent cancer, heart disease, and other chronic health problems.
Orthopedically, coral is used as a substrate for growing new bone in areas damaged by trauma, maxillofacial reconstruction, cosmetic facial surgery, and damaged weight-bearing bones.

Safety
LIKELY SAFE ...when used surgically as a bone substitute (10736,10737,10738,10739,10741). There is insufficient reliable information available about the safety of the oral use of coral.
PREGNANCY AND LACTATION: Insufficient reliable information available; avoid using.

Effectiveness
LIKELY EFFECTIVE

Bone substitute. Coral can be used in place of allographic or autographic bone for spinal fusions and bone tumors; as well as in periodontal, craniofacial, orthopedic, and neurosurgery surgery (10736,10737,10738,10739,10741).

There is insufficient reliable information available about the effectiveness of coral for its other uses.

Mechanism of Action
Coral (calcium carbonate matrix) is derived form coral exoskeletons. The structure of coral is similar to that of cancellous (spongy) bone. Coral is advantageous over bone autographs because it causes less trauma. It is also advantageous over human bone allographs because it doesn't carry the risk of transmitting infections such as Acquired Immunodeficiency Syndrome (AIDS), Hepatitis C, and Creutzfeldt-Jakob disease. The local infection rate was 4% for coral grafts as compared to the bone allograph infection rate of 20%. Coral seems to act as an adequate carrier for bone growth factors. It seems to allow osteocyte attachment, growth, spreading, and differentiation (10741). New bone and fibrovascular tissue grow within the implanted coral. Over time, the calcium carbonate framework is resorbed (10737).

Adverse Reactions
Surgically, coral can cause infections (10741).

Interactions with Herbs & Other Dietary Supplements
None known.

Interactions with Drugs
None known.

Interactions with Foods
None known.

Interactions with Lab Tests
None known.

Interactions with Diseases or Conditions
None known.

Dosage and Administration
No typical dosage.

Comments
The Federal Trade Commission has charged the marketers of a coral supplement called "Coral Calcium Supreme" with making unsubstantiated health and medical claims about the product's ability to cure cancer or other diseases such as multiple sclerosis and heart disease (10742). There's no evidence that calcium from a coral source has any advantages over calcium from other sources. Some coral calcium products contain excess lead. In one independent laboratory analysis a coral calcium product contained 2.5 mcg of lead per 1 gram of calcium (9598).
Avoid confusion with coral root (Corallorhiza odontorhiza).

CORAL ROOT

Also Known As

Chicken Toe, Crawley, Crawley Root, Fever Root, Scaley Dragon's Claw, Turkey Claw.
CAUTION: See separate listing for Coral.

Scientific Names

Corallorhiza odontorhiza, synonym Cymbidium odontorhizum.
Family: Orchidaceae.

Comments

At the date of publication, this product was not a common ingredient used in brand name supplements marketed to consumers. Details about this product are available in the online version of *Natural Medicines Comprehensive Database.* See www.naturaldatabase.com.

CORDYCEPS

Also Known As

Caterpillar Fungus, Cs-4, Dong Chong Xia Cao, Dong Chong Zia Cao, Hsia Ts'Ao Tung Ch'Ung, Tochukaso, Vegetable Caterpillar.

Scientific Names

Cordyceps sinensis.
Family: Ascomycetes or Clavicipitaceae.

People Use This For

Orally, cordyceps is used for strengthening the immune system, improving athletic performance, reducing the effects of aging, promoting longevity, treating lethargy, and improving liver function in people with hepatitis B. It is also used to treat coughs, chronic bronchitis, respiratory disorders, kidney disorders, frequent nocturia, male sexual dysfunction, anemia, heart arrhythmias, high cholesterol, liver disorders, dizziness, weakness, tinnitus, wasting, and opium addiction. It is also used as a stimulant, a tonic, and as an adaptogen which is used to increase energy, enhance stamina, and reduce fatigue.

Safety

POSSIBLY SAFE ...when used orally and appropriately. Cordyceps and a specific cordyceps preparation (CordyMax Cs-4) appear to be safe when used orally, short-term (12,3417,3418,3419,3435,12095).
PREGNANCY AND LACTATION: Insufficient reliable information available; avoid using.

Effectiveness

POSSIBLY INEFFECTIVE

Athletic performance. Taking cordyceps orally doesn't seem to be effective for improving athletic performance. Endurance-trained cyclists who take a specific cordyceps preparation (CordyMax Cs-4) 3.15 grams/day for 5 weeks do not seem to have improved endurance time trials or improved aerobic capacity (VO2-peak) (12095).

INSUFFICIENT RELIABLE EVIDENCE to RATE

Aminoglycoside-induced nephrotoxicity. There is preliminary evidence that using cordyceps with amikacin might reduce amikacin-induced nephrotoxicity in older people (3419). It's not known if cordyceps helps for nephrotoxicity related to other aminoglycosides.

Chemotherapy. There is preliminary evidence that taking cordyceps orally following cancer chemotherapy might improve quality of life and cellular immunity (3417).

Cyclosporine-induced nephrotoxicity. There is preliminary evidence that taking cordyceps with cyclosporine can reduce cyclosporine-related nephrotoxicity in kidney-transplant recipients (3418).

Hepatitis B. There's preliminary evidence that taking cordyceps orally might improve liver function in hepatitis B patients (3435).

More evidence is needed to rate cordyceps for these uses.

Mechanism of Action

Cordyceps seems to have a beneficial effects on the immune, endocrine, cardiovascular, respiratory, renal, sexual, hepatic, immunologic, and nervous systems (3403,3404). Preliminary studies suggest cordyceps might stimulate immune function by increasing the number of T helper cells (3431); increasing the natural killer cell activity (3425,3427); stimulating the blood mononuclear cells (3414); increasing the levels of interferon-gamma, tumor necrosis factor-alpha, and interleukin-1 (3414); and prolonging the survival of lymphocytes (3432). Studies in animals with cancer suggest cordyceps improves immune response, reduces tumor size (3409,3431,3434), and lengthens survival time (3434,3437). Some evidence suggests cordyceps might be cytotoxic to cancer cells (3410,3416,3420), particularly lung carcinoma (3407) and melanoma (3427). Other evidence suggests that cordyceps might reduce the risk of renal toxicity from cyclosporine or aminoglycoside drugs (3411,3418,3419), and prove beneficial in chronic renal failure (3428). Cordyceps shows evidence that it can inhibit platelet aggregation and thrombus formation (3429). Other information suggests it might counteract or prevent arrhythmias, while decreasing heart rate and contractility (3436). Cordyceps polysaccharides show evidence that they might increase corticosterone production (3412). Other studies suggest they might reduce blood glucose (3415) without reducing plasma insulin levels (3415,3421), as well as reduce plasma triglycerides and cholesterol (3415). Preliminary animal studies suggest cordyceps could possibly be beneficial in treating systemic lupus erythematosus (3424). Limited human evidence suggests cordyceps can improve liver function in patients with chronic hepatitis B (3435).

Adverse Reactions

None reported.

Interactions with Herbs & Other Dietary Supplements

None known.

Interactions with Drugs

CYCLOPHOSPHAMIDE: Theoretically, cordyceps might reduce the immunosuppressive effects of cyclophosphamide (3427,3431).
PREDNISOLONE: Theoretically, cordyceps might reduce the immunosuppressive effects of prednisolone (3431,3437).

Interactions with Foods

None known.

Interactions with Lab Tests

LIVER FUNCTION TESTS: Cordyceps might improve liver function and test results in people with chronic hepatitis B (3435).

Interactions with Diseases or Conditions

HEPATITIS B: Based on limited human evidence, cordyceps might improve liver function and provide other benefits for people with chronic hepatitis B (3435).

Dosage and Administration

ORAL: A typical dosage of fermented Cordyceps sinensis is 3 grams per day (3403,3404).

Comments

Cordyceps sinensis is a fungus parasite that lives on caterpillars in high mountain regions of China (512). For commercial purposes, the cordyceps cells (Cs-4 strain) can be artificially propagated in the laboratory (512). Jinshuibao capsules are the commercially available form of fermented Cordyceps sinensis Cs-4 (3403).

CORIANDER

Also Known As

Chinese Parsley, Cilantro, Coriandri Fructus, Dhanyaka, Koriander, Kustumburi.

Scientific Names

Coriandrum sativum.
Family: Apiaceae/Umbelliferae.

People Use This For

Orally, coriander is used for dyspepsia, loss of appetite, nausea, diarrhea, as a stomach function stimulant, spasmolytic, antiflatulent, bactericide, fungicide, and to augment lactation.
Coriander is also used to treat measles, hernia, hemorrhoids, toothaches, worms, rheumatism, and joint pain.
In foods, coriander is used as a culinary spice and to prevent food poisoning.
In manufacturing, coriander is used as a flavoring agent in pharmaceutical preparations, as a fragrance component in cosmetics and soaps, and for flavoring tobacco.

Safety

LIKELY SAFE ...when used orally in amounts commonly found in foods. Coriander and coriander oil have Generally Recognized As Safe (GRAS) status in the US (4912).
POSSIBLY SAFE ...when used orally and appropriately for medicinal purposes (12).
PREGNANCY AND LACTATION: Insufficient reliable information available; avoid amounts in excess of those found in foods.

Effectiveness

There is insufficient reliable information available about the effectiveness of coriander.

Mechanism of Action

The applicable parts of coriander are the seed and leaves. Coriander is a rich source of vitamin C, calcium, magnesium, potassium, and iron (19). The odor and taste of coriander are due to the volatile oil, which consists mainly of linalool (60-70%) (7). In animals, coriander seems to have hypoglycemic activity (11). Coriander oil also has larvicidal properties (11).
There is interest in coriander to prevent food poisoning because constituents in coriander leaves seem to have bacteriocidal activity against the food-borne pathogen, salmonella (12031).

Adverse Reactions

Powdered coriander and especially the oil can cause allergic reactions and photosensitivity (8). Like other members of the Apiaceae/Umbelliferae (carrot family), coriander can cause contact dermatitis (19). Coriander has been associated with endocrine toxicity. A case report describes severe diarrhea, stomach pain, skin darkness, depressed mood, amenorrhea, and dehydration following consumption of 200 mL of a 10% coriander extract for 7 days (10635).

Interactions with Herbs & Other Dietary Supplements

None known.

Interactions with Drugs

None known.

Interactions with Foods

None known.

Interactions with Lab Tests

None known.

Interactions with Diseases or Conditions

None known.

Dosage and Administration

No typical dosage.

CORIOLUS MUSHROOM

Also Known As

Coriolus, Kawaratake, Krestin, Polysaccharide-K, Polysaccharide Krestin, Polysaccharide Peptide, PSK, PSP, Turkey Tail, Yun-Zhi (cloud mushroom).

Scientific Names

Coriolus versicolor, synonyms Trametes versicolor, Polyporus versicolor, Boletus versicolor, Polystictus versicolor.
Family: Polyporaceae.

People Use This For

Orally, coriolus mushroom or its derivatives are used for stimulating the immune system; treating herpes, chronic fatigue syndrome, hepatitis, and pulmonary disorders; reducing phlegm; improving body building; increasing energy; curing ringworm and impetigo; treating upper respiratory, urinary, and digestive tract infections; curing liver disorders including hepatitis; ameliorating the toxic effects and pain of chemotherapy and radiation therapy; promoting curative effect of chemotherapy; prolonging life and raising the quality of life; increasing appetite; and improving the effectiveness of cancer chemotherapy.

Safety

POSSIBLY SAFE ...when coriolus mushroom is used orally and appropriately (5477). ...when isolated PSK and PSP are used orally and appropriately (1635,1636,1640,1641,1648,1649,1650,1651,1652,1653,1654,1655,1656,1657,1658,1659,1660,1661,1662).

PREGNANCY AND LACTATION: Insufficient reliable information available; avoid using.

Effectiveness

POSSIBLY EFFECTIVE

Cancer. Taking polysaccharide krestin (PSK), a constituent of coriolus mushroom, orally may improve response and survival in some patients with cancer. It is given as a biologic response modifier (such as interferon or interleukin-2) as an adjunct to standard chemotherapy. It has been used in Japan for several decades for breast cancer, esophageal cancer, gastric cancer, lung cancer, hepatic cancer, colorectal cancer, and nasopharyngeal cancer (1640,1648,1649,1650,1651,1652,1653,1654,1655,1656,1657,1658,1659,1660,1661).

There is insufficient reliable information available about the effectiveness of coriolus mushroom for its other uses.

Mechanism of Action

The applicable parts of coriolus mushroom are the fruiting body and mycelium (5494).

Coriolus mushrooms have a long history in folk medicine, but researchers are just beginning to isolate and identify substances in coriolus that have pharmacological activity (5477,1635). Coriolus contains several polysaccharides, including polysaccharide peptide (PSP) and polysaccharide krestin (PSK), shown to have antitumor and immunomodulating effects (1600,1635,1636,1637,1638,1639,1640,1641,1642,1648,1649,1650,5484,5494).

PSK has been used in Japan as a biological response modifier in cancer chemotherapy regimens with varying results (1640,1641,1651,1652,1653,1654,1655,1656,1657,1658,1659,1660,1661,1662).

Early evidence suggests that PSP may have activity against lung cancers, leukemia, and gastric cancers (1635). When given with cyclophosphamide, PSP seems to improve immune function by increasing white cell, natural killer cell, and antibody levels (10291). These effects suggest that PSP might be a useful adjuvant in cancer therapy.

Coriolus might also have activity against the human immunodeficiency virus (HIV) (1643,1644).

Preliminary evidence suggests that coriolus might have analgesic activity and protect against acetaminophen-induced hepatotoxicity (1645,1646,1647).

Adverse Reactions

There have been no adverse reports for coriolus mushroom (1635,1636). Patients receiving PSK as an adjunct to chemotherapy experienced nausea, leukopenia, and liver function impairment (1651); however, this may have been due to the chemotherapy.

Interactions with Herbs & Other Dietary Supplements

None known.

Interactions with Drugs

None known.

Interactions with Foods

None known.

Interactions with Lab Tests

None known.

Interactions with Diseases or Conditions

None known.

Dosage and Administration

ORAL: A typical dose of tea is prepared from 20 grams of dried coriolus fruiting bodies three times daily, or take capsules containing up to 5 grams per day of the dried fruiting bodies. As an adjuvant to cancer chemotherapy, 3 grams of PSK is taken daily (1650,1654,1656,1658).

CORKWOOD TREE

Also Known As
Pituri.
CAUTION: See separate listing for Phellodendron.

Scientific Names
Duboisia myoporoides.
Family: Solanaceae.

People Use This For
Orally, corkwood quids (cured and rolled leaves) are chewed to ward off hunger, pain, and tiredness.
Alkaloids derived from the plant are used as a therapeutic substitute for atropine.

Safety
LIKELY UNSAFE ...when used orally. Corkwood tree leaves contain tropane alkaloids that are potent anticholinergics (6). Large doses of scopolamine and related alkaloids can be fatal (6).
PREGNANCY AND LACTATION: LIKELY UNSAFE ...when used orally (6); avoid using.

Effectiveness
There is insufficient reliable information available about the effectiveness of corkwood tree.

Mechanism of Action
The applicable part of corkwood tree is the leaf.
Researchers document tropane alkaloids (atropine, scopolamine, etc.) as constituents (6).
Stimulant and hallucinogenic properties are due to anticholinergic effects (6).

Adverse Reactions
Orally, corkwood tree can cause central nervous system disturbances (6).

Interactions with Herbs & Other Dietary Supplements
None known.

Interactions with Drugs
None known.

Interactions with Foods
None known.

Interactions with Lab Tests
None known.

Interactions with Diseases or Conditions
None known.

Dosage and Administration
ORAL: Leaves are cured and rolled into a quid which Australian natives chew (6).

Comments
Although at one time used as a source of scopolamine, other sources are more commercially viable (6).

CORN COCKLE

Also Known As
Cockle, Corn Campion, Corn Rose, Crown-of-the-Field, Purple Cockle.

Scientific Names
Agrostemma githago.
Family: Caryophyllaceae.

People Use This For

Orally, corn cockle is used as a diuretic, expectorant, menstrual stimulant, poison, vermifuge, and for jaundice. Topically, corn cockle seeds are used for treating cancers, hard tumors, warts, hard swelling of the uterus, and to induce inflammation of the conjunctiva and cornea. The root is used topically for exanthemata (acute skin eruptions signifying a viral or coccal infection), and hemorrhoids.

Safety

LIKELY UNSAFE ...when used orally, due to toxicity (6).
There is insufficient reliable information available about the safety of the topical use of corn cockle.
PREGNANCY AND LACTATION: LIKELY UNSAFE ...when used orally (6); avoid using.

Effectiveness

There is insufficient reliable information available about the effectiveness of corn cockle.

Mechanism of Action

The applicable parts of corn cockle are the root and seed. Poisonous constituents, githagin and agrostemmic acid, are reportedly absorbed from the GI tract causing GI irritation, severe muscle pain and twitching, depression, and coma (6).

Adverse Reactions

Orally, corn cockle can cause GI irritation, severe muscle pain and twitching, depression, and coma (6). Acute poisoning symptoms include: diarrhea, salivation, vertigo, vomiting, paralysis, and respiratory depression (6). Repeated poisoning by small doses is referred to as "githagism" (6).

Interactions with Herbs & Other Dietary Supplements

None known.

Interactions with Drugs

None known.

Interactions with Foods

None known.

Interactions with Lab Tests

None known.

Interactions with Diseases or Conditions

None known.

Dosage and Administration

No typical dosage.

CORN POPPY

Also Known As

Copperose, Corn Rose, Cup-Puppy, Headache, Headwark, Rakta Khakasa, Rakta-Posta, Red Poppy, Rhoeados Flos.
CAUTION: See separate listing for California Poppy.

Scientific Names

Papaver rhoeas.
Family: Papaveraceae.

People Use This For

Orally, corn poppy is used for respiratory tract diseases and discomforts, cough, disturbed sleep, and pain relief. For food uses, corn poppy is an ingredient in some "metabolic" teas. In other teas, it is used as a brightening agent.

Safety

POSSIBLY SAFE ...when the dried corn poppy flower petals are used orally and appropriately in medicinal amounts (2,18).
CHILDREN: POSSIBLY UNSAFE ...when the fresh leaves or blossoms are eaten because this can cause poisoning (18). There is insufficient reliable information available for the safety of dried corn poppy flower petals used in children.
PREGNANCY AND LACTATION: Insufficient reliable information available; avoid using.

Effectiveness
There is insufficient reliable information available about the effectiveness of corn poppy.

Mechanism of Action
The applicable part of corn poppy is the flower. There is insufficient reliable information available about the possible mechanism of action and active ingredients.

Adverse Reactions
No adverse effects in adults have been reported (2). However, poisonings have been reported in children who consumed the fresh leaves and blossoms. Symptoms include vomiting and stomach pain (18).

Interactions with Herbs & Other Dietary Supplements
None known.

Interactions with Drugs
None known.

Interactions with Foods
None known.

Interactions with Lab Tests
None known.

Interactions with Diseases or Conditions
None known.

Dosage and Administration
ORAL: For bronchial irritation, one cup tea (2 teaspoons dried petals in boiling water for 5-10 minutes) 2 to 3 times daily (may be sweetened with honey) has been used (18).

CORN SILK

Also Known As
Cornsilk, Indian Corn, Maidis Stigma, Maize Silk, Stigma Maydis, Zea.

Scientific Names
Zea mays.
Family: Poaceae/Gramineae.

People Use This For
Orally, corn silk is used for cystitis, urethritis, nocturnal enuresis, prostatitis, acute chronic inflammation of the urinary system, as a diuretic for congestive heart failure, to treat diabetes, and for hypertension.

Safety
LIKELY SAFE ...when used orally in amounts commonly found in foods. Corn silk, corn silk extract, and corn silk oil has Generally Recognized As Safe (GRAS) status in the US (4912).
POSSIBLY SAFE ...when used orally and appropriately in medicinal amounts (12).
PREGNANCY: POSSIBLY SAFE ...when consumed in food. LIKELY UNSAFE ...when used orally in larger amounts because it might have uterine stimulant effects (4); avoid using.
LACTATION: Insufficient reliable information available; avoid using.

Effectiveness
There is insufficient reliable information available about the effectiveness of corn silk.

Mechanism of Action
Corn silk contains tannins, which are astringent, and cryptoxanthin, which has vitamin A activity (4).

Adverse Reactions
Orally, prolonged use may cause hypokalemia (4).
Topically, allergy to cornsilk, corn pollen, or cornstarch may result in contact dermatitis or urticaria (4).

Interactions with Herbs & Other Dietary Supplements
None known.

Interactions with Drugs

ANTIDIABETES DRUGS: Theoretically, because some evidence suggests corn silk can reduce blood glucose levels, excessive amounts might interfere with diabetes therapy (4).
ANTIHYPERTENSIVE DRUGS: Theoretically, excessive doses of corn silk might cause hypotension and interfere with drugs used to treat hypertension or hypotension (4).
CORTICOSTEROIDS: Theoretically, prolonged use of corn silk might have additive effects with drugs that deplete potassium, including corticosteroids (4).
DIURETIC DRUGS: Overuse of corn silk might compound diuretic-induced potassium loss (4). There is some concern that people taking corn silk along with potassium depleting diuretics might have an increased risk for hypokalemia. Initiation of potassium supplementation or an increase in potassium supplement dose may be necessary for some patients. Some diuretics that can deplete potassium include chlorothiazide (Diuril), chlorthalidone (Thalitone), furosemide (Lasix), hydrochlorothiazide (HCTZ, Hydrodiuril, Microzide), and others.
WARFARIN (Coumadin): Corn silk contains vitamin K. Individuals taking warfarin should consume a consistent daily amount to maintain consistent anticoagulation (19).

Interactions with Foods

None known.

Interactions with Lab Tests

None known.

Interactions with Diseases or Conditions

DIABETES: Theoretically, excessive doses might reduce blood glucose level (4), interfering with control.
HYPERTENSION, HYPOTENSION: Theoretically, excessive doses might interfere with control of these conditions (4).
POTASSIUM DEPLETION: Theoretically, excessive doses might exacerbate this condition (4).

Dosage and Administration

ORAL: No typical dosage. However, traditionally, 4-8 grams dried style/stigma three times daily, or one cup tea (0.5 grams dried corn silk in 150 mL boiling water) several times daily (4,8). Liquid extract of maize stigmas, 4-8 mL (4). Tincture (1:5 in 25% alcohol), 5-15 mL three times daily (4).
Syrup of maize stigmas, 8-15 mL (4).

Comments

Corn silk is the so-called "silk" of an ear of ordinary Indian corn or maize.

CORNFLOWER

Also Known As

Bachelor's Buttons, Blue Cap, Blue Centaury, Bluebonnet, Bluebottle, Bluebow, Corn Flower, Cyani Blossoms, Cyani Flos, Cyani Flowers, Cyani Petals, Hurtsickle.
CAUTION: See separate listings for Buttercup and Feverfew.

Scientific Names

Centaurea cyanus, synonym Centaurea segetum.
Family: Asteraceae/Compositae.

People Use This For

Orally, cornflower is used for fever, menstrual disorders, vaginal candidiasis; and as a laxative, diuretic, expectorant, tonic, bitter, and as a liver and gallbladder stimulant.
Topically, cornflower is used for eye irritation or discomfort.
In foods, cornflower is utilized in herbal teas as a coloring agent.

Safety

LIKELY SAFE ...when used as a coloring agent in herbal teas (2).
There is insufficient reliable information available about the safety of cornflower for its other uses.
PREGNANCY AND LACTATION: Insufficient reliable information available; avoid using.

Effectiveness

There is insufficient reliable information available about the effectiveness of cornflower.

Mechanism of Action

The applicable part of cornflower is the dried flower. The color is due to anthocyanin constituents (1502).

Adverse Reactions
Cornflower may cause an allergic reaction in individuals sensitive to the Asteraceae/Compositae family. Members of this family include ragweed, chrysanthemums, marigolds, daisies, and many other herbs.

Interactions with Herbs & Other Dietary Supplements
None known.

Interactions with Drugs
None known.

Interactions with Foods
None known.

Interactions with Lab Tests
None known.

Interactions with Diseases or Conditions
CROSS-ALLERGENICITY: Cornflower may cause an allergic reaction in individuals sensitive to the Asteraceae/Compositae family. Members of this family include ragweed, chrysanthemums, marigolds, daisies, and many other herbs.

Dosage and Administration
ORAL: People typically use the crushed dried flowers as a tea. The tea is prepared by adding 1 gram of cornflower per cup of water (5252).
TOPICAL: No typical dosage.

CORYDALIS

Also Known As
Early Fumitory, Squirrel Corn.

Scientific Names
Corydalis cava, synonym Corydalis tuberosa.
Family: Fumariaceae.

Comments
At the date of publication, there was very little scientific information available about this product. Our staff is continually analyzing the available information on natural medicines and will add data to the online version of *Natural Medicines Comprehensive Database* as it becomes available. See www.naturaldatabase.com.

COSTUS

Also Known As
Auckland Costus, Kushtha, Kuth, Mokko, Mu Xiang, Yun Mu Xiang.

Scientific Names
Saussurea costus, synonyms Saussurea lappa, Aucklandia costus, Aplotaxis lappa.
Family: Asteraceae/Compositae.

People Use This For
Orally, costus oil is used for asthma, cough, dysentery, cholera, and as a tonic, gastric stimulant, and antiflatulent, Costus root is used orally for nematode infections.
In foods and beverages, costus oil is used as a flavoring component.
In manufacturing, costus oil is used as a fixative and fragrance in cosmetics.

Safety

LIKELY SAFE ...when used in amounts commonly found in foods.
Costus oil has Generally Recognized As Safe status (GRAS) for use in foods in the US (4912).
POSSIBLY SAFE ...when costus root is used orally and appropriately (12).
UNSAFE ...when aristolochic acid-contaminated costus products are used orally. Costus root is commonly contaminated with aristolochic acid, which is nephrotoxic and carcinogenic. The FDA considers all products containing aristolochic acid to be unsafe and adulterated. Only products analytically verified to be aristolochic acid-free should be used (6118).
PREGNANCY AND LACTATION: Insufficient reliable information available; avoid using.

Effectiveness

INSUFFICIENT RELIABLE EVIDENCE to RATE

Nematodes. In children, costus root reduces the number of nematode fecal eggs per gram similarly to treatment with pyrantel pamoate (1516). More evidence is needed to rate costus for this use.

Mechanism of Action

The applicable parts of costus are the root and oil. Costus oil is the distilled, extracted oil from the root. Costus root seems to have an antinematode effect (1516). Costus oil is reported to inhibit bronchospasm and lower blood pressure in animals (11).

Adverse Reactions

Orally, costus might cause allergic reactions, including contact dermatitis (11). Costus can cause an allergic reaction in individuals sensitive to the Asteraceae/Compositae family (6118). Members of this family include ragweed, chrysanthemums, marigolds, daisies, and many other herbs.
Costus root is commonly contaminated with aristolochic acid which is nephrotoxic and carcinogenic (6118).

Interactions with Herbs & Other Dietary Supplements

None known.

Interactions with Drugs

None known.

Interactions with Foods

None known.

Interactions with Lab Tests

None known.

Interactions with Diseases or Conditions

CROSS-ALLERGENICITY: Costus can cause an allergic reaction in individuals sensitive to the Asteraceae/Compositae family. Members of this family include ragweed, chrysanthemums, marigolds, daisies, and many other herbs.

Dosage and Administration

ORAL: As an antinematodal, 50 mg/kg root (or equivalent amount of methanol extract of root) as a single dose has been used (1516).

Comments

The FDA intends to automatically detain, without physical examination, any product which contains plants known or suspected to contain aristolochic acid, or which might be adulterated with plants known to contain aristolochic acid. Each detained product will be released only after the responsible party provides direct analytical evidence that it is free of aristolochic acid (6118).

COTTON

Also Known As

Cotton Root, Karpasa.
CAUTION: See separate listing for Gossypol.

Scientific Names

Gossypium herbaceum; Gossypium hirsutum; other Gossypium species.
Family: Malvaceae.

People Use This For

Orally, cotton is used for amenorrhea; dysmenorrhea; irregular, painful, or profuse menstrual bleeding; climacteric complaints; poor lactation; nausea; fever; headache; diarrhea; dysentery; urethritis; nerve inflammation; hemorrhage; as an oxytocic; and to expel afterbirth.
Cotton has been used as an anti-fertility drug in males, as well as in topical, vaginal contraceptive preparations.

Safety

POSSIBLY SAFE ...when used orally in medicinal amounts (12). ...when preparations of the root bark are used in amounts found in foods. Canadian regulations limit use to less than 450 ppm of free gossypol (including cotton seed meal and oil) (12).
PREGNANCY: LIKELY UNSAFE ...when used orally because it is a possible abortifacient and uterine stimulant (12).
LACTATION: Insufficient reliable information available; avoid using.

Effectiveness

There is insufficient reliable information available about the effectiveness of cotton.

Mechanism of Action

The applicable part of cotton is the root bark. It is believed to stimulate menstrual flow, act as an oxytocic, and male contraceptive (18). Some evidence suggests cotton root can cause histamine release (18). The constituent, gossypol that is extracted from cotton seed is used as a male contraceptive (6).

Adverse Reactions

None reported. However, in animals, long-term feeding with cotton seed cakes has been linked to poisonings and deaths (18).

Interactions with Herbs & Other Dietary Supplements

None known.

Interactions with Drugs

None known.

Interactions with Foods

None known.

Interactions with Lab Tests

None known.

Interactions with Diseases or Conditions

UROGENITAL IRRITATION OR SENSITIVITY: Contraindicated (12).

Dosage and Administration

ORAL: People typically prepare cotton root bark using one teaspoon boiled in a covered container with 3 cups of water for 30 minutes. The liquid is cooled slowly in the closed container and taken cold, 1 to 2 cups per day (5254).

Comments

Avoid confusion with gossypol (cotton seed extract).
Cotton's use as a male contraceptive agent is in question because it may potentially cause irreversible sterility (6002).

COUNTRY MALLOW

Also Known As

Bala, Bariar, Heartleaf, Khareti, Malva-Branca, Malva-Branca-Sedosa, Silky White Mallow, Vatya, White Mallow.
CAUTION: See separate listings for Mallow and Marshmallow.

Scientific Names

Sida cordifolia.
Family: Malvaceae.

People Use This For

Orally, country mallow is used to treat bronchial asthma, tuberculosis, colds, flu, chills, lack of perspiration, headaches, nasal congestion, cough and wheezing, urinary infections, stomatitis, and edema. It is also used orally for heart disease, stroke, facial paralysis, chronic tissue inflammation, sciatica, insanity, neuralgia, nerve inflammation, chronic rheumatism, and emaciation. Country mallow is also used orally as a stimulant, analgesic, diuretic, tonic, and aphrodisiac. It is also used before and after cancer chemotherapy to aid recovery.

In herbal combinations country mallow is used orally for weight loss, to burn fat, to increase energy, for impotence, sinus, allergy, throat diseases, asthma and bronchitis, and to promote a strong skeletal system. In combination with ginger, country mallow root is used orally for intermittent fever. In combination with milk and sugar, country mallow root is used for urinary urgency and leukorrhea.

Topically, country mallow is used for numbness, nerve pain, muscle cramps, skin disorders, tumors, joint diseases, wounds, ulcers, scorpion sting, snake bite, and as a massage oil.

Safety

LIKELY UNSAFE ...when used orally. Country mallow contains the constituent ephedrine, similar to the herb ephedra. Ephedra, country mallow, and other ephedrine-containing herbs are banned in the US due to several case reports that have linked ephedra to serious side effects including hypertension, myocardial infarction (MI), seizure, stroke, psychosis, and others (1276,2729,6486,6998,9167,10689). Tell patients to avoid this and other products that contain ephedrine.

PREGNANCY AND LACTATION: LIKELY UNSAFE ...when used orally. The ephedrine constituent of country mallow has been linked to several cases of severe side effects (1276,2729,6486,6998,9167,10689).

Effectiveness

There is insufficient reliable information available about the effectiveness of country mallow.

Mechanism of Action

The applicable parts of country mallow are the root, leaves, and seeds. Country mallow contains the alkaloids cryptolepine, ephedrine, pseudoephedrine, vasocinone, and vasicine. Preliminary research suggests the extracts of the aerial and root parts have analgesic, anti-inflammatory, and hypoglycemic properties.

The analgesic and anti-inflammatory effects appear to result from cyclooxygenase (COX) inhibition (4299,12906).

Ephedrine and pseudoephedrine are both non-selective alpha- and beta-receptor agonists. The ephedrine and pseudoephedrine constituents can directly and indirectly stimulate the sympathetic nervous system (12813).

Ephedrine and pseudoephedrine can increase systolic and diastolic blood pressure, heart rate, and cardiac contractility, and cause peripheral vasoconstriction, bronchodilation, and central nervous system stimulation (8644).

Ephedrine, which was used in combination with theophylline and phenobarbital (Tedral) for many years to treat asthma, causes bronchodilation and increased oxygen consumption (8645).

Ephedrine is thought to stimulate thermogenesis and contribute to modest short-term weight loss, possibly by increasing norepinephrine release. Aspirin and caffeine might act synergistically with ephedrine by inhibiting prostaglandin, which also increases norepinephrine release (314,729,10003).

Ephedrine and related alkaloids have been linked to myocarditis and myocardial infarction. This has been attributed to coronary artery vasoconstriction and possibly vasospasm caused by ephedrine. Ephedrine might also cause cardiac arrhythmia due to adrenergic effects that shorten the cardiac refractory period, causing re-entrant arrhythmias (6486). A specific weight loss product (Metabolife 356), which contains ephedrine from the herb ephedra and caffeine in addition to 17 other ingredients, can prolong the QT interval by an average of 27 milliseconds in healthy volunteers (11355). A prolonged QT interval increases the risk of potentially serious ventricular arrhythmias such as torsades de pointes.

There's some evidence that ephedrine alone or in combination with caffeine can improve anaerobic exercise performance. Ephedrine causes catecholamine release and increases CNS stimulation, which may lead to better performance (8646).

Country mallow might have antibacterial effects. An aqueous extract shows evidence that it limits the virulence of dental bacteria, reducing the rate of plaque formation (4303). The country mallow constituent, cryptolepine, appears to have antibacterial activity against Proteus vulgaris (12905).

Adverse Reactions

Orally, side effects specifically for country mallow have not been reported. Since country mallow contains the ephedrine constituent there is concern that it might cause side effects that have occurred with other products that contain ephedrine such as ephedra. As a result of this concern, like ephedra, country mallow is banned in the US. Ephedrine-containing products have been associated with side effects such as dizziness, restlessness, anxiety, irritability, personality changes, difficulty concentrating, insomnia, headache, increased thirst, dry mouth, anorexia, nausea, vomiting, heartburn, flushing, tingling, difficulty urinating, tachycardia, heart palpitations, hyperthermia, and increased blood pressure (1276,3719,6008,6486,8647,10004,10382). Psychosis has also been reported in people taking ephedrine-containing products (1276,6998,10689). Long-term use or high doses of ephedrine have been associated with dependence and tolerance (1381).

There are also several reports of serious life-threatening or debilitating adverse effects associated with ephedrine

products. Ephedrine use has been associated with cardiomyopathy (1270), hypersensitivity myocarditis (1271,6487), chest tightness, myocardial infarction (6486), cardiac arrest and sudden death (1274,6486), and cardiac arrhythmias.
In healthy volunteers, ECG changes, including prolonged QT interval and premature atrial contractions, can occur with ingestion of recommended doses of ephedrine-containing products (11135,11708). Other reported events include stroke, transient ischemic attack, cerebral hemorrhage, seizure, and loss of consciousness (1275,1380,1381,2729,6486,8643).
There are also reports of myopathies, including myalgia, rhabdomyolysis, eosinophilia-myalgia syndrome (1270), and nephrolithiasis (1272). Other reported events include sudden hearing loss (10005).
Adverse effects are consistent with catecholamine excess (8643).
Large studies looking at the safety of ephedrine have not been performed. Since most of the adverse effect data are from case reports, it is impossible to determine the overall incidence of these adverse effects. It is also difficult to determine which patient groups might be most likely to experience an adverse event. Patients with a history of cardiovascular disease would be expected to be at a higher risk. However, there have been several reports of serious events in patients with no known pre-existing medical condition. In many of these cases, ephedrine was used in combination with another stimulant such as caffeine (10307). However, there are also reports of serious adverse effects when ephedrine has been used alone.
The safety of ephedrine and country mallow are controversial and highly debated. Some claim that ephedrine is only unsafe when used inappropriately and in excessive doses. The supplement industry maintains that it is safe when taken in doses recommended on labeling. However, there are several cases where severe life-threatening or debilitating effects occurred with short-term use of relatively low doses ranging from 20-60 mg ephedra alkaloids per day (6486). There is also considerable inter- and intra-product variability in labeled ephedra content, which adds to concern about ephedrine toxicity (8643,11336). Contaminants such as norpseudoephedrine, a schedule IV controlled substance, are also present in some products (8643). Until more is known, warn patients that the potential risks of using country mallow, and other ephedrine-containing products outweigh any potential benefit.

Interactions with Herbs & Other Dietary Supplements

ERGOT ALKALOID DERIVATIVES: Theoretically, concomitant use might cause excessive vasoconstriction and hypertension due to the ephedrine contained in country mallow (6009).
HERBS AND SUPPLEMENTS WITH STIMULANT PROPERTIES: Use of country mallow and other stimulant herbs, such as those containing caffeine, can increase the risk of common side effects such as insomnia, jitteriness, tremulousness, dizziness, etc. Using country mallow with other stimulants might also increase the risk of more serious adverse effects such as hypertension, myocardial infarction (MI), stroke, and death. There are several reports of serious life-threatening or debilitating adverse events in patients taking ephedrine-containing herbs in combination with caffeine and other stimulants (1275,1380,6486,10307). Some herbs and supplements with significant caffeine content include black tea, coffee, cola nut, green tea, guarana, mate, and others.
PANAX GINSENG: Panax ginseng can cause prolonged QT interval with initial use. It might have an additive effect with country mallow on the QT interval, increasing the risk for arrhythmias (4322,11355).

Interactions with Drugs

ANTIDIABETES DRUGS: The ephedrine constituent of country mallow might raise blood glucose levels and might decrease the effectiveness of drug therapy. Monitor blood glucose concentrations closely (12857).
Some antidiabetes drugs include glimepiride (Amaryl), glyburide (DiaBeta, Glynase PresTab, Micronase), insulin, pioglitazone (Actos), rosiglitazone (Avandia), and others.
DEXAMETHASONE (Decadron): Theoretically, concomitant use might reduce the effectiveness of dexamethasone, due to the ephedrine contained in country mallow. Ephedrine increases the clearance rate of dexamethasone (11462).
ERGOT DERIVATIVES: Theoretically, concomitant use of country mallow and ergot alkaloids might cause hypertension, due to the ephedrine contained in country mallow (6009).
METHYLXANTHINES: Use of ephedrine-containing herbs with caffeine or other methylxanthines such as theophylline might increase the risk of stimulatory adverse effects (8641). There is also some evidence that using ephedrine with caffeine might increase the risk of serious life-threatening or debilitating adverse effects such as hypertension, myocardial infarction (MI), stroke, seizures, and death (1275,1380,6486,10307).
Tell patients to avoid taking country mallow with caffeine and other stimulants.
MONOAMINE OXIDASE INHIBITORS (MAOIs): Concomitant use of country mallow with MAOIs might increase the risk of hypertension (6009).
QT INTERVAL-PROLONGING DRUGS: Country mallow contains the constituent ephedrine. Ephedrine from another herb, ephedra, has been linked to QT-interval prolongation (11355). Theoretically, country mallow might have an additive effect with drugs that prolong the QT interval. This might increase the risk of ventricular arrhythmias.
Drugs that prolong the QT interval include amiodarone (Cordarone), disopyramide (Norpace), dofetilide (Tikosyn), ibutilide (Corvert), procainamide (Pronestyl), quinidine, sotalol (Betapace), thioridazine (Mellaril), and many others.
STIMULANT DRUGS: Theoretically, drugs with CNS stimulant properties, such as phenylpropanolamine, pseudoephedrine, and diethylpropion, and many others might increase the risk of hypertension and adverse cardiovascular effects of country mallow due to its ephedrine content (4304).

Interactions with Foods

COFFEE, TEA: Theoretically, concomitant use of the country mallow constituent ephedrine and large amounts of caffeinated coffee or tea might increase the stimulatory effects and adverse effects of caffeine and ephedrine (12857).

Interactions with Lab Tests

AMPHETAMINE/METHAMPHETAMINE: Country mallow might cause false-positive urine amphetamine or methamphetamine test results. False-positive urine methamphetamine assays have been attributed to the use of herbal supplements containing ephedrine (1381,10688).

CATECHOLAMINE: Ephedrine, a constituent of country mallow, can increase plasma catecholamine levels (8646).

EPHEDRINE: Country mallow can cause a positive urine ephedrine test due to its ephedrine content. A case of an athlete whose urine tested positive for norpseudoephedrine was attributed to the use of an herbal supplement labeled to contain ephedra. However, the product might also have contained added norpseudoephedrine as an unlabeled ingredient (1259).

GLUCOSE: Ephedrine, a constituent of country mallow, can increase blood glucose levels and test results (8646). Monitor blood glucose levels in diabetes patients closely.

LACTATE: Ephedrine, a constituent of country mallow, can increase blood lactate levels (8646).

Interactions with Diseases or Conditions

ANGINA: Country mallow is contraindicated in people with angina; it might induce or exacerbate angina due its cardiac stimulant effects (8644,12813).

ANXIETY: Large doses of country mallow might cause or exacerbate anxiety due to central nervous system (CNS) stimulant effects (8644,12813).

ARRHYTHMIA: Country mallow might cause tachycardia or arrhythmias, due to its cardiac stimulant effects (11355,11708).

DIABETES: Country mallow might interfere with blood sugar control, and exacerbate high blood pressure and circulatory problems in people with diabetes (12857).

ESSENTIAL TREMOR: Country mallow might exacerbate essential tremor due to its stimulant effects (1715).

HYPERTENSION: Country mallow might exacerbate hypertension (11355); contraindicated in uncontrolled hypertension.

HYPERTHYROID, THYROTOXICOSIS: Theoretically, country mallow might stimulate the thyroid and exacerbate hyperthyroid symptoms; contraindicated (12858).

KIDNEY STONES (Nephrolithiasis): The country mallow constituent, ephedrine, might cause kidney stones (1272).

LONG QT INTERVAL SYNDROME: Ephedrine-containing herbs appear to prolong the QT interval (11355). This might increase the risk of ventricular arrhythmias in patients with long QT interval syndrome.

NARROW-ANGLE GLAUCOMA: Country mallow might exacerbate narrow-angle (angle-closure) glaucoma by causing mydriasis (12859).

PHEOCHROMOCYTOMA: Country mallow might exacerbate the symptoms of pheochromocytoma; contraindicated (8644,12813).

Dosage and Administration

ORAL: No typical dosage. Traditionally, a dose of powder (root, leaves, seeds) is 0.5-1 gram, twice daily. A typical dose of the fresh juice is 15-30 mL twice daily (4310)

TOPICAL: No typical dosage.

Comments

On December 30, 2003, the FDA announced that it will ban ephedra, country mallow, and other ephedrine-containing products in the US (10055). The ban went into effect in April 2004.

COWHAGE

Also Known As

Atmagupta, Couhage, Cowitch, Feijao macaco, HP 200, HP-200, Kapikachchhu, Kaunch, Kawanch, Kiwach, Mucuna, Mucuna prurient, Pica Pica, Pica-Pica, Velvet Bean.

Scientific Names

Mucuna pruriens; Mucuna pruriens var. hirsuta, synonyms Mucuna hirsuta, Stizolobium hirsutum.
Family: Fabaceae/Leguminosae.

People Use This For

Orally, cowhage is used for Parkinson's disease, anxiety, arthritis, hyperprolactinemia, and for parasitic infections. It's also used as an analgesic for pain, for fever, to induce vomiting, and as an aphrodisiac.
Cowhage is also used prophylactically as snakebite remedy.
Topically, cowhage is used as a rubefacient or counterirritant for rheumatic conditions, myalgias, to stimulate cutaneous blood flow in paralytic conditions, and to treat scorpion stings.

Safety

POSSIBLY SAFE ...when used orally and appropriately. Powdered formulations of cowhage seed have been used safely for up to 20 weeks (6899,7020,7203).
POSSIBLY UNSAFE ...when the hair of the cowhage bean pod is used orally or topically.
The bean pod hairs are strong irritants and can cause severe itching, burning, and inflammation (18).
PREGNANCY AND LACTATION: There is insufficient reliable information available about the safety of cowhage; avoid using.

Effectiveness

INSUFFICIENT RELIABLE EVIDENCE to RATE

Hyperprolactinemia. There is some evidence that cowhage might be useful for chlorpromazine-induced hyperprolactinemia in men (7207), but it does not appear to be effective for hyperprolactinemia of unknown cause in women (7206).

Parkinson's disease. There is preliminary evidence that some cowhage preparations might help improve symptoms of Parkinson's disease when used in combination with conventional drugs such as amantadine, selegiline, and anticholinergic agents. Cowhage contains 3-6% levodopa (L-dopa). Specific cowhage extracts standardized to 3.3% L-dopa (HP-200) and other powdered formulations providing 75 to 220 mg per day of L-dopa are being used for patients with Parkinson's (6899,7020,7203). There is also evidence that taking a single dose of 30 grams of power preparation containing 1000 mg L-dopa has a quicker onset of action, longer duration of action, and provides higher drug levels compared to 200 mg of conventional levodopa in combination with carbidopa (12232).

More evidence is needed to rate cowhage for these uses.

Mechanism of Action

The applicable parts of cowhage are the bean or seed and the hair on the bean pod. Cowhage is thought to work for Parkinson's disease because it contains a significant amount of levodopa (L-dopa). The whole cowhage bean contains about 3-6% L-dopa (7020,7021). The inner layer (endocarp) of the pericarp, which has also been studied in patients with Parkinson's disease, usually contains the highest amount of L-dopa, about 5.3% (7020). Symptoms of Parkinson's disease occur in patients due to a depletion of the neurotransmitter dopamine. L-dopa is a precursor to dopamine. To be effective for Parkinson's disease, L-dopa must cross the blood-brain barrier where it is then decarboxylated to dopamine. However, the majority of L-dopa is metabolized peripherally and probably less than 1% actually reaches the brain (15). Some powdered cowhage seed preparations containing L-dopa seem to lessen symptoms of Parkinson's disease at a relatively low dose, compared to conventional L-dopa products. So there is some speculation that constituents other than levodopa might have antiparkinson activity (7203).
Cowhage also contains prurieninin, which might slow heart rate, decrease blood pressure, and stimulate intestinal peristalsis (18). Cowhage has also been reported to have anthelmintic, antiflatulent, and cholesterol lowering properties (18), but these effects have not been verified in humans.
Animal studies show that cowhage might lower blood glucose levels (7221) and possibly slow the development of diabetic nephropathy (7220). Cowhage contains significant amounts of minerals, including calcium, magnesium, phosphorus, iron, manganese, zinc, and copper. Some researchers speculate that cowhage might exert its hypoglycemic effect due to trace element stimulation of insulin or possibly because of orally active insulin-like compounds in cowhage (7221).
There is interest in using cowhage for snakebite. Cowhage extract seems to have a procoagulant effect against the venom of the saw scaled viper (Echis carinatus), when given at least 24 hours prior to laboratory exposure to the venom (7222).
Cowhage also possesses counterirritant and rubefacient properties (18). The hairs (spicules) of the bean pod or seed cause severe itching, burning, and inflammation when they penetrate the epidermis (18,6898). Serotonin and protein constituents such as mucunain are released into the skin, causing blood vessel dilation, redness, and inflammation (18,6898). Repeated boiling of the bean is sometimes used to eliminate the pharmacologically and toxicologically active principles so that the bean can be consumed as food (7021,7205).

Adverse Reactions

Orally, cowhage seems to be fairly well tolerated when a standardized powdered formulation, known as HP-200, made from the inner portion (endocarp) of the bean wall (pericarp) is used. The most common side effects reported are nausea and a sensation of abdominal distention. Other side effects less frequently reported are vomiting, dyskinesias, and insomnia (7020). Adverse effects reported with other cowhage bean preparations include headache; palpitations; sweating; flatulence; diarrhea; dry mouth; rash and pruritus; changes in urine color; and symptoms of psychosis including confusion, giddiness, agitation, hallucinations, and paranoid delusions (7203,7021).
Cowhage-induced psychosis has been successfully treated with intravenous chlorpromazine (Thorazine) (7021).
Theoretically, due to the levodopa (L-dopa) constituent, cowhage is likely to cause the same adverse effects that have been attributed to the purified L-dopa prescription drug. Some of these side effects include elevated liver enzymes, respiratory disturbances, urinary retention, darkening of bodily fluids, muscle cramps, headache, and priapism (15). However, these effects have not yet been reported for cowhage. Ingestion of hairs from the bean pod or seed can result in significant mucosal irritation and should be avoided.
Topically, hairs from the cowhage bean pod or seed can cause severe itching, burning, inflammation, and erythematous macular rashes (18,6898). Symptoms resolve spontaneously within several hours, but may also be relieved with antihistamines (6898). The hairs can be removed from the skin by washing, but the hairs can also be retained, and transferred to other people, in fabrics and carpets. Clothing and other materials that come in contact with the cowhage hairs should also be thoroughly washed (6898).

Interactions with Herbs & Other Dietary Supplements

HERBS AND SUPPLEMENTS WITH HYPOGLYCEMIC EFFECTS: There is some evidence that cowhage might have hypoglycemic effects (7221). Theoretically, concomitant use with other herbs and supplements that decrease blood glucose levels might increase the risk of hypoglycemia.
Some of these products include bitter melon, ginger, goat's rue, fenugreek, kudzu, willow bark, and others.
KAVA: Theoretically, kava might reduce the effectiveness of cowhage. There is some evidence that kava might have antidopaminergic effects and possibly decrease the effects of levodopa (L-dopa) in cowhage (19).
VITAMIN B6 (Pyridoxine): Vitamin B6 can decrease the effectiveness of the cowhage constituent levodopa (L-dopa) in patients with Parkinson's disease. Vitamin B6 increases peripheral decarboxylation of L-dopa to dopamine (15). Tell patients taking cowhage for Parkinson's disease to avoid taking vitamin B6 supplements.

Interactions with Drugs

ANESTHESIA: Concomitant use of some anesthetics and the cowhage constituent, levodopa (L-dopa) has resulted in cardiac arrhythmia. This effect has only been associated with cyclopropane and the halogenated hydrocarbons. Other anesthetics have not been implicated (15). Use other anesthetics in patients taking cowhage or tell patients to stop taking cowhage at least 2 weeks before surgery.
ANTIDIABETES DRUGS: There is some evidence that cowhage might have hypoglycemic effects (7221). Theoretically, concomitant use with drugs that decrease blood glucose levels might increase the risk of hypoglycemia. Dosing adjustments for insulin or oral hypoglycemic agents may be necessary.
Oral hypoglycemic drugs include glimepiride (Amaryl), glipizide (Glucotrol), glyburide (Diabeta, Micronase), tolazamide (Tolinase), tolbutamide (Orinase), and others.
ANTIPSYCHOTIC DRUGS: Due to the antidopaminergic effects of antipsychotic medications, concomitant use of cowhage and these drugs might decrease the effectiveness of some antipsychotics (15).
Some of these drugs include chlorpromazine (Thorazine), clozapine (Clozaril), fluphenazine (Prolixin), haloperidol (Haldol), olanzapine (Zyprexa), perphenazine (Trilafon), prochlorperazine (Compazine), quetiapine (Seroquel), risperidone (Risperdal), thioridazine (Mellaril), and thiothixene (Navane).
GUANETHIDINE (Ismelin): Cowhage might have additive hypotensive effects when used concomitantly with guanethidine (15); avoid using.
METHYLDOPA (Aldomet): Cowhage might have additive hypotensive effects when used concomitantly with methyldopa. Furthermore, methyldopa can inhibit peripheral decarboxylation of the cowhage constituent levodopa (L-dopa). This could increase the amount of L-dopa reaching the central nervous system and potentially lead to toxicity (15).
MONOAMINE OXIDASE INHIBITORS (MAOIs): Due to the levodopa (L-dopa) content of cowhage, it should not be given with non-selective MAOIs such as phenelzine (Nardil) and tranylcypromine (Parnate). Concomitant use can cause hypertensive crisis. However, cowhage can be used concurrently with the MAO-B selective inhibitor selegiline (Deprenyl) (15).
TRICYCLIC ANTIDEPRESSANTS (TCAs): There is some concern that TCAs might decrease absorption of the active cowhage constituent, levodopa (L-dopa). TCAs can slow gastric emptying which can prevent L-dopa from being fully absorbed. There have also been rare reports of hypertension and dyskinesias in some patients taking both TCAs and L-dopa (15). Concomitant use of cowhage and TCAs should be done cautiously or avoided.
Some TCAs include amitriptyline (Elavil), clomipramine (Anafranil), desipramine (Norpramin), doxepin (Sinequan), imipramine (Tofranil), nortriptyline (Pamelor), and protriptyline (Vivactil).

Interactions with Foods
None known.

Interactions with Lab Tests
GLUCOSE: Due to the levodopa (L-dopa) content, cowhage might cause false-positive urine glucose tests when cupric sulfate reagents, such as Benedict's reagent or Clinitest tablets, are used. Cowhage might cause false-negatives when glucose oxidase tests such as Clinistix and Tes-Tape are used (15).
KETONES: Due to the levodopa (L-dopa) content, cowhage might cause a false positive urine ketones reaction when sodium nitroprusside reagents such as Acetest, Ketostix, and Labstix are used (15).
LIVER FUNCTION TESTS: Due to the levodopa content, cowhage might cause elevated liver function tests. L-dopa has caused transiently increased liver function tests including alkaline phosphatase, aspartate aminotransferase (AST or SGOT), alanine aminotransferase (ALT or SGPT), lactate dehydrogenase (LDH), and bilirubin (15). However, this effect has not yet been reported for cowhage.
URIC ACID: Due to the levodopa (L-dopa) content of cowhage, serum and urine uric acid levels might appear elevated when colorimetric tests are used. However, cowhage does not effect tests using uricase (15).

Interactions with Diseases or Conditions
CARDIOVASCULAR DISEASE: Due to the levodopa (L-dopa) content of cowhage, it should be avoided or used cautiously in patients with cardiovascular disease. L-dopa can frequently cause orthostatic hypotension, dizziness, and syncope. Much less frequently, L-dopa can also cause palpitations and cardiac arrhythmias (15).
DIABETES: There is some evidence that cowhage can lower blood glucose levels and might cause hypoglycemia (7221). Advise patients to increase blood glucose monitoring. Dosing adjustments to diabetes medications may be necessary.
HYPOGLYCEMIA: There is some evidence that cowhage can lower blood glucose levels and might exacerbate hypoglycemia (7221).
LIVER DISEASE: Due to the levodopa (L-dopa) content of cowhage, use cautiously in patients with liver disease. L-dopa has been reported to cause increased liver function tests (15).
MELANOMA: Since levodopa (L-dopa) in cowhage is a precursor to the skin pigment melanin, there is some concern that it might worsen melanoma (15). Tell patients with malignant melanoma, history of melanoma or a suspicious undiagnosed skin lesions to avoid cowhage.
PEPTIC ULCER DISEASE (PUD): Since cowhage contains levodopa (L-dopa), there is some concern that it might induce gastrointestinal bleeding in patients with peptic ulcer disease. L-dopa has been reported to cause gastrointestinal bleeding in patients with PUD (15). However, this has not yet been reported with cowhage.
PSYCHIATRIC DISEASE: Due to the levodopa (L-dopa) content, cowhage might worsen psychiatric disease in patients with an existing condition (15). Furthermore, patients with a history of mental illness might be more likely to experience a cowhage-induced psychiatric disturbance.

Dosage and Administration
ORAL: For Parkinson's disease, a powdered cowhage extract known as HP-200, standardized to contain 3.3% levodopa (L-dopa) has been used. Dosages ranged from 22.5 to 67.5 grams divided into 2 to 5 doses per day (7020). Nonstandardized ground cowhage preparations have also been used. These contain 4.5% to 5.5% levodopa (L-dopa) and have been taken in doses of 40 to 60 grams per day in 4 divided doses (7203).

Comments
Cowhage is a legume that grows wild in the tropics, including India and the Bahamas, and its range may extend to southern Florida (6898). It has been used since ancient times in Ayurvedic medicine for the treatment of Parkinson's disease (7223). Prior to commercial synthesis of levodopa from vanillin, cowhage was investigated as a potential source of the drug with efforts to increase the yield of levodopa from the seeds and leaves (7203,7204). The barbed spicules detach easily from the fruiting pods and have been sold commercially as itching powder (6898).

COWSLIP

Also Known As
Arthritica, Buckels, Butter Rose, Crewel, English Cowslip, Fairy Caps, Herb Perter, Key Flower, Key of Heaven, Mayflower, Our Lady's Keys, Paigle, Paigle Peggle, Palsywort, Password, Peagle, Peagles, Petty Mulleins, Plumrocks, Primrose, Primula.
CAUTION: See separate listing for Marsh Marigold.

Scientific Names
Primula veris, synonym Primula officinalis; Primula elatior.
Family: Primulaceae.

People Use This For

Orally, cowslip flower is used for respiratory tract mucous membrane inflammation, cough, bronchitis, insomnia, nervous excitability, headache, hysteria, neuralgia, tremors, hydroticum, as a diuretic, antispasmodic, as a heart tonic for sensations of dizziness and cardiac insufficiency, whooping cough, asthma, gout, and neurologic complaints.

In combination with gentian root, European elder flower, verbena, and sorrel, cowslip is used orally for maintaining healthy sinuses and treating sinusitis.

Safety

POSSIBLY SAFE ...when used orally and appropriately (2,12). ...when used orally with gentian root, European elder flower, verbena, and sorrel (Quanterra Sinus Defense, Sinupret) (7,374,379).

PREGNANCY AND LACTATION: Insufficient reliable information available; avoid using.

Effectiveness

POSSIBLY EFFECTIVE

Sinusitis. Taking cowslip orally in combination with gentian root, European elder flower, verbena, and sorrel (Quanterra Sinus Defense, Sinupret), seems to help improve symptoms and resolve acute or chronic sinusitis (7,374,379).

There is insufficient reliable information available about the effectiveness of cowslip for its other uses.

Mechanism of Action

The applicable parts of cowslip are the flower and root. Cowslip is a rich source of beta-carotene and vitamin C (19). Cowslip is reported to have antispasmodic, diuretic, expectorant, hypnotic, laxative, secretion-reducing, and sedative activities (2,4). Evidence suggests the saponin fraction might initially cause hypotension followed by long-lasting hypertension (4). Flavonoid constituents might have anti-inflammatory and antispasmodic effects. The tannin constituents have astringent effects (4).

Adverse Reactions

Orally, cowslip can cause gastric discomfort and nausea (2,4,12). It may cause an allergic reaction in sensitive individuals (4). Toxicity, when it occurs, seems to be associated with saponin constituents of the underground parts of the plant (4).

Interactions with Herbs & Other Dietary Supplements

None known.

Interactions with Drugs

CNS DEPRESSANTS: Cowslip may potentiate effects of sedatives (6002).

DIURETIC DRUGS: Cowslip may potentiate effects of diuretics (6002).

Interactions with Foods

None known.

Interactions with Lab Tests

None known.

Interactions with Diseases or Conditions

HYPERTENSION, HYPOTENSION: Theoretically, excessive doses may interfere with control of these conditions (4).

Dosage and Administration

ORAL (flower): One cup tea (1-2 grams dried flowers steeped in 150 mL of boiling water 5-10 minutes, strain) three times daily (4). Liquid extract (1:1 in 25% alcohol), 1-2 mL three times daily (4).

Tincture, 2.5-7.5 grams per day (2). For acute or chronic sinusitis, two Sinupret tablets three times daily for up to two weeks has been used in clinical trials (7,374,379), equivalent to gentian root 12 mg, European elder flower 36 mg, verbena 36 mg, cowslip flower 36 mg, and sorrel 36 mg three times daily.

ORAL (root): 0.5-1.5 grams dried root per day, or as prepared tea. Tincture, 1.5-3 grams per day (2).

CRAMP BARK

Also Known As

Common Guelder-Rose, Crampbark, Cranberry bush, European Cranberry-Bush, Guelder Rose, Guelder-Rose, High Bush Cranberry, High-Bush Cranberry, Snowball Bush.
CAUTION: See separate listings for Alpine Cranberry, Black Haw, Cranberry, and Uva Ursi.

Scientific Names

Viburnum opulus.
Family: Adoxaceae/Viburnaceae or Caprifoliaceae.

People Use This For

Orally, cramp bark is used to relieve cramps, including muscle spasms, menstrual cramps, and cramps during pregnancy. It is also used orally as a kidney stimulant in painful or spasmodic urinary conditions, cancer, hysteria, infection, nervous disorders, scurvy, and uteritis. Cramp bark is also used as a diuretic, emetic, purgative, and sedative.

Safety

There is insufficient reliable information available about the safety of cramp bark.
Pregnancy and Lactation: Insufficient reliable information available; avoid using.

Effectiveness

There is insufficient reliable information available about the effectiveness of cramp bark.

Mechanism of Action

The applicable parts of cramp bark are the bark and root bark. At least two active constituents have been identified, scopoletin and viopudial. These constituents appear to have smooth muscle antispasmodic effects in vitro. Viopudial appears to have cholinergic effects by inhibiting acetylcholinesterase. In animal models viopudial causes bradycardia, hypotension, and a decrease in myocardial contractility (12229).

Adverse Reactions

None reported.

Interactions with Herbs & Other Dietary Supplements

None known.

Interactions with Drugs

None known.

Interactions with Foods

None known.

Interactions with Lab Tests

None known.

Interactions with Diseases or Conditions

None known.

Dosage and Administration

No typical dosage.

Comments

Cramp bark is a native American plant that is currently considered a decorative plant (12229).
Historically, North American Indians have used cramp bark medically as a diuretic, for reducing swollen glands, mumps, and eye disorders. It was also smoked as a substitute for tobacco (12229). Avoid confusion with black haw (Vibernum prunifolium), which is sometimes referred to as cramp bark.

CRANBERRY

Also Known As

American Cranberry, Arandano Americano, Arandano Trepador, European Cranberry, Grosse Moosbeere, Kranbeere, Large Cranberry, Moosebeere, Mossberry, Ronce d'Amerique, Small Cranberry, Trailing Swamp Cranberry, Tsuru-kokemomo.
CAUTION: See separate listings for Alpine Cranberry, Cramp Bark (European Cranberry-Bush), and Uva Ursi (Mountain Cranberry).

Scientific Names

Vaccinium macrocarpon, synonym Oxycoccus macrocarpos; Vaccinium oxycoccos, synonyms Oxycoccus hagerupii, Oxycoccus microcarpus, Oxycoccus palustris, Oxycoccus quadripetalus, Vaccinium hagerupii, Vaccinium microcarpum, Vaccinium palustre.
Family: Ericaceae.

People Use This For

Orally, cranberry is used for prevention and treatment of urinary tract infections, neurogenic bladder, as a urinary deodorizer for people with incontinence, prevention of urinary catheter blockage, and to heal skin around urostomy stomas. Cranberry is also used for type 2 diabetes, scurvy, pleurisy, as a diuretic, antiseptic, antipyretic, and for cancer.
In foods, cranberry fruit is used in fruit juice, jelly, and sauce.

Safety

LIKELY SAFE ...when used orally and appropriately (6758,7008,8253,8995).
CHILDREN: LIKELY SAFE ...when used orally and appropriately (2811,6759).
PREGNANCY AND LACTATION: LIKELY SAFE ...when used orally in amounts commonly found in food (5). There is insufficient reliable information about the safety of cranberry when used therapeutically during pregnancy or lactation; avoid using.

Effectiveness

POSSIBLY EFFECTIVE

Urinary odor. Cranberry juice appears to reduce urinary odors when given orally on a regular basis to patients with urinary incontinence (3333,3334,8254).
Urinary tract infections (UTIs). Daily consumption of cranberry juice 10 oz (300 mL) seems to prevent recurrent UTIs in some young and elderly women (6758,7008,8253). A combination product containing cranberry juice plus alpine cranberry (Vaccinium vitis-idaea) also seems to be helpful for prevention (8253).
But neither cranberry juice nor cranberry extract seem to prevent UTI in adults or children related to neurogenic bladder (2811,6759,11980).
Tell patients not to try cranberry juice for treating UTIs. There's not enough evidence it works (8252,8995).
Some patients are trying encapsulated forms of concentrated cranberry. So far, there is little reliable evidence that these preparations offer the same benefits as the juice (6760). Tell women interested in trying cranberry for UTI prevention to stick with the juice.

POSSIBLY INEFFECTIVE

Diabetes. Taking cranberry supplements orally doesn't seem to improve fasting serum glucose, glycosylated hemoglobin (HbA1c), fructosamine, triglyceride, high-density lipoprotein (HDL) cholesterol, or low-density lipoprotein (LDL) cholesterol levels in patients with type 2 diabetes (11328).
There is insufficient reliable information available about the effectiveness of cranberry for its other uses.

Mechanism of Action

The applicable part of the cranberry plant is the fruit. The cranberry is acidic, but does not acidify the urine as previously thought. Cranberries contain proanthocyanidins, also known as condensed tannins, and a high-molecular weight compound that has not yet been identified. These constituents seem to interfere with bacterial adherence to the urinary tract epithelial cells (2812,2814,3335,3337,3339,6753,6755,6757). For example, proanthocyanidins seem to be capable of "wrapping" around Escherichia coli (E. coli), which is the cause of most urinary tract infections (UTIs), and preventing it from adhering to the urinary tract wall (3333,3338,6690). It probably also has this effect against other urinary tract pathogens (2815). Cranberry, however, does not seem to have the ability to release bacteria which are already adhered to the urinary tract epithelial cells (8252). Laboratory evidence suggests that fructose in cranberries might also contribute to the anti-infective activity (2813,3333,6757). Cranberry juice has shown antibacterial activity in culture medium against E. coli, Staphylococcus aureus, Klebsiella pneumoniae, Pseudomonas aeruginosa, and Proteus mirabilis (3333,3338,6753). Whether urinary concentrations of the active constituents reach bactericidal levels is currently a topic of research (6753).
Preliminary data suggest that a high molecular weight cranberry constituent might prevent adhesion of plaque bacteria that cause periodontal disease (2816). Cranberry compounds might also prevent adhesion of Helicobacter pylori (H. pylori) in the stomach (6690). Early evidence shows that cranberry juice might increase the antioxidant

capacity of plasma (6754). There is also preliminary evidence that the proanthocyanidin fraction of cranberry might have anticarcinogenic activity (888).

Cranberry, as well as many other fruits and vegetables, contains significant amounts of salicylic acid. Salicylic acid, the active metabolite of aspirin, has anti-inflammatory, antiplatelet, and antitumor effects. Cranberry juice contains about 7 mg of salicylic acid per liter. Drinking three 250 mL servings of cranberry juice daily for two weeks increases serum salicylate levels. It also increases excretion of salicylic and salicyluric acids (a salicylic acid metabolite) in the urine (12669,12670,12879).

Adverse Reactions

Orally, cranberry is usually well tolerated (6758,7008,8253,8995). However, in very large doses, for example 3-4 L per day of juice, cranberry can cause gastrointestinal upset and diarrhea. Consuming more than 1 L per day over a prolonged period of time might also increase the risk of uric acid kidney stone formation (3334).

Interactions with Herbs & Other Dietary Supplements

None known.

Interactions with Drugs

CYTOCHROME P450 2C9 (CYP2C9) SUBSTRATES: There's preliminary evidence that flavonoids in cranberry might inhibit cytochrome P450 2C9 (CYP2C9) enzymes (10452,11115). Some drugs metabolized by CYP2C9 include amitriptyline (Elavil), diazepam (Valium), zileuton (Zyflo), and others.

WARFARIN (Coumadin): Cranberry juice can cause increases in the international normalized ratio (INR) in patients taking warfarin, which has been associated with severe spontaneous bleeding and excessive post-surgical bleeding (10452,12189,12668). Flavonoids in cranberry might inhibit cytochrome P450 2C9 (CYP2C9) isoenzyme, which could reduce the metabolism of warfarin and increase the anticoagulant effect (11115). Another theoretical mechanism is the anti-platelet effect of the cranberry constituent, salicylic acid. Many vegetables, fruits, and berries, including cranberries contain a high concentration of salicylic acid (12669). In people with a high intake of food from plant sources, serum salicylate levels are about the same as those in patients taking low-dose (75 mg) aspirin (12670). Cranberry juice contains about 7 mg salicylic acid per liter. Two weeks of ingesting 750 mL of cranberry juice per day increases serum salicylate levels. Theoretically, chronic consumption of large amounts of cranberry juice could increase salicylate levels and have an additive effect on the anticoagulant activity of warfarin (12879).

Interactions with Foods

None known.

Interactions with Lab Tests

SALICYLATE: Ingesting 250 mL cranberry juice daily can increase serum and urine salicylate levels (12879).

Interactions with Diseases or Conditions

ASPIRIN ALLERGY: Cranberry juice, like many other fruits and berries, contains significant amounts of salicylic acid. Theoretically, large amounts of cranberry juice could trigger allergic reaction in people with aspirin allergy or asthma (12669,12670,12879).

ATROPHIC GASTRITIS: Cranberry juice might increase absorption of dietary vitamin B12 in people with atrophic gastritis due to its acidity (4485).

DIABETES: Caution patients with diabetes to avoid cranberry juice cocktail products sweetened with sugar and instead to use cranberry juice cocktail products sweetened with artificial sweeteners.

HYPOCHLORHYDRIA: Cranberry juice might increase absorption of dietary vitamin B12 in people with hypochlorhydria due to its acidity (4485).

KIDNEY STONES (Nephrolithiasis): There is some concern that cranberry juice and cranberry extracts might increase the risk of kidney stones because of its high oxalate content. Drinking cranberry juice 30 mL typically provides approximately 1.9 mg of oxalate. Concentrated cranberry extracts might contain higher amounts of oxalate. There is some evidence that some cranberry extract tablets can boost urinary oxalate concentration by as much as 43% (7074). Tell patients with a history of kidney stones to avoid cranberry extract products or excessive consumption of cranberry juice.

Dosage and Administration

ORAL: For preventing urinary tract infections (UTIs), cranberry juice 1-10 oz per day has been used (6758,7008,8995). However, the ideal dose has not yet been determined. Some people drink up to 10-32 oz per day of cranberry juice for treating UTIs (515). For preventing UTIs in children a dose of 15ml/kg daily as 30% cranberry concentrate has been used (6759). For use as a urinary deodorizer for incontinent patients, 3-6 oz per day of cranberry juice has been used (8254). For type 2 diabetes, six capsules (equivalent to 240 ml cranberry juice cocktail) daily for 12 weeks has been used (11328). Encapsulated formulations are often taken in doses of 300-400 mg twice daily (7010).

Approximately 1500 grams of fresh fruit produces 1 L of juice. Cranberry juice cocktail is approximately 26% to 33% pure cranberry juice, sweetened with fructose or artificial sweetener (515,3335).

CREATINE

Also Known As

Cr, Creatine Monohydrate, Creatine Pyruvate.

Scientific Names

N-amidinosarcosine; N-(aminoiminomethyl)-N methyl glycine.

People Use This For

Orally, creatine is used for improving exercise performance and increasing muscle mass in athletes and older adults. Creatine is also used orally for congestive heart failure (CHF), neuromuscular disease, mitochondrial cytopathies, gyrate atrophy of the choroid and retina, and hyperlipidemia. It is also used orally for slowing the progression of amyotrophic lateral sclerosis (ALS, Lou Gehrig's disease), rheumatoid arthritis, McArdle disease, and for various muscular dystrophies.

Intravenously, creatine is used in cardiac surgery and for congestive heart failure.

Safety

POSSIBLY SAFE ...when used orally and appropriately. Creatine supplementation appears generally to be safe when used in appropriate doses in healthy adults (1367,2100,2101,2103,3996,4569,6052,10062,10064). Creatine has been safely used daily for up to 5 years (3996).

POSSIBLY UNSAFE ...when used orally in high doses. There is some concern that very high doses of creatine might adversely affect renal, hepatic, or cardiac function and have other adverse effects, such as hypertension (1367,6052); however, a clear association between high dose creatine and significant adverse effects has not yet been established.

PREGNANCY AND LACTATION: Insufficient reliable information available; avoid using.

Effectiveness

POSSIBLY EFFECTIVE

Athletic performance. Taking creatine orally seems to enhance muscle performance during repeated bouts of brief, high-intensity exercise. Numerous studies suggest that creatine is beneficial for certain types of high-intensity exercises (2100,2101,2102,4591,4592,4593,4594,4601,4602,4604,4605,6015,10064,11331); however, for other exercises, creatine appears to offer no benefit (4582,4595,4596,4597,4606,6183). Creatine seems to be more effective for increasing muscular power in healthy young adults during repeated, short, maximal energy bursts than for single event performances (4593,4598,4599,4600,6052,10064,11331). It might also be beneficial for exercise of longer duration with the intensity alternating between anaerobic and aerobic metabolism (6926). Many variables seem to determine the effect of creatine on performance, including the subject's training status, the type of sport being tested, diet, age of the subject, and the dose regimen of creatine. Creatine does not seem to improve performance in aerobic exercises, or benefit older individuals. Additionally, creatine doesn't increase endurance or improve performance in highly trained athletes (2103,2105,2106,4607). It is possible that the benefit in certain sports is offset by weight gain from creatine supplementation (2106,4576,4601,4604,4605,6015,6052). Acute creatine loading may be more effective than chronic continuous use (4603). Most studies have used 20 grams daily for 5 days for creatine loading; however, various other regimens have been studied. One study used 9 grams daily for 5 days and was beneficial in weight lifters, while another study used 20 grams daily for 3 days and was not beneficial for single sprints in cyclists (4576,4599,6015). Due to the variety of study methodologies and some conflicting findings, it has yet to be determined exactly who can benefit from creatine supplementation and what dosing schedule might be most effective. All studies have been limited by small sample size; all have involved fewer than 40 subjects and most fewer than 25.

Congestive heart failure (CHF). Taking creatine orally seems to improve exercise tolerance, but does not affect ejection fraction in people with CHF (4562,4563). Intravenous creatine improves cardiac function, including ejection fraction, even in the presence of conventional pharmacologic therapy. Following an infusion of 6 grams of IV creatine, improvements in ejection fraction persist for more than 12 hours (1369).

Gyrate atrophy of the choroid and retina. Creatine supplementation seems to slow visual deterioration in patients with gyrate atrophy (4577,4578).

McArdle's disease. There is some preliminary clinical evidence that daily high-dose creatine supplementation can increase exercise capacity and decreases exercise-induced muscle pain in some patients with McArdle's disease (70).

Muscular dystrophy. Taking creatine orally short-term seems to improve muscle strength and daily-life activity in adults and children with various muscular dystrophies (6182). Creatine monohydrate daily for eight weeks seems to mildly improve muscle strength and daily-life activity in children and adults with facioscapulohumeral dystrophy, Becker dystrophy, Duchenne dystrophy, or sarcoglycan-deficient limb girdle muscular dystrophy (6182). Taking creatine orally also seems to improve refractory muscle pain in patients with myotonic dystrophy type 2/proximal myotonic myopathy (DM2/PROMM). Muscle strength and performance might also improve in these patients after three months of treatment (10654).

POSSIBLY INEFFECTIVE

Amyotrophic lateral sclerosis (ALS, Lou Gehrig's disease). Taking creatine orally doesn't seem to have any beneficial effect on disease progression or survival in patients with ALS (11332).

Rheumatoid arthritis (RA). Taking creatine orally doesn't seem to help symptoms of RA. Creatine supplementation can increase muscle creatine content and muscle strength, but has no significant effect on physical functional ability or disease activity (6929).

LIKELY INEFFECTIVE

Athletic conditioning. Taking creatine orally doesn't seem to improve isometric strength and body composition in adults over age 60 (4570,4571,4572). Creatine dosed at 20 grams per day for 5 days followed by lower maintenance doses has no beneficial effect on exercise except reducing muscle fatigue (4570,4571,4572). In one study it had no effect on quadriceps fatigue after repeated sets of explosive work (6183).

Mechanism of Action

Creatine is found primarily in skeletal muscle (95%), but is also found in heart, brain, testes, retina, and other tissues (3997,3998). The body synthesizes 1 to 2 grams of creatine a day, primarily in the liver, kidneys, and pancreas (3997). Dietary sources, such as fish and meats, supply an additional 1 to 2 grams. For example, one pound of fresh uncooked steak contains about 2 grams of creatine (4575). Intestinal absorption of creatine is nearly 100% (6052). Creatine is irreversibly converted to creatinine and excreted by the kidneys (3997). Creatine in skeletal muscles exists in dynamic equilibrium with phosphocreatine (3997). Body stores of phosphocreatine in skeletal muscle serve as a precursor to the energy molecule, adenosine triphosphate (ATP). Higher levels of creatine are thought to enhance the ability to renew ATP for short 10-20 second energy bursts and improve resynthesis of phosphocreatine during recovery from intense exercise. Creatine supplementation enhances both creatine and phosphocreatine concentrations, providing a larger total creatine pool in the skeletal muscle. Creatine hinders the creatine-creatine kinase-phosphocreatine circuit. However, there is some debate about whether increased phosphocreatine resynthesis actually occurs (2103,3997,4574,4576,4580,4583,6925,6927,11330).

People who have lower initial total creatine, such as vegetarians, are more likely to respond to supplemental creatine, while people with higher initial levels may not respond (4574). Repeated creatine dosing causes a reduction in creatine clearance. Skeletal muscle has a saturation point at which additional supplemental creatine will not increase intracellular creatine levels. This reduction may result from skeletal muscle saturation (10065), which occurs within the first few days of loading (3999,6052,10065). Excess supplementation increases urinary creatine and creatinine (4576). Exogenous creatine supplementation also appears to reduce endogenous creatine production; whether this has any clinically significant negative effect on metabolic regulation within the liver is unknown (6052). After discontinuing supplementation, endogenous creatine production and creatine levels typically return to baseline within 28 days (2101,4582,6052).

Although some laboratory evidence identifies creatine as a potential lean body mass builder, most clinical evidence supports increased cellular water retention as the primary cause of creatine-induced muscle gain (4569,4575,4576,4579,4588,6061,10062). The muscle enlargement due to increased water retention is short-term. This is compared to the muscle enlargement from strength training, which results in an increase in contractile and structural muscle proteins (6052). Creatine may allow athletes to train harder due to increased phosphocreatine resynthesis and subsequent energy production (6061). Creatine might also reduce lactate production (4604); however, this has not been consistently found in studies (4592). In patients with congestive heart failure (CHF), the cardiac creatine phosphate/adenosine triphosphate is lower than in people with normal cardiac function and correlates with the severity of heart failure (1369). Creatine phosphate appears to improve CHF by preserving intracellular high-energy phosphates in the myocardium, stabilizing the sarcolemma, preventing peroxidative damage, and improving microcirculation (1369). In patients with gyrate atrophy, an inherited metabolic disease in which phosphocreatine is depleted, supplemental creatine increased myofibrillar protein synthesis resulting in muscle accretion (4576,4587). In myophosphorylase deficiency, known as McArdle disease, a rare genetic metabolic disease in which ATP cannot be formed from glycogen in skeletal muscle, supplemental creatine is thought to serve as a source of energy (70). Creatine appears to also affect lipid metabolism. There is some preliminary evidence that it can modestly reduce total cholesterol and very low-density lipoprotein (VLDL) cholesterol (4573). Early laboratory evidence also suggests that creatine might be useful in diseases such as amyotrophic lateral sclerosis, Huntington's disease, and Parkinson's disease, possibly due to neuroprotective effects (4566,4567,4568). There is conflicting evidence on creatine and cancer. Some research suggests that creatine and its analogs, such as cyclocreatine, inhibit tumor growth (1393,1406,1432,1481). Creatine might alter energy production by the creatine kinase system, which appears to play a role in controlling some types of tumors such as breast tumors and neuroblastomas (1393,1406). Other research suggests that creatine or its metabolites can form mutagenic substances when combined at room temperature with sugars or heated (1486,1487), but this has not been verified.

Adverse Reactions

Orally, creatine can cause gastrointestinal pain, nausea, and diarrhea (2103,4576,6052). Case reports have found that 25% of male collegiate athletes taking creatine have muscle cramping (4584). A theoretical increase in risk of dehydration due to intracellular fluid shifts has led most creatine manufacturers to caution about adequate hydration with creatine supplementation (4576). Tell patients who are controlling their weight and engaging in strenuous exercise and/or exercising in hot environments to avoid creatine supplementation (6052). Creatine typically causes a weight gain of 0.5 to 1.6 kg that increases with prolonged supplementation (3997). This weight gain, most likely due to water retention, has been thought to also increase the risk for high blood pressure. However, a recent study showed no effect of 20 grams daily of creatine for 5 days on blood pressure (4569). Creatine might also cause renal dysfunction (184,2118), but this appears to be rare in people with healthy kidneys (1368,2120,3996). Most studies have not found alterations in renal function in people taking 5-20 grams of creatine daily for up to 5 years (3996,4569). However, there is one report of acute interstitial nephritis and focal tubular injury after four weeks of creatine at 5 grams four times daily (184). In another case, supplemental creatine, loaded at 15 grams per day for one week, then 2 grams per day, caused a significant decline in creatinine clearance in a man receiving cyclosporine for steroid-resistant focal segmental glomerulosclerosis (2118). Medical supervision is suggested for people who have kidney disease or have a high risk of kidney disease and use creatine (4569,6052). Renal failure with rhabdomyolysis has also been reported in patients taking creatine in addition to multiple performance enhancing supplements (12819,12820,12821) There is one report of ischemic stroke in an athlete who consumed a combination of 6 grams of creatine monohydrate, 400-600 mg of caffeine, 40-60 mg of ephedra, and a variety of other supplements daily for six weeks (1275).

Interactions with Herbs & Other Dietary Supplements

CAFFEINE: There is some concern that combining caffeine, ephedra, and creatine might increase the risk of serious adverse effects. There is a report of ischemic stroke in an athlete who consumed creatine monohydrate 6 grams, caffeine 400-600 mg, ephedra 40-60 mg, and a variety of other supplements daily for 6 weeks (1275). Caffeine might also decrease creatine's beneficial effects on athletic performance. Some researchers think caffeine can inhibit phosphocreatine resynthesis (2117,4575).

EPHEDRA: There is some concern that combining ephedra, caffeine, and creatine might increase the risk of serious adverse effects. There is a report of ischemic stroke in an athlete who consumed creatine monohydrate 6 grams, caffeine 400-600 mg, ephedra 40-60 mg, and a variety of other supplements daily for 6 weeks (1275).

Interactions with Drugs

NEPHROTOXIC DRUGS: There is some concern about using creatine with drugs that can be nephrotoxic. Since high doses of creatine might adversely affect renal function (6052), combining creatine with potentially nephrotoxic drugs might have additive harmful effects on kidney function. However, this effect has not yet been reported. Some potentially nephrotoxic drugs include cyclosporine (Neoral, Sandimmune); aminoglycosides including amikacin (Amikin), gentamicin (Garamycin, Gentak, others), and tobramycin (Nebcin, others); nonsteroidal anti-inflammatory drugs (NSAIDs) including ibuprofen (Advil, Motrin, Nuprin, others), indomethacin (Indocin), naproxen (Aleve, Anaprox, Naprelan, Naprosyn), piroxicam (Feldene); and numerous others.

Interactions with Foods

CARBOHYDRATES: Combining carbohydrates with creatine can increase muscle creatine levels more than creatine alone. Supplementing 5 grams of creatine with 93 grams of simple carbohydrates four times daily for 5 days can increase muscle creatine levels as much as 60% more than creatine alone (10063).

Interactions with Lab Tests

SERUM CREATININE (SCr): Creatine is metabolized to creatinine. Higher than normal serum creatinine levels can result in patients taking creatine, despite normal renal function (2100,2103).

Interactions with Diseases or Conditions

KIDNEY DYSFUNCTION: Creatine should be avoided by people with pre-existing renal disease or by people with diseases such as diabetes that increase the risk for renal dysfunction (4576). There is some concern that creatine might exacerbate renal dysfunction in these patients.

Dosage and Administration

ORAL: For improving physical performance, several dosing regimens have been tried. Creatine is typically acutely loaded with 20 grams per day (or 0.3 grams per kg) for 5 days followed by a maintenance dose of 2 or more grams (0.03 grams per kg) daily (4576,11331). Although 5 day loading is typical, 2 days of loading has also been used (4576). A loading dose of 9 grams per day for 6 days has also been used (6015). Some sources suggest that, instead of acutely loading, similar results can be obtained with 3 grams per day for 28 days (2104). During creatine supplementation, the water intake should be 64 ounces per day (2103,2104). For heart failure, 20 grams per day for 5-10 days has been used in clinical trials (4562,4563). For gyrate atrophy, 1.5 grams per day has been used (4577,4578). For McArdle disease, 150 mg/kg daily for 5 days followed by 60 mg/kg per day has been used (70). For muscular dystrophies, 10 grams per day has been used by adults and 5 grams per day has been used by children (6182). For myotonic dystrophy type 2/proximal myotonic myopathy, 10 grams per day has been used (10654). For amyotrophic lateral sclerosis (ALS, Lou Gehrig's disease), 10 grams daily for 12-16 months has been used (11332).

Comments

Creatine is allowed by the International Olympic Committee, National Collegiate Athletic Association (NCAA), and professional sports (3998,4575,4576). However, the NCAA no longer allows colleges and universities to supply creatine to their students with school funds. Students are permitted to buy creatine on their own and the NCAA has no plans to ban creatine unless sufficient medical evidence indicates that it is harmful (6140). With current testing methods, detection of supplemental creatine use would not be possible (4575). Creatine use is widespread among professional and amateur athletes and has been acknowledged by well-known athletes such as Mark McGuire, Sammy Sosa, and John Elway (3998). Following the finding that carbohydrate solution further increased muscle creatine levels more than creatine alone, creatine sports drinks have become popular (4576,4589). Annual consumption of creatine in the US is estimated to exceed 4 million kg (3998). California is considering legislation that would ban the sale of creatine and other supplements frequently used in sports performance-enhancing products to anyone under the age of 18. The bill, which received Senate approval and is now in the Assembly, would also require warning labels about the adverse effects of creatine (8639).

CROTON SEEDS

Also Known As

Croton, Tiglium, Tiglium Seeds.

Scientific Names

Croton tiglium.
Family: Euphorbiaceae.

People Use This For

Orally, croton seeds are used as a purgative, treat gallbladder colic, bowel obstruction, and malaria.
Topically croton seeds are used for rheumatism, gout, neuralgia, and bronchitis.

Safety

LIKELY UNSAFE ...when used orally. One drop of the oil can be toxic, and one mL (20 drops) of oil is considered lethal (18). Also, the phorbol esters in the oil are co-carcinogens (18). ...when used topically; avoid using (18).
PREGNANCY: UNSAFE ...when used orally due to abortifacient properties (19); avoid using.
LACTATION: UNSAFE ...when used orally (18); avoid using.

Effectiveness

There is insufficient reliable information available about the effectiveness of croton seeds.

Mechanism of Action

The applicable part of croton seeds is the oil from the seed. Croton seeds possess powerful, irritant, cathartic properties due to phorbol esters (3800). The diterpene, TPA, is carcinogenic, affecting prostaglandin metabolism (18).

Adverse Reactions

Orally, croton seeds can cause burning of mouth, vomiting, dizziness, stupor, painful bowel movements, and collapse (18).
Topically, croton seeds can cause itching, burning and blistering of skin (18).

Interactions with Herbs & Other Dietary Supplements

None known.

Interactions with Drugs

None known.

Interactions with Foods

None known.

Interactions with Lab Tests

None known.

Interactions with Diseases or Conditions

None known.

Dosage and Administration
No typical dosage.

CUBEBS

Also Known As
Cubeb, Cubeb Berries, Cubeba, Cubeba officinalis, Java Pepper, Tailed Chubebs, Tailed Pepper.

Scientific Names
Piper cubeba.
Family: Piperaceae.

People Use This For
Orally, cubebs is used as a diuretic, urinary antiseptic, for amoebic dysentery, as an antiflatulent, stimulating expectorant, for gonorrhea, and cancer.
In foods, cubebs oil is used as a flavoring ingredient.

Safety
LIKELY SAFE ...when used orally in amounts commonly found in foods. Cubebs has Generally Recognized As Safe status (GRAS) for use in foods in the US (4912).
POSSIBLY SAFE ...when used orally and appropriately in medicinal amounts (12).
PREGNANCY AND LACTATION: Insufficient reliable information available; avoid using.

Effectiveness
There is insufficient reliable information available about the effectiveness of cubebs.

Mechanism of Action
The applicable part of cubebs is the dried, fully grown but unripe fruit. Researchers think that the constituent cubebic acid is responsible for the stimulant effect on urinary and respiratory tract (11).

Adverse Reactions
None reported.

Interactions with Herbs & Other Dietary Supplements
None known.

Interactions with Drugs
ANTACIDS: Theoretically, due to reports that cubebs increases stomach acid, cubebs might decrease the effectiveness of antacids (19).
H2-BLOCKERS: Theoretically, due to reports that cubebs increases stomach acid, cubebs might decrease the effectiveness of H2-blockers (19). The H2 blockers include cimetidine (Tagamet), ranitidine (Zantac), nizatidine (Axid), and famotidine (Pepcid).
PROTON PUMP INHIBITORS (PPIs): Theoretically, due to reports that cubebs increases stomach acid, cubebs might decrease the effectiveness of PPIs (19). PPIs include omeprazole (Prilosec), lansoprazole (Prevacid), rabeprazole (Aciphex), pantoprazole (Protonix), and esomeprazole (Nexium).

Interactions with Foods
None known.

Interactions with Lab Tests
None known.

Interactions with Diseases or Conditions
GASTROINTESTINAL (GI) CONDITIONS: Cubebs may irritate the GI tract; contraindicated in individuals with infectious or inflammatory GI conditions (19).
NEPHRITIS: Cubebs is contraindicated in individuals with nephritis (12).

Dosage and Administration
ORAL: People typically use 2 to 4 grams of the powdered fruit or 2 to 4 mL of the liquid extract (223).

CUDWEED

Also Known As
Cotton Dawes, Cotton Weed, Dysentery Weed, Everlasting, Mouse Ear, Wartwort.
CAUTION: See separate listings for Cat's Foot and Mouse Ear.

Scientific Names
Gnaphalium uliginosum, synonym Filaginella uliginosa
Family: Asteraceae/Compositae.

People Use This For
Topically, cudweed is used as a gargle or rinse for diseases of the mouth or throat.

Safety
There is insufficient reliable information available about the safety of cudweed.
Pregnancy and Lactation: Insufficient reliable information available; avoid using.

Effectiveness
There is insufficient reliable information available about the effectiveness of cudweed.

Mechanism of Action
The applicable parts of cudweed are the above ground parts. Cudweed has astringent effects, and promotes and improves appetite (18). Unsubstantiated sources report it has antidepressant, aphrodisiac, and hypotensive effects (18).

Adverse Reactions
Topically, cudweed can cause an allergic reaction in individuals sensitive to the Asteraceae/Compositae family. Members of this family include ragweed, chrysanthemums, marigolds, daisies, and many other herbs.

Interactions with Herbs & Other Dietary Supplements
None known.

Interactions with Drugs
None known.

Interactions with Foods
None known.

Interactions with Lab Tests
None known.

Interactions with Diseases or Conditions
CROSS-ALLERGENICITY: Cudweed may cause an allergic reaction in individuals sensitive to the Asteraceae/Compositae family. Members of this family include ragweed, chrysanthemums, marigolds, daisies, and many other herbs.

Dosage and Administration
ORAL: People typically use 2 to 4 mL of the liquid extract (223).

Comments
Avoid confusion with Antennaria dioica, which is also referred to as cudweed. Avoid confusion with Pilosella officinarum, also known as mouse ear.

CUMIN

Also Known As
Cummin, Jeeraka, Svetajiraka, Zira.

Scientific Names
Cuminum cyminum, synonym Cuminum odorum.
Family: Apiaceae/Umbelliferae.

People Use This For
Orally, cumin is used as an antiflatulent, stimulant, antispasmodic, diuretic, aphrodisiac, for stimulating menstrual flow, treating diarrhea, colic, and flatulence.
In spices, foods, and beverages, cumin is used as a flavoring component.
In other manufacturing processes, cumin oil is used as a fragrance component in cosmetics (maximum use level 0.4% in perfumes).

Safety
LIKELY SAFE ...when used orally in amounts commonly found in foods. Cumin and cumin oil have Generally Recognized As Safe (GRAS) status in the US (4912).
POSSIBLY SAFE ...when used orally and appropriately in medicinal amounts (12).
PREGNANCY AND LACTATION: Insufficient reliable information available; avoid using in excess of food amounts.

Effectiveness
There is insufficient reliable information available about the effectiveness of cumin.

Mechanism of Action
The applicable part of cumin is the fruit/seed. Cumin is a rich source of iron (19). Cumin oil and constituent, cuminaldehyde, have been reported to exhibit strong larvicidal and antibacterial activity (6). Demonstrated phototoxic effects are reportedly not due to cuminaldehyde (11).

Adverse Reactions
Orally, use of undiluted cumin oil has phototoxic effects (6).

Interactions with Herbs & Other Dietary Supplements
None known.

Interactions with Drugs
ANTIDIABETES DRUGS: Monitor blood glucose levels closely due to claims that cumin has hypoglycemic effects (19).

Interactions with Foods
None known.

Interactions with Lab Tests
None known.

Interactions with Diseases or Conditions
None known.

Dosage and Administration
ORAL: The average single amount used is 5-10 fruits (18).

Comments
Fine grinding of the seed can cause loss of 50% of volatile oil, most within l hour (6).

CUP PLANT

Also Known As
Indian Gum, Pilot Plant, Polar Plant, Prairie Dock, Ragged Cup, Rosinweed, Turpentine Weed.
CAUTION: See separate listing for Rosinweed.

Scientific Names
Silphium perfoliatum.
Family: Asteraceae/Compositae.

Comments
At the date of publication, this product was not a common ingredient used in brand name supplements marketed to consumers. Details about this product are available in the online version of *Natural Medicines Comprehensive Database.* See www.naturaldatabase.com..

CUPMOSS

Also Known As
Chin Cups.

Scientific Names
Cladonia pyxidata.
Family: Cladoniaceae.

Comments
At the date of publication, this product was not a common ingredient used in brand name supplements marketed to consumers. Details about this product are available in the online version of *Natural Medicines Comprehensive Database.* See www.naturaldatabase.com.

CYCLAMEN

Also Known As
Groundbread, Ivy-Leafed Cyclamen, Sowbread, Swinebread.

Scientific Names
Cyclamen purpurascens, synonym Cyclamen europaeum.
Family: Primulaceae

People Use This For
Orally, cyclamen is used for menstrual complaints, "nervous emotional states," and digestive problems.

Safety
LIKELY UNSAFE ...when used orally. Doses as low as 300 mg can cause poisoning (18).
PREGNANCY AND LACTATION: LIKELY UNSAFE ...when used orally (18); avoid using.

Effectiveness
There is insufficient reliable information available about the effectiveness of cyclamen.

Mechanism of Action
The applicable parts of cyclamen are the rhizome and root. There is insufficient reliable information available about the possible mechanism of action and active ingredients.

Adverse Reactions
Orally, poisoning has been reported with doses as low as 300 mg; symptoms include stomach pain, nausea, vomiting, and diarrhea (18). High doses can cause severe poisoning; symptoms include spasm and asphyxiation (18,553).

Interactions with Herbs & Other Dietary Supplements
None known.

Interactions with Drugs
None known.

Interactions with Foods
None known.

Interactions with Lab Tests
None known.

Interactions with Diseases or Conditions
None known.

Dosage and Administration
ORAL: People typically use 20 to 40 grains (1300 to 2600 mg) of powdered cyclamen root (5267). Cyclamen should not be used without medical supervision (5263).

CYPRESS

Also Known As
None.

Scientific Names
Cupressus sempervirens.
Family: Cupressaceae.

Comments
At the date of publication, there was very little scientific information available about this product. Our staff is continually analyzing the available information on natural medicines and will add data to the online version of *Natural Medicines Comprehensive Database* as it becomes available. See www.naturaldatabase.com.

CYPRESS SPURGE

Also Known As
None.

Scientific Names
Euphorbia cyparissias.
Family: Euphorbiaceae.

People Use This For
Orally, cypress spurge is used for diseases of the respiratory organs, diarrhea, and skin diseases.

Safety
UNSAFE ...when used orally. The plant contains poisonous white latex (milky liquid) and cocarcinogenic agents (18). Both the fresh and dried latex are toxic (18).
PREGNANCY AND LACTATION: UNSAFE ...when used orally due to toxicity (18); avoid using.

Effectiveness
There is insufficient reliable information available about the effectiveness of cypress spurge.

Mechanism of Action
The applicable parts of cypress spurge are the flowering plant and root. Cypress spurge contains varied diterpenes and triterpenes. The ingenan esters are potent inflammatory and cocarcinogenic agents (18). Euphorbia species have topical irritant, GI irritant, emetic, and purgative effects (19).

Adverse Reactions
Orally, cypress spurge, which is part of the Euphorbia species, may cause GI irritation, nausea, vomiting, and diarrhea (19). Ingestion of the latex can cause burning of the mouth, vomiting, mydriasis, dizziness, painful bowel movements, stupor, cardiac arrhythmias, and collapse (18).
Topically, Euphorbia species may cause contact dermatitis (19). Skin contact with the latex causes reddening, itching, burning, and blisters (18). Eye contact can cause eyelid swelling, conjunctival inflammation, and corneal defects (18).

Interactions with Herbs & Other Dietary Supplements
None known.

Interactions with Drugs
None known.

Interactions with Foods
None known.

Interactions with Lab Tests
None known.

Interactions with Diseases or Conditions
DIARRHEA: Euphorbia species have purgative effects (19); avoid using.
GASTROINTESTINAL (GI) IRRITATION, INFLAMMATION: Euphorbia species have GI irritant effects (19); avoid using.
NAUSEA, VOMITING: Euphorbia species have emetic effects (19); avoid using.

Dosage and Administration
No typical dosage.

D-MANNOSE

Also Known As
Carubinose, Mannose, Seminose.

Scientific Names
D-Mannose.

People Use This For
Orally, d-mannose is used for urinary tract infections (UTIs) and for treating carbohydrate-deficient glycoprotein syndrome, an inherited metabolic disorder.

Safety
POSSIBLY SAFE ...when used orally and appropriately (13344,13345,13346,13348).
PREGNANCY AND LACTATION: Insufficient reliable information available; avoid using.

Effectiveness
INSUFFICIENT RELIABLE EVIDENCE to RATE

Carbohydrate-deficient glycoprotein syndrome type 1b. Anecdotal reports suggest that supplemental d-mannose improves protein loss, liver function, hypoglycemia, and coagulation disorders in people with carbohydrate-deficient glycoprotein syndrome type 1b, a rare autosomal recessive inherited metabolic disorder (13344,13345,13346,13348). More evidence is needed to rate d-mannose for this use.

Mechanism of Action
D-mannose is a 6-carbon sugar and an isomer of dextrose. It differs from dextrose only in the position of the hydroxyl group at the second carbon (13342). It is primarily derived from glucose via the enzyme phosphomannose isomerase (PMI). However, supplemental d-mannose is well absorbed from the gastrointestinal tract and is transported by mannose-specific transporters. The mannose content in foods and its bioavailability from foods has not been characterized. D-mannose is used by the body for glycosylation of proteins and fibroblast activity. It is present in small amounts in the blood, about 100 times less than glucose (13343,13347).
People with a rare genetic deficiency of PMI, known as carbohydrate-deficient glycoprotein syndrome type 1b, loss protein via the intestines, liver disease, hypoglycemia, and blood clotting disorders. PMI deficiency eliminates or decreases the synthesis of mannose 6-phosphate from fructose 6-phosphate. Supplemental d-mannose appears to overcome this deficiency (13346,13347).
Preliminary research suggests supplemental d-mannose might interfere with the adhesion of bacteria to the urinary tract, theoretically protecting from urinary tract infections (UTIs) (13342). Bacteria such as Escherichia coli produce lectins, which bind the organism to sugar residues, such as mannose, on host cells. Theoretically, giving supplemental mannose can bind the bacteria and prevent attachment to the urinary tract lining (13349,13350). This has not been demonstrated in humans.

Adverse Reactions
Orally, d-mannose can cause loose stools and abdominal bloating (13344). Excessive doses (toxic amounts unspecified) might be toxic to the kidneys (13348). Preliminary research suggests that d-mannose might be teratogenic; however, there are no reports of teratogenic or mutagenic effects in humans (13351).

Interactions with Herbs & Other Dietary Supplements
None known.

Interactions with Drugs
None known.

Interactions with Foods
None known.

Interactions with Lab Tests
CREATININE: Theoretically, large doses of d-mannose might adversely affect the kidneys and cause serum and urinary creatinine to increase (13348).
GLYCOSYLATED HEMOGLOBIN (HbA1c): Some clinical research suggests that d-mannose can increase glycosylated hemoglobin (13343).

Interactions with Diseases or Conditions

DIABETES: Some research suggests that d-mannose can increase glycosylated hemoglobin (HbA1c) (13343). Theoretically, d-mannose might worsen glucose control in patients with diabetes.

Dosage and Administration

No typical dosage.

DAFFODIL

Also Known As

Lent Lily.

Scientific Names

Narcissus pseudonarcissus.
Family: Amaryllidaceae.

People Use This For

Orally, daffodil is used to soothe mucous membrane irritation resulting from whooping cough, colds, asthma, bronchial catarrh, and as an emetic.
Topically, a plaster made from daffodil bulbs is used for wounds, burns, strains, and joint pain.

Safety

POSSIBLY UNSAFE ...when used topically. Severe cases of dermatitis have been reported (5004).
LIKELY UNSAFE ...when used orally (19). Merely chewing on the stem may be enough to cause a chill, shivering, and fainting. The constituent lycorine can cause salivation, vomiting, diarrhea at low doses, and paralysis and collapse at higher doses (271).
PREGNANCY AND LACTATION: LIKELY UNSAFE ...when used orally or topically (19); avoid using.

Effectiveness

There is insufficient reliable information available about the effectiveness of daffodil.

Mechanism of Action

The applicable parts of daffodil are the bulb, leaf, and flower. Daffodil contains numerous active constituents including alkaloids (lycorine and galanthamine) and chelidonic acid (18). In small amounts, lycorine causes salivation, vomiting, and diarrhea. At higher doses, it causes paralysis and collapse. Galanthamine is a cholinesterase inhibitor and analgesic (271), and it is being investigated for use in the treatment of Alzheimer's disease (5007). Lycorine, narciclasine, and other constituents are cytotoxic (271). The mucus and sap of daffodil plants and bulbs contain calcium oxalate crystals, which are most likely responsible for the skin irritation (5004). "Micro trauma" to the skin from the oxylate crystals allows penetration of other irritants and worsens dermatitis (5004).

Adverse Reactions

Orally, daffodil can cause irritation and swelling of the mouth, tongue, and throat (19), as well as vomiting, salivation, diarrhea, central nervous disorders, and respiratory or cardiovascular collapse and subsequent death (18). This is due to the lycorine component (6002).
Topically, daffodil use can cause dermatitis (5004,5005). People who simply handle daffodil plants or bulbs can get "Lily rash" or "daffodil itch" (18,5004).

Interactions with Herbs & Other Dietary Supplements

CALCIUM, IRON, ZINC: Concurrent use might decrease mineral absorption. Daffodil contains oxalate (5004), which can bind multivalent metal ions in the gastrointestinal tract and decrease mineral absorption.

Interactions with Drugs

None known.

Interactions with Foods

CALCIUM, IRON, ZINC: Concurrent use might decrease mineral absorption from foods. Daffodil contains oxalate (5004), which can bind multivalent metal ions in the gastrointestinal tract and decrease mineral absorption.

Interactions with Lab Tests

None known.

Interactions with Diseases or Conditions

None known.

Dosage and Administration

ORAL: Typically used as a powder and an extract (amount unspecified) (18).

DAMIANA

Also Known As

Damiana Aphrodisiaca, Damiana Herb, Damiana Leaf, Herba de la Pastora, Mexican Damiana, Mizibcoc, Old Woman's Broom, Turnerae diffusae folium, Turnerae Diffusae Herba.

Scientific Names

Turnera diffusa, synonym Turnera microphylla; Turnera diffusa var. aphrodisiaca.
Family: Turneraceae.

People Use This For

Orally, damiana is used to treat headache, bedwetting, depression, nervous dyspepsia, atonic constipation, for prophylaxis and treatment of sexual disturbances, strengthening and stimulation during exertion (overwork), boosting and maintaining mental and physical capacity, and as an aphrodisiac.
By inhalation, damiana is used for a subtle "high."

Safety

LIKELY SAFE ...when used orally in amounts commonly found in foods. Damiana has Generally Recognized As Safe status (GRAS) for use in foods in the US (4912).
POSSIBLY SAFE ...when used orally and appropriately in medicinal amounts (12).
PREGNANCY AND LACTATION: Insufficient reliable information available; avoid using.

Effectiveness

There is insufficient reliable information available about the effectiveness of damiana.

Mechanism of Action

The applicable parts of damiana are the leaf and stem. Ethanolic extracts are reported to exhibit CNS depressant activity (4). The quinone arbutin may be responsible for antibacterial properties (4).

Adverse Reactions

Orally, 200 grams of damiana extract has caused tetanus-like convulsions and paroxysms resulting in symptoms similar to rabies or strychnine poisoning (4).

Interactions with Herbs & Other Dietary Supplements

None known.

Interactions with Drugs

ANTIDIABETES DRUGS: Theoretically, damiana may interfere with diabetes therapy due to hypoglycemic activity (4).

Interactions with Foods

None known.

Interactions with Lab Tests

None known.

Interactions with Diseases or Conditions

DIABETES: Theoretically, damiana may interfere with blood glucose control (4).

Dosage and Administration

ORAL: Typical dosages are 2-4 grams dried leaf three times daily, or one cup tea (steep 2-4 grams dried leaf in 150 mL boiling water 5-10 minutes, strain) three times a day (4). Liquid extract of damiana, 2-4 mL has also been used (4).

DANDELION

Also Known As

Blowball, Cankerwort, Common Dandelion, Lion's Tooth, Pissenlit, Priest's Crown, Swine Snout, Taraxaci herba, Taraxacum, Wild Endive.

Scientific Names

Taraxacum officinale, synonyms Taraxacum vulgare, Leontodon taraxacum, Taraxacum dens-leonis.
Family: Asteraceae/Compositae.

People Use This For

Orally, dandelion is used for loss of appetite, dyspepsia, flatulence, gallstones, bile stimulation, for rheumatism, arthritic joints, muscle aches, eczema, bruises. Dandelion is also used as a laxative, diuretic, circulatory tonic, skin toner, blood tonic, and digestive tonic.
In foods, dandelion is used as a salad greens, in soups and wine, and the roasted root is used as a coffee substitute.

Safety

LIKELY SAFE ...when used orally in amounts commonly found in foods. Dandelion has Generally Recognized As Safe status (GRAS) in the US (4912).
POSSIBLY SAFE ...when used orally and appropriately in medicinal amounts (12).
PREGNANCY AND LACTATION: Insufficient reliable information available; avoid using amounts greater than those in foods.

Effectiveness

INSUFFICIENT RELIABLE EVIDENCE to RATE

Urinary tract infections (UTIs). A specific oral combination of dandelion root and uva ursi leaf extracts seems to help reduce the recurrence rate of UTIs in women (1932). In this combination uva ursi is used for its antibacterial properties and dandelion is used to increase urination. However, this combination should not be used long-term because is it not known if uva ursi is safe for extended use. More evidence is needed to rate dandelion for this use.

Mechanism of Action

The applicable parts of dandelion are the above ground parts and root. The sesquiterpene lactones are responsible for the diuretic effects and can contribute to dandelion's mild anti-inflammatory activity (6). Sesquiterpene lactone constituents are also thought to be associated with allergic reactions (4).
Dandelion also contains appetite-stimulating bitters identified as eudesmanolides, previously known as taraxacin (6). Dandelion can have a slight laxative effect (5). The bitter constituents in dandelion root are responsible for increasing bile flow (7).
The extracts seem to have diuretic effects in animals, and antitumor activity in vitro (4). The root extract has anti-inflammatory activity in animals (4).

Adverse Reactions

Orally, side effects have not been reported.
Topically, dandelion can cause contact dermatitis in sensitive individuals (6). Dandelion can cause an allergic reaction in individuals sensitive to the Asteraceae/Compositae family. Members of this family include ragweed, chrysanthemums, marigolds, daisies, and many other herbs.

Interactions with Herbs & Other Dietary Supplements

DIURETIC HERBS: Theoretically, dandelion can have additive effects with herbs that have diuretic properties. Herbs thought to have diuretic properties include agrimony, artichoke, broom, buchu, burdock, celery, cornsilk, couch grass, elder, guaiacum, juniper, pokeroot, shepherd's purse, squill, uva ursi, and yarrow.

Interactions with Drugs

ANTACIDS: Theoretically, due to reports that dandelion increases stomach acid, dandelion might decrease the effectiveness of antacids (19).
H2-BLOCKERS: Theoretically, due to reports that dandelion increases stomach acid, dandelion might decrease the effectiveness of H2-blockers (19). The H2 blockers include cimetidine (Tagamet), ranitidine (Zantac), nizatidine (Axid), and famotidine (Pepcid).
LITHIUM: Theoretically, concomitant use might cause lithium toxicity due to sodium depleting effects of dandelion (19).
POTASSIUM-SPARING DIURETICS: The above ground parts of dandelion contain large amounts of potassium (4). Concomitant use of potassium-spring diuretics with dandelion might increase the risk of hyperkalemia. Potassium-sparing diuretics include amiloride (Midamor), spironolactone (Aldactone), and triamterene (Dyrenium).
PROTON PUMP INHIBITORS (PPIs): Theoretically, due to reports that dandelion increases stomach acid,

dandelion might decrease the effectiveness of PPIs (19). PPIs include omeprazole (Prilosec), lansoprazole (Prevacid), rabeprazole (Aciphex), pantoprazole (Protonix), and esomeprazole (Nexium).

Interactions with Foods

None known.

Interactions with Lab Tests

None known.

Interactions with Diseases or Conditions

CROSS-ALLERGENICITY: Dandelion may cause an allergic reaction in individuals sensitive to the Asteraceae/Compositae family. Members of this family include ragweed, chrysanthemums, marigolds, daisies, and many other herbs.
GASTROINTESTINAL CONDITIONS: Dandelion plant is contraindicated in cases of acute gallbladder inflammation, bile duct obstruction, and intestinal blockage due to choleretic and laxative effects (5,7).

Dosage and Administration

ORAL: Traditionally dandelion leaf 4-10 grams or dandelion root 2-8 grams, in 150 mL of water has been three times a day (4). A root tincture (1:5 in 45% alcohol) 5-10 mL three times daily has also been used (4). The dose of the liquid extract of taraxacum is typically 2-8 mL (4).

Comments

Dandelions contain more vitamin A than carrots (6002).

DANSHEN

Also Known As

Ch'ih Shen, Chinese Salvia, Dan Shen, Dan-Shen, Huang Ken, Pin-Ma Ts'ao, Red Rooted Sage, Red Sage, Salvia Root, Shu-Wei Ts'ao, Tan-Shen, Tzu Tan-Ken.
CAUTION: See separate listing for Sage.

Scientific Names

Salvia bowleyana; Salvia miltiorrhiza; Salvia przewalskii; Salvia yunnanensis.
Family: Labiatae/Lamiaceae.

People Use This For

Orally, danshen is used for circulation problems, ischemic stroke, angina pectoris, and other cardiovascular diseases. It is also used orally for menstrual problems, chronic hepatitis, abdominal masses, insomnia due to palpitations and tight chest, acne, psoriasis, eczema, and other skin conditions. Danshen is also used orally to relieve bruising and to aid in wound healing.

Safety

POSSIBLY SAFE ...when used orally and appropriately (12).
PREGNANCY AND LACTATION: Insufficient reliable information available; avoid using.

Effectiveness

There is insufficient reliable information available about the effectiveness of danshen.

Mechanism of Action

The applicable part of danshen is the root. The constituents protocatechualdehyde and 3,4-dihydroxyphenyl-lactic acid may play a role in vasoactivity (6048). Other constituents, including the diterpenoids miltirone, Ro090680, and salvinone, as well as tanshinone derivatives, seem to have anticoagulant properties (7162,10649). Danshen appears to interfere with hemostasis by inhibiting platelet aggregation, interfering with extrinsic blood coagulation, mimicking the activity of antithrombin III, and promoting fibrinolytic activity (2237).
Danshen constituents and digoxin have some structural and pharmacological similarities. The tanshinone constituents of danshen have an aglycon ring that contains a common phenanthrene ring structure like digoxin and other cardiac glycosides (7311). Danshen is thought to work for cardiovascular diseases by dilating coronary arteries and affecting cardiac function. It appears to produce dose-dependent hypotensive effects, positive inotropic effects, and negative chronotropic effects (5884,6048,7311).

Adverse Reactions

Orally, danshen can cause pruritus, upset stomach, and reduced appetite (12).

Interactions with Herbs & Other Dietary Supplements

CARDIAC GLYCOSIDE-CONTAINING HERBS: Theoretically, using danshen with herbs containing cardiac glycosides might increase the risk cardiovascular effects and side effects such as arrhythmia. Danshen has structural and pharmacological similarities to cardiac glycosides (5884,6048,7311). Cardiac glycoside containing herbs include black hellebore, Canadian hemp roots, digitalis leaf, hedge mustard, figwort, lily-of-the-valley roots, motherwort, oleander leaf, pheasant's eye plant, pleurisy root, squill bulb leaf scales, and strophanthus seeds.
HERBS WITH ANTICOAGULANT/ANTIPLATELET POTENTIAL: Taking danshen with herbs that affect platelet aggregation could theoretically increase the risk of bleeding in some people (7162). These herbs include angelica, clove, feverfew, garlic, ginger, ginkgo, Panax ginseng, horse chestnut, red clover, turmeric, and others.
METHYL SALICYLATE OIL: There is one case report of increased international normalized ratio (INR) with concomitant use of topical methyl salicylate oil, oral danshen, and warfarin (612).

Interactions with Drugs

ANTICOAGULANT/ANTIPLATELET DRUGS: Concomitant use might increase the risk of bleeding due to decreased platelet aggregation. Danshen has been reported to have antithrombotic effects (6048); avoid concomitant use. Some of these drugs include aspirin, clopidogrel (Plavix), dalteparin (Fragmin), enoxaparin (Lovenox), heparin, ticlopidine (Ticlid), warfarin (Coumadin), and others.
DIGOXIN (Lanoxin): Theoretically, using danshen with digoxin might increase cardiovascular effects and side effects such as arrhythmia. Danshen has structural and pharmacological similarities to cardiac glycosides (5884,6048,7311).
WARFARIN (Coumadin): Concomitant use increases the anticoagulant effects of warfarin and the risk of bleeding (611,612). There have been several case reports of increased international normalized ratio (INR) after concomitant use of danshen and warfarin (611,612,2237,5883,5884). Elevations in INR have occurred as early as 3-5 days after start of danshen. Danshen might increase the rate of absorption and decrease the elimination rate of warfarin (5884,6048). Avoid concomitant use.

Interactions with Foods

None known.

Interactions with Lab Tests

DIGOXIN: Danshen can interfere with serum digoxin measurements. It falsely elevates serum digoxin concentrations when fluorescence polarization immunoassay (FPIA) is used. It falsely lowers digoxin concentrations when microparticle enzyme immunoassay (MEIA) is used. This interference is likely related to the structural similarity of danshen to digoxin. Danshen interference can be eliminated by monitoring the free digoxin concentration. This assay takes advantage of the stronger plasma protein binding of danshen than digoxin (7311).

Interactions with Diseases or Conditions

BLEEDING DISORDERS: Theoretically, danshen may increase the risk of bleeding (2237); avoid using.

Dosage and Administration

No typical dosage.

DATE PALM

Also Known As

Kharjura.

Scientific Names

Phoenix dactylifera.
Family: Arecaceae/Palmae.

Comments

At the date of publication, there was very little scientific information available about this product. Our staff is continually analyzing the available information on natural medicines and will add data to the online version of *Natural Medicines Comprehensive Database* as it becomes available. See www.naturaldatabase.com.

DEANOL

Also Known As
2-Dimethyl Aminoethanol, Deanol aceglumate, Deanol acetamidobenzoate, Deanol benzilate, Deanol bisorcate, Deanol cyclohexylpropionate, Deanol hemisuccinate, Deanol pidolate, Deanol tartrate, Dimethylaminoethanol, Dimethylethanolamine, DMAE.

Scientific Names
2-Dimethylaminoethanol.

People Use This For
Orally, deanol is used for treating attention deficit-hyperactivity disorder (ADHD), enhancing memory and mood, boosting cognitive function, treating Alzheimer's disease, increasing intelligence and physical energy, and improving athletic performance. It is also used for preventing aging or liver spots, improving red blood cell function, improving muscle reflexes, increasing oxygen efficiency, extending life span, treating autism, and treating tardive dyskinesia. Topically, deanol is used for signs of aging skin, particularly loose or sagging skin.

Safety
POSSIBLY SAFE ...when used orally or topically and appropriately (1668,1671,1672,1673,1674,1675,1676,1679,1680,1681,12023).
PREGNANCY AND LACTATION: Insufficient reliable information available; avoid using.

Effectiveness
POSSIBLY EFFECTIVE

Athletic performance. Taking deanol orally in combination with ginseng, vitamins, and minerals seems to improve exercise performance by increasing total work load and maximal oxygen consumption during exercise (1671).

LIKELY INEFFECTIVE

Alzheimer's disease. Taking deanol orally doesn't seem to improve symptoms of Alzheimer's disease (1680,1681).

Tardive dyskinesia. Taking deanol orally doesn't seem to improve tardive dyskinesia (1672,1673,1674,1675,1676,1803,1804).

INSUFFICIENT RELIABLE EVIDENCE to RATE

Aging skin. There's preliminary evidence that applying a 3% deanol gel to facial skin can decrease sagging skin by increasing skin tension (12023).

Attention deficit-hyperactivity disorder (ADHD). Clinical studies using deanol for treating ADHD have produced inconclusive results (1669,1677,1679).

More evidence is needed to rate deanol for these uses.

Mechanism of Action
Deanol is a precursor to choline and might enhance central acetylcholine formation (1669).
There is interest in deanol for Alzheimer's disease because it is thought to increase acetylcholine levels in the brain and potentially improve memory and cognitive function (1680,1681).
Deanol is also theorized to increase acetylcholine in tissues and therefore possible increase skin tone (12023). However, there is no reliable evidence that deanol increases acetylcholine levels in tissues when applied topically.
Deanol is often used in anti-aging preparations. But preliminary animal research suggests that it does not increase life span (1682,1683).
Deanol has been formulated in a variety of salts and esters including deanol aceglumate, deanol acetamidobenzoate, deanol bisorcate, deanol cyclohexylpropionate (cyprodenate, cyprodemanol), deanol hemisuccinate, deanol pidolate, and deanol tartrate. The hydrochloride salt of deanol benzilate (deanol diphenylglycoate, benzacine) has been included in antispasmodic preparations (9).

Adverse Reactions
Orally, deanol can cause constipation, urticaria, headache, drowsiness, insomnia, overstimulation, vivid dreams, confusion, depression, blood pressure elevation, hypomania, an increase in schizophrenia symptoms, and orofacial and respiratory tardive dyskinesia (1674,1680,1684,1685,1686,2706).

Interactions with Herbs & Other Dietary Supplements
None known.

Interactions with Drugs
ANTICHOLINERGIC DRUGS: Theoretically, concomitant use might decrease the effect of drugs with anticholinergic activity, due to the potential cholinergic activity of deanol (1669).

Interactions with Foods
None known.

Interactions with Lab Tests
None known.

Interactions with Diseases or Conditions
CLONIC-TONIC SEIZURES: Deanol is relatively contraindicated in people with clonic-tonic seizure disorders (2706).
DEPRESSION: Deanol might worsen depression. It is reported to cause depression as an adverse effect (1685).
SCHIZOPHRENIA: Deanol can worsen schizophrenia symptoms (1674); avoid using in patients with schizophrenia.

Dosage and Administration
ORAL: Doses have ranged from 300 to 2000 mg per day in clinical studies (1669,1672,1673).
TOPICAL: For aging skin, a 3% deanol gel has been used (12023).

Comments
Deanol was previously marketed as the prescription drug, Deaner, by Riker Laboratories for the management of children with behavior problems and learning difficulties (1669,2706). Deanol is not an approved food additive in the US, nor is it an orphan drug, as some supplement advertising suggests.

DEER VELVET

Also Known As
Cornu Cervi Parvum, Deer Antler, Deer Antler Velvet, Elk Antler, Elk Antler Velvet, Horns of Gold, Lu Rong, Nokyong, Rokujo, Velvet Antler, Velvet of Young Deer Horn.

Scientific Names
Cervus nippon; Cervus elaphus.

People Use This For
Orally, deer velvet is used to boost strength and endurance, for muscle aches and pains, to promote youthfulness, increase mental clarity, as an aphrodisiac, to treat sexual dysfunction, to boost estrogen and testosterone levels, to counter the effects of stress, to improve immune system functioning, and to promote rapid recovery from illness. It is used to improve fertility, for menstrual and menopause problems, to reduce hormone replacement therapy dose, to reduce cholesterol and high blood pressure, for liver and kidney disorders, to protect the liver from toxins, for migraines, asthma, indigestion, osteoporosis, and acne. It is also used for its anticancer and anti-inflammatory properties, as a source of growth factors IGR-1 & IGF-2, to stimulate production and circulation of blood, to increase blood count, and lower the level of free radicals. Deer velvet is also used to treat symptoms of impotence; cold extremities; soreness and weakness in the lower back and knees; leukorrhea; uterine bleeding; chronic skin ulcers; and frequent, copious, clear urination. It is also used as a tonic for children with failure to thrive, mental retardation, learning disabilities, insufficient growth, or skeletal deformities including rickets. It is also used at the onset of winter to ward off infections.
In herbal combinations, deer velvet is used to improve athletic performance, for an anti-aging effect, arthritis and osteoporosis, anemia, gonadotropic disorders, gynecological disorders, skin conditions, tissue and bone rejuvenation. It is also used to increase mental capacity and performance, increase blood circulation to the brain, reduce early stages of muscular degeneration, to improve eyesight and hearing, to help PMS, impotence, and reduce stress.

Safety
There is insufficient reliable information available about the safety of deer velvet.
Pregnancy and Lactation: Insufficient reliable information available; avoid using.

Effectiveness
There is insufficient reliable information available about the effectiveness of deer velvet.

Mechanism of Action
By weight, deer velvet is approximately 50% amino acids (5502). Deer velvet also contains vitamin A, estrone and estradiol, sphingomyelin, ganglioside, some prostaglandins (5502), and epidermal growth factor (5518). Deer velvet is believed to stimulate the growth of body tissues, particularly the reticuloendothelial cells and leukocytes. It also appears to stimulate wound healing. Deer velvet seems to reduce fatigue by improving sleep and stimulating appetite. It is believed to improve health, especially in children and the elderly (5502). Preliminary evidence suggests that athletes taking deer velvet experience increased muscular strength and endurance in training. They also seem to

recover faster from muscle tissue damage that results from exercise (5505). Other evidence suggests deer velvet extract might counteract certain effects of repeated doses of morphine, such as the development of tolerance (5503).

Adverse Reactions
None reported.

Interactions with Herbs & Other Dietary Supplements
None known.

Interactions with Drugs
None known.

Interactions with Foods
None known.

Interactions with Lab Tests
None known.

Interactions with Diseases or Conditions
ESTROGEN-SENSITIVE CONDITIONS: Theoretically, women with conditions sensitive to estrogen, i.e., history of breast or cervical cancer, should avoid using deer velvet.

Dosage and Administration
ORAL: A typical dose for treatment is 0.9-2.4 grams. Double-boiled, 3-4.5 grams are used. Alternately, it can be soaked in wine (5501) or prepared as a 20% tincture in wine (5502).

Comments
Deer velvet is the epidermis that covers the inner structure of the growing bone and cartilage that will become deer antlers (5504).

DEERTONGUE

Also Known As
Carolina Vanilla, Deer's Tongue, Hound's Tongue, Liatris, Vanilla Leaf, Vanilla Plant, Vanilla Trilisa, Wild Vanilla.
CAUTION: See separate listing for Hound's Tongue (Cyonglossum officinale).

Scientific Names
Trilisa odoratissima, synonyms Carphephorus odoratissimus.
Family: Asteraceae/Compositae.

People Use This For
Orally, deertongue is used for malaria.
In manufacturing, deertongue extracts are used to flavor tobacco, as a fragrance in cosmetics and soaps, and as a fixative in some products.

Safety
LIKELY UNSAFE ...when used orally for medicinal purposes. ...when used in amounts commonly found in foods. The use of deertongue is not permitted in foods in the US (11).
PREGNANCY AND LACTATION: LIKELY UNSAFE ...when used orally due to potential effects of coumarin constituents (11); avoid using.

Effectiveness
There is insufficient reliable information available about the effectiveness of deertongue.

Mechanism of Action
The applicable part of deertongue is the dried leaf. Coumarin constituents are reported to cause liver injury and hemorrhage (11).

Adverse Reactions
Liver injury and hemorrhage are possible due to coumarin content (11). Deertongue can cause an allergic reaction in individuals sensitive to the Asteraceae/Compositae family. Members of this family include ragweed, chrysanthemums, marigolds, daisies, and many other herbs.

Interactions with Herbs & Other Dietary Supplements

HERBS THAT AFFECT BLOOD CLOTTING: Theoretically, deertongue may enhance effects of other herbs that might also affect blood clotting. Some of these herbs include alfalfa, angelica, clove, feverfew, garlic, ginger, Panax ginseng, quassia, and red clover.

Interactions with Drugs

ANTICOAGULANT/ANTIPLATELET DRUGS: Theoretically, concomitant use may increase risk of bleeding.

Interactions with Foods

None known.

Interactions with Lab Tests

None known.

Interactions with Diseases or Conditions

CROSS-ALLERGENICITY: Deertongue may cause an allergic reaction in individuals sensitive to the Asteraceae/Compositae family. Members of this family include ragweed, chrysanthemums, marigolds, daisies, and many other herbs.

Dosage and Administration

No typical dosage.

DELPHINIUM

Also Known As

Delphinii Flos, Knight's Spur, Lark Heel, Larkspur, Lark's Claw, Lark's Toe, Rittersspornblüten, Staggerweed.

Scientific Names

Consolida regalis, synonym Delphinium consolida.
Family: Ranunculaceae.

People Use This For

Orally, delphinium is used as an anthelmintic, diuretic, sedative, and appetite stimulant.

Safety

LIKELY UNSAFE ...when used orally. Delphinium can be toxic to the heart and respiratory systems (17).
PREGNANCY AND LACTATION: LIKELY UNSAFE ...when used orally (17); avoid using.

Effectiveness

There is insufficient reliable information available about the effectiveness of delphinium.

Mechanism of Action

The applicable part of delphinium is the flower. Delphinium has a paralyzing effect on peripheral and motor nerve endings (18). The alkaloid constituents are thought to be cardiotoxic and seem to be responsible for the curare-like paralysis of the respiratory system (2).

Adverse Reactions

Orally, delphinium can cause bradycardia, hypotension, cardiac arrest, and respiratory failure (2). Animal deaths from poisoning are common (18).

Interactions with Herbs & Other Dietary Supplements

None known.

Interactions with Drugs

None known.

Interactions with Foods

None known.

Interactions with Lab Tests

None known.

Interactions with Diseases or Conditions

None known.

Dosage and Administration
No typical dosage.

Comments
Avoid confusion with Consolida orientalis (Delphinium orientale).

DEVIL'S CLAW

Also Known As
Grapple Plant, Griffe Du Diable, Harpagophyti Radix, Wood Spider.

Scientific Names
Harpagophytum procumbens, synonym Uncaria procumbens.
Family: Pedaliaceae.

People Use This For
Orally, devil's claw is used for arteriosclerosis, osteoarthritis, rheumatoid arthritis, gout, myalgia, fibrositis, lumbago, tendonitis, pleuritic chest pain, gastrointestinal (GI) upset or dyspepsia, fever, and migraine headache. It is also used for difficulties in childbirth, menstrual problems, allergic reactions, loss of appetite, kidney and bladder disease, and degenerative disorders of the locomotor system.
Topically, devil's claw is used for skin injuries and disorders.

Safety
POSSIBLY SAFE ...when used orally and appropriately, short-term. Devil's claw seems to be well tolerated when used daily for up to 16 weeks (6472).
There is insufficient reliable information available about the safety of topical or long-term oral use of devil's claw.
PREGNANCY: LIKELY UNSAFE ...when used orally. Devil's claw seems to have oxytocic effects (4); avoid using.
LACTATION: Insufficient reliable information available; avoid using.

Effectiveness
POSSIBLY EFFECTIVE

Back pain. Taking devil's claw orally seems to lessen nonspecific low-back pain. Some evidence suggests that an aqueous extract of devil's claw at doses of 50-100 mg harpagoside daily seems to decrease low back pain as well as 12.5 mg rofecoxib (Vioxx) (8608,12477).

Osteoarthritis. Taking devil's claw orally alone and in conjunction with nonsteroidal anti-inflammatory drugs (NSAIDs) seems to help decrease osteoarthritis-related pain (6472,8608,12477). Devil's claw seems to be comparable to diacerhein (a slow-acting drug for osteoarthritis; not available in the US) for improving osteoarthritis pain in the hip and knee after 16 weeks of treatment. Patients taking devil's claw also seem to be able to decrease use of NSAIDs for pain relief (6472). This study used a specific powdered devil's claw root product (Harpadol) containing 2% of the constituent harpagoside (9.5 mg per capsule) and 3% total iridoid glycosides (14.5 mg per capsule) (6472). Another specific devil's claw extract (Doleteffin) has been used in a dose of 60 mg harpagoside per day (8608).

INSUFFICIENT RELIABLE EVIDENCE to RATE

Rheumatoid arthritis (RA). Preliminary evidence suggests that taking devil's claw extract orally might not improve RA (8613). More evidence is needed to rate devil's claw for this use.

Mechanism of Action
The applicable part of devil's claw is the tuber. Devil's claw contains iridoid glycoside constituents primarily harpagoside, but also including harpagide, and procumbide; it appears that other compounds besides harpagoside contribute to its effect (8614,8616). It also contains the phenylethanol derivatives acteoside (verbascoside) and isoaceteoside, and the oligosaccharide stachyose (8616). People use devil's claw for osteoarthritis and other inflammatory conditions because the iridoid glycoside constituents seem to have an anti-inflammatory effect (6472). Some preliminary research suggests that harpagoside inhibits both the cyclooxygenase (COX) and lipoxygenase inflammatory pathways (8612). Devil's claw seems to inhibit COX-2 (but not COX-1) and nitric oxide synthetase, a modulator of inflammation (12478). Some evidence suggests that the anti-inflammatory effect is due to increased synthesis and release of tumor necrosis factor (TNF)-alpha by compounds other than harpagoside (8616). However, research in humans shows no effect of devil's claw on the arachidonic acid pathway (10642).
There is also some evidence that devil's claw products might be cardioactive due to a harpagide constituent. Low doses seem to slow the heart rate and increase the strength of contraction. High doses seem to weaken heart contraction and coronary blood flow (8609). Devil's claw extract and isolated harpagoside appear to have antiarrhythmic effects (8609,8610). Preliminary evidence suggests that devil's claw extract might be inactivated by stomach acid and might be more effective with parenteral or sublingual administration (8611,8614,8615,8617). However, this is somewhat controversial. Other researchers describe little effect of gastric pH on devil's claw (8612). There also

seems to be variability in harpagoside content among various commercial extracts, possibly because some products are prepared from a mixture of Harpagophytum procumbens and Harpagophytum zeyheri. These species are similar pharmacologically, but may have differing concentrations of harpagoside and related compounds (8615).

Adverse Reactions

Orally, devil's claw is generally well tolerated. The most common adverse effect is diarrhea, occurring in approximately 8% of patients in one study (6472). Other gastrointestinal complaints include nausea, vomiting, and abdominal pain. Devil's claw can cause allergic skin reactions. It might also cause dysmenorrhea and hemodynamic instability (8608). There is also a report of throbbing frontal headache, tinnitus, anorexia, and loss of taste associated with devil's claw (8613).

Interactions with Herbs & Other Dietary Supplements

None known.

Interactions with Drugs

ANTACIDS: Theoretically, due to reports that devil's claw increases stomach acid, devil's claw might decrease the effectiveness of antacids (19).

ANTIDIABETES DRUGS: Devil's claw might decrease blood glucose levels (4) and have additive effects with medications used for diabetes. Monitor blood glucose levels closely. Dose adjustments may be necessary.

ANTIHYPERTENSIVE DRUGS: Devil's claw might decrease blood pressure (4); use cautiously.

CYTOCHROME P450 2C9 (CYP2C9) SUBSTRATES: There's preliminary evidence that devil's claw might inhibit cytochrome P450 2C9 (CYP2C9) (12479). So far, this interaction has not been reported in humans. However, watch for an increase in the levels of drugs metabolized by CYP2C9 in patients taking devil's claw. Some drugs metabolized by CYP2C9 include nonsteroidal anti-inflammatory drugs (NSAIDs) such as diclofenac (Cataflam, Voltaren), ibuprofen (Motrin), meloxicam (Mobic), and piroxicam (Feldene); celecoxib (Celebrex); amitriptyline (Elavil); warfarin (Coumadin); glipizide (Glucotrol); losartan (Cozaar); and others. Use devil's claw cautiously or avoid in patients taking these drugs.

CYTOCHROME P450 2C19 (CYP2C19) SUBSTRATES: There's preliminary evidence that devil's claw might inhibit cytochrome P450 2C19 (CYP2C19) (12479). So far, this interaction has not been reported in humans. However, watch for an increase in the levels of drugs metabolized by CYP2C19 in patients taking devil's claw. Some drugs metabolized by CYP2C19 include proton pump inhibitors including omeprazole (Prilosec), lansoprazole (Prevacid), and pantoprazole (Protonix); diazepam (Valium); carisoprodol (Soma); nelfinavir (Viracept); and others.

CYTOCHROME P450 3A4 (CYP3A4) SUBSTRATES: There's preliminary evidence that devil's claw might inhibit cytochrome P450 3A4 (CYP3A4) enzyme (12479). So far, this interaction has not been reported in humans. However, watch for an increase in the levels of drugs metabolized by CYP3A4 in patients taking devil's claw. Some drugs metabolized by CYP3A4 include lovastatin (Mevacor), ketoconazole (Nizoral), itraconazole (Sporanox), fexofenadine (Allegra), triazolam (Halcion), and numerous others. Use devil's claw cautiously or avoid in patients taking these drugs.

H2-BLOCKERS: Theoretically, due to reports that devil's claw increases stomach acid, devil's claw might decrease the effectiveness of H2-blockers (19). The H2 blockers include cimetidine (Tagamet), ranitidine (Zantac), nizatidine (Axid), and famotidine (Pepcid).

PROTON PUMP INHIBITORS (PPIs): Theoretically, due to reports that devil's claw increases stomach acid, devil's claw might decrease the effectiveness of PPIs (19). PPIs include omeprazole (Prilosec), lansoprazole (Prevacid), rabeprazole (Aciphex), pantoprazole (Protonix), and esomeprazole (Nexium).

WARFARIN (Coumadin): Purpura has occurred in a patient taking warfarin and devil's claw concurrently, suggesting over-anticoagulation (613). Devil's claw should be avoided or used cautiously in patients taking warfarin. Warfarin dose adjustments may be necessary.

Interactions with Foods

None known.

Interactions with Lab Tests

None known.

Interactions with Diseases or Conditions

CARDIAC DISORDERS, HYPERTENSION, HYPOTENSION: Since devil's claw can affect heart rate, contractility of the heart, and blood pressure (4), it might adversely affect people with cardiovascular conditions; use cautiously.

DIABETES: Devil's claw might decrease blood glucose levels (4) and have additive effects with medications used for diabetes. Monitor blood glucose levels closely. Dose adjustments may be necessary.

GALLSTONES: Devil's claw might increase bile production and adversely affect people with gallstones (8); avoid using.

PEPTIC ULCER DISEASE (PUD): Since devil's claw might increase gastric acid secretion (19), it might adversely effect people with gastric or duodenal ulcer; avoid using.

Dosage and Administration

ORAL: For osteoarthritis, one clinical study used a specific powdered devil's claw root product (Harpadol) dosed at 2.6 grams per day. This dose provided a total of 57 mg of the harpagoside constituent and 87 mg of total iridoid glycosides daily. Each 435 mg capsule contained 2% harpagoside (9.5 mg per capsule) and 3% total iridoid glycosides (14.5 mg per capsule) (6472). For other uses, the usual dose is from 1-4.5 grams of the root per day (6472).

Comments

The botanical name Harpagophytum means "hook plant" in Greek. The plant, which is native to Africa, gets its name from the appearance of its fruit, which is covered with hooks meant to attach onto animals in order to spread the seeds (6002,8611).

DEVIL'S CLUB

Also Known As

Cukilanarpak, Devils Club, Devil's Root, Fatsia, Panax horridum.

Scientific Names

Oplopanax horridus; synonyms Echinopanax horridus, Fatsia horrida.
Family: Araliaceae.

People Use This For

Orally, devil's club is used for arthritis, as a purgative, an emetic, for wound healing, fever, tuberculosis, stomach trouble, cough, cold, sore throat, diabetes, hypoglycemia, and pneumonia.
Topically, devil's club is used as a treatment for swollen glands, boils, sores, and skin infections. The ashes have been used to treat burns.

Safety

There is insufficient reliable information available about the safety of devil's club.
Pregnancy and Lactation: Insufficient reliable information available; avoid using.

Effectiveness

There is insufficient reliable information available about the effectiveness of devil's club.

Mechanism of Action

The applicable part of devil's club is the inner bark of the root. Devil's club contains equinopanacene, equinopanacol, saponins, glycerides, tannins, and steroid-related compounds. It also contains nerolidol, which has sedative and spasmolytic activity, and stigmasterol and beta-sitosterol, which have antirheumatic and cholesterol-lowering properties (12704). Preliminary research suggests that devil's club extract might have activity against respiratory syncytial virus (12702). It also might have antifungal, antibacterial, and antimycobacterial activity (12705).

Adverse Reactions

None reported.

Interactions with Herbs & Other Dietary Supplements

None known.

Interactions with Drugs

None known.

Interactions with Foods

None known.

Interactions with Lab Tests

None known.

Interactions with Diseases or Conditions

None known.

Dosage and Administration

No typical dosage.

DHA (DOCOSAHEXAENOIC ACID)

Also Known As

DHA, Fish Oil Fatty Acid, N-3 Fatty Acid, Neuromins, Omega-3 Fatty Acids, W-3 Fatty Acid.
CAUTION: See separate listings for Cod Liver Oil, EPA (eicosapentaenoic acid), and Fish Oil.

Scientific Names

Docosahexaenoic acid.

People Use This For

Orally, docosahexanoic acid (DHA) is used as a supplement for preterm infants, as an ingredient in infant formula, during the first four months of life to enhance mental development. It is also used for treating type 2 diabetes, coronary artery disease (CAD), dementia, and attention deficit-hyperactivity disorder (ADHD). DHA is also used for enhancing vision, preventing age-related macular degeneration (AMD), preventing and treating depression, and reducing aggressive behavior in people under stressful situations.
In combination with eicosapentaenoic acid (EPA), DHA is used for a variety of conditions, including the prevention and reversal of heart disease, decreasing ectopic ventricular beats, asthma, cancer, painful menses, hay fever, lung diseases, lupus erythematosus, lupus nephritis, and IgA nephropathy. EPA and DHA are also used in combination for migraine headache prophylaxis in adolescents, atopic dermatitis, Behcet's syndrome, hyperlipidemia, hypertension, psoriasis, Raynaud's syndrome, rheumatoid arthritis, bipolar disorder, and ulcerative colitis. DHA is also used in combination with arachidonic acid during the first four to six months of life to enhance mental development of infants. It is also used orally in combination with evening primrose oil, thyme oil, and vitamin E (Efalex) to improve movement disorders in children with dyspraxia.

Safety

LIKELY SAFE ...when used orally and appropriately (1016,1043,11333). DHA has been used safely for four years (11333). Fish oil supplements containing DHA have been used safely for seven years (1016).
POSSIBLY SAFE ...when used intravenously and appropriately, short-term (1004).
POSSIBLY UNSAFE ...when used orally in high doses. Doses greater than 3 grams daily might decrease blood coagulation and increase the risk of bleeding (1313).
CHILDREN: POSSIBLY SAFE ...when used orally and appropriately (424,1045,5708,5941,7599).
PREGNANCY AND LACTATION: Insufficient reliable information available; avoid using.

Effectiveness

POSSIBLY EFFECTIVE

Age-related macular degeneration (AMD). Increased dietary consumption of DHA is associated with a decreased risk of AMD (10324).

Coronary artery disease. Increased dietary consumption of DHA may reduce the risk of death in patients with coronary artery disease (10322).

Psoriasis. DHA given intravenously in combination with eicosapentaenoic acid (EPA) appears to improve psoriatic lesions better than omega-6-lipid emulsion (1004).

POSSIBLY INEFFECTIVE

Attention deficit-hyperactivity disorder (ADHD). Low plasma levels of DHA are associated with ADHD in children (7599). However, taking DHA 345 mg orally per day doesn't seem to improve objective or subjective measures of ADHD symptoms (7599).

Depression. Taking DHA orally as monotherapy, does not seem to relieve symptoms of depression (10869).

Diabetes. Taking DHA orally does not seem to substantially improve cholesterol or other serum lipids or decrease blood sugar or hemoglobin A1c (HbA1c) in patients with type 2 diabetes (10321).

INSUFFICIENT RELIABLE EVIDENCE to RATE

Dyslexia. Taking DHA orally seems to improve night vision in children with dyslexia. Dyslexic children, who receive fish oils rich in DHA, developed significantly better dark adaptation when compared with controls (5708).

Dyspraxia. Taking DHA orally, in combination with evening primrose oil, thyme oil, and vitamin E (Efalex), seems to improve movement disorders in children with dyspraxia. One small clinical trial has shown that this combination significantly decreases movement disorders as determined by objective measures (5708).

More evidence is needed to rate DHA for these uses.

Mechanism of Action

DHA (docosahexanoic acid) is a long-chain n-3 polyunsaturated fatty acid that is found in the tissues of marine mammals and oily fish. DHA is also found in fish liver oils and in commercial fish oil products. DHA can be converted into EPA (eicosapentaenoic acid) in humans (1044). DHA competes with arachidonic acid for inclusion in cyclooxygenase and lipoxygenase pathways (8696). This may have an anti-inflammatory effect in diseases such as psoriasis (1004).

DHA may reduce cardiovascular mortality risk by several mechanisms. Its effects on lipids are mixed. Pure DHA reduces serum triglycerides in adults, and increases serum high-density lipoprotein (HDL) 2 cholesterol (1014,6143). It also increases low-density lipoprotein (LDL) cholesterol and LDL particle size, but has no effect on total cholesterol or fasting glucose in mildly hypercholesterolemic men (6143). DHA decreases blood viscosity and increases red blood cell deformability, which may protect against thrombosis (11111,11112). However, DHA does not significantly affect platelet function, clotting factors, fibrinogen concentrations, plasminogen activator inhibitor-1 or tissue plasminogen activator activity (10323,11112,11113).

Long-chain polyunsaturated fatty acids make up a third of all lipids in brain grey matter (425). DHA is thought to be important for normal neural function and might play a key role in the structural development of neural and synaptic membranes (424,425,8704,8705). There is preliminary evidence DHA might affect retinal, visual, learning, and memory function (8704,8705,8715). DHA accrues rapidly in the human brain during the third trimester of pregnancy and during the early postnatal period (8705). DHA is present in human breast milk, but not in standard infant formulas. Formula-fed infants have lower plasma and cerebral cortex DHA levels than breast milk-fed infants; the clinical significance of this, if any, is unknown. There is also concern pregnancy might cause long-term effects on the DHA stores in women. However, there is evidence that maternal DHA status probably normalizes within one year after pregnancy, and there is no evidence to suggest an association with the number of completed pregnancies and DHA stores (8716).

Adverse Reactions

Orally, DHA may cause nausea, flatulence, bruising, and prolonged bleeding (11333). Adverse reactions, however, are not commonly reported for DHA alone. For fish oils containing EPA and DHA, side effects can include fishy taste, belching, nosebleeds, nausea, and loose stools. High doses of fish oils might also decrease blood coagulation and increase the risk of bleeding (1313,8699,10007). Three people with pre-existing familial adenomatous polyposis were diagnosed with malignant lesions during the course of long-term fish oil use (999). There is also some evidence that increased serum levels of DHA might be associated with an increased risk for atrophic gastritis associated with Helicobacter pylori infection, but further research is needed to clarify this finding (8709).

Interactions with Herbs & Other Dietary Supplements

HERBS WITH ANTICOAGULANT/ANTIPLATELET POTENTIAL: DHA alone does not seem to affect blood clotting (11112,11113). However, when given in combination with EPA as fish oil, concomitant use with herbs that constituents that might affect platelet aggregation could theoretically increase the risk of bleeding in some people. These herbs include angelica, danshen, garlic, ginger, ginkgo, red clover, turmeric, willow, and others.

Interactions with Drugs

ANTICOAGULANT/ANTIPLATELET DRUGS: DHA alone does not seem to affect blood clotting (11112,11113). However, theoretically, when given in combination with EPA as fish oil, concomitant use with anticoagulant or antiplatelet drugs (including aspirin) might increase risk of bleeding.

ANTIHYPERTENSIVE DRUGS: Fish oils containing DHA can lower blood pressure and might have additive effects in patients treated with antihypertensives (1001,1020,1030,1033); use with caution.

Interactions with Foods

None known.

Interactions with Lab Tests

CHOLESTEROL: DHA can increase serum HDL2 cholesterol concentrations, LDL cholesterol concentrations, LDL particle size, and test results in mildly hypercholesterolemic patients (6143).

GLUCOSE: In people with type 2 diabetes, DHA seems to increase fasting blood glucose levels (10321).

INSULIN: DHA can increase fasting insulin concentrations and test results in mildly hypercholesterolemic patients (6143).

INTERNATIONAL NORMALIZED RATIO (INR)/PROTHROMBIN TIME (PT): DHA alone does not seem to affect blood clotting (11112,11113). However, when given in combination with EPA as fish oil, doses greater than 3 grams per day might decrease blood coagulation, increase INR and PT, and increase the risk of bleeding (1313).

PULMONARY FUNCTION TESTS: DHA might cause a decline in pulmonary function tests in aspirin-sensitive individuals (11869).

TRIGLYCERIDES: DHA can reduce serum triglyceride concentrations and test results in patients with hypercholesterolemia (6143).

Interactions with Diseases or Conditions

ASPIRIN-SENSITIVITY: Fish oils and other omega-3 fatty acids can lower pulmonary function tests in some aspirin-sensitive patients (10869).

HYPERTENSION: Fish oils containing DHA can lower blood pressure and might have additive effects in patients with high blood pressure who are treated with antihypertensives (1001,1020,1030,1033).

Dosage and Administration

ORAL: As a supplement in infant formula, 0.32% DHA has been used (424). For improving dark adaptation of vision in dyslexic individuals, a daily oral fish oil dose containing 480 mg DHA has been used (5708). For improving movement disorders in children with dyspraxia, a daily oral tuna fish oil dose containing 480 mg DHA, combined with 35 mg arachidonic acid, 96 mg gamma-alpha linoleic acid from evening primrose oil, 24 mg thyme oil, and 80 mg vitamin E (Efalex) has been used (5708).

INTRAVENOUS: For plaque psoriasis, DHA 4.2 grams and eicosapentaenoic acid (EPA) 4.2 grams per day has been used (1004).

Comments

Avoid confusing DHA with EPA (eicosapentaenoic acid).

DHEA

Also Known As

GL701, Prasterone.

CAUTION: See separate listing for 7-Keto-DHEA.

Scientific Names

Dehydroepiandrosterone; Prasterone.

People Use This For

Orally, DHEA is used for slowing or reversing aging, weight loss, metabolic syndrome, and increasing immune function. It is also used for increasing strength, energy, and muscle mass.

DHEA is also used for treating systemic lupus erythematosus (SLE), osteoporosis, multiple sclerosis (MS), Addison's disease, depression, schizophrenia, chronic fatigue syndrome (CFS), menopausal symptoms, and atrichia pubis. It is also used orally for improving cognitive function, and slowing the progression of Parkinson's and Alzheimer's diseases.

For people with HIV disease, DHEA is used to improve depressed mood and fatigue.

DHEA is also used orally by men for erectile dysfunction, and by healthy women and women who have adrenal or androgen insufficiency to improve well-being and sexuality. It is also used for preventing heart disease, breast cancer, diabetes, and metabolic syndrome.

Intravaginally, DHEA is used in postmenopausal women for vaginal atrophy and increasing bone mineral density.

Intravenously, DHEA is being investigated for improving skin graft-site healing.

Safety

POSSIBLY SAFE ...when used orally and appropriately, short-term. Most studies have been small and lasted from a few weeks to 6 months (793,2133,3231,4249,4251,4252,4253,4254,4255,9691,9692,10986,12215). Some studies have also used oral DHEA with apparent safety for up to 12 months (2113,6446,10406,11464,12561). ...when used intravaginally and appropriately. DHEA has been safely used intravaginally by postmenopausal women in a study lasting 12 months (4242).

POSSIBLY UNSAFE ...when used orally, long-term or in high doses. There is concern that long-term use or use of amounts that cause higher than normal physiological DHEA levels might increase the risk of prostate cancer (2111,2116), breast cancer, or other hormone-sensitive cancers (6445). In some cases, 50-100 mg daily can produce slightly higher than normal physiological DHEA levels (4249,4251).

PREGNANCY AND LACTATION: POSSIBLY UNSAFE ...when used orally. DHEA can cause higher than normal androgen levels (2133,4249,4251,4253), which might adversely affect pregnancy or a nursing infant.

Effectiveness

POSSIBLY EFFECTIVE

Adrenal insufficiency. Taking low-dose DHEA orally, 20-50 mg per day, seems to improve feelings of well-being, skin and hair, and sexuality in women with adrenal insufficiency or androgen deficiency due to hypopituitarism (3231,8593).

Aging skin. Taking DHEA orally seems to increase epidermal thickness, sebum production, skin hydration, and decrease facial skin pigmentation in elderly men and women (6446).

Erectile dysfunction (ED). Taking DHEA orally for 24 weeks seems to improve ED, orgasmic function, sexual desire, and overall sexual satisfaction in men with erectile dysfunction. DHEA seems to help men with erectile dysfunction secondary to hypertension or idiopathic erectile dysfunction, but doesn't seem to improve erectile dysfunction related to diabetes or neurological disorders (793,8596).

Menopausal symptoms. Taking DHEA orally 25 mg per day seems to improve subjective vasomotor symptoms such as hot flashes, as well as psychological symptoms throughout 12 months of therapy (11464).

Osteoporosis. Taking DHEA orally 50 to 100 mg per day seems to improve bone mineral density in older women and men with osteoporosis or osteopenia (12563,12564). It also may increase bone mineral density in young women with anorexia nervosa (12562).

Schizophrenia. Taking DHEA orally seems to improve both negative and positive symptoms in patients with schizophrenia. It may be more effective in women than in men (9692).

Systemic lupus erythematosus (SLE). Taking DHEA orally in conjunction with conventional treatment may help reduce SLE disease activity, frequency of flare-ups, and corticosteroid doses needed (2113,2114,2136,6447,6068,12561,12574). It may also help SLE symptoms such as muscle ache and oral ulcers (12561). DHEA also seems to improve bone mineral density in SLE patients being treated with high dose corticosteroids (6068,6097,6447).

POSSIBLY INEFFECTIVE

Alzheimer's disease. Taking DHEA orally for 6 months doesn't appear to be any more effective than placebo for improving symptoms of Alzheimer's disease (11334).

Cognitive function. Taking DHEA orally doesn't seem to improve cognitive function in healthy elderly people (3893). Muscle strength. Taking DHEA orally doesn't seem to improve muscle mass or muscle strength in elderly patients (10406).

Sexual arousal. Taking DHEA orally doesn't seem to influence response to sexual stimuli in sexually functional premenopausal women (8594). However, there is preliminary clinical evidence that suggests that a single 300 mg dose of DHEA might improve sexual response in postmenopausal women (9906). More evidence is needed.

INSUFFICIENT RELIABLE EVIDENCE to RATE

Addison's disease. Preliminary clinical evidence suggests that oral DHEA might improve symptoms of Addison's disease (8595).

Atrichia pubis. Preliminary clinical research suggests treatment with oral DHEA might stimulate growth of pubic hair and stimulate body growth in adolescent girls and young women with atrichia pubis (9691).

Chronic fatigue syndrome (CFS). Preliminary clinical evidence suggests that oral DHEA might improve symptoms of CFS (7559)

Depression. Some clinical research suggests that taking DHEA orally might improve symptoms of depression and dysthymia (3270,3892,4233).

HIV lipodystrophy. Supplemental DHEA given sublingually might help lipodystrophy in people with advanced HIV infection (8598).

Metabolic syndrome. There is preliminary evidence that DHEA might decrease risk factors associated with metabolic syndrome in overweight elderly men and women. Taking 50 mg/day for 6 months seems to significantly decrease weight, abdominal fat, and insulin levels (12215).

Vaginal atrophy. Applying DHEA vaginally seems to be effective for treating vaginal atrophy in elderly postmenopausal women (4242). It might also increase bone mineral density in these patients.

Weight loss. Preliminary evidence suggests that taking 50 mg/day for 6 months seems to reduce risk factors for metabolic syndrome including obesity in overweight elderly patients who are at risk for metabolic syndrome (12215). But it's not known if this potential benefit applies to younger patients when used specifically for weight loss

More evidence is needed to rate DHEA for these uses.

Mechanism of Action

DHEA is endogenously produced in the adrenal glands and liver in humans. In men, DHEA is also secreted by the testes. Additionally, the brain synthesizes minute quantities. DHEA and its sulfate ester, dehydroepiandrosterone sulfate (DHEA-S), are interconvertible. DHEA is initially converted to DHEA-S, which is considered the storage form of DHEA (5874,8592). Peripheral tissues and target organs convert DHEA-S back to DHEA, which is then metabolized to androstenedione, the major human precursor to androgens and estrogens (3232,6098). DHEA-S concentrations are 100 to 500 times higher than testosterone and 1000 to 10,000 times higher than estradiol. Although DHEA is a precursor to other hormones, it doesn't have estrogenic or androgenic activity (12559).
DHEA and DHEA-S levels are higher in men than in women. DHEA levels typically peak at about 20 years of age, but then decline rapidly after age 25 (12215). However, in about one-third of the population, DHEA-S levels

increase with age (4248,6013,6014,8597). DHEA-S levels don't seem to correlate with mortality in women. Mortality risk appears to be higher in men under 70 years old with very low DHEA-S levels. Men who smoke and have low DHEA-S levels seem to have a mortality risk more than 6 times greater than nonsmokers with high DHEA-S levels (8597). The cause of this increased risk and whether DHEA supplementation can lower mortality risk in men are unknown.

DHEA supplementation seems to change the circulating androgen/estrogen ratio in a gender-specific manner. That is, there appears to be significant increases in the levels of estrogens, but not as much of an increase in the amount of androgens in the blood of men given DHEA. Conversely, women given DHEA develop significant increases in the levels of androgens, but not as much of an increase in estrogen levels (6010,6011,9694,11465). For example, in elderly men, administration of DHEA 50 mg daily for 12 months increases DHEA-S to levels comparable with young adults; and testosterone levels don't significantly increase, but estradiol levels do significantly increase. In elderly women, administration of the same dose initially increases DHEA-S levels above those of young adults, but after 12 months of use levels fall back to the young adult range. Also, testosterone levels increase to levels comparable with young adults and estradiol levels increase, but not to levels as high as in young adults (6446). In both men and women, extended use seems to result in increased elimination of DHEA-S. After continuous oral administration of DHEA, DHEA-S levels seem to significantly increase after 6 months of use, but after 12 months of use, DHEA-S levels fall back some; however, DHEA-S levels remain higher than before supplementation began (6446). This suggests that the human body might have an adaptive mechanism, which limits the accumulation of DHEA-S and androgenic compounds (6446). The androgen-like or estrogen-like effects might be responsible for some of the benefits of DHEA (2115).

Researchers speculate that DHEA might have similar therapeutic benefits to estrogen-progestin hormone replacement therapy (HRT). In a low-estrogen environment such as menopause, DHEA has estrogenic effects. Some of the effects in postmenopausal women are similar to HRT including increasing estradiol, estrone, osteocalcin, growth hormone, and insulin-like growth factor 1 (IGF-1); however, unlike HRT, DHEA also increases androstenedione and testosterone (7327,11464). Conversion to estrogen doesn't seem to be necessary for its estrogenic activity. DHEA-S stimulates the growth of estrogen receptor-positive breast cancer cells. It can overcome the estrogen receptor blocking activity of drugs such as tamoxifen (Nolvadex) and fulvestrant (Faslodex). Some researchers think controlling DHEA-S serum levels may be useful in the treatment of breast cancer (10370).

Researchers have also suggested that replacing DHEA by supplementation might prevent some of the diseases and conditions associated with aging (6446). However, people whose DHEA-S levels increase with age don't seem to age any differently than people with declining DHEA-S levels. There does not appear to be an association between prematurely low DHEA-S levels and increased risk for diseases commonly seen with old age (6013,6014,8597). A correlation between DHEA-S levels and cognitive status or cognitive decline in elderly men has not been demonstrated (5874).

Some DHEA proponents suggest that DHEA supplements might be useful for metabolic syndrome. With aging, abdominal fat increases, increasing the risk of cardiovascular disease and mortality (12559). Abdominal obesity increases the risk for insulin resistance, diabetes, and atherosclerosis (12251). Although inactivity and overeating contribute to abdominal fat accumulation with aging, metabolic changes such as the decline in DHEA levels may also play a role. Obesity is associated with lower plasma free DHEA levels, but the relationship between DHEA-S levels and obesity are less clear; studies are conflicting (12559). The mechanism of DHEA in body fat distribution is not well understood. DHEA is a precursor to androgens and estrogens, which help regulate adipocyte physiology and the accumulation of adipose tissue. DHEA activates peroxisome proliferator-activated receptor (PPAR)-alpha, which seems to inhibit adipocyte differentiation into mature fat cells. PPAR may also upregulate the genetic expression of enzymes that regulate lipolysis and fatty acid oxidation in adipocytes, as well as suppressing enzymes that cause adipogenesis (12559,12560).

Endogenous DHEA levels are affected by certain activities and disease states. For example, exercising at maximal and submaximal levels and consuming food naturally increases endogenous DHEA levels. DHEA is decreased in anorexia nervosa, depression, end-stage renal disease, type 2 diabetes mellitus, schizophrenia, chronic fatigue syndrome (CFS), and systemic lupus erythematosus (SLE) (4248,5872,7558). Because decreased serum DHEA-S levels have been reported in men under age 60 with erectile dysfunction (5868), DHEA supplements are being used for erectile dysfunction. DHEA-S levels are also decreased in men with congestive heart failure (CHF), in proportion to its severity, possibly due to the effects of oxidative stress on electron transport required for DHEA synthesis (5871). DHEA is used for SLE because endogenous DHEA levels are decreased in SLE patients. It is thought that a high-estrogen, low-androgen state may contribute to the presence or activity of SLE, and that an increase in the level of androgens could help patients with this disease. DHEA has also been reported to correct defective interleukin-2 production in T-lymphocytes in people with SLE (5872,6098). The effects of DHEA on stimulation of bone formation in SLE patients has been attributed to the androgenic properties of DHEA (6447); however, the reduction in corticosteroid dose that DHEA permits might also be responsible for this effect. In women with adrenal insufficiency, DHEA does not seem to significantly affect measures of body composition including weight and bone mineral composition. The minor increase in osteocalcin in these patients does not appear to be clinically significant (9601).

In the brain, DHEA is concentrated in the limbic regions, and may function as an excitatory neuroregulator, antagonizing gamma-aminobutyric acid (GABA) transmission (5870). Low serum DHEA levels seem to be predictors of progression to AIDS in people with HIV infection (8598). DHEA has been used for HIV disease because of reports of modest antiviral effects of DHEA, possible immunomodulating effects, and findings that DHEA decreases with declining CD4 lymphocyte counts (3865,3866,3867); however, DHEA does not affect CD4 counts, even at doses as high as 2.25 grams per day (3865).

Research also suggests that DHEA might have beneficial effects on microvascular circulation and cardiovascular risk. Supplemental DHEA seems to inhibit synthesis of thromboxane A2 in platelets, increase serum levels of insulin-like growth factor 1 (IGF-1), and increase levels of cyclic guanosine monophosphate (GMP) and nitric oxide synthesis (8592). Some research also suggests DHEA might have a beneficial on lipid levels in postmenopausal women (10985). Endogenous DHEA is increased in some individuals taking diltiazem and alprazolam. Danazol, insulin, and morphine decrease DHEA levels (4248). Exogenous glucocorticoids also seem to suppress DHEA production. In vivo, glucocorticoids and DHEA are secreted concomitantly. Some researchers speculate that concurrent administration of DHEA with exogenous glucocorticoids might help combat the adverse effects of glucocorticoids (7328). Male sex hormones appear to have a harmful effect on organ function after trauma hemorrhage. DHEA attenuates depressed cardiac and hepatic function secondary to trauma hemorrhage in male rats, possibly due to estrogenic activity (6101). Estrogenic activity, together with nitric oxide release, may also be responsible for an antiatherosclerotic effect of DHEA observed in animal models (5869). Some preliminary animal research suggests that DHEA might have an additive anorexic effect when used with dexfenfluramine (Redux, no longer marketed in the US) (8599). The pharmacokinetics of DHEA are well defined. It has excellent absorption by the oral route. The elimination half-life of DHEA is 15 to 38 minutes; the half-life of DHEA-S is 7 to 22 hours. The kidneys eliminate 51 to 73% of DHEA-S and its metabolites (8592).

Adverse Reactions

Orally, DHEA adverse effects are generally mild at low doses such as 50 mg per day (12215). At doses of 200 mg per day, DHEA frequently causes adverse effects. Androgenic effects such as acne occur in about one-third of women taking DHEA 200 mg per day and hirsutism in about 16% (12561). DHEA can also cause hair loss, voice deepening, insulin resistance, changes in menstrual pattern, hepatic dysfunction, abdominal pain, and hypertension (2111,2116,6098). When used in very high doses it can cause mild insomnia (4248). In individuals with HIV, it is associated with nasal congestion, fatigue, and headache (4248). Doses up to 2.25 grams taken for four months were well tolerated with no serious adverse effects in people with mild HIV (3865). There are three cases of mania in men taking DHEA (5870,6102,7023). This has occurred in people with no history of psychiatric disease (6102) and in those with a history of mania (5870) and bipolar disorder (7023). Mania can occur with doses ranging from 50-300 mg per day. However, mania may not occur for 2-6 months after starting DHEA (6102,7023). There is some concern that DHEA might increase cancer risk when taken long-term. Some research suggests that it may increase the growth of malignant cells (6445,10370,10401,10403,12565). But, some preliminary research suggests DHEA might protect against cancer (12565,12566).

Interactions with Herbs & Other Dietary Supplements

SOY: Theoretically, soy might decrease the effects of DHEA. Soy consumption seems to decrease serum DHEA-S levels in premenopausal women (6445).

Interactions with Drugs

ANASTROZOLE (Arimidex): DHEA is a potent estrogen agonist. It may interfere with the anti-estrogen effects of anastrozole and other aromatase inhibitors (10401).

CORTICOSTEROIDS: Corticosteroid drugs can suppress endogenous DHEA production (7328). Some corticosteroid drugs include dexamethasone (Decadron), hydrocortisone (Cortef), methylprednisolone (Medrol), and prednisone (Deltasone). DHEA does not affect the pharmacokinetics of prednisolone or additively suppress excretion of endogenous corticosteroids when given with prednisolone (9693).

CYTOCHROME P450 3A4 (CYP3A4) SUBSTRATES: DHEA may increase levels of drugs metabolized by cytochrome P450 3A4 (CYP3A4) due to enzyme inhibition (1389); however, the clinical significance of these potential interactions is not known. Drugs that are substrates of CYP3A4 include alfentanil (Alfenta), alprazolam (Xanax), amitriptyline (Elavil), amiodarone (Cordarone), buspirone (BuSpar), cerivastatin (Baycol), citalopram (Celexa), felodipine (Plendil), fexofenadine (Allegra), itraconazole (Sporanox), ketoconazole (Nizoral), lansoprazole (Prevacid), losartan (Cozaar), lovastatin (Mevacor), midazolam (Versed), ondansetron (Zofran), prednisone (Deltasone, Orasone), sertraline (Zoloft), sibutramine (Meridia), sildenafil (Viagra), simvastatin (Zocor), verapamil (Calan, Covera-HS, Isoptin), and many others.

EXEMESTANE (Aromasin): DHEA is a potent estrogen agonist. It may interfere with the anti-estrogen effects of exemestane and other aromatase inhibitors (10401).

FULVESTRANT (Faslodex): DHEA is a potent estrogen agonist. It can overcome the estrogen receptor antagonist action of fulvestrant in estrogen-receptor positive cancer cells (10370). Patients with estrogen receptor positive cancers such as breast cancer, uterine cancer, and ovarian cancer should not take DHEA, even if they are being treated with fulvestrant.

INSULIN: Insulin can decrease levels of endogenous DHEA-S. Therefore, taking insulin might decrease the effectiveness of DHEA supplements which are converted to DHEA-S in the body (8592).

LETROZOLE (Femara): DHEA is a potent estrogen agonist. It may interfere with the anti-estrogen effects of letrozole and other aromatase inhibitors (10401).

TAMOXIFEN (Nolvadex): DHEA is a potent estrogen agonist. It can overcome the estrogen receptor antagonist activity of tamoxifen in estrogen-receptor positive cancer cells (10370,10403). Patients with estrogen receptor-positive cancers such as breast cancer, uterine cancer, and ovarian cancer should not take DHEA, even if they are being treated with tamoxifen.
TRIAZOLAM (Halcion): DHEA can increase plasma triazolam concentrations. Administration of DHEA 200 mg/day for two weeks was shown to inhibit cytochrome P450 3A4 (CYP3A4) metabolism of triazolam and is due to DHEA-S, rather than DHEA (1389).

Interactions with Foods

VEGETARIAN DIET: Strict vegetarians and lactovegetarians have higher serum DHEA levels than non-vegetarians. However, this difference is not apparent in postmenopausal vegetarians (6445). The clinical significance of these findings is not known.

Interactions with Lab Tests

CHOLESTEROL: DHEA can reduce total and high-density lipoprotein (HDL) cholesterol levels. Its effect on low-density lipoprotein (LDL) cholesterol is minimal (12561).
ESTRADIOL: DHEA can increase estradiol levels in postmenopausal women who do not take supplemental estrogen. In premenopausal women or in postmenopausal women taking estrogen, DHEA doesn't appear to significantly affect estradiol levels (12561).
TESTOSTERONE: DHEA can increase testosterone levels, particularly in postmenopausal women (12561).
TRIAZOLAM: DHEA can increase plasma triazolam concentrations and test results. DHEA-S, the activated form of DHEA, inhibits triazolam metabolism (1389).
TRIGLYCERIDES: DHEA can reduce triglyceride levels (12561).

Interactions with Diseases or Conditions

DIABETES: DHEA can increase insulin resistance or sensitivity. Monitor blood glucose level closely (2112,4249,4250).
HORMONE SENSITIVE CANCERS/HORMONE SENSITIVE CONDITIONS: DHEA is a potent estrogen receptor agonist. Theoretically, it might increase the risk of breast cancer and other hormone sensitive conditions. DHEA should be avoided in patients with hormone sensitive conditions such as breast cancer, uterine cancer, ovarian cancer, endometriosis, and uterine fibroids (6445,10370,10401,10403,12565).
HYPERLIPIDEMIA: DHEA may adversely affect lipid levels (12561). Preliminary research shows that DHEA may increase macrophage foam cell formation, a pro-atherogenic effect. This formation seems to involve the upregulation of lipoprotein-processing enzymes via the androgen receptor (11345). In humans given DHEA for at least 3 months, DHEA can lower high-density lipoprotein (HDL) cholesterol levels (12561).
LIVER DYSFUNCTION: DHEA can exacerbate liver dysfunction (2111,2116).
MOOD DISORDERS: There is some concern that patients with a history of depression and bipolar disorder might be at an increased risk of psychiatric adverse events associated with DHEA. DHEA has been found to cause hypomania, mania, irritability, sexual inappropriateness and psychosis in some patients with suspected mood disorders (4233,5870,7023).
POLYCYSTIC OVARY SYNDROME: DHEA may increase testosterone levels and worsen conditions of androgen excess such as polycystic ovary syndrome (12568).

Dosage and Administration

ORAL: In postmenopausal women and in elderly men, doses of 25-50 mg daily are commonly used (4249,4251,4252,4254,4255,11464). For depression, doses of DHEA 30-90 mg daily have been used, either alone or in combination with conventional antidepressant therapy (3270,4233). For treatment of schizophrenia, increasing doses of DHEA of 25 mg daily for 2 weeks, 25 mg two times daily for 2 weeks, and 50 mg two times daily for 2 weeks have been used (9692). For replacement therapy in individuals with adrenal suppression, clinical trials have used 25-50 mg, given daily as a single dose (2133,3231,4253,6012,11465). For systemic lupus erythematosus (SLE), the typical dose is 200 mg per day as an adjunct to conventional medical treatment (2113,2114,12561), but doses up to 600 mg per day have been used (5872). For improving bone mineral density in people with osteopenia or osteoporosis, 50 to 100 mg per day has been used (12562,12563,12564). For erectile dysfunction, 50 mg per day has been used (793). For treatment of atrichia pubis in adolescent girls and young women, DHEA 15 to 30 mg per meter squared has been used (9691). For Alzheimer's disease, 50 mg twice daily has been used (11334). For metabolic syndrome, 50 mg/day taken at bedtime has been used (12215).
VAGINAL: A 10% cream applied daily has been used (4242).

Comments

DHEA is a synthetic product that can be manufactured from natural sources such as soy and wild yam (which explains its ability to be marketed as a dietary supplement). Constituents, such as diosgenin, are converted in the laboratory to DHEA. However, diosgenin from ingested wild yam or soy cannot be converted to DHEA in the human body, as has been reported. Neither soy or wild yam taken orally has any effect on DHEA levels in humans (2112,7617,12571). People interested in taking DHEA should avoid wild yam and soy products labeled as "natural DHEA."

Like many dietary supplements, DHEA is plagued by quality control problems. DHEA content ranges from 0% to 150% of the labeled amount in tested products (12569,12570).

DHEA is banned by the National Collegiate Athletic Association (NCAA) (5041).

DHEA is being investigated as a prescription drug for treating systemic lupus erythematosus (SLE) and improving bone mineral density in women with lupus taking glucocorticoids. Its generic name is prasterone. Manufactured by Genelabs with the brand name Prastara, it received an approvable letter from the FDA in 2002 (12561,12573,12574).

DIACYLGLYCEROL

Also Known As

DAG, Diacylglycerol Oil, Dicylglycerol Oil, Diglyceride,.

Scientific Names

Diacylglycerol; 1,2-diglyceride; 1,3-diglyceride.

People Use This For

Orally, diacylglycerol is used for weight loss and hypertriglyceridemia.

In manufacturing, it is used as an emulsifier, stabilizer, thickener, and texturizer.

Safety

POSSIBLY SAFE ...when used orally and appropriately. Diacylglycerol seems to be safe when used orally for up to 24 weeks (9142,9143,9144).

PREGNANCY AND LACTATION: Insufficient reliable information available; avoid using.

Effectiveness

POSSIBLY EFFECTIVE

Obesity. Diacylglycerol incorporated into food products such as muffins, crackers, soup, cookies and granola bars might help modest weight loss when it is consumed as an alternative to dietary fat. Eating 2 to 5 servings per day with each serving containing 8 to 9 grams of diacylglycerol oil seems to cause a modest weight loss of 3.6% and body fat reduction of 8.3% in overweight and obese adults when used for 6 months (9142,9144).

INSUFFICIENT RELIABLE EVIDENCE to RATE

Diabetes. Some research suggests that diacylglycerol might be helpful in people with type 2 diabetes and hypertriglyceridemia. Diacylglycerol 10 grams per day in place of triglyceride fats seems to reduce triglycerides by about 40% and reduce hemoglobin A1C by about 10% (9143). More evidence is needed to rate diacylglycerol for this use.

Mechanism of Action

Diacylglycerol is a minor component of various edible oils and fats. It is synthesized commercially by enzyme-catalyzed esterification of glycerol with fatty acids from oils such as canola, soybean, corn, and olive oil to produce an 80% mixture of 1,3-diglyceride and 1,2-diglyceride in a 7 to 3 ratio. The main fatty acid constituents of diacylglycerol are oleic, linoleic, and linolenic acids (9142).

Diacylglycerol seems to induce weight loss by increasing fat oxidation and energy expenditure. Diacylglycerol contains approximately the same number of calories as triglyceride oils and seems to be digested to the same extent. However, the structural differences in diacylglycerol result in differences in metabolism. In the intestine, diacylglycerol is readily hydrolyzed to monoglycerides and fatty acids. Unlike triglyceride fats, diacylglycerol is not resynthesized and assembled into chylomicrons (9146). Triglyceride serum levels rise after ingestion of triglyceride fats, but not after ingestion of diacylglycerol (9142,9145). Diacylglycerol doesn't seem to affect fat-soluble vitamin absorption or serum lipid levels (9146).

Adverse Reactions

Orally, diacylglycerol can cause mild adverse effects such as gastrointestinal complaints, headache, taste disturbances, acne, and rash (9142).

Interactions with Herbs & Other Dietary Supplements

None known.

Interactions with Drugs
None known.

Interactions with Foods
None known.

Interactions with Lab Tests
None known.

Interactions with Diseases or Conditions
None known.

Dosage and Administration
ORAL: For weight loss and body fat reduction, 10 to 45 grams of diacylglycerol per day in foods in place of other fats has been used. Typically, each serving contains 8 to 9 grams of diacylglycerol oil, used in place of other dietary fats, in 2 to 5 servings per day (9142).

Comments
The FDA is reviewing the manufacturer's (Kao Corporation) application for Generally Recognized As Safe (GRAS) status for diacylglycerol. Currently, plant-derived oils that contain up to 15 percent diglycerides (compared with 80 percent in diacylglycerol) are considered GRAS (9140).

DIBENCOZIDE

Also Known As
Adenosylcobalamin, Cobalamin Enzyme, Cobamamide, Coenzyme B12, Co-enzyme B12, Coenzyme B-12, Co-enzyme B-12.
CAUTION: See separate listing for Vitamin B12.

Scientific Names
None.

People Use This For
Orally or sublingually, dibencozide is used as a preparation to stimulate protein metabolism; increase muscle mass and strength; increase mental concentration, and to treat depression, anxiety, and panic attacks.

Safety
LIKELY SAFE ...when used orally. There are no reports of toxicity from excessive amounts of cobalamins (272,5133). When tissue binding sites are saturated, excessive dibencozide is excreted in urine and bile (5133).
PREGNANCY AND LACTATION: Insufficient reliable information available; avoid using.

Effectiveness
There is insufficient reliable information available about the effectiveness of dibencozide.

Mechanism of Action
The term vitamin B12 refers to all cobalamins that are active as coenzymes in humans, including dibencozide (adenosylcobalamin), methylcobalamin, and hydroxocobalamin (5133). Cyanocobalamin, the most stable of the cobalamins, is metabolized in the body to an active coenzyme (5133). Vitamin B12 is involved in fat, protein, and carbohydrate metabolism. It is active in all cells, particularly in the bone marrow, CNS, and GI tract (272). Produced almost exclusively by microorganisms, vitamin B12 is found in animal protein and in some legumes in small amounts (272). Adults who eat meat in their diet usually ingest more than the RDA of 2.4 mcg (6243). Vitamin B12 is conserved by enterohepatic circulation. Deficiency takes about three years to develop in people with normal absorption (272). No benefit has been shown from taking large quantities of cobalamins unless an individual is deficient (272).

Adverse Reactions
None reported.

Interactions with Herbs & Other Dietary Supplements

VITAMIN C: Preliminary evidence suggests that vitamin C supplements can destroy dietary vitamin B12. However, other components of food, such as iron and nitrates, might counteract this effect (9511). It isn't clear whether this interaction is clinically significant, and it can likely be avoided if vitamin C supplements are taken at least 2 hours after meals.

Interactions with Drugs

CHLORAMPHENICOL: May impair hematopoietic response to vitamin B12 (15).

Drug Influences on Nutrient Levels and Depletion

SOME DRUGS CAN AFFECT DIBENCOZIDE LEVELS:

AMINOSALICYLIC ACID (para-aminosalicylic acid, PAS, Paser): Aminosalicylic acid can reduce oral vitamin B12 absorption, possibly by as much as 55%, as part of a general malabsorption syndrome (9574). Megaloblastic changes, and occasional cases of symptomatic anemia have occurred, usually after doses of 8 to 12 grams/day for several months (4558,9395,9397). Monitor vitamin B12 levels in people taking aminosalicylic acid for more than one month.

ANTIBIOTICS: Disruption of the normal gastrointestinal (GI) flora may interrupt enterohepatic recirculation of vitamin B12 and increase fecal excretion (4436). Vitamin B12 is also synthesized by the GI flora, but mainly in the colon where absorption is poor. The majority of bacterially synthesized vitamin B12 is therefore excreted in the feces and does not significantly contribute to the body's store of vitamin B12 (4437,9502). The effects of antibiotics on gastrointestinal bacteria are unlikely to have clinically significant effects on vitamin B12 levels. In people with bacterial overgrowth of the small bowel, antibiotics such as metronidazole (Flagyl) can actually improve vitamin B12 status. An increased bacterial load can bind significant amounts of vitamin B12 in the gut, preventing its absorption (4437,9502).

COBALT IRRADIATION: Cobalt irradiation of the small bowel can decrease gastrointestinal (GI) absorption of vitamin B12 (15).

COLCHICINE: Colchicine in doses of 1.9 to 3.9 mg/day can disrupt normal intestinal mucosal function, leading to malabsorption of several nutrients, including vitamin B12 (4543,4544,4545). Lower doses don't seem to have a significant effect on vitamin B12 absorption after 3 years of colchicine therapy (5921). The significance of this interaction isn't clear. Monitor vitamin B12 levels in people taking large doses of colchicine for prolonged periods.

COLESTIPOL (Colestid), CHOLESTYRAMINE (Questran): These resins can decrease gastrointestinal (GI) absorption of vitamin B12 by binding intrinsic factor and vitamin B12-intrinsic factor complexes (10542,10543). However, absorption isn't completely prevented (10542). It's unlikely that this interaction will deplete body stores of vitamin B12 unless there are other factors contributing to deficiency. In a group of children treated with cholestyramine for up to 2.5 years there wasn't any change in serum vitamin B12 levels (4455). Routine supplements aren't necessary.

H2-BLOCKERS: Reduced secretion of gastric acid and pepsin produced by H2-blockers can reduce absorption of protein-bound (dietary) vitamin B12, but not supplemental vitamin B12 (4539,4540,4541,9513,9514,9528). Gastric acid is needed to release vitamin B12 from protein for absorption (4541,9513,9514,9528). Clinically significant vitamin B12 deficiency and megaloblastic anemia are unlikely, unless H2-blocker therapy is prolonged (2 years or more), or the person's diet is poor (4539,9513,9514). It is also more likely if the person is rendered achlorhydric (4483), which occurs more frequently with proton pump inhibitors than H2-blockers. Monitor vitamin B12 levels in people taking high doses of H2 blockers for prolonged periods. The H2-blockers include cimetidine (Tagamet), ranitidine (Zantac), nizatidine (Axid), and famotidine (Pepcid).

METFORMIN (Glucophage): Metformin may reduce serum folic acid and vitamin B12 levels (32,4490,8834). These changes can lead to hyperhomocysteinemia, adding to the risk of cardiovascular disease in people with diabetes (32,4490). There are also rare reports of megaloblastic anemia in people who have taken metformin for 5 years or more (9520,9521,9522). Possible mechanisms for lowered vitamin B12 levels are decreased intrinsic factor secretion, reduced uptake of vitamin B12-intrinsic factor complexes, altered bowel motility, and bacterial overgrowth (32,9521). Reduced absorption of vitamin B12 can be measured with the Schilling test after a few weeks of metformin therapy. Reduced serum levels of vitamin B12 occur in up to 30% of people taking metformin chronically (4490,9520,9521,9523). However, clinically significant deficiency isn't likely to develop if dietary intake of vitamin B12 is adequate (9521). Deficiency can be corrected with vitamin B12 supplements even if metformin is continued (9520,9522). The metformin-induced malabsorption of vitamin B12 is reversible by oral calcium supplementation (8834,9523). A multivitamin preparation may also be valuable for some patients. Monitor for signs and symptoms of vitamin B12 and folic acid deficiency. Advise people taking metformin chronically to include adequate amounts of vitamin B12 in their diet, and have their serum vitamin B12 and homocysteine levels checked annually.

NEOMYCIN: Absorption of vitamin B12 can be reduced by neomycin, but prolonged use of large doses is needed to induce pernicious anemia (3046,8434). Supplements aren't needed with normal doses.

NITROUS OXIDE: Nitrous oxide inactivates the cobalamin form of vitamin B12 by oxidation. Symptoms of vitamin B12 deficiency, including sensory neuropathy, myelopathy, and encephalopathy, can occur within days or weeks of exposure to nitrous oxide anesthesia in people with subclinical vitamin B12 deficiency. Symptoms are treated with high doses of vitamin B12, but recovery can be slow and incomplete. People with normal vitamin B12 levels have sufficient vitamin B12 stores to make the effects of nitrous oxide insignificant, unless exposure is repeated and prolonged (nitrous oxide abuse) (9527,9532). In people with risk factors for vitamin B12 deficiency, check vitamin B12 levels prior to using nitrous oxide anesthesia.

ORAL CONTRACEPTIVES: The data regarding the effects of oral contraceptives on vitamin B12 serum levels are conflicting. Some studies have found reduced serum levels in oral contraceptive users (4547,9371,9373,9505), but others have found no effect despite use of oral contraceptives for up to 6 months (4498,7843,9372). When reduced serum levels are detected, vitamin B12 absorption, urinary excretion, tissue and erythrocyte levels, methylmalonic acid levels, and homocysteine are normal (9371,9373,9505,10123). When oral contraceptive use is stopped, normalization of vitamin B12 levels usually occurs (10123). It's suggested that oral contraceptives reduce production of transcobalamin I, the protein which transports vitamin B12 in the blood (4547,9373,9505). Thus more of the vitamin is available for tissue uptake and serum levels may be reduced. Vitamin B12 supplements don't seem to increase serum levels of vitamin B12 (9373). Lower vitamin B12 serum levels seen with oral contraceptives probably aren't clinically significant.

PHENYTOIN (Dilantin), PHENOBARBITAL, PRIMIDONE (Mysoline): These anticonvulsants have been associated with reduced vitamin B12 absorption, and reduced serum and cerebrospinal fluid levels in some patients. This may contribute to the megaloblastic anemia, primarily caused by folate deficiency, associated with these drugs (7843,10502,10503,10504). It's also suggested that reduced vitamin B12 levels may contribute to the neuropsychiatric side effects of these drugs (10504,10505). Encourage patients to maintain adequate dietary vitamin B12 intake, and check folate and vitamin B12 status if symptoms of anemia develop.

PROTON PUMP INHIBITORS (PPIs): The reduced secretion of gastric acid and pepsin produced by PPIs can reduce absorption of protein-bound (dietary) vitamin B12, but not supplemental vitamin B12 (4483,4484,4485,4486,9513,9528). Gastric acid is needed to release vitamin B12 from protein for absorption (4484,4486,9513,9528). Reduced vitamin B12 levels may be more common with PPIs than with H2-blockers, because they are more likely to produce achlorhydria (complete absence of gastric acid secretion) (4483,4486). However, clinically significant vitamin B12 deficiency is unlikely, unless PPI therapy is prolonged (2 years or more) or dietary vitamin intake is low (4483,4484,9513). Monitor vitamin B12 levels in people taking high doses of PPIs for prolonged periods. The PPIs include omeprazole (Prilosec, Losec), lansoprazole (Prevacid), rabeprazole (Aciphex), pantoprazole (Protonix, Pantoloc), and esomeprazole (Nexium).

ZIDOVUDINE (AZT, Combivir, Retrovir): Reduced serum vitamin B12 levels may occur when zidovudine therapy is started (30,10531). This adds to other factors that cause low vitamin B12 levels in people with HIV, and might contribute to the hematological toxicity associated with zidovudine (10531,10532). However, data suggests vitamin B12 supplements aren't helpful for people taking zidovudine (10532,10533).

Interactions with Foods

ALCOHOL (Ethanol): Excessive alcohol intake lasting longer than two weeks can decrease vitamin B12 absorption from the gastrointestinal tract (15).

Interactions with Lab Tests

None known.

Interactions with Diseases or Conditions

GI CONDITIONS: Ileal disease or resection, intrinsic factor deficiency can cause vitamin B12 malabsorption (272).

Dosage and Administration

No typical dosage.

Comments

Cyanocobalamin and hydroxocobalamin are the only forms of vitamin B12 stable for storage (5139).

DIGITALIS

Also Known As

Dead Man's Bells, Digitalis purpurea, Fairy Cap, Fairy Finger, Foxglove, Lady's Thimble, Lion's Mouth, Purple Foxglove, Scotch Mercury, Throatwort, Witch's Bells, Wolly Foxglove.

Scientific Names

Digitalis purpurea; Digitalis lanata.
Family: Scrophulariaceae.

People Use This For

Orally, digitalis is used for congestive heart failure, atrial fibrillation or flutter, for diureses in edema, asthma, as an emetic, for epilepsy, tuberculosis, constipation, headache, spasm, and wound and burn healing.

Safety

UNSAFE ...when used orally for self-medication. Use requires monitoring by a medical professional (12). Can cause heart arrhythmias and death (17). All parts of the plant are toxic (501). US regulations require labeling to inform consumers that digitalis is inappropriate for use as an anti-obesity agent (12). Canadian regulations prohibit digitalis in foods (12). Deaths have occurred when digitalis was mistaken for comfrey (501).
CHILDREN: LIKELY UNSAFE ...when used orally. Sucking on the flowers, ingesting seeds, or parts of the leaves has caused children to become ill (6).
PREGNANCY AND LACTATION: UNSAFE ...when used orally for self-medication (12); avoid using.

Effectiveness

LIKELY EFFECTIVE

Atrial fibrillation. Taking digitalis orally is effective for treating atrial fibrillation or flutter (6).
Congestive heart failure (CHF). Taking digitalis orally is effective for treating CHF and CHF-related edema (6).
There is insufficient reliable information available about the effectiveness of digitalis for its other uses.

Mechanism of Action

The applicable part of digitalis is the leaf. Digitalis contains varied glycosides, primarily glycoside A and glycoside B, which are precursors to digitoxin and gitoxin, respectively. Digitalis lanata contains lanatosides A,B,C,D, and E that yield digitoxin, gitoxin, digoxin, digitalin, and gitaloxin, respectively (6). Cardiac glycosides increase cardiac contractility, decrease heart rate and reduce AV node conduction, stabilize the heart rate, increase cardiac output, and relieve pulmonary congestion and peripheral edema (6).

Adverse Reactions

Orally, chronic use of digitalis can lead to intoxication symptoms including visual halos, yellow-green vision, and GI upset (6). Acute poisoning of digitalis includes GI upset, contracted pupils, blurred vision, strong slow pulse, nausea, vomiting, dizziness, excessive urination, fatigue, muscle weakness and tremors, stupor, confusion, convulsions, atrial arrhythmias, AV block, and death (6,159,501).

Interactions with Herbs & Other Dietary Supplements

CARDIAC GLYCOSIDE-CONTAINING HERBS: Contraindicated; concomitant use can increase the risk of cardiac glycoside toxicity. Cardiac glycoside containing herbs, including black hellebore, Canadian hemp roots, digitalis leaf, hedge mustard, figwort, lily-of-the-valley roots, motherwort, oleander leaf, pheasant's eye plant, pleurisy root, squill bulb leaf scales, and strophanthus seeds (19).
LICORICE/HORSETAIL: Theoretically, overuse/misuse of licorice rhizome or horsetail plant with cardiac glycoside-containing herbs increases the risk of toxicity due to potassium depletion (19).
OTHER CARDIOACTIVE HERBS: Avoid concomitant use with other cardioactive herbs due to unpredictability of effects and adverse effects. Other cardioactive herbs include calamus, cereus, cola, coltsfoot, devil's claw, European mistletoe, fenugreek, fumitory, ginger, Panax ginseng, hawthorn, white horehound, mate, parsley, quassia, scotch broom flower, shepherd's purse, and wild carrot (4).
STIMULANT LAXATIVE HERBS: Theoretically, overuse/misuse of stimulant laxatives with cardiac glycoside-containing herbs increases the risk of cardiac toxicity due to potassium depletion (19). Stimulant laxative herbs include aloe dried leaf sap, blue flag rhizome, alder buckthorn, European buckthorn, butternut bark, cascara bark, castor oil, colocynth fruit pulp, gamboge bark exudate, jalap root, black root, manna bark exudate, podophyllum root, rhubarb root, senna leaves and pods, wild cucumber fruit (Ecballium elaterium), and yellow dock root.

Interactions with Drugs

DIGOXIN (Lanoxin): Contraindicated; therapeutic duplication increases the risk of cardiac glycoside toxicity (2).
DIURETIC DRUGS: Theoretically, concomitant use of potassium depleting diuretics and digitalis can increase the risk of cardiac glycoside toxicity due to potassium depletion (506). Some diuretics that can deplete potassium include chlorothiazide (Diuril), chlorthalidone (Thalitone), furosemide (Lasix), hydrochlorothiazide (HCTZ, Hydrodiuril, Microzide), and others.
MACROLIDE ANTIBIOTICS: Theoretically, concomitant use may increase risk of cardiac glycoside toxicity (17).
QUININE: Use of quinine can with digitalis can increase the risk of digitalis toxicity (506).
STIMULANT LAXATIVES: Theoretically, overuse or misuse of stimulant laxative can increase risk of cardiac glycoside toxicity due to potassium depletion (506).
TETRACYCLINE ANTIBIOTICS: Theoretically, concomitant use may increase risk of cardiac glycoside toxicity (17).

Interactions with Foods

None known.

Interactions with Lab Tests

ELECTROCARDIOGRAM (ECG): Digitalis can normalize arrhythmias, and ECG readings, associated with atrial fibrillation or flutter in patients with congestive heart failure (15).

Interactions with Diseases or Conditions

HEART DISEASE: Self-use contraindicated; requires diagnosis, treatment, and monitoring (515,150).
RENAL DISEASE: May reduce excretion of digitalis, increasing the potential for toxicity (150).

Dosage and Administration

No typical dosage.

Comments

Digitalis is unsafe for self-medication. Digitalis lanata is the major source of digoxin in the US (6).

DIINDOLYLMETHANE

Also Known As

DIM.
CAUTION: See separate listing for Indole-3-Carbinol.

Scientific Names

3,3'-Diindolylmethane.

People Use This For

Orally, diindolylmethane is used for preventing breast, uterine, and colorectal cancer. It is also used orally to prevent benign prostatic hypertrophy (BPH) and treat premenstrual syndrome (PMS).

Safety

LIKELY SAFE ...when used orally in amounts typically found in foods. The typical diet supplies 2-24 mg of diindolylmethane (7170,7176,7664).
CHILDREN: LIKELY SAFE ...when used orally in amounts typically found in foods (7170,7176,7664).
PREGNANCY AND LACTATION: LIKELY SAFE ...when used orally in amounts typically consumed in foods (7170,7176,7664). There is insufficient reliable information available about the safety of diindolylmethane when used in amounts greater than those found in foods during pregnancy and lactation; avoid using.

Effectiveness

There is insufficient reliable information available about the effectiveness of diindolylmethane.

Mechanism of Action

Diindolylmethane is a major active metabolite of indole-3-carbinol (7664), which is a constituent of Cruciferous vegetables such as cabbage, Brussels sprouts, cauliflower, and broccoli. Indole-3-carbinol is thought to be one of the agents responsible for the cancer-protective properties of these vegetables (7664,7668). In stomach acid, indole-3-carbinol is unstable and readily converted to a variety of compounds including diindolylmethane (7669).
A typical diet provides 20-120 mg of indole-3-carbinol per day. Approximately 10% to 20% is converted to diindolylmethane, providing 2-24 mg daily (7170,7176,7664).
Researchers are interested in diindolylmethane due to potential activity against breast cancer cells (7664,7665,7666,7668,7669). Diindolylmethane has partial estrogen receptor agonist and antagonistic activity (7664,7669). There is preliminary evidence that diindolylmethane can inhibit the growth of mammary tumors in animal models (7666). Diindolylmethane induces apoptosis (programmed cell death) in human breast cancer cells in vitro (7668).

Adverse Reactions

None reported.

Interactions with Herbs & Other Dietary Supplements

None known.

Interactions with Drugs

CYTOCHROME P450 1A2 (CYP1A2) SUBSTRATES: There is some preliminary evidence that diindolylmethane can induce CYP1A2 (7667). Theoretically, diindolylmethane might increase metabolism of CYP1A2 substrates and lower serum concentrations. Some CYP1A2 substrates include clozapine (Clozaril), cyclobenzaprine (Flexeril), fluvoxamine (Luvox), haloperidol (Haldol), imipramine (Tofranil), mexilitine (Mexitil), olanzapine (Zyprexa), pentazocine (Talwin), propranolol (Inderal), tacrin (Cognex), theophylline, zileuton (Zyflo), zolmitriptan (Zomig), and others.

Interactions with Foods

None known.

Interactions with Lab Tests
None known.

Interactions with Diseases or Conditions
None known.

Dosage and Administration
No typical dosage.

DILL

Also Known As
American Dill, Anethi Fructus, Dillweed, Dilly, European Dill, Madhura, Satahva, Sotapa, Sowa.

Scientific Names
Anethum graveolens, synonyms Anethum sowa, Peucedanum graveolens.
Family: Apiaceae/Umbelliferae.

People Use This For
Orally, dill is used for gastrointestinal disorders, loss of appetite, kidney disease, flatulence, fever and colds, cough, bronchitis, infectious disease, liver and gallbladder complaints, urinary tract disorders, hemorrhoids, spasms, neuropathy, renal colic, dysuria, genital ulcers, dysmenorrhea, and insomnia and other sleep disorders.
Topically, dill seed is used for mouth and throat inflammation.
In foods, dill is used as a culinary spice.
In manufacturing, dill oil is used as a fragrance component in cosmetics, soaps, and perfumes.

Safety
LIKELY SAFE ...when used orally in amounts commonly found in foods. Dill has Generally Recognized As Safe (GRAS) status in the US (4912).
POSSIBLY SAFE ...when used orally and appropriately in medicinal amounts (12).
PREGNANCY: POSSIBLY UNSAFE ...when used in medicinal amounts. Dill seed is used to stimulate menstrual flow (19). Theoretically, dill seed might adversely affect pregnancy.
LACTATION: Insufficient reliable information available; avoid amounts greater than those found in foods.

Effectiveness
There is insufficient reliable information available about the effectiveness of dill.

Mechanism of Action
The applicable parts of dill are the seeds and above ground parts. Dill seed contains volatile oil rich in carvone (2).
Dill leaf is reported to be a rich source of beta-carotene, iron, and potassium (19).
Dill seed is thought to have antibacterial, sedative, and diuretic effects. It might also stimulate lactation (11). It is also a urinary irritant (19). An aqueous dill extract administered intravenously lowers blood pressure, dilates blood vessels, stimulates respiration, and slows heart rate in animals (11).
Dill seed oil has spasmolytic effects on smooth muscle (11).

Adverse Reactions
Topically, photodermatosis is possible after contact with juice from freshly harvested plants (19). Dill can also cause contact dermatitis (19).

Interactions with Herbs & Other Dietary Supplements
None known.

Interactions with Drugs
None known.

Interactions with Foods
None known.

Interactions with Lab Tests
None known.

Interactions with Diseases or Conditions

CROSS ALLERGENICITY: The use of dill above ground parts can cause allergic reactions in people who are allergic to plants in the carrot family plants (19). Some of these include asafoetida, caraway, celery, coriander, and fennel.

Dosage and Administration

ORAL: No typical dosage. However, traditionally the dried seeds 1-4 grams three times daily has been used (6002). As a tincture, up to teaspoon up to 3 times daily has been taken. Oil of dill is taken in doses of 100-300 mg (2-6 drops) daily (5252).

Comments

During the Middle Ages, people sometimes used dill as a charm against witchcraft and enchantments (6002).

DIMETHYLGLYCINE

Also Known As

Dimethyl Glycine, (Dimethylamino) acetic Acid, DMG, N,N-dimethylaminoacetic Acid, N-methylsarcosine.
CAUTION: Dimethylglycine is one of the compounds found in pangamic acid formulations.
See separate listing for Pangamic Acid.

Scientific Names

N,N-dimethylglycine.

People Use This For

Orally, dimethylglycine is used to improve speech and behavior in autism, for attention deficit-hyperactivity disorder (ADHD), to improve neurological function, and for epilepsy. It is also used to reduce physical and environmental stress, improve oxygen utilization, enhance liver function, and optimize athletic performance. Other uses include as an anti-inflammatory and for anti-aging effects. Dimethylglycine is used to improve the immune response; to treat tumors; and to enhance anti-viral, anti-bacterial, and anti-tumor defenses. It is also used for chronic fatigue syndrome, allergies, respiratory disorders, alcoholism, and drug addiction. Dimethylglycine is also used to lower blood cholesterol and triglycerides, and to help normalize blood pressure and blood glucose.

Safety

POSSIBLY UNSAFE ...when used orally. Dimethylglycine may react with nitrites in the gastrointestinal tract to form the potent carcinogen, dimethylnitrosamine (5827), although this has been questioned (5830).
PREGNANCY AND LACTATION: POSSIBLY UNSAFE ...when used orally (5827); avoid using.

Effectiveness

POSSIBLY INEFFECTIVE

Autism. Taking dimethylglycine orally doesn't seem to improve autism (5819).

Epilepsy. Taking dimethylglycine orally doesn't seem to be effective for the treatment of epilepsy (5823).

There is insufficient reliable information available about the effectiveness of dimethylglycine for its other uses.

Mechanism of Action

Dimethylglycine is the dimethylated form of the amino acid glycine, but it only exists in the body for seconds at a time, and in very small quantities (5827). It is formed from betaine during the methylation of homocysteine (5828). The effects of supplemental doses in excess of naturally occurring amounts are unknown. Preliminary evidence suggests that dimethylglycine enhances humoral and cell-mediated immune responses in humans and in some, but not all, animals (5820,5822,5825). Dimethylglycine has been reported to have anticonvulsant effects in animals (5828), including antagonizing strychnine- and penicillin-induced seizures (5824,5829). A single case report described a dramatic improvement in a person with mixed complex partial and grand mal seizures (5826), but a small study in people with generalized or akinetic/myoclonic seizures found no benefit with dimethylglycine 300 to 600 mg per day (5823). Several small studies in athletes have not found any benefit of dimethylglycine on athletic performance (5821); including maximal treadmill performance measured by maximal and recovery heart rates, treadmill time, and pre-test and post-test blood glucose and lactate levels (2645). A small study using low-dose dimethylglycine did not find any benefit in children with autism (5819).

Adverse Reactions

Orally, dimethylglycine may react with nitrites in the gastrointestinal tract to form carcinogenic substances (5827).

Interactions with Herbs & Other Dietary Supplements

None known.

Interactions with Drugs
None known.

Interactions with Foods
None known.

Interactions with Lab Tests
None known.

Interactions with Diseases or Conditions
None known.

Dosage and Administration
No typical dosage.

Comments
In the 1980s, a federal court in Chicago forbade interstate sale of a brand of dimethylglycine stating that it was an unsafe food additive (5827).

DIOSMIN

Also Known As
Citrus Bioflavonoid, Citrus Bioflavonoids, Flavonoid.
CAUTION: See separate listings for Chrysin, Hesperidin, Methoxylated Flavones, Quercetin, Rue, and Rutin.

Scientific Names
Diosmetin, Diosmin.

People Use This For
Orally, diosmin is used for treating acute internal hemorrhoids, preventing relapse of acute internal hemorrhoids, treating varicose veins, venous stasis, subconjunctival and retinal hemorrhage, lymphedema following breast cancer surgery, venous stasis, and gingival bleeding. Diosmin has also been used to protect against liver toxicity.

Safety
POSSIBLY SAFE ...when used orally and appropriately, short-term. Diosmin seems to be safe when used for up to 6 months (4861,4898,10227,10229).
There is insufficient reliable information available about the safety of diosmin when used for greater than 6 months.
PREGNANCY AND LACTATION: Insufficient reliable information available; avoid using.

Effectiveness
POSSIBLY EFFECTIVE

Hemorrhoids. The combination of diosmin 1350 mg plus hesperidin 150 mg twice daily for 4 days followed by diosmin 900 mg and hesperidin 100 mg twice daily for 3 days seems to significantly improve signs and symptoms of internal hemorrhoids. The combination can stop acute bleeding in up to 92% of patients after 4 days of treatment. It can also reduce symptoms such as anal discomfort, pain, discharge, and local lesions. Subjective symptoms can be relieved within 2 days of treatment. The combination also seems to reduce the duration and intensity of hemorrhoidal flare-ups (4861,4900). Some clinicians use diosmin in lower doses and in combination with bulk laxatives instead of hesperidin. Diosmin 600 mg three times daily for 4 days, then 300 mg twice daily for 10 more days plus the bulk laxative psyllium 11 grams daily does seem to slightly help after 4 days of treatment (4898). However, this combination does not seem to be as effective as the higher dose of diosmin plus hesperidin combination. Maintenance use of diosmin 450 mg plus hesperidin 50 mg twice daily for 3 months in patients following acute treatment for internal hemorrhoids seems to significantly decrease the relapse rate (4861).

Venous stasis ulcers. Diosmin, in combination with hesperidin and compression dressing, seems to improve healing of venous stasis ulcers less than 10 cm in size (10229).

POSSIBLY INEFFECTIVE

Lymphedema. Diosmin, in combination with hesperidin, may improve drainage of lymph from the arms of women after breast cancer surgery, but it does not reduce arm swelling or other clinical signs of lymphedema (10227).

Clinical trials have used specific brand name formulations of diosmin (Daflon 500 and Daflon, Les Laboratoires Servier, France). Each tablet of Daflon 500 contains a micronized formulation of diosmin 450 mg and hesperidin 50 mg extracted from rutaceae species. Each tablet of Daflon contains only diosmin 150 mg.

There is insufficient reliable information available about the effectiveness of diosmin for its other uses.

Mechanism of Action

Diosmin is one of over 4,000 flavonoids found in plants (4919,4959,5006). Diosmin is in a class of flavonoids primarily derived from citrus fruits and is known as a citrus bioflavonoid. It is closely related to other citrus bioflavonoids such as quercetin, rutin, and hesperidin. Diosmin alone, or in combination with other citrus bioflavonoids, is most often used for vascular conditions such as hemorrhoids and varicose veins. Diosmin seems to work by improving venous tone, reducing stasis, restoring normal capillary permeability, and improving lymphatic drainage. Diosmin might improve venous tone and reduce stasis by improving vasculature response to adrenergic stimulation. Diosmin's anti-inflammatory effects seem to help restore normal capillary permeability. Diosmin inhibits phosphodiesterase and increases intracellular cyclic adenosine monophosphate (cAMP), which causes decreased production of inflammatory prostaglandins E2 and F2 and thromboxane B2. Diosmin can also reduce the generation of free radicals (4861,4898,4900,4954). Some diosmin preparations use a micronized formulation. The smaller particle size seems to help increase absorption (4900). There is preliminary evidence that a diosmin metabolite, diosmetin, might also be hepatoprotective. Diosmetin might have direct antioxidant effects, increase glutathione (GSH) levels, and decrease lipid peroxidation (4954).

Adverse Reactions

Orally, diosmin can cause gastrointestinal side effects, including abdominal pain, diarrhea, and gastritis. Headache can also occur in some patients (4861,4898,4900).

Interactions with Herbs & Other Dietary Supplements

None known.

Interactions with Drugs

None known.

Interactions with Foods

None known.

Interactions with Lab Tests

None known.

Interactions with Diseases or Conditions

None known.

Dosage and Administration

ORAL: For the treatment of internal hemorrhoids, diosmin 1350 mg plus hesperidin 150 mg twice daily for 4 days followed by diosmin 900 mg and hesperidin 100 mg twice daily for 3 days has been used (4861,4900). Some clinicians also try diosmin 600 mg three times daily for 4 days, followed by 300 mg twice daily for 10 days, in combination with psyllium 11 grams daily (4898). However, this lower diosmin dose does not seem to be as effective. For prevention of relapse internal hemorrhoids, diosmin 450 mg plus hesperidin 50 mg twice daily for 3 months of therapy has been used (4861). For treating lymphedema following surgery for breast cancer, the combination of 900 mg diosmin and 100 mg hesperidin daily has been used for up to 6 months (10227). For the treatment of venous stasis ulcers, the combination of 900 mg diosmin and 100 mg hesperidin daily has been used for up to 2 months (10229).

DIVI-DIVI

Also Known As

Bonduc, Divi Divi, Gray Nicker, Nichol Seeds, Nikkar Nuts, Putikaranja, Udakiryaka.

Scientific Names

Caesalpinia bonduc, synonyms Caesalpinia bonducella, Caesalpinia crista, Guilandina bonduc, Guilandina bonducella.
Family: Fabaceae/Leguminosae.

Comments

At the date of publication, there was very little scientific information available about this product. Our staff is continually analyzing the available information on natural medicines and will add data to the online version of *Natural Medicines Comprehensive Database* as it becomes available. See www.naturaldatabase.com.

DIVINER'S SAGE

Also Known As
Divine Mexican Mint, Diviner's Mint, Diviners Sage, Divinorin, Divinorin A, Herb-of-the-Virgin, Herba de María, Hierba de la Virgen, Hojas de la Pastora, La Hembra, Leaves of the Virgin Shepherdess, Mexican Sage, Mexican Sage Incense, Pipiltzintzintli, Sadi, Salvia, Salvinorin, Salvinorin A, Sage of the Seers, Ska Maria, Ska Maria Pastora, Yerba de Maria.
CAUTION: See separate listings for Boneset, Clary Sage, Danshen, German Sarsaparilla, Purple Loosestrife, Sage, Spearmint, and Wood Sage.

Scientific Names
Salvia divinorum.
Family: Lamiaceae/Labiatae.

People Use This For
Orally and by inhalation, diviner's sage is used as a hallucinogen.
Orally, diviner's sage is used for diarrhea, headache, rheumatism, abdominal distension, and as a tonic and end-of-life remedy. It is also used orally to regulate urination and defecation.

Safety
There is insufficient reliable information available about the safety of diviner's sage.

Effectiveness
There is insufficient reliable information available about the effectiveness of diviner's sage.

Mechanism of Action
The applicable part of diviner's sage is the leaf. The leaves are chewed and swallowed, made into an infusion (tea), or smoked for hallucinogenic effects. The active constituent is the diterpene salvinorin A, which is also called divinorin A. Unlike other hallucinogens, salvinorin A is not an alkaloid (7350,7351,7352). Salvinorin A is the most potent hallucinogen known. It causes hallucinations in doses of 200 mcg to 500 mcg when vaporized and inhaled (7351). Salvinorin A is absorbed by the oral mucosa when chewed, but is inactivated by the gastrointestinal system when swallowed. It is absorbed and produces pharmacological activity when it is heated and the vapors are inhaled (7352). The onset of hallucinogenic activity occurs within 5 to 10 minutes when chewed and within 30 seconds when inhaled. The effects last about an hour when chewed and 20 to 30 minutes via inhalation (7352). However, the duration of effect appears to be dose-dependent (7351).
It's not clear how diviner's sage constituents cause hallucinations. Diviner's sage does not appear to affect receptor sites such as serotonin, dopamine, or monoamine oxidase that are often affected by other hallucinogens (7352).

Adverse Reactions
Orally, diviner's sage can cause nausea, dizziness, and slurred speech. It can also cause confusion and hallucinations (7350,7351).

Interactions with Herbs & Other Dietary Supplements
None known.

Interactions with Drugs
None known.

Interactions with Foods
None known.

Interactions with Lab Tests
None known.

Interactions with Diseases or Conditions
None known.

Dosage and Administration
No typical dosage.

Comments

Diviner's sage has been used for centuries in religious ceremonies by the Mazatec Indians, a native people who live in Oaxaca, Mexico. The Mazatecs believe it is an incarnation of the Virgin Mary (7350). Diviner's sage is widely available on the Internet. Its possession and use is legal in the US, but the Drug Enforcement Agency (DEA) is reviewing it for possible controlled substance regulation (7349).

DMSO (DIMETHYLSULFOXIDE)

Also Known As

Dimethyl Sulfoxide, Dimethyl Sulphoxide, Dimethylis sulfoxidum, Methyl sulphoxide, NSC-763, SQ-9453, Sulphinybismethane.

Scientific Names

Dimethylsulfoxide.

People Use This For

Orally, DMSO is used for the management of amyloidosis and related symptoms.

Topically, DMSO is used to decrease pain and speed the healing of wounds, burns, and acute musculoskeletal injuries. DMSO is also used topically to treat headache, inflammation, arthritis, tic douloureux, cataracts, glaucoma, retinal degeneration, bunions, calluses, fungus toenails, asthma, to flatten raised keloid scars, and for cancer. It is also used topically to prevent tissue necrosis after extravasation with antineoplastic agents, to treat osteoarthritis, rheumatoid arthritis, scleroderma, and amyloidosis. It is also used topically for reducing skin flap ischemia following surgery, complex regional pain syndromes, as a vehicle in combination with idoxuridine to decrease the development of inflammatory reactions and lesions associated with herpes zoster infection, and decrease the pain associated with postherpetic neuralgia.

Intravenously, DMSO is used to manage symptoms associated with secondary amyloidosis and to lower intracranial hypertension. DMSO is administered by intravesical instillation to treat symptoms of interstitial cystitis such as urinary frequency, urgency, nocturia and suprapubic pain. It is also used by intravesical instillation to treat symptoms associated with chronic inflammatory bladder disease. DMSO is infused alternatively with methyl-tert-butyl ether and a buffer solution of EDTA and sodium deoxycholate through a nasobiliary catheter for the dissolution of bile duct stones. DMSO is used for the cryopreservation of hematopoietic stem cells to be infused and transplanted at a later date.

In manufacturing, DMSO is used as an industrial solvent for herbicides, fungicides, antibiotics, and plant hormones.

Safety

LIKELY SAFE ... when used by intravesical instillation (5692,5694,5695,5696,5697). An aqueous 50% solution of DMSO is FDA approved for intravesical use in the treatment of interstitial cystitis (5692,5694).

POSSIBLY UNSAFE ...when used topically. It has been reported that industrial grade DMSO is being used topically for self-treatment of several disease conditions. Industrial grade DMSO is not of the same quality of that used for drug research purposes since it may contain impurities. DMSO readily penetrates the skin and enhances the absorption of impurities and other substances, which may be hazardous to health (6326).

PREGNANCY AND LACTATION: Insufficient reliable information available; avoid using.

Effectiveness

EFFECTIVE

Interstitial cystitis. Intravesical instillation of DMSO is effective for treatment of interstitial cystitis (5692,5694).

POSSIBLY EFFECTIVE

Amyloidosis. Applying DMSO topically seems to help treat amyloidosis (6304,6306).

Biliary stones. DMSO infused alternatively with methyl-tert-butyl ether and a buffer solution of EDTA and sodium deoxycholate through a nasobiliary catheter seems to dissolve bile duct stones (6315).

Extravasation. Applying DMSO topically seems to help prevent tissue necrosis after extravasation with antineoplastic agents (5698,5699).

Herpes zoster (shingles). Applying DMSO topically as a vehicle in combination with idoxuridine (40% idoxuridine in DMSO) seems to reduce the number of lesions and decrease the inflammatory reaction associated with herpes zoster infection (6308,6309,6311,6312).

Inflammatory bladder disease. DMSO used by intravesical instillation seems to decrease symptoms associated with chronic inflammatory bladder disease (5695,5696,5697).

Intracranial pressure. DMSO used intravenously seems to lower intracranial pressure (6300,6301).

Osteoarthritis. Applying DMSO topically seems to help decrease symptoms associated with osteoarthritis (6303,6304).

Postherpetic neuralgia. DMSO used topically as a vehicle in combination with idoxuridine (40% idoxuridine in DMSO) seems to decrease the pain associated with postherpetic neuralgia (6310,6311,6312). Trigeminal herpes zoster seems most responsive (6312).

Rheumatoid arthritis (RA). Applying DMSO topically seems to help decrease symptoms associated with RA (6303,6304).

Skin flap ischemia. Applying DMSO topically seems to reduce skin flap ischemia after surgery (6307).

POSSIBLY INEFFECTIVE

Scleroderma. Applying 2% or 70% DMSO topically does not seem to help treat symptoms of scleroderma such as open ulcers (6313). Open studies on DMSO for scleroderma have been conflicting (6304,6313,6314).

LIKELY INEFFECTIVE

Cancer. Applying DMSO topically is not effective for treating cancer (6327).

There is insufficient reliable information available about the effectiveness of DMSO for its other uses.

Mechanism of Action

DMSO is a highly polar solvent used for many organic and inorganic substances. It also interacts with other molecules such as proteins, carbohydrates, lipids, water and ethanol (6331).

DMSO easily penetrates the skin (6326), and distributes widely into body fluids and tissues after administration. DMSO is metabolized to dimethyl sulfone and dimethyl sulfide in the body. The dimethyl sulfide metabolite is thought to cause the distinctive odor associated with DMSO use.

Concentrated DMSO (80-100%) penetrates more effectively than concentrations of less than 70%. This is thought to be due to DMSOs ability to exchange and interchange water molecules in cell membranes (6326), and also its ability to interfere with and cause conformational changes in cell membrane phospholipids (6331,6330). DMSO facilitates topical penetration of many medications (6326,6330).

DMSO has been found to decrease skin adhesions by possibly dissolving collagen fibers and not elastic fibers (6330). DMSO also stabilizes lysosomal membranes and causes vasodilation (6330).

DMSO has free hydroxyl radical scavenging properties (6326,6330) which might contribute to DMSOs anti-inflammatory, cryopreservative, cryoprotective, anti-ischemic, and possible radioprotective activity (6326).

DMSO also demonstrates antimicrobial activity (6326,6330), possibly by changing the RNA structure necessary for bacterial protein synthesis (6330). Cardiovascular and vasoactive effects of DMSO such as lowered vagal threshold and increased response to nerve and muscle stimulation on skeletal, smooth, and cardiac muscle are thought to be due to inhibition of anticholinesterase activity (6326,6330).

In vitro, DMSO appears to protect against ischemic injury by increasing levels of prostaglandin-E1 (PGE1) which in turn increases cyclic-AMP levels and reduces platelet aggregation. DMSO also appears to protect against ischemic injury by decreasing the secretion of vasoactive substances such as fibrinogen and thromboxane A2 from platelets that can cause vasoconstriction, vasospasm, or obstruction of vessels (6302,6330). Evidence also suggests DMSO slows the conduction of C-type nerve fibers which might explain its analgesic effects (6329).

DMSO also causes histamine release from mast cells, which is thought to be responsible for the eosinophilia and hypersensitivity reactions associated with its use (6324).

DMSO might affect sensory nerves during bladder instillations by stimulating bladder afferent pathways, causing release of nitrogen oxide from afferent neurons (9,5693). Nitrogen oxide is thought to act as a peripheral neurotransmitter controlling the lower urinary tract function (5693). Some data suggests DMSO could help antineoplastic agents cross the blood-brain barrier (6327), but other results show DMSO doesn't significantly increase uptake of these compounds (6330).

There is also evidence that suggests DMSO may induce differentiation of tumor cells present in frozen cryopreserved marrow (6328). Preliminary evidence suggests DMSO may be effective in treating duodenal ulceration in patients infected with Helicobacter pylori (6321).

Adverse Reactions

Topically, DMSO can cause sedation, headache, dizziness, drowsiness, nausea, vomiting, diarrhea, constipation, anorexia, and eosinophilia, erythema, pruritus, burning, blistering, drying and scaling skin, dry or sore throat, cough, dry nasal passages, dyspnea, worsening of bronchial asthma, and an influenza-like syndrome (6303,6304,6306,6308,6309,6311,6312,6313).

Intravenously, DMSO can cause facial flushing, fluid overload, hypernatremia, electrolyte disturbances, diuresis, increased serum osmolality, eosinophilia, hemolysis, hematuria, weakness, confusion, lethargy, disorientation, agitation, dysarthria, hypoactive reflexes, decreased consciousness, vasodilation, hypotension, chest pains, sinus tachycardia, increased serum creatinine, and encephalopathy (6300,6301,6315,6325).

Intravesical instillation of DMSO may cause a chemical cystitis, bladder discomfort, and spasm (9). Infusion of hematopoietic stem cells cryopreserved with DMSO can cause rigors, nausea, vomiting (6318), hypertension with tachycardia, bradycardia, chest tightness, fever, chills, abdominal cramps, ventricular extrasystoles (6320), electrolyte disturbances, and decreased hemoglobin (5695,5696,5697). Garlic-like taste, breath, and garlic-onion-oyster body odor may be experienced with all routes of administration. Hypersensitivity reactions may be experienced by all routes of administration, rarely causing anaphylaxis. Headache and transient eye, nose, and throat irritations have been reported by individuals caring for patients with DMSO body odor (6323).

Interactions with Herbs & Other Dietary Supplements

None known.

Interactions with Drugs

ORAL DRUGS: Evidence from animal studies suggest DMSO may potentiate the action of numerous medications (6330).
TOPICAL DRUGS: Evidence from animal studies suggest DMSO may potentiate the action of numerous medications (6330).
INJECTABLE DRUGS: Evidence from animal studies suggest DMSO may potentiate the action of numerous medications (6330).

Interactions with Foods

None known.

Interactions with Lab Tests

None known.

Interactions with Diseases or Conditions

DIABETES: Topical administration of DMSO has been reported to potentiate the effects of insulin (6326); use with caution. Increased monitoring of blood glucose and insulin dosing adjustments may be necessary.
HEMATOLOGIC CONDITIONS: Hemolysis with intravenous use has been reported (9); use with caution.
INTRACRANIAL PRESSURE: Extreme serum hyperosmolality has been reported in patients with elevated intracranial pressure who were treated with DMSO (6325).
LIVER CONDITIONS: Liver function tests are recommended every 6 months (9). Hepatotoxicity with infusion of DMSO has been reported (9); use with caution.
RENAL CONDITIONS: Renal function tests are recommended every 6 months (9). Acute tubular necrosis has been reported (9); use with caution.

Dosage and Administration

ORAL: For symptoms of amyloidosis, 7-15 grams of DMSO daily has been used (6304).
TOPICAL: For prevention of tissue necrosis after extravasation with antineoplastic agents, 77-90% DMSO is typically applied every 3-8 hours for 10-14 days. For acute musculoskeletal injuries and inflammation, 60-90% DMSO solution or gel is typically applied to the affected area 1-3 times daily for 1-3 weeks (6304). For osteoarthritis, 60-90% DMSO is typically applied to the affected area daily (6304). For rheumatoid arthritis, 60-90% DMSO solution is typically applied to the affected area 2-4 times daily (6304,6313). For scleroderma, 50-90% DMSO solution is typically applied to the affected area or the affected area is immersed in solution twice daily (6304). For amyloidosis, 50-100% DMSO solution is typically applied twice weekly to the affected area (6304). For amyloid-produced itching, 50-100% DMSO solution has been applied to the affected area daily (6304). For surgical flaps, 60% DMSO has been applied to the flaps every 4 hours for 10 days (6307). For herpes zoster, 5-40% idoxuridine in DMSO has been started within 48 hours after the appearance of a rash and applied every 4 hours for 4 days (6308). For neuropathic pain, 50% DMSO solution has been used 4 times daily for up to 3 weeks (6317).
INTRAVENOUS: For intracranial hypertension, a 10% solution of DMSO has been infused rapidly at a dose of 1 g/kg or a 20% DMSO solution is infused and titrated against the intracranial pressure (6300). A 28% solution of DMSO has also been used by infusing rapidly at a dose of 1.12 g/kg (6301).
INTRAVESICAL INSTILLATION: For interstitial cystitis, typically 50 mL of aqueous 50% DMSO solution is instilled into the bladder, the catheter is removed and the patient is instructed to hold the medication in the bladder for 15-20 minutes before voiding (5692). 100 mg of hydrocortisone has been added to the solution before instillation for added anti-inflammatory action in patients who do not respond favorably (5694). For chronic inflammatory bladder disease, 50 mL of aqueous 50% DMSO solution is typically instilled every 2 weeks for 3 treatments and then once every 4 weeks until symptoms decrease or patient is symptom free. Patients are usually instructed to hold in the medication for 30 minutes after instillation before voiding (5695).
NASOBILIARY CATHETER: For dissolution of bile duct stones, a mixture of 70/30 DMSO/methyl tert-butyl ether and a mixture of 26 mM ethylene diamine tetraacetic acid with 40 mM sodium deoxycholate and 30% DMSO has been infused alternatively and continuously for 2 hours via a nasobiliary catheter in the common bile duct until disappearance of stones (6315).

DODDER

Also Known As

Beggarweed, Cuscutae, Devil's Guts, Dodder of Thyme, Hellweed, Lesser Dodder, Scaldweed, Strangle Tare, Tu Si Zi, Tu Sizi.

Scientific Names

Cuscuta epithymum; Cuscuta chinensis.
Family: Convolvulaceae.

Comments

At the date of publication, there was very little scientific information available about this product. Our staff is continually analyzing the available information on natural medicines and will add data to the online version of *Natural Medicines Comprehensive Database* as it becomes available. See www.naturaldatabase.com.

DOLOMITE

Also Known As

Dolomitic Limestone.
CAUTION: See separate listings for Calcium and Magnesium.

Scientific Names

None.

People Use This For

Orally, dolomite is used as a mineral supplement of calcium and magnesium.

Safety

POSSIBLY UNSAFE ...when used orally. Dolomite supplements may contain lead; safer supplements are available (997,11719).
CHILDREN: POSSIBLY UNSAFE ...when used orally long-term due to the presence of lead in some products. Children are more sensitive to lead than adults (152).
PREGNANCY AND LACTATION: POSSIBLY UNSAFE ...when used orally (997,11719); avoid using.

Effectiveness

There is insufficient reliable information available about the effectiveness of dolomite.

Mechanism of Action

Dolomite is a type of limestone. It is rich in magnesium and calcium carbonate, and has smaller amounts of several other minerals. Dolomite can be contaminated with heavy metals such as lead (997,11719).

Adverse Reactions

Orally, some dolomite products are contaminated with heavy metals including aluminum, arsenic, lead, mercury, nickel, and others that may cause heavy metal poisoning (997,11719). Contaminated products have induced seizure activity in otherwise well-controlled patients who have seizure disorders (997). Calcium used orally can cause gastrointestinal irritation and constipation (9). Calcium carbonate can cause acid rebound (9). Large amounts of calcium carbonate can cause hypercalcemia and alkalosis (9). Magnesium can cause gastrointestinal irritation, nausea, vomiting, and diarrhea (9,15). Larger amounts may cause hypermagnesemia (9) with symptoms including thirst, hypotension, drowsiness, confusion, loss of tendon reflexes, muscle weakness, respiratory depression, cardiac arrhythmias, coma, cardiac arrest, and death (9).

Interactions with Herbs & Other Dietary Supplements

BORON: Boron can increase serum magnesium levels (940).
CALCIUM: Theoretically, concomitant use with other calcium containing supplements can cause constipation.
MAGNESIUM: Theoretically, concomitant use with other magnesium containing supplements can cause diarrhea.
VITAMIN D: Concomitant use can increase active absorption of oral calcium (945).

Interactions with Drugs

BISPHOSPHONATES: Cations, including calcium and magnesium decrease absorption of bisphosphonates. Advise patients to take bisphosphonates at least 30 minutes before dolomite, but preferably at a different time of day (15). The bisphosphonates include alendronate (Fosamax), etidronate (Didronel), risedronate (Actonel), and tiludronate (Skelid).

ESTROGENS: Concomitant use of estrogen increases calcium absorption in postmenopausal women (995).

LEVOTHYROXINE (Synthroid, Levothroid, Levoxyl, and others): The calcium in dolomite reduces levothyroxine absorption, probably by forming insoluble complexes (5082). Calcium carbonate supplements reduce effectiveness of levothyroxine in patients with hypothyroid (5081,5082,6137). Advise patients to take levothyroxine and dolomite at least four hours apart.

POTASSIUM-SPARING DIURETICS: Potassium-sparing diuretics also have magnesium-sparing properties, which can counteract the magnesium losses associated with loop and thiazide diuretics (9613,9614,9622). Theoretically, dolomite might cause increased magnesium levels with concomitant use of potassium-sparing diuretics. Potassium-sparing diuretics include amiloride (Midamor), triamterene (Dyrenium), and spironolactone (Aldactone).

QUINOLONE ANTIBIOTICS: Taking dolomite at the same time as quinolones reduces quinolone absorption. Multivalent cations such as calcium and magnesium form insoluble complexes with quinolones (4412,10339). Advise patients to take these drugs at least 2 hours before, or four to six hours after dolomite (10339). Quinolones include ciprofloxacin (Cipro), levofloxacin (Levaquin), ofloxacin (Floxin), moxifloxacin (Avelox), gatifloxacin (Tequin), gemifloxacin (Factive), and others.

SOTALOL (Betapace): The calcium in dolomite appears to reduce the absorption of sotalol, probably by forming insoluble complexes (10018). Advise patients to separate doses by at least 2 hours before or four to six hours after dolomite.

TETRACYCLINE ANTIBIOTICS: Multivalent cations such as calcium and magnesium decrease the absorption of tetracyclines by forming insoluble complexes (9). Advise patients to take these drugs at least two hours before, or four to six hours after dolomite. Tetracyclines include demeclocycline (Declomycin), doxycycline (Vibramycin), and minocycline (Minocin).

THIAZIDE DIURETICS: Thiazides reduce calcium excretion by the kidneys (1902). Using thiazides along with moderately large amounts of dolomite increases the risk of milk-alkali syndrome (hypercalcemia, metabolic alkalosis, renal failure). These diuretics include chlorothiazide (Diuril), hydrochlorothiazide (HydroDIURIL, Esidrix), indapamide (Lozol), metolazone (Zaroxolyn), chlorthalidone (Hygroton), etc.

Drug Influences on Nutrient Levels and Depletion

SOME DRUGS CAN AFFECT DOLOMITE LEVELS:

CORTICOSTEROIDS: Corticosteroid use can decrease calcium absorption from dolomite and increase calcium excretion (15).

Interactions with Foods

DIETARY FIBER: Certain constituents of dietary fiber inhibit calcium absorption, including uronic acid and phytic acid, which is found in wheat bran (945).

FOOD: Concomitant ingestion with food, and food high in vitamin D, increases absorption of supplemental calcium (945).

IRON: Calcium carbonate taken with iron supplements and food might decrease supplemental iron absorption. Calcium carbonate taken with iron supplements on an empty stomach appears to have little effect on supplemental iron absorption (945).

Interactions with Lab Tests

ALKALINE PHOSPHATASE: The magnesium component might cause a false increase in serum alkaline phosphatase test results due to enzyme activation (275).

ANGIOTENSIN-CONVERTING ENZYME: The magnesium component might decrease serum ACE levels and test results (275).

CALCIUM: The magnesium component might cause a false increase in serum calcium test results in some procedures using edetate disodium (EDTA) (275).

DIAGNEX BLUE: The magnesium component might increase urine Diagnex blue excretion due to heavy metal displacement of Diagnex blue (275).

GASTRIN: The calcium component might cause a physiological increase in serum levels 30-75 minutes after using (275).

LIPASE: The calcium component might cause an analytical decrease in serum concentrations above 5 mmol/L on method of Tietz (275).

Interactions with Diseases or Conditions

HEART BLOCK: Magnesium is contraindicated in people with heart block (9).
HYPERPARATHYROIDISM: Primary hyperparathyroidism predisposes individuals to increased calcium absorption (945).
HYPOPARATHYROIDISM: Hypoparathyroidism redisposes individuals to reduced calcium absorption (945).
RENAL INSUFFICIENCY: Magnesium is contraindicated in people with severe renal disease. Use cautiously in individuals with reduced kidney function due to increased risk of hypermagnesemia (9). Calcium supplementation increases the risk of hypercalcemia and alkalosis in people with renal disease (9). Renal insufficiency predisposes individuals to reduced calcium absorption (945).
SARCOIDOSIS: Increases the risk of excessive calcium absorption and hypercalcemia (945).

Dosage and Administration

No typical dosage.

DONG QUAI

Also Known As

Angelicae gigantis radix, Chinese Angelica, Dang Gui, Ligustilides, Phytoestrogen, Radix angelicae gigantis, Tan Kue Bai Zhi, Tang Kuei.
CAUTION: See separate listing for Angelica.

Scientific Names

Angelica sinensis, synonym Angelica polymorpha var. sinensis.
Family: Apiaceae/Umbelliferae.

People Use This For

Orally, dong quai is used for dysmenorrhea, premenstrual syndrome (PMS), and symptoms of menopause. It is also used orally as a "blood purifier"; to manage hypertension, rheumatism, ulcers, anemia, and constipation; and in the prevention and treatment of allergic attacks. Dong quai is also used orally is for the treatment of skin depigmentation and psoriasis.
Topically, dong quai is used as part of a multi-ingredient preparation for treating premature ejaculation.

Safety

POSSIBLY SAFE ...when used orally and appropriately (10054). ...when used topically, short-term as part of a multi-ingredient preparation (SS Cream). This preparation was used safely for premature ejaculation in a clinical trial where the cream was applied and left on the glans penis for 1-hour (2537). More evidence is needed to determine its safety after prolonged, repetitive use.
POSSIBLY UNSAFE ...when used orally in large amounts. Dong quai contains several constituents that are carcinogenic (7162).
PREGNANCY: UNSAFE ...when used orally due to uterine stimulant and relaxant effects (8142).
LACTATION: Insufficient reliable information available; avoid using.

Effectiveness

POSSIBLY EFFECTIVE

Premature ejaculation. In one controlled clinical trial, a multi-ingredient cream preparation containing Panax ginseng root, dong quai, Cistanches deserticola, Zanthoxyl species, Torlidis seed, clove flower, Asiasari root, cinnamon bark, and toad venom (SS Cream) was applied to the glans penis 1-hour prior to intercourse and washed off immediately before intercourse. Men suffering from premature ejaculation who were treated with the cream had significantly improved ejaculatory latency compared to placebo (2537).

POSSIBLY INEFFECTIVE

Menopausal symptoms. Dong quai does not seem to have any effect on endometrial wall thickness or menopausal symptoms (738).

There is insufficient reliable information available about the effectiveness of dong quai for its other uses.

Mechanism of Action

The applicable part of dong quai is the root. Dong quai root has several coumarin constituents including osthol, psoralen, and bergapten, and contains 0.4% to 0.7% volatile oil (10054). Some coumarins can act as vasodilators and antispasmodics. Osthol appears to inhibit platelet aggregation and smooth muscle contraction, and cause hypotension (10057). Psoralen and bergapten are photosensitizing and can cause severe photodermatitis (10057). Bergapten and other dong quai constituents, such as safrole and isosafrole, are carcinogenic (7162). Dong quai also contains a low molecular weight polysaccharide that shows anti-tumor activity in animals (10056).
Limited research suggests that dong quai does not have estrogenic effects and therefore is not a phytoestrogen (738).

However, other research suggests estrogenic effects (6180). Dong quai might stimulate the growth of breast cancer cells (7860,10979).
A dong quai extract competitively inhibits estradiol binding to estrogen receptors and induces transcription activity in estrogen-responsive cells (6180).
Preliminary research suggests dong quai might protect against ischemia-reperfusion injury (9985).
A multi-ingredient preparation containing dong quai is thought to work in premature ejaculation by increasing the penile vibratory threshold and reducing the amplitude of penile somatosensory evoked potentials (2537).

Adverse Reactions

Orally, dong quai is well-tolerated (738). Dong quai contains constituents that are carcinogenic (7162). Whether these constituents are present in concentrations large enough to cause cancer with long-term or high-dose use is unknown. Dong quai also contains psoralens that may cause photosensitivity and photodermatitis (10054).

Interactions with Herbs & Other Dietary Supplements

HERBS WITH ANTICOAGULANT/ANTIPLATELET POTENTIAL: Concomitant use of herbs that have antiplatelet/anticoagulant effects could theoretically increase the risk of bleeding in some people (3526). These herbs include angelica, clove, danshen, garlic, ginger, ginkgo, panax ginseng, poplar, red clover, willow, and others.

Interactions with Drugs

ANTICOAGULANT/ANTIPLATELET DRUGS: Theoretically, dong quai might potentiate the therapeutic and adverse effects of these drugs. Dong quai has been reported to inhibit platelet aggregation (6048).
WARFARIN (Coumadin): Concomitant use increases the anticoagulant effects of warfarin and the risk of bleeding (3526,6048). In one case, after 4 weeks of dong quai 565 mg once or twice daily, INR increased to 4.9. INR normalized 4 weeks after discontinuation of dong quai. Dong quai is thought to inhibit platelet activation and aggregation (6048).

Interactions with Foods

None known.

Interactions with Lab Tests

PROTHROMBIN TIME (PT), INTERNATIONAL NORMALIZATION RATIO (INR): Dong quai can enhance the effects of warfarin, resulting in increased PT and INR test results (3526).

Interactions with Diseases or Conditions

HORMONE SENSITIVE CANCERS/CONDITIONS: Because dong quai has estrogenic effects, women with hormone sensitive conditions including breast cancer, uterine cancer, ovarian cancer, endometriosis, and uterine fibroids should avoid using dong quai (6180,7860).

Dosage and Administration

ORAL: For menopausal symptoms, 4.5 g of powdered Dong Quai root has been used daily (738).

DRAGON'S BLOOD

Also Known As

Draconis Resina, Dracorubin, Dragon's-Blood Palm, Dragons Blood, Sanguis Draconis, Xue Jie.
CAUTION: See separate listings for Herb Robert and Sangre de Grado.

Scientific Names

Daemonorops draco, synonym Calamus draco.
Family: Arecaceae/Palmae.

People Use This For

Orally, dragon's blood is used for diarrhea, digestive disorders and as a coloring agent.
Topically, dragon's blood is used as an astringent.

Safety

POSSIBLY SAFE ...when used orally (12).
There is insufficient reliable information available about the safety of dragon's blood for its other uses.
PREGNANCY AND LACTATION: Insufficient reliable information available; avoid using.

Effectiveness

There is insufficient reliable information available about the effectiveness of dragon's blood.

Mechanism of Action
The applicable part of dragon's blood is the fruit. There is insufficient reliable information available about the possible mechanism of action and active ingredients.

Adverse Reactions
None reported.

Interactions with Herbs & Other Dietary Supplements
None known.

Interactions with Drugs
None known.

Interactions with Foods
None known.

Interactions with Lab Tests
None known.

Interactions with Diseases or Conditions
None known.

Dosage and Administration
ORAL: Dragon's blood has been used as a powder (18).
TOPICAL: No typical dosage.

Comments
Dragon's blood is the red resin extracted from the fruit of Daemonorops draco (18).

DUCKWEED

Also Known As
None.

Scientific Names
Lemna minor.
Family: Lemnaceae.

Comments
At the date of publication, there was very little scientific information available about this product. Our staff is continually analyzing the available information on natural medicines and will add data to the online version of *Natural Medicines Comprehensive Database* as it becomes available. See www.naturaldatabase.com.

DUSTY MILLER

Also Known As
Silver Ragwort.

Scientific Names
Senecio cineraria, synonym Cineraria maritima.
Family: Asteraceae/Compositae.

People Use This For
Orally, dusty miller is used in preparations for eyesight problems (spots before the eyes), migraine, and to promote menstrual flow.
Topically, dusty miller is used as an eye wash for cataracts and blurred vision.

Safety

LIKELY UNSAFE ...when products containing hepatotoxic pyrrolizidine alkaloid (PA) constituents are used orally. Repeated exposure to low concentrations of hepatotoxic PAs can cause severe veno-occlusive disease. Hepatotoxic PAs might also be carcinogenic and mutagenic (12841,12842). Tell patients not to use dusty miller preparations that are not certified and labeled as hepatotoxic PA-free. ...when products containing hepatotoxic PAs are used topically on abraded or broken skin. Absorption of hepatotoxic PAs through broken skin can lead to systemic toxicities (12841). Tell patients not to use topical dusty miller preparations that are not certified and labeled as hepatotoxic PA-free. There is insufficient reliable information available about the safety of topical PA-free dusty miller on unbroken skin.
PREGNANCY: LIKELY UNSAFE ...when used orally. Dusty miller preparations containing hepatotoxic pyrrolizidine alkaloid (PA) constituents might be teratogenic and hepatotoxic (12841,12842). There is insufficient reliable information available about the safety of dusty miller products that do not contain hepatotoxic PAs when used during pregnancy.
LACTATION: LIKELY UNSAFE ...when used orally. Hepatotoxic pyrrolizidine alkaloid (PA) constituents in dusty miller are excreted in milk (12841,12842). There is insufficient reliable information available about the safety of dusty miller products that do not contain hepatotoxic PAs when used during lactation.

Effectiveness

There is insufficient reliable information available about the effectiveness of dusty miller.

Mechanism of Action

The applicable parts are the above ground parts. Dusty miller contains various pyrrolizidine alkaloids (PA), some of which are toxic. PAs are most concentrated in the plant roots, but may be found in all plant parts. PAs, particularly unsaturated PAs, can cause hepatotoxicity. Cyclic diesters such as retrorsine and senecionine are the most hepatotoxic. Liver toxicity may result from PA-enhanced oxidative stress, but the exact mechanism of toxicity is unknown. Single doses of 10-20 mg PAs or chronic ingestion of amounts less than 10 mcg can cause veno-occlusive disease. PAs are metabolized by cytochrome P450 3A4 (CYP3A4) to toxic dehydroalkaloids and pyrroles. Enzyme inducers such as phenobarbital seem to enhance toxicity (12841,12860). Pyrroles are excreted as N-acetyl cysteine conjugates. Some researchers speculate that early administration of N-acetylcysteine might reduce toxicity (11988). Metabolism is also affected by pregnane X receptor induction of CYP3A4. Genetic or drug induced variation in CYP3A4 or pregnane X receptor activity can affect the degree of PA toxicity by increasing or decreasing its metabolism (12841,12842). Hepatotoxic PAs are also toxic to the lungs. In animals, pneumotoxicity occurs as pulmonary hypertension and right ventricular hypertrophy. Hepatotoxic PAs are carcinogenic and mutagenic. There are sufficient amounts of hepatotoxic PAs in herbal products to cause toxicity (12841,12842).

Adverse Reactions

Orally, the major concern about dusty miller preparations is the hepatotoxic pyrrolizidine alkaloid (PA) content. These constituents are hepatotoxic, pneumotoxic, carcinogenic and mutagenic (12386,12841,12842). Chronic exposure to other plants containing hepatotoxic PA constituents is associated with veno-occlusive disease (4021). Subacute veno-occlusive disease causes vague symptoms with persistent liver enlargement (4021). Symptoms of acute veno-occlusive disease include colicky pains in epigastrium, vomiting and diarrhea, and ascites formation within several days. Enlargement and induration of the liver occurs within a few weeks (12842).
Dusty miller may cause an allergic reaction in individuals sensitive to the Asteraceae/Compositae family. Members of this family include ragweed, chrysanthemums, marigolds, daisies, and many other herbs.

Interactions with Herbs & Other Dietary Supplements

HEPATOTOXIC PYRROLIZIDINE ALKALOID (PA)-CONTAINING HERBS: Concomitant use is contraindicated due to the risk of additive toxicity. Herbs containing hepatotoxic PAs include alkanna, borage, butterbur, coltsfoot, comfrey, gravel root, groundsel, hemp agrimony, hound's tongue, and lungwort; and the Senecio species plants ragwort, groundsel, golden ragwort, and tansy ragwort (12841).
HERBS THAT INDUCE CYTOCHROME P450 3A4 (CYP3A4): Theoretically, herbs that induce CYP3A4 might increase the conversion of hepatotoxic PAs to toxic metabolites, enhancing toxicity (12841,12860). Herbs that induce CYP3A4 include St. John's wort and garlic.

Interactions with Drugs

CYTOCHROME P450 3A4 (CYP3A4) INDUCERS: Hepatotoxic pyrrolizidine alkaloids (PA) are substrates of cytochrome P450 3A4 (CYP3A4) (12841,12860). Theoretically, drugs that induce CYP3A4 might increase the conversion of PAs to toxic metabolites. Some drugs that induce CYP3A4 include carbamazepine (Tegretol), phenobarbital, phenytoin (Dilantin), rifampin, rifabutin (Mycobutin), and others.

Interactions with Foods

None known.

Interactions with Lab Tests

None known.

Interactions with Diseases or Conditions

CROSS-ALLERGENICITY: Dusty miller may cause an allergic reaction in individuals sensitive to the Asteraceae/Compositae family. Members of this family include ragweed, chrysanthemums, marigolds, daisies, and many other herbs.
LIVER DISEASE: Theoretically, pyrrolizidine alkaloids (PA) might exacerbate liver disease (12841,12842).

Dosage and Administration

No typical dosage.

Comments

None

DWARF ELDER

Also Known As

Blood Elder, Blood Hilder, Danewort, Walewort.
CAUTION: See separate listings for American Elder, Elderberry, and Elderflower.

Scientific Names

Sambucus ebulus.
Family: Adoxaceae/Sambucaceae or Caprifoliaceae.

People Use This For

Orally, dwarf elder is used for arthritis, weight reduction, and as a diuretic.

Safety

LIKELY UNSAFE ...when large quantities of any part of the plant are used orally. It can cause loss of consciousness and death (18).
There is insufficient reliable information available about the safety of the oral use of dwarf elder in small amounts.
PREGNANCY AND LACTATION: LIKELY UNSAFE ...when used orally in large quantities (18).

Effectiveness

There is insufficient reliable information available about the effectiveness of dwarf elder.

Mechanism of Action

Dwarf elder contains iridoide monoterpene glycosides. The constituents that cause nausea or purgative effects have not been identified (18).

Adverse Reactions

Orally, ingestion of large quantities of any plant part of dwarf elder may cause vomiting, bloody diarrhea, cyanosis, dizziness, headache and unconsciousness. Death has been reported (18). Cyanide poisoning can be caused by any plant part of dwarf elder. Sambunigrine, a cyanogenic glycoside, is present in the plant.

Interactions with Herbs & Other Dietary Supplements

None known.

Interactions with Drugs

None known.

Interactions with Foods

None known.

Interactions with Lab Tests

None known.

Interactions with Diseases or Conditions

None known.

Dosage and Administration

No typical dosage.

Comments

Dwarf elder is considered unsafe; avoid using. Dwarf elder is considered obsolete as a medicinal herb in many countries (18). Avoid confusion with Elderberry and American Elder, which are also members of the Sambucus genus (6002).

DWARF PINE NEEDLE

Also Known As

None.
CAUTION: See separate listings for Fir, Pine, and Poplar.

Scientific Names

Pinus mugo, synonym Pinus montana; Pinus mugo var. pumilio, synonym Pinus pumilio.
Family: Pinaceae.

People Use This For

Orally, dwarf pine needle is used as an expectorant.
Topically, dwarf pine needle is used in liniments and as an antiseptic.
In foods and beverages, dwarf pine needle is used as a flavoring agent.
In other manufacturing processes, dwarf pine needle is used as a flavoring and fragrance component in pharmaceutical preparations (cough and cold medicines, vaporizer fluids, nasal decongestants, analgesic ointments), and as a fragrance ingredient in soaps and cosmetics (maximum use level 1.2% in perfumes).

Safety

LIKELY SAFE ...when used orally in amounts commonly found in foods. Dwarf pine needle has Generally Recognized As Safe status (GRAS) for use in foods in the US (4912).
POSSIBLY SAFE ...when used topically. There is possible human skin irritation and demonstrated sensitizing in some individuals (11).
PREGNANCY AND LACTATION: Insufficient reliable information available; avoid using.

Effectiveness

There is insufficient reliable information available about the effectiveness of dwarf pine needle.

Mechanism of Action

The applicable part of dwarf pine needle is the oil. Constituents bornyl acetate, dipentene, and limonene are believed to have antibacterial and antiviral properties (11).

Adverse Reactions

Topically, dwarf pine needle can cause skin irritation (11). It also may be sensitizing in some individuals (11).

Interactions with Herbs & Other Dietary Supplements

None known.

Interactions with Drugs

None known.

Interactions with Foods

None known.

Interactions with Lab Tests

None known.

Interactions with Diseases or Conditions

ALLERGY: Avoid dwarf pine needle if allergic or sensitive to pine oil.

Dosage and Administration

No typical dosage.

Comments

Dwarf pine needle oil is produced by distillation of dwarf pine (Pinus mugo) needles and twigs. Avoid confusion with fir needle oil and scotch pine needle oil.

DYER'S BROOM

Also Known As

Broom Flower, Dyers Broom, Dyer's Greenwood, Dyer's Weed, Dyer's Whin, Furze, Green Broom, Greenweed, Wood Waxen.

Scientific Names

Genista tinctoria.
Family: Leguminosae or Fabaceae.

People Use This For

Orally, dyer's broom is used for digestive disorders, gout, as an emetic or purgative, and to remove bladder stones. It is also used orally to "detoxify" blood, to increase heart rate, strengthen blood vessels, stimulate blood flow to the kidneys, and to alter metabolism. It has been used to deepen breathing and alleviate pain in the lower back and pelvis.

Safety

POSSIBLY UNSAFE ...when above ground parts are used orally (12).
PREGNANCY: LIKELY UNSAFE ...when used orally because it could have uterine-stimulant activity (12).
LACTATION: POSSIBLY UNSAFE ...when used orally; avoid using.

Effectiveness

There is insufficient reliable information available about the effectiveness of dyer's broom.

Mechanism of Action

Dyer's broom contains quinolizidine alkaloids, including methylcytisine, anagyrine, isopsparteine, lupanine, tinctorin, and cysisine. It also contains flavonoids (including luteolin glycosides), isoflavonoids (including genistein and genistin), and lectins (18).

Adverse Reactions

Orally, dyer's broom may cause nausea and vomiting. Overuse of dyer's broom can lead to diarrhea (18).

Interactions with Herbs & Other Dietary Supplements

None known.

Interactions with Drugs

None known.

Interactions with Foods

None known.

Interactions with Lab Tests

None known.

Interactions with Diseases or Conditions

None known.

Dosage and Administration

No typical dosage.

ECDYSTERONE

Also Known As

Alfa-ecdysone, Beta-ecdysone, Ecdisten, Ecdysone, Hydroxyecdysterone, Isoinokosterone, Suma.
CAUTION: See separate listing for Suma.

Scientific Names

None.

People Use This For

Orally, ecdysterone is used to increase muscle mass and improve athletic performance.

Safety
There is insufficient reliable information available about the safety of ecdysterone.
Pregnancy and Lactation: Insufficient reliable information available.

Effectiveness
There is insufficient reliable information available about the effectiveness of ecdysterone.

Mechanism of Action
Ecdysterone is a chemical found in insects, some aquatic animals, and some plants. In insects and arthropods, ecdysterone promotes the act of molting (9903,10389).
Ecdysterone is chemically similar to testosterone, which has lead to the belief that it might possess anabolic properties. Animal research suggests that ecdysterone affects steroid receptors. It is unclear whether this effect is mediated by receptor or feedback loop regulation rather than bioconversion into steroids. Possible mechanisms include anticatabolic effects from blocking cortisol receptors and stimulation of anabolic or androgenic steroid receptors (9904,9905,10390). However, there is no research in humans demonstrating androgenic or myotrophic effect.
After oral administration, ecdysterone and its metabolites appear in the urine for approximately 68 hours. The primary metabolites are deoxyecdysterone and deoxyecdysone (9903).

Adverse Reactions
None reported.

Interactions with Herbs & Other Dietary Supplements
None known.

Interactions with Drugs
None known.

Interactions with Foods
None known.

Interactions with Lab Tests
None known.

Interactions with Diseases or Conditions
None known.

Dosage and Administration
No typical dosage.

ECHINACEA

Also Known As
American Cone Flower, Black Sampson, Black Susans, Brauneria Angustifolia, Brauneria Pallida, Comb Flower, Coneflower, Echinaceawurzel, Hedgehog, Igelkopfwurzel, Indian Head, Kansas Snakeroot, Narrow-leaved Purple Cone Flower, Pale Coneflower, Purple Cone Flower, Purpursonnenhutkraut, Purpursonnenhutwurzel, Racine d'echininacea, Red Sunflower, Rock-Up-Hat, Roter Sonnenhut, Schmallblaettrige Kegelblumenwurzel, Schmallblaettriger Sonnenhut, Scurvy Root, Snakeroot, Sonnenhutwurzel.

Scientific Names
Echinacea angustifolia; Echinacea pallida; Echinacea purpurea.
Family: Asteraceae/Compositae.

People Use This For
Orally, echinacea is used for treating and preventing the common cold and other upper respiratory infections. Echinacea is also used orally as an immunostimulant for fighting a variety of other infections, including urinary tract infections (UTIs), vaginal candidiasis (yeast infections), and genital herpes (HSV Type 1 and 2). Echinacea is also used orally for septicemia, nasopharyngeal catarrh, allergic rhinitis, pyorrhea, tonsillitis, streptococcus infections, syphilis, typhoid, malaria, and diphtheria. Other uses include rheumatism, migraines, dyspepsia, pain, dizziness, rattlesnake bites, and attention deficit-hyperactivity disorder (ADHD).
Topically, echinacea is used for boils, abscesses, skin wounds and ulcers, eczema, psoriasis, UV radiation skin damage, herpes simplex, bee stings, and hemorrhoids.

Intravenously, echinacea is used for recurrent vaginal candidiasis (yeast infections), and urinary tract infections (UTIs).
Intravenously and intramuscularly, echinacea is used to prolong survival time in patients with advanced hepatocellular carcinoma and colorectal cancer.

Safety

LIKELY SAFE ...when used orally and appropriately, short-term. Several formulations of echinacea have been used safely in trials lasting up to 12 weeks (1412,3279,3280,3281,3282,6417).
CHILDREN: POSSIBLY SAFE ...when used orally, short-term. There is some evidence that an Echinacea purpurea juice extract is safe in children aged 2-11 years when used for up to 10 days. However, echinacea might increase the risk of rash in some children (4989).
PREGNANCY: POSSIBLY SAFE ...when used orally, short-term. There is some evidence that mothers can safely use echinacea for 5-7 days during the first trimester of pregnancy without adversely affecting the fetus (7056). However, this evidence is preliminary. Tell pregnant patients not to use echinacea without the supervision of their healthcare provider.
LACTATION: Insufficient reliable information available; avoid using.

Effectiveness

POSSIBLY EFFECTIVE

Common cold. Taking echinacea orally might help reduce symptoms of the common cold in adults.
The majority of evidence suggests that echinacea modestly reduces symptom severity and duration by about 10% to 30% (1412,3281,6384,6385,6392,6417,10782,10802,12355). However, some studies show no benefit in adults (3282,10800,11970). Another study suggests that taking an Echinacea purpurea juice extract 7.5-10 mL/day to (Madaus AG, Germany) for up to 10 days does not decrease cold symptoms in children aged 2-11 years (4989).
Tell patients who try echinacea that it seems to be most effective if started when symptoms are first noticed and continued for 7-10 days. Explain to patients that echinacea does not seem to help when taken prophylactically to prevent the common cold (3281,3282,6386,6417,8228,10782,12354).
Most studies have used Echinacea purpurea species, but several other preparations have also been used including extracts of the herb, combination root and herb extracts, extracts of the root, as well as root extracts of Echinacea pallida and Echinacea angustifolia (1412,3280,3281,6417,8226). Echinacea teas and fixed combination herbal preparations containing echinacea have also been used (3281,6384,6392). Echinacea is inherently hard to study. The active constituent(s) has not been identified, so products are not standardized. Echinacea has a distinctively unpleasant taste, which makes blinding difficult (10800,12637).

Vaginal candidiasis. Taking echinacea orally in combination with a topical antifungal cream seems to be effective for preventing recurrent vaginal yeast infection. Herb juice of Echinacea purpurea in combination with topical econazole (Spectazole) lowers recurrence rate to 16.7% compared to 60.5% with econazole alone (13001).

POSSIBLY INEFFECTIVE

Herpes simplex virus (HSV). Taking echinacea orally doesn't seem to prevent or treat recurrent genital herpes infection. A specific Echinacea purpurea extract (Echinaforce by Bioforce AG) 800 mg twice daily for six months does not seem to prevent or reduce frequency or duration of recurrent genital herpes in patients with herpes simplex virus (HSV) type 1 or 2 (7087).
Clinical studies have used a wide variety of specific extracts and dosage forms of echinacea. Some of these include a Echinacea purpurea 95% herb and 5% root extract (Echinaforce, Bioforce); a fixed combination of Echinacea purpurea plus cedar and wild indigo extracts (Esberitox N, Enzymatic Therapy); and a tea containing a blend of Echinacea purpurea and Echinacea angustifolia leaves, stems, and flowers plus a dry extract of Echinacea purpurea root (Echinacea Plus, Traditional Medicinals).

INSUFFICIENT RELIABLE EVIDENCE to RATE

Influenza. Taking echinacea orally might modestly reduce some influenza symptoms. However, there is not enough specific evidence to know if echinacea is effective for influenza (3281,6384,6385,6386).
Leukopenia. An isolated polysaccharide fraction of Echinacea purpurea given intravenously might reduce leukopenia caused by chemotherapy (8523).
More evidence is needed to rate echinacea for these uses.

Mechanism of Action

The applicable parts of echinacea are the roots and the above ground parts. Echinacea is used for upper respiratory tract infections such as the common cold and influenza infections because it is reported to have antiviral and immune system stimulatory effects (3279). Echinacea increases phagocytosis and increases lymphocyte activity, possibly by promoting the release of tumor necrosis factor (TNF), interleukin-1 (IL-1), and interferon (3279,6388,6389). Several constituents of echinacea seem to be involved in stimulating this non-specific immune response. Some of these include high-molecular weight polysaccharides, such as heteroxylan and arabinogalactan; and lower molecular weight compounds, including alkylamides and caffeoyl conjugates such as chicoric acid and echinacosides (3279). Heteroxylan might activate phagocytosis, and arabinogalactan seems to induce macrophages to produce the cytokines TNF, IL-1, and interferon beta-2 (3279). Macrophages activated by arabinogalactan have been found to be cytotoxic against tumor cells and micro-organisms (6388). The chicoric acid and echinacosides constituents are thought to also play a role in enhancing phagocytosis (3279). Polysaccharides in echinacea also seem to have moderate effects on B-lymphocytes, but no apparent activity on T-lymphocytes (6389). However, echinacea doesn't seem to have any effect on the immune system of healthy volunteers (10797). Some researchers suggest that when echinacea is used for greater than eight weeks, the immunostimulatory effects might decline, making it less effective (6417,6418). To prevent this decline in activity, it is often recommended that a one-week drug holiday be taken after each eight-week treatment period (6418). However, there is no reliable evidence to support either of these claims.

Echinacea's effect on cold symptoms might result from anti-inflammatory activity. In vitro research suggests constituents of echinacea might inhibit cyclooxygenase and 5-lipogenase (10798,10799). Clinical research also suggests and anti-inflammatory effect. Serum ferritin, which appears to be an indicator of inflammatory cytokines, is lowered in people treated with echinacea (10797).

Echinacea is also reported to have antifungal properties, so people use it for yeast infections (vaginal candidiasis). Polyacetylenic compounds in echinacea, including ketoalkenes and ketoalkynes, seem to have antifungal activity, including activity against Candida yeast (6390).

For wound healing, echinacea seems to promote the formation of mesenchymal mucopolysaccharides, stimulate histogenic and hematogenic phagocytes, promote differentiation of fibrocytes from fibroblasts; and it also stimulates the anterior pituitary-adrenal cortex (11). Several conjugates isolated from echinacea have also been reported to inhibit tissue, and bacterial hyaluronidase and have anti-inflammatory activity (3279). The constituent echinacin has also been found to promote tissue granulation (3279). Preliminary information suggests that the caffeoyl constituents of echinacea might help treat or prevent UV radiation skin damage by protecting collagen from free radical damage (8227).

Preliminary research also suggests that high concentrations of Echinacea purpurea might reduce sperm and ova fertility (4239,4240). Initial research also shows that very high doses of echinacea do not seem to have genotoxic or carcinogenic effects (1413).

Adverse Reactions

Orally, echinacea is usually well-tolerated by most people (1412,3279,3280,3282,6387,11970). Some side effects that have been reported include allergic reactions, fever, nausea, vomiting, heartburn, constipation, abdominal pain, diarrhea, unpleasant taste, dry mouth, sore throat, tingling sensation and numbness of the tongue, mouth ulcers, headache, dizziness, insomnia, and disorientation (8225,11970,12354,12355).

Allergic reactions can include urticaria; erythema nodosum (7057); itchy, watery eyes; runny nose (8225); chest tightness; dyspnea; bronchospasm; acute asthma; facial and upper airway angioedema; and anaphylaxis (638,1358,8225).

In a study of children aged 2-11 years, about 7% of children experienced a rash after taking echinacea, which might have been caused by an allergic reaction (4989).

Allergic reactions seem to be uncommon, but some people are more likely to be sensitive. For example, atopic individuals, people with a genetic tendency toward allergic conditions, are at increased risk for allergic reactions to echinacea (1358,8225).

Individuals sensitive to the Asteraceae/Compositae plant family might also be more likely to experience an allergic reaction to echinacea (8225). Members of this family include ragweed, chrysanthemums, marigolds, daisies, and many other herbs.

Sjogren's syndrome has occurred in a patient taking herbal supplements including echinacea, St. John's wort, and kava. Laboratory, but not clinical, research suggests that echinacea has immunostimulant effects. Because Sjogren's syndrome is an autoimmune disorder, echinacea was suspected as the causative agent. However, the role of echinacea and the other herbal products in developing this syndrome is unclear (10319).

There is some preliminary evidence that suggests that high doses of echinacea might reduce male and female fertility (4239,4240). However, this effect has not yet been demonstrated in humans.

Parenterally, echinacea has been associated with shivering, muscle weakness, and slight reddening with transient pain at the injection site (6387).

Interactions with Herbs & Other Dietary Supplements

None known.

Interactions with Drugs

CYTOCHROME P450 3A4 (CYP3A4) SUBSTRATES: There's preliminary evidence that suggests that echinacea can inhibit the cytochrome P450 3A4 (CYP3A4) isoenzymes (6450,12155). Theoretically, echinacea might increase levels of drugs metabolized by CYP3A4. However, so far, this interaction has not been reported in humans. Some drugs metabolized by CYP3A4 include lovastatin (Mevacor), ketoconazole (Nizoral), itraconazole (Sporanox), fexofenadine (Allegra), triazolam (Halcion), and numerous others. Use echinacea cautiously or avoid in patients taking these drugs.

IMMUNOSUPPRESSANTS: Theoretically, echinacea may interfere with immunosuppressant therapy (3279) because of its immunostimulating activity. Echinacea stimulates phagocytosis and increases respiratory cellular activity and the mobility of leukocytes. Immunosuppressant drugs include azathioprine (Imuran), basiliximab (Simulect), cyclosporine (Neoral, Sandimmune), daclizumab (Zenapax), muromonab-CD3 (OKT3, Orthoclone OKT3), mycophenolate (CellCept), tacrolimus (FK506, Prograf), sirolimus (Rapamune), prednisone (Deltasone,

Orasone), and other corticosteroids (glucocorticoids).
MIDAZOLAM (Versed): Taking midazolam and echinacea together seems to increase midazolam availability. This suggests that echinacea inhibits cytochrome P450 3A4 (CYP3A4) (12155).

Interactions with Foods

None known.

Interactions with Lab Tests

None known.

Interactions with Diseases or Conditions

ATOPY: Individuals with atopy (a genetic tendency toward allergic conditions) may be more likely to experience an allergic reaction when taking echinacea. Case reports describe 23 cases of allergic reactions to echinacea consistent with IgE mediated hypersensitivity. Thirty-four percent of the reactions were in patients with atopy (1358). In a related study, 20% of 100 atopic patients tested who had never taken echinacea had positive skin test reactions to echinacea, indicating hypersensitivity without previous exposure (1358,8225).
PEMPHIGUS VULGARIS: In one case, a patient with well-controlled pemphigus vulgaris took echinacea and within 1 week developed a disease flare including blisters on his trunk, head, and oral mucosa. When echinacea was discontinued, symptoms decreased, but did not entirely resolve (12171). The immunostimulatory effects of echinacea are thought to exacerbate this and other autoimmune disorders.

Dosage and Administration

ORAL: For treatment of upper respiratory infections including the common cold and influenza, a wide variety of doses have been used depending on the formulation. A tablet containing 6.78 mg of Echinacea purpurea crude extract based on 95% herb and 5% root (Echinaforce, Bioforce AG) is dosed as two tablets given 3 times daily (1412). Freeze-dried echinacea juice extract capsules 100 mg three times daily have been used (11970). Echinacea purpurea herb juice has been used in a daily dose of 6-9 mL for up to a maximum of 8 weeks (3282). Echinacea purpurea herb juice has also been used in a dose of 20 drops every 2 hours for the first day followed by 20 drops three times daily until symptoms resolve. An echinacea pallida root tincture, equivalent to 900 mg herb daily, has also been used (3281). An echinacea herbal compound tea (Echinacea Plus, Traditional Medicinals), consisting of leaves, flowers, and stems of Echinacea purpurea and Echinacea angustifolia plus dried extract of Echinacea purpurea root, has been used by drinking 5-6 cups of tea on the first day of symptoms and titrating down to 1 cup per day over the next 5 days (6384). The tea is prepared by pouring 8 ounces of boiling water over one tea bag and steeping, covered, for 10-15 minutes (6384). Echinacea liquid (Echinagard) 20 drops every 2 hours for the first day of symptoms, then three times daily for up to 10 days has been used to decrease the duration of symptoms of the common cold (10320).
TOPICAL: No typical dosage.
INTRAVENOUS: No typical dosage.

Comments

There are three main Echinacea species of medicinal interest: Echinacea angustifolia, Echinacea pallida, and Echinacea purpurea. Echinacea species are native to North America and were used as traditional herbal remedies by the Great Plains Indian tribes, and were adopted for medicinal use by settlers (3279). Echinacea angustifolia and Echinacea pallida were official in the US National Formulary from 1916 to 1950 (12639). Conventional use of echinacea fell out of favor in the United States with the discovery of antibiotics and due to the lack of scientific data supporting its use, but it continued to be widely used in Europe (3279). The development of antibiotic resistance has contributed to the renewed interest in echinacea. Echinacea products have been commonly adulterated. The results from clinical studies performed prior to 1991 might be unreliable unless the plant material used was positively confirmed (1414,3279).
Identification of Echinacea is now confirmed by HPLC analysis (1414). Although some echinacea extract products are standardized for their echinacoside content, the active constituent(s) is unknown (12639). It has been suggested that Echinacea preparations could be standardized according to their alkamide content because alkamide levels have been found to vary significantly between the parts and commercial products of Echinacea purpurea (6391).
Despite the availability of methods to identify Echinacea species, echinacea products are frequently mislabeled or may contain no Echinacea. The claim "standardization" does not indicate accurate labeling (12638).

EDTA

Also Known As

Calcium Disodium Edathamil, Calcium Disodium Edetate, Calcium Disodium EDTA, Calcium Disodium Versenate, Calcium Edetate, Calcium EDTA, Disodium Edathamil, Disodium Edetate, Disodium EDTA, Disodium Tetraacetate, Iron EDTA, Sodium Edetate.

Scientific Names

Ethylenediamine tetraacetic acid; Disodium ethylenediamine tetraacetic acid; Trisodium ethylenediamine tetraacetic acid.

People Use This For

Topically, EDTA has been used as an ointment for skin irritations produced by metals such as chromium, nickel and copper.

Intravenously and intramuscularly, EDTA is used for acute and chronic lead poisoning and lead encephalopathy. Intravenous EDTA is also used in the calcium EDTA mobilization test which is used to evaluate a patient's response to chelation therapy for suspected lead poisoning. EDTA is also used intravenously to treat poisonings by radioactive products such as plutonium, thorium, uranium, and strontium. It is also used intravenously for removing copper in patients with Wilson's disease, hypercalcemia, cardiac glycoside-induced arrhythmias, atherosclerotic vascular disease, scleroderma, porphyria, hypercholesterolemia, and in the diagnosis of hypoparathyroidism. EDTA has also been used intravenously to treat essential hypertension, Raynaud's syndrome, intermittent claudication, gangrene, cancer, rheumatoid arthritis, osteoarthritis, decreased vision due to macular degeneration, diabetes, Alzheimer's disease, multiple sclerosis, Parkinson's disease, psoriasis, and angina.

Ophthalmically, EDTA is used for corneal calcium deposits in the eye.

In foods, EDTA is used as iron EDTA to fortify grain-based products such as breakfast cereals and cereal bars. EDTA is also used as calcium disodium EDTA and disodium EDTA as an additive to preserve food; and to promote the color, texture, and flavor of food.

In manufacturing, EDTA is used as disodium EDTA and trisodium EDTA to improve stability in pharmaceutical preparations, detergents, liquid soaps, shampoos, agricultural chemical sprays, oil emulsion devices, contact lens cleaners and cosmetics. It is also used in manufactured clinical laboratory evacuated blood collection tubes to anticoagulate blood specimens.

Safety

LIKELY SAFE ...when used orally in amounts commonly found in foods. EDTA has Generally Recognized As Safe status (GRAS) for use in foods in the US (4912,10266). ...when used intravenously or intramuscularly and appropriately, short-term. Parenteral EDTA in the disodium and calcium disodium forms are FDA-approved prescription products (15).

POSSIBLY SAFE ...when used ophthalmically and appropriately (5774). Solutions of 0.35-1.85% EDTA in the disodium form seem to be safe (5774).

LIKELY UNSAFE ...when used intravenously or intramuscularly in excessive doses or long-term. Doses exceeding 50 mg/kg/day or greater than 3 grams per day, or used longer than 5-7 days per treatment course are associated with severe toxicity including nephrotoxicity (5733). ...when used intravenously and infused at an excessive rate. Infusion of the disodium form of EDTA over less than 3 hours can cause severe, life-threatening adverse effects including hypocalcemia and death (5737).

PREGNANCY AND LACTATION: POSSIBLY SAFE ...when used orally and appropriately in amounts commonly found in foods (7705,10266). There is insufficient reliable information available for other forms of EDTA; avoid using.

Effectiveness

EFFECTIVE

Lead toxicity. Administering EDTA intravenously and intramuscularly is effective for treating acute and chronic lead poisoning and lead encephalopathy (15,5730,5731,5734,5735,5736). The calcium disodium form of EDTA is FDA approved for these uses (15). Calcium disodium EDTA is used when blood lead concentrations are 45 ug/dL or greater or when patients are symptomatic. Treatment of 3-5 days is usually required to lower blood lead levels below 40 ug/dL (15,5730,5733). A second treatment course can be required if blood lead concentrations rebound to 45 ug/dL or greater within 5-7 days after the initial treatment (15). Treatment with calcium disodium EDTA improves symptoms of lead poisoning such as abdominal pain, fatigue, constipation, and anorexia (5730). It also seems slow progression of renal dysfunction in patients who have had chronic lead poisoning (5732). Calcium disodium EDTA is preferred to disodium EDTA for lead poisoning because unlike calcium disodium EDTA, disodium EDTA can significantly lower serum calcium levels and cause hypocalcemia when used in doses necessary to treat lead poisoning (15). However, EDTA does not seem to be effective for diagnosing lead poisoning. Some clinicians use a diagnostic test known as the calcium EDTA mobilization test. Many experts consider the test obsolete due to technical inconsistencies in administering and interpreting the test (5733).

Treatment of lead poisoning should not be delayed for performance of this test if blood lead levels are 45 mcg/dL or greater (15).

LIKELY EFFECTIVE

Cardiac glycoside-induced ventricular arrhythmias. Administering EDTA intravenously is effective for emergency treatment of cardiac glycoside-induced ventricular arrhythmias. The disodium form of EDTA is approved by the FDA for this use. Disodium EDTA works rapidly to control ventricular arrhythmias, but it is very short acting (15,5761,5762). Clinicians do not consider it the preferred treatment (15). Other agents such as lidocaine or phenytoin (Dilantin) (505) are typically used because they are safer and more effective (15).

Hypercalcemia. Administering EDTA intravenously is effective for emergency treatment of hypercalcemia. The disodium form of EDTA is approved by the FDA for this use (15). Disodium EDTA can temporarily lower serum calcium to safe levels (15). However, clinicians generally prefer other methods of treatment such as forced diuresis with saline or use of pamidronate (Aredia), calcitonin (Miacalcin, others), or glucocorticoids (5775). These treatments more effectively lower serum calcium concentrations over longer periods of time than would be achieved with disodium EDTA and are less likely to cause renal side effects (15).

POSSIBLY EFFECTIVE

Corneal calcium deposits. A single ophthalmic application of the disodium form of EDTA can clear corneal calcium deposits, and improve eyesight (5773,5774). However, debridement of the corneal epithelium prior to application of EDTA is required (5773,5774).

POSSIBLY INEFFECTIVE

Scleroderma. Administering EDTA intravenously doesn't seem to be effective for treating localized and systemic scleroderma. Although there have been some anecdotal reports showing benefit (5757,5760), clinical studies show no significant changes or improvements in the skin or joints of scleroderma patients treated with disodium EDTA (5757,5758,5759,5760).

LIKELY INEFFECTIVE

Coronary heart disease. Administering EDTA intravenously isn't effective for treating coronary heart disease or peripheral arterial occlusive disease. The effectiveness of EDTA in chelation therapy is highly debated (5738,5739). Proponents often cite anecdotal reports or poorly controlled studies as evidence to support EDTA chelation therapy (5737,5738,5739,5740,5742,5743,5751,5770), but well-designed research shows that EDTA offers no significant benefit for these conditions (5737,5740,5742,5750,5752,5753,5754).

Mechanism of Action

Ethylenediaminetetraacetic acid (EDTA) is known as a chelating agent. It is a complex molecule with a claw-like structure, which binds and seizes divalent and trivalent metal ions such as calcium and aluminum to form a stable ring structure (5729,5749). EDTA binds and chelates metal ions in the following decreasing order: chromium, iron (ferric ion), mercury, copper, aluminum, nickel, zinc, calcium, cobalt, iron (ferrous ion), manganese, calcium, and magnesium (5737). After intravenous administration, accessible metal ions are chelated forming stable soluble complexes, which are then excreted in the urine (505). EDTA is not metabolized, but elimination is decreased with renal dysfunction (5737). Calcium disodium EDTA and disodium EDTA are the two forms of EDTA available for clinical use (15). Calcium disodium EDTA is the form of EDTA used primarily for lead poisoning (5730,5731,5732,5733,5734,5735,5736). The calcium in calcium disodium EDTA is displaced by metal ions such as lead to form a soluble complex that is then excreted in the urine (15). Unlike disodium EDTA, calcium disodium EDTA can be administered in large quantities without causing substantial changes in serum or total body calcium concentrations (15). Radioactive isotopes such as uranium and plutonium can also be chelated to a limited extent by calcium disodium EDTA (15).

Disodium EDTA antagonizes the ventricular inotropic and chronotropic effects of cardiac glycosides on the heart by decreasing the amount of extracellular calcium in the blood (5761,5762). Some researchers think that decreased extracellular calcium can increase potassium re-entry into myocardial cells which then counteracts with the intracellular potassium depletion caused by cardiac glycosides (5762).

Ophthalmically, disodium EDTA is used to dissolve corneal calcium deposits by binding with calcium in the eye (5774). EDTA can also disorganize the outer membrane of gram-negative bacteria, inhibit the coaggregation between pairs of microorganisms and is possibly an effective inhibitor of bacterial adhesins (5764).

Chelation therapy using disodium EDTA has been purported by many as being efficacious in the treatment of many disease conditions, including atherosclerosis (5738,5739,5743,5751,5768). Many biochemical mechanisms have been proposed to justify the use of disodium EDTA in the treatment of atherosclerotic vascular disease (5738,5741,5743). Mechanisms claimed include that EDTA chelation therapy can extract calcium out of atherosclerotic plaques and clear atherosclerotic arteries (5742,5749) or that calcium removed by chelation is replaced by calcium from the bone, causing secretion of parathyroid hormone (PTH) which then promotes a transfer of calcium from hardened arterial tissue and plaque to bone (5749).

Other mechanisms claimed also include that EDTA blocks production of free radicals involved in reactions causing atherosclerosis by reducing iron loads (5738), by binding toxic metals released when blood clots in occluded arteries (5749), or that disodium EDTA prevents damage and mutation of arterial cells caused by free radicals (5749). None of these proposed mechanisms have been scientifically proven (5749,5756), and controlled scientific clinical studies have been unable to confirm that EDTA can reverse peripheral arterial occlusive disease (5740,5742) or atherosclerotic vascular disease (5746,5750,5752,5753,5754,5769).

Severe nephrotoxicity is the major toxicity that can result when disodium EDTA and calcium disodium EDTA is used in excessively large doses (15). The degeneration of proximal tubular cells that results is proposed to be due to an interaction between EDTA and endogenous metals in the tubular cells (505). EDTA can also chelate and cause increased urinary excretion of magnesium (15), which may also result in decreased serum concentrations and increased excretion of potassium (15). Sudden decreases in calcium can occur if disodium EDTA is administered too rapidly, resulting in tetany, cardiac arrhythmias, and respiratory arrest (5763).

Disodium EDTA inhibits the growth of Candida albicans in vitro. EDTA binds the calcium that is required for growth of this fungal species (4621).

Adverse Reactions

Intravenously, EDTA can commonly cause abdominal cramps, anorexia, nausea, vomiting, diarrhea, headache (15), hypotension (5737), exfoliative dermatitis (15), and a burning sensation and pain at the site of infusion (5744).

EDTA can also sometimes cause fever, chills, fatigue, malaise, thirst, sneezing and nasal congestion (15), arrhythmias (5771,5772), thrombophlebitis (15), anemia (15), prolonged prothrombin time (PT) (5737), transient bone marrow depression (5737,5772), and urinary urgency and frequency (5772).

The calcium disodium form of EDTA can also cause zinc deficiency (5771,5772), hypercalcemia (5771,5772), mild elevations of serum alanine aminotransferase (ALT) and aspartate aminotransferase (AST) and decreased alkaline phosphatase levels (15).

The disodium form of EDTA can occasionally cause muscle cramps, back pains, muscle weakness, tremors, tingling, myalgias, paresthesias (15), decreased magnesium and potassium serum concentrations (5771,5772), and rarely cause histamine-like reactions and insulin shock (5737).

The most serious adverse effect of both forms of EDTA is nephrotoxicity (5772), which is dose dependent of greater than 3 grams per day (15). Both forms of EDTA can cause nocturia, hyperuricemia, polyuria, dysuria, oliguria, proteinuria, glycosuria, hematuria and distal tubule and glomeruli changes (15). Both forms of EDTA can also cause acute renal tubular necrosis, and renal insufficiency and failure (5772). Rapid infusion of disodium EDTA or when given in too concentrated a solution can cause hypocalcemia, tetany, convulsions, severe cardiac arrhythmias, respiratory arrest, and death (15). When used ophthalmically, disodium EDTA can cause transient chemosis and stromal edema (15). Inhalation of disodium EDTA contained in nebulizer solutions has been reported to cause dose-related bronchoconstriction (5765).

Interactions with Herbs & Other Dietary Supplements

MAGNESIUM: EDTA can bind to and cause increased urinary excretion of magnesium (15).

TRACE METALS (copper, iron, zinc, etc.): EDTA can bind to and cause increased urinary excretion of trace metals (15,5733).

Interactions with Drugs

DIURETIC DRUGS: EDTA can decrease serum potassium levels and increase excretion of potassium (15). There is some concern that people receiving EDTA along with potassium depleting diuretics might be at an increased risk for hypokalemia. Initiation of potassium supplementation or an increase in potassium supplement dose may be necessary for some patients. Some diuretics that can deplete potassium include chlorothiazide (Diuril), furosemide (Lasix), and hydrochlorothiazide (HCTZ, Hydrodiuril, Microzide).

INSULIN: Concomitant use of disodium EDTA with insulin can cause severe decreases in blood glucose concentrations (5737,5771). EDTA chelates zinc in insulin products (15) and might interfere with the designed onset and duration of activity of various insulin preparations.

WARFARIN (Coumadin): There is some concern that disodium EDTA can decrease the anticoagulant effects of warfarin. Disodium EDTA has been reported to decrease international normalized ratio (INR) in a patient taking warfarin (4611).

Interactions with Foods

None known.

Interactions with Lab Tests

ALANINE AMINOTRANSFERASE (ALT, SGPT): Calcium disodium EDTA can cause mild increases in serum ALT (15).

ALKALINE PHOSPHATASE: Disodium EDTA can decrease serum alkaline phosphatase concentrations (15,3314). Disodium EDTA can cause low magnesium serum concentrations, which decreases the activity of alkaline phosphatase (15).

ASPARTATE AMINOTRANSFERASE (AST, SGOT): Calcium disodium EDTA can cause mild increases in AST (15).

CALCIUM: Calcium serum concentrations cannot be determined by colorimetric methods in patients receiving disodium EDTA due to chelation of a calcium disodium complex. Oxalate and other precipitation methods may also give falsely decreased levels when disodium EDTA is present (15).

PROTHROMBIN TIME (PT): Disodium EDTA can increase prothrombin time (PT) in some patients (5737).

Interactions with Diseases or Conditions

ASTHMA: Nebulizer solutions containing disodium EDTA as a preservative can produce dose-related bronchoconstriction in some asthmatics (5765).
CARDIAC RHYTHM IRREGULARITIES: Calcium disodium EDTA can cause ECG changes such as T wave inversions (15). Disodium EDTA can have negative inotropic effects on the heart (15). Use with caution in patients with pre-existing cardiac rhythm irregularity conditions.
DIABETES: Use of disodium EDTA may result in poor control of glucose levels in diabetic patients due to disodium EDTA's interactions with insulin preparations and serum glucose lowering effect (15).
HYPOCALCEMIA: Disodium EDTA can decrease serum calcium levels. Disodium EDTA may exacerbate hypocalcemia in patients with existing low calcium levels (15); avoid using.
HYPOKALEMIA: EDTA can increase urinary excretion of potassium and reduce serum potassium concentrations (15). EDTA might exacerbate hypokalemia in patients with existing potassium deficiency; avoid using.
HYPOMAGNESEMIA: EDTA can chelate magnesium and cause increased urinary excretion of magnesium resulting in depletion of serum magnesium concentrations (15). EDTA might exacerbate hypomagnesemia in patients with existing magnesium depletion; avoid using.
LIVER DYSFUNCTION AND HEPATITIS: Calcium disodium EDTA can cause mild increases in serum ALT (SGPT) and AST (SGOT) (15). Theoretically, EDTA might exacerbate liver dysfunction in patients with liver dysfunction or hepatitis; avoid using.
RENAL DYSFUNCTION: EDTA is nephrotoxic and might exacerbate existing renal disease. Avoid using in patients with severe renal disease and renal failure. EDTA doses should be reduced in patients with renal insufficiency (15).
SEIZURE DISORDERS: There is some concern that disodium EDTA might increase the risk of seizure in people with epilepsy or those prone to seizure (15). Disodium can cause severe decreases in serum calcium which can induce seizure (15).
TUBERCULOSIS: Use of disodium EDTA is contraindicated in people with active tuberculosis or healed calcified tubercular lesions (15). Theoretically, use of EDTA may cause the chelation of calcium from calcified tubercular lesions, resulting in possible reactivation of the tuberculosis disease process.

Dosage and Administration

TOPICAL: For corneal calcium deposits, a 0.35% to 1.85% solution is prepared with sterile 0.9% sodium chloride and commercially available disodium EDTA preparations for injection (15). Debridement of the corneal epithelium must be done before application of the solution since EDTA does not penetrate the epithelium (5773,5774). The solution is applied as a corneal bath one time for 15-20 minutes (15) followed by debridement of the calcium (5774), or a cellulose sponge is soaked in disodium EDTA solution and wiped over the deposits until the calcium is removed (5774). The eye should be irrigated with 0.9% sodium chloride following application of disodium EDTA solution (15).
INTRAVENOUS: For acute and chronic lead poisoning and lead encephalopathy, a dose of calcium disodium EDTA 50 mg per kilogram body weight to a maximum daily dose of 3 grams (15) is diluted with 5% dextrose or 9% sodium chloride to a concentration of 2-4 mg/mL and given as a single infusion over 8-24 hours for up to 5 days (15). A minimal 2-day waiting period is suggested before starting a second 5-day course of chelation therapy to further minimize development of nephrotoxicity (15). For blood lead levels greater than 70 mcg/dL, it is recommended that dimercaprol (BAL, British Anti-Lewisite) be used in conjunction with calcium disodium EDTA (5731). For people exposed long-term to low levels of lead and with decreased renal function, 1 gram of calcium disodium EDTA has been used and mixed with 200 mL of 5% dextrose and infused over 2 hours once weekly for 2 months (5732). For hypercalcemia, a dose of disodium EDTA 50 mg/kg body weight up to a maximum daily dosage of 3 grams is diluted with 5% dextrose or 0.9 % sodium chloride to a concentration of 2-4 mg/mL and infused over 3 hours or more (15). For cardiac glycoside-induced ventricular arrhythmias, disodium EDTA is given in a dose of 15 mg/kg per hour to a maximum of 60 mg/kg infused in 5% dextrose (15). For the treatment of atherosclerotic vascular disease, people have used disodium EDTA in a dose of 50 mg/kg up to a maximum of 5 grams diluted in 500-1000 mL of a 150-osmolar carrier (5737). Heparin, sodium ascorbate, elemental magnesium, lidocaine, pyridoxine, and sodium bicarbonate is often added to the infusion with optional additives of adrenal cortex extract, cyanocobalamin, niacin, pantothenic acid, and vitamin-B complex (5737). People usually eat before treatment and bring snacks to eat during a 3-hour infusion (5738).
INTRAMUSCULAR: For acute and chronic lead poisoning and lead encephalopathy, the dosage of calcium disodium EDTA is the same as intravenous administration in divided doses every 8-12 hours (15). When given in conjunction with dimercaprol, the daily dosage is given in equally divided doses every 4 hours. To decrease pain at the injection site, 1 mL of 1% lidocaine HCl or 1 mL of 1% procaine HCl is added to each mL of calcium disodium EDTA to obtain a final lidocaine or procaine HCl concentration of 5 mg/mL (15).

Comments

The American College for Advancement of Medicine (ACAM) strongly supports using EDTA chelation therapy for cardiovascular conditions. ACAM has a standard chelation therapy protocol and has trained more than 6000 practitioners to administer chelation treatments for various conditions (5768). However, the majority of the medical community does not support chelation therapy due to the lack of supporting evidence (5747,5749,5756).

An iron-EDTA chelate is also used for iron fortification of grain-based foods. The established acceptable daily intake (ADI) for iron EDTA is 2.5 mg/kg/day. Iron EDTA has Generally Recognized As Safe (GRAS) status in the US (5728).

ELDERBERRY

Also Known As

Baccae, Baises De Sureau, Black-Berried Alder, Black Elder, Black Elderberry, Boor Tree, Bountry, Elder, Elder Berry, Elderberries, Ellanwood, Ellhorn, European Alder, European Elder Fruit, European Elderberry, Holunderbeeren, Sambuci Sambucus.

CAUTION: See separate listings for Elderflower, Dwarf Elder, and American Elder.

Scientific Names

Sambucus nigra.

Family: Adoxacaea/Sambucaceae or Caprifoliaceae.

People Use This For

Orally, elderberry juice-containing syrup is used for influenza ("the flu").

Elderberry fruit is also used as a laxative, diuretic, diaphoretic, to treat allergic rhinitis, sinusitis, sciatica, neuralgia, and cancer.

In manufacturing, elderberry fruit is used for making wine and as a food flavoring.

Safety

POSSIBLY SAFE ...when elderberry extract is used orally, short-term. A specific elderberry juice extract (Sambucol, Nature's Way) has been safely used for up to 5 days (5260,12235). ...when the cooked fruit is used orally (12).

POSSIBLY UNSAFE ...when the uncooked fruit is used. Uncooked or partially cooked elderberry fruit can cause nausea and vomiting (8,12).

PREGNANCY AND LACTATION: Insufficient reliable information available; avoid using.

Effectiveness

POSSIBLY EFFECTIVE

Influenza. A specific formulation of syrup containing elderberry juice (Sambucol, Nature's Way) taken orally seems to reduce the symptoms and duration of influenza infection when given within 48 hours of initial symptoms. Significant symptom relief seems to occur within 2 to 4 days of treatment for most patients (5260,12235). On average, elderberry extract seems to reduce the duration of symptoms by about 56% (12235).

There is insufficient reliable information available about the effectiveness of elderberry fruit for its other uses.

Mechanism of Action

Elderberries contain several flavonoids. The primary flavonoids are anthocyanidins called cyanidin 3-glucoside and cyaniding 3-sambubioside. Elderberries also contain rutin, isoquertin, and hyperoside (4,8).

Elderberry also contains 3% tannins and essential oil (4,8,12). The major protein of elder is a lectin called Sambucus nigra agglutinin IVf (4151).

The elderberry anthocyanidins are thought to have immunomodulating effects and possibly anti-inflammatory effects (12235). Elderberry extract has both antiviral and immunomodulating effects. Elderberry extract also inhibits hemagglutinin activity and replication of several strains of influenza viruses A and B (5260). Elderberry also seems to increase production of inflammatory cytokines, such as interleukins and tumor necrosis factor (10796).

Adverse Reactions

Orally, elderberry juice extract seems to be well tolerated when used for up to 5 days. No adverse effects have been reported in clinical trials in adults and children (5260,12235).

The raw and unripe fruit might can cause nausea, vomiting, or severe diarrhea (4,8,12). Weakness, dizziness, numbness, and stupor are reported following ingestion of elderberry juice (6).

Interactions with Herbs & Other Dietary Supplements

None known.

Interactions with Drugs

IMMUNOSUPPRESSANTS: Theoretically, elderberry might interfere with immunosuppressant therapy because of its immunostimulating activity. Elderberry stimulates production of cytokines including interleukin and tumor necrosis factor (10796). Immunosuppressant drugs include azathioprine (Imuran), basiliximab (Simulect), cyclosporine (Neoral, Sandimmune), daclizumab (Zenapax), muromonab-CD3 (OKT3, Orthoclone OKT3), mycophenolate (CellCept), tacrolimus (FK506, Prograf), sirolimus (Rapamune), prednisone (Deltasone, Orasone), and other corticosteroids (glucocorticoids).

Interactions with Foods

None known.

Interactions with Lab Tests

None known.

Interactions with Diseases or Conditions

None known.

Dosage and Administration

ORAL: For treating influenza, an adult dose of 15 mL (1 tablespoon) 4 times daily of a specific elderberry juice-containing syrup (Sambucol, Nature's Way) daily for 3-5 days has been used (5260,12235); a dose of 15 mL (1 tablespoon) twice daily for 3 days has been used in children (5260).

Comments

Avoid confusion with American elder (Sambucus canadensis).

ELDERFLOWER

Also Known As

Black-Berried Alder, Black Elder, Boor Tree, Bountry, Common Elder, Elder Flowers, Ellanwood, Ellhorn, European Alder, European Elder Flower, Sambucus, Sweet Elder.
CAUTION: See separate listings for American Elder, Dwarf Elder, and Elderberry.

Scientific Names

Sambucus nigra.
Family: Adoxaceae/Sambucaceae or Caprifoliaceae.

People Use This For

Orally, elderflower is used as a diuretic, laxative, and diaphoretic. It is also used orally to treat colds, flu, cough, and bronchitis.
Topically, elderflower preparations are used as a gargle and mouthwash for coughs, headcolds, laryngitis, flu, and shortness of breath. It is used on the skin as an astringent for rheumatism, swelling, and inflammation.
In combination with gentian root, verbena, cowslip flower, and sorrel, elderflower is used orally for maintaining healthy sinuses and treating sinusitis.
In foods and beverages, elderflowers are used as a flavoring component.
In manufacturing, elderflower extracts are used in perfumes. Elderflower water is used as a vehicle in eye and skin lotions.

Safety

LIKELY SAFE ...when used orally in amounts commonly found in foods. Elderflower has Generally Recognized As Safe (GRAS) status in the US (4912). ...when used orally and appropriately (2,4,12) in therapeutic amounts; no adverse effects have been reported (2,4,6,12).
POSSIBLY SAFE ...when used orally with gentian root, verbena, cowslip flower, and sorrel (Quanterra Sinus Defense, Sinupret) (7,374,379).
There is insufficient reliable information available about the safety of the topical use of elderflower.
PREGNANCY AND LACTATION: Insufficient reliable information available; avoid using.

Effectiveness

POSSIBLY EFFECTIVE

Sinusitis. Taking elderflower orally with gentian root, verbena, cowslip flower, and sorrel (Quanterra Sinus Defense, Sinupret) seems to be effective for treating acute or chronic sinusitis (7,374,379).

There is insufficient reliable information available about the effectiveness of elderflower for its other uses.

Mechanism of Action
Elderflower may have sweat-inducing, diuretic, and laxative effects. It also soothes mucous membranes and stimulates bronchial secretions (2,4,11). Compounds responsible for diuretic and laxative properties have not yet been isolated. Elderflower has demonstrated anti-inflammatory, antiviral, and diuretic effects in animals (4). Constituents of a related species, Sambucus formosana, appear to have a hepatoprotective activity against liver damage (6).

Adverse Reactions
None reported.

Interactions with Herbs & Other Dietary Supplements
None known.

Interactions with Drugs
None known.

Interactions with Foods
None known.

Interactions with Lab Tests
None known.

Interactions with Diseases or Conditions
None known.

Dosage and Administration
ORAL: People typically use one cup tea (steep 2-4 grams dried flowers in 250 mL boiling water 10-15 minutes, strain) three times daily (4); average daily dose 10-15 grams dried flowers (2). Liquid extract (1:1 in 25% alcohol), 2-4 mL three times daily has also been used (4). For acute or chronic sinusitis, two Sinupret tablets three times daily for up to two weeks has been used in clinical trials (7,374,379), equivalent to gentian root 12 mg, elderflower 36 mg, verbena 36 mg, cowslip flower 36 mg, and sorrel 36 mg three times daily.
TOPICAL: No typical dosage.

Comments
Avoid confusion with American elder (Sambucus canadensis). American elder (sambucus candadensis) and European elder (sambucus nigra) are discussed together despite the fact most of the information available pertains to American elder (11).

ELECAMPANE

Also Known As
Alant, Elfdock, Elfwort, Horse-Elder, Horseheal, Inula, Scabwort, Velvet Dock, Wild Sunflower, Yellow Starwort.

Scientific Names
Inula helenium, synonyms Helenium grandiflorum, Aster officinalis, Aster helenium.
Family: Asteraceae/Compositae.

People Use This For
Orally, elecampane is used as an expectorant, antitussive, and diaphoretic, for diseases of the respiratory tract, as an anthelmintic, for improving stomach function, as a diuretic, asthma, bronchitis, whooping cough, cough associated with tuberculosis, nausea, and diarrhea.
In foods and beverages, elecampane is used as a flavoring ingredient.
In other manufacturing processes, elecampane is used as a fragrance component in cosmetics and soaps.

Safety
LIKELY SAFE ...when used orally in amounts commonly found in foods. Elecampane has Generally Recognized As Safe status (GRAS) for use in foods in the US (4912).
POSSIBLY SAFE ...when the root and rhizome are used orally and appropriately in medicinal amounts (12).
POSSIBLY UNSAFE ...when used orally in large amounts. Elecampane can cause gastrointestinal upset and symptoms of paralysis (12).
PREGNANCY AND LACTATION: LIKELY UNSAFE ...when used orally (12); avoid using.

Effectiveness
There is insufficient reliable information available about the effectiveness of elecampane.

Mechanism of Action
The applicable parts of elecampane are the rhizome/root. Alantolactone and isoalantolactone, sesquiterpene alkaloids found in elecampane, show antibacterial and antifungal (11) activity in vitro and anthelmintic activity in humans (11). Alantolactone is used as an anthelmintic in Europe and the UK (11).

Adverse Reactions
Orally, large doses may cause vomiting, diarrhea, spasms, and symptoms of paralysis (12).
Topically, elecampane may cause allergic contact dermatitis (4).
It can cause an allergic reaction in individuals sensitive to the Asteraceae/Compositae family. Members of this family include ragweed, chrysanthemums, marigolds, daisies, and many other herbs.

Interactions with Herbs & Other Dietary Supplements
HERBS WITH SEDATIVE PROPERTIES: Theoretically, concomitant use with herbs that have sedative properties might enhance therapeutic and adverse effects. Some of these supplements include 5-HTP, calamus, California poppy, catnip, hops, Jamaican dogwood, kava, St. John's wort, scullcap, valerian, yerba mansa, and others.

Interactions with Drugs
CNS DEPRESSANTS: Theoretically, concomitant use with drugs with sedative properties may cause additive effects (4).

Interactions with Foods
None known.

Interactions with Lab Tests
None known.

Interactions with Diseases or Conditions
CROSS-ALLERGENICITY: Can cause an allergic reaction in individuals sensitive to the Asteraceae/Compositae family. Members of this family include ragweed, chrysanthemums, marigolds, daisies, and many other herbs.
DIABETES: Theoretically, elecampane may interfere with blood glucose control (4).
HYPERTENSION, HYPOTENSION: Theoretically, elecampane may interfere with blood pressure control (4).

Dosage and Administration
ORAL: Typically, 1.5-4 grams of rhizome/root three times daily, or one cup tea (simmer 1.5-4 grams of rhizome/root in 150 mL boiling water 5-10 minutes, strain) three times daily is used (4). Liquid extract (1:1 in 25% alcohol) 1.5-4 mL three times daily is also used (4). As an anthelmintic for adults, alantolactone 300 mg daily for 2 courses of 5 days, with an interval of 10 days, is used. For children, alantolactone 50-200 mg daily is used (4).

ELEMI

Also Known As
Elemi Oleoresin, Elemi Resin, Manila Elemi.

Scientific Names
Canarium luzonicum, synonym Pimela luzonica; Canarium indicum, synonym Canarium commune.
Family: Burseraceae.

People Use This For
Orally, elemi is used for improving stomach function, as an expectorant, and as a local stimulant.
In foods and beverages, elemi is used as a flavoring agent.
In other manufacturing processes, elemi is used as a fixative and fragrance in cosmetics and soaps.

Safety
LIKELY SAFE ...when used orally in amounts commonly found in foods. Elemi has Generally Recognized As Safe status (GRAS) for use in foods in the US (4912).
There is insufficient reliable information available about the safety of the oral use of elemi in amounts greater than those found in foods.
PREGNANCY AND LACTATION: Insufficient reliable information available; avoid using.

Effectiveness
There is insufficient reliable information available about the effectiveness of elemi.

Mechanism of Action
The applicable parts of elemi are the gum and oil. There is insufficient reliable information available about the possible mechanism of action and active ingredients.

Adverse Reactions
None reported.

Interactions with Herbs & Other Dietary Supplements
None known.

Interactions with Drugs
None known.

Interactions with Foods
None known.

Interactions with Lab Tests
None known.

Interactions with Diseases or Conditions
None known.

Dosage and Administration
No typical dosage.

Comments
Elemi gum is resin exuded by the elemi tree (Canarium luzonicum). Elemi oil is produced by distillation of elemi gum resin.

ELLAGIC ACID

Also Known As
None.

Scientific Names
3,4,3',4'-hydroxyl-benzopyranol[5,4,3-c,d,e][1]benzopyrn-6-6'-dione.

People Use This For
Orally, ellagic acid is used to prevent cancer, and as an antiviral and antibacterial.

Safety
There is insufficient reliable information available about the safety of ellagic acid.
Pregnancy and Lactation: Insufficient reliable information available.

Effectiveness
There is insufficient reliable information available about the effectiveness of ellagic acid.

Mechanism of Action
Ellagic acid is a naturally occurring complex hydrocarbon. The best dietary sources of ellagic acid are raspberries, blackberries, strawberries, and walnuts (8955). Researchers are interested in potential anticancer activity of ellagic acid. Ellagic acid has lipophilic antioxidant activity, free radical scavenging capability, and the ability to inhibit DNA topoisomerases (8955,10342,11335). These characteristics support the observation that ellagic acid inhibits lipid peroxidation at lower concentrations than vitamin E (11335). Ellagic acid also seems to have anti-inflammatory and antimutagenic activity (11335). Derivatives of ellagic acid have the ability to induce DNA damage and inhibit the growth of yeast cells that model the growth of cancer cells (10343). Some researchers have suggested that the hydroxyl groups and lactone rings in the chemical structure of ellagic acid may bind or inactivate carcinogens (10340). Preliminary evidence also suggests ellagic acid may have potential use against malaria, due to its antiplasmodial activity (11460). However, the clinical usefulness of ellagic acid may be limited by its poor absorption and rapid elimination from the body. Because the ability to inhibit carcinogenesis appears to be highly dependent upon its functional groups, alterations in the molecule to improve absorption or decrease the rate of elimination often

decrease the activity of ellagic acid (10340,10342). However, short-term freezing and storage does not appear to decrease the activity of ellagic acid and related compounds in red raspberries (10344).

Adverse Reactions
None reported.

Interactions with Herbs & Other Dietary Supplements
None known.

Interactions with Drugs
None known.

Interactions with Foods
None known.

Interactions with Lab Tests
None known.

Interactions with Diseases or Conditions
None known.

Dosage and Administration
No typical dosage.

ELM BARK

Also Known As
Smooth-Leaved Elm.

Scientific Names
Ulmus minor.
Family: Ulmaceae.

Comments
At the date of publication, this product was not a common ingredient used in brand name supplements marketed to consumers. Details about this product are available in the online version of *Natural Medicines Comprehensive Database.* See www.naturaldatabase.com.

EMU OIL

Also Known As
Emu.

Scientific Names
Dromiceius novahollandiae (Emu).

People Use This For
Orally, emu oil is used for improving cholesterol levels, as a source of polyunsaturated and monounsaturated fatty acids, for weight loss, and as a cough syrup for colds and flu.
Topically, emu oil is used for relief from sore muscles; aching joints, pain or inflammation; carpal tunnel syndrome; sciatica, shin splints; and gout. It is also used topically to improve healing of wounds, incisions, and burns from radiation therapy; to reduce bruises and stretch marks; to reduce scarring and keloids; to heal the donor site of skin grafting; to diminish acne inflammation; to soften dry cuticles and promote healthy nails; for skin cancers; athlete's foot; diaper rash; canker sores; chapped lips; circulation; dry skin, eczema, psoriasis, wrinkles or age spots; dry or damaged hair; dandruff; in massage therapy; for its anti-aging properties; to protect skin from sun damage; and to promote skin rejuvenation. Emu oil is also used topically to reduce pain and irritation from shingles, bedsores, hemorrhoids, diabetic neuropathy, insect bites, earaches, eye irritation, "growing pains," and frostbite. It is used for rashes, razor burn and nicks, rosacea, and roseola.
Intranasally, emu oil is used to treat colds and flu.
In combination, emu oil (7%) is used with glycolic acid (10%) for lowering cholesterol, triglycerides, and low density lipoprotein; preventing and treating allergies; preventing scarring; treating headaches, especially migraines; preventing nosebleeds; treating and preventing cold and flu symptoms; and relieving discomfort

associated with menstruation.
In veterinary practice, emu oil is used to reduce swelling in joints, prevent cracked or peeling paws, calm "hot spots," and reduce irritation of flea bites.
In manufacturing, emu oil is used to sharpen and oil industrial machinery, for polishing timber and leather, and for conditioning and waterproofing.

Safety
There is insufficient reliable information available about the safety of emu oil.
Pregnancy and Lactation: Insufficient reliable information available; avoid using.

Effectiveness
There is insufficient reliable information available about the effectiveness of emu oil.

Mechanism of Action
Emu oil is obtained from the fat of the emu, a large flightless bird native to Australia. Though not standardized, emu oil typically contains myristic, palmitic, palmitoleic, stearic, oleic, linoleic, and linolenic fatty acids (8278). Topical emu oil has moisturizing, cosmetic, and texture properties similar to those of topical mineral oil. It appears to penetrate the stratum corneum barrier of the skin (10643). Preliminary animal evidence suggests that a topical emu lotion (a combination of emu oil, vitamin E and botanical oil) has the ability to promote wound healing by exerting both anti-inflammatory and anti-catalytic effects on soft tissue (8277). Additional animal evidence suggests topical emu oil is more effective in acute inflammation than in chronic inflammation (5923).

Adverse Reactions
None reported.

Interactions with Herbs & Other Dietary Supplements
HERBS WITH ANTICOAGULANT/ANTIPLATELET POTENTIAL: Theoretically, concomitant use of herbs that have constituents or affect platelet aggregation could theoretically increase the risk of bleeding in some people. These herbs include angelica, clove, danshen, garlic, ginger, ginkgo, Panax ginseng, red clover, turmeric, and others.

Interactions with Drugs
None known.

Interactions with Foods
None known.

Interactions with Lab Tests
None known.

Interactions with Diseases or Conditions
None known.

Dosage and Administration
No typical dosage.

ENGLISH ADDER'S TONGUE

Also Known As
Christs Spear, Christ's Spear, English Adders Tongue, Green Oil of Charity, Serpents Tongue, Serpent's Tongue.
CAUTION: See separate listing for American Adder's Tongue.

Scientific Names
Ophioglossum vulgatum.
Family: Ophioglossaceae.

Comments
At the date of publication, this product was not a common ingredient used in brand name supplements marketed to consumers. Details about this product are available in the online version of *Natural Medicines Comprehensive Database.* See www.naturaldatabase.com.

ENGLISH HORSEMINT

Also Known As

Biblical Mint, Wild Mint.
CAUTION: See separate listing for Wild Mint.

Scientific Names

Mentha longifolia, synonym Mentha sylvestris.
Family: Lamiaceae/Labiatae.

Comments

At the date of publication, this product was not a common ingredient used in brand name supplements marketed to consumers. Details about this product are available in the online version of *Natural Medicines Comprehensive Database.* See www.naturaldatabase.com.

ENGLISH IVY

Also Known As

Gum Ivy, Hederae helicis folium, Ivy, True Ivy, Woodbind.

Scientific Names

Hedera helix, synonym Hedera taurica.
Family: Araliaceae.

People Use This For

Orally, English ivy is used for inflammation of mucous membranes in respiratory passages, symptomatic treatment of chronic inflammatory bronchial conditions, as an expectorant, as an antispasmodic, to improve lung function in children with chronic obstructive bronchitis, liver disorders, spleen disorders, gallbladder disorders, gout, rheumatism, and scrofulosis.
Topically, English ivy is used for burn wounds, calluses, cellulitis, inflammations, neuralgia, parasitic disorders, ulcers, rheumatic complaints, and for phlebitis.

Safety

POSSIBLY SAFE ...when used orally and appropriately (2).
There is insufficient reliable information available about the safety of English ivy for its other uses.
PREGNANCY AND LACTATION: Insufficient reliable information available; avoid using.

Effectiveness

POSSIBLY EFFECTIVE

Chronic obstructive bronchitis. There is some evidence that taking English ivy orally might help improve lung function in children with chronic obstructive bronchitis (3471).

There is insufficient reliable information available about the effectiveness of English ivy for its other uses.

Mechanism of Action

The applicable part of English ivy is the leaf. English ivy has expectorant and antispasmodic actions. It irritates skin and mucosa (2). Researchers think the ivy leaf acts on the gastric mucosa to cause stimulation of mucous glands in the bronchi via parasympathetic sensory pathways (7). Fresh leaves contain the contact allergen falcarinol (7). Preliminary evidence suggests ivy leaf dried extract may improve lung function (measured as forced expiratory volume in one second) in children with chronic obstructive bronchitis due to its secretolytic and spasmolytic effects (3471). Human studies are needed to determine whether ivy leaf dried extract is as effective or beneficial as conventional agents used prophylactically to improve and maintain lung function such as bronchodilators and corticosteroids.

Adverse Reactions

Orally, fresh English ivy leaves can cause skin irritation (7). Saponin constituents, hederacosides, and hederin monodesmosides have acrid and/or bitter taste (7).

Interactions with Herbs & Other Dietary Supplements

None known.

Interactions with Drugs

None known.

Interactions with Foods
None known.

Interactions with Lab Tests
None known.

Interactions with Diseases or Conditions
None known.

Dosage and Administration
ORAL: People have used 300-800 mg dried leaf per day (2,18), or one cup tea, steep 1 heaping teaspoon of dried leaf in 1/4 cup boiling water 10 minutes, strain, up to three times daily (18). For chronic obstructive bronchitis in children, 35 mg dried leaf extract three times a day or 14 mg dried leaf alcohol-based extract three times a day has been used (3471).
TOPICAL: Fresh leaves placed on festering wounds and burns have been used (18). For rheumatism, prepare tea, simmer 200 grams of fresh leaves in 1 L boiling water 5-10 minutes, strain (18).

Comments
English ivy is most often used in the form of an extract and seldom used as a prepared tea (7).

ENGLISH WALNUT

Also Known As
Akschota, Fructus Cortex, Juglandis, Juglandis Folium, Juglans, Nogal, Walnussblätter, Walnussfrüchtschalen, Walnut.
CAUTION: See separate listings for Alpha-linolenic Acid and Black Walnut.

Scientific Names
Juglans regia.
Family: Juglandaceae.

People Use This For
Orally, English walnut fruit is used as a part of the diet for lowering cholesterol. The hull of English walnut is used to treat gastrointestinal mucous membrane inflammation. English walnut hull is also used to treat "blood poisoning" and as a "blood purifier" to remove undesirable agents from the blood. The leaf is used orally for treating diarrhea. The leaf is also used for gastrointestinal mucous membrane inflammation, as an anthelmintic, and "blood-purifying" agent.
Topically, English walnut hull is used for skin diseases, abscesses, and eye lid inflammation. It is also used topically as hair dye and in sunless tanning products. The leaf is used topically for superficial inflammation of the skin; excessive hand and/or foot perspiration; and for skin conditions such as acne, eczema, tuberculous skin lesions, pyodermia, ulcers; and fungal, bacterial and viral skin infections.
In combination with other herbs, English walnut hull is used to treat diabetes mellitus, gastritis, and anemia.
In foods, English walnut is commonly consumed, usually as a snack, in baking and in salads.

Safety
LIKELY SAFE ...when the fruit, leaf, or hull is consumed in amounts normally found in foods (4912,6431,8476,8477).
There is insufficient reliable information available about the safety of using English walnut as medicine.
PREGNANCY AND LACTATION: LIKELY SAFE ...when the fruit, leaf, or hull is consumed in amounts normally found in foods (4912). There is insufficient reliable information available about the safety of using English walnut as medicine during pregnancy and lactation; avoid using.

Effectiveness
POSSIBLY EFFECTIVE
Coronary heart disease. Some research suggests that people who increase dietary consumption of walnuts and other nuts might have a lower risk of coronary heart disease and death due to coronary events (8477,8478,13299).
Hypercholesterolemia. Consuming walnuts as part of a low fat diet seems to lower cholesterol. Total cholesterol and lipoproteins are decreased when walnuts are substituted for other fatty foods and constitute up to 20% of the calories in the diet. When English walnuts are added to a low fat diet, total cholesterol may be decreased by 4% to 12% and low-density lipoprotein (LDL) may be decreased by 8% to 16% (6431,8476,8477). Substituting walnuts for other dietary fats also seems to improve high-density lipoprotein (HDL) cholesterol-to-total cholesterol ratios in patients with type 2 diabetes (13300).
There is insufficient reliable information available about the effectiveness of English walnut for its other uses.

Mechanism of Action

The applicable parts of English walnut are the fruit, hull, and leaf. English walnut fruit (the "nut") contains high amounts of the polyunsaturated fatty acids, linoleic acid (an omega-6 fatty acid) and alpha-linolenic acid (an omega-3 fatty acid). It also contains significant amounts of fiber (about 7%), phosphorus, potassium, and folate. It also contains the antioxidants vitamin E (primarily as gamma-tocopherol) and ellagic acid (8478,8955). English walnut hulls and leaves contain juglone and plumbagin, which have astringent, antibacterial, antiviral and antifungal properties. Preliminary research suggests these constituents might be cytotoxic to skin cells (12980,12981).

Some clinical research suggests English walnut fruit can lower the risk of cardiovascular disease by lowering total and low-density lipoprotein (LDL) cholesterol. Theoretically, other constituents such as fiber, vitamin E, and folate might contribute to the apparent beneficial effect on cardiovascular disease risk (8478,8955). Clinical research also suggests walnuts might improve endothelial function, which might be beneficial in preventing atherosclerosis. In addition to alpha-linolenic acid, walnuts contain significant amounts of arginine, a precursor amino acid of the endogenous vasodilator nitric oxide (NO) (13301).

English walnut leaf might have antiviral, anthelmintic, antimicrobial, antihyperglycemic, cytotoxic, hypotensive, vasorelaxant, and smooth muscle stimulant effects (12979).

Adverse Reactions

Orally, the fruit of English walnut is well tolerated (8476,8477); however, it can cause softening of stools and mild bloating (6431). Oral allergy syndrome may occur in people who are allergic to English walnuts. This is characterized by itching of the oral cavity immediately after consumption. Rarely this syndrome may cause swelling of the lips and tongue (angioedema) (8479).

English walnut fruit may cause weight gain if it is not substituted for other dietary fats. About 81 percent of the total calories of walnuts are derived from fat, which accounts for 58 percent of their weight. An ounce of walnuts contains 190 calories (8477).

Topically, English walnut preparations containing the juglone constituent can lead to yellow or brown discoloration of skin and mucous membranes. It can also cause contact dermatitis (12980).

Interactions with Herbs & Other Dietary Supplements

None known.

Interactions with Drugs

None known.

Interactions with Foods

None known.

Interactions with Lab Tests

CHOLESTEROL: English walnut fruit can decrease serum total cholesterol and low-density lipoprotein (LDL) cholesterol levels and increase high density lipoprotein (HDL) cholesterol levels (6431,8476,8477,13300).

Interactions with Diseases or Conditions

None known.

Dosage and Administration

ORAL: For lowering cholesterol, the fruit of approximately 8-11 English walnuts or 30-56 grams (about 1/4 to 1/2 cup) has been substituted for other dietary fats (6431,13300).

EPA (EICOSAPENTAENOIC ACID)

Also Known As

EPA, Ethyl Eicosapentaenoic Acid, Fish Oil Fatty Acid, N-3 Fatty Acid, Omega Fatty Acid, Omega-3 Fatty Acids, W-3 Fatty Acid.

CAUTION: See separate listings for Cod Liver Oil, DHA (docosahexaenoic acid), and Fish Oil.

Scientific Names

Eicosapentaenoic acid.

People Use This For

Orally, eicosapentaenoic acid (EPA) is used for treating the symptoms of cystic fibrosis, reducing the risk of intrauterine growth retardation, treating depression, treating pregnancy-induced hypertension in high-risk pregnancies, preventing age-related macular degeneration (AMD), treating coronary artery disease, treating schizophrenia, personality disorder, and treating diabetes.

In combination, EPA is used with docosahexaenoic acid (DHA) in fish oil preparations for a variety of conditions, including preventing and reversing heart disease, decreasing ectopic ventricular beats, asthma, cancer, dysmenorrhea, hay fever, lung diseases, lupus erythematosus, lupus nephritis, and IgA nephropathy. They are also used in combination for migraine headache prophylaxis in adolescents, atopic dermatitis, Behcet's syndrome, hyperlipidemia, hypertension, psoriasis, Raynaud's syndrome, rheumatoid arthritis, Crohn's disease, and ulcerative colitis. EPA is also used in combination with RNA and L-arginine in the perioperative period to reduce infections, improve wound healing, and shorten recovery time.

Safety

LIKELY SAFE ...when used orally or intravenously, and appropriately (1004,1016,7819).

POSSIBLY UNSAFE ...when used orally in high doses. Doses greater than 3 grams daily might decrease blood coagulation and increase the risk of bleeding (1313).

PREGNANCY AND LACTATION: Insufficient reliable information available; avoid using.

Effectiveness

POSSIBLY EFFECTIVE

Coronary artery disease. Increased dietary consumption of EPA may slightly decrease the risk of death in patients with coronary artery disease (10322).

Depression. Taking eicosapentaenoic acid (EPA) orally 1 gram twice daily with standard therapy seems to improve symptoms of recurrent major depression, such as depressed mood, guilt feelings, worthlessness, and insomnia after two weeks of treatment (10872). Some research suggests that the ethyl form of EPA, ethyl-eicosapentaenoate (ethyl-EPA), might also be helpful for treating depression. It appears that 1 gram per day of ethyl-EPA may be more effective for depression than 2 or 4 grams per day (10215). Personality disorder. Taking EPA (as ethyl eicosapentaenoic acid) orally provides modest improvement in aggressive behavior and depression in women with moderately severe borderline personality disorder (10348).

Psoriasis. Taking EPA in combination with low-dose (20 mg per day) etretinate (Tegison, no longer available in the US) seems to be more effective than etretinate alone for plaque psoriasis (1000). EPA given intravenously in combination with docosahexaenoic acid (DHA) appears to improve psoriatic lesions better than omega-6-lipid emulsion (1004).

Surgery. Supplementing the diet with EPA in combination with RNA and L-arginine before surgery or in the postoperative period appears to reduce the number of perioperative infections, improves wound healing, and shortens recovery time (5531,5532,5533,7819).

POSSIBLY INEFFECTIVE

Age-related macular degeneration (AMD). Increased dietary consumption of EPA does not appear to prevent AMD (10324).

Allergic rhinitis (hayfever). Taking EPA orally doesn't appear to relieve hayfever symptoms, including wheezing, cough, and nasal symptoms (1036).

Asthma. Taking EPA orally doesn't seem to have any effect on asthma symptoms when given for four weeks (1023).

Cystic fibrosis. Taking EPA orally as a single agent doesn't seem to improve symptoms of cystic fibrosis (1006,1027).

Diabetes. Taking EPA orally does not seem to substantially improve cholesterol or other serum lipids or decrease blood sugar or hemoglobin A1c (HbA1c) in patients with type 2 diabetes (10321).

Intrauterine growth. Taking EPA orally doesn't seem to reduce the risk of intrauterine growth (1027).

Pregnancy-induced hypertension. Taking EPA orally doesn't seem to improve pregnancy-induced hypertension in women with high-risk pregnancies (1027).

Schizophrenia. Taking EPA orally does not consistently improve positive or negative symptoms of schizophrenia when used in conjunction with standard antipsychotic therapy (8720,10347).

There is insufficient reliable information available about the effectiveness of EPA for its other uses.

Mechanism of Action

Eicosapentaenoic acid (EPA) is a long-chain n-3 polyunsaturated fatty acid that is found in the tissues of marine mammals and oily fish. EPA is also found in fish liver oils and in commercial fish oil products. EPA competes with arachidonic acid for inclusion in cyclooxygenase and lipoxygenase pathways (8696). This may have an anti-inflammatory effect in diseases such as psoriasis (1004).

EPA decreases blood viscosity and increases red blood cell deformability. It also decreases platelet aggregation (9930). However, EPA does not significantly affect clotting factors, fibrinogen concentrations, plasminogen activator inhibitor-1 or tissue plasminogen activator activity (10323). Pure EPA reduces serum triglyceride concentrations, increases fasting insulin and glucose concentrations, but has no effect on total and low-density lipoprotein (LDL) cholesterol in mildly hypercholesterolemic men (6143,10322). There is some evidence that higher ratios of EPA to arachidonic acid are associated with lower ratios of total to high-density lipoprotein (HDL) cholesterol. EPA can increase HDL cholesterol by approximately 12% (10321). There is preliminary evidence that EPA decreases natural killer (NK) cell activity. Researchers think this effect might be beneficial in preventing rejection after bone marrow and organ transplantation, but further research is needed (8718). There is evidence EPA might have an additive effect to standard treatment on symptoms associated with schizophrenia and recurrent unipolar depressive disorder, but it is unknown if EPA has any antipsychotic and antidepressant activity of its own (8720,10872). Some evidence suggests that supplemental EPA might slow weight loss in cachectic cancer patients, possibly by inhibiting lipolysis. Other research suggests EPA does not inhibit lipolysis or lipid oxidation, suggesting a different mechanism might be responsible for this effect (8717).

Adverse Reactions

Orally, adverse reactions have not been reported for eicosapentaenoic acid (EPA) alone. However, for fish oils containing EPA and DHA, side effects can include fishy taste, belching, nosebleeds, nausea, and loose stools (10007). Three people with pre-existing familial adenomatous polyposis were diagnosed with malignant lesions during the course of long-term fish oil use (999). High doses of fish oils might also decrease blood coagulation and increase the risk of bleeding (1313). There is preliminary evidence that EPA in fish oil decreases natural killer (NK) cell activity. Due to this effect, there is concern that increased intake of EPA might have some adverse immunologic effects and possibly increase the risk for viral infections and some cancers (8718).

Interactions with Herbs & Other Dietary Supplements

HERBS WITH ANTICOAGULANT/ANTIPLATELET POTENTIAL: Concomitant use of herbs that have constituents that might affect platelet aggregation could theoretically increase the risk of bleeding in some people (9930). These herbs include angelica, clove, danshen, garlic, ginger, ginkgo, Panax ginseng, red clover, turmeric, and others.

Interactions with Drugs

ANTICOAGULANT/ANTIPLATELET DRUGS: Theoretically, concomitant use of EPA with anticoagulant or antiplatelet drugs, including aspirin, can increase the risk of bleeding (9930).
ANTIHYPERTENSIVE DRUGS: Fish oils containing EPA can lower blood pressure and might have additive effects in patients treated with antihypertensives (1001,1020,1030,1033); use with caution.

Interactions with Foods

None known.

Interactions with Lab Tests

INSULIN: EPA can increase fasting insulin concentrations and test results in mildly hypercholesterolemic patients (6143).
INTERNATIONAL NORMALIZED RATIO (INR), PROTHROMBIN TIME (PT): High doses of greater than 3 grams per day might decrease blood coagulation, increase INR and PT, and increase the risk of bleeding (1313).
PULMONARY FUNCTION TESTS: EPA might cause a decline in pulmonary function tests in aspirin-sensitive individuals (11869).
TRIGLYCERIDES: EPA can reduce serum triglyceride concentrations and test results in patients with hypercholesterolemia (6143).

Interactions with Diseases or Conditions

ASPIRIN-SENSITIVITY: Fish oils and other omega-3 fatty acids can lower pulmonary function tests in some aspirin-sensitive patients (11869).
HYPERTENSION: Fish oils including EPA can lower blood pressure and might have additive effects in patients with high blood pressure who are treated with antihypertensives (1001,1020,1030,1033).

Dosage and Administration

ORAL: Eicosapentaenoic acid (EPA) is usually administered with DHA (docosahexaenoic acid) as fish oil. A wide range of doses has been used. A typical dose is 5 grams of fish oil containing 169-563 mg of EPA and 72-312 mg of DHA. As an adjunct to standard antidepressant therapy for recurrent unipolar depressive disorder, 1 gram EPA twice daily has been used (10872). As an adjunct to standard antipsychotic therapy for schizophrenia, a dose of 3 grams EPA daily, in 2 to 3 divided doses (as ethyl eicosapentaenoic acid), has been used for 12-16 weeks (8720). For treatment of borderline personality disorder, 1 gram of EPA daily (as ethyl eicosapentaenoic acid) has been used for up to 8 weeks (10348). For plaque psoriasis, EPA ethyl ester 1800 mg daily has been used (1000).
Many fish oil preparations also contain small amounts of vitamin E as an antioxidant.
INTRAVENOUS: For plaque psoriasis, EPA 4.2 grams and docosahexaenoic acid (DHA) 4.2 grams per day has been used (1004).

Comments

Avoid confusion with DHA (docosahexaenoic acid) and fish oils, which contain EPA and DHA. Most available data involving EPA are from research and clinical experience with fish oil products containing variable combinations of EPA and DHA. For more information, see the separate listing for Fish Oils.
Researchers are investigating oils containing stearidonic acid (SDA) from genetically modified plants as an alternative source of omega-3 fatty acids. SDA is metabolized to EPA and DHA in animals. However, further research is needed on the effects and safety of SDA in humans.

EPHEDRA

Also Known As

Cao Mahuang, Chinese Ephedra, Chinese Joint-Fir, Cao Ma-Huang, Desert Herb, Herbal Ecstasy, Indian Jointfir, Joint Fir, Ma Huang, Mahuanggen (ma huang root), Mongolian Ephedra, Muzei Ma Huang, Pakistani Ephedra, Popotillo, Sea Grape, Shuang Sui Ma Huang, Teamster's Tea, Yellow Astringent, Yellow Horse, Zhong Mahuang.
CAUTION: See separate listing for Mormon Tea.

Scientific Names

Ephedra distachya, synonym Ephedra vulgaris; Ephedra equisetina, synonym Ephedra shennungiana; Ephedra gerardiana; Ephedra intermedia; Ephedra sinica; and other Ephedra species.
Family: Ephedraceae.

People Use This For

Orally, ephedra is used for weight loss and obesity and to enhance athletic performance. It is also used for allergies and allergic rhinitis; nasal congestion; and respiratory tract conditions such as bronchospasm, asthma, and bronchitis. It is also used orally for colds, flu, fever, chills, headache, anhidrosis, joint and bone pain, and as a diuretic for edema.

Safety

LIKELY UNSAFE ...when used orally. Ephedra can cause severe life-threatening or disabling adverse effects in some people. Ephedra is banned in the US. Several case reports have linked ephedra to serious side effects including hypertension, myocardial infarction (MI), seizure, stroke, psychosis, and others (1276,2729,6486,6998,9167,10689). Prolonged use or use of high doses might increase the risk of serious adverse effects (2729). Some suggest that ephedra is only harmful when used inappropriately in excessive doses or for prolonged periods. However, there are several cases of significant adverse events in patients who used ephedra short-term in relatively low doses ranging from 20-60 mg of ephedra alkaloids (2729,6486). There is some evidence that people who take doses greater than 32 mg per day might have more than triple the risk of hemorrhagic stroke, including subarachnoid hemorrhage and intracerebral hemorrhage (9167). It is not possible to determine who is at the greatest risk. However, people with existing conditions such as cardiovascular disease or those using ephedra products in combination with other stimulants such as caffeine, might be at increased risk. Tell patients to avoid ephedra-containing products.
CHILDREN: LIKELY UNSAFE ...when used orally. Ephedra has been linked to several cases of severe side effects (6486).
PREGNANCY AND LACTATION: LIKELY UNSAFE ...when used orally. Ephedra has been linked to several cases of severe side effects (1276,2729,6486,6998,9167,10689).

Effectiveness

POSSIBLY EFFECTIVE

Obesity. Taking ephedra orally seems to produce weight loss of approximately 0.9 kg/month for up to 6 months. It is not known if weight loss can be sustained beyond this time frame or if weight returns after ephedra is discontinued. Caffeine may provide additional weight loss (9740,9741). The combination of ephedra, cola nut, and willow bark may also cause modest weight loss in overweight and obese people (12811). There is preliminary evidence that a specific combination product containing ephedra, guarana, and 17 other vitamins, minerals, and supplements (Metabolife 356) might help reduce weight by approximately 2.7 kg over 8 weeks when used with a low-fat diet and exercise (3719). Ephedra 90 mg in combination with caffeine from cola nut 192 mg per day for six months seems to cause a modest weight reduction (5.3 kg) in people with a body mass index (BMI) between 25 and 40 kg per meter squared. This combination, along with limiting fat intake to 30 percent of calories and moderate exercise, also seems to reduce body fat, decrease low-density lipoprotein (LDL) cholesterol, and increase high-density lipoprotein (HDL) cholesterol. Even in carefully screened and monitored otherwise healthy adults, ephedra combinations can cause small changes in blood pressure and heart rate (8647). There are serious concerns about the safety of these products since they combine significant amounts of the stimulants ephedra and caffeine and are often taken without monitoring for adverse effects. Tell patients to avoid ephedra-containing products.

There is insufficient reliable information available about the effectiveness of ephedra for its other uses.

Mechanism of Action

The applicable part of ephedra is the stem and leaf (12813). Ephedra in dietary supplements is usually either a formulation of powdered stems and aerial portions or a dried extract (6488). Dried extracts contain more ephedra alkaloids per unit weight of material, due to the extraction process. The principal alkaloid constituents are ephedrine, pseudoephedrine, and sometimes small amounts of phenylpropanolamine (6008,6009). Other constituents that have been isolated include norpseudoephedrine, methylephedrine, and norephedrine (8644).

Ephedrine and pseudoephedrine are both non-selective alpha- and beta-receptor agonists. The ephedrine and pseudoephedrine constituents can directly and indirectly stimulate the sympathetic nervous system (12813). Ephedrine and pseudoephedrine can increase systolic and diastolic blood pressure, heart rate, and cardiac contractility, and cause peripheral vasoconstriction, bronchodilation, and central nervous system stimulation (8644). Ephedrine, which was used in combination with theophylline and phenobarbital (Tedral) for many years to treat asthma, causes bronchodilation and increased oxygen consumption (8645). A single dose of ephedra in combination with caffeine can increase heart rate from 67 beats per minute to 82 beats per minute in young, healthy people. The combination also increases systolic blood pressure and to a lesser extent, diastolic pressure (8644,11355,12856). Ephedra plus caffeine increases resting energy expenditure (REE), but the increase in energy expenditure is negligible in terms of weight loss (12856). Ephedrine is thought to cause thermogenesis and modest short-term weight loss, possibly by stimulating norepinephrine release. Some evidence suggests that aspirin and caffeine might act synergistically with ephedrine for weight loss by inhibiting prostaglandin, which increases norepinephrine release (314,729,10003).

Ephedra alkaloids have been linked to myocarditis and myocardial infarction. This has been attributed to coronary artery vasoconstriction and possibly vasospasm caused by ephedra. Ephedra might also cause cardiac arrhythmia due to adrenergic effects that shorten the cardiac refractory period, causing re-entrant arrhythmias (6486). The weight loss product Metabolife 356, which contains ephedra and caffeine in addition to 17 other ingredients, prolongs the QT interval by an average of 27 milliseconds in healthy volunteers (11355). As an indicator of ventricular depolarization and repolarization, a prolonged QT interval increases the risk of potentially serious ventricular arrhythmias such as torsades de pointes. Atrial premature contractions have been demonstrated in healthy volunteers taking recommended doses of Metabolife 356 for 14 days (11708).

Cerebral hemorrhage associated with ephedra has been attributed primarily to hypertensive effects and possibly due to cerebral vasculitis, which has been reported with other adrenergic drugs. Ischemic stroke has been attributed to ephedra's vasoconstrictive effects on cerebral vasculature and possibly platelet aggregation effects due to adrenergic stimulation (6486).

There's some evidence that ephedrine alone or in combination with caffeine can improve anaerobic exercise performance. Ephedrine causes catecholamine release and increases CNS stimulation, which may lead to better performance (8646).

Ephedrine is absorbed faster if it is consumed as the powdered extract. However, onset of action and extent of absorption does not differ greatly between the powdered extract and the powdered herb (6008,6009). Some sources claim ephedra is safer than pure ephedrine and pseudoephedrine because ephedrine from ephedra is absorbed more slowly. However, pharmacokinetic studies have found no differences in the pharmacokinetics of ephedrine from ephedra versus the purified form (6488). The time to maximum concentration (t max) for ephedra is 2.4 hours. The half-life is 6.1 hours (8644).

Adverse Reactions

Orally, ephedra is frequently associated with adverse reactions. In some cases, adverse effects can be severe or life-threatening. Ephedra is banned in the US. Poison control center data indicates ephedra is the herb most frequently associated with reports of adverse effects. It is 100 times more likely than other herbs to generate an adverse reaction report. Ephedra accounts for less than 1% of herbal product sales, but causes 64% of herbal adverse reaction reports to poison control centers (9170).

Ephedra most commonly causes dizziness, restlessness, anxiety, irritability, personality changes, difficulty concentrating, insomnia, headache, increased thirst, dry mouth, anorexia, nausea, vomiting, heartburn, flushing, tingling, difficulty urinating, tachycardia, heart palpitations, hyperthermia, and increased blood pressure (1276,3719,6008,6486,8647,10004,10382). Psychosis can occur in some people and in some cases it is prolonged for several months after discontinuation (1276,6998,10689). Long-term use or use in high doses has also been associated with dependence and tolerance (1381).

There are also several reports of serious life-threatening or debilitating adverse effects associated with ephedra products. Ephedra use has been associated with cardiomyopathy (1270), hypersensitivity myocarditis (1271,6487), chest tightness, myocardial infarction (6486), cardiac arrest and sudden death (1274,6486), and cardiac arrhythmias. In healthy volunteers, EKG changes including prolonged QT interval and premature atrial contractions can occur with ingestion of recommended doses of ephedra containing products (11135,11708). Ephedra can cause seizures in otherwise healthy people, as well as in people with underlying seizure disorders. In a review of cases of seizures linked to dietary supplements that were reported to the FDA over 7 years, 27 of 33 cases involved ephedra (13304). Other reported events include stroke, transient ischemic attack, cerebral hemorrhage, and loss of consciousness (1275,1381,2729,6486,8643). In a review of 926 cases reported to the FDA of possible adverse effects of ephedra, 37 patients had serious or fatal adverse reactions. Ephedra use was temporally related to 16 strokes, 10 myocardial infarctions, and 11 sudden deaths. These effects occurred in people aged 30-56 years. There is some evidence that people who take doses greater than 32 mg per day might have more than triple the risk of hemorrhagic

stroke, including subarachnoid hemorrhage and intracerebral hemorrhage (9167).
There are also reports of myopathies, including myalgia, rhabdomyolysis, eosinophilia-myalgia syndrome (1270), nephrolithiasis (1272), and acute hepatitis (1273). However, the single case of hepatitis is more likely the result of product contamination than due to ephedra itself (1273). Other reported events include sudden hearing loss (10005). Adverse effects are consistent with catecholamine excess (8643). The use of ephedra causes a 2.2- to 3.6-fold increase in the risk of developing psychiatric, autonomic, or gastrointestinal (GI) symptoms; and cardiac palpitations (9740). Large studies looking at the safety of ephedra have not been performed. Since most of the adverse effect data are from case reports, it is impossible to determine the overall incidence of these adverse effects. It is also difficult to determine which patient groups might be most likely to experience an adverse event. Patients with a history of cardiovascular disease would be expected to be at a higher risk. However, there have been several reports of serious events in patients with no known pre-existing medical condition. In many of these cases, ephedra was used in combination with another stimulant such as caffeine (10307). However, there are also reports of serious adverse effects when ephedra has been used alone. The safety of ephedra is controversial and highly debated. Some claim that ephedra is only unsafe when it is used inappropriately and in excessive doses. The supplement industry maintains that ephedra is safe when taken in doses recommended on labeling. However, there are several cases where severe life-threatening or debilitating effects occurred with short-term use of relatively low doses ranging from 20-60 mg ephedra alkaloids per day (6486). There is also considerable inter- and intra-product variability in labeled ephedra content, which adds to concern about ephedra toxicity (8643,11336). Contaminants such as norpseudoephedrine, a schedule 4 controlled substance, are also present in some products (8643). Until more is known, warn patients that the potential risks of using ephedra outweigh any potential benefit. Advise patients against using products containing ephedra, especially in combination with other stimulants such as caffeine, or if they have a pre-existing condition such as cardiovascular disease.

Interactions with Herbs & Other Dietary Supplements

ERGOT ALKALOID DERIVATIVES: Theoretically, concomitant use might cause excessive vasoconstriction and hypertension due to the ephedrine contained in ephedra (6009).
HERBS AND SUPPLEMENTS WITH STIMULANT PROPERTIES: Use of ephedra and other stimulant herbs, such as those containing caffeine, can increase the risk of common side effects such as insomnia, jitteriness, tremulousness, dizziness, etc. Using ephedra with other stimulants might also increase the risk of more serious adverse effects such as hypertension, myocardial infarction (MI), stroke, and death. There are several reports of serious life-threatening or debilitating adverse events in patients taking ephedra in combination with caffeine and other stimulants (1275,6486,10307). Some herbs and supplements with significant caffeine content include black tea, coffee, cola nut, green tea, guarana, mate, and others.
PANAX GINSENG: Panax ginseng can cause prolonged QT interval with initial use. It might have an additive effect with ephedra on the QT interval, increasing the risk for arrhythmias (4322,11355).

Interactions with Drugs

ANTICONVULSANTS: Theoretically, concomitant use of ephedra might interfere with the effectiveness of anticonvulsant drugs. Ephedra is associated with seizure activity (13304). Some anticonvulsant drugs include phenobarbital, primidone (Mysoline), valproic acid (Depakene), gabapentin (Neurontin), carbamazepine (Tegretol), phenytoin (Dilantin), and others.
ANTIDIABETES DRUGS: Ephedra can raise blood glucose levels and might decrease the effectiveness of drug therapy. Monitor blood glucose concentrations closely (12857). Some antidiabetes drugs include glimepiride (Amaryl), glyburide (DiaBeta, Glynase PresTab, Micronase), insulin, pioglitazone (Actos), rosiglitazone (Avandia), and others.
DEXAMETHASONE (Decadron): Theoretically, concomitant use might reduce the effectiveness of dexamethasone, due to the ephedrine contained in ephedra. Ephedrine increases the clearance rate of dexamethasone (11462).
ERGOT DERIVATIVES: Theoretically, concomitant use of ephedra and ergot alkaloids might cause hypertension, due to the ephedrine contained in ephedra (6009).
METHYLXANTHINES: Use of ephedra with caffeine or other methylxanthines such as theophylline might increase the risk of stimulatory adverse effects (8641). There is also some evidence that using ephedra with caffeine might increase the risk of serious life-threatening or debilitating adverse effects such as hypertension, myocardial infarction (MI), stroke, seizures, and death (1275,6486,10307). Tell patients to avoid taking ephedra with caffeine and other stimulants.
MONOAMINE OXIDASE INHIBITORS (MAOIs): Concomitant use of ephedra with MAOIs might increase the risk of hypertension (6009).
QT INTERVAL-PROLONGING DRUGS: Ephedra may have an additive effect with drugs that prolong the QT interval. This may increase the risk of ventricular arrhythmias (11355). Drugs that prolong the QT interval include amiodarone (Cordarone), disopyramide (Norpace), dofetilide (Tikosyn), ibutilide (Corvert), procainamide (Pronestyl), quinidine, sotalol (Betapace), thioridazine (Mellaril), and many others.
STIMULANT DRUGS: Theoretically, drugs with CNS stimulant properties, such as phenylpropanolamine, pseudoephedrine, and diethylpropion, and many others might increase the risk of hypertension and adverse cardiovascular effects of ephedra due to its ephedra content (6009,6486).

Interactions with Foods

COFFEE, TEA: Theoretically, concomitant use of large amounts of caffeinated coffee or tea might increase the stimulatory effects and adverse effects of caffeine and the ephedrine-associated adverse effects of ephedra (12857).

Interactions with Lab Tests

AMPHETAMINE/METHAMPHETAMINE: Ephedra might cause false-positive urine amphetamine or methamphetamine test results. False-positive urine methamphetamine assays have been attributed to the use of herbal supplements containing ephedra (1381,10688).
CATECHOLAMINE: Ephedrine, a constituent of ephedra, can increase plasma catecholamine levels (8646).
EPHEDRINE: Ephedra can cause a positive urine ephedrine test due to its ephedrine content. A case of an athlete whose urine tested positive for norpseudoephedrine was attributed to the use of an herbal supplement labeled to contain ephedra. However, the product might also have contained added norpseudoephedrine as an unlabeled ingredient (1259).
GLUCOSE: Ephedra can increase blood glucose levels and test results (8646). Monitor blood glucose levels in diabetes patients closely.
LACTATE: Ephedrine, a constituent of ephedra, can increase blood lactate levels (8646).

Interactions with Diseases or Conditions

ANGINA: Ephedra is contraindicated in people with angina; it might induce or exacerbate angina due its cardiac stimulant effects (8644,12813).
ANXIETY: Large doses of ephedra might cause or exacerbate anxiety due to central nervous system (CNS) stimulant effects (8644,12813).
ARRHYTHMIA: Ephedra might exacerbate arrhythmia. Ephedra has been linked to tachycardia and arrhythmias, due to its cardiac stimulant effects (11355,11708).
DIABETES: Ephedra might interfere with blood sugar control, and exacerbate high blood pressure and circulatory problems in people with diabetes (12857).
ESSENTIAL TREMOR: Ephedra might exacerbate essential tremor (1715).
HYPERTENSION: Ephedra might exacerbate hypertension (11355); contraindicated in uncontrolled hypertension.
HYPERTHYROID, THYROTOXICOSIS: Theoretically, ephedra might stimulate the thyroid and exacerbate hyperthyroid symptoms; contraindicated (12858).
KIDNEY STONES (Nephrolithiasis): Ephedra and ephedrine can cause kidney stones (1272).
LONG QT INTERVAL SYNDROME: Ephedra appears to prolong the QT interval (11355). It might increase the risk of ventricular arrhythmias in patients with long QT interval syndrome.
NARROW-ANGLE GLAUCOMA: Ephedra might exacerbate narrow-angle (angle-closure) glaucoma by causing mydriasis (12859).
PHEOCHROMOCYTOMA: Ephedra might exacerbate the symptoms of pheochromocytoma; contraindicated (8644,12813).
SEIZURE DISORDERS: Ephedra might cause an exacerbation or precipitation of a seizure in patients with an underlying seizure disorder. In a review of cases of seizures linked to dietary supplements that were reported to the FDA over 7 years, 27 of 33 cases involved ephedra (13304).

Dosage and Administration

ORAL: For reducing weight in obese patients, ephedra 12 mg in combination with guarana 40 mg three times daily plus 17 other vitamins, minerals, and supplements (Metabolife 356) has been used (3719). Ephedra 90 mg plus caffeine 192 mg per day has also been used for weight loss (8647). Ephedra 60 mg per day plus cola nut and willow bark has also been used for weight loss (12811). The typical dose of ephedra is 15-20 mg of the ephedra alkaloids calculated as ephedrine taken up to three times daily (6486).

Comments

On December 30, 2003, the FDA announced the ban of ephedra products in the US, effective April 2004 (10055). There has been a lot of debate about the safety of ephedra and legal wrangling over its status (8640,8641). In June of 1997, the FDA proposed restrictions on the ephedrine content of dietary supplements, new warning labels for ephedra alkaloid-containing products, and a prohibition on combination products containing ephedra and other natural stimulants, such as guarana and cola nut, both of which contain significant amounts of caffeine (2729). These proposals were dropped after the link between ephedra use and serious adverse effects was challenged by the General Accounting Office (GAO) and the dietary supplement industry (1381). According to the Dietary Supplement Health and Education Act of 1994, FDA must prove a supplement is unsafe before it can be withdrawn from the market (8642). The FDA reviewed numerous adverse event reports involving ephedra alkaloid-containing products, with 140 of the reports receiving in-depth clinical review by FDA and outside experts (1381,5047,6486). Findings from experts outside the FDA support the FDA's initial finding that ephedra is likely the cause of many of the reports (6486).
In April 2005, the dietary supplement industry successfully challenged the FDA Ban on ephedra. A year after the ban on ephedra began, a federal judge in Utah stuck down the FDA's action saying that FDA didn't prove that low doses of ephedra are harmful. FDA is currently reviewing the Utah court decision and is interpreting the ruling as relevant

only to ephedra products that contain 10 mg or less of ephedra. Some supplement manufacturers infer a complete reversal of the ephedra ban. Ephedra products are now readily available on the Internet (12912,12913).
Ephedra use is banned by the National Collegiate Athletic Association, International Olympic Committee, and National Football League (8642).
Ephedra is sometimes marketed as a recreational drug "herbal ecstasy." The FDA has announced that ephedra products marketed as recreational drugs are unapproved and misbranded drugs subject to seizure and injunction (5047).
Mormon tea and ephedra are often confused. Mormon tea or American ephedra comes from Ephedra nevadensis, and ephedra or ma huang comes primarily from Ephedra sinica. Mormon tea is alkaloid-free and lacks both the therapeutic effects and the toxicity of ephedrine (10055).

EPIMEDIUM

Also Known As

Barrenwort, Herba Epimedii, Horny Goat Weed, Japanese Epimedium, Xian Ling Pi, Yin Yang Huo.

Scientific Names

Epimedium grandiflorum; Epimedium brevicornum; Epimedium sagittatum; Epimedium acuminatum; Epimedium grandiflorum f. flavescens, synonym Epimedium koreanum; Epimedium pubescens; Epimedium wushanense; other Epimedium species.
Family: Berberidaceae.

People Use This For

Orally, epimedium is used for impotence, involuntary ejaculation, weak back and knees, arthralgia, mental and physical fatigue, memory loss, hypertension, coronary heart disease, bronchitis, chronic hepatitis, polio, chronic leukopenia, viral myocarditis, and as a tonic and aphrodisiac.
Epimedium is included in some personal care products for its antimicrobial effects.

Safety

LIKELY UNSAFE ...when large amounts are used orally. Some species of epimedium can cause respiratory arrest (10346).
There is insufficient reliable information available about the safety of epimedium when typical or low doses are used.
PREGNANCY: POSSIBLY UNSAFE ...when used orally. Epimedium might have androgenic activity (10346); avoid using.
LACTATION: Insufficient reliable information available; avoid using.

Effectiveness

There is insufficient reliable information available about the effectiveness of epimedium.

Mechanism of Action

The applicable part of epimedium is the leaf. Researchers think flavonoids, icariin, polysaccharides, glycosides, ceryl alcohol, essential oils, and fatty acids are the active constituents. Epimedium causes vasodilation, possibly by blocking calcium channels. It also seems to have hypotensive effects, possibly by catecholamine blockade (10346). The glycosides in epimedium might have hormonal effects. Animal research suggests that epimedium promotes semen secretion and stimulates growth of prostate, testes, and anus rector muscles. Some researchers think it might increase testosterone secretion (10346). Preliminary research suggests epimedium increases coronary blood flow and decreases platelet aggregation. It may also have immunostimulatory activity and activity against HIV (1512,10346).

Adverse Reactions

Orally, extended use of epimedium may result in dizziness, vomiting, dry mouth, thirst, and nosebleed. Large doses of epimedium may cause respiratory arrest and exaggeration of tendon reflexes to the point of spasm (10346).
There is a case report of tachyarrhythmia and hypomania in a 66 year-old man with a history of cardiovascular disease following 2 weeks of ingesting a product labeled as horny goat weed (epimedium) for improving sexual function (13006). It is not clear if this product contained the single ingredient epimedium or a combination of ingredients. Therefore, it is not possible to assess whether epimedium is the cause of this adverse event.

Interactions with Herbs & Other Dietary Supplements

HERBS AND SUPPLEMENTS WITH HYPOTENSIVE EFFECTS: Epimedium might have hypotensive effects (10346). Theoretically, concurrent use of epimedium with other herbs and supplements that decrease blood pressure might increase risk of hypotension. Some of these products include danshen, ginger, Panax ginseng, turmeric, valerian, and others.

HERBS WITH ANTICOAGULANT/ANTIPLATELET POTENTIAL: Concomitant use of herbs with constituents that might affect platelet aggregation could theoretically increase the risk of bleeding in some people when taken with epimedium (10346). These herbs include angelica, clove, danshen, garlic, ginger, ginkgo, quassia, red clover, turmeric, willow, and others.

Interactions with Drugs

ANTICOAGULANT/ANTIPLATELET DRUGS: Theoretically, epimedium might potentiate the effects of anticoagulant and antiplatelet drugs and possibly increase the risk of bleeding (10346). However, this effect has not yet been demonstrated in humans. Until more is known, use cautiously in patients taking anticoagulant or antiplatelet drugs. Some of these drugs include aspirin, clopidogrel (Plavix), dalteparin (Fragmin), enoxaparin (Lovenox), heparin, ticlopidine (Ticlid), warfarin (Coumadin), and others.
ANTIHYPERTENSIVE DRUGS: Epimedium might have hypotensive effects (10346). Theoretically, concomitant use with antihypertensives might have additive effects on blood pressure and increase the risk of hypotension.

Interactions with Foods

None known.

Interactions with Lab Tests

None known.

Interactions with Diseases or Conditions

HYPOTENSION: Epimedium might have hypotensive effects (10346). Theoretically, use in people with existing low blood pressure might exacerbate hypotension and possibly lead to syncope.

Dosage and Administration

No typical dosage.

Comments

The leaf of Japanese epimedium (Epimedium grandiflora) is generally used (12). Leaf, petiole, and stem of other Epimedium species are also sometimes used (11). As many as 15 Epimedium species are interchangeable as "yin yang huo" (11).

ERGOT

Also Known As

Cockspur Rye, Hornseed, Mother of Rye, Secale cornutum, Smut Rye, Spurred Rye.

Scientific Names

Claviceps purpurea. Plant host: Rye (Secale cereale).
Family: Clavicipitaceae.

People Use This For

Orally, ergot is used for obstetric and gynecologic conditions, including hemorrhage, climacteric hemorrhage, menorrhagia, metrorrhagia (before and after miscarriage), expulsion of placenta, shortening of afterbirth period, and atonia of the uterus.

Safety

UNSAFE ...when used orally due to poisoning risk and interactions with many disease states (11163,11164).
PREGNANCY AND LACTATION: UNSAFE ...when used orally due to high level of risk (11163,11164); avoid using.

Effectiveness

There is insufficient reliable information available about the effectiveness of ergot.

Mechanism of Action

Ergot is a fungal growth that occurs on rye (Secale cereale), and to a lesser extent, other grasses such as wheat (Triticum aestivum). The fungus contains ergot alkaloids (ergolines). Derivatives of ergot including lysergic acid, ergocristine, ergotamine, ergonovine (ergometrine), and many others have been isolated. Ergot alkaloids have various pharmacologic activities. They act as serotonin agonists, which can cause arterial vasoconstriction. Ergot alkaloids also act as dopamine agonists. For example, bromocriptine (Parlodel) is an ergot derivative. Some act as alpha-adrenergic antagonists and cause vasoconstriction. Ergot alkaloids, particularly ergonovine, also cause uterine smooth-muscle contraction. Ergot also contains histamine, tyramine, and acetylcholine, but these are probably not significantly absorbed when ergot is taken orally (11163).

Adverse Reactions

Orally, ergot can cause gastrointestinal (GI) symptoms such as nausea and abdominal pain. Weakness, muscle pain of the extremities, and numbness and tingling of the fingers and toes may also occur (9). Symptoms of acute overdose include nausea, vomiting, diarrhea, extreme thirst, coldness, tingling and itching of the skin, a rapid and weak pulse, hypotension, shock, confusion, seizures, unconsciousness, and death (9). Chronic toxicity or ergotism rarely occurs after a single oral dose. It usually results from cumulative doses over a short period of time (11163). Symptoms of ergotism are related to circulatory disturbances. Numbness, coldness, and tingling of the extremities, particularly the feet and legs occur along with paleness or cyanosis. There may be no pulse in the affected area. This may develop into gangrene, especially in the toes (9,11163). A convulsive form of ergotism may also occur. Symptoms include muscle spasms in the trunk and limbs, painful involuntary flexion of the fingers and wrists, and either flexion or extension of the ankles. Central nervous system (CNS) adverse effects such as drowsiness, delirium, lethargy, mental changes, and visual disturbances can also occur. Sweating, fever, muscle stiffness, twitching and seizures have also been reported (9,11163). Ergotism from food is rare today. It is more common from overdoses of prescription ergot alkaloids (11164).

Interactions with Herbs & Other Dietary Supplements

HERBS AND SUPPLEMENTS WITH SEROTONERGIC PROPERTIES: Theoretically, ergot might increase the effects and adverse effects of products that increase serotonin levels, including 5-hydroxytryptophan, Hawaiian baby woodrose, l-tryptophan S-adenosylmethionine (SAMe), and St. John's wort (11163).
HERBS AND SUPPLEMENTS WITH SYMPATHOMIMETIC ACTIVITY: Theoretically, ergot might enhance the effects and adverse effects of herbs and supplements that have sympathomimetic activity, including bitter orange, caffeine, country mallow, guarana, and ephedra (11163).

Interactions with Drugs

ANTIDEPRESSANT DRUGS: Combining serotonergic antidepressants with ergot might increase the risk of serotonergic side effects including serotonin syndrome and cerebral vasoconstrictive disorders such as Call-Fleming syndrome (8056,11163). These drugs include the selective serotonin reuptake inhibitors (SSRIs) such as fluoxetine (Prozac), paroxetine (Paxil), sertraline (Zoloft), and others; and tricyclic and atypical antidepressants such as amitriptyline (Elavil), clomipramine (Anafranil), imipramine (Tofranil), and others.
CYTOCHROME P450 3A4 (CYP3A4) INHIBITORS: Ergotamine, a constituent of ergot, is a substrate of cytochrome P450 3A4 (CYP3A4) (11163). Theoretically, drugs that inhibit CYP3A4 might increase the risk of ergot toxicity. Some of these drugs include amiodarone (Cordarone), clarithromycin (Biaxin), diltiazem (Cardizem), erythromycin (E-mycin, Erythrocin), indinavir (Crixivan), ritonavir (Norvir), saquinavir (Fortovase, Invirase), and many others.
DEXTROMETHORPHAN (Robitussin DM, others): Combining serotonergic drugs such as dextromethorphan with ergot might increase the risk of serotonergic side effects including serotonin syndrome and cerebral vasoconstrictive disorders such as Call-Fleming syndrome (8056,11163).
ERGOT DERIVATIVES: Ergot alkaloids or derivatives may increase the risk of adverse effects (11163). Some of these include bromocriptine (Parlodel), dihydroergotamine (Migranal, DHE-45), ergotamine (Cafergot), and pergolide (Permax).
MEPERIDINE (Demerol): Combining serotonergic drugs such as meperidine with ergot might increase the risk of serotonergic side effects including serotonin syndrome and cerebral vasoconstrictive disorders such as Call-Fleming syndrome (8056,11163).
MONOAMINE OXIDASE INHIBITORS (MAOIs): Combining serotonergic drugs such as one of the MAOIs with ergot might increase the risk of serotonergic side effects including serotonin syndrome and cerebral vasoconstrictive disorders such as Call-Fleming syndrome (8056,11163).
PENTAZOCINE (Talwin): Combining serotonergic drugs such as pentazocin with ergot might increase the risk of serotonergic side effects including serotonin syndrome and cerebral vasoconstrictive disorders such as Call-Fleming syndrome (8056,11163).
STIMULANT DRUGS: Co-administration with ergot may increase the risk of vasoconstriction. Some sympathomimetics include albuterol (Proventil, Ventolin), diethylpropion (Tenuate), dopamine, epinephrine, phentermine (Ionamin), pseudoephedrine (Sudafed), and many others (11163).
TRAMADOL (Ultram): Combining serotonergic drugs such as tramadol with ergot might increase the risk of serotonergic side effects including serotonin syndrome and cerebral vasoconstrictive disorders such as Call-Fleming syndrome (8056,11163).

Interactions with Foods

None known.

Interactions with Lab Tests

None known.

Interactions with Diseases or Conditions
HEART DISEASE: Ergot can cause arterial constriction and may worsen coronary insufficiency (11163).
KIDNEY DISEASE: Reduced renal clearance of ergot may increase the risk of ergot poisoning (9).
LIVER DISEASE: Reduced hepatic clearance of ergot may increase the risk of ergot poisoning (9).
PERIPHERAL VASCULAR DISEASE: Ergot can cause vasoconstriction and may worsen peripheral vascular disease (9).

Dosage and Administration
No typical dosage.

Comments
Historically, ergot was used to speed labor, but its use was abandoned when increased risk of stillbirth was recognized (11163).
During the Middle Ages, ergotism was common from food contamination (such as rye bread) and was known as St. Anthony's fire. It was often cured by visiting the shrine of St. Anthony, which happened to be in an ergot-free region of France. Some historians think the Salem witchcraft trials of 1692 might have resulted from a convulsive form of ergotism (11164).

ERYNGO

Also Known As
Eringo, Eryngii Herba, Eryngii Radix, Sea Holly, Sea Holme, Sea Hulver.
CAUTION: See separate listing for Iceland Moss.

Scientific Names
Eryngium campestre, synonyms Eryngium maritimum, Eyrnigium planum, Eryngium yuccifolium.
Family: Apiaceae/Umbelliferae.

People Use This For
Orally, eryngo above ground parts are used for urinary tract infections and inflammation, prostatitis, and respiratory mucous membrane inflammation. Eryngo root is used for kidney and bladder stones, renal colic, kidney and urinary tract inflammation, urinary retention, edema, coughs, bronchitis, and skin and respiratory disorders.

Safety
There is insufficient reliable information available about the safety of eryngo.
Pregnancy and Lactation: Insufficient reliable information available; avoid using.

Effectiveness
There is insufficient reliable information available about the effectiveness of eryngo.

Mechanism of Action
The applicable parts of eryngo are the above ground parts and the root. Eryngo above ground parts are thought to have a diuretic effect. Eryngo root is thought to have expectorant and antispasmodic effects (18). However, there is very little scientific evidence available about the pharmacological properties of this plant.

Adverse Reactions
None reported.

Interactions with Herbs & Other Dietary Supplements
None known.

Interactions with Drugs
None known.

Interactions with Foods
None known.

Interactions with Lab Tests
None known.

Interactions with Diseases or Conditions
CROSS-ALLERGENICITY: Theoretically, eryngo might cause an allergic reaction in people who are sensitive to other plants in the Apiaceae family. These plants include celery, fennel, dill, and many others.

Dosage and Administration

ORAL: No typical dosage. However, traditionally as a tea, 1 teaspoon ground root in 150 mL of boiling water until cold; 3-4 cups have been used daily (18). As a decoction 2-3 cups, 4 teaspoons of ground root in 1 L water for 10 minutes, have been used daily (18); or 50-60 drops of tincture, 1:4 60% alcohol, divided into 3 or 4 doses daily has been used.

EUCALYPTUS

Also Known As

Blue Gum, Blue Mallee, Blue Mallee Oil, Eucalypti Folium, Fever Tree, Fieberbaumblatter, Gully Gum, Gum Tree, Red Gum, Stringy Bark Tree, Sugandhapatra, Tailapatra, Tasmanian Blue Gum.
CAUTION: See separate listing for Lemon Eucalyptus.

Scientific Names

Eucalyptus globulus; Eucalyptus bicostata; Eucalyptus smithii; Eucalyptus odorata, synonym Eucalyptus fruticetorum; Eucalyptus polybractea.
Family: Myrtaceae.

People Use This For

Orally, eucalyptus leaf is used for infections, fever, dyspepsia, and as an expectorant for coughs. The leaf is also used orally for treating respiratory tract infections, whooping cough, asthma, pulmonary tuberculosis, osteoarthritis, rheumatism, acne, wounds, poorly healing ulcers, burns, bacterial dysentery, ringworms, liver and gallbladder complaints, loss of appetite, stomatitis, bleeding gums, bladder diseases, gonorrhea, flu, diabetes, neuralgia, and cancer. Orally, eucalyptus oil is used for inflammation of respiratory tract mucous membranes, coughs, bronchitis, sinusitis, asthma, chronic obstructive pulmonary disease (COPD), and respiratory infections. It is also used as an expectorant, antiseptic, antipyretic, and in vaporizer fluids. Other uses include wounds, burns, ulcers, and cancer.
Topically, eucalyptus oil is used for inflammation of respiratory tract mucous membranes, rheumatic complaints, rheumatoid arthritis, athletic performance, genital herpes, and nasal stuffiness. It is also used as an insect repellant.
In dentistry, eucalyptus oil is a component of sealers and solvents for root canal fillings.
In foods, dried eucalyptus leaf is used as a flavoring agent.
In manufacturing, eucalyptus oil is used as a fragrance component in perfumes and cosmetics. It is also used as a mouthwash, antiseptic, liniment and ointment, and in toothpaste, cough drops, and gum lozenges.

Safety

LIKELY SAFE ...when used orally in amounts commonly found in foods. Eucalyptus has Generally Recognized As Safe status (GRAS) for use in foods in the US (4912).
POSSIBLY SAFE ...when eucalyptol, a constituent of eucalyptus oil, is used orally and appropriately. Eucalyptol appears to be safe for up to 12 weeks (13302).
POSSIBLY UNSAFE ...when the undiluted oil is used topically. Prolonged or widespread exposure has caused neurotoxicity (12869).
LIKELY UNSAFE ...when the undiluted oil is ingested orally. Ingesting 3.5 mL of undiluted oil can be fatal (12867). There is insufficient reliable information available about the safety of eucalyptus leaf in medicinal amounts; avoid using.
CHILDREN: LIKELY SAFE ...when used orally in amounts commonly found in foods. Eucalyptus has Generally Recognized As Safe status (GRAS) for use in foods in the US (4912). LIKELY UNSAFE ...when used topically in infants and young children because it can cause neurotoxicity (12868,12869). ...when the oil is used orally (12867). There is insufficient reliable information available about the safety of eucalyptus leaf in medicinal amounts; avoid using.
PREGNANCY AND LACTATION: LIKELY SAFE ...when used orally in amounts commonly found in foods (4912). There is insufficient reliable information available about the safety of medicinal amounts of eucalyptus oil; avoid using.

Effectiveness

INSUFFICIENT RELIABLE EVIDENCE to RATE

Asthma. Preliminary clinical research suggests that eucalyptol, a constituent of eucalyptus oil, has mucolytic properties. When used orally, it may allow dosage reduction of oral steroids in patients with severe asthma (13302). More evidence is needed to rate eucalyptus for this use.

Mechanism of Action

The applicable parts of eucalyptus are the leaf and oil. Eucalyptus leaf extracts seem to have antimicrobial and antifungal activity (12870).

An aqueous extract of eucalyptus leaf appears to have hypoglycemic activity. Preliminary research suggests it increases insulin secretion and enhances the uptake and metabolism of glucose by muscle (12871).

Eucalyptus oil, which is made from the leaves and branches of eucalyptus, contains 60% to 90% eucalyptol (1,8-cineole). Eucalyptol appears to have analgesic and anti-inflammatory effects (12866). Preliminary research suggests eucalyptol might block the production of arachidonic acid metabolites that mediate pain. It might also inhibit cyclooxygenase pathways (12866,13302). It also seems to inhibit the production of cytokines responsible for inflammation such as tumor necrosis factor (TNF)-alpha, interleukin (IL)-1beta, leukotriene B4, and thromboxane B2. This might explain its use in asthma (12866).

Eucalyptus oil also contains cineole, which can cause seizures when consumed in high doses (12868). Eucalyptus and eucalyptus oil also contain the very toxic hydrocyanic acid (13303).

Eucalyptus oil appears to inhibit cytochrome P450 enzymes, according to preliminary research (12479).

Adverse Reactions

Orally, eucalyptus leaf theoretically might cause gastrointestinal effects. Oral use of eucalyptus oil can cause nausea, vomiting, and diarrhea. Signs of eucalyptus oil poisoning include central nervous system depression, shallow respiration, rapid pulse, coma, and death. The ingestion of 3.5 mL of the oil can be fatal to adults (12867).

Topically, prolonged exposure or large amounts of eucalyptus oil can cause agitation, drowsiness, slurred speech, ataxia, muscle weakness, and seizures. The risk of toxicity may be greater in children (12868,12869). Eucalyptus pollen can cause contact dermatitis in sensitive people (13303).

Interactions with Herbs & Other Dietary Supplements

HEPATOTOXIC PYRROLIZIDINE ALKALOID (PA)-CONTAINING PLANTS: Eucalyptus can potentiate the toxicity of herbs that contain hepatotoxic pyrrolizidine alkaloids (PAs) (12865). Herbs containing hepatotoxic PAs include alkanna, borage, coltsfoot, comfrey, gravel root, hemp agrimony, hound's tongue, and lungwort, and the Senecio species plants dusty miller, alpine ragwort, groundsel, golden ragwort, and tansy ragwort.

Interactions with Drugs

ANTIDIABETES DRUGS: Preliminary research suggests eucalyptus leaf might have hypoglycemic activity, and might have additive effects when used with antidiabetes drugs (12871). This might increase the risk of hypoglycemia in some patients. Monitor blood glucose levels closely. Some antidiabetes drugs include glimepiride (Amaryl), glyburide (DiaBeta, Glynase PresTab, Micronase), insulin, metformin (Glucophage), pioglitazone (Actos), rosiglitazone (Avandia), and others.

CYTOCHROME P450 1A2 (CYP1A2) SUBSTRATES: There's preliminary evidence that eucalyptus oil might inhibit cytochrome P450 1A2 (CYP1A2) (12479). So far, this interaction has not been reported in humans. However, watch for an increase in the levels of drugs metabolized by CYP1A2 in patients taking eucalyptus oil. Some drugs metabolized by CYP1A2 include amitriptyline (Elavil), haloperidol (Haldol), ondansetron (Zofran), propranolol (Inderal), theophylline (Theo-Dur, others), verapamil (Calan, Isoptin, others), and others. Use eucalyptus oil cautiously or avoid in patients taking these drugs.

CYTOCHROME P450 2C19 (CYP2C19) SUBSTRATES: There's preliminary evidence that eucalyptus oil might inhibit cytochrome P450 2C19 (CYP2C19) (12479). So far, this interaction has not been reported in humans. However, watch for an increase in the levels of drugs metabolized by CYP2C19 in patients taking eucalyptus oil. Some drugs metabolized by CYP2C19 include proton pump inhibitors including omeprazole (Prilosec), lansoprazole (Prevacid), and pantoprazole (Protonix); diazepam (Valium); carisoprodol (Soma); nelfinavir (Viracept); and others.

CYTOCHROME P450 2C9 (CYP2C9) SUBSTRATES: There's preliminary evidence that eucalyptus oil might inhibit cytochrome P450 2C9 (CYP2C9) (12479). So far, this interaction has not been reported in humans. However, watch for an increase in the levels of drugs metabolized by CYP2C9 in patients taking eucalyptus oil. Some drugs metabolized by CYP2C9 include nonsteroidal anti-inflammatory drugs (NSAIDs) such as diclofenac (Cataflam, Voltaren), ibuprofen (Motrin), meloxicam (Mobic), and piroxicam (Feldene); celecoxib (Celebrex); amitriptyline (Elavil); warfarin (Coumadin); glipizide (Glucotrol); losartan (Cozaar); and others. Use eucalyptus oil cautiously or avoid in patients taking these drugs.

CYTOCHROME P450 3A4 (CYP3A4) SUBSTRATES: There's preliminary evidence that eucalyptus oil might inhibit cytochrome P450 3A4 (CYP3A4) enzyme (12479). So far, this interaction has not been reported in humans. However, watch for an increase in the levels of drugs metabolized by CYP3A4 in patients taking eucalyptus oil. Some drugs metabolized by CYP3A4 include lovastatin (Mevacor), ketoconazole (Nizoral), itraconazole (Sporanox), fexofenadine (Allegra), triazolam (Halcion), and numerous others. Use eucalyptus oil cautiously or avoid in patients taking these drugs.

Interactions with Foods

None known.

Interactions with Lab Tests

BLOOD GLUCOSE: Preliminary research suggests eucalyptus leaf might have hypoglycemic activity and theoretically might lower blood glucose and test results (12871).

Interactions with Diseases or Conditions

DIABETES: Preliminary research suggests eucalyptus leaf might have hypoglycemic activity and theoretically might have additive effects when used with antidiabetes drugs (12871). This might increase the risk of hypoglycemia in some patients. Monitor blood glucose levels closely.

Dosage and Administration

ORAL: For asthma, the eucalyptol constituent of eucalyptus oil has been given in doses of 200 mg three times daily (13302).

EUPHORBIA

Also Known As

Asthmaplant, Pillbearing Spurge, Snakeweed.

Scientific Names

Chamaesyce hirta, synonyms Euphorbia hirta, Euphorbia pilulifera; Euphorbia capitulata.
Family: Euphorbiaceae.

People Use This For

Orally, euphorbia is used for respiratory disorders including asthma, bronchitis, catarrh, laryngeal spasm, hay fever, and tumors, and as an expectorant and an emetic. It is also used orally for treating worms, dysentery, gonorrhea, and digestive problems in India.

Safety

There is insufficient reliable information available about the safety of euphorbia.
PREGNANCY AND LACTATION: POSSIBLY UNSAFE ...when used orally; avoid using.
Euphorbia is reported to cause smooth muscle contraction and relaxation (4).

Effectiveness

There is insufficient reliable information available about the effectiveness of euphorbia.

Mechanism of Action

The applicable parts of euphorbia are the above ground parts. It is reported to have antispasmodic, histamine potentiator, antitumor, and antibacterial activity against gram positive and gram negative organisms in animals (4). The constituent choline is reported to produce contraction of isolated pig ileum. The constituent shikimic acid produces relaxation (11).

Adverse Reactions

Orally, euphorbia may cause nausea and vomiting (12).
Topically, skin contact with fresh euphorbia can cause irritation or contact dermatitis (19).

Interactions with Herbs & Other Dietary Supplements

None known.

Interactions with Drugs

None known.

Interactions with Foods

None known.

Interactions with Lab Tests

None known.

Interactions with Diseases or Conditions

GI CONDITIONS: Euphorbia can irritate the gastrointestinal tract. Contraindicated in individuals with infectious or inflammatory gastrointestinal conditions (19).

Dosage and Administration

ORAL: Typical dose is one cup tea prepared by steeping 120-300 mg above ground parts in 150 mL boiling water 5-10 minutes and then straining (4). Liquid extract, concentration unspecified, 0.12-0.3 mL, and tincture, concentration unspecified, 0.6-2 mL have also been used (4). As and expectorant, 2 grams above ground parts has been used; emetic dose may be similar.

EUROPEAN BARBERRY

Also Known As

Agracejo, Berberidis cortex, Berberidis fructus, Berberidis radicis cortex, Berberidis radix, Berberitze, Berberry, Berbis, Common Barberry, Epine-Vinette, Espino Cambrón, Jaundice Berry, Mountain Grape, Oregon Grape, Pipperidge, Piprage, Sauerdorn, Sow Berry, Vinettier.
CAUTION: See separate listing for Oregon Grape.

Scientific Names

Berberis vulgaris, synonyms Berberis jacquinii, Berberis sanguinea.
Family: Berberidaceae.

People Use This For

Orally, the fruit of European barberry is used for kidney, urinary tract, and gastrointestinal tract discomforts such as heartburn, stomach cramps, constipation, lack of appetite, liver and spleen disease, for bronchial and lung discomforts, spasms, as a stimulant for circulation, for people susceptible to infection, and as a supplemental source of vitamin C. The bark, root, and root bark of European barberry are also used orally for ailments and complaints of the GI tract, liver, gallbladder, kidney and urinary tract, respiratory tract, heart and circulatory system, as an antipyretic, "blood purifier", and for narcotic withdrawal. European barberry root bark is used for liver dysfunction, gallbladder disease, jaundice, splenopathy, diarrhea, indigestion, hemorrhoids, renal and urinary tract diseases, gout, rheumatism, arthritis, mid and low back pain, malaria, and leishmaniasis.
In foods, European barberry fruit is used in making jam, jellies, and wine.
In manufacturing, the fruit syrup is used for masking tastes in pharmaceutical preparations.

Safety

LIKELY SAFE ...when the fruit is consumed in food amounts. The fruit is considered to contain only trace amounts of berberine (2,12).
POSSIBLY SAFE ...when the fruit, root, bark, or root bark are used orally and appropriately for medicinal uses. Amounts of less than 500 mg of berberine are usually considered safe (2,12,18).
LIKELY UNSAFE ...when more than 500 mg of berberine is consumed. Berberine is considered moderately toxic (12). The LD50 in humans is reported to be 27.5 mg/kg (12).
PREGNANCY: LIKELY UNSAFE ...when used orally because it can have uterine stimulant properties (11,12).
LACTATION: Insufficient reliable information is available; avoid using.

Effectiveness

There is insufficient reliable information available about the effectiveness of European barberry.

Mechanism of Action

The applicable parts of European barberry are the bark, fruit, root, and root bark. European barberry fruit contains vitamin C (18). Researchers think it has mild diuretic activity due to the acid content (18). The bark, root, and root bark of European barberry contain isoquinolone alkaloid constituents, including berberine, berbamine, columbamine, jatorrhizine, palmatine, and oxyacanthine (11,19). The constituents berberine, columbamine, and oxyacanthine show evidence of antibacterial activity (11). Berberine has anticonvulsant, sedative, hypotensive, antifibrillatory, and bile-stimulating effects. In low doses, it is a cardiac and respiratory stimulant. In high doses it is a depressant (11,12,515). Some evidence suggests berberine sulfate might be amebicidal and trypanocidal (11). Other information suggests the constituent berbamine might have antiarrhythmic, hypotensive, spasmolytic, and immunostimulating activity (11,515).

Adverse Reactions

Orally, ingestion of greater than 500 mg berberine, which is found in European barberry, can cause lethargy, nose bleed, skin and eye irritation, nephritis and kidney irritation (2). It might also cause dyspnea, hypotension, cardiac damage (12), nausea, vomiting, diarrhea, hemorrhagic nephritis, respiratory spasms and arrest, and death (2).

Interactions with Herbs & Other Dietary Supplements

BERBERINE-CONTAINING HERBS: Concomitant use can increase the risk of berberine toxicity. Berberine-containing herbs include: bloodroot, goldenseal, celandine, Chinese goldthread, goldthread, Oregon grape (Mahonia species), amur cork tree, and Chinese corktree (12).

Interactions with Drugs
None known.

Interactions with Foods
None known.

Interactions with Lab Tests
None known.

Interactions with Diseases or Conditions
GI IRRITATION: European barberry can irritate gastrointestinal tract. It is contraindicated in individuals with infectious or inflammatory gastrointestinal conditions (19).
KIDNEY DISEASE: Berberine, which is found in European barberry, can cause kidney irritation and nephritis (2).

Dosage and Administration
ORAL :A typical dose is one cup tea. To make tea, steep 1-2 teaspoons of whole or squashed berries in 150 mL boiling water 10-15 minutes and strain (18) or steep 2 grams of root bark in 250 mL boiling water 5-10 minutes and strain (18). Root bark is typically used as a tincture (1:10), 20-40 drops per day (18). Root tea is not recommended (2,18).

EUROPEAN BUCKTHORN

Also Known As
Buckthorn, Buckthorn Berry, Hartshorn, Highwaythorn, Kreuzdornbeeren, Ramsthorn, Rhamni cathartica fructus, Waythorn.
CAUTION: See separate listings for Alder Buckthorn, Sea Buckthorn, and Cascara (California Buckthorn).

Scientific Names
Rhamnus cathartica.
Family: Rhamnaceae.

People Use This For
Orally, European buckthorn is used for constipation.

Safety
POSSIBLY SAFE ...when the standardized preparations of the berry are used orally and appropriately for less than eight to ten days (12). It is important not to exceed recommended amounts (12).
POSSIBLY UNSAFE ...when standardized preparations are used more than ten days (12).
LIKELY UNSAFE ...when nonstandardized preparations are used orally (12).
CHILDREN: LIKELY UNSAFE ...when used orally in children younger than 12 years of age (12).
PREGNANCY AND LACTATION: LIKELY UNSAFE ...when used orally (12); avoid using.

Effectiveness
LIKELY EFFECTIVE

Constipation. Taking European buckthorn orally is effective as a stimulant laxative for constipation (3,4,7,12) and is comparable to the gentle, laxative effects of cascara (3).

Mechanism of Action
The applicable part of European buckthorn is the berry. The anthraquinones in the European buckthorn berry can increase intestinal GI motility by inhibiting stationary contractions and stimulating propulsive contractions (2). Stimulation of active chloride secretion increases the water and electrolytes in intestinal contents, increasing the risk of electrolyte loss with overuse or misuse of the berry (2). Anthroid laxative use is not associated with an increased risk of developing colorectal adenoma or carcinoma (6138).

Adverse Reactions
Orally, European buckthorn can cause abdominal pain, cramps, or watery diarrhea (12). Chronic use or abuse of the berry can lead to potassium depletion, albuminuria, and hematuria. Potassium depletion can lead to disturbed heart function and muscle weakness (2). Chronic use can cause pseudomelanosis coli (pigment spots in intestinal mucosa) which is harmless, usually reverses with discontinuation (2), and is not associated with an increased risk of developing colorectal ademoma or carcinoma (6138).

Interactions with Herbs & Other Dietary Supplements

CARDIAC GLYCOSIDE-CONTAINING HERBS: Theoretically, overuse or abuse of European buckthorn can increase the risk of cardiac glycoside toxicity. Cardiac glycoside containing herbs include black hellebore, Canadian hemp roots, digitalis leaf, hedge mustard, figwort, lily-of-the-valley root, motherwort, oleander leaf, pheasant's eye plant, pleurisy root, squill bulb leaf scales, and strophanthus seeds (19).

HORSETAIL/LICORICE: Theoretically, concomitant use of European buckthorn berry with horsetail plant or licorice rhizome increases the risk of potassium depletion (19).

STIMULANT LAXATIVE HERBS: Theoretically, concomitant use of European buckthorn with other stimulant laxative herbs can increase the risk of potassium depletion (19). Stimulant laxative herbs include aloe dried leaf sap, wild cucumber fruit (Ecballium elaterium), blue flag rhizome, alder buckthorn, butternut bark, cascara bark, castor oil, colocynth fruit pulp, gamboge bark exudate, jalap root, black root, manna bark exudate, podophyllum root, rhubarb root, senna leaves and pods, and yellow dock root.

Interactions with Drugs

DIGOXIN (Lanoxin): The overuse or abuse of European buckthorn can increase the toxicity of cardiac glycoside drugs (19).

DIURETIC DRUGS: Overuse of European buckthorn might compound diuretic-induced potassium loss (19). There is some concern that people taking European buckthorn along with potassium depleting diuretics might have an increased risk for hypokalemia. Initiation of potassium supplementation or an increase in potassium supplement dose may be necessary for some patients. Some diuretics that can deplete potassium include chlorothiazide (Diuril), chlorthalidone (Thalitone), furosemide (Lasix), hydrochlorothiazide (HCTZ, Hydrodiuril, Microzide), and others.

ORAL DRUGS: European buckthorn can decrease bowel transit time, reducing absorption of oral drugs (19).

Interactions with Foods

None known.

Interactions with Lab Tests

COLORIMETRIC TESTS: Due to its anthraquinone content, European buckthorn can discolor urine (pink, red, purple, orange, rust), interfering with diagnostic tests that depend on a color change (12,275).

POTASSIUM: Excessive use of European buckthorn can cause potassium depletion, reducing serum potassium concentrations and test results (12,19).

Interactions with Diseases or Conditions

GASTROINTESTINAL (GI) CONDITIONS: European buckthorn is contraindicated in individuals with intestinal obstruction; abdominal pain of unknown origin; and intestinal inflammation, including appendicitis, Crohn's disease, irritable bowel syndrome (IBS), and ulcerative colitis (12).

Dosage and Administration

ORAL: The typical dose of European buckthorn berry is 20-30 mg of the hydroxyanthracene derivative per day calculated as glucofrangulin A (2). One cup of the tea is commonly taken in the evening, and if needed, in the morning and afternoon (8,12). The tea is prepared by steeping 2-4 grams of the fruit in 150 mL boiling water for 10-15 minutes and then straining (8,12). Use the smallest amount necessary to achieve a soft stool (2) and discontinue in the event of diarrhea or watery stools (12). Limit the use of European buckthorn to a maximum of 8 to 10 days (12). This preparation should be used only if no effect can be obtained through a change of diet or use of bulk-forming laxative products (2).

Comments

Avoid confusion with alder buckthorn (Rhamus frangula). The American Herbal Products Association (AHPA) recommends the following label statement: "Do not use this product if you have abdominal pain or diarrhea. Consult a healthcare provider prior to use if you are pregnant or nursing. Discontinue use in the event of diarrhea or watery stools. Do not exceed dose. Not for long-term use" (12). Today, European buckthorn is primarily used as a dye.

EUROPEAN CHESTNUT

Also Known As

Castaneae Folium, Husked Nut, Jupiter's Nut, Kastanienblaetter, Sardian Nut, Spanish Chestnut, Sweet Chestnut.
CAUTION: See separate listing for American Chestnut leaf.

Scientific Names

Castanea sativa, synonyms Castanea vesca, Castanea vulgaris, Fagus castanea, Fagus procera.
Family: Fagaceae.

People Use This For

Orally, European chestnut is used for respiratory tract complaints including bronchitis and whooping cough, disorders affecting the legs and circulation, diarrhea, fever, the passage of bloody stools, hydrocele, infection, inflammation, kidney disorders, myalgias, nausea, paroxysm, sclerosis, inflammation of the lymph nodes due to tuberculosis infection, and stomach disorders.

Topically, European chestnut is used as a gargle for sore throat and for wounds.

Safety

POSSIBLY SAFE ...when used orally and appropriately (12).

There is insufficient reliable information available about the safety of European chestnut for its other uses.

PREGNANCY AND LACTATION: Insufficient reliable information available; avoid using.

Effectiveness

There is insufficient reliable information available about the effectiveness of European chestnut.

Mechanism of Action

The applicable part of European chestnut is the leaf. European chestnut contains 9% tannins, which exert an astringent effect on the mucosal tissue. This effect causes localized dehydration that turns the external cells into a protective layer (12). Plants with 10% tannins or more may cause gastrointestinal disturbances, kidney damage, and necrotic conditions of the liver (12). Some animal experiments show that tannins may cause cancer; others show that they may prevent it (12). Regular consumption of herbs with high tannin concentrations correlates with increased incidence of esophageal or nasal cancer (12).

Adverse Reactions

None reported.

Interactions with Herbs & Other Dietary Supplements

TANNIN-CONTAINING HERBS: Theoretically, herbs that contain high percentages of tannins (such as European chestnut) may cause precipitation of constituents of other herbs.

Interactions with Drugs

ORAL DRUGS: Theoretically, concomitant oral administration may cause precipitation of some drugs due to the high tannin content of European chestnut (19). Separate administration of oral drugs and tannin-containing herbs by the longest period of time practical (19).

Interactions with Foods

None known.

Interactions with Lab Tests

None known.

Interactions with Diseases or Conditions

None known.

Dosage and Administration

ORAL: People typically prepare European chestnut as a tea with 1 teaspoon of leaves and bark boiled in a covered container with 2 cups of water for 30 minutes. The liquid is cooled slowly in the closed container and taken cold, 1 to 2 cups per day (5254).

EUROPEAN FIVE-FINGER GRASS

Also Known As

Cinquefoil, European Five Finger Grass, Five Fingers, Five-Finger Blossom, Sunkfield, Synkfoyle.

Scientific Names

Potentilla reptans.

Family: Rosaceae.

Comments

At the date of publication, there was very little scientific information available about this product. Our staff is continually analyzing the available information on natural medicines and will add data to the online version of *Natural Medicines Comprehensive Database* as it becomes available. See www.naturaldatabase.com.

EUROPEAN MANDRAKE

Also Known As

Alraunwurzel, Mandragora, Mandragore, Mandrake, Satan's Apple.
CAUTION: See separate listings for Bryonia (English Mandrake) and Podophyllum (American Mandrake).

Scientific Names

Mandragora officinarum, synonym Mandragora vernalis.
Family: Solanaceae.

People Use This For

European mandrake root is used orally as an emetic, purgative, sedative, anesthetic, pain killer, and aphrodisiac. It has also been used orally for treating stomach ulcers, colic, asthma, hay fever, convulsions, rheumatism, and whooping cough.
Topically, European mandrake fresh leaves and leaf extracts are used for treating skin ulcers.

Safety

POSSIBLY UNSAFE ...when used orally. European mandrake contains several anticholinergic alkaloids, which can cause significant side effects when used in therapeutic doses (12). Excessive doses of anticholinergic alkaloids can cause respiratory and cardiac arrest and death (15,17).
CHILDREN: LIKELY UNSAFE ...when used orally. Children can be more susceptible to the adverse effects of anticholinergic alkaloid constituents of European mandrake (15); avoid using.
PREGNANCY AND LACTATION: LIKELY UNSAFE ...when used orally. European mandrake contains anticholinergic alkaloids that can cross the placenta and adversely effect the fetus (15); avoid using.

Effectiveness

There is insufficient reliable information available about the effectiveness of European mandrake.

Mechanism of Action

The applicable parts of European mandrake are the root and leaf. European mandrake contains atropine, belladonnine, hyoscyamine, mandragorine, scopolamine, and scopoletin (513,816). The root contains 0.4% tropane alkaloids, principally hyoscyamine (18). All plant parts contain tropane alkaloids, principally hyoscyamine and scopolamine (17). The tropane alkaloids have anticholinergic effects, which inhibit the actions of acetylcholine at muscarinic receptors (15). They reduce saliva and gastric acid production; inhibit gastrointestinal motility; decrease the tone and amplitude of contractions of the ureters and bladder; reduce bronchial secretions; produce bronchodilation; inhibit sweat gland secretions reducing the volume of perspiration; reduce the movement disorders associated with Parkinsonism; prevent motion-induced nausea and vomiting; and block the responses of the sphincter muscle of the iris and the ciliary muscle of the lens, producing mydriasis and cycloplegia (15). In large doses tropane alkaloids cause tachycardia (15).

Adverse Reactions

Orally, European mandrake most commonly causes anticholinergic side effects including confusion, drowsiness, dry mouth, tachycardia, mydriasis, blurred vision, photophobia, decreased urination, decreased sweating and overheating, and flushing (15,17,18). Although some adverse reactions can occur even with low doses, adverse effects are dose related. Large doses can cause severe adverse reactions including somnolence, central excitation (restlessness, hallucinations, delirium, manic episodes), exhaustion, respiratory and cardiac arrest, and death (17,18). All parts of the European mandrake plant including the root, leaves, and fruit contain anticholinergic alkaloids and can cause these effects (17). Elderly patients and children can be more susceptible to the adverse effects of anticholinergic constituents of European mandrake (15).
There is some evidence that subcutaneous injection may cause anaphylactic shock including swelling of lips and eyelids, nausea, tingling in palms and scalp, abdominal cramping, stool incontinence, and loss of consciousness. This reaction has occurred with a very low dose of 2 mL of a 3 mcg/mL solution of European mandrake extract. Although Immunoglobulin E (IgE) antibodies to European mandrake may not be detected, in vitro evaluation may find strong T lymphocyte proliferation. Skin patch tests with European mandrake root powder in sensitive individuals is likely to produce a delayed-type reaction with erythema resembling acute dermatitis (7022). Skin patch tests should be performed to rule-out hypersensitivity before administration of subcutaneous European mandrake.

Interactions with Herbs & Other Dietary Supplements

HERBS WITH ANTICHOLINERGIC EFFECTS: Theoretically, concurrent use might have additive effects and adverse effects. Anticholinergic herbs include belladonna, henbane, scopolia, and bittersweet nightshade (2).

Interactions with Drugs

ANTICHOLINERGIC DRUGS: Concurrent use may cause additive anticholinergic effects and adverse effects. Anticholinergic drugs include conventional medications containing tropane alkaloids such as atropine, as well as phenothiazines, amantadine, some antiparkinson drugs, glutethimide, meperidine, tricyclic antidepressants, antiarrhythmic agents, and antihistamines (15).

ORAL DRUGS: Theoretically, concurrent use might increase absorption of some drugs because of inhibited gastrointestinal (GI) motility caused by European mandrake (15).

Interactions with Foods

None known.

Interactions with Lab Tests

None known.

Interactions with Diseases or Conditions

CONGESTIVE HEART FAILURE: Avoid using European mandrake due to anticholinergic effects (12,513).

CORONARY ARTERY DISEASE: Avoid using European mandrake due to anticholinergic effects (12,513).

DOWN SYNDROME: Avoid using European mandrake in people with Down syndrome. They may be hypersensitive to antimuscarinic effects of anticholinergics (12,513).

GASTRIC ULCER: Avoid using European mandrake due to anticholinergic effects (12,513).

GI INFECTIONS: Avoid using European mandrake due to anticholinergic effects (12,513).

HEPATIC OR RENAL DYSFUNCTION: Avoid using European mandrake due to anticholinergic effects (12,513).

HIATAL HERNIA: Avoid using European mandrake due to anticholinergic effects (12,513).

HYPERTENSION: Avoid using European mandrake due to anticholinergic effects (12,513).

HYPERTHYROIDISM: Avoid using European mandrake due to anticholinergic effects (12,513).

MYASTHENIA GRAVIS: Contraindicated due to the anticholinergic effects of European mandrake (12,513).

NARROW/CLOSED-ANGLE GLAUCOMA: Contraindicated due to the anticholinergic effects of European mandrake (12,513).

OBSTRUCTIVE GASTROINTESTINAL DISEASE: Contraindicated due to the anticholinergic effects of European mandrake (12,513).

OBSTRUCTIVE UROPATHY: Contraindicated due to the anticholinergic effects of European mandrake (12,513).

PARALYTIC ILEUS or INTESTINAL ATONY: Contraindicated due to the anticholinergic effects of European mandrake (12,513).

PROSTATIC HYPERTROPHY: Avoid using European mandrake due to anticholinergic effects (12,513).

REFLUX ESOPHAGITIS: Contraindicated due to the anticholinergic effects of European mandrake (12,513).

SPASTIC PARALYSIS/BRAIN DAMAGE: Avoid using European mandrake in children with spastic paralysis or brain damage. They may be hypersensitive to antimuscarinic effects of anticholinergics (12,513).

TACHYARRHYTHMIAS: Avoid using European mandrake due to anticholinergic effects (12,513).

ULCERATIVE COLITIS OR TOXIC MEGACOLON: Contraindicated due to the anticholinergic effects of European mandrake (12,513).

UNSTABLE CARDIOVASCULAR STATUS IN ACUTE HEMORRHAGE OR THYROTOXICOSIS: Contraindicated due to the anticholinergic effects of European mandrake (12,513).

Dosage and Administration

No typical dosage.

Comments

European mandrake has had many superstitions associated with it and has been claimed to have magical properties.

EUROPEAN MISTLETOE

Also Known As

All-Heal, Birdlime Mistletoe, Devil's Fuge, Drudenfuss, Eurixor, Helixor, Hexenbesen, Iscador, Isorel, Leimmistel, Mistlekraut, Mistletein, Mistletoe, Mystyldene, Visci, Vogelmistel, Vysorel.

CAUTION: See separate listing for American Mistletoe.

Scientific Names

Viscum album.

Family: Viscaceae.

People Use This For

Orally, European mistletoe is used for cancer; reducing side effects of chemotherapy and radiation therapy; cardiovascular conditions including high blood pressure, internal bleeding, hemorrhoids, epilepsy and infantile convulsions; arteriosclerosis; gout; psychiatric conditions such as depression; sleep disorders; headache; amenorrhea; symptoms of menopause; and for "blood purifying." It is also used orally for treating mental and physical exhaustion, as a tranquilizer, for whooping cough, asthma, vertigo, diarrhea, chorea, and liver and gallbladder conditions. Subcutaneously, European mistletoe injections are used for cancer and for degenerative joint disease.

Safety

POSSIBLY SAFE ...when used orally or subcutaneously and appropriately. There is some evidence that European mistletoe extracts can be used safely (7039,9769). However, they have a narrow therapeutic range; high doses are not safe. Tell patients not to consume more than 3 mistletoe berries or 2 leaves (12). Advise patients not to use European mistletoe for self-medication.

LIKELY UNSAFE ...when used orally in high doses. Ingestion of high doses of mistletoe berry or leaf can cause serious adverse reactions. More than 3 berries or 2 leaves can cause seizures, slow heart rate, low blood pressure, and death in some patients (7039).

PREGNANCY: LIKELY UNSAFE ...when used orally or subcutaneously. European mistletoe might have uterine stimulant and abortifacient activity (19).

LACTATION: Insufficient reliable information available; avoid using.

Effectiveness

LIKELY INEFFECTIVE

Cancer. Administering European mistletoe subcutaneously doesn't improve survival in patients with any form of cancer. Most cancer studies have been poorly designed and have produced inconsistent results. Discourage patients from relying on European mistletoe for treating cancer (10672). European mistletoe extract doesn't seem to significantly improve rates of partial or complete remission in patients with stage IV pancreatic cancer (3707,7039,8848). European mistletoe doesn't seem to improve survival in patients with stage IV kidney cancer (7039). Combining European mistletoe extract plus surgery or radiation for glioma doesn't improve overall survival or disease-free survival (7039). European mistletoe extract does not seem to improve overall survival or disease-free survival in patients with stage I or stage IIB melanoma (7039). Combining European mistletoe extract with surgery or radiation for head and neck squamous cell carcinoma doesn't improve overall survival or disease-free survival (8842).

INSUFFICIENT RELIABLE EVIDENCE to RATE

Breast cancer, colorectal cancer, and gastric cancer. There is some preliminary clinical research that indicates European mistletoe extracts might improve survival in patients with solid tumors of the breast, colon, and stomach (7039,7044,7045), but more research with better-designed studies is needed. Tell patients there isn't enough reliable research to support using European mistletoe to improve survival in any type of cancer.

Hepatitis C. Subcutaneous injection of an aqueous extract of European mistletoe may decrease viral load and improve quality of life in some patients with chronic hepatitis C (9769).

More evidence is needed to rate European mistletoe for these uses.

Mechanism of Action

The applicable parts of European mistletoe are the berries, leaf, and stem. European mistletoe is a parasitic plant that grows on several different trees, including pine, oak, apple, maple, and numerous others. So, the chemical composition of mistletoe preparations can vary depending on the species of tree it grows on, the time of harvest, and other factors (7039,7106). European mistletoe has several active constituents, including the three main glycoprotein lectins: MLI, also known as viscumin, MLII, and MLIII; as well as viscotoxins, alkaloids, and monoterpene glucosides (7039,8840,8841,8849,9770).

European mistletoe is best known as a potential anticancer agent. Researchers think it might work as a biological response modifier that both stimulates the immune system and exerts cytotoxic effects (7039). There is good evidence that European mistletoe can stimulate the immune system in both animal models and humans. It seems to cause leukocytosis, increasing both the number and activity of neutrophils and natural killer cells (8843,8844). European mistletoe also seems to increase white blood cell (WBC) secretion of cytokines interleukin-1 (IL-1), IL-6, and tumor necrosis factor-alpha (TNF-alpha) (7039,8843,8844). Additional evidence suggests European mistletoe might possess a DNA stabilizing effect, restricted primarily to the mononuclear cells of the peripheral blood in vitro (8844). There is also some evidence that European mistletoe can be cytotoxic to tumor cells in vitro and in animals, possibly by inhibiting cellular protein synthesis (8841,8849). Some researchers think it might induce apoptosis in tumor cells (7039). The toxicity appears to be specific to tumor cells, sparing normal lymphocytes (8845,8846,8847). The toxic glycoprotein lectin, viscumin, known also as ML-I seems to be primarily responsible for many of these immune stimulating and cytotoxic effects (8840,8841,8846,8847,8849). However, there is some evidence that viscotoxins and alkaloids might also play a role (7039,8840). So far, evidence for cytotoxic or antitumor effects of these has been conflicting.

Although European mistletoe does seem to affect the immune system in humans and possibly has cytotoxic effects, the clinical benefits in humans are unproven. Clinical studies show that European mistletoe does not improve survival in patients with a variety of cancers. Researchers theorize that it might not work in humans for several reasons. Mistletoe lectins may not be able to bind to certain human cells. Human plasma proteins might interfere or break down active components of mistletoe; or humans may produce antibodies that destroy active constituents of mistletoe (7039). In addition to potential anticancer effects, European mistletoe might also have hypotensive, cardiac depressant, anti-inflammatory, and sedative effects (11).

Adverse Reactions

Orally, European mistletoe can be well tolerated when used in small amounts. Consumption of 3 berries or 2 leaves or less does not seem to cause significant adverse effects. Larger amounts can cause significant toxicity. Oral use can cause vomiting, diarrhea, intestinal cramps, hepatitis, hypotension, contraction of the pupil, uncontrollable eye movement, seizures, coma, and death (18).

European mistletoe was once associated with hepatitis in a patient taking a combination herbal product (3932). However, it is unlikely that mistletoe actually caused this adverse effect. It was most likely attributable to another ingredient, or product contamination. There have never been additional reports of hepatitis from European mistletoe.

Subcutaneously, European mistletoe can cause pain at the injection site, chills, high fever, headaches, angina, orthostatic circulatory disturbances, eosinophilia, and allergic reaction (2).

Intraperitoneal injection and injection directly into a tumor can cause pain at the injection site, nausea, and eosinophilia (7106). Necrosis can also occur at the site of injection (8).

Interactions with Herbs & Other Dietary Supplements

HAWTHORN: There is some evidence that European mistletoe might have cardiotoxic and negative inotropic effects (4). Theoretically, European mistletoe might decrease the effectiveness of positive inotropic agents such as hawthorn.

Interactions with Drugs

ANTIHYPERTENSIVE DRUGS: There is some evidence that European mistletoe can cause hypotension (4). Theoretically, it might have additive blood pressure lowering effects and increase the risk of hypotension; use cautiously.

IMMUNOSUPPRESSANTS: There is some concern that European mistletoe might decrease the effectiveness of immunosuppressants (4). European mistletoe has immunostimulant effects and might counteract the effects of immunosuppressants. Immunosuppressant drugs include azathioprine (Imuran), basiliximab (Simulect), cyclosporine (Neoral, Sandimmune), daclizumab (Zenapax), muromonab-CD3 (OKT3, Orthoclone OKT3), mycophenolate (CellCept), tacrolimus (FK506, Prograf), sirolimus (Rapamune), prednisone (Deltasone, Orasone), and other corticosteroids (glucocorticoids).

Interactions with Foods

None known.

Interactions with Lab Tests

EOSINOPHILIA: Subcutaneous, intraperitoneal, and intratumoral administration has been associated with eosinophilia. Intratumoral administration has caused hypereosinophilia, up to 43% of the white blood cell count (7106).

Interactions with Diseases or Conditions

CARDIOVASCULAR DISEASE: There is some evidence European mistletoe can have cardiotoxic and negative inotropic effects and might worsen cardiovascular conditions (4).

ORGAN TRANSPLANT: There is some concern that European mistletoe might decrease the effectiveness of immunosuppressants in organ transplant patients (4). European mistletoe has immunostimulant effects and might potentially contribute to transplant rejection.

Dosage and Administration

SUBCUTANEOUS: Aqueous extract of European mistletoe 1 mL, containing 5 mg of viscum album, given 3 times weekly, has been used to treat chronic hepatitis C (9769).

Comments

Interest in mistletoe for cancer is growing in North America. A lot of patients are asking about it since Suzanne Somers announced on Larry King Live that she is using it to treat her breast cancer. European mistletoe has been used for treating cancer since the 1920s, especially in Europe. Several brand name mistletoe extracts are available there: Iscador, Eurixor, Helixor, Isorel, Vysorel, and ABNOBAviscum (7039). So far these products are not readily available in North America. There is no proof they work for breast or other cancers. Advise patients to avoid these and stick with proven cancer treatments.

EVENING PRIMROSE OIL

Also Known As

EPO, Evening Primrose, Fever Plant, Gamma Linolenic Acid (GLA), Huile D'Onagre, King's Cureall, Linoleic Acid, Night Willow-Herb, Primrose, Scabish, Sun Drop.
CAUTION: See separate listings for Black Currant, Borage, Flaxseed Oil, Gamma Linolenic Acid, and Omega-6 Fatty Acids.

Scientific Names

Oenothera biennis, synonyms Oenothera muricata, Oenothera purpurata, Oenothera rubricaulis, Oenothera suaveolens, Onagra biennis; and other Oenothera species.
Family: Onagraceae.

People Use This For

Orally, evening primrose oil is used for premenstrual syndrome (PMS), mastalgia, endometriosis, and symptoms of menopause such as hot flashes. It is also used orally for atopic eczema, psoriasis, acne, rheumatoid arthritis, osteoporosis, Raynaud's syndrome, multiple sclerosis, and Sjogren's syndrome. Evening primrose oil is also used orally for cancer, hypercholesterolemia and coronary heart disease, dyspraxia in children, intermittent claudication, alcoholism, Alzheimer's disease, and schizophrenia. It is also used orally for chronic fatigue syndrome (CFS); asthma; diabetic neuropathy; neurodermatitis; hyperactivity in children and attention deficit-hyperactivity disorder (ADHD); obesity and weight loss; whooping cough; and gastrointestinal disorders including ulcerative colitis, irritable bowel syndrome, and peptic ulcer disease. Evening primrose oil has also been used orally in pregnancy for preventing pre-eclampsia, shortening the duration of labor, stimulating labor, and preventing post-date deliveries.
In foods, evening primrose oil is used as a dietary source of essential fatty acids.
In manufacturing, evening primrose oil is used in soaps and cosmetics.

Safety

LIKELY SAFE ...when used orally and appropriately. Evening primrose oil is generally considered safe and has been used in several studies without reports of significant side effects (1106,6034,6036,6406,6847,7565,7566,7567,9794).
CHILDREN: POSSIBLY SAFE ...when used orally and appropriately. Doses of 3 grams per day for 16 weeks have been used in children with apparent safety (6443,6462,7565,7568,7570).
PREGNANCY: POSSIBLY UNSAFE ...when used orally. Evening primrose oil might increase the risk for pregnancy complications, including delayed rupture of membranes, oxytocin augmentation, arrest of descent, and vacuum extraction (1411); avoid using.
LACTATION: POSSIBLY SAFE ...when used orally. Nursing mothers who supplement their diets with evening primrose oil secrete high levels of the constituent gamma linolenic acid into breast milk (1982); however, gamma linolenic acid is a fatty acid that is normally present in significant proportions in breast milk (11884).

Effectiveness

POSSIBLY EFFECTIVE

Mastalgia. There is some evidence that taking evening primrose oil orally can relieve cyclic mastalgia in 45% of patients and non-cyclic mastalgia in 27% of patients (6406,9794). It may not be effective for chronic severe breast pain (9156). Evening primrose oil seems to be less effective than danazol, but similarly effective as bromocriptine (6406).

Osteoporosis. Taking evening primrose oil orally, in combination with fish oils and calcium, seems to decrease bone turnover and increase spinal and femoral bone mineral density in elderly people with osteoporosis (7611).

POSSIBLY INEFFECTIVE

Atopic dermatitis (eczema). Taking evening primrose oil orally for 16 to 24 weeks doesn't seem to improve symptoms of atopic eczema in adults or children (7565,7566,7567). Most studies have used the brand product Epogam (Scotia Pharmaceuticals). Earlier studies, which lasted 12 weeks or less, showed effectiveness, but the positive results appear to be due to flawed study designs (2039,7568,7569,7570).

Attention deficit-hyperactivity disorder (ADHD). Taking evening primrose oil orally doesn't improve symptoms of ADHD in children. Evening primrose oil is comparable to placebo for most measures of improvement (6443,6462).

Menopausal symptoms. Taking evening primrose oil orally doesn't seem to improve menopausal vasomotor symptoms. Evening primrose oil 4 grams daily for 6 months doesn't seem to help hot flashes or night sweats (274).

Premenstrual syndrome (PMS). Taking evening primrose oil orally doesn't seem to relieve symptoms associated with PMS (1105,1106,6034,6847). Multiple small-scale studies have not demonstrated significant benefit when compared to placebo (1105,1106). However, some researchers suggest that studies should last at least six months to allow the placebo effect to wear off and the benefit of evening primrose oil to become apparent (8129); most studies published have lasted no more than four months (1105).
Most clinical studies have used Epogam (Scotia Pharmaceuticals), which contains 40 mg of gamma-linolenic acid and 10 mg of vitamin E. It is sold as a prescription product in some countries and is not available in the US.

INSUFFICIENT RELIABLE EVIDENCE to RATE

Chronic fatigue syndrome (CFS). There is preliminary evidence that a specific combination of evening primrose oil and fish oils (Efamol Marine) might reduce the symptoms of CFS; however, study results have not been consistent (7563,7564).

Pregnancy-related complications. Taking evening primrose oil doesn't seem to shorten the duration of labor (1409,1411), prevent pre-eclampsia (1409), or prevent post-date deliveries in pregnant women (1411).

Rheumatoid arthritis (RA). There is some preliminary evidence that suggests taking evening primrose oil supplements might reduce subjective symptoms of pain in patients with rheumatoid arthritis (6036,12036). However, there is also evidence that suggests no benefit (12035).

Sjogren's syndrome. There is preliminary evidence that taking evening primrose oil supplements does not improve symptoms of Sjogren's syndrome (12037,12038).

More evidence is needed to rate evening primrose oil for these uses.

Mechanism of Action

Evening primrose oil is obtained from the seed of Oenothera biennis. It contains 2-16% gamma-linolenic acid (GLA), 65-80% linoleic acid, and vitamin E (3908,6036).

Evening primrose oil is thought to help for rheumatoid arthritis, eczema, and other inflammatory conditions due its potential anti-inflammatory effects. GLA seems to be responsible for the anti-inflammatory effects of evening primrose oil. GLA reduces production of interleukin 1 (IL-1)-beta, which may be involved in inflammation in diseases such as rheumatoid arthritis (12470). GLA is rapidly metabolized to dihomogammalinolenic acid (DGLA). DGLA is a precursor of the prostaglandin-1 series (PGE1), which inhibits the inflammatory polymorphonuclear leukocyte cells. DGLA is also converted to 15-hydroxy-DGLA, which blocks the transformation of arachidonic acid into inflammatory leukotrienes. GLA and DGLA seem to improve the ratio of inflammatory and non-inflammatory prostaglandins and leukotrienes (2039,6036).

There is also interest in using evening primrose oil for conditions that might result from metabolic deficiencies. For example, patients with premenstrual syndrome (PMS) are thought to have lower levels of GLA, possibly due to a defect in the conversion of linoleic acid to GLA (6034). Some children with attention deficit-hyperactivity disorder (ADHD) might also have deficiencies in certain essential fatty acids, including DGLA (6462).

Evening primrose oil might have other pharmacological effects related to its GLA content. There is some evidence it might lower elevated plasma lipids and inhibit platelet aggregation (1979). There is also preliminary evidence from animal models that evening primrose oil might improve neuronal blood supply and possibly play a role in preventing diabetic neuropathy (3909).

Preliminary evidence suggests GLA might have an antiestrogenic effect and might hasten the response to tamoxifen (Nolvadex) in women with estrogen-sensitive breast cancer (5902). GLA also seems to modulate the sensitivity of breast cancer cells to paclitaxel (Taxol) and fulvestrant (Faslodex), enhancing malignant cell killing without adverse effects on normal cells (8133,11791). However, other research suggests that taking GLA alone might stimulate the growth of breast cancer cells at low concentrations and inhibit growth at higher concentrations (11339).

Adverse Reactions

Orally, evening primrose oil is generally well tolerated (1106,6034,6036,6847). There is one case report of nocturnal seizures associated with the use of evening primrose oil, black cohosh, and chasteberry (588). Evening primrose oil might increase the risk for pregnancy complications, including prolonged rupture of membranes, oxytocin augmentation, arrest of descent, and vacuum extraction (1411).

Interactions with Herbs & Other Dietary Supplements

HERBS WITH ANTICOAGULANT/ANTIPLATELET POTENTIAL: Concomitant use of herbs that have constituents that might affect platelet aggregation could theoretically increase the risk of bleeding in some people (1979). These herbs include angelica, clove, danshen, garlic, ginger, ginkgo, red clover, turmeric, and others.

Interactions with Drugs

ANESTHESIA: There is a report of seizure in a patient taking evening primrose oil and receiving anesthesia; however, the patient was also taking other drugs. It is unclear if evening primrose or the other drugs were the cause (613).

ANTICOAGULANT/ANTIPLATELET DRUGS: Evening primrose oil, which contains gamma-linolenic acid (GLA), could have anticoagulant effects (1979). Theoretically, taking evening primrose oil with other anticoagulant or antiplatelet drugs might increase the risk of bruising and bleeding. Some of these drugs include aspirin, clopidogrel (Plavix), nonsteroidal anti-inflammatory drugs (NSAIDs) such as diclofenac (Voltaren, Cataflam, others), ibuprofen (Advil, Motrin, others), naproxen (Anaprox, Naprosyn, others), dalteparin (Fragmin), enoxaparin (Lovenox), heparin, warfarin (Coumadin), and others.

PHENOTHIAZINES: Theoretically, products containing gamma linolenic acid (GLA) and vitamin E might increase the risk of seizures in people being treat concomitantly with phenothiazine drugs (11021); use with caution.

Interactions with Foods
None known.

Interactions with Lab Tests
BLEEDING TIME: There is some concern that evening primrose oil might prolong bleeding time. Evening primrose oil contains gamma linolenic acid (GLA), which can inhibit platelet aggregation (1979).
LIPID PROFILE: Evening primrose oil might affect cholesterol levels. Evening primrose oil contains gamma-linolenic acid (GLA), which can lower plasma triglycerides and increase high-density lipoprotein (HDL) cholesterol (1979).

Interactions with Diseases or Conditions
BLEEDING DISORDERS: There is some concern that evening primrose oil might prolong bleeding time and increase the risk of bruising and bleeding. Evening primrose oil contains gamma-linolenic acid (GLA), which can inhibit platelet aggregation (1979).
EPILEPSY/SEIZURE DISORDER: There is concern that evening primrose oil might lower the seizure threshold or unmask undiagnosed temporal lobe epilepsy. However, current reports have only identified seizure in association with phenothiazine (11021).
SCHIZOPHRENIA: Seizures have been reported in people with schizophrenia treated concomitantly with phenothiazine drugs, GLA, and vitamin E (11021); use with caution.

Dosage and Administration
ORAL: For mastalgia, 3-4 grams daily has been used (6034,6406,9156). For premenstrual syndrome (PMS), 2-4 grams daily has been used (6034). For rheumatoid arthritis, doses ranging from 540 mg daily to 2.8 grams daily have been used (6036). For improving movement disorders in children with dyspraxia, 24 mg thyme oil combined with fish oils providing DHA 480 mg and 35 mg arachidonic acid, 96 mg gamma-alpha linoleic acid from evening primrose oil, and 80 mg vitamin E (Efalex) have been used (5708). For atopic eczema, 4-6 grams daily has been used in adults (2039,7569) and 3 grams in children (7565,7568).

Comments
The Medicines Control Agency (MCA), the British equivalent of the Food and Drug Administration, recently withdrew the licenses for evening primrose oil products marketed as prescription drug products under the brand names of Epogam and Efamast. Epogam was authorized for the symptomatic relief of atopic eczema in children and adults and Efamast was licensed to treat mastalgia. The licenses were withdrawn because the agency concluded that there is not enough evidence that they are effective (9882). The manufacturer claims to have data to support the use of evening primrose oil for atopic eczema, but it has not been published. Studies using borage seed oil, which also contains gamma-linolenic acid, have found no effect on atopic dermatitis (11341,11342).

EYEBRIGHT

Also Known As
Augentrostkraut, Euphraisia Eye Bright, Euphrasiae herba, Eye Bright, Herbe d'Euphraise.
CAUTION: See separate listing for Clary Sage.

Scientific Names
Eurphrasia rostkoviana; Euphrasia officinalis.
Family: Scrophulariaceae.

People Use This For
Orally, eyebright is used to treat nasal mucous membrane inflammation, allergies, allergic rhinitis, common cold, bronchial conditions, and sinusitis. It is also used orally for cancers, coughs, conjunctivitis, earaches, epilepsy, headaches, hoarseness, inflammation, jaundice, ophthalmia, rhinitis, skin ailments, and sore throat.
Topically, eyebright is used as an ophthalmic in the form of a lotion, poultice, or eyebath for a variety of conditions including conjunctivitis; blepharitis; eye fatigue; inflammation of the blood vessels, eyelids and conjunctiva; and for "glued" and inflamed eyes. Eyebright is also used topically to prevent mucous and mucous membrane inflammation of the eyes.
In foods, eyebright is used as a flavoring ingredient.

Safety
POSSIBLY SAFE ...when used orally and appropriately (12). ...when used orally in amounts commonly found in foods. Eyebright is listed by the Council of Europe as a natural source of food flavoring (4).
POSSIBLY UNSAFE ...when used as an ophthalmic; avoid using due to hygienic concerns. Eye products may be subject to contamination (8,11).
PREGNANCY AND LACTATION: Insufficient reliable information available; avoid using.

Effectiveness
There is insufficient reliable information available about the effectiveness of eyebright.

Mechanism of Action
Tannin constituents may be responsible for astringent properties (4). The constituent caffeic acid has bacteriostatic activity (4). Constituents, aucubin and iridoid glycosides, have purgative activity (4).

Adverse Reactions
Orally or topically, 10-60 drops eyebright tincture may induce mental confusion, headache, increased eye pressure with lacrimation, itching, redness, swelling of eyelid margins, dim vision, photophobia, weakness, sneezing, nausea, toothache, constipation, cough, dyspnea, insomnia, polyuria, and sweating (4).

Interactions with Herbs & Other Dietary Supplements
None known.

Interactions with Drugs
None known.

Interactions with Foods
None known.

Interactions with Lab Tests
None known.

Interactions with Diseases or Conditions
None known.

Dosage and Administration
ORAL: 2-4 grams dried above ground parts three times daily (4), or one cup tea (steep 2-4 grams dried above ground parts in 150 mL boiling water 5-10 minutes, strain) three times daily (4). Liquid extract (1:1 in 25% alcohol), 2-4 mL three times daily (4). Tincture (1:5 in 45% alcohol), 2-6 mL three times daily (4).
TOPICAL: No typical dosage.

Comments
Avoid use of nonsterile solutions (including homemade products) in the eye(s), due to high risk of infection. Ophthalmic application of eyebright is not recommended. Historically, eyebright has been used in British Herbal Tobacco, which was smoked for chronic bronchial conditions and colds (5).

FALSE UNICORN

Also Known As
Blazing Star, Fairywand, Helonias, Starwort.

Scientific Names
Chamaelirium luteum, synonyms Chamaelirium carolianum, Helonias dioica, Helonias lutea, Veratrum luteum.
Family: Liliaceae or Melanthiaceae.

People Use This For
Orally, false unicorn is used for ovarian cysts, menstrual problems, menopause, threatened miscarriage, vomiting from pregnancy, infertility, digestive problems, and to normalize hormones after oral contraceptive use. It is also used orally as a diuretic and to rid the intestines of worms.

Safety
POSSIBLY SAFE ...when the root preparations are used orally and appropriately (12).
PREGNANCY: LIKELY UNSAFE ...when used orally because it is a potential uterine stimulant (12,18).
LACTATION: Insufficient reliable information available; avoid using.

Effectiveness
There is insufficient reliable information available about the effectiveness of false unicorn.

Mechanism of Action
The applicable parts of false unicorn are the rhizome and root. False unicorn reportedly has anthelmintic, diuretic (18), uterine stimulant, and menstruation stimulant activity (12).

Adverse Reactions
Orally, large doses of false unicorn may cause nausea and vomiting (4).

Interactions with Herbs & Other Dietary Supplements
None known.

Interactions with Drugs
None known.

Interactions with Foods
None known.

Interactions with Lab Tests
None known.

Interactions with Diseases or Conditions
GI CONDITIONS: Can irritate the gastrointestinal tract. Contraindicated in individuals with infectious or inflammatory gastrointestinal conditions (19).

Dosage and Administration
ORAL: 1-2 grams dried root 3 times per day, or one cup tea (steep 1-2 grams dried root in 150 mL boiling water 5-10 minutes, strain) 3 times daily (4) has been used. As a liquid extract (1:1 in 45% alcohol), 1-2 mL has been used 3 times daily (4). As a tincture (1:5 in 45% alcohol), 2-5 mL 3 times daily has been used (4).

FENNEL

Also Known As
Bari-Sanuf, Bitter Fennel, Carosella, Common Fennel, Finnochio, Florence Fennel, Foeniculi antheroleum, Garden Fennel, Large Fennel, Phytoestrogen, Sanuf, Shatapuspha, Sweet Fennel, Wild Fennel.
CAUTION: See separate listing for Water Fennel.

Scientific Names
Foeniculum vulgare, synonyms Anethum piperitum, Foeniculum piperitum; Foeniculum officinale; Foeniculum capillaceum; Anethum foeniculum.
Family: Apiaceae/Umbelliferae.

People Use This For
Orally, fennel is used for increasing lactation, promoting menstruation, facilitating birth, and increasing libido. It is also used for upper respiratory tract infections, coughs, bronchitis, cholera, backache, bedwetting, dyspepsia, flatulence, bloating, loss of appetite, visual problems, and for colic in infants.
Topically, fennel powder is used as a poultice for snake bites.
In foods and beverages, fennel oil is used as a flavoring agent.
In other manufacturing processes, fennel oil is used as a flavoring agent in certain laxatives, and as a fragrance component in soaps and cosmetics.

Safety
LIKELY SAFE ...when used orally in amounts commonly found in foods. Fennel has Generally Recognized As Safe (GRAS) status in the US (4912).
POSSIBLY SAFE ...when used orally and appropriately in medicinal amounts, short-term (12).
POSSIBLY UNSAFE ...when used orally in medicinal amounts, long-term. The fennel constituent, estragole, is a procarcinogen (12). Theoretically, long-term use might increase the chance of adverse effects.
PREGNANCY AND LACTATION: Insufficient reliable information available; avoid using.

Effectiveness
There is insufficient reliable information available about the effectiveness of fennel.

Mechanism of Action

The applicable parts of fennel are the fruit (seed) and oil. Fennel seed is a rich source of beta-carotene and vitamin C (19). It also contains significant amounts of calcium, magnesium, and iron, and lesser amounts of other metal cations (6135). The seed contains the volatile oil composed largely of trans-anethole, but also contains fenchone, estragole, and other constituents (6135). The constituents, anethole and fenchone, reduce upper respiratory tract secretions (11). Some evidence suggests the aqueous fennel extract might also increase mucociliary activity (11). The constituent anethole appears to be allergenic, insecticidal, and toxic. Polymers of anethole also seem to have estrogenic activity (11).

The constituent estragole is a procarcinogen but the carcinogenic risk is thought to be minimal. It is not directly hepatotoxic or hepatocarcinogenic but requires activation by liver enzymes to reach full toxicity. In the liver, other enzymes inactivate the carcinogenic metabolites, limiting possible damage to the liver (12).

Preliminary evidence suggests that fennel oil can inhibit contractions of uterine tissue induced by prostaglandin E2. However, it does not inhibit uterine contractions induced by oxytocin (10349).

Adverse Reactions

Orally, fennel can cause allergic reactions affecting the skin and respiratory system (2). It can also cause photodermatitis. Advise patients to avoid excessive sunlight or ultraviolet light exposure while using this product (19).

Allergic cross-sensitivity is possible in people with allergies to carrot, celery, mugwort, or other Apiaceae family plants (6).

Interactions with Herbs & Other Dietary Supplements

None known.

Interactions with Drugs

CIPROFLOXACIN (Cipro): Concomitant use of fennel and ciprofloxacin might reduce the effectiveness of ciprofloxacin. Preliminary evidence suggests that fennel reduces ciprofloxacin bioavailability by nearly 50%, possibly due to the metal cations such as calcium, iron, and magnesium contained in fennel. Evidence also suggests that fennel increases tissue distribution and slows elimination of ciprofloxacin (6135).

CONTRACEPTIVE DRUGS: Theoretically, concomitant use of large amounts of fennel might interfere with contraceptive drugs, due to competition for estrogen receptors (11).

ESTROGENS: Theoretically, concomitant use of large amounts of fennel might interfere with hormone replacement therapy, due to competition for estrogen receptors (11).

TAMOXIFEN (Nolvadex): Theoretically, large doses of fennel might decrease the antiestrogenic effect of tamoxifen, due to fennel's potential estrogenic effects (11).

Interactions with Foods

None known.

Interactions with Lab Tests

None known.

Interactions with Diseases or Conditions

CROSS-ALLERGENICITY: Fennel might cause an allergic reaction in people who are also sensitive to celery, carrot, or mugwort (6).

HORMONE SENSITIVE CANCERS/CONDITIONS: Fennel might have estrogenic effects (11). Patients with hormone sensitive conditions should avoid fennel. Some of these conditions include breast, uterine, and ovarian cancer, and endometriosis and uterine fibroids.

Dosage and Administration

ORAL: No typical dosage. However, traditionally a tea prepared from 1-2 grams of the crushed or ground fruit or seed in 150 mL boiling water has been used. The common dose of the tincture compound is 5-7.5 grams per day (2). Fennel should be used on a short-term basis (2). Fennel oil, 0.1-0.6 mL, which is equivalent to 100-600 mg of the dried fruit or seed has also been used. It should only be used up to two weeks without professional evaluation (2). The fennel honey syrup, which contains 500 mg fennel oil/kg, is usually dosed 10-20 grams per day (2).

FENUGREEK

Also Known As

Alholva, Bird's Foot, Bockshornklee, Bockshornsame, Chandrika, Foenugraeci Semen, Foenugreek, Greek Clover, Greek Hay, Greek Hay Seed, Hu Lu Ba, Medhika, Methi, Trigonella.

Scientific Names

Trigonella foenum-graecum; Trigonella foenugraecum.
Family: Fabaceae/Leguminosae.

People Use This For

Orally, fenugreek is used for lowering blood glucose in people with diabetes, loss of appetite, dyspepsia, gastritis, constipation, atherosclerosis, high serum cholesterol and triglycerides, and for promoting lactation. Fenugreek is used orally for kidney ailments, beriberi, hernia, impotence, and other male problems. Fenugreek is also used orally for fever, mouth ulcers, boils, bronchitis, cellulitis, tuberculosis, chronic coughs, chapped lips, baldness, and cancer.
Topically, fenugreek is used as a poultice for local inflammation, myalgia, lymphadenitis, gout, wounds, leg ulcers, and eczema.
In foods, fenugreek is included as an ingredient in spice blends. It is also used as a flavoring agent in imitation maple syrup, foods, beverages, and tobacco.
In manufacturing, fenugreek extracts are used in soaps and cosmetics.

Safety

LIKELY SAFE ...when used orally in amounts commonly found in foods. Fenugreek has Generally Recognized As Safe (GRAS) status in the US (4912).
POSSIBLY SAFE ...when used orally in medicinal amounts (7389,9783,10883,10284,12533).
CHILDREN: POSSIBLY UNSAFE ...when used orally; avoid using. Fenugreek tea has caused loss of consciousness and unusual body odor in children. The body odor may be confused with maple syrup disease (9782).
PREGNANCY: LIKELY UNSAFE ...when used orally in amounts greater than those found in foods because of its potential oxytocic and uterine stimulant activity (12531). Consumption of fenugreek just before delivery may cause the neonate to have an unusual body odor, which could be confused with maple syrup disease. It does not appear to cause long-term sequelae (9781).
LACTATION: Insufficient reliable information available; avoid using. Although fenugreek is used to promote lactation, there are no clinical studies testing its safety in mother or infant (12535).

Effectiveness

INSUFFICIENT RELIABLE EVIDENCE to RATE

Diabetes. Consuming fenugreek, mixed with food during a meal, seems to reduce postprandial blood glucose levels in patients with type 1 or type 2 diabetes. It may be given in combination with guar gum or by itself (10283,10284,12534). Muffins made from a batter consisting of foxtail and barnyard millet, in combination with legumes and fenugreek, do not produce a substantial increase in postprandial blood glucose in diabetic patients (9784).
Hypercholesterolemia. There is conflicting evidence about the use of fenugreek for lowering serum cholesterol (7389,9783,10284).
More evidence is needed to rate fenugreek for these uses.

Mechanism of Action

The applicable part of fenugreek is the seed. The active constituents include trigonelline, 4-hydroxyisoleucine, and sotolon (7162,12533). Fenugreek seeds have a distinctive bitter taste and odor. Sotolon is frequently used as a flavoring for artificial maple syrup (12533). Soaking fenugreek seeds overnight and washing the seeds in water can decrease some of the taste and odor (9783).
Fenugreek seeds contain about 50% dietary fiber and may affect gastrointestinal transit, slowing glucose absorption. About 80% of the total content of free amino acids in the seeds is present as 4-hydroxyisoleucine, which appears to directly stimulate insulin (8112,12532,12533). This effect is glucose dependent and only occurs in the presence of moderate to high glucose concentrations.
Some evidence suggests the seed consumption might decrease calcium oxalate deposition in the kidneys (720).
Fenugreek contains coumarins and other constituents that might affect platelet aggregation, but this might not be significant clinically (7162).
Preliminary research suggests fenugreek has stimulating effects on the uterus, intestine, and heart (12531).

Adverse Reactions

Orally, fenugreek can cause diarrhea and flatulence (622). With large doses, hypoglycemia is possible (164). Fenugreek can cause allergic reactions including nasal congestion, hoarseness, persistent coughing, wheezing, facial angioedema, and shock (719). The paste of fenugreek applied to the scalp can cause allergic symptoms, including head numbness, facial swelling, and wheezing (719). Consumption of fenugreek by pregnant women just before delivery may cause the neonate to have an unusual body odor, which may be confused with maple syrup disease. It does not appear to cause long-term sequelae (9781). This unusual body odor may occur in children drinking fenugreek tea. Loss of consciousness may also occur in children drinking tea made from fenugreek (9782).

Interactions with Herbs & Other Dietary Supplements

HERBS WITH ANTICOAGULANT/ANTIPLATELET POTENTIAL: Concomitant use of herbs that have constituents that might affect platelet aggregation could theoretically increase the risk of bleeding in some people (5191,7162,7389). These herbs include angelica, clove, danshen, garlic, ginger, ginkgo, red clover, turmeric, and others.

HERBS WITH HYPOGLYCEMIC POTENTIAL: Theoretically, fenugreek might have additive effects with herbs that decrease blood glucose levels (10283,10284). Herbs with hypoglycemic potential include devil's claw, fenugreek, guar gum, Panax ginseng, and Siberian ginseng.

Interactions with Drugs

ANTICOAGULANT/ANTIPLATELET DRUGS: There is some concern that fenugreek might have additive effects when used with anticoagulant or antiplatelet drugs, resulting in increased risk of bruising and bleeding. Some of the constituents in fenugreek have antiplatelet effects, although these might not be present in concentrations that are clinically significant (5191,7162,7389). Some drugs with anticoagulant or antiplatelet effects include aspirin, clopidogrel (Plavix), nonsteroidal anti-inflammatory drugs (NSAIDs) such as diclofenac (Voltaren, Cataflam, others), ibuprofen (Advil, Motrin, others), naproxen (Anaprox, Naprosyn, others), dalteparin (Fragmin), enoxaparin (Lovenox), heparin, and others.

ANTIDIABETES DRUGS: Fenugreek may reduce blood glucose levels (10283,10284) and might have additive effects on glucose levels when used with antidiabetes drugs. Monitor blood glucose levels closely. Medication dose adjustments may be necessary. Some antidiabetes drugs include glimepiride (Amaryl), glyburide (DiaBeta, Glynase PresTab, Micronase), insulin, pioglitazone (Actos), rosiglitazone (Avandia), and others.

WARFARIN (Coumadin): Fenugreek might have additive effects with warfarin and increase the international normalized ratio (INR). Some fenugreek constituents have antiplatelet effects, although these might not be present in concentrations that are clinically significant (7162,7389). Fenugreek in combination with boldo has been associated with increased INR in a patient taking warfarin (5191).

Interactions with Foods

ALLERGY TO FABACEAE: Chickpea, also a member of the Fabaceae family, has shown cross-reactivity in patients allergic to fenugreek. Theoretically, patients who are allergic to other Fabaceae plants including soybeans, peanuts, and green peas might also be allergic to fenugreek (719).

Interactions with Lab Tests

BLOOD GLUCOSE: Fenugreek can lower blood glucose and test results (10283,10284).
URINE ODOR: Fenugreek can cause a maple syrup odor in urine.
Avoid confusion with "maple syrup urine" disease (8111).

Interactions with Diseases or Conditions

DIABETES: Fenugreek can alter blood sugar control in people with diabetes (10283,10284). Blood glucose levels should be monitored closely.

KIDNEY STONES (Nephrolithiasis): Theoretically, fenugreek can decrease calcium oxalate deposition and stone formation (720).

Dosage and Administration

ORAL: For reducing postprandial blood glucose in patients with diabetes, fenugreek 10 to 15 grams per day, as a single dose or in divided doses, with meals has been used (10283,10284). A hydroalcoholic extract of fenugreek seeds 1 gram per day has also been used (12534). For treating hyperlipidemia, 0.6 to 2.5 grams of fenugreek 2 times daily with meals has been used. It may be used alone or in combination with guar gum and other plant fibers (7389,10284).

Comments

The taste and odor of fenugreek resembles maple syrup, and it has been used to mask the taste of medicines (8111). Fenugreek leaves are eaten in India as a vegetable (719).

FEVER BARK

Also Known As
Alstonia Bark, Australian Febrifuge, Australian Fever Bush, Australian Quinine, Bitterbark, Devil Tree, Devil's Bit, Dita Bark, Pale Mara, Pali-Mara.

Scientific Names
Alstonia constricta.
Family: Apocynaceae.

People Use This For
Orally, fever bark is used for treating fever, hypertension, diarrhea, rheumatism, and malaria.
It is also used as a stimulant and a uterine stimulant.

Safety
POSSIBLY UNSAFE ...when used orally. Fever bark contains reserpine and yohimbine constituents (18), which can cause severe adverse effects including depression, psychosis, and acute renal failure (5,6,11,17,18,19).
PREGNANCY AND LACTATION: Insufficient reliable information available; avoid using.

Effectiveness
There is insufficient reliable information available about the effectiveness of fever bark.

Mechanism of Action
Fever bark contains various alkaloids including yohimbe. The constituents reserpine and deserpidine are likely responsible for its antihypertensive effects. Fever bark might also have antipyretic and antispasmodic properties (18).

Adverse Reactions
Orally, the reserpine constituent of fever bark can cause lethargy, nasal congestion, or depression (17). The yohimbine constituent of fever bark can cause salivation, irritability, fluid retention, skin eruptions, eye dilation, allergy, acute renal failure, and lupus-like syndrome (2,5,6,11,18,19). Yohimbine is reported to trigger psychosis in people predisposed to it (2,5,6,11,18). Symptoms of yohimbine toxicity include paralysis, severe hypotension, cardiac conduction disorders, cardiac failure, and death (6,18).

Interactions with Herbs & Other Dietary Supplements
INDIAN SNAKEROOT: Theoretically, concomitant use of Indian snakeroot with fever root can cause additive effects and side effects due to reserpine and deserpidine content of both herbs.
ST. JOHN'S WORT: Theoretically, concomitant use of St. John's wort extract might antagonize effects of reserpine, a constituent of fever bark (19).
TURMERIC: Theoretically, concomitant use of tumeric might reduce the frequency of gastric and duodenal ulcers associated with reserpine, a constituent of fever bark (19).
YOHIMBE: Theoretically, concomitant use of fever bark with yohimbe can cause additive effects or adverse effects.

Interactions with Drugs
ANESTHESIA: Reserpine, a constituent of fever bark, can increase the risk of cardiovascular instability in individuals receiving general anesthesia (151).
NALOXONE (Narcan): Concomitant use of the fever bark constituent yohimbine and naloxone can cause synergistic effects and adverse reactions (19).
PHENOTHIAZINES: Theoretically, phenothiazines might increase the toxicity of yohimbine, a constituent of fever bark, due to alpha-two adrenoreceptor antagonism (19).
STIMULANT DRUGS: Reserpine, a constituent of fever bark, might increase or decrease effects of sympathomimetics (151).

Interactions with Foods
None known.

Interactions with Lab Tests

5-HYDROXYINDOLEACETIC ACID (5-HIAA): Reserpine can increase test results (275).
17-HYDROXYCORTICOSTEROIDS: Reserpine can decrease urine levels (275).
FFA: Reserpine can increase serum free fatty acids (275).
GUAIACOLA SPOT TEST: Reserpine can cause a false reading with urine screening test of Rogers (275).
HOMOVANILLIC ACID: Reserpine can increase urine levels of homovanillic acid; maximum on second day (275).
HYDROCHLORIC ACID: Reserpine can increase gastric hydrochloric acid levels (275).
NOREPINEPHRINE: Reserpine can decrease urine levels of norepinephrine (275). Yohimbine can increase plasma and cerebrospinal fluid norepinephrine levels and test results (275).
PEPSIN: Reserpine can increase gastric pepsin levels and test results (275).
PLATELETS: Reserpine can decrease blood platelet levels and test results (275).
PROLACTIN: Reserpine can increase plasma prolactin levels and test results (275).
PROTHROMBIN TIME: Reserpine can decrease plasma prothrombin time (275).
SEROTONIN: Reserpine can decrease plasma 5-HT and test results (275).
T-4: Reserpine can decrease thyroxine (T-4) serum levels and test results (275).
TYRAMINE: Reserpine can cause a false positive response to tyramine test (275).
VANILLYMANDELIC ACID: Reserpine can decrease urine levels and test results (275).

Interactions with Diseases or Conditions

MENTAL DEPRESSION: Theoretically, contraindicated in individuals with a history of mental depression due to reserpine constituent (17,18).
PEPTIC ULCER: Theoretically, contraindicated in individuals with active peptic ulcer due to reserpine constituent (17).
SCHIZOPHRENIA: Theoretically, contraindicated in individuals with schizophrenia because yohimbine constituent might induce psychotic episodes (19).

Dosage and Administration

ORAL: A typical dose is 15 to 20 mL of tea daily. Tea can be made by steeping one part ground bark to 20 parts boiling water for 10-15 minutes, strain. Alternatively, 2-4 mL tincture (1:8 or 1:10) daily; or 4-8 mL of liquid extract (1:1) daily has also been used (18).

Comments

Most of the information available for fever bark concerns its constituents.

FEVERFEW

Also Known As

Altamisa, Bachelor's Buttons, Featerfoiul, Featherfew, Featherfoil, Flirtwort Midsummer Daisy, Santa Maria, Tanaceti parthenii.
CAUTION: See separate listings for Buttercup and Cornflower.

Scientific Names

Tanacetum parthenium, synonyms Chrysanthemum parthenium, Chrysanthemum praealtum Leucanthemum parthenium, Matricaria eximia, Matricaria parthenium, Pyrethrum parthenium.
Family: Asteraceae/Compositae.

People Use This For

Orally, feverfew is used for fever, headaches, prevention of migraines, and menstrual irregularities. It is also used orally for arthritis, psoriasis, allergies, asthma, tinnitus, vertigo, nausea and vomiting. Feverfew is also used for infertility, anemia, cancer, common cold, earache, liver disease, prevention of miscarriage, muscular tension, orthopedic disorders, swollen feet, diarrhea, and dyspepsia including indigestion and flatulence.
Topically, feverfew is used for toothaches and as an antiseptic and insecticide. It is also used as a general stimulant and tonic and for intestinal parasites.

Safety

LIKELY SAFE ...when used orally and appropriately, short-term. Feverfew has been used safely in studies lasting up to 4 months (6959,6960,6961).
There is insufficient reliable information available about the safety of the long-term use of feverfew. Although no significant adverse effects have been reported with long-term use (6959,12153); long-term safety has not been sufficiently evaluated (12153).
PREGNANCY: POSSIBLY UNSAFE ...when used orally. Feverfew might cause uterine contractions and abortion (12); avoid using.
LACTATION: Insufficient reliable information available; avoid using.

Effectiveness

POSSIBLY EFFECTIVE

Migraine headache. There is some evidence that taking feverfew orally can reduce the frequency of migraine headaches and reduce symptoms of pain, nausea, vomiting, and sensitivity to light and noise (5080,6959,6960,6961,12384). It may be more effective in patients with more frequent migraine attacks (12384). But there is also evidence that feverfew does not improve migraine symptoms or reduce the occurrence of migraine headache (6938,12153,12384). These conflicting findings may reflect differences in the harvested feverfew plants, extracts used, or differences in bioavailability of commercially prepared feverfew products (12153). A combination product containing feverfew, riboflavin, and magnesium doesn't seem to reduce the frequency or severity of migraine any better than placebo. However, some problems with study design suggest that more research should be conducted on this combination (12389).

Most studies have used feverfew products standardized to contain 0.2% to 0.35% of the parthenolide constituent, but this standardization does not seem necessary for effectiveness (6935,6938).

POSSIBLY INEFFECTIVE

Rheumatoid arthritis (RA). Taking feverfew orally doesn't seem to reduce the symptoms of RA (6933).

There is insufficient reliable information available about the effectiveness of feverfew for its other uses.

Mechanism of Action

The applicable part of feverfew is the leaf. At least 39 constituents of feverfew have been identified (724). However, there has been controversy regarding which constituents were responsible for feverfew's pharmacological effects. It used to be widely believed that the sesquiterpene lactone, parthenolide, was the active constituent (6935). Parthenolide, seems to selectively inhibit cyclooxygenase-2 (COX-2) and the proinflammatory cytokines tumor necrosis factor (TNF)-alpha and interleukin (IL)-1 (12483). It was suggested that at least 0.2% of parthenolide was required for efficacy for migraine (6935,6937). However, a study using an alcoholic extract of feverfew standardized to 0.35% parthenolide was found ineffective for preventing migraine (6938), suggesting that parthenolide may not be the active ingredient and that other constituents are necessary for benefit in the prevention of migraine (49,6935,6938). It's not yet clear how feverfew works in the prevention of migraine. Laboratory evidence suggests that feverfew extracts might inhibit platelet aggregation and inhibit serotonin release from platelets and leucocytes (6935,6936,6942,6943,6944,6945); however, platelet studies in people have not found this effect (6951). Feverfew might also inhibit serum proteases and leukotrienes (6939,6946). Feverfew also appears to block prostaglandin synthesis by inhibiting phospholipase, which prevents the release of arachidonic acid (6943,6953,6954). Preliminary research shows that extracts of fresh feverfew leaves and parthenolide might cause irreversible inhibition of vascular muscle contraction (6948,6950). Chrysanthenyl acetate, an essential oil of feverfew, has been suggested as one active component (6938). Chrysanthenyl acetate inhibits prostaglandin synthetase and might have analgesic properties (6713,12153). Feverfew also contains melatonin which might contribute to its pharmacological effect (50). Fresh or dried leaves contain significantly more melatonin than commercially prepared standardized feverfew tablets (50). Migraine attacks have been associated with decreased melatonin excretion (6712). Other pharmacological effects of feverfew include cytostatic effect on tumor cell growth (6957), inhibition of inflammation and pain transmission (6947), and anti-inflammatory effects (6941).

Adverse Reactions

Orally, feverfew is well tolerated. It can cause gastrointestinal symptoms such as heartburn, nausea, diarrhea, constipation, abdominal pain and bloating, and flatulence. It can also cause nervousness, tension headache, insomnia, dizziness, stiffness in joints, tiredness, menstrual changes, palpitations, skin rash, and weight gain (12383). The traditional method of feverfew administration, chewing fresh feverfew leaves, can result in mouth ulceration, inflamed oral mucosa and tongue, swelling of the lips, and occasionally, loss of taste (6935,6959). Mouth ulceration might result from direct contact with feverfew leaves during chewing, possibly attributable to the sesquiterpene lactone constituent (6959). Some researchers suggest that mouth ulceration is a systemic effect, but one study using dried feverfew capsules reported a higher incidence of mouth ulcers in subjects taking placebo than feverfew (6935,6959,6960). "Post-feverfew syndrome," including anxiety, headaches, insomnia, and muscle and joint stiffness, has been described in people who have taken feverfew over long periods of time (6959). Topically, allergic contact dermatitis can occur (6958).

Overall, feverfew might be better tolerated than some conventional migraine drugs used for prophylaxis. For example, in clinical trials, feverfew did not affect blood pressure, heart rate, body weight, blood chemistry, or cytology; like some conventional drugs do such as ergot derivatives, serotonin agonists ("triptans"), beta-blockers, valproic acid, and analgesics (6959,6960,6961,6965,12153). Feverfew may cause an allergic reaction in individuals sensitive to the Asteraceae/Compositae family. Members of this family include ragweed, chrysanthemums, marigolds, daisies, and many other herbs.

Interactions with Herbs & Other Dietary Supplements

HERBS WITH ANTICOAGULANT/ANTIPLATELET POTENTIAL: Some evidence suggests that feverfew may inhibit platelet aggregation. However, this has not been demonstrated in humans (6935,6936,6942,6943,6944,6945,6951). Theoretically, concomitant use of feverfew and herbs that affect platelet aggregation could increase the risk of bleeding in some people. Some of these herbs include angelica, clove, danshen, garlic, ginger, ginkgo, Panax ginseng, horse chestnut, red clover, turmeric, and others.

Interactions with Drugs

ANTICOAGULANT/ANTIPLATELET DRUGS: Some evidence suggests that feverfew may inhibit platelet aggregation. However, this has not been demonstrated in humans (6935,6936,6942,6943,6944,6945,6951). Theoretically, feverfew might have additive effects and increase the risk of bleeding when used with these drugs.
CYTOCHROME P450 1A2 (CYP1A2) SUBSTRATES: There's preliminary evidence that feverfew might inhibit cytochrome P450 1A2 (CYP1A2) (12479). So far, this interaction has not been reported in humans. However, watch for an increase in the levels of drugs metabolized by CYP1A2 in patients taking feverfew. Some drugs metabolized by CYP1A2 include amitriptyline (Elavil), haloperidol (Haldol), ondansetron (Zofran), propranolol (Inderal), theophylline (Theo-Dur, others), verapamil (Calan, Isoptin, others), and others. Use feverfew cautiously or avoid in patients taking these drugs.
CYTOCHROME P450 2C19 (CYP2C19) SUBSTRATES: There's preliminary evidence that feverfew might inhibit cytochrome P450 2C19 (CYP2C19) (12479). So far, this interaction has not been reported in humans. However, watch for an increase in the levels of drugs metabolized by CYP2C19 in patients taking feverfew. Some drugs metabolized by CYP2C19 include proton pump inhibitors including omeprazole (Prilosec), lansoprazole (Prevacid), and pantoprazole (Protonix); diazepam (Valium); carisoprodol (Soma); nelfinavir (Viracept); and others.
CYTOCHROME P450 2C9 (CYP2C9) SUBSTRATES: There's preliminary evidence that feverfew might inhibit cytochrome P450 2C9 (CYP2C9) (12479). So far, this interaction has not been reported in humans. However, watch for an increase in the levels of drugs metabolized by CYP2C9 in patients taking feverfew. Some drugs metabolized by CYP2C9 include nonsteroidal anti-inflammatory drugs (NSAIDs) such as diclofenac (Cataflam, Voltaren), ibuprofen (Motrin), meloxicam (Mobic), and piroxicam (Feldene); celecoxib (Celebrex); amitriptyline (Elavil); warfarin (Coumadin); glipizide (Glucotrol); losartan (Cozaar); and others. Use feverfew cautiously or avoid in patients taking these drugs.
CYTOCHROME P450 3A4 (CYP3A4) SUBSTRATES: There's preliminary evidence that feverfew might inhibit cytochrome P450 3A4 (CYP3A4) enzyme (12479). So far, this interaction has not been reported in humans. However, watch for an increase in the levels of drugs metabolized by CYP3A4 in patients taking feverfew. Some drugs metabolized by CYP3A4 include lovastatin (Mevacor), ketoconazole (Nizoral), itraconazole (Sporanox), fexofenadine (Allegra), triazolam (Halcion), and numerous others. Use feverfew cautiously or avoid in patients taking these drugs.

Interactions with Foods

None known.

Interactions with Lab Tests

None known.

Interactions with Diseases or Conditions

CROSS-ALLERGENICITY: Feverfew may cause an allergic reaction in individuals sensitive to the Asteraceae/Compositae family. Members of this family include ragweed, chrysanthemums, marigolds, daisies, and many others.

Dosage and Administration

ORAL: For migraine headache prophylaxis, clinical studies have used 50-100 mg of feverfew extract daily. Although most extracts used in clinical studies were standardized to 0.2% to 0.35% parthenolide content, this standardization does not appear to be necessary for effectiveness (6935,6938,6959,6960,6961).
TOPICAL: No typical dosage.

Comments

Some feverfew tablet products can contain little or no feverfew. The Therapeutic Products Directorate of the Health Products and Food Branch of Health Canada issued a Drug Identification Number (DIN) to a feverfew leaf (capsules) product standardized to 0.2% parthenolide, with the labeling claim "used as a prophylactic against migraines" (724).

FICIN

Also Known As

Doctor Oje, Leche de Higueron, Leche de Oje, Oje.

Scientific Names

Ficus insipida, synonyms Ficus anthelminthica, Ficus glabrata, and Ficus laurfolia.
Family: Moraceae.

People Use This For

Orally, ficin is used as a digestive aid, and as an anthelmintic.
In medical procedures, ficin is used to clean and prepare intestinal submucosa for the production of sutures, to clean and prepare animal arteries for human implantation, and in serologic testing (e.g., for Rh factor determination).
In manufacturing, ficin is used in European anti-inflammatory preparations, cheese manufacturing, chillproofing beer, preparation of protein hydrolysates, edible collagen films, and sausage casings. Ficin is sometimes included in meat tenderizers, usually in combination with papain and/or bromelain.

Safety

LIKELY UNSAFE ...when used topically. Crude ficin is corrosive to skin and prolonged contact can cause bleeding (11).
There is insufficient reliable information available about the safety of the oral use of ficin.
PREGNANCY AND LACTATION: LIKELY UNSAFE ...when used topically (11). There is insufficient reliable information available about the safety of ficin for oral use during pregnancy or lactation; avoid using.

Effectiveness

There is insufficient reliable information available about the effectiveness of ficin.

Mechanism of Action

Ficin is a sulfhydryl proteinase and can hydrolyze proteins, amides, esters, and small peptides (11). Some evidence suggests ficin might be useful in treating helminthiasis (11,3766). Other evidence suggests ficin has anti-inflammatory activity (11).

Adverse Reactions

Orally, large amounts of ficin can cause catharsis (11).
Topically, crude ficin is corrosive to skin and can cause bleeding with prolonged contact (11). Ficin can also cause contact allergies (11).

Interactions with Herbs & Other Dietary Supplements

None known.

Interactions with Drugs

None known.

Interactions with Foods

None known.

Interactions with Lab Tests

None known.

Interactions with Diseases or Conditions

None known.

Dosage and Administration

ORAL: As an anthelmintic, 1.0 cc of prepared latex/kg per day for 3 days to be repeated every 3 months has been used (3766).

Comments

Ficin is the latex harvested from the trunk of felled Ficus insipida trees. Crude ficin consists of the latex combined with acetic acid to prevent coagulation and sodium benzoate as a preservative (11). Purified ficin is not pure ficin. Rather, it is a mixture of several proteases and small amounts of other enzymes and other constituents (11).

FIELD SCABIOUS

Also Known As
Bluebuttons, Gypsy's-Rose.

Scientific Names
Knautia arvensis, synonym Scabiosa arvensis.
Family: Dipsacaceae.

Comments
At the date of publication, this product was not a common ingredient used in brand name supplements marketed to consumers. Details about this product are available in the online version of *Natural Medicines Comprehensive Database.* See www.naturaldatabase.com.

FIG

Also Known As
Caricae Fructus, Feigen.

Scientific Names
Ficus carica.
Family: Moraceae.

People Use This For
Orally, fig fruit is used as a laxative. Fig leaf is also used orally for diabetes, hyperlipidemia, eczema, psoriasis, and vitiligo.
Topically, latex from the fruit is used to treat skin tumors and warts.

Safety
LIKELY SAFE ...when the fresh or dried fruit is used orally in amounts commonly found in foods.
POSSIBLY SAFE ...when the leaf is used orally for up to one month (12578).
PREGNANCY AND LACTATION: LIKELY SAFE ...when the fresh or dried fruit is used orally in amounts commonly found in foods. There is insufficient reliable information available about the safety of fig leaf or fruit used in medicinal amounts during pregnancy and lactation.

Effectiveness
INSUFFICIENT RELIABLE EVIDENCE to RATE

Diabetes. Preliminary clinical research suggests that a tea made from fig leaves may reduce insulin requirements in patients with type 1 diabetes. It also seems to lower postprandial hyperglycemia (12578). More evidence is needed to rate fig for this use.

Mechanism of Action
The applicable parts of fig are the fruit and leaf. The leaf contains psoralen, beta-sitosterol, bergapten, and taraxasterol (12579). The latex from the leaves contains ficin, a proteolytic enzyme that causes itching (12690). An aqueous leaf extract can cause hypoglycemic activity in animals and humans with type 1 diabetes (6625,12578). Fig leaf may improve glucose update by skeletal muscle (12578). Other preliminary research suggests it may also lower triglyceride levels by altering lipid metabolism (12839).
Latex from the fruit seems to have cytoxic activity and inhibits proliferation of some cancer cells (12579).

Adverse Reactions
Orally, fig fruit can cause allergy and rarely, anaphylaxis (8815,12580). Fig leaf contains psoralens and may cause photodermatitis (12579,12581). Avoid excessive sunlight or ultraviolet light exposure while using products containing fig leaf. Oral use of fig fruit is unlikely to cause photodermatitis (12581).
Topically, exposure to fig fruit and leaves can cause contact dermatitis (12689).

Interactions with Herbs & Other Dietary Supplements
HERBS WITH HYPOGLYCEMIC POTENTIAL: Theoretically, fig leaf might have additive effects with herbs that decrease blood glucose levels (12578). Herbs with hypoglycemic potential include devil's claw, fenugreek, guar gum, gymnema, Panax ginseng, Siberian ginseng, and others.

Interactions with Drugs

ANTIDIABETES DRUGS: Theoretically, fig leaf might enhance the blood glucose lowering effects of hypoglycemic drugs (12578). Monitor blood glucose levels closely.
INSULIN: Fig leaf can enhance the blood glucose lowering effects of insulin (12578); blood glucose levels should be monitored closely.

Interactions with Foods

None known.

Interactions with Lab Tests

BLOOD GLUCOSE: Fig leaf can reduce blood glucose levels and lab tests (12578).

Interactions with Diseases or Conditions

None known.

Dosage and Administration

No typical dosage.

FIGWORT

Also Known As

Carpenter's Square, Common Figwort, Heal-all, Rosenoble, Scrophula Plant, Scrophularia, Throatwort.

Scientific Names

Scrophularia marilandica; Scrophularia nodosa.
Family: Scrophulariaceae.

People Use This For

Orally, figwort is used as a diuretic.
Topically, figwort is used for chronic skin diseases such as eczema, itching, and psoriasis, and hemorrhoids, swelling, and eruptions.

Safety

There is insufficient reliable information available about the safety of figwort.
Pregnancy and Lactation: Insufficient reliable information available; avoid using.

Effectiveness

There is insufficient reliable information available about the effectiveness of figwort.

Mechanism of Action

The applicable parts of figwort are the above ground parts and root. It is reported to have diuretic and laxative effects (18). Constituents, aucubin and catalpol, exert purgative action in mice; harpagide may have cardioactive and anti-inflammatory activity (4).

Adverse Reactions

None reported.

Interactions with Herbs & Other Dietary Supplements

CARDIAC GLYCOSIDE-CONTAINING HERBS: Contraindicated, and concomitant use can increase the risk of cardiac glycoside toxicity. Cardiac glycoside-containing herbs include black hellebore, Canadian hemp roots, digitalis leaf, hedge mustard, lily-of-the-valley roots, motherwort, oleander leaf, pheasant's eye plant, pleurisy root, squill bulb leaf scales, strophanthus seeds, and uzara (19).

Interactions with Drugs

DIURETIC DRUGS: Theoretically, overuse of figwort might compound diuretic-induced potassium loss. There is some concern that people taking figwort along with potassium depleting diuretics might have an increased risk for hypokalemia. Initiation of potassium supplementation or an increase in potassium supplement dose may be necessary for some patients. Some diuretics that can deplete potassium include chlorothiazide (Diuril), chlorthalidone (Thalitone), furosemide (Lasix), hydrochlorothiazide (HCTZ, Hydrodiuril, Microzide), and others.

Interactions with Foods

None known.

Interactions with Lab Tests
None known.

Interactions with Diseases or Conditions
DIABETES: Theoretically, figwort may alter blood glucose control (4); monitor closely.
VENTRICULAR TACHYCARDIA: Contraindicated (4,12).

Dosage and Administration
ORAL: As a tea, use 2-8 grams dried above ground parts in 150 mL boiling water 5-10 minutes, steep (4). As a liquid extract (1:1 in 25% alcohol), 2-8 mL has been used (4). As a tincture (1:10 in 45% alcohol), 2-4 mL has been used (4).
TOPICAL: No typical dosage.

Comments
Figwort is stated to be a suitable substitute for devil's claw (due to similar chemical composition) (4).

FIR

Also Known As
Norway Spruce, Piceae turiones recentes, Spruce Fir.
CAUTION: See separate listings for Dwarf Pine Needle, Pine, and Poplar.

Scientific Names
Abies alba, synonyms Abies alba f. pendula, Abies alba f. pyramidalis.
Family: Pinaceae.

People Use This For
Orally, fir is used for respiratory tract inflammation, colds, cough, bronchitis, fever, inflammation of the mouth and pharynx, muscle and nerve pain, tendency toward infection, and tuberculosis.
Topically, fir is used for mild myalgia, neuralgia, rheumatic pain, and applied externally as a bath additive for mental illness.

Safety
There is insufficient reliable information about the safety of fir.
Pregnancy and Lactation: Insufficient reliable information available; avoid using.

Effectiveness
There is insufficient reliable information available about the effectiveness of fir.

Mechanism of Action
The applicable parts of fir are the shoot and oil. Fir shoot can reduce secretions, enhance local circulation, and act as a mild antiseptic (2). The essential oil can have secretory and antibacterial effects on bronchial mucous membranes (18). The essential oil also acts as a rubefacient (counterirritant) and improves circulation when applied externally (18).

Adverse Reactions
None reported.

Interactions with Herbs & Other Dietary Supplements
None known.

Interactions with Drugs
None known.

Interactions with Foods
None known.

Interactions with Lab Tests
None known.

Interactions with Diseases or Conditions
ASTHMA, PERTUSSIS (whooping cough): The fir shoot can exacerbate these conditions (18).
Contraindicated for use as a bath additive for individuals with extensive skin injuries, acute skin diseases, feverish or infectious diseases, cardiac insufficiency, or hypertonia (18).

Dosage and Administration

ORAL: The typical dose is 5-6 grams of the fresh fir shoots per day (2,18). The essential oil is usually given as 4 drops in water or on a sugar lump three times daily (18).
TOPICAL: Boil 200-300 grams of the shoots in 1 L water, steep for 5 minutes, strain, and add to a full bath (2,18).
INHALATION: Inhale the vapor of 2 grams of the essential oil in hot water several times per day (18).

FIREWEED

Also Known As

Blood Vine, Blooming Sally, Flowering Willow, French Willow, French-Willow, Great Willowherb, Persian Willow, Purple Rocket, Rose Bay Willow, Rosebay Willow, Tame Withy, Wickup, Wicopy, Willow Herb, Willowherb.

Scientific Names

Epilobium angustifolium, synonyms Chamaenerion angustifolium, Chamerion angustifolium, Epilobium spicatum.
Family: Onagraceae.

People Use This For

Orally, fireweed is used for inflammation, fevers, tumors, wounds, as an astringent, and as a tonic.

Safety

POSSIBLY SAFE ...when used orally (12).
PREGNANCY AND LACTATION: Insufficient reliable information available; avoid using.

Effectiveness

There is insufficient reliable information available about the effectiveness of fireweed.

Mechanism of Action

The applicable parts of fireweed are the above ground parts. Preliminary evidence suggests that aqueous extracts of fireweed might affect reproduction (858) and have anti-inflammatory effects (859,860).

Adverse Reactions

None reported.

Interactions with Herbs & Other Dietary Supplements

None known.

Interactions with Drugs

None known.

Interactions with Foods

None known.

Interactions with Lab Tests

None known.

Interactions with Diseases or Conditions

None known.

Dosage and Administration

No typical dosage.

Comments

Other Epilobium species are also referred to as willow herb (18).

FISH OIL

Also Known As

Cod Liver Oil, Marine Oils, Menhaden Oil, N-3 Fatty Acids, N3-polyunsaturated Fatty Acids, Omega-3 Fatty Acids, PUFA, Salmon Oil, W-3 Fatty Acids.
CAUTION: See separate listings for Cod Liver Oil, DHA, EPA, and Shark Liver Oil.

Scientific Names

None.

People Use This For

Orally, fish oils are used for hyperlipidemia, hypertriglyceridemia, coronary heart disease, hypertension, stroke, bipolar disorder, depression, rheumatoid arthritis (RA), osteoporosis, psoriasis, atopic dermatitis, ulcerative colitis, Behcet's syndrome, and Raynaud's syndrome. Fish oils are also used orally for weight loss, asthma, cancer, painful menses, lung diseases, allergic rhinitis, Crohn's disease, chronic fatigue syndrome, albuminuria associated with diabetic neuropathy, restenosis after angioplasty, miscarriage, preeclampsia, preterm labor, and intrauterine growth retardation. Fish oils are used for systemic lupus erythematosus, cystic fibrosis, gingivitis, renal impairment associated with cirrhosis, hyperglycemia associated with type 2 diabetes, and claudication. Fish oils are also used to treat attention deficit-hyperactivity disorder (ADHD), dyslexia, and dyspraxia. Other uses include preventing muscular soreness after exercise, preventing thrombosis after placement of a hemodialysis graft, renal impairment associated with IgA nephropathy; and high blood pressure and renal impairment associated with heart transplantation.
In combination with linoleic and gamma-linoleic acid, fish oils are used orally for treating post-viral fatigue syndrome. Fish oils are also used orally in combination with garlic to treat hypercholesterolemia.
Intravenously, fish oils are used to treat psoriasis.

Safety

LIKELY SAFE ...when used orally and appropriately. Doses of 3 grams per day and less can be safely used by most people. Fish oils have Generally Recognized As Safe (GRAS) status in the US (1313,4912).
POSSIBLY UNSAFE ...when used orally in large amounts. Doses greater than 3 grams per day can inhibit blood coagulation and potentially increase the risk of bleeding. Doses greater than 3 grams per day might also suppress immune response (1313,7384). ...when fish oils from dietary sources are consumed in large amounts. Fatty fish can contain significant amounts of toxins such as mercury, polychlorinated biphenyls (PCBs), dioxin, and dioxin-related compounds. Very frequent consumption of contaminated fish can cause adverse effects such as tremor, numbness and tingling, difficulty concentrating, and vision problems. Avoid frequent consumption of shark, swordfish, king mackerel, tilefish (also called golden bass or golden snapper), and farm-raised salmon (12964,12965,12966).
CHILDREN: POSSIBLY SAFE ...when used orally and appropriately (5708,5711). POSSIBLY UNSAFE ...when fish oil from dietary sources are consumed in large amounts. Fatty fish can contain significant amounts of toxins such as mercury, polychlorinated biphenyls (PCBs), dioxin, and dioxin-related compounds. Frequent consumption of contaminated fish can cause brain damage, mental retardation, blindness and seizures in children.
Lower levels can cause more subtle problems such as learning disabilities (12964). Young children should limit consumption to no more than 2 ounces/ week of fish (12867,12968).
PREGNANCY AND LACTATION: POSSIBLY SAFE ...when used orally and appropriately (1026,1027,1042,8706,12969,12970,12971,12972,12973). POSSIBLY UNSAFE ...when fish oil from dietary sources are consumed in large amounts. Fatty fish can contain significant amounts of toxins such as mercury, polychlorinated biphenyls (PCBs), dioxin, and dioxin-related compounds.
Women who are pregnant or who may become pregnant, and nursing mothers should avoid shark, swordfish, king mackerel, and tilefish (also called golden bass or golden snapper), which may contain high levels of methylmercury. They should also limit consumption of other fatty fish to 12 ounces per week or about 3-4 servings/week (12867,12968).

Effectiveness

EFFECTIVE

Hypertriglyceridemia. Fish oils from supplements or from dietary sources can reduce triglyceride levels by 20% to 50% (1024,2299,2300,2301,2302,2315,2317,5702,5705,5706,6394,6399,7368,7369,7380,12921,12922,13011,). This effect appears to be dose-dependent (5706,7380). However, fish oil supplements in doses of 4 grams/ day do not seem to be as effective as gemfibrozil (Lopid) 1200 mg per day (7377). For patients with hypertriglyceridemia associated with the atherogenic lipoprotein phenotype (ALP), which is thought to be a marker for cardiovascular disease, 6 grams of supplemental fish oils taken daily might reduce triglyceride levels by 35% (8683).
A specific fish oil preparation (Omacor, Reliant Pharmaceuticals), which contains 465 mg of eicosapentaenoic acid (EPA) and 375 mg of docosahexaenoic acid (DHA) in one gram capsules, is FDA-approved for treating hypertriglyceridemia (triglyceride levels of 500 mg/dL and above) in conjunction with dietary modifications (12982).

LIKELY EFFECTIVE

Cardiovascular disease. Consuming fish oil from dietary sources (fish), 2 servings of fatty fish/week, seems to reduce the risk of developing cardiovascular disease (primary prevention) (2309,8676,10006,10007,12915,12977). In people with existing heart disease (secondary prevention), consuming fish oils from dietary sources or taking fish oil supplements seems to reduce the risk of cardiovascular and all-cause mortality. Consuming 1 gram/day of fish oils from fish (about 3 ounces of fatty fish such as salmon) or fish oil supplements seems to decrease the risk of myocardial infarction, stroke, and progression of atherosclerosis (2307,7359,8673,8676,10007,12915). According to one analysis of the evidence, consuming dietary fish oils or taking fish oil supplements is associated with a 23% reduction in overall mortality and a 32% reduction in death from cardiovascular causes in people with or without cardiovascular disease. By comparison, statins lower overall mortality by 13% and cardiovascular mortality by 22% (12916). There is some controversy about the degree of protection provided by fish oils. Different analyses have found different degrees of protection (8673,12916,12917). Some research suggests fish oil supplements might not have additional protective effects in cardiovascular disease patients whose diet already includes fish oil (7361). Most epidemiological research on fish oil has not considered the methods of fish preparation. However, some research suggests broiled and baked fish have beneficial effects on cardiovascular disease risk, but fried fish and fish sandwiches increase risk (12976).

POSSIBLY EFFECTIVE

Age-related maculopathy. There is some evidence that people who ingest fish oils from dietary fish sources more than once per week have a reduced risk of developing age-related maculopathy (6260).

Angioplasty. Taking fish oils orally seems to prevent restenosis after percutaneous transluminal coronary angioplasty (PTCA) (8680). Fish oils appear to decrease restenosis rate (up to 26% reduction) when given for one month before PTCA and continued for one month thereafter. When given for less than one month before PTCA, fish oils don't seem to have any effect on restenosis (1028,1038,2320).

Antiphospholipid syndrome-associated miscarriage. Taking fish oils orally seems to prevent recurrent miscarriage and increase live birth rate in pregnant women with antiphospholipid syndrome (1032).

Asthma. Some research suggests that fish oil supplementation might improve peak flow, and reduce medication use and cough in children with asthma. In adults, fish oils don't seem to improve indicators of asthma such as forced expiratory volume in one second (FEV1), peak flow rate, asthma symptoms, asthma medication use or bronchial hyper-reactivity (12954,12963).

Atherosclerosis. Fish oil supplements, 6 grams per day for three months and then 3 grams per day for 21 months, might modestly slow the progression, or cause mild to moderate regression of atherosclerosis as measured by angiography in people with coronary artery disease. However, fish oils don't seem to improve luminal diameter (1022,2311) or decrease intima-media thickness of the carotid arteries in people with coronary artery disease (8681).

Bipolar disorder. Taking fish oils orally, with conventional therapies, seems to improve symptoms of depression and increase length of remission (7202). However, fish oils don't seem to have beneficial effects on manic symptoms in bipolar patients (5713,7202).

Cachexia. Taking a high-dose (7.5 grams per day) fish oil supplement seems to slow weight loss in some patients with cancer-related cachexia (11979). Lower doses (3 grams per day) don't seem to have any effect (10008). There is some preliminary evidence that a protein product supplemented with fish oils might help to improve appetite and increase lean body mass in patients with advanced pancreatic cancer (5701).

Cancer. Some, but not all, epidemiological research suggests fish oils from dietary sources seem to decrease the general risk of cancer. Intake of 1 gram/week of fish oils from dietary fish consumption seems to significantly lower the risk of several cancers including oral cancer, pharyngeal cancer, esophageal cancer, colon cancer, rectal cancer, breast cancer, ovarian cancer, and prostate cancer (10153,12958,12959,12961,12962). For colorectal cancer, there is a stronger association with reduced risk in men. In women, higher intake of fish and fish oils might reduce the progression of small adenomas to large adenomas (12960).

Cataracts. Epidemiological research suggests that women who eat fish three times a week have a modestly reduced risk of developing cataracts. Eating fish 3 times a week rather than once a month is associated with a 11% reduction in developing cataracts (12955).

Coronary artery bypass. Taking supplemental fish oils orally seems to decrease the incidence of coronary artery bypass graft occlusion following coronary artery bypass grafting (2314).

Cyclosporine-induced hypertension. Taking fish oils orally seems to prevent cyclosporine-induced hypertension following cardiac transplant. There is also some evidence that fish oils can maintain pre-cyclosporine blood pressure in patients taking cyclosporine (1012).

Cyclosporine-induced nephrotoxicity. Taking fish oils orally seems to prevent cyclosporine-induced nephrotoxicity, and significantly improve glomerular filtration rate (GFR) and renal blood flow in individuals taking cyclosporine (1021).

Depression. Taking fish oils orally seems to improve response to conventional antidepressants (10871). Low omega-3 levels in plasma and red blood cells are associated with depression (10859,10860). Epidemiological research suggests eating fish lowers the risk of depression and suicide (10867), and the prevalence of depression is lower in countries with higher fish consumption (10868).

Diabetic nephropathy. Taking fish oils orally seems to reduce albuminuria in individuals with diabetic nephropathy (1025).

Dyslexia. Taking fish oils orally seems to improve night vision in children with dyslexia. Dyslexic children who take fish oils seem to develop significantly better dark adaptation (5708).

Dyslipidemia. Taking 12 grams of fish oils orally in combination with garlic 900 mg daily seems to lower total cholesterol, triglycerides and the ratios of total cholesterol to high-density lipoprotein (HDL) and low-density lipoprotein (LDL) to HDL in patients with hypercholesterolemia (2318,2319). There is also some evidence that taking fish oils can decrease elevated triglyceride levels, decrease secretion of very low-density lipoproteins (VLDLs), increase VLDL apolipoprotein B secretion, and increase levels of HDL cholesterol in people with type 2 diabetes and dyslipidemia (8714,8807,12182). However, elevated levels of small, dense LDL cholesterol particles, are unaffected by fish oils in patients with type 2 diabetes (8714). There's also preliminary data that suggests fish oils, combined with pravastatin, might be helpful when used orally to correct the dyslipidemia associated with post-renal transplantation (8805).

Dysmenorrhea. Taking fish oils, alone or in combination with vitamin B12, seems to decrease pain and interference with daily activities in adolescent girls and women with dysmenorrhea (7574,7575).

Dyspraxia. Taking fish oils orally, in combination with evening primrose oil, thyme oil, and vitamin E (Efalex), seems to improve movement disorders in children with dyspraxia. One small clinical trial has shown that this combination significantly decreases movement disorders as determined by objective measures (5708).

Endometrial cancer. There is some evidence that women who regularly consume approximately two servings per week of fatty fish have a reduced risk for endometrial cancer (8690,9774).

Heart transplant. Taking fish oils orally seems to preserve renal function and reduce the long-term continuous rise in blood pressure after heart transplantation. There is evidence a dose of 4 grams of fish oils daily (46.5% EPA and 37.8% DHA) after heart transplantation prevents changes in systolic and diastolic blood pressures, glomerular filtration rate, and serum creatinine (8687).

Hemodialysis grafts. Taking fish oils orally seems to help prevent thrombosis in hemodialysis grafts. Fish oil supplements 4 grams daily started within two weeks of graft placement seems to prevent the development of access thrombosis in hemodialysis patients (8684).

Hypertension. Taking fish oils orally seems to produce modest, but significant reductions in systolic and diastolic blood pressure in patients with mild hypertension with or without type 2 diabetes (1001,1020,2301).

IgA nephropathy. Long-term use (two years) of fish oils 4-8 grams daily can slow the rate of renal function loss in high-risk patients with IgA nephropathy (8686,8711).

Obesity. There is some evidence that fish oils from dietary fish sources can improve weight loss and decrease blood glucose and insulin concentrations in overweight and hypertensive patients (2049).

Osteoporosis. Epidemiological research indicates increasing intake of foods including fish that are high in omega-3 fatty acids and decreasing intake of omega-6 fatty acids is associated with higher bone mineral density at the hip in both women and men (12956).Taking fish oils orally, in combination with evening primrose oil and calcium, seems to decrease bone turnover and increase spinal and femoral bone mineral density in elderly people with osteoporosis (7611,12925).

Prostate cancer. Population studies indicate that prostate cancer risk is significantly lower in men who regularly include fish oils in the diet. It appears that to significantly reduce the risk of prostate cancer at least 3 meals per week containing fish oil should be consumed (7378,9773,9774). Men who have higher serum levels of eicosapentaenoic acid (EPA) and docosahexaenoic acid (DHA), fatty acids that are in fish, seem to have a lower risk of developing prostate cancer (6395).

Psoriasis. There is some evidence that administering fish oils intravenously can decrease severity of symptoms in patients with acute, extended guttate psoriasis and chronic plaque psoriasis. Fish oils seem to be superior to omega-6 fatty acids for this use (1004,1034). However, fish oils taken orally don't seem to have any effect on psoriasis despite promising preliminary research (1035,8708).

Raynaud's syndrome. There's some evidence that taking fish oils orally can improve tolerance to cold and delay the onset of vasospasm in people with primary Raynaud's syndrome. People with Raynaud's syndrome caused by progressive systemic sclerosis don't seem to respond to fish oil supplements (7573).

Rheumatoid arthritis (RA). Taking fish oils orally, alone or in combination with naproxen (Naprosyn), seems to significantly decrease the duration of morning stiffness in patients with RA (1017,1039,1041,12924,12925). Use of fish oils might also reduce nonsteroidal anti-inflammatory drug (NSAID) requirements when used concomitantly (1031).

Stroke. Consuming fish oils from dietary sources at least once a week seems to reduce the risk of ischemic stroke by 27% (7373). Higher serum levels of fish oils are also associated with a decreased risk of stroke (7372). The method of preparing fish may be important. Eating tuna or other broiled or baked fish is associated with lower risk of ischemic stroke, while fried fish or fish sandwiches is associated with higher risk of ischemic stroke in elderly people (12923). Consumption of very high amounts of fish oils from dietary sources might increase the risk of stroke. People who eat more than 46 grams/day of fish or more than 660 mg per day of n-3 fatty acids appear to be nearly twice as likely to have an ischemic or hemorrhagic stroke. Tell patients that moderate consumption of fish (once or twice a week) is probably a good idea, but very high consumption of fish oils might be harmful (1313,7603,7610,8699). Dietary fish oils don't seem to further reduce ischemic stroke risk in people who already take aspirin (7373).

POSSIBLY INEFFECTIVE

Cirrhosis. Taking fish oils orally doesn't seem to help renal impairment associated with advanced cirrhosis (1013).

Claudication. Taking fish oils orally appears to have no effect on walking distance in patients with stable claudication (1002).

Gingivitis. Taking fish oils orally doesn't seem to improve gingivitis (1005).

Helicobacter pylori (H pylori). Taking fish oils orally, in combination with pantoprazole and clarithromycin (Biaxin), is inferior for eradicating H. pylori infection when compared with a combination of pantoprazole, clarithromycin, and metronidazole (8710).

Mastalgia. Taking fish oil orally isn't any more effective than placebo when 3 grams daily are taken for 6 months for severe chronic breast pain (9156).

Migraine headache. Taking fish oils orally doesn't appear to have any effect in decreasing the frequency or severity of migraine headaches in adolescents and adults (8712,8713).

Myalgia. Taking fish oils orally 1.8 grams per day taken orally for one month prior to and during physical exercise doesn't seem to prevent muscle soreness (8524).

LIKELY INEFFECTIVE

Diabetes. Taking fish oils orally has no effect on fasting plasma glucose levels or serum hemoglobin A1c in people with type 2 diabetes (2299,2300,2302,7368,7369,12182,12925,13011).

INSUFFICIENT RELIABLE EVIDENCE to RATE

Atopic dermatitis. Preliminary clinical research suggests maternal ingestion of fish oil supplements during pregnancy might reduce the severity of atopic dermatitis in infants at risk for atopy (12971).

Atrial fibrillation. Epidemiological and clinical research on the effects of fish oil on atrial function is conflicting. People aged 65 years and older who regularly consume tuna or other broiled or baked fish providing omega-3 fatty acids seem to have a lower risk of atrial fibrillation compared to those who eat fish less than once per month. People who consume fish 5 or more times per week have a 31% lower risk. People who consume fish 1 to 4 times per week have a 28% lower risk. However, consuming fried fish or fish sandwiches is not associated with a decreased risk of atrial fibrillation (12055). Interventional research suggests taking fish oil supplements might lower risk of atrial fibrillation after cardiac bypass surgery (12984). But contradictory epidemiological research suggests a diet high in fish doesn't affect risk for atrial fibrillation (12919).

Attention deficit-hyperactivity disorder (ADHD). There is preliminary evidence that taking fish oils orally might be helpful for ADHD (8800).

Chronic fatigue syndrome (CFS). There is some conflicting evidence about the use of a proprietary combination of fish oils and evening primrose oil (Efamol Marine) to reduce the symptoms CFS (7563,7564).

Chronic renal insufficiency. Preliminary clinical evidence suggests fish oils might reduce elevated levels of C-reactive protein (CRP) and increase hemoglobin, albumin levels, and urine output in patients on chronic hemodialysis (8685). However, fish oils don't appear to have any effect in healthy people with low CRP levels. Whether fish oils have any beneficial effects in patients with elevated CRP levels and conditions such as coronary artery disease is unknown (10155,12925).

Impaired glucose tolerance. Preliminary clinical evidence suggests fish oil supplements may reduce the risk of conversion from impaired glucose tolerance to type 2 diabetes. In patients with hypertriglyceridemia and impaired glucose tolerance, fish oil 2 grams per day lowers triglycerides with no deterioration in glucose tolerance over one year (7368).

Inflammatory bowel disease (IBD). There is some conflicting evidence suggesting fish oils might be helpful for IBD, but more evidence is needed (1037,1040,5709,6257,6258,6259,12925).

Pregnancy-associated complications. Some research suggests fish oils can prevent premature delivery when given during the third trimester of pregnancy (30 weeks and after) (8706,12972). However, fish oil doesn't seem to affect intrauterine growth retardation and pregnancy induced hypertension (1026,1027,1042,12972).

Schizophrenia. There is a case report of daily fish oils monotherapy (4 grams EPA and 2 grams DHA) improving symptoms of schizophrenia in a pregnant female (8702).

Systemic lupus erythematosus (SLE). Preliminary clinical research suggests fish oils might reduce SLE symptoms (7572,12925,12953). However other research shows no effect on disease activity or renal function (7571).

Ventricular arrhythmias. Evidence about the effect of fish oil on ventricular function is conflicting. Epidemiological research suggests eating a diet high in fish has no effect on risk for premature ventricular complexes (12920). Interventional clinical research suggests taking fish oil supplements might actually increase the risk of ventricular tachycardia and ventricular fibrillation in patients with implantable defibrillators (12986).

More information is needed to rate fish oils for these uses.

Mechanism of Action

Fish such as herring, kipper, mackerel, menhaden, pilchard, salmon, sardine, and trout contain oils with high amounts of long-chain, polyunsaturated fats called omega-3 fatty acids. These fish oils are especially high in the omega-3 fatty acids eicosapentaenoic acid (EPA) and docosahexaenoic acid (DHA). EPA and DHA seem to have different physiologic effects than their precursor alpha-linolenic acid, a plant-derived omega-3 fatty acid (10323,12918). Alpha-linolenic acid, even with long-term consumption, doesn't have the same effects as fish oils on triglyceride concentrations, on tissue DHA concentrations, or on in vitro susceptibility to oxidation of low-density lipoprotein (LDL) cholesterol (12918).

Omega-3 fatty acids from fish oils have anti-inflammatory and antithrombotic effects because they compete with arachidonic acid in the cyclooxygenase and lipoxygenase pathways. Fish oils inhibit the arachidonic acid synthesis of thromboxane A2, which causes platelet aggregation and vasodilation. Fish oils can also cause increased production of prostacyclin, a prostaglandin that causes vasodilation and reduces platelet aggregation (8671,8679,8696). Omega-3 fatty acids seem to suppress COX-2 expression and the inflammatory cytokines interleukin (IL)-1 alpha and tumor necrosis factor (TNF)-alpha (12471). Preliminary clinical evidence suggests that fish oils might have an additive or synergistic effect with aspirin on inhibiting synthesis of thromboxane A2 and the highly inflammatory leukotriene B4 (8701), but it's too early to recommend this combination.

Fish oils are used for cardiovascular conditions, including stroke and heart disease, due to anti-inflammatory and antithrombotic effects. Fish oils decrease blood viscosity, increase red blood cell deformability, and possibly provide protection against red cell hemolysis. Vasodilatory effects of omega-3 fatty acids in fish oils may also prevent increases in blood pressure and maintain renal function. Fish oils may have an antiarrhythmic effect. There is some evidence prostaglandins derived from arachidonic acid are proarrhythmic, whereas equivalent prostaglandins derived from EPA are not. Preclinical research suggests fish oils might have a membrane stabilizing effect (12987). Fish oils might regulate calcium movement through calcium channels in the heart and suppress intracellular calcium activity, which has been associated with arrhythmias. Increased dietary intake of omega-3 fatty acids increases the amount of EPA and DHA in cell membranes, which is thought to cause changes in enzyme and receptor function that secondarily leads to changes in calcium fluxes across cell membranes (8676). There's also some evidence fish oils might affect sodium channels and inhibit ischemia-induced arrhythmias (7362,7363,8671,8676,8677,8687). Regular consumption of fish seems to decrease heart rate, which might protect against cardiovascular events. Omega-3 fatty acids in fish oil, especially DHA, are associated with decreased heart rate Fish oils might also protect the heart by reducing inflammation and thrombosis, and inhibiting atherosclerosis (10154,11344,12919,12920).

In hypertriglyceridemia, fish oils are thought to lower triglycerides by decreasing secretion of very low-density lipoproteins (VLDLs), increasing VLDL apolipoprotein B secretion, possibly by increasing VLDL clearance, and reducing triglyceride transport (5707). In addition, fish oils appear to decrease synthesis of VLDL by inhibiting 1,2-diacylglycerol-sterol o-acyltransferase or phosphatidate phosphatase (6394). Fish oils may decrease chylomicron concentrations. More lipoprotein lipase becomes available due to decreased VLDL levels, which causes increased hydrolysis of chylomicrons (6394). Fish oils also increase fatty acid oxidation by peroxisomal and mitochondrial routes, reduce fatty acid synthesis, divert fatty acids into phospholipid synthesis, increase hepatic uptake of triglycerides, and down-regulate fatty acid esterifying enzymes (5707).

Fish oils may decrease cholesterol absorption from the gut and decrease cholesterol synthesis (5707).

There is evidence fish and fish oils increase high-density lipoproteins (HDL) and decrease the total cholesterol to HDL ratio (2318,5707,8674,8678,8698). Fish oils may increase low-density lipoprotein (LDL) concentrations (2299,2318,8678,8698) by increasing the size of LDL particles (9771). It is thought that fish oils might cause a more buoyant LDL to be formed, which might be less atherogenic (2299,8678). There is some evidence that vitamin B12 used with fish oils might have additive effects in lowering cholesterol, but the mechanism for this effect is unknown (8894). Fish oils also improve flow-mediated arterial dilation in people with hypercholesterolemia (5702). Unlike some other kinds of dietary fat, omega-3 fatty acids from fish oils do not seem to impair endothelial function, which is thought to be a precursor to atherogenesis (5702,7382). In some patients, fish oils appears to improve arterial compliance (1029,5707).

Fish oil can change the way dietary fatty acids are utilized. Omega-3 fatty acids found in fish oil compete metabolically with omega-6 fatty acids and omega-3 fatty acids in vegetable oils. Alpha linolenic acid and gamma linolenic acid are the primary omega-3 and omega-6 (respectively) fatty acids found in vegetable oils. Fish oil can modify the way these dietary fatty acids are incorporated into fatty acid chains and cell membranes and how they are used in other metabolic processes (7381,8693,9772). Omega-6 fatty acids, from fish oil, seem to inhibit the incorporation of omega-3 fatty acids into tissue lipids. In addition, omega-3 fatty acids inhibit the conversion of the omega-6 fatty acids into arachidonic acid. There is some concern that dietary vegetable oils in the diet might negate the beneficial cardiovascular effects of fish oils, but omega-3 fatty acids from fish oils seem to reduce cardiovascular risk factors despite concurrent omega-6 fatty acid ingestion (7381,8693). By increasing the intake of omega-3 fatty acids EPA and DHA, a corresponding increase of these fatty acids seems to occur in cell membranes and circulatory lipids along with a simultaneous reduction of omega-6 fatty acids (8677). The efficacy of omega-3 fatty acid containing products such as fish oils seems to be determined by an increased intake of omega-3 fatty-acids, a decreased intake of omega-6 fatty acids, and a decreased ratio of arachidonic acid to EPA and DHA (8671,8694). Omega-3s are metabolized to products that inhibit platelet aggregation or inactive metabolites. Some research suggests that EPA and DHA might block the inflammatory, vasoconstrictive, and thrombogenic effects of omega-6 fatty acids (10007,12914).

Fish oils can suppress mediators of immune function by reducing the production of cytokines such as interleukin-1(IL-1), interleukin-2 (IL-2), and tumor necrosis factor (TNF). Some researchers think fish oils might prevent weight loss in cancer patients by inhibiting cytokines, which cause muscle catabolism. Fish oils also suppress T- and B-cell proliferation and decrease delayed-type hypersensitivity skin response (DTH). They also decrease antibody production and increase free radical activity (1313,7383,7384,11979).

Due to fish oils' anti-inflammatory effects, they are tried for a variety of inflammatory conditions, including psoriasis, systemic lupus erythematosus (SLE), inflammatory bowel disease, and others. Fish oils seem to be beneficial in rheumatoid arthritis due to anti-inflammatory effects, and epidemiological data that suggests EPA levels are decreased in total plasma fatty acids and synovial fluid, and DHA is decreased in the synovial fluid of patients with rheumatoid arthritis (5710).

Preliminary clinical evidence suggest fish oil supplements might prolong pregnancy and depress levels of thromboxane A2 which is thought to cause vasoconstriction, platelet aggregation, and reduced uteroplacental blood flow associated with preeclampsia (8707).

Fish oils have been proposed as a treatment for attention deficit-hyperactivity disorder (ADHD) due to epidemiological data that suggests symptoms of ADHD might be inversely related to the omega 3-fatty acid phospholipid content (5711). In individuals with bipolar disorder, the fatty acids in fish oils are thought to have an effect similar to lithium or valproate, slowing nerve signaling (7202). In depression, omega-3s might normalize altered neuronal membrane microstructure and faulty neurotransmission in patients with depression. Omega-3s might also play a role in correcting defects in the arachidonic acid cascade, which is involved in second messenger processes that affect neurotransmitter uptake (10871). A diet deficient in omega-3 fatty acids may affect the fatty acid composition of cells in the central nervous system and alter neural function, including intellectual or cognitive development. DHA is thought to be important for normal neural function and might play a key role in the structural development of neural and synaptic membranes (8704,8705,8803). There is preliminary evidence that low levels of omega-3 fatty acids, especially DHA, might affect retinal, visual, learning, and memory function (8704,8705,8715).

Some researchers think fish oils might also help prevent some forms of cancer. People with high EPA and DHA levels in their erythrocytes seem to have decreased rates of prostate cancer (6395). EPA and DHA might compete with arachidonic acid as substrates for cyclooxygenases that produce prostaglandins that can enhance tumor growth (6385,7378). There is evidence fish oil supplementation decreases the expression of the enzyme cyclooxygenase-2 (COX-2) which has been found in prostate cancer tissue and is thought to play a role in promoting the growth of cancer cells (8689). There is also preliminary evidence that high levels of EPA and DHA can be beneficial for prolonging cancer remission. Fish oils might decrease production of lactic acid by tumor cells. Lactic acidosis is a marker of unfavorable metabolic conditions associated with many cancers (6398). There is also some evidence that fish oils might be cytotoxic to some cancer cells (1008). Preliminary evidence suggests that omega-3 fatty acids are first oxidized and then accumulate in tumor cell membranes, resulting in cell membrane perforation and eventually tumor cell death (8691).

Adverse Reactions

Orally, fish oils are generally well-tolerated at doses of 3 grams or less per day. Fish oil supplements can cause a fishy aftertaste or "fishy burp." Gastrointestinal adverse effects such as nausea occasionally occur. Taking supplements with meals or freezing them seems to help some patients (12975). Fish oils can also cause halitosis, heartburn, nausea, loose stools, and rash (6258,10007,12982).

Doses greater than 3 grams per day of fish oil or high dietary intake of fish can inhibit platelet aggregation, cause bleeding, and potentially increase the risk for hemorrhagic stroke (1313,8699). Very high consumption of fish (more than 46 grams per day) seems to increase the risk of both ischemic and hemorrhagic stroke (7603).

There's also some evidence that fish oils in doses greater than 3 grams per day might adversely affect immune function. Fish oils appear to suppress T- and B-cell function and to reduce the production of cytokines, which might be detrimental to elderly people and people with suppressed immune function such as patients with human immunodeficiency virus (HIV) infection (1313,7383,7384).

Fish oils don't seem to adversely affect low-density lipoprotein (LDL) cholesterol or cause development of atherosclerosis, despite earlier concerns that polyunsaturated fatty acids, such as omega-3 fatty acids, might increase the oxidation of LDL (1011,2323,7165,7366,9771). Supplemental fish oils do not seem to increase the susceptibility of LDL to oxidation (8695,8700). Although thiobarbituric acid reacting substances (TBARS) rise during fish oil supplementation, TBARS is now thought to inaccurately reflect LDL oxidation. More specific indicators of lipid peroxidation, such as F2-isoprostanes and malondialdehyde (MDA), suggest that fish oils are unlikely to have a negative effect on LDL and the risk for atherosclerosis (2323). There is also some evidence that fish oil supplements do not alter the serum concentrations of growth factors such as platelet-derived growth factor or transforming growth factor beta, which are also thought to play a role in the development of atherosclerotic plaques (8697).

Some fish oil preparations (e.g., cod liver oil) contain large amounts of vitamin A and vitamin D. If these preparations are used long-term or in large doses, there is a risk of vitamin A and D toxicity (see separate listing for cod liver oil) (6874).

Preliminary evidence suggests that increased serum levels of omega-3 fatty acids, especially DHA, might increase the risk for atrophic gastritis (8709).

There is some concern that fish or fish oil products might be contaminated with toxins or pesticides if the fish were caught in contaminated waters (6875). Heavy metals, especially mercury, are a particular concern (259). Consuming contaminated fish can result in accumulation of methylmercury and toxicity. High levels of methylmercury can cause symptoms such as tremor, numbness and tingling, difficulty concentrating, and vision problems. Methylmercury toxicity is most dangerous in very young children and women who are pregnant or likely to become pregnant. High methylmercury levels can cause brain damage, mental retardation, blindness and seizures. Lower levels can cause more subtle problems such as learning disabilities (12964). Methylmercury exposure has been associated with heart disease, particularly myocardial infarction. Some research suggests that methylmercury might antagonize the beneficial cardiovascular effects of omega-3s. Omega-3s might have antioxidant effects that are negated by the pro-oxidant effects of methylmercury (12973).

Other fish contaminants of concern are polychlorinated biphenyls (PCBs). PCBs are found in fish living in polluted waters and in some farmed fish such as salmon. Freshwater fish such as lake trout, smelt, and freshwater bluefish frequently contain high levels of PCBs. PCBs may be carcinogenic. They may also adversely affect the central nervous system, causing memory loss (12965).

Fish may also contain dioxin and dioxin-like compounds, which have carcinogenic, immunosuppressive, central nervous system (disturbances in learning and memory), and other adverse effects. Farmed fish, especially salmon, can be fed with fish feed that is contaminated with dioxin, making dioxin levels three to ten times higher in farmed than wild salmon. European farmed salmon contains more than American farmed salmon. Most salmon consumed in the US is farm-raised salmon; wild salmon is considerably more costly. To avoid toxic amounts of dioxin, consumers should limit American farmed salmon consumption to fewer than 10 times/month and European farmed salmon to fewer than 4 times/month (12966).

Women who are pregnant or who may become pregnant, and nursing mothers should avoid shark, swordfish, king mackerel, and tilefish (also called golden bass or golden snapper), which may contain high levels of methylmercury. They should also limit consumption of other fish to 12 ounces/week (about three to four servings/week). Young children should limit consumption to no more than two ounces of fish caught in sport fishing per week (12967,12968).

Fish oil supplements generally appear to be safe. Mercury accumulates in fish meat much more so than fish oils, which might explain the lack of detectable mercury in most fish oil supplements. Also, the manufacturing process used to deodorize fish oil supplements seems to lower levels of PCBs and other contaminants (12983). Laboratory analysis of fish oil supplements found no detectable levels of mercury or other toxins such as organochlorines in over 20 products tested (13009,13012). However, contaminants including organochlorines and PCBs have been reported in certain brands (13009,10007).

Fish oils also contribute to caloric intake and may cause weight gain if used long-term. One gram of fat or oil provides 9 kcal (6871). Fish oil capsules containing 500 mg omega-3 fatty acids in 1 gram of oil would supply about 13.5 kcal per capsule (6871,6874). Fish oil supplements also contain cholesterol in amounts from 1-6 mg per gram of fish oils (3022,6871).

Interactions with Herbs & Other Dietary Supplements

HERBS WITH ANTICOAGULANT/ANTIPLATELET POTENTIAL: Concomitant use of herbs that have antiplatelet/anticoagulant constituents could theoretically increase the risk of bleeding in some people (8671,8679,8696). These herbs include angelica, clove, danshen, garlic, ginger, ginkgo, Panax ginseng, red clover, turmeric, willow, and others.

VITAMIN E: Fish oils can reduce vitamin E levels. The mechanism is unknown, but might result from reduced vitamin E absorption or increased vitamin E utilization by tissues to reduce free radicals and prevent peroxidative damage (7384).

Interactions with Drugs

ANTICOAGULANT/ANTIPLATELET DRUGS: Fish oil has antiplatelet effects. Concomitant use with anticoagulant or antiplatelet drugs may increase the risk of bleeding (8671,8679,8696,11343). However, conflicting research suggests that 3 to 6 grams of fish oils per day does not significantly affect INR when use in patients taking warfarin (8801). Monitor patients taking fish oils and drugs that affect bleeding. Some of these drugs include aspirin, clopidogrel (Plavix), dalteparin (Fragmin), dipyridamole (Persantine), enoxaparin (Lovenox), heparin, ticlopidine (Ticlid), warfarin (Coumadin), and others.

ANTIHYPERTENSIVE DRUGS: Fish oils can lower blood pressure and might have additive effects in patients treated with antihypertensives (1001,1020,1030,1033); use with caution.

CONTRACEPTIVE DRUGS: There is some evidence that contraceptive drugs might interfere with the triglyceride lowering effects of fish oils (8694). Some of these drugs include ethinyl estradiol and levonorgestrel (Triphasil), ethinyl estradiol and norethindrone (Ortho-Novum 1/35, Ortho-Novum 7/7/7), and others.

Interactions with Foods

None known.

Interactions with Lab Tests

INTERNATIONAL NORMALIZED RATIO (INR), PROTHROMBIN TIME (PT): High doses of fish oils, greater than 3 grams per day, might decrease blood coagulation, increase INR and PT, and increase the risk of bleeding (1313).

Interactions with Diseases or Conditions

BIPOLAR DISORDER and DEPRESSION: Symptoms of hypomania can develop in patients taking fish oils who have bipolar (5713,7202) or major depressive disorders (6396).

CIRRHOSIS: Theoretically, use of fish oils may lower mean arterial pressure (MAP) to hypotensive levels, and may increase risk of bleeding (1013); use with caution.

DIABETES: There has been concern that doses of fish oil over 3 grams/day might worsen glucose control in diabetes patients (10007). However, there is no reliable scientific support for this concern. Doses from 2-18 grams/day do not seem to affect blood glucose or hemoglobin A1c (HbA1c) (2299,7368,7369,12182,13011,13013).

FAMILIAL ADENOMATOUS POLYPOSIS: Fish oils might further increase the risk of cancer in people with familial adenomatous polyposis. Three people, who had pre-existing familial adenomatous polyposis, were diagnosed with malignant lesions during the course of long-term use of fish oils (999).

HYPERTENSION: Fish oils can lower blood pressure and might have additive effects in patients treated with antihypertensives (1001,1020,1030,1033).

IMMUNODEFICIENCY: Higher doses of fish oils might cause suppression of immune and inflammatory response (1313,7383,7384). Tell immunocompromised patients (e.g., patients with HIV/AIDS) to avoid exceeding a dose of 3 grams per day.

IMPLANTABLE DEFIBRILLATORS: Some research suggests taking fish oil supplements can increase the risk of ventricular tachycardia and ventricular fibrillation in patients with implantable defibrillators (12986).

Dosage and Administration

ORAL: For hypertriglyceridemia, studies have used 1-4 grams of fish oils/day (5707,6394,6399). For a specific FDA-approved fish oil product (Omacor), 4 grams/day given in two divided doses or as single dose is recommended (12982). For hypertriglyceridemia in patients with the atherogenic lipoprotein phenotype (ALP), 6 grams per day has been used (8683).

For hypertension, studies have used either 4 grams of fish oils or fish oils providing eicosapentaenoic acid (EPA) 2.04 grams and docosahexaenoic acid (DHA) 1.4 grams daily (1001,1020).

For hypertension secondary to cyclosporine in heart transplant patients, 4 grams per day has been used (1012).

For atrial fibrillation, consuming tuna or baked or broiled fish providing omega-3 fatty acids (fish oils) one or more times per week seems to reduce the risk of atrial fibrillation in patients aged 65 or older compared to consuming fish once per month or less (12055). However, this benefit is not found with fried fish or fish sandwiches.

For cyclosporine nephrotoxicity, 12 grams per day containing 2.2 grams EPA and 1.4 grams DHA has been used (1021). For reducing overall mortality and sudden death in patients with coronary heart disease, a daily dose of fish oils providing EPA 0.3 to 6 grams with 0.6 to 3.7 grams DHA has been used (8673).

For treating asthma in children, 17 to 26.8 mg/kg EPA and 7.3 to 11.5 mg/kg DHA have been used (12954).

For preventing and reversing the progression of atherosclerosis in the coronary arteries, 6 grams of fish oil for the first three months, followed by 3 grams daily thereafter, has been used (2311).

For improving endothelial function in individuals with hypercholesterolemia, 4 grams per day has been used (5702).

For decreasing duration of morning stiffness secondary to rheumatoid arthritis, fish oils providing EPA 3.8 grams and DHA 2 grams per day have been used (1039).

For preventing miscarriage in women with antiphospholipid antibody syndrome and a history of recurrent miscarriage, 5.1 grams fish oils with a 1.5 EPA:DHA ratio has been used (1032).

For treating dysmenorrhea, a daily dose of EPA 1080 mg and DHA 720 mg has been (7574).

For treating primary Raynaud's syndrome, a total daily dose of 3.96 grams EPA and 2.64 grams DHA has been used (7573).

As an adjunct to standard therapy for bipolar disorder, fish oils providing EPA 6.2 grams and DHA 3.4 grams daily have been used (7202).

For weight loss, a daily serving of 2-7 ounces of fish containing approximately 3.65 grams omega-3 fatty acids (0.66 gram from EPA and 0.60 gram from DHA) has been used (2049).

For slowing weight loss in patients with cancer, 7.5 grams fish oils providing EPA 4.7 grams and DHA 2.8 grams daily have been used (11979).

For improving dark vision adaptation in dyslexic individuals, fish oils providing DHA 480 mg daily have been used (5708).

For improving movement disorders in children with dyspraxia, fish oils providing DHA 480 mg combined with 35 mg arachidonic acid and 96 mg gamma-alpha linoleic acid from evening primrose oil, 24 mg thyme oil, and 80 mg vitamin E (Efalex) have been used (5708).

For treatment of depression along with conventional antidepressants, fish oils 9.6 grams per day have been used (10871).

For decreasing the frequency of vein graft occlusion after coronary bypass grafting, 4 grams of fish oil per day containing EPA 2.04 grams and DHA 1.3 grams has been used (2314).

For preventing restenosis after percutaneous transluminal coronary angioplasty (PTCA), 6 grams daily of fish oil starting one month before PTCA and continuing one month after PTCA, followed by 3 grams of fish oil daily thereafter for six months, has been used (8680).

For reducing and preventing the long-term continuous rise in blood pressure and to preserve renal function after heart transplantation, 4 grams daily of fish oils (46.5% EPA and 37.8% DHA) has been used (8687).

For preventing thrombosis after placement of a hemodialysis graft, 6 grams of fish oils has been used daily (8684).
For preserving renal function in patients with severe IgA nephropathy, 4-8 grams daily of fish oil has been used (8686,8711).
For combined hypertriglyceridemia and hypercholesterolemia, fish oils providing EPA 1800-2160 mg and DHA 1200-1440 mg combined with garlic powder 900-1200 mg daily has been used to lower total cholesterol, LDL, triglycerides, and the ratios of total cholesterol to HDL, and LDL to HDL (2318,2319).
For preventing muscle soreness after physical exercise, fish oil 1.8 grams per day has been used (8524).
Fish oil supplements often contain small amounts of vitamin E as an antioxidant to prevent spoilage. They might also be combined with calcium, iron, or vitamins A, B1, B2, B3, C, or D. Fish that are good sources of omega-3 fatty acids, including mackerel, tuna, salmon, sturgeon, mullet, bluefish, anchovy, sardines, herring, trout, and menhaden, provide about 1 gram of omega-3 fatty acids per 3.5 ounces of fish.
INTRAVENOUS: For chronic plaque psoriasis, a daily 200 mL intravenous dose of parenteral fish oil-based lipid emulsion (Omegavenous), containing 4.2 grams EPA and 4.2 grams DHA, has been used for 14 days (1004).
For acute, extended guttate psoriasis, a daily intravenous dose of a parenteral fish oil product, containing 2.1 grams EPA and 21 grams DHA, has been used for 10 days (1034).

Comments

Fish oils come from a variety of marine life including mackerel, herring, tuna, halibut, salmon cod liver, whale blubber, and seal blubber. Products that are commercially available contain varying amounts and ratios of docosahexaenoic acid (DHA) and eicosapentaenoic acid (EPA).
Omega-3 fatty acids are also called n-3 fatty acids. These names refer to the hydrocarbon chains with a methyl group at one end (called the omega position) and a carboxyl group at the other. Omega-3 fatty acids have a double bond at the third carbon (n-3). EPA and DHA are called long-chain fatty acids. EPA is sometimes written C20:5 omega-3 (20 carbons, 5 double bonds with the first at the n-3 position). DHA is C22:6 omega-3 (22 carbons, 6 double bonds with the first at the n-3 position). "Omega-3" is sometimes used to specifically refer to EPA and DHA, but alpha-linolenic acid in plants is also an omega-3 fatty acid (12914).

FLAXSEED

Also Known As

Atasi, Graine De Lin, Leinsamen, Lini Semen, Linseed, Lint Bells, Linum, Phytoestrogen, Winterlien.
CAUTION: See separate listings for Alpha Linolenic Acid, Conjugated Linoleic Acid (CLA), Docosahexaenoic Acid (DHA), Eicosapentaenoic Acid (EPA), Fish Oil, and Flaxseed Oil.

Scientific Names

Linum usitatissimum, synonyms Linum crepitans, Linum humile.
Family: Linaceae.

People Use This For

Orally, flaxseed is used for chronic constipation, colon damage due to laxative abuse, diverticulitis, irritable bowel syndrome (IBS) or irritable colon, gastritis, and enteritis. It is also used for menopausal symptoms, bladder inflammation, hypercholesterolemia, hypertriglyceridemia, atherosclerosis, protection against cancer, osteoporosis, attention deficit-hyperactivity disorder (ADHD), and systemic lupus erythematosus (SLE) nephritis.
Topically, flaxseed is used as a poultice for skin inflammation.
Ophthalmically, flaxseed is used for the removal of foreign bodies from the eye.

Safety

LIKELY SAFE ...when used orally and appropriately (5899,6800,6802,6803,6808,8020). Flaxseed is well tolerated when taken with sufficient fluid. Tell patients to consume at least 150 mL of liquid for every 10 grams of whole or cracked flaxseed (12).
PREGNANCY AND LACTATION: Insufficient reliable information available.

Effectiveness

LIKELY EFFECTIVE

Constipation. Taking flaxseed orally as a bulk forming laxative is effective for relieving constipation (6803).
Hypercholesterolemia. Various flaxseed preparations, including raw, ground, partially defatted, and flaxseed bread and muffins seem to significantly reduce total cholesterol and low-density lipoprotein (LDL) cholesterol in people with normal cholesterol levels (5899,6803) and in people with hypercholesterolemia (6800,6808). Preparations providing flaxseed 40 to 50 grams per day seem to reduce total cholesterol by 5% to 9% and LDL cholesterol by 8% to 18% (5899,6800,6803,6808,10952), but flaxseed doesn't seem to have much effect on LDL in hypercholesteremic postmenopausal women (10952,10978). However, flaxseed does not affect high-density lipoprotein (HDL) cholesterol. Apolipoprotein A-1 and apolipoprotein B, which are indicators of the risk for coronary heart disease, may be decreased by 6 and 7.5%, respectively (10952). Most flaxseed preparations also do not affect triglyceride

levels, but partially defatted flaxseed (flaxseed without as much alpha-linolenic acid content) can increase triglycerides by approximately 10% (6808).

POSSIBLY EFFECTIVE

Menopausal symptoms. Taking flaxseed orally 40 grams per day seems to be similar to hormone therapy for improving mild menopausal symptoms (10978). Whether flaxseed is effective for moderate to severe menopausal symptoms is unknown.

Systemic lupus erythematosus (SLE) nephritis. Taking flaxseed orally seems to improve renal function in people with systemic lupus erythematosus (SLE) nephritis. There is evidence that daily use of flaxseed can lower serum creatinine (6802,8021).

INSUFFICIENT RELIABLE EVIDENCE to RATE

Osteoporosis. Consuming ground flaxseed 40 grams/day does not seem to affect markers of bone metabolism in women (10952). More evidence is needed to rate flaxseed for this use.

Mechanism of Action

Flaxseed is a bulk-forming fibrous product that stimulates intestinal peristalsis, producing a laxative effect (18). The soluble fiber in flaxseed is found primarily in the seed coat gum, which is a mixture of polysaccharides including glucuronic acids, rhamnose, arabinose, xylose, and galactose (6808). Ten grams of flaxseed typically provides approximately 44 kilocalories energy, 2 grams protein, 4 grams fat and 4 grams dietary fiber (6801). Flaxseed is a rich source of alpha-linolenic acid and long-chain n-3 polyunsaturated fatty acids. Supplementation with flaxseed significantly increases n-3 polyunsaturated fatty acids in plasma and erythrocytes (5899,6803). Flaxseed is used for atherosclerosis because it can reduce platelet aggregation and serum cholesterol and thereby might lower atherogenic risks (6,6808). In animal models, flaxseed supplementation seems to significantly reduce the risk of developing aortic atherosclerosis (6806,6807). The fiber content of flaxseed is thought to be important for flaxseed's lipid lowering effects. High fiber diets increase fecal elimination of bile acids, which increases primary bile acid synthesis (6800,6808). The alpha-linolenic acid content of flaxseed might also help lower serum cholesterol (6800). However, because partially defatted flaxseed also seems to lower cholesterol, other mechanisms are likely involved (6807,6808). Alpha-linolenic acid may also be involved in the beneficial effects on platelets (6800). Flaxseed might also have hypoglycemic effects. The postprandial glucose response to a 50 gram carbohydrate load given as flaxseed bread is 27% lower compared with regular white bread (5899). Flaxseed also seems to lower insulin levels in postmenopausal women (10978).

Flaxseed is also the most abundant indirect food source of lignans (5897,8026). Secoisolariciresinol diglycoside (SDG), a major lignan precursor, is found in high concentrations in flaxseed. SDG is converted by bacteria in the colon to the lignans enterolactone and enterodiol, which undergo enterohepatic circulation and then are excreted in the urine as glucuronide conjugates (5897,8022,8023,9592). The lignan precursor content of flaxseed can vary significantly depending on growing location and harvest year (5897). Serum concentrations and urinary excretion of lignans can increase in variable amounts when people consume large amounts of flaxseed and other lignan-containing foods (5894,6801,6803,8026). Lignans might have some beneficial effects. Lignans have weak estrogenic effects and possibly anti-estrogenic effects. There is preliminary evidence that flaxseed supplementation may decrease cellular proliferation in mammary glands (8022,8867,9593). Inhibition of mammary tumor growth by the lignans enterolactone and enterodiol has been reported in vitro (5895,8867). Preliminary evidence shows enterolactone and estradiol inhibit each other's proliferative effect on estrogen-dependent breast cancer cells. This competition might reduce endogenous estrogen binding to estrogen receptors, resulting in an anti-estrogen effect (8868,9593). Lignans have also been shown to stimulate sex hormone binding globulin production in the liver, and inhibit aromatase enzyme activity in preadipose cells. These effects may inhibit growth of hormone-dependent cancer cells such as breast cancer cells (6801,8024,9591,9592). In postmenopausal women, the urinary excretion of enterolactone and enterodiol seems to be lower in women with breast cancer than in women without breast cancer (8025,9592,9593). Supplementation with flaxseed also increases urinary excretion of certain estrogen metabolites, especially 2-hydroxyestrogen. This metabolite has been hypothesized to confer protective effects against breast cancer in premenopausal and postmenopausal women since it has little estrogenic activity and may even have antiestrogenic activity (5893,8020). There is preliminary evidence that flaxseed may also reduce insulin-like growth factor I (IGF-I) plasma level concentrations, a factor associated with increased breast cancer risk (8023).

Flaxseed and the constituent secoisolariciresinol diglycoside have also been reported to be protective against chemical-induced carcinogenesis in animal models (5897). Preliminary evidence shows secoisolariciresinol diglycoside seems to be effective against new tumor development and alpha-linolenic acid seems to be effective in reducing growth of established tumors (6805). Alpha-linolenic acid also seems to suppress the production of interleukin-1 (IL-1), tumor necrosis factor (TNF) and leukotriene B4, and production of oxygen free radicals by polymorphonuclear (PMN) leukocytes and monocytes (6806). Although both alpha-linolenic acid and lignans constituents have been reported to have antioxidant effects (6806), there is some evidence that partially defatted flaxseed might actually have pro-oxidant activity (6808). There is some evidence lignans may have platelet activating factor (PAF) receptor antagonist effects (6802,6806), stimulate production of sex-hormone binding globulin in the liver (6801), and inhibit angiogenesis (6803). Inhibition of colon tumor growth by the lignans enterolactone and enterodiol has also been reported in vitro (5895).

For systemic lupus erythematosus (SLE), flaxseed is thought to improve renal function by decreasing blood viscosity, reducing serum cholesterol, and reducing inflammatory response (6802).

Preliminary evidence suggests that flaxseed constituents such as alpha-linolenic acid and lignans might have a beneficial effect on bone, but thus far, clinical evidence does not support this (8504,10952).
Flaxseed also contains cyanogenic glycosides (linustatin, neolinustatin, and linamarin), which can increase blood levels and urinary excretion of thiocyanate in humans consuming raw flaxseed, and can cause toxicity in grazing animals (5899); however, these glycosides have not been detected after flaxseed is baked in muffins (5899).

Adverse Reactions

Orally, flaxseed can significantly increase the number of bowel movements and the risk for diarrhea (6803,8021). Doses greater than 45 grams per day may not be tolerated for this reason (6802). For every 10 grams of whole or cracked flaxseed, 150 mL or greater of liquid should be consumed to prevent intestinal blockage (12). Occasionally, allergic and anaphylactic reactions have been reported after ingestion of flaxseed and flaxseed oil. Individuals handling and processing flax products can develop a positive antigen test to flaxseed and may be more likely to be hypersensitive (6,6809).

Interactions with Herbs & Other Dietary Supplements

None known.

Interactions with Drugs

ANTICOAGULANT/ANTIPLATELET DRUGS: There is some evidence that flaxseed oil can decrease platelet aggregation and increase bleeding time (5898). Theoretically, using flaxseed oil in combination with anticoagulant or antiplatelet drugs might have additive effects and increase the risk of bleeding. Some of these drugs include aspirin, clopidogrel (Plavix), dalteparin (Fragmin), enoxaparin (Lovenox), heparin, ticlopidine (Ticlid), warfarin (Coumadin), and others.
ANTIDIABETES DRUGS: Flaxseed can lower blood glucose levels (5899,10978) and might have additive effects when used with antidiabetes drugs. This might increase the risk of hypoglycemia in some patients. Monitor blood glucose levels closely. Some antidiabetes drugs include glimepiride (Amaryl), glyburide (DiaBeta, Glynase PresTab, Micronase), insulin, metformin (Glucophage), pioglitazone (Actos), rosiglitazone (Avandia), and others.
ORAL DRUGS: The fiber in flaxseed can impair absorption of oral drugs (19).

Interactions with Foods

None known.

Interactions with Lab Tests

CHOLESTEROL: Flaxseed can lower total serum cholesterol and low-density lipoprotein cholesterol levels, and test results (5899,6800,6803).
GLUCOSE: Flaxseed might lower blood glucose concentrations (5899,10978).
TRIGLYCERIDES: Partially defatted flaxseed (flaxseed without as much alpha-linolenic acid content) can increase triglyceride levels, and test results (6808).

Interactions with Diseases or Conditions

BLEEDING DISORDERS: There is some evidence that flaxseed can decrease platelet aggregation and increase bleeding time (5898). Theoretically, flaxseed might increase the risk of severe bleeding in patients with bleeding disorders; use with caution.
DIABETES: Flaxseed can lower blood glucose levels and might have additive effects when used with antidiabetes drugs (5899,10978). This might increase the risk of hypoglycemia in some patients. Monitor blood glucose levels closely.
GASTROINTESTINAL OBSTRUCTION: People with bowel obstruction, esophageal stricture, and acute intestinal inflammation should avoid flaxseed. Flaxseed is a bulk forming laxative and might further contribute to obstruction (12).
HORMONE SENSITIVE CANCERS/CONDITIONS: Because flaxseed might have estrogenic effects (5893,8020), women with hormone sensitive conditions should avoid flaxseed. Some of these conditions include breast, uterine, and ovarian cancer; endometriosis; and uterine fibroids.
HYPERTRIGLYCERIDEMIA: Partially defatted flaxseed (flaxseed with less alpha linolenic acid content) might increase triglyceride levels (6808) and should be avoided in patients with hypertriglyceridemia.

Dosage and Administration

ORAL: For hypercholesterolemia, baked goods such as muffins containing flaxseed have been used to provide a daily dose of 50 grams of flaxseed per day (6803,6808). For improving renal function in patients with systemic lupus erythematosus (SLE) nephritis, 15 grams of ground flaxseed has been used twice daily with cereal, or tomato or orange juice (8021). For improving mild menopausal symptoms, 40 grams of crushed flaxseed daily has been used (10978).

FLAXSEED OIL

Also Known As
Atasi, Flax Oil, Flax Seed Oil, Graine De Lin, Linoleic Acid, Linseed Oil.
CAUTION: See separate listings for Alpha Linolenic Acid (ALA), Conjugated Linoleic Acid (CLA), Decosahexaenoic Acid (DHA), Eicosapentaenoic Acid (EPA), Evening Primrose Oil (EPO), Fish Oil, and Flaxseed.

Scientific Names
Linum usitatissimum, synonyms Linum crepitans, Linum humile.
Family: Linaceae.

People Use This For
Orally, flaxseed oil is used as a laxative for constipation, for arthritis, cancer, anxiety, benign prostatic hyperplasia (BPH), vaginitis, weight loss, hypertriglyceridemia, hypercholesterolemia, dry eyes, and to prevent heart attacks. Flaxseed oil is also used as a supplemental source of dietary alpha-linolenic acid.
Topically, flaxseed oil is used for its demulcent and emollient properties.
In foods, flaxseed oil is used as a cooking oil and in margarines.
In manufacturing, flaxseed oil is used as a component in paints, varnishes, linoleum, and soap; and as a waterproofing agent.

Safety
LIKELY SAFE ...when used orally in amounts found in foods.
POSSIBLY SAFE ...when used orally and appropriately for medicinal purposes, short-term. Flaxseed oil has been used safely in studies lasting up to 3 months (845,3912,5898).
There is insufficient reliable information available about the safety of topical use of flaxseed oil.
PREGNANCY: LIKELY SAFE ...when used orally in amounts found in foods. LIKELY UNSAFE ...when used orally in medicinal amounts. Flaxseed oil might affect menstruation (19); contraindicated.
LACTATION: LIKELY SAFE ...when used orally in amounts found in foods. There is insufficient reliable information available about the safety of flaxseed oil in breast-feeding women when used in medicinal amounts; avoid using.

Effectiveness
POSSIBLY INEFFECTIVE
Rheumatoid arthritis (RA). Taking flaxseed oil daily for 3 months does not seem to improve symptoms of pain and stiffness, and has no effect on laboratory measures of RA, such as C-reactive protein and erythrocyte sedimentation rate (ESR) (5898).
There is insufficient reliable information available about the effectiveness of flaxseed oil for its other uses.

Mechanism of Action
Flaxseed oil contains linolenic, linoleic, and oleic acids (6). It is among the best sources of alpha-linolenic acid (6). Linoleic acid and alpha-linolenic acid are required for the structural integrity of all cell membranes. Alpha-linolenic acid raises serum omega-3 polyunsaturated fatty acids, including eicosapentaenoic acid (EPA) and docosahexaenoic acid (DHA) (845,6803).
There is some evidence that flaxseed oil can lower triglyceride levels (3911). Flaxseed oil seems to have other potentially beneficial cardiovascular effects. There is also some preliminary evidence that a low fat diet plus the flaxseed oil can increase systemic arterial elasticity, which might improve circulatory function (5896).
Some researchers think flaxseed oil can also decrease platelet aggregation (845,6806), and increase the bleeding time (5898), but data are conflicting (3912). Higher serum levels of linoleic acid, an omega-6 fatty acid contained in flaxseed oil, seems to protect against ischemic stroke and lacunar infarction, possibly by lowering blood pressure and improving blood flow by reducing platelet aggregation and enhancing erythrocyte deformability (9562).
Flaxseed oil is used for rheumatoid arthritis because it might have anti-inflammatory effects. Alpha-linolenic acid contained in flaxseed oil is a precursor of eicosapentaenoic acid (EPA) and docosahexaenoic acid (DHA) which are converted to non- or anti-inflammatory prostaglandins and leukotrienes in the body. Supplementation with flaxseed oil or alpha-linolenic acid increases the ratio of EPA and DHA to the pro-inflammatory arachidonic acid (5898). Alpha-linolenic acid has also been reported to suppress the production of interleukin-1 (IL-1), tumor necrosis factor (TNF), leukotriene B4, and oxygen free radicals by polymorphonuclear (PMN) leukocytes and monocytes (6806).
There is some evidence that alpha-linolenic acid from flaxseed oil might have anti-tumor effects, possibly by increasing peroxidation of fatty acids in tumor cell membranes, or by altering the balance of prostaglandin production away from tumor promoting prostaglandins of the E2 series (6805). Flaxseed oil seems to reduce the volume of chemically-induced mammary tumors in animal models (6805).

Adverse Reactions
Orally, flaxseed oil is typically well-tolerated. However, doses of flaxseed oil of 30 grams per day and higher have been associated with loose stools and diarrhea (5898). Allergic and anaphylactic reactions have been reported with flaxseed oil ingestion and also in workers processing flaxseed products (6809).

Interactions with Herbs & Other Dietary Supplements
None known.

Interactions with Drugs
ANTICOAGULANT/ANTIPLATELET DRUGS: There is some evidence that flaxseed oil can decrease platelet aggregation and increase bleeding time (5898). Theoretically, using flaxseed oil in combination with anticoagulant or antiplatelet drugs might have additive effects and increase the risk of bleeding. Some of these drugs include aspirin, clopidogrel (Plavix), dalteparin (Fragmin), enoxaparin (Lovenox), heparin, ticlopidine (Ticlid), warfarin (Coumadin), and others.

Interactions with Foods
None known.

Interactions with Lab Tests
PROTHROMBIN TIME (PT): Flaxseed oil may affect platelet aggregation and prolong bleeding time and test results (5898).
TRIGLYCERIDES: Flaxseed oil might decrease serum triglyceride concentrations and test results in some patients with hyperlipoproteinemia (3911).

Interactions with Diseases or Conditions
BLEEDING DISORDERS: There is some evidence that flaxseed oil can decrease platelet aggregation and increase bleeding time (5898). Theoretically, flaxseed oil might increase the risk of severe bleeding in patients with bleeding disorders; use with caution.

Dosage and Administration
ORAL: A typical dose is 15-30 mL daily (3912).
TOPICAL: No typical dosage.

Comments
Specific deficiencies from inadequate intakes of essential fatty acids are rare except in individuals with severe, untreated fat malabsorption or those suffering from famine. Symptoms include dry, cracked, scaly and bleeding skin, excessive water loss from the skin, and impaired liver function resulting from the accumulation of lipid in the liver (i.e., fatty liver) (298).

FLUORIDE

Also Known As
Acidulated Phosphate Fluoride, Fluorophosphate, Hydrogen Fluoride, MFP, Monofluorophosphate, Sodium Fluoride, Sodium Monofluorophosphate, Stannous Fluoride.

Scientific Names
F; atomic number 9.

People Use This For
Orally, fluoride is used for treating osteoporosis and preventing dental caries. It is also used orally to prevent bone loss in people with rheumatoid arthritis and Crohn's disease.
Topically, fluoride is used for preventing dental caries.

Safety
LIKELY SAFE ...when used orally and appropriately. Fluoride is safe when used in doses below the tolerable upper intake level (UL) of 10 mg per day of elemental fluoride (7555). ...when used topically and appropriately. Fluoride is safe when used in quantities typically found in toothpastes, mouth rinses, and professionally applied fluoride dental treatments (8950).
POSSIBLY SAFE ...when used orally in higher doses of up to 20 mg per day of elemental fluoride. Monofluorophosphate containing 20 mg elemental fluoride taken daily has been used safely for up to 4 years (9124,9125). Sustained release sodium fluoride 11.3 mg containing elemental fluoride has been used safely for 42 weeks using a 12 months on, 3 months off cyclic regimen (9103).

POSSIBLY UNSAFE ...when used orally in high doses, long-term. Doses greater than 20 mg elemental fluoride for 9 months are associated with increased risk of fractures (8949). Long-term exposure to high doses above the daily upper intake level (UL) of 10 mg for greater than 10 years can cause skeletal fluorosis (7555).
CHILDREN: LIKELY SAFE ...when used orally and appropriately. Fluoride is safe when used in doses below the tolerable upper intake level (UL) of 10 mg per day of elemental fluoride for children age 8 years and older, 2.2 mg per day for children 4 to 8 years, 1.3 mg per day for children 1 to 3 years, 0.9 mg for infants 7 through 12 months, and 0.7 mg for infants 6 months and younger (7555). ...when used topically and appropriately. Fluoride is safe in quantities typically found in toothpastes, mouth rinses, and professionally applied fluoride dental treatments (8950,9100). POSSIBLY UNSAFE ...when used orally in high doses, long-term. Long-term exposure for greater than ten years to high doses above the daily upper intake level (UL) can cause skeletal fluorosis (7555).
PREGNANCY AND LACTATION: LIKELY SAFE ...when used orally and appropriately. Fluoride is safe when used in doses below the tolerable upper intake level (UL) of 10 mg per day of elemental fluoride (7555). ...when used topically and appropriately. Fluoride is safe in quantities typically found in toothpastes, mouth rinses, and professionally applied fluoride dental treatments (8950). POSSIBLY UNSAFE ...when used orally at high doses above the daily upper intake level (UL) of 10 mg for prolonged periods. Long-term exposure to high doses can cause skeletal fluorosis, but pregnancy or lactation doesn't seem to affect susceptibility to skeletal fluorosis (7555).

Effectiveness

EFFECTIVE

Dental caries. Fluoride added to drinking water and fluoride in toothpastes, mouthwashes, and other dental products can reduce dental caries (tooth decay) (7555,8950,9102,9128).

POSSIBLY EFFECTIVE

Osteoporosis. Elemental fluoride taken orally in daily doses, 11.3 mg to 20 mg, continuously or cyclicly might increase bone mineral density. Monofluorophosphate containing 20 mg elemental fluoride taken daily on a continuous basis for 96 weeks by postmenopausal women with osteopenia appears to increase spinal bone mineral density by 2.4%. In combination with hormone replacement therapy, monofluorophosphate may increase spinal bone mineral density by 11.8% (9125). In postmenopausal women with osteoporosis, monofluorophosphate containing 20 mg elemental fluoride taken daily for 4 years seems to increase spinal bone mineral density by 10% (9124). Monofluorophosphate containing 15 mg elemental fluoride taken daily on a cyclical basis (three months on, one month off) for 3 years by men with osteoporosis seems to spinal bone mineral density by 9% (8948). The effect on fractures is less clear. Sustained-release sodium fluoride 25 mg daily (equivalent to 11.3 mg elemental fluoride) given cyclicly for 12 months on followed by 2 months off for 42 months seems to reduce the risk for vertebral fracture by 32% in postmenopausal women with osteoporosis (9103). In postmenopausal women with osteoporosis, monofluorophosphate appears to reduce the risk of vertebral fracture from 10% in women taking only calcium to 2.4% in women taking fluoride plus calcium (9124).
In men with osteoporosis, fluoride treatment seems to reduce the risk of vertebral fracture by 30% and also to reduce back pain (8948). Other studies have found no effect on fractures (9132,9133). Studies have generally been small and have used various fluoride preparations including sodium fluoride, enteric-coated sodium fluoride, sustained-release sodium fluoride, and sodium monofluorophosphate (8948,8949,9103,9124,9125,9129,9132,9133). Some researchers suggest that staring fluoride early in the course of osteoarthritis and treating with 20 mg per day along with 800 to 1000 mg per day of calcium for at least 3 years is necessary for efficacy (9162). Long-term (20 years) exposure to fluorinated water seems to reduce the risk of hip fracture in older women by 31% and the risk of vertebral fracture by 27% (9102).

INSUFFICIENT RELIABLE EVIDENCE to RATE

Crohn's disease. Preliminary clinical evidence suggests fluoride might increase vertebral bone mass in Crohn's disease patients who have low bone mass (9134).
Rheumatoid arthritis (RA). Preliminary clinical evidence suggests fluoride might increase vertebral bone mass in RA patients who have low bone mass (9130).
More evidence is needed to rate fluoride for these uses.

Mechanism of Action

Fluoride is the ionic form of fluorine, a halogen and the most electronegative of the elements on the periodic table. Fluoride combines reversibly with hydrogen to form hydrogen fluoride. Diffusion of hydrogen fluoride accounts for much of its physiological behavior, including absorption from the stomach, distribution between extra- and intracellular-fluid compartments, and renal clearance (7555). Fluoride has a high affinity for calcium; more than 99% of calcium in the body is in calcified tissue.
Fluoride exerts a cariostatic (decay preventing) effect on the teeth by interfering with metabolism of bacteria in dental plaque and preserving tooth enamel. The fluoride concentration in plaque is dependent on exposure to fluoride concentrations in water, beverages, foods, and dental products, and the frequency of their use. Plaque is affected by topical exposure to fluoride and as well as fluoride secreted in saliva and gingival crevicular fluid after oral ingestion. Fluoride protects dental enamel by inhibiting bacterial enzymes that produce acid in plaque. It also reduces acid solubility of enamel, promotes remineralization of early enamel lesions, and prevents demineralization of plaque (7555).
Unlike most other drugs used for osteoporosis which prevent bone resorption, fluoride stimulates osteoblast activity.

Fluoride has been used on and off again for over 30 years as a treatment for osteoporosis. Although fluoride increases bone mineral density (BMD), there is a corresponding decrease in elasticity and strength of bone. Fluoride is also thought to alter the crystalline structure of bone (9129).

Preliminary evidence suggests that fluoride can inhibit the calcification of soft tissues, including the aorta. This suggests that adequate fluoridation of the water supply might reduce the risk of ischemic heart disease, but more research is needed (7555).

Most fluoride in the diet comes from fluorinated water, beverages, and dental products, but some foods and beverages such as marine fish and tea contain significant amounts of fluorine. Up to 80% of ingested fluoride is absorbed from gastrointestinal tract. Elimination is almost entirely via the kidneys with a variable degree of tubular resorption, depending on urinary pH (7555).

Adverse Reactions

Orally, fluoride can cause gastric pain and nausea, and lower extremity pain, particularly with long-term use (9129). Enteric-coated and sustained-release dosage forms of sodium phosphate and sodium monofluorophosphate may cause fewer adverse effects than plain sodium fluoride (9127,9129). Adverse effects appear to be dose related. Daily doses of 40 to 65 mg sodium fluoride can cause nausea, vomiting, GI bleeding, and stress fractures (15,9127). Fluoride at high doses for prolonged periods, over 10 mg per day for 10 or more years, can cause skeletal fluorosis. Skeletal fluorosis is characterized by joint stiffness and pain initially, followed by crippling due to calcification of ligaments, osteosclerosis, muscle wasting, and neurological defects due to hypercalcification of the vertebra. Crippling skeletal fluorosis is extremely rare in the US (7555).

Fluoride can cause enamel fluorosis, a condition in which the teeth of children who ingest excessive amounts of fluoride during development of permanent teeth may be discolored and pitted. This is a cosmetic adverse effect; tooth enamel may be stronger and more resistant to caries with enamel fluorosis (7555).

Fluoride can cause allergic reactions including urticaria, exfoliative dermatitis, atopic dermatitis, stomatitis, and gastrointestinal allergic reactions. Respiratory allergic reactions occur rarely (15).

Interactions with Herbs & Other Dietary Supplements

CALCIUM: Calcium can decrease the bioavailability of fluoride. Calcium can form insoluble compounds with fluoride and reduce absorption by 10 to 25% (7555).

Interactions with Drugs

None known.

Interactions with Foods

INFANT FORMULA: Infant formula rich in calcium and other divalent or trivalent ions can form insoluble compounds and reduce fluoride bioavailability by up to 25% (7555,9161).

MILK, CALCIUM-RICH FOODS: Foods rich in calcium can decrease the bioavailability of fluoride by up to 25% (7555,9161).

Interactions with Lab Tests

None known.

Interactions with Diseases or Conditions

None known.

Dosage and Administration

ORAL: In the US, municipal water is fluorinated to a concentration of 0.7 to 1.2 parts per million (ppm) (8950).

To prevent dental caries in areas where the fluoride ion level in drinking water is less than 0.3 ppm (such as in well water), children 6 months to 3 years should receive a fluoride supplement of 0.25 mg per day; children 3 to 6 years, 0.5 mg per day; and children 6 to 16 years, 1 mg per day. For children living in areas where the fluoride level is 0.3 to 0.6 ppm, children 3 to 6 years should receive 0.25 mg per day, and children 6 to 16 years, 0.5 mg per day. No supplement is needed in areas where the fluoride in drinking water exceeds 0.6 ppm (9101).

For treating osteoporosis, 15 to 20 mg per day of elemental fluoride has been used (8948,8949,9103,9125).

The daily Adequate Intakes (AI) for elemental fluoride from all sources including drinking water are: infants birth through 6 months, 0.01 mg; babies age 7 through 12 months, 0.5 mg; children 1 through 3 years, 0.7 mg; 4 through 8 years, 1 mg; 9 through 13 years, 2 mg; 14 through 18 years, 3 mg; men 19 years and older, 4 mg; women 14 years and older, including those pregnant or lactating, 3 mg.

The daily upper intake levels (UL) for fluoride are 0.7 mg for infants birth through 6 months; 0.9 mg for infants 7 through 12 months; 1.3 mg for children 1 through 3 years; 2.2 mg for children 4 through 8 years and 10 mg for children older than 8 years, adults, and pregnant and lactating women (7555).

Sodium fluoride contains 45% elemental fluoride. Monofluorophosphate contains 19% elemental fluoride (8948,8949).

Comments

Currently, the FDA requires this warning on all fluoride toothpastes: "If you accidentally swallow more than used for brushing, seek professional help or contact a poison control center." The warning is intended to reduce the risk of dental fluorosis, in which light spots form on developing permanent teeth. However, fluorosis develops with extended use, rather than following a single dose, causing some experts to question this warning (7555,9100). Toothpaste and fluoride rinses should not be routinely swallowed, particularly by children. Recommend limiting use of toothpaste to a pea-sized amount for children under six in case of accidental swallowing (9100).

FO-TI

Also Known As

Chinese Cornbind, Chinese Knotweed, Climbing Knotweed, Flowery Knotweed, Fo Ti, Fo-Ti-Tient, Foti, He Shou Wu, He-Shou-Wu, Heshouwu, Ho Shou Wu, Ho-Shou-Wu, Hoshouwu, Multiflora Preparata, Polygonum, Radix Polygoni Multiflori, Radix Polygoni Shen Min, Shen Min, Shou Wu, Shou-Wu, Shouwu, Shou-Wu-Pian, Zhihe Shou Wu, Zhihe-Shou-Wu, Zhiheshouwu, Zi Shou Wu, Zi-Shou-Wu, Zishouwu.

Scientific Names

Polygonum multiflorum.
Family: Polygonaceae.

People Use This For

Orally, fo-ti is used for treating lymph node tuberculosis, cancer, and constipation. It is also used orally as a liver and kidney tonic; as a blood and vital essence toner; and to fortify muscles, tendons, and bones. Fo-ti is also used orally for hyperlipidemia, insomnia, limb numbness, lower back and knee soreness or weakness, premature graying, and dizziness with tinnitus.
Topically, fo-ti is used for sores, carbuncles, skin eruptions, and itching.
In manufacturing, fo-ti extract is used as an ingredient in hair and skin care products.

Safety

POSSIBLY UNSAFE ...when used orally. Fo-ti may cause hepatitis in some patients (7626,7627).
There is insufficient reliable information available about the topical use of fo-ti.
PREGNANCY: POSSIBLY UNSAFE ...when used orally. Fo-ti contains anthraquinone constituents, which can exert a stimulant laxative effect. Bulk-forming or emollient laxatives are preferred in pregnancy (272). There is insufficient reliable information available about the topical use of fo-ti during pregnancy.
LACTATION: POSSIBLY UNSAFE ...when used orally. Anthraquinone constituents can cross into breast milk and might cause loose stools in some breast-fed infants (272). There is insufficient reliable information available about the topical use of fo-ti while nursing.

Effectiveness

There is insufficient reliable information available about the effectiveness of fo-ti.

Mechanism of Action

The applicable part of fo-ti is the rhizome. Fo-ti is either used raw (uncured) or processed (cured) by repeated steaming and sun drying. Raw fo-ti root contains the anthraquinone derivatives, chrysophanol and emodin, along with a small amount of rhein. These constituents have stimulant laxative effects, which probably accounts for fo-ti's use in constipation. Curing fo-ti reduces these constituents by 42-96% (5). Some evidence suggests that isolated stilbene glycoside constituents in the raw fo-ti root might have liver protectant effects, including inhibition of alanine aminotransferase (ALT, formerly SGOT) and aspartate aminotransferase (AST) (11). However, the anthraquinones in fo-ti are converted to highly reactive anthrones in the gastrointestinal tract, which may cause hepatitis (7626,7627).
Fo-ti reportedly has hypoglycemic effects (5,19). Cured fo-ti shows evidence it might increase the levels of superoxide dismutase (SOD), serotonin, norepinephrine, dopamine, and decrease levels of monoamine oxidase-B (MAO-B), lipid peroxide, and malonyl dialdehyde (MDA) (11); these are believed to be markers for anti-aging effects. Some evidence suggests fo-ti might also increase serum ceruloplasmin levels, reduce thymus gland atrophy, and inhibit atrophy of adrenal glands; enhancing nonspecific and cellular immunity, and antagonizing the immunosuppressive effects of prednisolone or hydrocortisone (11). Other evidence suggests the alcoholic extract might increase high-density lipoprotein (HDL) cholesterol, reduce total cholesterol, free cholesterol, triglycerides, and retard atherosclerosis (11). The aqueous extract appears to inhibit the replication of hepatitis B (11). Some evidence suggests fo-ti has approximately 0.3% of the estrogen activity of 17-beta-estradiol itself and is approximately equivalent to the estrogen activity found in soy and red clover (10143).

Adverse Reactions

Orally, fo-ti, particularly the raw root, may cause catharsis, diarrhea, abdominal pain, nausea, and vomiting (12). There is some concern that fo-ti can cause hepatitis in some patients. There have been 2 cases of hepatitis occurring 2 weeks after starting fo-ti in the usual recommended doses. It was characterized by symptoms including jaundice, dark urine, malaise, and increased liver function tests (LFT). The symptoms and increased LFTs resolved within a month after discontinuing fo-ti (7626,7627).

Interactions with Herbs & Other Dietary Supplements

None known.

Interactions with Drugs

ANTIDIABETES DRUGS: Theoretically, concomitant use of fo-ti with antidiabetic agents might increase the risk of hypoglycemia. Fo-ti reportedly has hypoglycemic effects (5,19). Dosing adjustments for insulin or oral hypoglycemic agents may be necessary. Oral hypoglycemic drugs include glimepiride (Amaryl), glipizide (Glucotrol), glyburide (Diabeta, Micronase), tolazamide (Tolinase), tolbutamide (Orinase), and others. Monitor blood glucose levels closely.

CYTOCHROME P450 1A2 (CYP1A2) SUBSTRATES: There's preliminary evidence that fo-ti might inhibit cytochrome P450 1A2 (CYP1A2) (12479). So far, this interaction has not been reported in humans. However, watch for an increase in the levels of drugs metabolized by CYP1A2 in patients taking fo-ti. Some drugs metabolized by CYP1A2 include amitriptyline (Elavil), haloperidol (Haldol), ondansetron (Zofran), propranolol (Inderal), theophylline (Theo-Dur, others), verapamil (Calan, Isoptin, others), and others. Use fo-ti cautiously or avoid in patients taking these drugs.

CYTOCHROME P450 2C19 (CYP2C19) SUBSTRATES: There's preliminary evidence that fo-ti might inhibit cytochrome P450 2C19 (CYP2C19) (12479). So far, this interaction has not been reported in humans. However, watch for an increase in the levels of drugs metabolized by CYP2C19 in patients taking fo-ti. Some drugs metabolized by CYP2C19 include proton pump inhibitors including omeprazole (Prilosec), lansoprazole (Prevacid), and pantoprazole (Protonix); diazepam (Valium); carisoprodol (Soma); nelfinavir (Viracept); and others.

CYTOCHROME P450 2C9 (CYP2C9) SUBSTRATES: There's preliminary evidence that fo-ti might inhibit cytochrome P450 2C9 (CYP2C9) (12479). So far, this interaction has not been reported in humans. However, watch for an increase in the levels of drugs metabolized by CYP2C9 in patients taking fo-ti. Some drugs metabolized by CYP2C9 include nonsteroidal anti-inflammatory drugs (NSAIDs) such as diclofenac (Cataflam, Voltaren), ibuprofen (Motrin), meloxicam (Mobic), and piroxicam (Feldene); celecoxib (Celebrex); amitriptyline (Elavil); warfarin (Coumadin); glipizide (Glucotrol); losartan (Cozaar); and others. Use fo-ti cautiously or avoid in patients taking these drugs.

CYTOCHROME P450 3A4 (CYP3A4) SUBSTRATES: There's preliminary evidence that fo-ti might inhibit cytochrome P450 3A4 (CYP3A4) enzyme (12479). So far, this interaction has not been reported in humans. However, watch for an increase in the levels of drugs metabolized by CYP3A4 in patients taking fo-ti. Some drugs metabolized by CYP3A4 include lovastatin (Mevacor), ketoconazole (Nizoral), itraconazole (Sporanox), fexofenadine (Allegra), triazolam (Halcion), and numerous others. Use fo-ti cautiously or avoid in patients taking these drugs.

DIGOXIN (Lanoxin): Theoretically, overuse of anthraquinone laxatives (e.g., fo-ti) might increase the risk of hypokalemia and digoxin cardiotoxicity (151,272).

DIURETIC DRUGS: Overuse of fo-ti might compound diuretic-induced potassium loss (151,272). There is some concern that people taking fo-ti along with potassium depleting diuretics might have an increased risk for hypokalemia. Initiation of potassium supplementation or an increase in potassium supplement dose may be necessary for some patients. Some diuretics that can deplete potassium include chlorothiazide (Diuril), chlorthalidone (Thalitone), furosemide (Lasix), hydrochlorothiazide (HCTZ, Hydrodiuril, Microzide), and others.

STIMULANT LAXATIVES: Theoretically, concomitant use of fo-ti with other laxatives can increase the risk of fluid and electrolyte depletion (151,272).

Interactions with Foods

None known.

Interactions with Lab Tests

CHOLESTEROL: Theoretically, cured fo-ti might reduce serum total cholesterol concentrations and test results (11).

COLORIMETRIC TESTS: Fo-ti might discolor urine (pink, red, purple, orange, rust), interfering with diagnostic tests that depend on a color change, due to its anthraquinone content (11,275).

GLUCOSE: Theoretically, fo-ti might decrease blood glucose concentrations and test results (5,6,19).

POTASSIUM: Excessive use of fo-ti might cause hypokalemia, reducing serum potassium concentrations and test results due to its anthraquinone content (11).

TRIGLYCERIDES: Theoretically, cured fo-ti might reduce serum triglyceride concentrations and test results (11).

Interactions with Diseases or Conditions

GASTROINTESTINAL DISEASE: Fo-ti exerts a stimulant effect on the intestinal tract (5). Avoid its use in diarrhea, intestinal obstruction, acute intestinal inflammation (Crohn's disease, ulcerative colitis, appendicitis), ulcer, abdominal pain of unknown origin, nausea, and vomiting.
HEART CONDITIONS: Theoretically, the laxative effect of fo-ti might cause hypokalemia with overuse/misuse, potentially decreasing cardiac function (15).
LIVER DISEASE: Fo-ti should be avoided in patients with a history of liver disease, because it has been associated with hepatitis in isolated cases (7626,7627).

Dosage and Administration

No typical dosage.

Comments

Avoid confusion with the commercial product Fo-ti-Teng which contains no fo-ti (6).

FOLIC ACID

Also Known As

B Complex Vitamin, Folacin, Folate, Vitamin B9.

Scientific Names

Pteroylglutamic acid; Pteroylmonoglutamic acid; Pteroylpolyglutamate.

People Use This For

Orally, folic acid is used for preventing and treating folate deficiency, megaloblastic anemia resulting from folate or vitamin B12 deficiency, megaloblastic anemia in sickle cell disease, and for folate deficiency in intestinal malabsorption or sprue. It is also used for preventing neural tube defects, reducing the risk of colorectal cancer, and preventing pregnancy loss. Folic acid is also used for hyperhomocysteinemia, coronary artery disease, fragile-X syndrome, gingival hyperplasia, memory deficit, Alzheimer's disease, vitiligo, osteoporosis, restless leg syndrome, insomnia, depression, peripheral neuropathy, myelopathy, and AIDS. It is also used for reducing lometrexol and methotrexate toxicity; and for preventing signs of aging, heart attack, and stroke. Folic acid is also used for other conditions commonly associated with folate deficiency, including ulcerative colitis; liver disease; alcoholism; renal dialysis; and drug-induced deficiency related to phenytoin, primidone, barbiturates, oral contraceptives, and nitrofurantoin.
Topically, folic acid is used for treating gingival hyperplasia and gingivitis.
Parenterally, folic acid is used intramuscularly, subcutaneously, or intravenously for treating folate deficiency, particularly in patients with malabsorption or those who cannot take oral treatment. Folic acid has also been used parenterally to treat chronic fatigue syndrome.

Safety

LIKELY SAFE ...when used orally or parenterally and appropriately. Folic acid is safe when used in doses less than 1000 mcg per day (6241). In cases of megaloblastic anemia resulting from folate deficiency or malabsorption disorders such as sprue, oral doses of 1-5 mg per day can also be used safely until hematologic recovery is documented if vitamin B12 levels are routinely measured (6241,7725,8739).
POSSIBLY UNSAFE ...when used orally in large doses. Doses above 1000 mcg per day should be avoided if possible to prevent precipitation or exacerbation of neuropathy related to vitamin B12 deficiency (6241,6242,6245). However, there is some evidence that doses of 5 mg per day orally for up to 4 months can be used safely if vitamin B12 levels are routinely measured (7725). Very high doses of 15 mg per day can cause significant central nervous system (CNS) and gastrointestinal side effects (505).
PREGNANCY AND LACTATION: LIKELY SAFE ...when used orally and appropriately. Folic acid 300-400 mcg is commonly used during pregnancy for prevention of neural tube defects (8739).

Effectiveness

EFFECTIVE

Folate deficiency. Administering folic acid orally or parenterally improves folate deficiency (505,8739).

LIKELY EFFECTIVE

End-stage renal disease (ESRD). Taking folic acid orally reduces homocysteine levels in people with ESRD, including those on hemodialysis. Over 85% of people with ESRD have hyperhomocysteinemia. Treatment of hyperhomocysteinemia in people with ESRD is often more difficult than in people with normal renal function (1489,3324,7289,9409,9413,9414,9416). The reasons for this aren't fully understood; renal uptake and metabolism of homocysteine may be reduced in severe renal failure, and hemodialysis may contribute to vitamin deficiencies (6884,9414,9417). Doses of 0.8 to 15 mg folic acid/day are generally used, but the degree of homocysteine reduction is very variable (between 12-50%), and normal homocysteine levels (<12 micromoles/L) cannot always be achieved (1489,6884,7289,7881,9322,9413,9414,9415,9416). Folic acid 2.5 to 5 mg three times weekly also reduces homocysteine levels in ESRD patients on dialysis (9417). Doses greater than 15 mg per day don't provide additional benefit. Doses of 30 to 60 mg seem to cause a rebound in homocysteine levels when treatment is stopped (9219). Folic acid supplementation also doesn't appear to improve endothelial function, suggesting folic acid does not prevent or treat vascular disease in patients with ESRD (9322). In most studies vitamin B12 (0.4 to 1 mg/day) and pyridoxine (20 to 50 mg/day) were taken with the folic acid (3324,6884,7881,9414,9415,9416). As in people with normal renal function, vitamin B12 probably has an additional homocysteine-lowering effect over folic acid alone, especially in people with low vitamin B12 levels (7289), and pyridoxine helps reduce post-methionine load homocysteine levels (1489).

Hyperhomocysteinemia. Taking folic acid orally 0.4 to 5 mg/day lowers fasting homocysteine levels by about 20% to 30% in people with normal renal function (3047,6366,9307,9400,9401,9405,9408,9409,9410,10350,11337,11338). However, 0.8-1 mg/day seems to provide maximal reduction of homocysteine levels (9307,9408). Doses greater than 1 mg/day do not seem to produce any greater benefit (2147,9307,9410), except in some people with certain gene mutations that cause homocysteine levels of 20 micromoles/L or higher (9408). In people with asymptomatic atherosclerosis, lowering homocysteine levels with folic acid reduces progression of the atherosclerosis and improves arterial blood flow (412,3886,3887,6236,7725). In patients with high coronary risk or atherosclerotic disease, there is preliminary evidence that 10 mg per day of folic acid for 2 months improves coagulation status, oxidative stress, and endothelial dysfunction (9319). The effects of folic acid increase with increasing pretreatment of homocysteine levels, and decreasing pretreatment of folate levels (2149,9400,9405,9409). Taking folic acid orally also seems to reduce increased homocysteine concentrations associated with nitrous oxide general anesthesia. A supplement containing 25 mg pyridoxine, with 2.5 mg of folic acid and 500 mcg of vitamin B12, taken daily was used (9481). Additional evidence suggests that the higher the initial homocysteine levels, the lower the folic acid dose needed to attain maximum reduction of homocysteine levels (9307). However, some reduction in the fasting homocysteine levels is seen when dietary folate and supplemental folic acid (including multivitamins) are increased in people who are not folate deficient and have normal homocysteine levels (<12 micromoles/L) (412,2146,2147,9302,9303,9304,9305,9306,9401). Increasing folic acid intake by supplements or folate-fortified cereal products is more effective for reducing homocysteine levels than increasing intake of folate-rich foods (6367). However, initial data suggest that the US Government-mandated fortification of cereals and flour with 140 mcg folic acid per 100 grams is reducing the mean homocysteine level in the general population by about 7% (7881,9404,9407). Consumption of at least 300 mcg per day of dietary folate seems to be associated with a 20% lower risk of stroke and a 13% lower risk of cardiovascular disease when compared with consumption of less than 136 mcg of folate per day (9318). Taking folic acid orally, in combination with pyridoxine, seems to reduce post-prandial hyperhomocysteinemia (indicated by elevated homocysteine levels after consuming a methionine load). Folic acid 0.5 to 5 mg/day alone reduces homocysteine levels by 27% to 30%, but addition of pyridoxine (50 to 250 mg/day) produces greater reductions and is generally recommended (1489,9406,9408). Adding vitamin B12 (mean dose, 0.5 mg/day) to folic acid therapy produces an additional decrease in homocysteine levels of about 7% on average (9400,9405,9409), but probably only in people with vitamin B12 deficiency (2147,3047). Some people recommend routine use of vitamin B12 in homocysteine-lowering regimens, to avoid the risk of neuropathy in people with undetected vitamin B12 deficiency (9405). Adding pyridoxine (vitamin B6) to the regimen doesn't produce any additional lowering of fasting homocysteine levels (2148,3047,9405). Elevated homocysteine levels are an independent risk factor for vascular disease. But elevated homocysteine levels may be a marker instead of a cause of vascular disease (11387,11388). Although folic acid lowers homocysteine levels, it's not yet known whether this reduces the risk of vascular disease (cardiac, peripheral, or cerebral). Preliminary data suggest it might. Large-scale clinical trials are currently underway to determine whether homocysteine-lowering therapy is of any benefit (9306,9308). However, folic acid supplementation alone or in combination with pyridoxine and vitamin B12 doesn't seem to help with secondary prevention of death or cardiovascular events such as stroke or myocardial infarction in people with existing coronary artery disease or prior stroke (11337,11387). There is also conflicting evidence that suggests supplemental folic acid might improve endothelial function, prevent nitric oxide synthase dysfunction induced by continuous nitroglycerin, and nitrate tolerance in patients with hyperhomocysteinemia (9313,9314,9315,9316). Large randomized controlled trials are needed to confirm or refute these findings. Until definitive data are available, the current recommendation is screening of 40 year old men and 50 year old women for hyperhomocysteinemia. For patients with homocysteine levels greater than 11 micromoles/L, supplement with folic acid and vitamin B12 (9308).

Methotrexate toxicity. Taking folic acid orally seems to reduce methotrexate toxicity symptoms such as nausea and vomiting in the treatment of rheumatoid arthritis (RA) and psoriasis (768,2162,2163,2164,4492,4493,4494,9369,9419).

Neural tube birth defects. Consuming a high dietary intake of folate and taking folic acid supplements orally reduces the risk of neural tube birth defects (3325,9309). High dietary intake of vegetables during pregnancy improves plasma and red blood cell folate concentrations and reduces the risk of folate deficiency (9309).

POSSIBLY EFFECTIVE

Breast cancer. Consuming dietary folate seems to decrease the risk of breast cancer, especially in women who also consume high amounts of dietary methionine, vitamin B12, or pyridoxine (vitamin B6) (9328).

Colorectal cancer. Taking folic acid orally from dietary and supplemental sources seems to reduce the risk of colon cancer (505,2140,2141,2142,2143,2144,2145,2250,9325,9326). Dietary intake of folate greater than 249 mcg per day in men and 400 mcg per day in women is associated with a reduced risk of colon cancer, especially in women with a family history of the disease (9325,9326). There is also evidence daily use of folic acid-containing multivitamins for greater than 5 years can decrease the risk of colon cancer by almost 50% in women with a family history of colon cancer (9326).

Depression. Taking folic acid orally with conventional antidepressants might improve treatment response (3657,10884,10887). However, limited clinical research suggests that folic acid is not effective as a replacement for conventional antidepressant therapy (10886).

Pancreatic cancer. Consuming greater than 280 mcg per day of dietary folate is associated with a decreased risk of exocrine pancreatic cancer (9327).

Phenytoin-induced gingival hyperplasia. Applying folic acid topically seems to inhibit gingival hyperplasia secondary to phenytoin therapy (2151). However, taking folic acid orally doesn't seem to improve gingival hyperplasia secondary to phenytoin therapy (2150,2151,2152).

Pregnancy-related gingivitis. Applying folic acid topically seems to improve gingivitis in pregnancy (2152).

Vitiligo. Taking folic acid orally seems to improve symptoms of vitiligo (2153,2154).

POSSIBLY INEFFECTIVE

Chronic fatigue syndrome (CFS). Daily injections of a combination of folic acid, bovine liver extract, and vitamin B12 for three weeks appear to have no effect on CFS symptoms (7561).

Coronary artery disease. Taking folic acid orally doesn't seem to be useful for secondary prevention in people with existing coronary artery disease. Supplementation with 0.5 mg folic acid daily, in addition to statin therapy, doesn't seem to affect risk for death or cardiovascular events such as stroke or myocardial infarction in people with existing CAD (11337).

Lometrexol toxicity. Taking folic acid orally doesn't seem to reduce lometrexol toxicity (2161).

Stroke. Taking folic acid orally doesn't seem to be useful for preventing stroke recurrence. In people with a history of stroke, neither high dose folic acid combinations containing 25 mg of pyridoxine, 0.4 mg of vitamin B12, and 2.5 mg of folic acid nor low dose combinations containing 200 mcg of pyridoxine, 6 mcg of vitamin B12, and 20 mcg of folic acid seem to affect risk of recurring stroke (11387).

LIKELY INEFFECTIVE

Fragile-X syndrome. Taking folic acid orally doesn't improve symptoms of fragile-X syndrome (2155,2156,2157,2158,2159,2160).

INSUFFICIENT RELIABLE EVIDENCE to RATE

Angioplasty. There are conflicting findings about the benefits of taking folic acid plus vitamin B6 and vitamin B12 following angioplasty. Some evidence suggests that folic acid 1 mg plus vitamin B12 400 mcg and pyridoxine 10 mg daily can decrease the rate of restenosis in patients treated with balloon angioplasty (8009,9412). But this combination does not seem to be as effective for reducing restenosis in patients after coronary stenting (8009). An intravenous loading dose of folic acid, vitamin B6 and vitamin B12 followed by oral administration of folic acid 1.2 mg plus vitamin B6 48 mg and vitamin B12 60 mcg taken daily after coronary stenting also does not seem to reduce restenosis and might actually increase restenosis (12150,12151). Due to the lack of evidence of benefit and potential for harm, this combination of vitamins should not be recommended for patients receiving coronary stents (12151).

Fenofibrate (Tricor)-associated hyperhomocysteinemia. There is some evidence 10 mg of folic acid taken every other day might reduce elevated plasma homocysteine levels (up to 59%) associated with fenofibrate (Tricor) administration (9321).

Infertility. Some research suggests that daily consumption of folic acid 5 mg plus zinc sulfate 66 mg can increase sperm count in subfertile men. Further study is required to determine the effect of this combination on infertility (9334).

Lung cancer. There does not appear to be a relationship between deficiency of folic acid and lung cancer (9454).

Restless leg syndrome. There are reports of folic acid reducing symptoms associated with restless leg syndrome such as numbness, cramps, and paresthesias. Whether restless leg syndrome is due to acquired or familial folate deficiency is unknown and requires further study (9332).

Sickle cell disease. Daily intake of 700 mcg of folic acid in combination with 4.2-6 mcg of vitamin B12 and 4.2-6.0 mg of pyridoxine (vitamin B6) might lower homocysteine levels, but it is unknown if this effect will reduce the risk of endothelial damage in patients with sickle cell disease (9324).

Ulcerative colitis-associated cancer. Preliminary clinical evidence suggests folate supplementation might protect against cancer in people with ulcerative colitis (6271).

More evidence is needed to rate folic acid for these uses.

Mechanism of Action

Folate is the general term that refers to a variety of chemical forms folic acid. Folic acid, or pteroylmonoglutamic acid, is the form used in vitamin supplements and fortified foods. Folate in food is pteroylpolyglutamate, which has a polyglutamate side chain with peptide linkages (6241). Folic acid is distributed in a wide variety of foods, but it is most abundant in green leafy vegetables (9518).

Folate in food is about 40-50% less bioavailable than synthetic folic acid, which is almost 100% bioavailable. Before folate from food can be absorbed, the polyglutamate side chain must undergo enzymatic deconjugation in the small intestine to form the absorbable monoglutamate form (6241,9300). Folate deconjugation occurs maximally at a pH of 6-7 (6241,9300). After folic acid is absorbed, it is reduced to tetrahydrofolate and then enters a methylation cycle (9317).

In humans, tetrahydrofolate-based coenzymes play a major role in intracellular metabolism. Tetrahydrofolate plays an indirect role in the rate-limiting step of DNA synthesis. Abnormalities in this process that occur with folic acid deficiency can cause megaloblastic anemia. Folic acid reduces damage to DNA and prevents replication errors (2139,2144). Folic acid deficiency disturbs cell cycling, induces cell apoptosis, and increases the rate of cell death (9329). In the bone marrow, abnormal cellular maturation and division caused by folic acid deficiency leads to the development of abnormal red blood cell precursors, which are known as megaloblasts. Megaloblasts are unable to mature into red blood cells properly and many of them are phagocytosed by macrophages in the bone marrow, which contributes to the development of megaloblastic anemia (9518).

Folic acid is also involved in the metabolism of homocysteine. Low folate levels are associated with increased plasma homocysteine levels. Hyperhomocysteinemia is a risk factor for coronary, cerebral, and peripheral atherosclerosis; recurrent thromboembolism; deep vein thrombosis; myocardial infarction; and ischemic stroke (1899,2147,3047,3323,9402,9405,9408,9409). Low serum folate levels (less than 9.9 nmol/L) and low dietary folate intake (less than 211 mcg per day) are also associated with an increased risk for acute coronary events and cardiovascular disease mortality (9311,9312). A 5 micromole increase in plasma homocysteine increases the risk of cerebrovascular disease by 50%, and the risk of coronary heart disease by 60% in men and 80% women (9407,9411). The best predictor of response to folic acid therapy is the baseline homocysteine plasma concentration. The higher the homocysteine level, the better the response is to folic acid therapy. Folic acid has little effect on normal homocysteine levels. Genetic variations in the enzyme 5,10-methylenetetrahydrofolate reductase can influence the effectiveness of folate in reducing homocysteine levels (9219). The mechanisms of the adverse effects of homocysteine isn't fully understood, but might include vascular endothelial cell damage, impaired endothelium dependent vasodilation due to reduced nitric oxide activity, arterial stiffening due to increased oxidation and arterial deposition of low-density lipoproteins (LDL), increased platelet adhesiveness, and activation of the clotting cascade (2147,3047,9310,9403,9408).

Homocysteine is metabolized via two pathways; remethylation or trans-sulfuration. Remethylation of homocysteine to methionine requires folate and vitamin B12 as cofactors (3047,9310,9320,9407,9409). The methyl donor is 5-methyltetrahydrofolate, and the enzymes involved are 5,10-methyltetrahydrofolate reductase (MTHFR), and 5-methyltetrahydrofolate-homocysteine-methyltransferase, which is vitamin B12-dependent (2148,9310). Impairment of this pathway leads to increased fasting homocysteine levels, and can occur in people with folate deficiency, vitamin B12 deficiency, or who are homozygous for the mutations of the gene for MTHFR (TT genotype) (1489,9301,9315,9409). Mutation of the MTHFR gene produces a variant of the enzyme that is thermolabile, less active, and it impairs the formation of 5-methyltetrahydrofolate (9301,9320). Folic acid supplements increase the activity of this pathway, which lowers homocysteine levels (412,2146,2147,2148,2149,3886,9301). Trans-sulfuration of homocysteine results in degradation to cystathionine and then to cysteine by the pyridoxine (vitamin B6) dependent enzymes cystathionine-beta-synthase and cystathionine-gamma-synthase (2148,3047,9310,9407,9409). This pathway is primarily active after ingesting a methionine load (animal protein). Deficiencies of pyridoxine or cystathionine-beta-synthase impair this pathway, raising post-methionine load homocysteine levels (1489,2148,9408). Elevation of these levels is a risk factor for cardiovascular disease, independent of elevated fasting homocysteine levels (1489).

Folic acid might also improve endothelial dysfunction and the coagulation and oxidative status in individuals with high coronary risk and atherosclerotic disease. There is preliminary evidence folic acid can decrease concentrations of von Willebrand factor, which is associated with endothelial dysfunction. Folic acid might also decrease fibrinogen concentrations, while increasing plasminogen, antithrombin III, glutathione peroxidase, red cell glutathione, and red cell superoxide dismutase concentrations (9319).

Folic acid might also prevent nitroglycerin-induced nitrate tolerance and cross tolerance to endothelial nitric oxide. Nitrate tolerance is associated with an increased vascular production of superoxide anions by NADPH oxidase and endothelial nitric oxide synthase. Folic acid is thought to deplete NADPH and decrease the activity of these enzymes (9317).

Folic acid also plays an important role in pregnancy. Low folate levels are associated with recurrent spontaneous pregnancy loss (6237). Folic acid supplementation also prevents neural tube defects in the fetus, but the exact role of folic acid in this process is not completely understood.

Folic acid might play a role in Alzheimer's disease. Preliminary evidence indicates that low folate concentrations might be related to atrophy of the cerebral cortex, particularly in people with neocortical lesions related to Alzheimer's disease (6234). Homocysteine is thought to be neurotoxic, causing DNA damage and cell apoptosis (9331). Low serum folate levels are strongly correlated with cerebral atrophy on autopsy (6234). Functional and mental deterioration is also sometimes associated with low folate levels and low intake of folate in elderly people (6238,9330).

Folic acid deficiency is common among people with depression (10879,10880,10881). Low folate levels have been linked to poor response to antidepressant treatment (6239,10880). In the general population, people with low folate status or lower dietary folate intake have a higher risk for depression (10882,10883). The exact role of folic acid in depression is unknown. It is required for the remethylation of homocysteine to methionine and for s-adenosylmethionine (SAMe) conversion (5232). Folate is also required for the methylation of tetrahydrobiopterin, an essential cofactor for the hydroxylase enzymes involved in the production of neurotransmitters such as serotonin (10884,10885).

Some patients with chronic fatigue syndrome (CFS) also have decreased folic acid levels (6082,6083), so some people

try folic acid supplements for chronic fatigue.
Crohn's disease has also been associated with decreased folate levels (6269). Folic acid is thought to prevent carcinogenesis. Folate and methionine are important factors in the methylation of DNA. There is evidence that folate deficiency might cause massive misincorporation of uracil into DNA and increased chromosomal breaks (9325,9236,9327,9328). Low red blood cell folate levels have been associated with the development of dysplasia and cancer in ulcerative colitis (6270).

Adverse Reactions

Orally, folic acid is well tolerated in amounts found in fortified foods and supplements in doses less than 1000 mcg per day (6243). Doses of 5 mg per day can cause abdominal cramps, diarrhea, and rash (7225). Folic acid 15 mg per day can sometimes cause altered sleep patterns, vivid dreaming, irritability, excitability, overactivity, confusion, impaired judgment, exacerbation of seizure frequency and psychotic behavior, nausea, abdominal distention, flatulence, bitter taste in the mouth, allergic skin reactions, and zinc depletion (15). Large doses of folic acid can also precipitate or exacerbate neuropathy in people deficient in vitamin B12 (6243).
Allergic reactions only rarely occur. Symptoms can include rash, erythema, itching, malaise, and bronchospasm. An anaphylactic reaction has been reported in one patient receiving intravenous folic acid. Use of folic acid for undiagnosed anemia has masked the symptoms of pernicious anemia, resulting in lack of treatment and eventual neurological damage (15). Patients should be warned not to self-treat suspected anemia.
There is some concern that consuming high amounts of folic acid from the diet and/or supplements might worsen cognitive decline in older people. A large-scale study suggests that people over 65 years of age who consume large amounts of folic acid (median of 742 mcg/day) have cognitive decline at a rate twice as fast as those consuming smaller amounts (median of 186 mcg/day). It's not known if this is directly attributable to folic acid. It is theorized that it could be due to folic acid masking a vitamin B12 deficiency. Vitamin B12 deficiency is associated with cognitive decline (13068). More evidence is needed to determine the significance of this finding. For now, suggest that most patients aim for the recommended folic acid intake of 400 mcg/day.
Some preliminary research has raised concerns that women who take folic acid 5 mg/day during and immediately after pregnancy might have an increase risk of all-cause mortality and mortality related to breast cancer (12227). However, these findings were not statistically significant and were likely due to chance (12228). Contrary evidence actually suggests folic acid is protective against breast cancer (9328). Women should continue to be encouraged to take folic acid during pregnancy to prevent neural tube defects.

Interactions with Herbs & Other Dietary Supplements

None known.

Interactions with Drugs

FOSPHENYTOIN (Cerebyx): Folic acid may be a cofactor in phenytoin metabolism (4471). Folic acid, in doses of 1 mg per day or more, can reduce serum levels of phenytoin in some patients (4471,4477,4531,4536). Increases in seizure frequency have been reported. If folic acid supplements are added to established phenytoin therapy, monitor serum phenytoin levels closely. If phenytoin and folic acid are started at the same time and continued together, adverse changes in phenytoin pharmacokinetics are avoided (4471,4472,4473,4531). Note that phenytoin also reduces serum folate levels.
METHOTREXATE (MTX, Rheumatrex): Methotrexate exerts its cytotoxic effects by preventing conversion of folic acid to the active form needed by cells. There is some evidence that folic acid supplements reduce the efficacy of methotrexate in the treatment of acute lymphoblastic leukemia, and theoretically they could reduce its efficacy in the treatment of other cancers (9420). Advise cancer patients to consult their oncologist before using folic acid supplements. In patients treated with long-term, low-dose methotrexate for rheumatoid arthritis (RA) or psoriasis, folic acid supplements can reduce the incidence of side effects, without reducing efficacy (768,2162,4492,4493,4494,4546,9369). Note that methotrexate can reduce serum folate levels.
PHENOBARBITAL (Luminal): Folic acid can have direct convulsant activity in some people, reversing the effects of phenobarbital and worsening seizure control (4427,9357,9358). Monitor closely for increased seizure activity. Note that phenobarbital also reduces serum folate levels.
PHENYTOIN (Dilantin): Folic acid may be a cofactor in phenytoin metabolism (4471). Folic acid, in doses of 1 mg per day or more, can reduce serum levels of phenytoin in some patients (4471,4477,4531,4536). Increases in seizure frequency have been reported. If folic acid supplements are added to established phenytoin therapy, monitor serum phenytoin levels closely. If phenytoin and folic acid are started at the same time and continued together, adverse changes in phenytoin pharmacokinetics are avoided (4471,4472,4473,4531). Note that phenytoin also reduces serum folate levels.
PRIMIDONE (Mysoline): Folic acid can have direct convulsant activity in some people, reversing the effects of primidone and worsening seizure control (4427,9357,9358). Monitor closely for increased seizure activity. Note that primidone also reduces serum folate levels.
PYRIMETHAMINE (Daraprim): Folic acid can antagonize the antiparasitic effects of pyrimethamine against Toxoplasmosis and Pneumocystis carinii pneumonia. Folic acid doesn't antagonize the effects of pyrimethamine in the treatment of malaria, because malarial parasites cannot use exogenous folic acid. Use folinic acid as an alternative to folic acid when indicated (9380). Note that pyrimethamine also reduces serum folate levels.

Drug Influences on Nutrient Levels and Depletion

SOME DRUGS CAN AFFECT FOLIC ACID LEVELS:

AMINOSALICYLIC ACID (para-aminosalicylic acid, PAS, Paser): Aminosalicylic acid can reduce dietary folate absorption, worsening folate deficiency often seen with active tuberculosis, or preventing reversal during treatment (9363,9388,9395,9396,9397). Megaloblastic anemia occurs rarely, and usually with other contributing factors such as concurrent vitamin B12 malabsorption (4559). Advise patients being treated for tuberculosis to take folic acid supplements if their dietary folate intake is low.

ANTACIDS: Folic acid absorption in the small intestine is optimal at pH 5.5 to 6 (8441). Chronic use of large doses of antacids can reduce folic acid absorption, but this is likely only significant if dietary folate intake is very low (2677,8441). Advise patients to maintain the recommended daily intake of folic acid in their diet.

ANTIBIOTICS: Antibiotic therapy can disrupt the normal gastrointestinal (GI) flora, interfering with enterohepatic recirculation (reabsorption) of folic acid (4436). The normal GI flora also synthesizes and consumes folic acid, which may also be disrupted by antibiotics (2677,4437,6243). Folic acid synthesized by GI bacteria can be absorbed in the large intestine, but the amount synthesized and absorbed is variable (4437,6243). For instance, it can depend on dietary fiber intake and gastric pH; hypochlorhydria causes bacterial overgrowth and increased folate synthesis (4437,9364). In most people it's unlikely that a course of antibiotics will reduce folic acid levels significantly, and therefore supplements are unnecessary.

ASPIRIN: Aspirin may decrease serum folate levels by reducing bindgin to plasma proteins, especially when large doses are taken regularly (e.g., for treatment of rheumatoid arthritis). But there doesn't seem to be an increase in urinary folate losses and red blood cell levels are normal (9351,9360). This suggests folate is just being redistributed in the body and deficiency isn't likely.

CARBAMAZEPINE (Tegretol): Carbamazepine can reduce serum folate levels, but megaloblastic anemia has not been reported (4426,4427,4428,4429,9359). Reduced folate levels might contribute to mild, asymptomatic reductions in nerve conduction velocities, and mental changes seen with carbamazepine (4427,4429). Possible mechanisms include reduced folic acid absorption, and increased metabolism by induced hepatic enzymes (4426,4428,4429). Pregnant women taking carbamazepine may be especially at risk from reduced folate levels (9355). Low folate levels during pregnancy may contribute to birth defects and pregnancy loss (9355,9356). However, folic acid supplements have worsened seizure control in some people with epilepsy (4427). Advise patients taking carbamazepine chronically to consult their physician before starting folic acid supplements.

CHOLESTYRAMINE (Questran): Cholestyramine reduces folic acid absorption. It can lower serum and red blood cell folate levels in children taking large doses (0.2 to 1.1 grams/kg/day) for several months (4455). There aren't any reports of deficiency in adults. Encourage patients to maintain a good dietary intake of folic acid.

COLESTIPOL (Colestid): Colestipol can interfere with absorption of folic acid, and reduce serum folate levels (4461). Encourage patients to maintain good dietary intake of folic acid.

CYCLOSERINE (Seromycin Pulvules): Cycloserine can reduce serum folate levels, rare cases of megaloblastic anemia have occurred (4531,4536,9363). The mechanism is uncertain, but may involve absorption and metabolism of folate (4531,4536). Advise patients receiving long-term treatment to maintain a good dietary intake of folic acid.

DIURETICS: Limited data suggests diuretics may increase excretion of folic acid. Reduced red blood cell folate levels, possibly contributing to increased homocysteine levels, were found in one group of people taking diuretics for six months or longer (1898). The need for folic acid supplementation during diuretic therapy hasn't been adequately studied. Advise patients to maintain a good dietary intake of folic acid.

ESTROGENS: Reduced serum and red blood cell folate levels can occur in some women taking conjugated estrogens (Premarin) or oral contraceptives, but this is unlikely in women with adequate dietary folate intake (4459,4498,7843,7844,9371,9373). There are rare reports of megaloblastic anemia associated with oral contraceptive use, usually in women with other conditions contributing to folate deficiency (9371,9372). Possible mechanisms by which estrogens contribute to folate deficiency include reduced absorption of dietary folate, increased excretion, induction of liver enzymes, and increased protein binding of folate in serum (4459,9371). There is some evidence that oral contraceptives can increase the rate of progression of cervical dysplasia to cervical cancer, and that folic acid can slow or reverse this dysplasia (9352,9370). Advise women taking oral contraceptives or other estrogens to maintain a good dietary intake of folate. Recommend supplements only for those women with inadequate dietary intake or other conditions that contribute to folate deficiency (4459,9371,9373), and for those diagnosed with, or at increased risk for, cervical dysplasia.

H2 BLOCKERS: Folic acid absorption from the small intestine is optimal at pH 5.5 to 6 (8441). The increased pH associated with use of H2 blockers may therefore reduce folic acid absorption, but this is probably only significant if dietary folate intake is very low (4483,8441). Advise patients to maintain the recommended daily dietary intake of folic acid. The H2 blockers include cimetidine (Tagamet), ranitidine (Zantac), nizatidine (Axid), and famotidine (Pepcid).

METFORMIN (Glucophage): Reduced vitamin B12 and, to a lesser extent, folate levels occur in some people with diabetes and can contribute to hyperhomocysteinemia, adding to their already increased risk of cardiovascular disease (32,4490,9366,9367). The reduced folate levels seen in diabetics have been linked to metformin use in some cases, possibly as a result of reduced folic acid absorption (32,9367,9368). Symptomatic folate deficiency is unlikely to occur with metformin, but people with diabetes may need folic acid supplements to reduce hyperhomocysteinemia (9367).

METHOTREXATE: Methotrexate is a folate antagonist which prevents conversion of folic acid to its active form, and lowers plasma and red blood cell folate levels (4492,4493,4494,4546). In patients treated with long-term, low-dose methotrexate for rheumatoid arthritis (RA) or psoriasis development of folate deficiency is associated with increased risk of certain side effects. These include gastrointestinal effects, stomatitis, alopecia, abnormal liver function tests, myelosuppression, megaloblastic anemia, and increased homocysteine levels (768,4492,4493,4494,4546). Folic acid supplements (1 to 5 mg/day) reduce these side effects without reducing the efficacy of methotrexate in treating RA or psoriasis (768,2162,4492,4493,4494,9369,9418). Advise patients taking methotrexate for these conditions to take a folic acid supplement (1 mg/day is probably sufficient), especially if their dietary folate intake is low and they are experiencing the side effects described (4494,4546,9369,9419). It's likely that people who have experienced side effects will need to continue taking folic acid for the duration of methotrexate therapy (9418). Advise patients being treated with methotrexate for cancer to avoid folic acid supplements, unless recommended by their oncologist. Folic acid could interfere with the anticancer effects of methotrexate (9420).

METHYLPREDNISOLONE: Reduced serum folate levels were noted in people with multiple sclerosis (MS) after treatment with methylprednisolone sodium succinate (Solu-Medrol) 1 gram daily for 10 days. The clinical significance of this change isn't known (9362).

NONSTEROIDAL ANTI-INFLAMMATORY DRUGS (NSAIDs): Folate-dependent enzymes are inhibited in vitro by NSAIDs with carboxylic acid-containing side chains. Some of these NSAIDS include ibuprofen (Advil, Motrin), naproxen (Anaprox, Aleve), indomethacin (Indocin), and sulindac (Clinoril). The clinical significance of isn't clear (2677,9361).

PANCREATIC ENZYMES, PANCRELIPASE, PANCREATIN: Reduced folate levels can occur in some people taking pancreatic extracts. This may be due to reduced absorption, since folate can form insoluble complexes with pancreatic extracts (9374). Advise patients to have their folate levels checked if they take pancreatic enzymes for prolonged periods, and to take a supplement if the level is low. These drugs include Pancrease, Cotazym, Viokase, Creon, Ultrase, and others.

PENTAMIDINE: Pentamidine is a weak folate antagonist which prevents conversion of folic acid to its active form, although this isn't thought to contribute significantly to its antiprotozoal activity (9378). Decreased serum folate levels and megaloblastic bone marrow changes can occur rarely with prolonged parenteral pentamidine therapy (9378). Most patients are unlikely to need folic acid supplements. These drugs include Pentacarinat, and Pentam 300.

PHENOBARBITAL (Luminal), PRIMIDONE (Mysoline): These drugs can reduce serum folate levels, occasionally leading to megaloblastic anemia (usually in people with low dietary folate intake), and possibly contributing to neurological side effects, mental changes, and cerebral atrophy (4427,4530,4536,9333,9357,9358,9359). Possible mechanisms include reduced folic acid absorption, increased metabolism, increased demand for folic acid as a coenzyme for induced hepatic enzymes, or competitive interaction between folate coenzymes and phenobarbital (9357). Pregnant women taking phenobarbital or primidone may be especially at risk from reduced folate levels (9354,9355). Low folate levels during pregnancy may contribute to birth defects and pregnancy loss (9355,9356). Folic acid therapy seems to reverse these neurological effects (9333). However, folic acid can worsen seizure control. Advise patients taking phenobarbital or primidone chronically to consult their physician before taking folic acid supplements.

PHENYTOIN (Dilantin), FOSPHENYTOIN (Cerebyx): Phenytoin can reduce serum folate levels, occasionally leading to megaloblastic anemia, and possibly contributing to neurological side effects and mental changes (4427,4536,9357,9358,9359). Possible mechanisms include reduced folic acid absorption, increased metabolism, increased demand for folic acid as a coenzyme for induced hepatic enzymes, or competitive interaction between folate coenzymes and phenytoin (9357). Folic acid supplements may reduce phenytoin side effects (4471,4477). Pregnant women taking phenytoin may be especially at risk from reduced folate levels (9354,9355). Low folate levels during pregnancy may contribute to birth defects and pregnancy loss (9355,9356). However, folic acid can reduce phenytoin serum levels and increase seizure frequency. Advise patients taking phenytoin chronically to consult their physician before taking folic acid supplements.

PROTON PUMP INHIBITORS (PPIs): Folic acid absorption in the small intestine is optimal at pH 5.5 to 6 (8441). The increased pH associated with use of PPIs could theoretically reduce folic acid absorption (8441), but preliminary data suggests use of PPIs for several years doesn't cause folate deficiency (4483). Advise patients to maintain the recommended dietary intake of folic acid. PPIs include omeprazole (Prilosec), lansoprazole (Prevacid), rabeprazole (Aciphex), pantoprazole (Protonix), and esomeprazole (Nexium).

PYRIMETHAMINE (Daraprim): Pyrimethamine is a folate antagonist that prevents conversion of folic acid to its active form (4425,4532). At high doses used to treat toxoplasmosis (50 to 75 mg/day), megaloblastic anemia may occur due to deficiency of active folate, and it's recommended that all patients receive folinic acid (leucovorin calcium, Wellcovorin, an active form of folic acid) to prevent this (4532). Folinic acid doesn't antagonize the therapeutic effect of pyrimethamine because Toxoplasma does not have a membrane transport system for exogenous folinic acid (9380). Advise patients to avoid folic acid supplements since they can antagonize the therapeutic effect of pyrimethamine against Toxoplasma and Pneumocystis carinii. Advise patients taking lower doses of pyrimethamine for prolonged periods to maintain the recommended dietary folate intake. Monitor for folate deficiency.

SULFASALAZINE (Azulfidine): Sulfasalazine competitively inhibits absorption of folic acid in the intestine (2677,4515,4560,9353). It also interferes with the breakdown of dietary folate to its absorbable form, and can cause hemolysis, which increases folate requirements for formation of new red blood cells (4515,4560).

Long-term sulfasalazine therapy can cause reduced serum and red blood cell folate levels and hyperhomocysteinemia, which is a risk factor for cardiovascular disease (4515,9377). Occasionally, megaloblastic anemia develops, usually with high doses of sulfasalazine (>2 grams/day), and when there are other factors contributing to folate deficiency (4515,4516,4517,4536,9376,9377). Reduced folate levels are often found in people with severe chronic ulcerative colitis, due to the disease and sulfasalazine therapy. Reduced folate levels might contribute to the increased risk of colon cancer and colonic mucosal dysplasia, seen in people with ulcerative colitis. Preliminary evidence suggests that folate supplements can reduce this risk (9379). Advise patients on chronic sulfasalazine therapy to increase their dietary folate intake, and to take a supplement if they have any other condition which could also contribute to deficiency (2677,9353,9379).

TRIAMTERENE (Dyrenium): Triamterene is a folate antagonist that prevents conversion of folic acid to its active form, and also reduces folate absorption (4425,4536,4537,9375). Reduced serum and red blood cell folate levels have occurred, and occasional cases of megaloblastic anemia, usually in people with other conditions contributing to folate deficiency (4537,9375). Advise patients on chronic triamterene therapy to maintain the recommended dietary folate intake, or to take a supplement if this is not possible.

TRIMETHOPRIM (Trimpex): Trimethoprim, including trimethoprim contained in the combination antibiotic trimethoprim/sulfamethoxazole (TMP/SMX, co-trimoxazole, Bactrim, Septra), inhibits the enzyme involved in conversion of folic acid to its active form (4468,4531). The bacterial and protozoal enzymes are 1000 to 10,000 times more sensitive to trimethoprim than human enzymes (2677,4468,9382). Therefore, low doses of trimethoprim (10 mg/kg/day) don't affect human enzymes and symptoms of folate deficiency aren't seen (9381,9383,9394). However, at high doses, trimethoprim inhibits the enzyme in human bone marrow and megaloblastic anemia can occur in people taking 1 gram or more daily (20 mg/kg/day) for 2 to 4 weeks, or 500 mg daily for several months (4468,9383,9384). The risk is higher with other conditions contributing to folate deficiency or megaloblastic anemia (9382,9394). Its generally agreed that if megaloblastic anemia occurs, trimethoprim should be stopped and treatment with folinic acid (an active form of folic acid) should be given (9382). Whether folic acid or folinic acid can be given concurrently with trimethoprim to prevent megaloblastic anemia is controversial. The practice may not be effective, especially in people with AIDS in whom immunologic reactions, as well as folate deficiency, probably contribute to hematologic changes (9385,9386,9398). There is a general belief that folic/folinic acid supplements don't interfere with the therapeutic effects of trimethoprim, because infecting organisms can't utilize exogenous folate sources (2677,9382,9384). However, this view has been challenged (4468,9386), and failure of trimethoprim therapy has occurred rarely when folinic acid is given concurrently (9387,9399). Advise patients taking low doses of trimethoprim (100 to 200 mg/day) for treatment or prophylaxis of urinary tract infections that they are unlikely to need folate supplements. Advise patients taking high doses of trimethoprim (20 mg/kg/day) to maintain good dietary folate intake, but to avoid folate supplements unless prescribed by their physician.

VALPROIC ACID, SODIUM VALPROATE, DIVALPROEX SODIUM (Depakene, Depakote): Valproate may reduce folate levels in some people, but symptomatic deficiency has not been reported (4428,9356,9359). Pregnant women taking valproate may be especially at risk from reduced folate levels (9355). Low folate levels during pregnancy may contribute to birth defects and pregnancy loss (9355,9356). However, folic acid supplements have worsened seizure control in some people with epilepsy (4427). Advise patients taking valproate chronically to consult their physician before taking folic acid supplements.

Interactions with Foods

FOOD: The absorption of supplemental folic acid is reduced slightly when taken with food (6241,6243). Bioavailability is around 85% with food, compared with nearly 100% when taken on an empty stomach, this difference is not clinically significant (6241,6243).

ZINC: The data on the effects of supplemental folic acid on dietary zinc absorption is conflicting (9389,9390,9391,9392,9393,9421). However, normal supplemental doses of folic acid are unlikely to have an adverse effect on zinc balance in people with adequate dietary zinc intake (7135,9391).

Interactions with Lab Tests

MEAN CORPUSCULAR VOLUME (MCV): Folic acid supplementation can normalize megaloblastic anemia in cases of folic acid and vitamin B12 deficiencies. In cases of vitamin B12 deficiency or pernicious anemia, treatment with folic acid will normalize hematological findings, but will not prevent neurological damage (7725).

Interactions with Diseases or Conditions

ANGIOPLASTY: An intravenous loading dose of folic acid, vitamin B6 and vitamin B12 followed by oral administration of folic acid 1.2 mg plus vitamin B6 48 mg and vitamin B12 60 mcg taken daily after coronary stenting might actually increase restenosis rates (12150). Due to the potential for harm this combination of vitamins should not be recommended for patients receiving coronary stents (12151).

PERNICIOUS ANEMIA: Folic acid can mask pernicious anemia by decreasing megaloblastic anemia. This can prevent appropriate treatment with vitamin B12 and result in neurological damage (6241,7725,8739). Patients should be warned to avoid treating undiagnosed anemia with folic acid.

SEIZURE DISORDERS: Supplemental folic acid might exacerbate seizures in people with seizure disorders, particularly in very high doses. Doses less than 1000 mcg have rarely been associated with increased seizure activity (9901).

Dosage and Administration

ORAL: For folate deficiency, the typical dose is 250-1000 mcg per day. For severe folate deficiency, such as in cases of megaloblastic anemia and malabsorption disorders, 1-5 mg per day is used until hematologic recovery is documented (8739). For preventing neural tube defects, at least 400 mcg folic acid per day from supplements or fortified food should be taken by women capable of becoming pregnant and continued through the first month of pregnancy (3325,6241,6243,8739). Women with a history of previous pregnancy complicated by such neural tube defects usually take 4 mg per day beginning one month before and continuing for three months after conception (8739). For reducing colon cancer risk, 400 mcg per day has been used (2250,9326). For treating hyperhomocysteinemia, 0.5 to 5 mg/day has been used (3047,6366,9307,9400,9401,9405,9408,9409,9410,10350), although 0.8 to 1 mg/day is appears to provide maximal reduction of homocysteine levels (9307,9408). In patients with high coronary risk or atherosclerotic disease, 10 mg per day of folic acid has been used to improve coagulation status, oxidative stress, and endothelial dysfunction (9319). In people with end-stage renal disease, hyperhomocysteinemia may be more resistant to treatment, and doses of 0.8 to 15 mg/day have been used (1489,6884,7289,7881,9322,9413,9414,9415,9416). Other regimens such as 2.5 to 5 mg 3 times weekly have also been used (9417). Doses higher than 15 mg daily do not seem provide additional homocysteine-lowering effect (9219). For preventing increases in homocysteine levels after nitrous oxide anesthesia, folate 2.5 mg in combination with pyridoxine 25 mg and vitamin B12 500 mcg has been used daily for 1 wk before surgery (9481). As adjunct treatment with conventional antidepressants, 200 to 500 mcg per day has been used (10884). For enhancing response to antidepressants, 500 mcg daily has been used (3657). For vitiligo, 5 mg is typically taken twice daily (2153). For reduction of toxicity associated with methotrexate therapy for rheumatoid arthritis (RA) or psoriasis, 1 mg/day is probably sufficient, but up to 5 mg/day may be used (768,2162,4492,4493,4494,9369,9418). The adequate intakes (AI) for infants are 65 mcg for infants 0-6 months and 80 mcg for infants 7-12 months of age (6243). The recommended dietary allowances (RDAs) for folate in DFE, including both food folate and folic acid from fortified foods and supplements are: Children 1-3 years, 150 mcg; Children 4-8 years, 200 mcg; Children 9-13 years, 300 mcg; Adults over 13 years, 400 mcg; Pregnant women 600 mcg; and Lactating women, 500 mcg (6243). The tolerable upper intake levels (UL) of folate are 300 mcg for children 1-3 years of age, 400 mcg for children 4-8 years, 600 mcg for children 9-13 years, 800 mcg for adolescents 14-18 years, and 1000 mcg for everyone over 18 years of age (6243).

TOPICAL: No typical dosage.

Comments

Beginning in 1998, the US government required folic acid fortification of all cold cereals and baking flour, which extends to breads, pastas, bakery items, cookies, crackers, etc (6241). Foods that are naturally high in folate content with 60% to 90% folic acid bioavailability include leafy vegetables (such as spinach, broccoli, and lettuce), okra, asparagus, fruits (such as bananas, melons, and lemons) legumes, yeast, mushrooms, animal protein (such as beef liver and kidney), orange juice, and tomato juice (6241,8739,9300). Folic acid is frequently used in combination with other B vitamins in vitamin B complex formulations. Vitamin B complex generally includes vitamin B1 (thiamine), vitamin B2 (riboflavin), vitamin B3 (niacin/niacinamide), vitamin B5 (pantothenic acid), vitamin B6 (pyridoxine), vitamin B12 (cyanocobalamin), and folic acid. However, some products do not contain all of these ingredients and some may include others, such as biotin, para-aminobenzoic acid (PABA), choline bitartrate, and inositol (3022).

FOOL'S PARSLEY

Also Known As

Dog Parsley, Dog Poison, Fool's-Cicely, Fools Parsley, Lesser Hemlock, Small Hemlock.
CAUTION: See separate listings for Parsley and Parsley Piert.

Scientific Names

Aethusa cynapium.
Family: Apiaceae/Umbelliferae.

People Use This For

Orally, fool's parsley is used for gastrointestinal complaints in children, infantile cholera, Summer diarrhea, and convulsions.

Safety

LIKELY UNSAFE ...when used orally; avoid using. Plant parts are considered poisonous and are associated with serious, potentially life-threatening poisonings (18).

PREGNANCY AND LACTATION: UNSAFE ...when used orally; contraindicated, due to potential for poisoning (18).

Effectiveness

There is insufficient reliable information available about the effectiveness of fool's parsley.

Mechanism of Action
Fool's parsley contains varied flavone glycosides (rutoside, narcissine, camphor oil-3-glucorhamnoside). Freshly harvested leaves (only) contain polyenes aethusin, aethusanol A, and asthusanol B (18).

Adverse Reactions
Orally, there are reports that fool's parsley caused deaths when it was mistaken for garden parsley; however, there is some evidence that the botanical to blame was actually spotted hemlock (18). Nevertheless, caution is warranted.

Interactions with Herbs & Other Dietary Supplements
None known.

Interactions with Drugs
None known.

Interactions with Foods
None known.

Interactions with Lab Tests
None known.

Interactions with Diseases or Conditions
None known.

Dosage and Administration
No typical dosage.

Comments
Fool's parsley is considered unsafe; avoid using. Fool's parsley looks a lot like young garden parsley; hence its name. Be careful not to confuse the two, since fool's parsley is poisonous (18).

FORGET-ME-NOT

Also Known As
Field Scorpion Grass, Forget Me Not.

Scientific Names
Myosotis arvensis.
Family: Boraginaceae.

People Use This For
Orally, forget-me-not is used for respiratory disorders and nose bleeds.

Safety
POSSIBLY UNSAFE ...when used orally in excessive amounts. Though the alkaloids have not been characterized, hepatotoxic pyrrolizidine alkaloids (PAs) are common in this genus (12842).
PREGNANCY AND LACTATION: POSSIBLY UNSAFE ...when used orally, due to possible hepatotoxic pyrrolizidine alkaloid content (12842); avoid using.

Effectiveness
There is insufficient reliable information available about the effectiveness of forget-me-not.

Mechanism of Action
The applicable part of forget-me-not is the whole flowering plant. Forget-me-not might contain hepatotoxic pyrrolizidine alkaloids (PA), which can also cause lung toxicity and are carcinogenic (12842).

Adverse Reactions
Orally, exposure to hepatotoxic pyrrolizidine alkaloids (PA) can cause veno-occlusive disease, lung toxicity, and cancer. Symptoms of acute veno-occlusive disease include colicky pains in epigastrium, vomiting and diarrhea, and ascites formation within several days. Enlargement and induration of the liver occurs within a few weeks (12842).

Interactions with Herbs & Other Dietary Supplements
None known.

Interactions with Drugs
None known.

Interactions with Foods
None known.

Interactions with Lab Tests
None known.

Interactions with Diseases or Conditions
None known.

Dosage and Administration
No typical dosage.

FORSKOLIN

Also Known As
Borforsin, Coleus barbatus, Coleus Forskohlii, Colforsin, Forskohlii, HL-362, L-75-1362B, Plectranthus barbatus.

Scientific Names
17beta-acetoxy-8,13-epoxy-1alpha,6beta,9alpha-trihydroxylabd-14-en-11-one.

People Use This For
Orally, forskolin is used for asthma, allergies, eczema, psoriasis, obesity, dysmenorrhea, irritable bowel syndrome (IBS), urinary tract infections (UTI), bladder infections, hypertension, angina, metastatic cancer, thrombosis, impotence, insomnia, and convulsions.
Intravenously, forskolin is used for idiopathic congestive cardiomyopathy and congestive heart failure (CHF).
By inhalation, forskolin is used for asthma and bronchospasm.
Ophthalmologically, forskolin is used for glaucoma.

Safety
POSSIBLY SAFE ...when used intravenously and appropriately, short-term. Intravenous forskolin seems to be safe and well tolerated when given at an appropriate rate of 0.5 mcg/kg/minute and increased at 15 minute intervals to 1.0, 2.0, and 3.0 mcg/kg/minute up to 1 hour (7278,7279). ...when used by inhalation and appropriately. Single-dose inhalation of forskolin powder (10 mg) from a Spinhaler inhalator seems to be safe and well tolerated (7281). ...when used ophthalmologically and appropriately. Forskolin suspension eye drops (1%) seem and well-tolerated (7282,7283,7284,7402,7403,7405).
PREGNANCY AND LACTATION: Insufficient reliable information available; avoid using.

Effectiveness
POSSIBLY EFFECTIVE

Asthma. There is some evidence that a single-dose inhalation of forskolin powder 10 mg from a Spinhaler inhaler can significantly increase forced expiratory volume in 1 second (FEV1) in patients with asthma (7281).

Idiopathic congestive cardiomyopathy. There is some evidence that intravenous forskolin, starting at 0.5 mcg/kg/minute, increasing at 15 minute intervals to 1.0, 2.0, and 3.0 mcg/kg/minute, is effective in improving cardiac output and pulmonary vascular pressures in patients with idiopathic congestive cardiomyopathy (7278).

INSUFFICIENT RELIABLE EVIDENCE to RATE

Intraocular pressure. There is some preliminary evidence that forskolin suspension eye drops (1%) can significantly decrease intraocular pressure in healthy people without eye disease (7282,7283,7284,7402,7403,7405). Forskolin has not yet been tested in patients with glaucoma. More evidence is needed to rate forskolin for this use.

Mechanism of Action
Forskolin is a diterpene and the major active constituent found in the roots of the plant Plectranthus barbatus (Coleus forskohlii) (7277). Forskolin stimulates and activates the enzyme adenylate cyclase in the heart and smooth muscle. This causes increased production of cyclic AMP (cAMP), which causes calcium channels to open and intracellular calcium concentrations to increase, resulting in increased contractility of heart muscle and relaxation of smooth muscle (7277,7406,7407,7408,7409). Researchers speculate that forskolin might also activate adenylate cyclase in other cells of the body such as platelet cells and cells in the thyroid, pancreas, adrenal, or pituitary glands (7277). There is preliminary evidence that forskolin prevents platelet aggregation and adhesion (7410,7411); and may also block tumor cell-induced human platelet aggregation, prevent tumor cell growth, and prevent cancer metastasis (7412,7413).

Adverse Reactions

Intravenously, forskolin can cause flushing and hypotension (7279).
Inhalation of forskolin can cause throat and upper respiratory tract irritation, mild to moderate cough, tremor, and restlessness (7281).
Ophthalmologically, forskolin can cause stinging of the eyes and conjunctival hyperemia (7283).

Interactions with Herbs & Other Dietary Supplements

CARDIOACTIVE HERBS: Theoretically, concomitant use of forskolin and cardioactive herbs could potentiate the cardiac effects and adverse effects (7278,7279). Some cardioactive herbs include calamus, cereus, cola, coltsfoot, devil's claw, European mistletoe, fenugreek, fumitory, ginger, Panax ginseng, white horehound, mate, parsley, quassia, scotch broom flower, shepherd's purse, wild carrot, and some cardiac glycoside-containing herbs such as digitalis leaf or lily-of-the-valley roots.
HERBS WITH ANTICOAGULANT/ANTIPLATELET POTENTIAL: Theoretically, concomitant use of forskolin with herbs that affect platelet aggregation could potentially increase the risk of bruising and bleeding. Some of these herbs include angelica, anise, arnica, asafetida, bogbean, boldo, capsicum, celery, chamomile, clove, danshen, fenugreek, feverfew, garlic, ginger, ginkgo, Panax ginseng, horseradish, licorice, meadowsweet, prickly ash, onion, papain, passionflower, poplar, quassia, red clover, turmeric, wild carrot, wild lettuce, willow, and others.

Interactions with Drugs

ANTICOAGULANT/ANTIPLATELET DRUGS: Theoretically, concomitant use of forskolin and anticoagulant or antiplatelet agents might increase the risk of bruising and bleeding. There is some evidence forskolin can inhibit platelet aggregation and adhesion (7410,7411). Some anticoagulant and antiplatelet drugs include abciximab (ReoPro), anagrelide (Agrylin), antithrombin III (Thrombate III), ardeparin (Normiflo), cilostazol (Pletal), clopidogrel (Plavix), dalteparin (Fragmin), danaparoid (Orgaran), dicumarol, dipyridamole (Persantine), enoxaparin (Lovenox), eptifibatide (Integrilin), heparin, lepirudin (Refludan), tirofiban (Aggrastat), and warfarin (Coumadin).
CALCIUM CHANNEL BLOCKERS: Using forskolin with calcium channel blockers such as verapamil (Calan, Covera-HS, Verelan), nifedipine (Procardia), and diltiazem (Cardizem, Dilacor, Tiazac) might cause additive coronary vasodilatory effects (7278,7279).
NITRATES: Using forskolin with nitrates such as nitroglycerin (Nitro-Bid, Nitro-Dur, Nitrostat) and isosorbide (Imdur, Isordil, Sorbitrate) might cause additive coronary vasodilatory effects (7278,7279).

Interactions with Foods

None known.

Interactions with Lab Tests

BLEEDING TIME: Theoretically, forskolin might increase measures of bleeding time and increase tests results for prothrombin time (PT) and international normalized ratio (INR). There is some evidence that forskolin inhibits platelet aggregation and adhesion (7410,7411).

Interactions with Diseases or Conditions

BLEEDING DISORDERS: Theoretically, forskolin may increase the risk of bleeding. There is some evidence that forskolin inhibits platelet aggregation and adhesion (7278,7279).
CARDIOVASCULAR DISEASE: There is some concern that forskolin might interfere with treatment for cardiovascular disease and potentially worsen cardiovascular conditions. Forskolin can cause vasodilation and significantly lower blood pressure (7278,7279). Use forskolin with caution in patients with cardiovascular conditions.

Dosage and Administration

INHALATION: For asthma, 10 mg of forskolin powder, using a Spinhaler inhalator, has been used (7281).
INTRAVENOUS: For idiopathic congestive cardiomyopathy, intravenous forskolin has been infused at 0.5 mcg/kg/min and increased at 15 minute intervals as tolerated up to 1.0, 2.0, and 3.0 mcg/kg/minute for up to 1 hour (7278,7279).
OPHTHALMIC: For lowering intraocular pressure, 50 microliters of forskolin suspension eye drops (1%), applied topically to the cornea, has been used in healthy people (7282,7283,7284,7402,7403,7405). An appropriate dose for patients with glaucoma is not known.
ORAL: No typical dosage.

Comments

Forskolin comes from Coleus forskohlii, an herb that has been used since ancient times to treat heart and respiratory disorders. Herbal product manufacturers are now producing Coleus forskohlii extracts with elevated levels of the constituent forskolin. These preparations are being promoted for the same conditions for which forskolin has been used. However, there is no reliable scientific information that shows Coleus forskolii extracts offer any therapeutic benefit.

FORSYTHIA

Also Known As
Forsythia Fructus, Golden Bell, Lian Qiao, Lien Chiao, Rengyo, Weeping Golden Bell.

Scientific Names
Forsythia suspensa, synonym Syringa suspensa; Forsythia viridissima; Forsythia viridissima var. koreana, synonym Forsythia koreana.
Family: Oleaceae.

People Use This For
Orally, forsythia is used for bronchiolitis, tonsillitis, pharyngitis, fever, gonorrhea, erysipelas, and inflammation. Parenterally, forsythia, in combination with other herbs, is used for bronchiolitis.

Safety
POSSIBLY SAFE ...when used by injection, short-term. An intravenous preparation that includes forsythia, honeysuckle, and Baikal skullcap has been used with apparent safety in children for up to 7 days (12613).
There is insufficient reliable information about the safety of forsythia when used orally or long-term.
PREGNANCY AND LACTATION: Insufficient reliable information available; avoid using.

Effectiveness
INSUFFICIENT RELIABLE EVIDENCE to RATE

Bronchiolitis. Preliminary clinical research suggests a combination of forsythia, honeysuckle, and Baikal skullcap given intravenously might decrease the duration of symptoms of bronchiolitis in children with respiratory syncytial virus infection (12613). More evidence is needed to rate forsythia for this use.

Mechanism of Action
The applicable part of forsythia is the fruit. Forsythia contains flavonoids, lignans, triterpenes, oleanolic acid, rutin, and other compounds (12658). Preliminary research suggests constituents of forsythia may have anti-inflammatory and analgesic effects (12656,12657). Forsythia extracts may exert anti-inflammatory activity by inhibiting 5-lipoxygenase and human leukocyte elastase (12615).
Other research suggests it might inhibit the release of tumor necrosis factor (TNF) from mast cells (12617). It also seems to inhibit leukotriene B4, which suggests it might be useful for treating skin conditions such as psoriasis (12615). Other preliminary research suggests forsythia extracts inhibit itching induced by substance P without causing sedation. Substance P is increased in patients with skin disorders such as atopic dermatitis and psoriasis (12623).
Forsythia contains tannic acid which seems to have antitumor and anti-inflammatory properties (12616).
Triterpene constituents may also contribute to anti-inflammatory activity (12618). Preliminary research suggests that forsythia might inhibit platelet activating factor (12619).
Preliminary research suggests forsythia has activity against the respiratory syncytial virus (RSV) (12614). Forsythia may also have antibacterial activity (12616).
Other research suggests it may reduce fever and stimulate bile flow (12656,12657).

Adverse Reactions
None reported.

Interactions with Herbs & Other Dietary Supplements
None known.

Interactions with Drugs
ANTICOAGULANT/ANTIPLATELET DRUGS: Theoretically, taking forsythia with anticoagulant or antiplatelet drugs might increase the risk of bleeding due to decreased platelet aggregation. Forsythia might reduce platelet aggregation by inhibiting platelet activating factor (12619). Some of these drugs include aspirin, clopidogrel (Plavix), dalteparin (Fragmin), enoxaparin (Lovenox), heparin, ticlopidine (Ticlid), warfarin (Coumadin), and others.

Interactions with Foods
None known.

Interactions with Lab Tests
None known.

Interactions with Diseases or Conditions
None known.

Dosage and Administration
No typical dosage.

FRANKINCENSE

Also Known As
Bible Frankincense, Olibanum.
CAUTION: See separate listing for Indian Frankincense.

Scientific Names
Boswellia sacra, synonym Boswellia carteri.
Family: Burseraceae.

People Use This For
Orally, frankincense is used for colic and flatulence.
Topically, frankincense is used in hand cream. The essential oil of frankincense is used topically and by inhalation as an analgesic.

Safety
POSSIBLY SAFE ...when used orally (12). ...when the frankincense essential oil is used topically and by inhalation (7107).
PREGNANCY AND LACTATION: Insufficient reliable information available; avoid using.

Effectiveness
There is insufficient reliable information available about the effectiveness of frankincense.

Mechanism of Action
The applicable part of frankincense is the resin. There is insufficient reliable information available about the possible mechanism of action and active ingredients.

Adverse Reactions
Topically, frankincense can cause mild irritation (18).

Interactions with Herbs & Other Dietary Supplements
None known.

Interactions with Drugs
None known.

Interactions with Foods
None known.

Interactions with Lab Tests
None known.

Interactions with Diseases or Conditions
None known.

Dosage and Administration
No typical dosage.

Comments
Frankincense is the hardened gum resin extruded from incisions made in the trunk of Boswellia carteri. Olibanum is a term which refers to the oleogum resin exuded from incisions in the bark of several Boswellia species, including Boswellia serrata (Indian frankincense), Boswellia sacra (Bible frankincense), Boswellia frereana (African elemi), and Boswellia bhau-dajiana (11). The black kohl used by Egyptian women to paint their eyelids is an ingredient from charred frankincense. Frankincense is considered obsolete as a medicinal herb (18).

FRINGETREE

Also Known As

Chionanthus, Fringe Tree, Gray Beard Tree, Old Man's Beard, Poison Ash, Snowdrop Tree, Snowflower, White Fringe.
CAUTION: See separate listings for Traveler's Joy, Usnea, and Woodbine.

Scientific Names

Chionanthus virginicus.
Family: Oleaceae.

Comments

At the date of publication, there was very little scientific information available about this product. Our staff is continually analyzing the available information on natural medicines and will add data to the online version of *Natural Medicines Comprehensive Database* as it becomes available. See www.naturaldatabase.com..

FROSTWORT

Also Known As

Frost Plant, Frostweed, Rock-Rose, Sun Rose.

Scientific Names

Helianthemum canadense, synonym Cistus canadensis.
Family: Cistaceae.

Comments

At the date of publication, there was very little scientific information available about this product. Our staff is continually analyzing the available information on natural medicines and will add data to the online version of *Natural Medicines Comprehensive Database* as it becomes available. See www.naturaldatabase.com.

FRUCTO-OLIGOSACCHARIDES

Also Known As

Beta-D-fructofuranosidase, Chicory Inulin Hydrolysate, FOS, Fructo Oligo Saccharides, Fructooligosaccharides, Inulin Hydrolysate, Oligofructose, Oligosaccharides, Prebiotic, SC-FOS, Short Chain Fructo-Oligosaccharides.
CAUTION: See separate listing for Inulin.

Scientific Names

Beta-D-fructofuranosidase.

People Use This For

Orally, fructo-oligosaccharides are used for constipation, traveler's diarrhea, increasing fecal mass, and reducing serum cholesterol. Fructo-oligosaccharides are also used as prebiotics.
In foods, fructo-oligosaccharides are used as a sweetener.

Safety

POSSIBLY SAFE ...when used orally and appropriately in amounts less than 30 grams per day (741,745,8505).
PREGNANCY AND LACTATION: Insufficient reliable information available; avoid using.

Effectiveness

POSSIBLY INEFFECTIVE

Traveler's diarrhea. Taking fructo-oligosaccharides orally doesn't seem to reduce the incidence of traveler's diarrhea (10373).

INSUFFICIENT RELIABLE EVIDENCE to RATE

Constipation. Some evidence suggests that fructo-oligosaccharides may relieve constipation by increasing fecal mass (8505). More evidence is needed to rate fructo-oligosaccharides for this use.

Mechanism of Action

Fructo-oligosaccharides (FOS) are plant sugars that occur in a wide variety of fruits, vegetables, and cereals. Chemically, fructo-oligosaccharides are made up of a glucose molecule joined to fructose molecules. They are produced commercially from sucrose using an enzymatic process, or they can be produced by partial hydrolysis of chicory inulin (750,8507,8563).

Fructo-oligosaccharides have prebiotic activity. Prebiotics are substances that selectively promote the growth and activity of specific species of bacteria in the gut. Fructo-oligosaccharides pass undigested through the small intestine. Colonic bacteria that produce acids, such as bifidobacteria and lactobacilli, are symbiotic with fructo-oligosaccharides. In the colon, fructo-oligosaccharides specifically promote the growth of beneficial bacteria, which in turn produce enzymes that metabolize fructo-oligosaccharides (750,8505,8507,8508,8509,8563). Fructo-oligosaccharides are not hydrolyzed by human digestive enzymes (746), and they are not recoverable in the feces. This suggests complete metabolism by colonic microflora (747).

Colonic fermentation leads to increased fecal biomass, decreased ceco-colonic pH, and production of short chain fatty acids. The short chain fatty acids exert systemic effects on lipid metabolism similarly to dietary fiber (744).

Preliminary evidence suggests that fructo-oligosaccharides might protect against colon cancer (748). In experimental models of colon cancer, fructo-oligosaccharides seem to stimulate local immune surveillance to inhibit tumor formation (8506).

FOS are derived from asparagus, Jerusalem artichokes, and soybeans, or produced synthetically (746,8563). FOS pass undigested through the small intestine and are fermented in the colon.

Adverse Reactions

Orally, the use of fructo-oligosaccharides can cause flatulence, belching, abdominal pain, intestinal sounds, and bloating (740,750,8609). These symptoms occur commonly but are generally mild at lower doses (less than 10 grams per day) (745,750,8509).

Interactions with Herbs & Other Dietary Supplements

BIFIDOBACTERIA: Concomitant use of fructo-oligosaccharides can promote the growth of supplemental bifidobacteria.

Interactions with Drugs

None known.

Interactions with Foods

None known.

Interactions with Lab Tests

None known.

Interactions with Diseases or Conditions

None known.

Dosage and Administration

ORAL: For treating constipation, a dose of 10 grams per day has been used (8505). For prebiotic effect (to increase fecal bifidobacteria), the typical dose is 4 to 10 grams per day (749,750).

Comments

Fructo-oligosaccharides are used as prebiotics, food constituents that increase the number of beneficial bacteria in the intestine. Don't confuse prebiotics with probiotics such as lactobacillus, bifidobacteria, and saccharomyces, which are live organisms used to re-colonize beneficial intestinal microorganisms (8509).

FUMITORY

Also Known As

Beggary, Earth Smoke, Fumiterry, Fumus, Hedge Fumitory, Herba fumariae, Vapor, Wax Dolls.

Scientific Names

Fumaria officinalis.
Family: Fumariaceae.

People Use This For

Orally, fumitory is used for GI spasms and as a bile flow stimulant.

Historically, fumitory has been used for skin eruptions, eczema, conjunctivitis, cardiovascular disorders, as a diuretic, and a laxative.

Safety

POSSIBLY SAFE ...when above ground parts are used orally and appropriately. No significant toxicity usually occurs in standard doses (4,6).
POSSIBLY UNSAFE ...when used orally in large amounts because it contains the alkaloid protopine. Other Fumariaceae species that contain alkaloids including protopine can cause convulsions and death when large amounts are ingested (6). ...when homemade, non-sterile products are used for ophthalmic use (4).
PREGNANCY AND LACTATION: Insufficient reliable information available; avoid using (4).

Effectiveness

INSUFFICIENT RELIABLE EVIDENCE to RATE

Biliary disorders. There's anecdotal evidence that fumitory might help reduce colicky pain associated with biliary disorders (280). More evidence is needed to rate fumitory for this use.

Mechanism of Action

The applicable parts of fumitory are the above ground parts. Fumitory can have weak antispasmodic effects on the smooth muscle of the bile duct and upper GI tract (2,4,18). The major alkaloid constituent, protopine, has antihistamine, hypotensive, bradycardic, and sedative activity in small doses, and it causes excitation and convulsions in large doses (4). Fumitory can exhibit bactericidal activity against gram-positive organisms, including Bacillus anthracis and Staphylococcus (4).

Adverse Reactions

Orally, adverse reactions to fumitory are not common; however, large quantities of alkaloids in other members of this family (Fumariaceae) have caused trembling, convulsions, and death (2).

Interactions with Herbs & Other Dietary Supplements

None known.

Interactions with Drugs

None known.

Interactions with Foods

None known.

Interactions with Lab Tests

None known.

Interactions with Diseases or Conditions

None known.

Dosage and Administration

ORAL: The typical dose of fumitory is 2-4 grams of the above ground parts per day or as a tea 3 times daily (4). The tea is prepared by steeping the herb in 150 mL boiling water for 5-10 minutes and then straining. The usual dose of the liquid extract (1:1 in 25% alcohol) is 2-4 mL 3 times daily, and the tincture (1:5 in 45% alcohol) is commonly dosed 1-4 mL 3 times daily (4).
INHALATION: Nebulizers have been used to administer the extract; no typical dosage (6).

Comments

The fumitory plant is a low shrub with gray pointed leaves, and from a distance the plant can have the wispy appearance of smoke, because of this it received the name "earth smoke" (6).

GABA (GAMMA-AMINOBUTYRIC ACID)

Also Known As

GABA, Gamma Amino Butyric Acid.

Scientific Names

Gamma-aminobutyric acid.

People Use This For

Orally, GABA is used for relieving anxiety, elevating mood, relieving premenstrual syndrome (PMS), and treating attention deficit-hyperactivity disorder (ADHD). It is also used for promoting lean muscle growth, burning fat, stabilizing blood pressure, and relieving pain.
Sublingually, GABA is used for increasing feeling of well being, relieving injuries, improving exercise tolerance, decreasing body fat, and increasing lean body weight.

Safety

There is insufficient reliable information available about the safety of GABA.
Pregnancy and Lactation: Insufficient reliable information available; avoid using.

Effectiveness

There is insufficient reliable information available about the effectiveness of GABA.

Mechanism of Action

In the central nervous system, GABA is the primary inhibitory neurotransmitter. It is synthesized in the brain by the decarboxylation of glutamate (5109,5110). GABA exerts anticonvulsant, sedative, and anxiolytic effects at the cellular level (5109,5110). Single, oral doses of GABA given to people with photo-convulsant epilepsy had no effect (5113). Single, oral doses of 5 or 10 grams of GABA caused a rise in C-peptide, insulin, and glucagon; but did not effect serum glucose in healthy people (5114). GABA given intravenously can cause dysphoria and dose-related increases in blood pressure and pulse (5116). In healthy volunteers, a single 5 gram dose of GABA increased growth hormone, but chronic four-day administration of 18 grams of GABA decreased growth hormone and increased serum prolactin (5115).

Adverse Reactions

Intravenously GABA can cause dysphoria and dose-related increases in blood pressure and pulse (5116).

Interactions with Herbs & Other Dietary Supplements

None known.

Interactions with Drugs

None known.

Interactions with Foods

None known.

Interactions with Lab Tests

None known.

Interactions with Diseases or Conditions

None known.

Dosage and Administration

No typical dosage.

GALBANUM

Also Known As

Galbanum Gum, Galbanum Gum Resin, Galbanum Oleogum Resin, Galbanum Oleoresin, Galbanum Resin.

Scientific Names

Ferula gummosa, synonym Ferula galbaniflua.
Family: Apiaceae/Umbelliferae.

People Use This For

Orally, galbanum is used for digestive disorders and flatulence, as an appetite stimulant, expectorant, and antispasmodic.
Topically, galbanum is used for wound treatment.
In food and beverages, galbanum oil and resin are used as flavor components.
In manufacturing, galbanum oil and resin are used as fragrance components in cosmetics. Galbanum is rarely used in pharmaceuticals.

Safety

LIKELY SAFE ...when used orally in amounts commonly found in foods. Galganum has Generally Recognized As Safe status (GRAS) for use in foods in the US (4912).
POSSIBLY SAFE ...when used topically (11).
There is insufficient reliable information available about the safety of the oral use of galbanum in medicinal amounts.
PREGNANCY AND LACTATION: There is insufficient reliable information available about the safety of the oral use of galbanum in medicinal amounts during pregnancy and lactation.

Effectiveness

There is insufficient reliable information available about the effectiveness of galbanum.

Mechanism of Action

The applicable part of galbanum is the gum resin from the roots and trunk. In vitro data suggest antimicrobial activity, particularly against Staphylococcus aureus. Galbanum may also be effective as an emulsion preservative. Emulsions containing galbanum were stable for up to 6 months (11).

Adverse Reactions

None reported.

Interactions with Herbs & Other Dietary Supplements

None known.

Interactions with Drugs

None known.

Interactions with Foods

None known.

Interactions with Lab Tests

None known.

Interactions with Diseases or Conditions

None known.

Dosage and Administration

No typical dosage.

GAMBOGE

Also Known As

Camboge, Gambodia, Gummigutta, Gutta Cambodia, Gutta Gamba, Guttagamba, Tom Rong.
CAUTION: See separate listing for Garcinia.

Scientific Names

Garcinia hanburyi.
Family: Clusiaceae.

People Use This For

Orally, gamboge is used for constipation, generally in combination with other laxatives, and for the evacuation of intestinal worms.

Safety

POSSIBLY UNSAFE ...when used orally. Deaths have been reported with ingestion of 4 grams (18).
PREGNANCY AND LACTATION: POSSIBLY UNSAFE ...when used orally (18); avoid using.

Effectiveness

There is insufficient reliable information available about the effectiveness of gamboge.

Mechanism of Action

The applicable part of gamboge is the resin. It contains resins (benzophenones and xanthones) and mucilages. Gamboge reportedly has strong laxative effect (18).

Adverse Reactions

Orally, abdominal pain and vomiting has been reported with as little as 200 mg; deaths were reported with ingestion of 4 grams (18).

Interactions with Herbs & Other Dietary Supplements

DIGITALIS: Theoretically, overuse/misuse may cause potassium depletion and increase risk of cardiotoxicity (19).
POTASSIUM DEPLETING HERBS: Theoretically, concomitant use with horsetail plant or licorice rhizome increases the risk of potassium depletion (19).
STIMULANT LAXATIVE HERBS: Theoretically, concomitant use with other stimulant laxative herbs may increase the risk of potassium depletion (19). Stimulant laxative herbs include aloe dried leaf sap, wild cucumber fruit (Ecballium elaterium), blue flag rhizome, alder buckthorn, European buckthorn, butternut bark, cascara bark, castor oil, colocynth fruit pulp, jalap root, black root, manna bark exudate, podophyllum root, rhubarb root, senna leaves and pods, and yellow dock root.

Interactions with Drugs

CORTICOSTEROIDS: Theoretically, prolonged use might have additive effects with drugs that deplete potassium, including corticosteroids (18,19).
DIGOXIN (Lanoxin): Theoretically, overuse of gamboge could decrease potassium levels, increasing the risk of toxicity for cardiac glycoside drugs such as digoxin (Lanoxin) (19).
DIURETIC DRUGS: Overuse of gamboge might compound diuretic-induced potassium loss (19). There is some concern that people taking gamboge along with potassium depleting diuretics might have an increased risk for hypokalemia. Initiation of potassium supplementation or an increase in potassium supplement dose may be necessary for some patients. Some diuretics that can deplete potassium include chlorothiazide (Diuril), chlorthalidone (Thalitone), furosemide (Lasix), and hydrochlorothiazide (HCTZ, Hydrodiuril, Microzide), and others.
STIMULANT LAXATIVES: Concomitant use of gamboge with stimulant laxatives may increase the risk of fluid and electrolyte loss (19).

Interactions with Foods

None known.

Interactions with Lab Tests

None known.

Interactions with Diseases or Conditions

HEART CONDITIONS: Theoretically, overuse/misuse may cause potassium depletion and exacerbate condition.
Gamboge is contraindicated in intestinal obstruction, acute intestinal inflammation (Crohn's disease, ulcerative colitis, appendicitis), ulcer, abdominal pain of unknown origin, nausea, and vomiting.

Dosage and Administration

No typical dosage.

Comments

The resin is extracted from Garcinia hanburyi. Avoid confusion with garcinia (Garcinia cambogia).
Gamboge may be adulterated with rice and wheat starches, sand, and vegetable fragments. These adulterated products are usually coarser and hard (215).

GAMMA BUTYROLACTONE (GBL)

Also Known As

1,2-Butanolide, 2(3H)-Furanone Dihydro, 3-Hydroxybutyric Acid Lactone, 4-Butanolide, 4-Butyrolactone, 4-Hydroxybutanoic Acid Lactone, Dihydro-2(3H)-Furanone, Gamma Butyrolactone, Gamma Hydroxybutyric Acid Lactone, GBL.
CAUTION: See seprate listings for Gamma Hydroxybutyrate (GHB) and Butanediol (BD).

Scientific Names

2,3 dihydro furanone; synonyms 2(3H) furanone dihydro, butyrolactone gamma, 2(3H)-furanone dihydro, butyrolactone, 4-butyrolactone, dihydro-2(3H)-furanone, 4-butanolide, tetrahydro-2-furanone.

People Use This For

Orally, gamma butyrolactone is used for relaxation, calming, increased mental clarity, fat loss, as a body or muscle "builder", recreational drug, for releasing growth hormone, improving athletic performance, inducing and improving sleep, relieving depression and stress, prolonging life, and improving sexual performance and pleasure.

Safety

UNSAFE ...when used orally. The use of GBL or the closely related substances gamma hydroxybutyrate (GHB) and butanediol (BD) has been linked to at least 3 deaths and 122 serious adverse effects (3678,3679). GBL can cause dangerously low respiratory rates and heart rates, seizures, and coma (4259).
PREGNANCY AND LACTATION: UNSAFE ...when used orally (3678,3679); avoid using.

Effectiveness

There is insufficient reliable information available about the effectiveness of gamma butyrolactone (GBL).

Mechanism of Action

Gamma butyrolactone (GBL) is metabolized in the body to gamma hydroxybutyrate (GHB) (see separate listing for GHB) (1430). However, it is more rapidly absorbed than GHB, has greater lipid solubility, and may avoid first-pass metabolism due to its lactone structure (5813). This can lead to higher serum concentrations and more marked hypnotic activity than with similar doses of GHB (5813). GHB can be converted in the brain to the neurotransmitter gamma aminobutyric acid (GABA) (3699), and specific GHB uptake systems, transport systems and receptors have also been identified (713,3699,5800,5801). Stimulation of GHB receptors reduces dopamine release in the brain (713,3699,5801), which may be the mechanism for GBL-induced reductions in dopamine neuronal impulse flow (5811). GBL has been reported to inhibit stereotyped behavior induced by dopamine agonists (5810,5811). The indirect dopamine agonist amphetamine has been reported to partially reverse effects of GBL (5810). GBL may also have some direct GABA agonist activity (5802), although the GABA antagonist bicuculline only partially reverses GBL-induced inhibition of apomorphine activity (5810). GBL, possibly through conversion to GHB, also affects the endogenous opioid system, and the opiate antagonists naloxone and naltrexone attenuate or abolish the electrical seizure activity, behavioral abnormalities, and increased striatal dopamine content produced by GBL (5812). GHB induces REM and non-REM sleep, hypothermia, abnormalities on the EEG similar to those seen in petit mal epilepsy (5800,5803), and it stimulates growth hormone secretion (5804).

Adverse Reactions

Orally, GBL has been associated with a minimum of 55 cases of adverse effects (at least five cases involving children), including involuntary muscle movements, fainting and seizures, bowel incontinence, vomiting, slow breathing, respiratory depression, apnea, slow heart rate, mental changes, severe central nervous system depression, agitation, combativeness, and amnesia. One death, two cases of respiratory arrest, and one case of cardiac arrest have been reported. Nineteen of the 55 cases involved unconsciousness or coma, and in some cases intubation was required for assisted breathing (665,682,1430). Withdrawal symptoms, including insomnia, tremor, anxiety, tachycardia, hypertension, hallucinations, and delirium can occur in chronic users of GBL and GHB (1430,10375,10376).

Interactions with Herbs & Other Dietary Supplements

HERBS AND SUPPLEMENTS WITH SEDATIVE PROPERTIES: Concomitant use is likely to cause additive sedation with GBL, increasing the risk of serious adverse effects.

Interactions with Drugs

ALCOHOL (Ethanol): Concomitant use with GBL and its metabolite GHB may increase the risk of serious CNS and respiratory depression (1430,3678).
AMPHETAMINES: Concomitant use with GHB (a metabolite of GBL) has been associated with severe side effects. Theoretically, concomitant use may also antagonize the effects of GHB (3682).
ANTICONVULSANTS: Theoretically, GHB (a metabolite of GBL) may antagonize the effects of GHB (3682).
ANTIPSYCHOTIC DRUGS: Concomitant use with GHB (a metabolite of GBL) has been associated with severe side effects. Antipsychotics can potentiate the effects of GHB (3682).
BENZODIAZEPINES: Concomitant use with GHB (a metabolite of GBL) has been associated with severe side effects Benzodiazepines can potentiate the effects of GHB (3682).
CNS DEPRESSANTS: Concomitant use with GHB (a metabolite of GBL) has been associated with severe side effects. Additive sedative effects with GBL may occur (3682,3679).
HALOPERIDOL (Haldol): Theoretically, Haloperidol may antagonize the effects of GHB (a metabolite of GBL) (3682).
NALOXONE (Narcan): Theoretically, concomitant use with GHB (a metabolite of GBL) may antagonize the effects of GHB (3682).
NARCOTIC DRUGS: Concomitant use with GHB (a metabolite of GBL) has been associated with severe side effects. Concomitant use of GHB with narcotic drugs can potentiate the therapeutic and adverse effects of narcotic analgesics (3682,3679).
RITONAVIR (Norvir): Concomitant use of the protease inhibitor-type antiretroviral drugs ritonavir and saquinavir with GHB (a metabolite of GBL) reportedly caused a near-fatal reaction, probably due to inhibition of GHB metabolism (1431).
SAQUINAVIR (Fortovase, Invirase): Concomitant use of the protease inhibitor-type antiretroviral drugs ritonavir and saquinavir with GHB (a metabolite of GBL) reportedly caused a near-fatal reaction, probably due to inhibition of GHB metabolism (1431).

SKELETAL MUSCLE RELAXANTS: Concomitant use with GHB (a metabolite of GBL) has been associated with severe side effects. Concomitant use with GHB can potentiate the therapeutic and adverse effects of skeletal muscle relaxants (3682).

Interactions with Foods

ALCOHOL: GHB (a metabolite of GBL) acts synergistically with alcohol to produce CNS and respiratory depression (1430).

Interactions with Lab Tests

None known.

Interactions with Diseases or Conditions

BRADYCARDIA: GHB and GBL should be avoided since they can cause bradycardia (4259).
EPILEPSY: GHB and GBL should be avoided due to their possible capacity to induce seizures (10658).
HYPERTENSION: GHB and GBL should be avoided since they may increase blood pressure (10658).

Dosage and Administration

No typical dosage.

Comments

FDA WARNING: Avoid all gamma butyrolactone containing products due to safety concerns (682). GBL has been marketed as an alternative to gamma hydroxybutyrate (GHB), but it is illegal to manufacture or market GBL or the related products GHB and butanediol (BD) (3678). Publication of a Federal Register notice on 3/13/00 brought into effect the Hillory J. Farias and Samantha Reid Date-Rape Drug Prohibition Act of 2000, which effected changes to the Controlled Substances Act, making GHB a schedule 1 controlled substance (like heroin), and GBL a list 1 chemical (3681). GBL, GHB and BD are associated with at least 122 reports of serious adverse effects including dangerously low respiratory rates (intubation might be required), unconsciousness/coma, vomiting, seizures, slowed heart rate, and death (4259).

GAMMA LINOLENIC ACID

Also Known As

Gamolenic Acid, GLA.
CAUTION: See separate listings for Black Currant, Borage, Evening Primrose Oil, and Omega-6 Oils.

Scientific Names

(Z,Z,Z)-Octadeca-6,9,12-trienoic acid.

People Use This For

Orally, gamma linolenic acid (GLA) is used for rheumatoid arthritis, oral mucoceles (mucous polyps), hyperlipidemia, heart disease, Syndrome-X, systemic sclerosis, diabetic neuropathy, cancer prevention, and to hasten the response to tamoxifen in people with breast cancer. It is also used for attention deficit-hyperactivity disorder (ADHD), depression, postpartum depression, chronic fatigue syndrome, allergic rhinitis, psoriasis, and eczema.

Safety

POSSIBLY SAFE ...when used orally and appropriately. Gamma linolenic acid appears to be safe when taken in oral doses of 2.8 grams per day or less for up to a year (1983,7701,7702,8926).
PREGNANCY AND LACTATION: Insufficient reliable information available; avoid using.

Effectiveness

POSSIBLY EFFECTIVE

Diabetic neuropathy. Taking gamma linolenic acid orally for 6 months to 1 year seems to reduce symptoms and prevent neurological deterioration in neuropathy patients who have type 1 or type 2 diabetes (1980,1981,1984,8926). It seems to be more effective in patients with better glucose control compared to patients with poor glucose control (8926).

POSSIBLY INEFFECTIVE

Scleroderma. Taking gamma linolenic acid orally doesn't seem to be effective for reducing symptoms of scleroderma (1977).

INSUFFICIENT RELIABLE EVIDENCE to RATE

Breast cancer. There is preliminary evidence that taking gamma linolenic acid orally seems to improve the response to tamoxifen in patients with breast cancer (5902). More evidence is needed to rate gamma linolenic acid for this use.

Mechanism of Action

Gamma linolenic acid (GLA) is an omega-6 fatty acid, derived from the seeds of plants such as evening primrose and borage (7701). GLA can be converted to compounds that have anti-inflammatory and antiproliferative properties (1975), including prostaglandins with vasoactive properties. Some research suggests that dihomogammalinolenic acid, a metabolite of GLA and precursor of prostaglandin E1, might act directly on T-cells to modulate immune response in diseases such as rheumatoid arthritis (RA) (7701). There is also some evidence that GLA might reduce interleukin-1-beta (IL-1-beta) auto induction, which is thought to be the cause of synovitis in patients with RA (8134). Preliminary evidence suggests GLA can hasten the response to tamoxifen (Nolvadex) in individuals with estrogen-sensitive primary breast cancer (5902). GLA might have an antiestrogenic effect. It seems to modulate the sensitivity of breast cancer cells to paclitaxel (Taxol) and fulvestrant (Faslodex), enhancing malignant cell killing without adverse effects on normal cells (8133,11791). However, other research suggests that GLA alone can stimulate the growth of breast cancer cells at low concentrations and inhibit growth at higher concentrations (11339).

GLA is believed to benefit individuals who have ischemic lesions associated with systemic sclerosis (1977) and individuals with diabetic neuropathy (1980,1981). Some evidence suggests that gamma linolenic acid might lower plasma triglycerides, increase HDL cholesterol, and prolong bleeding time (1979). Epidemiological research suggests that increased serum levels of GLA might be related to decreased risk for atrophic gastritis associated with Helicobacter pylori (H. pylori) infection. Further study is needed to confirm this observation and to determine a mechanism of action (8709).

Adverse Reactions

Orally, gamma linolenic acid (GLA) can cause mild gastrointestinal effects such as nausea, vomiting, soft stools, diarrhea, flatulence, and belching (7701,7702,8926). GLA might prolong bleeding time (1979).

Interactions with Herbs & Other Dietary Supplements

None known.

Interactions with Drugs

ANTICOAGULANT/ANTIPLATELET DRUGS: Gamma-linolenic acid (GLA) appears to have anticoagulant effects (1979). Theoretically, taking GLA with other anticoagulant or antiplatelet drugs might increase the risk of bruising and bleeding. Some of these drugs include aspirin, clopidogrel (Plavix), nonsteroidal anti-inflammatory drugs (NSAIDs) such as diclofenac (Voltaren, Cataflam, others), ibuprofen (Advil, Motrin, others), naproxen (Anaprox, Naprosyn, others), dalteparin (Fragmin), enoxaparin (Lovenox), heparin, warfarin (Coumadin), and others.

PHENOTHIAZINES: Theoretically, products containing gamma linolenic acid (GLA) and vitamin E might increase the risk of seizures in people being treat concomitantly with phenothiazine drugs (11021); use with caution.

Interactions with Foods

None known.

Interactions with Lab Tests

BLEEDING TIME: Gamma linolenic acid inhibits platelet aggregation and prolongs bleeding time and lab assay results (1979).

LIPID PROFILE: Gamma linolenic acid might lower plasma triglycerides and increase high-density lipoprotein (HDL) cholesterol (1979).

Interactions with Diseases or Conditions

BLEEDING DISORDERS: There is some concern that gamma linolenic acid (GLA) might prolong bleeding time and increase the risk of bruising and bleeding. GLA has platelet inhibiting effects (1979).

Dosage and Administration

ORAL: For rheumatoid arthritis, gamma linolenic acid (GLA) 1.1 grams per day has been used (1985). For diabetic neuropathy, 360 to 480 mg per day has been used (1984,8926). For hyperlipidemia, 1.5-6 grams per day has been used (1976,1979).

GAMMA ORYZANOL

Also Known As

Gamma-Oryzanol, Gamma-OZ, Oryzanol.

Scientific Names

Gamma oryzanol.

People Use This For

Orally, gamma oryzanol is used for hypercholesterolemia and dyslipidemia, increasing testosterone and human growth hormone levels, improving strength during resistance exercise training, and for treating symptoms associated with menopause and aging.

Safety

POSSIBLY SAFE ...when used orally and appropriately (751,752,753,754,755).
PREGNANCY AND LACTATION: Insufficient reliable information available; avoid using.

Effectiveness

POSSIBLY EFFECTIVE

Dyslipidemia. There is some preliminary clinical evidence that gamma oryzanol can significantly decrease total cholesterol, low-density lipoprotein (LDL) cholesterol, and triglyceride levels. Effects on high-density lipoprotein (HDL) cholesterol levels are conflicting (752,757).

There is insufficient reliable information available about the effectiveness of gamma oryzanol for its other uses.

Mechanism of Action

Gamma oryzanol is a group of constituents derived primarily from rice bran oil. It is also found in wheat bran and some fruits and vegetables. Gamma oryzanol itself is poorly absorbed from the gut (755). Researchers think it might help lower cholesterol by decreasing cholesterol absorption from the gut (756). Gamma oryzanol is also often promoted for treating menopause, but it is unclear how it would work for this use. Some researchers suspect it might be helpful due to effects on luteinizing hormone (LH) (755). However, this effect has not been verified in humans. Some people use gamma oryzanol for increasing testosterone and growth hormone levels. However, gamma oryzanol appears to have no effect on these hormone levels (751). Animal studies using parenteral administration actually show gamma oryzanol can be anti-anabolic by suppressing the release of LH and increasing the release of catecholamines, dopamine, and norepinephrine in the brain (755). If this occurs in humans, gamma oryzanol might actually reduce testosterone production (755). There is some evidence gamma oryzanol can reduce elevated serum TSH levels in hypothyroid patients. Some researchers think gamma-oryzanol inhibits serum TSH levels by a direct action at the hypothalamus rather than the pituitary (753).

Adverse Reactions

None reported.

Interactions with Herbs & Other Dietary Supplements

None known.

Interactions with Drugs

None known.

Interactions with Foods

None known.

Interactions with Lab Tests

CHOLESTEROL: Gamma oryzanol can reduce serum total cholesterol (752,757) and low-density lipoprotein (LDL) cholesterol (752) concentrations and test results. Gamma oryzanol might also increase serum high-density lipoprotein (HDL) cholesterol concentrations in some patients (757).
THYROID STIMULATING HORMONE (TSH): Gamma oryzanol can reduce serum TSH concentrations in patients with hypothyroidism (753).
TRIGLYCERIDES: Gamma oryzanol can reduce serum triglyceride concentrations and test results (757).

Interactions with Diseases or Conditions

PRIMARY HYPOTHYROIDISM: Gamma oryzanol can decrease TSH serum levels (753).

Dosage and Administration

ORAL: For reducing serum cholesterol, the usual dose of gamma oryzanol is 300 mg daily (752,757). In one study, 100 mg three times daily was used (752).

Comments

Gamma oryzanol is an extraction product from rice bran oil.

GAMMA-HYDROXYBUTYRATE (GHB)

Also Known As

4-Hydroxy Butyrate, Gamma Hydrate, Gamma Hydroxybutyrate Sodium, Gamma Hydroxybutyric Acid, Gamma-OH, GHB, Sodium Gamma-Hydroxybutyrate, Sodium Oxybate, Sodium Oxybutyrate.
CAUTION: See separate listings for Gamma Butyrolactone (GBL) and Butanediol (BD).

Scientific Names

Gamma hydroxybutyrate; 4-hydroxybutyric acid; Sodium 4-hydroxybutyrate.

People Use This For

Orally, gamma hydroxybutyrate (GHB) is used for reducing weight, enhancing muscle growth, as an aphrodisiac, as an hypnotic, for management of opiate withdrawal and alcohol dependence and withdrawal, and for posthypoxic cerebral edema. It is also used for improving pain, fatigue, and the alpha sleep anomaly in patients with fibromyalgia. GHB is also used orally as a sedative alternative to the dietary supplement L-tryptophan.
As an orphan drug, GHB has been approved by the FDA for treatment of narcolepsy (improving nighttime sleep, and the auxiliary symptoms of cataplexy, sleep paralysis, hypnagogic hallucinations, and automatic behavior).
Intravenously, GHB has been used as part of an anesthetic regimen, and to reduce intracranial pressure associated with trauma.

Safety

POSSIBLY SAFE ...when used orally and appropriately. GHB has FDA orphan drug status (4261).
UNSAFE ...when used orally without medical supervision. GHB can cause serious side effects including dangerously low respiratory rates, tonic-clonic seizure, coma, and death if used inappropriately (3678,3679,3680,3688,4259,10657,10658). GHB can also cause dependence requiring in-patient detoxification (6612,6613,10656).
There is insufficient reliable information available about the safety of GHB for its other uses.
PREGNANCY AND LACTATION: UNSAFE ...when used orally. GHB has been associated with life-threatening toxicities (3678,3679,3680,3688,4259); contraindicated.

Effectiveness

POSSIBLY EFFECTIVE

Alcoholism. Taking GHB orally might reduce alcohol withdrawal symptoms in alcoholics. It also appears to be useful for treating alcohol dependence (3684,3686,3696).
Fibromyalgia. Taking GHB orally seems to help reduce fibromyalgia-associated pain, fatigue, and alpha sleep anomaly (711).
Narcolepsy. Taking GHB orally seems to improve overnight sleep quality and reduce cataplexy in people with narcolepsy (3683,3689,3690,3691,3692). GHB has FDA orphan drug status for treatment of narcolepsy and associated symptoms (4261).
Opiate withdrawal. Taking GHB orally seems to suppress withdrawal symptoms in heroin addicted and methadone-maintained patients (3694,3695).
There is insufficient reliable information available about the effectiveness of GHB for its other uses.

Mechanism of Action

GHB occurs naturally in several areas of the brain, with the highest concentrations found in the basal ganglia. It is also found in other tissues including kidneys, liver, heart, and skeletal muscle and brown fat (3699,3682,10658). In the brain, it is formed as a metabolite of the neurotransmitter gamma aminobutyric acid (GABA), and can also be converted back to GABA during metabolism (3699,10658). Specific uptake and transport systems have been identified for GHB in the brain (3699,5800), and specific GHB receptors have been identified. Stimulation of GHB receptors results in a reduction in dopamine release in the basal ganglia (713,5801,10658), and it also influences dopamine release in the substantia nigra (3699). Some authors suggest that GHB interacts with GABA(B) receptors (713), but others report that GABA formed from GHB is likely involved and that GHB itself is not a GABA agonist (5801,5802). Another GHB metabolite, gamma butyrolactone (GBL) may have some GABA agonist activity (5802). GHB has also been reported to affect the endogenous opioid system, raising dynorphin levels (3682,5803).
GHB induces REM and non-REM sleep, hypothermia, and abnormalities on the EEG similar to those seen in petit mal epilepsy (5800,5803). It stimulates growth hormone secretion which occurs during slow wave sleep (5804); this has led to claims of anabolic effects (3688). It is also involved in preventing the production of, and scavenging, oxygen-derived free radicals in the brain (3682,5805). It decreases brain glucose utilization (3683), lowers cerebral energy requirements, and it may play a neuroprotective role, protecting against the effects of anoxia or excessive metabolic demand (3682,5800,5803). It has been suggested that the natural function of GHB may be to induce and maintain physiological states such as sleep and hibernation in which energy utilization is depressed (5803). Some of the effects of GHB are antagonized by the opiate antagonist, naloxone and anticonvulsant drugs (5800); but the stimulation of growth hormone release is antagonized by flumazenil (a benzodiazepine antagonist) and metergoline (a serotonin receptor antagonist) (5806).

The effects of GHB on sleep have been used to improve nighttime sleep quality, sleep continuity, stage 3 and 4 sleep, and cataplexy in people with narcolepsy, with some studies also reporting a reduction in the number of daytime sleep attacks (3689,3690,3691,3692).
Studies in rats indicate that a cross-tolerance can develop between GHB and ethanol with chronic exposure, leading to investigations of GHB for management of ethanol dependence and withdrawal (3686). Efficacy has also been reported in the management of opiate withdrawal (3694,3695).

Adverse Reactions

Orally, GHB can cause headaches, hallucinations, dizziness, confusion, nausea, vomiting, drowsiness, agitation, and diarrhea. It can also cause sexual arousal, numbing of legs, loss of peripheral vision, tightness of chest, slowed heart rate, depressed respiration, nystagmus, ataxia, eosinophilia-myalgia syndrome, and seizure-like activity (6016,10658). The symptoms usually occur within 15 to 60 minutes and subside within 2 to 96 hours (6016,10658), although dizziness can continue for up to 14 days. Doses of GHB greater than 10 mg/kg can cause amnesia and reduced muscle tone (6016). GHB and the chemically-related products, gamma butyrolactone (GBL) and 1,4 butanediol, have been associated with at least 122 reports of serious adverse reactions including dangerously low respiratory rates, some requiring intubation; unconsciousness and coma; vomiting, seizures; bradycardia; and multiple deaths (3680,4259,10657,10658). At least two deaths involved the use of GHB and alcohol. Death occurred in less than 24 hours after ingestion and was due to circulatory and respiratory collapse. The amount of GHB consumed in these two cases is not known; however, the GHB levels in blood and urine were significantly elevated (6016). GHB can cause dependence requiring in-patient detoxification. Withdrawal syndrome symptoms include nausea, vomiting, diarrhea, diaphoresis, tachycardia, hypertension, delirium with auditory and visual hallucinations; insomnia, panic, terror, anxiety, and tremor (6612,6613,10656,10658).

Interactions with Herbs & Other Dietary Supplements

PRODUCTS WITH SEDATIVE PROPERTIES: Theoretically, concomitant use with herbs that have sedative properties might enhance therapeutic and adverse effects. Some of these supplements include 5-HTP, calamus, California poppy, catnip, hops, Jamaican dogwood, kava, melatonin, St. John's wort, scullcap, valerian, yerba mansa, and others.

Interactions with Drugs

ALCOHOL (Ethanol): Concomitant use may increase the risk of serious CNS and respiratory depression (3678).
AMPHETAMINES: Concomitant use with GHB has been associated with severe side effects. Theoretically, concomitant use may also antagonize the effects of GHB (3682).
ANTICONVULSANTS: Theoretically, GHB may antagonize the effects of GHB (3682).
ANTIPSYCHOTIC DRUGS: Concomitant use with GHB has been associated with severe side effects. Antipsychotics can potentiate the effects of GHB (3682).
BENZODIAZEPINES: Concomitant use with GHB has been associated with severe side effects. Benzodiazepines can potentiate the effects of GHB (3682).
CNS DEPRESSANTS: Concomitant use with GHB has been associated with severe side effects. Additive sedative effects with GBL may occur (3682,3679).
HALOPERIDOL (Haldol): Theoretically, Haloperidol may antagonize the effects of GHB (3682).
NALOXONE (Narcan): Theoretically, concomitant use with GHB may antagonize the effects of GHB (3682).
NARCOTIC DRUGS: Concomitant use with GHB can potentiate the therapeutic and adverse effects of narcotic analgesics. Although GHB has been used with apparent safety to treat narcotic addiction, there is a case report of a fatality with concurrent use of GHB and heroin (3694,3695,5807).
RITONAVIR (Norvir): Concomitant use of the protease inhibitor-type antiretroviral drugs ritonavir and saquinavir with GHB reportedly caused a near-fatal reaction, probably due to inhibition of GHB metabolism (1431).
SAQUINAVIR (Fortovase, Invirase): Concomitant use of the protease inhibitor-type antiretroviral drugs ritonavir and saquinavir with GHB reportedly caused a near-fatal reaction, probably due to inhibition of GHB metabolism (1431).
SKELETAL MUSCLE RELAXANTS: Concomitant use with GHB has been associated with severe side effects. Concomitant use with GHB can potentiate the therapeutic and adverse effects of skeletal muscle relaxants (3682).

Interactions with Foods

ALCOHOL: Concomitant use with GHB can potentiate the CNS and respiratory depression effects of alcohol and GHB (3682).

Interactions with Lab Tests

None known.

Interactions with Diseases or Conditions

BRADYCARDIA: GHB should be avoided since they can cause bradycardia (4259).
EPILEPSY: GHB should be avoided due to their possible capacity to induce seizures (10658).
HYPERTENSION: GHB should be avoided since they may increase blood pressure (10658).

Dosage and Administration

ORAL: For narcolepsy and associate symptoms, a dose of 25 mg/kg at bedtime, repeated 3 hours later has been used (3689,3690). For treating alcohol dependence, 50 to 150 mg/kg divided into 3 to 6 doses per day has been used (3684,3696). As a hypnotic, 75-100 mg/kg has been used (3693).

Comments

Gamma butyrolactone (GBL) and butanediol (BD) are closely related to GHB and produce similar adverse effects (3678,3679). Due to reports of serious adverse effects, the FDA removed GHB from the market in 1990, but clandestine manufacture continued, with the drug being widely available on the Internet, and being implicated as a date rape agent (3687). Publication of a Federal Register notice on 3/13/00 brought into effect the Hillory J. Farias and Samantha Reid Date-Rape Drug Prohibition Act of 2000, which effected changes to the Controlled Substances Act, making GHB a schedule I controlled substance (like heroin), which it is illegal to produce, sell or possess, except for medical use (3680,3681). GHB is available under the generic name sodium oxybate and trade name Xyrem (Orphan Medical), for the treatment of cataplexy associated with narcolepsy. It is a Schedule III Controlled Substance (4261).

GARCINIA

Also Known As

Brindal Berry, Brindle Berry, Gorikapuli, HCA, Hydroxycitrate, Hydroxycitric Acid, Kankusta, Malabar Tamarind, Vrikshamla.
CAUTION: See separate listings for Gamboge, Malabar Nut, Mangosteen, and Tamarind.

Scientific Names

Garcinia gummi-guta, synonyms Cambogia gummi-guta, Garcinia cambogia, Mangostana cambogia.
Family: Clusiaceae/Guttiferae.

People Use This For

Orally, garcinia is used for weight loss, rheumatism, dysentery, as a purgative, and for treating worms and parasites. In foods, garcinia is used as a condiment in Thai and Indian cuisine.

Safety

POSSIBLY SAFE ...when used orally and appropriately for 12 weeks or less (728,11977).
There is insufficient reliable information available about the safety of the long-term use of garcinia.
PREGNANCY AND LACTATION: Insufficient reliable information available; avoid using.

Effectiveness

POSSIBLY INEFFECTIVE

Obesity. Taking garcinia fruit rind extract orally doesn't seem to help decrease weight, satiety, fat oxidation, or energy expenditure in obese people (728,8572,11407). There is some mixed evidence that garcinia might reduce food intake while sustaining satiety, but it's too early to recommend it for this use (8572).

There is insufficient reliable information available about the effectiveness of garcinia for its other uses.

Mechanism of Action

The applicable parts of garcinia are the fruit and rind. Garcinia fruit rind extract, reported to contain 50% hydroxycitrate acid (HCA), is theorized to interfere with lipogenesis (728). The active ingredient HCA is believed to be a competitive inhibitor of ATP-citrate-lyase, the enzyme responsible for converting citrate into acetyl-coenzyme A (acetyl-CoA). This conversion into acetyl-CoA occurs when the energy consumed exceeds the energy requirements of the body (4476,4478,4480). Other researchers think that garcinia inhibits the supply of fatty acids without affecting adipose conversion. Preliminary research suggests that garcinia inhibits the accumulation of lipid droplets in fat cells and thereby reduces lipid levels and decreases lipid accumulation in the liver (8571). The HCA found in garcinia is also theorized to improve exercise endurance by increasing lipid oxidation and decreasing carbohydrate utilization (4487). Some animal research suggests that HCA might suppress appetite (11977).

Adverse Reactions

Orally, garcinia can cause nausea, GI discomfort, and headache (11977).

Interactions with Herbs & Other Dietary Supplements

None known.

Interactions with Drugs

None known.

Interactions with Foods
None known.

Interactions with Lab Tests
None known.

Interactions with Diseases or Conditions
None known.

Dosage and Administration
ORAL: For weight loss, an extract containing 50% hydroxycitric acid, 1000 mg three times daily has been used (728). Hydroxycitric acid, 500 mg four times daily has also been used for weight loss (11407).

Comments
Avoid confusion with gamboge resin (Garcinia hanburyi).

GARDEN CRESS

Also Known As
None.

Scientific Names
Lepidium sativum.
Family: Brassicaceae/Cruciferae.

Comments
At the date of publication, there was very little scientific information available about this product. Our staff is continually analyzing the available information on natural medicines and will add data to the online version of *Natural Medicines Comprehensive Database* as it becomes available. See www.naturaldatabase.com.

GARDEN VIOLET

Also Known As
None.
CAUTION: See separate listing for Sweet Violet.

Scientific Names
Viola odorata.
Family: Violaceae.

Comments
At the date of publication, there was very little scientific information available about this product. Our staff is continually analyzing the available information on natural medicines and will add data to the online version of *Natural Medicines Comprehensive Database* as it becomes available. See www.naturaldatabase.com.

GARLIC

Also Known As
Aged Garlic Extract, Ail, Ajo, Allii Sativi Bulbus, Allium, Camphor of the Poor, Clove Garlic, Lasuna, Nectar of the Gods, Poor Man's Treacle, Rust Treacle, Stinking Rose.

Scientific Names
Allium sativum.
Family: Alliaceae or Liliaceae.

People Use This For

Orally, garlic is used for hypertension, hyperlipidemia, preventing coronary heart disease, preventing age-related vascular changes and atherosclerosis, reducing reinfarction and mortality rate post-myocardial infarction, earaches, and menstrual disorders. Garlic is also used orally for HIV-drug induced lipid disorders, and to treat Helicobacter pylori infection. Garlic is used to prevent colorectal cancer, gastric cancer, breast cancer, lung cancer, to treat and prevent prostate cancer, and to treat bladder cancer. Other uses include treatment of benign prostatic hyperplasia (BPH), diabetes, arthritis, allergies, traveler's diarrhea, colds and flu. It is also used for immune system stimulation, prevention of tick bites, and prevention and treatment of bacterial and fungal infections. Garlic is also used for diarrhea, amoebic and bacterial dysentery, tuberculosis, bloody urine, diphtheria, whooping cough, scalp ringworm, hypersensitive teeth, and vaginal trichomoniasis. Other uses include treatment of fever, coughs, headache, stomachache, sinus congestion, athlete's foot, gout, rheumatism, hemorrhoids, asthma, bronchitis, shortness of breath, arteriosclerosis, low blood pressure, hypoglycemia, hyperglycemia, and snakebites. It is also used as a diuretic, stimulant, cathartic, aphrodisiac, for enhancing circulation, fighting stress and fatigue, and maintaining healthy liver function.

Topically, garlic oil is used for tinea pedis, tinea corporis, tinea cruris, and onychomycosis.

Intravaginally, garlic is used alone or in combination with yogurt for vaginitis.

In foods and beverages, fresh garlic, garlic powder, and garlic oil are used as flavor components.

Safety

LIKELY SAFE ...when used orally and appropriately. Garlic has been used safely in clinical studies lasting up to four years without reports of significant toxicity (1873,4782,4783,4784,4785,4786,4787,4789,4790,4797,4798,6457,6897).

POSSIBLY UNSAFE ...when used topically (585). Garlic applied topically might cause severe skin irritation.

CHILDREN: POSSIBLY SAFE ...when used orally and appropriately, short-term. In one study, garlic extract 300 mg three times daily had side effects comparable to placebo when used in children ages 8-18 years for eight weeks (4796). POSSIBLY UNSAFE ...when used orally in large amounts. Some sources suggest that high doses of garlic could be dangerous or even fatal to children (12); however, the reason for this warning is not known. There are no case reports available of significant adverse events or mortality in children associated with ingestion of garlic.

PREGNANCY: LIKELY SAFE ...when used orally in amounts commonly found in foods (3319). POSSIBLY UNSAFE ...when used orally in medicinal amounts. Garlic is reported to have abortifacient activity (11020). One study also suggests that garlic constituents are distributed to the amniotic fluid after a single dose of garlic (4828). However, there are no published reports of garlic adversely affecting pregnancy. In one study, garlic 800 mg daily was used during the third trimester of pregnancy with no reported adverse outcomes (9201). There is insufficient reliable information available about the safety of topical garlic use during pregnancy.

LACTATION: POSSIBLY UNSAFE ...when used orally in amounts greater than those commonly found in foods. Several small studies suggest that garlic constituents are secreted in breast milk, and that nursing infants of mothers consuming garlic are prone to extended nursing and an altered flavor in breast milk (3319,4829,4830). There is insufficient reliable information available about the safety of topical garlic use during lactation.

Effectiveness

POSSIBLY EFFECTIVE

Atherosclerosis. Taking low doses of garlic powder orally, 300 mg per day, seems to lessen age-related decreases in aortic elasticity. Higher doses of 900 mg per day seem to slow development of atherosclerosis in both aortic and femoral arteries when used over a four-year period (3315,4797,4798).

Colorectal cancer. Several population studies suggest that increased dietary garlic consumption can decrease risk of developing colorectal cancer (3320,4770,4771,4772). However, garlic supplements do not seem to offer this benefit (4773).

Gastric cancer. There is some evidence from population studies that increasing dietary garlic consumption can decrease risk of developing stomach cancer (3320,4775,4776). It's not known if garlic supplements have this same benefit.

Hyperlipidemia. There is controversy over the effectiveness of taking garlic orally for hyperlipidemia. Some studies show no significant benefit (731,732,4792,4793,4794,4795,4807), but the majority of evidence suggests that garlic has modest benefit. It seems to decrease total cholesterol, low-density lipoprotein (LDL) cholesterol, and triglyceride levels (279,4782,4783,4784,4785,4786,4787,6457,6465,6897,9209). When used for 4-25 weeks, garlic seems to lower total cholesterol levels by about 4% to 12% (4786,6457). As a comparison, conventional "statin" drugs typically decrease cholesterol levels by 17% to 55% (6457). Garlic does not seem to affect high-density lipoprotein (HDL) cholesterol (6897). Because of the relatively minor cholesterol level reductions possible with garlic, some clinicians question its value in reducing cardiovascular disease. There is also some concern that garlic may not produce long-term benefits. Some studies show no significant benefit when used for 6 months or longer (6465,6897). Garlic alone is probably not appropriate for patients that require significant reductions in cholesterol levels. Most garlic preparations used in clinical studies were standardized based on the alliin constituent or the allicin yield. But there is also some evidence that aged garlic extracts (odorless garlic) standardized based on the S-allyl-L-cysteine constituent might also be beneficial (1873,1875,1876). Garlic is sometimes given in combination with fish oils (4789,4790) and ginkgo (4791); however, these combinations do not add substantially to the beneficial plasma lipid effects.

Hypertension. There is some evidence that taking garlic orally can modestly reduce blood pressure by 2% to 7% after 4 weeks of treatment (277,278,279,1873,6897).

Prostate cancer. Men who eat 2.14 grams of garlic (about one clove) per day seem to have a 50% decrease in the risk of developing prostate cancer (9876). There is preliminary evidence that suggests garlic supplements can also decrease the risk of developing prostate cancer (4777). There is also preliminary evidence that suggests a garlic extract might help improve urinary flow, decrease urinary frequency, and reduce other symptoms associated with prostate cancer (10374).

Tick bites. People consuming high doses of garlic (1200 mg daily) over a 20-week period seem to have a reduced number of tick bites when compared to controls (3318,8027).

Tinea corporis. Applying a garlic gel containing 0.6% ajoene seems to be as effective as terbinafine 1% cream for tinea corporis (4767).

Tinea cruris. Applying a garlic gel containing 0.6% ajoene seems to be as effective as terbinafine 1% cream for tinea cruris (4767).

Tinea pedis (athlete's foot). Applying a garlic gel containing 1% ajoene seems to be more effective than 0.6% ajoene gel, and seems to be as effective as 1% terbinafine (Lamisil) for tinea pedis infections. Sixty days after completing one week of treatment 1% ajoene produces 100% mycologic cure, 0.6 % produces 72% mycologic cure, and 1% terbinafine produces 94% mycologic cure (4766,8019).

POSSIBLY INEFFECTIVE

Breast cancer. Taking garlic orally does not seem to decrease the risk of developing breast cancer (4779).

Diabetes. Taking garlic orally has no significant effect on glucose in persons with or without diabetes (6465,6897).

Familial hypercholesterolemia. In children with familial hyperlipidemia, taking garlic powdered extract, standardized based on alliin content, orally does not seem to significantly improve total serum cholesterol, low-density lipoprotein (LDL) or high-density lipoprotein (HDL) cholesterol levels, triglycerides, lipoprotein (a), apolipoprotein B-100, homocysteine, fibrinogen, or blood pressure (4796).

Helicobacter pylori (H pylori). Taking garlic orally for H. pylori infection used to look promising due to laboratory and epidemiological evidence showing potential activity against H. pylori. However, when garlic cloves, powder, or oil is used in humans, it doesn't seem to have any beneficial effect for treating patients infected with H. pylori (3316,3322,4761,4762,4763,4764,4765,4774).

Lung cancer. Taking garlic orally does not seem to decrease the risk of developing lung cancer (4778).

Peripheral arterial disease. After 12 weeks of treatment, taking garlic orally does not seem to improve walking distance in patients with stage II peripheral arterial occlusive disease (4801,4809).

Most clinical studies have used the brand name product Kwai (Lichtwer Pharma), a dried garlic powder preparation standardized to contain 1.3% alliin. Some studies have used the brand name product Kyolic (Wakunaga of America), an aged garlic extract standardized based on the S-allyl-L-cysteine constituent.

INSUFFICIENT RELIABLE EVIDENCE to RATE

Benign prostatic hyperplasia (BPH). There is some preliminary evidence that taking garlic orally might be helpful for improving urinary flow, decreasing urinary frequency, and other symptoms associated with BPH (10374).

Common cold. Preliminary clinical research suggests garlic might reduce the frequency and number of colds when taken prophylactically (10787).

More evidence is needed to rate garlic for these uses.

Mechanism of Action

The applicable part of garlic is the bulb. Garlic is mostly used for its antihyperlipidemic, antihypertensive, and antifungal effects. However, it is also reported to have antibacterial, anthelmintic, antiviral, antispasmodic, diaphoretic, expectorant, immunostimulant, and antithrombotic effects (3234,4366,4768,8017,8018). Many of the pharmacological effects of garlic are attributed to the allicin, ajoene, and other organosulfur constituents such as S-allyl-L-cysteine (8017).

It's thought that the effectiveness of garlic products might to be determined by their ability to yield allicin, which in turn triggers production of other active constituents (3251). Intact garlic cells in fresh garlic contain the odorless amino acid, alliin. When intact cells are broken, alliin comes into contact with the enzyme allinase in garlic, producing allicin, an unstable, odiferous compound (3251,4768). Fresh garlic contains approximately 1% alliin. One milligram of alliin is converted to 0.458 mg allicin (4800). Further conversion yields ajoene. The amount of allicin in garlic preparations is dependent upon the method of preparation. Processes that involve maceration of the garlic clove increase the activity of allicinase. Freeze-dried garlic may contain little or no allicin. To improve effectiveness, garlic preparations may be enteric coated to protect the active constituents from degeneration by stomach acid (9203). Heat and steam distillation used to produce garlic oil from crushed garlic converts allicin to allyl sulfides which are also thought to have biological activity (3251). Garlic is aged to reduce the content of other sulfur compounds and the odor commonly associated with garlic. The process to produce odorless aged garlic extract reduces the alliin content to only 3% of what is typically contained in fresh garlic (4800). Aged garlic extract is usually standardized to S-allyl-L-cysteine, another major organosulfur constituent in garlic (3234).

In patients with hyperlipidemia, garlic might lower cholesterol levels by acting as a HMG-CoA reductase inhibitor (statin) (4810,4811). There is some evidence the constituent S-allyl-L-cysteine may be a potent inhibitor of hepatic cholesterol synthesis (8407).

For age-related vascular changes and atherosclerosis, garlic is thought to be beneficial and protect vascular endothelial cells from injury by reducing oxidative stress, inhibiting low-density lipoprotein (LDL) oxidation, and through antithrombotic effects (1880,4813,8017,8408). There is evidence that LDL oxidation may be inhibited by the constituents S-allyl cysteine, S-allyl mercaptocysteine, alliin, allixin, and by N-acetyl-S-allyl cysteine, a metabolite of S-allyl cysteine (8408). Garlic appears to prevent endothelial cell depletion of glutathione, which may be responsible for its antioxidant effects (1880).

Garlic powder and aged garlic preparations have been shown to have antiplatelet properties in both patients with cardiovascular disease and in healthy volunteers (1874,3234,4366,4802,4803). Garlic has been found to have antithrombotic properties and can increase fibrinolytic activity, decrease platelet aggregation and adhesion, increase the prothrombin time (PT), and inhibit metabolic enzymes in platelets responsible for the conversion of arachidonic acid into prostaglandins and other products (3234,4366,8017,12423). Raw garlic seems to have more potent antiplatelet properties than cooked garlic (4799,4804). Garlic oil does not appear to affect platelet aggregation (4805).

For hypertension, garlic is thought to reduce blood pressure by causing smooth muscle relaxation and vasodilation by activating production of endothelium-derived relaxation factor (EDRF, nitric oxide) (4812).

There is preliminary evidence that suggests garlic and aged garlic extract may have pharmacological effects that are similar to Bacillus Calmette-Guerin (BCG) vaccine in the treatment of bladder cancer (8018). Garlic also seems to have humoral and cellular immunostimulant activity. There is evidence garlic and aged garlic extract might stimulate T-cell proliferation; restore suppressed antibody responses; stimulate macrophage cytotoxicity and phagocytosis of tumor cells; and induce the release of interleukin-2 (IL-2), tumor necrosis factor-alpha (TNF-alpha), and gamma interferon (8018). The constituents in garlic S-allyl cysteine and S-allyl mercaptocysteine have been shown to have radical scavenging activity. S-allyl mercaptocysteine has also been shown to have activity against erythroleukemic cancer cells, breast cancer cells, and prostate cancer cells (1871,1877,1878,1879,1880,1881,1882). The constituent ajoene has been observed to induce apoptosis in human leukemia cells (8017). Laboratory evidence suggests garlic may induce detoxifying enzymes such as glutathione-S-transferase to remove harmful electrophiles from carcinogens (8017). Additionally, garlic might enhance selenium absorption and protect against tumorigenesis (4815).

The constituents allicin and ajoene are thought to be responsible for garlic's antifungal activity against tinea infections (8017,8019). Fresh garlic, but not aged garlic, has shown activity against Escherichia coli, methicillin-resistant Staph aureus, salmonella enteritidis, and Candida albicans in the laboratory; it has been suggested as a food additive to prevent food poisoning (4808). Preliminary evidence suggests that garlic compounds might have activity against viruses such as herpes simplex virus type 1, herpes simplex virus type 2, parainfluenza virus type 3, vaccinia virus, vesicular stomatitis virus, and human rhinovirus type 2 (4769).

S-allyl cysteine and S-allyl mercaptocysteine might protect the liver against acetaminophen and carbon tetrachloride, according to laboratory studies (9873). Other preliminary evidence suggests S-allyl cysteine might ameliorate doxorubicin-induced cardiac and hepatic toxicity (4780). Preliminary reports regarding possible hepatoprotective effects of aged garlic extract have been conflicting (1883,1884). Early evidence suggests a possible protective effect of aged garlic on intestinal toxicity induced by methotrexate (MTX) and fluorouracil (5FU) (1885,9208). Preliminary evidence suggests that garlic might interfere with the oral absorption of lead; the sulfur containing amino acids might chelate lead in the gastrointestinal tract (9202).

Preliminary clinical research suggests some compounds in garlic, such as S-methylcysteine sulfoxide and S-allylcysteine sulfoxide, might have some antidiabetic activity (9875). However, garlic doesn't seem to affect blood glucose in people without diabetes (9874). There are no reports of garlic affecting blood glucose in patients with diabetes.

Samgyetang, a soup made from chicken, jujube, panax ginseng, garlic, and chestnuts, appears to offer protection from experimentally induced peptic ulcers (10249).

There is some evidence that garlic might affect the cytochrome P450 (CYP450) enzyme system. In vitro evidence suggests that garlic might inhibit several CYP450 enzymes including CYP2C9, CYP2C19, and CYP3A4 (12198). Some findings indicate that garlic might mildly inhibit CYP2D6 activity by about 9% in humans (1303). This limited inhibition is not likely to produce clinically significant increases in drugs that are metabolized by the CYP2D6 isoenzyme. However, researchers suspect that garlic supplements containing allicin induce the CYP3A4 isoenzyme and can produce clinical significant decreases in levels of drugs metabolized by this enzyme (7027). An extract, containing alliin and alliinase, does not affect the activity of CYP2D6 or CYP3A4 (10335). The ability of garlic to induce or inhibit cytochrome P450 enzymes may depend upon the presence of other constituents in the preparation that is being used.

Adverse Reactions

Orally, garlic has dose-related adverse effects, which most commonly include breath and body odor, mouth and gastrointestinal burning or irritation, heartburn, flatulence, nausea, vomiting, and diarrhea. These effects can be more pronounced with consumption of raw garlic or in patients unaccustomed to eating garlic (3319,4783,4800). Oral use of garlic can also cause changes to the intestinal flora (3319,4800), which might result in gastrointestinal upset. Garlic's effect on platelet function is well known, and can possibly increase the risk of bleeding. Consumption of dietary garlic has caused platelet dysfunction, prolonged bleeding time, retrobulbar hemorrhage (bleeding behind the eye) postoperative bleeding, and spinal epidural hematoma (586,587,11325). Asthma has been reported in people working with garlic (4816,8017). Other allergic reactions associated with garlic include rhinitis, conjunctivitis, urticaria, anaphylaxis, and angioedema (6897). True IgE-mediated garlic allergy seems to be relatively rare, but can

occur more often in young people with pollen allergy (4816).
Topically, exposure and application of fresh garlic has caused dermatitis, eczema, blisters, and scarring (3317,4832,4833,8017). Application of a garlic poultice has caused ulcernecrotic lesions and burns that are similar in appearance to a second or third degree burn. Lesions usually heal without scarring within 3 weeks after discontinuation of the poultice (8017).

Interactions with Herbs & Other Dietary Supplements

EICOSAPENTAENOIC ACID (EPA, Fish Oils): Concomitant use of garlic can theoretically enhance antithrombotic effects (3234,4366,8017).
HERBS WITH ANTICOAGULANT/ANTIPLATELET POTENTIAL: Concomitant use of herbs that have constituents that might affect platelet aggregation could theoretically increase the risk of bleeding in some people. These herbs include angelica, clove, danshen, ginger, ginkgo, red clover, turmeric, vitamin E, willow, and others (1874,3234,4366,4802,4803).

Interactions with Drugs

ANTICOAGULANT/ANTIPLATELET DRUGS: Garlic might enhance the effects of warfarin (Coumadin) as measured by the International Normalized Ratio (INR) (616). Theoretically, garlic might also enhance the effects and adverse effects of other anticoagulant and antiplatelet drugs, including aspirin, clopidogrel (Plavix), enoxaparin (Lovenox), and others.
CONTRACEPTIVE DRUGS: The effect of garlic preparations on the metabolism of contraceptive drugs may vary. Some garlic preparations containing allicin might decrease the effectiveness of contraceptive drugs by increasing the activity of the cytochrome P450 3A4 (CYP3A4) isoenzyme (7027). However, other extracts, containing alliin and alliinase may not affect the activity of CYP3A4 (10335). Until more is known about this potential interaction, advise women taking garlic supplements and contraceptive drugs concurrently to use an additional or alternative form of birth control.
CYCLOSPORINE (Neoral, Sandimmune): The affect of garlic preparations on the metabolism of cyclosporine may vary. Some garlic preparations containing allicin might decrease the effectiveness of cyclosporine by increasing the activity of the cytochrome P450 3A4 (CYP3A4) isoenzyme (7027). However, other extracts, containing alliin and alliinase may not affect the activity of CYP3A4 (10335). Until more is known about this potential interaction, patients that are taking cyclosporine should avoid using garlic preparations.
CYTOCHROME P450 3A4 (CYP3A4) SUBSTRATES: It appears that some garlic preparations containing allicin may increase the activity of the cytochrome P450 3A4 (CYP3A4) isoenzymes (7027). However, other extracts, containing alliin and alliinase may not affect the activity of CYP3A4 (10335). Until more is known about this potential interaction, use caution when considering concomitant use of garlic and other drugs affected by this system. Drugs that might be affected include some calcium channel blockers (diltiazem, nicardipine, verapamil), chemotherapeutic agents (etoposide, paclitaxel, vinblastine, vincristine, vindesine), antifungals (ketoconazole, itraconazole), glucocorticoids, alfentanil (Alfenta), cisapride (Propulsid), fentanyl (Sublimaze), lidocaine (Xylocaine), losartan (Cozaar), fexofenadine (Allegra), midazolam (Versed), and others.
NON-NUCLEOSIDE REVERSE TRANSCRIPTASE INHIBITORS (NNRTIs): Some garlic preparations containing allicin may decrease plasma concentrations of the protease inhibitor saquinavir (Fortovase, Invirase) (7027). However, other extracts, containing alliin and alliinase may not affect the activity of CYP3A4 (10335). NNRTIs and protease inhibitors are metabolized through similar routes. Until more is known about this potential interaction, patients taking these medications should avoid using garlic. NNRTI-type antiretroviral drugs include nevirapine (Viramune), delavirdine (Rescriptor), and efavirenz (Sustiva).
SAQUINAVIR (Fortovase, Invirase): The effect of garlic preparations on the metabolism of saquinavir may vary. Some garlic preparations containing allicin might decrease area under the curve (AUC) of saquinavir by 51%. Peak concentrations of saquinavir might be decreased by 54% and mean levels decreased by 49%. These decreases are thought to be due to induction of the cytochrome P450 3A4 (CYP3A4) isoenzyme (7027). These subtherapeutic concentrations might cause therapeutic failure, increase development of viral resistance, and development of drug class resistance. However, other extracts, containing alliin and alliinase may not affect the activity of CYP3A4 (10335). Prolonged use (e.g., 10 days) of garlic supplements seems to be necessary for significant enzyme induction. Therefore, even occasional moderate to high consumption of garlic from dietary sources is not expected to cause a significant interaction. So far, this interaction has only been shown for saquinavir, but other protease inhibitors are also likely to be affected. Until more is known about this potential interaction, patients taking these medications should avoid taking garlic. Other protease inhibitors include amprenavir (Agenerase), nelfinavir (Viracept), and ritonavir (Norvir).
WARFARIN (Coumadin): Garlic might enhance the effects of warfarin (Coumadin) as measured by the International Normalized Ratio (INR) (616). Monitor patients using this combination closely. Dose adjustment may be necessary.

Interactions with Foods

None known.

Interactions with Lab Tests

BLOOD PRESSURE: Garlic can lower blood pressure and blood pressure readings (277,278,279).
CHOLESTEROL: Garlic can lower serum cholesterol concentrations and test results (277,278,279).
INTERNATIONAL NORMALIZED RATIO (INR), PROTHROMBIN TIME (PT): Garlic can increase INR in patients anticoagulated with warfarin (Coumadin). There are two case reports of increased INR associated with concomitant use of garlic products and warfarin (616).

Interactions with Diseases or Conditions

BLEEDING DISORDERS: Theoretically, garlic might increase the risk of bleeding (3234,4366,8017); contraindicated.
GASTROINTESTINAL (GI) IRRITATION: Garlic can irritate the GI tract; use with caution in individuals with infectious or inflammatory GI conditions (3319,4783,4800).
SURGERY: Garlic can prolong bleeding time and should be discontinued one to two weeks prior to scheduled surgery (587,4800,11325).

Dosage and Administration

ORAL: For hyperlipidemia and hypertension, garlic extract 600-1200 mg divided and given three times daily has been used in clinical trials. Most clinical studies have used a standardized garlic powder extract containing 1.3% alliin content (279,3321,4782,4783,4784,4785,4786,4787,4788,4789,4790,4791,6457,6465,6897). Aged garlic extract 600 mg to 7.2 grams per day has also been used. Aged garlic typically contains only 0.03% alliin (1874,1875,3319,3321). Fresh garlic 4 grams (approximately one clove) once daily has also been used. Fresh garlic typically contains 1% alliin (3319,4800). For prevention of colorectal and stomach cancer, fresh or cooked garlic 3.5-29 grams weekly has been used (3320). Garlic preparations are sometimes dosed based on the allicin constituent. For every milligram of alliin, 0.458 mg of allicin is typically generated. Therefore, a dose of garlic extract 600 mg that contains 1.3% alliin typically produces 3600 mcg allicin. A dose of fresh garlic 4 grams containing 1% alliin typically produces approximately 18,300 mcg of allicin.
TOPICAL: For tinea infections, clinical studies have used the garlic constituent ajoene as a 0.4% cream, 0.6% gel, and 1% gel applied twice daily for 1 week (4766,4767,8019).

Comments

There is some concern than marketed garlic preparations may not generate an adequate amount of the active ingredient allicin to be effective. There is a lot of variation among garlic products (9203). Some odorless garlic preparations may not contain active compounds at all (1877).

GELATIN

Also Known As

Collagen Hydrolysate, Denatured Collagen, Gelatine, Hydrolyzed Collagen Protein, Hydrolyzed Gelatin.

Scientific Names

Gelatin.

People Use This For

Orally, gelatin is used for osteoarthritis; osteoporosis; rheumatoid arthritis; weight loss; and strengthening bones, joints, and fingernails. It is also used for improving the quality of scalp hair and to shorten recovery after exercise and sports-related injury.
In manufacturing, gelatin is used for preparation of foods, cosmetics, and pharmaceuticals.

Safety

LIKELY SAFE ...when used orally in amounts commonly found in foods. Gelatin has Generally Recognized As Safe (GRAS) status in the US (4912).
POSSIBLY SAFE ...when used orally and appropriately in medicinal amounts (7704). There's some evidence that gelatin in doses up to 10 grams daily can be safely used for up to 6 months (7704). However, since gelatin is often derived from bovine bones and skin, there is some concern about contamination with diseased animal parts (1825). So far, there are no reports of disease transmission to humans due to use of contaminated gelatin preparations.
PREGNANCY AND LACTATION: There is insufficient reliable information available about the safety of gelatin during pregnancy and lactation when used in medicinal amounts.

Effectiveness

INSUFFICIENT RELIABLE EVIDENCE to RATE

Osteoarthritis. There is some clinical evidence that gelatin might relieve pain and improve joint function in patients with osteoarthritis (7704). More evidence is needed to rate gelatin for this use.

Mechanism of Action

Gelatin is a purified protein formed by hydrolysis of collagen obtained from the bones and hides of pigs and cows (7704). There is preliminary research in animal models of rheumatoid arthritis that suggests gelatin in combination with the antioxidant enzyme superoxide dismutase (SOD) might suppress joint inflammation. Oxygen radicals are thought to play a role in the joint damage caused by rheumatoid arthritis (7707).

There is preliminary research that gelatin might inhibit bone collagen breakdown in people with osteoporosis (7704). Gelatin may also cause increased production of collagen by chondrocytes. Chondrocytes are the cells responsible for maintenance of the connective tissue in the joints (10345).

Adverse Reactions

Orally, gelatin can cause unpleasant taste, sensation of heaviness in the stomach, bloating, dyspepsia, and belching (7704).

Gelatin can cause allergic reactions. Gelatin in foods can cause initial sensitization (7703).

Gelatin-containing medicines including oral medications, suppositories, vaccines, and injectable products can cause IgE-medicated allergic reactions, including urticaria, angioedema, wheezing, hypotension, and anaphylaxis (7708,7709,7710). In the US, gelatin is used as a stabilizer in some vaccines such as measles, mumps, and rubella (MMR), and diphtheria, pertussis, tetanus (DPT) (7711). Since gelatin is sometimes produced from bovine bones and skin, there is some concern about the potential risk of contamination with diseased animals and transmission of bovine spongiform encephalopathy (BSE, mad cow disease) and other diseases. Although bovine hide and bone tissue do not seem to carry a high risk of BSE disease infectivity, in some cases manufacturing methods might lead to contamination with other diseased animal tissues. So far there are no reports of BSE or other disease transmission to humans from dietary supplements containing animal materials and the risk of potential disease transmission is thought to be low. Although many manufacturers 'guarantee' the safety of their gelatin products, most manufacturers do not seem to take adequate measures to eliminate the risk of contamination.

Interactions with Herbs & Other Dietary Supplements

None known.

Interactions with Drugs

None known.

Interactions with Foods

None known.

Interactions with Lab Tests

None known.

Interactions with Diseases or Conditions

None known.

Dosage and Administration

ORAL: For osteoporosis, 10 grams daily has been used (7704).

Comments

Gelatin-chondroitin complexes have been investigated as intra-articular drug delivery systems to treat osteoporosis and rheumatoid arthritis (7706).

GELSEMIUM

Also Known As

Caroline Jasmine, Evening Trumpet Flower, False Jasmine, Gelsemii Rhizoma, Gelsemin, Gelsemiumwurzelstock Jessamine, Trumpet Flower, Woodbine, Yellow Jasmine, Yellow Jessamine Root.

CAUTION: See separate listings for Jasmine, American Ivy, Honeysuckle, and Woodbine.

Scientific Names

Gelsemium sempervirens, synonyms Gelsemium nitidum, Bignonia sempervirens.

Family: Loganiaceae or Gelsemiaceae.

People Use This For

Orally, gelsemium is used as an analgesic for trigeminal neuralgia and migraine headaches, and for asthma and in respiratory ailments.

Safety

UNSAFE ...when the rhizome or root are used orally. All parts of the plant contain toxic alkaloids. The adult lethal dose is 2-3 grams or 4 mL of the fluid extract (18).
CHILDREN: UNSAFE ...when used orally. The lethal dose is 500 mg (18).
PREGNANCY AND LACTATION: UNSAFE ...when used orally due to toxicity (6).

Effectiveness

There is insufficient reliable information available about the effectiveness of gelsemium.

Mechanism of Action

The applicable parts of gelsemium are the rhizome and root. Researchers think the active components in gelsemium are gelsamine alkaloids and related compounds (gelsemine, gelsemicine, gelsedine) (6). Gelsemium and the principal alkaloid, gelsemine, are reported to have CNS stimulant (6), CNS depressant (9), and analgesic effects (6).

Adverse Reactions

Orally, gelsemium can cause headache, drooping of the eyelid, double vision, difficulty swallowing, dizziness, muscle weakness or rigidity, seizures, dyspnea, and bradycardia. Death due to failure of respiratory muscles can occur (18).

Interactions with Herbs & Other Dietary Supplements

None known.

Interactions with Drugs

None known.

Interactions with Foods

None known.

Interactions with Lab Tests

None known.

Interactions with Diseases or Conditions

HEART DISEASE and WEAKNESS: Use of gelsemium is contraindicated in people with heart disease or weakness (18).

Dosage and Administration

ORAL: People typically use 0.3 to 1 mL gelsemium tincture (223).

Comments

There is a very narrow safety margin and medicinal preparations are considered obsolete (18). Avoid confusion with jasmine or woodbine (Clematis virginiana). Also, avoid confusing gelsemium with American ivy or honeysuckle, which are also known as woodbine.

GENISTEIN COMBINED POLYSACCHARIDE

Also Known As

Basidiomycetes Polysaccharide, Fermented Genistein, Fermented Isoflavone, Genistein Polysaccharide, GCP, Isoflavone Combined Polysaccharide, Soy Isoflavone Polysaccharide.
CAUTION: See separate listing for Soy.

Scientific Names

Genistein Combined Polysaccharide.

People Use This For

Orally, genistein combined polysaccharide is used for prostate cancer and breast cancer.

Safety

There is insufficient reliable information available about the safety of genistein combined polysaccharide.
Pregnancy and Lactation: Insufficient reliable information; avoid using.

Effectiveness

INSUFFICIENT RELIABLE EVIDENCE to RATE

Prostate cancer. There is anecdotal evidence that a patient with prostate cancer who took genistein combined polysaccharide had reduced prostate size and decreased PSA levels from 19.7 to 4.2 ng/mL after 6 weeks of treatment (12110). More evidence is needed to rate genistein combined polysaccharide for this use.

Mechanism of Action

Genistein combined polysaccharide is a soy-based product. It consists of a mixture of the soy isoflavone genistein and polysaccharide from the basidiomycetes, which are a variety of mushrooms. It is prepared by a fermentation in which a soy extract is fermented with basidiomycetes mushrooms (12110).

The fermentation process deglycosylates existing soy isoflavones in addition to forming novel isoflavones specific to this process (12110).

Both the genistein and polysaccharide components are thought to have pharmacological activity. Genistein is a phytoestrogen. It binds to beta-estrogen receptor more strongly that alpha-estrogen receptor. The beta-estrogen receptor predominates in the heart, vasculature, bone, and bladder. This might account for some of the beneficial effects attributed to phytoestrogens (3983).

Genistein seems to decrease expression of aromatase and 5-alpha reductase (12110). Some researchers suspect this might give genistein antiproliferative effects against hormone-dependent cancers such as breast cancer and prostate cancer. Genistein also seems to have antioxidant and antiangiogenic effects (3983).

In an animal model, genistein combined polysaccharide seems to inhibit breast cancer tumor proliferation by inducing apoptosis (12197).

Genistein is also an inhibitor of epidermal growth factor receptor tyrosine kinase (12110).

Polysaccharides from basidiomycetes are thought to have antiviral, antibacterial, antitumor, and immune modulating effects (12110).

Adverse Reactions

None reported.

Interactions with Herbs & Other Dietary Supplements

None known.

Interactions with Drugs

None known.

Interactions with Foods

None known.

Interactions with Lab Tests

None known.

Interactions with Diseases or Conditions

ESTROGEN SENSITIVE CANCERS/CONDITIONS: Genistein combined polysaccharide might have mild estrogenic effects (3983). Women with estrogen-sensitive conditions should avoid genistein combined polysaccharide. Some estrogen-sensitive conditions include breast cancer, uterine cancer, ovarian cancer, endometriosis, and uterine fibroids.

Dosage and Administration

ORAL: For prostate cancer, 1.5 grams/day has been used (12110).

GENTIAN

Also Known As

Bitter Root, Bitterwort, Gall Weed, Gentiana, Gentianae radix, Pale Gentian, Stemless Gentian, Yellow Gentian, Wild Gentian.

CAUTION: See separate listing for Canadian Hemp.

Scientific Names

Gentiana lutea; Gentiana acaulis, synonym Gentiana kochiana.

Family: Gentianaceae.

People Use This For

Orally, gentian is used for digestive disorders, such as loss of appetite, fullness, flatulence, diarrhea, gastritis, heartburn, and vomiting. It is used orally for fever, for hysteria, to stimulate menstrual flow, as an anthelmintic, and antiseptic.
Topically, gentian is used for treating wounds and cancer.
In combination with European elder flower, verbena, cowslip flower, and sorrel, gentian is used orally for maintaining healthy sinuses and treating sinusitis. It is used in combination with other products for malaria.
In foods and beverages, gentian is used as an ingredient.
In manufacturing, gentian is used in cosmetics.

Safety

LIKELY SAFE ...when the root preparations are used in amounts commonly found in foods. Gentian root has Generally Recognized As Safe status (GRAS) for use in foods in the US (4912).
POSSIBLY SAFE ...when used orally in therapeutic amounts (2). ...when gentian root is used orally with European elder flower, verbena, cowslip flower, and sorrel (Quanterra Sinus Defense, Sinupret) (7,374,379).
There is insufficient reliable information available about the safety of the topical use of gentian.
PREGNANCY: LIKELY UNSAFE ...when used orally; gentian is a potential mutagen and may effect the menstrual cycle (4).
LACTATION: Insufficient reliable information available; avoid using.

Effectiveness

POSSIBLY EFFECTIVE

Sinusitis. Taking gentian orally in a specific combination product that also contains elderflower, verbena, cowslip flower, and sorrel (Quanterra Sinus Defense, Sinupret) seems help treat acute or chronic sinusitis (374,379).

There is insufficient reliable information available about the effectiveness of gentian for its other uses.

Mechanism of Action

The applicable part of gentian is the root. The bitter constituents, gentiamarin, gentiopicrin, amarogentin, and swertiamarin, seem to increase saliva and digestive juice secretion (2,4). Some evidence suggests the constituent gentianine has anti-inflammatory activity (11). The constituents, gentisin and isogentisin, are both mutagenic (4). The constituent gentiopicrin is lethal to mosquito larvae (11).

Adverse Reactions

Orally, gentian root can cause gastrointestinal (GI) irritation, nausea, and vomiting (6). It can also cause headaches in individuals sensitive to bitter substances (12).

Interactions with Herbs & Other Dietary Supplements

None known.

Interactions with Drugs

ANTACIDS: Theoretically, due to reports that gentian increases stomach acid, gentian might decrease the effectiveness of antacids (19).
H2-BLOCKERS: Theoretically, due to reports that gentian increases stomach acid, gentian might decrease the effectiveness of H2-blockers (19). The H2 blockers include cimetidine (Tagamet), ranitidine (Zantac), nizatidine (Axid), and famotidine (Pepcid).
PROTON PUMP INHIBITORS (PPIs): Theoretically, due to reports that gentian increases stomach acid, gentian might decrease the effectiveness of PPIs (19). PPIs include omeprazole (Prilosec), lansoprazole (Prevacid), rabeprazole (Aciphex), pantoprazole (Protonix), and esomeprazole (Nexium).

Interactions with Foods

None known.

Interactions with Lab Tests

None known.

Interactions with Diseases or Conditions

DUODENAL AND GASTRIC ULCERS: Contraindicated due to bitter constituents (2).
GASTRIC IRRITATION OR INFLAMMATION: Contraindicated due to bitter constituents (12).
HYPERTENSION: Gentian root may not be well-tolerated in hypertensive individuals (5).

Dosage and Administration

ORAL: The typical dose of gentian is 0.6-2 grams of the dried root three times daily with a maximum of 4 grams per day. One cup of the tea is also taken three times daily (2,4,18). The tea is prepared by steeping 0.6-2 grams of the dried root in 150 mL boiling water for 5-10 minutes and then straining (2,4,18). The tea can be sweetened with honey. The common dose of the tincture (1:5 in 45% alcohol) is 1-3 grams daily (2) or 1-4 mL three times daily (4). The usual dose of the fluid extract is 2-4 grams daily (2). The irritating qualities of the gentian root are minimized in the tea and maximized in the tincture form (12).

For acute or chronic sinusitis, two Sinupret tablets three times daily for up to two weeks has been used in clinical trials (7,374,379), equivalent to gentian root 12 mg, European elder flower 36 mg, verbena 36 mg, cowslip flower 36 mg, and sorrel 36 mg three times daily.

TOPICAL: No typical dosage.

Comments

The highly toxic white hellebore (Veratrum album) can grow in proximity to gentian and has caused accidental poisoning when used in home-made preparations (11). A related Gentiana species is used in Chinese medicine for treating jaundice, headache, sores, inflammation, and rheumatoid arthritis (11). The gentian root is unrelated to the gentian violet dye.

GERMAN CHAMOMILE

Also Known As

Blue Chamomile, Camomilla, Camomille Allemande, Chamomilla, Echte Kamille, Feldkamille, Fleur de Camomile, Hungarian Chamomile, Kamillen, Kleine Kamille, Manzanilla, Matricaire, Matricariae Flos, Pin Heads, Sweet False Chamomile, True Chamomile, Wild Chamomile.

CAUTION: See separate listing for Roman Chamomile.

Scientific Names

Matricaria recutita, synonyms Chamomilla recutita, Matricaria chamomilla.

Family: Asteraceae/Compositae.

People Use This For

Orally, German chamomile is used for flatulence, travel sickness, nasal mucous membrane inflammation, allergic rhinitis, nervous diarrhea, attention deficit-hyperactivity disorder (ADHD), restlessness, and insomnia. It is also used for gastrointestinal (GI) spasms, inflammatory diseases of the GI tract, GI ulcers associated with nonsteroidal anti-inflammatory drugs (NSAIDs) and alcohol consumption, and as an antispasmodic for menstrual cramps.

Topically, German chamomile is used for hemorrhoids; mastitis; leg ulcers; skin, anogenital, and mucous membrane inflammation; and bacterial skin diseases, including those of the mouth and gums. It is also used topically for treating or preventing chemotherapy- or radiation-induced oral mucositis.

As an inhalant, German chamomile is used to treat inflammation and irritation of the respiratory tract.

In foods and beverages, German chamomile is used as flavor components.

In manufacturing, German chamomile is used in cosmetics, soaps, and mouthwashes.

Safety

LIKELY SAFE ...when used orally in amounts commonly found in foods. German chamomile has Generally Recognized As Safe (GRAS) status in the US (4912).

POSSIBLY SAFE ...when used orally, short-term. There is some evidence that German chamomile can be used safely for up to 8 weeks (6655,12724,12729). The long-term safety of German chamomile in medicinal doses is unknown. ...when used topically; avoid applying it near the eyes (10377).

PREGNANCY AND LACTATION: Insufficient reliable information available; avoid using.

Effectiveness

POSSIBLY EFFECTIVE

Dyspepsia. A specific combination product containing German chamomile (Iberogast, Enzymatic Therapy) seems to improve symptoms of dyspepsia. The combination includes German chamomile plus peppermint leaf, clown's mustard plant, caraway, licorice, milk thistle, celandine, angelica, and lemon balm (7049,12724). A meta-analysis of studies using this combination product suggests that taking 1 mL orally three times daily over a period of 4-weeks significantly reduces severity of acid reflux, epigastric pain, cramping, nausea, and vomiting compared to placebo (13089).

Oral mucositis. Using a German chamomile oral rinse (Kamillosan Liquidum) might help prevent or treat mucositis induced by radiation therapy and some types of chemotherapy (6655). German chamomile oral rinse seems to prevent or treat mucositis secondary to radiation therapy and some types of chemotherapy including asparaginase (Elspar), cisplatin (CDDP, Platinol-AQ), cyclophosphamide (Cytoxan, Neosar), daunorubicin (DaunoXome), doxorubicin (Adriamycin, Rubex), etoposide (VP-16, Etopophos, VePesid, Toposar), hydroxyurea

(Hydrea), mercaptopurine (6-MP, Purinethol), methotrexate (MTX, Rheumatrex), procarbazine (MIH, Mutlane), and vincristine (VCR, Oncovin, Vincasar) (6655). However, the rinse doesn't seem to be better than placebo for preventing fluorouracil (5-FU)-induced oral mucositis (6656).

POSSIBLY INEFFECTIVE

Dermatitis. Applying German chamomile cream topically does not seem to prevent dermatitis induced by cancer radiation therapy (9767).

Some clinical studies have used German chamomile extracts and flowers standardized to 1.2% apigenin.

There is insufficient reliable information available about the effectiveness of German chamomile for its other uses.

Mechanism of Action

The applicable part of German chamomile is the flowerhead. Active constituents of German chamomile include quercetin, apigenin, and coumarins, and the essential oils matricin, chamazulene, alpha bisaboloid, and bisaboloid oxides (10377).

German chamomile might have anti-inflammatory effects. Preliminary research suggests it can inhibit the enzymes cyclooxygenase and lipoxygenase, which reduces the production of prostaglandins and leukotrienes. Quercetin and apigenin can inhibit histamine release from mast cells that are antigen stimulated (10377,12729).

The constituent(s) responsible for the sedative activity of German chamomile are unclear. Some preliminary research suggests that apigenin can bind to gamma-aminobutyric acid (GABA) receptors. GABA receptors are the primary receptor sites of benzodiazepines in the central nervous system. However, other research suggests that apigenin doesn't affect GABA receptors, and other constituents of German chamomile are responsible for the sedative activity (9765,12725).

Preliminary research suggests that extracts of German chamomile might inhibit morphine dependence and withdrawal possibly by increasing cyclic adenosine monophosphate (c-AMP) levels (12726). Other preliminary research suggests that German chamomile flower extract taken orally might have an antipruritic effect (12727).

Extracts of German chamomile might have antiestrogen effects, according to preliminary research. It also seems to stimulate osteoblast activity (12728).

Adverse Reactions

Orally, German chamomile tea can cause allergic reactions including severe hypersensitivity reactions and anaphylaxis in some patients (567). Animal studies suggest no toxicity or teratogenicity of bisabolol, the main active constituent of German chamomile (8178). German chamomile can cause an allergic reaction in individuals sensitive to the Asteraceae/Compositae family. Members of this family include ragweed, chrysanthemums, marigolds, daisies, and many other herbs.

Topically, German chamomile may cause allergic dermatitis and eczema (9766,9768,10377). If used near the eyes, it can be irritating (10377).

Interactions with Herbs & Other Dietary Supplements

HERBS WITH SEDATIVE PROPERTIES: Theoretically, concomitant use with herbs that have sedative properties might enhance therapeutic and adverse effects (9765,12725). Some of these supplements include 5-HTP, calamus, California poppy, catnip, hops, Jamaican dogwood, kava, St. John's wort, scullcap, valerian, yerba mansa, and others.

Interactions with Drugs

BENZODIAZEPINES: Theoretically, concomitant use with benzodiazepines might cause additive effects and side effects (9765,12725). Some benzodiazepines are alprazolam (Xanax), clonazepam (Klonopin), diazepam (Valium), lorazepam (Ativan), midazolam (Versed), temazepam (Restoril), triazolam (Halcion), and others.

CNS DEPRESSANTS: Theoretically, concomitant use with drugs with sedative properties can cause additive effects and side effects (9765,12725). Some CNS depressants are benzodiazepines, pentobarbital (Nembutal), phenobarbital (Luminal), secobarbital (Seconal), fentanyl (Duragesic, Sublimaze), morphine, zolpidem (Ambien), and others.

CYTOCHROME P450 3A4 (CYP3A4) SUBSTRATES: There's preliminary evidence that suggests that German chamomile might inhibit the cytochrome P450 3A4 (CYP3A4) isoenzymes (6450). Theoretically, German chamomile might increase levels of drugs metabolized by CYP3A4. However, so far, this interaction has not been reported in humans. Some drugs metabolized by CYP3A4 include lovastatin (Mevacor), ketoconazole (Nizoral), itraconazole (Sporanox), fexofenadine (Allegra), triazolam (Halcion), and numerous others. Use German chamomile cautiously or avoid in patients taking these drugs.

Interactions with Foods

None known.

Interactions with Lab Tests

CREATININE: Chronic ingestion of German chamomile for two weeks can reduce urinary creatinine output. This effect may be prolonged for up to two weeks after discontinuing German chamomile. The mechanism for this effect is unclear (12729).

Interactions with Diseases or Conditions
CROSS-ALLERGENICITY: German chamomile may cause an allergic reaction in individuals sensitive to the Asteraceae/Compositae family. Members of this family include ragweed, chrysanthemums, marigolds, daisies, and many other herbs.

Dosage and Administration
ORAL: For dyspepsia, a specific combination product containing German chamomile (Iberogast, Enzymatic Therapy) and several other herbs has been used in a dose of 1 mL three times daily (7049,12724,13089).
TOPICAL: For chemotherapy- or radiation-induced oral mucositis, an oral rinse made with 10-15 drops of German chamomile liquid extract in 100 mL warm water has been used three times daily (6655).

Comments
Avoid confusion with Roman chamomile.

GERMAN IPECAC

Also Known As
Swallow wort.
CAUTION: See separate listing for Pleurisy Root.

Scientific Names
Vincetoxicum hirundinaria, synonyms Cynanchum vincetoxicum, Asclepias vincetoxicum, Vincetoxicum officinale.
Family: Apocynaceae or Asclepiadaceae.

People Use This For
Orally, German ipecac is used for digestive and kidney disorders, dysmenorrhea, edema, the plague, snake bite, as a diuretic, emetic, and diaphoretic.
Topically, German ipecac is used in poultices for healing swelling and bruising.

Safety
POSSIBLY UNSAFE ...when used orally (18).
There is insufficient reliable information available about the safety of German ipecac for its other uses.
PREGNANCY AND LACTATION: POSSIBLY UNSAFE ...when used orally (18); avoid using.

Effectiveness
There is insufficient reliable information available about the effectiveness of German ipecac.

Mechanism of Action
The applicable parts of German ipecac are the leaf and root/rhizome. There is insufficient reliable information available about the possible mechanism of action and active ingredients.

Adverse Reactions
Orally, high doses of German ipecac may cause vomiting, apnea, and cardiac arrest. Seed extracts may cause advancing paralysis of the central nervous system (18).

Interactions with Herbs & Other Dietary Supplements
None known.

Interactions with Drugs
None known.

Interactions with Foods
None known.

Interactions with Lab Tests
None known.

Interactions with Diseases or Conditions
None known.

Dosage and Administration
No typical dosage.

GERMAN SARSAPARILLA

Also Known As
Caricis rhizoma, Red Sage, Red Wheatgrass, Sand Sedge, Sandriedgraswurzelstock, Sea Sedge.
CAUTION: See separate listings for Sarsaparilla, Sage, and Wheatgrass.

Scientific Names
Carex arenaria.
Family: Cyperaceae.

Comments
At the date of publication, there was very little scientific information available about this product. Our staff is continually analyzing the available information on natural medicines and will add data to the online version of *Natural Medicines Comprehensive Database* as it becomes available. See www.naturaldatabase.com.

GERMANDER

Also Known As
Wall Germander, Wild Germander.

Scientific Names
Teucrium chamaedrys.
Family: Lamiaceae/Labiatae.

People Use This For
Orally, germander is used orally for treating gallbladder conditions, fever, stomachaches, mild diarrhea, as a digestive aid, an adjunct for weight loss, an antiseptic, and as "a rinse for gout."
Topically, germander is used as a mouthwash for oral hygiene.
In manufacturing, germander is used as a flavoring agent in alcoholic beverages.

Safety
LIKELY UNSAFE ...when used orally. Germander is associated with multiple cases of hepatitis and death (271,3741,3742,3743,3744). France has banned its sale (17). Canada does not allow germander to be included in oral products as a non-medicinal ingredient (12). However, the US still allows germander to be used in small amounts as a flavoring agent in alcoholic beverages (12).
PREGNANCY AND LACTATION: LIKELY UNSAFE ...when used orally (271,3741,3742,3743,3744).

Effectiveness
There is insufficient reliable information available about the effectiveness of germander.

Mechanism of Action
The applicable parts of germander are the above ground parts. Germander contains teucrin A, a diterpene, which causes hepatic necrosis in mice (3740).

Adverse Reactions
Orally, germander has been associated with hepatitis, liver cell necrosis, and death (271,3741,3742,3743,3744).

Interactions with Herbs & Other Dietary Supplements
None known.

Interactions with Drugs
None known.

Interactions with Foods
None known.

Interactions with Lab Tests
None known.

Interactions with Diseases or Conditions
None known.

Dosage and Administration
No typical dosage.

GERMANIUM

Also Known As
Carboxyethylgermanium Sesquioxide, Ge-132, GE-132, Ge-Oxy 132, Inorganic Germanium, Organic Germanium, Spirogermanium.

Scientific Names
Germanium; Ge; atomic number 32; Bis-carboxyethyl germanium sesquioxide; Germanium lactate citrate.

People Use This For
Orally, germanium is used for osteoarthritis, pain relief, osteoporosis, low energy, AIDS, cancer, high blood pressure, high cholesterol, heart disease, glaucoma, and cataracts. It is used orally for rheumatoid arthritis (RA), depression, hepatitis, cirrhosis, food allergies, candidiasis, chronic viral infections, and heavy metal poisoning (including mercury, cadmium). Germanium is also used orally for increasing circulation of blood to the brain, supporting the immune system, and as an antioxidant.

Safety
LIKELY UNSAFE ...when used orally; avoid using. There have been more than 30 reports of renal failure, hepatic steatosis, myopathy, lactic acidosis, or death caused by ingestion of 15-300 grams over 2 to 36 months (2360,10040,10041,10042,10043,10044,10052,10072,10073,10074).
PREGNANCY AND LACTATION: LIKELY UNSAFE ...when used orally due to reported toxicity (2360,10051); avoid using.

Effectiveness
INSUFFICIENT RELIABLE EVIDENCE to RATE

Cancer. Researchers are interested in germanium as an alternative or palliative treatment for various kinds of cancer including breast cancer, colon cancer, prostate cancer, ovary cancer, head and neck cancer, and lung cancer (10035,10037,10038,10039,10049,10050). One case report showed complete remission of pulmonary spindle cell carcinoma after treatment with oral germanium sesquioxide (10037). However, the majority of research in phase I and phase II trials suggests that germanium is unsafe for use due to various life-threatening side effects (10035,10038,10039,10072,10073,10074). More evidence is needed to rate the effectiveness of germanium for this use.

Mechanism of Action
Germanium is considered an ultra-trace element, with an atomic number of 32. Preliminary research suggests that germanium might have anti-viral, anti-inflammatory, and immunological properties. It may also have antioxidant properties. However, the exact mechanisms are poorly understood (10046,10048,10051). Animal studies indicate that germanium accumulates in the tissues of the body, especially in the nerves and kidneys, after long-term exposure (10034). Germanium deficiency might be a contributing factor in the etiology of Kashin-Beck disease (10047).

Adverse Reactions
Orally, germanium can cause renal tubular degeneration, renal failure, anemia, muscle weakness, myopathy, hepatic steatosis, peripheral neuropathy, lactic acidosis, and death (2360,10040,10041,10042,10043,10044,10045,10052,10072,10073,10074).

Interactions with Herbs & Other Dietary Supplements
None known.

Interactions with Drugs
FUROSEMIDE (Lasix): There is one case report of furosemide resistance associated with a ginseng product containing germanium (770).

Interactions with Foods
None known.

Interactions with Lab Tests
None known.

Interactions with Diseases or Conditions
None known.

Dosage and Administration

No typical dosage.

GINGER

Also Known As

African Ginger, Black Ginger, Cochin Ginger, Gingembre, Imber, Jamaica Ginger, Jiang, Kankyo, Kanshokyo, Race Ginger, Shoga, Shokyo, Sunthi, Zingiberis rhizoma.
CAUTION: See separate listings for Alpinia (Chinese Ginger), Asarabacca (Wild Ginger), Common Stonecrop (Wall Ginger), or Wormwood (Green Ginger).

Scientific Names

Zingiber officinale, synonym Amomum zingiber.
Family: Zingiberaceae.

People Use This For

Orally, ginger is used for motion sickness, morning sickness, colic, dyspepsia, flatulence, chemotherapy-induced nausea, rheumatoid arthritis (RA), osteoarthritis, loss of appetite, post-surgical nausea and vomiting, migraine headache, and for discontinuing selective serotonin reuptake inhibitor (SSRI) drug therapy. It is also used orally for anorexia, upper respiratory tract infections, cough, bronchitis, as a galactagogue, diaphoretic, diuretic, as a stimulant; and for treating stomachache, diarrhea, nausea, cholera, and bleeding. Fresh ginger is used orally for treating acute bacterial dysentery, baldness, malaria, orchitis, poisonous snake bites, rheumatism, and toothaches. Dried ginger is used for chest pain, low back pain, and stomach pain.
Topically, the fresh juice of ginger is used for treating thermal burns. The essential oil of ginger is used topically as an analgesic.
In foods and beverages, ginger is used as a flavoring agent.
In manufacturing, ginger is used as a fragrance component in soaps and cosmetics. The oleoresin of ginger is also used as an ingredient in digestive, laxative, antitussive, antiflatulent, and antacid preparations.

Safety

LIKELY SAFE ...when used orally in amounts commonly found in foods. Ginger, ginger extract, and ginger oil have Generally Recognized As Safe (GRAS) status in the US (4912). ...when used orally and appropriately in medicinal amounts (721,722,723,5343,7048,7084,7085,7400,7623,11346,12472,13080).
PREGNANCY: POSSIBLY SAFE ...when used orally for medicinal purposes. Using ginger during pregnancy is controversial (1921,7083). There is some concern due to preliminary evidence that ginger might affect fetal sex hormones (7083), and an anecdotal report of spontaneous abortion during week 12 of pregnancy in a patient who used ginger for morning sickness (721). However, studies in pregnant women suggest that ginger can be used safely for morning sickness without harm to the fetus. The risk for major malformations in infants of women taking ginger does not appear to be higher than the baseline rate of 1% to 3% (721,1922,5343,11346,13071,13080). As with any medication given during pregnancy, the potential benefit to risk must be weighed.
LACTATION: Insufficient reliable information available; avoid using amounts greater than those found in foods.

Effectiveness

POSSIBLY EFFECTIVE

Chemotherapy-induced nausea. There is some evidence that taking ginger orally might help prevent chemotherapy-induced nausea when given following administration of intravenous (IV) prochlorperazine (Compazine) (1919).
Morning sickness. Taking ginger orally seems to reduce the severity of nausea and vomiting in some pregnant patients with morning sickness. Ginger seems to be more effective than placebo and comparable to vitamin B6 (721,1922,5343,11346,13071). The decision to use ginger (or any drug) during pregnancy should be based on possible benefit compared to potential risk.
Postoperative nausea and vomiting. There is some evidence that taking ginger orally might be as effective as metoclopramide (Reglan) for reducing postsurgical nausea and vomiting in patients not concurrently receiving anesthesia or narcotic analgesia (722,723,1919). However, ginger doesn't prevent postoperative nausea and vomiting in the presence of narcotic anesthesia or analgesia (3452,3453).
Vertigo. Taking 1 gram of ginger orally seems to reduce symptoms of vertigo, including nausea; however, it does not seem to reduce nystagmus (7623).

POSSIBLY INEFFECTIVE

Motion sickness. Taking ginger orally, 500-1000 mg, up to 4 hours prior to travel does not seem to prevent motion sickness (7624,7625). Some patients report subjective feelings of improvement, but objective measures are not significantly affected by ginger (7400).

INSUFFICIENT RELIABLE EVIDENCE to RATE

Migraine headache. Anecdotal evidence suggests that ginger might reduce the severity and duration of migraine headache (7623).

Osteoarthritis. There is preliminary evidence that ginger might offer very modest benefits in osteoarthritis. Two studies have evaluated a specific ginger extract (Eurovita Extract 33; EV ext-33) taken orally 170 mg three times daily or 255 mg twice daily (510 mg total daily dose) for 3-6 weeks (7048,7084). Ginger might modestly improve pain after standing or walking and joint stiffness in some patients, but it does not seem to significantly improve functionality, quality of life, or use of relief analgesics (7084,7085). Ginger appears to reduce pain as well as ibuprofen 400 mg three times daily (7048). A third company-sponsored study using another ginger extract (Zintona EC) for knee osteoarthritis suggests it might take 3 months for ginger to be effective (12472).

Rheumatoid arthritis (RA). There is some preliminary evidence that ginger might be helpful for decreasing joint pain in patients with RA (7401).

More evidence is needed to rate ginger for these uses.

Mechanism of Action

The applicable parts of ginger are the rhizome and root. Ginger contains active constituents known as gingerol, gingerdione, and shogaol. The chemical constituents of ginger vary among fresh, semi-dry, and dry forms of ginger (12632).These constituents seem to have a variety of pharmacological properties including antipyretic, analgesic, antitussive, anti-inflammatory, sedative, antibiotic, weak antifungal, and other properties (7628,12632). However, all of these pharmacological effects may not occur when whole ginger preparations are used.

The mechanism by which ginger reduces nausea and vomiting might be due to the 6-gingerol constituent (1924). It was once thought that ginger might work by increasing gastrointestinal (GI) motility (1923), but more recent evidence shows that ginger does not influence GI emptying time (7621,7624). Other ginger constituents such as 6-shogaol and galanolactone seem to act on serotonin receptors (1924). Galanolactone seems to act primarily on 5-HT3 receptors in the ileum, which are the same receptors affected by some prescription antiemetics such as ondansetron (Zofran). The predominant antiemetic action of ginger is localized in the GI tract, but there is some evidence that ginger constituents may also have central nervous system (CNS) activity (1924).

Ginger is sometimes used for inflammatory conditions such as rheumatoid arthritis (RA). Some researchers speculate that certain constituents of ginger might inhibit cyclooxygenase (COX) and lipoxygenase pathways (7401). It may also inhibit tumor necrosis factor (TNF)-alpha (12473). It also seems to inhibit the synthesis of prostaglandin-E2 (PGE2) and thromboxane B2 (TXB2), which mediate inflammation (12634).

There is preliminary evidence that ginger may also have hypoglycemic, hypocholesterolemic, anthelmintic, gastroprotective, and antiplatelet effects (7628,12633,12636). In laboratory models of diabetes, ginger seems to increase the release of insulin and lower cholesterol levels (12636). The antiplatelet effect of ginger is exerted by its ability to inhibit platelet thromboxane (7622,12634).

Fresh ginger extract seems to have blood pressure-lowering effects, according to preliminary research. It seems to have calcium-channel blocking activity. It also has negative inotropic and chronotropic effects (12633).

There is very preliminary evidence that some extracts and constituents of ginger might have mutagenic properties. However, these constituents may only be mutagenic when in the presence of other mutagens. Other ginger constituents such as zingerone have the opposite effect and are antimutagenic. Whole ginger preparations may not have mutagenic effects (11299). Animal research hasn't shown any evidence of teratogenicity (11297,11298). However, one study did find evidence of embryo mortality (11298).

Ginger inhibits thromboxane synthetase. This could affect testosterone receptor binding in the fetus and theoretically affect sex steroid differentiation of the fetal brain (7083). However, this has not been seen in animals or humans.

Adverse Reactions

Orally, ginger is usually well tolerated when used in typical doses. However, higher doses of 5 grams per day increase the risk of side effects and decrease tolerability (7622). Common side effects of ginger include abdominal discomfort, heartburn, diarrhea, and a pepper-like irritant effect in the mouth and throat (5343,7400).

Topically, ginger can cause dermatitis in sensitive individuals (12635).

Interactions with Herbs & Other Dietary Supplements

HERBS WITH ANTICOAGULANT/ANTIPLATELET POTENTIAL: Concomitant use of herbs that have constituents that might affect platelet aggregation could theoretically increase the risk of bleeding in some people (7622,12634). These herbs include angelica, clove, danshen, garlic, ginkgo, Panax ginseng, red clover, turmeric, and others.

Interactions with Drugs

ANTICOAGULANT/ANTIPLATELET DRUGS: Theoretically, excessive amounts of ginger might increase the risk of bleeding. Ginger is thought to inhibit thromboxane synthetase and decrease in platelet aggregation (7622,12634). Some anticoagulant or antiplatelet drugs include aspirin, clopidogrel (Plavix), dalteparin (Fragmin), enoxaparin (Lovenox), heparin, ticlopidine (Ticlid), warfarin (Coumadin), and others.
ANTIDIABETES DRUGS: Preliminary research suggests ginger might increase insulin levels. Theoretically, it could have an additive effect with antidiabetes drugs and cause hypoglycemia (12636). Some antidiabetes drugs include glimepiride (Amaryl), glyburide (DiaBeta, Glynase PresTab, Micronase), insulin, metformin (Glucophage), pioglitazone (Actos), rosiglitazone (Avandia), and others.
CALCIUM CHANNEL BLOCKERS: Theoretically, ginger might have an additive effect with calcium channel blockers. Preliminary research suggests it might have hypotensive and calcium channel-blocking effects (12633). Calcium channel blockers include nifedipine (Adalat, Procardia), verapamil (Calan, Isoptin, Verelan), diltiazem (Cardizem), isradipine (DynaCirc), felodipine (Plendil), amlodipine (Norvasc), and others.
PHENPROCOUMON: Phenprocoumon, a warfarin-related anticoagulant used in Europe, might increase the international normalized ratio (INR) when taken with ginger. There is one case report of a 76 year old woman with a stable INR on phenprocoumon that increased to greater than 10 when she began consuming dried ginger and ginger tea (12880).
WARFARIN (Coumadin): Preliminary evidence suggests that ginger might inhibit thromboxane synthetase and decrease platelet aggregation (7622,12634). There is one case report that ginger increases the INR when taken with phenprocoumon, which has similar pharmacological effects as warfarin (12880). However, research in healthy people suggests that chronic ingestion of ginger has no effect on INR, or the pharmacokinetics or pharmacodynamics of warfarin (12881). Until more is known, monitor INRs closely in patients taking significant amounts of ginger.

Interactions with Foods

None known.

Interactions with Lab Tests

None known.

Interactions with Diseases or Conditions

BLEEDING CONDITIONS: Theoretically, excessive doses of ginger can interfere with these conditions and increase risk of bleeding (7622,12634).
DIABETES: Theoretically, excessive doses of ginger can cause hypoglycemia, necessitating a change in dose of diabetes medication (12636).
HEART CONDITIONS: Theoretically, excessive doses of ginger might worsen some heart conditions. Preliminary research suggests it has negative inotropic and chronotropic activity (12633).

Dosage and Administration

ORAL: For morning sickness, 250 mg ginger 4 times daily has been used (721,5343,13080). For motion sickness, 1 gram of dried powdered ginger root 30 minutes to 4 hours before travel has been used (1919,7400). For osteoarthritis, a specific ginger extract (Eurovita Extract 33; EV ext-33), 170 mg three times daily or 255 mg twice daily has been used (7048,7084). For nausea and disequilibrium resulting from selective serotonin reuptake inhibitor (SSRI) discontinuation or tapering, 550-1100 mg ginger 3 times daily has been used (3451). For preventing postoperative nausea and vomiting, 1 gram powdered ginger root 1 hour before induction of anesthesia has been used (722,723). For migraine headache, ginger 500 mg at the onset and repeated every 4 hours up to 1.5-2 grams per day for 3-4 days has been used (7623). For chemotherapy-induced nausea, powdered ginger 2-4 grams daily has been used (1920). A ginger tea has also been used and is typically prepared and taken on the day of chemotherapy and continued for as long as needed (1920).
As a general anti-emetic, powdered root 2 grams daily is typically used (1920).
It is generally recommended that doses not exceed 4 grams per day (1920).

Comments

Ginger is commonly found in the warmer climates, including India, Jamaica, and China. Its flowers are similar to orchids. The rhizome is used as the source for the dried, powder spice.

GINKGO

Also Known As

Adiantifolia, Bai Guo Ye, Baiguo, Fossil Tree, Ginkgo Folium, Japanese Silver Apricot, Kew Tree, Maidenhair Tree, Salisburia Adiantifolia, Yinhsing.

Scientific Names

Ginkgo biloba.
Family: Ginkgoaceae.

People Use This For

Orally, ginkgo leaf is used for dementia, including Alzheimer's, vascular, and mixed dementia. Ginkgo leaf is also used orally for conditions associated with cerebral vascular insufficiency, especially in the elderly, including memory loss, headache, tinnitus, vertigo, dizziness, difficulty concentrating, mood disturbances, and hearing disorders. It is also used orally for relief of walking pain associated with intermittent claudication, particularly in patients with Fontaine's stage IIa or IIb peripheral arterial occlusive disease. Ginkgo leaf is also used orally to treat sexual dysfunction and to reverse sexual dysfunction caused by SSRI antidepressants. It is also used orally for cognitive disorders secondary to depression; eye problems, including macular degeneration and glaucoma; attention deficit-hyperactivity disorder (ADHD); thrombosis; heart disease; arteriosclerosis; angina pectoris; hypercholesterolemia; cardiac reperfusion injury; premenstrual syndrome (PMS); dysentery and filariasis; and diabetic retinopathy. Ginkgo leaf is also used orally to improve cognitive behavior and sleep patterns in patients with depression, and for the prevention of winter depression. Ginkgo leaf is also used orally for preventing acute mountain sickness and aging, regulating gastric acidity, improving liver and gallbladder function, regulating bacterial flora, controlling blood pressure, and treating Raynaud's disease. It is also used orally to treat asthma, allergies, bronchitis, and for various disorders of the central nervous system.

Ginkgo seed is used for cough, asthma, bronchitis, genitourinary complaints, to aid digestion, and to prevent drunkenness.

Topically, ginkgo leaf is used to wash chilblains, which are lesions on the fingers, toes, heels, ears, and nose caused by exposure to extreme cold. It is also used topically in wound dressings to improve circulation in the skin. Ginkgo seed is used for scabies and skin sores.

Intravenously, ginkgo leaf is used to increase cerebral blood flow, improve cognition, for psychiatric conditions in the elderly, and for metastatic colorectal cancer.

In manufacturing, ginkgo leaf extract has been used in cosmetics.

In foods, roasted ginkgo seed, which has the pulp removed, is an edible delicacy in Japan and China.

Safety

LIKELY SAFE ...when used orally and appropriately. Standardized ginkgo leaf extracts have been used safely in trials lasting from several weeks to a year (1514,1515,3461,5717,5718,6211,6212,6213,6214,6215,6216,6222,6223,6224,6225,6490). Tell patients to avoid crude ginkgo plant parts; which can exceed concentrations of 5 ppm of the toxic ginkgolic acid constituents, and can cause severe allergic reactions (5714).

POSSIBLY SAFE ...when used intravenously. Ginkgo leaf extract EGb 761 given intravenously seems to be safe for short-term use for up to 10 days (9871,9872).

POSSIBLY UNSAFE ...when the roasted seed is used orally. Consuming more than 10 roasted seeds per day can cause difficulty breathing, weak pulse, seizures, loss of consciousness, and shock (8231,8232).

LIKELY UNSAFE ...when the fresh ginkgo seed is used orally. Fresh seeds are toxic and potentially deadly (11296). There is insufficient reliable information available about the safety of ginkgo when used topically.

CHILDREN: LIKELY UNSAFE ...when ginkgo seed is used orally. The fresh seeds have caused seizures and death in children (8231,11296). There is insufficient reliable information available about the safety of ginkgo leaf when used in children.

PREGNANCY AND LACTATION: Insufficient reliable information available; avoid using.

Effectiveness

POSSIBLY EFFECTIVE

Age-related memory impairment. Taking ginkgo leaf extract orally seems to improve cognitive function in some elderly people with mild to moderate age-related memory impairment. Ginkgo leaf extract might modestly improve some measures of cognitive function, particularly short-term visual memory and possibly speed of cognitive processing, in non-demented patients with age-related memory impairment (5717,6216).

But taking ginkgo leaf extract doesn't seem to improve memory in people over the age of 60 with normal mental function (5718,8586,8587,8588). Tell cognitively healthy older patients ginkgo probably won't help forgetfulness.

Cognitive function. Taking ginkgo leaf extract orally seems to improve some measures of cognitive function in healthy young to middle-aged people. Ginkgo might modestly improve memory and speed of cognitive processing, including increasing speed of performance on factors assessing attention in people with no complaints of memory impairment (6214,6215,8236,8544,8588,9759). Lower doses of 120-240 mg per day seem to be as effective or more effective than higher doses up to 600 mg per day (6214,8236,8588). Some evidence suggests a combination of

Panax ginseng and ginkgo is effective for enhancing memory and that the combination might be more effective than either product alone (1903,8591).

Dementia. Taking ginkgo leaf orally seems to modestly improve symptoms of Alzheimer's, vascular, or mixed dementias. Studies lasting from 3 months to a year show that ginkgo leaf extract can stabilize or improve some measures of cognitive function and social functioning in patients with multiple types of dementia (1514,1515,2665,2666,6222,6223,6225). Although there is one report with conflicting findings (5720), the majority of evidence indicates that ginkgo leaf extract can be modestly helpful. Some researchers suggest that the improvement with ginkgo leaf extract is roughly equivalent to a six-month delay in disease progression (1514). However, outcome studies have not yet verified ginkgo's effects on disease progression. Doses ranging from 120-240 mg daily have been beneficial after six to eight weeks of treatment. German practitioners consider ginkgo leaf extract the treatment of choice for dementia (6491). However, ginkgo leaf extract has not been directly compared to conventional medicines for dementia. Improvement appears to be less than that found with the prescription drugs donepezil (Aricept), tacrine (Cognex), and other cholinesterase inhibitors. Reserve ginkgo for patients who cannot take cholinesterase inhibitors (1514,1515,6224,6490,11981).

Diabetic retinopathy. There is some evidence that taking ginkgo leaf extract orally for six months can significantly improve measures of color vision in patients with early diabetic retinopathy (6175).

Glaucoma. Taking ginkgo leaf extract orally seems to improve pre-existing damage to the visual field in patients with normal tension glaucoma (10378).

Intermittent claudication. Taking ginkgo leaf orally seems to increase pain-free walking distance in patients with Fontaine's IIb peripheral arterial occlusive disease and intermittent claudication (3461,6211,6212,6213). Although significant benefit has been found with doses as low as 120-160 mg per day (6211), there is some evidence that a higher dose of 240 mg per day might be more beneficial in some patients (3461,6212).

Premenstrual syndrome (PMS). Taking ginkgo leaf extract orally seems to produce significant relief in breast tenderness and neuropsychological symptoms associated with PMS when started during the 16th day of the menstrual cycle and continued until the 5th day of the following cycle (6229).

Raynaud's syndrome. Taking ginkgo leaf extract orally seems to decrease the number of painful attacks per week in patients with Raynaud's syndrome (11363).

Vertigo. Taking ginkgo leaf orally seems to improve symptoms of vertigo and equilibrium disorders (6208,6220,6221). There is evidence from two clinical studies that ginkgo leaf extract is significantly more effective than placebo (6220) and possibly as effective as betahistine for improving vertigo and dizziness caused by vascular vestibular disorders and vestibular disorders of unknown origin (6220,6221).

POSSIBLY INEFFECTIVE

Altitude sickness. A small preliminary study suggested that a specific ginkgo extract (EGb 761, Tanakan) 80 mg twice daily significantly reduced the occurrence of symptoms of acute altitude sickness including headache, fatigue, dyspnea, nausea, and vomiting in climbers to an altitude of 5400 meters (6230). But a large-scale trial using a different ginkgo extract (GK 501, Pharmaton, Switzerland) 120 mg twice daily shows that ginkgo has no effect on preventing altitude sickness in climbers to an altitude of 4928 meters (11766).

Antidepressant-induced sexual dysfunction. Although some preliminary clinical research suggests taking ginkgo leaf extract orally might help sexual dysfunction caused by antidepressant therapy (3965,3967), subsequent research indicates that it is probably ineffective (207,3966,3969,10893).

Seasonal affective disorder (SAD). Taking ginkgo leaf extract orally doesn't seem to prevent winter depression symptoms in patients with SAD (8233).

Tinnitus. Taking ginkgo leaf extract orally doesn't seem to improve symptoms of tinnitus. Some studies have shown benefit, but the majority of evidence indicates that ginkgo leaf extract is not consistently effective for patients with tinnitus (221,910,6208,6218,6219,9871).

Most of the clinical studies on the effectiveness of ginkgo leaf have used the standardized extracts EGb 761 (Tanakan) and LI 1370 (Lichtwer Pharma). These two extracts are similar and prepared to contain approximately 24% to 25% flavone glycosides and 6% terpene lactones. Products with similar ingredients include Ginkai (Lichtwer Pharma), Ginkgo 5 (Pharmline), Ginkgold and Ginkgo (Nature's Way), and Quanterra Mental Sharpness (Warner-Lambert).

INSUFFICIENT RELIABLE EVIDENCE to RATE

Age-related macular degeneration (AMD). Preliminary clinical research suggests that taking ginkgo leaf extract orally might improve symptoms of AMD (6227,6228,11797). There is limited evidence that ginkgo leaf extract might significantly improve distance vision in patients with AMD (6227).

Attention deficit-hyperactivity disorder (ADHD). There is preliminary evidence that ginkgo leaf extract, in combination with American ginseng (Panax quinquefolius), might help improve symptoms in children with ADHD (8235).

Colorectal cancer. Preliminary clinical research suggests the intravenous ginkgo extract (EGb 761) in combination with 5-fluorouracil might be useful for metastatic colorectal cancer (9872).

Hearing loss. There is preliminary evidence that ginkgo leaf extract 120 mg twice daily might help short-term idiopathic hearing loss (8543), but because many of these patients recover spontaneously, evaluating its effectiveness for this use is difficult.

More evidence is needed to rate ginkgo for these uses.

Mechanism of Action

The applicable parts of ginkgo are the leaf and the seed. Ginkgo leaf is the most commonly used form of ginkgo, usually as an extract.

Ginkgo leaf and its extracts contain several active constituents including flavonoids, terpenoids, and organic acids. Many ginkgo leaf extracts are standardized to contain 24% to 25% flavonoid glycosides and 6% terpenoids. The major flavonoids are primarily derived from the flavonol rutin and include isorhamnetin, quercetin, kaempferol, and proanthocyanidins. The primary terpenoids are ginkgolides A, B, C, M, and J, and bilobalide (1515). Although many of ginkgo's constituents have intrinsic pharmacological effects individually, there is evidence that the constituents work synergistically to produce more potent pharmacological effects than any individual constituent (1514,6494).

Although the mechanism of action of ginkgo leaf is only partially understood, there are several theories about how it might work for various disease states. One theory is that ginkgo leaf might work by protecting tissues from oxidative damage. Ginkgo leaf flavonoids have antioxidant and free radical scavenging properties (2660,5715,5717,5719). The flavonoids seem to prevent or reduce cell membrane lipid peroxidation (1515), and decrease oxidative damage to erythrocytes (5717). Ginkgo's flavonoids also protect neurons and retinal tissue from oxidative stress (1515,5719), and injury following ischemic episodes (1515,2660). Protecting neurons and other tissues from oxidative damage might prevent progression of tissue degeneration in patients with dementia and other conditions. Central nervous system (CNS) disorders, such as dementia, and other conditions including peripheral arterial disease, hypersensitivity disorders, allergies, asthma, and bronchitis might benefit from ginkgo's anti-inflammatory effects.

Ginkgolides in the leaf competitively inhibit platelet activating factor (PAF) binding at the membrane receptors of numerous cells (5719,9760). PAF inhibition decreases platelet aggregation (5717), decreases phagocyte chemotaxis and smooth muscle contraction (1515), prevents degranulation of neutrophils, decreases free radical production (5716,5717), decreases damaging glycine production after brain injury, and reduces excitatory amino acid receptor function (2660). Inhibition of PAF might increase cardiac contractility and coronary blood flow. Preliminary research suggests that ginkgo leaf extract might also inhibit formation of platelet thromboxane A2, further reducing platelet aggregation (8583).

However, there is contradictory, but questionable, evidence that ginkgo leaf does not reduce platelet aggregation and blood clotting. In this study, healthy men who took the specific ginkgo leaf extract (EGb 761) 160 mg twice daily for 7 days did not have reduced prothrombin times (12114).

Ginkgo leaf products might benefit CNS and vascular conditions by improving circulation. Ginkgo leaf seems to improve blood flow to capillaries throughout the body including in the CNS, eyes, ears, extremities, and other tissues. Ginkgo leaf likely improves circulation by both decreasing blood viscosity and affecting vascular smooth muscle. Ginkgo leaf seems to restore the balance between prostacyclin and thromboxane A2, resulting in improved vasoregulation. Therefore, ginkgo leaf relaxes spasmodic contracting vasculature and contracts abnormally dilated vessels. It is not clear exactly how ginkgo causes vascular contraction and improves venous tone, but these effects might be due to phosphodiesterase inhibition, resulting in increased cAMP levels and release of catecholamines (6492). Some ginkgo constituents may also have a potent relaxing effect on vascular smooth muscle and improve blood flow to the corpus cavernosum; which is thought to be helpful for erectile dysfunction (213).

Overall, ginkgo leaf seems to increase cerebral and peripheral blood flow microcirculation, and reduce vascular permeability (5721,6492).

Ginkgo leaf extract might be helpful for Alzheimer's disease due to effects on beta-amyloid proteins.

There is preliminary evidence that ginkgo leaf extract can inhibit toxicity and cell death induced by beta-amyloid peptides (6494). However, this has not yet been demonstrated in vivo. Ginkgo might also influence certain neurotransmitter systems, such as the cholinergic system (6490), and seems to produce EEG changes similar to the acetylcholinesterase inhibitor tacrine (Cognex) (6067). There has been some speculation that ginkgo leaf inhibits monoamine oxidase A and B (5721), but so far studies have found conflicting results (6231,6232,6233). It is suggested that ginkgo leaf inhibits catechol-O-methyl transferase (COMT, an enzyme which breaks down adrenergic transmitters) and increases the number of alpha-adrenoreceptors in the brain; which would help reverse the decline in brain alpha-adrenoceptor activity that occurs with aging (2660).

There is some evidence that ginkgo flavonoids have GABA-ergic effects and might directly affect benzodiazepine receptors (6423). However, the clinical significance of this effect is not known.

The ginkgolides A and B seem to decrease glucocorticoid biosynthesis, which might also play a role in ginkgo's proposed anti-stress and neuroprotective effects (5723,5724,8236).

Ginkgo leaf might have some antimicrobial activity, including activity against Pneumocystis carinii and possibly some gram-positive bacteria and yeast (6069). There is also some preliminary evidence that ginkgo might have a role in fighting syndrome X.

In healthy volunteers, ginkgo leaf extract can increase pancreatic beta-cell function in response to glucose loading and seems to reduce blood pressure. Some researchers think it might decrease development of hyperinsulinemia associated with hypertension, which often precedes development of type 2 diabetes and atherosclerotic cardiovascular disease (5719).

Some crude extracts from ginkgo leaves contain the constituent ginkgolic acid. This constituent can have strong allergenic properties and might have possible mutagenic and carcinogenic properties. Standardized ginkgo leaf extracts such as EGb 761 contain no greater than 5 ppm in concentration of ginkgolic acids (5714,8584).

Ginkgo leaves and ginkgo leaf extracts also contain the neurotoxin ginkgotoxin (4'-O-methylpyridoxine, MPN), which might lead to seizures in susceptible people. Ginkgotoxin indirectly inhibits GABA. Ginkgotoxin antagonizes

the activity of pyridoxine, possibly by inhibiting enzymes such as pyridoxal kinase or glutamate decarboxylase in the brain. GABA is synthesized from glutamate by glutamate decarboxylase. By inhibiting glutamate decarboxylase, ginkgotoxin indirectly inhibits GABA (12183).
Ginkgotoxin is present in much higher amounts in ginkgo seeds than leaves. It is unclear whether it is present in ginkgo leaf extracts in high enough concentrations to cause toxicity (11296).
There is some preliminary evidence that ginkgo leaf extract can inhibit cytochrome P450 1A2 (CYP1A2) activity by approximately 13%, and CYP2D6 by approximately 9%. Ginkgo leaf extract seems to inhibit CYP2D6 more in males than females (1303). The effects of ginkgo leaf extract on CYP3A4 are unclear. There is some in vitro evidence that ginkgo leaf extract might inhibit CYP3A4 (6450); while in vivo, ginkgo leaf extract does not seem to inhibit CYP3A4 activity (1303). In addition, there is anecdotal evidence that suggests ginkgo leaf extract might actually induce CYP3A4 (6423), but this effect has not yet been verified. The ginkgo leaf extract EGb 761, which is the most common extract used in clinical studies, also seems to strongly inhibit CYP2C9 in vitro. The terpenoidic fraction (ginkgolides) only inhibits CYP2C9. The flavonoidic fraction (quercetin, keampferol, etc) seems to inhibit CYP2C9, CYP1A2, CYP3A4, and CYP2E1 (12061).
Ginkgo seeds seem to have antibacterial and antifungal effects (11701,11702). Ginkgo seeds also contain the neurotoxin ginkgotoxin (4'-O-methylpyridoxine). Ginkgotoxin can cause seizures and death in high doses. Ginkgotoxin indirectly inhibits GABA. Ginkgotoxin antagonizes the activity of pyridoxine, possibly by inhibiting enzymes such as pyridoxal kinase or glutamate decarboxylase in the brain. GABA is synthesized from glutamate by glutamate decarboxylase. By inhibiting glutamate decarboxylase, ginkgotoxin indirectly inhibits GABA (12183).
Ginkgotoxin is present in much larger amounts in ginkgo seeds than leaves. Boiling ginkgo seeds seems to reduce the ginkgotoxin content to safe levels (11296).

Adverse Reactions

Orally, ginkgo leaf extract is well tolerated in typical doses (11981). It can cause mild gastrointestinal (GI) upset, headache, dizziness, palpitations, constipation, and allergic skin reactions (5719,5721,6220). Large doses can cause restlessness, diarrhea, nausea, vomiting, lack of muscle tone, and weakness.
Spontaneous bleeding is one of the most concerning potential side effects associated with ginkgo. There are at least 15 published case reports linking ginkgo to episodes of minor to severe bleeding; however, not all case reports clearly establish ginkgo as the cause of bleeding. In most cases, other bleeding risk factors were also present including taking other medications, old age, liver cirrhosis, and other conditions. In most cases, bleeding occurred after several weeks or months of taking ginkgo (13135).
There are several case reports of intracerebral bleeding. Some of these cases resulted in permanent neurological damage and one case resulted in death (8581,13135).
There are at least 4 cases of ocular bleeding including spontaneous hyphema (bleeding from the iris into the anterior part of the eye) and retrobulbar hemorrhage associated with ginkgo use (579,10450,13135).
There are also cases of surgical and post-surgical complications in patients using ginkgo. Retrobulbar hemorrhage (bleeding behind the eye) during cataract surgery has been associated with ginkgo use (10450). Excessive postoperative bleeding requiring transfusion has also occurred following laparoscopic surgery in a patient who had been taking ginkgo leaf extract (887). There are also 2 cases of excessive bleeding during surgery and post-surgical hematoma in patients undergoing rhytidoplasty and blepharoplasty (13002).
In another case, an elderly man experienced nose bleeds and ecchymosis following use of ginkgo. These instances of bleeding stopped when ginkgo was discontinued, and recurred when the patient started taking ginkgo again (13135).
Ginkgo leaf extract can cause serious allergic skin reactions in some patients. There is one case of Stevens-Johnson syndrome following a second administration of a preparation containing ginkgo leaf extract, choline, vitamin B6, and vitamin B12 (208).
Fresh ginkgo seeds can cause stomachache, nausea, vomiting, diarrhea, restlessness, difficulty breathing, weak pulse, seizures, loss of consciousness, and shock. Ingesting roasted seeds in amounts larger than the normal food amounts of 8-10 seeds per day, or long-term, can also cause these same adverse reactions (8231,8232).
The fresh seeds contain large amounts of ginkgotoxin, which can cause seizures and death. The antidote for ginkgotoxin poisoning is pyridoxine (11296). Ginkgo leaf and ginkgo leaf extract contain small amounts of ginkgotoxin.
The small amount of ginkgotoxin in the leaves and leaf extract seems unlikely to cause toxicity (11296). However, there are anecdotal reports of seizure occurring after use of ginkgo leaf preparations both in patients without a history seizure disorder and in those with previously well-controlled epilepsy (7030,7090). There is not enough evidence to prove that ginkgo leaf is the sole cause of seizure in these patients. Until more is known, advise patients with seizure disorders and those taking drugs that lower the seizure threshold to avoid ginkgo leaf products.
There is some in vitro evidence that suggests high concentrations of ginkgo might reduce male and female fertility (4239,4240); however, this has not been demonstrated in humans.
Topically, ginkgo fruit and pulp can cause severe allergic skin reactions and irritation of mucous membranes and the gastrointestinal tract (12). Cross-reactivity is possible with ginkgo fruit in individuals allergic to poison ivy, poison oak, poison sumac, mango rind, and cashew shell oil (380).

Interactions with Herbs & Other Dietary Supplements

ANTICOAGULANT /ANTIPLATELET HERBS AND SUPPLEMENTS: Concomitant use of herbs and supplements that affect platelet aggregation could theoretically increase the risk of bleeding in some people due to ginkgo's effects on platelet aggregation (5717,5719). Some other herbs include angelica, clove, danshen, garlic, ginger, ginkgo, Panax ginseng, and others.

SEIZURE THRESHOLD LOWERING HERBS AND SUPPLEMENTS: Ginkgo seeds contain ginkgotoxin, which can cause seizures in high doses (11296). Theoretically, patients taking supplements that also lower the seizure threshold might be at greater risk. There are anecdotal reports of seizure occurring after use of ginkgo leaf both in patients without a history seizure disorder and in those with previously well-controlled epilepsy (7030,7090). Advise patients taking these supplements to avoid ginkgo products. Some of these supplements include butanediol (BD), cedar leaf, Chinese club moss, EDTA, folic acid, gamma butyrolactone (GBL), gamma hydroxybutyrate (GHB), glutamine, huperzine A, hydrazine sulfate, hyssop oil, juniper, L-carnitine, melatonin, rosemary, sage, wormwood, and others.

ST. JOHN'S WORT: Ginkgo in combination with buspirone (BuSpar), fluoxetine (Prozac), melatonin, and St. John's wort might cause hypomania in patients with depression (8582). Whether ginkgo alone, or in combination with St. John's wort, can cause hypomania is unknown.

Interactions with Drugs

ANTICOAGULANT/ANTIPLATELET DRUGS: Concomitant administration can increase the risk of bleeding. Ginkgo leaf has been shown to decrease platelet aggregation. It is thought that the ginkgo constituent, ginkgolide B, displaces platelet-activating factor (PAF) from its binding sites, decreasing blood coagulation (6048,9760). Some of these drugs include aspirin, clopidogrel (Plavix), dalteparin (Fragmin), enoxaparin (Lovenox), heparin, indomethacin (Indocin), ticlopidine (Ticlid), warfarin (Coumadin), and others.

ANTICONVULSANTS: Consumption of ginkgo seeds can cause seizures due to ginkgotoxin contained in the seeds. Large amounts of ginkgotoxin can cause neurotoxicity and seizure. Ginkgotoxin is present in much larger amounts in ginkgo seeds than leaves (8232). Ginkgo leaf extract contains trace amounts of ginkgotoxin. The amount of ginkgotoxin in ginkgo leaf and leaf extract seems unlikely to cause toxicity (11296). However, there are anecdotal reports of seizure occurring after use of ginkgo leaf both in patients without a history of seizure disorder and in those with previously well-controlled epilepsy (7030,7090). Theoretically, taking ginkgo might reduce the effectiveness of anticonvulsants for preventing seizure. Some anti-epileptic drugs include phenobarbital, primidone (Mysoline), valproic acid (Depakene), gabapentin (Neurontin), carbamazepine (Tegretol), phenytoin (Dilantin), and others.

BUSPIRONE (BuSpar): Ginkgo in combination with fluoxetine (Prozac), St. John's wort, melatonin, and buspirone might cause hypomania in patients with depression (8582). Whether ginkgo alone or in combination with buspirone can cause hypomania is unknown.

CYTOCHROME P450 1A2 (CYP1A2) SUBSTRATES: There is preliminary evidence that ginkgo leaf extract can mildly affect cytochrome P450 1A2 (CYP1A2) enzymes (1303,6423,6450). Since ginkgo leaf extract seems to only mildly affect these enzymes, it is not likely to produce clinically significant interactions; however, it might slightly increase levels of some drugs metabolized by these enzymes. Until more is known, use ginkgo cautiously in patients taking drugs metabolized by these enzymes. Some drugs metabolized by CYP1A2 include acetaminophen (Tylenol), amitriptyline (Elavil), clopidogrel (Plavix), clozapine (Clozaril), diazepam (Valium), estradiol, olanzapine (Zyprexa), ondansetron (Zofran), propranolol (Inderal), ropinirole (Requip), tacrine (Cognex), theophylline, verapamil (Calan, Covera-HS, Isoptin, Verelan), warfarin (Coumadin), and others.

CYTOCHROME P450 2C19 (CYP2C19) SUBSTRATES: There is some evidence that a specific ginkgo leaf extract (Remembrance, Herbs Product LTD, Hong Kong) 140 mg twice daily can induce CYP2C19 enzymes and potentially decrease levels of drugs metabolized by these enzymes (13108). Some drugs metabolized by CYP2C19 include amitriptyline (Elavil), carisoprodol (Soma), citalopram (Celexa), diazepam (Valium), lansoprazole (Prevacid), omeprazole (Prilosec), phenytoin (Dilantin), warfarin, and many others.

CYTOCHROME P450 2C9 (CYP2C9) SUBSTRATES: There is preliminary evidence that a specific standardized extract of ginkgo leaf (EGb 761) can strongly inhibit CYP2C9 (12061). The terpenoid (ginkgolides) and flavonoid (quercetin, keampferol, etc) constituents seem to be responsible for the enzyme inhibition. Most ginkgo extracts contain some amount of these constituents. Therefore, other ginkgo leaf extracts likely also inhibit the CYP2C9 enzyme. Ginkgo leaf extracts might increase levels of drugs metabolized by CYP2C9. Advise patients not to take ginkgo leaf or use it cautiously if they take any CYP2C9 substrate. Some of these drugs include warfarin (Coumadin), glyburide, glipizide, amitriptyline valdecoxib (Bextra), phenytoin (Dilantin), and many others.

CYTOCHROME P450 2D6 (CYP2D6) SUBSTRATES: There is preliminary evidence that ginkgo leaf extract can mildly affect CYP2D6 enzymes (1303,6423,6450). Since ginkgo leaf extract seems to only mildly affect these enzymes, it is not likely to produce clinically significant interactions; however, it might slightly increase levels of some drugs metabolized by these enzymes. Some drugs metabolized by CYP2D6 include amitriptyline (Elavil), clozapine (Clozaril), codeine, desipramine (Norpramin), donepezil (Aricept), fentanyl (Duragesic), flecainide (Tambocor), fluoxetine (Prozac), meperidine (Demerol), methadone (Dolophine), metoprolol (Lopressor, Toprol XL), olanzapine (Zyprexa), ondansetron (Zofran), tramadol (Ultram), trazodone (Desyrel), and others.

CYTOCHROME P450 3A4 (CYP3A4) SUBSTRATES: There is preliminary evidence that ginkgo leaf extract can affect cytochrome P450 3A4 enzymes (CYP3A4). However, there is conflicting evidence about whether it induces or inhibits CYP3A4 (1303,6423,6450). Until more is known, use ginkgo cautiously in patients taking drugs metabolized by these enzymes. Some drugs metabolized by CYP3A4 include lovastatin (Mevacor), ketoconazole (Nizoral), itraconazole (Sporanox), fexofenadine (Allegra), triazolam (Halcion), and others.

FLUOXETINE (Prozac): Ginkgo in combination with buspirone (BuSpar), St. John's wort, melatonin, and fluoxetine might cause hypomania in patients with depression (8582). Whether ginkgo alone or in combination with fluoxetine can cause hypomania is unknown.

INSULIN: Ginkgo leaf extract can alter insulin secretion and metabolism, and might affect blood glucose levels (5719). People taking insulin should monitor glucose levels closely. Insulin dose adjustments might be necessary.

OMEPRAZOLE (Prilosec): A specific ginkgo leaf extract (Remembrance, Herbs Product LTD, Hong Kong) 140 mg twice daily can induce CYP2C19 enzymes and decrease levels of omeprazole by about 27% to 42% (13108).

SEIZURE THRESHOLD LOWERING DRUGS: Consumption of ginkgo seeds can cause seizures due to ginkgotoxin contained in the seeds. Large amounts of ginkgotoxin can cause neurotoxicity and seizure. Ginkgotoxin is present in much larger amounts in ginkgo seeds than leaves (8232). Ginkgo leaf extract contains trace amounts of ginkgotoxin. The amount of ginkgotoxin in ginkgo leaf and leaf extract seems unlikely to cause toxicity (11296). However, there are anecdotal reports of seizure occurring after use of ginkgo leaf both in patients without a history of seizure disorder and in those with previously well-controlled epilepsy (7030,7090). Advise patients taking these drugs to avoid ginkgo leaf products. Some drugs that lower the seizure threshold include anesthetics (propofol, others), antiarrhythmics (mexiletine), antibiotics (amphotericin, penicillin, cephalosporins, imipenem), antidepressants (bupropion, others), antihistamines (cyproheptadine, others), immunosuppressants (cyclosporine), narcotics (fentanyl, others), stimulants (methylphenidate), theophylline, and others.

TRAZODONE (Desyrel): Use of ginkgo leaf extract with trazodone has been associated with coma. In one case, an Alzheimer's patient taking trazodone 20 mg twice daily and ginkgo leaf extract 80 mg twice daily for four doses became comatose. The coma was reversed by administration of flumazenil (Romazicon). Coma might have been induced by excessive GABA-ergic activity. Ginkgo flavonoids are thought to have GABA-ergic activity and act directly on benzodiazepine receptors. Ginkgo might also increase metabolism of trazodone to active GABA-ergic metabolites, possibly by inducing cytochrome P450 3A4 (CYP3A4) metabolism (6423).

WARFARIN (Coumadin): Ginkgo leaf might increase the anticoagulant effects of warfarin and risk of bleeding (576). Ginkgo is thought to have antiplatelet effects and might have additive effects when used with warfarin. There is also some evidence that ginkgo leaf extract can inhibit cytochrome P450 2C9, the enzyme that metabolizes warfarin, and therefore might increase warfarin levels (12061). However, research in healthy people suggests that chronic ingestion of ginkgo has no effect on INR, or the pharmacokinetics or pharmacodynamics of warfarin (12881). There is also some preliminary clinical research that suggests ginkgo might not significantly increase the effects of warfarin in patients that have a stable INR (11905); however, these contradictory findings are in small-scale, short-term studies that may not have the power to detect a small or moderate effect on bleeding risk. Until more is known, monitor INRs closely in patients taking ginkgo.

Interactions with Foods

None known.

Interactions with Lab Tests

None known.

Interactions with Diseases or Conditions

BLEEDING DISORDERS: Ginkgo leaf can decrease platelet aggregation by inhibiting platelet-activating factor (PAF) and may exacerbate bleeding disorders (6048,9760); use with caution.

DIABETES: Theoretically, ginkgo may interfere with the management of diabetes. Ginkgo has been reported to increase pancreatic beta-cell function in response to glucose and may also increase the metabolic clearance of insulin (5719). Monitor blood glucose levels closely. Diabetes medications might require dose adjustment.

EPILEPSY: Consumption of ginkgo seeds can cause seizures due to ginkgotoxin contained in the seeds. Large amounts of ginkgotoxin can cause neurotoxicity and seizure. Ginkgotoxin is present in much larger amounts in ginkgo seeds than leaves (8232). Ginkgo leaf and ginkgo leaf extract contain trace amounts of ginkgotoxin, which can cause seizures in high doses. The amount of ginkgotoxin in ginkgo leaf and leaf extract seems unlikely to cause toxicity (11296). However, there are several anecdotal reports of seizure occurring in patients taking combination products containing ginkgo and single ingredient ginkgo products. However, there is not yet enough evidence to prove that ginkgo can actually cause seizure in certain patients (7030). Until more is known, use cautiously or avoid in epileptic patients or patients prone to seizure.

INFERTILITY: Some evidence suggests that Ginkgo biloba might inhibit oocyte fertilization and should be avoided in couples attempting to conceive (4239,4240). This effect has not yet been demonstrated in humans; however, until more is known, use with caution in couples attempting to conceive and avoid use in couples having difficulty conceiving.

SURGERY: Ginkgo leaf extract has antiplatelet effects and can cause excessive bleeding if used prior to surgery (887,13002). Tell patients to discontinue ginkgo at least 2 weeks before elective surgical procedures.

Dosage and Administration

ORAL: For dementia syndromes, a dosage of 120-240 mg per day of ginkgo leaf extract, divided in two or three doses, has been used (1514,1515). To relieve walking pain in patients with intermittent claudication, a dosage of 120-240 mg per day of ginkgo leaf extract, divided into two or three doses, has been used; however, the higher dose may be more effective (3461). For reversing sexual dysfunction due to SSRIs, the typical starting dose is 60 mg twice daily of ginkgo leaf extract. This dose can be titrated up to 240 mg twice daily (212). For cognitive function improvement in healthy young people, dosages of 120-600 mg per day have been used (6214,6215,8236). For vertigo or tinnitus, dosages of 120-160 mg per day of ginkgo leaf extract, divided into two or three doses, have been used (221). For prevention of altitude sickness, 80 mg of ginkgo leaf extract twice daily has been used (6230). For premenstrual syndrome (PMS), 80 mg twice daily, starting on the sixteenth day of the menstrual cycle until the fifth day of the next cycle has been used (6229). For the treatment of attention deficit-hyperactivity disorder (ADHD), a dosage of 50 mg ginkgo leaf extract combined with 200 mg American ginseng twice daily has been used (8235).

For the treatment of normal tension glaucoma, ginkgo leaf extract 40 mg 3 times daily has been used for up to 4 weeks (10378). For Raynaud's disease, a dosage of 360 mg per day of ginkgo leaf extract, divided into three doses, has been used (11363). For all indications, start at a lower dose of not more 120 mg per day to avoid adverse gastrointestinal (GI) effects. Titrate to higher doses as needed. Dosing may vary depending on the specific formulation used. Most trials used specific standardized Ginkgo biloba leaf extracts. Some people take 0.5 mL of a standard 1:5 tincture of the crude ginkgo leaf three times daily (5011). Tell patients to avoid crude ginkgo plant parts; which can exceed concentrations of 5 ppm of the toxic ginkgolic acid constituents, and can cause severe allergic reactions (5714).

Comments

When people talk about Ginkgo biloba, they usually mean ginkgo leaf extract. However, traditionally only Ginkgo biloba fruit was used. "Ginkgo biloba" comes from the Chinese term Yin-Kuo, meaning "silver apricot," and biloba also describes its two-lobed, fan shaped leaves (6208). Ginkgo biloba is the longest living tree species in the world. Ginkgo trees can live as long as a thousand years. Using ginkgo for asthma and bronchitis was described in the first pharmacopoeia, Chen Noung Pen T'sao, dating to 2600 BC (6208). Ginkgo is the most frequently prescribed herbal medicine in Germany (6208) and is the preferred treatment for dementia (6491).

The National Center for Complementary and Alternative Medicine (NCCAM) is conducting a 5-year study of 3000 people aged 75 and older to determine if ginkgo, 240 mg daily, prevents dementia or Alzheimer's disease (6226). In isolated cases ginkgo has been contaminated with colchicine (8541). However, follow-up studies indicate that this contamination is not widespread (8542).

GINSENG, AMERICAN

Also Known As

American Ginseng, Anchi Ginseng, Canadian Ginseng, Ginseng, Ginseng Root, North American Ginseng, Occidental Ginseng, Ontario Ginseng, Panax quinquefolium, Red Berry, Ren Shen, Sang, Shang, Wisconsin Ginseng, Xi Yang Shen.

CAUTION: See separate listings for Blue Cohosh, Canaigre, Codonopsis, Ginseng Siberian, Ginseng Panax, Panax Pseudoginseng, and Ashwaganda.

Scientific Names

Panax quinquefolius.

Family: Araliaceae.

People Use This For

Orally, American ginseng is used as an adaptogen, for increasing resistance to environmental stress, as a general tonic, stimulant, diuretic, and digestive aid. It is also used for anemia, diabetes, insomnia, neurasthenia, gastritis, impotence, fever, hangover symptoms, stimulating immune function, attention deficit-hyperactivity disorder (ADHD), and for eradicating Pseudomonas infection in cystic fibrosis. American ginseng is also used for acute respiratory illness, improving stress resistance, preventing the effects of aging, improving stamina, blood and bleeding disorders, atherosclerosis, loss of appetite, vomiting, colitis, dysentery, cancer, insomnia, neuralgia, rheumatism, memory loss, dizziness, headaches, convulsions, and disorders of pregnancy and childbirth.

In food manufacturing, American ginseng is used in soft drinks.

In other manufacturing processes, American ginseng oil and extracts are used in soaps and cosmetics.

Safety

POSSIBLY SAFE ...when used orally and appropriately, short-term (8235,11351).

PREGNANCY: POSSIBLY UNSAFE ...when used orally. Ginsenoside Rb1, an active constituent of American ginseng, has teratogenic effects in animal models (10447); avoid using.

LACTATION: Insufficient reliable information available; avoid using.

Effectiveness

POSSIBLY EFFECTIVE

Diabetes. Taking American ginseng 3 grams orally, up to two hours before a meal, can significantly reduce postprandial glucose levels in patients with type 2 diabetes (1018,6461). However, doses greater than 3 grams do not seem to offer any additional benefit (6461). The glucose lowering effect may vary among preparations because of variations in the concentration of ginsenosides (9732).

INSUFFICIENT RELIABLE EVIDENCE to RATE

Attention deficit-hyperactivity disorder (ADHD). There is preliminary evidence that American ginseng in combination with Ginkgo biloba leaf extract might help improve symptoms in children with ADHD (8235).

Influenza. Preliminary evidence suggests that an American ginseng extract might reduce the risk of influenza in institutionalized elderly patients. Taking a specific extract CVT-E002 (Cold-FX, CV Technologies, Canada) 200 mg twice daily orally over a 12-week period during influenza season might reduce the risk of laboratory confirmed influenza or influenza and respiratory syncytial virus (RSV) infections. But it does not seem to reduce the appearance of influenza symptoms, symptom severity, or symptom duration (11351).

More evidence is needed to rate American ginseng for these uses.

Mechanism of Action

The applicable part of American ginseng is the root. The principle constituents of American ginseng are known as ginsenosides, panaxosides, or saponins (11). American ginseng contains primarily ginsenoside Rb-1, which reportedly lowers blood pressure; has antihemolytic, antipyretic, antipsychotic, CNS depressant, and ulcer protective activity; increases GI motility; and decreases islet insulin concentrations (4,11). At least 30 ginsenosides are known to exist in varying concentrations in the assorted species of ginseng (9735,12536). American ginseng contains higher amounts of Rb1, Re, Rc, and Rd relative to other ginsengs, and lesser amounts of Rb2 and Rg1. American ginseng also contains nonsaponin peptidoglycans called quinquefolans, which have hypoglycemic effects (12536).

For diabetes, ginsengosides and possibly other constituents are thought to reduce postprandial glucose levels. This effect might be due to either tissue insulin sensitization or direct stimulation of insulin release or both of these mechanisms (6461). The effect of various ginsengs on glucose appears to be related in part to the mix of ginsenosides. Other nonginsenoside constituents likely affect blood glucose as well. Panax ginseng and other ginsengs contain protopanaxadiol (PPD) ginsenosides, Rb1, Rb2, Rc, and Rd. They also contain protopanaxatriol (PPT) ginsenosides, Rg1, Re, and Rf. A higher ratio of PPD ginsenosides to PPT ginsenosides is related to greater blood glucose and insulin lowering potency of the ginseng product. Compared with Panax ginseng, American ginseng appears to have a higher PPD to PPT ratio and may have greater blood glucose and insulin lowering potency. There appears to be some differences in the PPD to PPT ratio between wild and cultivated American ginseng. The ginsenoside content also varies among batches, plant parts, and preparation methods (12536).

An American ginseng extract decreases LH (luteinizing hormone) levels and increases serum ceruloplasmin oxidase activity (a measure of estrogenic activity in the liver) in an animal model (6180). Preliminary research suggests that American ginseng extract might reduce breast cancer cell growth (389); however, this effect may be outweighed by its estrogenic action, which might increase the growth of breast cancer cells (7860).

American ginseng seems to have immunomodulating activity. Polysaccharides and oligosaccharides from ginseng are thought to be responsible for the immunomodulating effects (11351). American ginseng seems to activate monocytes, induce tumor necrosis factor (TNF)-alpha, and interferon-gamma (7602,11351). It also stimulates natural killer cell activity, interleukin-2 (IL-2), and other factors involved in cell-mediated immunity (11351).

Ginsenosides might improve memory by influencing the effect of acetylcholine in the central nervous system by an unknown mechanism. Ginsenosides do not appear to change metabolism, release, or reuptake of acetylcholine (9736). There's also some evidence that ginsenosides might cause an increase in sexual drive (11162).

Preliminary evidence suggests that saponins found in the stems and leaves of American ginseng can reduce oxidation of low density lipoprotein (LDL) cholesterol. These saponins might reverse the decrease in venous relaxation in response to acetylcholine that occurs in the presence of oxidized LDL (9733). A hot water extract of American ginseng root seems to decrease endothelial constriction by promoting the release of nitric oxide (9734).

Adverse Reactions

Orally, American ginseng can cause gastrointestinal, nervous and cardiovascular system adverse effects; however, these are similar to placebo (11351). Adverse reactions reported for the related species Panax ginseng include insomnia, mastalgia, vaginal bleeding, tachycardia, mania, cerebral arteritis, Stevens Johnson syndrome, cholestatic hepatitis (associated with a panax-containing, multi-ingredient product, Prostata), amenorrhea, decreased appetite, edema, hyperpyrexia, pruritus, rose spots, hypotension, palpitations, headache, vertigo, euphoria, and neonatal death (589,590,591,592,594,595,596,598). Diarrhea or allergic skin reactions can occur, especially with large amounts or prolonged use. There are reports of ginseng abuse syndrome, which includes hypertension, nervousness, insomnia, and increased libido; however, this is controversial and has not been verified by other reports (515).

Interactions with Herbs & Other Dietary Supplements

CAFFEINE, COFFEE, GUARANA, MATE, TEA: Concomitant use of American ginseng can potentiate the caffeine stimulant effects of these drugs (4,12).

Interactions with Drugs

ANTIDIABETES DRUGS: American ginseng may lower blood glucose (1018,6461). Theoretically, concomitant use with antidiabetes drugs might enhance blood glucose lowering effects and possibly cause hypoglycemia. Monitor blood glucose levels closely. Some antidiabetes drugs include glimepiride (Amaryl), glyburide (Diabeta, Glynase PresTab, Micronase), insulin, pioglitazone (Actos), rosiglitazone (Avandia), and others.
ANTIPSYCHOTIC DRUGS: Theoretically, American ginseng may interfere with antipsychotic drugs. Ginsenoside fractions of Panax ginseng seem to inhibit the uptake of several neurotransmitters in animals.
MONOAMINE OXIDASE INHIBITORS (MAOIs): Theoretically, American ginseng may interfere with MAOI therapy. There is one case report of insomnia, headache, and tremors with concomitant phenelzine (Nardil) and unspecified ginseng use (617). There is also one case report of hypomania with concomitant phenelzine (Nardil) and unspecified ginseng use (618).
STIMULANT DRUGS: Theoretically, concomitant use of American ginseng may potentiate the activity of stimulant drugs (4,12).
WARFARIN (Coumadin): American ginseng can decrease the effectiveness of warfarin therapy. Healthy patients receiving warfarin 5 mg daily, who also take American ginseng 1 gram twice daily, seem to have a significantly reduced international normalized ratio (INR) (619,12032). To avoid this potential interaction, advise patients who take warfarin not to take American ginseng.

Interactions with Foods

None known.

Interactions with Lab Tests

BLOOD GLUCOSE: American ginseng may decrease postprandial blood glucose levels and test results (1018,6461).
PROTHROMBIN TIME (PT): Theoretically, American ginseng may prolong thrombin time (TT) and activated partial thromboplastin time (aPTT), which is based on in vitro studies with the related species, Panax ginseng (1522).

Interactions with Diseases or Conditions

BLEEDING CONDITIONS: American ginseng has been reported to decrease blood coagulation (4); use with caution.
CARDIAC CONDITIONS: American ginseng is reported to have negative inotropic and chronotropic activity and hypotensive effects. Ginseng might adversely affect patients with cardiac disorders (4); use with caution.
DIABETES: American ginseng has hypoglycemic activity (4,1018,6461). Use in diabetics might increase the risk of hypoglycemic episodes; use with caution.
HORMONE SENSITIVE CANCERS OR CONDITIONS: Because American ginseng might have estrogenic effects, women with hormone sensitive conditions should avoid American ginseng. Some of these conditions include breast cancer, uterine cancer, ovarian cancer, endometriosis, and uterine fibroids (6180,7860).
INSOMNIA: High doses of American ginseng have been associated with insomnia (597). Theoretically, use in patients with insomnia might worsen the condition; use with caution.
SCHIZOPHRENIA: High doses of American ginseng have been associated with insomnia and agitation in schizophrenic patients (597); use with caution.

Dosage and Administration

ORAL: For reducing postprandial glucose levels in patients with type 2 diabetes, 3-9 grams up to two hours before a meal has been used (1018,6461). However, there is no added benefit to taking more than 3 grams (6461). American ginseng should be taken within two hours of a meal to avoid potential hypoglycemia (1018,6461). For preventing acute respiratory illness (ARI) in elderly patients, American ginseng extract 200 mg twice daily for 8-12 weeks has been used (11351). In children with attention deficit-hyperactivity disorder (ADHD), American ginseng 200 mg two times daily has been used for four weeks, in combination with Ginkgo biloba (8235).

Comments

Avoid confusion with Eleutherococcus senticosus, referred to as Siberian ginseng; and Panax ginseng, referred to as Asian ginseng. Wild American ginseng is so extensively sought that it has been declared an endangered species in the US (515).

GINSENG, PANAX

Also Known As

Asian Ginseng, Asiatic Ginseng, Chinese Ginseng, Ginseng, Ginseng Asiatique, Ginseng Radix Alba, Ginseng Root, Guigai, Hong Shen, Japanese Ginseng, Jen-Shen, Jinsao, Jintsam, Insam, Korean Ginseng, Korean Panax Ginseng, Korean Red Ginseng, Ninjin, Oriental Ginseng, Radix Ginseng Rubra, Red Ginseng, Ren Shen, Renshen, Renxian, Sheng Shai Shen, White Ginseng.
CAUTION: See separate listings for Blue Cohosh, Canaigre, Codonopsis, Ginseng American, Ginseng Siberian, Panax Pseudoginseng, and Ashwaganda.

Scientific Names

Panax ginseng, synonym Panax schinseng.
Family: Araliaceae.

People Use This For

Orally, Panax ginseng is used as a so-called "adaptogen" for increasing resistance to environmental stress and as a general tonic for improving well-being. It is also used for stimulating immune function, improving physical and athletic stamina, improving cognitive function, concentration, memory, and work efficiency. It is also used orally for depression, anxiety, Pseudomonas infection in cystic fibrosis, chronic bronchitis, irritated or inflamed tissues, and as a diuretic. Panax ginseng is also used orally for anemia, diabetes, gastritis, neurasthenia, erectile dysfunction, impotence and male fertility, fever, hangover, and asthma. It is also used orally for bleeding disorders, loss of appetite, vomiting, colitis, dysentery, cancer, insomnia, neuralgia, rheumatism, dizziness, headache, convulsions, disorders of pregnancy and childbirth, hot flashes due to menopause, and to slow the aging process.
Topically, Panax ginseng is used as part of a multi-ingredient preparation for treating premature ejaculation.
In manufacturing, Panax ginseng is used to make soaps, cosmetics, and as a flavoring in beverages.

Safety

POSSIBLY SAFE ...when used orally and appropriately, short-term. Panax ginseng seems to be safe when used for less than 3 months (8813,8814). ...when used topically, short-term as part of a multi-ingredient preparation (SS Cream). This preparation seems to be safe when applied and left on the glans penis for one hour (2537). Further evaluation is needed to determine its safety after prolonged, repetitive topical use.
POSSIBLY UNSAFE ...when used orally, long-term. There is some concern about the long-term safety due to potential hormone-like effects, which might cause adverse effects with prolonged use (12537). Tell patients to limit continuous use to less than 3 months.
CHILDREN: LIKELY UNSAFE ...when used orally in infants. Use of Panax ginseng in newborns is associated with intoxication that can lead to death (12). There is insufficient reliable information about use in older children; avoid using.
PREGNANCY: POSSIBLY UNSAFE ...when used orally. Ginsenoside Rb1, an active constituent of Panax ginseng, has teratogenic effects in animal models (10447); avoid using.
LACTATION: Insufficient reliable information available; avoid using.

Effectiveness

POSSIBLY EFFECTIVE

Cognitive function. Taking Panax ginseng orally might improve abstract thinking, mental arithmetic skills, and reaction times in healthy, middle-aged people (2064). Panax ginseng alone does not seem to improve memory (2064), but there is some evidence that a combination of Panax ginseng and ginkgo leaf extract can improve memory in otherwise healthy people ages 38 to 66 years (1903,8591).

Diabetes. There is some evidence that taking Panax ginseng orally, 200 mg daily, can decrease fasting blood glucose levels and hemoglobin A1c (HbA1c) in patients with type 2 diabetes (4225).

Erectile dysfunction (ED). Taking Panax ginseng orally seems to improve sexual function in men with erectile dysfunction (8813).

Premature ejaculation. Applying a multi-ingredient cream preparation containing Panax ginseng, angelica root, Cistanches deserticola, Zanthoxyl species, torlidis seed, clove flower, asiasari root, cinnamon bark, and toad venom (SS Cream) to the glans penis one hour prior to intercourse and washing off immediately before intercourse seems to improve ejaculatory latency in men with premature ejaculation (2537).

POSSIBLY INEFFECTIVE

Athletic performance. Taking Panax ginseng orally doesn't seem to improve aerobic exercise performance (1427,4230,4231,4236).

Menopausal symptoms. Taking Panax ginseng orally doesn't seem to help vasomotor symptoms such as hot flashes in postmenopausal women (10981). In postmenopausal women, some preliminary clinical research suggests that panax ginseng might improve quality of life, and menopausal symptoms such as fatigue, insomnia, and depression (3863,10981).

Quality of life. Taking Panax ginseng orally doesn't seem to be helpful for improving mood, sense of well being and overall quality of life. Although some research suggests that Panax ginseng might improve self-rated quality of life (6254), other studies show no benefit (8601,10314). Tell patients not to rely on Panax ginseng to improve mood or sense of well being.

INSUFFICIENT RELIABLE EVIDENCE to RATE

Bronchitis. Taking a specific Panax ginseng extract (G115) orally might be beneficial when used adjunctively for treating acute exacerbations of chronic bronchitis. Panax ginseng, combined with antibiotic therapy, might reduce bronchial bacterial counts more than antibiotic therapy alone (8814).

Cancer. Epidemiological data suggests that taking ginseng orally might decrease the incidence of cancer, specifically stomach cancer, lung cancer, liver cancer, ovarian cancer, and skin cancer (2063,3122).

Common cold. There is some evidence that taking a specific Panax ginseng extract (G115) orally can decrease the chance of catching a cold (589).

Congestive heart failure (CHF). An intravenous formulation of ginseng seems to increase ejection fraction in patients with congestive heart failure. Ginseng might improve hemodynamics and might work synergistically with digoxin (4243,8604).

Influenza. There is some preliminary evidence that suggests taking a specific Panax ginseng extract (G115) orally four weeks prior to influenza vaccination and continued for eight more weeks can decrease the risk of getting the flu (589).

More evidence is needed to rate Panax ginseng for these uses.

Mechanism of Action

The applicable part of Panax ginseng is the root. Panax ginseng contains several active constituents. The constituents thought to be of most importance are triterpenoid saponins referred to collectively as ginsenosides or panaxosides. Ginsenosides is the term developed by Asian researchers, and the term panaxosides was developed by early Russian researchers. Numerous subtypes of ginsenosides have been identified. Other constituents include pectin, B vitamins, and various flavonoids (11). Panax ginseng also contains the peptidoglycans, panaxans, which have hypoglycemic effects (12536). The ginsenosides have a wide range of pharmacological activity and effects. In some cases, these isolated constituents seem to counteract each other's activity. For example, ginsenoside Rg1, raises blood pressure and acts as a central nervous system (CNS) stimulant. Ginsenoside Rb1 lowers blood pressure and acts as a CNS depressant (11). They also seem to interfere with platelet aggregation and coagulation (1522). Ginsenosides also potentiate nerve growth factor (11) and might confer neuroprotection through nicotinic activity (3109). There is also evidence that ginsenosides can relax human bronchial smooth muscle by stimulating the release of nitrous oxide from airway epithelium which may account for the potential anti-asthmatic effect of Panax ginseng (11007). However, research on related ginseng species, Panax pseudoginseng, suggests these ginsenosides may not be pharmacologically significant. Rb1 has a low oral bioavailability, and Rg1 is rapidly eliminated from the blood in animal models (11153).

Ginseng is widely used as a general tonic or "adaptogen" for fighting stress. There is some evidence that it might work against stress by affecting the hypothalamic-pituitary-adrenal (HPA) axis. Panax ginseng saponins seem to increase serum cortisol concentrations (3256,3257) and stimulate adrenal function (13). Panax ginseng might also increase dehydroepiandrosterone sulfate (DHEA-S) levels in women (3863).

Panax ginseng might affect immune function and might have anticancer effects. Panax ginseng appears to stimulate natural-killer cell activity and possibly other immune-system activity. It might also have some antitumor activity (3122). Extracts of Panax ginseng decrease the production of tumor necrosis factor (TNF), diminish DNA strand breakage, and inhibit the formation of induced skin tumors (11006). There is conflicting research about the antioxidant and free radical scavenging activity of panax ginseng (4227,8602). Ginsenosides have been shown to inhibit tumor cell invasion and suppress sister chromatid exchanges in human lymphocytes (11006). Panax ginseng also contains water insoluble polyacetylenic constituents such as panaxynol, panaxydol, and panaxytriol. Panaxydol seems to have antiproliferative effects on various types of cancer cells by inhibiting cancer cell growth at the cell cycle G1 to S transition phase (11005). In peptic ulceration, Panax ginseng has shown inhibitory activity on Helicobacter pylori-induced hemagglutination (3121). Samgyetang, a soup made from chicken, panax ginseng, garlic, jujube, and chestnuts, appears to offer protection from experimentally induced peptic ulcers (10249).

Panax ginseng may lower serum cholesterol and triglycerides, possibly by increasing lipoprotein lipase activity, which enhances lipid metabolism (12538). However, panax ginseng appears to have negligible effects on cardiovascular function (4322).

Panax ginseng may affect blood glucose. Preliminary evidence that Panax ginseng might reduce tissue insulin resistance and changes in gene expression in Type II diabetes (8605). Ginsenosides in Panax ginseng might also directly stimulate insulin release (6461). The effect of various ginsengs on glucose appears to be related in part to the mix of ginsenosides. Other nonginsenoside constituents likely affect blood glucose as well. Panax ginseng and other ginsengs contain protopanaxadiol (PPD) ginsenosides, Rb1, Rb2, Rc, and Rd. They also contain protopanaxatriol (PPT) ginsenosides, Rg1, Re, and Rf. A higher ratio of PPD ginsenosides to PPT ginsenosides is related to greater blood glucose and insulin lowering potency of the ginseng product. Compared with American ginseng, panax ginseng appears to have a lower PPD to PPT ratio and may have less blood glucose. Some research suggests Panax ginseng may actually increase postprandial blood glucose and lower preprandial insulin levels. However, ginsenoside content varies among batches, plant parts, and preparation methods (12536).

The estrogenic effects of ginseng are controversial. Some clinical evidence suggests it doesn't have estrogen-mediated effects such as increasing follicle-stimulating hormone (FSH), estradiol levels, or endometrial thickness (10981). However, case reports of ginseng side effects such as postmenopausal vaginal bleeding suggest estrogen activity (590,591,592,10982,10983). Panax ginseng extract has been shown to increase serum ceruloplasmin oxidase activity (a measure of estrogenic activity in the liver) in animal models when ovaries are removed (6180). In vitro research also shows estrogen activity. Studies on human breast cancer cells indicate that ginseng, specifically its constituent ginsonside-Rb1, acts as a phytoestrogen (10984).

Panaxagin, a protein isolated from unprocessed ginseng root, seems to have antiviral and antifungal activity, according to preliminary research. It appears to inhibit HIV reverse transcriptase and ribosomal activity of some fungi (8603).

A multi-ingredient cream preparation containing Panax ginseng is thought to work in premature ejaculation by increasing the penile vibratory threshold and reducing the amplitude of penile somatosensory evoked potentials (2537). Some people try ginseng for cystic fibrosis because there is preliminary evidence that it has activity against Pseudomonas aeruginosa lung infections, but this effect has not yet been demonstrated in humans (3095,3096). There is some evidence that a Panax ginseng root extract can mildly inhibit cytochrome P450 2D6 (CYP2D6) activity by approximately 6% in humans. However, it appears to have no effect on CYP3A4 activity (1303).

Adverse Reactions

Orally, Panax ginseng is usually well tolerated, but some patients can experience side effects. The most common side effect is insomnia (589). Less commonly patients can experience mastalgia (590), vaginal bleeding (591,592,3354), amenorrhea, tachycardia and palpitations, hypertension, hypotension, edema, decreased appetite, diarrhea, hyperpyrexia, pruritus, rose spots, headache, vertigo, euphoria, and mania (594).

Uncommon side effects can include cerebral arteritis (595), Stevens-Johnson syndrome (596), cholestatic hepatitis (associated with a Panax ginseng-containing, multi-ingredient product, Prostata) (598), and anaphylaxis (11971).

There is a lot of controversy about the existence of a "ginseng abuse syndrome". In the late 1970s one author reported the existence of this syndrome that occurred after long-term use of ginseng. Symptoms included one or more of the following- hypertension, nervousness, insomnia, increased libido, estrogenic effects, skin eruptions, edema, and diarrhea (3353). Experts now agree there is not a ginseng abuse syndrome (515). However, many of these individual side effects can occur in some patients, even after short-term use of Panax ginseng.

There is a case report of menometrorrhagia and tachyarrhythmia in a 39-year-old woman who took Panax ginseng 1000-1500 mg/day orally and also applied a facial cream topically that contained Panax ginseng. Upon evaluation for menometrorrhagia, the patient also reported a history of palpitations. It was discovered that she had sinus tachycardia on ECG. However, the patient was a habitual consumer of coffee 4-6 cups/day and at the time of evaluation was also mildly anemic. The patient was advised to discontinue taking Panax ginseng. During the 6 month period following discontinuation the patient did not have any more episodes of menometrorrhagia or tachyarrhythmia (13030).

Topically, when a specific multi-ingredient cream preparation (SS Cream) has been applied to the glans penis, sporadic erectile dysfunction, excessively delayed ejaculation, mild pain, and local irritation and burning has occurred (2537).

Interactions with Herbs & Other Dietary Supplements

BITTER ORANGE: Theoretically, comitant use might prolong the QT interval due to its sympathomimetic effects. Ephedra, another herb with sympathomimetic effects, has been reported to have an additive effect with Panax ginseng and increase the risk of life-threatening ventricular arrhythmias (4322,11355).

COFFEE, GUARANA, TEA: Theoretically, concomitant use may potentiate therapeutic and adverse effects due to the caffeine content of coffee, guarana, or tea (589,594).

COUNTRY MALLOW: Theoretically, comitant use might prolong the QT interval due to its ephedrine content. Ephedra, which also contains ephedrine, has been reported to have an additive effect with Panax ginseng and increase the risk of life-threatening ventricular arrhythmias (4322,11355).

EPHEDRA: Ephedra-containing supplements may prolong the QT interval. This might have an additive effect with Panax ginseng and increase the risk of life-threatening ventricular arrhythmias (4322,11355).

HERBS AND SUPPLEMENTS WITH HYPOGLYCEMIC EFFECTS: There is some evidence that Panax ginseng might lower blood glucose (4225). Theoretically, concomitant use with other herbs and supplements that decrease blood glucose levels might increase the risk of hypoglycemia. Some of these products include bitter melon, ginger, goat's rue, fenugreek, kudzu, willow bark, and others.

Interactions with Drugs

ALCOHOL (Ethanol): Taking Panax ginseng 3 grams/65 kg body weight before drinking alcohol seems to significantly increase the clearance of alcohol. People taking Panax ginseng have blood alcohol levels about 35% lower compared to people not taking Panax ginseng while drinking alcohol. It is thought that Panax ginseng might lower alcohol levels by increasing activity of alcohol and aldehyde dehydrogenase (12191).

ANTICOAGULANT/ANTIPLATELET DRUGS: In vitro evidence suggests that ginsenoside constituents in Panax ginseng might decrease platelet aggregation (1522,11891). However, research in humans suggests that ginseng does not affect platelet aggregation (11890). Animal research indicates low oral bioavailability of Rb1 and rapid elimination of Rg1, which might explain the discrepancy between in vitro and human research (11153). Until more is known, use with caution in patients concurrently taking anticoagulant or antiplatelet drugs. Some antiplatelet and anticoagulant drugs include aspirin, cilostazol (Pletal), clopidogrel (Plavix), dalteparin (Fragmin), enoxaparin

(Lovenox), heparin, ticlopidine (Ticlid), and others.
ANTIDIABETES DRUGS: Theoretically, concomitant use might enhance blood glucose lowering effects (4225). Monitor blood glucose levels closely. Some antidiabetes drugs include glimepiride (Amaryl), glyburide (DiaBeta, Glynase PresTab, Micronase), insulin, pioglitazone (Actos), rosiglitazone (Avandia), and others.
CAFFEINE: Theoretically, caffeine might have an additive effect on the stimulant effects of panax ginseng (589,594).
CYTOCHROME P450 2D6 (CYP2D6) SUBSTRATES: There is some evidence that Panax ginseng can inhibit the cytochrome P450 2D6 (CYP2D6) enzyme by approximately 6% (1303). Although this effect is unlikely to produce clinically significant interactions, it might cause slightly elevated levels of drugs metabolized by the CYP2D6 enzyme. Some of these drugs include amitriptyline (Elavil), clozapine (Clozaril), codeine, desipramine (Norpramin), donepezil (Aricept), fentanyl (Duragesic), flecainide (Tambocor), fluoxetine (Prozac), meperidine (Demerol), methadone (Dolophine), metoprolol (Lopressor, Toprol XL), olanzapine (Zyprexa), ondansetron (Zofran), tramadol (Ultram), trazodone (Desyrel), and others.
FUROSEMIDE (Lasix): There is some concern that Panax ginseng might contribute to diuretic resistance. There is one case of resistance to furosemide diuresis in a patient taking a germanium-containing ginseng product (770).
IMMUNOSUPPRESSANTS: Theoretically, concurrent use might interfere with immunosuppressive therapy. Panax ginseng might have immune system stimulating properties (3122). Immunosuppressant drugs include azathioprine (Imuran), basiliximab (Simulect), cyclosporine (Neoral, Sandimmune), daclizumab (Zenapax), muromonab-CD3 (OKT3, Orthoclone OKT3), mycophenolate (CellCept), tacrolimus (FK506, Prograf), sirolimus (Rapamune), prednisone (Deltasone, Orasone), and other corticosteroids (glucocorticoids).
INSULIN: There is some concern that Panax ginseng might have additive hypoglycemic effects when used with insulin. Insulin dose adjustments might be necessary in patients taking Panax ginseng (4225); use with caution.
MONOAMINE OXIDASE INHIBITORS (MAOIs): Theoretically, Panax ginseng can interfere with MAOI therapy. Concomitant use with phenelzine (Nardil) is associated with insomnia, headache, tremors (617), and hypomania (618).
STIMULANT DRUGS: Theoretically, panax ginseng might have an additive effect when used with stimulant drugs (589,594).
WARFARIN (Coumadin): There has been a single case report of decreased effectiveness of warfarin in a patient who also took Panax ginseng (619). However, it's questionable whether Panax ginseng was the cause of this decrease in warfarin effectiveness. Research in humans and animals suggests that Panax ginseng does not affect the pharmacokinetics of warfarin (2531,11890).

Interactions with Foods

ALCOHOL: Taking Panax ginseng 3 grams/65 kg body weight before drinking alcohol seems to significantly increase the clearance of alcohol. People taking Panax ginseng have blood alcohol levels about 35% lower compared to people not taking Panax ginseng while drinking alcohol. It is thought that Panax ginseng might lower alcohol levels by increasing activity of alcohol and aldehyde dehydrogenase (12191).
COFFEE, TEA: Theoretically, panax ginseng might have an additive stimulant effect with the caffeine in coffee and tea (589,594).

Interactions with Lab Tests

ACTIVATED PARTIAL THROMBOPLASTIN TIME (aPTT), THROMBIN TIME (TT): Theoretically, Panax ginseng might prolong aPTT, TT, and increase test results (1522).
GLUCOSE: The effect of Panax ginseng on blood glucose may vary with batches, plant parts, and preparation methods (12536). Panax ginseng might reduce or increase fasting blood glucose concentrations and test results (4225,12536).
GLYCOSYLATED HEMOGLOBIN (HbA1c): Panax ginseng might improve glucose control and reduce HbA1c values in patients with type 2 diabetes (4225).

Interactions with Diseases or Conditions

BLEEDING CONDITIONS: Ginseng has been reported to decrease blood coagulation (3122); contraindicated in cases of hemorrhage or thrombosis.
CARDIAC CONDITIONS: Ginseng can slightly increase the QT interval and slightly decrease diastolic blood pressure in healthy adults on the first day of therapy. However, there are no changes with prolonged use (4322). Ginseng has not been studied in people with cardiovascular disease. Use with caution.
DIABETES: Ginseng is reported to have hypoglycemic activity (4225). Use in diabetics might increase the risk of hypoglycemic episodes; use with caution.
HORMONE SENSITIVE CANCERS/CONDITIONS: Because ginseng seems to have estrogenic effects (6180,10984), women with hormone sensitive conditions should avoid ginseng. Some of these conditions include breast cancer, uterine cancer, ovarian cancer, endometriosis, and uterine fibroids.
INSOMNIA: High doses of ginseng have been associated with insomnia (597). Theoretically, use in patients with insomnia might worsen the condition; use with caution.
ORGAN TRANSPLANT RECIPIENTS: Theoretically, concurrent use might interfere with immunosuppressive therapy. Panax ginseng might have immune system stimulating properties (3122); avoid concurrent use.

SCHIZOPHRENIA: High doses of ginseng have been associated with insomnia and agitation in schizophrenic patients (597); use with caution.

Dosage and Administration

ORAL: For reducing the risk of getting the common cold or flu, Panax ginseng 100 mg daily started four weeks prior to influenza vaccination and continued for eight weeks thereafter has been used (589). For use in an acute attack of chronic bronchitis, Panax ginseng 100 mg twice daily for 9 days combined with antibiotic therapy has been used (8814). For erectile dysfunction, Panax ginseng 900 mg three times daily has been used (8813). For treating type 2 diabetes, 200 mg daily has been used (4225).
TOPICAL: For premature ejaculation, a cream containing panax ginseng and other ingredients has been applied to the glans penis 1 hour before intercourse and washed off before intercourse (2537).

Comments

Ginseng has been used for medicinal purposes for over two thousand years. Approximately six million Americans use it regularly. Some consider the age of the ginseng roots important. In 1976, a four hundred year old root of Manchurian ginseng from the mountains of China reportedly sold for $10,000 per ounce. The contents of commercial preparations labeled as containing Panax ginseng can vary greatly; many contain little or no Panax ginseng (6,13). Sometimes you will hear people refer to ginseng as red or white ginseng. This distinguishes how some ginseng roots are prepared. For example, red ginseng is produced by steam-curing the root. Heat treatment of ginseng at a temperature and pressure higher than what is conventionally used to prepare red ginseng has been found to cause increased production of the ginsenosides Rg3, Rg5, Rg6, Rh2, Rh3, Rh4, and Rs3 which are usually absent or present in only small amounts in preparations of white or red ginseng (11006). In contrast to the usual promotion of ginseng as a stimulant, ginseng is used in Traditional Chinese Medicine (TCM) as a calming and sedative agent. It is also widely used in China as a cardiovascular agent. Typically, higher doses are used in TCM than Western medicine (8600,8604).

GINSENG, SIBERIAN

Also Known As

Ci Wu Jia, Ciwujia, Devil's Bush, Devil's Shrub, Eleuthero Ginseng, Eleutherococci Radix, Eleutherococcus, Ginseng, Ginseng Root, Phytoestrogen, Prickly Eleutherococcus, Russian Root, Shigoka, Siberian Ginseng, Thorny Bearer of Free Berries, Touch-Me-Not, Untouchable, Ussuri, Ussurian Thorny Pepperbrush, Wild Pepper, Wu Jia Pi, Wu-jia.
CAUTION: See separate listings for American Ginseng, Ashwaganda, Blue Cohosh, Canaigre, Codonopsis, Panax Ginseng, and Panax Pseudoginseng.

Scientific Names

Eleutherococcus senticosus, synonym Acanthopanax senticosus, Hedera senticosa.
Family: Araliaceae.

People Use This For

Orally, people use Siberian ginseng as an adaptogen, for increasing resistance to environmental stress. It is also used orally for normalizing high or low blood pressure, atherosclerosis, pyelonephritis, craniocerebral trauma, rheumatic heart disease, neuroses, insomnia, and increasing work capacity. Other oral uses include Alzheimer's disease, attention deficit-hyperactivity disorder (ADHD), chronic fatigue syndrome, diabetes, fibromyalgia, rheumatoid arthritis, influenza, chronic bronchitis, tuberculosis, improving athletic performance, reducing toxicity of chemotherapy, and symptomatic treatment of herpes simplex type II infections. It is also used orally as a general stimulant, diuretic, appetite stimulant, immune system stimulant, and for preventing colds and flu. In manufacturing, Siberian ginseng is added to skin care products.

Safety

POSSIBLY SAFE ...when used orally and appropriately, short-term. Siberian ginseng root extract has been used safely for up to 6 weeks (7522).
PREGNANCY AND LACTATION: Insufficient reliable information available; avoid using.

Effectiveness

POSSIBLY EFFECTIVE

Herpes simplex virus type 2 (HSV-2). Taking a specific Siberian ginseng extract, standardized to contain eleutheroside 0.3% (Elagen), orally seems to reduce the frequency, severity, and duration of herpes simplex type II infections (730,1427).

POSSIBLY INEFFECTIVE

Athletic performance. Taking Siberian ginseng orally doesn't seem to increase speed, quality, and capacity for physical work. A specific Siberian ginseng root liquid extract standardized to eleutherosides B and E content 3.4 mL daily doesn't seem to have any effect on endurance; performance; or psychological, cardiac, or respiratory parameters in trained distance runners (7522,7593). In trained endurance cyclists, Siberian ginseng 1200 mg per day (Endurox) doesn't seem to have any effect on glycogen, fat utilization, or cycling performance time (2335). It also doesn't seem to improve respiration; reduce lactate production; or hasten heart rate recovery during stair-stepping exercise, treadmill, or cyclic ergometry (7600,7601,8994).

INSUFFICIENT RELIABLE EVIDENCE to RATE

Cognitive performance. There is preliminary evidence that suggests Siberian ginseng might improve memory and feelings of well-being in middle-aged people (2574).

Heart disease. There is preliminary evidence that suggests administering Siberian ginseng intravenously might be useful for hyperlipidemia, and arrhythmias (7523,7524).

Ischemic stroke. There is preliminary evidence that suggests administering Siberian ginseng intravenously might be useful for treating acute cerebral infarction (7529).

More evidence is needed to rate Siberian ginseng for these uses.

Mechanism of Action

The applicable parts of Siberian ginseng are the root and leaf. The root, which is most commonly used, contains active compounds referred to as eleutherosides A through M (1954). Eleutheroside B (syringin) and eleutheroside E (syringaresinol) are the most plentiful and are used as marker compounds for Siberian ginseng products (7533). The eleutherosides include a variety of diverse compounds including saponins (daucosterol, beta-sitosterol, hederasaponin B), coumarins (isofraxidin), lignans (sesamin, syringaresinol), phenylpropanoids (syringin, caffeic acid, sinapyl alcohol, coniferyl aldehyde, protocatechuic acid), betulinic acid, vitamin E, and provitamins like beta-carotene (1954). Several constituents including syringin, syringoresinol, sesamin, beta sitosterol, caffeic acid, and coniferyl aldehyde are thought to have antioxidant and possible anticancer effects (1954). In addition, there is some evidence that the constituent coniferyl aldehyde protects DNA against breakage caused by ultraviolet light (1954). Siberian ginseng root extracts seem to have an antiproliferative effect on leukemia cells and appear to potentiate the effect of antimetabolites such as cytarabine (7525). There's also preliminary evidence that suggests it might act as an antioxidant and prevent damage in ischemic stroke (7529). Siberian ginseng root, the lignan constituent sesamin, and the phenylpropanoid syringin seem to have immunostimulatory effects (1954). Siberian ginseng increases lymphocyte counts and phagocyte activity (6206).

Eleutherosides A through G, particularly eleutheroside G, appear to have hypoglycemic activity (7591,12536). However, some research suggests that Siberian ginseng may actually increase postprandial blood glucose (12536).

Siberian ginseng constituents have a variety of other pharmacological effects. Protocatechuic acid seems to inhibit platelet aggregation (7592). Other constituents are also thought to be anti-inflammatory, sedative, diuretic, gonadotropic, estrogenic, protein-anabolic, and stimulate the pituitary-adrenocortical system (7531).

Siberian ginseng root extract seems to inhibit RNA-type viruses including human rhinovirus, respiratory syncytial virus (RSV), and influenza A virus, but has no effect on DNA viruses such as adenovirus or herpes simplex type 1 virus (HSV-1) (7526). Polysaccharide derivatives of Siberian ginseng appear to inhibit growth of the tuberculosis bacterium (7530).

The possible pharmacologic effects of Siberian ginseng leaves are also a current area of research. The leaves contain saponins that might have hypoglycemic effects and antihistaminic effects (7527,7592). There's also preliminary evidence that leaf saponins, given intravenously, might reduce myocardial infarct (MI) size (7528).

Whole plant extracts, as well as root extracts, seem to have an inhibitory effect on cytochrome P450 (CYP450) enzymes. Preliminary evidence suggests that Siberian ginseng might inhibit CYP1A2, CYP2C9, CYP2D6, and CYP3A4 (7531,7532). However, Siberian ginseng does not appear to inhibit drug metabolism by CYP2D6 and CYP3A4 in humans (7532,10400).

Adverse Reactions

Orally, Siberian ginseng can cause slight drowsiness, anxiety, irritability, and melancholy. Mastalgia can also occur. These adverse effects are more likely with higher than normal doses. Siberian ginseng should be used cautiously in patients with cardiovascular disorders (e.g., atherosclerotic or rheumatic heart disease), because it can cause palpitations, tachycardia, and hypertension (6500). Headache and pericardial pain can also occur in patients with rheumatic heart disease. Long-term use of Siberian ginseng is associated with inflamed nerves, often the sciatic nerve, which can then cause muscle spasms. There is one case report of neonatal androgenization following maternal use of Siberian ginseng (593,6500). However, it was later discovered that the androgenization was not due to Siberian ginseng, but due to silk vine (Periploca sepium) bark contamination (850,6500).

Interactions with Herbs & Other Dietary Supplements

ANTICOAGULANT, ANTIPLATELET HERBS AND SUPPLEMENTS: Concomitant use with herbs and supplements that affect platelet aggregation could theoretically increase the risk of bleeding in some people due to Siberian ginseng's possible effect on platelet aggregation (7592). Some of these herbs and supplements include angelica, clove, danshen, fish oil, garlic, ginger, Panax ginseng, red clover, turmeric, vitamin E, others.
HERBS AND SUPPLEMENTS WITH HYPOGLYCEMIC EFFECTS: There is preliminary evidence that suggests Siberian ginseng might have hypoglycemic effects (7591). Theoretically, concomitant use with other herbs and supplements that decrease blood glucose levels might increase the risk of hypoglycemia. Some of these products include bitter melon, ginger, goat's rue, fenugreek, kudzu, gymnema, and others.
HERBS WITH SEDATIVE PROPERTIES: There is preliminary evidence that Siberian ginseng root extract might cause dose-dependent sedation (7531). Theoretically, concomitant use with herbs that have sedative properties might enhance therapeutic and adverse effects. These include calamus, California poppy, catnip, German chamomile, gotu kola, hops, Jamaican dogwood, kava, lemon balm, sage, St. John's wort, sassafras, scullcap, valerian, wild carrot, wild lettuce, and others.

Interactions with Drugs

ALCOHOL (Ethanol): There is preliminary evidence that suggests that Siberian ginseng root extract might have sedative effects (7531). Theoretically, it might have an additive sedative effect with alcohol.
ANTICOAGULANT/ANTIPLATELET DRUGS: A constituent of Siberian ginseng, dihydroxybenzoic acid, appears to inhibit platelet aggregation (7592). Concomitant use with anticoagulant or antiplatelet drugs might increase the risk of bleeding.
ANTIDIABETES DRUGS: Certain constituents of Siberian ginseng appear to have hypoglycemic activity (7591). Monitor blood glucose levels closely. Some antidiabetes drugs include glimepiride (Amaryl), glyburide (DiaBeta, Glynase PresTab, Micronase), insulin, pioglitazone (Actos), rosiglitazone (Avandia), and others.
CNS DEPRESSANTS: There is preliminary evidence that suggests that Siberian ginseng root extract may have sedative properties (7531). Theoretically, concomitant use with drugs with sedative properties may cause additive effects and side effects.
CYTOCHROME P450 1A2 (CYP1A2) SUBSTRATES: Preliminary evidence suggests that standardized extracts of Siberian ginseng might inhibit cytochrome P450 1A2 (CYP1A2) in vitro and in animal models (7532). Until more is known about the effect on CYP1A2 Siberian ginseng should be used cautiously in patients taking drugs that are metabolized by these CYP450 enzymes. Some drugs metabolized by CYP1A2 include clozapine (Clozaril), cyclobenzaprine (Flexeril), fluvoxamine (Luvox), haloperidol (Haldol), imipramine (Tofranil), mexiletine (Mexitil), olanzapine (Zyprexa), Pentazocine (Talwin), propranolol (Inderal), tacrine (Cognex), theophylline (Slo-bid, Theo-Dur, others), zileuton (Zyflo), Zolmitriptan (Zomig), and others.
CYTOCHROME P450 2C9 (CYP2C9) SUBSTRATES: Preliminary evidence suggests that standardized extracts of Siberian ginseng might inhibit cytochrome P450 2C9 (CYP2C9) in vitro and in animal models (7532). Until more is known about the effect on CYP2C9, Siberian ginseng should be used cautiously in patients taking drugs that are metabolized by these CYP450 enzymes. Some drugs metabolized by CYP2C9 include amitriptyline (Elavil), diazepam (Valium), estradiol (Estrace), tacrine (Cognex), verapamil (Calan), warfarin (Coumadin), zileuton (Zyflo), and others.
CYTOCHROME P450 2D6 (CYP2D6) SUBSTRATES: Preliminary evidence suggests that standardized extracts of Siberian ginseng might inhibit cytochrome P450 2D6 (CYP2D6) in vitro and in animal models. However, Siberian ginseng does not appear to inhibit drug metabolism by CYP2D6 in humans (7532,10400).
CYTOCHROME P450 3A4 (CYP3A4) SUBSTRATES: Preliminary evidence suggests that standardized extracts of Siberian ginseng might inhibit cytochrome P450 3A4 (CYP3A4) in vitro and in animal models. However, Siberian ginseng does not appear to inhibit drug metabolism by CYP3A4 in humans (7532,10400).
DIGOXIN (Lanoxin): One case report associated Siberian ginseng with elevated serum digoxin levels, without symptoms of toxicity (543). However, it is not clear if this was due to an interaction or whether the product ingested in this case actually contained cardiac glycoside-like constituents. The product was found to be free of digoxin and digitoxin (543), but was not tested for the presence of eleutherosides (797). It is unclear whether the product actually contained Eleutherococcus. It has been postulated that it may have contained silk vine (Periploca sepium) which is reported to contain cardiac glycosides, and silk vine is a common adulterant of Eleutherococcus senticosus (797).

Interactions with Foods

None known.

Interactions with Lab Tests

BLOOD GLUCOSE: The effect of Siberian ginseng on blood glucose may vary (12536). Some research suggests it might have hypoglycemic activity (7591). Other research suggests it might increase blood glucose (12536).

Interactions with Diseases or Conditions

CARDIOVASCULAR CONDITIONS: Siberian ginseng can cause palpitations, tachycardia, and hypertension and should be used cautiously in patients with cardiovascular disorders (e.g. atherosclerotic or rheumatic heart disease). It can also cause headache and pericardial pain in patients with rheumatic heart disease (6500).
DIABETES: Some research suggests that Siberian ginseng might increase postprandial glucose levels (12536). However, some constituents of Siberian ginseng might have blood glucose lowering effects (7591). Monitor blood glucose closely.
HORMONE SENSITIVE CANCERS/CONDITIONS: Because Siberian ginseng might have estrogenic effects (6180), women with hormone sensitive conditions should avoid Siberian ginseng. Some of these conditions include breast cancer, uterine cancer, ovarian cancer, endometriosis, and uterine fibroids.
HYPERTENSION: Siberian ginseng is contraindicated in individuals with blood pressure exceeding 180/90. Siberian ginseng can potentially exacerbate hypertension (12).
MYOCARDIAL INFARCTION (MI): Theoretically, Siberian ginseng may exacerbate MI (4); use with caution.
PSYCHIATRIC CONDITIONS: Theoretically, Siberian ginseng may exacerbate some psychiatric conditions including hysteria, mania, and schizophrenia (4); use with caution.

Dosage and Administration

ORAL: For herpes simplex type II infections, Siberian ginseng extract standardized to contain eleutheroside E 0.3% in doses of 400 mg per day has been used (1427).

Comments

"Adaptogen" is a non-medical term used to suggest that a substance can act to strengthen the body and increase general resistance. It is often used to describe the purported activity of Siberian ginseng (1954). The chemical content and potency of various Siberian ginseng products can vary (7533). Siberian ginseng is often misidentified or adulterated. Siberian ginseng is a completely different herb than American or Panax ginseng. American and Panax ginseng can be considerably more expensive. It is said that the Soviet Union wanted to provide its athletes with the advantage offered by ginseng but wanted a less expensive version. Therefore Siberian ginseng became popular, and this is why most studies on Siberian ginseng have been done in Russia. Exercise caution in differentiating ginseng products. Silk vine is a common adulterant of Siberian ginseng (797).

GLOBE FLOWER

Also Known As

Globe Crowfoot, Globe Ranunculus, Globe Trollius.

Scientific Names

Trollius europaeus.
Family: Ranunculaceae.

People Use This For

Orally, globe flower is used for scurvy.

Safety

LIKELY UNSAFE ...when any part of the fresh plant is used orally or topically because it can cause severe local irritation (18).
There is insufficient reliable information available about the safety of the dried, cut globe flower plant.
PREGNANCY AND LACTATION: LIKELY UNSAFE ...when any part of the fresh plant is used orally or topically (18). There is insufficient reliable information available about the safety of the dried, cut globe flower plant during pregnancy and lactation.

Effectiveness

There is insufficient reliable information available about the effectiveness of globe flower.

Mechanism of Action

The applicable part is the whole fresh plant. When the fresh plant is crushed or cut into small pieces, the glycoside ranunculin is enzymatically changed into a severely irritating protoanemonin, which, in turn, rapidly degrades into the less toxic anemonin (18). Both protoanemonin and ranunculin are destroyed to an unknown extent during the drying process (2).

Adverse Reactions

Orally, ingestion of globe flower can cause severe irritation of the gastrointestinal tract, with colic and diarrhea. Irritation of the urinary tract can also occur.
Topically, skin contact can cause blisters and burns that are difficult to heal (18).

Interactions with Herbs & Other Dietary Supplements
None known.

Interactions with Drugs
None known.

Interactions with Foods
None known.

Interactions with Lab Tests
None known.

Interactions with Diseases or Conditions
None known.

Dosage and Administration
No typical dosage.

GLOSSY PRIVET

Also Known As
Chinese Privet, Dongqingzi, Ligustro, Ligustrum, Ligustrum Fruit, Nu Zhen, Nu Zhen Zi, Nuzhenzi, Privet, To-Nezumimochi, Troène De Chine, Trueno, White Waxtree.

Scientific Names
Ligustrum lucidum.
Family: Oleaceae.

People Use This For
Orally, glossy privet is used for promoting growth and darkening of hair, reducing facial dark spots, palpitations, rheumatism, swelling, tumors, vertigo, common cold, congestion, constipation, deafness, debility, fever, headache, hepatitis, insomnia, rejuvenation and longevity. It is also used as a diaphoretic and tonic, for improving immune function, and reducing the side effects of chemotherapy. Glossy privet is also used for blurred vision, invigorating the liver and kidney, for dizziness, tinnitus, and for sore back and knees.

Safety
POSSIBLY SAFE ...when used orally and appropriately (12).
PREGNANCY AND LACTATION: Insufficient reliable information available; avoid using.

Effectiveness
There is insufficient reliable information available about the effectiveness of glossy privet.

Mechanism of Action
The applicable part of glossy privet is the ripe fruit (11). It contains triterpenoids, including oleanolic acid (ligustrin), acetyloleanolic acid, and ursolic acid; glycosides (including ligustroside, oleuropein, 4-hydroxy-beta-phenylethyl-beta-D-glucoside); mannitol; fatty oil, consisting mainly of linoleic, linolenic, oleic and palmitic acids; and a volatile oil consisting primarily of esters, alcohols, thioketones and hydrocarbons (11). Ligustrum is used clinically in China for treating leukopenia, although data involving experimentally-induced leukopenia did not show any effect (418). Ligustrum might also have immunomodulatory and antitumor effects (11). Preliminary evidence suggests that glossy privet fruit might inhibit growth of renal cell carcinoma, possibly via augmentation of phagocyte and lymphokine-activated killer cell activity (419). Glossy privet extracts inhibit mutagenicity in bacteria (420), stimulate T-cell function in cancer tissue (423), and reverse tumor-induced macrophage suppression (421). Preliminary evidence suggests that glossy privet fruit, and the ingredient ligustrin, might have anti-inflammatory, anti-allergic, mild cardiotonic, diuretic, sedative, lipid-lowering, blood flow enhancing, blood glucose lowering, and liver protectant effects (11).

Adverse Reactions
None reported. However, respiratory allergies (allergic rhinitis, asthma) and cross-allergenicity have been reported with the pollen of other Oleaceae species including common privet (Ligustrum vulgare), olive, ash, and lilac (416,417).

Interactions with Herbs & Other Dietary Supplements
None known.

Interactions with Drugs
None known.

Interactions with Foods
None known.

Interactions with Lab Tests
None known.

Interactions with Diseases or Conditions
None known.

Dosage and Administration
No typical dosage.

Comments
Avoid confusion with other species of privet such as Japanese privet (Ligustrum japonicum), border privet (Ligustrum obtusifolium), Chinese privet (Ligustrum sinense), privet (Ligustrum tschonoskii), common privet (Ligustrum vulgare), and golden privet (Ligustrum x vicaryi). The fruits of glossy privet (Ligustrum lucidum) and Ilex chinensis are both referred to by the Chinese name dongqingzi (11).

GLUCOMANNAN

Also Known As
Konjac, Konjac Mannan.

Scientific Names
Amorphophallus konjac, synonym Amorphophallus rivieri.
Family: Araceae.

People Use This For
Orally, glucomannan is used for constipation, weight loss in adults and children, type 2 diabetes, blood glucose control, and reducing serum cholesterol.
In foods, glucomannan is used in food preparation.

Safety
LIKELY SAFE ...when used orally as food (11358,11359). Glucomannan powder or flour is often used to enrich noodles in traditional Japanese foods.
POSSIBLY SAFE ...when used orally in powdered or encapsulated form. Glucomannan has been safely used in studies lasting up to 4 months (179,180,180,182,11357).
POSSIBLY UNSAFE ...when used orally in tablet form. There have been reports of esophageal and gastrointestinal obstruction (11293). Advise patients to use glucomannan in powdered or capsule form.
CHILDREN: POSSIBLY SAFE ...when used orally and appropriately in powdered or encapsulated form. Glucomannan has been safely used in children for up to 4 months (179,180). LIKELY UNSAFE ...when used orally in tablet form. There have been reports of esophageal and gastrointestinal obstruction (11293).
PREGNANCY AND LACTATION: Insufficient reliable information available; avoid using.

Effectiveness
POSSIBLY EFFECTIVE

Diabetes. Taking glucomannan orally seems to reduce serum cholesterol and blood glucose levels in patients with type 2 diabetes (183,11357,11359). Glucomannan may improve serum total cholesterol, low-density lipoprotein (LDL) levels, glycemic control, and systolic blood pressure in patients with type 2 diabetes and hyperlipidemia. Glucomannan also seems to improve insulin resistance syndrome, a prediabetic metabolic condition. The positive effect on insulin resistance syndrome appears to occur when glucomannan is mixed and consumed with carbohydrate foods (11358).

INSUFFICIENT RELIABLE EVIDENCE to RATE

Constipation. Preliminary clinical research suggests that taking glucomannan orally might relieve constipation. As a nonabsorbable dietary fiber, glucomannan may have a bulk laxative effect (11294,11295).
Obesity. There is preliminary evidence that taking glucomannan orally might help reduce weight in obese children and adults (180,181,182,183). But some research shows no effect (179).
More evidence is needed to rate glucomannan for these uses.

Mechanism of Action

Glucomannan is an unabsorbable polysaccharide composed of glucose and mannose that is derived from konjac (Amorphophallus konjac) root (11361). Glucomannan contains insoluble fiber that may increase water absorption by the stools (11294,11295).

Glucomannan seems to reduce serum total cholesterol and low-density lipoprotein (LDL) cholesterol levels in healthy men (178) and in adults with type 2 diabetes (11357). Glucomannan appears to improve lipid profiles by enhancing fecal excretion of cholesterol and bile acid (11357). Glucomannan may improve glycemic control in people with type 2 diabetes (11357,11359), possibly by slowing gastric emptying and increasing the viscosity of gastrointestinal contents (11361). Glucomannan also seems to improve systolic blood pressure in people with type 2 diabetes (11359).

Adverse Reactions

Orally, esophageal and gastrointestinal obstructions have been reported when the tablet form has been used (11293). Advise patients to use glucomannan in powdered or capsule form.

Interactions with Herbs & Other Dietary Supplements

HERBS AND SUPPLEMENTS WITH HYPOGLYCEMIC EFFECTS: There is some evidence that glucomannan might have hypoglycemic effects (183,11357,11359). Theoretically, concomitant use with other herbs and supplements that decrease blood glucose levels might increase the risk of hypoglycemia. Some of these products include bitter melon, cowhage, ginger, goat's rue, fenugreek, kudzu, willow bark, and others.

VITAMIN E, VITAMIN A, VITAMIN K, VITAMIN D: Glucomannan may reduce absorption of vitamin E and other fat soluble vitamins, possibly because it increases excretion of bile acids, which facilitate the transport and absorption of fat soluble vitamins. It doesn't seem to affect water-soluble vitamins (12539).

Interactions with Drugs

ANTIDIABETES DRUGS: Glucomannan can reduce blood glucose levels in patients with type 2 diabetes (11357,11359) and might have additive effects on glucose levels when used with antidiabetes drug therapy. Monitor blood glucose levels closely. Medication dose adjustments may be necessary. Some antidiabetes drugs include glimepiride (Amaryl), glyburide (DiaBeta, Glynase PresTab, Micronase), insulin, pioglitazone (Actos), rosiglitazone (Avandia), and others.

ORAL DRUGS: Glucomannan may decrease absorption of drugs taken orally, including sulfonylurea medications (11360). Some sulfonylurea drugs include chlorpropamide (Diabinese), glimepiride (Amaryl), glipizide (Glucotrol), glyburide (DiaBeta, Glynase PresTab, Micronase), and others. Take oral drugs one hour before or four hours after glucomannan to avoid decreased or delayed absorption.

Interactions with Foods

None known.

Interactions with Lab Tests

CHOLESTEROL: Glucomannan might reduce serum total cholesterol, LDL cholesterol, and test results in obese adults and adults with type 2 diabetes (181,182,183,11357,11359).

GLUCOSE: Glucomannan might reduce blood glucose concentrations and test results in patients with type 2 diabetes (11357,11359).

TRIGLYCERIDES: Glucomannan might reduce serum triglycerides and test results in obese adults (181,182).

Interactions with Diseases or Conditions

DIABETES: Glucomannan may interfere with blood sugar control (11357,11359), monitor closely.

Dosage and Administration

ORAL: For adult weight loss, 1 gram three times daily (1 hour before each meal) (182), has been used. For child weight loss, 2 to 3 grams per day has been used (180). For type 2 diabetes with hyperlipidemia, 3.6 to 10.6 grams per day has been used (11357,11359). For insulin resistance syndrome, 8 to 13 grams per day has been used (11358).

GLUCOSAMINE HYDROCHLORIDE

Also Known As

2-amino-2-deoxy-beta-D-glucopyranose, Amino Monosaccharide, Chitosamine, D-Glucosamine HCL, Glucosamine HCL, Glucose-6-Phosphate.

CAUTION: See separate listings for Glucosamine Sulfate and N-Acetyl Glucosamine.

Scientific Names

2-amino-2-deoxyglucose hydrochloride.

People Use This For

Orally, glucosamine hydrochloride is used for osteoarthritis and glaucoma.

Safety

POSSIBLY SAFE ...when used orally and appropriately, short-term. Glucosamine hydrochloride has been used safely in studies lasting up to 16 weeks (1520,4237).

There is insufficient reliable information available about the safety of long-term use of glucosamine hydrochloride.

PREGNANCY AND LACTATION: Insufficient reliable information available; avoid using.

Effectiveness

POSSIBLY EFFECTIVE

Osteoarthritis. Glucosamine hydrochloride seems to reduce subjective pain levels in some patients with osteoarthritis of the knee (1520,10312). The majority of evidence supporting glucosamine hydrochloride involves a specific combination product, which contains glucosamine hydrochloride, chondroitin sulfate, and manganese ascorbate (Cosamin-DS). This combination seems to improve both objective and subjective measures of pain in patients with osteoarthritis of the knee (4237,7169). It is not known if this benefit is due to glucosamine hydrochloride or the other ingredients. There is significantly more evidence supporting glucosamine sulfate for osteoarthritis. Encourage patients interested in trying glucosamine to use the glucosamine sulfate formulation.

There is insufficient reliable information available about the effectiveness of glucosamine hydrochloride for its other uses.

Mechanism of Action

Glucosamine hydrochloride is one of the salt forms of the amino sugar glucosamine, which is a constituent of cartilage proteoglycans. Other salt forms are also available including glucosamine sulfate and N-acetyl glucosamine. Although glucosamine is administered in a salt form, the salt is likely cleaved off in the stomach. Glucosamine base is completely ionized in the stomach. Laboratory data suggests that glucosamine base, glucosamine hydrochloride, and glucosamine sulfate may be equally active, but there are no head-to-head clinical studies (8128). Glucosamine is usually derived from marine exoskeletons or produced synthetically. Glucosamine is required for the synthesis of glycoproteins, glycolipids, and glycosaminoglycans (also known as mucopolysaccharides); these carbohydrate-containing compounds are found in tendons, ligaments, cartilage, synovial fluid, mucous membranes, structures in the eye, blood vessels, and heart valves. Glucosamine stimulates metabolism of chondrocytes in the articular cartilage and synovial cells in the synovial tissues. Glucosamine is also a component of biologically active compounds such as heparin, but it does not react with heparin-induced thrombocytopenia (HIT) antibodies (7640,7641,11831).

There has been a lot of concern about the effect of glucosamine on glucose metabolism. Preliminary evidence suggests glucosamine might decrease glucose-induced insulin secretion by inhibiting pancreatic glucokinase in the beta cells of the islet of Langerhans (371,372,3406). Other preliminary research suggests that glucosamine might also impair insulin-mediated glucose uptake and metabolism in skeletal muscle (372,3406). Animal research suggests glucosamine might increase glucose metabolism through the hexosamine pathway, a pattern of change in glucose metabolism similar to that seen in type 2 diabetes (3405,3406). However, animals may handle glucosamine differently than humans. Most of the research in humans suggests that glucosamine doesn't affect the pharmacokinetics of glucose. Research in people with normal glucose metabolism suggests glucosamine doesn't affect insulin sensitivity or plasma glucose (7637,7638). Clinical research in people with type 2 diabetes and people without diabetes suggests that glucosamine doesn't have any significant effect on blood glucose when given for up to 3 years (7026,10311,10317). Preliminary clinical research suggests that endogenous glucosamine and insulin levels are elevated in nondiabetic patients with ischemic heart disease (7640,7641). Some researchers think that increased glucosamine production might contribute to endothelial cell dysfunction (8944). Some glucosamine preparations are provided as topical creams. It is not known if glucosamine is absorbed transdermally.

Some researchers think the sulfate moiety in glucosamine sulfate might be responsible for its effect on osteoarthritis. Sulfate is required for articular cartilage glycosaminoglycan synthesis. Glucosamine might increase the absorption of sulfate. Glucosamine sulfate increases serum and synovial sulfate levels. Acetaminophen given concurrently with glucosamine sulfate, decreases sulfate levels, suggesting that use of acetaminophen in clinical trials might alter results. If the sulfate is the active moiety of glucosamine sulfate, theoretically glucosamine hydrochloride would be less effective (10313), but there are no head-to-head clinical studies of the sulfate and hydrochloride salts of glucosamine. More research is needed to determine the role of sulfate in the efficacy of glucosamine sulfate.

Adverse Reactions

Orally, glucosamine hydrochloride can cause mild gastrointestinal (GI) symptoms such as gas, abdominal bloating, and cramps (1520). Anecdotal reports have associated glucosamine with renal toxicity, but changes in renal function have not been reported in long-term studies (7026,8942,10408,10409).

Elevated blood glucose levels in patients with diabetes have been reported (22). However, 90 days of glucosamine therapy does not seem to affect hemoglobin A1C levels in people with type 2 diabetes (10311,10317). There is some concern that it might increase the risk of metabolic disturbances resulting in increased cholesterol levels and blood pressure. However, glucosamine hydrochloride does not appear to increase the risk of these adverse effects (7075).

In people older than 45, who have taken glucosamine for 3 years, there doesn't seem to be any adverse effects on blood glucose metabolism, lipid metabolism, or any other disturbances in metabolism (7026,8942).
Tell patients to look out for glucosamine plus chondroitin combination products that also contain manganese (e.g., Cosamin-DS). Remind patients to adhere to product directions. When taken at doses slightly higher than the recommended dose, these products can sometimes supply greater than the tolerable upper limit (UL) for manganese (11 mg per day). Ingestion of more than 11 mg per day of manganese might cause significant central nervous system toxicity (7135).

Interactions with Herbs & Other Dietary Supplements

None known.

Interactions with Drugs

ANTIDIABETES DRUGS: Preliminary research suggests that glucosamine might increase insulin resistance, or decrease insulin production, and potentially worsen diabetes control (371,372,3406,7637,7638). But there is some clinical evidence that suggests that taking glucosamine for 3 months does not increase hemoglobin A1c (HbA1c) in people with type 2 diabetes who have well-controlled glucose levels (10311,10317). Until more is known, advise patients with diabetes who take glucosamine to monitor their blood glucose levels closely. Some antidiabetes drugs include glimepiride (Amaryl), glyburide (DiaBeta, Glynase PresTab, Micronase), insulin, pioglitazone (Actos), rosiglitazone (Avandia), and others.
ANTIMITOTIC CHEMOTHERAPY: Theoretically, glucosamine might induce resistance to etoposide (VP16, VePesid) and doxorubicin (Adriamycin) by reducing the drugs' inhibition of topoisomerase II, an enzyme required for DNA replication in tumor cells (7639).
WARFARIN (Coumadin): There's some concern that high-dose glucosamine (3000 mg per day), combined with high-dose chondroitin sulfate (2400 mg per day), may enhance the effects of warfarin (Coumadin) as measured by the INR (11389). Chondroitin is a small component of a heparinoid and might have weak anticoagulant activity. Glucosamine is also a small component of heparin, but is does not seem to have anticoagulant activity. It's not known if glucosamine contributes to this potential interaction. Interactions with warfarin have not been reported at recommended dosages of glucosamine or chondroitin.

Interactions with Foods

None known.

Interactions with Lab Tests

BLOOD GLUCOSE: Glucosamine doesn't seem to adversely affect blood glucose control in people with type 2 diabetes, as measured by hemoglobin A1C (10311,10317). It also doesn't seem to affect blood glucose in nondiabetic people older than 45, who have taken glucosamine for osteoarthritis for 3 years (7026,8942). Some preliminary research raised concerns that glucosamine might exacerbate diabetes by increasing insulin resistance and/or decreasing insulin production, resulting in elevated blood glucose levels (5059). However, other research has shown no effect (7637,7638). There are also anecdotal reports of reduced blood glucose control in people with diabetes who take glucosamine (22,1203,1204,3405,3406). However, clinical studies indicate that glucosamine has little or no effect blood glucose (7026,8942,10311,10317).
INTERNATIONAL NORMALIZED RATIO (INR)/PROTHROMBIN TIME (PT): High dose glucosamine (3000 mg per day), combined with high dose chondroitin sulfate (2400 mg per day), may increase the INR in patients taking warfarin (Coumadin). There is one case report of an increased INR associated with concomitant use of warfarin a glucosamine-chondroitin supplement taken above recommended dosages (11389).

Interactions with Diseases or Conditions

ASTHMA: Glucosamine might exacerbate asthma by an unidentified allergic mechanism. Use glucosamine hydrochloride cautiously in patients with asthma (10002).
DIABETES: Glucosamine doesn't seem to adversely affect blood glucose control in people with type 2 diabetes, as measured by hemoglobin A1C (10311,10317). Some preliminary research raised concerns that glucosamine might exacerbate diabetes by increasing insulin resistance and/or decreasing insulin production, resulting in elevated blood glucose levels (5059). However, other research has shown no effect on insulin sensitivity or plasma glucose (7637,7638). There are also anecdotal reports of reduced blood glucose control in people with diabetes who take glucosamine (22,1203,1204,3405,3406). However, clinical studies indicate that glucosamine seems to be safe in people with type 2 diabetes (10311,10317).
SHELLFISH ALLERGY: There is concern that glucosamine products might cause allergic reactions in people who are sensitive to shellfish. Glucosamine is derived from the exoskeletons of shrimp, lobster, and crabs. But allergic reactions in people with shellfish allergy are caused by IgE antibodies to antigens in the meat of shellfish, not to antigens in the shell. There are no documented reports of allergic reaction to glucosamine in shellfish allergic patients. There is also some evidence that patients with shellfish allergy can safely take glucosamine products (12210).

Dosage and Administration

ORAL: For osteoarthritis, one study used glucosamine hydrochloride 500 mg three times daily (1520). A combination of glucosamine hydrochloride, 1500 mg/day, chondroitin sulfate, 1200 mg/day, and manganese ascorbate, 228 mg/day (Cosamin-DS, Nutramax Laboratories) has also been used (4237).

Comments

Read glucosamine product labels carefully for content. Avoid confusion with glucosamine sulfate and N-acetyl glucosamine. These products may not be interchangeable. Glucosamine sulfate has been studied the most for osteoarthritis. However, there is no clinical evidence to support the use of N-acetyl glucosamine for osteoarthritis. There is great variability among glucosamine and glucosamine plus chondroitin products. Actual content versus label claim varies from 25% to 115% (8128). Some products in the US that are labeled glucosamine sulfate are actually glucosamine hydrochloride with added sulfate (12464).

GLUCOSAMINE SULFATE

Also Known As

2-amino-2-deoxy-beta-D-glucopyranose, Amino Monosaccharide, Chitosamine, D-Glucosamine, G6S, Glucosamine, Glucosamine Sulphate, Glucose-6-phosphate, Glucose-6-sulfate, Glucose-6-sulphate, GS, Mono-Sulfated Saccharide, Sulfated Monosaccharide, Sulfated Saccharide, Sulphated Monosaccharide.
CAUTION: See separate listings for Glucosamine Hydrochloride and N-Acetyl Glucosamine.

Scientific Names

2-amino-2-deoxyglucose sulfate.

People Use This For

Orally, glucosamine sulfate is used for osteoarthritis, glaucoma, temporomandibular joint (TMJ) arthritis, and weight loss. Glucosamine sulfate is also used orally in combination with other products, including chondroitin sulfate, glucosamine hydrochloride, or N-acetyl glucosamine.
Topically, glucosamine sulfate is used in combination with chondroitin sulfate, shark cartilage, and camphor for osteoarthritis.
Parenterally, glucosamine sulfate is used short-term for reducing the symptoms of osteoarthritis.

Safety

LIKELY SAFE ...when used orally and appropriately. Glucosamine has been used safely in multiple clinical trials lasting from 4 weeks to 3 years (2533,2600,2602,2603,2604,2606,7026,8942,11340,12461,12465).
POSSIBLY SAFE ...when used intramuscularly and appropriately, short-term. Intramuscular glucosamine seems to be well tolerated when given twice weekly for up to six weeks (2605). ...when used topically and appropriately, short-term. Glucosamine sulfate in combination with chondroitin sulfate, shark cartilage, and camphor appears to be safe when applied topically on an as-needed basis for up to eight weeks (10327).
PREGNANCY AND LACTATION: Insufficient reliable information available; avoid using.

Effectiveness

LIKELY EFFECTIVE

Osteoarthritis. Taking glucosamine sulfate orally significantly improves symptoms of pain and functionality in patients with osteoarthritis of the knee in studies lasting up to 3 years (2533,2600,2602,2603,2604,2606,7026,8942,10310,10312,12461,12465). Some evidence suggests that glucosamine sulfate is comparable to the nonsteroidal anti-inflammatory drugs (NSAIDs) ibuprofen (2602,2604) and piroxicam (Feldene) for symptom relief (2606); however, NSAIDs appear to relieve symptoms within 2 weeks compared to 4 to 8 weeks with glucosamine sulfate (2602,2604,2606).
But not all research has been positive (12462,12463). Glucosamine sulfate might not be very effective for more severe, long-standing osteoarthritis (1330,11459); and osteoarthritis in older and heavier patients (1330). Product variation or differences in patient populations and study design might explain these conflicting findings (12464).
Preliminary evidence suggests that glucosamine might not prevent disease flare-ups (9118). But due to poor study design more evidence is needed to determine how effective glucosamine is for preventing disease flare-ups.
Glucosamine might have disease-modifying activity and slow joint degeneration in patients with osteoarthritis. Patients taking glucosamine for up to 3 years seem to have significantly less knee joint degeneration, less joint space narrowing, and significant symptom improvement when compared with placebo (7026,8942,12466).
Most studies have only evaluated glucosamine sulfate for osteoarthritis of the knee. It also might help hip osteoarthritis (12466). There is preliminary clinical evidence that glucosamine sulfate might also be helpful for osteoarthritis of the lumbar spine (1316). Intramuscular glucosamine sulfate also seems to help. When given twice per week for 6 weeks it reduces the severity of symptoms of knee osteoarthritis in patients with mild to moderately severe disease (radiological stage I-III) compared to placebo (2605).
There is a report that a topical preparation of glucosamine sulfate in combination with chondroitin sulfate, shark

cartilage, and camphor reduces osteoarthritis symptoms. But any symptom relief is most likely due to the counterirritant effect of camphor and not the other ingredients (10327). There are problems with study design and blinding, which limits the reliability of this research (12467). There's no research showing that glucosamine is absorbed topically. Don't recommend topical glucosamine products.

Most clinical trials have used a specific patented oral formulation of glucosamine sulfate (Dona, Viartril-S, Rottapharm, Italy) (11340).

Glucosamine sulfate is often combined with chondroitin, but it's not known if this combination is any more effective than the individual ingredients.

POSSIBLY EFFECTIVE

Temporomandibular joint (TMJ) arthritis. Taking glucosamine sulfate orally appears to be at least as effective as analgesic doses of ibuprofen for relieving pain and improving TMJ function such as chewing, yawning, talking, and laughing. In some patients pain relief persists for up to 90 days after glucosamine sulfate is discontinued (3714).

There is insufficient reliable information available about the effectiveness of glucosamine sulfate for its other uses.

Mechanism of Action

Glucosamine is an amino sugar, which is a constituent of cartilage proteoglycans. It is derived from marine exoskeletons or produced synthetically. Glucosamine is required for the synthesis of glycoproteins, glycolipids, and glycosaminoglycans (also known as mucopolysaccharides). These carbohydrate-containing compounds are found in tendons, ligaments, cartilage, synovial fluid, mucous membranes, structures in the eye, blood vessels, and heart valves. Glucosamine is also a component of biologically active compounds such as heparin, but it does not react with heparin-induced thrombocytopenia (HIT) antibodies (7640,7641,11831).

In osteoarthritis, glucosamine stimulates metabolism of chondrocytes in the articular cartilage and of synovial cells in the synovial tissues. There is evidence that suggests that glucosamine might have a disease-modifying effect, stopping or slowing the progression of osteoarthritis (7026). Preliminary research suggests that glucosamine inhibits protein N-glycosylation and cytokine-stimulated production of mediators of inflammation and cartilage degradation (9119). Glucosamine seems to inhibit interleukin 1-beta, IL-1beta, which stimulates the gene expression and protein synthesis of cyclooxygenase-2 (COX-2) (9121). Glucosamine doesn't seem to directly affect cyclooxygenase, which is responsible for anti-inflammatory and analgesic effects of nonsteroidal anti-inflammatory drugs (NSAIDs), as well as adverse gastrointestinal effects (2604).

There has been a lot of concern about the effect of glucosamine on glucose metabolism. Preliminary evidence suggests glucosamine might decrease glucose-induced insulin secretion by inhibiting pancreatic glucokinase in the beta cells of the islet of Langerhans (371,372,3406). Other preliminary research suggests that glucosamine might also impair insulin-mediated glucose uptake and metabolism in skeletal muscle (372,3406). Animal research suggests glucosamine might increase glucose metabolism through the hexosamine pathway, a pattern of change in glucose metabolism similar to that seen in type 2 diabetes (3405,3406). However, animals may handle glucosamine differently than humans. Most of the research in humans suggests that glucosamine doesn't affect the pharmacokinetics of glucose. Research in people with normal glucose metabolism suggests glucosamine doesn't affect insulin sensitivity or plasma glucose (7637,7638). Clinical research in people with type 2 diabetes and people without diabetes suggests glucosamine doesn't have any significant effect on blood glucose when given for up to 3 years (7026,8942,10311,10317).

Preliminary clinical research suggests that endogenous glucosamine and insulin levels are elevated in nondiabetic patients with ischemic heart disease (7640,7641). Some researchers think that increased glucosamine production might contribute to endothelial cell dysfunction (8944). However, preliminary evidence suggests that glucosamine might have a protective effect against atherosclerosis. It seems to prevent oxidation of lipoproteins by scavenging reactive carbonyl intermediates produced by oxidized lipoproteins (9122).

Glucosamine might have activity against human immunodeficiency virus (HIV). Preliminary evidence suggests that it might inhibit the intracellular viral movement and block viral replication (7642).

Glucosamine sulfate is absorbed 90% after oral administration. The bioavailability is approximately 26% to 44% after first-pass metabolism (2608,10316). Although the plasma concentration of glucosamine doesn't increase substantially after oral glucosamine sulfate, radiolabeling techniques demonstrate that it is significantly absorbed. The plasma half-life of glucosamine is about one hour. However, glucosamine is incorporated into plasma proteins and tissues and therefore stays in the body much longer. The half-life of elimination is about 95 hours (2607,10316).

Although glucosamine is administered in a salt form, most commonly as the hydrochloride or sulfate, the salt is likely cleaved off in the stomach. Glucosamine base is completely ionized in the stomach (10327).

Some glucosamine preparations are provided as topical creams. It is not known if glucosamine is absorbed transdermally (10327).

Some researchers think the sulfate moiety in glucosamine sulfate might be responsible for its effect on osteoarthritis. Sulfate is required for articular cartilage glycosaminoglycan synthesis. Glucosamine might increase the absorption of sulfate. Glucosamine sulfate increases serum and synovial sulfate levels. Acetaminophen given concurrently with glucosamine sulfate, decreases sulfate levels, suggesting that use of acetaminophen in clinical trials might alter results. If the sulfate is the active moiety of glucosamine sulfate, theoretically glucosamine hydrochloride would be less effective (10313). However, there are no head-to-head clinical studies of the sulfate and hydrochloride salts of glucosamine. More research is needed to determine the role of sulfate in the efficacy of glucosamine sulfate.

Adverse Reactions

Orally, glucosamine sulfate can commonly cause mild gastrointestinal (GI) problems including nausea, heartburn, diarrhea, and constipation. Drowsiness, skin reactions, and headache have also been reported (2608). However, adverse effects in clinical studies have generally been comparable to placebo (7026). Glucosamine sulfate 1500 mg per day is tolerated at least as well as the nonsteroidal anti-inflammatory drug (NSAID) ibuprofen 1200 mg per day, and it is better tolerated than piroxicam (Feldene) 20 mg daily (2602,2604,2606).

Anecdotal reports have associated glucosamine with renal toxicity, but changes in renal function have not been reported in long-term studies (7026,8942,10408,10409).

Elevated blood glucose levels in patients with diabetes have also been reported (22). However, 80-90 days of glucosamine therapy does not seem to affect hemoglobin A1C or blood glucose levels in people with type 2 diabetes or healthy people (10311,10317,12107).

There is some concern that it might increase the risk of metabolic disturbances resulting in increased cholesterol levels and blood pressure. However, glucosamine does not appear to increase the risk of these adverse effects (7075). In people older than 45, taking glucosamine sulfate for 3 years doesn't seem to have any adverse effects on blood glucose metabolism, lipid metabolism, or any other disturbances in metabolism (7026,8942).

There is concern that glucosamine products might cause allergic reactions in people who are sensitive to shellfish. Glucosamine is derived from the exoskeletons of shrimp, lobster, and crabs. But allergic reactions in people with shellfish allergy are caused by IgE antibodies to antigens in the meat of shellfish, not to antigens in the shell. There are no documented reports of allergic reaction to glucosamine in shellfish allergic patients. There is also some evidence that patients with shellfish allergy can safely take glucosamine products (12210).

Interactions with Herbs & Other Dietary Supplements

None known.

Interactions with Drugs

ACETAMINOPHEN (Tylenol, others): Very preliminary research suggests that the sulfate portion of glucosamine sulfate may contribute to its effect in osteoarthritis. Since acetaminophen metabolism requires sulfur and reduces serum sulfate concentrations, it may theoretically interfere with the action of glucosamine sulfate. Conversely, the administration of sulfate may theoretically decrease the effectiveness of acetaminophen in sulfate-deficient people by increasing its clearance (10313).

ANTIDIABETES DRUGS: Glucosamine sulfate seems to have little or no effect on control of blood glucose in patients with type 2 diabetes (10311,10317). Preliminary research suggests that glucosamine might increase insulin resistance or decrease insulin production (371,372,3406,7637,7638). However, clinical research suggests that glucosamine doesn't adversely affect diabetes treatment (10311,10317). Some antidiabetes drugs include glimepiride (Amaryl), glyburide (DiaBeta, Glynase PresTab, Micronase), insulin, pioglitazone (Actos), rosiglitazone (Avandia), and others.

ANTIMITOTIC CHEMOTHERAPY: Theoretically, glucosamine might induce resistance to etoposide (VP16, VePesid), teniposide (VM26), and doxorubicin (Adriamycin). Glucosamine sulfate might contribute to the development of chemotherapeutic resistance by reducing the drugs' inhibition of topoisomerase II, an enzyme required for DNA replication in tumor cells (7639,9559).

WARFARIN (Coumadin): There's some concern that high-dose glucosamine (3000 mg per day), combined with high-dose chondroitin sulfate (2400 mg per day), may enhance the effects of warfarin (Coumadin) as measured by the INR (11389). Chondroitin is a small component of a heparinoid and might have weak anticoagulant activity. Glucosamine is also a small component of heparin, but it does not seem to have anticoagulant activity. It's not known if glucosamine contributes to this potential interaction. Interactions with warfarin have not been reported at recommended dosages of glucosamine or chondroitin.

Interactions with Foods

None known.

Interactions with Lab Tests

BLOOD GLUCOSE: Glucosamine doesn't seem to adversely affect blood glucose control in people with type 2 diabetes, as measured by hemoglobin A1C (10311,10317). It also doesn't seem to affect blood glucose in nondiabetic people older than 45, taking glucosamine for osteoarthritis for 3 years (7026,8942). Some preliminary research raised concerns that glucosamine sulfate might exacerbate diabetes by increasing insulin resistance and/or decreasing insulin production, resulting in elevated blood glucose levels (5059), but other research has shown no effect (7637,7638). There are also anecdotal reports of reduced blood glucose control in people with diabetes who take glucosamine (22,1203,1204,3405,3406). However, clinical studies indicate that glucosamine sulfate has little or no effect blood glucose (7026,8942,10311,10317).

INTERNATIONAL NORMALIZED RATIO (INR)/PROTHROMBIN TIME (PT): High dose glucosamine (3000 mg per day), combined with high dose chondroitin sulfate (2400 mg per day), may increase the INR in patients taking warfarin (Coumadin). There is one case report of an increased INR associated with concomitant use of warfarin a glucosamine-chondroitin supplement taken above recommended dosages (11389).

Interactions with Diseases or Conditions

ASTHMA: Glucosamine might exacerbate asthma by an unidentified allergic mechanism. Use cautiously in patients with asthma (10002).

DIABETES: Glucosamine doesn't seem to adversely affect blood glucose control in people with type 2 diabetes, as measured by hemoglobin A1C (10311,10317). Some preliminary research raised concerns that glucosamine sulfate might exacerbate diabetes by increasing insulin resistance and/or decreasing insulin production, resulting in elevated blood glucose levels (5059), but other research has shown no effect on insulin sensitivity or plasma glucose (7637,7638,12107). There are also anecdotal reports of reduced blood glucose control in people with diabetes who take glucosamine (22,1203,1204,3405,3406). However, clinical studies indicate that glucosamine sulfate seems to be safe in people with type 2 diabetes (10311,10317).

HYPERLIPIDEMIA: Glucosamine doesn't seem to adversely affect lipid levels in people over age 45 who have taken glucosamine sulfate for 3 years (7026,8942). There was some concern that glucosamine sulfate might increase cholesterol and triglyceride levels. There is preliminary evidence that glucosamine sulfate can increase insulin levels. Hyperinsulinemia is associated with elevated triglycerides and cholesterol (5059,7075). However, glucosamine appears to have little or no effect on insulin, lipids, or triglycerides in humans (7026,8942).

HYPERTENSION: Glucosamine doesn't seem to adversely affect blood pressure in people older than 45 who have taken glucosamine sulfate for 3 years (7026,8942). There is some concern that glucosamine sulfate might increase blood pressure. Preliminary evidence suggested that glucosamine sulfate might increase insulin levels. Hyperinsulinemia is associated with increased blood pressure levels (7075). However, glucosamine appears to have little or no effect on insulin or blood pressure in humans (7026,8942).

SHELLFISH ALLERGY: There is concern that glucosamine products might cause allergic reactions in people who are sensitive to shellfish. Glucosamine is derived from the exoskeletons of shrimp, lobster, and crabs. But allergic reactions in people with shellfish allergy are caused by IgE antibodies to antigens in the meat of shellfish, not to antigens in the shell. There are no documented reports of allergic reaction to glucosamine in shellfish allergic patients. There is also some evidence that patients with shellfish allergy can safely take glucosamine products (12210).

Dosage and Administration

ORAL: For osteoarthritis, the typical dose is 1500 mg once daily or in 3 divided doses (2600,2602,2603,2606,7026,8942). For temporomandibular joint (TMJ) osteoarthritis, 500 mg 3 times daily has been used (3714).

TOPICAL: For osteoarthritis, topical administration of a cream containing glucosamine sulfate, 30 mg/g; chondroitin sulfate, 50 mg/g; shark cartilage, 140 mg/g; and camphor, 32 mg/g; has been used as needed on sore joints for up to 8 weeks (10327).

PARENTERAL: In other countries, intravenous, intramuscular, and intra-articular products are used (2601); however, these products are not available in the US. In one trial, glucosamine sulfate 400 mg intramuscularly twice per week was used (2605).

Comments

Although chondroitin sulfate and glucosamine sulfate are frequently marketed together in combination products, there is no evidence that the combination has greater benefit than either product alone. There is great variability among glucosamine and glucosamine plus chondroitin products. Actual content versus label claim varies from 0% to 115% (11340). Some products in the US that are labeled glucosamine sulfate are actually glucosamine hydrochloride with added sulfate (12464).

The National Institutes of Health (NIH) is sponsoring its first clinical trial of glucosamine sulfate in combination with chondroitin sulfate. The 24 week, parallel group, double-blind randomized controlled trial (RCT) includes five separate treatment arms, in which patients will ingest: placebo, glucosamine sulfate 500 mg three times per day, chondroitin 400 mg three times per day, a combination of glucosamine sulfate and chondroitin, or celecoxib (Celebrex) (11012).

GLUTAMINE

Also Known As

GLN, Glutamate, Glutamic Acid, Glutaminate, Levoglutamide, Levoglutamine, L-Glutamic Acid, L-Glutamic Acid 5-Amide, L-Glutamine, Q.

Scientific Names

L-(+)-2-Aminoglutaramic acid.

People Use This For

Orally, glutamine is used for depression, moodiness, irritability, anxiety, insomnia, short bowel syndrome, Crohn's disease, and enhancing exercise performance. Glutamine is also used orally for HIV wasting, abnormal intestinal permeability in people with HIV, chemotherapy-induced mucositis, chemotherapy-induced diarrhea, chemotherapy-induced neuropathy, and protection of immune and gut barrier function in people with esophageal cancer undergoing radiochemotherapy. It is also used for attention deficit-hyperactivity disorder (ADHD), cystinuria, peptic ulcer, ulcerative colitis, sickle cell anemia, improving recovery after bone marrow transplant, and for alcohol withdrawal support. It is also used orally as enteral nutrition, for preventing morbidity in trauma patients, preventing infectious complications in critically ill patients, and for paclitaxel-induced myalgia and arthralgia.

Intravenously, glutamine is administered for improving recovery after surgery and after bone marrow transplant, and preventing chemotherapy-induced mucositis.

Safety

POSSIBLY SAFE ...when used orally and appropriately. Glutamine seems to be safe in doses up to 40 grams per day (2334,2337,2338,2364,2365,5029,5462,7233,7288,7293). ...when used intravenously. Glutamine seems to be safe in doses up to 570 mg/kg/day when incorporated into parenteral nutrition (2363,2366,5448,5452,5453,5454,5458,7293).

CHILDREN: POSSIBLY SAFE ...when used orally and appropriately. Glutamine seems safe in amounts that do not exceed 0.65 grams per kg per day in children 3 to 18 years (11364). There is insufficient reliable information available about the safety of glutamine in higher amounts when used in children.

PREGNANCY AND LACTATION: Insufficient reliable information available; avoid using.

Effectiveness

POSSIBLY EFFECTIVE

Critical illness (trauma). Administering glutamine enterally in nutrition formulas seems to help prevent morbidity in trauma patients and infectious complications in critically ill patients. Glutamine seems to improve nutritional and immunologic status, and to reduce complications in critically ill (5450) and multiple-trauma patients (5449,7309). Preliminary evidence suggests glutamine might help prevent bacterial translocation from the intestine and subsequent infection when administered enterally after trauma or major surgery (7731,8184). There is also some preliminary evidence that suggests parenteral glutamine might lessen protein breakdown and branched-chain amino acid catabolism in critical illness such as sepsis, cancer, trauma, and burn injury (8182). Additionally, some preliminary research suggests that glutamine administered in parenteral nutrition with growth hormone and insulin-like growth factor might improve nitrogen balance in critically ill patients (8186).

HIV/AIDS-related wasting. Taking glutamine orally seems to enhance intestinal absorption of nutrients, decrease intestinal permeability, and increase weight gain in people with HIV/AIDS. Doses of 40 grams per day seem to produce the best effect (2337,2702,5461,7729). Lower doses (14 grams per day) might also be effective when used in combination with arginine and beta-hydroxy-beta-methylbutyrate (a leucine metabolite) (7310).

Oral mucositis. Taking glutamine orally seems to help reduce chemotherapy-induced mucositis (stomatitis). Glutamine appears to decrease the incidence, severity, and duration of mouth pain in some patients undergoing cancer chemotherapy or bone marrow transplant (2336,2364,2368,2704,5029), but glutamine is not effective for all patients (2365,5451,5462,7296). It's not clear which patients are most likely to benefit. However, some researchers speculate that those cancer patients with glutamine deficiency may benefit most (2368). Upcoming clinical trials will help clarify the best way to use glutamine and which patients are most likely to benefit (7288).

Surgery. Administering glutamine intravenously seems to improve recovery after bone marrow transplant and abdominal surgery. Most patients receiving glutamine-supplemented parenteral nutrition after bone marrow transplantation seem to have improved nitrogen balance, a diminished incidence of clinical infection, lower rates of microbial colonization, shortened hospital stay, and increased hepatic function and lymphocyte recovery compared with patients receiving standard parenteral nutrition (2366,5452,5453,5454). However, not all bone marrow transplant patients seem to benefit (5451). Glutamine-fortified parenteral nutrition appears to preserve intestinal mucosal structure and permeability, improve nitrogen balance, improve immune function, and shorten hospital stay in patients recovering from major abdominal surgery and other major surgeries (2363,5448,7299,7300,7732).

POSSIBLY INEFFECTIVE

Athletic performance. Taking glutamine orally doesn't seem to enhance exercise performance (2341,2342,5455,5456,5464,5465,5466).

Crohn's disease. Taking glutamine orally doesn't seem to improve symptoms of Crohn's disease (2338,6256). Neither supplemental glutamine 7 grams three times daily nor a glutamine-enriched diet seems to have any benefit in patients with Crohn's disease (2338,6256,7297).

Cystinuria. Taking glutamine orally doesn't seem to help improve cystinuria (2339).

Diarrhea. Taking glutamine orally doesn't seem to help improve acute diarrhea in infants. Glutamine administered in the standard World Health Organization (WHO) glucose-electrolyte solution doesn't seem to have any effect on diarrheal stool output, duration of diarrhea, or volume of rehydration solution required to achieve and maintain hydration (7298).

INSUFFICIENT RELIABLE EVIDENCE to RATE

Chemotherapy-induced diarrhea. There is preliminary evidence that glutamine might reduce the occurrence of chemotherapy-induced diarrhea (7235,7285), but so far research findings have been inconsistent (7233,7295).

Chemotherapy-induced lymphocytopenia. There is conflicting evidence regarding the potential benefits of glutamine for preventing chemotherapy-induced reduction of lymphocytes (2705,7295).

Paclitaxel-induced myalgia and arthralgia. There is early evidence that glutamine might help reduce paclitaxel-induced myalgia and arthralgia (6433).

Short bowel syndrome. Research findings are inconsistent for the combination of glutamine and growth hormone in the treatment of short bowel syndrome (8185). Glutamine plus growth hormone seems to decrease dependence on parenteral nutrition in some patients (2334,2361,2362,2703), but glutamine alone doesn't appear to be effective (7730). Glutamine currently has orphan drug status for this use (1691).

More evidence is needed to rate glutamine for these uses.

Mechanism of Action

Glutamine is the most abundant free amino acid in the body (7739). It is produced primarily in skeletal muscle and then released into the circulation. Tissues that require glutamine such as the immune system, gastrointestinal tract, kidneys, and liver obtain glutamine as needed from the blood (7729). Glutamine acts as an inter-organ nitrogen and carbon transporter (5467). Although traditionally classified as a non-essential amino acid, glutamine is essential for maintaining intestinal function, immune response, and amino acid homeostasis during times of severe stress, suggesting that it is more appropriately called a conditionally essential amino acid (5468,7736).

The rapidly growing fetus and premature infant seem to require glutamine for growth and normal physiologic functions (7740). Glutamine is metabolized in the mitochondria and is important for providing metabolic fuel to lymphocytes, macrophages, and fibroblasts (5468,5469,7739).

Glutamine can enhance the function of stimulated immune cells. It seems to affect lymphocyte proliferation, cytokine production, bacterial killing by neutrophils, and phagocytic and secretory activities of macrophages (7734). In patients with cancer, some research suggests it might restore natural killer cell function in healthy cells and improve protein metabolism (7739). Neutrophils and monocytes are dependent upon glutamine to maintain phagocytic action (10225).

Glutamine also functions as a precursor for other amino acids, glucose, purines and pyrimidines, glutathione, and glutamate (5468,5469,5470,7292,7740).

Following surgery or accidental injury, about one third of the nitrogen mobilized for wound repair and vital organ function is from glutamine (7735). During physical stress the body consumes more glutamine than the skeletal muscle can produce. Progressive muscle breakdown (wasting) can occur as the body tries to meet glutamine requirements (7729). Decreased glutamine concentrations following surgery seems to impair the function of neutrophils and monocytes, which might increase the risk of infection (10225).

The intestinal mucosa can also synthesize glutamine, but not enough to compensate for the body's needs during severe physiologic stress (7733). There's some evidence suggesting that glutamine, in addition to serving as a metabolic fuel for enterocytes, might play a regulatory role in the intestine, affecting cell proliferation and differentiation (7733). The gastrointestinal tract is one of the largest utilizers of glutamine in the body (5469). Depletion of glutamine can result in atrophy, ulceration, and necrosis of intestinal epithelium.

Some cancer patients may have reduced levels of glutamine (2368). Since gastrointestinal cells are rapidly dividing, they are highly susceptible to the cytotoxic effects of chemotherapy. Glutamine treatment is thought to help prevent chemotherapy and radiation-induced gastrointestinal toxicity by maintaining viability of gastrointestinal tissues (2368).

Preliminary evidence suggests that glutamine might protect the heart from ischemia and EKG changes in patients with chronic stable angina (8183).

Adverse Reactions

Orally and intravenously glutamine seems to be well tolerated (7293). Some patients find the grittiness of glutamine administered in water unacceptable (11364). Significant side effects have not been reported in clinical studies (2336,2364,2365,2368,2704,5029,5451,5462,7233,7235,7285,7288). However, glutamine is metabolized to glutamate and ammonia, both of which might have neurological effects in people with neurological and psychiatric diseases (7293). Mania has been reported in people with bipolar disorder and supplementation with glutamine (7291).

There is also some concern that glutamine might be used by rapidly growing tumors and possibly stimulate tumor growth. Although tumors may utilize glutamine and other amino acids, preliminary research shows that glutamine supplementation does not increase tumor growth (5469,7233,7738). In fact, there is preliminary evidence that glutamine might actually reduce tumor growth (5469).

Interactions with Herbs & Other Dietary Supplements

None known.

Interactions with Drugs

ANTICONVULSANTS: Theoretically, glutamine, which is metabolized to the excitatory neurotransmitter glutamate, might antagonize the anticonvulsant effects of medications taken for epilepsy (7292,7293,7294). Some anti-epileptic drugs include phenobarbital, primidone (Mysoline), valproic acid (Depakene), gabapentin (Neurontin), carbamazepine (Tegretol), phenytoin (Dilantin), and others.
CHEMOTHERAPY: There has been concern that glutamine might alter the pharmacokinetics of chemotherapeutic drugs or reduce effectiveness by enhancing tumor growth. However, available clinical data suggests that glutamine does not adversely affect outcomes when used concurrently with chemotherapy (7738).
LACTULOSE: Theoretically, glutamine might antagonize the anti-ammonia effects of lactulose. Glutamine is metabolized to ammonia (7293).

Interactions with Foods

None known.

Interactions with Lab Tests

AMMONIA SERUM LEVELS: Glutamine is partially metabolized to ammonia. In higher doses, it can increase serum ammonia levels (7293,11364).
GLUTAMATE SERUM LEVELS: Glutamine is partially metabolized to glutamate. In higher doses, it can increase serum glutamate levels (7293,11364).

Interactions with Diseases or Conditions

HEPATIC ENCEPHALOPATHY: Theoretically, glutamine, which is metabolized to ammonia, might worsen hepatic encephalopathy (7293).
MANIA, HYPOMANIA: Glutamine might cause affective changes in people with mania or hypomania (7291). Glutamine is a precursor of the excitatory neurotransmitter glutamate (7292).
MONOSODIUM GLUTAMATE (MSG) HYPERSENSITIVITY: People who are sensitive to MSG, also known as "Chinese Restaurant Syndrome," might be sensitive to glutamine. Glutamine is metabolized to glutamate in the body (5469,7291).
SEIZURE DISORDERS: Theoretically excess amounts of glutamine and its metabolite, glutamate, might lower the seizure threshold (7292,7293).

Dosage and Administration

ORAL: For reducing chemotherapy-induced mucositis (stomatitis), a variety of dosage regimens have been used. Most often glutamine suspension 4 grams swish and swallow every four hours around the clock starting with the first dose of chemotherapy and continued until discharge or resolution of symptoms has been used (5029). In some cases, 4 grams swish and swallow twice daily from day one of chemotherapy for 28 days, or for four days past the resolution of symptoms, has been used (2364). Other successful regimens include 2 grams per meter squared swish and swallow twice daily (2336) or 1 gram per meter squared swish and swallow 4 times daily (2368) on days of chemotherapy administration and for at least 14 additional days, or 500 mg/kg per day (2704). For children receiving chemotherapy, 0.35 to 0.65 grams per kilogram per day has been used (11364). For chemotherapy-induced diarrhea, 6 grams mixed in water three times daily beginning five days before chemotherapy for 15 consecutive days has been used (7285). For short bowel syndrome, 630 mg/kg per day has been used (2334). For HIV wasting, 8-40 grams per day has been used. However, 40 grams daily may be the most beneficial (2335,2702,5461). For preventing drops in lymphocyte counts and attenuating gut permeability in people with esophageal cancer during radiochemotherapy, 30 grams per day has been used (2705). For Crohn's disease, 7 grams three times daily has been used (2338). For treating paclitaxel-induced myalgia and arthralgia, 10 grams three times daily starting 24 hours after paclitaxel infusion has been used (6433).
INTRAVENOUS: For improving recovery after bone marrow transplantation, 570 mg/kg/day has been used (2366). For improving recovery after major surgery, doses of 20 grams and 300 mg/kg/day have been added to parenteral nutrition (2363,5448). When glutamine dipeptide is used following major surgery, 18 to 30 grams of glutamine dipeptides per day (equivalent to 13 to 20 grams of glutamine) is typically used in a 60 to 70 kg patient. Higher doses are used for severely stressed patients with multiple injuries, burns, sepsis, and immune deficiency (7737).

Comments

Glutamine powder can be ordered through most wholesale drug suppliers. Glutamine for commercial use is produced by a fermentation process with glutamine-producing bacteria (7736). Glutamine has low solubility and limited stability in parenteral amino acid solutions. Synthetic glutamine dipeptides, such as l-alanyl-l-glutamine, are sometimes used to overcome these problems. The glutamine dipeptide is cleaved in vivo (7732,7737).

GLUTATHIONE

Also Known As

gamma-Glutamylcysteinylglycine, gamma-L-Glutamyl-L-cysteinylglycine, GSH =, L-Glutathione.

Scientific Names

N-(N-L-gamma-Glutamyl-L-cysteinyl)glycine.

People Use This For

Orally, glutathione is used for treating cataracts, glaucoma, preventing aging, treating or preventing alcoholism, asthma, cancer, heart disease (atherosclerosis and hypercholesterolemia), hepatitis, liver disease, immunosuppression (including AIDS and chronic fatigue syndrome), maintaining immune function, memory loss, Alzheimer's disease, osteoarthritis, Parkinson's disease, and detoxifying metal and drugs.
Inhaled, glutathione is used for treating lung diseases, including idiopathic pulmonary fibrosis, cystic fibrosis, and lung disease in individuals with HIV disease.
Intramuscularly, glutathione is used for preventing toxicity of chemotherapy and for treating male infertility.
Intravenously, glutathione is used for preventing anemia in patients undergoing hemodialysis, preventing renal dysfunction after coronary bypass surgery, treating Parkinson's disease, improving blood flow and decreasing clotting in individuals with atherosclerosis, treating diabetes, and preventing toxicity of chemotherapy.

Safety

POSSIBLY SAFE ...when used orally (5361,5362). ...when used by inhalation (9,5367,5368,5369). ...when used intramuscularly (5374,5375,5384). ...when used as an intravenous injection (5344,5354,5357,5358,5359,5360,5373,5374,5375,5376,5377,5378,5379,5380,5381,5382,5383).
PREGNANCY AND LACTATION: Insufficient reliable information available; avoid using.

Effectiveness

POSSIBLY EFFECTIVE

Chemotherapy toxicity. Administering glutathione by intravenous injection seems to help prevent chemotherapy toxicity (5373,5374,5375,5376,5377,5378,5379,5380,5381,5382,5383).

There is insufficient reliable information available about the effectiveness of glutathione for its other uses.

Mechanism of Action

Glutathione is primarily synthesized in the liver (5387,5388). It is involved in DNA synthesis and repair, protein and prostaglandin synthesis, amino acid transport, metabolism of toxins and carcinogens, immune system function, prevention of oxidative cell damage, and enzyme activation (5344,5386). Cellular glutathione levels increase during exercise (5398,5386). Glutathione deficiency is associated with aging, age-related macular degeneration (AMD), diabetes, lung and gastrointestinal disease, pre-eclampsia, Parkinson's disease and other neurodegenerative disorders, and poor prognosis in AIDS (5344,5346,5347,5348,5349,5350,5351,5352,5353,5354,5393,5394,5395,5396,5397). Although glutathione is present in fruits, vegetables, and meats, the levels in the body do not seem to correlate to dietary intake. This suggests that oral glutathione might be inactivated by peptidases in the gut (5344). Despite evidence that suggests that glutathione is bioavailable in rodents (5363,5364), oral doses of 3 grams cause negligible increases in human plasma levels (5362). Preliminary evidence suggests glutathione intake from fruits and vegetables might be associated with a reduced risk of pharyngeal cancer (5345). In individuals with cirrhosis, oral glutathione has no effect on liver function tests (5361).
Glutathione may inhibit the activity of enzymes that help the flu virus colonize cells lining the mouth and throat. Flu-infected mice fed glutathione-enriched drinking water have lower tissue virus levels than untreated mice. Human studies are needed to determine the effects of glutathione on flu infection (5061).
Currently, researchers are investigating whether administering glutathione precursors, such as glutamine and n-acetylcysteine, might increase glutathione levels (5344,5389,5392).

Adverse Reactions

None reported.

Interactions with Herbs & Other Dietary Supplements

None known.

Interactions with Drugs

None known.

Drug Influences on Nutrient Levels and Depletion

SOME DRUGS CAN AFFECT GLUTATHIONE LEVELS:
ACETAMINOPHEN: Drugs that deplete glutathione, such as acetaminophen, might decrease the therapeutic effects of glutathione (5394).
ALCOHOL (Ethanol): Drugs that deplete glutathione, such as alcohol, might decrease the therapeutic effects of glutathione (5394).

Interactions with Foods

None known.

Interactions with Lab Tests

None known.

Interactions with Diseases or Conditions

ASTHMA: Inhaled (nebulized) glutathione can cause bronchospasm in individuals with asthma (5372).

Dosage and Administration

ORAL: Supplemental doses range from 50-600 mg per day, with a typical dose of 250 mg daily; however, orally administered glutathione is probably not bioavailable (5362).
INHALATION: A common dose is 600 mg, aerosolized twice daily (5367,5368,5369).
INTRAMUSCULAR: For infertility, 600 mg every other day for 2 months has been used (5384). As a chemotherapy adjunct, 600 mg on days 2 through 5 of chemotherapy has been used (5374,5375).
INTRAVENOUS: As a chemotherapy adjunct, 2.5 grams or 1.5 grams/meter squared immediately prior to chemotherapy has been used (5373,5374,5375,5376,5377,5378,5379,5380,5381,5382,5383).

Comments

The role of glutathione is being studied in the wasting of AIDS, heavy metal poisoning, sepsis, myocardial ischemia, renal dysfunction and nephrotoxicity, liver disorders, corneal disorders, and eczema (9,5344,5345).

GLYCEROL

Also Known As

Glicerol, Glucerite, Glycerin, Glycerolum, Glyceryl Alcohol.

Scientific Names

Glycerol; 1,2,3-propanetriol.

People Use This For

Orally, glycerol is used for weight loss, enhancing exercise performance, improving rehydration during acute gastrointestinal disease, and reducing intraocular pressure. Glycerol is also used by athletes as an aid to hydration.
Intravenously, glycerol is used for reducing intra-cranial pressure in various conditions including stroke, meningitis, encephalitis, Reye's syndrome, pseudotumor cerebri, central nervous system (CNS) trauma, and CNS tumors or space-occupying lesions; for reducing brain volume for neurosurgical procedures; and for postural syncope.
Topically, glycerol is used as a humectant to moisturize the skin.
Ophthalmically, glycerol is an ingredient for reducing corneal edema to facilitate ophthalmic exams.
Rectally, glycerol is used as a laxative.

Safety

LIKELY SAFE ...when used rectally, ophthalmically, or topically and appropriately (15,272). ...when used orally for glaucoma; glycerol is an FDA-approved prescription product for this use.
POSSIBLY SAFE ...when used orally (2474,2475).
POSSIBLY UNSAFE ...when used intravenously. In one study, hemolysis was reported in 98% of people treated for acute ischemic stroke (2482).
There is insufficient reliable information available about the safety of glycerol for its other uses.
PREGNANCY AND LACTATION: Insufficient reliable information available; avoid using.

Effectiveness

LIKELY EFFECTIVE

Constipation. Use of glycerol rectal suppositories have a laxative effect and decrease constipation (15).

POSSIBLY INEFFECTIVE

Weight loss. Taking glycerol orally doesn't seem to be effective for losing weight (2485).

LIKELY INEFFECTIVE

Athletic performance. Taking glycerol orally doesn't seem to improve physical exercise performance (2474,2475).

Stroke. Intravenous use of glycerol doesn't seem to improve symptoms of acute stroke (2480,2481,2482,2484,2486).

There is insufficient reliable information available about the effectiveness of glycerol for its other uses.

Mechanism of Action

Supplemental glycerol increases serum osmolality (2477). It also has hyperosmotic laxative activity (15). Glycerol consumption failed to enhance human exercise performance (2476,2492) or reduce water loss in underwater divers (2478). However, one study reported that following glycerol ingestion, participants had improved exercise tolerance and reduced heart rate during stationary cycling (2479). Intravenous glycerol failed to improve acute ischemic stroke survival in several clinical trials (2480,2481,2482,2484,2486). However, one study of elderly people with acute ischemic stroke found glycerol improved initial survival (2483).

Adverse Reactions

Orally, the use of glycerol can cause mild headache, dizziness, bloating, nausea, vomiting, thirst, and diarrhea (15,2475).

Intravenously, the use of glycerol has caused hemolysis in people treated for acute ischemic stroke (2480,2482).

Interactions with Herbs & Other Dietary Supplements

None known.

Interactions with Drugs

None known.

Interactions with Foods

None known.

Interactions with Lab Tests

None known.

Interactions with Diseases or Conditions

None known.

Dosage and Administration

ORAL: For enhancing exercise performance, the usual dose of glycerol is 1 gram/kg with 1.5 L fluid 60-120 minutes before competition (2475). For weight loss, 7.5 grams in a 25% solution is typically taken before meals (2485).

RECTAL: As an adult laxative, the common dose is a 2-3 grams suppository or a 5-15 mL enema (15). For children younger than six years old, the dose is a 1-1.7 grams suppository or a 2-5 mL enema (15).

OPHTHALMIC: Glycerol is an FDA-approved prescription product for reducing intraocular pressure.

INTRAVENOUS: No typical dosage.

GLYCINE

Also Known As

Athenon, Free Base Glycine, G Salt, Glycocoll, Glycosthene, Iconyl, L-Glycine, Monazol.

Scientific Names

Aminoacetic Acid.

People Use This For

Orally, glycine is used for schizophrenia, strokes, memory enhancement, benign prostatic hyperplasia (BPH), protection of the liver and kidneys, and cancer prevention. It is also used for 3-phosphoglycerate dehydrogenase deficiency and isovaleric acidemia.

Topically, glycine is used to treat leg ulcers and for wound healing.

Safety

POSSIBLY SAFE ...when used orally and appropriately (10250,10251,10252). ...when used topically and appropriately (10255).
PREGNANCY AND LACTATION: Insufficient information available; avoid using.

Effectiveness

POSSIBLY EFFECTIVE

Leg ulcers. Applying a cream containing glycine, l-cysteine, and dl-threonine seems to reduce pain and slightly improve healing of leg ulcers (10255).
Schizophrenia. Taking glycine orally in addition to conventional treatment seems to reduce negative symptoms of schizophrenia in patients that are resistant to monotherapy with conventional antipsychotics such as thioridazine (Mellaril), haloperidol (Haldol), and perphenazine (Trilafon). However, when used with the atypical neuroleptic agent clozapine (Clozaril), glycine appears to have a negligible effect or worsen symptoms of schizophrenia (10253,11321). Additionally, glycine does not seem to improve positive symptoms of schizophrenia (10250,10251,10252).
Stroke. Taking glycine sublingually may have neuroprotective effects if started within 6 hours after the onset of acute ischemic stroke (11320).

INSUFFICIENT RELIABLE EVIDENCE to RATE

3-phosphoglycerate dehydrogenase (3-PGDH) deficiency. There is preliminary evidence that suggests that oral glycine might reduce seizures in patients with 3-PGDH deficiency. 3-PGDH deficiency is a rare condition in which serine is not synthesized properly (10254).
Cognitive performance. Preliminary evidence suggests oral glycine may improve memory (11322).
Isovaleric acidemia. Glycine has been used orally with l-carnitine to treat isovaleric acidemia, which is caused by a defective enzyme needed for metabolism of leucine (10256).
More evidence is needed to rate glycine for these uses.

Mechanism of Action

Glycine is an amino acid. It is not considered an essential amino acid because the body makes glycine from serine. A typical diet contains about 2 grams of glycine daily. The primary sources are protein rich foods including meat, fish, dairy, and legumes (10252).
In the central nervous system (CNS) glycine acts as an agonist at the glutamate receptor N-methyl-D-aspartate (NMDA). NMDA receptors are associated with negative and positive symptoms of schizophrenia (10257). NMDA receptors also seem to be associated with memory and learning processes (11322). The concentration of glycine in the brain is fairly stable due to the dietary consumption of glycine. However, addition of supplements can increase CNS concentrations of glycine (10252).
Preliminary evidence suggests that glycine can protect the kidneys from damage induced by cyclosporine, possibly by reducing cyclosporine-induced hypoxia and free radicals (10258,10259).
Glycine may also help improve recovery of the liver after alcohol-induced damage. Glycine might reduce the production of tumor necrosis factor-alpha (TNF-alpha) by Kupffer cells. This effect leads to a reduction in inflammation, necrosis, and steatosis in alcohol-induced hepatitis (10260).
There is also evidence that glycine may inhibit the growth of certain types of cancer. It may decrease the growth of melanoma cells by inhibiting vascularization (10261). A similar effect may inhibit the growth of liver tumors (10262).

Adverse Reactions

Orally and topically, glycine is generally well tolerated. Nausea, vomiting, upper gastrointestinal (GI) tract discomfort, and mild sedation have occurred rarely with oral use of glycine. These symptoms resolve rapidly with discontinuation of glycine (10252,11320).

Interactions with Herbs & Other Dietary Supplements

None known.

Interactions with Drugs

CLOZAPINE (Clozaril): Glycine can make symptoms worse when given with clozapine (Clozaril) in patients with schizophrenia (10253). Although this effect has not been reported with other atypical antipsychotic agents, glycine should be used cautiously with all atypical antipsychotics.

Interactions with Foods

None known.

Interactions with Lab Tests

None known.

Interactions with Diseases or Conditions

None known.

Dosage and Administration

ORAL: In the treatment of schizophrenia, glycine has been used in doses ranging from 0.4 to 0.8 g/kg daily in divided doses. It is usually started at 4 g daily and increased by 4 g per day until the therapeutic dosage is obtained (10250,10251,10252,10253). For treating seizures induced by 3-PGDH deficiency, glycine 200 mg/kg daily has been used in combination with serine supplements (10254). In the treatment of isovaleric acidemia, glycine 250 mg/kg daily has been used; it may be given with or without l-carnitine (10256).
SUBLINGUAL: For neuroprotection after the onset of acute ischemic stroke, 1-2 grams glycine per day started within 6 hours after stroke onset has been used (11320).
TOPICAL: For treating leg ulcers a cream containing 10 mg glycine, 2 mg l-cysteine, and 1 mg dl-threonine per gram of cream has been used. The cream was applied at each wound cleaning and dressing change once daily, every other day, or twice daily (10255).

GOA POWDER

Also Known As

Araoba, Bahia Powder, Brazil Powder, Chrysatobine, Crude Chrysarobin, Ringworm Powder.

Scientific Names

Vataireopsis araroba, synonym Andira araroba.
Family: Fabaceae/Leguminosae.

People Use This For

Topically, goa powder is used for psoriasis and fungal infections of the skin.

Safety

POSSIBLY UNSAFE ...when used topically. Goa powder is severely irritating to skin and mucous membranes. It can also be absorbed through the skin with adverse effects. As little as 10 mg absorbed is associated with vomiting, diarrhea, and kidney inflammation (18).
PREGNANCY AND LACTATION: Insufficient reliable information available; avoid using.

Effectiveness

There is insufficient reliable information available about the effectiveness of goa powder.

Mechanism of Action

The applicable part of goa powder is the latex. Goa powder contains anthrone derivatives including chrysophanolanthrone. The powder is a strong reducing agent and inhibits glucose-6-phosphated-dehydrogenization in psoriatic skin conditions. It is considered a potent irritant to skin and mucous membranes and is easily absorbed through the skin (18).

Adverse Reactions

Orally, vomiting, diarrhea, and kidney inflammation can follow if ingested (18).
Topically, application of goa powder can cause redness, swelling, pustules, and conjunctivitis.

Interactions with Herbs & Other Dietary Supplements

None known.

Interactions with Drugs

None known.

Interactions with Foods

None known.

Interactions with Lab Tests

None known.

Interactions with Diseases or Conditions

None known.

Dosage and Administration

TOPICAL: People typically use a 2% goa powder ointment.

Comments

Goa powder has been replaced by synthetic anthranol (18). Goa should not be used internally (223).

GOAT'S RUE

Also Known As

French Honeysuckle, French Lilac, Galegae officinalis herba, Geissrautenkraut, Italian Fitch.
CAUTION: See separate listing for Rue.

Scientific Names

Galega officinalis, synonyms Galega bicolor, Galega patula.
Family: Fabaceae/Leguminosae.

People Use This For

Orally, goat's rue is used as supportive therapy for diabetes and as a diuretic.
In combination with other herbs, goat's rue is used for adrenal gland and pancreas stimulation, for glandular disturbances, blood purification, purifying the mesenchyma, digestive fluid secretion disturbances, fermentative dyspepsia, Roemheld syndrome, diarrhea, abnormal colonic bacterial flora, status lymphaticus and exudative diathesis, for stimulating lactation, as a tonic, and as a liver-protectant.

Safety

There is insufficient reliable information available about the safety of goat's rue.
Pregnancy and Lactation: Insufficient reliable information available; avoid using.

Effectiveness

There is insufficient reliable information available about the effectiveness of goat's rue.

Mechanism of Action

The applicable parts of goat's rue are the above ground parts. In vitro, the constituent galegine has hypoglycemic effects (2,18,4006), but these effects have not been demonstrated with goat's rue (2,18). In experimental rats, an intravenously administered aqueous extract suppresses platelet aggregation (4007). Fatal poisonings have been reported in grazing animals. Toxicity may involve galegine (4008).

Adverse Reactions

None reported in humans. However, fatal poisonings have been reported in grazing animals following ingestion of large amounts of goat's rue (2,18); poisoning symptoms in sheep include salivation, spasms, paralysis, and asphyxiation (2,18).

Interactions with Herbs & Other Dietary Supplements

HYPOGLYCEMIC HERBS: Theoretically, concomitant use could potentiate effects of other herbs that cause hypoglycemia (2,4006).

Interactions with Drugs

ANTIDIABETES DRUGS: Theoretically, concomitant use could potentiate hypoglycemic drug effects. Monitor closely (2,4006).

Interactions with Foods

None known.

Interactions with Lab Tests

BLOOD GLUCOSE: Theoretically, could cause a true decrease in blood glucose levels and test results (2,4006).

Interactions with Diseases or Conditions

DIABETES: Goat's rue may interfere with effective diabetes treatment; avoid using.

Dosage and Administration

ORAL: As prepared tea (steep 2 grams finely cut above ground parts in 150 mL boiling water 5-10 minutes, strain); frequency of use not specified (18).

Comments

Avoid confusion with rue (Ruta graveolens). Goat's rue is not recommended for diabetes mellitus therapy because its effectiveness is uncertain.

GOLDEN RAGWORT

Also Known As

Cocash Weed, Coughweed, False Valerian, Female Regulator, Golden Groundsel, Golden Senecio, Grundy Swallow, Life Root, Liferoot, Ragwort, Squaw Weed, Squawweed.
CAUTION: See separate listings for Alpine Ragwort and Tansy Ragwort.

Scientific Names

Senecio aureus.
Family: Asteraceae/Compositae.

People Use This For

Orally, golden ragwort is used for diabetes mellitus, high blood pressure, spasms, as a uterine stimulant, to minimize bleeding, and as a diuretic and mild expectorant.
Golden ragwort is also used orally for treating conditions involving the female reproductive tract, including functional amenorrhea, menopausal neurosis, dysmenorrhea, pain associated with childbirth, and for inducing uterine contractions.
Topically, golden ragwort is used to treat bleeding after tooth extraction and as a douche for leukorrhea.

Safety

LIKELY UNSAFE ...when products containing hepatotoxic pyrrolizidine alkaloid (PA) constituents are used orally. Repeated exposure to low concentrations of hepatotoxic PAs can cause severe veno-occlusive disease. Hepatotoxic PAs might also be carcinogenic and mutagenic (12841,12842). Tell patients not to use golden ragwort preparations that are not certified and labeled as hepatotoxic PA-free. ...when products containing hepatotoxic PAs are used topically on abraded or broken skin. Absorption of hepatotoxic PAs through broken skin can lead to systemic toxicities (12841). Tell patients not to use topical golden ragwort preparations that are not certified and labeled as hepatotoxic PA-free. There is insufficient reliable information available about the safety of using topical PA-free golden ragwort on unbroken skin.
PREGNANCY: LIKELY UNSAFE ...when used orally. Golden ragwort preparations containing hepatotoxic pyrrolizidine alkaloid (PA) constituents might be teratogenic and hepatotoxic (12841,12842). There is insufficient reliable information available about the safety of using golden ragwort products that do not contain hepatotoxic PAs during pregnancy.
LACTATION: LIKELY UNSAFE ...when used orally. Hepatotoxic pyrrolizidine alkaloid (PA) constituents in golden ragwort are excreted in breast-milk (12841,12842). There is insufficient reliable information available about the safety of using golden ragwort products that are PA-free during lactation; avoid using.

Effectiveness

There is insufficient reliable information available about the effectiveness of golden ragwort.

Mechanism of Action

Golden ragwort contains various pyrrolizidine alkaloids (PA), some of which are toxic. PAs are most concentrated in the plant roots, but may be found in all plant parts. PAs, particularly unsaturated PAs, can cause hepatotoxicity. Cyclic diesters such as retrorsine and senecionine are the most hepatotoxic. Liver toxicity may result from PA-enhanced oxidative stress, but the exact mechanism of toxicity is unknown. Single doses of 10 to 20 mg PAs or chronic ingestion of amounts less than 10 mcg can cause veno-occlusive disease. PAs are metabolized by cytochrome P450 3A4 (CYP3A4) to toxic dehydroalkaloids and pyrroles. Enzyme inducers such as phenobarbital seem to enhance toxicity (12841,12860). Pyrroles are excreted as N-acetyl cysteine conjugates. Some researchers speculate that early administration of N-acetylcysteine might reduce toxicity (11988).
Metabolism is also affected by pregnane X receptor induction of CYP3A4. Genetic or drug induced variation in CYP3A4 or pregnane X receptor activity can affect the degree of PA toxicity by increasing or decreasing its metabolism (12841,12842). Hepatotoxic PAs are also toxic to the lungs. Pneumotoxicity occurs as pulmonary hypertension and right ventricular hypertrophy. Hepatotoxic PAs are carcinogenic and mutagenic. There are sufficient amounts of hepatotoxic PAs in herbal products to cause toxicity (12841,12842).

Adverse Reactions

Orally, golden ragwort might cause toxicity. The major concern about golden ragwort preparations is the hepatotoxic pyrrolizidine alkaloid (PA) content. These constituents are hepatotoxic, pneumotoxic, carcinogenic, and mutagenic (12841,12842). Chronic exposure to other plants containing hepatotoxic PA constituents is associated with veno-occlusive disease (4021). Subacute veno-occlusive disease causes vague symptoms with persistent liver enlargement (4021). Symptoms of acute veno-occlusive disease include colicky pains in epigastrium, vomiting and diarrhea, and ascites formation within several days. Enlargement and induration of the liver occur within a few weeks (12842).

Interactions with Herbs & Other Dietary Supplements

HEPATOTOXIC PYRROLIZIDINE ALKALOID (PA)-CONTAINING HERBS: Concomitant use is contraindicated due to the risk of additive toxicity. Herbs containing hepatotoxic PAs include alkanna, borage, butterbur, coltsfoot, comfrey, gravel root, groundsel, hemp agrimony, and hound's tongue; and the Senecio species plants dusty miller, alpine ragwort, groundsel, and tansy ragwort (12841).

HERBS THAT INDUCE CYTOCHROME P450 3A4 (CYP3A4): Theoretically herbs that induce CYP3A4 might increase the conversion of hepatotoxic PAs to toxic metabolites, enhancing toxicity (12841,12860). Herbs that induce CYP3A4 include St. John's wort and garlic.

Interactions with Drugs

CYTOCHROME P450 3A4 (CYP3A4) INDUCERS: Hepatotoxic pyrrolizidine alkaloids (PA) are substrates of cytochrome P450 3A4 (CYP3A4) (12841,12860). Theoretically, drugs that induce CYP3A4 might increase the conversion of PAs to toxic metabolites. Some drugs that induce CYP3A4 include carbamazepine (Tegretol), phenobarbital, phenytoin (Dilantin), rifampin, rifabutin (Mycobutin), and others.

Interactions with Foods

None known.

Interactions with Lab Tests

None known.

Interactions with Diseases or Conditions

CROSS-ALLERGENICITY: Theoretically, golden ragwort might cause an allergic reaction in individuals sensitive to the Asteraceae/Compositae family (12842). Members of this family include ragweed, chrysanthemums, marigolds, daisies, and many other herbs.

LIVER DISEASE: Theoretically, hepatotoxic pyrrolizidine alkaloids (PA) might exacerbate liver disease (12841,12842).

Dosage and Administration

No typical dosage.

GOLDENROD

Also Known As

Aaron's Rod, Canadian Goldenrod, Early Goldenrod, European Goldenrod, Woundwort.

Scientific Names

Solidago virgaurea (European goldenrod); Solidago canadensis (Canadian goldenrod), synonym Solidago longifolia; Solidago gigantea (Early goldenrod), synonym Solidago serotina.

Family: Asteraceae/Compositae.

People Use This For

Orally, goldenrod is used as a diuretic, anti-inflammatory, and antispasmodic. It is also used orally for gout, rheumatism, arthritis, eczema, and other skin conditions. Goldenrod is also used for acute exacerbations of pulmonary tuberculosis, diabetes, enlargement of the liver, hemorrhoids, internal bleeding, allergic rhinitis, asthma, and prostatic hypertrophy. It is also used as "irrigation therapy" where it is taken with copious amounts of fluids to increase urine flow to treat inflammatory diseases of the lower urinary tract, urinary calculi, and kidney gravel. As "irrigation therapy," it is also used as prophylaxis for urinary calculi and kidney gravel.

Topically, goldenrod is used as a mouth rinse for inflammation of the mouth and throat and externally for poorly healing wounds.

Safety

There is insufficient reliable information available about the safety of goldenrod.

Pregnancy and Lactation: Insufficient reliable information available; avoid using.

Effectiveness

There is insufficient reliable information available about the effectiveness of goldenrod.

Mechanism of Action

The applicable parts of goldenrod are the above ground parts. Goldenrod is classified as an aquaretic, a compound that increases urine volume (water loss) but not electrolyte excretion (512). The anti-inflammatory and aquaretic effects of goldenrod may be due to the saponin and flavonoid constituents (8,512). Goldenrod might also have bacteriostatic activity (512).

Adverse Reactions
Orally, goldenrod may cause an allergic reaction in individuals sensitive to the Asteraceae/Compositae family. Members of this family include ragweed, chrysanthemums, marigolds, daisies, and many other herbs.

Interactions with Herbs & Other Dietary Supplements
None known.

Interactions with Drugs
DIURETIC DRUGS: Theoretically, goldenrod might interfere with diuretic therapy (512).

Interactions with Foods
None known.

Interactions with Lab Tests
None known.

Interactions with Diseases or Conditions
CROSS-ALLERGENICITY: Goldenrod may cause an allergic reaction in individuals sensitive to the Asteraceae/Compositae family. Members of this family include ragweed, chrysanthemums, marigolds, daisies, and many other herbs.
EDEMA DUE TO HEART OR KIDNEY CONDITIONS: "Irrigation therapy," where goldenrod is taken with copious amounts of fluids to increase urine flow, is contraindicated in these conditions with edema (2).
HYPERTENSION: Theoretically, goldenrod might increase sodium retention and worsen hypertension (512).
URINARY TRACT INFECTIONS (UTIs): Herbal "irrigation therapy" can be insufficient and require the addition of antibacterial agent. "Irrigation therapy" should be monitored closely (8).

Dosage and Administration
ORAL: The typical dose of goldenrod is one cup of the tea two to four times daily between meals (18). The tea is prepared by steeping 1-2 teaspoons, 3-5 grams, of the dried herb in 150 mL boiling water for 5-10 minutes and then straining. The usual dose ranges from 6-12 grams of the herb per day (2). The common dose of the liquid extract, 1:1 in 25% ethanol, is 0.5-2 mL two to three times daily (18). The typical dose of the tincture, 1:5 in 45% ethanol, is 0.5-1 mL two to three times daily (18). Drink plenty of water, at least 2 liters per day, with the use of goldenrod (18).

Comments
Avoid confusion with mullein (Verbascum densiflorum; also referred to as goldenrod). Early goldenrod, European goldenrod, and Canadian goldenrod are used interchangeably.

GOLDENSEAL

Also Known As
Eye Balm, Eye Root, Golden Seal, Goldenroot, Goldsiegel, Ground Raspberry, Hydrastis, Hydrastis Canadensis, Indian Dye, Indian Plant, Indian Tumeric, Jaundice Root, Orange Root, Sceau D'Or, Turmeric Root, Warnera, Wild Curcuma, Yellow Indian Paint, Yellow Paint, Yellow Puccoon, Yellow Root.
CAUTION: See separate listings for Barberry, Goldthread, Javanese Turmeric, Oregon Grape, Ox-Eye Daisy, and Turmeric.

Scientific Names
Hydrastis canadensis.
Family: Ranunculaceae.

People Use This For
Orally, goldenseal is used for the common cold and other upper respiratory tract infections, nasal congestion, allergic rhinitis, gastritis, peptic ulcers, colitis, diarrhea, constipation, flatulence, inflammation of vaginal and uretal mucous membranes, urinary tract infections (UTIs), menorrhagia, and dysmenorrhea. It is also used orally for hemorrhoids, anal fissures, internal hemorrhage, liver disorders, cancer, to mask urine tests for illicit drugs, jaundice, gonorrhea, child birth, post-partum hemorrhage, fever, pneumonia, malaria, whooping cough, and anorexia.
Topically, goldenseal is used as a mouthwash for sore gums and mouth. It is also used topically for skin rashes, skin ulcers, wound infections, itching, eczema, acne, dandruff, ringworm, herpes blisters, and herpes labialis.
Ophthalmically, goldenseal is used as an eyewash for eye inflammation and conjunctivitis.
Otologically, goldenseal is used for ringing of the ears, earache, and catarrhal deafness.

Safety

POSSIBLY SAFE ...when used orally and appropriately, short-term (12).
LIKELY UNSAFE ...when used orally in high doses or long-term. Doses providing more than 500 mg of the constituent berberine can cause significant toxicity. This may correspond to 8-100 grams of dry root, depending on the concentration of berberine (12). Overdoses of goldenseal can cause cardiac damage, spasms, and death (4). The LD50 of the berberine constituent in humans is thought to be 27.5 mg/kg (12). Prolonged use has also been associated with significant side effects, including digestive disorders and hallucinations (18).
CHILDREN: LIKELY UNSAFE ...when used orally in newborns. The berberine constituent of goldenseal can cause kernicterus in newborns, particularly preterm neonates with hyperbilirubinemia (2589).
PREGNANCY: LIKELY UNSAFE ...when used orally. Goldenseal is thought to affect menstruation and have oxytocic effects (4,12). Berberine and other constituents are also thought to cross the placenta and may cause harm to the fetus. Kernicterus has developed in newborn infants exposed to goldenseal (2589).
LACTATION: LIKELY UNSAFE ...when used orally. Berberine and other harmful constituents can be transferred to the infant through breast milk (2589).

Effectiveness

POSSIBLY INEFFECTIVE

Urine drug tests. Goldenseal is often promoted to mask illicit drugs in the urine, but taking goldenseal orally doesn't seem to cause a false negative immunoassay (EMIT and TDx) for marijuana, cocaine, or for Microgenics CEDIA DAU assay for amphetamines, barbiturates, benzodiazepines, cocaine, opiates, phencyclidine, and tetrahydrocannabinol. Drinking one gallon of water with goldenseal didn't increase the number of false negatives over water alone (260,261). Some people also claim that goldenseal can cause a false positive on a drug screen. But goldenseal does not seem to cause false positives for the fluorescent polarization immunoassay (FPIA) or thin-layer chromatography (TLC) assays for amphetamines, opiates, cocaine metabolites, methadone, or their metabolites (2590).

There is insufficient reliable information available about the effectiveness of goldenseal for its other uses.

Mechanism of Action

The applicable parts of goldenseal are the dried rhizome and root. The alkaloids hydrastine, berberine, canadine, and canadaline are the principle active constituents in goldenseal (7265,8012). However, these alkaloids are poorly absorbed when given orally (2591) and might not reach adequate concentrations to have significant pharmacological activity in humans. The isolated constituents have a variety of pharmacological effects. The berberine constituent has antimicrobial effects including antibacterial, antifungal, and some antimycobacterial and antiprotozoal activity (7258,7259). Berberine has activity against Staphylococcus aureus, Streptococcus pyogenes, Escherícha coli, Shigella boydii, Vibrio cholerae, Mycobacterium tuberculosis, Candida albicans, Candida tropicalis, Trichophyton mentagrophytes, Microsporum gypseum, Cryptococcus neoformans, Sporotrichum schenkii, Entamoeba histolytica, and Giardia lamblia (2530,2587,2588,7258,7259,8012). The constituents canadine and canadaline have activity against Pseudomonas aeruginosa. Both berberine and canadaline have similar activity against Escherichia coli, but canadaline has been shown to have more activity against gram-positive organisms than berberine (8012). These effects have not been demonstrated specifically for goldenseal. Due to the poor oral absorption of these alkaloids, goldenseal preparations might not be capable of achieving alkaloid serum concentrations high enough to be effective in humans. However, berberine from goldenseal is thought to concentrate in the bladder. Theoretically, goldenseal could potentially have activity against the binding of urinary tract pathogens, such as Escherichia coli, to bladder walls (2583). There is also preliminary evidence that the berberine constituent might have antitumor properties (7260). Isolated berberine and hydrastine seem to have cardiovascular effects. Berberine seems to increase coronary blood flow and stimulates the heart, although higher doses or long-term use are thought to inhibit cardiac activity (4,12). Berberine has antimuscarinic and antihistaminic activity (4). Hydrastine, in low doses, has hypotensive effects (4); however, at higher doses, hydrastine constricts peripheral blood vessels, potentially leading to hypertensive effects (4). There is preliminary evidence goldenseal might stimulate immunoglobulin M (IgM) antibody production (2530).

Adverse Reactions

Orally, prolonged use of goldenseal can cause digestive disorders, constipation, excitatory states, hallucinations, and occasionally delirium (18). Overdoses can cause stomach upset, nausea, vomiting, nervousness, depression, dyspnea, bradycardia, cardiac damage, hypotension, seizures, paralysis, spasms, and death (4,6). High doses of the constituent hydrastine can cause exaggerated reflexes, convulsions, paralysis, and death from respiratory failure (4). The fresh plant can cause mucosal irritation (12). Using goldenseal vaginally as a douche can cause ulceration (4). Use of goldenseal during pregnancy, lactation, or in newborn infants can cause kernicterus, and several resulting fatalities have been reported (2589). The LD50 of the berberine constituent in humans is reported to be 27.5 mg/kg (12).

Interactions with Herbs & Other Dietary Supplements

B VITAMINS: Theoretically, prolonged use of goldenseal can decrease B vitamin absorption (4).
HERBS WITH SEDATIVE PROPERTIES: Theoretically, concomitant use with herbs that have sedative properties might enhance therapeutic and adverse effects. Some of these supplements include 5-HTP, calamus, California poppy, catnip, hops, Jamaican dogwood, kava, St. John's wort, scullcap, valerian, yerba mansa, and others.

Interactions with Drugs

ANTACIDS: Theoretically, due to reports that goldenseal increases stomach acid, goldenseal might decrease the effectiveness of antacids (19).
ANTIHYPERTENSIVE DRUGS: Theoretically, large amounts of goldenseal might interfere with blood pressure control due to vasoconstrictive action of constituent hydrastine (4).
CNS DEPRESSANTS: Theoretically, concomitant use with drugs with sedative properties might cause additive effects and side effects (4).
CYTOCHROME P450 3A4 (CYP3A4) SUBSTRATES: There's conflicting research on the effect of goldenseal on cytochrome P450 3A4 (CYP3A4) enzymes (6450). Preliminary research suggests that goldenseal might inhibit CYP3A4 and increase levels of CYP3A4 substrates. However, goldenseal given in combination with indinavir (Crixivan), which is metabolized by CYP3A4, doesn't seem to affect peak concentration or oral clearance of indinavir in healthy volunteers (10690). Use goldenseal cautiously in patients taking drugs metabolized by CYP3A4. Some drugs metabolized by CYP3A4 include lovastatin (Mevacor), ketoconazole (Nizoral), itraconazole (Sporanox), fexofenadine (Allegra), triazolam (Halcion), and numerous others.
H2-BLOCKERS: Theoretically, due to reports that goldenseal increases stomach acid, goldenseal might decrease the effectiveness of H2-blockers (19). The H2 blockers include cimetidine (Tagamet), ranitidine (Zantac), nizatidine (Axid), and famotidine (Pepcid).
PROTON PUMP INHIBITORS (PPIs): Theoretically, due to reports that goldenseal increases stomach acid, goldenseal might decrease the effectiveness of PPIs (19). PPIs include omeprazole (Prilosec), lansoprazole (Prevacid), rabeprazole (Aciphex), pantoprazole (Protonix), and esomeprazole (Nexium).

Interactions with Foods

None known.

Interactions with Lab Tests

BILIRUBIN: Theoretically, goldenseal might increase bilirubin levels. This has been demonstrated with isolated berberine constituent, but not specifically with goldenseal. Berberine can cause a true increase in total and unbound bilirubin concentrations because it displaces bilirubin from albumin (2589).

Interactions with Diseases or Conditions

CARDIOVASCULAR DISEASE: Theoretically, low doses can increase coronary blood flow and stimulate the heart, while large doses can inhibit cardiac function (4).
GASTROINTESTINAL IRRITATION: Goldenseal might irritate gastrointestinal tract. Contraindicated in individuals with infectious or inflammatory gastrointestinal conditions (19).
HYPERBILIRUBINEMIA: The berberine in goldenseal can cause kernicterus in newborns, particularly preterm neonates with hyperbilirubinemia (2589); contraindicated in newborns.
HYPERTENSION: Vasoconstrictive action of the constituent hydrastine might interfere with blood pressure control (4); use with caution.

Dosage and Administration

ORAL: Doses of 0.5-1 gram three times daily of the dried root or rhizome or as a tea have been used. The tea is prepared by simmering 0.5-1 gram dried root or rhizome in 150 mL of boiling water for 5-10 minutes and then straining (4,12). 0.3-1.0 mL of the liquid extract, 1:1 in 60% ethanol, has been used three times daily (12). 2-4 mL of the tincture, 1:10 in 60% ethanol, has been used times daily (12).
TOPICAL: Goldenseal is used as a mouthwash 3-4 times daily. The mouthwash is prepared by steeping 2 teaspoons, 6 grams, of dried herb in 150 mL boiling water for 5-10 minutes, strain and allow to cool (3).

Comments

Goldenseal is commonly found in the deep woods from Vermont to Arkansas and received its name from the golden-yellow scars on the base of the stem. When the stem is broken, the scar resembles a gold wax letter seal. In the 1900s, goldenseal was immensely popular and has become endangered due to over-harvesting (13). In 1997, goldenseal became listed under Appendix II of the Convention on International Trade in Endangered Species of Wild Flora and Fauna (CITIES), which controls export of the root to other countries. Goldenseal is now being cultivated in many states as cash crop. Because it is so expensive, it is often adulterated. Common adulterants include Coptis and Xanthorrhiza (6). The concept of using goldenseal as an adulterant in drug screens came from the novel Stringtown on the Pike by the pharmacist John Uri Lloyd, but goldenseal caused a false positive for strychnine poisoning in this fictional situation (6).

GOLDTHREAD

Also Known As
Cankerroot, Chinese Goldthread, Coptide, Coptis, Coptis Chinesis, Gold Thread, Goldenthread, Huang Lian, Mouth Root, Yellowroot.

Scientific Names
Coptis chinensis; Coptis deltoidea; Coptis teeta, synonym Coptis teetoides; Coptis trifolia, synonyms Coptis groenlandica, Anemone groenlandica.
Family: Ranunculaceae.

People Use This For
Orally, goldthread is used for digestive disorders.

Safety
POSSIBLY SAFE ...when used orally and appropriately (12).
PREGNANCY: LIKELY UNSAFE ...when used orally; avoid using. Goldthread may induce menstruation and uterine contractions (12,19).
LACTATION: Insufficient reliable information available; avoid using.

Effectiveness
There is insufficient reliable information available about the effectiveness of goldthread.

Mechanism of Action
The applicable part of goldthread is the rhizome. Goldthread contains the bitter berberine, which stimulates bile secretion (12). Berberine also has antimicrobial, diuretic, smooth muscle relaxant, and cardiac depressant activities (12). Small doses stimulate the cardiac and respiratory systems and decrease intestinal peristalsis (12). High doses stimulate smooth muscle in the intestines and uterus, and depress respiration and cardiac function (12). In animal studies, berberine depresses cardiac function by dilating blood vessels and stimulating the vagal nerve (12).

Adverse Reactions
Orally, purified berberine can cause lethargy, nosebleed, dyspnea, skin and eye irritation, kidney irritation, nephritis, nausea, vomiting, and diarrhea (2).

Interactions with Herbs & Other Dietary Supplements
None known.

Interactions with Drugs
ANTACIDS: Theoretically, due to reports that goldthread increases stomach acid, goldthread might decrease the effectiveness of antacids (19).
H2-BLOCKERS: Theoretically, due to reports that goldthread increases stomach acid, goldthread might decrease the effectiveness of H2-blockers (19). The H2 blockers include cimetidine (Tagamet), ranitidine (Zantac), nizatidine (Axid), and famotidine (Pepcid).
PROTON PUMP INHIBITORS (PPIs): Theoretically, due to reports that goldthread increases stomach acid, goldthread might decrease the effectiveness of PPIs (19). PPIs include omeprazole (Prilosec), lansoprazole (Prevacid), rabeprazole (Aciphex), pantoprazole (Protonix), and esomeprazole (Nexium).

Interactions with Foods
None known.

Interactions with Lab Tests
None known.

Interactions with Diseases or Conditions
PEPTIC ULCER DISEASE: Contraindicated. Goldthread might increase stomach acid (19).

Dosage and Administration
ORAL: People typically use 0.5 to 1.2 grams of the powdered rhizome (223). As a liquid, 1 teaspoon is boiled with 1 cup water, and dosed 1 tablespoon 3 to 6 times daily. The liquid is sometimes used as a mouthwash or gargle. The tincture is taken 5 to 10 drops at a time (5263).

GOSSYPOL

Also Known As
Cottonseed Oil, Karpasa.
CAUTION: See separate listing for Cotton.

Scientific Names
Gossypium hirsutum; Gossypium herbaceum; other Gossypium species.
Family: Malvaceae.

People Use This For
Orally, gossypol is used as a male contraceptive. Gossypol is also used in treating uterine myoma, endometriosis, dysfunctional uterine bleeding, metastatic carcinoma of the endometrium or ovary, and HIV disease.
Topically, gossypol is used as a spermicidal cream or gel.

Safety
POSSIBLY UNSAFE ...when used orally (5914,8290,8463). The inhibitory effects on spermatogenesis are not predictably reversible, although sperm counts usually return to normal within three months to two years after discontinuation. In approximately 10% of men, the sperm counts remain suppressed for more than 4.5 years, following chronic use (8463). Gossypol might also be cytotoxic to endometrial cells (6).
There is insufficient reliable information available about the safety of the topical use of gossypol.
PREGNANCY: LIKELY UNSAFE ...when used orally; gossypol seems to have abortifacient and uterine stimulant effects, avoid using (6,12).
LACTATION: POSSIBLY UNSAFE ...when used orally; avoid using.

Effectiveness
POSSIBLY EFFECTIVE

Contraception. Taking gossypol orally seems to effectively inhibit sperm motility and production after 12-16 weeks of treatment in about 60% of men. A dose of 15 mg per day is given for 12-16 weeks to achieve spermatogenesis suppression, followed by a maintenance dose of 7.5-10 mg per day. Normalization of sperm function returns within three months to two years after discontinuation of treatment in about 50% of men (8290). There is also preliminary evidence that a topical gossypol preparation might also be effective as a spermicide (8906).

There is insufficient reliable information available about the effectiveness of gossypol for its other uses.

Mechanism of Action
Gossypol is a polyphenolic extract of the seed of the cotton plant. The cottonseed oil, stem, and roots of the cotton plant are extracted (5914).
Gossypol seems to suppress sperm independent of serum concentration, but recovery of spermatogenesis seems to be concentration dependent (8290). During continued treatment, sperm counts drop dramatically in the first two months and continues to be suppressed for at least six months (8463). The contraceptive action of gossypol results from the reduction of total cellular and microtubular tubulin content in sperm and spermatogenetic cells. Although the exact molecular mechanism of this reduction is not completely understood, evidence suggests that it is a result of inhibition of the enzyme lactate dehydrogenase X. This enzyme is crucial to energy metabolism in sperm and spermatogenic cells (8287,8290). Gossypol might also reduce the rate of tubulin synthesis or prevent the tubulin from assembling into microtubules (8287). Other research suggests that gossypol might damage spermatozoa by decreasing glucose uptake and increasing peroxidation of the cell membrane (7877). The contraceptive effect might also be mediated through inhibition of prostaglandin synthesis (17).
Gossypol is not toxic to genetic material and doesn't cause DNA changes (8464).
When used topically as a spermicidal agent, gossypol significantly reduces sperm motility, by decreasing intracellular concentration of cyclic adenosine monophosphate (cAMP) by decreasing its formation or increasing its breakdown. It also promotes damage to the cell membrane of spermatocytes. Topical gossypol concentrations of at least 20 mcg/mL reduce sperm motility (3586).
In women who consume gossypol, the uterus may decrease in size and amenorrhea may occur. During gossypol therapy, estrogen and progesterone levels drop and follicle stimulating hormone (FSH) and leuteinizing hormone (LH) levels increase. This is the basis for the use of gossypol in uterine myoma, endometriosis, dysfunctional uterine bleeding and other gynecologic disorders. However, the effects are not long lasting, requiring hysterectomy following gossypol (8463).
There is also interest in using gossypol to treat cancer. Early evidence suggests gossypol exhibits cytotoxic and anti-tumor properties on a large number of cytosolic and mitochondrial enzyme systems. These enzyme systems are necessary for tumor cell growth in preliminary studies using cellular and animal models. Gossypol is cytotoxic toward a variety of tumor cell lines including melanoma, endometrial, colon, lung, prostate, breast, brain, and adrenocortical cancer cells (5915,8289,8291,8292,8294,8295,8463).
Gossypol might have antiviral activity. It has shown activity against herpes simplex type 2 viruses and the human

immunodeficiency virus (HIV) (8462). Gossypol also seems to increase interferon levels (8463). The average half-life of gossypol is 286 hours (8463). The serum concentration of gossypol needed to reduce the sperm count is about 132 ng/mL (5914).

Adverse Reactions

Orally, gossypol can cause fatigue, changes in appetite, and gastrointestinal effects including diarrhea, mucosal sloughing, mucosal necrosis, ileus, and intestinal hemorrhage (6,9,17,21,8290).

Gossypol can cause persistent oligospermia. It can also cause a reduction in testicular volume, which is usually reversible (5914). The inhibitory effects on spermatogenesis are not predictably reversible, although reversibility seems to be better at lower doses. Sperm counts usually return to normal within 12 months after discontinuation (8290). In approximately 10% of men, the sperm counts remain suppressed for over 4.5 years, following chronic use (8463). Chronic use can cause sterility (12). Animal data suggest that gossypol might reduce libido in males, but this has not been observed in humans (8466,8290).

Gossypol can cause hypokalemia, which is more common in people with potassium deficient diets (5914,8288,8290). This hypokalemia can be caused by renal loss of potassium and may be resistant to potassium supplementation or potassium-sparing diuretics (9,21,8463).

High doses (100 to 700 times the contraceptive dose) may cause, hair discoloration, malnutrition, circulatory problems, and heart failure (6). Gossypol can cause amenorrhea and decreased uterine size. Gossypol can cause a photosensitivity reaction known as "burning fever," in which skin that is exposed to the sun develops a burning sensation, accompanied by generalized fatigue (8463).

Topically, gossypol might cause a burning sensation on the face and hands (9,17).

Interactions with Herbs & Other Dietary Supplements

CARDIAC GLYCOSIDE-CONTAINING HERBS: Theoretically, concomitant use might increase the risk of cardiac glycoside toxicity due to the potassium depleting effects of gossypol. Cardiac glycoside-containing herbs include black hellebore, Canadian hemp roots, digitalis leaf, hedge mustard, figwort, lily-of-the-valley roots, motherwort, oleander leaf, pheasant's eye plant, pleurisy root, squill bulb leaf scales, and strophanthus seeds (19).

LICORICE/HORSETAIL: Theoretically, overuse/misuse of licorice rhizome or horsetail plant with gossypol might increase the risk of potassium depletion (19).

STIMULANT LAXATIVE HERBS: Theoretically, overuse or misuse of stimulant laxatives with gossypol might increase the risk of potassium depletion. Stimulant laxative herbs include aloe dried leaf sap, blue flag rhizome, alder buckthorn, European buckthorn, butternut bark, cascara bark, castor oil, colocynth fruit pulp, gamboge bark exudate, jalap root, black root, manna bark exudate, podophyllum root, rhubarb root, senna leaves and pods, wild cucumber fruit (Ecballium elaterium), and yellow dock root (19).

Interactions with Drugs

DIGOXIN (Lanoxin): Theoretically, concomitant use with gossypol might increase the risk of cardiac glycoside drug toxicity due to the potassium-depleting effects of gossypol (9).

DIURETIC DRUGS: Overuse of gossypol might compound diuretic-induced potassium loss (9). There is some concern that people taking gossypol along with potassium depleting diuretics might have an increased risk for hypokalemia. Initiation of potassium supplementation or an increase in potassium supplement dose may be necessary for some patients. Some diuretics that can deplete potassium include chlorothiazide (Diuril), chlorthalidone (Thalitone), furosemide (Lasix), hydrochlorothiazide (HCTZ, Hydrodiuril, Microzide), and others.

NONSTEROIDAL ANTI-INFLAMMATORY DRUGS (NSAIDs): Concomitant use might increase the risk of gastrointestinal side effects (21). Some of these drugs include diclofenac (Voltaren, Cataflam, others), ibuprofen (Advil, Motrin, others), and naproxen (Anaprox, Naprosyn).

STIMULANT LAXATIVES: Theoretically, overuse or misuse of stimulant laxatives with gossypol might increase the risk of potassium depletion (19). Some of these drugs include cascara, bisacodyl (Dulcolax), and senna (Senkot).

THEOPHYLLINE: Theoretically, concomitant use might reduce the ability of gossypol to decrease sperm motility (3586).

Interactions with Foods

ALCOHOL: Preliminary evidence indicates that gossypol can inhibit alcohol dehydrogenase and aldehyde dehydrogenase, which may permit blood levels of ethanol and acetaldehyde to accumulate. Patients should avoid alcoholic beverages while taking gossypol (8461).

Interactions with Lab Tests

None known.

Interactions with Diseases or Conditions

HYPOKALEMIA: Gossypol may induce or exacerbate hypokalemia (8288).

UROGENITAL IRRITATION OR SENSITIVITY: Contraindicated (12).

Dosage and Administration

ORAL: For male contraception, 15-20 mg is typically used daily for 12-16 weeks, followed by a maintenance dose of 7.5-10 mg per day (8290).
TOPICAL: No typical dosage.

Comments

Gossypol is considered unsafe for self-medication due to toxic potential; administration requires monitoring.
Gossypol is found in cotton root, root bark, seed, and stem, but is commercially extracted from cotton seed (6).

GOTU KOLA

Also Known As

Brahma-Buti, Brahma-Manduki, Brahmi, Centella, Centellase, Gotu Cola, Hydrocotyle, Hydrocotyle Asiatique, Indischer Wassernabel, Idrocotyle, Indian Pennywort, Indian Water Navelwort, Luei Gong Gen, Madecassol, Mandukaparni, Manduk Parani, Marsh Penny, Talepetrako, Thick-Leaved Pennywort, Tsubo-kusa, Tungchian, White Rot.
CAUTION: See separate listings for Brahmi and Cola Nut.

Scientific Names

Centella asiatica, synonym Hydrocotyle asiatica; Centella coriacea.
Family: Apiaceae/Umbelliferae.

People Use This For

Orally, gotu kola is used for reducing fatigue, improving memory and intelligence, venous insufficiency including varicose veins, wound healing, and increasing longevity. It is also used for the common cold and influenza (flu), sunstroke, tonsillitis, pleurisy, urinary tract infection (UTI), hepatitis, jaundice, abdominal pain, diarrhea, indigestion, gastritis, peptic ulcer disease, dysentery, trauma, shingles, leprosy, cholera, syphilis, psychiatric disorders, epilepsy, asthma, anemia, diabetes, and hypertension. Gotu kola is also used for contraception, amenorrhea, elephantiasis, systemic lupus erythematosus (SLE), tuberculosis, memory loss, and as an aphrodisiac.
Topically, gotu kola is used for wound healing and reducing scars.
Parenterally, gotu kola is used for bladder lesions associated with schistosomiasis.

Safety

POSSIBLY SAFE ...when used orally or topically and appropriately (6887).
PREGNANCY: POSSIBLY UNSAFE ...when used orally. Gotu kola might be an abortifacient (4); avoid using.
LACTATION: Insufficient reliable information available; avoid using.

Effectiveness

POSSIBLY EFFECTIVE

Schistosomiasis. Using gotu kola parenterally seems to help bladder lesions of schistosomiasis (bilharzial infections) (9785).
Venous insufficiency. Taking gotu kola orally seems to help treat chronic venous insufficiency (6887). Triterpenes from gotu kola may reduce ankle edema and improve lower leg circulation in venous insufficiency (9786).

INSUFFICIENT RELIABLE EVIDENCE to RATE

Keloids. There is some evidence that applying gotu kola topically can help prevent keloids and hypertrophic scarring (4).
Psoriasis. Applying gotu kola topically seems to help treat psoriasis (6887).
Wound healing. Applying gotu kola topically seems to help improve wound healing (6887).
More evidence is needed to rate gotu kola for these uses.

Mechanism of Action

The applicable parts of gotu kola are the above ground parts. The primary constituents responsible for the pharmacological effects are thought to be the saponin-containing triterpene acids, 1% to 8%, and their sugar esters, including asiatic acid, madecassic acid, asiaticoside, asiaticoside A (madecassoside), and asiaticoside B. Gotu kola also contains essential oils, flavonoids, flavone derivatives including quercetin and kaempferol, sesquiterpenes, stigmasterol, sitosterol, and isothankuniside (6887,10276).
The triterpenoid saponins (e.g., asiaticoside, madecassoside) seem to be involved in wound healing and decreasing venous pressure in venous insufficiency (780,2700,9786); asiaticoside and madecassoside have anti-inflammatory activity (11). There is also some evidence that asiaticosides might promote wound healing by stimulating collagen and glycosaminoglycan synthesis (1890,2700).
Topical application of gotu kola extracts increases collagen synthesis, intracellular fibronectin content, and mitotic activity in the germ layer, and enlarges kerato-hyaline granules in scar tissue.
There's preliminary evidence that asiaticosides might also have preventive and therapeutic effects on gastrointestinal

ulcers (6887,7691). Anti-ulcer mechanisms may be due to strengthening action on gastric mucosal lining and suppression of damaging effects of free radicals (7691).

The asiaticosides have several other pharmacological effects, including elevating blood glucose, triglycerides, and cholesterol levels. They also seem to decrease blood urea nitrogen (BUN) and acid phosphatase levels.

Early evidence suggests that purified isothankuniside may decrease fertility. However, a crude extract of Centella asiatica does not reduce fertility (10276).

Some researchers think the asiaticoside derivatives, asiatic acid, asiaticoside 6, and SM2, might have a role in Alzheimer's disease. There is some early evidence that they might protect neurons from beta-amyloid toxicity (1889).

There is preliminary evidence that gotu kola extracts might have sedative, anticonvulsant, and analgesic effects, possibly mediated in part via increased levels of the inhibitory transmitter, GABA (6887). The terpenoid constituents brahmoside and brahminoside might be responsible for sedative effects (4).

Gotu kola extracts also seem to have antibacterial activity in vitro against Pseudomonas pyocyaneus, Trichoderma mentagrophytes, and Entamoeba histolytica, and antiviral activity against Herpes simplex type II (6887).

There is some interest in using gotu kola to treat cancer. Dried powder extracts of gotu kola exhibit cytotoxic and anti-tumor properties in preliminary studies. Normal lymphocytes are not harmed, which suggests gotu kola exerts selective toxicity towards tumor cells (7692).

Adverse Reactions

Orally, gotu kola is usually well tolerated when used in typical doses. However, in some patients it can cause gastrointestinal upset and nausea (6887), widespread pruritus, and photosensitivity (4). Caution patients using gotu kola to use sunscreen and wear adequate clothing to prevent sunburn. Large doses of gotu kola might increase blood pressure, glucose, and cholesterol levels (4). There is also some concern that large doses of gotu kola might cause sedation and drowsiness (4).

Topically, gotu kola can cause allergic contact dermatitis, characterized by erythema, itching, papules, and a burning sensation (4,6887,9789). Gotu kola may also cause eczema when applied topically (10277,10278).

Subcutaneous injection of gotu kola can cause pain and discoloration at injection site (6). This can be prevented by using intramuscular injections (6).

Interactions with Herbs & Other Dietary Supplements

HERBS WITH SEDATIVE PROPERTIES: Theoretically, concomitant use with herbs that have sedative properties might enhance therapeutic and adverse effects. Some of these supplements include 5-HTP, calamus, California poppy, catnip, hops, Jamaican dogwood, kava, St. John's wort, scullcap, valerian, yerba mansa, and others.

Interactions with Drugs

CNS DEPRESSANTS: Theoretically, concomitant use with drugs with sedative properties might cause additive effects and side effects (4). The constituents brahmoside and brahminoside might have CNS depressant action (4).

Interactions with Foods

None known.

Interactions with Lab Tests

None known.

Interactions with Diseases or Conditions

DIABETES: The asiaticoside constituent of Gotu kola might elevate blood glucose levels (4).
HYPERLIPIDEMIAS: The asiaticoside constituent of Gotu kola might elevate triglyceride and cholesterol levels (4).

Dosage and Administration

ORAL: Typical dosages are 600 mg dried leaves three times per day (18), or one cup tea (steep 600 mg dried leaves in 150 mL boiling water 5-10 minutes, strain) three times per day (18). Clinical trials for venous insufficiency used 60-120 mg titrated extract per day for two months (780).
TOPICAL: For wound healing, 1% gotu kola creams have been used (6887).
PARENTERAL: No typical dosage.

Comments

Avoid confusion with cola nut (Cola acuminata). Also avoid confusion with swamp pennywort (Centella cordifolia). Centella cordifolia is often misidentified as Centella asiatica (gotu kola).

GOUTWEED

Also Known As

Achweed, Ashweed, Bishop's Elder, Bishopsweed, Bishopswort, Eltroot, English Goatweed, Gout Herb, Goutwort, Ground Elder, Herb Gerard, Jack-Jump-About, Masterwort, Pigweed, Weyl Ash, White Ash.
CAUTION: See separate listings for Bishop's Weed and Masterwort.

Scientific Names

Aegopodium podagraria.
Family: Apiaceae/Umbelliferae.

Comments

At the date of publication, this product was not a common ingredient used in brand name supplements marketed to consumers. Details about this product are available in the online version of *Natural Medicines Comprehensive Database.* See www.naturaldatabase.com.

GRAINS OF PARADISE

Also Known As

Guinea Grains, Mallaguetta Pepper, Melegueta Pepper.
CAUTION: See separate listing for Capsicum.

Scientific Names

Aframomum melegueta, synonym Amomum melegueta.
Family: Zingiberaceae.

People Use This For

Orally, grains of paradise fruit and seeds are used as a stimulant.

Safety

POSSIBLY SAFE ...when used orally and appropriately (12).
PREGNANCY AND LACTATION: Insufficient reliable information available; avoid using.

Effectiveness

There is insufficient reliable information available about the effectiveness of grains of paradise.

Mechanism of Action

The applicable parts of grains of paradise are the fruit and seed. Grains of paradise contains a volatile oil and the constituents hydroxyphenylalkanones and hydroxyphenylalkanoles. The seed is said to be a stimulant (18).

Adverse Reactions

Theoretically, oral use of grains of paradise may cause GI and lower urinary tract irritation (18).

Interactions with Herbs & Other Dietary Supplements

None known.

Interactions with Drugs

None known.

Interactions with Foods

None known.

Interactions with Lab Tests

None known.

Interactions with Diseases or Conditions

None known.

Dosage and Administration

ORAL: People typically use 4 to 6 grams added to 3 to 4 cups of water and boiled until the volume is reduced by one-half. The cooled liquid is taken in 3 doses on an empty stomach (5251).

Comments

Avoid confusion with capsicum (Capsicum annuum), also known as grains of paradise.

GRAPE

Also Known As

Activin, Black Grape Raisins, Calzin, Draksha, Enocianina, Extrait De Pepins De Raisin, Flame Seedless, Folia Vitis Viniferae, Leucoanthocyanin, Muskat, Oligomeric Proanthocyanidins, Oligomeric Procyanidins, OPCs, PCOs, Petite Sirah, Proanthodyn, Procyanidolic Oligomers, Raisins, Red Globe, Red Malaga, Red Vine Leaf AS 195, Red Vine Leaf Extract, Sultanas, Table Grapes, Thompson Seedless, Wine Grapes.
CAUTION: See separate listings for Grapefruit, Pycnogenol, Resveratrol, and Wine.

Scientific Names

Vitis vinifera.
Family: Vitaceae.

People Use This For

Orally, grape is used for preventing cardiovascular disease, varicose veins, hemorrhoids, atherosclerosis, hypertension, peripheral vascular disease, edema associated with injury or surgery, and myocardial or cerebral infarction. Grape is also used and as a mild laxative for constipation. Grape "fasts" have been used for "detoxification."
Grape seed is used for diabetes complications such as neuropathy or retinopathy, improving wound healing, preventing dental caries, cancer prevention, macular degeneration, poor night vision, liver cirrhosis, allergic rhinitis, and prevention of collagen breakdown.
Dried grapes, raisins or sultanas, are used as an expectorant for cough.
Grape leaf is used orally for attention deficit-hyperactivity disorder (ADHD), diarrhea, heavy menstrual bleeding, uterine hemorrhage, and canker sores.
Intravaginally, grape leaf infusions are used as a douche.
Grape leaf is used as a food, particularly in Greek cooking.

Safety

LIKELY SAFE ...when used orally in amounts commonly found in foods. Grapes and grape skin extracts have Generally Recognized As Safe status (GRAS) for use in foods in the US (4912).
POSSIBLY SAFE ...when used orally and appropriately in medicinal amounts. Grape seed extracts have been safely used for up to 8 weeks in clinical studies (2541,3580,9182). Grape leaf extract has been safely used for up to 12 weeks in a clinical study (2538).
PREGNANCY AND LACTATION: There is insufficient reliable information about the safety of medicinal amounts of grape during pregnancy and breast-feeding; avoid using.

Effectiveness

POSSIBLY EFFECTIVE

Chronic venous insufficiency. Taking grape seed extract or its proanthocyanidin constituents orally seems to reduce subjective symptoms of chronic venous insufficiency and improve venous tone (2541). Additionally, in one clinical trial, a specific grape leaf extract, known as red vine leaf extract (AS 195, Antistax, Boehringer Ingelheim), was given orally to patients with stage I and stage II chronic venous insufficiency. Leg edema significantly decreased after 6 weeks of treatment compared to placebo. Doses of 360 mg and 720 mg daily were both effective, but the higher dose produced a slightly greater effect. Patients also reported significant decreases in subjective complaints such as tired or heavy legs, tension, and tingling and pain after 12 weeks of treatment (2538).

Ocular stress. Taking grape seed extract containing proanthocyanidin constituents orally might help decrease ocular stress from glare (2541).

POSSIBLY INEFFECTIVE

Allergic rhinitis (hayfever). Grape seed extract taken for 8 weeks before ragweed pollen season doesn't seem to decrease seasonal allergic rhinitis symptoms or antihistamine usage (9182).

INSUFFICIENT RELIABLE EVIDENCE to RATE

Cardiovascular disease. There is preliminary evidence that consumption of purple grape products, such as purple grape juice and red wine, might improve endothelium-dependent vasodilation, prevent LDL oxidation, and suppress platelet-mediated thrombosis. Theoretically, chronic ingestion of these products might reduce the risk of cardiovascular disease (8745,8746).

Night vision. Preliminary research suggests grape seed extract containing proanthocyanidins might also be beneficial for improving night vision (3580).

More evidence is needed to rate grape for these uses.

Mechanism of Action

The applicable parts of grape are the fruit, fruit skin, seed, and leaf.
Grape products contain phenolic compounds including oligomeric proanthocyanidins (OPCs), proanthocyanidins, flavonols, and polyflavan-3-ols.
Proanthocyanidins are responsible for producing the red color of grapes (3579). Red grape varieties provide more antioxidant protection than white or blush grape varieties (3579). Red wine contains approximately 10 times the amount flavonoids of white wine (8745). A significant correlation appears to exist between total phenol content, proanthocyanidin content, and the antioxidant activity of grape products (3579,8745).
Grape flavonoids have a wide variety of effects including antioxidant, vasodilating, anti-lipoperoxidant activity, and antiplatelet properties that might prevent heart disease (8476,8745,10156).
Specific flavonoids in grape products include quercetin, catechin, myricetin, and kaemferol. Quercetin has antioxidant effects, catechins can inhibit low-density lipoprotein (LDL) oxidation, and grape tannins have endothelium-dependent vasodilating activity. Intake of myricetin, kaemferol, and quercetin has been associated with reduced risk of coronary heart disease (8746). Preliminary research also suggests that catechins might inhibit allergen-induced histamine release from mast cells (9182).
The flavonoids also appear to decrease superoxide production, increase nitric oxide release from platelets, modestly increase the levels of antioxidants such as alpha-tocopherol, and decrease platelet protein-kinase C (PKC) activity (8745).
Preliminary evidence suggests that the proanthocyanidins delphinidin and delphinidin/cyanidin dimer might induce chromosomal damage (4074).
The red vine grape extract AS 195 (Antistax, Boehringer Ingelheim) used in one clinical trial primarily contains the flavonoids quercetin-3-O-beta-glucuronide and isoquercitrin (2538).
A grape seed extract (Leucoselect) containing an equivalent of 300 mg of grape seed proanthocyanidins seems to increase serum total antioxidant activity in healthy people (10156).
Some evidence suggests that proanthocyanidins from grape seeds can decrease reperfusion injury after cardiac ischemia by removing free radicals. This might also decrease the incidence of cardiac arrhythmias that sometimes occurs in cardiac reperfusion injury (10223). Preliminary evidence also suggests grape seed proanthocyanidins may provide greater protection against reactive oxygen species, free radical-induced lipid peroxidation, and DNA damage than the combination of vitamin E, vitamin C, and beta-carotene or a combination of vitamin E and vitamin C (10157).
Grape seed proanthocyanidins seem to inhibit the cytochrome P450 2E1 (CYP2E1) enzyme, which might protect normal cells against drug and chemical-induced toxicity (10157). Proanthocyanidins might also protect against tobacco-induced and chemotherapy drug-induced damage to normal cells, and minimize liver and kidney damage after overdosage of acetaminophen (10157).
Grape seed proanthocyanidins seem to decrease the proliferation of gastric adenocarcinoma, breast cancer, lung cancer, and prostate cancer cells by inhibiting cell growth and increasing cell death (10224, 10157).
OPCs are also thought to inhibit the proteolytic enzymes collagenase, elastase, hyaluronidase, and beta glucuronidase, which are involved in the breakdown of structural components of the vasculature and skin (3900).
Grape leaf is reported to have anti-inflammatory and astringent properties. These properties are reported to be greatest in the red leaves (4201).
Grape fruit are also reported to have laxative and expectorant properties (4201).

Adverse Reactions

Orally, grape seed extract is well tolerated. Headache, abdominal pain, sore throat, nausea, and cough have been reported with used of grape seed, but these effects occur at rates similar to placebo (9182).
Excessive consumption of grapes, dried grapes, raisins, or sultanas might cause diarrhea due to laxative effects (4201).
There is one report of an anaphylactic reaction to grape skin extract, which included urticaria and angioedema (4073).
Grape leaves have been reported to cause gastrointestinal discomfort, diarrhea, dyspepsia, dry mouth, and retching. Other adverse effects included infections, headache, and musculoskeletal disorders. One case of leg hematoma following a minor trauma was also reported in a person using grape leaf extract (2538).

Interactions with Herbs & Other Dietary Supplements

LACTOBACILLUS ACIDOPHILUS: Grape anthocyanins might inhibit the growth of Lactobacillus acidophilus. Theoretically, concurrent administration might prevent Lactobacillus acidophilus colonization of the gastrointestinal tract (11); avoid concurrent use.

Interactions with Drugs

CYTOCHROME P450 1A2 (CYP1A2) SUBSTRATES: Grape juice is thought to induce cytochrome P450 1A2 (CYP1A2) metabolism and may decrease plasma levels of CYP1A2 substrates (2539). Drugs metabolized by CYP1A2 include amitriptyline (Elavil), caffeine, chlordiazepoxide (Librium), clomipramine (Anafranil), clopidogrel (Plavix), clozapine (Clozaril), cyclobenzaprine (Flexaril), desipramine (Norpramin), diazepam (Valium), estradiol (Estrace, others), flutamide (Eulexin), fluvoxamine (Luvox), grepafloxacin (Raxar), haloperidol (Haldol), imipramine (Tofranil), mexiletine (Mexitil), mirtazapine (Remeron), naproxen (Naprosyn), nortriptyline (Pamelor), olanzapine (Zyprexa), ondansetron (Zofran), propafenone (Rythmol), propranolol (Inderal), riluzole (Rilutek), ropinirole (Requip), ropivacaine (Naropin), tacrine (Cognex), theophylline (Theo-Dur, others), verapamil (Calan, Covera-HS, others), warfarin (Coumadin), and zileuton (Zyflo).
PHENACETIN: Grape juice decreases phenacetin, but not acetaminophen plasma levels. It may decrease levels by inducing cytochrome P450 1A2 (CYP1A2) metabolism (2539).
WARFARIN (Coumadin): Theoretically, due to the tocopherol content of grape seed oil, concomitant use with warfarin might increase warfarin's effects and the risk of bleeding (272); use with caution.

Interactions with Foods

None known.

Interactions with Lab Tests

None known.

Interactions with Diseases or Conditions

None known.

Dosage and Administration

ORAL: For chronic venous insufficiency, one clinical trial used a standardized red vine grape extract AS 195 (Antistax, Boehringer Ingelheim). The dose used was 360 mg or 720 mg once daily (2538). Grape seed extract as tablets or capsules dosed at 75-300 mg daily for three weeks followed by a maintenance dose of 40-80 mg daily has been suggested by some sources (3900). For chronic venous insufficiency, grape seed extract proanthocyanidin doses of 150-300 mg per day have been used (2541). For reducing ocular stress due to glare, grape seed extract proanthocyanidin doses of 200-300 mg per day have been used (2541).

Comments

Grape seeds are typically obtained as a by-product of the manufacturing of wine (10156). Pycnogenol (pinebark extract) is similar to the grape seed extract in active ingredients and medicinal uses (272). Both pycnogenol and grape seed contain oligomeric proanthocyanidins (OPCs). Several other natural medicines contain constituents that are similar to the OPCs, including wine, cranberries, bilberries, green and black teas, black currant, onions, legumes, parsley, and hawthorn.

GRAPEFRUIT

Also Known As

Bioflavonoid Concentrate, Citrus Grandis Extract, Citrus Seed Extract, Cold-Pressed Grapefruit Oil, CSE, Expressed Grapefruit Oil, GSE, Paradisapfel, Pomelo, Shaddock Oil, Standardized Extract of Grapefruit, Toronja.

Scientific Names

Citrus paradisi; Citrus maxima, synonym Citrus decumana.
Family: Rutaceae.

People Use This For

Orally, grapefruit is used for hyperlipidemia, atherosclerosis, reducing hematocrit counts, cancer, psoriasis, and for weight loss and obesity.
Grapefruit seed extract is used orally for bacterial, viral, and fungal infections including yeast infections, Giardia lamblia and Entamoeba histolytica.
Topically, grapefruit oil is used for muscle fatigue, hair growth, toning the skin, and for acne and oily skin. It is also used for the common cold and flu (influenza). Grapefruit seed extract is used topically as a facial cleanser, first-aid treatment, as a treatment for mild skin irritations, and as a vaginal douche for vaginal candidiasis (yeast infection). It is also used as an ear or nasal rinse for preventing and treating infections; as a gargle for sore throats; and a dental rinse for preventing gingivitis, promoting healthy gums, and as a breath freshener.
By inhalation, grapefruit vapors are used to help the body retain water, for headache, stress, and depression. Grapeseed extract has also been nebulized for the treatment of lung infections.
In food and beverages, grapefruit is consumed as a fruit, juice, and is used as a flavoring component.
In manufacturing, grapefruit oil and seed extract are used as a fragrance component in soaps and cosmetics; and as a

household cleaner for fruits, vegetables, meats, kitchen surfaces, dishes, etc.
In agriculture, grapefruit seed extract is used as a bactericide and fungicide, a mold inhibitor, an antiparasitic for animal feeds, a food preservative and antioxidant, and a water disinfectant.

Safety

LIKELY SAFE ...when used orally in amounts commonly found in foods. Grapefruit has Generally Recognized As Safe status (GRAS) in the US (4912).
There is insufficient reliable information available about the safety of using grapefruit for medicinal purposes.
PREGNANCY AND LACTATION: There is insufficient reliable information about the safety of using medicinal amounts of grapefruit during pregnancy and lactation; avoid using.

Effectiveness

INSUFFICIENT RELIABLE EVIDENCE to RATE

Asthma. There is some evidence that consumption of vitamin C-rich citrus fruits, including grapefruit and others, might improve lung function in people with asthma. Intake of citrus fruits 1-2 times per week has produced this benefit in some studies (6049,6055,6056). However, other studies have not found this benefit (6057,6058).
Atopic dermatitis (eczema). There is preliminary evidence that suggests a citrus seed extract (ParaMycrocidin) can decrease complaints of constipation, flatulence, and abdominal discomfort possibly due to changes in intestinal microflora, in people with atopic eczema (5866).
More evidence is needed to rate grapefruit for these uses.

Mechanism of Action

The applicable parts of grapefruit are the fruit, juice, oil from the peel, and seed extract.
Grapefruit is high in fiber, and also contains significant amounts of potassium, vitamin C, pectin, and other nutrients. In addition to these nutrients, active constituents include flavonoids such as naringin and furanocoumarins including bergamottin (3769,7778,13031).
Grapefruit seeds contain numerous constituents including naringin, nomilin, deacetyl-nomilin, nomilinic-acid-17-O-beta-D-glucoside, deacetyl-nomilinic-acid-17-O-beta-D-glucoside, limonol, deoxy-limonol, 7-obacunol, obacunone, epi-iso-obacunoic-acid-17-O-beta-D-glucoside, iso-obacunoic-acid-17-O-beta-D-glucoside, and trans-obacunoic-acid-17-O-beta-D-glucoside (513).
Due to their flavonoid content, grapefruit and other citrus fruits are being investigated for preventing cardiovascular disease. Healthy volunteers who consume grapefruit juice seem to have a transient prolongation of the QT interval on electrocardiogram (ECG) compared to the normal daytime diurnal decrease in QT interval in control subjects. Grapefruit flavonoids are thought to antagonize cardiac potassium channels and therefore decrease cardiac repolarization. This suggests a possible antiarrhythmic effect of grapefruit juice with a mechanism similar to class III antiarrhythmic drugs (13031).
The potential benefits of grapefruit in asthma might be due to antioxidant properties of vitamin C or other fruit constituents (6049,6054,6055).
Naringin might induce red blood cell aggregation in vitro (6).
A commercial citrus seed extract used at a concentration of 0.5% has been reported to inhibit the in vitro growth of some bacteria, yeasts, and molds (Streptococcus species, Staph. aureus, enterococci, Enterobacter, E. coli, Candida, Geotrichum, Aspergillus, and Penicillium species) (5866). Grapefruit seed extracts have been reported to reduce counts of Salmonella typhimurium when sprayed on chicken skins (5862), but to have no effect in controlling fungal growth on unshelled peanuts (5864,5865).
When examined by HPLC, a commercial grapefruit seed extract was found to contain significant amounts of the preservatives methyl-p-hydroxybenzoate and triclosan, which were not present in an ethanol extract of grapefruit seeds (5863). In another study, five of six commercial grapefruit seed extracts tested contained significant amounts of the preservative benzethonium chloride, and three of these also contained triclosan and methyl-p-hydroxybenzoate. These five extracts had significant antibacterial activity, as measured by in vitro tests, but a sixth commercial extract which was preservative-free had no in vitro antibacterial activity (5867). It has therefore been hypothesized that the reported antimicrobial activity of grapefruit seed extract products is due to the preservative content (5867).
The effect of grapefruit juice on drugs is difficult to predict because the uptake of compounds such as naringenin and other constituents varies greatly among individuals (3775,7777,7779,11273).
Grapefruit juice flavonoids include naringin, naringenin, limonin, quercetin, kaempferol, and obacunone, which inhibit human hepatic microsomes (7778). Grapefruit juice furanocoumarins, including bergamottin and dihydroxybergamottin, inhibit cytochrome P450 3A4 (CYP3A4) (3769,5070,5071,11273). In addition, bergamottin inhibits CYP1A2, CYP2A6, CYP2C9, CYP2C19, CYP2D6, and CYP2E1 (5072).
It is likely that multiple constituents of grapefruit juice are responsible for its inhibition of CYP3A4 (11276).
Grapefruit juice selectively inhibits gut wall CYP3A4 and increases bioavailability and plasma concentrations of numerous drugs (1386). In higher doses, it may also inhibit hepatic CYP3A4 (7776,11275). Human research indicates that blended grapefruit segments, and an extract of grapefruit core and peel, also inhibit CYP3A4 activity (1388). Research on triazolam suggests that single doses of grapefruit juice increase plasma concentrations by inhibiting intestinal CYP3A4 during first pass metabolism. Repeated consumption of grapefruit juice inhibits hepatic CYP3A4 and prolongs elimination half-life (7776). Grapefruit juice appears to irreversibly inhibit CYP3A4, possibly leading to a

down-regulation of CYP3A4. Within 4 hours, grapefruit juice reduces intestinal CYP3A4 by 47% (11273). The maximum effect on drug metabolism appears to be within 24 hours of grapefruit consumption, but reduced drug metabolism can occur to a lesser degree for 3-7 days (7778,7782,11362). Research on midazolam suggests that recovery of gut wall CYP3A4 function occurs in 3 days after single exposure of grapefruit juice (10159). For some drugs, such as felodipine and nisoldipine, it may be necessary to allow a 3-day interval between grapefruit juice and drug administration to avoid interactions (5068,5069).

There is conflicting research about the effect of grapefruit on the drug transporter P-glucoprotein (1390,11270,11278,11362). However, research in humans using digoxin as a specific probe for P-glycoprotein activity suggests that grapefruit juice has little effect on P-glycoprotein (11277,11282).

Preliminary research suggests that grapefruit juice inhibits organic anion transporting polypeptides (OATPs), which could reduce the bioavailability of some oral drugs (11278).

Adverse Reactions

Orally, grapefruit seems to be well-tolerated. One study suggests that grapefruit can decrease hematocrit counts (531). Grapefruit products containing a preservative can cause vomiting, collapse, convulsions, and coma to occur (3082). Topically, contact dermatitis and phototoxic reactions, including skin blisters, have occurred with the use of other furocoumarin-containing herbs following sun exposure (11).

Interactions with Herbs & Other Dietary Supplements

RED YEAST (Cholestin): Concomitant use of grapefruit with red yeast increases the serum levels of lovastatin, a constituent of red yeast (527). This effect is likely caused by inhibition of cytochrome P450 (CYP450) enzymes by grapefruit.

Interactions with Drugs

ARTEMETHER (Artenam, Paluther): Grapefruit juice increases the oral bioavailability of artemether in healthy men by 90% to 250% (5065,5066).

BENZODIAZEPINES: Grapefruit juice can increase plasma triazolam (Halcion) concentrations. Repeated consumption of grapefruit juice greatly increases triazolam concentrations and prolongs the half-life, probably due to inhibition of cytochrome P450 3A4 (CYP3A4) (7776). Some studies suggest that grapefruit juice, particularly when taken in large quantities, reduces the clearance and increases the maximum blood levels, area under the plasma concentration curve (AUC), and duration of effect of midazolam (Versed). Other studies suggest there is no effect (4300,10159,11275). Grapefruit juice increases the maximum blood levels and duration of effect of diazepam (Valium), but the clinical significance of this is not known (3228).

BUSPIRONE (BuSpar): Grapefruit juice increases absorption and plasma concentrations of buspirone (3771).

CAFFEINE: Some studies suggest grapefruit juice decreases caffeine clearance, possibly increasing the effects and adverse effects of caffeine (4300).

CALCIUM CHANNEL BLOCKERS: Grapefruit juice increases absorption and plasma concentrations of amlodipine (Norvasc) (523), nifedipine (Procardia, Adalat) (528), nisoldipine (Sular) (529), felodipine (Plendil), nimodipine (Nimotop), nicardipine (Cardene), diltiazem (Cardizem) (524,528,1388,4300,7780), and verapamil (Calan, Isoptin, Verelan) (7779,8285). This interaction is likely the result of the inhibition of intestinal metabolism by CYP3A4 (7779,7780). Extensive intake of grapefruit juice (1 liter per day) can increase steady state concentrations of verapamil by as much as 50% (8285). Some references dispute the clinical relevance of the interactions with amlodipine, diltiazem, and verapamil (3230,4300). However, there is considerable interindividual variability in the effect of grapefruit juice on drug metabolism, which might account for inconsistent study results (7777,7779,8285). In healthy older adults, the hemodynamic response to felodipine (Plendil) plus grapefruit juice might be influenced by altered autonomic regulation. In older healthy adults, a single dose of grapefruit juice and felodipine enhanced the blood pressure lowering effects of felodipine. However, after a week of grapefruit juice and felodipine (steady state), the hypotensive activity was reduced, possibly due to compensatory tachycardia (1392).

Research indicates it is necessary to withhold grapefruit juice for three days to avoid interactions with felodipine and nisoldipine (5068,5069,6453).

CARBAMAZEPINE (Tegretol): Grapefruit juice increases absorption and plasma concentrations of carbamazepine (524).

CARVEDILOL (Coreg): Grapefruit juice is reported to increase the bioavailability of a single dose of carvedilol by 16% (5071).

CISAPRIDE (Propulsid): Grapefruit juice increases absorption and plasma concentrations of cisapride (1383,3226).

CLOMIPRAMINE (Anafranil): Grapefruit juice increases blood levels of clomipramine. Two cases are reported in which trough clomipramine blood levels increased significantly after adding grapefruit juice to the therapeutic regimen (5064).

CYCLOSPORINE (Neoral, Sandimmune): Grapefruit juice increases absorption and plasma concentrations of cyclosporine (522,11270). The mechanism of action is unclear. Advise patients taking cyclosporine to avoid grapefruit.

CYTOCHROME P450 1A2 (CYP1A2) SUBSTRATES: There's preliminary evidence that grapefruit juice might inhibit cytochrome P450 1A2 (CYP1A2) (12479). So far, this interaction has not been reported in humans. However, watch for an increase in the levels of drugs metabolized by CYP1A2 in patients taking grapefruit juice. Some drugs metabolized by CYP1A2 include amitriptyline (Elavil), haloperidol (Haldol), ondansetron (Zofran), propranolol

(Inderal), theophylline (Theo-Dur, others), verapamil (Calan, Isoptin, others), and others. Use grapefruit juice cautiously or avoid in patients taking these drugs.

CYTOCHROME P450 2C19 (CYP2C19) SUBSTRATES: There's preliminary evidence that grapefruit juice might inhibit cytochrome P450 2C19 (CYP2C19) (12479). So far, this interaction has not been reported in humans. However, watch for an increase in the levels of drugs metabolized by CYP2C19 in patients taking grapefruit juice. Some drugs metabolized by CYP2C19 include proton pump inhibitors including omeprazole (Prilosec), lansoprazole (Prevacid), and pantoprazole (Protonix); diazepam (Valium); carisoprodol (Soma); nelfinavir (Viracept); and others.

CYTOCHROME P450 2C9 (CYP2C9) SUBSTRATES: There's preliminary evidence that grapefruit juice might inhibit cytochrome P450 2C9 (CYP2C9) (12479). So far, this interaction has not been reported in humans. However, watch for an increase in the levels of drugs metabolized by CYP2C9 in patients taking grapefruit juice. Some drugs metabolized by CYP2C9 include nonsteroidal anti-inflammatory drugs (NSAIDs) such as diclofenac (Cataflam, Voltaren), ibuprofen (Motrin), meloxicam (Mobic), and piroxicam (Feldene); celecoxib (Celebrex); amitriptyline (Elavil); warfarin (Coumadin); glipizide (Glucotrol); losartan (Cozaar); and others. Use grapefruit juice cautiously or avoid in patients taking these drugs.

CYTOCHROME P450 3A4 (CYP3A4) SUBSTRATES: Grapefruit juice can inhibit CYP3A4 metabolism of drugs, causing increased drug levels and potentially increasing the risk of adverse effects (3227,3774,8283,8285,8286). Some drugs metabolized by CYP3A4 that might be affected include amitriptyline (Elavil), amiodarone (Cordarone), citalopram (Celexa), felodipine (Plendil), lansoprazole (Prevacid), ondansetron (Zofran), prednisone (Deltasone, Orasone), sertraline (Zoloft), sibutramine (Meridia), and many others.

DEXTROMETHORPHAN (Robitussin DM, others): Grapefruit juice can inhibit CYP3A4 metabolism (11362), causing increased dextromethorphan levels and potentially increasing the risk of adverse effects.

ERYTHROMYCIN: Concomitant use of erythromycin with grapefruit can inhibit CYP3A4 metabolism of erythromycin, increasing absorption and plasma concentrations (8286). Plasma concentrations of erythromycin can increase by 35% when administered with grapefruit juice.

ESTROGENS: Grapefruit juice increases absorption and plasma concentrations of 17-beta-estradiol (526) and ethinyl-estradiol (525).

ETOPOSIDE (VePesid): Grapefruit juice may decrease the absorption and plasma concentrations of etoposide. There is some evidence that grapefruit juice coadministered with oral etoposide can reduce the area under the concentration-time curve (AUC) of etoposide on average by 26.2% (8744).

FEXOFENADINE (Allegra): Grapefruit juice can significantly decrease oral absorption and blood levels of fexofenadine when taken together. Quarter-strength grapefruit juice decreases bioavailability of fexofenadine by about 24% and full strength by 67%. Grapefruit juice seems to inhibit organic anion transporting polypeptide (OATP), which is a drug transporter in the gut, liver, and kidney (7046). It's not yet known how long grapefruit juice inhibits OATP. Separating administration times might not prevent this interaction. Tell patients it's best to take their medications with a plain glass of water.

HMG-CoA REDUCTASE INHIBITORS ("Statins"): Grapefruit juice inhibits metabolism and increases absorption and plasma concentrations of lovastatin (Mevacor) (527,11274), simvastatin (Zocor) (3774,7782), and atorvastatin (Lipitor) (3227,12179). It does not affect pravastatin (3227,12179). There is considerable interindividual variability in the effect of grapefruit juice on drug metabolism, so individual patient response is difficult to predict (7777,7781).

ITRACONAZOLE (Sporanox): Grapefruit juice impairs itraconazole absorption (310).

LOSARTAN (Cozaar): Concomitant use of grapefruit juice and losartan might reduce losartan effectiveness, but this requires further study. Losartan is an inactive prodrug which must be metabolized to its active form, E-3174, to be effective. In one human study, grapefruit juice reduced losartan metabolism, increased losartan AUC, and reduced the AUC of the major active losartan metabolite, E-3174 (1391).

METHYLPREDNISOLONE: Grapefruit juice can increase plasma concentration of orally administered methylprednisolone. Grapefruit juice 200 mL three times daily given with methylprednisolone 16 mg increased methylprednisolone half-life by 35%, peak plasma concentration by 27%, and total area under the curve by 75% (3123). In some patients, consumption of large amounts of grapefruit juice with methylprednisolone might increase the risk of adverse effects; use cautiously. Some of these drugs include Adlone, A-Methapred, depMedalone, Depoject, Medrol, and Solu-Medrol.

PRAZIQUANTEL (Biltricide): Grapefruit juice can inhibit CYP3A4 metabolism of praziquantel, increasing plasma concentrations (8282). Plasma concentrations of praziquantel can increase by as much as 160% when administered with 250 mL of commercially squeezed grapefruit juice.

QUINIDINE: Grapefruit juice decreases quinidine clearance and prolongs the half-life by about 20% (5067). The clinical effect of this interaction is unknown.

SAQUINAVIR (Fortovase, Invirase): Grapefruit juice increases absorption and plasma concentrations of the protease inhibitor (PI)-type antiretroviral drug saquinavir (3773). However, grapefruit juice does not seem to significantly affect indinavir (Crixivan) pharmacokinetics (11269,11280).

SCOPOLAMINE: Grapefruit juice can inhibit CYP3A4 metabolism of scopolamine, increasing absorption and plasma concentrations (8284). Oral bioavailability of scopolamine can increase by 30% when administered with 150 mL of grapefruit juice.

SILDENAFIL (Viagra): Grapefruit juice can inhibit CYP3A4 metabolism of sildenafil, increasing absorption and plasma concentrations (8283). Oral bioavailability of sildenafil can increase by 23% when administered

with 500 mL of commercial grapefruit juice.
TERFENADINE (Seldane): Grapefruit juice increases absorption and plasma concentrations of terfenadine (530).
THEOPHYLLINE: Grapefruit juice seems to modestly decrease theophylline levels when given concurrently with sustained-release theophylline (11013). The mechanism of this interaction is unknown.
WARFARIN (Coumadin): Grapefruit juice might increase warfarin effects. One case is reported of significantly increased international normalized ratio (INR) associated with consumption of 50 ounces of grapefruit juice daily (12061). But smaller amounts of grapefruit juice might not be a problem. In a small clinical trial, consumption of 24 ounces of grapefruit juice daily for one week had no effect on INR in a group of men anticoagulated with warfarin (12063).

Interactions with Foods

TONIC WATER: Grapefruit's inhibitory effect on cytochrome P450 (CYP450) isoenzymes might interfere with the metabolism of quinine in tonic water. Grapefruit in combination with tonic water containing quinine should be avoided in people with cardiac rhythm disorders such as long QT syndrome that may worsen with quinine (10158).
WINE: Red wine, in combination with grapefruit juice, appears to have an additive inhibitory effect on CYP3A4, theoretically increasing the risk for interactions with other drugs. White wine does not appear to affect CYP3A4 (7778).

Interactions with Lab Tests

DRUG ASSAYS: Grapefruit juice decreases metabolism, and increases plasma concentrations and test results of amlodipine (Norvasc) (523), nifedipine (Procardia, Adalat) (528), nisoldipine (Sular) (529), felodipine (Plendil), nimodipine (Nimotop), nicardipine (Cardene), diltiazem (Cardizem, Dilacor XR, Tiazac) (524,528,1388,4300), verapamil (Calan, Isoptin, Verelan) (3229), buspirone (BuSpar) (3771), losartan (Cozaar) (1391), midazolam (Versed) and triazolam (Halcion) (4300), diazepam (Valium) (3228), carbamazepine (Tegretol) (524), cisapride (Propulsid) (3226), cyclosporine (Sandimmune, Neoral) (522), 17-beta-estradiol (526), ethinyl-estradiol (525), lovastatin (Mevacor) (527), saquinavir (Fortovase, Invirase) (3773), simvastatin (Zocor) (3774), atorvastatin (Lipitor) (3227), and terfenadine (530).
HEMATOCRIT: Some clinical research suggests that grapefruit may lower hematocrit count in people with an elevated hematocrit. However, in people with a low hematocrit, it may increase hematocrit. The effect appears to be the same with one-half or a whole grapefruit daily. The grapefruit constituent naringin may be responsible for this effect (531).

Interactions with Diseases or Conditions

SMOKING: Smoking can have an antagonistic effect on grapefruit-drug interactions. Smokers taking calcium channel blockers and grapefruit juice, or other drugs that interact with grapefruit juice, require special dosing considerations (8285).

Dosage and Administration

No typical dosage.

Comments

Drug interactions with grapefruit juice are well documented. The chemistry of the grapefruit varies by the species, the growing conditions, and the process used to extract the juice. Because grapefruit juice is not standardized, use as an adjunct to drug therapy is not recommended (3775). Grapefruit seed extract is processed from grapefruit seeds and pulp obtained as a byproduct from grapefruit juice production. Vegetable glycerin is added to the final product to reduce acidity and bitterness.

GRAVEL ROOT

Also Known As

Joe Pye, Kidney Root, Purple Boneset, Queen of the Meadow, Roter Wasserhanf, Trumpet Weed.
CAUTION: See separate listing for Boneset.

Scientific Names

Eupatorium purpureum, synonym Eupatoriadelphus purpureus.
Family: Asteraceae/Compositae.

People Use This For

Orally, gravel root is used for urinary calculus, renal or vesicular calculi, cystitis, painful urination, urethritis, prostatitis, rheumatism, and gout. It is also used orally for fever from malaria, dengue virus, fever, typhus; and as an antacid, aperitif, diuretic, emetic, stimulant, tonic, and for inducing sweating.

Safety

LIKELY UNSAFE ...when products containing hepatotoxic pyrrolizidine alkaloid (PA) constituents are used orally. Repeated exposure to low concentrations of hepatotoxic PAs can cause severe veno-occlusive disease. Hepatotoxic PAs might also be carcinogenic and mutagenic (12841,12842). Tell patients not to use gravel root preparations that are not certified and labeled as hepatotoxic PA-free. ...when products containing hepatotoxic PAs are used topically on abraded or broken skin. Absorption of hepatotoxic PAs through broken skin can lead to systemic toxicities (12841). Tell patients not to use topical gravel root preparations that are not certified and labeled as hepatotoxic PA-free. There is insufficient reliable information available about the safety of using topical UPA-free gravel root on unbroken skin.

PREGNANCY: LIKELY UNSAFE ...when used orally. Gravel root preparations containing hepatotoxic pyrrolizidine alkaloid (PA) constituents might be teratogenic and hepatotoxic (12841,12842). There is insufficient reliable information available about the safety of using gravel root products that do not contain hepatotoxic PAs during pregnancy.

LACTATION: LIKELY UNSAFE ...when used orally. Hepatotoxic pyrrolizidine alkaloid (PA) constituents in gravel root are excreted in milk (12841,12842). There is insufficient reliable information available about the safety of using gravel root products that do not contain hepatotoxic PAs during lactation.

Effectiveness

There is insufficient reliable information available about the effectiveness of gravel root.

Mechanism of Action

The applicable parts of gravel root are the above ground parts, rhizome, and roots. Although people think gravel root has antilithic, diuretic, and antirheumatic properties, this has not been studied. Some evidence suggests an ethanolic extract might have anti-inflammatory activity (4020).

Gravel root contains various pyrrolizidine alkaloids (PA), some of which are toxic. PAs are most concentrated in the plant roots, but may be found in all plant parts. PAs, particularly unsaturated PAs, can cause hepatotoxicity. Cyclic diesters such as retrorsine and senecionine are the most hepatotoxic. Liver toxicity may result from PA-enhanced oxidative stress, but the exact mechanism of toxicity is unknown. Single doses of 10-20 mg PAs or chronic ingestion of amounts less than 10 mcg can cause veno-occlusive disease. PAs are metabolized by cytochrome P450 3A4 (CYP3A4) to toxic dehydroalkaloids and pyrroles. Enzyme inducers such as phenobarbital seem to enhance toxicity (12841,12860). Pyrroles are excreted as N-acetyl cysteine conjugates. Some researchers speculate that early administration of N-acetylcysteine might reduce toxicity (11988).

Metabolism is also affected by pregnane X receptor induction of CYP3A4. Genetic or drug-induced variation in CYP3A4 or pregnane X receptor activity can affect the degree of PA toxicity by increasing or decreasing its metabolism (12841,12842). Hepatotoxic PAs are also toxic to the lungs. In animals, pneumotoxicity occurs as pulmonary hypertension and right ventricular hypertrophy. Hepatotoxic PAs are carcinogenic and mutagenic. There are sufficient amounts of hepatotoxic PAs in herbal products to cause toxicity (12841,12842).

Adverse Reactions

Orally, gravel root might cause toxicity. The major concern about gravel root preparations is the hepatotoxic pyrrolizidine alkaloid (PA) content. These constituents are hepatotoxic, pneumotoxic, carcinogenic and mutagenic (12841,12842). Chronic exposure to other plants containing hepatotoxic PA constituents is associated with veno-occlusive disease (4021). Subacute veno-occlusive disease causes vague symptoms with persistent liver enlargement (4021). Symptoms of acute veno-occlusive disease include colicky pains in epigastrium, vomiting and diarrhea, and ascites formation within several days. Enlargement and induration of the liver occurs within a few weeks (12842). Dietary supplement products sold in the US are not required to include the amount of PAs they may contain; therefore, all preparations used orally containing gravel root should be considered potentially unsafe (3484). Gravel root can cause an allergic reaction in individuals sensitive to the Asteraceae/Compositae family (4020). Members of this family include ragweed, chrysanthemums, marigolds, daisies, and many other herbs.

Interactions with Herbs & Other Dietary Supplements

HEPATOTOXIC PYRROLIZIDINE ALKALOID (PA)-CONTAINING HERBS: Concomitant use is contraindicated due to the risk of additive toxicity. Herbs containing hepatotoxic PAs include alkanna, alpine ragwort, borage, butterbur, coltsfoot, comfrey, European buckthorn, gravel root, groundsel, hemp agrimony, and hound's tongue; and the Senecio species plants dusty miller, groundsel, golden ragwort, and tansy ragwort (12841).

HERBS THAT INDUCE CYTOCHROME P450 3A4 (CYP3A4): Theoretically herbs that induce CYP3A4 might increase the conversion of hepatotoxic PAs to toxic metabolites, enhancing toxicity (12841,12860). Herbs that induce CYP3A4 include St. John's wort and garlic.

Interactions with Drugs

CYTOCHROME P450 3A4 (CYP3A4) INDUCERS: Hepatotoxic pyrrolizidine alkaloids (PA) are substrates of cytochrome P450 3A4 (CYP3A4) (12841,12860). Theoretically, drugs that induce CYP3A4 might increase the conversion of PAs to toxic metabolites. Some drugs that induce CYP3A4 include carbamazepine (Tegretol), phenobarbital, phenytoin (Dilantin), rifampin, rifabutin (Mycobutin), and others.

Interactions with Foods
None known.

Interactions with Lab Tests
None known.

Interactions with Diseases or Conditions
CROSS-ALLERGENICITY: Theoretically, gravel root might cause an allergic reaction in individuals sensitive to the Asteraceae/Compositae family (4020). Members of this family include ragweed, chrysanthemums, marigolds, daisies, and many other herbs.
LIVER DISEASE: Theoretically, hepatotoxic pyrrolizidine alkaloids (PA) might exacerbate liver disease (12841,12842).

Dosage and Administration
No typical dosage.

GRAVIOLA

Also Known As
Brazilian Cherimoya, Brazilian Paw Paw, Corossolier, Corossol epineux, Durian Benggala, Guanabana, Guanavana, Nangka Blanda, Nangka Londa, Soursop, Sour Sop, Toge-Banreisi.

Scientific Names
Annona muricata, synonym Annona macrocarpa; Annona cherimola.
Family: Annonaceae.

People Use This For
Orally, graviola is used as an antibiotic, sedative, antiparasitic, cathartic, emetic; and for coughs, catarrh, herpes, leshmaniasis, and cancer.
Topically, graviola is used for arthritis.
In foods, graviola is used in cooking and beverages.

Safety
LIKELY UNSAFE ...when used orally. Consumption of graviola fruit may cause movement disorders, similar to Parkinson's disease (7854). Tea made from the leaves and stems of graviola is associated with neurotoxicity (7856).
PREGNANCY AND LACTATION: LIKELY UNSAFE ...when used orally (7856).

Effectiveness
There is insufficient reliable information available about the effectiveness of graviola.

Mechanism of Action
The applicable parts of graviola are the fruit, seeds, leaves, and bark. Many active constituents have been identified, with acetogenins being the most important class of chemicals. Over 220 types of acetogenins have been isolated from graviola (7857). In vitro, the acetogenins have antimicrobial activity against Leishmania species (7858). Graviola also contains isoquinolone compounds which contribute to the neurotoxicity caused by preparations containing this plant (7856).
The alkaloids contained in graviola are toxic to dopaminergic and GABAnergic neurons in extremely low concentrations. The chloroform extract, which contains all of the alkaloids found in graviola, is toxic to dopaminergic neurons at a concentration of 10 mcg/mL. This is the mechanism by which graviola causes movement disorders (7876).
In multidrug resistant (MDR) cancer cells, acetogenins block the production of adenosine triphosphate (ATP), which inhibits the pump that removes cancer drugs from the cell. This permits chemotherapy to be more effective. Certain types of acetogenins are directly cytotoxic to cancer cells, by lowering the concentration of ATP (7857).
The ethanol extract of the bark of the graviola plant has in vitro activity against Herpes simplex virus-1 (HSV1) with a minimum inhibitory concentration of 1 mg/mL. This extract does not exhibit toxicity toward uninfected cells in culture (7855). Extracts of the leaf, root, stem, and bark of graviola are toxic to snails in concentrations of 60 to 100 parts per million. This action may be useful for controlling a vector for schistosomiasis (10379).

Adverse Reactions
Orally, graviola may cause movement disorders and myeloneuropathy. The symptoms of these disorders are similar to Parkinson's disease (7854). Consumption of tea made from the leaves of graviola may cause myeloneuropathy of the optic nerve (7856).

Interactions with Herbs & Other Dietary Supplements
None known.

Interactions with Drugs
None known.

Interactions with Foods
None known.

Interactions with Lab Tests
None known.

Interactions with Diseases or Conditions
PARKINSON'S DISEASE: There is some concern that graviola might exacerbate Parkinson's symptoms because acetogenin constituents are neurotoxins (7854,7856).

Dosage and Administration
No typical dosage.

GREAT PLANTAIN

Also Known As
Common Plantain, General Plantain, Greater Plantain, Plantain.
CAUTION: See separate listings for Black Psyllium, Blond Psyllium, Buckhorn Plantain, and Water Plantain.

Scientific Names
Plantago major.
Family: Plantaginaceae.

People Use This For
Orally, great plantain has been used for cystitis with hematuria, bronchitis, colds, and for irritated or bleeding hemorrhoids. Topically, great plantain is used for dermatological conditions, and eye irritation or discomfort.

Safety
POSSIBLY SAFE ...when the leaf is used orally and appropriately (12).
POSSIBLY UNSAFE ...when used topically. Great plantain can cause allergic contact dermatitis (4).
PREGNANCY: LIKELY UNSAFE ...when used orally because it can increase uterine tone (4).
LACTATION: Insufficient reliable information available; avoid using.

Effectiveness
INSUFFICIENT RELIABLE EVIDENCE to RATE

Bronchitis. There is preliminary evidence that suggests taking great plantain orally might be beneficial for treating chronic bronchitis (4).

Common cold. There is preliminary evidence that suggests taking great plantain orally might help reduce the symptoms of the common cold (4).

More evidence is needed to rate great plantain for these uses.

Mechanism of Action
The applicable part of great plantain is the leaf. Great plantain contains low levels of tannins (4), and relatively high concentrations of vitamin K, beta-carotene, and calcium (19). It also contains a variety of acids, amino acids, carbohydrates, and iridoids (4). The anti-inflammatory and wound-healing effects demonstrated in animal studies are attributed to the constituents chlorogenic acid and neochlorogenic acid (4). Studies in humans show great plantain is beneficial in treating chronic bronchitis and the common cold (4). In guinea pigs, an aqueous extract had bronchodilator effects; however, effects were less and had shorter duration than salbutamol or atropine (4). In animals, great plantain extract also lowers blood pressure, and decreases total plasma lipids, cholesterol, and triglycerides (4). In vitro, an aqueous extract increases animal uterine tissue tone (4), and fresh juice has antibacterial activity (4). Great plantain inhibits carcinogenesis and mammary tumor formation in experimental animals (6).

Adverse Reactions
Orally, excessive amounts of great plantain may have laxative and hypotensive effects (4).
Topically, application can cause allergic contact dermatitis (4).

Interactions with Herbs & Other Dietary Supplements

HERBS WITH CLOTTING POTENTIAL: Excessive use of herbs that contain vitamin K, an essential coagulation factor, can increase the risk of clotting in people using anticoagulants. These herbs include alfalfa, parsley, nettle, plantain, and others.

Interactions with Drugs

WARFARIN (Coumadin): Theoretically, consumption of large amounts of great plantain may antagonize drug effects due to vitamin K content. Individuals using anticoagulants should consume a consistent daily amount to maintain effect of anticoagulation therapy (19).

Interactions with Foods

None known.

Interactions with Lab Tests

BLOOD CLOTTING TESTS: Theoretically, consumption of large amounts of great plantain may reduce clotting time and test results due to vitamin K content (19).

Interactions with Diseases or Conditions

MELON ALLERGY: Plantago species pollen may cause cross-reactivity in people allergic to melon (4075).
PLANTAIN HYPERSENSITIVITY: Contraindicated.

Dosage and Administration

ORAL: People typically used 2-4 grams dried leaf three times daily, or one cup tea (steep 2-4 grams dried leaf in 150 mL boiling water 5-10 minutes, strain) three times daily (4). Liquid extract (1:1 in 25% in ethanol) 2-4 mL three times daily. Tincture (1:5 in 45% in ethanol) 2-4 mL three times daily (4).

Comments

Avoid confusion with Buckhorn plantain (Plantago lanceolata), Blond psyllium (Plantago ovata), and Black psyllium (Plantago psyllium).

GREATER BINDWEED

Also Known As

Bearbind, Bear's-Bind, Devil's Vine, Hedge Bindweed, Hedge Convolvulus, Hedge Lily, Lady's Nightcap, Old Man's Night Cap, Rutland Beauty.

Scientific Names

Calystegia sepium.
Family: Convolvulaceae.

People Use This For

Orally, greater bindweed is used for fever, urinary tract diseases, as a purgative for constipation, and for increasing bile production.

Safety

POSSIBLY UNSAFE ...when the whole plant is used orally because it has strong contact cathartic effects (271).
PREGNANCY AND LACTATION: POSSIBLY UNSAFE ...when used orally (271); avoid using.

Effectiveness

There is insufficient reliable information available about the effectiveness of greater bindweed.

Mechanism of Action

Greater bindweed is said to be a potent smooth muscle stimulant and to increase bile production (18). Constituent gluco-resins (glycoretins) are contact cathartics which cause an increase in water elimination and peristalsis (271).

Adverse Reactions

Theoretically, large amounts of greater bindweed may cause intestinal and stomach pain (18).

Interactions with Herbs & Other Dietary Supplements

CARDIAC GLYCOSIDE-CONTAINING HERBS: Concomitant use may increase the risk of cardiac glycoside toxicity. Cardiac glycoside-containing herbs include black hellebore, Canadian hemp roots, digitalis leaf, hedge mustard, figwort, lily-of-the-valley roots, motherwort, oleander leaf, pheasant's eye plant, pleurisy root, squill bulb leaf scales, and strophanthus seeds (19).

LICORICE/HORSETAIL: Theoretically, overuse/misuse of licorice rhizome or horsetail plant with cardiac glycoside-containing herbs increases the risk of cardiac toxicity due to potassium depletion (19).

STIMULANT LAXATIVE HERBS: Theoretically, concomitant use with other stimulant laxative herbs may increase the risk of potassium depletion. Stimulant laxative herbs include aloe dried leaf sap, blue flag rhizome, alder buckthorn, European buckthorn, butternut bark, cascara bark, castor oil, colocynth fruit pulp, gamboge bark exudate, jalap root, black root, manna bark exudate, podophyllum root, rhubarb root, senna leaves and pods, wild cucumber fruit (Ecballium elaterium), and yellow dock root (19).

Interactions with Drugs

DIGOXIN (Lanoxin): Theoretically, overuse or abuse of greater bindweed might increase the risk of adverse effects of cardiac glycoside drugs.

DIURETIC DRUGS: Overuse of Greater bindweed might compound diuretic-induced potassium loss (271). There is some concern that people taking greater bindweed along with potassium depleting diuretics might have an increased risk for hypokalemia. Initiation of potassium supplementation or an increase in potassium supplement dose may be necessary for some patients. Some diuretics that can deplete potassium include chlorothiazide (Diuril), chlorthalidone (Thalitone), furosemide (Lasix), hydrochlorothiazide (HCTZ, Hydrodiuril, Microzide), and others.

Interactions with Foods

None known.

Interactions with Lab Tests

None known.

Interactions with Diseases or Conditions

GI CONDITIONS: Contraindicated in individuals with intestinal obstruction, abdominal pain of unknown origin, or any inflammatory condition of intestines including appendicitis, colitis, Crohn's disease, irritable bowel syndrome (IBS), and others (12).

Dosage and Administration

ORAL: People typically use one level teaspoon of the powdered root once or twice daily. A liquid is prepared by boiling 1 teaspoon of the flowering plant in 1 cup of water. This is taken 1 tablespoon at a time, as needed.

GREATER BURNET

Also Known As

Garden Burnet, Sanguisorba.

Scientific Names

Sanguisorba officinalis, synonyms Poterium officinale, Sanguisorba carnea, Sanguisorba polygama.
Family: Rosaceae.

Comments

At the date of publication, there was very little scientific information available about this product. Our staff is continually analyzing the available information on natural medicines and will add data to the online version of *Natural Medicines Comprehensive Database* as it becomes available. See www.naturaldatabase.com.

GREATER CELANDINE

Also Known As

Bai Qu Cai, Celandine, Chelidonii Herba, Schollkraut, Tetterwort.
CAUTION: See separate listings for Jewelweed and Lesser Celandine.

Scientific Names

Chelidonium majus.
Family: Papaveraceae.

People Use This For

Orally, greater celandine is used for dyspepsia, gastroenteritis, cramps, loss of appetite, dysmenorrhea, cough, pain, liver and gallbladder disorders, stomach cancer, intestinal polyps, breast lumps, angina, edema, arteriosclerosis, hypertension, asthma, gout, and osteoarthritis.

Topically, greater celandine is used for warts, rashes, scabies, tooth pain, and to ease tooth extraction. The fresh root is also chewed to relieve toothache.

Safety

POSSIBLY UNSAFE ...when used orally. Greater celandine has been implicated in at least 10 cases of hepatitis involving five different brand products manufactured in Germany (363).

There is insufficient reliable information available about the safety of greater celandine when used topically.

CHILDREN: LIKELY UNSAFE ...when used orally (12); avoid using.

PREGNANCY: LIKELY UNSAFE ...when used orally. The berberine content of greater celandine might stimulate uterine contractions (12).

LACTATION: Insufficient reliable information available; avoid using.

Effectiveness

POSSIBLY EFFECTIVE

Dyspepsia. A specific combination product containing greater celandine (Iberogast, Enzymatic Therapy) seems to improve symptoms of dyspepsia. The combination includes greater celandine plus peppermint leaf, German chamomile, caraway, licorice, clown's mustard plant, lemon balm, angelica, and milk thistle (7049,12724). A meta-analysis of studies using this combination product suggests that taking 1 mL orally three times daily over a period of 4-weeks significantly reduces severity of acid reflux, epigastric pain, cramping, nausea and vomiting compared to placebo (13089).

Mechanism of Action

The applicable parts of greater celandine are the dried above ground parts and to a lesser extent the rhizome and root. The above ground parts contain 0.1% to 1% isoquinoline alkaloids (7,12), including chelidonine. Chelidonine is thought to act as an antispasmodic and weak central analgesic (7,8).

An alcoholic extract of greater celandine seems to increase bile flow (7), and might have hepatoprotective effects (8). The above ground parts contain small amounts of berberine, which is a uterine stimulant. In large amounts, berberine can depress cardiac function (12).

Adverse Reactions

Orally, greater celandine has been implicated in at least 10 cases of hepatitis (363). Large amounts of greater celandine can cause stomach pain, intestinal colic, urinary urgency, and hematuria accompanied by dizziness and stupor (7).

Interactions with Herbs & Other Dietary Supplements

None known.

Interactions with Drugs

None known.

Interactions with Foods

None known.

Interactions with Lab Tests

LIVER FUNCTION TESTS (LFTs): Greater celandine might increase levels of liver enzymes. Greater celandine has been linked to at least 10 cases of hepatitis (363).

Interactions with Diseases or Conditions

BILE TRACT OBSTRUCTION: Greater celandine is thought to stimulate bile flow. Theoretically, this might exacerbate bile tract obstruction (7).

HEPATITIS / LIVER DISEASE: Greater celandine taken orally has been implicated in causing hepatitis (363); avoid using in people with liver disease.

Dosage and Administration

ORAL: For dyspepsia, a specific combination product containing greater celandine (Iberogast, Enzymatic Therapy) and several other herbs has been used in a dose of 1 mL three times daily (7049,12724,13089).

Traditionally, dried herb or herb powder 2-5 grams per day (equivalent to 12-30 mg total alkaloids calculated as chelidonine) has been used (2). Fluid extract 1-2 mL three times daily has also been used (18). Greater celandine tea preparations are difficult to dose properly and are not recommended (7).

TOPICAL: No typical dosage.

Comments
Avoid confusion with lesser celandine (Family: Ranunculus ficaria).

GREEK SAGE

Also Known As
Greek Oregano, Three-Lobe Sage.

Scientific Names
Salvia fruticosa, synonym Salvia triloba.
Family: Lamiaceae/Labiatae.

People Use This For
Orally, Greek sage is used for inflammation of the mouth and throat.

Safety
There is insufficient reliable information available about the safety of Greek sage.
Pregnancy and Lactation: Insufficient reliable information available; avoid using.

Effectiveness
There is insufficient reliable information available about the effectiveness of Greek sage.

Mechanism of Action
Greek sage contains 2-3% volatile oil. Of the volatile oil, 60% is cineole, 5% is thujone (8). Greek sage can inhibit smooth-muscle contractions induced by acetylcholine, histamine, serotonin and $BaCl_2$ (4152). Constituents of the leaf can prolong hexobarbital sleep (4152). Some evidence suggests an aqueous extract of Greek sage might have a blood pressure-lowering effect (4152).

Adverse Reactions
None reported.

Interactions with Herbs & Other Dietary Supplements
None known.

Interactions with Drugs
HEXOBARBITAL: Greek sage can prolong the effects of hexobarbital (4152).

Interactions with Foods
None known.

Interactions with Lab Tests
None known.

Interactions with Diseases or Conditions
None known.

Dosage and Administration
ORAL: Greek sage is used as a tea. The tea is prepared by pouring boiling water over 3 grams of finely chopped leaf. After 10 minutes, strain (8).

Comments
Greek sage is very rare but sometimes it is found as an adulterant of Salvia officinalis (4,5).

GREEN TEA

Also Known As

EGCG, Epigallo Catechin Gallate, Epigallocatechin Gallate, Japanese Tea, Tea, Tea Green.
CAUTION: See separate listings for Black Tea, Oolong Tea, Coffee, Mate, Cocoa, Cola Nut, Guarana, Mate, and Caffeine.

Scientific Names

Camellia sinensis, synonyms Camellia thea, Camellia theifera, Thea bohea, Thea sinensis, Thea viridis.
Family: Theaceae.

People Use This For

Orally, green tea is used to improve cognitive performance, and mental alertness. It is also used to treat stomach disorders, vomiting, diarrhea, and headaches. Green tea is also used as a diuretic and in combination products for weight loss. Green tea is also used to treat solid tumor cancers, and to reduce the risk of breast cancer, prostate cancer, colon cancer, gastric cancer, cancer related to ultraviolet (UV) radiation (e.g., sunburn), and other environmental causes. It is also used to maintain remission in people with Crohn's disease, to prevent Parkinson's disease, heart disease, hypotension, dental caries, kidney stones, and skin damage.
Topically, green tea bags are used as a wash to soothe sunburn, as a poultice for bags under the eyes, as a compress for headache or tired eyes, and to stop the bleeding of tooth sockets. Green tea in chewable candy is used for gingivitis. Green tea is also used topically to prevent skin damage and cancer related to ultraviolet (UV) radiation (e.g., sunburn) and other environmental causes.
In foods, green tea is consumed as a beverage.

Safety

LIKELY SAFE ...when used orally in moderate amounts (733,6031,9222,9223,9225,9226,9227,9228). Green tea is often consumed daily in Asian cultures and has not been associated with significant adverse effects (6031).
POSSIBLY SAFE ...when green tea extract is used orally. Green tea extract containing 7% caffeine has been used safely for six months (8117). ...when used topically and appropriately (6065,11310).
POSSIBLY UNSAFE ...when used orally long-term in high doses. Green tea contains a significant amount of caffeine. Chronic use, especially in large amounts, can produce tolerance, habituation, psychological dependence, and other significant adverse effects. Doses greater than 250-300 mg per day have been associated with significant adverse effects such as tachyarrhythmias and sleep disturbances (11832). These effects would not be expected to occur with the consumption of decaffeinated green tea.
LIKELY UNSAFE ...when used orally in very high doses. The fatal acute oral dose of caffeine in green tea is estimated to be 10-14 grams (150-200 mg per kilogram). Serious toxicity can occur at lower doses depending on variables in caffeine sensitivity such as smoking, age, prior caffeine use, etc (11832).
CHILDREN: POSSIBLY SAFE ...when used in amounts commonly found in foods and beverages (7705,11833).
PREGNANCY: POSSIBLY SAFE ...when used orally in moderate amounts. Due to the caffeine content of green tea, mothers should closely monitor their intake to ensure moderate consumption. Fetal blood concentrations of caffeine approximate maternal concentrations (4260). Use of caffeine in pregnancy is controversial; however, moderate consumption has not been associated with clinically important adverse fetal effects (2708,2709,2710,2711,9606). Caffeine crosses the human placenta, but is not considered a teratogen. Mothers should keep caffeine consumption below 300 mg per day. This is similar to the amount of caffeine found in about 3 cups of coffee or tea (2708).
POSSIBLY UNSAFE ...when used orally in large amounts. Caffeine crosses the placenta, producing fetal blood concentrations similar to maternal levels (4260). Mothers should avoid consuming more than 300 mg of caffeine daily or more than 3 cups of tea or coffee per day (2708). High maternal doses of caffeine throughout pregnancy have resulted in symptoms of caffeine withdrawal in newborn infants (9891). High doses of caffeine have been associated with spontaneous abortion, premature delivery, and low birth weight (2709,2711). Fetal birth weight is reduced by 28 grams for every 100 mg per day of caffeine consumed during pregnancy. But this is unlikely to be clinically important except for women consuming more than 600 mg of caffeine daily (9606).
LACTATION: POSSIBLY SAFE ...when used orally in moderate amounts. Due to the caffeine content of green tea, nursing mothers should closely monitor caffeine intake. Breast milk concentrations of caffeine are thought to be approximately 50% of maternal serum concentrations. Minimal consumption would likely result in limited exposure to a nursing infant (9892). POSSIBLY UNSAFE ...when used orally in large amounts. Consumption of green tea might cause irritability and increased bowel activity in nursing infants (6026). Large doses or excessive intake of green tea should be avoided during lactation.

Effectiveness

LIKELY EFFECTIVE

Mental alertness. Consumption of green tea and other caffeinated beverages seems to prevent a decline in alertness and cognitive capacity when consumed throughout the day (4221,4224).

POSSIBLY EFFECTIVE

Bladder cancer, esophageal cancer, and pancreatic cancer. Drinking green tea seems to reduce the risk of bladder cancer, esophageal cancer, and pancreatic cancer (733,1457,1458,1459,6031).

Breast cancer. Drinking green tea seems to help reduce the risk of recurrence of breast cancer (3926,4218).

Cervical dysplasia. Green tea as an oral or topical preparation seems to reduce cervical dysplasia caused by human papilloma virus (HPV) infection (11310).

Gastric cancer. Drinking green tea seems to reduce the risk of stomach cancer. This effect appears to be dose related, with the most protection occurring in people drinking 10 or more cups of green tea daily (8903,9222,9225,9226,9227). Consuming less that 10 cups daily doesn't consistently provide protection (7033,9223).

Hyperlipidemia. Green tea taken orally seems to lower cholesterol and triglycerides. A theaflavin-enriched green tea extract, 375 mg daily for 12 weeks, seems to cause mild reductions in low-density lipoprotein (LDL) levels (11308). Epidemiological evidence suggests that higher consumption of green tea is associated with significantly lowered serum total cholesterol, triglycerides, LDL, and increased high-density lipoprotein (HDL) levels (6403).

Hypertension. Consumption of green tea 120 mL or more per day for one year may reduce the risk of hypertension. Epidemiological research in Chinese people suggests drinking 120-599 mL green or oolong tea per day can lower the risk for developing hypertension by 46% compared with nonhabitual tea drinkers. Drinking more than 600 mL per day may reduce risk by 65% (12518).

Hypotension. Consuming caffeinated beverages seems to increase blood pressure in elderly people with postprandial hypotension (11834,11835).

Oral leukoplakia. Drinking green tea orally seems to decrease the size of lesions in patients with oral leukoplakia (4213).

Ovarian cancer. Drinking at least one cup of green tea each week seems to reduce the risk of ovarian cancer (9228).

Parkinson's disease. Consuming green tea orally seems to help prevent or delay the onset of Parkinson's disease. There is some evidence from large-scale epidemiological studies that people who consume caffeinated beverages such as coffee, tea, and cola have a decreased risk of Parkinson's disease. For men, the effects seem to be dose related. Men consuming a total of 421-2716 mg of caffeine (approximately 5-33 cups of tea) from any source daily seem to have the greatest reduction in risk. However, there seems to be a significant reduction in risk even with consumption of as little as 124-208 mg caffeine per day (approximately one to three cups tea) (6022). In women, the effects do not seem to be dose related. Moderate consumption of approximately one to four cups daily seems to provide the most reduction in risk (1238).

POSSIBLY INEFFECTIVE

Colorectal cancer. Epidemiological evidence suggests that consuming green tea doesn't have any effect on colon cancer risk (9222,9223).

INSUFFICIENT RELIABLE EVIDENCE to RATE

Cardiovascular disease. Epidemiological studies suggest that consuming green tea might protect against ischemic heart disease and death after myocardial infarction; however, most of the tea drinkers consumed black tea. Whether green tea has a similar beneficial effect is unknown (8119,8120,8121).

Gingivitis. Green tea extract in chewable candy appears to reduce plaque accumulation and gingival inflammation (7594).

Obesity. Preliminary clinical information suggests that a specific green tea extract (AR25, Exolise) standardized to 25% epigallocatechin gallate (EGCG) might help reduce weight in moderately obese patients (8114).

Prostate cancer. Preliminary clinical research suggests that green tea doesn't have any effect on androgen-independent prostate cancer (11366).

More information is needed to rate green tea extract for these uses.

Mechanism of Action

The applicable parts of green tea are the leaf bud, leaf, and stem. Green tea is different than black and oolong teas because it is not fermented. Black tea is fully fermented and oolong tea is partially fermented. Green tea is produced by steaming fresh leaves at high temperatures. This process inactivates certain oxidizing enzymes, but doesn't decrease polyphenols. Polyphenols such as flavanols, flavandiols, flavonoids, and phenolic acids are abundant in green tea. Flavanols including epigallocatechin gallate (EGCG), epigallocatechin (EGC), epicatechin gallate (ECG), and epicatechin (EC), are all referred to as catechins. These seem to be responsible for many of the proposed benefits of green tea (6031,8118,11310).

Catechins in green tea might have anti-inflammatory activity. Catechins derived from green tea are a laboratory standard for COX-1 inhibition (12849). Catechins from green tea also might inhibit the production of leukotriene-B4 and the activity of 5-lipoxygenase (12850). EGCG inhibits IL-1 beta-induced COX-2 and nitric oxide synthetase activity (12485). EGCG and other catechins in green tea might also reduce inflammation and protect cartilage by inhibiting proteoglycan and collagen breakdown (12486). Green tea polyphenols seem to lessen joint degeneration in laboratory models of rheumatoid arthritis (12487).

It's often thought that green tea has more polyphenols, and therefore greater potential health benefits, than black tea. But there is some evidence that suggests there is no difference in quantity and quality of polyphenols between green and black teas (12087).

Green tea also contains 2% to 4% caffeine (519) or 10-80 mg caffeine per cup (4218). The caffeine in green tea stimulates the central nervous system (CNS), heart, muscles, and possibly the pressor centers that control blood pressure (2722). Possible mechanisms include adenosine receptor blockade and phosphodiesterase inhibition (2722). By blocking adenosine receptors, caffeine is thought to increase the release of neurotransmitters such as dopamine (6370). Caffeine also decreases airway resistance and stimulates respiration, via adenosine receptor blockade and phosphodiesterase inhibition (11836). It has also been proposed that caffeine may decrease GABA and serotonin signaling (6370). Caffeine stimulates gastric acid secretion, and increases plasma catecholamine levels (11837). Caffeine can have positive inotropic and chronotropic effects on the heart (11836). Caffeine can also acutely elevate both diastolic and systolic blood pressure, but might not have this effect in habitual users (2722).

Caffeine exerts a diuretic effect, with water losses estimated at 1.17 mL per milligram of caffeine (2712). Tachyphylaxis to the diuretic effect develops rapidly, diminishing fluid losses associated with caffeine intake (10206). Caffeine-containing beverages consumed during moderate endurance exercise do not appear to compromise bodily hydration status (2713). Caffeine doesn't substantially affect the fluid status of people who drink caffeinated beverages on a regular basis (10206). The caffeine content is also thought to be responsible for green tea's effects on cognitive performance (4221).

Some preliminary studies show that flavonoids found in green tea might reduce lipoprotein oxidation (6032,6033,9232). In vitro tests indicate that catechins in green tea reduce proliferation of vascular smooth muscle that occurs with high concentrations of low-density lipoproteins (9229). There is some evidence green tea suppresses thromboxane formation during blood clotting by inhibiting the release of arachidonic acid from platelets (8028).

However, when used in humans, green tea doesn't consistently exhibit useful effects on cardiovascular risk factors. Green tea doesn't reduce inflammation, vascular reactivity, or lipid oxidation. This may be due to low bioavailability of polyphenols (9230,9231).

Caffeine has been reported to cause increases and decreases in blood glucose. In people with type 2 diabetes, acute administration of caffeine impairs postprandial glucose metabolism, while acute abstention from caffeine reduces postprandial glucose levels by 21%. Whether these effects also occur with caffeinated beverages and herbs is unknown (12374). Other research in obese people suggests that caffeine ingestion may contribute to insulin resistance (12375). However, one study found that type 1 diabetics taking 200 mg of caffeine twice daily had increased frequency and intensity of warning signs of hypoglycemia. This may be due to a reduction in blood flow to the brain and an increase in glucose utilization by the brain (6024).

Green tea may protect against some kinds of cancer. Polyphenols in tea appear to have antimutagenic effects and may protect DNA (12523). Preliminary animal research suggests EGCG might prevent new blood vessel growth (angiogenesis) in tumors. EGCG may also inhibit tumor cell proliferation, causing cell cycle arrest or apoptosis (1454,1455,1456,8117,11309). ECG appears to induce apoptosis in cancer cells by reactive oxygen species formation and mitochondrial depolarization (8118). Green tea may also reduce oxidative DNA damage, lipid peroxidation, and free radical generation (4212); and might reduce mutagenic activity in smokers (4217). There is preliminary evidence that green tea might enhance the effects of doxorubicin (Adriamycin) on tumor cells (3940). Some research suggests that constituents of green tea may increase the activity of doxorubicin (Adriamycin). Caffeine, theanine, and EGCG appear to increase the concentration of doxorubicin inside tumor cells by inhibiting the efflux mechanisms that remove doxorubicin from the cell (7690).

The polyphenols in green tea appear to reduce the cellular adhesiveness of bacteria associated with dental disease (7594). Some evidence suggests that EGCG and EGC might inhibit 5 alpha-reductase and might potentially be useful in androgen-mediated skin disorders such as androgenic alopecia, hirsutism, and acne (8113).

Green tea is thought to be beneficial for preventing skin damage and cancer from ultraviolet (UV) radiation due to the antioxidant effects of polyphenols in green tea. Polyphenolic extracts of green tea, specifically EGCG and epicatechin-3-gallate, seem to produce dose-dependent topical protection against UVA and UVB sunburn. Areas of skin where green tea extracts were applied had fewer sunburned cells and less damage to epidermal Langerhans cells, which are responsible for cutaneous immune response. Green tea extracts also seem to prevent UV radiation-induced DNA damage (1359). Animal models indicate that green tea extracts reduce oxidative skin damage, skin inflammation, and epidermal hyperplasia due to UV radiation and other causes (6065). Unlike conventional sunscreens, green tea extracts do not absorb significant amounts of light in the UV range (1359).

Green tea is also used for weight loss. Early evidence indicates that a green tea extract rich in EGCG can increase calorie and fat metabolism. The caffeine, catechin, and theanine constituents of green tea might contribute to this effect (1453,8115,11960). There is also some evidence that EGCG might suppress appetite. However, there is some question about how well EGCG is absorbed orally (3922). The impact of EGCG and green tea on weight loss remains to be determined with well-designed studies in obese people.

Tannins in green tea can produce antidiarrheal effects. The polyphenols in green tea might increase the level of lactobacilli and bifidobacteria and reduce the population of enterobacteria (3941).

For prevention of Parkinson's disease, caffeine in green tea may prevent adenosine's inhibition of dopaminergic transmission. This may result in a reduction in the clinical expression of Parkinsonism (6022). Preliminary evidence suggests that EGCG may prevent oxidation and apoptosis of neurons, which may protect people from developing Alzheimer's disease (9224). Epidemiological research suggests that drinking green tea for at least ten years increases bone mineral density. The exact mechanism for the effects on bone is unknown, but several possibilities have been suggested. Tea leaves contain fluoride, which might slow osteoporosis. Tea also contains flavonoids and phytoestrogens, which might affect bone mineral density. Other proposed mechanisms include inhibition of bone resorption and effects on mineral metabolism by polyphenols and tannins (8116).

Adverse Reactions

Orally, green tea can cause nausea, vomiting, abdominal bloating and pain, dyspepsia, flatulence, and diarrhea. It can also cause central nervous system stimulation and adverse effects such as dizziness, insomnia, fatigue, agitation, tremors, restlessness and confusion. These effects are more common with higher doses of green tea or green tea extract, equivalent to 5 to 6 liters of tea per day (8117,11366). Although acute administration of green tea can cause increased blood pressure, regular consumption doesn't seem to increase either blood pressure or pulse when consumed on a regular basis, even in mildly hypertensive patients (1451,1452). Caffeine in green tea may exacerbate sleep disturbances in patients with acquired immunodeficiency syndrome (AIDS) (10204).

Allergic reactions to green tea include cough, dyspnea, loss of consciousness, and asthma. Occupational exposure to green tea dust can also cause sensitization, which may include nasal and asthmatic symptoms (11365). Caffeine in green tea can cause anaphylaxis in sensitive individuals, although true IgE-mediated caffeine allergy seems to be relatively rare (11315).

Although tolerance to caffeine is a widely held belief, there is little supportive clinical evidence. If it exists, it appears to be of little clinical significance (11839). Withdrawal symptoms such as irritability, sleepiness, delirium, nausea, vomiting, rhinorrhea, nervousness, restlessness, anxiety, muscle tension, muscle pains, and flushed face have been described. However, these symptoms may be from nonpharmacological factors related to knowledge and expectation of effects. Clinically significant symptoms caused by caffeine withdrawal may be uncommon (2723,11839).

Some evidence shows caffeine in green tea is associated with fibrocystic breast disease, breast cancer, and endometriosis in women; however, this is controversial since findings are conflicting (8043). Restricting caffeine in women with fibrocystic breast conditions doesn't seem to affect breast nodularity, swelling, or pain (8996).

Epidemiological evidence regarding the relationship between caffeinated beverages such as green tea and the risk for osteoporosis is contradictory. Caffeine can increase urinary excretion of calcium (2669,10202,11317). Women identified with a genetic variant of the vitamin D receptor appear to be at an increased risk for the detrimental effect of caffeine on bone mass (2669). However, moderate caffeine intake, less than 300 mg per day, doesn't seem to significantly increase osteoporosis risk in most postmenopausal women with normal calcium intake (2669,6025,10202,11317).

Combining ephedra with caffeine can increase the risk of adverse effects. Jitteriness, hypertension, seizures, temporary loss of consciousness, and hospitalization requiring life support has been associated with the combined use of ephedra and caffeine (2729). There is also a report of ischemic stroke in an athlete who consumed ephedra 40-60 mg, creatine monohydrate 6 grams, caffeine 400-600 mg, and a variety of other supplements daily for six weeks (1275).

Topically, green tea ointment can cause cervical and vaginal inflammation, vaginal irritation, and vulval burning (11310).

Interactions with Herbs & Other Dietary Supplements

CAFFEINE-CONTAINING HERBS/SUPPLEMENTS: Concomitant use can have additive effects with the caffeine in green tea, and can increase the risk of adverse effects. Some natural products that contain caffeine include coffee, black tea, guarana, mate, cola, and others.

CREATINE: There is some concern that combining caffeine, ephedra, and creatine might increase the risk of serious adverse effects. There is a report of ischemic stroke in an athlete who consumed creatine monohydrate 6 grams, caffeine 400-600 mg, ephedra 40-60 mg, and a variety of other supplements daily for 6 weeks (1275). Caffeine might also decrease creatine's possible beneficial effects on athletic performance. Some researchers think caffeine can inhibit phosphocreatine resynthesis (2117,4575).

EPHEDRA (Ma Huang): Use of ephedra with green tea can increase the risk of stimulatory adverse effects due to its caffeine content. There is evidence that using ephedra with caffeine might increase the risk of serious life-threatening or debilitating adverse effects such as hypertension, myocardial infarction, stroke, seizures, and death (6486,10307). Tell patients to avoid taking green tea with ephedra and other stimulants.

IRON: Green tea appears to reduce absorption of non-heme iron from foods (8110,8904). Infants given tea to drink seem to have an increased risk of microcytic anemia (631). However, a study of iron-deficient elderly patients suggests that concomitant use doesn't alter iron absorption in this population (185). Theoretically, green tea might reduce the absorption of iron supplements. For most patients, this effect will not be clinically significant. Advise patients with iron deficiency to consume tea between meals rather than with meals to lessen this interaction (8904).

Interactions with Drugs

ADENOSINE (Adenocard): The caffeine in green tea is a competitive inhibitor of adenosine at the cellular level. However, caffeine doesn't seem to affect supplemental adenosine because high interstitial levels of adenosine overcome the antagonistic effects of caffeine (11771). It is recommended that methylxanthines and methylxanthine-containing products be stopped 24 hours prior to pharmacological stress tests (11770). However, methylxanthines appear more likely to interfere with dipyridamole (Persantine) than adenosine-induced stress testing (11771).
ALCOHOL (Ethanol): Concomitant use of alcohol can increase caffeine serum concentrations and the risk of caffeine adverse effects. Alcohol reduces caffeine metabolism (6370).
AMPHETAMINES: Theoretically, the caffeine in green tea might increase the risk of additive CNS effects (2719).
ANTICOAGULANT/ANTIPLATELET DRUGS: Catechins in green tea and caffeine are reported to have antiplatelet activity (733,8028,8029,12882). Theoretically, green tea might increase the risk of bleeding when used with antiplatelet or anticoagulant drugs. This interaction has not been reported in humans; however a contradictory case report suggest that green tea might actually decrease the anticoagulant effect of warfarin. This could be due to vitamin K or other constituents contained in green tea (1460,1461,1463). Antiplatelet agents include aspirin, clopidogrel (Plavix), dipyridamole (Persantine), ticlopidine (Ticlid), and others. Anticoagulant agents include ardeparin (Normiflo), dalteparin (Fragmin), enoxaparin (Lovenox), heparin, and warfarin (Coumadin).
ANTIDIABETES DRUGS: Theoretically, concomitant use of green tea and diabetes drugs might interfere with blood glucose control due to the caffeine in green tea. The data are conflicting. Reports claim that caffeine might increase or decrease blood sugar (6024,8646).
CIMETIDINE (Tagamet): Concomitant use might increase the effects and adverse effects of caffeine in green tea. Cimetidine can reduce caffeine clearance by 31% to 42% (11736).
CLOZAPINE (Clozaril): Theoretically, concomitant administration might cause acute exacerbation of psychotic symptoms due to the caffeine in green tea. Caffeine can increase the effects and toxicity of clozapine. Caffeine doses of 400-1000 mg per day inhibit clozapine metabolism (5051).
COCAINE: Theoretically, the caffeine in green tea might increase the risk of additive CNS effects (2719).
CONTRACEPTIVE DRUGS: Concomitant use might increase the effects and adverse effects of caffeine in green tea. Oral contraceptives can decrease caffeine clearance by 40-65% (8644).
DIPYRIDAMOLE (Persantine): The caffeine in green tea might inhibit dipyridamole-induced vasodilation (11770,11772). It is recommended that methylxanthines and methylxanthine-containing products be stopped 24 hours prior to pharmacological stress tests (11770). Methylxanthines appear more likely to interfere with dipyridamole (Persantine) than adenosine-induced stress testing (11771).
DISULFIRAM (Antabuse): Concomitant use might increase the risk of adverse effects of caffeine in green tea. Disulfiram decreases the clearance and increases the half-life of caffeine (11840).
EPHEDRINE: Use of ephedrine with caffeine-containing products can increase the risk of stimulatory adverse effects. There is evidence that using ephedrine with caffeine might increase the risk of serious life-threatening or debilitating adverse effects such as hypertension, myocardial infarction, stroke, seizures, and death (6486,10307). Tell patients to avoid taking caffeine with ephedrine or other stimulants.
ESTROGENS: Concomitant use can increase serum concentrations of caffeine and the risk of caffeine adverse effects. Estrogen inhibits caffeine metabolism (2714).
FLUCONAZOLE (Diflucan): Concomitant use might increase the effects of caffeine in green tea. Fluconazole decreases caffeine clearance by approximately 25% (11022).
FLUVOXAMINE (Luvox): Concomitant use can increase serum concentrations of caffeine and the risk of caffeine adverse effects. Fluvoxamine reduces caffeine metabolism (6370).
LITHIUM: Abrupt caffeine withdrawal can increase serum lithium levels (609). Two cases of lithium tremor which worsened with abrupt coffee withdrawal have been reported (610).
MEXILETINE (Mexitil): Concomitant use might increase the effects and adverse effects of caffeine in green tea. Mexiletine can decrease caffeine elimination by 50% (1260).
MONOAMINE OXIDASE INHIBITORS (MAOIs): Theoretically, concomitant intake of large amounts of green tea with MAOIs might precipitate a hypertensive crisis, due to the caffeine contained in green tea. This is based on the claim that intake of large amounts of caffeine with MAOIs might precipitate a hypertensive crisis (15).
NICOTINE: Theoretically, the caffeine in green tea might increase the risk of additive CNS effects (2719).
PHENYLPROPANOLAMINE: Concomitant use of phenylpropanolamine and green tea might cause an additive increase in blood pressure due to the caffeine in green tea (11738).
QUINOLONE ANTIBIOTICS: Concomitant use might increase the effects and risk of adverse effects of caffeine in green tea. Quinolones decrease caffeine clearance (606,607,608). Quinolones include ciprofloxacin (Cipro), enoxacin (Penetrex), norfloxacin (Chibroxin, Noroxin), sparfloxacin (Zagam), trovafloxacin (Trovan), and grepafloxacin (Raxar).
RILUZOLE (Rilutek): Theoretically, concomitant use of riluzole and caffeinated beverages such as green tea might increase serum caffeine and riluzole concentrations and the risk of adverse effects of both caffeine and riluzole, due to the caffeine contained in green tea. Caffeine and riluzole are both metabolized by cytochrome P450 1A2, and concomitant use might reduce metabolism of one or both agents (11739).
TERBINAFINE (Lamisil): Concomitant use can increase serum caffeine concentrations and the risk of caffeine adverse effects. Terbinafine decreases the clearance of intravenous caffeine by 19% (11740).
THEOPHYLLINE: Concomitant use might increase the effects and adverse effects of theophylline due to the

caffeine in green tea. Caffeine can reduce theophylline clearance, increase elimination half-life, and increase serum levels (11862).
VERAPAMIL (Calan, Covera, Isoptin, Verelan): Theoretically, concomitant use of verapamil and caffeinated beverages such as green tea might increase plasma caffeine concentrations and the risk of adverse effects, due to the caffeine contained in green tea. Verapamil increases plasma caffeine concentrations by 25% (11741).
WARFARIN (Coumadin): In one case, consumption of large amounts of green tea is reported to decrease the effects of warfarin. This has been attributed to the vitamin K1 in green tea (4211). But, there is so little vitamin K1 in green tea (0.03 +/- 0.1 mcg/mL) that the interaction might be due to other constituents (1460,1461,1463). Contradictory evidence suggests that catechins and caffeine in green tea have antiplatelet activity (733,8028,8029,12882). Theoretically, this could increase the risk of bleeding in warfarin patients; however, this interaction has never been reported. Monitor international normalized ratios (INR) carefully.

Interactions with Foods

IRON: Green tea appears to reduce absorption of non-heme iron from foods (631,8110,9237).
MILK: When taken together, milk might bind the antioxidants in tea and reduce their beneficial effects (220); however, in one study this interaction did not occur (6032).

Interactions with Lab Tests

5-HYDROXYINDOLEACETIC ACID: Green tea might increase urine 5-hydroxyindoleacetic acid concentrations and test results, due to its caffeine content. Caffeine can increase urine catecholamine concentrations (15).
BLEEDING TIME: Theoretically, green tea might increase bleeding time. Caffeine theoretically can prolong bleeding time and increase the results of a bleeding time test, but this has not been reported in humans (1701). Caffeine is reported to have antiplatelet activity (8028,8029).
CATECHOLAMINE: The caffeine in green tea can increase plasma catecholamine levels (8646).
CREATINE: The caffeine in green tea can increase urine creatine levels (1701).
DIPYRIDAMOLE THALLIUM IMAGING: Green tea might interfere with dipyridamole thallium imaging studies, due to its caffeine content. Caffeine attenuates the characteristic cardiovascular responses to dipyridamole and has altered test results (11742).
FERRITIN: Drinking green tea may cause a reduction in serum ferritin in iron-deficient people (9237).
GLUCOSE: Caffeine has been reported to cause increases and decreases in blood glucose (8646).
HEMOGLOBIN: Drinking green tea may cause a reduction in hemoglobin in iron-deficient people (9237).
IRON: In people with iron deficiency, green tea may further reduce the concentration of serum iron (9237).
LACTATE: The combination of ephedrine, a constituent of ephedra, and the caffeine in green tea can increase blood lactate levels (8646).
NEUROBLASTOMA TESTS: Green tea (due to its caffeine content) might cause false-positive diagnosis of neuroblastoma, when diagnosis is based on tests of urine vanillylmandelic acid (VMA) or catecholamine concentrations. Caffeine can increase urine catecholamine and VMA concentrations (15).
PHARMACOLOGICAL STRESS TESTS: The caffeine in green tea is a competitive antagonist for adenosine receptors (11771). It is recommended that caffeine and caffeine-containing products be stopped 24 hours prior to pharmacological stress tests (11770). However, caffeine appears more likely to interfere with dipyridamole (Persantine) than adenosine (Adenocard) stress testing (11771). The interaction between caffeine and dipyridamole is unlikely to be significant in stress testing if the heart rate increase is greater than 5% after dipyridamole infusion (11772).
PHEOCHROMOCYTOMA TESTS: Green tea (due to its caffeine content) might cause false-positive diagnosis of pheochromocytoma, when diagnosis is based on tests of urine vanillylmandelic acid (VMA) or catecholamine concentrations. Caffeine can increase urine catecholamine and VMA concentrations (15).
PULMONARY FUNCTION TESTS: People may need to avoid caffeine and caffeinated beverages such as green tea for at least four hours prior to lung function testing. Forced expiratory volume in one minute (FEV1) seems to show a small improvement up to two hours after caffeine use. Mid-expiratory flow rates may also improve with caffeine for up to four hours (9607).
URATE: Green tea might falsely increase serum urate test results determined by the Bittner method, due to its caffeine content. Caffeine causes false elevations in serum urate test results determined by the Bittner method (11844).
URINARY CALCIUM: The caffeine in green tea can increase urinary calcium levels (11317).
VANILLYLMANDELIC ACID (VMA): Green tea might increase urine VMA concentrations and test results, due to its caffeine content. Caffeine can increase urine VMA concentrations (15).

Interactions with Diseases or Conditions

ANEMIA: Drinking green tea may worsen anemia in people with iron deficiency (9237).
ANXIETY DISORDERS: The caffeine in green tea might aggravate anxiety disorders (11743).
BLEEDING DISORDERS: Theoretically, caffeine in green tea might aggravate these conditions. Caffeine is reported to have antiplatelet activity (8028,8029); however, this interaction has not been reported in humans (1701). Caffeine can prolong bleeding time and increase the results of a bleeding time test (1701).
CARDIAC CONDITIONS: Caffeine in green tea can induce cardiac arrhythmias in sensitive individuals (11845); use with caution.
DIABETES: Some research suggests that caffeine may impair postprandial glucose metabolism in people with diabetes and contribute to insulin resistance. The effect of caffeinated beverages and herbs has not been studied (12374,12375). Caffeine in green tea may enhance the frequency and intensity of hypoglycemic warning symptoms in type 1 diabetics. This may increase the ability of diabetics to detect and treat hypoglycemia early. However, it might also increase the frequency of hypoglycemic events (6024). Caffeine has been reported to cause increases and decreases in blood glucose (8646); use with caution.
GLAUCOMA: Drinking caffeinated green tea increases intraocular pressure. The increase occurs within 30 minutes and persists for at least 90 minutes (8540).
HYPERTENSION: The caffeine in green tea might increase blood pressure in people with high blood pressure. However, this doesn't seem to occur in people who regularly consume green tea or other caffeinated products (1451,1452,2722).
OSTEOPOROSIS: Consuming caffeinated green tea can increase urinary excretion of calcium. Caffeine consumption should be limited to less than 300 mg per day (approximately 2-3 cups of green tea). Adequate calcium supplementation may partially compensate for calcium losses (2669,10202,11317). Postmenopausal women identified with a genetic variant of the vitamin D receptor should use caffeine with caution (2669).

Dosage and Administration

ORAL: Doses of green tea vary significantly, but usually range between 1-10 cups daily. The commonly used dose of green tea is based on the amount typically consumed in Asian countries, which is about 3 cups per day, providing 240-320 mg of polyphenols. The typical dose of caffeine for headache or restoring mental alertness is up to 250 mg per day (2718,11743). For improving cognitive performance, tea providing 60 mg of caffeine, or approximately one cup, has been used (4221). For reducing cholesterol, 10 or greater cups per day has been associated with decreased cholesterol levels (6403). Theaflavin-enriched green tea extract, 375 mg daily for 12 weeks, has also been used for cholesterol reduction (11308). For preventing breast cancer or breast cancer recurrence, three or more cups of green tea per day have been used (3926). For human papilloma virus (HPV) infected cervical lesions, green tea extract, 200 mg daily alone or in combination with topical green tea ointment, for 8-12 weeks has been used (11310). For preventing Parkinson's disease, men consuming 421-2716 mg total caffeine (approximately 5-33 cups of green tea) daily have the lowest risk of developing Parkinson's disease. However, a significantly lower risk is also associated with consumption of as little as 124-208 mg of caffeine (approximately 1-3 cups of green tea) daily (6022). In women, more moderate caffeine consumption seems to be best, equivalent to approximately 1-4 cups of green tea per day (1238). To make tea, people typically use 1 teaspoon of tea leaves in 8 ounces boiling water.
TOPICAL: For human papillomavirus (HPV)-infected cervical lesions, green tea ointment in an unspecified concentration has been used alone or in combination with oral green tea extract, twice weekly for 8-12 weeks (11310).

Comments

Camellia sinensis leaves and stems are used to manufacture green tea (non-fermented), oolong tea (partially fermented), and black tea (fermented) (4218). Leaves used for green tea are prepared immediately after harvest to limit enzymatic changes.

GROUND IVY

Also Known As

Alehoof, Catsfoot, Cat's-Paw, Creeping Charlie, Gill-Go-By-The-Hedge, Gill-Go-Over-The-Ground, Haymaids, Hedgemaids, Lizzy-Run-Up-The-Hedge, Nepeta hederacea, Robin-Run-In-The-Hedge, Tun-Hoof, Turnhoof.
CAUTION: See separate listing for Cat's Foot.

Scientific Names

Glechoma hederacea.
Family: Lamiaceae/Labiatae.

People Use This For

Orally, ground ivy is used for mild upper respiratory complaints, coughs, arthritis, rheumatism, as a diuretic in individuals with bladder and kidney stones, for menstrual irregularities, bronchitis, chronic bronchial inflammation, tinnitus, diarrhea, intestinal inflammation, hemorrhoids, cystitis, and gastritis.

Topically ground ivy is used for poorly healing wounds, ulcers, and other skin conditions.

In food manufacturing, ground ivy is used as a flavoring agent.

Safety

POSSIBLY SAFE ...when preparations of the above ground parts are consumed in amounts found in foods; listed by the Council of Europe as natural source of food flavoring (4). ...when used orally in medicinal amounts (4,18).

PREGNANCY: LIKELY UNSAFE ...when used orally because of abortifacient activity (4); avoid using.

LACTATION: Insufficient reliable information available; avoid using.

Effectiveness

There is insufficient reliable information available about the effectiveness of ground ivy.

Mechanism of Action

Ground ivy contains rosmarinic acid, which may be an astringent (4). It also contains the volatile oil pulegone, which has hepatotoxic, abortifacient, and irritant properties. The concentration of pulegone in ground ivy is low (4). Fatal poisonings have occurred in animals (18).

Adverse Reactions

Orally, ground ivy in excessive doses may irritate the GI mucosa and kidneys (4).

Interactions with Herbs & Other Dietary Supplements

PENNYROYAL: Avoid concomitant use, both herbs contain potentially hepatotoxic constituent, pulegone (4).

Interactions with Drugs

None known.

Interactions with Foods

None known.

Interactions with Lab Tests

None known.

Interactions with Diseases or Conditions

KIDNEY DISEASE: The volatile oil is contraindicated due to potential for kidney irritation (4).

LIVER DISEASE: Contraindicated, due to presence of hepatotoxic pulegone (4).

SEIZURE DISORDERS: Contraindicated (4).

Dosage and Administration

ORAL: 2-4 grams dried plant three times daily (4), or one cup tea (steep 2-4 grams dried plant in 150 mL boiling water 5-10 minutes, strain) three times daily (4). Liquid extract (1:1 in 25% alcohol), 2-4 mL three times daily (4).

TOPICAL: Apply crushed leaves to affected area(s) (18).

Comments

Ground ivy is a rich plant source of potassium and iron (19).

GROUND PINE

Also Known As

Bugle, Yellow Bugle.

Scientific Names

Ajuga chamaepitys, synonym Teucrium chamaepitys.

Family: Lamiaceae/Labiatae.

Comments

At the date of publication, this product was not a common ingredient used in brand name supplements marketed to consumers. Details about this product are available in the online version of *Natural Medicines Comprehensive Database.* See www.naturaldatabase.com.

GROUNDSEL

Also Known As
Common Groundsel, Ground Glutton, Grundy Swallow, Simson.

Scientific Names
Senecio vulgaris.
Family: Asteraceae/Compositae.

People Use This For
Orally, groundsel is used for worm infestations and colic. The pressed juice is used orally in the treatment of dysmenorrhea and epilepsy.
Topically, groundsel pressed juice is used as a dental styptic.

Safety
LIKELY UNSAFE ...when products containing hepatotoxic pyrrolizidine alkaloid (PA) constituents are used orally. Repeated exposure to low concentrations of hepatotoxic PAs can cause severe veno-occlusive disease. Hepatotoxic PAs might also be carcinogenic and mutagenic (12841,12842). Tell patients not to use groundsel preparations that are not certified and labeled as hepatotoxic PA-free. ...when products containing hepatotoxic PAs are used topically on abraded or broken skin. Absorption of hepatotoxic PAs through broken skin can lead to systemic toxicities (12841). Tell patients not to use topical groundsel preparations that are not certified and labeled as hepatotoxic PA-free. There is insufficient reliable information available about the safety of using topical PA-free groundsel on unbroken skin.
PREGNANCY: LIKELY UNSAFE ...when used orally. Groundsel preparations containing hepatotoxic pyrrolizidine alkaloid (PA) constituents might be teratogenic and hepatotoxic (12841,12842). There is insufficient reliable information available about the safety of using groundsel products that do not contain hepatotoxic PAs during pregnancy.
LACTATION: LIKELY UNSAFE ...when used orally. Hepatotoxic pyrrolizidine alkaloid (PA) constituents in groundsel are excreted in milk (12841,12842). There is insufficient reliable information available about the safety of using groundsel products that do not contain hepatotoxic PAs during lactation.

Effectiveness
There is insufficient reliable information available about the effectiveness of groundsel.

Mechanism of Action
The applicable part of groundsel is the whole flowering plant. Groundsel contains various pyrrolizidine alkaloids (PA), some of which are toxic. PAs are most concentrated in the plant roots, but may be found in all plant parts. PAs, particularly unsaturated PAs, can cause hepatotoxicity. Cyclic diesters such as retrorsine and senecionine are the most hepatotoxic. Liver toxicity may result from PA-enhanced oxidative stress, but the exact mechanism of toxicity is unknown. Single doses of 10-20 mg PAs or chronic ingestion of amounts less than 10 mcg can cause veno-occlusive disease. PAs are metabolized by cytochrome P450 3A4 (CYP3A4) to toxic dehydroalkaloids and pyrroles. Enzyme inducers such as phenobarbital seem to enhance toxicity (12841,12860). Pyrroles are excreted as N-acetyl cysteine conjugates. Some researchers speculate that early administration of N-acetylcysteine might reduce toxicity (11988).
Metabolism is also affected by pregnane X receptor induction of CYP3A4. Genetic or drug induced variation in CYP3A4 or pregnane X receptor activity can affect the degree of PA toxicity by increasing or decreasing its metabolism (12841,12842). Hepatotoxic PAs are also toxic to the lungs. In animals, pneumotoxicity occurs as pulmonary hypertension and right ventricular hypertrophy. Hepatotoxic PAs are carcinogenic and mutagenic. There are sufficient amounts of hepatotoxic PAs in herbal products to cause toxicity (12841,12842).

Adverse Reactions
Orally, the major concern about groundsel preparations is the hepatotoxic pyrrolizidine alkaloid (PA) content. These constituents are hepatotoxic, pneumotoxic, carcinogenic and mutagenic (12841,12842). Chronic exposure to other plants containing hepatotoxic PA constituents is associated with veno-occlusive disease (4021). Subacute veno-occlusive disease causes vague symptoms with persistent liver enlargement (4021). Symptoms of acute veno-occlusive disease include colicky pains in epigastrium, vomiting and diarrhea, and ascites formation within several days. Enlargement and induration of the liver occurs within a few weeks (12842). There is one case report of fatal hepatic veno-occlusive disease in an infant resulting from groundsel tea consumption (5606). Dietary supplements sold in the US are not required to include the amount of PAs they contain (3484); therefore, all preparations used orally containing groundsel should be considered potentially unsafe.
Theoretically, groundsel might cause an allergic reaction in individuals sensitive to the Asteraceae/Compositae family (12842). Members of this family include ragweed, chrysanthemums, marigolds, daisies, and many other herbs.

Interactions with Herbs & Other Dietary Supplements

HEPATOTOXIC PYRROLIZIDINE ALKALOID (PA)-CONTAINING HERBS: Concomitant use is contraindicated due to the risk of additive toxicity. Herbs containing hepatotoxic PAs include alkanna, borage, butterbur, coltsfoot, comfrey, gravel root, groundsel, hemp agrimony, and hound's tongue; and the Senecio species plants dusty miller, ragwort, golden ragwort, and tansy ragwort (12841).
HERBS THAT INDUCE CYTOCHROME P450 3A4 (CYP3A4): Theoretically, herbs that induce CYP3A4 might increase the conversion of hepatotoxic PAs to toxic metabolites, enhancing toxicity (12841,12860). Herbs that induce CYP3A4 include St. John's wort and garlic.

Interactions with Drugs

CYTOCHROME P450 3A4 (CYP3A4) INDUCERS: Hepatotoxic pyrrolizidine alkaloids (PA) are substrates of cytochrome P450 3A4 (CYP3A4) (12841,12860). Theoretically, drugs that induce CYP3A4 might increase the conversion of PAs to toxic metabolites. Some drugs that induce CYP3A4 include carbamazepine (Tegretol), phenobarbital, phenytoin (Dilantin), rifampin, rifabutin (Mycobutin), and others.

Interactions with Foods

None known.

Interactions with Lab Tests

None known.

Interactions with Diseases or Conditions

CROSS-ALLERGENICITY: Theoretically, groundsel might cause an allergic reaction in individuals sensitive to the Asteraceae/Compositae family (12842). Members of this family include ragweed, chrysanthemums, marigolds, daisies, and many other herbs.
LIVER DISEASE: Theoretically, pyrrolizidine alkaloids (PA) might exacerbate liver disease (12841,12842).

Dosage and Administration

No typical dosage.

GUAIAC WOOD resin, wood

Also Known As

Guaiac, Guaiac Heartwood, Guaiacum, Guajaci Lignum, Lingum Vitae, Pockwood.
CAUTION: See separate listing for Guaiac Wood Oil.

Scientific Names

Guaiacum officinale; Guaiacum sanctum, synonym Guaiacum guatemalense.
Family: Zygophyllaceae.

People Use This For

Orally, guaiac wood is used for subacute and chronic rheumatism, chronic rheumatoid arthritis, preventing gout, respiratory complaints, skin disorders, and syphilis.
Topically, guaiac wood is used as a bacteriostatic agent in mouthwashes.
In lab tests, guaiac resin is used as a diagnostic reagent in tests for occult blood.
As a flavoring agent, guaiac wood is used in foods and in edible oils and fats.

Safety

POSSIBLY SAFE ...when used orally in amounts commonly found in foods. Guaiac wood has Generally Recognized As Safe (GRAS) status in the US (4912). ...when used orally and appropriately for medicinal purposes. The resin can have low toxicity (4).
There is insufficient reliable information available about the safety of guaiac wood/resin for its other uses.
PREGNANCY AND LACTATION: Insufficient reliable information available; avoid using.

Effectiveness

There is insufficient reliable information available about the effectiveness of guaiac wood/resin.

Mechanism of Action

Guaiac wood/resin can have antirheumatic, anti-inflammatory, diuretic, mild laxative, diaphoretic, and fungistatic activity (4,18).

Adverse Reactions
Orally, guaiac wood/resin can cause skin rashes (18). High doses can cause diarrhea, gastroenteritis, or intestinal colic (18).

Interactions with Herbs & Other Dietary Supplements
None known.

Interactions with Drugs
None known.

Interactions with Foods
None known.

Interactions with Lab Tests
None known.

Interactions with Diseases or Conditions
ACUTE INFLAMMATORY CONDITIONS: The use of guaiac wood/resin is contraindicated in acute inflammatory conditions and individuals allergic or hypersensitive to the product (4).

Dosage and Administration
ORAL: The typical dose of guaiac wood is one cup of the tea three times daily (2,4,18). The tea is prepared by simmering 1.5 grams of the wood or resin in 150 mL boiling water for 5-10 minutes and then straining. The usual dose of the liquid extract (1:1 in 80% alcohol) is 1-2 mL per dose. The common dose of the tincture is 1-4 mL, which is about 20-40 drops (4,18).
TOPICAL: No typical dosage.

Comments
Avoid confusion with guaiac wood oil.

GUAR GUM

Also Known As
Dietary Fiber, Guar Flour, Indian Cluster Bean, Indian Guar Plant, Jaguar Gum.
CAUTION: See separate listing for Guarana.

Scientific Names
Cyamopsis tetragonoloba, synonyms Cyamopsis psoraloides, Dolichos psoraloides, Psoralea tetragonoloba.
Family: Fabaceae/Leguminosae.

People Use This For
Orally, guar gum is used as a bulk laxative. It is also used for treating diarrhea, irritable bowel syndrome (IBS), obesity, and diabetes; and for reducing serum cholesterol and preventing atherosclerosis.
In foods and beverages, guar gum is used as a thickening, stabilizing, suspending, and binding agent.
In manufacturing, guar gum is used as a binding and disintegrating agent in tablets, and as a thickening agent in lotions and creams.

Safety
LIKELY SAFE ...when used orally and appropriately (8305,10325,10326). Guar gum has Generally Recognized As Safe (GRAS) status in the US (4912).
PREGNANCY: POSSIBLY SAFE ...when used orally and appropriately in medicinal amounts (10895).
LACTATION: There is insufficient reliable information available about the safety of using medicinal amounts of guar gum in breast-feeding women; avoid using.

Effectiveness
POSSIBLY EFFECTIVE

Constipation. Taking guar gum orally seems to relieve constipation due to its bulk laxative effects (12548).
Diabetes. Taking guar gum orally with meals seems to lower post-prandial glucose levels in patients with type 1 diabetes (10896,12545). Guar gum administered with food also seems to lower blood glucose in patients with type 2 diabetes (12540,12541,12542,12543,12544). By slowing gastric emptying, guar gum may also lessen postprandial drops in blood pressure that occur frequently in patients with diabetes (12540).
Diarrhea. Adding guar gum to the enteral feeding formula may decrease the duration of diarrhea from about 30 days to about 8 days in critical care patients (10325).

Hypercholesterolemia. Taking guar gum orally seems to lower cholesterol levels in people with hypercholesterolemia (10897). Guar gum and pectin, taken with small amounts of insoluble fiber, also lower total and low-density lipoprotein (LDL) cholesterol, but don't affect high-density lipoprotein (HDL) cholesterol or triglycerides (12547).

Irritable bowel syndrome (IBS). Taking guar gum orally might reduce abdominal pain and improve bowel function in some patients with mild to moderate IBS. It may be more effective than wheat bran (10326).

POSSIBLY INEFFECTIVE

Weight loss. Taking guar gum orally doesn't seem to be beneficial for losing weight (8305).

There is insufficient reliable information available about the effectiveness of guar gum for its other uses.

Mechanism of Action

Guar gum is a soluble dietary fiber produced from the seed of the guar plant. It works as a bulk laxative. When ingested, it expands in the presence of water and tends to normalize bowel function. Like other fibers, it adsorbs glucose and lipids in the gut and decreases their absorption. Guar gum also seems to lower blood glucose by slowing the delivery of carbohydrate to the small intestine and may also increase hepatic extraction of insulin (12540,12541,12542).

The bulk forming properties may also cause a sense of fullness and cause decreased appetite (8305,10898).

Guar gum and pectin, taken with small amounts of insoluble fiber, don't appear to affect iron, ferritin, vitamin A, or vitamin E absorption when taken for 51 weeks (12547).

Adverse Reactions

Orally, guar gum can cause gastrointestinal adverse effects such as diarrhea, gas, and loose stools (12547). Gastrointestinal side effects can be minimized by starting with small doses and titrating up. When guar gum is consumed with inadequate amounts of fluids, it can also cause severe esophageal and small bowel obstruction. Tell patients to take guar gum with at least 8 ounces (250 mL) of water (602).

Asthma may result from occupational exposure (600,601).

Interactions with Herbs & Other Dietary Supplements

None known.

Interactions with Drugs

ANTIDIABETES DRUGS: There is some concern that guar gum can decrease glucose levels and might have additive effects with insulin and other diabetes medications (10897). Monitor blood glucose levels closely. Dose adjustments may be necessary.

DIGOXIN (Lanoxin): Use of guar gum with digoxin results in a decreased rate of digoxin absorption, but no change in extent of absorption (533).

ETHINYL ESTRADIOL (Oral Contraceptives): Concurrent use of guar gum with ethinyl estradiol results in a decrease in ethinyl estradiol absorption (12421). Ethinyl estradiol is in some oral contraceptives. Theoretically, guar gum might reduce the absorption of other estrogens.

METFORMIN (Glucophage): Concurrent use of guar gum with metformin may decrease metformin absorption and lower antidiabetic activity (12546).

PENICILLIN (Penicillin VK, Pen VK, Veetids): Concurrent use of guar gum with penicillin results in decreased penicillin absorption and reduced penicillin levels (533).

Interactions with Foods

None known.

Interactions with Lab Tests

CHOLESTEROL: Guar gum can reduce serum total cholesterol and low-density lipoprotein (LDL) cholesterol levels and test results (10897,12547).

GLUCOSE: Guar gum can reduce postprandial serum glucose concentrations and test results (10896).

Interactions with Diseases or Conditions

GASTROINTESTINAL (GI) OBSTRUCTION: Guar gum is contraindicated in cases of GI obstruction or narrowing, anatomical predisposition to luminal obstruction (602).

Dosage and Administration

ORAL: For constipation, 12 grams per day has been used. Recommend starting with a small dose of 4 grams per day and titrating to reduce occurrence of gastrointestinal side effects (12548). For diabetes, 15 grams per day has been used (12541,12544). For hypercholesterolemia, 15 grams per day of guar gum plus pectin in combination with 5 grams insoluble fiber has been used (12547). Adding 22 grams of guar gum per liter of enteral feeding formula has been used to treat diarrhea in critical care patients (10325). For irritable bowel syndrome, 5 grams of partially hydrolyzed guar gum has been used (10326).

GUARANA

Also Known As

Brazilian Cocoa, Paullinia, Zoom.

CAUTION: See separate listings for Caffeine, Cola Nut, Green Tea, Black Tea, Oolong Tea, Coffee, Cocoa, Mate, and Guar Gum.

Scientific Names

Paullinia cupana, synonym Paullinia sorbilis.

Family: Sapindaceae.

People Use This For

Orally, guarana is used for weight loss, to enhance athletic performance, to reduce mental and physical fatigue, as a stimulant, tonic, aphrodisiac, diuretic, and astringent. It is also used orally to prevent malaria and dysentery, and for chronic diarrhea, fever, heart problems, headache, rheumatism, lumbago, and heat stress.

In food manufacturing, guarana has been used as a flavoring ingredient in beverages and candy.

Safety

LIKELY SAFE ...when consumed in amounts typically found in foods. Guarana's usage in foods is approved in the US (4912).

POSSIBLY SAFE ...when used orally and appropriately short-term (12).

POSSIBLY UNSAFE ...when used orally long-term in high doses. Guarana contains a significant amount of caffeine. Chronic use, especially in large amounts, can produce tolerance, habituation, psychological dependence, and other significant adverse effects. Doses greater than 250-300 mg per day have been associated with significant adverse effects such as tachyarrhythmias and sleep disturbances (11832). These effects would not be expected to occur with the consumption of decaffeinated guarana.

LIKELY UNSAFE ...when used orally in very high doses. The fatal acute oral dose of caffeine is estimated to be 10-14 grams (150-200 mg per kilogram). Serious toxicity can occur at lower doses depending on variables in caffeine sensitivity such as smoking, age, prior caffeine use, etc (11832).

CHILDREN: POSSIBLY SAFE ...when consumed in amounts commonly found in foods (4912,11833).

PREGNANCY: POSSIBLY SAFE ...when consumed in amounts commonly found in foods. Due to the caffeine content of guarana, mothers should closely monitor their intake to ensure moderate consumption. Fetal blood concentrations of caffeine approximate maternal concentrations (4260). Use of caffeine in pregnancy is controversial; however, moderate consumption has not been associated with clinically important adverse fetal effects (2708,2709,2710,2711,9606). Caffeine crosses the human placenta, but is not considered a teratogen. Mothers should keep caffeine consumption below 200 mg per day. This is similar to the amount of caffeine found in about 3 cups of coffee or tea (2708). POSSIBLY UNSAFE ...when used orally in large amounts. Caffeine crosses the placenta, producing fetal blood concentrations similar to maternal levels (4260). Mothers should avoid consuming more than 300 mg of caffeine daily or more than 3 cups of tea or coffee per day (2708). High maternal doses of caffeine throughout pregnancy have resulted in symptoms of caffeine withdrawal in newborn infants (9891). High doses of caffeine have been associated with spontaneous abortion, premature delivery, and low birth weight (2709,2711). Fetal birth weight is reduced by 28 grams for every 100 mg per day of caffeine consumed during pregnancy. But this is unlikely to be clinically important except for women consuming more than 600 mg of caffeine daily (9606).

LACTATION: POSSIBLY SAFE ...when used orally in amounts commonly found in foods. Due to the caffeine content of guarana, nursing mothers should closely monitor caffeine intake. Breast milk concentrations of caffeine are thought to be approximately 50% of maternal serum concentrations. Minimal consumption would likely result in limited exposure to a nursing infant (9892). POSSIBLY UNSAFE ...when used orally in large amounts. Consumption of guarana might cause irritability and increased bowel activity in nursing infants (6026). Large doses or excessive intake of guarana should be avoided during lactation.

Effectiveness

INSUFFICIENT RELIABLE EVIDENCE to RATE

Obesity. Guarana taken orally might cause weight loss when used in combination with mate and damiana (11866). There is also preliminary evidence that a specific combination product containing guarana, ephedra, and 17 other vitamins, minerals, and supplements (Metabolife-356) might help reduce weight by approximately 2.7 kg over eight weeks when used with a low-fat diet and exercise (3719). More evidence is needed to rate guarana for this use.

Mechanism of Action

The applicable part of guarana is the seed. Guarana contains 3.6% to 5.8% caffeine (compared to 1% to 2% in coffee) (11845). Caffeine is responsible for the pharmacologic effects of guarana.

Caffeine is a methylxanthine compound and is structurally related to theophylline, theobromine, and uric acid (6372). It is 100% bioavailable after oral administration and is metabolized principally in the liver to paraxanthine, theophylline, and theobromine (6370). The half-life of caffeine is about six hours (8644).

Caffeine stimulates the central nervous system (CNS), heart, muscles, and possibly the pressor centers that control blood pressure (2722). Possible mechanisms include adenosine receptor blockade and phosphodiesterase inhibition (2722). By blocking adenosine receptors, caffeine is thought to increase the release of neurotransmitters such as dopamine (6370). Caffeine also decreases airway resistance and stimulates respiration via adenosine receptor blockade and phosphodiesterase inhibition (11836). It has also been proposed that caffeine may decrease GABA and serotonin signaling (6370). Caffeine stimulates gastric acid secretion, and increases plasma catecholamine levels (11837). Caffeine can have positive inotropic and chronotropic effects on the heart (11836). Caffeine can also acutely elevate both diastolic and systolic blood pressure, but might not have this effect in habitual users (2722).

Caffeine exerts a diuretic effect, with water losses estimated at 1.17 mL per milligram of caffeine (2712). Tachyphylaxis to the diuretic effect develops rapidly, diminishing fluid losses associated with caffeine intake (10206). Caffeine-containing beverages consumed during moderate endurance exercise do not appear to compromise bodily hydration status (2713). Caffeine does not substantially affect the fluid status of people who drink caffeinated beverages on a regular basis (10206). Caffeine's CNS stimulant effects are thought to improve vigilance and psychomotor performance (2720,10205). For improving athletic performance, caffeine has been shown to decrease perceived levels of exertion, which enables the athlete to feel less tired and increase their performance (6370). Caffeine alone or in combination with ephedrine can improve anaerobic exercise performance. Caffeine seems to enhance muscle metabolism and increases time to exhaustion and oxygen deficit, which may lead to better performance (8646). Studies have also suggested caffeine possibly influences cardiovascular stress reactivity, either by potentiating the stress response itself or adding to the level reached during stress (6372). Caffeine may cause a slight decrease in heart rate after consumption and appears to raise blood pressure during psychological stress (6372). Large amounts of caffeine, >10 mg/kg/day, can also produce tachycardia and premature ventricular contractions (6372).

Caffeine has been reported to cause increases and decreases in blood glucose. In people with type 2 diabetes, acute administration of caffeine impairs postprandial glucose metabolism, while acute abstention from caffeine reduces postprandial glucose levels by 21%. Whether these effects also occur with caffeinated beverages and herbs is unknown (12374). Other research in obese people suggests that caffeine ingestion may contribute to insulin resistance (12375). However, one study found that type 1 diabetics taking 200 mg of caffeine twice daily had increased frequency and intensity of warning signs of hypoglycemia. This may be due to a reduction in blood flow to the brain and an increase in glucose utilization by the brain (6024). For preventing Parkinson's disease, caffeine may protect dopaminergic neurons in the brain. This effect appears to be related to modulation of adenosine receptors (10201). This may result in a reduction in the clinical expression of Parkinsonism (6022). Evidence suggests that tolerance to caffeine's neuroendocrine and cardiovascular effects may develop during consumption throughout the day, but tolerance appears to be lost during overnight abstinence of caffeine (6372). Preliminary evidence also suggests caffeine may increase plasma levels of cortisol and adrenocorticotrophic hormone (ACTH), decrease levels of extracellular potassium, and increase levels of intracellular calcium in skeletal muscle; but the mechanisms are poorly understood (6370). Caffeine may be beneficial in the prevention of cardiovascular disease. There is evidence caffeine inhibits platelet aggregation and suppresses thromboxane formation during blood clotting (8028,8029). There is also evidence caffeine might be associated with decreased levels of testosterone and increased levels of estrone and sex-hormone binding globulin. These findings might explain why some studies have reported associations between caffeine and hormone-dependent conditions such as fibrocystic disease, osteoporosis, breast cancer, and endometriosis (8043). Caffeine is often used in combination with ephedra for weight loss and seems to have additive pharmacodynamic effects. A single dose of ephedra in combination with caffeine can increase heart rate from 67 beats per minute to 82 beats per minute in young, healthy people. The combination also increases systolic blood pressure and to a lesser extent, diastolic pressure (8644). Caffeine in combination with ephedra also increases oxygen consumption. Whether the increased oxygen consumption is an indication of a significant increase in metabolism and contributes to weight loss is unknown (8645).

Adverse Reactions

Orally, guarana can cause symptoms of caffeine toxicity. Caffeine can cause insomnia, nervousness, restlessness, gastric irritation, nausea, vomiting, tachycardia, quickened respiration, tremors, delirium, convulsions, and diuresis. Large doses can produce headache, anxiety, agitation, ringing in the ears, premature heartbeat, and arrhythmia (11832,11838). In fatal caffeine overdose, the cause of death is usually ventricular fibrillation (11838,11845). Insomnia is a frequent adverse effect in children (10755). Caffeine may cause feeding intolerance and gastrointestinal irritation in infants (6023). Caffeine may exacerbate sleep disturbances in patients with acquired immunodeficiency syndrome (AIDS) (10204).

Some evidence shows caffeine is associated with fibrocystic breast disease, breast cancer, and endometriosis in women; however, this is controversial since findings are conflicting (8043). Restricting caffeine in women with fibrocystic breast conditions doesn't seem to affect breast nodularity, swelling, or pain (8996).

Although acute administration of caffeine can cause increased blood pressure, regular consumption does not seem to

increase either blood pressure or pulse, even in mildly hypertensive patients (1451,1452,2722).
Tolerance to caffeine is a widely held belief, but there is little supportive clinical evidence. If it exists, it appears to be of little clinical significance (11839). Withdrawal symptoms such as irritability, sleepiness, delirium, nausea, vomiting, rhinorrhea, nervousness, restlessness, anxiety, muscle tension, muscle pains, and flushed face have been described. However, these symptoms may be from nonpharmacological factors related to knowledge and expectation of effects. Clinically significant symptoms caused by caffeine withdrawal may be uncommon (2723,11839).
Epidemiological evidence regarding the relationship between caffeine use and the risk for osteoporosis is contradictory. Caffeine can increase urinary excretion of calcium (2669,10202,11317). Women identified with a genetic variant of the vitamin D receptor appear to be at an increased risk for the detrimental effect of caffeine on bone mass (2669). However, moderate caffeine intake, less than 300 mg per day, does not seem to significantly increase osteoporosis risk in most postmenopausal women with normal calcium intake (2669,6025,10202,11317).
Combining ephedra with caffeine can increase the risk of adverse effects. Jitteriness, hypertension, seizures, temporary loss of consciousness, and hospitalization requiring life support has been associated with the combined use of ephedra and caffeine (2729). There is also a report of ischemic stroke in an athlete who consumed ephedra 40-60 mg, creatine monohydrate 6 grams, caffeine 400-600 mg, and a variety of other supplements daily for six weeks (1275).
Caffeine can cause anaphylaxis in sensitive individuals, although true IgE-mediated caffeine allergy seems to be relatively rare (11315).

Interactions with Herbs & Other Dietary Supplements

CAFFEINE CONTAINING HERBS/SUPPLEMENTS: Concomitant use of guarana and caffeine-containing herbs/supplements constitutes therapeutic duplication (due to the caffeine contained in guarana) which increases the risk of caffeine-related adverse effects. Other natural products which contain caffeine include black tea, cocoa, coffee, cola nut, and mate.
CALCIUM: High caffeine intake from foods, beverages, and herbs including guarana increases urinary calcium excretion (2570).
CREATINE: There is some concern that combining caffeine, ephedra, and creatine might increase the risk of serious adverse effects. There is a report of ischemic stroke in an athlete who consumed creatine monohydrate 6 grams, caffeine 400-600 mg, ephedra 40-60 mg, and a variety of other supplements daily for 6 weeks (1275). Caffeine might also decrease creatine's possible beneficial effects on athletic performance. Some researchers think caffeine can inhibit phosphocreatine resynthesis (2117,4575).
EPHEDRA (Ma Huang): Concomitant use can increase the risk of stimulatory adverse effects, due to the caffeine contained in guarana (7). One unpublished report associated jitteriness, hypertension, seizures, temporary loss of consciousness, and hospitalization requiring life support with the use of a combination ephedra and guarana (caffeine) product (1380).

Interactions with Drugs

ADENOSINE (Adenocard): The caffeine in guarana is a competitive inhibitor of adenosine at the cellular level. However, caffeine doesn't seem to affect supplemental adenosine because high interstitial levels of adenosine overcome the antagonistic effects of caffeine (11771).
ALCOHOL (Ethanol): Concomitant use of alcohol can increase caffeine serum concentrations and the risk of caffeine adverse effects. Alcohol reduces caffeine metabolism (6370).
AMPHETAMINES: Theoretically, the caffeine in guarana might increase the risk of additive CNS effects (2719).
ANTICOAGULANT/ANTIPLATELET DRUGS: Theoretically, the caffeine in guarana might increase the risk of bleeding when used concomitantly with these agents. Caffeine is reported to have antiplatelet activity (8028,8029); however, this interaction has not been reported in humans. Antiplatelet agents include aspirin, clopidogrel (Plavix), dipyridamole (Persantine), ticlopidine (Ticlid), and others. Anticoagulant agents include heparin and warfarin (Coumadin).
ANTIDIABETES DRUGS: Theoretically, concomitant use of caffeine, a constituent of guarana, and diabetes drugs might interfere with blood glucose control. Data are conflicting. Reports claim that caffeine might increase or decrease blood sugar (6024,8646).
CIMETIDINE (Tagamet): Theoretically, concomitant use might increase serum caffeine concentrations and the risk of adverse effects, due to the caffeine contained in guarana. Cimetidine decreases the rate of caffeine clearance by 30% to 50% (11736).
CLOZAPINE (Clozaril): Theoretically, co-administration might acutely exacerbate psychotic symptoms, due to the caffeine contained in guarana. Caffeine can increase the effects and toxicity of clozapine (151). Caffeine doses of 400-1000 mg per day inhibit clozapine metabolism (5051).
COCAINE: Theoretically, the caffeine in guarana might increase the risk of additive CNS effects (2719).
CONTRACEPTIVE DRUGS: Theoretically, concomitant use might increase caffeine concentrations and the risk adverse effects, due to the caffeine contained in guarana. Oral contraceptives decrease the rate of caffeine clearance by 40-65% (2714,11737).
DIPYRIDAMOLE (Persantine): The caffeine in guarana might inhibit dipyridamole-induced vasodilation (11770,11772).
DISULFIRAM (Antabuse): Theoretically, concomitant use might increase serum caffeine concentrations and the

risk of adverse effects, due to the caffeine contained in guarana. Disulfiram decreases the rate of caffeine clearance (15).
EPHEDRINE: Use of ephedrine with caffeine, a constituent of guarana, can increase the risk of stimulatory adverse effects. There is evidence that using ephedrine with caffeine might increase the risk of serious life-threatening or debilitating adverse effects such as hypertension, myocardial infarction, stroke, seizures, and death (1275,6486,10307). Tell patients to avoid taking caffeine with ephedrine and other stimulants.
ESTROGENS: Theoretically, concomitant use might increase serum caffeine concentrations and the risk of adverse effects, due to the caffeine contained in guarana. Estrogen inhibits caffeine metabolism (2714).
FLUCONAZOLE (Diflucan): Concomitant use might increase the effects of caffeine in guarana. Fluconazole decreases caffeine clearance by approximately 25% (11022).
FLUVOXAMINE (Luvox): Concomitant use of fluvoxamine with caffeine or caffeine-containing herbs such as guarana can increase caffeine serum concentrations, and the risk of caffeine adverse effects. Fluvoxamine reduces caffeine metabolism (6370).
LITHIUM: Theoretically, abrupt guarana withdrawal might increase serum lithium levels, due to the caffeine contained in guarana. There are two case reports of lithium tremor that worsened upon abrupt coffee withdrawal (609,610).
MEXILETINE (Mexitil): Concomitant use might increase the effects and adverse effects of caffeine in guarana. Mexiletine can decrease caffeine elimination by 50% (1260,11741).
MONOAMINE OXIDASE INHIBITORS (MAOIs): Theoretically, concomitant intake of large amounts of guarana with MAOIs might precipitate a hypertensive crisis, due to the caffeine contained in guarana. This is based on the claim that intake of large amounts of caffeine with MAOIs might precipitate a hypertensive crisis (15).
NICOTINE: Theoretically, the caffeine in guarana might increase the risk of additive CNS effects (2719).
PHENYLPROPANOLAMINE: Concomitant use of phenylpropanolamine and guarana might cause an additive increase in blood pressure due to the caffeine in guarana (11738).
QUINOLONE ANTIBIOTICS: Theoretically, concomitant use might increase serum caffeine concentrations and the risk of adverse effects, due to the caffeine contained in guarana. Quinolones decrease caffeine clearance (606,607,608). Quinolones (also referred to as fluoroquinolones) include ciprofloxacin (Cipro), enoxacin (Penetrex), gatifloxacin (Tequin), levofloxacin (Levaquin), lomefloxacin (Maxaquin), moxifloxacin (Avelox), norfloxacin (Noroxin), ofloxacin (Floxin), sparfloxacin (Zagam), and trovafloxacin (Trovan).
RILUZOLE (Rilutek): Theoretically, concomitant use of riluzole with caffeine or caffeine-containing herbs such as guarana might increase serum caffeine and riluzole concentrations and the risk of adverse effects of both caffeine and riluzole, due to the caffeine contained in guarana. Caffeine and riluzole are both metabolized by cytochrome P450 1A2, and concomitant use might reduce metabolism of one or both agents (11739).
TERBINAFINE (Lamisil): Theoretically, concomitant use might increase serum caffeine concentrations and the risk of adverse effects, due to the caffeine contained in guarana. Terbinafine decreases the rate of caffeine clearance (11740).
THEOPHYLLINE: Theoretically, concomitant use of theophylline and large amounts of guarana might increase the risk of theophylline toxicity, due to guarana's caffeine content. Caffeine decreases theophylline clearance by 23% to 29% (11741).
VERAPAMIL (Calan, Covera, Isoptin, Verelan): Theoretically, concomitant use might increase plasma caffeine concentrations and the risk of adverse effects, due to the caffeine contained in guarana. Verapamil increases plasma caffeine concentrations by 25% (11741).

Interactions with Foods

None known.

Interactions with Lab Tests

5-HYDROXYINDOLEACETIC ACID: Guarana might increase urine 5-hydroxyindoleacetic acid concentrations and test results, due to its caffeine content. Caffeine can increase urine catecholamine concentrations (15).
BLEEDING TIME: Guarana might prolong bleeding time and increase test results, due to its caffeine content (1701).
CATECHOLAMINES: Guarana might increase urine catecholamine concentrations and test results, due to its caffeine content. Caffeine can increase urine catecholamine concentrations (15).
CREATINE: Guarana might increase urine creatine concentrations and test results, due to its caffeine content (1701).
DIPYRIDAMOLE THALLIUM IMAGING: Guarana might interfere with dipyridamole thallium imaging studies, due to its caffeine content. Caffeine attenuates the characteristic cardiovascular responses to dipyridamole and has altered test results (11742).
GLUCOSE: Caffeine has been reported to cause increases and decreases in blood glucose (8646).
LACTATE: The combination of ephedrine, a constituent of ephedra, and caffeine, a constituent of guarana, can increase blood lactate levels (8646).
NEUROBLASTOMA TESTS: Guarana (due to its caffeine content) might cause false-positive diagnosis of neuroblastoma, when diagnosis is based on tests of urine vanillylmandelic acid (VMA) or catecholamine concentrations. Caffeine can increase urine catecholamine and VMA concentrations (15).
PHARMACOLOGICAL STRESS TESTS: The caffeine in guarana is a competitive antagonist for adenosine receptors (11771). It is recommended that caffeine and caffeine-containing products be stopped 24 hours prior

to pharmacological stress tests (11770). However, caffeine appears more likely to interfere with dipyridamole (Persantine) than adenosine (Adenocard) stress testing (11771). The interaction between caffeine and dipyridamole is unlikely to be significant in stress testing if the heart rate increase is greater than 5% after dipyridamole infusion (11772).
PHEOCHROMOCYTOMA TESTS: Guarana (due to its caffeine content) might cause false-positive diagnosis of pheochromocytoma, when diagnosis is based on tests of urine vanillylmandelic acid (VMA) or catecholamine concentrations. Caffeine can increase urine catecholamine and VMA concentrations (15).
PULMONARY FUNCTION TESTS: People may need to avoid caffeine and caffeine-containing beverages and herbs for at least four hours prior to lung function testing. Forced expiratory volume in one minute (FEV1) seems to show a small improvement up to two hours after caffeine use. Mid-expiratory flow rates may also improve with caffeine for up to four hours (9607).
URATE: Guarana might falsely increase serum urate test results determined by the Bittner method, due to its caffeine content. Caffeine causes false elevations in serum urate test results determined by the Bittner method (15).
URINARY CALCIUM: Caffeine, a constituent of guarana, can increase urinary calcium levels (11317).
VANILLYLMANDELIC ACID (VMA): Guarana might increase urine VMA concentrations and test results, due to its caffeine content. Caffeine can increase urine VMA concentrations (15).

Interactions with Diseases or Conditions

ANXIETY DISORDERS: The caffeine in guarana might aggravate anxiety disorders (11743).
BLEEDING DISORDERS: Theoretically, caffeine in guarana might aggravate these conditions. Caffeine is reported to have antiplatelet activity (8028,8029); however, this interaction has not been reported in humans (1701). Caffeine can prolong bleeding time and increase the results of a bleeding time test (1701).
CARDIAC CONDITIONS: Caffeine in guarana can induce cardiac arrhythmias in sensitive individuals (11845); use with caution.
DIABETES: Some research suggests that caffeine, a constituent of guarana, may impair postprandial glucose metabolism in people with diabetes and contribute to insulin resistance. The effect of caffeinated beverages and herbs has not been studied (12374,12375). Caffeine in guarana may enhance the frequency and intensity of hypoglycemic warning symptoms in type 1 diabetics. This may increase the ability of diabetics to detect and treat hypoglycemia early. However, it might also increase the frequency of hypoglycemic events (6024). Caffeine has been reported to cause increases and decreases in blood glucose (8646); use with caution.
GLAUCOMA: Consuming guarana increases intraocular pressure due to its caffeine content. The increase occurs within 30 minutes and persists for at least 90 minutes (8540).
HYPERTENSION: The caffeine in guarana might increase blood pressure in people with high blood pressure. However, this doesn't seem to occur in people who regularly consume guarana or other caffeinated products (1451,1452,2722).
OSTEOPOROSIS: Consuming guarana can increase urinary excretion of calcium due to its caffeine content. Caffeine consumption should be limited to less than 300 mg per day. Adequate calcium supplementation may partially compensate for calcium losses (2669,10202,11317). Postmenopausal women identified with a genetic variant of the vitamin D receptor should use caffeine with caution (2669).

Dosage and Administration

ORAL: Guarana is often used along with other ingredients in weight loss products.

Comments

Guarana is named for the Guarani tribe in the Amazon, who used the seeds to brew a drink. Guarana is a frequent addition to energy and weight loss products (11845).

GUGGUL

Also Known As

Guggal, Guggul Gum Resin, Guggulipid, Guggulsterone, Guggulu, Guggulu Suddha, Gum Guggal, Gum Guggulu, Indian Bdellium-Tree, Mukul Myrrh Tree.
CAUTION: See separate listing for Indian Frankincense and Myrrh.

Scientific Names

Commiphora wightii, synonyms Commiphora mukul, Balsamodendrum wightii, Balsamodendrum mukul.
Family: Burseracaea.

People Use This For

Orally, guggul gum resin is used for arthritis, lowering high cholesterol, atherosclerosis, nodulocystic acne, skin diseases, and weight loss.

Safety

POSSIBLY SAFE ...when the prepared gum resin is used orally and appropriately. It has been used safely in clinical trials for up to 24 weeks (3267,3268,10371). Some evidence also suggests that long-term use up to 75 weeks may be safe (8158).
PREGNANCY: LIKELY UNSAFE ...when used orally; avoid using. Guggul gum resin appears to stimulate menstrual flow and the uterus (12).
LACTATION: Insufficient reliable information available; avoid using.

Effectiveness

POSSIBLY EFFECTIVE

Nodulocystic acne. Taking guggul orally is comparable to oral tetracycline in the treatment of nodulocystic acne. Both treatments decreased inflammation and the number of relapses (3268).

POSSIBLY INEFFECTIVE

Hypercholesterolemia. Taking guggul orally in doses of 3000 or 6000 mg per day doesn't seem to lower total cholesterol or triglycerides, or raise high density lipoprotein (HDL) cholesterol in people on Western diets. It seems to increase low density lipoprotein (LDL) cholesterol by 9% to 10% (10371). This is in contrast to studies of guggul in Indian populations, where guggul seems to lower total cholesterol, LDL, and triglycerides (366,3267,8158).

INSUFFICIENT RELIABLE EVIDENCE to RATE

Obesity. There's some clinical evidence that suggests that guggul in combination with phosphate, hydroxycitric acid, and L-tyrosine plus exercise and calorie restriction might result in modest weight loss (8152).
Osteoarthritis. Preliminary clinical evidence suggests that guggul (containing 3.5% guggulsterones) 500 mg three times daily might improve osteoarthritis pain (8150,8151).
More evidence is needed to rate guggul for these uses.

Mechanism of Action

Guggul is an extract of the gum resin of the Commiphora mukul tree, which is native to India. The ketonic steroids Z-guggulsterone and E-guggulsterone are found in guggul extracts, including guggulipid, which is the ethyl acetate extract of the gum resin (3267).
Guggulsterones can inhibit the synthesis of cholesterol in the liver and seem to have an antioxidant effect on lipids (3267,8156). Guggulsterones seem to antagonize the farnesoid X receptor (FXR), which reduces the production of bile acids (12444).
Guggulsterone also has thyroid-stimulating activity (8152,8153,8156). It seems to increase T3 synthesis by increasing conversion of T4 to T3 (8156).
Guggul extracts seem to have anti-inflammatory activity (8150). Guggul might also lower lipoprotein (a) and C-reactive protein (10371). Preliminary evidence also suggests guggul might have antiplatelet and anticoagulant activity (3267,9557).
Preliminary evidence suggests that guggulsterone also has protective effects against drug-induced myocardial necrosis (8154).
Guggulipid might reduce secretion of sebum and inhibit bacterial metabolism of triglycerides which induces acne (3268). Guggulsterones act as agonists of the pregnane X receptor (PXR), estrogen-alpha receptor, and progesterone receptor. The PXR induces the expression of the cytochrome P450 enzyme CYP3A4 (12444).

Adverse Reactions

Orally, guggul can cause headaches, nausea, vomiting, loose stools, diarrhea, belching, bloating, and hiccups (3267,8155,8158,10371). Guggul can also cause hypersensitivity reactions including rash and pruritus (10371).
There is one case of rhabdomyolysis reported in a patient who took guggul 300 mg three times daily. The patient developed hemoglobinuria within 2 weeks of starting guggul in addition to increased alanine aminotransferase (ALT), aspartate aminotransferase (AST), lactate dehydrogenase, creatine kinase, and myoglobinemia. The patient did not have any muscular symptoms. The patient's condition improved when guggul was discontinued. The patient had a history of developing elevated creatine kinase levels after taking simvastatin; however, the patient was not taking a statin at the time of this episode of rhabdomyolysis (13029).

Interactions with Herbs & Other Dietary Supplements

HERBS WITH ANTICOAGULANT/ANTIPLATELET POTENTIAL: Preliminary research suggests that guggul might have antiplatelet and anticoagulant activity (3267,9557). Concomitant use of herbs that have constituents that might affect platelet aggregation could theoretically increase the risk of bleeding in some people. These herbs include angelica, clove, danshen, garlic, ginger, ginkgo, red clover, turmeric, and others.
HERBS WITH ESTROGENIC ACTIVITY: Theoretically, guggulsterones could be additive or antagonistic with other herbs that have estrogenic activity (12444). Some of these herbs include alfalfa, black cohosh, chasteberry, flaxseed, hops, ipriflavone, kudzu, licorice, red clover, and soy.

Interactions with Drugs

ANTICOAGULANT/ANTIPLATELET DRUGS: Guggul might have antiplatelet and anticoagulant effects (3267,9557). Theoretically, taking guggul with other antiplatelet or anticoagulant drugs might increase the risk of bruising and bleeding. Some of these drugs include aspirin; clopidogrel (Plavix); nonsteroidal anti-inflammatory drugs (NSAIDs) such as diclofenac (Voltaren, Cataflam, others), ibuprofen (Advil, Motrin, others), and naproxen (Anaprox, Naprosyn, others); dalteparin (Fragmin); enoxaparin (Lovenox); heparin; warfarin (Coumadin), and others.
CONTRACEPTIVE DRUGS: Theoretically, concomitant use of large amounts of guggul might increase the adverse effects of contraceptive drugs through estrogen-alpha receptor agonist activity (12444).
CYTOCHROME P450 3A4 (CYP3A4) SUBSTRATES: Preliminary research suggests that guggulsterones induce cytochrome P450 3A4 (12444). Use caution when considering concomitant use of guggul and other drugs affected by these enzymes. HMG CoA reductase inhibitors that are substrates of CYP 3A4 include atorvastatin (Lipitor) and lovastatin (Lovastatin). Other drugs that might be affected include some calcium channel blockers (diltiazem, nicardipine, verapamil), chemotherapeutic agents (etoposide, paclitaxel, vinblastine, vincristine, vindesine), antifungals (ketoconazole, itraconazole), glucocorticoids, cisapride (Propulsid), alfentanil (Alfenta), fentanyl (Sublimaze), losartan (Cozaar), fluoxetine (Prozac), midazolam (Versed), omeprazole (Prilosec), ondansetron (Zofran), propranolol (Inderal), fexofenadine (Allegra), and numerous others.
DILTIAZEM (Cardizem, Dilacor, Tiazac): Concomitant oral administration can reduce diltiazem bioavailability and might reduce therapeutic effects (383).
ESTROGENS: Theoretically, concomitant use of large amounts of guggulsterones might increase the adverse effects of hormone replacement therapy through estrogen-alpha receptor agonist activity (12444).
PROPRANOLOL (Inderal): Concomitant oral administration can reduce propranolol bioavailability and might reduce therapeutic effects (383).
TAMOXIFEN (Nolvadex): Theoretically, concomitant use of large amounts of guggul might interfere with tamoxifen through estrogen-alpha receptor agonist activity (12444).
THYROID HORMONE: Theoretically, concomitant use might interfere with therapy to normalize thyroid function; monitor (8152,8153).

Interactions with Foods

None known.

Interactions with Lab Tests

SERUM CHOLESTEROL: Guggul can reduce serum total cholesterol and low-density lipoprotein (LDL) cholesterol concentrations and test results (366,3267).
SERUM TRIGLYCERIDES: Guggul can reduce serum triglycerides and test results (366,3267).
THYROID STIMULATING HORMONE (TSH): Theoretically, guggul can lower TSH by feedback from increased triiodothyronine (T3) (8156).
TRIIODOTHYRONINE (T3): Theoretically, guggul can increase T3 levels by stimulating T3 production (8156).

Interactions with Diseases or Conditions

HORMONE SENSITIVE CANCERS/CONDITIONS: Some preliminary research suggests that guggulsterones might have agonist effects on estrogen-alpha and progesterone receptors (12444). Women with hormone sensitive conditions should avoid guggulsterones. Some of these conditions include breast cancer, uterine cancer, ovarian cancer, endometriosis, and uterine fibroids.
THYROID DISORDERS: Theoretically, concomitant use might interfere with therapy for hyperthyroid or hypothyroid conditions; monitor use (8152,8153).

Dosage and Administration

ORAL: For hypercholesterolemia, a guggul extract (guggulipid), providing 75 to 150 mg of guggulsterones daily, has been given as 1000 to 2000 mg doses 2 to 3 times daily for up to 8 weeks (366,3267,10371). For nodulocystic acne, a dose of the guggulipid equivalent up to 25 mg guggulsterones twice a day has been used (3268).

Comments

Guggul is of the same genus as Commiphora myrrha, the myrrh of the bible. The plant has been used in Ayurvedic medicine for centuries (7161). It was cited in the Ayurvedic texts dating back to 600 BC for treating atherosclerosis. Gugulipid is commercially manufactured in India (3267).

GUMWEED

Also Known As

August Flower, Grindelia, Grindeliae herba, Gum Weed, Gumweed Herb, Rosin Weed, Tar Weed.

Scientific Names

Grindelia camporum, synonym Grindelia robusta; Grindelia squarrosa.
Family: Asteraceae/Compositae.

People Use This For

Orally, gumweed is used for cough, bronchitis, and inflammation of the upper respiratory tract mucous membrane.

Safety

POSSIBLY SAFE ...when used orally and appropriately (2,12).
PREGNANCY AND LACTATION: Insufficient reliable information; avoid using.

Effectiveness

There is insufficient reliable information available about the effectiveness of gumweed.

Mechanism of Action

The applicable parts of gumweed are the dried top and leaf. Gumweed can have antibacterial effects in vitro (2).

Adverse Reactions

Orally, gumweed can cause gastric mucosa irritation (2,12), diarrhea (18), and kidney irritation (12). Gumweed can cause an allergic reaction in individuals sensitive to the Asteraceae/Compositae family. Members of this family include ragweed, chrysanthemums, marigolds, daisies, and many other herbs.

Interactions with Herbs & Other Dietary Supplements

None known.

Interactions with Drugs

None known.

Interactions with Foods

None known.

Interactions with Lab Tests

None known.

Interactions with Diseases or Conditions

CROSS-ALLERGENICITY: Can cause an allergic reaction in individuals sensitive to the Asteraceae/Compositae family. Members of this family include ragweed, chrysanthemums, marigolds, daisies, and many other herbs.

Dosage and Administration

ORAL: The typical dose of gumweed is 4-6 grams of the dried top or leaf per day (2). The usual dose of the fluid extract is 3-6 grams per day (2). The common dose of the 1:10 tincture (60-80% ethanol) is 1.5-3 mL per day, and the usual dose of the 1:5 tincture (60-80% ethanol) is 1.5-3 mL per day (2).

GYMNEMA

Also Known As

Gur-Mar, Gurmar, Gurmarbooti, Gemnema melicida, Madhunashini, Merasingi, Meshashringi, Miracle Plant, Vishani.

Scientific Names

Gymnema sylvestre, synonym Periploca sylvestris.
Family: Apocynaceae.

People Use This For

Orally, gymnema is used to treat diabetes and coughs; and as a snake bite antidote, antimalarial, digestive stimulant, laxative, and diuretic.
In combination with other products, gymnema is used for metabolic control.

Safety

POSSIBLY SAFE ...when used orally and appropriately. Gymnema appears to be safe when used for up to 20 months (45,46).
PREGNANCY AND LACTATION: Insufficient reliable information available; avoid using.

Effectiveness

INSUFFICIENT RELIABLE EVIDENCE to RATE

Diabetes. Preliminary clinical research suggests that taking a specific gymnema extract (GS4) orally in combination with insulin or oral hypoglycemics can further reduce blood glucose and glycosylated hemoglobin in patients with type 1 or type 2 diabetes (45,46). More evidence is needed to rate gymnema for this use.

Mechanism of Action

The applicable part of gymnema is the leaf. For diabetes, gymnema may affect blood glucose in several ways. Gymnemic acids seem to reduce intestinal absorption of glucose and may stimulate pancreatic beta cell growth (47,48,11367). Other research suggests that constituents of gymnema have a direct effect on beta-cell function, increasing the release of insulin (12549). Gymnema can increase serum C-peptide levels, suggesting an increase in endogenous insulin secretion (45).
The constituents, gymnemic acid and gurmarin, inhibit the ability to taste bitter (quinine) or sweet (sugar) without affecting the ability to taste sour, astringent, or pungent flavors (11292).

Adverse Reactions

None reported.

Interactions with Herbs & Other Dietary Supplements

None known.

Interactions with Drugs

ANTIDIABETES DRUGS: Gymnema can enhance the blood glucose lowering effects of hypoglycemic drugs (46). Monitor blood glucose levels closely.
INSULIN: Gymnema can enhance the blood glucose lowering effects of insulin (45); blood glucose levels should be monitored closely.

Interactions with Foods

None known.

Interactions with Lab Tests

BLOOD GLUCOSE: Gymnema can lower blood sugar resulting in lower blood glucose test results (45,46).

Interactions with Diseases or Conditions

DIABETES: Gymnema can affect blood sugar control, and blood glucose levels should be monitored closely (45,46).

Dosage and Administration

ORAL: For diabetes, the gymnema extract GS4 400 mg daily has been used (45,46).

HARONGA

Also Known As

Harongablädder leaf, Harongarinde bark, Harunganae madagascariensis cortex bark, Harunganae madagascariensis folium leaf.

Scientific Names

Harungana madagascariensis, synonym Haronga madagascariensis.
Family: Clusiaceae/Guttiferae or Hypericaceae.

People Use This For

Orally, haronga is used for dyspepsia, mild exocrine pancreatic insufficiency, liver and gallbladder complaints, and loss of appetite.

Safety

POSSIBLY SAFE ...when used orally and appropriately (2). The recommended maximum safe duration of use is two months (2).
PREGNANCY AND LACTATION: Insufficient reliable information available; avoid using.

Effectiveness
There is insufficient reliable information available about the effectiveness of haronga.

Mechanism of Action
The applicable parts of haronga are the bark and leaf. Haronga can have gallbladder stimulating (2), liver protectant, pancreas stimulating, gastric juice secretion stimulating, and antimicrobial effects (18). It can also have possible anti-amoebic activity (1519).

Adverse Reactions
Photosensitivity is possible with the use of haronga, especially in fair-skinned people (2). Phototoxicity is theoretically possible with large doses (18).

Interactions with Herbs & Other Dietary Supplements
None known.

Interactions with Drugs
None known.

Interactions with Foods
None known.

Interactions with Lab Tests
None known.

Interactions with Diseases or Conditions
CONTRAINDICATIONS: The use of haronga is contraindicated in acute pancreatitis and exacerbations of chronic pancreatitis, severe liver dysfunction, gallstones, biliary obstruction, gallbladder empyema, or obstruction of the bowels (2,18).
FAIR-SKINNED INDIVIDUALS: Haronga can cause photosensitivity in fair-skinned individuals (2).

Dosage and Administration
ORAL: The typical dose of the haronga dry extract is 7.5-15 mg per day, which corresponds to 25-50 mg of the herb (2,18). The recommended maximum safe duration of use is two months (2).

HARTSTONGUE

Also Known As
Buttonhole, God's-Hair, Hind's Tongue, Horse Tongue.

Scientific Names
Asplenium scolopendrium, synonym Scolopendrium vulgare.
Family: Aspleniaceae.

Comments
At the date of publication, this product was not a common ingredient used in brand name supplements marketed to consumers. Details about this product are available in the online version of *Natural Medicines Comprehensive Database.* See www.naturaldatabase.com.

HAWAIIAN BABY WOODROSE

Also Known As
Baby Hawaiian Woodrose, Baby Woodrose, Elephant Creeper, Elephant-Climber, Silver-Morning-Glory, Vidhara, Vriddadaru, Wood-Rose, Woolly Morning Glory.

Scientific Names
Argyreia nervosa, synonyms, Argyreia speciosa, Convolvulus nervosus, Convolvulus speciosus, Lettsomia nervosa.
Family: Convolvulaceae.

People Use This For
Orally, Hawaiian baby woodrose is used for pain relief, promoting sweating, for sacramental rituals, and as a hallucinogen.

Safety

LIKELY UNSAFE ...when used orally (17,5301). The seeds of Hawaiian baby woodrose have effects similar to the hallucinogen lysergic acid diethylamide (LSD), including flashbacks (5301).
PREGNANCY AND LACTATION: LIKELY UNSAFE ...when used orally (17,5301); avoid using.

Effectiveness

There is insufficient reliable information available about the effectiveness of Hawaiian baby woodrose.

Mechanism of Action

The applicable part of Hawaiian baby woodrose is the seeds. Hawaiian baby woodrose, an ornamental plant, has seeds that contain hallucinogens including ergonovine, isoergine (isolysergic acid amide), and ergine (lysergic acid amide) (17,5301,5304). Four to eight seeds are equivalent to 10 to 100 mcg of lysergic acid diethylamide (LSD) (5301), a potent serotonin-1A (5-HT1A) agonist (17). The hallucinatory effects of Hawaiian baby woodrose are similar to alcohol intoxication with psychedelic visual effects such as enhanced colors. The effects last 6-8 hours (5301,5304).

Adverse Reactions

Orally, ingestion can cause nausea and vomiting, dizziness, auditory hallucinations, blurred vision, dilated pupils, involuntary, rapid, rhythmic movement of eyeballs, sweating, fast heart rate, and hypertension (5301).

Interactions with Herbs & Other Dietary Supplements

ST. JOHN'S WORT: Theoretically, Hawaiian baby woodrose might increase the effects and adverse effects of products that increase serotonin levels, including St. John's wort (17).

Interactions with Drugs

ANTIDEPRESSANT DRUGS: Theoretically, because Hawaiian baby woodrose contains chemicals related to LSD, it might interact with drugs that increase serotonin including sertraline (Zoloft), paroxetine (Paxil), fluoxetine (Prozac), and other antidepressants. Seizures have occurred in people taking the related compound, LSD, with fluoxetine (Prozac) (17). Individuals who have previously used LSD have developed flashbacks and hallucinations when treated with serotonin reuptake inhibitors (17). Combining serotonergic antidepressants with Hawaiian baby woodrose might increase the risk of serotonergic side effects including serotonin syndrome and cerebral vasoconstrictive disorders such as Call-Fleming syndrome (8056).
CLOZAPINE (Clozaril): Theoretically, because selective 5-HT2 receptor antagonists such as clozapine antagonize the effect of LSD, they might also decrease the effect of Hawaiian baby woodrose (17).
CYPROHEPTADINE: Theoretically, because selective 5-HT2 receptor antagonists such as cyproheptadine antagonize the effect of LSD, they might also decrease the effect of Hawaiian baby woodrose (17).
DEXTROMETHORPHAN (Robitussin DM, others): Theoretically, concurrent use might cause additive serotonergenic effects and increase the risk of serotonin syndrome. Also, concurrent use might also cause cerebral vasoconstriction disorders such as Call-Fleming syndrome (8056).
MEPERIDINE (Demerol): Combining serotonergic drugs such as meperidine with Hawaiian baby woodrose might increase the risk of serotonergic side effects including serotonin syndrome and cerebral vasoconstrictive disorders such as Call-Fleming syndrome (8056).
MONOAMINE OXIDASE INHIBITORS (MAOIs): Combining serotonergic drugs such as one of the MAOIs with Hawaiian baby woodrose might increase the risk of serotonergic side effects including serotonin syndrome and cerebral vasoconstrictive disorders such as Call-Fleming syndrome (8056).
PENTAZOCINE (Talwin): Combining serotonergic drugs such as pentazocin with Hawaiian baby woodrose might increase the risk of serotonergic side effects including serotonin syndrome and cerebral vasoconstrictive disorders such as Call-Fleming syndrome (8056).
RISPERIDONE (Risperdal): Theoretically, because selective 5-HT2 receptor antagonists such as risperidone antagonize the effect of LSD, they might also decrease the effect of Hawaiian baby woodrose (17).
TRAMADOL (Ultram): Combining serotonergic drugs such as tramadol with Hawaiian baby woodrose might increase the risk of serotonergic side effects including serotonin syndrome and cerebral vasoconstrictive disorders such as Call-Fleming syndrome (8056).

Interactions with Foods

None known.

Interactions with Lab Tests

None known.

Interactions with Diseases or Conditions

PSYCHOSIS: Theoretically, because Hawaiian baby woodrose has effects similar to LSD, individuals with psychotic tendencies might experience prolonged psychotic reactions (17).

Dosage and Administration

No typical dosage.

Comments

Hawaiian baby woodrose is likely unsafe for oral use; avoid using. Hawaiian baby woodrose, a relative of the morning glory, grows in Florida, California, and Hawaii (17). Touted as a "natural LSD" in Internet advertising, the seeds are legal, and easily purchased from Internet sources (5301).

HAWTHORN

Also Known As

Aubepine, Bianco Spino, Crataegi Flos, Crataegi Folium, Crataegi Folium Cum Flore, Crataegi Fructus, English Hawthorn, Epine Blanche, Epine de Mai, Haagdorn, Hagedorn, Harthorne, Haw, Hawthorne, Hedgethorn, LI 132, LI132, May, Maybush, Maythorn, Mehlbeebaum, Meidorn, Nan Shanzha, Oneseed Hawthorn, Shanzha, Weissdorn, Whitehorn, WS 1442, WS1442.

Scientific Names

Crataegus monogyna; Crataegus laevigata, synonyms Crataegus oxyacantha, Mespilus laevigata; Crataegus cuneata, synonym Crataegus kulingensis; Crataegus pinnatifida.
Family: Rosaceae.

People Use This For

Orally, hawthorn is used for cardiovascular conditions such as congestive heart failure (CHF), coronary circulation problems, angina, and arrhythmias. It is also used to increase cardiac output reduced by hypertension or pulmonary disease, to treat both hypotension and hypertension, atherosclerosis, hyperlipidemia, and Buerger's disease.
Hawthorn is also used as a sedative, anxiolytic, antispasmodic, astringent, and diuretic. It is also used for amenorrhea, gastrointestinal conditions such as indigestion, enteritis, epigastric distension, diarrhea, and abdominal pain. Hawthorn is also used orally to treat tapeworm infections and acute bacillary dysentery.
Topically, hawthorn is used as a poultice for boils, sores, and ulcers. Hawthorn preparations are used as a wash for sores, itching, and frost bite.
In manufacturing, hawthorn is used for making candied fruit slices, jam, jelly, and wine.

Safety

POSSIBLY SAFE ...when used orally and appropriately, short-term. Hawthorn preparations seem to be safe when used for up to 16 weeks. Although hawthorn might be safe for long-term use, current studies have not extended past 16 weeks (8279,8280,8281,10144).
There is insufficient reliable information about the safety of hawthorn for its other uses.
PREGNANCY AND LACTATION: Insufficient reliable information available; avoid using.

Effectiveness

POSSIBLY EFFECTIVE

Congestive heart failure (CHF). Taking hawthorn orally, as a specific standardized leaf and flower extract (LI 132 or WS 1442), seems to improve ejection fraction, exercise tolerance, and reduce subjective symptoms associated with New York Heart Association stage II heart failure. Maximum effect is usually seen after 6-12 weeks of treatment with 240-600 mg per day of a standardized hawthorn extract (8279,8280,10144,11449). In addition, hawthorn extract WS 1442 combined with pre-existing diuretic therapy can improve exercise tolerance and reduce subjective symptoms associated with New York Heart Association stage III heart failure. Maximum effect is usually seen after 16 weeks of combined diuretic therapy and 1800 mg per day standardized hawthorn extract WS 1442 (8281).

INSUFFICIENT RELIABLE EVIDENCE to RATE

Anxiety. Preliminary clinical research suggests hawthorn, combined with magnesium and California poppy (Sympathyl, not available in the US), might be useful in treating mild to moderate anxiety disorders (12583). More evidence is needed to rate hawthorn for this use.

Mechanism of Action

The applicable parts of hawthorn are the leaf, fruit, and flower. The constituents responsible for the pharmacological effects of hawthorn preparations include flavonoids such as vitexin, rutin, quercetin, and hyperoside; and oligomeric proanthocyanidins (OPCs) such as epicatechin and procyanidins. Some hawthorn products are standardized based on their flavonoid (2.2%) and OPC (18.75%) content (12595). Hawthorn preparations act on the myocardium by increasing force of contraction and lengthening the refractory period, increasing coronary blood flow and cardiac output, and reducing oxygen consumption (10144,11450,12595). Hawthorn's cardiotrophic properties are attributed to increased membrane permeability for calcium (11450), and phosphodiesterase inhibition, which increases intracellular cAMP. Increased cAMP leads to increased coronary blood flow, vasodilation, and positive inotropic effects (11450,12595). Preliminary research suggests that hawthorn also has antiarrhythmic activity (12595). Hawthorn also seems to have hypotensive activity, according to preliminary research. It seems to cause peripheral vasodilation and to induce endothelium-dependent arterial relaxation. The proantocyanidin constituents seem to

cause this effect (12595).
Preliminary research suggests hawthorn can lower serum cholesterol, low-density lipoprotein (LDL) cholesterol, and triglycerides. It seems to lower accumulation of lipids in the liver and aorta. Hawthorn fruit extract may lower cholesterol by increasing bile acid excretion, reducing cholesterol synthesis by the liver, and enhancing LDL-receptor activity. Hawthorn also seems to have antioxidant activity (12595).
Animal evidence suggests that hawthorn might have hypoglycemic activity in individuals with diabetes (11451).

Adverse Reactions
Orally, hawthorn is generally well tolerated with vertigo and dizziness being the most common adverse effects (10144). Hawthorn preparations can cause nausea, gastrointestinal complaints, fatigue, sweating, and a rash on hands. Hawthorn can also cause palpitations, headache, dyspnea, nosebleeds, sleeplessness, agitation, and circulatory disturbances (8281,10144).

Interactions with Herbs & Other Dietary Supplements
HERBS AND SUPPLEMENTS WITH HYPOTENSIVE EFFECTS: Hawthorn might have hypotensive effects (12595). Theoretically, concurrent use of hawthorn with other herbs and supplements that decrease blood pressure might increase the risk of hypotension. Some of these products include danshen, epimedium, ginger, Panax ginseng, turmeric, valerian, and others.
OTHER CARDIOACTIVE HERBS: Avoid concomitant use with other cardioactive herbs due to unpredictability of effects and adverse effects (406,10144,11450). Other cardioactive herbs include calamus, cereus, cola, coltsfoot, devil's claw, European mistletoe, fenugreek, fumitory, ginger, Panax ginseng, white horehound, mate, parsley, quassia, scotch broom flower, shepherd's purse, and wild carrot.

Interactions with Drugs
BETA-BLOCKERS: Theoretically, using hawthorn with beta-blockers such as atenolol (Tenormin), metoprolol (Lopressor, Toprol XL), nadolol (Corgard), and propranolol (Inderal) might cause additive effects on blood pressure and heart rate (12595).
CALCIUM CHANNEL BLOCKERS: Theoretically, using hawthorn with calcium channel blockers such as verapamil (Calan, Covera-HS, Verelan), nifedipine (Procardia), and diltiazem (Cardizem, Dilacor, Tiazac) might cause additive coronary vasodilatory effects (12595).
DIGOXIN (Lanoxin): Theoretically, concomitant use with hawthorn might potentiate the effects of digoxin requiring digoxin dose reduction (12595).
NITRATES: Using hawthorn with nitrates such as nitroglycerin (Nitro-Bid, Nitro-Dur, Nitrostat) and isosorbide (Imdur, Isordil, Sorbitrate) might cause additive coronary vasodilatory effects (12595).
PHOSPHODIETERASE-5 INHIBITORS: Theoretically, concurrent use of phosphodiesterase-5 (PDE-5) inhibitors and hawthorn might result in additive vasodilation and hypotension (12595). PDE-5 inhibitors include sildenafil (Viagra), tadalafil (Cialis), and vardenafil (Levitra) (12595).

Interactions with Foods
None known.

Interactions with Lab Tests
CHOLESTEROL: Theoretically, hawthorn might lower blood levels total and low density lipoprotein (LDL) cholesterol and test results (12595).

Interactions with Diseases or Conditions
CARDIOVASCULAR CONDITIONS: Concomitant use of hawthorn with conventional cardiovascular drug therapy might potentiate or interfere with the treatment of these conditions (12595).

Dosage and Administration
ORAL: For heart failure, standardized hawthorn leaf with flower extract (LI 132 or WS 1442) 160 to 1800 mg (3.5-39.6 mg of total flavonoids calculated as hyperoside or 30-338 mg of proantocyanidins) has been used in 2-3 divided doses daily (8279,8280,8281,10144,11449). It should be used for 4 to 8 weeks to determine benefit (12595).

HAZELNUT

Also Known As
Aveleira, Avelinier, Avellano, Cobnut, Coudrier, European Filbert, European Hazel, Haselnuss, Haselstrauch, Hazel, Hazel Nut, Noisetier.

Scientific Names
Corylus avellana; Corylus heterophylla
Family: Betulaceae or Corylaceae.

People Use This For
Orally, hazelnut oil is used to reduce cholesterol and as an antioxidant.
Hazelnuts are commonly consumed as food.

Safety
LIKELY SAFE ...when used in amounts commonly found in foods.
PREGNANCY AND LACTATION: LIKELY SAFE ...when used in amounts commonly found in foods. There is insufficient reliable information available about the safety of the use of hazelnut in larger amounts; avoid using.

Effectiveness
There is insufficient reliable information available about the effectiveness of hazelnut.

Mechanism of Action
Hazelnuts contain 54.6-63.2% oil, 14.3-18.2% protein, and 9.8%-13.2% fiber (5995). Preliminary information suggests hazelnut oil and beta-carotene together might increase aminopyrine-N-dimethylase activity in the cytochrome P-450 system (5599).

Adverse Reactions
Orally, hazelnut can cause an allergic reaction in sensitive individuals (5991). Hazelnut has been associated with exercise-induced anaphylactic reaction (5998) and one outbreak of botulism from contaminated yogurt (5999).

Interactions with Herbs & Other Dietary Supplements
None known.

Interactions with Drugs
None known.

Interactions with Foods
None known.

Interactions with Lab Tests
None known.

Interactions with Diseases or Conditions
CROSS-ALLERGENICITY: Hazelnut is believed to be cross reactive with peanuts (5991), mugwort pollen (5993), brazil nut (5994), birch pollen (5996), and macadamia nut (5997).

Dosage and Administration
No typical dosage.

HEART'S EASE

Also Known As
European Wild Pansy, Field Pansy, Hearts Ease, Heartsease, Johnny-Jump-Up, Ladies' Delight, Pansy, Pensee Sauvage, Viola, Violae Tricoloris Herba, Wild Pansy.

Scientific Names
Viola tricolor.
Family: Violaceae.

People Use This For
Orally, heart's ease is used for promoting metabolism, as a demulcent for respiratory disorders such as throat inflammation and whooping cough, and as a laxative.
Topically, heart's ease is used for mild seborrheic skin disorders, milk scall (seborrhea of the scalp) in children, warts, mild skin inflammation, acne, exanthema (skin eruption), eczema, impetigo, and itching of the female external genitalia.

Safety
POSSIBLY SAFE ...when orally and appropriately (12). ...when used topically and appropriately (12).
PREGNANCY AND LACTATION: Insufficient reliable information; avoid using.

Effectiveness
There is insufficient reliable information available about the effectiveness of heart's ease.

Mechanism of Action

The applicable parts of heart's ease are the above ground parts. Heart's ease can have anti-inflammatory and antioxidant properties (18).

Adverse Reactions

Orally, heart's ease has caused hemolysis in a nine-month-old infant with glucose-6-phosphate-dehydrogenase (G6PD) deficiency (11324).

Interactions with Herbs & Other Dietary Supplements

None known.

Interactions with Drugs

None known.

Interactions with Foods

None known.

Interactions with Lab Tests

None known.

Interactions with Diseases or Conditions

None known.

Dosage and Administration

ORAL: The typical dose of heart's ease is one cup of the tea three times per day (18). The tea is prepared by steeping 1.5 grams of the above ground parts in 150 mL boiling water for 5-10 minutes and then straining.
TOPICAL: Heart's ease is commonly applied externally three times per day as a poultice or the prepared tea (18).

Comments

Store heart's ease in a well-sealed container and away from light (18).

HEATHER

Also Known As

Callunae vulgaris herba, Calluna vulgaris flos, Ling, Scotch Heather.

Scientific Names

Calluna vulgaris, synonyms Erica vulgaris.
Family: Ericaceae.

People Use This For

Orally, heather is taken for ailments of the kidney and lower urinary tract, prostate enlargement, diuresis, gastrointestinal ailments and diseases, diarrhea, gastrointestinal spasm, colic, disease of the liver and gallbladder, gout, arthritis, sleep disorders, respiratory disorders, cough, colds, and diaphoresis.
Topically, heather is used for wounds and inflamed eyes.
In combination with other herbs, heather is used for diabetes, menstrual discomfort, menopause, stimulation of digestion, nervous exhaustion, and regulation of the circulatory system.

Safety

POSSIBLY SAFE ...when used orally or topically and appropriately (12).
PREGNANCY AND LACTATION: Insufficient reliable information available; avoid using.

Effectiveness

There is insufficient reliable information available about the effectiveness of heather.

Mechanism of Action

The applicable parts of heather are the flower, leaf, and plant top. There is insufficient reliable information available about the possible mechanism of action and active ingredients.

Adverse Reactions

None reported.

Interactions with Herbs & Other Dietary Supplements

None known.

Interactions with Drugs
None known.

Interactions with Foods
None known.

Interactions with Lab Tests
None known.

Interactions with Diseases or Conditions
None known.

Dosage and Administration
ORAL: A typical dosage is one cup of tea (simmer 1.5 grams of flower/leaf/plant top in 250 mL boiling water 3 minutes, strain) three times daily between meals (18).
TOPICAL: As a bath, 500 grams of flower/leaf/plant top has been used in a few liters of water; strain and add to full bath (18).

HEDGE MUSTARD

Also Known As
English Watercress, Erysimum, Singer's Plant, St. Barbara's Hedge Mustard, Thalictroc.
CAUTION: See separate listings for Black Mustard, Clown's Mustard Plant, and White Mustard.

Scientific Names
Sisymbrium officinale, synonym Erysimum officinale.
Family: Brassicaceae/Cruciferae.

People Use This For
Orally, hedge mustard is used to treat urinary tract diseases, coughs, chronic bronchitis, and inflammation of the gallbladder.
Topically, hedge mustard is used as a gargle or mouthwash.

Safety
LIKELY UNSAFE ...when the flowering above ground parts are used orally since they contain cardioactive glycosides (18).
There is insufficient reliable information available about the safety of hedge mustard for its other uses.
PREGNANCY AND LACTATION: LIKELY UNSAFE ...when used orally (18); avoid using.

Effectiveness
There is insufficient reliable information available about the effectiveness of hedge mustard.

Mechanism of Action
The applicable parts of hedge mustard are the above ground parts. The foliage contains vitamin C and 0.05% cardenolides (cardioactive glycosides) including sinigrin and gluconapin. Hedge mustard also contains the volatile mustard oil allyl isothiocyanate and 3-butenylisothiocyanate (18).

Adverse Reactions
Theoretically, digitalis-like effects (vomiting, diarrhea, headache, and cardiac rhythm disorders) are possible with the oral use of hedge mustard (18).

Interactions with Herbs & Other Dietary Supplements
CARDIAC GLYCOSIDE-CONTAINING HERBS: Contraindicated, and concomitant use can increase the risk of cardiac glycoside toxicity. Cardiac glycoside-containing herbs include black hellebore, Canadian hemp root, digitalis leaf, figwort, lily-of-the-valley root, motherwort, oleander leaf, pheasant's eye plant, pleurisy root, squill bulb leaf scale, strophanthus seed, and uzara (19).
LICORICE/HORSETAIL: Theoretically, overuse/misuse of licorice rhizome or horsetail plant with cardiac glycoside-containing herbs increases the risk of cardiac toxicity due to potassium depletion (19).
OTHER CARDIOACTIVE HERBS: Avoid concomitant use with other cardioactive herbs due to unpredictability of effects (4).
STIMULANT LAXATIVE HERBS: Theoretically, overuse or misuse of stimulant laxatives with cardiac glycoside-containing herbs increases the risk of cardiac toxicity due to potassium depletion (19).

Interactions with Drugs

DIGOXIN (Lanoxin): Contraindicated due to therapeutic duplication and an increased risk of cardiac glycoside toxicity (2).
DIURETIC DRUGS: Theoretically, concomitant use of potassium depleting diuretics and hedge mustard can increase the risk of cardiac glycoside toxicity due to potassium depletion (506). Some diuretics that can deplete potassium include chlorothiazide (Diuril), chlorthalidone (Thalitone), furosemide (Lasix), hydrochlorothiazide (HCTZ, Hydrodiuril, Microzide), and others.
MACROLIDE ANTIBIOTICS: Theoretically, concomitant use may increase risk of cardiac glycoside toxicity (17).
QUININE: Theoretically, concomitant use of hedge mustard with quinine may increase risk of cardiac toxicity (506).
STIMULANT LAXATIVES: Theoretically, overuse or misuse of stimulant laxatives may increase the risk of cardiac glycoside toxicity due to potassium depletion (2).
TETRACYCLINE ANTIBIOTICS: Theoretically, concomitant use with hedge mustard may increase risk of cardiac glycoside toxicity (17).

Interactions with Foods

None known.

Interactions with Lab Tests

None known.

Interactions with Diseases or Conditions

HEART DISEASE: Theoretically, cardiac glycosides contained in hedge mustard may exacerbate condition or interfere with existing drug therapy; contraindicated.

Dosage and Administration

ORAL: A typical dosage is one cup tea (preparation unspecified) 3-4 times daily (18); average amount is 0.5-1 grams above ground parts per day (18).
TOPICAL: Tea is commonly used as a mouthwash or gargle, several times daily (18).

Comments

Avoid confusion with black mustard (Brassica nigra) and white mustard (Sinapis alba).

HEDGE-HYSSOP

Also Known As

Gratiola, Hedge Hyssop.

Scientific Names

Gratiola officinalis.
Family: Scrophulariaceae.

People Use This For

Orally, hedge-hyssop is used orally for treating the liver, as an emetic, and to induce bowel evacuation. It is also used in the elimination of intestinal parasites, and to increase urination.

Safety

UNSAFE ...when used orally (18).
PREGNANCY AND LACTATION: UNSAFE ...when used orally due to toxic potential (18).

Effectiveness

There is insufficient reliable information available about the effectiveness of hedge-hyssop.

Mechanism of Action

The applicable parts of hedge-hyssop are the above ground parts. Hedge-hyssop contains cucurbitacin glycosides which are released in aqueous environments and are extremely irritating to mucous membranes (18).

Adverse Reactions

Orally, taken in toxic doses, hedge-hyssop may cause vomiting, bloody diarrhea, colic, and kidney irritation characterized by initial diuresis followed by anuria. When people ingest very large amounts, spasms, paralysis, and circulatory collapse occur. Death occurs rarely (18).

Interactions with Herbs & Other Dietary Supplements

None known.

Interactions with Drugs
None known.

Interactions with Foods
None known.

Interactions with Lab Tests
None known.

Interactions with Diseases or Conditions
None known.

Dosage and Administration
No typical dosage.

Comments
Hedge-hyssop is considered unsafe for oral use; avoid using (18).

HEMLOCK

Also Known As
California Fern, Carrot Weed, Conium, Conium maculata, Nebraska Fern, Poison Fool's Parsley, Poison-Hemlock, Spotted Hemlock, Wild Carrot.
CAUTION: See separate listings for Hemlock Spruce, Water Hemlock, and Hemlock Water Dropwort.

Scientific Names
Conium maculatum.
Family: Apiaceae/Umbelliferae.

People Use This For
Orally, hemlock is used as a sedative, antispasmodic, and paralyzer. It is also used orally for nervous motor excitability, teething in children, cramps, spasms of the larnyx and gullet, acute mania, bronchitis, whooping cough, asthma, and as an antidote to strychnine poisoning. It is also used orally for indolent tumors, swollen and painful joints, skin infections, epilepsy, Parkinson's disease, Sydenham's chorea, and acute cystitis.

Safety
UNSAFE ...when used orally (6338). All parts of hemlock including seeds, flowers, and fruits are considered poisonous (6338,6339). Death has resulted after ingestion of hemlock (6340). Prompt medical attention is advised after ingestion of hemlock (6341).
CHILDREN: UNSAFE ...when used orally (6340). Acute, sometimes lethal poisoning has resulted after ingestion of leaf material (6340) or when hollow stems are used as peashooters, flutes, or whistles (6338).
PREGNANCY AND LACTATION: UNSAFE ...when used orally because ingestion can be lethal (6338); avoid using.

Effectiveness
There is insufficient reliable information available about the effectiveness of hemlock.

Mechanism of Action
All plant parts of hemlock can cause toxicity. Coniceine and coniine are the alkaloids in hemlock which account for its toxicity (6338,6340,6341). The amount of poisonous alkaloids in hemlock increase as the plant and fruit ripens and is also dependent on the amount of solar exposure and soil moisture (6338). It is most toxic during early stages of growth in the spring (6338,6339). Green fruit contains larger amounts of toxic alkaloids than mature fruit and seeds.
The amount of toxic alkaloids in hemlock decreases as the plant reaches maturity (6338). Coniine predominates in the plant during sunny dry weather. During cloudy and rainy weather, coniine and coniceine are produced in equal amounts in hemlock (6339). Coniceine predominates during early growth periods of hemlock and coniine predominates in mature hemlock plants and seeds (6339). The alkaloid's effects occur at the neuromuscular junction of the autonomic ganglia (6341), stimulating and then paralyzing nicotinic receptors (6340). Larger doses of the alkaloids produce narcotic-like depressant activity (6340). Death usually occurs by respiratory failure (6341).

Adverse Reactions
Orally, hemlock can cause salivation, drowsiness, mydriasis, muscle pain, rapid swelling and stiffening of muscles, tachycardia followed by bradycardia, loss of speech, paralysis, rhabdomyolysis, unconsciousness, cardiovascular collapse, and death (6340,6341). It also causes burning of the mouth, throat, and abdomen (6341).

Interactions with Herbs & Other Dietary Supplements
None known.

Interactions with Drugs
None known.

Interactions with Foods
None known.

Interactions with Lab Tests
None known.

Interactions with Diseases or Conditions
None known.

Dosage and Administration
No typical dosage.

Comments
Hemlock is native to Europe and western Asia and was introduced into North America as an ornamental plant (6338,6339,6341). It is frequently found in the US and southern Canada (6338). Hemlock is found along fences, in modified soils, roadsides, ditches, abandoned construction sites, pastures, crops, and fields (6338,6341). Hemlock can remain in a vegetative state throughout the winter (6338,6339) and accidental ingestion occurs after mistaking the root for parsnip, leaves for parsley, and seeds for anise (6338,6344). Poisoning and death have been reported after human consumption of migratory wild birds that have eaten hemlock seeds (6338,6340).

HEMLOCK SPRUCE

Also Known As
Balm of Gilead Fir, Balsam Fir, Canada Balsam, Fir Needle Oil, Fir Tree, Norway Pine, Norway Spruce, Picea aetheroleum, Picea turiones recentes, Spruce Fir.
CAUTION: See separate listings for Hemlock, Hemlock Water Dropwort, and Water Hemlock.

Scientific Names
Picea abies, synonym Picea excelsa, Pinus abies, Pinus viminalis; Abies excelsa.
Family: Pinaceae.

People Use This For
Orally, hemlock spruce is used for coughs, the common cold, bronchitis, fever, inflammation of the mouth and pharynx, muscular and nerve pain, arthritis, as an antibacterial, and for tuberculosis.
Topically, hemlock spruce is used for inflammation of the respiratory tract, arthritis pain, nerve pain, and for feelings of tension. It is also used topically as a counterirritant and to improve circulation, and as a bath additive for individuals who are mentally ill.

Safety
There is insufficient reliable information available about the safety of hemlock spruce.
Pregnancy and Lactation: Insufficient reliable information available; avoid using.

Effectiveness
There is insufficient reliable information available about the effectiveness of hemlock spruce.

Mechanism of Action
The applicable parts of hemlock spruce are the needles and oil obtained by steam distillation of the needles, branch tips or branches and the fresh fir shoots of Picea abies. There is insufficient reliable information available about the possible mechanism of action and active ingredients.

Adverse Reactions
None reported.

Interactions with Herbs & Other Dietary Supplements
None known.

Interactions with Drugs
None known.

Interactions with Foods
None known.

Interactions with Lab Tests
None known.

Interactions with Diseases or Conditions
ASTHMA and WHOOPING COUGH: Hemlock spruce may theoretically worsen asthma and whooping cough (18).
CARDIAC INSUFFICIENCY: Avoid using of hemlock spruce (18).
BROKEN SKIN: Hemlock spruce should not be applied to broken skin (18).

Dosage and Administration
ORAL: The typical daily dose is 4 drops of oil on a lump of sugar taken three times daily. Alternately, 2 grams of oil can be added to hot water and inhaled several times daily (18).
TOPICAL: Hemlock spruce is used as a 10-50% semi-solid preparation. Several drops of this oil are rubbed into the affected area (18).

Comments
Hemlock spruce is very similar sounding to water hemlock and European water hemlock, which are entirely different plants. Be careful not to confuse hemlock spruce with either form of water hemlock, because the water hemlocks are very toxic (18).

HEMLOCK WATER DROPWORT

Also Known As
Dead Tongue, Five-Fingered Root, Horsebane, Yellow Water Dropwort.
CAUTION: See separate listings for Hemlock, Hemlock Spruce, and Water Hemlock.

Scientific Names
Oenanthe crocata.
Family: Apiaceae/Umbelliferae.

People Use This For
Topically, hemlock water dropwort is used as a poultice for skin eruptions.

Safety
UNSAFE ...when used orally (6334). Ingestion of very small amounts of root may be fatal (6335,6337). Accidental ingestion requires prompt medical attention (6334).
There is insufficient reliable information available about the safety of hemlock water dropwort when used topically.
CHILDREN: UNSAFE ...when used orally (6334). Poisoning has occurred after accidental ingestion of roots or tubers (6334).
PREGNANCY AND LACTATION: UNSAFE ...when used orally. Ingestion can be lethal (6334).

Effectiveness
There is insufficient reliable information available about the effectiveness of hemlock water dropwort.

Mechanism of Action
The applicable part of hemlock water dropwort is the root. Oenanthetoxin, a highly unsaturated alcohol (6334), is the active principle toxin found in hemlock water dropwort (6332). The roots of hemlock water dropwort are considered to be the most poisonous part of the plant and the toxin is contained in a yellowish staining juice of the root (6334). The toxin is unstable when exposed to air and is chemically similar to cicutoxin found in water hemlock (Cicuta virosa) (6334). The exact mechanism of action of the toxin is unknown, but animal studies suggest that oenanthetoxin has an antagonizing effect on nerve impulses in the brain stem (6334).

Adverse Reactions
Orally, hemlock water dropwort can cause nausea, dizziness, (6334), abdominal pain (6335), vomiting, sweating (6332), salivation, weakness, confusion, slurred speech, muscle spasms, tonic-clonic movements, glycosuria, hematuria, hyperventilation, cyanosis, exhaustion (6334), seizures, metabolic acidosis (6335), generalized convulsions (6332), unconsciousness (6334), dilated pupils, and death (6332).

Interactions with Herbs & Other Dietary Supplements
None known.

Interactions with Drugs
None known.

Interactions with Foods
None known.

Interactions with Lab Tests
None known.

Interactions with Diseases or Conditions
None known.

Dosage and Administration
No typical dosage.

Comments
Hemlock water dropwort is commonly found in ditches, watering places, and marshy areas and banks (6334,6337). It is considered to be the most poisonous plant in the British Isles (6334). Hemlock water dropwort has been accidentally ingested after mistaking the tuber for wild parsnip, sweet flag, or pignut (6334,6337).

HEMP AGRIMONY

Also Known As
Alpenkraut, Chanvrin, Donnerkraut, Dostenkraut, Drachenkraut, Dutch Agrimony, Dutch Eupatoire Commune, Eupatorium, Gemeiner Wasswedost, Herbe de Sainte Cunegonde, Hirshklee, Holy Rope, Kunigundendraut, Leberkraut, Origan De Marais, St. John's Herb, Sweet Mandulin, Sweet-Smelling Trefoil, Thoroughwort, Wasshanf, Waterhemp, Water Maudlin.
CAUTION: See separate listings for Agrimony and Canadian Hemp.

Scientific Names
Eupatorium cannabinum.
Family: Asteraceae/Compositae.

People Use This For
Orally, hemp agrimony is used for liver and gallbladder disorders, colds, and fever.
Topically, hemp agrimony is used for wounds and skin infections.

Safety
LIKELY UNSAFE ...when products containing hepatotoxic pyrrolizidine alkaloid (PA) constituents are used orally. Repeated exposure to low concentrations of hepatotoxic PAs can cause severe veno-occlusive disease. Hepatotoxic PAs might also be carcinogenic and mutagenic (12841,12842). Tell patients not to use hemp agrimony preparations that are not certified and labeled as hepatotoxic PA-free. ...when products containing hepatotoxic PAs are used topically on abraded or broken skin. Absorption of hepatotoxic PAs through broken skin can lead to systemic toxicities (12841). Tell patients not to use topical hemp agrimony preparations that are not certified and labeled as hepatotoxic PA-free. There is insufficient reliable information available about the safety of using topical PA-free hemp agrimony on unbroken skin.
PREGNANCY: LIKELY UNSAFE ...when used orally. Hemp agrimony preparations, containing hepatotoxic pyrrolizidine alkaloid (PA) constituents, might be teratogenic and hepatotoxic (12841,12842). There is insufficient reliable information available about the safety of using hemp agrimony products that do not contain hepatotoxic PAs during pregnancy.
LACTATION: LIKELY UNSAFE ...when used orally. Hepatotoxic pyrrolizidine alkaloid (PA) constituents in hemp agrimony are excreted in milk (12841,12842). There is insufficient reliable information available about the safety of using hemp agrimony products that do not contain hepatotoxic PAs during lactation.

Effectiveness
There is insufficient reliable information available about the effectiveness of hemp agrimony.

Mechanism of Action

The applicable part of hemp agrimony is the flowering herb. Hemp agrimony contains various pyrrolizidine alkaloids (PA), some of which are toxic. PAs are most concentrated in the plant roots, but may be found in all plant parts. PAs, particularly unsaturated PAs, can cause hepatotoxicity. Cyclic diesters such as retrorsine and senecionine are the most hepatotoxic. Liver toxicity may result from PA-enhanced oxidative stress, but the exact mechanism of toxicity is unknown. Single doses of 10-20 mg PAs or chronic ingestion of amounts less than 10 mcg can cause veno-occlusive disease. PAs are metabolized by cytochrome P450 3A4 (CYP3A4) to toxic dehydroalkaloids and pyrroles. Enzyme inducers such as phenobarbital seem to enhance toxicity (12841,12860). Pyrroles are excreted as N-acetyl cysteine conjugates. Some researchers speculate that early administration of N-acetylcysteine might reduce toxicity (11988).

Metabolism is also affected by pregnane X receptor induction of CYP3A4. Genetic or drug induced variation in CYP3A4 or pregnane X receptor activity can affect the degree of PA toxicity by increasing or decreasing its metabolism (12841,12842). Hepatotoxic PAs are also toxic to the lungs. In animals, pneumotoxicity occurs as pulmonary hypertension and right ventricular hypertrophy. Hepatotoxic PAs are carcinogenic and mutagenic. There are sufficient amounts of hepatotoxic PAs in herbal products to cause toxicity (12841,12842).

Adverse Reactions

Orally, the major concern about hemp agrimony preparations is the hepatotoxic pyrrolizidine alkaloid (PA) content. These constituents are hepatotoxic, pneumotoxic, carcinogenic, and mutagenic (12841,12842). Chronic exposure to other plants containing hepatotoxic PA constituents is associated with veno-occlusive disease (4021). Subacute veno-occlusive disease causes vague symptoms with persistent liver enlargement (4021). Symptoms of acute veno-occlusive disease include colicky pains in epigastrium, vomiting and diarrhea, and ascites formation within several days. Enlargement and induration of the liver occurs within a few weeks. (12842). Dietary supplements sold in the US are not required to include the amount of PAs they contain (3484); therefore, all preparations used orally containing hemp agrimony should be considered potentially unsafe.

Theoretically, hemp agrimony might cause an allergic reaction in individuals sensitive to the Asteraceae/Compositae family (12842). Members of this family include ragweed, chrysanthemums, marigolds, daisies, and many other herbs.

Interactions with Herbs & Other Dietary Supplements

HEPATOTOXIC PYRROLIZIDINE ALKALOID (PA)-CONTAINING HERBS: Concomitant use is contraindicated due to the risk of additive toxicity. Herbs containing hepatotoxic PAs include alkanna, borage, butterbur, coltsfoot, comfrey, gravel root, groundsel, hound's tongue, and lungwort; and the Senecio species plants dusty miller, ragwort, golden ragwort, and tansy ragwort (12841).

HERBS THAT INDUCE CYTOCHROME P450 3A4 (CYP3A4): Theoretically, herbs that induce CYP3A4 might increase the conversion of hepatotoxic PAs to toxic metabolites, enhancing toxicity (12841,12860). Herbs that induce CYP3A4 include St. John's wort and garlic.

Interactions with Drugs

CYTOCHROME P450 3A4 (CYP3A4) INDUCERS: Hepatotoxic pyrrolizidine alkaloids (PA) are substrates of cytochrome P450 3A4 (CYP3A4) (12841,12860). Theoretically, drugs that induce CYP3A4 might increase the conversion of PAs to toxic metabolites. Some drugs that induce CYP3A4 include carbamazepine (Tegretol), phenobarbital, phenytoin (Dilantin), rifampin, rifabutin (Mycobutin), and others.

Interactions with Foods

None known.

Interactions with Lab Tests

None known.

Interactions with Diseases or Conditions

CROSS-ALLERGENICITY: Theoretically, hemp agrimony might cause an allergic reaction in individuals sensitive to the Asteraceae/Compositae family (12842). Members of this family include ragweed, chrysanthemums, marigolds, daisies, and many other herbs.

LIVER DISEASE: Theoretically, pyrrolizidine alkaloids (PA) might exacerbate liver disease (12841,12842).

Dosage and Administration

No typical dosage.

HEMPNETTLE

Also Known As
Galeopsidis Herba.

Scientific Names
Galeopsis segetum, synonym Galeopsis ochroleuca.
Family: Lamiaceae/Labiatae.

People Use This For
Orally, hempnettle is used for mild respiratory tract inflammation, cough, bronchitis, and as a diuretic.

Safety
POSSIBLY SAFE ...when used orally and appropriately (2).
PREGNANCY AND LACTATION: Insufficient reliable information available; avoid using.

Effectiveness
There is insufficient reliable information available about the effectiveness of hempnettle.

Mechanism of Action
The applicable parts of hempnettle are the above ground parts. Hempnettle can have astringent and expectorant effects (18).

Adverse Reactions
None reported.

Interactions with Herbs & Other Dietary Supplements
None known.

Interactions with Drugs
None known.

Interactions with Foods
None known.

Interactions with Lab Tests
None known.

Interactions with Diseases or Conditions
None known.

Dosage and Administration
ORAL: The typical dose of hempnettle is 6 grams of the above ground parts per day or one cup of the tea up to three times daily. The tea is prepared by steeping 2 grams of the above ground parts in 150 mL boiling water for 5-10 minutes and then straining (18). The use of hempnettle in children requires a dosing adjustment; however, no additional information is available on the exact dosing adjustments (510).

HENBANE

Also Known As
Devil's Eye, Fetid Nightshade, Hen Bell, Hog Bean, Hyoscyami Folium, Jupiter's Bean, Khurasani-Ajavayan, Parasigaya, Poison Tobacco, Stinking Nightshade.
CAUTION: See separate listings for Belladonna and Bittersweet Nightshade.

Scientific Names
Hyoscyamus niger.
Family: Solanaceae.

People Use This For
Orally, henbane leaf is used for spasms of the gastrointestinal tract.
Topically, henbane leaf oil is used for treating scar tissue.

Safety

POSSIBLY SAFE ...when the leaf is used orally and appropriately short-term under medical supervision (2). Henbane contains hyoscyamine and scopolamine alkaloids (2).
LIKELY UNSAFE ...when used orally for self-medication. Hyoscyamine and scopolamine have a narrow range of safe use. Excessive doses can cause poisoning and death (18).
There is insufficient reliable information available about the safety of henbane for its other uses.
PREGNANCY AND LACTATION: LIKELY UNSAFE ...when used orally because of its risk of poisoning (18).

Effectiveness

There is insufficient reliable information available about the effectiveness of henbane.

Mechanism of Action

The applicable part of henbane is the leaf. The alkaloid constituents, which include hyoscyamine and scopolamine, competitively inhibit acetylcholine, causing anticholinergic and parasympathetic effects (18). With storage, hyoscyamine converts to atropine. The inhibition of acetylcholine affects the muscarinic action but not the nicotinic effects of acetylcholine on ganglia and motor endplates. Henbane causes smooth muscle relaxation particularly in the GI tract, relieves muscle tremors of CNS origin, and has a sedative effect (2).

Adverse Reactions

Orally, henbane can cause dry mouth, red skin, constipation, overheating, reduced sweating, vision disturbances, tachycardia, and difficulty with urinating (2,18). Overdose poisoning symptoms include somnolence followed by CNS stimulation described as restlessness, hallucinations, delirium, and manic episodes followed by exhaustion and sleep. Henbane can cause death by asphyxiation (18).

Interactions with Herbs & Other Dietary Supplements

ANTICHOLINERGIC CONTAINING HERBS: Theoretically, concomitant use of henbane with other anticholinergic alkaloid-containing herbs, including belladonna, deadly nightshade, and jimson weed, can have additive therapeutic and adverse effects.

Interactions with Drugs

ANTICHOLINERGIC DRUGS: Concomitant use of henbane can have additive anticholinergic effects and adverse effects with amantadine, antihistamines, atropine, belladonna alkaloids, hyoscyamine, phenothiazines, procainamide, scopolamine, and tricyclic antidepressants (2).

Interactions with Foods

None known.

Interactions with Lab Tests

None known.

Interactions with Diseases or Conditions

CONGESTIVE HEART FAILURE (CHF): Contraindicated; henbane might cause tachycardia and exacerbate CHF due to its hyoscyamine (atropine) and scopolamine content (15).
CONSTIPATION: Contraindicated; henbane might cause constipation due to its hyoscyamine (atropine) and scopolamine content (15).
DOWN SYNDROME: Caution, patients with Down syndrome might be hypersensitive to the antimuscarinic effects (mydriasis, positive chronotropic heart effects, etc.) of hyoscyamine (atropine) and scopolamine contained in henbane (15).
ESOPHAGEAL REFLUX: Contraindicated; henbane might delay gastric emptying and decrease lower esophageal pressure, promoting gastric retention and exacerbating reflux due to its hyoscyamine (atropine) and scopolamine content (15).
FEVER: Contraindicated; henbane might increase the risk of hyperthermia in patients with fever due to its hyoscyamine (atropine) and scopolamine content (15).
GASTRIC ULCER: Contraindicated; henbane might delay gastric emptying and exacerbate gastric ulcers due to its hyoscyamine (atropine) and scopolamine content (15).
GI INFECTIONS: Contraindicated; henbane might suppress GI motility causing retention of infecting organisms or toxins due to its hyoscyamine (atropine) and scopolamine content (15).
HIATAL HERNIA: Contraindicated; henbane might delay gastric emptying and decrease lower esophageal pressure, promoting gastric retention and exacerbating hiatal hernia due to its hyoscyamine (atropine) and scopolamine content (15).
NARROW-ANGLE GLAUCOMA: Contraindicated; henbane might increase ocular tension in patients with narrow-angle (angle-closure) glaucoma due to its hyoscyamine (atropine) and scopolamine content (2,15).
OBSTRUCTIVE GI TRACT DISEASE: Contraindicated; henbane might exacerbate obstructive GI tract diseases (including atony, paralytic ileus, and stenosis) due to its hyoscyamine (atropine) and scopolamine content (15).

TACHYARRHYTHMIAS: Contraindicated; henbane might cause tachycardia due to its hyoscyamine (atropine) and scopolamine content (2,15).
TOXIC MEGACOLON: Contraindicated; henbane might suppress intestinal motility, which might produce paralytic ileus and exacerbate toxic megacolon, due to its hyoscyamine (atropine) and scopolamine content (2,15).
ULCERATIVE COLITIS: Contraindicated; henbane might suppress intestinal motility, which might produce paralytic ileus and precipitate toxic megacolon, due to its hyoscyamine (atropine) and scopolamine content (15).
URINARY RETENTION: Contraindicated; henbane might increase urinary retention due to its hyoscyamine (atropine) and scopolamine content (2,15).

Dosage and Administration

ORAL: The average single dose of the standardized henbane powder is 500 mg, which corresponds to 250-350 mg of the total alkaloid (2). The maximum single dose of henbane is 1 gram, which corresponds to 500-700 mg of the total alkaloid (2). The maximum daily dosage is 3 grams, which corresponds to 1.5-2.1 grams of the total alkaloid calculated as hyoscyamine (2).
TOPICAL: No typical dosage.

Comments

Avoid confusion with bittersweet nightshade (Solanum dulcamara) and belladonna (deadly nightshade). The flowering branches, dried seeds, and whole, fresh flowering plant of henbane may have medicinal uses (18).

HENNA

Also Known As

Alcanna, Egyptian Privet, Hennae folium, Henne, Jamaica Mignonette, Mehndi, Mendee, Mignonette Tree, Reseda, Smooth Lawsonia.
CAUTION: See separate listing for Alkanna (Alkanna tinctoria).

Scientific Names

Lawsonia inermis, synonym Lawsonia alba.
Family: Lythraceae.

People Use This For

Orally, henna is used for gastrointestinal ulcers.
Topically, henna is used for dandruff, eczema, scabies, fungal infections, and ulcers. It is also used topically for applying decorative henna "tattoos."
Traditionally, henna has been used for amebic dysentery, cancer, enlarged spleen, headache, jaundice, and skin conditions.
In manufacturing, henna is used in cosmetics; hair dyes and hair care products; and as a dye for nails, hands, and clothing. Lawsone, a constituent, can be used as an indicator for titration of strong acids with weak bases.

Safety

LIKELY SAFE ...when the leaf is applied topically. It is approved for topical use as a color additive in hair cosmetics in the US (11). However, contact dermatitis and hypersensitivity reactions have been reported with topical use (1370,4146,4148,6144,6145,6146,6147,6148,6149,6150,6151).
UNSAFE ...when used orally (12).
CHILDREN: POSSIBLY UNSAFE ...when applied topically on children, and especially on infants (4147,6144,6149,6150,10381). Use is associated with hemolysis in infants deficient in glucose-6-phosphate dehydrogenase (G6PD) (4147,10381). UNSAFE ...when used orally (12).
PREGNANCY: UNSAFE ...when used orally. Henna is believed to have abortifacient properties (12).
LACTATION: UNSAFE ...when used orally (12).

Effectiveness

There is insufficient reliable information available about the effectiveness of henna.

Mechanism of Action

The applicable part of henna is the leaf. Henna leaf contains lawsone, gallic acid, and 5-10% tannin (11). It is thought to have astringent and diuretic properties (18). Some evidence suggests henna might have activity against Mycobacterium tuberculosis (4150). In female rats, henna leaves inhibit fertility (11). The constituents, lawsone and gallic acid, have antibacterial properties (11). Studies suggest that lawsone might also have antifungal, antitumor, antispasmodic and weak vitamin K activity (11). Evidence shows it might be able to decrease the formation of sickled cells in individuals with sickle cell anemia (4149). An ethanol extract containing luteolin, beta-sitosterol, and lawsone was claimed to have anti-inflammatory, antihyaluronidase, and analgesic activity (11).

Adverse Reactions

Orally, henna can cause an upset stomach, possibly due to tannin content (18).
Topically, henna can cause contact dermatitis, including redness, itching, burning, swelling, scaling, fissuring, papules, blisters, and scarring (1370,4146,6144,6145,6146,6147,6148,6149,6150). There are two reports of occupational exposure associated with immediate-type hypersensitivity involving urticaria, rhinitis, wheezing, and bronchial asthma (4148,6151). In infants with glucose 6-phosphate dehydrogenase (G6PD) deficiency, topical henna use has been associated with hemolysis, anemia, reticulocytosis, and indirect hyperbilirubinemia (4147,10381). Prolonged use on hair may turn the hair orange-red, unless mixed with other dyes to get different shades (11).

Interactions with Herbs & Other Dietary Supplements

None known.

Interactions with Drugs

None known.

Interactions with Foods

None known.

Interactions with Lab Tests

None known.

Interactions with Diseases or Conditions

GLUCOSE-6-PHOSPHATE DEHYDROGENASE (G6PD) DEFICIENCY: There are reports of hemolysis in infants with G6PD deficiency after topical exposure to henna (4147,10381).
HENNA HYPERSENSITIVITY: Avoid topical exposure by individuals with henna hypersensitivity.

Dosage and Administration

No typical dosage.

Comments

Henna should not be confused with henna root (Alkanna tinctoria), also referred to as alkanna root (6).

HERB PARIS

Also Known As

Einbeere, Herb-Paris, One Berry, Oneberry, Tilki Uzumu, Uva De Raposa, Wang Sun.

Scientific Names

Paris quadrifolia.
Family: Trilliaceae.

People Use This For

Traditionally, Herb Paris is used for headache; longevity; neuralgia; rheumatism; genital tumors; palpitation; spasms; and as an emetic, narcotic, poison, and purgative.

Safety

LIKELY UNSAFE ...when used orally. The plant and berry are poisonous (18).
PREGNANCY AND LACTATION: UNSAFE ...when used orally (18).

Effectiveness

There is insufficient reliable information available about the effectiveness of Herb Paris.

Mechanism of Action

The applicable part of Herb Paris is the whole plant with ripe fruit. Herb Paris contains triterpene saponins (pennogenintetra glycosides), also referred to as parissaponins, which cause local irritation, increasing absorption of the toxic constituent, paristyphnin (18). Paristyphnin causes miosis and respiratory paralysis (18).

Adverse Reactions

Orally, Herb Paris can cause nausea, vomiting, diarrhea, headache, miosis, and respiratory paralysis (18).

Interactions with Herbs & Other Dietary Supplements

None known.

Interactions with Drugs
None known.

Interactions with Foods
None known.

Interactions with Lab Tests
None known.

Interactions with Diseases or Conditions
None known.

Dosage and Administration
No typical dosage.

HERB ROBERT

Also Known As
Dragon's Blood, Mountain Geranium, Stinky Bob, Storkbill, Wild Crane's-Bill.
CAUTION: See separate listings for Dragon's Blood (Daemonorops draco) and Sangre de Grado.

Scientific Names
Geranium robertianum.
Family: Geraniaceae.

People Use This For
Orally, Herb Robert is used for diarrhea; to improve functioning of the liver and gallbladder; to reduce inflammation of the kidney, bladder, and gallbladder; and to prevent the formation of calculi.
Topically, Herb Robert is used as a mouthwash or gargle. The fresh leaves are chewed to relieve inflammation of the mouth and throat.

Safety
There is insufficient reliable information available about the safety of Herb Robert.
Pregnancy and Lactation: Insufficient reliable information is available; avoid using.

Effectiveness
There is insufficient reliable information available about the effectiveness of Herb Robert.

Mechanism of Action
The applicable parts of Herb Robert are the above ground parts. Herb Robert contains several flavonoids including rutin. Some evidence suggests an ethanolic extract can inhibit the growth of E. coli, P. aeruginosa, and S. aureus. Other evidence indicates the extract of the fresh herb, including the root, has a mild antiviral effect against the vesicular stomatitis virus (18). Although general reviews report Herb Robert has hypotensive effects, no specific information is available (18). Some data show a crystalline fraction can protect the tobacco plant from pathogenic viruses (18).

Adverse Reactions
None reported.

Interactions with Herbs & Other Dietary Supplements
None known.

Interactions with Drugs
None known.

Interactions with Foods
None known.

Interactions with Lab Tests
None known.

Interactions with Diseases or Conditions
None known.

Dosage and Administration

ORAL: Herb Robert is used as tea, 2 to 3 cups daily between meals (18). To make tea, 1 teaspoon of herb is added to 500 mL of cold water, brought to a boil, allowed to draw, and strained.
TOPICAL: The prepared tea is used as mouthwash or gargle (18). Fresh leaves are chewed to relieve mouth or throat inflammation (18).

Comments

Herb Robert is characterized by an unpleasant smell of goats or bugs (18).

HESPERIDIN

Also Known As

Citrus Bioflavonoid, Citrus Bioflavonoids, Flavonoid.
CAUTION: See separate listings for Chrysin, Diosmin, Methoxylated Flavones, Quercetin, Rue, and Rutin.

Scientific Names

Hesperidin.

People Use This For

Orally, hesperidin is used for treating acute internal hemorrhoids, preventing relapse of acute internal hemorrhoids, lymphedema following breast cancer surgery, and for treating varicose veins and venous stasis.

Safety

POSSIBLY SAFE ...when used orally and appropriately, short-term. Hesperidin seems to be safe when used for up to 6 months (4861,10227,10229). There is insufficient reliable information available about the safety of hesperidin when used for longer than 6 months.
PREGNANCY AND LACTATION: Insufficient reliable information available; avoid using.

Effectiveness

POSSIBLY EFFECTIVE

Internal hemorrhoids. The combination of hesperidin 150 mg plus diosmin 1350 mg twice daily for 4 days, followed by hesperidin 100 mg and diosmin 900 mg twice daily for 3 days, seems to significantly improve signs and symptoms of internal hemorrhoids. The combination can stop acute bleeding in up to 92% of patients after 4 days of treatment. It can also reduce symptoms such as anal discomfort, pain, discharge, and local lesions. Subjective symptoms can be relieved within 2 days of treatment. The combination also seems to reduce the duration and intensity of hemorrhoidal flare-ups (4861,4900). Maintenance use of hesperidin 50 mg plus diosmin 450 mg twice daily for 3 months in patients following acute treatment for hemorrhoids seems to significantly decrease the relapse rate (4861).

Venous stasis ulcers. Hesperidin, in combination with diosmin and compression dressing, seems to improve healing of venous stasis ulcers less than 10 cm in size (10229).

POSSIBLY INEFFECTIVE

Lymphedema. Hesperidin, in combination with diosmin, may improve drainage of lymph from the arms of women after breast cancer surgery, but it does not reduce arm swelling or other clinical signs of lymphedema (10227).

Clinical trials have used specific brand name formulations of hesperidin (Daflon 500, Les Laboratoires Servier, France). Each tablet of Daflon 500 contains hesperidin 50 mg and a micronized formulation of diosmin 450 mg extracted from rutaceae species.

There is insufficient reliable information available about the effectiveness of hesperidin for its other uses.

Mechanism of Action

Hesperidin is one of over 4,000 flavonoids found in plants (4919,4959,5006). Hesperidin is in a class of flavonoids primarily derived from citrus fruits and is known as a citrus bioflavonoid. It is closely related to other citrus bioflavonoids such as quercetin, rutin, and diosmin. Hesperidin alone, or in combination with other citrus bioflavonoids, is most often used for vascular conditions such as hemorrhoids and varicose veins. Hesperidin seems to work by improving venous tone, reducing stasis, restoring normal capillary permeability, and improving lymphatic drainage. Hesperidin might improve venous tone and reduce stasis by improving vasculature response to adrenergic stimulation. Hesperidin's anti-inflammatory effects seem to help restore normal capillary permeability. Hesperidin inhibits phosphodiesterase and increases intracellular cyclic adenosine monophosphate (cAMP), which causes decreased production of inflammatory prostaglandins E2 and F2 and thromboxane B2. Hesperidin's analgesic effect seems to work through peripheral rather than central mechanisms. Hesperidin can also reduce the generation of free radicals and inhibit tumor growth (4861,4900,4919,4956).

Adverse Reactions
Orally, hesperidin can cause gastrointestinal side effects, including abdominal pain, diarrhea, and gastritis. Headache can also occur in some patients (4861,4900).

Interactions with Herbs & Other Dietary Supplements
None known.

Interactions with Drugs
None known.

Interactions with Foods
None known.

Interactions with Lab Tests
None known.

Interactions with Diseases or Conditions
None known.

Dosage and Administration
ORAL: For the treatment of internal hemorrhoids, hesperidin 150 mg plus diosmin 1350 mg twice daily for 4 days, followed by hesperidin 100 mg and diosmin 900 mg twice daily for 3 days, has been used (4861,4900). For prevention of relapse internal hemorrhoids, hesperidin 50 mg plus diosmin 450 mg twice daily for 3 months of therapy has been used (4861). For the treatment of venous stasis ulcers, a combination of 100 mg hesperidin and 900 mg diosmin daily has been used for up to 2 months (10229). For treating lymphedema following surgery for breast cancer, a combination of 100 mg hesperidin and 900 mg diosmin daily has been used for up to 6 months (10227).

HIBISCUS

Also Known As
Guinea Sorrel, Jamaica Sorrel, Karkade, Red Tea, Roselle, Sudanese Tea.

Scientific Names
Hibiscus sabdariffa.
Family: Malvaceae.

People Use This For
Orally, hibiscus is used for loss of appetite, colds, heart and nerve diseases, upper respiratory tract and stomach mucous membrane inflammation, disorders of circulation, for dissolving phlegm, and as a gentle laxative and diuretic.
In foods and beverages, hibiscus is used as a flavoring. It is also used to improve the odor, flavor, or appearance of tea mixtures.

Safety
LIKELY SAFE ...when used orally in amounts commonly found in foods. Hibiscus has Generally Recognized As Safe status (GRAS) for use in foods in the US (4912).
POSSIBLY SAFE ...when used orally in medicinal amounts (2,12); there are no known risks (2).
PREGNANCY: LIKELY UNSAFE ...when used orally. Hibiscus is thought to be a menstrual stimulant, and might have abortifacient effects (19).
LACTATION: Insufficient reliable information available; avoid using.

Effectiveness
There is insufficient reliable information available about the effectiveness of hibiscus.

Mechanism of Action
The applicable part of hibiscus is the flower and calyx. People think the laxative effects of hibiscus are due to high content of poorly absorbable fruit acids (18). Extracts have intestinal and uterine muscle antispasmodic activity (11,18), hypotensive effects (11,18), anthelmintic properties (11), and in vitro antibacterial activity (11).

Adverse Reactions
None reported.

Interactions with Herbs & Other Dietary Supplements
None known.

Interactions with Drugs
ACETAMINOPHEN (Tylenol, others): There is some evidence that consuming a hibiscus beverage (Zobo drink) before taking acetaminophen can decrease the elimination half-life of acetaminophen. Hibiscus does not seem to decrease maximum concentration or area under the curve of acetaminophen (12184). The clinical significance of this is unknown.

Interactions with Foods
None known.

Interactions with Lab Tests
None known.

Interactions with Diseases or Conditions
None known.

Dosage and Administration
ORAL: To prepare tea, steep 1.5 grams of flowers in 150 mL boiling water 5-10 minutes, strain (18).

HISTIDINE

Also Known As
Levo-Histidine, L-Histidine.

Scientific Names
L-2-Amino-3-(1H-imidazol-4-yl) propionic acid; alpha-amino-4-imidazole propanoic acid.

People Use This For
Orally, histidine is used for rheumatoid arthritis, allergic diseases, ulcers, and anemia.

Safety
POSSIBLY SAFE ...when used orally and appropriately. Clinical studies note the absence of side effects at doses up to 4 grams per day (2347,2353).
PREGNANCY AND LACTATION: Insufficient reliable information available; avoid using.

Effectiveness
POSSIBLY INEFFECTIVE

Anemia. Taking histidine orally doesn't seem to be effective for treating anemia of uremia or anemia associated with chronic dialysis (2352,2353).

Rheumatoid arthritis (RA). Taking histidine orally doesn't seem to be effective for treating RA (2350,2351).

There is insufficient reliable information available about the effectiveness of histidine for its other uses.

Mechanism of Action
Histidine is an essential amino acid involved in a wide range of metabolic processes (2354).

Adverse Reactions
None reported.

Interactions with Herbs & Other Dietary Supplements
None known.

Interactions with Drugs
None known.

Interactions with Foods
None known.

Interactions with Lab Tests
URINE FORMIMINOGLUTAMIC ACID (FIGLU): Use of histidine in people with folic acid deficiency can cause accumulation of the metabolite formiminoglutamic (2355).

Interactions with Diseases or Conditions

FOLIC ACID DEFICIENCY: Use of histidine in individuals with folic acid deficiency can cause accumulation of the metabolite formiminoglutamic acid (FIGLU) (2355).

Dosage and Administration

ORAL: For rheumatoid arthritis, the usual dose of histidine is 3.7-4.5 grams daily (2347,2350,2351). For anemia of uremia or anemia associated with maintenance dialysis, the typical dose is 1-4 grams daily (2352,2353).

HOLLY

Also Known As

Christ's Thorn, Holm, Holme Chase, Holy Tree, Hulm, Hulver Bush, Hulver Tree.

Scientific Names

Ilex aquifolium; Ilex opaca; Ilex vomitoria.
Family: Aquifoliaceae.

People Use This For

Orally, preparations of holly leaf are used as a diuretic, for coughs, digestive disorders, and jaundice. Ilex aquifolium leaves are used orally for treating intermittent fevers and rheumatism, as an antipyretic, astringent, diuretic, and expectorant. Ilex opaca leaves are used as a diuretic, tonic, purgative, and cardiac stimulant. Other Ilex species are used for treating coronary heart disease, dizziness, and hypertension.

Historically, Ilex opaca fruit tea was used as a cardiac stimulant by American Indians. Ilex vomitoria was used as an emetic, and Youpon tea (mixed leaves of Ilex cassine, Ilex vomitoria, and Ilex dahoon) was used as a ceremonial "cleanser" in South America.

Safety

UNSAFE ...when the berries are ingested. Eating berries can be fatal (18).
There is insufficient reliable information available about the safety of holly leaves.
CHILDREN: UNSAFE ...when the berries are ingested. Eating berries can be fatal (6).
PREGNANCY AND LACTATION: UNSAFE ...when berries are ingested (6).
There is insufficient reliable information available about the safety of holly leaves; avoid using.

Effectiveness

There is insufficient reliable information available about the effectiveness of holly.

Mechanism of Action

The applicable parts of holly are the leaf and berry. The constituent saponins are thought to cause GI irritation and emetic effects (6). Holly also contains a cyanogenic glycoside (4).

Adverse Reactions

Orally, ingestion of the leaf can cause GI irritation, diarrhea, nausea, and vomiting (6,18). Leaf spines may tear or puncture skin or mucous membranes (6). Ingestion of as few as 2 berries can cause vomiting and diarrhea in small children (6). Ingestion of more than 5 berries can cause nausea, vomiting, diarrhea, and stupor (6,18). Ingestion of 20-30 berries can cause death (18).

Interactions with Herbs & Other Dietary Supplements

None known.

Interactions with Drugs

None known.

Interactions with Foods

None known.

Interactions with Lab Tests

None known.

Interactions with Diseases or Conditions

DEHYDRATION: In addition to toxic effects, berry ingestion may cause or exacerbate dehydration by inducing vomiting and diarrhea (6).
ELECTROLYTE IMBALANCE: Berry ingestion may cause or exacerbate electrolyte imbalance by inducing vomiting and diarrhea (6).

Dosage and Administration

ORAL: People typically use 3.9 grams of powdered leaves in a tea, taken to reduce the effects of intermittent fevers (5254).

Comments

Many other Ilex species are referred to as holly. English holly, Oregon holly, American holly are used as ornamental Christmas holly (6). Yaupon, Appalachian tea, cassena, deer berry, Indian holly and Indian black drink may be included in discussions of holly (6). Leaf spines may tear or puncture skin or mucous membranes (6).

HOLLYHOCK

Also Known As

Althea Rose, Hollyhock Flower, Malva, Malva Flower, Malvae arboreae flos, Rose Mallow.
CAUTION: See separate listing for Mallow.

Scientific Names

Alcea rosea, synonym Althaea rosea, Althaea ficifolia.
Family: Malvaceae.

Comments

At the date of publication, there was very little scientific information available about this product. Our staff is continually analyzing the available information on natural medicines and will add data to the online version of *Natural Medicines Comprehensive Database* as it becomes available. See www.naturaldatabase.com.

HOLY BASIL

Also Known As

Bai Gkaprow, Green Holy Basil, Hot Basil, Indian Basil, Kemangen, Krishna Tulsi, Rama Tulsi, Red Holy Basil, Sacred Basil, Sacred Purple Basil, Shyama Tulsi, Tulasi, Tulsi.
CAUTION: See separate listing for Basil.

Scientific Names

Ocimum tenuiflorum, synonym Ocimum sanctum.
Family: Lamiaceae/Labiatae.

People Use This For

Orally, holy basil is used for the common cold, influenza ("the flu"), diabetes, asthma, bronchitis, earache, headache, stomach upset, heart disease, fever, viral hepatitis, malaria, and tuberculosis. It is also used for mercury poisoning, to promoted longevity, as a mosquito repellent, and as an antidote to snake and scorpion bites.
Topically, holy basil is used for ringworm.

Safety

POSSIBLY SAFE ...when used orally, short-term. There is some evidence that a holy basil leaf extract can be used safely for up to 4 weeks (12242).
PREGNANCY AND LACTATION: Insufficient reliable information available; avoid using.

Effectiveness

INSUFFICIENT RELIABLE EVIDENCE to RATE

Diabetes. Preliminary evidence suggests that a holy basil leaf extract might decrease fasting and postprandial blood glucose by 17.6% and 7.3% respectively in patients with type 2 diabetes (12242). More evidence is needed to rate holy basil for this use.

Mechanism of Action

The applicable parts of holy basil are the leaves, stems, seeds, and oil. Active constituents of the leaves and stems are thought to be saponins, flavonoids, triterpenoids, and tannins (12236). The leaves contain an essential oil with constituents including eugenol, methyl eugenol, and caryophyllene (12239,12242). The seed oil of holy basil contains linoleic acid (52%), linolenic acid (17%), oleic acid (14%), palmitic acid (12%), and stearic acid (3%).
Holy basil is thought to have antiemetic, anticancer, hypoglycemic, hypotensive, sedative, antimicrobial, antiviral, anti-inflammatory, antipyretic, analgesic, and antiulcer activity (12239,12242,12246,12249).
In animal models, holy basil leaf or stem extracts in doses of 400-800 mg/kg seem to have anticonvulsant effects comparable to phenytoin (12236).

Holy basil is considered an antistress or adaptogenic remedy in Ayurvedic medicine. In animal models, there is some evidence that a specific combination product containing holy basil, ashwagandha, asparagus, and Indian gooseberry (EuMil) can reduce several measures of stress response (12237).

Holy basil is used for poisonings. There is preliminary evidence that an aqueous extract of holy basil leaves might decrease some measures of mercury toxicity in animal models (12238).

In animal models and in humans, there is preliminary evidence that holy basil leaf extract has hypoglycemic activity (12242,12249,12250).

Holy basil leaf extract seems to have analgesic and antipyretic activity in animal models (12246,12248). It is thought to have both central and peripheral analgesic activity. The eugenol constituent is thought to be partially responsible for the analgesic activity (12248).

Holy basil leaf essential oil seems to have antihelmintic activity in vitro. Eugenol contained in the essential oil is thought to be responsible (13252).

There is also preliminary evidence that the leaf extract and the seed oil of holy basil might reduce the inflammatory response in animals given an inflammatory stimulus (12239,12246). The linolenic acid component of the oil is thought to be responsible for the anti-inflammatory effect. Linolenic acid is thought to inhibit the cyclooxygenase (COX) and lipoxygenase pathways of arachidonic acid metabolism (12240,12241).

Seed oil from holy basil also seems to have immunomodulatory effects. There is preliminary evidence that the oil can decrease the humoral and cell-mediated immune response to stress in animal models (12247).

There is interest in using holy basil seed oil for cancer. Preliminary evidence suggests that the oil can delay progression and improve survival rate in animals with experimentally induced fibrosarcoma. This effect has been attributed to antioxidant effects of the oil (13253).

Holy basil seed oil seems to have protective effects against aspirin, indomethacin, alcohol, and stress-induced ulceration in animals. It is thought that the oil might protect against gastric ulceration due to antisecretory and antihistaminic effects and inhibition of lipoxygenase (13254).

The seed oil of holy basil also seems to have a hypotensive effect, possibly due to a vasodilatory effect, in animal models (13251).

Seed oil also seems to prolong bleeding time, possibly due to inhibition of platelet aggregation. Linolenic acid contained in the seed oil can be converted to eicosapentanoic acid (EPA). EPA can inhibit thromboxane A2 (TXA2), which results in decreased platelet aggregation (13251).

Holy basil seems to have a variety of central nervous system effects. It reduces the duration of convulsions in animals subjected to electroshock- or pharmacologically-induced seizure. Holy basil also seems to have some stimulatory effects in animal models. Holy basil has additive activity when combined with bromocryptine, suggesting that holy basil has dompamine-2 receptor agonist activity (13056).

In animals, holy basil seed oil prolongs pentobarbitone-induced sleeping time. It's thought that holy basil might inhibit cytochrome metabolism of pentobarbitone (13251).

Adverse Reactions

Orally, no side effects have been reported.

There is preliminary evidence from animal models that suggests holy basil might decrease sperm counts and possibly decrease fertility (12243,12244).

Interactions with Herbs & Other Dietary Supplements

None known.

Interactions with Drugs

ANTICOAGULANT/ANTIPLATELET DRUGS: Theoretically, holy basil seed oil might increase the risk of bleeding when combined with anticoagulant or antiplatelet drugs. In an animal model, holy basil seed oil prolongs bleeding time, possibly due to inhibition of platelet aggregation (13251). Anticoagulant and antiplatelet drugs that might interact with holy basil seed oil include aspirin, clopidogrel (Plavix), dalteparin (Fragmin), enoxaparin (Lovenox), heparin, ticlopidine (Ticlid), warfarin (Coumadin), and others.

PENTOBARBITONE: Theoretically, combining holy basil seed oil and pentobarbitone might increase the sedative effects of pentobarbitone. In an animal model, holy basil seed oil increases pentobarbitone-induced sleeping time (13251). It is not known if this occurs in humans or if this applies to other barbiturates or sedatives.

Interactions with Foods

None known.

Interactions with Lab Tests

None known.

Interactions with Diseases or Conditions

None known.

Dosage and Administration

No typical dosage.

Comments

Holy basil is originally from India and is used in Ayurvedic medicine. It is considered a sacred plant by the Hindus and is often planted around Hindu shrines. The Hindu name for holy basil, Tulsi, means "the incomparable one." Holy basil is sometimes called "hot basil" because of its peppery taste. It's often added to stir fry dishes and spicy soups.

HONEY

Also Known As

Clarified Honey, Honig, Mel, Miel Blanc, Purified Honey, Strained Honey.
CAUTION: See separate listings for Bee Pollen, Bee Venom, and Royal Jelly.

Scientific Names

Apis mellifera (honey bee).
Family: Apidae.

People Use This For

Orally, honey is used for cough, asthma, and as an expectorant. It is also used orally for diarrhea and gastric ulcer associated with Helicobacter pylori. Honey is also used orally as a source of carbohydrate during vigorous exercise.
Topically, honey is used to speed healing in mild sores, wounds, skin ulcerations including diabetic foot ulcers, and burns; and for treating cataracts and postherpetic corneal opacities.
In foods, honey is used as a sweetening agent.
In manufacturing, honey is used as a fragrance and a moisturizer in soaps and cosmetics.

Safety

POSSIBLY SAFE ...when used topically (395,396,397,398,399,7847,7849,13133).
CHILDREN: POSSIBLY UNSAFE ...when used orally in infants and young children. Ingestion of honey contaminated with Clostridium botulinum spores may cause botulism poisoning in infants and young children (6,11). This is not a danger for older children or adults.
PREGNANCY AND LACTATION: Insufficient reliable information.

Effectiveness

POSSIBLY EFFECTIVE

Burns. Honey applied directly in gauze applications seems to improve formation of granulation tissue and healing time in partial thickness burns. It appears to compare favorably with silver sulfadiazine and moisture permeable polyurethane dressing (OpSite) (395,396,397,398,399). However, surgical intervention with tangential excision and skin grafting is more effective than honey for moderate burns (7848).

INSUFFICIENT RELIABLE EVIDENCE to RATE

Athletic performance. Some preliminary clinical evidence suggests that honey might normalize blood sugar following exercise and improve performance when given during exercise (7851).

Diabetic foot ulcers. Anecdotal reports suggest that applying topical raw honey can speed healing of otherwise non-healing diabetic foot ulcers, even in the presence methicillin-resistant Staphylococcus aureas (MRSA), vancomycin-resistant Enterococcus (VRE), and Pseudomonas infection. In one report, previously non-healing ulceration completely healed after applying honey dressings for 6-12 months and lower-limb amputation was prevented (13133).

Skin ulceration. Preliminary evidence suggests that applying honey topically can improve healing of skin ulceration, wounds, and mild sores (7847,7849).

More evidence is needed to rate honey for these uses.

Mechanism of Action

Honey is produced by bees (Apis mellifera) from the nectar of several varieties of plants. Pharmacological activity can vary depending on the type of plant from which the nectar is obtained. For example, honey produced from poisonous plants can be poisonous (6). Honey improves wound healing by promoting the formation of granulation tissue. It promotes the growth of epithelial cells by providing a barrier to moisture which helps keep the wound hydrated. Enzymes and hydrogen peroxide in honey can aid in debridement (395,396,399,7849). In surgery for some types of malignant cancer, cells from the tumor can become seeded in the wound margins during excision, resulting in growth of the cancer in the wound. Preliminary evidence indicates that honey can reduce the growth of these tumors, by impeding the seeding or inhibiting the growth of these cancer cells (7852).
Honey has antibacterial and antifungal activity, which might offer benefit in preventing wound infection and Helicobacter pylori infection in peptic ulcer disease. Honey inhibits the growth of Pseudomonas pyocyanea, Pseudomonas aeruginosa, Escherichia coli, Staphylococcus aureus, Proteus mirabilis, coliform species, Klebsiella species, Streptococcus faecalis, and Streptococcus pyogenes (7847,7849). Antibacterial peptides (apidaecins and abaecin) have been isolated in honeybees (6). The high osmolality, low pH, and hydrogen peroxide in honey also

contribute to antimicrobial activity. High osmolality causes shrinkage of microbes, because of intracellular water loss. Hydrogen peroxide is formed by the action of glucose oxidase (396,1261,1428,7850).
Honey and solutions with similar sugar content (15% w/v) demonstrate similar effectiveness at inhibiting Helicobacter pylori (1428), and 2-4% v/v dilutions of various types of honey inhibit the growth of coagulase-positive Staphylococcus aureus isolated from infected wounds (1261).

Adverse Reactions

Orally, honey can cause allergic reactions. Some honey is contaminated with Clostridium botulinum spores, which poses a risk to infants, but not older children or adults (6,11). Botulinum spores can proliferate in the intestines of infants and cause botulism poisoning.
Honey from the Black Sea coast of Turkey has been linked with a unique form of poisoning. Honey from this region sometimes contains excessive concentrations of acetylandromedol which can cause nausea, vomiting, dizziness, sweating, weakness, bradycardia, atrioventricular (AV) block, and hypotension within a few minutes to several hours after consumption. Fatalities have not been reported. Patients typically respond with fluids and reversal of cardiac conduction abnormalities with atropine. Honey containing this poison is sometimes called "mad honey" (12220).
Topically, honey may cause excessive dryness of wounds, which could delay healing. This can be managed by application of saline packs as needed (7850).

Interactions with Herbs & Other Dietary Supplements

None known.

Interactions with Drugs

None known.

Interactions with Foods

None known.

Interactions with Lab Tests

None known.

Interactions with Diseases or Conditions

POLLEN ALLERGIES: Honey may cause allergic reactions (6).

Dosage and Administration

TOPICAL: For the treatment of burns, honey has been applied directly or as a dressing made from gauze impregnated with honey. The dressings have been left in place for up to 25 days, with wound inspection every 2 days (397,398). When used directly, 15 to 30 mL of honey has been applied every 1 to 2 days, and covered with a dry sterile gauze and bandage (396,399).
For diabetic foot ulcer, ordinary honey purchased from a supermarket has been used. It is applied in thick applications to a 4x4 gauze and placed on the ulceration and then wrapped (13133).

Comments

Avoid confusion with bee pollen, bee venom, and royal jelly. Honey for medicinal use should be collected from hives that are free from pathogens and not treated with antibiotics. The nectar should be from plants that have not been treated with pesticides (7847).

HONEYSUCKLE

Also Known As

Goat's Leaf, Japanese Honeysuckle, Jin Yin Hua, Jinyinhua, Lonicera, Madreselva, Nindo, Ren Dong, Suikazura, Woodbine.
CAUTION: See separate listings for American Ivy, Gelsemium, and Woodbine.

Scientific Names

Lonicera caprifolia; Lonicera japonica, synonym Lonicera aureoreticulata; Lonicera bournei; other Lonicera sp.
Family: Caprifoliaceae.

People Use This For

Orally, honeysuckle is used for digestive disorders, enteritis, dysentery, urinary disorders, headache, diabetes, rheumatoid arthritis, malignant tumors, and to promote sweating. It is also used as a laxative, for colds and other upper respiratory tract infections, influenza, pneumonia, encephalitis, fever, inflammation, swelling, boils, sores, and viral and bacterial infections. It is also used as a poisoning antidote and contraceptive.
Topically, honeysuckle is used for inflammation, itching, and as an astringent and antimicrobial.

Safety

There is insufficient reliable information available about the safety of honeysuckle. An intravenous preparation that includes honeysuckle and two other herbs has been used with apparent safety in children for up to 7 days (12613). But more evidence is needed to rate the safety of honeysuckle.
Pregnancy and Lactation: Insufficient reliable information available; avoid using.

Effectiveness

INSUFFICIENT RELIABLE EVIDENCE to RATE

Bronchiolitis. Preliminary clinical research suggests a combination of honeysuckle, Baikal skullcap, and forsythia given intravenously might decrease the duration of symptoms of bronchiolitis in children with respiratory syncytial virus infection (12613). More evidence is needed to rate honeysuckle for this use.

Mechanism of Action

The applicable parts of honeysuckle are the flower, seed, and leaf. Honeysuckle contains essential oils, saponins, terpenoids, flavones, phenolics, and other compounds (12604,12608). The honeysuckle flavonoid, luteolin, inhibits tumor necrosis factor (TNF)-alpha production of interleukin (IL)-8 in intestinal cells, suggesting it might be useful for intestinal inflammatory disorders (12605). An aqueous extract of honeysuckle also seems to have anti-inflammatory effects in animal models of inflammation (12606). The loniceroside saponins of honeysuckle appear to have anti-inflammatory activity (12607). Other preliminary research suggests honeysuckle might increase neutrophil activity and increase phagocytosis. It may also protect the liver from injury caused by carbon tetrachloride (12606). In vitro research suggests that tannins from honeysuckle might inhibit reverse transcriptase activity in the human immunodeficiency virus (HIV) (12609). Phenolic compounds in honeysuckle seem to inhibit platelet activation and platelet thromboxane synthesis (12610). Honeysuckle might have contraceptive activity by inhibiting implantation, similar to oral contraceptives (12612).

Adverse Reactions

Topically, honeysuckle can cause contact dermatitis (12611).

Interactions with Herbs & Other Dietary Supplements

None known.

Interactions with Drugs

ANTICOAGULANT/ANTIPLATELET DRUGS: Concomitant use might increase the risk of bleeding due to decreased platelet aggregation. Honeysuckle has been reported to reduce platelet aggregation (12610); avoid concomitant use. Some of these drugs include aspirin, clopidogrel (Plavix), dalteparin (Fragmin), enoxaparin (Lovenox), heparin, ticlopidine (Ticlid), warfarin (Coumadin), and others.

Interactions with Foods

None known.

Interactions with Lab Tests

None known.

Interactions with Diseases or Conditions

None known.

Dosage and Administration

No typical dosage.

Comments

Avoid confusion with woodbine (Clematis virginiana). Also, avoid confusing honeysuckle with American ivy or gelsemium, which are also known as woodbine.

HOODIA

Also Known As

Cactus, Hoodia Gordonii Cactus, Hoodia P57, Kalahari Cactus, Kalahari Diet, P57, Xhoba.

Scientific Names

Hoodia gordonii.
Family: Apocynaceae.

People Use This For
Orally, hoodia is used as an appetite suppressant for obesity and weight loss.

Safety
There is insufficient reliable information available about the safety of hoodia.
Pregnancy and Lactation: Insufficient reliable information available; avoid using.

Effectiveness
There is insufficient reliable information available about the effectiveness of hoodia.

Mechanism of Action
The applicable parts of hoodia are the stems and roots. Hoodia is a cactus that grows in the Kalahari Desert. It is claimed that the San bushmen eat the cactus to stave off hunger during long hunts.
A specific component of hoodia extract is thought to be responsible for appetite suppressant properties. This constituent has been dubbed P57 (12002). This substance is thought to act centrally to stimulate sensations of satiety. The precise mechanism is not known.
Preliminary unpublished evidence suggests that overweight men who consume P57 have significantly lower calorie intake than those on placebo (12004). More evidence is needed to determine if hoodia is effective for any clinical condition.

Adverse Reactions
None reported.

Interactions with Herbs & Other Dietary Supplements
None known.

Interactions with Drugs
None known.

Interactions with Foods
None known.

Interactions with Lab Tests
None known.

Interactions with Diseases or Conditions
None known.

Dosage and Administration
No typical dosage.

Comments
The constituent of the hoodia extract called P57 is under development by Phytopharm. The company indicates that it has completed a positive study on the benefits of P57 for weight loss, but this study has not yet been published (12004). P57 was at one time licensed to Pfizer for development. Pfizer discontinued clinical development of P57 in 2003 (12003).
News reports suggest that some samples of hoodia products sold on the Internet show no evidence of containing actual hoodia (12002). Advise patients that they might not be getting what's listed on the label.

HOPS

Also Known As
Common Hops, European Hops, Hop Strobile, Hop Strobili, Hopfenzapfen, Houblon, Lupuli Strobulus.

Scientific Names
Humulus lupulus.
Family: Cannabaceae.

People Use This For

Orally, hops are used for restlessness, anxiety, insomnia and other sleep disorders, tension, excitability, attention deficit-hyperactivity disorder (ADHD), nervousness, and irritability. It is also used orally as an appetite stimulant, diuretic, a bitter tonic, and for indigestion. Other uses include tuberculosis, cystitis, intestinal cramps, mucous colitis, neuralgia, and priapism.
Topically, hops are used for leg ulcers and as an anti-bacterial.
Foods and beverages, the extracts and oil are used as flavor components. The strobile is often used for brewing beer.
In manufacturing, the extract is used in skin creams and lotions.

Safety

LIKELY SAFE ...when consumed in amounts commonly found in foods. Hops and hops oil have Generally Recognized As Safe (GRAS) status in the US (4912).
POSSIBLY SAFE ...when used orally and appropriately for medicinal purposes (12).
PREGNANCY AND LACTATION: Insufficient reliable information available; avoid using.

Effectiveness

There is insufficient reliable information available about the effectiveness of hops.

Mechanism of Action

The applicable part of hops is the dried, female flowering part (strobile). Nine flavonoids have been isolated from hops (10683). Hops contains a potent flavonoid phytoestrogen, 8-prenylnaringenin (10684). The flavonoid is structurally similar to estradiol and selective estrogen-receptor modulators (SERMs). The phenolic ring allows hops to bind to both the alpha and beta estrogen receptors, but with a higher affinity for the beta estrogen receptor. An extract of hops competitively inhibits estradiol binding to estrogen receptors and induces transcription activity in estrogen-responsive cells (6180). The weak endocrine activity of hops is believed to be primarily due to the high estrogenic activity of 8-prenylnaringenin (10685). Preliminary evidence suggests hops may possess antiproliferative properties, indicating potential chemoprevention against breast cancer and ovarian cancer (10683). One mechanism suggested includes the inhibition of the P450 enzymes that activate carcinogens (10686). Hops can also decrease LH (luteinizing hormone) levels in female rats that have had their ovaries removed (6180).

Adverse Reactions

Topically, allergic reactions are possible through contact with the fresh plant and plant dust. Contact dermatitis is attributed to the pollen (4).

Interactions with Herbs & Other Dietary Supplements

HERBS WITH SEDATIVE PROPERTIES: Theoretically, concomitant use with herbs that have sedative properties might enhance therapeutic and adverse effects. Some of these supplements include 5-HTP, calamus, California poppy, catnip, Jamaican dogwood, kava, St. John's wort, scullcap, valerian, yerba mansa, and others.

Interactions with Drugs

ALCOHOL (Ethanol): Concomitant use of hops can potentiate the sedative effects of alcohol (4).
CNS DEPRESSANTS: Theoretically, concomitant use with drugs having sedative properties can cause additive therapeutic and adverse effects (4,19).

Interactions with Foods

ALCOHOL: Concomitant use of hops with alcohol can potentiate the sedative effects (4).

Interactions with Lab Tests

None known.

Interactions with Diseases or Conditions

DEPRESSION: Hops may contribute to depression (12).

Dosage and Administration

No typical dosage.

HORSE CHESTNUT

Also Known As

Buckeye, Chestnut, Escine, Hippocastani Cortex, Hippocastani Flos, Hippocastani folium, Hippocastani Semen, Marron European, Spanish Chestnut, Venastat, Venostat, Venostasin Retard.

Scientific Names

Aesculus hippocastanum.
Family: Hippocastanaceae.

People Use This For

Orally, horse chestnut seed and leaf are used for the treatment of varicose veins, hemorrhoids, and phlebitis. Horse chestnut seed is used for diarrhea, fever, and enlarged prostate. Standardized horse chestnut seed extract products are used orally for the treatment of chronic venous insufficiency. A specially prepared product made from horse chestnut seed is used orally for the treatment of varicose veins, hemorrhoids, phlebitis, diarrhea, fever, and enlarged prostate. Horse chestnut branch bark is used for malaria and dysentery. Horse chestnut leaf is used for eczema, menstrual spastic pain, soft tissue swelling from bone fracture and sprains, complaints after concussion, cough, arthritis, and rheumatism.

Topically, horse chestnut branch bark is used for lupus and skin ulcers.

Safety

LIKELY SAFE ...when used orally and appropriately, short-term. Standardized horse chestnut seed extracts seem to be safe when used for 2-12 weeks (281,282,283,284,285,12113). These extracts have removed the primary toxic constituent, esculin (6420).

UNSAFE ...when the raw seed, bark, flower, or leaf is used orally. Horse chestnut contains significant amounts of the toxin esculin, and can be lethal (17).

CHILDREN: UNSAFE ...when the raw seeds, bark, flower, or leaves are used orally. Poisoning has been reported from children drinking tea made with twigs and leaves (9).

PREGNANCY AND LACTATION: UNSAFE ...when used orally as the raw seed, bark, flower, or leaf. Horse chestnut preparations can be lethal (17); avoid using. There is insufficient reliable information available about the safety of horse chestnut seed extract when used during pregnancy and lactation; avoid using.

Effectiveness

LIKELY EFFECTIVE

Chronic venous insufficiency. Taking horse chestnut seed extract orally can reduce some symptoms of chronic venous insufficiency, such as varicose veins, pain, tiredness, tension, swelling in the legs, itching, and edema (281,282,283,284,285,12113).

Clinical studies investigating the effectiveness of horse chestnut seed have used extracts standardized to 16% to 20% aescin.

There is insufficient reliable information available about the effectiveness of horse chestnut for its other uses.

Mechanism of Action

The applicable parts of horse chestnut are the seed, bark, flower, and leaf. An extract of horse chestnut seed is most commonly used. Horse chestnut contains triterpene saponins referred to as aescin (escin) and the toxic glycoside aesculin (esculin) (11). Aesculin is a hydroxycoumarin which may increase bleeding time due to antithrombin activity (19). Aescin decreases the permeability of venous capillaries. In vitro, aescin constricts veins and reduces the capillary permeability induced by histamine or serotonin (7162). These properties of the saponin components are the basis for the cosmetic applications of horse chestnut seed extract (4). In some countries, an intravenous mixture containing aescin is used after surgery (9). Aescin also seems to have a weak diuretic activity (7162). Aescin binds to plasma proteins (4). Horse chestnut branch bark and flower also contains sterols, stigmasterol, alpha-spinasterol, and beta-sitosterol (11).

Adverse Reactions

Orally, horse chestnut seed extract with the toxic constituent esculin removed, seems to be well-tolerated.

Some people who take this extract can experience dizziness, nausea, headache, and pruritis (12113).

The horse chestnut seed and bark can cause GI irritation and toxic nephropathy (4).

Horse chestnut contains esculin which has antithrombotic effects and might increase the risk of bleeding or bruising (19).

Symptoms of horse chestnut poisoning include muscle twitching, weakness, loss of coordination, dilated pupils, vomiting, diarrhea, depression, paralysis, and stupor (9).

Pollen from the horse chestnut flower can cause allergic reactions in children (7775). Horse chestnut can also cause hypersensitivity reactions, which occur more commonly in people who are allergic to latex (7853,8418).

Rectally, horse chestnut may cause severe allergic contact dermatitis and proctitis (10383).

Intramuscularly, horse chestnut leaf extract has been associated with cholestatic liver damage (2).

Intravenously, administration of aescin can cause anaphylaxis (18). Isolated cases of kidney and liver toxicity have occurred after intravenous administration (512).

Interactions with Herbs & Other Dietary Supplements

HERBS WITH ANTICOAGULANT/ANTIPLATELET POTENTIAL: Concomitant use of herbs that have constituents that might affect platelet aggregation could theoretically increase the risk of bleeding in some people. These herbs include angelica, clove, danshen, garlic, ginger, ginkgo, Panax ginseng, red clover, and others.
HERBS WITH HYPOGLYCEMIC ACTIVITY: Theoretically, concomitant use with herbs having hypoglycemic activity could have additive effects and adverse effects. Some herbs and supplements with hypoglycemic effects include alpha-lipoic acid, chromium, devil's claw, fenugreek, garlic, guar gum, Panax ginseng, psyllium, Siberian ginseng, and others.

Interactions with Drugs

ANTICOAGULANT/ANTIPLATELET DRUGS: Horse chestnut might have antiplatelet effects (19). Theoretically, taking horse chestnut with other antiplatelet or anticoagulant drugs might increase the risk of bruising and bleeding. Some of these drugs include aspirin, clopidogrel (Plavix), nonsteroidal anti-inflammatory drugs (NSAIDs) such as diclofenac (Voltaren, Cataflam, others), ibuprofen (Advil, Motrin, others), naproxen (Anaprox, Naprosyn, others), dalteparin (Fragmin), enoxaparin (Lovenox), heparin, warfarin (Coumadin), and others.
ANTIDIABETES DRUGS: Monitor blood glucose levels closely due to claims that horse chestnut seeds and bark can have hypoglycemic effects (19).

Interactions with Foods

None known.

Interactions with Lab Tests

None known.

Interactions with Diseases or Conditions

DIABETES: Monitor blood glucose levels closely due to claims that horse chestnut seeds can have hypoglycemic effects (19).
GI IRRITATION: Horse chestnut seeds and bark can irritate gastrointestinal tract; contraindicated in individuals with infectious or inflammatory gastrointestinal conditions (19).
HEPATIC IMPAIRMENT: There is one report of liver injury associated with horse chestnut (4); avoid using.
LATEX ALLERGY: People that are allergic to latex should not take horse chestnut because cross hypersensitivity may occur (7853,8418).
RENAL IMPAIRMENT: Toxic nephropathy has been reported as an adverse effect (4); avoid using.

Dosage and Administration

ORAL: For chronic venous insufficiency, horse chestnut seed extract 300 mg containing 50 mg aescin has been used twice daily (281,283).

Comments

Sometimes buckeye is referred to as horse chestnut. Do not confuse horse chestnut with the related species, Aesculus californica and Aesculus glabra, known respectively as the California and Ohio buckeye.

HORSEMINT

Also Known As

Monarda Lutea, Spotted Monarda, Wild Bergamot.

Scientific Names

Monarda punctata.
Family: Lamiaceae/Labitae.

People Use This For

Orally, horsemint is used for digestive disorders, flatulence, and dysmenorrhea. It is also used orally to promote menstruation and as a stimulant.

Safety

There is insufficient reliable information available about the safety of horsemint.
PREGNANCY: UNSAFE ...when used orally due to menstruation promoting and uterine stimulant effects (12).
LACTATION: Insufficient reliable information available; avoid using.

Effectiveness
There is insufficient reliable information available about the effectiveness of horsemint.

Mechanism of Action
There is insufficient reliable information available about the possible mechanism of action and active ingredients.

Adverse Reactions
None reported.

Interactions with Herbs & Other Dietary Supplements
None known.

Interactions with Drugs
None known.

Interactions with Foods
None known.

Interactions with Lab Tests
None known.

Interactions with Diseases or Conditions
None known.

Dosage and Administration
ORAL: The average daily dose is 2-4 mL of syrup prepared from the herb (18).

Comments
Horsemint has a pungent, bitter taste, and has a scent reminiscent of thyme (18).

HORSERADISH

Also Known As
Amoraciae Rusticanae Radix, Great Raifort, Meerrettich, Mountain Radish, Pepperrot, Red Cole.

Scientific Names
Armoracia rusticana, synonyms Armoracia lopathifolia, Cochlearia armoracia, Nasturtium armoracia, Rorippa armoracia.
Family: Brassicaceae/Cruciferae.

People Use This For
Orally, horseradish is used for urinary tract infection, urinary stones, edematous conditions, cough, bronchitis, for expelling afterbirth, treating gout, rheumatism, gallbladder disorders, sciatica pain, relief of colic, increasing urination, and intestinal worms in children.
Topically, horseradish is used for inflamed joints or tissues and minor muscle aches.
In foods, horseradish is used as a flavoring agent.

Safety
LIKELY SAFE ...when the root is used orally in amounts commonly found in foods. Horseradish has Generally Recognized As Safe (GRAS) status in the US (4912).
POSSIBLY SAFE ...when used orally and appropriately in larger amounts (2,4,6,12,18). ...when topical preparations containing 2% mustard oil, or less are used (2). Mustard oil is a constituent of horseradish.
CHILDREN: LIKELY UNSAFE ...when used orally in children less than 4 years of age because it can cause gastrointestinal problems (2,12,19).
PREGNANCY AND LACTATION: LIKELY UNSAFE ...when used orally in excessive amounts. Horseradish contains toxic and irritating mustard oil constituents (4). ...when the tincture is used regularly and in large amounts, it is considered an abortifacient (19).

Effectiveness
There is insufficient reliable information available about the effectiveness of horseradish.

Mechanism of Action
The applicable part of horseradish is the root. Researchers state horseradish has antimicrobial efficacy against gram negative and gram positive bacteria. It also has antispasmodic properties. Horseradish shows evidence that it can stimulate local blood flow; it might also be carcinostatic (2,18). The toxic mustard oil constituents of horseradish are extremely irritating to mucous membranes (2,4) and the urinary tract (19).

Adverse Reactions
Orally, consuming large amounts of horseradish can cause gastrointestinal upset, bloody vomiting and diarrhea (2,6), and irritation of mucous membranes (2,4) and the urinary tract (19). Horseradish, and other members of the cabbage and mustard family are associated with depressed thyroid function (4).
Topically, skin contact with fresh horseradish can cause irritation (4,19) or allergic reaction (4).

Interactions with Herbs & Other Dietary Supplements
HERBS WITH ANTICOAGULANT/ANTIPLATELET POTENTIAL: Concomitant use of herbs that have constituents that might affect platelet aggregation could theoretically increase the risk of bleeding in some people. These herbs include angelica, clove, danshen, garlic, ginger, ginkgo, Panax ginseng, red clover, turmeric, and others.

Interactions with Drugs
LEVOTHYROXINE (Synthroid, Levothroid, Levoxyl, and others): Theoretically, concomitant use of horseradish can interfere with levothyroxine or hypothyroid therapy (4).

Interactions with Foods
None known.

Interactions with Lab Tests
None known.

Interactions with Diseases or Conditions
GI CONDITIONS: Horseradish can irritate gastrointestinal tract. Contraindicated in individuals with infectious or inflammatory gastrointestinal conditions, or stomach or intestinal ulcers (19).
HYPOTHYROIDISM: Theoretically, horseradish might exacerbate hypothyroidism or interfere with therapy (19).
KIDNEY DISORDERS: Theoretically, because it has a strong diuretic effect (19), horseradish is contraindicated in individuals with kidney inflammation (2,18,19).

Dosage and Administration
ORAL: The typical dose of horseradish is 6-20 grams per day of the root or equivalent preparations (4,6,18).
TOPICAL: Ointments with a maximum of 2% mustard oil content are commonly used (6,18).

Comments
Horseradish has been cultivated for more than two thousand years (6) and is sometimes added to toxic substances as a taste repellent for animals (6002).

HORSETAIL

Also Known As
Bottle Brush, Corn Horsetail, Dutch Rushes, Equisetum, Field Horsetail, Horse Willow, Paddock-Pipes, Pewterwort, Prele, Scouring Rush, Souring Rush, Shave Grass, Toadpipe.

Scientific Names
Equisetum arvense; Equisetum telmateia.
Family: Equisetaceae.

People Use This For
Orally, horsetail is used for diuresis, edema, kidney and bladder stones, urinary tract infections, incontinence, and general disturbances of the kidney and bladder. It is also used for alopecia, tuberculosis, brittle fingernails, rheumatic diseases, gout, frostbite, profuse menstruation, and nasal, pulmonary, and gastric hemorrhage.
Topically, horsetail is used for supportive treatment of wounds and burns.

Safety

POSSIBLY UNSAFE ...when used orally and appropriately short-term (6,12).
LIKELY UNSAFE ...when used orally long-term. It can cause thiamine deficiency. The inorganic silica content can cause toxicity similar to nicotine poisoning (12).
CHILDREN: LIKELY UNSAFE ...when used orally. Horsetail contains inorganic silica and the powdered herb can cause toxicity similar to nicotine poisonings. Poisoning has been reported in children who chewed on the stem (12).
PREGNANCY AND LACTATION: Insufficient reliable information available; avoid using.

Effectiveness

There is insufficient reliable information available about the effectiveness of horsetail.

Mechanism of Action

The applicable parts of horsetail are above ground parts. Evidence suggests horsetail has a mild diuretic action (18), which is likely due to the constituents, equisetonin and flavone glycosides (6). It also contains minute amounts of nicotine (6).

Adverse Reactions

Orally, horsetail may lead to thiamine deficiency, and Canadian products are required to be certified as free from thiaminase-like effect (12). Toxicity has occurred in children who chewed the stems and is similar to nicotine poisoning (12).
Topically, horsetail can cause seborrheic dermatitis (6).

Interactions with Herbs & Other Dietary Supplements

CARDIAC GLYCOSIDE-CONTAINING HERBS: Concomitant use may increase the risk of cardiac glycoside toxicity due to potassium depletion. Cardiac glycoside-containing herbs, include black hellebore, Canadian hemp roots, digitalis leaf, hedge mustard, figwort, lily-of-the-valley roots, motherwort, oleander leaf, pheasant's eye plant, pleurisy root, squill bulb leaf scales, and strophanthus seeds (18,500).
CHROMIUM-CONTAINING SUPPLEMENTS: Horsetail contains chromium (0.0006%) and could increase the risk of chromium toxicity when taken with chromium supplements or chromium-containing herbs such as cascara (Rhamus purshiana) (9141).
LICORICE: Theoretically, overuse/misuse of licorice rhizome with horsetail increases the risk of cardiac toxicity due to potassium depletion (19).
STIMULANT LAXATIVE HERBS: Theoretically, concomitant use increases the risk of potassium depletion. Stimulant laxative herbs include aloe dried leaf sap, blue flag rhizome, alder buckthorn, European buckthorn, butternut bark, cascara bark, castor oil, colocynth fruit pulp, gamboge bark exudate, jalap root, black root, manna bark exudate, podophyllum root, rhubarb root, senna leaves and pods, wild cucumber fruit (Ecballium elaterium), and yellow dock root (19).

Interactions with Drugs

CORTICOSTEROIDS: Theoretically, concomitant use of horsetail with corticosteroids with mineral corticoid activity increases the risk of hypokalemia (4,13).
DIGOXIN (Lanoxin): Increased digoxin toxicity might occur due to the loss of potassium associated with the diuretic effect of horsetail (19).
DIURETIC DRUGS: Overuse of horsetail might compound diuretic-induced potassium loss (4,13). There is some concern that people taking horsetail along with potassium depleting diuretics might have an increased risk for hypokalemia. Initiation of potassium supplementation or an increase in potassium supplement dose may be necessary for some patients. Some diuretics that can deplete potassium include chlorothiazide (Diuril), chlorthalidone (Thalitone), furosemide (Lasix), hydrochlorothiazide (HCTZ, Hydrodiuril, Microzide), and others.

Interactions with Foods

REGULAR DIET: Horsetail can breakdown thiamine and theoretically increases the risk of thiamine deficiency (19).

Interactions with Lab Tests

None known.

Interactions with Diseases or Conditions

IMPAIRED HEART OR KIDNEY FUNCTION: The diuretic effect of horsetail can cause an increased excretion of potassium (19); avoid using.
THIAMINE DEFICIENCY: Theoretically, the horsetail stem can cause or exacerbate thiamine deficiency (12).

Dosage and Administration

ORAL: The typical dose of horsetail is 6 grams of the dried stem per day with ample fluid intake (18). One cup of the tea is commonly taken several times per day between meals. The tea is prepared by steeping 1.5 grams of the dried stem in 150 mL boiling water for 10-15 minutes and then straining (18). The powdered stem should be used only on a short-term basis in adults. Avoid the use of the powdered stem in children due to its inorganic silica content (12). The usual dose of the liquid extract (1:1 in 25% alcohol) is 1-4 mL three times per day (18). Do not exceed 2 grams of the powdered extract per day (12).
TOPICAL: Horsetail is commonly used as a compress containing 10 grams of the dried stem per L of water (18).

Comments

Adulteration with Equisetum palustre, which contains the toxic alkaloid palustrine, has occurred. Palustrine can be toxic in cattle, but toxicity in humans has not yet been established (12).

HOUND'S TONGUE

Also Known As

Cynoglossi herba, Cynoglossi radix, Dog-Bur, Dog's Tongue, Gypsy Flower, Sheep-Lice, Woolmat.
CAUTION: See separate listing for Deertongue.

Scientific Names

Cynoglossum officinale.
Family: Boraginaceae.

People Use This For

Orally, hound's tongue is used for diarrhea and other GI tract complaints, infections, skin diseases, and bronchitis. It is also used orally as an analgesic, expectorant, and cough sedative.
Topically, hound's tongue is used for painful discomfort of extremities, myalgia, neuralgia, trauma, nervous diseases, wound healing, and for care of scar tissue.

Safety

LIKELY UNSAFE ...when products containing hepatotoxic pyrrolizidine alkaloid (PA) constituents are used orally. Repeated exposure to low concentrations of hepatotoxic PAs can cause severe veno-occlusive disease. Hepatotoxic PAs might also be carcinogenic and mutagenic (12841,12842). Tell patients not to use hound's tongue preparations that are not certified and labeled as hepatotoxic PA-free. ...when products containing hepatotoxic PAs are used topically on abraded or broken skin. Absorption of hepatotoxic PAs through broken skin can lead to systemic toxicities (12841). Tell patients not to use topical hound's tongue preparations that are not certified and labeled as hepatotoxic PA-free. There is insufficient reliable information available about the safety of topical PA-free hound's tongue on unbroken skin.
PREGNANCY: LIKELY UNSAFE ...when used orally. Hound's tongue preparations containing hepatotoxic pyrrolizidine alkaloid (PA) constituents might be teratogenic and hepatotoxic (12841,12842). There is insufficient reliable information available about the safety of using hound's tongue products that do not contain hepatotoxic PAs during pregnancy.
LACTATION: LIKELY UNSAFE ...when used orally. Hepatotoxic pyrrolizidine alkaloid (PA) constituents in hound's tongue are excreted in milk (12841,12842). There is insufficient reliable information available about the safety of using hound's tongue products that do not contain hepatotoxic PAs during lactation.

Effectiveness

There is insufficient reliable information available about the effectiveness of hound's tongue.

Mechanism of Action

The applicable parts are the leaf and root. Hound's tongue contains various pyrrolizidine alkaloids (PA), some of which are toxic. PAs are most concentrated in the plant roots, but may be found in all plant parts. PAs, particularly unsaturated PAs, can cause hepatotoxicity. Cyclic diesters such as retrorsine and senecionine are the most hepatotoxic. Liver toxicity may result from PA-enhanced oxidative stress, but the exact mechanism of toxicity is unknown. Single doses of 10-20 mg PAs or chronic ingestion of amounts less than 10 mcg can cause veno-occlusive disease. PAs are metabolized by cytochrome P450 3A4 (CYP3A4) to toxic dehydroalkaloids and pyrroles. Enzyme inducers such as phenobarbital seem to enhance toxicity (12841,12860). Pyrroles are excreted as N-acetyl cysteine conjugates. Some researchers speculate that early administration of N-acetylcysteine might reduce toxicity (11988). Metabolism is also affected by pregnane X receptor induction of CYP3A4. Genetic or drug-induced variation in CYP3A4 or pregnane X receptor activity can affect the degree of PA toxicity by increasing or decreasing its metabolism (12841,12842). Hepatotoxic PAs are also toxic to the lungs. In animals, pneumotoxicity occurs as pulmonary hypertension and right ventricular hypertrophy. Hepatotoxic PAs are carcinogenic and mutagenic. There are sufficient amounts of hepatotoxic PAs in herbal products to cause toxicity (12841,12842).

Adverse Reactions

Orally, the major concern about hound's tongue preparations is the hepatotoxic pyrrolizidine alkaloid (PA) content. These constituents are hepatotoxic, pneumotoxic, carcinogenic and mutagenic (12841,12842). Chronic exposure to other plants containing hepatotoxic PA constituents is associated with veno-occlusive disease (4021). Subacute veno-occlusive disease causes vague symptoms with persistent liver enlargement (4021). Symptoms of acute veno-occlusive disease include colicky pains in epigastrium, vomiting and diarrhea, and ascites formation within several days. Enlargement and induration of the liver occurs within a few weeks (12842). Dietary supplements sold in the US are not required to include the amount of PAs they contain (3484); therefore, all preparations used orally containing hound's tongue should be considered potentially unsafe.

Interactions with Herbs & Other Dietary Supplements

HEPATOTOXIC PYRROLIZIDINE ALKALOID (PA)-CONTAINING HERBS: Concomitant use is contraindicated due to the risk of additive toxicity. Herbs containing hepatotoxic PAs include alkanna, borage, butterbur, coltsfoot, comfrey, gravel root, and hemp agrimony; and the Senecio species plants dusty miller, ragwort, golden ragwort, groundsel, and tansy ragwort (12841).

HERBS THAT INDUCE CYTOCHROME P450 3A4 (CYP3A4): Theoretically, herbs that induce CYP3A4 might increase the conversion of hepatotoxic PAs to toxic metabolites, enhancing toxicity (12841,12860). Herbs that induce CYP3A4 include St. John's wort and garlic.

Interactions with Drugs

CYTOCHROME P450 3A4 (CYP3A4) INDUCERS: Hepatotoxic pyrrolizidine alkaloids (PA) are substrates of cytochrome P450 3A4 (CYP3A4) (12841,12860). Theoretically, drugs that induce CYP3A4 might increase the conversion of PAs to toxic metabolites. Some drugs that induce CYP3A4 include carbamazepine (Tegretol), phenobarbital, phenytoin (Dilantin), rifampin, rifabutin (Mycobutin), and others.

Interactions with Foods

None known.

Interactions with Lab Tests

None known.

Interactions with Diseases or Conditions

LIVER DISEASE: Theoretically, pyrrolizidine alkaloids (PAs) might exacerbate liver disease (12841,12842).

Dosage and Administration

No typical dosage.

HOUSELEEK

Also Known As

Aaron's Rod, Ayegreen, Ayron, Bullock's Eye, Hens and Chickens, Jupiter's Beard, Jupiter's Eye, Liveforever, Sengreen, Thor's Beard, Thunder Plant.

Scientific Names

Sempervivum tectorum.
Family: Crassulaceae.

Comments

At the date of publication, this product was not a common ingredient used in brand name supplements marketed to consumers. Details about this product are available in the online version of *Natural Medicines Comprehensive Database.* See www.naturaldatabase.com.

HU ZHANG

Also Known As

Fleece Flower, Fleeceflower, Hu zhang extract, Hu zhang root, Itadori, Japanese bamboo, Japanese knotweed, Mexican bamboo, PCWE, Polygonum cuspidatum water extract.

Scientific Names

Polygonum cuspidatum; synonyms Fallopia japonica, Reynoutria japonica.
Family: Polygonaceae.

People Use This For

Orally, hu zhang is used for constipation, dysmenorrhea, menopausal symptoms such as hot flashes, cardiovascular disease, atherosclerosis, hyperlipidemia, cancer, skin burns, osteomyelitis, hepatitis, gout, and gallstones.

Safety

There is insufficient reliable information available about the safety of hu zhang.
Pregnancy and Lactation: Insufficient reliable information available; avoid using.

Effectiveness

There is insufficient reliable information available about the effectiveness of hu zhang.

Mechanism of Action

The applicable part of hu zhang is the root. Hu zhang has several active constituents including emodin, resveratrol, emodin-8-O-D-glucoside, physcion, piceid, and others.
The hu zhang constituent, emodin, is an anthraquinone, which seems to be responsible for many of hu zhang's potential pharmacological activity.
Emodin, like other anthraquinones, is thought to have a laxative effect (13122).
Hu zhang appears to have several potential anticancer effects. The emodin constituent and other polyphenols such as resveratrol contained in hu zhang seem to have antimutagenic effects. In vitro, hu zhang extracts and emodin decrease the mutagenicity of benzo[a]pyrene and other mutagens in a dose-dependent manner (13122).
Several constituents of hu zhang seem to have a cytotoxic effect on HL-60 cells. Emodin appears to be the most cytotoxic (13125). The emodin constituent of hu zhang is also a strong inhibitor of protein tyrosine kinase (13126,13128). Tyrosine kinases have a role in regulation of cell growth. Tyrosine kinases are therefore a target for potential anticancer agents (13126). Preliminary evidence also suggests that a hu zhang root extract has antiangiogenesis activity (13129).
In vitro evidence suggests that a hu zhang extract can increase proliferation of estrogen-sensitive breast tissue cells, MCF-7. The emodin constituent is binds both estrogen receptor-alpha and estrogen receptor-beta and is thought to be a potent phytoestrogen (13124).
Hu zhang extract also decreases serum very low density lipoprotein (VLDL) cholesterol levels in animal models. Hu zhang seems inhibit acyl-coenzyme A-cholesterol acyltransferase (ACAT), which is involved in determining cholesterol levels. The resveratrol constituent of hu zhang is thought to be the constituent primarily responsible for inhibiting ACAT (13123).
Preliminary evidence shows that a hu zhang root extract can inhibit xanthine oxidase, suggesting that hu zhang might have a role in gout. However, the xanthine oxidase inhibition is about 38 times with hu zhang compared to allopurinol (13127).

Adverse Reactions

None reported.

Interactions with Herbs & Other Dietary Supplements

None known.

Interactions with Drugs

ESTROGENS: Hu zhang appears to have estrogenic activity (13124). Theoretically, hu zhang might competitively inhibit the effects of estrogen replacement therapy.

Interactions with Foods

None known.

Interactions with Lab Tests

None known.

Interactions with Diseases or Conditions

HORMONE-SENSITIVE CANCERS/CONDITIONS: There is preliminary evidence that hu zhang has estrogenic activity. Theoretically, hu zhang might worsen hormone sensitive conditions. Until more is known, women with hormone-sensitive conditions should avoid hu zhang. Some of these conditions include breast cancer, uterine cancer, ovarian cancer, endometriosis, and uterine fibroids.

Dosage and Administration

No typical dosage.

Comments

Hu zhang is the Chinese name given to Polygonum cuspidatum. North American varieties are often referred to as Mexican bamboo.

HUPERZINE A

Also Known As
HupA, Huperzine, Huperzine-A, Selagine.
CAUTION: See separate listing for Chinese Club Moss.

Scientific Names
Huperzine A.

People Use This For
Orally, huperzine A is used for Alzheimer's disease, memory and learning enhancement, age-related memory impairment, increasing alertness and energy, protection from neurotoxic agents including organophosphate nerve gases, glutamate toxicity, and for treating myasthenia gravis.

Safety
POSSIBLY SAFE ...when used orally and appropriately, short-term. Huperzine A has been used safely in clinical trials lasting from 1-3 months (3138,3140,3171,3561,4624,4626).
PREGNANCY AND LACTATION: Insufficient reliable information available; avoid using.

Effectiveness
POSSIBLY EFFECTIVE

Cognitive function. Taking huperzine A orally seems to improve memory function for healthy adolescents. In a small-scale, placebo controlled trial, Chinese middle school children complaining of poor memory had significant improvement in memory quotient scores after taking huperzine A for 4 weeks compared to placebo (4626).

Dementia. Taking huperzine A orally seems to improve memory, cognitive function, and behavioral function in patients with Alzheimer's, multi-infarct, and senile dementia (3138,3140,3171,4624). In one clinical trial, patients with Alzheimer's disease treated with huperzine A had significant improvement in memory, cognitive, and behavioral function scales compared to placebo after 8 weeks of treatment (3138). In a small-scale, placebo-controlled trial, multi-infarct and senile dementia patients treated with huperzine A had significant improvement in memory function after 2-4 weeks of treatment (3140). Long-term, large scale trials are necessary to confirm these findings and determine huperzine A's potential role in dementia.

Myasthenia gravis. Administering huperzine A intramuscularly seems to prevent muscle weakness in patients with myasthenia gravis. In a short-term, small-scale, open-label trial, stabilized patients with myasthenia gravis given huperzine A intramuscularly for 10 days maintained muscle strength as well as patients treated with intramuscular neostigmine alternating with intramuscular huperzine A. Huperzine A was reported to have a 7 hour duration of effect compared to 4 hours for neostigmine (3561). Well-controlled, large-scale trials are necessary to confirm huperzine A's potential benefit in myasthenia gravis.

There is insufficient reliable information available about the effectiveness of huperzine A for its other uses.

Mechanism of Action
Huperzine A is an alkaloid isolated from Chinese club moss, Huperzia serrata and from Lycopodium selago. It is an optically active stereoisomer. Only the levorotatory-isomer is pharmacologically active (3561). Huperzine A is thought to be beneficial in dementia, memory impairment, and myasthenia gravis due to its effects on acetylcholine levels (3133,3134,3135,3136,3172). It is a reversible inhibitor of acetylcholinesterase (AChE) for up to three hours, and crosses the blood-brain barrier. It produces a variable degree of acetylcholine elevation in different areas of the brain, with maximal values in the frontal and parietal cortex (125% and 105% respectively), and 22% to 65% in other brain regions (3141). It might be more specific for AChE and have a longer duration of action than AChE inhibitors such as tacrine (Cognex) or donepezil (Aricept), which are marketed as prescription drugs for Alzheimer's disease (3131,3132). In animal studies, huperzine A was found to be 64 times more potent than tacrine. It also is more bioavailable and penetrates the blood-brain barrier better than tacrine (3561). Huperzine A protects neurons against toxic levels of glutamate by blocking glutamate-induce neuronal calcium influx and cell death (3131,3561). Although it has low affinity, huperzine A is also a cerebral cortex N-methyl-D-aspartate (NMDA) receptor antagonist (3129,3137). It might also protect against seizures and neuropathological changes caused by exposure to organophosphate nerve agents such as soman, by protecting peripheral and central stores of acetylcholine (3137,3139).

Adverse Reactions
Orally, huperzine A can cause nausea, sweating, blurred vision, hyperactivity, anorexia, decreased heart rate, and fasciculations (3140,3172,3561,4625). It has been suggested that huperzine A might have fewer cholinergic side effects than tacrine (Cognex) and donepezil (Aricept), but this has not been confirmed in human trials (3131).

Interactions with Herbs & Other Dietary Supplements
None known.

Interactions with Drugs

ACETYLCHOLINESTERASE (AChE) INHIBITORS: Theoretically, concurrent use might have additive effects with drugs that promote acetylcholine activity because huperzine A has AChE inhibitor properties (3131). AChE inhibitors and cholinergic drugs include bethanechol (Urecholine), donepezil (Aricept), echothiophate (Phospholine Iodide), edrophonium (Enoln, Reversol, Tensilon), neostigmine (Prostigmin), physostigmine (Antilirium), pyridostigmine (Mestinon, Regonol), succinylcholine (Anectine, Quelicin), and tacrine (Cognex).
ANTICHOLINERGIC DRUGS: Theoretically, concurrent use of anticholinergic drugs and huperzine A might decrease the effectiveness of huperzine A or the anticholinergic agent. In an animal model, huperzine A reversed cognitive deficits induced by scopolamine (3135). Other anticholinergic drugs include atropine, benztropine (Cogentin), biperiden (Akineton), procyclidine (Kemadrin), and trihexyphenidyl (Artane).
CHOLINERGIC DRUGS: Theoretically, concurrent use might have additive effects with drugs that promote acetylcholine activity because huperzine A has AChE inhibitor properties (3131). AChE inhibitors and cholinergic drugs include bethanechol (Urecholine), donepezil (Aricept), echothiophate (Phospholine Iodide), edrophonium (Enoln, Reversol, Tensilon), neostigmine (Prostigmin), physostigmine (Antilirium), pyridostigmine (Mestinon, Regonol), succinylcholine (Anectine, Quelicin), and tacrine (Cognex).

Interactions with Foods

None known.

Interactions with Lab Tests

None known.

Interactions with Diseases or Conditions

BRADYCARDIA/CARDIOVASCULAR DISEASE: Huperzine A can cause decreased heart rate and might exacerbate bradycardia and other cardiac conditions sensitive to decreased heart rate (3561); use with caution.
EPILEPSY: Theoretically, huperzine A might exacerbate seizure disorders (3561); use with caution.
GASTROINTESTINAL TRACT OBSTRUCTION: Theoretically, huperzine A might exacerbate gastrointestinal obstruction due to its pro-secretory effects (3561); use with caution.
PEPTIC ULCER DISEASE: Theoretically, huperzine A might exacerbate peptic ulcer disease due to its pro-secretory effects (3561); use with caution.
PULMONARY CONDITIONS: Theoretically, huperzine A might exacerbate pulmonary conditions such as asthma and chronic obstructive pulmonary disease due to its pro-secretory effects (3561); use with caution.
UROGENITAL TRACT OBSTRUCTION: Theoretically, huperzine A might exacerbate urogenital tract obstruction due to its pro-secretory effects (3561); use with caution.

Dosage and Administration

ORAL: For Alzheimer's disease and multi-infarct dementia, doses of 50-200 mcg twice daily have been used (3138,3140,4625). For senile or presenile dementia, doses of 30 mcg twice daily have been used (3140). For improving memory in adolescents, doses of 100 mcg twice daily have been used (4626).
INTRAMUSCULAR: For prevention of muscle weakness in myasthenia gravis, doses of 400 mcg daily have been used (3561).

Comments

The Cerebra brand name used for huperzine A has been confused with the prescription drugs Celebrex, Celexa, and Cerebyx (3142). Huperzine A is also referred to as selagine. Avoid confusion with the prescription drug selegiline (Eldepryl). Huperzine A is a drug that stretches the guidelines of the Dietary Supplement Health and Education Act (DSHEA). Although derived from a plant, huperzine A is a laboratory-manipulated, highly purified drug, unlike herbs which typically contain hundreds of constituents. Chemical hybrids of huperzine A plus tacrine and huperzine A plus donepezil are being investigated (4625). The hybrid of huperzine A plus donepezil has been referred to as huprine X (4625). Laboratory studies indicate that these hybrids have substantially greater affinity for AChE than tacrine or donepezil and show potential for enhanced efficacy at lower doses, with fewer side effects (4625).

HYALURONIC ACID

Also Known As

Hyaluran, Hyaluronan, Hyaluronate, Hyaluronate Sodium, Sodium Hyaluronate.
CAUTION: See separate listings for Glucosamine Hydrochloride, Glucosamine Sulfate, and N-Acetyl Glucosamine.

Scientific Names

Glycoaminoglycan.

People Use This For

Orally, hyaluronic acid is used for various joint disorders, including osteoarthritis and preventing the effects of aging.
By injection, hyaluronic acid is used as an adjunct in cataract surgery, detached retina, corneal transplantation, and eye trauma. It is also used for treating osteoarthritis and as a lip filler in plastic surgery.
Topically, hyaluronic acid is used for healing wounds, burns, skin ulcers, stomatitis, and moisturizing the skin.
In the ear, hyaluronic acid is used in tympanostomy tubes (ear tubes).

Safety

LIKELY SAFE ...when used topically and appropriately (7889,9126). ...when used parenterally and appropriately (7885,7886,7887,9319). There is insufficient reliable information about the safety of oral use of hyaluronic acid.
PREGNANCY: POSSIBLY SAFE ...when used parenterally and appropriately (7890). There is insufficient reliable information about the safety of oral and topical use of hyaluronic acid; avoid using.
LACTATION: POSSIBLY UNSAFE ...when used parenterally. There is insufficient reliable information about the safety of oral and topical use of hyaluronic acid. It is not known if hyaluronic acid is excreted in breast milk, avoid using (7890).

Effectiveness

LIKELY EFFECTIVE

Cataracts. Injecting hyaluronic acid into the eye is effective as an adjunct to cataract surgery (9139). Hyaluronic acid is approved by the FDA for use as an adjunct to cataract surgery, corneal transplantation, lens implantation, and glaucoma filtering surgery (8923).

Oral mucositis. Applying hyaluronic acid topically is an effective treatment for oral mucositis (stomatitis) (7889). An oral gel preparation of hyaluronic acid is approved by the FDA for treating oral mucositis (7892).

POSSIBLY EFFECTIVE

Osteoarthritis. Despite being approved by the FDA for treatment of osteoarthritis by intra-articular injection, hyaluronic acid seems to be variably effective (7887,7888,7890,7891). Subjective symptoms of stiffness and joint pain decrease modestly with hyaluronic acid treatment, but the effect of treatment is often not clinically significant (7887,7888). Whether hyaluronic acid might delay or lessen progressive joint damage with long-term use is unknown (7886).

INSUFFICIENT RELIABLE EVIDENCE to RATE

Eye trauma. In ophthalmology, some research suggests hyaluronic acid might be used as an intraocular injection in detached retina and eye trauma (9126).

Wound healing. Preliminary evidence suggests topical hyaluronic acid might be useful for treating burns, wounds, and skin ulcers (8497,9126,9139).

More evidence is needed to rate hyaluronic acid for these uses.

Mechanism of Action

Hyaluronic acid is a polysaccharide chain of repeating disaccharide units. It is found throughout the body where it serves as part of the supporting structure in the extracellular space. It is found most abundantly in cartilage, synovial fluid, skin, and the aqueous humor in the eye (9139). The disaccharide moiety consists of sodium acetyl glucosamine and sodium glucuronate (8498). Hyaluronic acid is obtained from rooster combs and from bacterial fermentation. The source and preparation method determine the molecular weight, which varies between 90,000 and 5,000,000 daltons.
The primary therapeutic effects of hyaluronic acid are physical lubricating and cushioning. The viscosity of hyaluronic acid increases as the concentration, molecular weight, and polysaccharide chain length increase (9139).
In addition to its physiochemical properties, hyaluronic acid might act as an antioxidant and modulate the immune system. Some research suggests it might prevent the breakdown of natural cushioning barriers in joint (9134,9139).
Hyaluronic acid seems to bind to cellular receptors on located on the surface membrane of cartilage and other cell types, possibly modulating immune response and improving wound healing (7883,9126). In osteoarthritis, hyaluronic acid might inhibit the release of enzymes that contribute to the breakdown of cartilage. It seems to inhibit chemotactic factors and phagocytosis by mononuclear leukocytes. High molecular weight hyaluronic acid (greater than 500,000 daltons) is used for treating osteoarthritis. After intraarticular injection, hyaluronic acid is present for only a few days, but its effects last for about six months (7883,7884). In promoting wound healing, hyaluronic acid might improve blood flow, regulate inflammatory processes, and promote formation of granulation tissue (9126). In addition, hyaluronic acid improves hydration of the wound margins (8497).
Preliminary evidence indicates that hyaluronic acid can decrease adhesions to devices implanted during surgical procedures (7882). It does not improve healing in experimental models of tympanostomy tube (ear tube) placement (8493).
The half-life of hyaluronic acid in serum is 2.5 to 5.5 minutes. It is eliminated from circulation through uptake and biotransformation in the liver and spleen (9139). No information is available about the behavior of hyaluronic acid after oral administration. However, because of its pharmacokinetic characteristics, it would not be expected to achieve significant blood concentrations after oral administration.

Adverse Reactions

Injected intra-articularly, hyaluronic acid can cause redness and soreness at the site of injection. Hyaluronic acid may rarely cause allergic reactions. Anaphylaxis occurs extremely rarely (7884,7885,7894).
After intraocular injection during eye surgery, hyaluronic acid commonly causes increased intraocular pressure. Increased intraocular pressure peaks approximately 24 hours after injection and resolves within 48 to 72 hours (8494,8495,9139). Aspiration of residual hyaluronic acid following surgery does not completely prevent this increased pressure (8496). Timolol drops 0.5% may be used to reduce the intraocular pressure (7893).

Interactions with Herbs & Other Dietary Supplements

None known.

Interactions with Drugs

None known.

Interactions with Foods

None known.

Interactions with Lab Tests

None known.

Interactions with Diseases or Conditions

None known.

Dosage and Administration

INTRA-ARTICULAR INJECTION: For treating osteoarthritis, hyaluronic acid 20 mg once per week for three to five weeks has been used (7886,7887).

Comments

Hyaluronic acid has been touted as a "fountain of youth." However, there is no evidence to support the claim that oral or topical use can prevent changes associated with aging.

HYDRANGEA

Also Known As

Mountain Hydrangea, Seven Barks, Smooth Hydrangea, Wild Hydrangea.

Scientific Names

Hydrangea arborescens, synonyms Viburnum alnifolium, Viburnum americanum.
Family: Hydrangeaceae.

People Use This For

Orally, hydrangea is used for conditions of the urinary tract, such as cystitis, urethritis, prostatitis, enlarged prostate, and urinary calculi. It is also used orally for allergic rhinitis.

Safety

POSSIBLY SAFE ...when used orally and appropriately, short-term (12).
LIKELY UNSAFE ...when used orally in excessive amounts (over 2 grams of dried rhizome/root per dose) (4,12).
...when used orally long-term (4,12).
PREGNANCY AND LACTATION: Insufficient reliable information available; avoid using.

Effectiveness

There is insufficient reliable information available about the effectiveness of hydrangea.

Mechanism of Action

The applicable parts of hydrangea are the rhizome and root. Researchers think hydrangea possesses mild diuretic activity and properties that prevent the formation of stones or calculus (4). The cyanogenic glycoside constituent, hydrangin, may be responsible for some of the potential adverse effects (12).

Adverse Reactions

Orally, hydrangea can cause gastroenteritis (4). Overdose symptoms include vertigo and a feeling of tightness in the chest (4). There is one case report of cholestatic hepatitis associated with Prostata, a multi-ingredient product containing hydrangea (598).

Interactions with Herbs & Other Dietary Supplements
None known.

Interactions with Drugs
None known.

Interactions with Foods
None known.

Interactions with Lab Tests
None known.

Interactions with Diseases or Conditions
None known.

Dosage and Administration
ORAL: A typical dose is 2-4 grams dried rhizome and root three times daily or one cup tea (steep 2-4 grams dried rhizome and root in 150 mL boiling water 5-10 minutes, strain) three times daily (4,12). Liquid extract (1:1 in 25% alcohol), 2-4 mL three times daily has been used (4,12). Tincture (1:5 in 45% alcohol), 2-10 mL three times daily is commonly used (4).

HYDRAZINE SULFATE

Also Known As
Sehydrin.

Scientific Names
Hydrazine sulfate.

People Use This For
Orally, hydrazine sulfate is used for treating colorectal cancer, lung cancer, neuroblastoma, Hodgkin's disease, and other cancers. It is also used for the general weight loss and wasting (cachexia) associated with cancer.

Safety
POSSIBLY UNSAFE ...when used orally. Hydrazine has been linked to cases of significant adverse effects including hepatotoxicity, seizure, coma, and death (8005,10384,10385,12780).
PREGNANCY AND LACTATION: POSSIBLY UNSAFE ...when used orally. Hydrazine has been linked to cases of significant adverse effects including hepatotoxicity, seizure, coma, and death (8005,10384,10385,12780).

Effectiveness
POSSIBLY INEFFECTIVE

Colorectal cancer. Taking hydrazine sulfate orally as a single agent doesn't seem to improve metastatic colorectal cancer (8002).

LIKELY INEFFECTIVE

Lung cancer. Taking hydrazine sulfate orally as an adjunct to chemotherapy is not helpful for treating non-small cell lung cancer. Hydrazine doesn't significantly improve quality of life, tumor response, weight gain, or survival in these patients (8001,8003,11368).

INSUFFICIENT RELIABLE EVIDENCE to RATE

Cachexia. There is preliminary evidence that hydrazine sulfate might slow weight loss in some cancer patients (8004).

Cancer. Preliminary clinical research suggests hydrazine sulfate is ineffective for treating ovarian cancer, colorectal cancer, breast cancer, lung cancer, pancreatic cancer, endocervical cancer, prostate cancer, uterine cancer, melanoma, and other kinds of cancer (11767).

Neuroblastoma and Hodgkin's disease. There is some evidence that hydrazine sulfate might prevent the growth of neuroblastoma and advanced Hodgkin's disease (10385).

More evidence is needed to rate hydrazine sulfate for these uses.

Mechanism of Action
Hydrazine sulfate is an organic compound used in various industrial processes and as jet fuel (8000). It is also a metabolite of isoniazid (12779).

Hydrazine sulfate inhibits phosphoenolpyruvate kinase (8000), an enzyme involved in gluconeogenesis. Some researchers theorize that excessive gluconeogenesis might be partially responsible for the cachexia that occurs in cancer patients (8000,8005). By blocking gluconeogenesis, hydrazine sulfate might reduce cachexia (8000).

Adverse Reactions

Orally, hydrazine sulfate can cause gastrointestinal adverse effects including nausea, vomiting, anorexia, heartburn, and diarrhea or constipation. It also frequently causes neurologic adverse effects including paresthesias, dizziness, drowsiness, peripheral neuropathies, mood stimulation, excitement, weakness, confusion, headache, blurred vision, and taste disturbances.
Other adverse effects include rash, irregular breathing, hypoglycemia or hyperglycemia, and diaphoresis. Hydrazine has also caused cases of lethargy, violent behavior, restlessness, seizures, coma, renal toxicity, and hepatotoxicity (8005,10384,10385,11767). In one case, fatal hepatorenal failure occurred in a patient with cancer who was taking hydrazine 180 mg per day (10384).

Interactions with Herbs & Other Dietary Supplements

HERBS AND SUPPLEMENTS WITH HYPOGLYCEMIC EFFECTS: There is some evidence that hydrazine sulfate might have hypoglycemic effects (11767). Theoretically, concomitant use with other herbs and supplements that decrease blood glucose levels might increase the risk of hypoglycemia. Some of these products include bitter melon, cowhage, ginger, goat's rue, fenugreek, kudzu, willow bark, and others.
PYRIDOXINE (Vitamin B6): Hydrazine may antagonize the action of pyridoxine (10384).

Interactions with Drugs

ANTIDIABETES DRUGS: Hydrazine sulfate can reduce blood glucose levels and might have additive effects on glucose levels when used with antidiabetes drug therapy (11767). Monitor blood glucose levels closely. Medication dose adjustments may be necessary. Some antidiabetes drugs include glimepiride (Amaryl), glyburide (DiaBeta, Glynase PresTab, Micronase), insulin, pioglitazone (Actos), rosiglitazone (Avandia), and others.
CNS DEPRESSANTS: Concomitant use with alcohol, barbiturates, or benzodiazepines can increase the toxicity and decrease the effectiveness of hydrazine (8005).
ISONIAZID (INH): Hydrazine is a metabolite of isoniazid and might be responsible for isoniazid-induced hepatotoxicity (12779). Theoretically, concurrent use of isoniazid and hydrazine might increase the risk for liver damage.
MONOAMINE OXIDASE INHIBITORS (MAOIs): Theoretically, concomitant use might increase the effects and adverse effects associated with MAOIs (8005).

Interactions with Foods

TYRAMINE-CONTAINING FOODS: Avoid concomitant use, hydrazine sulfate may have monoamine oxidase inhibiting activity (8005). Tyramine-containing foods, include avocado, banana, brewer's yeast, broad beans, caviar, aged cheese, aged red wine, herring, liver, and pickled meats.

Interactions with Lab Tests

5-HYDROXYINDOLACETIC ADIC (5-HIAA): Hydrazine sulfate can decrease urine levels and test results (275).
ALANINE AMINOTRANSFERASE (ALT): Hydrazine sulfate can increase serum levels and test results secondary to hepatotoxicity (275).
ALKALINE PHOSPHATASE (Alk Phos): Hydrazine sulfate can increase serum levels and test results secondary to hepatotoxicity (11767).
ASPARTATE AMINOTRANSFERASE (AST): Hydrazine sulfate can increase serum levels and test results secondary to hepatotoxicity (11767).
BILE: Hydrazine sulfate can increase urine levels and test results secondary to hepatotoxicity (275).
BILIRUBIN: Hydrazine sulfate can increase serum levels and test results secondary to hepatotoxicity (11767).
BROMOSULFOPHTHALEIN (BSP) RETENTION: Hydrazine sulfate can increase serum levels and test results secondary to hepatotoxicity (275).
ERYTHROCYTE SEDIMENTATION RATE (ESR): Hydrazine sulfate can increase sedimentation rate results secondary to a SLE-type syndrome (275).
GLUCOSE: Hydrazine sulfate can decrease serum glucose and test results by potentiating insulin effects (11767).
LACTATE DEHYDROGENASE (LDH): Hydrazine sulfate can increase LDH levels (11767).
LUPUS ERYTHEMATOSUS (LE) CELLS: Hydrazine sulfate can cause a positive blood test result by activating LE (275).
LYMPHOCYTES: Hydrazine sulfate can decrease blood levels and test results with megadose supplementation (275).
METANEPHRINES (total): Hydrazine sulfate can increase urine levels and test results (275).
NORMETANEPHRINE: Hydrazine sulfate can increase urine levels and test results (275).
VANILLYLMANDELIC ACID: Hydrazine sulfate can increase urine levels and test results (275).

Interactions with Diseases or Conditions

DIABETES: Hydrazine sulfate might interfere with blood glucose control due to effects on gluconeogenesis (8000).
LIVER DISEASE: Hydrazine can cause hepatotoxicity (10384,12779,12780,). Avoid using hydrazine in patients with liver disease.

Dosage and Administration

ORAL: For cachexia in people with cancer on a chemotherapy regimen, a typical dose used is 60 mg three times daily for a cycle of 30-45 days followed by a rest period of 2-6 weeks (8004,8005,10385).

Comments

Although some information shows hydrazine sulfate might be useful in the general weight loss and wasting associated with cancer, information is very limited and inconclusive (12780).

HYDROXYMETHYLBUTYRATE (HMB)

Also Known As

B-Hydroxy B-Methylbutyrate Monohydrate, Beta-Hydroxy-Beta-Methylbutyric Acid, HMB, Hydroxymethyl Butyrate.

Scientific Names

Beta-hydroxy-beta-methylbutyrate.

People Use This For

Orally, HMB is used for increasing the benefits from weight training and exercise, and treating cardiovascular disease, hypercholesterolemia, and hypertension. In combination with arginine and glutamine, HMB is also used orally for treating weight loss in people with AIDS.

Safety

POSSIBLY SAFE ...when used orally and appropriately, short-term. Doses of 3 grams per day or less for up to eight weeks seem to be safe (1909,2167,2168,3374).

PREGNANCY AND LACTATION: Insufficient reliable information available; avoid using.

Effectiveness

POSSIBLY EFFECTIVE

AIDS-related wasting. Taking HMB orally in combination with arginine and glutamine seems to increase body weight and lean body mass, and possibly improve immune function when used over eight weeks to prevent wasting in patients with Acquired Immunodeficiency Syndrome (AIDS) (1909).

INSUFFICIENT RELIABLE EVIDENCE to RATE

Athletic conditioning. There is conflicting evidence about the usefulness of HMB for weight training. Some research suggests HMB might increase muscular strength and body composition, and reduce muscle damage; other research shows no effect (1929,2167,2168,8968). Additionally, there are data that suggest that HMB may be more effective in people who have not previously trained, than in well-trained individuals (11003).

Hypercholesterolemia. There is preliminary clinical evidence that HMB can lower cholesterol (3374).

Hypertension. There is preliminary clinical evidence that HMB can lower blood pressure (3374).

More evidence is needed to rate HMB for these uses.

Mechanism of Action

Hydroxymethylbutyrate (HMB) is a byproduct of metabolism of the amino acid leucine (2168). HMB is also a precursor to cholesterol. HMB found in the cytosol of liver and muscle cells is converted to beta-hydroxy-beta-methylglutarate-Co-A (HMG-CoA). HMG-CoA is used for the cellular synthesis of cholesterol, and might also promote muscle growth by reducing the catabolism of muscle protein (2168,3374). There is also some evidence that HMB lowers levels of creatine phosphokine (CK) and lactate dehydrogenase (LDH), and decreases the excretion of 3-methylhistidine (3-MH). This suggests that HMB might also prevent or decrease muscle membrane inflammation or injury, and prevent increased proteolysis that is often associated with intense exercise (1929,2168).

Adverse Reactions

None reported.

Interactions with Herbs & Other Dietary Supplements

None known.

Interactions with Drugs

None known.

Interactions with Foods

None known.

Interactions with Lab Tests
None known.

Interactions with Diseases or Conditions
None known.

Dosage and Administration
ORAL: For treatment of AIDS-related wasting, 3 grams HMB in combination with 14 grams each of arginine and glutamine administered in two divided doses daily has been used (1909). For lowering cholesterol and blood pressure, 3 grams daily has been used (3374). For muscle building and increasing body strength during weight training, doses of 1 gram three times daily (1929,2167) or 1.5 grams once or twice daily has been used (3374).

HYSSOP

Also Known As
Hissopo, Hysope Officinale, Jufa, Rabo De Gato, Ysop.

Scientific Names
Hyssopus officinalis.
Family: Lamiaceae/Labiatae.

People Use This For
Orally, hyssop is used for liver and gallbladder complaints, intestinal inflammation, coughs, colds, respiratory and chest ailments, sore throats, asthma, urinary tract inflammation, gas and colic, to stimulate appetite and circulation, as an expectorant, for menstrual complaints, and for digestive and intestinal problems.
Topically, hyssop is used as a gargle; in baths to induce sweating; and for treating skin irritations, burns, bruises, and frostbite.
In foods, hyssop oil and extract are used as a flavoring.
In manufacturing, hyssop oil is used as a fragrance in soaps and cosmetics.

Safety
LIKELY SAFE ...when used orally in amounts commonly found in foods. Hyssop, hyssop oil, and hyssop extract have Generally Recognized As Safe (GRAS) status in the US (4912).
POSSIBLY SAFE ...when used orally and appropriately in medicinal amounts (12).
POSSIBLY UNSAFE ...when the oil is used orally for medicinal purposes. There are reports that associate ingestion of the oil with tonic-clonic convulsions (2,18).
There is insufficient reliable information available about the safety of hyssop for its other uses.
CHILDREN: LIKELY UNSAFE ...when used orally because of a report that 2-3 drops of oil over several days caused tonic-clonic convulsions (2,18); avoid using.
PREGNANCY: LIKELY UNSAFE ...when used orally because it might cause uterine stimulant and menstrual stimulant effects (12).
LACTATION: Insufficient reliable information available; avoid using.

Effectiveness
There is insufficient reliable information available about the effectiveness of hyssop.

Mechanism of Action
The applicable parts of hyssop are the above ground parts. Constituent marrubiin (11) has cardioactive effects and stimulates bronchial secretions (4). Caffeic acid and tannins may be responsible for the effect of extracts of dried leaves. Extracts show antiviral activity against herpes simplex virus and HIV in vitro (6,11). Hyssop oil causes convulsions (of CNS origin) and death in experimental rats (6), thought due to constituents pincamphone and isopincamphone (6). Hyssop oil is associated with tonic-clonic convulsions in adults and children (2,18).

Adverse Reactions
Orally, hyssop was associated with tonic-clonic convulsions in two adults (10-30 drops) and in one child (2-3 drops for several days) (2,18).

Interactions with Herbs & Other Dietary Supplements
None known.

Interactions with Drugs
None known.

Interactions with Foods
None known.

Interactions with Lab Tests
None known.

Interactions with Diseases or Conditions
SEIZURE DISORDERS: Theoretically, hyssop oil may exacerbate seizure disorders.

Dosage and Administration
ORAL: Typically people take two 445 mg capsules containing the hyssop herb three times daily (5019). Some people take 10-15 drops of the hyssop extract (12-14% by volume) in water two to three times daily (5023). People also consume or gargle the hyssop tea three times daily (6002). The tea is prepared by steeping 1-2 teaspoons of the dried hyssop flower tops in 150 mL boiling water for 10-15 minutes and then straining. Avoid internal use of hyssop oil due to possible neurotoxicity.
TOPICAL: No typical dosage.

IBOGA

Also Known As
None.

Scientific Names
Tabernanthe iboga.
Family: Apocyanceae.

People Use This For
Orally, iboga is used as an aperitif, aphrodisiac, tonic, for convalescence, debility, fever, flu, hypertension, neurasthenia, and preventing fatigue and drowsiness.

Safety
There is insufficient reliable information available about the safety of iboga.
Pregnancy and Lactation: Insufficient reliable information available; avoid using.

Effectiveness
There is insufficient reliable information available about the effectiveness of iboga.

Mechanism of Action
The applicable part of iboga is the root. The hallucinogenic properties of iboga are due to the indole alkaloids, ibogaine, ibogamone, iboluteine, and tabernanthine (6,271). Ibogaine inhibits cholinesterase, leading to synaptic acetylcholine accumulation (6). The associated dose-dependent CNS stimulation ranges from mild excitation and euphoria to visual and auditory hallucinations (6,271). Ibogaine has kappa agonist effects; it is serotonergic; and it exhibits nicotinic and N-methyl-D-aspartate (NMDA) antagonism (813). Animal experiments suggest these effects may have value in treating human addictions to alcohol, nicotine, opioids, cocaine, and other stimulants (812,813). The constituent tabernanthine demonstrates cardiac conduction effects similar to those of calcium channel antagonists (6).

Adverse Reactions
Iboga taken orally may cause bradycardia, hypotension, convulsions, paralysis, and respiratory arrest (6).
Amounts large enough to induce hallucinations may also cause anxiety, apprehension, and death (6).

Interactions with Herbs & Other Dietary Supplements
None known.

Interactions with Drugs
ANTICHOLINERGIC DRUGS: Theoretically, concomitant use can antagonize anticholinergic effects.
CHOLINERGIC DRUGS: Theoretically, concomitant use may enhance effects and adverse effects.

Interactions with Foods
None known.

Interactions with Lab Tests
None known.

Interactions with Diseases or Conditions
None known.

Dosage and Administration
ORAL: Dry root bark powder or root is chewed (6).

Comments
Iboga is used for ritual and ceremonial purposes in some African cultures (6,271,812).

ICELAND MOSS

Also Known As
Centraria, Eryngo-leaved Liverwort, Iceland Lichen, Lichen Islandicus.
CAUTION: See separate listing for Eryngo.

Scientific Names
Cetraria islandica.
Family: Parmeliaceae.

People Use This For
Orally, Iceland moss is used for irritation of the oral and pharyngeal mucous membranes and associated dry cough, for loss of appetite, common cold, cough and bronchitis, dyspeptic complaints, fevers, and the tendency toward infection, lung disease, and kidney and bladder complaints.
Topically Iceland moss is used for poorly healing wounds.
In foods, Iceland moss is utilized as an emergency food source in Iceland.
In manufacturing, Iceland moss is utilized as a flavoring agent in alcoholic beverages.

Safety
POSSIBLY SAFE ...when the dried plant is used orally, short-term for medicinal use (3,12). The dried plant can be contaminated with lead (3).
POSSIBLY UNSAFE ...when consumed in larger amounts as a food source because lead contamination can occur in amounts of up to 30 mg/kg of its dry weight (3). It is regulated in the US and allowable only as a flavoring agent in alcoholic beverages (12).
PREGNANCY AND LACTATION: POSSIBLY UNSAFE ...when used orally; avoid Iceland moss due to the potential for lead contamination (3).

Effectiveness
There is insufficient reliable information available about the effectiveness of Iceland moss.

Mechanism of Action
The applicable part of Iceland moss is the dried plant body. Iceland moss has soothing and mild antimicrobial action (2). The mucilage constituents, lichenin and isolichenin, and the bitter principles can be responsible for its effects (2,3). The bitter organic acid constituents can be responsible for an antibiotic effect (18).

Adverse Reactions
Orally, Iceland moss can cause GI irritation (12). Sensitization to Iceland moss is rare (18). It can be contaminated with lead up to 30 mg/kg of its dry weight (3).

Interactions with Herbs & Other Dietary Supplements
None known.

Interactions with Drugs
ORAL DRUGS: The mucilage in Iceland moss can impair absorption of oral drugs (19).

Interactions with Foods
None known.

Interactions with Lab Tests
None known.

Interactions with Diseases or Conditions
GASTRODUODENAL ULCERS: The alcohol extract and powder of Iceland moss is contraindicated due to the potential for mucosal irritation (12).

Dosage and Administration

ORAL: The typical dose of Iceland moss is one cup of tea several times daily. The tea is prepared by steeping or simmering 1.5-3 grams of the dried plant in 150 mL boiling water for 5-10 minutes and then straining (3,7). The maximum dose of the moss is 4-6 grams per day of the dried plant or equivalent preparations (2).

Comments

Iceland moss is a lichen, or an algae and a fungus growing together in a symbiotic relationship (3). Iceland is one the least polluted countries in the world, which is important for lichens. Lichens derive their nutrients from the environment and are easily contaminated with radioactive or heavy metals. Most of the lichens in Europe were contaminated by the fallout from the Chernobyl accident, but Iceland only received negligible radioactive levels (6002).

IDEBENONE

Also Known As

Hydroxydecyl benzoquinone.

Scientific Names

2,3-dimethoxy-5-methyl-6-(10-hydroxydecyl)-1,4-benzoquinone.

People Use This For

Orally, idebenone is used for Alzheimer's disease, Leber's disease, liver disease, cerebrovascular disease, mitochondrial encephalomyopathies, and Friedreich's ataxia.

Safety

POSSIBLY SAFE ...when used orally and appropriately. Idebenone seems to be safe when used for up to 2 years (11410,11413,11421,11427).

PREGNANCY AND LACTATION: Insufficient reliable information available; avoid using.

Effectiveness

POSSIBLY EFFECTIVE

Alzheimer's disease. There's some evidence that taking idebenone orally slows cognitive function decline in patients with Alzheimer's disease. Idebenone appears most effective in patients with moderately severe Alzheimer's disease, based on standard Alzheimer's disease rating scales (11421,11427).

INSUFFICIENT RELIABLE EVIDENCE to RATE

Friedreich's ataxia. Some preliminary clinical evidence suggests that taking idebenone orally may help control cardiac hypertrophy associated with Friedreich's ataxia, a genetic degenerative neurological disorder (11410,11413,11416,11418). Other research has failed to show an effect (11415). However, idebenone does not appear to slow the progression of ataxia (11410,11411).

Mitochondrial encephalomyopathies. There is preliminary clinical research that suggests idebenone given orally might reduce symptoms in patients with mitochondrial dysfunction such as MELAS (myoclonic epilepsy with lactic acidosis and stroke-like episodes) syndrome (11422,11424,11426).

More evidence is needed to rate idebenone for these uses.

Mechanism of Action

Idebenone is a synthetic quinone, similar to coenzyme Q-10. It diffuses across cell membranes more readily than coenzyme Q-10 and reaches concentrations in the brain similar to the plasma. Idebenone also distributes into tissues, with highest concentrations found in the kidney, gut, and liver. After oral administration, the half-life of idebenone is approximately 18 hours (11414,11417).

Many of the therapeutic benefits of idebenone are attributed to its antioxidant effects. As an antioxidant, idebenone appears to protect a wide variety of cell membranes and mitochondria from oxidative stress by inhibiting lipid peroxidation. Idebenone also seems to maintain ATP formation in ischemic sites, possibly by functioning as a carrier within the electron transport chain. These properties seem to protect the central nervous system from nerve damage and ischemia (11412,11417,11419,11420,11423,11425). Idebenone may also slow cognitive function decline in patients with Alzheimer's disease, possibly by stimulating nerve growth factor (11417).

Adverse Reactions

Orally, idebenone is well tolerated. In clinical studies, there have been no reports of significant adverse effects (11410,11413,11416,11418,11421,11422,11424,11426,11427).

Interactions with Herbs & Other Dietary Supplements

None known.

Interactions with Drugs
None known.

Interactions with Foods
None known.

Interactions with Lab Tests
None known.

Interactions with Diseases or Conditions
None known.

Dosage and Administration
ORAL: For Alzheimer's disease, idebenone 90 to 120 mg three times daily has been used (11421,11427).
For Friedreich's ataxia, 5 to 10 mg per kg divided three times daily has been used (11409,11413).
For mitochondrial encephalomyopathies, 90 to 270 mg divided three times daily has been used (11422,11424,11426).

IGNATIUS BEAN

Also Known As
Lu Song Guo, Saint Ignatius-beans.

Scientific Names
Strychnos ignatii, synonym Strychnos tieute.
Family: Loganiaceae.

People Use This For
Orally, ignatius bean is used for faintness; as a bitter or tonic; and as an agent to invigorate, refresh, or restore body function.

Safety
UNSAFE ...when used orally due to its strychnine content (18). The FDA banned strychnine from nonprescription drug products in 1989.
PREGNANCY AND LACTATION: UNSAFE ...when used orally due to toxic effects (18).

Effectiveness
There is insufficient reliable information available about the effectiveness of ignatius bean.

Mechanism of Action
Ignatius bean contains the centrally-acting neurotoxins strychnine and brucine (18). Strychnine competitively antagonizes post-synaptic binding of the inhibitory transmitter glycine, leading to heightened reflex excitability of muscles and convulsions (505). Strychnine can selectively inhibit the spinal cord in subconvulsive amounts (2). However, strychnine accumulates with extended administration, particularly in individuals with liver damage. Chronic use of subconvulsive amounts can cause death after a period of weeks (18).

Adverse Reactions
Orally, 30-50 mg ignatius bean (5 mg strychnine) can cause restlessness, feelings of anxiety, heightening of sense perception, enhanced reflexes, equilibrium disorders, painful neck and back stiffness, followed later by twitching, tonic spasms of jaw and neck muscles, painful convulsions of the entire body triggered by visual or tactile stimulation with possible opisthotonos, muscle hypertonicity, and agitation. Dyspnea may follow spasm of respiratory muscles (18). Seizures occur within 15 minutes of ingestion (or 5 minutes of inhalation) and may result in hyperthermia, metabolic and respiratory acidosis, rhabdomyolysis, and myoglobinuric renal failure (17). 1-2 grams of ignatius bean (50 mg strychnine) can be fatal (18); most deaths occur 3-6 hours post-ingestion from respiratory and subsequent cardiac arrest, anoxic brain damage, or multiple organ failure secondary to hyperthermia (18,505). Strychnine accumulates with extended administration, particularly in individuals with liver damage. Chronic use of subconvulsive amounts can cause death after a period of weeks (18).

Interactions with Herbs & Other Dietary Supplements
None known.

Interactions with Drugs
None known.

Interactions with Foods
None known.

Interactions with Lab Tests
None known.

Interactions with Diseases or Conditions
LIVER DISEASE: Contraindicated; strychnine accumulates in individuals with liver damage. Also, strychnine accumulation can cause liver damage (18).

Dosage and Administration
No typical dose.

Comments
Strychnine may be detected by thin-layer chromatography (qualitative analysis) and high performance liquid chromatography (quantitative analysis). Urine and gastric aspirate are most useful in confirming poisoning (17).

IMMORTELLE

Also Known As
Common Shrubby Everlasting, Eternal Flower, Goldilocks, Yellow Chaste Weed.
CAUTION: See separate listing for Sandy Everlasting.

Scientific Names
Helichrysum arenarium.
Family: Compositae/Asteraceae.

People Use This For
Orally, immortelle is used for liver and gallbladder disorders, including chronic gallstones with accompanying cramps. It is also used orally for dyspepsia, loss of appetite, to stimulate bile flow, as a diuretic, and as an antimicrobial.

Safety
There is insufficient reliable information available about the safety of immortelle.
Pregnancy and Lactation: Insufficient reliable information available; avoid using.

Effectiveness
There is insufficient reliable information available about the effectiveness of immortelle.

Mechanism of Action
The applicable part of immortelle is the dried flower. There is insufficient reliable information available about the possible mechanism of action and active ingredients.

Adverse Reactions
When immortelle is used in people with gallstones, it may cause colic (18). Immortelle can cause an allergic reaction in individuals sensitive to the Asteraceae/Compositae family. Members of this family include ragweed, chrysanthemums, marigolds, daisies, and many other herbs.

Interactions with Herbs & Other Dietary Supplements
None known.

Interactions with Drugs
None known.

Interactions with Foods
None known.

Interactions with Lab Tests
None known.

Interactions with Diseases or Conditions

BILIARY OBSTRUCTION: Immortelle is contraindicated during biliary obstruction secondary to its possible stimulation of biliary flow.
CROSS-ALLERGENICITY: Can cause an allergic reaction in individuals sensitive to the Asteraceae/Compositae family. Members of this family include ragweed, chrysanthemums, marigolds, daisies, and many other herbs.

Dosage and Administration

ORAL: One cup of tea daily. The tea is prepared by steeping 3-4 grams dried flower in 150 mL of boiling water for 10 minutes and straining. The tea is sometimes drunk throughout the day, but must be made fresh each time. The average daily dose is 3 grams of immortelle (18).

Comments

Immortelle is a protected species. It can easily be confused with sandy everlasting (Helichrysum augustifolium, synonym Helichrysum italicum), or Helichrysum stoechas (18). Avoid confusion with immortal (Asclepias asperula) (11).

INDIAN FRANKINCENSE

Also Known As

Boswellia, Boswellin, Boswellin Serrata Resin, Gajabhakshya, Indian Olibanum, Salai Guggal, Sallaki Guggul, Shallaki.
CAUTION: See separate listings for Frankincense and Guggul.

Scientific Names

Boswellia serrata.
Family: Burseraceae.

People Use This For

Orally, Indian frankincense is used for osteoarthritis, rheumatoid arthritis (RA), rheumatism, bursitis, and tendonitis. Other uses include ulcerative colitis, abdominal pain, asthma, allergic rhinitis, sore throat, syphilis, painful menstruation, pimples, and cancer. It is also used as a stimulant, respiratory antiseptic, diuretic, and for stimulating menstrual flow.
In manufacturing, Indian frankincense resin oil and extracts are used in soaps, cosmetics, foods, and beverages.

Safety

LIKELY SAFE... when used orally in amounts commonly found in foods (4912).
POSSIBLY SAFE ...when used orally and appropriately in medicinal amounts, short-term.
Safety beyond 12 weeks is unknown (1708,1709,12432,12433,12434,12436,12438).
PREGNANCY AND LACTATION: LIKELY SAFE ...when used orally in amounts commonly found in foods (4912). There is insufficient reliable information available about the safety of Indian frankincense in medicinal amounts.

Effectiveness

INSUFFICIENT RELIABLE EVIDENCE to RATE

Asthma. There is some preliminary evidence that taking Indian frankincense extract orally might help asthma. It may improve force expiratory volume (FEV), reduce the number of asthma attacks, and decrease dyspnea and rhonchi (1708).
Inflammatory bowel disease (IBD). There is preliminary evidence that taking Indian frankincense extract orally might reduce symptoms of inflammatory bowel disease. It seems to work as well as mesalazine (Asacol, Pentasa) for Crohn's disease (12436). The evidence for ulcerative colitis is conflicting (1709,12438).
Osteoarthritis. There is some preliminary evidence that taking Indian frankincense extract orally might reduce osteoarthritis symptoms such as knee pain and swelling (12432).
Rheumatoid arthritis. There is conflicting research about the usefulness of Indian frankincense extract taken orally for rheumatoid arthritis (12433,12434).
More evidence is needed to rate Indian frankincense for these uses.

Mechanism of Action

The applicable part of Indian frankincense is the resin. The principle constituents of Indian frankincense are boswellic acid and alpha- and beta-boswellic acid, which have anti-inflammatory properties (1706).

In preliminary research, Indian frankincense extracts show anti-inflammatory and antiarthritis effects, but not all Indian frankincense-containing products have antiarthritis, anti-inflammatory, or antipyretic effects (12432). Boswellic acids inhibit 5-lipoxygenase and leukotriene synthesis, and inhibit leukocyte elastase, which are the likely mechanisms for its anti-inflammatory properties. Boswellic acids also might have disease modifying effect, decreasing glycosaminoglycan degradation and cartilage damage. Indian frankincense also might inhibit mediators of autoimmune disorders. It seems to reduce production of antibodies and cell-mediated immunity (12432,12435,12437,12438).

Indian frankincense might be useful in treating cancer. Preliminary research suggests that boswellic acids have an antiproliferative and apoptotic effect on cancer cells (12435).

Preliminary research suggests boswellic acids stabilize mast cells, which suggests usefulness for asthma (12439).

Other preliminary research suggests that boswellic acids might prevent organ rejection and ischemia/reperfusion injury (12440).

Indian frankincense has an elimination half-life of 6 hours (12441).

Adverse Reactions

Orally, Indian frankincense can cause gastrointestinal (GI) adverse effects such as epigastric pain, heartburn, nausea, and diarrhea (12432,12438).

Topically, Indian frankincense can cause contact dermatitis (12442).

Interactions with Herbs & Other Dietary Supplements

None known.

Interactions with Drugs

None known.

Interactions with Foods

None known.

Interactions with Lab Tests

None known.

Interactions with Diseases or Conditions

None known.

Dosage and Administration

ORAL: For osteoarthritis, Indian frankincense extract 333 mg three times daily has been used (12432). For rheumatoid arthritis, Indian frankincense extract 3600 mg daily has been used (12433). For ulcerative colitis, a gum resin preparation of 350 mg three times daily has been used (1709). For bronchial asthma, a dosage of 300 mg three times daily has been used (1708).

Comments

Olibanum is another word for frankincense. It refers to the oleogum resin exuded from incisions in the bark of several Boswellia species, including Boswellia serrata, Boswellia carterii, and Boswellia frereana. Of these, Boswellia serrata is most commonly used medicinally (12443).

INDIAN GOOSEBERRY

Also Known As

Aamalaki, Amalaki, Amblabaum, Amla, Aonla, Emblic, Emblic Myrobalan, Emblica, Groseillier de Ceylan, Indian-Gooseberry, Mirobalano, Myrobalan Emblic, Neli.

Scientific Names

Phyllanthus emblica, synonyms Emblica officinalis, Mirobalanus embilica.

Family: Euphorbiaceae.

People Use This For

Orally, Indian gooseberry is used for lowering cholesterol, treating atherosclerosis, diabetes, pancreatitis cancer, dyspepsia, eye problems, joint pain, diarrhea, dysentery, "organ restoration", and as an anti-inflammatory and antimicrobial. It is also used orally for obesity.

Safety

LIKELY SAFE ...when consumed in amounts commonly found in foods (6,2076).
There is insufficient reliable information available about the safety of Indian gooseberry when used medicinally.
PREGNANCY AND LACTATION: Insufficient reliable information available; avoid using.

Effectiveness

There is insufficient reliable information available about the effectiveness of Indian gooseberry.

Mechanism of Action

The applicable part of Indian gooseberry is primarily the fruit (2075), but extracts from the leaves have also been used (2078,2079). Preliminary evidence suggests that Indian gooseberry fruit and juice may lower total serum cholesterol, low-density lipoprotein (LDL), triglycerides, and phospholipids without affecting high-density lipoprotein (HDL) levels; and it may have positive effects on atherosclerosis (2077,8180). Indian gooseberry fruit juice may also have antimicrobial, antimutagenic, and antioxidant activity (2080,2081). The leaf extract might have anti-inflammatory activity (2078,2079).

Adverse Reactions

None reported.

Interactions with Herbs & Other Dietary Supplements

None known.

Interactions with Drugs

None known.

Interactions with Foods

None known.

Interactions with Lab Tests

None known.

Interactions with Diseases or Conditions

None known.

Dosage and Administration

No typical dosage.

Comments

Indian gooseberry is a native deciduous tree in India and the Middle East. Indian gooseberry has been used in Ayurvedic medicine for thousands of years. Reference to Indian gooseberry appeared in an Ayurvedic medicine text in the seventh century (3563).

INDIAN LONG PEPPER

Also Known As

Bi Bo, Jaborandi Pepper, Kana, Langer Pfeffer, Long Pepper, Magadhi, Pimenta-Longa, Pippali, Poivre Long, Ushana.
CAUTION: See separate listings for Black Pepper and White Pepper, and Capsicum.

Scientific Names

Piper longum.
Family: Piperaceae.

People Use This For

Orally, Indian long pepper is used to treat headache, toothache, asthma, beri-beri, bronchitis, mucous membrane inflammation, cholera, coma, cough, diarrhea, dysentery, epilepsy, fever, frigidity, stomachache, stroke, heartburn, indigestion, insomnia, leprosy, lethargy, enlarged spleen, muscle pain, nasal discharge, painful menses, paralysis, psoriasis, sterility in women, snake bites, tetanus, thirst, tuberculosis, and tumors. It is also used during childbirth, and during the 3-6 weeks following childbirth while the uterus returns to normal size. The fruit is used orally to stimulate menstrual flow, appetite, and bile flow; to improve digestion; induce sweating; and as an abortifacient, analgesic, antiflatulent, aphrodisiac, astringent, bactericide, diuretic, larvicide, sedative, stimulant, tonic, and vermifuge.
In foods, the fruit is used in cooking, both as an ingredient and a spice. It is used in fresh or dried form.

Safety
There is insufficient reliable information available about the safety of Indian long pepper.

Effectiveness
There is insufficient reliable information available about the effectiveness of Indian long pepper.

Mechanism of Action
The applicable part of Indian long pepper is the fruit. Piper longum contains piperine which can increase oral absorption of drugs and other substances, possibly by modulating intestinal membrane dynamics (3757). Some evidence suggests an ethanolic extract and isolated piperine might have amoebicidal activity (3758). An Ayurvedic herbal preparation containing Piper longum and Butea monosperma (Pippali rasayana) shows evidence that it is useful for managing giardiasis (3754,3755). In mice, an ethanolic extract of piper longum administered chronically increased weights of lung, spleen, and reproductive organs. It also increased sperm count and motility without demonstrating acute or chronic toxicity (3756).

Adverse Reactions
None reported.

Interactions with Herbs & Other Dietary Supplements
SCOTCH BROOM: Piperine increases the bioavailability of sparteine, a constituent of scotch broom (19).

Interactions with Drugs
PHENYTOIN (Dilantin): Concomitant administration speeds absorption and slows elimination of phenytoin (Dilantin) (537).
PROPRANOLOL (Inderal): Concomitant administration speeds and increases absorption, and increases serum concentrations of propranolol (538).
THEOPHYLLINE: Concomitant administration increases absorption and serum concentrations of theophylline (538).

Interactions with Foods
None known.

Interactions with Lab Tests
SERUM DRUG ASSAYS: Indian long pepper can increase phenytoin, propranolol, and theophylline serum concentrations and test results (537,538).

Interactions with Diseases or Conditions
None known.

Dosage and Administration
No typical dosage.

Comments
Piper nigrum, the source of black pepper and white pepper, also contains the constituent piperine. However, red pepper and cayenne do not.

INDIAN PHYSIC

Also Known As
American Ipecacuanha, Bowman's Root, Gillenia, Indian Hippo.
CAUTION: See separate listings for Black Root and Canadian Hemp.

Scientific Names
Gillenia trifoliata, synonyms Porteranthus trifoliatus, Spiraea trifoliata.
Family: Rosaceae.

Comments
At the date of publication, this product was not a common ingredient used in brand name supplements marketed to consumers. Details about this product are available in the online version of *Natural Medicines Comprehensive Database.* See www.naturaldatabase.com.

INDIAN SNAKEROOT

Also Known As
Ajmaline, Chandrika, Chota-Chand, Covanamilpori, Dhanburua, Pagla-Ka-Dawa, Patalagandhi, Rauwolfae radix, Rauwolfia, Rauwolfia Serpentina, Rauwolfiawurzel, Sarpagandha, Serpentine-Wood, She Gen Mu.

Scientific Names
Rauvolfia serpentina, synonym Ophioxylon serpentinum.
Family: Apocynaceae.

People Use This For
Orally, Indian snakeroot is used for mild essential hypertension, symptomatic relief in individuals with agitated psychosis unable to tolerate other agents, for nervousness, and insomnia. Indian snakeroot is also used orally for snake and reptile bites, insanity, fever, constipation, feverish intestinal diseases, liver ailments, rheumatism, dropsy (edema), as a tonic for general debilities, for mental illness, and epilepsy.
As a prescription product, it is used to treat mild to moderate hypertension, schizophrenia, and vasospastic attacks due to peripheral vascular disorders.

Safety
POSSIBLY SAFE ...when the prescription product is used orally (15). ...when the standardized extract is used orally under the supervision of a medical professional trained in the use of Indian snakeroot (18).
POSSIBLY UNSAFE ...when used orally for self-medication. Appropriate use of Indian snakeroot requires medical diagnosis and treatment. Large amounts or overdose can lead to CNS depression, convulsions, extrapyramidal effects, and coma (15). ...when used by individuals operating motor vehicles or machinery. Indian snakeroot can alter reaction time (2,15).
PREGNANCY: LIKELY UNSAFE ...when used orally (2,18); the reserpine alkaloid constituents cross the placenta and can be potentially teratogenic (15,4260).
LACTATION: POSSIBLY UNSAFE ...when used orally. The reserpine alkaloids are excreted in breast milk (4260); avoid using.

Effectiveness
INSUFFICIENT RELIABLE EVIDENCE to RATE

Insomnia. Early evidence indicates that Indian snakeroot in a specific combination with two other herbs might offer some benefit for insomnia (6051). More evidence is needed to rate the effectiveness for this use.

Mechanism of Action
The applicable part of Indian snakeroot is the root. The properties of the whole root of rauwolfia serpentina differ from those of reserpine. The whole root contains over 50 alkaloids (13). Rauwolfia serpentina demonstrates hypotensive, sedative, and tranquilizing effects (15). It also reduces heart rate (13), has anti-arrhythmic effects (18), and causes a general sense of euphoria (13). The active constituents of the whole root include the rauwolfia alkaloids, reserpine, rescinnamine, and deserpidine (11-desmethoxyreseroine) (13). Hypotensive effects are believed to be due to the depletion of both catecholamine and serotonin stores and to the prevention of reabsorption (13,18). The greater the proportion of alkaloids present, the greater the hypotensive activity (13). The sedative effects of Indian snakeroot can result from the depletion of amine stores in the central nervous system (CNS) (13).

Adverse Reactions
Orally, low amounts of Indian snakeroot may cause adverse reactions including nasal congestion, abdominal cramps, diarrhea, nausea, vomiting, anorexia, increased gastric acid secretion, drowsiness, fatigue, lethargy, slowed reflexes, sexual dysfunction, and bradycardia. In larger amounts, mental depression may slowly develop. After discontinuation of Indian snakeroot, mental depression may persist for several months. In extremely large amounts, Parkinson-like symptoms, extrapyramidal reactions, and convulsions may occur. Allergic reactions from the use of Indian snakeroot are rare, but it may precipitate asthma (15).

Interactions with Herbs & Other Dietary Supplements
CARDIOACTIVE GLYCOSIDE-CONTAINING HERBS: Theoretically, concomitant use of Indian snakeroot may increase the risk of bradycardia (2,18), angina-like symptoms, and arrhythmias (15). Cardioactive glycoside containing herbs include black hellebore, digitalis, lily-of-the-valley, oleander leaf, pheasant's eye, and squill (19).
EPHEDRA: Theoretically, concomitant use of ephedra with Indian snakeroot may decrease ephedrine effects (15).

Interactions with Drugs

ALCOHOL (Ethanol): Use Indian snakeroot and ethanol with caution; concomitant use may increase the risk of additive CNS-depressant effects (15).
ANTIPSYCHOTIC DRUGS: Concomitant use of neuroleptics with Indian snakeroot may potentiate the effects of these drugs and the rauwolfia alkaloids (2,18).
BARBITURATES: Concomitant use of barbiturates with Indian snakeroot may potentiate the effects of these drugs and the rauwolfia alkaloids (2,18). Some of these sedative medications include pentobarbital (Nembutal), phenobarbital (Luminal), secobarbital (Seconal), and others.
DIGOXIN (Lanoxin): Concomitant use of digoxin with Indian snakeroot may cause bradycardia (2,18), angina-like symptoms, and arrhythmias (15). Avoid large amounts of the rauwolfia alkaloids together with digitalis cardiac glycosides (15).
DIURETIC DRUGS: Concomitant use of diuretics with Indian snakeroot may potentiate the hypotensive effects of rauwolfia alkaloids (15).
EPHEDRINE: Concomitant use of ephedrine with Indian snakeroot may reduce indirect-sympathomimetic drug activity (15).
LEVODOPA: Avoid using Indian snakeroot with levodopa; concomitant use may reduce drug effectiveness and increase extrapyramidal motor symptoms (15,18).
MONOAMINE OXIDASE INHIBITORS (MAOIs): Avoid concomitant or overlapping use of Indian snakeroot and MAOIs within several days. The overlap may increase the risk of excitation and hypertension (15).
PROPRANOLOL (Inderal): Concomitant use of propranolol with Indian snakeroot may enhance beta-blockade due to the rauwolfia alkaloid catecholamine-depleting effects (15).
STIMULANT DRUGS: Concomitant use of sympathomimetic drugs with Indian snakeroot may cause an initial increase in blood pressure and enhance or prolong the pressor effects (15,18).
TRICYCLIC ANTIDEPRESSANTS (TCAs): Concomitant use of tricyclic antidepressants with Indian snakeroot may decrease the effectiveness of rauwolfia alkaloids (15).

Interactions with Foods

ALCOHOL (Ethanol): Concomitant use of Indian snakeroot with ethanol should be used with caution; concomitant use with alcohol may increase the risk of additive CNS-depressant effects (15).

Interactions with Lab Tests

17-HYDROXYCORTICOSTEROIDS: Indian snakeroot might reduce urinary 17-hydroxycorticosteroid concentrations and test results, possibly due to suppression of central 17-hydroxycorticosteroid synthesis by its rauwolfia alkaloid content. Indian snakeroot might interfere with colorimetric assays of urinary 17-hydroxycorticosteroid concentrations by the Glenn-Nelson technique, due to its rauwolfia alkaloid content. Theoretically, Indian snakeroot might interfere with colorimetric assays of urinary 17-hydroxycorticosteroid concentrations which rely on the Porter-Silber reaction, due to its reserpine content (15,275).
17-KETOSTEROIDS: Indian snakeroot might interfere with colorimetric assays of urinary 17-ketosteroids by the Holtorff Koch modification of the Zimmerman reaction, due to its rauwolfia alkaloid content (15).
4-HYDROXY-3-METHOXY PHENYLETHYLENE GLYCOL (HMPG): Theoretically, Indian snakeroot might increase or decrease urinary HMPG concentrations and test results, due to its reserpine content. Reserpine can increase urinary HMPG concentrations by causing release of stored norepinephrine. Long-term reserpine administration can decrease urinary HMPG concentrations (275).
5-HYDROXYINDOLEACETIC ACID (5-HIAA): Large doses of Indian snakeroot might increase urinary 5-HIAA excretion and test results. Large doses of rauwolfia alkaloids may release serotonin (5-HT) from brain tissues, resulting in increased urinary 5-HIAA excretion (15,275).
BILIRUBIN: Theoretically, large doses of Indian snakeroot might cause falsely high serum bilirubin test results, due to the resperpine content. Reserpine concentrations greater than 61 mg/L can cause falsely high serum bilirubin test results when measured by the Jendrassik and Grof method (275).
BLOOD PRESSURE: Indian snakeroot might lower blood pressure and blood pressure readings in patients with mild to moderate hypertension, due to the alkaloids (2,15).
CATECHOLAMINES: Overdose of Indian snakeroot might initially increase urinary catecholamine excretion and test results. Rauwolfia alkaloids release stored norepinephrine, resulting in increased urinary catecholamine excretion. Chronic use of Indian snakeroot might decrease urinary catecholamine excretion, due to its rauwolfia alkaloid content. Chronic use of rauwolfia alkaloids decreases urinary catecholamine excretion (15,275).
GLUCOSE: Theoretically, Indian snakeroot might increase blood glucose concentrations and test results, due to its reserpine content. Reserpine might increase blood glucose concentrations following administration (275).
GUAIACOLS SPOT TEST: Theoretically, Indian snakeroot might cause false-positive urine guaiacols spot test results, due to the reserpine content. Reserpine can cause a false-positive reaction for urinary guaiacols with the screening test of Rogers (275).
LUPUS ERYTHEMATOSUS (LE) CELLS: Theoretically, Indian snakeroot might trigger the presence of LE cells in the blood and positive LE cell test results, due to the reserpine content. Reserpine might cause systemic lupus erythematosus (SLE) and the presence of LE cells in the blood; however, this usually normalizes when reserpine is discontinued (275).

NOREPINEPHRINE: Theoretically, Indian snakeroot might decrease urinary norepinephrine concentrations, due to the reserpine content.
OCCULT BLOOD: Theoretically, Indian snakeroot might activate peptic ulcers, resulting in bleeding and positive fecal occult blood tests, due to the reserpine content (275).
PLATELETS: Theoretically, Indian snakeroot might cause thrombocytopenia, decreasing blood platelets and platelet counts. Reserpine might cause thrombocytopenia (275).
PROLACTIN: Theoretically, large doses of Indian snakeroot might increase plasma prolactin levels and test results in patients with hypertension, due to the reserpine content. Reserpine, in daily doses greater than 0.25 mg, may increase plasma prolactin levels in patients with hypertension (275).
THYROXINE (T4): Theoretically, Indian snakeroot might decrease serum T4 concentrations and test results, due to the reserpine content. Reserpine may decrease serum T4 concentrations by increasing hepatic T4 metabolism (275).
TYRAMINE: Theoretically, Indian snakeroot might cause false-negative tyramine test results, due to the reserpine content. Reserpine may inhibit patient responsiveness to tyramine tests (275).
VANILLYLMANDELIC ACID (VMA): Overdose of Indian snakeroot might initially increase urinary VMA excretion and test results. Rauwolfia alkaloids release stored norepinephrine, resulting in increased urinary VMA excretion. Chronic use of Indian snakeroot might decrease urinary VMA excretion, due to its rauwolfia alkaloid content. Chronic use of rauwolfia alkaloids decreases urinary VMA excretion (15,275).

Interactions with Diseases or Conditions

ELECTROCONVULSIVE THERAPY (ECT): Indian snakeroot is contraindicated during ECT (15), and one week should elapse between cessation of rauwolfia alkaloids and initiation of ECT (15).
GALLBLADDER DISEASE: Use cautiously in individuals with a history of gallstones; Indian snakeroot may precipitate biliary colic (15).
GASTROINTESTINAL (GI) CONDITIONS: Indian snakeroot is contraindicated in individuals with active peptic ulcer disease or ulcerative colitis (15). Use Indian snake root cautiously in individuals with a history of these diseases.
HYPERSENSITIVITY: Indian Snakeroot is contraindicated in individuals hypersensitive to rauwolfia alkaloids (15).
MENTAL DEPRESSION: Indian snakeroot is contraindicated, especially in individuals with a past history of depression or suicidal tendencies (15).
PHEOCHROMOCYTOMA: Contraindicated (18).

Dosage and Administration

ORAL: The average daily amount of Indian snakeroot is 600 mg of the powdered whole root, which is equivalent to 6 mg total alkaloids (2,18). Rauwolfia serpentina, deserpidine, and reserpine are available as FDA-approved prescription drugs (15).

Comments

Reserpine is commercially obtained from Rauvolfia serpentina and the related species, Rauvolfia micrantha, Rauvolfia tetraphylla, and Rauvolfia vomitoria (13). Spelling note: The genus, Rauvolfia, is correctly spelled with a "v", while Rauwolfia or Rauwolfia serpentina (names for the dried root of Rauvolfia serpentina) are correctly spelled with a "w" (2,13).

INDOLE-3-CARBINOL

Also Known As

I3C, 3-Hydroxymethyl Indole, 3 Hydroxymethyl Indole, Indole 3 Carbinol, 3-(hydroxymethyl), 3 (hydroxymethyl) Indole, 3-Indolylcarbinol, 3 Indolylcarbinol, 3-Indolylmethanol, 3 Indolylmethanol, Indole.
CAUTION: See separate listing for Diindolylmethane.

Scientific Names

Indole-3-methanol.

People Use This For

Orally, indole-3-carbinol is used for prevention of breast cancer, colon cancer, and other types of cancer. Indole-3-carbinol is also used orally for fibromyalgia, laryngeal papillomatosis, cervical dysplasia, and systemic lupus erythematosus (SLE). It is also used to balance hormone levels, detoxify the intestines and liver, and to support the immune system.

Safety

LIKELY SAFE ...when used orally in amounts typically found in the diet. Dietary consumption of indole-3-carbinol is typically 20-120 mg per day (7170,7176).

POSSIBLY SAFE ...when used orally and appropriately in medicinal amounts. Doses of 200-400 mg per day seem to be safe and well tolerated when used for up to 3 months (7173,7174,7175). There is also some evidence that lower doses of 100-200 mg per day can be used safely for up to 15 months (7172).

CHILDREN: LIKELY SAFE ...when used orally in amounts typically found in the diet (7170,7176). POSSIBLY SAFE ...when used orally and appropriately in medicinal amounts. There is some evidence that indole-3-carbinol can be safely used in children ages 2 to 12 years. Doses of 100-200 mg, based on body weight, seem to be safe and well tolerated when used for up to 15 months (7172).

PREGNANCY AND LACTATION: LIKELY SAFE ...when used in amounts typically consumed in foods (7170). There is insufficient reliable information available about the safety of indole-3-carbinol when used in amounts greater than those found in the diet during pregnancy and lactation; avoid using.

Effectiveness

POSSIBLY EFFECTIVE

Cervical dysplasia (cervical intraepithelial neoplasia, CIN). Treatment with indole-3-carbinol for 12 weeks seems to cause complete regression of CIN in 45-50% of patients with stage II-III CIN. Lower doses of 200 mg per day seem to be just as effective as higher doses of 400 mg per day (7173).

INSUFFICIENT RELIABLE EVIDENCE to RATE

Respiratory papillomatosis. There is some preliminary clinical evidence that long-term use of indole-3-carbinol might reduce papilloma growth in patients with recurrent respiratory papillomatosis (7172). More evidence is needed to rate indole-3-carbinol for this use.

Mechanism of Action

Indole-3-carbinol is a constituent of cruciferous vegetables of the Brassica genus. Some of these vegetables include broccoli, Brussels sprouts, cabbage, collards, cauliflower, kale, kohlrabi, mustard greens, rapeseed, and root vegetables such as turnips and rutabagas (7170,7176). One head of cabbage contains approximately 1200 mg of indole-3-carbinol (7173). Daily dietary intake of indole-3-carbinol is typically 20-120 mg (7170,7176). In plant cells, indole-3-carbinol exists in the form of 3-indolylmethyl glucosinolate, which is then converted to indole-3-carbinol when the plant is cut or chewed (7170). However, indole-3-carbinol is also produced synthetically (7170). Indole-3-carbinol itself is not active. When indole-3-carbinol comes in contact with stomach acid it is converted to active metabolites, diindolylmethane and indolylcarbazole. Therefore, parenterally administered indole-3-carbinol does not produce active metabolites (7188). Researchers are interested in indole-3-carbinol for cancer prevention, particularly breast, cervical and endometrial, and colorectal cancer. Their reason is that diets with higher amounts of fruit and vegetable consumption are associated with a decreased risk of developing cancer. Researchers suspect indole-3-carbinol is one of several vegetable components that might be cancer protective (7174,7180,7181,7182,7187). However, researchers are finding that indole-3-carbinol has a variety of effects on liver metabolism of toxins. Some effects on metabolism seem to be cancer protective while others might potentially increase cancer risk. Some researchers think indole-3-carbinol might be particularly helpful against hormone-dependent cancers such as breast cancer. Indole-3-carbinol induces cytochrome P450 1A1 (CYP1A1) and 1A2 (CYP1A2), which alters estrogen metabolism. Estradiol is normally metabolized to both 16-alpha-hydroxyestrone and 2-alpha-hydroxyestrone. The 16-alpha-hydroxysestrone metabolite has both genotoxic and tumorigenic effects and is thought to increase the risk of breast and cervical cancers. Indole-3-carbinol shifts metabolism of estradiol from 16-alpha-hydroxyestrone to the weaker estrogen and more benign 2-alpha-hydroxyestrone metabolite, possibly producing a protective effect against hormone-mediated cancers (7175,7177,7179,7180,7181,7182). Indole-3-carbinol also induces cytochrome P450 2B1, 2B2, 3A1, and 3A2, as well as phase II enzymes including glutathione S-transferase (GST), quinone reductase, and uridine diphosphate glucuronide transferase (7176,7187). The phase II enzyme induction seems to have a detoxifying effect by increasing water solubility and increasing excretion of carcinogenic toxins (7176). There is some evidence that indole-3-carbinol might have other protective effects including antioxidant properties (7178,7188) and might also cause cancer cell apoptosis and cell cycle arrest (7176,7188). The majority of evidence seems to indicate that indole-3-carbinol has a protective effect against cancer. However, there is some concern that it might enhance carcinogenicity in some cases (7170,7171,7184,7185,7186). Some of the effects of indole-3-carbinol on metabolism actually seem to increase carcinogenicity of certain toxins. Since indole-3-carbinol induces CYP1A1 metabolism, it can also increase conversion of procarcinogens to their active carcinogenic form (7170). Ultimately, whether indole-3-carbinol has a cancer preventive effect or increases cancer risk in humans probably depends on several factors, including dietary factors, and duration and timing of exposure to indole-3-carbinol. For example, in animal models, there is some evidence that indole-3-carbinol has a protective role if administered before or in conjunction with a carcinogenic agent. If indole-3-carbinol is given after carcinogen exposure during the initiation phase of tumor induction, it might act as a tumor promoting agent and increase the risk of developing a tumor (7184,7185,7186). However, there is some conflicting evidence (7189). Indole-3-carbinol seems be active against diseases that are related to the human papilloma virus, including cervical cancer and laryngeal papillomatosis (7172,7173,7183).

Indole-3-carbinol also seems to have immune modulating effects. In animal models, high doses of indole-3-carbinol seem to depress natural killer cell activity, but enhance delayed-type hypersensitivity in laboratory models (7190). Whether these immune system effects contribute to the effects of indole-3-carbinol on carcinogenicity is unknown (7190).

Adverse Reactions

Orally, indole-3-carbinol is usually well tolerated. However, some patients can experience skin rash and small increases in the liver enzyme alanine aminotransferase (ALT, SGPT) (7170,7174). However, this seems to rarely occur. In very high doses, greater than 400 mg per day, dysequilibrium symptoms, tremor, and nausea can occur (7172). There is some concern that certain patients might be at risk for tumor promoting effects of indole-3-carbinol. There is some preliminary evidence that indole-3-carbinol might promote tumorigenesis in patients who are in the initiation phase of tumor induction due to carcinogen exposure (7171). However, this potential risk is controversial and has never been documented in humans. Until more is known, it is not possible to determine if there is a real risk to humans or who might be susceptible to this risk.

Interactions with Herbs & Other Dietary Supplements

None known.

Interactions with Drugs

CYTOCHROME P450 1A2 (CYP1A2) SUBSTRATES: There is some evidence that indole-3-carbinol induces CYP1A2 isozymes (7187). Theoretically, indole-3-carbinol might increase the metabolism of CYP1A2 substrates and lower serum concentrations. Some substrates of CYP1A2 include clozapine (Clozaril), cyclobenzaprine (Flexeril), fluvoxamine (Luvox), haloperidol (Haldol), imipramine (Tofranil), mexiletine (Mexitil), olanzapine (Zyprexa), pentazocine (Talwin), propranolol (Inderal), tacrine (Cognex), theophylline, zileuton (Zyflo), zolmitriptan (Zomig), and others.

Interactions with Foods

None known.

Interactions with Lab Tests

ALANINE AMINOTRANSFERASE (ALT, SGPT): A mild increase in ALT can occur in some patients taking indole-3-carbinol (7174). However, this effect seems to rarely occur. Routine liver function tests are probably not necessary.

Interactions with Diseases or Conditions

None known.

Dosage and Administration

ORAL: For cervical dysplasia, 200-400 mg per day has been used. However, 200 mg seems to be as effective as the higher dose (7173). For breast cancer prevention, 300 mg per day has been used (7174). For adults with recurrent respiratory papillomatosis, 200 mg twice daily has been used (7172). For children with respiratory papillomatosis, dosing is weight based. For children weighing 6-10 kg, 50 mg twice daily has been used. For children weighing 11-19 kg, 75 mg twice daily has been used. For children weighing 20-29 kg, 100 mg twice daily has been used, etc. Children 60 kg and above have used the adult dose of 200 mg twice daily (7172).

Comments

Indole-3-carbinol is becoming a very popular dietary supplement. Usage of indole-3-carbinol is expected to grow by 3000% between the year 2000 and 2002 (7170,7176). The National Institutes of Health (NIH) has reviewed indole-3-carbinol as a possible cancer preventive agent and is now sponsoring clinical research for breast cancer prevention (7170).

INOSINE

Also Known As

Hypoxanthine Riboside, Hypoxanthosine.

Scientific Names

2,3-Diphosphoglycerate; 6,9-Dihydro-9-B-D-ribofuranosyl-1H-puin-6-one; 9-B-D-ribofuranosylhypoxanthine.

People Use This For

Orally, inosine is used for enhancing athletic performance.

Safety
There is insufficient reliable information available about the safety of inosine.
Pregnancy and Lactation: Insufficient reliable information available; avoid using.

Effectiveness
LIKELY INEFFECTIVE

Athletic performance. Taking inosine orally does not improve athletic performance (2369,2370).

Mechanism of Action
Preliminary evidence suggests inosine might stimulate axon growth from uninjured nerve cells to injured nerve cells of the central nervous system. Further studies in humans are needed to establish whether this finding has significance in restoring function after spinal cord injuries (370).

Adverse Reactions
None reported.

Interactions with Herbs & Other Dietary Supplements
None known.

Interactions with Drugs
None known.

Interactions with Foods
None known.

Interactions with Lab Tests
None known.

Interactions with Diseases or Conditions
GOUT: Excess purinesm such as inosine, can aggravate gout.

Dosage and Administration
ORAL: 5 to 6 grams per day have been used in clinical studies of effects on athletic performance (2369,2370).

INOSITOL

Also Known As
Antialopecia Factor, Cyclohexitol, Dambrose, Inose, Inosite, Inositol Monophosphate, Lipositol, Meso-inositol, Mouse Antialopecia Factor, Myo-inositol, Vitamin B8.
CAUTION: See separate listings for Inositol Nicotinate and IP-6.

Scientific Names
Hexahydroxycyclohexane, synonyms 1,2,3,4,5,6-Cyclohexanehexol, cis-1,2,3,5-trans-4,6-Cyclohexanehexol; D-chiro-inositol, synonym (+)-chiroinositol, 1,2,5/3,4,6-inositol, (1S)-inositol, (1S)-1,2,4/3,5,6-inositol.

People Use This For
Orally, inositol is used for diabetic neuropathy, conditions associated with disorders of fat transport and metabolism, panic disorder, high cholesterol, insomnia, cancer, depression, schizophrenia, Alzheimer's disease, attention deficit-hyperactivity disorder (ADHD), autism, treating lithium-induced side effects, psoriasis, and promoting hair growth. Inositol is also used orally for treating conditions associated with polycystic ovary syndrome, including anovulation, hypertension, hypertriglyceridemia, and elevated serum concentrations of testosterone.
Parenterally, inositol is used for treating respiratory distress syndrome in premature infants.

Safety
POSSIBLY SAFE ...when used orally and appropriately. Inositol has been used in amounts up to 12 grams per day for up to 4 weeks, and 6 grams daily for 10 weeks with no significant adverse effects (2184,2185,2187).
CHILDREN: POSSIBLY SAFE ...when used parenterally and appropriately for treating respiratory distress syndrome in premature infants (2191,2192).
PREGNANCY: Insufficient reliable information available; avoid using.
LACTATION: Insufficient reliable information available; avoid using. Breast milk is rich in endogenous inositol (2138); however, the effects of exogenously administered inositol are not known.

Effectiveness

POSSIBLY EFFECTIVE

Lithium-induced side effects. Taking inositol orally seems to improve psoriasis associated with lithium. But it doesn't seem to help psoriasis in patients who aren't taking lithium (11972). Additionally, preliminary evidence suggests that taking inositol orally is not beneficial for reducing lithium-induced adverse effects, including tremor, thirst, and thyroid and adrenal function (2027).

Obsessive-compulsive disorder (OCD). There is some evidence that OCD patients who receive inositol orally for 6 weeks have significant improvement, based on Yale-Brown Obsessive Compulsive Scale scores, compared to placebo (2186).

Panic disorder. Taking inositol orally seems to be helpful for treating panic disorder with or without agoraphobia. Inositol seems to significantly reduce the severity and rate of panic attacks and the severity of agoraphobia over 4 weeks of treatment (2184). Some research suggests that it may be as effective as fluvoxamine (Luvox) for treatment of panic disorder (10387). Large scale, long-term trials are needed to confirm inositol's potential benefit in panic disorders.

Polycystic ovary syndrome. Taking the inositol isomer D-chiro-inositol orally seems to decrease serum triglyceride and testosterone levels, modestly decreases blood pressure, and induces ovulation in obese women with polycystic ovary syndrome (2028).

Respiratory distress syndrome. Administering inositol parenterally as a nutritional supplement seems to improve survival and symptoms in premature infants with respiratory distress syndrome. Inositol seems to lower inspiratory oxygen requirements, mean airway pressure, and the incidence of bronchopulmonary dysplasia in premature infants not receiving surfactant when compared to placebo and glucose (2191,2192).

POSSIBLY INEFFECTIVE

Alzheimer's disease. Taking inositol orally doesn't seem to improve symptoms of Alzheimer's disease (2189).

Autism. Taking inositol orally doesn't seem to improve symptoms of autism (2190).

Depression. Although limited research suggests that depressed patients receiving inositol for 4 weeks may improve, patients initially responding to inositol seem to relapse rapidly upon discontinuation of treatment (2026,2185). Inositol given in combination with SSRIs doesn't improve the effectiveness of SSRIs or improve depression in SSRI treatment failures (2025,10851).

Schizophrenia. Taking inositol orally doesn't seem to improve symptoms of schizophrenia (2188).

LIKELY INEFFECTIVE

Diabetic neuropathy. Taking inositol orally doesn't improve the symptoms of diabetic neuropathy (2193,2194,2195).

INSUFFICIENT RELIABLE EVIDENCE to RATE

Attention deficit-hyperactivity disorder (ADHD). Preliminary evidence suggests inositol might not help improve ADHD symptoms (2187). More evidence is needed to rate inositol for this use.

Mechanism of Action

Endogenous inositol is an essential component of cell membrane phospholipids. It has weak lipotropic activity, and can move fat out of liver and intestine cells (2187). Inositol is a constituent of the intracellular phosphatidyl inositol second messenger system, which is linked to serotonin, norepinephrine, and cholinergic receptors (10850,11972). Inositol has a variety of stereoisomers, including myo-inositol and D-chiro-inositol. Myo-inositol is the most abundant form in the central nervous system (CNS). Biological function varies among the isomers (2047,2048). Inositol might reverse desensitization of serotonin receptors (2187). Limited clinical evidence suggests exogenous inositol may have benefits similar to selective-serotonin-reuptake inhibitors (SSRIs) in conditions such as panic disorder, depression, and obsessive-compulsive disorder. Researchers think that D-chiro-inositol isomer induces ovulation in women with polycystic ovary syndrome by improving insulin sensitivity. Reduced insulin resistance is also thought to be responsible for improving other symptoms associated with polycystic ovary syndrome, including hypertension, hyperlipidemia, type 2 diabetes, obesity, and increased serum testosterone concentrations (2028). Additionally, patients with insulin resistance, including those with impaired glucose tolerance and type 2 diabetes, might have D-chiro-inositol deficiency (2028).

Supplemental inositol seems to help psoriasis that is made worse or triggered by lithium. The mechanism is unknown, but lithium seems to cause a reduction of inositol in both the brain and other tissues. Supplementation with inositol doesn't seem to adversely affect the efficacy of lithium for bipolar disorder (11972).

Adverse Reactions

Orally, inositol is generally well tolerated. It can cause nausea, tiredness, headache, and dizziness (10387,11972).

Interactions with Herbs & Other Dietary Supplements

None known.

Interactions with Drugs

None known.

Interactions with Foods

MINERALS: Phytic acid, the form of inositol found in foods, may interfere with absorption of minerals, especially calcium, zinc, and iron (16).

Interactions with Lab Tests

None known.

Interactions with Diseases or Conditions

None known.

Dosage and Administration

ORAL: For depression, inositol 12 grams per day has been used (2185). For panic disorder, 12 to 18 grams per day has been used (2184,10387). For obsessive-compulsive disorder, inositol 18 grams per day has been used (2186). For treating symptoms associated with polycystic ovary syndrome, D-chiro-inositol 1200 mg per day has been used (2028). For treating lithium-related psoriasis, 6 grams daily has been used (11972).
PARENTERAL: For respiratory distress syndrome in premature infants, inositol 80 mg/kg parenterally per day has been used (2191).

INOSITOL NICOTINATE

Also Known As

Hexanicotinoyl Inositol, Inositol Hexaniacinate, Inositol Hexanicotinate, Inositol Niacinate, Meso-Inositol Hexanicotinate, No-Flush Niacin.
CAUTION: See separate listings for Inositol and Niacin and Niacinamide (Vitamin B3).

Scientific Names

Hexanicotinyl cis-1,2,3-5-trans-4,6-cyclohexane; Myo-inositol hexa-3-pyridine-carboxylate.

People Use This For

Orally, inositol nicotinate is used for improving circulation and for treating peripheral vascular disease, cerebral vascular disease, intermittent claudication, stasis dermatitis, and Raynaud's disease. It is also used for hypercholesterolemia, atherosclerosis-related migraines, scleroderma, supporting nervous system and brain function, improving sleep, lowering blood pressure, calming effects, restless leg syndrome, acne, dermatitis herpetiformis, exfoliative glossitis, psoriasis, and schizophrenia and other mental illnesses.

Safety

POSSIBLY SAFE ...when used orally and appropriately (496).
PREGNANCY AND LACTATION: Insufficient reliable information available; avoid using.

Effectiveness

POSSIBLY EFFECTIVE

Hyperlipidemia. Taking inositol nicotinate orally seems reduce serum lipid levels, especially in combination with clofibrate (496,499,1546).

Peripheral vascular disease. Taking inositol nicotinate orally seems to be effective for improving symptoms of peripheral vascular disorders, including intermittent claudication and Raynaud's syndrome (496,498,1544,1545). Several weeks of treatment may be necessary before the full beneficial effects are seen (1544,1545).

There is insufficient reliable information available about the effectiveness of inositol nicotinate for its other uses.

Mechanism of Action

Inositol nicotinate consists of six molecules of niacin (nicotinic acid) chemically linked to an inositol molecule. It is hydrolyzed in the body to free niacin and inositol, although this occurs slowly, with peak serum levels not occurring until approximately 10 hours after ingestion (496). It is theoretically possible that this slow conversion might reduce peak plasma levels and thereby reduce the incidence of side effects that have been associated with niacin such as flushing. The mechanism of action of inositol nicotinate is believed to be the same as that of niacin (496). Several weeks of treatment may be necessary before the full beneficial effects of inositol nicotinate are seen in peripheral vascular disorders such as Raynaud's disease, suggesting that fibrinolysis, lipid lowering, and vasodilatory action contribute to its beneficial effects (1544,1545).

Adverse Reactions

Adverse effects from the use of inositol nicotinate in usual doses appear to be rare (496). However, inositol nicotinate is metabolized to niacin which is associated with numerous side effects including flushing, pruritus, GI complaints, hepatotoxicity, hyperuricemia, and impaired glucose tolerance (496).

Interactions with Herbs & Other Dietary Supplements

None known.

Interactions with Drugs

ANTICOAGULANT/ANTIPLATELET DRUGS: Theoretically, concomitant use might increase the risk of bleeding, due to the fibrinolytic effects of inositol nicotinate (496).
ANTIDIABETES DRUGS: Concomitant use might interfere with blood glucose control. Inositol nicotinate is metabolized to niacin in the body (496). Niacin and niacinamide can interfere with blood glucose control requiring dosing adjustment of antidiabetic agents. Niacin and niacinamide can cause hyperglycemia, abnormal glucose tolerance, and glycosuria. Increased blood glucose monitoring may be necessary, particularly early in the course of treatment (4859,4860,12033).
HMG-CoA REDUCTASE INHIBITORS ("Statins"): Concomitant use of niacin and HMG-CoA reductase inhibitors increases the risk of myopathy. Inositol nicotinate is metabolized to niacin in the body (496). HMG-CoA reductase inhibitors include cerivastatin (Baycol), atorvastatin (Lipitor), lovastatin (Mevacor), pravastatin (Pravachol), and simvastatin (Zocor).
TRANSDERMAL NICOTINE (Nicoderm, Nicotrol): Concomitant use of niacin and transdermal nicotine increases the risk of flushing and dizziness. Inositol nicotinate is metabolized to niacin in the body (496).

Interactions with Foods

HOT DRINKS: Niacin-induced flushing can be magnified by concomitant ingestion of hot drinks. Inositol nicotinate is metabolized to niacin (6243).

Interactions with Lab Tests

CATECHOLAMINES: Niacin, a metabolite of inositol nicotinate, can produce fluorescent substances in the urine, which cause false elevations in some fluorometric tests of urinary catecholamines (15).
LIVER FUNCTION TESTS: Inositol nicotinate may increase levels of liver enzymes. Liver function should be monitored periodically when using doses of 2000 mg per day or more (496).

Interactions with Diseases or Conditions

ALLERGIES: Niacin, a metabolite of inositol nicotinate, might exacerbate allergies by causing histamine release (15,496).
CORONARY ARTERY DISEASE/UNSTABLE ANGINA: Large amounts of niacin, a metabolite of inositol nicotinate, can increase the risk of cardiac arrhythmias (15,496). One study showed an increased incidence of cardiac arrhythmias when niacin was used in patients with coronary artery disease (15); use with caution.
DIABETES: Niacin, a metabolite of inositol nicotinate, can interfere with blood glucose control requiring dosing adjustment of antidiabetic agents. Niacin and niacinamide can cause hyperglycemia, abnormal glucose tolerance, and glycosuria. Increased blood glucose monitoring may be necessary, particularly early in the course of treatment (4859,4860,12033).
GALLBLADDER DISEASE: Niacin, a metabolite of inositol nicotinate, might exacerbate gallbladder disease (15,496); use with caution.
GOUT: Large amounts of niacin or niacinamide might precipitate gout. Niacin and niacinamide can cause hyperuricemia (12033); use with caution.
HYPOTENSION: Niacin, a metabolite of inositol nicotinate, can cause hypotension (15,496).
KIDNEY DISEASE: Niacin, a metabolite of inositol nicotinate, is excreted unchanged in the urine and might accumulate in patients with kidney disease (15,496); use with caution.
LIVER DISEASE: Inositol nicotinate should be avoided in people with liver disease. Niacin and niacinamide have been associated with liver damage (12033).
NIACIN HYPERSENSITIVITY: Inositol nicotinate is metabolized to niacin (15,496).
PEPTIC ULCER DISEASE: Large amounts of niacin, a metabolite of inositol nicotinate, might activate peptic ulcer disease (15,496).

Dosage and Administration

ORAL: For hyperlipoproteinemia, the typical dosing range is 1500-4000 mg daily given in 2-4 divided doses (496). For peripheral vascular disorders, the typical dosing range is 1500-4000 mg daily given in 2-4 divided doses (496).

Comments

Inositol nicotinate has been used in conventional medical practice in Great Britain for improving symptoms of peripheral vascular disorders and treating hyperlipidemia for many years, although it is not considered an agent of first choice.

INULIN

Also Known As

Chicory Extract, Chicory Inulin, Dahlia Extract, Dahlia Inulin, Fructo-Oligosaccharides, Fructooligosaccharides, Long-chain Oligosaccharides, Oligosaccharides, Prebiotic.
CAUTION: See separate listings for Chicory and Fructo-Oligosaccharides.

Scientific Names

Beta(2-1)fructans.

People Use This For

Orally, inulin is used for hypercholesterolemia, hypertriglyceridemia, hyperlipidemia, obesity and weight loss, improving gastrointestinal function, and as a food additive.

Safety

POSSIBLY SAFE ...when used orally and appropriately, short-term. Doses of 8 to 14 grams daily have been safely used for up to eight weeks (7604,7605,7606,7607,8451).
PREGNANCY AND LACTATION: Insufficient reliable information available; avoid using.

Effectiveness

POSSIBLY EFFECTIVE

Constipation. Taking inulin orally seems to increase the number of stools from 1-2 per week to 8-9 per week in elderly patients (10415).
Hypertriglyceridemia. Taking inulin orally seems to reduce triglycerides by up to 19% after eight weeks of treatment (7604).

POSSIBLY INEFFECTIVE

Hypercholesterolemia. Taking inulin orally as a supplement does not seem to significantly decrease serum cholesterol (7604,8450,10412,10413).
Obesity. Taking inulin orally, in combination with chromium picolinate, capsicum, L-phenylalanine, and other nutrients, doesn't seem to significantly reduce weight in moderately obese patients (7607).

Mechanism of Action

Inulin is an oligosaccharide, composed of chains of 2 to 60 glucose and fructose molecules. The major source of inulin in the diet is in wheat, onions, bananas, leaks, artichokes, and asparagus (10412,10414). Although inulin is found in many fruits, vegetables, and herbs, it is usually obtained by hot water extraction from chicory root (7606). Because it contributes very little in dietary calories, inulin is used as a food additive to increase bulk and palatability (8449).
Inulin is related to short-chain oligosaccharides (SCO), which are often referred to as fructo-oligosaccharides. Partial hydrolysis of chicory inulin yields SCO, which are usually 2 to 7 sugar molecules in length and have many of the same effects as inulin (7606).
Inulin has a prebiotic effect, meaning that it is not digested or absorbed, and it promotes the growth of specific types of bacteria in the large intestine. Inulin preferentially promotes the growth of bifidobacteria. Fermentation of inulin decreases fecal pH and increases fecal volume (7605,8447,10414). The products of fermentation are short-chain fatty acids that are absorbed and metabolized (8449).
Inulin decreases serum triglycerides by decreasing fatty acid synthesis and reducing production of very low density lipoproteins (VLDL) (7604). Preliminary evidence indicates that SCO can reduce the formation of very low density lipoproteins (VLDL) (8448).

Adverse Reactions

Orally, inulin can commonly cause flatulence, bloating, gastrointestinal cramps, and intestinal noises. These symptoms become more bothersome at doses over 30 grams (7604,8450,8509). Some people can experience severe allergic reactions to inulin-containing foods. There is one report of anaphylaxis following consumption of foods with a high concentration of inulin including salsify, artichoke leaves, and margarine with inulin as a food additive (7608).

Interactions with Herbs & Other Dietary Supplements

None known.

Interactions with Drugs

None known.

Interactions with Foods

CALCIUM: Inulin appears to have no clinically significant effect on the absorption of dietary calcium. Inulin does not seem to affect ionized calcium, parathyroid hormone levels, or calcium excretion (8451,10274).

Interactions with Lab Tests
None known.

Interactions with Diseases or Conditions
None known.

Dosage and Administration
ORAL: For hypertriglyceridemia, the typical dose of inulin is 10-14 grams daily (7604). For treatment of hypercholesterolemia, inulin 6 grams three times daily has been used for up to 6 weeks (10412). For treatment of constipation in elderly, 20-40 grams per day for 19 days has been used (10415).

Comments
Inulin is used as an additive in many food products because it improves their palatability (7605).

IODINE

Also Known As
Potassium Iodide, Povidone Iodine.

Scientific Names
Iodine; I; atomic number 53.

People Use This For
Orally, iodine is used as an expectorant, for treating endemic goiter, thyroid storm, hyperthyroidism, treating radiation emergency associated with radioactive iodides, cutaneous sporotrichosis, and fibrocystic breast disease. Topically it is used as an antiseptic, for preventing mucositis from chemotherapy, and treating diabetic ulcers. Iodine is also used for water purification.

Safety
LIKELY SAFE ...when used orally and appropriately. Iodine is safe in amounts that do not exceed 1100 mcg per day, the Tolerable Upper Intake Level (UL) (7135). Higher doses can be safely used therapeutically with appropriate medical monitoring (2197,7080). Advise patients not to use doses greater than the UL without medical supervision. ...when used topically as a 2% solution (15). Iodine is an FDA-approved prescription product.
POSSIBLY UNSAFE ...when used orally in high doses. Tell patients to avoid prolonged use of doses exceeding the UL of 1100 mcg per day without proper medical supervision. Higher intake can increase the risk of side effects such as thyroid dysfunction (7135).
CHILDREN: LIKELY SAFE ...when used orally and appropriately (7135). Iodine is safe in amounts that do not exceed the UL of 200 mcg per day for children 1 to 3 years, 300 mcg per day for children 4 to 8 years, 600 mcg per day for children 9 to 13 years, and 900 mcg per day for adolescents (7135). ...when used topically as a 2% solution (15). Iodine is an FDA-approved prescription product. POSSIBLY UNSAFE ...when used orally in high doses. Tell patients to avoid prolonged use of doses exceeding the UL of 200 mcg per day for children 1 to 3 years, 300 mcg per day for children 4 to 8 years, 600 mcg per day for children 9 to 13 years, and 900 mcg per day for adolescents (7135). Higher intake can cause thyroid dysfunction (7135).
PREGNANCY AND LACTATION: LIKELY SAFE ...when used orally and appropriately. Iodine is safe in amounts that do not exceed the UL of 1100 mcg per day (7135). ...when used topically as a 2% solution (15). Iodine is an FDA-approved prescription product. POSSIBLY UNSAFE ...when used orally in high doses. Tell patients to avoid exceeding the UL of 1100 mcg per day or 900 mcg per day for pregnant women ages 14 to 18. Higher intake can cause thyroid dysfunction (7135).

Effectiveness
EFFECTIVE

Cutaneous sporotrichosis. Taking iodine orally improves cutaneous sporotrichosis (15).
Radiation. Iodine taken orally is effective for radiation emergency associated with radioactive iodides (7517,7518).
Respiratory congestion. Iodine taken orally is effective as an expectorant (15).
Skin infection. Iodine used topically is an effective antiseptic (15).
Thyroid conditions. Taking iodine orally can improve thyroid storm, hyperthyroidism, and endemic goiter (15).
Water purification. Adding iodine to water is effective for purification (15,16).

POSSIBLY EFFECTIVE

Diabetic foot ulcers. Topical use of iodine may be useful for treating diabetic foot ulcers (2200).
Fibrocystic breast disease. Taking iodine orally may improve fibrocystic breast disease (2197).
Oral mucositis. Topical use of iodine may prevent oral mucositis caused by chemotherapy (2198,2199).

There is insufficient reliable information available about the effectiveness of iodine for its other uses.

Mechanism of Action

Iodine is an essential nutrient in humans. About 90% of iodine, which is ingested in a variety of chemical forms, is absorbed (7135). The iodine content of most foods is low and is affected by agricultural factors such as soil quality and climate. Marine animals concentrate iodine from seawater and have a higher content than most other foods (7135). Processed foods may add to dietary iodine due to the addition of iodate to salt. The thyroid gland in humans concentrates iodine for thyroid synthesis. Lesser amounts of iodine are found in the salivary glands, breast, choroid plexus, and gastric mucosa. Iodine is excreted by the kidney (7135). Iodine comprises 65% of thyroxine (T4) and 59% of triiodothyronine (T3). These iodine-rich thyroid hormones control many biochemical reactions, particularly protein synthesis and enzymatic processes. In people with hyperthyroidism, iodine inhibits the release and synthesis of thyroid hormone (15). Iodine in the form of potassium iodide can block or reduce the accumulation of radioactive iodine and damage to the thyroid gland if taken prior to or immediately following exposure to radioactive iodine (7517,7518).

Iodine deficiency is most devastating on the developing brain (7135). Thyroid hormone is responsible for myelination of the developing central nervous system. Iodine deficiency is associated with mental retardation, and in extreme cases, cretinism (7135). Most developed countries, including the US and Canada, screen for hypothyroidism at birth (7135). The earliest clinical symptom of iodine deficiency is thyroid enlargement (goiter) (7135). Iodide salts, such as potassium iodide, might increase respiratory tract secretions and thereby decrease mucus viscosity, but there is limited supporting evidence for this effect (15).

When used topically, iodine oxidizes organic substrates, killing microorganisms (15).

Adverse Reactions

Orally, iodine can cause marked sensitivity. Symptoms of iodine hypersensitivity are angioedema, cutaneous and mucosal hemorrhage, fever, arthralgia, lymph node enlargement, eosinophilia, urticaria, thrombotic thrombocytopenic purpura, and fatal periarteritis (15). Large amounts or chronic use of iodine can cause metallic taste; soreness in teeth and gums; burning in mouth and throat; increased salivation; coryza; sneezing; eye irritation and eyelid swelling; headache; cough; pulmonary edema; swelling of parotid and submaxillary glands; inflammation of the pharynx, larynx and tonsils; acneform skin lesions; gastric upset; diarrhea; anorexia; and depression (15,2138). Prolonged use of iodides can cause thyroid gland hyperplasia, thyroid adenoma, goiter, and severe hypothyroidism (15).

Topically, iodine may stain skin, irritate tissues, and cause sensitization in some individuals (15). Iodine burns are associated with application of 7% hydroalcoholic solution (15).

Interactions with Herbs & Other Dietary Supplements

None known.

Interactions with Drugs

ACE INHIBITORS (ACEIs): Concomitant use of these drugs with potassium iodide increases the risk of hyperkalemia (15). The ACE inhibitors include benazepril (Lotensin), captopril (Capoten), enalapril (Vasotec), fosinopril (Monopril), lisinopril (Prinivil, Zestril), moexipril (Univasc), perindopril (Aceon), quinapril (Accupril), ramipril (Altace), and trandolapril (Mavik).

AMIODARONE (Cordarone): Amiodarone contains 37.3% iodine. Plasma iodide levels may be increased and additive with iodine supplements (15,7135). Monitor thyroid function.

ANTITHYROID DRUGS: Concomitant use may result in additive hypothyroid activity, and may cause hypothyroidism (2138).

ANGIOTENSIN RECEPTOR BLOCKERS (ARBs): Concomitant use of these drugs with potassium iodide increases the risk of hyperkalemia (15). The ARBs include losartan (Cozaar), valsartan (Diovan), irbesartan (Avapro), candesartan (Atacand), telmisartan (Micardis), and eprosartan (Teveten).

LITHIUM: Concomitant use may have additive or synergistic hypothyroid effects (15).

POTASSIUM-SPARING DIURETICS: Concomitant use of potassium iodide with potassium sparing diuretics increases the risk of hyperkalemia (15). Potassium-sparing diuretics include spironolactone (Aldactone), Triamterene (Dyrenium), and amiloride (Midamor).

Interactions with Foods

None known.

Interactions with Lab Tests

THYROID HORMONES: Excess iodine intake can lower serum thyroid hormone and result in elevated thyroid stimulating hormone (TSH) levels (7135).

Interactions with Diseases or Conditions

AUTOIMMUNE THYROID DISEASE (AITD): People with AITD may have increased sensitivity to adverse effects of iodine (7135).

THYROID DYSFUNCTION: Prolonged use or excessive amounts of iodides may cause or exacerbate thyroid gland hyperplasia, thyroid adenoma, goiter, and hypothyroidism (15).

Dosage and Administration

ORAL: For fibrocystic breast disease, 80 mcg/kg molecular iodine has been used (2197). For radiation emergencies, potassium iodide (KI) should be taken just prior to, or as soon as possible after, exposure. Radiation is most toxic to pregnant or lactating women and children, so KI is dosed according to amount of radiation exposure and age. For infants, babies, children, adolescents, and pregnant or lactating women, KI is given if radiation exposure is 5 centigrays (cGy) or more. For birth through 1 month, the dose is KI 16 mg; for babies and children over 1 month through 3 years, 32 mg; for children 3 to 12 years, 65 mg; for adolescents 12 through 18 years, 65 mg or 120 mg if the adolescent is approaching adult size; and pregnant or lactating women, 120 mg. For adults 18 to 40 years with exposure to 10 cGy or more, KI 130 mg is given. For adults over 40 years with exposure to 500 cGy or more, KI 130 mg is given (7518). Tablets can be crushed and mixed with fruit juice, jam, milk, etc (7517). The National Institute of Medicine has set Adequate Intake (AI) of iodine for infants: 0 to 6 months, 110 mcg/day; 7 to 12 months, 130 mcg/day (7135). For children and adults, Recommended Dietary Amounts (RDA) have been set: children 1 to 8 years, 90 mcg/day; 9 to 13 years, 120 mcg/day; people age 14 and older, 150 mcg/day (7135). For pregnant women, the RDA is 209 mcg/day, and breast-feeding women, 290 mcg/day (7135). Tolerable Upper Intake Levels (UL) for iodine intake have been set: children 1 to 3 years, 200 mcg/day; 4 to 8 years, 300 mcg/day; 9 to 13 years, 600 mcg/day; 14 to 18 years (including pregnancy and lactation), 900 mcg/day.
For adults older than age 19 including pregnant and breast-feeding women, the UL is 1100 mcg/day (7135).
TOPICAL: As an antiseptic, 2% aqueous solution applied to affected skin areas (15). For preventing mucositis from chemotherapy, rinse mouth with povidone iodine solution 4 times daily (2198,2199). To treat diabetic foot ulcers, 0.9% iodine ointment (2200) has been used. Avoid occluding skin areas treated with iodine to reduce risk of iodine burn (15).

Comments

Iodine deficiency is a common world health problem (7135). Early in the twentieth century, iodine deficiency was common in the US and Canada, but the addition of iodine to salt has improved public health. The addition of potassium iodide at 100 ppm, or 76 mg of iodine per kg of salt, is mandatory in Canada, and iodized salt is used optionally by half of the US population (7135). Potassium iodide tablets for use in a radiation emergency are available as FDA-approved products (Thyro-Block, Iostat) and on the Internet as food supplements. Tell patients that potassium iodide should only be used in a radiation emergency, not as prophylaxis in case of a radiation emergency.

IP-6

Also Known As

Fytic Acid, Phytic Acid.
Caution: See separate listings for Inositol, Inositol Nicotinate, and Vitamin B3.

Scientific Names

Inositol hexaphosphate.

People Use This For

Orally, IP-6 is used to treat and prevent cancer, increase white blood cell production, prevent heart attacks, prevent and treat kidney stones, enhance the immune system, and as an antioxidant.

Safety

LIKELY SAFE ...when consumed in amounts commonly found in foods (1854).
There is insufficient reliable information available about the safety of IP-6 when used in supplemental doses in amounts greater than those found in foods.
PREGNANCY AND LACTATION: LIKELY SAFE ...when consumed in amounts commonly found in foods (1854). There is insufficient reliable information available about the safety of IP-6 when used in amounts greater than those found in foods; avoid using.

Effectiveness

POSSIBLY EFFECTIVE

Kidney stones (nephrolithiasis). There is some evidence that people with high dietary intake of IP-6 have a decreased risk of developing kidney stones (10296).

There is insufficient reliable information available about the effectiveness of IP-6 for its other uses.

Mechanism of Action

Inositol hexaphosphate (IP-6), the hexaphosphate ester of inositol, is the major phosphorus storage compound in plants, comprising from 1-7% of the dry weight of most cereals, nuts, and legumes (1855,1858). IP-6 and other less phosphorylated forms (e.g., inositol triphosphate) are also endogenous to most mammalian cells in much smaller amounts (1857). Cellular functions include signal transduction and cellular proliferation and differentiation (1857). IP-6 chelates multivalent metal ions (particularly zinc, calcium, and iron) forming insoluble salts in the

gastrointestinal (GI) tract and decreasing mineral bioavailability (1858,1869,1870).
In the urine, IP-6 can reduce the formation of calcium and oxalate crystals (10297). IP-6 appears to reduce the concentration of calcium and the formation of calcium crystals in renal papillary tissue (10298).
Preliminary evidence suggests that the ability of IP-6 to chelate minerals might decrease iron-mediated colon cancer risk, and lower serum cholesterol and triglycerides (1858).
There is interest in using IP-6 for cancer. Preliminary research shows that IP-6 inhibits cancer cell proliferation and increases cancer cell differentiation, sometimes resulting in reversion to a normal phenotype, in vitro (1859). IP-6 has anticancer activity in models of breast, colon, liver, prostate, and hematological cancers (1860,1861,1862,1863,1864,1865,13042). IP-6 is thought to potentially have antiangiogenic activity. In vitro, IP-6 inhibits experimentally induced angiogenesis (13041).
Preliminary in vitro evidence also suggests that IP-6 has a synergistic effect when used in combination with adriamycin or tamoxifen for inhibiting growth of breast cancer cells (13256).
IP-6 might also inhibit platelet aggregation and lower serum cholesterol and triglycerides, according to preliminary studies (1867,1868).
As a natural antioxidant, IP-6 added to food reduces lipid peroxidation and retards spoilage (1855,1858).

Adverse Reactions

None reported.

Interactions with Herbs & Other Dietary Supplements

CALCIUM, IRON, ZINC: Concurrent use of IP-6 may decrease mineral absorption. IP-6 can chelate multivalent metal ions in the gastrointestinal tract, forming insoluble salts and decreasing mineral absorption (1858).
HERBS WITH ANTICOAGULANT/ANTIPLATELET POTENTIAL: Theoretically, concomitant use of IP-6 with herbs that affect platelet aggregation might increase the risk of bleeding. In vitro IP-6 can inhibit platelet aggregation (1867). This effect has not been demonstrated in humans. Herbs with potential anticoagulant or antiplatelet properties include angelica, clove, danshen, garlic, ginger, ginkgo, Panax ginseng, red clover, turmeric, and others.

Interactions with Drugs

ANTICOAGULANT/ANTIPLATELET DRUGS: Theoretically, concomitant use of IP-6 with drugs that affect platelet aggregation may increase the risk of bleeding. In vitro IP-6 can inhibit platelet aggregation (1867). This effect has not been demonstrated in humans.

Interactions with Foods

None known.

Interactions with Lab Tests

CHOLESTEROL/TRIGLYCERIDES: Theoretically, IP-6 may reduce serum cholesterol and triglyceride levels. Preliminary research suggests that IP-6 can lower cholesterol and triglyceride levels (1868). This effect has not been demonstrated in humans.

Interactions with Diseases or Conditions

CLOTTING DISORDERS: Theoretically, IP-6 may increase risk of bleeding (1867). In vitro, IP-6 can inhibit platelet aggregation (1867). This effect has not been demonstrated in humans.
IRON-DEFICIENCY ANEMIA: IP-6 might decrease dietary and supplemental iron absorption. IP-6 chelates multivalent metal ions in the gastrointestinal tract, preventing absorption (1858).
OSTEOPOROSIS/OSTEOPENIA (Paget's Disease): IP-6 may decrease dietary and supplemental calcium absorption. IP-6 chelates multivalent metal ions in the gastrointestinal tract, preventing absorption (1858).

Dosage and Administration

No typical dosage.

Comments

Preliminary studies of inositol hexaphosphate in cancer have been ongoing since 1988; however, to date, no studies in humans with cancer have been performed (1866). "IP-6, Nature's Revolutionary Cancer-Fighter," a book by prominent inositol hexaphosphate researcher, Abulkalam M. Shamsuddin, MD, PhD, has popularized inositol hexaphosphate (1854).

IPECAC

Also Known As

Brazil Root, Brazilian Ipecac, Cartagena Ipecac, Ipecacuanha, Matto Grosso Ipecac, Nicaragua Ipecac, Panama Ipecac, Rio Ipecac.

Scientific Names

Psychotria ipecacuanha, synonyms Callicocca ipecacuanha, Cephaelis acuminata, Cephaelis ipecacuanha; Uragoga ipecacuanha; Uragoga granatensis.
Family: Rubiaceae.

People Use This For

Orally, ipecac is used as an expectorant and emetic, for croupous bronchitis in children, amebic dysentery, as an appetite stimulant (small doses), and for treating cancer.
Intravenously, ipecac is used for amebic abscesses and hepatitis.

Safety

POSSIBLY SAFE ...when the rhizome or syrup of ipecac is used orally and appropriately short-term (12).
POSSIBLY UNSAFE ...when used orally long-term. Theoretically, prolonged use might blunt the emetic reflex (19). ...when in contact with skin or when inhaled. The constituent emetine is a skin irritant, and ipecac powder is a respiratory irritant (6,18).
LIKELY UNSAFE ...when used orally in large amounts. Misuse can lead to serious toxicity or death (6,12). ...when a total dose of more than 1 gram is injected, it can cause nervous system symptoms, blood in the urine, and circulatory collapse (6).
CHILDREN: LIKELY SAFE ...when used orally and appropriately as an emetic (272,11349). LIKELY UNSAFE ...when used orally in large doses and in infants under 1 year old (12,19). Children are more sensitive to large doses and effects on the nervous system than adults (19).
PREGNANCY: LIKELY UNSAFE ...when used orally; ipecac is a potential uterine stimulant (12,19).
LACTATION: Insufficient reliable information available; avoid using.

Effectiveness

POSSIBLY EFFECTIVE

Poisoning. Taking syrup of ipecac orally is an effective emetic (15). Ipecac is an FDA-approved prescription product. However, the efficacy in preventing pediatric deaths with routine use of ipecac at home has never been proven. The American Academy of Pediatrics recommended in 1983 that all households keep a 1-ounce bottle of syrup of ipecac at home. Ipecac could then be used on the advice of a physician, emergency department, or poison control center to induce vomiting. This recommendation has recently been reversed stating, "Syrup of ipecac should no longer be routinely used as a poison treatment intervention in the home" (11349).

There is insufficient reliable information available about the effectiveness of ipecac for its other uses.

Mechanism of Action

Ipecac contains the alkaloids, emetine and cephaeline (13). Ipecac produces emesis by irritating the GI mucosa and by stimulating the chemoreceptor trigger zone in the brain (6,13).

Adverse Reactions

Orally, ipecac causes nausea, vomiting (3,6,13,15,18), GI irritation, dizziness, hypotension, dyspnea, and tachycardia (11). Chronic use is associated with myopathies and death (6,18). Overdose is associated with erosion of GI tract mucous membranes, cardiac arrhythmias, disorders of respiratory function, convulsions, shock, and coma (18).
Topically, emetine is a skin irritant (6). Ipecac powder is a respiratory irritant.
Intravenously, emetine may cause inflammation of the muscle tissue at the injection site with chronic administration. In total doses over 1 gram, it can lead to gastrointestinal and nervous system symptoms, hematuria and circulatory collapse (6).

Interactions with Herbs & Other Dietary Supplements

PODOPHYLLUM: Ipecac reduces the intensity of the cathartic effect of podophyllum (19).

Interactions with Drugs

ACTIVATED CHARCOAL: Activated charcoal adsorbs and inactivates syrup of ipecac; avoid co-administration (506).

Interactions with Foods

None known.

Interactions with Lab Tests

None known.

Interactions with Diseases or Conditions

GI CONDITIONS: Ipecac can irritate gastrointestinal tract. Contraindicated in individuals with infectious or inflammatory gastrointestinal conditions (19).
HEART DISEASES: Use of ipecac is contraindicated (12), due to cardiotoxic potential of emetine (6), and its depressive effect on the heart (19).
POISONINGS: Ipecac is contraindicated in individuals poisoned with corrosives (risks re-exposure of esophageal tissue), petroleum distillates (risks aspiration pneumonia), strychnine (risk of convulsions) (12,19).
UNCONSCIOUSNESS: Contraindicated (12).

Dosage and Administration

ORAL: Expectorant (adults), 0.4-1.4 mL ipecac syrup (USP) (12). Emetic, 15 mL ipecac syrup (USP) followed by 1-2 glasses of water (12); may repeat once in 20 minutes if no results (12,13). Before using ipecac syrup to treat poisoning, call poison control for recommendation. Ipecac syrup is available both as a nonprescription product and as an FDA-approved prescription product.

IPORURU

Also Known As

Iporoni, Iporuro, Ipurosa, Ipururo, Macochihua, Niando.

Scientific Names

Alchornea castaneifolia.
Family: Euphorbiaceae.

Comments

At the date of publication, there was very little scientific information available about this product. Our staff is continually analyzing the available information on natural medicines and will add data to the online version of *Natural Medicines Comprehensive Database* as it becomes available. See www.naturaldatabase.com.

IPRIFLAVONE

Also Known As

7-Isopropoxy-Isoflavone, 7-Isopropoxy Isoflavone, FL-113, TC-80.
CAUTION: See separate listings for Red Clover and Soy.

Scientific Names

7-isopropoxyisoflavone.

People Use This For

Orally, ipriflavone is used for preventing and treating postmenopausal and senile osteoporosis, preventing drug-induced osteoporosis, relieving osteoporotic pain, treating Paget's disease and renal osteodystrophy, and for reducing bone loss in hemiplegic stroke patients. Ipriflavone is also used by bodybuilders as an anabolic agent.

Safety

LIKELY SAFE ...when used orally and appropriately. Ipriflavone seems to be safe when used for up to 3 years (427,428,430,431,432,433,1196,2169,2170,2171,2172,2173,2174,2175,4749,10228). However, there is concern that ipriflavone can cause subclinical (asymptomatic) lymphocytopenia in some patients taking it for greater than 6 months (1196). Monitor white blood cell (WBC) count in patients taking ipriflavone long-term. Tell patients not to take ipriflavone without proper medical supervision and monitoring.
PREGNANCY AND LACTATION: Insufficient reliable information available; avoid using.

Effectiveness

LIKELY EFFECTIVE

Osteoporosis. Taking ipriflavone orally in combination with calcium 1000 mg daily can prevent loss of bone mineral density (BMD) in postmenopausal women with osteoporosis or low bone mass (430,432,433,2169,2170,2175). There is some evidence that it might actually increase BMD in some of these patients (428,2173,2175,4756). Concurrent use of calcium in doses of at least 1000 mg per day might be necessary for greatest benefit. One study using ipriflavone with only 500 mg per day of calcium found no effect on BMD (1196). Ipriflavone can also significantly reduce osteoporotic pain and seems to be as effective as inhaled calcitonin (432,2175,4756,4757). Taking Ipriflavone plus calcium or vitamin D prophylactically also seems to help prevent osteoporosis in postmenopausal women (2171,2174). However, using ipriflavone in combination with low-dose estrogen seems to be more beneficial than ipriflavone alone for preventing osteoporosis. Ipriflavone plus conjugated estrogen 0.3 mg per day and calcium 500-1000 mg daily seems to consistently increase BMD in postmenopausal women (427,2171,2172). Ipriflavone in combination with conjugated estrogen 0.625 mg per day can also decreases loss of bone mineral density (BMD) better than estrogen or ipriflavone alone in oophorectomized women (4749). Ipriflavone also seems to prevent loss of bone mineral density (BMD) induced by the gonadotropin hormone-releasing hormone agonist, leuprolide (Lupron) (10228). Adding calcium provides further benefit (4746). Ipriflavone in combination with vitamin D, seems to prevent BMD loss significantly better than vitamin D alone in hemiplegic stroke patients with vitamin D deficiency (429).

POSSIBLY EFFECTIVE

Paget's disease. There is some evidence that ipriflavone 600 mg or 1200 mg given orally for 30 days can reduce serum alkaline phosphatase and hydroxyproline/creatinine excretion and decrease bone pain in patients with Paget's disease (2176).

Renal osteodystrophy. Taking ipriflavone orally seems to be beneficial for people with renal osteodystrophy (2177).

There is insufficient reliable information available about the effectiveness of ipriflavone for its other uses.

Mechanism of Action

Ipriflavone is a semisynthetic isoflavone manufactured in the laboratory from daidzein, a compound derived from soy (431). Ipriflavone enhances osteoblast function and inhibits bone resorption, mainly by inhibiting recruitment of osteoclasts (2173,2176,2179). Preliminary evidence suggests that ipriflavone prevents bone density loss without suppressing the rate of bone formation (unlike 17-beta-estradiol which suppresses the rate of bone formation) (426). Ipriflavone has no direct estrogenic activity in postmenopausal women, but might potentiate the effects of estrogen on bone, increase uterotropic activity of estrogen, and stimulate estrogen-induced calcitonin secretion (434,2179). Clinical evidence suggests that using ipriflavone in combination with conjugated estrogens for postmenopausal osteoporosis might allow for use of a lower estrogen dose (427,2171,2172). Ipriflavone, or its metabolite 7-hydroxy-isoflavone, might inhibit cytochrome P450 (CYP450) enzymes CYP1A2 and CYP2C9 (2178). Laboratory evidence suggests that isoflavones can inhibit oxidative and conjugative metabolism (4736). Isoflavones might also affect drug absorption and biliary excretion by interacting with drug transporters such as P-glycoprotein and the canalicular multispecific organic anion transporter (4736). Whether ipriflavone has similar activity is unknown.

Adverse Reactions

Orally, ipriflavone is usually well-tolerated. However, some patients taking ipriflavone can experience epigastric pain, diarrhea, and dizziness (432). There is some concern about ipriflavone causing lymphocytopenia. In one study, subclinical (asymptomatic) lymphocytopenia occurred in about 13% of patients. Decreased lymphocytes (less than 500/microliter) seems to be most likely to occur after 6 months of treatment, but may not occur until much later (1196). The clinical significance of this effect on lymphocytes is not known. Monitor white blood cell (WBC) counts in patients taking ipriflavone long-term. Consider discontinuing ipriflavone if lymphocytes drop below 1000 per microliter. Lymphocyte counts seem to normalize in most patients within 12 months after discontinuing ipriflavone (1196). Tell patients not to take ipriflavone without proper medical supervision and monitoring.

Interactions with Herbs & Other Dietary Supplements

CALCIUM: Concomitant use may enhance effects in preventing osteoporosis (2169,2170,2171,2173,2175).
VITAMIN D: Concomitant use may enhance effects in preventing osteoporosis (2174).

Interactions with Drugs

CYTOCHROME P450 1A2 (CYP1A2) SUBSTRATES: Ipriflavone is thought to competitively inhibit cytochrome P450 1A2 (CYP1A2) (2178). Theoretically, concurrent use of ipriflavone and drugs metabolized by these enzymes might result in decreased drug elimination, increased serum levels, and potential toxicity. Some drugs metabolized by CYP1A2 include clozapine (Clozaril), cyclobenzaprine (Flexeril), fluvoxamine (Luvox), haloperidol (Haldol), imipramine (Tofranil), mexiletine (Mexitil), olanzapine (Zyprexa), Pentazocine (Talwin), propranolol (Inderal), tacrine (Cognex), theophylline (Slo-bid, Theo-Dur, others), zileuton (Zyflo), Zolmitriptan (Zomig), and others.

CYTOCHROME P450 2C9 (CYP2C9) SUBSTRATES: Ipriflavone is thought to competitively inhibit cytochrome P450 2C9 (CYP2C9) (2178). Theoretically, concurrent use of ipriflavone and drugs metabolized by

these enzymes might result in decreased drug elimination, increased serum levels, and potential toxicity. Some drugs metabolized by CYP2C9 include amitriptyline (Elavil), diazepam (Valium), estradiol (Estrace), tacrine (Cognex), verapamil (Calan), warfarin (Coumadin), zileuton (Zyflo), and others.
IMMUNOSUPPRESSANTS: Concurrent use of ipriflavone and immunosuppressant drugs might have additive effects on inhibiting immune function. Some patients taking ipriflavone experience subclinical (asymptomatic) lymphocytopenia (1196); avoid concurrent use. Immunosuppressant drugs include azathioprine (Imuran), basiliximab (Simulect), cyclosporine (Neoral, Sandimmune), daclizumab (Zenapax), muromonab-CD3 (OKT3, Orthoclone OKT3), mycophenolate (CellCept), tacrolimus (FK506, Prograf), sirolimus (Rapamune), prednisone (Deltasone, Orasone), and other corticosteroids (glucocorticoids).
THEOPHYLLINE: Concomitant use of theophylline and ipriflavone can increase serum theophylline levels. Increased theophylline levels have occurred in two cases after patients started taking ipriflavone (2178,6604). Ipriflavone is thought to decrease theophylline metabolism through competitive inhibition of the cytochrome P450 1A2 (CYP1A2) enzyme (2178,6604).

Interactions with Foods

None known.

Interactions with Lab Tests

LYMPHOCYTES: Ipriflavone can decrease lymphocytes in some patients. Lymphocytes can often decrease by about 27% in patients after 6 months of use and then they stabilize. However, in a smaller number of patients, about 13% in one study, subclinical (asymptomatic) lymphocytopenia (less than 500/microliter) can occur (1196). White blood cell (WBC) count should be monitored in patients using ipriflavone long-term. Consider discontinuing ipriflavone if lymphocytes drop below 1000 per microliter. Lymphocyte counts seem to normalize in most patients within 12 months after discontinuing ipriflavone (1196).

Interactions with Diseases or Conditions

IMMUNOSUPPRESSION: Theoretically, ipriflavone might have additive immunosuppressive effects in patients with a compromised immune system. Ipriflavone can cause lymphocytopenia in some patients (1196); use with caution.
LYMPHOCYTOPENIA: Since ipriflavone has been reported to cause lymphocytopenia in some patients (1196), it might further decrease lymphocyte counts when used in patients with pre-existing lymphocytopenia; use with caution.

Dosage and Administration

ORAL: The typical dose for postmenopausal osteoporosis is 200 mg three times daily (2169,2170,2171,2172,2173,2175). For Paget's disease, ipriflavone 600-1200 mg daily has been used (2176). For treating renal osteodystrophy, 400-600 mg ipriflavone daily has been used (2177). For reducing drug-induced bone mineral loss, ipriflavone 600 mg daily has been used (10228).

Comments

Ipriflavone is used in Italy and Japan in the treatment of osteoporosis.

IRON

Also Known As

Elemental Iron, Fer, Ferrous Carbonate Anhydrous, Ferrous Fumarate, Ferrous Gluconate, Ferrous Pyrophosphate, Ferrous Sulfate.

Scientific Names

Iron; Fe; atomic number 26.

People Use This For

Orally, iron salts are used for preventing and treating iron deficiency and iron deficiency anemia. It is also used for attention deficit-hyperactivity disorder (ADHD), improving athletic performance, treating oral canker sores, Crohn's disease, depression, fatigue, female infertility, and menorrhagia.

Safety

LIKELY SAFE ...when used orally and appropriately. For people age 14 and older with adequate iron stores, iron supplements are safe when used in doses below the tolerable upper intake level (UL) of 45 mg per day of elemental iron. The UL is not meant to apply to those who receive iron under medical supervision (7135). To treat iron deficiency, most people can safely take up to 300 mg elemental iron per day (15).
LIKELY UNSAFE ...when used orally in excessive doses. Doses greater than the UL of 45 mg frequently cause gastrointestinal side effects such as constipation and nausea (7135). Doses of 30 mg/kg are associated with acute toxicity. Long-term use of high doses of iron can cause hemosiderosis and multiple organ damage. The estimated lethal dose of iron is 180-300 mg/kg; however, doses as low as 60 mg/kg have also been lethal (15).
CHILDREN: LIKELY SAFE ...when used orally and appropriately (7135). LIKELY UNSAFE ...when used orally in excessive amounts. Tell patients who are not iron-deficient not to use doses above the tolerable upper intake level (UL) of 40 mg per day of elemental iron for infants and children. Higher doses frequently cause gastrointestinal side effects such as constipation and nausea (7135). Iron is the most common cause of pediatric poisoning deaths. Doses as low as 60 mg/kg can be fatal (15).
PREGNANCY AND LACTATION: LIKELY SAFE ...when used orally and appropriately. Iron is safe for pregnant and breast-feeding women with adequate iron stores when used in doses below the tolerable upper intake level (UL) of 45 mg per day of elemental iron (7135). LIKELY UNSAFE ...when used orally in high doses. Tell patients who are not iron deficient to avoid exceeding the tolerable upper intake level (UL) of 45 mg per day of elemental iron. Higher doses frequently cause gastrointestinal side effects such as nausea and vomiting. High hemoglobin concentrations at the time of delivery are associated with adverse pregnancy outcomes (7135).

Effectiveness

EFFECTIVE

Anemia of chronic disease. Taking iron orally with epoetin alfa (erythropoietin, EPO, Epogen, Procrit) is effective for treating anemia associated with chronic renal failure and chemotherapy. Epoetin alfa is needed to ensure that the response is not limited by lack of iron for erythropoiesis (1087,1091).

Iron deficiency anemia. Taking iron orally is effective for treating iron deficiency anemia (1089,7135).

POSSIBLY EFFECTIVE

ACE inhibitor-associated cough. Taking iron orally seems to inhibit cough associated with angiotensin converting enzyme (ACE) inhibitors. Ferrous sulfate 256 mg daily might reduce or eliminate cough associated with ACE inhibitors such as captopril (Capoten), enalapril (Vasotec), Lisinopril (Prinivil, Zestril), and others (7307).

Cognitive function. Taking iron orally seems to improve cognitive function in iron-deficient children and adolescents. Supplemental iron seems to improve verbal learning and memory in non-anemic iron-deficient adolescent girls (1095). It might also reverse developmental and learning deficits in iron-deficient children (1104).

INSUFFICIENT RELIABLE EVIDENCE to RATE

Attention deficit-hyperactivity disorder (ADHD). Taking iron orally might improve symptoms of attention deficit-hyperactivity disorder (ADHD) (1093).

Fatigue. There is preliminary evidence that iron supplementation might improve unexplained fatigue in non-anemic women. Ferrous sulfate 80 mg daily may improve fatigue primarily in women with borderline or low serum ferritin concentrations (11406).

More evidence is needed to rate iron for these uses.

Mechanism of Action

Iron is a trace mineral found in two ionic forms in the body. It exists in a reduced state as ferrous iron and in an oxidized state as ferric iron. Most of the iron in the body is found in the hemoglobin of red blood cells and in the myoglobin of muscle cells where it is required for oxygen and carbon dioxide transport (1093).
Iron also functions in the electron transport chain as an electron carrier in cytochromes. It is also found in the functional groups of most enzymes in the Krebs cycle (945). Iron is an essential cofactor in the synthesis of neurotransmitters such as dopamine, norepinephrine, and serotonin.
Iron deficiency anemia in early life seems to negatively affect behavioral and neural development (1093,9962). Signs and symptoms of deficiency include microcytic and hypochromic anemia, lethargy, cognitive impairment, developmental delay, amenorrhea, hair loss, enlarged liver, and others (7135). Iron deficiency in pregnancy has been associated with adverse pregnancy outcomes and increased perinatal maternal mortality (7135).
The rate of iron absorption from food and supplements is variable. Absorption of iron from foods depends on the source. Meats, such as red meat, poultry, and fish provide iron in heme and non-heme forms. Meats contain about 40% heme iron and 60% non-heme iron. Heme iron is absorbed at a rate of 23% compared to 2% to 20% for non-heme iron. Iron from plant sources is only in the non-heme form. Iron bioavailability from a vegetarian diet is estimated to be 5% to 10%. Meats and fish seem to enhance the absorption of non-heme iron (7135).
Boiling, steaming, or stir-frying appears to enhance the bioavailability of iron contained in many vegetables including asparagus, broccoli, cabbage, red and green peppers, and tomatoes; but cold storage of cooked vegetables might greatly reduce the increases in iron bioavailability gained from cooking (5044). Overall, dietary iron

absorption is only 10% to 15%. However, this varies significantly depending on the person and the iron demand of the body (403).

Vegetarians and people who engage in intense physical exercise, particularly female athletes, may have increased iron requirements (7135). Blood loss and rapid growth also increase gastrointestinal absorption (1101). Iron is stored as ferritin or hemosiderin (7135).

Body iron is highly conserved. In the absence of bleeding (including menstruation) or pregnancy, the body loses only a small quantity of iron each day, mostly through the feces (7135).

There is interest in using iron to treat attention deficit-hyperactivity disorder (ADHD). Research suggests that children with ADHD are more likely to be iron deficient. The level of iron deficiency seems to be positively correlated with the severity of ADHD symptoms (10700).

Iron also seems to reduce nitric oxide production. This effect might be clinically useful in the suppression of cough associated with angiotensin converting enzyme (ACE) inhibitors. Iron might reduce the generation of nitric oxide, which is thought to be increased by ACE inhibitors (7303).

Adverse Reactions

Orally, iron can cause gastrointestinal irritation, abdominal pain, constipation or diarrhea, nausea, and vomiting. At doses below the tolerable upper intake level (UL) of 45 mg per day of elemental iron in adults with normal iron stores, gastrointestinal adverse effects are uncommon (7135). Higher doses can be taken safely in adults with iron deficiency, but gastrointestinal side effects may occur. Taking iron supplements with food seems to reduce gastrointestinal side effects (7135). Liquid oral preparations can blacken teeth (9). Long-term use of high doses of iron can cause hemosiderosis that clinically resembles hemochromatosis (15). Acute overdosage, 60 mg/kg and more, can cause vomiting and diarrhea, followed by cardiovascular or metabolic toxicity, and death (7135). There is a debate regarding the potential association between high levels of iron stores and cancer. So far, data are conflicting and inconclusive (1098,1099,1100,1102). There is also a debate regarding a potential association between coronary heart disease or myocardial infarction (MI) and high iron intake or high body iron stores; some studies have reported associations (1492,7135,9542,9544,9545). Some studies only found an association with high heme iron intake (1492,9546). However the majority of research has found no association (1097,1099,9543,9547,9548,9549,9550). The currently available data doesn't support a recommendation to reduce iron intake to reduce cardiovascular risks, especially considering the potential problems associated with iron deficiency (9543).

Interactions with Herbs & Other Dietary Supplements

ACACIA: Acacia forms an insoluble gel with ferric iron (16). It isn't known whether this leads to a significant interaction when the two are ingested together.

CALCIUM: Calcium inhibits the absorption of dietary heme- and non-heme iron (7135,7308,9573). However, in people with adequate iron stores, this doesn't appear to be clinically significant (1848,1849,1850,7135,7308). Advise people at risk for iron deficiency to take calcium supplements at bedtime, instead of with meals, to avoid inhibiting dietary iron absorption (7308). Calcium supplements can also inhibit absorption of iron supplements. However, the effect is very variable and depends on the salt form used, presence or absence of food, and the type of food (9586). The clinical significance is unclear, but advise patients to take calcium and iron supplements at different times of the day if possible.

RIBOFLAVIN (Vitamin B2): Riboflavin supplements may improve the hematological response to iron supplements in some people with anemia (9518). Riboflavin is thought to be involved in mobilization of iron for heme synthesis from the storage form, ferritin, and in globin synthesis (9518). This effect is probably only significant in people with riboflavin deficiency.

SOY: Soy protein reduces absorption of dietary non-heme (plant-derived) iron, probably due to binding of iron by phytate and calcium present in soy (5053,9573). Fermented soy products seem to inhibit of iron absorption less (9586). The clinical significance of these effects hasn't been determined.

VITAMIN A, BETA-CAROTENE: Vitamin A appears to be involved in mobilizing iron from tissue stores for delivery to developing red blood cells in the bone marrow. Improvements in hemoglobin levels can occur in people with anemia and low serum retinol levels when they are given vitamin A supplements (9586). Vitamin A may also be involved in the differentiation and proliferation of blood stem cells in the bone marrow, and in the synthesis of erythropoietin (9518). Preliminary evidence also suggests that vitamin A and beta-carotene may enhance non-heme iron absorption from iron-fortified wheat and corn flour, and rice. It's suggested that these vitamins bind to iron in the gut, improving its solubility and preventing binding by dietary polyphenols and phytate, which reduce iron absorption (9569). It's unlikely that vitamin A supplements would have significant effects on iron status in people without vitamin A deficiency.

VITAMIN C (Ascorbic acid): Supplemental or dietary vitamin C improves absorption of supplemental or dietary non-heme (plant-derived) iron ingested at the same time (9518,9571,9586). The amount of vitamin C in the diet is a factor in dietary iron absorption and iron status (9570,9572). Vitamin C can counteract the effects of substances which inhibit iron absorption such as dietary phytates, polyphenols, and tannins possibly by chemically reducing iron and preventing the formation of less soluble ferric compounds (9518,9573,9586). Taking a vitamin C supplement to improve absorption of dietary or supplemental iron probably isn't necessary for most people, especially if their diet contains plenty of vitamin C (9571).

ZINC: Under some circumstances iron and zinc can interfere with each other's absorption. When high supplemental doses of zinc are taken on an empty stomach there is a measurable reduction in iron absorption, and high supplemental doses of non-heme iron taken on an empty stomach can reduce zinc absorption, especially when dietary mineral intake is low (8856,9579,9580,9581,9582,9583,9584). This is probably because the carriers for iron and zinc in the gut become saturated at high doses, and the ions then compete for non-specific carriers. If one of the ions is present in excess, absorption of the other will be decreased (9580). When food is present, the ions become complexed with food components and don't compete for absorption (9579). Therefore, there isn't a significant interaction between dietary iron and zinc, or between supplemental iron and zinc when taken with food (8866,9579,9581). Advise patients to take these supplements with food.

Interactions with Drugs

BISPHOSPHONATES: Divalent cations, including iron, can decrease absorption of bisphosphonates by forming insoluble complexes (15). Advise patients that doses of bisphosphonates should be separated by at least two hours from doses of all other medications, including supplements such as iron. The bisphosphonates include alendronate (Fosamax), etidronate (Didronel), risedronate (Actonel), and tiludronate (Skelid).

CHLORAMPHENICOL: Chloramphenicol can reduce the response to iron therapy in iron deficiency anemia, because it interferes with erythrocyte maturation (15,3046). Since chloramphenicol isn't usually taken for prolonged periods, this isn't likely to be clinically significant.

LEVODOPA: There is some evidence in healthy people that iron forms chelates with levodopa, reducing the amount of levodopa absorbed by around 50% (9567). The clinical significance of this hasn't been determined. Advise patients to separate doses of levodopa and iron as much as possible.

LEVOTHYROXINE (Synthroid, Levothroid, Levoxyl, and others): Iron can decrease the absorption and efficacy of levothyroxine by forming insoluble complexes in the gastrointestinal tract (9568). Advise patients to separate levothyroxine and iron doses by at least two hours.

METHYLDOPA (Aldomet): Concomitant use can decrease absorption of methyldopa, resulting in increases in blood pressure (7900). Advise patients to separate iron and methyldopa doses by at least two hours.

MYCOPHENOLATE MOFETIL (CellCept): Oral iron supplements markedly reduce absorption of mycophenolate mofetil, probably by forming nonabsorbable chelates. If concurrent therapy is essential, advise patients to take iron four to six hours before, or two hours after mycophenolate mofetil (3046).

PENICILLAMINE: Oral iron supplements can reduce absorption of penicillamine by 30% to 70%, probably due to chelate formation. Efficacy of penicillamine is reduced in Wilson's Disease; the clinical significance in people with rheumatoid arthritis (RA) hasn't been determined (3046,3072). Advise patients to take penicillamine at least two hours before or after iron-containing supplements.

QUINOLONE ANTIBIOTICS: Iron decreases the absorption of quinolones due to formation of insoluble complexes (15). Advise patients to take these antibiotics at least 2 hours before or 2 hours after iron-containing supplements (3072). Quinolones include ciprofloxacin (Cipro), levofloxacin (Levaquin), ofloxacin (Floxin), and others.

TETRACYCLINE ANTIBIOTICS: Concomitant use can decrease absorption of tetracyclines by 50% to 90% (15). Advise patients to take tetracyclines at least two hours before or after iron-containing supplements. Some of these drugs include doxycycline (Vibramycin), minocycline (Minocin), tetracycline (Achromycin), and others.

Drug Influences on Nutrient Levels and Depletion

SOME DRUGS CAN AFFECT IRON LEVELS:

AMINOSALICYLIC ACID: Aminosalicylic acid sometimes causes a malabsorption syndrome, resulting in weight loss, iron depletion, and excessive fat in the stools (steatorrhea) (9574). Advise patients to consult their physician if these symptoms occur. Some of these drugs include para-aminosalicylic acid, PAS, and Paser.

ANTACIDS: Gastric acid is important for absorption of dietary, non-heme (plant-derived) iron (4539). Antacids may therefore reduce iron absorption by increasing gastric pH and reducing iron solubility (3072). This isn't likely to be clinically significant in most people with adequate dietary iron intake. However, antacids can reduce absorption of iron from supplements by 30% to 40%, and reduced efficacy has occurred occasionally (3046). Advise patients who need iron supplements to avoid antacids or separate the doses as much as possible.

ASPIRIN, NONSTEROIDAL ANTI-INFLAMMATORY DRUGS (NSAIDs): Aspirin and NSAIDs can cause mucosal damage and bleeding throughout the gastrointestinal (GI) tract. This may be asymptomatic and undetected. In people taking these drugs for prolonged periods, including those taking low-dose aspirin, this chronic blood loss may contribute to iron deficiency anemia (8888,9515,9576,9577). Advise patients to consult their physician promptly if they have symptoms of anemia, GI irritation, or blood in the stools. Since iron supplements may also irritate the GI tract, patients should not use them concurrently with NSAIDs unless recommended by a physician. Encourage patients to include iron-rich foods in their diet.

CHOLESTYRAMINE (Questran), COLESTIPOL (Colestid): Cholestyramine and colestipol may bind iron in the gut, reducing its absorption (9566). Clinically significant iron deficiency induced by these drugs hasn't been reported, and supplements aren't likely to be needed. If patients are taking iron supplements for other causes of deficiency, recommend they separate the iron and cholestyramine or colestipol doses by at least four hours.

H2-BLOCKERS: Gastric acid is important for the absorption of iron, particularly dietary non-heme (plant-derived) iron (4539). Dose-dependent reductions in dietary iron absorption have been noted with cimetidine, ranging from

28% to 65% with single doses of 300 to 900 mg (8876). However, long-term treatment, up to 18 years, with H2-blockers isn't associated with iron depletion or anemia in people with normal iron stores (4483,4539,9578). Advise people to maintain adequate dietary iron intake. Supplements aren't necessary unless people have other factors contributing to iron deficiency. The H2-blockers include cimetidine (Tagamet), ranitidine (Zantac), famotidine (Pepcid), and nizatidine (Axid).

PANCREATIC ENZYMES, PANCRELIPASE, PANCREATIN: There is some evidence that pancreatic enzyme supplements can reduce iron absorption, possibly by binding iron or altering pH (9575,9585). It's unlikely that this will be clinically significant, except in people with cystic fibrosis who need pancreatic enzyme supplements for prolonged periods, and have other factors contributing to iron deficiency (9575). Advise these patients to have their iron status checked regularly. Some of these drugs include Pancrease, Cotazym, Viokase, Creon, and Ultrase.

PENICILLAMINE (Cuprimine, Depen): Penicillamine chelates iron in the gastrointestinal tract and decreases absorption. If iron supplements are used, separate from penicillamine by at least 2 hours (9630).

PROTON PUMP INHIBITORS: Gastric acid is important for the absorption of iron, particularly dietary non-heme (plant-derived) iron (4539). However, long-term treatment, up to 12.5 years, with proton pump inhibitors isn't associated with iron depletion or anemia in people with normal iron stores (4483,8850,9578). Advise people to maintain adequate dietary iron intake. Supplements aren't necessary unless people have other factors contributing to iron deficiency. Proton pump inhibitors include lansoprazole (Prevacid), omeprazole (Prilosec), rabeprazole (Aciphex), pantoprazole (Protonix, Pantoloc), and others.

QUINOLONES: Quinolones form complexes with iron in the GI tract, which could reduce absorption of both the fluoroquinolone and iron if taken at the same time (2682). Significant effects on iron levels are unlikely when quinolones are taken at least two hours before, or four to six hours after iron supplements or iron-containing foods. Quinolones include ciprofloxacin (Cipro), levofloxacin (Levaquin), ofloxacin (Floxin), moxifloxacin (Avelox), gatifloxacin (Tequin), and others.

TETRACYCLINES: Tetracyclines form complexes with iron in the GI tract, reducing absorption of both the tetracycline and iron if taken at the same time (4412,4549,4550). Significant effects on iron levels are unlikely when tetracyclines are taken at least two hours before or after iron supplements or iron-containing foods. Tetracyclines include demeclocycline (Declomycin), doxycycline (Vibramycin and others), and minocycline (Minocin and others).

Interactions with Foods

COFFEE AND TEA: These beverages can reduce absorption of both dietary and supplemental iron when taken at the same time. This is likely due to binding of iron in the gut by polyphenols and tannins in tea and coffee (8887,9570,9571,9573). Body iron stores (measured by serum ferritin) are inversely related to coffee and tea intake (9571). These effects could potentially contribute to iron deficiency anemia, especially in people with other risk factors.

DAIRY PRODUCTS: Calcium in dairy products such as milk and cheese can reduce the absorption of dietary and supplemental iron (8875). This is unlikely to be clinically significant in people with adequate iron stores. Advise patients who need iron supplements to take them with a meal that is relatively low in dairy products whenever possible. Maximal absorption of iron supplements would occur when they are taken on an empty stomach, but this increases the risk of gastric irritation and shouldn't be recommended.

Interactions with Lab Tests

GUAIAC TEST: Iron may cause a false-positive reading for occult fecal blood. However, the benzidine test for occult fecal blood is not likely to be affected (15).

Interactions with Diseases or Conditions

ACHLORHYDRIA: Decreased stomach acidity may impair iron absorption (7135).

CHRONIC UNDERNUTRITION, MICRONUTRIENT DEFICIENCY: Supplemental iron can normalize serum ferritin, but may not raise low hemoglobin in chronic undernutrition and multiple micronutrient deficiency (6923).

HEMODIALYSIS: Supplemental iron absorption is decreased in people requiring chronic hemodialysis (1088,1090).

HEMOGLOBIN DISEASES: Iron overload is likely to occur in people with hemoglobinopathies or other refractory anemias erroneously diagnosed as iron deficiency anemia (15).

IRON DEFICIENCY: Iron absorption is increased (945).

MALABSORPTION SYNDROMES: Oral iron therapy may be ineffective in individuals with diarrhea, post-gastrectomy, or other malabsorption syndromes (945).

PEPTIC ULCER DISEASE, REGIONAL ENTERITIS, ULCERATIVE COLITIS: Iron can exacerbate these conditions (15); contraindicated.

PREMATURE INFANTS: Use of oral iron preparations in premature infants with low serum vitamin E levels may cause hemolysis and hemolytic anemia (15); vitamin E deficiency should be corrected before administering supplemental iron (15).

Dosage and Administration

ORAL: For treating iron deficiency anemia in adults, 50-100 mg elemental iron is given three times daily. For children with iron deficiency anemia, the dose is 4-6 mg/kg per day divided into three doses (15). Treatment is usually continued 6 months to replenish iron stores (15). Two to three months of treatment may reverse anemia without replenishing iron stores (945). Iron deficiency due to chronic, uncontrolled bleeding requires continuous iron therapy (945). For preventing iron deficiency in menstruating women who have undergone gastric bypass surgery, 320 mg twice daily has been used (1089). For improving unexplained fatigue in non-anemic women, ferrous sulfate 80 mg daily has been used (11406). For improving cognitive function in iron-deficient adolescents, 650 mg ferrous sulfate twice daily has been used (1095). For reducing angiotensin converting enzyme (ACE) inhibitor cough, 256 mg ferrous sulfate has been given daily (7307).

The adequate intake (AI) of iron for infants 6 months of age and less is 0.27 mg/day (7135).

For older infants and children, the recommended daily allowances (RDAs) for iron are: Infants 7 to 12 months, 11 mg/day; children 1 to 3 years, 7 mg/day; 4 to 8 years, 10 mg/day; 9 to 13 years, 8 mg/day; boys 14 to 18 years, 11 mg/day; girls 14 to 18 years, 15 mg/day. For adults, the RDA for iron is 8 mg/day for men ages 19 and older, and women ages 51 and older. For women 19 to 50 years, the RDA is 18 mg/day. For pregnant women, the RDA is 27 mg/day. For lactating women, the RDA is 10 mg/day for ages 14 to 18 years, and 9 mg/day for ages 19 to 50 (7135). Tolerable upper intake levels (UL) for iron are: infants and children birth to age 13, 40 mg/day; people age 14 and older (including pregnancy and lactation), 45 mg/day (7135). UL recommendations do not apply to people under medical supervision for iron deficiency (7135). All forms of iron are not equivalent; 1 gram of ferrous gluconate = 120 mg elemental iron (12% iron); 1 gram of ferrous sulfate = 200 mg elemental iron (20% iron); 1 gram of ferrous fumarate = 330 mg elemental iron (33% iron) (15).

Comments

Premenopausal women who have asymptomatic iron deficiency can improve their iron status by altering their diet to include more iron-rich foods, although changes are generally less than with iron supplements (9540,9541). High iron foods include beef, liver, and lamb. Medium iron foods include pork, ham, chicken, fish, and beans (9540).

ISATIS

Also Known As

Ban Lang Gen, Chinese Indigo, Da Qing Ye, Da Quing Ye, Dyer's Woad, Färberwaid, Folium Isatidis, Hierba Pastel, Indigo Woad, Pastel Des Teinturiers, Qing Dai, Radix Isatidis, Woad.

Scientific Names

Isatis tinctoria, synonym Isatis indigotica.
Family: Brassicaceae/Cruciferae.

People Use This For

Orally, isatis is used to treat acute parotitis, upper respiratory infection, encephalitis, hepatitis, lung abscess, dysentery, acute gastroenteritis, and HIV.

In combination with other herbs, isatis is used to treat prostate cancer.

In manufacturing, the above ground parts of isatis are used to make indigo dye.

Safety

There is insufficient reliable information available about the safety of isatis.

Effectiveness

There is insufficient reliable information available about the effectiveness of isatis.

Mechanism of Action

The applicable parts of isatis are the leaf and root. Tryptanthrin, an isatis leaf constituent that is produced during the drying process, inhibits cyclooxygenase-2 (COX-2) and 5-lipoxygenase, which are mediators of inflammatory activity (12641,12646,12647). Indirubin, a constituent of isatis root, might inhibit airway inflammation produced by the influenza virus, according to preliminary research (12640). Other isatis root constituents such as isaindigotone seem to be a superoxide scavenger and inhibit 5-lipoxygenase and leukotriene B4 production, which might also contribute to its anti-inflammatory effect (12645). Isatis root also contains salicylic acid (12643). Indirubin and its derivatives also seem to have an antiproliferative effect on leukemia and other cancer cells (12642). Other constituents appear to have antiviral, antibacterial, antifungal, analgesic, and antipyretic activity (12643,12644).

Adverse Reactions

None reported.

Interactions with Herbs & Other Dietary Supplements
None known.

Interactions with Drugs
None known.

Interactions with Foods
None known.

Interactions with Lab Tests
None known.

Interactions with Diseases or Conditions
ASPIRIN ALLERGY: Isatis contains unknown quantities of salicylate (12643). Theoretically, the salicylate constituents in isatis could trigger allergic reaction in people with aspirin allergy or aspirin-related asthma.

Dosage and Administration
No typical dosage.

Comments
Other herbs considered to be Qing Dai (indigo naturalis) are Baphicacanthus cusia (Acanthaceae), Polygonum tinctorium (Polygonaceae), Indigofera suffrutticosa (Fabaceae), and Indigofera tinctoria (Fabaceae) (12642).
In Traditional Chinese Medicine, Ban Lang Gen refers to the isatis root. Da Qing Ye refers to the leaf. Isatis has been used medicinally since ancient times and is mentioned in the writings of Galen and Pliny (12647).

IVY GOURD

Also Known As
Kovai, Little Gourd, Tela Kucha.
CAUTION: See separate listings for Levant Berry and Bitter Melon.

Scientific Names
Coccinia grandis, synonyms Coccinia indica, Coccinia ordifolia.
Family: Cucurbitaceae.

People Use This For
Orally, ivy gourd is used for diabetes, gonorrhea, and as a laxative.
Topically, ivy gourd leaves are used for treating skin lesions.

Safety
POSSIBLY SAFE ...when used orally and appropriately for up to six weeks (12693). The long-term safety of ivy gourd is unknown.
PREGNANCY AND LACTATION: Insufficient reliable information available; avoid using.

Effectiveness
INSUFFICIENT RELIABLE EVIDENCE to RATE

Diabetes. Preliminary clinical research suggests that ivy gourd might improve glucose control in patients with type 2 diabetes (12693). More evidence is needed to rate ivy gourd for this use.

Mechanism of Action
The applicable parts of ivy gourd are the roots, leaves, and fruit. All parts of ivy gourd seem to have hypoglycemic effects. Preliminary research suggests that pectin, a constituent of ivy gourd fruit, has hypoglycemic activity (12249,12694,12696). Ivy gourd leaf extracts seem to depress gluconeogenesis by inhibiting enzymes such as glucose-6-phosphatase (12697). Triterpene constituents of ivy gourd leaves seem to have antidiabetic activity and may also lower cholesterol and improve metabolic function (12698). Other preliminary research suggests ivy gourd leaf extract might stimulate insulin production and have antioxidant effects (12699).

Adverse Reactions
None reported.

Interactions with Herbs & Other Dietary Supplements

HERBS & SUPPLEMENTS WITH HYPOGLYCEMIC POTENTIAL: Ivy gourd can lower blood glucose levels (12693) and might have additive effects when used with other herbs and supplements that also lower glucose levels. This might increase the risk of hypoglycemia in some patients. Some herbs and supplements with hypoglycemic effects include alpha-lipoic acid, bitter melon, chromium, devil's claw, fenugreek, garlic, guar gum, horse chestnut seed, Panax ginseng, psyllium, Siberian ginseng, and others.

Interactions with Drugs

ANTIDIABETES DRUGS: Ivy gourd can lower blood glucose levels (12693) and might have additive effects when used with antidiabetes drugs. This might increase the risk of hypoglycemia in some patients. Monitor blood glucose levels closely. Some antidiabetes drugs include glimepiride (Amaryl), glyburide (DiaBeta, Glynase PresTab, Micronase), insulin, metformin (Glucophage), pioglitazone (Actos), rosiglitazone (Avandia), and others.

Interactions with Foods

None known.

Interactions with Lab Tests

BLOOD GLUCOSE: Ivy gourd can lower blood glucose and test results in patients with type 2 diabetes (12693).

Interactions with Diseases or Conditions

DIABETES: Ivy gourd can lower blood glucose levels (12693) and might have additive effects when used with antidiabetes drugs. This might increase the risk of hypoglycemia in some patients. Monitor blood glucose levels closely.

Dosage and Administration

No typical dose.

Comments

Ivy gourd fruit and leaves are used as a vegetable in India and other Asian countries (12694).

JABORANDI

Also Known As

Arruda Bravam, Arruda Do Mato, Jamguarandi, Juarandi, Maranhao Jaborandi.

Scientific Names

Pilocarpus microphyllus.
Family: Rutaceae.

People Use This For

Orally, jaborandi is used to treat diarrhea, and as a diaphoretic.
Topically, jaborandi is used for glaucoma.

Safety

UNSAFE ...when the leaf is used orally or topically, because it contains pilocarpine. The lethal dose of jaborandi is estimated to be 5-10 grams of leaf (18).
PREGNANCY: UNSAFE ...when used orally or topically because it has teratogenic and uterine stimulant effects and contains pilocarpine(19).
LACTATION: UNSAFE ...when used orally or topically because it contains pilocarpine (18).

Effectiveness

There is insufficient reliable information available about the effectiveness of jaborandi.

Mechanism of Action

The applicable part of jaborandi is the leaf. Jaborandi contains the parasympathetic system stimulant pilocarpine. Among its cholinergic effects are the stimulation of saliva secretion, sweat, and smooth muscle contraction in the gastrointestinal tract (18). It also causes ocular miosis (15).

Adverse Reactions

The lethal oral dose of the pilocarpine constituent in jaborandi is approximately 60 mg, corresponding to approximately 5-10 grams of jaborandi leaf. Symptoms of poisoning include bradycardia, bronchospasm, colic, cardiac collapse and possible arrest, convulsions, hypotension, dyspnea, nausea, severe salivation, strong secretion of sweat, and vomiting (18).

Interactions with Herbs & Other Dietary Supplements
None known.

Interactions with Drugs
None known.

Interactions with Foods
None known.

Interactions with Lab Tests
INTRAOCULAR PRESSURE: Jaborandi might reduce intraocular pressure due to its pilocarpine content (15,18).

Interactions with Diseases or Conditions
None known.

Dosage and Administration
TOPICAL: Pharmaceutical pilocarpine eye drops are a prescription only medication (15,18).

Comments
Jaborandi itself is obsolete as a medicinal herb, but it is used in the production of pilocarpine (18). Avoid confusing jaborandi with Pilocarpus jaborandi (Pernambuco jaborandi) (19) and Pilocarpus pennatifolius (Paraguay jaborandi).

JACOB'S LADDER

Also Known As
Charity, English Green Valerian, Jacobs Ladder.
CAUTION: See separate listings for Abscess Root and Lily-of-the-Valley.

Scientific Names
Polemonium caeruleum.
Family: Polemoniaceae.

Comments
At the date of publication, this product was not a common ingredient used in brand name supplements marketed to consumers. Details about this product are available in the online version of *Natural Medicines Comprehensive Database.* See www.naturaldatabase.com.

JALAP

Also Known As
Jalapa, Jalape, Mechoacán.
CAUTION: See separate listings for Mexican Scammony Root, Pokeweed.

Scientific Names
Ipomoea purga, synonym Exogonium purga; Convolvulus purga.
Family: Convolvulaceae.

People Use This For
Orally, jalap is used as a cathartic, purgative, and diuretic.

Safety
UNSAFE ...when used orally. Jalap has potent purgative effects (12).
PREGNANCY AND LACTATION: UNSAFE ...when used orally. Jalap can be a menstrual stimulant (19); avoid using.

Effectiveness
There is insufficient reliable information available about the effectiveness of jalap.

Mechanism of Action
The applicable part of jalap is the root. The roots of the jalap (ipomoea purga) plant contain gluco-resins that act as a cathartic. They increase water elimination and cause peristalsis (271).

Adverse Reactions

Orally, jalap has potent purgative effects (12).

Interactions with Herbs & Other Dietary Supplements

CARDIAC GLYCOSIDE-CONTAINING HERBS: Overuse/abuse of jalap may increase the risk of cardiac glycoside toxicity. Cardiac glycoside-containing herbs include black hellebore, Canadian hemp roots, digitalis leaf, hedge mustard, figwort, lily-of-the-valley roots, motherwort, oleander leaf, pheasant's eye plant, pleurisy root, squill bulb leaf scales, and strophanthus seeds (19). Jalap may increase risk of cardioglycoside toxicity due to increase risk of potassium loss.

HORSETAIL/LICORICE: Theoretically, concomitant use with horsetail plant or licorice rhizome increases the risk of potassium depletion (19).

STIMULANT LAXATIVE HERBS: Theoretically, concomitant use with other stimulant laxative herbs may increase the risk of potassium depletion. Stimulant laxative herbs include aloe dried leaf sap, blue flag rhizome, alder buckthorn, European buckthorn, butternut bark, cascara bark, castor oil, colocynth fruit pulp, gamboge bark exudate, black root, manna bark exudate, podophyllum root, rhubarb root, senna leaves and pods, wild cucumber fruit (Ecballium elaterium), and yellow dock root (19).

Interactions with Drugs

DIGOXIN (Lanoxin): Theoretically, overuse or abuse of jalap might increase the toxicity of cardiac glycoside drugs due to possible potassium loss.

DIURETIC DRUGS: Overuse of jalap might compound diuretic-induced potassium loss (19). There is some concern that people taking jalap along with potassium depleting diuretics might have an increased risk for hypokalemia. Initiation of potassium supplementation or an increase in potassium supplement dose may be necessary for some patients. Some diuretics that can deplete potassium include chlorothiazide (Diuril), chlorthalidone (Thalitone), furosemide (Lasix), hydrochlorothiazide (HCTZ, Hydrodiuril, Microzide), and others.

ORAL DRUGS: Theoretically, jalap may reduce absorption of drugs due to reduced transit time (19).

STIMULANT LAXATIVES: Concomitant use of jalap with other laxatives may lead to electrolyte and fluid depletion (19).

Interactions with Foods

None known.

Interactions with Lab Tests

None known.

Interactions with Diseases or Conditions

GASTROINTESTINAL (GI) CONDITIONS: Jalap may have GI irritant effects (19). Contraindicated in individuals with infectious or inflammatory gastrointestinal conditions (19). Stimulant laxatives are contraindicated in individuals with symptoms of appendicitis (abdominal pain, nausea, and vomiting) (272).

Dosage and Administration

ORAL: Jalap is typically prepared as a liquid, using 1 teaspoon root to 1 cup of water. The dose is 1 cup daily, a mouthful at a time (5263). The usual dose of the powdered root is 3 to 20 grains (195 to 1300 mg) (5267). The resin from the root is dosed 60 to 300 mg, and the tincture is taken 2 to 4 mL (223).

Comments

Avoid confusion with pokeweed (Phytolacca americana) or Mexican scammony root (Ipomoea orizabensis), also known as jalap.

JAMAICAN DOGWOOD

Also Known As

Fishfudle, Fish Poison Bark, Fish-Poison Tree, Jamaica Dogwood, West Indian Dogwood.
CAUTION: See separate listing for American Dogwood.

Scientific Names

Piscidia piscipula, synonyms Erythrina piscipula, Ichthyomethia piscipula, Piscidia erythrina; Piscidia communis.
Family: Fabaceae/Leguminosae.

People Use This For

Orally, Jamaican dogwood is used for anxiety and fear, as a daytime sedative, for neuralgia, migraine, insomnia (especially sleeplessness due to nervous tension), and dysmenorrhea.

Safety

LIKELY UNSAFE ...when the root bark is used orally for self-medication because it is considered toxic (4). The elderly are particularly sensitive to potent neuro-muscular depressant effects (19).
CHILDREN: LIKELY UNSAFE ...when used orally; avoid using. Children are particularly sensitive to potent, neuro-muscular depressant effects (19).
PREGNANCY: LIKELY UNSAFE ...when used orally; avoid using due to possible uterine depressant effects (4).
LACTATION: LIKELY UNSAFE ...when used orally (4); avoid using.

Effectiveness

There is insufficient reliable information available about the effectiveness of Jamaican dogwood.

Mechanism of Action

The applicable part of Jamaican dogwood is the root bark. Animal studies have shown that an extract of Jamaican dogwood has sedative effects, marked antitussive and antipyretic activities, and also anti-inflammatory and antispasmodic action on smooth muscles (4,11). In some in vitro tests, the extract's antispasmodic effects have been at least as strong as papaverine's (4). The constituent rotenone has shown some anticancer activity towards lymphocytic leukemia and human epidermoid carcinoma of the nasopharynx; yet, paradoxically, rotenone is also documented to be carcinogenic (4). Rotenone is toxic to fish and insects, and to animals when administered parenterally, but non-toxic when administered orally (4). Another constituent, ichtynone, is toxic to fish (4).

Adverse Reactions

Orally, Jamaican dogwood is an irritant and toxic to humans (4). Overdose symptoms include numbness, tremors, salivation, and sweating (4).

Interactions with Herbs & Other Dietary Supplements

HERBS WITH SEDATIVE PROPERTIES: Theoretically, concomitant use with herbs that have sedative properties might enhance therapeutic and adverse effects. Some of these supplements include 5-HTP, calamus, California poppy, catnip, hops, kava, St. John's wort, scullcap, valerian, yerba mansa, and others.

Interactions with Drugs

CNS DEPRESSANTS: Jamaican dogwood may potentiate sedative effects (4).

Interactions with Foods

None known.

Interactions with Lab Tests

None known.

Interactions with Diseases or Conditions

None known.

Dosage and Administration

No typical dosage.

Comments

Jamaican dogwood is likely unsafe and without any documented effectiveness; avoid using. Root bark and liquid extract are reportedly no longer used (18). Avoid confusion with American dogwood (Cornus florida).

JAMBOLAN

Also Known As

Badijamun, Jambu, Jambul, Jamum, Java Plum, Jumbul, Mahajambu, Phadena, Rajajambu, Rose Apple.

Scientific Names

Syzygium cumini, synonyms Eugenia cumini, Eugenia jambolana, Syzygium jambos, Syzygium jambolanum.
Family: Mytraceae.

People Use This For

Orally, jambolan is used for diabetes, flatulence, as an antispasmodic, for stimulating stomach function, as an aphrodisiac, and as a tonic. Jambolan is also used orally for acute diarrhea, bronchitis, asthma, and dysentery.
Topically, jambolan is used for mild inflammation of the oral-pharyngeal mucosa and skin and for ulcers.
In herbal combinations, jambolan seed is used for atonic and spastic constipation, diseases of the pancreas, gastric and pancreatic complaints, nervous disorders, depression, and exhaustion.

Safety

POSSIBLY SAFE ...when used orally or topically, and appropriately (12,13092).
PREGNANCY AND LACTATION: Insufficient reliable information available; avoid using.

Effectiveness

POSSIBLY INEFFECTIVE

Diabetes. There is some evidence that drinking jambolan tea prepared from 2 grams/liter of water does not improve fasting blood glucose in patients with type 2 diabetes (13092).

Mechanism of Action

The applicable parts of jambolan are the seed and bark. The bark seems to have an astringent effect due to the tannin constituents (2). Preliminary evidence also suggests that jambolan bark might have antibacterial, hypoglycemic, and CNS-depressant effects (4).

Adverse Reactions

None reported.

Interactions with Herbs & Other Dietary Supplements

None known.

Interactions with Drugs

None known.

Interactions with Foods

None known.

Interactions with Lab Tests

None known.

Interactions with Diseases or Conditions

DIABETES THERAPY: Jambolan seed is thought to have hypoglycemic effects. Monitor blood glucose levels closely (19).

Dosage and Administration

ORAL: No typical dosage. However, 0.3-2 grams of the powdered seeds has been used. A liquid extract of the seeds has also been used

JAPANESE MINT

Also Known As

American Corn Mint, Brook Mint, Canadian Mint, Chinese Mint, Chinese Mint Oil, Corn Mint, Cornmint Oil, Field Mint Oil, Mentha arvensis aetheroleum, Mint Oil, Minzol, Poleo, Pudina, Putiha.
CAUTION: See separate listing for Schizonepeta.

Scientific Names

Mentha canadensis, synonym Mentha arvensis var. piperascens.
Family: Lamiaceae/Labiatae.

People Use This For

Orally, Japanese mint is used for flatulence, improving gastrointestinal and gallbladder function, for gallstones, and irritable bowel syndrome (IBS) common cold, cough, bronchitis, fever, mouth and pharynx inflammation, pain, liver and gallbladder complaints, tendency to infection, for improving appetite and digestion, indigestion, nausea, sore throat, diarrhea, headaches, toothaches, cramps, earache, tumors, sores, cancer, a stimulant, an antiseptic, a local anesthetic, and an antispasmodic. Japanese mint is also used for functional cardiac complaints, breathing difficulties, and sensitivity to weather changes.
Topically, Japanese mint is used for myalgia, neuralgic ailments, pruritus, urticaria, oral mucosal inflammation, and rheumatic conditions.
When inhaled, Japanese mint is used for mucous membrane inflammation of the upper respiratory tract.
In manufacturing, Japanese mint is also used as a fragrance in toothpaste, mouthwash, gargles, soaps, detergents, creams, lotions, and perfumes. Commercially it is used as a source of menthol.

Safety
POSSIBLY SAFE ...when the oil is used orally and appropriately (2). ...when used topically and appropriately (2). There is insufficient reliable information available about the safety of Japanese mint for its other uses.
CHILDREN: LIKELY UNSAFE ...when the oil is used topically on the faces of infants and children, particularly in the nasal area, it can trigger glottal or bronchial spasm, asthma-like attacks, or even respiratory failure (2). There is insufficient reliable information about Japanese mint used for medicinal purposes; avoid using.
PREGNANCY AND LACTATION: Insufficient reliable information available; avoid using.

Effectiveness
There is insufficient reliable information available about the effectiveness of Japanese mint.

Mechanism of Action
Japanese mint oil is thought to have antiflatulent and cooling effects (2). It might also stimulate bile flow (2). Some evidence demonstrates that Japanese mint oil has cytotoxic properties. Other evidence suggests it might have antimicrobial activity (11). Japanese mint oil contains up to 95% menthol (11). Used topically it has the potential to cause sensitization (18). Processing removes some of the menthol in the Japanese mint oil that is commercially available (2,11).

Adverse Reactions
Orally, Japanese mint oil can cause stomach upset when taken orally (2).
Topically, contact dermatitis can result from use (11). In children, topical use on the face can trigger glottal or bronchial spasm, asthma-like attacks, or even respiratory failure (18).
By inhalation, the menthol content of Japanese mint oil can worsen bronchial asthma spasms (18). Menthol can also cause allergic reactions including flushing or headache (11).

Interactions with Herbs & Other Dietary Supplements
None known.

Interactions with Drugs
None known.

Interactions with Foods
None known.

Interactions with Lab Tests
None known.

Interactions with Diseases or Conditions
BRONCHIAL SPASMS: Theoretically, the menthol content of Japanese mint oil might worsen bronchial asthma spasms (18).
GALLBLADDER CONDITIONS: Use of Japanese mint is contraindicated in individuals with bile duct obstruction or gallbladder inflammation (2). Individuals with gallstones may experience pain and spasms (18).
LIVER DISEASE: Use of Japanese mint is contraindicated in individuals with severe liver damage (2).

Dosage and Administration
ORAL: A typical dose is 3-6 drops of oil daily (2).
TOPICAL: Rub several drops of oil or equivalent preparations into affected areas of skin (2). Japanese mint oil is also available as 5-20% oil and semi-solid preparations, in hydroalcoholic preparations of 5% to 10%, and as 1% to 5% essential oil in nasal ointments (2).
INHALATION: A typical dose is 3-4 drops of oil in hot water (2).

Comments
Japanese mint oil is the partially dementholated, distilled oil of the above ground parts of Japanese mint (Mentha canadensis) (2,11). There are more than 20 different species of Mentha with as many as 2300 named variations. Commercial varieties of mint oil can be distinguished by the relative amounts of menthol and carvone (11).

JASMINE

Also Known As
Catalonina Jasmine, Common Jasmine, Italian Jasmine, Jati, Poet's Jessamine, Royal Jasmine, Spanish Jasmine.
CAUTION: See separate listing for Gelsemium.

Scientific Names
Jasminum grandiflorum, synonym Jasminum officinale.
Family: Oleaceae.

People Use This For
Orally, jasmine has been used for pepatitis, hepatic pain due to cirrhosis, and abdominal pain due to dysentery.
Many Jasminum species have been used as a sedative, aphrodisiac, or in cancer treatment.
In foods, jasmine is utilized to flavor beverages, frozen dairy desserts, candy, baked goods, gelatins, and puddings.
In manufacturing, jasmine is used to add fragrance to creams, lotions, and perfumes.

Safety
LIKELY SAFE ...when used orally in the amounts commonly found in foods. Jasmine has Generally Recognized As Safe (GRAS) status in the US (4912).
There is insufficient reliable information available about the safety jasmine in medicinal amounts.
PREGNANCY AND LACTATION: Insufficient reliable information available; avoid using in amounts greater than those found in food.

Effectiveness
There is insufficient reliable information available about the effectiveness of jasmine.

Mechanism of Action
The applicable part of jasmine is the flower. There is insufficient reliable information available about the possible mechanism of action and active ingredients.

Adverse Reactions
Jasmine may possibly cause hypersensitivity (11).

Interactions with Herbs & Other Dietary Supplements
None known.

Interactions with Drugs
None known.

Interactions with Foods
None known.

Interactions with Lab Tests
None known.

Interactions with Diseases or Conditions
None known.

Dosage and Administration
ORAL: People typically prepare jasmine as a tea, adding 1 to 2 teaspoons of jasmine flowers to 1 cup of water. The dose is 1 cup daily (5263).

Comments
Concrétes are the fat-soluble abstracts of the flower. Absolutes, the alcoholic extracts of concrétes, are more commonly used as a fragrance (11).

JAVA TEA

Also Known As
Orthosiphon, Orthosiphonis folium.

Scientific Names
Orthosiphon aristatus, synonyms Orthosiphon stamineus, Clerodendranthus spicatus, Clerodendrum spicatum, Ocimum aristatum.
Family: Lamiaceae/Labiatae.

People Use This For
Orally, java tea is taken as "irrigation therapy" (where it is used as a mild diuretic along with copious fluid intake to increase urine flow), for bacterial and inflammatory diseases of the lower urinary tract, renal gravel, and liver and gallbladder complaints. It is also used orally for bladder and kidney disorders, gallstones, gout, and rheumatism.

Safety
There is insufficient reliable information available about the safety of java tea.
Pregnancy and Lactation: Insufficient reliable information available; avoid using.

Effectiveness
There is insufficient reliable information available about the effectiveness of java tea.

Mechanism of Action
The applicable parts of java tea are the leaf and stem tip. Java tea is stated to have diuretic, weak antispasmodic, and antimicrobial effects (2,18).

Adverse Reactions
None reported.

Interactions with Herbs & Other Dietary Supplements
None known.

Interactions with Drugs
None known.

Interactions with Foods
None known.

Interactions with Lab Tests
None known.

Interactions with Diseases or Conditions
EDEMA: Java tea is contraindicated for use as "irrigation therapy" in cases of edema due to limited heart or kidney function (2).

Dosage and Administration
ORAL: The typical dose of java tea is 6-12 grams of the dried leaf or stem tips per day or equivalent preparations, including the prepared tea (2,18). Adequate fluid intake is essential, at least 2 L per day (18).

JAVANESE TURMERIC

Also Known As
Curcuma, Curcumae xanthorrhizae rhizoma, Java Turmeric, Temu Lawak, Temu Lawas, Tewon Lawa.
CAUTION: See separate listings for Goldenseal, Turmeric, and Zedoary.

Scientific Names
Curcuma xanthorrhiza.
Family: Zingiberaceae.

People Use This For
Orally, Javanese turmeric is used for indigestion, feelings of fullness, bloating after meals, flatulence, peptic disorders, for improving appetite and digestion, and for liver and gallbladder complaints.

Safety
POSSIBLY SAFE ...when the dried rhizome is used orally and appropriately for short periods of time (2,8).
POSSIBLY UNSAFE ...when used orally in large amounts or for prolonged use. It can cause gastric irritation and nausea (2,8).
PREGNANCY AND LACTATION: Insufficient reliable information available; avoid using.

Effectiveness
There is insufficient reliable information available about the effectiveness of Javanese turmeric.

Mechanism of Action
The applicable part of Javanese turmeric is the root. Javanese turmeric root contains a volatile oil with the chief components of alpha-curcumene, xanthorrhizole, beta-curcumene, germacrene, furanodien, and furanodienone. The root also contains curcumin, demethoxycurcumin, and non-phenolic diarylheptanoids (18). Javanese turmeric is thought to stimulate bile production (2). It might also have antitumor effects (18).

Adverse Reactions
Orally, use of large amounts or for prolonged periods of time can cause gastric irritation and nausea (2,8).

Interactions with Herbs & Other Dietary Supplements
None known.

Interactions with Drugs
None known.

Interactions with Foods
None known.

Interactions with Lab Tests
None known.

Interactions with Diseases or Conditions
LIVER OR GALLBLADDER DISEASE: Javanese turmeric is contraindicated in people with acute bile duct inflammation, biliary tree inflammation (8), bile duct obstruction (2,8), or jaundice (8) due to bile stimulating effects (2). Individuals with gallstones should have medical evaluation before using (2).

Dosage and Administration
ORAL: To stimulate bile production, a typical oral dose is one cup tea several times daily between meals. To make tea, steep 0.5-1 grams coarsely powdered root in 150 mL boiling water for 5-10 minutes, and strain. The average daily amount used is 2 grams root or equivalent preparations (2).
For improving appetite, digestion, or for flatulence, a typical dose is one cup tea before or during meals. To make tea, steep 0.5-1 grams coarsely powdered root in 150 mL boiling water for 5-10 minutes, and strain (8). The average daily amount used is 2 grams root or equivalent preparations (2).

Comments
Javanese turmeric is indigenous to the forests of Indonesia and the Malaysian peninsula (18).

JEWELWEED

Also Known As
Balsam-Weed, Garden Balsam, Impatiens, Jewel Balsam Weed, Quick-In-The-Hand, Silverweed, Slipper Weed, Speckled Jewels, Spotted Touch-Me-Not, Touch-Me-Not, Wild Balsam, Wild Celandine, Wild Lady's Slipper.
CAUTION: See separate listings for Greater Celandine, Lesser Celandine, and Potentilla.

Scientific Names
Impatiens pallida; Impatiens balsamina, synonyms Balsamina foemina, Impatiens giorgii; Impatiens capensis, synonym Impatiens biflora.
Family: Balsaminaceae.

People Use This For
Orally, jewelweed is used for mild digestive disorders.
Orally and topically, jewelweed is used for poison ivy dermatitis.

Safety
POSSIBLY SAFE ...when used orally. ...when used topically. There are no published reports of significant toxicity for either route of administration (18).
PREGNANCY AND LACTATION: Insufficient reliable information available; avoid using.

Effectiveness
There is insufficient reliable information available about the effectiveness of jewelweed.

Mechanism of Action
The applicable parts of jewelweed are the above ground parts. Impatiens balsamina has digestive and diuretic effects (18). One constituent, 2-methoxynaphthoquinone, has antifungal activity (6).

Adverse Reactions
None reported.

Interactions with Herbs & Other Dietary Supplements
None known.

Interactions with Drugs
None known.

Interactions with Foods
None known.

Interactions with Lab Tests
None known.

Interactions with Diseases or Conditions
None known.

Dosage and Administration
No typical dosage.

Comments
Avoid confusion with potentilla (Potentillae anserinae), also known as silverweed.

JIAOGULAN

Also Known As
Adaptogen, Amachazuru, Dungkulcha, Fairy Herb, Gynostemma, Immortality Herb, Jiao Gu Lan, Miracle Grass, Penta Tea, Southern Ginseng, Xianxao.
CAUTION: See separate listings for Blue Cohosh, Canaigre, Codonopsis, Ginseng American, Ginseng Siberian, Ginseng Panax, Panax Pseudoginseng, and Ashwaganda.

Scientific Names
Gynostemma pentaphyllum, synonyms Gynostemma pedatum, Vitis pentaphylla.
Family: Cucurbitaceae.

People Use This For
Orally, jiaogulan is used for hyperlipidemia, hypertension, strengthening immune function, and increasing stamina and endurance. It is also used orally for appetite stimulation, chronic bronchitis, chronic gastritis, ulcers, constipation, gallstones, obesity, cancer, diabetes, insomnia, backache, and pain. Jiaogulan is also used orally for improving memory, improving coronary and cardiovascular functions, stress, preventing hair loss, and as an anti-aging agent. It is also used orally as an anti-inflammatory agent, antioxidant, detoxifying agent, decongestant and cough suppressant, and as an "adaptogen" for increasing resistance to environmental stress.

Safety
POSSIBLY SAFE ...when used orally and appropriately, short-term. There is preliminary evidence that jiaogulan can be safely used for up to 30 days (7069,7070).
PREGNANCY: POSSIBLY UNSAFE ...when used orally. Ginsenoside Rb1, which is identical to the jiaogulan constituent gypenoside 3, has teratogenic effects in animal models; avoid using (10447).
LACTATION: Insufficient reliable information available; avoid using.

Effectiveness
POSSIBLY EFFECTIVE

Hypercholesterolemia. There is some evidence that taking jiaogulan orally can decrease total cholesterol and increase the high-density lipoprotein (HDL)/total cholesterol ratio in patients with high cholesterol levels (7069,7070).

There is insufficient reliable information available about the effectiveness of jiaogulan for its other uses.

Mechanism of Action
The applicable part of jiaogulan is the leaf. The leaves of jiaogulan contain a large number of triterpene saponins referred to as gypenosides. Many of the gypenosides are identical to the ginsenosides found in Panax ginseng. For example, gypenoside 3 is identical to ginsenoside Rb1, gypenoside 4 is the same as ginsenoside Rb3, and gypenoside 8 is the same as ginsenoside Rd. The amount of saponins in the leaves of jiaogulan is similar to the amount found in ginseng roots. Due to the similar chemical make up between jiaogulan and ginseng, jiaogulan is often assumed to have the same effects as ginseng. Most jiaogulan products are standardized by the amount of saponins they contain. However, jiaogulan contains a wide variation of gypenosides which makes standardizing according to specific gypenosides difficult. Most of the evidence about the pharmacological effects of jiaogulan comes from preliminary animal or in vitro research (6).

There is some evidence that jiaogulan has antioxidant activity. There is also some evidence that the gypenoside constituents have several cardiovascular effects and may prevent the development of atherosclerosis and slow the aging process (9349).

Preliminary evidence suggests the gypenosides in jiaogulan have antilipid peroxidation activity and protect vascular endothelial cells and their membranes from oxidative damage (9349). In animal research, jiaogulan seems to lower blood pressure, heart rate, blood vessel resistance, increase coronary blood flow, inhibit platelet aggregation, and possibly protect against cerebral ischemic damage (7071). Evidence from human studies suggest that jiaogulan has cholesterol lowering effects (7069,7070).

There is also preliminary evidence a combination of jiaogulan with Nelumbo nucifera (Lotus flower or seed) and Crataegus cuneata (Hawthorn) might have both a cholesterol- and triglyceride-lowering effect. It is unclear whether these effects are due to an interaction among these agents or if one of the agents is primarily responsible (9348). There is preliminary evidence that jiaogulan may have immunostimulatory effects and possible anti-cancer activity (6).

Some research suggests that hot water extracts of jiaogulan contain a factor that induces platelet aggregation, but the effect occurs only with washed platelets and is not observed in platelet-rich plasma. This suggests the factor is unlikely to cause thrombosis in vivo. It is unknown if this factor might affect other cells or tissues. However, its discovery might help investigators better understand the mechanism of platelet activation (9350).

Adverse Reactions

Orally, use of jiaogulan might cause severe nausea and increased bowel movements (6).

Interactions with Herbs & Other Dietary Supplements

HERBS WITH ANTICOAGULANT/ANTIPLATELET POTENTIAL: Concomitant use of jiaogulan with herbs that inhibit platelet aggregation might increase the risk of bleeding in some people (7071). Some of these herbs include angelica, clove, danshen, garlic, ginger, ginkgo, Panax ginseng, horse chestnut, red clover, turmeric, and others.

Interactions with Drugs

ANTICOAGULANT/ANTIPLATELET DRUGS: Theoretically, using jiaogulan with drugs that have anticoagulant or antiplatelet effects might increase the risk of bruising and bleeding. Jiaogulan also seems to have antiplatelet effects (7071). Some of these drugs with anticoagulant or antiplatelet effects include aspirin, dalteparin (Fragmin), enoxaparin (Lovenox), heparin, indomethacin (Indocin), ticlopidine (Ticlid), warfarin (Coumadin), and others.

IMMUNOSUPPRESSANTS: Theoretically, concurrent use might interfere with immunosuppressive therapy (6); avoid concurrent use. Immunosuppressant drugs include azathioprine (Imuran), basiliximab (Simulect), cyclosporine (Neoral, Sandimmune), daclizumab (Zenapax), muromonab-CD3 (OKT3, Orthoclone OKT3), mycophenolate (CellCept), tacrolimus (FK506, Prograf), sirolimus (Rapamune), prednisone (Deltasone, Orasone), and other corticosteroids (glucocorticoids).

Interactions with Foods

None known.

Interactions with Lab Tests

BLEEDING TIME: Theoretically, jiaogulan might increase measures of bleeding time such as prothrombin time (PT) or international normalize ratio (INR) (7071).

BLOOD PRESSURE: Theoretically, jiaogulan might reduce blood pressure and blood pressure readings (6).

CHOLESTEROL: Jiaogulan might reduce serum total cholesterol concentrations and test results (6).

Interactions with Diseases or Conditions

BLEEDING DISORDERS: Theoretically, jiaogulan might increase the risk of bleeding due to its antiplatelet effects (7071).

Dosage and Administration

ORAL: For hypercholesterolemia, jiaogulan extract 10 mg three times daily has been used (7069).

Comments

Jiaogulan grows wild in China. It is sometimes referred to as Southern Ginseng because it grows in south central China and is used in similar ways as ginseng. Jiaogulan is a newcomer to traditional Chinese medicine.

Jiaogulan has reportedly been adulterated with Cayratia japonica.

JIMSON WEED

Also Known As

Angel Tulip, Datura, Devil's Apple, Devil's Trumpet, Jamestown Weed, Locoweed, Mad-Apple, Nightshade, Peru-Apple, Stinkweed, Stinkwort, Stramonium, Thorn-Apple.

Scientific Names

Datura stramonium, synonyms Datura inermis, Datura tatula.
Family: Solanaceae.

People Use This For

Orally, jimson weed is used to treat asthma, spastic or convulsive cough, pertussis during bronchitis and influenza, and as basic therapy for diseases of the autonomic nervous system. It is also used orally to induce hallucinations and euphoria.

Safety

UNSAFE ...when the leaf or seed are used orally, inhaled (13,5622). Although all parts of the plant contain belladonna alkaloids and are poisonous, the seeds contain the most (5623). Ingestion of jimson weed can cause acute anticholinergic poisoning and death (17,5621,5622). The lethal dose for adults is 15-100 grams of leaf or 15-25 grams of the seeds (equivalent to 100 mg atropine) (18).
CHILDREN: UNSAFE ...when the seed or leaf are used orally or inhaled. Children are more sensitive to the effects than adults, and the lethal dose is less (18).
PREGNANCY AND LACTATION: UNSAFE ...when used orally (2); avoid using.

Effectiveness

There is insufficient reliable information available about the effectiveness of jimson weed.

Mechanism of Action

The applicable parts of jimson weed are the leaf and seed. Jimson weed contains 0.1-0.6% alkaloids including atropine, l-hyoscyamine and l-scopolamine which are responsible for anticholinergic action and toxicity (2).

Adverse Reactions

Orally, ingestion of jimson weed can cause dilated pupils, dry mouth, dry skin, extreme thirst, dry mucous membranes, tachycardia, blurred vision, nausea and vomiting, decreased bowel sounds, difficulty swallowing and speaking, auditory and visual hallucinations, hyperthermia, hypertension, seizure, loss of consciousness, and coma (13,18,5623). Potential adverse effects also include confusion, emotional lability, reduced coordination, and headache (636). Death may result from central nervous system depression, circulatory collapse, and hypotension (18). Edema of the lungs and pectichial hemorrhages of the endocardium have been reported at autopsy (5622).

Interactions with Herbs & Other Dietary Supplements

None known.

Interactions with Drugs

ANTICHOLINERGIC DRUGS: Concomitant use with jimson weed may increase anticholinergic effects and adverse effects. Anticholinergic drugs include amantadine, atropine, belladonna alkaloids, phenothiazines, scopolamine, tricyclic antidepressants (506); avoid using.

Interactions with Foods

None known.

Interactions with Lab Tests

None known.

Interactions with Diseases or Conditions

CONGESTIVE HEART FAILURE (CHF): Contraindicated; jimson weed might cause tachycardia and exacerbate CHF due to its hyoscyamine (atropine) and scopolamine content (15).
CONSTIPATION: Contraindicated; jimson weed might cause constipation due to its hyoscyamine (atropine) and scopolamine content (15).
DOWN SYNDROME: Caution, patients with Down syndrome might be hypersensitive to the antimuscarinic effects (mydriasis, positive chronotropic heart effects, etc.) of hyoscyamine (atropine) and scopolamine contained in jimson weed (15).
ESOPHAGEAL REFLUX: Contraindicated; jimson weed might delay gastric emptying and decrease lower esophageal pressure, promoting gastric retention and exacerbating reflux due to its hyoscyamine (atropine) and scopolamine content (15).

FEVER: Contraindicated; jimson weed might increase the risk of hyperthermia in patients with fever due to its hyoscyamine (atropine) and scopolamine content (15).
GASTRIC ULCER: Contraindicated; jimson weed might delay gastric emptying and exacerbate gastric ulcers due to its hyoscyamine (atropine) and scopolamine content (15).
GASTROINTESTINAL (GI) INFECTIONS: Contraindicated; jimson weed might suppress GI motility causing retention of infecting organisms or toxins due to its hyoscyamine (atropine) and scopolamine content (15).
HIATAL HERNIA: Contraindicated; jimson weed might delay gastric emptying and decrease lower esophageal pressure, promoting gastric retention and exacerbating reflux due to its hyoscyamine (atropine) and scopolamine content (15).
NARROW-ANGLE GLAUCOMA: Contraindicated; jimson weed might increase ocular tension in patients with narrow-angle (angle-closure) glaucoma due to its hyoscyamine (atropine) and scopolamine content (2,15).
OBSTRUCTIVE GASTROINTESTINAL (GI) TRACT DISEASE: Contraindicated; jimson weed might exacerbate obstructive GI tract diseases (including atony, paralytic ileus, and stenosis) due to its hyoscyamine (atropine) and scopolamine content (15).
TACHYARRHYTHMIAS: Contraindicated; jimson weed might cause tachycardia due to its hyoscyamine (atropine) and scopolamine content (2,15).
TOXIC MEGACOLON: Contraindicated; jimson weed might suppress intestinal motility, which might produce paralytic ileus and exacerbate toxic megacolon, due to its hyoscyamine (atropine) and scopolamine content (2,15).
ULCERATIVE COLITIS: Contraindicated; jimson weed might suppress intestinal motility, which might produce paralytic ileus and precipitate toxic megacolon, due to its hyoscyamine (atropine) and scopolamine content (15).
URINARY RETENTION: Contraindicated; jimson weed might increase urinary retention due to its hyoscyamine (atropine) and scopolamine content (2,15).

Dosage and Administration

No typical dosage.

JOJOBA

Also Known As

Deernut, Goatnut, Pignut.

Scientific Names

Simmondsia chinensis, synonyms Buxus chinensis, Simmondsia californica.
Family: Simmondsiaceae.

People Use This For

Topically, jojoba is used for acne, psoriasis, sunburn, and chapped skin. It is also used topically as a hair restorer.
In manufacturing, jojoba is used as a component in shampoo; lipstick; makeup; cleansing products; and in face, hand, and body lotions.
In foods, roasted jojoba seeds are used as a coffee substitute.

Safety

LIKELY SAFE ...when used topically (6).
LIKELY UNSAFE ...when used orally because it contains 14% erucic acid, which can cause myocardial fibrosis (6); avoid using.
PREGNANCY AND LACTATION: LIKELY SAFE ...when used topically for hygienic uses (6).
LIKELY UNSAFE ...when used orally (6).

Effectiveness

There is insufficient reliable information available about the effectiveness of jojoba.

Mechanism of Action

The applicable parts of jojoba are the oil and wax. Jojoba seeds yield a colorless, odorless oil that is an emollient (11). Jojoba oil penetrates skin and skin oils easily, unclogging hair follicles and preventing sebum build up, which could lead to hair loss (6). Taken by mouth, jojoba wax passes through the body without being digested, but is stored in intestinal cells and the liver (18).

Adverse Reactions

Topically, contact dermatitis occurs with use of shampoos and hair conditioners containing jojoba oil (6).
Hypoallergenic sensitivity to jojoba wax may occur (6).

Interactions with Herbs & Other Dietary Supplements
None known.

Interactions with Drugs
None known.

Interactions with Foods
None known.

Interactions with Lab Tests
None known.

Interactions with Diseases or Conditions
None known.

Dosage and Administration
TOPICAL: Jojoba oil ingredient levels vary. In skin care products 5-10%; shampoos and conditioners 1% to 2%; bar soaps 0.5% to 3% (6).

Comments
Jojoba oil and wax are produced from the seeds of jojoba, a shrub native to arid regions of northern Mexico and the southwestern US (3901). Jojoba wax is unsuitable for food use (18).

JUJUBE

Also Known As
Black Date, Chinese Date, Chinese Jujube, Da Zao, Hei Zao, Hong Zao, Jujube Plum, Jujubi, Red Date, Zao, Zizyphus, Zyzyphus Jujube.

Scientific Names
Ziziphus jujuba, synonyms Ziziphus sativa, Ziziphus spinosa, Ziziphus vulgaris, Ziziphus zizyphus, Rhamnus zizyphus.
Family: Rhamnaceae.

People Use This For
Orally, jujube is used for improving muscular strength, as a prophylaxis for liver diseases and stress ulcers, as a sedative, and to neutralizing drug toxicities. Jujube is also used for dry and itchy skin, lack of appetite, fatigue, diarrhea, hysteria, anemia, hypertension, purpura, fever, wounds, ulcers, inflammation, asthma, and eye diseases.
In foods, jujube is used in a variety of recipes.
In manufacturing, jujube extracts are used in skin care products as an anti-inflammatory, antiwrinkle, moisturizer, and for relief from sunburn.

Safety
There is insufficient reliable information available about the safety of jujube.
Pregnancy and Lactation: Insufficient reliable information available; avoid using.

Effectiveness
There is insufficient reliable information available about the effectiveness of jujube.

Mechanism of Action
The applicable part of jujube is the fruit. Animal data suggests that jujube increases body weight, increases swimming endurance and protects against carbon tetrachloride-induced liver damage. Animal data also suggests that an ethanolic extract may have anti-inflammatory effects and inhibit growth of Bacillus subtilis. A methanolic extract containing oleanolic acid and ursolic acid inhibits dental cavity-producing activity of Streptococcus mutans in vitro (11).
Samgyetang, a soup made from chicken, jujube, panax ginseng, garlic, and chestnuts, appears to offer protection from experimentally induced peptic ulcers (10249).

Adverse Reactions
None reported.

Interactions with Herbs & Other Dietary Supplements
None known.

Interactions with Drugs
None known.

Interactions with Foods
None known.

Interactions with Lab Tests
None known.

Interactions with Diseases or Conditions
None known.

Dosage and Administration
No typical dosage.

JUNIPER

Also Known As
Common Juniper, Common Juniper Berry, Enebro, Extract of Juniper, Genievre, Ginepro, Juniper Berry, Juniper Berry Oil, Juniper Extract, Juniper Oil, Juniperi fructus, Juniperus communis Oil, Oil of Juniper, Wacholderbeeren, Zimbro.
CAUTION: See separate listing for Cade Oil.

Scientific Names
Juniperus communis.
Family: Cupressaceae.

People Use This For
Orally, juniper is used for dyspepsia, flatulence, heartburn, bloating, loss of appetite, urinary tract infections (UTIs), kidney and bladder stones, snakebite, intestinal worms, gastrointestinal infections, and cancer.
Topically, juniper is used for rheumatic pains in joints and muscles, inflammatory diseases, and wounds.
As an inhalant, the essential oil of juniper is used as an analgesic for pain and for bronchitis as an inhaled vapor.
In foods, the juniper berry is often used as a culinary condiment, a flavor component in gin and bitter preparations, and the extract and oil are used as a flavoring agent in foods and beverages.
In manufacturing, the juniper oil is used as a fragrance component in soaps and cosmetics.

Safety
LIKELY SAFE ...when used orally in amounts commonly found in foods. Juniper, juniper berry, and juniper extract has Generally Recognized As Safe (GRAS) status in the US (4912).
POSSIBLY SAFE ...when used orally and appropriately in medicinal amounts short-term (12). ...when used topically on limited areas of skin (12230). ...when the oil is used by inhalation and appropriately as aromatherapy (7107).
LIKELY UNSAFE ...when used orally in excessive amounts, long-term. Prolonged use of high doses can increase the potential for severe side effects such as convulsions or kidney damage (8,19). ...when used topically on large skin wounds or in individuals with acute skin conditions (18).
PREGNANCY: UNSAFE ...when used orally. Juniper can increase uterine tone, interfere with fertility and implantation, and cause abortion (4,19).
LACTATION: Insufficient reliable information available; avoid using.

Effectiveness
There is insufficient reliable information available about the effectiveness of juniper.

Mechanism of Action
The applicable part of juniper is the berry. The berry contains 0.5% to 1.55% essential oil. The oil contains about 20% alpha-pinene, 10% cadinene, 9% limonene, 8.5% myrcene, 8% borneol, 7.2% caryophyllene, 7% germacrene, and several other constituents in smaller concentrations (12230).
Juniper berry has aquaretic, antiseptic, antiflatulent, and antirheumatic effects. It also stimulates stomach function (4,512). Aquaretics increase urine volume (water loss) but not electrolyte excretion (512). The constituent terpinen-4-ol increases the glomerular filtration rate, but it can also irritate the kidneys (4).
The juniper berry oil stimulates uterine activity (4) and has GI antiseptic, and irritant effects (11). The oil seems to have antispasmodic effects in smooth muscle (11). In experimental animals, juniper berry extracts show abortifacient, antifertility, anti-inflammatory, anti-implantation, hypotensive, and hypertensive effects (4).
In vitro, juniper berry oil exhibits antiviral activity against the herpes simplex virus and has antibacterial and antifungal activity (4,10939).

Juniper berry extract seems to have a hypoglycemic effect in animal models. It seems to work primarily by increasing peripheral glucose uptake (10580).

Juniper oil is also thought to have tissue reparative effects and increase the rate of wound or burn healing in animal models (12230).

Adverse Reactions

Orally, excessive amounts of the juniper berry oil can cause kidney irritation (4). Overdose symptoms include kidney pain, diuresis, albuminuria, hematuria, purplish urine, tachycardia, hypertension, convulsions, metrorrhagia, and abortion (4).

Topically, juniper can cause skin irritation (4). Signs of topical poisoning include burning, erythema, inflammation with blisters, and edema (4). Repeated exposure to the juniper pollen can cause occupational allergies that affect the skin and respiratory tract (6).

Interactions with Herbs & Other Dietary Supplements

None known.

Interactions with Drugs

ANTIDIABETES DRUGS: Theoretically, juniper berry might potentiate diabetes therapy due to hypoglycemic activity (4).

DIURETIC DRUGS: Theoretically, juniper berry might interfere with diuretic therapy (4,512).

Interactions with Foods

None known.

Interactions with Lab Tests

URINE TESTS: The juniper berry can interfere with urine assays, and large amounts can cause purplish urine (4).

Interactions with Diseases or Conditions

DIABETES: Monitor blood glucose level closely due to claims that juniper has hypoglycemic effects (4,19).

GI CONDITIONS: Juniper berry can irritate the gastrointestinal tract (19). It is contraindicated in individuals with infectious or inflammatory gastrointestinal conditions (19).

HYPERTENSION, HYPOTENSION: Theoretically, juniper berry might interfere with blood pressure control (4,512).

KIDNEY DISEASE: Contraindicated (4,12).

SEIZURE DISORDERS: Theoretically, the juniper berry might exacerbate these conditions.

OTHER: Individuals with cardiac insufficiency, hypertonia, fever, acute skin disease, or large skin wounds should not use juniper berry (18).

Dosage and Administration

ORAL: The typical dose of juniper is 1-2 grams of the berry three times daily (4) or one cup of the tea three to four times daily (8). The tea is prepared by steeping 1 teaspoon of the crushed juniper berry, about 2-3 grams, in 150 mL boiling water for 10 minutes and then straining. Juniper should be used up to a maximum of 10 grams of the dried berry per day, corresponding to 20-100 mg of the essential oil (2). This dose should not be used longer than four weeks without physician consultation (8). The usual dose of the liquid extract (1:1 in 25% alcohol) is 2-4 mL three times daily (4). The common dose of the tincture (1:5 in 45% alcohol) is 1-2 mL three times daily (4).

The berry oil (1:5 in 45% alcohol) is typically taken as 0.03-0.2 mL three times daily (4).

CAUTION: The juniper berry oil should only be used under supervision (4).

TOPICAL: The juniper berry is commonly used in bath salts for treating rheumatism (18).

Comments

Avoid confusion with cade oil, which is distilled from juniper wood (Juniperus oxycedrus). Turpentine oil has been used to adulterate juniper berry oil (512).

Juniper is a short to medium height tree that is native to and grows wild in some parts of Europe, North America, and Asia. There are many varieties of juniper, but Juniperus communis is the most common in North America (12230).

Juniper extract and juniper oil are used in cosmetics including lipstick, foundation, hair conditioners, bath oils, bubble bath, eye shadow, and many other products (12230).

In the former Soviet Union, juniper berry oil was listed in the State Pharmacopoiea of the USSR as a diuretic (12230).

KAMALA

Also Known As
Kamcela, Kameela, Rottlera Tinctoria, Spoonwood.

Scientific Names
Mallotus philippensis.
Family: Euphorbiaceae.

Comments
At the date of publication, there was very little scientific information available about this product. Our staff is continually analyzing the available information on natural medicines and will add data to the online version of *Natural Medicines Comprehensive Database* as it becomes available. See www.naturaldatabase.com.

KAOLIN

Also Known As
Argilla, Bolus Alba, China Clay, Heavy Kaolin, Light Kaolin, Porcelain Clay, White Bole.

Scientific Names
Hydrated aluminum silicate.

People Use This For
Orally, kaolin is used for mild to moderate acute diarrhea, cholera, enteritis, and dysentery.
Topically, kaolin is used as a poultice, dusting powder, drying agent, and emollient.
In combination products, kaolin is used for symptomatic diarrhea control, in relief of radiation-induced mucositis, in the treatment of chronic ulcerative colitis, and to treat spontaneous pneumothorax.
Diagnostic uses of kaolin include, as a contrast media agent (C,D), automated testing for activated coagulation time (ACT), serodiagnosis of tuberculosis, and the kaolin agglutination test (KAT).
In manufacturing, kaolin is used as a diluent in tablet preparation, and a filtering or decolorizing agent.
Kaolin is also a food additive.

Safety
POSSIBLY SAFE ...when used orally in appropriate amounts (186,187).
PREGNANCY AND LACTATION: POSSIBLY SAFE ...when used orally in appropriate amounts.
Kaolin has a category B pregnancy designation by the FDA (12576).

Effectiveness
POSSIBLY EFFECTIVE

Oral mucositis. Kaolin taken orally seems to decrease the pain and severity of radiation-induced mucositis (186,187).

There is insufficient reliable information available about the effectiveness of kaolin for its other uses.

Mechanism of Action
Kaolin is hydrated aluminum silicate, which is purified for pharmaceutical use by treatment with hydrochloric acid or sulfuric acid, or both, then washed with water (9,16). Heavy kaolin (Kaolinum ponderosum) is the purified natural form of variable composition (9,16), and light kaolin is prepared from heavy kaolin by elutriation (separation of finer from coarser particles by suspension in water) (9,16).
In radiation-induced mucositis, kaolin may act as a protective coating to decrease the severity of pain (186).
Topically, kaolin acts as a drying agent adsorbing a wide variety of substances (9,16).

Adverse Reactions
Orally, kaolin can cause constipation, particularly in children and the elderly (15).
Occupational kalinosis (pulmonary disease) is reported in miners following inhalation (195,196,197).

Interactions with Herbs & Other Dietary Supplements
None known.

Interactions with Drugs

CLINDAMYCIN (CLEOCIN): Kaolin appears to slow the rate of clindamycin absorption, but doesn't affect the extent of absorption (253).
DIGOXIN (Lanoxin): Evidence is conflicting about the effect of kaolin on digoxin pharmacokinetics (198,251,252). To avoid a potential interaction, separate digoxin and kaolin doses by at least 2 hours.
QUINIDINE: Preliminary evidence suggests that kaolin might decrease quinidine absorption (250). To avoid a potential interaction, separate quinidine and kaolin doses by at least 2 hours.
TRIMETHOPRIM (PROLOPRIM): Kaolin may reduce the absorption of trimethoprim (199). To avoid a potential interaction, separate trimethoprim and kaolin doses by at least 2 hours.

Interactions with Foods

None known.

Interactions with Lab Tests

None known.

Interactions with Diseases or Conditions

None known.

Dosage and Administration

ORAL: For relief of radiation-induced mucositis, 15 ml (50% kaolin/pectin, a 50% diphenhydramine) solution is used as a rinse four times a day (186).

Comments

Kaolin has been used for years in combination with pectin (Kaopectate) for diarrhea. However in April 2003, the FDA found insufficient support for its use as an antidiarrheal. As of April 2004, kaolin is no longer permitted as an antidiarrhea agent in OTC products (12577). Note that Kaopectate no longer contains pectin and kaolin.

KARAYA GUM

Also Known As

Bassora Tragacanth, Indian Tragacanth, Kadaya, Kadira, Karaya, Katila, Kullo, Mucara, Sterculia Gum.

Scientific Names

Sterculia urens; Sterculia villosa; Sterculia tragacantha; other Sterculia species.
Family: Malvaceae or Sterculiaceae.

People Use This For

Orally, karaya gum is used as a bulk laxative and as an aphrodisiac.
In manufacturing, karaya gum is used as a thickener in pharmaceuticals and cosmetics; denture and ostomy adhesives; and a binder and stabilizer in foods and beverages.

Safety

LIKELY SAFE ...when used orally in amounts commonly found in foods. Karaya gum has Generally Recognized As Safe (GRAS) status in the US (4912). ...when used orally in medicinal amounts (6).
PREGNANCY AND LACTATION: Insufficient reliable information available.

Effectiveness

POSSIBLY EFFECTIVE

Constipation. Taking karaya gum orally seems to be effective for treating constipation when used as a bulk-forming laxative (6,11).

There is insufficient reliable information available about the effectiveness of karaya gum for its other uses.

Mechanism of Action

Karaya gum is not digested or absorbed but swells in the presence of water, forming a viscous colloidal solution that stimulates peristalsis in the GI tract (6,11).

Adverse Reactions

None reported.

Interactions with Herbs & Other Dietary Supplements

None known.

Interactions with Drugs

ORAL DRUGS: Co-administration of oral drugs with bulk forming laxatives may decrease the absorption of the drugs (12).

Interactions with Foods

None known.

Interactions with Lab Tests

None known.

Interactions with Diseases or Conditions

BOWEL OBSTRUCTION: In general, bulk laxatives are contraindicated in individuals with bowel obstruction (12).

Dosage and Administration

No typical dosage.

Comments

Karaya gum is exuded from Sterculia species trees, that are native to India, when charred or scarred (6,3901).
Adequate fluid intake is important with bulk forming laxatives.

KAVA

Also Known As

Ava, Ava Pepper, Ava Root, Awa, Gea, Gi, Intoxicating Long Pepper, Intoxicating Pepper, Kao, Kava Pepper, Kava Root, Kavain, Kavapipar, Kawa Kawa, Kawa Pepper, Kawapfeffer, Kew, Long Pepper, Maori Kava, Malohu, Maluk, Meruk, Milik, Rauschpfeffer, Rhizome Di Kava-Kava, Sakau, Tonga, Wurzelstock, Yagona, Yangona, Yaqona, Yongona.
CAUTION: See separate listing for Indian Long Pepper.

Scientific Names

Piper methysticum.
Family: Piperaceae.

People Use This For

Orally, kava is used to treat anxiety disorders, stress, attention deficit-hyperactivity disorder (ADHD), insomnia, and restlessness. It is also used orally for epilepsy, psychosis, depression, headaches including migraines, common cold and other respiratory tract infections, tuberculosis, cancer prevention, musculoskeletal pain, and bladder cancer. Kava is also used orally for urinary tract infection (UTI), uterine inflammation, venereal disease, menstrual discomfort, vaginal prolapse, and as an aphrodisiac.
Topically, kava is used for skin diseases including leprosy, to promote wound healing, and as an analgesic. It is also used topically as a poultice for otitis and abscesses, and as a mouthwash for canker sores and toothaches.
Ceremonially, kava is used as a beverage to induce relaxation.

Safety

POSSIBLY UNSAFE ...when used orally. There is concern that kava preparations can induce hepatotoxicity and liver failure in patients taking relatively normal doses, short-term. Kava extracts have been safely used under medical supervision for up to six months (2092,2093,2094,2095,4032,7325). However, there are at least 68 reported cases of liver toxicity following kava use. The use of kava for as little as one to three months has resulted in the need for liver transplants, and even death (7024,7068,7086,7096). However, some experts question the clinical validity of several of these cases (11369,11371). Kava has been banned from the market in Switzerland, Germany, Canada, and several other countries are considering similar action. Some patients may be more at risk than others. Patients who are "poor metabolizers" might be at greatest risk, but this has not been verified (7068). Until more is known, tell patients to avoid kava. Recommend routine liver function tests for patients who continue to use kava.
PREGNANCY: POSSIBLY UNSAFE ...when used orally. There is some concern that pyrone constituents in kava can cause loss of uterine tone (19); avoid using.
LACTATION: POSSIBLY UNSAFE ...when used orally. There is concern that the toxic pyrone constituents of kava can pass into breast milk (19); avoid using.

Effectiveness

LIKELY EFFECTIVE

Anxiety. Kava extracts standardized to 70% kava-lactones are superior to placebo (2093,2094,2095,7325,11372), and possibly comparable to low-dose benzodiazepines (2092). Treatment for 1-8 weeks may be necessary for significant improvement (2094,2095). Most clinical studies on the effectiveness of kava for anxiety disorders have used the standardized extract WS 1490 (W. Schwabe). This extract is standardized to contain 70% kava-lactones (also known as kavapyrones). This extract is more than twice as concentrated as most products that are commercially available.

POSSIBLY EFFECTIVE

Benzodiazepine withdrawal. There is some evidence that upwardly titrating kava over one week while tapering the benzodiazepine over two weeks can prevent withdrawal symptoms in some people with non-psychotic anxiety (7325).

Menopausal anxiety. Two small trials have shown that kava standardized to 15% or 70% kava-lactones is superior to placebo taken orally for short-term treatment of neurovegetative and anxiety symptoms related to climacteric. Significant improvement occurred after one week of treatment (2096).

INSUFFICIENT RELIABLE EVIDENCE to RATE

Cancer. Epidemiological evidence suggests that increasing kava consumption might lower incidence of cancer (8175).

Social anxiety. Preliminary clinical research in healthy volunteers suggests that taking kava orally might reduce physiological reactivity during stressful situations (9893).

More evidence is needed to rate kava for these uses.

Mechanism of Action

The applicable parts of kava are the rhizome, root, and stem. Pharmacological activity has largely been attributed to the kava-lactones (also known as kavapyrones), kawain (kavain), dihydrokawain, methysticin, dihydromethysticin, yangonin, and others (9920,9923). The dried herb typically contains at least 3.5% kava-lactones. Kava is traditionally prepared by water extraction from the fresh root. Kava is prepared commercially with ethanol, yielding 30% kava-lactones or acetone, yielding 70% kava-lactones (9920,9921).

Kava has been found to have a variety of pharmacological effects, including anxiolytic, sedative, anti-convulsant, local anesthetic, spasmolytic, anti-inflammatory, and analgesic activities; however, the exact mechanism for these effects is not known. Some evidence suggests the sedative effects may be due to an increase in the number of GABA binding sites (4037,8440,9923). Other preliminary evidence suggests the sedative effects might be the result of dopamine antagonism, particularly by the vangonin constituent (4055,7727,8415,8740). There is some evidence the kava pyrones (+)-methycystine, (+)-kavain, and (±)-kavain also inhibit the uptake of noradrenaline which might also contribute to the psychotropic actions of kava (8740). Kava is not, however, thought to affect benzodiazepine receptors (6401,4038,11373). Analgesia is not believed to occur by the opiate pathway because naloxone does not reverse the effects of kava. Furthermore, kava is thought to produce motor sedation without affecting respiratory processes (2095).

Kava doesn't seem to impair cognitive function (2097,2098,11373). Even at intoxicating doses, the only cognitive impairment observed with kava is a decline in accuracy of visual attention (11373).

Some research suggests that kava can produce muscle paralysis by a mechanism similar to local anesthetics such as cocaine (9924). When chewed, kava root reportedly numbs the mouth similar to cocaine (1740). Some evidence suggests kava may affect the limbic system (6002). People consuming kava have reported feeling more sociable, tranquil, and generally happy (1740). The kavapyrones desmethoxyyangonin and methysticin appear to competitively inhibit monoamine oxidase B (MAO-B) (2500). Kava is thought to work for a variety of inflammatory conditions by inhibiting both COX-1 and COX-2 enzymes, the enzymes responsible for converting arachidonic acid to prostaglandins (8413).

There is some evidence the kavapyrone (+)-kavain has antithrombotic activity. By inhibiting cyclooxygenase and decreasing the synthesis of thromboxane A2, (+)-kavain appears to decrease the aggregation of platelets (2501).

Adverse Reactions

Orally, kava can cause gastrointestinal (GI) upset, headache, dizziness, drowsiness, enlarged pupils and disturbances of oculomotor equilibrium and accommodation, dry mouth, and allergic skin reactions (4032,11370). It may also cause extrapyramidal side effects such as involuntary oral and lingual reflexes, and twisting movements of the head and trunk, possibly due to dopamine antagonism (4055,8415). Unlike benzodiazepines, kava is not thought to be associated with impaired cognitive function (2097,2098,11373). Use of normal doses of kava may affect the ability to drive or operate machinery. Driving under the influence (DUI) citations have been issued to individuals observed driving erratically after drinking large amounts of kava tea (535).

Hepatoxicity is a particular concern with kava. There are at least 68 reported cases of hepatotoxicity following use of kava products (7024,7068,7086,7096,11795). However, some experts question the clinical validity of several of these cases (11369,11371). In susceptible patients, symptoms can show up after as little as 3-4 weeks of kava use, including yellowed skin (jaundice), fatigue, and dark urine (7024,7068). Liver function tests can be elevated after 3-8 weeks of use, possibly followed by hepatomegaly and onset of encephalopathy (7024). Kava can also exacerbate hepatitis in patients with a history of recurrent hepatitis. Symptoms seem to resolve spontaneously after discontinuation of kava (390). Liver toxicity is more frequently associated with prolonged use of very high doses (6401). But there is some concern that even short-term use of kava in typical doses might cause acute hepatitis in some patients, including severe hepatocellular necrosis. Death or liver transplant has been required after as little as 1-3 months of kava use (7024,7068,7086,11795). Symptoms of liver toxicity may occur following a single occasion of alcohol consumption while taking kava (7068). Kava supplements have been banned in Switzerland, Germany, and Canada. Several other countries are considering removing kava from the market (7086).

Most patients taking kava have not experienced such severe adverse effects. Kava mixed with water is used in the Pacific Islands as a ceremonial and social beverage without reported hepatotoxicity (11794). It is unclear which patients might be susceptible to adverse liver effects. There is some speculation that so-called "poor metabolizers" or those patients with deficiency in the cytochrome P450 2D6 (CYP2D6) isoenzyme may be at increased risk for hepatotoxic effects of kava (7068). Up to 10% of people of European descent have a genetic deficiency of CYP2D6. This deficiency has not been found in Pacific Islanders. Some people speculate that the type of extraction method could be responsible. Alcohol and acetone extracts of kava have been linked to liver toxicity; water extracts have not. But there is no research to support the contention that water-extracted kava is safe (11794).Until more is known, tell patients to avoid kava. Advise patients who continue to use kava to routinely monitor liver function. In patients who develop symptoms, discontinue kava and monitor liver function tests. Liver function tests may normalize within eight weeks following discontinuation (7068).

Long-term use of very large amounts of kava, especially in high doses (400 mg kava pyrones daily) is also associated with overall poor health including symptoms of low body weight, reduced protein levels, puffy face, hematuria, increased red blood cell volume, decreased platelets and lymphocytes, and possibly pulmonary hypertension (4032,6402). Chronic use of high doses of kava has also been associated with kava dermopathy, which consists of reddened eyes; dry, scaly, flaky skin; and temporary yellow discoloration of the skin, hair, and nails (6401,8414,8417,11370). This pellagra-like syndrome is unresponsive to niacinamide treatment (6240,7728,11370). The cause is unknown, but may relate to interference with cholesterol metabolism (6240). Kava's adverse effects on liver function might also contribute to kava dermopathy (6401,8417). Kava dermopathy usually occurs within three months to one year of regular kava use, and resolves when the kava dose is decreased or discontinued (6401,8414). Kava dose should be decreased or discontinued if kava dermopathy occurs (6401).

Kava has been associated with severe, rapidly progressive, persistent Parkinsonism. In a previously healthy 45-year-old woman with a family history of essential tremor, Parkinsonian symptoms developed following ten days of taking 65 mg kava per day. Parkinsonian symptoms improved with administration of anticholinergics, but residual symptoms required chronic medication (7727).

Sjogren's syndrome has been associated with a herbal supplement containing kava, echinacea, and St. John's wort. Echinacea may have been the primary cause, because Sjogren's syndrome is an autoimmune disorder. The role of kava in this syndrome is unclear (10319).

Interactions with Herbs & Other Dietary Supplements

HEPATOTOXIC HERBS AND SUPPLEMENTS: There is some concern that kava can adversely affect the liver (7024,7068). Theoretically, concomitant use with other potentially hepatotoxic products might increase the risk of developing liver damage. Some of these products include androstenedione, chaparral, coenzyme Q10 (only in high doses), comfrey, DHEA, germander, niacin, pennyroyal oil, red yeast, and others.

HERBS AND SUPPLEMENTS WITH SEDATIVE PROPERTIES: Theoretically, concomitant use with herbs and supplements that have sedative properties might increase the risk of excessive drowsiness. Some of these supplements include 5-HTP, calamus, California poppy, catnip, hops, Jamaican dogwood, kava, St. John's wort, scullcap, valerian, yerba mansa, and others.

Interactions with Drugs

ALPRAZOLAM (Xanax): There is one report of an individual who was hospitalized due to lethargy and disorientation that occurred when alprazolam, cimetidine, terazosin, and kava were used concomitantly (536).

CNS DEPRESSANTS: Concomitant use of kava and alcohol, barbiturates, benzodiazepines, or other CNS depressants can increase the risk of drowsiness and motor reflex depression (2093,2098).

CYTOCHROME P450 1A2 (CYP1A2) SUBSTRATES: Preliminary evidence suggests that kava significantly inhibits cytochrome P450 1A2 (CYP1A2) (8743,12479). Some substrates of CYP1A2 include clozapine (Clozaril), cyclobenzaprine (Flexeril), fluvoxamine (Luvox), haloperidol (Haldol), imipramine (Tofranil), mexiletine (Mexitil), olanzapine (Zyprexa), pentazocine (Talwin), propranolol (Inderal), tacrine (Cognex), theophylline, zileuton (Zyflo), zolmitriptan (Zomig), and others. Use kava cautiously or avoid in patients taking these drugs.

CYTOCHROME P450 2C19 (CYP2C19) SUBSTRATES: Preliminary evidence suggests that kava significantly inhibits cytochrome P450 2C19 (CYP2C19) (8743,12479). Some substrates of CYP2C19 include amitriptyline (Elavil), clomipramine (Anafranil), cyclophosphamide (Cytoxan), diazepam (Valium), lansoprazole (Prevacid), omeprazole (Prilosec), lansoprazole (Protonix), phenytoin (Dilantin), phenobarbital (Luminal), progesterone, and others. Use kava cautiously or avoid in patients taking these drugs.

CYTOCHROME P450 2C9 (CYP2C9) SUBSTRATES: Preliminary evidence suggests that kava significantly inhibits cytochrome P450 2C9 (CYP2C9) (8743,12479). Some substrates of CYP2C9 include celecoxib (Celebrex), diclofenac (Voltaren), fluvastatin (Lescol), glipizide (Glucotrol), ibuprofen (Advil, Motrin), irbesartan (Avapro), losartan (Cozaar), phenytoin (Dilantin), piroxicam (Feldene), tamoxifen (Nolvadex), tolbutamide (Tolinase),

torsemide (Demadex), and warfarin (Coumadin). Use kava cautiously or avoid in patients taking these drugs.
CYTOCHROME P450 2D6 (CYP2D6) SUBSTRATES: Preliminary evidence suggests that kava significantly inhibits cytochrome P450 2D6 (CYP2D6) (8743,12479). Some drugs metabolized by CYP2D6 include amitriptyline (Elavil), codeine, desipramine (Norpramin), flecainide (Tambocor), haloperidol (Haldol), imipramine (Tofranil), metoprolol (Lopressor, Toprol XL), ondansetron (Zofran), paroxetine (Paxil), risperidone (Risperdal), tramadol (Ultram), venlafaxine (Effexor), and others. Use kava cautiously or avoid in patients taking these drugs.
CYTOCHROME P450 3A4 (CYP3A4) SUBSTRATES: Preliminary evidence suggests that kava significantly inhibits cytochrome P450 3A4 (CYP3A4) (8743,12479). Some drugs metabolized by CYP3A4 include alprazolam (Xanax), amlodipine (Norvasc), clarithromycin (Biaxin), cyclosporine (Sandimmune), erythromycin, lovastatin (Mevacor), ketoconazole (Nizoral), itraconazole (Sporanox), fexofenadine (Allegra), triazolam (Halcion), verapamil (Calan, Isoptin) and many others. Use kava cautiously or avoid in patients taking these drugs.
HEPATOTOXIC DRUGS: There is some concern that kava can adversely affect the liver (7024,7068). Theoretically, concomitant use with other potentially hepatotoxic drugs might increase the risk of developing liver damage. Some of these drugs include acarbose (Precose, Prandase), amiodarone (Cordarone), atorvastatin (Lipitor), azathioprine (Imuran), carbamazepine (Tegretol), cerivastatin (Baycol), diclofenac (Voltaren), felbamate (Felbatol), fenofibrate (Tricor), fluvastatin (Lescol), gemfibrozil (Lopid), isoniazid, itraconazole, (Sporanox), ketoconazole (Nizoral), leflunomide (Arava), lovastatin (Mevacor), methotrexate (Rheumatrex), nevirapine (Viramune), niacin, nitrofurantoin (Macrodantin), pioglitazone (Actos), pravastatin (Pravachol), pyrazinamide, rifampin (Rifadin), ritonavir (Norvir), rosiglitazone (Avandia), simvastatin (Zocor), tacrine (Cognex), tamoxifen, terbinafine (Lamisil), valproic acid, and zileuton (Zyflo).
LEVODOPA: There is some concern that kava might decrease the effectiveness of levodopa. In one case, kava seemed to reduce efficacy of levodopa. This effect might be due to dopamine antagonism by kava (7727).

Interactions with Foods

ALCOHOL: Concomitant use of kava with alcohol can increase the risk of side effects such as drowsiness and motor reflex depression (19). There is also some concern that concomitant use of kava and alcohol can increase the risk of developing hepatotoxicity (7068).

Interactions with Lab Tests

LIVER FUNCTION TESTS: There is some concern that kava can cause liver damage and increase liver function tests (LFTs) in some patients. Liver toxicity is primarily associated with prolonged use of high doses (6401). However, in some patients, short-term use (3-8 weeks) of typical doses might result in liver damage and increase liver function tests (390,7024,7068). Liver function tests affected include aspartate aminotransferase (AST), alanine aminotransferase (ALT), alkaline phosphatase, gamma-glutamyltransferase, lactate dehydrogenase (LDH), and total and conjugated bilirubin (7024,7068). Consider monitoring liver function tests in patients taking kava for more than one month or in patients symptoms of liver problems such as fatigue, yellowing of the skin (jaundice), or dark urine.

Interactions with Diseases or Conditions

DEPRESSION: There is some concern about using kava in depressed patients. Kava seems to have CNS depressant effects and theoretically might exacerbate depression in some patients (19); use with caution.
HEPATITIS: Kava might adversely affect the liver, especially when taken for prolonged periods or in high doses. Even when used short-term in typical doses, kava might exacerbate hepatitis in patients with a history of recurrent hepatitis (390). Tell patients with active hepatitis or a history of hepatitis to avoid kava.
PARKINSON'S DISEASE: There is some concern about using kava in patients with Parkinson's disease. Dopamine antagonism has been reported even when used in typical doses. Tell patients with Parkinson's disease to avoid kava (4032,8134,8415).

Dosage and Administration

ORAL: For anxiety disorders, most clinical trials have used kava extract standardized to 70% kava-lactone content. Doses of the kava extract were most commonly 100 mg (70 mg kava-lactones) three times daily (2092,2093,2094,2095,2096). For preventing benzodiazepine withdrawal, the 70% kava-lactone standardized extract has been used in doses increasing from 50 mg to 300 mg per day over one week, while the benzodiazepine is tapered over 2 weeks (7325). Because kava-lactone content varies substantially among products, appropriate dosing will also vary.

Comments

Kava was discovered by Captain Cook who named the plant, "intoxicating pepper" (6240). In the South Pacific, kava is a popular social drink, similar to alcohol in Western societies (9921). Kava is also prepared in a defined ritual manner and used for ceremonial purposes and has been used for thousands of years by Pacific Islanders (782,6240). The ban of kava in some countries has had a detrimental effect on the economies of Pacific Island countries that export kava (11794).

KEFIR

Also Known As

Fermented Dairy Product, Fermented Milk, Kefir Cheese, Kefir Grains, Kefir Yogurt.

Scientific Names

None.

People Use This For

Orally, kefir is used for improving digestion, lactose intolerance, and hyperlipidemia.

Safety

POSSIBLY SAFE ...when used orally and appropriately. Kefir appears safe when used for up to 6 months (7636,8452,8457,8480).
PREGNANCY AND LACTATION: ...Insufficient reliable information available; avoid using.

Effectiveness

LIKELY INEFFECTIVE

Hyperlipidemia. Taking kefir orally appears to have very little or no effect on total cholesterol and low-density lipoprotein (LDL) cholesterol (7636,8452,8457,8480).

There is insufficient reliable information available about the effectiveness of kefir for its other uses.

Mechanism of Action

Kefir consists of milk that has been fermented for 18 to 48 hours following the addition of kefir grain. After fermentation, kefir may have a pH as low as 4.5. It has a sour or effervescent taste and consistency. The primary active constituents of kefir include the polysaccharide, kefiran, and beta-galactosidase. Kefir grain is made up of a mixture of lactic acid bacteria, acetic acid bacteria, and yeast which is held together, in clumps, by polysaccharide links. When properly prepared, kefir grains resemble cooked cauliflower in color and texture. The composition of kefir grain varies with its origin, and as a result, there is considerable variation in the microbial content of the kefir after fermentation.

During fermentation, kefir becomes increasingly viscous due to the formation of additional kefiran polysaccharides by the lactic acid bacteria (8481,8482,8483,8484). Lactobacillus lactis, Lactobacillus casei, Lactobacillus helveticus, and other Lactobacillus species may be present in kefir. In addition, Streptococcus thermophilus and yeast species, including Kluyveromyces marxianus, Saccharomyces cerevisiae, and Candida species may be isolated (8485). Many of these species can survive transit through the stomach and inoculate the intestinal tract (8487).

The beta-galactosidase in kefir can facilitate the breakdown of lactose in the gastrointestinal tract, according to preliminary evidence. This action may increase the absorption of galactose and glucose after consuming milk (8485). The lactose found in milk decreases from 5% to about 3.6% during fermentation of kefir (8486).

Early evidence indicates that oral kefiran polysaccharide may increase both the intestinal and systemic immune response (8488,8489). This immune response may decrease the growth of carcinoma and sarcoma cells (8481,8482,8489).

Adverse Reactions

Orally, kefir can cause intestinal cramping and constipation, especially with initial use. These symptoms usually resolve after continued consumption of kefir (7636). Otherwise kefir appears to be well tolerated (7636,8452,8457,8480).

Interactions with Herbs & Other Dietary Supplements

None known.

Interactions with Drugs

IMMUNOSUPPRESSANTS: Kefir contains actively growing bacteria and yeast (8481,8482,8483,8484). Theoretically, patients taking immunosuppressant therapy might be more likely to develop an infection from the organisms. Use with caution in patients taking cyclosporine (Sandimmune, Neoral), azathioprine (Imuran), tacrolimus (FK506, Prograf), and others.

Interactions with Foods

None known.

Interactions with Lab Tests

None known.

Interactions with Diseases or Conditions

AIDS: Kefir contains actively growing bacteria and yeast (8481,8482,8483,8484). Theoretically, patients with an impaired immune system might be more likely to develop infections from these bacteria or yeast.
IMMUNOSUPPRESSION: There is some concern that immunocompromised patients taking kefir might be at an increased risk for fungemia or bacteriemia (8481,8482,8483,8484).

Dosage and Administration

ORAL: For hyperlipidemia, kefir 125 to 500 mL daily has been used for up to six months (7636,8452,8457,8480).

KHAT

Also Known As

Abyssinian Tea, Arabian-Tea, Chaat, Gat, Kat, Kus es Salahin, Miraa, Qut, Tchaad, Tohai, Tohat, Tschut.

Scientific Names

Catha edulis, synonym Celastrus edulis.
Family: Celastraceae.

People Use This For

Orally, khat leaf is used for depression, fatigue, obesity, gastric ulcers, and male infertility. The leaf and stem are chewed by people in East Africa and the Arabian countries as a euphoriant. It is also used to suppress the need for food and sleep, decrease sexual desires, and increase aggression.

Safety

POSSIBLY UNSAFE ...when used orally. Khat leaf is not physically addicting but is associated with psychological dependence (6). High doses of khat can cause paranoia, psychosis, and aggression (10120).
PREGNANCY: POSSIBLY UNSAFE ...when used orally. Khat may reduce infant birth weight (6).
LACTATION: POSSIBLY UNSAFE ...when used orally. Khat contains norpseudoephedrine, which passes into mother's milk (6); avoid using.

Effectiveness

There is insufficient reliable information available about the effectiveness of khat.

Mechanism of Action

The applicable parts of khat are the leaf and stem. Khat contains cathine, which has 1/10 the stimulant effect of d-amphetamine. It also contains cathinone, which is a more powerful stimulant than cathine and closely resembles ephedrine and amphetamine in chemical structure (10120). Both khat constituents decrease food intake and increase locomotor activity (6).

Adverse Reactions

Orally, consumption of Khat results in central stimulation including euphoria, increased alertness, excessive talkativeness, hyperactivity, excitement, aggressiveness, anxiety, elevated blood pressure, and manic behavior. Insomnia, malaise, and lack of concentration usually follow (6). Increased consumption can cause users to become paranoid and psychotic (10120). True psychotic reactions occur much less often than with amphetamines (6). Cardiovascular effects include tachycardia, palpitations, and increased blood pressure. Other effects include increased respiratory rate, hyperthermia, sweating, pupil dilation and decreased intraocular pressure, stomatitis, esophagitis, gastritis, periodontal disease, temporomandibular joint dysfunction and keratosis of buccal mucosa, and constipation (6). Chronic use in young people is linked to hypertension.
Severe adverse effects include migraine, cerebral hemorrhage, myocardial infarction (MI), pulmonary edema, and hepatic cirrhosis. Khat causes initial increase in men's libido followed by loss of sexual drive, spermatorrhea, and impotence (6). Females report increased sexual desire and improved performance (6).
There are also cases of infection with Fasciola hepatica following chewing khat leaves. Fasciola hepatica contamination might be most likely with freshly picked, damp leaves. Signs of Fasciola hepatica infection can include pain below the ribs, leukocytosis with eosinophilia, and large liver mass on CT examination (6464).

Interactions with Herbs & Other Dietary Supplements

None known.

Interactions with Drugs

None known.

Interactions with Foods

None known.

Interactions with Lab Tests

None known.

Interactions with Diseases or Conditions

DIABETES: Khat use suppresses appetite causing people to skip meals, decrease adherence to dietary advice, and increase consumption of sweetened beverages aggravating hyperglycemia (6).

Dosage and Administration

No typical dosage.

Comments

Khat is considered to be a dependence producing drug by the World Health Organization (WHO). In Somalia, civilian and military use of khat has been blamed for fueling civil conflict, draining the nation's economy, and thwarting international relief efforts (10120).

KHELLA

Also Known As

Ammi, Bischofskrautfruchte, Bishop's Weed, Bishop's Weed Fruit, Bishops Weed, Fruits de Khella, Khella Fruit, Khellin, Toothpick Ammi, Toothpick Plant, Visnaga, Visnaga Fruit, Visnagae, Visnagafruchte, Visnagin.
CAUTION: See separate listings for Goutweed and Bishop's Weed.

Scientific Names

Ammi visnaga, synonyms Ammi daucoides, Daucus visagna.
Family: Apiaceae/Umbelliferae.

People Use This For

Orally, khella is used for colic and abdominal cramps, kidney stones, menstrual pain, and premenstrual syndrome (PMS). Khella is also used for respiratory conditions including asthma, bronchitis, cough, and whooping cough. It is also used for cardiovascular disorders including hypertension, cardiac arrhythmias, congestive heart failure (CHF), angina, atherosclerosis, and hypercholesterolemia. It is also used for liver and gall bladder disorders, diabetes, and as a diuretic.
Topically, khella is used for vitiligo, psoriasis, wound healing, inflammation conditions, and poisonous bites.

Safety

POSSIBLY UNSAFE ...when used orally in high doses. High doses of khella can cause increases in liver enzymes and possible liver damage (2).
PREGNANCY: LIKELY UNSAFE ...when used orally. The active constituent, khellin, has uterine stimulant activity (19); contraindicated.
LACTATION: Insufficient reliable information available; avoid using.

Effectiveness

There is insufficient reliable information available about the effectiveness of khella.

Mechanism of Action

The applicable parts of khella are the dried, ripe fruits (7161). Khella has several constituents with known pharmacological activity, including visnadin, visnagin, and khellin. All of these constituents seem to have cardiovascular effects due to calcium channel blocking actions (8,2525). Visnadin is the most active. It can inhibit vascular smooth muscle contraction and seems to dilate peripheral and coronary vessels and increase coronary circulation (8,9,2523,2524). Visnagin also has negative chronotropic and inotropic effects and reduces peripheral vascular resistance (869). The khellin constituent also acts as a vasodilator and has bronchodilatory activity (9). There is some preliminary evidence that khellin might also increase high-density lipoprotein (HDL) levels without affecting total cholesterol or triglyceride concentrations (2522). A khella extract seems to have some antimicrobial activity. This might be attributable to both the khellin and visnagin constituents, which both seem to have antifungal, antibacterial, and antiviral activity (1907). Researchers are interested in khella for use in psoriasis. The khellin constituent is structurally similar to the psoralen nucleus and might be useful as a photosensitizer in patients with psoriasis (1908).

Adverse Reactions

Orally, prolonged use or use of high doses of khella can cause nausea, dizziness, constipation, lack of appetite, headache, itching, and insomnia. In some patients, khella can cause elevated liver transaminase and gamma-glutamyltransferase (GGT) levels (2), probably due to the khellin constituent, which is known to affect liver enzymes (6,2522). Liver dysfunction and jaundice is typically reversible when khella is discontinued (2). There is also some concern that khella might cause photosensitivity because of the constituents khellin and furocoumarin (2,7162).

Interactions with Herbs & Other Dietary Supplements

DIGITALIS: Theoretically, khella might decrease the effectiveness of digitalis. The visnagin constituent of khella has negative inotropic effects, which might counter the effects of digitalis (869).
HEPATOTOXIC HERBS: Khella might have additive effects with herbs that cause hepatotoxicity. Khella can cause increase liver enzymes and liver dysfunction in some patients. Other products that might affect the liver include borage, chaparral, uva ursi, and others (2,2522).
PHOTOSENSITIZING HERBS: Theoretically, khella might have an additive effects with products that increase sun sensitivity, such as St. John's wort (7162).

Interactions with Drugs

DIGOXIN (Lanoxin): Theoretically, khella might decrease the effectiveness of cardiac glycosides like digoxin. The khella constituent visnadin has negative inotropic effects that might counter the effects of cardiac glycosides (19,869).
HEPATOTOXIC DRUGS: Theoretically, khella might have additive adverse effects on the liver when used with hepatotoxic drugs. Khella can increase liver transaminases (2,2522). Some drugs that can adversely effect the liver include acetaminophen (Tylenol), amiodarone (Cordarone), carbamazepine (Tegretol), isoniazid (INH), methotrexate (Rheumatrex), methyldopa (Aldomet), and many others.
PHOTOSENSITIZING DRUGS: Theoretically, concomitant use might result in increased photosensitivity. Khella constituents can cause photosensitivity (2521,7162). Some drugs that cause photosensitivity include amitriptyline (Elavil), quinolones (Ciprofloxacin, others), sulfa drugs (Septra, Bactrim, others), and tetracycline.

Interactions with Foods

None known.

Interactions with Lab Tests

HIGH-DENSITY LIPOPROTEIN (HDL): Theoretically, khella might increase HDL levels. The isolated khella constituent khellin seems to increase in HDL levels without affecting total cholesterol or triglycerides (2522).
LIVER FUNCTION TESTS: In some patients, khella can cause elevated liver transaminase and gamma-glutamyltransferase (GGT) levels (2), probably due to the khellin constituent, which is known to affect liver enzymes (6,2522). Liver dysfunction is typically reversible when khella is discontinued (2).

Interactions with Diseases or Conditions

LIVER DISEASE: Khella might exacerbate liver dysfunction in patients with liver disease. Khella can increase liver enzymes in some patients, probably due to the khellin constituent (2,2522).

Dosage and Administration

ORAL: Khella is typically given as an extract standardized based on khellin content. Extracts are usually standardized to 12% khellin (6002). A typical dose of khella is an amount that provides 20 mg of the khellin constituent per day (8). For angina, khella in an amount providing doses of 30-300 mg of the khellin constituent has also been used (6002). Khella is sometimes used as a tea. The tea is usually prepared by pouring boiling water over powdered fruit, steeping 10-15 minutes, and straining (8).

Comments

Several conventional drugs including amiodarone, nifedipine, and cromolyn, have been developed from khella (9,7161). Khella is sometimes confused with its less used relative, bishop's weed (Ammi majus). The two species have some common chemical constituents and pharmacological effects, but khella is more commonly used for cardiac and pulmonary conditions, and bishop's weed is more commonly used for dermatological conditions (7161). Isolated khellin, a constituent of khella and bishop's weed, is used for angina pectoris; asthma; and in conjunction with phototherapy for vitiligo, psoriasis, and alopecia areata (9,560,849,868).

KINETIN

Also Known As

Kinerase, Kinetase, Kn.

Scientific Names

N-(2-furanylmethyl)-1H-purin-6-amine; N(6)furfuryladenine; 6-furfurylaminopurine.

People Use This For
Topically, kinetin is used to reduce the effects of skin aging; to reduce skin roughness; fine wrinkles; telangiectasias; and mottled, excessive pigmentation.
In combination, kinetin is used topically with retinol palmitate to treat signs of aging.

Safety
There is insufficient reliable information about the safety of kinetin.
Pregnancy and Lactation: Insufficient reliable information available; avoid using.

Effectiveness
There is insufficient reliable information available about the effectiveness of kinetin.

Mechanism of Action
Kinetin is a cytokinin, a plant growth factor. In plants, it seems to work to prevent or slow the aging process (12022). Effects in animals are not well understood. There is some evidence that kinetin acts as an antioxidant and might protect DNA from oxidative damage (4278). There is also some in vitro evidence kinetin might decrease some of the morphological changes that normally occur in human fibroblast cells as they age. However, kinetin doesn't not seem to increase the overall lifespan of these fibroblasts (12022).

Adverse Reactions
None reported.

Interactions with Herbs & Other Dietary Supplements
None known.

Interactions with Drugs
None known.

Interactions with Foods
None known.

Interactions with Lab Tests
None known.

Interactions with Diseases or Conditions
None known.

Dosage and Administration
TOPICAL: A typical dose is 0.05% cream or lotion or 0.1% cream or lotion applied twice daily (4284).

KIWI

Also Known As
China Gooseberry, Chinese Gooseberry, Kiwi Fruit.

Scientific Names
Actinidia chinensis.
Family: Actinidiaceae.

People Use This For
For food use, kiwi is eaten as a food, used as a meat tenderizer, and is a component in some sports drinks.

Safety
LIKELY SAFE ...when used in food amounts (6).
PREGNANCY AND LACTATION: LIKELY SAFE ...when used in food amounts (6).

Effectiveness
INSUFFICIENT RELIABLE EVIDENCE to RATE

Asthma. There is some evidence that consumption of vitamin C-rich citrus fruits, including kiwi and others, might improve lung function in people with asthma. Intake of citrus fruits 1-2 times per week has produced this benefit in some studies (6049,6055,6056). However, other studies have not found this benefit (6057,6058). More evidence is needed to rate the kiwi for this use.

Mechanism of Action
The applicable part of kiwi is the fruit. Kiwi fruit contains high concentrations of vitamin C and serotonin (6). The potential benefits of kiwi in asthma might be due to antioxidant properties of vitamin C or other fruit constituents (6049,6054,6055). The constituent, actinidin, is an enzyme with proteolytic activity similar to papain (6). Enzymatic components may be responsible for adverse effects (6).

Adverse Reactions
Orally, eating kiwi fruit or drinking the juice can lead to hypersensitivity reactions of the mouth, including dysphagia, urticaria, and vomiting immediately following ingestion (6).
Topically, use can cause contact urticaria (6). Kiwi may cause hypersensitivity reactions, which are more common in patients who are allergic to latex (6197,7853).

Interactions with Herbs & Other Dietary Supplements
None known.

Interactions with Drugs
None known.

Interactions with Foods
None known.

Interactions with Lab Tests
URINE TESTS: Kiwi may elevate urine levels of 5-hydroxyindoleacetic acid and interfere with lab tests for this serotonin metabolite (6).

Interactions with Diseases or Conditions
LATEX ALLERGY: People who are allergic to latex should avoid eating kiwi or taking products containing kiwi because of the possibility of cross hypersensitivity between kiwi and latex (6197,7853).

Dosage and Administration
No typical dosage.

KNOTWEED

Also Known As
Allseed Nine-Joints, Armstrong, Beggarweed, Bird's Tongue, Birdweed, Centinode, Cow Grass, Crawlgrass, Doorweed, Hogweed, Knot Grass, Knotgrass, Knotweed Herb, Mexican Sanguinaria, Ninety-Knot, Pigrush, Pigweed, Polygoni Avicularis Herba, Red Robin, Sparrow Tongue, Swine's Grass, Swynel Grass, Vogelknoeterichkraut.

Scientific Names
Polygonum aviculare.
Family: Polygonaceae.

People Use This For
Orally, knotweed is used for bronchitis, cough, gingivitis, and inflammation of the mouth and pharynx. It is also used for supportive treatment of pulmonary diseases, skin disorders, to suppress perspiration associated with tuberculosis, as a diuretic, and to stop bleeding.

Safety
POSSIBLY SAFE ...when used orally or topically (2,18,9347).
PREGNANCY AND LACTATION: Insufficient reliable information available; avoid using.

Effectiveness
INSUFFICIENT RELIABLE EVIDENCE to RATE

Gingivitis. Preliminary clinical research suggests a root extract of knotweed might be useful as a mouth rinse to treat gingivitis. It seems to decrease bleeding and inflammation of the gums associated with gingivitis. Some evidence suggests it might also interfere with the aggregation and adherence of plaque to teeth (9347). More evidence is needed to rate knotweed for this use.

Mechanism of Action

The applicable part of knotweed is the whole flowering plant. Knotweed might have astringent, anti-inflammatory, antihemorrhagic, antiglycolytic, and anticholinergic activity (2,18,9347). Knotweed contains flavonoids (avicularin, kaempferol, quercetin, myrecitin) and gallic acid. In addition to the astringent properties of knotweed, the flavonoids it contains might decrease capillary fragility and have a cortisone-like effect on gingival tissues. Its antiglycolytic activity might disrupt the aggregation and adherence of dental plaque to teeth (9347).

Adverse Reactions

None reported.

Interactions with Herbs & Other Dietary Supplements

None known.

Interactions with Drugs

None known.

Interactions with Foods

None known.

Interactions with Lab Tests

None known.

Interactions with Diseases or Conditions

None known.

Dosage and Administration

ORAL: One cup of tea (simmer 1.4 grams dried ground herb in 150 mL of boiling water for 10-15 minutes, strain) is typically taken orally 3 to 5 times daily. A daily oral dose of 4-6 grams dried ground herb has also been used (2,18). For gingivitis, twice daily use of an oral rinse containing sterilized water and root extract of knotweed (1mg/mL) has been used (9347).

KOMBUCHA TEA

Also Known As

Champagne Of Life, Combucha Tea, Dr. Sklenar's Kombucha Mushroom Infusion, Fungus Japonicus, Kargasok Tea, Kombucha Mushroom Tea, Kwassan, Manchurian Fungus, Manchurian Mushroom Tea, Spumonto, T'Chai from the Sea, Tschambucco.

Scientific Names

None.

People Use This For

Orally, kombucha tea is used for memory loss, premenstrual syndrome, rheumatism, aging, anorexia, AIDS, cancer, hypertension, increasing T-cell counts, strengthening the immune system and metabolism, constipation, arthritis, and hair regrowth.
Topically, it is used for analgesia.

Safety

POSSIBLY UNSAFE ...when used orally because non-sterile home preparations have a high risk of contamination (2650,2651,2652,2653).
LIKELY UNSAFE ...when used orally by individuals with compromised immunity, including HIV/AIDS, due to the risk of transmission of opportunistic pathogens (2652,2653), including Aspergillus (2652,2653) and anthrax (Bacillus anthracis) (2651). ...when kombucha tea prepared in a lead-glazed ceramic container is used orally. Lead poisoning was reported in two people who consumed kombucha tea prepared in a lead-glazed ceramic pot for six months (1366).
PREGNANCY AND LACTATION: POSSIBLY UNSAFE ...when used orally; avoid using.

Effectiveness

There is insufficient reliable information available about the effectiveness of kombucha tea.

Mechanism of Action

Kombucha tea can contain up to 1.5% alcohol, vinegar (acetic acid), and a variety of other metabolites (2655). The product contains high levels of B vitamins (2653). No clinically relevant pharmacology has been defined for the kombucha symbiot or its products (6). Caffeine (black tea) and sugar are theorized to account for the increased energy claimed by some tea users (2654). Kombucha tea has the potential to incubate pathogenic organisms, including Aspergillus and anthrax, during its preparation, which is commonly ten days of fermentation at room temperature (2651,2652,2653). Due to the vinegar and ethanol content, it also has the potential to leach lead and other toxic chemicals from the walls of the preparation and storage containers (2650).

Adverse Reactions

Orally, use of kombucha tea can cause stomach problems, yeast infections (2652), allergic reactions, jaundice, nausea, vomiting, head and neck pain (2656), anthrax (2651), and possibly death (2655). Symptomatic lead poisoning requiring chelation decontamination therapy was reported in two people who consumed kombucha tea prepared in a lead-glazed ceramic pot for six months (1366).

Interactions with Herbs & Other Dietary Supplements

None known.

Interactions with Drugs

DISULFIRAM (Antabuse): Theoretically, concomitant use with kombucha tea can cause a disulfiram reaction due to the alcohol contained in the fermented tea (2650).

Interactions with Foods

None known.

Interactions with Lab Tests

LIVER FUNCTION TESTS: There is one report of increased liver function tests after three weeks of consumption of kombucha tea (6).

Interactions with Diseases or Conditions

ALCOHOLISM: Kombucha tea is contraindicated in people with stabilized or therapeutically-controlled alcoholism, because the alcohol content of the tea can aggravate this condition (2650).
COMPROMISED IMMUNITY: Contraindicated because kombucha tea can harbor or culture organisms that cause opportunistic infections (2652,2653).

Dosage and Administration

No typical dosage.

Comments

The kombucha "mushroom" is a yeast or bacteria fungal symbiot and not an actual mushroom. It is derived from the fermentation of yeasts and bacteria with black tea, sugar, and other ingredients (6,2650). The resulting liquid is called kombucha tea. Although advocates of kombucha tea have attributed many therapeutic effects to the drink in the popular press, there is no scientific evidence to support any therapeutic claims (6,2650,2652,2654,2655). An outbreak of anthrax in twenty people in Iran confirmed the tea is a good culture medium for Bacillus anthracis (2651).

KOUSSO

Also Known As

Cossoo, Kooso, Kosso.

Scientific Names

Hagenia abyssinica, synonym Banksia abyssinica; Brayera anthelmintica.
Family: Rosaceae.

People Use This For

Orally, kousso is used orally for tapeworm infestations.

Safety

LIKELY UNSAFE ...when used orally (18).
PREGNANCY: UNSAFE ...when used orally due to abortifacient activity (19).
LACTATION: UNSAFE ...when used orally due to its potential for toxicity (18).

Effectiveness
There is insufficient reliable information available about the effectiveness of kousso.

Mechanism of Action
There is insufficient reliable information available about the possible mechanism of action or active ingredients.

Adverse Reactions
Orally, kousso can cause gastrointestinal irritation with accompanying salivation, headache, and general weakness. With overdose, people experience syncope and vision disorders. It can also cause colic, spasms, acidosis, and shock (18).

Interactions with Herbs & Other Dietary Supplements
None known.

Interactions with Drugs
None known.

Interactions with Foods
None known.

Interactions with Lab Tests
None known.

Interactions with Diseases or Conditions
GASTROINTESTINAL (GI) CONDITIONS: Kousso can irritate the GI tract. Contraindicated in individuals with infectious or inflammatory GI conditions (19).

Dosage and Administration
No typical dosage.

KUDZU

Also Known As
Daidzein, Fen Ke, Fenge, Gange, Ge Gen, Gegen, Isoflavones, Japanese Arrowroot, Kakkon, Kudsu, Kudzu Vine, Kwaao Khruea, Mealy Kudzu, Pueraria, Pueraria Root, Radix Puerariae, Yege.

Scientific Names
Pueraria montana var. lobata, synonyms Pueraria lobata, Pueraria thunbergiana, Pueraria pseudohirsuta, Dolichos lobatus, Dolichos hirsutus, Neustanthus chinensis, Pachyrhizus thunbergianus, Pueraria hirsuta, Pueraria lobata var. chinensis; Pueraria montana var. thomsonii, synonym Pueraria thomsonii; Pueraria candollei, synonym Pueraria mirifica; Pueraria tuberosa, synonym Hedysarum tuberosum.
Family: Fabaceae/Leguminosae.

People Use This For
Orally, kudzu is used for alcohol hangover, such as headache, upset stomach, dizziness, and vomiting, and for alcoholism and drunkenness. Kudzu is also used orally for menopause, myalgia, measles, dysentery, gastritis, fever, diarrhea, thirst, allergic rhinitis, cold, flu (influenza), neck stiffness, and as a diaphoretic. Other oral uses include for polio myelitis, encephalitis, hypertension, angina pectoris, arrhythmia, migraine, deafness, diabetes, traumatic injuries, sinusitis, urticaria, pruritus, and psoriasis.

Safety
POSSIBLY SAFE ...when used orally and appropriately. Kudzu appears to be safe for up to 4 months (10386,11386). The long-term safety of kudzu is unknown.
PREGNANCY AND LACTATION: Insufficient reliable information available; avoid using.

Effectiveness

INSUFFICIENT RELIABLE EVIDENCE to RATE

Alcoholism. Preliminary research suggests that heavy drinkers who take kudzu extract for 7 days consume less beer when given an opportunity to drink (13085). Kudzu does not seem to decrease the craving for alcohol (10386,13085). Kudzu extract also does not seem to improve sobriety in chronic alcoholics (10386).

Angina. Preliminary clinical research suggests oral and intravenous forms of the kudzu derivative, puerarin, might improve signs and symptoms of unstable angina. These products are not available in North America (13277,13279,13287).

Menopausal symptoms. Preliminary clinical research suggests kudzu taken orally does not affect menopausal changes. It doesn't significantly change lipid profiles, sex hormone levels, menopausal symptoms, or bone turnover markers. Kudzu may, however, have a positive effect on cognitive function in postmenopausal women (11386).

More evidence is needed to rate kudzu for these uses.

Mechanism of Action

The applicable parts of kudzu are the root, flower, and leaf. Kudzu contains isoflavone constituents including daidzin, daidzein, puerarin, genistin, and genistein (11711,13295).

Kudzu extracts or individual isoflavones such as daidzin consistently suppress voluntary alcohol intake in rodent models of alcoholism (1523,1524,13289,13290). Kudzu extract, daidzein, and daidzin decrease alcohol consumption and shorten alcohol-induced sleep in alcohol-craving animals. Preclinical research suggests kudzu causes later and lower peak blood alcohol levels, and a flattened dose response curve (13297). Kudzu might decrease peak blood alcohol levels due to delayed gastric emptying, exposing alcohol to a longer time for first-pass metabolism in the stomach (1523,1524). Slowed gastric emptying might prolong the effects of alcohol. Other research suggests kudzu might have antioxidant effects and speed up the metabolism of toxic alcohol metabolites (13294). Preliminary research suggests the kudzu constituent puerarin might lessen feelings of anxiety associated with alcohol withdrawal (13293).

Isoflavone constituents have both estrogenic and antiestrogenic activity, similar to selective estrogen receptor modulators (11386,13295). These phytoestrogens might have additive or synergistic effects with each other (13295).

Kudzu might also have effects on the cardiovascular system. Preliminary research suggests kudzu has a protective effect against myocardial ischemia (13282). Puerarin seems to reduce both systolic and diastolic blood pressure, and diminish myocardial oxygen consumption (13279). Puerarin also might have vasorelaxant properties, possibly by blocking beta-adrenergic receptors (13283). There is also some evidence that puerarin might decrease plasma renin and angiotensin II activity, and platelet aggregation (13278,13280,13291). The kudzu constituent daidzein might also have antiarrhythmic properties (13284).

Kudzu or its constituents might have hypoglycemic, hypocholesterolemic, and antioxidant activity (13285,13286,13288,13292). Kudzu also might have antipyretic effects, possibly through the effect of puerarin on serotonin receptors (13281,13282).

Preliminary research also suggests that kudzu and puerarin both inhibit and induce cytochrome P450 isoenzymes. However, it is unclear which CYP isoenzymes are affected and to what degree (13288).

Adverse Reactions

Orally, no side effects have been reported in clinical studies. There is one case report of allergic reaction following use of a combination herbal product containing kudzu (Kakkonto) involving a maculopapular eruption starting on the thighs and spreading over the entire body (13111).

Intravenously, the kudzu derivative, puerarin, has caused intravascular hemolysis (13298).

Interactions with Herbs & Other Dietary Supplements

HERBS & SUPPLEMENTS WITH HYPOGLYCEMIC POTENTIAL: Theoretically, kudzu might lower blood glucose levels (13285,13292), and have additive effects when used with other herbs and supplements that also lower glucose levels. This might increase the risk of hypoglycemia in some patients. Some herbs and supplements with hypoglycemic effects include alpha-lipoic acid, bitter melon, cassia cinnamon, chromium, devil's claw, fenugreek, garlic, guar gum, horse chestnut, Panax ginseng, psyllium, Siberian ginseng, and others.

HERBS WITH ANTICOAGULANT/ANTIPLATELET POTENTIAL: Theoretically, concomitant use of kudzu with herbs that might affect platelet aggregation might increase the risk of bleeding in some people (13278,13291). These herbs include angelica, clove, danshen, fenugreek, feverfew, garlic, ginger, ginkgo, Panax ginseng, poplar, red clover, turmeric, and others.

HERBS WITH ESTROGENIC ACTIVITY: Theoretically, kudzu might have additive or antagonistic effects with other herbs that have estrogenic activity (11386). These herbs include alfalfa, black cohosh, chasteberry, flaxseed, hops, ipriflavone, licorice, red clover, and soy.

Interactions with Drugs

ANTICOAGULANT/ANTIPLATELET DRUGS: Kudzu isoflavones are reported to have antiplatelet activity (13278,13291). Theoretically, kudzu might increase the risk of bleeding when used concomitantly with other drugs that have antiplatelet or anticoagulant effects. Antiplatelet agents include aspirin, clopidogrel (Plavix), dipyridamole (Persantine), ticlopidine (Ticlid), and others. Anticoagulant agents include heparin and warfarin (Coumadin).
ANTIDIABETES DRUGS: Kudzu might lower blood glucose levels and have additive effects in patients treated with antidiabetic agents (13285,13292). The dose of diabetes medications might need to be adjusted. Some antidiabetes drugs include glimepiride (Amaryl), glyburide (DiaBeta, Glynase PresTab, Micronase), insulin, metformin (Glucophage), pioglitazone (Actos), rosiglitazone (Avandia), and others.
CONTRACEPTIVE DRUGS: Theoretically, kudzu might competitively inhibit the effects of oral contraceptives (11386).
ESTROGENS: Theoretically, kudzu might competitively inhibit the effects of estrogen therapy (11386).
METHOTREXATE (Rheumatrex): Preclinical research suggests that kudzu extract greatly reduces the elimination and increases the toxicity of methotrexate. Kudzu might inhibit organic anion transporters (OATs) that are responsible for hepatobiliary and renal excretion of anions, similar to the interaction between methotrexate and NSAIDs (13296).
TAMOXIFEN (Nolvadex): Theoretically, kudzu might interfere with tamoxifen because of its potential estrogenic effects. Tell patients taking tamoxifen to avoid kudzu (11386).

Interactions with Foods

None known.

Interactions with Lab Tests

BLOOD GLUCOSE: Theoretically, kudzu might decrease blood glucose levels and test results. Constituents of kudzu have hypoglycemic activity in animals (13285,13292).
SERUM CHOLESTEROL: Theoretically, kudzu might decrease serum cholesterol levels and test results. Constituents of kudzu reduce serum cholesterol levels in animals (13285,13286).

Interactions with Diseases or Conditions

BLEEDING DISORDERS: Kudzu isoflavones are reported to have antiplatelet activity (13278,13291). Theoretically, kudzu might interfere with anticoagulant therapies.
CARDIOVASCULAR CONDITIONS: Theoretically, kudzu might interfere with cardiovascular treatments. Kudzu extracts have vasodilatory, hypotensive, and antiarrhythmic effects in animals (13280,13283,13284).
DIABETES: Theoretically, kudzu might interfere with blood glucose control requiring dosing adjustment of diabetes drug therapy. Kudzu constituents have hypoglycemic activity in animals (13285,13292).
HORMONE SENSITIVE CANCERS/CONDITIONS: Kudzu might have estrogenic effects (11386). Women with hormone sensitive conditions should avoid kudzu. Some of these conditions include breast cancer, uterine cancer, ovarian cancer, endometriosis, and uterine fibroids.

Dosage and Administration

ORAL: For alcoholism, kudzu root extract 1.2 grams twice daily has been used (10386). A specific kudzu extract (NPI-031, Natural Pharmacia Int.) in a dose of 500 mg three times daily has also been used. This extract is standardized to contain 19% puerarin, 4% daidzin, and 2% daidzein (13085). For menopausal symptoms, kudzu powder (containing 100 mg isoflavones) dissolved in water once daily has been used for 3 months (11386).

Comments

Kudzu was introduced in North America in 1876 in the southeastern US. It was initially used to prevent soil erosion. Kudzu spread quickly and overtook several farms and buildings. Some have referred to kudzu as "the vine that ate the South" (13085).

L-ARGININE

Also Known As

Arg, Arginine, Arginine HCl, Arginine Hydrochloride, L Arginine, L-Arginine HCl, L-Arginine-HCl, L-Arginine Hydrochloride.

Scientific Names

2-Amino-5-guanidinopentanoic acid.

People Use This For

Orally, L-arginine is used for cardiovascular conditions including congestive heart failure (CHF), angina pectoris, hypertension, and coronary artery disease. L-arginine is also used for intermittent claudication, senile dementia, erectile dysfunction, and male infertility. Furthermore, L-arginine is used for prevention of the common cold, interstitial cystitis, cyclosporine nephrotoxicity, pre-eclampsia, improving athletic performance, improving immune function, and preventing necrotizing enterocolitis in premature infants.

In combination with ibuprofen, L-arginine is used orally for migraine headaches, and as an adjunct to chemotherapy in breast cancer. In combination with hydroxymethylbutyrate (HMB) and glutamine, L-arginine is used orally for treating weight loss in people with AIDS. In the perioperative period, to reduce infections, improve wound healing, and shorten recovery time, L-arginine is used orally in combination with RNA and EPA.

Topically, L-arginine is used as an aid in wound healing, for treating cold hands and feet, and for male and female sexual dysfunction.

Intravenously, L-arginine is used for intermittent claudication, for detecting growth hormone deficiency, nutritional supplementation for the critically ill, metabolic acidosis, and persistent pulmonary hypertension in newborns.

Safety

LIKELY SAFE ...when used orally and appropriately. L-arginine is generally considered safe and has only been associated with minor side effects in clinical studies lasting a few days to six months (114,3330,3331,3460,3593,3595,3596,5531,5532,5533,6028,7813,7815,7816,7819,7822,8014,8473). ...when used intravenously and appropriately. Parenteral L-arginine is an FDA-approved prescription product (15).

There is insufficient reliable information available about the safety of the topical use of L-arginine.

CHILDREN: POSSIBLY SAFE ...when used orally in premature infants (8474).

PREGNANCY: POSSIBLY SAFE ...when used orally and appropriately, short-term. L-arginine 12 grams per day for 2 days has been used with apparent safety in women with gestational length of 28 to 36 weeks (11828). There is insufficient reliable information available about the safety of L-arginine for longer-term use in pregnant women.

LACTATION: Insufficient reliable information available; avoid using.

Effectiveness

POSSIBLY EFFECTIVE

AIDS-related wasting. Taking L-arginine orally, in combination with hydroxymethylbutyrate (HMB) and glutamine, seems to increase body weight, particularly lean body mass, and positively affect immune status when used for 8 weeks in patients with HIV/AIDS (1909).

Angina. Taking L-arginine orally seems to decrease symptoms and improve exercise tolerance and quality of life in patients with class II, III, and IV angina (3593,7815,7816). Some patients with class IV angina who have frequent attacks at rest despite treatment with standard antianginal agents might also benefit from L-arginine (3593). However, L-arginine does not seem to improve objective measures of blood vessel dilation or increase circulating concentrations of nitric oxide (7817).

Congestive heart failure (CHF). Taking L-arginine orally, in combination with conventional treatment, seems to improve glomerular filtration rate (GFR), creatinine clearance, and sodium and water elimination after saline loading (3596). However, improvements in exercise tolerance, quality of life, and peripheral vascular resistance are not consistently obtained (3595,6028,7813,8014). Tell patients that L-arginine should not be substituted for conventional treatment.

Erectile dysfunction (ED). Taking L-arginine orally in high doses, 5 grams daily, seems to improve subjective assessment of sexual function in men with organic ED (222). But taking lower doses might not be effective. L-arginine 500 mg 3 times daily in men with mixed-type impotence doesn't seem to be effective (2038). There is also some preliminary clinical evidence that adding pycnogenol 40 mg 3 times daily might improve the effectiveness of low-dose (1.7 grams/day) L-arginine for ED (10416).

Interstitial cystitis. Taking L-arginine orally seems to reduce symptoms, especially pain associated with interstitial cystitis (107,114,3460). Evidence suggests that patients with interstitial cystitis having a bladder capacity greater than 800 mL and/or a history of recurrent genitourinary infections might respond more favorably to L-arginine than patients with bladder capacity less than 800 mL and/or no history of recurrent genitourinary infections. Three months of treatment may be necessary before significant improvement occurs (3460).

Necrotizing enterocolitis (NEC). Taking L-arginine orally seems to be effective for preventing NEC in premature infants. L-arginine supplements added to formula may reduce the incidence of NEC by about 75% (8474).

Nitrate tolerance. Taking L-arginine orally 700 mg four times daily seems to prevent tolerance to transdermal nitrate, and theoretically to other nitrates, in patients with angina (8475).

Peripheral arterial disease. Using L-arginine intravenously or orally seems to improve symptoms of intermittent claudication associated with peripheral arterial disease (3465,7822).

Post-surgery recovery. Taking L-arginine enterally or orally, with RNA and eicosapentaenoic acid (EPA), seems to help reduce the recovery time after surgery or serious illness. Supplementing the diet of patients after surgery with RNA, L-arginine, and EPA appears to reduce the number of perioperative infections, improve wound healing, and shorten recovery time. Dietary supplementation may take place before surgery or in the postoperative period (5531,5532,5533,7819).

Renal transplant. Taking L-arginine orally seems to improve renal vasodilation and sodium excretion in renal transplant patients treated with cyclosporine (112).

POSSIBLY INEFFECTIVE

Pre-eclampsia. Taking L-arginine orally doesn't seem to lower diastolic blood pressure in women with pre-eclampsia at a gestational length of 28 to 36 weeks (11828).

LIKELY INEFFECTIVE

Coronary heart disease. Population studies indicate that intake of L-arginine does not reduce acute coronary events such as myocardial infarction or coronary heart disease-related mortality (3332,6896,7821,7822,10637).

INSUFFICIENT RELIABLE EVIDENCE to RATE

Dementia. Preliminary research suggests that L-arginine might improve senile dementia (8473).

Head and neck cancer. There is some interest in using L-arginine to enhance immune function in patients undergoing surgery for head and neck cancer. However, enteral nutrition supplemented with L-arginine does not seem to have any beneficial effects on markers of immune function such as interleukin-6 (IL-6) and tumor necrosis factor-alpha (TNF-alpha) (10160).

Hypertension. There is some preliminary evidence that oral administration of L-arginine can slightly reduce systolic and diastolic blood pressure in healthy people and mildly hypertensive patients with type 2 diabetes (7818,10636). It may also improve the effect of angiotensin converting enzyme (ACE) inhibitors in treating hypertension (7822).

Migraine headache. Taking L-arginine orally, in combination with ibuprofen, might be effective for treating migraine headache. Limited clinical research suggests the combination might reduce pain intensity within 30 minutes of administration. However, the contribution of L-arginine is unclear since ibuprofen alone relieves migraine pain in some patients (109).

Sickle cell disease. Preliminary research suggests that L-arginine, 0.1 grams per kg three times daily for five days, might be useful for patients with pulmonary hypertension in sickle cell disease (11428).

More evidence is needed to rate L-arginine for these uses.

Mechanism of Action

L-arginine is an amino acid necessary for protein synthesis. It is found naturally in foods such as red meat, poultry, fish, and dairy products (3330). L-arginine is best known for its effects on the vascular system. L-arginine is a substrate for the nitric oxide synthase (NOS) enzyme. NOS in vascular endothelial cells converts L-arginine to nitric oxide (NO), also known as endothelium-derived relaxation factor (EDRF), which causes vasodilation. L-arginine can improve coronary endothelial function and brachial artery endothelium-dependent dilation and reduce monocyte/endothelial cell adhesion in patients with coronary artery disease (CAD) or hypercholesterolemia, resulting in increased coronary blood flow (110,116,1362,1363,3330). The production of NO from L-arginine may be responsible for mildly reducing blood pressure (10636). Some evidence is available indicating the effect on coronary blood flow is larger in African-Americans than in Caucasians (8472). L-arginine seems to prevent nitrate tolerance by improving nitric acid bioavailability and may act as an antioxidant, decreasing production of vascular superoxide (8475). Intravenous L-arginine can have many beneficial hemodynamic effects in heart failure, including decreased heart rate (8 beats/minute), decreased mean arterial pressure (14 mmHg), increased cardiac output (0.7 l/minute), and increased stroke volume (14 mL) (8444). The production of NO from L-arginine substrate is impaired in patients with severe congestive heart failure (CHF) (8016). The beneficial effect of L-arginine on NO may help patients with pulmonary hypertension secondary to sickle cell disease. During times of sickle cell crisis, NO, a potent vasodilator, is deficient, and pulmonary hypertension may occur. L-arginine donates nitrogen for NO synthesis. L-arginine also decreases levels of circulating plasma endothelin-1, a potent vasoconstrictor (11428). In most people with a normal diet, the concentration of L-arginine inside the cells of the body is adequate to ensure that the NOS enzyme is producing NO at maximal capacity. As a result, L-arginine supplementation is likely to be more effective in patients who have a deficiency of L-arginine (7820,7822).

Besides its effect on the systemic cardiovascular system, NO also increases the relaxation of urinary tract smooth muscle (3259,3460) and is involved in erectile function. Although L-arginine appears to be helpful for erectile dysfunction, L-arginine may not affect the hemodynamics of the corpus cavernosum (222).

Nitric oxide might also be involved in host inflammatory and microbial killing responses (3460).

L-arginine is a precursor for collagen synthesis and together with fibroblast NO production might be important for wound healing (3259,3260).

L-arginine has actions on the cardiovascular system and other systems that are independent of the conversion to NO. Among other actions, L-arginine can directly reduce blood viscosity, reduce the activity of angiotensin converting enzyme, and reduce lipid peroxidation. Other physiologic actions include stimulating the release of growth hormone (GH), prolactin, glucagon, and insulin (7820). L-arginine also increases gastrin concentrations and inhibits tubular reabsorption of protein (3331,3460,8015).

There is interest in L-arginine for adjunctive use in treating breast cancer. There is some evidence that L-arginine modifies immune system function and might potentiate tumor cell response to anti-cancer drugs and possibly reduce the immunosuppressive effects of chemotherapy agents. L-arginine seems to increase lymphocyte reactivity to polyclonal mitogenic agents and might also enhance natural cytotoxicity (3331). However, L-arginine also promotes the growth of tumors by providing a source of nitrogen. In some situations the nutritional value of L-arginine may outweigh its antitumor effects (7814).

L-arginine has an oral bioavailability of 68% and an elimination half-life of approximately 80 minutes (108).

Adverse Reactions

Orally, L-arginine can cause abdominal pain and bloating, diarrhea, and gout (3331,3595). It can also cause allergic response or airway inflammation and exacerbation of airway inflammation in asthma (117,121).

Intravenous administration can cause allergic reactions including urticaria, periorbital edema, and pruritus (11830). Excessively rapid infusion of L-arginine has caused flushing, nausea and vomiting, local venous irritation, numbness, and headache. Extravasation has caused necrosis and superficial phlebitis (3330).

Interactions with Herbs & Other Dietary Supplements

XYLITOL: Concomitant use can reduce the glucagon response to L-arginine (15).

Interactions with Drugs

ANTIHYPERTENSIVE DRUGS: Theoretically, concomitant use might cause additive hypotensive effects; use with caution (7822,10636).

NITRATES: Theoretically, concomitant use might cause additive vasodilation and have a hypotensive effect; use with caution (7822,10636).

SILDENAFIL (Viagra): Theoretically, concurrent use of sildenafil and L-arginine might result in additive vasodilation and cause hypotension (7822,10636). However, this interaction has not been reported. Until more is known, use with caution or avoid using in combination.

Interactions with Foods

None known.

Interactions with Lab Tests

None known.

Interactions with Diseases or Conditions

ALLERGIC TENDENCIES/ASTHMA: L-arginine can cause an allergic response or aggravate airway inflammation (117), and inhaled L-arginine can amplify the inflammatory airway response in people with asthma (121); use with caution.

CIRRHOSIS OF THE LIVER: L-arginine-containing infusions can lead to a hyperdynamic circulatory state related to an elevation of the plasma level of nitrous oxide by L-arginine (122); use with caution.

HERPES VIRUS: Theoretically, L-arginine might exacerbate this condition. Preliminary evidence suggests that L-arginine may be necessary for viral replication (118,119).

HYPOTENSION: Theoretically, L-arginine might exacerbate hypotension (7822,10636).

Dosage and Administration

ORAL: For congestive heart failure, doses ranging from 6-20 grams per day, often as three divided doses, have been used in clinical studies (3595,3596,6028).

For angina pectoris associated with coronary artery disease, 3-6 grams three times per day has been used for up to one month (110,3593,7816,7817).

For preventing nitrate tolerance in angina patients, 700 mg four times daily has been used (8475).

For hypertension, hyperlipidemia, and congestive heart failure, L-arginine 6 grams daily has been given in combination with protein, vitamin C, vitamin E, folic acid, and other vitamins and minerals (7815,7822).

In patients with diabetes, to reduce low density lipoprotein (LDL) cholesterol, 7 grams 2 times a day for six weeks has been used (7821).

For interstitial cystitis, 500 mg-1.5 grams per day has been used (114,3330,3460).

For organic erectile dysfunction, 5 grams per day has been used (222). But taking lower doses might not be effective.

For senile dementia, 1.6 grams daily for three months has been used (8473).

For stimulation of host defenses in breast cancer patients undergoing chemotherapy, an oral dose of 10 grams three times per day for three days has been used (3331).

For preventing necrotizing enterocolitis in premature infants, 261 mg/kg has been added to oral feedings daily for the first 28 days of life (8474).

INTRAVENOUS: For intermittent claudication associated with peripheral arterial occlusive disease, 8 grams two times a day for three weeks has been used (3465).

Comments

Arginine butyrate has orphan drug status for beta-hemoglobinopathy, beta-thalassemia, and sickle cell disease (1691).

L-CARNITINE

Also Known As

B(t) Factor, Carnitine, Carnitor, D-Carnitine, DL-Carnitine, Levocarnitine, Vitacarn, Vitamin B(t).
CAUTION: See separate listings for Acetyl-L-Carnitine and Propionyl-L-Carnitine.

Scientific Names

3-carboxy-2-hydroxy-N,N,N-trimethyl-1-propanaminium inner salt; (3-carboxy2-hydroxypropyl) trimethylammonium hydroxide inner salt; B-hydroxy-N-trimethyl aminobutyric acid; beta-hydroxy-gamma-trimethylammonium butyrate; L-3-hydroxy-4-(trimethylammonium)-butyrate; (R)-(3-carboxy-2-hydroxypropyl) trimethylammonium hydroxide; (R)-3-hydroxy-4-trimethylammonio-butyrate; 3-hydroxy-4-N-trimethylaminobutyrate.

People Use This For

Orally, L-carnitine is used for treating primary L-carnitine deficiency, secondary L-carnitine deficiency due to inborn errors of metabolism, and L-carnitine deficiency in people requiring hemodialysis. It is also used orally for treating drug-induced L-carnitine deficiency and for treating valproate-induced toxicity. L-carnitine is also used orally for myopathies associated with zidovudine and isotretinoin, myocarditis associated with diphtheria, male infertility, Rett Syndrome, chronic stable angina pectoris, congestive heart failure (CHF), and myocardial infarction. It is also used orally as a supplement in low birthweight and preterm infants, in strict vegetarians or vegans, and in dieters.
L-carnitine is also used for anorexia, chronic fatigue syndrome, diabetes, hyperlipidemia, hyperthyroidism, attention deficit-hyperactivity disorder (ADHD), peripheral vascular disease and intermittent claudication, leg ulcers, and to enhance athletic performance and endurance.
Intravenously, L-carnitine is used to treat secondary L-carnitine deficiencies in people with inborn errors of metabolism who require hemodialysis; and to treat severe valproic acid-induced hepatotoxicity, especially in patients treated for overdose or accidental ingestion of valproic acid. It is also used intravenously for increasing CD4 cell counts in people with HIV/AIDS, acute myocardial infarction, and as a supplement in people receiving total parenteral nutrition.

Safety

LIKELY SAFE ...when used orally and appropriately (8047). ...when used parenterally as an FDA-approved prescription medicine. Avoid using D-carnitine and DL-carnitine, because they can act as competitive inhibitors of L-carnitine and cause symptoms of L-carnitine deficiency (1946).
PREGNANCY: Insufficient reliable information available; avoid using.
LACTATION: POSSIBLY SAFE ...when used orally. Supplemental doses of L-carnitine have been given to infants in breast milk and formula with no reported adverse effects. The effects of large doses used while nursing are unknown, but L-carnitine is secreted in the breast milk (3616).

Effectiveness

EFFECTIVE

End-stage renal disease (ESRD). Administering L-carnitine orally or intravenously can improve red blood cell count and hemoglobin during hemodialysis. However, it does not improve serum lipids or cholesterol (9790). Use of intravenous L-carnitine for prevention and treatment of L-carnitine deficiency in people with ESRD who are undergoing hemodialysis is an FDA-approved indication for L-carnitine.

L-carnitine deficiency. Administering L-carnitine orally or intravenously is effective for acute or chronic treatment of primary L-carnitine deficiency or secondary L-carnitine deficiency due to inborn errors of metabolism. This is an FDA-approved indication for L-carnitine (4949).

POSSIBLY EFFECTIVE

Angina. Taking L-carnitine orally seems to improve exercise tolerance in people with chronic stable angina (3623,3624).

Congestive heart failure (CHF). Taking L-carnitine orally seems to improve symptoms in people with congestive heart failure (3625,3626).

Hyperthyroidism. Taking 2-4 grams per day of L-carnitine seems to significantly improve symptoms associated with hyperthyroidism such as palpitations, nervousness, and asthenia. It also seems to reduce elevated serum levels of alanine aminotransferase (ALT), aspartate aminotransferase (AST), gamma-glutamyl transpeptidase (GGT), and ferritin elicited by thyroid hormone (8047).

Infertility. Taking L-carnitine orally, in combination with acetyl-L-carnitine for 6 months seems to increase sperm motility in men with infertility (12352). Some pregnancies occurred after taking these carnitines, but not enough to be statistically significant (12352). Taking L-carnitine orally, in combination with acetyl-L-carnitine and nonsteroidal anti-inflammatory drugs, seems to increase sperm count and motility in men with infertility caused by abacterial prostatovesiculoepididymitis; an inflammation of the prostate gland, seminal vesicles, and epididymis. L-carnitine supplementation should follow 2 months of treatment with nonsteroidal anti-inflammatory drugs (9791).

Low birth weight. Administering L-carnitine orally or intravenously seems to improve fat utilization in preterm infants on total parenteral nutrition (3633,3634,3635,3636,3637).

Myocardial infarction (MI). Taking L-carnitine orally after MI seems to reduce complications and mortality (3627,3628,3629).

Myocarditis. Taking L-carnitine orally seems to reduce the morbidity and mortality of myocarditis associated with diphtheria (3620,3621).

Valproic acid-induced toxicities. There is evidence that patients taking valproic acid orally or intravenously, who have neurologic or hepatic deterioration or hyperammonemia, seem to have improved neurologic and hepatic function and plasma ammonia levels within normal limits when L-carnitine is supplemented (1438,1914,1915,1916,1917,4523,5798,5799). Valproic acid toxicities are often associated with L-carnitine deficiency. There is also some evidence that intravenous L-carnitine can prevent the development of severe valproic acid-induced hepatotoxicity when given to patients being treated for overdose and accidental ingestion of valproic acid (1438,4528,5798,5799), especially if treatment is initiated early (4528).

LIKELY INEFFECTIVE

Athletic performance. Taking L-carnitine orally doesn't enhance athletic performance or endurance (1947,3639). Maximal exercise in trained athletes has been associated with a fall in plasma L-carnitine levels (3648). Although increases in maximum oxygen uptake and power output have been reported with L-carnitine supplements in some studies (3649,3650), there is no evidence that L-carnitine supplementation will improve exercise performance in individuals including trained athletes (1947,3639).

INSUFFICIENT RELIABLE EVIDENCE to RATE

Attention deficit-hyperactivity disorder (ADHD). Preliminary clinical research suggests L-carnitine might reduce ADHD symptoms (9956).

Peripheral vascular disease. Preliminary evidence suggests that L-carnitine may improve walking distances in people with peripheral vascular disease (3631).

Rett syndrome. Preliminary clinical research suggests that L-carnitine might improve well-being and motor skills in girls with Rett syndrome (1433,3622).

More evidence is needed to rate L-carnitine for these uses.

Mechanism of Action

L-carnitine is naturally found in the body. Endogenous carnitines exist as a "carnitine pool" consisting of L-carnitine, acetyl-L-carnitine, propionyl-L-carnitine, and several other acyl-carnitine esters. Intracellular enzymes and cell membrane transporters can rapidly interconvert the carnitines to the needed form and transport them between the tissues and extracellular space. The body obtains some carnitine from the diet, primarily from red meats and dairy products. The body can also synthesize carnitines from the amino acids, lysine and methionine. The kidney aids in keeping carnitine levels stable. Normally, greater than 90% of filtered carnitine is reabsorbed. If dietary intake of carnitines decreases, carnitine reabsorption becomes even more efficient (12744). Most L-carnitine in the body is found in cardiac and skeletal muscle. The highest concentration of L-carnitine is in the epididymal fluid (12352).

L-carnitine plays a key role in cellular energy production. It is essential for beta-oxidation of long-chain fatty acids in the mitochondria. To enter the mitochondria, fatty acids must bind to coenzyme A, forming fatty acyl-CoA. Long-chain fatty acyl-CoA molecules are too large to cross the internal mitochondrial membrane and rely on enzymatic transportation that requires L-carnitine. In the mitochondria, fatty acids undergo beta-oxidation to adenosine triphosphate (ATP) and L-acetyl-carnitine is excreted to begin a new transport cycle (12352).

L-carnitine may have antioxidant properties (12352). However, some preliminary research suggests that acetyl-L-carnitine might lessen oxidative stress and prevent oxidative damage in the brain better than L-carnitine (12688).

Primary tissue deficiency of L-carnitine can arise from hepatic synthesis failure, membrane transport failure, or disorders of reabsorption by the kidney. It is characterized by low concentrations of L-carnitine in plasma, red blood cells and tissues (3616). L-carnitine deficiency can also occur due to other disorders, such as inborn errors of metabolism, cirrhosis, and hypopituitarism. Carnitine deficiency most often presents with symptoms of progressive cardiomyopathy and skeletal muscle weakness, and less frequently with fasting hypoglycemic coma (12748).

Muscle L-carnitine deficiency has been reported in children with Duchenne muscular dystrophy (3640), and in people with myopathies due to zidovudine (3618) or isotretinoin (3619). Increased urinary losses of L-carnitine have been reported with ifosfamide and cisplatin therapy (3641,3642). Low serum L-carnitine levels can occur in patients taking valproic acid therapy (1910,1911,1912,1913,4526,4528), in pregnant women (3643), in people with chronic fatigue syndrome (3630), HIV/AIDS (3617), and in patients with hyperthyroidism (8047). However, the relationship between serum and tissue L-carnitine levels is not fully understood, and it is not known whether or not low serum levels necessarily lead to symptomatic deficiency (4528,4529,5798).

Symptomatic deficiency is unlikely to arise from insufficient dietary intake since the body is usually able to synthesize adequate quantities. However, preterm neonates have a reduced capacity to synthesize L-carnitine and they may become deficient, especially if receiving total parenteral nutrition without L-carnitine supplements (3633). Breast milk and some formulas contain L-carnitine; those that do not, generally do not induce symptomatic deficiencies in healthy full-term infants unless a metabolic disorder is also present, although utilization of fats may be impaired (3644).

Hemodialysis is associated with significant losses of L-carnitine (3616,3645); which may contribute to malaise, muscle weakness, cardiomyopathy, and cardiac arrhythmias (3616). L-carnitine supplements, usually given intravenously after dialysis may improve exercise performance, reduce muscle cramps and hypotension, improve erythrocyte survival time, and decrease dose requirements for erythropoietin used to treat anemia (3645,3646,3647).

In people with angina, a reduction in tissue L-carnitine levels has been observed during myocardial ischemia. L-carnitine can be decreased by as much as 50% in failing myocardium (8048). Preliminary studies have reported that daily infusions of L-carnitine may improve CD4 cell counts in people with HIV infection and reduce the percentage of CD4 and CD8 cells undergoing apoptosis. There is some evidence L-carnitine inhibits the enzyme activity of acidic sphingomyelinase and prevents sphingomyelin breakdown in these cells (798,3632,8049).

Carnitine levels are lower in people with complications of diabetes (12746). Preliminary studies also suggest that intravenous infusions of L-carnitine may produce short-term improvements in insulin sensitivity in people with type 2 diabetes (3651,3652). Additionally, preliminary clinical research suggests that L-carnitine might also improve glucose utilization, possibly by increasing expression of glycolytic and gluconeogenic enzymes (12754).

In hyperthyroidism, L-carnitine seems to reduce symptoms by blocking entry of thyroid hormone into the nucleus of hepatocytes, neurons, and fibroblasts (8047).

L-carnitine and acetyl-L-carnitine are present in human sperm and seminal fluid (3607). Their levels increase in sperm during the maturation process in the epididymis and coincide with the acquisition of progressive motility (3608,3609). An increase in sperm motility is seen in vitro when L-carnitine or acetyl-L-carnitine is added to the semen sample (3612).

In patients with alcohol-induced cirrhosis, serum levels of L-carnitine and its esters are sometimes increased, possibly due to increased L-carnitine biosynthesis (1931,1948).

Adverse Reactions

L-carnitine used orally or intravenously has been associated with nausea, vomiting, abdominal cramps, heartburn, gastritis, diarrhea, body odor, and seizures (3616). One of its metabolites can cause the urine, breath, and sweat to have a fishy odor (12756).

DL-carnitine, but not L-carnitine, has been associated with myasthenia syndrome with severe weakness, muscle wasting, and discolored urine possibly due to myoglobinuria. This may be due to competitive inhibition of L-carnitine by D-carnitine, leading to symptoms of L-carnitine deficiency (1946).

Interactions with Herbs & Other Dietary Supplements

D-CARNITINE: D-carnitine might compete with L-carnitine in active transport systems. Taking D-carnitine might cause symptoms of L-carnitine deficiency (1946,12760); avoid using.

Interactions with Drugs

ACENOCOUMAROL (Sintrom): Taking L-carnitine 1 gram/day seems to significantly increase the anticoagulant effects of acenocoumarol. This drug is an oral anticoagulant similar to warfarin, but shorter-acting (9878,12165). In one case, INR was stable in the normal range of 1.99-2.94 and then increased to 4.65 after L-carnitine was started and continued for 10 weeks. INR normalized after discontinuation of L-carnitine (12165).

WARFARIN (Coumadin): Taking L-carnitine 1 gram/day seems to potentiate acenocoumarol, a shorter acting anticoagulant drug similar to warfarin (9878,12165). There isn't enough information to know whether this interaction occurs with L-carnitine and warfarin.

ZIDOVUDINE (AZT, Retrovir): Zidovudine appears to inhibit cellular transport of L-carnitine (9885). Low serum carnitine levels are found in some people with HIV infection (3617). Consider zidovudine supplementation as the clinical situation warrants.

Drug Influences on Nutrient Levels and Depletion

SOME DRUGS CAN AFFECT L-CARNITINE LEVELS:

CARBAMAZEPINE (Tegretol): Carbamazepine can reduce carnitine levels. Whether this reduction is clinically important is unknown. The reduction in carnitine levels might be more significant when other factors are present that also lower carnitine levels such as other drugs that deplete carnitine, vegetarianism, or diabetes (1911,12758).

CEFDITOREN PIVOXIL (Spectracef): Taking cefditoren chronically can induce carnitine deficiency because of its pivalate content. Using cefditoren short-term is unlikely to have any clinically significant effect on carnitine (12759).

PHENOBARBITAL (Luminal): Phenobarbital can reduce carnitine levels. Whether this reduction is clinically important is unknown. The reduction in carnitine levels might be more significant when other factors are present that also lower carnitine levels such as other drugs that deplete carnitine, vegetarianism, or diabetes (1911,12758).

PHENYTOIN (Dilantin): Phenytoin can reduce carnitine levels. Whether this reduction is clinically important is unknown. The reduction in carnitine levels might be more significant when other factors are present that also lower carnitine levels such as other drugs that deplete carnitine, vegetarianism, or diabetes (1911,12758).

PIVAMPICILLIN (Pondocillin): Taking pivampicillin chronically can induce carnitine deficiency because of its pivalate content. Using pivampicillin short-term is unlikely to have any clinically significant effect on carnitine (12759).

VALPROIC ACID (VPA, valproate, Depakene, Depakote): Valproic acid can induce L-carnitine deficiency by altering carnitine metabolism and synthesis (4528,4529,5798). However, carnitine blood levels seem to be more dependent on nutritional status than valproic acid concentration. L-carnitine supplementation is not necessary for patients who have adequate nutritional intake (9612).

Interactions with Foods

None known.

Interactions with Lab Tests

CD4/CD8 COUNTS: L-carnitine infusions can increase CD4 and CD8 lymphocyte counts in some individuals with HIV-1 infection who have not been treated with antiretroviral therapy (798,8049).
HIGH-DENSITY LIPOPROTEIN (HDL) CHOLESTEROL: Intravenous L-carnitine supplementation can increase serum HDL cholesterol concentrations and test results in children on hemodialysis with type IV hyperlipoproteinemia (275).
TRIGLYCERIDES: Intravenous L-carnitine supplementation can decrease serum triglyceride concentrations and test results in children on hemodialysis with type IV hyperlipoproteinemia (275).

Interactions with Diseases or Conditions

HEMODIALYSIS/ANURIA/UREMIA: Avoid DL-carnitine; it is reported to cause myasthenia-like symptoms when administered by IV after dialysis (L-carnitine has not been reported to have this effect) (1946).
HYPOTHYROIDISM: Avoid using L-carnitine in patients with hypothyroidism. L-carnitine seems to inhibit the activity of thyroid hormone in target tissues (12761).
SEIZURES: An increase in seizure frequency or severity has been reported in people with a history of seizures who have used L-carnitine orally or intravenously (3616).

Dosage and Administration

ORAL: For primary or secondary L-carnitine deficiencies in adults, 990 mg two to three times per day in tablets or as an oral solution is used (3616). For valproate-induced toxicities often associated with L-carnitine deficiency, 50 to 100 mg/kg/day in three or four divided doses, to a maximum of 3 grams/day is used (3616,4528,5798). For chronic stable angina and congestive heart failure (CHF), 1 gram twice daily has been used (3623,3624,3625,3626). Following myocardial infarction, 2 to 6 grams daily have been used (3627,3628,3629). For peripheral vascular disease, a dose of 2 grams of L-carnitine twice daily has been used (3631). People on hemodialysis have used 2 to 4 grams per day in divided doses (1933). For Rett syndrome, 100 mg/kg/day L-carnitine in three divided doses has been used (1433). For myocarditis associated with diphtheria, DL-carnitine 100 mg/kg/day for 4 days has been used (3620,3621). For hyperthyroidism, 1-2 grams twice daily has been used (8047). For male infertility, 2 grams of L-carnitine plus 1 gram of L-acetyl-carnitine daily has been used (12352). For male infertility secondary to abacterial prostatovesiculoepididymitis, carnitine 1 gram plus acetyl-L-carnitine 500 mg every 12 hours has been used following 2 months of treatment with nonsteroidal anti-inflammatory drugs (9791).
INTRAVENOUS: For inborn error of metabolism resulting in secondary L-carnitine deficiency, 50 mg/kg given as a slow (2 to 3 minute) bolus injection or by infusion followed by 50 mg/kg administered in divided doses every 3 to 4 hours over the next 24 hours is used. Subsequent daily maintenance doses are usually in the range of 50 mg/kg (3616). For people with L-carnitine deficiency secondary to hemodialysis, 10 to 20 mg/kg adjusted according to plasma L-carnitine levels is used (3616). For treating and preventing valproic acid-induced hepatotoxicity in patients being treated for accidental ingestion or overdose of valproic acid, 150-500 mg/kg/day up to 3 grams/day is used (4528,5798). A dose of 10 mg/kg has been used to improve fat utilization in premature infants on total parenteral nutrition (3637).

Comments

The body can convert L-carnitine to acetyl-L-carnitine and propionyl-L-carnitine. But, no one knows whether the benefits of carnitines are interchangeable. For now, tell patients not to substitute one form of carnitine for another (12744).

L-TRYPTOPHAN

Also Known As

L-trypt, Tryptophan.
CAUTION: See separate listing for 5-HTP.

Scientific Names

L-2-amino-3-(indole-3-yl) propionic acid.

People Use This For

Orally, L-tryptophan is used for insomnia, depression, myofascial pain, premenstrual syndrome (PMS), smoking cessation, bruxism, grinding teeth during sleep, attention deficit-hyperactivity disorder (ADHD), Tourette's syndrome, and to improve athletic performance.

Safety

LIKELY UNSAFE ...when used orally. L-tryptophan has been linked to eosinophilia-myalgia syndrome (EMS) and death (7067,8053,10085,11474,11478). In 1990, L-tryptophan was recalled from the market due to these safety concerns (7067). However, under the Dietary Supplement Health and Education Act (DHSEA) of 1994 it is currently available and marketed as a dietary supplement.
PREGNANCY: UNSAFE ...when used orally because it can cause respiratory depression in utero (1142); avoid using.
LACTATION: Insufficient reliable information available; avoid using.

Effectiveness

POSSIBLY EFFECTIVE

Premenstrual dysphoric disorder (PMDD). Taking L-tryptophan orally 6 grams per day seems to decrease mood swings, tension, and irritability in women with PMDD (6246).
Smoking cessation. Taking L-tryptophan orally seems to help as adjunct treatment for smoking cessation (1138).

POSSIBLY INEFFECTIVE

Athletic performance. Taking L-tryptophan orally doesn't seem to improve athletic performance (1135).
Bruxism. Taking L-tryptophan orally doesn't seem help treat bruxism (1139).
Myofascial pain. Taking L-tryptophan orally doesn't seem to reduce myofascial pain (1140,1145).

INSUFFICIENT RELIABLE EVIDENCE to RATE

Attention deficit-hyperactivity disorder (ADHD). Preliminary clinical research suggests L-tryptophan levels are lower in children with ADHD, but oral L-tryptophan supplements don't appear to help ADHD symptoms (9948,9952).
Depression. Some preliminary clinical research suggests that L-tryptophan might improve the effectiveness of conventional antidepressants (6245,10856).
Seasonal affective disorder (SAD). Preliminary clinical evidence suggests L-tryptophan might be helpful in SAD (6247).
Sleep apnea. There is preliminary evidence that taking L-tryptophan orally might improve sleep in patients with obstructive sleep apnea. It does not appear to be beneficial in patients with central sleep apnea (1144,1146).
More evidence is needed to rate L-tryptophan for these uses.

Mechanism of Action

L-tryptophan is an essential amino acid present in concentrations of 1-2% in many plant and animal proteins (5). The body absorbs tryptophan from dietary protein sources, converts it to 5-hyrdoxytryptophan (5-HTP), then to serotonin (5-hydroxytryptamine). Both L-tryptophan and 5-HTP can penetrate the blood-brain barrier (10853,10857). L-tryptophan has sedative effects (1143).
Tryptophan depletion can cause a relapse in treated depression and precipitate depressive symptoms in patients with a history or family history of depression, as well as in healthy volunteers (10854,10855).
Additionally, dietary tryptophan depletion has been associated with bulimia relapse (1133) and deterioration of schizophrenia symptoms (1134), but it does not seem to worsen symptoms in people with untreated depression (1136).

Adverse Reactions

Orally, L-tryptophan can cause gastrointestinal (GI) side effects such as heartburn, stomach pain, belching and flatulence, nausea, vomiting, diarrhea, headache, lightheadedness, dry mouth, visual blurring, ataxia, drowsiness, and anorexia (10853).
In 1989, more than 1500 cases of eosinophilia-myalgia syndrome (EMS) and 37 deaths were associated with L-tryptophan use in the US. About 95% of all EMS cases were traced to L-tryptophan produced by a single manufacturer in Japan. In 1990, L-tryptophan was recalled in the U.S. and an FDA alert was put into force limiting the importation of all over-the-counter L-tryptophan products (7067,11477,11478). After the limitation of L-tryptophan products, the incidence of EMS dropped abruptly (11474). Under the Dietary Supplement Health and Education Act (DHSEA) of 1994 L-tryptophan is currently available and marketed as a dietary supplement.
Symptoms of EMS associated with L-tryptophan use include intense eosinophilia; fatigue; incapacitating myalgia; neuropathy; sclerodermiform skin changes; alopecia; rash; and inflammatory disorders affecting the joints, connective tissue, lungs, heart, and liver (8053,11477). Symptoms tend to improve over time, however some individuals may still experience symptoms up to 2 years after the onset of EMS and complete resolution of symptoms may not occur (8053,10287). There is some evidence suggesting that daily use of a multivitamin or B-complex vitamin supplement prior to the onset of EMS may have decreased the severity of symptoms in some cases (8052). The exact cause of EMS in patients taking L-tryptophan is unknown, but some evidence suggests it may be due to contaminated L-tryptophan products (8050,8051,11477,11478). Some experts disagree with the hypothesis that contaminated L-tryptophan products are the cause of EMS. These experts suggest the true cause of EMS has not yet been identified (11475,11476). There are 5 contaminants that have been associated with EMS after taking L-tryptophan, but other causal factors cannot be ruled out (8054,10288,10289). There are also cases of EMS following L-tryptophan use that have not been linked to apparent contamination. There is also some evidence of an association between L-tryptophan-related EMS and the occurrence of chronic B-cell lymphocytic leukemia (8055).

Interactions with Herbs & Other Dietary Supplements

HERBS AND SUPPLEMENTS WITH SEDATIVE PROPERTIES: L-tryptophan can cause drowsiness and sedation (1143). Theoretically, concomitant use with herbs that have sedative properties might enhance therapeutic and adverse effects. Some of these supplements include 5-HTP, calamus, California poppy, catnip, hops, Jamaican dogwood, kava, St. John's wort, scullcap, valerian, yerba mansa, and others.
HERBS AND SUPPLEMENTS WITH SEROTONERGIC PROPERTIES: Theoretically, L-tryptophan might increase the effects and adverse effects of products that increase serotonin levels, including 5-hydroxytryptophan, Hawaiian baby woodrose, S-adenosylmethionine (SAMe), and St. John's wort (1141).

Interactions with Drugs

ANTIDEPRESSANT DRUGS: Combining serotonergic antidepressants with L-tryptophan might increase the risk of serotonergic side effects including serotonin syndrome, and cerebral vasoconstrictive disorders such as Call-Fleming syndrome (1141,8056). These drugs include the selective serotonin reuptake inhibitors (SSRIs) such as fluoxetine (Prozac), paroxetine (Paxil), sertraline (Zoloft), and others; and tricyclic and atypical antidepressants such as amitriptyline (Elavil), clomipramine (Anafranil), imipramine (Tofranil), and others.
BENZODIAZEPINES: Concomitant use of L-tryptophan with benzodiazepines can cause sexual disinhibition, reversible dyskinesias, and reversible Parkinsonian-like rigidity (9). Benzodiazepines include clonazepam (Klonopin), diazepam (Valium), lorazepam (Ativan), and others.
CNS DEPRESSANTS: Theoretically, concomitant use with medications that cause sedation may have additive effects when taken with medications that cause sedation such as clonazepam (Klonopin), lorazepam (Ativan), phenobarbital (Donnatal), zolpidem (Ambien), and others. L-tryptophan can cause fatigue and drowsiness (1143).
DEXTROMETHORPHAN (Robitussin DM, others): Theoretically, concurrent use might cause additive serotonergic effects and increase the risk of serotonin syndrome (1141). Also, concurrent use might theoretically cause cerebral vasoconstriction disorders such as Call-Fleming syndrome (8056).
MEPERIDINE (Demerol): Theoretically, concurrent use with meperidine might cause additive serotonergic effects, and increase the risk of serotonin syndrome (1141). Also, concurrent use might theoretically cause cerebral vasoconstriction disorders such as Call-Fleming syndrome (8056).
MONOAMINE OXIDASE INHIBITORS (MAOIs): Combining serotonergic drugs such as MAOIs with L-tryptophan might increase the risk of serotonergic side effects including serotonin syndrome and cerebral vasoconstrictive disorders such as Call-Fleming syndrome (8056).
PENTAZOCINE (Talwin): Theoretically, concurrent use with pentazocine might cause additive serotonergic effects and increase the risk of serotonin syndrome (1141). Also, concurrent use might theoretically cause cerebral vasoconstriction disorders such as Call-Fleming syndrome (8056).
PHENOTHIAZINES: Concomitant use of L-tryptophan with phenothiazines can cause sexual disinhibition, reversible dyskinesias, and reversible Parkinsonian-like rigidity (9). Phenothiazines include chlorpromazine (Thorazine), prochlorperazine (Compazine), and others.
TRAMADOL (Ultram): Theoretically, concurrent with use tramadol might cause additive serotonergic effects and increase the risk of serotonin syndrome (1141). Also, concurrent use might theoretically cause cerebral vasoconstriction disorders such as Call-Fleming syndrome (8056).

Interactions with Foods

None known.

Interactions with Lab Tests

EOSINOPHIL COUNT: In cases of eosinophilia myalgia syndrome, L-tryptophan can increase serum eosinophil counts and test results (8053).
LIVER FUNCTION TESTS: In cases of eosinophilia myalgia syndrome, L-tryptophan can increase serum liver enzyme levels and test results (8053).

Interactions with Diseases or Conditions

EOSINOPHILIA: Theoretically, L-tryptophan may exacerbate this condition. L-tryptophan use has been associated with the development of eosinophilia-myalgia syndrome (EMS) (7067).
KIDNEY OR LIVER DYSFUNCTION: Theoretically, L-tryptophan may exacerbate these conditions since its use has been associated with the development of eosinophilia-myalgia syndrome (EMS) (7067).

Dosage and Administration

ORAL: Clinical studies for sleep disorders have used doses from 1 to 2.5 grams (1144,1146).
For depression, 300 mg daily in combination with antidepressants has been used (6245).
For premenstrual syndrome, 6 grams daily was used in one study (6246).
High dose L-tryptophan (50 mg/kg/day) has been used as adjunct therapy for smoking cessation (1138).

Comments

L-tryptophan is not available as a dietary supplement in the US. It is unclear whether supplement manufacturers are able to produce contaminant-free, pure L-tryptophan products (7067). L-tryptophan in the United States is limited for use under medical supervision in special dietary products such as infant formulas, enteral products, and approved parenteral drug products (7067). Older people may require lower amounts (9).

LABDANUM

Also Known As

Ambreine, Ciste, Cyste, Rockrose.

Scientific Names

Cistus ladanifer, synonym Cistus ladaniferus; Cistus creticus, synonyms Cistus incanus, Cistus villosus; Cistus polymorphus; and other Cistus species.
Family: Cistaceae.

People Use This For

Orally, labdanum is used for inflammation of the respiratory tract mucous membrane, bronchitis, diarrhea, edema, hernia, tumors, leprosy, and spleen sclerosis. Labdanum is also used orally for its expectorant, stimulant, purgative, and cleansing properties.
Topically, labdanum is used for its astringent and hemostatic properties.
In foods and beverages, the absolute, oleoresin, and oil are used as flavoring agents.
In cosmetics, labdanum absolute and oil are used as fixative and fragrance components.
In addition, people use labdanum as a fumigant and insecticide.

Safety

LIKELY SAFE ...when used orally in amounts commonly found in foods. Labdanum has Generally Recognized As Safe status (GRAS) for use in foods in the US (4912).
POSSIBLY SAFE ...when used topically for medicinal purposes. It is nontoxic and nonirritating to human skin (11). There is insufficient reliable information available about the safety of labdanum for its other uses.
PREGNANCY AND LACTATION: Insufficient reliable information available; avoid using.

Effectiveness

There is insufficient reliable information available about the effectiveness of labdanum.

Mechanism of Action

The applicable parts of labdanum are the above ground parts. Beta-pinene, eugenol, eucalyptol (cineole), and benzaldehyde are thought to be the most active constituents of labdanum (11). Some evidence suggests the essential oil of labdanum and resin might have antibacterial and antifungal activity (11). Other evidence indicates an aqueous extract of Cistus incanus might protect against gastric lesions (4050). One study in experimental animals found that a non-alkaloid substance extracted by alcohol but not water caused liver changes (11), which might indicate some safety risks.

Adverse Reactions

None reported.

Interactions with Herbs & Other Dietary Supplements

None known.

Interactions with Drugs

None known.

Interactions with Foods

None known.

Interactions with Lab Tests

None known.

Interactions with Diseases or Conditions

None known.

Dosage and Administration

No typical dosage.

Comments

Labdanum oleoresin (gum, gum cistus) is obtained by boiling the above ground parts of labdanum (Cistus ladanifer) in water and separating the resin layer (11). Labdanum oil is distilled from the above ground parts of labdanum (Cistus ladanifer). Labdanum absolute (cyste absolute) is obtained by evaporation of the alcohol extract of fat soluble portions of labdanum (Cistus ladanifer) after removal of alcohol insoluble substances (11).

LABRADOR TEA

Also Known As

Continental Tea, St. James' Tea.
CAUTION: See separate listing for Marsh Tea.

Scientific Names

Rhododendron groenlandicum, synonyms Ledum groenlandicum, Ledum latifolium.
Family: Ericaceae.

People Use This For

Orally, labrador tea is used as an expectorant, abortifacient, for "female disorders", sore throats, coughs, pulmonary infections and other chest ailments, dysentery, diarrhea, kidney problems, rheumatism, headache, and cancer.
Topically or in a bath, labrador tea is used for skin problems.
As a beverage, labrador tea is used as beverage or to make beer more intoxicating by adding leaves.

Safety

POSSIBLY SAFE ...when the leaves or flowering shoots are used orally as weak tea or in small amounts (6).
LIKELY UNSAFE ...when used orally in concentrated solutions or in large amounts. It can cause delirium, paralysis, and death (6).
PREGNANCY: UNSAFE ...when used orally because it might induce abortion (18).
LACTATION: Insufficient reliable information available; avoid using.

Effectiveness

There is insufficient reliable information available about the effectiveness of labrador tea.

Mechanism of Action

The applicable parts of labrador tea are the leaf and flowering shoots. Labrador tea has expectorant activity (18) and narcotic properties (6). The constituent ledol (ledum camphor) can cause gastrointestinal (GI) irritation (vomiting, gastroenteritis, diarrhea) and central nervous system (CNS) excitation, spasms, and paralysis (18). The constituent grayanotoxin (andromedotoxin), can cause bradycardia, hypotension, loss of coordination, convulsions, paralysis, and death (6).

Adverse Reactions

Orally, labrador tea can cause gastrointestinal irritation (vomiting, gastroenteritis, diarrhea); and central nervous system excitation, spasms, paralysis, and death (6,18).

Interactions with Herbs & Other Dietary Supplements

None known.

Interactions with Drugs

None known.

Interactions with Foods

None known.

Interactions with Lab Tests

None known.

Interactions with Diseases or Conditions

None known.

Dosage and Administration

No typical dosage.

Comments

Medicinal uses of labrador tea are now largely obsolete (18).

LABURNUM

Also Known As
Bean Trifoil, Golden Chain, Legume, Pea Tree.

Scientific Names
Laburnum anagyroides, synonyms Cytisus laburnum, Cytisus alschingeri.
Family: Fabaceae/Leguminosae.

People Use This For
Orally, laburnum is used as an emetic and purgative.
In manufacturing, laburnum is used as a pesticide.

Safety
UNSAFE ...when used orally (18).
PREGNANCY AND LACTATION: UNSAFE ...when used orally (18).

Effectiveness
There is insufficient reliable information available about the effectiveness of laburnum.

Mechanism of Action
The applicable part of laburnum is the seed. There is insufficient reliable information available about the possible mechanism of action and active ingredients.

Adverse Reactions
Orally, the fatal adult dose of laburnum is 20 seeds or 3-4 unripe berries. Symptoms of laburnum poisoning include nausea, dizziness, salivation, and pain in the mouth, throat and stomach. This is accompanied by sweating, headaches, and extended, severe, and occasionally bloody vomiting. The centrally-stimulating effects of laburnum lead to tonic-clonic spasms followed by paralysis. Some patients experience anuria or uremia. Death occurs by asphyxiation (18).

Interactions with Herbs & Other Dietary Supplements
None known.

Interactions with Drugs
None known.

Interactions with Foods
None known.

Interactions with Lab Tests
None known.

Interactions with Diseases or Conditions
None known.

Dosage and Administration
No typical dosage.

Comments
Laburnum is spelled very similarly to labdanum, but they are very different plants. The similar spelling could cause confusion.

LACTASE

Also Known As
None.

Scientific Names
Beta-galactosidase.

People Use This For
Orally, lactase is used for preventing symptoms of lactose intolerance, of which symptoms include cramps, diarrhea, and gas.

Safety
LIKELY SAFE ...when used orally and appropriately. There is an absence of adverse effects up to 9,900 IU of lactase (2371,2372,2373). It is an FDA-approved, nonprescription product available in the US.
PREGNANCY AND LACTATION: Insufficient reliable information available; avoid using.

Effectiveness
LIKELY EFFECTIVE

Lactose intolerance. Taking lactase orally is effective for reducing GI symptoms in lactose-intolerant people when used before the consumption of lactose or when added to milk prior to consumption (2371,2372,2373).

Mechanism of Action
Lactase is a sugar-splitting enzyme that hydrolyzes lactose, a milk sugar, to produce glucose and galactose (9,511).

Adverse Reactions
None reported.

Interactions with Herbs & Other Dietary Supplements
None known.

Interactions with Drugs
None known.

Interactions with Foods
None known.

Interactions with Lab Tests
None known.

Interactions with Diseases or Conditions
None known.

Dosage and Administration
ORAL: The typical dose of lactase is 6000-9000 IU tablets chewed and swallowed at the start of a lactose-containing meal (2374) or 2000 IU of the solution added to 500 mL of milk immediately before consumption (2375).

Comments
Lactase deficiency can be one of several factors that predispose an individual to the development of osteoporosis, possibly through diminished calcium intake (2376,2377).

LACTOBACILLUS

Also Known As
Acidophilus, L. acidophilus, L. amylovorus, L. brevis, L. bulgaricus, L. casei, L. crispatus, L. delbrueckii, L. fermentum, L. gallinarum, L. johnsonii, L. johnsonii LC-1, L. plantarum, L. reuteri, L. salivarius, L. sporogenes, LC-1, Lacto Bacillus, Lactobacilli, Lactobacillus GG, Lactobacillus rhamnosus GG, Probiotics.
CAUTION: See separate listings for Bifidobacteria, Saccharomyces boulardii, and Yogurt.

Scientific Names
Lactobacillus acidophilus; Lactobacillus amylovorus; Lactobacillus brevis; Lactobacillus bulgaricus; Lactobacillus casei; Lactobacillus casei sp. rhamnosus; Lactobacillus crispatus; Lactobacillus delbrueckii; Lactobacillus fermentum; Lactobacillus gallinarum; Lactobacillus johnsonii; Lactobacillus plantarum; Lactobacillus reuteri; Lactobacillus rhamnosus; Lactobacillus salivarius; Lactobacillus sporogenes.
Family: Lactobacillaceae.

People Use This For

Orally, lactobacillus is used for treating and preventing diarrhea, including infectious types such as rotaviral diarrhea in children and traveler's diarrhea. It is used orally to prevent and treat antibiotic-associated diarrhea. It is used to prevent respiratory infections in children attending day-care centers. Lactobacillus is also used orally for general digestion problems, irritable bowel syndrome (IBS), inflammatory bowel syndrome (IBD, Crohn's disease, ulcerative colitis), relapsing Clostridium difficile colitis, bacterial overgrowth in short bowel syndrome, and Helicobacter pylori infection. It is also used orally for lactose intolerance, urinary tract infections, vaginal and Candida-related (yeast) infections, high cholesterol levels, hives, fever blisters, canker sores, and adolescent acne. Lactobacillus is used to treat and prevent atopic allergy in infants. It is also used orally to prevent cancer or the formation of carcinogens, to stimulate the immune system, and as a vaccine adjuvant.

Intravaginally, lactobacillus is used to treat vaginitis and urinary tract infections.

Safety

LIKELY SAFE ...when used orally and appropriately. Several species of lactobacillus, including Lactobacillus acidophilus, Lactobacillus bulgaricus, Lactobacillus casei, Lactobacillus delbrueckii, Lactobacillus rhamnosus, and Lactobacillus plantarum have been safely used in studies lasting up to nine months (4367,4380,6087,12108).

POSSIBLY SAFE ...when used intravaginally and appropriately. Several species of lactobacillus including Lactobacillus casei sp. rhamnosus and Lactobacillus fermentum have been used safely in studies lasting from ten weeks to six months (4397,6094,6095,12108).

CHILDREN: LIKELY SAFE ...when used orally and appropriately. Lactobacillus GG, a specific strain of Lactobacillus rhamnosus, has been used safely in studies lasting from seven days to 15 months (4369,4372,4373,4377,7741,8565,8566,8567,8568). Lactobacillus reuteri has been used safely for up to five days (7751,8566,8567). Lactobacillus sporogenes has been used safely in newborn infants for 12 months (7742,8515). The safety of other Lactobacillus species in children is not known.

PREGNANCY: POSSIBLY SAFE ...when used orally and appropriately. Lactobacillus GG, a specific strain of Lactobacillus rhamnosus, has been used with apparent safety during pregnancy starting 2 to 4 weeks before delivery (7743,8515). The safety of other Lactobacillus species in pregnant women is not known.

LACTATION: POSSIBLY SAFE ...when used orally and appropriately. Lactobacillus GG, a specific strain of Lactobacillus rhamnosus, has been used with apparent safety in lactating women for up to six months (7743,8515). The safety of other Lactobacillus species in lactating women is not known.

Effectiveness

LIKELY EFFECTIVE

Rotaviral diarrhea. Lactobacillus GG, a specific strain of Lactobacillus rhamnosus, can reduce the duration of the diarrheal phase of rotavirus infection by 1-3 days in infants and young children (4369,4377). Lactobacillus reuteri also seems to reduce the duration of acute diarrhea (mostly rotavirus) in hospitalized infants and young children (7751). Lactobacillus casei also seems to shorten the course of acute diarrhea in infants and young children (1253). For babies and children ages 6 to 36 months, a daily dose of 10 billion live, freeze-dried Lactobacillus reuteri reduces the duration of diarrhea (7753). A combination of Lactobacillus rhamnosus and Lactobacillus reuteri seems to reduce the diarrhea phase of rotaviral infection in hospitalized babies and children ages 6 to 36 months by 20% and also seems to reduce the duration of rotavirus excretion. Combination treatment seems to be similarly effective to single-strain Lactobacillus treatments. In patients with diarrhea for less than 60 hours before the start of treatment (early intervention), probiotic treatment can reduce hospital stay by 48% (8567). The combination of Lactobacillus rhamnosus and Lactobacillus reuteri also seems to reduce the duration of diarrhea in babies and children ages 9 to 44 months attending day-care centers. Early intervention reduces recovery time by about 43% (8566). Overall, Lactobacillus seems to reduce the duration of diarrhea by 0.7 days and diarrheal stools by 1.6 stools on day 2 of treatment (8568). Effectiveness appears to be dose dependent, at least 10 billion colony-forming units during the first 48 hours should be used.

POSSIBLY EFFECTIVE

Antibiotic-associated diarrhea. Concurrent oral treatment with Lactobacillus GG, a specific strain of Lactobacillus rhamnosus, and antibiotics significantly decreases stool frequency and improves stool consistency compared to treatment with antibiotics alone in children (4371,8511). Lactobacillus GG seems to reduce the rate of antibiotic-associated diarrhea by approximately 11% (4372). However, Lactobacillus GG does not seem to reduce the occurrence of antibiotic-associated diarrhea in hospitalized adults (7306).

Atopic dermatitis (eczema). There is some evidence that taking Lactobacillus GG orally can reduce symptoms of atopic eczema in infants allergic to cow's milk (4369). A combination of lyophilized Lactobacillus rhamnosus and Lactobacillus reuteri seems to reduce atopic dermatitis symptoms in children ages 1 to 13 years. The treatment seems to be more effective in allergic patients with a positive skin prick test response and increased IgE levels (12773). Lactobacillus seems to decrease markers of hypersensitivity reactions and intestinal inflammation, such as tumor necrosis factor (TNF), and alpha 1-antitrypsin (4369,11383). Lactobacilli also seem to stimulate the production of transforming growth factor-beta (TGF-beta), which protects against allergy (7743).

Atopic disease. Lactobacillus GG taken orally two to four weeks before delivery and continued for the first three to six months of breast-feeding seems to prevent atopic allergies (asthma, allergic rhinitis, and eczema) in infants with a family history of atopy. It appears to be equally effective when taken by the breast-feeding woman or by the bottle-feeding infant (7743,8515,11381). This preventive effect of lactobacillus in at-risk infants appears to extend up to 4 years of age (11381).

Chronic pouchitis. Continuous oral treatment for one year with a specific concentrated formulation of Lactobacillus, Bifidobacterium, and Streptococcus (VSL#3) can maintain remission in 85% of patients (6087,12769).

Clostridium difficile diarrhea. Patients treated with metronidazole and vancomycin for Clostridium difficile diarrhea have a 20% chance for developing a secondary or recurring Clostridium difficile infection when antibiotic therapy is stopped. Taking Lactobacillus GG, a specific strain of Lactobacillus rhamnosus, orally during conventional antibiotic therapy seems to reduce the recurrence rate of Clostridium difficile diarrhea after antibiotics are stopped; and also seems to improve some symptoms of an active Clostridium difficile infection, including cramping and diarrhea (4392,4394). Preliminary evidence suggests another strain, Lactobacillus plantarum 299v, may also prevent recurrent episodes of Clostridium difficile diarrhea (11378).

Diarrhea. Lactobacillus GG given prophylactically on hospital admission seems to reduce the risk of non-rotaviral diarrhea and nosocomial rotavirus gastroenteritis in infants and children ages 1 to 36 months (7741). Lactobacillus GG, a specific strain of Lactobacillus rhamnosus, can significantly reduce the occurrence of diarrhea from all causes in undernourished children (4373). Lactobacillus sporogenes seems to reduce the incidence and duration of diarrhea in newborns in rural areas of developing countries (7742).

Helicobacter pylori (H pylori). Taking Lactobacillus johnsonii or gasseri seems to reduce inflammation and gastritis associated with Helicobacter infection (12764,12765). Lactobacillus species, alone or in combination with bifidobacteria, and the probiotic yeast Saccharomyces boulardii seem to be equivalent for reducing the adverse effects of Helicobacter therapy, but none seem to improve compliance (12763). Most research suggests that Lactobacillus doesn't help eradicate Helicobacter pylori (12764,12766); however, results are conflicting (8562).

Respiratory infections. Children ages 1 to 6 years who attend day-care centers seem to get fewer and less severe respiratory infections when given milk with Lactobacillus GG. Children receiving milk with lactobacilli also seem to have fewer days of illness-related absence (8565).

Travelers' diarrhea. Taking Lactobacillus GG orally seems to reduce the occurrence of diarrhea in travelers (4374,10216). The effectiveness of Lactobacillus GG can vary significantly based upon the destination of travel. Destinations in the same country can have different results, probably because of differences in bacteria and other microorganisms at different locations (10216).

POSSIBLY INEFFECTIVE

Intestinal bacterial overgrowth. Lactobacillus fermentum 100 to 300 billion cells given orally twice daily for two weeks doesn't seem to improve symptoms such as abdominal pain and bloating, or stool frequency in adults with overgrowth of intestinal bacteria such as Klebsiella, Bacteroides, Escherichia coli, Enterococcus, or Proteus mirabilis. It also doesn't lower breath hydrogen concentration, a measure of intestinal bacterial overgrowth (8514).

Lactose intolerance. Consuming Lactobacillus acidophilus milk seems to produce the same symptoms of intolerance as regular cow's milk in people with lactose intolerance (123).

Vulvovaginitis. A combination of Lactobacillus rhamnosus plus Bifidobacterium longum (Lactobac) given orally or a combination of Lactobacillus rhamnosus, Lactobacillus delbruekii, Lactobacillus acidophilus, and Streptococcus thermophilus (Femilac) given vaginally doesn't seem to reduce the chance of vaginal candidiasis infection following use of antibiotics (12108).

INSUFFICIENT RELIABLE EVIDENCE to RATE

Bacterial vaginosis. Preliminary clinical evidence suggests that eating yogurt enriched with lactobacillus acidophilus daily may slightly decrease the incidence of bacterial vaginosis. However, it does not appear to reduce candidal vaginitis (1245).

Crohn's disease. Lactobacillus GG doesn't seem to prevent recurrence of Crohn's disease after surgery (12767). However, preliminary clinical research suggests a combination of four Lactobacillus species plus other probiotics might help (12768).

Irritable bowel syndrome (IBS). There is contradictory evidence about the effectiveness of lactobacillus for IBS. Heat-killed Lactobacillus acidophilus given in capsule form or as a Lactobacillus plantarum beverage seems to improve abdominal pain, bloating, number and quality of stools, and general physical state (7744,10419). A specific lactobacillus combination probiotic containing viable lyophilized bacteria species including lactobacillus, bifidobacteria, and streptococcus (VSL#3) also appears to improve IBS symptoms (11379). However, other research suggests that taking Lactobacillus GG or Lactobacillus plantarum doesn't help IBS symptoms (12770,12771). Consuming Lactobacillus salivarius one billion cells daily in a malted milk drink for 8 weeks also does not seem to reduce the symptoms of IBS (13054).

The placebo response rate in patients with IBS may be as high as 50% with benefits persisting for 3 months (12772).

Substitution of Lactobacillus acidophilus milk for regular cow's milk seems to have no effect on symptoms of IBS (123).

Urinary tract infections (UTIs). There is some preliminary evidence that intravaginal use of some Lactobacillus species might be helpful for preventing UTIs, but there have been some conflicting findings in studies (4581,6094,6095).

More evidence is needed to rate lactobacillus for these uses.

Mechanism of Action

Lactobacillus refers to a group of lactic acid producing, gram-positive rods that are obligate and facultative anaerobes (7755,7760). The name lactobacillus refers to the ability bacterium's ability to produce lactic acid, not to the ability to digest lactose (12762). Most are non-spore-forming with the exception of Lactobacillus sporogenes (8563). Lactobacilli are symbiotic and make up some of the 400 normal flora in the human gastrointestinal and genitourinary tracts (6089,6094,6096,7754,7755). They are also found in some fermented food products such as yogurt as well as in capsule form (6099). Some of the specific lactobacillus species include Lactobacillus acidophilus, Lactobacillus bulgaricus, Lactobacillus casei sp. rhamnosus, Lactobacillus delbrueckii, Lactobacillus fermentum, Lactobacillus plantarum, Lactobacillus reuteri, Lactobacillus rhamnosus, and Lactobacillus sporogenes. Of these, Lactobacillus reuteri is the most commonly occurring species in the gastrointestinal tract. It is also found in breast milk (7751,7755). Lactobacilli are used therapeutically as probiotics, the opposite of antibiotics. They are considered "friendly" bacteria and are taken for the purpose of re-colonizing areas of the body where they normally would occur. The human body relies on the normal flora for several functions including metabolizing foods and certain drugs, absorbing nutrients, and preventing colonization by pathogenic bacteria. Lactobacilli seem to provide nutritional benefits including inducing growth factors and increasing the bioavailability of minerals (7754). Lactobacilli also stabilize the mucosal barrier and decrease intestinal permeability (7751,7755). Probiotics such as lactobacillus are typically used in cases when a disease occurs or might occur due to depleted normal flora. For example, treatment with antibiotics can kill off pathogenic bacteria and also the normal flora of the gastrointestinal and genitourinary tracts. Altering the normal flora allows for potential colonization by pathogenic organisms (6088), which can result in side effects such as diarrhea, cramping, and less commonly pseudomembranous colitis caused by Clostridium difficile.

The theory is that taking lactobacillus probiotics during antibiotic treatment can prevent or minimize normal flora depletion and pathogenic bacteria colonization. There is some evidence to support this theory (5500,11382). When taken orally, lactobacilli pass through the gut and attach to the intestinal mucosa where they can persist for at least one week (5500). When probiotic lactobacilli latch on to and colonize the intestinal and urogenital mucosa, it seems to prevent epithelial attachment by pathogenic bacteria (4369,4378,6086,6089,6091,6092). Lactobacilli seem to have this effect by increasing epithelial mucus production and competing with pathogens for mucosal binding sites, possibly through steric hindrance (4388,6086,6089,6091,6092,7755,8562). Lactobacilli also inhibit bacterial pathogens by producing lactic acid, and many lactobacilli also produce hydrogen peroxide (6089,6090,6096). Hydrogen-peroxide producing lactobacilli are bacteriocidal to the vaginal pathogen Gardnerella vaginalis, and their presence in the vagina has been associated with decreased frequencies of bacterial vaginosis and trichomoniasis (7745). In the vagina, lactic acid from lactobacilli lowers vaginal pH, which can prevent pathogen growth. Lactobacilli might also produce substances called bacteriocins that can inhibit growth of some bacteria and fungi, and biosurfactants that can prevent some bacteria from adhering to the epithelium (6089,6090,6091,6096,8514). Lactobacilli might also inhibit the translocation of bacteria across the intestinal mucosa by strengthening the epithelial barrier and by promoting accelerated epithelial repair (8516). Some researchers think lactobacilli and other probiotics might have immunomodulating effects (4368,4369,8512). Lactobacilli seem to modulate non-specific cellular and humoral immunity possibly by stimulating lymphocyte and macrophage activity (6089,8565) and modulating cytokine production by mononuclear cells (4379,8512).

They also appear to enhance synthesis of antibodies in response to microbial pathogens, particularly secretory immunoglobulin A (7754). However, the way lactobacilli affect immune function may differ depending on the health status of the patient. In people with an immune system hypersensitivity, lactobacilli seem to down-regulate immune function. In healthy people without an immune system hypersensitivity, lactobacilli seem to stimulate the immune system (4399). In healthy children attending day-care centers, lactobacilli seem to have an immunostimulatory effect (8565). Due to these immunomodulating effects, some researchers think lactobacillus and other probiotics might not only fight intestinal and urogenital pathogens, but might also be helpful for conditions such as inflammatory bowel disease, pouchitis, food allergy, and for use as an adjuvant to vaccination (4368,4379,4393,4399).

Clinical research suggests that Lactobacillus rhamnosus taken orally might enhance natural immunity in healthy adults. It appears to increase the phagocytic activity in polymorphonuclear cells and monocytes, and enhance natural killer cell tumor killing activity (7756,7757). Orally administered lactobacillus brevis seems to increase the production of interferon-alpha (7758). Whether lactobacilli administration can increase resistance to disease is unknown. Some preliminary research suggests that lactobacilli and other probiotics might inhibit pathogens such as Candida albicans and prolong survival in immune deficiency states (7746). Other preliminary research suggests that Lactobacillus reuteri might prevent infection with Cryptosporidium parvum in immunodeficient patients. Lactobacillus reuteri is known to secrete reuterin, which has activity against Salmonella, Listeria, Clostridium, and Escherichia species and other pathogens (7749,7755). Fermentation of milk products with lactobacilli might increase the content of vitamins such as folic acid, niacin, riboflavin, thiamine, pyridoxine, and cyanocobalamin (8564). There is also some preliminary evidence that lactobacilli and other probiotics might help protect against cancer. In animal models, lactobacillus has been shown to bind dietary carcinogens (4376) and decrease development of tumors in the colon after carcinogen challenge (4382,4387,8564). Preliminary research also suggests that lactobacilli, especially Lactobacillus plantarum, can reduce the severity of chemotherapy-induced enterocolitis. There is also some preliminary research that suggests the ability of lactobacilli to reduce adherence of pathogenic bacteria to the colonic mucosa, and to reduce bacterial translocation, which might make it useful in the treatment of conditions such as Crohn's disease (7747,7750,7754). Additional preliminary evidence suggests lactobacillus GG milk products might be useful as a vehicle for antibodies against human cariogenic bacteria (11380). Other preliminary research suggests that Lactobacillus bulgaricus and Lactobacillus sporogenes might have hypolipidemic and antiatherosclerotic effects. Limited clinical evidence suggests that it can reduce total and low-density lipoprotein (LDL) cholesterol with no effect on high-density lipoprotein (HDL) (7759,8563). Fermented dairy products, such as yogurt and acidophilus milk also seem to have a beneficial effect on cholesterol. Lactobacilli and other probiotic bacteria seem to bind bile acids to cholesterol, resulting in increased bile acid-cholesterol excretion. They also seem to increase fatty acid production in the intestine, which decreases circulatory fatty acid concentrations either by inhibiting hepatic cholesterol synthesis or redistributing cholesterol from the plasma to the liver. To be clinically useful, fermented dairy products would likely have to be taken daily (8559).

Most researchers agree that the effectiveness of lactobacilli and other probiotics for all indications depends on their ability to colonize an area of tissue. To do this, lactobacillus preparations must contain live and viable organisms. Products stored for long periods of time or stored improperly may contain few live and active organisms.

For oral preparations, bacteria must also remain viable after passing through the gut and then they must be able to latch on to the intestinal epithelium. Lactobacilli strains might vary in their effectiveness due to differences in their ability to adhere to the epithelial cells (4373,6091,6094). Some strains might also have differing activity against specific pathogens (6094). Host factors such as hormone levels can also influence adherence and effectiveness. The ability of lactobacilli to attach to epithelial cells can change during a woman's menstrual cycle in response to changing hormone levels. In post-menopausal women, correcting low estrogen levels can help restore lactobacillus colonization without supplementation (6089,6094). There is some evidence that Lactobacillus GG, a strain of Lactobacillus rhamnosus, attaches to intestinal epithelial cells better than Lactobacillus acidophilus (4373). Lactobacillus casei may adhere better to urogenital cells than other lactobacillus species (6091). Lactobacilli, even strains of the same species, might not act similarly at the same site. Lactobacillus rhamnosus GR-1 seems to have anti-yeast and antiviral effects in the vagina that persist for at least 14 days after vaginal administration, while the effects of Lactobacillus rhamnosus GG diminish quickly (8560). Probiotic strains may also differ in specific metabolic activities, and not all lactobacilli species inhibit a wide range of pathogenic bacteria (6093). Therefore, some researchers theorize that probiotic preparations containing several species might offer more benefit than a single species (6087,6094). However, this theory has not yet been evaluated in studies.

Adverse Reactions

Orally, lactobacillus species are usually well-tolerated (6087,8565,8566,8567,8568). The most common side effect is flatulence; however; it is usually mild and subsides as therapy continues.

Since lactobacillus preparations contain live and active microorganisms, there is some concern that they might cause pathological infection in some patients. Lactobacillus bacteremia and sepsis has been reported in severely ill and/or immunocompromised patients (4380,8561,13008). Fatal Lactobacillus rhamnosus septicemia has been reported in an immunocompromised patient consuming yogurt and taking prolonged courses of multiple broad spectrum antibiotics (8561). There is a case report of lactobacillus sepsis in a severely ill 6-week-old infant following use of Lactobacillus rhamnosus GG (Culturelle) for antibiotic-associated diarrhea. There is also a report of Lactobacillus sepsis in a 6-year-old child with cerebral palsy following use of lactobacillus rhamnosus GG (Culturelle) for intermittent diarrhea (13008). In another case, an 11-month old infant with short bowel syndrome developed bacteremia after receiving Lactobacillus rhamnosus for 5-weeks through a gastrostomy tube for rotaviral diarrhea (13070).

Although there are a few cases of pathogenic lactobacillus infection in ill or immunocompromised patients, this is a very rare finding. The risks are considered negligible. There are no reports of pathogenic colonization in relatively healthy patients with intact immune systems (4380,4389,4390,4391,4393,4398).

Adults infected with HIV have taken 10 billion live Lactobacillus reuteri orally daily for 21 days without safety or tolerance problems (7752).

Intravaginally, Lactobacillus species are usually well tolerated (6094).

Interactions with Herbs & Other Dietary Supplements

None known.

Interactions with Drugs

ANTIBIOTIC DRUGS: There is some concern that concomitant administration of antibiotics might decrease the effectiveness of lactobacillus. Since lactobacillus preparations usually contain live and active organisms, simultaneously taking antibiotics might kill a significant number of the organisms (1740). Tell patients to separate administration of antibiotics and lactobacillus preparations by at least two hours.

IMMUNOSUPPRESSANTS: Theoretically, lactobacillus could cause infection in patients taking medications that suppress the immune system. These include cyclosporine (Neoral, Sandimmune), tacrolimus (Prograf), azathioprine (Imuran), and cancer chemotherapeutic agents like cyclophosphamide (Cytoxan) and cisplatin (Platinol-AQ) (4380,4391,4393,4398).

Interactions with Foods

None known.

Interactions with Lab Tests

None known.

Interactions with Diseases or Conditions

IMMUNODEFICIENCY: There is some concern that lactobacillus preparations might cause pathogenic colonization, especially in patients who are immunocompromised. Although lactobacilli have caused bacteremia and other pathogenic infections, it rarely occurs. Pathogenic colonization is more likely to occur in severely immunocompromised patients (4380,4391,4393,4398). Adults infected with HIV have taken 10 billion live Lactobacillus reuteri orally daily for 21 days without safety or tolerance problems (7752). The risk of longer-term treatment or in very severely compromised patients is unknown.

SHORT BOWEL SYNDROME: Patients with short bowel syndrome might be predisposed to pathogenic infection from lactobacillus. There is a case of bactermia in an 11-month old infant with short bowel syndrome who developed bacteremia after receiving Lactobacillus rhamnosus for 5-weeks thought a gastrostomy tube for rotaviral diarrhea (13070). This might be due to impaired gut integrity in patients with short-bowel syndrome. Use lactobacillus with caution in patients with this condition.

Dosage and Administration

ORAL: The strength of lactobacillus preparations is usually quantified by the number of living organisms per capsule. Typical doses usually range from 1 to 10 billion viable organisms taken daily in 3-4 divided doses (6002). For children with diarrhea, 5-10 billion live Lactobacillus GG in a rehydrating solution has been used (4369,4370). For babies and children with diarrhea, 10 to 100 billion live Lactobacillus reuteri daily for up to 5 days has been used (7751,7753). Lower doses may not be effective (7753). Also, combination of Lactobacillus rhamnosus and Lactobacillus reuteri, 10 billion live cells of each strain, has been used twice daily for 5 days for babies and children with diarrhea (8567). For preventing antibiotic-associated diarrhea in children, 20 billion live Lactobacillus GG daily was used throughout the conventional antimicrobial treatment period (4372). For preventing diarrhea in hospitalized infants and children ages 1 to 36 months, 6 billion live Lactobacillus GG has been used twice daily (7741). For preventing and shortening the duration of diarrhea in newborns within the first year of life in rural areas of developing countries, 100 million live Lactobacillus sporogenes have been given daily for one year (7742). For preventing respiratory infections in children attending day-care centers, milk with 500,000 to 1 million colony-forming units of Lactobacillus GG per ml has been used; average milk consumption was 260 ml (8565). For recurrent Clostridium difficile, 1.25 billion live Lactobacillus GG in two divided doses for 2 weeks has been used (4394). For milk hypersensitivity, 2600 million Lactobacillus GG daily has been used (4399). For preventing atopic allergies in infants with a family history of atopy, 20 billion live Lactobacillus GG daily has been given to pregnant women for 2 to 4 weeks prior to delivery, and then for the first 3 to 6 months to the breast-feeding women or bottle-feeding infants (7743,8515). For chronic pouchitis, 3 grams twice daily of a specific concentrated formula containing 300 billion viable bacteria per gram of several strains of Lactobacillus, Bifidobacterium, and Streptococcus has been used (6087). For preventing traveler's diarrhea Lactobacillus GG, 2 billion organisms daily, has been used (10216). For treating irritable bowel syndrome (IBS), 10 billion heat-killed Lactobacillus acidophilus given orally twice daily in capsule form, 450 billion viable lyophilized Lactobacillus (VSL#3) powder divided twice daily in capsule form, or 20 billion colony-forming units of Lactobacillus plantarum given daily as a beverage have been used for 4 to 6 weeks (7744,10419,11379).

INTRAVAGINAL: For bacterial vaginitis, vaginal suppositories containing 1 billion live Lactobacillus GG twice daily for 7 days has been used (4397). For reducing the risk of recurrent urinary tract infection's (UTI's), lactobacillus suppositories containing 0.5 gram (1.6 billion organisms) of L. casei var rhamnosus and L. fermentum has been used twice weekly for two weeks, then once a month for two months (6095). A vaginal solution containing 100 billion viable bacteria/mL in a dose of 1 mL twice weekly has also been used (6094).

Comments

Some products labeled to contain Lactobacillus acidophilus have been found to actually contain little or no Lactobacillus acidophilus. Products may also contain other strains of lactobacillus, including Lactobacillus bulgaricus. Some products have been found to also contain contaminants, including Enterococcus faecium, Clostridium sporogenes, and Pseudomonas species. Lactobacilli, when prepared properly, seem to be stable in pharmaceutical preparations. Various strains of Lactobacillus remain viable after freeze-drying and 1-year of storage when anaerobic conditions are maintained (7745,7755). Cultivation at a pH of 5 seems in improve survival of Lactobacillus reuteri when subjected to freeze-drying (7748). Lactobacillus products are used as functional foods (7755).

Lactobacillus rhamnosus GG gets its name from the scientists, Gorbach and Goldin, who isolated it from human intestinal flora (12762).

LACTOFERRIN

Also Known As

Bovine Lactoferrin, Human Lactoferrin, Lactoferrins, Recombinant Human Lactoferrin.
CAUTION: See separate listings for Bovine Colostrum, Whey Protein

Scientific Names

Lactoferrin.

People Use This For

Orally, lactoferrin is used for treating peptic ulcer disease (PUD) and Helicobacter pylori infection, diarrhea, and hepatitis C. It is also used as an antioxidant, antibacterial, and antiviral agent. Other uses include stimulating the immune system, preventing tissue damage related to aging, promoting healthy intestinal flora, preventing cancer, and regulating iron metabolism.

In industrial agriculture, lactoferrin is used as an antibacterial in meat processing.

Safety

LIKELY SAFE ...when used orally in amounts commonly found in foods. Lactoferrin has Generally Regarded As Safe (GRAS) status in the US (13312).

POSSIBLY SAFE ...when used orally in medicinal amounts. Bovine lactoferrin has been safely used for up to 12 months (13313,13314,13315,13316,13320,13321,13322,13323). Recombinant human lactoferrin has been safely used for up to 14 days (13317,13318,13319).

PREGNANCY AND LACTATION: LIKELY SAFE ...when used orally in amounts commonly found in foods. Lactoferrin has Generally Regarded as Safe (GRAS) status in the US (13312). There is insufficient reliable information available about the safety of lactoferrin when used medicinally during pregnancy or lactation; avoid using.

Effectiveness

POSSIBLY EFFECTIVE

Hepatitis C. Some patients with hepatitis C seem to respond to oral bovine lactoferrin. Lactoferrin seems to decrease serum levels of hepatitic C virus RNA and alanine aminotransferase (ALT) levels (13320,13321). Lactoferrin doses of 1.8 or 3.6 grams/day appear to be necessary for efficacy (13323,13324). Lower doses don't seem to have any effect (13313,13314).

INSUFFICIENT RELIABLE EVIDENCE to RATE

Helicobacter pylori (H pylori). There is conflicting clinical research about the effectiveness of adding bovine lactoferrin to standard 3-drug Helicobacter pylori eradication regimens. Some studies suggest lactoferrin improves efficacy when added to a rabeprazole (AcipHex), clarithromycin (Biaxin), and tinidazole (Tindamax) regimen (13316,13332). However, other research that used lactoferrin with esomeprazole (Nexium), clarithromycin, and amoxicillin found no difference in Helicobacter pylori eradication rates. It is possible that lactoferrin activity on the bacterial cell wall interferes with the cell wall activity of amoxicillin (13315). Monotherapy with human recombinant lactoferrin, even at high doses (5 g/day), doesn't suppress or eradicate H. pylori infection (13317). More evidence is needed to rate lactoferrin for this use.

Mechanism of Action

Lactoferrin is an iron-binding glycoprotein in the transferrin family that is in human and bovine milk. Lactoferrin is the major whey protein in human milk. Human colostrum (the first postpartum milk produced) contains high levels of lactoferrin, up to 7 mg/mL. Mature milk has a lactoferrin content of about 1 mg/mL. Lactoferrin is produced by exocrine glands and is found in high concentrations in mucosal secretions including those of the eye, nose, throat, respiratory tract, and vagina. It is also in seminal fluid, saliva, and intestinal mucus. Lactoferrin is also produced and stored in some neutrophil granules. It is released during neutrophil activation and degranulation in sites of infection or inflammation (13324,13327,13328,13329,13330).

In the stomach, lactoferrin is metabolized to lactoferricin (13328). Some research suggests that lactoferrin supplements are completely degraded before reaching the colon and that lactoferrin in the colon is likely from endogenous production (13318).

Lactoferrin has many physiological functions in the body. It helps regulate intestinal iron absorption, promotes intestinal cell growth, and protects against microbial infection. Lactoferrin also seems to be involved with regulation of bone marrow function (myelopoiesis) and systemic immune responses (13330). It also seems to have antioxidant properties (13318).

Lactoferrin has antibacterial activity through several mechanisms. It exerts a bacteriostatic effect by sequestering iron, which is essential for bacterial growth. Lactoferrin also has bacteriocidal effects by binding to bacterial cell surfaces and causing cell lysis. It may also inhibit the adhesion and invasion of bacteria in host cells.

Other preliminary research suggests a peptide in lactoferrin (LF-33) can neutralize bacterial endotoxin.

Lactoferrin also might inhibit bacterial aggregation and biofilm development of Pseudomonas aeruginosa and Streptococcus mutans (13327,13327,13333). Some evidence suggests that lactoferrin has activity against Helicobacter pylori (13316,13317,13332,13336).

In vitro, lactoferricin B, a peptide derived from lactoferrin, has antibacterial activity against a wide range of gram positive and gram negative bacteria (2491). The lactoferrin constituent, lactoferricin, has activity against Escherichia coli, Helicobacter pylori, and staphylococcus aureus. Bovine lactoferricin appears to be more active that human, mouse, or goat lactoferricin (13328).

Lactoferrin appears to confer antibacterial defense to breast-fed neonates (13324,13325). Lactoferrin is in amniotic fluid and greatly increases with intrauterine infection (13326). Lactoferrin has antiviral activity against herpes simplex virus (HSV) 1 and 2, cytomegalovirus, human immunodeficiency virus (HIV), human papillomavirus, hepatitis B virus, hepatitis C virus, respiratory syncytial virus, hantavirus, rotavirus, poliovirus, adenovirus and enterovirus 71 (13324,13327,13334,13335,13340). Lactoferrin, which is normally present in tiny amounts in serum, appears to be lower in patients with HIV infection (13341).

Lactoferrin also appears to have antifungal activity. Preliminary research suggests that it is active against Candida and Trichophyton species (13327).

Lactoferrin also plays a role in immune system function. Its production is upregulated in response to inflammatory stimuli. It seems to bind with epithelial cells at the site of infection and inhibits inflammatory cytokine production (13330,13339). Preliminary evidence suggests that lactoferrin supplementation might increase the phagocytic activity of polymorphonuclear leukocytes and the proportion of natural killer cells in the host defense system (2490).

Preliminary research suggests the small intestines have lactoferrin receptors. Binding of lactoferrin to its receptors might increase production of interleukin-18 (IL-18), interferon (IFN)-gamma, and caspase-1. In patients with hepatitis C, oral bovine lactoferrin is associated with increased levels of IL-18, and IFN-gamma, and IL-4 (13324).

Animal research suggests that lactoferrin protects the intestinal tract by blocking inflammation. Several mechanisms are proposed including lactoferrin's ability to sequester iron, bind bacterial endotoxin, inhibit cytokine release and reduce hydroxy radical production (13331). Other preliminary research suggests that lactoferrin might protect the small intestine from methotrexate toxicity by inhibiting epithelial cell proliferation (13332). In healthy volunteers, orally administered lactoferrin seems to lessen indomethacin-induced enteropathy, possibly through an antioxidant effect (13319).

Adverse Reactions

Orally, bovine and human recombinant lactoferrin are well tolerated (13315,13316,13317,13320,13323,13332). Diarrhea has occurred in some patients. At higher doses (7.2 grams/day), skin rash, anorexia, fatigue, chills, and constipation have been reported (13323).

Interactions with Herbs & Other Dietary Supplements

None known.

Interactions with Drugs

None known.

Interactions with Foods

None known.

Interactions with Lab Tests

None known.

Interactions with Diseases or Conditions

None known.

Dosage and Administration

ORAL: For treating hepatitis C, bovine lactoferrin 1.8 to 3.6 grams/day has been used. Some experts recommend starting lactoferrin 1 to 3 months before starting interferon to identify lactoferrin responders (13321,13322,13323,13324).

Comments

The risk for contamination of lactoferrin with the bovine spongiform encephalopathy prion appears to be negligible (13337). Recombinant human lactoferrin can be extracted from rice in high volumes at low cost. Some researchers suggest it might play a role in global health problems such as iron deficiency and acute diarrhea (13338).

LADY FERN

Also Known As
Brake Root, Common Polypod, Oak Fern, Rock Brake, Rock of Polypody.

Scientific Names
Athyrium filix-femina, synonym Polypodium filix-femina.
Family: Dryopteridaceae.

Comments
At the date of publication, this product was not a common ingredient used in brand name supplements marketed to consumers. Details about this product are available in the online version of *Natural Medicines Comprehensive Database.* See www.naturaldatabase.com.

LADY'S BEDSTRAW

Also Known As
Cheese Rennet, Cheese Renning, Curdwort, Ladys Bedstraw, Maid's Hair, Petty Mugget, Yellow Cleavers, Yellow Galium.

Scientific Names
Galium verum.
Family: Rubiaceae.

People Use This For
Orally, lady's bedstraw is used for treating swollen ankles, as a diuretic for bladder and kidney mucous discharge, for cancer, epilepsy, hysteria, spasms, tumors, and for relief of chest and lung ailments. It is also used orally to induce sweating; as a tonic; to stimulate appetite; as an aphrodisiac; and for astringent, cleansing, and purgative effects.
Topically, lady's bedstraw is used for poorly healing wounds and to stop bleeding.

Safety
There is insufficient reliable information available about the safety of lady's bedstraw.
Pregnancy and Lactation: Insufficient reliable information available; avoid using.

Effectiveness
There is insufficient reliable information available about the effectiveness of lady's bedstraw.

Mechanism of Action
The applicable parts of lady's bedstraw are the above ground parts. There is insufficient reliable information available about the possible mechanism of action and active ingredients.

Adverse Reactions
None reported.

Interactions with Herbs & Other Dietary Supplements
None known.

Interactions with Drugs
None known.

Interactions with Foods
None known.

Interactions with Lab Tests
None known.

Interactions with Diseases or Conditions
None known.

Dosage and Administration

ORAL: Typically, lady's bedstraw is used as a tea (18).
TOPICAL: Lady's bedstraw is used as a poultice. To prepare, pour 250 mL cold water over 2 heaping teaspoons of above ground parts, bring to simmer, and allow to steep (18).

LAMINARIA

Also Known As

Brown Algae, Kelp, Kombu, Makombu Thallus, Sea Girdles, Seagirdle Thallus.
CAUTION: See separate listings for Algin and Bladderwrack.

Scientific Names

Laminaria digitata; Laminaria japonica.
Family: Laminariaceae.

People Use This For

Orally, laminaria is used for weight loss, preventing cancer, hypertension, as a bulk laxative for constipation, and for treating radioactive intoxication.
Topically, laminaria is used as a "tent" placed into the cervix to cause cervical dilation prior to D & C, for removal of intrauterine devices, diagnostic procedures, for relief of cervical stenosis, and to facilitate uterine placement of therapeutic radium. Laminaria tents are also used in pregnancy for near-term or term cervical ripening particularly for a first pregnancy, to facilitate labor, alone or as adjunct to prostaglandins, and for inducing first-trimester abortions.

Safety

POSSIBLY UNSAFE ...when used orally. The average laminaria-based supplement might contain as much as 1000 mcg iodine. Ingesting more than 150 mcg iodine per day can cause hypothyroidism, hyperthyroidism, or exacerbate existing hyperthyroidism (9556). In addition, some laminaria supplements may contain arsenic (645,10275). There is insufficient reliable information available about the safety of laminaria for its other uses.
PREGNANCY: POSSIBLY UNSAFE ...when used topically for cervical ripening; there is an increased risk of maternal and neonatal infection (8945). LIKELY UNSAFE ...when used topically to induce labor because use is associated with maternal endometriosis, neonatal sepsis, fetal hypoxia, and intrauterine death (6). UNSAFE ...when used orally because of potential hormonal effects (19); avoid using.
LACTATION: LIKELY UNSAFE ...when used orally because of potential toxicity (19).

Effectiveness

POSSIBLY INEFFECTIVE

Parturition. Applying laminaria topically doesn't seem to be effective for cervical ripening. Although laminaria might reduce the duration of induction, it doesn't seem to reduce the incidence of birth by cesarian section. It also increases maternal and fetal infectious complications (8945).

There is insufficient reliable information available about the effectiveness of laminaria for its other uses.

Mechanism of Action

Laminaria is a seaweed that is native to Japan (8945). Laminaria contains iodine (9556), and is considered to be a rich source of iron and potassium (19). Iodine, which is the essential substrate for the thyroid hormone, is present in concentrations from 0.03-1.0% in laminaria (18). The constituents of laminaria include alginate, lamine, and laminarin (6).
Much of the utility of laminaria relates to its ability to form a viscous colloidal solution of gel in water. This allows laminaria to function as a bulk laxative. It also allows laminaria to be used to dilate the cervix for procedures or to ripen the cervix and hasten the onset of labor. For these uses, laminaria "tents" are inserted cervically. They absorb ambient moisture, gradually swelling to a diameter of 1/2 inch over 4-6 hours. This swelling causes cervical dilation that can induce labor (6).
The mechanism of cervical "ripening" might be similar to that of a foreign body that disrupts the normal chorioamniotic balance and initiates prostaglandin synthesis. That, in turn, causes myometrial contractions and cervical ripening. An alternative theory is that laminaria causes ripening because it contains high levels of the prostaglandin precursor, arachidonic acid. Still another theory is that laminaria causes partial detachment of the placenta and induces cervical dilation. Although laminaria can reduce the duration of labor induction, it is associated with an increased risk for maternal endometritis and neonatal sepsis (6).
Some other laminaria constituents might also have medical uses. The polysaccharide constituent of laminaria, laminarin, has antilipemic activity when partially sulfated and anticoagulant activity similar to heparin when more extensively sulfated. The basal portion of the blades is used as a hypotensive agent; the constituents histamine and lamine may be responsible for hypotensive effects (6). The constituent algin (sodium alginate) has bulk laxative and demulcent (soothing) effects (272). Alginate-containing kelp reduces absorption of radioactive strontium in animals

and humans and it has been used for managing radioactive intoxication (6). Preliminary evidence also suggests that alginate-containing kelp extracts might have antiviral effects, possibly by inhibiting viral enzyme activity (9554). However, the risk of adverse effects resulting from laminaria's iodine content may outweigh the benefits of its use as a routine preventative measure (515).

Adverse Reactions

Orally, laminaria can induce or exacerbate acne (9555). Oral use may also cause hypothyroidism or hyperthyroidism, or exacerbate existing hyperthyroidism (9556). Iodine can cause idiosyncratic or allergic reactions (18). Arsenic poisoning is a risk with laminaria, because the plant concentrates arsenic from the ocean. The concentration of arsenic in laminaria may vary depending upon the part of the world where it was harvested. The concentration of arsenic has been reported to be higher in laminaria preparations in Australia than in Great Britain (645,10275).
Topically, laminaria used for cervical ripening can cause pelvic cramps and cervical bleeding. Its use for cervical ripening is associated with neonatal and maternal infection (8945); however, in a small study of "tent" use with manufacturer recommended procedures, no infection occurred. Manufacturer recommendation included prior swabbing of the cervical canal with a suitable lubricant and antibacterial agent, then packing the canal with antibacterial gel. Uterine contractions associated with laminaria use have been implicated in fetal hypoxia and subsequent intrauterine death. Tent use is also associated with possible rupture of the cervical wall and subsequent infection (6).

Interactions with Herbs & Other Dietary Supplements

POTASSIUM SUPPLEMENTS: Theoretically, due to the potassium content of laminaria, concomitant use can increase the risk of hyperkalemia (19).

Interactions with Drugs

ACE INHIBITORS (ACEIs): Theoretically, due to the potassium content of laminaria, concomitant use might increase the risk of hyperkalemia (19).
DIGOXIN (Lanoxin): Theoretically, due to the potassium content laminaria may cause hyperkalemia in susceptible individuals and potentiate digoxin effects and adverse effects (19). Use with caution.
POTASSIUM SUPPLEMENTS: Theoretically, due to the potassium content of laminaria, concomitant use can increase the risk of hyperkalemia (19).
POTASSIUM-SPARING DIURETICS: Theoretically, due to the potassium content of laminaria, concomitant use may cause hyperkalemia (19).
THYROID HORMONE: Theoretically, due to the significant iodine content laminaria might interfere with drugs for hyper or hypothyroidism (9556).

Interactions with Foods

None known.

Interactions with Lab Tests

POTASSIUM: Theoretically, laminaria may increase serum potassium levels and test results (19).
THYROID HORMONES: Theoretically, the iodine in laminaria might elevate thyroid stimulating hormone (TSH) levels (9556).

Interactions with Diseases or Conditions

RENAL INSUFFICIENCY: Theoretically, laminaria may induce hyperkalemia in people with renal insufficiency on a potassium restricted diet (19). Laminaria also contains significant amounts of iodine (9556). Use with caution.
THYROID DISEASE: Laminaria contains significant amounts of iodine, which might exacerbate hyper- or hypothyroidism (9556).

Dosage and Administration

ORAL: People typically use capsules or tablets containing 500 to 650 mg of ground laminaria once daily (6002).
TOPICAL: No typical dosage.

LARCH ARABINOGALACTAN

Also Known As

AG, Ara-6, Arabinogalactan, Dietary Fiber, Larch, Larch Gum, Larix, Mongolian Larch, Mongolian Larchwood, Stractan, Western Larch, Wood Gum, Wood Sugar.
CAUTION: See separate listing for Larch Turpentine.

Scientific Names

Larix occidentalis; Larix gmelinii var. gmelinii, synonyms Larix dahurica, Abies gmelinii.
Family: Pinaceae.

People Use This For

Orally, larch arabinogalactan is used for the common cold, flu, metastatic liver disease, pediatric otitis media, HIV/AIDS, adjunctive therapy during cancer chemotherapy, as a dietary fiber supplement, immunostimulant, anti-inflammatory agent, and for hepatic encephalopathy.

In foods, Larch arabinogalactan is used as a stabilizer, emulsifier, binder, and sweetener.

Safety

LIKELY SAFE ...when used in amounts found in foods. Larch arabinogalactan is approved by the FDA for use in foods (3529).

POSSIBLY SAFE ...when used orally, appropriately, and short-term in therapeutic amounts (6,3529,3530).

There is insufficient reliable information available about the safety of the long-term use of larch arabinogalactan.

PREGNANCY AND LACTATION: Insufficient reliable information available; avoid using.

Effectiveness

There is insufficient reliable information available about the effectiveness of larch arabinogalactan.

Mechanism of Action

Larch arabinogalactan is a polysaccharide produced from the bark of the Larch tree. Arabinogalactans are found throughout nature and are found in other plants with immunostimulatory activity, including echinacea. Larch arabinogalactan is thought to have immunostimulatory effects by increasing release of interferon gamma, tumor necrosis fact alpha, interleukin-1 and interleukin-6 and stimulating phagocytosis and natural killer cell activity. Larch arabinogalactan is a fibrous product which ferments in the gut. It increases gut microflora, e.g., Lactobacillus, increases short-chain fatty acid production, and minimizes ammonia production and absorption. These effects suggest it may be beneficial as a dietary fiber supplement for improving gastrointestinal health and as an adjunct for treating hepatic encephalopathy. Larch arabinogalactan has been shown to concentrate in the liver. Some people think it might block hepatic receptors for metastatic cells and decrease liver metastases (3529,3530).

Adverse Reactions

Orally, bloating and flatulence have been reported (3530).

Interactions with Herbs & Other Dietary Supplements

None known.

Interactions with Drugs

IMMUNOSUPPRESSANTS: Theoretically, larch arabinogalactan might interfere with immunosuppression therapy due its immunostimulatory activity (3529). Immunosuppressant drugs include azathioprine (Imuran), basiliximab (Simulect), cyclosporine (Neoral, Sandimmune), daclizumab (Zenapax), muromonab-CD3 (OKT3, Orthoclone OKT3), mycophenolate (CellCept), tacrolimus (FK506, Prograf), sirolimus (Rapamune), prednisone (Deltasone, Orasone), and other corticosteroids (glucocorticoids).

ORAL DRUGS: Theoretically, concurrent administration might decrease the absorption of some oral drugs due to the fibrous nature of larch arabinogalactan.

Interactions with Foods

None known.

Interactions with Lab Tests

None known.

Interactions with Diseases or Conditions

TRANSPLANT RECIPIENTS: Theoretically, larch arabinogalactan might interfere with immunosuppression therapy.

Dosage and Administration

ORAL: For colds and the flu, one teaspoon of larch arabinogalactan powder in juice or water is usually taken 2-3 times daily until symptoms are relieved (3531).

Comments

Larch arabinogalactan specifically concentrates in hepatocytes and might have future application as a diagnostic tool or as a vehicle for delivering drugs to the liver (3529,3530).

LARCH TURPENTINE

Also Known As
Terebinthina Laricina, Terebinthina Veneta, Venetian Turpentine.
CAUTION: See separate listing for Larch Arabinogalactan.

Scientific Names
Larix decidua, synonyms Larix europaea, Pinus larix.
Family: Pinaceae.

People Use This For
Topically, larch turpentine is used for treating neuralgia, rheumatic discomfort, furuncles, fevers, colds, cough, bronchitis, tendency toward infection, blood pressure problems, and inflammation of the mouth and pharynx.

Safety
POSSIBLY SAFE ...when used topically and appropriately on intact skin (2).
POSSIBLY UNSAFE ...when used orally (18). ...when used topically on damaged skin, particularly if used on large areas (18). Skin damage allows systemic absorption, which can cause kidney and central nervous system toxicity (18). ...when inhaled, because it can cause acute airway inflammation (18).
PREGNANCY AND LACTATION: Insufficient reliable information available; avoid using.

Effectiveness
There is insufficient reliable information available about the effectiveness of larch turpentine.

Mechanism of Action
Larch turpentine is an oily exudate obtained by drilling into the trunks of Larix decidua trees. It contains up to 20% volatile oil (2). When topically applied, it increases local blood flow and can have an antiseptic effect (2).

Adverse Reactions
Topically, larch turpentine can cause allergic skin reactions (2).
When taken orally or applied to large areas of skin or damaged skin, it can cause kidney and central nervous system damage (18).
Inhalation can cause acute respiratory tract inflammation (18).

Interactions with Herbs & Other Dietary Supplements
None known.

Interactions with Drugs
None known.

Interactions with Foods
None known.

Interactions with Lab Tests
None known.

Interactions with Diseases or Conditions
BRONCHITIS: Inhalation of larch turpentine is contraindicated because it may worsen respiratory tract inflammation (2).

Dosage and Administration
TOPICAL: The ointments, gels, emulsions, and oils commonly contain 10 to 20 percent larch turpentine as liniments for external application (2).

LATHYRUS

Also Known As
Caley Pea, Chickling Vetch, Chick-Pea, Everlasting Pea, Flat-Podded Vetch, Singletary Pea, Spanish Vetchling, Sweet Pea, Wild Pea.

Scientific Names
Lathyrus cicera; Lathyrus clymenum; Lathyrus hirsutus; Lathyrus incanus; Lathyrus odoratus; Lathyrus pusillus; Lathyrus sativus; Lathyrus sylvestris.
Family: Fabaceae/Leguminosae.

People Use This For
In foods, Lathyrus sativus is used in unleavened Indian bread. Lathyrus seeds are eaten as food and used as animal fodder throughout the world.
The flowers of sweet pea (Lathyrus odoratus) are cultivated for their color and fragrance.

Safety
LIKELY UNSAFE ...when used orally. The seeds of Lathyrus can be neurotoxic (6).
PREGNANCY AND LACTATION: LIKELY UNSAFE ...when used orally (6); avoid using.

Effectiveness
There is insufficient reliable information available about the effectiveness of lathyrus.

Mechanism of Action
Lathyrus seeds contain multiple constituents including phytates, divicine, and a mixture of alkaloids (6). The toxicity of lathyrus results from several compounds. The neurotoxic effects are linked to constituent beta-N-oxalyl-L-alpha, beta-diaminopropionic acid (ODAP). Constituent beta-aminopropionitrile (BAPN) causes skeletal abnormalities and damage to blood vessels (6).

Adverse Reactions
Orally, lathyrus can cause neurotoxic manifestations including muscular rigidity, spasticity, weakness, paralysis of leg muscles, weak pulse, shallow breathing, convulsions, or death (6). Prolonged neurotoxicity is characterized by poor central motor coordination and reduced nerve conduction in the lower limbs (6).

Interactions with Herbs & Other Dietary Supplements
None known.

Interactions with Drugs
None known.

Interactions with Foods
None known.

Interactions with Lab Tests
None known.

Interactions with Diseases or Conditions
None known.

Dosage and Administration
No typical dosage.

Comments
Neurolathyrism and its complications are rare in western countries, yet they have been documented for more than a century in Europe, Africa, and Asia. Despite the attempt to ban the sale of Lathyrus sativus in several states of India, distribution continues. To deactivate the toxin, several methods have been tried. Typically they involve soaking the seeds in water followed by steaming or sun drying. Roasting the seeds at high temperatures for twenty minutes also helps to destroy the neurotoxic constituent. However, these methods are only 80-85% effective (6).

LAURELWOOD

Also Known As
Alexandrian-laurel, Alexandrinischer Lorbeer, Borneo-mahogany, Calanolide, Calophyllum Tree, Indian-laurel, Kamani Punna, Mahogany, Oleum Calophyllum, Palo de Santa Maria, Palo Maria, Punnanga, Undi.

Scientific Names
Calophyllum inophyllum.
Family: Clusiaceae/Guttiferae.

People Use This For
Orally, the laurelwood constituent (+)-calanolide A is used for HIV infection. Laurelwood is also used orally for leprosy, piles, scabies, gonorrhea, vaginitis, and chicken pox.
Topically, tamanu oil from the nut of the laurelwood is used for skin ailments including sunburn, rashes, burns, psoriasis, dermatitis, scratches, skin blemishes, acne, skin allergies, bedsores, rosacea, and hemorrhoids; and for infant skin care.

Safety
POSSIBLY SAFE ...when the laurelwood constituent (+)-calanolide A is used orally by HIV-negative individuals (4290).
There is insufficient reliable information available about the safety of laurelwood for its other uses.
PREGNANCY AND LACTATION: Insufficient reliable information available; avoid using.

Effectiveness
There is insufficient reliable information available about the effectiveness of laurelwood.

Mechanism of Action
Laurelwood is one of many species of Calophyllum that contains constituents that seem to have activity against the HIV virus. Recent interest has centered on the calanolide compounds, particularly (+)-calanolide A. This constituent, now in phase I testing, appears to be a unique and specific non-nucleoside inhibitor of the reverse transcriptase of the HIV-1 virus (4292,4293). It does not appear to have activity against HIV-2 (4295). Some evidence suggests calanolide A might have synergistic effects with zidovudine (Retrovir), lamivudine (Epivir), nelfinavir (Viracept) (4290), and nevirapine (Viramune) (4294). At least two isomers of calanolide A known as costatolide and dihydrocostatolide possess similar properties (4291,4292). Calanolide A also shows evidence of antituberculosis effects (4290).

Adverse Reactions
Orally, the use of the laurelwood constituent, (+)- calanolide A, by healthy individuals can cause dizziness, oily aftertaste, headache, and nausea (4290).
Topically, there are no reported adverse reactions when tamanu oil from the nut of laurelwood is used.

Interactions with Herbs & Other Dietary Supplements
None known.

Interactions with Drugs
None known.

Interactions with Foods
None known.

Interactions with Lab Tests
None known.

Interactions with Diseases or Conditions
None known.

Dosage and Administration
No typical dosage.

Comments

The laurelwood constituent (+)-canolide A is in Phase IB testing as an anti-HIV agent. The purpose of the current study is to determine its safety and its effect on development of resistance, CD4 count and viral load (4289). Phase IA testing in 94 healthy HIV-negative individuals showed it was well tolerated (4290). Sarawak MediChem Pharmaceuticals Inc. (Lemont, Illinois) is the agency supporting testing (4289). Avoid confusing laurelwood (Caulophyllum inophyllum) with blue cohosh (Caulophyllum thalictroides).

LAVENDER

Also Known As

Alhucema, Common Lavender, English Lavender, French Lavender, Garden Lavender, Ostokhoddous, Spanish Lavender, Spike Lavender, True Lavender.
CAUTION: See separate listing for Lavender Cotton.

Scientific Names

Lavandula angustifolia, synonyms Lavandula officinalis, Lavandula vera, Lavandula spica; Lavandula dentata; Lavandula latifolia; Lavandula pubescens; Lavandula stoechas.
Family: Lamiaceae/Labiatae.

People Use This For

Orally, lavender is used for restlessness, insomnia, nervousness, depression, meteorism (abdominal swelling from gas in the intestinal or peritoneal cavity), and loss of appetite. Lavender is also used orally for flatulence, upset stomach, giddiness, migraine headaches, toothaches, sprains, neuralgia, rheumatism, acne, sores, nausea, vomiting, to promote menstruation, and to treat cancer.
Topically, lavender is used for alopecia areata, pain, and in baths for circulation disorders. It is also used topically as a mosquito repellent and insect repellent.
By inhalation, lavender is used as aromatherapy for insomnia, pain, and agitation related to dementia.
In foods and beverages, lavender is used as a flavor component.
In manufacturing, lavender is utilized in pharmaceutical products and as a fragrance ingredient in soaps and cosmetics. Lavender is also used as an insect repellent.

Safety

LIKELY SAFE ...when used orally in amounts commonly found in foods. Lavender has Generally Recognized As Safe (GRAS) status for food use in the US (4912).
POSSIBLY SAFE ...when used orally and appropriately (9792). ...when used topically and appropriately (5177). Lavender oil has been used safely for up to 7 months (5177). ...when the essential oil is inhaled as a part of aromatherapy (7107,12213).
PREGNANCY AND LACTATION: Insufficient reliable information available; avoid using.

Effectiveness

POSSIBLY EFFECTIVE

Alopecia areata. There is some evidence that applying lavender oil in combination with the essential oils from thyme, rosemary, and cedarwood might improve hair growth by as much as 44% after 7 months of treatment (5177).

INSUFFICIENT RELIABLE EVIDENCE to RATE

Agitation. Preliminary evidence suggests that lavender aromatherapy does not reduce agitation in severely demented nursing home patients (12213).

Depression. In mild to moderate depression, tincture of lavender appears to be slightly less effective than imipramine (Tofranil). Lavender might have some additive antidepressant effect with imipramine (9792).
More evidence is needed to rate lavender for these uses.

Mechanism of Action

The applicable parts of lavender are the flowers, leaves, and oil. Lavender contains several potential active constituents including cineole from the essential oil and borneol and camphor from the leaves (12219). Lavender preparations and the isolated constituents have several pharmacological effects in vitro and in animals. However, the effects in humans are less well known.
Lavender seems to induce relaxation and sedation. Lavender decreases EEG potentials and decreases alertness in humans (7).
There is some evidence that lavender has spasmolytic effects on smooth muscle (6) and might have analgesic effects (7107).
There is also some evidence from animal models that lavender might have anticonvulsant effects and possibly potentiate chloral hydrate and pentobarbital effects (7).

In animal models, lavender leaf extract and essential oils seem to have analgesic and anti-inflammatory properties (12219).
There is some interest in lavender as an anticancer agent. The constituent perillyl alcohol seems to have some anticancer activity in vitro and in animal models (6).
Theoretically, lavender might potentiate the effects of HMG CoA reductase inhibitors due to the perillyl alcohol content (6).
Lavender might also have stimulant effects on hair growth (5177); however, the mechanism of this effect is not known.

Adverse Reactions

Orally, tincture of lavender may cause constipation, headache, and increased appetite (9792).
Topically, use of lavender rarely can cause contact dermatitis (6).

Interactions with Herbs & Other Dietary Supplements

None known.

Interactions with Drugs

BARBITURATES: Theoretically, lavender can potentiate the therapeutic effects of barbiturates (7). Some of these sedative medications include pentobarbital (Nembutal), phenobarbital (Luminal), secobarbital (Seconal), and others.
CHLORAL HYDRATE: Theoretically, lavender can potentiate the therapeutic effects of chloral hydrate (7).
CNS DEPRESSANTS: Theoretically, lavender can enhance the therapeutic and adverse effects of CNS depressants (7).

Interactions with Foods

None known.

Interactions with Lab Tests

SERUM CHOLESTEROL: Theoretically, lavender can decrease serum cholesterol levels and test results (6).

Interactions with Diseases or Conditions

None known.

Dosage and Administration

ORAL: For depression, tincture of lavender (1:5 in 50% alcohol) 60 drops per day has been used for 4 weeks (9792).
TOPICAL: For alopecia areata, one study used a combination of essential oils including lavender 3 drops (108 mg), rosemary 3 drops (114 mg), thyme 2 drops (88 mg), and cedarwood 2 drops (94 mg), all mixed with 3 mL jojoba oil and 20 mL grapeseed oil. Each night, the mixture is massaged into the scalp for 2 minutes with a warm towel placed around the head to increase absorption (5177).

Comments

Lavender is a popular component in perfumes, potpourri, and decorations (6002). Lavender is commonly adulterated with related species, including Lavandula hybrida, which is a cross between Lavandula angustifolia and Lavandula latifolia, from which lavandin oil is obtained (8).

LAVENDER COTTON

Also Known As

Santolina.
CAUTION: See separate listing for Lavender.

Scientific Names

Santolina chamaecyparissus.
Family: Asteraceae/Compositae.

People Use This For

Orally, lavender cotton is used for digestive disorders, premenstrual syndrome (PMS), worm infestations, jaundice, and as a spasmolytic. It is also used as an anti-inflammatory.
Topically, lavender cotton is used as an insect repellent.

Safety

There is insufficient reliable information available about the safety of lavender cotton.
Pregnancy and Lactation: Insufficient reliable information available; avoid using.

Effectiveness
There is insufficient reliable information available about the effectiveness of lavender cotton.

Mechanism of Action
The applicable parts of lavender cotton are the above ground parts and root bark. There is insufficient reliable information available about the possible mechanism of action and active ingredients.

Adverse Reactions
Lavender cotton may cause an allergic reaction in individuals sensitive to the Asteraceae/Compositae family. Members of this family include ragweed, chrysanthemums, marigolds, daisies, and many other herbs.

Interactions with Herbs & Other Dietary Supplements
None known.

Interactions with Drugs
None known.

Interactions with Foods
None known.

Interactions with Lab Tests
None known.

Interactions with Diseases or Conditions
CROSS-ALLERGENICITY: Lavender cotton may cause an allergic reaction in individuals sensitive to the Asteraceae/Compositae family. Members of this family include ragweed, chrysanthemums, marigolds, daisies, and many other herbs.

Dosage and Administration
ORAL: People typically prepare lavender cotton root bark using one teaspoon boiled in a covered container with 3 cups of water for 30 minutes. The liquid is cooled slowly in the closed container and taken cold, 1 to 2 cups per day (5254).

Comments
The whole lavender cotton plant is used externally as a moth and insect repellent due to its strong smell (18). Lavender cotton is unrelated to lavender and its scent is distinctly different from that of lavender (513).

LECITHIN

Also Known As
Egg Lecithin, Ovolecithin, Soy Bean Lecithin, Soy Lecithin, Soya Lecithin, Soybean Lecithin, Vegilecithin, Vitellin. CAUTION: See separate listings for Alpha-GPC, Choline, Phosphatidylcholine, Phosphatidylserine, and Soy.

Scientific Names
None.

People Use This For
Orally, lecithin is used for treating dementia and Alzheimer's disease, for extrapyramidal disorders, reducing hepatic steatosis (fat accumulation) in long-term parenteral nutrition patients, treating gallbladder disease, aiding ultrafiltration in peritoneal dialysis, treating liver disease, treating manic-depressive illness, improving memory, treating hypercholesterolemia, for anxiety, and eczema. It is also used as a source of choline, inositol, phosphorus, and linoleic and linolenic acids.

Topically, lecithin is used as a moisturizing agent for dermatitis and dry skin.

As a pharmaceutical and food additive, lecithin is used for emulsifying and stabilizing water-based products, and as an antioxidant in foods and pharmaceutical preparations. In the manufacture of preparations for intravenous and subcutaneous use, lecithin is used both as an emulsifying agent and a stabilizing agent.

Safety

LIKELY SAFE ...when used orally in amounts found in foods. Lecithin has Generally Recognized As Safe (GRAS) status in the US (4912). ...when used orally and appropriately for medicinal purposes (2619,4914). ...when used topically (4914). ...when used intravenously or subcutaneously and appropriately (16,4914).
PREGNANCY AND LACTATION: Insufficient reliable information available; avoid using in amounts greater than found in foods.

Effectiveness

LIKELY EFFECTIVE

Dermatitis. Applying lecithin topically seems to improve dermatitis (272).
Dry skin. Applying lecithin topically seems to reduce dry skin (272).

POSSIBLY EFFECTIVE

Hepatic steatosis. Taking lecithin orally seems to reduce hepatic steatosis in patients on long-term parenteral nutrition (5140).

POSSIBLY INEFFECTIVE

Gallbladder disease. Taking lecithin orally doesn't seem to resolve gallbladder disease (5142,5155).
Hypercholesterolemia. Taking lecithin orally doesn't seem to lower cholesterol levels (5147,5148).

LIKELY INEFFECTIVE

Alzheimer's disease and dementia. Taking lecithin orally doesn't improve symptoms of dementia and Alzheimer's disease (5149,5150,5151,5152).
Extrapyramidal disorders. Taking lecithin orally doesn't help extrapyramidal disorders (5139,6243).

There is insufficient reliable information available about the effectiveness of lecithin for its other uses.

Mechanism of Action

Lecithin is a phospholipid composed of phosphatidyl esters (phosphatides), chiefly consisting of phosphatidylcholine, phosphatidylethanolamine, phosphatidylserine and phosphatidylinositol, and varying amounts of other substances such as triglycerides, fatty acids, and carbohydrates, depending on source (9). For example, egg lecithin contains 69% phosphatidylcholine and 24% phosphatidylethanolamine, while soybean lecithin contains 24% phosphatidylcholine, 22% phosphatidylethanolamine, and 19% phosphatidylinositol. Lecithin is a precursor to acetylcholine (5156).

Adverse Reactions

Orally, lecithin can cause diarrhea, nausea, abdominal pain, or fullness (5140,6243).

Interactions with Herbs & Other Dietary Supplements

None known.

Interactions with Drugs

None known.

Interactions with Foods

None known.

Interactions with Lab Tests

None known.

Interactions with Diseases or Conditions

None known.

Dosage and Administration

ORAL: A typical oral dose is 1.2-2.4 grams/day (5153). For reducing cholesterol, 20-30 grams daily has been used in studies (5147,5148). For improving memory and Alzheimer's disease, 20-45 grams daily has been tried (5146,5149,5151,5152).

Comments

Unlike choline, lecithin does not cause unpleasant body and breath odor (5153). Lecithin contains phosphatidylcholine, which contains choline (16). Although closely related, these terms are not synonymous.

LEMON

Also Known As
Limon, Nimbaka, Nimbuka.

Scientific Names
Citrus limon, synonym Citrus limonum.
Family: Rutaceae.

People Use This For
Orally, lemon is used as a source of vitamin C in the treatment of scurvy, low resistance, and colds. It is also used as a digestive aid, an anti-inflammatory, diuretic, and to improve vascular permeability.
In foods, lemon is used as a food and flavoring agent.

Safety
LIKELY SAFE ...when used in amounts commonly found in foods. Lemon has Generally Recognized As Safe (GRAS) status in the US (4912).
POSSIBLY SAFE ...when used orally in medicinal amounts (12).
PREGNANCY AND LACTATION: Avoid using in amounts greater than those typically found in foods.

Effectiveness
There is insufficient reliable information available about the effectiveness of lemon.

Mechanism of Action
The applicable parts of lemon are the fruit, juice, and peel. Limonene is the most abundant monoterpene in lemon juice (4946). The furocoumarins bergapten and oxypeucedanin in lemon oil are photosensitizing (11019).

Adverse Reactions
Topically, photosensitivity can occur especially in fair-skinned people (11909).

Interactions with Herbs & Other Dietary Supplements
None known.

Interactions with Drugs
None known.

Interactions with Foods
None known.

Interactions with Lab Tests
None known.

Interactions with Diseases or Conditions
None known.

Dosage and Administration
ORAL: Lemon is taken as an oil, tincture, or fresh fruit (18).

LEMON BALM

Also Known As
Balm, Cure-All, Dropsy Plant, Honey Plant, Melissa, Melissae folium, Melissenblatt, Sweet Balm, Sweet Mary.

Scientific Names
Melissa officinalis.
Family: Lamiaceae/Labiatae.

People Use This For

Orally, lemon balm is used for anxiety, insomnia, dyspepsia, bloating, flatulence, and for attention deficit-hyperactivity disorder (ADHD). Lemon balm is also used for Graves' disease, dysmenorrhea, cramps, headache, toothache, sores, tumors, and insect bites. It is also used orally for Alzheimer's disease, hysteria and melancholia, chronic bronchial mucous membrane inflammation, nervous palpitations, vomiting, and high blood pressure.
As an inhalant, lemon balm is used as aroma therapy for Alzheimer's disease.
Topically, lemon balm is used for cold sores (herpes labialis).
In foods and beverages, the extract and oil of lemon balm are used for flavoring.

Safety

LIKELY SAFE ...when used orally in amounts commonly found in foods. Lemon balm has Generally Recognized As Safe (GRAS) status in the US (4912).
POSSIBLY SAFE ...when used appropriately for oral or topical medicinal purposes on a short-term basis (790,9993,9994,9995,12724). Oral lemon balm has been used with apparent safety for up to 4 months (9993). The safety of long-term use is unknown.
PREGNANCY AND LACTATION: Insufficient reliable information available; avoid using.

Effectiveness

POSSIBLY EFFECTIVE

Alzheimer's disease. Taking a standardized extract of lemon balm orally, daily for 4 months, seems to reduce agitation and improve symptoms of mild to moderate Alzheimer's disease on standard Alzheimer's disease rating scales (9993).

Dyspepsia. A specific combination product containing lemon balm (Iberogast, Enzymatic Therapy) seems to improve symptoms of dyspepsia. The combination includes lemon balm plus peppermint leaf, German chamomile, caraway, licorice, clown's mustard plant, celandine, angelica, and milk thistle (7049,12724).
A meta-analysis of studies using this combination product suggests that taking 1 mL orally three times daily over a period of 4-weeks significantly reduces severity of acid reflux, epigastric pain, cramping, nausea, and vomiting compared to placebo (13089).

Herpes labialis (cold sores). Applying a lip balm containing 1% lemon balm extract seems to shorten healing time, prevent infection spread, and reduce symptoms of recurring herpes labialis (790,9995).

Sleep. Taking lemon balm orally, in combination with valerian, appears to improve the quality and quantity of sleep in healthy people (10423).

Mechanism of Action

The applicable part of lemon balm is the leaf and leaf oil. Lemon balm seems to have sedative, antioxidant, and antiviral effects (790,9993,9994,9995). Lemon balm contains citronellal, neral, and geranial monoterpenoid aldehydes; flavonoids and polyphenolic compounds (including rosmarinic acid); and monoterpene glycosides. These substances may contribute to the behavioral effects of lemon balm dried leaf and essential oil (9994). Some research suggests lemon balm might have acetylcholine receptor activity with both nicotinic and muscarinic binding properties (9994). Clinical research suggests that lemon balm induces a calming effect and reduces alertness (9994).
Lemon balm is used in aroma therapy. The essential oil of lemon balm contains terpenes, which are rapidly absorbed through the lungs and cross the blood-brain barrier. In addition, these may possess cholinergic activity or act on gamma-aminobutyric acid (GABA) receptors (10422).

Adverse Reactions

Orally, lemon balm is well tolerated. It can cause nausea, vomiting, abdominal pain, dizziness, and wheezing (9993).
Topically, there is one report of irritation and one report of exacerbation of herpes symptoms when lemon balm was applied (790).

Interactions with Herbs & Other Dietary Supplements

HERBS WITH SEDATIVE PROPERTIES: Theoretically, concomitant use with herbs that have sedative properties might enhance therapeutic and adverse effects (9994). Some of these supplements include 5-HTP, calamus, California poppy, catnip, hops, Jamaican dogwood, kava, St. John's wort, scullcap, valerian, yerba mansa, and others.

Interactions with Drugs

CNS DEPRESSANTS: Theoretically, concomitant use of lemon balm with drugs with sedative properties may cause additive effects and side effects (9994).

Interactions with Foods

ETHANOL: Theoretically, lemon balm might increase the sedative effects of ethanol (9994).

Interactions with Lab Tests

None known.

Interactions with Diseases or Conditions
None known.

Dosage and Administration
ORAL: For mild to moderate Alzheimer's disease, 60 drops per day of a standardized lemon balm extract, prepared 1:1 in 45% alcohol, has been used (9993).
For sleep, lemon balm extract 80 mg, with valerian extract 120 mg 3 times daily, has been used for up to 30 days (10423).
For dyspepsia, a specific combination product containing lemon balm (Iberogast, Enzymatic Therapy) and several other herbs has been used in a dose of 1 mL three times daily (7049,12724,13089).
TOPICAL: For herpes labialis (cold sores), the cream or ointment containing 1% of a 70:1 lyophilized aqueous extract is usually applied two to four times daily from first sign of prodrome to a few days after the lesions have healed (790,9995).

LEMON EUCALYPTUS

Also Known As
Citron-Scent Gum, Lemon Scented Gum, Oil of Lemon Eucalyptus, OLE, P-menthane Diol, P-menthane-3,8-Diol, Para-menthane-3,8-diol, PMD, Quwenling, Spotted Gum, Wild Eucalyptus Citriodora.
CAUTION: See separate listings for Eucalyptus, Lemon, Lemon Balm, Lemon Verbena, and Lemongrass.

Scientific Names
Corymbia citriodora, synonym Eucalyptus citriodora.
Family: Myrtaceae.

People Use This For
Topically, lemon eucalyptus oil is used for preventing mosquito and deer tick bites, osteoarthritis and other joint pain, and as a smooth muscle spasmolytic.

Safety
LIKELY SAFE ...when used topically, short-term. Lemon eucalyptus oil seems to be safe when applied in concentrations of 30% to 75%, short-term (13065,13074,13076,13081,13115,13117,13118). The US Environmental Protection Agency (EPA) has approved lemon eucalyptus oil as a safe insecticide for human use (13075). The Centers for Disease Control (CDC) considers topical application of lemon eucalyptus oil as a safe alternative to low concentrations of DEET for use as a mosquito repellent; however, there is less experience using lemon eucalyptus oil compared to DEET (13063).
PREGNANCY AND LACTATION: Insufficient reliable information available; avoid using.

Effectiveness
LIKELY EFFECTIVE

Mosquito repellent. Lemon eucalyptus oil in concentrations of 40% to 75% seems to be comparable to 20% to 40% DEET for preventing mosquito bites (13065,13074,13117). The 75% lemon eucalyptus oil preparation does not appear to be more effective than the lower 40% concentration (13065).
Lemon eucalyptus oil in a concentration of 30% seems to be comparable to DEET 15% (13076).
A towelette wipe providing 0.574 grams of lemon eucalyptus oil also seems to be comparable to DEET 15% lotion (13081).
DEET might provide a longer duration of protection than lemon eucalyptus oil. Lemon eucalyptus oil in 30%, 40%, or 50% concentrations seems to provide 97% to 100% protection for a duration of about 1-5 hours (13074,13076,13117,13118). DEET 20% to 25% seems to provide 100% protection for up to about 5-6 hours (13074,13117); however, in another study, DEET 15% provided only 85% protection for 4 hours (13076).
The Centers for Disease Control (CDC) now considers topical application of lemon eucalyptus oil as an effective alternative to low concentrations of DEET; however, there is less experience using lemon eucalyptus oil compared to DEET (13063).

POSSIBLY EFFECTIVE

Tick repellent. Applying a specific 30% lemon eucalyptus oil extract (Citriodiol) significantly decreases the number of tick attachments when applied up to three times daily to people living in tick-infested areas (13115).
This specific extract is used in commercial products such as Mosi-guard and Repel Oil of Lemon Eucalyptus.

There is insufficient reliable information available about the effectiveness of lemon eucalyptus for other uses.

Mechanism of Action

The applicable parts of lemon eucalyptus are the leaves and the oil. Constituents isolated from lemon eucalyptus include eucalytptin, beta-sitosterol, and triterpenoids (13064).
The primary active constituent of the oil is p-menthane-3,8-diol (PMD), which has mosquito repellent activity. Commercial lemon eucalyptus oil-based mosquito repellents contain this constituent (13065). PMD consists of four stereoisomers. Each stereoisomer appears to have equal insect repellant activity (13116).
PMD is also contained in the waste distillate of lemon eucalyptus called quwenling (13065).
Lemon eucalyptus oil also has significant in vitro antifungal activity (13064).

Adverse Reactions

Topically, some people can be sensitive to lemon eucalyptus oil and develop skin reactions (13077).

Interactions with Herbs & Other Dietary Supplements

None known.

Interactions with Drugs

None known.

Interactions with Foods

None known.

Interactions with Lab Tests

None known.

Interactions with Diseases or Conditions

None known.

Dosage and Administration

TOPICAL: For preventing mosquito bites, a 30%, 40%, or 75% lemon eucalyptus oil has been used (13065,13074,13076); however, the higher concentration does not appear to be more effective than the lower concentration (13065).
For preventing tick bites and attachments, a specific 30% lemon eucalyptus oil extract (Citriodiol) has been applied up to three times daily when exposed to tick infested areas (13115). This specific extract is used in commercial products such as Mosi-guard and Repel Oil of Lemon Eucalyptus.
Commercial products available in the US (e.g., Repel Lemon Eucalyptus) contain 10% to 30% lemon eucalyptus oil. Commercial product directions suggest applying the oil no more than twice per day. Advise patients to wash their hands thoroughly after applying the oil.

LEMON VERBENA

Also Known As

Herb Louisa, Lemon-Scented Verbena, Louisa, Verveine Citronelle.
CAUTION: See separate listing for Verbena.

Scientific Names

Aloysia citrodora, synonyms Aloysia triphylla, Lippia citrodora, Lippia triphylla, Verbena triphylla, Zappania citrodora.
Family: Verbenaceae.

People Use This For

Orally, lemon verbena is used for digestive disorders, agitation, insomnia, asthma, cold, fever, flatulence, colic, diarrhea, indigestion, febrile hemorrhoids, varicose veins, skin conditions, chills, and constipation.
In foods and manufacturing, lemon verbena is used as an ingredient in herbal teas, as a fragrance component in perfumes, and also as an ingredient in alcoholic beverages.

Safety

LIKELY SAFE ...when used orally in amounts commonly found in foods. Lemon verbena has Generally Recognized As Safe (GRAS) status in the US (4912).
POSSIBLY SAFE ...when used orally and appropriately in medicinal amounts (12).
There is insufficient reliable information available about the safety of lemon verbena when used topically.
PREGNANCY AND LACTATION: Insufficient reliable information available; avoid using.

Effectiveness

There is insufficient reliable information available about the effectiveness of lemon verbena.

Mechanism of Action

The applicable parts of lemon verbena are the leaf and flowering tops. Oil of verbena (the essential oil distilled from lemon verbena leaf) may be acaricidal and bactericidal (6). Terpene-rich volatile oils in the plant are considered irritants (4).

Adverse Reactions

Orally, volatile oils may irritate the kidneys during excretion (4).
Topically, contact dermatitis may occur (6).

Interactions with Herbs & Other Dietary Supplements

None known.

Interactions with Drugs

None known.

Interactions with Foods

None known.

Interactions with Lab Tests

None known.

Interactions with Diseases or Conditions

KIDNEY DISEASE: Avoid excessive amounts due to possible kidney irritation (4).

Dosage and Administration

ORAL: One cup tea has been used two to five times daily (18). The tea is prepared by steeping 5-29 grams of the leaf in 1 L of boiling water for 10-15 minutes then straining (18).
TOPICAL: No typical dosage.

LEMONGRASS

Also Known As

British Indian Lemongrass, Capim-Cidrao, Ceylon Citronella Grass, Citronella, Cochin Lemongrass, East Indian Lemongrass, Fever Grass, Guatemala Lemongrass, Lemon Grass, Madagascar Lemongrass, West Indian Lemongrass.
CAUTION: See separate listings for Citronella Oil, Lemon Eucalyptus, and Stone Root.

Scientific Names

Cymbopogon citratus, synonym Andropogon citratus; Cymbopogon flexuosus, synonym Andropogon flexuosus.
Family: Poaceae/Gramineae.

People Use This For

Orally, lemongrass is used for treating gastrointestinal spasms, stomachache, hypertension, convulsions, pain and neuralgia, vomiting, cough, rheumatism, fever, common cold, and exhaustion. It is also used orally as an antiseptic and as a mild astringent.
Topically, lemongrass and its essential oil are used for headache, stomachache, abdominal pain, and musculoskeletal pain.
By inhalation, the essential oil of lemongrass is used as aromatherapy for musculoskeletal pain.
In food and beverages, lemongrass is used as a flavoring.
In manufacturing, lemongrass is used as a fragrance in soaps and cosmetics. Lemongrass is also used in synthesizing vitamin A and natural citral.

Safety

LIKELY SAFE ...when used orally in amounts commonly found in foods. Lemongrass has Generally Recognized As Safe (GRAS) status in the US (4912).
POSSIBLY SAFE ...when used orally or topically, short-term for medicinal purposes. Lemongrass has been safely used in studies lasting up to 2 weeks (6,12,2612,7107). ...when the essential oil of lemongrass is used by inhalation as a component of aromatherapy (7107).
PREGNANCY: LIKELY UNSAFE ...when used orally. Lemongrass seems to have uterine and menstrual flow stimulating effects (12); avoid using.
LACTATION: Insufficient reliable information available; avoid using.

Effectiveness

There is insufficient reliable information available about the effectiveness of lemongrass.

Mechanism of Action

The applicable part of lemongrass is the leaf and oil. The lemongrass leaves are commonly used as "lemon" flavoring in herbal teas. The essential oil from lemongrass contains geraniol, limonene, alpha-pinene, and alpha-terpineole, which have antimicrobial properties (2130,7162). The oil has in vitro antimicrobial activity against a variety of common gram positive and gram negative organisms, including Acinetobacter calcoacetica, Enterococcus faecalis, Escherichia coli, Klebsiella pneumoniae, Pseudomonas aeruginosa, Salmonella species, Serratia marcescens, Staphylococcus aureus, and the yeast Candida albicans (2131). Lemongrass oil also contains citral, 65-85%. Although citral is a central nervous system (CNS) depressant (11,7162), lemongrass does not seem to have significant CNS effects (2612). Lemongrass is also thought to have analgesic, antipyretic, and antioxidant properties (11), as well as uterine and menstrual flow stimulating effects (12).

Adverse Reactions

Orally, there is a single report of fatal poisoning after a child ingested a lemongrass oil-based insect repellent (2).
Topically, rare allergic reactions have occurred following use (2,18).
By inhalation, there have been two cases of toxic alveolitis associated with an unknown quantity of lemongrass oil (2).

Interactions with Herbs & Other Dietary Supplements

None known.

Interactions with Drugs

None known.

Interactions with Foods

None known.

Interactions with Lab Tests

AMYLASE, BILIRUBIN: Lemongrass may cause elevations in serum bilirubin (direct) and amylase levels (2612).

Interactions with Diseases or Conditions

None known.

Dosage and Administration

ORAL: People typically use 1 to 2 teaspoons of lemongrass in 6 oz boiling water as a tea (6006).
TOPICAL: No typical dosage.

Comments

Avoid confusion with citronella oil (Cymbopogon nardus).

LENTINAN

Also Known As

None.
CAUTION: See separate listing for Shiitake Mushroom.

Scientific Names

Polysaccharide derived from Lentinus edodes, synonyms Lenticus edodes, Lentinan edodes, Lentinula edodes, Tricholomopsis edodes.
Family: Polyporaceae.

People Use This For
Lentinan is given by intravenous, intramuscular, and intraperitoneal injection as an adjunctive treatment for cancer and HIV infection.

Safety
There is insufficient reliable information available about the safety of lentinan.
Pregnancy and Lactation: Insufficient reliable information available; avoid using.

Effectiveness
POSSIBLY EFFECTIVE

Breast cancer. Administering lentinan by injection as adjunctive treatment seems to help improve response in patients being treated for breast cancer (1112).

Gastric cancer. Administering lentinan by injection as adjunctive treatment seems to help improve response in patients being treated for gastric cancer (1108,1113).

HIV/AIDS. Administering lentinan by injection as adjunctive treatment in combination with didanosine (ddI) seems to increase CD4 counts compared to ddI alone (1107).

Prostate cancer. Administering lentinan by injection as adjunctive treatment seems to help improve response in patients being treated for prostate cancer (1109).

Mechanism of Action
Lentinan is not directly cytotoxic, but may augment natural killer cell activity, activate macrophages and may enhance T-helper cell function (6). It may enhance the anti-HIV effects of zidovudine (6).

Adverse Reactions
Mild thrombocytopenia (6); minor adverse effects (unspecified) were reported in clinical trials (one case report) (6). Rapid intravenous infusion of lentinan is reported to cause "oppression" of the anterior chest and dryness of the throat; these symptoms disappeared with slow drip infusion (1111).

Interactions with Herbs & Other Dietary Supplements
None known.

Interactions with Drugs
None known.

Interactions with Foods
None known.

Interactions with Lab Tests
CD4 COUNTS: Intravenously administered lentinan, combined with didanosine (ddI, Videx), might enhance drug-induced increases in CD4 concentrations and test results in some HIV+ patients with low CD4 counts (1107).

Interactions with Diseases or Conditions
MALNUTRITION: In one clinical trial, gastric cancer patients with low serum protein levels (consistent with poor nutritional status) did not respond to lentinan therapy, while patients with normal serum protein levels (consistent with adequate nutritional status) had favorable responses to lentinan (1110).

Dosage and Administration
ORAL: No typical dosage.
INJECTION: 1-4 mg per week have been used in clinical trials (6,1108,1111).

Comments
Lentinan is a polysaccharide derived from shiitake mushroom (Lenticus edode).

LESSER CELANDINE

Also Known As
Ficaria, Figwort, Pilewort, Ranunculus, Smallwort.
CAUTION: See separate listings for Amaranth, Bulbous Buttercup, Greater Celandine, and Jewelweed.

Scientific Names
Ranunculus ficaria.
Family: Ranunculaceae.

People Use This For

Orally, lesser celandine is used for scurvy.

Topically, lesser celandine is used for bleeding wounds and gums, swollen joints, warts, scratches, and hemorrhoids (internal or prolapsed piles, with or without hemorrhage).

For food uses, fresh leaf sheaths of lesser celandine are sometimes used in salads.

Safety

POSSIBLY SAFE ...when small amounts of fresh leaf sheaths are eaten (18).

POSSIBLY UNSAFE ...when used topically (4,18). Extended contact with the fresh, bruised plant can cause blisters (18).

LIKELY UNSAFE ...when used orally (4,18); avoid using.

PREGNANCY AND LACTATION: LIKELY UNSAFE ...when used orally (4); avoid using.

Effectiveness

There is insufficient reliable information available about the effectiveness of lesser celandine.

Mechanism of Action

The applicable parts of lesser celandine are the above ground parts. Lesser celandine contains large amounts of vitamin C (18). It also has astringent and demulcent effects (4). Protoanemonin, a constituent, is believed to be an acrid skin irritant (4). However, when the above ground parts are dried or prepared, protoanemonin changes into a pungent, volatile intermediate that quickly dimerizes to a form that does not irritate the mucous membrane (18). Some studies suggest the constituents, anemonin and protoanemonin, might have antibacterial and antifungal activity (4). The saponin constituents show some evidence of antihemorrhoidal activity (4). Large amounts of protoanemonin-forming plants have caused death of experimental animals by asphyxiation (18).

Adverse Reactions

Orally, use is associated with severe GI irritation, colic, diarrhea, and irritation of the urinary tract (18).

One report associates the use of lesser celandine with a case of recurrent, acute hepatitis (390).

Topically, use can cause mucous membrane and skin irritation (18). Extended contact with fresh, bruised plant can cause blisters (18). Some Ranunculus species also cause photodermatitis (19).

Interactions with Herbs & Other Dietary Supplements

None known.

Interactions with Drugs

None known.

Interactions with Foods

None known.

Interactions with Lab Tests

None known.

Interactions with Diseases or Conditions

GI CONDITIONS: Lesser celadine can irritate gastrointestinal tract. Contraindicated in individuals with infectious or inflammatory gastrointestinal conditions (19).

Dosage and Administration

ORAL: No typical dosage.

TOPICAL: Liquid extract (1:1 in 25% alcohol), 2-5 mL 3 times daily (4). Ointment (3%) or Pilewort Ointment (30% fresh herb in benzoinated lard) (4). Liquid extract can be added to baths for hemorrhoids, warts, or scratches (18).

Comments

Avoid confusion with greater celandine (Chelidonium majus). Scrophularia nodosa (Family: Scrophulariaceae) is also referred to as figwort (4). Amaranth and bulbous buttercup are also referred to as pilewort.

LEVANT BERRY

Also Known As

Cocculus, Cocculus Indicus, Coculus Fructus, Fish Berries, Fish Killer, Hockle Elderberry, Indian Berry, Levant Nut, Louseberry, Poisonberry.
CAUTION: See separate listings for Chenopodium Oil, Ivy Gourd, Mugwort, Wormseed, Wormwood, and Wormwood Oil.

Scientific Names

Anamirta cocculus, synonyms Anamirta paniculata, Menispermum cocculus, Menispermum lacunosum; Cocculus suberosus; Cocculus lacunosus.
Family: Menispermaceae.

People Use This For

Orally, levant berry is used for peripheral and vestibular nystagmus and peripherally-based dizziness. The constituent, picrotoxin, is used orally for treating epilepsy, night sweats, and as a stimulant for barbituric acid poisoning.
Topically, it is used as a powder to treat scabies.
In India, the leaves are inhaled as snuff to relieve malaria; whole fruits are used for paralyzing fish and killing birds or dogs; picrotoxin is applied to arrow tips for hunting by jungle tribes, and was formerly used to paralyze fish in the fishing industry; extracts are applied topically for lice.

Safety

POSSIBLY UNSAFE ...when used topically; avoid application to broken skin (6).
LIKELY UNSAFE ...when used orally due to toxic potential (6). Picrotoxin 30 mg/kg or 2-3 cocculus kernels can cause death (6,18).
PREGNANCY AND LACTATION: LIKELY UNSAFE ...when used orally or topically (6); avoid using.

Effectiveness

There is insufficient reliable information available about the effectiveness of levant berry.

Mechanism of Action

The applicable parts of levant berry are the dried fruit and seed. The seed contains highly toxic picrotoxin (6,18), which stimulates the central nervous system via parasympathetic nerves, is a GI irritant, stimulates the medulla oblongata resulting in changes in respiration rate, slows heart rate due to vagal nerve stimulation, and increases blood pressure (6,18).

Adverse Reactions

Picrotoxin is a GI irritant and central nervous system stimulant (6). Mild poisoning can lead to headache, dizziness, nausea, coordination disturbances, depression, and spasms or twitching (18). Larger amounts can cause salivation, vomiting, purging, rapid shallow breathing, drowsiness, palpitations or bradycardia, tonic-clonic spasms, stupor, loss of consciousness, and death (6). The lethal dose is stated to be 30 mg/kg (6) or 2-3 Cocculus kernels (seeds) (18).

Interactions with Herbs & Other Dietary Supplements

None known.

Interactions with Drugs

None known.

Interactions with Foods

None known.

Interactions with Lab Tests

None known.

Interactions with Diseases or Conditions

None known.

Dosage and Administration

No typical dosage.

Comments

Although picrotoxin is used experimentally, medicinal use has been abandoned in the US and Europe (6).

LICORICE

Also Known As
Alcacuz, Alcazuz, Chinese Licorice, Gan Cao, Gan Zao, Glycyrrhiza, Isoflavone, Jethi-Madh, Mulhathi, Lakritze, Liquiritiae radix, Liquirizia, Liquorice, Orozuz, Phytoestrogen, Reglisse, Regliz, Russian Licorice, Spanish Licorice, Subholz, Sweet Root, Yashti-Madhu, Yashti-Madhuka.

Scientific Names
Glycyrrhiza glabra; Glycyrrhiza glabra var. glandulifera; Glycyrrhiza uralensis.
Family: Fabaceae/Leguminosae.

People Use This For
Orally, licorice is used for gastric and duodenal ulcers, sore throat, bronchitis, chronic gastritis, dyspepsia, colic, primary adrenocortical insufficiency, cough, osteoarthritis, systemic lupus erythematosus (SLE), and for bacterial and viral infections. It is also used orally for cholestatic liver disorders, hypokalemia, hypertonia, malaria, tuberculosis, abscesses, food poisoning, diabetes insipidus, and contact dermatitis.

In combination with Panax ginseng and Bupleurum falcatum, licorice is used orally to help stimulate adrenal gland function, particularly in patients with a history of long-term corticosteroid use. As a component of the herbal formula, Shakuyaku-Kanzo-To, licorice is used to increase fertility in women with polycystic ovary syndrome. In combination with other herbs, licorice is used to treat prostate cancer and atopic dermatitis (eczema).

Topically, licorice is used as a shampoo to reduce sebum secretion.

Intravenously, licorice components are used for treating hepatitis B and C.

Licorice is used as a flavoring in foods, beverages, and tobacco.

Safety
LIKELY SAFE ...when used orally in amounts commonly found in foods. Licorice has Generally Recognized As Safe (GRAS) status in the US (4912).

POSSIBLY SAFE ...when used orally and appropriately for medicinal purposes, short-term (3247,3250,3251,6196,11312,11313). Long-term use increases the risk of adverse effects such as hypertension and hypokalemia (7620).

PREGNANCY: UNSAFE ...when used orally. Licorice has abortifacient, estrogenic, and steroid effects; and can cause uterine stimulation. Heavy consumption of licorice, 500 mg per week or more, during pregnancy seems to increase the risk of delivering before gestational age of 38 weeks (7619,10618); avoid using.

LACTATION: Insufficient reliable information available; avoid using.

Effectiveness
POSSIBLY EFFECTIVE

Dyspepsia. A specific combination product containing licorice (Iberogast, Enzymatic Therapy) seems to improve symptoms of dyspepsia. The combination includes licorice plus peppermint leaf, German chamomile, caraway, lemon balm, clown's mustard plant, celandine, angelica, and milk thistle (7049,12724). A meta-analysis of studies using this combination product suggests that taking 1 mL orally three times daily over a period of 4-weeks significantly reduces severity of acid reflux, epigastric pain, cramping, nausea, and vomiting compared to placebo (13089).

INSUFFICIENT RELIABLE EVIDENCE to RATE

Atopic dermatitis (eczema). Licorice given orally in combination with 9 other herbs (Zemaphyte) might reduce redness and skin lesions in adults and children with nonexudative atopic eczema (12627,12628,12629). However, other research shows no effect (12630).

Hepatitis. Preliminary evidence suggests that isolated constituents of licorice may be effective for treating hepatitis B and C. Glycyrrhizin- and glycyrrhizic acid-containing intravenous preparations (Stronger Neominophagen C and Remefa S) show activity against hepatitis B and hepatitis C in humans, but the trials are too small to draw any definitive conclusions (3247,3250,3251).

Peptic ulcers. There is some evidence that deglycyrrhizinated licorice (DGL) might accelerate the healing of peptic ulcers (11312,11313).

Weight loss. There is conflicting information about the use of licorice for weight loss. Licorice has been shown to reduce body fat, however accompanying fluid retention offsets any change in body weight (6196).

More evidence is needed to rate licorice for these uses.

Mechanism of Action

The applicable part of licorice is the root. Licorice has antispasmodic, anti-inflammatory, laxative, and soothing properties. The constituents glycyrrhizin and glycyrrhetinic acid inhibit 11-beta-hydroxysteroid dehydrogenase, an enzyme located in the aldosterone receptor cells of the cortical collecting duct (10619). Glycyrrhizin may contribute to licorice-associated mineralocorticoid side effects, including hypertension and hypokalemia, by both binding directly to mineralocorticoid receptors and by decreasing the conversion of active cortisol to inactive cortisone (3252,3253,7620,10619). Panax ginseng appears to compliment licorice by increasing serum cortisol concentrations (3257).

Licorice appears to block metabolism of prostaglandins E and F2 alpha, which suggests a possible beneficial effect on peptic ulcer. Preliminary information suggests deglycyrrhizinated licorice (DGL) may accelerate the healing of peptic ulcers. DGL seems to be similar to carbenoxolone for ulcer reduction without the fluid retention or electrolyte imbalance of carbenoxolone. Carbenoxolone is a semisynthetic derivative of glycyrrhetic acid that is used outside the US for treating gastric and duodenal ulcer disease (11311,11312,11313).

Licorice appears to have anti-estrogenic and estrogenic action. Preliminary research indicates that licorice does not stimulate the growth of estrogen dependent breast cancer cells (7860). However, the estrogenic effects of licorice might be concentration dependent. Glabridin, an isoflavone constituent of licorice, seems to have an estrogen receptor-dependent growth-promoting effect at low concentrations. At higher concentrations, it seems to have an estrogen receptor-independent antiproliferative effect (10617). Licorice has been shown to reduce body fat, however accompanying fluid retention offsets any change in body weight (6196).

Licorice also decreases testosterone production in men who eat licorice (3246,13072). This is likely due to the licorice constituent, glycyrrhetinic acid, inhibiting the enzyme 17-hydroxysteroid dehydrogenase, which converts androstenedione to testosterone. Glycyrrhetinic acid also seems to inhibit 17-20 lyase which converts 17-hydroxyprogesterone to androstenedione (13072).

Glycyrrhizin- and glycyrrhizic acid-containing intravenous preparations (Stronger Neominophagen C and Remefa S) show activity against hepatitis B and C in humans, but the trials are too small to draw any definitive conclusions (3247,3250,3251). In vitro data suggests that glycyrrhizin suppresses the production and expression of hepatitis B surface antigen (HbS-Ag) (3248,3249). Preliminary evidence suggests that glycyrrhizin may inhibit the growth of the coronavirus, which is associated with severe acute respiratory syndrome (SARS). The exact mechanism of the antiviral effect of glycyrrhizin is not known (10299).

Adverse Reactions

Orally, licorice may cause hypertension, sodium and water retention, edema, lethargy, amenorrhea, and headache with consumption of 50 grams per day or chronic use longer than six weeks. Higher levels of consumption may cause hypokalemia, hypokalemic myopathy, rhabdomyolysis, myoglobinuria, severe congestive heart failure (CHF), pulmonary edema, lower extremity weakness, hypertensive encephalopathy, and quadriplegia due to pseudoaldosteronism and hypermineralocorticoidism (781,7620,10393,10619). Hypokalemia caused by licorice can cause muscle weakness and dropped head syndrome (DHS) (10393). Because licorice can decrease serum testosterone and increase 17-hydroxyprogesterone, it might cause decreased libido and sexual dysfunction in men (3246).

Chewing tobacco flavored with licorice has also been associated with toxicity. Chewing licorice-flavored tobacco has been associated with hypertension and suppressed renin and aldosterone levels (12671,12837).

Interactions with Herbs & Other Dietary Supplements

HERBS WITH CARDIAC ACTIVITY: Theoretically, the overuse or misuse of licorice can increase the risk of cardiotoxicity due to potassium depletion (10393). Cardioactive herbs include digitalis, lily-of-the-valley, pheasant's eye, and squill.

STIMULANT LAXATIVE HERBS: Theoretically, concomitant overuse or misuse of licorice with stimulant laxatives can increase the risk of potassium depletion (10393). Stimulant laxative herbs include aloe vera, alder buckthorn, European buckthorn, cascara sagrada, castor oil, rhubarb, and senna.

Interactions with Drugs

ANTIHYPERTENSIVE DRUGS: Theoretically, licorice might reduce the effect of antihypertensive drug therapy. Licorice increases blood pressure in a dose dependent manner (7620).

CORTICOSTEROIDS: Theoretically, concomitant use might potentiate the duration of activity of corticosteroids, e.g., hydrocortisone (12672). Concomitant use of licorice and corticosteroids might also increase potassium loss and increase the risk of potassium depletion. Overuse or misuse of licorice can cause potassium depletion (10393).

CYTOCHROME P450 2B6 (CYP2B6) SUBSTRATES: There's preliminary evidence that licorice can inhibit the cytochrome P450 2B6 (CYP2B6) isoenzymes (10300). Theoretically, licorice might increase levels of drugs metabolized by CYP2B6; however, as of yet, these interactions have not been reported in humans. Some drugs that are metabolized by CYP2B6 include ketamine (Ketalar), phenobarbital, orphenadrine (Norflex), secobarbital (Seconal), and dexamethasone (Decadron). Use licorice cautiously or avoid in patients taking these drugs.

CYTOCHROME P450 3A4 (CYP3A4) SUBSTRATES: There's preliminary evidence that licorice can inhibit the cytochrome P450 3A4 (CYP3A4) isoenzymes (6450,10300). Theoretically, licorice might increase levels of drugs metabolized by CYP3A4; however, as of yet, these interactions have not been reported in humans. Some drugs metabolized by CYP3A4 include lovastatin (Mevacor), ketoconazole (Nizoral), itraconazole (Sporanox), fexofenadine (Allegra), triazolam (Halcion), and numerous others.

DIGOXIN (Lanoxin): Overuse or misuse of licorice with cardiac glycoside therapy might increase the risk of cardiac toxicity due to potassium loss (10393).

DIURETIC DRUGS: Overuse of licorice might compound diuretic-induced potassium loss (10393). There is some concern that people taking licorice along with potassium depleting diuretics might have an increased risk for hypokalemia. Initiation of potassium supplementation or an increase in potassium supplement dose may be necessary for some patients. Some diuretics that can deplete potassium include chlorothiazide (Diuril), chlorthalidone (Thalitone), furosemide (Lasix), hydrochlorothiazide (HCTZ, Hydrodiuril, Microzide), and others.

ESTROGENS: Theoretically, licorice might interfere with hormone therapy due to estrogenic and anti-estrogenic effects (7860).

ETHACRYNIC ACID (Edecrin): Theoretically, ethacrynic acid might enhance the mineralocorticoid effects of licorice by inhibiting the enzyme that converts cortisol to cortisone; however, bumetanide (Bumex) does not appear to have this effect (3255).

FUROSEMIDE (Lasix): Theoretically, furosemide might enhance the mineralocorticoid effects of licorice by inhibiting the enzyme that converts cortisol to cortisone; however, bumetanide (Bumex) does not appear to have this effect (3255).

Interactions with Foods

GRAPEFRUIT JUICE: Theoretically, grapefruit juice and its component naringenin might enhance the mineralocorticoid activities of licorice, by blocking the conversion of cortisol to cortisone (3254,3255).

Interactions with Lab Tests

17-HYDROXYPROGESTERONE: Licorice can increase serum 17-hydroxyprogesterone concentrations and test results in healthy volunteers who consume 7 grams of licorice per day (3246,13072).

BLOOD PRESSURE: Excessive use of licorice can cause hypertension and increase blood pressure readings (1372).

POTASSIUM: Excessive use of licorice can cause hypokalemia, reducing serum potassium levels and test results (10393).

TESTOSTERONE: Licorice can decrease serum testosterone concentrations and test results in healthy volunteers who consume 7 grams of licorice per day (3246,13072).

Interactions with Diseases or Conditions

HEART DISEASE: The mineralocorticoid effects of licorice can induce fluid retention and worsen congestive heart failure (12672). Licorice can also cause hypokalemia and increase the risk of arrhythmias. Advise patients with heart disease to avoid licorice.

HORMONE SENSITIVE CANCERS/CONDITIONS: Licorice might have estrogenic effects (6180). Women with hormone sensitive conditions should avoid using licorice. Some of these conditions include breast cancer, uterine cancer, ovarian cancer, endometriosis, and uterine fibroids.

HYPERTENSION: The mineralocorticoid effects of licorice increase blood pressure. Advise patients with hypertension to avoid licorice (1372).

HYPERTONIA: Licorice-induced hypokalemia may worsen hypertonia (10393).

HYPOKALEMIA: Licorice can cause hypokalemia (10393).

KIDNEY INSUFFICIENCY: The mineralocorticoid effects of licorice may worsen renal function. Advise patients with severe renal insufficiency to avoid licorice (12672).

SEXUAL DYSFUNCTION: Theoretically, licorice might decrease libido and worsen erectile dysfunction by decreasing testosterone and increasing 17-hydroxyprogesterone serum concentrations (3246).

Dosage and Administration

ORAL: For dyspepsia, a specific combination product containing licorice (Iberogast, Enzymatic Therapy) and several other herbs has been used in a dose of 1 mL three times daily (7049,12724,13089).

Comments

Many "licorice" products manufactured in the US actually don't contain any licorice. Instead, they contain anise oil, which has the characteristic smell and taste called "black licorice".

LILY-OF-THE-VALLEY

Also Known As

Constancy, Convallaria, Convallaria herba, Convall-Lily, Jacob's Ladder, Ladder-To-Heaven, Lily, May Bells, May Lily, Muguet, Our Lady's Tears.
CAUTION: See separate listings for Abscess Root and Jacob's Ladder.

Scientific Names

Convallaria majalis.
Family: Liliaceae or Convallariaceae.

People Use This For

Orally, lily-of-the-valley is used for mild cardiac insufficiency, heart insufficiency due to old age, chronic cor pulmonale, arrhythmias, urinary tract infections (UTIs), kidney stones, weak contractions in labor, epilepsy, edema, strokes and ensuing paralysis, conjunctivitis, and leprosy.

Safety

POSSIBLY SAFE ...when the standardized extract is used orally under medical supervision (2,12). Poor oral absorption of its cardiac glycosides can reduce the risk of poisoning (18), but the number of glycosides and their varied properties makes controlled use difficult (7).
LIKELY UNSAFE ...when the standardized extract is used orally for self-medication (12).
PREGNANCY AND LACTATION: UNSAFE ...when used orally for self-medication (12).

Effectiveness

There is insufficient reliable information available about the effectiveness of lily-of-the-valley.

Mechanism of Action

The applicable parts of lily-of-the-valley are the root, rhizome, and dried flowering tops. Lily-of-the-valley contains over 40 cardioactive glycosides, principally convallatoxin; and other minor glycosides, including canvallatoxol and convalloside (13). The cardiac glycosides exert positive inotropic, negative chronotropic, negative dromotropic (conduction), and positive bathmotropic (excitability) effects (7). They can lower elevated left-ventricular diastolic pressure as well as pathologically elevated venous pressure (2). Diuretic, natriuretic, and dose-dependent vasoconstrictive effects have been observed in experimental animals (18).

Adverse Reactions

Orally, lily-of-the-valley can cause nausea, vomiting, cardiac arrhythmias (2), headache, and stupor (18). Visual color disturbances can also occur (18).

Interactions with Herbs & Other Dietary Supplements

CARDIAC GLYCOSIDE-CONTAINING HERBS: Contraindicated. Concomitant use can increase the risk of cardiac glycoside toxicity. Cardiac glycoside-containing herbs include black hellebore, Canadian hemp root, digitalis leaf, hedge mustard, figwort, motherwort, oleander leaf, pheasant's eye plant, pleurisy root, squill bulb leaf scales, strophanthus seeds, and uzara (2,18,19,500).
LICORICE/HORSETAIL: Theoretically, the overuse or misuse of licorice rhizomes or horsetail plant with cardiac glycoside-containing herbs increases the risk of cardiac toxicity due to potassium depletion (19).
OTHER CARDIOACTIVE HERBS: Avoid concomitant use with other cardioactive herbs due to the unpredictability of therapeutic and adverse effects. Other cardioactive herbs include calamus, cereus, cola, coltsfoot, devil's claw, European mistletoe, fenugreek, fumitory, ginger, Panax ginseng, hawthorn, white horehound, mate, parsley, quassia, scotch broom flower, shepherd's purse, and wild carrot (4).
STIMULANT LAXATIVE HERBS: Theoretically, the overuse or misuse of stimulant laxatives with cardiac glycoside-containing herbs increases the risk of cardiac toxicity due to potassium depletion. Stimulant laxative herbs include aloe dried leaf sap, blue flag rhizome, alder buckthorn, European buckthorn, butternut bark, cascara bark, castor oil, colocynth fruit pulp, gamboge bark exudate, jalap root, black root, manna bark exudate, podophyllum root, rhubarb root, senna leaves and pods, wild cucumber fruit (Ecballium elaterium), and yellow dock root (19).

Interactions with Drugs

CALCIUM SUPPLEMENTS: Calcium salts can enhance the therapeutic and adverse effects of lily-of-the-valley (18).
CORTICOSTEROIDS: Theoretically, concomitant, long-term corticosteroid use can increase the risk of cardiac glycoside toxicity due to potassium depletion (2).
DIGOXIN (Lanoxin): Contraindicated; therapeutic duplication increases the risk of cardiac glycoside toxicity (2).
DIURETIC DRUGS: Concomitant use of potassium depleting diuretics and lily-of-the-valley can increase the risk of cardiac glycoside toxicity due to potassium depletion (506). Some diuretics that can deplete potassium include

chlorothiazide (Diuril), chlorthalidone (Thalitone), furosemide (Lasix), hydrochlorothiazide (HCTZ, Hydrodiuril, Microzide), and others.
MACROLIDE ANTIBIOTICS: Theoretically, concomitant use may increase risk of cardiac glycoside toxicity (17).
QUININE: Theoretically, concomitant use of lily-of-the-valley and quinine can increase the risk of cardiac toxicity (506).
STIMULANT LAXATIVES: Theoretically, the overuse or misuse of stimulant laxatives can increase the risk of cardiac glycoside toxicity due to potassium depletion (19).
TETRACYCLINE ANTIBIOTICS: Theoretically, concomitant use may increase the risk of cardiac glycoside toxicity (17).

Interactions with Foods
None known.

Interactions with Lab Tests
None known.

Interactions with Diseases or Conditions
HEART DISEASE: Self-medication with lily-of-the-valley is contraindicated; treatment requires diagnosis, treatment, and monitoring (515).
POTASSIUM DEFICIENCY: Contraindicated (2).

Dosage and Administration
ORAL: The average daily amount is 600 mg of the standardized lily-of-the-valley powder (0.2-0.3% cardioactive glycosides) or equivalent preparations (2).

Comments
The large number of cardiac glycosides in lily-of-the-valley makes monitoring and therapeutic control more difficult than digitalis or digoxin therapy (7). Lily-of-the-valley has a short duration of action. This correlates with lower absorption rates and makes treatment more difficult to control than with isolated cardiac glycosides, especially due to the narrow therapeutic range of these constituents (7). When indicated, digoxin of standard potency and purity is a safer alternative than nonstandardized lily-of-the-valley (7). Store lily-of-the-valley in well-sealed containers and protect from light (18).

LIME

Also Known As
Adam's Apple, Bara Nimbu, Bijapura, Italian Limetta, Key Lime, Limette, Turanj.
CAUTION: See separate listing for Linden.

Scientific Names
Citrus aurantifolia, synonyms Citrus medica var. acida, Citrus acida, Citrus lima, Citrus limetta var. aromatica, Limonia aurantiifolia.
Family: Rutaceae.

People Use This For
Orally, lime juice is used for dysentery.
Topically, lime oil is used as a stimulant, antiseptic, and for nausea.
In cosmetics, expressed lime oil is used as a fragrance component. Distilled lime oil is used as a fixative in cosmetics.

Safety
LIKELY SAFE ...when used orally in amounts commonly found in foods. Lime has Generally Recognized As Safe status (GRAS) for use in foods in the US (4912).
POSSIBLY SAFE ...when lime peel is used orally in medicinal amounts (12).
POSSIBLY UNSAFE ...when used topically. Lime oil contains photosensitizing constituents (11019).
PREGNANCY AND LACTATION: Insufficient reliable information available; avoid using in amounts greater than those typically found in foods.

Effectiveness
There is insufficient reliable information available about the effectiveness of lime.

Mechanism of Action

The applicable parts of lime are the peel, fruit, and juice. The furocoumarins bergapten and oxypeucedanin in lime oil are photosensitizing (11019). Some evidence suggests expressed and distilled lime oils might promote tumors in the presence of carcinogenic chemicals (11).

Lime juice contains bergamottin, which competitively inhibits cytochrome P450 3A4 (CYP3A4) activity (11976).

Adverse Reactions

Topically, lime oil can cause hypersensitivity (4058). Photosensitivity might occur, especially in fair-skinned people (11019).

Interactions with Herbs & Other Dietary Supplements

None known.

Interactions with Drugs

CYTOCHROME P450 3A4 (CYP3A4) SUBSTRATES: Lime juice inhibits cytochrome P450 3A4, causing increased drug levels and potentially increasing the risk of adverse effects (11976). Some drugs metabolized by CYP3A4 that might be affected are some benzodiazepines such as alprazolam (Xanax), diazepam (Valium), midazolam (Versed), triazolam (Halcion); calcium channel blockers such as amlodipine (Norvasc), diltiazem (Cardizem, Dilacor, others), felodipine (Plendil), verapamil (Calan, Verelan, others); cyclosporine (Neoral, Sandimmune); some HIV antivirals such as indinavir (Crixivan), ritonavir (Norvir), saquinavir (Fortovase, Invirase); some HMG CoA reductase inhibitors such as atorvastatin (Lipitor), lovastatin (Mevacor); some macrolide antibiotics such as erythromycin and clarithromycin (Biaxin); quinidine; and many others.

PHOTOSENSITIZING DRUGS: Theoretically, concomitant use of lime oil with photosensitizing drugs may increase the risk of phototoxicity (11019).

Interactions with Foods

None known.

Interactions with Lab Tests

None known.

Interactions with Diseases or Conditions

None known.

Dosage and Administration

No typical dosage.

Comments

Distilled lime oil is made from the whole crushed fruit of the lime tree. Expressed lime oil is obtained from unripe lime peel.

LIMONENE

Also Known As

Alpha-Limonene, Dipentene, D-Limonene, L-Limonene, R-Limonene, S-Limonene.

Scientific Names

Limonene.

People Use This For

Orally, limonene is used for weight loss, cancer prevention and treatment, and bronchitis.

In foods, limonene is used as a flavoring agent for foods, beverages, and chewing gum.

In pharmaceuticals, limonene is used as a penetration enhancer in transdermal delivery systems.

In manufacturing, limonene is used as a fragrance, solvent, and as an ingredient in water-free hand cleansers.

Safety

LIKELY SAFE ...when consumed in amounts commonly found in foods. Limonene has Generally Recognized As Safe (GRAS) status in the US (4912).

POSSIBLY SAFE ...when used orally and appropriately in medicinal amounts. Limonene has been safely used in one trial for up to a year (12709).

PREGNANCY AND LACTATION: LIKELY SAFE ...when consumed in amounts commonly found in foods. Limonene has Generally Recognized As Safe (GRAS) status in the US (4912). There is insufficient reliable information available about using limonene in medicinal amounts during pregnancy or breast-feeding; avoid using.

Effectiveness

INSUFFICIENT RELIABLE EVIDENCE to RATE

Cancer. D-limonene taken orally in 21-day cycles seems to concentrate in tumor tissue in patients with advanced cancer and may slow disease progression, but its effect on survival is uncertain (12709). More evidence is needed to rate limonene for this use.

Mechanism of Action

Limonene is classified chemically as a monoterpene. It exists naturally as two enantiomers. D-limonene is the main constituent of the oil in citrus fruits and the essential oil of caraway. L-limonene is found in many trees such as pine and in herbs in the Mentha family. Plants may produce limonene to prevent dehydration and inhibit the growth microbes, especially fungi (12712,12713).

Preliminary research on cancer cells indicates that limonene may prevent lymphoma, breast, skin, liver, lung, colon, and gastric cancer. It might also cause regression of malignant tumors in animals. Limonene might help reduce the risk of cancer by inducing phase I and phase II cytochrome P450 (CYP450) hepatic enzymes that metabolize carcinogens to harmless products. Limonene may induce CYP2B1, CYP2C, glutathione-S-transferase, and UDP-glucuronyl transferase. It might also prevent tumor cell proliferation. Limonene inhibits protein isoprenylation, which might preferentially cause cancer cell death (12714). However, other preliminary research suggests that limonene causes nephropathy and renal tumors in male, but not female, rats. However, it does not appear to be mutagenic (12710).

Preliminary research suggests that limonene stimulates immune system activity (12711).

Topically, limonene appears to enhance the ability of ethanol as a vehicle for percutaneous absorption of lipophilic drugs (12719).

Limonene has high oral bioavailability and is metabolized to active and inactive metabolites by phase I enzymes CYP2C9 and CYP2C19, and by phase II metabolism. Excretion occurs primarily via the urine (12714,12718).

Adverse Reactions

Orally, limonene can cause nausea, vomiting, and diarrhea (12709).

Topically, limonene can cause contact dermatitis (12715,12716).

Preliminary research suggests high exposure (1000 ppm) by inhalation to limonene can cause mild bronchoconstriction (12712). Very high concentrations are toxic to human lung cells (12717).

Interactions with Herbs & Other Dietary Supplements

None known.

Interactions with Drugs

CYTOCHROME P450 2C19 (CYP2C19) INDUCERS: There's preliminary evidence that limonene might be a substrate for cytochrome P450 2C19 (CYP2C19) (12714,12718). CYP2C19 inducers might decrease the effects of limonene. So far, this interaction has not been reported in humans. Inducers of CYP2C19 include carbamazepine (Tegretol), prednisone (Deltasone), and rifampin (Rifadin, Rimactane).

CYTOCHROME P450 2C19 (CYP2C19) INHIBITORS: There's preliminary evidence that limonene might be a substrate for cytochrome P450 2C19 (CYP2C19) (12714,12718). So far, this interaction has not been reported in humans. However, watch for an increase in the limonene levels when it is taken with drugs that inhibit CYP2C19. Some drugs that inhibit CYP2C19 include cimetidine (Tagamet), fluvoxamine (Luvox), omeprazole (Prilosec); ticlopidine (Ticlid), topiramate (Topamax), and others.

CYTOCHROME P450 2C9 (CYP2C9) INDUCERS: There's preliminary evidence that limonene might be a substrate for cytochrome P450 2C9 (CYP2C9) (12714,12718). Inducers of CYP2C9 might decrease limonene levels. Inducers of CYP2C9 include rifampin (Rifadin, Rimactane) and secobarbital (Seconal).

CYTOCHROME P450 2C9 (CYP2C9) INHIBITORS: There's preliminary evidence that limonene might be a substrate for cytochrome P450 2C9 (CYP2C9) (12714,12718). So far, this interaction has not been reported in humans. However, watch for side effects in patients taking limonene and CYP2C9 inhibitors. Some CYP2C9 inhibitors include amiodarone (Cordarone), fluconazole (Diflucan), lovastatin (Mevacor), paroxetine (Paxil), zafirlukast (Accolate), and many others.

CYTOCHROME P450 2C9 (CYP2C9) SUBSTRATES: There's preliminary evidence that limonene might be a substrate for cytochrome P450 2C9 (CYP2C9), as well causing its induction (12714,12718). So far, this interaction has not been reported in humans. However, watch for a decrease in the levels of drugs metabolized by CYP2C9 in patients taking limonene. Some drugs metabolized by CYP2C9 include nonsteroidal anti-inflammatory drugs (NSAIDs) such as diclofenac (Cataflam, Voltaren), ibuprofen (Motrin), meloxicam (Mobic), and piroxicam (Feldene); celecoxib (Celebrex); amitriptyline (Elavil); warfarin (Coumadin); glipizide (Glucotrol); losartan (Cozaar); and others.

Interactions with Foods

None known.

Interactions with Lab Tests
None known.

Interactions with Diseases or Conditions
None known.

Dosage and Administration
No typical dosage.

Comments
In industry, limonene is used as a solvent, replacing chlorinated hydrocarbon and chloroflurocarbon cleaners (12717).

LINDEN

Also Known As
Basswood, European Linden, Hungarian Silver Linden, Lime Flower, Lime Tree, Linden Charcoal, Silver Lime, Silver Linden, Tiliae Folium, Tiliae Flos, Tiliae Lignum.
CAUTION: See separate listing for Lime.

Scientific Names
Tilia europaea, synonym Tilia vulgaris; Tilia cordata, synonyms Tilia parvifolia, Tilia ulmifolia; Tilia tomentosa, synonym Tilia argentea; Tilia platyphyllos, synonyms Tilia grandifolia, Tilia rubra.
Family: Malvaceae or Tiliaceae.

People Use This For
Orally, linden leaf is used for colds, nasal congestion, throat irritation, palpitations, hypertension, headaches, insomnia, sinus headache, migraine headache, incontinence, hemorrhage, hysteria, arteriosclerotic hypertension, fever, and nervous tension. It is also used as a diaphoretic, diuretic, antispasmodic, and as an expectorant for coughs. Linden sapwood is used orally for liver disease and gallbladder disease, and for cellulitis. Linden charcoal is used orally for intestinal disorders.
Topically, linden is used for itchy skin, rheumatism, and lower leg abscesses (ulcus cruris).

Safety
POSSIBLY SAFE ...when used orally and appropriately (12).
PREGNANCY AND LACTATION: Insufficient reliable information available; avoid using.

Effectiveness
There is insufficient reliable information available about the effectiveness of linden.

Mechanism of Action
The applicable parts of linden are the dried leaf, flower, and wood (sapwood).
Charcoal from the wood is also used.
Linden has antispasmodic, diaphoretic, diuretic, sedative, mild astringent, and antifungal activity (4,6).
In vitro, its antispasmodic activity is attributed to p-coumaric acid and the flavonoid constituents (4).
Diaphoretic effects are thought to be due to kaempferol, p-coumaric acid, and quercetin constituents (6).
The volatile oils, including citral, citronellal, citronellol, eugenol, and limonene, exert sedative and antispasmodic effects (4,6).
A diuretic effect may be due to the irritant action of terpenoid on the kidneys (4).

Adverse Reactions
Orally, frequent consumption of linden tea is thought to be associated with cardiac damage, but this seems to be rare (6).
Topically, linden dried flower can cause contact urticaria (6).

Interactions with Herbs & Other Dietary Supplements
None known.

Interactions with Drugs
None known.

Interactions with Foods
None known.

Interactions with Lab Tests
None known.

Interactions with Diseases or Conditions
CARDIOVASCULAR DISEASE: Frequent use of linden tea has been associated with cardiac damage; use with caution in individuals with existing heart disease (4,6).

Dosage and Administration
ORAL: No typical dosage. However, traditionally 1-2 cups of the tea has been used. The tea is prepared by steeping 2 grams of linden in 150 mL boiling water (8). Additionally, 2-4 mL of the tincture (1:5 in 45% alcohol), and 1-2 mL of the liquid extract (1:1 in 25% alcohol) is 1-2 mL has also been used (4).

Comments
There is very little scientific information about this product. Our staff is continually analyzing the available information on natural medicines and will add data here as it becomes available.

LIPASE

Also Known As
None.

Scientific Names
Triacylglycerol lipase.

People Use This For
Orally, lipase is used for indigestion, heartburn, celiac disease, Crohn's disease, and cystic fibrosis.

Safety
LIKELY SAFE ...when used orally and appropriately (12721,12722,12723).
PREGNANCY AND LACTATION: Insufficient reliable information available; avoid using.

Effectiveness
EFFECTIVE

Pancreatic insufficiency. Taking lipase in combination with amylase and protease reduces steatorrhea and improves nutritional status in patients with pancreatic insufficiency associated with cystic fibrosis (12721,12722,12723).

Mechanism of Action
Lipase is a digestive enzyme that is widely distributed in the plant world, in milk, milk products, bacteria, molds, and animal tissues (2383). Castor beans and hulled oats are also plant sources of acid-stable lipases (2383). Lipase and other pancreatic enzymes aid in fat digestion by hydrolyzing fat in the small intestine. Lipase and other pancreatic enzymes are destroyed by pepsin and gastric acid, so most products are microencapsulated and enteric coated to make them more acid resistant (12721).
Commonly used prescription and OTC products include combination pancreatic enzymes, lipase plus protease and amylase, rather than lipase as a single ingredient. This combination of enzymes is called pancrelipase (Cotazym, Creon, Ultrase, Viokase, Zymase). Potency is usually expressed in terms of lipase content (12721,12722,12723).

Adverse Reactions
Orally, taking large amounts of lipase in combination with other pancreatic enzymes can cause diarrhea, abdominal pain, flatulence, and nausea. To improve fat absorption and reduce steatorrhea, patients often must take many capsules of pancreatic enzymes per day, which may reduce adherence (12722,12723).

Interactions with Herbs & Other Dietary Supplements
None known.

Interactions with Drugs
None known.

Interactions with Foods
None known.

Interactions with Lab Tests
None known.

Interactions with Diseases or Conditions

CYSTIC FIBROSIS: High doses of lipase appear to increase the risk of fibrosing colonopathy and colonic strictures in individuals with cystic fibrosis (2379,2380,2381,2382).

Dosage and Administration

ORAL: For pancreatic insufficiency associated with cystic fibrosis, a typical dose for adults is 4500 units per kilogram of lipase (included in pancrelipase) per day. For children, a typical dose is 5100 units per kilogram per day. Dose is titrated to effect and may vary widely (12723).

LITHIUM

Also Known As

Lithium Carbonate, Lithium Citrate, Lithium Orotate.

Scientific Names

Lithium; Li; atomic number 3.

People Use This For

Orally, lithium is used for bipolar disorder, depression, schizophrenia, anorexia nervosa, bulimia, headache and alcoholism. Other uses include neutropenia, epilepsy anemia, diabetes, liver disease, kidney disorders, arthritis, seborrhea, and hyperthyroidism. It is also used for syndrome of inappropriate antidiuretic hormone (SIADH), asthma, Huntington chorea, Graves' disease, herpes simplex, drug-induced tardive dyskinesia, Tourette syndrome, cyclical vomiting, Meniere's disease, paresthesias, control of levodopa side effects, and ulcerative colitis in patients with affective disorders.

Safety

LIKELY SAFE ...when used orally and appropriately. Lithium carbonate and lithium citrate are FDA-approved drugs (15).

CHILDREN: POSSIBLY SAFE ...when lithium carbonate and lithium citrate are used orally and appropriately (15).

PREGNANCY: POSSIBLY SAFE ...when lithium carbonate and lithium citrate are used orally (15). Lithium can cause fetal toxicity and increases the risk for cardiac and other abnormalities, but it may be given with careful monitoring when the potential maternal benefits outweigh the possible risk to the fetus (15,9166).

LACTATION: UNSAFE ...when used orally. Lithium is secreted into breast milk and may cause adverse effects in the nursing infant (15).

There is insufficient reliable information about the safety of lithium orotate.

Effectiveness

EFFECTIVE

Bipolar disorder. Taking lithium orally is FDA-approved for treatment of mania in mixed bipolar disorder and prevention of recurrence of bipolar episodes (15).

LIKELY EFFECTIVE

Depression. Taking lithium orally appears to be effective in some patients with major depression (15).

POSSIBLY EFFECTIVE

Attention deficit-hyperactivity disorder (ADHD). Preliminary evidence suggests that lithium might be effective for impulsive aggressive behavior, aggression associated with ADHD (15).

Schizophrenia. Lithium is typically used in combination with antipsychotic drugs when it is used for schizophrenia or schizoaffective disorders. In some cases, lithium is beneficial as monotherapy for these patients (15).

There is insufficient reliable information available about the effectiveness of lithium for its other uses.

Mechanism of Action

Lithium is the lightest of the alkali metal elements. It is a monovalent cation and has some chemical properties of calcium and magnesium (15). Lithium is normally present in all organs and tissues with highest concentrations in the brain and kidneys. Lithium is uniformly distributed in body water; there is only a small difference between extracellular and intracellular levels. It does not bind to plasma proteins (15,9163). Lithium salts are virtually 100% absorbed from the small intestine via the sodium channels and are excreted primarily by the kidneys. Lithium appears to be an essential micronutrient; however, defined human lithium deficiency diseases have not been observed. Primary dietary sources include grains and vegetables with smaller amounts obtained from animal-derived foods. The average daily intake of an American 70 kg adult ranges from 650-3100 mcg. In some geographical areas, drinking water may contribute significantly to lithium intake (9163). Epidemiological evidence suggests that areas with lower lithium content in tap water have higher rates of mental hospital admissions, suicides, homicides, and other crimes, suggesting that lithium intake might affect behavior (9163). Animal studies suggest that lithium deficiency can adversely affect mortality and reproduction. Lithium appears to be essential for fetal development,

particularly during the first trimester of gestation. It appears to have a role in fetal blood cell development.
Lithium is involved with many physiological functions. It works with other elements, drugs, enzymes, hormones, vitamins, and growth and transforming factors. Theoretically, many of the biological actions of lithium are caused by the powerful polarizing effect caused by its small atomic radius, allowing it to displace sodium, potassium, magnesium, and calcium from membrane or enzyme binding sites (9163).
The exact mechanism of action of lithium in psychological and behavioral disorders is unknown. It appears to affect dopamine and serotonin activity (15). Lithium might increase monoamine oxidase (MAO) activity. It also enhances folate and vitamin B12 transport into brain cells, which might affect mood (9163).
Lithium stimulates the production of colony-stimulating factor by monocytes. It produces neutrophilia and may also increase erythrocyte and platelet counts, and decrease lymphocyte counts. The increase in neutrophils is usually seen 3-7 days after initiation of lithium and rapidly reverses 1-2 weeks after lithium is discontinued (15).
Lithium causes changes in renal function, often producing a mild nephrogenic diabetes insipidus. The drug decreases renal concentrating ability and water reabsorption. Initially, sodium and potassium excretion increases. Some of these effects improve with physiologic compensation; others may persist. Glomerular filtration rate (GFR) may decrease with prolonged therapy (15).
Lithium is excreted unchanged, predominately in the urine. The elimination half-life is 20-24 hours with normal renal function, but increases with decreasing renal function. The half-life in elderly patients may increase to 36 hours. In renal impairment, the half-life can increase to 40-50 hours.
Lithium has a narrow therapeutic window and must be monitored to avoid toxicity. Lithium levels should be drawn 12 hours after the last dose of lithium after steady state concentrations have been attained (4-7 days).
For depression and schizoaffective disorders, therapeutic levels are 0.4-1.3 mEq/L. For acute mania, therapeutic levels are 1.0-1.3 mEq/L. Toxicity is most common at levels of 1.5 mEq/L, although some patients develop toxicity at levels less than 1 mEq/L, especially children and older patients (15).
The onset of activity is slow, often requiring 10-21 days to achieve full therapeutic effect (15).

Adverse Reactions

Orally, lithium can cause nausea, diarrhea, vertigo, muscle weakness, lethargy, fatigue, and a dazed feeling. These adverse effects often improve with continued use. Fine tremor, polyuria, and polydipsia can occur and may persist with continued use. Weight gain and edema, which should not be treated with diuretics, are also seen. Lithium can also cause or exacerbate skin disorders such as acne, psoriasis, and rashes. Long-term effects include hypothyroidism, goiter, (rarely hyperthyroidism), and mild cognitive and memory impairment (9,15).
Signs of lithium toxicity include increasing diarrhea, vomiting, anorexia, muscle weakness, lethargy, giddiness with ataxia, lack of coordination, choreoathetosis, tinnitus, blurred vision, coarse tremor of the extremities and lower jaw, muscle hyperirritability, dysarthria, and drowsiness. Severe toxicity can cause toxic psychosis, syncope, renal failure, dehydration, circulatory failure, coma, and occasionally death (9).
Abrupt drops in serum lithium levels can precipitate recurrence of bipolar symptoms (9165).
Preclinical studies suggest that lithium orotate might be more likely to cause nephrotoxicity than lithium carbonate (9164).

Interactions with Herbs & Other Dietary Supplements

CAFFEINE CONTAINING HERBS/SUPPLEMENTS: Concomitant use can increase lithium clearance (9,15). Natural products that contain caffeine include black tea, coffee, green tea, guarana, mate, and cola nut.
DIURETIC HERBS: Theoretically, herbs having diuretic properties might reduce the clearance of lithium (9,15). Herbs thought to have diuretic properties include agrimony, artichoke, broom, buchu, burdock, celery, cornsilk, couch grass, elder, guaiac wood, juniper, pokeroot, shepherd's purse, squill, uva ursi, and yarrow.
HERBS/SUPPLEMENTS WITH SEROTONERGIC ACTIVITY: Theoretically, lithium might increase the effects and adverse effects of products that increase serotonin levels, including 5-hydroxytryptophan, Hawaiian baby woodrose, L-tryptophan, S-adenosylmethionine, and St. John's wort (9,15).

Interactions with Drugs

ACE INHIBITORS (ACEIs): Concomitant administration may increase lithium concentrations. Lithium dosage reductions may be necessary (9,15). Some ACE inhibitors are captopril (Capoten), enalapril (Vasotec), lisinopril (Prinivil, Zestril), ramipril (Altace), and others.
ANTICONVULSANTS: Drugs such as carbamazepine (Tegretol) and phenytoin (Dilantin) might increase the risk of neurotoxicity (9,15).
ANTIDEPRESSANT DRUGS: Combining serotonergic antidepressants with lithium might increase the risk of serotonergic side effects including serotonin syndrome and cerebral vasoconstrictive disorders such as Call-Fleming syndrome (8056). These drugs include the selective serotonin reuptake inhibitors (SSRIs) such as fluoxetine (Prozac), paroxetine (Paxil), sertraline (Zoloft), and others; and tricyclic and atypical antidepressants such as amitriptyline (Elavil), clomipramine (Anafranil), imipramine (Tofranil), and others.
CALCIUM CHANNEL BLOCKERS: Calcium channel blockers might reduce lithium concentrations. Monitor lithium levels with concurrent use. Calcium channel blockers might also increase adverse neurological and gastrointestinal adverse effects (9,15). Calcium channel blockers include nifedipine (Adalat, Procardia), verapamil

(Calan, Isoptin, Verelan), diltiazem (Cardizem), isradipine (DynaCirc), felodipine (Plendil), amlodipine (Norvasc), and others.
DEXTROMETHORPHAN (Robitussin DM, others): Combining serotonergic drugs such as dextromethorphan with lithium might increase the risk of serotonergic side effects including serotonin syndrome and cerebral vasoconstrictive disorders such as Call-Fleming syndrome (8056).
LOOP DIURETICS: Loop diuretics might reduce lithium excretion, particularly in sodium-restricted patients. Monitor lithium levels (9,15). Loop diuretics include bumetanide (Bumex), ethacrynic acid (Edecrin), and furosemide (Lasix).
MEPERIDINE (Demerol): Combining serotonergic drugs such as meperidine with lithium might increase the risk of serotonergic side effects including serotonin syndrome and cerebral vasoconstrictive disorders such as Call-Fleming syndrome (8056).
METHYLDOPA (Aldomet): Concurrent use of methyldopa increases the risk of lithium toxicity (9).
METHYLXANTHINES: Xanthines such as aminophylline, caffeine, and theophylline (Theo-Dur, Theo-24, others) might increase the clearance of lithium. Monitor lithium levels (9,15).
MONOAMINE OXIDASE INHIBITORS (MAOIs): Combining serotonergic drugs such as one of the MAOIs with lithium might increase the risk of serotonergic side effects including serotonin syndrome and cerebral vasoconstrictive disorders such as Call-Fleming syndrome (8056).
NONSTEROIDAL ANTI-INFLAMMATORY DRUGS (NSAIDs): NSAIDs can decrease the renal clearance of lithium levels and increase lithium levels (9,15). NSAIDs include diclofenac (Voltaren, Cataflam, others), ibuprofen (Advil, Motrin, others), naproxen (Anaprox, Naprosyn, others), and others.
PENTAZOCINE (Talwin): Combining serotonergic drugs such as pentazocine with lithium might increase the risk of serotonergic side effects including serotonin syndrome and cerebral vasoconstrictive disorders such as Call-Fleming syndrome (8056).
PHENOTHIAZINES: Concomitant use of lithium with phenothiazines might reduce lithium concentrations. Lithium might also reduce phenothiazine concentrations, making the pharmacokinetic effect unpredictable (9,15). Some phenothiazines are fluphenazine (Permitil, Prolixin), chlorpromazine (Thorazine), prochlorperazine (Compazine), thioridazine (Mellaril), trifluoperazine (Stelazine), and others.
SKELETAL MUSCLE RELAXANTS: Lithium might prolong neuromuscular blockade. Monitor carefully with concurrent use (9,15). Neuromuscular blockers include atracurium (Tracrium), pancuronium (Pavulon), succinylcholine (Anectine), and others.
THIAZIDE DIURETICS: Thiazide diuretics reduce lithium excretion and increase lithium levels. Reduce lithium dose by 50 per cent and monitor lithium levels (9,15). Thiazides include chlorothiazide (Diuril), hydrochlorothiazide (HydroDIURIL, Esidrix), indapamide (Lozol), metolazone (Zaroxolyn), and chlorthalidone (Hygroton).
TRAMADOL (Ultram): Combining serotonergic drugs such as tramadol with lithium might increase the risk of serotonergic side effects including serotonin syndrome and cerebral vasoconstrictive disorders such as Call-Fleming syndrome (8056).

Interactions with Foods

None known.

Interactions with Lab Tests

ERYTHROCYTES: Lithium can increase erythrocyte counts (15).
LEUKOCYTES: Lithium usually causes a reversible leukocytosis with leukocyte counts of 10,000 to 15,000 per cubic millimeter (15).
PLATELETS: Lithium can increase platelet counts (15).
THYROID FUNCTION TESTS (LFTs): Lithium can cause hypothyroidism, and less frequently, hyperthyroidism (15).

Interactions with Diseases or Conditions

CARDIOVASCULAR DISEASE: Lithium may cause arrhythmias. Cardiovascular disease may increase the risk for toxicity (15).
RENAL IMPAIRMENT: Lithium is excreted renally. Dosage reductions may be required depending on the severity of renal dysfunction (9).
THYROID DISEASE: Lithium may worsen thyroid disease (15).

Dosage and Administration

ORAL: For acute manic episodes, lithium carbonate 1.8 g or 20 to 30 mg per kg per day in 2 to 3 divided doses is used. Some clinicians begin therapy at 600 to 900 mg per day and titrate up. For bipolar disorder and other psychiatric conditions, the usual adult maintenance dose is 900 mg to 1.2 g per day in 2 to 4 divided doses. Lithium citrate solution 24 to 32 mEq given in 2 to 4 divided doses daily has also been used. Maintenance doses usually should not exceed 2.4 g of lithium carbonate or 65 mEq lithium citrate daily. For children, 15 to 60 mg per kg (0.4 to 1.6 mEq per kg) per day in divided doses has been used (9,15).
Lithium may be administered as a single daily dose, but is usually given in divided doses to lessen side effects (15). Abrupt discontinuation of lithium therapy increases the risk for relapse of bipolar disorder. Lithium should be tapered gradually over at least 14 days (9165).

There is no recommended dietary allowance (RDA) for lithium. A provisional RDA of 1 mg per day for a 70 kg adult has been suggested (9163).

Comments

Lithium gets its name from the Greek word for stone, lithos, because it is present in trace amounts in virtually all rocks (9163).

LIVER EXTRACT

Also Known As

Aqueous Liver Extract, Hydrolyzed Liver Extract, Liquid Liver Extract, Liver, Liver Concentrate, Liver Factors, Liver Fractions, Liver Hydrolysate, Liver Substance, Raw Liver.
CAUTION: See separate listing for Shark Liver Oil.

Scientific Names

None.

People Use This For

Orally, liver extract is used for improving liver function, treating chronic liver diseases, preventing liver damage, and regenerating liver tissue. It is also used for allergies; enhancing muscle development in bodybuilders; improving stamina, strength, and physical endurance; enhancing detoxification; and as an aid to recovery from chemical addiction or poisoning.

Safety

There is insufficient reliable information available about the safety of liver extract. However, since some preparations are derived from animals, there is concern about contamination with diseased animal parts (1825). So far, there are no reports of disease transmission to humans due to use of contaminated liver extract.
Pregnancy and Lactation: Insufficient reliable information available; avoid using.

Effectiveness

There is insufficient reliable information available about the effectiveness of liver extract.

Mechanism of Action

Liver extract is a concentrated product derived from animal liver, most commonly from cattle. It contains vitamin B12, folic acid, and up to 3-4 mg of heme iron per gram of product (6614). Liver extract increases liver weight and shows evidence of stimulating liver cell proliferation in experimental animals after partial hepatectomy (6650). However, information about pharmacological effects in humans is not available.

Adverse Reactions

Adverse reactions have not been reported. However, there is some concern about the possibility of contamination. Liver extract is derived from raw animal liver gathered from slaughterhouses, possibly from sick or diseased animals (6616). Products made from contaminated or diseased organs might present a human health hazard. There is also concern that liver extracts produced from cows in countries where bovine spongiform encephalitis (BSE) has been reported might be contaminated with diseased tissue. Countries where BSE has been reported include Great Britain, France, The Netherlands, Portugal, Luxembourg, Ireland, Switzerland, Oman, and Belgium (1825). However, there have been no reports of BSE transfer to humans from contaminated liver extract products. Until more is known, tell patients to avoid these products unless the country of origin can be determined. Patients should avoid products that are produced in countries where BSE has been found.

Interactions with Herbs & Other Dietary Supplements

IRON: Concomitant use might increase the risk of iron overload. Liver extract can contain 3-4 mg heme iron per gram of product (6614).

Interactions with Drugs

None known.

Interactions with Foods

None known.

Interactions with Lab Tests

HEMOGLOBIN: Liver extract might increase hemoglobin concentrations and test results due to its iron content (6614).
IRON: Liver extract might increase iron concentrations and test results due to its iron content (6614).

Interactions with Diseases or Conditions

IRON METABOLISM DISORDERS: Liver extract contains 3-4 mg of heme iron and might adversely affect people with iron metabolism disorders, including hemochromatosis (6614); contraindicated.

Dosage and Administration

No typical dosage.

LIVERWORT

Also Known As

American Liverleaf, Anémone à Lobes Aigus, Anémone d'Amérique, Hepatici noblis herba, Hépatique à Lobes Aigus, Hépatique d'Amérique, Herb Trinity, Kidney Wort, Leberbluemchenkraut, Liverleaf, Liverweed, Liverwort-Leaf, Round-Leaved Hepatica, Round-Lobe Hepatica, Sharp-Lobe Hepatica, Trefoil.
CAUTION: See separate listings for Agrimony and Red Clover.

Scientific Names

Anemone acutiloba, synonym Hepatica nobilis var. acuta; Anemone americana, synonym Hepatica nobilis var. obtusa; Anemone hepatica.
Family: Ranunculaceae.

People Use This For

Orally, liverwort is used for liver diseases, jaundice, liver enlargement, congestion, portal vein problems, hepatitis, and liver cirrhosis. It is also used orally for gastric and digestive discomfort, stimulating appetite, relieving sensation of fullness, for treating gallstones and gravel, for regulating bowel function, stimulating pancreatic function, regulating blood lipid levels, for varicose veins, stimulating systemic and cardiac circulation, increasing myocardium blood supply, strengthening nerves, "purifying" blood, stimulating metabolism, relief of menopausal symptoms, and as a general tonic or sedative.
Topically, liverwort is used for hemorrhoids or as an external rinse.

Safety

LIKELY UNSAFE ...when the fresh above ground parts are used orally or topically (2).
There is insufficient reliable information available about the safety of dried liverwort.
PREGNANCY: LIKELY UNSAFE ...when used orally or topically (2).
LACTATION: LIKELY UNSAFE ...when the fresh above ground parts are used orally or topically (2). There is insufficient reliable information available about the safety of dried liverwort while breast-feeding; avoid using.

Effectiveness

There is insufficient reliable information available about the effectiveness of liverwort.

Mechanism of Action

The applicable parts of liverwort are the fresh or dried above ground parts (2). Liverwort contains ranunculin (18), which hydrolyzes to toxic, unstable protoanemonin, which readily dimerizes to nontoxic anemonin (4). Some evidence suggests anemonin might be cytotoxic (4). Other evidence indicates anemonin and protoanemonin might have sedative and antipyretic activity (4). Protoanemonin has antimicrobial activity (2). It causes central nervous system stimulation, then paralysis in experimental animals (2). Kidney and urinary tract irritation might be due to the alkylating action of protoanemonin (2).

Adverse Reactions

Orally, fresh liverwort can cause colic, diarrhea, gastrointestinal irritation (18), and kidney and urinary tract irritation (2).
Topically, skin contact with fresh liverwort can cause irritation, mucous membrane irritation, itching, and pustule formation known a ranunculus dermatitis (2).
Inhalation of protoanemonin-containing volatile oil can cause nasal mucosal and conjunctival irritation (4).

Interactions with Herbs & Other Dietary Supplements

None known.

Interactions with Drugs

None known.

Interactions with Foods

None known.

Interactions with Lab Tests
None known.

Interactions with Diseases or Conditions
None known.

Dosage and Administration
No typical dosage.

LOBELIA

Also Known As
Asthma Weed, Bladderpod, Emetic Herb, Gagroot, Indian Tobacco, Lobelie, Pukeweed, Vomit Wort, Wild Tobacco.

Scientific Names
Lobelia inflata.
Family: Campanulaceae or Lobeliaceae.

People Use This For
Orally, lobelia is used for asthma, bronchitis, whooping cough, inducing sweating, and as a sedative.
Lobelia is also used as an ingredient in smoking cessation products and for treating apnea in newborn infants.
Topically, lobelia is used for muscle inflammation, rheumatic nodules, bruises, sprains, insect bites, poison ivy, and ringworm.
In manufacturing, lobelia is used in cough preparations and counterirritant products.

Safety
LIKELY UNSAFE ...when used orally (3,11). 0.6-1 gram of the leaf is said to be toxic and 4 grams may be fatal (18).
There is insufficient reliable information available about the safety of the topical use of lobelia.
PREGNANCY AND LACTATION: LIKELY UNSAFE ...when used orally because it has emetic effects (4,12).
There is insufficient reliable information available about the safety of lobelia for topical use during pregnancy and lactation.

Effectiveness
LIKELY INEFFECTIVE

Smoking cessation. Taking lobeline, a constituent of lobelia, is not effective when used orally for smoking cessation (13).

There is insufficient reliable information available about the effectiveness of lobelia for its other uses.

Mechanism of Action
The applicable parts of lobelia are the above ground parts. Lobelia has some anti-asthmatic, antispasmodic, emetic, expectorant, and respiratory stimulant effects (4,13). The primary constituent, (-)-lobeline, is known as alpha lobeline, to distinguish it from the mixture of lobelia alkaloids formerly called lobeline. Like nicotine but weaker, alpha lobeline exhibits effects on the peripheral circulation, neuromuscular system and central nervous system (CNS) (4,13). Small amounts of lobeline stimulate respiration and have expectorant activity (11,18). Larger amounts have emetic, purgative, and diuretic effects (11). Lobeline first causes CNS stimulation then CNS and respiratory depression (505).

Adverse Reactions
Orally, lobelia can cause nausea, vomiting, diarrhea, coughing, dizziness, and tremors (4). Overdose may cause sweating, tachycardia, convulsions, hypothermia, hypotension, coma, and possibly death (4,11).

Interactions with Herbs & Other Dietary Supplements
TOBACCO: Concomitant use with lobelia may enhance nicotine effects and adverse effects (505).

Interactions with Drugs
None known.

Interactions with Foods
None known.

Interactions with Lab Tests
None known.

Interactions with Diseases or Conditions
GASTROINTESTINAL (GI) CONDITIONS: Lobelia can irritate the GI tract. It is contraindicated in individuals with infectious or inflammatory GI conditions (19).
HEART DISEASE: Caution; dose-dependent cardiac activity is reported with lobelia (12).

Dosage and Administration
ORAL: A typical dose as an expectorant is 100 mg of leaf, 0.6-2.0 mL of the tincture (12). The dosage of specific products varies widely from 375 mg once daily to 820 mg three times daily. One supplier warns not to exceed 50 mg of the dried lobelia. An extract of lobelia is used in a dose of 2 to 5 drops three to four times daily. The extract contains alcohol (6006).

Comments
Clinical research was unable to demonstrate lobeline efficacy greater than placebo in smoking cessation (13) and it was disallowed as an ingredient in anti-smoking products in the US in 1993 (11).

LOGWOOD

Also Known As
Bloodwood, Peachwood.

Scientific Names
Haematoxylum campechianum; Haematoxylum lignum.
Family: Fabaceae/Leguminosae.

Comments
At the date of publication, this product was not a common ingredient used in brand name supplements marketed to consumers. Details about this product are available in the online version of *Natural Medicines Comprehensive Database.* See www.naturaldatabase.com.

LOOSESTRIFE

Also Known As
Yellow Willowherb.
CAUTION: See separate listing for Purple Loosestrife.

Scientific Names
Lysimachia vulgaris.
Family: Primulaceae.

Comments
At the date of publication, this product was not a common ingredient used in brand name supplements marketed to consumers. Details about this product are available in the online version of *Natural Medicines Comprehensive Database.* See www.naturaldatabase.com.

LORENZO'S OIL

Also Known As
Lorenzos Oil, Glycerol Trierucate Oil, Glycerol Trioleate Oil.

Scientific Names
13-Docosenoic acid (erucic acid); cis-9-Octadecenoic acid (oleic acid).

People Use This For
Orally, Lorenzo's oil is used as a treatment for two related genetic neurological syndromes: adrenoleukodystrophy, which occurs in children, and adrenomyeloneuropathy, which occurs in adults.

Safety
There is insufficient reliable information available about the safety of Lorenzo's oil.
Pregnancy and Lactation: Insufficient reliable information available; avoid using.

Effectiveness
LIKELY INEFFECTIVE

Adrenoleukodystrophy and adrenomyeloneuropathy. Taking Lorenzo's oil orally doesn't seem to be effective for treating adrenoleukodystrophy and adrenomyeloneuropathy (920,921,922,923,924,930). There is one case report of modest clinical benefit in a child with symptomatic adrenoleukodystrophy (929).

Mechanism of Action
Adrenoleukodystrophy and adrenomyeloneuropathy are rare genetic disorders that result in an impaired ability to oxidize saturated, very-long chain fatty acids. Buildup of these acids is thought to cause neurologic symptoms associated with the disorder (6). Monounsaturated fatty acids have been shown to inhibit production of very-long-chain fatty acids (6). However, when Lorenzo's oil is given to patients with adrenoleukodystrophy, eruric acid does not enter the brain in a significant quantity, which may be a factor in the negative results (931).

Adverse Reactions
Orally, Lorenzo's oil can cause asymptomatic thrombocytopenia (924,927) and asymptomatic neutropenia (6). One case report of purpura, petechia, and bleeding (926). May cause decrease in plasma docosahexanoic acid levels without essential fatty acid deficiency (individuals studied were also taking supplemental safflower and fish oils) (6).

Interactions with Herbs & Other Dietary Supplements
ESSENTIAL FATTY ACIDS: Supplemental essential fatty acids taken concomitantly may not prevent decreased plasma levels of docosahexaenoic acid (6).

Interactions with Drugs
None known.

Interactions with Foods
None known.

Interactions with Lab Tests
PLATELET COUNTS: Lorenzo's oil may cause false low platelet counts (927). High monounsaturated fat diets may cause true thrombocytopenia (925,927). A hand-count of platelets is recommended in individuals taking Lorenzo's oil (927).

Interactions with Diseases or Conditions
THROMBOCYTOPENIA and NEUTROPENIA: Theoretically, Lorenzo's oil may worsen existing conditions.

Dosage and Administration
ORAL: People typically use a mixture of approximately 20% erucic acid and 80% oleic acid (5278).
One clinical study used 0.3 gram per kg per day of erucic acid and 1.7 grams per kg of oleic acid per day (5277).

Comments
Lorenzo's oil is a combination of erucic acid and oleic acid in a 1:4 ratio.

LOTUS

Also Known As
Lian Fang, Lian Xu, Lian Zi, Semen Nelumbinis.

Scientific Names
Nelumbo nucifera, synonyms Nelumbo caspica, Nelumbo komarovii, Nelumbo nelumbo, Nelumbo speciosum, Nymphaea nelumbo.
Family: Nelumbonaceae.

Comments
At the date of publication, there was very little scientific information available about this product. Our staff is continually analyzing the available information on natural medicines and will add data to the online version of *Natural Medicines Comprehensive Database* as it becomes available. See www.naturaldatabase.com.

LOVAGE

Also Known As

Lavose, Levistici radix, Love Parsley, Maggi Plant, Sea Parsley, Smallage, Smellage.

Scientific Names

Levisticum officinale, synonyms Angelica levisticum, Hipposelinum levisticum, Ligusticum levisticum.
Family: Apiaceae/Umbelliferae.

People Use This For

Orally, lovage is used as "irrigation therapy" for inflammation of the lower urinary tract, for prevention of kidney gravel, and as a diuretic for urinary tract infections or pedal edema. Lovage is also used orally for indigestion, heartburn, stomach distention, flatulence, as an expectorant, to loosen secretions in respiratory conditions, for menstrual irregularities, sore throat, boils, jaundice, malaria, pleurisy, gout, rheumatism, and migraines.
In foods and beverages, lovage is used as a flavor component.
In manufacturing, lovage is used as a fragrance component in soaps and cosmetics.

Safety

LIKELY SAFE ...when used orally in amounts commonly found in foods. Lovage has Generally Recognized As Safe status (GRAS) for use in foods in the US (4912).
POSSIBLY SAFE ...when used orally and appropriately (12).
PREGNANCY: LIKELY UNSAFE ...when used orally; lovage is reported to have uterine and menstrual stimulant effects (12).
LACTATION: Insufficient reliable information available; avoid using.

Effectiveness

There is insufficient reliable information available about the effectiveness of lovage.

Mechanism of Action

The applicable parts of lovage are the rhizome and root. Lovage contains 0.2-2% volatile oil (5,6,8,11).
Its principal constituents are lactone derivatives known as phthalides. Of these, ligustilide has sedative (6,8,11), antispasmodic (6,8,11), and aquaretic (5,6,8,11,512) effects in experimental animals. Aquaretics increase urine volume (water loss) but not electrolyte excretion (512). It can also have varied actions including cholinergic and antimicrobial activity (18), increased uterine tone (12), and increased gastrointestinal blood flow (6). The bitter taste and aroma of lovage can increase the production of saliva and gastric juices (6,8,18). The furanocoumarin constituents might cause phototoxic reactions including photosensitivity dermatitis (2,5,6,8,11,12).

Adverse Reactions

Orally, long-term use may result in an increased risk of phototoxic reactions, including photosensitivity dermatitis (2,5,6,8,11,12). Avoid excessive exposure to the sun or UV light if using lovage (2,12).

Interactions with Herbs & Other Dietary Supplements

None known.

Interactions with Drugs

DIURETIC DRUGS: Theoretically, lovage root might interfere with diuretic therapy due to the aquaretic effects of lovage (512).

Interactions with Foods

None known.

Interactions with Lab Tests

None known.

Interactions with Diseases or Conditions

EDEMA: "Irrigation therapy," which is the use of a mild diuretic and copious fluid intake to increase urine flow, is contraindicated in cases of edema that are due to limited heart or kidney function (2).
HYPERTENSION: Theoretically, lovage root might increase sodium retention and worsen hypertension (512).
RENAL DISEASE: Lovage is contraindicated in acute kidney inflammation (2,8,12) or impaired kidney function (2,12).

Dosage and Administration

ORAL: The typical dose of lovage is one cup of the tea two to three times per day (8). The tea is prepared by steeping 1.5-3 grams of the dried root in 150 mL boiling water for 10-15 minutes and then straining. Lovage should only be used up to 4-8 grams of the dried root per day (2,7). Ample fluid intake is essential when used for "irrigation therapy" (18). For stomach complaints, one cup of the tea is commonly taken 30 minutes before meals (8). Avoid excessive sun or UV light exposure with prolonged use of lovage due to its phototoxic adverse effects.

LUFFA

Also Known As

Angled Loofah, Dishcloth Sponge, Loofa, Loofah, Luffaschwamm, Sigualuo, Silky Loofah, Smooth Loofah, Sponge Cucumber, Vegetable Sponge, Water Gourd.

Scientific Names

Luffa aegyptiaca; Luffa acutangula; Luffa cylindrica.
Family: Cucurbitaceae.

People Use This For

Orally, luffa is used for treating and preventing colds, nasal inflammation, sinusitis, suppuration of the sinuses, for arthritis pain, muscle pain, chest pain, amenorrhea, and to promote lactation.
Topically, luffa sponge is used to remove dead skin and stimulate the skin. Luffa charcoal is used topically for shingles in the face and eye region.
In foods, young luffa fruits are eaten as vegetables.
In cosmetics, powdered luffa is used in skin care products as an anti-inflammatory and detoxicant.

Safety

LIKELY SAFE ...when used topically as a sponge for exfoliation (11).
POSSIBLY SAFE ...when used orally in amounts found in foods (11).
There is insufficient reliable information available about the safety of luffa for its other uses.
PREGNANCY AND LACTATION: POSSIBLY SAFE ...when used orally in amounts found in foods (11).

Effectiveness

There is insufficient reliable information available about the effectiveness of luffa.

Mechanism of Action

The applicable part of luffa is the dried fiber structure from the ripe fruit. The toxicity of luffa is low.

Adverse Reactions

None reported.

Interactions with Herbs & Other Dietary Supplements

None known.

Interactions with Drugs

None known.

Interactions with Foods

None known.

Interactions with Lab Tests

None known.

Interactions with Diseases or Conditions

None known.

Dosage and Administration

ORAL: No typical dosage.
TOPICAL: Luffa is powdered and used in skin care products. The intact sponge is also used to remove dead skin (11).

LUNGMOSS

Also Known As
Lungwort, Oak Lungs.
CAUTION: See separate listing for Lungwort.

Scientific Names
Lobaria pulmonaria.
Family: Lobariaceae.

Comments
At the date of publication, there was very little scientific information available about this product. Our staff is continually analyzing the available information on natural medicines and will add data to the online version of *Natural Medicines Comprehensive Database* as it becomes available. See www.naturaldatabase.com.

LUNGWORT

Also Known As
Dage of Jerusalem, Lungenkraut, Pulmonariae herba.
CAUTION: See separate listing for Lungmoss.

Scientific Names
Pulmonaria officinalis.
Family: Boraginaceae.

People Use This For
Orally, lungwort is used to treat conditions of the respiratory tract, gastrointestinal (GI) tract, kidney tract, and urinary tract. Lungwort is also used orally in irritant-relieving cough medicines, as a diuretic, and to treat lung diseases such as tuberculosis.
Topically, it is used as an astringent and to treat wounds.

Safety
There is insufficient reliable information available about the safety of lungwort.
Pregnancy and Lactation: Insufficient reliable information available; avoid using.

Effectiveness
There is insufficient reliable information available about the effectiveness of lungwort.

Mechanism of Action
The applicable parts of lungwort are the above ground parts. Most plants in this family contain hepatotoxic pyrrolizidine alkaloids, but lungwort doesn't appear to contain these toxins (12842).

Adverse Reactions
None reported.

Interactions with Herbs & Other Dietary Supplements
None known.

Interactions with Drugs
None known.

Interactions with Foods
None known.

Interactions with Lab Tests
None known.

Interactions with Diseases or Conditions
None known.

Dosage and Administration
No typical dosage.

LUTEIN

Also Known As
Xanthophyll, Zeaxanthin.

Scientific Names
Beta,epsilon-carotene-3,3'-diol.

People Use This For
Orally, lutein is used for preventing age-related macular degeneration (AMD), cataracts, retinitis pigmentosa, and colon cancer.

Safety
LIKELY SAFE ...when used orally (219,3219,3220).
PREGNANCY AND LACTATION: LIKELY SAFE ...when used orally (219,3219,3220).

Effectiveness
POSSIBLY EFFECTIVE

Age-related macular degeneration (AMD). There is some epidemiological evidence that people who consume higher amounts of lutein in their diet have a reduced risk of developing AMD (219,2394). Preliminary clinical research suggests that taking lutein supplements 10 mg per day for 12 months can improve some symptoms of AMD such as macular pigment optical density and glare recovery, near vision acuity, and contrast sensitivity. But lutein supplements don't seem to affect the progression of AMD. It's not known whether lutein supplements can decrease the risk of AMD as effectively as dietary lutein (11798).

Cataracts. There are epidemiological studies that suggest a reduced risk of developing severe cataracts that require surgical removal in people consuming higher amounts of lutein in their diet (2395,3219,3220). It is not known if supplemental lutein offers the same benefit.

Colorectal cancer. There is epidemiological evidence that suggests a reduced risk of developing colon cancer in people consuming higher amounts of lutein in their diet (3962). It is not known if supplemental lutein offers the same benefit.

INSUFFICIENT RELIABLE EVIDENCE to RATE

Retinitis pigmentosa. Preliminary clinical evidence suggests that oral lutein might be helpful in the treatment of retinitis pigmentosa (10279). More evidence is needed to rate lutein for this use.

Mechanism of Action
Lutein is a carotenoid that is typically found in combination with its stereoisomer, zeaxanthin. Lutein makes up about 11% of the total carotenoids in serum and about 20% of the carotenoids in adipose tissue. Serum and adipose tissue levels are affected by dietary intake. Lutein levels in breast adipose tissue seem to be affected by diet, which could explain the lower incidence of breast cancer with increased fruit and vegetable intake (10243). Additionally, there is some evidence of an inverse association between serum lutein levels and breast cancer risk (10132). Lutein and zeaxanthin are the two major carotenoid pigments in the human macula and retina (2388,3225). They are thought to function as antioxidants and as blue light filters, protecting underlying ocular tissues from photodamage.
Epidemiological evidence has associated high dietary lutein intake with reduced risk of developing age-related macular degeneration (AMD) and cataracts (2394,2395,3219,3220). Increasing dietary lutein intake increases serum lutein levels and macular pigment density (2389,10245). Low dietary lutein intake is associated with males, smokers, and people who drink alcohol (more than 2 drinks per week); while higher dietary lutein intake is associated with females, increasing age, and people with hypertension (2398). Foods containing high concentrations of lutein such as broccoli, spinach, and kale, are associated with the greatest eye health benefits (3219,3220). Other carotenoids and antioxidants such as vitamin A, lycopene, alpha- or beta-carotene, vitamin C, and vitamin E have not been associated with this benefit (3219,3220,3221,3222,3223). Epidemiologic studies have shown that carotenoids might be inversely associated with cancer (3963,3964).

Adverse Reactions
None reported.

Interactions with Herbs & Other Dietary Supplements
BETA-CAROTENE: Concomitant administration may reduce bioavailability of lutein and may reduce or increase bioavailability of beta-carotene (2390,2391).

Interactions with Drugs
None known.

Interactions with Foods

OLESTRA: Theoretically, use of Olestra may interfere with supplemental lutein activity. Olestra (fat substitute) lowers serum lutein concentrations in healthy people (2392).

Interactions with Lab Tests

None known.

Interactions with Diseases or Conditions

None known.

Dosage and Administration

ORAL: For reducing the risk of cataracts and age-related macular degeneration (AMD), 6 mg of lutein per day, either through diet or supplementation has been suggested. People consuming 6.9-11.7 mg of lutein per day through diet had the lowest risk of developing AMD and cataracts (3219,3220). For reducing symptoms of AMD, 10 mg per day of lutein supplements have been used (11798). There is 44 mg of lutein per cup of cooked kale, 26 mg/cup of cooked spinach, and 3 mg/cup of broccoli (219,3219,3220). Commercial products containing 6 mg or 20 mg of lutein are available (5020). Supplemental esterified lutein is better absorbed when taken with high fat (36 grams fat) meals compared to low-fat (3 grams fat) meals (6133).

Comments

Centrum and Centrum Silver now contain lutein 0.25 mg per tablet, but probably not enough to provide much benefit (219,3219,3220). Avoid confusion with lutein extract (dried powdered hog corpora lutea) formerly used as a source of progesterone (511). Although dark green leafy vegetables contain 15-47% lutein, they have a very low zeaxanthin content (0-3%). Corn is richest in lutein (60% of total carotenoids), and orange pepper is richest in zeaxanthin (37% of total). Substantial amounts of lutein and zeaxanthin (30-50%) are also present in kiwi fruit, grapes, spinach, orange juice, zucchini, and different kinds of squash (3224).

LYCIUM

Also Known As

Barberry Matrimony Vine, Chinese Boxthorn, Chinese Wolfberry, Di Gu Pi, Digupi, Fructus Lycii, Fructus Lycii Berry, Goji, Goji Berry, Goji Juice, Gou Qi Zi, Gouqizi, Lycii Berries, Matrimony Vine, Ning Xia Gou Qi, Wolfberry.

Scientific Names

Lycium chinense; Lycium barbarum.
Family: Solanaceae.

People Use This For

Orally, lycium is used for diabetes, hypertension, fever, malaria, and cancer. It's also used for improving circulation, erectile dysfunction, dizziness, tinnitus; and as an eye tonic for blurred vision, macular degeneration, and other ophthalmic disorders. Lycium is also used orally to strengthen muscles and bone, and as a blood, liver, and kidney tonic. It is used orally to reduce fever, sweating, irritability, thirst, nosebleeds, hemoptysis, cough, and wheezing. In foods, the berries are eaten raw and used in cooking.

Safety

POSSIBLY SAFE ...when used orally and appropriately (12,7126).
PREGNANCY AND LACTATION: LIKELY UNSAFE ...when used orally. Lycium contains betaine, which is an emmenagogue and abortifacient (12,7123); avoid using.

Effectiveness

There is insufficient reliable information available about the effectiveness of lycium.

Mechanism of Action

The applicable parts of lycium are the dried berries and root bark. Both the root bark and berries contain pharmacologically active constituents. Both contain beta-sitosterol which can reduce cholesterol levels by preventing cholesterol absorption in the gastrointestinal tract (5814,7123,7126). The root bark also contains the constituent kukoamine, which might also have cholesterol lowering effects and antihypertensive effects (7123,7126). Lycium root bark also seems to have hypoglycemic effects. Peak blood glucose lowering effects are thought to occur after 3-4 hours and last for 7-8 hours. Lycium root bark is also thought to have antibacterial, antipyretic, and antihypersensitivity properties (7126). Both the root bark and berry contain betaine, which has uterine stimulant properties (7123,7126). The berries also contain beta-carotene, niacin, pyridoxine, and ascorbic acid (7123). There is some preliminary evidence that a cerebroside constituent found in lycium berry might also have hepatoprotective properties (7125).

Adverse Reactions

Orally, the dried root bark has been associated with nausea and vomiting (7126).

Interactions with Herbs & Other Dietary Supplements

HERBS AND SUPPLEMENTS WITH HYPOGLYCEMIC EFFECTS: Lycium root bark might have hypoglycemic effects (7126). Theoretically, concomitant use with other herbs and supplements that decrease blood glucose levels might increase the risk of hypoglycemia. Some of these products include bitter melon, ginger, goat's rue, fenugreek, kudzu, willow bark, and others.

HERBS AND SUPPLEMENTS WITH HYPOTENSIVE EFFECTS: Lycium root bark might have antihypertensive effects (7126). Theoretically, concurrent use of lycium root bark with other herbs and supplements that decrease blood pressure might increase risk of hypotension. Some of these products include danshen, ginger, Panax ginseng, turmeric, valerian, and others.

Interactions with Drugs

ANTIDIABETES DRUGS: Lycium root bark might have hypoglycemic effects (7126). Theoretically, concomitant use with drugs used for diabetes might enhance blood glucose lowering effects and increase the risk of hypoglycemia. Monitor blood glucose levels closely. Some antidiabetes drugs include glimepiride (Amaryl), glyburide (Diabeta, Glynase PresTab, Micronase), insulin, pioglitazone (Actos), rosiglitazone (Avandia), and others.

ANTIHYPERTENSIVE DRUGS: Lycium root bark might have hypotensive effects (7126). Theoretically, concomitant use with antihypertensives might have additive effects on blood pressure and increase the risk of hypotension.

CYTOCHROME P450 2C9 (CYP2C9) SUBSTRATES: There is some evidence that lycium can inhibit CYP2C9 (7158). Watch for an increase in the levels of drugs metabolized by CYP2C9 in patients taking lycium. Some drugs metabolized by CYP2C9 include amitriptyline (Elavil), diazepam (Valium), estradiol (Estrace), tacrine (Cognex), verapamil (Calan), warfarin (Coumadin), zileuton (Zyflo), and others.

WARFARIN (Coumadin): There is some evidence that lycium can increase the effects of warfarin and possibly increase the risk of bleeding. International normalized ratio (INR) can increase in patients stabilized on warfarin who begin taking lycium. Researchers think that lycium inhibits cytochrome P450 2C9 (CYP2C9) metabolism of warfarin and increases warfarin levels (7158). Use with caution. Warfarin dose adjustments may be necessary.

Interactions with Foods

None known.

Interactions with Lab Tests

BLOOD GLUCOSE: Lycium root bark might lower blood glucose levels in some patients (7126).

WHITE BLOOD CELL COUNT (WBC): Lycium berries might increase leukocyte and lymphocyte counts in some patients (7126).

Interactions with Diseases or Conditions

DIABETES: Lycium root bark might have hypoglycemic effects (7126). Theoretically, use in patients treated with antidiabetes medications might enhance blood glucose lowering effects and increase the risk of hypoglycemia. Monitor blood glucose levels closely (7126).

HYPERTENSION: Lycium root bark might have hypotensive effects (7126). Theoretically, concomitant use in patients treated with antihypertensives might have additive effects on blood pressure and potentially increase the risk of hypotension.

HYPOTENSION: Lycium root bark might have hypotensive effects (7126). Theoretically, use in people with existing low blood pressure might exacerbate hypotension and possibly lead to syncope.

Dosage and Administration

ORAL: Lycium is usually taken as a tea. A typical dose is one or more cups of tea daily; however, the strength of the tea can vary depending on the condition being treated. Typically the tea is made by boiling 20 grams of berries or root bark in 3 cups of water and simmered until the volume is reduced to 2 cups. For fever, one cup daily of this preparation is commonly used (7122). For diabetes, 6 to 12 grams is commonly boiled and consumed as a tea. For hypertension, 30 grams of the root bark boiled in 100 mL is commonly used. For treating malaria, 30 grams of the root bark is commonly boiled and consumed as a tea (7126).

Comments

Lycium is a native Chinese deciduous shrub with bright red berries. The use of lycium was first described in the first century AD in Chinese literature. Traditionally, lycium has been used to promote longevity. Legend reports that one herbalist who used lycium in combination with other tonic herbs lived 252 years (7122).

LYCOPENE

Also Known As
Lycopenes.

Scientific Names
All-Trans Lycopene, Psi-Psi-Carotene.

People Use This For
Orally, lycopene is used for preventing atherosclerosis, cardiovascular disease, and cancer. Lycopene is also used to treat prostate cancer, human papilloma virus (HPV) infection, and asthma.

Safety
LIKELY SAFE ...when consumed in amounts commonly found in foods (2406,7772,7773).
POSSIBLY SAFE ...when used orally in medicinal amounts. Lycopene supplements 30 mg daily have been used safely for eight weeks (7771,7898,7899).
PREGNANCY AND LACTATION: LIKELY SAFE ...when consumed in amounts commonly found in foods. There is insufficient reliable information available about the safety of lycopene supplements used during pregnancy and lactation; avoid using in amounts greater than those typically found in foods.

Effectiveness
POSSIBLY EFFECTIVE

Asthma. Taking a specific tomato extract containing lycopene (Lyc-o-mato) orally seems to reduce exercise-induced asthma. Lycopene seems to prevent decreases in forced expiratory volume (FEV1) in response to exercise in some people with exercise-induced asthma (7898).

Lung cancer. There is epidemiological evidence that consuming lycopene from foods (12 mg per day or more for men, and 6.5 mg per day or more for women) decreases the risk of lung cancer in nonsmoking men aged 40 to 75, and non-smoking women aged 30 to 55 (2595).

Ovarian cancer. There is some evidence a diet rich in carotenoids, including lycopene, can decrease the risk of ovarian cancer in premenopausal women (10133).

Prostate cancer. Men who consume 6 mg per day or more of lycopene from foods such as tomatoes and tomato products seem to have a significantly reduced risk of developing prostate cancer (2406,7772,7773,7895,12878). Men with high lycopene plasma levels seem to have an 83% lower risk of prostate cancer compared to men with low plasma lycopene levels (7773). Lycopene supplements haven't been studied for prostate cancer prevention. Recommend a diet high in tomatoes and tomato products, particularly tomato sauce, to men concerned about prostate cancer prevention (7772). However, there is preliminary evidence that lycopene supplements might help for prostate cancer treatment. Taking lycopene supplements, 15 mg twice daily, for three weeks before radical prostatectomy might decrease tumor growth (7771).

POSSIBLY INEFFECTIVE

Bladder cancer. Consuming dietary lycopene doesn't seem to reduce the risk of bladder cancer. Epidemiological research shows no association between dietary lycopene intake or serum lycopene levels and the risk of bladder cancer (2407).

Cardiovascular disease. Epidemiologic evidence in women without heart disease suggests that there is no association between dietary lycopene intake and the risk of myocardial infarction, stroke, and other cardiovascular events (10418). Epidemiologic evidence in men at low risk for heart disease suggests dietary intake of lycopene doesn't prevent myocardial infarction (9594).

Colorectal cancer. Epidemiological research shows no association between dietary lycopene intake and the risk of colon cancer (3962).

INSUFFICIENT RELIABLE EVIDENCE to RATE

Atherosclerosis. Epidemiological studies of dietary lycopene intake and prevention of atherosclerosis are inconclusive (1446,1449).

Breast cancer. Preliminary research suggests that higher serum levels of lycopene might be protective against breast cancer (10132).

Human papilloma virus (HPV). Preliminary evidence suggests that women with higher plasma levels of lycopene have a faster rate of oncogenic HPV clearance compared to women with lower levels of plasma lycopene. Women with higher levels of lycopene cleared oncogenic HPV in an average of 8.5 months compared to 11-12 months in women with lower levels (12177).

More evidence is needed to rate lycopene for these uses.

Mechanism of Action

Lycopene is a carotenoid, but contains no vitamin A activity (1928,7771,7895,7896). It is the pigment that gives some fruits and vegetables, such as tomatoes, their red color (1928,2401). It is also found in watermelons, pink grapefruits, apricots, and pink guavas.

In North America, 85% of dietary lycopene comes from tomato-derived products such as tomato juice or paste. One cup (240 mL) of tomato juice provides about 23 mg of lycopene (1499). Lycopene exists naturally in fresh fruits and vegetables in the trans configuration, which is poorly absorbed (1928). Heat processing of raw foods into products such as tomato paste, juice, ketchup, and others induces the isomerization of lycopene from the trans- to the cis-configuration. The cis isomer has better bioavailability (1928,1497). Serum concentrations and adipose tissue concentrations of lycopene are influenced by dietary intake (10243). Lycopene supplements seem to have a similar bioavailability to foods; lycopene supplements can provide serum lycopene levels similar to tomato juice when ingested in equivalent amounts (1498).

Lycopene is a predominant carotenoid in blood and tissues (7773,10243). It is highly lipophilic and is commonly found within cellular membranes. Lycopene has the most potent antioxidant activity of any common carotenoid; it might reduce cancer risk by scavenging free radicals and quenching singlet oxygen, which prevents oxidative damage to DNA (2401,7773). Some researchers are interested in lycopene as a prevention of cancer, atherosclerosis, and other conditions. In vitro, lycopene seems to inhibit the oxidation of low density lipoproteins (LDL) (1928). Like other carotenoid substances, lycopene is transported in the blood and on LDL cholesterol, making it readily available to act as an antioxidant. Preliminary evidence suggests that lycopene may decrease cholesterol synthesis and increase removal of LDL cholesterol from circulation (7896). Lower tissue levels of lycopene have been associated with increased risk of myocardial infarction (MI), but epidemiological studies have found no correlation between lycopene intake and MI risk (7897,9594,10418).

In vitro, lycopene inhibits the proliferation of breast cancer, lung cancer, and prostate cancer (1928). There is also some evidence that decreased serum or tissue lycopene concentrations might increase the risk of developing prostate cancer (1447,1496,2405,2406,2407). Lycopene seems to have some direct effects within the prostate, specifically up-regulating tumor suppressor genes (7771). However, some preliminary research in human prostate cancer cells suggests lycopene might worsen established prostate cancer. It doesn't seem to inhibit cancer cell proliferation, but might increase bone metastasis. It also doesn't seem to increase expression of the cancer-suppressing protein, connexin (12895). However, limited clinical research suggests lycopene might be useful for treating prostate cancer in combination with surgery (7771).

Animal research suggests lycopene alone might not affect prostate cancer risk. Tomato products, which contain lycopene, inhibit experimentally induced prostate cancer; lycopene alone does not (11304,11305). Lycopene supplements for prostate cancer have not been studied in humans.

Lycopene seems to reduce proliferation of prostatic epithelial cells (11237). But there's no credible clinical research to support using lycopene supplements to treat or prevent benign prostatic hyperplasia (BPH).

Adverse Reactions

None reported.

Interactions with Herbs & Other Dietary Supplements

BETA-CAROTENE: Concomitant ingestion may increase lycopene absorption (2403).

Interactions with Drugs

None known.

Interactions with Foods

None known.

Interactions with Lab Tests

PROSTATE-SPECIFIC ANTIGEN (PSA): Lycopene seems to reduce plasma PSA levels in men with prostate cancer (7771,7774).

Interactions with Diseases or Conditions

PROSTATE CANCER: Preliminary research suggests lycopene might worsen established prostate cancer by increasing metastasis without having any effect on cancer cell proliferation (12895). Until more is known, avoid lycopene use in men with established prostate cancer.

Dosage and Administration

ORAL: For decreasing the growth of prostate cancer, lycopene 15 mg twice daily has been used (7771). For reducing the risk of prostate cancer, at least 6 mg of lycopene per day from foods is needed (2406). Suggest eating one serving per day or five servings per week of tomato products (12883). For reducing the risk of lung cancer in non-smoking men, at least 12 mg of lycopene per day from foods is needed (2595). For reducing the risk of lung cancer in non-smoking women, at least 6.5 mg of lycopene per day from foods is needed (2595). For preventing exercise-induced asthma, lycopene 30 mg daily has been used (7898).

LYSINE

Also Known As
L-Lysine, Lys, Lysine Hydrochloride, Lysine Monohydrochloride.

Scientific Names
L-2,6-diaminohexanoic acid.

People Use This For
Orally, lysine is used for preventing and treating clinical symptoms of recurrent herpes simplex labialis. It is also used as an aid to improving athletic performance.
Lysine monohydrochloride is used to treat metabolic alkalosis.

Safety
POSSIBLY SAFE ...when used orally and appropriately for up to one year (1114,1120).
PREGNANCY AND LACTATION: Insufficient reliable information available; avoid using.

Effectiveness
POSSIBLY EFFECTIVE

Herpes labialis (cold sores). Taking lysine orally seems to reduce recurrences of herpes simplex labialis infections (1114,1115,1116,1118,1120), and reduce the severity and healing time of herpes simplex labialis infections (1119,1120).

There is insufficient reliable information available about the effectiveness of lysine for its other uses.

Mechanism of Action
Lysine is required for collagen synthesis and it may be important to bone health (1124,1130). Lysine antagonizes herpes simplex virus (HSV) growth in vitro and this effect may be important clinically (119).

Adverse Reactions
Orally, diarrhea and abdominal pain occur have been reported (1114,1115,1116,1118,1120). There is one case report of supplemental lysine use associated with tubulointerstitial nephritis progressing to chronic renal failure (1121).

Interactions with Herbs & Other Dietary Supplements
CALCIUM SUPPLEMENTS: Concomitant use may increase supplemental calcium absorption and decrease urine calcium loss (1131).

Interactions with Drugs
CALCIUM SUPPLEMENTS: Concomitant use may increase supplemental calcium absorption and decrease urine calcium loss (1131).

Interactions with Foods
None known.

Interactions with Lab Tests
None known.

Interactions with Diseases or Conditions
KIDNEY DISEASES: There is one case report of supplemental lysine associated with tubulointerstitial nephritis progressing to chronic renal failure (1121).
OSTEOPOROSIS: Concomitant use of lysine and calcium supplements may increase supplemental calcium absorption and decrease urine calcium loss (1131).

Dosage and Administration
ORAL: Recurrent herpes simplex labialis infections, 1000 mg daily for twelve months and 1000 mg three times daily for six months reported in clinical trials (1114,1120).

MACA

Also Known As
Ayak Chichira, Ayuk Willku, Maca Maca, Maino, Maka, Peruvian Ginseng.

Scientific Names
Lepidium meyenii, synonym Lepidium peruvianum.
Family: Brassicaceae/Cruciferae.

People Use This For
Orally, maca is used for anemia; chronic fatigue syndrome; and enhancing energy, stamina, athletic performance, and memory. It is also used for female hormone imbalance, menstrual irregularities, enhancing fertility, menopause symptoms, depression, stomach cancer, leukemia, AIDS, tuberculosis, as an aphrodisiac, for impotence, and as an immunostimulant.
In foods, maca is eaten baked or roasted, prepared as a soup, and used for making a fermented drink, maca chicha.

Safety
LIKELY SAFE ...when maca is consumed in food amounts (9926).
POSSIBLY SAFE ...when used orally and appropriately, short-term. Maca appears to be safe in doses up to 3 grams daily for 12 weeks (10218).
PREGNANCY AND LACTATION: There is insufficient reliable information available about the safety of maca in medicinal amounts during pregnancy and lactation; avoid using.

Effectiveness
POSSIBLY EFFECTIVE

Sexual desire. Taking maca orally 1.5 to 3 grams per day seems to increase subjective feelings of sexual desire in healthy men (9928).

There is insufficient reliable information available about the effectiveness of maca for its other uses.

Mechanism of Action
The applicable part of maca is the root. Dried maca root contains 59% carbohydrates; 10.2% protein; 8.5% fiber; and 2.2% lipids including linolenic, palmitic, and oleic acids. It contains sterols such as campesterol, stigmasterol, and beta-sitosterol. It also contains significant amounts of minerals including iron, calcium, and copper (9929). Two polyunsaturated fatty acids, macaene and macamide, are used as marker compounds for maca (9926). Lipid extracts of macaene and macamide seem to increase sexual activity and correct erectile dysfunction in experimental animals. The mechanism for this activity is unknown (10218). Maca does not appear to significantly affect serum concentrations of reproductive hormones including testosterone, estradiol, and 17-hydroxyprogesterone in healthy men (10219).
Maca also contains glucosinolates, which might have cancer-protecting properties and central nervous system effects (9927,9929).

Adverse Reactions
None reported.

Interactions with Herbs & Other Dietary Supplements
None known.

Interactions with Drugs
None known.

Interactions with Foods
None known.

Interactions with Lab Tests
None known.

Interactions with Diseases or Conditions
None known.

Dosage and Administration
ORAL: For enhancing sexual desire in men, 1500 to 3000 mg daily in 3 divided doses has been used. The 1500 mg dose appears to be as effective as the 3000 mg dose (9928).

Comments
Maca grows in central Peru in the high plateaus of the Andes mountains. It has been cultivated as a vegetable crop in the Andes mountains of Peru for at least 3000 years. Maca is a relative of the radish and has an odor similar to butterscotch. It was also used to enhance the fertility of humans and livestock (9925,9926).

MACADAMIA NUT

Also Known As
Australian Nut, Bopple Nut, Bush Nut, Queensland Nut.

Scientific Names
Macadamia integrifolia; Macadamia tetraphylla.
Family: Proteaceae.

People Use This For
Orally, macadamia nuts are used to lower cholesterol.
In foods, macadamia nuts are used as a roasted snack.

Safety
LIKELY SAFE ...when used as food (12598,12599).
POSSIBLY SAFE ...when used in medicinal amounts (12598,12599).
PREGNANCY and LACTATION: LIKELY SAFE ...when used as food (12598,12599). There is insufficient reliable information available about the safety of using macadamia nuts in medicinal amounts during pregnancy; avoid using.

Effectiveness
POSSIBLY EFFECTIVE

Hypercholesterolemia. Eating macadamia nuts as part of a healthy diet seems to modestly lower total and low-density lipoprotein (LDL) cholesterol, and to raise high-density lipoprotein (HDL) cholesterol (12598,12599). In hypercholesterolemic men, eating 40 to 90 grams (about 17 to 37 nuts) per day of macadamia nuts for 4 weeks, total cholesterol is decreased by 3% and LDL by 5.3% while HDL increased by 7.9% (12598).

Mechanism of Action
The applicable part of the macadamia nuts are the hulled seed (nut). Macadamia nuts are about 75% fat by weight with 85% of its energy from fat. Macadamia nuts contain the highest amount of monounsaturated fatty acids (MUFA) of any food. It contains oleic acid as well as a substantial amount of palmitoleic acid (do not confuse with palmitic acid). Macadamia nuts also contain plant sterols. Both MUFA and plant sterols can lower cholesterol. Macadamia nuts also contain carbohydrates, fiber, and vitamins and minerals (12598,12599).

Adverse Reactions
Orally, macadamia nuts are well tolerated (12598,12599). Rarely, eating macadamia nuts can cause allergy including anaphylaxis (12600,12601). Processing methods may affect allergenicity of nuts (12602). Dermatitis has been associated with occupational exposure to macadamia nut shells (12603).

Interactions with Herbs & Other Dietary Supplements
None known.

Interactions with Drugs
None known.

Interactions with Foods
None known.

Interactions with Lab Tests
CHOLESTEROL: Macadamia nuts seem to reduce serum total cholesterol and low-density lipoprotein (LDL) cholesterol and increase high-density lipoprotein (HDL) cholesterol concentrations and test results (12598,12599).

Interactions with Diseases or Conditions
None known.

Dosage and Administration
ORAL: For reducing cholesterol, 40 to 90 grams (about 17 to 37 nuts) per day has been used (12598).

Comments

Macadamia nuts are native to Australia. They are grown commercially in Hawaii, and to a much smaller extent in California and Florida (12601,12603).

MADAGASCAR PERIWINKLE

Also Known As

Cape Periwinkle, Catharanthus, Church-Flower, Magdalena, Myrtle, Old Maid, Periwinkle, Ram-Goat Rose, Red Periwinkle.
CAUTION: See separate listing for Periwinkle.

Scientific Names

Catharanthus roseus, synonyms Vinca rosea, Lochnera rosea, Ammocallis rosea.
Family: Apocynaceae.

People Use This For

Orally, Madagascar periwinkle is used for diabetes, cancer, as a cough remedy, for easing lung congestion, throat inflammation, and as a diuretic.
Topically, it is used as a hemostatic, for insect bites, wasp stings, eye irritation, infection, and inflammation.

Safety

LIKELY UNSAFE ...when the plant or root are used orally. Madagascar periwinkle contains vinca alkaloids which can cause death (6).
There is insufficient reliable information available about the safety of the topical use of Madagascar periwinkle.
PREGNANCY: LIKELY UNSAFE ...when used orally because it has abortifacient and teratogenic properties (19).
LACTATION: LIKELY UNSAFE ...when used orally (6); avoid using.

Effectiveness

There is insufficient reliable information available about the effectiveness of Madagascar periwinkle.

Mechanism of Action

The applicable parts of Madagascar periwinkle are the above ground parts. The vinca alkaloids, vincristine and vinblastine, block cell mitosis, have immunosuppressive effects, and in high concentrations, exert effects on nucleic acid and protein synthesis (6,15). The constituent, catharanthine, demonstrates diuretic properties (6). Hypotensive constituents, reserpine and alstonine, have also been isolated from Madagascar periwinkle root (6). The constituent, ajmalicine, may improve cerebral blood flow; it has been combined with rauwolfia alkaloids for treating high blood pressure (6). Concentrated extracts are reported to lower blood glucose (6), but studies by one pharmaceutical company found the plant had no effect on blood glucose levels (6).

Adverse Reactions

Orally, the plant is an hallucinogen, and has caused seizures, GI upset, hepatotoxicity, and alopecia (17). Adverse effects of Vinca alkaloids include nausea, vomiting, alopecia, dizziness, nystagmus, vertigo, hearing impairment, leukopenia, thrombocytopenia, bleeding, hyperuricemia, neurotoxicity, and possibly death (6,15).

Interactions with Herbs & Other Dietary Supplements

None known.

Interactions with Drugs

ANTIDIABETES DRUGS: Madagascar periwinkle may cause hypoglycemia (6,19); monitor blood glucose control closely.

Interactions with Foods

None known.

Interactions with Lab Tests

BLOOD GLUCOSE: Madagascar periwinkle may lower blood glucose. There is conflicting information about possible hypoglycemic activity (6,19).

Interactions with Diseases or Conditions

DIABETES: Madagascar periwinkle may cause hypoglycemia (6,19).

Dosage and Administration

No typical dosage.

Comments
Madagascar periwinkle is considered likely unsafe; avoid, due to presence of toxic vinca alkaloids. The vinca alkaloids, vinblastine and vincristine, isolated from Madagascar periwinkle, are FDA approved for use as chemotherapeutic agents to treat cancers, including Hodgkin's disease, leukemia, Kaposi's sarcoma, malignant lymphomas, mycosis fungoides neuroblastoma, and Wilm's tumor (6).

MADDER

Also Known As
Dyer's Madder, Farberrote, Garance, Robbia, Rubia, Rubiae tinctorum radix.

Scientific Names
Rubia tinctorum.
Family: Rubiaceae.

People Use This For
Orally, madder is used for preventing kidney stones, for disintegrating kidney stones, and for general menstrual and urinary disorders.

Safety
LIKELY UNSAFE ...when used orally. It is potentially carcinogenic and mutagenic (2,18,19).
PREGNANCY: UNSAFE ...when used orally because it may be a potential menstrual stimulant and a genotoxin (2,19).
LACTATION: UNSAFE ...when used orally because it is a potential genotoxin (2,19). It also can cause red-colored breast milk (2).

Effectiveness
There is insufficient reliable information available about the effectiveness of madder.

Mechanism of Action
The applicable part of madder is the root. Madder contains lucidin, which is an anthracene derivative. The Ames test shows that anthracene has genotoxic activity, and causes dose-dependent increases in benign and malignant liver and kidney tumors in experimental rats (3718). Madder also seems to decrease calcium oxalate crystallization in the kidney, which potentially could induce kidney or bladder stones (2).

Adverse Reactions
Orally, madder can cause red colored urine, saliva, perspiration, and breast milk (2). There is some concern that madder can stain contact lenses. Advise patients to be cautious (6002).

Interactions with Herbs & Other Dietary Supplements
None known.

Interactions with Drugs
None known.

Interactions with Foods
None known.

Interactions with Lab Tests
COLORIMETRIC TESTS: Theoretically, madder might interfere with colorimetric tests involving urine, saliva, perspiration, and breast milk due to red coloring of these body fluids (2).

Interactions with Diseases or Conditions
None known.

Dosage and Administration
ORAL: People typically prepare madder bark using one teaspoon boiled in a covered container with 3 cups of water for 30 minutes. The liquid is cooled slowly in the closed container and taken cold, 1 to 2 cups per day (5254).

MAGNESIUM

Also Known As

Chelated Magnesium, Epsom Salts, Magnesia, Magnesium Aspartate, Magnesium Carbonate, Magnesium Chloride, Magnesium Citrate, Magnesium Gluconate, Magnesium Hydroxide, Magnesium Lactate, Magnesium Orotate, Magnesium Oxide, Magnesium Sulfate, Magnesium Trisilicate, Milk of Magnesia.
CAUTION: See separate listings for Chelated Minerals and Dolomite.

Scientific Names

Magnesium; Mg; atomic number 12.

People Use This For

Orally, magnesium is used for treating and preventing hypomagnesemia. It is also used orally as a laxative for constipation and for preparation of the bowel for surgical or diagnostic procedures. Magnesium is also used orally for treating symptoms of asthma and allergic rhinitis; for cardiovascular diseases including angina, arrhythmias, hypertension, coronary heart disease and hyperlipidemia, low high-density lipoprotein (HDL) levels, mitral valve prolapse, vasospastic angina, myocardial infarction, multiple sclerosis; and as an antacid for symptoms of gastric hyperacidity. It is also used orally for treating attention deficit-hyperactivity disorder (ADHD), chronic fatigue syndrome (CFS), fibromyalgia, pregnancy-induced leg cramps, diabetes, kidney stones, migraine headaches, osteoporosis, premenstrual syndrome, altitude sickness, urinary incontinence, kidney stones, erythromelalgia, restless leg syndrome, and for preventing hearing loss. Magnesium is also used orally by athletes to increase energy and endurance.

Topically, magnesium is used for treating infected skin ulcers, boils, and carbuncles; and for speeding wound healing. It is also used topically as a cold compress in the treatment of erysipelas and as a hot compress for deep-seated skin infections.

Parenterally, magnesium is used for acute hypomagnesemia occurring in conditions such as pancreatitis, malabsorption disorders, and cirrhosis, and for treating pre-eclampsia and eclampsia. It is also used as an additive to total parenteral nutrition (TPN) for prevention of hypomagnesemia. Intravenously, magnesium is used for controlling seizures associated with epilepsy, glomerulonephritis, or hypothyroidism when low serum magnesium levels are present. It is also used intravenously in the treatment of atrial and ventricular arrhythmias, including torsades de pointes, for preventing arrhythmias after myocardial infarction, and for cardiac arrest. Magnesium is also used intravenously for treating acute exacerbations of asthma and chronic obstructive pulmonary disease (COPD), for migraine headaches, neuropathic pain and postoperative pain, as an osmotic agent for cerebral edema, and for tetanus.

Safety

LIKELY SAFE ...when used orally and appropriately. Oral magnesium is safe when used in doses below the tolerable upper intake level (UL) of 350 mg per day (7555). ...when used parenterally and appropriately. Parenteral magnesium sulfate is an FDA-approved prescription product (9495).

POSSIBLY UNSAFE ...when used orally in excessive doses. Doses greater than the tolerable upper intake level (UL) of 350 mg frequently cause loose stools and diarrhea (7555). ...when magnesium sulfate is used topically, long-term. Prolonged use may damage the skin (9).

CHILDREN: LIKELY SAFE ...when used orally and appropriately. Magnesium is safe when used in doses below the tolerable upper intake level (UL) of 65 mg per day for children 1 to 3 years, 110 mg per day for children 4 to 8 years, and 350 mg per day for children older than 8 years (7555). ...when used parenterally and appropriately (9496). LIKELY UNSAFE ...when used orally in excessive doses. Tell patients not to use doses above the tolerable upper intake level (UL). Higher doses can cause diarrhea and symptomatic hypermagnesemia including hypotension, nausea, vomiting, and bradycardia (7555,8095).

PREGNANCY AND LACTATION: LIKELY SAFE ...when used orally and appropriately. Magnesium is safe for pregnant and breast-feeding women when used in doses below the tolerable upper intake level (UL) of 350 mg per day (7555). POSSIBLY SAFE ...when given intramuscularly prior to delivery (15). POSSIBLY UNSAFE ...when used orally in excessive doses. Tell patients to avoid exceeding the tolerable upper intake level (UL) of 350 mg per day. Higher doses frequently can cause diarrhea (7555). LIKELY UNSAFE ...when used intravenously less than two hours before delivery. Intravenous infusions of magnesium sulfate can cause neonatal respiratory depression when given to toxemic mothers (15).

Effectiveness

EFFECTIVE

Constipation. Taking magnesium orally is helpful as a laxative for constipation and for preparation of the bowel for surgical or diagnostic procedures. Magnesium citrate, sulfate, and hydroxide salts are typically used for this indication. The magnesium sulfate salt is the most potent (6430).

Gastroesophageal reflux disease (GERD). Taking magnesium orally as an antacid reduces symptoms of gastric hyperacidity or GERD. Typically, magnesium carbonate, hydroxide, oxide, or trisilicate salts are used. Magnesium hydroxide has the fastest onset of action. Magnesium carbonate is slower due to its crystal structure.

Magnesium trisilicate has the slowest onset and longest duration due to poor solubility (6844).

Hypomagnesemia. Taking magnesium orally or parenterally is helpful for treating and preventing hypomagnesemia. Magnesium deficiency typically occurs in certain disease states such as alcoholism and cirrhosis of the liver, congestive heart failure, severe or prolonged diarrhea or vomiting, kidney dysfunction, inflammatory bowel disease (IBS), pancreatitis, and various malabsorption syndromes (6280,6281,8088,8089). Hypomagnesemia is often associated with other electrolyte disorders such as hypokalemia, hyponatremia, hypophosphatemia, and hypocalcemia (8088). Magnesium deficiency can also negatively affect insulin sensitivity and metabolic control in type 2 diabetes (10664). There is some controversy regarding whether parenteral or oral magnesium replacement is better. Because higher oral doses of magnesium might result in diarrhea, some suggest parenteral administration is better. However, oral magnesium can be used carefully in adequate doses for replacement without causing diarrhea. Magnesium gluconate or chloride are preferred for oral replacement because they cause diarrhea less often (6430). Oral magnesium chloride solution has also been used for replacement purposes (10664). Magnesium oxide should be avoided due to greater risk of diarrhea. Magnesium carbonate may not be soluble enough to adequately replace magnesium levels and should also be avoided. Magnesium-rich mineral water (Hepar) has also been used for dietary supplementation (8099).

LIKELY EFFECTIVE

Pre-eclampsia and eclampsia. Administering magnesium parenterally is helpful for preventing and managing pre-eclampsia and eclampsia (9473). Intravenous or intramuscular magnesium sulfate is considered the agent of choice for pre-eclampsia and eclampsia (15).

Torsade de pointes. Administering magnesium intravenously is helpful for treating torsade de pointes. Magnesium sulfate is first-line therapy for torsade de pointes (6844).

POSSIBLY EFFECTIVE

Acute myocardial infarction (MI). Administering magnesium intravenously seems to reduce arrhythmia and mortality after an acute MI. Intravenous magnesium appears to reduce the incidence of complex ventricular arrhythmias after myocardial infarction (9497). However, intravenous magnesium therapy in an acute MI is controversial (8999), and oral magnesium supplementation seems to be ineffective for this use (1198,6844).

Arrhythmias. Administering magnesium intravenously seems to be helpful for treating atrial tachycardia, ventricular fibrillation and tachycardia, and supraventricular tachycardia (15).

Asthma. Administering magnesium intravenously seems to improve acute asthma attacks. A single dose of magnesium seems to improve pulmonary function in asthma exacerbation (9495,9496). However, magnesium supplementation doesn't seem to improve forced expiratory volume in one second (FEV1) or reduce the need for bronchodilator use in patients with chronic asthma (1173).

Cancer-associated neuropathic pain. Administering magnesium intravenously seems to relieve neuropathic pain associated with cancer. Single 500 mg to 1 gram doses of magnesium sulfate seem to relieve neuropathic pain for up to four hours (6846).

Chronic fatigue syndrome (CFS). Administering magnesium intramuscularly seems to improve symptoms for CFS. There is some controversy about the clinical benefits of magnesium for CFS. In people with low red blood cell magnesium, there is some evidence that weekly intramuscular injections of 1 gram magnesium sulfate might improve CFS symptoms (7556). However, there is additional evidence that most patients with CFS have normal magnesium stores (7557,8084,8086,8087). Also, measurement of red cell magnesium is considered to be a poor indicator of body magnesium (8085).

Chronic obstructive pulmonary disease (COPD). Administering magnesium intravenously seems to be helpful for treating acute exacerbation of COPD (1208).

Cluster headache. Administering magnesium intravenously seems to improve cluster headaches (1184,1185).

Coronary artery disease. Taking magnesium orally seems to reduce anginal attacks in people with coronary artery disease (1181).

Diabetes. Higher dietary magnesium intake seems to lower the risk of developing type 2 diabetes, especially in overweight middle-aged women (11352). However, magnesium doesn't seem to improve glycemic control in type 2 diabetes (1171,1172).

Hearing loss. Taking magnesium orally seems to prevent hearing loss in individuals exposed to loud noise (1205).

Hypercholesterolemia. There is some evidence that taking magnesium chloride and magnesium oxide orally can produce small decreases in low-density lipoprotein (LDL) and total cholesterol levels, and small increases in high-density lipoprotein (HDL) levels. However, magnesium does not seem to improve lipoprotein (a) levels (1193).

Hypertension. Taking magnesium orally can reduce blood pressure to a small extent in people with mild to moderate hypertension. The effect appears to be dose related, requiring doses of 600 to 1000 mg daily (1192,1199,9465). However, significantly lower doses do not seem to have this effect (1180,1195,1197,8098).

Kidney stones (nephrolithiasis). Taking magnesium orally seems to prevent the recurrence of kidney stones. Prophylactic treatment with magnesium hydroxide might decrease the recurrence rate of calcium stone formation (2007). Magnesium in combination with pyridoxine (vitamin B6) also seems to decrease urinary oxalate levels in people with hyperoxaluria who have previously had kidney stones (1201). However, it's unclear if this effect on urinary oxalate levels translates into a reduced incidence of kidney stones. There is also evidence that treatment with other medications such as chlorthalidone (Hygroton) may be more effective than magnesium hydroxide in preventing kidney stone formation (8097).

Migraine headache. Taking high-dose magnesium citrate or trimagnesium dicitrate orally seems to reduce the frequency and severity of migraine headaches (4891,9498). However, other research suggests that magnesium doesn't have any effect (10661). In children, treatment with magnesium oxide may also reduce the frequency and severity of migraine headaches (10663). Although some patients with normal magnesium levels can respond to intravenous magnesium for acute migraine, most patients who benefit seem to have low magnesium levels (6844). A combination product containing magnesium, riboflavin, and feverfew doesn't seem to reduce the frequency or severity of migraine any better than placebo. However, some problems with study design suggest that more research should be conducted on this combination (12389).

Mitral valve prolapse. Taking magnesium orally seems to reduce symptoms of mitral valve prolapse in people with low serum magnesium levels (1191).

Osteoporosis. There is preliminary evidence that suggests taking magnesium orally might prevent bone loss in postmenopausal osteoporosis (9104). In another study of postmenopausal women who were also taking estrogen, magnesium 600 mg plus calcium 500 mg and a multivitamin supplement daily increased bone mass better than estrogen alone (12506). What effect magnesium has with this combination is speculative. Epidemiological research suggests that magnesium intake is related to bone mineral density (12501,12502,12503,12504) although not all studies have found an association (12505).

Post-hysterectomy pain. Administering magnesium intravenously seems to be helpful for pain control after hysterectomy. There is some evidence that a high magnesium dose of 3 grams followed by a 500 mg per hour infusion can reduce discomfort and analgesic requirements in patients post-hysterectomy. However, lower doses of 200 mg followed by an infusion of 200 mg per hour are not effective and might actually increase pain in some patients (6846).

Pregnancy-induced leg cramps. Taking magnesium orally seems to be helpful for treating pregnancy-induced leg cramps (1194).

Premenstrual syndrome (PMS). Taking magnesium orally seems to relieve symptoms of PMS. There is some evidence that magnesium supplementation can improve symptoms including mood changes and fluid retention in some patients with PMS (1187,1188,6847). Taking magnesium orally also seems to prevent premenstrual migraine (1186,6847).

Preterm labor. Administering magnesium intravenously seems to be helpful for acute prevention of uterine contractions in preterm labor (tocolysis) (9,15). The use of magnesium for tocolysis is controversial. Not all experts agree it is beneficial (6844). However, most clinicians consider magnesium and beta-adrenergic agonists first-line therapy when tocolysis is indicated. Intravenous magnesium sulfate seems to be effective for delaying delivery for 24 to 48 hours (9,15). Oral magnesium therapy is not effective because it cannot achieve sufficiently high magnesium plasma levels (15).

Stroke. There is some evidence that increasing dietary magnesium intake might decrease the relative risk of stroke in men. However, there is no proof that taking magnesium supplements has this same effect (9001,9002). There is also preliminary clinical evidence that suggests intravenous magnesium may act as a neuroprotective agent in patients diagnosed with acute stroke (9000,9003).

Vasospastic angina. Administering magnesium intravenously seems to prevent coronary spasm in patients with vasospastic angina. There is evidence that administration of intravenous magnesium (0.27 mmol/kg body weight over 20 minutes) dilates coronary arteries and suppresses acetylcholine-induced coronary spasms in patients with vasospastic angina (8091).

Wound healing. Applying magnesium topically seems to speed wound healing including skin ulcers and inflammatory conditions such as boils and carbuncles (9).

POSSIBLY INEFFECTIVE

Athletic performance. Taking magnesium orally doesn't seem to increase energy and endurance during athletic activity. Magnesium oxide, aspartate, and orotate salts don't seem to improve exercise performance when used alone or in combination with potassium (2825,2826,2827,2828,2829,2830).

Cardiac arrest. Administering magnesium intravenously doesn't seem to improve successful resuscitation in people with cardiac arrest (1190).

Cerebral palsy. Administering magnesium intravenously doesn't seem to decrease the risk of cerebral palsy in premature infants. Earlier evidence suggested that treatment with magnesium sulfate for tocolysis might also be protective against cerebral palsy. However, there is no additional evidence to confirm that such an association exists (8093).

INSUFFICIENT RELIABLE EVIDENCE to RATE

Attention deficit-hyperactivity disorder (ADHD). Children with ADHD seem to have lower magnesium levels (9969); preliminary clinical research suggests that magnesium might be useful for ADHD in children with low magnesium levels (1189).

Fibromyalgia. Taking magnesium hydroxide plus malic acid (Super Malic tablets) orally seems to decrease fibromyalgia-related pain and tenderness in some patients (3262).

Multiple sclerosis (MS). There is some evidence that magnesium may reduce the spasticity associated with MS (9499).

Restless leg syndrome. Preliminary clinical research suggests that taking magnesium orally might be useful for treating restless leg syndrome (periodic limb movement during sleep). In some patients, magnesium treatment may decrease the amount of movement and increase the amount of sleep in patients with restless leg syndrome or

periodic limb movement during sleep (9466). However, both magnesium deficiency and high magnesium blood levels have been observed in patients with restless leg syndrome (8096,9472).
More evidence is needed to rate magnesium for these uses.

Mechanism of Action

Magnesium is the second most plentiful cation in the intracellular fluid and the most plentiful cation in the body. Magnesium is involved with more than 300 enzyme systems. The body contains about 25 grams of magnesium, which is divided in roughly equal portions between the skeleton and soft tissue. About a third of skeletal magnesium is on the surface of the bone and acts as a reservoir to maintain the extracellular magnesium concentration. The remaining two-thirds of magnesium in bone is a constituent of bone crystals and is not readily available as a magnesium source (7555,12499,12507). Extracellular magnesium makes up only 1% of total body magnesium. In plasma, 55% is ionized or free, about 30% is bound to plasma proteins, and 15% complexed to anions (12507).
Magnesium is important for normal bone structure (272), and plays an essential role in more than 300 cellular reactions (945). Magnesium is required for the formation of cyclic AMP (cAMP) and is involved in ion movements across cell membranes (945). It is involved in protein synthesis and carbohydrate metabolism (272). Extracellular magnesium is critical to both maintaining nerve and muscle electrical potentials and transmitting impulses across neuromuscular junctions (272).
Dietary sources of magnesium include legumes, whole grains, vegetables (especially broccoli, squash, and green leafy vegetables), animal proteins, seeds, and nuts. Other sources include dairy products, meats, chocolate, and coffee. Water with a high mineral content, or "hard" water, is also a source of magnesium. Dietary intake of magnesium may be low, particularly among women (8088,12505). Magnesium deficiency is not uncommon in the US. It's particularly prevalent among African Americans and the elderly. Low intake and impaired absorption of magnesium have also been associated with the development of various disease states such as osteoporosis, hypertension, atherosclerotic vascular disease, cardiomyopathy, diabetes, and stroke (8088,8099,8998,9001,12510,12511).
Hypomagnesemia is usually asymptomatic. The serum magnesium level is the most commonly used test to assess magnesium status. However, it is also known that the serum magnesium level is depressed only in cases of severe magnesium deficiency and that it poorly correlates with body magnesium (8089). The body preserves serum magnesium at the expense of magnesium in cells and bone, so serum levels may appear normal in magnesium deficiency (12510,12511). Red cell and urine magnesium levels also have been used but they are also poor indicators of body magnesium (8085,8089). The intravenous magnesium loading test is considered to be a more reliable test to measure magnesium status; but the test is cumbersome and requires full participation from the patient. It is known that serum magnesium actually consists of three fractions. They are protein-bound, complexed, and free ionic magnesium. It is the free ionic magnesium that is biologically active. Despite whether the serum magnesium level is low or normal, free ionic magnesium levels have been shown to vary consistently with many disorders such as cardiac disease, stroke, diabetes, and migraines. In recent years, instruments have become available that measure free ionic magnesium, allowing for a more accurate assessment of body magnesium (8090). Symptoms of severe magnesium deficiency include convulsions, confusion, muscle weakness, abnormal muscle movements, and others (403).
As antacids, magnesium salts work by reacting with gastric acid to form magnesium chloride. Magnesium hydroxide has the fastest onset of action, magnesium carbonate is slower due to its crystal structure, and magnesium trisilicate has the slowest onset and longest duration due to its poor solubility (6844).
The laxative effects and diarrhea produced by magnesium salts are due to the osmotic effects of unabsorbed salts in the intestine and colon, and stimulation of gastric motility due to the release of gastrin and cholecystokinin (6844). The inhibitory effect of magnesium on preterm labor contractions (tocolysis) is attributed to antagonism of calcium-mediated myometrial contractions (6844).
The mechanism of action for magnesium in pre-eclampsia and eclampsia is not clear. There is some evidence that magnesium dilates blood vessels in the central nervous system (CNS) to reduce ischemia. Contrary to this view are indications that magnesium may decrease CNS blood flow (9473). Additionally, magnesium may have anticonvulsant actions in eclampsia due to depression of neuromuscular transmission, direct depressant effect on smooth muscle, and CNS depression (6844). There is some evidence that magnesium is important in regulating blood pressure (1170,1182). Magnesium deficiency has been found to cause intracellular concentrations of sodium and potassium to increase, which can lead to increased peripheral resistance and vasospasm (8088). In cell membranes, a decreased concentration of magnesium and increased calcium to magnesium ratio has also been associated with hypertension (8092). There is also some evidence that hypertensive patients with hypomagnesemia usually require more antihypertensive medications than hypertensive patients with normal magnesium levels (8088).
There is some evidence that serum magnesium deficiency might play a role in both ischemic and hemorrhagic stroke (8998). Preliminary information shows magnesium may act as a neuroprotective agent in patients diagnosed with acute stroke. Several possible mechanisms of neuroprotection exist, including noncompetitive N-methyl-D-aspartate (NMDA) antagonism and calcium channel antagonism (9000,9003).
In patients with congestive heart failure, there is evidence magnesium reduces coronary vascular resistance, increases coronary artery blood flow, has antiarrhythmic effects, and improves cardiac indexes (8088).
There is some evidence that low magnesium levels play a role in diabetes (1168,1183). Magnesium seems to affect glucose control and insulin homeostasis. Magnesium blood levels might play a role in insulin resistance (1168,6844,11352). There is also some evidence that low dietary intake of magnesium increases the risk of

developing type 2 diabetes (6845,11352).
Magnesium might play a role in migraine headache. Low levels of magnesium may induce cerebral arterial vasoconstriction, increase platelet aggregation and promote serotonin release, and potentiate the vasoactive properties of serotonin (6844,12388).
Magnesium deficiency may affect the integrity of bone. Magnesium deficiency leads to impairment of osteoblast (bone-building cells) function, according to preliminary research. There's also evidence that magnesium deficiency increases the formation and activity of osteoclasts (bone resorbing cells). Magnesium deficiency causes increases in substance P and tumor necrosis factor (TNF)-alpha in bone, which increase osteoclastic bone resorption. Increased bone resorption causes release of magnesium as well as calcium from bone. Since magnesium is an essential nutrient, the body may sacrifice bone in times of deficiency as a magnesium source to maintain homeostasis (12499,12500).
Magnesium deficiency might be a risk factor for postmenopausal osteoporosis, but its exact role is unknown (7555).
Magnesium, like calcium, is regulated by parathyroid hormone (PTH). In humans, severe to moderate magnesium deficiency commonly causes hypocalcemia. Normally, magnesium deficiency increases PTH activity. PTH increases renal calcium reabsorption, increases phosphate excretion, and increases renal magnesium reabsorption. Impaired parathyroid hormone (PTH) activity and impaired response to PTH seem to be the predominant reasons that magnesium-deficient people are also hypocalcemic (12499).
In women with premenstrual syndrome, intracellular levels of magnesium, measured in erythrocytes and leukocytes, have been found to be lower than women without PMS. It is thought that magnesium might be beneficial for improving some symptoms of PMS due to magnesium's role in the activity of serotonin and other neurotransmitters. Magnesium is also involved in vascular contraction, neuromuscular function, and cell membrane stability and fluidity. These factors could also contribute to magnesium's effects in PMS (6847).
Magnesium is reported to be an antagonist at N-methyl-D-aspartate (NMDA) receptors, which are involved in the potentiation of pain. This effect and magnesium's depressant effects on nerves and smooth muscle are thought to contribute to the possible effects of magnesium in relieving symptoms associated with migraine headaches, postoperative pain, neuropathic pain, erythromelalgia, Raynaud's Phenomenon, and other vascular disorders and pain syndromes (6846,6848,8094).
There is some evidence that magnesium metabolism is a factor in renal stone formation and prevention (2006,2007).
There is preliminary evidence that magnesium can reduce hypertension and nephrotoxicity induced by cyclosporine. Magnesium supplementation appears to reduce the thickening of the renal vascular walls that may occur with cyclosporine therapy; potassium supplementation may increase the effectiveness of magnesium for this use (9500).
In asthma, intravenous administration of magnesium might cause bronchodilation (2003).

Adverse Reactions

Orally, magnesium can cause gastrointestinal irritation, nausea, vomiting, and diarrhea (4891,10661,10663). Although rare, larger amounts might cause hypermagnesemia with symptoms including thirst, hypotension, drowsiness, confusion, loss of tendon reflexes, muscle weakness, respiratory depression, cardiac arrhythmias, coma, cardiac arrest, and death (8095). There are two reports of fatal hypermagnesemia. One report involved a 28 month-old child treated with 800 mg of oral magnesium oxide per day for constipation, then given 2400 mg magnesium oxide for several days before hospital admission (serum magnesium 20.3 mg/dL) (1360). Another report involved a patient who gargled with Epsom salts over several weeks. Epsom salts are almost 100% magnesium sulfate. The patient used an entire box two days prior to hospital admission (serum magnesium 23.6 mg/dL) (8095).
Topically, prolonged use of magnesium sulfate in the treatment of boils and carbuncles can cause damage to surrounding skin (9). Intravenously, urticaria has been reported (9). Chronic use of magnesium-containing antacids, especially those that do not contain aluminum, can cause diarrhea leading to fluid and electrolyte imbalances (15).

Interactions with Herbs & Other Dietary Supplements

BORON: Boron supplements can reduce urinary excretion of magnesium and increase serum levels in women (940,9623,9529). In young women, age 18 to 25 years, the effect appears to be greater in sedentary than athletic women (940). In postmenopausal women, the effect is more marked in women with low dietary magnesium intake (9623). The clinical significance of these effects, and whether they occur in men, isn't known.
CALCIUM: Calcium supplements can decrease the absorption of dietary magnesium, but only at very high, supra-therapeutic doses (2600 mg per day). However, in people with adequate magnesium stores, calcium doesn't have any clinically significant effect on long-term magnesium balance. Advise patients at high risk for magnesium deficiency to take calcium supplements at bedtime, instead of with meals, to avoid inhibiting dietary magnesium absorption (4623,7555,11159).
MALIC ACID: Malic acid is used with magnesium hydroxide for reducing pain and tenderness associated with fibromyalgia (3262). The mechanism of the effect and any interactions between the two isn't known.
VITAMIN D: One intestinal route of magnesium absorption is thought to be vitamin D dependent (9634). Various forms of vitamin D, including ergocalciferol, 25-hydroxyergocalciferol, 25-hydroxycholecalciferol (calcifediol), and 1,25-dihydroxycholecalciferol (calcitriol) increase magnesium absorption; especially when taken in high doses (9634,9635,9636,9637). This effect has been used to treat hypomagnesemia in people with malabsorption syndromes (9635,9636,9516).
ZINC: Supplementation with high doses of zinc, 142 mg/day, appears to decrease magnesium absorption and magnesium balance in healthy adult males (9624). Also, moderately high dietary zinc intake (53 mg per day) seems to

increase magnesium excretion without affecting copper metabolism in postmenopausal women. This might adversely affect bone health. Zinc may compete with magnesium for ion exchange transport in the intestine (12424). More research on the clinical importance of these observations is needed.

Interactions with Drugs

AMINOGLYCOSIDE ANTIBIOTICS: Use of an aminoglycoside antibiotic and magnesium concurrently can lead to neuromuscular weakness and possible paralysis. Both agents reduce presynaptic acetylcholine release, which can lead to neuromuscular blockade. This is most likely to occur with high doses of magnesium given intravenously (15). The aminoglycosides include amikacin (Amikin), gentamicin (Garamycin), kanamycin (Kantrex), streptomycin, and tobramycin (Nebcin).
BISPHOSPHONATES: Cations, including magnesium, can decrease bisphosphonate absorption. Advise patients to separate doses of magnesium and these drugs by at least 2 hours (9). The bisphosphonates include alendronate (Fosamax), etidronate (Didronel), tiludronate (Skelid), and risedronate (Actonel).
CALCIUM CHANNEL BLOCKERS: Magnesium inhibits calcium entry into smooth muscle cells and may therefore have additive effects with calcium channel blockers. Severe hypotension and neuromuscular blockades can occur when nifedipine is used with intravenous magnesium (3046). High doses of magnesium could theoretically have additive effects with other calcium channel blockers. These drugs include nifedipine (Adalat, Procardia), nicardipine (Cardene), isradipine (DynaCirc), amlodipine (Norvasc), and others.
POTASSIUM-SPARING DIURETICS: Potassium-sparing diuretics also have magnesium-sparing properties, which can counteract the magnesium losses associated with loop and thiazide diuretics (9613,9614,9622). Theoretically, increased magnesium levels could result from concomitant use of potassium-sparing diuretics and magnesium supplements. The potassium-sparing diuretics include amiloride (Midamor), triamterene (Dyrenium), and spironolactone (Aldactone).
QUINOLONE ANTIBIOTICS: Magnesium can form insoluble complexes with quinolones and decrease their absorption (3046). Advise patients to take these drugs at least 2 hours before, or 4 to 6 hours after, magnesium supplements. Quinolones include ciprofloxacin (Cipro), levofloxacin (Levaquin), ofloxacin (Floxin), moxifloxacin (Avelox), gatifloxacin (Tequin), and others.
SKELETAL MUSCLE RELAXANTS: Parenteral magnesium can potentiate the effects of skeletal muscle relaxants by decreasing acetylcholine release from motor nerve terminals (3046). These drugs include atracurium (Tracrium), cisatracurium (Nimbex), mivacurium (Mivacron), rapacuronium (Raplon), rocuronium (Zemuron), pancuronium (Pavulon), vecuronium (Norcuron), and others.
TETRACYCLINE ANTIBIOTICS: Magnesium can form insoluble complexes with tetracyclines and decrease their absorption (9). Advise patients to take these drugs at least 2 hours before, or 4 to 6 hours after, magnesium supplements. Tetracyclines include demeclocycline (Declomycin), doxycycline (Vibramycin), minocycline (Minocin), and tetracycline (Achromycin, Sumycin).

Drug Influences on Nutrient Levels and Depletion

SOME DRUGS CAN AFFECT MAGNESIUM LEVELS:
ALDESLEUKIN (interleukin-2, IL-2, Proleukin): Asymptomatic hypomagnesemia can occur with aldesleukin therapy, probably due to an intracellular shift of magnesium. There isn't any increase in urinary magnesium, and serum levels normalize a few days after the drug is stopped (8874).
AMIFOSTINE (Ethyol, WR-2721): Amifostine reduces serum magnesium levels by reducing renal tubular reabsorption of magnesium and increasing urinary losses (9625). This effect seems to occur acutely after a single dose, and levels may return to normal within 24 hours (9625). The clinical significance therefore isn't clear.
AMINOGLYCOSIDES: Nephrotoxicity caused by aminoglycosides may lead to increased urinary losses of various electrolytes, including magnesium. Monitor patients closely to detect declining renal function and electrolyte disturbances. The aminoglycoside may need to be discontinued and intravenous electrolyte replacement given (15). Some aminoglycosides include amikacin (Amikin), gentamicin (Garamycin), kanamycin (Kantrex), streptomycin, and tobramycin (Nebcin).
AMPHOTERICIN-B (Abelcet, Amphotec, AmBisome, Amphocin, Fungizone): Electrolyte disturbances, including low serum magnesium levels, develop in a large proportion of patients receiving amphotericin-B. Lipid-based formulations might have a lesser effect than the conventional formulations (15). This disturbance has been association with nephrotoxicity, and may necessitate stopping the drug and giving intravenous electrolyte replacement.
BETA-2 AGONISTS: Beta-2 agonists promote movement of magnesium from the extracellular to the intracellular space, and increase magnesium excretion in the urine (2644,9517,9641). Reduced serum magnesium levels occur after a single dose of albuterol or terbutaline orally, by IV infusion, SC injection, or by inhalation (2644,6203,6205,6209,6217,8882,9517). The reductions are generally small, about 4.5-9%, or 0.04 to 0.06 mmol/L compared with the normal serum magnesium range of 0.65 to 1.1 mmol/L (6205,6217). However, it's been suggested that these acute changes could contribute to ECG changes, including prolonged QT intervals (2644,8882). With chronic use of beta-2 agonists, it appears that serum magnesium levels return to normal, but muscle magnesium levels remain low (6209,6210,9507). The clinical significance of this is not clear. It's unlikely that people using regular doses of beta-2 agonists for treatment of asthma will need magnesium supplements, unless they have other factors contributing to magnesium deficiency. The beta-2 agonists include albuterol (salbutamol, Proventil, Ventolin), bitolterol (Tornalate),

isoetharine, levalbuterol (Xopenex), metaproterenol (Alupent), pirbuterol (Maxair), salmeterol (Serevent), and terbutaline (Brethine).

CARBOPLATIN (Paraplatin), CISPLATIN (Platinol-AQ): Carboplatin and cisplatin can cause hypomagnesemia due to renal tubular damage, which increases urinary magnesium losses (9626). With carboplatin, hypomagnesemia is rarely symptomatic and usually doesn't require magnesium supplements. Hypomagnesemia is usually more severe with cisplatin and worsens with progressive courses of treatment. Most patients who receive cumulative doses of cisplatin above 400 mg/m2 will develop hypomagnesemia (9626). Intravenous or oral magnesium supplements reduce the severity of this hypomagnesemia (9626). Monitor patients closely.

CHOLESTYRAMINE (Questran): Preliminary evidence suggests that cholestyramine may slightly increase urinary magnesium excretion, possibly by binding vitamin D and leading to reduced magnesium absorption (9566,9627). Clinically significant magnesium deficiency hasn't been reported, and supplements aren't likely to be needed.

CORTICOSTEROIDS (glucocorticoids): Chronic use of corticosteroids increases the amount of magnesium excreted in the urine. This is thought to be due to catabolism of bone which releases magnesium and increases the amount available for excretion (9628,9629). However, there doesn't seem to be a significant effect on serum levels (9507,9508,9509). Monitor magnesium levels in patients with other conditions that could contribute to magnesium deficiency.

CYCLOSPORINE (Neoral, Sandimmune): Cyclosporine can cause significant loss of magnesium in the urine, probably by reducing tubular reabsorption and causing tubular damage (9117,9632,9633). Hypomagnesemia may contribute to seizures and neurotoxicity associated with cyclosporine (9117,9632). Monitor magnesium levels carefully. If hypomagnesemia occurs magnesium supplements may be needed, and/or dosage reduction or discontinuation of cyclosporine.

DIGOXIN (Lanoxin, Lanoxicaps): Digoxin decreases renal tubular reabsorption of magnesium, increasing excretion in the urine (4556,9631). People taking digoxin for heart failure may also be taking loop or thiazide diuretics, increasing the potential for hypomagnesemia (9613,9631). Low magnesium levels increase the risk of arrhythmias associated with high digoxin levels (9631). Monitor patients carefully.

DIURETICS: Loop diuretics and, to a lesser extent thiazide diuretics, interfere with magnesium reabsorption in the kidneys, which increases urinary losses and reduces serum magnesium levels (4412,9613,9614,9622). Some patients taking these diuretics chronically may also be taking digoxin, and may be at risk for cardiac arrhythmias. Low serum magnesium levels increases the risk of digoxin toxicity and arrhythmias (9613,9614). Potassium-sparing diuretics, such as amiloride, triamterene, or spironolactone, are also magnesium-sparing, and can therefore counteract the magnesium losses seen with loop diuretics and thiazides (9613,9614,9622). Monitor patients closely and use magnesium supplements or potassium-sparing diuretics when needed. The loop diuretics include furosemide (Lasix), bumetanide (Bumex), ethacrynic acid (Edecrin), and torsemide (Demadex). The thiazides include hydrochlorothiazide (Esidrix, HydroDiuril), chlorothiazide (Diuril), and others.

ESTROGENS and ESTROGEN-CONTAINING ORAL CONTRACEPTIVES: Estrogens enhance magnesium uptake by soft tissues and bones, lowering serum levels (9621,9639). There appears to be an inverse relationship between estrogen levels and magnesium serum levels (9638,9639,9640). Estrogen therapy, including the use of oral contraceptives, lowers serum magnesium levels and can cause hypomagnesemia, especially in people with low dietary magnesium intake or other factors contributing to magnesium loss (9639,9640). It's likely that hypomagnesemia can contribute to the thromboembolic complications associated with estrogens (9621,9639). Monitor magnesium levels in patients.

FLUOROQUINOLONES: Fluoroquinolones form complexes with magnesium in the GI tract (3046). This could theoretically reduce absorption of both the fluoroquinolone and magnesium if taken at the same time. Significant effects on magnesium levels are unlikely when fluoroquinolones are taken at least 2 hours before, or 4 to 6 hours after magnesium supplements. Fluoroquinolones include ciprofloxacin (Cipro), levofloxacin (Levaquin), ofloxacin (Floxin), moxifloxacin (Avelox), gatifloxacin (Tequin), and others.

FOSCARNET (Foscavir): Foscarnet can cause various electrolyte disturbances, including symptomatic hypomagnesemia (8869,9617). This may be due to chelation of magnesium and increased elimination (8869). Monitor magnesium levels. Magnesium supplements may be needed, especially if foscarnet can't be discontinued (8869,9617).

PENICILLAMINE (Cuprimine): Penicillamine chelates magnesium, although with lower affinity than other metals such as copper, iron, and zinc (9630). It can potentially contribute to hypomagnesemia, especially in people with other factors which lower serum magnesium (4534). Magnesium supplements should be taken several hours apart from penicillamine to avoid forming nonabsorbable chelates in the gut.

PENTAMIDINE (NebuPent, Pentacarinat, Pentam 300): Symptomatic hypomagnesemia can occur with pentamidine, especially when given intravenously. This is likely due to renal tubular injury, leading to increased urinary losses of magnesium. Hypomagnesemia usually requires treatment with intravenous, followed by oral, magnesium supplements. Supplementation may need to be continued after pentamidine is stopped since the drug effects remain for six to eight weeks (8872,9618,9619). It isn't known whether magnesium given prophylactically with pentamidine can prevent hypomagnesemia. Monitor patients closely.

SODIUM PHOSPHATES (monobasic sodium phosphate and dibasic sodium phosphate, Fleet Phospho-soda): Use of high doses of sodium phosphates, such as those used for bowel cleansing before surgery, can cause hypomagnesemia (9615,9616). Advise people to avoid using high doses of these products for self-treatment of constipation.

TACROLIMUS (FK506, Prograf): Tacrolimus reduces renal tubular reabsorption of magnesium, producing increased magnesium wasting (8900,9620). This leads to hypomagnesemia in a significant proportion of people treated with tacrolimus (9620). Monitor magnesium levels.
TETRACYCLINES: Tetracyclines form complexes with magnesium in the GI tract, which could reduce absorption of both the tetracycline and magnesium when taken at the same time (9). Significant effects on calcium levels are unlikely when tetracyclines are taken at least 2 hours before, or 4 to 6 hours after, magnesium supplements. Tetracyclines include demeclocycline (Declomycin), doxycycline (Vibramycin), minocycline (Minocin), and tetracycline (Achromycin, Sumycin).

Interactions with Foods

None known.

Interactions with Lab Tests

ALKALINE PHOSPHATASE (ALK PHOS): Magnesium salts can cause a false increase in serum alkaline phosphatase test results due to the activation of enzymes used in lab procedures (275).
ANGIOTENSIN-CONVERTING ENZYME (ACE): Magnesium sulfate can reduce serum ACE concentrations and test results (275).
BLOOD PRESSURE: Orally, magnesium can lower blood pressure and reduce blood pressure readings in patients with mild to moderate hypertension (1192,1199).
CALCIUM: Magnesium salts can cause a false increase in serum calcium test results in some procedures using edetate disodium (EDTA) (275).
CORTISOL: Intravenous magnesium sulfate can decrease plasma cortisol concentrations and test results (275).
DIAGNEX BLUE: Magnesium salts can increase urine diagnex blue concentrations and test results by heavy metal displacement of diagnex blue (275).
ELECTROCARDIOGRAM (ECG): Orally, magnesium can normalize arrhythmias and ECG readings in some patients with angina (1181). Intravenous magnesium can normalize arrhythmias and ECG readings in some people with atrial fibrillation or ventricular tachydysrhythmias (1202,3314).
PARATHYROID HORMONE: Decreased magnesium serum levels increase stimulation of PTH secretion. Paradoxically, a more profound decrease in serum magnesium can actually decrease PTH secretion. In severe magnesium deficiency, PTH secretion is impaired, but serum PTH increases within minutes of intravenous magnesium administration (12509).
TESTOSTERONE: Intravenous magnesium sulfate can reduce serum testosterone concentrations and test results (275).

Interactions with Diseases or Conditions

ALCOHOLISM: Alcohol abuse increases the risk for magnesium deficiency. Alcohol impairs the ability of the kidney to conserve magnesium (12507).
DIABETES: Diabetes increases the risk for magnesium deficiency. Poorly controlled diabetes leading to glycosuria leads to reduced renal reabsorption of magnesium (12507).
ELDERLY: The elderly are at an increased risk for hypomagnesemia. They are more prone to decreased magnesium absorption, increased urinary loss, and disease states associated with abnormal magnesium status (1167).
HEART BLOCK: Hypermagnesemia can cause heart block. Intravenous magnesium is contraindicated in people with heart block (9,15).
MALABSORPTION SYNDROMES: Intestinal magnesium absorption can be decreased in bile insufficiency states, gastrointestinal infections, gluten enteropathy, immune diseases with villous atrophy, inflammatory bowel disease, intestinal fistulas, lymphectasia, primary idiopathic hypomagnesemia, radiation enteritis, sprue, and others (6280,6281).
RENAL DISEASE: Use cautiously in individuals with reduced kidney function due to an increased risk of hypermagnesemia (12507).
RESTLESS LEG SYNDROME: High magnesium levels were reported in association with restless leg syndrome, but a causal relationship was not established (8096). Magnesium deficiency may also be associated with restless leg syndrome (9472).

Dosage and Administration

ORAL: For preventing migraine headaches, magnesium citrate 1830 mg given in three divided doses has been used for up to 3 months (9498). Trimagnesium dicitrate 600 mg (24 mmol) daily for up to 3 months has also been used (4891). For preventing migraine headaches in children, magnesium oxide 9 mg/kg in three divided doses has been used for up to 16 weeks (10663). A combination product providing magnesium 300 mg, riboflavin 400 mg, and feverfew 100 mg daily has also been used. However, this product was not found to be effective (12389).
For treatment of hypomagnesemia in patients with type 2 diabetes, a dose of 50 mL magnesium chloride solution (containing 50 grams magnesium chloride per 1000 mL of solution) daily for 16 weeks has been used (10664).
For premenstrual syndrome (PMS), 200-360 mg/day has been used; however, 360 mg/day seems to be more effective than 200 mg/day (6847).
PARENTERAL: For treatment of hypomagnesemia, doses must be individualized according to serum magnesium levels, but a typical starting dose for mild deficiency is 1 gram intramuscularly (IM) every 6 hours for 4 doses. For

more severe deficiency, 5 grams may be given in a 1 liter intravenous (IV) infusion over 3 hours (15).
As part of total parenteral nutrition (TPN), adults typically receive 500 mg to 3 grams magnesium sulfate daily (15).
For treatment of severe pre-eclampsia or eclampsia, a typical initial dose is 4 grams by IV infusion, followed by 4-5 grams IM every 4 hours, or 1-3 grams per hour by constant IV infusion. Doses should be adjusted according to serum levels and urinary excretion, and should not exceed 30-40 grams daily (15).
As a tocolytic in preterm labor, an initial dose of 4-6 grams infused IV over 20 minutes has been used, followed by a maintenance infusion of 2-4 grams per hour, adjusted according to the response (15).
For treatment of life-threatening ventricular arrhythmias such as torsades de pointes, 1-6 grams is given IV over several minutes, followed by an IV infusion, and for atrial tachycardia, 3-4 grams is given over 30 seconds. These IV push doses should be given with extreme caution (15).
For vasospastic angina, a dose of 0.27 mmol/kg body weight infused over 20 minutes has been used to reduce coronary spasm (8091).
For reducing cardiovascular morbidity and mortality after a myocardial infarction, magnesium is started within 6 hours of symptoms. A dose of 2 grams IV over 5-15 minutes has been used, followed by an IV infusion of 18 grams over 24 hours (15).
For reducing the frequency of ventricular arrhythmias after myocardial infarction, 8 grams of magnesium sulfate infused IV over 12 hours has been used (9497).
For treatment of acute stroke, 8-16 mmol magnesium sulfate in 100 mL normal saline, given IV over 15 minutes, has been used. This is followed by 65 mmol magnesium sulfate in 100 mL normal saline IV over 24 hours (9000,9003).
For neuropathic pain associated with cancer, single 500 mg or 1 gram doses have been used (6846).
For cluster headaches and acute migraine, 1 gram IV doses have been used (6844).
As an adjunct to analgesics for pain after hysterectomy, a 3 grams bolus dose followed by an infusion of 0.5 g/hour has been used (6848).
For adjunctive treatment of acute asthmatic attacks, doses of 1-2 grams infused IV over 15-30 minutes have been used (6844). For treatment of acute asthma in children, magnesium sulfate 40 mg/kg infused IV over 20 minutes has been used (9496).
Acute exacerbations of COPD have also been treated with 1.2 grams magnesium sulfate IV (6844).
For treatment of chronic fatigue syndrome (CFS) in patients with low red blood cell magnesium levels, weekly 1 gram intramuscular injections have been used (7556).

Comments

Supplement manufacturers of magnesium/calcium combination products promote a 2:1 or 3:1 ratio as being ideal for absorption of these elements. However, there is no credible research to support this claim. Products such as coral calcium that claim to have ideal combinations of magnesium and calcium to cure a variety of diseases and conditions have come under scrutiny of the FDA and FTC (12508).

MAGNOLIA

Also Known As

Beaver Tree, Flos Magnoliae, Holly Bay, Ho-No-Ki, Hou Po, Hou Po Hua, Houpu, Indian Bark, Japanese Whitebark Magnolia, Red Bay, Swamp Laurel, Swamp Sassafras, Sweet Bay, White Bay, White Laurel.

Scientific Names

Magnolia biondii, synonym Magnolia fargesii; Magnolia denudata, synonyms Magnolia conspicua, Magnolia yulan; Magnolia heptaperta; Magnolia virginiana, synonym Magnolia glauca; Magnolia obovata, synonym Magnolia hypoleuca; Magnolia officinalis; Magnolia sprengeri; Magnolia sargentiana; Magnolia emargenata; Magnolia wilsonii, synonyms Magnolia nicholsoniana, Magnolia taliensis; Magnolia salicifolia, synonyms Buergeria salicifolia, Magnolia proctoriana; other Magnolia species.
Family: Magnoliaceae.

People Use This For

Orally, magnolia bark is used for digestive disorders, as a laxative, an anti-inflammatory, a stimulant, and to promote sweating. It is also used for anxiety, stress, depression, weight loss, fever, headache, stroke, and asthma. Magnolia flower bud is used orally for nasal congestion, runny nose, common cold, sinusitis, allergic rhinitis, headache, and facial dark spots.
Topically, magnolia flower bud is used for toothaches.
In skin care products, magnolia flower bud extract is used topically as a skin whitener and to minimize or counteract irritant effects of other ingredients.

Safety

POSSIBLY SAFE ...when the bark or flower bud is used orally and appropriately (12). There is insufficient reliable information available about the topical use of magnolia.
PREGNANCY: UNSAFE ...when the flower bud is used orally due to reports of uterine stimulant activity (11953).

There is insufficient reliable information available about the safety of using magnolia bark; avoid using.
LACTATION: Insufficient reliable information available; avoid using.

Effectiveness

There is insufficient reliable information available about the effectiveness of magnolia.

Mechanism of Action

The applicable parts of magnolia are the bark and flower bud. Magnolia bark contains the active constituents magnolol, dihydroxydihdromagnolol, honokiol, and dihydrohonokiol (11945,11946,11947,11948).
Magnolol seems to have central nervous system effects, antiplatelet effects, anti-inflammatory effects, and smooth muscle relaxant effects. Magnolol also suppresses the conversion of cortisol to cortisone by blocking hydroxysteroid dehydrogenase. It increases the production of corticosterone, a glucocorticoid similar to cortisol. This may explain magnolia's use for asthma. Magnolol may also lower cholesterol production (11945). Other preliminary research suggests that magnolol might have anti-leukemic properties (11949). Magnolol and dihydroxydihydromagnolol seem to have antidepressant effects (11950).
Honokiol and dihydrohonokiol seem to have anxiolytic effects in animals, possibly by interacting with gamma-aminobutyric acid-A (GABA-A) receptors (11946,11947). However, dihydrohonokiol doesn't seem to cause motor dysfunction, CNS depression, amnesia, or physical dependence at doses that produce an anxiolytic effect (11948).
At high doses, magnolia bark seems to have CNS depressant effects. Honokiol seems to inhibit catecholamine secretion (11952).
Magnolol and honokiol might enhance cholinergic function, which could be useful in diseases such as Alzheimer's. At high doses, these compounds increase acetylcholine release in the hippocampus of the brain and have a neurotrophic effect, theoretically improving neuronal function (11951).
Magnolia flower bud seems to have uterine stimulating, hypotensive, antifungal, and skeletal muscle contracting effects. Its constituents, especially magnone, may also have platelet-activating factor antagonist activity, which might explain its use in nasal congestion and rhinitis (11953).

Adverse Reactions

Theoretically, magnolia bark might cause central nervous system depressant effects at high doses (11952).

Interactions with Herbs & Other Dietary Supplements

HERBS AND SUPPLEMENTS WITH SEDATIVE PROPERTIES: Theoretically, concomitant use with herbs and supplements that have sedative properties might increase the risk of excessive drowsiness. Some of these supplements include 5-HTP, calamus, California poppy, catnip, hops, Jamaican dogwood, kava, St. John's wort, scullcap, valerian, yerba mansa, and others (11952).

Interactions with Drugs

ALCOHOL (Ethanol): Theoretically, concomitant use of large doses of magnolia bark and alcohol might increase the risk of drowsiness and motor reflex depression (11952).
BARBITURATES: Theoretically, concomitant use of large doses of magnolia bark and barbiturates might increase the risk of drowsiness and motor reflex depression (11952). Some of these sedative medications include pentobarbital (Nembutal), phenobarbital (Luminal), secobarbital (Seconal), and others.
BENZODIAZEPINES: Theoretically, concomitant use of large doses of magnolia bark and benzodiazepines might increase the risk of drowsiness and motor reflex depression (11952).
CNS DEPRESSANTS: Theoretically, concomitant use of large doses of magnolia bark and CNS depressants might increase the risk of drowsiness and motor reflex depression (11952).

Interactions with Foods

None known.

Interactions with Lab Tests

None known.

Interactions with Diseases or Conditions

None known.

Dosage and Administration

No typical dosage.

Comments

Magnolia bark is an ingredient in the traditional Chinese and Japanese (Kampo) medicines Hange-koboku-to, which is composed of 5 plant extracts, and Saiboku-to, which is composed of 10 plant extracts. These are used to decrease anxiety and nervous tension and to improve sleep. Honokiol, a constituent of magnolia bark, appears to cause these effects (11946).
Some weight loss products include magnolia bark with claims that it reduces cortisol levels. There is no evidence

that magnolia bark causes weight loss or reduces cortisol levels. In fact, it appears to increase levels of corticosterone, a glucocorticoid similar to cortisol (11945).

MAIDENHAIR FERN

Also Known As

Five-Finger Fern, Hair of Venus, Maiden Fern, Rock Fern, Venus' Hair.

Scientific Names

Adiantum pedatum; Adiantum capillus-veneris.
Family: Adiantiaceae or Pteridaceae.

People Use This For

Orally, maidenhair fern is used for bronchitis, coughs, whooping cough, and painful and excessive menstruation. It is also used orally as an expectorant, demulcent, severe coughs.
Topically, maidenhair fern is used for hair loss and to promote dark hair color.

Safety

POSSIBLY SAFE ...when used orally in amounts found in foods.
There is insufficient reliable information available about the safety of maidenhair fern for its other uses.
PREGNANCY: UNSAFE ...when used orally; contraindicated, most likely due to its emetic effects at higher doses (12).
LACTATION: Insufficient reliable information available; avoid using.

Effectiveness

There is insufficient reliable information available about the effectiveness of maidenhair fern.

Mechanism of Action

There is insufficient reliable information available about the possible mechanism of action and active ingredients.

Adverse Reactions

Orally, people using large amounts may experience emesis (12).

Interactions with Herbs & Other Dietary Supplements

None known.

Interactions with Drugs

None known.

Interactions with Foods

None known.

Interactions with Lab Tests

None known.

Interactions with Diseases or Conditions

None known.

Dosage and Administration

ORAL: Maidenhair fern is usually taken as a tea. A single dose is equivalent to 1.5 grams ground or powdered herb. The tea is prepared by steeping 1.5 grams dried herb in 150 mL of boiling water for 10-15 minutes and straining (18).

Comments

Maidenhair tree is another name for Ginkgo biloba, and is distinct from maidenhair fern (18).

MAITAKE MUSHROOM

Also Known As
Dancing Mushroom, Grifola, Hen Of The Woods, King Of Mushrooms, Maitake, Monkey's Bench, Shelf Fungi.

Scientific Names
Grifola frondosa.
Family: Polyporaceae.

People Use This For
Orally, maitake mushroom is used for cancer, HIV/AIDS, chronic fatigue syndrome (CFS), hepatitis, hay fever, diabetes, high blood pressure, hyperlipidemia, weight loss or control, and chemotherapy support.
For food uses, maitake mushroom is edible and has been consumed in Asia for thousands of years.

Safety
POSSIBLY SAFE ...when used orally and appropriately (12).
PREGNANCY AND LACTATION: Insufficient reliable information available; avoid using.

Effectiveness
INSUFFICIENT RELIABLE EVIDENCE to RATE

Diabetes. Preliminary clinical evidence suggests that maitake mushroom polysaccharides (MMP) might lower blood glucose in people with type 2 diabetes (8188). More evidence is needed to rate maitake mushroom for this use.

Mechanism of Action
The applicable parts of maitake mushroom are the fruiting body and mycelium. Maitake mushroom contains beta-glucan, which has been shown to possess antitumor activity. The "D-fraction" of beta-glucan appears to be the most active and potent form. Maitake mushroom has immunostimulant effects and activates natural killer cells, cytotoxic T-cells, interleukin-1, and superoxide anions. Preliminary research suggests that maitake mushroom can prevent metastasis of experimentally induced tumors as well as prevent tumor occurrence in normal cells. Researchers are particularly interested in maitake mushroom and its extracts because they appear to be active orally (8189,8190,8191). Other research suggests that maitake mushroom can lower blood pressure (1213,1214), and improve the lipid profile in experimental hyperlipidemia (1211). Polysaccharides from the fruiting bodies in maitake mushroom appear to have a hypoglycemic effect, possibly by activating insulin receptors (1212,8188). Maitake mushroom also appears to cause weight loss (8188).

Adverse Reactions
None reported.

Interactions with Herbs & Other Dietary Supplements
HERBS & SUPPLEMENTS WITH HYPOGLYCEMIC POTENTIAL: Maitake mushroom might lower blood glucose levels and might have additive effects when used with other herbs and supplements that also lower glucose levels (19,1212,8188). This might increase the risk of hypoglycemia in some patients. Some herbs and supplements with hypoglycemic effects include alpha-lipoic acid, bitter melon, chromium, devil's claw, fenugreek, garlic, guar gum, horse chestnut seed, Panax ginseng, psyllium, Siberian ginseng, and others.

Interactions with Drugs
ANTIDIABETES DRUGS: Monitor blood glucose levels closely. Maitake mushroom appears to have hypoglycemic effects (19,1212,8188).

Interactions with Foods
None known.

Interactions with Lab Tests
BLOOD GLUCOSE: Maitake mushroom might lower blood glucose and test results in patients with type 2 diabetes (19,1212,8188).

Interactions with Diseases or Conditions
None known.

Dosage and Administration
No typical dosage.

Comments
Warn patients about the importance of positive identification of maitake mushroom to avoid confusion with poisonous mushrooms.

MALABAR NUT

Also Known As
Adulsa, Arusa.
CAUTION: See separate listing for Garcinia.

Scientific Names
Justicia Adhatoda.
Family: Acanthaceae.

People Use This For
Orally, malabar nut is used as an expectorant and secretory agent. It is also used as a bronchodilatory agent and mild spasmolytic.

Safety
There is insufficient reliable information available about the safety of malabar nut.
PREGNANCY: UNSAFE ...when used orally (18); contraindicated.
LACTATION: Insufficient reliable information available; avoid using.

Effectiveness
There is insufficient reliable information available about the effectiveness of malabar nut.

Mechanism of Action
The applicable part of malabar nut is the leaf. The quinazoline alkaloid vasicine has excitatory activity when taken in large amounts (18).

Adverse Reactions
None reported.

Interactions with Herbs & Other Dietary Supplements
None known.

Interactions with Drugs
None known.

Interactions with Foods
None known.

Interactions with Lab Tests
None known.

Interactions with Diseases or Conditions
None known.

Dosage and Administration
No typical dosage.

Comments
Vasicine was formerly used as the starting substance for production of mucolytics Bromhexin and Ambroxol. Neither of these products are available in the US (18).

MALE FERN

Also Known As
American Aspidium, Bear's Paw, European Aspidium, Knotty Brake, Marginal Fern, Shield Fern.

Scientific Names
Dryopteris Filix-Mas.
Family: Dryopteridaceae.

People Use This For
Orally, male fern is used to treat recurrent nose bleeds, heavy menstrual bleeding, wounds, tumors, and as an anthelmintic.
In veterinary medicine, male fern is used as an anthelmintic.

Safety
LIKELY UNSAFE ...when used orally. Male fern can be a violent poison (2,11). For this reason, it should no longer be used internally (2). Canada requires that it be labeled "For external use only" (12).
There is insufficient reliable information available about the safety of male fern for its other uses.
PREGNANCY AND LACTATION: LIKELY UNSAFE ...when used orally (12); contraindicated. There is insufficient reliable information available about the safety of male fern used topically; avoid using.

Effectiveness
There is insufficient reliable information available about the effectiveness of male fern.

Mechanism of Action
The applicable parts of male fern are the above ground parts, leaf, and rhizome. Male fern contains filicin and filmarone. These are active anthelmintics and act as a vermifuge to kill worms. Active constituents are soluble derivatives of phloroglucinol. These constituents are inactivated in an alkaline environment. Male fern also contains volatile oils, tannin, albaspidin, and desaspidin. All of these compounds together are called filicin, and work together to kill tapeworms. It is important to remember that once the tapeworm has been killed, a simultaneously administered saline laxative is used expel the worm (6).

Adverse Reactions
Orally, male fern may cause headaches, dyspnea, nausea, diarrhea, vertigo, tremors, convulsions, cardiac and respiratory failure, and optic neuritis (6). Death has occurred with severe poisoning. Symptoms of toxicity include muscular weakness, coma, temporary or permanent blindness (11).

Interactions with Herbs & Other Dietary Supplements
CASTOR OIL: Taking castor oil enhances the absorption and toxic potential of male fern (6).

Interactions with Drugs
None known.

Interactions with Foods
FATS, OILS, AND ALCOHOL: Increases absorption and side effects (2).

Interactions with Lab Tests
None known.

Interactions with Diseases or Conditions
GASTROINTESTINAL (GI) CONDITIONS: Theoretically, damaged GI mucosa or conditions which prolong GI transit may increase absorption and the risk of side effects.

Dosage and Administration
ORAL: Adults in a fasting state usually receive 3-6 mL orally. Children up to age two receive up to 2 mL in divided doses. Children over age two are given 0.25-0.5 mL per year of age up to a total of 4 mL in divided doses. The dose is typically given with a purgative (saline laxative) to aid expulsion of tapeworms (6,11).

Comments
High toxicity potential precludes use (2,6). Treatment of overdose consists of giving saline cathartic followed by demulcent fluids. It is important to avoid fats and oils. If seizures occur, benzodiazepines may be used, and assisting respiration may be required. Since there are other products available that are effective and safer than male fern, it should not be used (6002).

MALLOW

Also Known As
Blue Mallow Flower, Cheeseflower, Dwarf Mallow, Gul-Khair, High Mallow, Malvae flos, Malvae folium, Mauls.
CAUTION: See separate listings for Country Mallow and Marshmallow.

Scientific Names
Malva sylvestris, synonym Malva mauritiana; Malva neglecta, synonym Malva rotundifolia.
Family: Malvaceae.

People Use This For
Orally, mallow is used for irritation of the oral and pharyngeal mucosa, dry cough, bronchitis, as a mild astringent for gastroenteritis, and for bladder complaints.
Topically, mallow is used as a poultice or bath additive for wounds.
In foods, mallow is used as a food-coloring agent.

Safety
There is insufficient reliable information available about the safety of mallow.
Pregnancy and Lactation: Insufficient reliable information available; avoid using.

Effectiveness
There is insufficient reliable information available about the effectiveness of mallow.

Mechanism of Action
Mallow contains mucilage which protects and soothes mucous membranes. The mucilage has been shown in vitro to inactivate the serum complement, which is a component in the host defense system (1526). The anthocyanins constituents are a source of color (8).

Adverse Reactions
None reported.

Interactions with Herbs & Other Dietary Supplements
None known.

Interactions with Drugs
None known.

Interactions with Foods
None known.

Interactions with Lab Tests
None known.

Interactions with Diseases or Conditions
None known.

Dosage and Administration
ORAL: No typical dosage. However, traditionally one cup of tea prepared by steeping 1.5-2 grams of the dried flowers in 150 mL boiling water has been used. A tea from the leaves is prepared by steeping 3-5 grams of the dried leaves in 150 mL boiling water for 10-15 minutes (6). The maximum use of mallow leaf or flower is 5 grams of the dried leaves per day (8).

MANACA

Also Known As
Pohl, Vegetable Mercury.

Scientific Names
Brunfelsia uniflora, synonym Brunfelsia hopeana.
Family: Solanaceae.

Comments
At the date of publication, there was very little scientific information available about this product. Our staff is continually analyzing the available information on natural medicines and will add data to the online version of *Natural Medicines Comprehensive Database* as it becomes available. See www.naturaldatabase.com.

MANGANESE

Also Known As
Manganese Amino Acid Chelate, Manganese Aminoate, Manganese Ascorbate, Manganese Aspartate Complex, Manganese Chloride, Manganese Chloridetetrahydrate, Manganese Dioxide, Manganese Gluconate, Manganese Sulfate, Manganese Sulfate Monohydrate, Manganese Sulfate Tetrahydrate, Manganum.

Scientific Names
Manganese; Mn; atomic number 25.

People Use This For
Orally, manganese is used for prevention and treatment of manganese deficiency, osteoporosis, microcytic anemia, and symptoms of premenstrual syndrome (PMS).
In combination, Manganese is used with chondroitin sulfate and glucosamine hydrochloride for osteoarthritis.
Intravenously, manganese is used as a trace element in total parenteral nutrition (TPN) preparations.

Safety
LIKELY SAFE ...when used orally and appropriately. Manganese is usually safe in doses up to 11 mg per day for adults 19 years and older (7135).
POSSIBLY UNSAFE ...when used orally in high doses. Doses exceeding 11 mg per day can cause significant adverse effects (7135).
CHILDREN: LIKELY SAFE ...when used orally and appropriately. Manganese is usually safe in children when used in daily doses less than the tolerable upper intake level (UL) of 2 mg in children 1 to 3 years, 3 mg in children 4 to 8 years, 6 mg in children 9 to 13 years, 9 mg in children 14 to 18 years (7135). POSSIBLY UNSAFE ...when used orally in excessive doses. Daily doses greater than the tolerable upper intake level (UL) are associated with a greater risk of toxicity (7135).
PREGNANCY AND LACTATION: LIKELY SAFE ...when used orally and appropriately. Manganese is usually safe in pregnant or lactating adult women aged 19 or older when used in doses of less than 11 mg per day. However, pregnant and lactating women under age 19 should limit doses to less than 9 mg per day (7135). POSSIBLY UNSAFE ...when used orally in excessive doses. Doses over 11 mg per day are associated with a greater risk of toxicity (7135).

Effectiveness
EFFECTIVE

Manganese deficiency. Taking manganese orally or intravenously is effective for preventing or treating manganese deficiency (15).

POSSIBLY EFFECTIVE

Osteoporosis. Taking manganese orally in combination with calcium, zinc, and copper seems to help reduce spinal bone loss in postmenopausal women (1994).

INSUFFICIENT RELIABLE EVIDENCE to RATE

Premenstrual syndrome (PMS). Preliminary evidence suggests that taking manganese orally in combination with calcium seems to help improve symptoms of PMS including crying, loneliness, anxiety, restlessness, irritability, mood swings, depression, and tension (2004). It's not known if this potential benefit is due to calcium or manganese. More evidence is needed to rate manganese for this use.

Mechanism of Action
Manganese is an essential nutrient that acts as a cofactor in several metabolic and enzymatic reactions (2003,7135). Manganese is found in several foods including nuts, legumes, seeds, tea, whole grains, and leafy green vegetables (2005,2008,7135). However, typically less than 5% of dietary manganese is absorbed. Manganese deficiency

has not been clinically recognized in humans (12468). It's not known if absorption of manganese from supplements is better or worse than manganese from dietary sources. Men seem to absorb less manganese than women. The reason for this is not known, but it might be due to higher serum ferritin concentrations in men. Ferritin is associated with decreased manganese absorption (7135). Manganese is involved in amino acid, cholesterol, and carbohydrate metabolism (7135). Manganese metalloenzymes include arginase, glutamine synthetase, phosphoenolpyruvate decarboxylase, and manganese superoxide (7135).

Researchers think manganese might have a role in osteoporosis. Decreased plasma manganese concentrations have been linked to osteoporosis, and bone mineral density seems to improve when trace minerals including manganese are added to calcium supplementation (7135).

In patients with premenstrual syndrome (PMS), low dietary manganese has been associated with altered mood and increased pain (7135).

Manganese is cleared hepatically and chronic liver disease can cause manganese accumulation and toxicity (1992). Manganese accumulation seems to play a role in Parkinsonian symptoms and encephalopathy associated with chronic liver disease (1992,10666). Some researchers believe neurotoxicity of manganese may result from the depletion of dopamine and production of dopamine quinone and hydrogen peroxide (10665). Manganese is transported by transferrin. The globus pallidus and substantia nigra, areas of the brain associated with the extrapyramidal system, are high in transferrin receptor density, which may result in concentration of manganese (7135). Other research suggests that manganese neurotoxicity results from degenerative processes related to the mitochondria and oxidative stress that cause dysfunction in the basal ganglia (12468).

Adverse Reactions

Orally, manganese is usually well tolerated when used in doses below 11 mg per day (7135). There is some concern that higher doses might increase risk of neurotoxicity, including Parkinsonian-like extrapyramidal symptoms (7135,10665,10666). Symptomatic neurotoxicity caused by manganese is called manganism (12468). People with impaired manganese excretion can also experience these effects even with very low manganese intake. Manganese accumulation due to chronic liver disease seems to cause Parkinsonian-like extrapyramidal symptoms, encephalopathy, and psychosis (1992,7135). Chronic occupational exposure to manganese dust or fumes can also cause extrapyramidal reactions, orthostatic hypotension, decreased heart rate, mood disturbance, and dementia (1990,7135).

Interactions with Herbs & Other Dietary Supplements

CALCIUM: Concomitant administration can decrease manganese absorption (2000).

IP-6 (Phytic Acid): IP-6 found in foods, such as cereals, nuts, and beans, and in supplements can decrease manganese absorption (7135). IP-6 chelates multivalent metal ions in the gastrointestinal tract and prevents absorption (1858). Suggest that patients separate intake of manganese and IP-6 by at least two hours.

IRON: Concomitant administration can decrease manganese absorption (2004).

ZINC: Concomitant administration can increase manganese absorption and plasma levels (2000).

Interactions with Drugs

QUINOLONE ANTIBIOTICS: Theoretically, manganese might reduce the absorption of quinolones. Interactions occur with other multivalent cations, such as calcium and iron (488). Quinolones include ciprofloxacin (Cipro), levofloxacin (Levaquin), gatifloxacin (Tequin), sparfloxacin (Zagam), and others.

TETRACYCLINE ANTIBIOTICS: Theoretically, manganese might reduce the absorption of tetracyclines. Interactions occur with other multivalent cations, such as calcium and iron (488). Tetracyclines include demeclocycline (Declomycin), minocycline (Minocin), and tetracycline (Achromycin).

Interactions with Foods

None known.

Interactions with Lab Tests

ALKALINE PHOSPHATASE: Manganese salts can cause a false increase in serum alkaline phosphatase test results due to enzyme activation in the laboratory procedure (275).

BONE MINERAL DENSITY (BMD): Manganese (in combination with calcium, zinc, and copper) might improve BMD and BMD test results in patients with osteoporosis (1994).

STOOL COLOR: Manganese dioxide might cause stools to turn dark brown to black (275).

Interactions with Diseases or Conditions

CHRONIC LIVER DISEASE: Chronic liver disease can lead to manganese accumulation and toxicity (1992,2001); use manganese cautiously.

IRON-DEFICIENCY ANEMIA: Individuals with iron-deficiency anemia might have enhanced manganese absorption (2002).

PARENTERAL NUTRITION: Patients receiving parenteral nutrition are at increased risk of manganese toxicity. Toxicity has been reported at doses of 0.1 mg manganese per day. Manganese toxicity has been reported in people receiving parenteral nutrition, either as a result of added manganese or as an unintended contaminant (12468).

Dosage and Administration

ORAL: For osteoporosis, 5 mg per day combined with 1000 mg elemental calcium, 15 mg zinc, and 2.5 mg copper has been used (1994). For premenstrual syndrome (PMS), 1 mg or 5.6 mg daily of manganese in combination with calcium 587 mg or 1336 mg daily has been used (2004).

No recommended dietary allowances (RDA) for manganese have been established. The daily Adequate Intake (AI) levels for manganese are: infants birth to 6 months, 3 mcg; 7 to 12 months, 600 mcg; children 1 to 3 years, 1.2 mg; 4 to 8 years 1.5 mg; boys 9 to 13 years, 1.9 mg; 14 to 18 years, 2.2 mg; girls 9 to 18 years, 1.6 mg; men age 19 and older, 2.3 mg; women 19 and older, 1.8 mg; pregnancy age 14 to 50, 2 mg; lactation, 2.6 mg (7135). Tolerable Upper Intake Levels (UL) for manganese have been established (7135). The daily ULs for manganese are: children 1 to 3 years, 2 mg; 4 to 8 years, 3 mg; 9 to 13 years, 6 mg; 14 to 18 years (including pregnancy and lactation), 9 mg; for adults 19 years and older (including pregnancy and lactation), 11 mg (7135).

INTRAVENOUS: In parenteral nutrition, manganese is administered in doses of 150-800 mcg per day for adults and 2 -10 mcg/kg per day for children (157).

Comments

Tell patients to look out for manganese hidden in some supplements. Certain supplements, including those commonly used for osteoarthritis (e.g., Cosamin-DS), contain manganese. Remind patients to adhere to product directions. When taken at doses slightly higher than the recommended dose, these products provide more than the tolerable upper limit (UL) of 11 mg per day.

MANGOSTEEN

Also Known As

Amibiasine, Mang Cut, Manggis, Manggistan, Mangosta, Mangostan, Mangostana, Mangostanier, Mangostao, Mangostier, Mangoustanier, Mangouste, Manguita, Meseter, Queen of Fruits, Sementah, Semetah, Xango, Xango Juice.

CAUTION: See separate listing for Garcinia.

Scientific Names

Garcinia mangostana.

Family: Clusiaceae.

People Use This For

Orally, mangosteen is used for dysentery, diarrhea, urinary tract infections (UTI), gonorrhea, thrush, tuberculosis, menstrual disorders, stimulating the immune system, cancer, osteoarthritis, and improving mental health.

Topically, mangosteen is used for eczema and other skin conditions.

Safety

There is insufficient reliable information available about the safety of mangosteen.

Pregnancy and Lactation: Insufficient reliable information available; avoid using.

Effectiveness

There is insufficient reliable information available about the effectiveness of mangosteen.

Mechanism of Action

The applicable parts of mangosteen are the fruit, juice, rind, bark, and twigs. The fruit and juice are consumed as a healthful and medicinal food and drink. The dried and powdered rind is most commonly used for medicinal purposes. The bark extract, called Amibiasine, is used for amebic dysentery.

Mangosteen fruit, rind, and bark seem to contain several pharmacologically active constituents. The activity of some of these isolated constituents has been characterized. But there is no reliable information about the effects of eating the whole fruit or taking the powdered rind or bark extracts.

The mangosteen rind reportedly contains tannins. Tannins can have an astringent effect on mucosal tissue and can reduce secretions. This astringent effect might reduce diarrhea.

Mangosteen also contains xanthones that have antioxidant and other effects. The specific xanthones include alpha-mangostins, beta-mangostins, and gamma-mangostins (12016). Alpha- and beta-mangostins appear to have in vitro activity against the human leukemia cell line HL60 (12013) and Mycobacterium tuberculosis (12014). Mangosteen also contains the xanthone derivatives garcinone B and garcinone E. These constituents also appear to have in vitro activity against Mycobacterium tuberculosis (12014). Garcinone E also has in vitro cytotoxic activity against hepatocellular carcinomas (12015).

The alpha- and gamma-mangostins also appear to have serotonin and histamine receptor blocking effects (12017).

Adverse Reactions

None reported.

Interactions with Herbs & Other Dietary Supplements
None known.

Interactions with Drugs
None known.

Interactions with Foods
None known.

Interactions with Lab Tests
None known.

Interactions with Diseases or Conditions
None known.

Dosage and Administration
No typical dosage.

Comments
Mangosteen is a tropical fruit. Its fruit is sourly sweet. It's often consumed as a dessert fruit or made into jams. It was thought to be Queen Victoria's favorite fruit.
Mangosteen juice is becoming a popular healthful and medicinal drink. It is usually marketed with the name xango juice. Some marketers claim that xango juice can treat diarrhea, menstrual problems, urinary tract infections, tuberculosis, and a variety of other conditions. There is no reliable scientific evidence to support these claims.

MANNA

Also Known As
Flake Manna, Flowering Ash, Manna Ash.

Scientific Names
Fraxinus ornus.
Family: Oleaceae.

People Use This For
Orally, the dried sap of manna is used as a laxative for constipation and a stool softener for anal fissure, hemorrhoids, and after anorectal surgery.

Safety
POSSIBLY SAFE ...when used orally and appropriately on a short-term basis (2); avoid extended use of manna (2,18).
PREGNANCY AND LACTATION: Insufficient reliable information available; avoid using.

Effectiveness
There is insufficient reliable information available about the effectiveness of manna.

Mechanism of Action
Manna consists of the dried sap collected from the splits in branches and trunk of Fraxinus ornus. The manna bark contains coumarins which can inactivate the serum complement, a component in the host defense system (1527). Manna contains 40-90% mannitol (9,18), which acts as an osmotic laxative (2,18).

Adverse Reactions
Orally, manna can cause nausea or flatulence (2,18).

Interactions with Herbs & Other Dietary Supplements
POTASSIUM DEPLETING HERBS: Theoretically, due to manna's laxative effect, concomitant use of manna with horsetail plant or the licorice rhizome increases the risk of potassium depletion.
STIMULANT LAXATIVE HERBS: Theoretically, concomitant use of manna with stimulant laxatives might increase the risk of potassium depletion. Stimulant laxative herbs include aloe latex, wild cucumber fruit (Ecballium elaterium), blue flag rhizome, alder buckthorn, European buckthorn, butternut bark, cascara bark, castor oil, colocynth fruit pulp, gamboge bark exudate, jalap root, black root, podophyllum root, rhubarb root, senna leaves and pods, and yellow dock root (19).

Interactions with Drugs

DIGOXIN (Lanoxin): Theoretically, the overuse or abuse of manna might increases the risk of adverse effects of cardiac glycoside drugs. Manna contains mannitol, which acts as an osmotic laxative (19).
DIURETIC DRUGS: Overuse of manna might compound diuretic-induced potassium loss (19). There is some concern that people taking manna along with potassium depleting diuretics might have an increased risk for hypokalemia. Initiation of potassium supplementation or an increase in potassium supplement dose may be necessary for some patients. Some diuretics that can deplete potassium include chlorothiazide (Diuril), chlorthalidone (Thalitone), furosemide (Lasix), hydrochlorothiazide (HCTZ, Hydrodiuril, Microzide), and others.

Interactions with Foods

None known.

Interactions with Lab Tests

None known.

Interactions with Diseases or Conditions

GI OBSTRUCTION: Manna is contraindicated in cases of bowel obstruction or ileus (2,18).

Dosage and Administration

ORAL: For adults, the typical dose of manna is 20-30 grams per day or equivalent preparations (2,18). For children, the common dose is 2-16 grams per day (2,18). Manna should not be taken for prolonged use (2,18).

MARIJUANA

Also Known As

Anashca, Banji, Bhang, Blunt, Bud, Cannabis, Charas, Dope, Esrar, Gaga, Ganga, Grass, Hash, Hashish, Hemp, Joint, Kif, Mariguana, Marihuana, Mary Jane, Pot, Sawi, Sinsemilla, Weed.

Scientific Names

Cannabis sativa.
Family: Cannabaceae.

People Use This For

Orally, marijuana is used recreationally as a euphoriant. A cannabinoid from marijuana is used in the prescription-only product dronabinol (Marinol) for the treatment of anorexia or appetite loss associated with AIDS and for cancer chemotherapy induced nausea and vomiting unresponsive to traditional medications. Cannabinoid constituents from marijuana have also been used orally to treat pain and multiple sclerosis (MS).
As an inhalant, marijuana is smoked for nausea, glaucoma, appetite stimulation, and recreationally for altering senses (psychoactivity) and euphoria. Marijuana is also smoked for mucous membrane inflammation, leprosy, fever, dandruff, hemorrhoids, obesity, asthma, urinary tract infections, cough, anorexia associated with weight loss in AIDS patients, pain, multiple sclerosis, and for producing immunosuppression after renal transplantation.

Safety

LIKELY SAFE ...when the cannabinoid constituent dronabinol is used orally and appropriately. Dronabinol (Marinol) is an FDA-approved prescription product (6606,10241).
POSSIBLY UNSAFE ...when marijuana is used orally or inhaled (1395,1396).
PREGNANCY: UNSAFE ...when used orally or inhaled; marijuana passes through the placenta and can reduce fetal growth. Marijuana use during pregnancy is also associated with childhood leukemia (4260).
LACTATION: LIKELY UNSAFE ...when used orally or inhaled because dronabinol (THC) is concentrated and excreted in breast milk (2619,2620).

Effectiveness

POSSIBLY EFFECTIVE

Glaucoma. Smoking marijuana seems to reduce intraocular pressure in patients with glaucoma (1268). There is some evidence marijuana can decrease intraocular pressure, but it also seems to decrease blood flow to the optic nerve. So far, it is not known if it can improve visual function (1268).

HIV/AIDS-related weight loss. Smoking marijuana seems to stimulate the appetite of patients with AIDS. Marijuana cigarettes can increase caloric intake and weight gain in HIV positive patients also taking indinavir (Crixivan) or nelfinavir (Viracept) without affecting viral load (6606,11166).

Multiple sclerosis (MS). Marijuana seems to be effective when smoked, or when the cannabinoids are taken orally for the treatment of spasticity and tremor associated with MS (11167,11168).

There is insufficient reliable information available about the effectiveness of marijuana for its other uses.

Mechanism of Action

The applicable parts of marijuana are the flower and leaf. Marijuana contains cannabinoids, including tetrahydrocannabinol (THC, dronabinol), that act on the central nervous system (CNS) (13). The THC concentration is highest in the flowers and leaves and lowest in the stems, roots, and seeds (6). THC can interact with cell-wall lipids or affect prostaglandin biosynthesis (18). It can act via cannabinoid receptors in neural tissues (2619) or opiate receptors in the forebrain, leading to indirect inhibition of the emetic center in the medulla oblongata (13).
Two types of cannabinoid receptors have been identified in animals: CB1, which is found predominantly in the CNS and is thought to be responsible for the psychoactive effects, and CB2 which is found in high levels on immune system cells including leukocytes, and to a lesser extent in the brain (5887,5888,5889). Endogenous substances which bind to these receptors have been identified (5887,5888).
Tetrahydrocannabinol is a partial CB1 receptor agonist and has limited CB2 agonist activity (5889). While short-term inhalation increases bronchodilation and reduces bronchospasm, long-term use impairs lung function, which can result in constrictive lung disease. The cannabinoids in marijuana are allergenic in animal models (6).
THC is absorbed orally or by inhalation, is rapidly distributed throughout the body, and has a high affinity for fat tissues (6). The metabolites appear in the urine for ten days or more after a single exposure and for several weeks after chronic exposure (6). In an animal model of multiple sclerosis, tetrahydrocannabinol has been reported to reduce tremor and spasticity, possibly through its activity at CB1 receptors in the brain (5889).
THC seems to suppress the immune function by its action at the CB2 receptors. It increases the activity of interleukin-10 (IL-10) and IL-4, and other cytokines that inhibit immune function. This effect might reduce resistance to infections (10239,10240).
Research on the effect of cannabinoids on cancer is conflicting. The effect of THC on IL-10, IL-4, and other cytokines suggests it might promote the growth of cancer cells (10239,10240). However, cannabinoids seem to inhibit human breast cancer cell proliferation in vitro. When THC is infused directly into the tumor mass, it seems to produce tumor eradication or improvements in survival in animals with experimentally induced malignant gliomas (a type of brain tumor). THC induces tumor cell apoptosis via CB1 and CB2 receptors expressed on the glioma cells (5887).

Adverse Reactions

The use of marijuana can cause xerostomia (dry mouth), nausea, vomiting, and a characteristic reddening of the eyes. Cardiovascular effects can include tachycardia, hypotension or hypertension, syncope, palpitations, and vasodilation (13,2619).
Intoxicating doses of marijuana impair reaction time, motor coordination, and visual perceptions, and can also produce panic reactions, hallucinations, flashbacks, depression, and other emotional disturbances. An individual's driving ability can be impaired up to 8 hours (18). Long-term use of marijuana can cause cognitive impairment that lasts longer than the period of acute intoxication. These cognitive impairments develop slowly and worsen as the years of marijuana use increase, becoming clinically significant after about 2 decades of use (10242).
The chronic use of marijuana can cause laryngitis, bronchitis, apathy, psychic decline, sexual dysfunction, and abnormal menstruation (18), and has been associated with several cases of an unusual pattern of bullous emphysema (1395). Signs of acute poisoning from marijuana include nausea, vomiting, lacrimation, hacking cough, disturbed cardiac function, and limb numbness (18). Marijuana has a high abuse potential (6). Regular smoking of 3-4 marijuana cigarettes per day is reported to produce as many symptoms as an average of 22 tobacco cigarettes per day, and comparable airway histological effects as 20 tobacco cigarettes per day (1395).
Regular use of marijuana in middle-aged persons has been associated with an increased risk of myocardial infarction. Unpublished evidence indicates that there is a 4.8 fold increase in relative risk of myocardial infarction within the first hour following smoking marijuana. Regular marijuana smoking was defined as smoking marijuana less than once a month to daily (1356).

Interactions with Herbs & Other Dietary Supplements

SUPPLEMENTS WITH SEDATIVE PROPERTIES: Theoretically, concomitant use of marijuana with supplements that have sedative properties might increase the risk of excessive drowsiness (2619). Some of these supplements include 5-HTP, calamus, California poppy, catnip, hops, Jamaican dogwood, kava, St. John's wort, scullcap, valerian, yerba mansa, and others.

Interactions with Drugs

BARBITURATES: Marijuana can decrease barbiturate clearance rate (2619). Some of these sedative medications include pentobarbital (Nembutal), phenobarbital (Luminal), secobarbital (Seconal), and others.
CNS DEPRESSANTS: Use of dronabinol can have additive or synergistic effects drugs such as narcotics, antihistamines, benzodiazepines and other CNS depressants (2619).
DISULFIRAM (Antabuse): Concomitant use with marijuana can cause transient hypomanic episodes (2619).
FLUOXETINE (Prozac): Concomitant use with marijuana can cause transient hypomanic episodes (2619).
THEOPHYLLINE: Concomitant use with marijuana can increase theophylline metabolism (2619).

Interactions with Foods

ALCOHOL: Concomitant use of alcohol with dronabinol can have additive or synergistic CNS effects (2619).

Interactions with Lab Tests

INTRAOCULAR PRESSURE: Marijuana smoking reduces intraocular pressure and test results in some patients with glaucoma (1268).

Interactions with Diseases or Conditions

CARDIOVASCULAR DISEASES: Marijuana has the potential to cause tachycardia and transient hypertension (6).
COMPROMISED IMMUNE FUNCTION: Cannabinoids in marijuana can decrease immune function, which might reduce resistance to infections (10239,10240).
RESPIRATORY DISEASES: Long-term use of marijuana can exacerbate respiratory conditions (6). Chronic marijuana use has been associated with several cases of an unusual pattern of bullous emphysema (1395).
SEIZURE DISORDERS: Marijuana might exacerbate, or help control, seizure disorders in some individuals (6).

Dosage and Administration

ORAL: People typically use 5 to 15 drops of marijuana tincture or 1 to 3 drops of fluid extract. The prescription product dronabinol (Marinol) is used in doses of 5 to 15 mg/m2 every 2 for 4 hours for cancer chemotherapy-induced nausea and vomiting, and 2.5 to 10 mg twice daily for appetite stimulation in people with AIDS (6606,11166).
INHALATION: People typically use 1 to 3 grains (65 to 195 mg) of cannabis for smoking. Hashish, the plant resin, is smoked in a dose of up to 1 grain (16 to 65 mg). Potency may vary. The drug deteriorates rapidly, requiring ascending doses to produce its effect (5267).

Comments

Avoid confusion with hemp, a distinct variety of Cannabis sativa cultivated for its fiber and seeds, which contains less than 1% THC. Marijuana is classified as a Schedule I controlled substance, making possession illegal. The cannabinoid constituent of marijuana, dronabinol (Marinol), is an FDA-approved prescription product. It's approved for AIDS-related anorexia and chemotherapy induced nausea and vomiting (6606,10241,11166). Cannabinoids are at least as effective as prochlorperazine (Compazine), metoclopramide (Reglan), chlorpromazine (Compazine), thiethylperazine (Torecan), and other conventional antiemetic drugs (6606,10241).
Cannabinoids from marijuana also appear to be similar to codeine for treatment of pain. However, excessive sedation and other central nervous system effects make cannabinoids undesirable as analgesics (10235).

MARJORAM

Also Known As

Garden Marjoram, Gartenmajoran, Knotted Marjoram, Majoran, Majorana Aetheroleum Oil, Majorana Herb, Marjolaine, Mejorana, Sweet Marjoram.
CAUTION: See separate listing for Oregano.

Scientific Names

Origanum majorana, synonyms Majorana hortensis, Majorana majorana.
Family: Lamiaceae/Labiatae.

People Use This For

Orally, marjoram is used for rhinitis and colds in infants and toddlers, gastritis, stimulating appetite, as a digestive aid, antispasmodic, antiflatulent, astringent, ulcus ventriculi, to promote circulation, healthy sleep, and treat mood swings. Marjoram is also used orally for liver disease, gallstones, dry and irritating coughs, swellings of the nasal and pharyngeal mucosa, inflammation of the ears, headaches, reducing blood glucose levels, promoting lactation, urogenital bleeding, climacteric complaints, as a nerve tonic, heart tonic, and sprains, bruises, lumbago.
Marjoram oil is used for coughs, gall bladder complaints, gastrointestinal cramps and disorders, depression, dizziness, migraines, nervous headaches, neurasthenia, paralysis, paroxysmal coughs, rhinitis, and as a diuretic.
In foods, marjoram is a culinary spice and commonly used in foods. The oil and oleoresin are used as flavor ingredients in foods and beverages.
In manufacturing, the oil is used as a fragrance component in soaps and cosmetics.

Safety

LIKELY SAFE ...when used in amounts commonly found in foods. Marjoram has Generally Recognized As Safe (GRAS) status in the US (4912).
POSSIBLY SAFE ...when the leaf is used orally for medicinal purposes (12) on a short-term basis (2). ...when marjoram oil is used orally and appropriately (11).
POSSIBLY UNSAFE ...when the flower, leaf, and oil are used long-term because marjoram contains arbutin and hydroxyquinone. Some information suggests hydroxyquinone might cause cancer (2). ...when using fresh marjoram topically because it can cause eye and skin inflammation (11).
CHILDREN: POSSIBLY UNSAFE ...when excessive amounts are used in children; avoid using (2).
PREGNANCY: POSSIBLY UNSAFE ...when used in medicinal amounts; marjoram has the potential for

stimulating menstruation (19).
LACTATION: Insufficient reliable information available; avoid using in amounts larger than those found in foods.

Effectiveness

There is insufficient reliable information available about the effectiveness of marjoram.

Mechanism of Action

The applicable parts of marjoram are the flower, leaf and oil. Marjoram has antiflatulent, antispasmodic, diaphoretic, and diuretic properties (11). The volatile oil demonstrates antimicrobial and insecticidal activity (18). There is some evidence that marjoram has antibacterial activity and antiviral activity against the herpes simplex virus (11). The constituents of marjoram include small amounts of arbutin and hydroxyquinone (2). Arbutin, an antibacterial principle, is poorly absorbed from the gastrointestinal tract (7). Marjoram is a rich source of calcium and iron (19).

Adverse Reactions

Topically, fresh marjoram can cause eye and skin inflammation (11). Hydroxyquinone can cause skin depigmentation (2); however, this adverse effect has not been reported with the use of the marjoram ointment (2).

Interactions with Herbs & Other Dietary Supplements

None known.

Interactions with Drugs

None known.

Interactions with Foods

None known.

Interactions with Lab Tests

None known.

Interactions with Diseases or Conditions

CROSS-ALLERGENICITY: Marjoram can cause allergic reactions in people allergic to the Lamiaceae family plants, which include basil, hyssop, lavender, mint, oregano, and sage (3705).

Dosage and Administration

ORAL: The typical dose of marjoram is one to two cups of the tea throughout the day (18). The tea is prepared by steeping 1-2 teaspoons of the flower or leaf in 250 mL boiling water for 5 minutes and then straining.
TOPICAL: Marjoram is commonly used as a poultice or mouthwash (18).

Comments

In early Greek mythology, the goddess of love, Aphrodite, was believed to have grown marjoram, and marjoram has since been used in various love potions (6002). Avoid confusion with oregano (Origanum vulgare), also referred to as wild marjoram and winter marjoram (2,18).

MARSH BLAZING STAR

Also Known As

Backache Root, Blazing-Star, Button Snakeroot, Colic Root, Devil's Bite Prairie-Pine, Gay-Feather.

Scientific Names

Liatris spicata, synonyms Laciniaria spicata, Liatris callilepis, Serratula spicata.
Family: Asteraceae/Compositae.

People Use This For

Orally, marsh blazing star is used for kidney disorders, dysmenorrhea, gonorrhea, and as a diuretic.

Safety

There is insufficient reliable information available about the safety of marsh blazing star.
Pregnancy and Lactation: Insufficient reliable information available; avoid using.

Effectiveness

There is insufficient reliable information available about the effectiveness of marsh blazing star.

Mechanism of Action

The applicable part of marsh blazing star is the root. Marsh blazing star contains coumarin as its active principle (18). However, coumarin itself is not an anticoagulant. It has only 0.1%-0.02% of the anticoagulant effect of bishydroxycoumarin (295). Some studies suggest coumarin might be effective in reducing edemas and inflammations by increasing venous and lymphatic return (295).

Adverse Reactions

Orally, marsh blazing star, which contains coumarin, can be associated with nausea and vomiting (286), diarrhea, dizziness, insomnia (287), asymptomatic SGOT elevations (286), and liver toxicity (6,18).
Topically, handling the plant can cause contact dermatitis (3837).
Marsh blazing star can cause an allergic reaction in individuals sensitive to the Asteraceae/Compositae family. Members of this family include ragweed, chrysanthemums, marigolds, daisies, and many other herbs.

Interactions with Herbs & Other Dietary Supplements

None known.

Interactions with Drugs

None known.

Interactions with Foods

None known.

Interactions with Lab Tests

None known.

Interactions with Diseases or Conditions

CROSS-ALLERGENICITY: Can cause an allergic reaction in individuals sensitive to the Asteraceae/Compositae family. Members of this family include ragweed, chrysanthemums, marigolds, daisies, and many other herbs.

Dosage and Administration

ORAL: The ground root is used as tea (6).

MARSH MARIGOLD

Also Known As

Bull's Eyes, Cowslip, Horse Blobs, Kingcups, Leopard's Foot, Meadow Routs, Palsy Root, Solsequia, Sponsa Solis, Verrucaria, Water Blobs, Water Dragon.
CAUTION: See separate listing for Cowslip.

Scientific Names

Caltha palustris, synonym Caltha palustris.
Family: Ranunculaceae.

People Use This For

Orally, marsh marigold is used to stop pain and cramps, for menstrual disorders, bronchial inflammation, jaundice, and liver and biliary disorders. Marsh marigold is also used orally as a laxative, diuretic, and to lower cholesterol levels and raise blood sugar.
Topically, marsh marigold is used for cleaning skin lesions and sores.

Safety

LIKELY UNSAFE ...when the fresh above ground parts are used orally or topically because they cause severe local irritation (18).
There is insufficient reliable information about the safety of the medicinal use of the dried above ground parts.
PREGNANCY AND LACTATION: LIKELY UNSAFE ...when the fresh above ground parts are used orally or topically (18). There is insufficient reliable information available about the safety of the dried above ground parts during pregnancy and lactation.

Effectiveness

There is insufficient reliable information available about the effectiveness of marsh marigold.

Mechanism of Action

The applicable parts of marsh marigold are the above ground parts of the flowering plant. When the fresh plant is crushed or cut into small pieces, the glycoside ranunculin is enzymatically changed into a severely irritating protoanemonin, which in turn, rapidly degrades into the less toxic anemonin (18). Both protoanemonin and ranunculin are destroyed to an unknown extent during the drying process (2).

Adverse Reactions

Orally, ingestion of marsh marigold can cause severe irritation of the gastrointestinal tract with colic and diarrhea. Irritation of the urinary tract can also occur.
Topically, skin contact with the fresh plant can cause blisters and burns that are difficult to heal (18).

Interactions with Herbs & Other Dietary Supplements

None known.

Interactions with Drugs

None known.

Interactions with Foods

None known.

Interactions with Lab Tests

None known.

Interactions with Diseases or Conditions

None known.

Dosage and Administration

No typical dosage.

MARSH TEA

Also Known As

James' Tea, Ledi palustris herba, Marsh Citrus, Moth Herb, Romarin Sauvage, Sumpfporst, Swamp Tea, Wild Rosemary.
CAUTION: See separate listing for Labrador Tea.

Scientific Names

Rhododendron tomentosum var. tomentosum, synonyms Ledum palustre, Rhododendron palustre.
Family: Ericaceae

People Use This For

Orally, marsh tea is used for rheumatic discomforts, whooping cough, for bronchitis, cold, cough, whitlow (herpes infection of the finger), relieving chest and lung ailments, stimulating milk flow, as a diaphoretic, diuretic, abortifacient, expectorant, and narcotic.

Safety

LIKELY UNSAFE ...when large amounts are used orally to try to cause abortion (2). The essential oil of marsh tea causes severe gastrointestinal (GI) tract irritation, kidneys and urinary tract damage, and central nervous system (CNS) excitation followed by paralysis (2).
There is insufficient reliable information available about the safety of marsh tea for its other uses.
PREGNANCY: LIKELY UNSAFE ...when used orally; avoid using (2,19). Marsh tea is considered to be a potential uterine stimulant (19).
LACTATION: Insufficient reliable information available; avoid using.

Effectiveness

There is insufficient reliable information available about the effectiveness of marsh tea.

Mechanism of Action

Some evidence suggests marsh tea might have antitussive and anti-inflammatory activity. It might also inhibit motility (2) and stimulate uterine activity (19).

Adverse Reactions

Orally, ingestion of large amounts of marsh tea can cause poisoning (2). The essential oil of marsh tea can cause severe irritation of the gastrointestinal (GI) tract, vomiting, diarrhea, irritation and damage to the kidneys and urinary tract, heavy perspiration, myalgias, arthralgias, and central nervous system excitation with narcotic intoxication, followed by paralysis (2).

Interactions with Herbs & Other Dietary Supplements
None known.

Interactions with Drugs
CNS DEPRESSANTS: Marsh tea can potentiate effects of barbiturates and alcohol (2).

Interactions with Foods
None known.

Interactions with Lab Tests
None known.

Interactions with Diseases or Conditions
GASTROINTESTINAL (GI) IRRITATION: Theoretically, might exacerbate gastrointestinal tract inflammation or irritation (2).
KIDNEY DYSFUNCTION: Contraindicated in individuals with kidney dysfunction (2).
URINARY TRACT IRRITATION: Theoretically, might exacerbate urinary tract irritation and inflammation (2).

Dosage and Administration
No typical dosage.

MARSHMALLOW

Also Known As
Alteia, Althaeae folium, Althaeae radi, Althea, Herba Malvae, Mallards, Mortification Root, Racine De Guimauve, Sweet Weed, Wymote.
CAUTION: See separate listings for Country Mallow and Mallow.

Scientific Names
Althaea officinalis, synonym Althaea taurinensis.
Family: Malvaceae.

People Use This For
Orally, marshmallow leaf and root are used for respiratory tract mucous membrane inflammation, dry cough, inflammation of the gastric mucosa, diarrhea, peptic ulcers, constipation, urinary tract inflammation, and urinary calculus.
Topically, marshmallow leaf and root are used for abscesses, for varicose and thrombotic ulcers, as a poultice for skin inflammation or burns, and for other wounds. Marshmallow leaf is used topically as a poultice for insect bites. Marshmallow root is used topically in ointments for chapped skin and chilblains.
For foods, marshmallow leaf is used as a flavoring agent.
In manufacturing, the marshmallow root is used in foods and beverages.

Safety
LIKELY SAFE ...when used in amounts commonly found in foods. Marshmallow root has Generally Recognized As Safe status (GRAS) for use in foods in the US (4912). ...when used orally in medicinal amounts (4,12).
POSSIBLY SAFE ...when used topically (4).
PREGNANCY AND LACTATION: Insufficient reliable information available.

Effectiveness
There is insufficient reliable information available about the effectiveness of marshmallow.

Mechanism of Action
The applicable parts of marshmallow are the leaves and the root. Marshmallow leaf and root contain mucilage polysaccharides that can soothe and protect mucous membranes from local irritation by forming a protective layer (1,4,6,7,9,18). The mucilage can inhibit mucociliary transport (1,6,18), stimulate phagocytosis (1,18), suppress cough (1,6,8,11), increase the anti-inflammatory effects of topical dexamethasone (1,6,18), and have hypoglycemic activity (1,4). The mucilage can also have antimicrobial, spasmolytic, antisecretory, diuretic, antilithic, and wound-healing effects (4,6).

Adverse Reactions
Orally, marshmallow can cause hypoglycemia (4,11,18).

Interactions with Herbs & Other Dietary Supplements
HERBS AND SUPPLEMENTS: Concomitant use of marshmallow can retard the absorption of other herbs or supplements (1,11,12).

Interactions with Drugs
ANTIDIABETES DRUGS: Theoretically, due to claims of hypoglycemic effects, marshmallow might interfere with hypoglycemic therapy (4).
ORAL DRUGS: The mucilage in marshmallow might impair absorption of oral drugs (1,11,12,19).

Interactions with Foods
None known.

Interactions with Lab Tests
BLOOD GLUCOSE: Theoretically, marshmallow could lower blood glucose and test results (4,11,18).

Interactions with Diseases or Conditions
DIABETES: Theoretically, marshmallow could interfere with blood sugar control (4).

Dosage and Administration
ORAL: For irritation of the mouth or pharynx and associated dry cough, the typical dose of marshmallow is 2-5 grams of the dried leaf, 5 grams of the dried root or one cup of either leaf or root tea three times daily (4). The leaf tea is prepared by steeping 2-5 grams of the dried leaf in 150 mL boiling water for 5-10 minutes and then straining. The root tea is prepared by steeping 2-5 grams of the dried root in 150 mL cold water for 1-1.5 hours, straining, and then warming before consumption. The usual dose of the liquid leaf or root extract (1:1 in 25% alcohol) is 2-5 mL three times daily (4). For irritation of oral or pharyngeal mucosa and the associated cough, the common dose of the marshmallow root syrup is 2-10 mL up to three times daily (1,4).
TOPICAL: The 5% powdered leaf in an ointment base is commonly applied three times daily (4).

Comments
Avoid confusion with the mallow (Malva sylvestris) flower and leaf.

MARTAGON

Also Known As
Purple Turk's Cap Lily, Turk's Cap.

Scientific Names
Lilium martagon.
Family: Liliaceae

Comments
At the date of publication, this product was not a common ingredient used in brand name supplements marketed to consumers. Details about this product are available in the online version of *Natural Medicines Comprehensive Database.* See www.naturaldatabase.com.

MASTERWORT

Also Known As
Cow Cabbage, Cow Parsnip, Hogweed, Madnep, Radix Pimpinelle Franconiae, Woolly Parsnip, Youthwort.
CAUTION: See separate listing for Goutweed.

Scientific Names
Heracleum sphondylium, Heracleum sphondylium subsp. montanum, synonyms Heracleum lanatum, Heracleum maximum, Heracleum montanum.
Family: Apiaceae/Umbelliferae.

People Use This For
Orally, masterwort is used for relief of muscle cramps, stomach disorders, digestive problems, diarrhea, and mucous membrane inflammation of the GI tract.

Safety
POSSIBLY UNSAFE ...when used orally. Masterwort can cause phototoxicity (19), and some of the furocoumarin constituents can be carcinogenic (4).
PREGNANCY: LIKELY UNSAFE ...when used orally; contraindicated for use in early pregnancy, due to the reported ability to stimulate menstruation (19).
LACTATION: POSSIBLY UNSAFE ...when used orally (4); avoid using.

Effectiveness
There is insufficient reliable information available about the effectiveness of masterwort.

Mechanism of Action
Masterwort is considered to be a mild expectorant, although this effect remains unproven (18). It contains furocoumarins (bergapten, isopimpinellin, pimpinellin, isoberapten, spondin) and a volatile oil containing n-octylacetate (18). Bergapten, also known as 5-methoxypysoralen, is phototoxic and may also be carcinogenic (4).

Adverse Reactions
Orally, use increases skin sensitivity to UV light and can lead to phototoxicity (19).
Topically, application of the fresh plant can cause photodermatitis (3835).
Masterwort may also be carcinogenic.

Interactions with Herbs & Other Dietary Supplements
None known.

Interactions with Drugs
PHOTOSENSITIZING DRUGS: Contraindicated due to additive photosensitizing effect (19).

Interactions with Foods
None known.

Interactions with Lab Tests
None known.

Interactions with Diseases or Conditions
ULTRAVIOLET LIGHT THERAPY: Contraindicated due to photosensitizing effect (19); avoid excessive periods in sun (19).

Dosage and Administration
No typical dosage.

Comments
Masterwort is reportedly used as a replacement/adulterant for greater burnet-saxifrage (Pimpinella major) (7).

MASTIC

Also Known As
Lentisk, Mastich, Mastix.

Scientific Names
Pistacia lentiscus.
Family: Anacardiaceae.

People Use This For
Orally, mastic is used for gastric and duodenal ulcers, respiratory conditions, muscle aches, and to improve circulation. It is also used for bacterial and fungal infections.
Topically, mastic is used as skin care for cuts, as an insect repellent, to improve adhesive strength in surgical tapes, and as a drug releasing vehicle.
In dentistry, mastic resin is used as a material for fillings. The masticated resin releases substances that freshen the breath and tighten the gums.
In manufacturing, mastic resin is used in the food and drink industries and in the production of chewing gum.

Safety
POSSIBLY SAFE ...when used orally (18).
PREGNANCY AND LACTATION: Insufficient reliable information available; avoid using.

Effectiveness
There is insufficient reliable information available about the effectiveness of mastic.

Mechanism of Action
The applicable part of mastic is the resin. Mastic tree contains resins including the triterpenes mastic acid, isomastic acid, oleanlic acid, and tirucallol. It also contains a volatile oil containing alpha-pinene as a constituent. The volatile oil and the resin are both thought to have astringent and aromatic effects (18). For prevention of gastric and duodenal ulcers, some researchers think mastic might have antisecretory and possibly cytoprotective effects. Animal models show that it seems to help protect the gastric mucosa during aspirin, phenylbutazone, or reserpine therapy (4142). This effect has not yet been found in humans. There is some in vitro evidence that mastic extract has antimicrobial and antifungal activity (4141). There is also preliminary evidence that mastic might have hypotensive and antioxidant effects (6).

Adverse Reactions
Children who ingest mastic tree resin might develop diarrhea (18). The pollen of mastic tree is allergenic (4140). Exposure to mastic tree can cause allergic reactions in individuals allergic to Schinus terebintifolious and other Pistacia species (4140).

Interactions with Herbs & Other Dietary Supplements
CROSS-ALLERGENICITY: Individuals allergic to mastic tree might also have an allergic reaction to Schinus terebintifolious and other Pistacia species (4140).

Interactions with Drugs
None known.

Interactions with Foods
None known.

Interactions with Lab Tests
None known.

Interactions with Diseases or Conditions
None known.

Dosage and Administration
No typical dosage.

Comments
Mastic resin is the resin from the trunk of Pistacia lentiscus.

MATE

Also Known As
Chimarrao, Hervea, Ilex, Jesuit's Tea, Maté Folium, Paraguay Tea, St. Bartholemew's Tea, Yerba Maté.
CAUTION: See separate listings for Caffeine, Green Tea, Black Tea, Oolong Tea, Cocoa, Cola Nut, Guarana, Mate.

Scientific Names
Ilex paraguariensis.
Family: Aquifoliaceae.

People Use This For
Orally, mate is used as a stimulant to relieve mental and physical fatigue. It's also used as a diuretic, for modifying mood or affective disorders, as a mild analgesic for headache and rheumatic pains, and as a laxative in large amounts. It is also used orally for depression, weight loss, urinary tract infection, cardiac insufficiency, arrhythmias, hypotension, nervous heart complaints, kidney and bladder stones, and to promote cleansing and excretion of waste. In foods, the use of mate includes a tea-like beverage.

Safety
POSSIBLY SAFE ...when used orally and appropriately on a short-term basis (11866).
POSSIBLY UNSAFE ...when mate is used orally in large amounts or for prolonged periods of time. Mate is associated with an increased risk of mouth cancer, esophageal cancer, laryngeal cancer, kidney cancer, bladder cancer, and lung cancer (1528,1529,1530,1531,11863,11864).
LIKELY UNSAFE ...when used orally in very high doses. Mate contains caffeine. The fatal acute oral dose of

caffeine is estimated to be 10-14 grams (150-200 mg per kilogram). Serious toxicity can occur at lower doses depending on variables in caffeine sensitivity such as smoking, age, prior caffeine use, etc. (11832).

CHILDREN: POSSIBLY UNSAFE ...when used orally. Mate is associated with an increased risk of mouth cancer, esophageal cancer, laryngeal cancer, kidney cancer, bladder cancer, and lung cancer (1528,1529,1530,1531,11863,11864).

PREGNANCY: POSSIBLY UNSAFE ...when used orally. Mate is associated with an increased risk of mouth cancer, esophageal cancer, laryngeal cancer, kidney cancer, bladder cancer, and lung cancer (1528,1529,1530,1531,11863,11864). Teratogenic studies have not been performed. Mate contains caffeine. Caffeine crosses the placenta, producing fetal blood concentrations similar to maternal levels. It is generally recommended that mothers should avoid consuming more than 300 mg of caffeine daily or more than 3 cups of tea or coffee per day (2708). High maternal doses of caffeine throughout pregnancy have resulted in symptoms of caffeine withdrawal in newborn infants (9891). High doses of caffeine have also been associated with spontaneous abortion, premature delivery, and low birth weight (2709,2711); however, one retrospective study of mothers consuming mate tea during pregnancy found no significant association between mate consumption and preterm or small for gestational age births (13113). But this study did not consider the amount of mate or caffeine consumption, only the frequency of consumption.

LACTATION: POSSIBLY UNSAFE ...when used orally. Mate is associated with an increased risk of mouth cancer, esophageal cancer, laryngeal cancer, kidney cancer, bladder cancer, and lung cancer (1528,1529,1530,1531,11863,11864). Whether carcinogenic constituents of mate are transferred via breast milk is unknown. Mate contains caffeine. Consumption of mate might cause irritability and increased bowel activity in nursing infants (6026).

Effectiveness

INSUFFICIENT RELIABLE EVIDENCE to RATE

Obesity. Mate taken orally might cause weight loss when used in combination with guarana and damiana (11866). More evidence is needed to rate mate for this use.

Mechanism of Action

The applicable parts of mate are the leaf and leaf stem. It contains caffeine, theobromine, theophylline, phytol, stigmasterol, and squalene. The concentrations of these constituents vary with growing conditions, harvesting, and preparation methods (11865,11867). Mate also contains various minerals including phosphorus, iron, calcium, thiamine, riboflavin, vitamin C, and vitamin E. Other constituents include tannins and N-nitroso compounds that are potential carcinogens (11863,11865).

The usual concentration of caffeine in mate is 0.5% to 0.8% (compared to 1-2% in coffee) (11865,11867). The caffeine in mate stimulates the central nervous system (CNS), heart, muscles, and possibly the pressor centers that control blood pressure (2722). Possible mechanisms include adenosine receptor blockade and phosphodiesterase inhibition (2722). By blocking adenosine receptors, caffeine is thought to increase the release of neurotransmitters such as dopamine (6370). Caffeine also decreases airway resistance and stimulates respiration, via adenosine receptor blockade and phosphodiesterase inhibition (11836). It has also been proposed that caffeine may decrease GABA and serotonin signaling (6370). Caffeine stimulates gastric acid secretion, and increases plasma catecholamine levels (11837). Caffeine can have positive inotropic and chronotropic effects on the heart (11836). Caffeine can also acutely elevate both diastolic and systolic blood pressure, but might not have this effect in habitual users (2722). Caffeine exerts a diuretic effect, with water losses estimated at 1.17 mL per milligram of caffeine (2712). Tachyphylaxis to the diuretic effect develops rapidly, diminishing fluid losses associated with caffeine intake (10206). Caffeine-containing beverages consumed during moderate endurance exercise do not appear to compromise bodily hydration status (2713). Caffeine does not substantially affect the fluid status of people who drink caffeinated beverages on a regular basis (10206).

Caffeine, a constituent of mate, has been reported to cause increases and decreases in blood glucose. In people with type 2 diabetes, acute administration of caffeine impairs postprandial glucose metabolism, while acute abstention from caffeine reduces postprandial glucose levels by 21%. Whether these effects also occur with caffeinated beverages and herbs is unknown (12374). Other research in obese people suggests that caffeine ingestion may contribute to insulin resistance (12375). However, one study found that type 1 diabetics taking 200 mg of caffeine twice daily had increased frequency and intensity of warning signs of hypoglycemia. This may be due to a reduction in blood flow to the brain and an increase in glucose utilization by the brain (6024).

In vitro and epidemiological research suggests that mate may be carcinogenic. Carcinogenesis may result from thermal injury; mate is consumed as a hot beverage in South America. Because smoking in combination with mate greatly increases cancer risk, some researchers think that mate might act as a solvent for carcinogens in tobacco.

Adverse Reactions

Orally, the prolonged use of mate is associated with an increased risk of mouth cancer, esophageal cancer, laryngeal cancer, kidney cancer, bladder cancer, and lung cancer (1528,1529,1530,1531,11863,11864). The effect seems to be cumulative-dose dependent. The risk of cancer with mate use seems to increase if it is taken as a warm beverage. Tobacco and alcohol use can increase risk 7-fold (11863). There is one report of venous occlusive disease associated with excessive, long-term mate consumption (5614).

The caffeine constituent of mate can cause insomnia, nervousness, restlessness, gastric irritation, nausea and

vomiting, as well as tachycardia, quickened respiration, tremors, delirium, convulsions, and diuresis (11832,11838).
Caffeine may exacerbate sleep disturbances in patients with acquired immunodeficiency syndrome (AIDS) (10204).
Caffeine can cause anaphylaxis in sensitive individuals, although true IgE-mediated caffeine allergy seems to be relatively rare (11315).

Large doses of caffeine can produce headache, anxiety, agitation, ringing in the ears, premature heartbeat, and arrhythmia (11832,11838). In fatal overdose, the cause of death is usually ventricular fibrillation (11838). High doses of mate providing 250 mg of caffeine can also increase blood pressure. This doesn't seem to occur in people who habitually consume caffeine products (2722). Although tolerance to caffeine is a widely held belief, there is little supportive clinical evidence. If it exists, it appears to be of little clinical significance (11839). Withdrawal symptoms such as irritability, sleepiness, delirium, nausea, vomiting, rhinorrhea, nervousness, restlessness, anxiety, muscle tension, muscle pains, and flushed face have been described. However, these symptoms may be from nonpharmacological factors related to knowledge and expectation of effects. Clinically significant symptoms caused by caffeine withdrawal may be uncommon (2723,11839).

Some evidence shows caffeine is associated with fibrocystic breast disease, breast cancer, and endometriosis in women; however, this is controversial since findings are conflicting (8043). Restricting caffeine in women with fibrocystic breast conditions doesn't seem to affect breast nodularity, swelling, or pain (8996).

Epidemiological evidence regarding the relationship between caffeine use and the risk for osteoporosis is contradictory. Caffeine can increase urinary excretion of calcium (2669,10202,11317). Women identified with a genetic variant of the vitamin D receptor appear to be at an increased risk for the detrimental effect of caffeine on bone mass (2669). However, moderate caffeine intake, less than 300 mg per day, does not seem to significantly increase osteoporosis risk in most postmenopausal women with normal calcium intake (2669,6025,10202,11317).

Combining ephedra with mate increases the risk of adverse effects, due to the caffeine contained in mate (2729).
One unpublished report associated jitteriness, hypertension, seizures, temporary loss of consciousness, and hospitalization requiring life support with the use of a combination ephedra and guarana (caffeine) product (1380).
There is one report of ischemic stroke in an athlete who consumed ephedra 40-60 mg, creatine monohydrate 6 grams, caffeine 400-600 mg, and a variety of other supplements daily for six weeks (1275). Some evidence shows caffeine is associated with fibrocystic breast disease, breast cancer, and endometriosis in women; however, this is controversial since findings are conflicting (8043).

Interactions with Herbs & Other Dietary Supplements

CAFFEINE-CONTAINING HERBS/SUPPLEMENTS: Concomitant use of mate and caffeine-containing herbs/supplements constitutes therapeutic duplication (due to the caffeine contained in mate) which increases the risk of caffeine-related adverse effects. Other natural products which contain caffeine include cocoa, coffee, cola nut, black tea, and guarana.

CALCIUM: High caffeine intake from foods and beverages including mate increases urinary calcium excretion (2570).

CREATINE: There is some concern that combining caffeine, a constituent of mate, with ephedra and creatine might increase the risk of serious adverse effects. There is a report of ischemic stroke in an athlete who consumed creatine monohydrate 6 grams, caffeine 400-600 mg, ephedra 40-60 mg, and a variety of other supplements daily for 6 weeks (1275). Caffeine might also decrease creatine's possible beneficial effects on athletic performance. Some researchers think caffeine can inhibit phosphocreatine resynthesis (2117,4575).

EPHEDRA (Ma Huang): Use of ephedra with mate can increase the risk of stimulatory adverse effects due to its caffeine content. There is evidence that using ephedra with caffeine might increase the risk of serious life-threatening or debilitating adverse effects such as hypertension, myocardial infarction, stroke, seizures, and death (6486,10307). Tell patients to avoid taking mate with ephedra and other stimulants such as bitter orange.

Interactions with Drugs

ADENOSINE (Adenocard): The caffeine in mate is a competitive inhibitor of adenosine at the cellular level. However, caffeine doesn't seem to affect supplemental adenosine because high interstitial levels of adenosine overcome the antagonistic effects of caffeine (11771).

ALCOHOL (Ethanol): Concomitant use of alcohol can increase caffeine serum concentrations and the risk of caffeine adverse effects. Alcohol reduces caffeine metabolism (6370).

AMPHETAMINES: Theoretically, the caffeine in mate might increase the risk of additive CNS effects (2719).

ANTICOAGULANT/ANTIPLATELET DRUGS: Theoretically, the caffeine in mate might increase the risk of bleeding when used concomitantly with these agents. Caffeine is reported to have antiplatelet activity (8028,8029); however, this interaction has not been reported in humans. Antiplatelet agents include aspirin, clopidogrel (Plavix), dipyridamole (Persantine), ticlopidine (Ticlid), and others. Anticoagulant agents include heparin and warfarin (Coumadin).

ANTIDIABETES DRUGS: Theoretically, concomitant use of caffeine, a constituent of mate, and diabetes drugs might interfere with blood glucose control. Data are conflicting. Reports claim that caffeine might increase or decrease blood sugar (6024,8646).

CIMETIDINE (Tagamet): Theoretically, concomitant use might increase serum caffeine concentrations and the risk of adverse effects, due to the caffeine contained in mate. Cimetidine decreases the rate of caffeine clearance by 30% to 50% (11736).

CLOZAPINE (Clozaril): Theoretically, co-administration might acutely exacerbate psychotic symptoms, due to the caffeine contained in mate. Caffeine can increase the effects and toxicity of clozapine (151). Caffeine doses of 400-1000 mg per day inhibit clozapine metabolism (5051).
COCAINE: Theoretically, the caffeine in mate might increase the risk of additive CNS effects (2719).
CONTRACEPTIVE DRUGS: Theoretically, concomitant use might increase caffeine concentrations and the risk adverse effects, due to the caffeine contained in mate. Oral contraceptives decrease the rate of caffeine clearance by 40% to 65% (2714,11737).
DIPYRIDAMOLE (Persantine): The caffeine in mate might inhibit dipyridamole-induced vasodilation (11770,11772).
DISULFIRAM (Antabuse): Theoretically, concomitant use might increase serum caffeine concentrations and the risk of adverse effects, due to the caffeine contained in mate. Disulfiram decreases the rate of caffeine clearance (15).
EPHEDRINE: Use of ephedrine with caffeine, a constituent of mate, can increase the risk of stimulatory adverse effects. There is evidence that using ephedrine with caffeine might increase the risk of serious life-threatening or debilitating adverse effects such as hypertension, myocardial infarction, stroke, seizures, and death (1275,6486,10307). Tell patients to avoid taking caffeine with ephedrine and other stimulants.
ESTROGENS: Theoretically, concomitant use might increase serum caffeine concentrations and the risk of adverse effects, due to the caffeine contained in mate. Estrogen inhibits caffeine metabolism (2714).
FLUCONAZOLE (Diflucan): Concomitant use might increase the effects of caffeine in mate. Fluconazole decreases caffeine clearance by approximately 25% (11022).
FLUVOXAMINE (Luvox): Concomitant use of fluvoxamine with caffeine or caffeine-containing herbs such as mate can increase caffeine serum concentrations, and the risk of caffeine adverse effects. Fluvoxamine reduces caffeine metabolism (6370).
LITHIUM: Theoretically, abrupt mate withdrawal might increase serum lithium levels, due to the caffeine contained in mate. There are two case reports of lithium tremor that worsened upon abrupt coffee withdrawal (609,610).
MEXILETINE (Mexitil): Concomitant use might increase the effects and adverse effects of caffeine in mate. Mexiletine can decrease caffeine elimination by 50% (1260,11741).
MONOAMINE OXIDASE INHIBITORS (MAOIs): Theoretically, concomitant intake of large amounts of mate with MAOIs might precipitate a hypertensive crisis, due to the caffeine contained in mate. This is based on the claim that intake of large amounts of caffeine with MAOIs might precipitate a hypertensive crisis (15).
NICOTINE: Theoretically, the caffeine in mate might increase the risk of additive CNS effects (2719).
PHENYLPROPANOLAMINE: Concomitant use of phenylpropanolamine and mate might cause an additive increase in blood pressure due to the caffeine in mate (11738).
QUINOLONE ANTIBIOTICS: Theoretically, concomitant use might increase serum caffeine concentrations and the risk of adverse effects, due to the caffeine contained in mate. Quinolones decrease caffeine clearance (606,607,608). Quinolones (also referred to as fluoroquinolones) include ciprofloxacin (Cipro), enoxacin (Penetrex), gatifloxacin (Tequin), levofloxacin (Levaquin), lomefloxacin (Maxaquin), moxifloxacin (Avelox), norfloxacin (Noroxin), ofloxacin (Floxin), sparfloxacin (Zagam), and trovafloxacin (Trovan).
RILUZOLE (Rilutek): Theoretically, concomitant use might increase serum caffeine and riluzole concentrations and the risk of adverse effects of both caffeine and riluzole, due to the caffeine contained in mate. Caffeine and riluzole are both metabolized by cytochrome P450 1A2, and concomitant use might reduce metabolism of one or both agents (11739).
TERBINAFINE (Lamisil): Theoretically, concomitant use might increase serum caffeine concentrations and the risk of adverse effects, due to the caffeine contained in mate. Terbinafine decreases the rate of caffeine clearance (11740).
THEOPHYLLINE: Theoretically, concomitant use of theophylline and large amounts of mate might increase the risk of theophylline toxicity, due to mate's caffeine content. Caffeine decreases theophylline clearance 23% to 29% (11741).
VERAPAMIL (Calan, Covera, Isoptin, Verelan): Theoretically, concomitant use might increase plasma caffeine concentrations and the risk of adverse effects, due to the caffeine contained in mate. Verapamil increases plasma caffeine concentrations by 25% (11741).

Interactions with Foods

None known.

Interactions with Lab Tests

5-HYDROXYINDOLEACETIC ACID: Mate might increase urine 5-hydroxyindoleacetic acid concentrations and test results, due to its caffeine content. Caffeine can increase urine catecholamine concentrations (15).
BLEEDING TIME: Mate might prolong bleeding time and increase test results, due to its caffeine content (1701).
CATECHOLAMINES: Mate might increase urine catecholamine concentrations and test results, due to its caffeine content. Caffeine can increase urine catecholamine concentrations (8646).
CREATINE: Mate might increase urine creatine concentrations and test results, due to its caffeine content (1701).
DIPYRIDAMOLE THALLIUM IMAGING: Mate might interfere with dipyridamole thallium imaging studies, due to its caffeine content. Caffeine attenuates the characteristic cardiovascular responses to dipyridamole and has altered test results (11742).

GLUCOSE: Caffeine, a constituent of mate, has been reported to cause increases and decreases in blood glucose (8646).
LACTATE: The combination of ephedrine, a constituent of ephedra, and caffeine, a constituent of mate, can increase blood lactate levels (8646).
NEUROBLASTOMA TESTS: Mate (due to its caffeine content) might cause false-positive diagnosis of neuroblastoma, when diagnosis is based on tests of urine vanillylmandelic acid (VMA) or catecholamine concentrations. Caffeine can increase urine catecholamine and VMA concentrations (15).
PHARMACOLOGICAL STRESS TESTS: The caffeine in mate is a competitive antagonist for adenosine receptors (11771). It is recommended that caffeine and caffeine-containing products be stopped 24 hours prior to pharmacological stress tests (11770). However, caffeine appears more likely to interfere with dipyridamole (Persantine) than adenosine (Adenocard) stress testing (11771). The interaction between caffeine and dipyridamole is unlikely to be significant in stress testing if the heart rate increase is greater than 5% after dipyridamole infusion (11772).
PHEOCHROMOCYTOMA TESTS: Mate (due to its caffeine content) might cause false-positive diagnosis of pheochromocytoma, when diagnosis is based on tests of urine vanillylmandelic acid (VMA) or catecholamine concentrations. Caffeine can increase urine catecholamine and VMA concentrations (15).
PULMONARY FUNCTION TESTS: People may need to avoid caffeine and caffeine-containing herbs such as mate for at least four hours prior to lung function testing. Forced expiratory volume in one minute (FEV1) seems to show a small improvement up to two hours after caffeine use. Mid-expiratory flow rates may also improve with caffeine for up to four hours (9607).
URATE: Mate might falsely increase serum urate test results determined by the Bittner method, due to its caffeine content. Caffeine causes false elevations in serum urate test results determined by the Bittner method (11844).
URINARY CALCIUM: Caffeine, a constituent of mate, can increase urinary calcium levels (11317).
VANILLYLMANDELIC ACID (VMA): Mate might increase urine VMA concentrations and test results, due to its caffeine content. Caffeine can increase urine VMA concentrations (15).

Interactions with Diseases or Conditions

ALCOHOLISM: Heavy alcohol with long-time mate consumption increases the risk of cancer from 3-fold to 7-fold (11864).
ANXIETY DISORDERS: The caffeine in mate might aggravate anxiety disorders (11743).
BLEEDING DISORDERS: Theoretically, caffeine in mate might aggravate these conditions. Caffeine is reported to have antiplatelet activity (8028,8029); however, this interaction has not been reported in humans.
CARDIAC CONDITIONS: Caffeine in mate can induce cardiac arrhythmias in sensitive individuals (11845); use with caution.
DIABETES: Some research suggests that caffeine, a constituent of mate, may impair postprandial glucose metabolism in people with diabetes and contribute to insulin resistance. The effect of caffeinated beverages and herbs has not been studied (12374,12375). Caffeine in mate may enhance the frequency and intensity of hypoglycemic warning symptoms in type 1 diabetics. This may increase the ability of diabetics to detect and treat hypoglycemia early. However, it might also increase the frequency of hypoglycemic events (6024); use with caution. Caffeine has been reported to cause increases and decreases in blood glucose (8646); use with caution.
GLAUCOMA: Consuming mate increases intraocular pressure due to the caffeine content. The increase occurs within 30 minutes and persists for at least 90 minutes (8540).
HYPERTENSION: The caffeine in mate might increase blood pressure in people with high blood pressure. Consumption of 250 mg caffeine can increase blood pressure in healthy people, but this doesn't seem to occur in people who habitually consume caffeine products (2722).
OSTEOPOROSIS: Consuming mate can increase urinary excretion of calcium due to its caffeine content. Caffeine consumption should be limited to less than 300 mg per day (approximately 2-3 cups of mate). Adequate calcium supplementation may partially compensate for calcium losses (2669,10202,11317). Postmenopausal women identified with a genetic variant of the vitamin D receptor should use caffeine with caution (2669).
SMOKING: The risk of cancer increases from 3-fold to 7-fold in people who smoke and consume mate for extended periods of time (11864).

Dosage and Administration

No typical dosage.

Comments

Mate, also known as Yerba Maté, is a popular beverage, much like coffee or tea, in Brazil, Paraguay, and Argentina (6002). The beverage is often prepared from leaves of Ilex paraguariensis, also referred to as Jesuit's tea, Jesuit's Brazil tea, Paraguay tea, and St. Bartholemew's tea. The herbal tea has caused multiple anticholinergic poisonings. However, belladonna alkaloids were identified and the poisonings were traced to a single contaminated lot of imported herbs (785).

MEADOWSWEET

Also Known As
Bridewort, Dolloff, Dropwort, Filipendula, Lady Of The Meadow, Meadow Queen, Meadow-Wart, Queen Of The Meadow, Spiraeae flos, Spireae herba.

Scientific Names
Filipendula ulmaria, synonym Spiraea ulmaria.
Family: Rosaceae.

People Use This For
Orally, meadowsweet is used for colds, bronchitis, dyspepsia, heartburn, peptic ulcer disease, and rheumatic disorders including gout. It is also used orally as a diuretic and urinary antiseptic for acute cystitis.

Safety
POSSIBLY SAFE ...when used orally and appropriately (12).
POSSIBLY UNSAFE ...when an aqueous extract (tea) is used in large amounts or for prolonged periods of time because meadowsweet contains high amounts of tannins (4).
PREGNANCY: LIKELY UNSAFE ...when used orally. Some evidence suggests meadowsweet might stimulate uterine activity (4).
LACTATION: Insufficient reliable information available; avoid using.

Effectiveness
There is insufficient reliable information available about the effectiveness of meadowsweet.

Mechanism of Action
The applicable parts of meadowsweet are the above ground parts. Meadowsweet has stomachic, mild urinary antiseptic, antirheumatic, astringent, and antacid activities (4). It contains tannins and salicin, a plant salicylate (7,12). In animals, the above ground parts of meadowsweet decrease motor activity, lower temperature, induce muscle relaxation, and potentiate the effect of narcotics (4). In animals, the flower extract increases life expectancy; decreases vascular permeability; increases bronchial, intestinal, and uterine tone; and promotes uric acid excretion. In vitro, it has bacteriostatic activity (4). Meadowsweet aqueous extracts contain high concentrations of tannins with strong astringent effects (4).

Adverse Reactions
Orally, meadowsweet can cause nausea and other stomach complaints (18). Bronchospastic activity has occurred with use (4). Meadowsweet contains salicylate constituents. There is insufficient reliable information available to know if the side effects and toxicity normally associated with salicylates could occur. The adverse reactions associated with salicylates include gastric and renal irritation, hypersensitivity, blood in stool, tinnitus, nausea, and vomiting. Salicin has been associated with skin rashes (4).

Interactions with Herbs & Other Dietary Supplements
None known.

Interactions with Drugs
ASPIRIN: Meadowsweet contains salicin, a plant salicylate. Theoretically, meadowsweet might have an additive effect with other salicylate-containing drugs such as aspirin. Salicin doesn't seem to have the antiplatelet effects of aspirin (12).
CHOLINE MAGNESIUM TRISALICYLATE (Trilisate): Meadowsweet contains salicin, a plant salicylate. Theoretically, meadowsweet might have an additive effect with other salicylate-containing drugs such as choline magnesium trisalicylate (12).
NARCOTIC DRUGS: Theoretically, meadowsweet can potentiate narcotic effects (4).
SALSALATE (Disalcid): Meadowsweet contains salicin, a plant salicylate. Theoretically, meadowsweet might have an additive effect with other salicylate-containing drugs such as salsalate (12).

Interactions with Foods
None known.

Interactions with Lab Tests
None known.

Interactions with Diseases or Conditions
ASPIRIN ALLERGY: Use meadowsweet cautiously in individuals with aspirin allergy; it contains salicylate constituents.

ASTHMA: Theoretically, meadowsweet might exacerbate asthma due to bronchospastic effects. Use cautiously in individuals with asthma (4).

Dosage and Administration

ORAL: For adults, the typical dose is one cup of the tea several times per day (8). The tea is prepared by steeping 2.5-3.5 grams of the dried flower or 4-5 grams of the above ground parts in 150 mL boiling water for 10 minutes and then straining. The usual dose of the liquid extract (1:1 in 25% alcohol) is 1.5-6 mL three times per day (4). The common dose of the tincture (1:5 in 45% alcohol) is 2-4 mL three times per day (4).

MEDIUM CHAIN TRIGLYCERIDES (MCT)

Also Known As

MCT, MCT's, MCTs, Medium-Chain Triglycerides.

Scientific Names

Medium chain triglycerides.

People Use This For

Orally, medium chain triglycerides (MCTs) are used as adjunctive therapy for malabsorption syndromes including diarrhea, steatorrhea (fat indigestion), gastrectomy, lymphatic abnormalities, celiac disease, hepatic disease, and intestinal resection (short bowel syndrome). MCTs are also used for chyluria and chylothorax; gallbladder disease; AIDS; cystic fibrosis; and for seizures in children, including akinetic, clonic, and petit mal. MCTs are also used for nutritional support of athletic training, and decreasing body fat and increasing lean muscle mass.
Intravenously, MCTs are used as a source of fat in total parenteral nutrition.

Safety

LIKELY SAFE ...when used orally and appropriately (2273,2274). ...when used parenterally and appropriately (2275,2276,2278).
PREGNANCY AND LACTATION: LIKELY SAFE ...when used orally and appropriately (15).

Effectiveness

POSSIBLY EFFECTIVE

Cachexia. Intravenous MCTs can provide calories in critically ill patients, but don't seem to offer any advantages over long chain triglycerides (2275,2276,2278).

Seizures. Using MCTs orally seems to help reduce seizures in children, including akinetic, clonic, and petit mal types (2273,2274).

POSSIBLY INEFFECTIVE

AIDS-related wasting. Using MCTs orally doesn't seem to be any better than multivitamins and minerals alone for prevention of weight loss associated with AIDS (11730).

INSUFFICIENT RELIABLE EVIDENCE to RATE

Chylothorax. Using MCTs orally or in parenteral nutrition might prevent malnutrition and immunocompromise in pediatric and adult patients with chylothorax, according to preliminary clinical research (11726,11727,11728,11729). More evidence is needed to rate MCTs for this use.

Mechanism of Action

Medium chain triglycerides (MCTs) are semi-synthetic lipids composed of fatty acids, mostly lauric acid, with a chain length of six to twelve carbon atoms. MCTs are made from hydrolyzed coconut oil or palm kernel oils. The resulting fatty acids are fractionated and esterified to produce MCTs (11724,11725).
MCTs are efficiently absorbed. At physiological pH, MCTs are weak electrolytes and highly ionized, which increases their solubility (11724). Unlike long chain triglycerides (dietary fat), MCTs don't require the intestinal lymphatic system or bile salts for absorption (11723). They are usually used in patients who can't absorb conventional long chain fatty acids. MCTs do not contain essential fatty acids, and therefore they are normally only substituted for 50-70% of dietary fat. Some evidence suggests that absorption of long chain triglycerides may improve if combined with MCTs (11723). MCTs are metabolized primarily in the liver (11724).
MCTs are absorbed by the portal system rather than by the intestinal lymph system. MCTs have been tried for chylothorax, an effusion of a milky fluid (chyle) into the pleural space, due to trauma or a defect of the thoracic duct. Administering MCTs may decrease lymph flow in the thoracic duct will diminish and allow the thoracic duct defect to heal (11726,11727,11728,11729).
There has been some interest in using MCTs for injured and stressed patients since it causes mild ketosis and may decrease skeletal muscle catabolism (11725). However, clinical trials have not shown any clear advantage of MCTs over long chain triglycerides (2275,2276,2278).
In healthy people, single doses of MCT oil can reduce blood triglyceride levels (834). Some preliminary evidence suggests that MCT may increase metabolic rate and energy expenditures by the body when substituted in the diet for

other types of fat. MCT may induce satiety, leading to decreased consumption of calories. Increased metabolic rate and decreased caloric intake may lead to a slight decrease in body fat; however, these effects have not been rigorously tested in humans (10421,11724). MCTs contain 6 to 8.5 kcal per gram (11724).

Adverse Reactions

Orally, MCTs can cause diarrhea, vomiting, irritability, nausea, abdominal discomfort, intestinal gas noises, and essential fatty acid deficiency (2274,11723). MCT oil contains 6 to 8.5 calories per gram, and one tablespoon provides about 14 grams and about 115 calories (11724). Excessive consumption could result in weight gain.

Interactions with Herbs & Other Dietary Supplements

None known.

Interactions with Drugs

None known.

Interactions with Foods

FOOD: Co-administration of MCTs with food can reduce the adverse effects associated with MCTs (2273).

Interactions with Lab Tests

TRIGLYCERIDES: MCTs can lower blood triglyceride levels and test results (834).

Interactions with Diseases or Conditions

DIABETES: MCTs can cause ketosis; use with caution (11724).
HEPATIC ENCEPHALOPATHY, CIRRHOSIS: MCTs are primarily metabolized in the liver. MCTs can cause narcosis and coma in patients with hepatic cirrhosis; use with caution (11724).

Dosage and Administration

ORAL: For improving seizure control in children, MCT oil is used as 60% of the caloric intake (2274).
INTRAVENOUS (IV): As a fat source in total parenteral nutrition formulations, a fat mixture containing 50% MCT and 50% long chain triglycerides is commonly used (2275,2276,2278).

Comments

Ingesting MCTs with food reduces the adverse effects (2273).

MELANOTAN-II

Also Known As

Melanotan II, MT-II.
CAUTION: See separate listing for Melatonin.

Scientific Names

Melanotan-II.

People Use This For

Subcutaneously, melanotan-II has been used to evaluate its effects on psychogenic erectile dysfunction, organic erectile dysfunction, and its effects after unilateral nerve-sparing radical prostatectomy. It has also been used subcutaneously to evaluate its effects on tanning of the skin and for the prevention of sunlight-induced skin cancers.

Safety

POSSIBLY SAFE ...when used subcutaneously to initiate penile erections in men with psychogenic or organic erectile dysfunction (5687,5688). Controlled clinical studies suggest mild to moderate adverse effects such as decreased appetite, facial flushing, and nausea might occur with a dosage of 0.025 mg/kg (5685,5687,5688).
There is insufficient reliable information available about the safety of melanotan-II for its other uses or at other dosages.
PREGNANCY AND LACTATION: Insufficient reliable information available; avoid using.

Effectiveness

POSSIBLY EFFECTIVE

Erectile dysfunction (ED). Preliminary clinical trials have shown melanotan-II used subcutaneously is superior to placebo in men with psychogenic or organic erectile dysfunction for initiating spontaneous sustained penile erections (5685,5687,5688).

Tanning skin. Using melanotan-II subcutaneously seems to be effective for visible tanning of the skin (5685).
A controlled clinical pilot study demonstrated melanotan-II caused increased pigmentation in the

face, upper body, and buttocks (5685).
There is insufficient reliable information available about the effectiveness of melanotan-II for its other uses.

Mechanism of Action

Melanotan-I and Melanotan-II are two alpha-melanocyte-stimulating-hormone analogues currently being extensively studied (5686). Both analogues have the ability to darken and tan the skin (5686) and were developed to not only promote skin pigmentation but also to possibly prevent sunlight-induced skin cancers (5683,5686). Compared to alpha-melanocyte-stimulating-hormone, melanotan-I and melanotan-II have increased melanotropic potency (26-100-fold) and increased resistance to degradation by plasma enzymes due to two amino acid substitutions (norleucine for methionine at position 4 and racemization of D-phenylalanine at position 7) in the alpha-melanocyte-stimulating-hormone peptide sequence (5685,5686). Melanotan-II is a cyclic heptapeptide containing a lactam bridge between the amino acids lysine and aspartic acid, enabling it to have even greater melanotropic potency than melanotan-I, a linear tridecapeptide (5685,5686). During a pilot phase-I clinical study, it was discovered by observers that melanotan-II not only caused increased visible tanning but also spontaneous penile erections with use (5685). Subsequent controlled clinical trials have shown melanotan-II initiates erections in men with psychogenic and organic dysfunction (5687,5688). The exact mechanism of action is unknown, but it is hypothesized that melanotan-II acts on pro-erectile pathways at the level of the central nervous system (5687). There are distinct melanocortin receptors found primarily in the brain (5686) and animal data suggests melanotropic peptides act in the hypothalamic regions surrounding the third ventricle (5687). Since dopamine agonists also induce penile erections (and yawning), evidence suggests the central mechanism involves a dopamine-oxytocin pathway (5687).

Adverse Reactions

Subcutaneously, melanotan-II can cause gastrointestinal cramping (5685), nausea (5685,5687,5688), decreased appetite (5687), facial flushing (5685,5688), fatigue, somnolence (5685), yawning, stretching, and spontaneous penile erections (5685,5687,5688). It can also cause increased pigmentation of the face, upper body, and buttocks (5685).

Interactions with Herbs & Other Dietary Supplements

None known.

Interactions with Drugs

None known.

Interactions with Foods

None known.

Interactions with Lab Tests

None known.

Interactions with Diseases or Conditions

None known.

Dosage and Administration

SUBCUTANEOUS: The typical dosage is 0.025 mg/kg (5685,5687,5688).

Comments

Commercial dosage forms of melanotan-II such as a nasal spray or as an eyedrop are being investigated (5684,5687).

MELATONIN

Also Known As

MEL, MLT, Pineal Hormone.
CAUTION: See separate listing for Melanotan-II.

Scientific Names

N-acetyl-5-methoxytryptamine.

People Use This For

Orally, melatonin is used for jet lag, insomnia, shift-work disorder, circadian rhythm disorders in the blind, and benzodiazepine and nicotine withdrawal. Melatonin is also used orally for Alzheimer's disease, tinnitus, depression, delayed sleep phase syndrome (DSPS), chronic fatigue syndrome (CFS), fibromyalgia, migraine and cluster headaches, idiopathic stabbing headache, and insomnia associated with attention deficit-hyperactivity disorder (ADHD), and irritable bowel syndrome (IBS). Other uses include hypertension, hyperpigmentation, osteoporosis, breast cancer, brain cancer, lung cancer, prostate cancer, head cancer, neck cancer, and gastrointestinal cancer. It is also used for thrombocytopenia, cachexia, neuropathy, and asthenia associated with cancer chemotherapy. Melatonin

is also used orally for epilepsy, as an antiaging agent, for menopause, as preanesthetic medication, and for birth control.
Transbuccal and sublingual forms of melatonin are also used for insomnia, shift-work disorder, and as preanesthetic medication.
Topically, melatonin is used as a skin protectant against ultraviolet (UV) light and sunburn.
Intramuscularly, melatonin is used for treating cancer.

Safety

LIKELY SAFE ...when used orally or parenterally and appropriately, short-term. Melatonin seems to be safe when used for up to two months (1049,1068,1077,1085,1738,1754,5854,5855,5857,12226). ...when used topically and appropriately (1066,1768,1769,4713,4714).
POSSIBLY SAFE ...when used orally and appropriately, long-term. There is some evidence melatonin can be used safely for up to nine months in some patients (7040,7043).
CHILDREN: POSSIBLY UNSAFE ...when used orally or parenterally. Melatonin supplementation might adversely affect children. Young people up to the age of 20 years produce melatonin endogenously in high levels (1740). Melatonin levels are inversely related to gonadal development (1739,1742,1743). Theoretically, exogenously administered melatonin might adversely affect gonadal development; use with caution.
PREGNANCY: POSSIBLY UNSAFE ...when used orally or parenterally. High doses might inhibit ovulation, causing a contraceptive effect (1740,6002,8271). It is not known if lower doses cause this effect. Until more is known about the safety of melatonin, advise pregnant patients and patients wishing to become pregnant to avoid using melatonin at any dose.
LACTATION: Insufficient reliable information available; avoid using.

Effectiveness

LIKELY EFFECTIVE

Circadian rhythm sleep disorders. Taking melatonin orally helps improve circadian rhythm sleep disorders in blind children and adults. Melatonin has FDA orphan drug status for this indication (1082,1691,1744,1749,6585).

Sleep-wake cycle disturbances. Taking melatonin orally is helpful for sleep-wake cycle disturbances in children and adolescents with mental retardation, autism, and other central nervous system disorders (1056,1745,1746,1747,1771). Melatonin also appears to improve the time to fall asleep in children with developmental disabilities, including cerebral palsy, autism, and mental retardation (9707). Melatonin treatment seems to subjectively improve secondary insomnia associated with various sleep-wake cycle disturbances (1053,1729,8240,8245).

POSSIBLY EFFECTIVE

Benzodiazepine withdrawal. Taking melatonin orally seems to be beneficial for facilitating benzodiazepine withdrawal in elderly people with insomnia. This benefit has only been demonstrated with a controlled-release formulation of melatonin (349,1751).

Cluster headache. Taking melatonin orally 10 mg every evening might reduce the frequency of episodic cluster headaches (1127). However, 2 mg at bedtime doesn't seem to be effective (9702).

Delayed sleep phase syndrome (DSPS). Taking melatonin orally seems to improve insomnia and other quality of life factors such as mental health, vitality, and bodily pain in young adults with DSPS (8244,12226).

Insomnia. Melatonin supplementation seems to be most beneficial for elderly patients with insomnia related to melatonin deficiency (1072,1729,1738,1754,7081). Melatonin might also improve subjective quality of sleep in non-elderly patients, but probably will not improve objective measures such as the time it takes to fall asleep (sleep latency) or total sleep time (1068,1070,1083,12226). In children with insomnia due to delayed onset of sleep, melatonin seems to shorten the time that it takes to fall asleep and increase the duration of sleep (9708). Melatonin also seems to improve secondary insomnia related to depression (1053,1729), schizophrenia (8245), Alzheimer's disease (1729), hospitalization (9709), and insomnia termed "ICU syndrome" referring to sleep disturbances while in the intensive care unit (8240). Sustained-release melatonin preparations seem to be better for improving sleep maintenance (1738,1754), and immediate-release preparations seem to be more beneficial for decreasing sleep latency (1738).

Jet lag. Taking melatonin orally seems to reduce symptoms of jet lag, although some researchers have found no effect (6496). However, the majority of evidence shows that melatonin can modestly improve certain symptoms of jet lag such as alertness and psychomotor performance. Melatonin can also improve, to a lesser extent, other jet lag symptoms such as daytime sleepiness and fatigue (12226). Doses between 0.5 mg and 5 mg appear to be equally effective, but higher doses produce a greater hypnotic effect. Travelers traveling eastward through five or more time zones may find 2 mg to 3 mg of melatonin useful when taken at local bedtime on the day of arrival and for 2-5 nights thereafter. Taking melatonin in advance of travel doesn't help prevent jet lag. The usefulness of melatonin for westward travel or over fewer time zones is less clear (1049,1077,1079,1085,1722,8273,9181,9750). Taking melatonin in advance of travel doesn't help prevent jet lag.

Nicotine withdrawal. A single oral dose of melatonin 0.3 mg 3.5 hours after nicotine withdrawal in smokers seems to reduce subjective symptoms of anxiety, restlessness, irritability, depression, and cigarette craving over the next 10 hours (2424).

Preoperative anxiety and sedation. Melatonin used sublingually seems to help reduce preoperative anxiety and improve sedation. Sublingual melatonin in doses of 0.05, 0.1, or 0.2 mg per kilogram appears to be as effective as comparable doses of midazolam as a preanesthetic agent (1125). In some cases, melatonin might be preferable to midazolam because melatonin doesn't seem to cause anterograde amnesia or impair cognitive and psychomotor skills (1125).

Prostate cancer. Taking melatonin orally, in combination with the luteinizing hormone-releasing hormone (LHRH) analogue triptorelin, might be beneficial for metastatic prostate cancer. There is evidence that 20 mg of oral melatonin used daily in combination with 37.5 mg of intramuscular triptorelin injected every 28 days can significantly decrease levels of prostate-specific antigen (PSA) and growth factors for prostate cancer, prolactin (PRL), and insulin-like growth factor-1 (IGF-1) (7255).

Solid tumors. There is some evidence that taking combined high-dose melatonin with conventional chemotherapy or with interleukin-2 (IL-2) might improve tumor regression rate in patients with breast cancer, lung cancer, kidney cancer, liver cancer, pancreatic cancer, stomach cancer, or colon cancer (1692,5854,5855,5857,7040,7043,8268). Melatonin plus chemotherapy in patients with metastatic solid tumors seems to increase regression rate and one-year survival rate by approximately 50% compared to chemotherapy alone (7040). The addition of melatonin also seems to help reduce chemotherapy toxicities, including hematologic complications, cachexia, asthenia, and neuropathy (8268). There is also some preliminary evidence that melatonin alone, orally or intramuscularly, might improve stabilization rate and possibly one-year survival rate in patients with resistant or untreatable lung neoplasms, liver neoplasms, pancreas neoplasms, colon neoplasms, breast neoplasms, and brain neoplasms (1080,1688,1693,2566).

Sunburn. Applying melatonin topically seems to prevent erythema (sunburn) from ultraviolet (UV) light exposure. When applied prior to UV light exposure, melatonin seems to significantly decrease erythema (1066,1768,1769). In one study, topically applied vitamin E in combination with vitamin C and melatonin, provided modest photoprotective effect when used prior to UV exposure, but had no effect when used during or after UV exposure (4713,4714).

Tardive dyskinesia. Taking melatonin orally 10 mg daily seems to decrease symptoms by 24-30% in some patients with TD after six weeks of treatment (7082).

Thrombocytopenia. There is some evidence that taking melatonin orally can improve thrombocytopenia associated with cancer, cancer treatment, and other disorders. There is also some evidence melatonin can prevent thrombocytopenia induced by chemotherapy or interleukin-2 (IL-2) (1694,1695,1696,1697,2564,8268).

POSSIBLY INEFFECTIVE

Chronic fatigue syndrome (CFS). Taking melatonin orally 5 mg every evening doesn't seem to relieve CFS symptoms (9705).

Rotating shift work. Taking melatonin orally doesn't seem to improve sleep and adjustment to rotating shift work (1052,1054,1721).

LIKELY INEFFECTIVE

Depression. Although melatonin might help improve insomnia in some patients with depression, it does not seem to improve objective measures of depression (1053,1764,1766). There is also some concern that oral melatonin can worsen symptoms in some patients (1764). Some preliminary clinical research suggests melatonin may decrease winter depression symptoms in patients with seasonal affective disorder (SAD) (10670). Until more is known, tell patients with depression to avoid melatonin.

INSUFFICIENT RELIABLE EVIDENCE to RATE

Attention deficit-hyperactivity disorder (ADHD). Preliminary clinical research suggests melatonin might be useful for treating insomnia in children with ADHD (9980).

Beta-blocker-induced insomnia. Beta-blockers such as atenolol and propranolol seem to decrease endogenous melatonin levels. This might result in insomnia as a side effect. There is preliminary evidence that taking a melatonin supplement might decrease the insomnia caused by beta-blockers (1062,1780).

Fibromyalgia. Melatonin may decrease the severity of pain and the number of painful joints in people with fibromyalgia (9701).

Irritable bowel syndrome (IBS). Preliminary evidence suggests that patients with irritable bowel syndrome who also complain of poor sleep have decreased symptoms of IBS-related abdominal pain after taking melatonin 3 mg at bedtime for 2 weeks. Melatonin also seems to increase the rectal pain threshold. But melatonin does not seem to influence stool frequency or consistency; decrease bloating; or affect mood, sleep, or overall quality of life (13112).

Menopausal symptoms. Preliminary clinical research suggests that taking melatonin orally is ineffective for relieving menopausal symptoms. Melatonin in combination with soy isoflavones might help psychological symptoms associated with menopause (11806).

Migraine headache. There is preliminary evidence that patients with episodic migraine headache who take melatonin prophylactically, 3 mg every evening before bed, have significantly reduced migraine frequency, decreased migraine intensity, and decreased migraine duration (12149). Some research suggests that melatonin production might be altered in people with migraine (6712).

Seizures. There is some evidence that melatonin 3 mg at bedtime may reduce the frequency and duration of both nocturnal and daytime seizures in children with epilepsy (9699,9745,9746). It should be used cautiously, because melatonin may increase the frequency of seizures in some patients (8248,9744).

Stabbing headache. Case reports suggest that melatonin 3 to 12 mg per day may prevent idiopathic stabbing headache (11806).
More evidence is needed to rate melatonin for these uses.

Mechanism of Action

Melatonin is a hormone synthesized endogenously in the pineal gland (1123), collected by the venous capillary system, then secreted into the cerebrospinal fluid and the venous systemic circulation (1123,8239). It is produced from tryptophan, which is converted to 5-hydroxytryptophan, then to serotonin, then to N-acetylserotonin, and finally to melatonin (1773). In the brain, melatonin appears to increase the binding of gamma-aminobenzoic acid (GABA) to its receptors, by affecting membrane characteristics, not by increasing the number of receptors. Melatonin may decrease neurotransmission by a direct effect on nerve cells (9695).

Melatonin's primary role seems to be regulation of the body's circadian rhythm, endocrine secretions, and sleep patterns (1773,7043). Melatonin production is influenced by day/night cycles. Light inhibits melatonin secretion and darkness stimulates secretion (1773). For example, people who suffer from an insufficient amount of environmental light often have decreased endogenous melatonin secretion (8247). Endogenous melatonin is involved in several other functions including growth hormone secretion and sexual maturation (1776,1777,1778,6497,8246), pain control, balance, and sexual activity (1776,1777,1778,6497). However, it does not appear to directly affect heart function or blood pressure (9714). Excretion of melatonin is similar in males and females (9747). Some research suggests that meditation techniques might increase endogenous melatonin concentrations (9748). Melatonin release peaks between one to three years of age. Nocturnal serum melatonin levels naturally decline with increasing pubertal stages (1781,8246,8263). Melatonin suppression by light is not affected by age (1775). However, there is good evidence that melatonin levels can be abnormally low in certain conditions or disease states. For example, infants with low melatonin production are more likely to experience a life-threatening event (ALTE) (8262). Insomniacs of all ages can also have decreased melatonin levels. Patients with sleep disorders related to other conditions, such as fibromyalgia and depression, can also have low levels (6498). Recent information also shows that music therapy can improve endogenous serum melatonin levels in patients with Alzheimer's disease, possibly a contributing factor to patients' relaxed and calm mood (8241). In other conditions, melatonin's response to light can be altered. For example, in patients with bipolar I disorder, melatonin response to light appears to be abnormal, but is not affected in less severe bipolar II disorder or unipolar depression (1123).

When exogenous melatonin is administered, it has a rapid, transient, and mild sleep-inducing effect. Orally administered melatonin has the ability to shift the circadian rhythm. Taking melatonin can delay the rhythm when given in the morning and advance the rhythm when administered in the evening (8274). It can lower alertness, body temperature, blood pressure, and performance for three to four hours after oral administration. However, there is not usually a "hangover" effect the following day (1068,1132,1753,1756,1757,1758,1759,1774,8272). People with jet lag and insomnia use melatonin primarily for its effects on circadian rhythm (8272,8274).

People use melatonin for cluster headache due to its effects on body temperature. Those with cluster headache seem to have a rise in body heat, and melatonin can lower core body temperature (1128,1129,1132). However, there is no clear relationship between pain perception and urinary concentrations of melatonin metabolites (9700).

Melatonin has been tried for idiopathic stabbing headache due to its structural similarity to indomethacin (Indocin), one of the few effective treatments for this condition. The mechanism of action for both melatonin and indomethacin for idiopathic stabbing headache is unknown (11806).

Some research suggests that melatonin production might be altered in people with migraine (6712). The production of melatonin is increased in patients with uncontrolled epilepsy. This observation may be explained in two contradictory ways. The brain may be attempting to reduce epileptic nerve transmissions by increasing the concentration of melatonin (9696). In contrast, it may be that melatonin has proconvulsant activity. Concentrations of melatonin are increased at night and there is also an increased incidence of seizures during the night (9697). It is thought that melatonin might increase seizure activity by affecting the activity of dopamine in the brain (9744). However, many people with seizures have low endogenous melatonin levels, which increase after a seizure occurs. This suggests that melatonin levels increase to compensate for the increased nerve activity that occurs during a seizure (8249). In addition, some anticonvulsant medications increase concentrations of endogenous melatonin (9698), and exogenous melatonin may be used to treat some types of epilepsy (9699). Until more is known about the potential for melatonin to increase seizure activity, it should be avoided in people with seizure disorders (9744).

Melatonin is a potent antioxidant. It is thought to be 6-10 times more active than vitamin E as an antioxidant (7082). It may act as an oxygen free radical scavenger and by preventing several enzymatic reactions that generate reactive oxygen species (ROS). The antioxidant activity of melatonin may be useful in preventing oxidative injury in shock, inflammation, and reperfusion damage following coronary revascularization procedures (9712).

There is a lot of interest in using melatonin for patients with cancer. This area of research started due to the "Melatonin Hypothesis" which suggests that people with decreased pineal gland function are at an increased risk for developing cancer. Some researchers predicted that increased exposure to light would lower melatonin production and increase risk for some cancers (7042). Population studies have in fact found that blind patients and people living in arctic regions have relatively lower rates of breast cancer (7041,7042). There is also evidence that patients with advanced cancer have pineal gland hypofunction and low melatonin levels. Researchers now think supplemental melatonin might help prevent and treat certain cancers due to several pharmacological effects including antioxidant, immunomodulatory, and oncostatic effects. Cancer prevention may be the result of reduced cell proliferation, reduced cellular transformation, and DNA synthesis changes (8238). Melatonin seems to have very potent antioxidant effects. It might reduce chemotherapy toxicity by scavenging free radicals produced by treatment. Preliminary data suggest that melatonin may decrease oxidative renal damage caused by cisplatin (9749). Melatonin seems to also affect immune function by activating monocytes and increasing interleukin 2 (IL-2) activity. It appears to enhance IL-2-induced lymphocytosis (2568). Melatonin might improve survival in patients with cancer by preventing the immunosuppression caused by chemotherapy (7040). It may also help prevent thrombocytopenia associated with cancer chemotherapy by preventing chemotherapy-induced apoptosis of bone marrow cells, and acting synergistically with cytokines to stimulate platelet generation (2564). Other pineal hormones, such as 5-methoxytryptamine, may also contribute to the thrombopoietic effects of melatonin (2565). Melatonin also seems to have oncostatic effects. Melatonin slows growth of breast cancer cells in vitro and inhibits melanoma cell growth in vitro and in animal models (1064,5856,9751). Researchers think it has direct oncostatic effects, possibly by controlling oncogene expression and inducing cancer cell apoptosis (7040). Melatonin can also affect hormones that influence cancer cell growth. For example, it seems to reduce levels of insulin-like growth factor 1 (IGF-1) and prolactin (PRL), which have a role in breast cancer and prostate cell proliferation (1064,5854,5855,5857,7043,7255). In breast cancer cells, melatonin seems to reduce the number and activity of estrogen receptors (9711).

Melatonin has a variety of other effects. Melatonin is thought to be 6-10 times more effective than vitamin E as an antioxidant. Some researchers are interested in using melatonin for tardive dyskinesia (TD). Melatonin is theorized to work in TD due to a potential antioxidant effect on dopaminergic neurons. There is also some evidence that patients with TD have pineal gland calcification and low endogenous melatonin levels (7082).

Animal research suggests melatonin may reduce the volume of cerebral infarction when used within 2 hours of stroke onset (10671).

In addition to the pineal gland, melatonin is also produced endogenously in the gut. Melatonin is involved in regulation of gastrointestinal motility. Melatonin is thought to be potentially beneficial for irritable bowel syndrome (IBS) by decreasing gut visceral hypersensitivity. Some evidence suggests that melatonin decreases the rectal pain threshold in IBS patients when measured by rectal manometry (13112).

Melatonin seems to promote osteoblast differentiation and matrix mineralization in bone (3265). There is preliminary evidence that very high melatonin doses plus norethisterone can have additive or synergistic effects on inhibiting ovarian function in women and possibly act as a contraceptive (769,1740).

There is also interest in using melatonin for menopausal symptoms. Melatonin seems to reverse or reduce menopause related changes in thyroid hormone, luteinizing hormone (LH), and follicle stimulating hormone (FSH) in menopausal women (2425). However, it does not significantly alter catecholamine levels or cardiovascular responses in postmenopausal women (9704).

In vitro evidence suggests that melatonin may inhibit the biochemical processes involved with the development of myeloid plaques found in the brains of patients with Alzheimer's disease. The clinical significance of these findings is not established (9710). There is some interest in melatonin for its antimicrobial effects. Preliminary evidence shows that melatonin alone or in combination with isoniazid (INH) is active against some Mycobacterium species (330).

Some people use melatonin for improving sexual performance. In animal models, melatonin has dose dependent effects on sexual function. Repeated high doses seem to decrease sexual behavior. However, a single low dose of melatonin does seem to increase sexual behavior (6497).

Exogenous melatonin undergoes extensive and rapid first-pass metabolism (1773,6498,8239). After a typical oral dosage, an average of 30-60 % of the melatonin is rapidly metabolized by this first pass effect (8239). It is first hydroxylated and then undergoes sulphate conjugation (1773,6498). There is also some evidence that cytochrome P450 1A2 and 2C19 catalyze melatonin hydroxylation (6498).

Orally, melatonin has an absolute bioavailability of 15% for doses of 2 and 4 mg (1126). Half-life is about 30-60 minutes in humans (1385,1772). Melatonin can be absorbed transdermally, but time to peak levels is delayed (1058).

The timing of melatonin administration is important for best therapeutic effect. For jet lag and insomnia, evening doses are best because melatonin has the ability to advance the circadian rhythm (7081,8269,8273,8274).

For cancer, researchers theorize that evening doses are best because melatonin might have the greatest activity in the evening (1064). In otherwise healthy people, melatonin given at bedtime doesn't seem to affect nocturnal sleep. When given in the early evening (presumably in the absence of endogenous melatonin), it appears to be similar to temazepam (Restoril) in hypnotic effect (9706).

Adverse Reactions

Orally, melatonin is well-tolerated. The most common side effects include daytime drowsiness (20%) headache (7.8%), and dizziness (4%). But these don't seem to occur any more frequently than with placebo (12226). Other side effects that have been reported include transient depressive symptoms, mild tremor, mild anxiety, abdominal cramps, irritability (169,1078,8272,8273,9701), reduced alertness (1078), confusion, nausea, vomiting (8273), and hypotension (8272).

In perimenopausal women, melatonin has caused a resumption of spotting or menstrual flow (11806).

People should not drive or use machinery for 4 to 5 hours after taking melatonin (1772). Aircraft crew undergoing multiple time zone travel might experience further disruption in circadian rhythms (1722). Melatonin has exacerbated dysphoria in depressed patients (1764). Whether chronic administration of melatonin suppresses endogenous production of melatonin by the pineal gland is unknown (1772).

Not all melatonin products are safe. Some preparations of melatonin contain contaminants that are associated with eosinophilia-myalgia syndrome (9715,9716). Most commercial melatonin is synthesized in the laboratory. However, in rare cases it can be derived from animal pineal gland. Melatonin from animal sources should be avoided due to the possibility of contamination (1772,8266).

Interactions with Herbs & Other Dietary Supplements

HERBS WITH ANTICOAGULANT/ANTIPLATELET POTENTIAL: Theoretically, melatonin might increase the effect of herbs that have antiplatelet/anticoagulant constituents and might theoretically increase the risk of bleeding in some people (9181). These herbs include angelica, clove, danshen, garlic, ginger, ginkgo, Panax ginseng, red clover, willow, and others.

HERBS/SUPPLEMENTS WITH SEDATIVE PROPERTIES: Theoretically, concomitant use with herbs that have sedative properties might enhance therapeutic and adverse effects (1772). Some of these supplements include 5-HTP, calamus, California poppy, catnip, hops, Jamaican dogwood, kava, St. John's wort, scullcap, valerian, yerba mansa, and others.

Interactions with Drugs

ANTICOAGULANT/ANTIPLATELET DRUGS: There are isolated case reports of minor bleeding and decreased prothrombin activity in people taking melatonin with warfarin (Coumadin). The mechanism, if any, of this interaction is unknown. Theoretically, melatonin might increase the effect of anticoagulant or antiplatelet drugs (9181). Some drugs with anticoagulant or antiplatelet effects include aspirin, clopidogrel (Plavix), nonsteroidal anti-inflammatory drugs (NSAIDs) such as diclofenac (Voltaren, Cataflam, others), ibuprofen (Advil, Motrin, others), naproxen (Anaprox, Naprosyn, others), dalteparin (Fragmin), enoxaparin (Lovenox), heparin, and others.

ANTIDIABETES DRUGS: Melatonin might impair glucose utilization and increase insulin resistance (9713). Although the clinical significance is not known, melatonin may theoretically decrease the ability of hypoglycemic drugs to reduce blood glucose. Hypoglycemic drugs include insulin, glyburide (Micronase, DiaBeta), glipizide (Glucotrol), chlorpropamide (Diabinese), and tolbutamide (Orinase).

BENZODIAZEPINES: Theoretically, chronic benzodiazepine administration might decrease endogenous melatonin levels (8270).

CAFFEINE: Caffeine consumption can decrease endogenous melatonin levels. Theoretically, caffeine use may decrease the effectiveness of oral melatonin (8265).

CNS DEPRESSANTS: Theoretically, concomitant use of melatonin with alcohol, benzodiazepines, or other sedative drugs might cause additive sedation.

CONTRACEPTIVE DRUGS: Contraceptive drugs can increase the levels of endogenous melatonin. Theoretically, it may increase the effects and adverse effects of oral melatonin use (8265).

FLUMAZENIL (Romazicon): Preliminary evidence suggests that flumazenil may inhibit the effect of melatonin (9703).

FLUVOXAMINE (Luvox): Fluvoxamine can significantly increase melatonin levels. In some cases, fluvoxamine might increase bioavailability of exogenously administered melatonin by up to 20 times (5038,6499,8251). Some researchers think this might be a beneficial interaction and be potentially useful for cases of refractory insomnia (6499). However, this interaction might also cause unwanted excessive drowsiness and possibly other adverse effects. Fluvoxamine is known to increase endogenous melatonin secretion (6498). It seems to increase serum levels of exogenously administered melatonin possibly by decreasing melatonin metabolism by inhibiting cytochrome P450 (CYP450) 1A2 and 2C19 or by inhibiting melatonin elimination. This effect has been found in healthy people taking fluvoxamine 50-75 mg and melatonin 5 mg (5038,6498,6499,8251).

IMMUNOSUPPRESSANTS: Melatonin can stimulate immune function and might interfere with immunosuppressive therapy (7040); avoid using. Immunosuppressant drugs include azathioprine (Imuran), basiliximab (Simulect), cyclosporine (Neoral, Sandimmune), daclizumab (Zenapax), muromonab-CD3 (OKT3, Orthoclone OKT3), mycophenolate (CellCept), tacrolimus (FK506, Prograf), sirolimus (Rapamune), prednisone (Deltasone, Orasone), and other corticosteroids (glucocorticoids).

NIFEDIPINE GITS (Procardia XL): Melatonin can decrease the effectiveness of nifedipine GITS. Immediate-release melatonin 5 mg at night in combination with nifedipine GITS 30-60 mg daily increases systolic blood pressure an average of 6.5 mmHg and diastolic by an average of 4.9 mmHg. Concomitant use with melatonin also increases heart rate by 3.9 bpm (6436). The mechanism of this interaction is not known.

VERAPAMIL (Calan, Covera, Isoptin, Verelan): Concomitant use can increase melatonin excretion (1063).

Interactions with Foods

None known.

Interactions with Lab Tests

BLOOD PRESSURE: Melatonin can increase blood pressure in patients treated with antihypertensive medications. Immediate-release melatonin 5 mg at night in combination with nifedipine GITS (Procardia XL) increases systolic blood pressure an average of 6.5 mmHg and diastolic by an average of 4.9 mmHg (6436).

HEART RATE: Melatonin in combination with antihypertensive medications can increase heart rate. Immediate-release melatonin 5 mg at night in combination with nifedipine GITS (Procardia XL) increases heart rate by an average of 3.9 bpm (6436).

HUMAN GROWTH HORMONE: Melatonin supplementation can increase human growth hormone serum levels and test results (1076,1779).

LUTEINIZING HORMONE: Melatonin supplementation can decrease serum luteinizing hormone levels and test results (1741).
OXYTOCIN: Melatonin can produce dose-dependent changes in plasma oxytocin concentrations and test results. A 500 mcg melatonin dose increases oxytocin levels; a 5 mg melatonin dose reduces oxytocin levels (1779).
VASOPRESSIN: Melatonin can produce dose-dependent changes in plasma vasopressin concentrations and test results. A 500 mcg melatonin dose increases vasopressin levels; a 5 mg melatonin dose reduces vasopressin levels (1779).

Interactions with Diseases or Conditions

CANCER: Melatonin can decrease the incidence of cytokine (interleukin II and tumor necrosis factor) induced hypotension in cancer patients (1069).
DEPRESSION: Melatonin can worsen dysphoria in some people with depression (1764).
DIABETES: Melatonin may decrease glucose utilization and increase insulin resistance (9713). It may theoretically increase blood glucose concentrations in people with diabetes.
HYPERTENSION: Melatonin can worsen blood pressure in patients who are taking antihypertensive medications. Immediate-release melatonin 5 mg at night in combination with nifedipine GITS (Procardia XL) increases systolic blood pressure an average of 6.5 mmHg, diastolic blood pressure by an average of 4.9 mmHg, and increases heart rate by 3.9 bpm (6436). The mechanism of this interaction is not known.
SEIZURE DISORDERS: Exogenous melatonin may increase the incidence of seizures (9744). Children with multiple neurological disorders, including seizure activity, might have an increase in seizure activity after treatment with oral melatonin for sleep disorders (8248); use with caution.

Dosage and Administration

ORAL: For insomnia, a typical dose of 0.3-5 mg at bedtime has been used (1072,1729,1738,1754,7081). In children with insomnia due to delayed sleep onset, melatonin 5 mg at 6:00 PM daily has been used (9708). Melatonin 5 mg at 8:00 PM daily has been used to treat insomnia in children with developmental disorders, including cerebral palsy, autism, and mental retardation (9707). Both immediate-release and sustained-release preparations have been used.
For jet lag, 0.5-5 mg at bedtime is commonly taken on the arrival day at the destination, continuing for 2-5 days. Low doses of 0.5-3 mg are often used to avoid the hypnotic properties of the higher 4-5 mg doses (1049,1077,1079,1085,1722,8269,8273).
For tardive dyskinesia, 10 mg daily of a controlled-release formulation has been used (7082). As adjunctive treatment for solid tumors, 10-50 mg in combination with radiotherapy, chemotherapy, or interleukin 2 (IL-2) has been used in clinical studies. Melatonin is typically started 7 days prior to start of chemotherapy and continued throughout full treatment course (1773,7040,7043,8268).
For irritable bowel syndrome (IBS), 3 mg at bedtime has been used (13112).
For treatment of metastatic prostate cancer resistant to triptorelin used alone, 20 mg taken daily has been used in combination with 3.75 mg of triptorelin injected intramuscularly every 28 days (7255).
For prevention and treatment of thrombocytopenia associated with cancer chemotherapy, a dose of 20 mg each evening has been used (2564).
For benzodiazepine withdrawal in elderly people with insomnia, 2 mg of controlled-release melatonin taken at bedtime for 6 weeks (the benzodiazepine dosage is reduced 50% during the second week, 75% during weeks 3 and 4, and stopped during weeks 5 and 6) and continued up to 6 months, has been used (349).
For treatment of winter depression, 0.125 mg twice daily has been used (10670).
For prevention of cluster headache, an evening dose of 10 mg has been used (1127).
For preventing migraine headaches, 3 mg every evening before bed has been used (12149).
For prevention of idiopathic stabbing headache, 3 to 12 mg at bedtime has been used (11806). As premedication for surgery in adults, 0.05 mg/kg sublingually has been used (1125,1768,1769). For reducing the symptoms of acute nicotine withdrawal, 0.3 mg orally 3.5 hours after stopping smoking has been used (2424).
TOPICAL: No typical dosage.

Comments

The controlled-released product, Circadin (not available in the US), is undergoing a multi-center Phase III clinical study in France for the indication of sleep. The manufacturer, Neurim Pharmaceutical Labs (Israel), has applied for approval of Circadin as a prescription drug in Canada and Europe.

MENTZELIA

Also Known As
Anguraté.

Scientific Names
Mentzelia cordifolia.
Family: Loasaceae.

Comments
At the date of publication, this product was not a common ingredient used in brand name supplements marketed to consumers. Details about this product are available in the online version of *Natural Medicines Comprehensive Database.* See www.naturaldatabase.com.

MERCURY HERB

Also Known As
None.

Scientific Names
Mercurialis annua.
Family: Euphorbiaceae.

People Use This For
Orally, mercury herb is used for inflammation with pus, as a laxative, a diuretic, and as an adjuvant treatment for gastrointestinal and urinary tract disease.

Safety
LIKELY UNSAFE ...when the fresh plant, particularly the root and rhizome are used orally (18). Small amounts might cause symptoms no worse than diarrhea.
PREGNANCY AND LACTATION: LIKELY UNSAFE ...when used orally (18); avoid using.

Effectiveness
There is insufficient reliable information available about the effectiveness of mercury herb.

Mechanism of Action
Mercury herb contains saponins, a small amount of cyanogenic glycosides, pyridone derivatives including hermidin, amines including methylamine, and flavonoids including rutin, narcissin, and isorhamnetin (18). The root and stock of mercury herb act as strong laxatives (18). There is no information regarding the toxic compound in the plant (18). The insignificant amount of cyanogenic glycosides cannot account for the plant's toxicity (18).

Adverse Reactions
Orally, ingestion might cause diarrhea and overactive bladder (18). Symptoms of poisoning might include nerve paralysis, liver and kidney failure, as well as death (18). The pollen has shown to be allergenic (4143,4144), and may be responsible for rhinitis and asthmatic symptoms (4143). Mercury herb might also cause allergic reactions in individuals allergic to Olea europaea, Fraxinus elatior, Ricinus communis, Salsola kali, Parietaria judaica, and Artemisia vulgaris (4143).

Interactions with Herbs & Other Dietary Supplements
CROSS-ALLERGENICITY: Individuals allergic to mercury herb might also be allergic to Mercurialis annua and Olea europaea, Fraxinus elatior, Ricinus communis, Salsola kali, Parietaria judaica, and Artemisia vulgaris (4143).

Interactions with Drugs
None known.

Interactions with Foods
None known.

Interactions with Lab Tests
None known.

Interactions with Diseases or Conditions
None known.

Dosage and Administration

ORAL: Mercury herb is typically administered as an extract or in juice (18).

MESOGLYCAN

Also Known As

Aortic GAGs, Aortic Glycosaminoglycans, Glycosaminoglycans, Heparinoid Fraction, Heparinoids, Mucopolysaccharide, Sulfomucopolysaccharide.
CAUTION: See separate listing for Chondroitin Sulfate.

Scientific Names

None.

People Use This For

Orally, mesoglycan is used for treating atherosclerosis, varicose veins, hemorrhoids, phlebitis, thrombophlebitis, lower limb ischemia, deep vein thrombosis, hyperlipidemia, peripheral obliterative arterial disease, venous insufficiency, venous stasis ulcers, cerebrovascular disease, and stroke.
Topically, mesoglycan is used for treating leg ulcers.
Intramuscularly, mesoglycan is used for treating venous insufficiency, venous stasis ulcers, cerebrovascular disease, stroke, and cutaneous necrotizing venulitis.
Intravenously, mesoglycan is used for treating lower limb ischemia.

Safety

POSSIBLY SAFE ...when used orally or parenterally and appropriately (6630,6635,6637,6638,6639,6644,6645). Since these products are derived from animals there are concerns about contamination with diseased animal parts (1825). However, there are no reports of disease transmission to humans due to use of contaminated mesoglycan.
There is insufficient reliable information available about the safety of mesoglycan when used topically or intravenously.
PREGNANCY AND LACTATION: Insufficient reliable information available; avoid using.

Effectiveness

POSSIBLY EFFECTIVE

Cerebrovascular disease. Taking mesoglycan orally seems to reduce ischemic events, improve quality of life, and provide subjective improvement when used over a 6 month period in patients with cerebrovascular disease (6635,6637,6639). There is some evidence that mesoglycan might be comparable to standard antiplatelet drug therapy (6639).
Hypertriglyceridemia. There is some evidence that taking mesoglycan orally seems to reduce total and VLDL triglycerides in patients with hypertriglyceridemia (6646).
Peripheral arterial disease. Alternating intravenous and oral mesoglycan seems to improve walking distance in patients with intermittent claudication due to peripheral arterial disease (6629).
Venous insufficiency. There is some evidence from uncontrolled trials that administering mesoglycan orally or parenterally may improve the subjective and objective symptoms associated with various venous conditions including varicose syndromes, post-phlebitic syndromes, and thrombophlebitis when used over a 1-3 month period (6630,6638,6644,6645). Applying mesoglycan topically also seems to be helpful for treating leg ulcers in patients with chronic venous insufficiency (6627).
Venous stasis ulcers. Administering a combination of intramuscular and oral mesoglycan as an adjunct to traditional chronic venous stasis ulcer therapy seems to improve the rate of healing compared to traditional therapy alone (11479).

POSSIBLY INEFFECTIVE

Deep vein thrombosis (DVT). Oral mesoglycan plus compression stockings appears to be no better than placebo, following standard DVT therapy, for preventing recurrent DVT and/or pulmonary embolism during a follow-up period ranging from 5 to 48 months (6640).
Stroke. There seems to be no difference in outcome in patients treated for acute ischemic stroke with intravenous dexamethasone alone, or in combination with intramuscular mesoglycan for 5 days followed by 25 days of oral mesoglycan (6641).

INSUFFICIENT RELIABLE EVIDENCE to RATE

Atherosclerosis. There is some early evidence that mesoglycan might slow the progression of atherosclerosis by decreasing the rate of carotid and femoral artery intima-media thickening (6628).
Cutaneous necrotizing venulitis. There is some preliminary evidence that intramuscular mesoglycan might be useful for treating cutaneous necrotizing venulitis in patients with reduced fibrinolytic activity (6634). More evidence is needed to rate mesoglycan for these uses.

Mechanism of Action

Mesoglycan belongs to a broad class of compounds called glycosaminoglycans (GAG). GAGs, also called mucopolysaccharides, are amino hexose polysaccharides contained in mucoproteins, glycoproteins, and blood group substances. GAGs are a heparinoid (non-heparin) byproduct of heparin extraction from cow lung tissue or aorta, and pig intestinal mucosa (15). Mesoglycan specifically is composed of dermatan sulfate and heparan sulfate, with smaller concentrations of chondroitin sulfate, hyaluronic acid, and related hexosaminoglycans (6614). The concentrations of these substances can vary depending on the origin of the product. People try it for vascular conditions because it seems to have numerous pharmacological effects on the vascular system. Mesoglycan exhibits profibrinolytic activity without influencing hemaglutination in humans after oral administration (6631,6642). It seems to also decrease plasma fibrinogen concentrations without affecting prothrombin time, partial thromboplastin time, or antithrombin III (6633). Mesoglycan might restore normal fibrinolysis in patients with reduced cutaneous fibrinolytic activity (6634). However, mesoglycan has been shown to prolong activated partial thromboplastin time (aPTT) (6629). Mesoglycan seems to reduce pericapillary connective tissue edema, and capillary and venule dilation, in patients with primary venous insufficiency (6630). It also improves arterial wall elasticity, trancutaneous oxygen perfusion, and blood flow (6643,6644). Mesoglycan reduces total and VLDL triglyceride concentrations and increases lipoprotein lipase activity in patients with hypertriglyceridemia (6646). It reduces total cholesterol and triglyceride concentrations, and increases HDL cholesterol concentrations in patients recovering from cerebral ischemic episode (6633).

Adverse Reactions

Orally, nausea, vomiting, epigastric pain, heartburn, headache, diarrhea, and local cutaneous reactions have been reported (6629).

There is some concern about potential contamination. Mesoglycan is derived from raw animal tissues gathered from slaughterhouses, possibly from sick or diseased animals. Products made from contaminated or diseased organs might present a human health hazard. There is also concern that mesoglycan produced from cows in countries where bovine spongiform encephalitis (BSE) has been reported might be contaminated with diseased tissue. Countries where BSE has been reported include Great Britain, France, The Netherlands, Portugal, Luxembourg, Ireland, Switzerland, Oman, and Belgium (1825). However, there have been no reports of BSE transfer to humans from contaminated mesoglycan products. Until more is known, tell patients to avoid these products unless country of origin can be determined. Patients should avoid products that are produced in countries where BSE has been found.

Interactions with Herbs & Other Dietary Supplements

None known.

Interactions with Drugs

ANTICOAGULANT/ANTIPLATELET DRUGS: Theoretically, combined use might increase bleeding risk. However, human evidence suggests that mesoglycan has profibrinolytic activity without affecting coagulation (6631,6642). These agents include aspirin, clopidogrel (Plavix), dalteparin (Fragmin), enoxaparin (Lovenox), heparin, ticlopidine (Ticlid), warfarin (Coumadin), and others.

THROMBOLYTIC DRUGS: Theoretically, combined use might increase bleeding risk (6629). These drugs include alteplase (Activase), anistreplase (Eminase), reteplase (Retevase), streptokinase (Streptase), and urokinase (Abbokinase).

Interactions with Foods

None known.

Interactions with Lab Tests

ACTIVATED PARTIAL THROMBOPLASTIN TIME (aPTT): Intravenous mesoglycan prolongs activated partial thromboplastin time (6629).

CHOLESTEROL: Intramuscular mesoglycan reduces total cholesterol and increases HDL cholesterol concentrations and test results (6633).

FIBRINOGEN: Intramuscular mesoglycan decreases plasma fibrinogen concentrations and test results (6633).

TRIGLYCERIDES: Intramuscular mesoglycan decreases plasma triglyceride concentrations and test results (6633).

Interactions with Diseases or Conditions

COAGULATION DISORDERS: Mesoglycan might cause bleeding in people with coagulation disorders (6633).

HEPARINOID HYPERSENSITIVITY: Mesoglycan might cause allergic reactions in people hypersensitive to heparin or heparinoid derivatives (15).

Dosage and Administration

ORAL: A typical dose is 100 mg per day (6614). For cerebrovascular disease, 100-144 mg per day has been used (6635,6639,6641). For deep vein thrombosis (DVT), 72 mg per day has been used (6640). For hypertriglyceridemia, 96 mg per day has been used (6646). For venous insufficiency, 50 mg three times daily has been used (6638).

INTRAMUSCULAR: For cerebrovascular disease, 30 mg once or twice daily has been used (6635,6637,6639). For venous insufficiency, 30 mg per day has been used (6630,6638,6644,6645). For venous stasis ulcers, as an adjunct to

traditional chronic venous ulcer therapy, 30 mg intramuscular mesoglycan per day has been used for three weeks followed by 100 mg oral mesoglycan per day for up to 21 weeks (11479).
TOPICAL: No typical dosage.

METHIONINE

Also Known As

DL-Methionine, DL Methionine, L-Methionine.

Scientific Names

L-2-amino-4-(methylthio)butyric acid.

People Use This For

Orally, methionine is used to prevent liver damage in acetaminophen poisoning and to test individuals for hyperhomocysteinemia. It is also used orally for lowering urinary pH, treating liver disorders, and improving wound healing. Methionine is also used orally for treating depression, alcoholism, allergies, asthma, copper toxicity, radiation side effects, schizophrenia, drug withdrawal, and Parkinson's disease.

Safety

POSSIBLY SAFE ...when used orally or intravenously, and appropriately (2410,2411,2413).
POSSIBLY UNSAFE ...when used orally or intravenously in excessive doses. Doses larger than 100 mg/kg should be avoided to prevent severe and potentially lethal cerebral effects (9339).
CHILDREN: POSSIBLY SAFE ...when used orally or intravenously, and appropriately. POSSIBLY UNSAFE ...when used intravenously in infants receiving parenteral nutrition. In infants, blood methionine concentration can increase due to lower enzyme activity and inability to metabolize methionine. High levels of methionine can cause liver toxicity (9338).
PREGNANCY AND LACTATION: Insufficient reliable information available; avoid using.

Effectiveness

POSSIBLY EFFECTIVE

Acetaminophen poisoning. Taking methionine orally or intravenously seems to be effective for treating acetaminophen poisoning (2413). Methionine 2.5 grams every 4 hours for 4 doses seems to be as effective as acetylcysteine in preventing liver damage and death after an acetaminophen overdose if methionine is given within 10 hours of acetaminophen ingestion (2413).

INSUFFICIENT RELIABLE EVIDENCE to RATE

Cobalamin deficiency. There is some evidence methionine administered preoperatively might prevent the adverse effects mimicking those of cobalamin deficiency due to prolonged exposure to nitrous oxide (2414).
Colorectal cancer. There is some evidence a high dietary intake of methionine and folate might have a synergistic effect in decreasing the risk of colon cancer, especially in individuals with a family history of colon cancer and those who consume large amounts of alcohol (9325,9326).
More evidence is needed to rate methionine for these uses.

Mechanism of Action

Methionine is a sulfur-containing essential amino acid found in animal protein (9,9343). Methionine plays a role in many cellular functions. It is used for protein synthesis, and methylation of DNA, RNA, and other molecules (9336,9342).
To be metabolized, methionine enters the methionine cycle and is transformed into S-adenosylmethionine (SAMe). After donating its methyl group, SAMe is hydrolyzed to homocysteine, and then either remethylated to methionine or transsulfurated, which leads to the formation of cysteine, taurine, and glutathione (9336,9338). As an antioxidant, glutathione prevents free radical injury to the liver and taurine plays a role in bile acid conjugation (9338).
Failure to maintain the homeostasis of the methionine cycle is thought to result in liver injury. Patients with alcohol-induced liver disease often exhibit hypermethioninemia, which is thought to be caused by decreased metabolism of methionine to SAMe. With low levels of glutathione, the liver is at an increased risk of damage from free radicals (9336,9338).
Toxic levels of methionine can be corrected with glycine. Glycine seems to enhance the degradation of methionine through transsulfuration by acting as a receptor for methyl groups. Excessive methionine competes for glycine and limits the availability of glycine for other metabolic interactions, such as the synthesis of glutathione (2415).
In acetaminophen poisoning, methionine seems to prevent liver damage and necrosis by promoting glutathione synthesis. The toxic metabolite of acetaminophen (N-acetyl-p-benzquinoneimine) will then bind to glutathione instead of liver cells (9340).
Dietary methionine usually has no effect on homocysteine levels. Levels can increase and possibly cause hyperhomocysteinemia if enzymes used for the metabolism of homocysteine are defective and/or there is a deficiency in folate, vitamin B12, or vitamin B6 (9343). Hyperhomocysteinemia might cause endothelial damage and

increase the risk for vascular disease (2410,2411). Hyperhomocysteinemia that is unresponsive to vitamin supplementation sometimes responds to dietary restriction of methionine (9345).
Methionine might play a role in preventing adverse effects caused by prolonged nitrous oxide exposure. Nitrous oxide toxicity resembles cobalamin deficiency. Preliminary evidence suggests nitrous oxide can selectively impair the function of cobalamin-dependent methionine synthase. Administering methionine preoperatively might prevent the inactivation of methionine synthase and prevent cobalamin inactivation in patients undergoing nitrous oxide anesthesia (2414).
Many amino acids are known to stimulate growth hormone. There is preliminary evidence that methionine also potentiates the secretion of basal growth hormone and growth hormone induced by growth hormone releasing hormone (GHRH) (2412).
Methionine might act synergistically with folate to decrease the risk of colon cancer (9325,9326). However, there is also evidence a high dietary intake of methionine with salt and nitrates might increase the risk of gastric cancer (2409).
Rates of methylation are much higher in tumor than in normal tissue (9342). Most tumors are dependent on exogenous, preformed methionine for growth (9341). Preliminary clinical evidence suggests restriction of dietary methionine in cancer patients might inhibit tumor growth and improve cancer treatment outcomes (9341,9342).

Adverse Reactions

Orally or intravenously, methionine can cause nausea, vomiting, dizziness, drowsiness, hypotension, and irritability (9339,9340). Methionine may aggravate existing liver damage and should be used with caution in patients with severe liver disease (9336,9338,9340). A single dose of 8 grams methionine can cause hepatic encephalopathy to occur in patients with cirrhosis (9340). Methionine may cause decreased serum folate levels, leucocytosis, and increased urinary calcium excretion at dosages of 8 to 13.9 g/day for 4 to 5 days (9340).
Methionine can cause changes in the serum pH and should not be used in patients with acidosis (9340).
Cerebral effects such as cerebral edema can occur when plasma methionine levels rise above 3000 umol/L (9339).
In schizophrenic patients, large doses of methionine (e.g., 20 g/day for 5 days) can cause confusion, disorientation, delirium, agitation, listlessness, and other similar symptoms (9339,9340).
Long-term use of methionine-containing parenteral nutrition solution has been linked to liver toxicity in infants (9338).

Interactions with Herbs & Other Dietary Supplements

None known.

Interactions with Drugs

None known.

Interactions with Foods

SALT and NITRITE: Some evidence suggests that a diet rich in methionine, salt, and nitrite might increase the risk of gastric cancer (2409).

Interactions with Lab Tests

BLOOD pH: Methionine can lower serum pH by increasing sulfuric acid formation (9344).
HOMOCYSTEINE: Methionine might increase plasma homocysteine levels and test results (2410,2411). Patients who are deficient in folate, vitamin B12, or vitamin B6; or patients who have disorders of homocysteine metabolism are particularly sensitive to methionine (2410,9343).

Interactions with Diseases or Conditions

ACIDOSIS: Methionine can cause changes in the serum pH and should not be used in patients with acidosis (9340). Metabolism of methionine can result in the formation of sulfuric acid (9344).
ATHEROSCLEROSIS: Theoretically, methionine might promote or exacerbate atherosclerosis (2410). Dietary or supplemental methionine can increase homocysteine levels (2410,2411), especially in patients who are deficient in folate, vitamin B12, or B6, or patients who have disorders of homocysteine metabolism (9343). Hyperhomocysteinemia is associated with an increased risk for vascular disease (2410,2411).
CANCER: Most tumors are dependent on exogenous, preformed methionine for growth (9341). There is some evidence restriction of dietary methionine in cancer patients might inhibit tumor growth and improve cancer treatment outcomes (9341,9342).
LIVER DISEASE AND CIRROHSIS: Methionine may aggravate existing damage in the liver in patients with liver disease (9).
METHYLENETETRAHYDROFOLATE REDUCTASE (MTHFR) DEFICIENCY: Patients with a genetic mutation, MTHFR C677T, which results in homocysteine metabolic deficiency, should avoid methionine supplements. Theoretically, methionine in patients with this genotype could increase the risk for the adverse vascular effects of hyperhomocysteinemia (11014,11709).
SCHIZOPHRENIA: Large doses of methionine (e.g., 20 g/day for 5 days) might cause confusion, disorientation, delirium, agitation, listlessness, and other similar symptoms in patients with schizophrenia (9339,9340).

Dosage and Administration

ORAL: For acetaminophen poisoning, methionine 2.5 grams every 4 hours for 4 doses has been used to prevent liver damage and death (2413). For testing for hyperhomocysteinemia, an oral loading dose of 50-100 mg/kg is usually used (2410,2411).

Comments

Methionine is possibly unsafe, and should only be used by emergency room personnel for medical emergencies.

METHOXYLATED FLAVONES

Also Known As

Citrus Bioflavones, Citrus Bioflavonoids, Citrus Flavones, Citrus Flavonoids, Citrus Polymethoxylated Flavones, Flavonoids, Gardenin D, Heptamethoxyflavones, Hexamethoxyflavones, Methoxyflavones, Nobiletin, Pentamethoxyflavones, PMF, Polymethoxylated Flavones, Sinensetin, Tangeretin, Tetramethoxyflavones.
CAUTION: See separate listings for Chrysin, Diosmin, Hesperidin, Quercetin, and Rutin.

Scientific Names

5,6,7,8,4'-pentamethoxyflavone (Tangeretin); 5,6,7,3',4'-pentamethoxyflavone (Sinensetin); 5,6,7,8,3',4'-hexamethoxyflavone (nobiletin); 3,5,6,7,8,3',4'-heptamethoxyflavone (heptamethoxyflavone).

People Use This For

Orally, methoxylated flavones are used for venous insufficiency, varicose veins, cardiovascular disease, hyperlipidemia, and cancer.

Safety

LIKELY SAFE ...when consumed orally in amounts typically found in foods (12078).
There is insufficient reliable information available about the safety of methoxylated flavones when used in amounts greater than those in foods or when taken as a dietary supplement.
PREGNANCY AND LACTATION: LIKELY SAFE ...when consumed orally in amounts typically found in foods (12078). There is insufficient reliable information about the safety of methoxylated flavones when used in amounts greater than those found in foods during pregnancy or breast-feeding; avoid using.

Effectiveness

There is insufficient reliable information available about the effectiveness of methoxylated flavones.

Mechanism of Action

Methoxylated flavones are one group in the huge class of flavonoids. Flavonoids are plant pigments found in every vascular plant. These pigments give flowers and foods their yellow, orange, or red color (12078).
Methoxylated flavones occur in many foods. Citrus foods are a predominant source. Orange juice contains 2-7 ppm of the methoxylated flavones sinensetin, tangeretin, nobiletin, and heptamethoxylated flavone (12079).
Methoxylated flavones might be more stable than some other flavonoids. For example, quercetin is readily broken down through oxidative metabolism. Due to the methylation of phenolic groups of methoxylated flavones, they are thought to resist oxidative breakdown (12078).
Flavonoids, including the methoxylated flavones, are thought to be beneficial for cardiovascular disease. There is some evidence that methoxylated flavones can decrease platelet aggregation and erythrocyte sedimentation rate in animals and in vitro (12079,12080,12082,12083). There is also evidence that nobiletin can prevent experimentally induced thrombosis to a greater extent than heparin (12081). The antiplatelet effects of the methoxylated flavones seem to be greater than the flavonoids quercetin, rutin or hesperidin. Within the methoxylated flavone group, tangeretin seems to have the least antiplatelet effect and sinensetin has the greatest effect. Nobiletin and heptamethoxyflavone fall in the middle (12079,12082). These effects on platelet adhesion could theoretically play a role in prevention cardiovascular disease.
Dietary consumption of methoxylated flavones might reduce lipid levels. In animal models of hyperlipidemia, a diet consisting of 1% tangeretin or 1% tangeretin plus nobiletin significantly reduces total cholesterol, low-density lipoprotein (LDL) cholesterol, and triglycerides. But a diet consisting of a smaller concentration of these methoxylated flavones, 0.25%, does not seem to significantly reduce cholesterol levels. It's thought that methoxylated flavones might alter lipid metabolism in the liver (12112).
Methoxylated flavones seem to have some effect on immune function. Tangeretin, a polymethoxylated flavonoid, seems to reduce expression of class II histocompatibility antigens in human blood monocytes. But neither tangeretin nor another polymethoxylated flavone, nobiletin, seem to decrease antigen-induced histamine release (12078).
Methoxylated flavones, like many other flavonoids, have antioxidant capabilities and seem to decrease lipid peroxidation (12078).
There is interest in flavonoids including methoxylated flavones for preventing cancer due to their antioxidant effects and other potential protective effects. Tangeretin seems to induce apoptosis of HL-60 cells. Nobiletin and tangeretin

seem to induce liver metabolism and detoxification of some hydrocarbon carcinogens. They also inhibit growth of squamous cell carcinoma and gliosarcoma cells in culture. But these flavonoids don't seem to inhibit proliferation of normal cells, which suggests that they have a specific action against tumor cells (12078). Methoxylated flavones have also been shown to have in vitro activity against six human cancer cell lines including melanoma, prostate, colon, and lung cancer cells (12084).

Nobiletin has anti-inflammatory effects which are estimated to have a potency of about 68% of hydrocortisone (12081). Tetramethoxyflavones seem to have antiviral activity against the rhinovirus in vitro (12081).

Tangeretin is thought to be demethoxylated via cytochrome P450 (CYP450) metabolism. Tangeretin might also induce cytochrome P450 1A2 (CYP1A2), possibly by increasing gene transcription (12078).

Adverse Reactions
None reported.

Interactions with Herbs & Other Dietary Supplements
None known.

Interactions with Drugs
CYTOCHROME P450 1A2 (CYP1A2) SUBSTRATES: There is preliminary evidence that methoxylated flavones might induce CYP1A2 (12078). Theoretically, concurrent use of methoxylated flavones and drugs metabolized by these enzymes might result in increased drug elimination, decreased serum levels, and decreased effectiveness. Some drugs metabolized by CYP1A2 include clozapine (Clozaril), cyclobenzaprine (Flexeril), fluvoxamine (Luvox), haloperidol (Haldol), imipramine (Tofranil), mexiletine (Mexitil), olanzapine (Zyprexa), Pentazocine (Talwin), propranolol (Inderal), tacrine (Cognex), theophylline (Slo-bid, Theo-Dur, others), zileuton (Zyflo), Zolmitriptan (Zomig), and others.

Interactions with Foods
None known.

Interactions with Lab Tests
None known.

Interactions with Diseases or Conditions
None known.

Dosage and Administration
No typical dosage.

Comments
In 1936, it was proposed that flavonoids be recognized as vitamins. It was thought that they were necessary to prevent abnormal capillary permeability and capillary fragility. But there was not adequate evidence to establish flavonoids as vitamins (12079).

Flavonoids are plant pigments found in all vascular plants. They are responsible for many of the yellow, red, and orange colors in plants. Common food sources include red wine, stems, flowers, fruits, vegetables, nuts, seeds, herbs, spices, coffee, and teas. They are prominent components of citrus fruits (12078). Flavonoids are grouped based on slight differences in structure. These subdivisions include flavanols, anthocyanidins, flavones, flavanones, and chalcones (12078).

There have been over 4000 unique flavonoids identified from plant sources (12078).

MEXICAN SCAMMONY ROOT

Also Known As
Ipomoea, Orizaba Jalap.

CAUTION: See separate listings for Jalap, Pokeweed.

Scientific Names
Ipomoea orizabensis, synonyms Convolvulus orizabensis, Convolvulus superbus, Ipomoea superba, Ipomoea tyrianthina.

Family: Convolvulaceae.

People Use This For
Orally, Mexican scammony root is used as a purgative.

Safety
There is insufficient reliable information available about the safety of Mexican scammony root.
PREGNANCY: LIKELY UNSAFE ...when used orally (18); avoid using.
LACTATION: There is insufficient reliable information available about the safety of Mexican scammony root during pregnancy; avoid using.

Effectiveness
There is insufficient reliable information available about the effectiveness of Mexican scammony root.

Mechanism of Action
Mexican scammony root exerts a potent stimulant laxative effect on the intestines. It contains 12-15% resinous polymeric ester glycosides (18).

Adverse Reactions
Orally, it can cause intestinal colic, and in large amounts, vomiting (18).

Interactions with Herbs & Other Dietary Supplements
CARDIAC GLYCOSIDE-CONTAINING HERBS: Overuse or abuse of Mexican scammony root may increase the risk of cardiac glycoside toxicity (19).
HORSETAIL/LICORICE: Theoretically, concomitant use of Mexican scammony root with horsetail plant or licorice rhizome increases the risk of potassium depletion (19).
STIMULANT LAXATIVE HERBS: Theoretically, concomitant use with other stimulant laxative herbs may increase the risk of potassium depletion (19).

Interactions with Drugs
DIGOXIN (Lanoxin): Theoretically, overuse or abuse of Mexican scammony root might increase the risk of adverse effects of cardiac glycoside drugs.
DIURETIC DRUGS: Overuse of Mexican scammony might compound diuretic-induced potassium loss (18). There is some concern that people taking Mexican scammony along with potassium depleting diuretics might have an increased risk for hypokalemia. Initiation of potassium supplementation or an increase in potassium supplement dose may be necessary for some patients. Some diuretics that can deplete potassium include chlorothiazide (Diuril), chlorthalidone (Thalitone), furosemide (Lasix), hydrochlorothiazide (HCTZ, Hydrodiuril, Microzide), and others.
ORAL DRUGS: Theoretically, Mexican scammony may reduce absorption of drugs due to reduced transit time (19).
STIMULANT LAXATIVES: Concomitant use of Mexican scammony and laxatives may lead to electrolyte and fluid depletion (19).

Interactions with Foods
None known.

Interactions with Lab Tests
None known.

Interactions with Diseases or Conditions
GI CONDITIONS: Contraindicated; may have GI irritant effects (19). Stimulant laxatives are contraindicated in individuals with symptoms of appendicitis (abdominal pain, nausea and vomiting) (272).

Dosage and Administration
ORAL: People typically take 3 to 12 grains (195 to 780 mg) of the powdered root. The powdered resin from the root is dosed 3 to 8 grains (195 to 520 mg) (5267).

Comments
Ipomoea orizabensis is no longer used as a purgative because of the adverse effect of vomiting.

MEZEREON

Also Known As
Camolea, Daphne, Dwarf Bay, Spurge Flax, Spurge Laurel, Spurge Olive, Wild Pepper.

Scientific Names
Daphne mezereum.
Family: Thymelaeaceae.

People Use This For
Orally, mezereon is used to relieve headaches and toothaches.
Topically, mezereon is used for joint pains and to increase circulation in rheumatic conditions.

Safety
POSSIBLY UNSAFE ...when used topically (18). Prolonged skin contact can lead to necrosis (18).
LIKELY UNSAFE ...when used orally. The plant is poisonous and can cause death (18).
PREGNANCY AND LACTATION: LIKELY UNSAFE ...when used orally or topically (18); avoid using.

Effectiveness
There is insufficient reliable information available about the effectiveness of mezereon.

Mechanism of Action
The applicable part of mezereon is the bark. Mezereon contains diterpenes including mezerein and daphnetoxin. It possesses powerful skin stimulating effects and can be hallucinogenic (18).

Adverse Reactions
Orally, mezereon can cause reddening and swelling of the oral mucous membranes, salivation, thirst, stomach pains, vomiting, and severe diarrhea (18). Symptoms can also include headache, dizziness, stupor, tachycardia, spasms, and death through circulatory collapse (18).
Topically, mezereon can cause red, painful swelling of the skin, blister formation, and shedding of the epidermis (18). Extended exposure can cause necrosis (18). Contact with the eyes can cause severe conjunctivitis (18).

Interactions with Herbs & Other Dietary Supplements
None known.

Interactions with Drugs
None known.

Interactions with Foods
None known.

Interactions with Lab Tests
None known.

Interactions with Diseases or Conditions
None known.

Dosage and Administration
TOPICAL: Mezereon was typically used as a 20% ointment (18).

Comments
Mezereon is a protected species (18). It is seldom used medicinally today (18).

MGN-3

Also Known As
Biobran, Hemicellulose Complex with Arabinoxylane.

Scientific Names
None.

People Use This For
Orally, MGN-3 is used for boosting immune function, preventing and treating cancer, treating AIDS, hepatitis, diabetes, chronic fatigue syndrome and other immunodeficiency disorders.

Safety
There is insufficient reliable information available about the safety of MGN-3.
Pregnancy and Lactation: Insufficient reliable information available; avoid using.

Effectiveness
There is insufficient reliable information available about the effectiveness of MGN-3.

Mechanism of Action
MGN-3 is a hemicellulose complex containing arabinoxylane as a major component. It is produced by hydrolyzing rice bran using enzymes from mycelia of Shiitake, Kawaratake, and Suehirotake mushrooms. Some studies suggest it might improve immunity by enhancing natural killer cell activity, increasing interferon-gamma production by peripheral blood mononuclear cells, and acting synergistically with interleukin-2 (aldesleukin) to increase natural killer cell activity and production of tumor necrosis factor alpha (3116,3117). Other evidence suggests that MGN-3 has activity against HIV (3113). Results from three small studies of healthy individuals and individuals with cancer suggest that MGN-3 also enhances natural killer cell activity (3118,3119,3120).

Adverse Reactions
None reported.

Interactions with Herbs & Other Dietary Supplements
None known.

Interactions with Drugs
None known.

Interactions with Foods
None known.

Interactions with Lab Tests
None known.

Interactions with Diseases or Conditions
None known.

Dosage and Administration
ORAL: A dose of 3 grams per day has been used in cancer patients (3119,3120).

Comments
The FDA is seeking a permanent injunction against the marketing of MGN-3 by Lane Labs. The complaint charges that MGN-3 is an unapproved drug product promoted as treatment for cancer and HIV infection (387).

MILK THISTLE

Also Known As
Blessed Milk Thistle, Cardui mariae fructus, Cardui Mariae Herba, Holy Thistle, Lady's Thistle, Legalon, Marian Thistle, Mariendistel, Mary Thistle, Our Lady's Thistle, Silybin, Silybum, Silymarin, St. Mary Thistle.
CAUTION: See separate listing for Blessed Thistle.

Scientific Names
Silybum marianum, synonym Carduus marianus.
Family: Asteraceae/Compositae.

People Use This For
Orally, milk thistle is used for liver disorders including toxic liver damage caused by chemicals, Amanita phalloides mushroom poisoning, jaundice, chronic inflammatory liver disease, hepatic cirrhosis, and chronic hepatitis. It is also used orally for loss of appetite, dyspepsia and gallbladder complaints, hangover, and diseases of the spleen. Milk thistle is used orally for prostate cancer, pleurisy, malaria, depression, uterine complaints, stimulating breast milk flow, and stimulating menstrual flow.
Intravenously, milk thistle is used as a supportive treatment for Amanita phalloides mushroom poisoning.
In foods, the milk thistle leaves and flowers are eaten as a vegetable and seeds are roasted for use as a coffee substitute.

Safety
POSSIBLY SAFE ...when used orally and appropriately. Milk thistle extracts standardized to contain 70-80% of the silymarin constituent seems to be safe when used for up to 41 months (2614,2616).
There is insufficient reliable information available about the safety of intravenous formulations of milk thistle and its constituents.
PREGNANCY AND LACTATION: Insufficient reliable information available; avoid using.

Effectiveness

POSSIBLY EFFECTIVE

Dyspepsia. A specific combination product containing milk thistle (Iberogast, Enzymatic Therapy) seems to improve symptoms of dyspepsia. The combination includes milk thistle plus peppermint leaf, German chamomile, caraway, licorice, clown's mustard plant, celandine, angelica, and lemon balm (7049,12724). A meta-analysis of studies using this combination product suggests that taking 1 mL orally three times daily over a period of 4-weeks significantly reduces severity of acid reflux, epigastric pain, cramping, nausea, and vomiting compared to placebo (13089).

INSUFFICIENT RELIABLE EVIDENCE to RATE

Alcohol-related liver disease. Preliminary clinical research suggests that milk thistle taken orally might be helpful for treating alcoholic liver disease (2613,2616,2618,7321,7322,7355).

Amanita mushroom poisoning. Administering silibinin, a constituent of milk thistle, intravenously (IV) may lessen liver damage due to Amanita phalloides mushroom (death cap) poisoning (2615). Silibinin is not readily available in the US.

Diabetes. Preliminary clinical evidence suggests that the milk thistle constituent silymarin can reduce insulin resistance in people with coexisting diabetes and alcoholic cirrhosis (2617).

Hepatitis B or Hepatitis C. Preliminary clinical research suggests a specific oral preparation of silibinin, an active constituent extracted from milk thistle, complexed with phosphatidylcholine (Silipide), may improve liver function tests (LFTs) in patients with chronic active hepatitis. Silibinin is complexed with phosphatidylcholine to theoretically improve the bioavailability of silibinin (7356).

Toxin-induced liver damage. Some research suggests milk thistle may limit liver damage after exposure to industrial toxicants such as toluene and xylene (2614).

Most clinical studies of milk thistle's effectiveness have used a specific extract standardized to 70-80% silymarin (Legalon). In the US, this formulation is found in the brand name product Thisilyn (Nature's Way).

More evidence is needed to rate milk thistle for these uses.

Mechanism of Action

The applicable parts of milk thistle are the seed and above ground parts. The seed is most commonly used medicinally. Silymarin, the active constituent of the milk thistle seed, consists of four flavonolignans called silibinin (silybin), isosilybinin, silichristin (silychristin), and silidianin. Silibinin makes up about 70% of silymarin (7318,8956). When ingested, silymarin undergoes enterohepatic recirculation and has higher concentrations in liver cells.

Silymarin is a potent inhibitor of tumor necrosis factor (TNF). The cytotoxicity, inflammation, and apoptosis induced by TNF are effectively blocked by silymarin. Although the mechanism of this effect is not clear, it probably involves intracellular signaling (7859). Silybin is an antioxidant, a free radical scavenger, and an inhibitor of lipid peroxidation (8957). In vitro silybin has shown an affinity for binding to p-glycoprotein, a transporter thought to be involved in the drug resistance of cancer cells (11481).

Several activities seem to contribute to the therapeutic effect of silymarin in liver disease. Silymarin seems to cause an alteration of the outer hepatocyte cell membrane that prevents toxin penetration. It also stimulates nucleolar polymerase A, resulting in increased ribosomal protein synthesis, which can stimulate liver regeneration and the formation of new hepatocytes. There is also some evidence that suggests that silymarin might have antifibrotic, anti-inflammatory, and immunomodulating effects that could also be beneficial in liver disease (6879). Silymarin and silybin inhibit beta-glucuronidase, which might help protect against hepatic injury and possibly colon cancer. Inhibition of beta-glucuronidase is thought to reduce the hydrolysis of glucuronides into toxic metabolites in the liver and intestine (7354).

Preliminary evidence indicates that milk thistle constituents might protect against kidney damage. In vitro, silibinin and silicristin can protect the kidney cells from nephrotoxic drugs such as acetaminophen, cisplatin, and vincristine. Silibinin and silicristin also appear to have a regenerative effect on kidney cells, similar to the effects on hepatic cells (7320).

There is some interest in using milk thistle for prostate cancer. In vitro research shows that silymarin and silibinin have antiproliferative effects on androgen-responsive prostate cancer cells (7319).

The above ground parts seem to have some estrogenic activity. A milk thistle plant extract appears to enhance estradiol binding to estrogen receptors, induce transcription activity in estrogen-responsive cells, and enhance estradiol-induced transcription activity in estrogen-responsive cells (6180). There is also preliminary evidence that suggests that milk thistle might affect drug metabolism. In vitro, silymarin and its flavonolignan, silibinin, inhibit cytochrome P450 2C9 (CYP2C9) and cytochrome P450 3A4 (CYP3A4), the major phase 1 hepatic enzyme. However, silymarin does not seem to affect the metabolism of indinavir (Crixivan), a CYP3A4 substrate, in healthy volunteers (10427). In vitro, silymarin and silibinin also inhibit uridine diphosphoglucuronosyl transferase (UGT), the major phase 2 enzyme that is responsible for glucuronidation (6450,7089,7318).

Adverse Reactions

Orally, milk thistle is usually well-tolerated (6879,8956). It can cause an occasional laxative effect (8956). Other less common gastrointestinal (GI) effects include nausea, diarrhea, dyspepsia, flatulence, abdominal bloating, fullness or pain, and anorexia (6879). There is one case of a woman who experienced intermittent episodes of sweating, nausea, abdominal pain, vomiting, diarrhea, weakness, and collapse, requiring hospitalization (3525).

Some patients may have allergic reactions to milk thistle including pruritus, rash, urticaria, eczema, and anaphylaxis (6879,8956). Allergic reactions may be more likely to occur in patients sensitive to the Asteraceae/Compositae family. Members of this family include ragweed, chrysanthemums, marigolds, daisies, and many other herbs.

Interactions with Herbs & Other Dietary Supplements

None known.

Interactions with Drugs

CYTOCHROME P450 2C9 (CYP2C9) SUBSTRATES: There's preliminary evidence that milk thistle might inhibit cytochrome P450 2C9 (CYP2C9) (7089,8234). So far, this interaction has not been reported in humans. However, watch for an increase in the levels of drugs metabolized by CYP2C9 in patients taking milk thistle. Some drugs metabolized by CYP2C9 include amitriptyline (Elavil), diazepam (Valium), verapamil (Calan), warfarin (Coumadin), zileuton (Zyflo), and others. Use milk thistle cautiously or avoid in patients taking these drugs.
CYTOCHROME P450 3A4 (CYP3A4) SUBSTRATES: There's preliminary evidence that milk thistle might inhibit cytochrome P450 3A4 (CYP3A4) enzyme (6450,7089,7318,8234). So far, this interaction has not been reported in humans. Milk thistle does not affect plasma concentrations of the CYP3A4 substrate indinavir in healthy volunteers, so interactions with drugs metabolized by CYP3A4 are not likely clinically significant (10427).
ESTROGENS: Theoretically, silymarin, an active constituent of milk thistle, might increase the clearance of estrogen by inhibiting beta-glucuronidase (6879).
GLUCURONIDATED DRUGS: Theoretically, silymarin, an active constituent of milk thistle, might increase the clearance of drugs that undergo glucuronidation. Some of these drugs include acetaminophen, atorvastatin (Lipitor), diazepam (Valium), digoxin, entacapone (Comtan), irinotecan (Camptosar), lamotrigine (Lamictal), lorazepam (Ativan), lovastatin (Mevacor), meprobamate, morphine, oxazepam (Serax), and others (7318,7354).
INDINAVIR (Crixivan): Milk thistle does not appear to affect the metabolism of indinavir in healthy volunteers (10427). Although preclinical research suggested milk thistle might inhibit CYP3A4 and potentially increase indinavir levels (7318), milk thistle does not appear to affect the pharmacokinetics of indinavir in humans.

Interactions with Foods

None known.

Interactions with Lab Tests

None known.

Interactions with Diseases or Conditions

CROSS-ALLERGENICITY: Milk thistle may cause an allergic reaction in individuals sensitive to the Asteraceae/Compositae family. Members of this family include ragweed, chrysanthemums, marigolds, daisies, and many other herbs.
HORMONE SENSITIVE CANCERS/CONDITIONS: Because milk thistle plant extract might have estrogenic effects (6180), women with hormone sensitive conditions should avoid milk thistle above ground parts. Some of these conditions include breast cancer, uterine cancer, ovarian cancer, endometriosis, and uterine fibroids. The more commonly used milk thistle seed extracts are not known to have estrogenic effects.

Dosage and Administration

ORAL: For hepatic cirrhosis, a milk thistle extract containing 70% to 80% silymarin (Legalon), 420 mg per day has been used (2616).
For chronic active hepatitis, a milk thistle constituent, silibinin (Silibide), 240 mg twice daily as been used (7356).
Some people make a milk thistle tea, but the active ingredients are not very soluble in water (515).
For dyspepsia, a specific combination product containing milk thistle (Iberogast, Enzymatic Therapy) and several other herbs has been used in a dose of 1 mL three times daily (7049,12724,13089).
INTRAVENOUS: For Amanita phalloides mushroom poisoning, the common dose is 20-50 mg/kg over 24 hours, divided into four infusions, each administered over a two hour period. This is usually started within 48 hours after mushroom ingestion (2615). Intravenous silibinin is not available in the US.

Comments

The broken leaves of the milk thistle plant exude a milky sap. The leaves have distinctive white markings which, according to legend, were the Virgin Mary's milk (7161). Milk thistle is grown as a vegetable for salads and as a substitute for spinach. Avoid confusion with blessed thistle (Cnicus benedictus).

MONEYWORT

Also Known As

Creeping Jenny, Creeping Joan, Herb Two-Pence, Meadow Runagates, Running Jenny, Serpentaria, String Of Sovereigns, Twopenny Grass, Wandering Jenny, Wandering Tailor.

Scientific Names

Lysimachia nummularia.
Family: Primulaceae.

Comments

At the date of publication, this product was not a common ingredient used in brand name supplements marketed to consumers. Details about this product are available in the online version of *Natural Medicines Comprehensive Database.* See www.naturaldatabase.com.

MORINDA

Also Known As

Ba Ji Tian, Bois Douleur, Canarywood, Cheese Fruit, Hai Ba Ji, Hog Apple, Indian Mulberry, Luoling, Mengkudu, Menkoedoe, Mora De La India, Mulberry, Nhau, Noni, Nono, Nonu, Pau-Azeitona, Rotten Cheese Fruit, Ruibarbo Caribe, Tahitian Noni Juice, Ura, Wild Pine, Wu Ning.
CAUTION: See separate listing for Ba Ji Tian.

Scientific Names

Morinda citrifolia.
Family: Rubiaceae.

People Use This For

Orally, morinda is used for colic, convulsions, cough, diabetes, dysuria, stimulating menstrual flow, fever, hepatosis, constipation, leukorrhea, malarial fever, and nausea. It is also used for smallpox, splenomegaly, swelling, asthma, arthritis and other bone and joint problems, cancer, cataracts, colds, depression, digestive problems, and gastric ulcers. Other uses include high blood pressure, infections, kidney disorders, migraine, premenstrual syndrome, stroke, pain, and sedation. The fruit juice is used for arthritis, diabetes, high blood pressure, muscle aches and pains, menstrual difficulties, headaches, heart disease, AIDS, cancers, gastric ulcers, sprains, depression, senility, poor digestion, atherosclerosis, circulation problems, and drug addiction. The leaves have been used in medicines for rheumatic aches and swelling of the joints, stomachache, dysentery, and swelling caused filariasis. The bark has been used in a preparation to aid childbirth.

Topically, morinda is used as an emollient and to reduce signs of aging. The leaves are used topically for arthritis by wrapping around the affected joint, for headache by applying to the forehead, and for direct application to burns, sores, wounds, and leprotic lesions. A mixture of leaves and fruit is applied to abscesses, and preparations of the root are used on stonefish and sting-ray wounds, and as a smallpox salve.

In foods, the fruits, leaves, roots, seeds, and bark are eaten.

Safety

POSSIBLY SAFE ...when used orally or topically and appropriately for medicinal purposes (11944). ...when the fruit is consumed as food (11944).

PREGNANCY: POSSIBLY UNSAFE ...when used orally. Historically, morinda has been used as an abortifacient (11964).

LACTATION: Insufficient reliable information available; avoid using.

Effectiveness

There is insufficient reliable information available about the effectiveness of morinda.

Mechanism of Action

The applicable parts of morinda are the fruits, leaves, flowers, stems, bark, and roots. Morinda contains potassium, vitamin C, anthraquinones, beta-sitosterol, carotene, vitamin A, flavone glycosides, linoleic acid, caproic acid (which may explain its foul odor), ursolic acid, rutin, and other constituents (11944). The fruit juice also contains a significant amount of potassium, approximately 56 mEq/L (1298).

Preliminary research suggests that constituents in the fruit and roots of morinda might have antibacterial, antiviral (including HIV), and antihelmintic effects. Other preliminary research suggests that morinda might have analgesic, hypotensive, and immunological activity (11944,11964).

The fruit juice contains a polysaccharide-rich substance which increases survival in mice with Lewis lung carcinoma, possibly by activating the host immune system (441). Damnacanthal, an anthraquinone isolated from the roots of morinda, may affect second messenger signaling and reverse mutagenicity of cancer cells (442,443). It also seems to promote capillary degeneration and death in experimental tumor tissue (11965). Other very preliminary research suggests that morinda may inhibit cancer cell proliferation (11964). In mice, lyophilized aqueous extracts of morinda roots have sedative and central analgesic effects, the latter blocked by naloxone (444). Animal research suggests morinda root extract might have antidepressant activity (11966).

A report has been published in a botanical journal about 2 constituents of morinda, xeronine and proxeronine, that are touted in advertising about morinda. However, these compounds have not been chemically identified or described in medical literature and are currently regarded as questionable (11964).

There is no reliable published clinical research on morinda.

Adverse Reactions

Orally, no side effects have been reported in studies of morinda; however, there is one case report of hepatotoxicity in an otherwise healthy patient who consumed morinda tea. The patients developed symptoms beginning a week after consuming the tea daily including malaise, nausea, abnormal fatigue, and shortness of breath while exercising. Hepatotoxicity was diagnosed after 3 weeks of ingesting the tea and liver function tests were found to be elevated. Liver function tests declined within 2 days of discontinuing the morinda tea and were normalized within a month (13107). From this single case report, it is not possible to prove that morinda was the cause of hepatotoxicity in this case. Potential product contamination was not ruled out. However, researchers theorize that anthraquinones contained in morinda could potentially cause hepatotoxicity. Other products containing anthraquinones, such as senna, have been linked to cases of hepatotoxicity. More evidence is needed to determine if morinda causes hepatotoxicity.

Interactions with Herbs & Other Dietary Supplements

None known.

Interactions with Drugs

ACE INHIBITORS (ACEIs): Morinda juice contains significant amounts of potassium, about 56 mEq/L (1298). ACE inhibitors can also increase potassium levels. Theoretically, combining morinda and ACE inhibitors might increase the risk of hyperkalemia. The ACE inhibitors include benazepril (Lotensin), captopril (Capoten), enalapril (Vasotec), fosinopril (Monopril), lisinopril (Prinivil, Zestril), moexipril (Univasc), perindopril (Aceon), quinapril (Accupril), ramipril (Altace), and trandolapril (Mavik).

ANGIOTENSIN RECEPTOR BLOCKERS (ARBs): Morinda juice contains significant amounts of potassium, about 56 mEq/L (1298). ARBs can also increase potassium levels. Theoretically, combining morinda and ARBs might increase the risk of hyperkalemia. The ARBs include losartan (Cozaar), valsartan (Diovan), irbesartan (Avapro), candesartan (Atacand), telmisartan (Micardis), and eprosartan (Teveten).

POTASSIUM-SPARING DIURETICS: Morinda juice contains significant amounts of potassium, about 56 mEq/L (1298). Potassium-sparing diuretics also increase potassium levels. Theoretically, combing morinda and a potassium-sparing diuretic might increase the risk of hyperkalemia.

Interactions with Foods

None known.

Interactions with Lab Tests

URINE COLOR: The anthraquinone constituents can discolor urine from pink to rust and interfere with diagnostic tests, due to anthraquinone content (275).

Interactions with Diseases or Conditions

CHRONIC RENAL INSUFFICIENCY: Consuming morinda fruit juice might increase the risk of hyperkalemia in patients with renal insufficiency. There is one published case report of hyperkalemia in a patient with chronic renal insufficiency who consumed morinda juice. Morinda fruit juice contains approximately 56 mEq/L of potassium (1298).

HYPERKALEMIA: Consuming morinda fruit juice might increase potassium levels and exacerbate hyperkalemia. Morinda fruit juice contains approximately 56 mEq/L of potassium (1298).

Dosage and Administration

No typical dosage.

Comments

Morinda is a small evergreen tree in the Pacific Islands, Southeast Asia, Australia, and India that often grows among lava flows. Morinda's most common traditional use is topical. Morinda roots and bark have been used to make a red or yellow dye for clothing. The smell and taste of some Morinda citrifolia fruit and juice (noni juice) are unpleasant. The FDA has issued multiple warnings to morinda manufacturers about unsubstantiated claims (11944,11964).

The National Center for Complimentary and Alternative Medicine is sponsoring a Phase I study on the use of morinda freeze-dried noni fruit extract. Study results have not been published (11967).

MORMON TEA

Also Known As

Brigham Tea, Desert Tea, Gray Ephedra, Nevada Ephedra, Popotillo, Squaw Tea, Teamster's Tea.
CAUTION: See separate listing for Ephedra.

Scientific Names

Ephedra nevadensis.
Family: Ephedraceae.

People Use This For

Orally, Mormon tea is used for syphilis, gonorrhea, colds, kidney disorders, and as a "spring" tonic.
Mormon tea is consumed as a beverage.

Safety

LIKELY SAFE ...when consumed in food amounts (12).
There is insufficient reliable information about the safety of Mormon tea for medicinal use.
PREGNANCY AND LACTATION: Insufficient reliable information available; avoid using in amounts greater than those commonly found in foods.

Effectiveness

There is insufficient reliable information available about the effectiveness of Mormon tea.

Mechanism of Action

Mormon tea contains large amounts of tannins (515). Tannin constituents exert an astringent effect on the mucosal tissue. This effect dehydrates the tissue, reducing internal secretions, and binding external cells into a protective layer (12). Plants with at least 10% tannins can cause gastrointestinal disturbances, kidney damage, and necrotic conditions of the liver (12). Some animal experiments show that tannins might cause cancer. Others show they might prevent it (12). Regular consumption of herbs with high tannin concentrations correlates to an increase in esophageal or nasal cancer (12). Despite being in the Ephedra genus, Mormon tea contains no ephedrine or other alkaloids (515). An aqueous extract demonstrates mild diuresis and constipation (515).

Adverse Reactions

None reported.

Interactions with Herbs & Other Dietary Supplements

TANNIN-CONTAINING HERBS: Theoretically, herbs that contain high percentages of tannins might cause precipitation of constituents of other herbs (19).

Interactions with Drugs

ORAL DRUGS: Theoretically, concomitant oral administration may cause precipitation of some drugs due to the high tannin content of Mormon tea (19). Separate administration of oral drugs and tannin-containing herbs by the longest period of time practical (19).

Interactions with Foods

None known.

Interactions with Lab Tests

None known.

Interactions with Diseases or Conditions

None known.

Dosage and Administration

ORAL: Mormon tea is typically prepared by steeping the dried branches in 150 mL boiling water for five to ten minutes and then straining (6002).

MOTHERWORT

Also Known As
Leonuri cardiacae herba, Leonurus, Lion's Ear, Lion's Tail, Roman Motherwort, Throw-Wort.

Scientific Names
Leonurus cardiaca.
Family: Lamiaceae/Labiatae.

People Use This For
Orally, motherwort is used for cardiac symptoms of neurosis, cardiac insufficiency, fast heart rate or other arrhythmias, amenorrhea, flatulence, and hyperthyroidism.
Topically, motherwort is used for itching and shingles. The seeds of Leonurus artemisia or Leonurus heterophyllus are used to improve eyesight and as a general tonic.

Safety
POSSIBLY SAFE ...when used orally and appropriately (12).
PREGNANCY: LIKELY UNSAFE ...when used orally because it might have uterine-stimulating effects (4,12,19).
LACTATION: Insufficient reliable information available; avoid using.

Effectiveness
There is insufficient reliable information available about the effectiveness of motherwort.

Mechanism of Action
The applicable parts of motherwort are the above ground parts. Motherwort has sedative (4,18), negative chronotropic, hypotonic (18), cardiac-inhibitory, and antispasmodic effects (4). Constituents include leonurine and stachydrine, which can stimulate uterine tone and blood flow (4,12,19). Ursolic acid can have antiviral, tumor-inhibiting, and cytotoxic activity (4). The intravenous administration of a Leonurus heterophyllus extract can decrease blood viscosity by decreasing platelet aggregation, decreasing fibrinogen, and increasing erythrocyte deformability (1533).

Adverse Reactions
Orally, use of motherwort in amounts greater than 3 grams can cause diarrhea, stomach irritation, and uterine bleeding (12). The leaves can cause contact dermatitis, and the oil can cause photosensitivity (4). Motherwort can also cause allergic reactions in sensitive individuals (4).

Interactions with Herbs & Other Dietary Supplements
CARDIAC GLYCOSIDE-CONTAINING HERBS: Contraindicated; concomitant use can increase the risk of cardiac glycoside toxicity (19). Cardiac glycoside-containing herbs include black hellebore, Canadian hemp roots, digitalis leaf, hedge mustard, figwort, lily-of-the-valley roots, oleander leaf, pheasant's eye plant, pleurisy root, squill bulb leaf scales, strophanthus seeds, and uzara.

Interactions with Drugs
CNS DEPRESSANTS: Concomitant use of motherwort can potentiate the sedative and tranquilizing effects of these drugs, including the sedative effects of antihistamines (19).

Interactions with Foods
None known.

Interactions with Lab Tests
THYROID FUNCTION: Motherwort might improve thyroid function and thyroid function test results in patients with thyroid hyperfunction (2).

Interactions with Diseases or Conditions
CARDIAC DISORDERS: Excessive use of motherwort can interfere with the treatment of cardiac disorders (4).
UTERINE BLEEDING CONDITIONS: Theoretically, it can exacerbate uterine bleeding due to its possible stimulation of uterine blood flow (4,12,19).

Dosage and Administration
ORAL: The typical dose of motherwort is 2 grams of the dried above ground parts or 1 cup of the tea 3 times per day (4). To prepare tea steep 2 grams of the dried above ground parts in 150 mL boiling water for 5-10 minutes, then strain. The average amount used is 4.5 grams per day (2).

MOUNTAIN ASH

Also Known As
Eberesche, Ebereschenbeeren, European Mountain-Ash, Quickbeam, Rowan Tree, Sorb Apple, Sorbi acupariae fructus, Witchen.

Scientific Names
Sorbus aucuparia, synonym Pyrus aucuparia.
Family: Rosaceae.

People Use This For
Orally, mountain ash is used for kidney diseases, diabetes, arthritis, disorders of uric acid metabolism, dissolution of uric acid deposits, mucous membrane inflammation, internal inflammations, vitamin C deficiency, alkalizing the blood, increasing metabolism, purifying the blood, and for menstrual complaints. It is also used orally for diarrhea and lung conditions, especially those associated with fever.
In manufacturing, mountain ash is used as an ingredient in marmalade, stewed fruit, juice, liqueur, vinegar, and in tea mixtures.

Safety
POSSIBLY UNSAFE ...when large amounts of fresh berries are ingested. The constituent, parasorbic acid, is an irritant and large amounts can cause gastric irritation and kidney damage (18).
There is insufficient reliable information available about the safety of the oral use of dried or cooked berries.
PREGNANCY AND LACTATION: POSSIBLY UNSAFE ...when large amounts of fresh berries are ingested (18). There is insufficient reliable information available about the safety of dried or cooked berries; avoid using.

Effectiveness
There is insufficient reliable information available about the effectiveness of mountain ash.

Mechanism of Action
The applicable part of mountain ash is the berry used fresh, dried, or cooked then dried. Mountain ash berry contains parasorbic acid, cyanogenic glycosides, fruit acids (malic acid, tartaric acid), tannins, and vitamin C (18). The parasorbic acid that is contained in the fresh berry can cause local irritation. However, the compound is partially degraded by drying and completely destroyed by cooking (2).

Adverse Reactions
Orally, large amounts of fresh berries may cause gastroenteritis, vomiting, queasiness, gastric pain, diarrhea, kidney damage (albuminuria, glycosuria), and polymorphic xanthomas due to parasorbic acid (18).

Interactions with Herbs & Other Dietary Supplements
None known.

Interactions with Drugs
None known.

Interactions with Foods
None known.

Interactions with Lab Tests
None known.

Interactions with Diseases or Conditions
None known.

Dosage and Administration
No typical dosage.

MOUNTAIN FLAX

Also Known As
Dwarf Flax, Fairy Flax, Mill Mountain, Purging Flax.

Scientific Names
Linum catharticum.
Family: Linaceae.

People Use This For
Orally, mountain flax is used as an emetic and purgative to cause bowel elimination.

Safety
POSSIBLY UNSAFE ...when used orally, particularly with long-term use (18).
PREGNANCY AND LACTATION: UNSAFE ...when used orally due to possible emetic effects (18).

Effectiveness
There is insufficient reliable information available about the effectiveness of mountain flax.

Mechanism of Action
The applicable parts of mountain flax are the above ground flowering parts. Mountain flax is thought to have laxative effects at 0.5 grams. It contains the lignan achromatin, tannins, and a volatile oil (18).

Adverse Reactions
Orally, mountain flax can cause vomiting, gastrointestinal tract inflammation and diarrhea (18).

Interactions with Herbs & Other Dietary Supplements
None known.

Interactions with Drugs
None known.

Interactions with Foods
None known.

Interactions with Lab Tests
None known.

Interactions with Diseases or Conditions
None known.

Dosage and Administration
No typical dosage.

MOUNTAIN LAUREL

Also Known As
Broad-Leafed Laurel, Calico Bush, Lambkill, Laurel, Mountain Ivy, Rose Laurel, Sheep Laurel, Spoon Laurel.

Scientific Names
Kalmia latifolia.
Family: Ericaceae.

People Use This For
Topically, mountain laurel is used for tinea capitis, psoriasis, herpes, and secondary syphilis.

Safety
UNSAFE ...when used orally. Mountain laurel leaf is not only an irritant, but can also lead to cardiac arrest, respiratory failure and death (18).
There is insufficient reliable information available about safety of the topical use of mountain laurel.
PREGNANCY AND LACTATION: UNSAFE ...when used orally (18). There is insufficient reliable information available about safety of mountain laurel for topical use; avoid using.

Effectiveness
There is insufficient reliable information available about the effectiveness of mountain laurel.

Mechanism of Action
The applicable part of mountain laurel is the fresh or dried leaf. Mountain laurel contains andromedan derivatives, flavonoids, and acylphloroglucinols (18). Andromedan derivatives act on the sodium channels, inhibiting conduction by preventing closure of the excitable cells (18). The andromedan derivative Grayanotoxin I and the acylphloroglucinol constituents can be cytotoxic (4145).

Adverse Reactions
Orally, mountain laurel can result in painful oral and gastric mucous membranes, increased salivation, cold sweat, nausea, vomiting, diarrhea, and paresthesias (18). Dizziness; headache; fever attacks; and intoxicated states with temporary loss of vision, muscle weakness, coordination disorders, and spasms can also develop. Bradycardia, cardiac arrhythmias, drop in blood pressure, eventual cardiac arrest, and respiratory failure can lead to death (18).

Interactions with Herbs & Other Dietary Supplements
None known.

Interactions with Drugs
None known.

Interactions with Foods
None known.

Interactions with Lab Tests
None known.

Interactions with Diseases or Conditions
None known.

Dosage and Administration
TOPICAL: Mountain laurel is only available in homeopathic preparations (18).

MOUSE EAR

Also Known As
Hawkweed.
CAUTION: See separate listing for Cudweed.

Scientific Names
Hieracium pilosella, synonym Pilosella officinarum.
Family: Asteraceae/Compositae.

People Use This For
Orally, mouse ear is used for asthma, bronchitis, coughs and whooping cough. It is also used orally as a diuretic, to promote sweating, and to relieve flatulence and colic.
Topically, mouse ear is used for wounds.

Safety
There is insufficient reliable information available about the safety of mouse ear.
Pregnancy and Lactation: Insufficient reliable information available; avoid using.

Effectiveness
There is insufficient reliable information available about the effectiveness of mouse ear.

Mechanism of Action
The applicable parts of mouse ear are the above ground flowering plant parts. There is insufficient reliable information available about the possible mechanism of action and active ingredients.

Adverse Reactions
Mouse ear can cause an allergic reaction in individuals sensitive to the Asteraceae/Compositae family. Members of this family include ragweed, chrysanthemums, marigolds, daisies, and many other herbs.

Interactions with Herbs & Other Dietary Supplements
None known.

Interactions with Drugs
None known.

Interactions with Foods
None known.

Interactions with Lab Tests
None known.

Interactions with Diseases or Conditions
CROSS-ALLERGENICITY: Can cause an allergic reaction in individuals sensitive to the Asteraceae/Compositae family. Members of this family include ragweed, chrysanthemums, marigolds, daisies, and many other herbs.

Dosage and Administration
ORAL: Mouse ear is used as a liquid extract (18).
TOPICAL: It is used as a liquid extract (18).

MSM (METHYLSULFONYLMETHANE)

Also Known As
Crystalline DMSO, Dimethyl Sulfone, DMSO2, Methyl-Sulfonyl-Methane, Methyl Sulfone, MSM, Sulfonyl Sulfur.

Scientific Names
Methylsulfonylmethane; Dimethylsulfone.

People Use This For
Orally and topically, MSM is used for chronic pain, arthritis, joint inflammation, rheumatoid arthritis, osteoporosis, bursitis, tendinitis, tenosynovitis, musculoskeletal pain, muscle cramps, scleroderma, scar tissue, stretch marks, wrinkles, protection against sun/wind burn, eye inflammation, oral hygiene, periodontal disease, wounds, cuts, and abrasions/accelerated wound healing. Orally, MSM is also used for relief of allergies (allergic rhinitis, allergic sinusitis, allergy-induced asthma, inhalant allergens, environmental allergens), drug hypersensitivity, gastrointestinal upset, chronic constipation, gastric hyperacidity, ulcers, diverticulosis, premenstrual syndrome (PMS), mood elevation, obesity, poor circulation, hypertension, and elevated serum cholesterol. It is also used orally for diabetes mellitus type 2 (NIDDM), interstitial cystitis, hepatic dysfunction, Alzheimer's disease, snoring, lung dysfunction including emphysema and pneumonia, chronic fatigue syndrome, auto-immune disorders (systemic lupus erythematous), HIV infection and AIDS, and cancer (breast cancer and colon cancer). Other oral uses of MSM include eye inflammation, mucous membrane inflammation, myositis ossificans generalis, temporomandibular joint dysfunction, leg cramps, connective tissue disorders, migraine, headaches, hangover, parasitic infections of the intestinal and urogenital tracts including Trichomonas vaginalis and Giardia, Candida albicans and other yeast infections, insect bites, radiation poisoning, and as an immunostimulant.

Safety
POSSIBLY SAFE ...when used orally and appropriately short-term. MSM 2600 mg per day has been used safely for up to 30 days (8574).
There is insufficient reliable information available about the safety of topical use of MSM.
PREGNANCY AND LACTATION: Insufficient reliable information available; avoid using.

Effectiveness
INSUFFICIENT RELIABLE EVIDENCE to RATE

Allergic rhinitis (hayfever). Preliminary clinical evidence suggests MSM given orally might relieve some symptoms of seasonal allergic rhinitis (8574). However, this study has been criticized for lack of information on pollen counts and severity of symptoms (12000).

Osteoarthritis. Preliminary clinical research suggests that MSM taken orally alone or in combination with glucosamine might reduce osteoarthritis symptoms. The study, which lasted only 12 weeks, suggests that MSM might reduce pain and swelling, and improve joint function (12469).

More evidence is needed to rate MSM for these uses.

Mechanism of Action
MSM is a naturally occurring compound found in green plants such as field horsetail (Equisetum arvense), certain species of algae, fruits, vegetables, grains, and both bovine and human adrenal glands, milk, and urine (8574). It is an

odorless metabolite of dimethyl sulfoxide (DMSO) (10625). MSM is a source of sulfur for cysteine and methionine. Incorporation of MSM-derived sulfur into methionine is regulated by a limiting step involving micro-organisms in the intestinal lumen (3501). Supplemental MSM crosses the blood-brain barrier (12351).

Preliminary research suggests MSM might inhibit degenerative changes in arthritis (8576). MSM delays chemically-induced colon cancer tumor onset in animals (3502). A 4% MSM solution delays the latency period between induction and onset of chemically-induced mammary tumors or cancers in rats (3503). MSM does not affect expression of autoimmune diabetes in spontaneously diabetic mice (3504).

There is little reliable clinical research on the use of MSM in humans.

Adverse Reactions

Orally, MSM can cause nausea, diarrhea, and headache in some patients. It can also cause pruritus and increased allergy symptoms (8574).

Interactions with Herbs & Other Dietary Supplements

None known.

Interactions with Drugs

None known.

Interactions with Foods

None known.

Interactions with Lab Tests

None known.

Interactions with Diseases or Conditions

None known.

Dosage and Administration

ORAL: For allergic rhinitis, 2600 mg per day has been used (8574).

TOPICAL: No typical dosage.

Comments

MSM has been popularized by the book, The Miracle of MSM: The Natural Solution for Pain (8575). There is little published scientific research to support its use. Contrary to some MSM promotional literature, there is no Recommended Dietary Allowance (RDA) for sulfur or MSM. Sulfur deficiency has not been described in the medical literature. Directions for compounding MSM nose drops for snoring have been published, but there's no evidence that MSM has any effect on snoring (8577).

MUGWORT

Also Known As

Armoise Commune, Artemisia, Artemisiae vulgaris herba, Artemisiae vulgaris radix, Carline Thistle, Felon Herb, Gemeiner Beifuss, Hierba de San Juan, Nagadamni, Sailor's Tobacco, St. John's Plant, Wild Wormwood.

CAUTION: See separate listings for Tarragon, Wormseed, and Wormwood.

Scientific Names

Artemisia vulgaris.

Family: Asteraceae/Compositae.

People Use This For

Orally, mugwort above ground parts are used for gastrointestinal (GI) problems such as colic, diarrhea, constipation, cramps, weak digestion, worm infestations, and persistent vomiting. It is also used to stimulate gastric juice and bile secretion, as a laxative in cases of obesity, as a liver tonic; and for hysteria, epilepsy, convulsions in children, menstrual problems, irregular periods, to promote circulation, and as a sedative.

Orally, mugwort root is used as a tonic in individuals with diminished strength and energy.

In combination with other ingredients, mugwort root is used for psychoneuroses, neurasthenia, depression, hypochondria, autonomic neuroses, general irritability, restlessness, insomnia, and anxiety.

Safety

There is insufficient reliable information available about the safety of mugwort.

PREGNANCY: LIKELY UNSAFE ...when used orally. Mugwort is said to be an abortifacient and a menstrual and uterine stimulant (2,12).

LACTATION: Insufficient reliable information available; avoid using.

Effectiveness
There is insufficient reliable information available about the effectiveness of mugwort.

Mechanism of Action
The applicable parts of mugwort are the above ground parts and root. Mugwort contains sesquiterpene lactones, lipophilic flavonoids, polyenes, umbelliferone and aesculetin. It also contains a complex volatile oil with constituents of 1,8 cineole, camphor, linalool or thujone (18). Some evidence suggests mugwort can stimulate uterine activity (19), possibly due to the thujone content (19). Other evidence suggests the aqueous extract and the volatile oil have antimicrobial properties (18).

Adverse Reactions
Orally, mugwort may cause an allergic reaction in individuals sensitive to the Asteraceae/Compositae family. Members of this family include ragweed, chrysanthemums, marigolds, daisies, and many other herbs.
Mugwort is also more likely to cause an allergic reaction in people who are sensitive to birch, celery, or wild carrot. This has been called the "celery-carrot-mugwort-spice syndrome" (12192).
Mugwort pollen may cause reactions in people who are allergic to tobacco (3716). Theoretically, mugwort might cause allergic reaction in people allergic to honey or royal jelly (3717).

Interactions with Herbs & Other Dietary Supplements
None known.

Interactions with Drugs
None known.

Interactions with Foods
None known.

Interactions with Lab Tests
None known.

Interactions with Diseases or Conditions
CROSS-ALLERGENICITY: Mugwort may cause an allergic reaction in individuals sensitive to the Asteraceae/Compositae family. Members of this family include ragweed, chrysanthemums, marigolds, daisies, and many other herbs. Mugwort might also cause an allergic reaction in people who are sensitive to birch, celery, or wild carrot. This has been called the "celery-carrot-mugwort-spice syndrome" (12192). Theoretically, mugwort might cause allergic reactions in individuals with allergies to honey or royal jelly (3717). Mugwort pollen might cause reactions in people allergic to tobacco (3716).

Dosage and Administration
ORAL: People use 5 mL of mugwort tincture 30 minutes before bedtime or 1-4 mL of the tincture up to three times daily (6002). Some people use 10 to 25 drops of the tincture, 1:5, 50% alcohol (5013). Two to three cups of tea is taken daily before meals (6002). The tea is prepared by steeping 15 grams of the dried herb in 500 mL of boiling water and straining (6002).

Comments
Mugwort has a pleasant, tangy taste. The plant is indigenous to Asia, North America, and Northern Europe (18).

MUIRA PUAMA

Also Known As
Muira-Puama, Muirapuama, Potency Wood, Ptychopetali lignum.

Scientific Names
Ptychopetalum olacoides; Ptychopetalum uncinatum.
Family: Olacaceae.

People Use This For
Orally, muira puama is used for preventing sexual disorders, and as an aphrodisiac. It is also used orally as a nerve stimulant, for dyspepsia, menstrual irregularities, rheumatism, paralysis caused by poliomyelitis, a general tonic, and as an appetite stimulant.
Topically, it is used as an aphrodisiac, for rheumatism, and muscle paralysis.
In combination with other herbs, muira puama is used as a remedy for sexual impotence.

Safety
There is insufficient reliable information available about the safety of muira puama.
Pregnancy and Lactation: Insufficient reliable information available; avoid using.

Effectiveness
There is insufficient reliable information available about the effectiveness of muira puama.

Mechanism of Action
The applicable parts of muira puama are the wood and root. No constituents in muira puama are known to exhibit any pronounced physiological activity (5).

Adverse Reactions
None reported.

Interactions with Herbs & Other Dietary Supplements
None known.

Interactions with Drugs
None known.

Interactions with Foods
None known.

Interactions with Lab Tests
None known.

Interactions with Diseases or Conditions
None known.

Dosage and Administration
ORAL: People typically use 1 to 2 mL of the muira puama extract in water two to three times daily. The number of drops recommended varies among products. The labeling on one product says one dropperful equals 1 mL and contains 500 mg muira puama. Other products do not specify the concentration of the active ingredient. Shake well before using; contains alcohol (6006).
TOPICAL: No typical dosage.

Comments
Previously, Liriosma ovata and Acanthea virilis were each thought to be the source of muira puama. They continue to be sold as muira puama in the herb trade (5).

MULLEIN

Also Known As
Aaron's Rod, Adam's Flannel, American Mullein, Beggar's Blanket, Blanket Herb, Blanket Leaf, Bouillon Blanc, Candleflower, Candlewick, Clot-Bur, Clown's Lungwort, Cuddy's Lungs, Duffle, European Mullein, Feltwort, Flannelflower, Fluffweed, Hag's Taper, Hare's Beard, Hedge Taper, Higtaper, Jacob's Staff, Longwort, Orange Mullein, Our Lady's Flannel, Rag Paper, Shepherd's Club, Shepherd's Staff, Torch Weed, Torches, Velvet Plant, Verbasci flos, Wild Ice Leaf, Woolen, Wooly Mullein.

Scientific Names
Verbascum densiflorum; Verbascum phlomides; Verbascum thapiforme; Verbascum thapsus.
Family: Scrophulariaceae.

People Use This For
Orally, mullein is used for respiratory tract mucous membrane inflammation, cough, whooping cough, tuberculosis, bronchitis, hoarseness, pneumonia, earaches, colds, chills and flu, fever, allergies, tonsillitis, and tracheitis. Other uses include asthma, diarrhea, colic, gastrointestinal bleeding, migraines, and gout. It is also used as a sedative, narcotic, diuretic, and antirheumatic. The root is used for croup.
Topically, mullein is used for wounds, burns, hemorrhoids, bruises, frostbite, erysipelas, and inflamed mucosa. The leaves are used topically to soften and protect the skin.
In manufacturing, mullein is used as a flavoring component in alcoholic beverages.

Safety
There is insufficient reliable information available about the safety of mullein.
Pregnancy and Lactation: Insufficient reliable information available; avoid using.

Effectiveness
There is insufficient reliable information available about the effectiveness of mullein.

Mechanism of Action
The applicable parts of mullein are the flower, leaf, and root. Mullein contains harpagoside, harpagide, aucubin, hesperidin, verbascoside, saponins, and volatile oils (12703). Preliminary research suggests that a flower extract may have activity against influenza and herpes simplex viruses (1534). Other preliminary research suggests that a leaf extract might have activity against herpes simplex virus type 1 (12702). Leaf extracts might also have antibacterial activity against Klebsiella pneumonia, Staphylococcus aureus, Staphylococcus epidermidis, and Escherichia coli. It might also have antitumor effects. Preliminary research suggests it might be toxic in excessive doses (12703).

Adverse Reactions
None reported.

Interactions with Herbs & Other Dietary Supplements
None known.

Interactions with Drugs
None known.

Interactions with Foods
None known.

Interactions with Lab Tests
None known.

Interactions with Diseases or Conditions
None known.

Dosage and Administration
No typical dosage.

Comments
Avoid confusion with goldenrod (Solidago species), also known as Aaron's rod. There is confusion as to which Verbascum species are associated with the name American mullein and which are associated with the name European mullein.

MUSK

Also Known As
Deer Musk, Tonquin Musk.

Scientific Names
Moschus moschiferus (Musk Deer).
Family: Moschidae.

Comments
At the date of publication, there was very little scientific information available about this product. Our staff is continually analyzing the available information on natural medicines and will add data to the online version of *Natural Medicines Comprehensive Database* as it becomes available. See www.naturaldatabase.com.

MYRRH

Also Known As
Abyssinian Myrrh, African Myrrh, Arabian Myrrh, Bal, Balsamodendron Myrrha, Bdellium, Bol, Bola, Commiphora, Didin, Didthin, Gum Myrrh, Heerabol, Opopanax, Somalien Myrrh, Yemen Myrrh.

Scientific Names
Commiphora myrrha, synonyms Commiphora molmol, Balsamodendrum myrrha; Commiphora habessinica, synonyms Commiphora abyssinica, Balsamodendrum habessinicum; Commiphora madagascariensis; Commiphora kataf, synonyms Commiphora erythraea, Amyris kataf, Hemprichia erythraea; other Commiphora species.
Family: Burseraceae.

People Use This For
Orally, myrrh is used for indigestion, ulcers, colds, cough, asthma, bronchial congestion, arthritic pain, cancer, leprosy, and syphilis. It is also used orally as a stimulant, antispasmodic, and to increase menstrual flow.
Topically, myrrh is used for mild inflammation of the oral and pharyngeal mucosa, aphthous ulcers, gingivitis, chapped lips, hemorrhoids, bedsores, wounds, abrasions, furunculosis, bad breath, and loose teeth.
In foods and beverages, myrrh is used as a flavoring component.
In manufacturing, myrrh is used as a fragrance and fixative in cosmetics.
It is also used in embalming and as incense.

Safety
LIKELY SAFE ...when consumed in amounts commonly found in food (11). Myrrh is approved for use in foods in the US (11).
POSSIBLY SAFE ...when used orally and appropriately (12). ...when used topically and appropriately (2,4,5,11,18).
POSSIBLY UNSAFE ...when used orally in excessive doses (12).
PREGNANCY: LIKELY UNSAFE ...when used orally because myrrh stimulates uterine tone and blood flow, and possibly has an abortifacient effect (4,12,19). There is insufficient reliable information available about the safety of the topical use of myrrh during pregnancy.
LACTATION: Insufficient reliable information available; avoid using.

Effectiveness
There is insufficient reliable information available about the effectiveness of myrrh.

Mechanism of Action
The applicable part of myrrh is resin. Myrrh resin contains a volatile oil and mucilage that have antimicrobial (4,6), deodorizing (8), anti-inflammatory (4,8), antitumor (1536), and astringent effects (4,6). In animals, it exhibits antipyretic and hypoglycemic effects (4), as well as protects against the development of gastric ulcers (1535). Myrrh can stimulate smooth muscle (6,12) and possibly peristalsis (6). It stimulates uterine tone (6,12) and promotes uterine blood flow (12,19).

Adverse Reactions
Topically, dermatitis has been reported with the use of myrrh (6).
Orally, amounts greater than 2-4 grams can cause kidney irritation and diarrhea (12). Large amounts can affect the heart rate (19).

Interactions with Herbs & Other Dietary Supplements
None known.

Interactions with Drugs
ANTIDIABETES DRUGS: Myrrh extract might interfere with diabetic therapy due to hypoglycemic effects (4).

Interactions with Foods
None known.

Interactions with Lab Tests
BLOOD GLUCOSE: Theoretically, myrrh can lower blood glucose and test results.

Interactions with Diseases or Conditions
DIABETES: Theoretically, myrrh can interfere with diabetes therapy (4).
HEART CONDITIONS: Use myrrh with caution in individuals with heart conditions, because large amounts can affect the heart rate (19).
OTHER: Use myrrh with caution because it can exacerbate uterine bleeding (12,19), fever, and systemic inflammation (19).

Dosage and Administration

TOPICAL: For mild mouth and throat irritation, dab the undiluted tincture of myrrh on affected areas two to three times daily. Myrrh is also commonly used as a rinse or gargle with 5-10 drops in a glass of water (2,8). A typical mouthwash can contain 30-60 drops in a glass of water also (8). The tooth powder contains 10% powdered resin (2,18).

Comments

Myrrh is the oleo-gum resin exuded from fissures or cuts in the bark of Commiphora species trees. Commiphora mukul, a related species, is not a source of myrrh (8).

MYRTLE

Also Known As

Myrti aetherolum, Myrti folium.

Scientific Names

Myrtus communis.
Family: Myrtaceae.

People Use This For

Orally, myrtle is used for treating acute and chronic respiratory infections including bronchitis, whooping cough, tuberculosis, bladder conditions, diarrhea, and worm infestation.

Safety

LIKELY UNSAFE ...when the undiluted oil is used orally because it contains cineole. Ingesting more than 10 grams of cineole can result in respiratory failure and collapse (18).
There is insufficient reliable information available about the safety of myrtle leaf and branch.
CHILDREN: LIKELY UNSAFE ...when used orally. Avoid facial contact with myrtle oil preparations which may cause glottal spasm, bronchospasm, asthma-like attacks, or respiratory failure in infants or small children (18).
PREGNANCY AND LACTATION: LIKELY UNSAFE ...when used orally (18); avoid using.

Effectiveness

There is insufficient reliable information available about the effectiveness of myrtle.

Mechanism of Action

The applicable parts of myrtle are the leaf and branch. Myrtle contains a volatile oil, tannins, and acylphloroglucinols. Myrtol, a volatile oil, stimulates mucous membranes of the stomach and deodorizes the breath. It might also have fungicidal, disinfectant, and antibacterial properties (18). The volatile oil contains between 15-45% of 1,8-cineole, a constituent responsible for toxicity (18).

Adverse Reactions

Orally, myrtle can cause nausea, vomiting, and diarrhea (18). Consumption of large amounts might lead to low blood pressure, circulatory disorders, respiratory failure, and collapse (18).
Topically, facial contact with myrtle oil preparations may cause glottal or bronchial spasm, asthma-like attacks, or respiratory failure in infants and children (18).

Interactions with Herbs & Other Dietary Supplements

None known.

Interactions with Drugs

None known.

Interactions with Foods

None known.

Interactions with Lab Tests

None known.

Interactions with Diseases or Conditions

None known.

Dosage and Administration

ORAL: A typical dose is 200 mg one time only (18).

Comments
Myrtle leaves resemble the leaves of Bux semper-virens and Vaccinium vitisidaea (18).

N-ACETYL CYSTEINE

Also Known As
Acetylcysteine, L-Cysteine, NAC, N-Acetyl L-Cysteine, N-Acetyl-B-Cysteine, N-Acetylcysteine, N-Acetyl-Cysteine.

Scientific Names
N-acetyl-L-cysteine.

People Use This For
Orally, N-acetyl cysteine is used as an antidote for acetaminophen and carbon monoxide poisoning. It is also used for unstable angina, common bile duct obstruction in infants, lysosomal storage disorders, amyotrophic lateral sclerosis (ALS, Lou Gehrig's disease), Alzheimer's disease, phenytoin-induced hypersensitivity, and keratoconjunctivitis. It is also used for reducing lipoprotein (a) levels, reducing homocysteine levels, reducing risk of cardiovascular events in patients with end-stage renal disease, chronic bronchitis, chronic obstructive pulmonary disease (COPD), allergic rhinitis, fibrosing alveolitis, head and neck cancer, and lung cancer. N-acetyl cysteine is also used orally for myoclonus epilepsy; otitis media; hemodialysis-related pseudoporphyria; Sjogren's syndrome; preventing sports injury complications; radiation therapy; increasing immunity to flu; and for detoxifying heavy metals such as mercury, lead, and cadmium. It is also used orally for preventing alcoholic liver damage; for protecting against environmental pollutants including carbon monoxide, chloroform, urethanes and certain herbicides; for reducing toxicity of ifosfamide and doxorubicin; as a hangover remedy; for preventing nonionic low-osmolality contrast agent-induced reduction of renal function in patients with renal insufficiency; and for human immunodeficiency virus (HIV).

Topically, N-acetyl cysteine is used for reducing dental plaque.

Intravenously, N-acetyl cysteine is used for acetaminophen overdose, acrylonitrile poisoning, amyotrophic lateral sclerosis (ALS, Lou Gehrig's disease), for hepatorenal syndrome, for decreasing mortality rate due to multisystem organ failure, for unstable angina in combination with nitroglycerin, and for acute myocardial infarction with nitroglycerin and streptokinase.

Rectally, N-acetyl cysteine is used for meconium ileus and meconium ileus equivalent.

By inhalation or intratracheal installation, N-acetyl cysteine is used as a mucolytic agent in acute and chronic lung disorders such as pneumonia, bronchitis, emphysema, cystic fibrosis, and others.

Safety
LIKELY SAFE ...when used orally, intravenously, intratracheally, by inhalation, and appropriately. N-acetyl cysteine is an FDA-approved prescription drug (832,1539,1705,1710,2245,2246,2252,2253,2254,2256,2258,2259,2260) (5808,6176,6611,7868,10270,10271).

PREGNANCY: POSSIBLY SAFE ...when used orally, intratracheally, or by inhalation. N-acetyl cysteine crosses the placenta, but has not been associated with adverse effects to the fetus or mothers (1711). However, N-acetyl cysteine should only be used in pregnant women when clearly indicated, such as in cases of acetaminophen toxicity.

LACTATION: Insufficient reliable information available; avoid using.

Effectiveness
EFFECTIVE

Acetaminophen poisoning. Administering N-acetyl cysteine orally or intravenously is equally effective in decreasing mortality rate and preventing the permanent sequelae of acetaminophen poisoning (17).

Atelectasis. N-acetyl cysteine is helpful for atelectasis caused by mucus obstruction (15).

Bronchial diagnostic studies. N-acetyl cysteine is helpful when used for preparing people for bronchial diagnostic studies (15).

Bronchopulmonary disorders. Administering N-acetyl cysteine by inhalation is effective as a mucolytic for adjunctive treatment of acute and chronic bronchopulmonary disorders (15).

Cystic fibrosis. N-acetyl cysteine is effective for cystic fibrosis (15).

Tracheostomy care. N-acetyl cysteine is effective when used as an adjunct for preventing endotracheal crusting in tracheostomy care (15).

POSSIBLY EFFECTIVE

Angina. Administering N-acetyl cysteine orally or intravenously seems to improve unstable angina pectoris in combination with nitroglycerin (2245,2246). Concurrent intravenous administration of N-acetyl cysteine also seems to reduce development of nitroglycerin tolerance (832,2245). However, severe headache can occur when N-acetyl cysteine and nitroglycerin are administered together and may limit feasibility of concomitant use (2245).

Bronchitis. Taking N-acetyl cysteine orally seems to reduce the risk of acute exacerbations of chronic bronchitis when used over a three to six month period (6176).

Chronic obstructive pulmonary disease (COPD). In patients with moderate to severe COPD, taking N-acetyl cysteine orally can decrease the number of acute exacerbations by about 40% when used in addition to standard therapy (10429).

Contrast agent-induced nephropathy. Taking N-acetyl cysteine orally seems to prevent nonionic low-osmolality contrast agent-induced nephropathy in patients with renal insufficiency. Oral N-acetyl cysteine, with hydration with intravenous saline, seems to prevent acute renal damage in patients with chronic renal insufficiency (serum creatinine greater than 2.4 mg/dL) receiving iopromide (Ultravist-300) administration for elective computed tomography (CT) or coronary angiography (6611,10428). However, in patients with reduced renal function (serum creatinine greater than 1.2 ml/dL, but less than 2.4 ml/dL), oral N-acetyl cysteine doesn't seem to reduce the risk of contrast agent-induced renal damage after coronary angiography (11430).

End-stage renal disease (ESRD). Taking N-acetyl cysteine orally seems to reduce the incidence of cardiovascular events such as ischemic stroke and myocardial infarction by about 40% in patients with ESRD. However, the risk of total mortality or mortality from cardiovascular causes is not decreased (10430).

Epilepsy. Taking N-acetyl cysteine orally seems to be helpful for treating myoclonus epilepsy (2259).

Fibrosing alveolitis. Taking N-acetyl cysteine orally seems to improve pulmonary function tests and decrease biochemical markers of disease in patients with fibrosing alveolitis (7868).

Hyperhomocysteinemia. Taking N-acetyl cysteine orally seems to reduce homocysteine levels (2256,2258).

Ifosfamide (Ifex) toxicity. Taking N-acetyl cysteine orally seems to reduce ifosfamide-induced bladder toxicity (5808,10270). However, mesna (Mesnex) seems to be more effective for preventing ifosfamide toxicity than N-acetyl cysteine (10748).

Influenza. Taking N-acetyl cysteine orally seems to reduce symptoms of influenza (2260).

POSSIBLY INEFFECTIVE

Amyotrophic lateral sclerosis (ALS, Lou Gehrig's disease). Administering N-acetyl cysteine intravenously doesn't seem to improve symptoms of ALS (2254).

Doxorubicin-induced cardiac toxicity. Taking N-acetyl cysteine orally doesn't seem to prevent or reverse doxorubicin-induced cardiac toxicity (2252,2253).

LIKELY INEFFECTIVE

Alzheimer's disease. Taking N-acetyl cysteine orally doesn't improve symptoms of Alzheimer's disease (7870).

Head and neck cancer or lung cancer. Taking N-acetyl cysteine orally in patients with head and neck cancer or lung cancer doesn't prevent second primary tumors (1710). N-acetyl cysteine alone, or in combination with retinyl palmitate, has no effect on mortality or event-free survival in patients with head and neck cancer or lung cancer (1705,1710).

Multisystem organ failure. Administering N-acetyl cysteine intravenously, greater than 24 hours after hospital admission, might increase mortality rate due to multisystem organ failure. The effect of N-acetyl cysteine given within 24 hours of hospital admission requires further study (7871).

Nitrate tolerance. Taking N-acetyl cysteine orally doesn't reduce nitroglycerin tolerance (2281,2282).

INSUFFICIENT RELIABLE EVIDENCE to RATE

Colorectal cancer. Oral N-acetyl cysteine may reduce the likelihood of colorectal cancer in patients with a history of adenomatous colon polyps (7873).

Hepatorenal syndrome. There is some preliminary clinical evidence that intravenous N-acetyl cysteine might improve renal function in hepatorenal syndrome (1752).

Lamellar ichthyosis. There is some evidence that topical N-acetyl cysteine might be useful for lamellar ichthyosis, a congenital skin disease (3974,3975).

Myocardial infarction (MI). Early evidence shows that intravenous N-acetyl cysteine, when given with nitroglycerin and streptokinase, in patients with evolving MI, may preserve left ventricular function and reduce oxidative stress (7872).

More evidence is needed to rate N-acetyl cysteine for these uses.

Mechanism of Action

N-acetyl cysteine is the N-acetyl derivative of the amino acid L-cysteine (1705). N-acetyl cysteine is a precursor of glutathione, which is a potent antioxidant. Glutathione can not cross the cell membrane, but N-acetyl cysteine easily crosses the cell membrane where it is converted to cysteine and, subsequently, glutathione. Reactive oxygen species (ROS) such as hydrogen peroxide and hydroxyl-free radicals reduce intracellular and extracellular concentrations of glutathione. N-acetyl cysteine is a very efficient way to replenish glutathione and reduce damage caused by ROS (7874,1761).

The antioxidant effects of N-acetyl cysteine may explain its apparent ability to prevent adverse effects caused by toxic chemicals, drug reactions, and nonionic low-osmolality contrast agents (1762,6611). The antioxidant and free radical properties might also make N-acetyl cysteine useful in the treatment of pulmonary and cardiac disease (1705,1765). N-acetyl cysteine also appears to reduce cellular production of pro-inflammatory mediators such as tumor necrosis factor-alpha, TNF-alpha, and interleukin 1, IL-1 (1763).

N-acetyl cysteine is effective for acetaminophen hepatotoxicity because it restores glutathione levels in the liver and acts as an alternative substrate for conjugation of toxic acetaminophen metabolites (15). N-acetyl cysteine might be helpful in the congenital skin disease lamellar ichthyosis due to antiproliferative effects on skin cells (3975).

N-acetyl cysteine may also have anticarcinogenic properties by inhibiting the invasive activity of tumor cells and

angiogenesis of tumor cells (1767).
N-acetyl cysteine might decrease bladder toxicity caused by ifosfamide. The exact mechanism is not understood, but it probably involves binding of the thiol-sulfhydryl groups in N-acetyl cysteine to ifosfamide and its metabolite acrolein. N-acetyl cysteine does not appear to affect the anticancer activity of ifosfamide (10269,10268).
Preliminary evidence indicates that N-acetyl cysteine can impair platelet aggregation. N-acetyl cysteine appears to increase synthesis of nitric oxide, a potent inhibitor of platelet function (10272).
In patients with human immunodeficiency virus (HIV) disease, N-acetyl cysteine can increase levels of glutathione. Increased concentration of glutathione seems to reduce oxidative stress associated with HIV disease and to improve the number and activity of CD4 T-lymphocytes (1539).
Assessing the pharmacokinetics of N-acetyl cysteine is difficult because it binds to cysteine and other sulfhydryl molecules. Because these compounds are widely available in tissues, N-acetyl cysteine is rapidly removed from plasma. After oral administration of N-acetyl cysteine, the time to maximum plasma concentration (Tmax) is approximately 0.72 hours. With a dose of 250 mg/m2, the maximum plasma concentration (Cmax) is about 1.75 mcg/mL. The half life (T1/2) of N-acetyl cysteine is about 2 hours (10268).

Adverse Reactions

Orally, N-acetyl cysteine can cause gastrointestinal adverse effects including nausea, abdominal pain, vomiting, constipation, and diarrhea, particularly when used in high doses (1539,10270,10271,11430). N-acetyl cysteine has an unpleasant odor that sometimes makes it difficult for patients to take orally. Using a straw to drink N-acetyl cysteine solutions can improve tolerability (17). In some cases, placement of a nasogastric or duodenal tube and administration of metoclopramide or ondansetron can also be helpful for patients unable to tolerate oral N-acetyl cysteine (17).
Rarely, generalized urticaria with mild fever, sulfhemoglobinemia, headache, hypotension, rash, and hepatotoxicity has occurred (17).
Intravenously, N-acetyl cysteine can sometimes cause allergic reactions including anaphylactoid reactions (1716). For less severe allergic reactions, diphenhydramine can be administered and the N-acetyl cysteine infusion can be continued. For more severe reactions (e.g., angioedema, respiratory symptoms), the infusion should be temporarily discontinued and resumed an hour after diphenhydramine administration (1716).
By inhalation, N-acetyl cysteine has been associated with stomatitis, nausea, vomiting, drowsiness, clamminess, and severe rhinorrhea (15). Fever, chills, chest tightness, and bronchoconstriction have been reported rarely (15).
Sensitization and dermal eruptions have also been reported. However, sensitization has not been confirmed by patch testing (15).
In cases of N-acetyl cysteine overdose, symptoms typically resemble a severe anaphylactoid reaction (17).

Interactions with Herbs & Other Dietary Supplements

None known.

Interactions with Drugs

ACTIVATED CHARCOAL: N-acetyl cysteine appears to reduce the capacity of charcoal to adsorb acetaminophen and salicylic acid (7869). But concomitant use of activated charcoal does not seem to reduce the effectiveness of N-acetyl cysteine (1755).
NITROGLYCERIN: Concomitant administration of N-acetyl cysteine and intravenous nitroglycerin can cause severe hypotension (2246) and intolerable headaches (2245,2280).

Interactions with Foods

None known.

Interactions with Lab Tests

BLOOD PRESSURE: Concomitant administration of intravenous NAC and nitroglycerin can lower blood pressure and reduce blood pressure readings (2246).
CHLORIDE: NAC can cause false-positive serum chloride test results measured with the Beckman Synchron CX3 analyzer (275).
CREATININE: Intravenous NAC can cause falsely low serum creatinine test results when measured by single-slide method on Kodak Ektachem systems (275).
CYSTEINE (FREE): Intravenous NAC can increase free cysteine plasma concentrations and test results (275).
GOLD: Intravenous NAC can increase urinary gold excretion (concentration) and test results in patients previously given gold (275).
KETONES: NAC can cause false-positive urine ketone test results when measured with Chemstrips (Boehringer Mannheim) or Multistix (Miles) (275).
LIPOPROTEIN A: Used orally, NAC might reduce serum lipoprotein A concentrations and test results in some patients (275).
LITHIUM: Very high serum NAC concentrations might cause falsely low serum lithium test results when measured with Kodak Ektachem systems (275).
LIVER FUNCTION TESTS: NAC might increase liver enzyme (AST, ALT) concentrations and test results. Liver function tests were markedly elevated on two occasions in a child with cystic fibrosis after receiving large NAC doses by rectal and naso-gastric tube administration (15).

PROTHROMBIN TIME (PT): Intravenous NAC can decrease PT and test results (1341).
SALICYLATE: Serum NAC concentrations of 50 mg/dL (occurring with intravenous NAC administration) can cause falsely low serum salicylate test results when measured with Kodak Ektachem systems. Serum NAC concentrations of 10 mg/dL (occurring with oral NAC administration) do not interfere with serum salicylate results measured with Kodak Ektachem systems (275).

Interactions with Diseases or Conditions

ALLERGY: Contraindicated in individuals with acetylcysteine allergy (15).
ASTHMA: Oral NAC inhalation or intratracheal administration might cause bronchospasm, monitor closely (15).
HEMODIALYSIS-ASSOCIATED PSEUDOPORPHYRIA: NAC might improve pseudoporphyria skin lesions associated with hemodialysis. Two cases are reported in which pseudoporphyria skin lesions healed with oral NAC administration in patients on chronic hemodialysis (5052).

Dosage and Administration

ORAL: For acetaminophen overdose, an oral loading dose of 140 mg/kg of a 5% solution should be administered. The commercially available 10% and 20% solutions may be diluted with water, carbonated, or non-carbonated beverages, and administered through a straw to lessen the disagreeable odor of N-acetyl cysteine. Seventeen additional doses of 70 mg/kg as a 5% solution should be given every 4 hours, for a total dose of 1330 mg/kg over 72 hours (17). A typical dose for unstable angina is 600 mg three times daily with transdermal nitroglycerin (2245). For preventing acute exacerbations of chronic bronchitis, doses of 200 mg twice daily, 200 mg three times daily, 300 mg slow-release twice daily, and 600 mg controlled-release twice daily have been used (6176). For treating chronic obstructive pulmonary disease (COPD), N-acetyl cysteine 600 mg once daily, in addition to standard care, has been used for up to 6 months (10429). For treating fibrosing alveolitis, N-acetyl cysteine 600 mg 3 times daily has been used (7868). For prophylaxis of urinary bladder toxicity due to ifosfamide, 1 to 2 grams every 6 hours has been used (5808,10268,10269,10270,10271). For reducing plasma homocysteine levels, 1.2 grams daily has been used (2258). For myoclonus epilepsy, 4-6 grams daily has been used (2259). For reducing symptoms of influenza, 600 mg twice daily has been used (2260). For reducing the risk of cardiovascular events in patients with end-stage renal disease, 600 mg twice daily has been used (10430). For hemodialysis-associated pseudoporphyria skin lesions, 200 mg four times daily or 600 mg twice daily has been used (5052). For preventing iopromide (Ultravist-300)-induced reduction of renal function in patients with chronic renal insufficiency, 400 to 600 mg N-acetyl cysteine twice daily on the day before and on the day of iopromide administration, with IV saline (0.45%) 1 mL/kg body weight per hour for 12 hours before and 12 hours after iopromide administration, has been used (6611,10428). In Alzheimer's disease, N-acetyl cysteine 50 mg/kg/day has been used (7870).
INTRAVENOUS: There are 2 dosage regimens for intravenous N-acetyl cysteine. For patients presenting 10 to 24 hours after acetaminophen ingestion, particularly if large doses were taken, the following 48-hour regimen should be used (17). Administer a loading dose of 140 mg IV N-acetyl cysteine as a 3% solution over 1 hour. The 3% solution is prepared by diluting the 20% IV solution with 5% dextrose. Twelve additional doses of 70 mg/kg IV N-acetyl cysteine should be administered over 1 hour every 4 hours thereafter. The alternative 20-hour regimen consists of IV administration of 150 mg/kg N-acetyl cysteine in 200 ml of 5% dextrose solution, administered over 15 minutes. Follow this dose with 50 mg/kg N-acetyl cysteine in 500 mL 5% dextrose over 4 hours and 100 mg/kg in 1 liter 5% dextrose over 16 hours. The total dose is 300 mg/kg over 20 hours. This regimen is most effective if begun within 8 hours of acetaminophen ingestion (17). In evolving acute myocardial infarction (MI), N-acetyl cysteine 20 mg/minute for 1 hour followed by 10 mg/minute for 23 hours, for a total of 15 grams/24 hours, has been used. Intravenous nitroglycerin and streptokinase were also given (7872). For reducing mortality rate due to multisystem organ disease, N-acetyl cysteine 150 mg/kg bolus, followed by a continuous infusion of 12 mg/kg/hr for 3 to 5 days has been used; however, mortality rate was not significantly reduced (7871).

N-ACETYL GLUCOSAMINE

Also Known As

Acetylglucosamine, Glucosamine N-Acetyl, N-Acetyl D-Glucosamine, NAG, N-A-G, Poly-NAG.
CAUTION: See separate listings for Glucosamine Sulfate and Glucosamine Hydrochloride.

Scientific Names

2-acetamido-2-deoxyglucose.

People Use This For

Orally, N-acetyl glucosamine is used for osteoarthritis and inflammatory bowel disease (IBD), including ulcerative colitis and Crohn's disease.

Safety

There is insufficient reliable information available about the safety of N-acetyl glucosamine.
Pregnancy and Lactation: Insufficient reliable information available; avoid using.

Effectiveness

INSUFFICIENT RELIABLE EVIDENCE to RATE

Inflammatory bowel disease (IBD). There is preliminary evidence that oral or rectal N-acetyl glucosamine might decrease symptoms of IBD in children with Crohn's disease or ulcerative colitis (10234). More evidence is needed to rate N-acetyl glucosamine for this use.

Mechanism of Action

N-acetyl glucosamine is the acetylated derivative of the amino sugar glucosamine, which is a constituent of cartilage proteoglycans. It is derived from marine exoskeletons or produced synthetically. Glucosamine is required for the synthesis of glycoproteins, glycolipids, and glycosaminoglycans (also known as mucopolysaccharides); these carbohydrate-containing compounds are found in tendons, ligaments, cartilage, synovial fluid, mucous membranes, structures in the eye, blood vessels, and heart valves. Glucosamine is also a component of biologically active compounds such as heparin, but it does not react with heparin-induced thrombocytopenia (HIT) antibodies (7640,7641,11831). In osteoarthritis, glucosamine stimulates metabolism of chondrocytes in the articular cartilage and synovial cells in the synovial tissues. There is some evidence that suggests that glucosamine might have a disease-modifying effect, therefore stopping or slowing the progression of osteoarthritis (7026). Glucosamine doesn't seem to directly affect cyclooxygenase, which is responsible for anti-inflammatory and analgesic effects of nonsteroidal anti-inflammatory drugs (NSAIDs), as well as adverse gastrointestinal (GI) effects (2604). In inflammatory bowel disease (IBD), N-acetylation of glucosamine is relatively deficient, possibly reducing the synthesis of the gastric and intestinal mucosa's protective glycoprotein cover (2609). Theoretically, supplementation with N-acetyl glucosamine could remedy this deficiency and restore the glycoprotein cover (2609). However, there aren't any human studies that have evaluated this claim.

There has been a lot of concern about the effect of glucosamine on glucose metabolism. Preliminary evidence suggests that glucosamine might decrease glucose-induced insulin secretion by inhibiting pancreatic glucokinase in the beta cells of the islet of Langerhans (371,372,3406). Other preliminary research suggests that glucosamine might also impair insulin-mediated glucose uptake and metabolism in skeletal muscle (372,3406). Animal research suggests glucosamine might increase glucose metabolism through the hexosamine pathway, a pattern of change in glucose metabolism similar to that seen in type 2 diabetes (3405,3406). However, animals may handle glucosamine differently than humans. Most of the research in humans suggests that glucosamine doesn't affect the pharmacokinetics of glucose. Research in people with normal glucose metabolism suggests glucosamine doesn't affect insulin sensitivity or plasma glucose (7637,7638). Clinical research in people with type 2 diabetes and people without diabetes suggests glucosamine doesn't have any significant effect on blood glucose when given for up to 3 years (7026,8942,10311,10317). Preliminary clinical research suggests that endogenous glucosamine and insulin levels are elevated in nondiabetic patients with ischemic heart disease (7640,7641). Some researchers think that increased glucosamine production might contribute to endothelial cell dysfunction (8944). Glucosamine is absorbed 90% after oral administration. The bioavailability is approximately 26% after first pass metabolism (2608). Glucosamine is incorporated into plasma proteins during first-pass metabolism, and unbound glucosamine is concentrated in the articular cartilage (2608). Free glucosamine is undetectable in the plasma (2607).

Adverse Reactions

Orally, N-acetyl glucosamine might cause mild gastrointestinal (GI) problems, including nausea, heartburn, diarrhea, and constipation; similar to the effects seen with glucosamine sulfate. Drowsiness, skin reactions, and headaches have also been reported (2608). Anecdotal reports have associated glucosamine with renal toxicity, but changes in renal function have not been reported in long-term studies (7026,8942,10408,10409).

Elevated blood glucose levels in patients with diabetes have also been reported (22). Some research suggests that glucosamine sulfate can also increase insulin levels in non-diabetic people, but glucosamine doesn't seem to cause hyperglycemia or diabetes in otherwise healthy patients taking 1500 mg per day for three years. Also, glucosamine doesn't seem to cause any adverse effects on blood glucose metabolism, lipid metabolism, or any other disturbances in metabolism (3406,5059,7026,8942).

There is concern that use of N-acetyl glucosamine products derived from marine exoskeletons might cause reactions in people allergic to shellfish, although no reactions have been reported. Until more is known, and because the source of N-acetyl glucosamine products is not listed on product labels, use N-acetyl glucosamine with caution in people with shellfish allergy.

Interactions with Herbs & Other Dietary Supplements

None known.

Interactions with Drugs

ANTIDIABETES DRUGS: Preliminary research suggests that glucosamine might increase insulin resistance, or decrease insulin production, and potentially worsen diabetes control (371,372,3406,7637,7638). But there is some clinical evidence that suggests that taking glucosamine for 3 months does not increase hemoglobin A1c (HbA1c) in people with type 2 diabetes who have well-controlled glucose levels (10311,10317). Until more is known, advise patients with diabetes who take glucosamine to monitor their blood glucose levels closely. Some antidiabetes drugs include glimepiride (Amaryl), glyburide (DiaBeta, Glynase PresTab, Micronase), insulin, pioglitazone (Actos),

rosiglitazone (Avandia), and others.
CHEMOTHERAPY: Theoretically, glucosamine might induce resistance to etoposide (VP16, VePesid) and doxorubicin (Adriamycin) by reducing the drugs' inhibition of topoisomerase II, an enzyme required for DNA replication in tumor cells (7639).
WARFARIN (Coumadin): There's some concern that high-dose glucosamine (3000 mg per day), combined with high-dose chondroitin sulfate (2400 mg per day), may enhance the effects of warfarin (Coumadin) as measured by the INR (11389). Chondroitin is a small component of a heparinoid and might have weak anticoagulant activity. Glucosamine is also a small component of heparin, but is does not seem to have anticoagulant activity. It's not known if glucosamine contributes to this potential interaction. Interactions with warfarin have not been reported at recommended dosages of glucosamine or chondroitin.

Interactions with Foods

None known.

Interactions with Lab Tests

BLOOD GLUCOSE: Glucosamine doesn't seem to adversely affect blood glucose control in people with type 2 diabetes, as measured by hemoglobin A1C (10311,10317). It also doesn't seem to affect blood glucose in nondiabetic people older than 45 who have taken glucosamine for osteoarthritis for 3 years (7026,8942). Some preliminary research raised concerns that glucosamine might exacerbate diabetes by increasing insulin resistance and/or decreasing insulin production, resulting in elevated blood glucose levels (5059), but other research showed no effect (7637,7638). There are also anecdotal reports of reduced blood glucose control in people with diabetes who take glucosamine (22,1203,1204,3405,3406). However, clinical studies indicate that glucosamine has little or no effect on blood glucose (7026,8942,10311,10317).
INTERNATIONAL NORMALIZED RATIO (INR)/PROTHROMBIN TIME (PT): High dose glucosamine (3000 mg per day), combined with high dose chondroitin sulfate (2400 mg per day), may increase the INR in patients taking warfarin (Coumadin). There is one case report of an increased INR associated with concomitant use of warfarin a glucosamine-chondroitin supplement taken above recommended dosages (11389).

Interactions with Diseases or Conditions

ASTHMA: Glucosamine might exacerbate asthma by an unidentified mechanism. Use N-acetyl glucosamine cautiously in patients with asthma (10002).
DIABETES: Glucosamine doesn't seem to adversely affect blood glucose control in people with type 2 diabetes, as measured by hemoglobin A1C (10311,10317). Some preliminary research raised concerns that glucosamine might exacerbate diabetes by increasing insulin resistance and/or decreasing insulin production, resulting in elevated blood glucose levels (5059), but other research showed no effect on insulin sensitivity or plasma glucose (7637,7638). There are also anecdotal reports of reduced blood glucose control in people with diabetes who take glucosamine (22,1203,1204,3405,3406). However, clinical studies indicate that glucosamine seems to be safe in people with type 2 diabetes (10311,10317).
SHELLFISH ALLERGY: There is concern that glucosamine products might cause reactions in people who are sensitive to shellfish. Glucosamine is derived from the exoskeletons of shrimp, lobster, and crab. But allergic reactions in people with shellfish allergy are caused by IgE antibodies to antigens in the meat of shellfish, not to the antigens in the shell. There are no documented reports of allergic reaction to glucosamine in shellfish allergic patients. There is also some evidence that patients with shellfish allergy can safely take glucosamine products (12210).

Dosage and Administration

ORAL: For inflammatory bowel disease in children, N-acetyl glucosamine 3 to 6 grams per day in 3 divided doses has been used (10234).
RECTAL: For inflammatory bowel disease in children, N-acetyl glucosamine 3 to 4 grams per day in 2 divided doses has been used (10234).

Comments

Avoid confusion with glucosamine sulfate and glucosamine hydrochloride. Read glucosamine product labels carefully for their content. Although glucosamine sulfate and glucosamine hydrochloride are marketed together in combination products with N-acetyl glucosamine, there haven't been any human studies that have evaluated these combinations for treating osteoarthritis. Chitosan is the deacylated polymer of N-acetyl glucosamine.

NADH

Also Known As

B-DPNH, BNADH, Coenzyme 1, Enada, NAD, Reduced DPN, Reduced Nicotinamide Adenine Dinucleotide.

Scientific Names

Nicotinamide Adenine Dinucleotide Hydrate.

People Use This For

Orally, NADH is used for improving mental clarity, alertness, and concentration; improving memory; cellular energy; for antioxidant effects; chronic fatigue syndrome (CFS); depression; jet lag; hypertension; Alzheimer's disease; Parkinson's disease; improving athletic endurance; enhancing energy; improving DNA repair; enhancing immune function; reducing aging; protecting the liver from alcohol damage; preventing alcohol-induced inhibition of testosterone; lowering cholesterol levels; and protecting against zidovudine (AZT) toxicity.
Intravenously, NADH is used as an IM or IV injection for Parkinson's disease and depression.

Safety

POSSIBLY SAFE ...when used orally and appropriately (8267,8275). NADH is generally considered safe and has been used for up to 12 weeks without reports of side effects.
PREGNANCY AND LACTATION: Insufficient reliable information available; avoid using.

Effectiveness

POSSIBLY INEFFECTIVE

Dementia. Taking NADH orally seems to be ineffective for mild to moderate dementia of the Alzheimer's, vascular, or fronto-temporal type (8275). Dementia patients treated with 10 mg per day NADH had no significant improvement in memory, cognitive, and behavioral function scales after 12 weeks of treatment.

INSUFFICIENT RELIABLE EVIDENCE to RATE

Chronic fatigue syndrome (CFS). There is preliminary clinical evidence that NADH might reduce the symptoms of CFS when used as an adjunctive therapy to traditional medications (8267).

Parkinson's disease. There is conflicting preliminary research about the usefulness of NADH for Parkinson's disease (3086,3089,3090).

More evidence is needed to rate NADH for these uses.

Mechanism of Action

NADH is the reduced form of NAD (nicotinamide adenine dinucleotide), a coenzyme necessary to dehydrogenate primary and secondary alcohols (3082). In dehydrogenation, NAD acts as a hydrogen acceptor, forming NADH. NADH, in turn, serves as a hydrogen donor in the respiratory chain. NADH is an essential intermediate in the cellular processes that generate energy from glucose in the form of ATP. Some evidence suggests oral NADH reduces blood pressure, total cholesterol, and low-density lipoprotein (LDL) (3083). Preliminary evidence suggests that NADH might help people with chronic fatigue syndrome (CFS) by triggering energy production through ATP generation (8267). Preliminary research suggests that NADH might protect against age-related hypertension, possibly by lowering lipid peroxidation and free radical formation (8260). NADH has been proposed as a therapeutic agent for people with Parkinson's disease because evidence suggests it might increase tyrosine hydroxylase activity and dopamine production (3085,3086,3088,3091).

Adverse Reactions

None reported.

Interactions with Herbs & Other Dietary Supplements

None known.

Interactions with Drugs

None known.

Interactions with Foods

None known.

Interactions with Lab Tests

None known.

Interactions with Diseases or Conditions

None known.

Dosage and Administration

ORAL: For nutrition and energy enhancement, a typical dose is 2.5-5 mg daily or every other day (3462).
For therapeutic support of Alzheimer's disease (3462,8275), Parkinson's disease and chronic fatigue syndrome (CFS) (3462,8267), a typical dose is 10-15 mg daily or every other day. Some people recommend the disodium salt form of NADH, taken with water either 30 minutes before or two hours after meals (3462).

NASTURTIUM

Also Known As
Indian Cress.
CAUTION: See separate listing for Watercress.

Scientific Names
Tropaeolum majus.
Family: Tropaeolaceae.

People Use This For
Orally and in combination with other herbs, nasturtium is used for urinary tract infection, respiratory tract mucous membrane inflammation, and cough and bronchitis.
Topically, nasturtium is used in combination with other herbs for mild muscular pain.

Safety
POSSIBLY SAFE ...when used topically (2). ...when used orally in combination with other herbs (2).
There is insufficient reliable information available about the safety of nasturtium used orally as a single entity.
CHILDREN: LIKELY UNSAFE ...when used orally in combination with other herbs. Contraindicated (2,18).There is insufficient reliable information about the safety of the topical use of nasturtium by children.
PREGNANCY AND LACTATION: Insufficient reliable information available; avoid using nasturtium by itself or in combination with other herbs.

Effectiveness
There is insufficient reliable information available about the effectiveness of nasturtium.

Mechanism of Action
The applicable parts of nasturtium are the above ground parts. Nasturtium contains 300 mg vitamin C per 100 grams of fresh plant (18). Benzyl mustard oil (benzyl isothiocyanate), the principal active constituent of nasturtium, may have bacteriostatic, virustatic, antimycotic (2,18), and antitumor (1537) activity. It is accumulated and excreted mainly in the respiratory and the urinary tracts (2,18). Applied topically, benzyl mustard oil has rubifacient activity (2,18).

Adverse Reactions
Orally, large amounts of nasturtium or benzyl mustard oil can cause GI tract irritation (2,18); one case of urticarial exanthema is reported (2). Large amounts of nasturtium can cause albuminuria due to glomerular and tubular damage (2).
Topically, long-term intensive contact with the plant can cause skin irritation (18); benzyl mustard oil can cause skin and mucosal irritation (2). Benzyl mustard oil is a contact allergen if applied to the skin (2).

Interactions with Herbs & Other Dietary Supplements
None known.

Interactions with Drugs
None known.

Interactions with Foods
None known.

Interactions with Lab Tests
None known.

Interactions with Diseases or Conditions
GI ULCERS: Contraindicated in individuals with gastric or intestinal ulcers (2,18).
KIDNEY DISEASE: Contraindicated in individuals with kidney disease.

Dosage and Administration
ORAL: No typical dosage.
TOPICAL: When used in combination with other herbs, the dose varies according to the combination (2).

NATTOKINASE

Also Known As

BSP, Fermented Soybeans, Natto Extract, NK, Subtilisin NAT.
CAUTION: See separate listing for Soy.

Scientific Names

Nattokinase.

People Use This For

Orally, nattokinase is used for cardiovascular disease, stroke, angina, deep vein thrombosis (DVT), atherosclerosis, hemorrhoids, venous stasis, varicose veins, peripheral vascular disease, claudication, pain, fibromyalgia, chronic fatigue syndrome, endometriosis, uterine fibroids, muscle spasms, hypertension, infertility, cancer, and beriberi.

Safety

LIKELY SAFE ...when used orally in amounts commonly found in foods. Nattokinase is a natural component of the soy food natto. It has been routinely consumed in Japanese cultures for hundreds of years (12072,12073).
POSSIBLY SAFE ...when used orally in two doses. There is preliminary evidence that taking two doses separated by 6 hours of a specific combination product containing nattokinase (Flite Tabs) seems to be safe (12075). There is not enough evidence to know if taking multiple doses of nattokinase supplements is safe.
PREGNANCY AND LACTATION: Insufficient information available; avoid using.

Effectiveness

INSUFFICIENT RELIABLE EVIDENCE to RATE

Deep vein thrombosis (DVT). There is some evidence that taking a specific combination product (Flite Tabs) might decrease the risk of DVT during long-haul plane flights. The product combines a blend of 150 mg of nattokinase plus pycnogenol. Two capsules are taken 2 hours before the flight and then again 6 hours later (12075). More evidence is needed to rate nattokinase for this use.

Mechanism of Action

Nattokinase is a fibrinolytic enzyme derived from a Japanese food called natto. Natto is boiled soybeans fermented with the bacteria Bacillus natto (12072,12090). Nattokinase is thought to be produced through this specific fermentation process. Therefore, nattokinase isn't a component of other soy foods.
Nattokinase works by inactivating plasminogen activator inhibitor 1 (PAI-1) (12070,12091). Nattokinase has fibrinolytic activity that is 4-times more potent than plasmin (12074). Its average activity is about 40 CU (plasmin units) /gram (12072).
Nattokinase is thought to help for atherosclerosis due to its fibrinolytic activity at the blood vessel wall. There is preliminary evidence from animal models that taking a natto extract containing nattokinase can reduce vessel wall thickening following endothelial injury. Nattokinase also seems to cause lysis of thrombi that form at the vessel wall (12070,12071).
Nattokinase seems to be orally available when administered to humans. Taking enteric-coated nattokinase capsules 1.3 grams three times daily seems to significantly increase measures of fibrinolytic activity for 2 to 8 hours (12073).

Adverse Reactions

None reported.

Interactions with Herbs & Other Dietary Supplements

SUPPLEMENTS WITH ANTICOAGULANT/ANTIPLATELET POTENTIAL: Nattokinase has thrombolytic activity (12070). Taking nattokinase along with other supplements that might have antiplatelet or anticoagulant effects might increase the risk of bruising and bleeding. Some supplements that might have antiplatelet or anticoagulant activity include angelica, clove, danshen, garlic, ginger, ginkgo, fish oil, turmeric, vitamin E, willow, and others.

Interactions with Drugs

ANTICOAGULANT/ANTIPLATELET DRUGS: Nattokinase has thrombolytic activity (12070). Theoretically, taking nattokinase with drugs that have antiplatelet or anticoagulant effects might increase the risk of bruising and bleeding. Some of these drugs include aspirin, clopidogrel (Plavix), diclofenac (Voltaren, Cataflam, others), ibuprofen (Advil, Motrin, others), naproxen (Anaprox, Naprosyn, others), dalteparin (Fragmin), enoxaparin (Lovenox), heparin, warfarin (Coumadin), and others.

Interactions with Foods

None known.

Interactions with Lab Tests

None known.

Interactions with Diseases or Conditions

BLEEDING DISORDERS: Nattokinase has thrombolytic effects (12070) and may exacerbate bleeding disorders; use with caution.

Dosage and Administration

ORAL: For preventing deep vein thrombosis (DVT) during long-haul flights, a specific product (Flite Tabs) containing a 150 mg blend of nattokinase plus pycnogenol has been used. Two capsules are taken 2 hours before the flight and 2 capsules are taken 6 hours later (12075).

Comments

Nattokinase was discovered by a University of Chicago researcher, Dr. Hiroyuki Sumi. He referred to it as "The Enzyme of Enzymes." Natto, which nattokinase is derived from, has been a popular food in the Japanese culture for hundreds of years. It has also been used as a folk remedy for cardiovascular diseases.

NEEM

Also Known As

Arishta, Arishtha, Bead Tree, Holy Tree, Indian Lilac, Indian Neem, Margosa, Nim, Nimb, Nimba, Persian Lilac, Pride of China.

Scientific Names

Azadirachta indica, synonyms Antelaea azadirachta, Melia azadirachta.
Family: Meliaceae.

People Use This For

Orally, neem leaf is used for leprosy, eye disorders, epistaxis, intestinal worms, abdominal upset, anorexia, skin ulcers, cardiovascular disease, contraception, abortion, fever, diabetes, gingivitis, and hepatic dysfunction. The bark is used for malaria, peptic ulcer, skin diseases, pain, and fever. The flower is used for bile suppression, intestinal worms, and phlegm. The fruit is used for hemorrhoids, intestinal worms, urinary disorders, epistaxis, phlegm, eye disorders, diabetes, wounds, and leprosy. Neem twigs are used for cough, asthma, hemorrhoids, intestinal worms, spermatorrhea, urinary disorders, and diabetes. The seed and seed oil are used for leprosy, abortion, contraception, and intestinal worms. The stem, root bark, and fruit are used as a tonic and astringent.
Topically, neem is used to treat head lice, for skin diseases, wounds, skin ulcers, and as a mosquito repellent and an emollient.
Intravaginally, neem is used as a contraceptive.
Neem is also used as an insecticide.

Safety

POSSIBLY SAFE ...when neem bark extract is used orally and appropriately for up to 10 weeks (12822). ...when neem leaf extract gel is used intraorally for up to 6 weeks (12824).
POSSIBLY UNSAFE ...when neem is used orally in large amounts or long-term. Preliminary clinical research suggests neem might be toxic to the kidneys or liver with high-dose or chronic use (12835).
CHILDREN: LIKELY UNSAFE ...when the oil or seeds are used orally. There are reports of infants who were severely poisoned and died (3473,3474,3476).
PREGNANCY: LIKELY UNSAFE ...when neem oil or leaf is used orally. Neem oil and leaf have been used as abortifacients (12825,12835).
LACTATION: Insufficient reliable information available; avoid using.

Effectiveness

INSUFFICIENT RELIABLE EVIDENCE to RATE

Dental plaque. Applying neem leaf extract gel to the teeth and gums twice daily for 6 weeks might reduce plaque formation, according to preliminary clinical research. It also might reduce bacterial counts of Streptococcus mutans and Lactobacilli species, which have been associated with plaque formation (12824).
Peptic ulcers. Taking neem bark extract orally 30-60 mg twice daily for 10 weeks seems to aid in the healing of gastroduodenal ulcers, according to preliminary clinical research (12822).
More evidence is needed to rate neem for these uses.

Mechanism of Action

The applicable parts of neem are the bark, leaf, seed, seed oil, and less frequently, the root, flower, and fruit. More than 135 compounds have been isolated from neem. Neem contains isoprenoids, proteins, polysaccharides, flavonoids, dihydrochalcone, coumarin, tannins, and other compounds. Nimibidin is a constituent of neem seed oil. Preliminary research suggests it might have anti-inflammatory, antiarthritic, antipyretic, hypoglycemic, antiulcer, and diuretic effects. It also seems to have antifungal and antibacterial activity. Nimibidin and another neem seed oil constituent, nimbin, have spermicidal activity. The seed oil constituent nimbolide, seems to have antimalarial and antibacterial activity. Gedunin appears to have activity against fungal and malarial microbes. Azadirachtin also has antimalarial activity and is used as an insecticide. Mahmoodin has antibacterial activity (12823,12836). Neem seed oil also might have immunostimulant effects. It seems to stimulate cellular immune response. Preliminary clinical research suggests it might be useful as a long-term vaginal contraceptive, an effect that may be caused by a local cell-mediated immune response to the allogenic sperm and embryo (12825). A single intravaginal dose of neem seed extract provides long-term, reversible contraception in animals (12827).

Neem bark contains tannins and polysaccharides that might have anti-inflammatory activity. Other neem bark polysaccharides seem to have antitumor effects. Margolone, margolonone, and isomargolonone appear to be active against bacteria such as Klebsiella, Staphylococcus, and Serratia species (12823). An aqueous extract of neem bark seems to have antisecretory and antiulcer activity (12822). An aqueous extract of neem root bark might have hypoglycemic effects (12829).

Sulfur-containing neem leaf extracts seem to have antifungal effects. An aqueous extract of neem leaves seems to have hypoglycemic activity (12823). Neem leaf extract seems to have antispermatogenic and antiandrogenic properties. It seems to adversely affect sperm mobility and viability (12826,12828). Other preliminary research suggests that neem leaf extract might protect the liver from the hepatotoxic effects of acetaminophen (12831,12832).

An extract of neem fruit seems to have antiulcer activity (12823).

Neem oil is toxic to infants and children, but the toxic constituent is unknown (3473,3475). Researchers speculate that a long-chain monounsaturated free acid may be responsible (3475).

Adverse Reactions

Orally, severe poisoning in infants and small children characterized by vomiting, loose stools, drowsiness, metabolic acidosis, anemia, polymorphonuclear leukocytosis, seizure, loss of consciousness, coma, cerebral edema, Reye's syndrome-like symptoms and death have been reported to occur within hours after ingestion of neem oil (3473,3474,3476). Liver and renal biopsy reports have revealed pathologic findings seen typically in Reye's syndrome (3473,3474,3475). Preliminary research suggests that neem leaf might also have hepatotoxic and nephrotoxic effects (12833,12834). Oliguria, anuria, jaundice, anemia, acute tubular necrosis, hemolysis, hepatotoxicity, and nephrotoxicity have been reported in humans taking neem leaf (12835).

Interactions with Herbs & Other Dietary Supplements

HERBS WITH HYPOGLYCEMIC POTENTIAL: Theoretically, neem might have additive effects with herbs that decrease blood glucose levels (12823). Herbs with hypoglycemic potential include devil's claw, fenugreek, garlic, guar gum, horse chestnut, Panax ginseng, psyllium, and Siberian ginseng.

Interactions with Drugs

ANTIDIABETES DRUGS: There is some evidence that neem might have hypoglycemic effects (12823). Theoretically, concomitant use with drugs that decrease blood glucose levels might increase the risk of hypoglycemia. Dosing adjustments for insulin or oral hypoglycemic agents may be necessary. Oral hypoglycemic drugs include glimepiride (Amaryl), glipizide (Glucotrol), glyburide (DiaBeta, Micronase), tolazamide (Tolinase), tolbutamide (Orinase), and others.

IMMUNOSUPPRESSANTS: Theoretically, neem might decrease the effectiveness of immunosuppressants (12825). Preliminary research suggests neem might have immunostimulant effects and might counteract the effects of immunosuppressants. Immunosuppressant drugs include azathioprine (Imuran), basiliximab (Simulect), cyclosporine (Neoral, Sandimmune), daclizumab (Zenapax), muromonab-CD3 (OKT3, Orthoclone OKT3), mycophenolate (CellCept), tacrolimus (FK506, Prograf), sirolimus (Rapamune), prednisone (Deltasone, Orasone), and other corticosteroids (glucocorticoids).

Interactions with Foods

None known.

Interactions with Lab Tests

None known.

Interactions with Diseases or Conditions

AUTOIMMUNE DISEASES: Theoretically, neem might adversely affect patients with autoimmune disorders because of its possible immune stimulating effects (12825). Avoid using in patients with multiple sclerosis, systemic lupus erythematosus (SLE), or other autoimmune disorders.

DIABETES: There is some evidence that neem can lower blood glucose levels and might cause hypoglycemia (12823). Advise patients to increase blood glucose monitoring. Dosing adjustments to diabetes medications may be necessary.

INFERTILITY: Theoretically, neem might have detrimental effects on male and female fertility. It might cause an allergic response to sperm and embryos. (12825). Other preliminary research suggests neem oil can cause morphological changes in sperm, and neem leaf can adversely affect sperm motility and viability (12826,12828). Avoid in couples with infertility.

ORGAN TRANSPLANT: Theoretically, neem might decrease the effectiveness of immunosuppressants in organ transplant patients (12825). Preliminary research suggests neem might have immunostimulant effects and might potentially contribute to transplant rejection.

Dosage and Administration

No typical dosage.

Comments

Neem twigs, which are used as chewing sticks in lieu of toothbrushes in the tropics, are often contaminated with fungi within 2 weeks of harvest and should be avoided (12830).

Neem seed oil is approved by the Environmental Protection Agency for pesticide use in the US (12836).

NERVE ROOT

Also Known As

American Valerian, Bleeding Heart, Cypripedium, Lady's Slipper, Moccasin Flower, Monkey Flower, Noah's Ark, Shoe, Slipper Root, Venus' Shoe, Yellows.

Scientific Names

Cypripedium parviflorum, synonym Cypripedium pubescens; Cypripedium calceolus.
Family: Orchidaceae.

People Use This For

Orally, nerve root is used for menorrhagia and diarrhea. Nerve root is also used orally for insomnia; emotional tension; hysteria; anxiety states; agitation; nervousness; and specifically, anxiety states associated with insomnia.

Topically, nerve root is used to treat pruritus vulvae.

Safety

POSSIBLY UNSAFE ...when the root or rhizome is used orally. Nerve root is reported to cause hallucinations (4).
PREGNANCY AND LACTATION: POSSIBLY UNSAFE ...when used orally (4); avoid using.

Effectiveness

There is insufficient reliable information available about the effectiveness of nerve root.

Mechanism of Action

The applicable parts of nerve root are the rhizome and root. Nerve root contains tannins, glycosides, resins, quinones, and a volatile oil (4,18), and is said to have astringent and styptic properties (18). The quinone constituent of nerve root is thought to be responsible for its sensitizing properties (4).

Adverse Reactions

Orally, nerve root can cause hallucinations (4). Large doses are associated with giddiness, restlessness, headache, mental excitement and visual hallucinations (4).

Topically, it can cause contact dermatitis (4).

Interactions with Herbs & Other Dietary Supplements

None known.

Interactions with Drugs

None known.

Interactions with Foods

None known.

Interactions with Lab Tests

None known.

Interactions with Diseases or Conditions

None known.

Dosage and Administration

ORAL: A typical dose is 2-4 grams dried rhizome/root or as tea (steep 2-4 grams dried rhizome/root in 150 mL of boiling water for 5-10 minutes, strain), three times daily (4). A liquid extract (1:1 in 45% alcohol) 2-4 mL is typically used three times daily (4).

Comments
Avoid confusion with Calypso bulbosa (Cypripedium bulbosum) and Cypripedium parviflorum, related species also known as lady's slipper.

NEW JERSEY TEA

Also Known As
Jersey Tea, Mountain-Sweet, Red Root, Redroot, Walpole Tea, Wild Snowball.

Scientific Names
Ceanothus americanus, synonym Ceanothus intermedius.
Family: Rhamnaceae.

People Use This For
Orally, New Jersey tea has been used orally as an expectorant, antispasmodic, clotting agent, an astringent, to treat gonorrhea, syphilis, colds, fever, chills, pelvic cysts, and as a lymphagogue.

Safety
LIKELY SAFE ...when used as an oral medicinal (12,18).
PREGNANCY AND LACTATION: Insufficient reliable information available; avoid using.

Effectiveness
There is insufficient reliable information available about the effectiveness of New Jersey tea.

Mechanism of Action
The applicable parts of New Jersey tea are the root, root bark, and leaf. New Jersey tea contains cyclic peptide alkaloids and triterpenes (18). An aqueous-ethanol extract of New Jersey tea is said to reduce the blood-clotting time by 25% in blood taken from young rats (18).

Adverse Reactions
None reported.

Interactions with Herbs & Other Dietary Supplements
None known.

Interactions with Drugs
None known.

Interactions with Foods
None known.

Interactions with Lab Tests
None known.

Interactions with Diseases or Conditions
None known.

Dosage and Administration
ORAL: New Jersey tea is typically used as an extract (18).

NEW ZEALAND GREEN-LIPPED MUSSEL

Also Known As
Green Lipped Mussel, New Zealand Green Lipped Mussel, NZGLM.

Scientific Names
Perna canaliculus.
Family: Mytilidae.

People Use This For
Orally, New Zealand green-lipped mussel is used for symptoms of rheumatoid arthritis and osteoarthritis.

Safety
POSSIBLY SAFE ...when used orally. There is only limited information available (6).
PREGNANCY: POSSIBLY UNSAFE ...when used orally; avoid using. It may cause retarded fetal development and delay in parturition (936).
LACTATION: Insufficient reliable information available; avoid using.

Effectiveness
POSSIBLY INEFFECTIVE

Rheumatoid arthritis (RA). Taking New Zealand green-lipped mussel orally doesn't seem to help RA (6,935). There is insufficient reliable information available about the effectiveness of New Zealand green-lipped mussel for its other uses.

Mechanism of Action
The dried New Zealand green-lipped mussels may contain a prostaglandin inhibitor that exerts an anti-inflammatory effect (932,933). Researchers report that an extract of New Zealand green-lipped mussel reduced symptoms in dogs with advanced arthritis. The results of this unpublished study were presented at the Experimental Biology 2000 conference (5055).

Adverse Reactions
Orally, New Zealand green-lipped mussel can cause diarrhea, nausea, and flatulence (6). One case was reported of reversible, granulomatous hepatitis associated with New Zealand green-lipped mussel (6).

Interactions with Herbs & Other Dietary Supplements
None known.

Interactions with Drugs
None known.

Interactions with Foods
None known.

Interactions with Lab Tests
None known.

Interactions with Diseases or Conditions
None known.

Dosage and Administration
ORAL: New Zealand green-lipped mussel extract 300-350 mg three times per day was used in human studies for rheumatoid arthritis; except for one early trial, studies found New Zealand green-lipped mussels ineffective (6,935).

Comments
New Zealand green-lipped mussels are available commercially as a freeze dried, ground, and encapsulated product.

NIACIN AND NIACINAMIDE (VITAMIN B3)

Also Known As
3-Pyridine Carboxamide, Anti-Blacktongue Factor, Antipellagra Factor, B Complex Vitamin, Niacin-Niacinamide, Niacin/Niacinamide, Nicamid, Nicosedine, Nicotinamide, Nicotinic Acid Amide, Nicotylamidum, Pellagra Preventing Factor, Vitamin B-3, Vitamin PP.
CAUTION: See separate listings for Inositol Nicotinate (Inositol Hexaniacinate) and Tryptophan.

Scientific Names
Niacin; Niacinamide; Nicotinic acid; Vitamin B3.

People Use This For
Orally, niacin is used for hyperlipidemia. It is also used in conjunction with other therapies for peripheral vascular disease, vascular spasm, migraine headache, Meniere's syndrome, vertigo, and to reduce the diarrhea associated with cholera. Orally, niacin or niacinamide is also used for preventing vitamin B3 deficiency, treating pellagra, schizophrenia, drug-induced hallucinations, Alzheimer's disease and age-related cognitive decline, chronic brain syndrome, hyperkinesis, depression, motion sickness, alcohol dependence, vasculitis associated with skin lesions, and edema. Niacin or niacinamide is also used for acne, leprosy, attention deficit-hyperactivity disorder (ADHD), preventing premenstrual headache, improving digestion, for protection from toxins and pollutants, for reducing the

effects of aging, memory loss, arthritis, lowering blood pressure, improving circulation, promoting relaxation, improving orgasm, and preventing cataracts. Niacinamide is also used orally treating diabetes, and the skin conditions bullous pemphigoid and granuloma annulare.
Topically, niacinamide is used for treating inflammatory acne vulgaris.

Safety

LIKELY SAFE ...when used orally and appropriately. Niacin and niacinamide are FDA-approved products (12033).
POSSIBLY SAFE ...when niacinamide is used topically and appropriately up to 12 weeks (5940).
PREGNANCY AND LACTATION: LIKELY SAFE ...when used orally in amounts that do not exceed the recommended dietary allowance (RDA). The RDA for pregnant and lactating women, 14-18 years is 30 mg. For pregnant and lactating women older than 18 years the RDA is 35 mg (6243). There is insufficient reliable information available about the safety of larger oral doses of niacin, niacinamide, or topical niacinamide when used during pregnancy or lactation; avoid using.

Effectiveness

EFFECTIVE

Hyperlipidemia. Some niacin products are FDA-approved prescription products for treating hyperlipidemia. These prescription niacin products typically come in high strengths of 500 mg or higher. Dietary supplement forms of niacin usually come in strengths of 250 mg or less. Since very high doses of niacin are required for hyperlipidemia, dietary supplement niacin usually isn't appropriate.
Prescription niacin is generally considered a second-line therapy for patients who mainly need to decrease low-density lipoprotein (LDL) cholesterol. But niacin is often considered first-line for patients with mixed hyperlipidemia or patients who need to increase high-density lipoprotein (HDL) cholesterol. Niacin only reduces LDL cholesterol by about 5% to 25%, compared to 18% to 55% with statins. But niacin can decrease triglycerides by 20% to 50% and increase HDL by 15% to 35% (4818,4867,4886,4887,4888,4889,4890,12033). Niacin is also commonly combined with other cholesterol-lowering drugs when diet and single-drug therapy are not adequately effective (4867). Concurrent use of statins with 1 or 2 grams of sustained release niacin daily can additionally reduce total cholesterol by 8% or 21%, LDL by 8% or 31%, triglycerides by 24% or 27%, and increase HDL by 23% or 27% (8545).
The effects of niacin are dose-dependent. The most pronounce increases in HDL and decreases in triglycerides occur at 1200-1500 mg/day. Niacin's greatest effects on LDL occur at 2000-3000 mg/day (12033). A very low dose of niacin, 50 mg daily, can modestly increase HDL cholesterol by 2.1 mg/dL, but appears to have no effect on total cholesterol, LDL cholesterol, or triglycerides when added to statin therapy (8546). Niacin also seems to be effective for isolated hypoalphalipoproteinemia (4817). Niacinamide has no effect on lipid levels in patients with hyperlipidemia.
Niacin deficiency and pellagra. Both niacin and niacinamide are FDA-approved for the prevention and treatment of niacin deficiency and pellagra. Niacinamide is sometimes preferred for this indication because it lacks the vasodilating effects of niacin (15,6243).

POSSIBLY EFFECTIVE

Alzheimer's disease. There is some evidence that people who consume higher amounts of niacin (17-45 mg/day) from food and multivitamin sources have a lower risk of developing Alzheimer's disease compared to people who consume less niacin (14 mg/day) (12077). Food sources high in niacin include meat, fish, beans, nuts, coffee, and fortified grains and cereals. Explain to patients that there is no reliable evidence that taking a stand-alone niacin supplement is beneficial for reducing the risk of Alzheimer's disease.
Atherosclerosis. Taking niacin orally, in combination with a bile acid sequestrant, seems to reduce atherosclerosis in high-risk men with existing cardiovascular disease. In a large-scale trial, niacin plus colestipol significantly decreased coronary atherosclerosis progression; increased frequency of atherosclerosis regression; and decreased incidence of cardiovascular events including death, myocardial infarction, and revascularization procedures (4848).
Cardiovascular disease. Taking niacin orally, in combination with simvastatin (Zocor), seems to reduce cardiovascular disease risk in people with coronary disease and low high-density lipoprotein (HDL) cholesterol. Patients titrated up to 2-4 grams of sustained-release niacin and 10-20 mg simvastatin daily seem to have a reduced risk of a first cardiovascular event such as death, myocardial infarction (MIs), or stroke. This combination also seems to cause regression of coronary stenosis (7388). Taking niacin alone also seems to reduce the risk of secondary MIs. In a large scale, long-term study, high-dose niacin significantly reduced the risk of a second heart attack in men; however, there was not a significant decrease in overall or cause-specific mortality (4847).
Cataracts. Taking niacin orally seems to reduce the occurrence of cataracts. A large-scale population-based study found high dietary intake of niacin is associated with a reduced risk of nuclear cataracts (6378).
Cholera. Taking niacin orally seems to control fluid loss due to cholera (4868). In a randomized controlled study, divided doses of 2 grams of nicotinic acid daily reduced diarrhea in adults with cholera (4868). Laboratory evidence supports the use of nicotinic acid, but not niacinamide, to reduce intestinal secretion induced by cholera toxin (4869).
Diabetes. Taking high-dose niacinamide orally seems to help reduce the risk of type 1 diabetes in high-risk

children (4874). Following the success of this trial, a very large, multinational, long-term study was begun to determine whether regular use of niacinamide can prevent diabetes (4876). Preliminary results released by a German group found no protective effect, but the authors cautioned that their findings did not exclude the possibility that niacinamide might be effective (4875). There is also evidence that suggests niacinamide might reserve residual beta-cell function in newly diagnosed type 1 diabetes (4877,4878,4879,4880). Clinical trials, including one placebo-controlled trial and one vitamin E-comparison study showed niacinamide might prolong the "honeymoon period" in newly-diagnosed type 1 diabetes when the pancreas is still capable of producing some insulin (4877,4878,4879,4880). The clinical studies to date have been performed by one group of Italian investigators. Concerns about potential concurrent induction of insulin resistance have been raised (4881). Niacinamide is also useful when used orally for protecting residual beta-cell function and improving glycemic control in adults with type 2 diabetes (4882). In a small, placebo-controlled, single-blind study, niacinamide increased C-peptide release and improved insulin secretion in lean diabetics who had failed sulfonylurea therapy (4882).

Osteoarthritis. Taking niacinamide orally, 3 grams daily in divided doses, seems to improve joint flexibility and reduce inflammation, and might allow for a reduction in standard anti-inflammatory drug doses (4883).

INSUFFICIENT RELIABLE EVIDENCE to RATE

Attention deficit-hyperactivity disorder (ADHD). There is conflicting preliminary clinical evidence regarding the usefulness of niacinamide in combination with other megadose vitamins for the treatment of ADHD (3351,9957). More evidence is needed to rate niacinamide for this use.

Mechanism of Action

Vitamin B3 includes niacin (nicotinic acid) and niacinamide (nicotinamide) (6243). The term niacin refers specifically to nicotinic acid, but is also used collectively to refer to both nicotinic acid and nicotinamide (niacinamide). Niacin is converted to niacinamide when ingested in amounts that do not exceed physiological requirements. The pharmacological effects of niacin and niacinamide are indistinguishable. Niacin is a water-soluble vitamin which is well absorbed when used orally (6243). Dietary sources include meats, beans, and various niacin-fortified foods. In addition, dietary tryptophan is biosynthetically converted to niacin (60 mg tryptophan equals 1 mg of niacin or one niacin equivalent) (6243). Niacinamide is required for lipid metabolism, tissue respiration, and glycogenolysis. Niacinamide is incorporated into the coenzymes, nicotinamide adenine dinucleotide (NAD), and nicotinamide adenine dinucleotide phosphate (NADP). These coenzymes act as hydrogen-carrier molecules.

Niacin deficiency causes pellagra, a condition that affects the gastrointestinal tract, skin, and central nervous system (6243). Pellagra was common in the early twentieth century, but niacin-fortified foods have virtually eliminated this deficiency disease except in conditions such as chronic alcoholism (4850). Some researchers think that sleep deprivation-induced dermatitis might be caused by niacin depletion because of similarities between this condition and pellagra (1350). Causes of niacin deficiency include poor diet, isoniazid therapy, carcinoid tumors that decrease endogenous production, and Hartnup disease, an autosomal recessive disorder that interferes with tryptophan absorption (6243). Conditions that increase niacin requirements, such as hyperthyroidism, diabetes mellitus, liver cirrhosis, pregnancy, and lactation, rarely cause deficiency (4969).

When doses of niacin or niacinamide greater than 300-800 mg daily are administered different pharmacological effects occur. Niacin 1000 mg or more per day can decrease total cholesterol by 8 to 21%, low-density lipoprotein (LDL) cholesterol by 8 to 25%, triglycerides by 20 to 50%, and increase high-density lipoprotein (HDL) concentrations by 15 to 35% (4867,8545). The exact mechanism for the beneficial effects on serum lipids is unknown, but niacin inhibits free fatty acid release from adipose tissue; and inhibits cyclic AMP accumulation which controls the activity of triglyceride lipase and hence lipolysis. It also decreases the rate of liver synthesis of LDL and VLDL; and increases the rate of chylomicron triglyceride removal from plasma secondary to increased lipoprotein lipase activity (6243). Niacin produces vasodilation of cutaneous blood vessels of the face, neck, and chest, probably mediated by prostaglandins, such as prostacyclin. In most individuals, tolerance to these effects occurs within two weeks (15). Preliminary clinical data suggest that some people with schizophrenia do not experience the characteristic vasodilatory response to niacin, suggesting an impaired response to phospholipid-dependent signaling (4870). Niacin also causes the release of histamine, which increases gastric motility and acid secretion (15). Niacin in combination with riboflavin might reduce the incidence of cataract development in older people (4885). Niacin might have beneficial effects on coagulation in people at risk for cardiovascular disease. Preliminary clinical research indicates that niacin reduces fibrinogen concentrations in plasma and stimulates fibrinolysis in hyperlipidemic men (4871). In patients with peripheral arterial disease niacin lowers fibrinogen and F1.2, a marker of thrombin conversion (8547). Large amounts of niacin can decrease uric acid excretion (15).

Niacinamide has no beneficial effect on lipids and should not be used for treating hyperlipidemia (6243). Niacinamide does not cause the vasodilation associated with niacin (6243). High-dose niacinamide prevents or delays insulin deficiency in laboratory models of type 1 diabetes and protects islet cells from cytotoxic actions (4872,4873). Niacinamide is a free radical scavenger and might alter the auto-immune processes in type 1 diabetes that cause beta-cell destruction (4872,4873). Niacinamide is hypothesized to inhibit induction of nitric oxide synthase by interleukin 1 in chondrocytes, leading researchers to speculate about its potential use in destructive joint diseases (4884).

Adverse Reactions

Orally, small amounts of niacin and niacinamide typically found in dietary supplements are well-tolerated and cause minor adverse reactions. But doses of niacin as low as 30 mg/day can sometimes cause flushing, burning, tingling, and itching sensations as well as erythema on the face, arms, and chest (6243). Flushing may be accompanied by itching, headache, increased intracranial blood flow, and occasionally, pain (6243). Onset is highly variable, from within 30 minutes to as long as 6 weeks after the initial dose (6243). Higher doses of niacin are more likely to cause these side effects. Slow dose titration, pretreatment with 325 mg aspirin, and taking niacin with meals or the sustained release product at bedtime may reduce flushing (4852,4853,4854,4858). Flushing tends to decrease over time, despite dosage elevation (4864).

At higher doses, side effects distinguish niacin and niacinamide (6243). Niacinamide in large amounts is associated with headache, dizziness, nausea and vomiting, diarrhea, blurred vision, hepatotoxicity, hyperglycemia, abnormal prothrombin times, and hypoalbuminemia (15).

Niacin in large amounts is associated with flushing, pruritus, burning sensations, stinging or tingling of the skin, nausea, bloating, flatulence, hunger pains, vomiting, heartburn, diarrhea, increased sebaceous gland activity, hypotension, dizziness, tachycardia, arrhythmias, syncope, vasovagal attacks, headache, and blurred vision (15). Dental and gingival pain have also been reported (4862). In most people taking niacin, flushing and other skin sensations, increased sebaceous gland activity, and increased gastrointestinal motility disappear within two weeks; however, adverse effects have been reported to appear up to 2 years after initiation of therapy (4851).

Immediate-release niacin products are more likely to cause flushing and other vasodilatory side effects. Extended-release formulations may reduce the occurrence of these side effects (4857). But extended release or sustained release niacin products seem to increase the risk of hepatotoxicity (4855,4856,12026).

Niacin, particularly at doses of 3 to 9 grams per day, might cause jaundice and elevated serum transaminases (6243). The drug should be discontinued if liver function tests rise to three times the upper limit of normal (4863). Severe hepatotoxicity with fulminant hepatitis and subsequent liver transplant has been reported (6243).

Chronic use of large amounts of niacin have been associated with rash, hyperpigmentation resembling acanthosis nigricans, dry skin, xerostomia, hyperuricemia, gout, peptic ulcer, amblyopia, proptosis, loss of central vision secondary to an atypical form of cystoid macular edema, nervousness, panic, hyperglycemia, abnormal glucose tolerance and glycosuria, hepatotoxicity, abnormal prothrombin times and hypoalbuminemia (15). Niacin in higher doses can significantly raise homocysteine levels; 17% increase with 1000 mg niacin per day and 55% with 3000 mg per day (1733). Elevated homocysteine levels are an independent risk factor for arterial occlusive disease (490); however, the clinical significance of the effect of niacin on homocysteine is not yet known.

Interactions with Herbs & Other Dietary Supplements

ANTIOXIDANTS: Concurrent use of the antioxidants vitamins C and E, beta-carotene, and selenium seems to blunt the positive effect of niacin on high-density lipoprotein (HDL) cholesterol. Antioxidant supplements also appear to antagonize the beneficial effect of the combination of simvastatin (Zocor) and sustained-release niacin on cardiovascular disease risk (7388). This combination of antioxidants reduces the HDL-2-raising effects of niacin and HMG-CoA reductase inhibitors by more than 50% in people with heart disease (7388).

HEPATOTOXIC HERBS AND SUPPLEMENTS: Niacin can adversely affect the liver (4863). Theoretically, concomitant use with other potentially hepatotoxic products might increase the risk of developing liver damage. Some of these products include androstenedione, borage leaf, chaparral, coenzyme Q-10 (only in high doses), comfrey, dehydroepiandrosterone (DHEA), germander, pennyroyal oil, red yeast, and others.

Interactions with Drugs

ANTIDIABETES DRUGS: Niacin and niacinamide can interfere with blood glucose control requiring dosing adjustment of antidiabetic agents. Niacin and niacinamide can cause hyperglycemia, abnormal glucose tolerance, and glycosuria. Increased blood glucose monitoring may be necessary, particularly early in the course of treatment (4859,4860,12033). Monitor blood glucose levels carefully.

HMG-CoA REDUCTASE INHIBITORS ("Statins"): Concomitant use of niacin with HMG-CoA reductase inhibitors can increase the risk of myopathy. HMG-CoA reductase inhibitors include atorvastatin (Lipitor), cerivastatin (Baycol), fluvastatin (Lescol), lovastatin (Mevacor), pravastatin (Pravachol), and simvastatin (Zocor). NCEP guidelines suggest combination therapy only when diet and single drug therapy is not sufficiently effective (4867).

TRANSDERMAL NICOTINE (Nicoderm, Nicotrol): Concomitant use with niacin can increase the risk of flushing and dizziness (15).

Drug Influences on Nutrient Levels and Depletion

SOME DRUGS CAN AFFECT NIACIN AND NIACINAMIDE LEVELS:

ANTIBIOTICS: Destruction of normal gastrointestinal flora by antibiotics can cause decreased production of B vitamins. The clinical significance of this decreased production is not known. Consider supplementation only if clinical judgment warrants it (4434,4435,4436,4437,4438,4439,4440,4441,4442,4443).

BILE ACID SEQUESTRANTS: Cholestyramine (Questran) and colestipol (Colestid) reduce niacin absorption (15).

ISONIAZID (INH): Isoniazid inhibits the conversion of tryptophan to niacin and might induce pellagra, particularly in poorly nourished patients (4865,4866).

Interactions with Foods

HOT DRINKS: Concomitant ingestion of niacin and hot drinks can magnify niacin-induced flushing (6243).

Interactions with Lab Tests

CATECHOLAMINES: Niacin can falsely increase some urinary catecholamine fluorometric assay results. Niacin produces fluorescent substances in the urine, which can falsely elevate test results (15).
GLUCOSE: Niacin can cause a false-positive reactions with urine glucose tests which rely on cupric sulfate solution (Benedict's reagent) (15).
HOMOCYSTEINE: At higher doses, niacin can increase homocysteine levels. Doses of 1000 mg and 3000 mg per day reportedly increase homocysteine levels by 17% and 55% respectively (1733).
LIVER FUNCTION TESTS: Both niacin and niacinamide can increase serum bilirubin, alanine aminotransferase (ALT), aspartate aminotransferase (AST), and lactate dehydrogenase (LDH) concentrations and test results. Liver function tests should be monitored regularly, particularly early in the course of therapy and in patients receiving long-term treatment with high doses of niacin or niacinamide. Niacin should be discontinued if liver function tests rise to three times the upper limit of normal (4863).

Interactions with Diseases or Conditions

ALLERGIES: Niacin and niacinamide might exacerbate allergies by causing histamine release (15).
CORONARY ARTERY DISEASE/UNSTABLE ANGINA: Large amounts of niacin can increase the risk of cardiac arrhythmias. One study showed an increased incidence of cardiac arrhythmias when niacin was used in patients with coronary artery disease (15); use with caution.
CROHN'S DISEASE: Nicotinic acid (niacin) serum levels decrease with increases in the Crohn's disease activity index in patients who do not receive nutritional treatments (6269).
DIABETES: Niacin and niacinamide can interfere with blood glucose control requiring dosing adjustment of antidiabetic agents. Niacin and niacinamide can cause hyperglycemia, abnormal glucose tolerance, and glycosuria. Increased blood glucose monitoring may be necessary, particularly early in the course of treatment (4859,4860,12033).
GALLBLADDER DISEASE: Niacin or niacinamide might exacerbate gallbladder disease (15); use with caution.
GOUT: Large amounts of niacin or niacinamide might precipitate gout. Niacin and niacinamide can cause hyperuricemia (12033); use with caution.
KIDNEY DISEASE: Niacin is excreted unchanged in the urine and might accumulate in patients with kidney disease (15); use with caution.
LIVER DISEASE: Contraindicated; niacin and niacinamide have been associated with liver damage. Avoid large amounts in patients with a history of liver disease (12026,12033).
PEPTIC ULCER DISEASE: Contraindicated in patients with active peptic ulcer disease. Large amounts of niacin or niacinamide might activate peptic ulcer disease (15); use with caution in patients with a history of peptic ulcer disease.
SEVERE HYPOTENSION: Contraindicated; niacin can cause hypotension (15).

Dosage and Administration

ORAL: For hyperlipidemia the effects of niacin are dose-dependent. The most pronounce increases in HDL and decreases in triglycerides occur at 1200-1500 mg/day. Niacin's greatest effects on LDL occur at 2000-3000 mg/day (12033). To prevent coronary events in people with hyperlipidemia, niacin 4 grams daily has been used (4848). For preventing and treating vitamin B3 deficiency, doses of nicotinic acid and niacinamide are considered equivalent. For mild vitamin B3 deficiency, niacin or niacinamide 50-100 mg per day is used. For pellagra in adults, niacin or niacinamide 300-500 mg daily is given in divided doses. For pellagra in children, niacin or niacinamide 100-300 mg daily is given in divided doses. For Hartnup disease, niacin or niacinamide 50-200 mg daily is used (15). For reducing fluid loss induced by cholera toxin, niacin 2 grams daily has been used (4868). To prevent type 1 diabetes in high-risk children, sustained-release niacinamide 1.2 grams/m2 (body surface area) per day has been used (4875). To slow disease progression of newly diagnosed type 1 diabetes, niacinamide 25 mg/kg daily has been used (4878). For treating osteoarthritis, niacinamide 3 grams per day in divided doses has been used (4883). A daily dietary intake of approximately 44 mg of niacin has been associated with reduced risk of nuclear cataracts (6378).
The daily recommended dietary allowances (RDAs) of niacin are: Infants 0-6 months, 2 mg; Infants 7-12 months, 4 mg; Children 1-3 years, 6 mg; Children 4-8 years, 8 mg; Children 9-13 years, 12 mg; Men 14 years and older, 16 mg; Women 14 years and older, 14 mg; Pregnant women, 18 mg; and Lactating women, 17 mg (6243). The maximum daily dose of niacin is: Children 1-3 years, 10 mg; Children 4-8 years, 15 mg; Children 9-13 years, 20 mg; Adults, including Pregnant and Lactating women, 14-18 years, 30 mg; and Adults, including pregnant and lactating women, older than 18 years, 35 mg (6243).

Comments

Vitamin B3 is present in many foods including yeast, meat, fish, milk, eggs, green vegetables, and cereal grains. The term niacin is used to refer specifically to nicotinic acid, but is also used collectively to refer to both nicotinic acid and nicotinamide (niacinamide). Niacin and niacinamide are frequently used in combination with other B vitamins in vitamin B complex formulations. Vitamin B complex generally includes vitamin B1 (Thiamine), vitamin B2 (Riboflavin), vitamin B3 (Niacin/Niacinamide), vitamin B5 (pantothenic acid), vitamin B6 (pyridoxine), vitamin B12 (cyanocobalamin), and folic acid. However, some products do not contain all of these ingredients and some may include others, such as biotin para-aminobenzoic acid (PABA), choline bitartrate, and inositol.

NIAULI OIL

Also Known As
Caje Oil, Niauli Aetheroleum.
CAUTION: See separate listings for Cajeput Oil and Tea Tree Oil.

Scientific Names
Melaleuca viridiflora.
Family: Myrtaceae.

People Use This For
Orally and topically, niauli oil is used for upper respiratory tract mucous membrane inflammation, cough, and bronchitis.

Safety
POSSIBLY SAFE ...when used orally and appropriately (2,18). ...when used topically and appropriately (12,18).
LIKELY UNSAFE ...when greater than 10 grams of oil is ingested orally. Can cause hypotension, circulatory disorders, and respiratory failure (18).
CHILDREN: LIKELY UNSAFE ...when used topically in the nasal and facial areas because it could cause bronchospasm, asthma-like symptoms, and respiratory failure (2,18).
PREGNANCY AND LACTATION: Insufficient reliable information available; avoid using.

Effectiveness
There is insufficient reliable information available about the effectiveness of niauli oil.

Mechanism of Action
Niauli oil contains cineole (7,9), which has in vitro antibacterial activity and stimulates circulation (2,18). Cineole has actions similar to that of eucalyptus oil (9). Cineole induces liver enzymes involved with drug metabolism (18).

Adverse Reactions
Orally, niauli oil can cause nausea, vomiting, and diarrhea (2). The consumption of amounts greater than 10 grams can cause hypotension, circulatory disorders, collapse, and respiratory failure (18).
Topically, it can cause glottal spasm, bronchospasm, and respiratory failure when applied to facial and nasal areas of infants and small children (2,18).

Interactions with Herbs & Other Dietary Supplements
None known.

Interactions with Drugs
None known.

Interactions with Foods
None known.

Interactions with Lab Tests
None known.

Interactions with Diseases or Conditions
GI TRACT DISEASE: Niauli oil is contraindicated in individuals with inflammatory diseases of the GI tract.
LIVER DISEASE: Contraindicated in individuals with severe liver disease or bile duct inflammation (2,18).

Dosage and Administration
ORAL: The typical dose of niauli oil is 200 mg per administration, up to 2 grams per day (2,18).
TOPICAL: Niauli oil is commonly used as oily nose drops, consisting of 2-5% niauli oil in vegetable oil (2,18). Other topical preparations contain 10-30% niauli oil in an oil base (2,18).

Comments
Niauli oil consists of the essential oil distilled from leaves of Melaleuca viridiflora. Avoid confusion with tea tree oil (Maleleuca alternifolia) and cajeput oil (Melaleuca leucodendra and Melaleuca quinquenervia).

NORTHERN PRICKLY ASH

Also Known As
Angelica Tree, Pepper Wood, Prickly Ash, Toothache Bark, Xanthoxylum, Yellow Wood, Zanthoxylum.
CAUTION: See separate listings for Ash and Southern Prickly Ash.

Scientific Names
Zanthoxylum americanum.
Family: Rutaceae.

People Use This For
Orally, northern prickly ash is used for cramps, intermittent claudication, Raynaud's syndrome, chronic rheumatic conditions, peripheral circulatory insufficiency associated with rheumatic symptoms, for low blood pressure, fever, inflammation, as a tonic, stimulant, for toothache, sores, ulcers, as a diaphoretic in fever, and cancer (as an ingredient in Hoxsey cure).
In manufacturing, northern prickly ash is used as a flavoring agent in foods and beverages.

Safety
POSSIBLY SAFE ...when the bark is used orally and appropriately in medicinal amounts (12).
There is insufficient reliable information available about the safety of the oral use of northern prickly ash berry.
PREGNANCY: POSSIBLY UNSAFE ...when the bark is used orally (12); avoid using. There is insufficient reliable information available about the safety of the berry during pregnancy; avoid using.
LACTATION: insufficient reliable information available; avoid using.

Effectiveness
There is insufficient reliable information available about the effectiveness of northern prickly ash.

Mechanism of Action
The applicable parts of northern prickly ash are the bark and berry. There is insufficient reliable information available about the possible mechanism of action and active ingredients. Northern prickley ash contains alkaloids, coumarins, resin, acid volatile oil, and tannins, which may be pharmacologically active (4).

Adverse Reactions
None reported.

Interactions with Herbs & Other Dietary Supplements
HERBS WITH ANTICOAGULANT/ANTIPLATELET POTENTIAL: Concomitant use of herbs that have constituents that might affect platelet aggregation could theoretically increase the risk of bleeding in some people. These herbs include angelica, danshen, garlic, ginger, ginkgo, Panax ginseng, horse chestnut, red clover, turmeric, and others.

Interactions with Drugs
ANTACIDS: Theoretically, due to reports that northern prickly ash increases stomach acid, northern prickly ash might decrease the effectiveness of antacids (19).
H2-BLOCKERS: Theoretically, due to reports that northern prickly ash increases stomach acid, northern prickly ash might decrease the effectiveness of H2-blockers (19). The H2 blockers include cimetidine (Tagamet), ranitidine (Zantac), nizatidine (Axid), and famotidine (Pepcid).
PROTON PUMP INHIBITORS (PPIs): Theoretically, due to reports that northern prickly ash increases stomach acid, northern prickly ash might decrease the effectiveness of PPIs (19). PPIs include omeprazole (Prilosec), lansoprazole (Prevacid), rabeprazole (Aciphex), pantoprazole (Protonix), and esomeprazole (Nexium).

Interactions with Foods
None known.

Interactions with Lab Tests
None known.

Interactions with Diseases or Conditions
GASTROINTESTINAL ULCERS: Contraindicated. Northern prickly ash can stimulate gastrointestinal secretions (19).
GI CONDITIONS: Northern prickly ash can irritate the gastrointestinal tract. It is contraindicated in individuals with infectious or inflammatory gastrointestinal conditions (19).

Dosage and Administration

ORAL, Bark: 1-3 grams dried bark, or drink as decoction (boil 1-3 grams dry bark 10-15 minutes, strain), three times daily; liquid bark extract (1:1 in 45% alcohol) 1-3 mL three times daily; bark tincture (1:5 in 45% alcohol) 2-5 mL three times daily (4).
ORAL, Berry: Liquid berry extract (1:1 in 45% alcohol) 0.5-1.5 mL (4).

NUTMEG AND MACE

Also Known As

Jaatipatree, Jatikosha, Jatipatra, Jatipatri, Jatiphala, Jatiphalam, Mace, Macis, Muscadier, Muskatbuam, Muskatnuss, Myristica, Myristicae Aril, Myristicae Semen, Noix Muscade, Nuez Moscada, Nutmeg, Nux Moschata.

Scientific Names

Myristica fragrans, synonym Myristica officinalis.
Family: Myristicaceae.

People Use This For

Orally, nutmeg and mace are used for diarrhea, nausea, gastric spasms, flatulence, and gastric mucosal inflammation. They are also used for cancer, kidney disease, insomnia, increasing menstrual flow, inducing abortion, as a hallucinogen, and a general tonic.
Topically, nutmeg and mace are used as an analgesic, especially for rheumatism, mouth sores, and toothache.
In foods, nutmeg and mace are used as culinary spices. In foods and beverages, nutmeg, nutmeg oil, mace, and mace oil are used as flavor components.
In manufacturing, nutmeg oil is used as a fragrance component in soaps and cosmetics.

Safety

LIKELY SAFE ...when used orally in amounts commonly found in foods. Nutmeg, mace, nutmeg oil and mace oil have Generally Recognized As Safe (GRAS) status in the US (4912).
LIKELY UNSAFE ...when used orally for self-medication in medicinal amounts (12). There is insufficient reliable information available about the safety of the topical use of nutmeg and mace.
PREGNANCY: POSSIBLY UNSAFE ...when used orally in medicinal amounts. Nutmeg and mace might have abortifacient activity, and safrole content might be mutagenic (12).
LACTATION: There is insufficient reliable information available about the safety of nutmeg and mace during lactation; avoid using.

Effectiveness

There is insufficient reliable information available for the effectiveness of nutmeg and mace.

Mechanism of Action

Both nutmeg and mace contain volatile oils with constituents that include myristicin, elemicin, eugenol, isoeugenol, gerinol, pinese, cineole, borneol, and safrole (2563). Volatile oil constituents of nutmeg and mace have a variety of individual pharmacological effects, some of which oppose others. For example, the volatile oil borneol is thought to be responsible for CNS stimulant effects, whereas several others such as methyleugenol, isoeugenol, safrole, myristicin, 1,8-cineole, geranyl acetate, and 1,8-p-methadiene seem to have sedative effects (2563). Alpha- and beta-pinene, and 1,8-cineole seem to have convulsant activity, whereas safrole, eugenol, and methyleugenol have anticonvulsant activity (2563). Nutmeg also has psychoactive effects and can cause hallucinations, feelings of unreality, euphoria, and delusions (2563). The constituents myristicin and elemicin are thought to be metabolized to amphetamine-related compounds (6), but this has not yet been verified (2563). Myristicin and elemicin might also have effects on serotonergic systems and possibly have an antidepressant effect (2563). Some constituents have anesthetic activity such as myristicin, methyleugenol, methylisoeugenol, safrole, and 1,8-cineole (2563). Antihistaminic effects have been found with elemicin and methylisoeugenol (2563). High doses of nutmeg can cause anticholinergic side effects, but the constituents 1,8-cineole and alpha-terpinene are reported to have anticholinesterase activity (2563). Nutmeg and mace and their oils have a variety of other effects including antispasmodic (2,6), antioxidant (11), hypotensive (2563), emetic (6), antibacterial, antifungal (6) and larvicidal effects (11). Calcium antagonist activity has been reported with myristicin, eugenol, and safrole (2563). Myristicin, eugenol, and isoeugenol inhibit prostaglandin activity and might have anti-inflammatory properties (6). Safrole found in nutmeg oil promotes liver carcinomas in mice (6). Animal studies suggest myristicin acts as an inducer of cytochrome P-450 enzyme systems (3492,3493) and may inhibit tumor formation (3492).

Adverse Reactions

Orally, nutmeg and mace can cause significant side effects when used in amounts greater than those found in foods. Anticholinergic effects can occur with doses of 9 teaspoons of nutmeg powder such as flushing, tachycardia, and dry mouth (2563). Higher doses can cause more significant side effects. For example, ingestion of 5 grams or more of

powdered nutmeg or mace can cause thirst, dry mouth, nausea and vomiting, burning epigastric pain, urgency, weak pulse, tachycardia, hypotension, flushing, feeling of pressure in the chest or lower abdomen, hot and cold sensations, sweating, hypothermia, dizziness, blurred vision, double and triple vision, miosis, nystagmus, headache, numbness, weakness, unsteady gait, drowsiness, stupor, disorientation, euphoria, anxiety, panic, mild to intense visual hallucinations, often with sensation of limb loss and fear of impending death, auditory hallucinations, agitation, hyperactivity, aimless wandering, incoherent and irrelevant speech, combativeness, seizures, shock, coma, and occasionally death (9,12,2492,2563,3492,3494). Many of these symptoms are attributed to excessive anticholinergic activity. Symptoms generally occur 2-6 hours after ingestion and recovery usually occurs within 24 hours, but can take several days, depending on the dose used (3492).
In pregnant women, large amounts can also cause abortion (2).
Topically, nutmeg can cause allergic dermatitis (6,18).

Interactions with Herbs & Other Dietary Supplements

SAFROLE-CONTAINING HERBS: Avoid concomitant use with other safrole-containing herbs due to potential for additive toxicity (12). Other herbs that contain safrole include basil, camphor, and cinnamon (12).

Interactions with Drugs

CYTOCHROME P450 1A1 (CYP1A1) SUBSTRATES: Theoretically, concomitant use may affect drugs metabolized by cytochrome P450 1A1(CYP1A1) enzyme system (3493). Some of these drugs include chlorzoxazone, theophylline, and bufuralol.
CYTOCHROME P450 1A2 (CYP1A2) SUBSTRATES: Theoretically, concomitant use may affect drugs metabolized by cytochrome P450 1A2 (CYP1A2) enzyme system (3493).
CYTOCHROME P450 2B1 (CYP2B1) SUBSTRATES: Theoretically, concomitant use may affect drugs metabolized by cytochrome P450 2B1 (CPY2B1) enzyme system (3493).
CYTOCHROME P450 2B2 (CYP2B2) SUBSTRATES: Theoretically, concomitant use may affect drugs metabolized by cytochrome P450 2B2 (CYP2B2) enzyme system (3493).
PHENOBARBITAL (Luminal): Theoretically, concomitant use may decrease the therapeutic effects of phenobarbital (3492). Studies suggest myristicin, a constituent of nutmeg and mace, acts as an inducer of cytochrome P450 enzyme systems (3492,3493).

Interactions with Foods

None known.

Interactions with Lab Tests

None known.

Interactions with Diseases or Conditions

None known.

Dosage and Administration

ORAL: Typical dose for antiflatulent effect is 0.03 mL nutmeg oil (17). For nausea, gastric upset, or chronic diarrhea, the common dose is 3-5 drops of the essential oil on a sugar lump or in honey (6002). For diarrhea, 4-6 tablespoons of the powder has been used daily (6002).
TOPICAL: For toothache, 1 to 2 drops of essential oil are applied to the surrounding gum (6002).

Comments

Nutmeg is the shelled, dried seed of Myristica fragrans (11). Nutmeg oil is distilled from worm-eaten nutmeg seeds; the worms remove much of the starch and fat leaving portions of the seed rich in volatile oil (11). Mace is the dried aril (netlike covering) surrounding the shell of the seed of Myristica fragrans (11). Ingestion of 5-20 grams of nutmeg powder (1-3 whole seeds) might cause psychoactive effects (6). Because nutmeg and mace are so similar, high doses of mace might also have psychoactive effects but as yet this has not been proven (6).

NUX VOMICA

Also Known As

Brechnusssamen, Poison Nut, Quaker Buttons, Shudha Kupilu, Strychni Semen, Strychnos Seed, Vishamushti.

Scientific Names

Strychnos nux-vomica.
Family: Loganiaceae.

People Use This For

Orally, nux vomica is used for impotence and for glycine encephalopathy. It is also used in combination for diseases of the gastrointestinal tract, organic and functional disorders of the heart and circulatory system, diseases of the eye, nervous conditions, depression, migraine, climacteric complaints, facial neuralgias (Sympatalgien), and Raynaud's disease. Nux vomica is also used as an oral tonic and as an appetite-stimulant. It is also used for diseases of the respiratory tract, anemia, and geriatric complaints.

Nux vomica contains strychnine and brucine and has, therefore, been used in manufacturing. It is used as a rodenticide.

Safety

UNSAFE ...when used orally (2,13,18,505). Nux vomica in doses of 30-50 mg contains approximately 5 mg of strychnine, and can cause severe adverse effects. 1-2 grams of nux vomica contains 60-90 mg of strychnine, and can be fatal (13,18). Chronic ingestion of lesser amounts can cause death after a period of weeks (18).

PREGNANCY AND LACTATION: UNSAFE ...when used orally (2,13,18,505); avoid using.

Effectiveness

There is insufficient reliable information available about the effectiveness of nux vomica.

Mechanism of Action

The applicable part of nux vomica is the seed. Nux vomica contains strychnine and brucine (13). These are centrally-acting neurotoxins. Strychnine competitively antagonizes post-synaptic binding of the inhibitory transmitter glycine, which leads to heightened reflex excitability of muscles. External irritations or centrally-acting stimulants can trigger convulsions (2,505). Nux vomica can selectively inhibit the spinal cord in subconvulsive amounts (2). However, strychnine accumulates with extended administration, particularly in individuals with liver damage (2). Chronic use of subconvulsive amounts can cause death after a period of weeks (18). Strychnine causes convulsions by leading to a full contraction of all voluntary muscles. Death is secondary to impaired respiration or exhaustion (13,18,505).

Adverse Reactions

Orally, 30-50 mg nux vomica (5 mg strychnine) can cause restlessness, feelings of anxiety, heightening of sense perception, enhanced reflexes, equilibrium disorders, painful neck and back stiffness, followed later by twitching, tonic spasms of jaw and neck muscles, painful convulsions of the entire body triggered by visual or tactile stimulation with possible opisthotonos, muscle hypertonicity and agitation. Dyspnea may follow spasm of the respiratory muscles (18). Seizures occur within 15 minutes of ingestion (or 5 minutes of inhalation) and may result in hyperthermia, metabolic and respiratory acidosis, rhabdomyolysis, and myoglobinuric renal failure (17). 1-2 grams of nux vomica (60-90 mg strychnine) can be fatal (13,505); most deaths occur 3-6 hours post-ingestion from respiratory and subsequent cardiac arrest, anoxic brain damage, or multiple organ failure secondary to hyperthermia (18,505). Strychnine accumulates with extended administration, particularly in individuals with liver damage (2). Chronic use of subconvulsive amounts can cause death after a period of weeks (18).

Interactions with Herbs & Other Dietary Supplements

None known.

Interactions with Drugs

None known.

Interactions with Foods

None known.

Interactions with Lab Tests

None known.

Interactions with Diseases or Conditions

LIVER DISEASE: Contraindicated. Strychnine accumulates in individuals with liver damage (2). Also, strychnine accumulation can cause liver damage (18).

Dosage and Administration

Toxic, avoid using.

Comments

Strychnine may be detected by thin-layer chromatography (qualitative analysis) and high performance liquid chromatography (quantitative analysis). Urine and gastric aspirate are most useful in confirming poisoning (17).

Nux vomica powder may be confused with the powder of date nuts, olive stones, and by-products of stone-nut processing (18).

OAK bark

Also Known As
Common Oak, Durmast Oak, Eichenrinde, English Oak, Pedunculate Oak, Quercus cortex, Sessile Oak, Stave Oak, Stone Oak, Tanner's Bark, Tanner's Oak.

Scientific Names
Quercus robur, synonym Quercus pedunculata; Quercus petraea, synonym Quercus sessiliflora; Quercus alba.
Family: Fagaceae.

People Use This For
Orally, oak bark is used for diarrhea, colds, fever, cough and bronchitis, and for stimulating appetite and improving digestion.
Topically, oak bark is used for inflammatory skin conditions; mild inflammation of the mouth, throat, genital, and anal region; and for chilblains.

Safety
POSSIBLY SAFE ...when used orally (2,12) for up to 3-4 days for treating diarrhea (7). ...when used topically up to 2-3 weeks on intact skin (2).
LIKELY UNSAFE ...when used topically on extensive areas of damaged skin or for longer than 2-3 weeks (2).
PREGNANCY AND LACTATION: Insufficient reliable information available; avoid using.

Effectiveness
There is insufficient reliable information about the effectiveness of oak bark.

Mechanism of Action
Oak bark contains 8-20% tannins, including gallotannins (7,8). Gallotannins are extensively hydrolyzed in the upper small intestine and are unlikely to produce astringent activity in the colon (7,3901). Some studies suggest tannins might have antiviral and antimicrobial effects, and CNS depressant and cariostatic effects (11). Other studies suggest they can depress growth. Tannins exert an astringent effect on mucosal tissue. This effect dehydrates the tissue, internally reducing secretions, and externally forming a protective layer of harder, constricted cells (12). Plants with at least 10% tannins can cause gastrointestinal disturbances, kidney damage, and necrotic conditions of the liver (12). Some evidence suggests that tannins might cause cancer. Others information suggests they might prevent it (12). Regular consumption of herbs with high tannin concentrations correlates to an increased incidence of esophageal or nasal cancer (12).

Adverse Reactions
Orally, oak bark can cause gastrointestinal disturbances, kidney damage, and necrotic conditions of the liver (12).

Interactions with Herbs & Other Dietary Supplements
IRON: Theoretically, concomitant administration might precipitate iron salts due to tannin content (19).
TANNIN-CONTAINING HERBS: Theoretically, herbs that contain high percentages of tannins such as oak bark may cause precipitation of alkaloids and other constituents of herbs (19).

Interactions with Drugs
None known.

Interactions with Foods
None known.

Interactions with Lab Tests
None known.

Interactions with Diseases or Conditions
CARDIAC CONDITIONS: Oak bark baths are contraindicated in individuals with cardiac insufficiency (2).
ECZEMA: Oak bark baths are contraindicated in individuals with weeping eczema or large areas of skin damage (2).
HYPERTONIA: Oak bark baths are contraindicated in individuals with hypertonia (2).
INFECTION: Oak bark baths are contraindicated in individuals with febrile or infectious diseases (2).
KIDNEY DYSFUNCTION: Theoretically, oral use of oak bark might worsen kidney dysfunction (12).
LIVER DYSFUNCTION: Theoretically, oral use of oak bark might worsen liver dysfunction (12).

Dosage and Administration
ORAL: A typical dose of oak bark for diarrhea is one cup tea up to three times a day for up to 3-4 days. To make tea, add 1 gram coarsely powdered bark to 150 mL cold water, boil for a short period of time, strain (8).

TOPICAL: For rinses, compresses, poultices, and gargles, prepare with 20 grams bark in 1 L of water (18). For baths, prepare with 5 grams of bark in 1 L of water, added to bath water (18). Oak bark should not be used topically longer than 2-3 weeks (2).

OAK MOSS

Also Known As

Lichen Oak Moss, Tree Moss.
CAUTION: See separate listing for Usnea.

Scientific Names

Evernia prunastri.
Family: Usneaceae.

People Use This For

Orally, oak moss is used as an intestinal tonic.
In manufacturing, it is used as a fragrance component in perfumes.

Safety

POSSIBLY SAFE ...when used orally in prepared teas or aqueous forms for short periods of time (12). Although water extracts of oak moss contain the constituent thujone that is known to cause adverse effects, the amount of thujone is low (2).
LIKELY UNSAFE ...when used orally long-term, in large amounts of tea, or as a hot alcoholic extract (12) because enough thujone might be consumed to cause renal damage (4,12).
There is insufficient reliable information available about the safety of oak moss for its other uses.
PREGNANCY AND LACTATION: POSSIBLY UNSAFE ...when used orally. The constituent thujone shows evidence of uterine stimulant activity (19).

Effectiveness

There is insufficient reliable information available about the effectiveness of oak moss.

Mechanism of Action

Oak moss contains thujone, a ketone that shows evidence of neurotoxicity. Thujone intoxication causes psychoactivity resembling that of cannabinoid intoxication (12). Some data suggest thujone-containing volatile oils have uterine stimulant effects (19). Other information suggests thujone might exacerbate liver conditions, e.g., porphyria (12).

Adverse Reactions

Orally, large amounts or long-term use of thujone-containing products can cause restlessness, vomiting, vertigo, tremors, renal damage, and convulsions (12).
Topically, use of oak moss can cause contact sensitivity (4034,4039) and allergic reaction in people with lichen and moss allergy (4023,4033).

Interactions with Herbs & Other Dietary Supplements

THUJONE CONTAINING HERBS: Avoid; concomitant use may increase the risk of thujone toxicity. Thujone-containing herbs include oriental arborvitae, sage, tansy, thuja (cedar), tree moss, and wormwood (2,4,11,12).

Interactions with Drugs

None known.

Interactions with Foods

None known.

Interactions with Lab Tests

None known.

Interactions with Diseases or Conditions

CROSS-ALLERGENICITY: Oak moss may cause reaction in people allergic to lichens and mosses (4023,4033).
PORPHYRIA: Oak moss may exacerbate porphyria in patients with underlying defects in hepatic heme synthesis (12).
RENAL DYSFUNCTION: Oak moss may exacerbate renal dysfunction (12).

Dosage and Administration

No typical dosage.

Comments

Avoid confusing oak moss (Evernia prunastri) with other usnea species. Many, including oak moss, are referred to as tree moss.

OATS

Also Known As

Avena Fructus, Avenae herba, Avenae stramentum, Cereal Fiber, Dietary Fiber, Groats, Oat Bran, Oat Straw, Oatmeal, Whole Oats, Wild Oat Herb, Straw.
CAUTION: See separate listings for Beta-Glucans and Wheat Bran.

Scientific Names

Avena sativa, synonyms Avena byzantina, Avena orientalis, Avena volgensis.
Family: Poaceae/Gramineae.

People Use This For

Orally, oat bran and whole oats are used for hypercholesterolemia, diabetes, gallstones, irritable bowel syndrome (IBS), diverticulosis, inflammatory bowel disease (IBD), hypertension, and preventing colon cancer and gastric cancer. Oats are also used for constipation, diarrhea, rheumatism, fat redistribution syndrome, fatigue, neurasthenia syndrome, opioid and nicotine withdrawal, and lowering uric acid levels. Oats are also used for acute or chronic anxiety, excitation and stress, weak bladder, connective tissue disorders, gout, kidney ailments, skin diseases, and as a tonic. Oat straw is used for the flu, coughs, abdominal fatigue, bladder and rheumatic disorders, eye ailments, frostbite, gout, impetigo, and metabolic diseases.
Topically, oats are used for skin injury, pruritus, seborrhea, dry and itchy skin, weeping eczema, contact dermatitis, chickenpox, osteoarthritis, liver disorders, and in foot baths for chronically cold or tired feet.
In foods, oats are used as a grain or cereal.
In manufacturing, oats are a component of bath products and soaps.

Safety

LIKELY SAFE ...when used orally and appropriately (4960,4969,5792,5797). Oat bran has Generally Recognized As Safe (GRAS) status in the US (4912).
POSSIBLY SAFE ...when used topically and appropriately (12).
PREGNANCY AND LACTATION: LIKELY SAFE ...when used orally (5792,5797).

Effectiveness

LIKELY EFFECTIVE

Cardiovascular disease. A diet that includes foods high in fiber, such as oat bran, reduces the risk of heart disease and death from cardiovascular disease when consumed as part of a diet low in saturated fat and cholesterol (2737,4960,4962,4963,4964,4965,4966,4967,4968).
Hypercholesterolemia. Oats, oat bran, and other soluble fibers can modestly reduce total and low-density lipoprotein (LDL) cholesterol when consumed as part of a diet low in saturated fat. Consuming 56-150 grams of whole oat products such as oatmeal and oat bran, containing 3.6-10 grams of soluble fiber, can significantly lower total and low density lipoprotein (LDL) cholesterol levels 1.42 mg/dL (0.037 mmol/L) and 1.23 mg/dL (0.032 mmol/L) respectively per gram of soluble fiber (5786,5787,5788,5792,5794,5795,5796,8521); however, doses of soluble fiber greater than 10 grams/ day don't seem to increase effectiveness (5788).
Eating three bowls of oatmeal (28 gram servings) daily can decrease total cholesterol by about 5 mg/dL (4972,4973,4974,4975,4976,4977,5786,5788,6188). Oat bran products (oat bran muffins, oat bran flakes, oat bran Os, etc.) may vary in their ability to lower cholesterol, depending on the total soluble fiber content and other dietary variables (6188). Whole oat products might be more effective in lowering LDL and total cholesterol than foods containing oat bran plus beta-glucan soluble fiber (10145).

POSSIBLY EFFECTIVE

Diabetes. Consuming oats and oat bran for 6 weeks significantly decreases preprandial blood glucose, 24-hour plasma glucose, and insulin levels in people with type 2 diabetes (4980,4982,6266). There is some evidence that consuming 50 grams daily, containing 25 grams of soluble fiber, might be more effective than the moderate fiber diet of 24 grams daily recommended by the American Diabetes Association (ADA).
Gastric cancer. Epidemiologic evidence suggests that consuming a diet that includes dietary cereal fiber, including oats and oat bran, might reduce the incidence of stomach cancer (10435).

POSSIBLY INEFFECTIVE

Colorectal cancer. Consuming oat bran or oats orally doesn't seem to reduce the risk of colon cancer. Fiber, including oat-bran fiber, does not prevent the recurrence of colorectal adenomas (4820,5104).
Hypertension. Consumption of oats as oat meal and oat cereal does not seem to reduce diastolic or systolic blood pressure in men with minor elevations in blood pressure (2956).

INSUFFICIENT RELIABLE EVIDENCE to RATE

Fat redistribution syndrome. Consumption of a high fiber diet, including oats, with adequate energy and protein might prevent fat deposition in patients with HIV. A one-gram increase in total dietary fiber may decrease the risk of fat deposition by 7% (12517). More evidence is needed to rate oats for this use.

Mechanism of Action

The applicable parts of oats are the seeds, straw, and bran. Oat bran is milled from the outer layer of hulled whole oats. Oats consumed as part of the diet are a good source of protein, fat, and fiber. Oats contain both soluble and insoluble fiber, but a greater proportion of soluble fiber than any other grain (4960,4961,4963,4970).

Oat bran decreases serum cholesterol, decreases absorption of cholesterol or fatty acids, and decreases absorption of biliary cholesterol or bile acids (4974,4960,4963).

Oats contain beta-glucan, also known as oat gum, a water soluble polysaccharide fiber (4961,4981). Beta-glucan is thought to be responsible for the cholesterol-lowering effects of oats. Soluble fibers, such as beta-glucan, lower cholesterol levels by binding with bile acids in the gut and increasing fecal bile acid excretion (4974,5786,5787,5789). This decreases enterohepatic circulation of bile acids, which increases hepatic conversion of cholesterol to bile acids, increases up-regulation of low-density lipoprotein (LDL)-receptors, and increases clearance of LDL cholesterol (4984,5786,5787).

Beta-glucan might also decrease cholesterol absorption by inhibiting the formation of micelles, which are necessary for fat absorption (5786). There is also some evidence that soluble fibers, such as beta-glucan, ferment to short-chain fatty acids in the gut, including acetate, propionate, and butyrate. Absorption of these short-chain fatty acids might inhibit cholesterol synthesis in the liver (5786,5787,5788).

Beta-glucan, increases the viscosity of food in the small intestine and delays absorption, thereby reducing peak postprandial plasma glucose and insulin levels both in people with and without diabetes (4961,4980,4981,4982,4983,5796). Beta-glucan might help control appetite by slowing stomach emptying, prolonging the feeling of fullness and stabilizing blood sugar (11135). Because of the high fiber content, oats can increase stool weight and accelerate colonic transit time (12513).

Although earlier studies did not differentiate between types of fiber (5105,5106,5108), later studies indicate that oat bran, unlike wheat bran, does not protect against colon cancer (5104,5107).

Oats also contain alpha-tocotrienols, an isomer of vitamin E. There is some preliminary evidence that alpha-tocotrienols can inhibit hepatic hydroxymethylglutaryl coenzyme A (HMG-CoA) reductase, which is the rate-limiting enzyme required for cholesterol synthesis (5786).

Adverse Reactions

Orally, oats are usually very well tolerated. Increasing fiber in the diet can cause flatulence, bloating, abdominal distention, and unpleasant taste. To minimize side effects, doses should be slowly titrated to the desired level. Adverse effects usually subside with continued use (12514). Oat bran may cause bezoars (concretions) and intestinal obstruction, especially in people who have difficulty chewing or swallowing food, or have conditions that decrease small bowel motility (4979,4985,12550).

Topically, oat-containing preparations can cause contact dermatitis in some patients (12515).

Interactions with Herbs & Other Dietary Supplements

None known.

Interactions with Drugs

MORPHINE: Theoretically, concomitant use of oats and morphine might antagonize morphine (19).

Interactions with Foods

None known.

Interactions with Lab Tests

BLOOD GLUCOSE: Oat bran lowers postprandial blood glucose and test results (4961).

CHOLESTEROL: Oat bran lowers blood levels total and low density lipoprotein (LDL) cholesterol and test results (5788).

INSULIN: Oat bran lowers postprandial insulin levels and test results (4961).

Interactions with Diseases or Conditions

CELIAC DISEASE: Oats and oat bran have been excluded from gluten-free diets. However, oat products that are not contaminated with wheat, rye, or barley do not appear to cause adverse effects in nutrition, intestinal histology, or serology in adults with celiac disease in remission (12516).

GASTROINTESTINAL (GI) DYSFUNCTION: Oats and oat bran can cause GI obstruction, particularly in people who have difficulty chewing or swallowing food or have conditions that decrease small bowel motility (4979,4985,12550).

Dosage and Administration

ORAL: For hypercholesterolemia, 56-150 grams of whole oat products such as oat bran or oatmeal, containing 3.6-10 grams of soluble fiber, is used daily as part of a low-fat diet (5786,5787,5788,5792,5794,5795,5796,10145). For lowering blood glucose levels in patients with type 2 diabetes, high fiber foods such as whole oat products containing 25 grams of soluble fiber are used daily (6266). 38 grams of oat bran or 75 grams of dry oatmeal contains about 3 grams of beta-glucan (4961,5788). Traditionally milky oat pods are also used as a tincture and tea.
TOPICAL: No typical dosage.

Comments

Current FDA regulations and guidelines allow food products containing whole oats to be labeled with the health claim that the product may reduce the risk of heart disease if they contain at least 750 mg of soluble fiber per serving, when included as part of a diet low in saturated fat and cholesterol (5792,5797). The FDA also recommends that approximately 3 grams of soluble fiber taken daily is needed to lower blood cholesterol levels (5792,5797); however, evidence from controlled clinical studies show at least 3.6 grams of soluble fiber daily is needed (5786,5787,5788,5794,5795,5796).

OCTACOSANOL

Also Known As

Hexacosanol (26-C), Tetracosanol (24-C), Triacontanol (30-C).
CAUTION: See separate listing for Policosanol.

Scientific Names

1-Octacosanol; N-octacosanol; Octacosyl alcohol.

People Use This For

Orally, octacosanol is used for exercise performance including strength, stamina and reaction time; for herpes; inflammatory skin diseases; Parkinson's disease; amyotrophic lateral sclerosis (ALS, Lou Gehrig's disease); hyperlipidemia; and atherosclerosis.

Safety

There is insufficient reliable information available about the safety of octacosanol.
Pregnancy and Lactation: Insufficient reliable information available; avoid using.

Effectiveness

INSUFFICIENT RELIABLE EVIDENCE to RATE

Amyotrophic lateral sclerosis (ALS, Lou Gehrig's disease). Preliminary evidence suggests that octacosanol does not improve objective symptoms of ALS (12156).

Parkinson's disease. Preliminary evidence suggests that some patients with Parkinson's disease who take octacosanol might have improved symptoms (11901).

More evidence is needed to rate octacosanol for these uses.

Mechanism of Action

Octacosanol is a 28-carbon alcohol that can be extracted from a variety of plant sources including sugar cane and wheat germ oil. It is related in structure to vitamin E. Octacosanol products are sometimes a mixture of 24- to 36-carbon alcohols, including tetracosanol (24-C), hexacosanol (26-C), and triacontanol (30-C). Octacosanol is not a normal component of the diet (12156).

It is hypothesized that octacosanol could improve oxygen utilization during anaerobic glycolysis and aid in lactic acid removal by increasing the efficiency of the tricarboxylic acid cycle (17).

In rats, octacosanol suppresses lipid accumulation in adipose tissue and increases the mobilization of free fatty acids from the fat cells in muscle (2924,2925).

There is interest in using octacosanol for various central nervous system disorders. Even though octacosanol is not a typical component of the diet, it is present in the central nervous system (12156).

Adverse Reactions

None reported.

Interactions with Herbs & Other Dietary Supplements

None known.

Interactions with Drugs

LEVODOPA/CARBIDOPA (Sinemet): Octacosanol might worsen dyskinesias and increase nervous tension in patients being treated with levodopa/carbidopa (11901).

Interactions with Foods
None known.

Interactions with Lab Tests
None known.

Interactions with Diseases or Conditions
PARKINSON'S DISEASE: Octacosanol might worsen dyskinesias associated with the levodopa/carbidopa treatment of Parkinson's disease (11901).

Dosage and Administration
ORAL: For Parkinson's disease, the typical dose of octacosanol is 5 mg three times a day with meals (11901). For amyotrophic lateral sclerosis (ALS, Lou Gehrig's disease), the usual dose is 40 mg per day (2921,12156).

Comments
Avoid confusion with policosanol.

OLEANDER

Also Known As
Common Oleander, Oleanderblatter, Oleandri folium, Rose Bay, Rose Laurel, Yellow Oleander.

Scientific Names
Nerium oleander, synonyms Nerium indicum, Nerium odorum; Thevetia peruviana, synonyms Cascabela thevetia, Cerbera thevetia, Thevetia neriifolia.
Family: Apocynaceae.

People Use This For
Orally, oleander is used for cardiac conditions, asthma, epilepsy, cancer, dysmenorrhea, eprosy, malaria, ringworm, indigestion, venereal disease, and as an abortifacient. A fixed combination of oleander leaf powdered extract, pheasant's eye fluid extract, lily-of-the-valley fluid extract, and squill powdered extract has been used for treating mild limited heart failure with circulatory instability.
Topically, oleander is used to treat skin eruptions and warts.

Safety
LIKELY UNSAFE ...when used orally. Ingestion of oleander leaf, oleander leaf tea, and oleander seeds has led to fatal poisonings (9,3495).
There is insufficient reliable information available about the safety of the topical use of oleander.
PREGNANCY AND LACTATION: LIKELY UNSAFE ...when used orally. Oleander has been reported to have abortifacient properties (5000). There is insufficient reliable information available about the safety of topical use of oleander during pregnancy and lactation; avoid using.

Effectiveness
There is insufficient reliable information available about the effectiveness of oleander.

Mechanism of Action
All parts of the oleander plant contain the cardiac glycosides oleandrin, oleandroside, nerioside, digitoxigenin, which have positive inotropic and negative chronotropic actions (3495). They bind to sodium- and potassium-sensitive membrane-bound enzymes called ATPases and inhibit enzyme activities, resulting in increased intracellular sodium ions and calcium ions and increased extracellular potassium levels (3477,5000). At toxic levels, the sodium and calcium ions depolarize the cell after repolarization, causing late afterdepolarization and increased automaticity. Severe toxicity produces bradycardia and heart block (3477). Oleander leaf also contains other biologically active constituents that have antimitotic and insecticidal properties (5000). Oleander is also reported to have emetogenic, cathartic, insecticidic, parasiticidic, anthelmintic, menstrual stimulant, and abortifacient activities (6002).

Adverse Reactions
Orally, oleander can cause bitter taste, burning sensation in mouth, nausea, vomiting, diarrhea, weakness, headache, stupor (17,18,3495), mucus membrane irritation, increased salivation, abdominal pain, buccal erythema, visual disturbances, mydriasis, peripheral neuritis (3495,5000), malignant dysrhythmias, ventricular ectopy, cardiovascular collapse, cardiac arrest (17), hyperkalemia (2532,3495) and death (3495). Oleander poisoning resembles digitoxin poisoning. Predominant symptoms are nausea and vomiting (onset in several hours), and cardiac toxicity, with conduction delays lasting for 3-6 days (17). Yellow oleander toxicity has been reported to be reversed with anti-digoxin Fab fragments. The majority of patients with yellow oleander toxicity who received anti-digoxin Fab

fragments converted from an oleander-induced arrhythmia to normal sinus rhythm within 8 hours. A dose of 800 mg anti-digoxin Fab fragments was used intravenously. Associated hyperkalemia reversed within the first two hours (2532). A recurrence of arrhythmia can occur 48 hours post-exposure from any seed fragments remaining in the gastrointestinal tract (2532).

Interactions with Herbs & Other Dietary Supplements

CALCIUM: Calcium supplements may enhance the therapeutic effects of oleander (18).
CARDIAC GLYCOSIDE-CONTAINING HERBS: Contraindicated, and concomitant use can increase the risk of cardiac glycoside toxicity. Cardiac glycoside-containing herbs include black hellebore, Canadian hemp roots, digitalis leaf, hedge mustard, figwort, lily-of-the-valley roots, motherwort, pheasant's eye plant, pleurisy root, squill bulb leaf scales, strophanthus seeds, and uzara (19).
LICORICE/HORSETAIL: Theoretically, overuse/misuse of licorice rhizome or horsetail plant with cardiac glycoside-containing herbs increases the risk of cardiac toxicity due to potassium depletion (19).
OTHER CARDIOACTIVE HERBS: Avoid concomitant use with other cardioactive herbs due to unpredictability of effects (4).
STIMULANT LAXATIVE HERBS: Theoretically, overuse or misuse of stimulant laxatives with cardiac glycoside-containing herbs increases the risk of cardiac toxicity due to potassium depletion (19).

Interactions with Drugs

CALCIUM SUPPLEMENTS: Calcium salts may enhance the therapeutic effects of oleander (18).
DIGOXIN (Lanoxin): Contraindicated; therapeutic duplication increases risk of cardiac glycoside toxicity (2).
DIURETIC DRUGS: Theoretically, concomitant use of potassium depleting diuretics and oleander can increase the risk of cardiac glycoside toxicity due to potassium depletion (506). Some diuretics that can deplete potassium include chlorothiazide (Diuril), chlorthalidone (Thalitone), furosemide (Lasix), hydrochlorothiazide (HCTZ, Hydrodiuril, Microzide), and others.
MACROLIDE ANTIBIOTICS: Theoretically, concomitant use may increase risk of cardiac glycoside toxicity (17).
QUININE: Theoretically, concomitant use of quinine and oleander may increase the risk of cardiac toxicity (506).
STIMULANT LAXATIVES: Theoretically, overuse or misuse or stimulant laxatives may increase the risk of cardiac glycoside toxicity due to potassium depletion (2).
TETRACYCLINE ANTIBIOTICS: Theoretically, concomitant use may increase risk of cardiac glycoside toxicity (17).

Interactions with Foods

None known.

Interactions with Lab Tests

None known.

Interactions with Diseases or Conditions

ELECTROLYTE IMBALANCE: Theoretically, based on digitalis glycosides (15), contraindicated in individuals with potassium deficiency states and hypercalcemia.
HEART DISEASE: Self-use contraindicated; requires diagnosis, treatment, and monitoring (515).

Dosage and Administration

No typical dosage.

Comments

The annual incidence of oleander poisoning in Sri Lanka exceeds 150 per 100,000. Approximately 10% of these ingestions are fatal (2532). Abbott TDx Digoxin II assay can be used for rapid confirmation of the ingestion of oleander (17).

OLIVE

Also Known As

Extra Virgin Olive Oil, Green Olive, Monounsaturated Fatty Acid, n-9 Fatty Acid, Oleae Folium, Olivae Oleum, Omega-9 Fatty Acids, Salad Oil, Sweet Oil, Unsaturated Fatty Acid, Virgin Olive Oil.

Scientific Names

Olea europaea.
Family: Oleaceae.

People Use This For

Orally, olive oil is used for cardiovascular disease, hypertension, hypercholesterolemia, and diabetes. Olive oil is also used orally for breast cancer, rheumatoid arthritis (RA), migraine headache, firming the breasts, treating bile duct and gallbladder inflammation, gallstones, jaundice, flatulence, and meteorism (swelling of the abdomen due to intestinal or peritoneal gas). It is also used orally for preventing colorectal cancer, as a mild laxative for constipation, and for Roemheld's syndrome. Some people also use olive oil to boost bacteria in the gut and as a "cleanser" or "purifier."

Orally, olive leaf is used for treatment of viral, bacterial and protozoal conditions including influenza, the common cold, meningitis, Epstein-Barr Virus (EBV), encephalitis, herpes, shingles, HIV/ARC/AIDS, chronic fatigue, and hepatitis B. Olive leaf is also used for pneumonia; tuberculosis (TB); gonorrhea; malaria; dengue; bacteremia; severe diarrhea; blood poisoning; and infections including dental, ear, urinary tract, and surgical infections. Other uses include hypertension, diabetes, allergic rhinitis, improving renal and digestive function, and as a diuretic and antipyretic.

Topically, olive oil is used for softening earwax, treating ringing and pain in the ears, as nose drops, for wound dressing, treating minor burns and psoriasis, preventing and treating stretch marks due to pregnancy, and for protecting the skin from ultraviolet (UV) damage after sun exposure.

In foods, olive oil is used as a cooking and salad oil.

In manufacturing, olive oil is used to make soaps, in commercial plasters and liniments, and as a setting-retardant in dental cements.

Safety

LIKELY SAFE ...when used orally and appropriately. Olive oil can be used safely as 14% of total daily calories, or approximately 2 tablespoons (28 grams) daily (2219,2220,2221,2222,2223,3285,3286,3287,3288,3289,3362,12211). ...when used topically and appropriately (3276).

There is insufficient reliable information available about the safety of olive leaf.

PREGNANCY AND LACTATION: Insufficient reliable information, avoid using in amounts greater then those commonly found in foods.

Effectiveness

LIKELY EFFECTIVE

Constipation. Taking olive oil orally is effective as a mild laxative for reducing constipation (16).

POSSIBLY EFFECTIVE

Breast cancer. People who have higher dietary intake of olive oil seem to have a lower risk of developing breast cancer (2221,2222,2223).

Cardiovascular disease. Replacing dietary saturated fats with olive oil can reduce risk factors for cardiovascular disease, including reducing blood pressure and cholesterol (2219,2220). Including olive oil in the diet is associated with a reduced risk of first myocardial infarction (MI). A high dietary intake of olive oil (54 grams/day) was shown to cause an 82% relative reduction in risk of first MI compared with a low intake of 7 grams or less per day (8131).

The FDA now allows olive oil and olive oil-containing food labels to state that limited, but not conclusive evidence, suggests that consuming 23 grams/day (about 2 tablespoons) of olive oil instead of saturated fats may reduce the risk of heart disease (12211).

Colorectal cancer. There is some evidence that people with higher intakes of dietary olive oil have a decreased risk of developing colorectal cancer. Olive oil intake also seems to reduce colorectal mucosal changes and polyp formation, which are two factors involved in the sequence of developing colorectal cancer (3362).

Hypercholesterolemia. Increasing dietary olive oil consumption, in place of saturated fat in the diet, can significantly reduce total serum cholesterol levels (2219,2220,3285,3286,3287,3288,3289,3290). However, some research suggests other dietary oils such as sunflower and rapeseed (canola) might reduce low-density lipoprotein (LDL) cholesterol and apolipoprotein B better than olive oil (9780).

Hypertension. Consuming a modified diet including high amounts of extra virgin olive oil over 6 months, in conjunction with conventional treatments for hypertension, can significantly improve blood pressure. In some cases, patients with mild to moderate hypertension can decrease doses or discontinue use of antihypertensive medications (2219,2220,3289,5091). Taking olive leaf extract orally also seems to lower blood pressure in patients with hypertension (1540).

Rheumatoid arthritis (RA). There is some evidence that people consuming high amounts of dietary olive oil have a decreased risk of developing RA (3454).

POSSIBLY INEFFECTIVE

Earwax. Applying olive oil topically doesn't seem to soften earwax (3274).

Otitis media. Applying olive oil topically doesn't seem to be effective for treating ear pain in children with acute otitis media (3276).

INSUFFICIENT RELIABLE EVIDENCE to RATE

Diabetes. Olive oil in a Mediterranean-type diet seems to reduce chylomicron remnant particles compared with a polyunsaturated diet in diabetes patients, suggesting that it might reduce the risk of atherosclerosis (8132). Olive oil, rather than polyunsaturated oils such as sunflower oil, might be a better choice for patients with diabetes.

Migraine headache. Taking olive oil containing oleic acid (1,382 mg daily over a 2-month period) seems to reduce frequency, duration, and severity of migraine headaches in adolescents. Olive oil was used as a placebo to test the effectiveness of fish for migraines. More research is needed to tell whether olive oil actually helps migraine or whether the effect was simply a placebo response (5097).
More evidence is needed to rate olive for these uses.

Mechanism of Action

The applicable parts of olive are the oil and the leaf. Olive oil contains the monounsaturated fatty acid oleic acid (56% to 83%), palmitic acid (8% to 20%), and linoleic acid (4% to 20%) (2224,12211).
People use olive oil to prevent cardiovascular disease and atherogenesis because it seems to lower certain cardiac risk factors (2219,2220,2224,10673). Phenolic compounds present in olive oil seem to possess antioxidant, vasodilating, and antiplatelet properties. The compounds act as free radical scavengers, inhibiting platelet aggregation and thromboxane release (10673).
Olive oil seems to increase low-density lipoprotein (LDL) cholesterol resistance to oxidation and therefore possibly decreases its contribution to atherogenesis (2219,2220,2224). It also seems to improve the function of endothelial tissue in patients with hypercholesterolemia. Olive oil seems to lower blood pressure and decrease postprandial factor VII clotting activity (8131).
Olive oil might also have anti-inflammatory effects by decreasing pro-inflammatory omega-6 fatty acid concentrations and increasing anti-inflammatory omega-3 fatty acid concentrations (3289). The metabolites of oleic acid, an omega-9 monounsaturated fatty acid, in olive oil seem to competitively inhibit the production of inflammatory omega-6 fatty acid prostaglandins and leukotrienes. Oleic acid metabolites might also suppress production of inflammatory cytokines (3454).
Some researchers think olive oil might have a role in preventing colon cancer. Consumption of olive oil seems to reduce production of deoxycholic acid, a bile acid thought to be involved in the development of mucosal changes and polyp formation preceding colorectal cancer (3362). Other compounds in olive oil called secoiridoides (oleuropein and derivatives) have broad-spectrum antimicrobial activity in vitro (3284).
The leaf constituent, oleuropein, has bacteriostatic (1541) and antioxidant (271) activity. An aqueous olive leaf extract reduced blood pressure in one small, uncontrolled trial of people with hypertension (1540).

Adverse Reactions

Orally, olive oil is well tolerated. Olive leaf hasn't been associated with adverse effects (1540).
Topically, delayed hypersensitivity and contact dermatitis have been reported after using olive oil (289,3275). Olive tree pollen can cause seasonal respiratory allergy (1543).

Interactions with Herbs & Other Dietary Supplements

HERBS WITH HYPOGLYCEMIC POTENTIAL: Theoretically, olive leaf might have additive effects with herbs that decrease blood glucose levels (1540). Herbs with hypoglycemic potential include devil's claw, fenugreek, garlic, guar gum, horse chestnut, Panax ginseng, psyllium, and Siberian ginseng.

Interactions with Drugs

ANTIDIABETES DRUGS: Theoretically, concomitant use with olive might enhance blood glucose lowering effects (1540). Monitor blood glucose levels closely. Some antidiabetes drugs include glimepiride (Amaryl), glyburide (DiaBeta, Glynase PresTab, Micronase), insulin, pioglitazone (Actos), rosiglitazone (Avandia), and others.
ANTIHYPERTENSIVE DRUGS: Theoretically, concomitant with olive use may enhance blood pressure-lowering effects (1540,2219,2220,3289,5091).

Interactions with Foods

None known.

Interactions with Lab Tests

BLOOD PRESSURE: Olive might reduce blood pressure and blood pressure readings (1540).
CALCIUM: Olive leaf might reduce serum calcium levels and test results (1540).
GLUCOSE: Olive leaf might reduce blood glucose levels and test results (1540).

Interactions with Diseases or Conditions

DIABETES: Olive leaf might lower blood glucose (1540). Monitor glucose levels and adjust therapy accordingly.

Dosage and Administration

ORAL: For constipation, 30 mL has been used (16). For hypertension, 30-40 grams per day of extra-virgin olive oil has been used as part of the diet (5091). Olive leaf extract 400 mg four times daily has also been used for hypertension (1540). For reducing the risk of myocardial infarction, consuming 54 grams per day has been associated with a reduced risk of first myocardial infarction (8132). For hyperlipidemia and to decrease cardiovascular disease risk, olive oil 23 grams/day (about 2 tablespoons) providing 17.5 grams mono unsaturated fatty acids in place of saturated fats in the diet has been used (12211).
TOPICAL: No typical dosage.

Comments

Olive oil is classified, in part, according to acid content, measured as free oleic acid. Extra virgin olive oil contains a maximum of 1% free oleic acid, virgin olive oil contains 2%, and ordinary olive oil contains 3.3%. Unrefined olive oils with more than 3.3% free oleic acid are considered "unfit for human consumption" (3273).

Ozonated olive oil is promoted for everything from bee stings and insect bites to bacterial and fungal skin infections to cancer. The Food and Drug Administration allows the use of ozone as an antimicrobial agent on food, including meat and poultry, but the food industry has been slow to adopt it (8187). Ozone is extremely unstable and must be produced on site. Topical olive oil products purported to contain ozone are unlikely to remain stable during shipping. There are no clinically proven medical uses of ozone or ozonated olive oil. Tell patients other topical anti-infectives are a better choice.

OMEGA-6 FATTY ACIDS

Also Known As

N-6 Essential Fatty Acids, Omega 6 Fatty Acids, Omega 6 Oils, Polyunsaturated Fatty Acids, PUFAs.
CAUTION: See separate listings for Gamma Linolenic Acid, Evening Primrose Oil, Borage, and Black Currant.

Scientific Names

Omega-6 polyunsaturated fatty acids.

People Use This For

Orally, omega-6 fatty acids are used for reducing the risk of coronary heart disease, lowering total cholesterol and LDL cholesterol levels, increasing HDL cholesterol levels, and reducing cancer risk.

Arachidonic acid, an omega-6 fatty acid, is used as a supplement in infant formulas.

Safety

There is insufficient reliable information available about the safety of omega-6 fatty acids.

Pregnancy and Lactation: Insufficient reliable information available; avoid using.

Effectiveness

POSSIBLY INEFFECTIVE

Enhancing infant development. Taking arachidonic acid (an omega-6 fatty acid) orally as a supplement in infant formula doesn't seem to be effective for improving cognitive and mental development or growth up to 18 months of age (424).

There is insufficient reliable information available about the effectiveness of omega-6 fatty acids for its other uses.

Mechanism of Action

Omega-6 fatty acids are essential polyunsaturated fatty acids (PUFA) with a double bond at the 6 position of the carbon chain. Some omega-6 fatty acids include linoleic acid, gamma-linolenic acid and arachidonic acid. Linoleic acid is found in vegetable oils, including corn, evening primrose seed, safflower, and soybean oils. Gamma-linolenic acid is found in black currant seed, borage seed, and evening primrose oils (7701).

Omega-6 fatty acids are components of cell membrane structure and play a role in cell signaling pathways and epithelial cell function (11120). Preliminary studies suggest that omega-6 fatty acids might play a role in breast cancer development (3508); however, it is unclear whether omega-6 fatty acids are associated with breast cancer in humans (3508,3511). A low-fat diet with reduced omega-6 fatty acid content can decrease sex steroid hormone levels, alter eicosanoid biosynthesis, and play a role in preventing and treating breast and prostate cancers (3510). Long-chain polyunsaturated fatty acids, such as arachidonic acid, make up a third of all lipids in the brain's grey matter (425). Arachidonic acid is a membrane component in the central nervous system, and may have a role as a neurotransmitter (424,425). Arachidonic acid is present in human breast milk but not in standard infant formulas. Formula-fed infants have lower plasma arachidonic acid levels than breast milk-fed infants; the clinical significance of this, if any, is unknown (424).

Adverse Reactions

Orally, omega-6 fatty acids can elevate triglycerides (3509).

Interactions with Herbs & Other Dietary Supplements

None known.

Interactions with Drugs

None known.

Interactions with Foods

None known.

Interactions with Lab Tests
None known.

Interactions with Diseases or Conditions
HYPERTRIGLYCERIDEMIA: Omega-6 fatty acids can elevate triglyceride levels (3509); avoid using.

Dosage and Administration
No typical dosage.

Comments
Information on omega-6 fatty acid dietary supplementation derives from studies using specific omega-6 fatty acids or plant oils containing omega-6 fatty acids. See separate listings for black currant seed oil, borage seed oil, and evening primrose oil.

ONION

Also Known As
Allii cepae bulbus, Green Onion, Onions, Shallot.

Scientific Names
Allium cepa.
Family: Alliaceae or Liliaceae.

People Use This For
Orally, onion is used for loss of appetite, preventing atherosclerosis, for treating dyspepsia, fever, colds, cough, bronchitis, hypertension, tendency toward infection, inflammation of the mouth and pharynx, whooping cough, asthma, angina, stimulation of gallbladder, dehydration, and as a menstruation aid. It is also used orally for hypertension, diabetes, as an antiflatulent, anthelmintic, and diuretic.
Topically, onion is used for insect bites, wounds, light burns, furuncles, warts, and bruises.
In foods, onion is considered a culinary food and condiment.
In manufacturing, the oil is used as a flavoring agent in foods.

Safety
LIKELY SAFE ...when consumed in amounts commonly found in foods. Onion has Generally Recognized As Safe (GRAS) status in the US (4912).
POSSIBLY SAFE ...when used orally and appropriately (2). A maximum of 35 mg of the diphenylamine constituent is recommended per day if onion preparations are used over several months (2).
There is insufficient reliable information available about the safety of onion for its other uses.
PREGNANCY AND LACTATION: Insufficient reliable information available; avoid using in amounts greater than used in foods.

Effectiveness
There is insufficient reliable information available about the effectiveness of onion.

Mechanism of Action
The applicable part of the onion is the bulb. Onion contains essential oils (2), sulfur compounds, and cysteine sulfoxide compounds. One of the sulfur compounds, thiosulphinate, exhibits antimicrobial effects (18). The methyl and propyl compounds of cysteine sulfoxide are primarily responsible for onion flavor and lacrimation (7,11). Diphenylamine is also a constituent of onion (513). Diphenylamine is referred to as a dose standard (2). The mechanism of the diuretic effect of onion is unknown. In people with asthma, an ethanolic onion extract significantly reduced bronchial constriction (18). In sensitized guinea pigs, onion juice provided protection from asthma attacks (18). In humans, eating onions reversed the effect of a fatty meal, restoring fibrinolytic activity (7). In humans, onion also inhibits platelet aggregation (7). Onions show hypoglycemic actions, and in animals, both cholesterol lowering effects and antifungal activities have been noted (11).

Adverse Reactions
The consumption of large quantities of onions can cause stomach distress (18). Hand eczema can occur with frequent contact (18).

Interactions with Herbs & Other Dietary Supplements

HERBS WITH ANTICOAGULANT/ANTIPLATELET POTENTIAL: Concomitant use of herbs that have constituents that might affect platelet aggregation could theoretically increase the risk of bleeding in some people. These herbs include angelica, clove, danshen, garlic, ginger, ginkgo, Panax ginseng, horse chestnut, red clover, turmeric, and others.

Interactions with Drugs

ANTICOAGULANT/ANTIPLATELET DRUGS: Theoretically, concomitant use with onion might enhance antiplatelet drug activity and increase bleeding risk (19).
ANTIDIABETES DRUGS: Theoretically, concomitant use with onion might enhance antidiabetes drug effects and alter blood sugar control (19).
ASPIRIN: Concomitant intake might augment onion allergy. One case is reported of severe urticaria and swelling in a person with a known mild onion allergy after consuming onion and aspirin (5054).

Interactions with Foods

None known.

Interactions with Lab Tests

BLOOD GLUCOSE: Onions can decrease blood glucose levels and test results (19).

Interactions with Diseases or Conditions

DIABETES: Theoretically, therapeutic amounts of onions can interfere with blood sugar control. Monitor blood sugar carefully when using onion for medicinal purposes (19).

Dosage and Administration

ORAL: The typical dose is 50 grams of fresh onion per day. The juice of 50 grams fresh onion or 20 grams dried onion is also used per day (2). A maximum of 35 mg diphenylamine per day is recommended if onion preparations are used over several months (2).
TOPICAL: An onion slice is typically placed on the skin, or the juice is used as a poultice (18).

Comments

Onions are rich in vitamin C (19) and in folk medicine, were cooked in milk and used as a mucolytic to clear congested airways (7).

OOLONG TEA

Also Known As

Brown Tea, EGCG, Epigallo Catechin Gallate, Epigallocatechin Gallate, Tea Oolong.
CAUTION: See separate listings for Black Tea, Green Tea, and Caffeine.

Scientific Names

Camellia sinensis, synonyms Camellia thea, Camellia theifera, Thea bohea, Thea sinensis, Thea viridis.
Family: Theaceae.

People Use This For

Orally, oolong tea is used to improve cognitive performance, and to improve mental alertness. It is also used to prevent cancer, tooth decay, and cardiovascular disease. It is also used orally to treat atopic dermatitis, obesity, diabetes, atherosclerosis, and hyperlipidemia, and to improve resistance to disease.

Safety

LIKELY SAFE ...when used orally in moderate amounts. Oolong tea is often consumed daily in Asian cultures and has not been associated with significant adverse effects (12518).
POSSIBLY UNSAFE ...when used orally long-term in high doses. Oolong tea contains a significant amount of caffeine. Chronic use, especially in large amounts, can produce tolerance, habituation, psychological dependence, and other significant adverse effects. Doses of caffeine greater than 250-300 mg per day have been associated with significant adverse effects such as tachyarrhythmias and sleep disturbances (11832). These effects would not be expected to occur with the consumption of decaffeinated oolong tea.
LIKELY UNSAFE ...when used orally in very high doses. The fatal acute oral dose of caffeine in oolong tea is estimated to be 10-14 grams (150-200 mg per kilogram). Serious toxicity can occur at lower doses depending on variables in caffeine sensitivity such as smoking, age, prior caffeine use, etc (11832).
CHILDREN: POSSIBLY SAFE ...when used in amounts commonly found in foods and beverages (11833).
PREGNANCY: POSSIBLY SAFE ...when used orally in moderate amounts. Due to the caffeine content of oolong tea, mothers should closely monitor their intake to ensure moderate consumption. Fetal blood concentrations of

caffeine approximate maternal concentrations (4260). Use of caffeine in pregnancy is controversial; however, moderate consumption has not been associated with clinically important adverse fetal effects (2708,2709,2710,2711,9606). Caffeine crosses the human placenta, but is not considered a teratogen. Mothers should keep caffeine consumption below 300 mg per day. This is similar to the amount of caffeine found in about 3 cups of coffee or tea (2708). POSSIBLY UNSAFE ...when used orally in large amounts. Caffeine crosses the placenta, producing fetal blood concentrations similar to maternal levels (4260). Mothers should avoid consuming more than 300 mg of caffeine daily or more than 3 cups of tea or coffee per day (2708). High maternal doses of caffeine throughout pregnancy have resulted in symptoms of caffeine withdrawal in newborn infants (9891). High doses of caffeine have been associated with spontaneous abortion, premature delivery, and low birth weight (2709,2711). Fetal birth weight is reduced by 28 grams for every 100 mg per day of caffeine consumed during pregnancy. But this is unlikely to be clinically important except for women consuming more than 600 mg of caffeine daily (9606).

LACTATION: POSSIBLY SAFE ...when used orally in moderate amounts. Due to the caffeine content of oolong tea, nursing mothers should closely monitor caffeine intake. Breast milk concentrations of caffeine are thought to be approximately 50% of maternal serum concentrations. Minimal consumption would likely result in limited exposure to a nursing infant (9892). POSSIBLY UNSAFE ...when used orally in large amounts. Consumption of oolong tea might cause irritability and increased bowel activity in nursing infants (6026). Large doses or excessive intake of oolong tea should be avoided during lactation.

Effectiveness

LIKELY EFFECTIVE

Mental alertness. Consumption of oolong tea and other caffeinated beverages seems to prevent a decline in alertness and cognitive capacity when consumed throughout the day (4221,4224).

POSSIBLY EFFECTIVE

Hypertension. Consumption of oolong tea 120 mL or more per day for one year may reduce the risk of hypertension. Epidemiological research in Chinese people suggests drinking 120-599 mL oolong or green tea per day can lower the risk for developing hypertension by 46% compared with nonhabitual tea drinkers. Drinking more than 600 mL per day may reduce risk by 65% (12518).

INSUFFICIENT RELIABLE EVIDENCE to RATE

Atopic dermatitis. Preliminary clinical research suggests that drinking 1000 mL oolong tea per day in 3 divided doses improves treatment-resistant atopic dermatitis. A beneficial effect may appear within 1 to 2 weeks of initiation of treatment (12520).

Diabetes. Consumption of oolong tea 1500 mL per day for 30 days seems to lower blood glucose in patients with type 2 diabetes, according to preliminary clinical research (12519).

More information is needed to rate oolong tea for these uses.

Mechanism of Action

The applicable parts of oolong tea are the leaf bud, leaf, and stem. Oolong tea is partially fermented. Black tea is fully fermented, and green tea is unfermented. Flavanols including epigallocatechin gallate (EGCG), epigallocatechin (EGC), epicatechin gallate (ECG), epicatechin (EC), and gallocatechin gallate (GCG) are all referred to as catechins. Green tea contains 26.7% catechins, oolong tea 23.2%, and black tea 4.3% (12522). When tea is oxidized, polyphenols such as bisflavonols, theaflavins, and thearubigins are formed. Oolong contains these polyphenols in smaller amounts than black tea because oolong tea is only partly oxidized (12523). Oolong tea is more closely related to green tea than it is to black tea (12524).

The caffeine content of oolong tea is variable, as with green and black teas. Oolong tea also contains 50-60 mg caffeine per cup (12525). The caffeine in oolong tea stimulates the central nervous system (CNS), heart, muscles, and possibly the pressor centers that control blood pressure (2722). Possible mechanisms include adenosine receptor blockade and phosphodiesterase inhibition (2722). By blocking adenosine receptors, caffeine is thought to increase the release of neurotransmitters such as dopamine (6370). Caffeine also decreases airway resistance and stimulates respiration, via adenosine receptor blockade and phosphodiesterase inhibition (11836). It has also been proposed that caffeine may decrease GABA and serotonin signaling (6370). Caffeine stimulates gastric acid secretion, and increases plasma catecholamine levels (11837). Caffeine can have positive inotropic and chronotropic effects on the heart (11836). Caffeine can also acutely elevate both diastolic and systolic blood pressure, but might not have this effect in habitual users (2722).

Caffeine exerts a diuretic effect, with water losses estimated at 1.17 mL per milligram of caffeine (2712).

Tachyphylaxis to the diuretic effect develops rapidly, diminishing fluid losses associated with caffeine intake (10206). Caffeine-containing beverages consumed during moderate endurance exercise do not appear to compromise bodily hydration status (2713). Caffeine does not substantially affect the fluid status of people who drink caffeinated beverages on a regular basis (10206). The caffeine content is also thought to be responsible for oolong tea's effects on cognitive performance (4221).

Oolong tea seems to have antioxidant properties (12522). It seems to suppress the oxidation low-density lipoprotein (LDL) cholesterol. Oxidized LDL may contribute to atherosclerosis (12525). In patients with coronary artery disease, oolong tea 1000 mL per day seems to lower hemoglobin A1c levels and to increase plasma adiponectin and low-density lipoprotein particle size, which may reduce the progression of atherosclerosis (12521).

Caffeine, a constituent of oolong tea, has been reported to cause increases and decreases in blood glucose. In people with type 2 diabetes, acute administration of caffeine impairs postprandial glucose metabolism, while acute abstention from caffeine reduces postprandial glucose levels by 21%. Whether these effects also occur with caffeinated beverages and herbs is unknown (12374). Other research in obese people suggests that caffeine ingestion may contribute to insulin resistance (12375). However, one study found that type 1 diabetics taking 200 mg of caffeine twice daily had increased frequency and intensity of warning signs of hypoglycemia. This may be due to a reduction in blood flow to the brain and an increase in glucose utilization by the brain (6024).

Oolong tea is also used for weight loss. The caffeine in oolong tea may contribute to this effect, but other as yet unidentified constituents also seem to cause weight loss by inhibiting the activity of pancreatic lipase, which breaks down fat. Preliminary research suggests that oolong tea has an antiobesity effect in a high-fat diet (12526). Preliminary clinical research suggests that oolong tea increases the metabolic rate and fat oxidation (12527).

Oolong tea may also have antiallergic properties. Catechins in oolong tea, particularly gallocatechin gallate (GCG) and epigallocatechin gallate (EGCG), seem to inhibit histamine release (12528).

Adverse Reactions

Orally, oolong tea can cause symptoms of caffeine toxicity. Caffeine can cause insomnia, nervousness, restlessness, gastric irritation, nausea, vomiting, tachycardia, quickened respiration, tremors, delirium, convulsions, and diuresis. Large doses can produce headache, anxiety, agitation, ringing in the ears, premature heartbeat, and arrhythmia (11832,11838). In fatal caffeine overdose, the cause of death is usually ventricular fibrillation (11838,11845). Insomnia is a frequent adverse effect in children (10755). Caffeine may cause feeding intolerance and gastrointestinal irritation in infants (6023). Caffeine may exacerbate sleep disturbances in patients with acquired immunodeficiency syndrome (AIDS) (10204).

Some evidence shows caffeine is associated with fibrocystic breast disease, breast cancer, and endometriosis in women; however, this is controversial since findings are conflicting (8043). Restricting caffeine in women with fibrocystic breast conditions doesn't seem to affect breast nodularity, swelling, or pain (8996).

Although acute administration of caffeine can cause increased blood pressure, regular consumption does not seem to increase either blood pressure or pulse, even in mildly hypertensive patients (1451,1452,2722). Some evidence suggests chronic consumption may reduce the risk of hypertension (12518).

Tolerance to caffeine is a widely held belief, but there is little supportive clinical evidence. If it exists, it appears to be of little clinical significance (11839). Withdrawal symptoms such as irritability, sleepiness, delirium, nausea, vomiting, rhinorrhea, nervousness, restlessness, anxiety, muscle tension, muscle pains, and flushed face have been described. However, these symptoms may be from nonpharmacological factors related to knowledge and expectation of effects. Clinically significant symptoms caused by caffeine withdrawal may be uncommon (2723,11839).

Epidemiological evidence regarding the relationship between caffeine use and the risk for osteoporosis is contradictory. Caffeine can increase urinary excretion of calcium (2669,10202,11317). Women identified with a genetic variant of the vitamin D receptor appear to be at an increased risk for the detrimental effect of caffeine on bone mass (2669). However, moderate caffeine intake, less than 300 mg per day, does not seem to significantly increase osteoporosis risk in most postmenopausal women with normal calcium intake (2669,6025,10202,11317).

Combining ephedra with caffeine can increase the risk of adverse effects. Jitteriness, hypertension, seizures, temporary loss of consciousness, and hospitalization requiring life support has been associated with the combined use of ephedra and caffeine (2729). There is also a report of ischemic stroke in an athlete who consumed ephedra 40-60 mg, creatine monohydrate 6 grams, caffeine 400-600 mg, and a variety of other supplements daily for six weeks (1275).

Caffeine can cause anaphylaxis in sensitive individuals, although true IgE-mediated caffeine allergy seems to be relatively rare (11315).

Interactions with Herbs & Other Dietary Supplements

CAFFEINE-CONTAINING HERBS/SUPPLEMENTS: Concomitant use can have additive effects with the caffeine in oolong tea, and can increase the risk of adverse effects. Some natural products that contain caffeine include coffee, black tea, green tea, oolong tea, mate, cola, and others.

CREATINE: There is some concern that combining caffeine, ephedra, and creatine might increase the risk of serious adverse effects. There is a report of ischemic stroke in an athlete who consumed creatine monohydrate 6 grams, caffeine 400-600 mg, ephedra 40-60 mg, and a variety of other supplements daily for 6 weeks (1275). Caffeine might also decrease creatine's possible beneficial effects on athletic performance. Some researchers think caffeine can inhibit phosphocreatine resynthesis (2117,4575).

EPHEDRA (Ma Huang): Use of ephedra with oolong tea can increase the risk of stimulatory adverse effects due to its caffeine content. There is evidence that using ephedra with caffeine might increase the risk of serious life-threatening or debilitating adverse effects such as hypertension, myocardial infarction, stroke, seizures, and death (6486,10307). Tell patients to avoid taking oolong tea with ephedra and other stimulants.

IRON: Oolong tea appears to reduce absorption of non-heme iron from foods (8110,8904). Infants given tea to drink seem to have an increased risk of microcytic anemia (631). However, a study of iron-deficient elderly patients suggests that concomitant use does not alter iron absorption in this population (185). Theoretically, oolong tea might reduce the absorption of iron supplements. For most patients, this effect will not be clinically significant. Advise patients with iron deficiency to consume tea between meals rather than with meals to lessen this interaction (8904).

Interactions with Drugs

ADENOSINE (Adenocard): The caffeine in oolong tea is a competitive inhibitor of adenosine at the cellular level. However, caffeine doesn't seem to affect supplemental adenosine because high interstitial levels of adenosine overcome the antagonistic effects of caffeine (11771).

ALCOHOL (Ethanol): Concomitant use of alcohol can increase caffeine serum concentrations and the risk of caffeine adverse effects. Alcohol reduces caffeine metabolism (6370).

AMPHETAMINES: Theoretically, the caffeine in oolong tea might increase the risk of additive CNS effects (2719).

ANTICOAGULANT/ANTIPLATELET DRUGS: Theoretically, the caffeine in oolong tea might increase the risk of bleeding when used concomitantly with these agents. Caffeine is reported to have antiplatelet activity (8028,8029); however, this interaction has not been reported in humans. Antiplatelet agents include aspirin, clopidogrel (Plavix), dipyridamole (Persantine), ticlopidine (Ticlid), and others. Anticoagulant agents include heparin and warfarin (Coumadin).

ANTIDIABETES DRUGS: Theoretically, concomitant use of caffeine, a constituent of oolong tea, and diabetes drugs might interfere with blood glucose control. Data are conflicting. Reports claim that caffeine might increase or decrease blood sugar (6024,8646).

CIMETIDINE (Tagamet): Theoretically, concomitant use might increase serum caffeine concentrations and the risk of adverse effects, due to the caffeine contained in oolong tea. Cimetidine decreases the rate of caffeine clearance by 30% to 50% (11736).

CLOZAPINE (Clozaril): Theoretically, co-administration might acutely exacerbate psychotic symptoms, due to the caffeine contained in oolong tea. Caffeine can increase the effects and toxicity of clozapine. Caffeine doses of 400-1000 mg per day inhibit clozapine metabolism (5051).

COCAINE: Theoretically, the caffeine in oolong tea might increase the risk of additive CNS effects (2719).

CONTRACEPTIVE DRUGS: Theoretically, concomitant use might increase caffeine concentrations and the risk adverse effects, due to the caffeine contained in oolong tea. Oral contraceptives decrease the rate of caffeine clearance by 40% to 65% (2714,11737).

DIPYRIDAMOLE (Persantine): The caffeine in oolong tea might inhibit dipyridamole-induced vasodilation (11770,11772).

DISULFIRAM (Antabuse): Theoretically, concomitant use might increase serum caffeine concentrations and the risk of adverse effects, due to the caffeine contained in oolong tea. Disulfiram decreases the rate of caffeine clearance (15).

EPHEDRINE: Use of ephedrine with caffeine, a constituent of oolong tea, can increase the risk of stimulatory adverse effects. There is evidence that using ephedrine with caffeine might increase the risk of serious life-threatening or debilitating adverse effects such as hypertension, myocardial infarction, stroke, seizures, and death (1275,6486,10307). Tell patients to avoid taking caffeine with ephedrine and other stimulants.

ESTROGENS: Theoretically, concomitant use might increase serum caffeine concentrations and the risk of adverse effects, due to the caffeine contained in oolong tea. Estrogen inhibits caffeine metabolism (2714).

FLUCONAZOLE (Diflucan): Concomitant use might increase the effects of caffeine in oolong tea. Fluconazole decreases caffeine clearance by approximately 25% (11022).

FLUVOXAMINE (Luvox): Concomitant use of fluvoxamine with caffeine or caffeine-containing herbs such as oolong tea can increase caffeine serum concentrations, and the risk of caffeine adverse effects. Fluvoxamine reduces caffeine metabolism (6370).

LITHIUM: Theoretically, abrupt oolong tea withdrawal might increase serum lithium levels, due to the caffeine contained in oolong tea. There are two case reports of lithium tremor that worsened upon abrupt coffee withdrawal (609,610).

MEXILETINE (Mexitil): Concomitant use might increase the effects and adverse effects of caffeine in oolong tea. Mexiletine can decrease caffeine elimination by 50% (1260,11741).

MONOAMINE OXIDASE INHIBITORS (MAOIs): Theoretically, concomitant intake of large amounts of oolong tea with MAOIs might precipitate a hypertensive crisis, due to the caffeine contained in oolong tea. This is based on the claim that intake of large amounts of caffeine with MAOIs might precipitate a hypertensive crisis (15).

NICOTINE: Theoretically, the caffeine in oolong tea might increase the risk of additive CNS effects (2719).

PHENYLPROPANOLAMINE: Concomitant use of phenylpropanolamine and oolong tea might cause an additive increase in blood pressure due to the caffeine in oolong tea (11738).

QUINOLONE ANTIBIOTICS: Theoretically, concomitant use might increase serum caffeine concentrations and the risk of adverse effects, due to the caffeine contained in oolong tea. Quinolones decrease caffeine clearance (606,607,608). Quinolones (also referred to as fluoroquinolones) include ciprofloxacin (Cipro), enoxacin (Penetrex), gatifloxacin (Tequin), levofloxacin (Levaquin), lomefloxacin (Maxaquin), moxifloxacin (Avelox), norfloxacin (Noroxin), ofloxacin (Floxin), sparfloxacin (Zagam), and trovafloxacin (Trovan).

RILUZOLE (Rilutek): Theoretically, concomitant use of riluzole with caffeine or caffeine-containing herbs such as oolong tea might increase serum caffeine and riluzole concentrations and the risk of adverse effects of both caffeine and riluzole, due to the caffeine contained in oolong tea. Caffeine and riluzole are both metabolized by cytochrome P450 1A2 (CYP1A2), and concomitant use might reduce metabolism of one or both agents (11739).

TERBINAFINE (Lamisil): Theoretically, concomitant use might increase serum caffeine concentrations and the risk of adverse effects, due to the caffeine contained in oolong tea. Terbinafine decreases the rate of caffeine clearance (11740).

THEOPHYLLINE: Theoretically, concomitant use of theophylline and large amounts of oolong tea might increase the risk of theophylline toxicity, due to oolong tea's caffeine content. Caffeine decreases theophylline clearance 23% to 29% (11741).

VERAPAMIL (Calan, Covera, Isoptin, Verelan): Theoretically, concomitant use might increase plasma caffeine concentrations and the risk of adverse effects, due to the caffeine contained in oolong tea. Verapamil increases plasma caffeine concentrations by 25% (11741).

Interactions with Foods

IRON: Theoretically, oolong tea might reduce absorption of non-heme iron from foods (631,8110,9237).

MILK: When taken together, milk might bind the antioxidants in tea and reduce their beneficial effects (220); however, in one study this interaction did not occur (6032).

Interactions with Lab Tests

5-HYDROXYINDOLEACETIC ACID: Oolong tea might increase urine 5-hydroxyindoleacetic acid concentrations and test results, due to its caffeine content. Caffeine can increase urine catecholamine concentrations (15).

BLEEDING TIME: Oolong tea might prolong bleeding time and increase test results, due to its caffeine content (1701).

CATECHOLAMINES: Oolong tea might increase urine catecholamine concentrations and test results, due to its caffeine content. Caffeine can increase urine catecholamine concentrations (15).

CREATINE: Oolong tea might increase urine creatine concentrations and test results, due to its caffeine content (1701).

DIPYRIDAMOLE THALLIUM IMAGING: Oolong tea might interfere with dipyridamole thallium imaging studies, due to its caffeine content. Caffeine attenuates the characteristic cardiovascular responses to dipyridamole and has altered test results (11742).

GLUCOSE: Caffeine has been reported to cause increases and decreases in blood glucose (8646).

LACTATE: The combination of ephedrine, a constituent of ephedra, and caffeine, a constituent of oolong tea, can increase blood lactate levels (8646).

NEUROBLASTOMA TESTS: Oolong tea (due to its caffeine content) might cause false-positive diagnosis of neuroblastoma, when diagnosis is based on tests of urine vanillylmandelic acid (VMA) or catecholamine concentrations. Caffeine can increase urine catecholamine and VMA concentrations (15).

PHARMACOLOGICAL STRESS TESTS: The caffeine in oolong tea is a competitive antagonist for adenosine receptors (11771). It is recommended that caffeine and caffeine-containing products be stopped 24 hours prior to pharmacological stress tests (11770). However, caffeine appears more likely to interfere with dipyridamole (Persantine) than adenosine (Adenocard) stress testing (11771). The interaction between caffeine and dipyridamole is unlikely to be significant in stress testing if the heart rate increase is greater than 5% after dipyridamole infusion (11772).

PHEOCHROMOCYTOMA TESTS: Oolong tea (due to its caffeine content) might cause false-positive diagnosis of pheochromocytoma, when diagnosis is based on tests of urine vanillylmandelic acid (VMA) or catecholamine concentrations. Caffeine can increase urine catecholamine and VMA concentrations (15).

PULMONARY FUNCTION TESTS: People may need to avoid caffeine and caffeine-containing beverages and herbs for at least four hours prior to lung function testing. Forced expiratory volume in one minute (FEV1) seems to show a small improvement up to two hours after caffeine use. Mid-expiratory flow rates may also improve with caffeine for up to four hours (9607).

URATE: Oolong tea might falsely increase serum urate test results determined by the Bittner method, due to its caffeine content. Caffeine causes false elevations in serum urate test results determined by the Bittner method (15).

URINARY CALCIUM: Caffeine, a constituent of oolong tea, can increase urinary calcium levels (11317).

VANILLYLMANDELIC ACID (VMA): Oolong tea might increase urine VMA concentrations and test results, due to its caffeine content. Caffeine can increase urine VMA concentrations (15).

Interactions with Diseases or Conditions

ANXIETY DISORDERS: The caffeine in oolong tea might aggravate anxiety disorders (11743).

BLEEDING DISORDERS: Theoretically, caffeine in oolong tea might aggravate these conditions. Caffeine is reported to have antiplatelet activity (8028,8029); however, this interaction has not been reported in humans (1701). Caffeine can prolong bleeding time and increase the results of a bleeding time test (1701).

CARDIAC CONDITIONS: Caffeine in oolong tea can induce cardiac arrhythmias in sensitive individuals (11845); use with caution.

DIABETES: Some research suggests that caffeine, a constituent of oolong tea, may impair postprandial glucose metabolism in people with diabetes and contribute to insulin resistance. The effect of caffeinated beverages and herbs has not been studied (12374,12375). Caffeine in oolong tea may enhance the frequency and intensity of hypoglycemic warning symptoms in type 1 diabetics. This may increase the ability of diabetics to detect and treat hypoglycemia early. However, it might also increase the frequency of hypoglycemic events (6024). Caffeine has been reported to cause increases and decreases in blood glucose (8646); use with caution.

GLAUCOMA: Consuming oolong tea increases intraocular pressure due to its caffeine content. The increase occurs

within 30 minutes and persists for at least 90 minutes (8540).
HYPERTENSION: The caffeine in oolong tea might increase blood pressure in people with high blood pressure. However, this doesn't seem to occur in people who regularly consume oolong tea or other caffeinated products (1451,1452,2722).
OSTEOPOROSIS: Consuming oolong tea can increase urinary excretion of calcium due to its caffeine content. Caffeine consumption should be limited to less than 300 mg per day. Adequate calcium supplementation may partially compensate for calcium losses (2669,10202,11317). Postmenopausal women identified with a genetic variant of the vitamin D receptor should use caffeine with caution (2669).

Dosage and Administration

ORAL: Doses of oolong tea vary significantly, but usually range between 1-10 cups daily. For preventing hypertension, doses ranging from 120 mL to more than 600 mL of oolong tea per day have been used (12518). The typical dose of caffeine for headache or restoring mental alertness is up to 250 mg per day (2718,11743).

OPIUM ANTIDOTE

Also Known As

Combretum, Jungle Weed.

Scientific Names

Combretum micranthum.
Family: Combretaceae.

Comments

At the date of publication, this product was not a common ingredient used in brand name supplements marketed to consumers. Details about this product are available in the online version of *Natural Medicines Comprehensive Database*. See www.naturaldatabase.com.

ORCHIC EXTRACT

Also Known As

Bovine Orchic Extract, Bovine Testicle Extract, Bull Balls Extract, Orchic, Orchic Concentrate, Orchic Factors, Orchic Substance.

Scientific Names

None.

People Use This For

Orally, men use orchic extract to maintain healthy testicular function.

Safety

There is insufficient reliable information available about the safety of orchic extract. However, since orchic extract preparations are derived from animals, there is concern about contamination with diseased animal parts (1825). So far, there are no reports of disease transmission to humans due to use of contaminated orchic extract.
Pregnancy and Lactation: Insufficient reliable information available; avoid using.

Effectiveness

There is insufficient reliable information available about the effectiveness of orchic extract.

Mechanism of Action

Orchic extract is obtained from bovine testicles (1319). Marketers imply that orchic extracts are a good source of testosterone. However, there is no evidence to support this claim.

Adverse Reactions

Adverse effects for orchic extract have not been reported. However, there are concerns about possible product contamination. Orchic extract is derived from raw bovine testes gathered from slaughterhouses, possibly from sick or diseased animals (1319). Products made from contaminated or diseased organs might present a human health hazard. There is also concern that orchic extracts produced from cows in countries where bovine spongiform encephalitis (BSE) has been reported might be contaminated with diseased tissue. Countries where BSE has been reported include Great Britain, France, The Netherlands, Portugal, Luxembourg, Ireland, Switzerland, Oman, and Belgium (1825). However, there have been no reports of BSE transfer to humans from contaminated orchic extract products. Until more is known, tell patients to avoid these products unless country of origin can be determined. Patients should avoid products that are produced in countries where BSE has been found.

Interactions with Herbs & Other Dietary Supplements
None known.

Interactions with Drugs
None known.

Interactions with Foods
None known.

Interactions with Lab Tests
ANABOLIC STEROIDS: Theoretically, orchic extract might cause a positive anabolic steroid screening test result (1320). However, this effect has not been demonstrated.

Interactions with Diseases or Conditions
None known.

Dosage and Administration
No typical dosage.

OREGANO

Also Known As
Carvacrol, Dostenkraut, European Oregano, Mediterranean Oregano, Mountain Mint, Oil of Oregano, Oregano Oil, Organy, Origani vulgaris herba, Origano, Origanum, Phytoprogestin, Wild Marjoram, Winter Marjoram, Wintersweet.
CAUTION: See separate listing for Marjoram.

Scientific Names
Origanum vulgare.
Family: Lamiaceae/Labiatae.

People Use This For
Orally, oregano is used for respiratory tract disorders such as coughs, asthma, croup, and bronchitis. Oregano is also used orally for gastrointestinal disorders, such as dyspepsia and bloating. It is also used orally for dysmenorrhea, rheumatoid arthritis, urinary tract disorders including urinary tract infections (UTIs), headaches, and heart conditions. The oil of oregano is also used orally for intestinal parasites, allergies, sinusitis, arthritis, cold and flu, earaches, and fatigue.
Topically, oregano oil is used for acne, athlete's foot, dandruff, insect and spider bites, canker sores, gum disease, toothaches, psoriasis, seborrhea, ringworm, rosacea, muscle pain, varicose veins, and warts. It is also used topically as an insect repellent.
In foods and beverages, oregano is used as a culinary spice and a food preservative.

Safety
LIKELY SAFE ...when used orally in amounts commonly found in foods. Oregano leaf and oil have Generally Recognized As Safe (GRAS) status in the US (4912).
POSSIBLY SAFE ...when used orally or topically and appropriately in medicinal amounts (12).
There is insufficient reliable information available about the safety of oregano oil when used in medicinal amounts.
PREGNANCY: POSSIBLY UNSAFE ...when used orally in medicinal amounts. Oregano is thought to have abortifacient and emmenagogue effects (19,7122).
LACTATION: There is insufficient reliable information available about the safety of oregano when used in medicinal amounts while nursing.

Effectiveness
POSSIBLY EFFECTIVE

Intestinal parasitic infection. Taking the emulsified oil of oregano orally 200 mg three times daily for 6 weeks can eradicate the parasites Blastocystis hominis, Entamoeba hartmanni, and Endolimax nana from the stools of infected patients (6878).

There is insufficient reliable information available about the effectiveness of oregano for its other uses.

Mechanism of Action

The applicable part of oregano is the leaf and oil. Oregano contains the constituents carvacrol and thymol which have anthelmintic, fungicidal, and irritant properties (2129). The essential oil is thought to have diuretic, expectorant, and antispasmodic properties. It might also stimulate bile production (11). Oregano oil also has in vitro activity against a variety of common gram positive and gram negative organisms, including Acinetobacter calcoacetica, Enterococcus faecalis, Escherichia coli, Klebsiella pneumoniae, Pseudomonas aeruginosa, Salmonella species, Serratia marcescens, Staphylococcus aureus, and the yeast Candida albicans (316,2129,2130,3702,3703,3704). The carvacrol and thymol constituents also inhibit bacterial growth, with additive or possibly synergistic activity in oregano oil (2130). Carvacrol has a bacteriocidal effect on Bacillus cereus, a common food pathogen, by altering bacterial membrane permeability (165). Oregano oil seems to inhibit the growth intestinal parasites in vivo (6878). There is preliminary evidence that oregano may contain phytoprogestins that bind the progesterone receptor (3701).

Adverse Reactions

Orally, large amounts of oregano can cause gastrointestinal upset. Concentrated, non-emulsified oil of oregano can cause localized irritation of the gastrointestinal tract (6878). Oregano might also cause systemic allergic reactions (3705). Individuals allergic to Lamiaceae family plants including basil, hyssop, lavender, marjoram, mint, and sage, might also demonstrate an allergic reaction to oregano (3705).

Interactions with Herbs & Other Dietary Supplements

None known.

Interactions with Drugs

None known.

Interactions with Foods

None known.

Interactions with Lab Tests

None known.

Interactions with Diseases or Conditions

CROSS-ALLERGENICITY: Oregano can cause reactions in people allergic to Lamiaceae family plants, including basil, hyssop, lavender, marjoram, mint, and sage (3705).

Dosage and Administration

ORAL: For intestinal parasitic infection, emulsified oil of oregano has been used in a dose of 200 mg three times daily for 6 weeks (6878). Traditionally, a typical dose is one cup of tea. To make tea, steep 1 heaping teaspoon of leaf in 250 mL boiling water 10 minutes, strain. Tea may be sweetened with honey (18).

TOPICAL: No typical dosage. Traditionally, unsweetened tea is used as a gargle or mouthwash (18). To use oregano as a bath additive, steep 100 grams dried leaf in 1 L water for 10 minutes, strain, and add to a full bath (18).

Comments

Oregano oil has been tested as an insect repellent for Culicodoides imicola, a pathogen-bearing species of insects commonly known as no-see-ums or biting midges. Oregano oil is not as effective as DEET for protecting horses (and presumably, people) from C. imicola (2119).

OREGON FIR BALSAM

Also Known As

Balsam, Balsam Fir Oregon, Balsam Oregon, Coastal Douglas Fir, Douglas Fir, Douglas Spruce, Oregon Balsam, Red Fir.

Scientific Names

Pseudotsuga menziesii, synonym Pseudotsuga douglasii; Pseudotsuga mucronata; Pseudotsuga taxifolia.
Family: Pinaceae.

Comments

At the date of publication, there was very little scientific information available about this product. Our staff is continually analyzing the available information on natural medicines and will add data to the online version of *Natural Medicines Comprehensive Database* as it becomes available. See www.naturaldatabase.com.

OREGON GRAPE

Also Known As

Barberry, Blue Barberry, Creeping Barberry, Holly Barberry, Holly-Leaved Berberis, Holly Mahonia, Mountain-Grape, Oregon Barberry, Oregon-Grape, Oregon Grape-Holly, Scraperoot, Trailing Mahonia, Water-Holly.
CAUTION: See separate listing for European Barberry.

Scientific Names

Mahonia aquifolium, synonyms Berberis aquifolium, Berberis diversifolia, Mahonia diversifolia; Mahonia nervosa, synonym Berberis nervosa; Mahonia repens, synonyms Berberis repens, Berberis sonnei, Mahonia sonnei.
Family: Beberidaceae.

People Use This For

Orally, Oregon grape is used for ulcers, heartburn, stomach problems, as a bitter tonic, as a cathartic, and to treat infections. The American Indians used Oregon grape for general debility and as an appetite stimulant.
Topically, Oregon grape is used for psoriasis, as a disinfectant.

Safety

POSSIBLY SAFE ...when used topically and appropriately (854,857). Canada has approved a Mahonia aquifolium product for topical use based on safety data (856). ...when used orally. Amounts of less than 500 mg per day of berberine, a constituent of Oregon grape, are usually considered safe (12).
LIKELY UNSAFE ...when more than 500 mg per day berberine is consumed (12). Berberine is considered moderately toxic (12). The human LD50 for berberine is reported to be 27.5 mg/kg (12).
PREGNANCY: LIKELY UNSAFE ...when used orally (12) due to potential uterine stimulant activity of berberine (19).
LACTATION: Insufficient reliable information available; avoid using.

Effectiveness

INSUFFICIENT RELIABLE EVIDENCE to RATE

Psoriasis. There is some evidence that Oregon grape, applied topically, may be useful for treating psoriasis (854,857). More evidence is needed to rate Oregon grape for this use.

Mechanism of Action

The applicable parts of Oregon grape are the rhizome and root. Oregon grape root contains 2.4-4.5% of isoquinoline alkaloid constituents including berberine, berbamine, and oxyacanthine (515). Berberine and oxyacanthine show evidence of antibacterial activity (11). Berberine has anticonvulsant, sedative, hypotensive, antifibrillatory, bile-stimulating, and anti-inflammatory effects. In low doses, it is a cardiac and respiratory stimulant. In high doses, it is a depressant (515,10377). Some evidence suggests berberine sulfate might be amebicidal and trypanocidal (11). Other information suggests the constituent berbamine might have antiarrhythmic, hypotensive, spasmolytic, and immunostimulating activity (515).

Adverse Reactions

No reports of adverse effects associated with Oregon grape. Ingesting more than 500 mg berberine, a constituent of Oregon grape, can cause lethargy, nosebleed, skin and eye irritation, kidney irritation (12), hemorrhagic nephritis (2), dyspnea, hypotension, cardiac damage (12), nausea, vomiting, diarrhea, respiratory spasms and arrest, and death (2).
When used topically, Oregon grape can cause itching, burning, skin irritation, and allergic reactions (854).

Interactions with Herbs & Other Dietary Supplements

BERBERINE-CONTAINING HERBS: Concomitant use can increase the risk of berberine toxicity. Berberine-containing herbs include bloodroot, goldenseal, celandine, Chinese goldthread, goldthread, amur cork tree, Chinese corktree (12).

Interactions with Drugs

None known.

Interactions with Foods

None known.

Interactions with Lab Tests

None known.

Interactions with Diseases or Conditions

KIDNEY IRRITATION: CAUTION, berberine may exacerbate kidney irritation. It can cause kidney irritation and nephritis (2).

Dosage and Administration

ORAL: The common dose of the tincture is 2-4 mL three times daily, and the usual dose of the powder is 0.5 to 1 gram three times daily (6002).
TOPICAL: For psoriasis, 10% Mahonia aquifolium bark extract ointment is typically applied to affected areas two to three times daily. Mahonia aquifolium 10% root extract cream is typically massaged into affected areas three times daily or as directed by physician (854).

Comments

A Mahonia aquifolium root extract product, Prime Relief, received a Drug Identification Number (DIN) from Health Canada. The DIN allows this product to be labeled and marketed for treating psoriasis in Canada (856).

ORIENTAL ARBORVITAE

Also Known As

Biota orientalis, Ce Bai, Chinese Arborvitae.

Scientific Names

Platycladus orientalis, synonyms Retinispora juniperoides, Thuja orientalis.
Family: Cupressaceae.

People Use This For

Orally, oriental arborvitae is used orally for headache, apprehension, calming nervous disorders and excitement, for cancer, constipation, convulsions, dysmenorrhea, ejaculation problems, narrowing of intestine, fever, vomiting blood, bloody stools, blood in urine, hemorrhage, insomnia, painful menses, heavy menstrual flow, irregular and variable menstrual bleeding, nausea, neurasthenia, palpitation, perspiration, rheumatism, tumors, and as a tonic. It is also used orally for diuretic, laxative, menstrual-stimulant, pain-reliever, parasiticide, and sedative effects.
Topically, oriental arborvitae is used for nosebleed, piles, for burns and scalds, and as a hair tonic. It is also used topically for its astringent and antiperspirant properties.

Safety

POSSIBLY SAFE ...when the seed is used orally (12). ...when the leafy twigs are used orally in tea. It is important to use it short-term and not to exceed the usual dose (12).
There is insufficient reliable information available about the safety of oriental arborvitae for its other uses.
PREGNANCY AND LACTATION: POSSIBLY UNSAFE ...when used orally because it contains thujone (12) which shows some evidence of uterine stimulant activity (19); avoid using.

Effectiveness

There is insufficient reliable information is available about the effectiveness of oriental arborvitae.

Mechanism of Action

The applicable parts of oriental arborvitae are the seed and the cacumen (leafy twigs) (12). Oriental arborvitae contains thujone in the volatile oil. Alcoholic extracts and essential oils containing thujone can cause neurotoxicity including convulsions and hallucinations (12). Some evidence suggests Thuja orientalis might have antibacterial activity (4041).

Adverse Reactions

Thujone intoxication can cause psychoactivity similar to tetrahydrocannibinol, the active constituent in marijuana. Long-term or high dosages of plants containing thujone can cause restlessness, vomiting, dizziness, tremors, renal damage, and convulsions (12).

Interactions with Herbs & Other Dietary Supplements

THUJONE CONTAINING HERBS: Avoid; concomitant use may increase the risk of thujone toxicity.
Thujone-containing herbs include oak moss (12), sage (2,4,12), tansy (2,4,12), thuja (cedar) (11,12), tree moss (12), and wormwood (2,12).

Interactions with Drugs

None known.

Interactions with Foods

None known.

Interactions with Lab Tests

None known.

Interactions with Diseases or Conditions

PORPHYRIA: Can exacerbate porphyria in patients with underlying defects in hepatic heme synthesis (12).
RENAL DYSFUNCTION: Can exacerbate this condition (12).

Dosage and Administration

ORAL: A standard dose for the leafy twigs is 5-15 grams of raw or charred, daily as tea (12).
TOPICAL: No typical dosage.

ORNITHINE

Also Known As

L-Ornithine.
CAUTION: See separate listing for Ornithine Ketoglutarate.

Scientific Names

L-5-aminorvaline; L-2,5-diaminovaleric acid.

People Use This For

Orally, ornithine is used for improving athletic performance, reducing glutamine toxicity in the treatment of hepatic encephalopathy, and for wound healing.

Safety

There is insufficient reliable information available about the safety of ornithine.
Pregnancy and Lactation: Insufficient reliable information available; avoid using.

Effectiveness

POSSIBLY INEFFECTIVE

Athletic performance. Taking ornithine orally doesn't seem to enhance athletic performance (2417,2418).

INSUFFICIENT RELIABLE EVIDENCE to RATE

Hepatic encephalopathy. Preliminary clinical research suggests an L-ornithine-L-aspartate infusion might reduce the harmful effects of glutamine in the treatment of hepatic encephalopathy (10655). More evidence is needed to rate ornithine for this use.

Mechanism of Action

Ornithine is a non-essential amino acid produced in the body by hydrolysis of arginine. By supplementing ornithine, people believe they can increase their anabolic hormone levels, reducing skeletal muscle hypertrophy (2417). However, supplemental ornithine has no effect on insulin secretion (2417,2418) or serum human growth hormone (hGH) levels in bodybuilders (2418).

Adverse Reactions

None reported.

Interactions with Herbs & Other Dietary Supplements

None known.

Interactions with Drugs

None known.

Interactions with Foods

None known.

Interactions with Lab Tests

None known.

Interactions with Diseases or Conditions

None known.

Dosage and Administration

ORAL: The typical dose is one 500 mg capsule containing L-ornithine daily on an empty stomach before bedtime (5020).

Comments
Avoid confusion with ornithine alpha-ketoglutarate (OKG).
There is very little scientific information about this product. Our staff is continually analyzing the available information on natural medicines and will add data here as it becomes available.

ORNITHINE KETOGLUTARATE

Also Known As
L-Ornithine Alpha-Ketoglutarate, OKG, Ornicetil, Ornithine Alpha Ketoglutarate, Ornithine Alphaketoglutarate,.
CAUTION: See separate listing for Ornithine.

Scientific Names
L(+)-ornithine alpha-ketoglutarate.

People Use This For
Orally, ornithine ketoglutarate is used for enhancing athletic performance and wound healing.
Intravenously, it is used as a component in total parenteral nutrition for preventing growth retardation in children receiving long-term total parenteral nutrition. It is also used intravenously for improving skeletal muscle protein synthesis after surgery, preventing decreases in muscle free glutamine concentrations, and preserving protein synthesis after total hip replacement or stroke.

Safety
POSSIBLY SAFE ...when use intravenously and appropriately (2444,2445,2446,2448).
There is insufficient reliable information available about the safety of the oral use of ornithine ketoglutarate.
PREGNANCY AND LACTATION: Insufficient reliable information available; avoid using.

Effectiveness
POSSIBLY EFFECTIVE

Burns. Taking ornithine ketoglutarate orally seems to improve wound healing in burn patients (2443).

POSSIBLY INEFFECTIVE

Athletic performance. Taking ornithine ketoglutarate orally doesn't seem to enhance athletic performance (2452).

LIKELY INEFFECTIVE

Hepatic encephalopathy. Administering ornithine ketoglutarate intravenously isn't effective for treating encephalopathy in patients with acute and chronic liver disease (2449,2450).

INSUFFICIENT RELIABLE EVIDENCE to RATE

Growth retardation. Preliminary clinical research suggests ornithine ketoglutarate might prevent growth retardation in children receiving long-term total parenteral nutrition (2444).

Surgery related myoatrophy. Preliminary clinical research suggests ornithine ketoglutarate might improve skeletal muscle protein synthesis after surgery (2446,2448).

More evidence is needed to rate ornithine ketoglutarate for these uses.

Mechanism of Action
Ornithine ketoglutarate modifies amino acid metabolism and increases blood insulin and glucagon levels in healthy people (2415).

Adverse Reactions
None reported.

Interactions with Herbs & Other Dietary Supplements
None known.

Interactions with Drugs
None known.

Interactions with Foods
None known.

Interactions with Lab Tests
None known.

Interactions with Diseases or Conditions
None known.

Dosage and Administration

ORAL: For the healing of burn wounds, 30 grams is taken daily as an enteral bolus (2443).
INTRAVENOUS: For preventing growth retardation in children receiving long-term total parenteral nutrition (TPN), 15 grams of ornithine ketoglutarate is typically added to the daily TPN (2444). For improving skeletal muscle protein synthesis after surgery, 350 mg/kg per day is added to the TPN (2446). For preventing decreases in muscle free glutamine concentrations and preserving protein synthesis after total hip replacement, 280 mg/kg per day is added to the TPN (2448).

Comments

Avoid confusion with ornithine.

ORRIS

Also Known As

Blue Flag, Daggers, Flag Lily, Flaggon, Fliggers, Florentine Iris, Gladyne, Iris, Jacob's Sword, Liver Lily, Myrtle Flower, Poison Flag, Rhizoma Iridis, Segg, Sheggs, Snake Lily, Water Flag, White Dragon Flower, Wild Iris, Yellow Flag, Yellow Iris.
CAUTION: See separate listing for Blue Flag.

Scientific Names

Iris pallida, synonym Iris junonia; Iris germanica; Iris germanica var. florentina, synonym Iris florentina.
Family: Iridaceae.

People Use This For

Orally, orris root is used for "blood-purifying", "gland-stimulating", increasing kidney activity, skin diseases, bronchitis, cold, cancer, stimulating appetite and digestion, stimulating bile flow, sciatica, sclerosis, splenitis. It is also used as a diuretic, emetic, laxative, purgative, and sedative. Orris root is also used orally for headache, toothache, muscle and joint pain, migraine, bowel sluggishness, bloating, diabetes, urinary tract inflammation, and skin diseases.
Topically, orris root is used for halitosis, nasal polyps, teething, tumors, uric acid sedimentation, kyphosis, keloid formation, rheumatic disorders, burns, and cuts.

Safety

POSSIBLY SAFE ...when used orally (12). Orris root must be carefully peeled and dried before using (2). Fresh root and juice can cause severe mucosal and skin irritation (12).
There is insufficient reliable information available about the safety of the topical use of orris.
PREGNANCY AND LACTATION: Insufficient reliable information available; avoid using.

Effectiveness

There is insufficient reliable information available about the effectiveness of orris.

Mechanism of Action

The applicable parts of orris are the rhizome and root. Orris root contains triterpenes, including irigermanal, and isoflavonoids, including irilon, irisolone, irigenine, and tectoridine. It also contains C-glucosylxanthones and a volatile oil. The chief constituents of the volatile oil are irones, particularly alpha-, beta-, and gamma-irone. Some think orris root has mild expectorant effects (18).

Adverse Reactions

No adverse effects are reported when orris root has been carefully peeled and dried. However, taken orally the fresh plant juice or root can cause severe mucosal irritation, abdominal pain, vomiting, and bloody diarrhea (18).
Topically, the fresh plant juice or root can cause severe skin and mucosal irritation (12,18).

Interactions with Herbs & Other Dietary Supplements

None known.

Interactions with Drugs

None known.

Interactions with Foods

None known.

Interactions with Lab Tests

None known.

Interactions with Diseases or Conditions
None known.

Dosage and Administration
No typical dosage.

Comments
Orris root is generally used in combination with other herbs and can be found in homeopathic dilutions and tea preparations (18). Historically, orris root was highly prized in the perfume industry. Upon drying, the root develops a pleasant violet-like scent. This scent continues to improve in storage, reaching its peak in about three years. Orris root was widely used in face powders and other cosmetics until it was determined to cause allergic reactions. Orris root powder is still used extensively in potpourris, sachets, and pomanders. It is one of the most effective fixatives and it prolongs the scent of the more transient volatile oils. Of the two orris species, Iris germanica var. florentina root is considered superior to Iris pallida (4081).

OSCILLOCOCCINUM

Also Known As
Anas Barbariae, Avian Heart and Liver, Avian Liver Extract, Canard de Barbarie, Duck Liver Extract, Muscovy Duck, Oscillo.

Scientific Names
Cairina moschata; Anas barbaria; Anas moschata.

People Use This For
Orally, oscillococcinum is used for symptoms of influenza infections ("the flu").

Safety
POSSIBLY SAFE ...when used orally. Oscillococcinum has been safely used in clinical trials (10804). This is a homeopathic product and contains no measurable amount of active ingredient. Therefore this product is not expected to cause any beneficial or adverse effect.
PREGNANCY AND LACTATION: Insufficient reliable information available. This product has not been studied in these patients. However, it is a homeopathic product and contains no measurable amount of active ingredient. Therefore this product is not expected to cause any beneficial or adverse effect.

Effectiveness
INSUFFICIENT RELIABLE EVIDENCE to RATE

Influenza. Oscillococcinum does not seem to help prevent influenza illness. However, there is preliminary evidence that oscillococcinum might reduce the duration of influenza symptoms by 0.28 days (10804,12245). This small decrease in duration may not be clinically meaningful. The credibility of this finding is questioned due to the methodological flaws of the study. More evidence is needed to rate oscillococcinum for this use.

Mechanism of Action
Oscillococcinum is a homeopathic dilution of duck liver and heart extract. Homeopathy is a system of medicine established in the 19th century by a German physician named Samuel Hahnemann. Its basic principles are that "like treats like" and "potentiation through dilution." For example, in homeopathy, influenza would be treated with an extreme dilution of a substance that normally causes influenza when taken in high doses.
A French physician discovered a substance he called "oscillococci" while investigating the Spanish flu in 1917. But he was mistaken that his oscillococci were the cause of the flu (12011).
Practitioners of homeopathy believe that more diluted preparations are more potent. Many homeopathic preparations are so diluted that they contain little or no active ingredient. Therefore, most homeopathic products are not expected to have any pharmacological effects, drug interactions, or other harmful effects. Any beneficial effects are controversial and cannot be explained by current scientific methods.
Dilutions of 1 to 10 are designated by an "X." So, a 1X dilution = 1:10; 3X = 1:1000; 6X = 1:1,000,000. Dilutions of 1 to 100 are designated by a "C." A 1C dilution = 1:100; 3C = 1:1,000,000. Dilutions of 24X or 12C or more contain zero molecules of the original active ingredient. Oscillococcinum is usually diluted from 9C to 200C and therefore usually contains no measurable active ingredient (12011).

Adverse Reactions
None reported. Oscillococcinum is a homeopathic product and contains no active ingredient. Therefore, it is not expected to cause any adverse effects.

Interactions with Herbs & Other Dietary Supplements
None known.

Interactions with Drugs
None known.

Interactions with Foods
None known.

Interactions with Lab Tests
None known.

Interactions with Diseases or Conditions
None known.

Dosage and Administration
ORAL: For influenza, one manufacturer (Boiron) recommends taking the contents of one tube up to 3 times per day.

Comments
Oscillococcinum is a brand name homeopathic product manufactured by Boiron. Similar homeopathic products are found in other brands. Boiron claims that their Oscillococcinum is the number one over-the-counter medicine for flu in France and the number one homeopathic remedy for flu in the US.

Homeopathic products are permitted for sale in the US due to legislation passed in 1938 sponsored by a homeopathic physician who was also a Senator. The law still requires that the FDA allow the sale of products listed in the Homeopathic Pharmacopeia of the United States. However, homeopathic preparations are not held to the same safety and effectiveness standards as conventional medicines.

OSHA

Also Known As
Bear Root, Chuchupate, Colorado Cough Root, Indian Parsley, Mountain Lovage, Porter's Licorice Root, Wild Celery Root.

CAUTION: See separate listings for Lovage and Licorice.

Scientific Names
Ligusticum porteri.

Family: Apiaceae/Umbelliferae.

People Use This For
Orally, osha is used for sore throat, bronchitis, cough, common cold, influenza, pneumonia, and indigestion. It is also used orally to treat other viral infections including herpes and AIDS/HIV.

Topically, osha is used to prevent infections of skin wounds.

Traditionally, osha has also been used by Native American and Hispanic cultures for pneumonia, colds, bronchitis, influenza, tuberculosis, hay fever, and coughs.

Safety
POSSIBLY SAFE ...when used orally and appropriately (12).

PREGNANCY: LIKELY UNSAFE ...when used orally. Osha has been used to stimulate menstruation and is reported to have abortifacient activity (12,19); contraindicated.

LACTATION: Insufficient reliable information available; avoid using.

Effectiveness
There is insufficient reliable information available about the effectiveness of osha.

Mechanism of Action
The applicable part of osha is the root (12). Osha contains the compound ligustilide, which might have antimicrobial and antiviral activities (6734,6736). Preliminary evidence indicates that osha might have viral protease inhibitory effects. It might also inhibit the influenza virus (6733). To date, there are no studies published of osha use in humans or animals.

Adverse Reactions
None reported.

Interactions with Herbs & Other Dietary Supplements
None known.

Interactions with Drugs
None known.

Interactions with Foods
None known.

Interactions with Lab Tests
None known.

Interactions with Diseases or Conditions
None known.

Dosage and Administration
ORAL: As a tincture, osha is commonly taken as 20-60 drops up to 5 times daily. These are usually prepared as a 1:2 tincture with the fresh root or 1:5 tincture with the dried root (6729). Osha is often combined with other herbs and supplements and sold as a multi-ingredient product.

Comments
The leaves of osha are similar in appearance to the very toxic poison hemlock. Osha must be identified by the root, which is described as malodorous with a strong celery-like odor, or should be obtained from reputable commercial sources. Osha, which grows at higher elevations in the western US, is difficult to cultivate. The popularity of Osha has led to over harvesting of the wild plant (6735). Osha has been designated an endangered plant by conservationists (6735).

OSTRICH FERN

Also Known As
Fiddlehead Fern, Garden Fern, Hardy Fern.

Scientific Names
Matteuccia struthiopteris, synonym Osmunda struthiopteris.
Family: Dryopteridaceae.

People Use This For
Orally, ostrich fern is used as a gargle for sore throat.
Topically, ostrich fern is used for wounds and boils.
Ostrich fern is used for food. It is regarded as a seasonal delicacy.

Safety
LIKELY SAFE ...when used as a food if prepared appropriately (6,5002).
LIKELY UNSAFE ...when not cooked properly (6); may cause severe food poisoning.
PREGNANCY AND LACTATION: Insufficient reliable information available; avoid using.

Effectiveness
There is insufficient reliable information available about the effectiveness of ostrich fern.

Mechanism of Action
The applicable part of ostrich fern is the young shoot top. One field guide states wild ostrich fern greens have laxative properties (6). Toxins responsible for poisonings have not been identified, but they are believed deactivated by boiling. The CDC recommends thorough cooking (e.g., boiling for 10 minutes) before eating (5002).

Adverse Reactions
Centers for Disease Control and Prevention (CDC) links outbreaks of severe food poisoning to consumption of raw or lightly cooked ostrich ferns (6,5002). Ostrich fern can cause nausea, vomiting, abdominal cramping (6), diarrhea, and headaches after ingestion (5002).

Interactions with Herbs & Other Dietary Supplements
None known.

Interactions with Drugs
None known.

Interactions with Foods
None known.

Interactions with Lab Tests
None known.

Interactions with Diseases or Conditions
None known.

Dosage and Administration
ORAL: Cook young shoots of ostrich fern (fiddleheads) thoroughly (e.g., boiling for 10 minutes) before eating (5002).

Comments
The tops of the young shoots of ostrich fern, known as fiddleheads, are regarded as a seasonal delicacy. They are available canned, frozen, or fresh (6). Boil at least 10 minutes before eating.

OSWEGO TEA

Also Known As
Bee Balm, Blue Balm, High Balm, Low Balm, Monarda, Mountain Balm, Mountain Mint, Scarlet Monarda.
CAUTION: See separate listing for Horsemint.

Scientific Names
Monarda didyma.
Family: Lamiaceae/Labiatae.

People Use This For
Orally, oswego tea is used for digestive disorders including flatulence and premenstrual syndrome. It is also used as an antispasmodic and diuretic.
In Europe, oswego tea is used for decreasing fever and as a fragrance.

Safety
There is insufficient reliable information available about the safety of oswego tea.
PREGNANCY: UNSAFE ...when used orally because it may possibly promote menstruation and stimulate menstrual flow (12).
LACTATION: Insufficient reliable information available; avoid using.

Effectiveness
There is insufficient reliable information available about the effectiveness of oswego tea.

Mechanism of Action
There is insufficient reliable information available about the possible mechanism of action and active ingredients.

Adverse Reactions
None reported.

Interactions with Herbs & Other Dietary Supplements
None known.

Interactions with Drugs
None known.

Interactions with Foods
None known.

Interactions with Lab Tests
None known.

Interactions with Diseases or Conditions
None known.

Dosage and Administration
ORAL: Oswego tea is taken as tea prepared from the powdered herb (18).

Comments
Oswego tea got the alternate name bergamot because of the similarity of its pleasant scent to that of the oil of bergamot oranges (see separate listing). During the period of the Boston tea party, it was drunk in place of black tea. Lemon balm is also known as bee balm, a common name for oswego tea, and may be confused with it.

OX-EYE DAISY

Also Known As
Butter Daisy, Dun Daisy, Golden Daisy, Goldenseal, Great Ox-Eye, Herb Margaret, Horse Daisy, Horse Gowan, Marguerite, Maudlin Daisy, Maudlinwort, Moon Daisy, Moon Flower, Moon Penny, Ox Eye Daisy, Poverty Weed, White Daisy, White Weed.
CAUTION: See separate listing for Goldenseal (Hydrastis canadensis).

Scientific Names
Chrysanthemum leucanthemum.
Family: Compositae.

People Use This For
Orally, ox-eye daisy is used for indications similar to German chamomile. These uses include the common cold, cough, bronchitis, fever, mouth and pharynx inflammation, liver and gallbladder complaints, loss of appetite, and susceptibility to infection. It is also used as an antispasmodic, diuretic, and tonic.
Topically, ox-eye daisy is used for skin inflammation, wounds, and burns.

Safety
There is insufficient reliable information available about the safety of ox-eye daisy.
Pregnancy and Lactation: Insufficient reliable information available; avoid using.

Effectiveness
There is insufficient reliable information available about the effectiveness of ox-eye daisy.

Mechanism of Action
The applicable parts of ox-eye daisy are the above ground flowering parts. There is insufficient reliable information available about the possible mechanism of action and active ingredients.

Adverse Reactions
Ox-eye daisy can cause an allergic reaction in individuals sensitive to the Asteraceae/Compositae family. Members of this family include ragweed, chrysanthemums, marigolds, daisies, and many other herbs.

Interactions with Herbs & Other Dietary Supplements
None known.

Interactions with Drugs
None known.

Interactions with Foods
None known.

Interactions with Lab Tests
None known.

Interactions with Diseases or Conditions
CROSS-ALLERGENICITY: Can cause an allergic reaction in individuals sensitive to the Asteraceae/Compositae family. Members of this family include ragweed, chrysanthemums, marigolds, daisies, and many other herbs.

Dosage and Administration
ORAL: The daily dose is equivalent to 10-15 grams dried herb, taken as tea. The tea is prepared by steeping 3 grams dried leaf in 150 mL of boiling water for 10-15 minutes and straining (18).
TOPICAL: A tea is prepared by steeping 2 teaspoons of dried leaf in 1 cup of boiling water for 15 minutes, straining and applied topically. As a bath additive, 50 grams of dried herb is added to 1 L bath water (18).

Comments
Ox-eye daisy is alternately known as goldenseal, but it is unrelated to the more commonly known goldenseal (Hydrastis canadensis).

PAGODA TREE

Also Known As
Chinese Scholartree, Japanese Pagoda Tree.

Scientific Names
Styphnolobium japonicum, synonym Sophora japonica.
Family: Fabaceae/Leguminosae.

People Use This For
Orally, pagoda tree is used in dilutions for dysentery.

Safety
POSSIBLY UNSAFE ...when the seeds are used orally (18). Regular use of seed meal can cause facial edema or even death. High doses could cause cystine poisoning (18).
PREGNANCY AND LACTATION: POSSIBLY UNSAFE ...when used orally (18); avoid using.

Effectiveness
There is insufficient reliable information available about the effectiveness of pagoda tree.

Mechanism of Action
The applicable parts of the pagoda tree are the seeds. Cystine poisoning may occur with high dosages (18).

Adverse Reactions
None reported with short-term use. Using pagoda tree seed long-term may cause edema and death (18).

Interactions with Herbs & Other Dietary Supplements
None known.

Interactions with Drugs
None known.

Interactions with Foods
None known.

Interactions with Lab Tests
None known.

Interactions with Diseases or Conditions
None known.

Dosage and Administration
No typical dosage.

PANAX PSEUDOGINSENG

Also Known As
Chai-Jen-Shen, Field Seven, Himalayan Ginseng, Jia Renshen, Nepal Ginseng, Notoginseng, Pseudoginseng Root, Samch'il, San Qi, San-Qi Ginseng, San Qui, Sanqi, Sanqi Powder, Sanchi, Sanshichi, Three Seven, Tian Qi, Tienchi, Tienchi Ginseng.
CAUTION: See separate listing for Ginseng, Panax.

Scientific Names
Panax pseudoginseng, synonyms Panax notoginseng, Aralia pseuodoginseng.
Family: Araliaceae.

People Use This For
Orally, panax pseudoginseng is used as a hemostatic for conditions including vomiting and coughing up blood, blood in the urine or stool, nosebleed, and hemorrhagic disease. It is also used to relieve pain; and to reduce swelling, blood cholesterol, and blood pressure. Panax pseudoginseng is also used for angina, dizziness, and acute sore throat.
Topically, Panax pseudoginseng is used to stop bleeding.
In combination with seven other herbs (PC-SPES), Panax pseudoginseng is used to treat prostate cancer.

Safety
There is insufficient reliable information available about the safety of Panax pseudoginseng.
PREGNANCY AND LACTATION: LIKELY UNSAFE ...when used orally; contraindicated (5559). Ginsenoside Rb1, an active constituent of Panax pseudoginseng, has teratogenic effects in animal models (10447).

Effectiveness
There is insufficient reliable information available about the effectiveness of Panax pseudoginseng.

Mechanism of Action
Panax pseudoginseng root contains 12% saponins; the most important are triterpenoid saponins referred to collectively as ginsenosides or panaxosides. Ginsenosides is the term developed by Asian researchers, and the term panaxosides was developed by Russian researchers. Numerous subtypes of ginsenosides have been identified. Like Panax ginseng, Panax pseudoginseng contains the ginsenosides Rb1 and Rg1, and lesser amounts of Rd and Re. Rb1 has a low oral bioavailability, and Rg1 is rapidly eliminated from the blood in animal models, which limits its pharmacologic effects (11153,12536). Panax pseudoginseng is believed to dilate the coronary vessels, reduce vascular resistance, and improve the coronary collateral circulation. This could increase blood flow while reducing blood pressure. It would also reduce the heart metabolic rate and oxygen consumption. Evidence also suggests Panax pseudoginseng has an antiarrhythmic effect (5558). Animal evidence suggests orally administered Panax pseudoginseng root can reduce fibrinogenaemia, an increased level of fibrinogen in the blood (11487). Evidence also suggests oral administration can decrease plasma lipid levels by reducing total cholesterol and triglycerides (11487). Trilinolein, a triacylglycerol purified from Panax pseudoginseng, might have antioxidant activity (6289). When applied topically, however, preliminary information suggests the dried root of panax pseudoginseng may be useful as a hemostatic agent because it appears to shorten bleeding time (4056). In vitro research shows estrogen-like activity. Studies on human breast cancer cells indicate that Panax pseudoginseng root, specifically its constituent ginsenonside-Rg1, acts as a phytoestrogen by stimulating human breast cancer cell proliferation (11488). Pananotin, a protein isolated from Panax pseudoginseng root, seems to have antiviral and antifungal activity, according to preliminary research. It appears to inhibit HIV reverse transcriptase in vitro (11485,11486).
Unlike some other ginsengs, Panax pseudoginseng doesn't appear to affect blood glucose levels (12536).

Adverse Reactions
Orally, Panax pseudoginseng can cause dry mouth, flushed skin, nervousness, insomnia, nausea, and vomiting (5558).

Interactions with Herbs & Other Dietary Supplements
None known.

Interactions with Drugs
None known.

Interactions with Foods
None known.

Interactions with Lab Tests
None known.

Interactions with Diseases or Conditions
HORMONE SENSITIVE CANCERS/CONDITIONS: Because Panax pseudoginseng seems to have estrogenic effects, women with hormone sensitive conditions including breast cancer, uterine cancer, ovarian cancer, endometriosis, and uterine fibroids should avoid using panax pseudoginseng (11488).

Dosage and Administration
ORAL: A typical dose is 1-1.5 grams divided into three doses per day (5558).
TOPICAL: No typical dosage.

PANCREATIN

Also Known As
Pancreatinum, Pancreatis pulvis.

Scientific Names
Pancreatin.

People Use This For

Orally, pancreatin is used to treat malabsorption syndromes associated with pancreatic insufficiency in cystic fibrosis, chronic pancreatitis, or pancreas removal. It is also used orally for flatulence or as a digestive aid.

Safety

LIKELY SAFE ...when used orally and appropriately for replacement therapy by individuals with pancreatic insufficiency (15). Some pancreatin products contaminated by Salmonella have caused illness (9). Use only products from reputable manufacturers.

PREGNANCY AND LACTATION: Insufficient reliable information available; avoid using unless essential for replacement therapy (15).

Effectiveness

EFFECTIVE

Pancreatic insufficiency. Taking pancreatin orally is effective as replacement therapy in pancreatic insufficiency due to cystic fibrosis, chronic pancreatitis, or pancreas removal (15).

LIKELY INEFFECTIVE

Digestive disorders. Taking pancreatin orally isn't effective for treating digestive disorders not related to pancreatic insufficiency, including flatulence (15,16).

Mechanism of Action

Pancreatin contains digestive enzymes, including lipase, protease, and amylase. These enzymes are usually obtained from pork or beef pancreas (15). These enzymes catalyze the hydrolysis of fats, peptides, and starches in the small intestine. Pancreatin is inactivated when acid, including gastric acid, is present in more than trace amounts (15,506).

Adverse Reactions

Orally, excessive doses of pancreatin can cause nausea, vomiting, diarrhea, or other transient intestinal upset, and perianal soreness. Extremely high doses have been associated with high uric acid level in blood and urine, and colon strictures (15).

Topically, pancreatin preparations that are held in the mouth prior to swallowing can cause irritation of the mucosa, including ulceration and stomatitis (15). Pancreatin powder is irritating to the skin, eyes, mucus membranes, and respiratory tract. Hypersensitivity reactions, e.g., sneezing, lacrimation, and skin rash, have been reported (15). Inhalation of dust containing pancreatin has been associated with pulmonary hypersensitivity reactions, allergic rhinitis, bronchospasm, and asthma (11768,11769).

Interactions with Herbs & Other Dietary Supplements

FOLIC ACID: Pancreatin can decrease absorption of folic acid (9).

Interactions with Drugs

ACARBOSE (Precose, Prandase): Enzymes present in pancreatin can decrease the efficacy of acarbose (9).

Interactions with Foods

ACIDIC FOODS: Concomitant intake of acidic foods or fruit juices can break down pancreatin enzymes, reducing the activity of pancreatin preparations that are not enteric-coated (15).

ALKALINE FOODS: Mixing enteric-coated granules into alkaline foods, e.g., chicken, veal, or green beans, might destroy the coating (15).

Interactions with Lab Tests

URIC ACID: Pancreatin, particularly at high doses, can cause an increase in serum and urine uric acid levels (15).

Interactions with Diseases or Conditions

None known.

Dosage and Administration

ORAL: For pancreatic replacement therapy, the initial dose of pancreatin is usually 8,000 to 24,000 USP units of lipase activity taken before or with each meal or snack. To control steatorrhea, dose can be increased as needed or until nausea, vomiting, or diarrhea occurs (15). Pancreatin is available as enteric-coated tablets, powder, or capsules containing the powder or enteric-coated granules (506).

Comments

Each mg of pancreatin contains not less than 25 USP units of amylase activity, not less than 2 USP units of lipase activity, and not less than 25 USP units of protease activity (15,16). Pancreatin that is more potent is labeled as a multiple of these three minimum activities, e.g., pancreatin 4X (10,16).

PANGAMIC ACID

Also Known As
Calcium Pangamate, Calgam, Di-isopropylamine Dichloroacetate, Vitamin B15.
CAUTION: See separate listing for Dimethylglycine.

Scientific Names
None.

People Use This For
Orally, pangamic acid is used for detoxifying the body; treating asthma and allied diseases; conditions of the skin and respiratory tract; painful nerve and joint afflictions; cell proliferation like cancer; eczema; arthritis; neuritis; and improving the oxygenation of the heart, brain, and other vital organs. It is also used orally for alcoholism, hangovers, fatigue, protecting against urban air pollutants, extending cell life, stimulating increased immune system response, lowering blood cholesterol levels, and assisting in hormone regulation.

Safety
POSSIBLY UNSAFE ...when used orally (5,2623). There is no standard chemical identity for pangamic acid. Dichloroacetate, present in some formulations, is mutagenic, possibly carcinogenic. Dimethylglycine, present in some formulations, can react with nitrites in the intestines to form the potent carcinogen, dimethylnitrosamine (5).
PREGNANCY AND LACTATION: POSSIBLY UNSAFE ...when used orally; avoid using because it is difficult to know what constituents are present. Dichloroacetate, present in some formulations, is mutagenic according to the Ames test (5).

Effectiveness
POSSIBLY INEFFECTIVE

Athletic performance. Taking pangamic acid orally doesn't seem to improve exercise endurance (2645).
There is insufficient reliable information available about the effectiveness of pangamic acid for its other uses.

Mechanism of Action
There is no standard chemical identity for pangamic acid. Formulations can include one or more of the following: sodium gluconate, calcium gluconate, glycine, diisopropylamine dichloroacetate, dimethylglycine, calcium chloride, dicalcium phosphate, stearic acid, cellulose, or other constituents (5). Diisopropylamine acts on the smooth muscle to reduce blood pressure (5). In the intestines, dimethylglycine reacts with nitrates to form the potent carcinogen, dimethylnitrosamine (5).

Adverse Reactions
Orally, use of pangamic acid can be potentially carcinogenic (2623).

Interactions with Herbs & Other Dietary Supplements
CARDIAC GLYCOSIDE-CONTAINING HERBS: Theoretically, concomitant use of these herbs with large amounts of calcium salts, including calcium chloride and dicalcium phosphate, can increase the inotropic effects of cardiac glycosides and the risk of arrhythmias. Cardiac glycoside-containing herbs include black hellebore, Canadian hemp, digitalis, figwort, lily-of-the-valley, motherwort, oleander, pheasant's eye, pleurisy root, squill, and strophanthus (4,19).

Interactions with Drugs
CALCIUM CHANNEL BLOCKERS: Theoretically, concomitant use of calcium channel blockers with calcium salts, including calcium chloride and dicalcium phosphate, can decrease the drug's effects (506). Calcium channel blockers include nifedipine (Adalat, Procardia), verapamil (Calan, Isoptin, Verelan), diltiazem (Cardizem), isradipine (DynaCirc), felodipine (Plendil), amlodipine (Norvasc), and others.
DIGOXIN (Lanoxin): Theoretically, concomitant use of digoxin with large amounts of calcium salts, such as calcium chloride and dicalcium phosphate, can increase the inotropic effects of digoxin and the risk of arrhythmias (15).
THIAZIDE DIURETICS: Theoretically, concomitant use of these diuretics with calcium salts like calcium chloride and dicalcium phosphate can result in hypercalcemia (15).

Interactions with Foods
None known.

Interactions with Lab Tests
None known.

Interactions with Diseases or Conditions
KIDNEY DYSFUNCTION: Use pangamic acid with caution, because it can cause oxalate stones and other kidney problems (5).

Dosage and Administration
No typical dosage.

Comments
There is no standard chemical identity for pangamic acid. Pangamic acid is the name given to a product originally claimed to contain D-gluconodimethyl aminoacetic acid, which was obtained from apricot kernels and later from rice bran (5). It is also referred to as vitamin B15, but pangamic acid is not generally recognized as a vitamin (2623). Research by Soviet sports scientists focused attention on pangamic acid, but little, if any, research has been conducted in the US. The claims of pangamic acid's effectiveness are controversial (5). Natural sources for D-gluconodimethyl aminoacetic acid include brewer's yeast, whole brown rice, sesame seeds, and pumpkin seeds.

PANTETHINE

Also Known As
Bis-pantothenamidoethyl Disulfide, D-Pantethine, Pantetina, Pantomin, Pantosin.
CAUTION: See separate listings for Pantothenic Acid and Coenzyme Q10.

Scientific Names
D-bis-(N-Pantothenyl-B-aminoethyl)-disulfide.

People Use This For
Orally, pantethine is used for lowering cholesterol, preventing inflammation, boosting immune function, treating cystinosis, treating gastrointestinal diseases, and improving athletic performance. It is also used orally for improving energy, lowering cardiovascular risk, improving adrenal function, protecting against mental and physical stress, and preventing allergy symptoms in people allergic to formaldehyde.

Safety
POSSIBLY SAFE ...when used orally and appropriately. Pantethine appears to be safe for up to 12 months (8313,8314,8315,10237,10238).
PREGNANCY AND LACTATION: Insufficient reliable information available; avoid using.

Effectiveness
POSSIBLY EFFECTIVE

Hyperlipoproteinemia. A clinically significant effect of pantethine on hyperlipoproteinemia appears to be modest. Taking pantethine orally might slightly lower triglycerides, total cholesterol, and low-density lipoprotein (LDL) cholesterol; and raise high-density lipoprotein (HDL) cholesterol (8313,8314,8317,8318,8319,9123,10238). The lipoprotein lowering effect seems to be maintained with continued treatment for up to one year (10238). Pantethine also appears to correct lipoprotein abnormalities that often occur in patients with renal failure undergoing hemodialysis (10237). Other investigators have found no effect (8315,8316). Pantethine seems to be less effective than gemfibrozil (Lopid) for lowering lipids and triglycerides (9123).

INSUFFICIENT RELIABLE EVIDENCE to RATE

Athletic performance. Some clinical research suggests that pantethine in combination with pantothenic acid and thiamine (given as allithiamin) does not improve muscular strength or endurance in well-trained athletes (10432).
Cystinosis. Preliminary evidence suggests that pantethine might be beneficial for cystinosis, an autosomal recessive genetic disease (8860).
More evidence is needed to rate pantethine for these uses.

Mechanism of Action
Pantethine is a vitamin-like dietary supplement. In the body, it is converted to pantetheine, which is a precursor and component of coenzyme A. Pantethine is related to pantothenic acid (vitamin B5), but seems to have different physiological effects (8318,8320). Pantethine seems to have a beneficial effect on triglyceride and lipoprotein levels by producing cystamine. The hydrolysis product cystamine inhibits acetyl-CoA carboxylase, which in turn reduces triglyceride synthesis. Pantethine might also reduce cholesterol synthesis by inhibiting HMG-CoA reductase (8320,8321,8861,8863), by inhibiting the conversion of lanosterol to cholesterol (8865), and by inhibiting the lipid peroxidation of low-density lipoproteins (LDL) (8861,8864). Preliminary research suggests that pantethine might reduce atherosclerosis (8322). Some clinical evidence indicates pantethine might decrease platelet aggregation (9123). By producing cystamine that can deplete the cystinotic fibroblasts of cystine, pantethine might be beneficial for cystinosis, an autosomal recessive genetic disease (8860). Preliminary evidence also suggests pantethine might prevent the hypersecretion of cortisol associated with high mental and physical stress conditions, but the mechanisms are

poorly understood (8859).
Pantethine seems to slow formation of experimentally induced cataracts, but in mice that develop age-related cataracts, pantethine doesn't seem to provide any protective effect (8323,8324,8325).

Adverse Reactions
Orally, pantethine seems to be well-tolerated (8313,8314,8316,8317,8318,8319). It can cause minor gastrointestinal complaints such as nausea, diarrhea, and epigastric discomfort (8315).

Interactions with Herbs & Other Dietary Supplements
ANTICOAGULANT, ANTIPLATELET HERBS AND SUPPLEMENTS: Concomitant use of herbs and supplements that affect platelet aggregation could theoretically increase the risk of bleeding in some people due to the possible effects of pantethine on platelet aggregation (9123). Some of these herbs and supplements include angelica, clove, danshen, fenugreek, feverfew, fish oils, garlic, ginger, horse chestnut, Panax ginseng, red clover, turmeric, vitamin E, and others.

Interactions with Drugs
ANTICOAGULANT/ANTIPLATELET DRUGS: Concomitant administration might increase the risk of bleeding. Some evidence suggests that pantethine reduces platelet aggregation (9123). When taken concurrently with drugs that affect platelets or coagulation, it might have an additive effect. Some of these drugs include aspirin, clopidogrel (Plavix), dalteparin (Fragmin), enoxaparin (Lovenox), heparin, indomethacin (Indocin), ticlopidine (Ticlid), warfarin (Coumadin), and others.

Interactions with Foods
None known.

Interactions with Lab Tests
None known.

Interactions with Diseases or Conditions
BLEEDING DISORDERS: There is some evidence that pantethine can decrease platelet aggregation (9123). Theoretically, pantethine might increase the risk of severe bleeding in patients with bleeding disorders; use with caution.

Dosage and Administration
ORAL: For treating hyperlipoproteinemia, 300 mg has been used 3 to 4 times daily (8313,8314,8315,8316,8317,8318,8319,8862,9123). For treating lipoprotein abnormalities in patients with renal failure undergoing hemodialysis, 600 to 1200 mg pantethine daily has been used (10237).

PANTOTHENIC ACID (VITAMIN B5)

Also Known As
B Complex Vitamin, Calcii Pantothenas, Calcium Pantothenate, D-Calcium Pantothenate, D-Panthenol, D-Pantothenyl Alcohol, Dexpanthenol, Dexpanthenolum, Panthenol, Pantothenol, Pantothenylol, Vitamin B-5, Vitamin B5.
CAUTION: See separate listing for Pantethine.

Scientific Names
D-pantothenic acid; Pantothenic acid.

People Use This For
Orally, pantothenic acid is used for treating dietary deficiencies, acne, alcoholism, allergies, alopecia, asthma, attention deficit-hyperactivity disorder (ADHD), autism, burning feet syndrome, candidiasis, cardiac failure, carpal tunnel syndrome, respiratory disorders, celiac disease, colitis, conjunctivitis, convulsions, and cystitis. It is also used orally for dandruff, depression, diabetic neuropathy, enhancing immune function, improving athletic performance, glossitis, gray hair, headache, hyperactivity, hypoglycemia, insomnia, irritability, low blood pressure, multiple sclerosis, muscular dystrophy, muscular cramps in the legs associated with pregnancy or alcoholism, neuralgia, and obesity. Pantothenic acid is also used orally for osteoarthritis, rheumatoid arthritis, Parkinson's disease, peripheral neuritis, premenstrual syndrome (PMS), prostatitis, protection against mental and physical stress and anxiety, reducing adverse effects of thyroid therapy in congenital hypothyroidism, reducing signs of aging, reducing susceptibility to colds and other infections, retarded growth, shingles, skin disorders, stimulating adrenal glands, stomatitis, chronic fatigue syndrome, salicylate toxicity, streptomycin neurotoxicity, vertigo, and wound healing.
Topically, dexpanthenol, an analog of pantothenic acid, is used for itching, promoting healing of mild eczemas and dermatoses, insect stings, bites, poison ivy, diaper rash, acne, and preventing and treating acute

radiotherapy skin reactions.
Intramuscularly or by intravenous infusion, dexpanthenol is used for stimulating intestinal peristalsis, to minimize the possibility of paralytic ileus after major abdominal surgery, for intestinal atony causing abdominal distension, postoperative or postpartum flatus, for postoperative delay in resumption of intestinal motility, and for treating paralytic ileus.

Safety

LIKELY SAFE ...when used orally and appropriately. Amounts up to 10 grams have been ingested without significant adverse effects (15).
PREGNANCY: LIKELY SAFE ...when used orally in amounts not exceeding the recommended daily allowance (RDA). The RDA during pregnancy is 6 mg (3094). There is insufficient reliable information about the safety of using pantothenic acid in amounts exceeding the RDA during pregnancy; avoid using.
LACTATION: LIKELY SAFE ...when used orally in amounts not exceeding the recommended daily allowance (RDA). The RDA during lactation is 7 mg (3094). There is insufficient reliable information available about the safety of using pantothenic acid in amounts exceeding the RDA during lactation; avoid using.

Effectiveness

EFFECTIVE

Pantothenic acid deficiency. Taking pantothenic acid orally is effective for treating and preventing pantothenic acid deficiency (15).

POSSIBLY INEFFECTIVE

Irradiated skin. Twice daily topical application of dexpanthenol, an analog of pantothenic acid, to areas of irradiated skin does not seem to reduce erythema, desquamation, itching, or pain following radiation treatment (7192).

INSUFFICIENT RELIABLE EVIDENCE to RATE

Athletic performance. Some clinical research suggests that pantothenic acid in combination with pantethine and thiamine (given as allithiamin) does not improve muscular strength or endurance in well-trained athletes (10432).
Attention deficit-hyperactivity disorder (ADHD). There is conflicting preliminary clinical evidence regarding the usefulness of pantothenic acid in combination with other megadose vitamins for the treatment of ADHD (3351,9957).
Osteoarthritis and rheumatoid arthritis. Preliminary clinical research suggests pantothenic acid (given as calcium pantothenate) does not significantly reduce the symptoms of arthritis in patients with rheumatoid arthritis, osteoarthritis, or other forms of arthritis (10433).
More evidence is needed to rate pantothenic acid for these uses.

Mechanism of Action

Pantothenic acid is required for intermediary metabolism of carbohydrates, proteins, and lipids (15). Dexpanthenol is converted in the body to pantothenic acid. Pantothenic acid is a precursor of coenzyme A, which is required in the acetylation reactions in gluconeogenesis; in the release of energy from carbohydrates; in the synthesis and degradation of fatty acids; and in the synthesis of sterols, steroid hormones, porphyrins, acetylcholine, and other compounds (15). Pantothenic acid also appears to be essential to normal epithelial function (15). Dietary deficiency of pantothenic acid has not been identified, but experimentally-induced deficiency has been associated with somnolence, fatigue, headache, paresthesia of the hands and feet followed by hyperreflexia and muscle weakness in the legs, cardiovascular instability, gastrointestinal (GI) complaints, changes in disposition, and increased susceptibility to infections (15). In large parenteral doses, dexpanthenol has been reported to increase GI peristalsis by stimulating acetylation of choline to acetylcholine, but efficacy has not been proven (15).

Adverse Reactions

Orally, large amounts of pantothenic acid can cause diarrhea. There is also one case of eosinophilic pleuro-pericardial effusion in a patient taking pantothenic acid 300 mg per day in combination with biotin 10 mg per day for 2 months (3914).

Interactions with Herbs & Other Dietary Supplements

None known.

Interactions with Drugs

None known.

Drug Influences on Nutrient Levels and Depletion

SOME DRUGS CAN AFFECT PANTOTHENIC ACID LEVELS:
ANTIBIOTICS: Destruction of normal gastrointestinal flora by antibiotics can cause decreased production of B vitamins. The clinical significance of this decreased production is not known. Consider supplementation only if clinical judgment warrants it (4434,4435,4436,4437,4438,4439,4440,4441,4442,4443).

Interactions with Foods
None known.

Interactions with Lab Tests
None known.

Interactions with Diseases or Conditions
GI OBSTRUCTION: Dexpanthenol, an alcohol analog of pantothenic acid, injection is contraindicated in individuals with gastrointestinal obstruction (15).
HEMOPHILIA: Dexpanthenol may prolong bleeding time (15).

Dosage and Administration
ORAL: As a dietary supplement, 5-10 mg pantothenic acid has been used (15). Recommended daily intakes for vitamin B5 are as follows: Infants 0-6 months, 1.7 mg; Infants 7-12 months, 1.8 mg; Children 1-3 years, 2 mg; Children 4-8 years, 3 mg; Children 9-13 years, 4 mg; Men and women 14 years and older, 5 mg (3094); Pregnant women, 6 mg; and Lactating women, 7 mg (3094).
TOPICAL: Dexpanthenol 2% as a cream applied to the affected areas once or twice daily (15).
INJECTION: Dexpanthenol as an injection is an FDA-approved prescription drug.

Comments
Only the dextrorotatory isomer of pantothenic acid has biologic activity (15). Vitamin B5 is commercially available as D-pantothenic acid and the synthetic derivatives, dexpanthenol and calcium pantothenate (15). Pantothenic acid is widely distributed in plant and animal tissues; rich sources include meat, vegetables, cereal grains, legumes, eggs, and milk (15). Calcium pantothenate 10 mg is equivalent to pantothenic acid 9.2 mg (15). Pantothenic acid is frequently used in combination with other B vitamins in vitamin B complex formulations. Vitamin B complex generally includes vitamin B1 (thiamine), vitamin B2 (riboflavin), vitamin B3 (niacin/niacinamide), vitamin B5 (pantothenic acid), vitamin B6 (pyridoxine), vitamin B12 (cyanocobalamin), and folic acid. However, some products do not contain all of these ingredients and some may include others, such as biotin, para-aminobenzoic acid (PABA), choline bitartrate, and inositol (3022).

PAPAIN

Also Known As
Papainum Crudum, Plant Protease Concentrate, Vegetable Pepsin.
CAUTION: See separate listings for Bromelain, Papaya, and American Pawpaw.

Scientific Names
Carica papaya.
Family: Caricacea.

People Use This For
Orally, papain is used for inflammation and edema following trauma and surgery, as a digestive aid, for treating parasitic worms, inflammation of the throat and pharynx, herpes zoster symptoms, chronic diarrhea, hay fever, nasal drainage, and psoriasis. Papain is also used as an adjuvant treatment for tumors.
Topically, it is used to treat infected wounds, sores, and ulcers.
In manufacturing, papain is a component of cosmetics, dentifrices, enzymatic soft contact lens cleaners, meat tenderizers, and meat products. It is also used for stabilizing and chillproofing beer.

Safety
LIKELY SAFE ...when used orally in amounts commonly found in foods. Papain has Generally Recognized As Safe (GRAS) status in the US (4912).
POSSIBLY SAFE ...when used orally and appropriately for medicinal purposes (964,968,969).
POSSIBLY UNSAFE ...when used orally in large amounts. In excessive doses, papain can cause significant side effects including esophageal perforation (6) ...when raw papain is used topically. Raw papain or papaya latex is a severe irritant and vesicant (6).
PREGNANCY: POSSIBLY UNSAFE ...when used orally. There is some concern that crude papain is teratogenic and embryotoxic (6).
LACTATION: Insufficient reliable information available; avoid using.

Effectiveness
POSSIBLY EFFECTIVE

Herpes zoster (shingles). Taking papain orally may improve the symptoms of herpes zoster (965).
Pharyngitis. Taking papain orally, in combination with other agents, may relieve pharyngeal

inflammation and swelling (964,968,969).
There is insufficient reliable information available about the effectiveness of papain for its other uses.

Mechanism of Action

Papain is actually a mixture of the proteolytic enzymes papain, chymopapain A, chymopapain B, and papaya peptidase A isolated from the fruit of Carica papaya. Chymopapain A and B have a similar proteolytic spectrum to papain but are less potent (6). There is some evidence that a multi-enzyme preparation containing papain can increase the release of reactive oxygen species (ROS) by polymorphonuclear cells (PMNs). ROS are thought to have tumoricidal effects (962). The multi-enzyme preparation also seems to induce the cytokines tumor necrosis factor (TNF)-alpha, interleukin-1 (IL-1)-beta, and interleukin-6 (IL-6) in a time and dose dependent manner (1364).

Adverse Reactions

Orally, large amounts of papain can cause esophageal perforation (6). Ingestion of papaya latex (raw papain) can cause severe gastritis.
Topically, papaya latex can cause severe irritation and blisters (6). Topical use of papain can cause itching (966).
Severe allergic reactions have been reported in sensitive individuals (6,967). One case report suggests that there may be cross-sensitivity between papain, fig, and kiwi (963).

Interactions with Herbs & Other Dietary Supplements

HERBS WITH ANTICOAGULANT/ANTIPLATELET POTENTIAL: Concomitant use of herbs that have constituents that might affect platelet aggregation could theoretically increase the risk of bleeding in some people. These herbs include angelica, clove, danshen, garlic, ginger, ginkgo, Panax ginseng, red clover, turmeric, and others.

Interactions with Drugs

None known.

Interactions with Foods

FIG, KIWI: Cross sensitivity to papain may occur in individuals sensitive to fig and kiwi (963).
POTATO PROTEIN: May inhibit papain proteolytic activity (958).

Interactions with Lab Tests

INTERNATIONAL NORMALIZATION RATIO (INR): Concomitant use of papaya extract (papain) and warfarin may increase INR (613).

Interactions with Diseases or Conditions

CLOTTING DISORDERS: Theoretically, may increase bleeding risk (2); avoid using.

Dosage and Administration

ORAL: Clinical trials have used 1500 mg (2520 FIP units) per day to treat inflammation and swelling following trauma and surgery (2).
TOPICAL: No typical dosage.

PAPAYA

Also Known As

Caricae papayae folium, Chirbhita, Erandachirbhita, Mamaerie, Melon Tree, Melonenbaumblaetter, Papaw, Papayas.
CAUTION: See separate listings for Papain and American Pawpaw.

Scientific Names

Carica papaya, synonyms Papaya carica, Carica peltata, Carica posoposa.
Family: Caricaceae.

People Use This For

Orally, papaya is used orally for preventing and treating gastrointestinal tract disorders, intestinal parasite infections, and as a sedative and diuretic.
Topically, papaya is used for nervous pains and elephantoid growths.

Safety

LIKELY SAFE ...when used orally in amounts commonly found in foods. Papaya has Generally Recognized As Safe (GRAS) status in the US (4912).
POSSIBLY SAFE ...when used orally and appropriately in medicinal amounts (6).
POSSIBLY UNSAFE ...when used orally in excessive amounts; papaya may cause esophageal perforation (6).
...when used topically; papaya latex (raw papain) is a severe irritant and vesicant (6).
PREGNANCY: POSSIBLY UNSAFE ...when used orally; avoid using. Crude papain shows evidence that it is

teratogenic and embryotoxic (6); however, this might be due to extraneous substances rather than papain (11).
LACTATION: Insufficient reliable information available; avoid using.

Effectiveness
There is insufficient reliable information available about the effectiveness of papaya.

Mechanism of Action
The applicable part of papaya is the leaf. Papaya leaf contains 2% papain and carpain (6). Papain is a mixture of enzymes that degrade protein, carbohydrates, and fats (515). Papain is unstable in digestive juices, which raises questions about whether it can be effective when used orally (515). Carpain is thought to be amebicidal. It might cause bradycardia (4009) or have central nervous system depressant or paralytic effects.

Adverse Reactions
Ingestion of large amounts of papain might cause esophageal perforation. Severe allergic reactions can occur in individuals sensitive to papain (6,515). Papaya may cause hypersensitivity reactions, which occur more commonly in people who are allergic to latex (6197,7853).

Interactions with Herbs & Other Dietary Supplements
PAPAIN: Concomitant use of papain and papaya can increase the effects and adverse effects of papain.

Interactions with Drugs
WARFARIN (Coumadin): Concomitant use might potentiate the effects of warfarin increasing the international normalization ratio (INR) (613).

Interactions with Foods
None known.

Interactions with Lab Tests
INTERNATIONAL NORMALIZATION RATIO (INR): Papain, which is in papaya leaf, can increase INR in people maintained on warfarin (Coumadin) (613).

Interactions with Diseases or Conditions
LATEX ALLERGY: People who are allergic to latex should avoid eating papaya or taking papaya-containing products because of the possibility of cross hypersensitivity between latex and papaya (6197,7853).

Dosage and Administration
ORAL: People typically use papaya with enzyme chewable tablets which contain 250 mg of papaya powder, 150 mg of dried pineapple juice powder, and 10 mg of papain (5024). One tablet is chewed up to three times daily, preferably after a meal (5024).
TOPICAL: No typical dosage.

Comments
Fermenting papaya leaves may make more potent, richer brewed teas (515).

PARA-AMINOBENZOIC ACID (PABA)

Also Known As
ABA, Aminobenzoate Potassium, Aminobenzoic Acid, Ethyl Dihydroxypropyl Aminobenzoate, Glyceryl Paraaminobenzoate, Octyl Diemthyl PABA, PABA, Padamate O, P-Aminobenzoic Acid, Vitamin B10, Vitamin H.

Scientific Names
Para-aminobenzoic acid; 4-aminobenzoic acid.

People Use This For
Orally, PABA is used for vitiligo, pemphigus, dermatomyositis, morphea, scleroderma, and Peyronie's disease. PABA is also used orally to treat female infertility, arthritis, anemia, rheumatic fever, constipation, disseminated systemic lupus erythematosus, lymphoblastoma cutis, and headaches. It is also used orally to darken gray hair, prevent hair loss, rejuvenate the skin, and prevent phototoxic reactions.
Topically, PABA is used as a sunscreen.

Safety
LIKELY SAFE ...when used topically and appropriately. PABA is FDA approved for topical use and there have not been reports of significant toxicity (266,272).
POSSIBLY SAFE ...when used orally and appropriately (10). PABA is an FDA-approved drug, but some potentially

serious side effects have been reported (10).
POSSIBLY UNSAFE ...when used orally in high doses. Doses greater than 12 grams per day have been associated with leukopenia (1061).
CHILDREN: LIKELY SAFE ...when used topically and appropriately (266,272). POSSIBLY SAFE ...when used orally and appropriately (10). PABA is an FDA-approved drug for use in children, but serious side effects have been reported (10). POSSIBLY UNSAFE ...when used orally in high doses. Doses greater than 220 mg/kg/day have been associated with fatal toxic effects (1061).
PREGNANCY AND LACTATION: LIKELY SAFE ...when used topically and appropriately (266,272). There is insufficient reliable information available about the safety of the oral use of PABA during pregnancy and breast-feeding; avoid using.

Effectiveness

EFFECTIVE

Sunburn. PABA is an FDA-approved sunscreen (266,8952). PABA seems to be effective during sweating, but not when skin is immersed in water (272).

POSSIBLY INEFFECTIVE

Scleroderma. Although PABA is FDA-approved for scleroderma, evidence supporting using PABA orally for scleroderma is limited. Some retrospective studies suggest it might help for some symptoms of scleroderma, but the most convincing evidence shows that it does not help (1071,1073,1074,1075).

INSUFFICIENT RELIABLE EVIDENCE to RATE

Dermatomyositis. PABA is FDA-approved for use in dermatomyositis, but there is limited evidence to support this use (10).
Morphea. PABA is FDA-approved for use in morphea, but there is limited evidence to support this use (10).
Pemphigus. PABA is FDA-approved for use in pemphigus, but there is limited evidence to support this use (10).
Peyronie's disease. PABA is FDA-approved for use in Peyronie's disease, but there is very limited evidence to support this use (1067,8951).
Vitiligo. PABA is FDA-approved for use in vitiligo, but there is limited evidence to support this use (10).
More evidence is needed to rate PABA for these uses.

Mechanism of Action

Para-aminobenzoic Acid (PABA) is a part of the folic acid molecule (16) and is found naturally in several foods including grains, eggs, milk, and meat (266). PABA was once considered to be a B vitamin, but is now considered a nonessential nutrient (16,8954). Interestingly, pathogenic bacteria require PABA to synthesize folic acid. Sulfonamide antibiotics exert their antibacterial effect by inhibiting folic acid synthesis from PABA (16). Although blood, urine, sweat, and spinal fluid contain detectable amounts of PABA, deficiency of PABA has not been described in humans (266). Endogenous PABA seems to be involved in a number of biologic processes, but its precise role is not known (10,266). The bioavailability of PABA may decline with age. Factors such as bacterial overgrowth due to chronic atrophic gastritis and reduced secretion of gastric acid that may occur with aging might limit the absorption of PABA (12460).
PABA is exogenously administered for fibrotic diseases such as dermatomyositis, morphea, pemphigus, Peyronie's disease, and scleroderma. Fibrosis might be caused by a long-term imbalance of serotonin and monoamine oxidase (MAO) activity at the tissue level. MAO requires significant tissue oxygenation to function properly. PABA may enhance MAO activity by increasing tissue oxygenation (10,266,8951).
PABA is also taken orally to darken gray hair. Although the exact mechanism is unknown, PABA appears to have an effect on melanin metabolism (8953,8954). PABA may act synergistically with cortisone in the treatment of rheumatoid arthritis. Although the mechanism is not completely understood, it is theorized that the metabolism of cortisone by the liver is decreased when oral PABA and intramuscular cortisone are given simultaneously (4488).
Topically, PABA is used as a sunscreen because it can act as a filter to block the penetration of ultraviolet (UV) radiation to the cells of the epidermis. PABA primarily blocks UVB sunlight, but may give some protection against UVA radiation at higher concentrations (272,8952).

Adverse Reactions

Orally, nausea, vomiting, dyspepsia, diarrhea, and anorexia are the most common side effects of PABA (10,1074). PABA should be discontinued if adverse effects prevent the patient from eating (10). In one report up to 25% of patients discontinued PABA due to intolerance of side effects (1074). Allergic reactions including fever and skin rash have also occurred (10,1074). Liver toxicity, including fatal hepatitis has been reported in patients taking high doses (12-48 grams per day) (1061,1094). In one case 12 grams per day for 2 months caused liver toxicity (1094). Although PABA is sometimes used to treat vitiligo, it has also been reported to cause vitiligo (1086). High dose PABA (up to 48 grams per day) can cause decreased white blood count below 4,000 mm3 in approximately 30% of patients (1061). Death has been reported in 3 children treated with 24 grams of PABA per day for rheumatic fever or arthritis. At autopsy, all had fatty changes in the liver, kidney, and myocardium (1061).
Topically, PABA can cause contact dermatitis and sometimes paradoxical photosensitivity (272). Some forms of PABA may stain clothing with a yellow discoloration (266).

Interactions with Herbs & Other Dietary Supplements
None known.

Interactions with Drugs
CORTISONE (Cortisone Acetate): PABA might decrease the metabolism of cortisone when oral PABA and intramuscular cortisone are given simultaneously, possibly increasing both the effects and side-effects of cortisone (4488). Dosage adjustments of cortisone may be necessary.
DAPSONE (Avlosulfon): PABA might inhibit the antibacterial effects of dapsone; avoid concurrent use (266).
SULFONAMIDE ANTIBIOTICS: PABA inhibits the antimicrobial activity of sulfonamide antibiotics. Sulfonamide antibiotics exert antibacterial effect by competitively inhibiting folic acid synthesis from PABA. Excess PABA may overcome the folate depleting effect of the sulfonamides (10). Avoid using PABA concurrently with sulfonamide antibiotics. Sulfonamide antibiotics include sulfadiazine, sulfisoxazole (Gantrisin), sulfamethoxazole (Gantanol), sulfamethizole (Thiosulfil Forte), sulfasalazine (Azulfidine), and co-trimoxazole (trimethoprim-sulfamethoxazole, Bactrim, Septra).

Interactions with Foods
None known.

Interactions with Lab Tests
LEUKOPENIA: White blood cell count might be transiently reduced when PABA is initiated, especially with high doses, but normalizes with continued administration (10).
LIVER FUNCTION TESTS: PABA has been reported to elevate liver function tests (1084). Monitor liver function tests at baseline, one month after initiating PABA therapy, and every 3 to 6 months thereafter (1084).

Interactions with Diseases or Conditions
RENAL DISEASE: PABA is renally excreted and might accumulate in patients with renal dysfunction (10); use cautiously. Dose adjustments may be necessary.

Dosage and Administration
ORAL: For vitiligo, pemphigus, dermatomyositis, morphea, scleroderma, and Peyronie's disease, the FDA approved dose for adults is 12 grams daily in 4 to 6 divided doses of the potassium salt of PABA (10). In children, the FDA approved dose is 220 mg/kg per day in 4 to 6 divided doses. PABA should be taken with meals or a snack to avoid stomach upset (10). Since PABA is renally excreted, dosage adjustments might be necessary in renal dysfunction.
TOPICAL: PABA sunscreens come in concentrations of 1% to 15% (272).

Comments
PABA appears to have fallen into disuse due to lack of proven efficacy and fears of significant toxicity (1061,1065,1084).

PAREIRA

Also Known As
Ice Vine, Pereira Brava, Velvet Leaf.
CAUTION: See separate listing for Abuta.

Scientific Names
Chondrodendron tomentosum.
Family: Menispermaceae.

People Use This For
Orally, pareira is used as a diuretic and to promote menstruation.
Parenterally, the component tubocurarine is used as a neuromuscular blocking agent.

Safety
There is insufficient reliable information available about the safety of pareira.
PREGNANCY: UNSAFE ...when used orally or parenterally because it may promote menstruation (19).
LACTATION: Insufficient reliable information available; avoid using.

Effectiveness
There is insufficient reliable information available about the effectiveness of pareira.

Mechanism of Action

The applicable part of pareira is the root. Pareira contains tubocurarine, which is used in modern anesthetics. It competitively inhibits acetylcholine binding at the nicotinic receptors at the neuromuscular junction, resulting in skeletal muscle paralysis. Tubocurarine and the other curare-like alkaloids contained in pareira are quaternary alkaloids and carry a positive charge that is not altered by pH. For this reason, they are poorly absorbed when taken orally and therefore have little neuromuscular blocking activity (505).

Adverse Reactions

None reported when pareira is used orally (18). Tubocurarine can cause hypotension due to histamine release and ganglionic blockade if IV administration is too rapid. The histamine release can also cause increased salivation, and bronchospasm. The ganglionic blockade can cause decreased GI motility and tone. Tubocurarine can also cause allergic reactions in susceptible patients (15).

Interactions with Herbs & Other Dietary Supplements

None known.

Interactions with Drugs

None known.

Interactions with Foods

None known.

Interactions with Lab Tests

None known.

Interactions with Diseases or Conditions

None known.

Dosage and Administration

No typical dosage.

Comments

Tubocurarine, a constituent of pareira, is unsafe for parenteral self-medication (15,505).

PARSLEY

Also Known As

Common Parsley, Garden Parsley, Hamburg Parsley, Persely, Persil, Petersylinge, Petroselini fructus, Petroselini herba, Petrosilini radix, Rock Parsley.
CAUTION: See separate listings for Fool's Parsley and Parsley Piert.

Scientific Names

Petroselinum crispum, synonyms Apium petroselinum, Apium crispum, Carum petroselinum, Petroselinum hortense, Petroselinum sativum, Petroselinum vulgare.
Family: Apiaceae/Umbelliferae.

People Use This For

Orally, parsley is used for urinary tract infections (UTIs), kidney stones (nephrolithiasis), gastrointestinal (GI) disorders, constipation, jaundice, flatulence, indigestion, colic, cough, asthma, edema, osteoarthritis, anemia, hypotension, prostate conditions, and spleen conditions. It is also used orally to promote menstrual flow, induce abortion, as an aphrodisiac, and as a breath freshener.
Topically, parsley is used for cracked or chapped skin, bruises, tumors, insect bites, lice, parasites, and to stimulate hair growth.
In foods and beverages, parsley is widely used as a garnish, condiment, food, and flavoring.
In manufacturing, parsley seed oil is used as a fragrance in soaps, cosmetics, and perfumes.

Safety

LIKELY SAFE ...when used orally in amounts commonly found in foods. Parsley has Generally Recognized As Safe (GRAS) status in the US (4912).
POSSIBLY SAFE ...when used orally and appropriately in medicinal amounts (12).
LIKELY UNSAFE ...when used orally in very large doses (i.e., 200 grams); the apiole constituent might cause toxicity. Apiole can cause blood dyscrasias, kidney toxicity, and liver toxicity (4). Parsley oil contains significant amounts of the potentially toxic constituents, apiole and myristicin (11). Myristicin can cause giddiness and

hallucinations (4). ...when parsley seed oil is used topically, it can cause photodermatitis upon sun exposure (4). There is insufficient reliable information available about the safety of the topical use of parsley leaf and root.
PREGNANCY: LIKELY UNSAFE ...when used orally in medicinal amounts. Parsley has been used orally as an abortifacient and to stimulate menstrual flow (4,12,515).
LACTATION: Insufficient reliable information available; avoid using.

Effectiveness

There is insufficient reliable information available about the effectiveness of parsley.

Mechanism of Action

The applicable parts of parsley are the leaf, seed, and root. Parsley contains volatile oils, carotene, vitamin B1, vitamin B2, and vitamin C (515). Parsley leaf also contains significant amounts of vitamin K (11285).
The volatile oil contains apiole, myristicin, and photosensitizing furanocoumarins (psoralens) (512). The volatile oil might stimulate appetite and improve digestion, and have a laxative effect (515,8812).
Parsley might cause a laxative effect by inhibition of the Na-K pump and by stimulation of the NaKCL2 transporter (8812).
The apiole constituent appears to be associated with antispasmodic and vasodilatory effects. Both apiole and myristicin appear to be responsible for the uterine stimulant effects (11,512). Apiole can also increase smooth muscle contractibility in the bladder and intestines (11).
Parsley seems to have an antiflatulent, antispasmodic, antirheumatic, expectorant, antimicrobial, and aquaretic effects (6,512). Aquaretics increase urine volume (water loss) but not electrolyte excretion (512). Both the apiole and myristicin constituents are believed to have aquaretic and uterine stimulant effects (512). The mechanism of aquaresis is thought to be that parsley irritates the kidney epithelium which increases renal blood flow and glomerular filtration rate (512).

Adverse Reactions

Orally, adverse effects specifically associated with more than 10 grams of the constituent, apiole, include hemolytic anemia, thrombocytopenia purpura, nephrosis, hepatic dysfunction, and kidney irritation (4). Adverse effects specifically associated with the constituent myristicin include giddiness, deafness, hallucinations, hypotension, bradycardia, paralysis, and fatty degeneration of the liver and kidneys (4). Parsley oil can cause contact photodermatitis with sun exposure (4).
Topically, parsley can cause contact photodermatitis (4).

Interactions with Herbs & Other Dietary Supplements

None known.

Interactions with Drugs

ASPIRIN: Concomitant intake with parsley might augment parsley allergy. There is one case report of severe urticaria and swelling in a person with a known mild parsley allergy after consuming parsley and aspirin (5054).
DIURETIC DRUGS: Theoretically, parsley leaf and root might interfere with diuretic therapy due to aquaretic effects (512).
WARFARIN (Coumadin): Theoretically, large amounts of parsley leaf and root might interfere with oral anticoagulant therapy with warfarin, due to vitamin K contained in parsley (19).

Interactions with Foods

None known.

Interactions with Lab Tests

INTERNATIONAL NORMALIZED RATIO (INR)/PROTHROMBIN TIME (PT): Theoretically, parsley leaf might decrease coagulation test results due to high vitamin K content (11285).

Interactions with Diseases or Conditions

EDEMA: Theoretically, parsley might increase sodium retention and worsen edema (512).
HYPERTENSION: Theoretically, parsley might increase sodium retention and worsen hypertension (512).
KIDNEY DISEASE: Parsley is contraindicated in individuals with kidney disease or inflammation. Parsley contains constituents that can aggravate these conditions (4,19).

Dosage and Administration

No typical dosage.

PARSLEY PIERT

Also Known As

Field Lady's Mantle, Parsley Breakstone, Parsley Piercestone.
CAUTION: See separate listings for Fool's Parsley, Parsley, Alpine Lady's Mantle, and Alchemilla.

Scientific Names

Aphanes arvensis, synonyms Alchemilla arvensis, Alchemilla occidentalis.
Family: Rosaceae.

Comments

At the date of publication, this product was not a common ingredient used in brand name supplements marketed to consumers. Details about this product are available in the online version of *Natural Medicines Comprehensive Database.* See www.naturaldatabase.com.

PARSNIP

Also Known As

Pastinacae herba, Pastinacae Radix.

Scientific Names

Pastinaca sativa.
Family: Apiaceae/Umbelliferae.

Comments

At the date of publication, there was very little scientific information available about this product. Our staff is continually analyzing the available information on natural medicines and will add data to the online version of *Natural Medicines Comprehensive Database* as it becomes available. See www.naturaldatabase.com.

PASSIONFLOWER

Also Known As

Apricot Vine, Corona De Cristo, Fleischfarbige, Fleur De La Passion, Flor De Passion, Madre Selva, Maracuja, Maypop, Maypop Passion Flower, Passiflora, Passiflorae herba, Passiflore, Passiflorina, Passion Flower, Passion Vine, Passionaria, Passionblume, Passionflower Herb, Passionsblumenkraut, Purple Passion Flower, Water Lemon, Wild Passion Flower.

Scientific Names

Passiflora incarnata.
Family: Passifloraceae.

People Use This For

Orally, passionflower is used for insomnia, gastrointestinal (GI) upset related to anxiety or nervousness, generalized anxiety disorder (GAD), and symptoms of opiate withdrawal. Passionflower is also used orally for neuralgia, generalized seizures, hysteria, spasmodic asthma, climacteric (menopausal) symptoms, attention deficit-hyperactivity disorder (ADHD), nervousness and excitability, palpitations, cardiac rhythm abnormalities, high blood pressure, and pain relief.
Topically, passionflower is used in bath preparations, for hemorrhoids, burns, and inflammation.
In foods and beverages, passionflower extract is used as a flavoring.

Safety

LIKELY SAFE ...when used orally in amounts commonly found in foods. Passionflower has Generally Recognized As Safe status (GRAS) for use in foods in the US (4912).
POSSIBLY SAFE ...when used orally and appropriately, short-term for medicinal purposes. There is some evidence that passionflower liquid extracts can be safely used for up to one month (12,2303,8007).
POSSIBLY UNSAFE ...when used orally in excessive amounts (4).
There is insufficient reliable information available about the safety of the topical use of passionflower.
PREGNANCY: UNSAFE ...when used orally. Some passionflower constituents show evidence of uterine stimulation (4,6).
LACTATION: Insufficient reliable information available; avoid using.

Effectiveness

POSSIBLY EFFECTIVE

Adjustment disorder with anxious mood. A specific six-ingredient combination product (Euphytose, EUP) that includes passionflower seems to relieve some symptoms of adjustment disorder with anxious mood. However, it's not known which ingredient or ingredients are responsible for the beneficial effects. Other herbs in the product are crataegus, ballota, and valerian, which have mild sedative effects, and cola and paullinia with stimulant properties (6250).

Generalized anxiety disorder (GAD). There is some evidence that passionflower liquid extract 45 drops can be comparable to oxazepam (Serax) 30 mg for treating symptoms of GAD in some patients (8007).

Opiate withdrawal. Passionflower liquid extract 60 drops in combination with clonidine 0.8 mg daily seems to be significantly better than clonidine alone when used for reducing symptoms such as anxiety, irritability, insomnia, and agitation. However, the combination is no better than clonidine alone for physical symptoms such as tremor and nausea (2303).

There is insufficient reliable information available about the effectiveness of passionflower for its other uses.

Mechanism of Action

The applicable parts of passionflower are the above ground parts. Passionflower contains several active constituents, including the flavonoids apigenin, luteolin, quercetin, kaempferol, and vitexin. The harman (harmala) alkaloids identified in passionflower include harmine, harmaline, harmalol, harman, and harmin (8811,9558). Experts do not agree about whether passionflower contains the cyanogenic glycoside gynocardine (11,19,9558). Passionflower has sedative, hypnotic, anxiolytic, and antispasmodic effects (8811,9558). It also relieves pain (4). Some evidence suggests the passionflower constituent apigenin binds to central benzodiazepine receptors (4001), possibly causing anxiolytic effects without impairing memory or motor skills (4001). Other evidence suggests passionflower extracts might reduce amphetamine-induced hypermotility, aggressiveness, and restlessness; and raise the pain threshold (1,4,11). Although animal data suggest the constituents maltol and ethylmaltol can reduce spontaneous motor activity, prolong barbiturate-induced sleep time, and show anticonvulsant activity (1,4), not enough maltol is found in passionflower preparations to cause these effects (1). Some evidence suggests the harman alkaloids have central nervous system (CNS) stimulant activity via a monoamine oxidase mechanism (4,4002); however, the sedative effects of maltol and ethylmaltol can mask these effects. The constituent passicol shows some evidence of antibacterial and antifungal activity (4).

Adverse Reactions

Orally, passionflower can cause dizziness, confusion, and ataxia in some patients (8007).

There are some reports of more severe side effects. Vasculitis and altered consciousness have been reported with use of a specific herbal product (Relaxir) produced mainly from the fruits of passionflower (6). There is also a case report involving a 34-year-old woman who developed severe nausea, vomiting, drowsiness, prolonged QT interval, and episodes of nonsustained ventricular tachycardia, requiring hospitalization for IV hydration and cardiac monitoring following use of therapeutic doses of passionflower (6251).

There is some debate about whether passionflower contains cyanogenic glycosides. Several related Passiflora species do contain them (3), including Passiflora edulis, which is associated with liver and pancreas toxicity (7).

Interactions with Herbs & Other Dietary Supplements

HERBS WITH ANTICOAGULANT/ANTIPLATELET POTENTIAL: Concomitant use of herbs that have constituents that might affect platelet aggregation could theoretically increase the risk of bleeding in some people. These herbs include angelica, clove, danshen, garlic, ginger, ginkgo, Panax ginseng, horse chestnut, red clover, turmeric, and others.

HERBS WITH SEDATIVE PROPERTIES: Theoretically, concomitant use with herbs that have sedative properties might enhance therapeutic and adverse effects. Some of these supplements include 5-HTP, calamus, California poppy, catnip, hops, Jamaican dogwood, kava, St. John's wort, scullcap, valerian, yerba mansa, and others.

Interactions with Drugs

BARBITURATES: Theoretically, concomitant use can increase drug-induced sleep time (1). Some of these sedative medications include pentobarbital (Nembutal), phenobarbital (Luminal), secobarbital (Seconal), and others.

CNS DEPRESSANTS: Theoretically, concomitant use can potentiate the effects of these drugs, including the sedative effects of antihistamines (19).

Interactions with Foods

None known.

Interactions with Lab Tests

None known.

Interactions with Diseases or Conditions

None known.

Dosage and Administration

ORAL: For generalized anxiety disorder (GAD), 45 drops of passionflower liquid extract has been used daily (8007). For reducing symptoms associated with opiate withdrawal, 60 drops of passionflower liquid extract in combination with 0.8 mg of clonidine has been used daily (2303).

The typical dose of crude passionflower herb is 0.25-2 grams of the dried above ground parts three times daily or one cup of the tea two to three times daily and 30 minutes before bedtime (1,4). The tea is prepared by steeping 0.25-2 grams of the dried above ground parts in 150 mL boiling water for 10-15 minutes and then straining. The average amount of passionflower is 4-8 grams per day. The usual dose of the liquid extract (1:1 in 25% alcohol) is 0.5-1.0 mL three times daily. The common dose of the tincture (1:8 in 45% alcohol) is 0.5-2 mL three times daily (4).

TOPICAL: Passionflower is typically used as a hemorrhoid rinse, which is prepared by simmering 20 grams of the dried above ground parts in 200 mL water, straining, and cooling before use (18).

Comments

In 1569, Spanish explorers discovered passionflower in Peru. They believed the flowers symbolized Christ's passion and indicated his approval for their exploration (6). Passionflower is found in combination herbal sedative products, some of which include German chamomile, hops, kava, scullcap, and valerian. Passionflower was formerly approved as an OTC sedative and sleep aid in the US, but it was taken off the market in 1978 because safety and effectiveness had not been proven (11,515).

PATCHOULY OIL

Also Known As

Huo xiang, Patchouli, Patchouly, Putcha-Pat.

Scientific Names

Pogostemon cablin, synonyms Mentha cablin, Pogostemon patchouly; Pogostemon heyneanus.
Family: Lamiaceae/Labiatae.

People Use This For

Orally, patchouly oil is used for colds, tumors, headaches, nausea, vomiting, diarrhea, and abdominal pain. It is also used to treat bad breath, particularly when it is associated with alcohol ingestion.

In foods and beverages, patchouly oil is used as a flavor ingredient.

In manufacturing, patchouly oil is used in perfumes and cosmetics.

Safety

LIKELY SAFE ...when used orally in amounts commonly found in foods. Patchouly oil has Generally Recognized As Safe status (GRAS) for use in foods in the US (4912).

There is insufficient reliable information available about the safety of patchouly oil in medicinal amounts.

PREGNANCY AND LACTATION: Insufficient reliable information available; avoid using.

Effectiveness

There is insufficient reliable information available about the effectiveness of patchouly oil.

Mechanism of Action

Patchouly oil is the oil distilled from the dried leaf, young leaves, and shoots. Animal data suggests that patchouly oil is nontoxic with short-term oral use. Patchouly oil may have bactericidal activity, and the component pogostone appears to have antibacterial and antifungal activities. The components eugenol, cinnamaldehyde, and benzaldehyde may have insecticidal activity against insects in stored grain (11).

Adverse Reactions

None reported.

Interactions with Herbs & Other Dietary Supplements

None known.

Interactions with Drugs

None known.

Interactions with Foods

None known.

Interactions with Lab Tests

None known.

Interactions with Diseases or Conditions
None known.

Dosage and Administration
No typical dosage.

Comments
Patchouly oil can be adulterated with other oils, including gurjun balsam oil, copaiba balsam oil, and cedarwood oil (11).

PAU D'ARCO

Also Known As
Ipe, Ipe Roxo, Ipes, Lapacho, Lapacho Colorado, Lapacho Morado, Pau dArco, Pau de Arco, Purple Lapacho, Red Lapacho, Taheebo, Taheebo Tea, Trumpet Bush.

Scientific Names
Tabebuia impetiginosa, synonyms Tabebuia avellanedae, Tabebuia palmeri, Tecoma impetiginosa; Tabebuia heptaphylla, synonyms Bignonia heptaphylla, Tabebuia ipe, Tecoma ipe.
Family: Bignoniaceae.

People Use This For
Orally, pau d'arco is used for Candida yeast infections, infectious diarrhea, bladder infections, parasitic infections, cancer, diabetes, ulcers, gastritis, liver ailments, asthma, bronchitis, cystitis, prostatitis, ringworm, rheumatism, hernias, gonorrhea, syphilis, chlorosis, boils, wounds, as a "tonic and blood builder", and for viral respiratory infections including the common cold and flu
Topically, pau d'arco is used for Candida infections.

Safety
POSSIBLY UNSAFE ...when used orally in typical doses. Significant evaluation of the safety of pau d'arco in typical doses has not been conducted; however, serious toxicities have been found with higher doses (6,515). Pau d'arco should be used with caution.
LIKELY UNSAFE ...when used orally in large doses. In studies in cancer patients, when doses were elevated to provide therapeutic plasma levels of the active constituent lapachol, patients experienced significant toxicities, including increased risk of bleeding (6,515). Doses of pau d'arco providing greater than 1.5 grams per day of the lapachol constituent have been associated with the most risk (6).
There is insufficient reliable information available about the safety of pau d'arco for its other uses.
PREGNANCY: POSSIBLY UNSAFE ...when used orally in typical doses; avoid using. LIKELY UNSAFE ...when used orally in large doses; contraindicated. Significant evaluation of the safety of pau d'arco in typical doses has not been conducted; however, serious toxicities have been found with higher doses (6,515).
There is insufficient reliable information available about the safety of pau d'arco used topically in pregnancy.
LACTATION: Insufficient reliable information; avoid using.

Effectiveness
There is insufficient reliable information available about the effectiveness of pau d'arco.

Mechanism of Action
The applicable parts of pau d'arco are the bark and the wood. The active constituents are thought to be a naphthoquinone derivative, lapachol, and its derivatives. The wood contains lapachol and the bark contains mostly lapachol derivatives. Lapachol and its derivatives are thought to have similar pharmacological activities (515). Lapachol is thought to be responsible for increasing the risk of bleeding by prolonging prothrombin time. Its effects on clotting are reversible by vitamin K (6). Preliminary data suggests that lapachol also has anti-inflammatory, antimalarial, antibacterial, antifungal, antiparasitic, and immunomodulatory activity (6,515). Some evidence suggests that lapachol is active against sarcomas, but at potentially effective levels, adverse effects are severe enough to prevent its use for that indication (515).

Adverse Reactions
Orally, pau d'arco causes severe nausea, vomiting, diarrhea, dizziness, anemia, and increases the risk of bleeding when used in high doses (515). Doses of pau d'arco providing greater than 1.5 grams per day of the lapachol constituent have been associated with the most risk (6).

Interactions with Herbs & Other Dietary Supplements

HERBS WITH ANTICOAGULANT/ANTIPLATELET POTENTIAL: Theoretically, concomitant use with herbs that have constituents that might affect platelet aggregation could theoretically increase the chance of bleeding in some people. These herbs include alfalfa, angelica, clove, danshen, horse chestnut, red clover, turmeric, and others.

Interactions with Drugs

ANTICOAGULANT/ANTIPLATELET DRUGS: Theoretically, concomitant use with pau d'arco might increase clotting time and increase the risk for bleeding (515).

Interactions with Foods

None known.

Interactions with Lab Tests

PROTHROMBIN TIME (PT)/INTERNATIONAL NORMALIZED RATION (INR): Pau d'arco can increase PT and INR test results and increase the risk of bleeding (6,515).

Interactions with Diseases or Conditions

COAGULATION DISORDERS: Pau d'arco can increase bleeding time and might interfere with therapy in patients with coagulation disorders (6,515); use with caution.

Dosage and Administration

ORAL: People typically use 1 to 4 grams daily in 2 to 3 divided doses. One manufacturer warns that the product should not be used for more than 7 days; however, the reason for this warning is not known. The contents of pau d'arco capsules may also be emptied and prepared as a tea. A tincture in the amount of 0.5 to 1 mL and a glycerin-based liquid in the amount of 1 to 3 mL are used 3 times daily (6006).

Comments

Pau d'arco wood is extremely hard and almost indestructible (515). In South America, the Indians used the tree to make bows for hunting. Pau d'arco is the Spanish name for "bow stick" (6002). Teas, labeled as pau d'arco or lapacho, do not always contain the Tabebuia species; in some cases they have contained the related species, Tecoma curialis (515). Some report that the inner-bark preparations of pau d'arco are preferred because they are the most effective. Some products may use the outer-bark and mislabel the product as true inner-bark pau d'arco (3564). The anticancer activity of the pau d'arco constituent lapachol was extensively researched in the 1960s. The research was abandoned due to its toxicity (6).

PEANUT OIL

Also Known As

Arachis, Earth-Nut, Groundnuts, Monkey Nuts.

Scientific Names

Arachis hypogaea.
Family: Fabaceae/Leguminosae.

People Use This For

Orally, peanut oil is used to lower cholesterol and prevent heart disease. It is also used orally to aid in weight loss and decrease appetite, and to help prevent cancer.
Topically, peanut oil is used for arthritis and joint pain, scalp crusting and scaling without hair loss, dry skin, eczema, and ichthyosis (noninflammatory skin disorders that cause scaling).
Rectally, peanut oil is used in ointments and medicinal oils for treating constipation.
It is also used as a vehicle for external, enteral, and parenteral pharmaceutical formulations.
In manufacturing, peanut oil is used in skin care products and baby care products.

Safety

LIKELY SAFE ...when used orally in amounts commonly found in foods. Peanut oil has Generally Recognized As Safe status (GRAS) for use in foods in the US (4912). ...when used orally, topically, or rectally in medicinal amounts.
PREGNANCY AND LACTATION: There is insufficient reliable information about the safety of medicinal amounts of peanut oil during pregnancy and breast-feeding; avoid using.

Effectiveness

There is insufficient reliable information available about the effectiveness of peanut oil.

Mechanism of Action

Peanuts contain beta-sitosterol and resveratrol, which may contribute to cardioprotective and cancer protective activity (4263,4267). The high monounsaturated, low saturated fat content of peanut oil is thought to prevent heart disease and lower cholesterol. Population studies suggest people who eat nuts have a lower risk of developing heart disease (4264). This benefit must be weighed against animal evidence that suggests peanut oil is atherogenic, perhaps due to the triglyceride content or the presence of a lectin (4265,4266).

Adverse Reactions

Peanut oil can cause a severe allergic reaction in individuals allergic to the Fabaceae family. Members of this family include peanuts and soybeans (4079,4080).

Interactions with Herbs & Other Dietary Supplements

None known.

Interactions with Drugs

None known.

Interactions with Foods

None known.

Interactions with Lab Tests

None known.

Interactions with Diseases or Conditions

CROSS-ALLERGENICITY: Peanut oil can cause a severe allergic reaction in individuals sensitive to the Fabaceae family. Members of this family include peanuts and soybeans (4079,4080).

Dosage and Administration

ORAL: No typical dosage.
TOPICAL: For bath use, 4 mL peanut oil is added to 10 L water. Adults bathe for 15-20 minutes 2-3 times daily. Children bathe for a few minutes 2-3 times weekly (18).
RECTAL: As an enema, 130 mL of room temperature peanut oil has been used.

Comments

Sometimes the less expensive soya oil is added to peanut oil (18).

PEAR

Also Known As

Pears.

Scientific Names

Pyrus communis, synonyms Pyrus asiae-mediae, Pyrus balansae, Pyrus bourgaeana, Pyrus domestica, Pyrus elata, Pyrus medvedevii.
Family: Rosaceae.

People Use This For

Orally, pear fruit is used for mild digestive disorders, cholera, colic, diarrhea, nausea, liver sclerosis, spasms, tumors, and for reducing fevers. It is used orally for its laxative, bactericidal, calmative, and diuretic properties.
Topically, pear fruit is used as an astringent.
In foods, pears are eaten as fresh fruit, preserved fruit, and used in cooking.

Safety

LIKELY SAFE ...when used orally (18).
There is insufficient reliable information available about the safety of pear fruit for its other uses.
PREGNANCY AND LACTATION: LIKELY SAFE ...when consumed in amounts commonly found in foods (18).

Effectiveness

There is insufficient reliable information available about the effectiveness of pear.

Mechanism of Action

The applicable part of the pear is the fruit. Pear fruit contains pectin (18) that might contribute to antidiarrheal activity (7).

Adverse Reactions
None reported.

Interactions with Herbs & Other Dietary Supplements
None known.

Interactions with Drugs
None known.

Interactions with Foods
None known.

Interactions with Lab Tests
None known.

Interactions with Diseases or Conditions
None known.

Dosage and Administration
No typical dosage.

PECTIN

Also Known As
Pectinic Acid.

Scientific Names
Pectin.

People Use This For
Orally, pectin is used as an adsorbent, for reducing high cholesterol and triglycerides, for reducing the risk of colon cancer, for reducing damage from radiation, for treating diabetes, for treating gastro-esophageal reflux disease (GERD), and as an antibacterial.
Topically, pectin is used for protecting raw or ulcerated mouth and throat sores.
In combination with kaolin (Kaopectate) or paregoric (Parepectolin), pectin is used to treat diarrhea.
In food manufacturing, pectin is used as a thickening agent in cooking and baking.
In manufacturing, pectin is used as a denture adhesive component.

Safety
LIKELY SAFE ...when used in amounts commonly found in foods. Pectin has Generally Recognized As Safe (GRAS) status in the US (4912).
POSSIBLY SAFE ...when used orally in medicinal amounts (12547).
CHILDREN: LIKELY SAFE...when used in amounts commonly found in foods. Pectin has Generally Recognized As Safe (GRAS) status in the US (4912). POSSIBLY SAFE ...when used orally in medicinal amounts (12575).
PREGNANCY AND LACTATION: LIKELY SAFE ...when used in amounts commonly found in foods. Pectin has Generally Recognized As Safe (GRAS) status in the US (4912).
POSSIBLY SAFE ...when used orally in medicinal amounts. Pectin is has a category B pregnancy designation by the FDA (12577).

Effectiveness
POSSIBLY EFFECTIVE

Hypercholesterolemia. Taking pectin orally seems to lower cholesterol (2214,2215,2216,2217). Pectin and guar gum, taken with small amounts of insoluble fiber, also lower total and low-density lipoprotein (LDL) cholesterol, but don't affect high-density lipoprotein (HDL) cholesterol or triglycerides (12547).

INSUFFICIENT RELIABLE EVIDENCE to RATE

Diarrhea. In children age 5 to 12 months, pectin 4 grams per kilogram seems to reduce the duration of diarrhea and vomiting, and reduce consumption of oral rehydration solution and intravenous fluid in children with persistent diarrhea and in developing nations (12577). More evidence is needed to rate pectin for this use.

Mechanism of Action
Pectin is a soluble fiber (polysaccharide) in fruits. It is a starch that is resistant to amylase. It is found in the cell walls of plant tissue and helps give plants rigidity (12575).
Pectin is metabolized by intestinal bacteria to short-chain fatty acids in the colon. Pectin may relieve diarrhea by

increasing the absorption of salt and water. It may also act as an energy source, increase protein synthesis, and improve oxygen use by the colonic mucosa. Dietary fiber such as pectin may also slow gut motility and increase gastrointestinal transit time (12575).

Pectin might reduce the amount of stomach contents refluxed into the esophagus. Like alginic acid (Gaviscon), it floats on top of the stomach contents and may serve as a barrier between the stomach acid and the esophagus. Pectin does not affect the pH in the stomach. It might be useful for treating gastro-esophageal reflux disease (GERD), but more clinical research is needed before pectin can be recommended for this use (10431).

Pectin and guar gum, taken with small amounts of insoluble fiber, don't appear to affect iron, ferritin, vitamin A, or vitamin E absorption when taken for 51 weeks (12547).

Adverse Reactions

Orally, pectin in combination with guar gum and insoluble fiber can cause gastrointestinal adverse effects such as diarrhea, gas, and loose stools (12547).

The occupational inhalation of pectin dust can cause asthma (580,581,582,583,584).

Interactions with Herbs & Other Dietary Supplements

BETA-CAROTENE: Concomitant use of pectin can significantly reduce beta-carotene absorption (2225).

Interactions with Drugs

DIGOXIN (Lanoxin): Concomitant use of pectin can interfere with the intestinal absorption of digoxin (2212).

LOVASTATIN (Mevacor): Concomitant use of pectin can interfere with the intestinal absorption of lovastatin (615).

TETRACYCLINE ANTIBIOTICS: Concomitant use of pectin can interfere with the intestinal absorption of tetracyclines (2213).

Interactions with Foods

None known.

Interactions with Lab Tests

CHOLESTEROL: Pectin can decrease serum cholesterol and test results (275).

Interactions with Diseases or Conditions

None known.

Dosage and Administration

ORAL: For hypercholesterolemia, 15 grams per day has been used (2214). For persistent diarrhea in children, 4 grams per kilogram of body weight per day has been used (12575).

TOPICAL: No typical dosage.

Comments

Pectin has been used for years in combination with kaolin (Kaopectate). However in April 2003, the FDA found insufficient support for its use as an antidiarrheal. As of April 2004, pectin is no longer permitted as an antidiarrhea agent in OTC products (12577). Note that Kaopectate no longer contains pectin and kaolin.

PELLITORY

Also Known As

Akarakarabha.

CAUTION: See separate listing for Pellitory-of-the-Wall.

Scientific Names

Anacyclus pyrethrum, synonym Anthemis pyrethrum.

Family: Asteraceae/Compositae.

People Use This For

Orally, pellitory is used for arthritis and as a digestive aid.

Topically, pellitory is used for toothaches and as an insecticide.

Safety

There is insufficient reliable information available about the safety of pellitory.

Pregnancy and Lactation: Insufficient reliable information available; avoid using.

Effectiveness

There is insufficient reliable information available about the effectiveness of pellitory.

Mechanism of Action
The applicable part of pellitory is the root. Application of pellitory to skin may stimulate nerve endings and result in redness and irritation, which is felt as a hot, burning sensation. Alkylamines may possibly contribute, since they may stimulate mucous membranes (18).

Adverse Reactions
Signs of skin irritation may occur with overuse (18). Pellitory can cause an allergic reaction in individuals sensitive to the Asteraceae/Compositae family. Members of this family include ragweed, chrysanthemums, marigolds, daisies, and many other herbs.

Interactions with Herbs & Other Dietary Supplements
None known.

Interactions with Drugs
None known.

Interactions with Foods
None known.

Interactions with Lab Tests
None known.

Interactions with Diseases or Conditions
CROSS-ALLERGENICITY: Can cause an allergic reaction in individuals sensitive to the Asteraceae/Compositae family. Members of this family include ragweed, chrysanthemums, marigolds, daisies, and many other herbs.

Dosage and Administration
No typical dosage.

Comments
Avoid confusing with the similar sounding pellitory-of-the-wall.

PELLITORY-OF-THE-WALL

Also Known As
Lichwort, Pellitory of the Wall.
CAUTION: See separate listing for Pellitory.

Scientific Names
Parietaria officinalis.
Family: Urticaceae.

People Use This For
Orally, pellitory-of-the-wall is used as a diuretic, laxative, and as a demulcent. It is also used for chronic cough and for a variety of kidney disorders including urinary tract infections (UTIs) and pyelonephritis, renal pain, and kidney stones.
Topically, pellitory-of-the-wall is used for treating burns and wounds.

Safety
POSSIBLY SAFE ...when used orally (12).
PREGNANCY AND LACTATION: Insufficient reliable information available; avoid using.

Effectiveness
There is insufficient reliable information available about the effectiveness of pellitory-of-the-wall.

Mechanism of Action
The applicable parts of pellitory-of-the-wall are the aerial parts. It contains flavonoids and tannins (7161).

Adverse Reactions
Pellitory-of-the-wall pollen has been associated with seasonal allergy (7161).

Interactions with Herbs & Other Dietary Supplements
None known.

Interactions with Drugs
None known.

Interactions with Foods
None known.

Interactions with Lab Tests
None known.

Interactions with Diseases or Conditions
None known.

Dosage and Administration
No typical dosage.

Comments
The name pellitory-of-the-wall comes from its habit of growing in old walls and dry, stony areas (7161). Avoid confusion between pellitory-of-the-wall and the similar sounding pellitory.

PENNYROYAL

Also Known As
American Pennyroyal, European Pennyroyal, Lurk-In-The-Ditch, Mosquito Plant, Piliolerial, Pudding Grass, Pulegium, Run-By-The-Ground, Squaw Balm, Squawmint, Stinking Balm, Tickweed.

Scientific Names
Mentha pulegium, synonym Pulegium vulgare; Hedeoma pulegioides, synonym Melissa pulegioides.
Family: Lamiaceae/Labiatae.

People Use This For
Orally, pennyroyal is used as an antispasmodic, antiflatulent, diaphoretic, stimulant, and as a diuretic. It is also used for pneumonia, colds, respiratory ailments, stomach pains, and weakness. It is also used orally as an abortifacient; as a menstrual stimulant or regulator; and for intestinal disorders, digestive disorders, and liver and gallbladder disorders.
Topically, pennyroyal oil is used as an antiseptic, insect repellent, and for skin diseases. It is also used topically for tactile hallucinations, gout, venomous bites, mouth sores, as a flea-killing bath, and as a counterirritant.
In foods, pennyroyal is used as a flavoring agent.
In manufacturing, pennyroyal oil is used as a dog and cat flea repellent, and a fragrance for detergents, perfumes, and soaps.

Safety
LIKELY UNSAFE ...when used orally or topically (4). Neurologic injury has been reported in adults consuming 2.5-5.0 mL of pennyroyal oil (5,6,9). Nephrotoxicity, hepatotoxicity, and death have been reported after ingestion of 15-30 mL (12,5601). Repeated use of an alcoholic pennyroyal leaf extract over a period of 2 weeks has also been linked to a death (650).
There is insufficient reliable information available about the safety of using pennyroyal leaf as a tea.
CHILDREN: LIKELY UNSAFE ...when used orally. There is a report of 2 infants developing severe hepatic and neurologic injuries and one infant death after use of pennyroyal (291).
PREGNANCY: LIKELY UNSAFE ...when used orally or topically. Pennyroyal oil is thought to act as an abortifacient (4). Pennyroyal leaf tea is reported to cause onset of menses (650). Pennyroyal can also cause serious adverse effects when applied topically or taken orally (5,6,9,12,650,5601).
LACTATION: LIKELY UNSAFE ...when used orally or topically (4); avoid using.

Effectiveness
There is insufficient reliable information available about the effectiveness of pennyroyal.

Mechanism of Action
The applicable parts of pennyroyal are the leaves and oil.
Pennyroyal leaves contain 1% to 2% of essential oil, tannins, and flavonoids (12). The volatile oil, pulegone and its metabolite, menthofuran, or methofuran's metabolites might be responsible for pennyroyal's toxic effects including hepatotoxicity, neurotoxicity, and bronchiolar epithelial cell destruction (650).
The oxidative metabolites of pulegone and menthofuran may cause cell damage by binding to target proteins (650), depleting hepatic glutathione levels (292,650), and by direct cellular damage similar to acetaminophen toxicity (291).

Pennyroyal is thought to have abortifacient effects, which might be due to uterine contractions triggered by genitourinary tract irritation (4,6,19). Large doses required for the abortifacient effect can cause irreversible kidney damage, hepatic damage, and death (6).
In the American species of pennyroyal, pulegone is 30% less concentrated than in the European species (62% to 97%) (12).

Adverse Reactions

Orally, pennyroyal can cause abdominal pain and tenderness, nausea, vomiting (possibly bloody), burning of the throat, fever, lethargy alternating with agitation, confusion, delirium, restlessness, seizures, dizziness, auditory and visual hallucinations, elevated blood pressure and pulse rate, bilateral lung congestion, acidosis, disseminated intravascular coagulation, abortion, hepatic failure, renal failure, respiratory failure, shock, and death (5601).
Topically, pennyroyal can cause a urticarial rash (5601) and dermatitis (6).

Interactions with Herbs & Other Dietary Supplements

None known.

Interactions with Drugs

None known.

Interactions with Foods

None known.

Interactions with Lab Tests

None known.

Interactions with Diseases or Conditions

KIDNEY DISEASE: The volatile oil in pennyroyal can cause kidney irritation and might worsen existing kidney disease (19).
LIVER DISEASE: The volatile oil in pennyroyal can cause hepatotoxicity and might worsen existing liver disease (5601).

Dosage and Administration

No typical dosage.

Comments

American pennyroyal and European pennyroyal are historically interchangeable as a source of pennyroyal oil (12).
About 50-100 grams of leaves are required to produce 1 mL of pennyroyal oil (4).

PEONY

Also Known As

Common Peony, Coral Peony, European Peony, Paeoniae Flos, Paeoniae Radix, Piney.

Scientific Names

Paeonia mascula, synonym Paeonia caucasica; Paeonia officinalis.
Family: Paeoniaceae.

People Use This For

Orally, peony is used for gout, osteoarthritis, respiratory tract ailments, and for cough. Peony is also used orally for epilepsy, dyspepsia, to induce vomiting, and for inducing menstruation or miscarriage. Peony is also used orally for spasms, whooping cough (pertussis), neuralgia, migraine headache, and for chronic fatigue syndrome (CFS).
Topically, peony is used for skin and mucous membrane diseases, and for healing fissures, especially anal fissures associated with hemorrhoids.

Safety

There is insufficient reliable information available about the safety of peony.
PREGNANCY: POSSIBLY UNSAFE ...when used orally due to historical use as an abortifacient and menstruation-inducing agent (19).
LACTATION: Insufficient reliable information available; avoid using.

Effectiveness

There is insufficient reliable information available about the effectiveness of peony.

Mechanism of Action

The applicable parts of peony are the flowers and root.
Peony root extract exhibits neuroprotective activity and prevents experimentally induced brain neuron spike discharges in rats (3818). Researchers attribute neuroprotection to the gallotannin and paeoniflorin constituents (3818).

Adverse Reactions

Orally, overdose with peony has reportedly led to gastroenteritis with vomiting, colic, and diarrhea (8).

Interactions with Herbs & Other Dietary Supplements

None known.

Interactions with Drugs

PHENYTOIN (Dilantin): Peony root might reduce levels of phenytoin and potentially reduce the therapeutic effectiveness of phenytoin (8657). It's theorized that peony root might affect cytochrome P450 2C9 (CYP2C) enzymes, which metabolizes phenytoin. But there is evidence that peony root does not alter levels of losartan (Cozaar), which is also metabolized by CYP2C9 (11480). More evidence is needed to determine if peony root significantly affects other drugs metabolized by CYP2C9.

Interactions with Foods

None known.

Interactions with Lab Tests

None known.

Interactions with Diseases or Conditions

None known.

Dosage and Administration

ORAL: No typical dosage. However, traditionally one cup of tea (steep one gram flowers in 150 mL boiling water 5-10 minutes, strain) has been used daily (8).
TOPICAL: No typical dosage.

PEPPERMINT

Also Known As

Brandy Mint, Lamb Mint, Menthae Piperitae Aetheroleum, Menthae Piperitae Folium, Menthe Poivree, Paparaminta, Peppermint Leaf, Peppermint Oil.

Scientific Names

Mentha piperita, synonym Mentha lavanduliodora.
Family: Lamiaceae/Labiatae.

People Use This For

Orally, peppermint is used for the common cold, cough, inflammation of the mouth and pharynx, sinusitis, fever, liver and gallbladder complaints, irritable bowel syndrome (IBS), cramps of the upper gastrointestinal (GI) tract and bile ducts, dyspepsia, fever, flatulence, and for tension headache. It is also used for nausea, vomiting, morning sickness, respiratory infections, dysmenorrhea, diarrhea, small intestinal bacterial overgrowth, and as a stimulant.
Topically, peppermint oil is used for headache, myalgias, neuralgias, toothache, oral mucosa inflammation, rheumatic conditions, pruritus, urticaria, bacterial and viral infections, as an antispasmodic in barium enemas, and for repelling mosquitoes.
As an inhalant, peppermint oil is used as an aromatic, for symptomatic treatment of cough and colds, and as an analgesic for pain.
In foods and beverages, peppermint is a common flavoring agent.
In manufacturing, peppermint oil is used as a fragrance component in soaps and cosmetics, and as a flavoring agent in pharmaceuticals.

Safety

LIKELY SAFE ...when used orally in amounts commonly found in foods. Peppermint has Generally Recognized As Safe (GRAS) status in the US (4912).
POSSIBLY SAFE ...when peppermint oil is used orally, topically, or rectally and appropriately in medicinal amounts (3801,3804,6190,6740,6741,10075,12009). ...when peppermint leaf is used orally and appropriately, short-term. There is some evidence that peppermint leaf can be used safely for up to 8 weeks (12724). The long-term safety of peppermint leaf in medicinal doses is unknown. ...when peppermint oil is used by inhalation as aromatherapy (7107).

LIKELY UNSAFE ...when peppermint oil is used orally in large amounts. High doses of peppermint oil have been associated with interstitial nephritis and acute renal failure (7). Menthol, a major constituent, is considered lethal at a dose of 2-9 grams (7).
CHILDREN: POSSIBLY SAFE ...when used orally in medicinal amounts in children 8 years of age and older. Enteric-coated peppermint oil capsules seem to be safe when used under medical supervision in children 8 years of age and older (4469). LIKELY UNSAFE ...when used orally in medicinal amounts in infants and small children. Oral peppermint oil has caused tongue spasms and respiratory arrest in infants and small children (4800). ...when applied topically to the facial, nasal, and chest areas of infants and small children. Peppermint oil can cause bronchospasm, spasms of the tongue, or respiratory arrest (4800). ...when inhaled for medicinal purposes by small children (502).
PREGNANCY: LIKELY UNSAFE ...when used orally in medicinal amounts. High doses of peppermint oil can induce menstruation (19).
LACTATION: Insufficient reliable information available; avoid using.

Effectiveness

POSSIBLY EFFECTIVE

Barium enema-related colonic spasm. Rectal use of peppermint oil, added as an ingredient in barium enema preparations, seems to relax the colon during barium enema radiologic examination (6739,6749,12009). Adding peppermint oil to the barium enema seems to be at least as effective as using systemic scopolamine (Buscopan) for decreasing colon spasms. Adding peppermint oil to the barium solution does not seem to impair image quality (12009).
Dyspepsia. Taking peppermint oil orally in combination with caraway oil seems to reduce symptoms of non-ulcerative dyspepsia including feelings of fullness and mild gastrointestinal (GI) spasms. The combination of enteric-coated peppermint oil 90 mg and caraway oil 50 mg, which is not available in the US, appears to be comparable to cisapride for relieving dyspepsia (6740,6741,10075). A specific combination product containing peppermint leaf (Iberogast, Enzymatic Therapy) also seems to improve symptoms of dyspepsia. The combination includes peppermint leaf plus clown's mustard plant, German chamomile, caraway, licorice, milk thistle, angelica, celandine, and lemon balm (7049,12724). A meta-analysis of studies using this combination product suggests that taking 1 mL orally three times daily over a period of 4-weeks significantly reduces severity of acid reflux, epigastric pain, cramping, nausea, and vomiting compared to placebo (13089).
Postoperative nausea. Taking peppermint oil orally seems to help reduce postoperative nausea (3804).
Tension headache. Applying peppermint oil topically seems to help relieve tension headaches (3801,6190).

INSUFFICIENT RELIABLE EVIDENCE to RATE

Irritable bowel syndrome (IBS). Taking enteric-coated peppermint oil capsules orally seems to reduce abdominal pain, distention, flatulence, and bowel movements in some patients with IBS (3802,3804,4469,11778,11779). However, other research using equal doses of enteric-coated peppermint oil has shown no effect (3803,11777,11789).
Postherpetic neuralgia. Preliminary clinical information suggests that peppermint oil applied topically might provide temporary relief from postherpetic pain (11781).
More evidence is needed to rate peppermint for these uses.

Mechanism of Action

The applicable parts of peppermint are the aerial parts and oil. Peppermint oil is obtained by distilling the aerial parts of peppermint. Peppermint oil is a complex mixture of compounds, including 28-29% menthol, 20-31% menthone, and 3-10% menthyl acetate (3582). However, pharmaceutical grade peppermint oil is typically standardized to contain at least 44% menthol.
Peppermint leaf contains menthol, narirutin, hesperidin, diosmin, rosmarinic acid, luteolin-7-O-rutinoside, and other compounds (12730).
Peppermint oil is thought to be helpful for respiratory tract symptoms associated with the common cold by increasing salivation which increases the swallowing reflex and suppresses the cough reflex (3,7), reduces bronchial secretions, and can have nasal decongestant activity (1).
Peppermint oil is used for irritable bowel syndrome (IBS) due to its antispasmodic effects. The antispasmodic activity appears to result from direct relaxing effects on the gastrointestinal (GI) tract smooth muscle, characteristic of calcium antagonist action. Peppermint oil may also inhibit potassium depolarization-induced responses in the intestine (6744,11775). This is thought to prevent the hypercontractility that is commonly found in patients with IBS.
Peppermint oil is thought to be helpful for gaseousness and flatulence by relaxing the lower esophageal sphincter and equalizing the intraluminal pressures between the stomach and esophagus, which increases belching (512,3582).
Preliminary evidence suggests that peppermint oil in combination with caraway oil can reduce gastroduodenal motility when administered orally in enteric-coated capsules (6742).
Menthol and other peppermint oil constituents are rapidly absorbed in the proximal intestine resulting in upper gastrointestinal effects such as relaxation of the lower esophageal sphincter. For peppermint oil to exert effects on the lower intestine, it must pass through the upper gastrointestinal tract unmetabolized. Enteric coated peppermint oil formulations prevent upper gastrointestinal tract metabolism (11780). Preliminary research suggests that administering menthol-beta-D-glucuronide orally as a prodrug might deliver menthol to the large intestine. In the intestine, menthol-beta-D-glucuronide is hydrolyzed by bacterial beta-D-glucuronidases to menthol, possibly increasing its usefulness in treating diseases such as ulcerative colitis and Crohn's disease (11776).

For pain in myalgias and neuralgias, topical peppermint oil is thought to have counterirritant effects (3582).
Peppermint oil has antimicrobial and antiviral activities in vitro (11).
Preliminary research suggests that luteolin-7-O-rutinoside from peppermint leaf can inhibit histamine release (12730).
Laboratory models of allergic rhinitis suggest that peppermint leaf extract might relieve nasal symptoms (12733).
Preliminary research suggests that peppermint leaf might be hepatotoxic in high doses (12731). Other preliminary research suggests that peppermint leaf tea might lower testosterone levels and decrease spermatogenesis in male animals (12732).

Adverse Reactions

Orally, peppermint oil can cause heartburn, nausea and vomiting, and allergic reactions, including flushing and headache. Enteric-coated capsules help reduce the incidence of heartburn (3582,3802,4469,6740,11777). Enteric-coated capsules can cause anal burning in conditions where bowel transit time is decreased (11782). Oral peppermint oil has also been associated with burning mouth syndrome and chronic mouth ulceration in people with contact sensitivity to peppermint (6743).
Excessive consumption of mint candies containing peppermint oil has been linked to cases of stomatitis (13114).
Peppermint oil, when used in combination with caraway oil, may cause a substernal burning sensation, belching, heartburn, nausea, vomiting, and diarrhea (6740,6741,6742,10075).
Topically, peppermint oil can cause skin irritation and contact dermatitis (11781). Application of the oil to facial, nasal, or chest areas of babies and small children can cause laryngeal and bronchial spasms and instant respiratory collapse (1,6). When inhaled, peppermint oil can cause flushing and headache (6).

Interactions with Herbs & Other Dietary Supplements

None known.

Interactions with Drugs

ANTACIDS: Drugs that decrease stomach acid and raise gastric pH can cause premature dissolution of enteric-coated peppermint oil (787). Separate dose administration times by at least 2 hours.
CYCLOSPORINE (Neoral, Sandimmune): Preliminary research suggests that peppermint oil inhibits cyclosporine metabolism and may increase cyclosporine levels. Inhibition of CYP3A4 may be partially responsible for this interaction (11784). An interaction between peppermint oil and cyclosporine has not been reported in humans.
CYTOCHROME P450 1A2 (CYP1A2) SUBSTRATES: There's preliminary evidence that peppermint oil and leaf might inhibit cytochrome P450 1A2 (CYP1A2) (12479,12734). So far, this interaction has not been reported in humans. However, watch for an increase in the levels of drugs metabolized by CYP1A2 in patients taking peppermint oil. Some drugs metabolized by CYP1A2 include amitriptyline (Elavil), haloperidol (Haldol), ondansetron (Zofran), propranolol (Inderal), theophylline (Theo-Dur, others), verapamil (Calan, Isoptin, others), and others. Use peppermint oil cautiously or avoid in patients taking these drugs.
CYTOCHROME P450 2C19 (CYP2C19) SUBSTRATES: There's preliminary evidence that peppermint oil might inhibit cytochrome P450 2C19 (CYP2C19) (12479). So far, this interaction has not been reported in humans. However, watch for an increase in the levels of drugs metabolized by CYP2C19 in patients taking peppermint oil. Some drugs metabolized by CYP2C19 include proton pump inhibitors including omeprazole (Prilosec), lansoprazole (Prevacid), and pantoprazole (Protonix); diazepam (Valium); carisoprodol (Soma); nelfinavir (Viracept); and others.
CYTOCHROME P450 2C9 (CYP2C9) SUBSTRATES: There's preliminary evidence that peppermint oil might inhibit cytochrome P450 2C9 (CYP2C9) (12479). So far, this interaction has not been reported in humans. However, watch for an increase in the levels of drugs metabolized by CYP2C9 in patients taking peppermint oil. Some drugs metabolized by CYP2C9 include nonsteroidal anti-inflammatory drugs (NSAIDs) such as diclofenac (Cataflam, Voltaren), ibuprofen (Motrin), meloxicam (Mobic), and piroxicam (Feldene); celecoxib (Celebrex); amitriptyline (Elavil); warfarin (Coumadin); glipizide (Glucotrol); losartan (Cozaar); and others. Use peppermint oil cautiously or avoid in patients taking these drugs.
CYTOCHROME P450 3A4 (CYP3A4) SUBSTRATES: There's preliminary evidence that peppermint oil can inhibit cytochrome P450 3A4 (CYP3A4) enzymes (11783). Peppermint oil might increase levels of drugs metabolized by CYP3A4. However, other preliminary research suggests peppermint oil inhibits CYP3A4 only at very high concentrations (12479). Some drugs metabolized by CYP3A4 include lovastatin (Mevacor), ketoconazole (Nizoral), itraconazole (Sporanox), fexofenadine (Allegra), triazolam (Halcion), and numerous others. Use peppermint oil cautiously or avoid in patients taking these drugs.
H2-BLOCKERS: Drugs that decrease stomach acid and raise gastric pH can cause premature dissolution of enteric-coated peppermint oil (787). The H2 blockers include cimetidine (Tagamet), ranitidine (Zantac), nizatidine (Axid), and famotidine (Pepcid).
PROTON PUMP INHIBITORS (PPIs): Drugs that decrease stomach acid and raise gastric pH can cause premature dissolution of enteric-coated peppermint oil (787). PPIs include omeprazole (Prilosec), lansoprazole (Prevacid), rabeprazole (Aciphex), pantoprazole (Protonix), and esomeprazole (Nexium).

Interactions with Foods

FOOD: Enteric-coated peppermint oil capsules should be taken between meals (787).

Interactions with Lab Tests

FOLLICLE-STIMULATING HORMONE (FSH): Preliminary research suggests peppermint leaf might increase FSH levels in male animals (12732).
LUTEINIZING HORMONE (LH): Preliminary research suggests peppermint leaf might increase LH levels in male animals (12732).
TESTOSTERONE: Preliminary research suggests peppermint leaf might reduce testosterone levels in male animals. Whether this occurs in humans is unknown, although anecdotal reports suggest reduced libido in men consuming large quantities (4 cups per day) of peppermint tea (12732).

Interactions with Diseases or Conditions

ACHLORHYDRIA: Enteric-coated peppermint oil should not be used when the stomach is not producing hydrochloric acid. Achlorhydria increases gastric pH and may cause premature dissolution of the enteric coating (787).
DIARRHEA: Conditions that greatly increase intestinal motility interfere with the absorption of enteric coated peppermint formulations. Insufficient absorption may cause high concentrations of unabsorbed menthol in anal mucosa and cause anal burning (11782).
GASTROESOPHAGEAL REFLUX DISEASE (GERD): Theoretically, peppermint oil might exacerbate the heartburn in people with GERD due to its relaxation of gastrointestinal (GI) smooth muscle.
HERNIA: Theoretically, peppermint oil might worsen the heartburn symptoms of a hiatal hernia due to its relaxation of gastrointestinal (GI) smooth muscle.

Dosage and Administration

ORAL: For irritable bowel syndrome (IBS), the usual dose is 0.2-0.4 mL three times daily in enteric-coated capsules (3802,11778,11779). For children 8 years of age and older with IBS, the usual dose is 0.1-0.2 mL three times daily in enteric-coated capsules (4469).
For dyspepsia, peppermint oil 90 mg per day has been used in combination with caraway oil (6740,6741,10075). A specific combination product containing peppermint leaf and several other herbs (Iberogast, Enzymatic Therapy) has been used in a dose of 1 mL three times daily (7049,12724,13089).
TOPICAL: For tension headaches, 10% peppermint oil in ethanol solution applied across the forehead and temples, repeated after 15 and 30 minutes, has been used (6190). To decrease colonic spasms during barium enema, 8 mL of peppermint oil was added 100 mL water along with a surface active agent, Tween 80. The insoluble fraction was removed, then 30 mL of the remaining peppermint solution was added to 300 mL of the barium solution (12009).
INHALATION: A typical dose is 3-4 drops of the oil in hot water. A lozenge containing 2-10 mg is also used (1).

Comments

In 1990, the FDA banned the sale of peppermint oil as an over-the-counter drug for use as a digestive aid due to lack of proof of efficacy.

PERILLA

Also Known As

Beefsteak Plant, Wild Coleus.
CAUTION: See separate listing for Alpha-Linolenic Acid.

Scientific Names

Perilla frutescens, synonyms Dentidia nankinensis, Ocimum frutescens, Perilla arguta, Perilla nankinensis, Perilla ocymoides.
Family: Lamiaceae/Labiatae.

People Use This For

Orally, perilla is used for treating asthma. It is also used orally for nausea, sunstroke, inducing sweating, and as an antispasmodic.
In foods, perilla is used as a flavoring.
In manufacturing, perilla seed oil is used commercially in the production of varnishes, dyes, and inks.

Safety

POSSIBLY SAFE ...when used orally and appropriately. There is some evidence perilla can be safely used for up to 4 weeks (1338).
PREGNANCY AND LACTATION: Insufficient reliable information available; avoid using.

Effectiveness

INSUFFICIENT RELIABLE EVIDENCE to RATE

Asthma. There is preliminary evidence that perilla seed oil might improve pulmonary function in people with asthma (1338). More evidence is needed to rate perilla for this use.

Mechanism of Action

The applicable parts of perilla are the leaf and seed. Perilla contains multiple flavones. The major flavones apigenin and luteolin are found in the leaves and seeds, along with other flavones including shishonin (6). Perilla seed oil is also high in the fatty acid alpha-linolenic acid. Alpha-linolenic acid is thought to decrease serum cholesterol and triglyceride levels, increase the concentration of the fatty acids eicosapentaenoic acid and arachidonic acid, and inhibit production of inflammatory leukotrienes. Perilla seed oil is thought to help asthma because of the alpha-linolenic acid effects on leukotrienes (1338). Animal and in vitro studies suggest perilla oil may have antitumor effects (6). Perilla extract may have an immunosuppressant effect by preferentially attenuating IgE production (6). Patch testing suggests 1-perillaldehyde and perillalcohol contained in perilla oil are responsible for the occurrence of dermatitis (6). Cell studies have shown luteolin to have anti-proliferative activity (5003). Animals grazing on perilla have developed pulmonary edema and respiratory distress. Animal studies show the oil constituent, perilla ketone, induces pulmonary edema. Aldehyde antioxide contained in perilla oil may be toxic (6).

Adverse Reactions

Topically, perilla may cause contact dermatitis (6).

Interactions with Herbs & Other Dietary Supplements

None known.

Interactions with Drugs

None known.

Interactions with Foods

None known.

Interactions with Lab Tests

None known.

Interactions with Diseases or Conditions

None known.

Dosage and Administration

ORAL: For asthma, perilla seed oil 10 to 20 grams per day has been used (1338).

PERIWINKLE

Also Known As

Common Periwinkle, Earlyflowering, Evergreen, Lesser Periwinkle, Myrtle, Periwinkle, Small Periwinkle, Vincae minoris herba, Wintergreen.

CAUTION: See separate listing for Madagascar Periwinkle and Wintergreen.

Scientific Names

Vinca minor.

Family: Apocynaceae.

People Use This For

Orally, periwinkle is used for "brain health" (increasing cerebral circulation, supporting brain metabolism, increasing mental productivity, preventing memory and concentration impairment and feebleness, improving memory and thinking capacity, preventing premature aging of brain cells, and geriatric support). It also is used orally for mucous membrane inflammation, diarrhea, vaginal discharge, "blood-purification", throat ailments, tonsillitis, angina, sore throat, intestinal inflammation, toothache, edema, promoting wound healing, improving immune function, as a diuretic, sedative, antihypertensive, and hemostatic remedy.

Safety

UNSAFE ...when used orally (2,17). Periwinkle contains pharmacologically active toxic alkaloids that can cause nerve, liver, and kidney damage (17).

PREGNANCY AND LACTATION: UNSAFE ...when used orally (2,17); avoid using.

Effectiveness

There is insufficient reliable information available about the effectiveness of periwinkle.

Mechanism of Action

The applicable parts of periwinkle are the above ground parts. Periwinkle contains pharmacologically active, toxic alkaloids, including vincristine, which have cytotoxic and neurological actions and can injure liver and kidneys (513). Periwinkle may have astringent activity (19). The constituent, vincamine, has hypotensive activity (19). In animals, periwinkle causes leukocytopenia, lymphocytopenia, and lowers alpha-1, alpha-2, and gamma-globulin levels presumably due to immune suppression (2).

Adverse Reactions

Orally, periwinkle may cause cytotoxic, neurologic, liver, and kidney damage due to vinca alkaloid constituents (17). Periwinkle may also potentially cause GI complaints and skin flushing (18). Consuming large amounts may cause severe drop in blood pressure (18).

Interactions with Herbs & Other Dietary Supplements

None known.

Interactions with Drugs

ANTIHYPERTENSIVE DRUGS: Theoretically, concomitant use may increase therapeutic effects of antihypertensive therapy due to hypotensive activity of vincamine, a constituent of periwinkle (12,19).

Interactions with Foods

None known.

Interactions with Lab Tests

None known.

Interactions with Diseases or Conditions

CONSTIPATION: Use of periwinkle is contraindicated due to astringent activity (12,19).
HYPOTENSION: Use of periwinkle is contraindicated due to potential hypotensive effects (12,19).

Dosage and Administration

ORAL: People typically add 3 to 10 drops of the extract to water and use two to three times daily. Periwinkle extract contains glycerin and alcohol (6006).

Comments

The periwinkle constituent, vincamine, can be converted in the laboratory to the compound vinpocetine which is marketed as a dietary supplement (1799) (see separate listing for Vinpocetine). Avoid confusing periwinkle with Madagascar periwinkle (Catharanthus roseus).

PERU BALSAM

Also Known As

Balsam, Balsam of Peru, Balsam Peru, Balsamum Peruvianum, Black Balsam, Indian Balsam, Peruvian Balsam.
CAUTION: See separate listing for Tolu Balsam.

Scientific Names

Myroxylon balsamum var. pereirae, synonyms Myrospermum pereirae, Myroxylon pereirae, Toluifera pereirae.
Family: Fabaceae/Leguminosae.

People Use This For

Orally, Peru balsam is used for cancer, as a diuretic, and to expel worms.
Topically, Peru balsam is used for infected and poorly healing wounds, burns, decubitus ulcers (bed sores), frost bite, ulcus cruris, bruises caused by prosthetics, hemorrhoids, anal pruritus, diaper rash, intertrigo, and bleeding.
In dentistry, Peru balsam is a component of dental preparations for treating dry socket and as an ingredient in some dental impression materials. It is also used in toothpaste and toothpowder.
In manufacturing, Peru balsam is utilized as a fixative or fragrance in soaps and cosmetics and as a food flavoring agent.

Safety

POSSIBLY SAFE ...when Peru balsam preparations are used topically for less than 1 week (2). In some individuals, peru balsam is a contact allergen (11).

LIKELY UNSAFE ...when used orally; avoid using. Peru balsam is for external use only (2,6). Kidney damage can occur with internal consumption of large doses (18).
PREGNANCY: Insufficient reliable information available; avoid using.
LACTATION: POSSIBLY UNSAFE ...when used topically because systemic toxicity to babies can occur following application of Peru balsam to the nipples of nursing mothers (6).

Effectiveness
There is insufficient reliable information available about the effectiveness of Peru balsam.

Mechanism of Action
The applicable part of peru balsam is the oleo resin. Peru balsam's volatile oil consists mainly of benzoic and cinnamic acid esters, including benzyl benzoate (11). Benzyl benzoate is an effective scabicide (19). Peru balsam also has mild antiseptic and antibacterial properties and is believed to promote epithelial cell growth (11).

Adverse Reactions
Orally, Peru balsam can cause kidney damage with consumption of large amounts (18).
Topically, Peru balsam can cause allergic skin reactions and contact dermatitis, including urticaria, recurring aphthoid oral ulcers, Quincke's disease, and diffuse purpurea (2,18). It has the potential to cause photodermatitis and phototoxicity (18). Kidney damage can also occur with the external use of large amounts (18).

Interactions with Herbs & Other Dietary Supplements
None known.

Interactions with Drugs
None known.

Interactions with Foods
None known.

Interactions with Lab Tests
None known.

Interactions with Diseases or Conditions
KIDNEY DISEASE: Use Peru balsam with caution or avoid due to its potential to cause kidney damage.

Dosage and Administration
TOPICAL: Preparations of Peru balsam usually contain 5-20% Peruvian balsam (2). The maximum concentration for extensive surface application is 10% Peruvian balsam (2).

Comments
Avoid confusion with tolu balsam, which is the oleo resin exuded from scorched tree stems of Myroxylon balsamum.

PEYOTE

Also Known As
Devil's Root, Dumpling Cactus, Mescal Buttons, Mescaline, Pellote, Sacred Mushroom.

Scientific Names
Lophophora williamsii.
Family: Cactaceae.

People Use This For
Orally, peyote is used for treating fevers, rheumatism, and paralysis.
Topically, peyote is used for treating fractures, wounds, and snake bite.
Recreationally, peyote is used as a hallucinogen.

Safety
UNSAFE ...when used orally. Peyote is illegal in the US. It is an FDA schedule I controlled substance (9,17,11757).
PREGNANCY AND LACTATION: UNSAFE ...when used orally. The active constituent of peyote, mescaline, may be teratogenic (11758).

Effectiveness
There is insufficient reliable information available about the effectiveness of peyote.

Mechanism of Action

The applicable parts of peyote, which is a small cactus, are the above ground parts. The cactus crown has disc-shaped buttons that are cut from the plant, sliced, and dried. The dried buttons may be chewed, or soaked in water and the resulting liquid used (11757).
The clinical effects of peyote are due to mescaline. Mescaline has sympathomimetic and hallucinogenic activity similar to LSD. Mescaline is less potent than LSD. Its effects last up to 12 hours (9).

Adverse Reactions

Orally, ingestion of peyote can cause mild gastrointestinal effects, nausea, vomiting, and rarely diarrhea, which may occur during the first 30 to 60 minutes of ingestion. Sympathomimetic effects including mydriasis, mild tachycardia and hypertension, sweating, and tremor may follow. Psychic effects and visual hallucinations similar to LSD peak between 4 to 6 hours of ingestion. An average mescaline dose of 5 mg per kilogram causes psychic effects and visual hallucinations. Anxiety, paranoia, fear, and emotional instability can cause self-inflicted or accidental injury. At high doses (greater than 20 mg per kilogram of mescaline), hypertension, bradycardia, respiratory depression, and rarely death can occur. Symptoms usually subside in about 12 hours after ingestion (9,17).

Interactions with Herbs & Other Dietary Supplements

None known.

Interactions with Drugs

STIMULANT DRUGS: Concomitant use may increase the risk of adverse CNS effects (9,17). Some CNS stimulants include nicotine, cocaine, sympathomimetic amines, and amphetamines.

Interactions with Foods

None known.

Interactions with Lab Tests

None known.

Interactions with Diseases or Conditions

None known.

Dosage and Administration

No typical dosage.

PHEASANT'S EYE

Also Known As

Adonis herba, False Hellebore, Oxeye, Red Morocco, Rose-A-Rubie, Sweet Vernal, Yellow Pheasant's Eye, Yellow Pheasants Eye.
CAUTION: See separate listings for American Hellebore, Black Hellebore, and White Hellebore.

Scientific Names

Adonis vernalis.
Family: Ranunculaceae.

People Use This For

Orally, pheasant's eye is used for mild heart failure, arrhythmia, nervous heart complaints, cramps, fever, and menstrual disorders.

Safety

POSSIBLY SAFE ...when the standardized extract is used orally under the supervision of a medical professional trained in the appropriate use of pheasant's eye (2).
LIKELY UNSAFE ...when the standardized extract is used orally without appropriate medical supervision (18,512). Pheasant's eye contains cardiac glycosides and monitoring is required to minimize serious adverse effects.
UNSAFE ...when the plant is ingested. Pheasant's eye is highly poisonous (18).
PREGNANCY AND LACTATION: LIKELY UNSAFE ...when used orally for self-medication (512).

Effectiveness

There is insufficient reliable information available about the effectiveness of pheasant's eye.

Mechanism of Action

The applicable parts of pheasant's eye are the above ground parts. Pheasant's eye contains cardioactive glycosides (7,18). It has cardiac effects similar to digoxin, including positive inotropic and negative chronotropic effects (7). In experimental animals, pheasant's eye demonstrates a tonic effect on veins (2).

Adverse Reactions

Orally, symptoms of pheasant's eye overdose include nausea, vomiting, and arrhythmias (2).

Interactions with Herbs & Other Dietary Supplements

CALCIUM: Concomitant use with calcium can increase the risk of cardiac toxicity (3805).
CARDIAC GLYCOSIDE-CONTAINING HERBS: Contraindicated. Concomitant use can increase the risk of cardiac glycoside toxicity. Cardiac glycoside-containing herbs include black hellebore, Canadian hemp roots, digitalis leaf, hedge mustard, figwort, lily-of-the-valley roots, motherwort, oleander leaf, pleurisy root, squill bulb leaf scales, strophanthus seeds, and uzara (19).
CARDIOACTIVE HERBS: Avoid concomitant use with cardioactive herbs due to unpredictability of effects and adverse effects. These include calamus, cereus, cola, coltsfoot, devil's claw, European mistletoe, fenugreek, fumitory, ginger, Panax ginseng, hawthorn, white horehound, mate, parsley, quassia, scotch broom flower, shepherd's purse, and wild carrot (4).
LICORICE/HORSETAIL: The overuse or misuse of licorice rhizome or horsetail plant increases the risk of cardiac toxicity due to potassium depletion (19).
STIMULANT LAXATIVE HERBS: The overuse or misuse of stimulant laxatives increases the risk of cardiac toxicity due to potassium depletion. Stimulant laxative herbs include aloe dried leaf sap, blue flag rhizome, alder buckthorn, European buckthorn, butternut bark, cascara bark, castor oil, colocynth fruit pulp, gamboge bark exudate, jalap root, black root, manna bark exudate, podophyllum root, rhubarb root, senna leaves and pods, wild cucumber fruit (Ecballium elaterium), and yellow dock root (19).

Interactions with Drugs

CALCIUM SUPPLEMENTS: Concomitant use of pheasant's eye with calcium can increase the risk of cardiac glycoside arrhythmias (3805).
CORTICOSTEROIDS: Concomitant use with pheasant's eye can increase the therapeutic and adverse effects of long-term corticosteroid use (2).
DIGOXIN (Lanoxin): Concomitant use of pheasant's eye is contraindicated due to an increased risk of cardiac glycoside toxicity (4).
DIURETIC DRUGS: Theoretically, concomitant use of potassium depleting diuretics and pheasant's eye can increase the risk of cardiac glycoside toxicity due to potassium depletion (506). Some diuretics that can deplete potassium include chlorothiazide (Diuril), chlorthalidone (Thalitone), furosemide (Lasix), hydrochlorothiazide (HCTZ, Hydrodiuril, Microzide), and others.
QUINIDINE: Concomitant use with pheasant's eye can increase cardiac effects and adverse effects (2).
STIMULANT LAXATIVES: Concomitant use of stimulant laxatives with pheasant's eye can increase the risk of cardiac glycoside toxicity due to potassium loss (2).

Interactions with Foods

None known.

Interactions with Lab Tests

None known.

Interactions with Diseases or Conditions

HYPERCALCEMIA: Using pheasant's eye in people with hypercalcemia is contraindicated (3805).
HYPOKALEMIA: Using pheasant's eye in people with hypokalemia is contraindicated (3805).

Dosage and Administration

No typical dosage.

Comments

Pheasant's eye is considered a poisonous plant (18).

PHELLODENDRON

Also Known As
Amur Cork Tree, Corktree, Huang Bai, Phellodendri Cortex.
CAUTION: See separate listing for Corkwood Tree.

Scientific Names
Phellodendron amurense.
Family: Rutaceae.

People Use This For
Orally, phellodendron is used for diarrhea, peptic ulcers, diabetes, meningitis, pneumonia, eye infections, tuberculosis, and hepatic cirrhosis.
Topically, phellodendron is used as an antibacterial and anti-inflammatory agent.

Safety
There is insufficient reliable information available about the safety of phellodendron.
Pregnancy and Lactation: Insufficient reliable information available; avoid using.

Effectiveness
There is insufficient reliable information available about the effectiveness of phellodendron.

Mechanism of Action
The applicable part of phellodendron is the bark. Phellodendron contains berberine, palmitine, and phellodendrine, and other alkaloids. Berberine has anti-inflammatory, antiproliferative, antisecretory, fungicidal, antimycotic, antileishmanial, and cardiovascular effects (12426,12427,12488). Preliminary research suggests berberine selectively inhibits cyclooxygenase (COX)-2 expression (12488). Palmitine may have antifungal effects (12428). Phellodendrine may have immunosuppressant effects (12429). Phellodendron seems to have anti-inflammatory properties, even when administered as a berberine free extract (12430). Topically applied phellodendron also seems to have anti-inflammatory activity (12431). It also may have antiulcer activity (12430). Phellodendron extract in combination with extract from Aralia elata seems to protect the kidneys in laboratory models of diabetes (12427).
There is no reliable research about the use of phellodendron in humans.

Adverse Reactions
None reported.

Interactions with Herbs & Other Dietary Supplements
None known.

Interactions with Drugs
None known.

Interactions with Foods
None known.

Interactions with Lab Tests
None known.

Interactions with Diseases or Conditions
None known.

Dosage and Administration
No typical dosage.

Comments
Do not confuse phellodendron with the unrelated houseplant philodendron.

PHENYLALANINE

Also Known As
DLPA, D-Phenylalanine, DL-Phenylalanine, L-Phenylalanine.

Scientific Names
Alpha-aminohydrocinnamic acid; Beta-phenyl-alanine.

People Use This For
Orally, phenylalanine is used for depression, attention deficit-hyperactivity disorder (ADHD), Parkinson's disease, chronic pain, osteoarthritis, rheumatoid arthritis, alcohol withdrawal symptoms, and vitiligo.
Topically, it is used for vitiligo.

Safety
LIKELY SAFE ...when L-phenylalanine is consumed in amounts typically found in foods (11120).
POSSIBLY SAFE ...when L-phenylalanine is used orally for therapeutic purposes (2455,2456,2461,2463,2465,2466,2467,2468,2469).
There is insufficient reliable information available about the safety of D-phenylalanine.
PREGNANCY: LIKELY SAFE ...when L-phenylalanine is consumed in amounts typically found in foods by pregnant women with normal phenylalanine metabolism and serum levels (2020,11120). UNSAFE ...when L-phenylalanine is consumed in amounts typically found in foods by pregnant women with high serum phenylalanine concentrations or when L-phenylalanine is taken in high doses. Serum levels of phenylalanine greater than 360 micromol/L increases the risk of birth defects (1402,11468). The risk for facial defects is highest at gestation weeks 10-14, neurological and growth abnormalities between 3-16 weeks, and cardiovascular defects at 3-8 weeks. Experts recommend that women with high phenylalanine serum concentrations follow a low phenylalanine diet for at least 20 weeks prior to conception to decrease the risk for birth defects (1402). In addition, some experts recommend screening in women not tested for phenylketonuria (PKU) at birth (1401).
There is insufficient reliable information available about the safety of oral, therapeutic amounts of L-phenylalanine in pregnant women with normal phenylalanine metabolism and serum concentrations; avoid using.
There is insufficient reliable information available about the safety of oral D-phenylalanine in pregnant women; avoid using.
LACTATION: LIKELY SAFE ...when L-phenylalanine is consumed in amounts typically found in foods by breast-feeding women with normal phenylalanine metabolism (2020,11120). There is insufficient reliable information available about the safety of oral, therapeutic amounts of L-phenylalanine in breast-feeding women with normal phenylalanine metabolism; avoid using. There is insufficient reliable information available about the safety of oral D-phenylalanine during lactation; avoid using.

Effectiveness
POSSIBLY EFFECTIVE

Vitiligo. Taking L-phenylalanine orally in combination with UVA exposure or applying L-phenylalanine topically in combination with UVA exposure seems to be effective for treating vitiligo in adults (2461,2463,2464,2466) and in children (2467).

POSSIBLY INEFFECTIVE

Attention deficit-hyperactivity disorder (ADHD). Taking phenylalanine orally doesn't seem to have any effect on ADHD. Some research suggests that patients with ADHD have lower levels of amino acids such as phenylalanine (9948), but neither D-phenylalanine nor DL-phenylalanine appear to have any sustained effect on ADHD symptoms (9950,9951).

Pain. Taking D-phenylalanine orally doesn't seem to improve chronic pain of varied etiology (2459).

INSUFFICIENT RELIABLE EVIDENCE to RATE

Acupuncture anesthesia. Preliminary clinical research suggests that oral D-phenylalanine might enhance acupuncture anesthesia during tooth extraction (2456). However, it doesn't seem to enhance acupuncture anesthesia for chronic low back pain (2456).

Depression. Limited clinical research performed over 2 decades ago suggests L-phenylalanine or DL-phenylalanine might be useful for depression (2468,2469), but this research needs to be replicated with up-to-date study methods.

Parkinson's disease. Limited clinical research suggests taking D-phenylalanine orally might decrease symptoms of Parkinson's disease (2455). However, taking DL-phenylalanine orally doesn't seem to be effective for treating Parkinson's disease (2454).

Phenylalanine deficiency. Preliminary clinical research suggests administering phenylalanine orally might improve phenylalanine deficiency in children who have tyrosinemia, while maintaining tyrosine levels at less than 600 micromol/L. Phenylalanine deficiency is a necessary consequence of an effective treatment regimen for tyrosinemia (11469).

More evidence is needed to rate phenylalanine for these uses.

Mechanism of Action

Phenylalanine exists as two enantiomers, D-phenylalanine and L-phenylalanine. The racemic mix DL-phenylalanine (50% D-, 50% L-phenylalanine) is produced by laboratory synthesis. D-phenylalanine is non-nutritive (not an essential human amino acid), and its role in humans is not currently understood. Human data suggests that about one-third of a 25 mg/kg dose of D-phenylalanine is converted to L-phenylalanine (2052). L-phenylalanine is an essential human amino acid, and is the only form of phenylalanine found in proteins. Major dietary sources of L-phenylalanine include meat, fish, eggs, cheese, and milk (2023). L-phenylalanine is normally metabolized to tyrosine (2052,9949).

L-phenylalanine exacerbates tardive dyskinesia in people with schizophrenia (2457) and can contribute to the development and severity of tardive dyskinesia in people with unipolar depression treated with neuroleptics (2458). L-phenylalanine does not alter pain tolerance to burns in healthy people (2460). D-phenylalanine increases the pain threshold in animals, inducing a naloxone-reversible analgesia by blocking enzymatic degradation of enkephalin (2459). Large neutral amino acids (LNAAs) including DL-phenylalanine, leucine, and isoleucine can exacerbate tremor, rigidity, and the "on-off" syndrome in people with Parkinson's disease who have used levodopa for more than 5-10 years (2454,3291). The amount of dietary LNAAs appears to affect the severity of "on-off" symptoms and may be independent of dietary protein-induced alterations in oral levodopa bioavailability (3291,3292,3293,3294). DL-phenylalanine and other LNAAs might worsen symptoms by decreasing the amount of levodopa that crosses the blood-brain barrier (3291,3294). Preliminary evidence suggests that L-phenylalanine, given with the non-selective monoamine oxidase (MAO-A/MOA-B) inhibitor pargyline, might prevent the elimination of tyramine, increasing the risk of hypertensive crisis (2021). However, hypertensive crisis was not reported in a small number of patients who used L-phenylalanine with the partially selective monoamine oxidase B (MAO-B) inhibitor, selegiline (Eldepryl) (2469).

Adverse Reactions

Orally, L-phenylalanine can exacerbate tardive dyskinesia in people with schizophrenia (2457). Large neutral amino acids (LNAAs; including DL-phenylalanine, leucine and isoleucine) exacerbate tremor, rigidity, and the "on-off" syndrome in patients with Parkinson's disease using levodopa (2454,3291,3292,3293,3294).

Interactions with Herbs & Other Dietary Supplements

None known.

Interactions with Drugs

ANTIPSYCHOTIC DRUGS: Concomitant use of L-phenylalanine and neuroleptics can contribute to the development and severity of tardive dyskinesia in patients with neuroleptic-treated unipolar depression (2458).

LEVODOPA: Concomitant use of DL-phenylalanine and levodopa can exacerbate tremor, rigidity, and the "on-off" syndrome in patients with Parkinson's disease (2454,3291,3292,3293,3294).

MONOAMINE OXIDASE INIHIBTORS (MAOIs): Theoretically, concomitant use of L-phenylalanine and non-selective MAOI drugs might increase the risk of hypertensive crisis. Some evidence suggests that L-phenylalanine, given with the non-selective MAOI drug pargyline, might prevent the elimination of tyramine, increasing the risk of hypertensive crisis (2021).

Interactions with Foods

None known.

Interactions with Lab Tests

None known.

Interactions with Diseases or Conditions

HYPERPHENYLALANINEMIA: Phenylalanine should be avoided in people with inherited disorders of phenylalanine metabolism. Hyperphenylalaninemia is the result of impaired metabolism of phenylalanine due to a deficiency of the liver enzyme phenylalanine hydroxylase. People with the genetic disorder known as phenylketonuria (PKU) have an absence or lack of this enzyme activity, and normally show high levels of blood phenylalanine, and build up phenylketones (10754,11468). Warn patients that phenylalanine consumption may cause mental retardation, hypertension, stroke, and many other adverse effects in people with an inability to properly metabolize phenylalanine (2084,10754,11468).

SCHIZOPHRENIA: Use with caution. L-phenylalanine can exacerbate tardive dyskinesia in people with schizophrenia (2457).

Dosage and Administration

ORAL: For Parkinson's disease, the dose of D-phenylalanine is typically 200 to 500 mg per day (2455). As an adjunct to acupuncture anesthesia or analgesia in tooth extraction, 4 grams of D-phenylalanine is usually taken 30 minutes before acupuncture (2456). For unipolar depression, the usual dose of L-phenylalanine is 250 mg with 5-10 mg L-deprenyl per day (2469), and the common dose of DL-phenylalanine is 150 to 200 mg per day (2468). For vitiligo in adults, 50-100 mg/kg of L-phenylalanine is typically used per day along with UVA exposure (2461,2463,2464,2465,2466).

For phenylalanine deficiency in tyrosinemia, phenylalanine 30-40 mg/kg per day has been used in children (11469).
TOPICAL: A 10% L-phenylalanine cream along with UVA exposure is commonly used for vitiligo (2461).

PHOSPHATE SALTS

Also Known As

Bone Phosphate, Calcium Orthophosphate, Calcium Phosphate-Bone Ash, Calcium Phosphate Dibasic Anhydrous, Calcium Phosphate Dibasic Dihydrate, Calcium Phosphate Tribasic, Di-Calcium Phosphate, Dicalcium Phosphate, Dicalcium Phosphates, Neutral Calcium Phosphate, Precipitated Calcium Phosphate, Tertiary Calcium Phosphate, Tricalcium Phosphate, Whitlockite, Potassium Phosphate, Dipotassium Hydrogen Orthophosphate, Dipotassium Monophosphate, Dipotassium Phosphate, Monobasic Potassium Phosphate, Potassium Acid Phosphate, Potassium Biphosphate, Potassium Dihydrogen Orthophosphate, Sodium Phosphate, Anhydrous Sodium Phosphate, Dibasic Sodium Phosphate, Disodium Hydrogen Orthophosphate, Disodium Hydrogen Orthophosphate Dodecahydrate, Disodium Hydrogen Phosphate, Disodium Phosphate, Phosphate of Soda, Sodium Orthophosphate.
CAUTION: Do not confuse Phosphate Salts with toxic substances such as Organophosphates, or with Tribasic Sodium Phosphates and Tribasic Potassium Phosphates which are strongly alkaline.

Scientific Names

Aluminum phosphate; Calcium phosphate; Potassium phosphate; Sodium phosphate.

People Use This For

Orally, phosphate salts are used for treating hypophosphatemia and hypercalcemia, hypophosphatemic rickets or osteomalacia, and for prevention of recurrent nephrolithiasis (kidney stones). Phosphate salts are also used orally for enhancing exercise performance, as an antacid for gastroesophageal reflux disease (GERD), and as a laxative for presurgical bowel preparation.
Topically, phosphate salts are used with calcium in dentistry for sensitive teeth.
Rectally, phosphate salts are used as a laxative for presurgical bowel preparation.
Intravenously, potassium phosphate is used for hypophosphatemia and hypokalemia, preventing hypophosphatemia in people receiving parenteral nutrition, and treating hypercalcemia.

Safety

LIKELY SAFE ...when sodium, potassium, aluminum, and calcium phosphates are used orally and appropriately short-term (15). ...when sodium phosphate is used rectally and appropriately short-term (15). Long-term use or high doses used orally or rectally require monitoring of serum electrolytes (2494,2495,2496,2497,2498,3092). ...when used intravenously, potassium phosphate is an FDA-approved prescription drug (15).
POSSIBLY UNSAFE ...when phosphate (expressed as phosphorus) intake exceeds the tolerable upper intake level (UL). Hyperphosphatemia, resulting in electrolyte disturbances, alterations in calcium homeostasis, and calcification of nonskeletal tissues, may occur. The UL for adults under age 70 is 4 grams per day. For adults older than age 70, the UL is 3 grams per day (7555).
CHILDREN: LIKELY SAFE ...when used orally and appropriately at recommended dietary allowances (RDAs). The daily RDAs are: children 1-3 years, 460 mg; children 4-8 years, 500 mg; males and females 9-18 years, 1250 mg (7555). ...when sodium phosphate is used rectally and appropriately short-term (15). ...when used intravenously, potassium phosphate is an FDA-approved prescription drug (15). POSSIBLY UNSAFE ...when phosphate (expressed as phosphorus) intake exceeds the tolerable upper intake level (UL). Hyperphosphatemia, resulting in electrolyte disturbances, alterations in calcium homeostasis, and calcification of nonskeletal tissues, may occur. The ULs are: children 1-8 years, 3 grams per day; children 9 years and older, 4 grams per day (7555).
PREGNANCY AND LACTATION: LIKELY SAFE ...when used orally and appropriately at recommended dietary allowances (RDAs) of 1250 mg daily for women 14-18 years of age and 700 mg daily for those over 18 years of age (7555). ...when sodium phosphate is used rectally and appropriately short-term (15). ...when used intravenously, potassium phosphate is an FDA-approved prescription drug (15). POSSIBLY UNSAFE ...when phosphate (expressed as phosphorus) intake exceeds the tolerable upper intake level (UL). Hyperphosphatemia, resulting in electrolyte disturbances, alterations in calcium homeostasis, and calcification of nonskeletal tissues, may occur. The UL for pregnant women age 14-50 is 3.5 grams per day. For lactating women age 14-50, the UL is 4 grams per day (7555).

Effectiveness

EFFECTIVE

Hypophosphatemia. Taking sodium and potassium phosphates orally is effective for preventing and treating hypophosphatemia (15). The FDA-approved IV product is also used for the correction of hypophosphatemia (8302,8303).

LIKELY EFFECTIVE

Hypercalcemia. Taking sodium and calcium phosphates orally is effective for treating hypercalcemia (15).

POSSIBLY EFFECTIVE

Kidney stones (nephrolithiasis). Taking potassium and sodium phosphate salts orally may help prevent kidney stones in patients with hypercalciuria (2209,6470).

LIKELY INEFFECTIVE

Athletic performance. Taking phosphates orally doesn't improve exercise performance (2499,8300,8301).

There is insufficient reliable information available about the effectiveness of phosphate salts for their other uses.

Mechanism of Action

Phosphate is the most common form of phosphorus (7555). It is the most abundant intracellular anion in the body. It is critical for membrane structure, transport, and energy storage (3092). In adults, phosphorus makes up from 0.65 % to 1.1% of the body. Eighty-five per cent is in bone. Normal plasma concentrations range from 0.8-1.6 mmol/L, or 2.5-5 mg/dL (0.032 mmol phosphate = 1 mg). Phosphate plays an important role in buffering body fluids, and plays a primary role in the renal excretion of hydrogen ions. It is present in carbohydrates, proteins, lipids and various enzymes involved in energy transfer (7555). Vitamin D3 and its metabolites influence phosphate absorption from the gut and also affect renal tubular reabsorption of phosphate (3092,3372,8821). Inadequate dietary phosphate lowers serum phosphate levels, which are inversely related to serum calcium levels (3372,8821). Hypophosphatemia causes an increase in intestinal calcium absorption and increased calcium in the blood, which can inhibit formation of new bone (3372,8821), and potentially lead to a greater risk of renal calcium stone formation (3372). Hyperphosphatemia can occur with excessive intake of vitamin D (3092). Sodium phosphates are used as saline laxatives. They cause influx of fluids in the intestine by an osmotic action and increase peristalsis (15). Aluminum phosphate used orally neutralizes gastric acid (15). Oral ingestion of large amounts of sodium dihydrogen phosphate can lower urine pH (1).

Adverse Reactions

Orally, phosphate salts can cause gastrointestinal irritation, fluid and electrolyte disturbances including hyperphosphatemia and hypocalcemia, and extraskeletal calcification. Potassium phosphates can cause hyperkalemia. Sodium phosphates can cause hypernatremia and hypokalemia (15,2494,2495,2496,2497). Sodium and potassium phosphates can cause diarrhea (15). Aluminum phosphate can cause constipation (15). Rectally, phosphate salts can cause fluid and electrolyte disturbances including hyperphosphatemia and hypocalcemia (15).

Interactions with Herbs & Other Dietary Supplements

None known.

Interactions with Drugs

ANTACIDS: Antacids containing aluminum, calcium, or magnesium can bind phosphate in the gut and prevent its absorption (3371). Some patients with phosphate depletion due to chronic antacid abuse might also present with recurrent nephrolithiasis and ureter obstruction (3371).

CHOLESTYRAMINE (Questran): Concomitant administration of bile acid sequestrants and phosphate can decrease oral absorption of phosphate supplements (15).

COLESTIPOL (Colestid): Concomitant administration of bile acid sequestrants and phosphate can decrease oral absorption of phosphate supplements (15).

Drug Influences on Nutrient Levels and Depletion

SOME DRUGS CAN AFFECT PHOSPHATE LEVELS:

ALUMINUM SALTS: Use of aluminum salts can bind phosphate in the gut and reduce serum phosphate levels. Avoid prolonged administration of large doses of aluminum-containing drugs, which might lead to hypophosphatemia (3371,4400).

Interactions with Foods

None known.

Interactions with Lab Tests

ACID PHOSPHATASE: Phosphates can cause a false-decrease in serum test results. High substrate concentrations can inhibit the analytic reaction (275).

ALKALINE PHOSPHATASE: Phosphates can cause a false-decrease in serum test results. High substrate concentrations can inhibit the analytic reaction (275).

AMMONIA: Phosphates can cause a false-decrease in plasma test results by inhibiting formation of indophenol color in Berthelot reaction (275).

CALCIUM: Phosphates can increase fecal levels and test results (275). Phosphates can cause a false-decrease in serum and urine test results by inhibiting emission in some flame methods and by competing with EDTA for calcium (275).

LIPID GLYCEROL: Phosphates can cause a false-decrease in serum test results by inhibiting phospholipase with method of Horney (275).

MAGNESIUM: Phosphates can decrease urine levels and test results by reducing increased excretion with bed rest (275).

PARATHYROID HORMONE: Phosphates can increase plasma levels and test results (275).

PHOSPHATE: Phosphates increase fecal, serum, and urine levels and test results (275).

POTASSIUM: Phosphates (except potassium phosphate) can decrease serum levels and test results (275).

PYRUVATE KINASE: Phosphates can cause a false-increase in red blood cell test results by activating analytic enzyme (275).

Interactions with Diseases or Conditions

CARDIAC DISEASE: Use sodium-containing phosphates cautiously in people with cardiac disease (15).
EDEMA: Use sodium-containing phosphates with caution in people with cirrhosis, heart failure, or other edematous conditions (15).
HYPERCALCEMIA: Use cautiously in individuals with high serum calcium levels. The product of serum phosphate and calcium levels should not exceed 60 to prevent precipitation of calcium phosphate and soft tissue calcification (6479).
HYPERPHOSPHATEMIA: People with Addison's disease, severe cardiopulmonary, renal disease, or hepatic disease are at risk for hyperphosphatemia and hypocalcemia when taking phosphates (2497). Hyperphosphatemia might also occur in people with renal insufficiency, hypoparathyroidism, severe hyperthyroidism, untreated adrenal insufficiency (due to volume contraction, metabolic acidosis and reduced glomerular permeability), metabolic, lactic or respiratory acidosis, rhabdomyolysis, infarction, hemolysis, or tumor lysis syndrome (3092).
HYPOPHOSPHATEMIA: Low phosphate levels can be associated with many conditions, including poor oral intake or absorption, reduced renal tubular reabsorption, respiratory alkalosis, excessive insulin use, certain malignancies, diabetic ketoacidosis, and chronic alcoholism (3092).
KIDNEY DYSFUNCTION: Closely monitor serum electrolytes when phosphates are used by people with mild to moderate renal impairment (15).

Dosage and Administration

ORAL: For bowel preparation for diagnostic tests, a typical dose is dibasic sodium phosphate 3.42 to 7.56 grams and monobasic sodium phosphate 9.1-20.2 grams daily given as a single dose (15). Phosphate laxative preparations should be taken with plenty of water (15). Treating hypophosphatemia or hypercalcemia with oral phosphates requires monitoring of serum electrolyte levels (15). For kidney stones, potassium and sodium phosphate salts providing 1200-1500 mg of elemental phosphate have been used (2209,6470).
As a supplement, the recommended daily dietary allowances (RDAs) of phosphate (expressed as phosphorus) are: Children 1-3 years, 460 mg; Children 4-8 years, 500 mg; Males and females 9-18 years, 1250 mg; Males and females over 18 years, 700 mg (3094). The adequate intakes (AI) for infants are: 100 mg for infants 0-6 months old and 275 mg for infants 7-12 months of age (7555). Tolerable upper intake levels for phosphate (expressed as phosphorus) per day are: children 1-8 years, 3 grams per day; children and adults 9-70 years, 4 grams; adults older than 70 years, 3 grams; pregnant 14-50 years, 3.5 grams; and lactating women 14-50 years, 4 grams (7555).
RECTAL: For bowel preparation for diagnostic tests, a typical dose is dibasic sodium phosphate 6.84-7.56 grams and monobasic sodium phosphate 18.24-20.16 grams daily, administered as a single dose. Treating hypophosphatemia with rectal phosphates requires monitoring of serum electrolyte levels (15).
INTRAVENOUS: Injectable potassium phosphate is an FDA-approved prescription product.

Comments

Foods high in phosphate include dairy products, whole grain cereals, nuts, and some meats (7555). Phosphates present in dairy products and meats are soluble and readily absorbed, whereas those in cereal grains are bound and insoluble, and may be poorly absorbed (3092). Cola drinks contain significant amounts of phosphate, and excessive intake can result in hyperphosphatemia and hypocalcemia (7555).

PHOSPHATIDYLCHOLINE

Also Known As

Phosphatidyl Choline.
CAUTION: See separate listings for Alpha-GPC, Choline, Lecithin, Phosphatidylserine, and Soy.

Scientific Names

None.

People Use This For

Orally, phosphatidylcholine is used for treating anxiety, eczema, gallbladder disease, hepatitis, manic-depressive illness, peripheral vascular disorders, hyperlipidemias, improving ultrafiltration in peritoneal dialysis, tardive dyskinesia, premenstrual syndrome, memory loss, Alzheimer's disease, immunodepression, and preventing aging.

Safety

POSSIBLY SAFE ...when used orally and appropriately. Large doses up to 30 grams per day for 6 weeks have been well tolerated (5223). Lecithin, which contains a substantial amount of phosphatidylcholine, has Generally Recognized As Safe (GRAS) status in the US (4912).
PREGNANCY AND LACTATION: Insufficient reliable information available; avoid using.

Effectiveness

POSSIBLY EFFECTIVE

Hepatitis C. Taking the polyunsaturated form of phosphatidylcholine orally, in combination with interferon, seems to help reduce liver enzymes in patients with chronic hepatitis C (5226).

POSSIBLY INEFFECTIVE

Hepatitis A. Taking phosphatidylcholine orally doesn't seem to reduce serum bilirubin or liver enzyme levels in patients with hepatitis A (5225).

Peritoneal dialysis. Taking phosphatidylcholine orally doesn't seem to improve ultrafiltration in peritoneal dialysis (5222).

Tardive dyskinesia. Taking phosphatidylcholine orally doesn't seem to improve tardive dyskinesia (5223).

INSUFFICIENT RELIABLE EVIDENCE to RATE

Hepatitis B. Studies regarding hepatitis B show conflicting results (5224,5226).

Memory. There is preliminary evidence that taking a single dose of phosphatidylcholine 25 grams (PC-55, TwinLab) can improve some measures of memory in healthy college students (5228).

More evidence is needed to rate phosphatidylcholine for these uses.

Mechanism of Action

Phosphatidylcholine is a phospholipid and a major constituent of lecithin. Egg lecithin contains 69% phosphatidylcholine, while soybean lecithin contains 24% phosphatidylcholine (4914).

Choline is a component of phosphatidylcholine. Choline is a precursor to acetylcholine (5228).

Acetylcholine is thought to be involved in memory. Since phosphatidylcholine might increase acetylcholine, there is interest in using it for improving memory and for conditions such as Alzheimer's disease.

The hydrolysis of phosphatidylcholine by pancreatic phospholipase A2 appears to play a direct role in regulating the absorption of certain lipids and lipid-soluble vitamins (8808). Polyunsaturated phosphatidylcholine may also provide protection against liver fibrosis and alcohol induced oxidative stress, although the exact mechanisms are not completely understood (8809).

Adverse Reactions

Orally, phosphatidylcholine can increase sweating (5229). Ingesting large amounts (30 grams per day) can cause gastrointestinal upset and diarrhea (5223).

Interactions with Herbs & Other Dietary Supplements

None known.

Interactions with Drugs

None known.

Interactions with Foods

None known.

Interactions with Lab Tests

None known.

Interactions with Diseases or Conditions

None known.

Dosage and Administration

ORAL: For hepatitis C, 1.8 grams of lecithin used daily with hepatitis C interferon (5226).

Comments

The term "phosphatidylcholine" is sometimes used interchangeably with "lecithin" although the two are different. Choline is a component of phosphatidylcholine, which is a component of lecithin. Although closely related, these terms are not synonymous. However, in clinical literature, they are often confused.

PHOSPHATIDYLSERINE

Also Known As

BC-PS, Bovine Cortex Phosphatidylserine, LECI-PS, Lecithin Phosphatidylserine, PS, PtdSer, Soy-PS, Soy Phosphatidylserine.

CAUTION: See separate listings for Choline, Lecithin, Phosphatidylcholine, and Soy.

Scientific Names

Phosphatidylserine.

People Use This For

Orally, phosphatidylserine is used for Alzheimer's disease and other dementias, age-related decline in mental function, improving cognitive function in young people, attention deficit-hyperactivity disorder (ADHD), depression, preventing exercise-induced stress, and improving athletic performance.

Safety

POSSIBLY SAFE ...when used orally and appropriately. Phosphatidylserine seems to be safe when used for up to 6 months (2255,2437,2438,2439,2440,2441,7118). Most studies have used bovine cortex derived phosphatidylserine. Since these preparations are derived from animals, there is some concern about contamination with diseased animal parts (1825). So far, there are no reports of disease transmission to humans due to use of contaminated phosphatidylserine preparations. Most manufacturers now only produce soy or cabbage derived phosphatidylserine (1825,7115).
CHILDREN: POSSIBLY SAFE ...when used orally and appropriately (7117).
PREGNANCY AND LACTATION: Insufficient reliable information available; avoid using.

Effectiveness

POSSIBLY EFFECTIVE

Age-related cognitive impairment. Phosphatidylserine seems to improve attention, arousal, verbal fluency, and memory in aging people with cognitive deterioration (2440,2441,7119,7120).

Alzheimer's disease. Taking phosphatidylserine orally can increase cognitive function, global improvement rating scales, and improve behavioral rating scales over 6-12 weeks of treatment (2255,2437,2438,2439,7114,7118).
Phosphatidylserine seems to be most effective in patients with less severe symptoms (2437,2439).
Phosphatidylserine might lose its effectiveness with extended use. After 16 weeks of treatment, progression of Alzheimer's disease seems to overcome any benefit of phosphatidylserine (2255).
Most clinical studies have used phosphatidylserine derived from bovine cortex. However, most supplements now use soy or cabbage derived phosphatidylserine. Clinical studies have not yet evaluated phosphatidylserine from soy or other sources. It is not known if phosphatidylserine from soy and other sources is as effective as bovine-derived products.

INSUFFICIENT RELIABLE EVIDENCE to RATE

Depression. There is some preliminary evidence that phosphatidylserine might improve depression in geriatric patients (7113).

Exercise-induced stress. There is some evidence that athletes taking phosphatidylserine orally during over-training might have the perception of well being and reduced muscle soreness (2264). Some research also suggests that non-athletically trained healthy men might benefit from both acute and chronic phosphatidylserine administration (8851,8852).
More evidence is needed to rate phosphatidylserine for these uses.

Mechanism of Action

Phosphatidylserine is a fat-soluble phospholipid that occurs endogenously in humans. It is the most abundant phospholipid in the human brain and is important in neuronal membrane functions such as maintenance of the cell's internal environment, signal transduction, secretory vesicle release, cell-to-cell communication, and cell growth regulation (2437,7115). Phosphatidylserine is also a component of the mitochondrial membrane, where it might function as a metabolic reservoir for other phospholipids (7121). Although the body is able to synthesize phosphatidylserine through an elaborate series of reactions and substantial energy expenditure, the body obtains most phosphatidylserine from dietary sources. Phosphatidylserine is present in small quantities in most foods (7116).
It is not clear how phosphatidylserine works for dementia such as Alzheimer's disease and age-related memory impairment. However, one theory is that patients with dementia or age-related memory impairment have structural or functional abnormalities in neuronal membranes that cause changes in neurotransmitter functioning. People with cognitive dysfunction often have changes in acetylcholine, norepinephrine, and serotonin levels. Some researchers think the abnormal neuronal function can be attributed to changes in lipid composition of the brain. It is thought that exogenous administration of phosphatidylserine might then normalize brain lipid content and return neuronal function to normal (2441). Phosphatidylserine has been shown to increase acetylcholine, norepinephrine, serotonin, and dopamine levels in animal models and patients with Alzheimer's disease (2437,8857,8858). In animal models, phosphatidylserine improves spatial memory and passive avoidance (8858). It also appears to minimize age-related neuronal dendrite loss and atrophy of cholinergic neurons (2437,8857). The fatty acid docosahexaenoic acid (DHA), which is readily present in neuronal cells, appears to further promote the accumulation of phosphatidylserine in cell membranes, which in turn prevents apoptotic cell death (8857).
Evidence shows that high levels of procoagulant endothelial particles containing phosphatidylserine are present in patients with acute coronary syndromes. Although these increased levels are hypothesized to contribute to plaque disruption and thrombosis, the exact mechanisms are not yet understood (8855).
There is also interest in phosphatidylserine for decreasing exercise-induced stress. Some preliminary evidence shows that phosphatidylserine might blunt the rise in cortisol and adrenocorticotropin following strenuous training (2264,8851,8852). Very preliminary clinical laboratory research suggests that phosphatidylserine 300 mg per day might improve mood and subjective feelings of stress (11963).

In animal models of multiple sclerosis, phosphatidylserine reduces tremor, spasticity, and urinary incontinence, possibly by suppressing the release of the cytokine tumor necrosis factor (8853,8854).

Adverse Reactions

Orally, phosphatidylserine is typically well tolerated. Some patients can experience gastrointestinal upset or insomnia. These side effects are more likely to occur with higher doses, 300 mg for gastrointestinal upset and 600 mg for insomnia (7116,7121). Most phosphatidylserine supplements used to be derived from bovine cortex, so there has been some concern about possible contamination from sick or diseased animals, including those harboring bovine spongiform encephalopathy (BSE, mad cow disease). Using supplements produced from diseased animals might present a human health hazard. So far there are no reports of BSE or other disease transmission to humans from dietary supplements containing animal materials and the risk of potential disease transmission is thought to be low. However, because of this concern most manufacturers now only produce soy or cabbage derived phosphatidylserine.

Interactions with Herbs & Other Dietary Supplements

None known.

Interactions with Drugs

None known.

Interactions with Foods

None known.

Interactions with Lab Tests

ALANINE AMINOTRANSFERASE (ALT, SGPT): Phosphatidylserine 300 mg daily can reduce alanine aminotransferase levels (7116).
URIC ACID: Phosphatidylserine 300 mg daily can reduce uric acid levels (7116).

Interactions with Diseases or Conditions

None known.

Dosage and Administration

ORAL: For Alzheimer's disease, senile dementia, and age-related cognitive or memory impairment, 100 mg three times daily has been used in clinical studies (2437,2438,2440,2441). For treatment of attention deficit-hyperactivity disorder (ADHD) in children, people typically use 200 to 300 mg daily (7117).

Comments

Cephalin (synonym kephalin) is the term formerly used to refer to what are now known as phosphatidylserine and phosphatidylethanolamine.

PICRORHIZA

Also Known As

Hu Huang Lian, Katki, Katuka, Katuko, Katurohini, Katvi, Kuru, Kutki, Xi Zang Hu Huang Lian.

Scientific Names

Picrorhiza kurroa; Neopicrorhiza scrophulariiflora, synonym Picrorhiza scrophulariiflora.
Family: Scrophulariacae.

People Use This For

Orally, picrorhiza is used for jaundice, acute viral hepatitis, indigestion, constipation, fever, allergy, and asthma. Other uses include vitiligo, eczema, infection, scorpion stings, chronic diarrhea, epilepsy, malaria, and rheumatoid arthritis.

Safety

POSSIBLY SAFE ...when used orally and appropriately. Picrorhiza seems to be safe when used for up to 1 year (11493,11848,11858).
PREGNANCY AND LACTATION: Insufficient reliable information available; avoid using.

Effectiveness

POSSIBLY EFFECTIVE

Vitiligo. Taking picrorhiza orally for up to 1 year, in combination with oral and topical methoxsalen, seems to help treat vitiligo in adults and children (11493).

POSSIBLY INEFFECTIVE

Asthma. Taking picrorhiza orally for up to 12 weeks doesn't seem to help asthma symptoms or improve measurements of lung function (11858).

INSUFFICIENT RELIABLE EVIDENCE to RATE

Viral hepatitis. Preliminary clinical research suggests that picrorhiza given orally for 2 weeks might help acute viral hepatitis. It seems to improve symptoms such as anorexia, nausea, malaise, and lower bilirubin and transaminase levels (11848). Picrorhiza has not been tested in patients with hepatitis B. More evidence is needed to rate picrorhiza for this use.

Mechanism of Action

The applicable parts of picrorhiza are the leaves and rhizome. There is preliminary evidence that the constituent picroside might protect against liver injury (11848). Picroliv, a combination of picroside, kutkoside, cucurbitacin glycosides, and other unidentified constituents, also appears to have hepatoprotective activity. Picroliv seems to protect the liver from hepatotoxic agents, such as ethanol and the Amanita mushroom (11850,11852,11856). This protective effect against liver damage might be due to the prevention of lipid peroxidation and generation of free radicals, decreasing the formation of reactive metabolites (11491,11494).

Picroliv also appears to have anticarcinogenic activity when used orally or topically in experimentally-induced liver and skin cancer. Picroliv might also inhibit topoisomerase I and II, which might inhibit cancer cell proliferation (11849,11851).

Picrorhiza has been used traditionally for asthma, but human research has been negative (11858). Picroliv might have immunostimulant and antiallergic activity, possibly by stabilizing mast cells (11853). The picrorhiza constituent androsin may contribute to the antiallergic effect by inhibiting platelet-activating factor (11857).

Animal data suggests both the leaves and rhizomes of picrorhiza have immunostimulatory activity (11492).

The immunostimulatory actions of picrorhiza might also be involved in improving vitiligo (11493). The picrorhiza constituent apocynin may have anti-inflammatory activity. Research in animals suggests it may have anti-arthritic activity (11847,11859,11860).

Picroliv also appears to have activity against parasites such as Leishmania donovani, which causes leishmaniasis, and Plasmodium berghei, which causes malaria (11854,11855).

Adverse Reactions

Orally, picrorhiza can cause vomiting, rash, anorexia, diarrhea, itching, and giddiness (11858).

Interactions with Herbs & Other Dietary Supplements

None known.

Interactions with Drugs

IMMUNOSUPPRESSANTS: Theoretically, picrorhiza may interfere with immunosuppressant therapy. Picrorhiza seems to have immunostimulating activity (11492,11853). Immunosuppressant drugs include azathioprine (Imuran), basiliximab (Simulect), cyclosporine (Neoral, Sandimmune), daclizumab (Zenapax), muromonab-CD3 (OKT3, Orthoclone OKT3), mycophenolate (CellCept), tacrolimus (FK506, Prograf), sirolimus (Rapamune), prednisone (Deltasone, Orasone), and other corticosteroids (glucocorticoids).

Interactions with Foods

None known.

Interactions with Lab Tests

None known.

Interactions with Diseases or Conditions

AUTOIMMUNE DISEASES: There is some concern that picrorhiza might adversely affect patients with autoimmune disorders because of its immune stimulating effects (11492,11853). Avoid using in patients with multiple sclerosis (MS), systemic lupus erythematosus (SLE), rheumatoid arthritis (RA), or other autoimmune disorders.

Dosage and Administration

ORAL: For vitiligo, picrorhiza rhizome powder 200 mg orally two times a day has been used, in combination with oral and topical methoxsalen therapy (11493). For acute viral hepatitis, picrorhiza root powder 375 mg orally three times a day has been used (11848).

Comments

Picrorhiza grows in the Himalayan mountains. It has been harvested to near extinction. It is a constituent of many Ayurvedic medicines (11848).

PIMPINELLA

Also Known As

Bibernellkraut, Burnet Saxifrage, Greater Burnet-Saxifrage, Pimpernell, Pimpinellae Herba, Pimpinellae Radix, Saxifrage.

Scientific Names

Pimpinella saxifraga; Pimpinella major, synonyms Pimpinella magna.
Family: Apiaceae/Umbelliferae.

People Use This For

Orally, pimpinella is used for upper respiratory tract infections, urinary tract infections (UTIs), bladder and kidney stones (nephrolithiasis), edema, and to stimulate gastrointestinal activity.
Topically, pimpinella is used for inflammation of the oral and pharyngeal mucous membranes, as a bath additive for poorly healing wounds, and for varicose veins.

Safety

There is insufficient reliable information available about the safety of pimpinella.
Pregnancy and Lactation: Insufficient reliable information available; avoid using.

Effectiveness

There is insufficient reliable information available about the effectiveness of pimpinella.

Mechanism of Action

The applicable parts of pimpinella are the above ground parts and root. Pimpinella root is thought to loosen and aid in moving bronchial secretions (18); however, there is no scientific support for this.

Adverse Reactions

None reported.

Interactions with Herbs & Other Dietary Supplements

None known.

Interactions with Drugs

None known.

Interactions with Foods

None known.

Interactions with Lab Tests

None known.

Interactions with Diseases or Conditions

None known.

Dosage and Administration

ORAL: No typical dosage. However, traditionally, one cup tea, 3 grams finely cut root in 150 mL boiling water, has been used 3-4 times daily (8). The tincture (1:5), 6-15 mL per day has also been used (8).
TOPICAL: No typical dosage.

Comments

Pimpinella root is often adulterated with other herbs including Hercaleum sphondylium, Heracleum mantegazianum, and Pastinaca sativa (8).

PINE

Also Known As

Dwarf-Pine, Monteray Pine, Pine Needle Oil, Pine Oils, Pini Atheroleum, Pini Turiones, Pix Liquida, Pumilio Pine, Scotch Fir, Scotch Pine, Swiss Mountain Pine.
CAUTION: See separate listings for Dwarf Pine Needle, Fir, and Poplar.

Scientific Names

Pinus sylvestris; Pinus radiata.
Family: Pinaceae.

People Use This For

Orally, pine is used for upper and lower respiratory tract infections, blood pressure problems, common cold, cough or bronchitis, fevers, tendency towards infection, to treat uncomplicated coughs and acute bronchial disease, nasal congestion, and hoarseness.
Topically, pine is used for mild muscular pain and neuralgia.

Safety

There is insufficient reliable information available about the safety of pine.
Pregnancy and Lactation: Insufficient reliable information available; avoid using.

Effectiveness

There is insufficient reliable information available about the effectiveness of pine.

Mechanism of Action

The applicable parts of pine are the sprout, bark, and oil from the needles. Pine bark contains constituents that might inhibit the proinflammatory mediators nitro-oxide and prostaglandin E2 (12707). Oils from pine needles contain pinene, limonene, beta-caryophylene, borneol, and other compounds (12708). Pine oil seems to have activity against bacteria, yeast, and fungi (12708).

Adverse Reactions

None reported.

Interactions with Herbs & Other Dietary Supplements

None known.

Interactions with Drugs

None known.

Interactions with Foods

None known.

Interactions with Lab Tests

None known.

Interactions with Diseases or Conditions

ASTHMA, ALLERGY: Pine pollen can cause an increase in allergic symptoms, even in people who test negatively to pine skin tests (12706).

Dosage and Administration

No typical dosage.

Comments

Avoid confusion with fir shoots (Picea abies or Abies alba) or synthetic "pine oil."

PINELLIA TERNATA

Also Known As
Ban Xia, Banha, P. Ternata, Pinellia tuber.

Scientific Names
Pinellia ternata, synonyms Arisaema cochinchinense, Arum dracontium, Arum ternatum, Pinellia cochinchinense, Pinellia tuberifera, Pinellia wawrae.
Family: Araceae.

People Use This For
Orally, Pinellia ternata is used for nausea, morning sickness, cough, birth control, influenza (flu), and inflammation.

Safety
POSSIBLY UNSAFE ...when used orally. Pinellia ternata contains ephedrine alkaloids and is banned in the US (12147). There is no reliable evidence available about the safety of Pinellia ternata in humans. Because it contains ephedrine alkaloids, it is likely that Pinellia ternata might potentially cause the adverse effects reported with ephedra, including heart attack, stroke, seizure, and other serious side effects.
PREGNANCY AND LACTATION: Insufficient reliable information; avoid using.

Effectiveness
There is insufficient reliable information available about the effectiveness of Pinellia ternata.

Mechanism of Action
The applicable part of Pinellia ternata is the tuber. Tuber extracts are thought to have antiemetic, anti-inflammatory, antitussive, sedative, and anti-implantation effects (12143).
Pinellia ternata is also a plant source of ephedrine alkaloids (12147). The tuber contains approximately 0.002% L-ephedrine (12172).
The constituent responsible of the antiemetic effect seems to be present in an ethanol extract of the Pinellia ternata tuber (12143).
In an animal model, an aqueous extract of Pinellia ternata seems suppress gastric emptying (12144).
There is interest in Pinellia ternata for the flu (influenza). Pinellic acid from the Pinellia ternata tuber seems to increase IgA and IgG antibody titers in mice when used in conjunction with influenza vaccine (12146).
Pinellia ternata might have antimicrobial effects. The constituent pinelloside has in vitro activity against Bacillus subtillis, Staphylococcus aureus, Aspergillus niger, and Candida albicans (12200).

Adverse Reactions
Orally, there is no reliable evidence available about the safety or side effects associated with Pinellia ternata in humans. Because it contains ephedrine alkaloids, it is likely that Pinellia ternata might potentially cause the adverse effects reported with ephedra, including heart attack, stroke, seizure, and other serious side effects (12147).
Inhaled, Pinellia ternata can cause IgE-mediated occupational asthma (12145).

Interactions with Herbs & Other Dietary Supplements
None known.

Interactions with Drugs
None known.

Interactions with Foods
None known.

Interactions with Lab Tests
None known.

Interactions with Diseases or Conditions
None known.

Dosage and Administration
No typical dosage.

Comments

On December 30, 2003, the FDA announced that it will ban dietary supplements containing ephedrine alkaloids. This includes Pinellia ternata, ephedra, and heart leaf (country mallow) (10055). The ban went into effect in April 2004 (12147).

Pinellia ternata is a common component in Traditional Chinese Medicine formulations. Many of these formulations are used for morning sickness. Pinellia ternata, along with ginger, is an ingredient in the herbal formulation Xiao-Ban-Xia-Tang (XBXT), which is used as an antiemetic (12144). Pinellia ternata is also used in Japanese Kampo medicine. It is an ingredient in Sho-seiryu-to (SST) (12146), which is used for the flu.

PINK ROOT

Also Known As

American Wormgrass, Carolina Pink, Indian Pink, Maryland Pink, Pinkroot, Starbloom, Wormgrass.

Scientific Names

Spigelia marilandica, synonym Lonicera marilandica.
Family: Loganiaceae.

People Use This For

Orally, pink root is used to treat worm infestation.

Safety

POSSIBLY SAFE ...when used orally and appropriately, short-term (12).
POSSIBLY UNSAFE ...when fresh root is used or when use is not accompanied by catharsis (12).
PREGNANCY: LIKELY UNSAFE ...when used orally. For pink root to be effective, it must be used along with a purgative laxative. However, purgative laxative use is contraindicated during pregnancy (272). For this reason, pink root should not be used in pregnancy.
LACTATION: Insufficient reliable information available; avoid using.

Effectiveness

There is insufficient reliable information available about the effectiveness of pink root.

Mechanism of Action

The applicable parts of pink root are the dried rhizome and root. Pink root has anthelmintic actions (18). Although there has been no recent research involving pink root, older sources identify the chief constituents as acidic resins, volatile oil, tannins, waxes, and a volatile base (presumably identical to isoquinoline) (18).

Adverse Reactions

Pink root allegedly contains a toxin that can paralyze the spinal marrow and lead to death by asphyxiation (18). Theoretically, prolonged use of pink root can cause depressive effects on the heart (19).

Interactions with Herbs & Other Dietary Supplements

None known.

Interactions with Drugs

None known.

Interactions with Foods

None known.

Interactions with Lab Tests

None known.

Interactions with Diseases or Conditions

None known.

Dosage and Administration

ORAL: A typical adult dose is 2-5 grams twice daily (12). A common dose for children over 4 years is 0.5-4 grams twice daily (12). A strong purgative laxative (e.g., senna) should always be used with pink root (12).

Comments

As late as 1955, pink root was commonly used throughout the country as an anthelmintic. Various unpleasant symptoms have been reported from use of the fresh root or when use is not accompanied by catharsis (12).

PINUS BARK

Also Known As

Canada Pitch, Canadian Hemlock, Eastern Hemlock, Hemlock Bark, Hemlock Gum, Hemlock Spruce, Hemlocktanne, Pruche de l'Est.

Scientific Names

Tsuga canadensis.
Family: Pinaceae or Abietaceae.

People Use This For

Orally, pinus bark is used for digestive disorders, diarrhea, scurvy, and diseases of the mouth and throat.

Safety

There is insufficient reliable information available about the safety of pinus bark.
Pregnancy and Lactation: Insufficient reliable information available; avoid using.

Effectiveness

There is insufficient reliable information available about the effectiveness of pinus bark.

Mechanism of Action

Pinus bark is reputed to have astringent, anti-inflammatory, and diuretic properties. It is also thought to induce sweating. The astringent effects of pinus bark are attributed to its tannin content (18). Tannins dehydrate the mucous membrane tissue, reducing internal secretions and causing external cells to form a protective layer. Plants with at least 10% tannins may cause gastrointestinal disturbances, kidney damage, and necrotic conditions of the liver. Some animal experiments show that tannins may cause cancer; others show they may prevent it. Regular consumption of herbs with high tannin concentrations correlates with increased incidence of esophageal or nasal cancer (12).

Adverse Reactions

None reported.

Interactions with Herbs & Other Dietary Supplements

TANNIN-CONTAINING HERBS: Theoretically, herbs that contain high percentages of tannins (such as pinus bark) may cause precipitation of constituents of other herbs (19).

Interactions with Drugs

ORAL DRUGS: Theoretically, concomitant oral administration may cause precipitation of some drugs due to the high tannin content of pinus bark (19). Separate administration of oral drugs and tannin-containing herbs by the longest period of time practical (19).

Interactions with Foods

None known.

Interactions with Lab Tests

None known.

Interactions with Diseases or Conditions

None known.

Dosage and Administration

No typical dosage.

Comments

Pinus bark is seldom used (18).

PIPSISSEWA

Also Known As

Bitter Winter, Bitter Wintergreen, Chimaphila, Ground Holly, Holly, King's Cure, King's Cureall, Love in Winter, Prince's Pine, Rheumatism Weed, Spotted Wintergreen, Umbellate Wintergreen.

Scientific Names

Chimaphila umbellata synonym Chimaphila corymbosa.
Family: Ericaceae.

People Use This For

Orally, pipsissewa is used as a urinary antiseptic. It is also used orally as a diuretic, astringent, mild disinfectant, antispasmodic, for bladder stones, epilepsy, nervous disorders, and cancer.
Topically, pipsissewa is used for treating ulcerous sores and blisters.
In food and beverages, pipsissewa extracts are used as flavor components.

Safety

LIKELY SAFE ...when used in amounts commonly found in foods. Pipsissewa leaf extract has Generally Recognized As Safe (GRAS) status in the US (4912).
POSSIBLY SAFE ...when used orally short-term (12).
POSSIBLY UNSAFE ...when used orally long-term because it can cause hydroquinone toxicity (18).
There is insufficient reliable information available about the topical use of pipsissewa.
PREGNANCY AND LACTATION: Insufficient reliable information.

Effectiveness

There is insufficient reliable information available about the effectiveness of pipsissewa.

Mechanism of Action

The applicable parts of pipsissewa are the above ground plant parts. The component chimaphilin has a weak sensitizing effect. It is not suitable for long-term use due to its hydroquinone glycoside content (18). Chimaphilin may have urinary antiseptic, bacteriostatic, and astringent activity (11). Animal data suggests pipsissewa may elicit hypoglycemia. Arbutin may have urinary antiseptic properties due to hydrolysis to its hydroquinone by the intestinal flora (7,11).

Adverse Reactions

Orally, chronic use may lead to hydroquinone toxicity. Symptoms of toxicity include tinnitus, vomiting, delirium, convulsions, and collapse (11).

Interactions with Herbs & Other Dietary Supplements

None known.

Interactions with Drugs

None known.

Interactions with Foods

None known.

Interactions with Lab Tests

None known.

Interactions with Diseases or Conditions

None known.

Dosage and Administration

No typical dosage.

Comments

Pipsissewa is used similarly to uva ursi (18).

PITCHER PLANT

Also Known As

Eve's Cups, Fly-Catcher, Fly-Trap, Huntsman's Cup, Purple Pitcher Plant, Purple Side-Saddle Flower, Sarapin, Side-Saddle Plant, Smallpox Plant, Water-cup.

Scientific Names

Sarracenia purpurea.
Family: Sarraceniaceae.

People Use This For

Orally, pitcher plant is used for digestive disorders, particularly constipation, urinary tract diseases, as a diuretic, a cure for smallpox, and to prevent scar formation.
By injection, pitcher plant extract (Sarapin) is used as a trigger point injection to treat pain including sciatic pain, intercostal pain, alcoholic or occipital neuritis, brachial plexus neuralgia, meralgia paresthetica, and lumbar or trigeminal neuralgia. Pitcher plant extract (Sarapin) has been used by injection in combination with bupivacaine hydrochloride 0.5% (Marcaine) and gamma globulin to treat the omohyoideus myofascial pain syndrome. It has been used in combinations by injection (extract triamcinolone and lidocaine with adrenalin) to treat migraine cephalagia, for diagnosis and treatment of forms of sciatic pain including piriformis syndrome (extract and lidocaine), quadratus lumborum syndrome (extract and corticosteroid), and in combination with physiotherapy and an intraoral splint to treat the Ernest Syndrome that is often mistaken for temporomandibular joint problems. It is also used in prolotherapy (phenol and extract) to cause inflammation at the site where the ligaments and tendons attach to the bone to stimulate the body to proliferate stronger, shorter, and less painful ligaments and/or tendons.

Safety

LIKELY SAFE ...when the extract of pitcher plant, Sarapin (a prescription product), is used appropriately by injection by a qualified health professional (5971).
There is insufficient reliable information available about the safety of the oral use of pitcher plant.
POSSIBLY UNSAFE ...when the extract of pitcher plant, Sarapin (a prescription product), is injected in areas of inflammation (5971).
PREGNANCY AND LACTATION: Insufficient reliable information available; avoid using.

Effectiveness

There is insufficient reliable information available about the effectiveness of pitcher plant.

Mechanism of Action

The pitcher plant leaf and root contain sarracenia acid, tannin, resin, and the alkaloid sarracenin (5944). The extract has an effect on sensory nerves without changing skin sensation or affecting motor nerves. Some evidence suggests that pitcher plant extract affects only C nerve fibers, perhaps containing a biological antagonist that potentiates the action of the ammonium ion (5975). This could be beneficial in chronic neuropathic pain.

Adverse Reactions

Used by injection, pitcher plant extract can cause a local sensation of heaviness. Some individuals experience a local sensation of heat or aggravation of symptoms.

Interactions with Herbs & Other Dietary Supplements

None known.

Interactions with Drugs

None known.

Interactions with Foods

None known.

Interactions with Lab Tests

None known.

Interactions with Diseases or Conditions

None known.

Dosage and Administration

INJECTION: Pitcher plant extract (Sarapin) is given by nerve block or local infiltration. Doses are as follows: 2-3 mL cervical, 5-10 mL dorsal, 5-10 mL lumbar, 3-5 mL sacral, 10 mL caudal canal, 10 mL sciatic nerve, 5-10 mL local infiltration. Following injection, patients should be maintained in recumbent position for 15 minutes (5971).

For use in migraine, 4 mg triamcinolone, 0.75 mL Sarapin and 0.15 mL lidocaine with adrenalin drawn into a syringe in that order have been administered at the trigger points in both temples using a 28 gauge, 5/8 inch needle (5973). Sarapin is an FDA-approved prescription product. For additional information, contact the manufacturer, High Chemical Company, 1-800-447-8792.

PLEURISY ROOT

Also Known As

Butterfly Weed, Canada Root, Flux Root, Orange Milkweed, Orange Swallow Wort, Pleurisy, Swallow-Wort, Tuber Root, White Root, Wind Root.
CAUTION: See separate listing for Amaranth.

Scientific Names

Asclepias tuberosa.
Family: Asclepiadaceae or Apocynaceae.

People Use This For

Orally, pleurisy root is used for coughs, pleurisy, uterine disorders, to ease breathing, as an analgesic, expectorant, antispasmodic, and to promote sweating. It is also used orally for bronchitis, pneumonitis, and influenza.

Safety

POSSIBLY UNSAFE ...when the root is used orally because it contains digitalis-like cardenolide glycosides (4). It can cause vomiting (12). Canadian regulations do not allow pleurisy root as a non-medicinal ingredient for oral use products (12).
PREGNANCY: UNSAFE ...when used orally (12) because it might have uterine stimulant and estrogenic activity (19).
LACTATION: POSSIBLY UNSAFE ...when used orally (12); avoid using.

Effectiveness

There is insufficient reliable information available about the effectiveness of pleurisy root.

Mechanism of Action

Pleurisy root contains digitalis-like cardenolide glycosides (18). Animal data suggest that pleurisy root does not affect blood pressure, respiration, or heart muscle (4).

Adverse Reactions

Pleurisy root may cause dermatitis. It is also a gastrointestinal irritant and emetic, and can cause nausea and vomiting (19). At higher doses, it may cause digitalis-like poisoning symptoms (18).

Interactions with Herbs & Other Dietary Supplements

CARDIAC GLYCOSIDE-CONTAINING HERBS: Contraindicated. Concomitant use can increase the risk of cardiac glycoside toxicity. Cardiac glycoside-containing herbs include black hellebore, Canadian hemp roots, digitalis leaf, hedge mustard, figwort, lily-of-the-valley roots, motherwort, oleander leaf, pheasant's eye plant, squill bulb leaf scales, strophanthus seeds, and uzara (19).

Interactions with Drugs

DIGOXIN (Lanoxin): Because pleurisy root contains cardenolide glycosides, it could have additive effects with digoxin (19).
DIURETIC DRUGS: Theoretically, concomitant use of potassium-depleting diuretics and pleurisy root can increase the risk of cardiac glycoside toxicity due to potassium depletion (19). Some diuretics that can deplete potassium include chlorothiazide (Diuril), chlorthalidone (Thalitone), furosemide (Lasix), hydrochlorothiazide (HCTZ, Hydrodiuril, Microzide), and others.
ESTROGENS: Theoretically, excessive amounts of pleurisy root might interfere with hormone drug therapy (4).

Interactions with Foods

None known.

Interactions with Lab Tests

None known.

Interactions with Diseases or Conditions

CARDIAC CONDITIONS: Pleurisy root may worsen or interfere with cardiac drug therapy (4).

Dosage and Administration
No typical dosage.

PODOPHYLLUM

Also Known As
American Mandrake, Devil's Apple, Duck's Foot, Ground Lemon, Himalayan Mayapple, Hog Apple, Indian Apple, Indian Podophyllum, Mandrake, Mayapple, Podophylli pelati rhizoma/resina, Podophyllin, Raccoon Berry, Umbrella Plant, Vegetable Calomel, Vegetable Mercury, Wild Lemon, Wild Mandrake.
CAUTION: See separate listings for Bryonia (English Mandrake) and European Mandrake.

Scientific Names
Podophyllum hexandrum, synonyms Podophyllum emodi, and Sinopodophyllum emodi; Podophyllum peltatum.
Family: Berberidaceae.

People Use This For
Orally, podophyllum is used as a cathartic, for jaundice and liver ailments, fever, syphilis, and cancer. It is also used as an anthelmintic, antidote for snake bites, abortifacient, and for hearing loss.
Topically, podophyllum is used for removal of topical warts, including plantar warts, condyloma acuminata (venereal warts), and other papillomas. It is also used for treating oral hairy leukoplakia.
Intravaginally, podophyllum is used to treat gynecologic infections.

Safety
POSSIBLY SAFE ...when used topically and appropriately. Treatment areas should be limited to 10 cm2 and the volume to 0.5 mL Podophyllum resin is potentially carcinogenic and mutagenic. Risk of systemic toxicity increases if applied to large areas, open lesions, normal skin or mucous membranes. Podophyllotoxin, another podophyllum constituent, is safer and has largely replaced podophyllum (12897,12902,12903,12904).
LIKELY UNSAFE ...when used orally. Podophyllum is potentially lethal. Fatalities have been reported from oral ingestion and topical application (5617,12898,12900).
PREGNANCY: LIKELY UNSAFE ...when used orally or topically for self-medication; avoid using. Podophyllum is considered potentially embryotoxic and teratogenic (12898,12899). Fetal intrauterine death and multiple birth deformities associated with oral and topical podophyllum use have been reported (5618).
LACTATION: LIKELY UNSAFE ...when used orally or topically for self-medication (5617); avoid using.

Effectiveness
LIKELY EFFECTIVE

Genital warts (condylomata acuminata). Applying podophyllum resin, also called podophyllin, as a 10% to 25% suspension in tincture of benzoin topically is effective for removal of anogenital warts caused by human papillomavirus. However, the podophyllum constituent podophyllotoxin is usually used because it is less toxic. Podophyllotoxin (podofilox, Condylox) is an FDA-approved drug (12902,12903). Podophyllotoxin might be more effective than podophyllum (12904).

INSUFFICIENT RELIABLE EVIDENCE to RATE

Hairy leukoplakia. Preliminary clinical research suggests that a single topical application of 25% podophyllum resin in tincture of benzoin can cause remission of lesions of oral hairy leukoplakia (12897).

Mechanism of Action
The applicable parts of podophyllum are the root, rhizome, and resin. Podophyllin resin is obtained from the rhizome. The major active constituents in podophyllum resin are podophyllotoxin, quercetin, and kampherol (12896,12902). Podophyllum seems to be cytotoxic by interrupting cellular mitosis at metaphase (5617,12897,12899). Podophyllum seems to increase the incorporation of amino acids into proteins, and inhibit purine synthesis and incorporation of purines into RNA. It also seems to inhibit mitochondrial function (5617). The oncologic drugs etoposide (VePesid, VP-16, Etophophos) and teniposide (Vumon) are a semisynthetic derivative of podophyllotoxin (12898). The flavonoids quercetin and kampherol are mutagenic (12902). Preliminary research suggests that an aqueous extract of podophyllum, quercetin, and podophyllotoxin might have antioxidant effects and protect against radiation damage. These podophyllum constituents also seem to increase apoptosis (cell death) and phagocytosis of cells damaged by radiation, making way for new cells (12896,12901). Podophyllum also contains the toxin podophylloresin and alpha- and beta-peltatin. The entire plant, except the fruit, is poisonous (12900). Significant absorption occurs through the skin and gastrointestinal (GI) tract (5617).

Adverse Reactions
Orally, podophyllum resin can cause nausea, severe vomiting, diarrhea, abdominal pain, tachycardia, hypertension or hypotension, tachypnea and dyspnea, bone marrow depression, cardiotoxicity, polyneuropathy, hallucinations, renal failure, hepatotoxicity, ileus, loss of reflexes, paralysis, coma, and death (5617,12898,12900). Death has occurred with

ingestion of 350 mg; however, survival has been reported after ingestion of 2.8 grams (5617). Extensive topical use can cause similar effects. Topical application of 5 mL of a 20% solution has caused severe poisoning (12898,12900). Symptoms of toxicity usually do not appear for a period of time, ranging from a few to 13 hours after ingestion or absorption (5617). Podophyllum toxicity has been successfully treated using charcoal hemoperfusion (5617).
Chronic use as a cathartic can cause hypokalemia and metabolic alkalosis (5617). Oral or topical use of podophyllum in pregnant women can cause fetal congenital malformations and death (5618).
Topically, podophyllum resin applied to the tongue or oral mucosa can cause transient loss of taste and local irritation (12897). Podophyllum can cause severe local irritation and severe ulcerations or persistent neuropathies (12900). Podophyllotoxin (podophilox) causes fewer and milder adverse effects. Topical application can cause erythema, erosions, burning, pain, itching, and tenderness associated with wart necrosis (12902,12903).

Interactions with Herbs & Other Dietary Supplements
None known.

Interactions with Drugs
None known.

Interactions with Foods
None known.

Interactions with Lab Tests
LEUKOCYTES, PLATELETS: Podophyllum resin can cause leukopenia, thrombocytopenia, and pancytopenia (12900).
LIVER FUNCTION TESTS: Podophyllum resin can cause increased liver function tests including alkaline phosphatase (Alk Phos), alanine aminotransferase (ALT), aspartate aminotransferase (AST), lactate dehydrogenase (LDH), total bilirubin, and prothrombin time (PT) test results (12900).

Interactions with Diseases or Conditions
None known.

Dosage and Administration
TOPICAL: Podophyllum resin, as a 10% to 25% suspension in tincture of benzoin, is applied to an area no more than 10 square cm, with protection of surrounding skin to minimize toxicity. It should be washed off four to six hours after application (12902,12903,12904). Podophyllum should not be used for self-treatment. Podophyllotoxin 0.5% gel is applied twice daily for three consecutive days and repeated for two to four cycles. It is considered safe for patient application (12902,12903,12904).

Comments
Podophyllum resin is sometimes called podophyllin.
Podophyllum has been used as a laxative. (It was an ingredient in Carter's Little Liver Pills.) But it has been removed from the market due to safety concerns (12902).

POINSETTIA

Also Known As
Christmas Flower, Easter Flower, Lobster Flower Plant, Lobsterplant, Mexican Flame Leaf, Paintedleaf, Papagallo.

Scientific Names
Euphorbia pulcherrima, synonym Poinsettia pulcherrima; Euphorbia poinsettia.
Family: Euphorbiaceae.

People Use This For
Orally, poinsettia is used as an antipyretic, to stimulate milk production, and as an abortifacient. The latex is used orally as an analgesic, antibacterial, and emetic.
Topically, poinsettia latex is used as a depilatory, skin remedy, for warts, and for toothaches.

Safety
POSSIBLY UNSAFE ...when used orally or topically, but toxicity is limited to local irritation, contact dermatitis, mucosal burns, and keratoconjunctivitis (17).
CHILDREN: POSSIBLY UNSAFE ...when used orally or topically. Poinsettia was implicated in the poisoning death of a 2 year old child (6).
PREGNANCY AND LACTATION: POSSIBLY UNSAFE ...when used orally or topically (17); avoid using.

Effectiveness
There is insufficient reliable information available about the effectiveness of poinsettia.

Mechanism of Action
The applicable parts of poinsettia are the whole plant and latex. There is insufficient reliable information available about the possible mechanism of action and active ingredients.

Adverse Reactions
Toxicity is limited to local irritation, contact dermatitis, mucosal burns, and keratoconjunctivitis (17).

Interactions with Herbs & Other Dietary Supplements
None known.

Interactions with Drugs
None known.

Interactions with Foods
None known.

Interactions with Lab Tests
None known.

Interactions with Diseases or Conditions
GI IRRITATION, INFLAMMATION: Euphorbia species are said to have GI irritant effects (19); avoid using.

Dosage and Administration
No typical dosage.

Comments
Recent studies indicate that the plant is less toxic than once believed (6). American Association of Poison Control Centers reported 22,793 cases of poisoning with no fatalities and 92.4% with no toxicity (3838).

POISON IVY

Also Known As
Markweed, Poison Vine, Three-Leafed Ivy.

Scientific Names
Toxicodendron radicans, synonym Rhus radicans; Toxicodendron pubescens, synonyms Rhus toxicodendron, Toxicodendron quercifolium, Toxicodendron toxicarium.
Family: Anacardiaceae.

People Use This For
Orally, poison ivy is used to treat pain.

Safety
LIKELY UNSAFE ...when used orally or topically (6).
PREGNANCY AND LACTATION: LIKELY UNSAFE ...when used orally or topically (6); avoid using.

Effectiveness
There is insufficient reliable information available about the effectiveness of poison ivy.

Mechanism of Action
Poison ivy is a severe skin irritant that stimulates the immune system (18). Contact sensitivity is due to the urushiols, which bind to skin proteins, sensitizing the individual (6). Once sensitized, re-exposure leads to allergic reactions (6).

Adverse Reactions
Orally, the plant can cause severe mucous membrane irritation, nausea, vomiting, intestinal colic, diarrhea, dizziness, stupor, nephritis, hematuria, fever, and unconsciousness (18).
Topically, the plant can cause contact dermatitis, reddening, swelling, herpes-like blisters (18), and erythema multiforme (3839). Eye contact can cause severe conjunctivitis, corneal inflammations, or loss of sight (18).
Inhalation due to burning of the plant can result in fever, major lung infection, and death from throat swelling (6).

Interactions with Herbs & Other Dietary Supplements

GINKGO BILOBA: Fruit pulp can cause cross-reactivity in people allergic to poison ivy (6).

Interactions with Drugs

None known.

Interactions with Foods

CASHEW: Nut shell oil can cause cross-reactivity in people allergic to poison ivy (6,735).
MANGO: Fruit skin can cause cross-reactivity in people allergic to poison ivy (6,735).

Interactions with Lab Tests

None known.

Interactions with Diseases or Conditions

None known.

Dosage and Administration

No typical dosage.

Comments

To prevent poison ivy from causing skin irritation, wash exposed area with water within 5 to 10 minutes (6). Use soap and water first, then ether or alcohol (18).

POISONOUS BUTTERCUP

Also Known As

Celery-Leafed Crowfoot, Cursed Crowfoot.
CAUTION: See separate listings for Buttercup and Bulbous Buttercup.

Scientific Names

Ranunculus sceleratus.
Family: Ranunculaceae.

People Use This For

Topically, poisonous buttercup is used as a stimulant for skin diseases (e.g., scabies) and leucoderma.

Safety

LIKELY UNSAFE ...when the above ground parts are used orally or topically. The fresh plant causes severe local irritation (18).
There is insufficient reliable information about the safety of the oral or topical use of the dried, cut leaf.
PREGNANCY AND LACTATION: LIKELY UNSAFE ...when used orally or topically (18,19). Oral use might possibly stimulate uterine activity (19).

Effectiveness

There is insufficient reliable information available about the effectiveness of poisonous buttercup.

Mechanism of Action

The applicable parts of poisonous buttercup are the above ground parts. Poisonous buttercup contains ranunculin, anemonin, and protoanemonin. Protoanemonin is a potent topical irritant (18). It causes pain and burning sensations, severe tongue inflammation, and increases salivation. When the freshly harvested plant is cut into small pieces or perhaps when it is dried, protoanemonin changes into a pungent, volatile intermediate that quickly dimerizes to a form that does not irritate the mucous membrane. In vitro, leaf extracts have shown a wide fungicidal spectrum of activity (3836).

Adverse Reactions

Topically, extended contact with fresh or bruised plant can lead to blisters and burns that are difficult to heal (18). Some species of Ranunculus can cause photodermatitis. Avoid excessive sunlight or ultraviolet light exposure while using this product (19).

Interactions with Herbs & Other Dietary Supplements

None known.

Interactions with Drugs

None known.

Interactions with Foods
None known.

Interactions with Lab Tests
None known.

Interactions with Diseases or Conditions
None known.

Dosage and Administration
TOPICAL: Poisonous buttercup is used as a tincture (18).

POKEWEED

Also Known As
American Nightshade, American Spinach, Bear's Grape, Branching Phytolacca, Cancer Jalap, Chongras, Coakum, Coakum-Chorngras, Cokan, Crowberry, Fitolaca, Garget, Hierba Carmín, Inkberry, Jalap, Kermesbeere, Phytolacca Berry, Pigeonberry, Pocan, Poke, Pokeberry, Raisin d'Amérique, Red Plant, Red Weed, Red-Ink Plant, Scoke, Skoke, Teinturière, Virginian Poke.
CAUTION: See separate listings for Jalap and Mexican Scammony Root.

Scientific Names
Phytolacca americana, synonym Phytolacca decandra.
Family: Phytolaccaceae.

People Use This For
Orally, pokeweed root is used as an emetic, for rheumatism, mucous membrane inflammation of upper and lower respiratory tract, tonsillitis, laryngitis, adenitis, mastitis, mumps, skin infections (scabies, tinea, sycosis, ringworm, acne), mammary abscesses, edema, skin cancers, dysmenorrhea, and syphilis.
In foods, pokeweed berry is used as red food coloring and as a wine coloring agent.
In manufacturing, pokeweed berry is used to make ink and dye.

Safety
LIKELY UNSAFE ...when pokeweed is ingested or applied to the skin. All parts of the pokeweed plant, especially the root, are considered to be toxic (3477,3479,3483). Severe poisoning has been reported from ingesting tea brewed from pokeweed root (3478) and pokeweed leaves (3480). Poisoning also has resulted from ingestion of pokeberry wine and pokeberry pancakes (3479). Consuming just 10 berries can be toxic to an adult (6). Green berries are considered more toxic than mature, red berries (4). The Herb Trade Association recommends against selling pokeweed as an herbal beverage or food (3478). Skin contact can cause hematological changes (3477,3481,3482). Protective gloves should be used to handle the plant (3477).
CHILDREN: UNSAFE ...when used orally. Consumption of even one berry can be toxic. Children have died after ingesting pokeweed berries (3479,3483).
PREGNANCY AND LACTATION: LIKELY UNSAFE ...when pokeweed is ingested or applied topically; avoid using. Evidence suggests the berry has uterine stimulant and abortifacient effects (4,19). Pokeweed is generally considered unsafe for any use.

Effectiveness
There is insufficient reliable information available about the effectiveness of pokeweed.

Mechanism of Action
The applicable parts of pokeweed are the root, leaves, and berries. Pokeweed contains saponin glycosides, proteinaceous mitogens (3477,3478), tannins, and resin (6).
The toxicity of pokeweed is attributed to proteinaceous mitogens and the saponin glycosides which include phytolaccatoxin and phytolaccagenin. The saponin glycosides cause gastrointestinal irritation and the proteinaceous mitogens are thought to affect thymus-dependent (T) cells and thymus-independent (B) lymphocytes (3477,3478).

Adverse Reactions
Orally, all parts of the pokeweed plant can cause nausea, vomiting, cramping, abdominal pain, diarrhea, burning sensation in mouth and throat, weakness, bloody emesis, hypotension, bloody diarrhea, tachycardia, difficulty in breathing, salivation, urinary incontinence, spasm, convulsion (3477,3478,3479), severe thirst, somnolence, transient blindness, respiratory failure (3477,3479), and death (3477,3483). Plasmacytosis, mitotic changes in peripheral blood cells, eosinophilia, thrombocytopenia, abnormal platelet morphology, and other hematologic abnormalities may result from topical exposure (especially in individuals with cuts or abrasions on hands or other extremities) and ingestion of

pokeweed plant, berries, or root (3477,3478,3481,3482).
Topically, pokeweed can cause hematological changes after contact with the skin (3477,3481,3482). Protective gloves should be used to handle the plant (3477).

Interactions with Herbs & Other Dietary Supplements
None known.

Interactions with Drugs
None known.

Interactions with Foods
None known.

Interactions with Lab Tests
None known.

Interactions with Diseases or Conditions
None known.

Dosage and Administration
No typical dosage.

Comments
All parts of the pokeweed plant are considered toxic except the above ground leaves grown in early spring (6). The immature leaves are canned and marketed as the food product, "poke salad" (6). Ongoing research is investigating the use of pokeweed in flu, HSV-1, and polio (4,18). The United Kingdom allows pokeweed in medicinal products provided toxic constituents are absent and the product adheres to mandated limits (4).

POLICOSANOL

Also Known As
32-C, Dotriacontanol, Heptacosanol, Hexacosanol, Nonacosanol, Octacosanol, Tetracosanol, Tetratriacontanol, Triacontanol.
CAUTION: See separate listing for Octacosanol.

Scientific Names
Policosanol.

People Use This For
Orally, policosanol is used for hyperlipidemia, intermittent claudication, decreasing myocardial ischemia in patients with coronary heart disease, and as an anti-plaque agent.

Safety
POSSIBLY SAFE ...when used orally and appropriately. Policosanol seems to be safe when used in doses of 10-20 mg per day for up to 2 years (2927,2928,2929,2930,2931,2943,2944,12166).
PREGNANCY AND LACTATION: Insufficient reliable information available; avoid using.

Effectiveness
POSSIBLY EFFECTIVE

Hypercholesterolemia. Taking policosanol orally 10-20 mg/day seems to significantly decrease total cholesterol and low-density lipoprotein (LDL) cholesterol, and increase high-density lipoprotein (HDL) cholesterol. Policosanol seems to decrease LDL cholesterol by 11% to 31% and increase HDL cholesterol by 7% to 9% (2927,2928,2929,2930,2943,2944). Policosanol 10 mg/day seems to be comparable to fluvastatin (Lescol) 20 mg/day and simvastatin (Zocor) 10 mg/day in cholesterol-lowering ability (8147,12190). Most of these studies have used policosanol derived from sugar cane. It is not known if policosanol from other plant sources is effective. There is some evidence that wheat germ-derived policosanol 20 mg/day does not significantly lower cholesterol after 4 weeks of treatment (12166). The reason for this potential difference is unclear since wheat germ derived policosanol is almost identical to sugar cane derived policosanol. More evidence is needed to determine the effectiveness of non-sugar cane derived policosanol.

Intermittent claudication. Taking policosanol orally seems to significantly improve walking distance in patients with intermittent claudication (2931).

Mechanism of Action

Policosanol is a mixture of waxy alcohols derived from a variety of plant sources including sugar cane and wheat germ oil. It refers to a mixture of 24-34 carbon alcohols comprised primarily of octacosanol (28-C) and also including tetracosanol (24-C), hexacosanol (26-C), heptacosanol (27-C), nonacosanol (29-C), triacosanol (30-C), dotriacontanol (32-C), and tetratriacontanol (268,269,270).

Sugar cane derived policosanol contains 66% to 67% octacosanol, 12% to 14% triacosanol, 7% to 8% hexacosanol, and 11% to 15% of other carbon alcohols. Wheat germ derived policosanol contains about 68% octacosanol, 12.6% triacosanol, 8% hexacosanol, and about 11% of other carbon alcohols (12166).

Policosanol seems to lower cholesterol levels by inhibiting hepatic cholesterol synthesis (2934,2939), and increasing the degradation of low-density lipoprotein (LDL) cholesterol (2939).

Policosanol also decreases arachidonic acid and collagen-induced platelet aggregation (2933,2935,2936,2937,2938).

Policosanol 20 mg per day reduces platelet aggregation about as much as aspirin 100 mg per day (2937), but it does not seem to significantly affect coagulation time (2935,2937).

Adverse Reactions

Orally, policosanol is usually well-tolerated (2927,2928,2929,2930,2931,2943,2944,12166). In some patients it can cause erythema (2929), migraines, insomnia, somnolence, irritability, dizziness, upset stomach, polyphagia, dysuria, weight loss, skin rash, and nose and gum bleeding (2937).

Interactions with Herbs & Other Dietary Supplements

None known.

Interactions with Drugs

ANTICOAGULANT/ANTIPLATELET DRUGS: Policosanol can inhibit platelet aggregation (2936,2937,2938). Theoretically, taking policosanol with other antiplatelet or anticoagulant drugs might increase the risk of bruising and bleeding. Some of these drugs include aspirin, clopidogrel (Plavix), nonsteroidal anti-inflammatory drugs (NSAIDs) such as diclofenac (Voltaren, Cataflam, others), ibuprofen (Advil, Motrin, others), naproxen (Anaprox, Naprosyn, others), dalteparin (Fragmin), enoxaparin (Lovenox), heparin, warfarin (Coumadin), and others.

Interactions with Foods

None known.

Interactions with Lab Tests

CHOLESTEROL: Policosanol can decrease serum total cholesterol and low-density lipoprotein (LDL) cholesterol levels and increase high density lipoprotein (HDL) cholesterol levels (2927,2928,2943).

Interactions with Diseases or Conditions

None known.

Dosage and Administration

ORAL: For hypercholesterolemia, the typical dose of policosanol is 5-10 mg twice daily (2927,2928,2929,2930). For intermittent claudication, 10 mg twice daily has been used (2931).

POMEGRANATE

Also Known As

Dadima, Granada, Grenadier, Shi Liu Gen Pi, Shi Liu Pi.

Scientific Names

Punica granatum.
Family: Lythraceae or Punicaceae.

People Use This For

Orally, pomegranate is used for hypertension, congestive heart failure (CHF), atherosclerosis, tapeworm infestations, and opportunistic intestinal worms. It is also used as an astringent, for diarrhea and dysentery, and as an abortive. Topically, pomegranate is used as a gargle for sore throat and to treat hemorrhoids.

Safety

LIKELY SAFE ...when the fruit juice is consumed orally and appropriately. Concentrated pomegranate juice has been safely used in studies lasting up to 1 year (8310,13022,13023).

LIKELY UNSAFE ...when the root is used orally. The root contains the toxic alkaloid pelletierine (12).

There is insufficient reliable information available about the topical safety of pomegranate bark and root.

PREGNANCY: LIKELY UNSAFE ...when used orally. The bark, root, and fruit rind can stimulate menstruation or

uterine contractions (12,19).
LACTATION: LIKELY UNSAFE ...when the bark or root is used orally (12).
There is insufficient reliable information available about the safety of pomegranate during pregnancy and breast-feeding when used topically; avoid using.

Effectiveness

INSUFFICIENT RELIABLE EVIDENCE to RATE

Atherosclerosis. Preliminary evidence suggests that patients who consume 50 mL/day of concentrated pomegranate juice have reduced intima-media thickness of the carotid artery by up to 35% after one year. These patients also seem to have modestly reduced blood pressure after a year of juice consumption (13023).
Hyperlipidemia. There is preliminary evidence that drinking concentrated pomegranate juice 40 grams/day can significantly reduce total cholesterol and low-density lipoprotein (LDL) cholesterol in patients with hyperlipidemia and type 2 diabetes. Pomegranate doesn't seem to affect triglycerides or high-density lipoprotein (HDL) cholesterol (13023).
Hypertension. There is preliminary evidence that drinking pomegranate juice 50 mL/day can reduce systolic blood pressure about 5% (8310).
More evidence is needed to rate pomegranate for these uses.

Mechanism of Action

The applicable parts of the pomegranate are the bark, rind, root, seed, stem, fruit, and fruit juice (1287).
The seed oil contains polyphenols and fatty acids, including punicic acid, palmitic acid, stearic acid, oleic acid, and linoleic acid (1287).
Pomegranate bark, leaf, and fruit husk also contain significant amounts of ellagitannins and gallotannins (13024).
Pomegranate juice typically contains 0.2% to 1.0% polyphenols. These polyphenols primarily include anthocyanidins such as delphinidin, cyanidin, pelargonidin, and catechins, ellagic and gallic acids, and tannins (13022). Pomegranate juice has more polyphenols than red wine, blueberry, cranberry, green tea, or orange juice (13025).
Pomegranate polyphenols have antioxidant activity (1287,8308). The antioxidant activity of pomegranate juice can be as much as three times higher than red wine or green tea (13024).
In addition to polyphenols, pomegranate juice also contains citric acid and ascorbic acid (13024).
Estrone and other nonsteroidal estrogenic substances are found in pomegranate seeds (8311).
Pomegranate root and stem contain the piperidine alkaloids isopelletierine, N-methyliospelletierine, and pseudopelletierin.
The root contains up to 25% tannins, and the fruit rind contains up to 28% tannins (18). Tannins can exert an astringent effect on mucosal tissues, dehydrating the tissue, reducing internal secretions and forming a hardened, external protective layer of cells. Some preliminary data suggest that tannins might cause cancer; other data suggest tannins may prevent it (12).
Preliminary data suggests pomegranate juice may slow the progression of atherosclerosis. The antioxidant effects may contribute to decreased macrophage activity in atherosclerotic plaques and reduced lipid peroxidation of low-density lipoproteins (LDL) (8309).
Pomegranate juice might reduce cholesterol due to its polyphenol constituents. It is thought that polyphenols might decrease cholesterol synthesis in the liver (13022).
Pomegranate juice can reduce the activity of angiotensin converting enzyme (ACE) and reduce blood pressure in patients with hypertension. The serum activity of ACE is reduced approximately 36%, with incremental decreases occurring in patients already taking angiotensin converting enzyme inhibitors (ACEI) (8310).

Adverse Reactions

Orally, pomegranate fruit or seeds may cause allergic reactions. These allergic reactions occur more commonly in people who are allergic to other plants (7674). After oral ingestion of the fruit, pomegranate may rarely cause angioedema. Angioedema seems to occur without warning and in people who have eaten pomegranate for many years. Patients should be told to stop eating pomegranate if swelling of the tongue or face develops (7673).
Pomegranate can cause gastrointestinal disturbances, kidney damage, and necrotic conditions of the liver, due to the high concentration of tannins. Regular consumption of herbs with high tannin concentrations correlates with increased incidence of esophageal or nasal cancer (12).
Pomegranate root and stem contain pelletierine. Orally, overdoses can cause strychnine-like effects in the form of heightened reflex arousal that can escalate to paralysis. At amounts greater than 80 grams, people experience vomiting including bloody emesis, followed by dizziness, chills, vision disorders, collapse, and possibly death due to respiratory failure. Total blindness can occur within a few hours to a few days after ingestion, and resolves after several weeks (18).
Topically, pomegranate may cause contact hypersensitivity characterized by urticaria, angioedema, rhinorrhea, red itchy eyes, and dyspnea arising within a few minutes of exposure (8445).

Interactions with Herbs & Other Dietary Supplements

HERBS AND SUPPLEMENTS WITH HYPOTENSIVE EFFECTS: Pomegranate juice might have antihypertensive effects (8310). Theoretically, concurrent use of pomegranate juice with other herbs and supplements that decrease blood pressure might increase risk of hypotension. Some of these products include danshen, ginger, Panax ginseng, turmeric, valerian, and others.
TANNIN-CONTAINING HERBS: Theoretically, herbs that contain high percentages of tannins (such as pomegranate) may cause precipitation of constituents of other herbs (19).

Interactions with Drugs

ACE INHIBITORS (ACEIs): Pomegranate juice might have additive ACE inhibitor effects (8310). Monitor blood pressure and potassium levels. ACE inhibitors include captopril (Capoten), enalapril (Vasotec), lisinopril (Prinivil, Zestril), ramipril (Altace), and others.
ANTIHYPERTENSIVE DRUGS: Theoretically, concomitant use with pomegranate juice might cause additive hypotensive effects; use with caution (8310).
ORAL DRUGS: Theoretically, concomitant oral administration may cause precipitation of some drugs due to the high tannin content of pomegranate (19). Separate administration of oral drugs and tannin-containing herbs by the longest period of time practical (19).

Interactions with Foods

None known.

Interactions with Lab Tests

None known.

Interactions with Diseases or Conditions

HYPERTENSION: Pomegranate juice might have hypotensive effects (8310). Theoretically, concomitant use in patients treated with antihypertensives might have additive effects on blood pressure and potentially increase the risk of hypotension.
HYPOTENSION: Pomegranate juice might have hypotensive effects (8310). Theoretically, use in people with existing low blood pressure might exacerbate hypotension and possibly lead to syncope.
PLANT ALLERGIES: People with plant allergies seem to be at greater risk for allergic reactions to pomegranate (7674).

Dosage and Administration

ORAL: For hypertension, pomegranate juice 50 mL/day has been used (8310). For hyperlipidemia, concentrated pomegranate juice 40 grams/day has been used (13022). For atherosclerosis, concentrated pomegranate juice 50 mL/day has been used (13023).

Comments

The root and stem bark are unsafe for self-medication (12). When used to treat parasites, the fruit rind should not be taken with fats or oils (12).

POPLAR

Also Known As

Balm of Gilead, Balsam Poplar Buds, Jia Yang, Pappelknospen, Populi Gemma.
CAUTION: See separate listings for Dwarf Pine Needle, Fir, and Pine.

Scientific Names

Populus canadensis, synonyms Populus euramericana, Populus marilandica, Populus serotina; Populus balsamifera subsp. balsamifera, synonyms Populus tacamahacca, Populus candicans.
Family: Salicaceae.

People Use This For

Orally, poplar is used as an ingredient in herbal cough preparations. It is also used orally as a stimulant and expectorant.
Topically, poplar is used for sores, bruises, cuts, pimples, external hemorrhoids, frostbite, and sunburn.

Safety

LIKELY SAFE ...when applied topically and used appropriately (2,12).
There is insufficient reliable information available about the safety of poplar for its other uses.
PREGNANCY AND LACTATION: Insufficient reliable information available; avoid using.

Effectiveness
There is insufficient reliable information available about the effectiveness of poplar.

Mechanism of Action
The applicable parts of the poplar are the dried unopened leaf buds. Poplar contains salicin (11).

Adverse Reactions
Topically, occasional allergic skin reactions can occur with the use of poplar (2).
There are no reports of aspirin-type allergic reactions with the use of salicin-rich plants (12).

Interactions with Herbs & Other Dietary Supplements
None known.

Interactions with Drugs
None known.

Interactions with Foods
None known.

Interactions with Lab Tests
None known.

Interactions with Diseases or Conditions
ALLERGIES: Contraindicated in people allergic to poplar buds, propolis, Peru balsam, or salicylates (2,18).

Dosage and Administration
ORAL: No typical dosage.
TOPICAL: The common application of poplar is 5 grams of the dried buds per day or semi-solid preparations equivalent to 20-30% dried buds per day (2,18).

Comments
Available information supports only the external use of poplar. Avoid confusion with spruce (Picea abies) and Canada balsam (Abies balsamea), also known as balm of Gilead.

PORIA MUSHROOM

Also Known As
Fu Ling, FuShen, Hoelen, Indian Bread, Matsuhodo, Polyporus, Poria, Sclerotium Poriae Cocos, Tuckahoe.

Scientific Names
Wolfiporia cocos, synonym Poria cocos.
Family: Polyporaceae.

People Use This For
Traditionally, poria mushroom filaments have been used for amnesia, anxiety, restlessness, fatigue, tension, nervousness, dizziness, dysuria and urination problems, edema, insomnia, splenitis, stomach problems, diarrhea, tumors, and as an antitussive. In herbal combinations, poria filaments have been used as a component of various herbal combinations for treating diarrhea, chronic glomerulonephritis, tinnitus, and for decreasing upper gastrointestinal tract bleeding.

Safety
POSSIBLY SAFE ...when used orally (12).
PREGNANCY AND LACTATION: Insufficient reliable information available; avoid using.

Effectiveness
There is insufficient reliable information available about the effectiveness of poria mushroom.

Mechanism of Action

The applicable part of poria mushroom is the sclerotium (filament). Poria contains pachyman which prevents urinary protein excretion, serum cholesterol elevation, and reduces the degree of histopathological changes in nephritic rats (3727). Some evidence suggests a hydroalcoholic extract (3728) and isolated triterpene constituents (3729,3736,3737) might have anti-inflammatory activity. Poria may inhibit 5-lipoxygenase, and human leukocyte elastase. It also seems to inhibit leukotriene B4, which suggests it might be useful for treating skin conditions such as psoriasis (12615). Other evidence suggests poria extracts might also have immunosuppressive effects (3726).
In addition, isolated triterpene constituents show evidence that they might have antitumor (3729) and anti-emetic effects (3730).

Adverse Reactions

None reported.

Interactions with Herbs & Other Dietary Supplements

None known.

Interactions with Drugs

None known.

Interactions with Foods

None known.

Interactions with Lab Tests

None known.

Interactions with Diseases or Conditions

None known.

Dosage and Administration

No typical dosage.

Comments

Various combination herbal mixtures containing poria are reported to be effective for treating diarrhea (3731,3732), chronic glomerulonephritis (3733), tinnitus (3734), and decreasing upper gastrointestinal tract bleeding (3735).
Further studies are needed to verify these results.

POTASSIUM

Also Known As

Potassium Acetate, Potassium Bicarbonate, Potassium Chloride, Potassium Citrate, Potassium Gluconate, Potassium Phosphate.

Scientific Names

Potassium; K; atomic number 19.

People Use This For

Orally, potassium is used for treating and preventing hypokalemia, hypertension, Menière's disease, thallium poisoning, hypercalciuria, insulin resistance, myocardial infarction, stroke prevention, symptoms of menopause, and infant colic. It is also used orally for allergies, headaches, acne, alcoholism, Alzheimer's disease, arthritis, blurred vision, cancer, chronic fatigue syndrome, colitis, confusion, constipation, dermatitis, edema, fever, gout, insomnia, irritability, mononucleosis, muscle weakness, muscular dystrophy, stress, and as an adjunct for treating myasthenia gravis.
Intravenously, potassium is used for treating and preventing hypokalemia, cardiac arrhythmias including atrial tachycardia and ventricular arrhythmias, and myocardial infarction.

Safety

LIKELY SAFE ...when used orally in amounts up to 80-90 mEq total potassium (supplements and diet) per day (15,16). Larger amounts increase the risk of hyperkalemia (15). ...when used intravenously (IV). Parental potassium is an FDA-approved prescription product (15).
UNSAFE ...when use in excessive amounts. Doses that increase potassium blood levels above 7 mEq/L are potentially life-threatening (15).
PREGNANCY AND LACTATION: LIKELY SAFE ...when used orally in dietary amounts of 40-80 mEq per day (15).

Effectiveness

EFFECTIVE

Hypokalemia. Administering potassium orally or intravenously is effective for treating and preventing hypokalemia (15).

POSSIBLY EFFECTIVE

Hypercalciuria. Taking potassium orally seems to decrease calcium in the urine (2208,2209).

Hypertension. Taking potassium orally seems to reduce systolic blood pressure by about 2-4 mm Hg and diastolic blood pressure by about 0.5-3.5 mm Hg (3385). Potassium seems to be most effective for people with low potassium levels, high daily sodium intake, and for African Americans (3384,3385,3386). Consuming potassium from dietary sources also seems to decrease the risk of developing hypertension. Foods that provide at least 350 mg of potassium per serving and that are low in sodium, saturated fat, and cholesterol might help reduce the risk of developing high blood pressure (1310,8817). However, there is no proof that taking potassium supplements can help prevent hypertension.

Stroke. Consuming potassium from dietary sources seems to decrease the risk of stroke. There is some evidence that foods providing at least 350 mg of potassium per serving and that are low in sodium, saturated fat, and cholesterol might help reduce the risk stroke (1310,8817). However, there is no proof that taking potassium supplements can decrease the risk of stroke.

There is insufficient reliable information available about the effectiveness of potassium for its other uses.

Mechanism of Action

The potassium mineral plays a role in many body functions including acid-base balance, electrodynamic characteristics of the cell, isotonicity, and various enzymatic reactions (15). It is essential in physiological processes including nerve impulse transmission; cardiac, smooth, and skeletal muscle contraction; gastric secretion; renal function; tissue synthesis; and carbohydrate synthesis (15). Inadequate dietary intake of potassium might play a role in the development of hypertension, stroke, and cardiovascular disease. It is likely that potassium works together with other nutrients to produce beneficial physiological effects (1310,8817).

Adverse Reactions

Orally or intravenously (IV), potassium can cause stomach upset, nausea, diarrhea, vomiting, belching, flatulence, and ulcerations (15,16,3385). Hyperkalemia, typically serum potassium above 5 mEq/L, can cause paresthesia, generalized weakness, flaccid paralysis, listlessness, vertigo, mental confusion, hypotension, blood in the stool, cardiac arrhythmias, heart block, and death (15,16,3385).

Interactions with Herbs & Other Dietary Supplements

VITAMIN B12 (cyanocobalamin, hydroxocobalamin): Transient hypokalemia can occur when severe megaloblastic anemia is treated with parenteral vitamin B12. The increase in red blood cell production creates new intracellular sites that can drain extracellular sites of potassium. The resulting hypokalemia is usually temporary and corrected by normal homeostatic mechanisms (9519). Monitor serum potassium levels in people with other risk factors for hypokalamia.

Interactions with Drugs

ACE INHIBITORS (ACEIs): Concomitant use of these drugs with potassium supplements increases the risk of hyperkalemia (15). The ACE inhibitors include benazepril (Lotensin), captopril (Capoten), enalapril (Vasotec), fosinopril (Monopril), lisinopril (Prinivil, Zestril), moexipril (Univasc), perindopril (Aceon), quinapril (Accupril), ramipril (Altace), and trandolapril (Mavik).

ANGIOTENSIN RECEPTOR BLOCKERS (ARBs): Concomitant use of these drugs with potassium supplements increases the risk of hyperkalemia (15). The ARBs include losartan (Cozaar), valsartan (Diovan), irbesartan (Avapro), candesartan (Atacand), telmisartan (Micardis), and eprosartan (Teveten).

POTASSIUM-SPARING DIURETICS: Concomitant use of these drugs with potassium supplements increases the risk of hyperkalemia (15). Potassium-sparing diuretics include amiloride (Midamor), spironolactone (Aldactone), and triamterene (Dyrenium).

Drug Influences on Nutrient Levels and Depletion

SOME DRUGS CAN AFFECT POTASSIUM LEVELS:

AMINOGLYCOSIDES: Nephrotoxicity caused by aminoglycosides may lead to increased urinary losses of various electrolytes, including potassium (9519). Monitor patients closely for declining renal function and electrolyte disturbances. Aminoglycosides may need to be discontinued, and intravenous electrolyte replacement given (15). Aminoglycosides include amikacin (Amikin), gentamicin (Garamycin), kanamycin (Kantrex), streptomycin, and tobramycin (Nebcin).

AMPHOTERICIN-B (Abelcet, Amphotec, AmBisome, Amphocin, Fungizone): Amphotericin-B increases urinary potassium losses due to toxic effects on renal tubular epithelium. Hypokalemia can occur in up to 50% of patients (9519). Monitor serum potassium and give supplements when necessary. If hypokalemia is associated with worsening renal function, amphotericin-B may need to be discontinued.

BETA-2 AGONISTS: Binding of agonists to beta-2 receptors stimulates adenylate cyclase, increasing intracellular cyclic-AMP and activating membrane Na/K-ATPase pumps. This increases cellular potassium uptake, potentially leading to hypokalemia (8880,8886). Reduced serum potassium levels can occur with oral, parenteral, or inhaled beta-2 agonists, especially during acute use of high doses (6217,7001,8880,8881,8882,8883,8884,8885,8886,8889,8890,9534,9599). Occasionally, ventricular ectopy, prolonged QTc intervals, and arrhythmias have been associated with beta-2 agonists induced hypokalemia (7001,8880,8883,8891,9534). This usually occurs in people with low baseline serum potassium levels, heart disease, digoxin therapy, or concomitant use of other potassium-lowering drugs (8882,8883,8890,9534,9599). Tachyphylaxis to the hypokalemic effect occurs, i.e., serum potassium levels return to baseline despite continued use of the beta-2 agonist (8880,8882,8883,8886,8890,8891). Monitor serum potassium levels in people receiving acute high dose beta-2 agonists (acute asthma attacks or preterm labor), and in those with other risk factors for hypokalemia; potassium supplements may be necessary if symptomatic hypokalemia develops (8880). Beta-2 agonists include albuterol (salbutamol, Proventil, Ventolin), bitolterol (Tornalate), isoetharine, levalbuterol (Xopenex), metaproterenol (Alupent), pirbuterol (Maxair), salmeterol (Serevent), and terbutaline (Brethine).
DIURETICS, LOOP and THIAZIDE: Loop and thiazide diuretics increase urinary potassium excretion. Monitor serum potassium levels and give potassium supplements when necessary (4412,4425,4449). Loop diuretics include furosemide (Lasix), bumetanide (Bumex), ethacrynic acid (Edecrin), and torsemide (Demadex). Thiazide diuretics include chlorothiazide (Diuril), hydrochlorothiazide (HydroDiuril, Esidrix), indapamide (Lozol), metolazone (Zaroxolyn), chlorthalidone (Hygroton), and others.
FLUCONAZOLE (Diflucan): Fluconazole can increase urinary potassium losses, possibly due to toxic effects on the renal tubular epithelium (9519). Monitor serum potassium in people with additional risk factors for hypokalemia, and those taking fluconazole for prolonged periods.
GLUCOCORTICOIDS, MINERALOCOTICOIDS: Mineralocorticoids and some glucocorticoids (corticosteroids) cause sodium retention, resulting in compensatory renal potassium excretion and hypokalemia. This effect is dose-related and depends on mineralocorticoid potency. It is most common with hydrocortisone (Cortef, Hydrocortone, Solu-Cortef), cortisone (Cortone), and fludrocortisone (Florinef), followed by prednisone (Deltasone) and prednisolone (Delta-Cortef). Glucocorticoids without significant salt-retaining activity include betamethasone (Celestone), dexamethasone (Decadron), methylprednisolone (Medrol, Depo-Medrol, Solu-Medrol), and triamcinolone (Aristocort, Kenalog) (4425). Monitor serum potassium regularly. If levels become low, change to a glucocorticoid with less mineralocorticoid activity, or give potassium supplements.
LAXATIVES, STIMULANT: Long-term use of stimulant laxatives, or acute use of high doses (e.g., in bowel-cleansing regimens), can result in potassium loss and hypokalemia. Advise people to limit stimulant laxative to short-term use of recommended doses (4411,4412,4425). Some stimulant laxatives include cascara (CitraMax Plus), senna (Senokot), bisacodyl (Dulcolax), and others.
LEVODOPA (L-DOPA, Larodopa, Dopar): Increased urinary potassium losses occur in some people treated with levodopa. The mechanism isn't clear, but the effect doesn't occur when a peripheral decarboxylase inhibitor, such as carbidopa, is used with levodopa (as in Sinemet) (7201). This interaction is therefore unlikely to be clinically significant.
METHYLXANTHINES: Theophylline and related drugs can reduce serum potassium levels, possibly by increasing intracellular uptake of potassium. Hypokalemia is most likely to occur after acute overdose of these drugs (17). However, reduced potassium levels can occur with therapeutic doses, and the incidence and degree of hypokalemia increases with increasing serum theophylline levels (9534,9537,9538,9539). Monitor potassium levels in people with other risk factors for hypokalemia.
PENICILLINS: Penicillins which are formulated as sodium salts present a large sodium load to the kidneys. Increased amounts of sodium are reabsorbed, and the penicillin moiety acts as a non-reabsorbable anion, promoting urinary potassium excretion (9519). Penicillins associated with hypokalemia include penicillin G sodium (Pfizerpen), mezlocillin (Mezlin), carbenicillin (Geocillin), ticarcillin (Ticar), and piperacillin (Pipracil). Monitor serum potassium levels and give potassium supplements, or switch to an alternative antibiotic, as necessary.
SODIUM PHOSPHATES (monobasic sodium phosphate and dibasic sodium phosphate, Fleet Phospho-soda): Use of high doses (> 45 mL in 24 hours), such as those used for bowel cleansing before surgery, can lead to serious electrolyte disturbances, including hypokalemia. Avoid large doses, especially in the elderly and people with other risk factors for electrolyte disturbances (8877,9531). Advise people to avoid using high doses of these products for self-treatment of constipation.
TETRACYCLINES: Use of outdated tetracyclines can lead to nephropathy and electrolyte disturbances, including hypokalemia. This is due to toxic effects of a degradation product (4425). Advise people to complete courses of tetracyclines as prescribed, and not to save them for later use.

Interactions with Foods

POTASSIUM-CONTAINING FOODS: Theoretically, concomitant use can increase potassium levels and the risk of adverse effects, especially in individuals with renal dysfunction, ACE inhibitor or potassium-sparing diuretic therapy. Potassium-containing foods include fruits (especially dried), cereals, beans, milk, and vegetables (16).
POTASSIUM-CONTAINING SALT SUBSTITUTES: Theoretically, concomitant use can increase potassium levels and the risk of adverse effects, especially in individuals with renal dysfunction, ACE inhibitor, or potassium-sparing diuretic therapy.

Interactions with Lab Tests

BLOOD PRESSURE: Potassium taken orally can reduce blood pressure and blood pressure readings (3385).

Interactions with Diseases or Conditions

ASPIRIN OR TARTRAZINE SENSITIVITY: Avoid oral potassium products that contain tartrazine (15).
GI MOTILITY CONDITIONS: Oral potassium tablets and capsules are contraindicated in individuals with gastrointestinal motility conditions (15).

Dosage and Administration

ORAL: Potassium supplementation must be individualized and based on the person's serum potassium level, which should be maintained between 3.5-5 mEq/L. The normal adult daily requirement and usual dietary intake is 40-80 mEq daily (15). For preventing hypokalemia, 20 mEq is typically taken daily (15). The common dose of potassium for treating hypokalemia is 40-100 mEq or more daily, in two to four divided amounts (15).
For hypercalciuria, 1 mEq/kg is taken daily (2208,2209) or four tablets of Urophos-K are taken twice a day (2209).
The typical dose for hypertension is 48-90 mEq daily (3385). For preventing stroke, dietary intake of approximately 75 mEq (about 3.5 g of elemental potassium) daily may reduce risk. Foods that contain at least 350 mg potassium can be labeled "Diets containing foods that are good sources of potassium and low in sodium may reduce the risk of high blood pressure and stroke (1310,8817).

POTATO

Also Known As

Irish Potato, White Potato.
CAUTION: See separate listing for African Wild Potato.

Scientific Names

Solanum tuberosum.
Family: Solanaceae.

People Use This For

Orally, raw potato juice is used for gastritis, stomach disorders, and edema. A purified protein extract from potato is used as an appetite suppressant for weight loss.
Topically, raw potato is used as a poultice for arthritis, infections, boils, burns, and sore eyes.
In foods, potato is eaten, used as a source of starch, and fermented into alcohol.

Safety

LIKELY SAFE ...when unblemished, ripe potatoes are used as food (6).
POSSIBLY SAFE ...when unblemished, ripe potatoes are used orally for medicinal purposes (6).
LIKELY UNSAFE ...when damaged, green potatoes and sprouts are consumed. These contain toxic solanum alkaloids that cannot be destroyed by cooking and can cause serious adverse effects (6).
There is insufficient reliable information available about the safety of potato for its other uses.
PREGNANCY AND LACTATION: LIKELY SAFE ...when unblemished, ripe potatoes are used orally in food amounts. There is insufficient reliable information available about the safety of medicinal use of potato in pregnancy and lactation.

Effectiveness

There is insufficient reliable information available about the effectiveness of potato.

Mechanism of Action

The applicable part of the potato is the tuber. Potatoes are a source of vitamin C, iron, riboflavin, and are rich in carbohydrates (6). A proteinase inhibitor isolated from potatoes is claimed to increase the effects of cholecystokinin (CCK), by blocking the effects of the enzymes chymotrypsin and trypsin, which break down CCK. CCK produces satiety and has been shown to play a role in the short-term inhibition of food intake (476,477,6255). It has been reported by the manufacturer of a purified protein extract from potato (Satietrol), which contains this proteinase inhibitor and other nutrients and minerals claimed to affect CCK, that the product reduced feelings of hunger by 30% to 32% 3.5 hours after a fixed calorie meal. These effects were also found in a group of people who lost weight on a calorie-controlled diet (473). Damaged green potatoes and sprouts contain toxic solanum alkaloids that cannot be destroyed by cooking. Researchers report that a potato peel extract inhibited bacterial adhesion to host cells without killing the bacteria. They believe this activity might be due to polyphenol oxidase, a compound known to have anti-adhesive properties (6107).

Adverse Reactions

Adverse reactions have not been reported with unblemished, ripe potatoes. Solanum glycosides found in damaged, green potatoes and sprouts can cause headache, flushing, nausea, vomiting, diarrhea, abdominal pain, thirst, and restlessness. Deaths have been reported in malnourished individuals who may not have received adequate medical care (17). Twenty mg solanine per 100 grams potato is the maximum concentration considered safe. Solanum glycosides cannot be destroyed by cooking (6). Exposure to potato dust is associated with a high-incidence of respiratory symptoms due to bacterial and fungal contaminants (6).

Interactions with Herbs & Other Dietary Supplements

None known.

Interactions with Drugs

THROMBOLYTIC DRUGS: Theoretically, concomitant use of potato may enhance thrombolytic effects. A carboxypeptidase inhibitor isolated from potato tubers may have inhibitory effects on thrombin-activatable thrombolysis inhibitor, and thereby enhance the activity of thrombolytic agents (474,475).

Interactions with Foods

None known.

Interactions with Lab Tests

None known.

Interactions with Diseases or Conditions

DIABETES: Potatoes can affect blood sugar control. They should be consumed as appropriate carbohydrate equivalents (6).

Dosage and Administration

ORAL: For appetite suppression and weight loss, a purified protein extract from potato (Satietrol) containing a proteinase inhibitor, is marketed as a powder to be mixed with 8 ounces of water and taken 15 minutes before meals (473). There is no typical dosage of potato juice.
TOPICAL: Raw potato is used as a poultice (6).

Comments

The potato is one of the main food crops of the world (6).

POTENTILLA

Also Known As

Crampweed, Goose Grass, Goose Tansy, Goosewort, Moor Grass, Prince's Feather, Silverweed, Trailing Tansy, Wild Agrimony.
CAUTION: See separate listings for Agrimony, Amaranth, Clivers, Tormentil, and Jewelweed.

Scientific Names

Potentilla anserina.
Family: Rosacea.

People Use This For

Orally, potentilla flower and leaf are used for premenstrual syndrome (PMS), mild dysmenorrhea, and diarrhea.
Topically, potentilla flower and leaf are used for the local treatment of oropharyngeal inflammation.

Safety

POSSIBLY SAFE ...when used orally and appropriately (2).
PREGNANCY AND LACTATION: Insufficient reliable information available; avoid using.

Effectiveness

There is insufficient reliable information available about the effectiveness of potentilla.

Mechanism of Action

The applicable parts of potentilla are the flower and leaf. The tannin constituents of potentilla have astringent effects (2) and are likely responsible for antidiarrheal and local anti-inflammatory activity. Potentilla also increases tonus and the contraction frequency of isolated animal uterus (2,7).

Adverse Reactions
Orally, potentilla can cause stomach irritation (7,12).

Interactions with Herbs & Other Dietary Supplements
None known.

Interactions with Drugs
None known.

Interactions with Foods
None known.

Interactions with Lab Tests
None known.

Interactions with Diseases or Conditions
None known.

Dosage and Administration
ORAL: For premenstrual syndrome (PMS), dysmenorrhea, and acute diarrhea, the typical dose is 4-6 grams per day (2,18). Potentilla is often prepared as a tea and given in a dose of one cup 2-3 times daily. The tea is prepared by steeping 2 grams of the finely cut flower or leaf in 150 mL boiling water for 10 minutes and then straining (18).
TOPICAL: No typical dosage.

Comments
Avoid confusion with agrimony (Agrimonia eupratoria) and tormentil (Potentilla erecta), also referred to as potentilla. Avoid confusion with jewelweed, also known as silverweed.

PRECATORY BEAN

Also Known As
Bead Vine, Black-Eyed Susan, Buddhist Rosary Bead, Crab's Eye, Indian Bead, Jequirity Bean, Jequirity Seed, Legume, Love Bean, Lucky Bean, Ojo De Pajaro, Prayer Beads, Prayer Head, Rosary Pea, Seminole Bead, Weather Plant.

Scientific Names
Abrus precatorius, synonym Glycine abrus.
Family: Fabaceae/Leguminosae.

People Use This For
Orally, precatory bean is used orally to quicken labor, as an abortifacient, oral contraceptive, and as an analgesic in terminally-ill patients. The whole plant is used for ophthalmic inflammations.

Safety
LIKELY UNSAFE ...when used orally. Ingesting 5 mg of abrin, a constituent of precatory bean, is toxic to humans (6). Significant precatory bean ingestion causes severe gastroenteritis, followed by diarrhea and vomiting that can become bloody. Symptoms may not appear for several days (3499). Fatalities can occur after 3-4 days of persistent gastroenteritis (17,3499).
CHILDREN: UNSAFE ...when used orally. Ingestion of one seed in young children can be fatal (3499,5607). Older children aged 9-13 years have been reported to experience severe abdominal pain, vomiting, bloody stools (5607,11473), and pulmonary edema after ingesting just one or more seeds (11473).
PREGNANCY AND LACTATION: LIKELY UNSAFE ...when used orally (6); avoid using.

Effectiveness
There is insufficient reliable information available about the effectiveness of precatory bean.

Mechanism of Action
The precatory bean plant contains the indole alkaloids abrine, abrus agglutinin, hyaphorine, and precatorine (6). Abrin, isolated from the seeds, is a potent inhibitor of protein synthesis and moderate inhibitor of DNA synthesis. In vitro, ethanol extracts of the seeds causes irreversible impairment in human sperm motility (3842), and aqueous extracts of the seeds agglutinate human red blood corpuscles (6369). Some isoflavanquinone constituents isolated from the root inhibit platelet aggregation; others possess potent anti-inflammatory and antiallergic effects (3841).

Adverse Reactions
Orally, seeds that are chewed or have cracked shells can cause stomach cramping, nausea, vomiting, severe diarrhea (possibly bloody), cold sweat, fever, drowsiness, weakness, and tachycardia. Pulmonary edema, kidney failure, liver toxicity, coma, circulatory collapse, cerebral edema, and death (3499,5608,11473). Signs of toxicity, including gastroenteritis, may sometimes occur several hours after ingestion of the seeds, followed by the development of bloody diarrhea. More often, however, there can be a latent period of approximately 3-4 days after ingestion of the seeds, prior to the development of toxic symptoms. Symptoms, including death, may occur up to 10-14 days after ingestion of the seeds (11473).
Topically, the seeds can cause dermatitis when used as a necklace (6). Eye contact with the seed's contents can cause necrotizing conjunctivitis (3499).
TOXICITY MANAGEMENT: There is no known antidote. There is no method for enhancing elimination. Patients seen within 4 hours of seed ingestion should be treated with usual decontamination methods including lavage, charcoal, and cathartics. In cases of diarrhea, the need for cathartics may be unnecessary (17).

Interactions with Herbs & Other Dietary Supplements
None known.

Interactions with Drugs
None known.

Interactions with Foods
None known.

Interactions with Lab Tests
None known.

Interactions with Diseases or Conditions
None known.

Dosage and Administration
No typical dosage.

Comments
Children are attracted to the bright colors of the seed (17). The hard coat of a mature seed may resist digestion when swallowed but treatment for suspected poisoning should begin as soon as possible (3499). Abrin, a constituent of precatory bean, is being investigated for the treatment of experimental cancers and is used as a "molecular probe" to investigate cell function (6).

PREGNENOLONE

Also Known As
None.
CAUTION: See separate listings for Progesterone and Wild Yam.

Scientific Names
Pregnenolone; (3 beta)-3-hydroxypregn-5-en-20-one; delta 5-pregnen-3 beta-ol-20-one; 17 beta-(1-ketoethyl)- delta 5-androsten-3 beta-ol.

People Use This For
Orally, pregnenolone is used for slowing or reversing aging, for arthritis, depression, endometriosis, fatigue, fibrocystic breast disease, memory enhancement, menopause, premenstrual syndrome (PMS), stress, increasing energy, and improving immunity. It is also used for strengthening the heart, Alzheimer's disease, allergic reactions, detoxification, lupus, multiple sclerosis (MS), prostate disorders, psoriasis, scleroderma, seizures, trauma, and injuries.

Safety
There is insufficient reliable information available about the safety of pregnenolone.
Pregnancy and Lactation: Insufficient reliable information available; avoid using.

Effectiveness
There is insufficient reliable information available about the effectiveness of pregnenolone.

Mechanism of Action
Pregnenolone is synthesized in the body from cholesterol and is the precursor for all the steroid hormones, including progesterone, aldosterone, cortisol, dehydroepiandrosterone (DHEA), testosterone, and estrogens (3008). Lower cerebrospinal fluid (CSF) pregnenolone levels have been reported in people with affective disorders, particularly episodes of active depression (3005). Pregnenolone has antagonist activity at GABA-A receptors in the brain and induces changes in the sleep EEG by increasing the time spent in slow wave sleep (3007). Higher pregnenolone serum concentrations during the luteal phase are associated with more severe PMS symptoms (3006). Reliable information on the effects of exogenously administered pregnenolone is not available (3005).

Adverse Reactions
Orally, supplemental pregnenolone may cause steroid-related adverse effects (3008).

Interactions with Herbs & Other Dietary Supplements
DEHYDROEPIANDROSTERONE (DHEA): Theoretically, pregnenolone can enhance the effects of steroid hormone drugs including DHEA (3008).

Interactions with Drugs
ESTROGENS: Theoretically, pregnenolone can enhance the effects of steroid hormone drugs including estrogens (3008).
PROGESTIN: Theoretically, pregnenolone can enhance the effects of steroid hormone drugs including progestin (3008).
TESTOSTERONE: Theoretically, pregnenolone can enhance the effects of steroid hormone drugs including testosterone (3008).

Interactions with Foods
None known.

Interactions with Lab Tests
None known.

Interactions with Diseases or Conditions
HORMONE SENSITIVE CANCERS/CONDITIONS: Because pregnenolone is converted to estrogens (3008), women with hormone sensitive conditions should avoid pregnenolone. Some of these conditions include breast cancer, uterine cancer, ovarian cancer, endometriosis, and uterine fibroids.

Dosage and Administration
No typical dosage.

Comments
Pregnenolone was studied for stress, fatigue, and arthritis in the 1940s before synthetic hormones became available.

PREMORSE

Also Known As
Devil's Bit, Ofbit, Premorse Scaboius.

Scientific Names
Scabiosa succisa.
Family: Dipsacaceae.

Comments
At the date of publication, this product was not a common ingredient used in brand name supplements marketed to consumers. Details about this product are available in the online version of *Natural Medicines Comprehensive Database.* See www.naturaldatabase.com.

PRICKLY PEAR CACTUS

Also Known As

Barbary-fig Cactus, Cactus Flowers, Cactus Fruit, Cactus Pear Fruit, Gracemere-Pear, Indian-fig Prickly Pear Cactus, OPI, Opuntia, Opuntia ficus, Nopal, Nopol, Tuna Cardona, Westwood-Pear.

Scientific Names

Opuntia ficus-indica; Opuntia fuliginosa; Opuntia hyptiacantha; Opuntia lasciacantha; Opuntia macrocentra, synonym Opuntia violacea; Opuntia megacantha; Opuntia puberula; Opuntia streptacantha, synonym Opuntia cardona; Opuntia velutina.
Family: Cactaceae.

People Use This For

Orally, prickly pear cactus is used for diabetes, hypercholesterolemia, obesity, alcohol-induced hangover (veisalgia), and as an antiviral agent. It is also used for colitis, diarrhea, and benign prostatic hypertrophy (BPH).
In foods, the prickly pear juice is used in jellies and candies.

Safety

LIKELY SAFE ...when used orally as a food (5969).
POSSIBLY SAFE ...when the leaves, stems, or standardized extracts from the prickly pear cactus are used orally short-term (5959,5960,5963,12085,12086). Single doses of prickly pear cactus extract or fruit seem to be safe (5959,5960,5963,12085). There is also evidence that taking 250 grams of fresh prickly pear cactus fruit pulp twice daily for 2 weeks might be safe (12086). ...when flowers of prickly pear cactus are used orally. Preliminary evidence suggests that powdered prickly pear cactus flowers 1500 mg/day can be safely used for up to 8 months (12175).
PREGNANCY AND LACTATION: Insufficient reliable information available; avoid using.

Effectiveness

POSSIBLY EFFECTIVE

Diabetes. There is some preliminary clinical evidence that prickly pear cactus used orally can decrease blood glucose levels in patients with type 2 diabetes. Single doses can decrease blood glucose levels by 17% to 46% in some patients (5959,5961,5962,5964). However, it is not known if extended daily use can consistently lower blood glucose levels and decrease HbA1c levels. Only the broiled stems of the specific species Opuntia streptacantha seem to be beneficial. Raw or crude stems do not seem to decrease glucose levels (5961). Other prickly pear cactus species do not seem to significantly lower blood glucose levels either (5970,7028).

Hangover. There is some evidence that taking a specific prickly pear cactus fruit extract (Tex-OE, Extracts Plus, Inc.) might reduce symptoms of alcohol-induced hangover. Taking 1600 IU of the extract 5 hours prior to binge alcohol consumption seems to reduce the chance of having a severe hangover the following day by about 50%. It also seems to significantly reduce some specific symptoms of hangover such as nausea, anorexia, and dry mouth. But it does not seem to reduce other symptoms such as headache, dizziness, diarrhea, or soreness (12085).

INSUFFICIENT RELIABLE EVIDENCE to RATE

Benign prostatic hypertrophy (BPH). Preliminary evidence suggests that some patients who take powdered prickly pear cactus flowers 500 mg 3 times daily for 2-8 months have subjective improvements in symptoms such as urgency and feelings of fullness in the bladder (12175). More evidence is needed to rate prickly pear cactus for this use.

Mechanism of Action

The applicable parts of prickly pear cactus are the leaves, flowers, stems, and fruit. Prickly pear cactus is often consumed as part of the diet. Ingesting 500 grams of prickly pear cactus provides 14.3 grams carbohydrate, 8.25 grams protein, 1.05 grams lipids, 18.85 grams cellulose (fibrous polysaccharide), 455.75 grams water, and 99.75 kilocalories (7028).
Some species of prickly pear cactus can lower blood glucose and lipid levels (5958,5959,5960,5963). This effect is often attributed to the high fibrous polysaccharide content, including pectin (5958). Fiber can slow carbohydrate absorption and decrease lipid absorption from the gut. However, some researchers suspect prickly pear might also have an insulin sensitizing effect (7028). In experimental diabetes in animals, prickly pear cactus stem extract seems to improve glucose utilization at the cellular level, mimicking the action of insulin. The extract seems to be effective at low doses (1 mg/kg) for lowering hemoglobin A1c levels alone or in combination with insulin (5955).
Broiled stems seem to be more effective for reducing blood glucose levels than raw stems (5961,5964). The reason for this difference is not known. The hypoglycemic effects of prickly pear cactus peak 3-4 hours after ingestion and can last for up to 6 hours.
There is also some evidence that the pectin component of prickly pear cactus can also alter the liver metabolism of cholesterol and affect cholesterol levels (5958). Prickly pear cactus fruit also seems to improve platelet function in people with familial hypercholesterolemia, which may prevent initiation and progression of atherosclerosis (12391).
Prickly pear cactus is thought to reduce symptoms of alcohol-induced hangovers by decreasing inflammation. Alcohol-induced hangovers are associated with an inflammatory response. Alcohols containing high amounts of

impurities known as congeners (tequila, bourbon, scotch) are associated with increased inflammatory response and increased severity of hangover. People with an alcohol induced hangover have increase levels of the inflammatory markers C-reactive protein (CRP) and cortisol. People who take a specific prickly pear cactus extract seem to have lower CRP and cortisol levels, suggesting that prickly pear cactus might have anti-inflammatory effects (12085).
Prickly pear cactus also has antioxidant effects. Consuming prickly pear cactus fruit pulp for 2 weeks seems to decrease pro-oxidants, decrease oxidation of lipids, and improve antioxidant status. This may be due to the vitamin C and the plant pigments called betanin and indicaxanthin contained in prickly pear cactus (12086).
There is some preliminary evidence that prickly pear cactus has antiviral activity against the herpes simplex virus (HSV), respiratory syncytial virus (RSV), and human immunodeficiency virus (HIV) (5956).

Adverse Reactions

Orally, prickly pear cactus is usually well-tolerated. However, prickly pear cactus can cause some side effects including mild diarrhea, nausea, increased stool volume, increased stool frequency, abdominal fullness, and headache (7028). Although the prickly pear cactus reduces blood glucose levels in people with diabetes, it does not seem to cause hypoglycemia (5959,5960,5963).

Interactions with Herbs & Other Dietary Supplements

None known.

Interactions with Drugs

CHLORPROPAMIDE (Diabinese): Using chlorpropamide and prickly pear cactus together can have additive effects on blood glucose and insulin levels in patients with type 2 diabetes (5968). There is some concern that people taking both chlorpropamide or other hypoglycemic drugs and prickly pear cactus might be at an increased risk for hypoglycemia. Advise patients to monitor glucose levels closely. Dose adjustments may be necessary. Other hypoglycemic drugs include glimepiride (Amaryl), glipizide (Glucotrol), glyburide (Diabeta, Micronase), tolazamide (Tolinase), tolbutamide (Orinase), and others.

Interactions with Foods

None known.

Interactions with Lab Tests

BLOOD GLUCOSE: Prickly pear cactus can reduce blood glucose levels and lab tests (5957).
CHOLESTEROL: There is some evidence that prickly pear cactus might reduce total and low-density lipoprotein (LDL) cholesterol levels (5958).

Interactions with Diseases or Conditions

DIABETES: Prickly pear cactus can reduce blood glucose in patients with type 2 diabetes (5957). Prickly pear cactus might have additive effects with diabetes medications and potentially cause hypoglycemia. Advise patients to closely monitor glucose levels after starting prickly pear cactus. Dose adjustments to diabetes medications may be necessary.

Dosage and Administration

ORAL: For diabetes, broiled stems 100-500 grams daily is typically used (5964). Doses are often divided and given three times daily.
For alcohol-induced hangover, 1600 IU of a specific prickly pear cactus extract (Tex-OE, Extracts Plus, Inc.) taken 5 hours before alcohol ingestion has been used (12085).
For benign prostatic hypertrophy (BPH), dried powdered flowers of prickly pear cactus, 500 mg three times daily, has been used (12175).

Comments

Prickly pear cactus is primarily used in Mexican and Mexican-American cultures as a part of the diet and as a treatment for type 2 diabetes (12551). Most research on this product has been performed in Mexico by one research group. The immature form of prickly pear cactus is used. Mature stems are fibrous and tough and not appropriate for consumption (7028).

PROCAINE

Also Known As

Gero-Vita, Gerovital, Gerovital-H3, GH-3, KH-3, Procaine Hydrochloride.

Scientific Names

2-Diethylaminoethyl p-aminobenzoate monohydrochloride.

People Use This For

Orally or parenterally, procaine is used for arthritis, cerebral atherosclerosis, dementia, depression, hair loss, hypertension, sexual dysfunction, and an overall rejuvenating effect.
Parenterally, prescription-only procaine is used for local anesthesia.

Safety

LIKELY SAFE ...when the prescription-only product is used parenterally as a local anesthetic (15).
There is insufficient reliable information available about the safety of the oral use of procaine.
PREGNANCY: LIKELY UNSAFE ...when used for self-medication; avoid using (6).
LACTATION: There is insufficient reliable information available about the safety of procaine for self-medication; avoid using.

Effectiveness

EFFECTIVE

Pain. Procaine injection is an FDA-approved prescription product used as a local anesthetic (15).

Mechanism of Action

Procaine has poor oral absorption, and there is no evidence that pharmacologic levels are achieved with oral administration (6). Hematoporphyrin is added to some oral preparations to increase procaine absorption (6), although no evidence supports this effect.

Adverse Reactions

Orally, procaine can cause heartburn, migraines, and systemic lupus erythematosus (SLE) (6).

Interactions with Herbs & Other Dietary Supplements

DIGITALIS: Intravenous use of procaine hydrochloride is contraindicated with concurrent use of digitalis (15).

Interactions with Drugs

AMINOSALICYLIC ACID: A metabolite of procaine, aminobenzoic acid, can antagonize the effect of aminosalicylic acid. Theoretically, procaine might also reduce aminosalicylic activity (15).
DIGOXIN (Lanoxin): Intravenous use of procaine hydrochloride is contraindicated (15).
SKELETAL MUSCLE RELAXANTS: Intravenous use of procaine hydrochloride is contraindicated (15).
SUCCINYLCHOLINE: Intravenous use of procaine hydrochloride is contraindicated (15).
SULFONAMIDE ANTIBIOTICS: A metabolite of procaine, aminobenzoic acid, can antagonize the effect of sulfonamides. Theoretically, procaine might also reduce sulfonamide activity (15). Some sulfonamides include sulfamethoxazole (Gantanol), sulfasalazine (Azulfidine), sulfisoxazole (Gantrisin), and trimethoprim/sulfamethoxazole (Bactrim, Septra).

Interactions with Foods

None known.

Interactions with Lab Tests

None known.

Interactions with Diseases or Conditions

MYASTHENIA GRAVIS: The intravenous use of procaine is contraindicated in individuals with myasthenia gravis, which is progressive muscular weakness (15).
PSEUDOCHOLINESTERASE DEFICIENCY: Contraindicated (6).
SYSTEMIC LUPUS ERYTHEMATOSUS (SLE): Contraindicated. Theoretically, procaine might exacerbate this condition (6).

Dosage and Administration

ORAL: People typically take procaine in a cyclical regimen: 200 mg procaine once or twice daily for 25 days, then no drug for 5 days, then repeat the cycle (5274).

PROGESTERONE

Also Known As

Corpus Luteum Hormone, Luteal Hormone, Luteohormone, Lutine, NSC-9704, Pregnancy Hormone, Pregnanedione, Progestational Hormone, Progesteronum.
CAUTION: See separate listings for Pregnenolone and Wild Yam.

Scientific Names

Progesterone; 4-Pregnene-3; 20-Dione.

People Use This For

Orally, progesterone is used for treating secondary amenorrhea, abnormal uterine bleeding associated with hormonal imbalance, treating severe symptoms of premenstrual syndrome (PMS), and treating benzodiazepine dependence and withdrawal. Oral progesterone preparations are also used in combination with estrogens as part of hormone replacement therapy to prevent irregular bleeding and the increased risk of endometrial carcinoma associated with estrogen monotherapy.
Topically, progesterone is used as an alternative to oral treatment as a component of hormone replacement therapy and for treating menopausal vasomotor symptoms. Topical progesterone is also used for treating or preventing hormone-mediated allergies, bloating, breast tenderness, decreased sex drive, depression, fatigue, fibrocystic breasts, headaches, hypoglycemia, increased blood clotting, infertility, irritability, memory loss, miscarriages, osteoporosis, premenopausal bone loss, symptoms of premenstrual syndrome, thyroid dysfunction, unclear thinking, uterine cancer, uterine fibroids, water retention, weight gain, and treating vulval lichen sclerosis.
Intravaginally, progesterone is used for cervical ripening, mastodynia in women with benign breast disease, and to prevent and treat endometrial hyperplasia. Progesterone is also used intravaginally or intramuscularly for treating infertility in women, anovulatory bleeding, and treating symptoms of premenstrual syndrome (PMS).

Safety

LIKELY SAFE ...when used orally and appropriately. Micronized progesterone (Prometrium) is an FDA-approved prescription product. Micronized progesterone (Prometrium) has been safely used in multiple clinical trials lasting up to 3 years (226,228,1216,1220,1221,1224). ...when used intravaginally and appropriately, short-term (1225,2031,2032,2033,2034). Progesterone intravaginal gel (Crinone) is an FDA-approved prescription product. Progesterone intravaginal gel (Crinone) has been safely used in trials lasting up to 3 months (1225,2031,2033,2034,2041). ...when used intramuscularly and appropriately, short-term (227,1218,1225,2034). Progesterone oil for intramuscular injection is an FDA-approved prescription product (227,1218,1225,2034). ...when used transdermally and appropriately. Transdermal progesterone has been used safely in clinical trials lasting up to a year (224,1229).
There is insufficient reliable information available about the safety of other progesterone preparations.
PREGNANCY: LIKELY SAFE ...when used intravaginally and appropriately as part of infertility treatment. Intravaginal progesterone gel (Crinone 8%) is FDA-approved for use in conjunction with infertility treatment (1225). LIKELY UNSAFE ...when used orally, intramuscularly, intravaginally, or transdermally for purposes other than medically supervised adjunctive treatment for infertility; contraindicated (15).
LACTATION: Insufficient reliable information available; avoid using.

Effectiveness

LIKELY EFFECTIVE

Amenorrhea. Taking progesterone orally and applying progesterone gel intravaginally is effective for treating secondary amenorrhea in premenopausal women. Micronized progesterone is FDA-approved for the treatment of secondary amenorrhea (15). Intravaginal progesterone gel (Crinone 4%) is FDA-approved for the treatment of secondary amenorrhea. Several open-label clinical trials have shown intravaginal progesterone gel (Crinone 4%) to be effective for restoring menses when used in conjunction with estrogen replacement therapy (2041,2091).

Hormone replacement therapy (HRT). Micronized progesterone (Prometrium) is FDA-approved for use with estrogen as a component of HRT. Micronized progesterone (Prometrium) has been shown to provide the same protection against the effects of unopposed estrogen therapy as medroxyprogesterone in women with a uterus (226,228,1216,1217,1226,1230,8144). In one trial, micronized progesterone (Prometrium) did not reduce the beneficial lipid effects of estrogen therapy as much as medroxyprogesterone (226); however, this effect was not seen in another trial (1216).

Infertility. Intravaginal progesterone gel (Crinone 8%) is FDA-approved for use as a component of infertility treatment in women. Clinical trials suggest that both intravaginal and intramuscular progesterone achieves pregnancy rates comparable to oral progesterone in infertile women due to various etiologies (227,1225,2032,2091). Clinical trials comparing intravaginal progesterone to intramuscular progesterone have shown varying relative efficacy results (1218,2086,2089).

POSSIBLY EFFECTIVE

Endometrial hyperplasia. Intravaginal progesterone (Crinone) seems to prevent endometrial hyperplasia in women with an intact uterus taking estrogen replacement therapy (2031). Also, one short-term, open label clinical trial has shown that a specific intravaginal progesterone cream may help reverse endometrial hyperplasia and decrease vaginal bleeding in premenopausal women with benign endometrial hyperplasia (2033).

Mastodynia. Intravaginal progesterone gel (Crinone) seems to reduce breast pain and tenderness in women with benign breast disease (1223).

Menopausal symptoms. One clinical trial has shown that topical progesterone cream (Progest) is superior to placebo for reducing vasomotor symptoms such as hot flashes in menopausal women (224).

POSSIBLY INEFFECTIVE

Benzodiazepine withdrawal. Oral micronized progesterone is comparable to placebo for relieving symptoms of withdrawal and for helping patients remain drug-free from diazepam (1221).

Osteoporosis. Topical progesterone is comparable to placebo for increasing bone mineral density in postmenopausal women (224).

Premenstrual syndrome (PMS). Taking progesterone orally doesn't seem to have any effect on the behavioral or physical symptoms of PMS (1220,10332).

Vulval lichen sclerosis. One clinical trial has shown that topical progesterone is comparable to placebo and inferior to clobetasol (Temovate) for treating the signs and symptoms of vulval lichen sclerosis (225).

INSUFFICIENT RELIABLE EVIDENCE to RATE

Cardiovascular disease. Preliminary evidence suggests that progesterone vaginal gel might be beneficial for cardiovascular disease. It can increase exercise time to myocardial ischemia compared with oral medroxyprogesterone in women with coronary artery disease or previous myocardial infarction (8146). More evidence is needed to rate progesterone for this use.

Mechanism of Action

Progesterone is an endogenous progestin secreted by the corpus luteum. The hormone is not available from any natural source without extraction and synthesis. Products marketed as natural progesterone are those products that are structurally identical to endogenous progesterone. "Natural progesterones," including the prescription products Crinone and Prometrium, are synthesized from the constituent diosgenin, isolated from wild yam or soy. In the laboratory, this constituent is converted to pregnenolone and then to progesterone. The human body is not capable of synthesizing progesterone from diosgenin in vivo (8143).

Progesterone is primarily secreted during the luteal phase of the menstrual cycle, but small amounts are also secreted during the follicular phase (15). The normal physiological effects of progesterone are responsible for its therapeutic benefit when administered exogenously. Progesterone transforms proliferative endometrium into a secreting endometrium. This effect is beneficial in preventing and treating endometrial hyperplasia. It may also be beneficial in infertility because progesterone is necessary for implantation of the fertilized ovum and for maintaining pregnancy (15). In premenstrual syndrome (PMS), progesterone has been proposed as a therapy because the symptoms of PMS are thought to correlate with physiological fluctuations in endogenous progesterone (1220).

It was thought to be beneficial for preventing benzodiazepine withdrawal because metabolites of progesterone have been found to have sedative-hypnotic properties (1221).

Other effects of progesterone include growth of mammary tissue and uterine smooth muscle relaxation. Progesterone also has mild estrogenic and androgenic effects (15). Micronized progesterone seems to have effects similar to medroxyprogesterone on endothelium-dependent vasodilator responsiveness and markers of inflammation, hemostasis, and fibrinolysis inhibition, suggesting a possible protective effect for atherosclerosis (8145). Intravaginal, topical, and intramuscular administration of progesterone may be advantageous over oral dosing because it avoids first-pass effect and may achieve greater concentrations in the uterus (2033,2034).

Adverse Reactions

Orally, progesterone can cause gastrointestinal (GI) disturbances, changes in appetite, weight gain, fluid retention and edema, fatigue acne, drowsiness or insomnia, allergic skin rashes, hives, fever, headache, depression, breast discomfort or enlargement, PMS-like syndrome, altered menstrual cycles, and irregular bleeding (506,1224).

Topically, progesterone can cause vaginal spotting (224).

Interactions with Herbs & Other Dietary Supplements

None known.

Interactions with Drugs

ESTROGENS: Concomitant use can cause breast tenderness (228). Use of conjugated equine estrogens with oral micronized progesterone in postmenopausal women may blunt the beneficial effects of estrogen on the lipoprotein profile (1216), although it might not affect estrogen-induced reduction in plasma lipoprotein (a) (1217).

Interactions with Foods

None known.

Interactions with Lab Tests

16-ALPHA-HYDROXYPROGESTERONE: Progesterone can cause increase in plasma test results (275).
17-HYDROXYCORTICOSTEROIDS: Progesterone can decrease urine level and test results (275).
ALANINE AMINOTRANSFERASE (ALT): Progesterone can increase serum levels and test results due to hepatotoxicity (275).
ALBUMIN: May increase serum levels and test results (275).
ALKALINE PHOSPHATASE (Alk Phos): Progesterone can increase serum levels and test results due to hepatotoxicity (275).
ASPARTATE AMINOTRANSFERASE (AST): Progesterone can decrease serum levels and test results in healthy people or increase serum levels and test results due to hepatotoxicity (275).
BILE: Progesterone can increase urine levels and test results due to hepatotoxicity (275).
BILIRUBIN: Progesterone can increase serum levels and test results due to hepatotoxicity (275).
CHOLESTEROL: Progesterone might decrease serum levels and test results (275).
GAMMA-GLOBULIN: Progesterone can increase serum levels and test results (275).
GLOBULIN: Progesterone can decrease serum levels and test results (275).
GLUCARIC ACID: Progesterone can increase urine level and test results (275).
LUTEINIZING HORMONE (LH): Progesterone can decrease peak plasma level and test results (275).
MAGNESIUM: Progesterone can increase serum level and test results (275).
PREGNANEDIOL: Progesterone can decrease urine level and test results (275).
PROSTAGLANDIN: Progesterone can decrease urine levels and test results (275).
PROTEIN: Progesterone can increase serum levels and test results (275).
SODIUM: Progesterone can increase serum and test results due to sodium retention (275). Large doses of progesterone can increase urine levels and test results (275).
THYROXINE (T4) BINDING GLOBULIN: Progesterone can increase serum levels and test results due to increased synthesis (275).

Interactions with Diseases or Conditions

ARTERIAL DISEASE: Contraindicated in individuals with high risk arterial disease (9).
BREAST CANCER: Should be avoided except as part of the management of breast cancer (9).
DEPRESSION: Use cautiously in individuals with a history of major depression (9).
LIVER DISEASE: Progesterone has been associated with attacks of acute porphyria (9); contraindicated.
VAGINAL BLEEDING: Contraindicated in women who have undiagnosed vaginal bleeding (9).

Dosage and Administration

ORAL: For hormone replacement therapy, 200 mg micronized progesterone (Prometrium) orally per day is typically used for 12 days of a 25 day cycle with 0.625 mg conjugated estrogens (1215,1217).
TOPICAL: For menopausal vasomotor symptoms, 20 mg progesterone cream (equivalent to 1/4 teaspoon Progest cream) is typically applied daily to rotating sites including upper arms, thighs, or breasts (224).
INTRAMUSCULAR: As a component of in vitro fertilization, 50 mg is commonly used intramuscularly (227,1218,1225,2034).
INTRAVAGINAL: For mastodynia associated with benign breast disease, a typical dose of 4 grams of vaginal cream containing 2.5% natural progesterone is placed intravaginally from the 19th to the 25th day of a 28 day cycle (1223). As a component of in vitro fertilization, one applicator (90 mg) of progesterone gel (Crinone 8%) is placed intravaginally 1-2 times daily (2032,2036). For secondary amenorrhea, one applicator (90 mg) of progesterone gel (Crinone 4% or 8%) is typically placed intravaginally every other day for 6 days per month (2041). For hormone replacement therapy, one applicator (90 mg) of progesterone gel (Crinone 4% or 8%) is typically placed intravaginally on days 17, 19, 21, 23, 25, and 27 of a 28 day cycle with 0.625 mg conjugated equine estrogens (2031). For reducing intravaginal bleeding and reversal of hyperplasia in premenopausal women with benign endometrial hyperplasia, a dose of 100 mg progesterone cream placed intravaginally daily from day 10 to day 25 of a 28 day cycle has been used (2033).

Comments

Progestin is a general term for a substance that causes some or all of the biologic effects of progesterone. The term "progestin" is sometimes used to specifically refer to the synthetic derivatives of progesterone in oral contraceptives and hormone replacement therapy (8143). However, all progesterone and progestin products are synthetic. The term "natural progesterone" is really a misnomer. OTC progesterone products may not contain progesterone concentrations as labeled. According to a British report, two-ounce jars of Progest cream used in a clinical trial contained 100 mg progesterone per ounce rather than the 465 mg claimed by the manufacturer (1228,1231). Topical progesterone products marketed as cosmetics require no FDA approval prior to marketing. There is currently no limit on the amount of progesterone allowed in cosmetic products. In 1993 the FDA proposed, but never finalized, a rule limiting progesterone-containing cosmetic products to a maximum level of 5 mg/oz with the product label specifying consumer usage not to exceed 2 oz per month (365).

PROPIONYL-L-CARNITINE

Also Known As
L-Carnitine Propionyl, LPC, PLC.
CAUTION: See separate listings for Acetyl-L-Carnitine and L-Carnitine.

Scientific Names
Propionyl-L-carnitine.

People Use This For
Orally, propionyl-L-carnitine is used for treating peripheral vascular disease (PVD), atherosclerotic and diabetic angiopathies, intermittent claudication, and congestive heart failure (CHF).
In combination with acetyl-L-carnitine, propionyl-L-carnitine is used orally for treating chronic fatigue syndrome (CFS) and symptoms of age-related testosterone deficiency.
Intravenously, propionyl-L-carnitine is used for treating peripheral vascular disease and intermittent claudication; to improve healing of ulcerative lesions in people with peripheral vascular disease; and to treat ischemic heart disease, angina, and congestive heart failure.

Safety
LIKELY SAFE ...when used orally and appropriately (1434,1435,1436,1437). ...when single intravenous doses are used under appropriate medical supervision (1571,1572,1573,1575).
PREGNANCY AND LACTATION: Insufficient reliable information available; avoid using.

Effectiveness
POSSIBLY EFFECTIVE

Age-related testosterone deficiency. Taking propionyl-L-carnitine orally, in combination with acetyl-L-carnitine, seems to help symptoms of androgen decline in older men. The combination taken for 6 months seems to be similar to testosterone for improving sexual dysfunction, depression, and fatigue (12353).

Angina. Taking propionyl-L-carnitine orally seems to produce small improvements in myocardial ischemia and exercise capacity in patients with chronic, stable angina (1579,1580,1581).

Chronic ischemic heart disease. In patients with chronic myocardial ischemia, intravenous administration of propionyl-L-carnitine may improve left ventricular function and cardiac output, as well as decrease myocardial ischemia (1571,1572,1573).

Congestive heart failure (CHF). Taking propionyl-L-carnitine orally seems to improve left ventricular function and exercise capacity in people with class II or III congestive heart failure (1575,1582,1583).

Erectile dysfunction (ED). In men with diabetes and erectile dysfunction, combination therapy with propionyl-L-carnitine and sildenafil (Viagra) may improve erectile function better than sildenafil alone. In men unresponsive to 8 uses of sildenafil, adding propionyl-L-carnitine 2 grams daily to continued twice weekly doses of sildenafil 50 mg seems to improve erections and successful intercourse attempts more than treatment with sildenafil alone (12682).

Intermittent claudication. Administering propionyl-L-carnitine orally or intravenously may help some patients with intermittent claudication and peripheral vascular disease. In patients with peripheral vascular disease and intermittent claudication that restricts walking distance to less than 250 meters, propionyl-L-carnitine may increase walking distance and time. Propionyl-L-carnitine doesn't seem to help milder peripheral vascular disease (1434,1435,1436,1437,1576,10456).

Peyronie's disease. Combining propionyl-L-carnitine with injectable verapamil seems to be more effective than injectable verapamil plus oral tamoxifen for men with advanced or resistant Peyronie's disease. The combination of propionyl-L-carnitine and intraplaque injection of verapamil seems to improve erectile function, slow disease progression, and reduce the need for surgery (12683).

INSUFFICIENT RELIABLE EVIDENCE to RATE

Chronic fatigue syndrome (CFS). Preliminary clinical research suggests that propionyl-L-carnitine might improve general fatigue in patients with CFS. The combination of propionyl-L-carnitine and acetyl-L-carnitine appears to be less effective than either supplement alone (11788). More evidence is needed to rate propionyl-L-carnitine for this use.

Mechanism of Action
Propionyl-L-carnitine is found naturally in most cells in the body. Endogenous carnitines exist as a "carnitine pool" consisting of L-carnitine, acetyl-l-carnitine, propionyl-L-carnitine, and several other acyl-carnitine esters. Intracellular enzymes and cell membrane transporters can rapidly interconvert the carnitines to the needed form and transport them between the tissues and extracellular space. The body obtains some carnitine from the diet, primarily from red meats and dairy products. The body can also synthesize carnitines from the amino acids, lysine and methionine. The kidneys aid in keeping carnitine levels stable. Normally, greater than 90% of filtered carnitine is reabsorbed. If dietary intake of carnitines decreases, carnitine reabsorption becomes even more efficient (12683,12744). There may be altered homeostasis and reduced levels of L-carnitine in peripheral vascular disease, myocardial

ischemia, and heart failure (1572). Carnitine deficiency most often presents with symptoms of progressive cardiomyopathy and skeletal muscle weakness, and less frequently with fasting hypoglycemic coma (12748). In patients with alcohol induced cirrhois, serum levels of L-carnitine and its esters are sometimes increased, possibly due to increased L-carnitine biosynthesis (1931,1948).

Within cells, propionyl-L-carnitine helps to maintain mitochondrial acyl-CoA/CoA ratios which are increased in L-carnitine deficient states, leading to deficient metabolism of fatty acids and urea synthesis (1439). Propionyl-L-carnitine also increases pyruvate flux into the Krebs Cycle, stimulates pyruvate dehydrogenase activity, has free radical scavenging activity, improves homeostasis in the coagulation cascade, and has positive effects on blood viscosity (1578). Compared with L-carnitine, propionyl-L-carnitine may produce greater increases in cellular L-carnitine concentrations, possibly by being transported into muscle fibers easier, and may provide additional substrates for muscle-cell energy production. Heart tissues may be able to utilize exogenous propionyl-L-carnitine to stimulate the tricarboxylic acid cycle and protect against ischemia (1439).

Intravenous and oral treatment may improve physical functioning in some people with peripheral vascular disease (1434,1435,1436,1437,1576), but a study suggesting that propionyl-L-carnitine was superior to L-carnitine in this regard used only single intravenous doses, and the clinical significance of the difference was questionable (1437).

Propionyl-L-carnitine improves energy, metabolism, and myocardial contractility in experimental models of heart failure (1577). Small studies suggest that propionyl-L-carnitine may have a positive inotropic effect and improve ventricular function and cardiac output in chronic heart failure (1571,1572,1573). It reduces myocardial ischemia, as measured by ST segment depression, in people with angina (1573,1579).

Carnitines, including propionyl-L-carnitine, are increased by male and female sex hormones (12353). Theoretically, propionyl-L-carnitine improves vasodilation and enhances penile blood flow, resulting in improved erectile function (12682). Preliminary research suggests propionyl-L-carnitine might have anti-inflammatory effects, which might be responsible for its effect in Peyronie's disease (12683,12684,12685).

Adverse Reactions

Orally, nausea, vomiting, gastric pain, asthenia, and angina have been reported with propionyl-L-carnitine use (1579,1580,1581,1582,1583,12682). One of its metabolites can cause the urine, breath, and sweat to have a fishy odor (12756).

Propionyl-L-carnitine is used for age-related testosterone deficiency. Unlike testosterone, it doesn't cause prostate enlargement or increase prostate-specific antigen when taken orally for 6 months (12353).

Interactions with Herbs & Other Dietary Supplements

D-CARNITINE: D-carnitine might compete with L-carnitine in active transport systems. Taking D-carnitine might cause symptoms of L-carnitine deficiency, and theoretically propionyl-L-carnitine deficiency (1946,12760); avoid using.

Interactions with Drugs

ACENOCOUMAROL (Sintrom): Taking L-carnitine 1 gram/day seems to significantly increase the anticoagulant effects of acenocoumarol. Acenocoumarol is an oral anticoagulant similar to warfarin, but shorter-acting (9878,12165). In one case, INR was stable in the normal range of 1.99-2.94 and then increased to 4.65 after L-carnitine was started and continued for 10 weeks. INR normalized after discontinuation of L-carnitine (12165). This interaction has only been reported with L-carnitine, but theoretically could occur with propionyl-L-carnitine.

WARFARIN (Coumadin): Use propionyl-L-carnitine cautiously in patients taking warfarin. L-carnitine can significantly increase the anticoagulant effects acenocoumarol, a shorter-acting oral anticoagulant similar to warfarin (9878,12165).

ZIDOVUDINE (AZT, Retrovir): Zidovudine inhibits the transport of L-carnitine into muscle. This might cause the muscle weakness seen in patients treated with zidovudine. Whether propionyl-L-carnitine can reverse or prevent this effect is unknown. Low serum carnitine levels are found in some people with HIV infection (3617).

Drug Influences on Nutrient Levels and Depletion

SOME DRUGS CAN AFFECT PROPIONYL-L-CARNITINE LEVELS:

CARBAMAZEPINE (Tegretol): Carbamazepine can reduce carnitine levels. Whether this reduction is clinically important is unknown. The reduction in carnitine levels might be more significant when other factors are present that also lower carnitine levels such as other drugs that deplete carnitine, vegetarianism, or diabetes (1911,12758).

CEFDITOREN PIVOXIL (Spectracef): Taking cefditoren chronically can induce carnitine deficiency because of its pivalate content. Using cefditoren short-term is unlikely to have any clinically significant effect on carnitine levels (12759).

PHENOBARBITAL (Luminal): Phenobarbital can reduce carnitine levels. Whether this reduction is clinically important is unknown. The reduction in carnitine levels might be more significant when other factors are present that also lower carnitine levels such as other drugs that deplete carnitine, vegetarianism, or diabetes (1911,12758).

PHENYTOIN (Dilantin): Phenytoin can reduce carnitine levels. Whether this reduction is clinically important is unknown. The reduction in carnitine levels might be more significant when other factors are present that also lower carnitine levels such as other drugs that deplete carnitine, vegetarianism, or diabetes (1911,12758).

PIVAMPICILLIN (Pondocillin): Taking pivampicillin chronically can induce carnitine deficiency because of its pivalate content. Using pivampicillin short-term is unlikely to have any clinically significant effect on carnitine (12759).

VALPROIC ACID (Depakote): Valproic acid can reduce carnitine levels. Whether this reduction is clinically important is unknown. The reduction in carnitine levels might be more significant when other factors are present that also lower carnitine levels such as other drugs that deplete carnitine, vegetarianism, or diabetes (1911,12758).

Interactions with Foods

None known.

Interactions with Lab Tests

None known.

Interactions with Diseases or Conditions

HYPOTHYROIDISM: Avoid using propionyl-L-carnitine in patients with hypothyroidism. L-carnitine seems to inhibit the activity of thyroid hormone in target tissues (12761). Theoretically this might occur with proprionyl-L-carnitine.

SEIZURES: An increase in seizure frequency or severity has been reported in people with a history of seizures who have used L-carnitine orally or intravenously (3616). Theoretically, this might occur with propionyl-L-carnitine.

Dosage and Administration

ORAL: For peripheral vascular disease (PVD), atherosclerotic or diabetic arteriopathies, and intermittent claudication, 500-1500 mg propionyl-L-carnitine twice daily has been used (1434,1435,1436,10456). One study in peripheral vascular disease used 1000 mg three times daily (1576). A dose of 500 mg three times daily has been used in congestive heart failure and stable angina (1579,1580,1581,1583). For symptoms of age-related testosterone deficiency, 2 grams of acetyl-L-carnitine plus 2 grams of propionyl-L-carnitine daily has been used (12353). For erectile dysfunction, propionyl-L-carnitine 2 grams daily has been used in combination with sildenafil (12682). For Peyronie's disease, propionyl-L-carnitine 2 grams daily has been used in combination with intraplaque injections with verapamil (12683).

INTRAVENOUS: A 1500 mg bolus followed by 1 mg/kg/minute infused for 30 minutes has been used to restore muscle L-carnitine levels in people with peripheral vascular disease (1434,1435,1436,1437,1576,10456). Single 600 mg bolus doses have also been tested in people with peripheral vascular disease (1437), and infusions of 2000 mg twice daily have been used to improve healing of ulcerative lesions in people with peripheral vascular disease (1574).

Single doses of 15 to 30 mg/kg have been used in people with chronic ischemic heart disease or congestive heart failure (1571,1572,1573,1575).

Comments

The body can convert L-carnitine to propionyl-L-carnitine and acetyl-L-carnitine. But, no one knows whether the benefits of carnitines are interchangeable. For now, tell patients not to substitute one form of carnitine for another (12744).

PROPOLIS

Also Known As

Bee Glue, Bee Propolis, Hive Dross, Propolis Balsam, Propolis Resin, Propolis Wax, Russian Penicillin.

Scientific Names

Propolis.

People Use This For

Orally, propolis is used for tuberculosis, bacterial and fungal infections, protozoal infections, nasopharyngeal carcinoma, treating the common cold, and improving immune response. Propolis is also used orally for treating gastrointestinal disturbances including Helicobacter pylori infection in peptic ulcer disease. It is also used as an antioxidant and anti-inflammatory agent.

Topically, propolis is used for wound cleansing, genital herpes, as a mouth rinse for enhancing healing following oral surgery, and for the treatment of minor burns.

In manufacturing, propolis is used as an ingredient in cosmetics.

Safety

There is insufficient reliable information available about the safety of propolis.

Pregnancy and Lactation: Insufficient reliable information available; avoid using.

Effectiveness

POSSIBLY EFFECTIVE

Herpes simplex virus type 2 (HSV-2). A 3% propolis ointment seems to significantly improve healing of recurrent genital lesions caused by herpes simplex virus type 2 (HSV-2). There is some evidence that it might help heal lesions faster and more completely than 5% acyclovir ointment (1926).

Sulcoplasty. Propolis mouth rinse following sulcoplasty seems to improve healing and reduce pain and inflammation (799).

INSUFFICIENT RELIABLE EVIDENCE to RATE

Common cold. There is some evidence that propolis might be helpful for treating the common cold. Propolis might decrease the duration of cold symptoms by 2.5 times compared with placebo in patients with rhinovirus infection (6602).

Minor burns. Propolis used topically might help in the treatment of minor burns. There is some evidence propolis skin cream compared with silver sulfadiazine might be as effective in preventing infection. It might also be more effective in the re-epithelization and healing of minor burn wounds such as superficial second degree burns (8663).

More evidence is needed to rate propolis for these uses.

Mechanism of Action

Propolis is a resinous material from poplar and conifer buds. Bees use it for maintaining their hives. Since propolis is incorporated into beehives, harvesting the pure product is difficult. Many propolis preparations are frequently contaminated with beehive by-products (3574).

Therapeutic uses of propolis are primarily attributed to antiviral, antibacterial, and antimycotic effects. Propolis contains flavonoids including pinocembrin, galangin, pinobanksin, and pinobanksin-3-acetate, which are thought to be responsible for its antimicrobial effects (5,1926). Propolis extracts that contain the constituents pinocembrim and galagin have been shown to inhibit the growth and enzyme activity of Streptococcus mutans, an organism that causes dental caries (2631). Propolis also seems to have in vitro activity against a variety of bacteria that cause periodontal disease such as Porphyromonas gingivalis, Prevotella intermedia, Actinobacillus actinomycetemcomitans, and Fusobacterium nucleatum (8664).

Propolis might also have anti-inflammatory effects. There is preliminary evidence that it might suppress the lipoxygenase pathway of arachidonic acid metabolism and decrease the synthesis of prostaglandins and leukotrienes involved in inflammation (2630).

Topically applied propolis seems to help accelerate epithelial repair in animal models (800). Propolis also contains caffeic acid phenethyl esters (CAPE), which might have cancer chemopreventative properties (2629). These same constituents seem to also be contact allergens (2633). Propolis also has weak free radical scavenging properties (6).

Adverse Reactions

Orally, propolis can cause allergic reactions (6,2632) and acute oral mucositis with ulceration from the use of the propolis-containing lozenges (2632). Patients allergic to bees or bee products may be more likely to experience allergic reactions.

Topically, propolis-containing products, including some cosmetics can cause eczematous contact dermatitis (6,2632).

Interactions with Herbs & Other Dietary Supplements

None known.

Interactions with Drugs

None known.

Interactions with Foods

None known.

Interactions with Lab Tests

None known.

Interactions with Diseases or Conditions

ASTHMA: Some sources suggest allergens in propolis may worsen asthma (3574); avoid using.

HYPERSENSITIVITY: Avoid using propolis in people hypersensitive to bee by-products including honey, conifers, poplars, Peruvian balsam, and salicylates (19).

Dosage and Administration

ORAL: No typical dosage.

TOPICAL: As a mouth rinse after sulcoplasty, a 5% aqueous alcohol solution of propolis is commonly used (799). For herpetic lesions, 3% propolis ointment applied to the lesions 4 times daily has been used (1926).

Comments
Propolis has a long history of medicinal use, dating back to 350 B.C., the time of Aristotle. Greeks have used propolis for abscesses; Assyrians have used it for healing wounds and tumors; and Egyptians have used it for mummification (3574).

PUFF BALL

Also Known As
Bovista, Deer Balls, Hart's Truffle Puffball.

Scientific Names
Lycoperdon sp.
Family: Gasteromycetes.

People Use This For
Orally, puff ball is used for nosebleeds and skin disorders.
For food uses, young puff ball mushrooms are edible.

Safety
LIKELY SAFE ...when young puff ball mushrooms are consumed as food (18).
There is insufficient reliable information available about the safety of the oral use of puff ball for medicinal purposes.
PREGNANCY AND LACTATION: Insufficient reliable information available; avoid using.

Effectiveness
There is insufficient reliable information available about the effectiveness of puff ball.

Mechanism of Action
The applicable parts of puff ball are the aerial parts and spores. Puff ball contains amino acids, glucosamine, sterol, enzymes, and approximately 3% urea (18).

Adverse Reactions
Inhaling the spores can cause respiratory illness, pneumonia-like symptoms, and widespread lung densities (3846,3847).

Interactions with Herbs & Other Dietary Supplements
None known.

Interactions with Drugs
None known.

Interactions with Foods
None known.

Interactions with Lab Tests
None known.

Interactions with Diseases or Conditions
None known.

Dosage and Administration
ORAL: Puff ball is used in pulverized form or in alcoholic extracts (18).

PULSATILLA

Also Known As
Easter Flower, European Pasqueflower, Meadow Anenome, Meadow Windflower, Pasque Flower, Pasqueflower, Passe Flower, Wind Flower.

Scientific Names
Anemone pulsatilla, synonym Pulsatilla vulgaris, Anemone serotina; Anemone pratensis, synonym Anemone nigricans, Pulsatilla nigricans, Pulsatilla pratensis.
Family: Ranunculacaeae.

People Use This For

Orally, pulsatilla is used for painful conditions of the male or female reproductive system, such as dysmenorrhea, orchitis, ovaralgia, or epididymitis. Pulsatilla is also used for tension headache, hyperactive states, insomnia, boils, asthma and pulmonary disease, earache, migraines, neuralgia, general restlessness, diseases and functional disorders of the gastrointestinal GI and urinary tract.

Topically, pulsatilla is used for boils, skin eruptions associated with bacterial infection, and inflammatory and infectious diseases of the skin and mucosa.

Safety

LIKELY UNSAFE ...when fresh above ground parts are used orally or topically; pulsatilla is a severe local irritant (4).

There is insufficient reliable information available about the safety of the use of dried pulsatilla.

PREGNANCY: LIKELY UNSAFE ...when used orally. The fresh or dried above ground parts are contraindicated due to abortifacient and teratogenic effects (2). ...when the fresh above ground parts are used topically.

There is insufficient reliable information available about the safety of topical dried pulsatilla during pregnancy.

LACTATION: LIKELY UNSAFE ...when the fresh above ground parts are used for oral or topical use (19).

There is insufficient reliable information available about the safety of dried pulsatilla during breast-feeding.

Effectiveness

There is insufficient reliable information available about the effectiveness of pulsatilla.

Mechanism of Action

The applicable parts of pulsatilla are the above ground parts. Pulsatilla has analgesic, antispasmodic, sedative, and antibacterial properties. It exhibits both uterine stimulant and depressant activities. Pulsatilla contains ranunculin. Ranunculin hydrolyzes to a toxic unstable compound called protoanemonin, which readily dimerizes to nontoxic anemonin (4). Protoanemonin causes central nervous system (CNS) stimulation, then paralysis in experimental animals. It also has antimicrobial activity (2). Both anemonin and protoanemonin show some evidence of sedative and antipyretic activity (4). Irritation of the kidney and urinary tract might be due to the alkylating action of protoanemonin (2). Some evidence suggests anemonin might be cytotoxic (4).

Adverse Reactions

Orally, fresh pulsatilla is a toxic gastrointestinal (GI) irritant (4,19). It can also cause kidney and urinary tract irritation (2).

Topically, contact with the fresh plant can cause skin irritation, mucous membrane irritation, itching, and pustule formation known as ranunculus dermatitis (2).

Inhalation of protoanemonin-containing volatile oil may cause nasal mucosal and conjunctival irritation (4). Allergic reactions have been documented with patch tests (4).

Interactions with Herbs & Other Dietary Supplements

None known.

Interactions with Drugs

None known.

Interactions with Foods

None known.

Interactions with Lab Tests

None known.

Interactions with Diseases or Conditions

None known.

Dosage and Administration

ORAL: A typical oral dose is 120-300 mg dried above ground parts three times daily. Alternatively one cup tea consumed three times daily. To make tea, steep or simmer 120-300 mg dried above ground parts in 150 mL water 5-10 minutes, strain (4). 0.12-0.3 mL of the liquid extract, 1:1 in 25% alcohol, has been used three times daily (4). 0.3-1 mL of the tincture, 1:10 in 40% alcohol, has been used three times daily (4).

TOPICAL: No typical dosage.

PUMPKIN

Also Known As
Cucurbitea Peponis Semen, Field Pumpkin, Pepo.

Scientific Names
Cucurbita pepo, synonyms Cucumis pepo, Cucurbita galeottii, Cucurbita mammeata.
Family: Cucurbitaceae.

People Use This For
Orally, pumpkin is used for dysuria secondary to benign prostatic hyperplasia (BPH), bladder irritation, treating intestinal worms, and treating pyelonephritis.
In combination, pumpkin is used in an herbal combination to treat symptoms of BPH.
The roasted pumpkins seeds are considered a snack food.

Safety
POSSIBLY SAFE ...when used orally and appropriately (2,7,18).
PREGNANCY AND LACTATION: Insufficient reliable information available; avoid using amounts greater than those found in food.

Effectiveness
POSSIBLY EFFECTIVE

Benign prostatic hyperplasia (BPH). Taking pumpkin seed oil extract orally alone, or with saw palmetto, may help BPH symptoms (6777,11231). An herbal product containing pumpkin seed oil extract 160 mg, saw palmetto lipoidal extract 106 mg, nettle root extract 80 mg, lemon bioflavonoid extract 33 mg, and vitamin A (100% as beta-carotene) 190 IU used three times daily for six months may shrink the prostate epithelium, although it may not significantly improve symptoms in some men (5093).

There is insufficient reliable information available about the effectiveness of pumpkin for its other uses.

Mechanism of Action
The applicable part of pumpkin is the seed. Pumpkin seeds contain as much as 35% fatty oil, 38% protein, and 37% carbohydrate content (8257). Pumpkin seeds are also rich in carotenoids, including lutein, carotene, and beta-carotene (515). The seed oil is rich in unsaturated fatty acids, including 47% linoleic acid, 29% oleic acid, 14% palmitic acid, and 8% stearic acid (8257). The oil is also rich in vitamin E, including both gamma-tocopherol and alpha-tocopherol (3 mg/100 g) (8257). The enzyme acyl-coenzyme A oxidase (ACOX) is present in the pumpkin seed. The ACOX enzyme catalyzes fatty acid oxidation, specifically the oxidation of fatty acid CoA esters with 4 to 10 carbon atoms (8256). Pumpkin seed oil can exhibit a diuretic effect, which can relieve bladder discomfort, causing the perception of reduced prostate gland swelling without reducing the gland size. The phytosterol constituents are also believed to affect urine flow (515). Animal research suggests it might improve bladder and urethral function, which might help BPH symptoms (11233).
Another constituent, cucurbitin, has anthelmintic effects. Concentration of cucurbitin varies significantly among Cucurbita species (515).

Adverse Reactions
One case is reported of decreased ejaculatory volume associated with an herbal blend product containing pumpkin seed oil extract, saw palmetto extract, nettle root extract, lemon bioflavonoid extract, and beta-carotene (5093).

Interactions with Herbs & Other Dietary Supplements
None known.

Interactions with Drugs
None known.

Interactions with Foods
None known.

Interactions with Lab Tests
None known.

Interactions with Diseases or Conditions
None known.

Dosage and Administration

ORAL: For benign prostatic hyperplasia, pumpkin seed oil extract 480 mg per day in 3 divided doses in combination with saw palmetto and other herbs has been used (5093,6777).

Comments

Seeds of autumn squash (Cucurbita maxima) and Canadian pumpkin (crooked neck squash, Cucurbita moschata) have properties similar to Cucurbita pepo seed (515).

PUNCTURE VINE

Also Known As

Abrojos, al-Gutub, Caltrop, Cat's-Head, Common Dubbletjie, Devil's-Thorn, Devil's-Weed, Espigón, Goathead, Gokhru, Gokshura, Nature's Viagra, Puncture Weed, Qutiba, Tribule Terrestre, Tribulis Terrestris, Tribulus Terrestris.

Scientific Names

Tribulus terrestris.
Family: Zygophyllaceae.

People Use This For

Orally, puncture vine is used for enhancing athletic performance, male impotence, spermatorrhea, gonorrhea, kidney stones, and painful urination. It is also used for angina pectoris, hypertension, hypercholesterolemia, treating anemia, Bright's disease, cancer, stomatitis, hepatitis, inflammation, nasal tumors, atopic dermatitis (eczema), psoriasis, rheumatism, leprosy, and scabies. Other uses include improving digestion, treating flatulence, colic, coughs, sore throat, headache, vertigo, and chronic fatigue syndrome. It is also used as a laxative, for stimulating appetite and milk flow, childbirth, as an abortifacient, aphrodisiac, astringent, diuretic, tonic, mood enhancer, and vermifuge.

Safety

POSSIBLY SAFE... when puncture vine is used orally and appropriately, short-term. Puncture vine has been safely used in studies for up to eight 8 weeks (7514,13255). The long-term safety of puncture vine is unknown.
LIKELY UNSAFE ...when the spine-covered fruit is used orally. There has been one report of a bilateral pneumothorax adverse effect (818).
PREGNANCY: POSSIBLY UNSAFE ...when used orally; avoid using. Animal research suggests puncture vine might adversely affect fetal development (12674); avoid using..
LACTATION: Insufficient reliable information available; avoid using.

Effectiveness

POSSIBLY INEFFECTIVE

Athletic performance. Taking puncture vine orally, alone or in combination with other herbs and supplements such as androstenedione, doesn't seem to enhance body composition or exercise performance in athletes (7514,13255).

INSUFFICIENT RELIABLE EVIDENCE to RATE

Angina pectoris. Preliminary clinical research suggests a puncture vine extract taken orally might reduce symptoms of angina (3931).

Atopic dermatitis (eczema). Puncture vine taken orally in combination with 9 other herbs (Zemaphyte) might reduce redness and skin lesions in adults and children with nonexudative atopic eczema (12627,12628,12629). However, other research shows no effect (12630).

More evidence is needed to rate puncture vine for these uses.

Mechanism of Action

The applicable parts of puncture vine are the leaf, fruit, and root. Puncture vine contains saponins such as diosgenin and protodioscin, flavonoids, and alkaloids (3929,12673,12675,12676).

Preliminary research suggests that puncture vine increases levels of testosterone, luteinizing hormone (LH), dehydroepiandrosterone (DHEA), and dihydrotestosterone. It may also have aphrodisiac activity. These effects are attributed to the protodioscin constituent of puncture vine (12675,12677). However, clinical research suggests puncture vine in combination with androstenedione, DHEA, chrysin, indole-3-carbinol, and saw palmetto raises only androstenedione levels. LH, estradiol, free testosterone, total testosterone, and other sex hormones are not affected (7514). Clinical research also suggests that puncture vine doesn't affect mood, body weight, body fat, muscle mass, or muscle strength in athletes (13255).

Preliminary clinical research suggests puncture vine might have anti-anginal activity. It seems to dilate coronary arteries and improve coronary circulation (3931). It also may lower blood pressure by inhibiting angiotensin-converting enzyme (ACE) (12673). Extracts from the fruit and leaves seem to have a diuretic effects, which may explain the traditional use of puncture vine for kidney stones and other urinary problems (12681).

Other preliminary research suggests puncture vine might have anti-inflammatory activity as a cyclooxygenase (COX)-2 inhibitor (12678). In animal models of diabetes, puncture vine lowers blood glucose (12679). Constituents of puncture vine also seem to have antihelmintic activity (12680).

Adverse Reactions

Orally, puncture vine supplement products have not been associated with adverse effects (3931,7514). There is one case report of bilateral pneumothorax following the removal of a puncture vine fruit (818).

Interactions with Herbs & Other Dietary Supplements

None known.

Interactions with Drugs

ANTIDIABETES DRUGS: Theoretically, puncture vine might enhance the blood glucose-lowering effects of hypoglycemic drugs (12679). Monitor blood glucose levels closely. Some antidiabetes drugs include glimepiride (Amaryl), glyburide (Diabeta, Glynase PresTabs, Micronase), insulin, metformin (Glucophage), pioglitazone (Actos), rosiglitazone (Avandia), and others.

Interactions with Foods

None known.

Interactions with Lab Tests

BLOOD GLUCOSE: Theoretically puncture vine might lower blood glucose and test results (12679).

Interactions with Diseases or Conditions

BENIGN PROSTATIC HYPERTROPHY (BPH): Theoretically, puncture vine might aggravate prostate conditions such as benign prostate hypertrophy (BPH). Preliminary research suggests that puncture vine can increase prostate weight (12677).

PROSTATE CANCER/CONDITIONS: Theoretically, puncture vine might aggravate prostate conditions such as benign prostate hypertrophy (BPH) or prostate cancer. Preliminary research suggests that puncture vine can increase prostate weight (12677).

Dosage and Administration

ORAL: For athletic performance, approximately 250 mg per day (3.21 mg per kg) has been used (7514,13255).

Comments

Puncture vine was so named because its spine-covered fruit can flatten bicycle tires (818).

PURPLE LOOSESTRIFE

Also Known As

Blooming Sally, Flowering Sally, Long Purples, Loosestrife, Lythrum, Milk Willow-Herb, Purple Willow-Herb, Rainbow Weed, Salicare, Soldiers, Spiked Loosestrife, Willow Sage.

CAUTION: See separate listings for Loosestrife and Sage.

Scientific Names

Lythrum salicaria.

Family: Lythraceae.

Comments

At the date of publication, this product was not a common ingredient used in brand name supplements marketed to consumers. Details about this product are available in the online version of *Natural Medicines Comprehensive Database.* See www.naturaldatabase.com.

PYCNOGENOL

Also Known As

Condensed Tannins, French Marine Pine Bark Extract, Leucoanthocyanidins, Oligomeric Proanthocyanidins, OPCs, PCOs, Pine Bark Extract, Procyandiol Oligomers, Procyanidin Oligomers, Procyanodolic Oligomers, Pygenol.

Scientific Names

Pinus pinaster, synonym Pinus maritima.
Family: Pinaceae.

People Use This For

Orally, pycnogenol is used for treating chronic venous insufficiency, allergies, asthma, hypertension, muscle soreness, pain, osteoarthritis, diabetes, attention deficit-hyperactivity disorder (ADHD), endometriosis, dysmenorrhea, erectile dysfunction, and retinopathy. It is also used orally for preventing stroke, preventing vascular conditions such as heart disease and varicose veins, slowing the aging process, maintaining skin health, improving athletic endurance, and improving sperm morphology in subfertile men.
Topically, pycnogenol is used as a component of "anti-aging" creams.

Safety

POSSIBLY SAFE ...when used orally and appropriately. Pycnogenol has been safely used in doses of 120-450 mg daily for up to three months (2435,2451,2462,2553,2554,2556,7693,10214,10416,12012).
There is insufficient reliable information available about the safety of pycnogenol when used topically.
CHILDREN: POSSIBLY SAFE ...when used orally and appropriately, short-term. Pycnogenol in a dose of 1 mg/lb body weight daily has been safely used in a clinical study of children aged 6-18 years for up to three months (13120).
PREGNANCY AND LACTATION: Insufficient reliable information available; avoid using.

Effectiveness

POSSIBLY EFFECTIVE

Asthma. Taking pycnogenol 1 mg/lb body weight daily in addition to conventional asthma medications seems to increase peak expiratory flow, decrease asthma symptoms, and decrease the need for rescue medications in children aged 6-18 years with mild-to-moderate asthma (13120).

Athletic performance. Taking pycnogenol orally 200 mg daily for 30 days seems to improve treadmill exercise capacity in recreational athletes aged 20-35 years (2554).

Chronic venous insufficiency. Taking pycnogenol orally seems to significantly reduce symptoms of leg pain and heaviness, and edema in people with chronic venous insufficiency (CVI) when used for 3-12 weeks. The dose of pycnogenol used most often is 100-120 mg three times daily (2451,2462,2493,7693), but a lower dose of 45 mg to 90 mg once daily also seems to be effective (2435). Some people also use horse chestnut seed extract to treat CVI, but pycnogenol alone appears to be more effective (7693).

Hypertension. In patients with mild hypertension (systolic 140-159 mm Hg; diastolic 90-99 mm Hg), taking pycnogenol orally may reduce systolic blood pressure to approximately 133 mm Hg. Diastolic blood pressure is not significantly reduced (10214).

Retinopathy. Taking pycnogenol 50 mg three times daily for two months seems to slow or prevent further deterioration of retinal function in patients with retinopathy caused by diabetes, atherosclerosis, or central venous thrombosis. Patients can have some improvement in visual acuity and retinal vascularization (2536).

POSSIBLY INEFFECTIVE

Attention deficit-hyperactivity disorder (ADHD). Taking pycnogenol orally doesn't seem to help ADHD symptoms in adults (9984). There are anecdotal reports that pycnogenol helps ADHD in children, but there isn't any research to support this claim (6558).

INSUFFICIENT RELIABLE EVIDENCE to RATE

Coronary artery disease. There is some evidence that pycnogenol 150 mg three times daily for 4 weeks might improve certain factors such as microcirculation, myocardial ischemia, and the potential for platelet aggregation in patients with coronary artery disease (2553).

Deep vein thrombosis (DVT). There is some evidence that taking a specific combination product (Flite Tabs) might decrease the risk of DVT during long-haul plane flights. The product combines a blend of 150 mg of pycnogenol plus nattokinase. Two capsules are taken 2 hours before the flight and then again 6 hours later (12075).

Erectile dysfunction (ED). Preliminary clinical research suggests pycnogenol, used alone (12012) or in combination with L-arginine (10416), might improve sexual function in men with erectile dysfunction. It seems to take up to 3 months of treatment for significant improvement.

Hypercholesterolemia. There is also some evidence that pycnogenol 120 mg three times daily lowers low-density lipoprotein (LDL) cholesterol (7693).

Pelvic pain. There is preliminary evidence that pycnogenol might help reduce pelvic pain in women with endometriosis or dysmenorrhea (2555).

More evidence is needed to rate pycnogenol for these uses.

Mechanism of Action

Pycnogenol is an extract from the bark of the French maritime pine tree (2431). Pycnogenol contains several active constituents including flavonoid monomers such as catechin, epicatechin, and taxifolin. It also contains condensed procyanidins (also called flavonoids or proanthocyanidins) such as procyanidin B1, B3, B6, and B7 which are dimers, oligomers, and polymers of catechin and epicatechin (2431,2433). Pycnogenol also contains phenolic acids including gallic, ferulic, caffeic, vanillic, p-coumaric, protocatechuic, and p-hydroxybenzoic acids, and their glucosides and glucose esters (2431,2433,2435,2543).

In chronic venous insufficiency (CVI, varicose veins) procyanidins in pycnogenol reduce capillary permeability, which contributes to edema and microbleeding, by cross-linking capillary wall proteins such as collagen and elastin (2435,2544). There is also some evidence that procyanidins make elastin more resistant to degradation by elastase (2451,2635), and that pycnogenol might inhibit elastase and collagenase released by activated macrophages (2462). Pycnogenol might also help prevent capillary permeability due to the antioxidant effects of several of its constituents (2433,2435,2636,2542,2451). Pycnogenol also seems to recycle ascorbyl and tocopheryl radicals, helping to maintain vitamin C and E levels (2542,7698). Benefits for other uses, including diabetic retinopathy and improving athletic performance, are also thought to be due to the antioxidant effects of pycnogenol (2536,2554).

Some research suggests that pycnogenol might be useful in the prevention of cardiovascular disease. In vitro, pycnogenol prevents oxidation of low-density lipoprotein (LDL) cholesterol and protects DNA from damage by free radicals (2433). It also seems to prevent free-radical induced endothelial damage in vitro (2433). Pycnogenol inhibits epinephrine-induced platelet aggregation, such as that seen in smokers (2435,3285), but pycnogenol does not appear to increase bleeding risk or affect smoking-related increases in blood pressure or heart rate (3283). In non-smokers, it decreases serum thromboxane B2 and reduces systolic blood pressure (10214). Pycnogenol inhibits angiotensin converting enzyme (ACE) in vitro, but is unlikely to have clinically significant hypotensive effects when used orally in humans (2435). Pycnogenol might also increase production of nitric oxide from vascular endothelial cells by stimulating nitric oxide synthetase. This can lead to vasodilatation and possibly reduce the potential for atherogenesis and thrombus formation (2433,2451,2545,2637). Increased nitric oxide production might also be the mechanism for the possible benefit of pycnogenol in erectile dysfunction (10416,12012).

Some people think pycnogenol may be beneficial for cardiovascular disease because of its anti-inflammatory effects. However, the anti-inflammatory effects of pycnogenol are controversial. Pycnogenol appears to have no effect on levels of inflammatory markers including C-reactive protein (CRP), interleukin-1 (IL-1), or interleukin-6 (IL-6) (7694). An increased risk of cardiovascular disease may be associated with increases in these inflammatory markers.

For asthma, pycnogenol is thought to be beneficial due to its anti-inflammatory and antioxidant effects. In children with asthma taking pycnogenol decreases urinary levels of leukotrienes compared to placebo (13120).

There is also interest in using pycnogenol to protect against sunburn. Skin exposure to ultraviolet radiation has been shown to increase levels of free radicals that can damage the skin. It is theorized that pycnogenol may counteract the damaging effects of ultraviolet radiation through its antioxidant effects. Oral supplementation with pycnogenol at doses of 1.10 mg/kg/day for 4 weeks followed by 1.66 mg/kg/day for an additional 4 weeks increases the amount of ultraviolet radiation, both UVA and UVB, required to cause erythema and pinkness of the skin in human volunteers. The higher dose appears more protective than the lower dose since a greater amount of ultraviolet radiation is required to cause erythema when the higher dose is taken (7696). Some research suggests that topical pycnogenol might be useful for skin diseases related to increased cell adhesion and inflammation such as psoriasis, atopic dermatitis, and lupus erythematosus. Preclinical research suggests that it reduces inflammation in keratinocytes (10213).

Preliminary evidence suggests that pycnogenol might stimulate the immune system. It seems to boost natural killer cell activity (2435) and improves T- and B-cell function in animal models (2636). Pycnogenol also increase tumor necrosis factor-alpha (TNF-alpha) secretion and natural factor-KB (NF-KB) activity also increase (7697). Pycnogenol appears to slow the development of immune dysfunction in animal models infected with a retrovirus similar to human immunodeficiency virus (HIV) by restoring imbalanced T-helper 1 and T-helper 2 cytokine secretion (7695).

Pycnogenol might have some activity in Alzheimer's disease. In vitro, pycnogenol protects animal brain cells from the toxic effects of high levels of glutamate, and also from the toxic effects of amyloid-beta-protein, which is found in the plaques characteristic of Alzheimer's Disease (2435,7699).

There is a developing interest in using pycnogenol to prevent obesity. In vitro, pycnogenol appears to inhibit insulin-induced lipogenesis and may stimulate lipolysis (8307).

Constituents of pycnogenol are metabolized through glucuronide and sulfate conjugation. Ferulic acid and taxifolin conjugates are excreted in the urine within 18-24 hours. Conjugated metabolites of the procyanidin fraction are excreted within 28-34 hours (2431,2543,10212).

Adverse Reactions

None reported.

Interactions with Herbs & Other Dietary Supplements

None known.

Interactions with Drugs
IMMUNOSUPPRESSANTS: Theoretically, pycnogenol may interfere with immunosuppressant therapy because of its immunostimulating activity (2435,2636). Immunosuppressant drugs include azathioprine (Imuran), basiliximab (Simulect), cyclosporine (Neoral, Sandimmune), daclixímab (Zenapax), muromonab-CD3 (OKT3, Orthoclone OKT3), mycophenolate (CellCept), tacrolimus (FK506, Prograf), sirolimus (Rapamune), prednisone (Deltasone, Orasone), and other corticosteroids (glucocorticoids).

Interactions with Foods
None known.

Interactions with Lab Tests
None known.

Interactions with Diseases or Conditions
AUTOIMMUNE DISEASES: There is some concern that pycnogenol might adversely affect patients with autoimmune disorders because of its immune stimulating effects (2435,2636). Avoid using in patients with multiple sclerosis, systemic lupus erythematosus (SLE), rheumatoid arthritis, or other autoimmune disorders.

Dosage and Administration
ORAL: For chronic venous insufficiency, 45-360 mg daily, or 100 mg three times daily have been used (2435,2451,2462,2493).
For diabetic and other retinopathies, 50 mg three times daily has been used (2536).
For coronary artery disease, 150 mg three times daily has been used (2553).
For erectile dysfunction, 120 mg daily has been used (10416,12012).
For hypercholesterolemia, a dose of 120 mg three times daily has been used (7693).
For mild hypertension, 200 mg of pycnogenol daily has been used (10214).
For asthma in children, 1 mg/lb body given in two divided doses has been used (13120).
To improve exercise capacity in athletes, 200 mg daily has been used (2554).
For chronic pelvic pain, dysmenorrhea, and endometriosis in women, 30 to 60 mg daily has been used (2555).
To improve sperm morphology in subfertile men, 200 mg daily has been used (2556).
For protection against sunburn, doses of 1.10 and 1.66 mg/kg/day have been used (7696).
TOPICAL: No typical dosage.

Comments
Pycnogenol is the US registered trademark for an extract derived from French Maritime Pine Bark (Pinus pinaster) which contains procyanidins, a group of bioflavonoids. Originally, the term "pycnogenol" was used as a generic term for procyanidins. Procyanidins are also referred to as condensed tannins, leucoanthocyanidins, proanthocyanidins, oligomeric proanthocyanidins (OPCs), and procyandiol oligomers (PCOs). They are derived from various other sources besides French maritime pine bark, including peanut skins (Arachis hypogaea), grape seed (Vitis vinifera) (515), and witch hazel bark (Hamamelis virginiana) (2641).

PYGEUM

Also Known As
African Plum Tree.

Scientific Names
Prunus africana, synonym Pygeum africanum.
Family: Rosaceae.

People Use This For
Orally, pygeum is used for treating functional symptoms of benign prostatic hyperplasia (BPH) (nocturia, dysuria, pollakiuria micturitional disorders, and bladder fullness) and prostatic adenoma.
Traditionally, pygeum is used orally for inflammation, kidney disease, urinary problems, malaria, stomachache, fever, difficult urination, fever, madness, prostate gland inflammation, and as an aphrodisiac.

Safety
LIKELY SAFE ...when used orally and appropriately (3902,3903,6368,10425,10426).
PREGNANCY AND LACTATION: Insufficient reliable information available; avoid using.

Effectiveness

LIKELY EFFECTIVE

Benign prostatic hyperplasia (BPH). Taking pygeum orally reduces the functional symptoms of BPH. Pygeum decreases nocturia by 19%, increases peak urine flow by 23%, and reduces residual urine volume by 24% in men with BPH (3902,3903,3904,4302,6368,10425,10426).

Mechanism of Action

The applicable part of pygeum is the bark. There is evidence that suggests pygeum extracts have antiproliferative effects on prostatic fibroblasts and epithelial cells. Pygeum might inhibit growth factors such as basic fibroblast growth factor (bFGF), epidermal growth factor (EGF), and insulin-like growth factor (IGF), which might inhibit prostate growth and cellular hyperplasia (4301,6769,11226). Preclinical research suggests that pygeum improves bladder contractility. It seems to affect adrenal androgens and to restore the secretory activity of prostate epithelium. It also decreases production of leukotrienes and other 5-lipoxygenase metabolites, which suggests possible anti-inflammatory activity (6769,10425,10426).

Adverse Reactions

Orally, pygeum bark is generally well tolerated. It can cause nausea and abdominal pain (10425,10426).

Interactions with Herbs & Other Dietary Supplements

None known.

Interactions with Drugs

None known.

Interactions with Foods

None known.

Interactions with Lab Tests

None known.

Interactions with Diseases or Conditions

None known.

Dosage and Administration

ORAL: For functional symptoms of benign prostatic hyperplasia (BPH), 75-200 mg standardized lipophilic extract (14% triterpenes, 0.5% n-docosanol) per day has been used (10425,10426). Some research suggests once or twice daily dosing is equally effective (6368).

PYRETHRUM

Also Known As

Dalmation Insect Flowers, Dalmation Pellitory.

Scientific Names

Tanacetum cinerariifolium, synonyms Chrysanthemum cinerariifolium, Pyrethrum cinerariifolium.
Family: Asteraceae/Compositae.

People Use This For

Topically, pyrethrum is used as an insecticide, particularly for head lice, crab lice and their nits, and as an antiscabies agent.

Safety

LIKELY SAFE ...when the commercially available combination of pyrethrins (0.17% to 0.33) and piperonyl butoxide (2% to 4%) are used topically and appropriately in a nonaerosol preparation (272).
POSSIBLY SAFE ...when pyrethrins are used topically in amounts less than 2 grams (18).
CHILDREN: POSSIBLY UNSAFE ...when used in children under the age of 2 years (4084).
PREGNANCY AND LACTATION: Insufficient reliable information available; avoid using.

Effectiveness

EFFECTIVE

Lice. Applying pyrethrins topically and appropriately in concentrations of 0.17-.0.33% for 12-24 hours is effective for treating head lice and crab lice. They are usually combined with piperonyl butoxide (2-4%) (272).

INEFFECTIVE

Scabies. Applying pyrethrum flowers topically is not effective for treating scabies (4084).

Mechanism of Action

The applicable part of pyrethrum is the flower head. Pyrethrum is also the name of the crude extract obtained from flowers of Chrysanthemum cinerariifolium. Pyrethrin refers to more refined extract containing several naturally occurring pyrethrins (505). The active constituents, the pyrethrins, are toxic to insect nervous systems (18).

Adverse Reactions

Pyrethrum has limited toxicity. The symptoms of overdose include headache, tinnitus, nausea, tingling of fingers and toes, respiratory disturbances, and other symptoms of neurotoxicity (18). The pyrethrum flower or derivatives of it might cause an allergic reaction in individuals sensitive to the Asteraceae/Compositae family. Members of this family include ragweed, chrysanthemums, marigolds, daisies, and many other herbs.

Interactions with Herbs & Other Dietary Supplements

None known.

Interactions with Drugs

None known.

Interactions with Foods

None known.

Interactions with Lab Tests

None known.

Interactions with Diseases or Conditions

ASTHMA: Exposure to pyrethrin might severely exacerbate asthma; avoid using. There is one case report of fatal asthma in a child with a history of asthma after bathing a pet dog with a 0.2% pyrethrin shampoo. There is speculation that this might have been due to allergenic impurities from the pyrethrin extraction process (6654).

CROSS-ALLERGENICITY: Can cause an allergic reaction in individuals sensitive to the Asteraceae/Compositae family. Members of this family include ragweed, chrysanthemums, marigolds, daisies, and many other herbs.

Dosage and Administration

TOPICAL: Externally as a liquid extract, rinse after use (18). In general, the OTC combination of pyrethrins (0.17% to 0.33%) and piperonyl butoxide (2% to 4%) are applied to the infested area and allowed to remain for not less than 10 minutes. It is then thoroughly washed off with warm water (272).

Comments

To treat lice, the OTC combination products with piperonyl butoxide are preferred for safety and effectiveness (272).

PYRIDOXINE (VITAMIN B6)

Also Known As

Adermine Hydrochloride, B Complex Vitamin, B6, Pyridoxal, Pyridoxal Phosphate, Pyridoxal-5-Phosphate, Pyridoxamine, Pyridoxine HCl, Pyridoxine Hydrochloride.

Scientific Names

Pyridoxine; Vitamin B6.

People Use This For

Orally, pyridoxine is used most commonly for treating premenstrual syndrome (PMS), vitamin B6 deficiency, "morning sickness" in pregnancy, depression associated with pregnancy or oral contraceptive use, primary homocystinuria, hyperhomocysteinemia, and preventing neuritis associated with isoniazid or penicillamine. Pyridoxine is also used orally for boosting immunity, muscle cramps, protection against cancer, diuresis, conjunctivitis, cystitis, primary hyperoxaluria, preventing kidney stones, carpal tunnel syndrome (CTS), night leg cramps, arthritis, and allergies. It is used for attention deficit-hyperactivity disorder (ADHD), Down syndrome, migraine headaches, asthma, pyridoxine-responsive sideroblastic anemia, sickle cell anemia, preventing anemia due to pyridoxine deficiency, xanthurenic aciduria, primary cystathioninuria, acne, various skin conditions, stimulating appetite, hyperlipidemia, heart disease, radiation sickness, menopausal symptoms, infertility, amenorrhea-galactorrhea syndrome, suppressing postpartum lactation, and to improve dream recall. Pyridoxine is also used orally for dizziness, motion sickness, psychosis, autism, hyperkinesis, acute chorea, chronic progressive hereditary chorea, tardive dyskinesia, absence (petit mal) seizures, febrile convulsions, gyrate atrophy of the choroid and retina, diabetes, diabetic neuropathy, alcohol intoxication, preventing leukopenia secondary to mitomycin, reversing procarbazine neurotoxicity, preventing seizures associated with cycloserine, fluorouracil-induced erythrodysesthesia, and acute hydrazine toxicity. It is also used orally to decrease the rate of restenosis after coronary angioplasty.

Intravenously, pyridoxine is used for seizures in infants unresponsive to other therapies, acute toxicity due to isoniazid, cycloserine or hydrazine overdose, and acute poisoning from mushrooms of the genus Gyromitra.

Safety

LIKELY SAFE ...when used orally and appropriately (15). ...when used parenterally and appropriately. Injectable pyridoxine is an FDA-approved prescription product (15).

POSSIBLY SAFE ...when used orally and appropriately in amounts exceeding the recommended dietary allowance (8558).

POSSIBLY UNSAFE ...when used orally in excessive doses, long-term. Doses exceeding 1000 mg daily or total doses of 1000 grams or more pose the most risk, although neuropathy can occur with lower daily or total doses (8195).

CHILDREN: LIKELY SAFE ...when used orally and appropriately (3094). POSSIBLY SAFE ...when used orally and appropriately in amounts exceeding the recommended dietary allowance (5049,8579). POSSIBLY UNSAFE ...when used orally in excessive doses, long-term (3094).

PREGNANCY: LIKELY SAFE ...when used orally in doses not exceeding the recommended dietary allowance (RDA). The RDA for pregnant women is 1.9 mg per day (3094). POSSIBLY SAFE ...when used orally and appropriately in amounts exceeding the recommended dietary allowance. A special sustained-release product providing pyridoxine 75 mg per day is FDA-approved for use in pregnancy. However, it should not be used long-term or without medical supervision and close monitoring. POSSIBLY UNSAFE ...when used orally in excessive doses. There is some concern that high-dose maternal pyridoxine can cause neonatal seizures (4609,6397,8197).

LACTATION: LIKELY SAFE ...when used orally in doses not exceeding the recommended dietary allowance (RDA) (3094). The RDA in lactating women is 2 mg per day. There is insufficient reliable information about the safety of pyridoxine when used in higher doses in lactating women.

Effectiveness

EFFECTIVE

Hereditary sideroblastic anemia. Taking pyridoxine orally is effective for treating hereditary sideroblastic anemia (15).

Pyridoxine-dependent seizures. Refractory seizures in neonates that are caused by pyridoxine dependence are typically controlled within minutes of intravenous administration of pyridoxine. Pyridoxine-dependent seizures can be due to genetic (autosomal recessive) pyridoxine dependency, or more commonly, the result of the use of high-dose pyridoxine in pregnancy (8197,8198).

Pyridoxine deficiency. Taking pyridoxine orally is effective for preventing and treating pyridoxine deficiency (15).

LIKELY EFFECTIVE

Hyperhomocysteinemia. Taking pyridoxine orally alone or in combination with folic acid is effective for treating postprandial hyperhomocysteinemia. Pyridoxine 50 to 200 mg/day reduces postprandial homocysteine levels by 32% to 35% (9406,10350). Pyridoxine doesn't seem to lower homocysteine concentrations unless folic acid and vitamin B12 are at physiologic levels, but it appears to reduce homocysteine concentrations when given with folic acid and vitamin B12 supplements (3047,9451). A combination of pyridoxine 100 mg and folic acid 0.5 mg/day seems to lower homocysteine levels by about 35% (9406). A combination of these vitamins is generally recommended for people with postprandial hyperhomocysteinemia (1489,9406,9408). Pyridoxine in doses up to 200 mg/day has no effect on fasting homocysteine levels (2149,9406,9408), and doesn't add to the effect of folic acid alone on fasting homocysteine levels in healthy people (9400,9405,9409). However, pyridoxine does seem to reduce homocysteine levels in patients with end-stage renal disease (ESRD), renal transplant patients (1489,6884,9414,9415), and patients who receive general anesthesia with nitrous oxide (9481). Hyperhomocysteinemia is a risk factor for coronary, cerebral and peripheral atherosclerosis; recurrent thromboembolism; deep vein thrombosis; myocardial infarction; and ischemic stroke (1899,2147,3047,3323,9402,9405,9408,9409). But elevated homocysteine levels may be a marker instead of a cause of vascular disease (11387,11388). A 5 micromole increase in plasma homocysteine increases the risk of cerebrovascular disease by 50%, and the risk of coronary heart disease by 60% in women and 80% in men (9407,9411). However, it's not clear if lowering homocysteine levels results in reduced cardiovascular morbidity and mortality (1489,6883,6884,9308,9400,9405,9409). Folic acid, pyridoxine (vitamin B6), and vitamin B12 supplementation can reduce total homocysteine from 13.4 to 11.0 micromoles per liter. However, this reduction doesn't seem to help with secondary prevention of death or cardiovascular events such as stroke or myocardial infarction in people with prior stroke (11387). More evidence is needed to fully explain the association of total homocysteine levels with vascular risk. Until definitive data is available, the current recommendation is screening of 40-year-old men and 50-year-old women for hyperhomocysteinemia (9308).

POSSIBLY EFFECTIVE

Hyperkinetic cerebral dysfunction syndrome. There is preliminary evidence that taking pyridoxine orally may have a beneficial effect on hyperkinetic children who have low levels of blood serotonin (3351).

Kidney stones (nephrolithiasis). There is some evidence that taking pyridoxine orally, alone, or in combination with magnesium, can decrease urinary oxalate levels in people with type I primary hyperoxaluria, a hereditary disorder (1201,6437,6438,6439,6440,8548,8549,8550). However, it doesn't appear to help people with other kinds of kidney stones (8551). There is preliminary evidence that higher pyridoxine intake in women is associated with decreased risk of kidney stone formation in women with no history of stone formation (6441), but this association has not been found in men (6442).

Lung cancer. Taking pyridoxine orally seems to decrease the risk of lung cancer. Epidemiological research suggests that male smokers with higher serum levels of pyridoxine have a lower risk of lung cancer (9454).

Pregnancy-induced nausea and vomiting. Taking pyridoxine orally 25 mg every eight hours for 72 hours decreases vomiting and severe nausea in pregnancy. However, it doesn't seem to improve mild to moderate nausea (6168). Lower doses, pyridoxine 10 mg every eight hours, improves nausea, but not vomiting in pregnancy (6167).

Premenstrual syndrome (PMS). There is some evidence that taking pyridoxine orally can improve symptoms of PMS such as breast pain or tenderness (mastalgia) and PMS-related depression in some patients. Pyridoxine 50 mg per day plus magnesium oxide 200 mg per day seems to relieve PMS-related anxiety (8555). Although some clinicians advocate higher doses of pyridoxine for PMS, such as 200-500 mg per day, lower doses of 50-100 mg per day seem to work just as well. There is no apparent dose-response curve for PMS, so the lowest effective dose should be used. Higher doses might increase the risk of side effects (3093).

Tardive dyskinesia. Pyridoxine 400 mg per day seems to improve Parkinsonian, dystonic, and dyskinetic symptoms in patients taking neuroleptic drugs for schizophrenia (8558).

POSSIBLY INEFFECTIVE

Autism. A moderate dose of 200 mg per day, and a high dose of 600 mg per day, of pyridoxine in combination with magnesium given for ten to 35 weeks doesn't seem to improve autistic behaviors in children (5049,8579).

Carpal tunnel syndrome. Most research suggests that people with carpal tunnel syndrome are not generally pyridoxine deficient and do not benefit from pyridoxine supplements (8203,8937,9448,9450,9453,9478,9482). Although early studies by a single group of researchers, and anecdotal reports, suggest pyridoxine may relieve carpal tunnel symptoms, more reliable research does not support pyridoxine for this use (8200,8201,8202,8204,9445,9446,9447,9449,9483). Some researchers have identified pyridoxine deficiency in people with carpal tunnel syndrome (8199). People who have peripheral neuropathy, as opposed to carpal tunnel syndrome, may benefit from pyridoxine (9453).

Stroke. Taking pyridoxine orally doesn't seem to be useful for preventing stroke recurrence. In people with a history of stroke, neither high dose pyridoxine combinations containing 25 mg of pyridoxine, 0.4 mg of vitamin B12, and 2.5 mg of folic acid nor low dose combinations containing 200 mcg of pyridoxine, 6 mcg of vitamin B12, and 20 mcg of folic acid seem to affect risk of recurring stroke (11387).

INSUFFICIENT RELIABLE EVIDENCE to RATE

Angioplasty. There are conflicting findings about the benefits of taking folic acid plus vitamin B6 and vitamin B12 following angioplasty. Some evidence suggests that folic acid 1 mg plus vitamin B12 400 mcg and pyridoxine 10 mg daily can decrease the rate of restenosis in patients treated with balloon angioplasty (8009,9412). But this combination does not seem to be as effective for reducing restenosis in patients after coronary stenting (8009). An intravenous loading dose of folic acid, vitamin B6, and vitamin B12 followed by oral administration of folic acid 1.2 mcg plus vitamin B6 48 mg and vitamin B12 60 mcg taken daily after coronary stenting also does not seem to reduce restenosis and might actually increase restenosis (12150,12151). Due to the lack of evidence of benefit and potential for harm, this combination of vitamins should not be recommended for patients receiving coronary stents (12151).

Asthma. There is some interest in using pyridoxine for asthma in patients who take theophylline. Some research suggests that children with severe asthma might inadequately metabolize tryptophan, indicating inadequate pyridoxine status (8552). Theophylline seems to lower pyridoxine levels (4522,7066,9503). Some clinicians are trying pyridoxine 200-300 mg daily to see if it improves symptoms, but the effectiveness of supplementation is questionable; many patients don't seem to benefit, and studies show conflicting results (7064,7065).

Attention deficit-hyperactivity disorder (ADHD). Preliminary clinical research suggests oral pyridoxine might help ADHD, alone or in combination with high doses of other B vitamins (41,9960). However, research using megadose pyridoxine in combination with other megadose vitamins seems to have no effect on ADHD symptoms (9957).

More evidence is needed to rate pyridoxine for these uses.

Mechanism of Action

Pyridoxine is required for amino acid metabolism. It is also involved in carbohydrate and lipid metabolism (15). In the body, pyridoxine is converted to coenzymes pyridoxal phosphate and pyridoxamine phosphate, in a wide variety of metabolic reactions. These reactions include transamination of amino acids, conversion of tryptophan to niacin, synthesis of gamma-aminobutyric acid (GABA) in the CNS, metabolism of serotonin, norepinephrine and dopamine, metabolism of polyunsaturated fatty acids and phospholipids, and the synthesis of the heme component of hemoglobin (15). Pyridoxine deficiency in adults principally affects the peripheral nerves, skin, mucous membranes, and hematopoietic system. In children, the CNS is also affected. Deficiency can occur in people with uremia, alcoholism, cirrhosis, hyperthyroidism, malabsorption syndromes, congestive heart failure (CHF), and in those receiving certain drugs (15). Pyridoxine is a cofactor for enzymes involved in one of the two pathways for the metabolism of homocysteine. Remethylation of homocysteine to methionine requires folate and vitamin B12 (3047,9407,9409). Folic acid supplements increase the activity of this pathway, lowering fasting homocysteine levels. Pyridoxine is not involved in this pathway and therefore doesn't affect fasting homocysteine levels (3047,9400,9406). Trans-sulfuration of homocysteine to form cystathionine is catalyzed by cystathione-beta-synthase, which is pyridoxine (vitamin B6) dependent (2148,3047,9407,9409). This pathway is primarily active after ingesting a methionine load (i.e., after a meal). Deficiencies of pyridoxine or cystathione-beta-synthase impair this pathway, raising post-methionine load homocysteine levels (1489,2148,9408). Pyridoxine supplements can lower post-methionine load homocysteine levels (1489,3047,7881). Evidence suggests elevated homocysteine levels might cause vascular endothelial cell damage, impaired endothelium dependent vasodilation due to reduced nitric oxide activity, increased oxidation and arterial deposition of low-density lipoproteins (LDL), increased platelet adhesiveness, and activation of the clotting cascade (2147,3047,9403,9408).

Decreased pyridoxine concentrations are associated with increased plasma levels of C-reactive protein (CRP). CRP is an indicator of inflammation that is implicated in increased cardiovascular morbidity (9452).

Pyridoxine has some antioxidant and free radical scavenging activities, which might explain its beneficial effects on tardive dyskinesia (8558). For kidney stones, pyridoxine is thought to be beneficial by decreasing urinary excretion of oxalate in some patients. Most kidney stones are composed of calcium oxalate, and high urinary oxalate has been associated with development and recurrence of kidney stones. In patients with type I primary hyperoxaluria, pyridoxine seems to reduce stone formation by shifting the breakdown of the oxalic acid precursor, glyoxalic acid, to glycine as opposed to oxalic acid (6437,6438,6439,6440,6441,6442,8205). In attention deficit-hyperactivity disorder (ADHD), some kids can have low serotonin levels (41); however, this is controversial (6444). It's thought that pyridoxine can increase serotonin levels and might improve symptoms in some kids with low serotonin levels (41). Some researchers think pyridoxine supplementation might also be useful for some dysphoric mental states because it increases the production of serotonin and GABA, but the evidence is still preliminary (8554). It has been suggested that large doses of vitamin B6 may be useful in carpal tunnel syndrome, based on an observation of low vitamin B6 tissue levels in autopsy specimens from people who had the syndrome (6885). However, tissue levels decline in dead or infarcted tissue and the existence of vitamin B6 deficiency during life cannot be deduced from these observations (6885).

Adverse Reactions

Orally or by injection, pyridoxine can cause nausea, vomiting, abdominal pain, loss of appetite, headache, paresthesia, somnolence, increased serum aspartate transaminase (AST, SGOT), decreased serum folic acid concentrations, skin and other allergic reactions, breast soreness or enlargement, and photosensitivity (8195,9479).

Pyridoxine can cause sensory neuropathy, which is related to daily dose and duration of intake. Doses exceeding 1000 mg daily or total doses of 1000 grams or more pose the most risk, although neuropathy can occur with lower daily or total doses as well (8195). The mechanism of the neurotoxicity is unknown, but is thought to occur when the liver's capacity to phosphorylate pyridoxine, via the active coenzyme pyridoxal phosphate, is exceeded (8204). Some researchers recommend pyridoxal phosphate to avoid pyridoxine neuropathy, but its safety is unknown (8204).

Pyridoxine neuropathy is characterized by numbness and impairment of the sense of position and vibration of the distal limbs, and a gradual progressive sensory ataxia (8196,10439). The syndrome is usually reversible with discontinuation of pyridoxine at the first appearance of neurologic symptoms. Residual symptoms have been reported in patients taking more than 2 grams daily for extended periods (8195,8196). Tell patients daily doses of 100 mg or less are unlikely to cause problems (3094).

High-dose pyridoxine (80 mg/day) and vitamin B12 (20 micrograms/day) may cause rosacea fulminans characterized by intense erythema with nodules, papules, and pustules. Symptoms may persist for up to 4 months after the supplement is stopped, and may require treatment with systemic corticosteroids and topical therapy (10998).

There is some concern that long-term dietary pyridoxine intake in small amounts ranging from 3.56-6.59 mg daily can increase the risk of developing ulcerative colitis (3350). However, this concern is preliminary. It is too soon to suggest that patients cut back on pyridoxine intake.

Interactions with Herbs & Other Dietary Supplements

None known.

Interactions with Drugs

AMIODARONE (Cordarone): Preliminary research suggests that pyridoxine could exacerbate amiodarone-induced photosensitivity. Other research suggests a protective effect (8892,8893).

LEVODOPA: Pyridoxine enhances the metabolism of levodopa, reducing its anti-parkinsonism effects. However, this interaction doesn't occur when carbidopa is used concurrently with levodopa (Sinemet), therefore it isn't likely to be a problem in most people (3046).

PHENOBARBITAL (Luminal): Preliminary data suggests that pyridoxine 200 mg/day can reduce plasma levels of phenobarbital, possibly by increasing metabolism. It isn't known whether lower doses have any effect. Advise people taking phenobarbital drugs to avoid high doses of pyridoxine (3046,10801).

PHENYTOIN (Dilantin): Preliminary data suggests that pyridoxine 200 mg/day can reduce plasma levels of phenytoin, possibly by increasing metabolism. It isn't known whether lower doses have any effect. Advise people taking phenytoin to avoid high doses of pyridoxine (3046,10801).

Drug Influences on Nutrient Levels and Depletion

SOME DRUGS CAN AFFECT PYRIDOXINE LEVELS:

ANTIBIOTICS: Destruction of normal gastrointestinal flora by antibiotics can cause decreased production of B vitamins. The clinical significance of this decreased production is not known. Consider supplementation only if clinical judgment warrants it (4434,4435,4436,4437,4438,4439,4440,4441,4442,4443).

ESTROGENS and ESTROGEN-CONTAINING ORAL CONTRACEPTIVES: Use of estrogens and estrogen-containing oral contraceptives can interfere with pyridoxine metabolism, reducing serum pyridoxine levels. The need for pyridoxine supplementation has not been adequately studied (4459,4498,4547).

HYDRALAZINE (Apresoline): Hydralazine can increase pyridoxine requirements. The need for pyridoxine supplementation has not been adequately studied (4453,4531,4533).

ISONIAZID (INH, Rifamate): Isoniazid can increase pyridoxine requirements. Patients receiving more than 10 mg/kg/day of INH should be supplemented with 50-100 mg of pyridoxine per day (4481,4482).

PENICILLAMINE (Cuprimine): Penicillamine can increase pyridoxine requirements. The need for pyridoxine supplementation has not been adequately studied (4453,4531).

THEOPHYLLINE (Theo-Dur): Theophylline interferes with pyridoxine metabolism (4522,7066). Theophylline can inhibit pyridoxal kinase, which decreases the conversion of pyridoxine into its physiologically active forms (4522,9480,9503). However, the clinical significance of this is not known. Some clinicians try supplementing with pyridoxine 200-300 mg daily in asthmatic patients taking theophylline (7064,7065), but the effectiveness of supplementation is questionable. Many patients don't seem to benefit, and outcomes with pyridoxine supplementation are not consistent (7064,7065).

Interactions with Foods

None known.

Interactions with Lab Tests

UROBILINOGEN: Pyridoxine can cause a false positive result in the spot test with Ehrlich's reagent (15).

Interactions with Diseases or Conditions

ANGIOPLASTY: An intravenous loading dose of folic acid, vitamin B6, and vitamin B12 followed by oral administration of folic acid 1.2 mcg plus vitamin B6 48 mg and vitamin B12 60 mcg taken daily after coronary stenting might actually increase restenosis rates (12150). Due to the potential for harm this combination of vitamins should not be recommended for patients receiving coronary stents (12151).

Dosage and Administration

ORAL: For vitamin B6 deficiency in adults, the typical dose is 2.5-25 mg daily for three weeks, then 1.5-2.5 mg per day as maintenance therapy (15). For vitamin B6 deficiency in women taking oral contraceptives, the dose is 25-30 mg per day (15). For symptoms associated with premenstrual syndrome (PMS), the daily dose is 50-100 mg. Doses as high as 500 mg per day have been used, but daily doses over 100 mg don't appear to have additional benefit, and may increase the risk for adverse effects (3093). For hereditary sideroblastic anemia, initially 200-600 mg per day is used, decreasing to 30-50 mg daily after an adequate response (15). For metabolic disorders, including xanthurenic aciduria, primary cystathioninuria, or primary homocystinuria, 100-500 mg daily is generally effective (15). For post-prandial hyperhomocysteinemia, 50 to 200 mg of pyridoxine used alone or a combination of pyridoxine 100 mg and folic acid 0.5 mg has been used daily (1489,9406,10350). For kidney stones, 25-500 mg daily has been used (6437,6439). For primary hyperoxaluria, 2 to 200 mg has been used (6439,6440). When used with magnesium for preventing kidney stones, pyridoxine 10 mg daily has been used in combination with magnesium 300 mg daily (1201). For preventing anemia due to pyridoxine deficiency or neuritis in people receiving isoniazid or penicillamine, the typical dose is 10-50 mg daily (15). For treating tardive dyskinesia, 100 mg per day has been titrated weekly up to 400 mg per day, given in two divided doses (8558). For preventing seizures in people receiving cycloserine, 100-300 mg is taken daily in divided doses (15). For nausea during pregnancy, 10-25 mg pyridoxine every eight hours has been used (6167,6168); alternatively, 75 mg of sustained-release pyridoxine combined with 12 mcg vitamin B12 (cyanocobalamin), 1 mg folic acid, and 200 mg calcium (PremesisRx) is used daily as an FDA-approved prescription supplement for nausea during pregnancy (23). For hyperkinetic cerebral dysfunction syndrome in children, 300 mg daily has been used in a clinical trial. However, some children can require larger dosages ranging from 500 mg to 2 grams daily (3351). To decrease the rate of restenosis after coronary angioplasty, a combination of pyridoxine 10 mg plus vitamin B12 400 mcg and folic acid 1 mg taken daily has been used (8008). The daily recommended dietary allowances (RDAs) of vitamin B6 are: Infants 0-6 months, 0.1 mg; Infants 7-12 months, 0.3 mg; Children 1-3 years, 0.5 mg; Children 4-8 years, 0.6 mg; Children 9-13 years, 1 mg; Males 14-50 years, 1.3 mg; Males over 50 years, 1.7 mg; Females 14-18 years, 1.2 mg; Females 19-50 years, 1.3 mg; Females over 50 years, 1.5 mg; Pregnant women, 1.9 mg; and Lactating women, 2 mg (3094). Some researchers think the RDA for women 19-50 years should be increased to 1.5-1.7 mg per day (8556). The recommended maximum daily intake is: Children 1-3 years, 30 mg; Children 4-8 years, 40 mg; Children 9-13 years, 60 mg; Adults, pregnant and lactating women, 14-18 years, 80 mg; and Adults, pregnant and lactating women, over 18 years, 100 mg (3094).

INJECTION: This is an FDA-approved prescription product that is available as a 100 mg/mL injection. For seizures in neonates and infants, 10 to 100 mg pyridoxine IV or IM is recommended (15).

Comments

Pyridoxine is present in many foods including cereal grains, legumes, vegetables, liver, meat, and eggs (15).
Pyridoxine is frequently used in combination with other B vitamins in vitamin B complex formulations. Vitamin B complex generally includes vitamin B1 (thiamine), vitamin B2 (riboflavin), vitamin B3 (niacin/niacinamide), vitamin B5 (pantothenic acid), vitamin B6 (pyridoxine), vitamin B12 (cyanocobalamin), and folic acid. However, some products do not contain all of these ingredients and some may include others, such as biotin, para-aminobenzoic acid (PABA), choline bitartrate, and inositol (3022). Pyridoxine and the sedative antihistamine doxylamine were ingredients in Bendectin, a widely-prescribed antinausea product for use in pregnancy. The product was removed from the US market in 1983 due to litigation costs. A similar product, Diclectin, has remained available in Canada. Animal studies have disclosed no teratogenic potential or pyridoxine or Bendectin. Following removal of Bendectin from the market, there was no reduction in birth defects, but a doubling in hospitalization rates for pregnancy-related nausea and vomiting (8195).

PYRUVATE

Also Known As

2-Oxypropanoic Acid, Acetylformic Acid, Alpha-Keto Acid, Alpha-Ketopropionic Acid, Calcium Pyruvate, Creatine Pyruvate, Magnesium Pyruvate, Potassium Pyruvate, Proacemic Acid, Pyruvic Acid, Sodium Pyruvate.

Scientific Names

2-Oxopropanoate (pyruvate); 2-oxopropanoic acid (pyruvic acid).

People Use This For

Orally, pyruvate is used for weight loss, improving exercise endurance, and inhibiting tumor growth.
Topically, pyruvic acid is used for signs of aging skin such as wrinkles.

Safety

POSSIBLY SAFE ...when used orally and appropriately, short-term. There is some evidence that pyruvate can be safely used for up to 6 weeks (2472,2474). ...when used topically and appropriately. There is some evidence that a 50% pyruvic acid skin peel can be safely applied by a health professional (12020).
PREGNANCY AND LACTATION: Insufficient reliable information available; avoid using.

Effectiveness

POSSIBLY EFFECTIVE

Aging skin. Applying a 50% pyruvic acid skin peel once a week for 4 weeks seems to smooth skin, decrease fine wrinkles, and decrease hyperpigmentation associated with photoaging (12020).

Weight loss. Taking pyruvate orally in place of a portion of dietary carbohydrates and in combination with a low calorie diet seems to help increase weight loss (2472,2474).

Mechanism of Action

Pyruvic acid is an alpha-keto acid which is converted to the alpha-hydroxy acid lactic acid. It seems to be helpful for aging skin by exfoliating the surface layers of skin (12020).
Some evidence suggests that pyruvate reduces free radical production (2487), increases lipid oxidation, and decreases carbohydrate oxidation (2488).
Very small clinical trials suggest dietary supplementation with dihydroxyacetone and pyruvate increases arm and leg exercise endurance (807,808).
Very preliminary evidence also suggests a liquid diet supplemented with pyruvate might inhibit tumor growth (806).

Adverse Reactions

Intravenously, one death was associated with pyruvate use in a child with restrictive cardiomyopathy (2473).
Topically, applying pyruvic acid as a facial peel can cause an intense burning sensation. It should only be applied over small areas. Vapors have been reported to cause respiratory irritation and should only be applied in a room with adequate ventilation (12020).

Interactions with Herbs & Other Dietary Supplements

None known.

Interactions with Drugs

None known.

Interactions with Foods
None known.

Interactions with Lab Tests
None known.

Interactions with Diseases or Conditions
CARDIOMYOPATHY: One death was associated with intravenous use in a child with restrictive cardiomyopathy (2473).

Dosage and Administration
ORAL: For weight loss 22 to 44 grams per day, as an adjunct to a low-cholesterol, low-fat diet has been used (2474).
TOPICAL: For aging skin, a 50% pyruvic acid peel applied once weekly for 4 weeks has been used (12020).

QUASSIA

Also Known As
Amargo, Bitter-Ash, Bitter Wood, Jamaican Quassia, Picrasma, Ruda, Surinam Quassia, Surinam Wood.

Scientific Names
Quassia amara; Picrasma excelsa.
Family: Simaroubaceae.

People Use This For
Orally, quassia is used for anorexia; indigestion; constipation; fever; as an anthelmintic for thread worms, nematodes, and ascaris; as a tonic or purgative; and as a mouthwash.
Topically, quassia is used for pediculosis.
Rectally, quassia is used for nematode infestation.
In manufacturing, quassia is used as a flavoring agent in foods, beverages, pastilles, lozenges, and laxatives. The bark and wood have been used as an insecticide.

Safety
POSSIBLY SAFE ...when used in amounts commonly found in foods. Quassia has Generally Recognized As Safe (GRAS) status in the US (4912).
POSSIBLY UNSAFE ...when used orally in therapeutic amounts. Quassia wood contains cardioactive glycosides (4), but toxicity is likely limited by emetic effects of large doses (4).
There is insufficient reliable information available about the safety of the topical or rectal use of quassia.
PREGNANCY AND LACTATION: LIKELY UNSAFE ...when used orally; avoid using. Quassia has cytotoxic and emetic properties (4,18,19). There is insufficient reliable information available about the safety of rectal or topical use during pregnancy or lactation; avoid using.

Effectiveness
POSSIBLY EFFECTIVE
Lice. Applying quassia tincture topically to the scalp seems to be an effective treatment for head lice (4).
There is insufficient reliable information available about the effectiveness of quassia for its other uses.

Mechanism of Action
The applicable part of quassia is the wood (4,8,11). Quassia leaves are also reportedly used (6). Quassia contains quassinoids that have potent bitter properties (11). Quassia also contains beta-carboline alkaloids, quassin, quassimarin, canthin-6-one (4), and small amounts of the coumarin scopoletin (4). The quassinoid constituents increase gastric acid and bile secretions, perhaps accounting for appetite stimulant and digestive effects (18,19,4). There is evidence that the beta-carboline alkaloids might have positive inotropic activity (4). The constituent canthin-6-one is reported to have antibacterial, antifungal, and cytotoxic activity (4). Quassimarin demonstrates evidence of antileukemic (11) and antitumor effects (18,4). Quassin demonstrates antilarval activity against Culex quinquefasciatus (mosquito) (3302).

Adverse Reactions
Quassia can cause mucous membrane irritation, nausea, and vomiting (4,18). Long-term use can cause vision changes and blindness (18).

Interactions with Herbs & Other Dietary Supplements

CARDIOACTIVE GLYCOSIDE-CONTAINING HERBS: Theoretically, concomitant use with other cardiac glycoside-containing herbs might increase risk of cardiac toxicity. Cardiac glycoside-containing herbs include black hellebore, Canadian hemp roots, digitalis leaf, hedge mustard, figwort, lily-of-the-valley roots, motherwort, oleander leaf, pheasant's eye plant, pleurisy root, squill bulb leaf scales, and strophanthus seeds (19).
CARDIOACTIVE HERBS: Avoid concomitant use with other cardioactive herbs due to unpredictability of effects and adverse effects. Other cardioactive herbs include calamus, cereus, cola, coltsfoot, devil's claw, European mistletoe, fenugreek, fumitory, ginger, Panax ginseng, hawthorn, white horehound, mate, parsley, scotch broom flower, shepherd's purse, and wild carrot (4).
HORSETAIL/LICORICE: Theoretically, abuse of licorice or horsetail might increase risk of cardiac toxicity due to potassium loss (4).
STIMULANT LAXATIVE HERBS: Theoretically, abuse might increase risk of cardiac toxicity due to potassium depletion. Stimulant laxative herbs include aloe dried leaf sap, blue flag rhizome, alder buckthorn, European buckthorn, butternut bark, cascara bark, castor oil, colocynth fruit pulp, gamboge bark exudate, jalap root, black root, manna bark exudate, podophyllum root, rhubarb root, senna leaves and pods, wild cucumber fruit (Ecballium elaterium), and yellow dock root (19).

Interactions with Drugs

ANTACIDS: Theoretically, due to reports that quassia increases stomach acid, quassia might decrease the effectiveness of antacids (19).
DIGOXIN (Lanoxin): Theoretically, concomitant use with cardiac medications might increase the risk of therapeutic and adverse effects (4).
DIURETIC DRUGS: Overuse of quassia might compound diuretic-induced potassium loss (13). There is some concern that people taking quassia along with potassium depleting diuretics might have an increased risk for hypokalemia. Initiation of potassium supplementation or an increase in potassium supplement dose may be necessary for some patients. Some diuretics that can deplete potassium include chlorothiazide (Diuril), chlorthalidone (Thalitone), furosemide (Lasix), and hydrochlorothiazide (HCTZ, Hydrodiuril, Microzide), and others.
H2-BLOCKERS: Theoretically, due to reports that quassia increases stomach acid, quassia might decrease the effectiveness of H2-blockers (19). The H2 blockers include cimetidine (Tagamet), ranitidine (Zantac), nizatidine (Axid), and famotidine (Pepcid).
PROTON PUMP INHIBITORS (PPIs): Theoretically, due to reports that quassia increases stomach acid, quassia might decrease the effectiveness of PPIs (19). PPIs include omeprazole (Prilosec), lansoprazole (Prevacid), rabeprazole (Aciphex), pantoprazole (Protonix), and esomeprazole (Nexium).

Interactions with Foods

None known.

Interactions with Lab Tests

None known.

Interactions with Diseases or Conditions

GI IRRITATION AND INFLAMMATION: In large amounts quassia can irritate the gastrointestinal tract; avoid using (8).

Dosage and Administration

ORAL: A typical dose is one cup tea 2-3 times daily (12). To make tea, simmer 1-2 grams of wood in 150 mL boiling water 10-15 minutes, strain (12).
RECTAL: As an enema (1:20), 150 mL is typically used rectally every morning for 3 days with 16 gram magnesium sulfate orally (4).
TOPICAL: No typical dosage.

Comments

Quassia bark has been used as an insecticide (11).

QUEBRACHO

Also Known As

Quebracho Blanco, White Quebracho.

Scientific Names

Aspidosperma quebracho-blanco.
Family: Apocynaceae.

People Use This For

Orally, quebracho is used for asthma and conditions of the lower respiratory tract. It is also used as an expectorant and respiratory tract stimulant. Sometimes it is used to lower blood pressure (particularly arterial hypertension), as a spasmolytic, diuretic, peripheral vasoconstrictor, uterine sedative, local anesthetic, to decrease fever, and as an aphrodisiac.

In foods and beverages, it is used as a flavoring agent.

Safety

LIKELY SAFE ...when used in amounts commonly found in foods. Quebracho has Generally Recognized As Safe status (GRAS) for use in foods in the US (4912).

There is insufficient reliable information available about the safety of quebracho bark in medicinal amounts.

PREGNANCY AND LACTATION: There is insufficient reliable information about the safety of medicinal amounts of quebracho during pregnancy and breast-feeding; avoid using.

Effectiveness

There is insufficient reliable information available about the effectiveness of quebracho.

Mechanism of Action

The applicable part of quebracho is the bark. There is insufficient reliable information available about the possible mechanism of action and active ingredients.

Adverse Reactions

Orally, people who take quebracho bark may experience side effects including salivation, headache, outbreaks of sweating, vertigo, stupor, and sleepiness. In large doses, it can cause nausea and vomiting (18).

Interactions with Herbs & Other Dietary Supplements

None known.

Interactions with Drugs

None known.

Interactions with Foods

None known.

Interactions with Lab Tests

None known.

Interactions with Diseases or Conditions

None known.

Dosage and Administration

ORAL: It is used as an extract or powder and in combination bronchial preparations (18).

Comments

The bark is odorless and has a bitter taste. Quebracho Colorado or red quebracho is also known as quebracho, but is chemically distinct from white quebracho. Be careful not to confuse these two plants (11).

QUEEN'S DELIGHT

Also Known As

Cockup Hat, Marcory, Queens Delight, Queen's Root, Queens Root, Silver Leaf, Stillingia, Yaw Root.

Scientific Names

Stillingia sylvatica, synonym Stillingia tenuis.

Family: Euphorbiaceae.

People Use This For

Orally, queen's delight is used as a "blood purifier"; for digestive disorders; treatment of hepatic, gallbladder, and skin diseases; and as an emetic and laxative. Queen's delight is also used orally for bronchitis, laryngitis, laryngismus stridulus, and constipation.

Topically, queen's delight is used for cutaneous eruptions, hemorrhoids, and exudative skin eruptions with lymphatic involvement.

Safety

POSSIBLY UNSAFE ...when used orally in medicinal amounts; the dried root preparations contain diterpene esters that are highly irritating (4,12). Queen's delight might activate latent viruses, and it might be carcinogenic (18). ...when the dried or fresh root preparations are used topically (4).
LIKELY UNSAFE ...when the fresh root is used orally; it contains a caustic white latex that is highly irritating to mucous membranes (12).
PREGNANCY: POSSIBLY UNSAFE ...when the dried root preparations are used orally. ...when the dried or fresh root is used topically; avoid using (4). LIKELY UNSAFE ...when the fresh root preparations are used orally (12).
LACTATION: POSSIBLY UNSAFE ...when the dried or fresh root are used topically. LIKELY UNSAFE ...when used orally; contraindicated (4,12,19).

Effectiveness

There is insufficient reliable information available about the effectiveness of queen's delight.

Mechanism of Action

The applicable part of queen's delight is the root. Queen's delight contains a volatile oil and diterpenes including prostatin, gnidilatidin, and others (18). Diterpene esters, isolated in the latex (or milky juice) of the fresh or green root, are potent irritants that cause swelling of the skin and mucous membranes (4,18). Diterpenes may also be carcinogenic agents; they are believed able to activate latent viruses (18).

Adverse Reactions

Orally, queen's delight can cause vomiting, diarrhea, and nausea (18,19). In large amounts, it may cause a burning sensation of the mouth, throat, diarrhea, nausea, vomiting, dysuria, aches and pains, pruritus, skin eruptions, cough, depression, fatigue, and perspiration (4).
Topically, it may cause inflammation, swelling, and contact dermatitis (18,19).

Interactions with Herbs & Other Dietary Supplements

None known.

Interactions with Drugs

None known.

Interactions with Foods

None known.

Interactions with Lab Tests

None known.

Interactions with Diseases or Conditions

GASTROINTESTINAL (GI) CONDITIONS: Queen's delight is contraindicated in individuals with GI irritation, inflammation, nausea or vomiting (19).

Dosage and Administration

ORAL: People typically prepare queen's delight as a liquid, boiling 1 teaspoon of the dried root with one cup of water. The suggested dose is a cup a day, taken a mouthful at a time. As a tincture, queen's delight is taken in a dose of 5 to 20 drops (5263).

QUERCETIN

Also Known As

Citrus Bioflavonoid, Citrus Bioflavonoids, Flavonoid, Meletin, Sophretin.
CAUTION: See separate listings for Chrysin, Diosmin, Hesperidin, Methoxylated Flavones, and Rutin.

Scientific Names

3,3',4'5,7-Penthydroxyflavone.

People Use This For

Orally, quercetin is used for treating atherosclerosis; hypercholesterolemia; coronary heart disease; vascular insufficiency; diabetes; cataracts; allergies; allergic rhinitis; peptic ulcer; schizophrenia; inflammation; asthma; gout; viral infections; preventing cancer; and for treating chronic, bacterial prostatitis.
Intravenously and intraperitoneally, quercetin is used for treating cancer.

Safety

POSSIBLY SAFE ...when used orally in amounts up to 500 mg twice daily for up to one month (481). ...when used intravenously in amounts less than 945 mg/m2 (9564).
LIKELY UNSAFE ...when used intravenously in amounts greater that 945 mg/m2 which are reported to cause nephrotoxicity (9564).
There is insufficient reliable information available about the safety of intraperitoneal quercetin, or quercetin used orally in larger doses or long-term.
PREGNANCY AND LACTATION: Insufficient reliable information available; avoid using.

Effectiveness

POSSIBLY EFFECTIVE

Prostatitis. Taking quercetin orally seems to reduce pain and improve quality of life, but does not seem to affect voiding dysfunction in patients with chronic, nonbacterial prostatitis (481).

INSUFFICIENT RELIABLE EVIDENCE to RATE

Coronary heart disease. There is preliminary evidence that increasing dietary intake of quercetin might reduce the risk of coronary heart disease mortality in elderly men (7726).

Hypercholesterolemia. Short-term use of quercetin supplements for 1 month does not appear to reduce low-density lipoprotein (LDL) cholesterol, total cholesterol, or increase high-density lipoprotein (HDL) cholesterol (1998,1999).

More evidence is needed to rate quercetin for these uses.

Mechanism of Action

Quercetin is a dietary flavonoid found in many plants (481,483,1995). Buckwheat tea has a high concentration of quercetin. The most common form of quercetin is rutin, in which quercetin is bound to a glucose-rhamnose moiety. Quercetin is also found bound to one or two glucose molecules (monoglycoside and diglycoside forms) (9442,9443). Quercetin has antioxidant, anti-inflammatory, nitric oxide inhibitor, and tyrosine kinase inhibitor (leading to inhibition of the division and growth of T-cells and some cancer cells) activity (481,1995). The anti-inflammatory effects of quercetin might be due to inhibition of the production and activity of leukotrienes and prostaglandins, and inhibition of histamine release by basophils and mast cells (483). Preliminary research suggests it might slow cyclooxygenase (COX)-2 production, but this may not occur in vivo (12489). Preliminary evidence suggests that quercetin might work similarly to cromolyn, inhibiting antigen-stimulated histamine release from mast cells of patients with allergic rhinitis (9176). Quercetin also appears to reduce capillary fragility, and it might offer some protection against diabetic cataracts, possibly by inhibiting aldose reductase in the lens (483,9563). The anti-inflammatory and antioxidant effects might be responsible for the observed benefits in men with chronic, nonbacterial prostatitis (481).

Quercetin might reduce cancer risk by inactivating malignant precursors or by inhibiting carcinogenesis (9563). Preliminary studies suggest it might have inhibitory effects on various cancer types, including breast, leukemia, colon, ovary, oral squamous cell, endometrial, gastric, and non-small-cell lung (483,485). Quercetin has antiestrogenic effects in cultures of breast cancer cells (484). It also inhibits estrone sulfatase and estrogen synthesis in liver cells (489). Existing evidence suggests quercetin alters intestinal cell homeostasis of copper, iron, and manganese (1997). Although researchers believe quercetin might protect against heart disease (1995), short-term supplementation does not show affect on any of the known risk factors for heart disease (1998,1999). Preliminary evidence suggests that quercetin might inhibit collagen- and ADP-induced platelet aggregation, but at concentrations much higher than those achieved with typical oral dosing (1999). Quercetin seems to inhibit the ability of monocytes to attach to vascular endothelial cells, which may reduce atherosclerosis (9444).

Evidence also suggests that quercetin might benefit some people with schizophrenia when used in combination with other antioxidants, intestinal adsorbents, and conventional therapy (1996). Quercetin demonstrates activity against retroviruses, Herpes simplex, polio, parainfluenza, and respiratory syncytial viruses (483).

The oral absorption of quercetin is highly variable, depending on the source (481,486,487).

These glycoside forms of quercetin are not absorbed from the gastrointestinal tract and must be hydrolyzed, permitting absorption of the aglycone form of quercetin. The hydrolysis of quercetin glycosides occurs efficiently and completely, resulting in 64 to 80% bioavailability of quercetin (9442).

The time to maximum plasma concentration (Tmax) after oral administration of aglycone quercetin is dose-dependent. After an oral dose of 8, 20, or 50 mg, the Tmax is 1.9, 2.7, or 4.9 hours, respectively. The half-life of quercetin is 15 to 17 hours. However, it appears that quercetin is conjugated in the intestine (9174). In plasma, quercetin is found primarily as glucuronide or sulfate form (9175,9442). In vitro research has been done with unconjugated quercetin. It is questionable whether free quercetin absorption is sufficient to exert a pharmacologic effect. Research in humans suggests that quercetin taken orally doesn't reach serum concentrations at which in vitro activity has been seen (9174). Plasma protein binding might also affect the activity of quercetin (481,486,487).

Plasma concentrations of quercetin glucuronide, sulfate, or unconjugated quercetin aglycone from the glycoside rutin appear to be higher in women than men. When administered as quercetin aglycone, however, there are no bioavailability differences between men and women. Quercetin is absorbed from different parts of the intestines when given as quercetin aglycone or rutin, but the sex differences in bioavailability are not completely understood (9442).

Adverse Reactions

Orally, quercetin can cause headache and tingling of the extremities (481).
Intravenous administration of quercetin is associated with flushing, sweating, dyspnea, nausea, and vomiting (9564).
Injection pain can be minimized by premedicating patient with 10 mg of morphine and administering amounts greater than 945 mg/m2 over 5 minutes (9564). Nephrotoxicity has been reported with use of amounts greater than 945 mg/m2 (9563,9564).

Interactions with Herbs & Other Dietary Supplements

None known.

Interactions with Drugs

QUINOLONE ANTIBIOTICS: Quercetin might competitively inhibit quinolone antibiotics by binding to the DNA gyrase site on bacteria (481).

Interactions with Foods

None known.

Interactions with Lab Tests

None known.

Interactions with Diseases or Conditions

KIDNEY DYSFUNCTION: Theoretically, intravenous quercetin may exacerbate kidney dysfunction (9563,9564).

Dosage and Administration

ORAL: A common dose is 400-500 mg three times daily (483). For prostatitis, 500 mg twice daily has been used (481).
INTRAVENOUS: For treating cancer, 420-1400 mg/m2 by IV bolus weekly or in 3-week intervals has been used (9564).
INTRAPERITONEAL: No typical dosage.

Comments

Quercetin is a dietary flavonoid that occurs abundantly in red wine, tea, onions, green tea, apples, berries, and brassica vegetables (481,483,1995,7726). Quercetin is also found in Ginkgo biloba, St. John's Wort (Hypericum perforatum) and American Elder (Sambucus canadensis) (483).

QUILLAIA

Also Known As

China Bark, Murillo Bark, Panama Bark, Quillaja, Soap Tree, Soap Tree Bark, Soapbark.

Scientific Names

Quillaja saponaria.
Family: Rosaceae.

People Use This For

Orally, quillaia inner bark is used for cough, bronchitis, and pulmonary ailments.
Topically, quillaia extract is used to treat skin sores, athletes' foot, itchy scalp, in shampoos for dandruff, in hair tonic preparations, in douches, and for leukorrhea.
In foods, quillaia is used in frozen dairy desserts, candy, baked goods, gelatins, and puddings.
In manufacturing, quillaia extracts are used in dermatological creams, as foaming agents in root beer, in beverages, and cocktails. Quillaia is also used as a foaming agent in fire extinguishers.

Safety

LIKELY SAFE ...when used in amounts commonly found in foods. Quillaia has Generally Recognized As Safe status (GRAS) for use in foods in the US (4912).
POSSIBLY UNSAFE ...when used orally in medicinal amounts. Quillaia is a gastrointestinal tract irritant that contains oxalates and tannins. Large amounts can cause liver damage, respiratory failure, convulsions, and coma (12).
There is insufficient reliable information available about the safety of the topical or vaginal use of quillaia.
PREGNANCY AND LACTATION: POSSIBLY UNSAFE ...when used in medicinal amounts (12); avoid using.

Effectiveness

There is insufficient reliable information available about the effectiveness of quillaia.

Mechanism of Action

The applicable part of quillaia is the inner bark. Quillaia contains tannins, oxalates, and saponins. Tannins possess strong astringent properties (7,12). Upon contact, they dehydrate the external layer of tissue, reducing internal secretions, and forming external cells into a protective layer (12). Plants with at least 10% tannins, like quillaia (19), can cause gastrointestinal disturbances, kidney damage, and necrotic conditions of the liver (12). Some evidence suggests that tannins might cause cancer; other evidence shows they might prevent it (12). Regular consumption of herbs with high tannin concentrations correlates with increased incidence of esophageal or nasal cancer (12). When ingested, oxalates combine with calcium in the blood forming insoluble oxalates and depleting available calcium, potentially to deficiency levels. Insoluble calcium oxalate, deposited in the kidneys, can cause mechanical damage. Precipitation of calcium oxalate in renal tubules can result in acute renal failure (12). Some evidence suggests saponins might cause red blood cell hemolysis and GI irritation (11). Other evidence suggests they might have anti-inflammatory, antimicrobial, and cytotoxic effects (11). They also possess expectorant properties, can induce sneezing, and can depress cardiac and respiratory activity (6,11). Preliminary information suggests quillaia saponins can reduce the rate of absorption of bile salts (3850), suggesting they might be effective in reducing cholesterol levels (11). QS-21, an isolated saponin from the bark, appears to be a potent immuno-stimulatory complex adjuvant when administered with vaccines (6). It shows evidence that it might augment both antibody and cell-mediated immune responses (3851), significantly increasing antibody levels (6). For this reason it is being evaluated in HIV patients (11). Another purified saponin, DS-1, is being investigated as a pharmaceutical excipient in nasal and ocular delivery of insulin (3852), and also as a transmucosal delivery agent for the aminoglycoside antibiotics (3853).

Adverse Reactions

Orally, large amounts of quillaia are associated with liver damage, diarrhea, respiratory failure, stomach pain, convulsions, coma (12), red blood cell hemolysis (11), and renal failure (12).
If inhaled, the powder can cause sneezing (6). It also can be caustic to mucosa (12).

Interactions with Herbs & Other Dietary Supplements

CALCIUM, IRON, ZINC: Concurrent use might decrease mineral absorption. Quillaia contains oxalate (7,12), which can bind multivalent metal ions in the gastrointestinal tract and decrease mineral absorption.

Interactions with Drugs

METFORMIN (Glucophage): Quillaia might reduce efficacy of metformin (Glucophage) (7). Quillaia contains tannins that might decrease the absorption of metformin by forming insoluble complexes.
ORAL DRUGS: Theoretically, the tannin content might delay absorption of sedatives, hypnotics, antidepressants, and tranquilizers due to tannin content (7,19).

Interactions with Foods

CALCIUM, IRON, ZINC: Concurrent use might decrease mineral absorption from foods. Quillaia contains oxalate (7,12), which can bind multivalent metal ions in the gastrointestinal tract and decrease mineral absorption.

Interactions with Lab Tests

None known.

Interactions with Diseases or Conditions

GI CONDITIONS: Contraindicated in individuals with gastrointestinal inflammation or irritation due to irritant properties (18).
KIDNEY DISEASE: Contraindicated in individuals with kidney disease or a history of kidney stones due to oxalate content (12,19).

Dosage and Administration

ORAL: A typical dose is 200 mg prepared as tea (12).
TOPICAL: No typical dosage.

Comments

In South America, quillaia bark is used to wash clothes (6).

QUINCE

Also Known As

Cognassier, Coing, Marmelo, Membrillo, Quitte, Quittenbaum.

Scientific Names

Cydonia oblongata, synonyms Cydonia vulgaris, Pyrus cydonia.
Family: Rosaceae.

People Use This For
Orally, quince is used for digestive disorders, diarrhea, coughs, and gastrointestinal inflammation.
Topically, quince is used as a compress or poultice for injuries, inflammation of the joints, injuries of the nipples, and gashed or deeply cut fingers. A topical lotion is used to soothe the eyes.

Safety
There is insufficient reliable information available about the safety of quince.
Pregnancy and Lactation: Insufficient reliable information available; avoid using.

Effectiveness
There is insufficient reliable information available about the effectiveness of quince.

Mechanism of Action
The applicable part of quince is the seed. The seeds contain cyanogenic glycosides as amygdalin at 0.4% to 1.5%, or 27-75 mg cyanide per 100 grams of seeds, suggesting potential toxicity (18).

Adverse Reactions
None reported.

Interactions with Herbs & Other Dietary Supplements
None known.

Interactions with Drugs
ORAL DRUGS: Quince may impair absorption of concomitantly administered medications due to the high mucilage fiber in quince seeds (19).

Interactions with Foods
NUTRIENTS: Quince may reduce serum nutrient levels due to possible binding by the high water-soluble fiber content of quince seed (19).

Interactions with Lab Tests
None known.

Interactions with Diseases or Conditions
None known.

Dosage and Administration
ORAL: Quince seed is taken as a powder, extract, or tea. The tea is prepared by steeping 1 teaspoon of whole seeds in 150 mL of boiling water for 10-15 minutes and straining (18).
TOPICAL: A viscous poultice is prepared from the ground seeds (18).

RADISH

Also Known As
Radis, Raphani sativi radix, Small Radish, Turnip Radish.

Scientific Names
Raphanus sativus.
Family: Brassicaceae/Cruciferae.

People Use This For
Orally, radish is used for peptic disorders, dyskinesia of the bile ducts, loss of appetite, inflammation of the mouth and pharynx, tendency towards infections, inflammation or excessive mucus of the respiratory tract, bronchitis, fever, colds, and cough.

Safety
LIKELY SAFE ...when used orally in moderate amounts (18). Large amounts may lead to gastrointestinal irritation (18).
PREGNANCY AND LACTATION: Insufficient reliable information available; avoid very large doses.

Effectiveness
There is insufficient reliable information available about the effectiveness of radish.

Mechanism of Action
The applicable part of radish is the root. Radish root stimulates secretions in the upper GI tract, promotes motility, stimulates bile flow, and has antimicrobial effects (2,18).

Adverse Reactions
Orally, large amounts of radish may cause irritation of the gastrointestinal mucus membrane (18).

Interactions with Herbs & Other Dietary Supplements
None known.

Interactions with Drugs
None known.

Interactions with Foods
None known.

Interactions with Lab Tests
None known.

Interactions with Diseases or Conditions
CHOLELITHIASIS: Radish is contraindicated, because it might cause biliary colic (18).

Dosage and Administration
ORAL: A typical dosage is 0.5 tablespoons pressed root juice, several times daily; up to 50-100 mL per day (18).

RASPBERRY leaf

Also Known As
Framboise, Red Raspberry, Rubi idaei folium, Rubus.
CAUTION: See separate listing for Blackberry leaf.

Scientific Names
Rubus idaeus, synonym Rubus buschii; Rubus strigosus.
Family: Rosaceae.

People Use This For
Orally, raspberry leaf is used for GI tract disorders, upper and lower respiratory tract disorders, cardiovascular system disorders, influenza, fever, diabetes, vitamin deficiency, as a diaphoretic or diuretic, for stimulating bile production, "purification of skin and blood", diarrhea, dysmenorrhea, menorrhagia, morning sickness associated with pregnancy, preventing miscarriage, and facilitating labor and delivery.
Topically, raspberry leaf is used for inflammation of the mouth and throat, and skin rash and inflammation.
In foods, raspberry leaf in small quantities is a source of natural flavoring in Europe.

Safety
LIKELY SAFE ...when used orally in amounts commonly found in foods.
POSSIBLY SAFE ...when used orally or topically and appropriately in medicinal amounts (12).
PREGNANCY: POSSIBLY SAFE ...when used orally and appropriately in medicinal amounts during late pregnancy and under the supervision of a healthcare provider. Raspberry leaf is commonly used by nurse midwives to facilitate delivery. There is some evidence that raspberry leaf can be safely used for this purpose (6481,9796). Make sure patients do not use raspberry leaf without the guidance of a health care professional. LIKELY UNSAFE ...when used orally in medicinal amounts throughout pregnancy or for self-treatment. Raspberry leaf can cause uterine contractions (19) and might have estrogenic effects (6180). These effects can adversely affect pregnancy. Tell pregnant patients not to use raspberry leaf at any time during pregnancy without the close supervision of a healthcare provider.
LACTATION: There is insufficient reliable information available about the safety of raspberry leaf in medicinal amounts while breast-feeding; avoid using.

Effectiveness
POSSIBLY INEFFECTIVE

Labor facilitation. Taking raspberry leaf orally does not seem to reduce the length of labor or decrease the need for analgesics in the perinatal time period (9796).

There is insufficient reliable information available about the effectiveness of raspberry leaf for its other uses.

Mechanism of Action

Raspberry leaf contains a high tannin content (13-15%), which is responsible for its astringent properties (4). When applied topically to skin or mucous membranes tannins cause capillary vasoconstriction, decreased vascular permeability, and a local anti-inflammatory effect (7). The effects of raspberry leaf on smooth muscle, such as that found in the uterus seems to be variable. Different constituents found in raspberry leaf seem to either stimulate or contract uterine smooth muscle. When used in humans, raspberry leaf might have either stimulatory or spasmolytic effects. There is some evidence that these effects might be dose and tissue dependent. For example, in low doses raspberry leaf might cause more contraction, while higher doses might have spasmolytic effects and decrease contraction. Also, raspberry might decrease contraction of tonic tissues and increase contraction of relaxed tissues (1096,1122). Raspberry leaf might also have some estrogenic effects. In an animal model, raspberry leaf seems to increase serum ceruloplasmin oxidase activity, which is a measure of estrogenic activity in the liver (6180).

Adverse Reactions

None reported.

Interactions with Herbs & Other Dietary Supplements

IRON, CALCIUM, MAGNESIUM: Theoretically, concomitant use may decrease mineral absorption due to tannin content (7).

Interactions with Drugs

METFORMIN (Glucophage): Raspberry leaf might reduce efficacy of metformin (Glucophage) (7). Raspberry leaf contains tannins that might decrease the absorption of metformin by forming insoluble complexes.
ORAL DRUGS: Theoretically, the tannin content of raspberry leaf may modify absorption of sedatives, hypnotics, antidepressants, and tranquilizers (19).

Interactions with Foods

None known.

Interactions with Lab Tests

None known.

Interactions with Diseases or Conditions

HORMONE SENSITIVE CANCERS/CONDITIONS: Because raspberry leaf might have estrogenic effects (6180), women with hormone sensitive conditions should avoid raspberry leaf. Some of these conditions include breast, uterine, and ovarian cancer, and endometriosis and uterine fibroids.

Dosage and Administration

ORAL: For facilitating labor, midwives typically prescribe raspberry leaf tea prepared by steeping 2 grams dried leaf in 240 mL of boiling water for 5 minutes and then straining (1122). Doses for other uses are typically one cup of tea up to 6 times daily. The tea is prepared by steeping 1.5 grams (approximately 2 teaspoons) of finely cut leaves in 150 mL boiling water 5 minutes and then straining (18). Alternatively, soak finely cut leaves in cold water for 2 hours and then strain (3). A liquid extract (1:1 in 25% alcohol) is also often used and dosed as 4-8 mL three times daily (4). Raspberry leaf tablets 2.4 grams per day have been used for reducing labor pains, starting at 32 weeks gestation through labor (9796).

Comments

Raspberry leaf extract has been used in Europe for centuries. The therapeutic use of raspberry leaf was first described in 1597 in The Herbal, or a General History of Plants (1096).

RED BUSH TEA

Also Known As

Kaffree Tea, Red Bush, Rooibos, Rooibos Tea.

Scientific Names

Aspalathus linearis, synonyms Aspalathus contaminatus, Borbonia pinifolia, Psoralea linearis.
Family: Fabaceae/Leguminosae.

People Use This For

Orally, red bush tea is used for HIV infection, preventing cancer, and improving cognitive function.
In foods, red bush tea is used as a beverage.

Safety

LIKELY SAFE ...when used orally as a beverage (6,4120).
PREGNANCY AND LACTATION: Insufficient reliable information available; avoid using.

Effectiveness

There is insufficient reliable information available for the effectiveness of red bush tea.

Mechanism of Action

Red bush tea contains polysaccharides (4120,4121), flavonoids (6,4122), a low amount of tannins (less than 5%) (5,6), and a relatively high amount of vitamin C (9.4%) (6). Some evidence suggests daily intake of acid polysaccharides found in the extracts of red bush tea might suppress HIV infection (4120,4121). Other information suggests the tea could prevent age-related changes to the central nervous system (4123) or suppress mutagenic activity (6).

Adverse Reactions

Orally, one report of salmonella contamination has occurred, possibly from lizard origin (6).

Interactions with Herbs & Other Dietary Supplements

None known.

Interactions with Drugs

None known.

Interactions with Foods

None known.

Interactions with Lab Tests

None known.

Interactions with Diseases or Conditions

None known.

Dosage and Administration

No typical dosage.

Comments

Tea is made from the branches and twigs of Aspalathus linearis. The fragrant, caffeine-free tea is the national drink of South Africa (5,6,7).

RED CLOVER

Also Known As

Beebread, Clovone, Cow Clover, Daidzein, Genistein, Isoflavone, Meadow Clover, Phytoestrogen, Purple Clover, Trefoil, Trifolium, Wild Clover.
CAUTION: See separate listings for Liverwort, Soy, and Sweet Clover.

Scientific Names

Trifolium pratense.
Family: Fabaceae/Leguminosae.

People Use This For

Orally, red clover is used for menopausal symptoms and hot flashes, cyclic breast pain or tenderness (mastalgia), premenstrual syndrome (PMS), cancer prevention, indigestion, whooping cough, cough, asthma, bronchitis, and sexually transmitted diseases (STDs).
Topically, red clover is used for cancerous growths, skin sores, burns, sore eyes, and chronic skin diseases including eczema and psoriasis.
In foods and beverages, the solid extract of red clover is used as a flavoring ingredient.

Safety

LIKELY SAFE ...when used orally in amounts commonly used in foods. Red clover has Generally Recognized As Safe status (GRAS) for use in foods in the US (4912,9553,10372).
POSSIBLY SAFE ...when used orally and appropriately in medicinal amounts. Red clover extracts seem to be safe when used for up to one year (3375,6127,8925).
There is insufficient reliable information available about the safety of the topical use of red clover.

PREGNANCY AND LACTATION: LIKELY SAFE ...when used orally in amounts commonly used in foods (4912).
LIKELY UNSAFE ...when used orally in medicinal amounts. Red clover has estrogenic activity (9553); avoid using. There is insufficient reliable information available about the safety of the topical use of red clover during pregnancy and lactation.

Effectiveness

POSSIBLY INEFFECTIVE

Hypercholesterolemia. Taking red clover extract orally for 12 weeks does not seem to significantly lower cholesterol in postmenopausal women with moderately elevated cholesterol levels (3375).

Menopausal symptoms. Taking red clover extract orally for 12 weeks does not seem to reduce menopausal symptoms such as hot flashes (8925,10975,10976,10991). One specific supplement that contains a high proportion of biochanin A and genistein (Promensil) might relieve hot flashes more quickly, but not more frequently that placebo (10991). Tell women red clover is unlikely to have much, if any, effect on hot flashes.

INSUFFICIENT RELIABLE EVIDENCE to RATE

Benign prostatic hyperplasia (BPH). Research suggests that red clover isoflavones 40-80 mg daily for three months might improve BPH. It seems to decrease nocturnal urinary frequency, international prostate symptom scores (IPSS), and to improve the quality of life in men with BPH. However, red clover isoflavones do not seem to affect urine flow rate, prostatic-specific antigen (PSA) values, or prostate size (6128).

Mastalgia. Preliminary evidence suggests that red clover might relieve cyclic mastalgia. Red clover isoflavones 40-80 mg daily seem to reduce breast pain and tenderness in 45% of patients (9552).

Osteoporosis. Preliminary evidence suggests that red clover isoflavones 40 mg daily for one year can significantly reduce the loss of spinal bone mineral density and bone mineral content (BMC) in pre- and perimenopausal women; however, red clover isoflavones don't seem to have this effect in postmenopausal women. Red clover also does not seem to affect hip bone density or mineral content (6127).

More evidence is needed to rate red clover for these uses.

Mechanism of Action

The applicable parts of red clover are the flowering tops. The flowering tops contain more than 100 different chemicals. Red clover contains isoflavones, a class of phytoestrogens, which are structurally similar to estrogens. The principal isoflavones found in red clover are biochanin A and formononetin. When ingested, biochanin A and formononetin are metabolized to the isoflavones genistein and daidzein, respectively (3375,3376). A substantial portion of the isoflavones are hydrolyzed by beta-glucosidases in the jejunum, releasing genistein and daidzein (3982).
A small amount of unhydrolyzed isoflavones still in the methyl form remains in circulation. The health effects of these methylated isoflavones have not been evaluated (9346). Red clover isoflavone constituents might act as selective estrogen-receptor modulators (SERMs), although genistein seems to act as a weak estrogen agonist (3376,8192). In premenopausal women with normal endogenous estrogen levels, isoflavones may have an anti-estrogen effect. In postmenopausal women with low endogenous estrogens, isoflavones are likely to act as weak estrogens (3387,3988,3989,3990,3994,6029). Isoflavones have a higher affinity for the beta estrogen receptor than the classical alpha estrogen receptor (3376,3983,3992,6029). The beta estrogen receptor predominates in the heart, vasculature, bone, and bladder, which may account for some of red clover's beneficial effects (7344,9346).
Osteoporosis in postmenopausal women is related to declining estrogen levels. Red clover is thought to be beneficial for preventing osteoporosis due to its weak estrogenic effects (3376,6029,6127). The isoflavone genistein also appears to directly inhibit osteoclast activity (9346).
Dietary phytoestrogens are associated with a reduced risk of endometrial cancer. Besides their effects on estrogen, phytoestrogenic substances in red clover might inhibit aromatase, which converts androstenedione to estrone. Increased estrone is associated with endometrial cancer (10372).
Red clover isoflavones might also have anticarcinogenic activity (4740,4742), possibly due to both estrogenic and nonestrogenic mechanisms (4741). The antiproliferative effects of the isoflavone genistein don't seem to be mediated by the estrogen receptors (ER) themselves since these effects occur both in ER-positive and ER-negative cell lines (9346).
Dietary intake of phytoestrogens among Western-culture middle-aged women doesn't seem to affect breast cancer risk, positively or negatively (11391). There is also evidence that taking a specific red clover extract (Promensil) 1 tablet/day for a year does not significantly affect breast tissue density based on mammography (13027).
For lowering cholesterol, the estrogenic effects of red clover isoflavones might be involved in modulating lipid metabolism. Red clover can also increase bile acid excretion and might up-regulate low-density lipoprotein (LDL) receptors (6029,6030,4738). Some researchers think red clover may play a role in preventing cardiovascular disease due to its potential effects on cholesterol levels, and associated preliminary evidence suggests that it might improve systemic arterial compliance (836,3375,9346). Research is conflicting regarding the effects of red clover on high-density lipoprotein (HDL) levels (9346).
Preliminary research suggests that red clover might affect the prostate. Animal research suggests that red clover might reduce prostate size by an anti-androgenic effect (11239). But preliminary clinical research hasn't shown any effect on prostate size (6128). Red clover seems to increase apoptosis (death) of prostate cells rather than affecting cell proliferation (11240). Laboratory research suggests that genistein, a red clover metabolite, decreases the growth of

both benign prostatic hyperplasia (BPH) and prostate cancer tissue (11238).
Red clover also contains the constituent coumestrol, which seems to have activity similar to diethylstilbestrol (DES) (4743). The coumarin constituents contained in red clover can have anticoagulant effects (10977).
There is some evidence that red clover isoflavones can inhibit oxidative and conjugative metabolism (4736). Isoflavones might also affect drug absorption and biliary excretion by interacting with multi-drug transporters such as the P-glycoproteins (4736). Given the wide range of drugs and metabolites whose pharmacokinetics depend on these mechanisms, drug interactions with isoflavones might be more common than literature reports suggest.
Genistein and daidzein are widely distributed in the body with peak concentrations at four to eight hours after short-term administration and excreted within 24 hours (3982). Chronic administration of supplemental red clover isoflavones results in a half-life of 13 to 16 hours, suggesting once daily dosing (8193). The absorption of isoflavones from food may be saturable, suggesting improved effect if ingested throughout the day (3982). Supplemental isoflavone bioavailability does not seem to be affected by foods source of isoflavones or other foods in the diet (3982).

Adverse Reactions

Orally, red clover is generally well tolerated (8925). It can cause rash-like reactions, myalgia, headache, nausea, and vaginal spotting (8194).
The ingestion of phytoestrogens in dietary amounts, 1 to 3 mg isoflavones per day, doesn't seem to increase the risk of endometrial cancer (10372).

Interactions with Herbs & Other Dietary Supplements

HERBS WITH ANTICOAGULANT/ANTIPLATELET POTENTIAL: Concomitant use of herbs that have constituents that might affect platelet aggregation could theoretically increase the risk of bleeding in some people (10977). Some of these herbs include angelica, clove, danshen, garlic, ginger, ginkgo, Panax ginseng, horse chestnut, turmeric, and others.
HERBS WITH ESTROGENIC ACTIVITY: Theoretically, red clover could be additive or antagonistic with other herbs that have estrogenic activity (3387,3988,3989,3990,3994,6029). These herbs include alfalfa, black cohosh, chasteberry, flaxseed, hops, ipriflavone, kudzu, licorice, and soy.

Interactions with Drugs

ANTICOAGULANT/ANTIPLATELET DRUGS: Theoretically, concomitant use with large amounts of red clover can increase the anticoagulant effects and bleeding risk due to its coumarin content (9553).
CONTRACEPTIVE DRUGS: Theoretically, concomitant use with large amounts of red clover might interfere with contraceptive drugs due to competition for estrogen receptors (4737,4743,9553).
CYTOCHROME P450 1A2 (CYP1A2) SUBSTRATES: There's preliminary evidence that red clover might inhibit cytochrome P450 1A2 (CYP1A2) (12479). So far, this interaction has not been reported in humans. However, watch for an increase in the levels of drugs metabolized by CYP1A2 in patients taking red clover. Some drugs metabolized by CYP1A2 include amitriptyline (Elavil), haloperidol (Haldol), ondansetron (Zofran), propranolol (Inderal), theophylline (Theo-Dur, others), verapamil (Calan, Isoptin, others), and others. Use red clover cautiously or avoid in patients taking these drugs.
CYTOCHROME P450 2C19 (CYP2C19) SUBSTRATES: There's preliminary evidence that red clover might inhibit cytochrome P450 2C19 (CYP2C19) (12479). So far, this interaction has not been reported in humans. However, watch for an increase in the levels of drugs metabolized by CYP2C19 in patients taking red clover. Some drugs metabolized by CYP2C19 include proton pump inhibitors including omeprazole (Prilosec), lansoprazole (Prevacid), and pantoprazole (Protonix); diazepam (Valium); carisoprodol (Soma); nelfinavir (Viracept); and others.
CYTOCHROME P450 2C9 (CYP2C9) SUBSTRATES: There's preliminary evidence that red clover might inhibit cytochrome P450 2C9 (CYP2C9) (12479). So far, this interaction has not been reported in humans. However, watch for an increase in the levels of drugs metabolized by CYP2C9 in patients taking red clover. Some drugs metabolized by CYP2C9 include nonsteroidal anti-inflammatory drugs (NSAIDs) such as diclofenac (Cataflam, Voltaren), ibuprofen (Motrin), meloxicam (Mobic), and piroxicam (Feldene); celecoxib (Celebrex); amitriptyline (Elavil); warfarin (Coumadin); glipizide (Glucotrol); losartan (Cozaar); and others. Use red clover cautiously or avoid in patients taking these drugs.
CYTOCHROME P450 3A4 (CYP3A4) SUBSTRATES: There's preliminary evidence that suggests that red clover may inhibit the cytochrome P450 3A4 (CYP3A4) isoenzymes (6450,9553,12479). Theoretically, red clover might increase the levels of drugs metabolized by CYP3A4. However, so far, this interaction has not been reported in humans. Some drugs metabolized by CYP3A4 include lovastatin (Mevacor), ketoconazole (Nizoral), itraconazole (Sporanox), fexofenadine (Allegra), triazolam (Halcion), and numerous others. Use red clover cautiously or avoid use in patients taking these drugs.
ESTROGENS: Theoretically, concomitant use of large amounts of red clover might interfere with hormone replacement therapy through competition for estrogen receptors (4737,4743,9553).
TAMOXIFEN (Nolvadex): There is some concern that red clover might interfere with tamoxifen because of its potential estrogenic effects. There is preliminary evidence that genistein, a constituent of red clover, might antagonize the antitumor effects of tamoxifen (8192). Tell patients taking tamoxifen to avoid red clover.

Interactions with Foods
None known.

Interactions with Lab Tests
None known.

Interactions with Diseases or Conditions
BREAST CANCER: There is some concern that red clover might increase the risk of breast cancer due to estrogenic isoflavone constituents. However, dietary intake of phytoestrogens among Western-culture middle-aged women doesn't seem to affect breast cancer risk, positively or negatively (11391). There is also evidence that taking a specific red clover extract (Promensil) 1 tablet/day for a year does not significantly affect breast tissue density based on mammography (13027).
COAGULATION DISORDERS: Use red clover with caution and avoid large amounts due to its coumarin content, which might increase the risk of bleeding (9553).
HORMONE SENSITIVE CANCERS/CONDITIONS: Because the isoflavones in red clover have estrogenic effects (4741,8192,9553), women with hormone sensitive conditions should avoid red clover. Some of these conditions include breast cancer, uterine cancer, ovarian cancer, endometriosis, and uterine fibroids.

Dosage and Administration
ORAL: For reducing hot flashes in postmenopausal women, a red clover isoflavone extract (Promensil) 40-160 mg per day has been used (8925,9553). For cyclic mastalgia, red clover isoflavones 40-80 mg daily has been used (9552).
TOPICAL: No typical dosage.

Comments
Red clover in large quantities induces sterility in livestock (4743). The cheetah population in zoos was threatened by reproductive failure and liver disease, thought to be caused by diets high in isoflavones (4735).

RED MAPLE

Also Known As
Bird's Eye Maple, Sugar Maple, Swamp Maple.

Scientific Names
Acer rubrum.
Family: Aceraceae.

Comments
At the date of publication, there was very little scientific information available about this product. Our staff is continually analyzing the available information on natural medicines and will add data to the online version of *Natural Medicines Comprehensive Database* as it becomes available. See www.naturaldatabase.com.

RED SANDALWOOD

Also Known As
Red Sanderswood, Red Saunders, Rubywood, Sandalwood Padauk, Santali lignum rubrum, Sappan.
CAUTION: See separate listings for White Sandalwood Oil and White Sandalwood wood.

Scientific Names
Pterocarpus santalinus.
Family: Fabaceae/Leguminosae.

Comments
At the date of publication, there was very little scientific information available about this product. Our staff is continually analyzing the available information on natural medicines and will add data to the online version of *Natural Medicines Comprehensive Database* as it becomes available. See www.naturaldatabase.com.

RED SOAPWORT

Also Known As

Bouncing-Bet, Saponariae rubrae radix, Soapwort.
CAUTION: See separate listing for White Soapwort.

Scientific Names

Saponaria officinalis.
Family: Caryophyllaceae.

People Use This For

Orally, red soapwort is used for inflammation of mucous membranes in the upper and lower respiratory tract.
Topically, red soapwort is used as a remedy for poison ivy, acne, psoriasis, eczema, and boils.
In manufacturing, red soapwort is used as an ingredient in soaps, herbal shampoos, and detergents.
It is used as a foaming agent in beer.

Safety

LIKELY SAFE ...when used topically. Red soapwort is widely used in soaps and shampoos (6) without reports of adverse effects.
POSSIBLY SAFE ...when used orally (2).
PREGNANCY AND LACTATION: Insufficient reliable information available; avoid using.

Effectiveness

There is insufficient reliable information available about the effectiveness of red soapwort.

Mechanism of Action

The applicable part of red soapwort is the root. The root contains saponin constituents that have expectorant effects. Saponins irritate the gastric mucosa, which then stimulate bronchial mucous secretion via the parasympathetic sensory pathways (7). In large amounts, red soapwort is cytotoxic (2).

Adverse Reactions

Orally, red soapwort can cause stomach irritation (2), nausea, and vomiting (7).

Interactions with Herbs & Other Dietary Supplements

None known.

Interactions with Drugs

None known.

Interactions with Foods

None known.

Interactions with Lab Tests

None known.

Interactions with Diseases or Conditions

GI MUCOSAL IRRITATION (e.g. ulcers, etc.): Red soapwort is contraindicated, because it can exacerbate existing GI mucosal irritation due to its saponin content (6).

Dosage and Administration

ORAL: The typical dose of red soapwort is 1.5 grams of the dried root per day as a tea or equivalent preparation (2).
TOPICAL: No typical dosage.

Comments

In the Middle Ages, Franciscan and Dominican monks viewed soapwort as a divine gift that was meant to keep them clean (6). Avoid confusion with white soapwort root.

RED YEAST

Also Known As

Hong Qu, Monascus, Red Rice Yeast, Red Yeast Rice, Xue Zhi Kang, Zhi Tai.
CAUTION: See separate listing for Beta-Sitosterol.

Scientific Names

Monascus purpureus; other Monascus species.
Family: Monascaceae.

People Use This For

Orally, red yeast is used for maintaining desirable cholesterol levels in healthy people, reducing cholesterol in people with hyperlipidemia, for indigestion, diarrhea, improving blood circulation, and for spleen and stomach health.
In foods, red yeast is used as a food coloring for Peking duck and other foods.

Safety

POSSIBLY SAFE ...when used orally and appropriately, short-term. Red yeast has been safely used in studies lasting up to 12 weeks (512,2624,6988,6990,6995,6996).
There is insufficient reliable information available about the safety of red yeast when used orally, long-term.
CHILDREN: POSSIBLY UNSAFE ...when used orally. Safety has not been established in children under 18 years of age and questions remain about the benefit of lowering cholesterol in children (512).
PREGNANCY: LIKELY UNSAFE ...when used orally. The red yeast constituent, lovastatin, has induced fetal skeletal malformations in animals (2619); avoid using.
LACTATION: Insufficient reliable information available; avoid using.

Effectiveness

LIKELY EFFECTIVE

Hypercholesterolemia. Taking red yeast orally can significantly lower total and low-density lipoprotein (LDL) cholesterol levels, and triglycerides when used for 8-12 weeks (2624,6990). The dose used most commonly is 2.4 grams per day, but a dose of 1.2 grams per day provides some benefit (6988). Some research suggests that red yeast might be as effective as simvastatin (Zocor) for improving lipid profiles (6993). Most studies used a specific proprietary red yeast product (Cholestin, Pharmanex).

POSSIBLY EFFECTIVE

HIV/AIDS. Taking red yeast orally seems to reduce lipids with dyslipidemia related to HIV infection (9475).

There is insufficient reliable information available about the effectiveness of red yeast for its other uses.

Mechanism of Action

Red yeast is the product of rice fermented with Monascus purpureus yeast (512). Red yeast supplements are different than red yeast rice sold in Chinese grocery stores (6994). Supplements are manufactured by culturing M. purpureus on rice at carefully-controlled temperature and growing conditions to increase the concentration of mevinic acids (6994). Red yeast contains ten mevinic acids, also known as monacolins, the highest concentration of which is constituted by lovastatin (also referred to as monacolin K or mevinolin) (512,2624,6988,9588). These compounds, which constitute about 0.4% of red rice, competitively inhibit 3-hydroxy-3-methyl-glutaryl-coenzyme A (HMG-CoA) reductase, blocking cholesterol biosynthesis (512,2624). Red yeast also contains sterols, including beta-sitosterol, campesterol, stigmasterol, and sapogenin; isoflavones and isoflavone glycosides; and monounsaturated fatty acids (2624,6988). Although the cholesterol lowering effect is likely partially caused by the lovastatin content, it is unclear to what extent. The overall cholesterol-lowering effect of red yeast is likely also the result of the combination of lovastatin, mevinic acids, and other constituents.
Red yeast that is not fermented correctly may contain citrinin. Citrinin is a toxin that may cause kidney failure (9588).

Adverse Reactions

Orally, red yeast can cause gastritis, abdominal discomfort, and elevated liver enzymes (512). In clinical studies, heartburn, flatulence, and dizziness were reported infrequently and did not result in study withdrawal (6988).
Anaphylaxis following inhalation of red yeast has also been reported (6997).
Like HMG-CoA reductase inhibitor (statins) drugs, red yeast may cause rhabdomyolysis, which is related to the mevinic acids that it contains (9587).
The contaminant citrinin may be found in some products containing red yeast. Citrinin is a nephrotoxin that results from incorrect rice fermentation processes (9588).

Interactions with Herbs & Other Dietary Supplements

CHOLESTEROL LOWERING HERBS/SUPPLEMENTS: Theoretically, red yeast might enhance the effects of herbs and supplements that also lower cholesterol. Some of these herbs and supplements include chromium, flaxseed, garlic, guar gum, niacin, oat bran, psyllium, and others.

COENZYME Q10 (CoQ10, Ubiquinone): Theoretically, red yeast can lower coenzyme Q10 levels. Red yeast contains the constituent lovastatin and related compounds, which can lower coenzyme Q10 levels (6983,6984,6985,6986).

GRAPEFRUIT: Concomitant use of red yeast (Cholestin) and grapefruit products can increase the serum levels of lovastatin, a constituent of red yeast. Grapefruit and grapefruit seed extract products can inhibit cytochrome P450 metabolism of lovastatin (527).

HEPATOTOXIC HERBS & SUPPLEMENTS: Theoretically, red yeast might enhance the adverse effects of potentially hepatotoxic herbs and supplements such as borage, chaparral, niacin, valerian, and uva ursi; avoid concurrent use.

HERBS/SUPPLEMENTS WITH THYROID ACTIVITY: Theoretically, red yeast might interfere with effects of herbs and supplements that affect thyroid function, including bugleweed, balm leaf, tiratricol, and wild thyme. Concomitant use of levothyroxine with the red yeast constituent lovastatin can also cause thyroid function abnormalities (15); avoid concurrent use.

ST. JOHN'S WORT: Theoretically, St. John's wort might reduce serum levels of red yeast. St. John's wort induces cytochrome P450 3A4 enzyme that can lower serum levels of the lovastatin constituent (1290).

Interactions with Drugs

ALCOHOL (Ethanol): Theoretically, alcohol may adversely affect liver function in patients taking red yeast, due to the lovastatin constituent (15).

CYCLOSPORINE (Neoral, Sandimmune): Theoretically, red yeast in combination with cyclosporine might increase the risk of myopathy due to the red yeast lovastatin constituent (15); use with caution.

CYTOCHROME P450 3A4 (CYP3A4) INHIBITORS: Theoretically, drugs that inhibit the cytochrome P450 3A4 (CYP3A4) enzymes might increase serum levels of red yeast constituents, such as lovastatin, and increase the risk of adverse effects. Drugs with this interaction include clarithromycin, erythromycin, itraconazole, ketoconazole, cimetidine, nefazodone, protease inhibitors, and others (6987).

GEMFIBROZIL (Lopid): Theoretically, red yeast in combination with gemfibrozil might increase the risk of myopathy due to the red yeast lovastatin constituent (15).

HMG-CoA REDUCTASE INHIBITORS ("Statins"): Using red yeast with these drugs might increase the risk of adverse effects without necessarily improving therapeutic benefit; avoid concomitant use. HMG-CoA reductase inhibitors include atorvastatin (Lipitor), cerivastatin (Baycol), fluvastatin (Lescol), lovastatin (Mevacor), pravastatin (Pravachol), and simvastatin (Zocor) (15).

LEVOTHYROXINE (Synthroid, Levothroid, Levoxyl, and others): Theoretically, concomitant use of levothyroxine with red yeast might cause thyroid function abnormalities due to the red yeast lovastatin constituent (15).

NIACIN: Theoretically, red yeast in combination with high-dose niacin might increase the risk of myopathy due to the red yeast lovastatin constituent (15).

Interactions with Foods

ALCOHOL: Theoretically, alcohol may adversely affect liver function in patients taking red yeast due to the lovastatin constituent (15).

FOOD: Food enhances the bioavailability of lovastatin (15), a constituent of red yeast.

GRAPEFRUIT JUICE: Concomitant use of grapefruit juice and lovastatin, a constituent of red yeast, can increase serum lovastatin levels and the risk of adverse effects (527).

Interactions with Lab Tests

CREATINE KINASE (CK): Red yeast might increase serum creatine kinase concentrations and test results due its lovastatin content. Lovastatin can increase serum creatine kinase concentrations and test results (15).

LIVER ENZYMES: Red yeast might increase serum liver transaminase concentrations and test results due to its lovastatin content. Lovastatin can increase serum liver transaminase concentrations and test results (15).

SERUM CHOLESTEROL: Red yeast can reduce serum cholesterol concentrations and test results. Red yeast contains a mixture of lovastatin and other HMG-CoA reductase inhibitors (2624).

Interactions with Diseases or Conditions

LIVER DYSFUNCTION: Red yeast is contraindicated in people with liver dysfunction, risk of liver dysfunction, or abnormal liver function test results (2619).

THYROID DYSFUNCTION: Concomitant use of lovastatin with levothyroxine can interfere with thyroid therapy (15).

Dosage and Administration

ORAL: Most clinical studies have used a specific brand product (Cholestin). However, most other red yeast brands contain a similar amount of red yeast, 600 mg. For hypercholesterolemia, a typical dose of red yeast is 1200 mg two times daily with food (2624). A total daily dose of 2400 mg red yeast contains approximately 9.6 mg total statins, of which 7.2 mg is lovastatin (2624). For dyslipidemia related to HIV infection, 1200 mg twice daily has been used (9475).

Comments

Red yeast is the product of rice fermented with the Monascus purpureus yeast that contains monacolin K (lovastatin, mevinolin) and other HMG-CoA reductase inhibiting compounds (512). Cholestin (Pharmanex) was one of the most widely studied red yeast products. But the FDA now considers red yeast to be an unapproved drug because it contains a prescription-only statin (6610). Cholestin has been reformulated and now contains policosanol as the active ingredient.

Red yeast should be treated as an HMG-CoA reductase inhibitor, with all the possible side effects, drug interactions, and precautions associated with this drug class. The American Heart Association has cautioned against using red yeast pending the results of long-term studies (6991).

Chemical assay indicates that red yeast products vary considerably in content and concentration of monacolin K and other monocolins (9588).

RED-SPUR VALERIAN

Also Known As

Bouncing Bess, Bovis and Soldier, Delicate Bess, Drunken Sailor, Fox's-Brush, Jupiter's Beard, Pretty Betsy, Red Spur Valerian, Red Valerian.

Scientific Names

Centranthus ruber, synonym Valeriana rubra.
Family: Valerianaceae.

Comments

At the date of publication, this product was not a common ingredient used in brand name supplements marketed to consumers. Details about this product are available in the online version of *Natural Medicines Comprehensive Database.* See www.naturaldatabase.com.

REED HERB

Also Known As

Common Reed, Ditch Reed, Giant Reed, Phragmites, Reed, Roseau Commun, Schilf.

Scientific Names

Phragmites australis, synonyms Phragmites communis, Arundo phragmites, Arundo vulgaris, Phragmites longivalvis, Phragmites vulgaris.
Family: Poaceae/Gramineae.

Comments

At the date of publication, there was very little scientific information available about this product. Our staff is continually analyzing the available information on natural medicines and will add data to the online version of *Natural Medicines Comprehensive Database* as it becomes available. See www.naturaldatabase.com.

REISHI MUSHROOM

Also Known As

Ling Chih, Ling Zhi, Mannentake, Mushroom of Immortality, Mushroom of Spiritual Potency, Rei-Shi, Reishi, Spirit Plant.

Scientific Names

Ganoderma lucidum.
Family: Ganodermataceae.

People Use This For

Orally, reishi mushroom is used for enhancing the immune system, lowering blood pressure and cholesterol, treating and preventing viral infections and tumors, treating inflammatory disease, cardiovascular disease, asthma and bronchial diseases. It is also used orally for reducing stress, as a kidney tonic, treating hepatitis and liver disease, supporting HIV disease, treating or preventing altitude sickness, and supporting chemotherapy. Other oral uses include preventing fatigue, treating insomnia, gastric ulcers, neurasthenia, poisoning, post-herpetic neuralgia, and herpes zoster pain.

In combination with other herbs, reishi mushroom is used to treat prostate cancer.

Safety

POSSIBLY SAFE ...when used orally and appropriately (12).

PREGNANCY AND LACTATION: Insufficient reliable information available; avoid using.

Effectiveness

There is insufficient reliable information available about the effectiveness of reishi mushroom.

Mechanism of Action

The applicable parts of reishi mushrooms are the fruiting body and mycelium (12). Reishi mushrooms have a long history in folk medicine, but researchers are just beginning to isolate and identify medicinal substances in reishi that have antitumor, immune modulating, anti-aging, cardiovascular, anticoagulant, cholesterol lowering, hypoglycemic, hepatoprotective, antiviral, and antibacterial effects (5476,5477,5481,5482,5483,5484,5485,5486,5487,5488,5489,5490,5491,5492). Protease inhibitors and other anti-HIV substances have been found in reishi mushrooms (5479,5480). Studies of these compounds have not been performed in humans. Reishi mushroom extracts contain high levels of adenosine (5478).

Adverse Reactions

Orally, reishi mushroom can cause dryness of the mouth, throat, and nasal area; itchiness; stomach upset; nosebleed; and bloody stools, which have occurred with extended oral use, 3 to 6 months (12). Also, a rash with the consumption of reishi wine and respiratory allergy to reishi spores can occur (12,5479).

Interactions with Herbs & Other Dietary Supplements

HERBS WITH ANTICOAGULANT/ANTIPLATELET POTENTIAL: Concomitant use of with herbs that have anticoagulant or antiplatelet activity could theoretically increase the risk of bleeding in some people (5476). These herbs include angelica, anise, arnica, clove, danshen, garlic, ginger, ginkgo, Panax ginseng, horse chestnut, red clover, turmeric, and others.

HERBS/SUPPLEMENTS WITH HYPOTENSIVE ACTIVITY: Theoretically, concurrent use might increase risk of hypotension with herbs that lower blood pressure (5488), including black cohosh, celery seed, Panax ginseng, and others.

Interactions with Drugs

ANTICOAGULANT/ANTIPLATELET DRUGS: Reishi may have anticoagulant effects (5476). Theoretically, taking reishi with other anticoagulant or antiplatelet drugs might increase the risk of bruising and bleeding. Some of these drugs include aspirin; clopidogrel (Plavix); nonsteroidal anti-inflammatory drugs (NSAIDs) such as diclofenac (Voltaren, Cataflam, others), ibuprofen (Advil, Motrin, others), naproxen (Anaprox, Naprosyn, others); dalteparin (Fragmin); enoxaparin (Lovenox); heparin, warfarin (Coumadin); and others.

ANTIHYPERTENSIVE DRUGS: Theoretically, concurrent use might increase risk of hypotension with drugs that lower blood pressure (5488). These include captopril (Capoten), enalapril (Vasotec), losartan (Cozaar), valsartan (Diovan), diltiazem (Cardizem), Amlodipine (Norvasc), hydrochlorothiazide (HydroDiuril), furosemide (Lasix), and many others.

Interactions with Foods

None known.

Interactions with Lab Tests

BLEEDING TIME: Theoretically, reishi mushroom use might prolong coagulation and bleeding time results (5476).

Interactions with Diseases or Conditions

HYPOTENSION: Theoretically, reishi mushroom use might worsen hypotension or interfere with drug therapy to increase blood pressure (5488).

THROMBOCYTOPENIA: Theoretically, reishi mushroom use might increase the risk of bleeding in people with thrombocytopenia (5476).

Dosage and Administration

ORAL: People typically use 1.5-9 grams orally per day of the crude dried mushroom, 1-1.5 grams per day of reishi powder, or 1 mL per day of reishi tincture (5473). Reishi tea is also used therapeutically (5473).

Comments

The flesh of Reishi is described as "tough" and "woody" with a bitter taste.

RESVERATROL

Also Known As

Cis-Resveratrol, Kojo-Kon, Phytoestrogen, Protykin, Resveratrols, Trans-Resveratrol.
CAUTION: See separate listings for Grape, Quercetin, and Wine.

Scientific Names

3,4',5-stilbenetriol; 3,5,4' -trihydroxystilbene; 3,4',5-trihydroxystilbene.

People Use This For

Orally, resveratrol is used for atherosclerosis, lowering cholesterol levels, increasing HDL cholesterol levels, and preventing cancer.

Safety

LIKELY SAFE ...when consumed in amounts found in foods (2030).
There is insufficient reliable information available about the safety of resveratrol when used in supplemental doses in amounts greater than those found in foods.
PREGNANCY AND LACTATION: LIKELY SAFE ...when used in amounts found in some foods (2030).
Resveratrol is found in grape skins, grape juice, wine, and other food sources. Wine should not be used as a source of resveratrol during pregnancy and lactation.

Effectiveness

There is insufficient reliable information available about the effectiveness of resveratrol.

Mechanism of Action

Resveratrol is a polyphenolic compound that exists in nature as cis- and trans- stereoisomers. Resveratrol is primarily found in red wine, red grape skins, purple grape juice, mulberries, and in smaller amounts in peanuts (513,2030,2956). Other sources include eucalyptus (Eucalyptus wandoo, Eucalyptus sideroxylon), spruce (Picea excelsa), and Bauhinia racemosa (2030). Polygonum cuspidatum, the roots of which are used in Chinese and Japanese traditional medicine, is considered to be one of the richest sources of trans-resveratrol (2030).
The trans-resveratrol content of wine is highly dependent on grape type, climate, and practices used to make the wine (9). White wines have very low trans-resveratrol concentrations. Pinot Noir consistently has the highest concentrations of trans-resveratrol, regardless of climate. Other red wines, including Cabernet Sauvignon, produced in cold, humid climates, such as Bordeaux and Canada, have higher trans-resveratrol content than those produced in hot, dry climates (2030). Unfermented grape juice does not contain resveratrol. Resveratrol is not found in significant quantities in fermented grape beverages that are stored in oak barrels, such as cognac (7864).
Resveratrol is rapidly absorbed with peak concentrations occurring within 30 minutes. Resveratrol is conjugated in the intestine and absorbed as the conjugated form. In plasma, resveratrol is found primarily as glucuronide or sulfate form. In vitro research has been done with unconjugated resveratrol. It is questionable whether free resveratrol absorption is sufficient to exert a pharmacologic effect. Research in humans suggests that quercetin taken orally doesn't reach serum concentrations at which in vitro activity has been seen (9174).
Resveratrol is a weak phytoestrogen (2960). It binds to both alpha and beta estrogen receptors, but its affinity for these receptors is about 7,000 times less than estrogen (7865).
Resveratrol decreases the activity of inflammatory cytokines, which suggests a mechanism for reducing mortality in cardiovascular diseases and cancer (6126). Early research suggests resveratrol might reduce the risk of cancer (2948,2959). Biological activity in humans has not yet been described (2030). Preliminary evidence suggests that trans-resveratrol has antioxidant and antimutagenic activity (2948). It may also inhibit tumor growth and promote apoptosis (2958,2959,12482). Preliminary evidence suggests that trans-resveratrol interferes with blood coagulation by inhibiting cyclooxygenases 1 and 2 (COX-1 and COX-2), hydroperoxidases, 5-lipoxygenase (2030,2948), and platelet aggregation (2949,2950,2951,2952,2961). It also causes blood vessel dilation (2954).
The anti-inflammatory effects of resveratrol also suggest potential usefulness for inflammatory diseases such as arthritis. Preliminary evidence suggests resveratrol is a more potent anti-inflammatory agent than either aspirin or ibuprofen (12483); resveratrol seems to inhibit COX-1 and COX-2 (12482,12484).
Resveratrol inhibits formation of cholesterol in certain strains of bacteria (7863), but it is not known if this contributes significantly to cholesterol lowering in humans. In human colon cancer cells, resveratrol inhibits cell division and function of RNA and DNA. These effects are reversible and cell growth resumes 40 hours after exposure (7861).
Preliminary data suggest that resveratrol may prevent liver cancer cells from invading local tissues (7862). Resveratrol inhibits the replication of herpes simplex virus. Although the mechanism of this action is not fully known, exposure to resveratrol within one hour of cellular infection appears to be most effective in arresting viral growth. This suggests that resveratrol reduces production of proteins needed to regulate viral proliferation (7866).

The activity of cytochrome P450 (CYP450) enzymes is inhibited by resveratrol in hepatocytes (7864). Whether this action interferes with metabolism of drugs in humans is not known.

Adverse Reactions

None reported.

Interactions with Herbs & Other Dietary Supplements

HERBS WITH ANTICOAGULANT/ANTIPLATELET POTENTIAL: Theoretically, concomitant use of resveratrol with herbs that have anticoagulant or antiplatelet activity could increase the risk of bleeding in some people (2949,2950,2951,2952,2961). These herbs include angelica, clove, danshen, feverfew, garlic, ginger, ginkgo, ginseng Panax, horse chestnut, red clover, turmeric, and others.

Interactions with Drugs

ANTICOAGULANT/ANTIPLATELET DRUGS: Resveratrol seems to have antiplatelet effects (2949,2950,2951,2952,2961). Theoretically, taking resveratrol with other antiplatelet or anticoagulant drugs might increase the risk of bruising and bleeding. Some of these drugs include aspirin; clopidogrel (Plavix); nonsteroidal anti-inflammatory drugs (NSAIDs) such as diclofenac (Voltaren, Cataflam, others), ibuprofen (Advil, Motrin, others), naproxen (Anaprox, Naprosyn, others); dalteparin (Fragmin); enoxaparin (Lovenox); heparin; warfarin (Coumadin); and others.

CYTOCHROME P450 3A4 (CYP3A4) SUBSTRATES: Preliminary evidence shows that resveratrol might inhibit the cytochrome P450 enzymes, CYP3A, CYP1A, and CYP2E1 (7864). Theoretically, it might increase levels of drugs metabolized by these enzymes. However, this interaction has not been reported in humans. Some drugs metabolized by CYP3A include lovastatin (Mevacor), ketoconazole (Nizoral), itraconazole (Sporanox), fexofenadine (Allegra), triazolam (Halcion), and numerous others. Use resveratrol cautiously or avoid in patients taking these drugs.

Interactions with Foods

None known.

Interactions with Lab Tests

None known.

Interactions with Diseases or Conditions

HORMONE SENSITIVE CANCERS/CONDITIONS: Because resveratrol might have estrogenic effects (2960), women with hormone sensitive conditions should avoid resveratrol. Some of these conditions include breast, uterine, and ovarian cancer, and endometriosis and uterine fibroids.

Dosage and Administration

No typical dosage.

RHATANY

Also Known As

Brazilian Rhatany, Krameria, Mapato, Peruvian Rhatany, Pumacuchu, Raiz Para Los Dientes, Ratanhiae radix, Ratanhiawurzel, Red Rhatany, Rhatanhia, Rhatania.

Scientific Names

Krameria lappacea, synonyms Krameria triandra, Krameria iluca; Krameria argentea.
Family: Krameriaceae.

People Use This For

Orally, rhatany is used as an antidiarrheal agent for enteritis and angina.
Topically, rhatany is used for mild inflammation of the oral and pharyngeal mucosa, inflammation of the gums, fissures of the tongue, stomatitis, pharyngitis, non-infectious canker sores, chilblains, and leg ulcers.

Safety

POSSIBLY SAFE ...when used topically short-term (2,12). Use should be limited to two weeks unless medical evaluation determines that there is no problem and use can continue (2).
There is insufficient reliable information available about the safety of rhatany for its other uses.
PREGNANCY AND LACTATION: Insufficient reliable information available; avoid using.

Effectiveness

There is insufficient reliable information available about the effectiveness of rhatany.

Mechanism of Action

The applicable part of rhatany is the root. Rhatany contains high concentrations of proanthocyanidin tannins (10% to 15%), which are responsible for the observed astringent properties (2,3,18,4100). The alcohol in the tincture preparation may enhance astringent effects (272). Astringents precipitate the surface proteins of cells decreasing the cell size (4101) and secretions from the inflamed tissues (272), diminishing inflammation. Astringents also have the ability to alleviate inflammation by constricting the blood vessels and reducing the supply of blood to the affected area (272).

Adverse Reactions

Orally, rhatany can cause digestive complaints (18).
Topically, allergic mucous membrane reactions have occurred rarely with rhatany (2,18).

Interactions with Herbs & Other Dietary Supplements

None known.

Interactions with Drugs

ORAL DRUGS: Theoretically, concomitant oral administration may cause precipitation of some drugs due to the high tannin content of rhatany. Separate administration of oral drugs and tannin-containing herbs by the longest period of time practical (19).

Interactions with Foods

None known.

Interactions with Lab Tests

None known.

Interactions with Diseases or Conditions

ALLERGY: Contraindicated in people with rhatany allergy.

Dosage and Administration

ORAL: Rhatany is sometimes taken as a decoction of 1 gram of the herb in 1 cup of water or as 5-10 drops of the tincture in one glass of water (6002).
TOPICAL: As mouth wash or gargle (simmer 1-1.5 grams of powdered root in 150 mL boiling water 10-15 minutes, strain) two to three times daily (8). As mouth wash or gargle, 5-10 drops of rhatany tincture in one glass of water two to three times daily (8). Undiluted rhatany tincture (oral paint) used directly on the affected area two to three times daily (2). Limit rhatany use to maximum two weeks without medical evaluation (2).

Comments

Avoid confusion with roots of other Krameria species (18). Rhatany (Krameria triandra) root is difficult to find and adulteration is common with other Krameria species (8).

RHUBARB

Also Known As

Chinese Rhubarb, Da Huang, Garden Rhubarb, Himalayan Rhubarb, Indian Rhubarb, Medicinal Rhubarb, Rhei, Rhei radix, Rheum, Turkey Rhubarb.

Scientific Names

Rheum officinale; Rheum palmatum; Rheum tanguticum; Rheum australe, synonym Rheum emodi; Rheum hybridum, synonyms Rheum cultorum, Rheum rhabarbarum, Rheum rhaponticum.
Family: Polygonaceae.

People Use This For

Orally, rhubarb is used for constipation, diarrhea, dyspepsia, gastritis, gastrointestinal (GI) bleeding, preparation for GI diagnostic procedures after recto-anal surgery, for bowel movement relief when anal fissures are present, and for hemorrhoids.
Topically, rhubarb is used for herpes labialis (cold sores).
In foods, rhubarb stems are edible. Rhubarb is also used as a flavoring agent.

Safety

LIKELY SAFE ...when the root is used in amounts commonly found in foods. Chinese and garden rhubarb have Generally Recognized As Safe status (GRAS) for use in foods in the US (4912).
POSSIBLY SAFE ...when used orally and appropriately in medicinal amounts for less than eight days (10436).
...when used topically, and appropriately (10437).
CHILDREN: POSSIBLY UNSAFE ...when used orally. Rhubarb root or rhizome should not be used in children under age 12 (12). There is one report of a 4-year-old who ingested rhubarb leaves (containing oxalic acid) and died (17).
PREGNANCY AND LACTATION: POSSIBLY UNSAFE ...when used in medicinal amounts, rhubarb is a stimulant laxative; avoid using (12).

Effectiveness

POSSIBLY EFFECTIVE

Herpes labialis (cold sores). Applying rhubarb topically in combination with sage (Salvia officinalis) seems to improve herpes labialis (cold sores). Treatment of herpes labialis with a cream containing rhubarb and sage may be about as effective as acyclovir (Zovirax) cream. Acyclovir cream heals lesions in about 6.3 days; the rhubarb and sage cream heals lesions in about 7.2 days (10437).

INSUFFICIENT RELIABLE EVIDENCE to RATE

Gastrointestinal bleeding. Preliminary clinical evidence suggests that oral rhubarb powder might be useful for treating gastrointestinal bleeding (10436). More evidence is needed to rate rhubarb for this use.

Mechanism of Action

The applicable parts of rhubarb are the rhizome and root. The active constituents include hydroxyanthracene derivatives, anthraquinones, tannins, and calcium oxalate (18,10437). At low doses, the tannin effects predominate and have an astringent effect on the gastrointestinal (GI) tract that relieves diarrhea (7). At higher doses, anthraquinone effects seem to predominate, producing a stimulant laxative effect that relieves constipation (7).

Adverse Reactions

Orally, rhubarb can cause cramp-like or spasmodic gastrointestinal (GI) discomfort, watery diarrhea, and uterine contractions; there is also one report of anaphylaxis with short-term use (18). Chronic use or abuse of rhubarb can cause electrolyte loss (especially potassium), hyperaldosteronism, accelerated bone deterioration, albuminuria, hematuria, dehydration, inhibition of gastric motility, pseudomelanosis coli (pigment spots in intestinal mucosa), arrhythmias, muscular weakness, nephropathies, and edema (12). Chronic use of anthroid laxatives can cause pseudomelanosis coli, which is harmless, usually reverses with discontinuation, and is not associated with an increased risk of developing colorectal ademoma or carcinoma (6138).

Interactions with Herbs & Other Dietary Supplements

CALCIUM, IRON, ZINC: Concurrent use might decrease mineral absorption. Rhubarb contains oxalates, which can bind multivalent metal ions in the gastrointestinal (GI) tract and decrease mineral absorption (12).
CARDIAC GLYCOSIDE-CONTAINING HERBS: Overuse of rhubarb might cause potassium depletion, increasing the risk of cardiac toxicity (500). Cardiac glycoside-containing herbs include black hellebore, Canadian hemp root, digitalis leaf, hedge mustard, figwort, lily-of-the-valley roots, motherwort, oleander leaf, pheasant's eye plant, pleurisy root, squill bulb leaf scales, and strophanthus seeds.
CARDIOACTIVE HERBS: Overuse of rhubarb might cause potassium depletion, increasing risk of toxicity of cardioactive herbs (4). These include calamus, cereus, cola, coltsfoot, devil's claw, European mistletoe, fenugreek, fumitory, ginger, Panax ginseng, hawthorn, mate, parsley, quassia, scotch broom flower, shepherd's purse, white horehound, and wild carrot.
LICORICE/HORSETAIL: Theoretically, concomitant use with horsetail plant or licorice rhizome increases the risk of potassium depletion (19).
STIMULANT LAXATIVE HERBS: Theoretically, concomitant use with other stimulant laxative herbs may increase the risk of potassium depletion (19). Stimulant laxative herbs include aloe dried leaf sap, blue flag rhizome, alder buckthorn, European buckthorn, butternut bark, cascara bark, castor oil, colocynth fruit pulp, gamboge bark exudate, jalap root, black root, manna bark exudate, podophyllum root, senna leaves and pods, wild cucumber fruit (Ecballium elaterium), and yellow dock root.

Interactions with Drugs

CORTICOSTEROIDS: Overuse of rhubarb might compound corticosteroid-induced potassium loss (2).
DIGOXIN (Lanoxin): Overuse of rhubarb might cause potassium depletion, increasing the risk of digoxin toxicity (19).
DIURETIC DRUGS: Overuse of rhubarb might compound diuretic-induced potassium loss (19). There is concern that people receiving rhubarb along with potassium depleting diuretics might be at an increased risk for hypokalemia. Initiation of potassium supplementation or an increase in potassium supplement dose may be necessary for some patients. Some diuretics that can deplete potassium include chlorothiazide (Diuril), chlorthalidone (Thalitone), furosemide (Lasix), and hydrochlorothiazide (HCTZ, Hydrodiuril, Microzide), and others.

ORAL DRUGS: Concomitant use might reduce absorption of drugs due to reduced gastrointestinal transit time (500).
STIMULANT LAXATIVES: Concomitant use might compound fluid and electrolyte loss.

Interactions with Foods

CALCIUM, IRON, ZINC: Concurrent use might decrease mineral absorption from foods. Rhubarb contains oxalates (7,12), which can bind multivalent metal ions in the gastrointestinal tract and decrease mineral absorption.

Interactions with Lab Tests

URINE TESTS: Rhubarb might discolor urine and interfere with diagnostic tests (2).

Interactions with Diseases or Conditions

CONSTIPATION, DIARRHEA: Rhubarb can exacerbate diarrhea or constipation depending on the preparation used (12).
GASTROINTESTINAL (GI) CONDITIONS: Rhubarb is contraindicated in cases of intestinal obstruction; appendicitis; abdominal pain of unknown origin; and inflammatory conditions of the intestines including Crohn's disease, colitis, and irritable bowel syndrome (IBS) (12).
KIDNEY STONES (Nephrolithiasis): Rhubarb contains calcium oxalate. Use it with caution in people with a history of kidney stones (12).

Dosage and Administration

ORAL: Rhubarb is used short-term only, ideally for less than eight days (12). For constipation, 1-4 grams of the dried root has been used daily (7). For diarrhea, 100-300 mg of the dried root has been used daily (7).
TOPICAL: For treatment of herpes labialis (cold sores), a cream containing 23 mg/gram each of rhubarb extract and sage extract has been applied every 2 to 4 hours while awake, with treatment starting within one day of symptoms and continuing for 10 to 14 days (10437).

RIBOFLAVIN (VITAMIN B2)

Also Known As

B Complex Vitamin, Flavin, Flavine, Lactoflavin, Riboflavin 5' Phosphate, Vitamin B2, Vitamin G.

Scientific Names

Riboflavin; Vitamin B2.

People Use This For

Orally, riboflavin is used for preventing riboflavin deficiency, treating ariboflavinosis, preventing migraine headaches, treating acne, congenital methemoglobinemia, muscle cramps, burning feet syndrome, carpal tunnel syndrome, red blood cell aplasia, multiple acylcoenzyme A dehydrogenase deficiency, eye fatigue, cataracts, and glaucoma. It is also used orally for increasing energy levels; boosting immune system function; maintaining healthy hair, skin, mucous membranes, and nails; for slowing aging; canker sores; memory loss including Alzheimer's disease; ulcers; boosting athletic performance; promoting healthy reproductive function; burns; alcoholism; liver disease; sickle cell anemia; and for treating lactic acidosis induced by nucleoside analog reverse transcriptase inhibitor (NRTI) drugs.

Safety

LIKELY SAFE ...when used orally. No toxic effects have been reported (1396,1397,1398).
PREGNANCY: LIKELY SAFE ...when used orally at the recommended dietary allowance (RDA) of 1.4 mg per day (3094). There is insufficient reliable information about the safety of using larger amounts during pregnancy.
LACTATION: LIKELY SAFE ...when used orally at the recommended dietary allowance (RDA) of 1.6 mg per day (3094). There is insufficient reliable information about the safety of using larger amounts during lactation.

Effectiveness

EFFECTIVE

Ariboflavinosis. Taking riboflavin orally prevents riboflavin deficiency and improves ariboflavinosis (15).

POSSIBLY EFFECTIVE

Cataracts. Taking riboflavin orally seems to reduce the occurrence of cataracts. A large-scale population-based study found that high dietary intake of riboflavin is associated with a reduced risk of nuclear cataracts (6378).

Migraine headache. Taking high dose riboflavin 400 mg/day seems to significantly reduce the frequency of migraine headache attacks (1397,1398,12387). Some evidence suggests that riboflavin might be as effective for reducing migraine headache frequency as the beta-blockers, bisoprolol (Zebeta) and metoprolol (Lopressor) (1396). However, there is some conflicting evidence. Taking a specific combination product providing riboflavin 400 mg, magnesium 300 mg, and feverfew 100 mg does not seem to reduce the frequency or severity of migraine any better than placebo. However, study design problems suggest that more research is needed on this combination (12389).

Taking riboflavin does not appear to reduce the severity or duration of an acute migraine headache (1398).

INSUFFICIENT RELIABLE EVIDENCE to RATE

AIDS-related lactic acidosis. There is preliminary clinical evidence that riboflavin may be useful for treating lactic acidosis in patients with acquired immunodeficiency syndrome (AIDS) caused by nucleoside analog reverse transcriptase inhibitors (NRTI) (2024,10468). More evidence is needed to rate riboflavin for this use.

Mechanism of Action

Riboflavin is an essential B vitamins (vitamin B2). It is required for tissue respiration. It is converted to the coenzyme riboflavin 5-phosphate (flavin mononucleotide, FMN) and then to the coenzyme flavin adenine dinucleotide (FAD). These act as hydrogen carriers for several enzymes known as flavoproteins, which are involved in oxidation-reduction reactions of organic substrates and in intermediary metabolism (15). It is also indirectly involved in maintaining erythrocyte integrity. Riboflavin deficiency, or ariboflavinosis, is characterized by cheilosis, angular stomatitis, glossitis, sore throat, keratitis, scrotal skin changes, neuropathy, and seborrheic dermatitis. In severe cases there is a normocytic and normochromic anemia (15).

Riboflavin deficiency can occur in people with long-standing infections such as HIV, liver disease, alcoholism, and malignancy (15). Researchers think that riboflavin deficiency might contribute to lactic acidosis that can occur in HIV patients taking stavudine (d4T, Zerit), zidovudine (AZT, Retrovir) and similar nucleoside analog reverse transcriptase inhibitor (NRTI) drugs (2024). Although NRTI-induced lactic acidosis has been considered irreversible and fatal, riboflavin reportedly can reverse this condition in some patients (2024).

Adverse Reactions

Orally, large doses of riboflavin (400 mg per day) might cause diarrhea and polyuria (1398). Riboflavin can cause a yellow-orange discoloration of the urine (15).

Interactions with Herbs & Other Dietary Supplements

IRON: Riboflavin supplements may improve the hematological response to iron supplements in some people with anemia. Riboflavin is thought to be involved in mobilizing iron from the storage form ferritin, for heme and globin synthesis (9518). This effect is probably only significant in people with riboflavin deficiency.

Interactions with Drugs

ANTICHOLINERGIC DRUGS: The rate of supplemental riboflavin absorption is decreased, but the total amount of the vitamin absorbed is increased, by drugs with anticholinergic effects. These drugs reduce gut motility, increasing the time the vitamin is present at absorption sites in the intestine (10513,10514). This has been demonstrated with propantheline (Pro-Banthine), but could theoretically occur with any drug that has anticholinergic effects. The clinical significance isn't known.

PHENOBARBITAL (Luminal): Phenobarbital induces metabolism of riboflavin in the liver. Levels of the active form of riboflavin, flavin adenine dinucleotide (FAD), are increased in the liver and levels of a hydroxylated metabolite are increased in the urine (10534,10535). The clinical significance of this isn't clear.

PROBENECID (Benemid): Probenecid reduces renal tubular secretion and total urinary excretion of both supplemental and dietary riboflavin (10515,10516,10517). It may also reduce the active intestinal absorption mechanism for riboflavin (10516). After single doses of probenecid, the effect on renal excretion predominates and plasma riboflavin levels are increased (10516,10517). The effect of prolonged probenecid therapy on riboflavin balance, and therefore the clinical significance, isn't known.

PSYLLIUM: Psyllium reduces absorption of supplemental riboflavin in healthy women (10094). It isn't clear whether this occurs with dietary riboflavin, or whether it's clinically significant. Products containing psyllium include Metamucil, Konsyl, and Perdiem.

TRICYCLIC ANTIDEPRESSANTS: Tricyclic antidepressants have structural similarities to riboflavin and can interfere with its conversion to the active form flavin adenine dinucleotide (FAD) (10518). In animal models, very high doses of amitriptyline and imipramine (50 mg/kg/day) decrease FAD levels in the liver, heart and brain. Lower doses (10 mg/kg/day) only affect the heart (10519). Since these doses are higher than those used therapeutically in humans, it's unlikely that the effect is clinically significant, or that supplements are necessary.

Drug Influences on Nutrient Levels and Depletion

SOME DRUGS CAN AFFECT RIBOFLAVIN LEVELS:

ANTIBIOTICS: Interference with the normal gastrointestinal flora by antibiotics may reduce bacterial synthesis of riboflavin (4437). However, this synthesis doesn't seem to significantly contribute to the body's supply of riboflavin, which is primarily obtained from dietary sources in the small intestine (6243,9530). Riboflavin supplements aren't necessary during antibiotic therapy.

CHLORPROMAZINE (Thorazine): Chlorpromazine has structural similarities to riboflavin and can interfere with its conversion to the active form, flavin adenine dinucleotide (FAD) (10518). In rats, chlorpromazine decreases FAD levels in the liver, kidneys, heart and skeletal muscle, increases urinary riboflavin excretion, and produces changes in erythrocyte enzyme activity consistent with riboflavin deficiency (10518,10519,10520,10521). Chlorpromazine also inhibits renal tubular secretion and reabsorption of riboflavin (10515). Although these effects occur in rats at similar doses to those used in humans, data in humans are lacking. There isn't enough evidence to recommend use of riboflavin supplements with chlorpromazine or other phenothiazines.

DOXORUBICIN (Adriamycin, Rubex): Preliminary evidence indicates that doxorubicin interacts with riboflavin by forming complexes, competing for tissue binding sites, reducing conversion to flavin adenine dinucleotide (FAD, the active form of riboflavin), and increasing urinary excretion (9533,10528,10529,10530). These effects may contribute to cardiac and muscle toxicity associated with doxorubicin, but data in humans are lacking.

ORAL CONTRACEPTIVES: Oral contraceptives may interfere with the absorption of riboflavin, or its conversion to active coenzyme forms (9505,10525). However, studies are conflicting. Some have found reduced levels of flavin adenine dinucleotide (FAD, the active form of riboflavin), reduced urinary riboflavin excretion, or reduced erythrocyte glutathione reductase activity consistent with riboflavin deficiency, in women taking oral contraceptives (4548,10523,10524,10525). However, many of these studies involved women with marginal or deficient dietary riboflavin intake, who used high-dose oral contraceptives (50 mcg ethinyl estradiol/day). When dietary riboflavin intake is adequate, no interaction with oral contraceptives is found (9373,10526,10527,10536). Routine riboflavin supplementation isn't necessary in women taking oral contraceptives.

QUINACRINE: Quinacrine has structural similarities to riboflavin and can interfere with its conversion to the active form flavin adenine dinucleotide (FAD) (505,10521). It's suggested that this could lead to riboflavin deficiency in humans, but it may also contribute to the therapeutic effects of quinacrine against malaria (10522). The clinical significance isn't known.

Interactions with Foods

FOOD: Absorption of riboflavin supplements may be increased when taken with food because bile salts facilitate intestinal uptake of riboflavin (9530). However, the absorption mechanism for riboflavin is saturable; therefore, the clinical significance isn't clear.

Interactions with Lab Tests

ACETOACETATE DECARBOXYLASE: Riboflavin can falsely increase serum acetoacetate decarboxylase test results due to enzyme activation (275).

CATECHOLAMINES: Riboflavin can falsely elevate plasma and urine fluorometric catecholamine test results due to fluorescent metabolites in the plasma and urine (275).

COLORIMETRIC TESTS: Large amounts of riboflavin can interfere with urinalysis based on spectrometry or color reactions. Large amounts of riboflavin cause bright yellow urine (275).

DIAGNEX BLUE EXCRETION: Riboflavin can falsely increase urine Diagnex blue excretion test results, by color interference (275).

DRUGS-OF-ABUSE ASSAYS: Large doses of riboflavin (200 mg twice daily) cause errors in Abbott TDx drugs-of-abuse urine assays. Riboflavin produces a fluorophore that competes with the fluorescein-labeled antibody used in the assay (1266).

UROBILINOGEN: Riboflavin can falsely increase plasma and urine fluorometric urobilinogen test results, due to fluorescent metabolites in the plasma and urine (275).

Interactions with Diseases or Conditions

HEPATITIS, CIRRHOSIS, BILIARY OBSTRUCTION: Riboflavin absorption is decreased in these conditions (15).

Dosage and Administration

ORAL: As a dietary supplement, 1-4 mg a day is generally sufficient (15). For riboflavin deficiency in adults, 5-30 mg is taken daily in divided doses (15). For preventing migraine headaches, a dose of 400 mg per day has been used (1396,1397,1398), and maximum benefit might take up to three months to achieve (1398). A daily dietary intake of approximately 2.6 mg of riboflavin has been associated with reduced risk of nuclear cataracts (6378).

The daily recommended dietary allowances (RDAs) of riboflavin are: Infants 0-6 months, 0.3 mg; Infants 7-12 months, 0.4 mg; Children 1-3 years, 0.5 mg; Children 4-8 years, 0.6 mg; Children 9-13 years, 0.9 mg; Men 14 years or older, 1.3 mg; Women 14-18 years, 1 mg; Women over 18 years, 1.1 mg; Pregnant women, 1.4 mg; and Lactating women, 1.6 mg (3094). For treating stavudine or zidovudine-induced lactic acidosis, 50 mg per day has been used (2024,6132).

Comments

Riboflavin is found in many foods including milk, meat, eggs, nuts, enriched flour, and green vegetables (15).

Riboflavin is frequently used in combination with other B vitamins in vitamin B complex formulations. Vitamin B complex generally includes vitamin B1 (thiamine), vitamin B2 (riboflavin), vitamin B3 (niacin/niacinamide), vitamin B5 (pantothenic acid), vitamin B6 (pyridoxine), vitamin B12 (cyanocobalamin), and folic acid. However, some products do not contain all of these ingredients and some may include others, such as biotin, para-aminobenzoic acid (PABA), choline bitartrate, and inositol (3022).

RIBOSE

Also Known As
D-ribose.

Scientific Names
Beta-D-ribofuranose.

People Use This For
Orally, ribose is used to increase muscle function, recovery, athletic performance, boost muscle tissue energy, and enhance effectiveness of creatine, maximize ribose production, replenish ATP stores, and improve or maintain nucleotide salvage and/or synthesis in heart and skeletal muscles following high intensity exercise. It has also been used to improve exercise tolerance, maintain or increase energy stores in the heart or muscle cells, and improve quality of life in individuals with reduced myocardial blood flow such as improving the heart's tolerance to ischemia in patients with coronary artery disease. Oral ribose has been used to prevent symptoms such as cramping, pain, and stiffness after exercise in patients with myoadenylate deaminase deficiency (MAD), also known as AMP deaminase deficiency (AMPD deficiency). Ribose has also been used orally to improve exercise tolerance in patients with McArdle's disease.

Intravenously, ribose has been used to facilitate thallium-201 redistribution and improve imaging of ischemic myocardium in patients with coronary artery disease. It has also been used intravenously in patients with MAD to prevent symptoms such as cramping, pain, and stiffness.

Safety
POSSIBLY SAFE ...when used orally or intravenously and appropriately, short-term (5662,5663,5664,5676,5677,5679,5680). There is insufficient reliable information available about the safety of ribose for its other uses.

PREGNANCY AND LACTATION: Insufficient reliable information available; avoid using.

Effectiveness
POSSIBLY EFFECTIVE

Coronary artery disease. Taking ribose orally seems to be effective for improving the heart's tolerance to ischemia in patients with coronary artery disease. A small randomized and placebo controlled study showed increased time to onset of moderate angina and time to ST depression during treadmill walking exercise testing in patients with coronary artery disease (5664).

Myoadenylate deaminase deficiency (MAD). Taking ribose orally or intravenously seems to be effective for preventing symptoms such as cramping, pain and stiffness after exercise in patients with MAD, also known as AMP deaminase deficiency (AMPD deficiency). One case report and a small clinical study suggest symptoms can be prevented with administration of ribose before and during exercise (5677,5679).

LIKELY INEFFECTIVE

McArdle's disease. Taking ribose orally doesn't improve exercise tolerance in patients with McArdle's disease (5678).

There is insufficient reliable information available about the effectiveness of ribose for its other uses.

Mechanism of Action
Ribose, a pentose sugar which is usually supplied by the oxidative pentose phosphate pathway (PPP) (also known as the hexose monophosphate shunt), is rapidly taken up by cells and phosphorylated to ribose-5-phosphate (5653). Ribose is rate-limiting in the production of phosphoribosyl-pyrophosphate (PRPP) (5652,5653,5682), a precursor for the salvage and de-novo adenine nucleotide synthetic pathways which maintain adenine, ADP, and AMP levels for the resynthesis of ATP (5651,5652,5665,5682). High energy bonds of ATP are the direct source for myocardial contractions (5652). During ischemia, the levels of ATP in the myocardium fall as the rate of oxidative phosphorylation decreases (5651,5653) and do not recover if the period of no perfusion is too long (5651). ADP and AMP levels rise transiently during ischemia but decrease as they are dephosphorylated into metabolites (adenine, inosine, and hypoxanthine), which easily diffuse through the cell membrane and are washed out of the myocardium during reperfusion (5652,5653). Since the metabolites, which use the salvage synthetic pathway are no longer available as precursors for ATP resynthesis, the de-novo synthetic pathway is activated (5652). Restoration of ATP levels via this pathway is slow in comparison to the salvage pathway (5652,5664) due to the short supply of PRPP, which is usually supplied by the oxidative pentose phosphate pathway (5664). Studies suggest that this also occurs during ischemic events after high intensity exercise in skeletal muscle (5656,5657,5658). Evidence suggests exogenous ribose bypasses the PPP when it is converted to ribose-5-phosphate, increasing the amount of PRPP available for the de-novo synthetic pathway and ultimately resulting in the repletion of ATP levels in the myocardium (5652). Animal studies suggest exogenous ribose with adenine improves myocardial ATP, ADP, and adenine nucleotide recovery after moderate periods of ischemia and improves recovery of contractile myocardial function (5652,5653). Other animal studies suggest exogenous ribose given during both periods of ischemia and reperfusion significantly increases ATP levels (5659) and may shorten ATP recovery time (5654,5659,5660). There have been no human studies done to confirm these findings. Laboratory evidence also suggests ribose may have a role in preserving hearts for transplantation by

maintaining ATP levels (5666). Controlled human studies have established that infusion of ribose facilitates the distribution and accelerates the clearance of thallium-201 from normal (nonischemic) regions of the coronary artery, leaving only thallium-201 in ischemic myocardium (5662,5663). The mechanism of action on how this occurs is unknown (5662). A small, randomized, placebo study controlled reported oral ribose given to patients with coronary artery disease may improve their tolerance to ischemia during exercise (5664). Other studies suggest oral ribose may prevent exercise-induced muscle pain and stiffness in patients with myoadenylate deaminase deficiency (5677,5676,5679,5680). Randomized, prospective controlled human studies are needed to establish the mechanism of action and the effectiveness of exogenous ribose when used to improve tolerance to exercise-induced ischemia in healthy individuals and patients with unstable cardiac condition such as coronary artery disease.

Adverse Reactions

Orally, ribose can cause diarrhea (5676), decreased blood glucose levels (5667), gastrointestinal discomfort, nausea and headache (5664). Hypoglycemia (5650,5662,5676), slightly increased serum insulin levels (5663) and decreased serum phosphate (5650) have been reported after infusion of ribose.

Interactions with Herbs & Other Dietary Supplements

None known.

Interactions with Drugs

ALCOHOL (Ethanol): Theoretically, ribose may increase the hypoglycemic effect of ethanol (5667).
ANTIDIABETES DRUGS: Theoretically, ribose may increase the hypoglycemic effect of oral antihyperglycemic agents such as the sulfonylureas, biguanides, alfa-glucosidase inhibitors, thiazolidinediones, and meglitinides (5667).
ASPIRIN: Theoretically, ribose may enhance the hypoglycemic effects of salicylate drugs such as aspirin (5667).
CHOLINE MAGNESIUM TRISALICYLATE (Trilisate): Theoretically, ribose may enhance the hypoglycemic effects of salicylate-containing drugs such as choline magnesium trisalicylate (5667).
INSULIN: Theoretically, ribose may increase the hypoglycemic effect of insulin and should be avoided by people taking insulin (5667).
PROPRANOLOL (Inderal): Theoretically, ribose may increase the hypoglycemic effect of propranolol (5667).
SALSALATE (Disalcid): Theoretically, ribose may enhance the hypoglycemic effects of salicylate-containing drugs such as salsalate (5667).

Interactions with Foods

None known.

Interactions with Lab Tests

GLUCOSE: Ribose may decrease serum glucose levels (5650,5662,5667,5676).
INSULIN: Ribose may increase serum insulin levels (5663).
PHOSPHATE: Ribose may decrease serum phosphate levels (5650).

Interactions with Diseases or Conditions

DIABETES: Theoretically, ribose should be avoided in patients with diabetes since it may interfere and enhance the glucose lowering effects of insulin or any oral antihyperglycemic agents.
HYPOGLYCEMIA: Theoretically, ribose should be avoided in patients who have hypoglycemia, or diseases or conditions that may increase their risk for hypoglycemia.

Dosage and Administration

ORAL: To improve exercise tolerance in patients with coronary artery disease, 15 grams four times per day has been used (5664). Beginning 1 hour before exercise until the end of the exercise session, 3 grams every 10 minutes has been used to reduce exercise-induced symptoms such as muscle stiffness and cramps associated with myoadenylate deaminase deficiency (5679).
INTRAVENOUS: For imaging of coronary arteries using thallium-201, a 30 minute 3.3 mg/kg/minute infusion of ribose as a 10% solution has been used (5662,5663).

RICE BRAN

Also Known As

Cereal Fiber, Dietary Fiber, Rice Bran Oil, Ricebran Oil, Stabilized Rice Bran.
CAUTION: See separate listings for Oat Bran and Wheat Bran.

Scientific Names

Oryza sativa.

People Use This For

Orally, rice bran is used for diabetes, hypertension, hyperlipidemia, alcoholism, weight loss, AIDS, preventing cancer, strengthening the immune system, increasing energy, enhancing athletic performance, aiding and improving liver function, preventing cardiovascular disease, and as an antioxidant. Rice bran oil is also used orally for hyperlipidemia.

Topically, rice bran is used for ectopic dermatitis.

Safety

LIKELY SAFE ...when used orally and appropriately. Rice bran and rice bran oil have been used safely in studies lasting up to 5 years (865,876,877,880,1354).

POSSIBLY SAFE ...when used as a bath additive. There is some evidence that a therapeutic bath containing rice bran broth can be safely used (872).

PREGNANCY AND LACTATION: LIKELY SAFE ...when used orally in amounts commonly found in foods. There is insufficient reliable information available about the safety of rice brand when used for medicinal purposes during pregnancy and lactation; avoid using.

Effectiveness

POSSIBLY EFFECTIVE

Atopic dermatitis (eczema). Applying rice bran broth topically seems to help reduce atopic dermatitis (872).

Gastric cancer. Consuming dietary cereal fiber, including rice bran, may decrease the incidence of stomach cancer (10435).

Hypercalciuria. Taking rice bran orally seems to reduce kidney stone (nephrolithiasis) recurrence, urine calcium excretion, and stone formation in people with hypercalciuria. Defatted rice bran 10 grams twice daily for 3 to 5 years seems to reduce urine calcium excretion and the incidence of kidney stone recurrence in people with hypercalcemia (876,878,880,881,882).

Hypercholesterolemia. Taking rice bran orally seems to lower cholesterol (865,877). Full-fat rice bran 85 grams per day, when added to a reduced-fat diet, seems to lower total cholesterol by 8% and low-density lipoprotein (LDL) cholesterol by 14%. Rice bran does not seem to affect triglycerides or high-density lipoprotein (HDL) cholesterol (865). Rice bran in a reduced-fat form at 11.8 grams per day appears to produce only a modest effect on cholesterol (877). Both full-fat and reduced-fat rice bran have comparable effects to oat bran for reducing cholesterol (865,877). Rice bran oil also seems to be effective for hypercholesterolemia.

There is some evidence that rice bran oil can reduce total cholesterol by 14%, LDL by 20%, triglycerides by 20%, and increase HDL by 41% (1354).

POSSIBLY INEFFECTIVE

Colorectal cancer. Consuming dietary cereal fiber, including rice bran, doesn't seem to reduce the risk of colorectal cancer (160,4819,4820,4821,5104).

There is insufficient reliable information available about the effectiveness of rice bran for its other uses.

Mechanism of Action

Rice bran is obtained from the outer hull of the rice Oryza sativa. It contains 21% fiber, 21% lipids, 13% amino acids, and a wide variety of vitamins and minerals (884,885). It also contains inositol and IP-6 (7598).

Most of the fiber in rice bran is insoluble. Rice bran contains a relatively high percentage of oil compared with most other brans (865). Although whole rice bran seems to have some antihypercholesterolemic properties, rice bran oil is likely responsible for the most significant effect. The oil contains beta-sitosterol and other phytosterols that are used to reduce cholesterol absorption (7520). Defatted rice bran oil does not appear to affect cholesterol (865,7520,7521). It also contains alpha-linolenic acid, which might increase the concentration of fatty acids such as eicosapentaenoic and docosahexaenoic acids (7520,7521).

Other constituents of rice bran oil are gamma oryzanol and tocotrienols, which might lower cholesterol by altering cholesterol absorption and excretion (7521,7598).

Rice bran also contains lipase, which causes a rapid deterioration of rice bran oil unless the lipase is promptly stabilized by heat or other treatments (865).

Rice bran can increase stool size by several mechanisms, including water retention (871,879). Scientists think increased fecal bulk reduces risk of cancer because it dilutes carcinogens, especially tumor promoters such as secondary bile acids (871). Diets high in fiber have resulted in lower insulin levels, less weight gain, and a reduction in cardiovascular disease risk factors such as hypertension (2737). Rice bran reduces the risk of recurrent urinary stone disease, perhaps because the phytin in rice bran reduces calcium absorption (881). Healthy women on a calcium-rich diet, who added rice bran to their diets decreased renal excretion of calcium and increased renal excretion of oxalic acid (874). A rice bran isolate designated as Compound X shows evidence of antihistamine activity. It also inhibits bacterial growth (884). A modified rice bran isolate, MGN-3 (see separate listing), exhibits anti-HIV activity (866).

Adverse Reactions

Orally, increasing the amount of bran in the diet can cause erratic bowel habits, flatulence, and abdominal discomfort during the first few weeks (272).
Topical use of rice bran broth baths can cause itching and skin redness (872). Rash and itching from rice bran has been associated in rare cases from contact infestation with Pyemotes tritici, an arthropod commonly called straw itch mite (2284).

Interactions with Herbs & Other Dietary Supplements

CALCIUM: Rice bran might reduce absorption of calcium in the intestine (881).
HERBS AND SUPPLEMENTS: Theoretically, rice bran might delay or impair the absorption of herbs and supplements due to the fiber contained in rice bran.
IRON: The fiber in rice bran might inhibit dietary iron absorption (156).

Interactions with Drugs

ORAL DRUGS: Theoretically, a diet high in rice bran might slow or reduce the absorption of some oral drugs.

Interactions with Foods

None known.

Interactions with Lab Tests

None known.

Interactions with Diseases or Conditions

GASTROINTESTINAL CONDITIONS: Contraindicated in people with intestinal ulcerations, stenosis, disabling adhesions, cathartic colon, or other conditions that may result in intestinal or esophageal obstruction due to the fiber contained in rice bran (272). Use with caution or avoid in people with difficulty chewing or swallowing food, or conditions that decrease small bowel motility.

Dosage and Administration

ORAL: For reducing cholesterol, 12-84 grams rice bran per day (865,877), or 4.8 grams rice bran oil (providing 312 mg tocotrienols, 360 mg tocopherols, and 2.4 grams other non-saponifiables) per day has been used (1354). For reducing the risk of kidney stones, 10 grams rice bran twice daily has been used (881,882). For decontamination of ingested polychlorinated biphenyl (PCB) and polychlorinated dibenzofuran (PCDF), 10 grams rice bran with a dietary fiber content 50% and 4 grams cholestyramine (Questran) three times a day has been used (870).

Comments

Rice bran oil is a popular "healthy oil" in Japan, Asia, and particularly India (7521).

RNA AND DNA

Also Known As

DNA, DeoxyNucleic Acid, Nuclei Acids, Nucleic, Nucleic Acid, Nucleic Acids, Nucleotides, Purines, Pyrimidines, RNA, RNA-DNA, RNA/DNA.

Scientific Names

Deoxyribonucleic Acid; Ribonucleic Acid.

People Use This For

Orally, RNA/DNA combinations are used to improve memory and mental sharpness, to treat or prevent Alzheimer's disease, to treat depression, increase energy, tighten skin, increase sex drive, and to counteract the effects of aging.
Enterally, RNA is used in nutrition formulations that include omega-3 fatty acids and arginine for reducing the time needed for recovery after surgery, to boost immune response, and to improve outcomes of burn patients and intensive care patients.
As an injection, RNA is used to treat eczema, psoriasis, hives, and shingles.

Safety

LIKELY SAFE ...when RNA and DNA are consumed in food. ...when RNA is used in enteral nutrition along with omega-3 fatty acids and L-arginine (5531,5533,5534,5535,5536,7819).
POSSIBLY SAFE ...when RNA is injected subcutaneously (5538).
There is insufficient reliable information available about the safety of oral RNA/DNA supplement combinations.
LIKELY SAFE ...when RNA is used in enteral nutrition along with omega-3 fatty acids and L-arginine (5531,5533,5534,5535,5536,7819).
POSSIBLY SAFE ...when RNA is injected subcutaneously (5538).

CHILDREN: LIKELY SAFE ...when infant formulas contain nucleotide supplements (5900).
PREGNANCY AND LACTATION: POSSIBLY UNSAFE ...when used orally as supplements. Some evidence suggests some orally ingested DNA might cross the placenta and be mutagenic (5539).

Effectiveness

POSSIBLY EFFECTIVE

Surgical recovery. Supplementing the diet of patients undergoing major surgery with enteral or oral RNA, L-arginine, and eicosapentaenoic acid might improve recovery. This combination administered in the perioperative period appears to boost immune response, reduce perioperative infections, improve wound healing, and shorten recovery time (5531,5532,5533,7819).

POSSIBLY INEFFECTIVE

Burns. Taking RNA and DNA enterally doesn't seem to produce a better outcome in burn patients than standard nutritional formulas (5535).

There is insufficient reliable information available about the effectiveness of RNA and DNA for their other uses.

Mechanism of Action

Although most organisms can synthesize nucleotides (5900), dietary nucleotides (derived from DNA and RNA) appear to be essential under conditions of rapid growth such as intestinal development, liver resection or injury and also during challenges to the immune system. When preformed nucleotides are consumed, they are degraded to free bases in the intestine before absorption. Experimental evidence shows they are incorporated into the hepatic pyrimidine nucleotide pool (5900) and that they affect the hepatic RNA content. The hepatic RNA content, in turn, affects the recovery time from liver injury. In protein-deprived animals, dietary nucleotides appear to benefit the intestinal tract. They can also restore immune function, while restoring the nitrogen balance (protein intake) does not (5543). In the absence of nucleotides, normal T-lymphocyte maturation is blocked (5543). A Crohn's disease model in rats shows RNA has a highly significant effect upon the healing intestinal ulcerations (5900). Supplementing an enteral diet with arginine, RNA, and omega-3 fatty acids can reduce concentrations of tumor necrosis factor alpha, and interleukin-6 and accelerate the recovery in the concentration of interleukin-1 beta and interleukin-2 alpha receptor (5532).

Adverse Reactions

Subcutaneously, an injection of RNA can cause itching, redness, and swelling at the injection site (5538).

Interactions with Herbs & Other Dietary Supplements

None known.

Interactions with Drugs

None known.

Interactions with Foods

None known.

Interactions with Lab Tests

None known.

Interactions with Diseases or Conditions

None known.

Dosage and Administration

ORAL: No typical dosage.
ENTERAL: A typical enteral dose of RNA is 30 mg/kg/day along with arginine and omega-3 fatty acids (5533,5534).
INJECTION: A typical dose is 10 mg injectable RNA every other day for 2-4 weeks (5538).

ROMAN CHAMOMILE

Also Known As

Chamomile, Chamomilla, Chamomillae ramane flos, English Chamomile, Fleur De Camomille Romaine, Flores Anthemidis, Garden Chamomile, Grosse Kamille, Ground Apple, Low Chamomile, Manzanilla, Römische Kamille, Sweet Chamomile, Whig Plant.
CAUTION: See separate listing for German Chamomile.

Scientific Names

Chamaemelum nobile, synonyms Anthemis nobilis, Ormenis nobilis.
Family: Asteraceae/Compositae.

People Use This For

Orally, Roman chamomile is used for indigestion, nausea and vomiting, anorexia, morning sickness, painful menstrual periods, flatulent indigestion associated with mental stress, mucous membrane inflammation, sinusitis, and rheumatic disorders.

Topically, Roman chamomile is used for eczema, wounds, and inflammation; and as an antiseptic in ointments, creams, and gels to treat cracked nipples, sore gums, and irritation of the skin and mucosa. It is also used topically for wounds, burns, frostbite, diaper rash, decubitus ulcers, and hemorrhoids.

In oral herbal combinations, Roman chamomile is used for liver and gallbladder disease, gallstones, fatty liver, chronic heartburn, loss of appetite, digestive disturbances, Roemheld's syndrome, indigestion in infants, and in spastic constipation. It is used as a "blood purifier", general female tonic, a preventative for menstrual discomforts, and for irregular periods.

In herbal inhalation therapy, Roman chamomile is used in steam baths for sinus inflammation, hay fever, pharyngeal swelling, ear inflammation, and as an analgesic.

In foods and beverages, the essential oil and extract are used as flavor components.

In manufacturing, the volatile oil of Roman chamomile is used as a fragrance component in soaps, cosmetics, and perfumes; and to flavor cigarette tobacco. The extract is also used in cosmetics and soaps. Teas have been used as a hair tint, conditioner, and to treat parasitic worm infections.

Safety

LIKELY SAFE ...when used orally in amounts commonly found in foods. Roman chamomile has Generally Recognized As Safe (GRAS) status in the US (4912).

POSSIBLY SAFE ...when used orally and appropriately in medicinal amounts (2,12). ...when the essential oil is inhaled or used topically as aromatherapy (7107).

PREGNANCY: LIKELY UNSAFE ...when used orally in medicinal amounts. Roman chamomile is believed to be an abortifacient (4). There is insufficient reliable information available about the safety of the topical use of Roman chamomile during pregnancy; avoid using.

LACTATION: Insufficient reliable information available; avoid using (4).

Effectiveness

There is insufficient reliable information available about the effectiveness of Roman chamomile.

Mechanism of Action

The applicable part of Roman chamomile is the flowerhead. Roman chamomile possesses antiflatulent, antispasmodic, and sedative properties (4). Large amounts of Roman chamomile can act as an emetic while small amounts act as an anti-emetic (4). In cosmetics, Roman chamomile is considered a deodorant and a stimulant to skin metabolism (11). Roman chamomile contains the coumarin scopoletin-7-glucoside and varied flavonoids, their glycosides (including rutin and volatile oils), as well as other constituents (4). Some evidence suggests azulene constituents contained in volatile oils exert anti-allergy and anti-inflammatory effects by inhibiting histamine release. However, the constituent nobilin, a sesquiterpene lactone, is thought to trigger allergy in sensitive individuals (4). Some evidence suggests Roman chamomile acts on the central nervous system, possibly reducing aggressive behavior (18). Experimental evidence suggests the volatile oil could have anti-inflammatory, antidiuretic, and sedative effects (4). The essential oil is active against gram-positive bacteria and dermatomyces (18). The sesquiterpinoids nobilin, 1,10-epoxynobilin, and 3-dehydronobilin show some evidence of antitumor activity (4). Although the constituents of Roman chamomile are not identical to those of German chamomile both plants are similarly used (512).

Adverse Reactions

Orally, large amounts of Roman chamomile might cause vomiting (11), although this is disputed (12).

Topically, Roman chamomile can cause contact dermatitis (4,567). Allergic skin reactions occur in up to 20% of individuals (19). It can cause an allergic reaction in individuals sensitive to the Asteraceae/Compositae family. Members of this family include ragweed, chrysanthemums, marigolds, daisies, and many other herbs.

Interactions with Herbs & Other Dietary Supplements

None known.

Interactions with Drugs

None known.

Interactions with Foods

None known.

Interactions with Lab Tests

None known.

Interactions with Diseases or Conditions

ASTHMA: May exacerbate asthma (4).
CROSS-ALLERGENICITY: Use of Roman chamomile can cause an allergic reaction in individuals sensitive to the Asteraceae/Compositae family. Members of this family include ragweed, chrysanthemums, marigolds, daisies, and many other herbs.

Dosage and Administration

ORAL: A typical dose is 1-4 grams dried flowerheads three times daily, or one cup tea.
To make tea, steep 1-4 grams dried flowerheads in 150 mL of boiling water for 5-10 minutes, strain (4).
Liquid extract (1:1 in 70% alcohol), 1-4 mL three times daily (4).
TOPICAL: A 3% steeped tea is prepared for topical use (8).

Comments

Most of the existing information on Roman chamomile concerns German chamomile (4,7), but it is extrapolated to Roman chamomile.

ROSE GERANIUM OIL

Also Known As

Aetheroleum Pelargonii, Algerian Geranium Oil, Bourbon Geranium Oil, Moroccan Geranium Oil, Oleum Geranii, Pelargonium Oil.

Scientific Names

Pelargonium graveolens.
Family: Geraniaceae.

People Use This For

Orally, rose geranium oil is used orally for neuropathic pain and diarrhea.
Topically, rose geranium oil is used as an astringent.
In foods and beverages, rose geranium oil is used as a flavoring agent.
In manufacturing, rose geranium oil is used as an inexpensive substitute for rose oil. It is also used as a fragrance component in soaps, cosmetics, and perfumes.

Safety

LIKELY SAFE ...when used in amounts commonly found in foods. Rose geranium oil has Generally Recognized As Safe (GRAS) status in the US (4912).
There is insufficient reliable information available about the safety of rose geranium oil for its other uses.
PREGNANCY AND LACTATION: Insufficient reliable information; avoid amounts greater than those found in foods.

Effectiveness

There is insufficient reliable information available about the effectiveness of rose geranium oil.

Mechanism of Action

The applicable part of rose geranium is the oil that is distilled from the stem and leaf. The geranium oil constituents citronellol, citronellyl acetate, citronellyl formate, and geraniol exhibit marginal antitumor activity (3751). The essential oils from Pelargonium species show some indication of antibacterial and antifungal activity (3752,3753).

Adverse Reactions

Topically, rose geranium oil has been associated with dermatitis in hypersensitive individuals (11); however, rose geranium oil is generally considered to be nonsensitizing, nonirritating, and nonphototoxic to human skin (11).

Interactions with Herbs & Other Dietary Supplements

None known.

Interactions with Drugs

None known.

Interactions with Foods

None known.

Interactions with Lab Tests

None known.

Interactions with Diseases or Conditions
None known.

Dosage and Administration
No typical dosage.

Comments
Avoid confusing rose geranium oil with East Indian or Turkish geranium oil (known as palmorosa oil) that is derived from a different plant (11).

ROSE HIP

Also Known As
Apothecary Rose, Cynosbatos, Dog Rose, Heps, Hip, Hip Fruit, Hip Sweet, Hipberry, Hop Fruit, Rosa de castillo, Rosae pseudofructus cum semen, Rose Hip with seed, Rose Hips, Rosehips, Satapatri, Satapatrika, Wild Boar Fruit.
CAUTION: See separate listings for Acerola, Vitamin C, and Cherokee Rosehip.

Scientific Names
Rosa canina, synonym Rosa lutetiana; Rosa alba; Rosa centifolia; Rosa damascena; Rosa gallica, synonym Rosa provincialis; Rosa rugosa; Rosa villosa, synonym Rosa pomifera; other Rosa species.
Family: Rosaceae.

People Use This For
Orally, rose hip is used as a supplemental source of dietary vitamin C, for preventing and treating colds, influenza-like infections, infectious diseases, vitamin C deficiencies, fever, increasing immune function during exhaustion, gastric spasms, gastric acid deficiency, preventing gastric mucosal inflammation and gastric ulcers, and as a "stomach tonic" for intestinal diseases. It is also used orally for diarrhea, gallstones, gallbladder ailments, lower urinary tract and kidney disorders, dropsy (edema), gout, disorders of uric acid metabolism, arthritis, sciatica, diabetes, increasing peripheral circulation, for reducing thirst, as a laxative and diuretic, and to treat chest ailments.
In foods and in manufacturing, it is used for rose hip tea, jam and soup, and as a natural source of vitamin C.

Safety
LIKELY SAFE ...when used in amounts commonly found in foods. Rose hips extract has Generally Recognized As Safe (GRAS) status in the US (4912).
POSSIBLY SAFE ...when used orally and appropriately for medicinal purposes (12).
PREGNANCY AND LACTATION: Insufficient reliable information available; avoid using in amounts greater than those found in foods.

Effectiveness
There is insufficient reliable information available about the effectiveness of rose hip.

Mechanism of Action
Rose hip contains pectin, citric acid, and malic acid, which can have laxative and diuretic activities (5,18).
The diuretic activity is controversial (8). Fresh rose hip contains between 0.5-1.7% vitamin C (5,8) and is estimated to contain 1250 mg vitamin C per 100 grams of rose hip (6). However, much of the vitamin C is destroyed during drying and processing (11), and declines rapidly with storage (2). Vitamin C is required for collagen formation and tissue repair (15). It is an enzyme cofactor in the synthesis of collagen, carnitine, norepinephrine, and peptide hormones, and in tyrosine metabolism (3042). Vitamin C is also involved in oxidation-reduction reactions, conversion of folic acid to folinic acid, carbohydrate metabolism, synthesis of lipids and proteins, iron metabolism, resistance to infections, and cellular respiration (15). It acts as an antioxidant, decreasing oxidants in gastric juice, decreasing lipid peroxidation, and decreasing oxidative DNA and protein damage (3042). Vitamin C deficiency that lasts for three to five months results in symptomatic scurvy that affects collagenous structures, bones, and blood vessels (15). Vitamin C enhances the absorption of soluble non-heme iron, either by reducing it (converting ferric to ferrous) or by preventing chelation by phytates or other food ligands (3042).

Adverse Reactions
Orally, the adverse effects of vitamin C are related to the amount of vitamin C actually contained in the rose hip product. The adverse reactions include nausea; vomiting; esophagitis; heartburn; abdominal cramps; GI obstruction; fatigue; flushing; headache; insomnia; sleepiness; diarrhea; hyperoxaluria; and precipitation of urate, oxalate, or cysteine stones or drugs in the urinary tract (15). Large amounts are associated with deep vein thrombosis (15). The inhalation of the rose hip dust is reportedly a respiratory allergen in production workers. It can cause mild to moderate anaphylaxis (6).
Topically, the rose hip dust ("itching powder") can cause itching by mechanical irritation (6).

Interactions with Herbs & Other Dietary Supplements

IRON: Concomitant use interacts with the vitamin C in rose hip; 200 mg of vitamin C per 30 mg of elemental iron increases oral iron absorption, especially ferric iron (3042).

Interactions with Drugs

ALUMINUM: Concomitant use interacts with the vitamin C in rose hip and can increase aluminum absorption, but the clinical significance of this is unknown (3046). Administer rose hip with vitamin C two hours before or four hours after antacids (3046).
ASPIRIN: The vitamin C in rose hip can increase urinary excretion of ascorbic acid and decrease excretion of salicylates, but this may not have a clinically significant effect on salicylate plasma levels (3046).
CHOLINE MAGNESIUM TRISALICYLATE (Trilisate): The vitamin C in rose hip can increase urinary excretion of ascorbic acid and decrease excretion of salicylates such as choline magnesium trisalicylate. But this may not have a clinically significant effect on salicylate plasma levels (3046).
ESTROGENS: Theoretically, the vitamin C in large amounts of rose hip might increase absorption and effects of estrogen (129,130).
FLUPHENAZINE (Prolixin): Concomitant use with rose hip decreases blood levels due to vitamin C content (15).
SALSALATE (Disalcid): The vitamin C in rose hip can increase urinary excretion of ascorbic acid and decrease excretion of salicylates such as salsalate. But this may not have a clinically significant effect on salicylate plasma levels (3046).
WARFARIN (Coumadin): Concomitant use interacts with the vitamin C in rose hip. Large amounts of vitamin C can impair the warfarin response (3046).

Interactions with Foods

IRON: Concomitant use interacts with the vitamin C in rose hip and can increase the absorption of dietary (ferric) iron (3042).

Interactions with Lab Tests

ACETAMINOPHEN: The vitamin C in rose hip can cause false negative urine results with methods based on hydrolysis and formation of an indophenol blue chromagen (275).
ASPARTATE AMINOTRANSFERASE (AST, SGOT): Large amounts of the vitamin C in rose hip can cause a false increase in results of serum tests relying on color reactions (Redox reactions) and Technicon SMA 12/60 (275).
BILIRUBIN: Large amounts of the vitamin C in rose hip can cause a false increase in serum test results measured by Technicon SMA 12/60 or colorimetric methods (275).
CALCIUM/SODIUM: 3-6 grams of vitamin C daily can cause a true increase in urinary calcium and test results (15) and a true decrease in urinary sodium and test results.
CARBAMAZEPINE (Tegretol): Large amounts of the vitamin C in rose hip can cause falsely increased serum assay results measured by Ames ARIS method (275).
CREATININE: The vitamin C in rose hip can cause a false increase in serum creatinine or urine test results (275).
GLUCOSE: Large amounts of the vitamin C in rose hip can cause false increases in urine test results measured by copper reduction methods (e.g., Clinitest) and false decreases in results measured by glucose oxidase methods (e.g., Clinistix, Tes-Tape) (15).
LDH: The vitamin C in rose hip can cause a false decrease measured by Technicon SMA 12/60 and Abbott 100 methods (275).
OCCULT BLOOD: The vitamin C in rose hip may cause false negative guaiac results to occur with 250 mg or more of vitamin C per day (3042).
THEOPHYLLINE: Large amounts of the vitamin C in rose hip can cause falsely decreased serum assay results when measured by the ARIS system or Ames Seralyzer photometer (275).
URIC ACID: Large amounts of the vitamin C in rose hip can cause a true decrease in serum uric acid concentrations and test results with enzymatic method assays (15).

Interactions with Diseases or Conditions

DIABETES: The vitamin C in rose hip might affect glycogenolysis and the control of diabetes, but not all experts agree on this (15).
GLUCOSE-6-PHOSPHATE DEHYDROGENASE DEFICIENCY: Large amounts of the vitamin C in rose hip might increase the risk of oxalate stone formation (15).
HEMOCHROMATOSIS, THALASSEMIA, SIDEROBLASTIC ANEMIA: Use rose hip with caution, because the vitamin C content can increase iron absorption, which could worsen this condition (15).
INCREASED NEEDS: Vitamin C requirements increase in pregnancy, lactation, hyperthyroidism, stress, fever, infection, trauma, burns, smoking, and cold exposure (15).
SICKLE CELL DISEASE: The vitamin C in rose hip rarely can decrease the blood pH, precipitating sickle cell crisis (15).

Dosage and Administration

ORAL: The typical dose of rose hips is as a tea, which is prepared by steeping 2-2.5 grams of the crushed rose hips in 150 mL boiling water for 10-15 minutes and then straining (8).

Comments

Rose hip with seed is the ripe, dried receptacle (hip) with fruit (seed) of various Rosa species, including dog rose (Rosa canina), white rose (Rosa alba), provence rose (Rosa centifolia), and damask rose (Rosa damascena). Avoid confusion with Cherokee rosehip, rose flower, and vitamin C. CAUTION: Sometimes rose hip seeds or plain rose hip receptacles without seeds are sold. These are different than rose hip with seed. Fresh rose hips contain a high concentration of vitamin C; however, much of the vitamin C is destroyed during drying and processing (11) and declines rapidly with storage (2). Many rose hip-derived "natural" vitamin C products are supplemented with synthetic vitamin C (6,11), but may not be clearly labeled accordingly (6).

ROSEMARY

Also Known As

Compass Plant, Compass Weed, Old Man, Polar Plant, Rusmari.
CAUTION: See separate listing for Rosinweed.

Scientific Names

Rosmarinus officinalis.
Family: Lamiaceae/Labiatae.

People Use This For

Orally, rosemary is used for dyspepsia, flatulence, inducing abortion, increasing menstrual flow, gout, cough, headache, liver and gallbladder complaints, loss of appetite, and for cardiovascular conditions such as high blood pressure.
Topically, rosemary is used for preventing baldness; alopecia areata; circulatory disturbances; toothache; eczema; joint or musculoskeletal pain such as myalgia, sciatica and intercostal neuralgia; balneotherapy; wound healing; and as an insect repellent.
In foods, rosemary is used as a spice. The leaf and oil are used in foods, and the oil in beverages.
In manufacturing, rosemary oil is used as a fragrant component in soaps and perfumes.

Safety

LIKELY SAFE ...when used orally in amounts typically found in foods. Rosemary has Generally Recognized As Safe (GRAS) status in the US (4912).
POSSIBLY SAFE ...when used orally and appropriately in medicinal amounts (18). ...when used topically and appropriately (5177). Rosemary oil has been used safely for up to 7 months (5177). ...when used by inhalation as aromatherapy (7107).
LIKELY UNSAFE ...when the essential oil is ingested. Ingestion of undiluted oil from rosemary can cause significant adverse effects (515).
PREGNANCY: POSSIBLY UNSAFE ...when used orally in medicinal amounts. Rosemary might have uterine and menstrual flow stimulant effects (4,12,18); avoid using. There is insufficient reliable information available about the safety of the topical use of rosemary during pregnancy.
LACTATION: There is insufficient reliable information available about the safety of using rosemary in medicinal amounts during lactation; avoid using.

Effectiveness

POSSIBLY EFFECTIVE

Alopecia areata. Rosemary oil in combination with the essential oils from thyme, lavender, and cedarwood seem to improve hair growth by 44% after 7 months of treatment for alopecia areata (5177).

POSSIBLY INEFFECTIVE

Abortion. Taking rosemary orally doesn't seem to be effective for use as an abortifacient (5,6).

There is insufficient reliable information available about the effectiveness of rosemary for its other uses.

Mechanism of Action

The applicable part of rosemary is the leaf. The active constituent of rosemary leaves is the essential oil.
Dried leaves contain from 1-2.5% of the essential oil (4,5). The oil consists primarily of cineole, borneol, camphor, and pinenes (4,6). The essential oil might have a spasmolytic effect on smooth muscle of the gastrointestinal tract and in the ducts of the gallbladder (4). Rosemary might also have a positive inotropic effect on the heart and increases coronary blood flow (2). It's not clear how rosemary oil works in alopecia areata (5177). However, there is some evidence that topical use of rosemary might irritate the skin and increase blood circulation (2). Rosemary also seems to have antibacterial, antifungal (4), and antioxidant properties (4,6).

Adverse Reactions

Orally, large amounts of leaves containing rosemary oil might cause deep coma, spasm, vomiting, gastroenteritis, uterine bleeding, kidney irritation, pulmonary edema, and death (18). Ingestion of undiluted oil might cause stomach and intestinal irritation, kidney damage, and seizures (5,6). The camphor constituent can sometimes lead to seizures (4).

Topically, rosemary use can lead to photosensitivity, erythema, and dermatitis in hypersensitive individuals (4,6). Asthma due to repeated occupational exposure (occupational asthma) can occur (783).

Interactions with Herbs & Other Dietary Supplements

None known.

Interactions with Drugs

None known.

Interactions with Foods

None known.

Interactions with Lab Tests

None known.

Interactions with Diseases or Conditions

SEIZURE DISORDERS: Theoretically, rosemary might potentiate seizure activity (7107); avoid using.

Dosage and Administration

ORAL: A typical dose is 1-2 grams of crude leaf. Rosemary is often prepared as a tea. A typical dose is one cup tea three times daily, prepared by steeping 1-2 grams leaf in 150 mL boiling water for 5-10 minutes then straining (2,4). A liquid extract (1:1 in 45% alcohol) has also been used in a dose of 2-4 mL three times daily (4).

TOPICAL: Typically, semi-solid or liquid preparations containing 6-10% of the essential oil are used (2). For a rosemary bath, 50 grams crude leaf in 1 L hot water is commonly added to bath water (18). For the treatment of alopecia areata, a combination of the essential oils including rosemary 3 drops or 114 mg, thyme 2 drops or 88 mg, lavender 3 drops or 108 mg, and cedarwood 2 drops or 94 mg, all mixed with 3 mL jojoba oil and 20 mL grapeseed oil has been used. Each night, the mixture is massaged into the scalp for 2 minutes with a warm towel placed around the head to increase absorption (5177).

ROSEROOT

Also Known As

Arctic Root, Golden Root, King's Crown, Lignum rhodium, Rhodiola, Rodia riza, Rosenroot.

Scientific Names

Rhodiola rosea, synonyms Sedum rhodiola, Sedum rosea.
Family: Crassulaceae.

People Use This For

Orally, roseroot is used for increasing energy, stamina, strength and mental capacity; and as a so-called "adaptogen" to help the body adapt to and resist physical, chemical, and environmental stress. It is also used for improving athletic performance, improving sexual function, depression, cardiac disorders such as arrhythmias, and hyperlipidemia. Roseroot is also used for treating cancer, tuberculosis, and diabetes; preventing cold and flu, aging, and liver damage; improving hearing; strengthening the nervous system; enhancing immunity; and shortening recovery time after prolonged workouts.

Safety

POSSIBLY SAFE ...when used orally and appropriately, short-term. There is some evidence that a roseroot extract 200 mg/day can be safely used for up to 4 weeks (13109).

PREGNANCY AND LACTATION: Insufficient reliable information available; avoid using.

Effectiveness

INSUFFICIENT RELIABLE EVIDENCE to RATE

Athletic performance. Preliminary evidence suggests that a single dose of roseroot extract 200 mg might modestly increase time to exhaustion, peak oxygen consumption (VO2), peak carbon dioxide output (VCO2), and pulmonary ventilation in healthy volunteers undergoing endurance exercise testing. However, roseroot extract does not seem to affect muscle strength, speed of limb movement, reaction times, or attention span (13109).

Fatigue. There is preliminary evidence that a standardized roseroot extract 170 mg daily might help for fatigue

in night shift workers. Roseroot extract seems to improve cognitive performance after the first treatment, but its effects don't seem to continue after the second treatment (6877).
More evidence is needed to rate roseroot for these uses.

Mechanism of Action

The applicable part of roseroot is the root. Roseroot contains a phenylpropanoid glycoside called salidroside. This constituent is also sometimes referred to as rhodioloside or rhodosine (13028). This constituent is thought to be responsible for roseroot's stimulant, anti-stress, and adaptogenic actions (increasing resistance to the harmful effects of stressors) (6877,13028).
Other constituents isolated from roseroot include rhodioniside, rhodiolin, rosin, rosavin, rosarin, rosiridin, rosiridol, and lotaustralin (13028,13059). It is thought that these constituents might also be involved in roseroot's adaptogenic effects (13028).
Some roseroot products are standardized based on rosavin content. Rosavin is specific to Rhodiola rosea and distinguishes it from other species in the Rhodiola genus (13028). Roseroot also contains the tannins gallic acid and caffeic acid, as well as chlorogenic acid and flavonoids such as catechins and proanthocyanidins (13028,13059). These compounds are likely responsible for the antioxidant activity of roseroot extracts (13028).
Animal studies are reported to show protection from stressors such as cold and radiation, increased work capacity, decreased fatigue and improved learning and memory (6877). Roseroot extracts demonstrate antiarrhythmic properties and protection against reperfusion injury after ischemia. These effects can be abolished by naloxone infusion, suggesting that the mechanism might involve an increase in endogenous opioids (3191,3192,3195).
Roseroot extracts might also prevent stress-induced cardiac damage by preventing rises in cardiac catecholamines and cyclic-AMP (3193).
Some evidence suggests that roseroot extract has an anti-inflammatory effect and can decrease C-reactive protein (CRP) levels. Healthy volunteers, who took a specific roseroot extract (Rhodax, Phoenix Labs) for several days before and after exhausting exercise, had lower C-reactive protein levels compared to people who took placebo (13109). The clinical significance of this finding is not known.
Roseroot extract reduces experimentally induced mutations, possibly by increasing the efficiency of intracellular DNA repair mechanisms (3190). Roseroot extracts also demonstrate hepatoprotective and myeloprotective effects (3196,3197). Roseroot extracts also demonstrate potential for improving learning and memory (3198,6877).
Preliminary research in a small number of patients with superficial bladder cancer suggests that roseroot extract might improve cell characteristics and reduce relapses (3194).

Adverse Reactions

None reported.

Interactions with Herbs & Other Dietary Supplements

None known.

Interactions with Drugs

None known.

Interactions with Foods

None known.

Interactions with Lab Tests

None known.

Interactions with Diseases or Conditions

None known.

Dosage and Administration

ORAL: For athletic performance, a specific roseroot extract 200 mg as a single dose or 100 mg twice daily has been used (13109). For improving well-being and psychomotor function during stress, roseroot extract 50 mg twice daily has been used (1927).

Comments

Roseroot is native to the arctic regions of Europe, Asia, and Alaska (13028). It has a long history of use as a medicinal plant in Iceland, Sweden, France, Russia, and Greece. It is mentioned by Dioscorides as early as the first century A.D. (6877). Roseroot is often promoted as an "adaptogen". Adaptogen is a non-medical term used to suggest that a substance can act to strengthen the body and increase general resistance (13028). The green aerial parts of the plant have been used as a food ingredient (6877).

ROSINWEED

Also Known As

Compass Weed, Pilot Weed, Polar Plant.
CAUTION: See separate listings for Cup Plant and Rosemary.

Scientific Names

Silphium laciniatum.
Family: Asteraceae/Compositae.

Comments

At the date of publication, this product was not a common ingredient used in brand name supplements marketed to consumers. Details about this product are available in the online version of *Natural Medicines Comprehensive Database.* See www.naturaldatabase.com.

ROYAL JELLY

Also Known As

Bee Saliva, Bee Spit, Honey Bee Milk.
CAUTION: See separate listings for Bee Pollen, Bee Venom, and Honey.

Scientific Names

Apis mellifera (Honey Bee).
Family: Apidae.

People Use This For

Orally, royal jelly is used for asthma, allergic rhinitis, liver disease, pancreatitis, insomnia, premenstrual syndrome (PMS), stomach ulcers, kidney disease, bone fractures, skin disorders, and hyperlipidemia. It is also used as a general health tonic, for rejuvenation, and potentiating the immune system.

Topically, royal jelly is used as a skin tonic and hair growth stimulant.

Safety

POSSIBLY SAFE ...when used orally and appropriately, short-term. Taking 2 tablets twice daily of a specific combination product containing royal jelly 6 mg, bee pollen extract 36 mg, and bee pollen plus pistil extract 120 mg (Femal, Natumin Pharma) per tablet for up to 2 months seems to be safe (12008). It's not known if other royal jelly doses and formulations are safe.

PREGNANCY AND LACTATION: Insufficient reliable information available; avoid using.

Effectiveness

INSUFFICIENT RELIABLE EVIDENCE to RATE

Hyperlipidemia. There is preliminary evidence that royal jelly might lower cholesterol levels in people with hyperlipidemia (3515).

Premenstrual syndrome (PMS). Preliminary evidence suggests that a specific combination product (Femal, Natumin Pharma) seems to decrease some symptoms of PMS including irritability, weight increases, and edema when given over a period of 2 menstrual cycles. This product contains royal jelly 6 mg, bee pollen extract 36 mg, and bee pollen plus pistil extract 120 mg per tablet. It is given as 2 tablets twice daily (12008).

More evidence is needed to rate royal jelly for these uses.

Mechanism of Action

Royal jelly is a milky secretion produced by glands in the heads of nurse honey bees (Apis mellifera). The composition of royal jelly varies with geographical areas and climatic conditions. It typically contains about 60% to 70% water, 12% to 15% crude proteins, 10% to 16% sugar, 3% to 6% lipids, and 2% to 3% low molecular weight compounds such as vitamins, salts, and free amino acids (7313). Royal jelly is used for the development and nurturing of queen bees (6). There is very little scientific information available about its effects in humans.

In animal models, royal jelly seems to have some antitumor activity (6) and antiatherogenic activity (3515).

Adverse Reactions

Orally, royal jelly appears to cause few side effects in nonallergic people (7314). There is one report of dizziness in a patient who took a combination product containing royal jelly, bee pollen extract, and a bee pollen plus pistil extract (12008).
In people with a history of atopy or asthma, royal jelly appears to cause a high rate of allergic symptoms including pruritus, urticaria, eczema, eyelid and facial edema, conjunctivitis, rhinorrhea, dyspnea, and asthma (7314,7315,7316,10623). In severe cases, royal jelly can cause status asthmaticus, anaphylaxis, and death (792,7315,7316,10623,10624). Allergic symptoms are associated with IgE-mediated hypersensitivity reactions (3513,10623). Tell people with a history of allergy or asthma not to use royal jelly.
There is also one case report of hemorrhagic colitis with abdominal pain, bloody diarrhea with concomitant hemorrhagic and edematous mucosa of the sigmoid colon after ingestion of royal jelly. Symptoms resolved within 2 weeks following discontinuation of royal jelly and conservative treatment (3516).
Topically, skin irritation, exacerbation of dermatitis, or contact dermatitis may occur (791).

Interactions with Herbs & Other Dietary Supplements

None known.

Interactions with Drugs

None known.

Interactions with Foods

None known.

Interactions with Lab Tests

None known.

Interactions with Diseases or Conditions

ASTHMA: In patients with asthma or atopy, royal jelly causes a high rate of allergic symptoms including pruritus, urticaria, eczema, eyelid and facial edema, conjunctivitis, rhinorrhea, dyspnea, and asthma (7314,7315,7316,10623). In severe cases, royal jelly can cause status asthmaticus, anaphylaxis, and death (792,7315,7316,10623,10624). Allergic symptoms have been associated with IgE-mediated hypersensitivity reactions (3513,10623). Advise people with asthma or allergies not to use royal jelly.
ATOPY: In patients with asthma or atopy, royal jelly causes a high rate of allergic symptoms including pruritus, urticaria, eczema, eyelid and facial edema, conjunctivitis, rhinorrhea, dyspnea, and asthma (7314,7315,7316,10623). In severe cases, royal jelly can cause status asthmaticus, anaphylaxis, and death (792,7315,7316,10623,10624). Allergic symptoms have been associated with IgE-mediated hypersensitivity reactions (3513,10623). Advise people with asthma or allergies not to use royal jelly.
DERMATITIS: Royal jelly might exacerbate dermatitis; avoid using (791).

Dosage and Administration

ORAL: For hyperlipidemia, 50-100 mg per day has been used (3515). For premenstrual syndrome (PMS), two tablets twice daily of a specific combination containing royal jelly 6 mg, bee pollen extract 36 mg, and bee pollen plus pistil extract 120 mg (Femal, Natumin Pharma) per tablet for 2 menstrual cycles has been used (12008).

Comments

Avoid confusion with bee pollen and bee venom.

RUE

Also Known As

Common Rue, Garden Rue, German Rue, Herb-of-Grace, Herbygrass, Raute, Ruda, Rue Officinale, Ruta graveolens, Rutae folium, Rutae herba.
CAUTION: See separate listing for Goat's Rue.

Scientific Names

Ruta graveolens.
Family: Rutaceae.

People Use This For

Orally, the above ground parts of rue are used for menstrual disorders and discomforts, as a uterine stimulant and abortifacient, for loss of appetite, dyspepsia, circulatory disorders, arteriosclerosis, heart palpitations, nervousness, hysteria, fever, feverish infectious diseases, cramps, hepatitis, diarrhea, pleurisy, headaches, neuralgic afflictions, and weakness of the eyes. It is also used orally for respiratory complaints, arthritis, intestinal worm infestations, epilepsy, multiple sclerosis, Bell's palsy, and cancer of the mouth. Rue is also used orally as an antispasmodic, diuretic, antibacterial, antifungal, hemostatic, and as a contraceptive agent.

Topically, rue is used for arthritis, dislocations, sprains, injuries of the bone, inflammation of the skin, oral and pharyngeal cavities, earaches, toothaches, headaches, tumors, warts, and as an insect repellent.

In foods and beverages, rue and its oil are used as flavor components.

In manufacturing, rue oil is used as a fragrance ingredient in soaps and cosmetics.

Safety

LIKELY SAFE ...when used orally in amounts commonly found in foods. Rue and rue oil have Generally Recognized As Safe (GRAS) status in the US (4912).

LIKELY UNSAFE ...when fresh rue is used orally for medicinal purposes (2). Fresh rue can cause severe kidney and liver damage (2). ...when more than 120 grams of leaves or 100 mL of oil are ingested. Rue can cause severe gastrointestinal upset, systemic complications, and death (2,6). Dried rue leaves contain less volatile oil than fresh rue, and has milder effects (515). Canadian regulations prohibit the use of rue as a non-medicinal ingredient in oral products (12). ...when fresh rue is applied topically (2); rue can cause contact dermatitis and severe photodermatitis (2,6,11,19).

PREGNANCY: LIKELY UNSAFE ...when used orally. Rue might have uterine stimulant and abortifacient effects (12); avoid using. Deaths have been reported in women who used rue as an abortifacient (2).

LACTATION: LIKELY UNSAFE ...when used orally in medicinal amounts.

Effectiveness

There is insufficient reliable information available about the effectiveness of rue.

Mechanism of Action

The applicable parts of rue are the above ground parts. Rue contains the alkaloids arborine, arborinine, and gamma-fagarine; and the furocoumarins rutamarin, bergapten, and xanthotoxin. The alkaloids and the furocoumarins have shown evidence of reversible spasmolytic activity, and anti-inflammatory and antihistaminic properties (6,11,515). The furocoumarins may also have photosensitizing, phototoxic, and mutagenic effects (2); and are responsible for adverse skin reactions (6,11,19,515). The constituent chalepensin may have antifertility and anti-implantation effects. The rutin constituent may have antispasmodic activity, and it might also decrease capillary permeability and fragility.

Rue oil has anthelmintic activities, possibly due to the constituent 2-undecanone; this constituent can also cause abortions (11). Although rue oil has caused fatal adrenal gland, liver, and kidney hemorrhage in animals, 30 mg per day for three months did not affect liver function in humans (11). The effects of rue extract on neuromuscular conditions are thought to result from potassium channel-blocking in myelinated nerve cells (6).

Adverse Reactions

Orally, rue can cause GI irritation (12), melancholic mood, sleep disorders, tiredness, dizziness, spasms, and severe kidney and liver damage (2). The fresh leaf juice can cause painful stomach and intestinal irritation, fainting, lethargy, bradycardia, abortion, swelling of the tongue, and clammy skin (2). Rue oil causes severe stomach pain, vomiting, exhaustion, confusion, and convulsions (11). Large amounts, over 100 mL of the oil or 120 grams of the leaf, can cause vomiting, violent gastric pain, systemic complications, and death (2,6). Contact dermatitis (2) and phototoxic reactions including skin blisters have occurred with topical exposure to the fresh plant and rue-containing products followed by exposure to sunlight (2,6). There is one case report of increased phototoxic response to PUVA (psoralen plus ultraviolet A) therapy associated with ingestion of a rue remedy (6177).

Interactions with Herbs & Other Dietary Supplements

GOLDENSEAL: The reports regarding overcoming the effects of large amounts of rue by administration of goldenseal are unsubstantiated (515).

Interactions with Drugs

PHOTOSENSITIZING DRUGS: Rue might increase the phototoxic response to PUVA therapy due to its 5-methoxypsoralen content. There is one case report of increased phototoxic response to PUVA therapy associated with ingestion of a rue remedy (6177). Drugs used in PUVA therapy include methoxsalen (8-methoxypsoralen, 8-MOP, Oxsoralen) and Trioxsalen (Trisoralen). Rue might also increase of the risk of phototoxicity when used with other drugs that cause photosensitivity. Some other drugs that cause photosensitivity include amitriptyline (Elavil), quinolones (Ciprofloxacin, others), sulfa drugs (Septra, Bactrim, others), and tetracycline.

Interactions with Foods

None known.

Interactions with Lab Tests
None known.

Interactions with Diseases or Conditions
GASTROINTESTINAL TRACT PROBLEMS: Rue can exacerbate pre-existing inflammation or irritation of the gastrointestinal tract (19).
KIDNEY OR LIVER DYSFUNCTION: Contraindicated (2,12).
URINARY TRACT PROBLEMS: Rue can exacerbate kidney inflammation and urinary tract discomfort (19).

Dosage and Administration
ORAL: People typically use 500 mg crushed rue. A maximum dose of 1 gram per day has been recommended. As a tea, 1 cup of boiling water is poured over 1 teaspoon of the herb. The tea is taken cold, 1 cup per day (5252,5254).
TOPICAL: No typical dosage.

Comments
Avoid confusion with goat's rue (Galega officinalis) and meadow rue (Thalictrum species).

RUPTUREWORT

Also Known As
Bruchkraut, Flax weed, Herniariae herba, Herniary.

Scientific Names
Herniaria glabra; Herniaria hirsuta.
Family: Rutaceae.

Comments
At the date of publication, this product was not a common ingredient used in brand name supplements marketed to consumers. Details about this product are available in the online version of *Natural Medicines Comprehensive Database.* See www.naturaldatabase.com.

RUSTY-LEAVED RHODODENDRON

Also Known As
Rhododendri Ferruginei Folium, Rosebay, Rust-Red Rhododendron, Rusty Leaved Rhododendron, Snow Rose.

Scientific Names
Rhododendron ferrugineum.
Family: Ericaceae.

People Use This For
In combination with other herbs, rusty-leaved rhododendron is used for extreme tension of the muscles or arteries (hypertonia), muscle and joint rheumatism, joint disease, hardening of muscles, muscular pain, weak connective tissue, neuralgia, sensitivity to weather change, sciatica, trigeminal neuralgia, migraine, headaches, intercostal neuralgia, gout, biliary or urinary stones, hypertension, and geriatric and aging disorders.

Safety
LIKELY UNSAFE ...when used orally (2). The entire plant is considered poisonous (2,7,18,3477,3496). Hydroquinone toxicity is also a potential risk with long-term use (2). Most poisonings result from the consumption of honey made from rhododendron nectar (3477).
PREGNANCY AND LACTATION: LIKELY UNSAFE ...when used orally; avoid using.

Effectiveness
There is insufficient reliable information available about the effectiveness of rusty-leaved rhododendron.

Mechanism of Action
The applicable part of rusty-leaved rhododendron is the leaf. Rusty-leaved rhododendron contains grayanotoxins and arbutin (2). Grayanotoxins lower blood pressure (7). Grayanotoxins also prevent nerve conduction by inhibiting the closure of sodium channels on cell membranes, which increases sodium conductance and causes cellular depolarization (18,3477). Grayanotoxin toxicity includes muscular and respiratory paralysis (7). Arbutin is hydrolyzed to hydroquinone by the intestinal flora (7). As a result, long-term use may to lead to hydroquinone toxicity (2).

Adverse Reactions

Orally, the adverse effects of rusty-leaved rhododendron include weakness, dizziness, nausea, vomiting, hypotension, bradycardia, transient A-V dissociation and blurred vision (17,3496). Symptoms of poisoning due to the constituent grayanotoxin include sweating, impaired consciousness, chills, fainting, shock, seizure, cardiac and respiratory arrest, severe stupor, and possibly death (2,18,3477,3496).
Chronic use may lead to hydroquinone toxicity (2). Hydroquinone toxicity is characterized by a gastroenteritis-like syndrome (17).

Interactions with Herbs & Other Dietary Supplements

None known.

Interactions with Drugs

None known.

Interactions with Foods

None known.

Interactions with Lab Tests

None known.

Interactions with Diseases or Conditions

None known.

Dosage and Administration

No typical dosage.

Comments

Rusty-leaved rhododendron is considered likely unsafe; avoid using. Rusty-leaved rhododendron is considered a poisonous plant (2,7,18). Rhododendron honey is also known as "mad honey" (3477,3496).

RUTIN

Also Known As

Citrus Bioflavonoid, Citrus Bioflavonoids, Eldrin, Flavonoid, Oxerutin, Quercetin-3-rhamnoglucoside, Quercetin-3-rutinoside, Rutine, Rutinum, Rutosid, Rutosidum, Sclerutin, Sophorin.
CAUTION: See separate listings for Chrysin, Diosmin, Hesperidin, Methoxylated Flavones, and Quercetin.

Scientific Names

Rutin, rutoside.

People Use This For

Orally, rutin is used as a vascular protectant, reducing capillary permeability and fragility, varicose veins, internal bleeding, hemorrhoids, to prevent strokes, and for prophylaxis of mucositis associated with cancer treatments.
In combination with trypsin and bromelain, rutin is used orally for osteoarthritis.

Safety

LIKELY SAFE ...when used orally in amounts present in fruits and vegetables.
POSSIBLY UNSAFE ...when used orally in medicinal amounts. Although rutin is generally considered nontoxic, there are reports of rutin forming an obstructive mass in the gastrointestinal tract (11). There is also concern that flavonoids, including rutin, could become mutagenic and play a role in the etiology of gastric cancer (3106).
PREGNANCY AND LACTATION: Insufficient reliable information available; avoid using amounts greater than those found in foods.

Effectiveness

POSSIBLY EFFECTIVE

Osteoarthritis. Taking rutin orally in combination with trypsin and bromelain seems to be effective for treating osteoarthritis (6252). In a double-blind trial, 73 patients with painful osteoarthritis of the knee were randomly assigned the combination enzyme product (Phlogenzym) or diclofenac (Voltaren) 50 mg three times daily during the first week and then twice daily in weeks 2 and 3. The enzyme product was similar to diclofenac in relieving pain and improving knee function (6252).

There is insufficient reliable information available about the effectiveness of rutin for its other uses.

Mechanism of Action

Rutin is a flavonoid. Rutin is thought to be an antioxidant, a free radical scavenger, and an iron-chelator (209,3100). It has been reported to decrease capillary fragility and permeability, although the existing evidence is inconclusive (11). Some studies suggest rutin might offer protection from damage induced by asbestos (209,3103), cytotoxic effects of oxidized low density lipoproteins (11,3105), and gastric injury from ethanol (3107). Other evidence suggests it might be beneficial in inflammatory bowel disease (3101,3102). When added to the diet, rutin appears to offer some protection against DNA damage caused by hepatocarcinogens (3104). However, limited preliminary evidence suggests rutin might worsen the progression of melanoma (211).

After oral administration, rutin is hydrolyzed in the gastrointestinal tract to release quercetin, which is responsible for many of the actions of rutin. It appears that quercetin from rutin is absorbed better in women than in men, although the gender related differences in bioavailability are not completely understood (9442).

Adverse Reactions

Orally, rutin may cause headache, flushing, rashes, or mild gastrointestinal disturbance (313).

Interactions with Herbs & Other Dietary Supplements

IRON: Some information suggests that rutin might have iron-chelating properties (209).

Interactions with Drugs

None known.

Interactions with Foods

None known.

Interactions with Lab Tests

None known.

Interactions with Diseases or Conditions

None known.

Dosage and Administration

ORAL: For relieving symptoms of edema associated with chronic venous insufficiency, a typical dose is 500 mg twice daily (313). For osteoarthritis, a combination enzyme product (Phlogenzym), which contains rutin 100 mg, trypsin 48 mg, and bromelain 90 mg, 2 tablets 3 times daily has been used (6252).

Comments

Rutin (rutoside) is a flavonoid present in numerous plants. The major sources of rutin for medical use include buckwheat, Japanese pagoda tree, and Eucalyptus macrorhyncha. Other sources of rutin include the leaves of several species of eucalyptus, lime tree flowers, elder flowers, hawthorn leaves and flowers, rue, St. John's Wort, Ginkgo biloba, apples, and other fruits and vegetables.

RYE GRASS

Also Known As

Grass Pollen, Grass Pollen Extract, Rye, Rye Grass Pollen, Rye Grass Pollen Extract, Rye Pollen Extract.

Scientific Names

Secale cereale.
Family: Poaceae/Gramineae.

People Use This For

Orally, rye grass is used for benign prostatic hyperplasia (BPH), prostate pain, and chronic prostatitis.

Safety

LIKELY SAFE ...when used orally and appropriately. Rye grass pollen extract appears to be safe when used for up to 24 weeks (5292,5293,5294,5296,8176,8177,8520). Long-term effects are unknown.
PREGNANCY AND LACTATION: Insufficient reliable information available; avoid using.

Effectiveness

POSSIBLY EFFECTIVE

Benign prostatic hyperplasia (BPH). Taking rye grass extracts orally seem to improve symptoms such as frequency, nocturia, urgency, decreased urine flow rate, dribbling, and painful urination in patients with mild to moderate BPH (5292,5293,5294). Some researchers report decreased prostate size, improved urinary flow, and decreased residual urine volume (5292,8520); others report no effect on objective BPH measures (8176). Studies have used a specific rye grass pollen extract (Cernilton) (5292,5293,5294,8176,8520). It is not known if rye grass pollen extract is comparable to finasteride (Proscar) or alpha-blockers. However, rye grass is comparable to Pygeum and Paraprost, a Japanese prostate remedy containing L-glutamic acid, L-alanine, and aminoacetic acid (8176,8177).

INSUFFICIENT RELIABLE EVIDENCE to RATE

Prostatitis and prostatodynia. Preliminary clinical evidence suggests that rye grass pollen extract might relieve chronic prostatitis and prostatodynia (5296). More evidence is needed to rate rye grass for these uses.

Mechanism of Action

The applicable part of rye grass is the pollen extract. Some rye grass pollen extracts are prepared by microbial digestion of the pollen, followed by water and acetone extraction (5290,5295). The extract contains beta-sterols. It seems to relax urethral smooth muscle tone and increase bladder muscle contraction. Some evidence suggests that it might affect alpha-adrenergic receptors and relax the internal and external bladder sphincter muscles (8176). The extract does not affect luteinizing hormone, follicle-stimulating hormone, testosterone, or dihydrotestosterone (5292).
Some evidence suggests that rye grass pollen extract might inhibit prostate cancer cell growth (5297).
Other evidence suggests that it might interfere with inflammation by inhibiting the biosynthesis of prostaglandins and leukotrienes (5298).

Adverse Reactions

Orally, rye grass can cause abdominal distention, heartburn, and nausea (5293).

Interactions with Herbs & Other Dietary Supplements

None known.

Interactions with Drugs

None known.

Interactions with Foods

None known.

Interactions with Lab Tests

None known.

Interactions with Diseases or Conditions

None known.

Dosage and Administration

ORAL: For benign prostatic hyperplasia (BPH), a specific rye grass pollen extract 126 mg three times daily has been used (5294,8176).

Comments

Rye grass pollen extract (Cernilton) is a registered pharmaceutical product in Western Europe, Japan, Korea, and Argentina (8176).

SACCHAROMYCES BOULARDII

Also Known As

Brewer's Yeast (Hansen CBS 5926), Probiotics, Saccharomyces, Saccharomyces cerevisiae Hansen CBS 5926, S. boulardii.
CAUTION: See separate listings for Brewer's Yeast (Saccharomyces cerevisiae), Bifidobacteria, and Lactobacillus.

Scientific Names

Saccharomyces boulardii.
Family: Saccharomycetaceae.

People Use This For

Orally, Saccharomyces boulardii is used for treating and preventing diarrhea, including infectious types such as rotaviral diarrhea in children, diarrhea caused by bacterial overgrowth in adults, traveler's diarrhea, and diarrhea associated with enteral tube feedings. It is also used orally to prevent and treat antibiotic-associated diarrhea. Saccharomyces boulardii is also used orally for general digestion problems, irritable bowel syndrome (IBS), inflammatory bowel syndrome (IBD, Crohn's disease, ulcerative colitis), relapsing Clostridium difficile colitis, and bacterial overgrowth in short bowel syndrome. It is also used orally for lactose intolerance, urinary tract infections (UTIs), vaginal and Candida-related (yeast) infections, high cholesterol levels, hives, fever blisters, canker sores, and adolescent acne.

Safety

LIKELY SAFE ...when used orally and appropriately (4353).
CHILDREN: POSSIBLY SAFE ...when used orally and appropriately (4347,4356).
PREGNANCY AND LACTATION: Insufficient reliable information available; avoid using.

Effectiveness

POSSIBLY EFFECTIVE

Acne. Taking Saccharomyces boulardii orally seems to help reduce chronic acne as adjuvant treatment (7140).
Antibiotic-associated diarrhea. Although there is a conflicting report (4350,4351), the majority of evidence shows that taking Saccharomyces boulardii orally can be useful for preventing antibiotic-associated diarrhea (4353,4355).
Clostridium difficile diarrhea. Taking Saccharomyces boulardii orally in combination with vancomycin or metronidazole, reduces the risk of recurrence of Clostridium difficile diarrhea (4352,4354). However, for people with an initial episode, Saccharomyces boulardii doesn't seem to be any more effective than the antibiotics alone (4352).
Crohn's disease. Taking Saccharomyces boulardii orally seems to reduce the frequency of bowel movements in patients with Crohn's disease (7646).
Diarrhea. Administering Saccharomyces boulardii in tube feedings seems to prevent diarrhea (4349). Taking Saccharomyces boulardii orally seems to be effective for treating acute diarrhea in infants (4347).
Helicobacter pylori (H pylori). Saccharomyces boulardii seems to reduce the adverse effects of Helicobacter therapy, but doesn't seem to improve compliance (12763).
HIV-related diarrhea. Taking Saccharomyces boulardii orally seems to help reduce HIV-related diarrhea (4347).
Traveler's diarrhea. Taking Saccharomyces boulardii orally seems to help prevent traveler's diarrhea (155).

INSUFFICIENT RELIABLE EVIDENCE to RATE

Cystic fibrosis. Taking Saccharomyces boulardii orally doesn't seem to decrease Candida albicans gastrointestinal colonization in patients with cystic fibrosis (7652). More evidence is needed to rate Saccharomyces boulardii for this use.

Mechanism of Action

Saccharomyces boulardii is typically a non-pathogenic yeast (4363). Saccharomyces boulardii is used as a probiotic agent to help colonize the gastrointestinal tract. It is used therapeutically in cases where disease is thought to occur due to depleted normal intestinal flora or colonization by pathogenic organisms. Saccharomyces boulardii typically reaches a maximum steady state in 3 days when taken orally. It does not multiply in the gut. Less than 1% of the ingested dose is recovered from stools (4363).

Saccharomyces boulardii is thought to help for Clostridium difficile infection by producing proteases that might decrease the toxicity of Clostridium difficile toxins A and B (4348,4361). Individuals who have low stool concentrations of Saccharomyces boulardii after repeated use are most likely to have Clostridium difficile recurrence (4360). In addition to its effect on Clostridium difficile, Saccharomyces boulardii also shows evidence of interaction with cholera toxin (4363).

In Crohn's disease, Saccharomyces boulardii increases secretory immune globulin A (IgA) in the intestine (7646). Saccharomyces boulardii might cause an increase in the intestinal chloride resorption, which also may play a role in the treatment of Crohn's disease (4362,7646).

Adverse Reactions

Orally, Saccharomyces boulardii can cause flatulence. Elevated sedimentation rate may occur when Saccharomyces boulardii is used to treat Crohn's disease (7646), but this effect may be part of the disease process.

Rarely, oral use has been associated with fungemia in both immunocompromised and immunocompetent people (1247,4357,4358,4360,7329). Thirty cases of Saccharomyces fungemia have been reported, all in very ill intensive care unit (ICU) patients with indwelling catheters. Most infections have occurred when packets of Saccharomyces were used or Saccharomyces capsules were opened at bedside (12776,12777).

The true incidence of fungemia is difficult to determine with Saccharomyces boulardii. Most clinical laboratories are unable to differentiate between Saccharomyces boulardii and Saccharomyces cerevisiae which might come from other sources (7353).

Interactions with Herbs & Other Dietary Supplements

None known.

Interactions with Drugs

ANTIFUNGALS: Theoretically, since Saccharomyces boulardii is a yeast, antifungals might decrease its effectiveness (4363).

Interactions with Foods

None known.

Interactions with Lab Tests

SACCHAROMYCES CEREVISIAE: In patients who experience fungemia following use of Saccharomyces boulardii, cultures can indicate fungemia from Saccharomyces cerevisiae (7329). Most laboratories are unable to distinguish between Saccharomyces cerevisiae and Saccharomyces boulardii (7353).

Interactions with Diseases or Conditions

IMMUNODEFICIENCY: There is some concern that immunocompromised patients taking Saccaromyces boulardii might be at an increased risk for fungemia. Although Saccharomyces is generally a nonpathogenic organism, there have been cases of fungemia following its use (1247,4357,4358,4360).

YEAST ALLERGY: Patients with yeast allergy can be allergic to products containing Saccharomyces boulardii (4363).

Dosage and Administration

ORAL: A typical dose to prevent diarrhea is 250-500 mg two to four times a day (4355). A typical dose to treat recurrent diarrhea in adults is 1 gram daily for four weeks along with antibiotic therapy (4352). In the treatment of Crohn's disease, Saccharomyces boulardii 250 mg three times daily, has been used for up to 9 weeks (7646). For infants: 250 mg two to four times a day has been used according to age (4356). To prevent contamination of indwelling catheters, open packets or capsules with gloves, outside the patient's room (4359). As an adjunct in Helicobacter pylori treatment, a dose of 5 billion colony forming units (CFUs) of Saccharomyces boulardii has been given once daily (12763).

Comments

Saccharomyces boulardii was previously identified as a unique species of yeast, but is now believed to be a strain of Saccharomyces cerevisiae (baker's yeast) (1227,1251,1282,7353).

SAFFLOWER

Also Known As

American Saffron, Bastard Saffron, Benibana, Dyer's Saffron, Fake Saffron, False Saffron, Hing Hua, Honghua, Zaffer, Zafran.

Scientific Names

Carthamus tinctorius.

Family: Asteraceae/Compositae.

People Use This For

Orally, safflower seed oil is used for reducing the risk of cardiovascular disease and preventing atherosclerosis, hyperemia in women, and to promote hair growth. Safflower is also used orally for fever, tumors, coughs, bronchial conditions, blood stasis, pain, blood invigoration, amenorrhea, painful menses, stimulating menstruation, coronary heart disease, chest pain, traumatic injuries, inducing sweating, as a laxative, purgative, stimulant, antiperspirant, abortifacient, and expectorant.

In foods, safflower seed oil is used as a cooking oil.

In manufacturing, safflower flower is used to color cosmetics and dye fabrics. Safflower seed oil is used as a paint solvent.

Safety

LIKELY SAFE ...when safflower seed oil is used orally (6).

POSSIBLY SAFE ...when safflower flower is used orally and appropriately (6,12,18).

PREGNANCY: LIKELY UNSAFE ...when safflower flower is used because it has abortifacient, menstrual stimulant, and uterine stimulant effects (11,12).

LACTATION: There is insufficient reliable information available about the safety of safflower during lactation; avoid using.

Effectiveness

POSSIBLY EFFECTIVE

Hypercholesterolemia. Taking safflower oil orally as a dietary supplement seems to reduce total and low-density lipoprotein (LDL) cholesterol (6). However, it does not seem to lower triglycerides or increase high-density lipoprotein (HDL) cholesterol (6).

There is insufficient reliable information available about the effectiveness of safflower for its other uses.

Mechanism of Action

The applicable parts of safflower are the flower and seed oil. Safflower flower contains a complex mixture of red and yellow pigments (11,18). The constituent, safflower yellow, has immunosuppressive and anticoagulant activity (11). Safflower polysaccharide has immunopotentiating effects (11). Safflower extracts exhibit cardiac stimulant, vasodilating, hypolipemic, hypotensive, and uterine stimulant properties (11). Safflower seed oil is a rich source of the essential unsaturated fatty acid, linoleic acid (6). It also contains linolenic acid (18). Some evidence suggests essential fatty acids are necessary to maintain the integrity of the central nervous system (6). Other evidence suggests that diets high in unsaturated and polyunsaturated fatty acids reduce atherosclerosis and the risk of heart disease (6). A diet rich in safflower oil can increase platelet linoleic acid levels, reduce serum cholesterol, particularly low-density lipoprotein (LDL) cholesterol, and apolipoprotein B levels (6) without affecting serum triglyceride, high-density (HDL) lipoprotein cholesterol or apolipoprotein A-1 levels (6).

Adverse Reactions

Safflower can cause an allergic reaction in individuals sensitive to the Asteraceae/Compositae family. Members of this family include ragweed, chrysanthemums, marigolds, daisies, and many other herbs.

Interactions with Herbs & Other Dietary Supplements

HERBS WITH ANTICOAGULANT/ANTIPLATELET POTENTIAL: Concomitant use with herbs that have constituents that might affect platelet aggregation could theoretically increase the risk of bleeding in some people. These herbs include angelica, clove, danshen, garlic, ginger, ginkgo, Panax ginseng, red clover, turmeric, and others.

Interactions with Drugs

ANTICOAGULANT/ANTIPLATELET DRUGS: Theoretically, concomitant use with safflower might increase effects and adverse effects of anticoagulants.

Interactions with Foods

None known.

Interactions with Lab Tests

None known.

Interactions with Diseases or Conditions

BLEEDING DISORDERS: Contraindicated in people with hemorrhagic diseases, peptic ulcers, or clotting disorders. Safflower can prolong coagulation time (12).

CROSS-ALLERGENICITY: Safflower can cause an allergic reaction in individuals sensitive to the Asteraceae/Compositae family. Members of this family include ragweed, chrysanthemums, marigolds, daisies, and many other herbs.

Dosage and Administration

ORAL: A typical dose is one cup of tea up to three times daily. To make tea, simmer 1 gram dried flower in 150 mL boiling water, 5-10 minutes, strain (18).

Comments

Although safflower seed oil is a rich source of linoleic acid, some experts contend gamma-linolenic acid might be more useful as a physiologic source of essential fatty acids. To be useful in the body, linoleic acid must be converted to dihomo-gamma-linolenic acid (DHGA) and arachidonic acid (6). Gamma-linolenic acid does not require this conversion before it can be used in the body.

SAFFRON

Also Known As

Autumn Crocus, Azafron, Croci stigma, Indian Saffron, Kumkuma, Saffron Crocus, Safran, Spanish Saffron, True Saffron.
CAUTION: See separate listing for Autumn Crocus.

Scientific Names

Crocus sativus.
Family: Iridaceae.

People Use This For

Orally, saffron is used for asthma, insomnia, cancer, atherosclerosis, cough, whooping cough (pertussis), and flatulence. Saffron is also used for depression, fright, shock, spitting up blood (hemoptysis), pain, dysmenorrhea, dyspepsia, premature ejaculation, and dry skin. It is also used as an aphrodisiac, to induce sweating, and as an expectorant.
Topically, saffron is used for baldness (alopecia).
In foods, saffron is used as a culinary spice, yellow food coloring, and as a flavoring agent.
In manufacturing, saffron extracts are used as fragrance in perfumes and as a dye for cloth.

Safety

LIKELY SAFE ...when used orally in amounts commonly found in foods. Saffron has Generally Recognized As Safe (GRAS) status in the US (4912).
POSSIBLY SAFE ...when used orally and appropriately, short-term for medicinal purposes. A specific saffron extract 30 mg/day (Novin Zaferan Co, Iran) seems to be safe when used for up to 6 weeks (11024,13103).
LIKELY UNSAFE ...when used orally in high doses. Taking 5 grams or more of saffron can cause severe side effects (12). Doses of 12-20 grams can be lethal (18).
PREGNANCY: LIKELY UNSAFE ...when used orally in amounts exceeding those commonly found in foods. Larger amounts of saffron have uterine stimulant and abortifacient effects (2,18); avoid using.
LACTATION: Insufficient reliable information available; avoid using.

Effectiveness

POSSIBLY EFFECTIVE

Depression. Taking a specific saffron extract 30 mg/day (Novin Zaferan Co, Iran) orally seems to improve symptoms of major depression after 6 weeks of treatment (11024,13103). There is also some evidence that this saffron extract might be as effective as taking the conventional antidepressant imipramine 100 mg/day (11024); however, this dose of imipramine is considered subtherapeutic.

There is insufficient reliable information available about the effectiveness of saffron for its other uses.

Mechanism of Action

The applicable part of saffron is the stigma. Saffron constituents include crocin, picrocrocin, and crocetin (6,11). Picrocrocin is responsible for the characteristic bitter taste of saffron and crocin for the yellow-red color (11).
It is not known how saffron might work for depression.
Preliminary evidence suggests that crocetin might improve atherosclerosis by increasing plasma oxygen diffusion (6,11) and decreasing cholesterol and triglyceride levels (4110). In addition, crocetin binds to albumin (4109), potentially increasing oxygen diffusion and improving atherosclerosis (4109).
Small amounts of saffron stimulate gastric secretions (18); larger amounts appear to stimulate uterine smooth muscle, contributing to abortifacient affects (18). Saffron extracts limit the in vitro growth of experimental tumor colony cells by inhibiting cellular nucleic acid synthesis (4104,4105).

Adverse Reactions

Orally, saffron extract seems to be well-tolerated. In studies evaluating a specific extract (Novin Zaferan Co, Iran) reported side effects include anxiety, decreased or increased appetite, drowsiness, nausea, vomiting, and hypomania (13103); however, these side effects did not occur at a higher rate than placebo.
Saffron poisoning can occur with 5 grams (2,11), symptoms include yellow appearance of the skin, sclera, and mucous membranes (mimicking icterus); vomiting; vertigo; bloody diarrhea; hematuria; bleeding from the nose, lips, eyelids or uterus; numbness; uremic collapse; and thrombocytopenic purpura leading to severe necrosis of the nose (2,11). Ingesting 10 grams of saffron can induce abortion (2); 12-20 grams is reportedly lethal (12). Rhinoconjunctivitis and allergy induced asthma have been reported (4106). Anaphylactic reactions can occur within minutes of eating food prepared with saffron (4107).

Interactions with Herbs & Other Dietary Supplements

CROSS-SENSITIVITY: Cross-reactivity exists between saffron and Lolium, Olea (includes olive), and Salsola species plants (4106).

Interactions with Drugs
None known.

Interactions with Foods
None known.

Interactions with Lab Tests
None known.

Interactions with Diseases or Conditions
BIPOLAR DISORDER: Saffron is thought to have antidepressant effects and has caused hypomania in depressed patients (13103). Theoretically, saffron might induce mania or hypomania in patients with bipolar disorder.
CROSS-ALLERGENICITY: Cross-reactivity reported between saffron and Lolium, Olea (includes olive), and Salsola species plants (4106).

Dosage and Administration
ORAL: For depression, a specific ethanol saffron extract 30 mg/day (Novin Zaferan Co, Iran) has been used (11024,13103).

Comments
The dried stigmas of saffron are used to make saffron spice. It can take 75,000 saffron blossoms to produce a single pound of saffron spice. Due to the intense labor involved in harvesting, saffron is considered one of the World's most expensive spices.

SAGE

Also Known As
Common Sage, Dalmatian Sage, Garden Sage, Meadow Sage, Sauge, Scarlet Sage, Spanish Sage, True Sage.
CAUTION: See separate listings for Boneset, Clary Sage, Danshen, German Sarsaparilla, Purple Loosestrife, Spearmint, and Wood Sage.

Scientific Names
Salvia officinalis; Salvia lavandulaefolia.
Family: Lamiaceae/Labiatae.

People Use This For
Orally, sage is used for loss of appetite; excessive perspiration; dysmenorrhea; diarrhea; gastritis; galactorrhea; reduction of saliva secretion; and digestive problems including flatulence, bloating, and dyspepsia. It is also used for depression, cerebral ischemia, memory enhancement, and Alzheimer's disease.
Topically, sage is used for herpes labialis, laryngitis, pharyngitis, stomatitis, gingivitis, glossitis, minor oral injuries, and inflammation of the nasal mucosa.
As an inhalant, sage is used for asthma.
In foods, it is used as a culinary spice.
In manufacturing, sage is used as a fragrance component in soaps and cosmetics.

Safety
LIKELY SAFE ...when used orally in amounts commonly found in foods. Sage is approved for food use in the US (4912).
POSSIBLY SAFE ...when used orally in therapeutic doses, short-term. Sage seems to be safe when taken orally for up to 4 months (10334,10810). ...when used topically (10437).
POSSIBLY UNSAFE ...when used orally in high doses, or when used long-term (12). Some species of sage contain a thujone constituent that can be toxic if enough is consumed (12).
PREGNANCY: LIKELY UNSAFE ...when used orally because the constituent, thujone, can have menstrual stimulant and abortifacient effects (19).
LACTATION: POSSIBLY UNSAFE ...when used orally; sage is thought to reduce the mother's milk supply (19).

Effectiveness
POSSIBLY EFFECTIVE

Alzheimer's disease. Taking extracts of Salvia officinalis and Salvia lavandulaefolia orally seem to improve cognitive function in patients with mild to moderate Alzheimer's disease when used for up to 4 months (10334,10810).
Herpes labialis (cold sores). Topical treatment of herpes labialis with a cream containing sage and rhubarb (Rheum officinale and Rheum palmatum) may be about as effective as acyclovir (Zovirax) cream. Acyclovir

cream provides healing of lesions in 6.3 days; the sage and rhubarb cream provides healing of lesion in 7.2 days. The combination of sage and rhubarb appears to improve the time to healing and to reduce pain, compared with sage alone (10437).

INSUFFICIENT RELIABLE EVIDENCE to RATE

Memory. Single doses of Salvia lavandulaefolia might enhance memory in a dose-dependent manner in young adults (10811). More evidence is needed to rate sage for this use.

Mechanism of Action

The applicable part of sage is the leaf and volatile oil. Sage contains 1-2.8% of volatile oil that may be responsible for pharmacological activity. The volatile oil contains several active constituents that have in vitro pharmacological activity. Rosmarinic acid, carvacrol, and luteolin have antioxidant properties. Cirsiliol is a central nervous system (CNS) depressant. Linalool and alpha-terpineol have CNS depressant and anticholinesterase activity. Other constituents with anticholinesterase activity are 1,8-cineole, alpha-pinene, and caryophyllene epoxide. The constituent geraniol exerts estrogenic activity. Some constituents also seem to have anti-inflammatory activity. These constituents might act synergistically and be beneficial for Alzheimer's disease. Animal studies of sage show anticholinesterase activity (10334).

Preliminary research suggests that sage might have hypoglycemic activity (10813).

Sage also contains camphor, which has pro-oxidant effects and is associated with hepatotoxicity and neurotoxicity a high doses (10334). Salvia officinalis contains significant amounts of thujone, a convulsant.

The thujone concentration of the volatile oil varies from 17% to 58%, depending on growing conditions, season of harvest, and other variables (10812). Salvia lavandulaefolia contains only trace amounts of thujone (10334).

Adverse Reactions

Orally, sage can cause nausea, vomiting, abdominal pain, dizziness, agitation, and wheezing (10810). It may increase the blood pressure of hypertensive patients (10334). Thujone, which is found in salvia officinalis, is a neurotoxin and can cause seizures (10812). Camphor, which is present in both of these species of sage, can cause hepatotoxicity and neurotoxicity in high doses (10334).

Interactions with Herbs & Other Dietary Supplements

HERBS WITH HYPOGLYCEMIC POTENTIAL: Theoretically, sage may have additive effects with herbs that decrease blood glucose levels (10813). Herbs with hypoglycemic potential include devil's claw, fenugreek, garlic, guar gum, horse chestnut seed, Panax ginseng, psyllium, and Siberian ginseng.

HERBS WITH SEDATIVE PROPERTIES: Some constituents of sage have CNS depressant activity (10334). Theoretically, concomitant use with herbs that have sedative properties might enhance therapeutic and adverse effects. Some of these supplements include 5-HTP, calamus, California poppy, catnip, hops, Jamaican dogwood, kava, St. John's wort, scullcap, valerian, yerba mansa, and others.

Interactions with Drugs

ANTICONVULSANTS: Some species of sage can cause convulsions. Theoretically, sage might interfere with the effectiveness of anticonvulsant drugs (10812).

ANTIDIABETES DRUGS: Preliminary research suggests sage might have hypoglycemic activity (10813). Theoretically, sage might have additive therapeutic effects and adverse effects with hypoglycemic drugs.

CNS DEPRESSANTS: Some constituents of sage have CNS depressant activity (10334). Theoretically, concomitant use with drugs with sedative properties might cause additive effects and side effects.

Interactions with Foods

None known.

Interactions with Lab Tests

BLOOD GLUCOSE: Preliminary research suggests sage might have hypoglycemic activity (10813).

Interactions with Diseases or Conditions

DIABETES: Preliminary research suggests sage might have hypoglycemic activity (10813). Monitor blood sugar closely.

HYPERTENSION: Sage can increase blood pressure in some people with hypertension (10334). Monitor blood pressure.

SEIZURE DISORDERS: Salvia officinalis contains significant amounts of thujone, a convulsant. Avoid the use of sage in quantities greater than those in food (10812).

Dosage and Administration

ORAL: For treating Alzheimer's disease, a fixed dose of salvia officinalis hydroalcoholic extract, equivalent to 1 gram of sage per day, has been used (10810). An extract of salvia lavandulaefolia, titrated up to 2.5 mg three times daily, has also been used (10334).

TOPICAL: For treatment of herpes labialis (cold sores) a cream containing 23 mg/gram each of sage extract and rhubarb extract has been applied every 2 to 4 hours while awake, with treatment starting within 1 day of the first symptoms and continuing for 10 to 14 days (10437).

Comments

Sage is a rich source of beta-carotene (19).

SALACIA

Also Known As

Chundan, Ponkoranti, S. Oblonga, SO.

Scientific Names

Salacia oblonga.
Family: Celastraceae.

People Use This For

Orally, salacia is used for diabetes, gonorrhea, asthma, pruritus, and rheumatism.

Safety

POSSIBLY SAFE ...when used orally. There is some evidence that single doses of salacia can be consumed safely in doses up to 1000 mg (13032).

PREGNANCY AND LACTATION: Insufficient reliable information; avoid using.

Effectiveness

INSUFFICIENT RELIABLE EVIDENCE to RATE

Diabetes. Preliminary evidence suggests that consuming a single dose of salacia in combination with a meal can decrease post-prandial serum insulin levels and possibly decrease post-prandial blood glucose in healthy volunteers (13032). Salacia's effects in diabetes patients are not known. More evidence is needed to rate salacia for this use.

Mechanism of Action

The applicable parts of salacia are the roots and stems.

The water-soluble portion of a methanol extract of salacia yields active constituents salacinol and kotalanol. These constituents seem to inhibit alpha-glucosidase in the intestinal brush border and inhibit aldose reductase (13034).

Inhibition of alpha-glucosidase decreases breakdown of carbohydrates into absorbable monosaccharides and therefore decreases postprandial blood glucose levels (13032,13033).

In an animal model of diabetes, salacia extract seems to decrease cardiac fibrosis, which is a slow developing complication of diabetes (13033).

Salacia rootbark powder also seems to have anti-inflammatory effects in animal models (13035).

A safety evaluation in animal models suggests that salacia extract in doses 10 times what is suggested for humans for 14 days has no significant adverse effect on blood chemistry, hematology, or organ weights (13119).

Adverse Reactions

Orally, salacia can cause flatulence and distention. Flatulence is more significant with a 1000 mg dose compared to a 500 mg dose (13032).

Interactions with Herbs & Other Dietary Supplements

None known.

Interactions with Drugs

None known.

Interactions with Foods

None known.

Interactions with Lab Tests

None known.

Interactions with Diseases or Conditions
None known.

Dosage and Administration
ORAL: For diabetes, salacia 500-1000 mg in combination with a meal has been used (13032).

Comments
Salacia species are native to India and Sri Lanka. Salacia has a long history of use in traditional Indian medicine, Ayurveda, as a treatment for diabetes.

SALEP

Also Known As
Cuckoo Flower, Levant Salep, Orchid, Sahlep, Saloop, Satyrion.

Scientific Names
Orchis morio.
Family: Orchidaceae.

People Use This For
Orally, salep is used for diarrhea (particularly in children), heartburn, flatulence, and indigestion.

Safety
POSSIBLY SAFE ...when used orally (18).
PREGNANCY AND LACTATION: Insufficient reliable information available; avoid using.

Effectiveness
There is insufficient reliable information available about the effectiveness of salep.

Mechanism of Action
The applicable part of salep is the tuber. Salep contains up to 40% mucilage including glucans, glucomannans, starch, and protein (18).

Adverse Reactions
None reported.

Interactions with Herbs & Other Dietary Supplements
None known.

Interactions with Drugs
None known.

Interactions with Foods
None known.

Interactions with Lab Tests
None known.

Interactions with Diseases or Conditions
None known.

Dosage and Administration
ORAL: It is typically used as a powdered formulation in medicinal preparations; taken in water before or after meals (18).

SAMe

Also Known As

Ademetionine, Adenosylmethionine, S-Adenosyl Methionine, S-Adenosylmethionine, S-Adenosyl-Methionine, SAM-e, Sammy.

Scientific Names

S-adenosyl-L-methionine.

People Use This For

Orally, SAMe is used for depression, heart disease, fibromyalgia, osteoarthritis, bursitis, tendonitis, chronic lower back pain, dementia, Alzheimer's disease, slowing the aging process, improving intellectual performance, and Parkinson's disease. Other uses include premenstrual syndrome (PMS), premenstrual dysphoric disorder (PMDD), attention deficit-hyperactivity disorder (ADHD), multiple sclerosis, spinal cord injury, seizures, migraine headache, chronic lead poisoning, disorders of porphyrin, and bilirubin metabolism.

Intravenously, SAMe is used for treating depression, osteoarthritis, AIDS-related myelopathy, fibromyalgia, liver disease, cirrhosis, and intrahepatic cholestasis.

Intramuscularly, SAMe is injected for fibromyalgia, depression, and Alzheimer's disease.

Safety

LIKELY SAFE ...when used orally, intravenously, or intramuscularly and appropriately. Serious toxicity has not been reported in multiple clinical studies involving as many as 22,000 patients and lasting from a few days to 2 years (5231,5232,5189,5201,5202,5209,5219,5231,12231).

PREGNANCY: POSSIBLY SAFE ...when used intravenously short-term during the third trimester of pregnancy. In two small-scale trials, SAMe 800 mg daily was used intravenously for 14-20 days during the third trimester of pregnancy for intrahepatic cholestasis. No adverse effects in the mother or fetus were observed (5219,5231,5240). Large-scale trials are needed to confirm the safety of SAMe use in pregnancy. Use of SAMe in pregnancy should only be considered when benefits clearly outweigh the potential risks. There is insufficient reliable information available about the use of SAMe at higher doses, for extended periods of time, or during the earlier trimesters of pregnancy.

LACTATION: Insufficient reliable information available; avoid using.

Effectiveness

LIKELY EFFECTIVE

Depression. Administering SAMe intravenously or intramuscularly, short-term, is helpful for treatment of major depression. Several small-scale clinical trials have shown that parenterally administered SAMe is superior to placebo and possibly as effective as intravenous or oral tricyclic antidepressants in studies lasting up to 30 days (2082,3562,5184,5189,5200,5231,9109). In some trials, the antidepressant effect occurred rapidly, within 1-2 weeks of initiation of treatment (5200). This benefit is likely the result of the parenteral route of administration (3562). Parenteral SAMe has been used successfully in combination with an oral tricyclic antidepressant to speed the onset of antidepressant action (5193).

Taking SAMe orally also seems to reduce symptoms of major depression. Several studies have shown that orally administered SAMe is superior to placebo and possibly as effective as tricyclic antidepressants in trials lasting up to 42 days (2082,2083,5189,5190,5192,5195,5196,5231,9108,9109). But most studies are limited by small numbers of patients, inconsistent diagnostic criteria, short treatment periods, and flawed study designs (3562,5189,5231,9108). Well designed, large scale studies with placebo controls are needed to clarify the benefit of orally administered SAMe in major depression.

Osteoarthritis. Multiple clinical trials show that taking SAMe orally is superior to placebo and comparable to NSAIDs, including the COX-2 inhibitor celecoxib (Celebrex), for decreasing symptoms associated with osteoarthritis. SAMe is associated with fewer adverse effects than NSAIDs and is comparable in reducing pain and improving functional limitation (5188,5199,5203,5204,5205,5206,5207,5208,5209,5215,9108,9111,12054). Significant symptom relief with SAMe may require up to 30 days of treatment compared to only 15 days with NSAIDs. Some evidence suggests that intravenous loading doses of SAMe given over five days, followed by oral treatment, can speed symptom relief to 14 days (5188).

POSSIBLY EFFECTIVE

AIDS-related myelopathy. Administering SAMe intravenously seems to improve AIDS-related myelopathy. SAMe has investigational orphan drug status for this use (1691,5217,5218).

Fibromyalgia. Taking SAMe orally seems to improve fibromyalgia. Two clinical trials demonstrated significant improvement in symptoms of fibromyalgia compared to placebo (5211,5241). But administering SAMe intravenously doesn't seem to improve symptoms of fibromyalgia (5221).

Intrahepatic cholestasis. Administering SAMe orally or intravenously seems to be helpful for treating intrahepatic cholestasis associated with acute or chronic liver disease and pregnancy-related intrahepatic cholestasis. Multiple clinical trials have shown that short-term SAMe therapy is superior to placebo in decreasing pruritus, fatigue, alkaline phosphatase levels, and total and conjugated bilirubin (5219,5238,5239,5240,9108). Trials have more frequently used injectable dosage forms than oral formulations (5219).

Liver disease. Administering SAMe orally or intravenously seems to decrease signs and symptoms of chronic liver disease caused by medications, alcoholism, or lead poisoning. Multiple clinical trials have shown that SAMe can normalize liver enzymes, decrease bilirubin, and decrease symptoms associated with various forms of chronic liver disease. Most trials have enrolled small numbers of patients and have been short duration (1712,5198,5231,5235,5236,5238). Large-scale studies are needed to confirm SAMe's potential benefit in chronic liver disease.

INSUFFICIENT RELIABLE EVIDENCE to RATE

Attention deficit-hyperactivity disorder (ADHD). Preliminary research suggests SAMe might lessen ADHD symptoms in adults (9981). More evidence is needed to rate SAMe for this use.

Mechanism of Action

S-adenosylmethionine (SAMe) is a naturally occurring molecule that is distributed throughout virtually all body tissues and fluids (5231). Concentrations are highest in childhood and decrease with age (9114). SAMe plays an essential role in more than 100 biochemical reactions involving enzymatic transmethylation. It contributes to the synthesis, activation and/or metabolism of hormones, neurotransmitters, nucleic acids, proteins, phospholipids, and some drugs (5231,5232,9110). SAMe is produced endogenously by adenosine triphosphate (ATP) activation of methionine that is synthesized in the body or obtained from metabolism of dietary protein (9110). SAMe synthesis is closely linked to vitamin B12 and folate metabolism (5231). Deficiencies of these vitamins can result in decreased SAMe concentrations in the central nervous system (CNS) (5231).

The mechanism for the antidepressant effect is unknown, but SAMe is associated with increased serotonin turnover and elevated dopamine and norepinephrine levels (5196,5232,9110). SAMe supplementation may also work by altering cellular membrane fluidity. Changes in neuronal membrane fluidity might facilitate signal transduction across membranes and increase the efficiency of receptor-effector coupling (5196,9110). Neuroimaging studies indicate that SAMe affects the brain similarly to conventional antidepressants (9114).

SAMe supplementation may be beneficial in osteoarthritis due to analgesic and anti-inflammatory effects. After oral administration of 400 mg daily for seven days, SAMe levels in synovial fluid increase by 3 to 4 fold (9110). Preliminary evidence suggests SAMe might stimulate articular cartilage growth and repair, specifically chondrocyte proteoglycan synthesis and proliferation rate (5209,9110). SAMe might also protect against cytokine-induced cell damage by antagonizing the activity of tumor necrosis factor-alpha (TNF-alpha) on synovial cell proliferation and fibronectin mRNA expression (9110).

In liver disease, there appears to be a deficiency in hepatic SAMe. Exogenously administered SAMe might act as an essential nutrient by restoring biochemical factors that are depleted in people with liver dysfunction. People with acute or chronic liver disease lose the ability to synthesize SAMe from methionine, possibly due to low activity of methionine adenosyl transferase (MAP), the enzyme that converts methionine to SAMe (9115). This can lead to deficiencies in cysteine and choline. It can also lead to depletion of glutathione, which plays a major role in liver detoxification and antioxidant reactions. This depletion may in turn exacerbate liver disease (5198,5219,5236,9116).

In alcoholic liver disease, among other actions SAMe may restore levels of glutathione, decreasing inflammation, and increasing the methylation of DNA (10465). SAMe may also be beneficial in AIDS-related myelopathy, by replenishing depleted endogenous SAMe. Epidemiological data suggests that people with AIDS have a deficiency of SAMe in their cerebrospinal fluid (CSF), and this may lead to myelopathy by impairing SAMe dependent myelin and oligodendrocyte repair mechanisms (1691,5217,5218). Some evidence suggests that SAMe might also have a gastric cytoprotective effect (5213).

SAMe is metabolized to s-adenosylhomocysteine, which can be metabolized to homocysteine (5232). Homocysteine is remethylated to form methionine, which can then form more SAMe, or be converted via transsulfuration to the antioxidant glutathione (5232). These reactions require folate, cyanocobalamin (vitamin B12), and pyridoxine (vitamin B6) (5231). There has been some concern that taking SAMe might increase homocysteine levels. Elevated levels of homocysteine have been linked to cardiovascular and renal disease (1698). However, in a study lasting 4 weeks, administration of SAMe orally in doses titrated up to 1600 mg/day, there was no significant increase in homocysteine levels (12231). In another study, there also was no difference in cardiovascular mortality in people with cirrhosis taking SAMe 1200 mg daily for two years (1712).

Low levels of SAMe have actually been correlated with coronary artery disease (1714). Administration of SAMe to healthy people has shown a positive effect on 5-methyltetrahydrofolate, a key cofactor in homocysteine metabolism. SAMe supplementation has been suggested as a remedy for elevated homocysteine levels (1713). Some research suggests that adequate intracellular SAMe promotes remethylation and transsulfuration of homocysteine (9112).

Exogenously administered SAMe has low oral bioavailability, which is presumably the result of significant first-pass effect and rapid hepatic metabolism (5231). It achieves peak plasma concentrations 3 to 5 hours after ingestion of an enteric-coated tablet, has a half-life of about 100 minutes and is excreted in urine and feces (5231). SAMe crosses the blood-brain barrier (5231,9110).

SAMe can induce symptoms resembling Parkinson's disease in animal models. This effect may be related to the ability of SAMe to add methyl groups to L-dopa. L-dopa has been shown to deplete the concentration of SAMe, which might explain the depression sometimes seen with Parkinson's disease (10466).

Adverse Reactions

Orally, SAMe can cause flatulence, nausea, vomiting, diarrhea, constipation, dry mouth, headache, mild insomnia, anorexia, sweating, dizziness, and nervousness (347,9113,12231). These side effects are more common with higher doses (5231).

Anxiety has occurred in people with depression (5231) and hypomania in people with bipolar disorder (5231). A case of mania with suicidal ideation has also been reported in an otherwise healthy patient (12231).

There has been some concern that taking SAMe might increase homocysteine levels. SAMe is metabolized to s-adenosylhomocysteine, which can be metabolized to homocysteine (5232). Elevated levels of homocysteine have been linked to cardiovascular and renal disease (1698). However, in a study lasting 4 weeks, administration of SAMe orally in doses titrated up to 1600 mg/day, there was no significant increase in homocysteine levels (12231). In another study, there also was no difference in cardiovascular mortality in people with cirrhosis taking SAMe 1200 mg daily for two years (1712).

When used as an injection, SAMe has caused mania in people with bipolar disorder (5216,5231).

Interactions with Herbs & Other Dietary Supplements

HERBS AND SUPPLEMENTS WITH SEROTONERGIC PROPERTIES: Theoretically, SAMe might increase the effects and adverse effects of products that increase serotonin levels, including 5-hydroxytryptophan (5-HTP), Hawaiian baby woodrose, L-tryptophan, and St. John's wort (3521,5193).

Interactions with Drugs

ANTIDEPRESSANT DRUGS: Concurrent use might cause additive serotonergic effects and serotonin syndrome-like effects, including agitation, tremors, anxiety, tachycardia, tachypnea, diarrhea, hyperreflexia, shivering, and diaphoresis (3521,5193); or theoretically concurrent use might cause cerebral vasoconstriction disorders such as Call-Fleming syndrome (8056). In one case report, SAMe 100 mg intramuscularly was given daily along with clomipramine (Anafranil) 25 mg per day. The clomipramine dose was later increased to 75 mg per day, and 48-72 hours later the patient experienced side effects similar to serotonin syndrome, requiring hospitalization (3521). Theoretically, this may also occur when SAMe is used with other tricyclic antidepressants and with non-tricyclic antidepressants (5193) such as fluoxetine (Prozac), paroxetine (Paxil), sertraline (Zoloft), amitriptyline (Elavil), clomipramine (Anafranil), and others. Concurrent use of SAMe with imipramine (Tofranil) has resulted in a more rapid onset of antidepressant action (5193,5231).

DEXTROMETHORPHAN (Robitussin DM, others): Theoretically, concurrent use might cause additive serotonergic effects and increase the risk of serotonin syndrome (3521,5193). Also, concurrent use might theoretically cause cerebral vasoconstriction disorders such as Call-Fleming syndrome (8056).

LEVODOPA: SAMe methylates levodopa, which might worsen Parkinsonian symptoms. Theoretically, SAMe might reduce the effectiveness of levodopa given for Parkinson's disease (10466).

MEPERIDINE (Demerol): Theoretically, concurrent use with meperidine might cause additive serotonergic effects and increase the risk of serotonin syndrome (3521,5193). Also, concurrent use might theoretically cause cerebral vasoconstriction disorders such as Call-Fleming syndrome (8056).

MONOAMINE OXIDASE INHIBITORS (MAOIs): Theoretically, because the effects of SAMe on serotonin and other neurotransmitters is similar to that of conventional antidepressants (5196,5232); concomitant use might have additive adverse effects including hypertension, hyperthermia, agitation, confusion, coma, etc. SAMe should be avoided in patients taking MAOIs and for 2 weeks after discontinuing an MAOI.

PENTAZOCINE (Talwin): Theoretically, concurrent use with pentazocine might cause additive serotonergic effects and increase the risk of serotonin syndrome (3521,5193). Also, concurrent use might theoretically cause cerebral vasoconstriction disorders such as Call-Fleming syndrome (8056).

TRAMADOL (Ultram): Theoretically, concurrent use with tramadol might cause additive serotonergic effects and increase the risk of serotonin syndrome (3521,5193). Also, concurrent use might theoretically cause cerebral vasoconstriction disorders such as Call-Fleming syndrome (8056).

Interactions with Foods

None known.

Interactions with Lab Tests

None known.

Interactions with Diseases or Conditions

BIPOLAR DISORDER: Use of SAMe can cause patients to convert from a depressed state to a hypomanic or manic state (3523).

PARKINSON'S DISEASE: SAMe methylates levodopa, which could theoretically worsen Parkinsonian symptoms. However, this has not been reported in humans (10466).

Dosage and Administration

ORAL: For depression, an oral dose of 400-1600 mg per day has been used (5231). Doses of 1600 mg per day are the most commonly used in clinical trials (5189). For osteoarthritis, an oral dose of 200 mg three times daily is typically

used (5188). For alcoholic liver disease or cirrhosis, oral doses of 1200-1600 mg per day have been used (1712,5231,5238,5241). For intrahepatic cholestasis, an oral dose of 800 mg twice daily is typically used (5219,5231,5239). For fibromyalgia, an oral dose of 800 mg per day is typically used (5241).
PARENTERAL: For depression, an intravenous or intramuscular injection of 200-400 mg per day is typically used (5231). For speeding the onset of antidepressant effect in combination with a tricyclic antidepressant, SAMe 200 mg intramuscularly for the first 2 weeks of tricyclic antidepressant therapy has been used (5193). For osteoarthritis, an intravenous dose of 400 mg per day has been used (5188). For intrahepatic cholestasis, an intravenous dose of 800 mg per day is typically used (5219,5231). For intrahepatic cholestasis of pregnancy (ICP), an intravenous dose of 800 mg per day has been used (5219,5231,5240). For AIDS-related myelopathy, an intravenous dose of 800 mg daily for 14 days has been used (5217).

Comments

Early studies used parenteral SAMe before an oral formulation was available (5231). Currently, several oral salt forms of SAMe are available: sulfate, sulfate-p-toluenesulfonate (also labeled as tosylate), and butanedisulfonate (5231,5444). The oral bioavailability of the tosylate salt is 1%, and the oral bioavailability of the butanedisulfonate salt is 5%, presumably due to a large first pass effect (1896,1897). Concerns about the stability of the tosylate formulation have been expressed (5446). The butanedisulfonate salt is stable for 2 years at room temperature (1896,5444). SAMe has been available as a dietary supplement in the US since 1999, but it has been used as a prescription drug in Italy since 1979, in Spain since 1985, and Germany since 1989. The potential usefulness of SAMe for treating osteoarthritis was discovered when patients in clinical trials of SAMe for depression noted improvement in their osteoarthritis symptoms (9110).

SAMPHIRE

Also Known As

Crest Marine, Peter's Cress, Pierce-Stone, Sampier, Sea Fennel.

Scientific Names

Crithmum maritimum.
Family: Apiaceae/Umbelliferae.

Comments

At the date of publication, there was very little scientific information available about this product. Our staff is continually analyzing the available information on natural medicines and will add data to the online version of *Natural Medicines Comprehensive Database* as it becomes available. See www.naturaldatabase.com.

SANDY EVERLASTING

Also Known As

Common Shrubby Everlasting, Eternal Flower, Everlasting, Fleur de Pied de Chat, Goldilocks, Harnblumen, Helichrysum, Katzenpfotchenbluten, Yellow Chaste Weed.
CAUTION: See separate listing for Immortelle.

Scientific Names

Helichrysum italicum, synonyms Helichrysum angustifolium, Gnaphalium angustifolium, Gnaphalium italicum; Helichrysum orientale, synonyms Elichrysum orientale, Gnaphalium orientale; Helichrysum stoechas, synonyms Elichrysum stoechas, Gnaphalium stoechas.
Family: Asteraceae/Compositae.

People Use This For

Orally, sandy everlasting is used for dyspepsia, liver ailments, chronic cholecystitis, and gallbladder complaints with accompanying cramps. Sandy everlasting is also used orally as a diuretic, for chronic bronchitis, asthma, whooping cough, psoriasis, burns, rheumatism, headache, migraine, and allergies.
In foods, beverages, and tobacco, the extract is used as a flavoring component.
In manufacturing, it is used in perfumes, and before- and after-sun products.

Safety

LIKELY SAFE ...when used orally in amounts commonly found in foods. Sandy everlasting has Generally Recognized As Safe (GRAS) status in the US (4912).
POSSIBLY SAFE ...when used orally and appropriately (2).
PREGNANCY AND LACTATION: Insufficient reliable information available; avoid using in amounts greater than those generally found in foods and beverages.

Effectiveness
There is insufficient reliable information available about the effectiveness of sandy everlasting.

Mechanism of Action
The applicable part of sandy everlasting is the dried flower. Sandy everlasting contains flavonoids, quercitrin, kaempferol, naringenin, and isohelichrysin. These components might increase bile secretion. They have been shown to increase bile secretion in animals (11). The flavonoids also absorb UV light (11). Quercitrin increases the detoxifying function of the liver and exhibits anti-inflammatory activity (11). The constituent arenarin has antibacterial activity and promotes gastric and pancreatic secretions (8). The volatile oil of Helichrysum italicum flowers seems to have some antibacterial and antifungal activity (11).

Adverse Reactions
Sandy everlasting can cause an allergic reaction in individuals sensitive to the Asteraceae/Compositae family. Members of this family include ragweed, chrysanthemums, marigolds, daisies, and many other herbs.

Interactions with Herbs & Other Dietary Supplements
None known.

Interactions with Drugs
None known.

Interactions with Foods
None known.

Interactions with Lab Tests
None known.

Interactions with Diseases or Conditions
BILIARY OBSTRUCTION: Sandy everlasting is contraindicated, due to bile stimulating effects (2,18).
CROSS-ALLERGENICITY: Sandy everlasting can cause an allergic reaction in individuals sensitive to the Asteraceae/Compositae family. Members of this family include ragweed, chrysanthemums, marigolds, daisies, and many other herbs.
GALLSTONES: Sandy everlasting might complicate therapy (2,18).

Dosage and Administration
ORAL: One cup fresh tea (made by steeping 1 gram dried flower in 150 mL boiling water 5-10 minutes, strain) is typically taken several times per day (8,18); average amount 3 grams of dried flower per day (2).
TOPICAL: No typical dosage.

SANGRE DE GRADO

Also Known As
Blood of the Dragon, Drago, Dragon's Blood, Lan-Hiqui, Laniqui, Sangre de Drago, Sangre de Dragon, Sangue de Agua, Sangue de Drago, SP 303, SP-303, Taspine.
CAUTION: See also Dragon's Blood (Draconis resina) and Herb Robert (Geranium robertianum).

Scientific Names
Croton lechleri.
Family: Euphorbiaceae.

People Use This For
Orally, sangre de grado or its constituent, SP-303, is used for treating diarrhea associated with cholera, AIDS, traveling, cancer treatment, Clostridium difficile infection, and irritable bowel syndrome (IBS). It is also used orally for supporting the body's tissue repair mechanisms and treating viral respiratory infection. Additionally, sangre de grado is used orally for oropharyngeal and gastrointestinal ulcers, fever, hemorrhage, bleeding gums, fractures, wound healing, hemorrhoids, eczema, insect bites and stings, vaginitis, for vaginal baths before childbirth, and as a general tonic.
Topically, sangre de grado or its constituent, SP-303, is used for treating herpes simplex virus (types 1 and 2).

Safety

POSSIBLY SAFE ...when SP-303, a derivative of sangre de grado, is used orally or topically and appropriately (2784,2787,2788).

There is insufficient reliable information available about the safety of sangre de grado.

PREGNANCY AND LACTATION: Insufficient reliable information available; avoid using.

Effectiveness

POSSIBLY EFFECTIVE

AIDS-related diarrhea. Taking sangre de grado as part of a standardized resin extract containing SP-303 (SB-Normal Stool Formula, ShamanBotanicals.com) orally seems to reduce stool weight and frequency in people with AIDS-related diarrhea (2784).

Herpes simplex virus (HSV). Applying sangre de grado topically as part of a standardized resin extract containing SP-303, seems to be effective for treating genital and anal herpes simplex lesions in people with AIDS (2788). But it doesn't seem to be effective for treating acyclovir-unresponsive mucocutaneous herpes simplex lesions in these patients (2787).

Traveler's diarrhea. Taking sangre de grado as part of a standardized resin extract containing SP-303 seems to be effective for symptomatic treatment of traveler's diarrhea (2806).

INSUFFICIENT RELIABLE EVIDENCE to RATE

Insect bites and plant reactions. Applying sangre de grado resin alleviated the symptoms of insect bites (fire ants, wasps, bees) and plant reactions in a group of pest control workers (6114). More evidence is needed to rate sangre de grado for this use.

Mechanism of Action

Sangre de grado is a tree native to the Amazon regions of South America (2805,2784). The resin, a viscous red latex, and bark have a long history of oral and topical medicinal use (2784,2797). Sangre de grado is reported to have anti-inflammatory (2804,6114), antibacterial, anti-hemorrhagic, antiseptic, anti-tumor properties (2804). Topically, it has been shown to reduce vasodilation, swelling, and secretory response to irritants, promote mucosal healing, and prevent hyperalgesic responses in the laboratory (6114). Several active constituents of sangre de grado have been isolated, including SP-303 and tapsine (2786,2796). Preliminary evidence suggests that the constituent SP-303 might control diarrhea by inhibiting cyclic adenosine monophosphate (cAMP), which causes chloride and fluid secretion (2786). SP-303 shows activity against types 1 and 2 herpes simplex viruses, respiratory syncytial virus (RSV), and influenza A virus, possibly by inhibiting viral penetration of cells (2790,2791,2792,2793,2794). Tapsine demonstrates anti-inflammatory and wound healing properties when applied topically (2795,2796). Sangre de grado does not stimulate cell proliferation and has not shown carcinogenic activity after 17 months of treatment in experimental models (2796,2797,2798). Preliminary evidence suggests that sangre de grado resin is not cytotoxic, and has antibacterial and pro-oxidant activity (2798,2799).

Adverse Reactions

Orally, no serious adverse reactions or lab abnormalities have been reported in clinical studies using the sangre de grado derivative, SP-303 (2784,2806).

Topically, SP-303 can cause local pain and burning (2787).

Interactions with Herbs & Other Dietary Supplements

None known.

Interactions with Drugs

None known.

Interactions with Foods

None known.

Interactions with Lab Tests

None known.

Interactions with Diseases or Conditions

None known.

Dosage and Administration

ORAL: For treating AIDS-related diarrhea, a sangre de grado extract containing 500 mg of SP-303 (SB-Normal Stool Formula) every 6 hours has been used (2784). For treating traveler's diarrhea, a sangre de grado extract containing 125-500 mg SP-303 (SB-Normal Stool Formula) 4 times daily for 2 days has been used (2806).

Comments

SP-303 was in Phase III clinical trials with "fast track" designation for treatment of AIDS-related diarrhea and Phase II trials for traveler's diarrhea (2807). After the FDA rejected a new drug application and requested additional clinical testing, the manufacturer, Shaman Pharmaceuticals, became Shaman Botanicals and elected to market SP-303 as a dietary supplement, SB-Normal Stool Formula (2807).

SANICLE

Also Known As
European Sanicle, Poolroot, Saniculae herba, Self-Heal, Wood Sanicle.
CAUTION: See separate listing for Self-Heal.

Scientific Names
Sanicula europaea.
Family: Apiaceae/Umbelliferae.

People Use This For
Orally, sanicle is used for mild respiratory tract mucous membrane inflammation, cough, and bronchitis.

Safety
POSSIBLY SAFE ...when used orally and appropriately (2,12).
PREGNANCY AND LACTATION: Insufficient reliable information available; avoid using.

Effectiveness
There is insufficient reliable information available about the effectiveness of sanicle.

Mechanism of Action
The applicable parts of sanicle are the above ground parts. Sanicle contains triterpene saponins, caffeine derivatives, and flavonoids such as rutin, isoquercitrin, astragalin. It seems to have astringent and expectorant effects (18). The expectorant effect seems to result from the irritation caused by the saponins on the gastric mucosa that reflexly stimulates the bronchial mucous glands via parasympathetic sensory pathways (7). Large amounts of saponins may cause stomach upset, nausea, and vomiting (7). In animals, sanicle demonstrates edema reduction (18).

Adverse Reactions
Orally, large amounts of sanicle may cause upset stomach, nausea, and vomiting due to saponin content (7).

Interactions with Herbs & Other Dietary Supplements
None known.

Interactions with Drugs
None known.

Interactions with Foods
None known.

Interactions with Lab Tests
None known.

Interactions with Diseases or Conditions
GI MUCOSAL IRRITATION (e.g., ulcers, etc.): Theoretically, sanicle may exacerbate existing GI mucosal irritation due to saponin content (6); contraindicated.

Dosage and Administration
ORAL: A typical dose is 4-6 grams dried above ground parts per day (2).

Comments
Avoid confusion with Prunella vulgaris, also referred to as self-heal. In commerce, sanicle may be mixed with leaves of Cardamine enneaphylos, and Astrantia major is sometimes labeled as sanicle (18).

SARSAPARILLA

Also Known As
Ecuadorian Sarsaparilla, Honduras Sarsaparilla, Jamaican Sarsaparilla, Mexican Sarsaparilla, Salsaparilha, Salsepareille, Sarsa, Sarsaparillae radix, Sarsaparillewurzel, Smilax, Smilax aristolochiaefolii.
CAUTION: See separate listings for German Sarsaparilla.

Scientific Names
Smilax febrifuga; Smilax aristolochiifolia (Mexican Sarsaparilla), synonym Smilax medica; Smilax regelii (Honduran Sarsaparilla), synonym Smilax ornata; Smilax officinalis; other Smilax species.
Family: Smilacaceae.

People Use This For
Orally, sarsaparilla is used for psoriasis and other skin diseases, rheumatoid arthritis (RA), kidney disease, as an anabolic for performance enhancement or body-building in athletes, gout, and as a diuretic and diaphoretic.
Sarsaparilla is also used as an adjunct for treating leprosy and for syphilis.
Mexican and Honduran sarsaparilla are used for treating gonorrhea, fevers, and digestive disorders.
In manufacturing, sarsaparilla is used as a flavoring agent in foods, beverages, and pharmaceuticals.

Safety
LIKELY SAFE ...when used orally in amounts commonly found in foods. Sarsaparilla has Generally Recognized As Safe status (GRAS) for use in foods in the US (4912).
POSSIBLY SAFE ...when used orally and appropriately for medicinal purposes (12).
POSSIBLY UNSAFE ...when used in excessive amounts; gastrointestinal (GI) irritation may occur due to its saponin constituents (4).
PREGNANCY AND LACTATION: Insufficient reliable information available; avoid using.

Effectiveness
There is insufficient reliable information available about the effectiveness of sarsaparilla.

Mechanism of Action
The applicable part of sarsaparilla is the root. Sarsaparilla can have antirheumatic, antiseptic, and antipruritic activity (4). It contains about 2% saponins and other varied constituents, including quercetin and phytosterols (beta-sitosterol, stigmasterol, pollinastanol). The saponins, including sarsasapogenin and smilagenin (3,4,5,11), may have diuretic, diaphoretic, expectorant, and laxative effects (5). The sterols contained in sarsaparilla are not anabolic steroids nor are they converted in vivo to anabolic steroids (3,11). Testosterone has never been detected in any plant, including sarsaparilla (3,5). Sarsaparilla may improve appetite and digestion (4), and its extracts may improve psoriasis symptoms (4). Preliminary evidence suggests that sarsaparilla may have hepato-protective and anti-inflammatory activity (4).

Adverse Reactions
Orally, sarsaparilla may cause GI irritation or temporary kidney impairment when used in excessive amounts (11). Large doses can lead to European cholera, diuresis, and shock (18). Occupational exposure to sarsaparilla root dust can cause rhinitis and asthma symptoms (4111).

Interactions with Herbs & Other Dietary Supplements
DIGITALIS: Sarsaparilla may increase digitalis glycoside absorption (2,11).
OTHER HERBS: Theoretically, sarsaparilla may alter the absorption or elimination of simultaneously administered herbs (2).

Interactions with Drugs
DIGOXIN (Lanoxin): Sarsaparilla may increase digitalis glycoside absorption (2,11).

Interactions with Foods
None known.

Interactions with Lab Tests
None known.

Interactions with Diseases or Conditions
ASTHMA: Sarsaparilla root dust can cause the symptoms of asthma (4111).
KIDNEY DYSFUNCTION: Theoretically, sarsaparilla can exacerbate kidney impairment (2,11).

Dosage and Administration

ORAL: The typical oral dose of sarsaparilla is 1-4 grams of the dried root or one cup of the tea three times daily. The tea is prepared by simmering 1-4 grams of the dried root in boiling water for 5-10 minutes and then straining (4). The typical dose of the liquid extract, 1:1 in 20% alcohol or 10% glycerol, is 8-15 mL (4).

Comments

In the Old West of the United States, sarsaparilla was the most popular drink of the cowboys (6002). Avoid confusion with Indian or false sarsaparilla (Hemidesmus indicus, Family: Apocyanaceae), reportedly a widespread adulterant of sarsaparilla (3,5,11). False sarsaparilla contains none of the saponins or other principal constituents found in sarsaparilla (5).

SASSAFRAS

Also Known As

Ague Tree, Cinnamon Wood, Common Sassafras, Kuntze Saloop, Sassafrax, Saxifrax.

Scientific Names

Sassafras albidum, synonyms Sassafras officinale, Sassafras variifolium, Laurus albida.
Family: Lauraceae.

People Use This For

Orally, sassafras is used for urinary tract disorders, mucous membrane inflammation, syphilis, bronchitis, geriatric high blood pressure, gout, arthritis, skin problems, kidney disorders, cancers, and as a tonic and "blood purifier."
Topically, sassafras is used to treat skin eruptions, rheumatism, eye inflammation, sprains, swelling, and for relief of insect bites or stings. Sassafras oil is also used topically as an antiseptic and pediculicide.
In beverages and candy, a safrole-free bark extract has limited use as a flavoring agent.

Safety

POSSIBLY SAFE ...when used in amounts commonly found in foods. Safrole-free sassafras has Generally Recognized As Safe status (GRAS) for use in foods in the US (4912).
POSSIBLY UNSAFE ...when safrole-free sassafras is used in medicinal amounts. Some studies link even safrole-free sassafras extracts to tumors (515).
LIKELY UNSAFE ...when used orally as a medicinal agent; avoid using (3,4). Sassafras root bark and oil contain safrole and related compounds that are carcinogenic and hepatotoxic in animals (4,12,17). Consumption of 5 mL sassafras oil can be fatal in adults (4). ...when used topically; avoid external use due to toxic safrole content (4).
CHILDREN: LIKELY UNSAFE ...when used orally. A few drops of sassafras oil can be fatal (4).
PREGNANCY AND LACTATION: LIKELY UNSAFE ...when used orally (12); avoid using. Sassafras oil has abortifacient effects (4).

Effectiveness

There is insufficient reliable information available about the effectiveness of sassafras.

Mechanism of Action

The applicable part of sassafras is the root bark. The major constituent of the volatile oil, safrole, is carcinogenic (causes malignant liver tumors in experimental animals) (6,11). Safrole and its metabolite, L-hydroxysafrole, are neurotoxic (6).

Adverse Reactions

Orally, sassafras can cause diaphoresis and hot flashes (11). Consumption of large amounts of sassafras oil can cause hallucinations lasting for several days (4). In adults, 5 mL sassafras oil can cause shakes, vomiting, dilated pupils, hypertension, tachycardia, stupor, collapse, abortion, paralysis, liver cancer, and death (4,6). A few drops of sassafras oil may be fatal in children (4).
Topically, sassafras can result in contact dermatitis (6).

Interactions with Herbs & Other Dietary Supplements

HERBS WITH SEDATIVE PROPERTIES: Theoretically, concomitant use with herbs that have sedative properties might enhance therapeutic and adverse effects. Some of these supplements include 5-HTP, calamus, California poppy, catnip, hops, Jamaican dogwood, kava, St. John's wort, scullcap, valerian, yerba mansa, and others.
SAFROLE-CONTAINING HERBS: Avoid concomitant use with other safrole-containing herbs due to potential for additive toxicity (12). Other herbs that contain safrole include basil, camphor, cinnamon, and nutmeg (12).

Interactions with Drugs
CNS DEPRESSANTS: Theoretically, concomitant use with drugs with sedative properties may cause additive effects (19).

Interactions with Foods
None known.

Interactions with Lab Tests
PHENYTOIN: Sassafras oil may cause false-positive blood phenytoin test results (6).

Interactions with Diseases or Conditions
URINARY CONDITIONS: Sassafras can aggravate urinary irritation (19).

Dosage and Administration
No typical dosage.

Comments
Use only safrole-free extract and leaves. Sassafras was used in the past to flavor root beer (11). In 1976, the FDA banned marketing of sassafras as sassafras tea (4). One study estimates that safrole 0.66 mg/kg could be toxic. One cup of tea made with 2.5 grams of sassafras is estimated to contain 200 mg of safrole, approximately 3 mg/kg (4).

SAVIN TOPS

Also Known As
Sabina, Savin, Savine.

Scientific Names
Juniperus sabina.
Family: Cupressaceae.

People Use This For
Orally, savin tops are used to induce abortions.
Topically, savin tops are used as a powder to treat fig warts.

Safety
POSSIBLY UNSAFE ...when used topically. Savin tops can cause severe irritation of skin and mucous membranes (18).
UNSAFE ...when used orally. Savin tops may be fatal if ingested as a powder or tea; 6 drops of the volatile oil can cause death (18).
PREGNANCY AND LACTATION: UNSAFE ...when used orally or topically due to overall toxicity as well as ability to induce abortions (19); avoid using.

Effectiveness
There is insufficient reliable information available about the effectiveness of savin tops.

Mechanism of Action
The applicable parts of savin tops are the branches and leaves. Savin tops contains ligans (thujone, podophyllotoxin, and others), hydroxycoumarins, and volatile oil (3-5%) including sabinyl acetate and sabinene (18). The ligans may have antineoplastic and antiviral properties (18). Savin tops has powerful irritant properties that can cause inflammation of the skin and mucous membranes (18,19).

Adverse Reactions
Orally, symptoms of poisoning include queasiness, cardiac rhythm disorders, spasm, kidney damage, hematuria, central paralysis, unconsciousness, and death (18). Ingestion can also cause irritation of the mucous membranes resulting in gastroenteritis, hepatitis, pneumonitis, and nephritis (19).
Topically, the volatile oil can cause skin irritation, blisters, necroses, and resorbent poisoning (18).

Interactions with Herbs & Other Dietary Supplements
None known.

Interactions with Drugs
None known.

Interactions with Foods
None known.

Interactions with Lab Tests
None known.

Interactions with Diseases or Conditions
INFLAMMATION: Components of the essential oil (sabinene and sabinyl acetate) may increase irritation of the skin or mucous membranes (19).

Dosage and Administration
ORAL: No typical dosage.
TOPICAL: The powder is typically applied twice daily (amount unspecified); "put bandages into skin folds" (18).

Comments
Use only safrole-free extract and leaves. The toxicity of the oil depends on how long it has been stored. Toxicity of oil develops over time through terpene peroxide formation (18). The toxicity of fresh branch tips is apparently low.

SAW PALMETTO

Also Known As
American Dwarf Palm Tree, Cabbage Palm, Ju-Zhong, Palmier Nain, Sabal, Sabal Fructus, Saw Palmetto Berry.

Scientific Names
Serenoa repens, synonyms Serenoa serrulata, Sabal serrulata.
Family: Arecaceae/Palmae.

People Use This For
Orally, saw palmetto is used for symptoms of benign prostatic hyperplasia (BPH). It is also used orally as a mild diuretic, a sedative, an anti-inflammatory, and as an antiseptic. Saw palmetto is used to increase breast size, to improve sexual vigor, and as an aphrodisiac. It is also used to treat chronic nonbacterial prostatitis/chronic pelvic pain syndrome, colds, coughs, irritated mucous membranes, sore throat, asthma, chronic bronchitis, migraines, cancer, and to stimulate hair growth.
In combination with other herbs, saw palmetto is used to treat prostate cancer.
Vaginally, the powdered fruit is used as a uterine and vaginal tonic.

Safety
LIKELY SAFE ...when used orally and appropriately. Saw palmetto has been safely used in clinical studies lasting up to 52 weeks (2732,2735,11354).
PREGNANCY AND LACTATION: LIKELY UNSAFE ...when used orally. Saw palmetto has hormonal activity (6766); avoid using.

Effectiveness
LIKELY EFFECTIVE

Benign prostatic hyperplasia (BPH). Multiple clinical studies lasting up to 48 weeks have shown that saw palmetto significantly improves urinary symptoms such as frequent urination, painful urination, hesitancy, urgency, and perineal heaviness. It also decreases nocturia, improves peak and mean urinary flow, and lowers residual urine volume in patients with BPH (2732,5094,6750,6751,6752,6762,6764,6772,6773,6777,6778,8330). Some research suggests that saw palmetto might not be helpful in men with relatively mild BPH (11314). Saw palmetto seems to be comparable in efficacy to finasteride (Proscar), but saw palmetto might be better tolerated (6424). The combination of a specific brand formulation containing saw palmetto and stinging nettle root (PRO 160/120) also seems to be comparable to finasteride (Proscar) for relieving symptoms of BPH (6763). However, saw palmetto does not reduce prostate size or prostate-specific antigen (PSA) levels like finasteride (6424). Alpha-adrenergic blockers such as prazosin (Minipress) seem to be superior to saw palmetto for relieving symptoms of BPH (6775,6776). However, other preliminary research suggests that saw palmetto is similar in efficacy to tamsulosin (Flomax) after 12 months (11243). The addition of saw palmetto to an alpha-blocker such as tamsulosin doesn't seem to relieve symptoms any better than an alpha-blocker alone (8901). Treatment for one to two months with saw palmetto is usually necessary before significant symptomatic improvement occurs (2732,6750,6778). Most clinical studies have used a liposterolic extract of saw palmetto berry containing 80-90% fatty acids. This formulation is similar to Quanterra Prostate (Warner-Lambert), Super Saw Palmetto (Enzymatic Therapy), ProstaPro (Phytopharmica), Saw Palmetto (Centrum), Standardized Saw Palmetto Extract (Nature's Way), and others.
A different formulation which contains saw palmetto lipid extract 106 mg, nettle root extract 80 mg, pumpkin seed oil extract 160 mg, lemon bioflavonoid extract 33 mg, and beta-carotene 190 IU taken

three times daily for six months doesn't seem to be beneficial for men with BPH (5093).

INSUFFICIENT RELIABLE EVIDENCE to RATE

Prostatitis and chronic pelvic pain syndrome. Preliminary clinical research suggests that saw palmetto given orally for one year doesn't help nonbacterial prostatitis and chronic pelvic pain syndrome (11354). More evidence is needed to rate saw palmetto for these uses.

Mechanism of Action

The applicable part of saw palmetto is the ripe fruit. The lipid fraction contains volatile oils and fatty oils, which are active in treating benign prostatic hyperplasia (BPH). Many saw palmetto products are standardized based on the fatty acid content. The most effective saw palmetto products seem to be whole berries or berry extracts prepared with lipophilic nonpolar solvents. Water extraction, including brewed tea, probably does not adequately extract fat-soluble active constituents.

Saw palmetto has antiandrogenic, antiproliferative, and anti-inflammatory properties that seem to be responsible for improving symptoms of benign prostatic hyperplasia (BPH). Saw palmetto appears to noncompetitively inhibit 5 alpha-reductase types 1 and 2 and to prevent the conversion of testosterone to dihydrotestosterone (DHT) in vitro, which might reduce prostate growth (6765,6769,6770,6773). However, 5 alpha-reductase levels in prostatic tissue and serum testosterone, DHT, and PSA are not significantly reduced by saw palmetto in vivo (2735,6771). Saw palmetto does not seem to affect overall prostate size, but shrinks the inner prostatic epithelium (2736,5093). Saw palmetto, which appears to exert prostate-specific activity, might slow prostate cell proliferation by inhibiting fibroblast growth factor and epidermal growth factor and stimulating apoptosis (6765,6769,6770).

Inflammatory mediators appear to contribute to the etiology of BPH. In men with BPH, a liposterolic extract of saw palmetto berry seems to lower tumor necrosis factor (TNF)-alpha and interleukin (IL)-1beta, which are markers of inflammation in prostate tissue (11224). Laboratory evidence suggests that saw palmetto inhibits lipoxygenase and cyclooxygenase (COX), which are involved in inflammation (6769,6779).

Increased COX-2 expression is also associated with an increased incidence of prostate cancer. Preliminary research indicates that saw palmetto reduces the proliferation of experimental prostate cells, possibly by inhibiting COX-2 expression (8902).

Saw palmetto also seems to have antiestrogen, antispasmodic, and alpha-adrenergic inhibitory properties (5095,6766,6780). Laboratory fertility studies indicate that saw palmetto has no effect on oocytes or sperm motility, but it might induce metabolic changes in sperm (4239,4240).

Saw palmetto doesn't seem to affect the cytochrome P450 (CYP450) enzymes, 2D6 (CYP2D6) and 3A4 (CYP3A4), in healthy volunteers taking 320 mg per day (11225). Drug interactions involving these enzymes have not been reported.

Adverse Reactions

Orally, the adverse effects of saw palmetto are generally mild and comparable to placebo. Dizziness, headache, and gastrointestinal complaints such as nausea, vomiting, constipation, and diarrhea are the most frequently reported adverse effects (6751,6752,6762,11354). There is one case report of cholestatic hepatitis associated with the use of the multi-ingredient product that contains saw palmetto (Prostata) (598).

Some clinicians are concerned that saw palmetto might cause erectile dysfunction, ejaculatory disturbance, or altered libido because of its potential effects on 5-alpha-reductase. There is one case report of decreased ejaculatory volume associated with an herbal blend product containing saw palmetto extract, nettle root extract, pumpkin seed oil extract, lemon bioflavonoid extract, and beta-carotene (5093). However, clinical studies indicate that the occurrence of impotence in men taking saw palmetto is similar to placebo and significantly less than finasteride (Proscar) (2732,6424,6762).

There is also concern that saw palmetto might have antiplatelet effects and potentially increase the risk of bleeding in some patients. There is one report of excessive intraoperative bleeding in a patient who took saw palmetto prior to surgery. Bleeding time normalized when saw palmetto was discontinued (8659). To date, there are no documented cases of spontaneous bleeding in patients taking saw palmetto.

Interactions with Herbs & Other Dietary Supplements

None known.

Interactions with Drugs

ANTICOAGULANT/ANTIPLATELET DRUGS: Theoretically, saw palmetto might increase the risk of bleeding when used concomitantly with these agents. Saw palmetto is reported to prolong bleeding time (8659). Some of these drugs include aspirin; clopidogrel (Plavix); nonsteroidal anti-inflammatory drugs (NSAIDs) such as diclofenac (Voltaren, Cataflam, others), ibuprofen (Advil, Motrin, others), naproxen (Anaprox, Naprosyn, others); dalteparin (Fragmin); enoxaparin (Lovenox); heparin; warfarin (Coumadin); and others.

CONTRACEPTIVE DRUGS: Theoretically, concomitant use with saw palmetto might interfere with contraceptive drugs. Saw palmetto might have antiestrogenic effects (6766).

ESTROGENS: Theoretically, concomitant use with saw palmetto might interfere with hormone therapy. Saw palmetto might have antiestrogenic effects (6766).

Interactions with Foods
None known.

Interactions with Lab Tests
BLEEDING TIME: Saw palmetto can prolong bleeding time and increase the results of bleeding time tests (8659).
PROSTATE-SPECIFIC ANTIGEN: Contrary to earlier concerns, saw palmetto extract appears to have no significant effect on serum prostate-specific antigen (PSA) levels (764).

Interactions with Diseases or Conditions
SURGERY: There is concern that saw palmetto might have antiplatelet effects and could potentially cause excessive bleeding during surgery. Excessive intraoperative bleeding has been reported in one case in a patient who took saw palmetto before surgery (8659). Advise patients to discontinue saw palmetto at least 2 weeks prior to elective surgery.

Dosage and Administration
ORAL: For benign prostatic hyperplasia (BPH), 160 mg twice daily or 320 mg once daily of a lipophilic extract containing 80% to 90% fatty acids has been used in clinical trials (2732,5094,6750,6751,6752,6762,6764,6772,6773,6777) (6778,8330).

Comments
In the first half of the twentieth century, saw palmetto tea was included in the United States Pharmacopeia and the National Formulary.

SCARLET PIMPERNEL

Also Known As
Adder's Eyes, Poor Man's Weatherglass, Red Chickweed, Red Pimpernel, Shepherd's Barometer.

Scientific Names
Anagallis arvensis.
Family: Primulaceae.

People Use This For
Orally, scarlet pimpernel is used for depression, mucous membrane disorders, liver disorders, herpes, and as supportive therapy for carcinomas. It is also used orally for painful kidney disorders, particularly those with inflammation and an increase in urination.
Topically, scarlet pimpernel is used for poorly healing wounds and pruritus.
It is used both orally and topically to treat painful joints.

Safety
POSSIBLY UNSAFE ...when used orally or topically long-term (18).
There is insufficient reliable information available about the safety of scarlet pimpernel for short-term oral or topical use.
PREGNANCY: LIKELY UNSAFE ... when used orally or topically long-term. Scarlet pimpernel shows evidence of uterine stimulant activity (18).
LACTATION: POSSIBLY UNSAFE ...when used orally or topically long-term; avoid using.

Effectiveness
There is insufficient reliable information available about the effectiveness of scarlet pimpernel.

Mechanism of Action
The applicable parts of scarlet pimpernel are the above ground flowering plant parts. In vitro data suggests that the aqueous extract has fungitoxic activity, and the isolated components triterpenglycoside, anagalloside and aglycon anagalligenone have bacteriostatic activity. Animal and human tissue data suggests uterine contracting activity. Triterepene saponins isolated from scarlet pimpernel may have activity against human sperm and may have estrogenic activity. A methanolic extract has hemolytic activity in human blood, and has activity against herpes simplex I, adenovirus type II, and polio type II. The gastrointeritis and nephritis that occurs with large doses or long-term administration is probably due to the cucurbitacins that are present in scarlet pimpernel (18).

Adverse Reactions
Orally, gastrointeritis and nephritis may occur with large doses or long-term administration (18).

Interactions with Herbs & Other Dietary Supplements
None known.

Interactions with Drugs
None known.

Interactions with Foods
None known.

Interactions with Lab Tests
None known.

Interactions with Diseases or Conditions
HORMONE SENSITIVE CANCERS/CONDITIONS: Because scarlet pimpernel might have estrogenic effects (18), women with hormone sensitive conditions should not use scarlet pimpernel. Some of these conditions include breast, uterine, and ovarian cancer, and endometriosis and uterine fibroids.
INFERTILITY: Scarlet pimpernel might have activity against sperm (18). Use cautiously or avoid in women trying to conceive and in men with fertility problems.

Dosage and Administration
ORAL: One cup of tea is commonly taken throughout the day. The tea is prepared by steeping teaspoons of dried plant in 150 mL of boiling water for 10 minutes and straining. The usual daily dosage can be up to 1.8 grams 4 times daily (18).
TOPICAL: No typical dosage.

SCHISANDRA

Also Known As
Bac Ngu Vi Tu, Bei Wu Wei Zi, Beiwuweizi, Chinesischer Limonenbaum, Chosen-Gomischi, Five-Flavor-Fruit, Five-Flavor-Seed, Gomishi, Hoku-Gomishi, Kita-Gomishi, Limonnik Kitajskij, M Mei Gee, Magnolia Vine, Matsbouza, Nanwuweizi, Ngu Mei Gee, Northern Schisandra, Omicha, Schisandra Berry, Schisandrae, Schizandra, Schizandrae, Shisandra, Southern Schisandra, Western Shisandra, Wu Wei Zi, Wu-Wei-Zi, Wuweizi, Xiwuweizi.

Scientific Names
Schisandra chinensis, synonym Kadsura chinensis; Schisandra splenanthera, synonym Schisandra chinensis var. rubriflora; other Schisandra species.
Family: Schisandraceae.

People Use This For
Orally, schisandra is used as an adaptogen for increasing resistance to disease and stress, increasing energy, and increasing physical performance and endurance. Schisandra is also used orally for improving vision, boosting muscular activity, improving cellular energy, for hepatitis, liver protection, preventing premature aging, increasing lifespan, for premenstrual syndrome (PMS), stimulating the immune system, speeding recovery after surgery, protecting against radiation, counteracting the effects of sugar, preventing motion sickness, normalizing blood sugar and blood pressure, reducing high cholesterol, preventing infection, improving adrenal health, and energizing RNA-DNA to rebuild cells. Schisandra is also used for coughs, asthma, insomnia, neurasthenia, chronic diarrhea, dysentery, night sweats, spontaneous sweating, involuntary seminal discharge, thirst, impotence, physical exhaustion, excessive urination, depression, irritability, and memory loss.
Schisandra fruit is eaten as a food.

Safety
POSSIBLY SAFE ...when used orally and appropriately (12,3559).
PREGNANCY: POSSIBLY UNSAFE ...when used orally; avoid using. Some evidence suggests schisandra fruit is a uterine stimulant (11,3559).
LACTATION: Insufficient reliable information; avoid using.

Effectiveness
POSSIBLY EFFECTIVE

Concentration, coordination, and endurance. Taking schisandra fruit extract orally seems to improve concentration, coordination, and endurance (3559).

Hepatitis. Taking schisandra fruit extract orally seems to improve liver function in patients with hepatitis. Schisandra fruit extracts reduce serum glutamic-pyruvic transaminase (SGPT) levels in patients with viral or drug-induced hepatitis (3559).

There is insufficient reliable information available about the effectiveness of schisandra for its other uses.

Mechanism of Action

The applicable part of schisandra is the fruit. A variety of active constituents including schizandrins, schizandrols, gomisins, schizandrers, schisantherins, wuweizisus, and many others, collectively known as lignans, have been isolated from schisandra (11,3559). Some schisandra extracts are standardized based on specific lignan content (3559). Schisandra improves liver function by increasing hepatic glutathione, glucose-6-phosphate, and glutathione-reductase activity. It might also have a hepatoprotective effect by inhibiting lipid peroxidation, increasing liver glycogen production, inducing cytochrome P450 (CYP450) enzymes, and promoting hepatocyte growth (11,3559). Schisandra is referred to as an adaptogen; it seems to increase concentration, coordination, and endurance (3559). The mechanisms for these effects is not yet known. Schisandra also seems to have antioxidant and anti-inflammatory properties (3559). Other reported properties of various schisandra lignans include antitussive (6), anticonvulsant, antidepressant, antifatigue, tranquilizing, respiratory stimulant (11), and platelet activating factor (PAF) inhibition (3767). Some evidence suggests that nigranoic acid, isolated from the stem of Schisandra sphaerandra, might be useful in HIV therapy. In vitro it exhibits anti-HIV reverse transcriptase and polymerase activity (3768).

Adverse Reactions

Orally, schisandra can cause heartburn, acid indigestion, decreased appetite, stomach pain, allergic skin rashes, and urticaria in some patients (11,3559).

Interactions with Herbs & Other Dietary Supplements

None known.

Interactions with Drugs

None known.

Interactions with Foods

None known.

Interactions with Lab Tests

SERUM GLUTAMIC-PYRUVIC TRANSAMINASE (SGPT)/ALANINE AMINOTRANSFERASE (ALT): Schisandra might lower serum SGPT/ALT levels and test results (11,3559).

Interactions with Diseases or Conditions

EPILEPSY: One source recommends to avoid use in patients with epilepsy (3559). The reason for this warning is not clear, but it may be due to schisandra's potential CNS stimulating effects (6).
GASTROESOPHAGEAL REFLUX DISEASE (GERD), PEPTIC ULCER DISEASE (PUD): Schisandra might exacerbate GERD or PUD by increasing gastric acidity (3559).
HIGH INTRACRANIAL PRESSURE: One source recommends to avoid use in patients with high intracranial pressure (3559). The reason for this warning is not clear, but it may be due to schisandra's potential CNS stimulating effects (6).

Dosage and Administration

ORAL: For hepatitis, schisandra extract standardized to 20 mg lignan content (equivalent to 1.5 grams crude schisandra) given daily has been used (3559). For improving mental and physical performance, schisandra extract 500 mg to 2 grams daily or crude schisandra 1.5-6 grams daily have been used (3559); Crude schisandra decoction (boiled tea) 5-15 grams daily has also been used (3559). People have also taken schisandra extract 100 mg twice daily (6002). Appropriate dosing may vary depending on extract type and standardization.

Comments

An antihepatotoxic drug known as DBD has been developed in China derived from the schisandra constituent schisandrin C (3559).

SCHIZONEPETA

Also Known As

Japanese Catnip, Japanese Mint, Jing Jie, Tenuifolia.
CAUTION: See separate listings for Catnip and Japanese Mint.

Scientific Names

Schizonepeta tenuifolia; Schizonepeta multifida, synonym Nepeta multifida.
Family: Lamiaceae/Labiatae.

People Use This For

Orally, schizonepeta is used for the common cold, fever, sore throat, allergic dermatitis, eczema, psoriasis, metrorrhagia, and to stop bleeding.

Safety

POSSIBLY SAFE ...when used orally and appropriately. Schizonepeta has been used safely in studies lasting up to a year (12627,12628,12629).
POSSIBLY UNSAFE ...when used orally in excessive amounts. Schizonepeta contains pulegone, a known hepatotoxin. High doses of schizonepeta might cause hepatotoxicity (12620,12626).
PREGNANCY AND LACTATION: Insufficient reliable information available; avoid using.

Effectiveness

INSUFFICIENT RELIABLE EVIDENCE to RATE

Atopic dermatitis (eczema). Schizonepeta given orally in combination with 9 other herbs (Zemaphyte) might reduce redness and skin lesions in adults and children with nonexudative atopic eczema (12627,12628,12629). However, other research shows no effect (12630). More evidence is needed to rate schizonepeta for this use.

Mechanism of Action

The applicable parts of schizonepeta are the above ground parts. Schizonepeta is processed by either allowing it to sun dry or by carbonizing it. Carbonization involves stir-frying at a high temperature until the surface of the leaves and stems become blackish-brown and the interior surface becomes dark yellow. Schizonepeta contains volatile oils including menthol, pulegone, and d-limonene. It also contains flavonoids such as hesperetin and luteolin. The amounts of these constituents vary with plant parts and processing methods (12620,12625).
Preliminary research suggests that schizonepeta has superoxide scavenging activity, which might explain its use for psoriasis and eczema (12621). However, other research suggests it can increase production of tumor necrosis factor (TNF)-alpha. Schizonepeta might exert an anti-allergic effect by reducing histamine release (12622). It seems to inhibit substance-P-induced itching in animals (12623).
The carbonized form of schizonepeta seems to exert hemostatic effects by inhibiting fibrinolysis and promoting coagulation (12624).

Adverse Reactions

Orally, in combination with other herbs, schizonepeta can cause nausea, vomiting, mild diarrhea, dizziness, urticaria, photosensitivity, an exacerbation of eczema, night diuresis, and discoloration of teeth (12629).

Interactions with Herbs & Other Dietary Supplements

None known.

Interactions with Drugs

None known.

Interactions with Foods

None known.

Interactions with Lab Tests

LIVER FUNCTION TESTS: Schizonepeta in combination with other herbs is associated with reversible increases in liver function tests (12629). Schizonepeta contains variable quantities of pulegone, which is hepatotoxic (12620,12626). Monitor liver function tests including alkaline phosphatase, aspartic acid transaminase (AST,SGOT), alanine aminotransferase (ALT, SGPT), total bilirubin, gamma-glutamyltransferase, and lactate dehydrogenase.

Interactions with Diseases or Conditions

LIVER DISEASE: Theoretically, schizonepeta might exacerbate liver dysfunction in patients with liver disease (12629).

Dosage and Administration

ORAL: For eczema, approximately 5.625 and 7.5 grams of schizonepeta taken as a tea has been used per day (12631).

SCOPOLIA

Also Known As

Belladonna, Belladonna Scopola, Glockenbilsenkraut, Japanese Belladonna, Russian Krainer Tollkraut, Scopola, Scopoliae Rhizoma.
CAUTION: See separate listing for Belladonna.

Scientific Names

Scopolia carniolica.
Family: Solanaceae.

People Use This For

Orally, scopolia is used for spasms of the gastrointestinal (GI) tract, bile ducts, and urinary tract, and for liver and gallbladder complaints. Scopolia is also used orally as a diuretic, sedative, hypnotic, narcotic, for dilating pupils, and pain relief.

Safety

LIKELY UNSAFE ...when used orally for self-medication (12). Use of scopolia requires monitoring (12). The lethal adult dose is considered to be 100 mg of atropine which is approximately 20-50 grams of scopolia root or rhizome depending on its alkaloid content (18).
PREGNANCY AND LACTATION: LIKELY UNSAFE ...when used orally for self-medication (12); avoid using.

Effectiveness

There is insufficient reliable information available about the effectiveness of scopolia.

Mechanism of Action

The applicable parts of scopolia are the rhizome and root. Scopolia root or rhizome contains 0.3-0.8% alkaloids, primarily L-hyoscyamine and lesser amounts of atropine and scopolamine (2). L-Hyoscyamine, the levorotatory isomer of atropine, is considered the active principle (2). Scopolia root has parasympatholytic activity. It is a competitive antagonist of acetylcholine, acting preferentially at the muscarinic receptors (2). Scopolia has antispasmodic effects, relaxing the smooth muscle of the gastrointestinal tract and bile ducts (2). Scopolia root can eliminate muscular tremors and muscular rigidity caused by central nervous impulses. It also has positive chronotropic and dromotropic effects (2).

Adverse Reactions

Orally, scopolia root can cause dry mouth, dry and reddened skin, hyperthermia, disturbance of ocular accommodation, tachycardia, difficulty urinating, glaucoma attacks (2), and constipation (18). Early symptoms of poisoning include reddened skin, dry mouth, and tachycardiac arrhythmias (18). Ingestion of large amounts can cause central excitation including restlessness, compulsive speech, hallucinations, delirium, manic episodes, followed by exhaustion and sleep, and asphyxiation (18).

Interactions with Herbs & Other Dietary Supplements

ANTICHOLINERGIC HERBS: Scopolia can potentiate the effects and adverse effects of other herbs with anticholinergic activity including belladonna, henbane, mandrake, and jimson weed (12).

Interactions with Drugs

ANTICHOLINERGIC DRUGS: The alkaloid constituents, hyoscyamine, scopolamine, and atropine could potentiate the effects and adverse effects of anticholinergic drugs (15).
QUINIDINE: Concomitant use with scopolia might increase effects (2).
TRICYCLIC ANTIDEPRESSANTS (TCAs): Concomitant use with scopolia can potentiate anticholinergic effects and adverse effects (2).

Interactions with Foods

None known.

Interactions with Lab Tests

None known.

Interactions with Diseases or Conditions

CONGESTIVE HEART FAILURE (CHF): Contraindicated; scopolia might cause tachycardia and exacerbate CHF due to its hyoscyamine (atropine) and scopolamine content (15).
CONSTIPATION: Contraindicated; scopolia might cause constipation due to its hyoscyamine (atropine) and scopolamine content (15).
DOWN SYNDROME: Caution, patients with Down syndrome might be hypersensitive to the antimuscarinic effects

(mydriasis, positive chronotropic heart effects, etc.) of hyoscyamine (atropine) and scopolamine contained in scopolia (15).
ESOPHAGEAL REFLUX: Contraindicated; scopolia might delay gastric emptying and decrease lower esophageal pressure, promoting gastric retention and exacerbating reflux due to its hyoscyamine (atropine) and scopolamine content (15).
FEVER: Contraindicated; scopolia might increase the risk of hyperthermia in patients with fever due to its hyoscyamine (atropine) and scopolamine content (15).
GASTRIC ULCER: Contraindicated; scopolia might delay gastric emptying and exacerbate gastric ulcers due to its hyoscyamine (atropine) and scopolamine content (15).
GI INFECTIONS: Contraindicated; scopolia might suppress GI motility causing retention of infecting organisms or toxins due to its hyoscyamine (atropine) and scopolamine content (15).
HIATAL HERNIA: Contraindicated; scopolia might delay gastric emptying and decrease lower esophageal pressure, promoting gastric retention and exacerbating reflux due to its hyoscyamine (atropine) and scopolamine content (15).
NARROW-ANGLE GLAUCOMA: Contraindicated; scopolia might increase ocular tension in patients with narrow-angle (angle-closure) glaucoma due to its hyoscyamine (atropine) and scopolamine content (2,15).
OBSTRUCTIVE GI TRACT DISEASE: Contraindicated; scopolia might exacerbate obstructive GI tract diseases (including atony, paralytic ileus, and stenosis) due to its hyoscyamine (atropine) and scopolamine content (15).
TACHYARRHYTHMIAS: Contraindicated; scopolia might cause tachycardia due to its hyoscyamine (atropine) and scopolamine content (2,15).
TOXIC MEGACOLON: Contraindicated; scopolia might suppress intestinal motility, which might produce paralytic ileus and exacerbate toxic megacolon, due to its hyoscyamine (atropine) and scopolamine content (2,15).
ULCERATIVE COLITIS: Contraindicated; scopolia might suppress intestinal motility, which might produce paralytic ileus and precipitate toxic megacolon, due to its hyoscyamine (atropine) and scopolamine content (15).
URINARY RETENTION: Contraindicated; scopolia might increase urinary retention due to its hyoscyamine (atropine) and scopolamine content (2,15).

Dosage and Administration

ORAL: The average daily dose is 0.25 mg total alkaloids calculated as hyoscyamine (2). The maximum single dose is 1 mg total alkaloids calculated as hyoscyamine (2). The maximum daily dose is 3 mg total alkaloids calculated as hyoscyamine. Scopolia is administered as pulverized root, powder, or other preparations (2).

SCOTCH BROOM

Also Known As

Bannal, Basam, Besenginaterkraut, Besom, Bizzom, Breeam, Broom Tops, Browme, Brum, Butcher's-Broom, Genet a Balais, Ginsterkraut, Herbe de Hogweed, Hogweed, Irish Broom Tops, Scoparium, Scoparius.
CAUTION: See separate listings for Butcher's Broom and Spanish Broom.

Scientific Names

Cytisus scoparius, synonyms Sarothamnus scoparius, Sarothamnus vulgaris, Spartium scoparium, Genista andreana.
Family: Fabaceae/Leguminosae.

People Use This For

Orally, scotch broom is used for edema, improving circulation, cardiac dropsy, cardiac arrhythmia, tachycardia, low blood pressure, hemorrhaging after giving birth, and profuse menstruation. It is also used as a cathartic and emetic. Scotch broom is also used for bleeding gums, hemophilia, gout, rheumatism, sciatica, gallbladder and kidney stones (nephrolithiasis), splenomegaly, jaundice, bronchial conditions, and snake bites.
Topically, scotch broom is used for sore muscles, abscesses, and swelling. It is also used in hair rinses to lighten and brighten hair.

Safety

LIKELY UNSAFE ...when used orally (4,12). Scotch broom contains sparteine, an alkaloid with cardiac depressant activities similar to quinidine (4).
PREGNANCY: LIKELY UNSAFE ...when used orally; scotch broom appears to be an abortifacient (5,9,12).
LACTATION: LIKELY UNSAFE ...when used orally (4,12); avoid using.

Effectiveness

There is insufficient reliable information available about the effectiveness of scotch broom.

Mechanism of Action

The applicable parts of scotch broom are the flower and above ground parts. Scotch broom contains sparteine, an alkaloid, which has curare-like properties and mimics quinidine's anti-arrhythmic effect (4). Sparteine extends diastole without a positive inotropic effect (8). Scotch broom is thought to have a diuretic effect due to the flavone glycoside, scoparoside (5). Scotch broom also contains tyramine (6,11).

Adverse Reactions

Orally, toxicity from the sparteine constituent of scotch broom can occur with doses greater than 300 mg of sparteine, which is roughly equivalent to 30 grams of scotch broom. Symptoms of this toxicity include dizziness, headache, palpitations, prickling in the extremities, a feeling of weakness in the legs, sweating, sleepiness, pupil dilation, and ocular palsy (18). Scotch broom may cause nausea, diarrhea, vertigo, stupor, tachycardia with circulatory collapse, and respiratory arrest (4). Smoking scotch broom cigarettes may cause headaches and uterine stimulation (6), and may risk contracting pulmonary aspergillosis (5,6).

Interactions with Herbs & Other Dietary Supplements

None known.

Interactions with Drugs

HALOPERIDOL (Haldol): Haloperidol (Haldol) inhibits sparteine metabolism, increasing the risk of adverse effects including circulatory collapse (17).
MONOAMINE OXIDASE INHIBITORS (MAOIs): Scotch broom flower contains tyramine. Combined use with MAOI's might cause a hypertensive crisis (2).
QUINIDINE: Quinidine (Quinidex) inhibits sparteine metabolism, which is found in scotch broom, increasing the risk of adverse effects including circulatory collapse (17).

Interactions with Foods

None known.

Interactions with Lab Tests

None known.

Interactions with Diseases or Conditions

CARDIAC DISEASE: Contraindicated due to negative inotropic and negative chronotropic effects (2,4).
HYPERTENSION: Contraindicated due to vasoconstrictive effect (2,4).
KIDNEY DISORDERS: The component, scoparin, might have diuretic activity which could aggravate kidney disorders (19).

Dosage and Administration

ORAL: No typical dosage. However, scotch broom has traditionally been used as a tea, 1-2 grams in boiling water, three times daily (4,7); a liquid extract (1:1 in 25% alcohol), 1-2 mL (4); or a tincture (1:5 in 45% alcohol), 0.5-2 mL (4).

Comments

Scotch broom seeds used as a coffee substitute are dangerous (6).

SCOTCH THISTLE

Also Known As

Woolly Thistle.

Scientific Names

Onopordum acanthium.
Family: Asteraceae.

Comments

At the date of publication, this product was not a common ingredient used in brand name supplements marketed to consumers. Details about this product are available in the online version of *Natural Medicines Comprehensive Database.* See www.naturaldatabase.com.

SCURVY GRASS

Also Known As

Scrubby Grass, Spoonwort.
CAUTION: See separate listing for Watercress.

Scientific Names

Cochlearia officinalis.
Family: Brassicaceae/Cruciferae.

People Use This For

Orally, scurvy grass is used for vitamin C deficiency, gout, arthritis, stomachache, as a diuretic, and as a blood purifier.
Topically, scurvy grass is used for skin irritations, canker sores, and gum disease.

Safety

There is insufficient reliable information available about the safety of scurvy grass.
Pregnancy and Lactation: Insufficient reliable information available; avoid using.

Effectiveness

There is insufficient reliable information available about the effectiveness of scurvy grass.

Mechanism of Action

The applicable parts of scurvy grass are the leaves and aerial parts or pressed juice. Alcohol extracts of scurvy grass are used topically. Scurvy grass contains glucosilinates, an unidentified volatile oil and bitter principle, tannin, and vitamin C. It might have antiseptic, diuretic, and mild laxative actions (7122). The mustard oils in scurvy grass can irritate the mucous membranes (18).

Adverse Reactions

Orally, large amounts of scurvy grass can cause symptoms of gastrointestinal irritation.
Topically, skin irritation may occur with topical application of scurvy grass.

Interactions with Herbs & Other Dietary Supplements

None known.

Interactions with Drugs

None known.

Interactions with Foods

None known.

Interactions with Lab Tests

None known.

Interactions with Diseases or Conditions

None known.

Dosage and Administration

No typical dosage.

Comments

Scurvy grass was once used by sailors to prevent scurvy (7122). Scurvy grass is also known as watercress (see separate listing). Be careful not to confuse these two plants. The scurvy grass flowers have a strong fragrance and taste when they are rubbed (18).

SEA BUCKTHORN

Also Known As

Argasse, Argousier, Buckthorn, Dhar-Bu, Espino Armarillo, Espino Falso, Finbar, Grisset, Meerdorn, Oblepikha, Purging Thorn, Rokitnik, Sallow Thorn, Sanddorn, Sceitbezien, Sea Buckhorn, Seabuckthorn, Sea-Buckthorn, Seedorn, Star-Bu, Tindved.

CAUTION: See separate listings for Alder Buckthorn, European Buckthorn, and Cascara (California Buckthorn).

Scientific Names

Hippophae rhamnoides.

Family: Elaeagnaceae.

People Use This For

Orally, sea buckthorn leaves and flowers are used for treating arthritis, gastrointestinal ulcers, gout, and exanthemata. A tea containing sea buckthorn leaves is used as a source of vitamins, flavones, amino acids, fatty acids and minerals; for improving blood pressure and blood lipids; preventing and controlling blood vessel diseases; removing free radicals; and boosting immunity.

Orally, sea buckthorn berries are used for preventing infections, improving sight, and inhibiting sclerosis and aging. Orally, sea buckthorn seed or berry oil is used as an expectorant, for treating asthma, cardiac disorders including angina, for lowering cholesterol, preventing atheroma, and as an antioxidant. It is also used orally for postponing senility; reducing cancer morbidity and the toxicity of chemotherapy; balancing the immune system; stomach and intestinal diseases including ulcers and reflux esophagitis; treating night blindness; and as a supplemental source of vitamins C, A, and E, beta-carotene, flavonoids, superoxide dismutase, minerals, amino acids, and fatty acids.

Topically, sea buckthorn berries, berry concentrate, and berry or seed oil are used as a sunscreen, for treating radiation damage from x-rays and sunburns; healing wounds including bedsores, burns, and cuts; for acne, dermatitis, dry skin, eczema, skin ulcers, postpartum pigmentation, and for protecting mucus membranes.

In foods, sea buckthorn berries are used to make jellies, juices, purees, and sauces.

In manufacturing, sea buckthorn is used in cosmetics and anti-aging preparations.

Safety

LIKELY SAFE ...when consumed in amounts found in foods (9898). There is insufficient reliable information available about the safety of medicinal use of sea buckthorn.

PREGNANCY AND LACTATION: LIKELY SAFE ...when used in amounts commonly found in foods. Insufficient reliable information available about medicinal use; avoid using in amounts greater than those found in foods.

Effectiveness

There is insufficient reliable information available about the effectiveness of sea buckthorn.

Mechanism of Action

The applicable parts of sea buckthorn are the flowers, fruit, seeds, and leaves. Sea buckthorn fruit, which is used to make jams and jellies, contains fruit acids including malic acid, acetic acid, and quinic acid; as well as volatile oil, sitosterol, and flavonoids. It also contains carotenoids including beta-carotene, gamma-carotene, and lycopene; and fatty oils including oleic acid, isolinol acid, linolenic acid, stearic acid, and palmitoleic acid. The fruit also contains vitamins A, B1, B2, B6, C, and tocopherols (4504,9898).

Preliminary evidence suggests that sea buckthorn extract (plant part not specified) and two constituents of the seed oil (beta-sitosterol-beta-D-glucoside and aglycone) might have activity against gastric ulcers (466,472). The fruit juice reduces the incidence and growth of experimentally-induced tumors (468). The seed oil might protect against carbon tetrachloride, ethyl alcohol and acetaminophen-induced liver damage (469,470). Some data suggest that sea buckthorn extract (plant part not specified) might protect cells against lipid peroxidation injury (471) and might increase the rate and extent of wound tissue epithelialization and granulation (467). Preliminary human evidence indicates that sea buckthorn seed oil might reduce the toxicity of chemotherapy on the blood, gastrointestinal tract and immune system (478), improve symptoms of reflux esophagitis (479), and improve the symptoms and cure rate of peptic ulcers (480). Sea buckthorn berry oil can inhibit aggregation of platelets (10208).

Adverse Reactions

None reported.

Interactions with Herbs & Other Dietary Supplements

HERBS WITH ANTICOAGULANT/ANTIPLATELET POTENTIAL: Concomitant use of herbs that effect platelet aggregation could theoretically increase the risk of bleeding because sea buckthorn berry oil can decrease platelet aggregation (10208). Some of these herbs and supplements include angelica, clove, danshen, feverfew, fish oil, garlic, ginger, ginkgo, Panax ginseng, horse chestnut, red clover, turmeric, vitamin E, and others.

Interactions with Drugs

ANTICOAGULANT/ANTIPLATELET DRUGS: Sea buckthorn berry oil can inhibit platelet aggregation (10208). Theoretically, using sea buckthorn berry oil in combination with anticoagulant or antiplatelet drugs might have additive effects and increase the risk of bleeding. Some of these drugs include aspirin, clopidogrel (Plavix), dalteparin (Fragmin), enoxaparin (Lovenox), heparin, ticlopidine (Ticlid), warfarin (Coumadin), and others.

Interactions with Foods

None known.

Interactions with Lab Tests

None known.

Interactions with Diseases or Conditions

None known.

Dosage and Administration

ORAL: 1-2 cups of a tea prepared from the leaves is typically consumed daily (461). 1-3 seed oil capsules (500 mg per capsule) are commonly used three times daily (462). 3-5 mL of the seed oil is commonly used three times daily (478,479). Up to 2 dropperfuls of the berry oil is commonly used three times daily (463).
TOPICAL: The berry or seed oil is typically applied three or four times per day (462,463).

Comments

Avoid confusion with alder buckthorn (Rhamnus frangula). The fatty oil of sea buckthorn seeds and berries is harvested from August until the first snow of December (18). The fruit juices and purees are popular due to their flavor (4504).

SECRETIN

Also Known As

None.

Scientific Names

Secretin; Oxykrinin.

People Use This For

Sublingually, secretin is used for treating autism.
Intravenously, secretin is used for autism and pervasive developmental disorder, diagnosing Zollinger-Ellison syndrome, pancreatic dysfunction, hyperparathyroidism, preventing stress ulcers, treating duodenal ulcers, gastrointestinal bleeding, pancreatitis, and cardiac failure.

Safety

LIKELY SAFE ...when used parenterally and appropriately. Secretin is an FDA-approved, prescription product (2917,6136).
There is insufficient reliable information available about the safety of secretin when used sublingually.
PREGNANCY AND LACTATION: Insufficient reliable information available; avoid using.

Effectiveness

LIKELY INEFFECTIVE

Autism or pervasive developmental disorder. Administering secretin intravenously doesn't improve symptoms of autism or pervasive developmental disorder. The use of secretin for autism is controversial. There have been some anecdotal and preliminary reports showing subjective improvement in gastrointestinal function, social and behavioral function, and language skills after single infusions of secretin (2917,6632). However, the majority of evidence shows that secretin, both synthetic human and porcine-derived preparations, is no better than placebo for any outcome measure when given in single or repeated doses (5247,6136,7052).

INSUFFICIENT RELIABLE EVIDENCE to RATE

Pancreatitis. There is preliminary evidence secretin might help symptoms of chronic recurrent pancreatitis (2918).
Post-surgical stress ulcers. There is some preliminary evidence that secretin might help prevent post-surgical stress ulcers (2912,2913).
More evidence is needed to rate secretin for these uses.

Mechanism of Action

Secretin is an endogenously occurring gastrointestinal hormone in humans. Secretin is in a family of hormones that also includes glucagon, glucose-dependent insulin releasing peptide (GIP), vasoactive intestinal polypeptide (VIP), and others. Normal fasting serum levels are 3-15 pg/mL. Secretin is released from S cells in the duodenum and proximal jejunum when duodenal pH falls below 4.5. Serum levels can increase to 30 pg/mL after stimulation. The primary action of secretin is to stimulate release of bicarbonate and water from the pancreas. Intravenous administration of secretin in physiological doses has the same effect. The concurrent presence of cholecystokinin (CCK) potentiates the action of secretin on the pancreas. Administration in pharmacological doses also causes decreased release of meal-stimulated gastrin and decreases gastric acid secretion (7053). Secretin is given intravenously because orally administered secretin is inactivated by proteolytic enzymes (15). Synthetic secretin appears to be as effective as secretin of porcine origin (10226).

Many people use secretin for autism, but a potential mechanism of action in autism is not known. Secretin began being used for autism based on anecdotal cases showing improvement in symptoms (2917,6632). Some researchers have speculated that certain autistic patients might have abnormally low secretin levels, but this has not been verified. Reliable clinical evidence now shows that secretin probably does not have a viable role in treating autism (5247,6136,7052).

Adverse Reactions

Intravenously, the most common adverse reaction is flushing of the face, neck, and chest immediately after infusion (6007,7052). Less common potential adverse effects are vomiting (6007,7052), diarrhea, fainting, venous thrombosis (15), fever, and tachycardia (7052). Some patients can have allergic reactions including urticaria, erythema, and anaphylaxis (7052). Because of the potential for these hypersensitivity reactions, a 0.1 mL test dose is often administered prior to giving a full dose (7052).

Interactions with Herbs & Other Dietary Supplements

None known.

Interactions with Drugs

None known.

Interactions with Foods

None known.

Interactions with Lab Tests

None known.

Interactions with Diseases or Conditions

None known.

Dosage and Administration

INTRAVENOUS: For autism, a wide variety of doses have been used. Due to the potential for hypersensitivity reactions, a 0.1 CU test dose is often given prior to administration of the full dose. Clinical studies have used either single infusions or repeated infusions for 2 or more doses separated by 6 weeks or more. Doses are most often 2 CU/kg (5247,7052), but clinicians use a wide range of doses (6007). So far, clinical research does not support the use of secretin for autism. No dosage regimen has yet been proven to improve the symptoms of autism.

Comments

Secretin products are available in the forms of purified porcine secretin and synthetic human secretin (6136).

SELENIUM

Also Known As

L-Selenomethionine, Selenite, Selenium Dioxide, Selenized Yeast, Selenomethionine.

Scientific Names

Selenium; Se; atomic number 34.

People Use This For

Orally, selenium is used for treating HIV/AIDS, heart disease, hypothyroidism, osteoarthritis, rheumatoid arthritis (RA), abnormal pap smears, atherosclerosis, macular degeneration, allergic rhinitis, infertility, gray hair, Osgood-Schlatter disease, Keshan disease, mood disorders, preventing cancer, and preventing miscarriage.

Safety

LIKELY SAFE ...when used orally and appropriately. Selenium is safe in amounts that do not exceed the tolerable upper intake level (UL) of 400 mcg per day (4844,7830,7831,7841,7836,9724).

LIKELY UNSAFE ...when used orally in excessive doses. Doses above 400 mcg may cause significant toxicity (4844,7825).

CHILDREN: LIKELY SAFE ...when used orally and appropriately. Selenium is safe when used in doses below the tolerable upper intake level (UL) of 45 mcg per day for infants up to age 6 months, 60 mcg per day for infants 7 to 12 months, 90 mcg per day for children 1 to 3 years, 150 mcg per day for children 4 to 8 years, 280 mcg per day for children 9 to 13 years, and 400 mcg per day for children age 14 years and older (4844). POSSIBLY SAFE ...when used via a nasogastric tube in premature infants (7835,9764).

PREGNANCY: LIKELY SAFE ...when used orally and appropriately. Selenium is safe in amounts that do not exceed the tolerable upper intake level (UL) of 400 mcg per day (4844). LIKELY UNSAFE ...when used orally in excessive doses. Doses above 400 mcg may cause significant toxicity (4844).

LACTATION: LIKELY SAFE ...when used orally and appropriately. Selenium is safe in amounts that do not exceed the tolerable upper intake level (UL) of 400 mcg per day (4844). LIKELY UNSAFE ...when used orally in excessive doses. Doses above 400 mcg may cause significant toxicity (4844,7838).

Effectiveness

POSSIBLY EFFECTIVE

Prostate cancer. Increased intake of dietary selenium seems to reduce the risk of prostate cancer, as measured by selenium levels in serum, plasma, and toenails (2667,8734,8735,8736). Taking selenized yeast supplements might also help decrease the risk of prostate cancer. Selenized yeast is brewer's yeast that has been grown in selenium rich broth and then used as a selenium supplement (7831,13259). The greatest benefit is obtained in patients who have a selenium deficiency before supplementation (9722,13259). There is also some evidence that adequate dietary vitamin E intake might be important along with adequate selenium for prevention of prostate cancer (10263).

POSSIBLY INEFFECTIVE

Cardiovascular disease. In people with coronary heart disease, selenium 100 mcg daily in combination with beta-carotene and vitamin C and vitamin E doesn't seem to protect against cardiovascular disease progression and related events such as myocardial infarction (MI). There is some evidence that this antioxidant combination might lower high-density lipoprotein 2 (HDL2), which is considered to be the most cardioprotective component of HDL (7388).

Lung cancer. Epidemiologic studies suggest no decrease in the risk of lung cancer as dietary selenium increases, although a small benefit may occur in people that are selenium deficient (9722,9798).

Rheumatoid arthritis (RA). Selenized yeast, providing 200 micrograms daily does not seem to improve objective measures of RA. There might be small improvements in quality of life measures (9763).

Skin cancer. Taking selenium orally 200 mcg daily does not seem to protect against the development of basal cell carcinoma (2664,10687). In addition, daily selenium supplementation may increase the risk of squamous cell carcinoma and total nonmelanoma skin cancer (10687).

INSUFFICIENT RELIABLE EVIDENCE to RATE

Arsenic poisoning. Selenized yeast seems to decrease the concentration of arsenic in Chinese people environmentally exposed to high concentrations of arsenic; however, the effect on clinical signs of arsenic toxicity is not known (7831).

Colorectal cancer. Evidence is conflicting about the effect of selenium on colorectal cancer (2664,2667,9722,12185).

Esophageal cancer. Taking selenium supplements does not seem to significantly decrease the risk of esophageal cancer.

Human immunodeficiency virus (HIV). Preliminary evidence suggests that L-selenomethionine, an organic form of selenium, has no effect on clinical outcome in patients infected with HIV (7830).

Hypothyroidism. In areas of the world that are deficient in iodine, selenium can decrease the concentration of thyroid peroxidase autoantibodies; however, the effect on hypothyroidism is not clear (9797).

Stroke and cancer mortality. There is some evidence that selenized yeast 50 mcg in combination with beta carotene 15 mg and vitamin E (alpha tocopherol) 60 mg used daily might decrease stroke mortality, cancer mortality, and total mortality (2673).

More evidence is needed to rate selenium for these uses.

Mechanism of Action

Selenium is a metallic substance that is available in a variety of chemical compounds. Often selenium is attached to an organic molecule as in selenocysteine, selenomethionine, and kappa-selenocageenan. In broccoli, garlic, onions, and other selenium-accumulating plants it is found as Se-methylselenocysteine or selenocysathionine (7833,7836). In dietary supplements selenium is commonly provided as selenomethionine or in a selenite or selenate salt form (7841). Often selenium is given as selenized yeast, which is common brewer's yeast that has been grown in selenium-rich media (7838). After ingestion as a selenate salt, selenite salt, or as one of the organic forms, selenium must be reduced or metabolized to form hydrogen selenide, an important intermediary form. Selenide is essential for the activity of selenoproteins, such as the glutathione peroxidase enzyme (GSH-Px). The primary organic forms of selenium are the amino acid-based selenocysteine and selenomethionine. Selenomethionine is incorporated directly into proteins, because RNA does not differentiate it from methionine (7832,9718). Selenomethionine serves as a storage form, releasing selenium as the proteins containing it are catabolized (7834,9718). Although the various organic forms of selenium appear to have similar bioavailability after oral consumption (6485), there are substantial differences in the disposition and biologic action of these various forms (7832,7833). Selenomethionine results in high concentrations of selenium in hair and urine, but it does not have the biologic activity of other selenium compounds (7832,7833).

Administration of selenomethionine results in plasma selenium concentrations twice as high as equivalent doses of the selenate form (9762). Of the inorganic salt forms, the bioavailability of the selenate salt is 2 to 3 times higher than the selenite salt, but selenate is more rapidly metabolized. The difference in bioavailability doesn't seem to be significant nutritionally (9717,9761).

The dietary content of selenium required for health falls into a narrow range. Diets containing less than 0.1 mcg/gram of food often result in deficiency, whereas diets containing more than 1 mcg/gram of food may cause toxicity. Consumption of plants that are selenium accumulators, such as Astragalus species (loco weed), can cause significant selenium toxicity if they are grown in selenium-rich soil (7832). Approximately 40 to 100 mcg/day of dietary selenium is needed to maintain a selenium plasma concentration of 70 to 135 nanograms/mL. This is the concentration range needed for maximal activity of selenium dependent enzymes (1665,9718). The content of selenium in the diet is primarily dependent upon the concentration of selenium in the soil. Canada, Japan, Norway, and the United States are the only four countries in the world where the dietary content of selenium is adequate (9718). Dietary selenium is superior to supplements in maintaining adequate plasma concentrations (9721).

At plasma concentrations below 1000 mcg/L, selenium activates glutathione peroxidase (GSH-Px), which reduces oxidative stress by handling free radicals and hydrogen peroxide. At concentrations above 2000 mcg/L selenium paradoxically increases cellular oxidation by promoting the formation of reactive oxygen species (ROS), such as hydroxyl free radicals and superoxide. At higher concentrations selenium also promotes the intracellular formation of nitric oxide, which is converted to toxic nitrous oxide (2664,7825,7826,7827,7828,7829). To reduce the effect of ROS formation, selenium is often given with other antioxidants, such as vitamin E or vitamin C. However, vitamin E might actually increase the cytotoxic effects of high selenium levels, whereas vitamin C appears to reduce the cytotoxicity of selenium (7841). Selenium plays a major role in the synthesis and metabolism of thyroid hormones. The thyroid gland has a higher concentration of selenium than any other organ in the body. Iodothyronine dehydrogenase is at least partially dependent upon selenium for its activity (1665,9724). A deficiency of selenium can exacerbate hypothyroidism in iodine deficiency (1664,9724). In addition, selenium may be able to prevent alterations in thyroid hormone levels that are sometimes observed in patients after trauma (9725). Selenium appears to increase cancer cell death by causing apoptosis and by reducing the formation of ROS. The magnitude of the anticancer effects varies substantially among selenium compounds. Selenite has a high potency to cause apoptosis and selenocystamine is lower. Kappa-selenocageenan also has the ability to induce apoptosis. Selenomethionine has almost no effect on apoptosis (7827,7828). Se-methylselenocysteine found in broccoli, garlic, and onions may be better than supplemental selenite in preventing colonic cancer (7833). Epidemiological evidence indicates that lower blood selenium concentrations increases the likelihood of prostate cancer (8734,8735,8736). Higher levels of selenium may slow prostate cancer tumor progression (13257). Selenium seems to accumulate in the prostate, and protect against DNA damage and increase apoptosis in cancer cells (13258). Lower selenium blood concentrations have also been associated with colorectal cancer (9726). However, supplementing the diet with selenium does not appear to reduce the risk for colorectal cancer (9722). However, early data suggests that there may be more effective and less toxic forms of organic selenium, for preventing colorectal cancer, than those used previously (9737). Preliminary data suggests that supplementing the diet with selenium can reduce the risk for developing breast cancer, but no benefit has been shown in humans (9690,9723). The urinary excretion of selenium is increased during cervical cancer, but the clinical significance of this observation is not known (9727). Selenium improves immunologic function by increasing the activity of interleukin-2 (IL-2) and promoting the normal growth and development of T helper cells. These actions may be important in treating acquired immunodeficiency syndrome (AIDS) because selenium deficiency is common in this condition (7829). There is preliminary experimental evidence selenium inhibits reverse transcriptase and replication of human immunodeficiency virus (HIV). However, there is also some evidence that selenium may improve subjective feelings of well-being in patients infected with HIV, but it does not appear to affect overall outcomes (3341,7830,9719). Selenium deficiency is associated with increased viral shedding in women infected with HIV. Supplementing the diet of these women with selenium may decrease the transmission of AIDS (9720). In cardiovascular disease, selenium may prevent the oxidative modification of low-density lipoproteins (LDLs). Selenium deficiency has been implicated in the etiology of Keshan disease, an endemic cardiomyopathy observed in China, and congestive cardiomyopathy in people on artificial nutrition (2676,3341). In children with severe deficiency, Keshan disease may also occur (9718).

Selenium is used for arthritis due to its antioxidant effects. It may reduce inflammation by reducing the cellular concentration of reactive oxygen species (ROS) (2662). There is also evidence that suggests that deficiency of selenium may increase inflammatory lung damage caused during influenza virus infection (9728). In liver transplant, ROS are generated when the organ is reperfused with blood following a period of extended warm ischemia. Preliminary evidence suggests that the antioxidant action of selenium can decrease liver damage and improve microcirculation (7839). Selenium may act as part of a defense mechanism, decreasing oxidative stress in peptic ulcer disease (7840). Selenium also might protect patients infected with hepatitis B or C from developing liver cancer (3341). Selenium is required for testosterone biosynthesis and the formation and development of sperm. Low selenium levels have been linked to decreased male fertility. Low selenium levels also appear to be associated with first trimester or recurrent miscarriages, suggesting selenium possibly prevents early pregnancy loss (3341). During pregnancy, the concentration of selenium in blood usually increases. Supplementing the diet with low doses of iron seems to prevent this increase (10217). At the start of breast feeding, the concentration of selenium in blood increases, but the concentration in milk decreases as breast feeding continues (1239). Low levels of selenium appear to be associated with a greater incidence of depression, anxiety, confusion, and hostility. Some researchers think a high dietary or supplemental intake of selenium might improve mood (3341). With severe deficiency, Kaschin-Beck disease, a cartilage abnormality (chondrodystrophy) might occur (9718).

Adverse Reactions

Orally, selenium can cause symptoms of acute toxicity including nausea, vomiting, nail changes, fatigue, irritability, and weight loss (7834). At doses above the tolerable upper intake level (UL) of 400 mcg per day for adults, hair and nail brittleness and loss occur (4844). Chronic toxicity resembles arsenic toxicity, with symptoms including hair loss, white horizontal streaking on fingernails, paronychia, fatigue, irritability, hyperreflexia, nausea, vomiting, garlic odor on breath, and a metallic taste. Muscle tenderness, tremor, lightheadedness, and facial flushing are also observed in selenium poisoning (4844). Selenium can cause thrombocytopenia and moderate hepatorenal dysfunction (4844).
Blood selenium levels can be used to assess the degree of toxicity. Levels below 1000 mcg/L are not usually associated with serious damage, whereas levels above 2000 mcg/L are predictive of serious damage (4844,7825).
Selenium ingestion has been linked to increased incidence of skin cancer, but research is conflicting. Accidental introduction of inorganic selenium (selenite) in a municipal water supply for 11 years has been associated with a quadruple risk of developing melanoma (3343). However, other research suggests higher plasma selenium levels have no effect on skin cancer risk (11114). Selenium supplementation, 200 mcg per day, has been studied as a prophylactic measure in patients with a history of skin cancer. Selenium supplementation for 6 years seems to have no effect on skin cancer risk (2664). But longer-term supplementation for up to 13 years might slightly increase the risk of squamous cell carcinoma and nonmelanoma skin cancer (10687). More research is needed to establish the effect of long-term selenium supplementation on skin cancer recurrence.
Diets that are high in selenium may cause decreased sperm motility. The impact on male fertility is not known (9729).

Interactions with Herbs & Other Dietary Supplements

IRON: Supplementing the diet with iron, 18 mg daily, may prevent the increased selenium serum concentration that occurs during pregnancy (10217).

Interactions with Drugs

HMG-CoA REDUCTASE INHIBITORS ("Statins"): Concomitant use of selenium in combination with beta-carotene and vitamins C and E appears to decrease the effectiveness of the combination of simvastatin (Zocor) and niacin (7388). Theoretically, selenium could reduce the effectiveness of other HMG-CoA reductase inhibitors such as atorvastatin (Lipitor), fluvastatin (Lescol), lovastatin (Mevacor), and pravastatin (Pravachol).
NIACIN: Concomitant use of selenium in combination with beta-carotene, vitamin C, and vitamin E appears to decrease the effectiveness of the combination of niacin and simvastatin (Zocor) (7388).

Interactions with Foods

None known.

Interactions with Lab Tests

BLOOD SELENIUM ASSAYS: Avoid powdered gloves when drawing blood for selenium and other trace element assays due to the potential for sample contamination (2663).
CREATININE KINASE: Selenium toxicity can elevate serum creatinine kinase levels (17).
ELECTROCARDIOGRAM (ECG): Selenium toxicity can elevate the ST segment and cause T-wave changes characteristic of myocardial infarction (MI) (4844).
HIGH-DENSITY LIPOPROTEIN 2 (HDL2): Selenium in combination with beta-carotene, vitamin C, and vitamin E seems to lower HDL2 levels (7388).
SPERM MOTILITY: Diets that are high in selenium may cause a decrease in sperm motility. The impact on male fertility is not known (9729).

Interactions with Diseases or Conditions

HEMODIALYSIS: Blood selenium levels may be low in patients undergoing hemodialysis. Selenium levels may increase somewhat after hemodialysis, but concentrations remain below normal (1805).
HYPOTHYROIDISM: Selenium deficiency can worsen iodine-deficient hypothyroidism (1664,9724).
IMPAIRED MALE FERTILITY: A diet that is high in selenium may decrease the motility of sperm (9729). This effect could theoretically decrease male fertility.
SKIN CANCER: Long-term use of selenium supplements might slightly increase the risk of skin cancer recurrence, but this is controversial (10687). Tell patients with a history of skin cancer that selenium supplements don't protect against skin cancer recurrence. Until more is known about the possible increase in skin cancer risk, patients with a history of skin cancer should avoid long-term use of selenium supplements.

Dosage and Administration

ORAL: For cancer prevention or to reduce the risk of cancer mortality, 200 mcg of selenium supplied as a 0.5 gram high-selenium brewer's yeast tablet taken daily has been used (2664,2667). In humans, 30 mcg per day is considered necessary to prevent Keshan disease, which is associated with selenium deficiency (2671). For patients infected with human immunodeficiency virus (HIV), 250 mcg of L-selenomethionine daily has been used for 12 months (7830).
For people environmentally exposed to arsenic, 100 to 200 mcg of selenized yeast daily has been used for

14 months (7831). To treat selenium deficiency in premature infants, 5 mcg per day of selenized yeast has been given by a nasogastric tube (9764).
The daily recommended dietary allowances (RDAs) of selenium are: Children 1-3 years, 20 mcg; Children 4-8 years, 30 mcg; Children 9-13 years, 40 mcg; People over 13 years, 55 mcg; Pregnant women, 60 mcg; and Lactating women, 70 mcg (3341,4844). Due to the demands of the fetus on the mother, the dietary need for selenium increases during pregnancy (7837).
The RDA for infants has not been determined. For infants up to 6 months old, 2.1 mcg/kg is adequate intake (AI). The AI for infants 7-12 months is 2.2 mcg/kg per day (4844).
The tolerable upper limit for adults is 400 mcg per day for adults and adolescents 14 years and older. The tolerable upper intake level (UL) for infants up to age 6 months is 45 mcg per day; for infants 7 to 12 months, 60 mcg per day; for children 1 to 3 years, 90 mcg per day; for children 4 to 8 years, 150 mcg per day; for children 9 to 13 years, 280 mcg per day (4844,7830,7831,7835,7841).

Comments
Most of the selenium in the body is obtained via the diet. The amount of selenium in food depends on where it is grown or raised. Crab, liver, fish, poultry, and wheat are generally good selenium sources; however, natural selenium levels in the soil are highly variable throughout the world (2671,3341,7834,9718). In the US, the Eastern Coastal Plain, and the Pacific Northwest have the lowest selenium levels, and people in these regions naturally ingest about 60 to 90 mcg per day, which is adequate (2671,9718). The average daily intake in the US is 125 mcg, ranging from 60 to 200 mcg (2671,7834,9718).

SELF-HEAL

Also Known As
All-Heal, Blue Curls, Brownwort, Carpenter's Herb, Carpenter's Weed, Heal-All, Heart of the Earth, Hercules Woundwort, Hock-Heal, Prunella, Self Heal, Sicklewort, Siclewort, Slough-Heal, Woundwort.
CAUTION: See other listing for Sanicle.

Scientific Names
Prunella vulgaris.
Family: Labiatae/Lamiaceae.

People Use This For
Orally, self-heal is used for inflammatory bowel disease (Crohn's disease and ulcerative colitis), HIV/AIDS, fever, headache, colic, vertigo, liver disease, spasm, diarrhea, gastroenteritis, as an antiseptic, expectorant, and astringent. It is also used for mouth and throat ulcers, sore throat, and internal hemorrhaging.
Topically, self-heal is used for leukorrhea, gynecological disorders, wounds and bruises.

Safety
POSSIBLY SAFE ...when used orally (12).
PREGNANCY AND LACTATION: Insufficient reliable information available; avoid using.

Effectiveness
There is insufficient reliable information available about the effectiveness of self-heal.

Mechanism of Action
Self-heal contains entacyclic triterpenes, tannins, caffeic and rosmarinic acids, thiamine, and vitamins C and K. It has antioxidant and astringent properties (7122). Laboratory evidence suggests that an aqueous extract of self-heal has activity against HIV and might work synergistically with zidovudine (AZT, Retrovir) and didanosine (ddI, Videx) (7234,7286).

Adverse Reactions
None reported.

Interactions with Herbs & Other Dietary Supplements
None known.

Interactions with Drugs
None known.

Interactions with Foods
None known.

Interactions with Lab Tests
None known.

Interactions with Diseases or Conditions
None known.

Dosage and Administration
ORAL: One cup of tea is commonly used. The tea is prepared by simmering one teaspoon of the dried plant in 150 mL of boiling water for 10-15 minutes and straining. For a gargle, the tea is simmered for 9 minutes (18).

Comments
Sanicle is also less commonly known as self-heal. Be careful not to confuse these two plants.

SENEGA

Also Known As
Chinese Senega, Flax, Klapperschlangen, Milkwort, Mountain Polygala, Polygala glomerata, Polygala reinii, Polygalae radix, Rattlesnake Root, Senaga Snakeroot, Seneca, Seneca Snakeroot, Senega Snakeroot, Seneka, Snake Root.
CAUTION: See separate listings for Asarabacca and Bitter Milkwort.

Scientific Names
Polygala japonica; Polygala senega; Polygala tenuifolia.
Family: Polygalaceae.

People Use This For
Orally, senega is used for respiratory tract mucous membrane inflammation, bronchial asthma, chronic bronchitis, emphysema, rattlesnake bite, for inducing sweating, increasing saliva, as an expectorant, and an emetic.
Topically, senega is used as a gargle for pharyngitis.

Safety
POSSIBLY SAFE ...when used orally and appropriately short-term (12).
LIKELY UNSAFE ...when used orally, long-term. Prolonged use can cause gastrointestinal (GI) irritation (12).
There is insufficient reliable information available about the safety of the topical use of senega.
PREGNANCY: LIKELY UNSAFE ...when used orally; senega appears to have uterine and menstrual flow stimulant effects (12,19). There is insufficient reliable information available about the safety of the topical use of senega during pregnancy.
LACTATION: Insufficient reliable information available; avoid using.

Effectiveness
There is insufficient reliable information available about the effectiveness of senega.

Mechanism of Action
The applicable part of senega is the root. Senega root contains salicylic acid, methyl salicylate, and a saponin mixture referred to as senegin (4). People claim senega has expectorant and emetic activity, and that it can stimulate sweating and saliva (2,4,515). The active expectorant principles are triterpenoid saponins (515). Researchers think the saponins irritate the gastrointestinal (GI) tract mucosa and cause reflex secretion of mucous in the bronchioles (515). A French patent based on human studies states that a triterpenic acid extract has anti-inflammatory activity, and is effective against graft rejection, eczema, psoriasis, and multiple sclerosis (4).

Adverse Reactions
Orally, prolonged use of senega can cause gastrointestinal (GI) irritation (2). Large amounts can cause diarrhea, dizziness (8), queasiness (18), vomiting, and purging (4).

Interactions with Herbs & Other Dietary Supplements
None known.

Interactions with Drugs
None known.

Interactions with Foods
None known.

Interactions with Lab Tests

None known.

Interactions with Diseases or Conditions

FEVER: Contraindicated due to CNS depressant effects (19).
GASTROINTESTINAL (GI) CONDITIONS: Senega is contraindicated in individuals with gastrointestinal (GI) conditions including inflammation and gastritis or gastric ulcers (4,12) due to local stimulant activity and intestinal irritant effects (19).

Dosage and Administration

ORAL: A typical dose is 0.5-1 grams dried root or 1 cup of tea three times daily. To make tea, steep 0.5-1 grams dried root in 150 mL boiling water 5-10 minutes, and strain (4).
TOPICAL: No typical dosage.

Comments

Avoid confusion with Polygala sibirica, also referred to as polygala.

SENNA

Also Known As

Alexandrian Senna, Alexandrinische Senna, Casse, Indian Senna, Khartoum Senna, Sena Alejandrina, Séné d'Egypte, Sennae folium, Sennae fructus, Sennae fructus acutifoliae, Sennae fructus angustifolia, Tinnevelly Senna, True Senna.

Scientific Names

Senna alexandrina, synonyms Cassia acutifolia, Cassia angustifolia, Cassia senna, Cassia lanceolata.
Family: Fabaceae/Leguminosae

People Use This For

Orally, senna used as a laxative for constipation, after anorectal surgery, for hemorrhoids, evacuating the GI tract to facilitate diagnostic tests, evacuation relief in individuals with anal fissures, and in "slimming" and "cleansing" teas.

Safety

LIKELY SAFE ...when used orally and appropriately, short-term (12,272).
POSSIBLY UNSAFE ...when used orally long-term or in high doses. Long-term, frequent use, or use of high doses has been linked to serious side effects including laxative dependence and liver toxicity (6,12,272,13057,13095).
PREGNANCY: POSSIBLY UNSAFE ...when used orally. Constipation in pregnancy should not be self-medicated (6,12).
LACTATION: POSSIBLY UNSAFE ...when used orally. Anthraquinone constituents cross into breast milk and can cause loose stools in some breast-fed infants (272).

Effectiveness

LIKELY EFFECTIVE
Constipation. Taking senna orally is effective as a laxative for reducing constipation (6,272).
There is insufficient reliable information available about the effectiveness of senna for its other uses.

Mechanism of Action

The applicable parts of senna are the leaf and fruit. Senna leaf and fruit are stimulant laxatives (272). The cathartic properties of the leaf are greater than the fruit (4). Senna contains anthraquinones including dianthrone that consists mostly of sennosides A and B and minor amounts of sennosides C and D (6,11). Senna also contains small amounts of free anthraquinones. The dianthrone glycosides are not present in the fresh leaf, but appear to form during the drying process (11). Although it is not known exactly how the anthraquinone laxatives work, the cathartic action is limited primarily to the colon (272). Sennosides irritate the lining of the large intestine, causing contraction. Sennosides A and B also seem to induce fluid secretion in the colon. Prostaglandins might be involved in the laxative effect (6).
Anthraquinone laxatives produce an effect 8-12 hours after administration, though sometimes up to 24 hours can be required (272).
When taken orally, sennosides are metabolized to rhein anthrone by bacteria in the colon. Rhein anthrone is absorbed and thought to be responsible for the toxic effects of senna (13057).
Anthroid laxative does not seem to be associated with an increased risk of developing colorectal ademoma or carcinoma (6138).

Adverse Reactions

Orally, senna can cause abdominal pain and discomfort, cramps, and diarrhea (4). Excessive use can cause potassium depletion and other electrolyte abnormalities. Excessive use of senna has also been linked to finger clubbing, development of cachexia, decreased serum globulin concentrations, heart function disorders, muscular weakness, osteomalacia, arthropathy, hepatitis, coma, neuropathy, asthma, allergy symptoms, and rhinoconjunctivitis (4,6).
There is a case report of hepatitis in a woman who consumed moderate amounts of senna tea. In this case, the patient was a poor metabolizer of cytochrome P450 2D6 (CYP2D6). It's thought that moderate doses of senna in this patient led to toxic hepatitis due to the patient's reduced ability to metabolize and eliminate the rhein anthrone metabolites of senna, which are thought to cause systemic toxicity (13057).
There is also a case of liver failure, encephalopathy, and renal insufficiency in a woman who consumed excessive amounts of senna tea. In this case, liver failure and renal insufficiency developed after over 3 years of consuming 1 liter/day of senna tea prepared from 70 grams of dried senna fruit (13095).
Chronic use can cause pseudomelanosis coli (pigment spots in intestinal mucosa) which is harmless, usually reverses with discontinuation, and is not associated with an increased risk of developing colorectal adenoma or carcinoma (6138).
There is some concern that prolonged senna use can cause "laxative-dependency syndrome" characterized by poor gastric motility, non-functioning colon, and laxative-induced diarrhea (4,6). But there is not much scientific support for this concern. Increased use of the laxative is more likely to be associated with worsening constipation rather than laxative dependency (13096).
Occupational exposure has been linked to asthma and allergy symptoms, including rhinoconjunctivitis (6).

Interactions with Herbs & Other Dietary Supplements

HORSETAIL/LICORICE: Theoretically, concomitant use with horsetail plant or licorice rhizome increases the risk of potassium depletion (19).
STIMULANT LAXATIVE HERBS: Theoretically, concomitant use with other stimulant laxative herbs increases the risk of potassium depletion (19). Stimulant laxative herbs include aloe dried leaf sap, wild cucumber fruit (Ecballium elaterium), blue flag rhizome, alder buckthorn, European buckthorn, butternut bark, cascara bark, castor oil, colocynth fruit pulp, gamboge bark exudate, jalap root, black root, manna bark exudate, podophyllum root, rhubarb root, and yellow dock root.

Interactions with Drugs

DIGOXIN (Lanoxin): Theoretically, overuse/abuse of this product increases the risk of adverse effects of cardiac glycoside drugs.
DIURETIC DRUGS: Overuse of senna might compound diuretic-induced potassium loss (19). There is some concern that people taking senna along with potassium depleting diuretics might have an increased risk for hypokalemia. Initiation of potassium supplementation or an increase in potassium supplement dose may be necessary for some patients. Some diuretics that can deplete potassium include chlorothiazide (Diuril), chlorthalidone (Thalitone), furosemide (Lasix), and hydrochlorothiazide (HCTZ, Hydrodiuril, Microzide), and others.

Interactions with Foods

None known.

Interactions with Lab Tests

COLORIMETRIC TESTS: Senna can discolor urine (pink, red, purple, orange, rust), interfering with diagnostic tests that depend on a color change, due to its anthraquinone content (1,4,12,275).
POTASSIUM: Excessive use of senna can cause potassium depletion, reducing serum potassium concentrations and test results (1,4,12,19).

Interactions with Diseases or Conditions

ELECTROLYTE DISTURBANCES, POTASSIUM DEFICIENCY: Overuse of senna can exacerbate these conditions (2).
FLUID DEPLETION: Senna is contraindicated in individuals with dehydration, diarrhea, or loose stools. It can exacerbate these conditions.
GASTROINTESTINAL (GI) CONDITIONS: Senna is contraindicated in people with abdominal pain, intestinal obstruction, and acute intestinal inflammation including Crohn's disease, ulcerative colitis, appendicitis, stomach inflammation, anal prolapse, hemorrhoids, or undiagnosed abdominal pain (4,19).
HEART DISEASE: Senna can cause electrolyte disturbances and exacerbate these conditions (2).

Dosage and Administration

ORAL: A typical dose is 15-30 mg hydroxyanthracene derivatives daily, calculated as sennoside B (1,2). Senna leaf is used as a tea, one cup in the morning and/or at bedtime. To make tea, steep 0.5-2 grams finely chopped leaf in warm but not boiling water for 10 minutes, and strain (8). Alternatively, a cold water tea might have less adverse GI effects. To make cold water tea, steep 0.5-2 grams finely chopped leaf in cold water for 10-12 hours, and strain (8). Liquid leaf extract (1:1 in 25% alcohol), 0.5-2.0 mL (frequency unspecified) (4). One cup of fruit tea is taken in the morning and/or at bedtime. To make tea, steep 1/2 flat teaspoon of senna fruit in 150 mL warm, but not boiling water, for ten minutes, and strain (8). Individualize senna dosing to the smallest amount necessary to maintain a soft stool (2). Senna leaf should not be used continuously for more than one to two weeks (2). Use of standardized OTC senna leaf preparations reduces variability and improves dosing control (4,515).

Comments

Because senna fruit is gentler than senna leaf, the American Herbal Products Association only warns against long-term use for senna leaf, not senna fruit (12). The AHPA recommends that senna leaf products be labeled "Do not use this product if you have abdominal pain or diarrhea. Consult a healthcare provider prior to use if you are pregnant or nursing. Discontinue use in the event of diarrhea or watery stools. Do not exceed recommended dose. Not for long-term use." (12).

SERRAPEPTASE

Also Known As

Butterfly Enzyme, SER, Serratiopeptidase, Silk Worm Enzyme, Silkworm Extract.

Scientific Names

Serratia peptidase.

People Use This For

Orally, serrapeptase is used for back pain, osteoarthritis, rheumatoid arthritis, osteoporosis, carpel tunnel syndrome, sinusitis, laryngitis, pharyngitis, diabetes, leg ulcers, migraine headache, tension headache, asthma, empyema, thrombophlebitis, fibromyalgia, fibrocystic breast disease, inflammatory bowel disease (IBD) including ulcerative colitis and Crohn's disease, breast engorgement, atherosclerosis, cardiovascular disease, post-operative swelling, and otitis media.

Safety

POSSIBLY SAFE ...when used orally and appropriately, short-term. Serrapeptase seems to be safe when used in clinical trials lasting up to 4 weeks (13151,13152,13153).
There is insufficient reliable information available about the safety of serrapeptase when used long-term.
PREGNANCY AND LACTATION: Insufficient reliable information; avoid using.

Effectiveness

POSSIBLY EFFECTIVE

Post-operative swelling. Patients undergoing maxillary antrotomy for empyema who take serrapeptase 10 mg orally three times on the day before surgery, once in evening after surgery, and three times daily for 5 days after surgery seem to have modestly reduced buccal swelling compared to placebo (13151)

INSUFFICIENT RELIABLE EVIDENCE to RATE

Bronchitis. Preliminary evidence suggests that patients with chronic bronchitis or bronchiectasis who take serrapeptase 30 mg daily for 4 weeks have significantly reduced frequency of cough and expectoration. These patients who took serrapeptase also seem to have decreased sputum viscosity and lower neutrophil counts in sputum samples (13153).

Laryngitis. Preliminary evidence suggests that patients with laryngitis who take serrapeptase 10 mg three times daily have significantly reduced pain, secretions, difficulty swallowing, and body temperature after 3-4 days of treatment (13152).

Pharyngitis. Preliminary evidence suggests that patients with pharyngitis who take serrapeptase 10 mg three times daily have significantly reduced pain, secretions, difficulty swallowing, and body temperature after 3-4 days of treatment (13152).

Sinusitis. Preliminary evidence suggests that patients with sinusitis who take serrapeptase 10 mg three times daily have significantly reduced pain, nasal secretions, nasal obstruction, and anosmia after 3-4 days of treatment (13152).

More evidence is needed to rate serrapeptase for these uses.

Mechanism of Action

Serrapeptase is a proteolytic enzyme isolated from the silk worm. It is thought to have anti-inflammatory, antiedemic, and fibrinolytic effects (13151,13152).
Serrapeptase is also thought to decrease pain by inhibiting release of bradykinin and other factors from inflamed or damaged tissue (13152).
Serrapeptase is thought to reduce inflammatory conditions such as post-operative swelling, pharyngitis, sinusitis, and others due to its anti-inflammatory effects (13151). Serrapeptase is also thought to help break down of proteinaceous secretions and therefore facility elimination of excessive secretions (13152).
Serrapeptase also seems to decrease sputum viscosity and decrease neutrophils in the sputum of patients with

chronic airway disease (13153).
Serrapeptase appears to be absorbed from the gastrointestinal tract when taken orally (13151).

Adverse Reactions

Orally, serrapeptase appears to be well-tolerated. Some patients have reported experiencing epigastric pain, gastrointestinal upset, and nausea (13152); however, these side effects appear to occur at the same rate as placebo. There is a case report of bullous pemphigoid, an autoimmune subepidermal dermatosis, in an elderly man who took serrapeptase (13154) .

Interactions with Herbs & Other Dietary Supplements

None known.

Interactions with Drugs

None known.

Interactions with Foods

None known.

Interactions with Lab Tests

None known.

Interactions with Diseases or Conditions

None known.

Dosage and Administration

ORAL: For post-operative buccal swelling following maxillary antrotomy, 10 mg three times on the daily be surgery, once on the night of the operation, and then 3-times daily for 5 days following surgery has been used (13151).
For laryngitis, 10 mg three times daily after meals has been used (13152).
For pharyngitis, 10 mg three times daily after meals has been used (13152).
For sinusitis, 10 mg three times daily after meals has been used (13152).
For bronchitis, 30 mg daily has been used (13153).

Comments

Serrapeptase is a commonly used drug in Japan and Europe. It is manufactured by Takeda Chemical Industries.

SHARK CARTILAGE

Also Known As

AE-941, MSI-1256F, Neovastat.
CAUTION: See separate listings for Bovine Cartilage, Chondroitin, Shark Liver Oil, and Squalamine.

Scientific Names

Squalus acanthias.

People Use This For

Orally, shark cartilage is used for preventing and treating cancer, arthritis, psoriasis, and wound healing. It is also used for enteritis, diabetic retinopathy, and cutaneous Kaposi sarcoma.
Topically, shark cartilage is used for arthritis and psoriasis.
Rectally, shark cartilage is used for cancer.

Safety

POSSIBLY SAFE ...when used orally and appropriately. Shark cartilage has been safely used for up to 20 weeks (2015,4938,6709,6716,6717,13086) in multiple trials and for up to 40 months in a phase II trial (10900). ...when used topically and appropriately, short-term. Shark cartilage, in combination with glucosamine, chondroitin, and camphor, appears to be safe when applied topically on an as-needed basis for up to 8 weeks (10327).
There is insufficient reliable information available about the safety of shark cartilage for its other uses.
PREGNANCY AND LACTATION: Insufficient reliable information available; avoid using.

Effectiveness

LIKELY INEFFECTIVE

Cancer. Taking shark cartilage orally appears to offer no benefit in people with advanced, previously-treated cancer, including breast cancer, colorectal cancer, lung cancer, prostate cancer, and brain cancer; and non-Hodgkin's lymphoma (2015,6716,6717,13086). However, studies of shark cartilage in people with less advanced cancer or in combination with other cancer treatments have not been published.

INSUFFICIENT RELIABLE EVIDENCE to RATE

Kaposi sarcoma. There is anecdotal evidence that shark cartilage might be beneficial for cutaneous Kaposi sarcoma and possibly decrease Kaposi sarcoma lesions and increase histological regression (4938).

Osteoarthritis. A topical preparation of shark cartilage, in combination with chondroitin sulfate, glucosamine sulfate, and camphor, reportedly reduces arthritis symptoms. However, any symptom relief is most likely due to the counterirritant effect of camphor and not the other ingredients (10327). There's no research showing that shark cartilage is absorbed topically. Don't recommend topical shark cartilage products.

Plaque psoriasis. Preliminary clinical evidence suggests that AE-941 taken orally might improve appearance and decrease itching of plaque psoriasis (10399).

Renal cell carcinoma. Taking AE-941 orally seems to increase survival in patients with advanced renal cell carcinoma (4894,10900). AE-941 (Neovastat), a derivative of shark cartilage, has FDA orphan drug status for renal cell carcinoma (10899).

More evidence is needed to rate shark cartilage for these uses.

Mechanism of Action

Shark cartilage is found in the skeletal structure of sharks. It is made up of about 40% proteins, 5% to 20% glycosaminoglycans, and calcium salts. Chondroitin, a glycosaminoglycan in cartilage, might be an active constituent (6714).

The use of shark cartilage attracted popular attention after some publications suggested that sharks don't get cancer and implied that shark cartilage could prevent cancer in humans (2014,6722). Since then renal cell carcinoma, lymphoma, and cartilage tumors have been identified in sharks (6714). However, there is still some preliminary evidence that shark cartilage might have some potential as an anticancer agent.

Shark cartilage might inhibit angiogenesis and prevent the new vessel growth required for solid tumor proliferation (2013). There is preliminary clinical evidence that shark cartilage given orally inhibits wound angiogenesis (6709). Topical shark cartilage also seems to inhibit local angiogenic activity. Because macrophages and T lymphocytes found at the sites of psoriasis lesions can produce angiogenic activity, shark cartilage might have potential as a treatment for psoriasis (4893). Preliminary laboratory research suggests that shark cartilage might also have antimutagenic, antioxidant, anti-inflammatory, and analgesic activity (6723,6724,6725).

AE-941 (Neovastat) is one of the components of shark cartilage that is well studied. It is a naturally occurring component of cartilage made up of a mixture of proteins with a molecular weight less than 500 kilodaltons. AE-941 inhibits angiogenesis, the outgrowth of new capillaries from pre-existing blood vessels. Angiogenesis is increased in highly vascularized cancers, suggesting possible usefulness of AE-941in treatment of some malignancies.

As an antiangiogenic agent, it interferes with binding of cytokines and other enzymes at their receptor sites. AE-941 competes for binding sites with fibroblast growth factor, tumor necrosis factor-alpha, vascular endothelial growth factor, and other cytokines. It also inhibits a matrix metalloproteinase (MMP), an enzyme that facilitates angiogenesis (10397,10398). In addition, AE-941 induces apoptosis of endothelial cells involved with growth of blood vessels. This action is mediated by activation of caspases, which are key mediators of programmed cell death in many types of cells. AE-941 appears to activate caspase-1 and caspase-2 that are specific mediators of apoptosis in blood vessel endothelial cells (10396).

Adverse Reactions

Orally, shark cartilage can cause taste disturbances, nausea, vomiting, dyspepsia, constipation, hypotension, dizziness, hyperglycemia, hypoglycemia, hypercalcemia, altered consciousness, decreased motor strength, decreased sensation, erythema, peripheral edema, generalized weakness, fatigue, and decreased performance (2014,2015,6716,10900). It might also cause signs of acute hepatitis, including low-grade fever, jaundice, yellowing of eyes, right upper quadrant tenderness, and elevated liver enzymes (2012). Some shark cartilage products have an offensive odor and taste (2014).

Interactions with Herbs & Other Dietary Supplements

CALCIUM: Shark cartilage might cause hypercalcemia (2015,6716). Theoretically, concomitant use with supplemental calcium might exacerbate this adverse effect.

Interactions with Drugs

None known.

Interactions with Foods

FRUIT JUICE: Acidic fruit juice such as orange, apple, grape, or tomato, can decrease potency of shark cartilage over time. If shark cartilage is added to a fruit juice, it should be mixed immediately prior to use (2014).

Interactions with Lab Tests

CALCIUM: Shark cartilage might increase serum calcium levels and test results (2015,6716).

Interactions with Diseases or Conditions

HYPERCALCEMIA: Shark cartilage is reported to cause hypercalcemia (2015,6716) and might exacerbate this condition; avoid using.

Dosage and Administration

ORAL: For refractory metastatic renal cell carcinoma, a specific water-soluble shark cartilage extract, AE-941 (Neovastat), 60-240 mL per day has been used (4894,10900). For the treatment of solid tumors, 30 to 240 mL daily has been used (10397). For the treatment of plaque psoriasis, 30 to 240 mL per day has been used for up to 12 weeks (10399). For cutaneous Kaposi Sarcoma, shark cartilage 3750 to 4500 mg per day has been used (4938). Commercial products typically suggest doses ranging from 500 mg to 4.5 grams given in 2-6 divided doses daily (6002).

Comments

Shark cartilage is typically obtained from sharks caught in the Pacific Ocean. The anti-tumor effects of numerous shark cartilage derivatives and extracts, including squalamine lactate, AE-941, and U-995, are currently being investigated in several preclinical and phase I to III clinical trials (6718,6719,6720,6721,6726,6727).

SHARK LIVER OIL

Also Known As

Basking Shark Liver Oil, Deep Sea Shark Liver Oil, Dog Fish Liver Oil.
CAUTION: See separate listings for Cod Liver Oil, Fish Oil, Liver Extract, Shark Cartilage, and Squalamine.

Scientific Names

Cetorhinus maximus; Centroporus squamosus; Squalus acanthias.

People Use This For

Orally, shark liver oil is used as an adjunctive treatment for leukemia and other cancers, to prevent radiation illness from cancer X-ray therapy, to prevent the common cold and flu, and for general immunostimulation. It is also used orally for increasing leukocyte and thrombocyte counts during chemotherapy.
Topically, shark liver oil is used for skin conditions, skin cancer, and as a topical protectant.

Safety

There is insufficient reliable information available about the safety of shark liver oil.
Pregnancy and Lactation: Insufficient reliable information available; avoid using.

Effectiveness

There is insufficient reliable information available about the effectiveness of shark liver oil.

Mechanism of Action

Shark liver oil is a major source of squalene and alkylglycerols. Shark liver oil is classified as a topical protectant (2551). Alkoxyglycerol derived from shark liver oil may decrease irradiation damage in patients undergoing treatment of uterine cancer (2552). It is thought that the radioprotective properties of alkoxyglycerol may stem from its incorporation into a pool of platelet-activating factors, and resulting in biosynthesis (2550). Alkoxyglycerol may also increase leukocyte and thrombocyte counts within specific dose ranges (2552). Shark liver oil has been shown in animals to have antiangiogenesis properties in certain cancers, including cutaneous lesions, kidney cancer and urinary bladder cancer including L-1 syngeneic (2549). However, other findings are contradictory (2552).

Adverse Reactions

Both shark liver oil and the constituent squalene have been associated with cases of aspiration and subsequent lipoid pneumonia (2546,2547,2548).

Interactions with Herbs & Other Dietary Supplements

None known.

Interactions with Drugs

None known.

Interactions with Foods

None known.

Interactions with Lab Tests

None known.

Interactions with Diseases or Conditions

None known.

Dosage and Administration
No typical dosage.

Comments
Shark liver oil is commercially derived from the livers of three species of shark: the deep sea shark (Centrophorus squamosus), the dogfish (Sqaulus acanthias), and the basking shark (Cetorhinus maximus). The liver constitutes 25% of the total shark body weight.

SHELLAC

Also Known As
Gommelaque, Lac, Lacca.

Scientific Names
Laccifer lacca (Scale insect).
Family: Coccidae.

People Use This For
In dentistry, shellac is used as a binding agent for dentures, restorations, moldings, and as a constituent in "artificial calculus" in dental schools.
In the pharmaceutical industry, shellac is used in tablet coating formulations, enteric coating, microencapsulation, matrix formulation, humidity tolerance, and for its binding ability.
In manufacturing, shellac is used as a finish for furniture, an ingredient in hair spray and in other cosmetics.

Safety
LIKELY SAFE ...when used orally in amounts commonly found in foods. Purified shellac and shellac wax have Generally Recognized As Safe (GRAS) status in the US (4912).
PREGNANCY AND LACTATION: Insufficient reliable information available.

Effectiveness
There is insufficient reliable information available about the effectiveness of shellac.

Mechanism of Action
Aleuretic acid, r-butolic acid, shellolic acid, and jalaric acid are the major constituents of shellac (6).

Adverse Reactions
There is one report of contact cheilitis associated with shellac (6).

Interactions with Herbs & Other Dietary Supplements
None known.

Interactions with Drugs
None known.

Interactions with Foods
None known.

Interactions with Lab Tests
None known.

Interactions with Diseases or Conditions
SHELLAC ALLERGY: Contraindicated.

Dosage and Administration
No typical dosage.

Comments
Shellac is derived from the secretions of the insect Laccifer. Although shellac has been used for years in pharmacy, dentistry, and as a finish for furniture, it has fallen into disfavor for some products because it ages over time (6).

SHEPHERD'S PURSE

Also Known As
Blind Weed, Bursae Pastoris Herba, Capsella, Caseweed, Cocowort, Lady's Purse, Mother's-Heart, Pepper-And-Salt, Pick-Pocket, Poor Man's Parmacettie, Rattle Pouches, Sanguinary, Shepherd's Heart, Shepherd's Scrip, Shepherd's Sprout, Shovelweed, St. James' Weed, Toywort, Witches' Pouches.

Scientific Names
Capsella bursa-pastoris, synonym Thlaspi bursa-pastoris.
Family: Brassicaceae/Cruciferae.

People Use This For
Orally, shepherd's purse is used for headache, mild cardiac insufficiency, hypotension, nervous heart complaints, premenstrual complaints, prolonged or painful menstrual periods, vomiting blood, blood in urine, diarrhea, and acute catarrhal cystitis.
Topically, it is used for nosebleeds, superficial burns, and bleeding skin injuries.

Safety
POSSIBLY SAFE ...when preparations of the above ground parts are used orally and appropriately (4,12). ...when used topically (4).
POSSIBLY UNSAFE ...when large amounts of shepherd's purse are ingested, it can cause heart palpitations (12).
PREGNANCY: LIKELY UNSAFE ...when used orally or topically, due to possible uterine stimulation, menstrual flow stimulation, and miscarriage (12).
LACTATION: Insufficient reliable information available; avoid excessive use (4).

Effectiveness
There is insufficient reliable information available about the effectiveness of shepherd's purse.

Mechanism of Action
The applicable parts of shepherd's purse are the above ground parts. Shepherd's purse has constituents that cause positive and negative inotropic effects, and positive and negative chronotropic effects. It also seems to cause hypertensive and sometimes antihypertensive effects. It stimulates smooth muscle and increases uterine contraction. It also has abortifacient effects, and antihemorrhagic and urinary antiseptic effects (4,18). One constituent in shepherd's purse is sinigrin, which can be broken down to allyl isothiocyanate. Allyl isothiocyanate is associated with abnormal thyroid function and goiter (4).

Adverse Reactions
Orally, shepherd's purse can cause sedation, hypertension, hypotension, abnormal thyroid function, abnormal menstruation (4), palpitations (12). Toxic doses in animals have caused sedation, paralysis, respiratory depression, and death (4).

Interactions with Herbs & Other Dietary Supplements
None known.

Interactions with Drugs
CNS DEPRESSANTS: Theoretically, concomitant use with drugs with sedative properties may cause additive effects and side effects (4).
THYROID HORMONE: Theoretically, concomitant use may interfere with thyroid dysfunction therapy (4).

Interactions with Foods
None known.

Interactions with Lab Tests
None known.

Interactions with Diseases or Conditions
CARDIOVASCULAR CONDITIONS: Use with caution, shepherd's purse may interfere with therapy (4).
KIDNEY STONES (Nephrolithiasis): Shepherd's purse contains oxalates, use with caution in people with a history of kidney stones (12).
THYROID CONDITIONS: Use with caution, shepherd's purse may interfere with therapy (4).

Dosage and Administration
ORAL: A typical dosage is 1-4 grams dried above ground parts three times daily, or one cup tea (steep 1-4 grams dried above ground parts in 150 mL boiling water 10-15 minutes, strain) three times daily (4). The liquid extract

(1:1 in 25% alcohol), is used in doses of 1-4 mL three times daily (4). Avoid excessive amounts (12).
TOPICAL: The tea is applied topically. The tea is prepared by steeping 3-5 grams dried above ground parts in 180 mL boiling water 10-15 minutes, strain (2).

SHIITAKE MUSHROOM

Also Known As
Forest Mushroom, Hua Gu, Lentinula, Pasania Fungus, Shiitake, Shitake, Snake Butter.
CAUTION: See separate listing for Lentinan.

Scientific Names
Lentinus edodes, synonyms Lenticus edodes, Lentinan edodes, Lentinula edodes, Tricholomopsis edodes.
Family: Polyporaceae.

People Use This For
Orally, shiitake mushroom is used for boosting the immune system, reducing serum cholesterol levels, as an anti-aging agent, and for prostate cancer.

Safety
LIKELY SAFE ...when consumed in food amounts (6).
POSSIBLY UNSAFE ...when used as an oral medicinal; ingestion of 4 grams shiitake powder daily for 10 weeks can cause eosinophilia (1149).
PREGNANCY AND LACTATION: Insufficient reliable information available; avoid consuming greater than food amounts.

Effectiveness
POSSIBLY INEFFECTIVE

Prostate cancer. Shiitake mushroom extract does not seem to prevent disease progression, as determined by prostate-specific antigen (PSA) levels (10451).

There is insufficient reliable information available about the effectiveness of shiitake mushroom for its other uses.

Mechanism of Action
Shiitake contains very low concentrations of lentinan (0.02%), which has antitumor effects (6). Shiitake may reduce plasma levels of free cholesterol, triglycerides, and phospholipids (1155).

Adverse Reactions
Orally, shiitake mushrooms can cause abdominal discomfort, eosinophilia (1149), "shiitake" dermatitis (1148,1152), and possibly photosensitivity (1148). There is one report of abdominal obstruction and death due to ingestion of a whole shiitake mushroom (1147). Ingestion of 4 grams shiitake powder daily for 10 weeks caused eosinophilia in 5 of 10 healthy humans (1149). An allergic contact dermatitis can be induced by shiitake hyphae (filaments) (1153). In mushroom workers, hypersensitivity pneumonitis due to shiitake spore inhalation has occurred (1150,1151).

Interactions with Herbs & Other Dietary Supplements
None known.

Interactions with Drugs
None known.

Interactions with Foods
None known.

Interactions with Lab Tests
None known.

Interactions with Diseases or Conditions
EOSINOPHILIA: Contraindicated, may exacerbate condition (1149).

Dosage and Administration
ORAL: For prostate cancer, shiitake mushroom extract 8 g daily has been used for up to 6 months (10451).

SILICON

Also Known As

Orthosilicic Acid, Phytolithic Silica, Silica, Silicium, Silicon Dioxide, Sodium Silicate.

Scientific Names

Silicon; Si; atomic number 14.

People Use This For

Orally, silicon is used for osteoporosis, cardiovascular disease, Alzheimer's disease, and improving hair and nail quality. It is also used for improving skin healing, treating sprains and strains, and digestive system disorders.

Safety

LIKELY SAFE ...when used orally in amounts commonly found in foods (7135,10470). There is insufficient reliable information available about the safety of silicone when used in medicinal amounts.
PREGNANCY AND LACTATION: LIKELY SAFE ...when used orally in amounts commonly found in foods (7135,10470). There is insufficient reliable information available about the safety of silicone when used in medicinal amounts; avoid using.

Effectiveness

POSSIBLY EFFECTIVE

Osteoporosis. Men and premenopausal women who have higher dietary intake of silicon seem to have higher bone mineral density, which could reduce the risk of osteoporosis.. But higher silicon intake does not seem to benefit postmenopausal women (10470,12425). Bone loss is postmenopausal women is primarily due to bone resorption. Silicon seems to affect only bone formation (12425).

There is insufficient reliable evidence about the effectiveness of silicon for its other uses.

Mechanism of Action

Silicon is a trace mineral that is found in the body as orthosilicic acid. Silicon dioxide, also known as silica, is present in foods such as vegetables, whole gains, and seafood (11556). A clear biological function of silicon in humans has not been established. There is some evidence, though, that it might have a role in bone and collagen formation. Most of the silicon in the body is contained in connective tissues such as in the aorta, trachea, bone, tendons, and skin. Silicon might also protect against atherogenesis (7135,12425). Coffee, beer, and unfiltered drinking water are the major sources of dietary silicon, followed by grains, grain products, fruits and vegetables, especially bananas, raisins, beans, and lentils. The average intake of silicon in adults is 14 to 21 mg per day. Foods from animal sources and silicate food additives (which prevent foaming and caking) are lesser sources. The bioavailability of silicate additives is low (7135,12425).

After oral consumption, silicon is converted to orthosilicic acid, which increases its absorption. The bioavailability of dietary silicon is about 40% and the primary route of excretion is in the urine. In the glomerulus, silicon is highly filtered and only slightly reabsorbed (10470). People with renal failure have higher serum levels of silicon than people with normal renal function (7135). Orthosilicic acid seems to stimulate osteoblasts in humans (12425). Preclinical research suggests that silicon supplementation might inhibit bone resorption and stimulate bone formation in laboratory models of estrogen deficiency (4988).

Adverse Reactions

Orally, silicon that occurs in food and water doesn't cause any known adverse effects. Long-term ingestion of magnesium trisilicate-containing antacids (Gaviscon tablets) can rarely cause silicon-containing kidney stones (11760,11861). Even more rarely, silica kidney stones can occur without magnesium trisilicate ingestion (11556).

Interactions with Herbs & Other Dietary Supplements

None known.

Interactions with Drugs

None known.

Interactions with Foods

None known.

Interactions with Lab Tests

None known.

Interactions with Diseases or Conditions

None known.

Dosage and Administration
ORAL: For osteoporosis, dietary intakes of 40 mg are associated with increased bone mineral density compared to lower intakes. There is no recommended dietary allowance (RDA) for silicon since an essential biological role for it has not been identified (7135).

Comments
Do not confuse silicon with silicone. Silicone is the name of a group of polymers that contain silicon, oxygen, and other organic groups. Silicone is used to make breast implants, medical tubing, and a variety of other medical devices.

SIMARUBA

Also Known As
Bitter Damson, Dysentery Bark, Mountain Damson, Simarouba, Slave Wood, Stave Wood, Sumaruba.

Scientific Names
Simarouba amara, synonym Quassia simarouba.
Family: Simaroubaceae.

People Use This For
Orally, simaruba is used to treat diarrhea, dysentery, malaria, water-retention, fever, unspecified gastrointestinal upset, as a tonic, and to cause abortion.

Safety
There is insufficient reliable information available about the safety of simaruba.
PREGNANCY AND LACTATION: LIKELY UNSAFE ...when used orally due to apparent abortifacient effects (18,4500); avoid using.

Effectiveness
There is insufficient reliable information available about the effectiveness of simaruba.

Mechanism of Action
The applicable part of simaruba is the bark. Simaruba contains the following active ingredients: 20-27% tannins, simarubin, essential oil, and fat (18,4500). It also contains the following bitter substances: quassinoids including simarolide, simarubidin, 13,18-dehydro-glaucarubinone; 0.1-0.2% 5-hydroxy-canthin-6-one a volatile oil; and unspecified alkaloids (18).

Adverse Reactions
Orally, ingesting large amounts of simaruba can cause vomiting (18).

Interactions with Herbs & Other Dietary Supplements
None known.

Interactions with Drugs
None known.

Interactions with Foods
None known.

Interactions with Lab Tests
None known.

Interactions with Diseases or Conditions
None known.

Dosage and Administration
ORAL: A typical dose is 1 gram (18).

Comments
Simaruba amara grows in the Caribbean islands and in the northern parts of South America (18).

SITOSTANOL

Also Known As

24-alpha-ethylcholestanol, Beta-sitostanol, Dihydro-beta-sitosterol, Fucostanol, Phytostanol, Plant Stanol, Plant Stanol Esters, Stigmastanol.
CAUTION: See separate listing for Beta-sitosterol.

Scientific Names

3-beta,5-alpha-stigmastan-3-ol.

People Use This For

Orally, sitostanol is used for prevention of heart disease and hypercholesterolemia.

Safety

LIKELY SAFE ...when used orally and appropriately. Sitostanol has been safely used in studies lasting up to one year (5336,5429,5430,5431,5432,5433,5434,5435,5436,5437,5438,5439,5441,5443,5814).
CHILDREN: LIKELY SAFE ...when used orally and appropriately, short-term. Sitostanol has been safely used in children in studies lasting for up to 3 months (3888,3889,5438,7193,7194). There is insufficient reliable information available about the safety of long-term use of sitostanol in children.
PREGNANCY AND LACTATION: Insufficient reliable information available; avoid using.

Effectiveness

LIKELY EFFECTIVE

Hypercholesterolemia. Taking sitostanol orally is effective for reducing cholesterol levels in adults with hypercholesterolemia (1886,3888,5336,5429,5430,5431,5432,5433,5434,5435,5437,5438,5439,5441,5443,7103). Sitostanol also seems to be effective for reducing cholesterol levels in healthy children (7193,7194). However, treating children is not recommended unless low-density lipoprotein (LDL) levels are greater that 190 mg/dL or greater that 160 mg/dL in the presence of other coronary risk factors. Sitostanol is usually taken as a component of a sitostanol-enriched food such as margarine. It is effective in about 88% of patients when used alone or in combination with a low-fat diet or HMG-CoA reductase inhibitor ("statin") for reducing total and low-density lipoprotein cholesterol (3888,5431,5433,5435,5437,5814,7195). Sitostanol alone can reduce total and LDL cholesterol levels by 10-15% (5443). Peak cholesterol lowering effects occur at about 2 grams per day. Higher doses do not seem to offer any additional benefit (5814,6185,7195). When added to a statin such as pravastatin (Pravachol) or simvastatin (Zocor), sitostanol reduces total cholesterol by an additional 3-11% and LDL cholesterol by another 7-16% (5431,5433). Treatment with sitostanol for 2-3 weeks is usually necessary before cholesterol levels decrease significantly. If sitostanol is discontinued, cholesterol levels tend to rise within 2-3 weeks (7105).

POSSIBLY EFFECTIVE

Familial hypercholesterolemia. Taking sitostanol orally seems to be effective for treating familial hypercholesterolemia in children (3888,3889,5438).

Mechanism of Action

Sitostanol is a saturated form of plant sterols that structurally resembles cholesterol. It is prepared commercially from vegetable oils or the oil from pine tree wood pulp and is then made fat-soluble with canola oil (5435,5430,5814). Sitostanol is unabsorbable and tasteless. It competitively inhibits both dietary and biliary cholesterol absorption by competing with cholesterol for the limited space in mixed micelles (5435,5439,5443,5814,7196). However, sitostanol doesn't have to be taken with meals to lower cholesterol blood levels. Some researchers think sitostanol remains in the intestinal lumen or in the enterocytes after ingestion. So administration of sitostanol at any time of day seems to be as effective as multiple daily doses with meals (7103). Cholesterol levels decrease within 2 to 3 weeks of initiation of sitostanol, and return to pretreament levels within 2 to 3 weeks of discontinuation (7105) which also suggests a prolonged effect. Sitostanol may not have the same effect in all people. Preliminary clinical evidence suggests that sitostanol might work better in people with apolipoprotein E4 alleles, a genetic predisposition to hypercholesterolemia (7105,7195). About 12% of patients do not respond to sitostanol. In certain patients, hepatic cholesterol synthesis might increase in response to decreased availability of cholesterol, resulting in no change in cholesterol levels (5430,5443). There is some concern that sitostanol might decrease absorption of some nutrients since it decreases fat absorption. Sitostanol does seem to reduce the absorption of dietary beta-carotene. However, when corrected for lower levels of LDL, the major carrier of beta-carotene, the reduction in beta-carotene levels may not be clinically significant (7103,7104,7105). Sitostanol does not seem to affect retinol, vitamin D, or lycopene (5434,7104,7105).

Adverse Reactions

Orally, sitostanol seems to be very well tolerated. Adverse effects have not been reported in clinical trials in adults or children (5336,5429,5430,5431,5432,5433,5434,5435,5436,5437,5438,5439,5441,5443,7103,7104,7105,7193,7194). However, because sitostanol decreases cholesterol absorption in the gut, it might be expected to produce some gastrointestinal symptoms like diarrhea and excess amounts of fat in the stool (steatorrhea).

Interactions with Herbs & Other Dietary Supplements

BETA-CAROTENE: Sitostanol can reduce absorption and blood levels of beta-carotene (3888,5434,5814,7103,7104,7105). Sitostanol lowers blood levels of low-density lipoprotein (LDL) cholesterol, which is a major carrier of fat-soluble antioxidants (7103,7104,7105). When corrected for lower LDL levels, the reduction in beta-carotene levels does not seem to be clinically significant (7103,7104,7105). Supplementation with beta-carotene is probably not necessary. Suggest that concerned patients increase dietary consumption of beta-carotene rich vegetables or take a multivitamin that contains beta-carotene (7104).

CHOLESTEROL LOWERING HERBS/SUPPLEMENTS: Sitostanol might enhance the effects of herbs and supplements that also lower cholesterol levels. Some of these herbs and supplements include chromium, flaxseed, garlic, guar gum, niacin, oat bran, psyllium, red yeast, and others.

Interactions with Drugs

None known.

Interactions with Foods

BETA-CAROTENE: Sitostanol can reduce absorption and blood levels of beta-carotene (3888,5434,5814,7103,7104,7105). Sitostanol lowers blood levels of low-density lipoprotein (LDL) cholesterol, which is a major carrier of fat-soluble antioxidants (7103,7104,7105). When corrected for lower LDL levels, the reduction in beta-carotene levels does not seem to be clinically significant (7103,7104,7105). Supplementation with beta-carotene is probably not necessary. Suggest that concerned patients increase dietary consumption of beta-carotene rich vegetables or take a multivitamin that contains beta-carotene (7104).

Interactions with Lab Tests

SERUM CHOLESTEROL: Sitostanol decreases total and low-density lipoprotein (LDL) cholesterol and test results (5336,5429,5431,5432,5433,5435,5437,5438,5439,5441).

Interactions with Diseases or Conditions

None known.

Dosage and Administration

ORAL: For hypercholesterolemia, clinical studies have used from 800 mg to 4 grams per day (5814). However, doses above 2 grams per day do not seem to provide additional benefit (7195). Effectiveness is not dependent on administration schedule. Single daily doses seem to be as effective as divided doses administered twice or three times daily (7195). For familial hypercholesterolemia in children, clinical studies have used 2-6 grams daily initially and then tapered down to 1.5 grams daily (3888,3889,5438).

Comments

Sitostanol is an ingredient in the functional food product Benecol margarine and in some salad dressings. The FDA authorized the use of labeling health claims for foods containing plant stanol esters, including sitostanol, for reducing the risk of coronary heart disease (CHD). This rule is based on the FDA's conclusion that plant stanol esters in conjunction with a diet low in saturated fat and cholesterol might reduce the risk of CHD by lowering blood cholesterol levels (6668). Although there is plenty of evidence that sitostanol does lower cholesterol levels, so far there is no proof that long-term use actually lowers the risk of developing CHD. Do not confuse sitostanol with beta-sitosterol, an unsaturated plant sterol in the cholesterol-lowering margarine Take Control (5443). Both sitostanol and beta-sitosterol are used for lower cholesterol levels in people with hypercholesterolemia and appear to be equally effective (7196).

SKIRRET

Also Known As

Chervis.

Scientific Names

Sium sisarum.
Family: Apiaceae/Umbelliferae.

Comments

At the date of publication, this product was not a common ingredient used in brand name supplements marketed to consumers. Details about this product are available in the online version of *Natural Medicines Comprehensive Database.* See www.naturaldatabase.com.

SKULLCAP

Also Known As
Blue Pimpernel, Blue Skullcap, Helmet Flower, Hoodwort, Mad Weed, Mad-Dog Skullcap, Quaker Bonnet, Scullcap, Scutelluria.
CAUTION: See separate listing for Baikal Skullcap.

Scientific Names
Scutellaria lateriflora.
Family: Lamiaceae/Labiatae.

People Use This For
Orally, skullcap is used for insomnia, anxiety, ischemic stroke, and paralysis caused by stroke. It is also used orally for fever, hyperlipidemia, atherosclerosis, rabies, chorea, epilepsy, nervous tension, allergies, dermatitis, inflammation, and spasms.

Safety
There is insufficient reliable information available about the safety of skullcap.
Pregnancy and Lactation: Insufficient reliable information available; avoid using.

Effectiveness
INSUFFICIENT RELIABLE EVIDENCE to RATE

Anxiety. Preliminary evidence suggests that healthy people who take a single dose of skullcap extract might feel more relaxed than tense. This effect appears to last for about 2 hours (12216). But it is not known if taking skullcap is effective for anxiety disorders or if extended use is beneficial. More evidence is needed to rate skullcap for this use.

Mechanism of Action
The applicable parts of skullcap are the above ground parts. The principle flavonoids of skullcap are baicalin and wogonin (12104,12216). Other flavonoids found in skullcap include scutellarin, methoxyflavone, and catalpol. Skullcap also contains lignins, resins, tannins, and volatile oils (12104).
It is thought that the flavonoid constituents of skullcap might act as GABA agonists and therefore have a sedating and anxiolytic effect (12216).
Constituents of skullcap seem to bind the serotonin receptor 5-HT7. But it's not known if these constituents have agonist or antagonist properties on the receptor (12104). Skullcap's effects on the serotonin receptor may be involved in potential sedative properties.

Adverse Reactions
Orally, single doses of skullcap extract appear to be well-tolerated. A single skullcap extract dose of 100 mg does not seem to affect cognition or cause significant sedation. But a higher dose of 200 mg might cause more sedation and cognitive impairment (12216). The effect of these typical doses in repeated doses is not known.
High doses of skullcap can cause giddiness, stupor, confusion, limb twitching, seizures (4,6), "intermission" of the pulse, and other symptoms consistent with epilepsy (6).
There are four reports of hepatotoxicity, one of which led to a fatality, associated with products thought to contain skullcap. However, it is uncertain whether the products actually contained skullcap. It is thought that the products might have been contaminated with an adulterant such as germander (515), which is known to cause liver damage.

Interactions with Herbs & Other Dietary Supplements
HERBS WITH SEDATIVE PROPERTIES: Theoretically, concomitant use with herbs that have sedative properties might enhance therapeutic and adverse effects. Some of these supplements include 5-HTP, calamus, California poppy, catnip, hops, Jamaican dogwood, kava, St. John's wort, valerian, yerba mansa, and others.

Interactions with Drugs
None known.

Interactions with Foods
None known.

Interactions with Lab Tests
None known.

Interactions with Diseases or Conditions
None known.

Dosage and Administration

ORAL: A typical dose is 1-2 grams or as a tea three times daily (4). To make tea, steep 1-2 grams above ground parts in 150 mL of boiling water for 5-10 minutes, strain. The extract is typically used 2-4 mL (1:1 in 25% alcohol) three times daily. The tincture is typically used 1-2 mL (1:5 in 45% alcohol) three times daily (4).

Comments

Skullcap has been commonly adulterated with germander and teucrium (12). There are over 200 members of the genus Scutellaria. Other species in this genus are often substituted for skullcap (Scuttelaria lateriflora). The most often substituted species are Western Skullcap (Scuttelaria canescens), Southern Skullcap (Scutellaria cordifolia), or Marsh Skullcap (Scutellaria galericulatum). However, these species have a different constituent profile, particularly with regard to flavonoid constituents, and therefore are not considered interchangeable (12216).

SKUNK CABBAGE

Also Known As

Dracontium, Meadow Cabbage, Polecatweed, Skunkweed, Spathyema Foetida, Swamp Cabbage.

Scientific Names

Symplocarpus foetidus, synonym Dracontium foetidum.
Family: Araceae.

People Use This For

Orally, skunk cabbage is used to treat bronchitis, asthma, whooping cough, catarrh, cancer, chorea, convulsions, cough, edema, epilepsy, headache, hemorrhage, hysteria, pregnancy, labor, worms, rheumatism, ringworm, scabies, snakebite, skin sores, spasms, splinters, swellings, toothache, and wounds. It is also used as a gastrointestinal (GI) stimulant.

As a food, the young leaves, roots, and stalks have been boiled and eaten.

Safety

POSSIBLY SAFE ...when used orally and appropriately; the young boiled leaves, roots, and stalks are used as food (4500,4502) without reports of serious adverse effects (4).

PREGNANCY AND LACTATION: POSSIBLY UNSAFE ...when used orally; avoid using. It may affect the menstrual cycle (4), and irritant properties may stimulate uterine contractions (4,12).

Effectiveness

There is insufficient reliable information available about the effectiveness of skunk cabbage.

Mechanism of Action

Skunk cabbage contains a variety of constituents, including an acrid principle, unspecified alkaloids, essential oil, fatty oil, phenolic compounds, and tannins (4,4502). The seeds are reported to contain a narcotic (4502). The root contains calcium oxalate which could irritate the kidney or promote kidney stones in sensitive individuals (12,4502). The leaves contain n-hydroxytryptamine (4).

Adverse Reactions

Orally, large amounts of skunk cabbage are reported to cause nausea, vomiting, headache, vertigo, and dimness of vision (18,4502). Excessive use of gastrointestinal (GI) irritants can cause abdominal cramps, burning, blistering in the mouth and throat, nausea, colic, and watery or bloody diarrhea (12).

Topically, the fresh plant can cause severe itching, inflammation, and blistering (4,4502).

Interactions with Herbs & Other Dietary Supplements

CALCIUM, IRON, ZINC: Concurrent use might decrease mineral absorption. Skunk cabbage contains oxalate (7,12), which can bind multivalent metal ions in the gastrointestinal (GI) tract and decrease mineral absorption.

Interactions with Drugs

None known.

Interactions with Foods

CALCIUM, IRON, ZINC: Skunk cabbage might decrease mineral absorption from foods. Skunk cabbage contains oxalates (7,12), which can bind multivalent metal ions in the gastrointestinal (GI) tract and decrease mineral absorption.

Interactions with Lab Tests

None known.

Interactions with Diseases or Conditions
GASTROINTESTINAL (GI) CONDITIONS: Skunk cabbage may aggravate GI ulcers, GI inflammation or cause GI irritation (12,19).
KIDNEY STONES (Nephrolithiasis): Individuals with a history of oxalate kidney stones should avoid skunk cabbage or use it cautiously (12,4502).

Dosage and Administration
ORAL: People typically use the powdered rhizome/root, 0.5-1 mg three times daily mixed with honey or by infusion or decoction (4). 0.5-1 mL the liquid extract, 1:1 in 25% alcohol, has been used three times daily (4). 2-4 mL of the tincture, 1:10 in 45% alcohol, has been used three times daily (4).

Comments
Skunk cabbage is also a common name for members of the toxic Veratrum family. Skunk cabbage gets its name from a volatile oil emitted by the plant that has a highly disagreeable odor (18).

SLIPPERY ELM

Also Known As
Indian Elm, Moose Elm, Red Elm, Sweet Elm.

Scientific Names
Ulmus rubra, synonym Ulmus fulva.
Family: Ulmaceae.

People Use This For
Orally, slippery elm is used for coughs, sore throat, colic, diarrhea, constipation, hemorrhoids, irritable bowel syndrome (IBS), cystitis, urinary inflammation, urinary tract infections, syphilis, herpes, and for expelling tapeworms. It is also used orally for protecting against stomach and duodenal ulcers, for colitis, diverticulitis, GI inflammation, and acidity. Slippery elm is used orally as an abortifacient.
Topically, slippery elm is used for wounds, burns, gout, rheumatism, cold sores, boils, abscesses, ulcers, toothaches, sore throat, and as a lubricant to ease labor.
In manufacturing, slippery elm is used in some baby foods and adult nutritionals, and in some oral lozenges used for soothing throat pain.

Safety
LIKELY SAFE ...when used orally and appropriately (4,12,512).
PREGNANCY: POSSIBLY SAFE ...when the inner bark is used orally in amounts used in foods (4). LIKELY UNSAFE ...when the whole bark is used. Use of the whole bark is contraindicated because it is an abortifacient (4,6).
LACTATION: Insufficient reliable information available; avoid using.

Effectiveness
POSSIBLY EFFECTIVE

Sore throat. Slippery elm has demulcent properties and, added to lozenges, can soothe sore throats (272,512,1740).
There is insufficient reliable information available about the effectiveness of slippery elm for its other uses.

Mechanism of Action
The applicable part of slippery elm is the inner bark rind. The mucilages are considered the principal constituent. They are responsible for slippery elm's demulcent and emollient effects (4,18). Used internally, slippery elm preparations cause reflex stimulation of nerve endings in the GI tract, leading to mucous secretion (6). This induced mucous may protect the GI tract against ulcers, excess acidity, etc. Tannin constituents have astringent properties (4). Oleoresins of some species are responsible for contact dermatitis (6).

Adverse Reactions
Orally, the whole bark is an abortifacient (4).
Topically, slippery elm extracts can cause contract dermatitis (6). The pollen is an allergen (6).

Interactions with Herbs & Other Dietary Supplements
None known.

Interactions with Drugs
ORAL DRUGS: Theoretically, may slow the absorption and reduce serum levels of orally administered drugs due to mucilage content (19).

Interactions with Foods
None known.

Interactions with Lab Tests
None known.

Interactions with Diseases or Conditions
None known.

Dosage and Administration
ORAL: People typically use the powdered inner bark (1:8 as a decoction), 4-16 mL three times daily (4). As a nutritional supplement, 4 grams powdered inner bark in 500 mL boiling water, three times daily (4) has been used. People typically use the alcohol extract (1:1 in 60% alcohol), 5 mL three times daily (4).
TOPICAL: As a poultice, people typically use the coarse powdered inner bark mixed with boiling water (4).

Comments
Avoid confusing whole bark with inner bark. Commercial lozenges containing slippery elm are preferred to the native herb when used for cough and sore throat, because they provide sustained release of mucilage to the throat (3).

SMARTWEED

Also Known As
Arsesmart, Smart Weed, Water Pepper.

Scientific Names
Polygonum hydropiper.

People Use This For
Orally, smartweed is used to treat bleeding of the womb, menstrual bleeding, bleeding hemorrhoids, and diarrhea. Topically, smartweed is used to wash bloody wounds.

Safety
There is insufficient reliable information available about the safety of smartweed.
Pregnancy and Lactation: Insufficient reliable information available; avoid using.

Effectiveness
There is insufficient reliable information available about the effectiveness of smartweed.

Mechanism of Action
The applicable parts of smartweed are the leaf, and the entire plant during flowering season. Smartweed contains tannins, hydropiperoside, sesquiterpenealdehydes, and flavonoids (18). Smartweed is reported to stop bleeding. It is also thought to influence the elimination of urine and to have some effect on rheumatic pain (18).

Adverse Reactions
Orally, smartweed can cause gastrointestinal irritation (19).
Topically, the fresh plant can cause inflammatory reactions due to chemical irritation (18).

Interactions with Herbs & Other Dietary Supplements
None known.

Interactions with Drugs
WARFARIN (Coumadin): Smartweed is high in vitamin K. Concomitant use can decrease the anticoagulant effects of warfarin (Coumadin) (19).

Interactions with Foods
None known.

Interactions with Lab Tests
None known.

Interactions with Diseases or Conditions
GASTROINTESTINAL DISORDERS: Smartweed can exacerbate inflammatory conditions by irritating the mucous membranes (19).

Dosage and Administration
ORAL: A small amount of the powdered drug three times a day or one cup tea (one teaspoon of the drug per cup, boil) three times per day (18).
TOPICAL: No typical dosage.

Comments
Smartweed has an extraordinary hot pepper-like taste (18).

SMOOTH ALDER

Also Known As
Hazel Alder, Tag Alder.

Scientific Names
Alnus serrulata.
Family: Betulaceae.

Comments
At the date of publication, this product was not a common ingredient used in brand name supplements marketed to consumers. Details about this product are available in the online version of *Natural Medicines Comprehensive Database.* See www.naturaldatabase.com.

SNEEZEWORT

Also Known As
Sneezeweed.

Scientific Names
Achillea ptarmica.
Family: Asteraceae/Compositae

People Use This For
Orally, sneezewort is used for rheumatic and painful disorders, toothache, diarrhea, nausea, vomiting, flatulence, tiredness, urinary tract complaints, and as an appetite stimulant.
Topically, sneezewort is used for toothache.

Safety
There is insufficient reliable information available about the safety of sneezewort.
Pregnancy and Lactation: Insufficient reliable information available; avoid using.

Effectiveness
There is insufficient reliable information available about the effectiveness of sneezewort.

Mechanism of Action
The applicable part of sneezewort is the dried root. Sneezewort contains alkamides, polyynes, and volatile oil (18).

Adverse Reactions
Orally, sneezewort may cause an allergic reaction (18).

Interactions with Herbs & Other Dietary Supplements
None known.

Interactions with Drugs
None known.

Interactions with Foods
None known.

Interactions with Lab Tests
None known.

Interactions with Diseases or Conditions
SNEEZEWORT ALLERGY: Contraindicated.

Dosage and Administration
ORAL: A typical dose is two cups of tea daily. To make tea, simmer 2 teaspoons of the cut root in 2 cups of water (18).
TOPICAL: The fresh root can be chewed (18).

SOLOMON'S SEAL

Also Known As
Dropberry, Ladys Seals, Lady's Seals, Sealroot, Sealwort, Solomons Seal, St Marys Seal, St. Mary's Seal.

Scientific Names
Polygonatum multiflorum.
Family: Liliaceae.

People Use This For
Orally, Solomon's seal is used for respiratory and lung disorders, and as an astringent and anti-inflammatory.
Topically, Solomon's seal is used for bruises, furuncles, ulcers or boils on the fingers, hemorrhoids, skin redness, edema, and hematoma.

Safety
POSSIBLY SAFE ...when used orally, short-term (12).
PREGNANCY AND LACTATION: Insufficient reliable information available; avoid using.

Effectiveness
There is insufficient reliable information available about the effectiveness of Solomon's seal.

Mechanism of Action
There is insufficient reliable information available about the possible mechanism of action and active ingredients. Solomon's seal may cause hypoglycemia (19).

Adverse Reactions
Long-term use may cause gastrointestinal irritation. Use of large doses or overdoses may cause nausea, diarrhea, gastric complaints, and nausea (18).

Interactions with Herbs & Other Dietary Supplements
HYPOGLYCEMIC HERBS: Theoretically, concomitant use with other hypoglycemic herbs may have additive effects (19).

Interactions with Drugs
ANTIDIABETES DRUGS: Theoretically, concomitant use may enhance hypoglycemic drug effects and alter blood glucose control (19). Monitor blood glucose.
CHLORPROPAMIDE (Diabinese): Concomitant use may cause additive hypoglycemic effects (19).
INSULIN: Insulin dosage adjustments may be necessary, due to the possible hypoglycemic effects of Solomon's seal (19).

Interactions with Foods
None known.

Interactions with Lab Tests
None known.

Interactions with Diseases or Conditions
DIABETES: Theoretically may interfere with blood glucose control (19).

Dosage and Administration
No typical dosage.

Comments
Solomon's seal is obsolete as a medicinal herb.

SORREL

Also Known As

Acedera Común, Azeda-Brava, Garden Sorrel, Sorrel Dock, Sour Dock, Wiesensauerampfer.
CAUTION: See separate listings for Wood Sorrel and Yellowdock.

Scientific Names

Rumex acetosa.
Family: Polygonaceae.

People Use This For

Orally, sorrel is used for acute and chronic inflammation of the nasal passages and respiratory tract, and as an adjunct to antibacterial therapy. It is also used as a diuretic and to stimulate secretions.
In combination with gentian root, European elder flower, verbena, and cowslip flower, sorrel is used orally for maintaining healthy sinuses and treating sinusitis.

Safety

POSSIBLY SAFE ...when used orally in amounts commonly found in foods. ...when used orally in combination with gentian root, European elder flower, verbena, and cowslip flower (Quanterra Sinus Defense, Sinupret) (374,379).
LIKELY UNSAFE ...when used in large amounts. A 53-year old died after ingesting 500 grams of sorrel in soup (17).
There is insufficient reliable information available about the safety of sorrel used in medicinal amounts.
CHILDREN: POSSIBLY UNSAFE ...when used orally because it contains oxalic acid. A four-year old child died after consuming rhubarb leaves, which are also a source of oxalic acid (17).
PREGNANCY AND LACTATION: There is insufficient reliable information available about the safety of sorrel in medicinal amounts during pregnancy and lactation; avoid using.

Effectiveness

POSSIBLY EFFECTIVE

Sinusitis. Taking sorrel orally in a specific combination product which also contains gentian root, European elder flower, verbena, and cowslip flower (Quanterra Sinus Defense, Sinupret) seems to help treat acute or chronic sinusitis (374,379).

There is insufficient reliable information available about the effectiveness of sorrel for its other uses.

Mechanism of Action

Sorrel contains 7-15% tannins (11), which exert an astringent effect on the mucosal tissue. This effect dehydrates the tissue, reducing internal secretions and forming the external cells into a protective layer. Plants with at least 10% tannins may cause gastrointestinal disturbances, kidney damage, and necrotic conditions of the liver. Some animal data show that tannins may cause cancer; other data show they may prevent it. Regular consumption of herbs with high tannin concentrations correlates with increased incidence of esophageal or nasal cancer (12). Sorrel leaf has a 0.3% oxalate content (12). Once absorbed, the oxalic acid reacts with calcium in plasma and resulting insoluble calcium oxalate may precipitate in the kidneys, blood vessels, heart, lungs, and liver. This may also cause hypocalcemia (12,17). Oxalate crystals damage mucosal tissue, resulting in severe irritation and possible damage. The systemic absorption of oxalates may result in kidney damage, both in people with pre-existing kidney disease and in healthy kidneys (19).

Adverse Reactions

Orally, excessive amounts of sorrel can cause diarrhea, nausea, polyuria (6), dermatitis (4) and gastrointestinal symptoms. Oxalic acid (constituent) poisoning affects skin, eyes, respiratory system, and kidneys. Oral symptoms of oxalate irritation include swelling of the mouth, tongue, and throat, with difficulty in speaking and suffocation. It has a corrosive effect on the digestive tract and can lead to oxalic acid crystals in the kidneys, blood vessels, heart, lungs, liver, and/or hypocalcemia (17).

Interactions with Herbs & Other Dietary Supplements

CALCIUM, IRON, ZINC: Concurrent use might decrease mineral absorption. Sorrel contains oxalate (7,12), which can bind multivalent metal ions in the gastrointestinal tract and decrease mineral absorption.
TANNIN-CONTAINING HERBS: Theoretically, herbs that contain high percentages of tannins (such as sorrel) may cause precipitation of constituents of other herbs (19).

Interactions with Drugs

ORAL DRUGS: Theoretically, concomitant oral administration may cause precipitation of some drugs due to the high tannin content of sorrel (19). Separate administration of oral drugs and tannin-containing herbs by the longest period of time practical (19).

Interactions with Foods

CALCIUM, IRON, ZINC: Concurrent use might decrease mineral absorption from foods. Sorrel contains oxalate (7,12), which can bind multivalent metal ions in the gastrointestinal tract and decrease mineral absorption.

Interactions with Lab Tests

None known.

Interactions with Diseases or Conditions

COAGULATION DISORDERS: Oxalate constituents can alter the calcium concentrations and decrease coagulation time (4,12).
GI CONDITIONS: Theoretically, sorrel can exacerbate stomach and intestinal ulcers due to mucosal irritant effect (19).
KIDNEY DISEASE: Can damage kidneys with formation of insoluble oxalate; use with caution or avoid in individuals with history of kidney stones (12,19).

Dosage and Administration

ORAL: For acute or chronic sinusitis, two Sinupret tablets three times daily for up to two weeks has been used in clinical trials (7,374,379), equivalent to gentian root 12 mg, European elder flower 36 mg, verbena 36 mg, cowslip flower 36 mg, and sorrel 36 mg three times daily.

Comments

Roselle (Hibiscus sabdariffa) is also known as Jamaica sorrel or Guinea sorrel. It could be confused with sorrel (11,18).

SOUR CHERRY

Also Known As

Cerezo Acido, Cerisier Acide, English Morello, Ginjeira, Griottier, Guindo, Montmorency Cherry, Morello Cherry, Pie Cherry, Red Cherry, Richmond, Sauerkirsche, Sauerkirschenbaum, Tart Cherry.

Scientific Names

Prunus cerasus, synonyms Cerasus vulgaris, Prunus vulgaris.
Family: Rosaceae.

People Use This For

Orally, sour cherry is used for arthritis, gout, to cause diuresis, and to facilitate digestion.
In foods, sour cherries are eaten as a food or flavoring.
In manufacturing, sour cherry is used to make cherry syrup USP for drugs with an unpleasant taste.

Safety

LIKELY SAFE ...when the fruit is used in amounts commonly found in foods. ...when the fruit is used in medicinal amounts (6).
There is insufficient reliable information available about the safety of the oral use of sour cherry stem.
PREGNANCY AND LACTATION: LIKELY SAFE ...when the fruit is consumed in typical food amounts. There is insufficient reliable information available about the safety of sour cherry stem use during pregnancy or lactation.

Effectiveness

There is insufficient reliable information available about the effectiveness of sour cherry.

Mechanism of Action

The applicable parts of sour cherry are the fruit and stem. Sour cherry fruit contains vitamin C, vitamin A, alpha-linolenic acid, and traces of vitamin E, beta-carotene, folacin thiamine, as well as other constituents (4282). It contains varied antioxidants including kaempferol and quercetin (4282,4283). A preliminary study at Michigan State University suggests compounds found in the sour cherry have anti-inflammatory effects that are ten times stronger than aspirin but without aspirin's side effects (6). The stem of the sour cherry contains an isoflavone constituent, prunetin 5-O-beta-D-glycopyranoside (4284).

Adverse Reactions

None reported.

Interactions with Herbs & Other Dietary Supplements

None known.

Interactions with Drugs
None known.

Interactions with Foods
None known.

Interactions with Lab Tests
None known.

Interactions with Diseases or Conditions
None known.

Dosage and Administration
No typical dosage.

Comments
Of the more than 270 varieties of sour cherry, only a few are important commercially. These include the Montmorency, Richmond, and English morello (6).

SOUTHERN PRICKLY ASH

Also Known As
Prickly Ash, Prickly Yellow Wood, Sea Ash, Toothache Tree, Xanthoxylum, Zanthoxylum.
CAUTION: See separate listings for Ash and Northern Prickly Ash.

Scientific Names
Zanthoxylum clava-herculis.
Family: Rutaceae.

People Use This For
Orally, southern prickly ash is used for cramps, intermittent claudication, Raynaud's syndrome, chronic rheumatic conditions, and peripheral circulatory insufficiency associated with rheumatic symptoms, as a tonic, stimulant, for toothache, sores, ulcers, as a diaphoretic in fever, and for cancer (as an ingredient in Hoxsey cure).

Safety
POSSIBLY SAFE ...when the bark is used orally in medicinal amounts (12).
There is insufficient reliable information about the safety of the oral use of the berry.
PREGNANCY: LIKELY UNSAFE ...when used orally (12) because it might have menstrual stimulant effects (19).
There is insufficient reliable information about the safety of the berry during pregnancy; avoid using.
LACTATION: LIKELY UNSAFE ...when used orally because it might cause colic in nursing infants (19).

Effectiveness
There is insufficient reliable information available about the effectiveness of southern prickly ash.

Mechanism of Action
The applicable parts of southern prickly ash are the bark and berry. Southern prickly ash contains nitidine (hypotensive, antileukemic, hepatic enzyme inhibitor), chelerythrine (anti-inflammatory, antibiotic against gram positive bacteria, potentiates barbiturate induced sleep, hepatic enzyme inhibitor), asarinin (antitubercular), and neoherculin (insecticidal, salivation stimulant) (4). Reports of death after ingestion by cattle, chickens, and fish attributed to the neuromuscular blocking properties of the bark (4).

Adverse Reactions
None reported.

Interactions with Herbs & Other Dietary Supplements
DIGITALIS: May interfere with cardiac glycoside therapy (4).

Interactions with Drugs
ANTACIDS: Theoretically, due to reports that southern prickly ash increases stomach acid, southern prickly ash might decrease the effectiveness of antacids (19).
H2-BLOCKERS: Theoretically, due to reports that southern prickly ash increases stomach acid, southern prickly ash might decrease the effectiveness of H2-blockers (19). The H2 blockers include cimetidine (Tagamet), ranitidine (Zantac), nizatidine (Axid), and famotidine (Pepcid).

PROTON PUMP INHIBITORS (PPIs): Theoretically, due to reports that southern prickly ash increases stomach acid, southern prickly ash might decrease the effectiveness of PPIs (19). PPIs include omeprazole (Prilosec), lansoprazole (Prevacid), rabeprazole (Aciphex), pantoprazole (Protonix), and esomeprazole (Nexium).

Interactions with Foods
None known.

Interactions with Lab Tests
None known.

Interactions with Diseases or Conditions
LIVER DISEASE: Theoretically, southern prickly ash may inhibit hepatic enzymes.

Dosage and Administration
ORAL: People typically use 1-3 grams dried bark, or drink as decoction (boil 1-3 grams dry bark 10-15 minutes, strain), three times daily; liquid bark extract (1:1 in 45% alcohol) 1-3 mL three times daily; or bark tincture (1:5 in 45% alcohol) 2-5 mL three times daily (4). People typically use 0.5-1.5 grams dried berry or liquid berry extract (1:1 in 45% alcohol) 0.5-1.5 mL (4).

SOY

Also Known As
Daidzein, Edamame, Frijol de Soya, Genistein, Haba Soya, Hydrolyzed Soy Protein, Isoflavone, Legume, Miso, Natto, Phytoestrogen, Plant Estrogen, Shoyu, Soja, Sojcomponentsabohne, Soy Fiber, Soy Milk, Soy Protein, Soya, Soybean, Soybean Curd, Tempeh, Texturized Vegetable Protein, Touchi, Tofu.
CAUTION: See separate listings for Alpha-GPC, Nattokinase, and Soybean Oil.

Scientific Names
Glycine max, synonyms Glycine soja, Dolichos soja, Glycine gracilis, Glycine hispida, Phaseolus max Soja hispida, Soja max.
Family: Fabaceae/Leguminosae.

People Use This For
Orally, soy is used for hyperlipidemia, menopausal symptoms, preventing osteoporosis, and preventing cardiovascular disease. It is also used orally for cyclic breast pain, preventing hot flashes in breast cancer survivors, premenstrual syndrome (PMS), hypertension, type 2 diabetes, constipation, diarrhea, and muscle soreness caused by exercise. Other uses include slowing the progression of kidney disease, decreasing urine protein excretion, improving memory, and preventing breast cancer, endometrial cancer, prostate cancer, and thyroid cancer.
In foods, soy is used as a milk substitute for infant feeding formulas, and as an alternative to cow's milk. Soybeans are eaten boiled or roasted. Soy flour is used as an ingredient in foods, beverages, and condiments.

Safety
LIKELY SAFE ...when soy protein is used orally and appropriately. Soy protein products in doses up to 60 grams per day providing up to 185 mg isoflavones have been safely used in studies lasting up to 16 weeks (842,2293,2294,2296,3025,3402,3977,4755,6412,8530,8531,10372,11805).
POSSIBLY SAFE ...when soy extracts are used orally and appropriately, short-term. Soy extracts containing concentrated isoflavones in doses of 35-110 mg/day seem to be safe when used for up to 6 months (4751,6455,12040,12048).
POSSIBLY UNSAFE ...when soy extracts are used orally in high doses, long-term. Postmenopausal women who consume soy isoflavone tablets 150 mg/day for 5 years seem to have an increased occurrence of endometrial hyperplasia (12105). However, there is no evidence that consuming a diet that is high in soy foods causes this potential adverse effect. People who consume a diet high in soy foods actually seem to have a reduced risk of endometrial cancer (7338,10372).
CHILDREN: LIKELY SAFE ...when consumed in amounts commonly found in foods (4912). Soy in amounts commonly found in food or as a component of infant formula seem to be safe (3400,7331). Exposure to soy formula in infancy does not appear to cause health or reproductive problems later in life (7331). However, soy milk that's not designed for infants is not a substitute for infant formula. Regular soy milk can lead to nutrient deficiencies (12045).
POSSIBLY UNSAFE ...when used orally as an alternative to cow's milk in children with severe milk allergy. Although soy protein-based infant formulas are often promoted for children with milk allergy, children with a severe allergy to cow's milk are also frequently sensitive to soy protein (9883). There is insufficient reliable information available about the safety of soy products when used in amounts higher than typical food quantities for children.
PREGNANCY: LIKELY SAFE ...when used orally in amounts commonly found in foods (4912).
POSSIBLY UNSAFE ...when used orally in medicinal amounts. Soy contains mildly estrogenic

constituents (3373,3988,3989,3990,3994,6029). Theoretically, therapeutic use of soy might adversely affect fetal development; avoid using.

LACTATION: LIKELY SAFE ...when used orally in amounts commonly found in foods (4912). A single 20 gram dose of roasted soybeans, containing 37 mg isoflavones, produces four to six times less isoflavones in breast milk than provided in a soy-based infant formula (2290). There is insufficient reliable information available about the safety of long-term use of therapeutic amounts of soy during lactation.

Effectiveness

LIKELY EFFECTIVE

Hyperlipidemia. Taking soy protein preparations orally reduces total cholesterol and low-density lipoprotein (LDL) levels in both hypercholesterolemic and normocholesterolemic men and women (842,2293,2294,2296,2585,3402,4755,6412,7346,7803,8528,8530). Replacement of dietary animal protein with soy protein decreases serum total cholesterol by 9%, LDL cholesterol by 13%, and triglycerides by 11% after one to two months. The effect on high-density lipoprotein (HDL) cholesterol is not consistent (2560,3401,7659,7804). Some of the beneficial effects might be attributed to the isoflavone content of soy protein, since preparations providing higher concentrations of isoflavones seem to produce more significant effects (3402,6413,10459). However, purified soy isoflavone supplements alone do not seem to decrease LDL cholesterol (8502).

The hormonal changes that occur in perimenopausal women might suppress the effect of soy protein on serum lipoproteins (9679). Soy protein may not reduce cholesterol levels in healthy postmenopausal women aged 60 to 75 years (12034).

Tell patients not to rely on concentrated soy extracts or purified isoflavone supplements for lowering lipids. They lack the fiber and beneficial fatty acids of soy protein and don't seem to be as effective as isoflavone rich foods like soy protein for lowering serum cholesterol concentrations (851,4738,7345,8502,10459). The FDA has approved labeling soy products for cholesterol reduction when used in combination with a diet low in saturated fat and cholesterol. To be eligible for this labeling, soy products must provide at least 6.25 grams of soy protein per serving, which is 25% of the effective amount of 25 grams per day (3977).

POSSIBLY EFFECTIVE

Breast cancer. There is some evidence from population studies that Asian women who eat a diet high in soy have a reduced risk of developing breast cancer (5939,7334,7335,7336). Soy food intake during adolescence seems to correlate with decreased incidence of breast cancer among Chinese women. This benefit persists even when Asian women immigrate to the Western cultures where soy is less likely to be a regular component of the diet (7335,7336,9674). This suggests that early exposure to soy might be important for protection against breast cancer later in life. The estrogenic effect of soy might also be more pronounced in Asian women, possibly because of an ethnic difference in response (7663). Some epidemiologic research in Japan suggests that miso (fermented soybean paste) soup and dietary isoflavone consumption reduces breast cancer risk, but other soy foods do not (11807). In Western-culture populations, an association between soy and breast cancer risk has not been established. Total dietary intake of phytoestrogens among Western-culture middle-aged women doesn't appear to be related, positively or negatively, to breast cancer risk (11391).

Diabetes. In postmenopausal women with type 2 diabetes, treatment with a soy product containing 30 grams of soy protein and 132 mg isoflavones daily for 12 weeks seems to lower fasting insulin levels, hemoglobin A1c, insulin resistance, and low-density lipoprotein (LDL) cholesterol (8531). Preliminary clinical research suggests that an extract of the fermented soybean product, touchi, acts as an alpha-glucosidase inhibitor. It seems to modestly lower blood glucose, hemoglobin A1c, and triglycerides in patients with type 2 diabetes (11762). There is also preliminary evidence that patients with type 2 diabetes who consume 26 grams of fibrous soy hulls might have lower blood glucose levels and improved glucose tolerance (13141). Consuming a fibrous soy polysaccharide product 10 grams daily with a meal seems to reduce postprandial glucose and triglyceride levels in type 2 diabetes patients (13142).

Diabetic nephropathy. Soy isoflavones may help prevent or treat diabetic nephropathy. Replacing animal protein in the diet with soy protein reduces urinary albumin excretion (7348,12555,12556).

Diarrhea. Giving soy fiber orally seems to reduce the duration of diarrhea in infants (2291,2292).

Galactosemia, hereditary lactase deficiency, or lactose intolerance. Giving isolated soy protein-based formula orally to infants seems to be helpful for treating galactosemia, hereditary lactase deficiency, or lactose intolerance (3400).

Hypertension. Taking soy protein seems to modestly reduce systolic blood pressure by about 4 mmHg and diastolic blood pressure by about 3 mmHg in patients with prehypertension or mild hypertension (13139). Soy protein combined with psyllium seems to reduce systolic blood pressure by about 8 mmHg and diastolic blood pressure by about 2 mmHg in adult men and women with hypertension (10458). In perimenopausal women without hypertension, soy protein also seems to modestly lower diastolic blood pressure by about 5 mmHg (2296).

Kidney disease. Taking soy protein orally seems to reduce proteinuria in people with kidney disease (2286,2287,2288).

Menopausal symptoms. Consuming a diet high in soy seems to help reduce hot flashes related to menopause. Ingesting various amounts of soy isoflavones seems to a have similar effects on vasomotor symptoms. Patient expectations also seem to be linked to the perceived effectiveness of soy (7801,7802,9916). Soy protein 20-60 grams providing 34-76 mg of isoflavones daily seems to modestly decrease the frequency and severity of hot flashes in some menopausal women (2296,2297,3978,3986,3987,7653,9917,11805). However, not all research has found that soy helps hot flashes, possibly due to a high placebo response (11806). Soy extracts, providing 35-100 mg of isoflavones daily, seem to have similar beneficial effects (4751,6455,10460,11805,11993). Genistein, a soy isoflavone, also seems to reduce hot flashes. A dose of 54 mg per day appears to be about half as effective as estrogen-progesterone supplementation (11994). Soy supplements appear to be helpful in about 30% of postmenopausal women (8499). The optimal dose and administration frequency of soy for menopausal symptoms have not been determined (11805). However, taking soy orally doesn't seem to prevent hot flashes in breast cancer survivors. There is also concern about possible stimulation of cancer cells by soy (3991,7658).

Osteoporosis. Most evidence suggests that soy protein can increase bone mineral density (BMD), or slow BMD loss, and improve biochemical markers of bone turnover in peri- and postmenopausal women (842,6449,9775,12044). The effect of soy protein on osteoporosis seems to be dependent upon the content of isoflavones. Taking isoflavones 80-90 mg, in 40 grams of soy protein, seems to be needed to improve BMD (842,6449,9775). Lower doses of isoflavones, between 4-56 mg, do not seem to be as effective in most women. Although, there is evidence that postmenopausal Japanese women who consume 54.3 mg isoflavones per day from dietary soy seem to have higher BMD than women who consume less (7342); this may be due to the increased sensitivity to the effect of soy isoflavones in Asian women.

There is also some conflicting evidence that suggests soy protein does not improve BMD in some postmenopausal women (4952,12034). The reasons for these inconsistent findings are not clear. However, different findings might be due to the variety of formulations of soy used, different age groups studied, and varying study designs (4950,4952). It's also thought that only "equol-producing" patients might have BMD benefits from soy. These are patients who can convert significant quantities of the daidzein isoflavone to equol, which is estrogenic. Only about 50% of people are "equol-producers" (4952).

Preliminary evidence also suggests that soy might have more pronounced effects on bone mineral content (BMC) in women who are in late postmenopause compared to early postmenopause, women with lower bodyweight compared to higher bodyweight, and women who consume less calcium compared to women who consume higher amounts of calcium (4951).

Soy doesn't seem to affect BMD in premenopausal women or bone turnover in adolescents (7660,8532,9684).

So far, there is no evidence that taking soy can reduce the risk of fractures in any patient population (4950).

POSSIBLY INEFFECTIVE

Cardiovascular disease. Higher dietary intake of phytoestrogens, including isoflavones from soy, does not seem to be associated with a reduced risk of primary cardiovascular events such as myocardial infarction or stroke in Western women (13040). However, the amount of phytoestrogens typically consumed in Western diets is significantly lower than the amount typically consumed in Asian diets. It is not known if higher levels of dietary phytoestrogen consumption would be associated with a decrease in cardiovascular events in this population.

Exercise-induced muscle soreness. Taking soy isoflavone extract orally for 30 days prior to exercise doesn't seem to ameliorate muscle soreness caused by exercise (8524).

INSUFFICIENT RELIABLE EVIDENCE to RATE

Cognitive function. There is conflicting evidence about the effect of soy on cognitive function. Some evidence suggests that college students who increase soy food consumption providing 100 mg/day of isoflavones have improved short- and long-term memory (12039). Postmenopausal women aged 50 to 65 years who take a soy extract supplement providing 60 mg/day of isoflavones also seem to have some improvement in some measures of cognitive function (12048). There is also evidence that older postmenopausal women aged 55 to 75 years that taking a soy extract supplement providing 110 mg/day of isoflavones might improve verbal memory scores (12040). However, another study in this patient population suggests that consuming 25.6 grams/day of soy protein providing 99 mg of isoflavones does not improve cognitive function (12034). Differing study designs and soy formulations used make comparisons of these findings difficult.

Endometrial cancer. There is some epidemiological evidence that increasing soy intake might lower the risk of endometrial cancer. Endometrial cancer incidence is lower in Japan, China, and other Asian countries where the typical diet is low in calories and high in soy and whole grain foods, vegetables, and fruits (7338).

Mastalgia. There is some preliminary evidence that soymilk (34 grams soy protein/day) might reduce cyclical breast pain in some women (2428).

Memory. Some research suggests that a high soy diet might slightly improve performance on memory tests (9671).

Prostate cancer. Epidemiological research about the effect of soy on prostate cancer risk has been mixed. Men consuming an Asian diet, which contains ten times more soy than the average American diet seem to have a lower risk of prostate cancer. However, it's unclear whether soy in the diets of Asian populations protects against prostate cancer or genetic differences or environmental factors such as fat ingestion are responsible (2298,12884,12886,12887). Soy protein containing 83 mg isoflavones taken daily for a year doesn't seem to affect PSA levels in otherwise healthy men aged 50 to 80 years (12888); however, there is some evidence that men with prostate cancer who consume a specific bread containing 50 grams of soy and providing 117 mg isoflavones have significantly reduced PSA levels after about 3 weeks of treatment (13140).

Thyroid cancer. Epidemiological research suggests that high dietary intake of soy might reduce the risk of thyroid cancer (7662,12041).

More evidence is needed to rate soy for these uses.

Mechanism of Action

The applicable part of soy is the bean. Soybeans are legumes that contain up to 50% protein; 24% carbohydrates; and 25% oil including stearic, linoleic, and palmitic acids. The active constituents of soybeans are the phytoestrogens, known as isoflavones (3387,3978,4753,6029), and phytosterols such as beta-sitosterol, campesterol, and stigmasterol (8528). Soybeans are also rich in calcium, iron, potassium, amino acids, vitamins, and fiber. Soy protein contains all of the essential amino acids in sufficient quantities to support human life (2426). Non-fortified soy beverages such as soymilk contain only about 10 mg of calcium per serving. But calcium-fortified soymilk can contain from 80-500 mg of calcium per serving in the form of tricalcium phosphate (6414). However, calcium from cow's milk is significantly better absorbed than calcium from fortified soymilk (6414). Fermented soy foods, such as soy sauce, miso, tempeh, and natto, have higher amounts of calcium and vitamin K2 (7342).

Soybeans and soy foods are the most significant dietary source of isoflavones (3387,3978,4753,6029). They contain the isoflavone glucosides genistein and daidzein in their inactive conjugated forms. In the gastrointestinal tract, genistein and daidzein are hydrolyzed by beta-glucosidases in the jejunum, releasing the isoflavone aglycone forms of genistein and daidzein (3982,5937,9346). Daidzein is further metabolized by gut flora to the estrogenic compound, equol. The extent of conversion of daidzein to equol varies among people due to differences in gut flora. Theoretically, people who do not convert significant amounts of daidzein to equol ("non-equol producers") might not experience the same pharmacological effects as people who do convert significant amounts ("equol producers") (12049). About 50% of the population does not produce equol (4952).

The amount of isoflavones varies among the forms of soy. Soy milk and soy powder have a lower concentration of isoflavones than other soy products (7655). Soy protein usually contains 1-3 mg of isoflavones per gram of protein (7333).

Soy isoflavones are heterocyclic phenols with structural similarity to estradiol and selective estrogen-receptor modulators (SERMs). Soy isoflavones bind to both the alpha- and beta-estrogen receptors. But they have a higher affinity for the beta-estrogen receptor (3983,3992,6029,7344,7657).

The beta-estrogen receptor predominates in the heart, vasculature, bone, and bladder; and may account for some of soy's beneficial effects. Actions at the cellular level depend on the target tissue, receptor status of the tissue, and the level of endogenous estrogen (7344).

Soy phytoestrogens might act as SERMs (3387,3990). In premenopausal women with normal endogenous estrogen levels, soy phytoestrogens may have an anti-estrogen effect since soy isoflavones can displace endogenous estrogen from receptors. Consuming soy protein might also lower circulating levels of estradiol in premenopausal women over the entire menstrual cycle (7805). In postmenopausal women with low endogenous estrogens, soy phytoestrogens have a weak estrogenic effect (3373,3988,3989,3990,3994,6029,8529).

Soy has several pharmacological effects that might be beneficial for preventing cardiovascular disease (6029). It may lower homocysteine levels by unknown mechanisms, possibly related to the folic acid found in soy protein. Soy may also inhibit platelet aggregation (3992,8530,9776). Soy seems to lower blood pressure, in particular the diastolic pressure (9346).

Soy might increase bile acid excretion and up-regulate low-density lipoprotein (LDL) receptors (2426,2594,6029,6030,7344). Phytosterols in soy also contribute to the lowering of LDL cholesterol by competitively inhibiting cholesterol absorption in the small bowel (2594,8528).

Some preliminary evidence suggests that soy might prevent progression of coronary artery atherosclerosis (7333). The isoflavones found in soy, particularly genistein, inhibit oxidation of LDL particles, a process thought to play a role in early atherosclerosis (2586,6029,7347,9560,9561). The isoflavones seem to inhibit LDL oxidation by acting as free radical scavengers and by inhibiting cyclooxygenase (COX) (9683). In addition to preventing LDL oxidation, genistein also seems to protect vascular cells from oxidized LDL (8527). Some evidence suggests that genistein may prevent vascular remodeling, which is an important component of atherosclerotic plaque formation (8503). Genistein might produce these effects by inhibiting tyrosine kinase activity, and reducing the production of proteolytic enzymes and the migration of endothelial cells (9346). Soy also seems to improve arterial compliance in perimenopausal women (851).

Unlike oral estrogen, phytoestrogens don't seem to elevate C-reactive protein (CRP) levels (9919). However, lipoprotein (a), which has been identified as an independent risk factor for coronary heart disease, does not seem to be affected by soy in postmenopausal women. In men, most research suggests that soy doesn't negatively affect lipoprotein (a) (7347,8530,8963,8964). The effect of soy on endothelial function, an early marker of vascular disease, is variable. In middle-aged men, soy might improve endothelial function. However, soy does not seem to affect endothelial function in postmenopausal women and might worsen endothelial function in older men (8963,8964).

For preventing postmenopausal osteoporosis, soy is thought to work due to its weak estrogenic effects on bone (5598,6029). Like estrogen, soy seems to have the most effect on the bone mineral density of the lumbar spine (7660). Soy seems to increase serum levels of osteocalcin, a marker of bone formation, in postmenopausal women (7659). The soy isoflavone genistein appears to directly inhibit osteoclast activity (9346). High intake of soy also seems to lower parathyroid hormone levels, which might lower bone turnover (7660). In vitro tests suggest that genistein may promote the proliferation of osteoblasts by inhibiting oxidative damage (9682). However, soy proteins and isoflavones do not seem to influence calcium absorption or calcium retention (7343).

Estrogenic effects of soy have also been attributed to benefit menopausal symptoms such as hot flashes. Genistein seems to relieve hot flashes in some women (11994). However, some research suggests that the incidence of hot flashes does not seem to correlate with serum levels of the phytoestrogens genistein, daidzein, and equol. Other

components of soy, in addition to phytoestrogens, may be responsible for reduction in hot flashes (4752).
In cancer, soy is thought to be beneficial due to preliminary evidence that suggests soy isoflavones have antioxidant, antiproliferative, and antiangiogenic activity (2296,3983). Soy also contains other anticarcinogenic compounds such as saponins, phytates, protease inhibitors, and phytosterols (9346).
There is a lot of controversy about soy and its potential role in breast cancer. Some researchers think that soy is protective against breast cancer. Asian women who eat a traditional diet high in soy seem to have a lower risk of developing breast cancer (4590,5939). This benefit persists even when Asian women immigrate to the western cultures where soy is less likely to be a regular component of the diet (9674). This suggests that exposure to soy early in life (i.e., before menopause), provides the most benefit against breast cancer. It is theorized that isoflavones found in soy enhance early cellular differentiation and maturation of mammary glands. More mature mammary glands seem to be less susceptible to carcinogens (4590). Animal models show that soy protein can prevent chemically induced breast cancer (3976). There is also some evidence that the soy isoflavone, genistein, can suppress breast cancer cell growth by stimulating apoptosis (3378). Other research suggests that genistein influences enzymes involved in signal transduction that regulate cell growth and replication (7337). Genistein seems to exert multiple antiproliferative effects on both estrogen receptor positive (ER+) as well as estrogen receptor negative (ER-) human breast cancer cells (9346,10461). The ability of genistein to inhibit the growth of precancerous dysplastic cells in breast tissue may significantly contribute to the prevention of breast cancer (8965).
There is also some evidence that soy isoflavones can prolong the menstrual cycle and suppress midcycle surges of luteinizing hormone (LH) and follicle stimulating hormone (FSH), which may also decrease the risk of breast cancer (9346). Some research suggests that soy consumption alters the ratios of various estrogen metabolites in the urine, reducing excretion of potentially carcinogenic estrogen metabolites. This suggests that soy might cause a shift in estrogen metabolism to produce more benign metabolites (2430). However, some researchers suggest that due to the estrogenic effects of soy, it might actually increase the risk of breast cancer (6030). There is also preliminary in vitro data suggesting that soy can stimulate proliferation of normal human breast tissue (3980,3981). Higher serum estradiol levels are associated with increased risk of breast cancer. There is evidence that drinking soymilk daily can reduce serum 17-beta-estradiol and progesterone levels in premenopausal women. However, other research shows only a very modest effect of a high soy isoflavone diet on plasma hormones (2429,7654,9676). Tell patients the effect of soy on breast cancer is unknown.
"Unopposed estrogen" from the estrogenic activity of soy and its effects on the uterus has been a concern. There doesn't seem to be any significant effects on vaginal cytology or endometrial biopsy in premenstrual or postmenopausal women (2429,7654,9676,9917). Dietary phytoestrogens are associated with a reduced risk of endometrial cancer. Besides their effect on estrogen, isoflavones and other phytoestrogenic substances in soy might inhibit aromatase, which converts androstenedione to estrone, and may in turn increase endometrial cancer risk (7338,10372).
In prostatic diseases, soy phytoestrogens are thought to be potentially beneficial due to estrogenic mechanisms as well as inhibition of 5-alpha-reductase and 17-beta-hydroxysteroid dehydrogenase (3984,3985). A diet high in soy foods seems to reduce serum estradiol levels and testosterone levels (7339,9683). However, soy does not significantly reduce prostate specific antigen (PSA) levels (9777). Laboratory research suggests that genistein decreases the growth of both benign prostatic hyperplasia (BPH) and prostate cancer tissue (11238). Other preliminary research suggests that genistein might change androgen receptor expression and transcriptional activity of androgen-sensitive prostate cancer cells (12885).
The soy isoflavones, genistein and daidzein, seem to be responsible for the effects on thyroid hormones. These isoflavones seem to block production of thyroid hormone by interfering with thyroid peroxidase catalyzed iodination of thyroglobulin. This can result in increased thyroid stimulating hormone (TSH) and goiter. However, these clinical results appear most likely to occur in people with low iodine levels (6466). The effect on thyroid function is not likely to be clinically significant in patients with adequate dietary iodine intake (7806).
Soy isoflavones have potential benefits on cognitive function. Preliminary evidence suggests that the effects of soy isoflavones seem to be equivalent to those of 17 beta-estradiol in up-regulating choline acetyl transferase and nerve growth factor. These chemical factors are thought to be essential for learning and memory. Soy also might decrease the phosphorylation of the brain protein tau. Phosphorylation of this protein is associated with the development of Alzheimer's disease (9346).
Tofu, a soybean product, seems to inhibit the absorption of lead and prevent its build-up in the body, possibly because of its phytic acid and calcium content (7656).
There is some evidence that isoflavones can inhibit oxidative and conjugative metabolism of drugs (4736).
Isoflavones might also affect drug absorption and biliary excretion by interacting with drug transporters such as P-glycoprotein and the canalicular multispecific organic anion transporter (4736). Given the wide range of drugs and metabolites whose pharmacokinetics depends on these mechanisms, drug interactions with isoflavones might be more common than literature reports suggest. Postmenopausal women with high dietary intake of the soy isoflavone genistein seem to have a lower body mass index, waist circumference, and fasting insulin levels than women with lower intake (7804). However, soy supplementation does not significantly increase leptin concentrations in postmenopausal women. Leptin is a protein that is associated with decreased appetite and weight loss (9681).
For diabetes, soy protein might reduce glucose levels due to its fiber content. There is also evidence that soy might improve glycemic control by inhibiting tyrosine kinase activity, improving insulin receptor affinity, improving glucose transport and increasing tissue sensitivity to insulin (8513).
Touchi, a traditional Chinese food used as a seasoning agent, is prepared by steaming and then fermenting soybeans

with the fungus Aspergillus. Touchi extract might be beneficial for diabetes patients because it seems to inhibit intestinal alpha-glucosidase and lower postprandial glucose levels in a dose-dependent manner. It may also lower triglyceride levels (11762).

Genistein and daidzein are widely distributed in the body and undergo enterohepatic recycling (7330). Peak concentrations appear at 4-8 hours after dietary intake, and excretion is within 24 hours (3982). They are found both free in serum and bound to plasma proteins. The elimination half-life of free genistein and free daidzein are 3.2 and 4.2 hours, respectively. The elimination half-life of total genistein and total daidzein are 9.2 and 8.2 hours, respectively (7661). Both genistein and daidzein are conjugated to sulfate and glucuronide compounds. In plasma, 48% of genistein and 33% of daidzein are present as a glucuronide and 8% of genistein and 26% of daidzein are present as a sulfate. The half-lives of genistein glucuronide and daidzein glucuronide are 3.2 and 8.4 hours, respectively. The half-lives of genistein sulfate and daidzein sulfate are 3.1 and 5.7 hours, respectively (9673).The absorption of isoflavones from food may be saturable, suggesting improved effect if ingested throughout the day, but there is considerable variation in absorption from person to person (3380,3982,7344). There is some variation in how isoflavones are absorbed from different soy products. Soy germ products result in higher plasma levels of daidzein and lower levels of genistein. Soy protein products result in higher levels of genistein. Soy foods such as tofu produce less dramatic rises of daidzein and genistein. Genistein from soy food sources appears to be more bioavailable than daidzein (7330). Isoflavone bioavailability is similar for most soy foods (4750).

Adverse Reactions

Orally, soy is very well tolerated. The most common side effects include gastrointestinal upset, such as constipation, bloating, and nausea (2297). Some people can also experience insomnia (9917).

Use of soy isoflavone supplements may rarely cause migraine headaches. This effect may be related to the estrogen-like activity of the isoflavones (9680).

Soy can cause allergic reactions such as skin rash and itching in some people (6412). But this does not seem to be common.

There is controversy about the role of soy in breast cancer. Population studies suggest that soy is protective against breast cancer. Asian women who eat a traditional diet high in soy seem to have a lower risk of developing breast cancer (4590,5939,9674). However, some researchers suggest that, due to the estrogenic effects of soy, it might increase the risk of breast cancer (6030). Preliminary research suggests that soy stimulates proliferation of normal human breast tissue (3980,3981). More research is needed to define the role of soy in breast cancer.

There is also some concern that soy might increase the risk of endometrial hyperplasia due to its estrogenic effects. But there is conflicting evidence. Some studies suggest that soy foods do not have a proliferative effect on endometrial cells (7358,2429,7654,9676,9917). Population studies suggest that consuming soy foods and phytoestrogens in the diet might actually reduce the risk of endometrial cancer (7338,10372). But there is clinical evidence that postmenopausal women who take soy isoflavone tablets for 5 years seem to have a higher occurrence of endometrial hyperplasia (12105).

Soy products have been associated with goiter and hypothyroidism in children taking soy formula (6466). There is also some evidence that soy seems to inhibit thyroid hormone synthesis resulting in increased secretion of TSH in some postmenopausal women (7806). However, this seems to only occur in people with iodine deficiency (6466). In postmenopausal women with normal levels of iodine, taking a soy extract for 6 months does not seem to significantly affect thyroid hormone levels (13010).

Epidemiologic data suggests that soy products may increase the risk for urinary bladder cancer. Total soy intake of greater than 92.5 grams/1000 Kcal seems to cause a 2.3-fold increase in the risk for bladder cancer compared with intake of less than 36.9 grams/1000 Kcal (9677).

Consumption of large amounts of fermented soy products (e.g., miso, tempeh) might increase the risk of stomach cancer. These associations might be confounded by the higher salt and N-nitroso content of some fermented soy foods or other dietary factors such as fruit and vegetable intake. However, there is also evidence that nonfermented forms of soy may reduce the risk of stomach cancer (7340,7341). More research is required to determine if soy products have any role in stomach cancer.

Some research suggests that dietary consumption of two or more servings per week of tofu during midlife might decrease cognitive function in later years. However, numerous other factors, such as lifestyle and health could be involved (6415,6416). These findings are too preliminary to be used as a basis for clinical recommendations.

The association of isoflavone consumption and infertility in animals has led to concerns about the effect of isoflavones in infants fed soy-based formulas (7332,7344). Reassure parents that adults who received soy formulas as infants do not experience adverse health or reproductive outcomes compared with people who received cow milk formulas as infants (7331).

Inhaled soy dust and soy hull aeroallergen can trigger symptoms of asthma (5084,5085,5086).

Advise patients to use whole soy foods if possible instead of soy supplements. Since these products and supplements contain differing amounts of isoflavones, high consumption and uncontrolled use of soy supplements could increase the risk of adverse effects (9346).

Interactions with Herbs & Other Dietary Supplements

None known.

Interactions with Drugs

ANTIBIOTIC DRUGS: Antibiotics may decrease the action of isoflavones in soy, because intestinal bacteria are responsible in part for converting the isoflavones into their active forms. Antibiotics may decrease the ability of intestinal bacteria to convert the isoflavones (7657).
ESTROGENS: Theoretically, soy might competitively inhibit the effects of estrogen replacement therapy (3860).
TAMOXIFEN (Nolvadex): There is some concern that soy might interfere with tamoxifen because of its potential estrogenic effects. There is preliminary evidence that soy isoflavones might antagonize the antitumor effects of tamoxifen (7072). Tell patients taking tamoxifen to avoid therapeutic use of soy products.
WARFARIN (Coumadin): Soy milk has been reported to decrease the international normalized ratio (INR) in a patient taking warfarin. The mechanism of this interaction is not known. Soy may also inhibit platelet aggregation (3992). Dosing adjustments for warfarin may be necessary (9672).

Interactions with Foods

PLANT-BASED FOODS: Soy protein isolate reduces the absorption of non-heme iron from foods (5053). Non-heme iron is found in plant-based foods.

Interactions with Lab Tests

PARATHYROID HORMONE: High intake of soy seems to lower parathyroid hormone levels in postmenopausal women (7660).
PROSTATE SPECIFIC ANTIGEN (PSA): There is some evidence that men with prostate cancer who consume a specific bread containing 50 grams of soy and providing 117 mg isoflavones have significantly reduced PSA levels after about 3 weeks of use (13140).
THYROID STIMULATING HORMONE (TSH): Theoretically, soy might increase TSH levels. Soy seems to inhibit thyroid hormone synthesis resulting in increased secretion of TSH in some postmenopausal women (7806). There are also cases of hypothyroidism and goiter in infants fed soy formula (6466). But this seems to occur primarily in people with low iodine levels (6466). In postmenopausal women with normal levels of iodine, taking a soy extract for 6 months does not seem to significantly affect thyroid hormone levels (13010).

Interactions with Diseases or Conditions

ALLERGIC RHINITIS: People with allergic rhinitis are at increased risk for soy hull allergy. The risk and severity of symptoms increase with increased exposure (5084).
ASTHMA: People with asthma are at increased risk for soy hull allergy. The risk and severity of symptoms increase with increased exposure (5084).
BREAST CANCER: Soy isoflavones have estrogenic properties. Some experts are concerned about the use of soy in women with breast cancer because estrogens can increase this risk. However, some preclinical studies show that soy may have protective effects for breast cancer (3976), while others suggest soy might increase breast cell proliferation (3980,3981). Because there is insufficient reliable information about the effects of soy preparations in patients with breast cancer, a history of breast cancer, or a family history of breast cancer, therapeutic use of soy should be done with caution in these patients (956,7072,7655,8192).
CYSTIC FIBROSIS: Children with cystic fibrosis may develop hypoproteinemia when fed soymilk (368).
ENDOMETRIAL CANCER: Long-term use of concentrated soy isoflavone tablets 150 mg/day might increase the occurrence of endometrial hyperplasia (12105). Theoretically, taking these supplements might have an adverse effect on patients with endometrial cancer. However, there is no evidence that consuming soy foods adversely affects endometrial tissue. In fact, there is some evidence that consuming a diet high in soy foods might decrease the risk of endometrial cancer (7338,10372). Advise patients with endometrial cancer to avoid taking concentrated soy isoflavone supplements.
HYPOTHYROIDISM: Theoretically, soy might worsen hypothyroidism. There is some evidence that soy might inhibit thyroid hormone synthesis and increase thyroid stimulating hormone (TSH) in some postmenopausal women (7806). There are also cases of hypothyroidism and goiter in infants fed soy formula (6466). But this seems to occur primarily in people with low iodine levels (6466). In postmenopausal women with normal levels of iodine, taking a soy extract for 6 months does not seem to significantly affect thyroid hormone levels (13010).
KIDNEY STONES (Nephrolithiasis): There is some concern that soy products might increase the risk of kidney stones because of its high oxalate content. Soy products can contain from 0.5 mg to 14 mg oxalate per gram or approximately 43 mg to 640 mg per soy serving, depending on soy food type (7073). Tell patients with a history of kidney stones to avoid excessive consumption of soy.
MILK ALLERGY: Children who are severely allergic to cow's milk are frequently sensitive to soy as well (9883); use with caution or avoid.
RENAL FAILURE: In patients with end-stage renal disease (ESRD) phytoestrogens in soy may reach higher plasma concentrations, increasing the risk for toxicity (8522).
URINARY BLADDER CANCER: Soy products might increase the risk for urinary bladder cancer. Soy foods should be avoided in patients who are at risk or have a history of bladder cancer (9677).

Dosage and Administration

ORAL: For hyperlipidemia, a typical dose is 20-50 grams per day of soy protein (2293,2295,2296,3401,6412,7346).
For preventing osteoporosis, 40 grams per day soy protein containing 2-2.25 mg isoflavones per gram has been used in clinical studies (842,6449).
For menopausal symptoms such as hot flashes, 20-60 grams per day of soy protein providing 34-76 mg isoflavones has been used in studies (2296,2297); soy extract tablets and capsules providing 50-60 mg soy isoflavones per day have also been used (4751,6455,11993). Genistein, a soy isoflavone, 54 mg per day has also been used for hot flashes (11994).
For reducing the risk of prostate cancer, two or more glasses of soymilk daily has been used (2298). For proteinuria, a diet limited to 700-800 mg/kg soy protein daily has been used (2287).
For reducing cyclical breast pain in premenopausal women, 34 grams soy protein daily (as soymilk) has been used (2428).
For diarrhea in infants, soy fiber fortified formula containing 18-20 grams of soy protein per liter has been used (2291,2292).
For type 2 diabetes, touchi extract 300 mg three times daily with meals has been used (11762). For type 2 diabetes in postmenopausal women, 30 grams of soy protein daily, containing 132 mg of phytoestrogens, has been used daily for up to 12 weeks (8531).
For hypertension, 40 grams daily or 10 grams soy protein providing 18 mg isoflavones twice daily has been used (2296,13139).
Soy foods contain variable amounts of isoflavones. Soy flour contains 2.6 mg isoflavones per gram of soy flour, fermented soybeans contain 1.3 mg per gram, boiled soybeans contain 0.6 mg per gram, soymilk contains 0.4 mg per gram, soybean curd contains 0.5 mg per gram, fried soybean curd contains 0.7 mg per gram, soybean paste contains 0.4 mg per gram, and soy sauce contains 0.016 mg per gram (7342).

SOYBEAN OIL

Also Known As

Intralipid, Legume, Soy Bean Oil, Soya Oil, Soyca, Travmulsion.
CAUTION: See separate listing for Soy.

Scientific Names

Glycine max, synonyms Glycine soja, Dolichos soja, Glycine gracilis, Glycine hispida, Phaseolus max Soja hispida, Soja max.
Family: Fabaceae/Leguminosae.

People Use This For

Orally, plant sterols, derived from soybean oil, are used to lower total and LDL cholesterol. Unsaponifiable fractions of soybean oil are used to treat osteoarthritis.
Topically, soybean oil is used as a mosquito repellent and insect repellent.
Parenterally, soybean oil is used in nutrient formulas. It is also used as a source of lecithin.

Safety

LIKELY SAFE ...when used orally in amounts found in foods. Hydrogenated soybean oil has generally recognized as safe (GRAS) status in the US (4912). ...when used topically and appropriately. Health Canada considers soybean oil to be a safe alternative to low-dose DEET products when used topically as a mosquito repellent (13083). ...when pharmaceutical grade soybean oil products are used parenterally. Soybean oil is listed in the United States Pharmacopeia (10).
POSSIBLY SAFE ...when used orally and appropriately in medicinal amounts. Unsaponifiable fractions of soybean oil appear to be safe for up to 6 months (10693).
PREGNANCY: LIKELY SAFE ...when used orally in amounts commonly found in foods. Avoid using in amounts greater than those typically found in foods. POSSIBLY SAFE ...when used parenterally. Theoretically, parenteral use of lipids like soybean oil during pregnancy might lead to hypertriglyceridemia, ketonemia, premature labor, and placental infection. However, women have used parenteral nutrition with lipids to treat severe morning sickness without any adverse effects (4084).
LACTATION: LIKELY SAFE ...when used orally in amounts commonly found in foods. Avoid using in amounts greater than those typically found in foods.

Effectiveness

LIKELY EFFECTIVE

Mosquito repellent. Applying a commercial 2% soybean oil product (Bite Blocker) provides complete protection against mosquitoes for up to about 1.5 hours. This is comparable to products containing 4.7% DEET; however, higher concentration DEET products have a significantly longer duration of action (13077). DEET 10% to 35% provides from 4-12 hours of protection depending on the product formulation (13077,13083).
Health Canada considers soybean oil to be an alternative to low concentration DEET for protection against

mosquitoes with the caveat that soybean oil is considerably shorter-acting (13083).

POSSIBLY EFFECTIVE

Hypercholesterolemia. Soybean oil plant sterols used in margarine seem to help lower total and LDL cholesterol without affecting HDL (5336). The FDA has approved such labeling for the products Take Control and Benecol as a structure/function claim under the Dietary Supplement Health Education Act, not as a drug (4087).

Osteoarthritis. Taking unsaponifiable fractions of soybean and avocado oils orally appears to significantly improve pain and overall disability. It seems to be more effective for osteoarthritis of the hip than the knee (10693).

Mechanism of Action

Soybean oil is obtained by cold pressing the seeds of the Glycine soja. Soybean oil is used in parenteral nutrition as a source of fatty acids (16). In a comparison between diets with 20% fat from butter or soybean oil, people using soybean oil demonstrated a 12% decrease in LDL and a 3% reduction in HDL (4085). People using a margarine containing plant sterols from soybean oil reduced total and LDL cholesterol by 8-13% compared to a control group (5336).

Unsaponifiable fractions of plant oils, which are the residual matter obtained after hydrolysis of fatty acids, consist of sterols, squalene, terpenes, and vitamins (11785). Unsaponifiable fractions of soybean and avocado oils may reduce the progression of joint space loss in patients with osteoarthritis who have advanced joint space narrowing of the hip (10694). Preliminary evidence suggests this combination can inhibit cartilage degradation and promote cartilage repair in osteoarthritic chondrocytes (10695).

Adverse Reactions

Soybean oil can cause an allergic reaction in individuals allergic to the Fabaceae/Leguminosea family. Members of this family include peanuts, soybeans, and others (4079,4080).

Interactions with Herbs & Other Dietary Supplements

None known.

Interactions with Drugs

None known.

Interactions with Foods

None known.

Interactions with Lab Tests

CHOLESTEROL: Soybean oil sterols reduce serum total cholesterol and LDL cholesterol concentrations, and test results (5336).

Interactions with Diseases or Conditions

CROSS-ALLERGENICITY: Soybean oil may cause an allergic reaction in individuals sensitive to the Fabaceae/Leguminosea family. Members of this family include peanuts and soybeans (4079,4080).

Dosage and Administration

ORAL: In the form of a plant sterol-enriched margarine, such as Take Control, a serving size is one tablespoon, or 14 grams. For osteoarthritis, 300 mg daily (a combination of one-third avocado and two-thirds soybean unsaponifiables) has been used (10693).

TOPICAL: For preventing mosquito bites, 2% soybean oil products have been used (13077). Some commercial product (Bite Blocker) directions suggest reapplying every 2 hours.

PARENTERAL: No typical dosage.

SPANISH BROOM

Also Known As

Genet, Weaver's Broom.

CAUTION: See separate listings for Butcher's Broom and Scotch Broom.

Scientific Names

Spartium junceum; Genista juncea.

Family: Fabaceae/Leguminosae.

People Use This For

Orally, Spanish broom is used as a laxative and diuretic.

In foods and beverages, Spanish broom extracts are used as flavor components.

In manufacturing, Spanish broom extract is used as a fragrance in soaps and cosmetics.

Safety
LIKELY SAFE ...when used orally in amounts commonly found in foods. Spanish broom has Generally Recognized As Safe status (GRAS) for use in foods in the US (4912).
PREGNANCY AND LACTATION: POSSIBLY UNSAFE ...when used orally because large amounts of the alkaloid constituent sparteine can stimulate menstrual flow (19). The most common Spanish broom extract, Genet absolute, should not contain alkaloids because of the extraction method used, however, other extracts might (11).

Effectiveness
There is insufficient reliable information available about the effectiveness of Spanish broom.

Mechanism of Action
The applicable part of Spanish broom is the flower. Sparteine seems to hasten childbirth (11).

Adverse Reactions
None reported.

Interactions with Herbs & Other Dietary Supplements
None known.

Interactions with Drugs
None known.

Interactions with Foods
None known.

Interactions with Lab Tests
None known.

Interactions with Diseases or Conditions
None known.

Dosage and Administration
No typical dosage.

Comments
Avoid confusion with butcher's broom, scotch broom flower, and scotch broom herb. Spanish broom stems have appeared as an adulterant to scotch broom (Cytisus scoparius).

SPANISH ORIGANUM OIL

Also Known As
Origanum Oil, Sicilian Thyme, Spanish Origanum, Spanish Thyme.
CAUTION: See separate listings for Thyme Oil, Thyme, and Wild Thyme.

Scientific Names
Coridothymus capitatus, synonyms Satureja capitata, Thymus capitatus.
Family: Lamiaceae/Labiatae.

People Use This For
Topically, Spanish origanum oil is used for burns and to prevent and treat infections.
In foods and beverages, Spanish origanum oil is used as a flavor component.
In manufacturing, it is used as a fragrance component in soaps, cosmetics, and perfumes.

Safety
LIKELY SAFE ...when used orally in amounts commonly found in foods. Spanish origanum oil has Generally Recognized As Safe status (GRAS) for use in foods in the US (4912).
There is insufficient reliable information available about the safety of Spanish origanum oil in medicinal amounts.
PREGNANCY AND LACTATION: There is insufficient reliable information available about the safety of Spanish origanum oil in medicinal amounts during pregnancy; avoid using.

Effectiveness
There is insufficient reliable information available about the effectiveness of Spanish origanum oil.

Mechanism of Action
Spanish origanum oil is characterized by its carvacrol content (11). It contains carvacrol and thymol (11) which show some evidence of anthelmintic (11), antifungal (4059,4060,4062,4063), and antibacterial (4064,4065,4066) activity. These constituents also demonstrate some evidence of antioxidant activity, including decreased Fe (III) catalyzed phospholipid liposome peroxidation and peroxy radical scavenging activity (4067).

Adverse Reactions
None reported.

Interactions with Herbs & Other Dietary Supplements
None known.

Interactions with Drugs
None known.

Interactions with Foods
None known.

Interactions with Lab Tests
None known.

Interactions with Diseases or Conditions
None known.

Dosage and Administration
No typical dosage.

Comments
Spanish origanum oil is distilled from the flowering tops of Thymus capitatus and carvacrol-rich Origanum species.

SPEARMINT

Also Known As
Curled Mint, Fish Mint, Garden Mint, Green Mint, Lamb Mint, Mackerel Mint, Our Lady's Mint, Pahari Pudina, Putiha, Sage of Bethlehem, Spire Mint, Yerba Buena.
CAUTION: See separate listing for Sage.

Scientific Names
Mentha spicata, synonyms Mentha viridis, Mentha cordifolia, Mentha crispa.
Family: Lamiaceae/Labiatae.

People Use This For
Orally, spearmint is used for digestive disorders, including flatulence, indigestion, nausea, sore throat, diarrhea, colds, headaches, toothaches, cramps, cancer, bile duct and gallbladder inflammation, gallstones, upper gastrointestinal tract spasms, irritable bowel syndrome (IBS), and inflammation of respiratory tract. It is also used as an aromatic, stimulant, antiseptic, local anesthetic, and antispasmodic.
Topically, spearmint is used for oral mucosal inflammation, arthritis, local muscle and nerve pain, and skin conditions including pruritus and urticaria.
In foods and beverages, spearmint is used as a flavoring agent.
In manufacturing, spearmint is used in health food products, cosmetics, and oral hygiene products such as mouthwash and toothpaste.

Safety
LIKELY SAFE ...when used in amounts commonly found in foods. Spearmint and spearmint oil have Generally Recognized As Safe (GRAS) status (4912).
POSSIBLY SAFE ...when used orally or topically for medicinal reasons (11,12).
PREGNANCY AND LACTATION: Insufficinet reliable information available; avoid using in amounts greater than those typically found in foods.

Effectiveness
There is insufficient reliable information available about the effectiveness of spearmint.

Mechanism of Action
The applicable parts of spearmint are the leaf and oil. There is insufficient reliable information available about the possible mechanism of action and active ingredients.

Adverse Reactions
None reported.

Interactions with Herbs & Other Dietary Supplements
None known.

Interactions with Drugs
None known.

Interactions with Foods
None known.

Interactions with Lab Tests
None known.

Interactions with Diseases or Conditions
None known.

Dosage and Administration
ORAL: Spearmint is used in tea, and is also available in tablets, capsules, tinctures, and other oral formulations (11).
TOPICAL: No typical dosage.

SPINACH

Also Known As
Spinaciae folium, Spinatblatter.

Scientific Names
Spinacia oleracea, synonyms Spinacia inermis, Spinacia spinosa.
Family: Chenopodiaceae.

People Use This For
Orally, spinach is used for gastrointestinal complaints and fatigue. It is also used as a blood-builder, an appetite stimulant, for stimulating growth in children, and during convalescence.
In foods, spinach is a commonly consumed vegetable.

Safety
LIKELY SAFE ...when used in amounts commonly found in foods.
CHILDREN: LIKELY UNSAFE ...when used orally in infants under 4 months old; the nitrate content can cause methemoglobinemia (18).
PREGNANCY AND LACTATION: LIKELY SAFE ...when used in amounts commonly found in foods; avoid medicinal amounts.

Effectiveness
There is insufficient reliable information available about the effectiveness of spinach.

Mechanism of Action
The applicable part of spinach is the leaf. Spinach contains vitamin C, vitamin E, vitamin K, magnesium, and nitrates (18,19,11285). It also contains triterpene saponins and oxalic acid (18). Spinach is thought to have hypoglycemic effects (19). Consumption of fresh spinach is associated with a decreased risk of stomach cancer in humans (4112). Preliminary research suggests that compounds contained in spinach might slow aging effects on the nervous system (1418,1419).

Adverse Reactions
Orally, spinach may cause methemoglobinemia in infants younger than 4 months old (18).

Interactions with Herbs & Other Dietary Supplements
CALCIUM, IRON, ZINC: Concurrent use might decrease mineral absorption. Spinach contains oxalate (7,12), which can bind multivalent metal ions in the gastrointestinal tract and decrease mineral absorption.

Interactions with Drugs
ANTIDIABETES DRUGS: Monitor blood glucose level closely due to claims that spinach leaves have hypoglycemic effects (19).
WARFARIN (Coumadin): Spinach contains vitamin K. Individuals using anticoagulants should consume a consistent daily amount to maintain the effect of anticoagulant therapy (19).

Interactions with Foods
CALCIUM, IRON, ZINC: Concurrent use might decrease mineral absorption from foods. Spinach contains oxalate (7,12), which can bind multivalent metal ions in the gastrointestinal tract and decrease mineral absorption.

Interactions with Lab Tests
INTERNATIONAL NORMALIZED RATIO (INR)/PROTHROMBIN TIME (PT): Theoretically, spinach might decrease coagulation test results due to high vitamin K content (11285).

Interactions with Diseases or Conditions
DIABETES: Theoretically, spinach may interfere with blood glucose control (19).
KIDNEY DISEASE: Spinach may cause formation of insoluble oxalate crystals in the kidneys causing further damage (19).

Dosage and Administration
No typical dosage.

SPINY RESTHARROW

Also Known As
Cammock, Ground Furze, Hauhechelwurzel, Land Whin, Ononidis radix, Petty Whin, Restharrow, Stay Plough, Stinking Tommy, Wild Liquorice.

Scientific Names
Ononis spinosa.
Family: Fabaceae/Leguminosae.

People Use This For
Orally, spiny restharrow is used for gout, kidney and bladder stones, rheumatic complaints, urinary tract infections, irrigation therapy for inflammatory disease of the lower urinary tract, and prevention and treatment of kidney gravel.

Safety
POSSIBLY SAFE ...when used orally and appropriately (2).
PREGNANCY AND LACTATION: Insufficient reliable information available; avoid using.

Effectiveness
There is insufficient reliable information available about the effectiveness of spiny restharrow.

Mechanism of Action
The applicable part of spiny restharrow is the root. It contains isoflavonoids including ononin (2,18), triterpenes including alphaonoceradiendiol (18), and volatile oil (18). The volatile oil contains anethole, carvone, and menthol (18). Spiny restharrow is reported to have a diuretic effect (2,18).

Adverse Reactions
None reported.

Interactions with Herbs & Other Dietary Supplements
None known.

Interactions with Drugs
None known.

Interactions with Foods
None known.

Interactions with Lab Tests
None known.

Interactions with Diseases or Conditions

EDEMA: Contraindicated in individuals with edema resulting from cardiac or kidney impairment (2,18).

Dosage and Administration

ORAL: A typical oral dose is 6-12 grams daily or as a tea (2,18). To prepare tea, pour boiling water over 2-2.5 grams of ground drug, strain after 20-30 minutes (18). Drink with plenty of liquid (2,18).

SPLEEN EXTRACT

Also Known As

Bovine Spleen, Hydrolyzed Spleen Extract, Predigested Spleen Extract, Raw Spleen, Spleen, Spleen Concentrate, Spleen Factors, Spleen Peptides, Spleen Polypeptides, Splenopentin, Tuftsin.

Scientific Names

None.

People Use This For

Orally, spleen extract is used as replacement therapy after splenectomy or in people with inadequate spleen function. It is also used orally for treating people with low white blood cell counts, enhancing general immune function and immune function in people with cancer, and for treating bacterial infections. Spleen extract is also used orally for treating celiac disease, dermatitis herpetiformis, glomerulonephritis, HIV-related bacterial infections, rheumatoid arthritis, systemic lupus erythematosus, thrombocytopenia, ulcerative colitis, and vasculitis.

Safety

There is insufficient reliable information available about the safety of spleen extract. However, since spleen extract preparations are derived from animals, there is concern about contamination with diseased animal parts (1825). So far, there are no reports of disease transmission to humans due to use of contaminated spleen extract.

Pregnancy and Lactation: Insufficient reliable information available; avoid using.

Effectiveness

There is insufficient reliable information available about the effectiveness of spleen extract.

Mechanism of Action

Spleen extract is derived from fresh animal spleens. Spleen extract contains the peptides tuftsin and splenopentin (6614). Tuftsin stimulates phagocytosis, motility, and immunogenic response of phagocytic cells, and has bactericidal and tumoricidal activities (6660). Tuftsin activity correlates inversely with splenic function (6662). Spleen extracts are tried in people with HIV disease because some patients have significantly lower tuftsin activity than healthy people (6662). There is preliminary evidence that spleen extract might protect against radiation. Spleen extract seems to shorten the time to regain normal immune response in animals exposed to sublethal doses of radiation (6661).

Adverse Reactions

Adverse reactions have not been reported. However, there is some concern about contamination. Spleen extract is derived from raw animal spleens gathered from slaughterhouses, possibly from sick or diseased animals. Products made from contaminated or diseased organs might present a human health hazard. There is also concern that spleen extracts produced from cows in countries where bovine spongiform encephalitis (BSE) has been reported might be contaminated with diseased tissue. Countries where BSE has been reported include Great Britain, France, The Netherlands, Portugal, Luxembourg, Ireland, Switzerland, Oman, and Belgium (1825). There have been no reports of BSE transfer to humans from contaminated spleen extract products. Until more is known, tell patients to avoid these products unless country of origin can be determined. Patients should avoid products that are produced in countries where BSE has been found.

Interactions with Herbs & Other Dietary Supplements

None known.

Interactions with Drugs

None known.

Interactions with Foods

None known.

Interactions with Lab Tests

None known.

Interactions with Diseases or Conditions
None known.

Dosage and Administration
ORAL: A typical dose is approximately 1.5 grams total spleen peptides (equivalent to 50 mg of tuftsin and splenopentin) per day (6614).

SQUALAMINE

Also Known As
Spiny Dogfish Shark.

Scientific Names
Squalus acanthias (Spiny dogfish).
Family: Squalidae.

People Use This For
Orally, squalamine is used as an antibiotic.
Topically, synthetic squalamine compounds have been used as antibiotics.
In combination with captopril, oral squalamine is being investigated as an anti-angiogenic therapy for diabetic retinopathy.
Squalamine is also being investigated as a possible treatment for pediatric solid tumors.

Safety
There is insufficient reliable information available about the safety of squalamine or its derivative SM-7.
Pregnancy and Lactation: Insufficient reliable information available.

Effectiveness
There is insufficient reliable information available about the effectiveness of squalamine or its derivative SM-7.

Mechanism of Action
Squalamine was first isolated from the spiny dogfish shark and later synthesized synthetically. It shows evidence that it might have fungicidal and antiprotozoal activity (4139). Squalamine has also demonstrated significant activity against gram (-) and gram (+) bacteria (4139). Some compounds that mimic the structure of squalamine show promise in their activity against gram (-) rods, gram (+) cocci including methicillin-resistant Staphylococcus aureus, vancomycin-resistant Enterococcus faecium, and fungi (4138). In addition to antibiotic activity, squalamine also shows promise in inhibiting angiogenesis, and preventing formation and growth of tumors (4137,5043). Squalamine has also demonstrated activity against breast cancer, lung cancer, and neuroblastoma cancer (5043).

Adverse Reactions
None reported.

Interactions with Herbs & Other Dietary Supplements
None known.

Interactions with Drugs
None known.

Interactions with Foods
None known.

Interactions with Lab Tests
None known.

Interactions with Diseases or Conditions
None known.

Dosage and Administration
No typical dosage.

Comments
Avoid confusion with shark cartilage, which is prepared from the cartilage of spiny dogfish shark, hammerhead shark (Sphyrna lewini), and other shark species. Squalamine has been isolated from the stomach and liver tissues of the spiny dogfish shark. Synthetic products that mimic the structure of squalamine appear to be good candidates for

further development as topical antimicrobial agents. They have broad spectrum antimicrobial activity, but their potential for systemic toxicity limits their use (4138).
Researchers at Georgetown University Medical Center plan a study of squalamine as an antiangiogenic therapy in combination with captopril for diabetic retinopathy (1269).
Magainin, the manufacturer of an investigational squalamine drug product plans a clinical study of squalamine in the treatment of pediatric solid tumors (5043).

SQUAWVINE

Also Known As
Checkerberry, Deerberry, Hive Vine, Noon Kie Oo Nah Yeah, One-Berry, Partridgeberry, Running Box, Squaw Berry, Squaw Vine, Twinberry, Two-Eyed Berry, Winter Clover.

Scientific Names
Mitchella repens.
Family: Rubiaceae.

People Use This For
Orally, squawvine is used for amenorrhea, anxiety, diarrhea, edema, excessive menstruation, fibrocystic disease of the breast, oliguria, painful menstruation, postpartum depression, varicose veins, to ease childbirth, improving lactation, insomnia, congestive heart failure, kidney failure, liver failure, chronic dysentery, spermatorrhea, as an emmenagogue, as an abortifacient, as an astringent for treating colitis, and to reduce mucous membrane and leukorrheal discharges.
Topically, squawvine is used for treating sore nipples.

Safety
POSSIBLY SAFE ...when used orally and appropriately (12).
There is insufficient reliable information about the safety of squawvine topically.
PREGNANCY: POSSIBLY UNSAFE ...when used orally due to reported abortifacient properties (12).
LACTATION: Insufficient reliable information available; avoid using.

Effectiveness
There is insufficient reliable information available about the effectiveness of squawvine.

Mechanism of Action
The applicable parts of squawvine are the above ground parts. Squawvine is reported to contain resin, wax, mucilages, dextrin, saponins, alkaloids, glycosides, and tannins (410).

Adverse Reactions
None reported.

Interactions with Herbs & Other Dietary Supplements
None known.

Interactions with Drugs
None known.

Interactions with Foods
None known.

Interactions with Lab Tests
None known.

Interactions with Diseases or Conditions
None known.

Dosage and Administration
ORAL: A typical dose is 20-50 mg.

SQUILL

Also Known As
European Squill, Indian Squill, Mediterranean Squill, Red Squill, Scilla, Sea Onion, Sea Squill Bulb, White Squill.

Scientific Names
Urginea indica, synonyms Drimia indica, Scilla indica; Urginea maritima, synonyms Drimia maritima, Scilla maritima, Urginea scilla.
Family: Liliaceae or Hyacinthaceae.

People Use This For
Orally, squill is used for mild heart failure, arrhythmias, nervous heart complaints, some venous conditions, edema, emetic, as an expectorant, for chronic bronchitis, asthma with bronchitis, and whooping cough. Squill is also used orally as a diuretic, abortifacient, heart tonic, and a rat poison.
In manufacturing, squill is used in pest control as a rodenticide (red squill).

Safety
UNSAFE ...when used orally (4,6,18,512). Squill contains cardiac glycosides that can cause adverse effects (512).
PREGNANCY: UNSAFE ...when used orally because it can have an abortifacient effect (4).
LACTATION: UNSAFE ...when used orally (4).

Effectiveness
There is insufficient reliable information available about the effectiveness of squill.

Mechanism of Action
Squill contains cardioactive glycosides, including bufadienolides, scillaren A, and proscillaridin A (4,6,18). Squill seems to have cardiac effects similar to digoxin, including positive inotropic and negative chronotropic effects (4,7). The aglycones in squill are poorly absorbed from the gastrointestinal tract and are therefore less potent than digitalis cardiac glycosides. Squill has additional cardiovascular properties that include reducing left ventricular diastolic pressure, and reducing pathologically elevated venous pressure (18). Large amounts of squill can induce vomiting due to gastric irritation and central action (4). In lesser amounts squill causes an expectorant-like effect (6).

Adverse Reactions
Orally, squill can cause gastric irritation, loss of appetite, diarrhea, vomiting, stomach disorders, headache, irregular pulse (18), and convulsions (6). Skin contact with the fresh bulb can cause dermatitis (18). Signs of overdose include restlessness, nausea, vomiting, life-threatening arrhythmias (ventricular tachycardia, atrial tachycardia with atrioventricular block, ventricular fibrillation), stupor, vision disorders, depression, confusion, hallucinations, psychosis, seizure, cardiac arrest, asphyxiation, and death (18,3488). A fatality has been reported after ingestion of squill bulb (3488).

Interactions with Herbs & Other Dietary Supplements
CARDIAC GLYCOSIDE-CONTAINING HERBS: Contraindicated, and concomitant use can increase the risk of cardiac glycoside toxicity. Cardiac glycoside-containing herbs include black hellebore, Canadian hemp roots, digitalis leaf, hedge mustard, figwort, lily-of-the-valley roots, motherwort, oleander leaf, pheasant's eye plant, pleurisy root, strophanthus seeds, and uzara (19).
LICORICE/HORSETAIL: Theoretically, overuse/misuse of licorice rhizome or horsetail plant with cardiac glycoside-containing herbs increases the risk of cardiac toxicity due to potassium depletion (19).
OTHER CARDIOACTIVE HERBS: Avoid concomitant use with other cardioactive herbs due to unpredictability of effects and adverse effects. Other cardioactive herbs include calamus, cereus, cola, coltsfoot, devil's claw, European mistletoe, fenugreek, fumitory, ginger, Panax ginseng, hawthorn, white horehound, mate, parsley, quassia, scotch broom flower, shepherd's purse, and wild carrot (4). See individual product listings.
STIMULANT LAXATIVE HERBS: Theoretically, overuse or misuse of stimulant laxatives with cardiac glycoside-containing herbs increases the risk of cardiac toxicity due to potassium depletion (19). Stimulant laxative herbs include aloe dried leaf sap, blue flag rhizome, alder buckthorn, European buckthorn, butternut bark, cascara bark, castor oil, colocynth fruit pulp, gamboge bark exudate, jalap root, black root, manna bark exudate, podophyllum root, rhubarb root, senna leaves and pods, wild cucumber fruit (Ecballium elaterium), and yellow dock root.

Interactions with Drugs
CALCIUM SUPPLEMENTS: Concomitant use of calcium may increase risk of cardiac toxicity (3805).
CORTICOSTEROIDS: Concomitant use may increase effects and adverse effects of long-term corticosteroid use (2).
DIGOXIN (Lanoxin): Concomitant use is contraindicated due to therapeutic duplication and increased risk of cardiac glycoside toxicity (4).

DIURETIC DRUGS: Theoretically, concomitant use of potassium-depleting diuretics and squill can increase the risk of cardiac glycoside toxicity due to potassium depletion (19). Some diuretics that can deplete potassium include chlorothiazide (Diuril), chlorthalidone (Thalitone), furosemide (Lasix), hydrochlorothiazide (HCTZ, Hydrodiuril, Microzide), and others.
QUINIDINE: Concomitant use may increase the risk of cardiac and adverse effects (2).
STIMULANT LAXATIVES: Concomitant use of squill and stimulant laxatives may increase risk of cardiac glycoside toxicity due to potassium loss (19).

Interactions with Foods

None known.

Interactions with Lab Tests

None known.

Interactions with Diseases or Conditions

CARDIAC CONDITIONS: Contraindicated in individuals with second or third degree atrioventricular block, hypertrophic cardiomyopathy, carotid sinus syndrome, ventricular tachycardia, or thoracic aortic aneurysm Wolff-Parkinson-White syndrome (18).
ELECTROLYTE IMBALANCE: Contraindicated in individuals with hypokalemia or hypercalcemia.
GI CONDITIONS: Can irritate gastrointestinal tract. Contraindicated in individuals with infectious or inflammatory gastrointestinal conditions (19).

Dosage and Administration

ORAL: Mild heart failure (NYHA stage I and II heart disease), 100-500 mg standardized squill bulb powder per day (7).

Comments

Squill is unsafe for self-medication (512). New York Heart Association (NYHA) stage I and II heart disease refers to people with heart disease who do not have limitations of physical activity. They are comfortable at rest, but ordinary physical activity results in fatigue, palpitation, trouble breathing, or anginal pain (2).

ST. JOHN'S WORT

Also Known As

Amber, Amber Touch-and-Heal, Demon Chaser, Fuga Daemonum, Goatweed, Hardhay, Hypereikon, Hyperici Herba, Hypericum, Klamath Weed, Millepertuis, Rosin Rose, Saynt Johannes Wort, SJW, Tipton Weed.

Scientific Names

Hypericum perforatum.
Family: Hypericaceae or Clusiaceae.

People Use This For

Orally, St. John's wort is used for depression, dysthymia, anxiety, heart palpitations, mood disturbances associated with menopause, attention deficit-hyperactivity disorder (ADHD), obsessive-compulsive disorder (OCD), and seasonal affective disorder (SAD). Other uses include exhaustion, fibromyalgia, fibrositis, headache, migraine headache, muscle pain, neuralgia, and sciatica. It is also used orally for secondary symptoms associated with depression such as fatigue, loss of appetite, insomnia, and anxiety. It is also used orally for cancer, vitiligo, HIV/AIDS, hepatitis C, and as a diuretic. Oily St. John's wort preparations are used orally for gastric indigestion.
Topically, oily St. John's wort preparations are used for treating bruises and abrasions, inflammation and muscle pain, first degree burns, wound healing, bug bites, hemorrhoids, vitiligo, and neuralgia.
In manufacturing, the hypericin-free extracts of St. John's wort are used in the making of alcoholic beverages.

Safety

LIKELY SAFE ...when used orally and appropriately, short-term. St. John's wort extracts seem to be safe when used for up to 8 weeks (3547,3548,3549,3550,3551,3552,4835,5087,5096,6400,6434,7047,13021).
POSSIBLY UNSAFE ...when used orally in large doses. St. John's wort extract can be unsafe due to the risk of severe phototoxic skin reactions. Taking 2-4 grams St. John's wort extract (5-10 mg hypericin) daily appears to increase the risk of photosensitivity (758,4631,7808).
There is insufficient reliable information available about the safety of St. John's wort when used topically.
CHILDREN: POSSIBLY SAFE ...when used orally, and appropriately, short-term. St. John's wort extracts seem to be safe when used in children under 12 years of age for up to 6 weeks (4538).
PREGNANCY: POSSIBLY UNSAFE ...when used orally. Preliminary research suggests that constituents of St. John's wort might have teratogenic effects (9687); avoid using.

LACTATION: POSSIBLY UNSAFE ...when used orally. Nursing infants can experience colic, drowsiness, and lethargy (1377); avoid using.

Effectiveness

LIKELY EFFECTIVE

Depression. St. John's wort extracts are more effective than placebo (203,204,205,376,3548,3549,3551,3552,4899,6428,9597), likely as effective as low-dose tricyclic antidepressants (3548,3549,3551,6434), and likely as effective as the selective serotonin reuptake inhibitors (SSRIs) fluoxetine (Prozac) (3550,4897), sertraline (Zoloft) (6400), and paroxetine (Paxil) (13021). Taking St. John's wort extracts improves mood, decreases anxiety and somatic symptoms, and decreases insomnia related to mild to severe major depression (203,204,205,376,3548,3549,3550,3551,3552) (4897,4899,6400,6428,9597,9597,13021). Most studies have used St. John's wort extracts based on hypericin content, but extracts standardized based on hyperforin also seem to be effective (761,4538,4630). Most studies have evaluated St. John's wort in adults, however, there is also some evidence it might be effective for depression in children 6 to 16 years old (4538,10844).

The effectiveness of St. John's wort for depression has been called into question based on equivocal findings of two studies in psychiatric care settings (5096,10843). But the overwhelming majority of evidence in primary care settings shows that St. John's wort is effective for most patients. Patients in primary care settings may have less severe depression than patients seeking psychiatric care (11154).

Clinical guidelines from the American College of Physicians-American Society of Internal Medicine suggest that St. John's wort can be considered an option along with conventional antidepressants for short-term treatment of mild depression (5087). However, since St. John's wort has not been shown to be more effective or significantly better tolerated than conventional antidepressants; and since St. John's wort causes many drug interactions, it might not be an appropriate choice for many patients, particularly those who take other conventional drugs.

Most clinical studies on the effectiveness of St. John's wort have used preparations containing the specific standardized extract Lichtwer LI 160, containing 0.3% hypericin (382,4538). LI 160 is contained in the product Kira (Lichtwer Pharma US, Inc.). Lichtwer LI 160 WS is the hyperforin stabilized version of LI 160. LI 160 WS is contained in the product Quanterra Emotional Balance (Warner-Lambert). Some studies have also used the extract ZE 117, containing 0.2% hypericin (4897,6434). ZE 117 is contained in the product Remotiv (Zeller). Some studies have also used the extract WS 5572, containing 5% hyperforin (761,4630,13021). WS 5572 is contained in the product Movana (Pharmaton).

POSSIBLY EFFECTIVE

Somatization disorder. Taking a specific standardized hypericum extract (LI 160, Lichtwer Pharma) orally seems to reduce symptoms of somatization disorder after 6 weeks of treatment (9476).

POSSIBLY INEFFECTIVE

Hepatitis C. Taking St. John's wort orally as an antiretroviral agent doesn't seem to be effective for treating adults with chronic Hepatitis C Virus (HCV) infection. St. John's wort does not appear to have any detectable antiviral activity in patients with chronic HCV infection (4631).

HIV/AIDS. Taking St. John's wort orally as an antiretroviral agent doesn't seem to be effective for treating HIV-infected adults (206).

Polyneuropathy. Taking St. John's wort orally doesn't seem to relieve most measures of pain in diabetic and non-diabetic patients with polyneuropathy (7047).

INSUFFICIENT RELIABLE EVIDENCE to RATE

Obsessive-compulsive disorder (OCD). Preliminary evidence suggests St. John's wort might be useful for OCD. An extended-release formulation of St. John's wort standardized to 0.3% hypericin taken for 12 weeks seems to significantly improve symptoms in some patients with OCD (5075).

Premenstrual syndrome (PMS). There is preliminary clinical evidence that St. John's wort might be beneficial for PMS. St. John's wort extract standardized to 0.3% hypericin seems to improve symptoms of PMS by approximately 50% in some women (6429).

Seasonal affective disorder (SAD). Preliminary clinical research suggests that St. John's wort might help SAD. St. John's wort appears to improve symptoms of anxiety, decreased libido, and sleep disturbances associated with SAD. It is useful alone or in combination with light therapy (9686).

More evidence is needed to rate St. John's wort for these uses.

Mechanism of Action

The applicable parts of St. John's wort are the flowers and to a lesser extent, the leaves. Several active constituents, including melatonin, have been isolated. Two constituents that play a significant role are hypericin and hyperforin (50,761). Although hypericin was formerly thought to be the component of St. John's wort principally responsible for its action, it is now understood that hyperforin, adhyperforin, and several other related compounds are the primary active constituents (762,763,4521,4629,7807,11408). Both hyperforin and adhyperforin appear to modulate the effects of serotonin, dopamine, and norepinephrine (763,3553,4521,6474,11408), and may inhibit reuptake of these neurotransmitters (763,6427,8936).

St. John's wort also seems to act as a serotonergic 5-HT3 and 5-HT4 receptor antagonist (762), and down-regulate beta-adrenergic, and serotonergic 5-HT1 and 5-HT2 receptors when used chronically in animals (763,4632).

These influences on neurotransmission appear to cause cortisol stimulation in a dose-dependent manner (11408).

Hyperforin also inhibits synaptosomal uptake of gamma-butyric acid (GABA) and L-glutamate (3553,4521). St. John's wort effects on serotonin may be primarily responsible for its antidepressant activity (8936). Many constituents appear to contribute to the antidepressant action (762,4520,4521). Hypericin inhibits catechol-O-methyl transferase (COMT) and monoamine oxidase (MAO) in vitro. However, hypericin does not reach adequate concentrations in human tissue to achieve these effects (167,759). Hypericin also has affinity for sigma receptors and acts as a receptor antagonist at adenosine, benzodiazepine, GABA-A, GABA-B, and inositol triphosphate receptors (759). Preclinical research suggests that a 50% ethanolic extract of St. John's wort might have anxiolytic activity (8932). When used in humans, St. John's wort is a potent inducer of some cytochrome P450 (CYP450) enzymes. This results in increased metabolism and reduced plasma concentrations of many drugs (1292,1293,1303,3570,3599,4835,6425,7808). It appears that the hyperforin constituent is responsible for interactions. Hypericin doesn't seem to have any effect on drug metabolism (11889). St. John's wort extract increases induction activity of CYP3A4 by 98% (1303). The effect on CYP3A4 seems to be greater in females than males (10830,10847,11889). It also induces CYP2C9 and CYP1A2 (11889,11890). St. John's wort does not affect or has a marginal effect on CYP2D6 (3599,4835,10830,10847,10848,11889). Some discrepancies in reports about the effect of St. John's wort on CYP isozymes may reflect variability in St. John's wort preparations (10849).

The hyperforin constituent in St. John's wort seems to bind to a nuclear receptor called the pregnane X receptor (PXR), which results in increased expression of CYP3A4 (6463,6475). St. John's wort also induces the intestinal P-glycoprotein/multi-drug resistance 1 (MDR-1) drug transporter (1340). Induction of both intestinal P-glycoprotein/MDR-1 and hepatic CYP3A4 decreases the intestinal absorption and increases hepatic first pass clearance of numerous drugs such as cyclosporine, indinavir, and amitriptyline (382,1340,7808,7810).

St. John's wort does not significantly affect N-acetyltransferase (NAT2) (3571). St. John's wort extracts can prolong narcotic-induced sleep time, decrease barbiturate-induced sleep time, and antagonize the effects of reserpine (758). There is preliminary evidence that St. John's wort can enhance the analgesic effect of morphine, but St. John's wort alone does not have analgesic effects (1279).

Topical preparations are thought to be beneficial for inflammatory skin conditions and superficial wounds by inhibiting epidermal inflammatory response. It is likely that both the hypericin and hyperforin contribute to this effect (6426).

Hypericin is photodynamically active and is thought to be the constituent responsible for phototoxic reactions (3547). However, the flavonoid component of St. John's wort, primarily quercitrin, appears to play a role in controlling the severity of the phototoxic reactions (11490). St. John's wort and its constituents, hypericin and pseudohypericin, have activity against viruses and bacteria, including influenza virus, herpes simplex virus types I and II, Sindbis virus, poliovirus, retrovirus, murine cytomegalovirus (CMV), hepatitis C, and Gram negative and Gram positive bacteria. Hyperforin can inhibit growth of penicillin- and methicillin-resistant Staphylococcus aureus and other Gram positive organisms, but not Gram negative organisms (3554).

Hyperforin might have activity against cancer cells. It seems to inhibit the growth of a variety of cancer cell types by inducing apoptosis (9205). It is not known if these effects will have clinical applicability. Several factors might influence product variability of St. John's wort. The constituents of St. John's wort seem to have seasonal and regional variations (8933,8934). The hyperforin and hypericin constituents appear to be sensitive to light; amber containers or opaque capsules don't seem to completely protect from light degradation. These constituents may also be sensitive to storage temperature and humidity (8935). Preclinical research suggests that hypericin is teratogenic in rat embryos (9687). The effect of hypericin and St. John's wort on the human embryo is unknown.

Adverse Reactions

Orally, St. John's wort is usually well tolerated. Side effects can include insomnia, vivid dreams, restlessness, anxiety, agitation, irritability, gastrointestinal (GI) discomfort, diarrhea, fatigue, dry mouth, dizziness, and headache (394,758,3547,3569,4518,7808,9881,10845,13021). St. John's wort can also cause skin rash, paresthesia, and hypoglycemia (4835,5073,7404). Insomnia can often be alleviated by decreasing the dose or taking St. John's wort in the morning (3569). In clinical trials, the incidence of adverse effects in patients treated with St. John's wort is similar to placebo and less than conventional antidepressants (4899,10845).

St. John's wort can induce hypomania in depressed patients (325,3524,3568) and mania in depressed patients with occult bipolar disorder (3555,10845). There is also a case of first-episode psychosis in a woman with no history of psychiatric illness after taking St. John's wort extract 1800 mg for one week. Symptoms resolved after discontinuing St. John's wort and receiving treatment with an antipsychotic for several weeks (13015).

Both topical use and chronic oral use of St. John's wort can cause significant photodermatitis (206,620,758,4631,6477). The average threshold dose range for an increased risk of photosensitivity appears to be 2-4 grams St. John's wort extract or 5-10 mg hypericin, daily. Lower doses might not cause this effect (4542,7808). For example, a single-dose of St. John's wort extract 1800 mg, 5.4 mg hypericin, followed by 900 mg (2.7 mg hypericin) daily does not seem to produce skin hypericin concentrations thought to be high enough to cause phototoxicity (3900,4542). Light or fair-skinned people should employ protective measures against direct sunlight when using St. John's wort either topically or orally (628). Total body erythroderma without exposure to sunlight, accompanied by burning sensation of the skin, has also been reported (8930).

In isolated cases, St. John's wort has been associated with a syndrome consisting of extreme anxiety, confusion, nausea, hypertension, and tachycardia. These symptoms may occur within two to three weeks after it is started. In one case, the symptoms began after consuming foods containing tyramine including aged cheese and red wine (7812). Cardiovascular collapse following induction of anesthesia has been reported in an otherwise healthy patient who had been taking St. John's wort for six months (8931).

St. John's wort can cause intermenstrual or abnormal menstrual bleeding (1292). However, this effect has occurred in patients who were also taking an oral contraceptive. Changes in menstrual bleeding might be the result of a drug interaction (1292).

Overall, St. John's wort extracts seem to be better tolerated than tricyclic antidepressants (3548,3549), but similarly or better tolerated than fluoxetine (Prozac) (3550) and sertraline (Zoloft) (4897,6400). Unlike tricyclic antidepressants, research in healthy volunteers suggests that St. John's wort does not affect heart rate variability. It also doesn't appear to affect cognitive function (11800).

Sexual dysfunction can occur with St. John's wort, but less frequently than with SSRIs (10843). There is one report of loss of sexual libido in a man who took St. John's wort for nine months (7312).

Some in vitro evidence suggests that high doses of St. John's wort might reduce male and female fertility (4239,4240). This effect has not been demonstrated in humans, and animal studies suggest that St. John's wort doesn't adversely affect fertility or gestation 10846.

Neuropathy can also occur with use of St. John's wort (621). There is some speculation that St. John's wort might be associated with a higher incidence of cataracts. The hypericin constituent is photoactive and, in the presence of light, may damage lens proteins, leading to cataracts (1296); however, this effect has not been verified in humans.

St. John's wort has been associated with withdrawal effects similar to those found with conventional antidepressants. Headache, nausea, anorexia, dry mouth, thirst, cold chills, weight loss, dizziness, insomnia, paresthesias, confusion, and fatigue have been reported. Withdrawal effects are most likely to occur within two days after discontinuation, but can occur one week or more after stopping treatment in some people. Occurrence of withdrawal symptoms may not be related to dose or duration of use (3569,11801). Photosensitivity might occur in individuals with light or fair skin, diseased or open-wounded skin, or after extended periods of direct sunlight when using St. John's wort topically (206,620,628,758,4628). Sjogren's syndrome has been reported in a patient taking herbal supplements including St. John's wort, echinacea, and kava. Echinacea may have been the primary cause, because Sjogren's syndrome is an autoimmune disorder. The role of St. John's wort in causing this syndrome is unclear (10319).

Interactions with Herbs & Other Dietary Supplements

DIGITALIS: Concomitant use might reduce the therapeutic effects of digitalis. The St. John's wort extract, LI 160, decreases digoxin serum levels in healthy people. St. John's wort seems to lower digoxin serum concentrations by approximately 25%. St. John's wort seems to induces the activity of the carrier protein P-glycoprotein, which increases the clearance of digitalis (382,6473,7808,7810,9204).

HERBS AND SUPPLEMENTS WITH SEROTONERGIC PROPERTIES: Theoretically, St. John's wort might increase the effects and adverse effects of products that increase serotonin levels; including 5-hydroxytryptophan (5-HTP), Hawaiian baby woodrose, L-tryptophan, and SAMe (763,6427,8936,9204).

Interactions with Drugs

5-HT1 AGONISTS (Triptans): Theoretically, concomitant use of St. John's wort with selective serotonin agonists can increase the risk of serotonergic adverse effects and possibly serotonin syndrome. Concomitant use should be avoided (9204). The "triptans" include frovatriptan (Frova), naratriptan (Amerge), rizatriptan (Maxalt), sumatriptan (Imitrex), and zolmitriptan (Zomig). Also, concurrent use might theoretically cause cerebral vasoconstriction disorders such as Call-Fleming syndrome (8056).

ALPRAZOLAM (Xanax): St. John's wort may decrease the effect of alprazolam. Alprazolam, which is used as a probe for cytochrome P450 3A4 (CYP3A4) activity, has a two-fold increase in clearance when given with St. John's wort. St. John's wort reduces the half-life of alprazolam from 12.4 hours to 6 hours (10830).

AMINOLEVULINIC ACID: Concomitant use with St. John's wort extract may cause synergistic phototoxicity. Delta-aminolevulinic acid (an investigational drug used in oncologic diagnostic procedures) can cause a burning erythematous rash and severe swelling of the face, neck, and hands when taken with St. John's wort (9474).

AMITRIPTYLINE (Elavil): Concomitant use can reduce serum concentrations of amitriptyline by 22% and its metabolite, nortriptyline, by 42% (1378,7808). St. John's wort induces intestinal and hepatic CYP3A4 and intestinal P-glycoprotein/MDR-1, a drug transporter, which increases amitriptyline clearance (1340).

ANTIDEPRESSANT DRUGS: Concomitant use can lead to increased adverse effects and increase the risk of serotonergic side effects, including serotonin syndrome (166,542,3569). Although this effect has only been reported with nefazodone (Serzone), paroxetine (Paxil), and sertraline (Zoloft), it might also occur with other antidepressants. Use of St. John's wort with other antidepressants should only be done with close supervision. Also, concurrent use might theoretically cause cerebral vasoconstriction disorders such as Call-Fleming syndrome (8056).

BARBITURATES: St. John's wort can decrease barbiturate-induced sleep time (758). Some of these sedative medications include pentobarbital (Nebutal), phenobarbital (Luminal), secobarbital (Seconal), and others.

CLOPIDOGREL (Plavix): Taking St. John's wort with clopidogrel seems to increase the activity of clopidogrel. In clopidogrel non-responders, taking St. John's wort seems to induce clopidogrel metabolism to its active metabolite and therefore increase clopidogrel's antiplatelet activity (13038). Theoretically, in clopidogrel responders, this might lead to an increased risk of bleeding.

CONTRACEPTIVE DRUGS: St. John's wort can decrease norethindrone and ethinyl estradiol levels by 13-15%, resulting in breakthrough bleeding, irregular menstrual bleeding, or unwanted pregnancy (11886,11887,13099). Bleeding irregularities usually occur within a week of starting St. John's wort and regular cycles usually return when St. John's wort is discontinued. Unwanted pregnancy has occurred with concurrent use of oral contraceptives and St. John's wort extract (9880). St. John's wort is thought to induce the cytochrome P450 1A2 (CYP1A2), 2C9 (CYP2C9), and 3A4 (CYP3A4) enzymes, which are responsible for metabolism of progestins and estrogens in contraceptives (1292,7809,9204). Women taking St. John's wort and oral contraceptives concurrently should use an additional or alternative form of birth control.

CYCLOSPORINE (Neoral, Sandimmune): Concomitant use can decrease plasma cyclosporine levels by 30-70% (1234,4826,4831,4834,7808,9596,10628). Using St. John's wort with cyclosporine in patients with heart, kidney, or liver transplants can cause subtherapeutic cyclosporine levels and acute transplant rejection (1234,1293,1301,6112,6435,7808,9596). This interaction has occurred with a St. John's wort extract standardized to 0.3% hypericin and dosed at 300-600 mg per day (6435,10628). Withdrawal of St. John's wort can result in increased cyclosporine levels by 64% (1234,4513,4826,4831,4834). St. John's wort induces cytochrome P450 3A4 (CYP3A4) and the multi-drug transporter, P-glycoprotein/MDR-1, which increases cyclosporine clearance (1293,1340,9204,9596).

CYTOCHROME P450 1A2 (CYP1A2) SUBSTRATES: St. John's wort induces cytochrome P450 1A2, but to a lesser extent than CYP3A4 (9204,10848). Some substrates of CYP1A2 include clozapine (Clozaril), cyclobenzaprine (Flexeril), fluvoxamine (Luvox), haloperidol (Haldol), imipramine (Tofranil), mexiletine (Mexitil), olanzapine (Zyprexa), pentazocine (Talwin), propranolol (Inderal), tacrine (Cognex), zileuton (Zyflo), zolmitriptan (Zomig), and others.

CYTOCHROME P450 2C9 (CYP2C9) SUBSTRATES: St. John's wort induces cytochrome P450 2C9, but to a lesser extent than CYP3A4 (9204,10848,11889). Some substrates of CYP2C9 include celecoxib (Celebrex), diclofenac (Voltaren), fluvastatin (Lescol), glipizide (Glucotrol), ibuprofen (Advil, Motrin), irbesartan (Avapro), losartan (Cozaar), phenytoin (Dilantin), piroxicam (Feldene), tamoxifen (Nolvadex), tolbutamide (Tolinase), torsemide (Demadex), and warfarin (Coumadin).

CYTOCHROME P450 3A4 (CYP3A4) SUBSTRATES: St. John's wort induces cytochrome P450 3A4 (9204,10830,10847,10848,11889). Use caution when considering concomitant use of St. John's wort and other drugs affected by these enzymes. Drugs that might be affected include some calcium channel blockers (diltiazem, nicardipine, verapamil), chemotherapeutic agents (etoposide, paclitaxel, vinblastine, vincristine, vindesine), antifungals (ketoconazole, itraconazole), glucocorticoids, cisapride (Propulsid), alfentanil (Alfenta), fentanyl (Sublimaze), losartan (Cozaar), fluoxetine (Prozac), midazolam (Versed), omeprazole (Prilosec), ondansetron (Zofran), propranolol (Inderal), fexofenadine (Allegra), and numerous others (1290,1292,1293,4835,6425,6473,7808,7810,9204,10830).

DEXTROMETHORPHAN (Robitussin DM, others): Theoretically, concurrent use might cause additive serotonergic effects and increase the risk of serotonin syndrome (763,6427,8936). Also, concurrent use might theoretically cause cerebral vasoconstriction disorders such as Call-Fleming syndrome (8056).

DIGOXIN (Lanoxin): Concomitant use can reduce serum levels and the therapeutic effects of digoxin, requiring dosing adjustments when St. John's wort is started or stopped. St. John's wort extract 900 mg daily can reduce serum digoxin levels by 25% after 10 days in healthy people. St. John's wort is thought to affect the multidrug transporter, P-glycoprotein, which mediates the absorption and elimination of digoxin and other drugs (382,6473,7808,7810,9204).

FENFLURAMINE (Pondimin): Concomitant use with St. John's wort can increase the risk of serotonergic side effects and serotonin syndrome-like symptoms. St. John's wort 600 mg per day with fenfluramine can cause nausea, headache, and anxiety (3569).

FEXOFENADINE (Allegra): A single dose of St. John's wort can decrease the clearance of fexofenadine, resulting in increased plasma concentration of fexofenadine. However, with continued dosing, more than 2 weeks, St. John's wort does not appear to affect fexofenadine levels (9685). Patients taking fexofenadine and who start taking St. John's wort should be monitored for possible fexofenadine toxicity.

IMATINIB (Gleevec): Taking St. John's wort 900 mg/day decreases serum levels of imatinib by 30% in healthy volunteers. This is most likely due to St. John's wort's inducing effect on cytochrome P450 3A4 (CYP3A4) (11888). Advise patients not to take St. John's wort if they are taking imatinib.

IRINOTECAN (Camptosar): Concomitant use with St. John's wort can decrease serum levels of irinotecan by at least 50%. Clearance of the active metabolite of irinotecan, SN-38, is increased resulting in a 42% decrease in the area under the concentration curve (9206). St. John's wort is thought to lower drug levels by inducing cytochrome P450 3A4 (CYP3A4) (7092).

MEPERIDINE (Demerol): Theoretically, concurrent use with meperidine might cause additive serotonergic effects and increase the risk of serotonin syndrome (763,6427,8936). Also, concurrent use might theoretically cause cerebral vasoconstriction disorders such as Call-Fleming syndrome (8056).

MONOAMINE OXIDASE INHIBITORS (MAOIs): Theoretically, because St. John's wort might affect serotonin similar to conventional antidepressants (763,3553). Concurrent use might cause additive adverse effects, including hypertension, hyperthermia, agitation, confusion, coma, etc. St. John's wort should be avoided in patients taking MAOIs and for 14 days after MAOI discontinuation.

NARCOTIC DRUGS: St. John's wort can increase narcotic-induced sleep time (758) and might also increase analgesic effects (1279).

NEFAZODONE (Serzone): Concomitant use has been associated with serotonergic side effects, including nausea, vomiting, and restlessness (5074).

NON-NUCLEOSIDE REVERSE TRANSCRIPTASE INHIBITORS (NNRTIs): Concomitant use can decrease serum levels of NNRTIs. St. John's wort can increase the oral clearance of nevirapine (Viramune) by 35%.

Subtherapeutic concentrations are associated with therapeutic failure, development of viral resistance, and development of drug class resistance. St. John's wort induces intestinal and hepatic cytochrome P450 3A4 (CYP3A4) and intestinal P-glycoprotein/MDR-1, a drug transporter (1290,1340,4837). Other NNRTIs include delavirdine (Rescriptor), and efavirenz (Sustiva).

NORTRIPTYLINE (Pamelor, Aventyl): Concomitant use can reduce serum concentrations of amitriptyline by 22% and its metabolite, nortriptyline, by 42% (1378,7808).

P-GLYCOPROTEIN SUBSTRATES: St. John's wort induces P-glycoprotein. P-glycoprotein is a carrier mechanism responsible for transporting drugs and other substances across cell membranes. When P-glycoprotein is induced in the gastrointestinal (GI) tract, it can prevent the absorption of some medications. In addition, induction of p-glycoprotein can decrease entry of drugs into the central nervous system (CNS) and decrease access to other sites of action. Drugs that might be affected include some chemotherapeutic agents (etoposide, paclitaxel, vinblastine, vincristine, vindesine), antifungals (ketoconazole, itraconazole), protease inhibitors (amprenavir, indinavir, nelfinavir, saquinavir), H2 antagonists (cimetidine, ranitidine), some calcium channel blockers (diltiazem, verapamil), corticosteroids, erythromycin, cisapride (Propulsid), fexofenadine (Allegra), cyclosporine, loperamide (Imodium), quinidine, and others (382,1340,7810,11722).

PAROXETINE (Paxil): Concomitant use with St. John's wort might increase the risk of adverse effects and serotonin syndrome-like symptoms. People taking St. John's wort and paroxetine together can experience nervousness, hyperactivity, diaphoresis, nausea, weakness, fatigue, lethargy, and incoherence (542,3569). Also, concurrent use might theoretically cause cerebral vasoconstriction disorders such as Call-Fleming syndrome (8056).

PENTAZOCINE (Talwin): Theoretically, concurrent use with pentazocine might cause additive serotonergic effects and increase the risk of serotonin syndrome (763,6427,8936). Also, concurrent use might theoretically cause cerebral vasoconstriction disorders such as Call-Fleming syndrome (8056).

PHENOBARBITAL (Luminal): St. John's wort may increase the metabolism of phenobarbital, resulting in loss of seizure control. Plasma concentrations of phenobarbital should be monitored carefully. The dose of phenobarbital may need to be increased when St. John's wort is started and decreased when it is stopped (9204).

PHENPROCOUMON: St. John's wort appears to increase the metabolism of phenprocoumon (an anticoagulant that is not available in the US) by increasing the activity of the cytochrome P450 2C9 (CYP2C9) enzyme. This may result in decreases in the anticoagulant effect and international normalized ratio (INR) (9204).

PHENYTOIN (Dilantin): St. John's wort may increase the metabolism of phenytoin, resulting in the loss of seizure control. Plasma concentrations of phenytoin should be monitored carefully. The dose of phenytoin may need to be increased when St. John's wort is started and decreased when it is stopped (9204).

PHOTOSENSITIZING DRUGS: Theoretically, concomitant use might increase the possibility of photosensitivity reactions (166). Some drugs that cause photosensitivity include amitriptyline, quinolones, sulfa drugs, and tetracycline.

PROTEASE INHIBITORS (PIs): Concomitant use can reduce serum concentrations of PIs. In healthy volunteers, St. John's wort can reduce the serum indinavir (Crixivan) area under the curve (AUC) by 57% and the extrapolated trough by 81%. Subtherapeutic concentrations are associated with therapeutic failure, development of viral resistance, and development of drug class resistance. St. John's wort induces cytochrome P450 enzymes and might also affect other PI-type antiretroviral drugs (1290,7808); including amprenavir (Agenerase), nelfinavir (Viracept), ritonavir (Norvir), and saquinavir (Fortovase, Invirase). St. John's wort also induces P-glycoprotein, which can result in decreased intracellular protease inhibitor concentrations and increased elimination (9204,9204).

RESERPINE: St. John's wort can antagonize the effects of reserpine (758).

SERTRALINE (Zoloft): Concomitant use can cause serotonergic side effects, including dizziness, nausea, vomiting, epigastric pain, headache, anxiety, confusion, and feelings of restlessness and irritability (5074).

SIMVASTATIN (Zocor): Concomitant use can reduce plasma concentrations of the simvastatin metabolite, simvastatin hydroxy acid, by 28%. St. John's wort induces intestinal and hepatic cytochrome P450 3A4 (CYP3A4) and intestinal P-glycoprotein/MDR-1, a drug transporter, which increases simvastatin clearance. St. John's wort does not appear to affect the plasma concentration of pravastatin (Pravachol) and fluvastatin (Lescol), which are not substrates of CYP3A4 or P-glycoprotein. Theoretically, St. John's wort could reduce the effectiveness of other HMG-CoA reductase inhibitors that are CYP3A4 substrates such as atorvastatin (Lipitor) and lovastatin (Mevacor) (10627).

TACROLIMUS (Prograf, Protopic): A St. John's wort extract (Jarsin) 600 mg daily significantly decreases tacrolimus serum levels. Dose increases of 60% may be required to maintain therapeutic tacrolimus levels in patients taking St. John's wort concomitantly. St. John's wort is thought to lower tacrolimus levels due to cytochrome P450 3A4 (CYP3A4) enzyme induction (7095,10329).

THEOPHYLLINE: St. John's wort doesn't seem to significantly affect theophylline pharmacokinetics (11802). There is a single case report of possible interaction with theophylline. A patient who smoked and was taking 11 other drugs experienced an increase in theophylline levels after discontinuation of St. John's wort. This increase has been attributed to a rebounding of theophylline serum levels after St. John's wort was no longer present to induce cytochrome P450 1A2 (CYP1A2) enzyme (3556,7808,9204). However, studies in healthy volunteers suggest that St. John's wort is unlikely to affect theophylline to any clinically significant degree (11802).

TRAMADOL (Ultram): Theoretically, concurrent use with tramadol might cause additive serotonergic effects and increase the risk of serotonin syndrome (763,6427,8936). Also, concurrent use might theoretically cause cerebral vasoconstriction disorders such as Call-Fleming syndrome (8056).

WARFARIN (Coumadin): Concomitant use might decrease the therapeutic effects of warfarin (1292). St. John's wort seems to significantly decrease International Normalized Ratio (INR) (1292). In healthy volunteers, St. John's wort increases the clearance of both S- and R-warfarin. This suggests it might induce CYP1A2 and CYP3A4, which metabolize R-warfarin and CYP2C9, which metabolizes L-warfarin (11890). In addition, warfarin physically interacts with hypericin and pseudohypericin, active constituents of St. John's wort. When the dried extract is mixed with warfarin in an aqueous medium, up to 30% of warfarin is bound to particles, reducing its absorption (10448). Taking warfarin at the same time as St. John's wort might reduce its bioavailability.

Interactions with Foods

None known.

Interactions with Lab Tests

PROTHROMBIN TIME (PT)/INTERNATIONAL NORMALIZED RATIO (INR): St. John's wort can decrease PT/INR test results in patients treated with warfarin (Coumadin) (1292).
THYROID STIMULATING HORMONE (TSH): Some preliminary research suggests that St. John's wort might elevate TSH levels (8569,8570).

Interactions with Diseases or Conditions

ALZHEIMER'S DISEASE: St. John's wort might induce psychosis in patients with Alzheimer's dementia. In one case, psychotic delirium developed in an elderly woman within three weeks of starting a low dose (75 mg per day) of St. John's wort extract standardized to 0.3% hypericin (St. John's wort, Pharmanex). Symptoms resolved within several days after discontinuing St. John's wort and starting medications for treatment of Alzheimer's disease. Although it is not clear if St. John's wort caused the delirium or contributed to the underlying dementia, there is concern that St. John's wort might contribute to dementia in patients with Alzheimer's disease (5249).
ANESTHESIA: St. John's wort might cause cardiovascular collapse during anesthesia. St. John's wort, used chronically for six months, appears to be the cause of severe hypotension following induction of anesthesia in an otherwise healthy patient. St. John's wort might cause adrenergic desensitization and decreased responsiveness to vasopressors, similar to the effects of antidepressants (8931).
BIPOLAR DISORDER: St. John's wort can induce hypomania or mania when used in patients with bipolar disorder or depressed patients with occult bipolar disorder (3555,3568). In some cases, mania occurred after two to eight weeks of treatment with St. John's wort and was effectively managed by decreasing the dose of St. John's wort and increasing the dose of mood stabilizers such as lithium (3568). Theoretically, like other antidepressants, St. John's wort may also induce rapid cycling between depression and mania in patients with bipolar disorder (3555).
DEPRESSION: St. John's wort can induce hypomania with typical doses in patients with major depression (325,3524,3568). In one case, hypomania occurred after four to eight weeks of treatment with St. John's wort and was effectively managed by decreasing the dose and initiating valproic acid (3568).
INFERTILITY: Preliminary evidence suggests that St. John's wort might inhibit oocyte fertilization and alter sperm DNA (4239,4240). This effect has not yet been demonstrated in humans, and animal studies suggest that St. John's wort doesn't adversely affect fertility or gestation (10846). However, until more is known, use with caution in couples attempting to conceive, and avoid use in couples having difficulty conceiving.
SCHIZOPHRENIA: St. John's wort might induce psychosis in patients with schizophrenia. There are two cases of relapse in non-medicated schizophrenia patients in remission who started taking St. John's wort. Psychotic symptoms resolved with readministration of antipsychotics and discontinuation of St. John's wort (6478).

Dosage and Administration

ORAL: For mild to moderate depression, most clinical trials have used St. John's wort extract standardized to 0.3% hypericin content. Doses are most commonly 300 mg three times daily (3548,3549). Doses of 1200 mg daily have also been used (5096). Some studies have also used a 0.2% hypericin extract dosed at 250 mg twice daily (4897,6434).
A St. John's wort extract standardized to 5% hyperforin and dosed at 300 mg three times daily has also been used (761,4630). For children under 12 years of age with depression, St. John's wort extract standardized to 0.3% hypericin 300 mg daily has been used (4538).
For obsessive-compulsive disorder (OCD), one study used an extended-release preparation of St. John's wort extract standardized to 0.3% hypericin content, dosed at 450 mg twice daily (5075). For premenstrual syndrome (PMS), one study used St. John's wort extract standardized to 0.3% hypericin dosed at 300 mg once daily (6429).
For somatic symptoms associated with depression, 300 mg three times daily of the standardized hypericin extract has been used (376).
For somatization disorder, a specific extract (LI 160, Lichtwer Pharma) 600 mg/day has been used (9476).
Advise patients to avoid abrupt discontinuation of St. John's wort due to the risk of adverse withdrawal effects (3569).
TOPICAL: No typical dosage.

Comments

St. John's wort is native to Europe but is commonly found in the US and Canada in the dry ground of roadsides, meadows, and woods. Although not indigenous to Australia and long considered a weed, St. John's wort is now grown as a cash crop and produces 20 percent of the world's supply (6200).
The use of St. John's wort dates back to the ancient Greeks. Hippocrates documented the medical use of

St. John's wort flowers. St. John's wort is so named because it blooms about June 24th, the birthday of John the Baptist. "Wort" is an old English word for plant (11804).
France has banned the use of St. John's wort products. The ban appears to be based on a report issued by the French Health Product Safety Agency warning of significant drug-herb interactions. Several other countries including Japan, the United Kingdom, and Canada are in the process of including drug-herb interaction cautionary language on St. John's wort products (4892).

STAR ANISE

Also Known As

Aniseed Stars, Anisi stellati fructus, Badiana, Chinese Anise, Chinese Star Anise, Eight-Horned Anise, Eight Horns, Illicium.
CAUTION: See separate listing for Anise.

Scientific Names

Illicium verum.
Family: Illiciaceae.

People Use This For

Orally, star anise is used for respiratory tract mucous membrane inflammation, peptic discomfort, flatulence, loss of appetite, infant colic, cough, and bronchitis. Star anise is also used orally for increasing milk secretion, promoting menstruation, facilitating childbirth, increasing libido, and treating symptoms of male climacteric.
As an inhalant, star anise is used for respiratory tract congestion.
In foods and beverages, star anise is considered a culinary spice; both the seed and oil are used as flavoring.
In manufacturing, the oil is used as a fragrance component in soaps, cosmetics, perfumes, and toothpaste, and to mask undesirable odors in drug products.

Safety

LIKELY SAFE ...when used orally in amounts commonly found in foods. Star anise has Generally Recognized As Safe (GRAS) status in the US (4912).
POSSIBLY SAFE ...when used orally and appropriately for medicinal purposes (12). However, star anise is sometimes contaminated with Japanese star anise (Illicium anisatum), which is toxic and should not be taken orally (10407).
There is insufficient reliable information available about the safety of star anise when used by inhalation.
CHILDREN: LIKELY UNSAFE ...when used orally in infants. Star anise is commonly used in infants and has a history of safe use. However, consumption of star anise tea in infants has been associated with adverse neurological reactions, including irritability, vomiting, and seizures. These symptoms are likely attributable to star anise which has been adulterated with Japanese star anise (Illicium anisatum), which is considered toxic (11384,13058). Unless it can be verified that star anise tea does not contain Japanese star anise, the tea should be avoided in infants.
There is insufficient reliable information available about the safety of star anise for older children.
PREGNANCY AND LACTATION: Insufficient reliable information available; avoid using.

Effectiveness

There is insufficient reliable information available about the effectiveness of star anise.

Mechanism of Action

The applicable part of star anise is the seed. Star anise seed contains a volatile oil, 75% of which is anethole (11384). Anethole has antiflatulent and expectorant effects. It also can have insecticidal and antifungal activity (11). At one time anethole was considered the active estrogenic agent in the essential oil. However, more recent information suggests the active estrogenic compounds are the anethole polymers, dianethole and photoanethole (11). Anethole might be mutagenic (11).

Adverse Reactions

Orally, star anise (Illicium verum) is usually well tolerated. However, some types of star anise have been contaminated with Japanese star anise (Illicium anisatum), which is toxic and should not be taken orally. Symptoms resulting from drinking tea made from contaminated star anise include seizures, vomiting, nervousness, rapid eye movements, and other serious neurological effects (10407,13058).
In infants aged 2 weeks to 3 months, star anise tea can cause acute onset irritability, jitteriness, clonus or myoclonus, increased deep tendon reflexes, nystagmus, vomiting, and seizures. It is unclear whether this toxicity is caused by star anise alone or by contamination with Japanese star anise (11384).
Topically, use of the constituent anethole can cause dermatitis, including erythema, scaling, and vesiculation (11). Sensitization rarely occurs (18).

Interactions with Herbs & Other Dietary Supplements
None known.

Interactions with Drugs
None known.

Interactions with Foods
None known.

Interactions with Lab Tests
None known.

Interactions with Diseases or Conditions
HORMONE SENSITIVE CANCERS/CONDITIONS: Star anise might have estrogenic effects (11), women with hormone sensitive conditions should avoid star anise. Some of these conditions include breast cancer, uterine cancer, ovarian cancer, endometriosis, and uterine fibroids.

Dosage and Administration
No typical dosage.

Comments
Star anise oil is the distilled oil of the seed (fruit) of star anise (Illicium verum). In the US, star anise oil (derived from Illicium verum) and anise oil (derived from Pimpinella anisum) are used interchangeably and both are recognized as "anise oil" in the USP (11).
Avoid confusing star anise with Japanese star anise (Illicium anisatum), a highly poisonous species. Japanese star anise is similar in appearance to Chinese star anise.
Some products described as "tea" have become contaminated with Japanese star anise, resulting in severe neurological toxicity. Until the safety of star anise tea can be determined, by chemical analysis, they should not be used (10407,13058).
Star anise tea is used to treat infant colic, particularly in Caribbean and Hispanic cultures. Star anise should not be given to infants. It can cause severe neurologic toxicity (11384,13058).

STAVESACRE

Also Known As
Lousewort.

Scientific Names
Delphinium staphisagria.
Family: Ranunculaceae.

People Use This For
Topically, stavesacre seeds are used to treat lice infestation and neuralgia.

Safety
LIKELY UNSAFE ...when used orally. The seeds are poisonous (18).
There is insufficient reliable information available about the safety of the topical use of stavesacre and the use of stavesacre extracts.
PREGNANCY AND LACTATION: LIKELY UNSAFE ...when used orally (18); avoid using.

Effectiveness
There is insufficient reliable information available about the effectiveness of stavesacre.

Mechanism of Action
Stavesacre contains diterpene alkaloids including delphinine, staphisine, and staphisagroine, which are reported to have effects similar to aconitine (18). Aconitine is a nor-diterpene alkaloid found in Monkshood, a highly toxic plant.

Adverse Reactions
Orally, stavesacre extract can cause inflammation of the alimentary tract (18,19), nausea, pruritus, urinary and stool urgency (18). Ingesting 2 teaspoons of seeds can cause weakened pulse, stomach pain, labored breathing, and collapse (18).
Topically, use of stavesacre can cause inflammation, eczema, and reddening of the skin (18).

Interactions with Herbs & Other Dietary Supplements
None known.

Interactions with Drugs
None known.

Interactions with Foods
None known.

Interactions with Lab Tests
None known.

Interactions with Diseases or Conditions
GASTROINTESTINAL IRRITATION: Can aggravate inflammation of the alimentary tract by irritating mucosal membranes (19).

Dosage and Administration
ORAL: No typical dosage.
TOPICAL: Washes and ointments are used to treat lice.

STEVIA

Also Known As
Azucacaa, Ca-A-Jhei, Ca-A-Yupi, Caa-He-É, Capim Doce, Eira-Caa, Erva Doce, Kaa Jhee, Paraguayan Sweet Herb, Stevioside, Sweet Herb of Paraguay, Sweet Leaf of Paraguay, Sweetleaf, Yerba Dulce.

Scientific Names
Stevia rebaudiana, synonym Eupatorium rebaudianum; Stevia eupatoria, synonyms Mustelia eupatoria, Stevia purpurea.
Family: Asteraceae/Compositae.

People Use This For
Orally, stevia is used as a weight loss aid, for treating diabetes, contraception, hypertension, heartburn, lowering uric acid levels, and as a cardiotonic and diuretic.
In foods, stevia is used as a non-caloric sweetener and flavor enhancer.

Safety
POSSIBLY SAFE ...when used orally in small amounts commonly found in foods and beverages as a sweetener. An acceptable daily dose is 25 mg per kg of body weight (11811). ...when stevioside, a constituent of stevia, is used orally. Doses up to 1500 mg per day for 2 years have been used (11809,11810).
There is insufficient reliable information about the safety of stevia used long-term. The FDA, regulatory agencies in Europe, and the World Health Organization have not approved stevia due to unanswered questions regarding chronic use and toxicity (5037).
PREGNANCY: POSSIBLY UNSAFE ...when used orally. There is preliminary evidence from animal studies that suggests a constituent of stevia called steviol might reduce birth weight of offspring (5036).
LACTATION: Insufficient reliable information available; avoid using.

Effectiveness
POSSIBLY EFFECTIVE

Hypertension. Taking stevioside, a constituent of stevia, orally seems to reduce blood pressure in people with hypertension. Doses of 750 or 1500 mg per day appear to reduce systolic blood pressure by 10-14 mmHg, and diastolic blood pressure by 6-14 mmHg. In patients with hypertension, the onset of decreased blood pressure begins within one week of initiation of treatment (11809,11811). Use of stevioside 1500 mg daily for 2 years might reduce the risk of left ventricular hypertrophy (11809).

INSUFFICIENT RELIABLE EVIDENCE to RATE

Diabetes. Preliminary clinical research suggests that stevioside, a constituent of stevia might reduce postprandial glucose levels by 18% in people with type 2 diabetes (11812). More evidence is needed to rate stevia for this use.

Mechanism of Action
The applicable part of stevia is the leaf. Stevia leaf contains the glycoside stevioside which is non-caloric, heat and acid stable, and 300 times sweeter than a 0.4% sucrose solution. Animal research suggests that stevioside is metabolized to steviol in the intestine, but significant amounts of steviol may not reach the blood stream (11809,11811). Stevia extract, and stevioside, seem to decrease blood pressure, according to human and animal studies (3745,3747).

Stevia extract has vasodilating and diuretic activity in rats (3746,3747). Stevioside might also act as a calcium channel blocker (11809,11811).

Preliminary evidence suggests that the stevia constituents, stevioside and steviol, might stimulate insulin secretion via a direct action on beta cells (5032). Additional evidence suggests that steviol might inhibit GI glucose absorption (5035). Other research suggests that stevioside increases insulin sensitivity and improves skeletal muscle glucose transport (11813). Stevioside increases hepatic glycogen synthesis in animal experiments (3750). An aqueous stevia leaf extract increased glucose tolerance and reduced plasma glucose levels in a small group of healthy people (3301).

A fermented aqueous extract of stevia is bactericidal against many food-borne pathogenic bacteria in vitro, including E. coli 0157:H7, the enterohemorrhagic E. coli responsible for outbreaks of severe food poisoning in recent years (3300). Stevioside has shown no evidence of mutagenic, genotoxic, antifertility, or teratogenic effects (11811). However, the stevia constituent steviol, and metabolized steviol, are mutagenic in vitro (3748,3749). Some evidence suggests that stevia might adversely affect reproduction. An aqueous stevia extract reduced sperm production and testis weight in male rats (5033). Steviol fed to female hamsters reduced the number and birth weight of offspring (5036).

Adverse Reactions

Orally, stevioside, a constituent of stevia, can cause gastrointestinal adverse effects such as abdominal fullness and nausea. It can also cause headache, dizziness, myalgia, and numbness (11809,11810). Theoretically, stevia might cause allergic reactions in individuals sensitive to Asteraceae/Compositae family plants (11811). Members of this family include ragweed, chrysanthemums, marigolds, daisies, and many other herbs.

Interactions with Herbs & Other Dietary Supplements

HERBS AND SUPPLEMENTS WITH HYPOGLYCEMIC POTENTIAL: Stevioside, a stevia derivative, can lower blood glucose levels (3301,11802) and might have additive effects when used with other herbs and supplements that also lower glucose levels. This might increase the risk of hypoglycemia in some patients. Some herbs and supplements with hypoglycemic effects include alpha-lipoic acid, bitter melon, chromium, devil's claw, fenugreek, garlic, guar gum, horse chestnut seed, Panax ginseng, psyllium, Siberian ginseng, and others.

HERBS AND SUPPLEMENTS WITH HYPOTENSIVE EFFECTS: Stevioside, a stevia derivative, might have hypotensive effects (11809,11810). Theoretically, concurrent use of stevia with other herbs and supplements that decrease blood pressure might increase risk of hypotension. Some of these products include danshen, ginger, Panax ginseng, turmeric, valerian, and others.

Interactions with Drugs

ANTIDIABETES DRUGS: Theoretically, stevia might enhance blood glucose control requiring dosing adjustment of diabetes drug therapy in patients with type 2 diabetes (3301,5032,5035,11812).

ANTIHYPERTENSIVE DRUGS: Concomitant use with stevia might cause additive hypotensive effects; use with caution (11809,11810). Some medications for high blood pressure include captopril (Capoten), enalapril (Vasotec), losartan (Cozaar), valsartan (Diovan), amlodipine (Norvasc), hydrochlorothiazide (HydroDiuril), furosemide (Lasix), and many others.

CALCIUM CHANNEL BLOCKERS: Stevioside, a constituent of stevia, might have calcium antagonist properties (11809,11811). Using stevia with calcium channel blockers such as verapamil (Calan, Covera-HS, Verelan), nifedipine (Procardia), diltiazem (Cardizem, Dilacor, Tiazac), and others might cause additive effects on blood pressure and the heart.

Interactions with Foods

None known.

Interactions with Lab Tests

BLOOD PRESSURE: Stevia might reduce blood pressure and blood pressure readings. Stevia extract and stevioside, contained in stevia, can lower blood pressure (3745,3747,5031,11809,11810).

GLUCOSE: Stevia might decrease blood glucose concentrations and test results (3301,5032,5035,11812).

Interactions with Diseases or Conditions

CROSS-ALLERGENICITY: Theoretically, stevia might cause allergic reactions in individuals sensitive to Asteraceae/Compositae family plants (11811). Members of this family include ragweed, chrysanthemums, marigolds, daisies, and many other herbs.

DIABETES: Stevia might reduce blood glucose and alter blood glucose control in patients with type 2 diabetes (3301,5032,5035,11812).

HYPOTENSION: Stevioside, a stevia derivative, has hypotensive effects (11809,11810). Theoretically, use in people with existing low blood pressure might exacerbate hypotension and possibly lead to syncope.

KIDNEY DISEASE: Theoretically, stevia might cause kidney damage. Preliminary evidence suggests that very large amounts of steviol, a metabolite of stevia, might cause acute renal damage (5034).

Dosage and Administration

Oral: For hypertension, stevioside, a constituent of stevia, 250 to 500 mg three times daily has been used (11809,11810).

Comments

The FDA classifies stevia as an "unsafe food additive." Stevia is considered "unsafe" because no one has ever provided FDA with adequate evidence that stevia is safe. Since stevia is not patentable, funding for safety studies seems unlikely (11808).

Dietary supplements are not regulated as food additives, so the FDA allows stevia to be imported "explicitly labeled as a dietary supplement or for use as a dietary ingredient of a dietary supplement" (11808). Canada and the European Community prohibit stevia as a food additive (5030). The FDA, regulatory agencies in Europe, and the World Health Organization have not approved stevia due to unanswered safety questions (5037). Stevia is approved for use in foods in Brazil, Japan, China, and other countries in Asia and South America (11811).

STINGING NETTLE

Also Known As

Common Nettle, Great Stinging Nettle, Nettle, Nettle Seed, Ortie, Small Nettle, Urtica, Urticae herba et folium, Urticae Radix.

CAUTION: See separate listings for White Dead Nettle.

Scientific Names

Urtica dioica; Urtica urens.

Family: Urticaceae.

People Use This For

Orally, stinging nettle root is used for urination disorders associated with benign prostatic hyperplasia (BPH), including nocturia, frequency, dysuria, urinary retention, and irritable bladder. Stinging nettle root is also used orally for joint ailments, as a diuretic, and an astringent.

Orally, stinging nettle above ground parts are used for allergies, allergic rhinitis, and musculoskeletal disease such as osteoarthritis. It is also used orally in conjunction with copious fluid intake in so-called "irrigation therapy" for urinary tract infections (UTI), and urinary tract inflammation, and kidney stones (nephrolithiasis). People also use the above ground parts of stinging nettle for internal bleeding, including uterine bleeding, epistaxis, and melena; anemia; poor circulation; splenomegaly; diabetes and other endocrine disorders; gastric hyperacidity; biliary complaints; diarrhea and dysentery; asthma; pulmonary congestion; rash and eczema; cancer; prevention of signs of aging; blood purification; wound-healing; and as a general tonic.

Topically, stinging nettle above ground parts are used for musculoskeletal aches and pains, scalp seborrhea and oily hair, and hair loss (alopecia).

In foods, young stinging nettle leaves are eaten as a cooked vegetable.

In manufacturing, stinging nettle extract is used as an ingredient in hair and skin products.

Safety

POSSIBLY SAFE ...when used orally and appropriately. Stinging nettle root has been used safely for up to six months (5093,11230). The long-term safety of stinging nettle root is unknown. ...when used orally or topically and appropriately (1,2,12,12490).

PREGNANCY: LIKELY UNSAFE ...when used orally due to possible abortifacient and uterine-stimulant effects (4,6,19).

LACTATION: Insufficient reliable information available; avoid using.

Effectiveness

POSSIBLY INEFFECTIVE

Benign prostatic hyperplasia (BPH). Taking an herbal blend containing stinging nettle root extract orally doesn't seem to be effective for treating symptoms of BPH. In a double-blind, placebo controlled trial, an herbal product containing stinging nettle root extract 80 mg, saw palmetto lipoidal extract 106 mg, pumpkin seed oil extract 160 mg, lemon bioflavonoid extract 33 mg, and vitamin A (100% as beta-carotene) 190 IU taken three times daily for six months failed to significantly improve symptoms in a group of men with BPH (5093).

INSUFFICIENT RELIABLE EVIDENCE to RATE

Allergic rhinitis (hayfever). There is preliminary evidence that stinging nettle above ground parts might improve symptoms of allergic rhinitis. Starting stinging nettle at the first sign of symptoms seems to provide subjective improvement (7035).

Osteoarthritis. There is evidence that oral or topical use of stinging nettle leaf extract might improve symptoms of pain in patients with osteoarthritis (1,6500). Some clinicians use stinging nettle leaf extract in combination with conventional nonsteroidal anti-inflammatory drugs (NSAIDs) or other analgesics. Evidence suggests that adding stinging nettle might allow for using lower analgesic doses in some patients (6500). Topically, stinging nettle leaf seems to improve pain and disability in patients with osteoarthritis of the thumb, according to preliminary research (12490).

More evidence is needed to rate stinging nettle for these uses.

Mechanism of Action

The applicable parts of stinging nettle are the above ground parts and root.

Stinging nettle root contains polysaccharides with immunomodulating and weak anti-inflammatory effects (1,7). The root seems to have an antiproliferative effect on prostatic epithelial and stromal cells (11227,11229); and may also lessen the effects of androgenic hormones by competitively blocking access to human sex hormone binding globulin (SHBG) (11228).

Stinging nettle leaves contain several nutrients and active constituents. The leaves are eaten as a food because of significant amounts carotene, vitamin C, vitamin K, potassium, and calcium (2,8,11,19). There is about as much vitamin C and carotene in stinging nettle leaves as in spinach and other greens (5). The leaves also contain beta-sitosterol and the flavonoids quercetin, rutin, kaempferol, and others. Stinging nettle tops seems to have a variety of pharmacological effects including analgesic (1,4), anti-inflammatory (19), local anesthetic (1), hemostatic (4), antibacterial (11), and antiviral (6). For osteoarthritis and other musculoskeletal conditions, stinging nettle above ground parts might work due to potential analgesic and anti-inflammatory effects. Some researchers think that stinging nettle might be beneficial for allergic rhinitis due to quercetin content. Quercetin is thought to have anti-inflammatory and mast-cell stabilizing effects. It decreases histamine release from basophils and mast cells (483). There is evidence that the above ground parts might inhibit adrenergic stimulation, tumor necrosis factor (TNF), and platelet activation factor (PAF) (1). Stinging nettle seems to also act as a diuretic. The leaf juice can increase urine output and slightly decrease systolic blood pressure and body weight in people with venous insufficiency (1,11). Because of these effects, some people use stinging nettle for urinary tract disorders, including urinary tract infections (UTIs) and kidney stones. Stinging nettle also seems to lower body temperature and have CNS depressant (4,6,11) and anti-seizure activity (4). Stinging nettle also seems to decrease blood pressure and heart rate (1,4).

Stinging nettle leaf is well known to cause skin irritation when touched. The stinging nettle hairs of the leaf contain histamine, acetylcholine, and serotonin that can cause local irritation. Preliminary evidence suggests applying the leaf topically might relieve arthritis pain by hyperstimulation, but the mechanism for this effect is unknown (12490).

Adverse Reactions

Orally, stinging nettle root can cause gastrointestinal complaints, sweating, and allergic skin reactions (1,7). One case is reported of decreased ejaculatory volume associated with an herbal blend product containing nettle root extract, saw palmetto extract, pumpkin seed oil extract, lemon bioflavonoid extract, and beta-carotene (5093).

Orally, stinging nettle above ground parts are well tolerated. Stinging nettle juice can sometimes cause diarrhea (1).

Topically, fresh stinging nettle leaves can cause localized rash, itching, and stinging (12490).

Interactions with Herbs & Other Dietary Supplements

HERBS WITH CLOTTING POTENTIAL: Excessive use of herbs that contain vitamin K can increase the risk of clotting in people using anticoagulants. These herbs include alfalfa, parsley, nettle leaves, plantain, and others.

Interactions with Drugs

ANTIDIABETES DRUGS: There is some evidence that stinging nettle can decrease blood glucose levels. Theoretically, concomitant use of excessive amounts of stinging nettle might interfere with blood glucose control (4).

ANTIHYPERTENSIVE DRUGS: There is some evidence that stinging nettle might have blood pressure lowering effects. Theoretically, concomitant use of excessive amounts of stinging nettle might have additive effects with antihypertensive drugs on blood pressure (4).

CNS DEPRESSANTS: There is some evidence that stinging nettle preparations might have CNS depressant activity. Theoretically, concomitant use of excessive amounts of stinging nettle might have additive effects with CNS depressant drugs (4).

WARFARIN (Coumadin): There is some concern that stinging nettle might decrease the effects of anticoagulant drugs such as warfarin (Coumadin). Stinging nettle contains a significant amount of vitamin K (19); use cautiously. Dose adjustment of anticoagulants may be needed.

Interactions with Foods

None known.

Interactions with Lab Tests

None known.

Interactions with Diseases or Conditions

DIABETES: There is some evidence stinging nettle above ground parts can increase blood glucose levels (4). Theoretically, stinging nettle might worsen blood glucose control in patients with diabetes; use with caution.

HYPERTENSION: There is some evidence that stinging nettle above ground parts might have blood pressure lowering effects (4). Theoretically, stinging nettle might have additive effects with medications used to treat high blood pressure; use with caution.

RENAL INSUFFICIENCY: The above ground parts of stinging nettle seem to have a diuretic effect (1,11); use with caution in people with kidney dysfunction.

Dosage and Administration

ORAL: For symptomatic treatment of benign prostatic hyperplasia (BPH), stinging nettle root extract 80 mg, in combination with saw palmetto lipoidal extract 106 mg, pumpkin seed oil extract 160 mg, lemon bioflavonoid extract 33 mg, and vitamin A (100% as beta-carotene) 190 IU taken three times daily has been used (5093). For osteoarthritis, people typically use crude stinging nettle leaf 9 grams daily (6500). For allergic rhinitis, people typically use stinging nettle leaf extract 300 mg three times daily. However, in some cases, 300 mg up to seven times daily has been used (7035).

TOPICAL: For osteoarthritis, fresh stinging nettle leaf has been applied to the painful joint once daily (12490).

Comments

Stinging nettle leaf has a long history of use. It was used primarily as a diuretic and laxative as early as the times of the Greek physicians Dioscorides and Galen. Avoid confusing stinging nettle (Uritica dioica) with white dead nettle (Lamium album).

STONE ROOT

Also Known As

Citronella, Colinsonia, Hardback, Hardhack, Heal-all, Horse Balm, Horseweed, Knob Grass, Knob Root, Knobweed, Richleaf, Rich Weed.

CAUTION: See separate listings for Citronella Oil and Lemongrass.

Scientific Names

Collinsonia canadensis.

Family: Lamiaceae/Labiatae.

People Use This For

Orally stone root is used to treat bladder inflammation, edema, gastrointestinal disorders, headaches, hyperuricuria, indigestion, kidney stones, urea "bladder semolina," urinary calculus, water retention, and as a tonic.

Safety

POSSIBLY SAFE ...when used orally and appropriately. There are no reports of serious adverse effects (4,12,18).

PREGNANCY AND LACTATION: Insufficient reliable information available; avoid using.

Effectiveness

There is insufficient reliable information available about the effectiveness of stone root.

Mechanism of Action

The applicable parts of stone root are the rhizome and root. Stone root rhizome or root contains a volatile oil, caffeic acid derivatives including rosmaric acid (18), saponins, tannin, mucilage, and resin (4). Constituents of the volatile oil include caryophyllene, germacrene D, limonene, alpha- and beta-pinenes (18). Although no pharmacologic data are documented (4), stone root is said to have diuretic effects (4,6), stimulate stomach function (18), cause sweating (4), and reduce occurrence of urinary stones and help rid the body of stones (4).

Adverse Reactions

Orally, ingesting large amounts of stone root can cause intestinal tract irritation and colic-like pain, dizziness, nausea, and painful urination (18).

Interactions with Herbs & Other Dietary Supplements

HERBS WITH DIURETIC PROPERTIES: Theoretically, due to the diuretic effects of stone root (4,6), there may be additive effects and side effects with herbs having diuretic activity.

Interactions with Drugs

DIURETIC DRUGS: Theoretically, due to the diuretic effects of stone root (4,6), there may be additive effects and side effects with drugs having diuretic activity.

Interactions with Foods

None known.

Interactions with Lab Tests

None known.

Interactions with Diseases or Conditions

None known.

Dosage and Administration

ORAL: A typical dose of dried root is 1-4 grams or as tea three times daily (4). To make tea, simmer 1-4 grams root or rhizome in 150 mL of boiling water for 5-10 minutes, strain. As liquid extract: (1:1 in 25% alcohol) 1-4 mL three times daily (4). Tincture, (1:5 in 40% alcohol) 2-8 mL three times daily (4); tincture of Collinsonia, 2-8 mL (4).

Comments

This aromatic perennial herb has a strong, unpleasant smell that is reported to be numbing in large amounts (18).

STORAX

Also Known As

American Storax, Balsam Styracis, Balsamum Styrax Liquidus, Copalm, Estoraque Liquido, Gum Tree, Levant Storax, Liquid Amber, Liquid Storax, Opossum Tree, Red Gum, Styrax, Sweet Gum, White Gum.

Scientific Names

Liquidambar orientalis; Liquidambar styraciflua, synonym Liquidambar macrophylla.
Family: Hamamelidaceae or Altingiaceae.

People Use This For

Orally, storax is used for cancer, coughs, colds, diarrhea, epilepsy, sore throats, and parasitic infections.
Topically, storax is used to protect wounds, for ulcers, and scabies. Storax is an ingredient in Compound Benzoin Tincture.
As an inhalant, storax is placed in a vaporizer and used to treat coughs and bronchitis.
In foods, storax is used as a flavoring component or fixative.
In manufacturing, storax is used as a fragrance component or fixative in soaps and perfumes. Storax is also used as a fumigant and imbedding material in microscopy.

Safety

LIKELY SAFE ...when used orally in amounts commonly found in foods. Storax has Generally Recognized As Safe status (GRAS) for use in foods in the US (4912).
POSSIBLY SAFE ...when used orally. There are no published reports of toxicity from oral use (6). ...when used topically. Storax should not be used topically on large, open wounds (18).
POSSIBLY UNSAFE ...when large amounts are ingested. ...when applied to large open wounds. Systemic absorption can cause poisoning including kidney damage, e.g., albuminuria and hemorrhagic nephritis (18).
PREGNANCY AND LACTATION: Insufficient reliable information available; avoid using.

Effectiveness

There is insufficient reliable information available about the effectiveness of storax.

Mechanism of Action

The applicable part of storax is the balsam. American storax balsam and Levant storax balsam are very similar chemically. Both contain aromatic alcohols (18), cinnamic acid (18,271), cinnamic acid esters (6,18), storesins (13), styrene (6,18,271), a volatile oil (11,13), vanillin (6,11,18) and triterpenes (18). However, the amount of constituents varies between the species. In Levant storax, the volatile oil is usually less than 1%. In American storax, it ranges from 7% to over 20% (11). Storax has stimulant, antiseptic, and expectorant properties (11,13). It is also reported to have antimicrobial and anti-inflammatory properties (11).

Adverse Reactions

Orally, storax balsam can cause diarrhea (18).
Topically, storax balsam can cause skin sensitization and contact allergies (9,18). When applied to large, open wounds, systemic absorption can cause kidney damage (e.g., albuminuria and hemorrhagic nephritis) (18).

Interactions with Herbs & Other Dietary Supplements

None known.

Interactions with Drugs

None known.

Interactions with Foods

None known.

Interactions with Lab Tests

None known.

Interactions with Diseases or Conditions
None known.

Dosage and Administration
ORAL: No typical dosage.
TOPICAL/INHALATION: Storax is applied topically and administered by inhalation via a vaporizer (6,18). It is available commercially in combination products.

Comments
Storax is a medicinal balsam obtained from the tree trunks of Liquidambar orientalis (Levant storax) or Liquidambar styraciflua (American storax) (13,271). It is obtained by traumatizing the bark of the tree in early summer and stripping the bark later, perhaps as late as autumn. The bark is pressed in cold water, alternating with boiling water, and the crude liquid storax is collected (6). Storax is considered to be similar to Peru balsam in its effects (9).

STRAWBERRY

Also Known As
Alpine Strawberry, Fragariae folium, Mountain Strawberry, Strawberries, Virginian Strawberry, Wild Strawberry, Wood Strawberry.

Scientific Names
Fragaria vesca, synonyms Fragaria insularis, Potentilla vesca; Fragaria virginiana, synonym Potentilla virginiana; Fragaria viridis, synonym Potentilla viridis, Fragaria collina.
Family: Rosaceae.

People Use This For
Orally, strawberry is used for GI tract mucous membrane inflammation, diarrhea, intestinal sluggishness, liver disease, jaundice, upper and lower respiratory tract mucous membrane inflammation, gout, arthritis, nervous tension, kidney ailments involving gravel and stones, diuretic, supportive for heart and circulatory ailments, fever, night sweats, blood purification, for stimulating metabolism, anemia, as a tonic, for inhibiting menstruation, and supporting "natural weight loss."
Topically, strawberry is used as a compress for rashes.

Safety
POSSIBLY SAFE ...when used orally and appropriately (12).
PREGNANCY AND LACTATION: Insufficient reliable information available; avoid using.

Effectiveness
There is insufficient reliable information available about the effectiveness of strawberry.

Mechanism of Action
The applicable part of strawberry is the leaf and fruit. Strawberry leaf contains ellagic acid tannins, oligomeric proanthocyanidins, and flavonoids including rutin and quercetin. People claim that strawberry leaf has astringent and diuretic activity (18); however, there are no data to support these claims (18). Strawberry leaves are rich in vitamin C (19). Preliminary research suggests that compounds contained in strawberry fruit might slow aging effects on the nervous system (1418,1419).

Adverse Reactions
Orally, allergic reactions may occur in people sensitive to strawberries (2).

Interactions with Herbs & Other Dietary Supplements
None known.

Interactions with Drugs
None known.

Interactions with Foods
None known.

Interactions with Lab Tests
None known.

Interactions with Diseases or Conditions

STRAWBERRY HYPERSENSITIVITY: Contraindicated (18).

Dosage and Administration

ORAL: Diarrhea, one cup tea (steep 1 gram dried leaf in 250 mL boiling water 5-10 minutes, strain); several cups daily (18).

STRONTIUM

Also Known As

Stable Strontium, Strontium Chloride, Strontium-89 Chloride, Strontium Citrate, Strontium Ranelate.

Scientific Names

Strontium; Sr; atomic number 38.

People Use This For

Orally, strontium is used for the prevention and treatment of osteoporosis. It is also used orally for metastatic cancer, bone pain, osteoarthritis, cough, seizures, sensitive teeth, and for preventing dental caries.
Intravenously, the strontium-89 isotope is used for skeletal metastases and prostate cancer.
Topically, strontium is used in toothpaste for sensitive teeth.

Safety

LIKELY SAFE ...when strontium-89 chloride is used intravenously, and appropriately. Strontium-89 chloride is an FDA-approved product (4948). ...when strontium chloride is used topically and appropriately as a toothpaste. Strontium chloride hexahydrate (Sensodyne-SC) is an FDA-approved product (9). The safety of strontium chloride when used orally is not known. Most dietary supplements with strontium contain the salt form of strontium chloride.
POSSIBLY SAFE ...when strontium ranelate is used orally and appropriately. Strontium ranelate seems to be safe when used for up to 3 years (11392,11393,11395).
There is insufficient reliable information about the safety of other strontium salts.
PREGNANCY AND LACTATION: LIKELY SAFE ...when strontium chloride is used topically and appropriately as a toothpaste (9). Strontium chloride hexahydrate (Sensodyne-SC) is an FDA approved product. Advise patients not to swallow the toothpaste.
Most dietary supplements with strontium contain the salt form of strontium chloride. The safety of using strontium chloride orally during pregnancy or lactation is not known; avoid using.

Effectiveness

EFFECTIVE

Dental hypersensitivity. Topical use of strontium chloride 10% in toothpaste relieves the pain of sensitive teeth (11745,11746). Best results are obtained with twice daily brushing (11756).

Painful bony metastases. Intravenous administration of strontium-89 chloride is effective for metastatic bone pain (11749,11750,11751,11752).

POSSIBLY EFFECTIVE

Osteoporosis. Taking strontium ranelate orally appears to reduce the risk of vertebral fractures by 40% in postmenopausal women with osteoporosis and a history of vertebral fracture. There is some evidence that it might actually increase bone mineral density (BMD) in these patients by 14% at the lumbar spine and 8% at the femoral neck (11392,11393,11395).

Prostate cancer. Intravenous administration of strontium-89 chloride seems to slow the progression of treatment-resistant prostate cancer and to relieve pain (11747,11748).

There is insufficient reliable information available about the effectiveness of strontium chloride, the form most commonly used in dietary supplements, when used orally for any condition.

Mechanism of Action

Strontium is an alkaline earth element, like calcium. It is physically and chemically similar to calcium. Ninety-nine percent of strontium is found in bone (11396,11753). Strontium is a silvery metal found naturally as a non-radioactive element. It has four known stable forms and twelve known radioactive isotopes (11399).
Strontium has a beneficial effect on bone. It seems to enhance the replication of preosteoblastic cells. It also appears to increase bone formation by stimulating preosteoblast replication. It may also reduce bone resorption by inhibiting osteoclast activity (11396,11399,11753). Animal research suggests that strontium doesn't have adverse effects on bone mineral profile, bone mineral chemistry, or bone matrix mineralization (11754).
Bone strontium levels rapidly decrease with withdrawal of treatment. Plasma levels seem to correlate well with bone strontium levels after 4 weeks of treatment (11753). Strontium is excreted renally (11394,11400,11755).
Most of the research studies on strontiums effects on bone have used the strontium ranelate salt (11753). Strontium ranelate consists of two atoms of stable strontium and an organic moiety called ranelic acid (11399). There is interest

in using strontium ranelate for osteoarthritis and bone pain due to metastatic cancer. Preliminary evidence suggests strontium ranelate may increase cartilage matrix formation, and remineralize bone lesions (11397,11402).

Strontium chloride is the most common salt form used in dietary supplements. But there isn't much research evaluating oral use of these formulations.

For cancer, radioactive strontium-89 is used. Strontium is preferentially taken up in areas of bone undergoing active bone turnover (11753,11755). This causes much greater concentrations of strontium-89 in tumorous bone than normal bone. Strontium-89 selectively irradiates metastatic bone with minimal effect on normal tissue (11755).

For dental hypersensitivity, strontium ions in toothpaste seem to relieve pain by blocking fluid flow in dentinal tubules, microscopic canals in the dentin (11756).

An inverse relationship also appears to exist between dental caries and content of stable strontium in drinking water (11402).

Adverse Reactions

Orally, strontium ranelate is usually well tolerated. However, strontium ranelate can cause epigastric pain and diarrhea (11392,11393,11395).

Intravenously, strontium-89 can cause a transient increase in bone pain. It can also cause bone marrow toxicity. In clinical studies, the nadir of platelet and white blood cell counts appears at approximately 4 to 8 weeks following injection, partially returning to baseline by 12 weeks (11752,11755). Patient should be given instructions about avoiding environmental radioactive contamination.

Interactions with Herbs & Other Dietary Supplements

None known.

Interactions with Drugs

None known.

Drug Influences on Nutrient Levels and Depletion

SOME DRUGS CAN AFFECT STRONTIUM LEVELS:

ANDROGENS: Androgens may decrease urinary excretion rates of strontium. Dosage adjustments may be necessary (11405).

CORTICOSTEROIDS: Corticosteroids may increase urinary excretion rates of strontium. Dosage adjustments may be necessary (11405).

ESTROGEN: Estrogens may decrease urinary excretion rates of strontium. Dosage adjustments may be necessary (11405).

Interactions with Foods

SODIUM: A sodium-poor diet increases the fecal elimination of calcium and may reduce the intestinal absorption of strontium (11403).

Interactions with Lab Tests

BLOOD CELL COUNTS: Strontium-89 depresses blood cell counts, particularly white cells and platelets. Monitor blood cell counts at least once every other week (11755).

CREATINE PHOSPHOKINASE: Strontium may cause a small rise in serum creatine phosphokinase. The clinical significance of this appears insignificant (11392,11395).

Interactions with Diseases or Conditions

BONE DISEASE: Delayed intestinal absorption of strontium may occur in patients with bone disease, such as postmenopausal osteoporosis or osteomalacia (11400,11404).

RENAL INSUFFICIENCY: Strontium is eliminated renally and, theoretically, might accumulate in patients with renal impairment (e.g., creatinine clearance less than 40 ml/minute) (11394,11400); use with caution.

Dosage and Administration

ORAL: For postmenopausal osteoporosis, strontium ranelate 2 grams daily has been used (11392,11395).

INTRAVENOUS: For treating bony metastases, 148MBq (MegaBequerel) strontium-89 chloride is given over 1 to 2 minutes. Or, a dose of 1.5 to 2.2 MBq per kilogram, 40 to 60 microCI (curie) per kilogram may be used (11755).

Comments

Strontium ranelate is being evaluated as a potential prescription treatment for osteoporosis. This is a different form than the strontium that is contained in most dietary supplements. Most supplements contain strontium chloride. But there isn't much scientific information about the oral use of strontium chloride in people. Advise patients against dietary supplements containing strontium chloride until more is known about long-term safety.

STROPHANTHUS

Also Known As
Kombe, Kombe-Strophanthus Seeds, Strophanthi Grati Semen, Strophanthi Kombe Semen, Strophanthus Seeds.

Scientific Names
Strophanthus gratus, synonym Roupellia grata; Strophanthus kombe.
Family: Apocynaceae.

People Use This For
Orally, strophanthus is used for arteriosclerosis, cardiac insufficiency, gastrocardial symptoms, hypertension, and neurodystonia.

Safety
UNSAFE ...when used orally for self-medication (12,4077).
PREGNANCY: UNSAFE ...when used orally due to possible uterine stimulating effects (19); avoid using.
LACTATION: UNSAFE ...when used orally; avoid using (4077).

Effectiveness
There is insufficient reliable information available about the effectiveness of strophanthus.

Mechanism of Action
The applicable part of strophanthus is the seed. Strophanthus gratus contains a cardiac glycoside strophanthin-G (ouabain) which has digitalis-like effects, but milder. The cardiac glycoside in Strophanthus kombe, strophanthin-K (strophoside), has milder effects than strophanthin-G (18,4077).

Adverse Reactions
Orally, side effects include nausea, vomiting, headache, stupor, disturbance of color vision, and cardiac arrhythmias, particularly when strophanthin-G is administered parenterally and during overdose (18).

Interactions with Herbs & Other Dietary Supplements
ANTHRAQUINONE-CONTAINING HERBS AND LAXATIVE HERBS: Anthraquinone-containing herbs such as aloe, alder buckthorn, European buckthorn, cascara sagrada, frangula, rhubarb, and senna; laxative herbs such as castor bean can worsen strophanthus seed toxicity, particularly with long-term use, due to electrolyte loss (19).
CARDIAC GLYCOSIDE-CONTAINING HERBS: Contraindicated, and concomitant use can increase the risk of cardiac glycoside toxicity. Cardiac glycoside-containing herbs include black hellebore, Canadian hemp roots, digitalis leaf, hedge mustard, figwort, lily-of-the-valley roots, motherwort, oleander leaf, pheasant's eye plant, pleurisy root, squill bulb leaf scales, and uzara (19).
CINCHONA and EPHEDRA: Use with strophanthus seed may increase risk of toxicity (19).
LICORICE: Can worsen effects of strophanthus seed due to hypokalemia (19).

Interactions with Drugs
CALCIUM SUPPLEMENTS: Calcium supplements may enhance the therapeutic effects of strophanthus (18).
CORTICOSTEROIDS: Use of corticosteroids may cause electrolyte depletion and increase the risk of strophanthus toxicity (19).
DIGOXIN (Lanoxin): Contraindicated; therapeutic duplication increases risk of cardiac glycoside toxicity (2).
DIURETIC DRUGS: Theoretically, concomitant use of potassium-depleting diuretics and strophanthus can increase the risk of cardiac glycoside toxicity due to potassium depletion (19). Some diuretics that can deplete potassium include chlorothiazide (Diuril), chlorthalidone (Thalitone), furosemide (Lasix), hydrochlorothiazide (HCTZ, Hydrodiuril, Microzide), and others.
QUINIDINE: Contraindicated; cardiac medications, including quinidine, may increase the risk of cardiac glycoside toxicity (18).
QUININE: Taking quinine with strophanthus may increase the risk of cardiac glycoside toxicity (18).
STIMULANT LAXATIVES: Overuse or misuse of laxatives may cause electrolyte depletion and increase risk of strophanthus toxicity (19).

Interactions with Foods
None known.

Interactions with Lab Tests
None known.

Interactions with Diseases or Conditions
CARDIAC CONDITIONS: CAUTION, strophanthus seed may cause arrhythmias (18).

Dosage and Administration

No typical dosage.

Comments

Strophanthus seeds can be confused with other African Strophanthus species (18). Strophanthus is used as an arrow poison in Africa (4077).

SULFORAPHANE

Also Known As

SFN, Sulforafane, Sulphorafane.

Scientific Names

1-isothiocyanate-4-methyl-sulfonyl butane.

People Use This For

Orally, sulforaphane is used for the prevention of prostate cancer and other types of cancer.

Safety

LIKELY SAFE ...when used orally in amounts found in foods (10264). There is insufficient reliable information available about the safety of sulforaphane in medicinal amounts.
CHILDREN: LIKELY SAFE ...when used orally in amounts found in foods (10264). There is insufficient reliable information available about the safety of sulforaphane in medicinal amounts.
PREGNANCY AND LACTATION: LIKELY SAFE ...when used orally in amounts found in foods (10264). There is insufficient reliable information available about the safety of sulforaphane in medicinal amounts.

Effectiveness

There is insufficient reliable information available about the effectiveness of sulforaphane.

Mechanism of Action

Sulforaphane, a sulfur-containing isothiocyanate, is a phytochemical found in cruciferous vegetables such as broccoli (particularly broccoli sprouts), cabbage, cauliflower, radish, and mustard (10264,10463,10681). After oral consumption, cruciferous vegetables containing glucosinolates are degraded to isothiocyanates. These isothiocyanates are conjugated to glutathione before excretion in the urine as an isothiocyanate mercapturic acid (10679). Cooking sulforaphane-containing vegetables seems to reduce the bioavailability of sulforaphane (10462).
Epidemiologic evidence suggests that consumption of cruciferous vegetables is inversely associated with various types of cancers, including leukemia, prostate cancer, and liver cancer (10264). Preliminary evidence suggests several theories of action, including the induction of carcinogen defense enzymes, inhibition of carcinogen-activating enzymes, induction of cell cycle arrest, and anti-inflammatory mechanisms (10265,10678,10681,10682). A combination of sulforaphane and selenium may also synergistically protect cells against oxidative damage. This synergy appears to occur at the levels of transcription and translation (10680). Sulforaphane seems to induce the enzyme thioredoxin reductase, which has antioxidant properties. Sulforaphane in combination with selenium causes greater induction of thioredoxin reductase than either compound alone (12700). Sulforaphane increases the action of phase 2 enzymes, which inactivate many carcinogens. Sulforaphane may also inhibit the activity of phase 1 enzymes, such as cytochrome P450 2E1 (CYP2E1) and CYP1A2, that increase the carcinogenic activity of some substances (10462,10463,12701).

Adverse Reactions

None reported.

Interactions with Herbs & Other Dietary Supplements

None known.

Interactions with Drugs

CYTOCHROME P450 1A2 (CYP1A2) SUBSTRATES: There is some preliminary evidence that sulforaphane inhibits CYP1A2 isozymes (12701). Theoretically, sulforaphane might decrease the metabolism of CYP1A2 substrates and increase serum concentrations. Some substrates of CYP1A2 include clozapine (Clozaril), cyclobenzaprine (Flexeril), fluvoxamine (Luvox), haloperidol (Haldol), imipramine (Tofranil), mexiletine (Mexitil), olanzapine (Zyprexa), pentazocine (Talwin), propranolol (Inderal), tacrine (Cognex), theophylline, zileuton (Zyflo), zolmitriptan (Zomig), and others.

Interactions with Foods

None known.

Interactions with Lab Tests
None known.

Interactions with Diseases or Conditions
None known.

Dosage and Administration
No typical dosage.

SUMA

Also Known As
Brazilian Ginseng, Pfaffia.

Scientific Names
Hebanthe eriantha, synonyms Pfaffia paniculata, Hebanthe paniculata, Gomphrena paniculata.
Family: Amaranthaceae.

People Use This For
Orally, suma is used as an immune enhancer or adaptogen to help the body adapt to all types of stress by enhancing or restoring the immune system. Suma is also used orally for cancer, diabetes, tumors, and as a tonic to restore body function.
Topically, suma is used for wounds and skin problems.

Safety
POSSIBLY SAFE ...when used orally short-term (12).
There is insufficient reliable information available about the safety using suma topically.
PREGNANCY AND LACTATION: Insufficient reliable information available; avoid using.

Effectiveness
There is insufficient reliable information available about the effectiveness of suma.

Mechanism of Action
The applicable part of suma is the root. Cell culture data suggests that the isolated constituents pfaffic acid, a nortriterpene, and saponin derivatives pfaffosiges A through F may inhibit melanoma growth. An ethanolic extract has been shown to have mild anti-inflammatory and analgesic effect, but did not relieve noninflammatory pain (515). At present, we don't know how these components relate to the uses of suma.

Adverse Reactions
Powdered suma root can cause occupational asthma during industrial exposure to the root powder (515).

Interactions with Herbs & Other Dietary Supplements
None known.

Interactions with Drugs
None known.

Interactions with Foods
None known.

Interactions with Lab Tests
None known.

Interactions with Diseases or Conditions
None known.

Dosage and Administration
No typical dosage.

Comments
Suma is called Brazilian ginseng, presumably to present the herb in terms that consumers understand. It is unrelated to the ginsengs (American Ginseng, Panax Ginseng, etc.) or other plants which use ginseng as an alternate common name as well (Blue Cohosh, Canaigre, Codonopsis, Siberian Ginseng, Ashwagandha) (515).

SUMBUL

Also Known As
Ferrula, Musk Root.

Scientific Names
Ferula sumbul.
Family: Apiaceae/Umbelliferae

Comments
At the date of publication, this product was not a common ingredient used in brand name supplements marketed to consumers. Details about this product are available in the online version of *Natural Medicines Comprehensive Database*. See www.naturaldatabase.com.

SUMMER SAVORY

Also Known As
Bean Herb, Bohnenkraut, Savory.
CAUTION: See separate listing for Winter Savory.

Scientific Names
Satureja hortensis, synonym Calamintha hortensis.
Family: Lamiaceae/Labiatae.

People Use This For
Orally, summer savory is used as an appetite stimulant or expectorant; for coughs; flatulence; intestinal disorders including cramps, indigestion, diarrhea, and nausea; and to relieve frequent thirst in people with diabetes. It is also used orally as a tea for sore throats, as a tonic, astringent, antiflatulent, and as an aphrodisiac.
Topically, summer savory is used for insect bites.
In foods, summer savory is used in cooking as a culinary spice. The oil is used as a flavoring agent.

Safety
LIKELY SAFE ...when used orally in amounts commonly found in foods. Summer savory has Generally Recognized As Safe (GRAS) status in the US (4912).
POSSIBLY SAFE ...when used orally and appropriately in medicinal amounts (5,6,18). ...when used topically as diluted oil (6,11), summer savory is nonirritating and nonsensitizing (11). Undiluted oil is a severe topical irritant (6).
PREGNANCY AND LACTATION: Insufficient reliable information available; avoid using amounts in excess of foods.

Effectiveness
There is insufficient reliable information available about the effectiveness of summer savory.

Mechanism of Action
The applicable parts of summer savory are the leaves and stem. Summer savory contains tannins (18), and a volatile oil (0.2-3.0 %) including thymol, carvacrol, p-cymene, limonene, and camphene (5,6,11,18). Other constituents also present include vitamin A, calcium, potassium, and proteins (11). Summer savory oil has antifungal, antibacterial, and spasmolytic properties (6,11). The mild antiseptic activity is due to cymene and carvacrol (5,18). A mild antidiarrheal effect is reportedly due to the astringent activity of the tannins (5,6,18).

Adverse Reactions
Topically, summer savory can cause skin eruptions (12). The concentrated oil of summer savory is strongly irritating (6).

Interactions with Herbs & Other Dietary Supplements
None known.

Interactions with Drugs
None known.

Interactions with Foods
None known.

Interactions with Lab Tests
None known.

Interactions with Diseases or Conditions
None known.

Dosage and Administration
ORAL: A typical dose is 3 teaspoons. In making the drink, do not boil. Allow plant to soak (18).
TOPICAL: No typical dosage.

SUNDEW

Also Known As
Dew Plant, Drosera, Lustwort, Red Rot, Round-Leafed Sundew, Youthwort.

Scientific Names
Drosera intermedia; Drosera anglica, synonym Drosera longifolia; Drosera ramentacea; Drosera rotundifolia.
Family: Droseraeae.

People Use This For
Orally, sundew is used for bronchitis, asthma, pertussis, tracheitis, gastric ulceration, cancer, coughing fits, and dry cough.

Safety
POSSIBLY SAFE ...when used orally and appropriately (2,4).
PREGNANCY AND LACTATION: Insufficient reliable information available; avoid using.

Effectiveness
There is insufficient reliable information available about the effectiveness of sundew.

Mechanism of Action
Sundew seems to cause antispasmodic, demulcent, and expectorant effects (4). Researchers wonder if the antitussive effect demonstrated in animals is due to naphthoquinone constituents (4). Antimicrobial activity is reported in vitro for naphthaquinone constituents (4).

Adverse Reactions
None reported.

Interactions with Herbs & Other Dietary Supplements
None known.

Interactions with Drugs
None known.

Interactions with Foods
None known.

Interactions with Lab Tests
None known.

Interactions with Diseases or Conditions
None known.

Dosage and Administration
ORAL: 1-2 grams dried plant three times daily, or one cup tea (made by steeping 1-2 grams dried plant in 150 mL boiling water 5-10 minutes, strain) three times daily (4); 3 grams dried plant is the average daily dose (2). Liquid extract (1:1 in 25% alcohol), 0.5-2 mL three times daily (4). Tincture (1:5 in 60% alcohol), 0.5-1 mL three times daily (4).

SUNFLOWER OIL

Also Known As
Corona Solis, Helianthi Annui Oleum, Marigold of Peru, Sunflower, Sunflower Oils, Sunflower Seed Oil.

Scientific Names
Helianthus annuus.
Family: Asteraceae/Compositae.

People Use This For
Orally, sunflower oil is used for constipation.
Topically, it is used for poorly healing wounds, skin lesions, psoriasis, arthritis, and as a massage oil.
In foods, sunflower oil is used as a cooking oil.

Safety
LIKELY SAFE ...when used orally and appropriately (9780).
There is insufficient reliable information available about the safety of topical medicinal uses for sunflower oil.
PREGNANCY AND LACTATION: Insufficient reliable information available; avoid using.

Effectiveness
INSUFFICIENT RELIABLE EVIDENCE to RATE

Hypercholesterolemia. There is evidence that using sunflower oil in the diet is more effective than olive oil for decreasing low density lipoprotein (LDL) cholesterol and apolipoprotein B (9780). More evidence is needed to rate sunflower oil for this use.

Mechanism of Action
Sunflower oil is cold pressed from the seeds of Helianthus annuus. Sunflower oil is high in linoleic acid and is used as a source of polyunsaturated fat in the diet (8132).

Adverse Reactions
Orally, sunflower oil seems to be well tolerated (8132). Sunflower oil can cause an allergic reaction in individuals sensitive to the Asteraceae/Compositae family. Members of this family include ragweed, chrysanthemums, marigolds, daisies, and many other herbs.

Interactions with Herbs & Other Dietary Supplements
None known.

Interactions with Drugs
None known.

Interactions with Foods
None known.

Interactions with Lab Tests
FASTING BLOOD GLUCOSE: A diet using sunflower oil as a fat source can cause increased fasting blood glucose levels in patients with type 2 diabetes (8132).
FASTING INSULIN: A diet using sunflower oil as a fat source can cause increased fasting insulin levels in patients with type 2 diabetes (8132).

Interactions with Diseases or Conditions
CROSS-ALLERGENICITY: Sunflower oil can cause an allergic reaction in individuals sensitive to the Asteraceae/Compositae family. Members of this family include ragweed, chrysanthemums, marigolds, daisies, and many other herbs.
DIABETES: A diet using sunflower oil as a fat source seems to increase fasting insulin and glucose levels.
It also seems to increase postprandial lipids, which might increase the risk of atherosclerosis in patients with type 2 diabetes (8132).

Dosage and Administration
No typical dosage.

SUPEROXIDE DISMUTASE

Also Known As
Orgotein, S.O.D., SOD, Super Dioxide Dismutase, Super-Oxide Dismutase.

Scientific Names
Superoxide dismutase.

People Use This For
Orally, superoxide dismutase is used for removing wrinkles, regenerating tissue, and extending the length of life.
As an injection, superoxide dismutase is used for inflammatory diseases including osteoarthritis, sports injuries, rheumatoid arthritis, radiation-induced or interstitial cystitis, hyperuricemic syndromes, acute paraquat poisoning, for improving tolerance to radiation therapy, treating cancer, improving rejection rates in kidney transplantation, managing reperfusion injury in acute myocardial infarction, and treating respiratory distress syndrome.

Safety
POSSIBLY SAFE ... when used parenterally, short-term. Intravenous, intramuscular, and local injections of superoxide dismutase (SOD) appear to be safe for short-term use (2230,2231,2232,2242,2233,2241,2243). However, since some SOD preparations are derived from animals, there is concern about contamination with diseased animal parts (1825). So far, there are no reports of disease transmission to humans due to use of contaminated SOD preparations.
PREGNANCY AND LACTATION: Insufficient reliable information available; avoid using.

Effectiveness
POSSIBLY EFFECTIVE

Bronchopulmonary dysplasia. Giving superoxide dismutase as an injection seems to reduce bronchopulmonary dysplasia in neonates with respiratory distress syndrome (2242).

Interstitial cystitis. Giving superoxide dismutase as an injection seems to be effective for treating interstitial cystitis (2233).

Osteoarthritis. Giving superoxide dismutase as an injection seems to be effective for treating osteoarthritis (2228,2229).

Rheumatoid arthritis (RA). Giving superoxide dismutase as an injection seems to be effective for treating RA (2230,2231,2232).

LIKELY INEFFECTIVE

Myocardial infarction (MI). Giving superoxide dismutase as an injection doesn't seem to be effective for managing reperfusion injury in acute MI (2241,2243).

Mechanism of Action
Superoxide dismutase (SOD) is an essential enzyme found in all living cells. Some cellular processes produce reactive oxygen species (ROS) such as superoxide radicals that can impair the function of cells and tissues. SOD catalyzes the conversion of superoxide to oxygen and hydrogen peroxide. SOD isoenzymes contain copper and zinc, and iron or manganese. Copper and zinc SOD is the most common. Researchers are interested in the role of SOD in a variety of diseases including familial amyotrophic lateral sclerosis, Parkinson's disease, Alzheimer's disease, dengue fever, cancer, Down's syndrome, cataract, and neurological disorders such as Creutzfeldt-Jakob disease (11157).
SOD is found in yeast, spinach, chicken liver, and bovine blood (11157). Commercially, it is typically obtained from bovine liver (11008).

Adverse Reactions
As an injection, SOD can cause pain or allergic reactions at injection site (2235). It can also cause anaphylactic shock, which may be caused by product impurities (11008).
SOD may be prepared from bovine liver. Products made from contaminated or diseased organs might present a human health hazard. There is also concern that spleen extracts produced from cows in countries where bovine spongiform encephalitis (BSE) has been reported might be contaminated with diseased tissue. Countries where BSE has been reported include Great Britain, France, The Netherlands, Portugal, Luxembourg, Ireland, Switzerland, Oman, and Belgium (1825). There have been no reports of BSE transfer to humans from contaminated SOD products. Until more is known, tell patients to avoid these products unless country of origin can be determined. Patients should avoid products that are produced in countries where BSE has been found.

Interactions with Herbs & Other Dietary Supplements
None known.

Interactions with Drugs
None known.

Interactions with Foods
None known.

Interactions with Lab Tests
None known.

Interactions with Diseases or Conditions
None known.

Dosage and Administration
ORAL: No typical dosage.
INJECTION: For osteoarthritis, 16 mg as an intra-articular injection is used every two weeks (2228,2229). For rheumatoid arthritis a typical dose is 4 mg as an intra-articular injection per week (2230,2232). A typical dose for interstitial or radiation-induced cystitis is 12 mg injected into the bladder wall, up to 6 times (2233). For radiation-induced cystitis, a typical dose is 8 mg injected intramuscularly per day (2234). For reducing rejection risk in kidney transplantation, a typical dose is 200 mg intravenously during surgery (2239). For reducing bronchopulmonary dysplasia in neonatal respiratory distress syndrome, 0.25 mg/kg subcutaneously twice daily until ventilator support is no longer required (2242).

Comments
Bovine or recombinant (rh-SOD) source parenteral SOD products are available (2238). There is no evidence that oral SOD products are absorbed.

SWAMP MILKWEED

Also Known As
Rose-Colored Silkweed, Swamp Silkweed.

Scientific Names
Asclepias incarnata.
Family: Asclepiadaceae or Apocynaceae.

People Use This For
Orally, swamp milkweed is used for digestive disorders.

Safety
LIKELY UNSAFE ...when used orally. It contains cardenolides, a type of cardioactive steroid. Digitalis-like poisonings are possible (18).
PREGNANCY AND LACTATION: LIKELY UNSAFE ...when used orally due to presence of cardioactive steroids (18); avoid using.

Effectiveness
There is insufficient reliable information available about the effectiveness of swamp milkweed.

Mechanism of Action
The applicable parts of swamp milkweed are the root and rhizome. Swamp milkweed contains cardioactive steroids known as cardenolides. In swamp milkweed, they have little therapeutic significance (18), but the concentration of the specific cardenolide present is not reported. In large amounts, swamp milkweed has an emetic effect (18).

Adverse Reactions
Orally, large amounts of swamp milkweed can cause vomiting (18).
Topically, the plant can cause local inflammation (19).

Interactions with Herbs & Other Dietary Supplements
CARDIAC GLYCOSIDE-CONTAINING HERBS: Contraindicated; concomitant use increases the risk of cardiac glycoside toxicity. Cardiac glycoside-containing herbs include black hellebore, Canadian hemp roots, digitalis leaf, hedge mustard, figwort, lily-of-the-valley roots, motherwort, oleander leaf, pheasant's eye plant, pleurisy root, squill bulb leaf scales, and strophanthus seeds (19).
LICORICE/HORSETAIL: Theoretically, overuse/misuse of licorice rhizome or horsetail plant with cardiac glycoside-containing herbs increases the risk of cardiac toxicity due to potassium depletion (19).
OTHER CARDIOACTIVE HERBS: Avoid concomitant use with other cardioactive herbs due to unpredictability of effects and adverse effects. Other cardioactive herbs include calamus, cereus, cola, coltsfoot, devil's claw, European mistletoe, fenugreek, fumitory, ginger, Panax ginseng, hawthorn, white horehound, mate, parsley, quassia,

scotch broom flower, shepherd's purse, and wild carrot (4).
STIMULANT LAXATIVE HERBS: Theoretically, overuse or misuse of stimulant laxatives with cardiac glycoside-containing herbs increases the risk of cardiac toxicity due to potassium depletion. Stimulant laxative herbs include aloe dried leaf sap, blue flag rhizome, alder buckthorn, European buckthorn, butternut bark, cascara bark, castor oil, colocynth fruit pulp, gamboge bark exudate, jalap root, black root, manna bark exudate, podophyllum root, rhubarb root, senna leaves and pods, wild cucumber fruit (Ecballium elaterium), and yellow dock root (19).

Interactions with Drugs

DIGOXIN (Lanoxin): Contraindicated; therapeutic duplication increases risk of cardiac glycoside toxicity (2).
DIURETIC DRUGS: Theoretically, concomitant use of potassium-depleting diuretics and swamp milkweed can increase the risk of cardiac glycoside toxicity due to potassium depletion (506). Some diuretics that can deplete potassium include chlorothiazide (Diuril), chlorthalidone (Thalitone), furosemide (Lasix), hydrochlorothiazide (HCTZ, Hydrodiuril, Microzide), and others.
MACROLIDE ANTIBIOTICS: Theoretically, concomitant use may increase risk of cardiac glycoside toxicity (17).
QUININE: Theoretically, concomitant use of swamp milkweed and quinine might increase risk of cardiac toxicity (506).
STIMULANT LAXATIVES: Theoretically, overuse or misuse of stimulant laxatives with swamp milkweed may increase risk of cardiac glycoside toxicity due to potassium depletion (19).
TETRACYCLINE ANTIBIOTICS: Theoretically, concomitant use may increase risk of cardiac glycoside toxicity (17).

Interactions with Foods

None known.

Interactions with Lab Tests

None known.

Interactions with Diseases or Conditions

HEART DISEASE: Contraindicated; theoretically the cardiac glycosides contained in swamp milkweed (18) might exacerbate the condition or interfere with existing drug therapy.

Dosage and Administration

No typical dosage.

SWEET ALMOND

Also Known As

Almond, Almond Oil, Almonds, Amygdala Dulcis, Expressed Almond Oil, Fixed Almond Oil, Sweet Almond Oil.
CAUTION: See separate listing for Bitter Almond.

Scientific Names

Prunus amygdalus dulcis.
Family: Rosaceae.

People Use This For

Orally, sweet almond is used as a mild laxative, and as a remedy for cancer of the bladder, breast, mouth, spleen, and uterus.
Topically, sweet almond is used as an emollient for chapped skin, to soothe mucous membranes (as a demulcent), and as a weak antibacterial.
Parenterally, sweet almond is also used as a solvent for injectable drugs.
Sweet almonds, themselves, are a familiar food.
In manufacturing, sweet almond is used widely in cosmetics.

Safety

LIKELY SAFE ...when used orally (11). Unlike bitter almond oil, sweet almond oil contains no benzaldehyde and no (or only trace) poisonous hydrocyanic acid HCN (11,12). ...when used topically. Almond oil is nonirritating and nonsensitizing to skin (11).
PREGNANCY AND LACTATION: Insufficient reliable information available; avoid using.

Effectiveness

POSSIBLY EFFECTIVE

Constipation. Taking sweet almond orally seems to relieve constipation due to its laxative effects (11).
Skin irritation. Applying sweet almond topically may act as an emollient and demulcent (11).

Mechanism of Action
The applicable part of sweet almond is the fixed oil. Researchers believe the effects of sweet almond oil are due to the presence of many triglycerides (largely triolein and dioleolinolein) and fatty acids (oleic, linoleic, palmitic, stearic, lauric, myristic and palmitoleic acids) (11). A Japanese patent claims isolation of low molecular weight peptides with analgesic and anti-inflammatory properties (11).

Adverse Reactions
None reported.

Interactions with Herbs & Other Dietary Supplements
None known.

Interactions with Drugs
None known.

Interactions with Foods
None known.

Interactions with Lab Tests
None known.

Interactions with Diseases or Conditions
None known.

Dosage and Administration
ORAL: As a laxative typical doses used are up to 30 mL (11).

Comments
Avoid confusion between volatile almond oil and fixed almond oil. Fixed almond oil (sweet almond oil) is prepared by pressing the kernels of both sweet almond and bitter almond. It does not contain benzaldehyde or hydrocyanic acid (HCN). Sweet almond does not yield a volatile oil. Volatile almond oil (bitter almond oil) contains 95% benzaldehyde and 2-4% poisonous HCN. It is made by water maceration and steam distillation of partially defatted bitter almond (Prunus dulcis amara), apricot (Prunus armeniaca), peach (Prunus persica), and plum (Prunus domestica) kernels (11).

SWEET ANNIE

Also Known As
Annual Mugwort, Annual Wormwood, Artemisia, Artemisinin, Chinese Wormwood, Ching-hao, Qing Hao, Qinghao, Qinghaosu, Sweet Wormwood.

Scientific Names
Artemisia annua.
Family: Asteraceae/Compositae.

People Use This For
Orally, sweet Annie is used for malaria, dysentery, dyspepsia, fever (antipyretic), jaundice, scabies, tuberculosis, cryptosporidiosis in people with AIDS, preventing pneumocystis carinii infections in people with AIDS, psoriasis, systemic lupus erythematosus and other auto-immune disorders, bacterial and fungal infections, inflammatory conditions, anorexia, circulatory disorders, common cold, constipation, gallbladder disorders, gastritis, nematode infestation, painful menstruation, and rheumatism.
Topically, sweet Annie is used for bacterial and fungal infections, arthritis, rheumatism, bruises, neuralgia, and sprains.

Safety
POSSIBLY SAFE ...when used orally and appropriately (12).
There is insufficient reliable information available about the safety of sweet Annie when used topically.
PREGNANCY: LIKELY UNSAFE ...when used orally; avoid using (12,19).
LACTATION: Insufficient reliable information available; avoid using.

Effectiveness
There is insufficient reliable information available about the effectiveness of sweet Annie.

Mechanism of Action

The applicable parts of sweet Annie are the above ground parts (12). The constituent, artemisinin (qinghaosu), is a sesquiterpene lactone with antimalarial activity. Preliminary evidence suggests that artemisinin and quercetagetin 6,7,3',4'-tetramethyl ether might have cytotoxic effects against some types of tumor cells (3183). Extracts of sweet Annie are reported to have antipyretic, anti-inflammatory, and bacteriostatic properties (3184). Evidence suggests that sweet Annie promotes cell-mediated immunity and inhibits antibody responses (3177). Preliminary research suggests that capsules containing sweet Annie herb might have antimalarial activity (3185).

Adverse Reactions

The use of artemether, the semisynthetic derivative of artemisinin, which is a constituent of sweet Annie, has been associated with hypoglycemia, prolongation of the QT interval on the electrocardiogram, abdominal pain, and local injection site pain (3180). Artesunate has been associated with prolonged ataxic gait and slurred speech (450). Sweet Annie might cause an allergic reaction in people sensitive to the Asteraceae/Compositae family. Members of this family include ragweed, chrysanthemums, marigolds, daisies, and many other herbs.

Interactions with Herbs & Other Dietary Supplements

None known.

Interactions with Drugs

None known.

Interactions with Foods

None known.

Interactions with Lab Tests

None known.

Interactions with Diseases or Conditions

CROSS-ALLERGENICITY: Sweet Annie might cause an allergic reaction in people sensitive to the Asteraceae/Compositae family. Members of this family include ragweed, chrysanthemums, marigolds, daisies, and many other herbs.

Dosage and Administration

ORAL: Daily doses of 3-9 grams of sweet Annie above ground parts have been used (3176,3177).

Comments

The semisynthetic derivatives of artemisinin (a constituent of sweet Annie), artemether, arteether, and artesunate, are used as prescription antimalarial drugs in Asia, Africa, and Europe (3181,3182).

SWEET BAY

Also Known As

Bay, Bay Laurel, Bay Leaf, Bay Tree, Daphne, Grecian Laurel, Laurel, Mediterranean Bay, Noble Laurel, Roman Laurel, True Bay.

Scientific Names

Laurus nobilis.
Family: Lauraceae.

People Use This For

Orally, sweet bay is used to treat cancer, and as a bile and general stimulant, antiflatulent, diaphoretic, and herb for foods.
Topically, sweet bay is used as an anti-dandruff agent, as a counterirritant, and to treat rheumatic conditions. The fruit essential and fatty oils of sweet bay are also used topically to treat furuncles, a localized infection of hair follicles.
In veterinary medicine, sweet bay is used as an udder ointment.
For food uses, sweet bay is used as a seasoning.
In food manufacturing, it is used as an herb and oil in processed foods.
In manufacturing, the oil is used in cosmetics, soaps, and detergents.

Safety

LIKELY SAFE ...when used orally in amounts found in foods (12). The highest levels of sweet bay used in food are 0.1% as a herb and 0.02% as an oil (11).

LIKELY UNSAFE ...when the whole, intact leaf is swallowed. The whole leaf is indigestible and can become lodged in the esophagus, hypopharynx (132,133,134,137), or perforate the intestinal lining (135,136).
PREGNANCY AND LACTATION: Insufficient reliable information available; avoid using in amounts exceeding those commonly found in foods.

Effectiveness
There is insufficient reliable information available about the effectiveness of sweet bay.

Mechanism of Action
The applicable part of sweet bay is the dried leaf. The sweet bay constituent, methyl eugenol, has sedative and narcotic properties in mice. The essential oil has bactericidal and fungicidal properties (11). The other constituents of sweet bay include proanthocyanidins, alkaloids, and plant acids (11).

Adverse Reactions
Sweet bay can cause allergic reactions, including contact dermatitis (11). The whole, intact leaf is indigestible and can become lodged in the esophagus and hypopharynx (132,133,134,137) and perforate the intestinal lining (135,136).

Interactions with Herbs & Other Dietary Supplements
None known.

Interactions with Drugs
CNS DEPRESSANTS: Because sweet bay theoretically can enhance the therapeutic and adverse effects of sedatives, concomitant use should be avoided.
NARCOTIC DRUGS: Theoretically, sweet bay can enhance the therapeutic and adverse effects of narcotics. Avoid concomitant use.

Interactions with Foods
None known.

Interactions with Lab Tests
None known.

Interactions with Diseases or Conditions
SWEET BAY ALLERGY: Because of contact dermatitis, sweet bay should be avoided in those having sensitivity to it.

Dosage and Administration
TOPICAL: An extract of sweet bay is typically used in baths and soaks (6002).
ORAL: No typical dosage.

Comments
The ancient Greeks and Romans crowned their victors with the leafy branches of sweet bay (11).

SWEET CICELY

Also Known As
British Myrrh, Shepherd's Needle, Sweet Bracken, Sweet Chervil, Sweet-Cus, Sweet-Fern, Sweet-Humlock, Sweets, The Roman Plant.

Scientific Names
Myrrhis odorata.
Family: Apiaceae/Umbelliferae.

Comments
At the date of publication, this product was not a common ingredient used in brand name supplements marketed to consumers. Details about this product are available in the online version of *Natural Medicines Comprehensive Database.* See www.naturaldatabase.com.

SWEET CLOVER

Also Known As
Common Melilot, Field Melilot, Hart's Tree, Hay Flower, King's Clover, Melilot, Meliloti herba, Melilotus, Sweet Lucerne, Sweet Melilot, Tall Melilot, Wild Laburnum, Yellow Melilot, Yellow Sweet Clover.
CAUTION: See separate listings for Red Clover.

Scientific Names
Melilotus altissimus, synonyms Melilotus macrorrhizus, Trifolium macrorrhizum; Melilotus officinalis, synonyms Melilotus arvensis, Melilotus vulgaris, Trifolium officinale.
Family: Fabaceae/Leguminosae.

People Use This For
Orally, sweet clover is used as a diuretic; and for symptoms of chronic venous insufficiency and varicose veins, including leg pain and heaviness, night cramps, pruritus and edema, supportive treatment of thrombophlebitis, hemorrhoids, post-thrombotic syndromes, and lymphatic congestion.
Topically, sweet clover is used for contusions and ecchymoses.

Safety
LIKELY SAFE ...when preparations of the flowering branch and leaf are used orally in moderate amounts (1,2,18).
LIKELY UNSAFE ...when excessive amounts are used orally because it can cause transient liver injury (18).
PREGNANCY: Insufficient reliable information available. A study of 30 second and third trimester pregnant women did not report any adverse effects (1).
LACTATION: Insufficient reliable information available; avoid using.

Effectiveness
POSSIBLY EFFECTIVE

Chronic venous insufficiency. Taking sweet clover orally seems to be effective for problems associated with chronic venous insufficiency such as varicose veins (1).

There is insufficient reliable information available about the effectiveness of sweet clover for its other uses.

Mechanism of Action
The applicable parts of sweet clover are the flowering branch and leaf. Fresh herb contains coumarinic acids (18), which are converted to free coumarins during drying (1,8,18). Dicoumarol, which has anticoagulant activity, can be formed if the fresh herb is allowed to spoil (1). There is some evidence to suggest that sweet clover aids wound healing (2,8), and a locally perfused sweet clover extract might eliminate adrenaline-induced vasoconstriction. This would indicate peripheral vasodilation (1). Coumarin isolated from sweet clover reduces experimentally-induced paw inflammation in rats (1). Intravenous administration decreases pain, edema, and improves wound healing in people with phlebitis, and relieves symptoms of varicose veins (1). Sweet clover seems to increase venous reflux and improve lymphatic kinetics, and therefore reduces edema (2).

Adverse Reactions
Orally, headaches are rare (1,2,18), and large amounts can cause stupor and transient liver injury in susceptible individuals (18). There was one case report of bleeding diathesis following two months ingestion of large amounts of a multi-herb, "seasonal tonic" tea containing melilot, sweet woodruff, and tonka bean (all coumarin-containing herbs) (809).

Interactions with Herbs & Other Dietary Supplements
HERBS WITH ANTICOAGULANT/ANTIPLATELET POTENTIAL: Concomitant use of herbs that have constituents that might affect platelet aggregation could theoretically increase the risk of bleeding in some people. These herbs include angelica, clove, danshen, garlic, ginger, ginkgo, Panax ginseng, horse chestnut, red clover, turmeric, and others.

Interactions with Drugs
ANTICOAGULANT/ANTIPLATELET DRUGS: Theoretically, concomitant use might increase bleeding risk (19).
HEPATOTOXIC DRUGS: Theoretically, concomitant use might increase risk of hepatotoxicity.

Interactions with Foods
None known.

Interactions with Lab Tests
LIVER ENZYMES: Sweet clover might cause an increase in liver enzymes and test results, indicating liver damage; monitor (18).

Interactions with Diseases or Conditions

LIVER DISEASE: Theoretically, sweet clover might exacerbate liver disease (see Adverse Reactions) (18); avoid using.

Dosage and Administration

ORAL: Average amount, sweet clover preparations equivalent to 3-30 mg coumarin per day (1,2). Phlebitis or varicose veins, one cup (made by steeping 1-2 teaspoons finely chopped sweet clover in 150 mL boiling water 5-10 minutes, strain) two to three cups per day (8,18); 6 mL Melilotus/rutin preparation (600 mg Melilotus extract containing 3 mg coumarin and 150 mg rutin) per day reported in one clinical trial (1). CAUTION: Monitor liver enzymes with oral use (18), especially in people at risk for liver damage.
TOPICAL: Sweet clover extract in semi-solid preparations containing 3-5 mg/g coumarin (2,8,18). As a poultice for sores and hemorrhoids, wrap sweet clover in linen, thoroughly soak with hot water, place on the affected area (8).
INJECTION: Liquid forms for parenteral use corresponding to 1-7.5 mg coumarin per day (2,8).

Comments

Avoid confusion with red clover (Trifolium pratense) and hay flower, the sieved flower and fruit from cut hay grass (Poaceae family) plants.

SWEET GALE

Also Known As

Bayberry, Bog Myrtle, Dutch Myrtle.
CAUTION: See separate listing for Bayberry.

Scientific Names

Myrica gale.
Family: Myricaceae.

People Use This For

Orally, sweet gale is used for digestive disorders.
In Sweden, a strong brew of sweet gale dried bark is used as an anthelmintic and to cure itching.

Safety

There is insufficient reliable information available about the safety of sweet gale. The volatile oil of sweet gale is considered toxic (18).
Pregnancy and Lactation: Insufficient reliable information available; avoid using.

Effectiveness

There is insufficient reliable information available about the effectiveness of sweet gale.

Mechanism of Action

The applicable parts of sweet gale are the leaf, branch, and wax from catkin. Sweet gale contains 0.4-0.7% of a volatile oil that contains alpha-pinene, delta-cadinene, gamma-cadinene, limonene, beta-myrcene, beta-phellandrene, and 1,8 cineole. It also contains flavonoids including myricitrin (18). Sweet gale is thought to have astringent and aromatic properties (18).

Adverse Reactions

Orally, the volatile oil is considered toxic.

Interactions with Herbs & Other Dietary Supplements

None known.

Interactions with Drugs

None known.

Interactions with Foods

None known.

Interactions with Lab Tests

None known.

Interactions with Diseases or Conditions

None known.

Dosage and Administration
No typical dosage.

Comments
In the Middle ages, sweet gale was mixed with beer, and is said to have led to periods of extreme excitation (18).

SWEET ORANGE

Also Known As
Citri Sinensis, Jaffa Orange, Navel Orange, Orange, Pericarpium, Valencia Orange.
CAUTION: See separate listings for Bergamot Oil, Oswego Tea, and Bitter Orange.

Scientific Names
Citrus sinensis, synonyms Citrus aurantium var. sinensis, Citrus macracantha, Citrus aurantium var. dulcis.
Family: Rutaceae.

People Use This For
Orally, the peel of sweet orange is used as an appetite stimulant. Sweet orange peel is also used to reduce phlegm, treat coughs, colds, anorexia, and malignant breast sores. It is also used as a tonic, antiflatulent, and for dyspepsia. In conjunction with other fruits and vegetables, sweet orange juice is used orally for the prevention of hypertension and stroke, and for the improvement of blood lipid profiles.

Safety
LIKELY SAFE ...when sweet orange juice or fruit is used orally in amounts commonly found in foods (1310,3340).
CHILDREN: LIKELY SAFE ...when sweet orange juice or fruit is used orally in amounts commonly found in foods. LIKELY UNSAFE ...when the sweet orange peel is used orally in excessive amounts. There are reports of intestinal colic, convulsions, and death in children given large amounts of sweet orange peel (11).
PREGNANCY AND LACTATION: LIKELY SAFE ...when sweet orange juice or fruit is used orally in amounts commonly found in foods (1310,3340).

Effectiveness
POSSIBLY EFFECTIVE

Hypercholesterolemia. Consuming sweet orange juice seems to help improve blood lipid profiles. Large amounts of orange juice (750 mL daily for four weeks) seems to increase high-density lipoprotein (HDL) cholesterol by 21%, and reduce the ratio of low-density lipoprotein (LDL) to HDL cholesterol by 16% in hypercholesterolemic patients. Because consumption of this large amount of juice daily consists of approximately 20% of the daily energy requirement, consuming a combination of fruits, vegetables, and orange juice in equivalent amounts to the 750 mL of orange juice on a daily basis is probably a more practical approach. However, this combination was not specifically studied (3340).

Hypertension and stroke. Consuming sweet orange juice seems to help lower the risk of hypertension and stroke. Sweet orange juice products that provide at least 350 mg of potassium per serving and are low in sodium, saturated fat, and cholesterol are permitted by the FDA to make labeling claims that they might reduce the risk of developing high blood pressure and stroke (1310).

INSUFFICIENT RELIABLE EVIDENCE to RATE

Asthma. There is some evidence that consumption of vitamin C-rich citrus fruits, including sweet orange and others, might improve lung function in people with asthma. However, this is controversial. Some studies show that intake of citrus fruits 1-2 times per week produces significant benefit (6049,6055,6056). However, other studies have not found this benefit (6057,6058). More evidence is needed to rate sweet orange for this use.

Mechanism of Action
The applicable parts of sweet orange are the peel, juice and fruit. Orange peel contains essential oil and bitter principles. Limonene is the most abundant monoterpene in sweet orange (4946). The flavonoid constituents naringin and nobiletin might have anti-inflammatory activity (1281). Potential benefits of sweet orange fruit in asthma have been attributed to antioxidant properties of vitamin C or other fruit constituents (6049,6054,6055). For preventing high blood pressure and stroke, sweet orange juice is thought to be beneficial due to high concentrations of potassium. Potassium consumption seems to reduce the risk of developing hypertension and stroke (1310).

There is conflicting data about the effects of sweet orange juice on P-glycoprotein. In animal models, an ethyl acetate extract of orange juice seems to inhibit drug efflux by P-glycoprotein. Theoretically, this would increase absorption of certain drugs that are transported by P-glycoprotein (12116). But in humans, drinking large amounts of sweet orange juice seems to decrease absorption and blood levels of celiprolol. This suggests that orange juice affects P-glycoprotein by actually inducing drug efflux by P-glycoprotein (12115). Other researchers speculate that sweet orange juice might inhibit the drug transporter organic anion transporting polypeptide (OATP) (7046). More

evidence is needed to determine sweet orange juice's effects on P-glycoprotein.
Sweet orange juice does not seem to affect cytochrome P450 3A4 (CYP3A4) (12116).

Adverse Reactions

There have been reports of intestinal colic, convulsions, and death in children following ingestion of large amounts of sweet orange peel (11).

Interactions with Herbs & Other Dietary Supplements

None known.

Interactions with Drugs

CELIPROLOL (Celicard): Sweet orange can decrease oral absorption and blood levels of celiprolol. Celiprolol levels, after a single dose of 100 mg, are decreased by about 80% to 90% in people who concurrently drink large amounts of sweet orange juice, 200 mL three times daily. It's not known if more moderate consumption of sweet orange juice affects celiprolol levels. Researchers theorize that this interaction might be due to sweet orange inhibiting the drug transporter in the gut, called organic anion transporting polypeptide (OATP), or inducing P-glycoprotein (12115).
FEXOFENADINE (Allegra): Sweet orange juice can significantly decrease oral absorption and blood levels of fexofenadine when used together. Sweet orange decreases bioavailability of fexofenadine by about 72%. Sweet orange juice seems to inhibit organic anion transporting polypeptide (OATP), which is a drug transporter in the gut, liver, and kidney (7046). It's not yet known how long sweet orange juice inhibits OATP. Separating administration times might not prevent this interaction. Tell patients it's best to take their medications with a plain glass of water.
IVERMECTIN: Taking ivermectin orally with sweet orange juice 750 mL over 4 hours seems to significantly reduce the bioavailability of ivermectin. This effect does not seem to be related to effects on p-glycoprotein. The effect on ivermectin is more pronounced in males compared to females (12154).

Interactions with Foods

None known.

Interactions with Lab Tests

None known.

Interactions with Diseases or Conditions

None known.

Dosage and Administration

ORAL: For improving lipid profiles, 750 mL sweet orange juice per day has been used (3340).
For appetite stimulation or as a digestive aid, 10-15 grams fresh or dry peel (free of white pulp layer) per day has been used (2). Peel may be used to prepare a tea (steep peel in boiling water 10-15 minutes, strain) or in other herbal preparations (2).

SWEET SUMACH

Also Known As

Aromatic Sumac, Fragrant Sumac, Polecatbush, Skunkbrush, Squawbush.

Scientific Names

Rhus aromatica, synonym Rhus canadensis.
Family: Anacardiaceae.

Comments

At the date of publication, there was very little scientific information available about this product. Our staff is continually analyzing the available information on natural medicines and will add data to the online version of *Natural Medicines Comprehensive Database* as it becomes available. See www.naturaldatabase.com.

SWEET VERNAL GRASS

Also Known As
Grass, Spring Grass.

Scientific Names
Anthoxanthum odoratum.
Family: Poaceae/Gramineae.

People Use This For
Orally, sweet vernal grass is used for headache, nausea, sleeplessness, and conditions of the urinary tract.
In Russia, sweet vernal grass is used as an ingredient in certain brandies.
In foods, sweet vernal grass is used as a flavoring agent.

Safety
LIKELY UNSAFE ...when used orally. Sweet vernal grass contains the constituent, dicoumarol that has anticoagulant properties (6,18).
There is insufficient reliable information available about the safety of the topical use of sweet vernal grass.
PREGNANCY AND LACTATION: LIKELY UNSAFE ...when used orally (6,18): avoid using.

Effectiveness
There is insufficient reliable information available about the effectiveness of sweet vernal grass.

Mechanism of Action
Sweet vernal grass contains hydroxycinnamic acid glycosides that form dicoumarol (up to 1.5%) when the harvested plant is dehydrated (18). After an outbreak of hemorrhagic diathesis in cattle fed sweet vernal grass hay, veterinary experiments identified dicumarol, a known anticoagulant, in the hay (6).

Adverse Reactions
Orally, use of high levels of sweet vernal grass can cause headaches and dizziness (18). Cattle poisoned by sweet vernal hay showed characteristically rapid onset of symptoms including progressive weakness, mucosal pallor, stiff gait, tachypnea, tachycardia, and hematomata, quickly resulting in death (6).

Interactions with Herbs & Other Dietary Supplements
HERBS WITH ANTICOAGULANT/ANTIPLATELET POTENTIAL: Concomitant use with herbs that have constituents that might affect platelet aggregation could theoretically increase the risk of bleeding in some people. These herbs include angelica, clove, danshen, garlic, ginger, ginkgo, Panax ginseng, horse chestnut, red clover, turmeric, and others.

Interactions with Drugs
ANTICOAGULANT/ANTIPLATELET DRUGS: Theoretically, sweet vernal grass might cause additive effects and side effects with drugs having anticoagulant or antiplatelet properties (19).

Interactions with Foods
None known.

Interactions with Lab Tests
None known.

Interactions with Diseases or Conditions
None known.

Dosage and Administration
ORAL: No typical dosage.
TOPICAL: Sweet vernal grass is sometimes used as an extract (18).

Comments
This aromatic plant has been used as a flavoring agent due to its vanilla-like aroma (6).

SWEET VIOLET

Also Known As
Banafshah, Garden Violet, Neelapushpa, Neelapuspha, Sweet Violet Herb, Sweet Violet Root, Violae Odoratae Rhizoma.
CAUTION: See separate listing for Garden Violet.

Scientific Names
Viola odorata.
Family: Violaceae.

People Use This For
Orally, sweet violet is used for calming and relaxing nerves, physical and mental exhaustion, physical and psychological symptoms associated with menopause (hot flashes), metabolic imbalances, and to "detoxify blood". It is also used orally for depression, irritability, anxiety, GI complaints, abdominal pain, gallbladder complaints, mucous membrane inflammation of the stomach and intestines, enteritis, duodenitis, digestion problems caused by improper diet, flatulence, heartburn, and loss of appetite , respiratory tract conditions, particularly dry mucous membrane inflammation, rheumatism of the minor joints, fever, skin diseases, inflammation of the oral mucosa, nervous strain, headache, and insomnia, coughs, hoarseness, tuberculosis, throat inflammation, bronchitis accompanied by fixed mucous, nervous strain, insomnia, and hysteria.
Topically, sweet violet is used for skin impurities and disorders, and as a skin cleanser.
In herbal combinations, sweet violet is used for acute and chronic bronchitis, bronchial asthma, acute and chronic mucous inflammations of the upper and lower respiratory tract, cold symptoms of the upper respiratory tract, hoarseness, cough, mucous congestion, bronchial inflammation, and late "flu" symptoms. It is also used for chesty, spastic and whooping coughs, emphysema, "dust-damaged" lung, urinary incontinence due to senility, irritable bladder, enuresis nocturna or prostate condition, insomnia, and improving deep sleep.

Safety
POSSIBLY SAFE ...when used orally in appropriate amounts (2,18).
There is insufficient reliable information available about the safety of the topical use of sweet violet.
PREGNANCY AND LACTATION: Insufficient reliable information available; avoid using.

Effectiveness
There is insufficient reliable information available about the effectiveness of sweet violet.

Mechanism of Action
The applicable parts of sweet violet are the root and above ground parts. Sweet violet contains saponins (2), which have expectorant properties, and in high doses irritate mucous membranes (2).

Adverse Reactions
None reported.

Interactions with Herbs & Other Dietary Supplements
None known.

Interactions with Drugs
None known.

Interactions with Foods
None known.

Interactions with Lab Tests
None known.

Interactions with Diseases or Conditions
None known.

Dosage and Administration
ORAL: The typical dose of sweet violet as an herb is one cup tea (steep 2 teaspoons herb in 250 mL boiling water 10-15 minutes, strain) 2-3 times daily (18). As a root (5% w/v), take 1 tablespoon 5-6 times daily (simmer 20 grams in boiling water for 10-15 minutes, and strain) (18).
TOPICAL: No typical dosage.

SWEET WOODRUFF

Also Known As
Galii odorati herba, Master of the Wood, Waldmeister, Woodruff, Wordward.

Scientific Names
Galium odorata, synonym Asperula odorata.
Family: Rubiaceae.

People Use This For
Orally, sweet woodruff is used for preventing and treating respiratory tract, gastrointestinal tract, liver, gallbladder, and urinary tract disorders; for blood purification; venous complaints; weak veins; hemorrhoids; vasodilation; spasms; abdominal discomforts; strengthening the nervous system; agitation; hysteria; nervous menstrual disorders; restlessness; insomnia; neuralgia; strengthening heart function; cardiac irregularity; stomachache; migraine; and bladder stones. Sweet woodruff is also used orally for inducing sweating, as an antispasmodic, diuretic, or expectorant.
Topically, sweet woodruff is used for skin diseases, treating wounds, venous conditions, hemorrhoids, and for reducing inflammation.
In foods and beverages, sweet woodruff is used as a flavoring component.
In manufacturing, the extracts of sweet woodruff above ground parts are used as fragrance components in perfumes.

Safety
LIKELY SAFE ...when used orally in amounts commonly found in foods. Sweet woodruff has Generally Recognized As Safe status (GRAS) for use in foods in the US (4912).
POSSIBLY SAFE ...when used orally and appropriately for medicinal uses on a short-term basis (12,18).
There is insufficient reliable information available about the safety of the topical use of sweet woodruff.
PREGNANCY AND LACTATION: Insufficient reliable information available; avoid using.

Effectiveness
There is insufficient reliable information available about the effectiveness of sweet woodruff.

Mechanism of Action
The applicable parts of sweet woodruff are the above ground parts. Sweet woodruff leaves and the constituent asperuloside show evidence of anti-inflammatory activity (11). Sweet woodruff also demonstrates antibacterial activity (4009). The fresh plant contains up to 1% coumarin as a bound glycoside. Coumarin is supposedly enzymatically released during dehydration (11). Interestingly, one investigation failed to detect any coumarins in sweet woodruff (11). The coumarin constituent is thought to have anti-inflammatory, anti-edema, spasmolytic, and lymphokinetic effects, but the levels found in sweet woodruff are so low that therapeutic effects are doubtful (18). Other constituents present in sweet woodruff include monotopein, tannins, anthracene and naphthalene derivatives, plus traces of nicotinic acid, a fixed oil, and a bitter principle (11).

Adverse Reactions
Orally, sweet woodruff above ground parts can be associated with headache (12), and in larger amounts, stupor (18). Long-term use can cause liver damage (18).

Interactions with Herbs & Other Dietary Supplements
None known.

Interactions with Drugs
None known.

Interactions with Foods
None known.

Interactions with Lab Tests
None known.

Interactions with Diseases or Conditions
None known.

Dosage and Administration
ORAL: A typical dose is one cup tea. To make tea, use 2 teaspoons (1.8 grams) in a glass of water (18). The average single-dose is 1 gram during the day or shortly before bedtime (18).
TOPICAL: No typical dosage.

Comments
Sweet woodruff root contains a red dye (6). Sweet woodruff is considered obsolete for medicinal use in many countries (18). Avoid confusing sweet woodruff, Galium odoratum, with Asperula odorata which is also referred to as woodruff.

TAGETES

Also Known As
African Marigold, Aztec Marigold, Big Marigold, Chinchilla Enana, Dwarf Marigold, French Marigold, Huacatay, Marigold, Mexican Marigold, Muster John Henry, Saffron Marigold, Stinking Roger.
CAUTION: See separate listing for Calendula.

Scientific Names
Tagetes erecta; Tagetes minuta, synonym Tagetes glandulifera; Tagetes patula.
Family: Asteraceae/Compositae.

People Use This For
Orally, tagetes is used as an anthelmintic, a menstrual flow stimulant, and for treating colic. Tagetes is also used orally for treating coughs, colds, mumps, mastitis, sore eyes, and dysentery.
Additionally, tagetes is used orally for improving digestion, inducing sweating, as an antiflatulent, sedative in gastric pain, bile flow and appetite stimulant, diuretic, and as an anti-abortifacient.
Topically, the leaves are used for treating sores and ulcers; and the flowers are used as a mosquito repellent. The juice of the leaves are used topically for eczema; and the oil is used for treating wound maggots.
In foods and beverages, tagetes is used as a flavor component.
In manufacturing, the oil is used as a fragrance in perfumes. The dried, ground flowers are used as chicken feed to enhance the characteristic yellow color of chicken skin and egg yolk.

Safety
LIKELY SAFE ...when used orally in amounts commonly found in foods. Tagetes has Generally Recognized As Safe (GRAS) status in the US (4912).
There is insufficient reliable information available about the safety of tagetes used in amounts greater than those found in foods.
PREGNANCY AND LACTATION: Insufficient reliable information available; avoid amounts greater than those commonly found in foods.

Effectiveness
There is insufficient reliable information available about the effectiveness of tagetes.

Mechanism of Action
The applicable parts of tagetes are the above ground parts. Some evidence suggests tagetes oil might have tranquilizing, hypotensive, bronchodilatory, spasmolytic, and anti-inflammatory properties (11). The constituent ocimenone demonstrates cidal activity against mosquito larvae (11). Alpha-terthienyl exhibits nematocidal and larvicidal activity (11). Patulin has demonstrated antispasmodic activity; and may reduce capillary permeability, and increase blood pressure (11).

Adverse Reactions
Topically, tagetes can cause contact dermatitis (11). Tagetes can also cause an allergic reaction in individuals sensitive to the Asteraceae/Compositae family. Members of this family include ragweed, chrysanthemums, marigolds, daisies, and many other herbs.

Interactions with Herbs & Other Dietary Supplements
None known.

Interactions with Drugs
None known.

Interactions with Foods
None known.

Interactions with Lab Tests
None known.

Interactions with Diseases or Conditions

CROSS-ALLERGENICITY: Tagetes can cause an allergic reaction in individuals sensitive to the Asteraceae/Compositae family. Members of this family include ragweed, chrysanthemums, marigolds, daisies, and many other herbs.

Dosage and Administration

No typical dosage.

Comments

Tagetes oil is distilled from the above ground parts of Tagetes erecta, minuta, and patula (11).

TAMARIND

Also Known As

Imlee, Tamarindo.
CAUTION: See separate listing for Garcinia.

Scientific Names

Tamarindus indica.
Family: Fabaceae/Leguminosae.

People Use This For

Orally, tamarind is used for chronic or acute constipation, liver and gallbladder disorders, to decrease fever, to treat pregnancy-related nausea, as an anthelmintic for children, for stomach disorders, and to treat colds.
Topically, a thick paste of the seeds is used as a cast for broken bones.
In foods and beverages, tamarind is used as a flavoring agent. It is also widely used in Asian cuisine for chutneys and curries.

Safety

LIKELY SAFE ...when used orally in amounts commonly found in foods. Tamarind has Generally Recognized As Safe (GRAS) status in the US (4912).
There is insufficient reliable information available about the safety of tamarind used in amounts greater than those found in food.
PREGNANCY AND LACTATION: Insufficient reliable information available; avoid using in amounts greater than those found in foods.

Effectiveness

There is insufficient reliable information available about the effectiveness of tamarind.

Mechanism of Action

The partially dried, fruit/pod of tamarind is used medicinally. It contains plant acids, largely d-tartaric acid, sugars, pectin, protein, vitamins, and minerals. The volatile oil contains over 60 compounds including methyl salicylate and safrole. The fruit pulp has mild laxative properties, but heat causes loss of this effect. Some evidence suggests an aqueous extract is highly toxic to the trematode Schistosoma mansoni, and the parasite-carrying snail Bulinus trucatus. Other evidence suggests that the tamarind constituent, tamarindienal might have antifungal activity against Aspergillus niger and Candida albicans, and antibacterial activity against Bacillus subtilis, Staphylococcus aureus, Escherichia coli, and Pseudomonas aeruginosa (11).

Adverse Reactions

None reported.

Interactions with Herbs & Other Dietary Supplements

None known.

Interactions with Drugs

ASPIRIN: Taking tamarind fruit extract as a component of the food millet porridge concurrently with aspirin seems to increase aspirin absorption and blood levels (12187). Theoretically, this could increase the risk of aspirin side effects.
IBUPROFEN: Taking tamarind fruit extract as a component of the food millet porridge concurrently with ibuprofen seems to increase ibuprofen absorption and blood levels (12093). Theoretically, this could increase the risk of ibuprofen side effects.

Interactions with Foods
None known.

Interactions with Lab Tests
None known.

Interactions with Diseases or Conditions
None known.

Dosage and Administration
ORAL: As a laxative, 10-50 grams of tamarind paste is used orally as fruit cubes (18). This is a paste prepared from the fermented fruit of Tamarindus indica (18).
TOPICAL: No typical dosage.

TANNIC ACID

Also Known As
None.

Scientific Names
Tannic acid.

People Use This For
Topically, tannic acid is used for cold sores and fever blisters, diaper rash and prickly heat, poison ivy, ingrown toenails, sore throat, inflamed tonsils, spongy or receding gums, acute dermatitis, and as a styptic. Tannic acid is used orally and topically for bleeding, chronic diarrhea, dysentery, bloody urine, painful joints, persistent coughs, and cancer.
Vaginally, tannic acid is used as a douche for leukorrhea. In foods and beverages, tannic acid is used as a flavoring agent.
In manufacturing, tannic acid is used in hemorrhoidal ointments and suppositories, for tanning hides and manufacturing ink, and to kill dust mites on furniture.

Safety
LIKELY SAFE ...when used orally in amounts commonly found in foods. Tannic acid has Generally Recognized As Safe (GRAS) status in the US (4912).
POSSIBLY UNSAFE ...when used topically to treat diaper rash and prickly heat (272), and minor burn or sunburn (272).
There is insufficient reliable information available about the safety of the topical use of tannic acid to treat cold sores and fever blisters. The FDA's concern about potential oral absorption and toxicity has prompted requests for further data (272).
PREGNANCY AND LACTATION: LIKELY UNSAFE ...when used topically on damaged skin or large areas of skin (2). There is insufficient reliable information available about the safety of the oral use of tannic acid during pregnancy and lactation; avoid using amounts greater than those found in foods.

Effectiveness
POSSIBLY INEFFECTIVE
Burns. Applying tannic acid doesn't seem to be effective for treating minor burn or sunburn (272).
Diaper rash. Applying tannic acid doesn't seem to be effective for treating diaper rash (272).
Herpes labialis (cold sores). Applying tannic acid doesn't seem to be effective for treating cold sores and fever blisters (272).
Prickly heat. Applying tannic acid doesn't seem to be effective for treating prickly heat (272).
There is insufficient reliable information available about the effectiveness of tannic acid for its other uses.

Mechanism of Action
Tannic acid is a mixture of glycosides of phenolics, mainly gallic acid (11). Pharmaceutical grade tannic acid is generally considered to be pentadigalloylglucose (11). Tannic acid has astringent effects (11,12). It dehydrates tissue, internally reducing secretions, and externally forming a protective layer of harder, constricted cells (12). Tannins show some evidence of antiviral, antimicrobial, CNS depressant, and cariostatic effects (11). Some evidence suggests that tannins might cause cancer, but other evidence shows tannins might prevent it (12). Regular consumption of herbs with high tannin concentrations correlates with increased incidence of esophageal or nasal cancer (12).

Adverse Reactions
Orally, large amounts of tannic acid can cause gastric irritation, nausea, and vomiting (11). Tannins have been associated with fatal liver damage from extensive use on burns or in enemas (11). However, the toxicity may be due to an impurity, digallic acid, rather than the tannins themselves (11).

Interactions with Herbs & Other Dietary Supplements
TANNIN-CONTAINING HERBS: Theoretically, herbs that contain high percentages of tannins (such as oak bark) might precipitate alkaloids and other alkaline constituents of herbs (19).

Interactions with Drugs
ORAL DRUGS: Theoretically, avoid concomitant administration due to potential of tannic acid to precipitate alkaloids and other basic drugs (19). Separate administration of oral drugs and tannic acid by the longest period of time practical (19).

Interactions with Foods
None known.

Interactions with Lab Tests
None known.

Interactions with Diseases or Conditions
KIDNEY DYSFUNCTION: Theoretically, oral use of tannic acid is contraindicated in individuals with kidney dysfunction. Tannic acid can cause kidney damage, potentially exacerbating a pre-existing condition (12).
LIVER DYSFUNCTION: Theoretically, oral use of tannic acid is contraindicated in individuals with liver dysfunction. Tannic acid can cause liver damage, potentially exacerbating a pre-existing condition (12).
PRE-EXISTING CONDITIONS: Theoretically, full baths are contraindicated in individuals with fever or infectious diseases, NYHA III and IV heart failure, or hypertonia stage IV (WHO) (2).
SKIN CONDITIONS: Full baths with tannic acid tea are contraindicated in individuals with weeping eczema and extensive skin damage (12).

Dosage and Administration
No typical dosage.

Comments
New York Heart Association (NYHA) stage I and II heart disease refers to people with heart disease without resulting limitations of physical activity and who are comfortable at rest and in whom ordinary physical activity results in fatigue, palpitation, trouble breathing, or anginal pain (2). Tannic acid is extracted from the nutgalls formed on twigs of certain oak trees by insects (Quercus infectoria and other Quercus species). The "universal antidote", formerly used for poisoning, contained tannic acid, activated charcoal, and magnesium oxide. These three ingredients in combination were believed to synergistically reduce the absorption of poisons. Unfortunately, tannic acid was instead adsorbed by activated charcoal, which diminished the benefit of the combination (272).

TANSY

Also Known As
Bitter Buttons, Buttons, Chrysanthemi vulgaris flos, Chrysanthemi vulgaris herba, Daisy, Hind Heal, Parsley Fern, Tansy Flower, Tansy Herb, Scented Fern, Stinking Willie.
CAUTION: See separate listing for Wood Sage.

Scientific Names
Tanacetum vulgare, synonyms Chrysanthemum vulgare, Tanacetum boreale.
Family: Asteraceae/Compositae.

People Use This For
Orally, tansy is used as an abortifacient, as an anthelmintic for roundworm or threadworm infestation in children, migraines, neuralgia, epilepsy, rheumatism, improving digestion and stimulating appetite, as an antispasmodic, for flatulence, bloating due to intestinal or peritoneal gas, stomach and duodenal ulcers, noninflammatory gallbladder conditions, palpitation, sciatica, stomachache, edema associated with weak heart, colds, fever, hysteria, calming nerves, gout, kidney problems, and tuberculosis. Tansy is also used as an antioxidant, antiseptic, bactericide, cordial, emmenagogue, diaphoretic, narcotic, pediculicide, tonic, and stimulant.
Topically, tansy is used for scabies, pruritus ani, bruises, sores, sprains, swelling, freckles, inflammation, leukorrhea, sunburn, swelling, toothache, tumors, and as an insect repellent.

In foods and manufacturing, tansy extracts are used in perfume, as a flavoring agent in foods and beverages, and a source of green dye.

Safety

POSSIBLY UNSAFE ...when used topically. Tansy can cause severe contact dermatitis (6,18,19).
LIKELY UNSAFE ...when varieties containing the toxic constituent thujone are used orally (2,6,515). Fatalities have been associated with ingestion of as little as 10 drops of tansy oil, although one individual recovered after ingesting 15 mL (6). Fatalities have also been reported from prepared teas or powdered forms (4,6). However, thujone concentration varies widely amongst tansy species (4,6,515).
PREGNANCY: LIKELY UNSAFE ...when used topically due to potential abortifacient, menstrual flow, and uterine stimulant effects (12,19).
LACTATION: POSSIBLY UNSAFE ...when used topically due to thujone content (2,6).

Effectiveness

There is insufficient reliable information available about the effectiveness of tansy.

Mechanism of Action

The applicable parts of tansy are the above ground parts. The activity and toxicity of the above ground parts of tansy vary greatly according to the subspecies (515). Thujone, a constituent with both activity and toxicity ranging from a concentration of 0-95% in the volatile oil (4,515). The thujone constituent causes an increase in salivation and an increase in blood flow to the mucous membranes and pelvic viscera (7). Researchers think thujone has a mind-altering effect similar to tetrahydrocannabinol (THC), the active principle in marijuana (515). Thujone also shows evidence of neurotoxicity (2), hepatotoxicity, and it might be harmful to individuals with defects in hepatic heme synthesis (4,12). Chronic thujone poisoning leads to seizures, delirium, and hallucinations (7). Tansy extracts have demonstrated effects in alleviating pain, stimulating bile, and increasing appetite in individuals with liver and gallbladder disorders (4). Some evidence suggests tansy extracts might also have antispasmodic activity (4). Other evidence suggests the constituent, caffeic acid, might have a role in the bile-stimulating effects (4). Tansy shows evidence that it might reduce serum lipid levels and has some hypoglycemic effects (4). Tansy demonstrates antifungal activity (4). Some evidence suggests tansy oil has antibacterial activity (6). In addition, tansy oil, ether extract, and the constituent beta-thujone show evidence of anthelmintic activity (4). Aqueous extracts of tansy can partially inactivate tick-borne encephalitis in vitro. They also induce resistance in experimental animals (6). Preliminary studies suggest tansy has some antitumor effects (4). The constituents believed to be responsible for allergic contact dermatitis are the sesquiterpene lactones (4,6,19).

Adverse Reactions

Orally, large amounts of thujone or using thujone-containing products long-term can cause restlessness, vomiting, vertigo, tremors, renal damage, and convulsions (12). Symptoms of toxicity include rapid, feeble pulse (4,6), severe gastroenteritis (2), severe spasms (4), convulsions (2,4), rapid breathing (2), vomiting, abdominal pain, facial flushing, loss of consciousness, irregular heartbeat, dilated pupils, pupillary rigidity, uterine bleeding, abortion, kidney damage, and liver damage (2,18). Death can occur 1-3.5 hours after ingestion (18).
Topically, tansy is associated with severe contact dermatitis (6,19) and local mucosal membrane irritation (19). It can cause an allergic reaction in individuals sensitive to the Asteraceae/Compositae family. Members of this family include ragweed, chrysanthemums, marigolds, daisies, and many other herbs.

Interactions with Herbs & Other Dietary Supplements

THUJONE-CONTAINING HERBS: Concomitant use of herbs containing thujone can increase the risk of thujone toxicity. Thujone-containing herbs include oak moss, oriental arborvitae, sage, wormwood, thuja (cedar), and tree moss (12); avoid using.

Interactions with Drugs

ALCOHOL (Ethanol): The constituent, thujone, heightens and alters the effect of alcohol (7).

Interactions with Foods

None known.

Interactions with Lab Tests

None known.

Interactions with Diseases or Conditions

CROSS-ALLERGENICITY: Tansy can cause an allergic reaction in individuals sensitive to the Asteraceae/Compositae family. Members of this family include ragweed, chrysanthemums, marigolds, daisies, and many other herbs.
PORPHYRIA: Theoretically, tansy can exacerbate porphyria in people with underlying defects in hepatic heme synthesis (12).

Dosage and Administration

No typical dosage.

Comments

The name tansy is derived from the Greek word, athanasia, for immortality. Tansy was thought to impart mortality and it was used for embalming (6). Avoid confusion with tansy ragwort (Senecio species) and other plants generically referred to as "tansy".

TANSY RAGWORT

Also Known As

Cankerwort, Common Ragwort, Dog Standard, European Ragwort, Ragweed, Ragwort, St. James' Wort, Staggerwort, Stammerwort, Stinking Nanny.
CAUTION: See separate listings for Alpine Ragwort, Golden Ragwort, and Tansy.

Scientific Names

Senecio jacobaea.
Family: Asteraceae/Compositae.

People Use This For

Orally, tansy ragwort is used for cancer, colic, wound-healing, spasms, as a laxative, to induce sweating and menstruation, and for "cleansing and purification."
Topically, tansy ragwort is used for muscle and joint pain.

Safety

LIKELY UNSAFE ...when products containing hepatotoxic pyrrolizidine alkaloid (PA) constituents are used orally. Repeated exposure to low concentrations of hepatotoxic PAs can cause severe veno-occlusive disease. Hepatotoxic PAs might also be carcinogenic and mutagenic (12841,12842). Tell patients not to use tansy ragwort preparations that are not certified and labeled as hepatotoxic PA-free. ...when products containing hepatotoxic PAs are used topically on abraded or broken skin. Absorption of hepatotoxic PAs through broken skin can lead to systemic toxicities (12841). Tell patients not to use topical tansy ragwort preparations that are not certified and labeled as hepatotoxic PA-free. There is insufficient reliable information available about the safety of using topical PA-free tansy ragwort on unbroken skin.
PREGNANCY: LIKELY UNSAFE ...when used orally. Tansy ragwort preparations containing hepatotoxic pyrrolizidine alkaloid (PA) constituents might be teratogenic and hepatotoxic (12841,12842). There is insufficient reliable information available about the safety of using tansy ragwort products that do not contain hepatotoxic PAs during pregnancy.
LACTATION: LIKELY UNSAFE ...when used orally. Hepatotoxic pyrrolizidine alkaloid (PA) constituents in tansy ragwort are excreted in milk (12841,12842). There is insufficient reliable information available about the safety of using tansy ragwort products that do not contain hepatotoxic PAs during lactation.

Effectiveness

There is insufficient reliable information available about the effectiveness of tansy ragwort.

Mechanism of Action

The applicable parts of tansy ragwort are the above ground flowering parts.
Tansy ragwort contains various pyrrolizidine alkaloids (PA), some of which are toxic. PAs are most concentrated in the plant roots, but may be found in all plant parts. PAs, particularly unsaturated PAs, can cause hepatotoxicity. Cyclic diesters such as retrorsine and senecionine are the most hepatotoxic. Liver toxicity may result from PA-enhanced oxidative stress, but the exact mechanism of toxicity is unknown. Single doses of 10-20 mg PAs or chronic ingestion of amounts less than 10 mcg can cause veno-occlusive disease. PAs are metabolized by cytochrome P450 3A4 (CYP3A4) to toxic dehydroalkaloids and pyrroles. Enzyme inducers such as phenobarbital seem to enhance toxicity (12841,12860). Pyrroles are excreted as N-acetyl cysteine conjugates. Some researchers speculate that early administration of N-acetylcysteine might reduce toxicity (11988).
Metabolism is also affected by pregnane X receptor induction of CYP3A4. Genetic or drug induced variation in CYP3A4 or pregnane X receptor activity can affect the degree of PA toxicity by increasing or decreasing its metabolism (12841,12842). Hepatotoxic PAs are also toxic to the lungs. In animals, pneumotoxicity occurs as pulmonary hypertension and right ventricular hypertrophy. Hepatotoxic PAs are carcinogenic and mutagenic. There are sufficient amounts of hepatotoxic PAs in herbal products to cause toxicity (12841,12842).

Adverse Reactions

Orally, the major concern about tansy ragwort preparations is the hepatotoxic pyrrolizidine alkaloid (PA) content. These constituents are hepatotoxic, pneumotoxic, carcinogenic and mutagenic (12841,12842). Chronic exposure to other

plants containing hepatotoxic PA constituents is associated with veno-occlusive disease (4021). Subacute veno-occlusive disease causes vague symptoms with persistent liver enlargement (4021). Symptoms of acute veno-occlusive disease include colicky pains in epigastrium, vomiting and diarrhea, and ascites formation within several days. Enlargement and induration of the liver occurs within a few weeks (12842). Dietary supplements sold in the US are not required to include the amount of PAs they contain (3484); therefore, all preparations used orally containing tansy ragwort should be considered potentially unsafe.
Theoretically, tansy ragwort might cause an allergic reaction in individuals sensitive to the Asteraceae/Compositae family (12842). Members of this family include ragweed, chrysanthemums, marigolds, daisies, and many other herbs.

Interactions with Herbs & Other Dietary Supplements

HEPATOTOXIC PYRROLIZIDINE ALKALOID (PA)-CONTAINING HERBS: Concomitant use is contraindicated due to the risk of additive toxicity. Herbs containing hepatotoxic PAs include alkanna, borage, butterbur, coltsfoot, comfrey, gravel root, groundsel, hound's tongue, and lungwort; and the Senecio species plants dusty miller, ragwort, golden ragwort, and tansy ragwort (12841).
HERBS THAT INDUCE CYTOCHROME P450 3A4 (CYP3A4): Theoretically herbs that induce CYP3A4 might increase the conversion of hepatotoxic PAs to toxic metabolites, enhancing toxicity (12841,12860). Herbs that induce CYP3A4 include St. John's wort and garlic.

Interactions with Drugs

CYTOCHROME P450 3A4 (CYP3A4) INDUCERS: Hepatotoxic pyrrolizidine alkaloids (PA) are substrates of cytochrome P450 3A4 (CYP3A4) (12841,12860). Theoretically, drugs that induce CYP3A4 might increase the conversion of PAs to toxic metabolites. Some drugs that induce CYP3A4 include carbamazepine (Tegretol), phenobarbital, phenytoin (Dilantin), rifampin, rifabutin (Mycobutin), and others.

Interactions with Foods

None known.

Interactions with Lab Tests

None known.

Interactions with Diseases or Conditions

CROSS-ALLERGENICITY: Theoretically, tansy ragwort might cause an allergic reaction in individuals sensitive to the Asteraceae/Compositae family (12842). Members of this family include ragweed, chrysanthemums, marigolds, daisies, and many other herbs.
LIVER DISEASE: Theoretically, pyrrolizidine alkaloids (PA) might exacerbate liver disease (12841,12842).

Dosage and Administration

No typical dosage.

TARRAGON

Also Known As

Estragon, Little Dragon, Mugwort.
CAUTION: See separate listing for Mugwort (Artemisia vulgaris).

Scientific Names

Artemisia dracunculus, synonym Artemisia glauca.
Family: Asteraceae/Compositae.

People Use This For

Orally, tarragon is used for digestive disorders, toothache, to promote menstruation, as a diuretic, appetite stimulant, and hypnotic.
In foods and beverages, tarragon is used as a culinary herb and a flavor component.
In manufacturing, tarragon is used as a fragrance component in soaps and cosmetics.

Safety

LIKELY SAFE ...when used orally in amounts commonly found in foods. Tarragon has Generally Recognized As Safe (GRAS) status in the US (4912).
POSSIBLY SAFE ...when used orally short-term in medicinal amounts (12).
POSSIBLY UNSAFE ...when used orally, long-term due to estragole, which can be carcinogenic (12).
PREGNANCY AND LACTATION: LIKELY UNSAFE ...when used in medicinal amounts due to possible menstrual promoting effects (11); avoid using.

Effectiveness
There is insufficient reliable information available about the effectiveness of tarragon.

Mechanism of Action
The applicable parts of tarragon are the above ground parts. Estragole is the main constituent of tarragon's essential oil (81%). The constituent estragole is a procarcinogen but the carcinogenic risk is minimal. It is not directly hepatotoxic or hepatocarcinogenic, but requires activation by liver enzymes to reach full toxicity. In the liver, other enzymes inactivate the carcinogenic metabolites, limiting possible damage to the liver (12). Tarragon shows evidence of antibacterial activity, but estragole does not appear to be responsible. Some information suggests undiluted tarragon oil can irritate the skin, but a concentration of 4% in petrolatum appears to be nonirritating and nonsensitizing (11).

Adverse Reactions
Tarragon can cause an allergic reaction in individuals sensitive to the Asteraceae/Compositae family. Members of this family include ragweed, chrysanthemums, marigolds, daisies, and many other herbs.

Interactions with Herbs & Other Dietary Supplements
None known.

Interactions with Drugs
None known.

Interactions with Foods
None known.

Interactions with Lab Tests
None known.

Interactions with Diseases or Conditions
CROSS-ALLERGENICITY: Can cause an allergic reaction in individuals sensitive to the Asteraceae/Compositae family. Members of this family include ragweed, chrysanthemums, marigolds, daisies, and many other herbs.

Dosage and Administration
No typical dosage.

Comments
Tarragon is also known as mugwort. Be careful not confuse it with mugwort (Artemisia vulgaris). Tarragon is a rich plant source of potassium (19). Adulteration of tarragon oil is common (11).

TAUMELLOOLCH

Also Known As
Bearded Darnel, Cheat, Darnel, Drake, Ray-Grass, Tare.

Scientific Names
Lolium temulentum.
Family: Poaceae/Gramineae.

People Use This For
Orally, taumelloolch is used for blood poisoning, cancer, cysts, dizziness, eczema, hemorrhage, idiocy, indurations, "knots", leprosy, gangrene, migraine, headache, nerve pain, nose bleeds, putrid flesh, sleeplessness, stomach cramps, involuntary dyskinetic movements, neuralgia, rheumatism, and sciatica, toothache, tumors, meningitis, urinary incontinence, and colic.
Topically, taumelloolch is used as a poultice for skin diseases, to draw out splinters, and for broken bones.

Safety
LIKELY UNSAFE ...when used orally. Symptoms of toxicity range from confusion and giddiness to weakness and death from respiratory failure (18,4502).
There is insufficient reliable information available about the safety of the topical use of taumelloolch.
PREGNANCY AND LACTATION: LIKELY UNSAFE ...when used orally (18,4502); avoid using.

Effectiveness
There is insufficient reliable information available about the effectiveness of taumelloolch.

Mechanism of Action

The applicable part of taumelloolch is the seed. The active agents of taumelloolch are temulentin, temultin acid, tannin, and glycoside (18). It has analgesic and narcotic properties, as well as toxicity (4502). Poisoning has been reported from ingestion of the grain, the berries mixed with grains, and the seed infected with a bacterial toxin (18,4502). To date, the toxic principle has not been identified (18,4502). No cases of poisonings have been reported in recent times, although the plant has become extremely rare through intensive seed-corn purification (18).

Adverse Reactions

Symptoms of taumelloolch toxicity include colic, confusion, giddiness, weakness, dizziness, dilated pupils, headache, confusion, staggering, somnolence, trembling, vision and speech disorders, vomiting, delirium, and death from respiratory failure (18,4502).

Interactions with Herbs & Other Dietary Supplements

None known.

Interactions with Drugs

None known.

Interactions with Foods

None known.

Interactions with Lab Tests

None known.

Interactions with Diseases or Conditions

None known.

Dosage and Administration

No typical dosage.

Comments

Taumelloolch is believed to be the tares of the biblical parable of the wheat and the tares (4502). Some information suggests that an ergot component extracted from the grass and seeds of taumelloolch is used by a mystic cult to induce religious ecstasy (4502).

TAURINE

Also Known As

Aminoethanesulfonate, L-Taurine.

Scientific Names

2-Aminoethane sulfonic acid.

People Use This For

Orally, taurine is used in the treatment of congestive heart failure (CHF), high blood pressure, hepatitis, high cholesterol (hypercholesterolemia), and cystic fibrosis. Other uses include seizure disorders (epilepsy), autism, attention deficit-hyperactivity disorder (ADHD), retinal degeneration, diabetes, and alcoholism. It is also used to improve mental performance and as an antioxidant.

Safety

POSSIBLY SAFE ...when used orally and appropriately. Taurine has been used safely in studies lasting up to one year (5248,5271,8217,8221).

CHILDREN: POSSIBLY SAFE ...when used orally and appropriately. Taurine has been given to children with apparent safety for up to 4 months (10455).

PREGNANCY AND LACTATION: Insufficient reliable information available; avoid using.

Effectiveness

POSSIBLY EFFECTIVE

Congestive heart failure (CHF). Taking taurine orally seems to improve left ventricular function (5248,5271,8221) and symptoms of heart failure (5271,5306,8221) in patients with New York Heart Association (NYHA) functional class II to IV. Some patients with severe heart failure rapidly improve from NYHA class IV to II after 4-8 weeks of treatment. Improvement seems to continue for as long as taurine treatment is continued, up to one year (5306,8217,8218,8221).

Hepatitis. Taking taurine orally might improve liver function in patients with acute hepatitis (10454).

INSUFFICIENT RELIABLE EVIDENCE to RATE

Cystic fibrosis. Taurine supplementation might be useful as adjunctive therapy to reduce steatorrhea in children with cystic fibrosis. However, it does not seem to improve growth, lung function, or other symptoms of cystic fibrosis (10455).

Mental performance. Preliminary clinical research suggests that taurine in combination with caffeine can produce minor improvements in mental performance. It might improve attention and verbal reasoning, but doesn't seem to have any effect on memory (9899).

More evidence is needed to rate taurine for these uses.

Mechanism of Action

Taurine is a conditionally essential amino sulfonic acid present in high amounts in meat and fish. The most abundant dietary source of taurine is human breast milk (3467). Large amounts of taurine are also found in the human brain, retina, heart, and platelets (8219,8220). Taurine is normally synthesized in the human body in adequate amounts from cysteine and hypotaurine (3467).

During prolonged times of insufficient intake, such as during parenteral nutrition, the body cannot maintain adequate levels of taurine and supplementation becomes necessary (3467). Supplementation is also necessary in non-breast-fed infants because their ability to synthesize taurine is undeveloped and cow's milk does not provide a sufficient amount (3467). Taurine is often added to human infant formulas, enteral products, and some parenteral nutritional solutions. Excess taurine is excreted by the kidneys (3467).

Taurine is involved in retinal photoreceptor activity, bile acid conjugation, white blood cell antioxidant activity, central nervous system neuromodulation, platelet aggregation, cardiac contractility, sperm motility, growth, insulin activity (8220), and osmoregulation (5280).

Taurine is thought to be beneficial in the treatment of congestive heart failure (CHF), although the exact mechanism of action remains unclear. The concentration of taurine increases in the left ventricle of patients with CHF; its function here is an area of active research (9900). Oral taurine alters intracellular calcium movement, increasing left ventricular function without any adverse changes in arterial pressure in patients with CHF (3467,5315,8222). Taurine might also improve heart failure because it seems to lower blood pressure and might normalize excessive sympathetic nervous system activity that often occurs in people with hypertension and CHF (3467,8219,8221,8222). Preliminary studies also suggest taurine might have natriuretic and diuretic activity. Taurine might also have a cholesterol-lowering effect. Taurine seems to stimulate bile acid synthesis. There is some evidence that taurine might also have antioxidant and free radical scavenging activity. Platelets normally have high levels of taurine, and can become more prone to aggregation during taurine depletion. However, it is unknown if taurine supplementation has any effect on platelet coagulation (3467).

Adverse Reactions

None reported.

Interactions with Herbs & Other Dietary Supplements

None known.

Interactions with Drugs

None known.

Interactions with Foods

None known.

Interactions with Lab Tests

None known.

Interactions with Diseases or Conditions

None known.

Dosage and Administration

ORAL: For the treatment of congestive heart failure, 2-6 grams per day in two or three divided doses has been used in clinical studies (3467,5248,5306,8217,8221). For the treatment of acute hepatitis, taurine 4 grams 3 times daily has been used for 6 weeks (10454). For treatment of steatorrhea in children with cystic fibrosis, taurine 30 mg/kg daily for 4 months in addition to pancreatic enzyme supplementation (10455).

TEA TREE OIL

Also Known As

Australian Tea Tree Oil, Melaleuca Oil, Oil of Melaleuca, Oleum Melaleucae.
CAUTION: See separate listings for Cajeput Oil and Niauli Oil.

Scientific Names

Melaleuca alternifolia.
Family: Myrtaceae.

People Use This For

Topically, tea tree oil is commonly used for skin and skin surface infections such as acne, onychomycosis, lice, scabies, athlete's foot, and ringworm. It is also used topically as a local antiseptic for cuts and abrasions, for burns, insect bites and stings, boils, vaginal infections, recurrent herpes labialis, toothache, infections of the mouth and nose, sore throat, and for ear infections such as otitis media and otitis externa.
It is also used as a bath additive to treat cough, bronchial congestion, and pulmonary inflammation.

Safety

POSSIBLY SAFE ...when used topically and appropriately (4028,4445,8573).
LIKELY UNSAFE ...when used orally. Like other essential oils, tea tree oil can cause significant toxicity if used orally (4028,10011).
CHILDREN: POSSIBLY SAFE ...when used topically and appropriately (8573). LIKELY UNSAFE ...when used orally. Ingestion of tea tree oil can be toxic (4030,10010,10013,11799).
PREGNANCY AND LACTATION: POSSIBLY SAFE ...when used topically and appropriately (512). LIKELY UNSAFE ...when used orally. Ingestion of tea tree oil can be toxic (515).

Effectiveness

POSSIBLY EFFECTIVE

Acne. Applying a 5% tea tree oil gel appears to be as effective as 5% benzoyl peroxide (Oxy-5, Benzac AC, and others) for treating acne. Tea tree oil might work more slowly than benzoyl peroxide, but seems to be less irritating to facial skin (8573).

Onychomycosis. Topical application of 100% tea tree oil solution twice daily for 6 months can produce a mycological cure in about 18% of patients with toenail infections. It can also improve nail appearance and symptoms in about 56% of patients after three months and 60% of patients after six months of treatment. It seems to be comparable to twice daily application of clotrimazole 1% solution (Fungoid, Lotrimin, Lotrimin AF) (7031). Lower concentrations of tea tree oil do not seem to be as effective. For example, there is some evidence that a 5% tea tree oil cream applied three times daily for two months has no beneficial effect (7032).

Tinea pedis (athlete's foot). Topical application of a 10% tea tree oil cream seems comparable to tolnaftate 1% cream (Genaspor, Tinactin, Ting, and others) for relieving symptoms of athlete's foot, including scaling, inflammation, itching, and burning. Application of 25% or 50% tea tree oil solution appears to produce both clinical improvement and a mycological cure in 48%-50% of patients after 4 weeks of treatment (10033). However, application of 10% tea tree oil cream appears no more effective than placebo in producing a mycological cure for tinea pedis (4031).

POSSIBLY INEFFECTIVE

Herpes labialis (cold sores). Application of 6% tea tree oil gel 5 times daily does not significantly improve recurrent herpes labialis (2035).

INSUFFICIENT RELIABLE EVIDENCE to RATE

Bacterial vaginosis. Preliminary evidence suggests tea tree oil may be beneficial for anaerobic bacterial vaginosis (10017).

Oropharyngeal candidiasis. There is preliminary evidence that tea tree oil might be beneficial for oropharyngeal candidiasis in patients with HIV/AIDS refractory to fluconazole. Swishing and expelling tea tree oil solution for two to four weeks seems to improve oral candidiasis (4445).

More evidence is needed to rate tea tree oil for these uses.

Mechanism of Action

Tea tree oil is obtained by the distillation of the leaves of the tea tree. The oil contains more than 100 monoterpenoid, sesquiterpenoid, and alcohol compounds. Up to 90% is made up of terpinen-4-ol, 1,8-cineole, alpha-terpineol, terpinolene, and alpha- and gamma-terpinene (4027,7111). The primary constituent terpinen-4-ol is active against numerous pathogenic bacteria and fungi but seems to spare normal skin flora. The constituents, alpha-terpineol and linalool, may also contribute to its antimicrobial activity (10012,10026). Tea tree oil appears to disrupt the permeability barrier of microbial cell membrane structures, causing loss of chemiosmotic control (10028).
Tea tree oil has been found to inhibit growth of the yeast Candida albicans (4445,4446,10012). The oil has in vitro activity against Enterococcus faecium and Enterococcus faecalis, including vancomycin-resistant strains, Klebsiella pneumoniae, including gentamicin-resistant strains, and Stenotrophomonas maltophilia (4448,4451,7111,10012,10026). Tea

tree oil also has in vitro activity against both methicillin-sensitive Staphylococcus aureus and methicillin-resistant Staphylococcus aureus (4448,4451,7111,10014,10027). The oil seems to have limited activity against Pseudomonas aeruginosa (7111,10012,10026). Oils produced with increased concentrations of terpinen-4-ol seem to have greater activity against these organisms (7111). Tea tree oil has also been found to inhibit in-vitro growth of the yeast species malassezia, commonly found on human skin (4450). It is also active against Propionibacterium acnes, Escherichia coli, Aspergillus flavus, Trichophyton mentagrophytes, and Trichophyton rubrum (8573). Additional evidence suggests tea tree oil may reduce histamine-induced skin inflammation caused by invading organisms. Tea tree oil applied to histamine-induced inflammation of the skin can decrease mean weal volume (10009). The constituents eucalyptol and limonene may be responsible for the adverse effect of contact eczema (10015,10029).

Adverse Reactions

Orally, tea tree oil and other essential oils can cause significant toxicity. Tea tree oil can cause confusion, inability to walk, disorientation, ataxia, systemic contact dermatitis (4028,10011,10016), and a eucalyptus-like odor on the breath (4028). There is at least one case of coma following ingestion of 120 mL of tea tree oil (4028). Ingestion of as little as 2.5 mL of tea tree oil can cause petechial body rash and neutrophil leukocytosis. It can take up to a week for symptoms to resolve (10011). In young children, ingestion of 10 mL or less of tea tree oil can cause significant ataxia, drowsiness, eucalyptus-like odor on the breath, respiratory failure, disorientation, and coma (4030,10010,11799). As a general rule, never use undiluted volatile oils internally.

Topically, tea tree oil is usually well tolerated; however, it can cause local irritation and inflammation, allergic contact eczema, and allergic contact dermatitis in some patients (658,4027,4029,10015,10029,10030,10031,10032). Tea tree oil can cause skin dryness, and less frequently pruritus, stinging, burning, and redness in patients with acne (8573). It may also cause mild oral mucosal burning (4445). There is some concern that topical use of tea tree oil in the middle ear for treatment of ear infections might cause ototoxicity. There is preliminary evidence that preparations of 100% tea tree oil can cause ototoxicity and impaired hearing. However, so far there are no reports of ototoxicity in humans. Until more is known, tell patients to avoid such highly concentrated tea tree oil preparations. Lower concentrations of 2% tea tree oil seem less likely to have this effect (7025).

Interactions with Herbs & Other Dietary Supplements

None known.

Interactions with Drugs

None known.

Interactions with Foods

None known.

Interactions with Lab Tests

None known.

Interactions with Diseases or Conditions

None known.

Dosage and Administration

TOPICAL: For onychomycosis, 100% tea tree oil solution applied twice daily for six months has been used (7031). For tinea pedis (athlete's foot), 25% or 50% tea tree oil solution applied twice daily for one month has been used (10033). Tea tree oil 10% cream applied twice daily for one month has also been used (4031). For acne, 5% tea tree oil gel applied daily has been used (8573). For oropharyngeal candidiasis, 15 ml tea tree oil solution swished and expelled four times daily for two to four weeks has been used (4445). For anaerobic bacterial vaginosis, 200 mg tea tree oil pessaries inserted vaginally once daily for 5 days have been used (10017).

Comments

Tea tree oil has the aroma of nutmeg (515). The tea tree was named by eighteenth century sailors who made an aromatic tea from the leaves of the tree growing on the swampy southeast Australian coast (515). Do not confuse the tea tree with the unrelated common tea plant that is used to make black and green teas. Avoid confusion with cajeput oil and niauli oil.

TEAZLE

Also Known As
Barber's Brush, Brushes and Combs, Card Thistle, Church Broom, Teasel, Venus' Basin.

Scientific Names
Dipsacus fullonum, synonym Dipsacus sylvestris.
Family: Dipsacaceae.

Comments
At the date of publication, this product was not a common ingredient used in brand name supplements marketed to consumers. Details about this product are available in the online version of *Natural Medicines Comprehensive Database*. See www.naturaldatabase.com.

TERMINALIA

Also Known As
Arjuna, Axjun Argun, Bahera, Bahira, Bala Harade, Balera, Behada, Beleric Myrobalan, Bihara, Chebulic Myrobalan, Hara, Harada, Haritaki, He Zi, Hirala, Indian Almond, Kalidruma, Karshaphala, Myrobalan, Tropical Almond, Vibhitaki.

Scientific Names
Terminalia arjuna, synonyms Pentaptera arjuna, Pentaptera glabra; Terminalia bellirica, synonym Myrobalanus bellirica; Terminalia chebula.
Family: Combretaceae.

People Use This For
Orally, Terminalia arjuna is used for cardiovascular conditions, including ischemic heart disease and angina, hypertension, and hyperlipidemia. It is also used orally as a diuretic, for earaches, dysentery, venereal and urogenital diseases, and as an aphrodisiac.
Orally, Terminalia belerica and Terminalia chebula are used for hyperlipidemia and digestive disorders, including both diarrhea and constipation, and indigestion. They have also been used for HIV infection. Terminalia belerica is also used orally as a hepatoprotectant and for respiratory conditions, including respiratory tract infections, cough, and sore throat. Terminalia chebula is also used orally for dysentery.
Topically, Terminalia belerica and Terminalia chebula are used as a lotion for sore eyes. Terminalia chebula is also used topically as a mouthwash and gargle.
Intravaginally, Terminalia chebula is used as a douche for treating vaginitis.
In traditional Ayurvedic medicine, Terminalia belerica has been used as a "health-harmonizer" in combination with Terminalia chebula and Emblica officinalis. This combination is also used to lower cholesterol and to prevent necrosis of cardiac tissue. In traditional Ayurvedic medicine, Terminalia arjuna has been used to balance the three humors, kapha, pitta, and vata. It has also been used for asthma, bile duct disorders, scorpion stings, and for poisonings.

Safety
POSSIBLY SAFE ...when used orally and appropriately, short-term. Several small studies have used the powdered bark of Terminalia arjuna safely in cardiac patients in trials lasting from 2 weeks to 3 months (2502,2503,2504); however, patients should avoid self-treatment with this product, due to the potentially significant cardiovascular effects. Further study is needed to determine the safety of Terminalia arjuna for long-term use.
There is insufficient reliable information available about the safety of Terminalia belerica and Terminalia chebula (6).
PREGNANCY: POSSIBLY UNSAFE ...when used orally. One source warns against using Terminalia belerica and Terminalia chebula during pregnancy; however, the reason for this warning is not described (33); avoid using.
There is insufficient reliable information available about the safety of Terminalia arjuna in pregnancy; avoid using.
LACTATION: Insufficient reliable information available; avoid using.

Effectiveness
POSSIBLY EFFECTIVE

Angina. Taking terminalia orally seems to be effective as a short-term adjunct to conventional therapy for treating postmyocardial infarction angina. In one small clinical trial, postmyocardial infarction patients with angina taking Terminalia experienced significantly less angina, improved left ventricular ejection fractions, and decreased left ventricular mass compared to patients receiving the standard therapy alone (2502,2503).

Congestive heart failure (CHF). Taking Terminalia orally as a short-term adjunct to conventional therapy seems to be effective for treating severe congestive heart failure. In a small cross-over trial, patients with severe, refractory congestive heart failure had significant reductions in symptoms and improved left ventricular function after 2 weeks of treatment (2504).

Large-scale, long-term trials are necessary to clarify Terminalia's potential role in the treatment of cardiovascular conditions.

There is insufficient reliable information available about the effectiveness of Terminalia for its other uses.

Mechanism of Action

There are three species of terminalia of medicinal interest: Terminalia arjuna, Terminalia belerica and Terminalia chebula (6,33). The applicable part of Terminalia arjuna is the bark. The bark contains several active constituents, including Terminalia arjuna gallic acid, ethyl gallate, and the flavone luteolin. Luteolin may have anticancer properties (2506). The bark of Terminalia arjuna is reported to be beneficial in cardiovascular conditions; however, the exact mechanism is not known. Terminalia arjuna is reported to lower serum cholesterol and low-density lipoprotein (LDL) levels (2505,2517,2519). It is also thought to have an antihypertensive effect and act as a cardiac stimulant. However, studies have been conflicting; some indicating that it may actually increase blood pressure (33).

The applicable part of Terminalia belerica and Terminalia chebula is the fruit (6). These species also have been reported to improve lipid profiles, but to a lesser degree than Terminalia arjuna. Terminalia chebula is reported to have a greater effect on lipids than Terminalia belerica (2517,2519). The astringent properties of Terminalia belerica and Terminalia chebula are attributed to their beneficial effects in bowel irregularity and indigestion (33). Terminalia belerica also contains gallic acid, and is thought to have hepatoprotective properties (2507). An ethanolic extract of Terminalia chebula containing gallic acid and its ethyl ester may have activity against methicillin-resistant Staphylococcus aureus (2508). Terminalia chebula may also have activity against cytomegalovirus (CMV), herpes simplex I, Streptococcus mutans, Salmonella sp., Shigella, and retroviral reverse transcriptase (2509,2510,2511,2512,2513,2514). Both Terminalia belerica and Terminalia chebula may have activity against HIV (2518). The gallic acid and chebulagic acid in Terminalia chebula may have immunosuppressive effects against cytotoxic T lymphocytes (2515).

Adverse Reactions

None reported in humans. In animal studies, Terminalia chebula has caused hepatic and renal lesions (2516).

Interactions with Herbs & Other Dietary Supplements

None known.

Interactions with Drugs

None known.

Interactions with Foods

None known.

Interactions with Lab Tests

None known.

Interactions with Diseases or Conditions

None known.

Dosage and Administration

ORAL: For improving left ventricular function, treating postmyocardial infarction anginal pain as an adjunct to conventional therapy, and congestive failure, a dose of the powdered bark of Terminalia arjuna 500 mg every 8 hours has been used (2502,2503,2504).

Comments

The bark of Terminalia arjuna has been used in India for more than 3000 years, primarily as a heart remedy. An Indian physician named Vagbhata has been credited as the first to use this product for heart conditions in the seventh century A.D. Research on Terminalia has been going on since the 1930s, but pharmacological studies have provided mixed results. Its role in heart disease remains unclear.

THEANINE

Also Known As

Gamma-glutamylethylamide, L-theanine.

CAUTION: See separate listings for Green Tea and Threonine.

Scientific Names

5-N-ethylglutamine.

People Use This For

Orally, theanine is used for anxiety, Alzheimer's disease, hypertension, and enhancing the effects of chemotherapy drugs.

Safety

POSSIBLY SAFE ...when used orally, short-term. There is some evidence that theanine 200 mg can be safely used when given once a week for 3 weeks (12188).
PREGNANCY AND LACTATION: Insufficient reliable information available; avoid using.

Effectiveness

INSUFFICIENT RELIABLE EVIDENCE to RATE

Anxiety. Preliminary evidence suggests that taking theanine 200 mg might induce subjective feelings of tranquility in healthy people. But theanine does not seem to reduce experimentally induced anticipatory anxiety (12188). More evidence is needed to rate theanine for this use.

Mechanism of Action

Theanine is the major amino acid found in green tea. Green tea contains 1% to 3% theanine (7685,7690). Theanine is also found in some mushrooms (12188).
Theanine has historically been used for it's relaxing and anti-anxiety effects. It's thought that theanine might work for anxiety by increasing levels of GABA and serotonin (12188).
There is interest in using theanine for dementia. Theanine is an analog of glutamate, which is an excitatory neurotransmitter. Levels of glutamate increase and cause neuronal death during periods of cerebral ischemia. Theanine demonstrates a protective effect by decreasing ischemic neuronal death in the forebrains of animal models (7685). The antagonistic effects of theanine on glutamate and N-methyl-D-aspartate (NMDA) receptors might provide neuroprotection (7685).
There is also interest in using theanine for hypertension. Theanine affects catecholamines that can cause vasoconstriction and lead to elevations in blood pressure. In animal models, theanine decreases norepinephrine levels (7686), decreases systolic and diastolic blood pressure (7687), and suppresses the stimulatory effects of caffeine (7685,8665). However, there is also some evidence that theanine might induce an excitatory effect when used in very small doses, suggesting the effects of theanine are dose dependent (8665).
Green tea might prevent atherosclerosis by inhibiting the proliferation of smooth muscle cells in blood vessel walls, but theanine doesn't seem to affect smooth muscle (8666). Additionally, there is evidence that suggests theanine might prevent the development of atherosclerosis by inhibiting lipid peroxidation of low-density lipoproteins (LDL) (8667).
There is also interest in using theanine adjunctively for cancer. In studies involving doxorubicin, theanine increases the concentration of doxorubicin and adriamycin in tumors by blocking efflux of the drug from tumor cells (7688,7690,8668,8669). Theanine seems to enhance the effects of doxorubicin and adriamycin on drug sensitive and multi-drug resistant tumors (7688,8668,8669). Theanine may also enhance the suppressive action of doxorubicin on metastatic tumors (8312). Theanine also inhibits the efflux of idarubicin from leukemia cells in animal models (7689). Additionally, theanine seems to decrease the toxicity of idarubicin by reversing adverse effects on leukocytes and bone marrow cells (7689).
There is also some evidence that theanine might decrease serotonin and 5-hydroxyindole acetic acid (5HIAA) concentrations in the brain. Theanine might enhance the degradation of serotonin, and it might also directly inhibit the enzyme responsible for serotonin synthesis (8670).
Animal research suggests theanine may act synergistically with caffeine and other constituents in green tea to cause weight loss (11960).

Adverse Reactions

None reported.

Interactions with Herbs & Other Dietary Supplements

None known.

Interactions with Drugs

ANTIHYPERTENSIVE DRUGS: Theoretically, concomitant use of theanine might potentiate the activity of antihypertensive medications (7687).
STIMULANT DRUGS: Theoretically, concomitant use of theanine might decrease the effects of stimulant drugs such as caffeine (7685,7686).

Interactions with Foods

None known.

Interactions with Lab Tests

None known.

Interactions with Diseases or Conditions
None known.

Dosage and Administration
ORAL: For anxiety, theanine 200 mg/day has been used (12188).

THIAMINE (VITAMIN B1)

Also Known As
Aneurine Hydrochloride, Antiberiberi Factor, Antiberiberi Vitamin, Antineuritic Factor, Antineuritic Vitamin, Anurine, B complex Vitamin, Thiamin Chloride, Thiamin Hydrochloride, Thiamine Chloride, Thiamine Hydrochloride, Thiaminium Chloride Hydrochloride.

Scientific Names
Thiamine; Thiamin; Vitamin B1; Vitamin B-1.

People Use This For
Orally, thiamine is used for thiamine deficiency syndromes, including beriberi, peripheral neuritis associated with pellagra, and neuritis of pregnancy. It is used for poor appetite, ulcerative colitis, chronic diarrhea, GI disorders, cerebellar syndrome, an insect repellent, diabetic neuropathy, AIDS, maintaining a positive mental attitude, enhancing learning abilities, heart disease, alcoholism, stress, improving athletic performance, and aging. Thiamine is also used orally for canker sores, immunodepression, memory loss including Alzheimer's disease, vision problems such as cataracts and glaucoma, motion sickness, and increasing energy.

By injection, thiamine is used for Wernicke's encephalopathy syndrome, other thiamine deficiency syndromes in critically ill people, acute alcohol withdrawal, and coma or hypothermia of unknown origin.

Safety
LIKELY SAFE ...when used orally and is generally considered nontoxic; although, rare hypersensitivity reactions have occurred (15). ...when used appropriately as the injectable FDA-approved prescription product.

PREGNANCY AND LACTATION: LIKELY SAFE ...when used orally at the recommended dietary allowance (RDA) of 1.4 mg per day (3094). There is insufficient reliable information available about the safety of using larger amounts during pregnancy or lactation.

Effectiveness
EFFECTIVE

Metabolic disorders. Taking thiamine orally helps to temporarily correct metabolic disorders associated with genetic diseases such as subacute necrotizing encephalopathy (SNE, Leigh's disease), maple syrup urine disease (branched-chain aminoacidopathy), and lactic acidosis associated with pyruvate carboxylase deficiency and hyperalaninemia (15).

Thiamine deficiency. Taking thiamine orally helps to prevent and treat thiamine deficiency syndromes including beriberi and peripheral neuritis associated with pellagra or neuritis of pregnancy. Thiamine deficiency can occur in people with malabsorption conditions such as alcoholism, cirrhosis, and gastrointestinal (GI) diseases; and in those with inadequate intake due to anorexia, nausea, and vomiting; and in those with increased requirements, including pregnancy, increased carbohydrate intake, increased physical activity, hyperthyroidism, infection, and hepatic disease; however, deficiency is rare with these conditions (15).

POSSIBLY EFFECTIVE

Cataracts. Taking thiamine orally seems to reduce the occurrence of cataracts. A large-scale population-based study found high dietary intake of thiamine was associated with a reduced risk of nuclear cataracts (6378).

INSUFFICIENT RELIABLE EVIDENCE to RATE

Athletic performance. Some clinical research suggests that thiamine (given as allithiamin), in combination with pantethine and pantothenic acid (vitamin B5) does not improve muscular strength or endurance in well-trained athletes (10432). More evidence is needed to rate thiamine for this use.

Mechanism of Action
Thiamine is required for carbohydrate metabolism. It combines with adenosine triphosphate (ATP) to form thiamine diphosphate, a coenzyme in carbohydrate metabolism, wherein the decarboxylation of pyruvic acid and alpha-ketoglutaric acid occurs. This coenzyme is also a part of transketolation reactions. Thiamine is also a coenzyme in the utilization of pentose in the hexose monophosphate shunt (15).

Thiamine deficiency leads to decreased transketolase activity in erythrocytes and increased pyruvic acid concentration in the blood (15). Pyruvic acid is converted to lactic acid. Therefore, lactic acidosis can also occur in patients with thiamine deficiency (15).

Thiamine might also be involved in neuromuscular transmission (10541).

Syndromes associated with thiamine deficiency are beriberi and Wernicke-Korsakoff syndrome (3041). Beriberi is characterized by anorexia; abdominal discomfort; constipation; peripheral neurologic changes; sleep disturbance; poor memory; and, sometimes, cardiovascular symptoms, including dyspnea, edema, palpitations, vasodilation, warm extremities, and high output cardiac failure. Wernicke-Korsakoff syndrome is characterized by confusion, aphonia, confabulation, nystagmus, ophthalmoplegia, and coma.

In Crohn's disease, decreased serum thiamine levels have been reported (6269). Preliminary animal data also suggests thiamine deficiency in diabetics may exacerbate the development of diabetic nephropathy (11467).

Adverse Reactions

Orally, thiamine is usually well tolerated, but in rare cases can cause dermatitis and other hypersensitivity reactions (15).

Injection of thiamine can cause feelings of warmth, tingling, pruritus, pain, urticaria, weakness, sweating, nausea, restlessness, tightness of the throat, angioedema, respiratory distress, cyanosis, pulmonary edema, GI bleeding, transient vasodilation and hypotension, vascular collapse, and death. Tenderness and induration can occur at IM injection sites (15).

Interactions with Herbs & Other Dietary Supplements

ARECA: Areca (betel) nuts reduce thiamine activity, probably by chemical inactivation (10538). Chronic, regular chewing of betel nuts may contribute to thiamine deficiency (10537,10538).

HORSETAIL: Horsetail (Equisetum) contains a thiaminase-like compound that can destroy thiamine in the stomach and theoretically cause symptomatic thiamine deficiency (10573). The Canadian Government requires that equisetum-containing products be certified free of thiaminase activity (10573). Avoid use of this herb in people at risk for thiamine deficiency.

Interactions with Drugs

None known.

Drug Influences on Nutrient Levels and Depletion

SOME DRUGS CAN AFFECT THIAMINE LEVELS:

ANTIBIOTICS: Interference with the normal gastrointestinal (GI) flora by antibiotics may reduce bacterial synthesis of thiamine. However, the majority of the daily thiamine requirement is obtained from the diet, rather than synthesis by the GI flora (9502). Therefore, this isn't likely to be clinically significant, and thiamine supplements aren't necessary.

CONTRACEPTIVE DRUGS: Some studies have reported a small reduction in activity of the thiamine-dependent enzyme erythrocyte transketolase in women taking oral contraceptives, suggesting mild thiamine deficiency (10548,10555). However, other studies have found no effect (10527,10556). Routine use of thiamine supplements with oral contraceptives isn't necessary.

DIURETICS: Increased urinary thiamine excretion and biochemical evidence of thiamine deficiency may occur in some people treated with diuretics, especially in high doses (e.g., >80 mg furosemide per day) for several months (1283,1284,1286,10507,10508). Although most case reports involve furosemide (Lasix), animal data suggest that the effect is related to increased urinary flow and may occur with any diuretic (10509). Diuretic-induced thiamine deficiency appears to be rare in people less than 60 years of age (10506). Most reports involve elderly people who may have inadequate dietary vitamin intake (1283,10507). The potential for thiamine deficiency in people taking diuretics is a concern because it could worsen heart failure (1284,1285,1286,10507). Limited research suggests that supplementation with thiamine 200 mg/day may improve left ventricular ejection fraction and functional capacity in some thiamine-deficient people treated with high doses of furosemide for heart failure (1284,1286,10508). However, other studies have found no improvement (1285). It's too soon to recommend routine thiamine supplementation for people on prolonged, high-dose diuretic therapy. Monitor for thiamine deficiency.

FLUOROURACIL (5-fluorouracil, 5-FU, Adrucil): People receiving fluorouracil-containing chemotherapy regimens may be at risk for thiamine deficiency. Fluorouracil might interfere with activation of thiamine or increase its breakdown (10552). However, there isn't enough research to recommend routine thiamine supplements. Thiamine deficiency has been reported with other chemotherapy regimens, but this is likely due to reduced dietary intake associated with cancer and its treatment (10553,10554).

METFORMIN (Glucophage): Theoretically, metformin might reduce thiamine activity. Thiamine is involved in the entrance of glycolytic pyruvate into the mitochondrial Kreb's cycle. Reducing thiamine activity might lead to increased amounts of pyruvate being converted to lactic acid. This effect might be responsible for some of the cases of lactic acidosis associated with Metformin. This theoretical effect is based on preclinical animal research with metformin's predecessor, phenformin (9536). This has not yet been substantiated in people taking metformin (11466).

PHENYTOIN (Dilantin): Some evidence suggests that chronic treatment with phenytoin might reduce levels of thiamine in plasma and cerebrospinal fluid, and reduce uptake of thiamine into nervous tissues (10510,10511,10512). Theoretically, this could contribute to side effects of phenytoin such as polyneuropathy and cerebellar ataxia (10510,10511). However it isn't clear whether the patients affected also have other factors contributing to thiamine deficiency, such as dietary insufficiency. There isn't enough evidence to recommend routine thiamine supplementation for all patients taking phenytoin.

Interactions with Foods

COFFEE, TEA: Polyphenols, such as tannins, in coffee and tea can react with thiamine, converting it to an unabsorbable and inactive form (9535,10539,10540,10544). Biochemical evidence of thiamine deficiency has been found in a rural Thai population consuming large quantities of tea (> 1 liter per day) or chewing fermented tea leaves chronically (10537,10538). However, this effect hasn't been found in Western populations, despite regular tea consumption (10539). The interaction isn't likely to be clinically significant, especially when the diet is adequate in thiamine and also ascorbic acid, which can prevent the reaction between thiamine and polyphenols (10538,10540).

SEAFOOD: Raw freshwater fish and shellfish contain thiaminase enzymes that destroy thiamine. Frequent ingestion of raw fish or shellfish can contribute to thiamine deficiency (9535,10537,10538). The enzymes are destroyed by cooking; therefore consumption of cooked seafood doesn't affect thiamine levels.

Interactions with Lab Tests

SERUM THEOPHYLLINE: Large amounts of thiamine can interfere with Schack and Waxler spectrophotometric determination of serum theophylline concentrations (15).

URIC ACID: Thiamine can cause false positive results in the phosphotungstate method for uric acid determination (15).

UROBILINOGEN: Thiamine can cause false positive results in the urine spot test with Ehrlich's reagent for urobilinogen (15).

Interactions with Diseases or Conditions

ALCOHOLISM, CIRRHOSIS, MALABSORPTION SYNDROMES: Thiamine absorption is decreased in these conditions (15).

Dosage and Administration

ORAL: As a dietary supplement in adults, 1-2 mg per day is commonly used. For mild thiamine deficiency syndromes in adults, the usual dose of thiamine is 5-30 mg daily in either a single dose or divided doses for one month (15). The typical dose for severe deficiency can be up to 300 mg per day (15). Parenteral thiamine is recommended for critically ill people (15). For genetic enzyme deficiency disorders, 10-20 mg daily is recommended, although 600-4000 mg daily in divided doses may be needed for Leigh's disease (15). A daily dietary intake of approximately 10 mg of thiamine has been associated with reducing the risk of nuclear cataracts (6378).

The daily recommended dietary allowances (RDAs) of thiamine are: Infants 0-6 months, 0.2 mg; Infants 7-12 months, 0.3 mg; Children 1-3 years, 0.5 mg; Children 4-8 years, 0.6 mg; Males 9-13 years, 0.9 mg; Males 14 years and older, 1.2 mg; Females 9-13 years, 0.9 mg; Women 14-18 years, 1 mg; Women over 18 years, 1.1 mg; Pregnant women, 1.4 mg; and Lactating women, 1.5 mg (3094).

Comments

Thiamine is frequently used in combination with other B vitamins in vitamin B complex formulations. Vitamin B complexes generally include vitamin B1 (thiamine), vitamin B2 (riboflavin), vitamin B3 (niacin/niacinamide), vitamin B5 (pantothenic acid), vitamin B6 (pyridoxine), vitamin B12 (cyanocobalamin), and folic acid. However, some products do not contain all of these ingredients and some may include others, such as biotin, para-aminobenzoic acid (PABA), choline bitartrate, and inositol.

THREONINE

Also Known As

None.

CAUTION: See separate listing for theanine.

Scientific Names

L-threonine.

People Use This For

Orally, threonine is used for spinal spasticity, multiple sclerosis, familiar spastic paraparesis, and amyotrophic lateral sclerosis (ALS, Lou Gehrig's disease).

Safety

POSSIBLY SAFE ...when used orally and appropriately. Taking threonine is doses of 2 grams to 4 grams daily for up to 12 months seems to be safe (681,12056,12057,12059).

PREGNANCY AND LACTATION: Insufficient reliable information; avoid using.

Effectiveness

POSSIBLY EFFECTIVE

Spinal spasticity. Taking threonine 6 grams/day orally seems to modestly decrease spasticity (12056).

POSSIBLY INEFFECTIVE

Amyotrophic lateral sclerosis (ALS, Lou Gehrig's disease). Taking threonine 2 grams to 4 grams daily for up to 12 months does not seem to slow the progression of ALS or reduce symptoms (681,12057). There is also concern that threonine might actually worsen pulmonary function in these patients. A significantly higher number of patients treated with threonine seem to have reduced pulmonary function compared to placebo (681).

INSUFFICIENT RELIABLE EVIDENCE to RATE

Familial spastic paraparesis (FSP). There is preliminary evidence that taking threonine 4.5 grams to 6 grams daily might improve some measures of motor impairment and spasticity. But the improvement does not seem to be clinically significant (12059).

Mechanism of Action

Threonine is a large neutral amino acid. Researchers are investigating threonine as a potential treatment for spasticity and amyotrophic lateral sclerosis (ALS) because it is a precursor to glycine. Glycine is the major inhibitory neurotransmitter in the spinal cord. But glycine itself poorly penetrates the central nervous system (CNS). Threonine has better penetration of the CNS. Threonine seems to boost glycine levels in the spinal cord (681,12056,12058). But it doesn't significantly increase glycine levels in the brain (12058).

In patients with spasticity, increasing glycine might reduce spasticity related to spinal cord injury (12056).

ALS is theorized to be cause by excess excitatory amino acids in the CNS such as glutamate. Increasing the inhibitory neurotransmitter, glycine, is thought to counter these excitatory amino acids (681,12057).

Following oral ingestion, plasma threonine levels rise rapidly. Fasting levels of threonine are approximately 113 mcgMol/L (681). After 2 weeks of taking 6 grams daily, plasma threonine levels rose to an average of 498 mcgMol/L (12056). Peak levels of threonine occur within 2 hours following administration (681).

Adverse Reactions

Orally, threonine seems to be well tolerated. Some patients can experience minor gastrointestinal upset including diarrhea (12056).

Other side effects reported in people who have taken threonine includes heachache, rhinorrhea, flatus, constipation, and skin rash. One patient had a two-fold increase in serum ammonia levels following administration of threonine 4 grams daily (681).

Interactions with Herbs & Other Dietary Supplements

ALANINE: Threonine might compete with other amino acids to cross the blood brain barrier into the central nervous system (CNS). Theoretically, high plasma levels of amino acids such as alanine might decrease how much threonine enters the CNS and therefore decrease the effectiveness of threonine (12058).

BRANCHED-CHAIN AMINO ACIDS: Threonine competes with other amino acids to cross the blood brain barrier into the central nervous system (CNS). Theoretically, high plasma levels of other amino acids might decrease how much threonine enters the CNS and therefore decrease the effectiveness of threonine (12058). The branch-chained amino acids include leucine, isoleucine, and valine.

PHENYLALANINE: Threonine might compete with other amino acids to cross the blood brain barrier into the central nervous system (CNS). Theoretically, high plasma levels of amino acids such as phenylalanine might decrease how much threonine enters the CNS and therefore decrease the effectiveness of threonine (12058).

SERINE: Threonine might compete with other amino acids to cross the blood brain barrier into the central nervous system (CNS). Theoretically, high plasma levels of amino acids such as serine might decrease how much threonine enters the CNS and therefore decrease the effectiveness of threonine (12058).

TRYPTOPHAN: Threonine might compete with other amino acids to cross the blood brain barrier into the central nervous system (CNS). Theoretically, high plasma levels of amino acids such as tryptophan might decrease how much threonine enters the CNS and therefore decrease the effectiveness of threonine (12058).

TYROSINE: Threonine might compete with other amino acids to cross the blood brain barrier into the central nervous system (CNS). Theoretically, high plasma levels of amino acids such as tyrosine might decrease how much threonine enters the CNS and therefore decrease the effectiveness of threonine (12058).

Interactions with Drugs

NMDA ANTAGONISTS: Threonine increases central nervous system (CNS) glycine levels (12058). Glycine seems to bind a site on NMDA receptors and enhance the activity of the receptor (681,12057). Theoretically, this might decrease the effects of NMDA receptor antagonists such as memantine (Namenda).

Interactions with Foods

None known.

Interactions with Lab Tests

None known.

Interactions with Diseases or Conditions

AMYOTROPHIC LATERAL SCLEROSIS (ALS, Lou Gehrig's disease): There is some concern that threonine might decrease pulmonary function in patients with ALS. In one study, ALS patients taking threonine 4 grams/day had significantly reduced forced vital capacity (FVC) compared to patients on placebo (681). More evidence is needed to determine if threonine was actually the cause of this adverse outcome.

Dosage and Administration

ORAL: For spinal spasticity, threonine 6 grams/day has been used (12056). For familial spastic paraparesis (FSP), threonine 4.5 gram to 6 grams daily has been used (12059).

THUNDER GOD VINE

Also Known As

Huang-T'eng Ken, Lei Gong Teng, Lei-Kung T'eng, Taso-Ho-Hua, Threewingnut, Yellow Vine.

Scientific Names

Tripterygium wilfordii.
Family: Celastraceae.

People Use This For

Orally, thunder god vine is used for rheumatoid arthritis, excessive menstrual periods, multiple sclerosis, and as a male contraceptive. It is also used for abscesses, boils, fever, inflammation, systemic lupus erythematosus (SLE), psoriasis, and Behcet's disease.
Topically, thunder god vine is used for rheumatoid arthritis.
Thunder god vine has also been used non-medicinally as an insecticide against maggots or larvae, and as a rat and bird poison.

Safety

POSSIBLY SAFE ...when used orally and appropriately (4046,10231,10674,10675,10676). Thunder god vine has been used with apparent safety for up to 5 years (10231). ...when used topically (10233).
PREGNANCY: LIKELY UNSAFE ...when used orally. Thunder god vine is thought to be teratogenic (4047); avoid using.
LACTATION: Insufficient reliable information available; avoid using.

Effectiveness

POSSIBLY EFFECTIVE

Rheumatoid arthritis (RA). Taking thunder god vine orally appears to produce symptom relief in patients with RA, including improvements in pain, tender and swollen joints, and physical function (10674,10675,10676). Additive symptom relief with nonsteroidal anti-inflammatory drugs (NSAIDs) has also been observed (4046). Applying a tincture of thunder god vine topically over affected joints seems to decrease joint tenderness, stiffness, and swelling (10233).

INSUFFICIENT RELIABLE EVIDENCE to RATE

Contraception. Taking thunder god vine orally might be effective as a male contraceptive. Normalization of sperm function seems to return six weeks after discontinuation of treatment (4046,11133).
Nephrotic syndrome. Preliminary evidence suggests thunder god vine may be effective for nephrotic syndrome in children (10677).
Systemic lupus erythematosus (SLE). There is preliminary evidence that thunder god vine may be effective for nephritis associated with SLE (10232).
More evidence is needed to rate thunder god vine for these uses.

Mechanism of Action

The applicable parts of thunder god vine are the leaf and root. The active constituents of thunder god vine are triterpenoids. At least 21 types of triterpenoids have been identified including tripchlorolide, triptolidenol, triptolide, tripdiolide, and 16-hydroxytriptolide (840,10230). Thunder god vine leaf and root seem to have antifertility effects in males by inhibiting sperm transformation, maturation, and mobility. Triptolide, tripdiolide, and possibly other compounds seem to be responsible for the contraceptive effect (11130,11131). Male fertility appears to return to normal six weeks after discontinuation (4046,11133).
Thunder god vine also seems to have immunosuppressive, anti-inflammatory, and anti-proliferative effects. The immunosuppressive effects of thunder god vine are attributed to the constituent triptolide. Triptolide inhibits lymphocyte activation and T-cell expression of interleukin-2 (5305,11132). An alcoholic extract, known as T2, that contains triptolide and tripdiolide, inhibits T-cell and B-cell proliferation, as well as immunoglobulin production by B-cells (1442). T2 also inhibits the release of prostaglandin 2 (PGE 2) from mononuclear leukocytes (5305). A water extract of thunder god vine inhibits the activity of cellular adhesion molecules of leukocytes and endothelial cells, including integrins and selectins (1206,8409).
An extract of the root of thunder god vine seems to exert anti-inflammatory activity by inhibiting cyclooxygenase 1 and 2 (COX-1 and COX-2), and 5-lipoygenase activity (12480).

The neotripterifordin, tripterifordin, and salaspermic acid constituents of thunder god vine exhibit potent anti-HIV replication activity in vitro (4048,4049).

Adverse Reactions

Orally, thunder god vine can cause gastrointestinal (GI) upset, diarrhea, headache, and hair loss (10675,10676). Infertility, lymphocyte suppression, menstrual changes, amenorrhea, and skin reactions may also occur (4046,10675,10676,11009). Decreased bone mineral content may occur in women taking thunder god vine for 5 or more years (10231). There is one report of a young male with some evidence of pre-existing heart damage who developed vomiting, diarrhea, leukopenia, renal failure, hypotension, and shock, and died three days after ingestion of thunder god vine (8658). There is also one report of an infant born with meningoencephalocele after the mother used thunder god vine for rheumatoid arthritis (RA) during pregnancy (4047). Thunder god vine extract may suppress immune function. However, this action only occurs at doses much higher than those typically used (10230).

Interactions with Herbs & Other Dietary Supplements

None known.

Interactions with Drugs

IMMUNOSUPPRESSANTS: Large doses of thunder god vine may suppress immune function (10230). Theoretically, concomitant use might enhance the effects of immunosuppressant drugs. Immunosuppressant drugs include azathioprine (Imuran), basiliximab (Simulect), cyclosporine (Neoral, Sandimmune), daclizumab (Zenapax), muromonab-CD3 (OKT3, Orthoclone OKT3), mycophenolate (CellCept), tacrolimus (FK506, Prograf), sirolimus (Rapamune), prednisone (Deltasone, Orasone), and other corticosteroids (glucocorticoids).

Interactions with Foods

None known.

Interactions with Lab Tests

None known.

Interactions with Diseases or Conditions

IMMUNE SYSTEM COMPROMISE: Large doses of thunder god vine may suppress immune function. Theoretically, thunder god vine might exacerbate these conditions (10230).
OSTEOPOROSIS: Thunder god vine can cause decreased bone mineral density. It should not be used by people with osteoporosis or people who are at risk for osteoporosis (10231).

Dosage and Administration

ORAL: For rheumatoid arthritis (RA), 180-570 mg thunder god vine extract per day has been used up to 20 weeks (10675,10676). For nephrotic syndrome in children, 1 mg per kg body weight daily has been used for up to 20 weeks (10677).
TOPICAL: For rheumatoid arthritis (RA), a tincture of thunder god vine applied over affected joints five to six times daily has been used (10232).

Comments

The National Institute of Arthritis and Musculoskeletal and Skin Diseases (NIAMS) is currently conducting a phase II trial to look at the effectiveness of thunder god vine for rheumatoid arthritis (12481).

THYME

Also Known As

Common Thyme, French Thyme, Garden Thyme, Oil of Thyme, Red Thyme Oil, Rubbed Thyme, Spanish Thyme, Thyme Aetheroleum, Thymi herba, White Thyme Oil.
CAUTION: See separate listing for Wild Thyme.

Scientific Names

Thymus vulgaris; Thymus zygis.
Family: Lamiaceae/Labiatae.

People Use This For

Orally, thyme is used for bronchitis, pertussis, sore throat, colic, arthritis, dyspepsia, gastritis, diarrhea, enuresis, dyspraxia, flatulence, skin disorders, as a diuretic, urinary disinfectant, anthelmintic, and as an appetite stimulant.
Topically, thyme is used for laryngitis, tonsillitis, stomatitis, and halitosis. Thyme oil is used topically as a counterirritant, an antiseptic in mouthwashes and liniments, and for alopecia areata.
Otically, thyme oil is used as an antibacterial and antifungal ingredient.

In foods, thyme is used as a flavoring agent.
In manufacturing, red thyme oil is used in perfumes. It is also used in soaps, cosmetics, and toothpastes.

Safety

LIKELY SAFE ...when used in amounts commonly found in foods. Thyme has Generally Recognized As Safe (GRAS) status in the US (4912).
POSSIBLY SAFE ...when used topically and appropriately (5177). Diluted thyme oil has been used safely for up to 7 months (5177).
There is insufficient reliable information available about the safety of thyme oil when used orally.
PREGNANCY: LIKELY UNSAFE ...when used in medicinal amounts; thyme has been used to induce menstruation (4,19); avoid using.
LACTATION: There is insufficient reliable information available about the safety of thyme in medicinal amounts during breast-feeding; avoid using.

Effectiveness

INSUFFICIENT RELIABLE EVIDENCE to RATE

Alopecia areata. Thyme oil applied topically in combination with the essential oils from rosemary, lavender, and cedarwood seem to improve hair growth by 44% after 7 months of treatment (5177).
Dyspraxia. Taking thyme oil in combination with evening primrose oil, fish oils, and vitamin E seems to improve movement disorders in children with dyspraxia (5708).
There is insufficient reliable information available about the effectiveness of thyme for its other uses.

Mechanism of Action

The applicable parts of thyme are the leaf, flower, and oil. Thyme contains thymol, carvacrol, and flavonoid constituents. These constituents are thought to have antispasmodic, antitussive, and expectorant effects (4).
The phenolic compounds of the volatile oil and flavonoids are associated with antispasmodic activity. This mechanism may involve blocking calcium channels. However, some scientists question whether the phenolic components are involved (4). The antibacterial and antifungal activity is associated with the thymol and carvacrol constituents (1). Thymol has fungicidal, antibacterial, anthelmintic (especially hookworms), and counterirritant properties (4,11).
The constituent, rosmarinic acid, reduces experimentally-induced edema, inhibits passive cutaneous anaphylaxis, and impairs experimental activation of macrophages in vivo (1).
Thyme extract seems to have analgesic and antipyretic effects (4). Thymus vulgaris is reported to have antithyrotropic activity (11). It's not clear how thyme oil works in alopecia areata (5177); however, it may be related to its effects as a counterirritant.

Adverse Reactions

Orally, thyme oil can cause nausea, vomiting, gastric pain, headache, dizziness, convulsions, coma, and cardiac and respiratory arrest (4).
Topically, thyme oil can cause irritation, cheilitis, and glossitis (4).

Interactions with Herbs & Other Dietary Supplements

None known.

Interactions with Drugs

None known.

Interactions with Foods

None known.

Interactions with Lab Tests

None known.

Interactions with Diseases or Conditions

CROSS-ALLERGENICITY: Cross-reactivity to oregano and other Lamiaceae species has been reported in an individual allergic to thyme (3808).
GASTROINTESTINAL (GI) IRRITATION: Thyme might exacerbate gastrointestinal conditions (19).

Dosage and Administration

ORAL: No typical dosage. However, 1-2 grams of dried leaf or flower has been used as a tea (1,18). As fluid extract, 1-2 grams up to three times daily has also been used (2).
TOPICAL: For the treatment of alopecia areata, a combination of the essential oils including thyme 2 drops or 88 mg, rosemary 3 drops or 114 mg, lavender 3 drops or 108 mg, and cedarwood 2 drops or 94 mg, all mixed with 3 mL jojoba oil and 20 mL grapeseed oil has been used. Each night, the mixture is massaged into the scalp for 2 minutes with a warm towel placed around the head to increase absorption (5177).

Comments

Thyme is a plant rich in iron (19). Thyme oil is obtained by distillation of the leaves and flowering tops of thyme. White thyme oil (redistilled red thyme oil) is often adulterated (11).

THYMUS EXTRACT

Also Known As

Predigested Thymus Extract, Pure Thymic Extract, Thymomodulin, Thymosin, Thymostimulin, Thymus, Thymus Acid Lysate Derivative, Thymus Complex, Thymus Concentrate, Thymus-Derived Polypeptides, Thymus Factors, Thymus Polypeptides, Thymus Substance.

Scientific Names

None.

People Use This For

Orally, thymus extract is used for infectious diseases including recurrent respiratory infections, colds, flu, hepatitis B, hepatitis C, Epstein-Barr virus (EBV), mononucleosis, herpes and shingles, sinusitis, and AIDS/HIV. It is also used orally for asthma, hay fever, food allergies, cancer, rheumatoid arthritis, chronic fatigue syndrome (CFS), and systemic lupus erythematosus (SLE). It is also used orally for maintaining white cell production in cancer patients treated with radiation or chemotherapy, and preventing the effects of aging.

Safety

POSSIBLY SAFE ...when used orally and appropriately. No adverse effects have been reported in human studies with purified thymus extract (938,1010,1175,1176,1177,1178,6691,6694,6696,6697,6698,6699). Although some evidence suggests these products are safe, since they are derived from animals, there is concern about contamination with diseased animal parts (1825). However, so far there are no reports of disease transmission to humans due to use of contaminated thymus extract.

PREGNANCY AND LACTATION: Insufficient reliable information available; avoid using.

Effectiveness

POSSIBLY EFFECTIVE

Allergic rhinitis (hayfever). There is some evidence that treatment for 4 months with thymomodulin (calf thymus extract) might reduce the frequency of allergic episodes in patients with allergic rhinitis (1010).

Asthma. Taking thymus extract orally may reduce acute asthma attacks in children with asthma. Thymomodulin (calf thymus extract) seems to improve immune function and reduce the number of asthma attacks up to one year after discontinuing intermittent treatment in children with asthma (6694).

Food allergies. Thymomodulin (calf thymus extract) plus an elimination diet might prevent allergic reactions to allergenic foods after completion of the elimination diet, compared to an elimination diet alone (1175,1176).

Respiratory infections. Taking thymus extract orally may be effective for treating adults and children with recurrent respiratory infections (938,6696,6697,6698,6699). Thymomodulin (calf thymus extract) treatment seems to reduce the number of infections or coughing attacks in patients with recurrent respiratory infections (6697,6698,6699). Thymomodulin (calf thymus extract) alone, or in combination with vaccine, seems to be more effective than vaccine alone or antibiotics in reducing the number and duration of infections in adults with recurrent respiratory infections (938).

There is insufficient reliable information available about the effectiveness of thymus extract for its other uses.

Mechanism of Action

Thymus extract is derived from bovine thymus glands (6614). Purified thymus extract induces immune response in spleen cells from athymic animals in vitro (6688). Preliminary human data suggests that a semipurified calf thymus extract might be useful for treating immunodeficiency conditions, bone marrow failure, auto-immune disorders, chronic skin diseases, recurrent viral and bacterial infections, and some cancers (6677).

Thymomodulin is a purified acid lysate derivative of calf thymus extract containing several polypeptides (6614,6689). It induces T-lymphocyte maturation, enhances the function of mature T-cells, and has indirect effects on B-cell and macrophage functions in vitro (6689). Thymomodulin improves immune function in patients with asthma, chronic bronchitis, recurrent respiratory infections, perennial allergic rhinnitis, food allergies, chronic active hepatitis B, and HIV infection (938,1010,1175,1176,1178,6694,6696,6697,6698,6699). It reduces airway hyperresponsiveness to methacholine in atopic patients with asthma (6695). Limited human data suggest that thymomodulin might be useful for treating chronic active hepatitis B (1015,1177) and improving symptoms in patients with HIV infection (1178). Thymomodulin demonstrates activity when administered orally in elderly patients (6691).

Thymosin is a polypeptide extracted from fetal calf thymus glands that stimulates in vitro T-cell proliferation when incubated with T-lymphocytes from people with low T-cell counts (511,6687).

Thymostimulin is a polypeptide extracted from bovine thymus glands (6680). Preliminary human evidence suggests that parenteral thymostimulin might be useful for improving immune function in infants with inadequate

B-lymphocyte or T-lymphocyte function (6682,6683), children with recurrent respiratory infections (6679,6684), and patients with primary immunodeficiencies (6685). Limited human evidence also suggests that parenteral thymostimulin might be useful for preventing recurrent herpes simplex labialis (HSL) episodes (6678), preventing exacerbations in patients with chronic obstructive pulmonary disease (COPD) (6681), and preventing cystitis, conjunctivitis, stomatomucositis, and myelotoxicity in women with breast cancer treated with chemotherapy (6680). Thymostimulin is not beneficial for treating patients with auto-immune chronic active hepatitis (6686).

Adverse Reactions

Adverse effects have not been reported. However, there is some concern about potential contamination. Thymus extract is derived from raw bovine thymus glands gathered from slaughterhouses, possibly from sick or diseased animals (6620). Products made from contaminated or diseased organs might present a human health hazard. There is also concern that thymus extract produced from cows in countries where bovine spongiform encephalitis (BSE) has been reported might be contaminated with diseased tissue. Countries where BSE has been reported include Great Britain, France, The Netherlands, Portugal, Luxembourg, Ireland, Switzerland, Oman, and Belgium (1825). However, there have been no reports of BSE transfer to humans from contaminated thymus extract products. Until more is known, tell patients to avoid these products unless country of origin can be determined. Patients should avoid products that are produced in countries where BSE has been found.

Interactions with Herbs & Other Dietary Supplements

None known.

Interactions with Drugs

IMMUNOSUPPRESSANTS: Patients using immunosuppressive drugs are cautioned to avoid thymus extract products, unless they are certified pathogen-free. Immunosuppressant drugs include azathioprine (Imuran), basiliximab (Simulect), cyclosporine (Neoral, Sandimmune), daclizumab (Zenapax), muromonab-CD3 (OKT3, Orthoclone OKT3), mycophenolate (CellCept), tacrolimus (FK506, Prograf), sirolimus (Rapamune), prednisone (Deltasone, Orasone), and other corticosteroids (glucocorticoids).

Interactions with Foods

None known.

Interactions with Lab Tests

None known.

Interactions with Diseases or Conditions

IMMUNE COMPROMISE, IMMUNOSUPPRESSION: Patients with compromised immune systems or using immunosuppressive drugs should be cautioned to avoid thymus extract products, unless they are certified pathogen-free, to reduce their risk of infection. This includes patients with HIV/AIDS and organ transplant recipients using immunosuppressive drugs.

Dosage and Administration

ORAL: A typical daily dose is 750 mg of crude thymus polypeptide fraction or 120 mg of pure thymus polypetides (thymomodulin) (6614).

Comments

The quality and potency of thymus extract products can vary greatly (6614).

TIRATRICOL

Also Known As

Triac, Triiodothyroacetic Acid.

Scientific Names

3,3',5-triiodothyroacetic acid.

People Use This For

Orally, tiratricol is used for treating pituitary resistance to thyroid hormone (PRTH), treating thyroid cancer (orphan drug designation), treating fetal hypothyroidism, increasing metabolic rate for weight loss, and reducing cellulite.

Safety

LIKELY SAFE ...when used orally under medical supervision for treating thyroid cancer (1616,1617,1618,1691).
...when used orally under medical supervision for treating pituitary resistance to thyroid hormone (PRTH) (1607,1608,1609,1610,1615).
POSSIBLY SAFE ...when used orally under medical supervision for treating fetal hypothyroidism (1613,1614).

POSSIBLY UNSAFE ...when used orally in the elderly, tiratricol might aggravate occult cardiac disease (15); avoid using.
LIKELY UNSAFE ...when used orally for increasing metabolic rate for weight loss or reducing cellulite (1620,1621,1622,1623,1624,1625). The FDA has issued a warning against tiratricol use for weight loss (1605).
PREGNANCY: POSSIBLY SAFE ...when used orally under medical supervision for treating fetal hypothyroidism (1613,1614). LIKELY UNSAFE ...when used orally for other purposes during pregnancy due to possible risk of fetal heart damage (1627,1628); avoid using.
LACTATION: Insufficient reliable information available; avoid using.

Effectiveness

LIKELY EFFECTIVE

Pituitary resistance to thyroid hormone (PRTH). Taking tiratricol orally is effective for treating pituitary resistance to thyroid hormone (PRTH) (1607,1608,1609,1610,1615).

POSSIBLY EFFECTIVE

Hypothyroidism. Taking tiratricol orally seems to be effective for treating fetal hypothyroidism (1613,1614).
Thyroid cancer. Taking tiratricol orally in combination with levo-thyroxine seems to be effective for treating thyroid cancer (1616,1617,1618). Tiratricol is an FDA designated orphan drug under study for use in combination with levo-thyroxine to suppress thyroid stimulating hormone (TSH) in patients with well-differentiated thyroid cancer who are intolerant to adequate doses of levo-thyroxine alone (1691).

LIKELY INEFFECTIVE

Weight loss. Taking tiratricol orally isn't effective for increasing metabolic rate for weight loss in people with normal thyroid function (1611,1612).

There is insufficient reliable information available about the effectiveness of tiratricol for its other uses.

Mechanism of Action

Tiratricol is a naturally occurring metabolite of T4 (thyroxine) and a structural analog of T3 (triiodothyronine) (1633,1634). Low concentrations of tiratricol are found in plasma, but tiratricol has no known role in thyroid physiology (1633). Tiratricol has a high affinity for T3 receptors and suppresses thyroid stimulating hormone (TSH) secretion at therapeutic doses without causing significant peripheral effects, such as increased basal metabolism rate and heart rate (1634). Tiratricol might lower total and LDL cholesterol, and stimulate bone formation (1632). About 67% of an oral dose of tiratricol is absorbed; the half-life is 6 hours (1631).

Adverse Reactions

Orally, tiratricol can cause severe diarrhea, fatigue, lethargy, and profound weight loss (1605). Heart attacks and strokes are possible, as well as symptoms of hyperthyroidism, including increased appetite, abdominal cramps, tremors, menstrual irregularities, nervousness, insomnia, sweating, intolerance to heat, fever, palpitations, tachycardia, increased pulse and blood pressure, chest pain, and cardiac arrhythmias (15,1605). Case reports have implicated tiratricol in centrally-mediated hypothyroidism, pseudohypothyroidism, internuclear ophthalmoplegia, and hepatotoxicity (1621,1623,1624,1625).

Interactions with Herbs & Other Dietary Supplements

HERBS AND SUPPLEMENTS WITH SYMPATHOMIMETIC ACTIVITY: Theoretically, large doses of tiratricol might enhance the effects and adverse effects of herbs and supplements that have sympathomimetic activity, including caffeine, guarana, and ephedra (15).
HERBS WITH THYROID ACTIVITY: Theoretically, tiratricol might enhance the effects and adverse effects of herbs that affect thyroid function, including bugleweed, balm leaf, and wild thyme.
VITAMIN K: Theoretically, tiratricol might antagonize the prothrombinemic effects of vitamin K by increasing catabolism of vitamin K-dependent clotting factors (15).

Interactions with Drugs

ANTICOAGULANT/ANTIPLATELET DRUGS: Theoretically, tiratricol might potentiate the hypoprothrombinemic effects of oral anticoagulants, including warfarin (Coumadin), by increasing catabolism of vitamin K-dependent clotting factors (15).
ANTIDIABETES DRUGS: Theoretically, tiratricol might interfere with blood glucose control requiring adjustment of diabetes drug therapy (15); monitor closely.
CHOLESTYRAMINE (Questran): Theoretically, cholestyramine might decrease tiratricol absorption (15).
STIMULANT DRUGS: Theoretically, large doses of tiratricol might enhance the effects and adverse effects of sympathomimetic drugs (15).
THYROID HORMONE: Concurrent use of tiratricol with thyroid hormones can have additive effects (1617); use only under medical supervision.

Interactions with Foods

None known.

Interactions with Lab Tests

PROTHROMBIN TIME (PT), INTERNATIONAL NORMALIZATION RATIO (INR): Theoretically, tiratricol might increase prothrombin time, increasing PT and INR test results, by increasing catabolism of vitamin K-dependent clotting factors (15).
THYROID FUNCTION TESTS: Abnormalities have been reported in people taking tiratricol (1691).
THYROID-STIMULATING HORMONE (TSH): Tiratricol reduces serum TSH levels, and test results (1631).
THYROTRPIN-RELEASING HORMONE (TRH) STIMULATION: Triatricol reduces TSH secretion, serum levels and test results, to exogenous TRH stimulation (1609,1611,1617,1623,1633).

Interactions with Diseases or Conditions

ADRENAL INSUFFICIENCY, DIABETES, HYPOPITUITARISM: Theoretically, tiratricol might unmask symptoms of these conditions in patients with untreated hypothyroidism (15).
ANGINA, CARDIOVASCULAR DISEASE, HYPERTENSION: Theoretically, tiratricol might aggravate symptoms of these conditions (15); avoid using.
DIABETES: Theoretically, tiratricol might interfere with blood glucose control requiring adjustment of diabetes drug therapy (15), monitor closely.
LIVER DISEASE: Tiratricol is potentially hepatotoxic and might worsen liver disease (1624); avoid using.
MYXEDEMA: Patients with myxedema might be particularly sensitive to thyroid agents, including tiratricol (15).
PROLONGED CLOTTING TIME: Theoretically, tiratricol might increase the risk of bleeding in people with prolonged clotting time by increasing catabolism of vitamin K-dependent clotting factors (15).

Dosage and Administration

ORAL: The dose for TSH suppression tests used in clinical trials is 10-24 mcg twice daily initially, titrated to a TSH concentration of less than 0.1 mU/L (1632,1633).

Comments

Tiratricol is a thyroid supplement and should not be used by anyone with normal thyroid function (1605). The drug, which is available by prescription in France, has been studied since the fifties, mostly for thyroid disease (1629,1630). The FDA has determined that the product Triax (TRIAC, tiratricol) is not a dietary supplement but an unapproved new drug containing a potent thyroid hormone, which may cause serious health consequences. The State of Missouri embargoed the product at its distributor (Syntrax) and the Utah-based manufacturer (Pharmatech) has agreed to stop distributing any product containing the ingredient TRIAC. The FDA has issued recalls for other tiratricol-containing products, including Tricana Metabolic Hormone Analogue, Tria-Cutz Thyroid Stimulator Dietary Supplement Capsules, and Sci-Fi-Tri-Cuts Dietary Supplement Capsules (6675).

TOLU BALSAM

Also Known As

Balsam, Balsam of Tolu, Balsam Tolu, Balsamum Tolutanum, Myroxylan balsamum, Myroxylan toluiferum, Opobalsam, Resin Tolu, Resina Tolutana, Thomas Balsam, Tolu, Toluiferum Balsamum.
CAUTION: See separate listing for Peru Balsam.

Scientific Names

Myroxylon balsamum; Myroxylon balsamum var. balsamum, synonym Toluifera balsamum.
Family: Fabaceae/Leguminosae.

People Use This For

Orally, tolu balsam is used for cough, bronchitis, inflammation of respiratory tract mucous membranes, as an expectorant, and for cancer.
Topically, tolu balsam is used to treat of bedsores, cracked nipples, lips, and minor skin cuts.
As an inhalant, tolu balsam is used to treat laryngitis and croup.
In foods, tolu balsam is also used to flavor chewing gum, foods, and beverages.
In manufacturing, tolu balsam is used as a fixative, as fragrances in soaps and cosmetics, and as a flavoring in cough medicines.

Safety

LIKELY SAFE ...when the oleo resin and extract are used orally in amounts commonly found in foods. Tolu balsam has Generally Recognized As Safe status (GRAS) for use in foods in the US (4912).
POSSIBLY SAFE ...when used orally and appropriately for medicinal purposes (2).
There is insufficient reliable information available about the safety of the topical use of tolu balsam.
PREGNANCY AND LACTATION: Insufficient reliable information available; avoid using.

Effectiveness
There is insufficient reliable information available about the effectiveness of tolu balsam.

Mechanism of Action
The applicable part of tolu balsam is the oleo resin. Tolu balsam has mild antiseptic action and expectorant properties (11).

Adverse Reactions
Orally, tolu balsam may cause kidney irritation (12).
Topically, it may cause allergic reactions (11).

Interactions with Herbs & Other Dietary Supplements
None known.

Interactions with Drugs
None known.

Interactions with Foods
None known.

Interactions with Lab Tests
None known.

Interactions with Diseases or Conditions
FEVER: Theoretically, tolu balsam is contraindicated in individuals with fever or inflammation (12,19).
KIDNEY DISEASE: Theoretically, tolu balsam might exacerbate kidney disease.
TOLU BALSAM ALLERGY: Avoid use of tolu balsam (11).

Dosage and Administration
ORAL: A typical dosage is 500-600 mg per day (2,18).
TOPICAL: No typical dosage.

Comments
Avoid confusion with Peru balsam. Tolu balsam is the oleo resin exuded from slits cut in the trunk of Myroxylon balsamum.

TOMATO

Also Known As
Love Apple.
CAUTION: See separate listing for Lycopene.

Scientific Names
Lycopersicon esculentum.
Family: Solanaceae.

People Use This For
Orally, tomato is used for reducing the risk of cancer, cardiovascular disease, and cataracts; and for treating arthritis, colds, chills, and digestive disorders.

Safety
LIKELY SAFE ...when the tomato fruit or its products are consumed in amounts found in foods (2406,9439,10418).
POSSIBLY UNSAFE ...when the leaf is used orally (18).
There is insufficient reliable information about the safety of the tomato vine.
PREGNANCY AND LACTATION: LIKELY SAFE ...when the tomato fruit or its products are consumed in typical food amounts. Avoid using amounts greater than those typically consumed in foods.

Effectiveness
POSSIBLY EFFECTIVE

Cardiovascular disease. Epidemiologic evidence suggests that increased consumption of tomato-based foods can decrease the risk myocardial infarction, stroke, and other cardiovascular events in women (10418).
Cataracts. Eating more than 3 servings of tomatoes each week may decrease the risk of developing cataracts (9439).

Prostate cancer. Consuming tomato fruit products seems to reduce the risk of prostate cancer. Epidemiological studies suggest that the risk of prostate cancer is decreased slightly in men who consume four or more weekly servings of tomato products, including tomatoes, tomato sauce, pizza, and tomato juice (2406,7895).

POSSIBLY INEFFECTIVE

Bladder cancer. Epidemiological studies have found no association between consuming tomatoes and tomato-based products, and the risk of bladder cancer (2407).

INSUFFICIENT RELIABLE EVIDENCE to RATE

Cancer. Epidemiological studies investigating consumption of tomatoes and tomato-based products, and the risk of breast cancer, cervical cancer, colon cancer, esophageal cancer, laryngeal cancer, lung cancer, oral cancer, ovarian cancer, pancreatic cancer, pleural cancer, rectal caner, and stomach cancer are inconclusive (1444,2404,2407). More evidence is needed to rate tomato for these uses.

Mechanism of Action

The applicable parts of tomato are the fruit, leaf, and vine. Tomatoes are the major dietary source of the carotenoid, lycopene. Lycopene is better absorbed from tomato products, such as tomato paste, than from fresh tomatoes (1497). Consumption of tomato juice can also significantly increase serum lycopene levels (1498,6607). One cup (240 mL) of tomato juice contains approximately 23 mg lycopene, depending on the brand (1499). Decreased serum or tissue lycopene concentrations are associated with an increased risk of prostate cancer (1447,1496,2405,2406,2407). Researchers have speculated that tomato products might stimulate immune function. However, there is evidence that long-term consumption of tomato juice has no effect on cell-mediated immune function (6607).

Adverse Reactions

Orally, symptoms of toxicity may include severe mucous membrane irritation, including vomiting, diarrhea, and colic. This is followed by dizziness, stupor, headache, bradycardia, respiratory disturbances, and mild spasms. In very severe cases, death by respiratory failure might occur (18). Signs of oral poisoning are not expected with ingestion of less than 100 grams of tomato leaves.

Interactions with Herbs & Other Dietary Supplements

None known.

Interactions with Drugs

None known.

Interactions with Foods

None known.

Interactions with Lab Tests

None known.

Interactions with Diseases or Conditions

None known.

Dosage and Administration

ORAL: For preventing prostate cancer, four or more servings of tomato products per week (equivalent to a dietary lycopene intake of greater than 6 mg daily) has been used (2406).

Comments

US Department of Agriculture (USDA) and Purdue University researchers are developing a tomato that contains more than twice as much lycopene and has a longer shelf life than currently available tomatoes (6671). The tomato, which is still in development, is modified with a yeast gene that slows the ripening process, allowing more time for lycopene to accumulate. Researchers think it will be several years before the tomato is commercially available.

TONKA BEAN

Also Known As

Cumaru, Dutch Tonka, English Tonka, Legume, Tonka, Tonka Seed, Tonquin Bean, Torquin Bean.

Scientific Names

Dipteryx odorata, synonym Coumarouna odorata.
Family: Fabaceae/Leguminosae.

People Use This For

Orally, tonka bean is used as a tonic, an aphrodisiac, to treat cachexia, cramps, lymphedema, nausea, cough, schistosomiasis, spasms, and tuberculosis.

Topically, tonka bean is used for mouth ulcers, earache, and sore throat.
In manufacturing, coumarin, one of the active constituents of tonka bean is used as a flavoring and fragrance in various products in the food, liquor, tobacco, soap, and cosmetic industries.
In foods, the seeds are used to make a nutty-flavored beverage.

Safety

LIKELY UNSAFE ...when used orally. The FDA deems any food containing tonka bean or tonka bean extract to be impure (6). Rarely, coumarin, a constituent, has been associated with hepatotoxicity ranging from elevated liver enzymes to severe hepatic damage (6,297).
There is insufficient reliable information available about the safety of the topical use of tonka bean.
PREGNANCY AND LACTATION: LIKELY UNSAFE ...when used orally (6,297); avoid using.

Effectiveness

There is insufficient reliable information available about the effectiveness of tonka bean.

Mechanism of Action

The applicable parts of tonka bean are the fruit and seed. Tonka bean seeds usually contain 1-3% coumarin but may contain up to 10% (6,4502). Tonka bean seeds also contain coumaric-acid-beta-glucoside, o-coumaric acid, linoleic acid, oleic-acid, sitosterol, stearic acid, stigmasterol, and umbelliferone (296). The fruit contains melilotoside-1-p-coumaryl-beta-d-glucose (296). There is some evidence that coumarin can reduce edema and inflammation by increasing venous and lymphatic return (295). Other information suggests tonka bean might have narcotic and spasmolytic properties (4502,18).

Adverse Reactions

Orally, coumarin can be associated with nausea, vomiting (286), diarrhea, dizziness, insomnia (287), asymptomatic SGOT elevations (286), and rarely, liver toxicity (6,297). Large doses of the extract can paralyze the heart (4502).

Interactions with Herbs & Other Dietary Supplements

None known.

Interactions with Drugs

None known.

Interactions with Foods

None known.

Interactions with Lab Tests

None known.

Interactions with Diseases or Conditions

LIVER DISEASE: Although it is rare, the tonka bean constituent, coumarin, can cause liver toxicity (298).

Dosage and Administration

ORAL: Some people use an amount of tonka bean based on its coumarin content, and the typical dose of coumarin used is 60 mg daily (6002).
TOPICAL: No typical dosage.

Comments

The term coumarin is derived from Coumarou, the Caribbean name for the tonka tree (13). In plants, more than 700 different coumarins have been identified. Coumarin, itself, is widely distributed and has the characteristic odor of new-mown hay (13). Do not confuse coumarin with the potent anticoagulants bishydroxycoumarin, dicumarol, (13,295) or warfarin (a derivative of 4-hydroxycoumarin) (16).

TORMENTIL

Also Known As

Biscuits, Bloodroot, Cinquefoil, Earthbank, English Sarsaparilla, Ewe Daisy, Flesh And Blood, Potentilla, Septfoil, Shepherd's Knapperty, Shepherd's Knot, Thormantle, Tormentilla, Tormentillae rhizoma.
CAUTION: See separate listings for German Sarsaparilla, Potentilla, and Sarsaparilla.

Scientific Names

Potentilla erecta, Potentilla tormentilla.
Family: Rosaceae.

People Use This For
Orally, tormentil is used to treat diarrhea, acute and subacute gastroenteritis, and fever.
Topically, tormentil is used for reducing superficial bleeding and treating mild inflammation of the oral and pharyngeal mucous membranes.

Safety
POSSIBLY SAFE ...when used orally and appropriately (12). ...when used topically and appropriately (12).
CHILDREN: POSSIBLY SAFE ...when used orally and appropriately up to 5 days (10667).
PREGNANCY AND LACTATION: Insufficient reliable information available; avoid using.

Effectiveness
There is insufficient reliable information available about the effectiveness of tormentil.

Mechanism of Action
The applicable part of tormentil is the root. It contains 17-22% tannins, proanthocyanidins, flavonoids, and triterpenes (18). The astringent effect of tannins relieves diarrhea and soothes mucus membrane inflammation. Tannins reduce superficial bleeding by causing skin and superficial capillary contraction. Tannins also show some evidence of antiviral, antimicrobial, CNS depressant, and cariostatic effects (11). Some evidence suggests that tannins might cause cancer but other evidence shows tannins might prevent it (12). Regular consumption of herbs with high tannin concentrations correlates with increased incidence of esophageal or nasal cancer (12).

Adverse Reactions
Orally, tormentil can cause nausea, vomiting (7,12,18), and stomach complaints (2). Tormentil contains 17-22% tannins and theoretically has the potential to cause kidney damage and necrotic conditions of the liver (12).

Interactions with Herbs & Other Dietary Supplements
None known.

Interactions with Drugs
None known.

Interactions with Foods
MILK: When added to tormentil tea, milk can bind to the tannins and decrease their astringent and adverse effects (12).

Interactions with Lab Tests
None known.

Interactions with Diseases or Conditions
None known.

Dosage and Administration
ORAL: For diarrhea, a typical dose is one cup of the tea 2-4 times daily between meals, up to 4-6 grams of root per day. The tea is prepared by steeping 2-3 grams of the finely cut or powdered root in 150 mL boiling water for 10-15 minutes and then straining (18). In children with rotavirus diarrhea, tormentil root 1:10 extract in a dose of 3 drops per year of life has been used three times daily for up to 5 days (10667).
TOPICAL: The usual daily dose of the tincture, 1:10, is 10-20 drops in one glass of water used as a mouth or throat rinse (18).

Comments
Avoid confusion with potentilla (Potentilla anserina).

TRAGACANTH

Also Known As
Goat's Thorn, Green Dragon, Gum Dragon, Gum Tragacanth, Gummi Tragacanthae, Hog Gum, Syrian Tragacanth, Tragacanth Gum.
CAUTION: See separate listing for Astragalus.

Scientific Names
Astragalus gummifer.
Family: Fabaceae/Leguminosae.

People Use This For

Orally, tragacanth is used both for diarrhea and as a laxative.
Topically, tragacanth is an ingredient in toothpastes, hand lotions, and vaginal creams and jellies.
In foods, tragacanth is important for stabilizing, thickening, and suspending ingredients in salad dressings, foods, and beverages.
In pharmaceutical preparations, tragacanth is used as an emulsifier, binding agent, and demulcent. It is also a component of denture adhesives.

Safety

LIKELY SAFE ...when used orally in amounts commonly found in foods. Tragacanth has Generally Recognized As Safe (GRAS) status in the US (4912). ...when used topically, in the amounts found in cosmetics. Tragacanth is not considered to be irritating, sensitizing, or phototoxic (4072).
POSSIBLY SAFE ...when used orally in medicinal amounts (4068). However, insufficient fluid intake with tragacanth might lead to esophageal closure or obstruction ileus (18).
PREGNANCY AND LACTATION: Insufficient reliable information available; avoid using amounts greater than those found in foods.

Effectiveness

There is insufficient reliable information available about the effectiveness of tragacanth.

Mechanism of Action

Tragacanth contains water-soluble tragacanthin and water-insoluble bassorin (11). When added to water, tragacanthin dissolves to form a viscous colloidal solution; bassorin swells to form a thick gel (11). Among plant gums, tragacanth produces the most viscous solution (11). When ingested, the bulk of tragacanth stretches the intestinal wall, increasing peristalsis (18). Although tragacanth increases stool weight and decreases GI transit time, it does not appear to affect cholesterol, triglyceride, or phospholipid levels as do other soluble fibers (6). Some preliminary data indicate that people with diabetes who ingest tragacanth along with a high sugar load have lower peak serum glucose and insulin levels (4069). However this effect has not been consistent (6). The mucilaginous, adhesive properties of tragacanth justify its use as a component in denture adhesives (6). Tragacanth appears to inhibit growth of cancer cells (11). Preliminary evidence suggests tragacanthin polysaccharides might offer some protection from hantavirus infections (4070). Tragacanth is highly susceptible to bacterial digestion, even in the presence of preservatives (11).

Adverse Reactions

Orally, use of tragacanth requires ample fluid intake. Insufficient fluid intake can lead to obstruction ileus and esophageal closure (18). Tragacanth can cause asthma symptoms in people who are sensitive to quillaia bark (6).

Interactions with Herbs & Other Dietary Supplements

HERBS AND SUPPLEMENTS: Theoretically, concomitant administration might reduce absorption of supplements and/or herbs due to hydrocolloidal fiber content of tragacanth (19).

Interactions with Drugs

ORAL DRUGS: Theoretically, concomitant administration of oral drugs might reduce drug absorption due to hydrocolloidal fiber content of tragacanth (19).

Interactions with Foods

NUTRIENTS: Theoretically, concomitant administration might impair nutrient absorption from foods due to hydrocolloidal fiber content of tragacanth (19).

Interactions with Lab Tests

None known.

Interactions with Diseases or Conditions

QUILLAIA ALLERGY: Tragacanth can cause asthma symptoms in individuals sensitive to quillaia bark (19).

Dosage and Administration

No typical dosage.

Comments

Karaya gum is a common adulterant in tragacanth (16). It is important to use any amount with adequate fluid intake to prevent esophageal closure or obstruction of the ileus (18).

TRAILING ARBUTUS

Also Known As
Gravel Plant, Ground Laurel, Mountain Pink, Water Pink, Winter Pink.

Scientific Names
Epigaea repens.
Family: Ericaceae.

People Use This For
Orally, trailing arbutus is used for urinary tract conditions, as an astringent, and a diuretic.

Safety
POSSIBLY SAFE ...when the leaves are used orally short-term (12).
UNSAFE ...when the fresh or dried leaves are used orally long-term because they could cause hydroquinone toxicity (18).
PREGNANCY AND LACTATION: Insufficient reliable information available; avoid using.

Effectiveness
There is insufficient reliable information available about the effectiveness of trailing arbutus.

Mechanism of Action
The applicable parts of trailing arbutus are the above ground parts. Trailing arbutus is not suitable for long-term use due to its hydroquinone glycoside content (18). Arbutin may have urinary antiseptic properties due to hydrolysis to its hydroquinone by the intestinal flora (7,11). As a result, long-term use is stated to lead to hydroquinone toxicity (18).

Adverse Reactions
Orally, chronic use of trailing arbutus may lead to hydroquinone toxicity. Symptoms of toxicity include tinnitus, vomiting, delirium, convulsions, and collapse (11). Liver damage, cachexia, hemolytic anemia, and hair depigmentation may also occur with long-term use (18). Overdosage could lead to inflammation of the mucous membranes of the bladder and urinary tract, and may be accompanied by bloody urine, difficulty with urination, and painful urination (18).

Interactions with Herbs & Other Dietary Supplements
None known.

Interactions with Drugs
None known.

Interactions with Foods
None known.

Interactions with Lab Tests
None known.

Interactions with Diseases or Conditions
None known.

Dosage and Administration
ORAL: Trailing arbutus is taken as a tea or extract (18).

Comments
Trailing arbutus's alternate name of gravel plant is similar to that of gravel root. Be careful not to confuse the two.

TRANSFER FACTOR

Also Known As
Bovine Dialyzable Leukocyte Extract, Bovine Dialyzable Transfer Factor, Bovine Transfer Factor, Dialyzable Leukocyte Extract, Dialyzable Transfer Factor, DLE, Human Dialyzable Leukocyte Extract, Human Transfer Factor, TF, TFd.
CAUTION: See separate listing for Bovine Colostrum.

Scientific Names
Transfer Factor

People Use This For
Orally and parenterally, transfer factor is used for infectious diseases in both immunocompetent and immunosuppressed patients, including cryptosporidiosis, septicemia, sinusitis and bronchitis, influenza, the common cold, herpes, varicella, hepatitis B, cytomegalovirus (CMV), Epstein-Barr virus, Pneumocystis carinii, Mycobacterium tuberculosis, Mycobacterium fortuitum, Mycobacterium avium, coccidioidomycosis, candidiasis, leishmaniasis, Cryptococcus, and lepromatous leprosy. Transfer factor is also used for diabetes, autism, infertility, systemic lupus erythematosus (SLE), fibromyalgia, chronic fatigue syndrome (CFS), Bechcet's syndrome, pemphigus vegetans, psoriasis, Wiskott-Aldrich syndrome, alopecia totalis, and Alzheimer's disease. It is also used for retinitis pigmentosa, chorioretinitis, amyotrophic lateral sclerosis (ALS, Lou Gehrig's disease), multiple sclerosis, osteosarcoma, bone metastasis, lung cancer, melanoma, epidermal dysplasia, food and chemical hypersensitivity, myasthenia gravis, subacute sclerosis panencephalitis, atopic dermatitis, and bronchial asthma.

Safety
POSSIBLY SAFE ...when used orally or parenterally and appropriately. Human-derived transfer factor has been used safely in studies lasting up to 2 years (3062,7562,7797,7798) and bovine-derived transfer factor has been safely used in small studies lasting up to 3 months (1445,1507). Some evidence suggests these products are safe; however, some preparations are derived from animals and there is concern about contamination with diseased animal parts (see Adverse Reactions) (1825). There are no reports of disease transmission to humans due to use of contaminated bovine transfer factor.
CHILDREN: POSSIBLY SAFE ...when used orally or parenterally and appropriately. Human-derived transfer factor administered subcutaneously has been used safely for up to 6 years (7794). Oral bovine transfer factor has been used safely for up to 6 months (350).
PREGNANCY AND LACTATION: Insufficient reliable information available; avoid using.

Effectiveness
POSSIBLY EFFECTIVE

Herpes zoster (shingles). Administering transfer factor subcutaneously seems to prevent varicella-zoster in children with leukemia. Human-derived transfer factor prepared from donors with varicella-zoster antibodies seems to protect nonimmune children with acute lymphocytic leukemia (384). However, administering human-derived transfer factor subcutaneously doesn't seem to prevent recurrent varicella-zoster infection or restore immunity in people receiving bone marrow transplant for leukemia (3278).

POSSIBLY INEFFECTIVE

Amyotrophic lateral sclerosis (ALS, Lou Gehrig's disease). Human-derived transfer factor from healthy donors doesn't seem to affect the course of ALS (7795).
Chronic fatigue syndrome (CFS). Administering transfer factor intramuscularly doesn't seem to improve CFS. Transfer factor, obtained from relatives or other human donors, doesn't seem to improve CFS symptoms when administered biweekly, either alone or in combination with cognitive behavioral therapy (7562).
Lung cancer. Administering human-derived transfer factor intramuscularly, in combination with lung resection and chemotherapy, doesn't seem to significantly affect survival (5447,7800).
Malignant melanoma. Administering human-derived transfer factor intramuscularly or subcutaneously, as adjuvant therapy, doesn't seem to affect disease progression or prolong survival when used for up to two years following surgery for Stage I and Stage II melanoma (3062,3063).

INSUFFICIENT RELIABLE EVIDENCE to RATE

AIDS-related cryptosporidiosis. There's some preliminary evidence that oral transfer factor might be beneficial for people with cryptosporidiosis related to AIDS. Transfer factor from bovine sources seems to improve stool frequency and help eradicate oocysts in some patients (1445,1480).
Hepatitis B. Transfer factor derived from patients with acute hepatitis B might be useful for treating chronic active hepatitis B infection (7797).
Leishmania lesions. There's some evidence that transfer factor obtained from patients with antibodies to leishmania can heal persistent cutaneous leishmania lesions (3930,8105).
Multiple sclerosis (MS). There's conflicting research about the use of human-derived transfer factor for MS. It might slow disease progression in people with mild to moderate symptoms. A positive effect is seen only after 18 months to 2 years of therapy (7798,7799).

Woskott-Aldrich syndrome. Some research suggests that human-derived transfer factor might prolong survival in people with Wiskott-Aldrich syndrome, an x-linked recessive genetic disorder (7794).
More evidence is needed to rate transfer factor for these uses.

Mechanism of Action

Transfer factor refers to a variety of dialyzable polypeptide molecules extracted from leukocytes of humans and animals, such as cows and mice (1493,1494). Bovine transfer factor is structurally similar to human-derived transfer factor (7788). Transfer factor contains more than 200 different substances (7790).
Transfer factors are products of T-lymphocytes that transfer the ability to express delayed-type hypersensitivity and cell-mediated immunity from sensitized donors to non-immune recipients (7793). Transfer factors are derived from sources that have developed immunity to certain infectious diseases. For example, bovine transfer factor for cryptosporidiosis is prepared by first inoculating calves with cryptosporidium and then harvesting of lymph nodes (1410,1420,1445,1480,7791). Human-derived transfer factor is prepared from blood of donors with antigen-specific immune responses (1476,1507). The theory is that use of transfer factor from sensitized donors, human or animal, can cause deficient recipients to express cell-mediated immunity (1493). This effect is antigen-specific and results in expression of delayed type hypersensitivity and production of lymphokines (1493,1495,1507,7788).
Animal studies indicate that transfer factor prepared from bovine lymphocytes or bovine colostrum confers cell-mediated immunity to specific antigens on recipients of different species (1475,1477,1478,7791,7792). The exact mechanism of action of transfer factors is unknown; however, a specific amino acid sequence in transfer factor has been identified, and antigen specificity is well-established (1475,1477,1478,7793). Although the recipient of transfer factor acquires the ability to express the cell-mediated immune responses of the donor, the serum of the recipient will not cause a similar response if used to inoculate an unsensitized individual. The production of transfer factor appears to be regulated by immune response genes, but the immunologic activities of transfer factor are not (7789). It is possible that transfer factors might cause an immune response by different mechanisms than active immunization (7793).
Research suggests that transfer factors specific to a variety of bacteria, viruses, protozoa, and other parasites might be useful for microbial diseases (7790). However, there is no evidence that non-specific transfer factor products, such as those marketed on the Internet, are effective for any indication.

Adverse Reactions

Orally or parenterally, transfer factor might cause fever in some patients (1507).
Parenterally, transfer factor is usually well tolerated (3062,3063,7562,7799). It can cause tenderness, pain, and swelling at the injection site (3062,7562,7799).
There is also some concern that bovine-derived transfer factor that is produced from cows in countries where bovine spongiform encephalitis (BSE) has been reported might be contaminated with diseased tissue. Countries where BSE has been reported include Great Britain, France, the Netherlands, Portugal, Luxembourg, Ireland, Switzerland, Oman, and Belgium (1825). However, there have been no reports of BSE transfer to humans from contaminated transfer factor products. Until more is known, tell patients to avoid these products unless country of origin can be determined. Patients should avoid products that are produced in countries where BSE has been found.

Interactions with Herbs & Other Dietary Supplements

None known.

Interactions with Drugs

None known.

Interactions with Foods

None known.

Interactions with Lab Tests

None known.

Interactions with Diseases or Conditions

None known.

Dosage and Administration

ORAL: For cryptosporidiosis, clinical studies used bovine transfer factor 1 unit (5 x 108 lymph node cell equivalents) weekly for 1-1/2 to 3 months (1420,1445).
SUBCUTANEOUS: For preventing varicella-zoster in nonimmune children with leukemia, a single dose of human-derived transfer factor, specific for varicella, of 100 million lymphocyte equivalents per 7 kg of body weight has been used (384).

Comments

Transfer factors thus far have been produced only in laboratories for experimental use. There's some evidence that they can be stored for 12 months and retain potency (7790).

TRAVELER'S JOY

Also Known As
Old Man's Beard, Travelers Joy.
CAUTION: See separate listings for Clematis, Fringetree, Usnea, and Woodbine.

Scientific Names
Clematis vitalba.
Family: Ranunculaceae.

People Use This For
Orally, traveler's joy is used for diseases of the male genitals and migraine headaches.
Topically, traveler's joy is used for poorly healing wounds and migraine headaches.

Safety
LIKELY UNSAFE ...when used orally or topically due to the constituent protoanemonin, which is a severe local irritant (18).
PREGNANCY AND LACTATION: LIKELY UNSAFE ...when used orally or topically (18).

Effectiveness
There is insufficient reliable information available about the effectiveness of traveler's joy.

Mechanism of Action
The applicable part of traveler's joy is the fresh leaf. When the fresh plant is crushed or cut into small pieces, the glycoside ranunculin is enzymatically changed into a severely irritating protoanemonin, which, in turn, rapidly degrades into the less toxic anemonin (18). Both protoanemonin and ranunculin are destroyed to an unknown extent during the drying process (2).

Adverse Reactions
Orally, traveler's joy can cause severe irritation of the gastrointestinal tract, including colic and diarrhea. Irritation of the urinary tract can also occur.
Topically, skin contact can cause blisters and burns that are difficult to heal (18).

Interactions with Herbs & Other Dietary Supplements
None known.

Interactions with Drugs
None known.

Interactions with Foods
None known.

Interactions with Lab Tests
None known.

Interactions with Diseases or Conditions
None known.

Dosage and Administration
No typical dosage.

TREE OF HEAVEN

Also Known As
A-Lan-Thus, Ailanto, Chinese Sumach, Copal Tree, Heaven Tree, Paradise Tree, Stinktree, Varnish Tree, Vernis de Japon.

Scientific Names
Ailanthus altissima, Ailanthus cacodendron, Ailanthus giraldii, Ailanthus glandulosa, Ailanthus vilmoriniana, Rhus cacodendron, Toxicodendron altissimum.
Family: Simaroubaceae.

People Use This For
Orally, tree of heaven is used for pathological leukorrhea, diarrhea, chronic diarrhea, chronic dysentery, dysmenorrhea, and asthma, cramps, epilepsy, fast heart rate, gonorrhea, malaria, and tapeworms. It has also been used as a bitter and a tonic.
In foods, the young leaves of the tree of heaven are eaten.
In manufacturing, tree of heaven is used as insecticide.

Safety
There is insufficient reliable information available about the safety of tree of heaven. However, fatal poisonings have been reported in animal experiments (18).
Pregnancy and Lactation: Insufficient reliable information available; avoid using.

Effectiveness
There is insufficient reliable information available about the effectiveness of tree of heaven.

Mechanism of Action
The applicable parts of tree of heaven are the dried trunk and root bark. The bark of the tree of heaven is said to have astringent, antipyretic, and antispasmodic properties (18). Some evidence suggests the quassionoid constituents, including ailanthone and quassin, have antiprotozoan, anthelmintic, antileukemic, and cytotoxic properties (18). The bark also contains tannins and indole alkaloids of the beta-carbolic type (18).

Adverse Reactions
Orally, large amounts of the tree of heaven bark can cause queasiness, dizziness, headache, limb tingling, and diarrhea (18).

Interactions with Herbs & Other Dietary Supplements
None known.

Interactions with Drugs
None known.

Interactions with Foods
None known.

Interactions with Lab Tests
None known.

Interactions with Diseases or Conditions
None known.

Dosage and Administration
ORAL: A typical dose is 6-9 grams (18).

Comments
Until recently, tree of heaven was used only in folk medicine. Currently, it is being investigated as a potential drug (18).

TRYPSIN

Also Known As
Proteinase, Proteolytic Enzyme, Tripsin.

Scientific Names
Trypsin.

People Use This For
Orally, trypsin is used for digestive enzyme supplementation in conjunction with lipase, amylase, and other proteases.
In combination with bromelain and rutin, trypsin is used for osteoarthritis.
Topically, trypsin is used for wound and ulcer cleansing to remove necrotic tissue and debris. Also, the prescription aerosol products containing trypsin, Peru balsam, and castor oil are applied topically for enzymatic debridement, promotion of normal wound healing, and promoting the healing of necrotic oral mucosa ulcers.

Safety

POSSIBLY SAFE ...when used topically by health care professionals trained in wound debridement (506). The topical combination containing trypsin, Peru balsam, and castor oil is an FDA-approved prescription aerosol product. There is insufficient reliable information available about the safety of trypsin for its other uses.
PREGNANCY AND LACTATION: Insufficient reliable information available; avoid using.

Effectiveness

POSSIBLY EFFECTIVE

Osteoarthritis. In a double-blind trial, 73 patients with painful osteoarthritis of the knee were randomly assigned the combination enzyme product (Phlogenzym) or diclofenac (Voltaren) 50 mg three times daily during the first week and then twice daily in weeks 2 and 3. The enzyme product was similar to diclofenac in relieving pain and improving knee function (6252).

Wound healing. Applying trypsin topically seems to be helpful for cleansing wounds of necrotic material and enhancing wound healing (715,716).

There is insufficient reliable information available about the effectiveness of trypsin for its other uses.

Mechanism of Action

Trypsin is a proteolytic enzyme formed in the small intestines by the action of enteropeptidase on trypsinogen (511). Trypsin supplements are derived from fungi or bacterial sources, pancreas of livestock, or from plant sources. It is used to remove dead tissue that remains after trauma, infections such as decubitus ulcers, and surgical procedures. The removal of dead cells allows the growth of healthy tissues (13). Some topical preparations that are available contain balsam of Peru and castor oil to protect the skin and prevent premature epithelial destruction (13). Evidence from in vitro studies of necroses and purulent exudates (2648) and a human study (2649) shows streptokinase-streptodornase can have better proteolytic activity than trypsin alone.

Adverse Reactions

Topically, trypsin can cause localized pain and transient burning (506).

Interactions with Herbs & Other Dietary Supplements

None known.

Interactions with Drugs

None known.

Interactions with Foods

None known.

Interactions with Lab Tests

None known.

Interactions with Diseases or Conditions

None known.

Dosage and Administration

ORAL: For osteoarthritis, a combination enzyme product (Phlogenzym), which contains rutin 100 mg, trypsin 48 mg, and bromelain 90 mg, has been given 2 tablets three times daily (6252).
TOPICAL: Wound debridement products (Dermuspray, Granulderm, Granulex, and GranuMed) containing trypsin, Peru balsam, and castor oil (506) are FDA-approved prescription products.

Comments

Commercial trypsin is prepared from animal sources, such as ox pancreas (13).

TUNG SEED

Also Known As

Balucanat, Candleberry, Candleberry Tree, Candlenut, China-Wood Oil, Country Walnut, Indian Walnut, Kukui, Otaheite Walnut, Tung, Varnish Tree.
CAUTION: See separate listing for Bayberry.

Scientific Names

Aleurites moluccanus, synonyms Aleurites javanicus, Aleurites pentaphyllus, Aleurites remyi, Aleurites trilobus, Jatropha moluccana; Vernicia cordata, synonym Aleurites cordatus.
Family: Euphorbiaceae.

People Use This For

Orally, tung seed is used for asthma, bloody diarrhea, dysentery, sprue, and as a bowel stimulant.
Topically, tung seed is used to stimulate hair growth and for constipation.
In manufacturing, the oil of tung seed is used in soaps, rubber substitutes, linoleum, and insulation. The seed cake of tung seed is used as a fertilizer. The seed is also the source of the oil that is widely used as a wood preservative and varnish.

Safety

LIKELY UNSAFE ...when used orally (6). Tung seed is believed to contain toxalbumin and hydrogen cyanide (6). Toxicity ranges from severe gastrointestinal irritation to death (6,4502). Even a single seed might cause severe poisoning (4502).
There is insufficient reliable information available about the safety of the topical use of tung seed.
PREGNANCY AND LACTATION: LIKELY UNSAFE ...when used orally (6,); avoid using.

Effectiveness

There is insufficient reliable information available about the effectiveness of tung seed.

Mechanism of Action

Tung seed contains an oil that consists of eleostearic acid, linolenic, linoleic, and oleic acid. It is also thought to contain a toxalbumin and hydrogen cyanide (6). Internally, tung seed has cathartic effects (6,4502). The kernels have laxative and stimulant effects. They also promote sweating (4502).

Adverse Reactions

Orally, tung seed can cause severe stomach pain, violent vomiting, debility, diarrhea, slowed reflexes, slowed breathing, and possibly death (6,4502). Skin contact with tung seed can cause acute dermatitis (4502).

Interactions with Herbs & Other Dietary Supplements

None known.

Interactions with Drugs

None known.

Interactions with Foods

None known.

Interactions with Lab Tests

None known.

Interactions with Diseases or Conditions

None known.

Dosage and Administration

No typical dosage.

Comments

The seeds of the fruit from this plant resemble a walnut, and the term walnut is applied to this species. Tung seed should never be confused with the common walnut. Unlike the walnut, if tung seeds are eaten raw they are toxic. When roasted, the kernels are reported to be edible (6). It is said that fishermen throw tung seeds into the water to stupefy the fish (6,4502).

TURKEY CORN

Also Known As

Bleeding Heart, Dutchman's Breeches, Squirrel Corn, Staggerweed.

Scientific Names

Dicentra cucullaria.
Family: Fumariaceae.

People Use This For

Orally, turkey corn is used for digestive and menstrual disorders, urinary tract diseases, and skin rashes.

Safety

POSSIBLY UNSAFE ...when used orally. Theoretically, the constituent bicuculline, an antagonist of gamma-aminobutyric acid (GABA), could cause poisoning (18).
PREGNANCY AND LACTATION: POSSIBLY UNSAFE ...when used orally (18); avoid using.

Effectiveness

There is insufficient reliable information available about the effectiveness of turkey corn.

Mechanism of Action

The applicable part of turkey corn is the dried tuber. Turkey corn is thought to have diuretic and tonic properties (18). It contains various isoquinoline alkaloids, including bicuculline, corlumine, protopine, cryptopine, and cularine. Bicuculline is a centrally-acting, spasmogenic antagonist of GABA (18).

Adverse Reactions

None reported.

Interactions with Herbs & Other Dietary Supplements

None known.

Interactions with Drugs

None known.

Interactions with Foods

None known.

Interactions with Lab Tests

None known.

Interactions with Diseases or Conditions

None known.

Dosage and Administration

ORAL: Turkey corn is used as a liquid extract (18).

TURMERIC

Also Known As

Curcumae Longae Rhizoma, Curcumin, Haridra, Indian Saffron, Nisha, Radix Curcumae, Rajani.
CAUTION: See separate listings for Javanese Turmeric, Zedoary, and Goldenseal.

Scientific Names

Curcuma longa, synonym Curcuma domestica; Curcuma aromatica.
Family: Zingiberaceae.

People Use This For

Orally, turmeric is used for dyspepsia, abdominal pain, hemorrhage, diarrhea, flatulence, abdominal bloating, loss of appetite, jaundice, hepatitis, and liver and gallbladder complaints. It is also used for headaches, bronchitis, colds, respiratory infections, fibromyalgia, leprosy, fever, amenorrhea, and cancer. Other uses include depression, edema, worms, kidney inflammation, and cystitis.
Topically, turmeric is used for analgesia, ringworm, bruising, leech bites, eye infections, inflammatory skin conditions, inflammation of the oral mucosa, and infected wounds.
In food and manufacturing, the essential oil is used in perfumes, and turmeric and its resin are used as a flavor and color component in foods. Turmeric is also a culinary spice and a major ingredient in curry powder.

Safety

LIKELY SAFE ...when used in amounts commonly found in foods. Turmeric has Generally Recognized As Safe (GRAS) status in the US (4912).
POSSIBLY SAFE ...when used orally or topically in medicinal amounts (10453,11144,11148,11149,11150).
PREGNANCY: LIKELY UNSAFE ...when used orally in medicinal amounts; turmeric might stimulate menstrual flow and the uterus (12).
LACTATION: There is insufficient reliable information available about the safety of turmeric in medicinal amounts during lactation.

Effectiveness

POSSIBLY EFFECTIVE

Dyspepsia. Taking turmeric orally seems to relieve dyspeptic symptoms (11144).

INSUFFICIENT RELIABLE EVIDENCE to RATE

Anterior uveitis. Clinical research suggests curcumin given orally might be useful for treating chronic anterior uveitis (11150).

Colorectal cancer. Preliminary clinical research suggests an extract of turmeric might stabilize colorectal cancer refractory to other treatments in some patients (10453).

Rheumatoid arthritis (RA). Curcumin, a constituent of turmeric, might relieve some symptoms of rheumatoid arthritis (RA) (11149).

Skin cancer. Other preliminary clinical research suggests that an ethanol extract of turmeric in combination with turmeric ointment might relieve odor and itching associated with skin cancers (11148).

More evidence is needed to rate turmeric for these uses.

Mechanism of Action

The applicable part of turmeric is the rhizome. Turmeric's major active constituents are curcuminoids including curcumin (diferuloylmethane), a yellow pigment. It seems to have anti-inflammatory activity, possibly by inhibiting cyclooxygenase-2 (COX-2), prostaglandins, and leukotrienes (11138,11139,11140,12482).

Turmeric also exhibits chemopreventive and growth inhibitory activity against several tumor cell lines. It seems to induce apoptosis in cancer cells and may inhibit angiogenesis (11141,11142,12482).

Curcumin might have antithrombotic effects. Preliminary research suggests it might inhibit platelet-activating factor and arachidonic acid platelet aggregation, possibly by interfering with thromboxane synthesis (11143).

Other preliminary research suggests that turmeric might also have antioxidant and immunostimulatory effects (11140,11147). It also seems to have activity against some bacteria, human immunodeficiency virus (HIV), and the protozoan Leishmania amazonensis (11140).

The bioavailability of curcumin is very low after oral administration (10453). Bromelain is sometimes recommended to enhance curcumin absorption, but there's no reliable evidence to support this.

Adverse Reactions

Orally, turmeric is generally well tolerated (10453,11144,11148,11149,11150). It can cause gastrointestinal (GI) adverse effects such as nausea and diarrhea (10453).

Topically, turmeric can cause allergic dermatitis (11146).

Interactions with Herbs & Other Dietary Supplements

HERBS WITH ANTICOAGULANT/ANTIPLATELET POTENTIAL: Concomitant use of turmeric with herbs might affect platelet aggregation could theoretically increase the risk of bleeding in some people (11143). These herbs include angelica, clove, danshen, garlic, ginger, ginkgo, Panax ginseng, red clover, willow, and others.

Interactions with Drugs

ANTICOAGULANT/ANTIPLATELET DRUGS: Concomitant use of turmeric with these drugs might increase the risk of bleeding due to decreased platelet aggregation. Turmeric has been reported to have antiplatelet effects (11143); avoid concomitant use. Some of these drugs include aspirin, clopidogrel (Plavix), dalteparin (Fragmin), enoxaparin (Lovenox), heparin, ticlopidine (Ticlid), warfarin (Coumadin), and others.

Interactions with Foods

None known.

Interactions with Lab Tests

None known.

Interactions with Diseases or Conditions

BILE DUCT OBSTRUCTION AND GALLSTONES: Turmeric can cause gallbladder contractions (11145). Use with caution in patients with gallstones or gallbladder disease.

Dosage and Administration

ORAL: For dyspepsia, 500 mg of turmeric four times daily has been used (11144). For colorectal cancer, curcuma extract 440 to 2200 mg, containing curcumin 36 to 180 mg, has been given daily for up to 4 months (10453).

TOPICAL: No typical dosage.

Comments

Turmeric has a warm, bitter taste and is frequently used to flavor or color curry powders, mustards, butters, and cheeses (6002). Avoid confusion with Javanese turmeric root (Curcuma zedoaria).

TURPENTINE OIL

Also Known As
Purified Turpentine Oil, Spirits Of Turpentine, Terebinthinae aetheroleum, Turpentine.

Scientific Names
Pinus palustris, synonym Pinus australis; Pinus pinaster; other Pinus species.
Family: Pinaceae.

People Use This For
Topically, turpentine oil is used for rheumatic and neuralgic ailments, muscle pain, toothaches, and disseminated sclerosis.
By inhalation, the vapors of turpentine oil are used to reduce the thickened secretions associated with chronic diseases of the bronchi.
In foods and beverages, distilled turpentine oil is used as a flavoring ingredient.
In manufacturing, turpentine oil is used as an ingredient in soap and cosmetics. Turpentine oil is also used as a paint solvent.

Safety
POSSIBLY SAFE ...when used topically and appropriately (2). ...when the vapors are inhaled appropriately (2).
POSSIBLY UNSAFE ...when applied topically to large areas (2).
LIKELY UNSAFE ...when used orally for medicinal purposes. 2 mL/kg of turpentine oil is considered toxic (17). 120-180 mL is potentially lethal in adults (17). Pulmonary aspiration can cause hemorrhagic pulmonary edema (17).
CHILDREN: LIKELY UNSAFE ...when used orally, 15 mL is potentially lethal (17). There is insufficient reliable information available about the safety of turpentine oil applied topically or inhaled as vapors in children.
PREGNANCY AND LACTATION: LIKELY UNSAFE ...when used orally. It might be an abortifacient (19). There is insufficient reliable information available about the safety of turpentine oil applied topically or inhaled as vapors during pregnancy and lactation.

Effectiveness
There is insufficient reliable information available about the effectiveness of turpentine oil.

Mechanism of Action
Turpentine oil is a central nervous system depressant and a pulmonary aspiration hazard. When applied topically, turpentine oil is irritating and exhibits rubefacient and counterirritant effects (6,11). When inhaled, turpentine oil can have a decongestant effect, possibly by stimulating the cold receptors, which results in reflex vasoconstriction (7).

Adverse Reactions
Orally, turpentine oil can cause headache, insomnia, coughing, vomiting, hematuria, albuminuria (6), urinary tract inflammation (17), coma (6), and death (17). Pulmonary aspiration produces hemorrhagic pulmonary edema (17). As inhalation therapy, it can cause mild respiratory tract inflammation (17). Turpentine oil can exacerbate bronchial spasms in people with asthma and whooping cough (7).
Topically, it can cause skin irritation, contact allergies, and hypersensitivity (6). Symptoms of poisoning can occur when turpentine oil is applied extensively, including kidney and central nervous system damage (2).

Interactions with Herbs & Other Dietary Supplements
None known.

Interactions with Drugs
None known.

Interactions with Foods
None known.

Interactions with Lab Tests
None known.

Interactions with Diseases or Conditions
ACUTE RESPIRATORY TRACT INFLAMMATION: Inhalation of turpentine is contraindicated (2).
ASTHMA, WHOOPING COUGH: Turpentine can exacerbate bronchial spasms (7).
HYPERSENSITIVITY: Contraindicated (2).

Dosage and Administration

TOPICAL: Several drops of the oil are typically rubbed onto the affected area. The liquid and semi-solid preparations are commonly made in concentrations of 10-50% (2). Application of turpentine should not exceed three to four times per day (3).
INHALATION: The vapors of turpentine are often inhaled as several drops of the oil in hot water (2).

Comments

Turpentine oil is obtained by the distillation of the oleoresin (gum turpentine) of longleaf pine (Pinus palustris) and other Pinus species. Terpin hydrate is a semi-synthetic derivative of turpentine (6). Turpentine oil has been used to adulterate juniper berry oil (512). Avoid confusion with gum turpentine, which is the oleoresin (6).

TURTLE HEAD

Also Known As

Balmony, Bitter Herb, Chelone, Hummingbird Tree, Salt-rheum Weed, Shellflower, Snakehead, Turtlebloom.

Scientific Names

Chelone glabra.
Family: Scrophulariaceae.

People Use This For

Orally, turtle head is used as a cathartic tonic.

Safety

POSSIBLY SAFE ...when used orally (12,18).
PREGNANCY AND LACTATION: Insufficient reliable information available; avoid using.

Effectiveness

There is insufficient reliable information available about the effectiveness of turtle head.

Mechanism of Action

The applicable parts of turtle head are the above ground parts and root. Turtle head contains iridoide monoterpenes including catalpol and a bitter-tasting resin (18).

Adverse Reactions

None reported.

Interactions with Herbs & Other Dietary Supplements

None known.

Interactions with Drugs

None known.

Interactions with Foods

None known.

Interactions with Lab Tests

None known.

Interactions with Diseases or Conditions

None known.

Dosage and Administration

No typical dosage.

Comments

Avoid confusion with Chelone obliqua which is commonly known as red turtle head (4500).

TYROSINE

Also Known As
L-tyrosine, Tyr, Tyrosinum.

Scientific Names
2-amino-3-(4-hydroxyphenyl)propionic acid.

People Use This For
Orally, tyrosine is used for depression, attention deficit disorder (ADD), attention deficit-hyperactivity disorder (ADHD), phenylketonuria (PKU), improving alertness following sleep deprivation. It is also used for stress, premenstrual syndrome (PMS), Parkinson's disease, chronic fatigue syndrome (CFS), narcolepsy, alcohol and cocaine withdrawal, Alzheimer's disease, cardiovascular disease, impotence, loss of libido, schizophrenia, and as a suntan agent and appetite suppressant.
Topically, tyrosine is used for signs of aging skin such as wrinkles.

Safety
LIKELY SAFE ...when used orally in amounts commonly found in foods. Tyrosine has Generally Recognized As Safe (GRAS) status in the US (4912).
POSSIBLY SAFE ...when used orally and appropriately, short-term. Tyrosine seems to be safe when used in doses up to 150 mg/kg per day for up to 3 months (7210,7211,7215). ...when used topically and appropriately (6155).
PREGNANCY AND LACTATION: There is insufficient reliable information available about the safety of tyrosine during pregnancy and lactation when used in medicinal amounts.

Effectiveness
EFFECTIVE

Phenylketonuria (PKU). Tyrosine is used as a component of protein supplements for people with phenylketonuria (PKU), a genetic disorder in which there is an inability to metabolize phenylalanine, a precursor of tyrosine (7212,7213,7232). The current recommendation for people with PKU is the incorporation of 6 grams of tyrosine per 100 grams of protein. However, additional separate supplementation with free tyrosine is not recommended because it can produce wide variations in tyrosine plasma concentrations and side effects (7212).

POSSIBLY EFFECTIVE

Sleep deprivation. Taking tyrosine orally seems to improve alertness following sleep deprivation (7215). Tyrosine 150 mg/kg seems to delay performance decline in psychomotor tests by about 3 hours after loss of a night's sleep (7215).

POSSIBLY INEFFECTIVE

Attention deficit disorder (ADD). Taking tyrosine orally doesn't seem to improve symptoms of adult ADD. Some patients might have transient improvement in symptoms after starting tyrosine, but adult patients quickly acquire tolerance (7210,7211).

Attention deficit-hyperactivity disorder (ADHD). Taking tyrosine orally doesn't seem to improve symptoms of childhood ADHD (7209).

Depression. Taking tyrosine orally doesn't seem to improve symptoms of moderate depression (7208).

INSUFFICIENT RELIABLE EVIDENCE to RATE

Wrinkled skin. A topical preparation containing 10% vitamin C as L-ascorbic acid, acetyl tyrosine, zinc sulfate, sodium hyaluronate, and bioflavonoids (Cellex-C High Potency Serum) applied for 3 months to photo-aged facial skin seems to improve fine and coarse wrinkling, yellowing and sallowness, roughness, and skin tone compared to placebo (6155). More evidence is needed to rate the effectiveness of tyrosine for this use.

Mechanism of Action
Tyrosine is a nonessential amino acid that the body synthesizes from phenylalanine. For people with phenylketonuria (PKU) who cannot synthesize tyrosine from phenylalanine, tyrosine is an essential amino acid (7212). Tyrosine can also be obtained from dietary proteins in dairy products, meats, fish, eggs, nuts, beans, oats, and wheat. When dietary intake of tyrosine is inadequate, phenylalanine is converted to tyrosine (7217). Dietary needs of tyrosine are dependent on phenylalanine intake. When phenylalanine intake is adequate (about 9 mg/kg/day), dietary tyrosine intake should be about 7 mg/kg/day (7214). Inadequate tyrosine intake is rare in developed nations. Tyrosine is incorporated into all proteins. Tyrosine is a precursor of thyroxine and melanin (7212); it is also a precursor for the synthesis of catecholamines, norepinephrine, epinephrine, and dopamine (7215,7217). Tyrosine is classified as a large neutral amino acid (LNAA) and is transported across the blood brain barrier by the LNAA transporter. Tyrosine competes with other LNAAs, such as tryptophan, to get into the brain (7217). There is interest in tyrosine for preventing the negative effects related to stress. Some scientists think that the brain may not be able to synthesize enough tyrosine from phenylalanine under stressful conditions (7217). Catecholamines like epinephrine, norepinephrine, and dopamine that are synthesized from tyrosine can become depleted during stress. There is speculation that increasing the availability of tyrosine to the brain allows increased catecholamine synthesis, and avoidance of the negative effects of stress. There is some evidence in animals and

humans that supplemental tyrosine might improve performance, memory, and learning, under extreme environmental conditions, intense exercise, or psychological stress (7215,7217).

Adverse Reactions

Orally, tyrosine can cause nausea, headache, fatigue, heartburn, and arthralgia (7211).

Interactions with Herbs & Other Dietary Supplements

None known.

Interactions with Drugs

LEVODOPA: There is some concern that tyrosine might decrease the effectiveness of L-dopa. Tyrosine and levodopa compete for absorption in the proximal duodenum by the large neutral amino acid (LNAA) transport system (2719). Advise patients to separate doses of tyrosine and L-dopa by at least 2 hours.
THYROID HORMONE: There is some concern that tyrosine might have additive effects with thyroid hormone medications. Tyrosine is a precursor to thyroid hormone and might boost levels (7212). These drugs include levothyroxine (Synthroid, Levoxyl) and liothyronine (Cytomel).

Interactions with Foods

None known.

Interactions with Lab Tests

THYROID STIMULATING HORMONE (TSH): Theoretically, tyrosine might decrease TSH levels. Tyrosine is a precursor of thyroxine and might boost thyroid hormone levels, which can decrease TSH results (7212).

Interactions with Diseases or Conditions

HYPERTHYROIDISM, GRAVES' DISEASE: Theoretically, tyrosine might exacerbate hyperthyroidism and Graves' disease. Tyrosine is a precursor of thyroxine and might boost thyroid hormone levels (7212). Tell patients with hyperthyroidism or Grave's disease not to take tyrosine supplements.

Dosage and Administration

ORAL: For improving alertness after sleep deprivation, 150 mg/kg/day of tyrosine has been used (7215).

USNEA

Also Known As

Beard Moss, Old Man's Beard, Sodium Usniate, Tree Moss, Tree's Dandruff, Usnea Lichen, Usnic Acid, Woman's Long Hair.
CAUTION: See separate listing for Oak Moss.

Scientific Names

Usnea barbata; Usnea florida; Usnea hirta; Usnea plicata.
Family: Usneaceae.

People Use This For

Orally, usnea is used for weight loss, pain relief, fever control, wound healing, and as an expectorant.
Topically, usnea is used for mild inflammation of the mouth and pharynx.

Safety

POSSIBLY SAFE ...when used topically and appropriately (12). There is insufficient reliable information available about the safety of usnea taken orally.
PREGNANCY AND LACTATION: Insufficient reliable information available; avoid using.

Effectiveness

There is insufficient reliable information available about the effectiveness of usnea.

Mechanism of Action

The applicable part of usnea is the plant body. Usnea contains a variety of lichen acids including usnic acid, thamnolic acid, lobaric acid, stictinic acid, evernic acid, barbatic acid, diffractaic acid, and protocetraric acid. However, the exact composition varies significantly among species (11720). The hydroalcoholic extracts of Usnea barbata and Usnea hirta have anti-inflammatory, analgesic, and antipyretic activity (852). The usnic acid constituent of usnea has antibacterial, antifungal, antiviral, and antiprotozoal activity. It also seems to have antipyretic, anti-inflammatory, and analgesic effects that may result from inhibition of prostaglandin synthesis. Preliminary research on leukemia cells suggests that usnic acid might also have antiproliferative activity (11720).

Adverse Reactions
Orally, usnic acid as an ingredient in the product LipoKinetix has been associated with hepatoxicity (7091). Topically, usnea can cause local irritation, contact dermatitis, and conjunctivitis (11720).

Interactions with Herbs & Other Dietary Supplements
None known.

Interactions with Drugs
None known.

Interactions with Foods
None known.

Interactions with Lab Tests
None known.

Interactions with Diseases or Conditions
None known.

Dosage and Administration
No typical dosage.

Comments
Sodium usniate (usnic acid) is a constituent of Usnea. Sodium usniate is also an ingredient of the brand named product LipoKinetix. There are serious concerns about the safety of LipoKinetix, which is marketed for weight loss. From July to December 2000 there were at least seven cases of acute hepatotoxicity in patients taking LipoKinetix. Symptoms including nausea, weakness and fatigue, abdominal pain, and yellowing of the skin usually develop from 2 weeks to 3 months after starting LipoKinetix. Symptoms resolve when it is discontinued (7091). It is unclear if the sodium usniate ingredient is the cause of these adverse events. Tell patients not to use this product.
Usnea species are whitish, reddish, or black lichens that grow on a variety of trees. Avoid confusion with oak moss (Evernia prunastri), also referred to as tree moss.

UVA URSI

Also Known As
Arberry, Bear's Grape, Bearberry, Beargrape, Common Bearberry, Hogberry, Kinnikinnik, Manzanita, Mountain Box, Mountain Cranberry, Ptarmigan Berry, Raisin D'Ours, Red Bearberry, Redberry, Rockberry, Sagackhomi, Sandberry, Uvae ursi folium.
CAUTION: See separate listings for Alpine Cranberry, Cramp Bark, and Cranberry.

Scientific Names
Arctostaphylos uva-ursi, synonym Arbutus uva-ursi.
Family: Ericacea.

People Use This For
Orally, uva ursi is used for urinary tract infections (UTIs), inflammatory conditions of the efferent urinary tract, cystitis, urethritis, diuresis, constipation, lithuria, dysuria, acidic urine, pyelonephritis, and bronchitis.
In combination, an herbal preparation containing uva ursi, hops, and peppermint is used to treat people with compulsive, strangury enuresis and painful urination.

Safety
POSSIBLY SAFE ...when used orally and appropriately, short-term (2,4,12).
POSSIBLY UNSAFE ...when used orally for extended periods. There is some concern about the safety of long-term use because of the hydroquinone constituent of uva ursi. Hydroquinone can have mutagenic and carcinogenic effects, and long-term use might result in significant adverse effects. Tell patients to avoid using uva ursi for more than one week or more than five times per year (2,7,18).
CHILDREN: LIKELY UNSAFE ...when used orally due to the risk of hepatotoxicity in children less than 12 years old (2,7,18).
PREGNANCY: LIKELY UNSAFE ...when used orally (2,4,6,7,12,18). Uva ursi can have oxytocic effects (19); avoid using.
LACTATION: Insufficient reliable information available; avoid using.

Effectiveness

INSUFFICIENT RELIABLE EVIDENCE to RATE

Urinary tract infections (UTIs). Preliminary evidence suggests that taking a combination product containing both uva ursi and dandelion orally seems to significantly reduce the recurrence rate of UTIs in women (1932). However, since it isn't clear if this kind of extended use is safe, tell patients not to use uva ursi for long-term prevention of UTIs. More evidence is needed to rate uva ursi for this use.

Mechanism of Action

The applicable part of uva ursi is the leaf. Uva ursi can have urinary antiseptic and astringent effects (4). Some references report diuretic activity, but others disagree (6,8). Its constituents include arbutin (a phenol), tannins, and hydroquinone (4,6,7). The tannins can be responsible for adverse gastrointestinal tract effects (5) and limit the duration of use (4). Uva ursi and the constituent, arbutin, exhibit antimicrobial activity in vitro (2,4). Arbutin is absorbed from the gastrointestinal tract unchanged and is hydrolyzed to hydroquinone in alkaline urine. There it can exert antiseptic and astringent effects (4,5,7). For this reason, urinary acidifying agents may decrease the effectiveness of uva ursi, and urinary alkalinizing agents may increase its effectiveness (19).

Hydroquinone is cytotoxic in vitro (4). Crude uva ursi extract can be more effective than the constituent arbutin as an astringent and antiseptic (4). In rats, uva ursi shows anti-inflammatory activity against experimentally-induced inflammation (4). Large amounts of uva ursi are reported to be oxytocic, although in vitro studies show no uteroactivity (4).

Adverse Reactions

Orally, uva ursi can cause nausea, vomiting (2), gastrointestinal discomfort, and a greenish-brown discoloration of the urine (4). Large amounts can be oxytocic, increasing the rapidity of labor (4). One gram of hydroquinone, equivalent to 6-20 grams of uva ursi, can cause tinnitus, nausea, vomiting, shortness of breath, cyanosis, convulsions, delirium, and collapse (4). Five grams of hydroquinone, equivalent to 30-100 grams of uva ursi, can cause death (4). Other adverse effects due to uva ursi include hepatotoxicity and irritation and inflammation of the urinary tract mucous membranes (18). Chronic use, especially in children (18), can cause liver impairment due to its tannin content (4).

Interactions with Herbs & Other Dietary Supplements

None known.

Interactions with Drugs

None known.

Interactions with Foods

None known.

Interactions with Lab Tests

COLORIMETRIC URINE TESTS: Theoretically, uva ursi can interfere with colorimetric urine tests and can turn urine greenish-brown (4).

Interactions with Diseases or Conditions

GI IRRITATION: Because excessive use of uva ursi can lead to stomach distress due to its tannin content, its use is contraindicated in patients with GI irritation (12,19).

KIDNEY DISORDERS: Contraindicated (12,19).

Dosage and Administration

ORAL: The typical dose of dried herb is 1.5-4 grams daily (4). It's also commonly used as a tea. The tea is prepared by steeping 3 grams of the dried leaf in 150 mL cold water for 12-24 hours and then straining. One cup of tea is usually taken up to 4 times daily (2,7,515). Uva ursi leaf teas should be prepared with cold water to minimize the tannin content (515). The hydroquinone derivative, calculated as water-free arbutin, is commonly dosed as 100-210 mg up to 4 times daily (2,7,515). The fluid extract (1:1 in 25% alcohol) is given 1.5-4 mL three times daily (4). Medical consultation is needed for urinary tract symptoms persisting longer than 48 hours (4). Uva ursi should not be used longer than one week without monitoring due to its potential risks (7). Limit its use to less than five times per year (7).

Comments

Bears are particularly fond of the fruit, which is implied in the Latin name "uva ursi", which means "bear's grape". Most authorities refer to Arctostaphylos uva-ursi as uva ursi. However, the related plants, Arctostaphylos adentricha and Arctostaphylos coactylis, have also been termed uva ursi by some authors (6).

UZARA

Also Known As
Uzarae radix.

Scientific Names
Xysmalobium undulatum.
Family: Asclepiadaceae.

People Use This For
Orally, uzara is used for diarrhea.

Safety
POSSIBLY SAFE ...when used orally for short-term use (2). Medical consultation is needed for diarrhea persisting more than three to four days (2).
LIKELY UNSAFE ...when used parenterally. Deaths have occurred after administration of uzara products (18).
PREGNANCY AND LACTATION: Insufficient reliable information available; avoid using.

Effectiveness
There is insufficient reliable information available about the effectiveness of uzara.

Mechanism of Action
The applicable part of uzara is the root. It inhibits intestinal motility (2), and in larger amounts, it can have digitalis-like effects on the heart (2). Uzara contains a cardiac glycoside mixture of cardenolides, which include uzarone, xysmalobin, and uzarin. The glycosides can be poorly absorbed (18).

Adverse Reactions
Orally, there have been no reports of adverse reactions associated with white uzara, but it is theoretically possible due to the cardiac glycoside content (18).
Parenterally, deaths have occurred after administration of uzara products (18).

Interactions with Herbs & Other Dietary Supplements
CARDIAC GLYCOSIDE-CONTAINING HERBS: Uzara is contraindicated with these herbs, and concomitant use can increase the risk of cardiac glycoside toxicity. Cardiac glycoside containing herbs include black hellebore, Canadian hemp roots, digitalis leaf, hedge mustard, figwort, lily-of-the-valley roots, motherwort, oleander leaf, pheasant's eye plant, pleurisy root, squill bulb leaf scales, and strophanthus seeds (19).
LICORICE/HORSETAIL: Theoretically, overuse or misuse of the licorice rhizome or horsetail plant with cardiac glycoside-containing herbs, like uzara, increases the risk of cardiac toxicity due to potassium depletion (19).
OTHER CARDIOACTIVE HERBS: Avoid concomitant use of uzara with other cardioactive herbs due to the unpredictability of therapeutic and adverse effects. Other cardioactive herbs include calamus, cereus, cola, coltsfoot, devil's claw, European mistletoe, fenugreek, fumitory, ginger, panax ginseng, hawthorn, white horehound, mate, parsley, quassia, scotch broom flower, shepherd's purse, and wild carrot (4).
STIMULANT LAXATIVE HERBS: Theoretically, overuse or misuse of stimulant laxatives with cardiac glycoside-containing herbs, like uzara, increases the risk of cardiac toxicity due to potassium depletion. Stimulant laxative herbs include the dried leaf sap of aloe, blue flag rhizome, alder buckthorn, European buckthorn, butternut bark, cascara bark, castor oil, colocynth fruit pulp, gamboge bark exudate, jalap root, black root, manna bark exudate, podophyllum root, rhubarb root, senna leaves and pods, wild cucumber fruit (Ecballium elaterium), and yellow dock root (19).

Interactions with Drugs
DIGOXIN (Lanoxin): Using uzara with digoxin is contraindicated due to therapeutic duplication and an increased risk of cardiac glycoside toxicity (2).
DIURETIC DRUGS: Theoretically, concomitant use of potassium-depleting diuretics and uzara can increase the risk of cardiac glycoside toxicity due to potassium depletion (506). Some diuretics that can deplete potassium include chlorothiazide (Diuril), chlorthalidone (Thalitone), furosemide (Lasix), hydrochlorothiazide (HCTZ, Hydrodiuril, Microzide), and others.
MACROLIDE ANTIBIOTICS: Theoretically, concomitant use may increase risk of cardiac glycoside toxicity (17).
QUININE: Theoretically, concomitant use of quinine and uzara can increase the risk of cardiac toxicity (506).
STIMULANT LAXATIVES: Theoretically, overuse or misuse of stimulant laxatives can increase the risk of cardiac glycoside toxicity due to potassium depletion (2).
TETRACYCLINE ANTIBIOTICS: Theoretically, concomitant use may increase risk of cardiac glycoside toxicity (17).

Interactions with Foods
None known.

Interactions with Lab Tests
None known.

Interactions with Diseases or Conditions
HEART DISEASE: Uzara is contraindicated in individuals with heart disease (18). Theoretically, the cardiac glycosides contained in uzara can exacerbate this condition or interfere with existing drug therapy.
HYPOKALEMIA: Theoretically, the use of uzara can increase the risk of cardiac toxicity in hypokalemic patients.

Dosage and Administration
ORAL: Uzara is commonly taken as liquid ethanol-water extracts or dry extracts obtained from methanol-water extractions (2). The initial dose is 75 mg of the total glycosides calculated as uzarin or the equivalent to 1 gram of the dried root (2). Then the dose is 45-90 mg per day of the total glycosides calculated as uzarin (2). Seek medical consultation for diarrhea persisting more than three to four days (2).

VALERIAN

Also Known As
Amantilla, All-Heal, Baldrian, Baldrianwurzel, Belgium Valerian, Common Valerian, Fragrant Valerian, Garden Heliotrope, Garden Valerian, Indian Valerian, Mexican Valerian, Pacific Valerian, Tagara, Valeriana, Valeriana rhizome, Valerianae radix, Valeriane.

Scientific Names
Valeriana officinalis; Valeriana edulis; Valeriana angustifolia; Valeriana jatamansii, synonym Valeriana wallichii; Valeriana sitchensis.
Family: Valerianaceae.

People Use This For
Orally, valerian is used as a sedative-hypnotic for insomnia and as an anxiolytic for restlessness and sleeping disorders associated with anxiety. It has also been used for mood disorders such as depression, infantile convulsions, mild tremors, epilepsy, and attention deficit-hyperactivity disorder (ADHD). It is also used orally for muscle and joint pain, and conditions associated with anxiety and psychological stress including nervous asthma, hysterical states, excitability, hypochondria, headaches, migraine, and stomach upset. Valerian is also used for menstrual cramps and symptoms associated with menopause, including hot flashes and anxiety.
Topically, valerian is used as a bath additive for restlessness and sleep disorders.
In manufacturing, the extracts and essential oil are used as flavoring in foods and beverages.

Safety
LIKELY SAFE ...when used in amounts commonly found in foods. Valerian has Generally Recognized As Safe (GRAS) status in the US (4912).
POSSIBLY SAFE ...when used orally and appropriately, short-term. Clinical studies have reported safe use of valerian for medicinal purposes in over 12,000 patients in trials lasting up to 28 days (2074,3484,3485,4032,6480). The safety of long-term use is unknown.
There is insufficient reliable information available about the safety of valerian when used topically.
CHILDREN: POSSIBLY SAFE ...when used orally and appropriately for up to 8 weeks (10207).
PREGNANCY AND LACTATION: Insufficient reliable information available; avoid using.

Effectiveness
POSSIBLY EFFECTIVE

Anxiety. Taking valerian orally seems to reduce self-reported stress in social anxiety and anxiety disorder (9893,9895,9896).

Insomnia. Taking valerian orally seems to reduce the time to sleep onset (sleep latency), and improve subjective sleep quality. The greatest benefit is usually seen in patients using 400-900 mg valerian extract up to two hours before bedtime (6248,6249,8250,8296). Valerian seems to improve the sleep quality of insomniacs who have recently withdrawn from benzodiazepines. After tapering the benzodiazepine over two weeks, 300 mg valerian extract in three divided daily doses might subjectively improve sleep quality (8006). Valerian does not always relieve insomnia as fast as benzodiazepines (6480). Continuous nightly use for several days to four weeks is required for significant effect (6249,10209). Some research suggests that valerian is inferior to temazepam (Restoril) and diphenhydramine (Benadryl) for causing sedation in elderly people (10424). A combination of valerian with lemon balm might improve the quality and quantity of sleep in healthy people (10423). There is also preliminary clinical research that suggests

valerian might help improve sleep in intellectually impaired children (10207).
There is insufficient reliable information available about the effectiveness of valerian for its other uses.

Mechanism of Action

The applicable part of valerian is the root. Valerian is reported to have sedative-hypnotic, anxiolytic, antidepressant, anticonvulsant, and antispasmodic effects (3484,3485). Valerian might also have hypotensive properties (9893). The pharmacological effects of valerian have primarily been attributed to valepotriates (iridoid esters), volatile oils, monoterpenes, and sesquiterpenes constituents. The primary monoterpene is berneol and the primary sesquiterpenes are valerenic acid, valerenone, and kessyl glycol (3484,3486). However, because valerian extracts without some of these constituents have similar effects, it is likely that multiple constituents are responsible for its pharmacological effects. Valepotriate constituents are known to have sedative-hypnotic and spasmolytic effects. Valepotriates have also been shown to decrease benzodiazepine withdrawal in an animal model and to bind dopamine receptors (3484,3486). The valepotriates might act as prodrugs. They are thought to rapidly decompose to homobaldrinal in the intestine after ingestion (3486). Valepotriates are highly unstable and rapidly decompose in acid or alkaline environments and at high temperatures. Although there are published reports of toxicity due to the valepotriate constituents, these constituents are poorly absorbed and quickly degraded to less toxic metabolites and are not likely to cause acute adverse reactions (3486). The presence of an epoxide group on the valepotriates has raised concern about possible cytotoxicity and carcinogenicity (3485,3486); however, in vivo studies to date have failed to show any carcinogenic effects (3486). The sesquiterpenes, valerenic acid and kessyl glycol, have been shown to cause sedation in animals (3486). Valerenic acid and other constituents of valerian are gamma-aminobutyric acid (GABA) agonists. Valerian constituents may inhibit the enzyme system responsible for the central catabolism of GABA, increasing GABA concentrations and decreasing central nervous system (CNS) activity (3486,12720). Valerian may also bind directly to GABA-A receptors and stimulate the release and reuptake of GABA (12720).
Valerian might also affect sleep regulation with activity on adenosine and 5-hydroxytryptamine-1 (12720). Valerian doesn't seem to have a negative impact on reaction time, alertness, and concentration the morning after intake (2074).
In healthy elderly people, valerian doesn't seem to affect psychomotor performance (10424).
In vitro and in vivo, valerian extract seems to inhibit the cytochrome P450 3A4 (CYP3A4) enzyme. It does not seem to significantly affect cytochrome P450 2D6 (CYP2D6) (13014).

Adverse Reactions

Orally, valerian can cause headache, excitability, uneasiness, cardiac disturbances, and insomnia (3484). Occasionally, valerian may cause gastric discomfort, dry mouth, vivid dreams (4032), and morning drowsiness (2074). Although residual morning effects on alertness and concentration appear uncommon, impaired alertness and information processing may sometimes occur (2074). Impairment is dose-dependent and peaks within the first few hours after an oral valerian dose (2074). Warn patients against driving or operating dangerous machinery after taking valerian.
There is little information regarding valerian overdose. In one individual, 20 times the normal dose caused fatigue, tight chest, abdominal cramping, and tremor of the hand and foot (659). Benzodiazepine-like withdrawal symptoms have been reported when treatment is discontinued (3487). Patients should taper doses slowly after extended use.
There have been several case reports of hepatotoxicity associated with the use of multi-ingredient preparations containing valerian. It is possible, however, that these preparations may have been adulterated with hepatotoxic agents (8243). Hepatotoxicity involving long-term use of single-ingredient valerian preparations has also been reported (3484). Because a variety of doses were used in these cases, and many people have used higher doses safely, these hepatotoxic reactions might have been idiosyncratic. Tell patients the long-term effect of valerian on liver function is unknown.

Interactions with Herbs & Other Dietary Supplements

HERBS AND SUPPLEMENTS WITH SEDATIVE PROPERTIES: Use of valerian with other herbs and supplements with sedative properties might enhance therapeutic and adverse effects (3496). Some of these products include calamus, California poppy, catnip, hops, Jamaican dogwood, kava, L-tryptophan, melatonin, sage, SAMe, St. John's wort, sassafras, scullcap, and others.

Interactions with Drugs

ALCOHOL (Ethanol): Theoretically, valerian might have an additive sedative effect with alcohol (9894).
ALPRAZOLAM (Xanax): Taking valerian extract 1000 mg/day (providing 10 mg valerenic acid) seems to increase alprazolam levels by about 19%. This is most likely due to valerien's inhibitory effects on cytochrome P450 3A4 (CYP3A4) (13014). Although this increase is statistically significant, it might not be clinical significant.
BENZODIAZEPINES: Theoretically, concomitant use with benzodiazepines may cause additive therapeutic and adverse effects (3486,12720). Some benzodiazepines are alprazolam (Xanax), clonazepam (Klonopin), diazepam (Valium), lorazepam (Ativan), midazolam (Versed), temazepam (Restoril), triazolam (Halcion), and others.
CNS DEPRESSANTS: Theoretically, concomitant use of valerian and drugs with sedative and anesthetic properties may cause additive therapeutic and adverse effects (3486,12720). Some CNS depressants are benzodiazepines, pentobarbital (Nembutal), phenobarbital (Luminal), secobarbital (Seconal), thiopental (Pentothal), fentanyl (Duragesic, Sublimaze), morphine, propofol (Diprivan), and others.
CYTOCHROME P450 3A4 (CYP3A4) SUBSTRATES: There is preliminary evidence that valerian may inhibit the cytochrome P450 3A4 (CYP3A4) enzyme (6450,12214). Theoretically, valerian might increase levels of drugs

metabolized by CYP3A4. However, so far, this interaction has not been reported in humans. Some drugs metabolized by CYP3A4 include lovastatin (Mevacor), ketoconazole (Nizoral), itraconazole (Sporanox), fexofenadine (Allegra), triazolam (Halcion), chemotherapeutic agents (etoposide, paclitaxel, vinblastine, vincristine, vindesine), and numerous others. Use valerian cautiously or avoid in patients taking these drugs.

Interactions with Foods

ALCOHOL: Theoretically, valerian might have an additive sedative effect with alcohol (9894).

Interactions with Lab Tests

None known.

Interactions with Diseases or Conditions

None known.

Dosage and Administration

ORAL: For decreasing sleep latency and improving sleep quality, most studies have used 400-900 mg valerian extract up to two hours before bedtime for as long as 28 days (2074,3484,6480,8006,8250,8296,10424). Other studies have used valerian extract 300-450 mg given in three divided doses (3484,8006). Valerian extract 120 mg, with lemon balm extract 80 mg, has been used 3 times daily for up to 30 days (10423). Valerian should be given 30 minutes to 2 hours before bedtime (9894).

VANADIUM

Also Known As

Metavanadate, Orthovanadate, Vanadate, Vanadium Pentoxide, Vanadyl, Vanadyl Sulfate.

Scientific Names

Vanadium; V; atomic number 23.

People Use This For

Orally, vanadium is used for diabetes, hypoglycemia, hyperlipidemia, heart disease, edema, improving athletic performance in weight training, and preventing cancer. Vanadium is also used for treating tuberculosis, diabetes, syphilis, and a form of microcytic anemia (chlorosis).

Safety

LIKELY SAFE ...when used orally and appropriately. Vanadium is safe when taken in amounts below the tolerable upper intake level (UL) of 1.8 mg per day (7135).
POSSIBLY UNSAFE ...when used orally in high doses. Taking more than the tolerable upper intake level (UL) of 1.8 mg per day can increase the risk of gastrointestinal side effects and theoretically, renal toxicity (7135). In some cases, patients with diabetes have used very high doses (100 mg per day) safely for up to 4 weeks (3055,3056,3057). However, there is concern that prolonged use of high doses might cause serious side effects including kidney damage (7135). Tell patients to avoid exceeding the UL.
CHILDREN: LIKELY SAFE ...when used orally in amounts found in foods (7135). There is insufficient reliable information available about the safety of vanadium when used in children in amounts greater than those typically found in foods.
PREGNANCY AND LACTATION: LIKELY SAFE ...when used orally in amounts found in foods (7135). There is insufficient reliable information available about the safety of vanadium when used in pregnant or breast-feeding women in amounts greater than those typically found in foods.

Effectiveness

INSUFFICIENT RELIABLE EVIDENCE to RATE

Diabetes. There is some evidence that high oral doses of vanadyl sulfate (100 mg daily, 31 mg elemental vanadium), can improve hepatic and peripheral insulin sensitivity in patients with type 2 diabetes and possibly reduce blood glucose levels (3055,3056,3057,12557,12558); however, prolonged use of these high doses might not be safe (7135). It's not known if lower doses have the same benefit. Clinical studies of vanadium have included a total of less than 40 patients. Until more is known, tell patients not to use vanadium for treating type 2 diabetes.

There is insufficient reliable information available about the effectiveness of vanadium for its other uses.

Mechanism of Action

Vanadium is a trace mineral. Good sources of dietary vanadium include mushrooms; shellfish; black pepper; parsley; dillseed; grains and grain products; and beverages such as beer, wine, and artificially sweetened drinks (7135). Drinking water can also contain trace amounts of vanadium (3011). Vanadyl sulfate contains 31% elemental vanadium. Sodium metavanadate contains 42% elemental vanadium. Sodium orthovanadate contains 28% elemental vanadium (16). The vanadium pentoxide form, which is considered toxic, is not found in foods or supplements. An average diet provides 6 to 18 mcg vanadium per day. Only about 5% of ingested vanadium is absorbed. In vivo, vanadium is converted to the vanadyl cation, which can form complexes with ferritin and transferrin. Highest concentrations are found in the liver, kidney, and bone (7135).

Vanadium appears to be important in normal bone growth and as a cofactor for various enzyme reactions. Vanadium inhibits ATPases, phosphatases, and phosphoryl-transfer enzymes (7135).

Vanadium also seems to have cardiovascular effects. There is some evidence that prolonged administration might be associated with dose-dependent increases in blood pressure (3012). Vanadium also inhibits cholesterol synthesis from mevalonic acid (3012).

Some evidence suggests that vanadium can mimic the actions of insulin, possibly by causing phosphorylation of insulin receptor proteins. Vanadium activates the receptor; stimulates glucose oxidation and transport; inhibits lipolysis in adipose tissue; stimulates glycogen synthesis in the liver; inhibits hepatic gluconeogenesis; inhibits intestinal glucose transport; and increases glucose uptake, utilization, and glycogen synthesis in skeletal muscle (3012,3013). It appears to augment the effects of insulin in insulin-resistant type 2 diabetes, but might not have an effect in type 1 diabetes (482). Preliminary evidence suggests that L-glutamic acid gamma-monohydroxamate might activate endogenous vanadium, facilitating glucose metabolism through conversion of intracellular vanadium into an active insulinomimetic compound (388).

There is also some evidence that vanadium might protect against dental caries (3012). A few preliminary studies suggest vanadium might offer protection against hematological toxicity and the development of hepatic carcinoma (3014,3016), but others suggest that vanadium is potentially mutagenic, carcinogenic (3019), and might interfere with mitosis and chromosome distribution (3051).

Adverse Reactions

Orally, vanadium most commonly causes mild gastrointestinal upset (7135). There is concern that taking doses exceeding the tolerable upper intake level (UL) of 1.8 mg per day can increase the risk of gastrointestinal side effects and possibly lead to more severe toxicity. At higher doses, vanadium frequently causes gastrointestinal effects including abdominal discomfort, diarrhea, nausea, and flatulence (3055,3056,3057,12557,12558).

In some cases, patients with diabetes have used very high doses (100 mg per day) safely for up to 4 weeks (3055,3056,3057). However, there is concern that prolonged use of high doses might cause serious side effects including kidney damage (7135). Doses of 22.5 mg daily for five months can cause cramps and diarrhea (3012). Vanadium has also been associated with green discoloration of tongue, fatigue, lethargy, and focal neurological lesions, which were unrelated to dose (7135).

Significant toxic effects have been observed in animal studies of vanadium including decreased weight gain, deterioration in health, pro-oxidant effects, alteration in renal function, increased serum urea and creatinine levels, tissue vanadium accumulation, and some deaths (3017,3018,3021). High body levels of vanadium have been associated with an increased incidence of renal stone disease, distal renal tubular acidosis, hypokalemic periodic paralysis, sudden unexplained nocturnal death, and malnutrition-related diabetes mellitus (3020).

Ingestion of vanadium pentoxide form of vanadium can cause significant toxicity. It has been associated with gastrointestinal disturbances, abnormalities of renal function tests, and nervous system effects (3011). Severe and chronic respiratory tract disorders have been reported from occupational exposure to vanadium dusts (17). This form of vanadium is not found in foods or vanadium supplements.

Interactions with Herbs & Other Dietary Supplements

None known.

Interactions with Drugs

ANTICOAGULANT/ANTIPLATELET DRUGS: Theoretically, the sodium orthovanadate form of vanadium might potentiate anticoagulant therapeutic and adverse effects (3054).

ANTIDIABETES DRUGS: The vanadyl sulfate form of vanadium might have additive effects with diabetes drug therapy. The vanadyl sulfate form of vanadium increases insulin sensitivity (3055,3056,3057) and might lower blood glucose (3057) in individuals with type 2 diabetes. Monitor carefully.

Interactions with Foods

None known.

Interactions with Lab Tests

BLOOD GLUCOSE: The vanadyl sulfate form of vanadium might lower blood glucose levels and test results in people with type 2 diabetes (3057).

SERUM CREATININE: There is preliminary evidence that vanadium might adversely affect renal function (7135). Theoretically, renal function tests might be altered in people taking high doses of vanadium for extended periods.

Interactions with Diseases or Conditions

DIABETES: The vanadyl sulfate form of vanadium might alter blood glucose control in patients with type 2 diabetes. The vanadyl sulfate form of vanadium increases insulin sensitivity (3055,3056,3057) and might lower blood glucose (3057) in individuals with type 2 diabetes. Monitor carefully.

RENAL DYSFUNCTION: There is preliminary evidence that vanadium might cause nephrotoxicity (7135). People with renal dysfunction should avoid vanadium supplements.

Dosage and Administration

ORAL: For type 2 diabetes, the vanadyl sulfate form of vanadium 50 mg twice daily has been used (3055,3056,3057). The National Institute of Medicine has set the tolerable upper intake level (UL) of vanadium at 1.8 mg per day of elemental vanadium for adults (7135). No UL has been set for infants, children, and pregnant or lactating women (7135). Vanadium intake should be limited to food or infant formula in these groups (7135). An average diet provides 6 to 18 mcg vanadium per day (7135). Vanadyl sulfate contains 31% elemental vanadium. Sodium metavanadate contains 42% elemental vanadium. Sodium orthovanadate contains 28% elemental vanadium (16).

Comments

Vanadium was named for the Norse goddess of beauty, Vanadis, because of its beautiful multicolored compounds.

VANILLA

Also Known As

Bourbon Vanilla, Common Vanilla, Madagascar Vanilla, Mexican Vanilla, Réunion Vanilla, Tahiti Vanilla, Tahitian Vanilla, Vanillin.

Scientific Names

Vanilla planifolia, synonyms Vanilla fragrans, Myrobroma fragrans; Vanilla tahitensis.
Family: Orchidaceae.

People Use This For

Orally, vanilla is used as an aphrodisiac, antiflatulent, antipyretic, and stimulant.
In foods and beverages, vanilla is used as a flavoring agent. It is added to foods to reduce the amount of sugar needed for sweetening and inhibit the development of dental caries.
In manufacturing, vanilla is used as a flavoring agent in syrups for pharmaceutical use. It is also used as a fragrance in perfumes.

Safety

LIKELY SAFE ...when used orally in amounts commonly found in foods. Vanilla has Generally Recognized As Safe (GRAS) status in the US (4912).
PREGNANCY AND LACTATION: Insufficient reliable information available; avoid amounts in excess of those found in foods.

Effectiveness

There is insufficient reliable information available about the effectiveness of vanilla.

Mechanism of Action

The applicable part of vanilla is the fruit. Although the constituent vanillin is primarily responsible for the flavor of vanilla (11), over 150 aromatic compounds contribute to its fragrance (11,6). The catechin content of vanilla shows evidence of an anti-caries effect (6). In controlled studies, meals flavored with vanilla provided a higher degree of satisfaction than identical meals without vanilla flavoring (6). Contact dermatitis associated with the vanilla plant is thought to be due to the calcium oxalate crystals in the plant (6).

Adverse Reactions

Orally and topically, vanilla has been associated with allergic responses including contact dermatitis (6,11). Workers preparing vanilla have reported headache, dermatitis, and insomnia, characterized as "vanillism."

Interactions with Herbs & Other Dietary Supplements

None known.

Interactions with Drugs

None known.

Interactions with Foods

None known.

Interactions with Lab Tests

None known.

Interactions with Diseases or Conditions
None known.

Dosage and Administration
No typical dosage.

Comments
Synthetically-produced vanillin is often used as a substitute for vanilla (6), even though the fragrance, rather than the vanillin content, determines the value of vanilla (11). Vanilla extracts have been extensively adulterated (11). Extracts of Mexican origin have been adulterated with coumarin, often due to tonka beans (6). Since 1954, the FDA has prohibited the use of coumarin in food (6).

VERBENA

Also Known As
Blue Vervain, Common Verbena, Common Vervain, Eisenkraut, Enchanter's Plant, European Vervain, Herb of Grace, Herb of the Cross, Holywort, Juno's Tears, Ma Bian Cao, Pigeon's Grass, Pigeonweed, Simpler's Joy, Turkey Grass, Verbenae herba, Vervain.
CAUTION: See separate listing for Lemon Verbena.

Scientific Names
Verbena officinalis.
Family: Verbenaceae.

People Use This For
Orally, verbena is used for sore throats and other oral and pharyngeal inflammation, respiratory tract diseases such as asthma and whooping cough, and angina. Verbena is also used orally for depression, melancholia, hysteria, generalized seizure, gallbladder pain, fever, debility of convalescence after fevers, pains, spasms, exhaustion, angina, nervous conditions, digestive disorders, liver and gallbladder diseases, jaundice, kidney and lower urinary tract ailments and diseases, menopausal complaints, irregular menstruation, for lactation during nursing, arthritic conditions, gout, metabolic disorders, anemia, and edema associated with weak heart.
Topically, verbena is used for poorly healing wounds, abscesses and burns, as a gargle for cold symptoms and oral/pharyngeal cavity diseases, arthritis, rheumatism, dislocations, contusions, itching, and minor burns.
In combination with gentian root, European elder flower, cowslip flower, and sorrel, verbena is used orally for maintaining healthy sinuses and treating sinusitis.
In manufacturing, verbena flowers are used as a flavoring agent in alcoholic beverages.

Safety
LIKELY SAFE ...when used orally in amounts commonly found in foods. Verbena has Generally Recognized As Safe status (GRAS) for use in foods in the US (4912).
POSSIBLY SAFE ...when used orally and appropriately in medicinal amounts (12). ...when verbena is used orally in a combination with gentian root, European elder flower, cowslip flower, and sorrel (Quanterra Sinus Defense, Sinupret) (7,374,379).
LIKELY UNSAFE ...when used orally in excessive amounts because the constituent, verbenalin, can cause stupor and convulsions (4).
There is insufficient reliable information available about the safety of the topical use of verbena.
PREGNANCY: LIKELY UNSAFE ...when used orally; verbena is believed to be an abortifacient and oxytoxic agent (4). There is insufficient reliable information available about the safety of the topical use of verbena during pregnancy.
LACTATION: Insufficient reliable information available; avoid using.

Effectiveness
POSSIBLY EFFECTIVE

Sinusitis. Taking verbena orally in combination with gentian root, European elder flower, cowslip flower, and sorrel (Quanterra Sinus Defense, Sinupret) seems to be effective for treating acute or chronic sinusitis (7,374,379).

There is insufficient reliable information available about the effectiveness of verbena for its other uses.

Mechanism of Action
The applicable parts of verbena are the above ground parts. They contain the iridoid glycosides verbascoside (acetoside), verbenalin, and verbenin (aucubin) (4). Verbena possesses weak parasympathetic properties and can cause a slight contraction of the uterus. The herb shows evidence of luteinizing activity, perhaps by inhibiting the gonadotrophic activity of the posterior pituitary (4). Some evidence indicates the iridoid glycosides have a mild laxative effect. Small amounts of the constituent, verbenin, appear to stimulate sympathetic activity. Larger amounts

of verbenin inhibit sympathetic activity (4). Preliminary evidence suggests verbenin might also stimulate milk secretion (4). The constituent, verbenalin, shows evidence of uterine stimulant activity (4). The constituent verbascoside shows evidence of analgesic and antihypertensive activity. Verbascoside also appears to enhance the antitremor action of levodopa (4).

Adverse Reactions

Orally, excessive amounts of the constituent, verbenalin, can cause CNS paralysis, stupor, and convulsions (4).

Interactions with Herbs & Other Dietary Supplements

None known.

Interactions with Drugs

ANTIHYPERTENSIVE DRUGS: Theoretically, excessive amounts of verbena can interfere with drug therapy for hypertension due to the antihypertensive effects of the constituent verbascoside (4).

Interactions with Foods

None known.

Interactions with Lab Tests

None known.

Interactions with Diseases or Conditions

HYPERTENSION: Theoretically, excessive amounts of verbena might reduce blood pressure (4).
HYPOTENSION: Theoretically, excessive amounts of verbena might exacerbate this condition (4).

Dosage and Administration

ORAL: A typical dose is one cup tea three times daily (4). To make tea, steep 2-4 grams dried above ground parts in 150 mL boiling water for 5 10 minutes and strain (4). 2-4 mL of the liquid extract, 1:1 in 25% ethanol, has been used three times daily (4). 5-10 mL of the tincture, 1:1 in 40% ethanol, has been used three times daily (4).
For acute or chronic sinusitis, two Sinupret tablets three times daily for up to two weeks has been used in clinical trials (7,374,379), equivalent to gentian root 12 mg, European elder flower 36 mg, verbena 36 mg, cowslip flower 36 mg, and sorrel 36 mg three times daily.
TOPICAL: No typical dosage.

VERONICA

Also Known As

Ehrenpreiskraut, Gypsy Weed, Speedwell, Veronica Herb, Veronicae herba.
CAUTION: See separate listings for Bugleweed; and for Black Root (Leptandra virginica) and Brooklime (Veronica beccabungo) which are both known also as Speedwell.

Scientific Names

Veronica officinalis.
Family: Scrophulariaceae.

People Use This For

Orally, veronica is used for diseases and discomforts of the respiratory tract, gastrointestinal tract, liver, kidney, and lower urinary tract. Veronica is also used orally for gout, arthritis, rheumatic complaints, diseases of the spleen, scrofulosis, as an appetite stimulant and tonic, to induce sweating, for nervous irritation, "blood purification," and promotion of metabolism.
Topically, veronica is used as a gargle for inflammation of the oral and pharyngeal mucosa, for perspiration of the feet, stimulation of wound healing, chronic skin conditions, and itching.

Safety

LIKELY SAFE ...when consumed in amounts commonly found in foods. Veronica has Generally Recognized As Safe status (GRAS) for use in foods in the US (4912).
POSSIBLY SAFE ...when used orally and appropriately in medicinal amounts (12).
There is insufficient reliable information available about the safety of the topical use of veronica.
PREGNANCY AND LACTATION: Insufficient reliable information available; avoid using.

Effectiveness

There is insufficient reliable information available about the effectiveness of veronica.

Mechanism of Action

The applicable parts of veronica are the above ground parts. Extracts of veronica may protect against ulcers induced by nonsteroidal anti-inflammatory drugs (NSAIDs). Veronica may enhance gastric mucosa regeneration (4010).

Adverse Reactions

None reported.

Interactions with Herbs & Other Dietary Supplements

None known.

Interactions with Drugs

None known.

Interactions with Foods

None known.

Interactions with Lab Tests

None known.

Interactions with Diseases or Conditions

GASTRIC ULCERS: Theoretically, veronica may enhance ulcer healing (4010).

Dosage and Administration

ORAL: As an expectorant, one cup tea (steep 1.5 grams finely cut above ground parts in 150 mL boiling water 10 minutes, strain) 2-3 times daily is commonly used (18).
TOPICAL: For lavages and compresses for eczema, ulcers, and wounds, boil one handful above ground parts in one L water for 10 minutes (18).

Comments

Avoid confusion with other Veronica species, including Veronica allionii and Veronica chamaedrys (18).

VETIVER

Also Known As

Chiendent Odorant, Cuscus, Cuscus Grass, Khas-khas, Khus Khus, Khus-khus Grass, Reshira, Sugandhimula, Ushira, Vétiver, Vetivergras, Zacate Violeta.

Scientific Names

Chrysopogon zizanioides, synonyms Vetiveria zizanioides, Anatherum zizanioides, Andropogon odoratus, Phalaris zizanioides.
Family: Poaceae/Gramineae.

People Use This For

Orally, vetiver is used as a uterine stimulant to promote menses and to cause abortion. It is also used orally for nervous and circulatory problems.
Topically, vetiver is used for stress relief, recovery from emotional traumas and shocks, treatment of lice, and as an insect repellent.
As an inhalant, vetiver is used for "aroma therapy" for nervousness, insomnia, rheumatism, and muscle relaxation.
In manufacturing, vetiver is used as a flavoring in alcoholic beverages.

Safety

LIKELY SAFE ...when used in amounts commonly found in foods. Vetiver has Generally Recognized As Safe status (GRAS) for use in foods in the US (4912).
POSSIBLY SAFE ...when used orally (12).
PREGNANCY: LIKELY UNSAFE ...when used orally because it is a potential abortifacient and it has menstrual and uterine stimulant effects (12).
LACTATION: Insufficient reliable information available: avoid using.

Effectiveness

There is insufficient reliable information available about the effectiveness of vetiver.

Mechanism of Action
The applicable part of vetiver is the root. Vetiver root contains numerous constituents including limonene, p-cymene, palmitic acid, benzoic acid, delta-3-carene (513). Vetiver may contain a volatile oil which accounts for its use as a repellent to flies, cockroaches, bedbugs, and clothes moths (5279).

Adverse Reactions
None reported.

Interactions with Herbs & Other Dietary Supplements
None known.

Interactions with Drugs
None known.

Interactions with Foods
None known.

Interactions with Lab Tests
None known.

Interactions with Diseases or Conditions
None known.

Dosage and Administration
No typical dosage.

VINPOCETINE

Also Known As
AY-27255, Cavinton, Ethyl Apovincaminate, Ethylapovincaminoate, RGH-4405, TCV-3b, Vinpocetin.

Scientific Names
Eburnamenine-14-carboxylic acid, Ethyl Ester.

People Use This For
Orally, vinpocetine is used for enhancing memory, improving cerebral blood flow, improving cerebral oxygen and glucose utilization, protecting against age-related cognitive decline and Alzheimer's disease, treating cerebrovascular disease, preventing post-stroke morbidity and mortality, treating organic psychosyndromes, treating intractable tumoral calcinosis in people undergoing hemodialysis, decreasing stroke risk, treating menopausal symptoms, seizure disorders, and preventing motion sickness.
Intravenously, vinpocetine is injected for treating seizure disorders and stroke.

Safety
POSSIBLY SAFE ...when used orally and appropriately (1784). No significant adverse effects were reported in a study of people with Alzheimer's disease treated with large doses of vinpocetine (60 mg per day) for one year (1784).
PREGNANCY AND LACTATION: Insufficient reliable information available; avoid using.

Effectiveness
POSSIBLY EFFECTIVE

Dementia. Vinpocetine is used to treat cognitive impairment due to vascular disease, Alzheimer's disease, and other kinds of dementias. It might have a modest effect on cognitive impairment from various causes, but most studies have lasted 6 months or less (1784,1787,1789). Most of the studies were published prior to 1990 and used a variety of terms and criteria for cognitive decline and dementia (10221,10827).

INSUFFICIENT RELIABLE EVIDENCE to RATE

Memory. Preliminary clinical research suggests vinpocetine might enhance memory in normal volunteers (1796,1797).

Stroke. Preliminary clinical research suggests vinpocetine might modestly reduce the residual effects of acute ischemic stroke (1785). There have been few clinical studies investigating the use of vinpocetine for stroke, and most have been published in languages other than English. Two meta-analyses of these studies found insufficient conclusive information to determine the effectiveness of vinpocetine for acute ischemic stroke (10222,10828).

More evidence is needed to rate vinpocetine for these uses.

Mechanism of Action

Vinpocetine is a synthetic derivative of apovincamine, a compound found in the periwinkle plant, Vinca minor. Vinpocetine appears to have many varied pharmacologic effects; but mechanisms of action are unclear and well-designed clinical studies to substantiate activity have not been published (10827). Some studies indicate that vinpocetine might enhance cerebral blood flow without affecting peripheral blood flow (1786,1793). Preliminary evidence indicates that vinpocetine stimulates cerebral metabolism and increases glucose and oxygen consumption by the brain (10827). Potential mechanisms for the nootropic-like effects of vinpocetine include indirect or direct cholinergic activity, augmented norepinephrine effects on cortical cyclic adenosine monophosphate (AMP), and increased turnover of brain catecholamines (1800). It might also improve microcirculation in the brain and increase cerebral blood flow by improving red blood cell deformability, reducing cerebral vascular resistance, and inhibiting platelet aggregation (10827). Vinpocetine inhibits drug-induced platelet aggregation (1801). Pharmacological effects that might be useful in treating stroke include a possible neuroprotective and anticonvulsant effect by blocking voltage-gated sodium channels. It also might protect neurons by enhancing the effect of adenosine in preventing hypoxia. Animal studies suggest that vinpocetine decreases neuronal death in ischemia and decreases the size of cerebral infarction in experimental strokes (10728). The bioavailability of vinpocetine varies from 7-57%; food significantly enhances absorption (1802).

Adverse Reactions

Orally, adverse effects include gastric discomfort, vertigo, anxiety, nausea, facial flushing, sleep disturbances, and headache (10221).

Interactions with Herbs & Other Dietary Supplements

HERBS WITH ANTICOAGULANT/ANTIPLATELET POTENTIAL: Theoretically, concomitant use with herbs that might affect platelet aggregation might increase the risk of bleeding in some people (1821). These herbs include angelica, clove, danshen, fenugreek, feverfew, garlic, ginger, ginkgo, Panax ginseng, poplar, red clover, turmeric, and others.

Interactions with Drugs

ANTICOAGULANT/ANTIPLATELET DRUGS: Vinpocetine seems to have antiplatelet effects (1801). Theoretically, taking vinpocetine with antiplatelet or anticoagulant drugs might increase the risk of bruising and bleeding. Some of these drugs include aspirin, clopidogrel (Plavix), nonsteroidal anti-inflammatory drugs (NSAIDs) such as diclofenac (Voltaren, Cataflam, others), ibuprofen (Advil, Motrin, others), naproxen (Anaprox, Naprosyn, others), dalteparin (Fragmin), enoxaparin (Lovenox), heparin, warfarin (Coumadin), and others.

WARFARIN (Coumadin): The combination of warfarin and vinpocetine leads to slight increases in the area under the concentration curve and prothrombin time. In most patients, this interaction is likely to be clinically insignificant (10829).

Interactions with Foods

FOODS: Administration of oral vinpocetine with food enhances its absorption (1802).

Interactions with Lab Tests

PROTHROMBIN TIME (PT)/ INTERNATIONAL NORMALIZATION RATIO (INR): Vinpocetine might increase PT and INR. It has been reported to modestly increase warfarin AUC, PT, and factor VII clotting time (10829).

Interactions with Diseases or Conditions

COAGULOPATHIES: Vinpocetine should not be used by people with blood-clotting disorders because it might increase the risk of bleeding (1801).

Dosage and Administration

ORAL: For treating cognitive impairment due to vascular disease, Alzheimer's disease, and other kinds of dementias, 5-10 mg three times daily has been used (1784,1787,1789).

Comments

Vinpocetine is a synthetic derivative of apovincamine which is found in periwinkle, Vinca minor (10827). Vinpocetine synthesis requires considerable laboratory manipulation, stretching the Dietary Supplement Health and Education Act (DSHEA) definition of a dietary supplement. Vinpocetine is sold by prescription in Germany under the brand name, Cavinton. It has also been referred to generically as cavinton. Although website advertising claims that "more than a hundred" safety and effectiveness studies have been funded by the Hungarian manufacturer Gedeon Richter, few double-blind controlled clinical studies have been published (1785).

VITAMIN A

Also Known As

3-Dehydroretinol, Antixerophthalmic Vitamin, Axerophtholum, Dehydroretinol, Oleovitamin A, Retinoids, Retinol, Retinol Acetate, Retinol Palmitate, Retinyl Acetate, Retinyl Palmitate, Vitamin A1, Vitamin A2, Vitaminum A.
CAUTION: See separate listings for Beta-Carotene and Lutein.

Scientific Names

Vitamin A.

People Use This For

Orally, vitamin A is used for vitamin A deficiency, improving vision, glaucoma, cataracts, infection, and improving immune function. It is also used orally for skin conditions including acne, eczema, psoriasis, cold sores, wounds and burns, sunburn, keratosis follicularis (Darier's disease), ichthyosis (noninflammatory skin scaling), lichen planus pigmentosus, and pityriasis rubra pilaris. Vitamin A is also used orally to prevent and treat vitamin A deficiency due to abnormal storage and transport of vitamin A in people with abetalipoproteinemia, protein deficiency, diabetes mellitus, hyperthyroidism, fever, liver disease, or cystic fibrosis with liver involvement. It is also used orally for heavy menses, premenstrual syndrome (PMS), atrophic vaginitis, candidiasis, fibrocystic breast disease, reduced sperm count, gastrointestinal ulcers, Crohn's disease, periodontal disease, diabetes, Hurler syndrome (mucopolysaccharidosis), sinusitis, allergic rhinitis, and urinary tract infections (UTIs). Vitamin A is also used for reducing complications of measles, shigellosis, atrophic rhinitis, loss of sense of smell, asthma, persistent headaches, kidney stones, hyperthyroidism, anemia, deafness, tinnitus, and leukoplakia. Other oral uses include preventing and treating cancer, degenerative diseases of the nervous system, protecting the heart and cardiovascular system (antioxidant effects), and slowing the aging process. Vitamin A is used orally to decrease morbidity associated with malaria in children, and to reduce morbidity and mortality from pneumonia and HIV in children with vitamin A deficiency. Vitamin A is also used orally to decrease the risk of HIV transmission to the fetus during pregnancy and transmission to the newborn during childbirth and early breast-feeding periods.

Topically, vitamin A is used to improve wound healing, reduce wrinkles, and to protect the skin against UV radiation.

Intramuscularly, vitamin A is used for preventing and treating the symptoms of vitamin A deficiency including xerophthalmia and night blindness, preventing vitamin A deficiency in people with malabsorption, preventing bronchopulmonary dysplasia in premature infants, and preventing stress ulcers in severely ill hospitalized patients.

Safety

LIKELY SAFE ...when used orally or intramuscularly and appropriately. Vitamin A is safe in adults when used in doses less than 10,000 units per day (7135).

POSSIBLY SAFE ...when used intravaginally and appropriately. All-trans-retinoic acid in concentrations up to 0.372% appears to be safe when used topically on the cervix (9199).

POSSIBLY UNSAFE ...when used orally in excessive doses. Prolonged use of excessive doses can cause significant side effects such as hypervitaminosis A. The risk for developing hypervitaminosis A is related to total cumulative dose of vitamin A rather than a specific daily dose (1467,1469). Tell patients to avoid extended use of doses greater than 10,000 units per day (7135).

CHILDREN: LIKELY SAFE ...when used orally or intramuscularly and appropriately. The amount of vitamin A that is safe depends on age. For children up to 3 years of age, doses less than 2000 units per day seem to be safe. For children ages 4 to 8, doses less than 3000 units per day seem to be safe. For children ages 9 to 13, doses less than 5700 units per day seem to be safe. For children 14 to 18, doses of 9300 units per day seem to be safe (7135).
POSSIBLY UNSAFE ...when used orally in excessive doses. For children up to 3 years of age, avoid doses greater than 2000 units per day. For children ages 4 to 8, avoid doses greater than 3000 units per day. For children ages 9 to 13, avoid doses greater than 5700 units per day. For children 14 to 18, avoid doses greater than 9300 units per day (7135). Higher doses of vitamin A supplementation have been associated with increased risk of side effects such as pneumonia and diarrhea (319). Long-term supplementation with low to moderate doses on a regular basis can cause severe, but usually reversible, liver damage (11978).

PREGNANCY AND LACTATION: LIKELY SAFE ...when used orally or intramuscularly and appropriately. Vitamin A is safe during pregnancy and lactation when used in doses less than 10,000 units per day (7135).
POSSIBLY UNSAFE ...when used orally or intramuscularly in excessive doses. Daily intake of greater than 10,000 units can cause fetal malformations (3066,7135). Excessive dietary intake of vitamin A has also been associated with teratogenicity (11978). The first trimester of pregnancy seems to be the critical period for susceptibility to vitamin A-associated birth defects such as craniofacial abnormalities and abnormalities of the central nervous system (7135). Pregnant women should monitor vitamin A intake from all sources. Forms of vitamin A are found in several foods including animal products, primarily liver, some fortified breakfast cereals, and dietary supplements (3066).

Effectiveness

EFFECTIVE

Vitamin A deficiency. Taking vitamin A orally is effective for preventing and improving symptoms of vitamin A deficiency, including xerophthalmia and night blindness. Vitamin A deficiency can occur due to abnormal storage and transport of vitamin A in people with abetalipoproteinemia, protein deficiency, diabetes mellitus, hyperthyroidism, fever, liver disease, and cystic fibrosis (7135).

POSSIBLY EFFECTIVE

Breast cancer. Epidemiological evidence shows an association between high dietary intake of vitamin A and a reduced risk of breast cancer among premenopausal women with a positive family history of breast cancer (1444). However, it's not known if supplemental vitamin A has a similar benefit.

Cataracts. A large-scale population-based study found high dietary intake of vitamin A was associated with a reduced risk of nuclear cataracts (6378).

HIV-related diarrhea. Taking vitamin A in combination with conventional medicines seems to decrease mortality rate from diarrhea in HIV-infected children with vitamin A deficiency (1465).

Malaria. Taking vitamin A orally seems to help decrease symptoms of malaria in children less than 3 years of age living in endemic malaria areas (1464).

Measles. Taking vitamin A orally seems to reduce the complications of measles in children with vitamin A deficiency (7135).

Photoreactive keratectomy. Taking vitamin A orally in combination with vitamin E seems to improve healing after photoreactive keratectomy. High dose (50,000 to 75,000 units) vitamin A in the form of retinol palmitate taken daily with 230 mg vitamin E (alpha-tocopheryl nicotinate) seems to accelerate re-epithelialization, reduce haze formation, and improve visual acuity in patients undergoing laser surgery for myopia (348).

Post-partum complications. Taking vitamin A orally seems to reduce the occurrence of post-partum diarrhea and fever in malnourished women. Retinyl acetate taken weekly before, during, and after pregnancy reduces, but does not eliminate, the occurrence of post partum diarrhea and fever (2581).

Pregnancy-related complications. Taking vitamin A orally seems to reduce pregnancy-related maternal mortality and night blindness in malnourished women. Retinyl acetate taken weekly before, during, and after pregnancy seems to reduce pregnancy-related mortality and night blindness (6153,6154). In one trial, 23,300 IU retinyl acetate reduced pregnancy-related mortality by 40% (6153). Some evidence suggests zinc supplements might potentiate the effects of vitamin A in restoring sight in zinc-deficient pregnant women affected by night-blindness (8630).

POSSIBLY INEFFECTIVE

Anemia. In developing nations with a high prevalence of anemia, taking 3,000 mcg retinol equivalent of vitamin A in combination with iron and folate orally doesn't seem to improve hemoglobin and erythropoietin concentrations any better than iron and folate alone (9188).

Chemotherapy-induced gastrointestinal (GI) adverse effects. Taking vitamin A orally by children receiving chemotherapy doesn't seem to prevent GI adverse effects. Vitamin A supplements don't seem to have any effect on the incidence or severity of symptoms such as diarrhea and mouth pain (9802).

Fetal and early infant mortality. Taking oral retinyl acetate 23,300 IU weekly before, during, and after pregnancy by malnourished women doesn't seem to reduce fetal and early infant mortality (6152).

HIV transmission. Taking vitamin A orally doesn't seem to decrease the risk of HIV transmission to the fetus during pregnancy, to newborns during delivery, or during the early breast-feeding periods (6376). Preliminary clinical research suggests vitamin A supplementation of pregnant women with HIV infection might increase the risk of HIV transmission to their babies through breast milk (9801).

LIKELY INEFFECTIVE

Head and neck cancer. Taking vitamin A orally doesn't reduce the risk of second primary tumors and tumor reoccurrence in patients with head and neck cancer. Vitamin A does not improve survival or event-free survival (1710).

Pneumonia. Taking vitamin A orally doesn't decrease the severity of pneumonia in children living in developing countries (1466).

INSUFFICIENT RELIABLE EVIDENCE to RATE

Cervical dysplasia. Preliminary clinical research suggests that a specific form of vitamin A, 13-cis-retinoic acid, taken orally might improve cervical dysplasia in women with human papillomavirus (HPV) infection (9198).

Cervical neoplasia. Research suggests that all-trans-retinoic acid, delivered topically with a collagen sponge or cervical cap can reduce mild to moderate cervical neoplasia (9199).

Colorectal cancer. Taking vitamin A in combination with beta-carotene does not seem to reduce the risk of colorectal cancer (12185).

Esophageal cancer. Taking vitamin A in combination with beta-carotene does not seem to reduce the risk of esophageal cancer (12185).

Gastric cancer. Taking vitamin A in combination with beta-carotene does not seem to reduce the risk of gastric cancer (12185).

Lung cancer. There is preliminary evidence that taking vitamin A orally might improve survival and reduce the reoccurrence of tumors in people with lung cancer (7875).

Ovarian cancer. Population research suggests that vitamin A consumption doesn't affect the risk of developing

ovarian cancer (9193).
Pancreatic cancer. Taking vitamin A in combination with beta-carotene does not seem to reduce the risk of pancreatic cancer (12185).
More evidence is needed to rate vitamin A for these uses.

Mechanism of Action

Vitamin A is a fat-soluble vitamin. Vitamin A includes a family of molecules containing a 20-carbon structure with various chemical groups at the 15 carbon position. Variations at the 15 carbon position yield different vitamin A forms, including retinol, retinal, retinoic acid, and retinyl ester. These different forms of vitamin A are often collectively referred to as "retinoids." The most potent form of vitamin A, all-trans retinol, is the form of retinol in the diet. It reverses signs and symptoms of vitamin A deficiency and is the standard for vitamin A activity (9191). The vitamin A family also includes provitamin A carotenoids, which are dietary precursors to retinol.
Vitamin A is found in foods in several forms. Retinol, also called preformed vitamin A, is present in esterified form in animal-derived products including eggs, whole milk, butter, fortified margarine, meat, and oily salt-water fish (7135). Animal liver contains the highest amount of dietary retinol. About two-thirds of vitamin A intake comes from dietary retinol (9189). Fresh water fish contain a form of vitamin A called 3-dehydroretinol, but have only 30% to 40% of the biologic activity of retinol (15). About a third of dietary vitamin A comes from plants, which synthesize carotenoids that are converted to vitamin A in the body (7135). Carotenoid pigments (including alpha-, beta-, and gamma-carotene and cryptoxanthin) are present in grains, oils, green and yellow vegetables, and especially in carrots and fruits (8044). The amount of carotenoids absorbed and converted to vitamin A depends upon the amount of carotenoids ingested, the individual's vitamin A status, and carotenoid body stores. Carotenoids provide approximately 50% of the vitamin A needed in the American diet (8044).
The liver seems to maintain vitamin A concentrations within a relatively narrow range by storage and release of vitamin A (9595). Dietary retinyl esters are hydrolyzed by pancreatic and intestinal enzymes. Unesterified retinol is directly absorbed intestinal cells, mostly by active transport at lower concentrations and by diffusion at higher concentrations (9186,9187). There seem to be differences in the absorption of various forms of vitamin A, but more research is needed to determine the clinical significance (9187). Ingested vitamin A is stored in the body as retinol, predominantly in the liver, but also in the retina, kidneys, lungs, adrenal glands, and intraperitoneal fat (1467). Retinol-binding protein (RBP) is required to transport retinol from the liver and accumulates in the liver during periods of vitamin A deficiency (6377). When vitamin A as retinol is available, it binds to accumulated RBP and is promptly released into the blood when needed (6377). A serum retinol level of 1.05 micromoles/liter or less is considered normal. Serum retinol levels increase with age (9197).
Transport protein levels can be reduced in people with protein malnutrition, causing signs of vitamin A deficiency. In alcoholism, vitamin A deficiency is common since alcohol accelerates the breakdown of retinol through induction of cytochrome isoenzymes and interferes with the conversion of beta-carotene to retinol (1488,7139). Serum retinol levels decrease transiently in acute response to infection, but overall vitamin A stores are not affected (9197).
The majority of vitamin A is excreted in the urine. Lesser amounts are lost through the breath and feces, as inactive metabolites (7135). In vitamin A excess, biliary excretion increases (7135).
Vitamin A is required for vision, growth and bone development, reproduction, cell proliferation and differentiation, immune function, and the integrity of mucosal and epithelial surfaces. All-trans retinol is converted in the body to all-trans retinoic acid by an unknown mechanism. All-trans retinoic acid is the active form of vitamin A in almost all biological processes. Retinoic acid regulates the expression of various genes that encode for structural proteins, such as keratins in the skin; enzymes, such as alcohol dehydrogenase; extracellular matrix proteins, such as the basement membrane protein laminin; and retinol binding proteins and receptors (7135,9189). Vitamin A acts as a cofactor in mucopolysaccharide synthesis, cholesterol synthesis, hydroxysteroid metabolism, and glycoprotein glycosylation (15). Vitamin A seems to have the opposite effect of steroids on wound healing. It stimulates the expression of transforming growth factor-beta (TGF-beta) and insulin-like growth factor (IGF), and increases collagen production, resulting in improved wound healing (320). Vitamin A is also important for immune function. Retinoic acid is required in maintaining sufficient levels of natural killer cells, and preliminary evidence suggests that retinoic acid might increase the production of cytokines, such as interleukin 1 (IL-1). Additionally, B lymphocyte growth, differentiation, and activation are dependent on retinol (7135). Retinol also seems to affect pulmonary function. Higher retinol levels have been associated with higher forced expiratory volume (FEV) and forced vital capacity (FVC) (9195).
Vitamin A is important for the normal utilization of iron and prevention of anemia. Deficiency of vitamin A impairs maturation of hematopoietic cells in the bone marrow. Vitamin A may facilitate mobilization of body stores of iron. Preliminary evidence also indicates that vitamin A and beta-carotene enhance non-heme iron absorption from iron-fortified wheat and corn flour, and rice. It's suggested that these vitamins bind to iron in the gut, improving its solubility and preventing binding by dietary polyphenols and phytate, which reduce iron absorption. In addition, vitamin A appears to be involved with production of erythropoietin by the liver and kidney (9518,9569,9586,).
In embryonic development, vitamin A plays an important role in neural development, and is also involved in the development of the limbs, lung, heart, eyes, and ears (7135,11978). Vitamin A deficiency seems to adversely affect fetal immune status. Maternal-fetal transmission of HIV is higher in the presence of low vitamin A status. However, excessive vitamin A is teratogenic, causing central nervous system, craniofacial, cardiovascular, and thymus malformations (11978).

In the retina, retinol is converted to cis-retinal, which combines with opsin to form rhodopsin, the visual pigment. Retinal is required by the eye for the transduction of light into the neural signals that produce vision. The most specific indicator of vitamin A deficiency is xerophthalmia, which is initially manifested by night blindness that progresses to complete visual loss if untreated. Vitamin A deficiency is also associated with follicular hyperkeratosis and increased risk of infectious morbidity and mortality (7135). Some research has linked retinol deficiency to development of cervical neoplasms in women with human immunodeficiency virus (HIV) infection (9800).

In vitro studies suggest retinoids might help prevent cancer by inducing tumor suppressor genes known as retinoic acid receptors (RAR). Tumor suppressor gene RAR-beta2 is absent in many malignant tumor cells, possibly due to methylation of the gene. When demethylated, the RAR-beta2 gene can be induced by retinoic acid to function and suppress growth of cancer cells (6380,6381). However, there is evidence that some forms of retinoic acid, such as all-trans-retinoic acid, do not use the RAR receptor to inhibit cancer growth and may use other mechanisms and pathways to inhibit growth (8045). There is also evidence that the inhibitory effect on cancer cell growth by certain statin drugs with a closed ring structure, such as mevastatin and lovastatin (Mevacor), may be enhanced when used with 13-cis retinoic acid (8046). Ethanol may compete with retinol for alcohol dehydrogenase and inhibit retinoic acid synthesis, interfering with normal retinoid signaling of RAR genes and cause malignant transformation of hepatic cells (6377). Preliminary evidence suggests that all-trans-retinoic acid applied topically might help protect the skin against UV radiation damage. UV radiation seems to cause a functional vitamin A deficiency in the skin (1468).

Based on cell culture and animal studies, it's been suggested that vitamin E affects the activity of vitamin A. These include preventing oxidation in the gut and increasing absorption, enhancing utilization, promoting liver storage, protecting against cell damage caused by high vitamin A levels, and reducing some of the symptoms of hypervitaminosis A (10545,10557,10558,10560). Supportive data in humans is very limited. There is some preliminary evidence that vitamin E increases the effects of vitamin A in the treatment of some skin conditions (10562). Small studies have reported increased vitamin A absorption and excretion, and both increases and decreases in vitamin A levels when vitamin E is taken concurrently (10559,10561,10563,10564). Despite the lack of good evidence of efficacy or necessity, vitamin E has been added to the intermittent, high doses of vitamin A sometimes used to treat deficiency in developing countries (10558,10560). Further research is needed to determine whether vitamin E affects the activity of vitamin A in humans.

Vitamin A toxicity can occur when vitamin A intake exceeds the storage capacity of the liver or when liver function is compromised. Vitamin A is released into the circulation as retinyl esters rather than bound to retinol-binding protein (RBP). The retinyl esters expose target tissues to free retinol, resulting in the damaging effects of hypervitaminosis A (9196).

Both human and animal studies suggest excessive vitamin A intake can have a negative effect on bone. It seems to suppress osteoblast activity, stimulate osteoclast formation, and antagonize the ability of vitamin D to maintain normal serum calcium levels (7712,9190,9191,9192). Some evidence suggests that older people can't metabolize vitamin A as well younger people, which could increase the risk of osteoporosis (9191).

Adverse Reactions

Orally, vitamin A is generally well tolerated at doses below the Tolerable Upper Intake Level (UL). For adults, the UL is 3,000 mcg per day (10,000 units). Acute toxicity following doses of 15,000 mcg (50,000 units) are characterized by nausea, vomiting, headache, increased cerebrospinal fluid pressure, vertigo, blurred vision, muscular incoordination, and bulging fontanelle in infants. These are usually transient effects involving single or short-term large doses (7135). Toxicity from a single ingestion of a large dose of vitamin A is more common in young children than adults (15). In children, approximately 25,000 units/kg can cause irritability, drowsiness, dizziness, delirium, coma, vomiting, diarrhea, increased intracranial pressure with bulging fontanelles in infants, headache, swelling of the optic disk, bulging eyeballs, and visual disturbances. Skin redness and generalized peeling of the skin occur a few days later and may last for several weeks (15).

Chronic toxicity is usually associated with ingestion of large doses greater than or equal to 30,000 mcg (100,000 units) for months or years. The liver is the main storage site and the primary target of vitamin A toxicity. Hepatotoxicity ranges from reversibly elevated liver enzymes, alanine aminotransferase (ALT, formerly SGPT) and aspartate aminotransferase (AST, formerly SGOT), to widespread fibrosis and cirrhosis and death (6377,7135). Chronic use of large amounts of vitamin A causes symptoms of vitamin A toxicity including fatigue, malaise, lethargy, irritability, psychiatric changes mimicking severe depression or schizophrenic disorder, anorexia, abdominal discomfort, nausea and vomiting, mild fever, and excessive sweating (7135). Other symptoms include dry skin and lips; cracking, scaling, and itchy skin; skin redness; hyperpigmentation; and massive skin peeling. Hypervitaminosis A can cause brittle nails, cheilitis, gingivitis, hair loss, reduced menstrual flow, spider angiomas, anemia, leukopenia, leukocytosis, and thrombocytopenia (15). Slow growth, premature epiphyseal closure, painful hyperostosis of the long bones, osteosclerosis, joint pain, muscle pain, hypercalcemia, and hypercalciuria have also been reported (15). Sometimes children fail to gain weight normally. Adults may lose weight (15). There is also some evidence that vitamin A supplementation might increase the risk of pneumonia and diarrhea in children. Although vitamin A can prevent diarrhea and reduce mortality in malnourished children, doses as low as 10,000 units weekly for 40 weeks have been associated with diarrhea and pneumonia in well-nourished children (319). Discourage vitamin A supplementation in healthy, well-nourished children.

Vitamin A can increase the risk for osteoporosis. Chronic, high intake of vitamin A 10,000 IU or more per day seems to increase the risk of osteoporosis and hip fracture in postmenopausal women (7712,7713) and overall risk of fracture

in middle-aged men (9190). High serum retinol levels also increase the risk of fracture in men. Men with high serum retinol levels are seven times more likely to fracture a hip than men with lower serum retinol levels (9190). Vitamin A damage to bone can occur subclinically, without signs or symptoms of hypervitaminosis A. Some researchers are concerned that consumption of vitamin A fortified foods such as margarine and low-fat dairy products in addition to in addition to vitamin A or multivitamin supplements might cause excessive serum retinol levels. Older people have higher levels of vitamin A and might be at increased risk for vitamin A induced osteoporosis. Recommendations for vitamin A intake are likely to be reassessed. For now, tell patients who eat a lot of low-fat dairy products, fruits, and vegetables that they don't need a vitamin A supplement (7712,9189,9190,9191,9192). Population research suggests high vitamin A intake might increase the risk of gastric carcinoma (9194).
Intravaginally, all-trans retinoic acid can cause vaginal discharge, itching, irritation, and burning (9199).

Interactions with Herbs & Other Dietary Supplements

IRON: Vitamin A may improve hemoglobin levels in people with anemia and low serum retinol levels.
It's unlikely that vitamin A supplements would have significant effects on iron status in people without vitamin A deficiency (9518,9569,9586).

Interactions with Drugs

HEPATOTOXIC DRUGS: Excessive doses of vitamin A can cause hepatotoxicity ranging from elevated liver enzymes to liver failure (7135). Taking high doses of vitamin A in combination with other potentially hepatotoxic drugs might increase the risk of liver disease. Advise patients against combining high doses of vitamin A with other hepatotoxic drugs. Some drugs that can adversely affect the liver include acetaminophen (Tylenol), amiodarone (Cordarone), carbamazepine (Tegretol), isoniazid (INH), methotrexate (Rheumatrex), methyldopa (Aldomet), and many others.
RETINOIDS: These vitamin A derivatives could have additive toxic effects with vitamin A supplements (3046). Advise patients taking retinoids to avoid vitamin A supplements. Some of these retinoids include acitretin (Soriatane), bexarotene (Targretin), etretinate (Tegison), and isotretinoin (Accutane), tretinoin (Retin-A, Renova), and tazarotene (Avage).
TETRACYCLINE ANTIBIOTICS: Benign intracranial hypertension (pseudotumor cerebri) can occur with tetracyclines and with vitamin A intoxication (either an acute overdose, or chronic accumulation from doses of 40,000 units/day or more). Case reports suggest that taking tetracyclines and vitamin A concurrently can increase the risk of this condition (10545,10546,10547). Avoid high doses of vitamin A in people taking tetracyclines chronically. Tetracyclines include demeclocycline (Declomycin), minocycline (Minocin), and tetracycline (Achromycin).
WARFARIN (Coumadin): Vitamin A toxicity is associated with hemorrhage and hypoprothrombinemia, possibly due to vitamin K antagonism (505). High doses of vitamin A could increase the risk of bleeding with warfarin. Advise patients taking warfarin to avoid doses of vitamin A above the Tolerable Upper Intake Level of 10,000 units/day for adults.

Drug Influences on Nutrient Levels and Depletion

SOME DRUGS CAN AFFECT VITAMIN A LEVELS:
BILE ACID SEQUESTRANTS: By reducing absorption of dietary fats, cholestyramine (Questran) and colestipol (Colestid) may also reduce absorption of fat-soluble vitamins such as vitamin A. Some studies have reported a fall in serum vitamin A levels, but they rarely fall below the normal range with therapy of up to 2 years' duration (4455,4457,4460). Since some of the vitamin A in plasma is carried on lipids, part of this fall in plasma vitamin A levels may be due to decreased plasma lipid levels (4457,4460). Other studies have reported no change in plasma vitamin A levels with colestipol, up to 30 grams/day for 6 months, or cholestyramine 12 to 24 grams/day for up to 10 years (4461,10566,10567,10568,10569). Routine vitamin A supplements aren't necessary in people taking bile acid sequestrants, but check vitamin A levels in people taking high doses for more than 2 years.
ESTROGENS, ORAL CONTRACEPTIVES: Women taking oral contraceptives have higher plasma levels of vitamin A than non-users, but may have reduced liver stores of the vitamin. It's thought that estrogens stimulate production of retinol binding protein which carries vitamin A in the blood, and may pull more vitamin A out of storage sites such as the liver (9373,9505,10523,10548). Supplementation with up to 5000 IU/day in women taking oral contraceptives doesn't significantly affect plasma vitamin A levels, but might maintain liver stores (9373,9505,10548). There isn't enough data to recommend routine use of vitamin A supplements.
MINERAL OIL: Mineral oil has been reported to reduce absorption of all fat-soluble vitamins (4454,4495). However, there was no change in serum vitamin A levels in children who used mineral oil for up to four months (4496). Mineral oil should not be used on a regular basis due to its side effects. Its effect on vitamin A levels with occasional use is unlikely to be clinically significant.
ORLISTAT (Xenical): Orlistat can decrease absorption of fat soluble vitamins including vitamin A, leading to low plasma levels in some patients (1730). Several studies suggest that vitamin A is not affected as much by orlistat as some other fat-soluble vitamins (1727,9595,10570,10571). However, the manufacturer of orlistat recommends that all patients take a multivitamin supplement containing all the fat soluble vitamins, separating the dosing time by at least 2 hours from orlistat (1730).
NEOMYCIN: Neomycin (Mycifradin, Neo-Fradin) can bind and precipitate fatty acids and bile acids in the gut, reducing fat absorption. There is limited evidence that this can affect fat-soluble vitamin absorption. Single doses of

neomycin reduced absorption of large doses (300,000 units) of vitamin A given concurrently (10565). However, there was no change in serum vitamin A levels in adults who took neomycin 1 to 2 grams/day for 18 weeks for treatment of hyperlipoproteinemia (10566). It's unlikely that neomycin, or the other oral aminoglycosides such as kanamycin (Kantrex), and paromomycin (Humatin), will cause clinically significant vitamin A depletion.

Interactions with Foods

FAT: Dietary fat increases vitamin A absorption (7135).

Interactions with Lab Tests

BILIRUBIN: Vitamin A can cause false increase in bilirubin test results using Ehrlich's reagent (15).
CHOLESTEROL: There are unsubstantiated reports that vitamin A can produce false increases in serum cholesterol test results measured by the Zlatkis-Zak reaction (15).

Interactions with Diseases or Conditions

ALCOHOLISM: Chronic alcohol ingestion might potentiate the adverse effects of vitamin A, particularly hepatotoxicity (7135,7139). There is some evidence that chronic and excessive ethanol intake induces cytochrome P450 2E1 (CYP2E1) metabolism of vitamin A, which can increase production of hepatotoxic and carcinogenic vitamin A metabolites (1488,7135,7139).
ANEMIA: Anemia may not be adequately treated by iron supplements alone in patients with vitamin A deficiency. Vitamin A deficiency impairs iron mobilization from body stores. Combining vitamin A with iron supplementation in anemic patients with concurrent vitamin A deficiency seems to improve hemoglobin concentrations better than iron alone (7135).
FAT MALABSORPTION DISORDERS: Oral vitamin A absorption is decreased in conditions where fat absorption is reduced, such as celiac disease, short gut syndrome, obstructive jaundice, cystic fibrosis, pancreatic disease, and cirrhosis of the liver (7135). Water-miscible oral vitamin A preparations should be used in patients with fat malabsorption disorders.
HYPERLIPIDEMIA: Type V hyperlipoproteinemia increases risk of vitamin A hypervitaminosis (7135).
INTESTINAL INFECTIONS AND INFESTATIONS: Ascariasis, giardiasis, hookworm, salmonellosis, schistosomiasis, and other intestinal infections and infestations can reduce oral vitamin A absorption (7135).
LIVER DISEASE: Patients with liver disease can have an increased risk of hypervitaminosis and hepatotoxicity, especially if they take excessive doses of vitamin A (7135).
MALNUTRITION: In severe protein energy malnutrition (marasmus and kwashiorkor), there is reduced release of retinol from the liver. Until nutrition status is normalized, there is increased risk of vitamin A hypervitaminosis (7135).
ZINC DEFICIENCY: Zinc is required in hepatic synthesis of retinol binding protein. Without adequate zinc, symptoms of vitamin A deficiency can appear, despite vitamin A supplementation (8630). Zinc in combination with vitamin A seems to improve measures of vitamin A adequacy in undernourished children better than vitamin A or zinc alone (8636).

Dosage and Administration

ORAL: Treatment of deficiency in adults without corneal changes is 10,000 to 25,000 units daily until clinical improvement occurs, usually 1-2 weeks. Individuals with fat malabsorption, low protein intake, or hepatic or pancreatic disease might benefit from water-miscible oral preparations. If oral absorption is still insufficient, parenteral administration may be necessary. For prevention of nuclear cataracts, 10,000 units per day has been used (6378). For accelerating re-epithelialization following photoreactive keratectomy, vitamin A (retinol palmitate) 25,000 units and 230 mg vitamin E (alpha-tocopheryl nicotinate) have been used 3 times daily for 30 days, followed by twice daily for 2 months (348). Adequate Intake (AI) levels of vitamin A for infants have been established: birth to 6 months, 400 mcg/day (1300 units); 7 to 12 months, 500 mcg/day (1700 units). Recommended Dietary Allowance (RDA) levels for children and adults have been established: children 1 to 3 years, 300 mcg/day (1000 units); 4 to 8 years, 400 mcg/day (1300 units); 9 to 13 years, 600 mcg/day (2000 units); men 14 years and older, 900 mcg/day (3000 units); women 14 years and older, 700 mcg/day (2300 units); pregnancy 14 to 18 years, 750 mcg/day (2500 units); 19 years and older, 770 mcg/day (2600 units); lactation 14 to 18 years, 1200 mcg/day (4000 units); 19 years and older 1300 mcg/day (4300 units) (7135). Tolerable Upper Intake Levels (UL) for vitamin A have also been established. The UL is the highest level of intake that is likely to pose no risk of adverse effects. The ULs for vitamin A are for preformed vitamin A (retinol) and do not include provitamin A carotenoids: infants and children from birth to 3 years, 600 mcg/day (2000 units); children 4 to 8 years, 900 mcg/day (3000 units); 9 to 13 years 1700 mcg/day (6000 units); 14 to 18 years (including pregnancy and lactation) 2800 mcg/day (9000 units); adults age 19 and older (including pregnancy and lactation) 3000 mcg/day (10,000 units). Vitamin A dosage is most commonly expressed in units, but dosage in micrograms is sometimes used. One mcg of vitamin A equals 3.33 units of vitamin A. Vitamin A recommendations are for retinol, or preformed vitamin A. Formerly, vitamin A RDA recommendations were expressed as retinol equivalents (RE) to account for the differences in bioconversion of the various vitamin A forms to retinol. Retinol activity equivalents (RAE) are now used: 1 mcg of retinol equals 1 RAE which equals 2 mcg supplemental beta-carotene, 12 mcg of dietary beta-carotene, and 24 mcg dietary alpha-carotene or beta-cryptoxanthin. Either preformed vitamin A from animal products (retinol) or provitamin A carotenoids from plant products is an acceptable vitamin A source, although provitamin A carotenoids must be consumed in larger quantities (7135). Consumption of 5 servings of fruits and vegetables per day supplies 5 to 6 mg per day of provitamin A carotenoids, which provides about 50-65% of the adult RDA for vitamin A (7135).

VITAMIN B12

Also Known As

B-12, B Complex, B Complex Vitamin, Bedumil, Cobalamin, Cobalamins, Cobamin, Cyanocobalaminum, Cycobemin, Hydroxocobalaminum, Hydroxocobemine, Idrossocobalamina, Vitadurin, Vitamin B-12.
CAUTION: See separate listing for Dibencozide.

Scientific Names

Vitamin B12; Cyanocobalamin; Hydroxocobalamin; Methylcobalamin.

People Use This For

Orally, vitamin B12 is used for treating pernicious anemia and preventing and treating vitamin B12 deficiency. It is also used orally for treating primary hyperhomocysteinemia, heart disease, male infertility, diabetes, memory loss, circadian rhythm sleep disorders, Alzheimer's disease, depression, psychiatric disorders, osteoporosis, tendonitis, immunosuppression, AIDS, inflammatory bowel disease, asthma, allergies, vitiligo, and seborrheic dermatitis. It is also used orally for thyrotoxicosis, amyotrophic lateral sclerosis (Lou Gehrig's disease), multiple sclerosis, periodontal disease, tinnitus, hemorrhage, malignancy, and liver and kidney disease. Vitamin B12 is also used orally for aging, improving concentration, mood elevation, boosting energy, maintaining fertility, and protection against the toxins and allergens from tobacco smoke.
Topically, a vitamin B12 nasal gel is applied for pernicious anemia and preventing and treating vitamin B12 deficiency.
Parenterally, vitamin B12 is used for pernicious anemia and preventing and treating vitamin B12 deficiency. It is also used parenterally for tremor associated with shaky-leg syndrome or orthostatic tremor. Vitamin B12 is also used parenterally to treat tiredness or fatigue, chronic fatigue syndrome, thyrotoxicosis, hemorrhage, malignancy, and liver and kidney disease.

Safety

LIKELY SAFE ...when used orally, intravenously, or intranasally and appropriately. Vitamin B12 is generally considered safe, even in large doses (15).
PREGNANCY: LIKELY SAFE ...when used orally in amounts that do not exceed the recommended dietary allowance (RDA). The RDA for vitamin B12 in pregnant women is 2.6 mcg per day (6243). There is insufficient reliable information available about the safety of larger amounts of vitamin B12 during pregnancy.
LACTATION: LIKELY SAFE ...when used orally in amounts that do not exceed the recommended dietary allowance (RDA). The RDA of vitamin B12 during lactation is 2.8 mcg per day (6243). There is insufficient reliable information available about the safety of larger amounts of vitamin B12 while nursing.

Effectiveness

EFFECTIVE

Imerslund-Grasbeck disease. Administering vitamin B12 intramuscularly is effective for treating familial selective vitamin B12 malabsorption (Imerslund-Grasbeck disease) (15).

Pernicious anemia. Administering vitamin B12 intramuscularly, intranasally, or orally is effective for treating pernicious anemia. Both the cyanocobalamin and hydroxocobalamin forms of vitamin B12 are used intramuscularly. Cyanocobalamin is also used for intranasal administration (15). Oral vitamin B12 is as effective as intramuscular administration provided that a large enough oral dose is used (2900,2902,2909,2910,3024). Some evidence suggests the most effective oral dose is between 647 mcg to 1032 mcg/day (13106). However, oral preparations should not be used in patients with diarrhea or vomiting, severe neurologic involvement, nor in patients likely to be nonadherent (2900).

Vitamin B12 deficiency. Administering vitamin B12 orally, intramuscularly, or intranasally is effective for preventing and treating vitamin B12 deficiency. It is commonly believed that only intramuscular vitamin B12 is effective for treating vitamin B12 deficiency. But oral therapy is as effective as intramuscular administration, even in patients with malabsorption disorders, if a high enough dose is given (2900,2901,2911,2915,9335). Some evidence suggests that the most effective oral dose is between 647 mcg to 1032 mcg/day (13106). However, in some situations oral treatment is not appropriate. Intramuscular vitamin B12 is more appropriate in severe cases of deficiency when there is neurological involvement and in patients with diarrhea or vomiting, and those patients likely to be nonadherent (2900).

Vitamin B12 deficiency is especially common in older adults, primarily due to lack of intrinsic factor and malabsorption (2915,2919,9335). Older adults who take oral vitamin B12 supplements in doses of 25 to 37.5 mcg/day are more likely to have normal vitamin B12 levels than those who don't take supplements (9335). However, some older adults with vitamin B12 deficiency might require daily supplementation of vitamin B12 in doses of 50-100 mcg/day in order to restore levels to normal (10126). Vitamin B12, in foods such as milk and fortified bread, is approximately 55% to 60% absorbed by people over 60 years of age (10124).

Other people at risk for vitamin B12 deficiency include strict vegetarians and people with increased vitamin B12 requirements associated with pregnancy, thyrotoxicosis, hemolytic anemia, hemorrhage, malignancy, and hepatic and renal disease. Moderate consumption of animal products may not be sufficient to restore and maintain vitamin B12 levels in adolescents (age 9-15 years) who have eaten a strict vegetarian diet with inadequate intake of vitamin B12 from infancy to six years of age. A higher dietary intake of vitamin B12 or supplements is usually needed in order to restore and maintain optimal vitamin B12 levels in these adolescents (10125).

LIKELY EFFECTIVE

Hyperhomocysteinemia. Taking vitamin B12 orally in combination with folic acid, and sometimes with pyridoxine (vitamin B6), can reduce serum concentrations of homocysteine. Folic acid 0.5 to 5 mg/day lowers fasting homocysteine levels by an average of 25% (9400,9405,9408,9409,9410). Adding vitamin B12 (mean dose, 0.5 mg/day) produces an additional decrease in homocysteine levels of about 7% on average (6883,9400,9401,9405,9409), but probably only in people with vitamin B12 deficiency (2147,3047). Vitamin B12 in combination with folic acid and other vitamins also seems to significantly reduce homocysteine levels in patients with end-stage renal disease (ESRD) (1489,6883,6884,7289,7881,9414,9415,9416). A supplement containing vitamin B12 500 mcg with folic acid 2.5 mg and pyridoxine 25 mg, taken daily, may reduce the increase in homocysteine concentrations associated with nitrous oxide general anesthesia (9481). Some researchers recommend routine use of vitamin B12 in homocysteine-lowering regimens to avoid the risk of neuropathy in people with undetected vitamin B12 deficiency (9405). There is also preliminary evidence that daily intake of 4.2-6.0 mcg of vitamin B12 in combination with 700 mcg of folic acid and 4.2-6.0 mg of pyridoxine (vitamin B6) might lower homocysteine levels in patients with sickle cell disease (SCD), but it is unknown if this effect will reduce endothelial damage in these patients (9324). Using vitamin B12 alone has a limited effect on homocysteine levels, and probably only in those people with vitamin B12 deficiency (2149,9410,9512). Hyperhomocysteinemia is a risk factor for coronary, cerebral, and peripheral atherosclerosis; recurrent thromboembolism; deep vein thrombosis; myocardial infarction; and ischemic stroke (1899,2147,3047,3323,9402,9405,9408,9409). But elevated homocysteine levels may be a marker instead of a cause of vascular disease (11387,11388). A 5 micromole increase in plasma homocysteine increases the risk of cerebrovascular disease by 50%, and the risk of coronary heart disease by 60% in men and 80% in women (9407,9411). However, it's not clear if lowering homocysteine levels results in reduced cardiovascular morbidity and mortality (1489,6883,6884,7229,9308,9400,9405,9409). Folic acid, pyridoxine (vitamin B6), and vitamin B12 supplementation can reduce total homocysteine from 13.4 to 11.0 micromoles per liter. However, this reduction doesn't seem to help with secondary prevention of death or cardiovascular events such as stroke or myocardial infarction in people with prior stroke (11387). More evidence is needed to fully explain the association of total homocysteine levels with vascular risk. Until definitive data are available, the current recommendation is screening of 40-year-old men and 50-year-old women for hyperhomocysteinemia. For patients with homocysteine levels greater than 11 micromoles/L, supplement with folic acid and vitamin B12 (9308).

POSSIBLY INEFFECTIVE

Circadian rhythm sleep disorders. Taking vitamin B12 orally, in methylcobalamin form, doesn't seem to be effective for treating delayed sleep phase syndrome. Methylcobalamin 0.5-1 mg three times daily, with or without bright light therapy, doesn't seem to help people with primary circadian rhythm sleep disorders (1344,1345,1346,1347,1348).

Stroke. Taking vitamin B12 orally doesn't seem to be useful for preventing stroke recurrence. In people with a history of stroke, neither high dose vitamin B12 combinations containing 25 mg of pyridoxine, 0.4 mg of vitamin B12, and 2.5 mg of folic acid nor low dose combinations containing 200 mcg of pyridoxine, 6 mcg of vitamin B12, and 20 mcg of folic acid seem to affect risk of recurring stroke (11387).

INSUFFICIENT RELIABLE EVIDENCE to RATE

Angioplasty. There are conflicting findings about the benefits of taking folic acid plus vitamin B6 and vitamin B12 following angioplasty. Some evidence suggests that folic acid 1 mg plus vitamin B12 400 mcg and pyridoxine 10 mg daily can decrease the rate of restenosis in patients treated with balloon angioplasty (8009,9412). But this combination does not seem to be as effective for reducing restenosis in patients after coronary stenting (8009). An intravenous loading dose of folic acid, vitamin B6 and vitamin B12 followed by oral administration of folic acid 1.2 mg plus vitamin B6 48 mg and vitamin B12 60 mcg taken daily after coronary stenting also does not seem to reduce restenosis and might actually increase restenosis (12150,12151). Due to the lack of evidence of benefit and potential for harm, this combination of vitamins should not be recommended for patients receiving coronary stents (12151).

Breast cancer. Higher dietary folate intake is associated with a reduced risk of breast cancer. The risk may even be further reduced in women who also consume high amounts of dietary vitamin B12 in combination with dietary pyridoxine and methionine. However, there is no evidence that dietary vitamin B12 alone reduces the risk of breast cancer (9328).

Fatigue. There is some evidence intramuscular injections of vitamin B12 5 mg given twice per week might improve the general well being and happiness of patients complaining of tiredness or fatigue (10127).

Hypertriglyceridemia. Some evidence suggests that 7.5 mcg of vitamin B12 in combination with 5 grams of fish oil might be superior to fish oil alone when used daily to reduce total serum cholesterol and triglycerides. This suggests vitamin B12 might have an independent effect in lowering serum cholesterol and triglycerides, but further investigation is needed to confirm this effect (8694).

Lung cancer. Preliminary evidence suggests that there is no relationship between vitamin B12 status and lung cancer (9454).
Shaky leg syndrome. There are some preliminary clinical reports that the cyanocobalamin form of vitamin B12 can help relieve tremor associated with shaky-leg syndrome (6358).
More evidence is needed to rate vitamin B12 for these uses.

Mechanism of Action

Vitamin B12 is a naturally occurring B complex vitamin that is formed by microorganisms. It is also found in some foods from animal origin (e.g., meat, fish, shellfish, liver) in coenzyme form, mainly adenosylcobalamin and methylcobalamin. Cyanocobalamin and hydroxocobalamin are synthetic forms of vitamin B12.
Vitamin B12 is required for nucleoprotein and myelin synthesis, cell reproduction, normal growth, and normal erythropoiesis. Synthetic vitamin B12 can be converted to coenzyme B12, which is essential for the conversion of methylmalonate to succinate, and the synthesis of methionine from homocysteine (15,9320). Vitamin B12 is involved in maintaining sulfhydryl groups in the reduced form required by enzymes involved in fat and carbohydrate metabolism and protein synthesis. Vitamin B12 is essential for folate utilization, and its absence results in a functional folate deficiency (15).
Vitamin B12 deficiency can take months to years to become symptomatic due to large body stores. Normal serum vitamin B12 levels range between 200-900 pg/mL. Serum concentrations less than 200 pg/mL indicate deficiency, and concentrations less than 100 pg/mL usually result in megaloblastic anemia or neurologic damage (15).
Vitamin B12 deficiency results in megaloblastic anemia, gastrointestinal lesions, and neurologic damage, beginning with an inability to produce myelin and progressing to degeneration of the axon and nerve head (15). Neurologic symptoms caused by vitamin B12 deficiency can include neuropsychiatric disorders such as depression (6357), paresthesias, ataxia, memory loss, weakness, and personality and mood changes without anemia (1484,1485,3235,5646). Some neurologic symptoms and elevated homocysteine levels can occur without any signs of B12 deficiency anemia (1484,1485,3235). Vitamin B12 deficiency is associated with impaired cognitive performance in adolescents (aged 10-16 years) who have been fed a strict vegetarian diet from infancy to 6 years of age. Consequences of low vitamin B12 intake during childhood and its effect on cognitive functioning in adulthood are unknown (10125).
Elevated methylmalonate or methylmalonic acid (MMA) levels occur early in vitamin B12 deficiency, and may precede other symptoms (1484,1485,5646). In combination with homocysteine levels, MMA levels can be used to diagnose vitamin B12 deficiency (5646).
Vitamin B12 is absorbed via an active transport mechanism in the terminal ileum. This requires the glycoprotein, intrinsic factor, which is produced by the stomach. At normal gastric pH, vitamin B12 is cleaved from proteins in food. It then binds to intrinsic factor and is absorbed by ileal transport. Absorption can be reduced by increased gastric pH such as in atrophic gastritis, use of acid-suppressing drugs, or partial gastrectomy. Reduced absorption also occurs with loss of intrinsic factor in conditions such as pernicious anemia (an autoimmune disorder in which the ability to produce intrinsic factor is lost) and total gastrectomy. Intramuscular administration is often used to avoid these absorption problems. However, there is also a lesser-known transport system for vitamin B12 that does not rely on either intrinsic factor or the terminal ileum. Absorption is more efficient by the intrinsic factor route (about 60%), but 1% of an oral dose of vitamin B12 can be absorbed without intrinsic factor or stomach acid. Large oral doses (300 to 1000 mcg) can be sufficiently absorbed to treat pernicious anemia and malabsorption from food (2900,2901,2909,9518). The risk for vitamin B12 deficiency is higher with increased age, male gender, and in people of Caucasian and Latin American descent. Deficiency in vitamin B12 results from insufficient intake, malabsorption from food, and other medical conditions (1484,1485). However, body stores of vitamin B12 are large, and it is widely available in food. Vitamin B12 deficiency is almost always caused by a disorder of absorption (9518).
Deficiency of vitamin B12 can be masked by folic acid, particularly in large doses. Folate will improve vitamin B12 associated anemia, but it will allow the neurologic abnormalities to progress. There is some concern that food fortified with folic acid can cause under-recognition of vitamin B12 deficiency, particularly in the elderly (5646).
Vitamin B12 is required in one of the pathways for homocysteine metabolism. Remethylation of homocysteine to methionine requires folate and the methylcobalamin form of vitamin B12 as a cofactor (3047,9407,9409). Some evidence suggests elevated homocysteine levels might cause vascular endothelial cell damage, impaired endothelium-dependent vasodilation due to reduced nitric oxide activity, increased oxidation and arterial deposition of low-density lipoproteins (LDL), increased platelet adhesiveness, and activation of the clotting cascade (2147,3047,9403,9408).
Vitamin B12 supplements have a small additive effect to folic acid in lowering fasting homocysteine levels, but probably only in people with vitamin B12 deficiency (2147,3047). Elevated homocysteine concentrations are possibly associated with other conditions such as decreased cognitive function, impaired memory, Alzheimer's disease, and vascular dementia (5646,9330,9331).
Low vitamin B12 levels are also associated with other conditions such as hearing loss in elderly women (1482) and possibly chronic fatigue syndrome (6082). Some researchers think that vitamin B12 supplements could help symptoms of chronic fatigue syndrome by correcting red blood cell abnormalities and improving oxygen delivery to tissues (6082). The methylcobalamin form of vitamin B12 might also influence melatonin levels. Methylcobalamin seems to improve alertness and reduce sleep time in humans with normal sleep patterns, possibly due to affects on melatonin (1349).

Adverse Reactions

Orally and intramuscularly, vitamin B12 does not usually cause adverse effects, even in large doses (6243). In some people, vitamin B12 can cause diarrhea, peripheral vascular thrombosis, itching, transitory exanthema, urticaria, feelings of swelling of the entire body, and anaphylaxis, possibly due to impurities in vitamin B12 preparations. Treatment of vitamin B12 deficiency can unmask polycythemia vera, which is an increase in blood volume and the number of red blood cells (15).

Vitamin B12 (20 micrograms/day) and pyridoxine (80 mg/day) may cause rosacea fulminans, characterized by intense erythema with nodules, papules, and pustules. Symptoms may persist for up to 4 months after the supplement is stopped, and may require treatment with systemic corticosteroids and topical therapy (10998).

Interactions with Herbs & Other Dietary Supplements

FOLIC ACID: Folic acid, particularly in large doses, can mask vitamin B12 deficiency (5646). In vitamin B12 deficiency, folic acid can produce hematologic improvement in megaloblastic anemia, while allowing potentially irreversible neurological damage to progress. Vitamin B12 status should be determined before folic acid is given as monotherapy (2677,3092,5646).

POTASSIUM: Potassium supplements can reduce absorption of vitamin B12 in some people (4511,4512). This might be due to acidification of the ileal contents, which reduces the activity of intrinsic factor (4512). This effect has been reported with potassium chloride and, to a lesser extent, with potassium citrate (10501). Potassium might contribute to vitamin B12 deficiency in some people with other risk factors, but routine supplements aren't necessary.

VITAMIN C: Preliminary evidence suggests that vitamin C supplements can destroy dietary vitamin B12. However, other components of food, such as iron and nitrates, might counteract this effect (9511). It isn't clear whether this interaction is clinically significant, and it can likely be avoided if vitamin C supplements are taken at least 2 hours after meals.

Interactions with Drugs

CHLORAMPHENICOL: Limited case reports suggest that chloramphenicol can delay or interrupt the reticulocyte response to supplemental vitamin B12 in some patients (3072). Monitor blood counts closely if this combination can't be avoided.

Drug Influences on Nutrient Levels and Depletion

SOME DRUGS CAN AFFECT VITAMIN B12 LEVELS:

AMINOSALICYLIC ACID (para-aminosalicylic acid, PAS, Paser): Aminosalicylic acid can reduce oral vitamin B12 absorption, possibly by as much as 55%, as part of a general malabsorption syndrome (9574). Megaloblastic changes, and occasional cases of symptomatic anemia have occurred, usually after doses of 8 to 12 grams/day for several months (4558,9395,9397). Monitor vitamin B12 levels in people taking aminosalicylic acid for more than one month.

ANTIBIOTICS: Disruption of the normal gastrointestinal (GI) flora may interrupt enterohepatic recirculation of vitamin B12 and increase fecal excretion (4436). Vitamin B12 is also synthesized by the GI flora, but mainly in the colon where absorption is poor. The majority of bacterially synthesized vitamin B12 is therefore excreted in the feces and does not significantly contribute to the body's store of vitamin B12 (4437,9502). The effects of antibiotics on gastrointestinal bacteria are unlikely to have clinically significant effects on vitamin B12 levels. In people with bacterial overgrowth of the small bowel, antibiotics such as metronidazole (Flagyl) can actually improve vitamin B12 status. An increased bacterial load can bind significant amounts of vitamin B12 in the gut, preventing its absorption (4437,9502).

COBALT IRRADIATION: Cobalt irradiation of the small bowel can decrease gastrointestinal (GI) absorption of vitamin B12 (15).

COLCHICINE: Colchicine in doses of 1.9 to 3.9 mg/day can disrupt normal intestinal mucosal function, leading to malabsorption of several nutrients, including vitamin B12 (4543,4544,4545). Lower doses don't seem to have a significant effect on vitamin B12 absorption after 3 years of colchicine therapy (5921). The significance of this interaction isn't clear. Monitor vitamin B12 levels in people taking large doses of colchicine for prolonged periods.

COLESTIPOL (Colestid), CHOLESTYRAMINE (Questran): These resins can decrease gastrointestinal (GI) absorption of vitamin B12 by binding intrinsic factor and vitamin B12-intrinsic factor complexes (10542,10543). However, absorption isn't completely prevented (10542). It's unlikely that this interaction will deplete body stores of vitamin B12 unless there are other factors contributing to deficiency. In a group of children treated with cholestyramine for up to 2.5 years there wasn't any change in serum vitamin B12 levels (4455). Routine supplements aren't necessary.

H2-BLOCKERS: Reduced secretion of gastric acid and pepsin produced by H2-blockers can reduce absorption of protein-bound (dietary) vitamin B12, but not supplemental vitamin B12 (4539,4540,4541,9513,9514,9528). Gastric acid is needed to release vitamin B12 from protein for absorption (4541,9513,9514,9528). Clinically significant vitamin B12 deficiency and megaloblastic anemia are unlikely, unless H2-blocker therapy is prolonged (2 years or more), or the person's diet is poor (4539,9513,9514). It is also more likely if the person is rendered achlorhydric (4483), which occurs more frequently with proton pump inhibitors than H2-blockers. Monitor vitamin B12 levels in people taking high doses of H2 blockers for prolonged periods. The H2-blockers include cimetidine (Tagamet), ranitidine (Zantac), nizatidine (Axid), and famotidine (Pepcid).

METFORMIN (Glucophage): Metformin may reduce serum folic acid and vitamin B12 levels (32,4490,8834). These changes can lead to hyperhomocysteinemia, adding to the risk of cardiovascular disease in people with diabetes (32,4490,7839). There are also rare reports of megaloblastic anemia in people who have taken metformin for 5 years or more (9520,9521,9522). Possible mechanisms for lowered vitamin B12 levels are decreased intrinsic factor secretion, reduced uptake of vitamin B12-intrinsic factor complexes, altered bowel motility, and bacterial overgrowth (32,9521). Reduced absorption of vitamin B12 can be measured with the Schilling test after a few weeks of metformin therapy (7841). Reduced serum levels of vitamin B12 occur in up to 30% of people taking metformin chronically (4490,9520,9521,9523). However, clinically significant deficiency isn't likely to develop if dietary intake of vitamin B12 is adequate (9521). Deficiency can be corrected with vitamin B12 supplements even if metformin is continued (9520,9522). The metformin-induced malabsorption of vitamin B12 is reversible by oral calcium supplementation (8834,9523). A multivitamin preparation may also be valuable for some patients. Monitor for signs and symptoms of vitamin B12 and folic acid deficiency. Advise people taking metformin chronically to include adequate amounts of vitamin B12 in their diet, and have their serum vitamin B12 and homocysteine levels checked annually.
NEOMYCIN: Absorption of vitamin B12 can be reduced by neomycin, but prolonged use of large doses is needed to induce pernicious anemia (3046,8434). Supplements aren't needed with normal doses.
NITROUS OXIDE: Nitrous oxide inactivates the cobalamin form of vitamin B12 by oxidation. Symptoms of vitamin B12 deficiency, including sensory neuropathy, myelopathy, and encephalopathy, can occur within days or weeks of exposure to nitrous oxide anesthesia in people with subclinical vitamin B12 deficiency. Symptoms are treated with high doses of vitamin B12, but recovery can be slow and incomplete. People with normal vitamin B12 levels have sufficient vitamin B12 stores to make the effects of nitrous oxide insignificant, unless exposure is repeated and prolonged (nitrous oxide abuse) (9527,9532). In people with risk factors for vitamin B12 deficiency, check vitamin B12 levels prior to using nitrous oxide anesthesia.
ORAL CONTRACEPTIVES: The data regarding the effects of oral contraceptives on vitamin B12 serum levels are conflicting. Some studies have found reduced serum levels in oral contraceptive users (4547,9371,9373,9505), but others have found no effect despite use of oral contraceptives for up to 6 months (4498,7843,9372). When reduced serum levels are detected, vitamin B12 absorption, urinary excretion, tissue and erythrocyte levels, methylmalonic acid levels, and homocysteine are normal (9371,9373,9505,10123). When oral contraceptive use is stopped, normalization of vitamin B12 levels usually occurs (10123). It's suggested that oral contraceptives reduce production of transcobalamin I, the protein which transports vitamin B12 in the blood (4547,9373,9505). Thus more of the vitamin is available for tissue uptake and serum levels may be reduced. Vitamin B12 supplements don't seem to increase serum levels of vitamin B12 (9373). Lower vitamin B12 serum levels seen with oral contraceptives probably aren't clinically significant.
PHENYTOIN (Dilantin), PHENOBARBITAL, PRIMIDONE (Mysoline): These anticonvulsants have been associated with reduced vitamin B12 absorption, and reduced serum and cerebrospinal fluid levels in some patients. This may contribute to the megaloblastic anemia, primarily caused by folate deficiency, associated with these drugs (7843,10502,10503,10504). It's also suggested that reduced vitamin B12 levels may contribute to the neuropsychiatric side effects of these drugs (10504,10505). Encourage patients to maintain adequate dietary vitamin B12 intake, and check folate and vitamin B12 status if symptoms of anemia develop.
PROTON PUMP INHIBITORS (PPIs): The reduced secretion of gastric acid and pepsin produced by PPIs can reduce absorption of protein-bound (dietary) vitamin B12, but not supplemental vitamin B12 (4483,4484,4485,4486,9513,9528). Gastric acid is needed to release vitamin B12 from protein for absorption (4484,4486,9513,9528). Reduced vitamin B12 levels may be more common with PPIs than with H2-blockers, because they are more likely to produce achlorhydria (complete absence of gastric acid secretion) (4483,4486). However, clinically significant vitamin B12 deficiency is unlikely, unless PPI therapy is prolonged (2 years or more) or dietary vitamin intake is low (4483,4484,9513). Monitor vitamin B12 levels in people taking high doses of PPIs for prolonged periods. The PPIs include omeprazole (Prilosec, Losec), lansoprazole (Prevacid), rabeprazole (Aciphex), pantoprazole (Protonix, Pantoloc), and esomeprazole (Nexium).
ZIDOVUDINE (AZT, Combivir, Retrovir): Reduced serum vitamin B12 levels may occur when zidovudine therapy is started (30,10531). This adds to other factors that cause low vitamin B12 levels in people with HIV, and might contribute to the hematological toxicity associated with zidovudine (10531,10532). However, data suggest vitamin B12 supplements aren't helpful for people taking zidovudine (10532,10533).

Interactions with Foods

ALCOHOL (Ethanol): Excessive alcohol intake lasting longer than two weeks can decrease vitamin B12 absorption from the gastrointestinal tract (15).

Interactions with Lab Tests

INTRINSIC FACTOR: Vitamin B12 can cause a false-positive test result for intrinsic factor antibodies (15).

Interactions with Diseases or Conditions

ANGIOPLASTY: An intravenous loading dose of folic acid, vitamin B6 and vitamin B12 followed by oral administration of folic acid 1.2 mg plus vitamin B6 48 mg and vitamin B12 60 mcg taken daily after coronary stenting might actually restenosis rates (12150). Due to the potential for harm, this combination of vitamins should not be recommended for patients receiving coronary stents (12151).

COBALAMIN OR COBALT HYPERSENSITIVITY: Contraindicated (15).
LEBER'S DISEASE: Vitamin B12 is contraindicated in early Leber's disease, which is hereditary optic nerve atrophy. Vitamin B12 can cause severe and swift optic atrophy (15).
MEGALOBLASTIC ANEMIA: The correction of megaloblastic anemia with vitamin B12 can result in fatal hypokalemia and gout in susceptible individuals, and it can obscure folate deficiency in megaloblastic anemia (15); use with caution.
POLYCYTHEMIA VERA: The treatment of vitamin B12 deficiency can unmask the symptoms of polycythemia vera (15).

Dosage and Administration

ORAL: For vitamin B12 deficiency or pernicious anemia, cyanocobalamin doses of 300-10,000 mcg daily have been used (2900,2901,2909); However, some evidence suggests that the most effective oral dose is between 647 mcg to 1032 mcg/day (13106).
For hyperhomocysteinemia, vitamin B12 500 mcg in combination with 0.5-5 mg folic acid and 16.5 mg pyridoxine has been used (9400,9405).
To decrease the rate of restenosis after coronary angioplasty, a combination of vitamin B12 400 mcg plus pyridoxine (vitamin B6) 10 mg and folic acid 1 mg taken daily has been used (8008).
For reducing increased homocysteine concentrations associated with nitrous oxide general anesthesia, a supplement containing vitamin B12 500 mcg with pyridoxine (vitamin B6) 25 mg and folic acid 2.5 mg taken daily for one week before surgery has been used (9481).
The typical general supplemental dose of vitamin B12 is 1-25 mcg per day (15). The recommended dietary allowances (RDAs) of vitamin B12 are: Infants 0-6 months, 0.4 mcg; Infants 7-12 months, 0.5 mcg; Children 1-3 years, 0.9 mcg; Children 4-8 years, 1.2 mcg; Children 9-13 years, 1.8 mcg; Older children and adults, 2.4 mcg; Pregnant women 2.6 mcg; and Lactating women, 2.8 mcg (3094). Because 10% to 30% of older people do not absorb food-bound vitamin B12 efficiently, those over 50 years should meet the RDA by eating foods fortified with B12 or by taking a vitamin B12 supplement (6243). Supplementation of 25-100 mcg per day has been used to maintain vitamin B12 levels in older people (2911,9335,10126).
INTRAMUSCULAR (IM): For treatment of vitamin B12 deficiency, the usual dose is 30 mcg daily for 5-10 days. For maintenance therapy, 100-200 mcg once monthly is commonly used. Both cyanocobalamin and hydroxocobalamin forms are used (15). For familial selective vitamin B12 malabsorption, cyanocobalamin 1000 mcg weekly for three weeks, followed by 250 mcg monthly is commonly used (15). For relief of tremor associated with shaky-leg syndrome, injections of 1000 mcg of the cyanocobalamin form of vitamin B12 daily for two weeks, then weekly for two months, and once a month thereafter has been used (6358). For decreasing homocysteine levels and normalizing B12 levels in adult vegetarians, cyanocobalamin 1000 mcg has been used (9512).

Comments

Vitamin B12 is frequently used in combination with other B vitamins in vitamin B complex formulations. Vitamin B complex generally includes vitamin B1 (Thiamine), vitamin B2 (Riboflavin), vitamin B3 (Niacin/Niacinamide), vitamin B5 (Pantothenic Acid), vitamin B6 (Pyridoxine), vitamin B12 (Cyanocobalamin), and folic acid. However, some products do not contain all of these ingredients and some may include others, such as biotin, para-aminobenzoic acid (PABA), choline bitartrate, and inositol (3022).

VITAMIN C (ASCORBIC ACID)

Also Known As

Antiscorbutic Vitamin, Ascorbate, Ascorbyl Palmitate, Calcium Ascorbate, Cevitamic Acid, Iso-Ascorbic Acid, L-Ascorbic Acid, Sodium Ascorbate.
CAUTION: See separate listings for Acerola, Cherokee Rosehip, and Rose Hip.

Scientific Names

Ascorbic acid.

People Use This For

Orally, vitamin C is used for preventing and treating scurvy; preventing deficiency in people with gastrointestinal diseases and those on chronic total parenteral nutrition or chronic hemodialysis; increasing iron absorption from the gastrointestinal tract; and increasing the healing rate of wounds, burns, fractures, ulcers, and pressure sores. It is used for urine acidification, treating idiopathic methemoglobinemia, correcting tyrosinemia in premature infants on high-protein diets, increasing iron excretion (in combination with deferoxamine), preventing and treating the common cold and other viral infections, bronchitis, human immunodeficiency virus (HIV) disease, Helicobacter pylori infection, tuberculosis, dysentery, furunculosis, hematuria, retinal hemorrhages, hemorrhagic states, and anemia. Vitamin C is also used orally for atherosclerosis, preventing vascular thrombosis, myocardial infarction, stroke, hypertension, lowering cholesterol, glaucoma, preventing cataracts, preventing gallbladder disease, dental caries, pyorrhea, gum infections, constipation, peptic ulcer, acne, dermatitis, improving immune function, hay fever, asthma, bronchitis, cystic fibrosis, cystitis, prostatitis, infertility, and diabetes. It is also used orally for mental depression, cognitive impairment, dementia, Alzheimer's disease, physical and mental stress, fatigue, attention deficit-hyperactivity disorder (ADHD), autism, collagen disorders, arthritis and bursitis, back pain and disc inflammation, cancer, osteogenesis imperfecta, and osteoporosis. Other uses include improving physical endurance, reducing aging, heat prostration, for counteracting the side effects of cortisone and related drugs, aiding drug withdrawal in addiction, and in the treatment of levodopa, succinylcholine, interferon, aspirin, and arsenic toxicity. Other uses include use as an adjunct to radiation therapy and treating chronic radiation proctitis. It is also used to prevent human immunodeficiency virus (HIV) transmission to breast-fed babies.

Topically, vitamin C is used for improving skin conditions, protecting against free radicals and pollutants, and for improving photo-aged skin. It is also applied topically for ulcerative mucositis associated with radiation therapy.

Parenterally, vitamin C is used for preventing and treating vitamin C deficiency and correcting tyrosinemia in premature infants on high-protein diets.

Safety

LIKELY SAFE ...when used orally, topically, intramuscularly, or intravenously and appropriately. Vitamin C is safe when taken orally in doses below the tolerable upper intake level (UL). Tell patients not to exceed the UL of 2000 mg per day (1959,4713,4714,4844). ...when used intravenously or intramuscularly and appropriately. Injectable vitamin C is an FDA-approved prescription product (15).

POSSIBLY UNSAFE ...when used orally in excessive doses. Doses greater than the tolerable upper intake level (UL) of 2000 mg per day can significantly increase the risk of adverse effects such as osmotic diarrhea and gastrointestinal upset (4844).

CHILDREN: LIKELY SAFE ...when used orally and appropriately (4844,10352). POSSIBLY UNSAFE ...when used orally in excessive amounts. Tell patients not to use doses above the tolerable upper intake level (UL) of 400 mg per day for children ages 1 to 3 years, 650 mg per day for children 4 to 8 years, 1200 mg per day for children 9 to 13 years, and 1800 mg per day for adolescents 14 to 18 years. Higher doses can cause osmotic diarrhea and gastrointestinal upset (4844).

PREGNANCY AND LACTATION: LIKELY SAFE ...when used orally and appropriately (4844). POSSIBLY UNSAFE ...when used orally in excessive doses. Tell patients not to use doses exceeding the UL of 2000 mg per day for pregnant or breast-feeding women over age 19; and 1800 mg per day for pregnant and breast-feeding women 14 to 18 years. Higher doses can cause osmotic diarrhea and gastrointestinal upset. Large doses of vitamin C during pregnancy can also cause newborn scurvy (4844); avoid using.

Effectiveness

EFFECTIVE

Vitamin C deficiency. Administering vitamin C orally or intramuscularly prevents and treats vitamin C deficiency, including scurvy. Vitamin C administration can reverse complications of scurvy within two days to three weeks (4844).

LIKELY EFFECTIVE

Iron absorption. Concurrent administration of at least 200 mg vitamin C per 30 mg iron increases iron absorption (3042,9518).

Tyrosinemia. Administering vitamin C orally or intramuscularly improves tyrosinemia in premature infants on high protein diets (15).

POSSIBLY EFFECTIVE

Age-related macular degeneration (AMD). Taking vitamin C 500 mg orally, in combination with elemental zinc 80 mg, vitamin E 400 IU, and beta-carotene 15 mg daily seems to provide a risk reduction of 27% for visual acuity loss and a risk reduction of 25% for progression of AMD in patients with advanced AMD (7303). Patients with monocular or binocular intermediate AMD or monocular advanced AMD are at high risk for advanced AMD. Theoretically, these patients may also benefit from vitamin C and antioxidant-zinc supplementation (11326). There isn't enough evidence to know if this combination is beneficial for people with less advanced macular disease or for preventing AMD. Vitamin C with other antioxidants, but without zinc, doesn't seem to have any effect on AMD (7303,7304). Epidemiological evidence suggests that increased vitamin C dietary intake and supplements might actually increase the risk of age-related maculopathy (9823).

Albuminuria. Taking vitamin C plus vitamin E can reduce the excretion of albumin by about 19% when given for 4 weeks in patients with type 2 diabetes. This might also reduce the risk of end-stage renal disease in patients with type 2 diabetes (10434).

Atherosclerosis and peripheral arterial disease. Taking vitamin C orally seems to decrease the risk of atherosclerosis and peripheral arterial disease. Patients with peripheral arterial disease, appear to have lower levels of vitamin C and higher levels of C-reactive protein, a marker of inflammation (9813). In women, there is some epidemiological evidence suggesting that dietary vitamin C can decrease the risk of peripheral arterial disease. However, it does not seem to have this effect in men (10130). However, other research suggests that slow release vitamin C 250 mg in combination with vitamin E 136 IU twice daily might slow the progression of atherosclerosis of the carotid artery. This combination appears to benefit both smoking and nonsmoking men, but has a marginal effect in postmenopausal women (1918,10473). Epidemiological evidence also suggests that dietary intake of vitamin C doesn't affect atherosclerotic markers such as carotid artery wall thickness or carotid artery plaque (9814). In children with familial hypercholesterolemia, vitamin C and vitamin E may increase flow mediated dilation, when used with a National Cholesterol Education Program Step II (NCEP-II) diet (10352). There's also some evidence that the combination of vitamin C and vitamin E might help prevent cardiac transplant-associated arteriosclerosis (5197). Overall, vitamin C appears to slow progression of atherosclerosis. The effects of dietary and supplemental vitamin C on atherosclerosis requires further study to determine if it is generally beneficial or more useful in specific patient populations (9815).

Cancer. Dietary vitamin C might decrease the risk of developing mouth cancer and other cancers (10819,10821). Some evidence suggests that a diet low in vitamin C might increase the risk of mortality due to cancer in men, but not in women (3910,5878). Research on the protective effects of vitamin C against developing breast cancer is mixed. Some research suggests that dietary vitamin C reduces breast cancer risk (1444,10823,10824); other research suggests no association between vitamin C intake and breast cancer risk (10825,10826). There is currently no evidence that vitamin C from supplements has any effect on breast cancer risk. Some researchers project that plasma ascorbic acid increases to theoretically protective levels against cancer with an increase of one serving of fruits and vegetables per day (3910). The use of high-dose vitamin C, as adjunctive therapy, in combination with other antioxidants to treat cancer is controversial. Some experts think these supplements might increase the sensitivity of tumor cells to radiation and reduce toxicity in normal cells. Other experts worry that antioxidants might protect cancer cells from the effects of radiation (9826). High dose oral vitamin C, 10 grams daily in patients with advanced cancer regardless of prior chemotherapy, does not seem to improve survival or decrease disease progression (4842,4843). Preliminary clinical evidence suggests high doses of vitamin C given intravenously might have a beneficial effect on survival rate in patients with terminal cancer. Thus far, this has not been tested in well-designed clinical trials (9809). Some observational research in children with lymphoblastic leukemia suggests that greater dietary vitamin C intake is associated with fewer delays in chemotherapy, less toxicity, and fewer hospitalization days (11997).

Common cold. There is a lot of controversy about the effectiveness of vitamin C for treating the common cold (1969,1989,7100,9835,9836). However, the majority of evidence shows that taking high doses of vitamin C orally might decrease the duration of cold symptoms by 1-1.5 days in some patients (1966,1967,1968,1987,6458,7102,9832). Other studies have found no effect with doses up to 3 grams daily (9833). Some research suggests vitamin C may be more effective for treating cold symptoms in children than in adults. There may also be a dose-dependent response, doses of at least 2 grams per day seems to work better than 1 gram doses (9834). Tell patients that the high doses used for treating the common cold, 1-3 grams daily, can increase the risk of side effects. Some patients might not think the modest benefit is worth the risk. Explain to patients that taking vitamin C supplements prophylactically does not decrease the risk of catching a cold (1966,1967,1968,1987,3042,6458,7101,9832). Dietary intake of vitamin C also doesn't seem to affect the risk of getting a cold (10780).

Contrast-mediated nephropathy. Taking vitamin C before and after coronary angiography seems to reduce the risk of developing contrast-mediated nephropathy compared to placebo (12234).

Erythema. There is some evidence that an aqueous formulation of topical vitamin C can decrease the degree and duration of erythema following cutaneous carbon dioxide laser resurfacing for scar and wrinkle removal (1959).

Exercise-induced respiratory infections. Some evidence suggests that prophylactic use of vitamin C in doses of 600 mg to 1 gram per day before heavy physical exercise, such as a marathon, might prevent upper respiratory infections that sometimes follow heavy exercise (9831).

Gallbladder disease. There is some evidence that vitamin C supplementation and increased vitamin C serum levels decreases the risk of developing gallbladder disease in women; however, it doesn't seem to have this effect in men (5877).

Helicobacter pylori (H pylori). Taking vitamin C orally seems to decrease gastritis associated with acid suppressive therapy in patients with H. pylori infection (10359). After H. pylori is eradicated, vitamin C appears to decrease the incidence of precancerous changes in stomach tissue (10360).

HIV transmission. Taking vitamin C orally during pregnancy and breast-feeding seems to reduce HIV transmission. Supplementation of mothers with HIV disease with vitamin B, vitamin C, and vitamin E seems to reduce child mortality and HIV transmission through breast milk (9801).

Hypertension. Taking vitamin C orally, added to a conventional antihypertensive medication regimen, appears to decrease both systolic and mean blood pressure, but does not seem to decrease diastolic pressure (2044). In patients with type 2 diabetes, vitamin C 500 mg taken daily for 4 weeks, in addition to antihypertensives, seems to reduce arterial blood pressure and improve arterial stiffness (9822). But supplemental vitamin C 500 mg per day taken without antihypertensives doesn't seem to reduce systolic or diastolic blood pressure (9821). Dietary restriction of vitamin C is associated with increases in both diastolic and systolic blood pressure (10354).

Lead toxicity. Consuming vitamin C from dietary sources seems to lower blood concentrations of lead (3097,3098,3099).

Nitrate tolerance. Taking vitamin C orally seems to prevent the development of nitrate tolerance in patients taking sublingual nitroglycerin. There is some evidence that short-term vitamin C supplementation can prevent attenuation of tolerance to the vasodilatory effects of nitrates (1441,1961).

Osteoarthritis. Consuming vitamin C from dietary sources seems to reduce the risk of cartilage loss and disease progression in people with osteoarthritis (5881).

Pre-eclampsia. Taking vitamin C orally with vitamin E seems to prevent pre-eclampsia in high-risk pregnancies (3236).

Reflex sympathetic dystrophy (RSD). Patients given vitamin C supplements for 50 days after a wrist fracture seem to be significantly less likely to develop RSD (2045).

Sunburn. Taking vitamin C orally in combination with vitamin E seems to prevent ultraviolet (UV) radiation-induced erythema (sunburn) (4715,4716). Vitamin C in combination with high dose oral RRR-alpha-tocopherol (natural vitamin E) seems to protect against skin inflammation after exposure to ultraviolet (UV) radiation (1416,4715). This effect is not found when vitamin C is used without vitamin E (1417). Applying vitamin C topically, in combination with vitamin E and melatonin, also seems to prevent ultraviolet (UV) radiation-induced erythema (sunburn). Topical vitamin C in combination with topical vitamin E and melatonin seems to provide modest photo-protective effects when used prior to UV exposure. However, it has no effect when used during or after UV exposure (4713,4714).

Wrinkled skin. Topical preparations containing 5-10% vitamin C seem to improve the appearance of wrinkled skin. In one trial, a topical preparation containing 10% vitamin C as L-ascorbic acid and acetyl tyrosine, zinc sulfate, sodium hyaluronate, and bioflavonoids (Cellex-C High Potency Serum) used for 3 months and applied to photo-aged facial skin improved fine and coarse wrinkling, yellowing and sallowness, roughness, and skin tone compared to placebo (6155).

POSSIBLY INEFFECTIVE

Acute bronchitis. Taking vitamin C orally 500 mg on day 1, then 250 mg on days 2 through 5 (similar to an azithromycin regimen) doesn't seem to have any effect on acute bronchitis duration or symptoms (9827).

Alzheimer's disease or vascular dementia. Consuming vitamin C from dietary sources, as a supplement alone, or in combination with vitamin E, doesn't seem to affect the risk of developing Alzheimer's disease or vascular dementia (4636,9824,10131). However, some epidemiological research suggests that long-term use of vitamin C and vitamin E supplements in combination, and in higher doses than typically found in multivitamins, is associated with a reduced prevalence and incidence of Alzheimer's disease (11390).

Attention deficit-hyperactivity disorder (ADHD). Taking megadose vitamins including vitamin C orally doesn't seem to help ADHD symptoms (9957,9958,9959).

Interferon-related retinopathy. Taking vitamin C 600 mg per day orally doesn't seem to reduce the risk of retinopathy associated with interferon therapy in patients with chronic hepatitis C (10355).

Radiation dermatitis. Applying a 10% vitamin C solution does not appear to have a protective effect when applied to the scalps of patients treated with radiation for intracranial tumors (789).

Stroke. Most population studies show that taking vitamin C orally doesn't seem to affect the risk of ischemic or hemorrhagic stroke (1449,1958,7390,7716). Lower plasma levels of vitamin C have been associated with increased stroke risk (1957,7714). Higher consumption of fruits and vegetables has been associated with reduced ischemic stroke risk (7394). Suggest a diet high in fruits and vegetables rather than vitamin C supplements to reduce stroke risk.

INSUFFICIENT RELIABLE EVIDENCE to RATE

Aspirin-associated gastric damage. Some clinical evidence suggests that vitamin C might prevent gastric damage associated with aspirin therapy by decreasing blood loss and preventing decreased gastric blood flow (10357).

Asthma. There is some evidence that low levels of vitamin C are associated with certain conditions. Vitamin C levels might be decreased in some asthmatics (5873). Some clinical evidence also suggests that oral vitamin C might decrease exercise-induced asthma (1443).

Bladder cancer. Epidemiological research suggests that supplemental vitamin C use does not affect mortality rate associated with bladder cancer (9839).

Cardiovascular disease. Using antioxidants such as vitamin C for preventing heart disease and cardiovascular events such as myocardial infarction (MI) is controversial. There have been lots of studies, but results have been mixed (11001). In populations with relatively low or deficient vitamin C intake, vitamin C seems to lower the risk of death from coronary heart disease, although not all studies have shown benefit (1958,7714,7715,10815,11001). Some large population studies have shown a reduction in mortality from coronary heart disease either from dietary sources or supplements (3910,7394,10358,10814,10816,10817,11003), but similar studies have shown no effect on mortality risk with increased vitamin C intake (1958,3933,3934,3938,7724). Interestingly, two of the positive studies found a 25-28% reduction of cardiovascular disease and cardiovascular disease mortality in women only who took vitamin C supplements (10358,11002). Some population studies that found benefit have been criticized for not considering concurrent vitamin E intake (7715,11002). Some research suggests that a combination of vitamin C and vitamin E might offer additional benefit for preventing coronary heart disease (3938). In people with coronary heart disease, the few studies that have been done haven't shown vitamin C to be beneficial (10817,10818,11000). Vitamin C in combination with selenium, beta-carotene, vitamin E also doesn't seem to protect against cardiovascular disease progression and related events such as MI (7388). Studies investigating serum vitamin C concentrations and cardiovascular mortality risk are inconclusive. One study found decreased mortality with increasing concentrations (3910); the other found no effect (5878). Tell patients more research is needed before supplemental vitamin C can be recommended for preventing coronary heart disease. Increasing fruit and vegetable intake by one serving per day in the average person could boost plasma ascorbic acid to theoretically protective levels (3910). A Science Advisory from the American Heart Association also states that the evidence does not justify use of antioxidants such as vitamin C for reducing the risk of cardiovascular disease (12142).

Cataracts. There is conflicting information about the use of vitamin C to prevent cataracts. Vitamin C plus vitamin E and beta-carotene doesn't seem to have any significant effect on age-related loss of vision due to cataracts in well-nourished people who took the supplement for an average of 6.3 years (7304). However, population research suggests that vitamin C use in multivitamins or any supplement containing vitamin C for 10 years appears to reduce the incidence of nuclear and cortical cataracts by 60%. Use of supplements for shorter periods doesn't appear to reduce the risk for cataract development (4208).

Chronic radiation proctitis. Preliminary clinical research suggests that vitamin C 500 mg plus vitamin E 400 IU three times daily might improve symptoms of chronic radiation proctitis (9825).

Colorectal cancer. Taking vitamin C in combination with beta-carotene plus vitamin E doesn't seem to reduce the risk of colorectal cancer (12185).

Esophageal cancer. Taking vitamin C in combination with beta-carotene plus vitamin E doesn't seem to reduce the risk of esophageal cancer (12185).

Gastric cancer. Taking vitamin C orally seems to promote regression of premalignant gastric lesions in people at high risk for gastric cancer. Vitamin C 1 gram twice daily seems to cause regression of intestinal metaplasia and multifocal nonmetaplastic atrophy (2579).There is conflicting epidemiological evidence regarding the effects of dietary and supplemental vitamin C on preventing gastric cancer (9194,9838,10819,10822). Taking vitamin C in combination with beta-carotene or beta-carotene plus vitamin E doesn't seem to reduce the risk of gastric cancer (12185).

HIV/AIDS. Taking vitamin C 250 mg daily in combination with vitamin A, beta-carotene, vitamin E, selenium, and coenzyme Q-10 seems to improve markers of oxidative defense and oxidative stress in men with human immunodeficiency virus (HIV) disease. However, higher doses of vitamin C, 1000 mg, and the other antioxidants don't seem to provide any additional effect. Neither high-dose nor low-dose antioxidants affect viral load (9830).

Infertility. There is preliminary evidence that women with infertility, due to luteal phase defect, might increase their progesterone levels by taking vitamin C 750 mg daily (12010). It's not currently known if vitamin C can significantly increase pregnancy rates.

Leukemia. There is some evidence that vitamin C might have a synergistic effect with arsenic trioxide (Trisenox) on myeloid leukemia cells. Preclinical evidence suggests that vitamin C might enhance the apoptotic effect of arsenic trioxide in patients with acute myeloid leukemia (9837).

Mental stress. Preliminary evidence suggests that vitamin C might reduce blood pressure and subjective symptoms during psychological or mental stress (10353).

Osteoporosis. Some evidence suggests that vitamin C intake might be related to bone mineral density in premenopausal women and men. In postmenopausal women who use estrogen and smoke, higher vitamin C levels might reduce fracture risk. However, in postmenopausal women without a history of smoking or estrogen use, higher serum vitamin C levels have been associated with lower bone mineral density. At present, there is not enough information to make recommendations about vitamin C and bone density (9828).

Ovarian cancer. Epidemiological research suggests that dietary vitamin C does not affect risk of developing ovarian cancer (9193).

Overall mortality. Some research suggests that plasma vitamin C levels are positively associated with a reduced risk of mortality from all causes (3910). However, in high-risk patients, vitamin C 250 mg in combination with vitamin E 600 mg and beta-carotene 20 mg daily doesn't seem to affect overall mortality risk. Additionally, this combination doesn't seem to reduce mortality rate or illness from vascular disease in people with diabetes, coronary disease, or occlusive arterial disease. This vitamin combination also doesn't seem to reduce the risk of cancer or hospitalization for any other nonvascular cause (9817).

Pancreatic cancer. Taking vitamin C in combination with beta-carotene plus vitamin E doesn't seem to reduce the risk of pancreatic cancer (12185).

Sickle cell disease. Vitamin C, in combination with aged garlic extract and vitamin E might be useful for sickle cell disease (5056).

More evidence is needed to rate vitamin C for these uses.

Mechanism of Action

Vitamin C is a commonly used water-soluble vitamin. Although many mammals can produce vitamin C, humans must obtain vitamin C from foods and other sources (1964). It's contained in the high concentration in fresh fruits and vegetables, especially the citrus fruits. Vitamin C is labile, and the amount in foods can decrease significantly with cooking and storage (3042). Vitamin C has a role in several physiological functions. It is involved in tyrosine metabolism and is a cofactor in the synthesis of carnitine, thyroxin, norepinephrine, dopamine, and tryptophan (3042). Vitamin C is also involved in a variety of metabolic processes including oxidation-reduction reactions and cellular respiration, carbohydrate metabolism, synthesis of lipids and proteins, catabolism of cholesterol to bile acids, conversion of folic acid to folinic acid, and iron metabolism (5877). Vitamin C is probably best known for its effects as an antioxidant and its role in maintaining proper immune function (15). Normal plasma vitamin C levels typically exceed 0.3 mg/dL. When plasma levels exceed 1.4 mg/dL, excretion of vitamin C greatly increases (1965,1969). Concentrations below 0.2 mg/dL indicate significant deficiency (1964).

Vitamin C deficiency can cause fatigue, personality changes, and decline in psychomotor performance and motivation within 84 to 97 days. Some evidence suggests that subclinical vitamin C deficiency is more common in healthy people than generally recognized (9810). Since the nonspecific symptom of fatigue is often the first symptom of deficiency, vitamin C depletion may go undiagnosed (9809). Sustained vitamin C deficiency over 3 to 5 months

results in symptomatic scurvy characterized by gingival swelling and bleeding, loosening of the teeth, hyperkeratosis, perifollicular hemorrhages, petechial hemorrhages in the viscera, and hemorrhages into the muscles of the arms, legs, and joints (1964). Severe scurvy may progress to neuritis, jaundice, fever, dyspnea, and death. In infants, vitamin C deficiency is initially manifested by listlessness, anorexia, irritability, and failure to thrive. Later symptoms result from hemorrhage and collagen deficiency, with seizures, shock, and death if left untreated (1965).
Because of vitamin C's role in maintaining normal immune function, a lot of people use it for treating and preventing infectious conditions such as the common cold. T-lymphocyte activity, phagocyte function, leukocyte mobility, and possibly antibody and interferon production seem to be increased by vitamin C (1963,1965). Vitamin C levels in phagocytes and lymphocytes are up to 100 times greater than in plasma (7101). Some researchers think that vitamin C levels in white blood cells decrease at the onset of a cold and that boosting vitamin C intake might be beneficial. There is some evidence vitamin C might have other effects in patients with the common cold. Vitamin C might protect normal tissues against reactive oxygen species that are produced by phagocytes during a viral infection. It might also enhance the proliferative responses of T-lymphocytes (1988). There is some evidence that vitamin C might also have weak antihistamine properties (1969). There is preliminary evidence vitamin C excretion might actually decrease during a cold, indicating that patients may retain vitamin C. However, absorption of vitamin C is unchanged during a cold (1986).
Other potentially beneficial effects of vitamin C are attributed primarily to its role as an antioxidant and free radical scavenging effects. Vitamin C readily undergoes reversible oxidation and reduction in the body (1963). Vitamin C decreases oxidants in gastric juice, lipid peroxidation, and oxidative DNA and protein damage (3042). Damage by reactive oxygen species are thought to be a contributing factor to a number of diseases, including dementia, asthma, hypertension, osteoarthritis, and cancer. Researchers theorized that antioxidants such as vitamin C might protect against some diseases associated with oxidative damage. For example, in hypertension, endothelium-derived nitric oxide (NO), which causes vasodilation, might be inhibited by superoxide anions. Vitamin C can scavenge the superoxide anions and theoretically might help patients with hypertension. However, in this case there is some evidence that oral doses might not reach concentrations high enough for this effect (5879). In people with chronic heart failure, intra-arterial vitamin C seems to improve endothelial dysfunction and flow-dependent dilation of the arteries. Vitamin C appears to prevent inactivation of NO-mediated vasodilation. Four weeks of oral vitamin C 1 gram twice daily appears to produce a similar effect (2434). There's also some evidence that vitamin C might suppress the apoptosis (death) of endothelial cells of patients with congestive heart failure, but the clinical relevance of this isn't known (9816). Intracoronary infusion of vitamin C has been shown to enhance the inotropic response to dobutamine (Dobutrex), possibly by reducing oxidative stress caused by beta-adrenergic stimulation of the ventricle (2432). Some researchers think vitamin C might prevent or slow atherosclerosis by inhibiting low-density lipoprotein (LDL) cholesterol; by impairing the products of reactive oxygen species from vascular cells; and by limiting the cellular responses to oxidized LDL, such as production of endothelium-derived NO (9812). In patients with coronary spastic angina, vitamin C seems to improve endothelial function when given by intravenous infusion as a single 2 gram dose (9819). Some research suggests that endothelial function may relate to insulin resistance in patients with hypertension. Single-dose intravenous vitamin C seems to improve endothelial function and restore insulin-mediated vasodilatation, but doesn't seem to improve glucose uptake (9820). Oral vitamin C seems to improve endothelial function in healthy young smokers, short-term; the improvements in endothelial function diminish within 8 weeks, even though vitamin C levels remain elevated (9818).
In smokers, a single 3 gram dose given by intravenous infusion appears to restore coronary microcirculatory responsiveness and impaired coronary flow reserve induced by the oxidant effects of smoking. Vitamin C might reduce oxidative stress caused by the large number of oxidants in cigarette smoke (1956). Whether these effects are sustained when vitamin C is taken chronically is unknown. Pulmonary function is also positively related to dietary vitamin C intake in smokers and nonsmokers (2400). For radiation-induced oral mucositis, the reduced form of vitamin C might be beneficial due to its antioxidant effect and role in maintaining connective tissue integrity (6103). Vitamin C may also reduce toxicity of reactive oxygen during radio-immunotherapy due to its antioxidant effects (5878).
Research in marathon runners suggests vitamin C might help post-race immune suppression. Vitamin C 1500 mg taken daily for 7 days before running seems to reduce post exercise serum cortisol and cytokines (11961).
Free radicals are also generated in the skin by exposure to ultraviolet light and cause photo-aging. Vitamin C in the skin is believed to play a key role in neutralizing these free radicals and reducing UV skin damage. Topical application of vitamin C is thought to prevent skin damage when applied prior to UV exposure due to vitamin C's antioxidant effects (6062,6155). Topical preparations are thought to help treat photo-aged and wrinkled skin due to vitamin C's antioxidant properties and by possibly by increasing collagen production and improving collagen organization (6155). Topical preparations containing 10% vitamin C might be most effective for increasing vitamin C concentrations in the skin. Because vitamin C is water soluble, oral supplementation of vitamin C might not produce high enough concentrations in the skin to treat photo-aged skin (6064,6155).
Vitamin C is well absorbed orally at lower doses, but absorption decreases as the dose increases. Approximately 87% of a 30 mg oral dose is absorbed, 80% of a 100 mg dose is absorbed, 63% of a 500 mg dose is absorbed, and less than 50% of a 1250 mg does is absorbed. Most of what is absorbed is excreted in the urine. Decreased bioavailability with increasing dosages and increased renal excretion limits the plasma levels attainable with oral vitamin C supplementation (9809).

Adverse Reactions

Orally, the adverse effects of vitamin C are dose-related (3042) and include nausea, vomiting, esophagitis, heartburn, abdominal cramps, gastrointestinal obstruction, fatigue, flushing, headache, insomnia, sleepiness, and diarrhea. Doses greater than the tolerable upper intake level (UL) of 2000 mg per day can increase the risk of significant adverse effects such as osmotic diarrhea and gastrointestinal upset (4844).

Vitamin C may also cause precipitation of urate, oxalate, or cysteine stones or drugs in the urinary tract (10356). Hyperoxaluria, hyperuricosuria, hematuria, and crystalluria have occurred in people taking 1 gram or more per day (3042). In people with a history of oxalate kidney stones (the most common type of nephrolithiasis), supplemental vitamin C 1 gram per day appears to increase stone risk by 40% (12653).

Large amounts of vitamin C are associated with deep vein thrombosis. Prolonged use of large amounts of vitamin C can also result in increased metabolism of vitamin C, and scurvy can occur when vitamin C intake is reduced (15).

High doses of vitamin C might not be safe for some people. In postmenopausal women with diabetes, supplemental vitamin C in doses greater than 300 mg per day is associated with increased risk of cardiovascular mortality (12498). Oral supplementation with vitamin C has also been associated with an increased rate of carotid inner wall thickening in men. There is preliminary evidence that supplemental intake of vitamin C 500 mg daily for 18 months can cause a 2.5-fold increased rate of carotid inner wall thickening in non-smoking men and a 5-fold increased rate in men who smoked. The men in this study were 40-60 years old. This effect was not associated with vitamin C from dietary sources (1355). There is also some concern that supplements of vitamin C 200 mg might increase production reactive oxygen molecules capable of damaging DNA. This is based on very preliminary in vitro evidence that vitamin C can induce decomposition of lipid hydroperoxides to reactive molecules. More evidence is needed to determine if this is clinically relevant in humans taking vitamin C supplements (7088).

Topically, vitamin C might cause tingling or irritation at the site of application (6166).

Interactions with Herbs & Other Dietary Supplements

ACEROLA: Acerola contains high concentrations of vitamin C (12651). Advise people to avoid taking large amounts of acerola along with vitamin C, which together could exceed the tolerable upper intake level of 2000 mg vitamin C per day for adults.

CHEROKEE ROSEHIP: Cherokee rosehip contains high concentrations of vitamin C (12652). Advise people to avoid taking large amounts of cherokee rosehip along with vitamin C, which together could exceed the tolerable upper intake level of 2000 mg vitamin C per day for adults.

CHROMIUM: Limited data suggests that vitamin C increases chromium absorption. The amount of chromium absorbed from a 1000 mcg dose approximately doubled when vitamin C 100 mg was given at the same time (10600). Advise people to avoid taking large doses of chromium and vitamin C together. It isn't known whether separating the doses by several hours avoids this interaction.

COPPER: High doses of vitamin C (1500 mg daily) can decrease serum levels of copper and the copper transport protein, ceruloplasmin, in young men. The acidity of vitamin C may convert copper in the gut to a less absorbable form, and vitamin C may directly interfere with transport of copper across the intestinal wall. It's also suggested that vitamin C can stimulate tissue copper utilization (710,11538). It's unlikely that this interaction is clinically significant unless dietary copper intake is low (710).

IRON: Supplemental or dietary vitamin C improves absorption of supplemental or dietary non-heme (plant-derived) iron when ingested at the same time (9518,9571,9586,11571). The amount of vitamin C in the diet is a factor in dietary iron absorption and iron status (9570,9572). Vitamin C can counteract the effects of substances which inhibit iron absorption such as dietary phytates, polyphenols, and tannins, possibly by chemically reducing iron and preventing the formation of less soluble ferric compounds (9518,9573,9586,11571). Taking a vitamin C supplement to improve absorption of dietary or supplemental iron probably isn't necessary for most people, especially if their diet contains plenty of vitamin C (9571).

ROSE HIP: Rose hips contain high concentrations of vitamin C (12652). Advise people to avoid taking large amounts of rosehip along with vitamin C, which together could exceed the tolerable upper intake level of 2000 mg vitamin C per day for adults.

VITAMIN B12: Preliminary evidence suggests that vitamin C supplements can destroy dietary vitamin B12. However, other components of food, such as iron and nitrates, might counteract this effect (9511). It isn't clear whether this interaction is clinically significant, and it can likely be avoided if vitamin C supplements are taken at least 2 hours after meals.

Interactions with Drugs

ACETAMINOPHEN (Tylenol): High doses of vitamin C (3 grams) competitively inhibits sulfate conjugation of acetaminophen. However, to compensate, elimination of acetaminophen glucuronide and unconjugated acetaminophen increases. Overall, the elimination rate is slightly slower, increasing the half-life from around 2.3 hours to 3.1 hours (6451). This isn't likely to be clinically significant.

ALUMINUM: Vitamin C can increase the amount of aluminum absorbed from aluminum compounds. It's thought that vitamin C chelates aluminum, keeping it in solution and available for absorption (10549,10550,10551). In people with normal renal function, urinary excretion of aluminum likely increases, making aluminum retention and toxicity unlikely (10549). Patients with renal failure who take aluminum-containing compounds chronically such as phosphate binders should avoid vitamin C supplements in doses above the recommended dietary allowances.

ASPIRIN: It's been suggested that acidification of the urine by vitamin C could increase reabsorption of salicylates by the renal tubules, and increase plasma salicylate levels (3046). However, short-term use of up to 6 grams/day of vitamin C doesn't seem to affect urinary pH or salicylate excretion (10588,10589), suggesting this interaction isn't clinically significant.

CHEMOTHERAPY: There's concern that antioxidants like vitamin C could reduce the activity of chemotherapy drugs which generate free radicals, such as cyclophosphamide, chlorambucil, carmustine, busulfan, thiotepa, and doxorubicin (391). Although it has been claimed this isn't a problem, there isn't any data on the effects of vitamin C on long-term outcomes of chemotherapy treatment. Advise patients to consult their oncologist before using vitamin C supplements, especially in high doses. Monitor response to chemotherapy closely if supplements are used.

CHOLINE MAGNESIUM TRISALICYLATE (Trilisate): It's been suggested that acidification of the urine by vitamin C could increase reabsorption of salicylates by the renal tubules, and increase plasma salicylate levels (3046,4531). However, short-term use of up to 6 grams/day of vitamin C doesn't seem to affect urinary pH or salicylate excretion (10588,10589), suggesting this interaction probably isn't clinically significant.

ESTROGENS: Increases in plasma estrogen levels of up to 55% occur under some circumstances when vitamin C is taken concurrently with oral contraceptives or hormone replacement therapy, including topical products (129,130,11161). It's suggested that vitamin C prevents oxidation of estrogen in the tissues, regenerates oxidized estrogen, and reduces sulfate conjugation of estrogen in the gut wall (129,11161). When tissue levels of vitamin C are high, these processes are already maximized and supplemental vitamin C doesn't have any effect on estrogen levels. Increases in plasma estrogen levels may occur when women who are deficient in vitamin C take supplements (11161). Monitor these patients for estrogen-related side effects.

FLUPHENAZINE (Prolixin): In one patient there was a clinically significant decrease in fluphenazine levels when vitamin C (500 mg twice daily) was started (11017). The mechanism isn't known and there's no further data to confirm this interaction.

HMG-CoA REDUCTASE INHIBITORS ("Statins"): A combination of simvastatin (Zocor) and niacin effectively raises HDL cholesterol ("good cholesterol") levels in people with coronary disease and low HDL levels. A combination of antioxidants (vitamin C, vitamin E, beta-carotene, and selenium) seems to blunt this rise in HDL, specifically the HDL-2 and apolipoprotein A1 fractions (7388,11537). HDL-2 is considered to be the most cardioprotective component of HDL (7388). It isn't known whether this adverse effect is due to a single antioxidant such as vitamin C, or to the combination. It also isn't known whether it will occur in other patient populations, or when antioxidant vitamins are combined with other lipid-altering regimens. Monitor lipid levels closely in people taking lipid-altering drugs and antioxidant vitamin supplements, including vitamin C. Other "statin" drugs include lovastatin (Mevacor), pravastatin (Pravachol), fluvastatin (Lescol), and atorvastatin (Lipitor).

NIACIN: A combination of niacin and simvastatin (Zocor) effectively raises HDL cholesterol ("good cholesterol") levels in people with coronary disease and low HDL levels. A combination of antioxidants (vitamin C, vitamin E, beta-carotene, and selenium) seems to blunt this rise in HDL, specifically the HDL-2 and apolipoprotein A1 fractions (7388,11537). HDL-2 is considered to be the most cardioprotective component of HDL (7388). It isn't known whether this adverse effect is due to a single antioxidant such as vitamin C, or to the combination. It also isn't known whether it will occur in other patient populations, or when antioxidant vitamins are combined with other lipid-altering regimens. Monitor lipid levels closely in people taking lipid-altering drugs and antioxidant vitamin supplements, including vitamin C.

NICARDIPINE (Cardene): Dihydropyridine calcium channel blockers (DCCBs) including nicardipine inhibit uptake of vitamin C by intestinal cells in vitro (9808). This likely occurs with other DCCBs such as amlodipine (Norvasc), felodipine (Plendil), isradipine (DynaCirc), and nisoldipine (Sular). Whether this causes a clinically significant reduction in vitamin C absorption in humans isn't known.

NIFEDIPINE (Adalat, Procardia): Dihydropyridine calcium channel blockers (DCCBs) including nifedipine inhibit uptake of vitamin C by intestinal cells in vitro (9808). This likely occurs with other DCCBs such as amlodipine (Norvasc), felodipine (Plendil), isradipine (DynaCirc), and nisoldipine (Sular). Whether this causes a clinically significant reduction in vitamin C absorption in humans isn't known.

PROTEASE INHIBITORS (PIs): Vitamin C seems to modestly reduce indinavir (Crixivan) levels. Vitamin C 1 gram daily for 7 days reduces the area under the concentration/time curve by 14%. The mechanism of this interaction is unknown, but it's unlikely to be clinically significant in most patients. However, the effect of higher doses of vitamin C is unknown (11300). It's also not known whether an interaction could occur with other protease inhibitors, such as amprenavir (Agenerase), nelfinavir (Viracept), ritonavir (Norvir), or saquinavir (Fortovase, Invirase).

SALSALATE (Disalcid): It's been suggested that acidification of the urine by vitamin C could increase reabsorption of salicylates by the renal tubules, and increase plasma salicylate levels (3046). However, short-term use of up to 6 grams/day vitamin C doesn't seem to affect urinary pH or salicylate excretion (10588,10589), suggesting this interaction probably isn't clinically significant.

WARFARIN (Coumadin): High doses of vitamin C may reduce the response to warfarin, possibly by causing diarrhea and reducing warfarin absorption (11566). This occurred in two people who took up to 16 grams/day of vitamin C (9804,9806). Lower doses of 5 to 10 grams/day can also reduce warfarin absorption, but this doesn't seem to be clinically significant (9805,9806,11566,11567).

Drug Influences on Nutrient Levels and Depletion

SOME DRUGS CAN AFFECT VITAMIN C LEVELS:

ASPIRIN: Aspirin increases elimination of vitamin C. It reduces tissue and leukocyte uptake of vitamin C, leaving more in the plasma to be filtered into the urine (10590,10591,10592). It may also reduce absorption of vitamin C from the gut (11526,11527). These effects are dose-related (10590,11526). Vitamin C supplementation has been suggested for people taking high-dose aspirin chronically, such as was used in the past for rheumatoid arthritis (10591). Supplements aren't needed with low doses of aspirin used for cardiovascular indications.

DIURETICS: In people with chronic renal failure, a 20 mg intravenous dose of furosemide (Lasix) increases urinary losses of vitamin C, probably due to increased water excretion (9525). Significant vitamin C depletion hasn't been reported with chronic oral use of furosemide or other diuretics.

ESTROGENS: Data regarding the effects of oral contraceptives and hormone replacement therapy on vitamin C levels is conflicting (10548,10583,10585,10586,11528,11875,11876). It's suggested that estrogens can reduce vitamin C absorption or increase its breakdown, and that vitamin C stores are used to prevent oxidation of estrogens in the tissues (10548,10583,10587,11161,11875). This probably only contributes to vitamin C depletion in women with very low intake of vitamin C (10548,11161,11528). Supplements aren't necessary for women on estrogens who have an adequate dietary intake of vitamin C.

PROTON PUMP INHIBITORS (PPIs): Preliminary data suggests omeprazole reduces vitamin C levels, possibly due to increased destruction of vitamin C at higher gastric pH levels (10572). It isn't known if this is clinically significant. Other proton pump inhibitors include lansoprazole (Prevacid), rabeprazole (Aciphex), pantoprazole (Protonix), and esomeprazole (Nexium).

Interactions with Foods

None known.

Interactions with Lab Tests

ACETAMINOPHEN: Vitamin C can cause false-negative urine results with methods based on hydrolysis and formation of an indophenol blue chromogen (275).

ASPARTATE AMINOTRANSFERASE (AST, SGOT): Large amounts of ascorbic acid can cause a false increase in results of serum tests relying on color reactions (Redox reactions) and Technicon SMA 12/60 (275).

BILIRUBIN: Large amounts of vitamin C can cause a false increase in serum test results measured by Technicon SMA 12/60 or colorimetric methods (275).

CALCIUM/SODIUM: Daily vitamin C 3-6 grams can cause an increase in urinary calcium and test results, and a decrease in urinary sodium and test results (15).

CARBAMAZEPINE (Tegretol): Large doses of vitamin C can cause falsely increased serum assay results measured by Ames ARIS method (275).

CREATININE: Vitamin C can cause a false increase in serum creatinine or urine test results (275).

GLUCOSE: Large amounts of vitamin C can cause false increases in urine test results measured by copper reduction methods (e.g., Clinitest), and false decreases in results measured by glucose oxidase methods (e.g., Clinistix, Tes-Tape) (15).

HIGH-DENSITY LIPOPROTEIN-2 (HDL-2): Vitamin C in combination with beta-carotene, selenium, and vitamin E seems to lower HDL-2 levels. This combination can lower HDL-2 levels by 15% in people with heart disease (7388).

IRON: Vitamin C can increase the absorption of iron and measures of iron status, such as serum iron and ferritin (9518).

LACTIC DEHYDROGENASE (LDH): Vitamin C can cause a false decrease in test results measured by Technicon SMA 12/60 and Abbott 100 methods (275).

OCCULT BLOOD: False-negative guaiac results occur with 250 mg or more of vitamin C per day (3042).

THEOPHYLLINE: Large amounts of vitamin C can cause a false decrease in serum assay results when measured by the ARIS system or Ames Seralyzer photometer (275).

URIC ACID: Large amounts of vitamin C can cause a decrease in serum uric acid concentrations and test results measured by enzymatic method assays (15).

VITAMIN B12: Large amounts of vitamin C can interfere with vitamin B12 assay, resulting in false decrease in vitamin B12 levels (1965).

Interactions with Diseases or Conditions

ANGIOPLASTY: There is some concern that when antioxidant vitamins, including vitamin C, are used in combination they might have harmful effects in patients after angioplasty. A combination of beta-carotene 30,000 IU, vitamin C 500 mg, and vitamin E 700 IU daily started 30 days before angioplasty, and continued for 6 months thereafter, seems to prevent beneficial vascular remodeling in patients by promoting fibrosis at the site of angioplastic intervention (11000). Tell patients to avoid taking supplements containing these vitamins immediately before and following angioplasty without the supervision of a health care professional.

CANCER: Cancerous cells accumulate high concentrations of vitamin C. Cancer cells uptake the oxidized form of vitamin C, dehydroascorbic acid, then convert it back to vitamin C (4838,4839,4840,4841). However, it is not yet known if this benefits growth of cancer cells or has any detrimental effect of cancer treatments. Until more is known, patients

with cancer should only use high doses of vitamin C under the direction of their oncologist.
DIABETES: Vitamin C can affect glycogenolysis and increase blood sugar, but this effect remains controversial (15). In postmenopausal women with diabetes, supplemental vitamin C in doses greater than 300 mg per day is associated with increased risk of cardiovascular mortality (12498).
GLUCOSE-6-PHOSPHATE DEHYDROGENASE DEFICIENCY: Large amounts of vitamin C can cause hemolysis in individuals with glucose-6-phosphate dehydrogenase deficiency (15).
IRON OVERLOAD, HEMOCHROMATOSIS, THALASSEMIA, SIDEROBLASTIC ANEMIA: Use vitamin C with caution, vitamin C can increase iron absorption, which could worsen these conditions (1960).
KIDNEY STONES (Nephrolithiasis): Large amounts of vitamin C can increase the risk of oxalate stone formation. Vitamin C is metabolized to oxalic acid, so increased consumption increases the urinary concentration of oxalic acid (10356). In people with a history of oxalate kidney stones (the most common type of nephrolithiasis), supplemental vitamin C 1 gram per day appears to increase stone risk by 40% (12653). Tell patients prone to kidney stone formation to avoid high doses of vitamin C.
MYOCARDIAL INFARCTION (MI): Vitamin C levels are significantly reduced during the acute phase after a MI. However, low plasma levels of vitamin C have not been associated with an increased risk of MI (5876).
SICKLE CELL DISEASE: Vitamin C can decrease blood pH, which can rarely precipitate sickle cell crisis (15).
NICOTINE and SMOKING: Smokers have lower plasma levels of vitamin C than nonsmokers with similar dietary intake of vitamin C. This is likely due to increased use of vitamin C to counteract oxidizing free radicals in cigarette smoke (5875,11501). Advise smokers to consume a diet rich in vitamin C, or recommend a supplement if this isn't possible. Smokers may need between 124 and 200 mg/day to maintain normal plasma levels (11546). There doesn't seem to be an effect of nicotine on vitamin C levels and depletion hasn't been reported with nicotine replacement products (e.g., patches, gum, etc.).
SMOKELESS TOBACCO USE: Users of chewing tobacco tend to have lower plasma levels of vitamin C than non-users with similar dietary intakes (11501). This may increase their risk of precancerous oral lesions, because the antioxidant effects of vitamin C are needed to prevent formation of carcinogenic nitrosamines from nitrates and nitrites in smokeless tobacco (11502). Advise tobacco users to consume a diet rich in vitamin C.

Dosage and Administration

ORAL: For scurvy, 100-250 mg once or twice daily for several days is commonly used (15). For treating the common cold, 1-3 grams daily has been used (6458).
For preventing the common cold, in people under physical stress, vitamin C 600-1000 mg daily has been used (9831).
During acute stress, vitamin C 1 gram 3 times daily, as a sustained release preparation, has been used for up to 14 days (10353).
For preventing contrast-mediated nephropathy, vitamin C 3 grams is given before coronary angiography and then 2 grams is given after the procedure in the evening and again the following morning (12234).
For chronic hemodialysis in adults, 100-200 mg per day is recommended (15).
For preventing nitrate tolerance, 3-6 grams of vitamin C daily has been used (1961).
For preventing sunburn, 2 grams of vitamin C in combination with RRR-alpha-tocopherol (natural vitamin E) 1000 IU has been used (4716).
For treatment of premalignant gastric lesions, vitamin C 1 gram twice daily has been used (2579).
For slowing progression of atherosclerosis, slow release vitamin C 250 mg in combination with 91 mg (136 IU) of vitamin E has been given twice daily for up to 6 years (1918,10473).
For treatment of familial hypercholesterolemia in children, vitamin C 500 mg daily and vitamin E 400 IU daily have been used for up to 6 months with a National Cholesterol Education Program Step II (NCEP-II) diet (10352).
For tyrosinemia in premature infants on high protein diets, 100 mg of vitamin C has been used (15).
For reducing albinuria in patients with type 2 diabetes, vitamin C 1250 mg with vitamin E 680 IU daily has been used for 4 weeks (10434).
For infertility associated with luteal phase defect, 750 mg per day has been used (12010).
The daily recommended dietary allowances (RDAs) are: Infants 0 to 12 months, human milk content (older recommendations specified 30-35 mg); Children 1 to 3 years, 15 mg; Children 4 to 8 years, 25 mg; Children 9 to 13 years, 45 mg; Adolescents 14 to 18 years, 75 mg for boys and 65 mg for girls; Adults age 19 and greater, 90 mg for men and 75 mg for women; Pregnancy and Lactation: age 18 or younger, 115 mg; ages 19 to 50 years 120 mg. People who use tobacco should take an additional 35 mg per day (4844).
The tolerable upper intake levels (UL) for vitamin C are 400 mg per day for children ages 1 to 3 years, 650 mg per day for children 4 to 8 years, 1200 mg per day for children 9 to 13 years, and 1800 mg per day for adolescents and pregnant and lactating women 14 to 18 years, and 2000 mg per day for adults and pregnant and lactating women (4844).
TOPICAL: Most topical preparations used for aged or wrinkled skin are applied daily. Studies have used creams containing 5% to 10% vitamin C (6155). In one study, a specific vitamin C formulation (Cellex-C High Potency Serum) used 3 drops applied daily to areas of facial skin (6155). Avoid application to eye area or eyelids. Also avoid contact with hair or clothes. It can cause discoloration (6166).

Comments

Most experts recommend getting antioxidants, including vitamin C, from a diet high in fruits, vegetables, and whole grains rather than taking supplements (1440,3042). Ready-to-drink orange juice contains 25% less active vitamin C than frozen orange juice. Oxidized vitamin C is not readily absorbed across the intestinal mucosa. Much, 51-76%, of the vitamin C in ready-to-drink orange juice is oxidized, compared with only 20% of vitamin C in frozen orange juice. Frozen orange juice consumed within one week of reconstitution is the most reliable source of vitamin C. Tell patients who prefer ready-to-drink orange juice that these products should be purchased 3 to 4 weeks before the expiration date and consumed within one week of opening (9811).

VITAMIN D

Also Known As

Alfacalcidol: 1-alpha-hydroxycholecalciferol, 1 alpha (OH)D3.
Calcifediol: 25-HCC, 25-hydroxycholecalciferol, 25-hydroxyvitamin D3, 25-OHCC, 25-OHD3.
Calcipotriene: Calcipotriol.
Calcitriol: 1,25-DHCC, 1,25-dihydroxycholecalciferol, 1,25-dihydroxyvitamin D3, 1,25-diOHC, 1,25(0H)2D3.
Cholecalciferol: Activated 7-dehydrocholesterol, colecalciferol, Vitamin D3.
Dihydrotachysterol: DHT, dihydrotachysterol 2, dichysterol.
Ergocalciferol: Activated ergosterol, Calciferol, Ergocalciferolum, Irradiated ergosterol, Viosterol, Vitamin D2.
Paricalcitol: 19-nor-1,25-dihydroxyvitamin D2, Paracalcin.

Scientific Names

1,25-dihydroxycholecalciferol; 25-hydroxycholecalciferol; Alfacalcidol; Calcifediol; Calcipotriene; Calcitriol; Cholecalciferol; Dihydrotachysterol; Ergocalciferol; Paricalcitol.

People Use This For

Orally, vitamin D is used for building bone mass and preventing bone loss, protecting against muscle weakness, promoting strong teeth, enhancing immune function, preventing auto-immune diseases, reducing risk of multiple sclerosis, rheumatoid arthritis, treating cancer, and reducing risk of colon, breast, and prostate cancer. It is also used orally for preventing and treating rickets, premenstrual syndrome (PMS), postmenopausal osteoporosis, to prevent falls and fractures in people at risk for osteoporosis, corticosteroid-induced osteoporosis, osteomalacia, anticonvulsant-induced osteomalacia, renal osteodystrophy, osteitis fibrosa in people on dialysis, hepatic osteodystrophy, and osteogenesis imperfecta. Vitamin D is also used for preventing and treating hypocalcemia and tetany in premature infants, hypocalcemic tetany, bone disorders in people with familial hypophosphatemia, hypophosphatemia associated with Fanconi syndrome, and hypocalcemia associated with postoperative or idiopathic hypoparathyroidism or pseudohypoparathyroidism. Other uses include plaque-type psoriasis, actinic keratoses, lupus vulgaris, squamous cell carcinomas, vitiligo, scleroderma, myelodysplastic syndrome, and preventing type 1 diabetes. Vitamin D is also used orally to treat severe proximal myopathy associated with vitamin D deficiency and to maintain bone density in prostatic cancer patients at risk for osteoporosis when treated with luteinizing hormone-releasing hormone analogue (LHRH-a).
Topically, vitamin D is used as calcitriol or calcipotriene for plaque-type psoriasis.
Intravenously, vitamin D, administered as calcitriol, is used for hypocalcemic tetany in premature infants, hypocalcemia and hyperparathyroidism in renal dialysis patients, and osteitis fibrosa.
Intramuscularly, vitamin D is administered as ergocalciferol for hepatic osteodystrophy, as an injectable source of vitamin D, and to treat severe proximal myopathy associated with vitamin D deficiency.

Safety

LIKELY SAFE ...when used orally and appropriately (7555). Vitamin D is safe when used in doses below the tolerable upper intake level (UL). Tell patients not to exceed the UL 50 mcg (2000 units) per day (7555).
POSSIBLY UNSAFE ...when used orally in excessive doses. Doses greater than the tolerable upper intake level (UL) of 50 mcg (2000 units) per day can increase the risk of hypercalcemia (7555).
CHILDREN: LIKELY SAFE ...when used orally and appropriately. Vitamin D is safe when used in doses below the tolerable upper intake level (UL). Children older than one year should not exceed the UL 50 mcg (2000 units) per day; children younger than one year should not exceed the UL 25 mcg (1000 units) per day (7555). POSSIBLY UNSAFE ...when used orally in excessive amounts. Tell patients not to use doses above the tolerable upper intake level (UL) of 50 mcg (2000 units) per day for children older than one year; children younger than one year should not exceed the UL 25 mcg (1000 units) per day. Higher doses can cause hypercalcemia (7555).
PREGNANCY: LIKELY SAFE ...when used orally and appropriately. Vitamin D is safe when used in doses below the tolerable upper intake level (UL) of 50 mcg (2000 units) per day (7555). POSSIBLY UNSAFE ...when used orally in excessive amounts. Tell patients not to use doses above the tolerable upper intake level (UL) of 50 mcg (2000 units) per day. Hypercalcemia during pregnancy due to excessive vitamin D intake can lead to suppression of parathyroid hormone, hypocalcemia, tetany, seizures, aortic valve stenosis, retinopathy, and mental and/or physical retardation in the infant (7555).

LACTATION: LIKELY SAFE ...when used orally and appropriately. Vitamin D is safe when used in doses below the tolerable upper intake level (UL) of 50 mcg (2000 units) per day (7555). POSSIBLY UNSAFE ...when used orally in excessive amounts. Tell patients not to use doses above the tolerable upper intake level (UL) of 50 mcg (2000 units) per day.

Effectiveness

EFFECTIVE

Familial hypophosphatemia. Taking calcitriol or dihydrotachysterol orally in conjunction with phosphate supplements is effective for treating bone disorders in people with familial hypophosphatemia (11818).

Fanconi syndrome. Taking ergocalciferol orally is effective for treating hypophosphatemia associated with Fanconi syndrome (11819).

Hypoparathyroidism. Taking dihydrotachysterol or calcitriol orally is effective for increasing serum calcium concentrations in people with hypoparathyroidism or pseudohypoparathyroidism. Ergocalciferol is effective in high doses for increasing serum calcium concentrations in people with hypoparathyroidism or pseudohypoparathyroidism (11820).

Osteomalacia. Taking cholecalciferol is effective for treating osteomalacia. Calcifediol orally is effective for treating osteomalacia secondary to liver disease (hepatic osteodystrophy), and anticonvulsant-induced osteomalacia. Ergocalciferol is effective for osteomalacia due to malabsorption syndromes and corticosteroid-induced osteomalacia (11821).

Psoriasis. Applying calcipotriene topically effectively treats plaque-type psoriasis in some patients (11822).

Renal osteodystrophy. Taking calcifediol orally manages hypocalcemia and prevents renal osteodystrophy in people with chronic renal failure undergoing dialysis (11823).

Rickets. Ergocalciferol is effective for treating rickets. Calcitriol should be used in patients with renal failure (11824).

LIKELY EFFECTIVE

Corticosteroid-induced osteoporosis. Taking calcifediol or cholecalciferol orally prevents corticosteroid-induced osteopenia and osteoporosis (7555).

Fall prevention. Vitamin D seems to reduce falls by 22% in older adults. To prevent one fall, 15 older adults would need to be given supplemental vitamin D. This risk reduction appears to be independent of calcium supplementation, but some experts think a combination of calcium and vitamin D may be important (11916). Vitamin D, in combination with calcium, but not calcium alone, may prevent falls by decreasing body sway and systolic blood pressure instead of increasing bone mass strength (6362,11939). Vitamin D deficiency is linked to increased risk of falls (11917,11918).

Osteoporosis. Taking vitamin D orally with calcium supplements can decrease postmenopausal bone loss and help prevent osteoporosis (7555,11827). Vitamin D with calcium seems to decrease the risk of non-vertebral fractures in elderly women (6362). Multiple clinical studies and meta-analyses suggest efficacy for calcium plus vitamin D for primary prevention (980,1836,8818,10932,12926,12930,12933,12934,12952). Oral vitamin D 700-800 IU daily seems to reduce fracture risk in ambulatory and institutionalized elderly people. The number needed to treat for vitamin D 800 IU taken daily for 2-5 years is 27 patients to prevent one nonvertebral fracture and 45 patients to prevent one hip fracture (12933). But taking vitamin D does not seem to prevent fractures in frail elderly people (10140).

There is also concern that calcium might not be effective for secondary prevention of fractures in elderly patients. Vitamin D 800 IU/day with or without calcium 1000 mg/day for 2-5 years does not significantly reduce fracture risk in elderly women or men who have had a previous fracture compared to placebo (13073). Another study also suggests that vitamin D 800 IU/day plus calcium 1000 mg/day might not prevent a second fracture in elderly patients, or prevent a first fracture in elderly patients with other risk factors such as low body weight (<58 kg, 127.6 pounds), smoking, family history of hip fracture, or fair or poor self-reported health (12929). However, these studies have been criticized for failing to measure vitamin D levels and low adherence to study protocol (12931). One of these studies did not use a placebo control (12929).

Giving vitamin D orally to breast-fed infants seems to help increase bone mineral density. In a retrospective study, prepubertal girls who received vitamin D in infancy had significantly greater bone mineral density at some skeletal sites compared to girls that did not receive vitamin D during infancy (3464).

Taking alfacalcidol orally seems to maintain bone density in prostatic carcinoma patients at risk for osteoporosis when treated with luteinizing hormone-releasing hormone analogue (LHRH-a). Alfacalcidol maintains but does not increase bone mineral density (6360).

POSSIBLY EFFECTIVE

Diabetes. Administering calcitriol orally to infants might help prevent the development of type 1 diabetes. Daily vitamin D supplementation in infants during the first year of life is associated with a reduced incidence of type 1 diabetes development later in life (10139).

Hyperparathyroidism-related bone loss. Taking cholecalciferol orally seems to help decrease secondary hyperparathyroidism and bone turnover in women. In one study, supplementation with cholecalciferol resulted in increased serum levels of 25-hydroxyvitamin D, reduced levels of parathyroid hormone, and decreased production of markers of bone turnover (3463).

Multiple sclerosis (MS). Population research suggests that long-term vitamin D supplementation decreases the risk of MS in women by up to 40%. The effect seems to be dose-dependent. Consumption of at least 400 IU per day, mainly in the form of a multivitamin supplement, appears to have the greatest protective effect (11356).

Osteogenesis imperfecta. Taking vitamin D orally seems to help treat osteogenesis imperfecta (11826).

Rheumatoid arthritis (RA). Population research suggests that older women who have a higher intake of vitamin D from foods or supplements tend to have a lower risk of developing RA (12206).

POSSIBLY INEFFECTIVE

Muscle strength. Oral cholecalciferol 1000 IU per day doesn't seem to increase muscle strength or improve physical performance in healthy older men who are not vitamin D deficient (11814).

Renal transplant-related bone loss. Calcitriol 0.25 mcg per day in combination with calcium carbonate 500 mg per day doesn't significantly decrease bone loss associated with long-term renal transplantation; however, calcitriol might reduce osteoclast suppression, help maintain trabecular bone volume and wall thickness, and improve axial bone mineral density (4823).

INSUFFICIENT RELIABLE EVIDENCE to RATE

Myelodysplastic syndrome. Taking calcitriol or calcifediol orally seems to help myelodysplastic syndrome (11825).

Premenstrual syndrome (PMS). There is some evidence that increasing total or dietary intake of vitamin D is associated with a decreased risk of developing PMS. Women with an average vitamin D intake of 706 mg/day seem to have about a 40% lower risk of developing PMS compared to women with an average vitamin D intake of 112 mg/day (13094); however, taking vitamin D supplements does not appear to be associated with the risk of developing PMS.

Proximal myopathy. Administering ergocalciferol intramuscularly or taking ergocalciferol orally seems to help treat severe proximal myopathy associated with severe vitamin D deficiency. Several case reports suggest vitamin D therapy can provide prompt relief of muscle weakness and restore mobility (11923).

More evidence is needed to rate vitamin D for these uses.

Mechanism of Action

Vitamin D is a fat-soluble vitamin. The term vitamin D refers to several forms of vitamin D. There are 2 forms that are physiologically important, ergocalciferol (vitamin D2) and cholecalciferol (vitamin D3). Ergocalciferol comes from ergosterol, a plant sterol, and yeast. Cholecalciferol is synthesized in the skin via 7-dehydrocholesterol, a cholesterol precursor. Both ergocalciferol and cholecalciferol are biologically inert and require hydroxylation in the body to form the active metabolite, calcitriol (7555). Some research suggests that vitamin cholecalciferol may be more efficient in raising 25-hydroxyvitamin D serum levels, the best measure of vitamin D status (11937,11938).

Very few foods naturally contain vitamin D. Dietary sources include eggs from hens that have been fed vitamin D and fatty fish such as herrings, mackerel, sardines, and tuna. In the US, Canada, and many other countries the main source of dietary vitamin D is fortified milk and other foods. But these are relatively minor sources of vitamin D (7555).

Brief exposure to sunlight (about 25% of the amount of time it would take to cause light pinkness to the skin) is the most efficient way to get vitamin D (11935). Skin exposure to the sun provides as much as 80% to 90% of the body's vitamin D stores (7133). Full-body sun exposure can lead to the synthesis of as much as 10,000 units of vitamin D per day (6855). Vitamin D is stored in body fat for use during periods without sun exposure. Conversely, excessive sun exposure causes photodegradation of vitamin D produced in the skin, limiting the risk of vitamin D toxicity from such exposure (11936).

Vitamin D insufficiency is common in the northern latitudes such as Canada and the northern half of the US. Prevalence of vitamin D insufficiency and deficiency among young, healthy people appears to be increasing, possibly because of overzealous use of sunscreens (12995).

Exposure to sunlight might not always be sufficient to cause vitamin D synthesis in the skin. Sunlight intensity is dependent on latitude, altitude, season, cloud cover, ozone levels and other factors. During winter in some northern latitudes (e.g., northern US and Canada), little, if any, vitamin D3 is produced in the skin. For example, in Boston there is insufficient UV-B energy for vitamin D production in the skin for 4 months of the year. In Edmonton, the skin can't produce vitamin D for 5 months of the year (12998,12999,13000).

Underway submariners, who get no sunlight for extended periods of time, have lowered 25-hydroxyvitamin D levels and evidence of bone resorption and turnover, even when supplemented with 400 IU daily of cholecalciferol. The capacity of UV-B mediated vitamin D synthesis is huge. Just 6 days of casual sunlight exposure without sunscreen can make up for 49 days of no sunlight exposure (12998).

Skin pigmentation affects vitamin D synthesis and 25-hydroxyvitamin D levels. A light-skinned person in a bathing suit who is not tanned would receive about 10,000 to 20,000 IU of cholecalciferol from 10-12 minutes of peak July summer sun in Boston. For a darker-skinned person, such as Asian Indian, getting this dose of vitamin D could take perhaps 30 min of exposure, and, for a very darkly pigmented African American, it could require 120 min of exposure (12997). The skin pigment melanin competes with vitamin D precursors in the skin for photons from UV-B light (6857). This also affects vitamin D in breast milk. For example, breast milk from African Americans is generally lower in vitamin D content than that from Caucasian women (35 units/L compared with 68 units/L, respectively) (6857). African American infants who are exclusively breast-fed are therefore at risk for vitamin D deficiency and rickets, even if they live in sunny climates such as the southern US (6857).

Sun exposure is an easy, reliable way for most patients to get vitamin D. Exposure of the hands, face, arms, and legs to sunlight two to three times a week for the amount of time equal to about 25% of what it would take to develop a mild sunburn will cause the skin to produce adequate vitamin D. Exposure time will vary with skin type, season, time of day, etc (12992).

Vitamin D supplements may be needed by elderly people with limited sun exposure, people living in northern latitudes, dark-skinned African Americans, Asian Indians living in the western hemisphere, as well as people with gastrointestinal diseases leading to malabsorption of vitamin D from the diet (6855,7133).

Vitamin D deficiency is particularly common in adults over age 50 years. More than 50% of North American women receiving therapy to prevent or treat osteoporosis have inadequate vitamin D stores (12996). Factors such as lack of exposure to sunlight, reduced skin synthesis of vitamin D, lower dietary intake, impaired intestinal absorption, and reduced metabolism to active forms of vitamin D by the kidneys increase with aging (11919). Also, vitamin D receptors seem to decrease with age (11921). The risk for vitamin D deficiency in elderly adults (>65 years) is very high (12995,12996).

Obese people (body mass index >30kg/m2) may have reduced serum vitamin D levels and reduced bioavailability of vitamin D from both cutaneous synthesis and gastrointestinal absorption. In response to similar UV-B exposures, the increase in serum vitamin D levels can be 57% less in obese people than in those who were slim. The content of vitamin D precursors in the skin are similar in both groups, suggesting that vitamin D synthesis is not affected in obese people, but that vitamin D is sequestered into body fat, reducing its availability (6856).

The main function of vitamin D is to regulate serum calcium and phosphorus concentrations. Vitamin D enhances the efficiency of the intestinal absorption of calcium, primarily in the duodenum and jejunum, and phosphorus, particularly in the jejunum and ilium. Vitamin D can increase serum calcium levels, but this effect is modest in healthy people in doses less than 1200 IU per day. If dietary intake of calcium is inadequate, calcitriol in combination with parathyroid hormone mobilizes calcium stores from bone. Calcitrol also appears to have effects in the brain, heart, pancreas, mononuclear cells, activated lymphocytes, and skin, but its exact physiologic role is unclear (7555).

The hydroxylation of vitamin D to calcitriol occurs in the kidneys. People with chronic renal failure may require forms of vitamin D such as calcitriol, dihydrotachysterol, or calcifediol that don't require renal hydroxylation (7555).

In people with granulomatous disorders such as tuberculosis, sarcoidosis, and histoplasmosis, vitamin D metabolism is disturbed. Vitamin D is converted to calcitriol by activated macrophages trapped in the pulmonary alveoli and granulomatous inflammation, in addition to the kidneys. This may increase the risk of hypercalcemia (7555,11881).

Since vitamin D is important for calcium homeostasis and for bone health, it is used to help prevent osteoporosis. Some researchers suggest that postmenopausal women need serum levels of 25-hydroxy-vitamin D (calcifediol) of at least 40 mmol/L for optimal bone health (6854). When intake of calcium is low in healthy elderly women, 25-hydroxy-vitamin D (calcifediol) seems to be more biologically active and a more important determinant of gut calcium absorption than calcitriol (10141). Osteopenia in elderly men also seems to correlate with circulating levels of vitamin D and vitamin K (7132). Vitamin D deficiency causes muscle pain and proximal muscle weakness with symptoms such as sensation of heaviness in the legs, rapid fatigue, and problems with climbing stairs and getting up from a chair. Some preliminary clinical research suggests that people with low vitamin D levels (less than or equal to 20 ng/mL) have more osteoarthritis pain and disability than people with adequate vitamin D stores. Vitamin D deficiency also increases postural sway and affects psychomotor function (11922,11923,11924,11925,12491).

Vitamin D may prevent falls by increasing muscle strength and neuromuscular function in addition to strengthening bone. It seems to increase muscle protein synthesis, possibly by activating second messengers and phosphorylation (11919,11922). The standard dose of 400 units that is found in most multivitamin tablets appears to be too low to prevent falls or reduce fracture risk, but the optimal dose is unknown (11926,11927,11928). Fractures were reduced in clinical trials using 700 to 800 units of vitamin D daily (980,11930,11931). Some research suggests that sufficient calcium intake along with vitamin D is necessary to prevent falls (11932).

Vitamin D also seems to have immunologic activity. In models of autoimmune disease, vitamin D seems to act as an immunosuppressant. This might explain why increased vitamin D intake is associated with a lower risk of rheumatoid arthritis (12206).

There is some epidemiological evidence that people with vitamin D deficiency might be at an increased risk of colon, breast, and prostate cancer, but more research is needed to know if vitamin D affects cancer risk (7555). Some researchers think vitamin D might have antiproliferative effects in these cancers (6855). Prostate cancer has been associated with decreased sun exposure and vitamin D receptor activity (12994).

Some evidence suggests vitamin D supplementation during infancy might prevent the development of type 1 diabetes later on in life. Type 1 diabetes is believed to be an autoimmune disease. Vitamin D supplementation might inhibit an autoimmune reaction that targets the beta cells of the pancreas (10139).

Adverse Reactions

Orally, vitamin D is well tolerated. Vitamin D intoxication can occur when vitamin D supplements are taken in excessive doses. Symptoms of vitamin D toxicity include hypercalcemia, azotemia, and anemia. Symptoms of hypercalcemia include weakness, fatigue, sleepiness, headache, loss of appetite, dry mouth, metallic taste, nausea, vomiting, abdominal cramps, constipation, diarrhea, dizziness, ringing in the ears, trouble walking, skin eruptions, hypotonia in infants, muscle pain, bone pain, and irritability. Advanced symptoms may include runny nose, itching, decreased libido, and kidney insufficiency due to precipitation of calcium phosphate in the tubules. Symptoms of renal impairment include frequency, nighttime awakening to urinate, thirst, inability to concentrate urine, and proteinuria. Renal impairment is usually reversible with discontinuation of vitamin D supplements (10142). Other symptoms of vitamin D toxicity include osteoporosis in adults, decreased growth in children, weight loss, anemia, calcific conjunctivitis, photophobia, metastatic calcification, pancreatitis, generalized vascular calcification, and seizures. Rarely, people develop hypertension and psychosis. Lab values of urinary calcium, phosphate, albumin, blood urea nitrogen, serum cholesterol, aspartate aminotransferase, and alanine aminotransferase concentrations might increase (10142). Serum alkaline phosphatase concentrations usually decrease in vitamin D deficiency (7555).

Interactions with Herbs & Other Dietary Supplements

MAGNESIUM: The protein which transports calcium across the intestinal wall can also bind and transport magnesium. This protein is stimulated by vitamin D, which may therefore increase magnesium absorption (11595,11598). In people with low vitamin D and magnesium levels, taking vitamin D may improve magnesium status (11599). In people with normal magnesium levels, this effect doesn't seem to be significant, possibly because urinary magnesium excretion also increases (11598).

Interactions with Drugs

ALUMINUM: The protein which transports calcium across the intestinal wall can also bind and transport aluminum. This protein is stimulated by vitamin D, which may therefore increase aluminum absorption (11595,11597). This mechanism may contribute to increased aluminum levels and toxicity in people with renal failure, when they take vitamin D and aluminum-containing phosphate binders chronically (11529,11596,11597).

CALCIPOTRIENE (Dovonex): Calcipotriene is a vitamin D analog used topically for psoriasis. It can be absorbed in sufficient amounts to cause systemic effects, including hypercalcemia (15). Theoretically, combining calcipotriene with vitamin D supplements might increase the risk of hypercalcemia. Tell patients not to take vitamin D supplements if they are taking calcipotriene.

CIMETIDINE (Tagamet): Cimetidine inhibits an enzyme involved in conversion of vitamin D to its active form in the liver. However, it doesn't affect formation of active vitamin D metabolites in the kidneys. Clinically significant vitamin D depletion isn't likely, except in people with other risk factors such as liver or kidney disease (11531,11532).

DIGOXIN (Lanoxin): High doses of vitamin D can cause hypercalcemia. Hypercalcemia increases the risk of fatal cardiac arrhythmias with digoxin (15). Avoid vitamin D doses above the tolerable upper intake level (50 mcg or 2000 units/day for adults) and monitor serum calcium levels in people taking vitamin D and digoxin concurrently.

DILTIAZEM (Cardizem, Dilacor, Tiazac): High doses of vitamin D can cause hypercalcemia. Hypercalcemia can reduce the effectiveness of verapamil in atrial fibrillation (10574). Theoretically this could also occur with diltiazem. Avoid vitamin D doses above the tolerable upper intake level (50 mcg or 2000 units/day for adults) and monitor serum calcium levels in people taking vitamin D and diltiazem concurrently.

HEPARIN: Unfractionated heparin is associated with reduced bone density and osteoporotic fractures, especially when doses of 15,000 units/day or more are used for 3 months or longer (10577,10594,10595,10596). This is primarily due to direct effects of heparin on bone (increased resorption and reduced bone formation), but metabolism of vitamin D to its active form is also reduced (10577,10593,10597). Although it's not clear whether vitamin D and calcium supplements prevent bone loss associated with heparin, recommend that people needing heparin therapy for several months maintain their recommended daily intakes of vitamin D and calcium, using supplements if necessary.

LOW MOLECULAR WEIGHT HEPARINS (LMWHs): Reduced bone density has been reported with LMWHs, but probably to a lesser extent than with unfractionated heparin (10593,10598,10599,11555). The effect is primarily due to direct effects of heparins on bone (increased resorption and reduced bone formation), but metabolism of vitamin D to its active form is also reduced (10577,10593,10597). Although it's not clear whether vitamin D and calcium supplements prevent bone loss associated with LMWH, recommend that people needing therapy for several months maintain their recommended daily intakes of vitamin D and calcium, using supplements if necessary. LMWHs include enoxaparin (Lovenox), dalteparin (Fragmin), and tinzaparin (Innohep).

THIAZIDE DIURETICS: Thiazide diuretics decrease urinary calcium excretion, which could lead to hypercalcemia if vitamin D supplements are taken concurrently (3072,11541). This has been reported in people being treated with vitamin D for hypoparathyroidism, and also in elderly people with normal parathyroid function who were taking a thiazide, vitamin D, and calcium-containing antacids daily (11539,11540). Use combinations of thiazides and vitamin D with caution and monitor serum calcium levels. Thiazide diuretics include chlorothiazide (Diuril), hydrochlorothiazide (HydroDIURIL, Esidrix), indapamide (Lozol), metolazone (Zaroxolyn), chlorthalidone (Hygroton), etc.

VERAPAMIL (Calan, Covera, Isoptin, Verelan): Hypercalcemia due to high doses of vitamin D can reduce the effectiveness of verapamil in atrial fibrillation (10574). Avoid vitamin D doses above the tolerable upper intake level (50 mcg or 2000 units/day for adults) and monitor serum calcium levels in people taking vitamin D and verapamil concurrently.

Drug Influences on Nutrient Levels and Depletion

SOME DRUGS CAN AFFECT VITAMIN D LEVELS:

CARBAMAZEPINE (Tegretol): Carbamazepine increases hepatic metabolism of vitamin D to inactive compounds, thereby reducing calcium absorption (2675,4430,4431). Hypocalcemia and osteomalacia have occurred, especially with prolonged therapy, concurrent use of other enzyme-inducing anticonvulsants, or when other risk factors for vitamin D deficiency are present (2675,4475,10578). Patients taking carbamazepine for 6 months or more may

need vitamin D and calcium supplements. Doses of vitamin D needed vary from 400 to 4000 units/day; therefore serum calcium and vitamin D levels should be monitored in high-risk patients (10578).
CHOLESTYRAMINE (Questran, LoCholest, Prevalite): Cholestyramine can reduce absorption of vitamin D. Occasionally this leads to osteomalacia, usually in patients receiving doses of cholestyramine over 32 grams/day, or prolonged therapy over 2 years, and with additional risk factors such as ileal resection or primary biliary cirrhosis, which deplete the bile acids needed for vitamin D absorption (4458,5655,5809,5838). Supplements of vitamin D, and sometimes calcium, are necessary in these patients. Use of cholestyramine (24 grams/day) for treatment of hyperlipidemia in otherwise healthy men doesn't seem to affect vitamin D and calcium levels, and supplements aren't necessary (2672).
COLESTIPOL (Colestid): Colestipol can reduce absorption of fat-soluble vitamins, including vitamin D. This doesn't seem to be clinically significant when up to 20 g/day is used for up to 2 years (4460,4461). Monitor serum levels of calcium and vitamin D in people receiving very high doses of colestipol for several years and give supplements if necessary.
CORTICOSTEROIDS: Corticosteroids, in daily doses equivalent to 7.5 mg or more of prednisone, cause significant bone loss, osteoporosis and increased risk of fractures. The severity increases with duration of therapy. Although this is due mainly to disturbances in calcium homeostasis and bone formation, rather than vitamin D depletion, supplements of vitamin D are helpful to improve calcium absorption. Advise people taking prednisone 7.5 mg/day or higher (or equivalent doses of other corticosteroids) for 6 months or longer to maintain a daily calcium intake of 1500 mg/day, and to take a supplement of 800 IU/day vitamin D. Serum calcium should be monitored regularly (1832).
MINERAL OIL: Mineral oil can reduce absorption of both vitamin D and calcium (4495). However, occasional or short-term use of mineral oil isn't likely to have a clinically significant effect.
ORLISTAT (Xenical): Orlistat decreases absorption of fat soluble vitamins including vitamin D, reducing plasma levels in some patients (1730,9595,10570). The manufacturer recommends that patients take a multivitamin supplement containing all the fat soluble vitamins, separating the dosing time by at least 2 hours from orlistat (1730).
PHENOBARBITAL: phenobarbital increases hepatic metabolism of vitamin D to inactive compounds, thereby reducing calcium absorption (2675,4430,4431). Hypocalcemia and osteomalacia have occurred, especially with prolonged therapy, concurrent use of other enzyme-inducing anticonvulsants, or when other risk factors for vitamin D deficiency are present (2675,4475,10578). Patients taking phenobarbital for 6 months or more may need vitamin D and calcium supplements. Doses of vitamin D needed vary from 400-4000 units/day; therefore serum calcium and vitamin D levels should be monitored in high-risk patients (10578).
PHENYTOIN (Dilantin), FOSPHENYTOIN (Cerebyx): phenytoin increases hepatic metabolism of vitamin D to inactive compounds, thereby reducing calcium absorption (2675,4430,4431). Hypocalcemia and osteomalacia have occurred, especially with prolonged therapy, concurrent use of other enzyme-inducing anticonvulsants, or when other risk factors for vitamin D deficiency are present (2675,4475,10578). Patients taking phenytoin for 6 months or more may need vitamin D and calcium supplements. Doses of vitamin D needed vary from 400-4000 units/day; therefore serum calcium and vitamin D levels should be monitored in high-risk patients (10578).
RIFAMPIN (rifampicin, Rifadin, Rimactane): Rifampin increases hepatic metabolism of 25-hydroxy-vitamin D, reducing its plasma levels (11561,11562,11563). This can contribute to osteomalacia after prolonged therapy (>1 year), especially if vitamin D intake is low (11562,11564). Monitor serum levels of calcium and vitamin D in people taking rifampin for prolonged periods and give supplements as necessary. If isoniazid (INH, Nydrazid) is taken concurrently with rifampin there doesn't seem to be any change in vitamin D status (11561,11563). Possibly this is because the enzyme-inducing effects on rifampin are canceled out by the enzyme-inhibiting effects of isoniazid (11563,11565).
STIMULANT LAXATIVES: Prolonged use of high doses of stimulant laxatives can reduce dietary vitamin D and calcium absorption, leading to hypocalcemia and osteomalacia (11530). Advise patients to limit stimulant laxatives to short-term use of recommended doses. Some stimulant laxatives include senna (Senokot), bisacodyl (Dulcolax), and others.
SUNSCREENS: Frequent and extensive application of sunscreens can reduce vitamin D synthesis in the skin and plasma levels (11507,11508,11509). There is increasing concern that overuse of sunscreen can contribute to vitamin D deficiency and increased risk of some kinds of cancer (12992,12993). Tell patients brief sun exposure is not likely dangerous and helps maintain adequate vitamin D levels. For longer exposure than a "dose" of dermal vitamin D, recommend use of a sunscreen with an SPF 15 or greater to protect the skin. Advise people to maintain the recommended dietary intake of vitamin D. Consider supplements for people with minimal sun exposure and poor dietary intake (12992).

Interactions with Foods

None known.

Interactions with Lab Tests

None known.

Interactions with Diseases or Conditions

ARTERIOSCLEROSIS: Hypercalcemia can contribute to arteriosclerosis, particularly in patients with kidney disease. Use supplemental vitamin D cautiously (11815,11816).

HISTOPLASMOSIS: Vitamin D may increase calcium levels in people with histoplasmosis. The metabolism to calcitriol is increased in people with histoplasmosis, which may cause hypercalcemia and complications such as kidney stones and calcified tissue. Use supplemental vitamin D cautiously (11881).

HYPERCALCEMIA: Vitamin D supplements may worsen hypercalcemia (11815).

HYPERPARATHYROIDISM: Vitamin D may increase calcium levels in people with hyperparathyroidism. Use supplemental vitamin D cautiously (11815).

LYMPHOMA: Vitamin D may increase calcium levels in people with lymphoma. In some kinds of lymphoma, vitamin D is more readily converted to calcitriol and may result in hypercalcemia and complications such as kidney stones and calcified tissue. Use supplemental vitamin D cautiously (11815,11881).

RENAL DISEASE: Vitamin D may increase calcium levels and increase the risk of arteriosclerosis in renal failure. This must be balanced with the need to prevent renal osteodystrophy. Monitor calcium levels carefully (11816).

SARCOIDOSIS: Vitamin D may increase calcium levels in people with sarcoidosis. The metabolism to calcitriol is increased in people with sarcoidosis, which may cause hypercalcemia and complications such as kidney stones and calcified tissue. Use supplemental vitamin D cautiously (11881).

TUBERCULOSIS: Vitamin D may increase calcium levels in people with tuberculosis. The metabolism to calcitriol is increased in people with tuberculosis, which may cause hypercalcemia and complications such as kidney stones and calcified tissue. Use supplemental vitamin D cautiously (11881).

Dosage and Administration

ORAL: Most vitamin supplements contain the equivalent of 10 mcg (400 units) vitamin D as calcifediol, calcitriol, cholecalciferol, and ergocalciferol. The National Academy of Sciences publishes an Adequate Intake (AI) recommendation which is an estimate of the amount of vitamin D that appears to sustain normal functioning. The current daily AI of vitamin D used as cholecalciferol or ergocalciferol to prevent rickets in healthy children and osteomalacia in adults is based on age. Birth through 50 years of age, 5 mcg (200 units); Adults (ages 51 to 70), 10 mcg (400 units); Adults (greater than 70 years of age), 15 mcg (600 units) daily (7555). Some authorities recommend 1000 units per day for older adults who are not exposed to sunlight (11933).

The upper intake levels (UL) for vitamin D are 25 mcg for infants 0 to 12 months and 50 mcg for everyone over one year of age (7555).

For preventing multiple sclerosis (MS), long-term consumption of at least 400 IU per day, mainly in the form of a multivitamin supplement, has been used (11356).

For preventing falls, 800 IU per day has been used in combination with calcium 1200 mg per day (11939).

For preventing fractures, some experts recommend 800-1000 IU per day for older adults (12933,13276).

Other vitamin D analogs and vitamin D products for other routes of administration are available as FDA-approved prescription drugs.

Comments

One unit of vitamin D equals the biologic activity of 25 nanograms of ergocalciferol or cholecalciferol (7555).

Canada recognizes the importance of vitamin D in the prevention of osteoporosis in its health claim for foods that contain calcium: "A healthy diet with adequate calcium and vitamin D, and regular physical activity, help to achieve strong bones and may reduce the risk of osteoporosis" (11940). The US version of this osteoporosis health claim does not yet include vitamin D.

VITAMIN E

Also Known As

All Rac-Alpha-Tocopherol, Alpha Tocopherol Acetate, Alpha Tocopheryl Acetate, d-Alpha-Tocopherol, d-Alpha-Tocopheryl, d-Alpha-Tocopheryl Acetate, d-Alpha-Tocopheryl Succinate, d-Beta-Tocopherol, d-Delta-Tocopherol, d-Gamma-Tocopherol, dl-Alpha-Tocopherol, dl-Alpha-Tocopheryl, dl-Alpha-Tocopheryl Acetate, d-Tocopherol, d-Tocopheryl Acetate, dl-Tocopherol, Mixed Tocopherols, RRR-Alpha-Tocopherol, Tocopherol, Tocopheryl Acetate, Tocopheryl Acid Succinate, Tocopheryl Succinate, Tocotrienol, Tocotrienol Concentrate.

Scientific Names

Alpha-tocopherol; alpha tocotrienol; beta-tocopherol; beta tocotrienol; delta-tocopherol; delta tocotrienol; gamma-tocopherol; gamma tocotrienol.

People Use This For

Orally, vitamin E is used for replacement therapy in vitamin E deficiency, treating and preventing cardiovascular disease, including slowing atherogenesis and preventing heart attacks. It is used orally for angina, thrombophlebitis, intermittent claudication, hypertension, and preventing ischemia-reperfusion injury after coronary artery bypass surgery. Vitamin E is also used orally for treating diabetes and its complications. Vitamin E is used orally for

preventing cancer, particularly lung and oral cancer in smokers; colorectal cancer and polyps; and gastric, prostate, and pancreatic cancer. Vitamin E is used orally for Alzheimer's disease and other dementias, Parkinson's disease, night cramps, restless leg syndrome, and as an adjunct in the treatment of epilepsy. Vitamin E is also used orally for preventing pre-eclampsia in high-risk women, for improving physical endurance, increasing energy, preventing allergies, for asthma and respiratory infections, for protecting against negative effects of air pollution, preventing aging, preventing cataracts, and improving healing after photoreactive keratectomy. It is also used orally for inflammatory skin disorders, aging skin, sunburns, cystic fibrosis, oral leukoplakia, premenstrual syndrome (PMS), dysmenorrhea, habitual abortion, menopausal syndrome, hot flashes associated with breast cancer, infertility, impotence, chronic cystic mastitis, mammary dysplasia, peptic ulcers, porphyria, tardive dyskinesia, neuromuscular disorders, Huntington's disease, chronic progressive hereditary chorea, and myotonic dystrophy. Additionally, vitamin E is used orally for preventing vitamin E deficiency in people with malabsorption syndromes or abetalipoproteinemia, treating hemolytic anemia caused by vitamin E deficiency in premature neonates, preventing retinopathy of prematurity, preventing bronchopulmonary dysplasia secondary to oxygen therapy in neonates, and preventing intraventricular hemorrhage in premature neonates. Vitamin E is used orally for correcting erythrocyte membrane abnormalities in people with beta-thalassemia, for hereditary spherocytosis, glucose-6-phosphate dehydrogenase deficiency or sickle-cell anemia, treating anemia in conjunction with erythropoietin in people on dialysis, reducing doxorubicin-induced hair loss, reducing amiodarone-induced pulmonary toxicity, and for radiation-induced fibrosis. Vitamin E is also used orally to treat retinitis pigmentosa, osteoarthritis, nonalcoholic steatohepatitis in children, reduce muscle damage after exercise, and improve muscle strength.
Topically, vitamin E is used for dermatitis, aging skin, granuloma annulare, and protecting against skin ulceration caused by extravasation of chemotherapy drugs.

Safety

LIKELY SAFE ...when used orally or topically and appropriately. Vitamin E is generally considered non-toxic, even at doses exceeding the recommended dietary allowance (RDA); however, adverse effects are more likely to occur with higher doses. The tolerable upper intake level (UL) in healthy people is 1000 mg/day, equivalent to 1100 IU of synthetic vitamin E and 1500 IU of natural vitamin E (4668,4681,4713,4714,4844). Advise non-healthy patients not to take doses of 400 IU/day or higher. There is concern that these patients who take doses of 400 IU/day or more might have an increased risk of adverse outcomes and increased mortality from all causes (12212,13036). This risk might increase as higher doses are used (12212).

POSSIBLY UNSAFE ...when used orally in high doses. Repeated doses exceeding the tolerable upper intake level (UL) of 1000 mg/day is associated with significant side effects in otherwise healthy people (4844). There is also concern that non-healthy people who take vitamin E in doses of 400 IU/day or more might have an increased risk of adverse outcomes and increased mortality from all causes (12212,13036). This risk might increase as higher doses are used (12212). Advise non-healthy patients not to take vitamin E in doses of 400 IU/day or higher. ...when used intravenously in large doses. Large repeated intravenous doses of all-rac-alpha-tocopherol (synthetic vitamin E) were associated with decreased activity of clotting factors and bleeding in one report (3074).

PREGNANCY: LIKELY SAFE ...when used orally in amounts that do not exceed the recommended dietary allowance (RDA); however, maternal supplementation is not generally recommended unless dietary vitamin E falls below the RDA (4260). POSSIBLY SAFE ...when used orally and appropriately in amounts exceeding the recommended dietary allowance (RDA). No adverse effects were reported with oral intake of 400 IU per day starting at weeks 18-22 of pregnancy in women at high risk for pre-eclampsia (3236), or with 600-900 IU daily during the last two months of pregnancy (4260).

LACTATION: LIKELY SAFE ...when used orally in amounts that do not exceed the recommended dietary allowance (RDA) (4844). There is insufficient reliable information about the safety of vitamin E supplementation in amounts greater than the RDA while nursing.

Effectiveness

EFFECTIVE

Vitamin E deficiency. Taking vitamin E orally is effective for preventing and treating vitamin E deficiency (4844). However, vitamin E deficiency is rare in humans. It most commonly occurs in people with malabsorption disorders such as abetalipoproteinemia; cystic fibrosis; gastrectomy; hepatitic-biliary tract disease including chronic cholestasis, hepatic cirrhosis, biliary atresia, and obstructive jaundice; in infants receiving formula with insufficient vitamin E; intestinal diseases including celiac and tropical sprue; and regional enteritis (4844).

POSSIBLY EFFECTIVE

Age-related macular degeneration (AMD). Taking vitamin E 400 IU orally, plus elemental zinc 80 mg, vitamin C 500 mg, and beta-carotene 15 mg daily seems to provide a risk reduction of 27% for visual acuity loss and a risk reduction of 25% for progression of AMD in patients with advanced AMD (7303). Patients with monocular or binocular intermediate AMD or monocular advanced AMD are at high risk for advanced AMD. Theoretically, these patients may also benefit from vitamin E and antioxidant-zinc supplementation (11326). There isn't enough evidence to know if this combination is beneficial for people with less advanced macular disease or for preventing AMD. Vitamin E with antioxidants, but without zinc, doesn't seem to have any effect on AMD (7303,7304). Vitamin E alone doesn't seem to prevent age-related maculopathy in men who smoke (4667).

Alzheimer's disease. There's some evidence that all-rac-alpha-tocopherol (synthetic vitamin E) 2000 IU per day is similar to selegiline (Eldepryl), and superior to placebo, for slowing cognitive function decline in patients with moderately severe Alzheimer's disease. But there doesn't appear to be an additive effect when vitamin E is used in combination with selegiline (Eldepryl) (4635). Retrospective data suggest that long-term combination therapy with donepezil (Aricept) 5 mg and vitamin E 1000 IU per day may help slow cognitive decline in patients with Alzheimer's disease (11472). But vitamin E does not seem to slow progression from mild cognitive impairment to a diagnosis of probable Alzheimer's disease. Patients with mild cognitive impairment who take vitamin E 2000 IU/day for 3 years progress to Alzheimer's disease at the same rate as those who take placebo (13060).

Anemia. Two small studies in adults and children on chronic hemodialysis have shown improved response to erythropoietin with vitamin E supplementation (4640,4647). In one study, children given vitamin E 15 mg/kg in combination with erythropoietin had significantly increased hemoglobin (Hgb) and hematocrit (Hct) levels after two weeks of combination treatment compared to eight and five weeks in patients without combination treatment (4640). In the other study of adults, concurrent supplementation with vitamin E 500 mg daily allowed dose reductions of erythropoietin from an average of 93 U/kg/week to 74 U/kg/week with the same results on Hgb levels (4647). However, vitamin E 50 IU daily does not appear to increase the response of preterm infants to erythropoietin and iron in anemia of prematurity (10362).

Beta-thalassemia. Taking vitamin E orally seems to be effective for correcting erythrocyte membrane abnormalities in children with beta-thalassemia and low vitamin E plasma concentrations (4642).

Bladder cancer. Taking vitamin E 200 IU orally for greater than 10 years seems to be associated with a reduced risk of bladder cancer mortality (9839).

Chemotherapy extravasation. Applying vitamin E topically, in combination with dimethylsulfoxide (DMSO), seems to be effective for treating chemotherapy extravasation (4668).

Cisplatin-induced neurotoxicity. Alpha-tocopherol administered before chemotherapy, and continued for 3 months after the completion of treatment, seems to reduce the incidence of peripheral neurotoxicity by 55% without affecting cisplatin efficacy (10366).

Dementia. A longitudinal cohort study of 3,385 elderly men aged 71 to 93 years found that men who consumed supplemental vitamin E and vitamin C had a decreased risk of developing vascular and mixed or other dementias; however, there was no protective effect for Alzheimer's dementia. This study did not distinguish between different forms of vitamin E (4636).

Dyspraxia. Taking vitamin E orally, in combination with evening primrose oil, thyme oil, and fish oils seems to improve movement disorders in children with dyspraxia (5708).

Glomerulosclerosis. There is some evidence that vitamin E taken orally might reduce proteinuria in children with focal segmental glomerulosclerosis who are refractory to standard medical management (4675).

Glucose-6-phosphate dehydrogenase (G6PD) deficiency. There is renewed interest in vitamin E taken orally for G6PD deficiency (4685). In two open studies, vitamin E 800 IU alone or in combination with selenium reduced hemolysis and reticulocytosis and increased red blood cell (RBC) half-life and vitamin E levels in patients with G6PD deficiency (4682,4683). In one study, vitamin E plus selenium 25 mcg daily offered significantly more improvement compared to vitamin E alone (4683). These findings are contrary to an earlier study that found no effect with vitamin E at 2000-2400 IU per day (4684).

Granuloma annulare. Topical vitamin E seems to clear granuloma annulare lesions within one to three weeks (4681).

Huntington's disease. RRR-alpha-tocopherol (natural vitamin E) can significantly improve symptoms in patients with early Huntington's disease, but this benefit is not seen in patients with more advanced disease (4686).

Infertility. In one study, males with asthenospermia or oligoasthenospermia, receiving oral vitamin E supplementation, achieved impregnation at a rate of 21% compared to none for similar patients receiving placebo (4695). In another study, males enrolled in an in vitro fertilization program who had previously had low fertilization rates were treated with oral vitamin E for three months. Fertilization rates increased significantly from 19% to 29% after one month of treatment (3583). In a crossover trial, males found to have elevated reactive oxygen species in their semen, which might be associated with infertility, were treated with oral vitamin E. After treatment, in vitro sperm binding to the zona pellucida was significantly increased (4693). Interestingly, high-dose vitamin E in combination with vitamin C does not seem to offer any benefit to sperm functionality (4696). Vitamin E plus selenium seems to improve sperm functionality, but doesn't improve fertilization rates (3585). Although vitamin E preparations used alone appear to offer some benefit in men with asthenospermia or oxidative damage to sperm, combining vitamin E with vitamin C or selenium does not appear to be beneficial. Studies did not differentiate between different forms of vitamin E.

Intracranial hemorrhage. Taking vitamin E orally seems to be effective for treating intracranial hemorrhage in premature neonates (4655).

Intraventricular hemorrhage. Taking vitamin E orally seems to be effective for treating intraventricular hemorrhage in premature neonates (4656).

Nitrate tolerance. There is some evidence that vitamin E 300-600 mg/day can help prevent nitrate tolerance (4705,11543). Nitrate tolerance might involve increased vascular superoxide anion production, and antioxidants may help prevent this (4705).

Parkinson's disease. Preliminary evidence suggests that dietary vitamin E intake might be associated with a decreased occurrence of Parkinson's disease (4712). But taking all-rac-alpha-tocopherol (synthetic vitamin E) 2000 IU supplements daily does not seem to have any benefit for patients who have Parkinson's disease (4709,4710,4711).

Photoreactive keratectomy. High dose (50,000-75,000 units) vitamin A in the form of retinol palmitate taken orally with 230 mg vitamin E (alpha-tocopheryl nicotinate) daily seems to accelerate re-epithelialization, reduce haze formation, and improve visual acuity in patients undergoing laser surgery for myopia (348).

Pre-eclampsia. Taking a combination of vitamin E 400 IU and vitamin C 1000 mg daily significantly reduced the risk of proteinuric hypertension in high-risk women when started in weeks 16 to 22 of pregnancy (3236). Other researchers using vitamin E in combination with vitamin C and allopurinol beginning at 24 to 32 weeks gestation found the combination similar to placebo (4718).

Premenstrual syndrome (PMS). Taking vitamin E orally seems to reduce symptoms of anxiety, craving, and depression in patients with PMS (4719,4720).

Radiation-induced fibrosis. Taking vitamin E 1000 IU orally with pentoxifylline 800 mg daily seems to reverse radiation-induced fibrosis (4672,4673). Regression of radiation-induced fibrosis becomes significant after three months of treatment and continues to improve thereafter. After 12 months of treatment, mean surface area of fibrosis can decrease by 66% (4672). However, vitamin E alone doesn't seem to be effective (10363).

Retrolental fibroplasia. Taking vitamin E orally seems to be effective for treating retrolental fibroplasia in premature neonates (10).

Rheumatoid arthritis (RA). Vitamin E taken orally in conjunction with standard therapy is superior to standard therapy alone for reducing pain, but not inflammation in patients with RA (4723).

Sunburn. High dose oral RRR-alpha-tocopherol (natural vitamin E) in combination with vitamin C protected against skin inflammation after exposure to ultraviolet (UV) radiation in two small, double-blind, placebo-controlled studies (4715,4716). Alpha-tocopherol acetate 400 IU alone does not seem to offer this benefit (4715). In one study, topically applied vitamin E in combination with topical vitamin C and melatonin provided modest photoprotective effect when used prior to UV exposure, but had no effect when used during or after UV exposure (4713,4714).

Tardive dyskinesia. Taking vitamin E orally seems to significantly improve Abnormal Involuntary Movement Scale (AIMS) scores in people with tardive dyskinesia. It seems to be more effective in higher doses and in people who have had tardive dyskinesia for less than five years (3942,3943,3944,3945,3946,3948). In the largest study to date, conflicting findings have been reported; however, this study has not yet been published, preventing further evaluation of its findings (3947). Both RRR-alpha-tocopherol (natural vitamin E) and unspecified forms were used in clinical trials.

Uveitis. Taking vitamin E orally with vitamin C seems to improve visual acuity in patients with acute anterior uveitis, but does not seem to decrease inflammation measured by laser flare (4730).

POSSIBLY INEFFECTIVE

Angina. Taking vitamin E orally may have some effect on endothelial dysfunction, but doesn't seem to help nonsmokers or smokers with angina (3896,4634,4649,4650,4651,4652).

Atherosclerosis. Taking RRR-alpha-tocopherol (natural vitamin E) orally doesn't appear to have any effect on atherosclerosis progression or mortality in patients with atherosclerosis (3899,3936). However, there is preliminary evidence that a combination of vitamin E and vitamin C, might help prevent the progression of atherosclerosis in men, particularly smokers and cardiac transplant patients (1918).

Breast cancer-related hot flashes. Taking vitamin E orally does not seem to significantly reduce hot flashes in women who have had breast cancer (454). There have been no clinical trials using vitamin E supplementation for postmenopausal symptoms.

Bronchopulmonary dysplasia. In one study, taking vitamin E orally had no benefit for treating bronchopulmonary dysplasia in premature infants weighing less than 1500 grams at birth (4657).

Colorectal cancer. The evidence for vitamin E and colorectal cancer is conflicting. Some evidence suggests that taking vitamin E orally in combination with vitamin A and vitamin C, or a multivitamin might have a protective effect in patients with previous colorectal adenomas (3954,3956). A retrospective study also links intake of vitamin E and multivitamins with a lower incidence of colorectal cancer (3958). But randomized, controlled trials show that taking vitamin E supplements alone, or in combination with beta-carotene or beta-carotene plus vitamin C does not prevent the development of colorectal adenomas, which are considered precursors to colon cancer (3953,3955,3957,12185). There is also evidence that patients with diabetes or cardiovascular disease who take RRR-alpha-tocopherol (natural vitamin E) 400 IU/day do not have a decreased risk of developing colon cancer (13036). In another large-scale study, women who take RRR-alpha-tocopherol (natural vitamin E) 600 IU every other day for up to 10 years also do not have a lower risk of developing colorectal cancer (13131).

Congestive heart failure (CHF). Taking vitamin E orally for 12 weeks doesn't seem to improve prognostic or functional indices of CHF or improve quality-of-life measurements (3906).

Duchenne muscular dystrophy. A double-blind study in 106 boys for 18 months found no difference between placebo and combination oral vitamin E and penicillamine for slowing disease progression (4703).

Head and neck cancer. Taking all-rac-alpha-tocopherol (synthetic vitamin E) 400 IU/day, during radiation therapy and for 3 years after the end of radiation therapy, does not seem to reduce the risk of recurrence of the first tumor or development of a second primary tumor. There is some concern that patients taking vitamin E seem to have an increased risk of tumor recurrence or a second primary tumor compared to patients taking placebo (13055). Advise patients with head and neck cancer to avoid taking vitamin E supplements in doses of 400 IU/day or more.

Hemolytic anemia. Vitamin E 25 IU per day given to premature infants for six weeks seems to have no beneficial effects on hemolytic anemia (4648).

Hypertension. Taking vitamin E orally for 3 to 4 years doesn't seem to lower blood pressure in patients already on hypertension treatment (5210).

Intermittent claudication. Taking all-rac-alpha-tocopherol (synthetic vitamin E) orally doesn't appear to have any effect when used alone or in combination with beta-carotene for treating symptoms or disease progression in male smokers (4732).

Myotonic dystrophy. A small study comparing placebo to combination vitamin E and selenium taken orally showed no difference in functional deterioration over two years (4704).

Oral mucosal lesions. Although there is some conflicting evidence (3951,4708), the largest and most significant controlled trial indicates that supplementation with all-rac-alpha-tocopherol (synthetic vitamin E) 50 mg daily for five to seven years has no effect on the incidence of oral lesions in male cigarette smokers (3951).

Osteoarthritis. Taking vitamin E 500 IU/day for 6 months does not seem to decrease symptoms of pain or stiffness in patients with osteoarthritis (5264,5881). Vitamin E 500 IU/day for up to 2 years also does not seem to slow cartilage loss (13066). Taking vitamin E also does not seem to reduce the risk of developing osteoarthritis (5881).

Pancreatic cancer. Taking vitamin E supplements alone or in combination with other antioxidants such as beta-carotene and vitamin C doesn't seem to reduce the risk of developing pancreatic cancer (12185). Taking all-rac-alpha-tocopherol (synthetic vitamin E) 50 mg daily supplements for 5 to 8 years by male smokers also does not seem to reduce the incidence or mortality of carcinoma of the pancreas (3961).

Respiratory infections. Taking oral vitamin E 200 mg daily, alone or in supplemental multivitamin form, does not appear to decrease the incidence, duration, or severity of upper or lower respiratory infections in elderly persons (10788,12094). But some evidence suggests that vitamin E might reduce the incidence of the common cold in elderly long-term care patients (12094). More evidence is needed to determine how effective vitamin E might be for reducing the incidence of the common cold.

Retinitis pigmentosa. Taking all-rac-alpha-tocopherol (synthetic vitamin E) orally does not appear to slow visual decline is people with retinitis pigmentosa and has been associated with more rapid loss of visual acuity, although the validity of the study with these findings has been questioned (83,84,85,86,87,88).

Scarring. Applying vitamin E topically doesn't seem to reduce surgical wound scarring (4721,4722).

LIKELY INEFFECTIVE

Benign breast disease. Taking vitamin E supplements does not seem to be effective for treating benign breast disease (4660,4661,4662).

Breast cancer. Increasing vitamin E intake from the diet or supplements does not seem to reduce the risk of developing breast cancer (4658,4659). However, some evidence suggests that higher serum levels of vitamin E might be associated with a reduced risk of breast cancer (10132). A large-scale randomized trial in patients with diabetes or cardiovascular disease shows that patients who take 400 IU/day of RRR-alpha-tocopherol (natural vitamin E) do not have a reduced risk of developing breast cancer (13036). In another large-scale study, women who take RRR-alpha-tocopherol (natural vitamin E) 600 IU every other day for up to 10 years also do not have a lower risk of developing breast cancer (13131).

Cardiovascular disease. Taking vitamin E supplements orally is not effective for preventing heart disease or adverse cardiovascular outcomes such as myocardial infarction (MI), stroke, hospitalizations for unstable angina, or cardiovascular death (12492,12493,13036). Observational studies have linked increased vitamin E intake with a decreased risk of cardiovascular events in men and women (3898,3933,3934) and decreased risk of peripheral arterial disease in men, but not in women (10130). But clinical trials using vitamin E supplements do not support this epidemiological evidence (10365). With few exceptions (3357,3936), large-scale controlled clinical trials show that vitamin E supplements offer no benefit for primary prevention in healthy or high risk patients (3907,3935,3937,13036,13131), or secondary prevention of heart disease and cardiovascular events such as MI, stroke, and death (3896,3899,13036). One large-scale trial in healthy women provides somewhat conflicting evidence. Women who take RRR-alpha-tocopherol (natural vitamin E) 600 IU every other day for up to 10 years also do not have a lower risk of major cardiovascular events such as myocardial infarction or ischemic or hemorrhagic stroke; however, they seem to have a 24% lower risk of cardiovascular death (13131). This finding is contradictory to previous findings.

There is debate about whether some forms of vitamin E might be more effective than others. Some people suggest that RRR-alpha-tocopherol (natural vitamin E) is more effective than all-rac-alpha-tocopherol (synthetic vitamin E). This has not been verified by studies. An analysis of vitamin E studies indicates that there is no significant difference in cardiovascular outcomes based on the form of vitamin E used (13132).

The FDA has refused to allow labeling claims for vitamin E supplements for prevention of cardiovascular disease (3939). A Science Advisory from the American Heart Association also states that the evidence does not justify use of antioxidants such as vitamin E for reducing the risk of cardiovascular disease (12142). Advise patients not to rely on vitamin E supplements for preventing heart disease. Recommend increasing dietary vitamin E consumption instead.

Lung cancer. Taking all-rac-alpha-tocopherol (synthetic vitamin E) 50 mg per day for 5 to 8 years is not associated with a lower risk of developing lung cancer for male smokers (3949). There is also some evidence that suggests patients with diabetes or cardiovascular disease who take RRR-alpha-tocopherol (natural vitamin E) 400 IU/day do not have a significantly lower risk of developing lung cancer (13036). In another large-scale study, women who take RRR-alpha-tocopherol (natural vitamin E) 600 IU every other day for up to 10 years also do not have a lower risk of developing lung cancer (13131).

INSUFFICIENT RELIABLE EVIDENCE to RATE

Cataracts. There is conflicting information about the use of vitamin E to prevent cataracts. Vitamin E alone or in combination with other vitamins does not seem to prevent the development and progression of age-related cataracts and vision loss (4666,7304). Vitamin E plus vitamin C and beta-carotene with zinc doesn't seem to have any significant effect on age-related loss of vision due to cataracts in well-nourished people when taken for an average of 6.3 years (7304), but most population research suggests a beneficial effect of vitamin E (2395,4208,4663,4664,4665,4759). Vitamin E use in multivitamins or any supplement containing vitamin E for ten years appears to reduce the incidence of nuclear and cortical cataracts by 60%, according to epidemiological research. Use of supplements for shorter periods doesn't appear to reduce the risk for cataract development (4208).

Chemotherapy-related infection. Observational research suggests that greater dietary intake of vitamin E may lower the incidence of infection in children undergoing chemotherapy for lymphoblastic leukemia (11997).

Diabetes. Vitamin E might be beneficial in diabetes and diabetic neuropathy, retinopathy, and nephropathy. Some evidence suggests it improves glucose disposal in type 2 diabetics (4726,4727), improves monocyte function, which lessens atherogenesis (95), improves nerve conduction in diabetic neuropathy (4724), improves retinal blood flow, and decreases creatinine clearance (4725). In type 1 diabetes, clinical research indicates that vitamin E might have a role in the management of early vascular disease by improving endothelial vasodilator function (94). One study has shown that 750 IU (503 mg) RRR-alpha-tocopherol daily for one year decreased lipoprotein susceptibility to copper oxidization in type 1 diabetics (3358).

Dysmenorrhea. Preliminary clinical research suggests vitamin E supplementation might reduce menstrual pain in teenaged girls with primary dysmenorrhea (10361).

Epilepsy. There is preliminary evidence that vitamin E might reduce seizure frequency in refractory epilepsy; however, trials have been few and contradictory (4670,4671,6066).

Esophageal cancer. Taking vitamin E supplements in combination with beta-carotene and vitamin C doesn't seem to reduce the risk of esophageal cancer (12185).

Gastric cancer. In a large-scale study of 29,584 people in China, the combination of oral vitamin E, beta-carotene, and selenium over 5.25 years significantly reduced total mortality, total cancer mortality, and stomach cancer mortality. However, this population has a high risk of gastric cancer, which is thought to be related to poor vitamin and mineral intake (4679). It is unknown if supplementation with these vitamins and minerals would be beneficial in people with adequate nutrition. Although there has been some conflicting evidence (4677), taking vitamin E supplements alone does not seem to offer this benefit (3960,4676,12185). Taking vitamin E plus beta-carotene or vitamin C and beta-carotene also does not seem to reduce the risk of gastric cancer (12185). There is preliminary evidence that increasing dietary consumption of vitamin E might slow progression of gastric carcinoma (3360).

Hyperlipidemia. Some preliminary clinical research suggests that vitamin E in combination with vitamin C might restore endothelial function in hyperlipidemic children, which might slow progression of atherosclerosis (10352).

Ischemic reperfusion injury. Taking vitamin E orally with vitamin C and allopurinol two days prior to coronary bypass surgery and one day postoperatively, patients had fewer perioperative infarctions and less creatine kinase-MB release (4699); however, this benefit was not found when using vitamin E alone or in combination with vitamin C without allopurinol (4697,4698).

Ischemic stroke. There is some evidence that all-rac-alpha-tocopherol (synthetic vitamin E) might reduce the risk of ischemic stroke in male smokers with hypertension and diabetes (3359).

Liver transplant. A water soluble form of vitamin E, tocopheryl succinate polyethylene glycol 10,000 (TPGS), may improve absorption of cyclosporine after liver transplant (10368).

Melanoma. There is some evidence from a large-scale trial that patients with diabetes or cardiovascular disease who take RRR-alpha-tocopherol (natural vitamin E) 400 IU/day orally do not have a reduced risk of developing melanoma (13036).

Nocturnal leg cramps. Limited evidence suggests vitamin E might offer some benefit for nocturnal leg cramps (4700,4701), but there is conflicting evidence (4702).

Pharyngeal cancer. There is some evidence from a large-scale trial that patients with diabetes or cardiovascular disease who take RRR-alpha-tocopherol (natural vitamin E) 400 IU/day orally do not have a reduced risk of developing oral or pharyngeal cancer (13036).

Prostate cancer. Some population studies suggest that increasing vitamin E consumption is associated with a reduced risk of prostate cancer (4644,4645,4646). However, others show no effect (12872). The Cancer Prevention Study II Nutrition Cohort followed the incidence of prostate cancer among 72,704 men. Use of supplemental vitamin E at least 4 times/week does not appear to be associated with a reduced risk of prostate cancer. Increasing doses of vitamin E also doesn't seem to have any effect (12873). Large-scale randomized, controlled trials also provide conflicting evidence. In a large-scale study of 29,133 smokers, patients taking 50 mg/day of all-rac-alpha-tocopherol (synthetic vitamin E) alone or in combination with beta-carotene had a significantly lower incidence of prostate cancer and mortality associated with prostate cancer (3959,11303). The cohort of patients from this study who developed prostate cancer tended to have lower levels of serum alpha-tocopherol and gamma-tocopherol compared to controls (13043). But another large-scale study in patients with diabetes or cardiovascular disease suggests that these patients who take 400 IU/day of RRR-alpha-tocopherol (natural vitamin E) do not have a decreased risk of developing prostate cancer (13036).

Sickle cell disease. Taking vitamin E orally with aged garlic extract and vitamin C might be useful for sickle cell anemia (5056).

Steatohepatitis. Preliminary clinical evidence indicates that vitamin E may be helpful in nonalcoholic steatohepatitis in children; however, long-term studies have not been performed (89).

More evidence is needed to rate vitamin E for these uses.

Mechanism of Action

Vitamin E is a fat-soluble vitamin. It is naturally occurring in many foods including vegetable oils, cereal grains, animal fats, meat, poultry, eggs, fruits, and vegetables (96). Wheat germ oil is a particularly rich source of vitamin E. Maximum vitamin E intake from diet alone typically reaches about 60 IU per day (97).

Vitamin E deficiency is rare and most typically seen in genetic abnormalities that prevent maintenance of normal blood concentrations of vitamin E or conditions that prevent absorption. Vitamin E deficiency does not cause specific disease in adults, although creatinuria, ceroid deposition, muscle weakness, and decreased erythrocyte survival are associated with low serum vitamin E concentrations. In adults, total body stores of vitamin E, found in adipose tissue, have been estimated to be 3-8 grams and are sufficient to meet the body's requirements for 4 or more years of a deficient diet. In premature infants, vitamin E deficiency can cause irritability, edema, thrombosis, and hemolytic anemia (15).

Vitamin E refers to 8 different forms including alpha-, beta-, gamma-, and delta-tocopherols and four tocotrienols. Most vitamin E in foods is gamma-tocopherol. Unlike most nutrients, vitamin E does not appear to have a specific role in a required metabolic process. The major function of vitamin E is probably that of a chain-breaking antioxidant that prevents the formation of free radicals. Vitamin E's therapeutic benefits have primarily been attributed to its antioxidant effects (4844,12494).

Supplemental vitamin E usually refers to alpha-tocopherol. For biological activity, vitamin E is dependent on hepatic alpha-tocopherol transfer protein (alpha-TTP) for distribution. Although the typical diet contains other forms of vitamin E (beta-, gamma-, and delta-tocopherols), these have very limited systemic bioavailability because they do not bind with alpha-TTP. Supplemental beta-, gamma-, and delta-tocopherols, and tocotrienols appear to have little in vivo activity in humans and do not contribute toward meeting established vitamin E requirements (4844). Only the alpha-tocopherol form of vitamin E is maintained in plasma and thought to be therapeutically useful. Alpha-tocopherol exists as eight stereoisomers. The RRR-alpha-tocopherol isomer, formerly called d-alpha-tocopherol, has the greatest affinity for alpha-TTP and the most biologic activity (4844). RRR-alpha-tocopherol is sometimes called natural vitamin E and occurs naturally in foods (4844). The racemic mixture of all eight alpha-tocopherol isomers, or all-rac-alpha-tocopherol, was formerly known as dl-alpha-tocopherol (4844). All-rac-alpha-tocopherol, sometimes called synthetic vitamin E, is found in vitamin E-fortified foods. Both forms of vitamin E, natural and synthetic, can be found in vitamin E supplements. All-rac-alpha-tocopherol has lower affinity for alpha-TTP and thus has less biologic activity than RRR-alpha-tocopherol (4627,4844). Based on weight, 15 mg of RRR-alpha tocopherol is approximately equivalent in potency to 30 mg of all-rac-alpha-tocopherol (99,200,218,4844).

Although higher bioavailability for the natural form is well-known, the relative potency of natural and synthetic vitamin E is controversial. Some researchers cite the potency of the natural to synthetic form as 1.36, rather than 2.0 (100,202,247,248). Clinical differences between natural and synthetic vitamin E at equivalent doses have not been shown. But some researchers speculate that natural vitamin E might have an anti-inflammatory effect and a potentially beneficial effect on atherosclerosis (12497).

Oxidative damage has been attributed to many conditions for which vitamin E is used, including lipid peroxidation in heart disease (6204). Some preliminary research suggests that vitamin E might inhibit the local inflammatory process and oxidation of low-density lipoprotein (LDL) cholesterol that is associated with atherosclerosis (97,249), but when this theory was tested in healthy adults without heart disease, RRR-alpha-tocopherol, even at 2000 IU/day, did not produce markers that indicate a reduction in lipid oxidation (13159). This appears to be another case where promising laboratory data turns out to be clinically irrelevant. Vitamin E also doesn't appear to improve endothelium-dependent vasodilation in older adults with hypercholesterolemia (11286).

Some researchers think the antioxidant activity of vitamin E may slow progression of renal disease. Oxidative metabolites may accumulate in renal dysfunction. Vitamin E could theoretically slow the rate of decline in chronic inflammatory kidney diseases such as IgA nephropathy, diabetic nephropathy, and glomerulosclerosis; and poisoning by nephrotoxic drugs and other compounds (10369).

In tardive dyskinesia, it is thought that some patients may have increased dopamine turnover resulting in increased production of free radicals and structural damage. Additionally, people with tardive dyskinesia may have decreased levels of vitamin E and vitamin C (3598). Oxidative damage has also been associated with diabetes and related complications.

Oxidative damage has also long been associated with the development of cancers. Vitamin E and other antioxidants are theorized to minimize this damage (5882). Several mechanisms have been theorized for reducing bladder carcinogenesis, including the neutralization of reactive oxygen species, the inhibition of the formation of nitrosamines, and enhancement of immune function (9839). Preliminary evidence also suggests vitamin E and other antioxidants can decrease oxidative damage associated with tumor-directed radio-immunotherapy (5882). Vitamin E is used for photo-aged skin and to prevent oxidative skin damage related to ultraviolet (UV) radiation (e.g., sunburn) due to its antioxidant effects. However, some researchers think that this benefit requires concomitant use with other antioxidants such as vitamin C to prevent degradation of vitamin E (6062,6064). Chemotherapy and radiation therapy also adversely affect vitamin E status (98).

Vitamin E status may also decline with standard parenteral nutrition formulas. Lipid emulsions and amino acid solutions appear to be susceptible to oxidative degradation with storage (98).

Vitamin E appears to slow the progression of Alzheimer's disease, possibly due to an interaction with free radicals and a disruption of cellular damage (11472). Preliminary data suggest vitamin E might improve cognitive function by decreasing beta-amyloid damage (4637,4638,4639).

Some evidence links asthma to increased oxidative stress and vitamin E deficiency (315,401,409,422,6058). Epidemiological and case-control studies have associated asthma with lower vitamin E intake, lower vitamin E serum levels, and lower vitamin levels in lung lining fluid, but clinical studies using vitamin E supplementation for asthma have not been performed (315,401,409,422,6058).

Lower vitamin E serum levels have also been associated with higher IgE levels and positive allergen skin tests (5275).

In addition to its antioxidant function, vitamin E inhibits protein kinase C activity, which is involved in cell proliferation and differentiation in several cell types, including smooth muscle, platelets, and monocytes (4844).

Preliminary research suggests that vitamin E might have an antiproliferative effect on benign hyperplastic prostate cells (11235).

Population studies suggest an association between low serum levels of alpha-tocopherol and higher risk of prostate cancer (12874). Vitamin E might have antiandrogen activity (12875,12876).

There is some concern that high doses of vitamin E might have a pro-oxidant rather than an antioxidant effect (12495,13036). High doses of vitamin E (alpha-tocopherol) alone might disrupt the normal antioxidant balance and decrease the effect of other vitamin E isomers such as gamma-tocopherol and other antioxidants (12496,13036). It might also lower the protective high-density lipoprotein (HDL) cholesterol. This potential pro-oxidant effect could result in adverse cardiovascular outcomes (13036).

Large amounts of vitamin E interfere with vitamin K-dependent clotting factor production, producing hypoprothrombinemic effects, especially in people with vitamin K deficiency or those who are taking oral anticoagulants (3073,3074). Mixed tocopherols seem to have a greater effect on platelet aggregation than alpha-tocopherol alone, which might explain the discrepancy between the effects of dietary vitamin E intake and supplemental vitamin E (alpha-tocopherol) in cardiovascular disease. Mixed tocopherols seem to increase nitric oxide (NO) release and superoxide dismutase (SOD) protein content in platelets, which may contribute to the effect on platelet aggregation (10364).

For immune function in the elderly, vitamin E supplementation might replenish an inapparent deficiency. Deficiency of vitamin E and other micronutrients are common in apparently well-nourished people over age 90 and might affect the number and function of natural killer cells in old age (4688). Most research suggests that vitamin E supplementation in healthy elderly people improves response to delayed-type hypersensitivity skin testing (DTH), an indicator of immune function, and antibody response to hepatitis B, tetanus and diphtheria, and pneumococcal vaccines (4676,4689,4690,4691). But whether vitamin E supplementation results in better health in elderly people is unknown.

In the treatment of epilepsy, vitamin E is primarily used because some patients taking anti-epileptic drugs have decreased blood levels of vitamin E. Vitamin E might also act as a membrane stabilizer and enzyme repressor in these patients (3356,6066).

Although biological activity of other forms is significantly less and current guidelines do not include forms of vitamin E other than alpha-tocopherol for meeting dietary requirements (4844), the other forms, such as gamma-tocopherol and the tocotrienols, have been associated with some pharmacological activity. For example, gamma-tocopherol appears to decrease the programmed death of human coronary artery endothelial cells, possibly by decreasing LDL oxidation (4092). Gamma-tocopherol inhibits prostate cancer cell growth in vitro (4089). Gamma-tocopherol also appears to prolong prothrombin and partial thromboplastin times and has caused hemorrhage in experimental animals (4098). Beta- and delta-tocopherol have also been shown to prolong prothrombin and partial thromboplastin times in laboratory animals (4098). RRR-alpha-tocopheryl succinate, known as vitamin E succinate (VES), is currently being researched for its chemotherapeutic and chemopreventive potential. VES has been shown to inhibit tumor cell growth, primarily by triggering apoptosis in human prostate carcinoma (3361). There is some evidence that the inhibitory effect on cancer cell growth by statin drugs with a closed ring structure, such as mevastatin and lovastatin (Mevacor), may be enhanced when used with alpha tocopheryl succinate (8046). The tocotrienols from rice and barley bran might lower total cholesterol and LDL, possibly by decreasing activity of HMG CoA reductase, but in a different way than "statin" drugs (3237,3238,3239,3240,3241). Tocotrienols might also be capable of decreasing carotid artery plaque size in some people, possibly by decreasing platelet aggregation (3239).

Some people think that taking vitamin E with a high fat meal is necessary to increase absorption. However, vitamin E (d-alpha-tocopherol) is similarly absorbed when taken with high-fat (36 grams) or low-fat (3 grams) meals (6133). In conditions with severe fat malabsorption such as short bowel syndrome, lipid soluble forms of vitamin E, such as those in food, may not be absorbed. A water soluble form of vitamin E such as tocopheryl succinate polyethylene glycol 10,000 (TPGS), may improve vitamin E status in these people (10367).

Adverse Reactions

Orally, vitamin E seldom causes adverse effects. In uncommon cases, vitamin E can cause nausea, diarrhea, intestinal cramps, fatigue, weakness, headache, blurred vision, rash, gonadal dysfunction, and creatinuria. It is unclear if vitamin E contributes to increased risk of hemorrhagic stroke. One study suggested a higher incidence of hemorrhagic stroke in male smokers taking all-rac-alpha-tocopherol (synthetic vitamin E), but several other studies lasting from 1.4 years to 4.5 years with study participants taking either all-rac-alpha-tocopherol (synthetic vitamin E) or RRR-alpha-tocopherol (natural vitamin E) showed no increased risk for stroke (2307,3896,3936,3949,4635).

High doses of vitamin E might increase the risk of bleeding due to antagonism of vitamin K-dependent clotting factors and platelet aggregation. Patients with vitamin K deficiencies or taking anticoagulant or antiplatelet drugs are at a greater risk for bleeding (4844,11999).

Non-healthy people should avoid vitamin E doses of 400 IU/day or more. There is evidence that these patients who take either all-rac-alpha-tocopherol (synthetic vitamin E) or RRR-alpha-tocopherol (natural vitamin E) in doses of 400 IU/day or higher might have increased adverse outcomes. In one analysis, non-healthy patients who took primarily all-rac-alpha-tocopherol (synthetic vitamin E) had an increased risk of mortality from all causes. The risk of mortality seems to increase when higher doses are used (12212). Results from a large-scale study suggest that patients with diabetes or cardiovascular disease who take RRR-alpha-tocopherol (natural vitamin E) have an increased risk of heart failure and heart failure-related hospitalization (13036). It is not known why vitamin E might be associated with these adverse outcomes. There is speculation that high-dose vitamin E might disrupt the normal antioxidant balance and result in pro-oxidant rather than antioxidant effects (13036).

There is some evidence that vitamin E in combination with simvastatin (Zocor), niacin, selenium, vitamin C, and beta-carotene might lower high density lipoprotein-2 (HDL-2) by 15%. HDL-2 is considered to be the most cardioprotective component of HDL (7388). However, vitamin E and a statin alone don't seem to negatively affect HDL (11286,11287). Although only certain isomers of vitamin E are included for determination of dietary requirements, all isomers are considered for determining safe intake levels. All the isomers are thought to potentially contribute to toxicity.

Topically, vitamin E has been associated with contact dermatitis, inflammatory reactions, and eczematous lesions (11998).

Interactions with Herbs & Other Dietary Supplements

BETA-CAROTENE: Some evidence suggests that vitamin E might reduce absorption of beta-carotene, due to competition for solubilization in micelles. Taking vitamin E 800 units daily seems to reduce plasma beta-carotene levels by 20%. It's thought that higher doses might further reduce beta-carotene levels (10561).

HERBS WITH ANTICOAGULANT/ANTIPLATELET POTENTIAL: Vitamin E inhibits platelet aggregation and adhesion (4844). Concomitant use with herbs that also affect platelet aggregation could theoretically increase the risk of bleeding in some people. These herbs include angelica, asafoetida, clove, danshen, garlic, ginger, ginkgo, Panax ginseng, horse chestnut, meadowsweet, poplar, quassia, red clover, willow, and others.

IRON: Limited data suggest excessive doses of vitamin E (>10 units/kg/day) can delay the red blood cell response to iron supplements in severely anemic infants (11547). Avoid high doses of vitamin E in infants. It isn't known whether this interaction occurs in adults.

OMEGA-6 FATTY ACIDS: Increased intake of omega-6 fatty acids may increase vitamin E requirements, particularly at higher doses (4844).

VITAMIN A: Based on cell culture and animal studies, it's been suggested that vitamin E affects the activity of vitamin A. These include preventing oxidation in the gut and increasing absorption, enhancing utilization, promoting liver storage, protecting against cell damage caused by high vitamin A levels, and reducing some of the symptoms of hypervitaminosis A (10545,10557,10558,10560).

VITAMIN K: Taking doses of vitamin E of 800 IU/day or more can decrease the effects of vitamin K. This might increase the risk of bleeding in people taking warfarin or other anticoagulants, especially in those patients with low vitamin K levels (93,7135). Vitamin E antagonizes vitamin K by decreasing its absorption and by binding to vitamin K dependent enzymes (7135,11512).

Interactions with Drugs

ANTICOAGULANT/ANTIPLATELET DRUGS: Concomitant use of vitamin E and anticoagulant or antiplatelet agents might increase the risk of bleeding. Vitamin E seems to inhibit of platelet aggregation and antagonize the effects of vitamin K-dependent clotting factors (4733,4844,11580,11582,11583,11584,11586). These effects appear to be dose-dependent, and are probably only likely to be clinically significant with 800 units/day or more (11582,11585). Mixed tocopherols, such as those found in food, might have a greater antiplatelet effect than alpha-tocopherol (10364). RRR alpha-tocopherol (natural vitamin E) 1000 IU per day antagonizes vitamin K dependent clotting factors (11999). Advise patients to avoid high doses of vitamin E, especially in people with low vitamin K intake or other risk factors for bleeding. Anticoagulant and antiplatelet drugs that might interact with vitamin E include aspirin, clopidogrel (Plavix), dalteparin (Fragmin), enoxaparin (Lovenox), heparin, ticlopidine (Ticlid), warfarin (Coumadin), and others.

CHEMOTHERAPY: There's concern that antioxidants like vitamin E could reduce the activity of chemotherapy drugs which generate free radicals, such as cyclophosphamide, chlorambucil, carmustine, busulfan, thiotepa, and doxorubicin (391). Although it has been claimed this isn't a problem, there isn't any data on the effects of vitamin E on long-term outcomes of chemotherapy treatment. Advise patients to consult their oncologist before using vitamin E

supplements, especially in high doses. Monitor response to chemotherapy closely if supplements are used.
CYCLOSPORINE (Neoral, Sandimmune): There is some evidence that one specific formulation of vitamin E (D-alpha-tocopheryl-polyethylene glycol-1000 succinate, TPGS, tocophersolan, Liqui-E) might increase absorption of cyclosporine. This vitamin E formulation forms micelles which seems to increase absorption of cyclosporine by 40% to 72% in some patients (10368). Monitor cyclosporine levels. Cyclosporine doses might need to be reduced to avoid toxicity. This interaction is unlikely to occur with the usual forms of vitamin E.
HMG-CoA REDUCTASE INHIBITORS ("Statins"): A combination of simvastatin (Zocor) and niacin effectively raises HDL (high density lipoprotein) cholesterol ("good cholesterol") in people with coronary disease and low HDL levels. A combination of antioxidants (vitamin C, vitamin E, beta-carotene, and selenium) seems to blunt this rise in HDL, specifically the HDL-2 and apolipoprotein A1 fractions (7388,11537). HDL-2 is considered to be the most cardioprotective component of HDL (7388). However, vitamin E alone combined with a statin doesn't seem to decrease HDL levels (11286,11287). It isn't known whether the adverse effect on HDL is due to one of the other antioxidants or to the combination. It also isn't known whether it will occur in other patient populations, or when antioxidant vitamins are combined with other lipid-altering regimens. Monitor lipid levels closely in people taking lipid-altering drugs and antioxidant vitamin supplements, including vitamin E. Other "statin" drugs include lovastatin (Mevacor), pravastatin (Pravachol), fluvastatin (Lescol), and atorvastatin (Lipitor).
NIACIN: A combination of niacin and simvastatin (Zocor) effectively raises HDL (high density lipoprotein) cholesterol ("good cholesterol") in people with coronary disease and low HDL levels. A combination of antioxidants (vitamin C, vitamin E, beta-carotene, and selenium) seems to blunt this rise in HDL, specifically the HDL-2 and apolipoprotein A1 fractions (7388,11537). HDL-2 is considered to be the most cardioprotective component of HDL (7388). However, vitamin E alone combined with a statin doesn't seem to decrease HDL levels (11286,11287). It isn't known whether the adverse effect on HDL is due to one of the other antioxidants or to the combination. It also isn't known whether it will occur in other patient populations, or when antioxidant vitamins are combined with other lipid-altering regimens. Monitor lipid levels closely in people taking lipid-altering drugs and antioxidant vitamin supplements, including vitamin E.
WARFARIN (Coumadin): Use of more than 400 IU of vitamin E per day with warfarin might prolong prothrombin time (PT), INR, and increase the risk of bleeding, due to interference with production of vitamin K-dependent clotting factors (91,92,93). At a dose of 1000 IU per day, vitamin E can antagonize vitamin K dependent clotting factors even in people not taking warfarin (11999). The risk for vitamin E interaction with warfarin is greater in people who are already deficient in vitamin K (91,92,93). Limited clinical evidence suggests that doses up to 1200 IU daily may be used safely by patients taking warfarin, but this may not be applicable in all patient populations (90). Monitor INR closely in patients taking warfarin who start vitamin E in doses of 400 IU or more.

Drug Influences on Nutrient Levels and Depletion

SOME DRUGS CAN AFFECT VITAMIN E LEVELS:
BILE ACID SEQUESTRANTS: Cholestyramine (Questran) and colestipol (Colestid) reduce absorption of dietary fat, so there is concern that they might reduce absorption of fat soluble vitamins, including vitamin E. Some studies suggest that the bile acid sequestrants lower vitamin E levels by 7% to 20%. But other studies have found no effect on vitamin E levels (4455,4456,4457,4460,4461,10566,10567). When decreases did occur, they were often in proportion to the lowering of LDL (on which vitamin E is transported), and did not fall below the lower limit of normal (5 micrograms/mL) with up to 2 years of treatment (4455,4457,4460,4461). Routine vitamin E supplements aren't necessary, but consider them for patients who take high doses of bile acid sequestrants for several years, or who have low serum vitamin E levels.
CARBAMAZEPINE (Tegretol): There is some evidence that children who take carbamazepine have serum vitamin E levels 9% to 26% lower than children with untreated epilepsy (11574,11575,11576,11577,11578). It's suggested more vitamin E is used to quench free radicals generated during metabolism of the anticonvulsant in the liver (11575,11577,11578). The clinical significance isn't clear. Vitamin E supplements don't seem to be harmful in children with epilepsy. They've been associated with either no effect on seizure control (11578), or improved seizure control (4671). Advise patients to maintain the recommended dietary intake of vitamin E. Consider supplements if plasma vitamin E levels are below 5 micrograms/mL.
CHEMOTHERAPY: Some chemotherapy drugs might reduce serum vitamin E levels, usually when used in high doses. These drugs include cisplatin, doxorubicin, etoposide, 5-fluorouracil, methotrexate, busulfan, cyclophosphamide, cytosine arabinoside, and thiotepa (98,10366,11588,11589). The clinical significance isn't clear, but there is some concern that low vitamin E levels might increase the risk of chemotherapy-associated toxicity (10366,11589). In some cases, vitamin E levels return to normal between chemotherapy cycles (11588). The role of supplements hasn't been established.
GEMFIBROZIL (Lopid): Data on the effects of gemfibrozil on vitamin E levels is conflicting. Some studies found decreased levels while others did not (4096,11548,11587). The clinical significance of any change isn't known.
MINERAL OIL: Mineral oil reduces absorption of all fat-soluble vitamins including vitamin E (4454,4495). However, serum vitamin E levels didn't change significantly in children who used mineral oil for up to four months (4496). Occasional or short-term use of mineral oil isn't likely to have a clinically significant effect on vitamin E levels.
ORLISTAT (Xenical): Orlistat decreases absorption of fat soluble vitamins including vitamin E (1727,1730). In most studies, vitamin E levels fall but remain within reference ranges, and only a few patients require supplements (9595,10570,10571). However, the manufacturer of orlistat recommends that all patients take a

multivitamin supplement containing all the fat soluble vitamins. Tell patients to separate the dose of the multivitamin by at least 2 hours from orlistat (1730).

PHENOBARBITAL: There is some evidence that children taking phenobarbital have serum vitamin E levels 9% to 26% lower than children with untreated epilepsy (11574,11575,11576,11577,11578). It's suggested that more vitamin E is used to quench free radicals generated during metabolism of the anticonvulsants in the liver (11575,11577,11578). The clinical significance isn't clear. Vitamin E supplements don't seem to be harmful in children with epilepsy. They've been associated with either no effect on seizure control (11578), or improved seizure control (4671). Advise patients to maintain the recommended dietary intake of vitamin E. Consider supplements if plasma vitamin E levels are low (below 5 micrograms/mL).

PHENYTOIN (Dilantin): There is some evidence that children who take phenytoin have serum vitamin E levels 9% to 26% lower than children with untreated epilepsy (11574,11575,11576,11577,11578). It's suggested that more vitamin E is used to quench free radicals generated during metabolism of the anticonvulsants in the liver (11575,11577,11578). The clinical significance isn't clear. Vitamin E supplements don't seem to be harmful in children with epilepsy. They've been associated with either no effect on seizure control (11578), or improved seizure control (4671). Advise patients to maintain the recommended dietary intake of vitamin E. Consider supplements if plasma vitamin E levels are low (below 5 micrograms/mL).

Interactions with Foods

FATTY FOODS: Fat is needed for vitamin E absorption, to allow solubilization and incorporation into micelles (4844). Therefore, it's been suggested that high-fat meals might increase vitamin E absorption. However, similar amounts of an alpha-tocopherol supplement were absorbed with a high-fat (36 grams) and a low-fat (3 grams) meal (6133). Tell patients that it isn't necessary to increase fat intake to ensure vitamin E absorption.

Interactions with Lab Tests

PROTHROMBIN TIME (PT)/INTERNATIONAL NORMALIZED RATIO (INR): High dose vitamin E might increase PT and INR in patients concurrently taking warfarin or other anticoagulant agents (4844). People with vitamin K deficiency are at greater risk for vitamin E interference with clotting and increased PT and INR (91,92,93).

TESTOSTERONE: Long-term vitamin E treatment can lower testosterone levels in older men (12876).

Interactions with Diseases or Conditions

ANGIOPLASTY: There is some concern that when antioxidant vitamins, including vitamin E, are used together they might have harmful effects in patients after angioplasty. A combination of beta-carotene 30,000 IU, vitamin C 500 mg, and vitamin E 700 IU daily started 30 days before angioplasty, and continued for 6 months thereafter, seems to prevent beneficial vascular remodeling in patients after angioplasty by promoting fibrosis at the site of angioplastic intervention (11000). Tell patients to avoid taking supplements of these vitamins immediately before and following angioplasty without the supervision of a healthcare professional.

BLEEDING DISORDERS: Vitamin E in doses of 1000 IU per day can decrease vitamin K-dependent clotting factors and may exacerbate bleeding disorders (11999); use with caution.

HEAD AND NECK CANCER: Some evidence suggests that patients with head and neck cancer who take all-rac-alpha-tocopherol (synthetic vitamin E) 400 IU/day during and for 3 years after radiation therapy have an increased risk of tumor recurrence or a second primary tumor compared to patients taking placebo (13055). Advise patients with head and neck cancer to avoid taking vitamin E supplements in doses of 400 IU/day or more.

RETINITIS PIGMENTOSA: All-rac-alpha-tocopherol (synthetic vitamin E) 400 IU has been associated with accelerated visual decline in people with retinitis pigmentosa. However, much lower doses (3 IU) does not seem to produce this effect (83).

VITAMIN K DEFICIENCY: Vitamin E might worsen coagulation defects in people with vitamin K deficiency (11999); use cautiously.

Dosage and Administration

ORAL: A typical dose for vitamin E deficiency in adults is RRR-alpha tocopherol (natural vitamin E) 60-75 IU per day (15). For tardive dyskinesia, most studies used RRR-alpha-tocopherol (natural vitamin E) 1600 IU daily (3942,3943,3944). For improving male fertility, vitamin E (type unspecified) 200-600 IU daily has been used (4693). For Alzheimer's disease, a typical dose is up to 2000 IU daily (4635). Combination therapy of donepezil (Aricept) 5 mg and vitamin E 1000 IU per day has been used for slowing cognitive decline in patients with Alzheimer's disease (11472). For early Huntington's chorea, one study used RRR-alpha-tocopherol (natural vitamin E) 3000 IU (4686). Rheumatoid arthritis pain has been treated with vitamin E (type unspecified) 600 IU twice daily (4723). For diabetic neuropathy, vitamin E (type unspecified) 900 mg daily has been used (4724). For preventing neurotoxicity caused by cisplatin, vitamin E (alpha-tocopherol) 300 mg daily has been used with each chemotherapy treatment and for up to 3 months after stopping cisplatin therapy (10366). For improving retinal blood flow and creatinine clearance in type 1 diabetes, vitamin E (type unspecified) 1800 IU has been used (4725). For enhancing immune function in elderly people, vitamin E (type unspecified) 100-200 mg daily has been used (4687,4689,4690). For preventing nitrate tolerance, vitamin E (type unspecified) 200 mg three times daily has been used (4705). For improving response to erythropoietin in people on dialysis, adults have received vitamin E (type unspecified) 300-500 mg daily, and children have received 15 mg per kg per day (4640,4641,4647). For children with focal segmental glomerulosclerosis, vitamin E (type unspecified) 200 IU has been used to reduce proteinuria (4675). For G6PD deficiency, vitamin E (type unspecified) 800 IU daily has been used (4682,4683). For children with familial hypercholesterolemia, vitamin E 200 IU, with vitamin C 250 mg, 2 times daily has been used for up to 6 months, with a National Cholesterol Education Program Step II (NCEP-II) diet (10352). For premenstrual syndrome (PMS), RRR-alpha-tocopherol (natural vitamin E) 400 IU daily has been used (4719). For treatment of dysmenorrhea, vitamin E 500 IU daily has been used starting 2 days before the menstrual period began and continuing through the first 3 days of bleeding (10361). For accelerating re-epithelialization following photoreactive keratectomy, 230 mg vitamin E (alpha-tocopheryl nicotinate) and vitamin A (retinol palmitate) 25,000 units have been used 3 times daily for 30 days, followed by twice daily for 2 months (348). In premature neonates, oral vitamin E (type unspecified) 15 to 30 IU per kg per day has been used to prevent retinopathy and bronchopulmonary dysplasia (15). For nocturnal leg cramps, vitamin E (type unspecified) 400 IU at bedtime has been used (4701). Radiation-induced fibrosis has been treated with vitamin E (type unspecified) 1000 IU daily in combination with pentoxifylline 800 mg (4672,4673). For beta-thalassemia, vitamin E 750 IU daily has been used (15). For preventing sunburn, RRR-alpha-tocopherol 1000 IU in combination with 2 grams of ascorbic acid has been used (4716). For preventing prostate cancer, vitamin E (type unspecified) 50-100 IU daily has been used (3959,4646,11303). For sickle cell anemia, 450 IU daily has been used (15). For preventing pre-eclampsia in high risk women, vitamin E 400 IU with vitamin C 1000 mg daily has been used (3236). The oral dose of palm oil tocotrienols (Palmvitee) used to reduce lipids is 200-260 mg per day (3238,3239,3240). For treatment of anemia of prematurity, 50 IU daily has been used for up to 6 weeks (10362).

The recommended daily intake of vitamin E for adults was recently increased. Both women and men should consume 15 mg of vitamin E from food (4844). This is equivalent to 22 IU of the RRR-alpha-tocopherol (natural vitamin E) or 33 IU of the all-rac-alpha-tocopherol (synthetic vitamin E) (4844). For Infants 7-12 months, 6 mg; Children 1-3 years, 7 mg; Children 4 -8 years, 11 mg; Older children and adults, 15 mg; Pregnant women, 15 mg; Lactating women, 19 mg (4844). The recommended upper dosage limit for all forms of supplemental alpha-tocopherol is 1000 mg (4844). Dosing for vitamin E can be confusing. Some sources and clinical studies choose to express vitamin E dosing based on mg or International Units (IU). Current guidelines have expressed recommended dietary allowance (RDA) and upper tolerable limits for vitamin E in milligrams. However most products are still labeled in IUs. It becomes important to understand how to convert between IUs and milligrams of vitamin E. The appropriate method for doing this depends of the formulation of vitamin E being considered and whether or not you are determining RDA or tolerable upper limit. For conversions related to RDA and to convert IUs of RRR-alpha-tocopherol (natural vitamin E) to milligrams of alpha-tocopherol, multiply by a factor of 0.67. For example, 30 IU of RRR-alpha-tocopherol is 20 mg RRR-alpha-tocopherol (natural vitamin E). To convert IUs of all-rac-tocopherol (synthetic vitamin E) to milligrams of alpha-tocopherol, multiply by a factor of 0.45. For example, 30 IU all-rac-tocopherol equals 13.5 mg of all-rac-alpha-tocopherol (synthetic vitamin E). The tolerable upper limit conversion factor for racemic and RRR-alpha tocopherol assumes that all isomers of vitamin E might contribute to toxicity so the conversion factor for all-rac-alpha tocopherol (synthetic vitamin E) is different. For conversions related to upper limit and to convert IUs all-rac-alpha tocopherol (synthetic vitamin E), multiply by a factor of 0.91. For example, 2000 IUs all-rac-alpha tocopherol (synthetic vitamin E) is equivalent to 1820 mg. The conversion factor of 0.67 is the same for calculating upper limit for RRR-alpha tocopherol (natural vitamin E). The same factors are used for either acetate or succinate salts because the content has been adjusted for the molecular weights of the salts (4844). Natural vitamin E (d-alpha-tocopherol) is similarly absorbed when taken with high-fat (36 grams) or low-fat (3 grams fat) meals (6133). Synthetic vitamin E (all-rac-alpha-tocopherol) should be taken with food for best absorption (6405).

TOPICAL: For treating chemotherapy extravasation, 10% vitamin E (type unspecified) has been used topically in combination with 90% dimethyl sulfoxide (DMSO) (4713).

Comments

The American Heart Association recommends obtaining antioxidants, including vitamin E, by eating a well-balanced diet high in fruits, vegetables, and whole grains rather than from supplements until more is known about the risks and benefits of supplementation (1440).

VITAMIN K

Also Known As

Vitamin K1: Methylphytyl Naphthoquinone, Phylloquinone, Phytomenadione, Phytonadione, 2-Methyl-3-Phytyl-1,4-Naphthoquinone.
Vitamin K2: Menaquinone, Menatetrenone, MK-1, MK-2, MK-4, MK-5, MK-6, MK-7, MK-8, MK-9, MK-10, MK-11, MK-12, MK-13.
Vitamin K3: Menadione, Menadione Sodium Bisulfite, 2-Methyl-1,4-Naphthoquinone.
Vitamin K4: Menadiol Diacetate, Menadiol Sodium Diphosphate, Menadiol Sodium Phosphate, Menadiolum Solubile Methylnaphthohydroquinone.
Vitamin K5: 4-Amino-2-Methyl-1-Naphthol.

Scientific Names

Phytonadione (K1); menaquinone (K2); menadione (K3); menadiol acetate (K4); 4-amino-2-methyl-1-naphthol (K5).

People Use This For

Orally, vitamin K1 (phytonadione) is used for preventing and treating hypoprothrombinemia caused by vitamin K deficiency; to counteract excessive doses of oral anticoagulants; to prevent hemorrhagic disease of the newborn; to treat hypoprothrombinemia induced by salicylates, sulfonamides, quinine, quinidine, or broad-spectrum antibiotic therapy; to prevent and treat osteoporosis; and relieve itching associated with primary biliary cirrhosis. Vitamin K2 (menaquinone) is used orally to treat osteoporosis and steroid-induced bone loss, and to lower total cholesterol in dialysis patients. Vitamin K3 (menadiol acetate) is used orally in combination with vitamin C for treating prostate and breast cancers. Vitamin K4 (menadiol sodium diphosphate) is used orally for treating hypoprothrombinemia resulting from impaired absorption or synthesis of vitamin K.

Topically, vitamin K1 (phytonadione) is used for eliminating spider veins, bruises, scars, stretch marks and burns, treating rosacea, speeding healing, and reducing postoperative bruising and swelling.

Parenterally, vitamin K1 (phytonadione) is used to prevent and treat hypoprothrombinemia caused by vitamin K deficiency, especially that associated with malabsorption syndromes or prolonged parenteral nutrition; to counteract excessive doses of oral anticoagulants; to prevent and treat hemorrhagic disease of the newborn; and to treat hypoprothrombinemia induced by salicylates, sulfonamides, quinine, quinidine, or broad-spectrum antibiotic therapy. Vitamin K4 (menadiol sodium diphosphate) is injected for treating hypoprothrombinemia resulting from impaired absorption or synthesis of vitamin K.

Safety

LIKELY SAFE ...when vitamin K1 is used orally or parenterally, and appropriately. Vitamin K1 (phytonadione) in oral and injectable form is an FDA-approved drug (15). A tolerable upper intake level for vitamin K has not been set (7135).

CHILDREN: LIKELY SAFE ...when vitamin K1 is used orally or parenterally and appropriately. Vitamin K1 (phytonadione) in oral and injectable form is FDA approved for use in children (15). A tolerable upper intake level for vitamin K in children has not been set (7135).

PREGNANCY AND LACTATION: LIKELY SAFE ...when used orally in amounts that do not exceed the recommended dietary allowance (RDA) (15). A tolerable upper intake level for vitamin K in pregnancy and lactation has not been set (7135).

Effectiveness

EFFECTIVE

Hemorrhagic disease. Vitamin K1 (phytonadione) administered orally can prevent hemorrhagic disease of newborns (15).

Hypoprothrombinemia. Vitamin K1 (phytonadione) used orally or parenterally can prevent and treat hypoprothrombinemia caused by vitamin K deficiency or induced by salicylates, sulfonamides, quinine, quinidine, or broad-spectrum antibiotic therapy (15).

Warfarin anticoagulation. Taking vitamin K1 (phytonadione) orally or parenterally will counteract excessive oral warfarin anticoagulation (15).

INSUFFICIENT RELIABLE EVIDENCE to RATE

Hypercholesterolemia. There is preliminary clinical evidence that vitamin K2 (menaquinone) might reduce serum cholesterol in patients on continuous ambulatory peritoneal dialysis with elevated cholesterol levels (59).

Osteoporosis. There is some preliminary clinical evidence that vitamin K2 (menaquinone) might help to treat osteoporosis by slowing bone loss and possibly decreasing fractures (54,55), but vitamin K2 (menaquinone) seems to be ineffective for preventing osteoporosis in postmenopausal women (58). Vitamin K2 (menaquinone) might also decrease steroid-induced osteoporosis (6799).

More evidence is needed to rate vitamin K for these uses.

Mechanism of Action

Vitamin K is a generic term for a group of related compounds. Vitamin K compounds have a common central ring structure, which results in similar activity. Varying side chains differentiate the compounds in terms of intestinal absorption, transport, tissue distribution, and bioavailability (57). Only small amounts of vitamin K are stored in body tissues (64). Vitamin K1 (phytonadione) is obtained from dietary sources, such as leafy green vegetables, broccoli, Brussels sprouts, plant oils, and margarine (57,7135). Vitamin K2 (menaquinone) is obtained from meat and cheeses and synthesis by bacteria in the colon (64). Vitamin K4 (menadiol sodium diphosphate) is a synthetic, water-soluble salt of vitamin K3 (menadione) and is converted to vitamin K3 in the liver. Bile salts are required for oral absorption of vitamin K1 (phytonadione) and vitamin K2 (menaquinone), but not vitamin K4 (menadiol sodium diphosphate) (15). Vitamin K is a coenzyme for the hepatic synthesis of blood coagulation factors II (prothrombin), VII (proconvertin), IX (Christmas factor or plasma thromboplastin component), and X (Stuart-Prower factor), and proteins C and S in the liver (57,7131,7135). Vitamin K is also involved in carboxylation of gamma-carboxyglutamate (Gla) proteins that facilitate binding of coagulation factors to platelets (57). In adequate doses, vitamin K reverses the inhibitory effects of coumarin and warfarin derivatives on the synthesis of clotting factors (15). Besides its classic role in blood coagulation, vitamin K is involved in other physiologic processes. People try supplementing vitamin K for osteoporosis because there is evidence that low vitamin K intake or serum levels are associated with reduced bone mineral density and fractures in people with osteoporosis (55,60,61,62,837,6193,7131). Osteopenia in elderly men seems to correlate with circulating levels of vitamins K and D (7132). Whether people taking vitamin K antagonists or oral anticoagulants are at increased risk of fracture is controversial (51,52,63,7134). Oral anticoagulants might have some effect on the bone mineral density of the radius of the arm, but no effect on the bones of the hip and back (7135). The most pronounced effects of vitamin K antagonists appear to be on rapidly growing bone (7133). Endogenous vitamin K is responsible for activation of osteocalcin (bone Gla protein) that provides calcium-attracting properties to bone (6797,7130). Supplementing vitamin K increases osteocalcin levels in postmenopausal women (56,6797,6798). Vitamin K is known to act as a cofactor for carboxylation of osteocalcin, leading to the suggestion that undercarboxylated osteocalcin (ucOC) levels could be used as an indicator of vitamin K nutritional status (7130,7131,7135). However, variations in testing methodology and inconsistent clinical findings indicate that the usefulness of ucOC levels is undecided (7135). Higher ucOC levels are seen in elderly women with hip fracture, and supplemental vitamin K1 normalizes ucOC levels and increases bone mass (7130). Preliminary evidence suggests that vitamin K may affect calcium balance, urinary calcium excretion, and the production of prostaglandin E2 and interleukin 6 (7131). Vitamin K might also play a role in prevention of atherosclerosis (53,57). Atherosclerosis has been linked to low serum vitamin K levels (53). Laboratory evidence suggests vitamin K supplementation might protect against atherosclerosis (65).

Adverse Reactions

Orally, oral vitamin K causes few adverse effects.
Intravenously, vitamin K can cause reactions that resemble hypersensitivity or anaphylaxis. These reactions are rare. It is unclear whether the adverse effect is caused by the drug or a component of the solution. There have been very rare cases of hyperbilirubinemia, particularly premature neonates, following large doses of vitamin K (15).

Interactions with Herbs & Other Dietary Supplements

COENZYME Q10: Coenzyme Q10 is chemically similar to vitamin K2 (menaquinone) and can have vitamin K-like effects, including antagonism of warfarin (2128,6048). Concomitant use of coenzyme Q10 and vitamin K might cause additive effects and increase the risk of clotting in people taking anticoagulants.
HERBS WITH CLOTTING POTENTIAL: Concomitant use of vitamin K with herbs that contain vitamin K can have additive effects and increase the risk of clotting in people using anticoagulants (57,7131,7135). Some of these herbs include alfalfa, cabbage, parsley, nettle, plantain, and others.
TIRATRICOL: Theoretically, tiratricol might antagonize the prothrombinemic effects of vitamin K by increasing catabolism of vitamin K-dependent clotting factors (15).
VITAMIN A: High doses of vitamin A antagonize effects of vitamin K in animals. However, it isn't known if this can occur in humans (7135,10560).
VITAMIN E: High doses of vitamin E (e.g., >800 units/day) can antagonize the effects of vitamin K, increasing the risk of bleeding in people who are taking warfarin or have low vitamin K intakes (93,7135). Vitamin E appears to reduce the absorption of vitamin K and to bind to vitamin K dependent enzymes, preventing their activity (7135,11512).

Interactions with Drugs

WARFARIN (Coumadin): Vitamin K antagonizes the effects of oral anticoagulants such as warfarin (Coumadin) (15). Excessive vitamin K intake, either from supplements or from changes in the diet, can reduce the anticoagulant effect (15).

Drug Influences on Nutrient Levels and Depletion

SOME DRUGS CAN AFFECT VITAMIN K LEVELS:
ANTIBIOTICS: Vitamin K produced by intestinal bacteria is absorbed from the ileum (4437,4439,9502). This contribution to overall vitamin K status is unclear, and likely varies (4439,7135). Destruction of vitamin K-producing bacteria by antibiotics can sometimes lead to vitamin K deficiency, prolonged clotting times, and bleeding (4439,9502,11513,11514,11515,11516). It's suggested that antibiotics such as cefamandole (Mandol) that are secreted into the bile in large amounts have a greater effect on vitamin K-producing bacteria (11514). Also, some cephalosporins have a methylthiotetrazole side chain that may interfere with vitamin K activity, directly inhibiting clotting factor production in the liver (4439,11516). These cephalosporins include cefamandole (Mandol), cefoperazone (Cefobid), cefmetazole (Zefazone), and cefotetan (Cefotan). This interaction is most likely to occur with prolonged antibiotic therapy (10 days or more) in people with poor dietary vitamin K intake (e.g., hospitalized patients with limited nutrient intake, or infants who have not built up stores of vitamin K) (11514,11515,11516). Vitamin K supplements aren't necessary for otherwise healthy people taking short courses of antibiotics.
ANTICONVULSANTS: When taken during pregnancy, anticonvulsants that induce hepatic enzymes (e.g., phenobarbital, phenytoin, carbamazepine) can reduce vitamin K levels in the fetus and increase the risk of intracranial hemorrhage soon after birth (11521,11522,11523,11524,11525). It's thought that liver enzyme induction by these drugs increases vitamin K metabolism (11521,11522,11523,11525). This has a significant effect on vitamin K levels in infants, who haven't built up stores of the vitamin (11525). Women who need these anticonvulsants during pregnancy should take vitamin K 10 to 20 mg/day orally for the last month of pregnancy, and the baby should receive vitamin K immediately after delivery (11522,11525). There's limited evidence that chronic carbamazepine or phenytoin therapy can cause subclinical reductions in vitamin K activity in adults. There are rare reports of prolonged clotting times and bleeding in people with additional risk factors for vitamin K deficiency, such as poor nutritional intake (10582,11533,11534). These anticonvulsants don't significantly affect vitamin K and clotting parameters in most children and adults.

BILE ACID SEQUESTRANTS: By reducing absorption of dietary fats, cholestyramine (Questran) and colestipol (Colestid) may also reduce absorption of fat-soluble vitamins such as vitamin K. Some studies have found no changes in vitamin K levels or prothrombin times with up to 2 years of cholestyramine or colestipol therapy (4455,4460,10566). However, there are a few case reports of hypoprothrombinemia and bleeding, usually in people with other risk factors (4458,11519). Monitor patients closely.
MINERAL OIL: Mineral oil can reduce absorption of fat soluble vitamins including vitamin K. Chronic use, both daily and intermittently, has been associated with prolonged clotting times (4495). Advise patients against regular or long-term use of mineral oil.
ORLISTAT (Xenical): Orlistat can reduce the absorption of some fat-soluble vitamins, although the extent of its effect on food-derived vitamin K hasn't been determined (1730). In healthy people, small decreases in plasma vitamin K levels can occur, but usually without any change in clotting times (9595,10570). However, prolonged clotting times might occur when orlistat is added to warfarin therapy. This may be due to both direct effects of orlistat on vitamin K absorption, and reduced intake of vitamin K-rich fatty foods that cause unpleasant side effects with orlistat (11520). The manufacturer of orlistat recommends that all patients take a multivitamin supplement containing all the fat soluble vitamins, separating the dosing time by at least 2 hours from orlistat (1730).
RIFAMPIN (Rifadin, Rimactane): There are occasional reports of vitamin K deficiency associated with rifampin therapy, leading to prolonged clotting times and, in one case, a cerebral bleed (11517,11518). Suggested mechanisms are reduced intestinal absorption of vitamin K, destruction of vitamin K-producing intestinal bacteria, and interference enzymes which regenerate vitamin K from its inactive metabolite. Symptomatic vitamin K deficiency is most likely to occur in people with poor dietary intake or other contributory factors (11517,11518). Monitor patients closely.

Interactions with Foods

None known.

Interactions with Lab Tests

17-HYDROXYCORTICOSTEROIDS: Might cause false increase in urine test results due to in vitro interference with Reddy method (275).
BILIRUBIN: Large amounts of vitamin K can increase serum bilirubin and test results in neonates or people with G-6-PD deficiency (275).
CALCIUM: Can reduce urinary calcium excretion and test results (275).
ERYTHROCYTES: Can decrease blood erythrocyte levels and test results (275).
HEMATOCRIT: Vitamin K3 and vitamin K4 might decrease hematocrit and test results, especially in people with G-6-PD deficiency (275).
HEMOGLOBIN: Vitamin K3 and vitamin K4 might decrease blood hemoglobin level and test results, especially in people with G-6-PD deficiency (275). Vitamin K can increase urine hemoglobin levels and test results (275).
HYDROXYPROLINE: Can decrease urine levels and test results (275).
LEUKOCYTES, PLATELETS: Vitamin K3 and vitamin K4 can decrease blood levels and test results due to pancytopenia (275).
OSTEOCALCIN: Can increase serum levels and test results in postmenopausal women (275).
PORPHYRINS: Can increase urine levels and test results (275).
PROTEIN: Can increase urine levels and test results (275).
PROTHROMBIN TIME (PT): Can decrease PT due to procoagulation effects of vitamin K (275).
UROBILINOGEN: May increase urine levels and test results due to hemolytic anemia in G-6-PD deficiency (275).

Interactions with Diseases or Conditions

HEMODIALYSIS: Excessive vitamin K intake has been associated with soft tissue calcification in patients receiving hemodialysis (11744).
LIVER DISEASE: Vitamin K is not effective for treating hypoprothrombinemia caused by severe liver disease. High doses may worsen coagulation defects (15).
REDUCED BILE SECRETION: People with decreased bile secretion may require co-administration of supplemental bile salts to ensure adequate vitamin K absorption (15).

Dosage and Administration

ORAL: There is no typical dose for vitamin K. Doses should be individualized and medically supervised (15). People with decreased bile secretion might require co-administration of supplemental bile salts to ensure adequate vitamin K absorption (15). Efficient absorption of vitamin K from the intestine requires dietary fat, although the amount needed for optimal absorption has not been determined (7135). For osteoporosis, clinical studies used vitamin K2 (menaquinone) 45 mg per day (54,55,59). Vitamin K2 (menaquinone) is not currently available in the US. There is insufficient information to determine recommended dietary allowances (RDAs) for vitamin K, so daily adequate intake (AI) recommendations have been formed: Infants 0-6 months, 2 mcg; Infants 6-12 months, 2.5 mcg; Children 1-3 years, 30 mcg; Children 4-8 years, 55 mcg; Children 9-13 years, 60 mcg; Adolescents 14-18 years (including those pregnant or lactating), 75 mcg; Men over 19 years, 120 mcg; Women over 19 years (including those pregnant and lactating), 90 mcg (7135).
PARENTERAL: Injectable vitamin K is an FDA-approved prescription product.

Comments
The name vitamin K comes from the German word Koagulationsvitamin (57). Vitamin K1 (phytonadione) is the only form of vitamin K available in the US. Vitamin K1 (phytonadione) is generally the preferred form of vitamin K, due to lower toxicity, rapid effects, greater potency, and superior efficacy in some indications, such as oral anticoagulant-induced hypoprothrombinemia (15,17). Vitamin K3 (menadione) is no longer used therapeutically because it has been linked to hepatic toxicity (7135). Vitamin K4 (menadiol), which was marketed as Synkayvite tablets and injection, is no longer available in the US. A specific form of vitamin K2 (menaquinone), MK-4, is an accepted treatment for osteoporotic osteopenia in Japan (57,58). An increased understanding of the physiologic role of vitamin K beyond blood coagulation has led some researchers to suggest that the guidelines for nutritional intake of vitamin K should be increased (57). The 2001 National Institute of Medicine Food and Nutrition Board slightly increased recommendations for adequate intake, but cited insufficient conclusive evidence for substantial increases (7135).

VITAMIN O

Also Known As
Liquid Oxygen, Stabilized Liquid Oxygen, Stabilized Oxygen.

Scientific Names
None.

People Use This For
Orally, vitamin O is used for increasing energy; improving immune function; eliminating bacteria, viruses, fungi and parasites; treating yeast infections; eliminating toxins and poisons from the body; and healing mouth sores. Vitamin O is also used for improving concentration, memory and alertness; calming the nervous system; easing depression, irritability, unexplained hostility and dizziness; relieving arthritis, muscle aches and pains, asthma, bronchial problems, emphysema and lung disease, sinus infection, diabetes, body weakness, chronic fatigue, and heart and circulation problems. Vitamin O has been used for obesity; constipation; gas and bloating; loss of appetite; poor digestion; stomach acid; premenstrual syndrome (PMS); menopause; sexual dysfunction; headaches; migraines; premature aging; rashes; skin problems; itchy ears, nose and anus; and tumors and deposit buildup.
Topically, it is used as an antiseptic.

Safety
There is insufficient reliable information available about the safety of vitamin O.
Pregnancy and Lactation: Insufficient reliable information available; avoid using.

Effectiveness
There is insufficient reliable information available about the effectiveness of vitamin O.

Mechanism of Action
The chemical formula of the oxygen compound in vitamin O is not disclosed in promotional information.
One supplier describes its product as a mildly buffered solution of deionized water and sodium chloride with a pH of 7.2 (5318). Another supplier lists magnesium peroxide as the active ingredient (5320). Still another claims the ingredients are secret (5321).

Adverse Reactions
None reported.

Interactions with Herbs & Other Dietary Supplements
None known.

Interactions with Drugs
None known.

Interactions with Foods
None known.

Interactions with Lab Tests
None known.

Interactions with Diseases or Conditions
None known.

Dosage and Administration

ORAL: In capsule form of unspecified strength, the dose is typically two capsules three times per day with water (5320). Various quantities, usually measured in drops, of solutions are recommended (e.g., 6 drops in 8 ounces of water, juice, milk, etc; 20 drops 3 times a day in a glass of water; 20 drops per gallon of water) (5321).

Comments

Although vitamin O is called liquid oxygen, remember that oxygen only exists in a liquid form at temperatures below -183 degrees C and that water, by weight, is about 88% oxygen (16). The FTC states that Vitamin O appears to be nothing more than saltwater (311).

In May 2000, Rose Creek Health Products agreed to pay $375,000 to settle Federal Trade Commission charges that they made false and unsubstantiated health claims in their advertising for "Vitamin O." The settlement prohibits the company from making unsupported representations that "Vitamin O" is an effective treatment for any life-threatening diseases, or that the effectiveness of "Vitamin O" is established by medical or scientific research or studies (5076).

WAFER ASH

Also Known As

Pickaway Anise, Prairie Grub, Scubby Trefoil, Stinking Prairie Bush, Swamp Dogwood, Three-Leaved Hop Tree, Wingseed.

Scientific Names

Ptelea trifoliata.
Family: Rutaceae.

Comments

At the date of publication, this product was not a common ingredient used in brand name supplements marketed to consumers. Details about this product are available in the online version of *Natural Medicines Comprehensive Database*. See www.naturaldatabase.com.

WAHOO

Also Known As

Arrowwood, Bitter Ash, Bleeding Heart, Burning Bush, Bursting Heart, Eastern Burning Bush, Fish Wood, Fusanum, Fusoria, Gadrose, Gatten, Gatter, Indian Arrowroot, Indian Arrowwood, Pegwood, Pigwood, Prickwood, Skewerwood, Spindle Tree, Strawberry Bush, Strawberry Tree.
CAUTION: See separate listing for Burning Bush.

Scientific Names

Euonymus atropurpureus.
Family: Celastraceae.

People Use This For

Orally, wahoo root bark is used orally for indigestion, to stimulate bile production, and as a laxative, diuretic, or tonic.

Safety

LIKELY UNSAFE ...when the bark, seeds or berries are used orally. Ingesting 36 berries can be fatal (18). The poisonous principle has not been identified (17).
PREGNANCY AND LACTATION: LIKELY UNSAFE ...when used orally (18).

Effectiveness

There is insufficient reliable information available about the effectiveness of wahoo.

Mechanism of Action

The applicable parts of wahoo are the trunk, root bark, and fruit. The seeds contain cardioactive steroids known as cardenolides. The trunk, root bark, and fruit also contain varied alkaloids, caffeine, and theobromine (18). Wahoo is thought to stimulate bile flow and have laxative effects. In larger amounts, it can affect the heart (18).

Adverse Reactions
Wahoo is considered poisonous (17). Several hours after ingesting wahoo seeds, people experience severe upset stomach, sometimes with bloody diarrhea, fever, shortness of breath, circulatory problems, signs of collapse, stupor increasing to unconsciousness, alternating with motor restlessness, severe tonic-clonic spasms with locked jaw muscles and coma.

Interactions with Herbs & Other Dietary Supplements
CARDIAC GLYCOSIDE-CONTAINING HERBS: Contraindicated; concomitant use increases the risk of cardiac glycoside toxicity. Cardiac glycoside-containing herbs include black hellebore, Canadian hemp roots, digitalis leaf, hedge mustard, figwort, lily-of-the-valley roots, motherwort, oleander leaf, pheasant's eye plant, pleurisy root, squill bulb leaf scales, and strophanthus seeds (19).
LICORICE/HORSETAIL: Theoretically, overuse/misuse of licorice rhizome or horsetail plant with wahoo increases the risk of cardiac toxicity due to potassium depletion (19).
OTHER CARDIOACTIVE HERBS: Avoid concomitant use with other cardioactive herbs due to unpredictability of effects and adverse effects. Other cardioactive herbs include calamus, cereus, cola, coltsfoot, devil's claw, European mistletoe, fenugreek, fumitory, ginger, Panax ginseng, hawthorn, white horehound, mate, parsley, quassia, scotch broom flower, shepherd's purse, and wild carrot (4).
STIMULANT LAXATIVE HERBS: Theoretically, use of stimulant laxatives can have additive effects and adverse effects. Use also increases the risk of cardiac toxicity due to potassium depletion. Stimulant laxative herbs include aloe dried leaf sap, blue flag rhizome, alder buckthorn, European buckthorn, butternut bark, cascara bark, castor oil, colocynth fruit pulp, gamboge bark exudate, jalap root, black root, manna bark exudate, podophyllum root, rhubarb root, senna leaves and pods, wild cucumber fruit (Ecballium elaterium), and yellow dock root (19).

Interactions with Drugs
DIGOXIN (Lanoxin): Contraindicated; using wahoo with digoxin increases risk of cardiac glycoside toxicity due to therapeutic duplication (2).
DIURETIC DRUGS: Theoretically, concomitant use of potassium-depleting diuretics with wahoo can increase the risk of cardiac glycoside toxicity due to potassium depletion (506). Some diuretics that can deplete potassium include chlorothiazide (Diuril), chlorthalidone (Thalitone), furosemide (Lasix), hydrochlorothiazide (HCTZ, Hydrodiuril, Microzide), and others.
MACROLIDE ANTIBIOTICS: Theoretically, concomitant use may increase risk of cardiac glycoside toxicity (17).
QUININE: Theoretically, concomitant use of quinine and wahoo might increase risk of cardiac toxicity (506).
STIMULANT LAXATIVES: Theoretically, use of stimulant laxatives with wahoo might have additive laxative effects, and can increase the risk of cardiac glycoside toxicity due to potassium depletion (2).
TETRACYCLINE ANTIBIOTICS: Theoretically, concomitant use may increase risk of cardiac glycoside toxicity (17).

Interactions with Foods
None known.

Interactions with Lab Tests
None known.

Interactions with Diseases or Conditions
GASTROINTESTINAL (GI) CONDITIONS: Theoretically, wahoo can increase gastric secretions and stimulate peristalsis. These effects might exacerbate GI irritation or inflammation (18).

Dosage and Administration
No typical dosage.

Comments
Avoid confusion with Euonymus europaeus (18).

WALLFLOWER

Also Known As
Beeflower, Gillyflower, Giroflier, Handflower, Keiri, Wallstock-Gillofer.

Scientific Names
Erysimum cheiri, synonym Cheiranthus cheiri.
Family: Brassicaceae/Cruciferae.

People Use This For
Orally, wallflower is used for cardiac insufficiency, to encourage menstruation, and as a laxative. It is also used orally for liver and gallbladder diseases because of its bitter taste.

Safety
POSSIBLY UNSAFE ...when used orally (18).
PREGNANCY AND LACTATION: POSSIBLY UNSAFE ...when used orally due to its possible toxic effects (18); avoid using.

Effectiveness
There is insufficient reliable information available about the effectiveness of wallflower.

Mechanism of Action
The applicable parts of wallflower are the above ground parts. It does contain cardiac glycosides, but they may be poorly absorbed when wallflower is taken orally (18).

Adverse Reactions
Poisoning may occur with parenteral administration, but is expected to be low with oral administration due to poor absorption of the cardiac glycosides (18).

Interactions with Herbs & Other Dietary Supplements
CARDIAC GLYCOSIDE-CONTAINING HERBS: Contraindicated, concomitant use may increase the risk of cardiac glycoside toxicity. Cardiac glycoside-containing herbs include black hellebore, Canadian hemp roots, digitalis leaf, hedge mustard, figwort, lily-of-the-valley roots, motherwort, oleander leaf, pheasant's eye plant, pleurisy root, squill bulb leaf scales, and strophanthus seeds (19).
CHINCHONA and EPHEDRA: Use with wallflower seed may increase risk of toxicity (19).
LICORICE/HORSETAIL: Theoretically, overuse/misuse of licorice rhizome or horsetail plant with cardiac glycoside-containing herbs increases the risk of cardiac toxicity due to potassium depletion (19).
OTHER CARDIOACTIVE HERBS: Avoid concomitant use with other cardioactive herbs due to unpredictability of effects and adverse effects. Other cardioactive herbs include calamus, cereus, cola, coltsfoot, devil's claw, European mistletoe, fenugreek, fumitory, ginger, Panax ginseng, hawthorn, white horehound, mate, parsley, quassia, scotch broom flower, shepherd's purse, and wild carrot (4).
STIMULANT LAXATIVE HERBS: Theoretically, overuse or misuse of stimulant laxatives with cardiac glycoside-containing herbs increases the risk of cardiac toxicity due to potassium depletion. Stimulant laxative herbs include aloe dried leaf sap, blue flag rhizome, alder buckthorn, European buckthorn, butternut bark, cascara bark, castor oil, colocynth fruit pulp, gamboge bark exudate, jalap root, black root, manna bark exudate, podophyllum root, rhubarb root, senna leaves and pods, wild cucumber fruit (Ecballium elaterium), and yellow dock root (19).

Interactions with Drugs
CALCIUM SUPPLEMENTS: Calcium supplements may enhance the therapeutic effects of wallflower (18).
CORTICOSTEROIDS: Use of corticosteroids may cause electrolyte depletion and increase risk of cardiac glycoside toxicity (19).
DIGOXIN (Lanoxin): Contraindicated; therapeutic duplication increases risk of cardiac glycoside toxicity (2).
DIURETIC DRUGS: Theoretically, concomitant use of potassium-depleting diuretics and wallflower can increase the risk of cardiac glycoside toxicity due to potassium depletion (506). Some diuretics that can deplete potassium include chlorothiazide (Diuril), chlorthalidone (Thalitone), furosemide (Lasix), hydrochlorothiazide (HCTZ, Hydrodiuril, Microzide), and others.
STIMULANT LAXATIVES: Overuse or misuse of stimulant laxatives may cause electrolyte depletion and increase the risk of cardiac glycoside toxicity (19).
QUINIDINE: Cardiac medications, including quinidine may increase the risk of cardiac glycoside toxicity; contraindicated (18).
QUININE: Taking quinine with wallflower may increase the risk of cardiac glycoside toxicity (18).

Interactions with Foods
None known.

Interactions with Lab Tests
None known.

Interactions with Diseases or Conditions
CARDIAC CONDITIONS: Wallflower may cause arrhythmias (18); use with caution.

Dosage and Administration
No typical dosage.

Comments
Canadian hemp is also known as wallflower (Cheiranthus cheiri). Wallflower is considered obsolete as a medicinal herb (18).

WATER AVENS

Also Known As
Chocolate Root, Cure All, Indian Chocolate, Throat Root, Water Chisch, Water Flower.

Scientific Names
Geum rivale.
Family: Rosaceae.

Comments
At the date of publication, this product was not a common ingredient used in brand name supplements marketed to consumers. Details about this product are available in the online version of *Natural Medicines Comprehensive Database*. See www.naturaldatabase.com.

WATER DOCK

Also Known As
None.

Scientific Names
Rumex aquaticus.
Family: Polygonaceae.

People Use This For
Orally, water dock is used for "blood purification" and constipation.
Topically, water dock is used for mouth ulcers, skin sores, scorbutic conditions, and for cleaning the teeth.
In foods, water dock leaves are used in salads.

Safety
There is insufficient reliable information available about the safety of water dock.
Pregnancy and Lactation: Insufficient reliable information is available; avoid using.

Effectiveness
There is insufficient reliable information available about the effectiveness of water dock.

Mechanism of Action
The applicable part of water dock is the dried root. Water dock contains anthracene derivatives, oxalic acid and calcium oxalate, and tannins (18), an essential oil, fat, protein, quercitrin, starch, and tannin. Water dock is considered to have digestive properties (18).

Adverse Reactions
None reported.

Interactions with Herbs & Other Dietary Supplements
CALCIUM, IRON, ZINC: Concurrent use might decrease mineral absorption. Water dock contains oxalate (7,12), which can bind multivalent metal ions in the gastrointestinal tract and decrease mineral absorption.

Interactions with Drugs
None known.

Interactions with Foods
CALCIUM, IRON, ZINC: Concurrent use might decrease mineral absorption from foods. Water dock contains oxalate (7,12), which can bind multivalent metal ions in the gastrointestinal tract and decrease mineral absorption.

Interactions with Lab Tests
None known.

Interactions with Diseases or Conditions

COAGULATION DISORDERS: Oxalate constituents can alter serum calcium concentrations, possibly decreasing coagulation time (12).

KIDNEY DISEASE: Use with caution in individuals with a history of kidney stones. Insoluble oxalate crystals may form in the kidneys, causing further damage (12).

Dosage and Administration

ORAL: Water dock is used orally or topically as a liquid extract or as a powder.

WATER FENNEL

Also Known As

Fine Leaf Water Dropwort, Horsebane, Water Dropwort, Water Hemlock.
CAUTION: See separate listing for Fennel and Hemlock Water Dropwort.

Scientific Names

Oenanthe aquatica.

Comments

At the date of publication, this product was not a common ingredient used in brand name supplements marketed to consumers. Details about this product are available in the online version of *Natural Medicines Comprehensive Database.* See www.naturaldatabase.com.

WATER GERMANDER

Also Known As

None.

Scientific Names

Teucrium scordium.
Family: Lamiaceae/Labiatae.

People Use This For

Orally, water germander is used for bronchial asthma, diarrhea, fever, intestinal parasites, hemorrhoids, and festering and inflamed wounds.

Safety

There is insufficient reliable information available about the safety of water germander.
Pregnancy and Lactation: Insufficient reliable information is available; avoid using.

Effectiveness

There is insufficient reliable information available about the effectiveness of water germander.

Mechanism of Action

The applicable parts of water germander are the above ground parts. There is insufficient reliable information available about the possible mechanism of action and active ingredients.

Adverse Reactions

None reported.

Interactions with Herbs & Other Dietary Supplements

None known.

Interactions with Drugs

None known.

Interactions with Foods

None known.

Interactions with Lab Tests

None known.

Interactions with Diseases or Conditions
None known.

Dosage and Administration
ORAL/TOPICAL: A typical dose is four teaspoons (7.2 grams) above ground parts per day, as a prepared tea (18). The same preparation can be used internally or externally (18).

Comments
There is very little scientific information about this product. Our staff is continually analyzing the available information on natural medicines and will add data here as it becomes available.

WATER HEMLOCK

Also Known As
Beaver Poison, Brook-Tongue, Carotte a Moreau, Children's Bane, Cique Vireuse, Cowbane, Death-of-Man, European Water Hemlock, False Parsley, Fever Root, Mockeel Root, Muskrat Weed, Musquash Root, Poison Parsnip, Snake Weed, Snakeroot, Spotted Cowbane, Spotted Hemlock, Spotted Parsley, Wasser-Schierling, Wild Carrot, Wild Dill, Wild Parsnip.
CAUTION: See separate listings for Hemlock, Hemlock Spruce, and Hemlock Water Dropwort.

Scientific Names
Cicuta virosa, synonym Cicuta mackenzieana; Cicuta maculata; Cicuta douglasii, synonyms Cicuta californica, Cicuta vagans, Sium douglasii; Cicuta occidentalis; Cicuta bulbifera.
Family: Apiaceae/Umbelliferae.

People Use This For
Orally, water hemlock is used for migraine headaches, painful menstruation, and worm infestations.
Topically, water hemlock is used for inflammation of the skin.

Safety
UNSAFE ...when used orally. Water hemlock is considered to be the most poisonous plant growing in North America (6349). Intoxication can result from chewing or ingestion any part of the plant (6348). The usual lethal adult dose is one rhizome (6347) or a 2-3 cm portion of root (6349). ...when used topically (6348). Death can result when hemlock is applied topically (6348,6349).
CHILDREN: UNSAFE ...when used orally or topically (6347,6351,6355). Fatalities have resulted when hollow stems of water hemlock are used as whistles (6347), when hemlock is ingested (6355), or when hemlock has been applied topically (6351).
PREGNANCY AND LACTATION: UNSAFE ...when used orally or topically. Water hemlock is toxic (6348,6349); avoid using.

Effectiveness
There is insufficient reliable information available about the effectiveness of water hemlock.

Mechanism of Action
All parts of water hemlock at all stages of growth, including leaves and stems, are considered poisonous and can be lethal if ingested (6346,6349). The freshly harvested root is considered most toxic in early spring (6346). All plant parts contain the toxin cicutoxin, but it is especially concentrated in the root (6350). Cicutoxin is a highly unsaturated aliphatic alcohol (6346,6347,6348) that is found in a yellow oily liquid of roots and stems (6354). Water hemlock poisoning consists of cholinergic effects such as salivation, perspiration, diaphoresis, abdominal discomfort, and nausea (6350); and occurs almost immediately after ingestion (6346). Convulsions, seizures, and spastic-tonic movements follow (6346,6350,6353) which are believed to be due to cholinergic stimulation of the brain stem (reticular formation) or the basal ganglia (6346,6350). Narrow pupils, most likely due to the cholinergic effects of the toxin, and dilated pupils, due to brain hypoxia or ischemia, have been reported (6346). Increases in creatine phosphokinase occur indicating the severity of muscle rigors, rigidity and convulsions, and increases in serum lactic dehydrogenase also may occur that indicate possible liver or skeletal muscle damage (6347). Cicutoxin can also be absorbed through the skin (6349). Death usually results from cyanosis, exhaustion, and respiratory paralysis (6347,6348,6350).

Adverse Reactions
Orally, toxic effects occur immediately (6350). Prompt medical attention is advised after ingestion of water hemlock (6346). Death can result 15 minutes to 8 hours after ingestion (6351,6353). The usual lethal adult dose is one rhizome (6347) or a 2-3 cm portion of root (6349). The first symptoms of water hemlock poisoning are nausea, vomiting, wheezing, salivation, sweating, dizziness, abdominal pain, flushing, lethargy, delirium, and defecation (6346,6347,6349,6350,6351). These symptoms are followed by respiratory distress, muscle spasms, restless

movements, bronchial secretions, convulsions, mydriasis, miosis, eyeball protrusion, glycosuria, proteinuria, abnormal EEG, metabolic acidosis, hypertension, supraventricular tachycardia, hypotension, bradycardia, muscle rigidity, tremors, grinding of teeth, tonic-clonic movements, grand-mal seizures, rhabdomyolysis, acute renal failure, cerebral edema, unconsciousness, and coma (6346,6347,6348,6349,6350,6351,6353). Elevated serum CPK, LDH, AST and alkaline phosphatase levels also occur (6346). Death can occur during convulsions and from respiratory paralysis, exhaustion, or heart failure (6347,6348,6350).

Interactions with Herbs & Other Dietary Supplements
None known.

Interactions with Drugs
None known.

Interactions with Foods
None known.

Interactions with Lab Tests
SERUM LIVER ENZYMES: Ingestion of water hemlock can cause elevations in serum liver enzymes such as lactic dehydrogenase (LDH), aspartate aminotransferase (AST), and alkaline phosphatase (6346,6347).
SERUM MUSCLE ENZYMES: Ingestion of water hemlock can cause elevations in serum muscle enzymes such as creatine phosphokinase (CPK) and lactic dehydrogenase (LDH isoenzyme fraction 5) levels (6346,6347).

Interactions with Diseases or Conditions
None known.

Dosage and Administration
No typical dosage.

Comments
Water hemlock is found in marshy, swampy areas of meadows, along banks of streams, pools, and rivers. Accidental ingestion usually occurs when water hemlock is mistaken for edible plants such as artichokes, celery, sweet potatoes, sweet anise, and wild parsnip (6346). There are approximately 20 species of water hemlock (Cicuta) and most are found in North America (6339). The most commonly encountered are Cicuta maculata in southern Missouri and the eastern US, Cicuta vagans in the Pacific Northwest, Cicuta bulbifera in the Middle Northwest, Cicuta occidentalis in the Rocky Mountain region (6351) and Cicuta virosa which is found throughout the US and is known as the common European water hemlock (6346,6347,6348). All species of water hemlock are considered poisonous (6351). The rhizome has an extremely unpleasant smell and is the most toxic portion of the plant.

WATER PLANTAIN

Also Known As
Alisma, Mad-Dog Weed, Plantain.
CAUTION: See separate listings for Great Plantain, Buckhorn Plantain, Blond Psyllium, Black Psyllium.

Scientific Names
Alisma plantago-aquatica; Alisma plantago-aquatica subsp. orientale, synonyms Alisma orientale, Alisma plantago-aquatica var. orientale.
Family: Alismataceae.

People Use This For
Orally, water plantain is used for bladder and urinary tract diseases.

Safety
POSSIBLY UNSAFE ...when used orally (18).
PREGNANCY AND LACTATION: POSSIBLY UNSAFE ...when used orally due to its toxic potential (18); avoid using.

Effectiveness
There is insufficient reliable information available about the effectiveness of water plantain.

Mechanism of Action
The applicable part of water plantain is the root/rhizome. The fresh rootstock is thought to be poisonous. It contains the cyanogenic chlorogenic acid sulfate (18).

Adverse Reactions
None reported.

Interactions with Herbs & Other Dietary Supplements
None known.

Interactions with Drugs
None known.

Interactions with Foods
None known.

Interactions with Lab Tests
None known.

Interactions with Diseases or Conditions
None known.

Dosage and Administration
No typical dosage.

Comments
Water plantain rootstock is said to be bitter in taste (18). It sounds similar to the common and species names of great plantain, and buckhorn plantain. Be careful not to confuse them.

WATERCRESS

Also Known As
Agrião, Berro, Berro Di Agua, Brunnenkresse, Crescione Di Fonte, Cresson au Poulet, Cresson D'eau, Cresson De Fontaine, Indian Cress, Mizu-Garashi, Nasilord, Nasturtii herba, Oranda-Garashi, Scurvy Grass, Selada-Air, Tall Nasturtium, Wasserkresse, Waterkres.
CAUTION: See separate listings for Nasturtium and Scurvy Grass.

Scientific Names
Nasturtium officinale, synonyms Radicula nasturtium, Rorippa nasturtium, Sisymbrium nasturtium.
Family: Brassicaceae/Cruciferae.

People Use This For
Orally, watercress is used for respiratory tract mucous membrane inflammation, coughs, bronchitis, as a spring tonic, an appetite stimulant, improving digestion, alopecia, cancer, flu, goiter, polyps, scurvy, tuberculosis, gland tumors, as an abortifacient, aphrodisiac, bactericide, laxative, restorative, stimulant, and anthelmintic.
Topically, watercress is used for arthritis, rheumatoid arthritis, earache, eczema, scabies, and warts.
In foods, watercress is widely used in leaf salads and as a culinary spice.

Safety
LIKELY SAFE ...when consumed in amounts commonly found in foods.
POSSIBLY SAFE ...when used orally in medicinal amounts, short-term (2,8,12).
POSSIBLY UNSAFE ...when used orally in excessive amounts (8,12,19). ...when used orally long-term (8,12,19).
Watercress can cause gastric mucosal irritation (8,12) or damage (19).
There is insufficient reliable information available about the safety of watercress for its other uses.
CHILDREN: LIKELY UNSAFE ...when used orally in medicinal amounts; avoid using in children younger than 4 years old (12,19).
PREGNANCY: LIKELY UNSAFE ...when used in medicinal amounts. Watercress might stimulate menstruation or have abortifacient effects (19).
LACTATION: Insufficient reliable information available; avoid using.

Effectiveness
There is insufficient reliable information available about the effectiveness of watercress.

Mechanism of Action
The applicable parts of watercress are the above ground parts. Watercress is thought to have antibiotic and diuretic activity (18). The above ground parts contain mustard oil (18), vitamin C, and beta-carotene, and vitamin K (19). Mustard oil is believed responsible for diuretic effects and gastrointestinal irritation after consumption of large

amounts of watercress (18). The constituent, phenethyl isothiocyanate, released by chewing watercress, might inhibit metabolic activation of a lung carcinogens (4019).

Adverse Reactions
Orally, large amounts of watercress can cause gastrointestinal irritation (18). Theoretically, excessive or prolonged use might cause kidney damage (19).

Interactions with Herbs & Other Dietary Supplements
None known.

Interactions with Drugs
CHLORZOXAZONE (Parafon Forte, Paraflex): Concomitant use with watercress may potentiate the effects of chlorzoxazone due to reduced metabolism and elimination (4018).
WARFARIN (Coumadin): Theoretically, consuming large amounts of watercress with high vitamin K content might antagonize the anticoagulant effects of warfarin (11285).

Interactions with Foods
None known.

Interactions with Lab Tests
INTERNATIONAL NORMALIZED RATIO (INR)/PROTHROMBIN TIME (PT): Theoretically, watercress might decrease coagulation test results due to high vitamin K content (11285).

Interactions with Diseases or Conditions
GASTRIC OR DUODENAL ULCERS: Watercress is contraindicated in people with gastric or duodenal ulcers (12,19).
INFLAMMATORY KIDNEY DISEASES: Watercress is contraindicated in people with inflammatory kidney disease (12,19).

Dosage and Administration
No typical dosage.

Comments
Avoid confusing watercress with nasturtium (Tropaeolum majus).

WHEAT BRAN

Also Known As
Bran, Cereal Fiber, Dietary Fiber.
CAUTION: See separate listings for Oat Bran and Rice Bran.

Scientific Names
Triticum aestivum.
Family: Poaceae/Gramineae.

People Use This For
Orally, wheat bran is used as a supplemental source of dietary fiber for preventing colon diseases (including cancer), preventing gastric cancer, treating irritable bowel syndrome (IBS), reducing the risk of hemorrhoids and hiatal hernia, hypercholesterolemia, hypertension, reducing the risk of breast cancer and gallbladder disease, and type 2 diabetes.

Safety
LIKELY SAFE ...when used orally and appropriately (10326,10328).
PREGNANCY AND LACTATION: LIKELY SAFE ...when used orally (5).

Effectiveness
POSSIBLY EFFECTIVE

Constipation. Taking wheat bran orally seems to be effective for treating mild constipation and restoring normal bowel function. Wheat bran seems to increase stool output and improve colonic transit, but does not soften normal-viscosity stool (6265,11004,11116,11117).
Gastric cancer. Epidemiologic evidence suggests that dietary cereal fiber can reduce the risk of gastric cancer (10435).
Hemorrhoids. Taking wheat bran orally seems to be effective for reducing the risk of hemorrhoids (11118,11119).
Hypertension. Taking wheat bran orally seems to produce modest, but significant reductions in systolic,

diastolic, and mean arterial blood pressures (4963,11463).

Irritable bowel syndrome (IBS). Taking wheat bran orally may reduce abdominal pain and improve bowel function in patients with mild to moderate IBS. However, it may not be as effective as guar gum (10326).

POSSIBLY INEFFECTIVE

Colorectal cancer. Several large well-designed studies showed that fiber, including wheat-bran fiber, does not prevent the recurrence of colorectal adenomas, despite earlier evidence that suggested a beneficial effect (160,4819,4820,4821).

Diabetes. Taking wheat bran orally does not seem to consistently improve indices of blood sugar control. It does not improve blood pressure, lipids, clotting factors, homocysteine, C-reactive protein, or other factors associated with cardiovascular disease in patients with type 2 diabetes (6266,10328).

There is insufficient reliable information available about the effectiveness of wheat bran for its other uses.

Mechanism of Action

The applicable part of wheat bran is the outer hull of the grain, which is largely composed of insoluble fiber (4963). The laxative effect of wheat bran is dependent on particle size; larger particles have a greater laxative effect than smaller particles (6265). Wheat bran has negligible water-holding capacity and no stool softening effect in people with normal stools (6265). Wheat bran increases colonic transit time, stool output, and bowel movement frequency (6265,11463). Preliminary evidence suggests consumption of wheat bran might move the digestion site of foods from the proximal to distal portion of the colon (375). In the distal colon, butyrate produced from digestion of grains and starches reduces ammonia produced by fermentation of foods high in fat and sugar, possibly preventing cell damage and reducing the risk of colon cancer (375).

Adverse Reactions

Orally, wheat bran may cause flatulence and GI discomfort, especially with initial use. One carefully controlled study designed to look at side effects noted no increase in GI symptoms in subjects taking 20 to 40 grams of wheat bran per day (6265).

Interactions with Herbs & Other Dietary Supplements

None known.

Interactions with Drugs

DIGOXIN (Lanoxin): Theoretically, wheat bran may interfere with absorption (156).

Interactions with Foods

IRON: Wheat bran inhibits dietary iron absorption (156).

Interactions with Lab Tests

BLOOD PRESSURE: Wheat bran might lower blood pressure and blood pressure readings in individuals with hypertension (4963).

Interactions with Diseases or Conditions

None known.

Dosage and Administration

ORAL: For laxative effects, 20 to 25 grams per day has been used (6265,11004,11116,11117). It appears that 40 grams per day is no more effective than 20 grams per day (6265). For the treatment of irritable bowel syndrome (IBS), wheat bran 30 grams per day has been used for up to 12 weeks (10326). For hypertension, 3-6 grams whole-wheat flour, wheat flakes, and brown rice, combined with a National Cholesterol Education Program (NCEP) step 1 diet has been used (11463).

Adequate intake (AI) levels for dietary fiber intake per day have been set. For children 1 to 3 years, the AI is 19 grams and 4 to 8 years, 25 grams. For boys 9 to 13 years, the AI is 31 grams, and 38 grams for boys 14 to 18 years. For girls 9 to 18 years, the AI is 26 grams. For men 19 to 50 years, the AI is 38 grams, and 30 grams for men older than 51 years. For women 19 to 50 years, the AI is 25 grams, and 21 grams for women older than 51 years. For pregnant women, the AI is 28 grams, and 29 grams for lactating women (11120). AI for children less than one year has not been set. A tolerable upper intake levels (UL) for fiber has not been set (11120).

Comments

Wheat bran is the outer grain hull of wheat (Triticum aestrivum).

WHEATGRASS

Also Known As

Agropyron, Couchgrass, Cutch, Dog Grass, Durfa Grass, Graminis rhizoma, Quack Grass, Quitch Grass, Scotch Quelch, Triticum, Twitchgrass, Witch Grass.

Scientific Names

Elytrigia repens, synonyms Agropyron repens, Agropyron firmum, Elymus repens, Triticum firmum, Triticum repens.
Family: Poaceae/Gramineae.

People Use This For

Orally, wheatgrass is primarily used as a concentrated source of nutrients. It is used therapeutically for increasing hemoglobin production, improving blood sugar disorders such as diabetes, preventing tooth decay, improving wound healing, and preventing bacterial infections. It is also used orally for removing deposits of drugs, heavy metals, and carcinogens from the body and neutralizing toxins, removing toxins from the liver and removing toxins from the blood stream. Additionally, wheatgrass is used orally for preventing gray hair, reducing high blood pressure, improving digestion, and blocking intestinal cholesterol absorption. It is used orally to treat cystitis, urethritis, prostatitis, benign prostatic hypertrophy (BPH), renal calculus (kidney stones), and in "irrigation therapy" (use of a mild diuretic and copious fluid intake to increase urine flow). It is also used orally for common cold, cough and bronchitis, fever and colds, inflammation of mouth and pharynx, tendency to infection, gout, liver disorders, ulcerative colitis, cancer, rheumatic pain, and chronic skin problems.
Wheatgrass is used for cancer and arthritis in alternative treatment programs.
In foods and beverages, wheatgrass extracts are used as a flavoring component.

Safety

LIKELY SAFE ...when consumed in amounts commonly found in foods (5286).
POSSIBLY SAFE ...when wheatgrass juice is taken orally, and appropriately, in medicinal amounts. Wheatgrass has been used safely for up to one month (11165).
There is insufficient reliable information available about the long-term safety of wheatgrass when used medicinally.
PREGNANCY AND LACTATION: Insufficient reliable information available; avoid using.

Effectiveness

INSUFFICIENT RELIABLE EVIDENCE to RATE

Ulcerative colitis. There is some evidence that wheatgrass juice taken orally might help active distal ulcerative colitis. Freshly extracted wheatgrass juice might reduce overall disease activity, and the severity of rectal bleeding (11165). More evidence is needed to rate wheatgrass for this use.

Mechanism of Action

The applicable parts of wheatgrass are the above ground parts, root, and rhizome. A constituent of wheatgrass, agropyrene, seems to have antibiotic activity (7162). The constituent, apigenin, may have antioxidant and anti-inflammatory activity, which might explain its use for ulcerative colitis (11165). Wheatgrass contains large amounts of chlorophyll. High-chlorophyll beverages are sometimes included in diets purported to treat diseases such as cancer and rheumatoid arthritis (5286,6982). It also contains vitamin A, vitamin C, and vitamin E, iron, calcium, magnesium and amino acids.
Wheatgrass juice is a popular health drink. It is thought to possess therapeutic qualities only when fresh and consumed on an empty stomach immediately after extraction. But there is no research to determine the effect of freshness on effectiveness or bioavailability of its constituents (11165).

Adverse Reactions

Orally, wheatgrass can cause nausea, anorexia, and constipation (11165).

Interactions with Herbs & Other Dietary Supplements

None known.

Interactions with Drugs

None known.

Interactions with Foods

None known.

Interactions with Lab Tests

None known.

Interactions with Diseases or Conditions

None known.

Dosage and Administration

ORAL: For treating ulcerative colitis, 100 mL of wheatgrass juice daily for 1 month has been used (11165).

WHEY PROTEIN

Also Known As

Bovine Whey Protein Concentrate.
CAUTION: See separate listing for Branched Chain Amino Acids.

Scientific Names

None.

People Use This For

Orally, whey protein is used as a food supplement, as an alternative to milk for people with lactose intolerance, for protein allergy, asthma, hyperlipidemia, obesity and weight loss, replacing or supplementing milk-based infant formulas, atopic disease in infants, treating metastatic carcinoma, colon cancer, and reversing weight loss and increasing glutathione (GSH) in people with HIV disease.

Safety

LIKELY SAFE ...when quality products are used orally and appropriately. There are no reports of toxicity in clinical trials (4926,4927,4929,4930,4932,4935,4936,4941).
PREGNANCY AND LACTATION: LIKELY SAFE ...when quality products are used orally and appropriately (4929).

Effectiveness

POSSIBLY EFFECTIVE

Atopic disease. Taking whey protein orally seems to decrease the risk of developing atopic disease in infants genetically predisposed to allergy (4927,4929).

HIV/AIDS-related weight loss. Taking whey protein orally seems to help reverse weight loss in patients with HIV (4926,4932,4935,4936).

INSUFFICIENT RELIABLE EVIDENCE to RATE

Cancer. There is preliminary evidence that taking whey protein orally might help produce tumor regression in some patients with metastatic carcinoma (4930). More evidence is needed to rate whey protein for this use.

Mechanism of Action

Whey is a by-product of cheese manufacturing which contains carbohydrates including lactose; minerals including calcium, sodium, phosphorus, and potassium (2640); proteins including alpha-lactalbumin, beta-lactoglobulin, lactoferrin, serum albumin, lysozyme, and immunoglobulins A, G, and M (2640); and cysteine (4937).
Whey protein may vary in the amount and activity of immunoglobulins and other proteins present, depending on the production methods used (2640). Whey protein typically contains 24% branched chain amino acids which are readily oxidized as an energy source during stress. Whey protein is also a source of gamma-glutamylcysteine, a precursor of glutathione (GSH), which acts as an intracellular antioxidant (2640). GSH is depleted by oxidative stress, which occurs during infections, trauma, or major surgery (2640). Low levels of GSH in patients with HIV have been associated with impaired T-cell function (2640). A specific whey protein formulation (Immunocal) might enhance the reduced-to-oxidized glutathione ratio (GSH/GSSG) in lymphocytes, a marker of oxidative stress in reactive oxygen species (ROS)-mediated diseases, including AIDS-related wasting (1382). Whey products also has anti-HIV and anti-apoptotic effects in vitro (4937).
In patients with HIV infection, whey protein increases body weight (4926,4935,4936), elevates GSH in mononuclear cells (4926), increases albumin, increases CD4 and CD8 counts (4935), and reduces diarrhea (4932,4936).
Whey protein also has immunomodulating activity (4939,4940). It's thought that immunoglobulins in whey protein may bind antigens in the gut and prevent their absorption (2640). Whey protein formulations can be produced that are high in specific immunoglobulins. For example, whey proteins derived from the milk of cows infected with Cryptosporidium may be a rich source of antibodies against Cryptosporidium (2640). These types of whey protein formulations can reduce gastrointestinal Cryptosporidium parvum infection in animal models (4934).
Some researchers are interested in using whey protein to prevent cancer. It's thought that whey protein might prevent cancer by providing GSH substrates and increasing tissue GSH levels (4943). Whey protein might exert antitumor effects by depleting tumor cells of GSH, making them more vulnerable to chemotherapy (2640,4930). Animal models of cancer indicated that whey protein diets might protect against certain cancers (3976,4928,4933).
Researchers are also interested in whey protein for cardiovascular conditions. There is preliminary evidence that a unique combination of hydrolyzed whey protein isolates inhibits angiotensin converting enzyme (ACE) (6171).

There is also interest in whey protein as a protein source in high-protein diets used for weight loss. In animal models, a whey protein diet seems to reduce weight and improve insulin sensitivity compared to red meat (12111).

Adverse Reactions

Orally, whey protein is usually well tolerated. High doses from 2.3 to 6.5 g/kg/day can cause increased stool frequency, nausea, thirst, bloating, cramps, reduced appetite, fatigue, and headache. Whey protein can also increase blood urea nitrogen (BUN) levels twofold (2640).

Interactions with Herbs & Other Dietary Supplements

None known.

Interactions with Drugs

ALENDRONATE (Fosamax): Theoretically, use of whey protein with alendronate might decrease absorption. Whey protein contains minerals that might bind alendronate in the gut (9).
LEVODOPA: Theoretically, concomitant use might decrease levodopa (Laradopa) absorption (4944).
QUINOLONE ANTIBIOTICS: Theoretically, use of whey protein with quinolones might decrease absorption. Whey protein contains minerals that might bind quinolones in the gut (9).
TETRACYCLINE ANTIBIOTICS: Theoretically, use of whey protein with tetracyclines might decrease absorption. Whey protein contains minerals that might bind tetracyclines in the gut (9).

Interactions with Foods

None known.

Interactions with Lab Tests

BLOOD UREA NITROGEN (BUN): Whey protein in amounts of 2.3 g/kg/day or more, in addition to a normal diet, can produce twofold increases in BUN concentrations (2640). However, whey protein does not change serum creatinine, indicating that the effect is due to protein loading, rather than reduced renal function (2640).

Interactions with Diseases or Conditions

MILK ALLERGY: Individuals allergic to bovine milk products should avoid using whey protein (4942).

Dosage and Administration

ORAL: A typical dose as a dietary supplement in people with HIV disease is 8.4-84 grams per day (4926,4935), or 2.4 g/kg per day in a calorie-enriched formula (4941), or 42-84 grams per day in a glutamine enriched formula (4935). A dose for treating metastatic carcinoma is 30 grams per day (4930).

Comments

Whey protein is the soluble protein contained in whey, the watery portion of milk that separates from the curds in the process of cheese making.

WHITE COHOSH

Also Known As

Baneberry, Coralberry, Doll's Eye, Red BaneBerry, Snakeberry, White Baneberry.
CAUTION: See separate listings for Black Cohosh, Blue Cohosh, and European Baneberry.

Scientific Names

Actaea pachypoda, synonym Actaea alba; Actaea rubra.
Family: Ranunculaceae.

People Use This For

Orally, white cohosh has been used to stimulate menstruation and to treat other female disorders. White cohosh is also used orally for colds and cough, urogenital disorders, stomach disorders, reviving those near death, as a purgative, in childbirth, and for curing itching.

Safety

LIKELY UNSAFE ...when used orally. The entire plant is toxic (6).
PREGNANCY AND LACTATION: LIKELY UNSAFE ...when used orally due to toxicity (6); avoid using.

Effectiveness

There is insufficient reliable information available about the effectiveness of white cohosh.

Mechanism of Action
The constituent protoanemonin is believed to cause irritant effects (6). The fruit and berries are especially toxic. They contain toxic glycosides and an essential oil (6).

Adverse Reactions
Orally, white cohosh can cause gastrointestinal (GI) irritation (19), acute stomach cramping, headache, tachycardia, vomiting, delirium, and circulatory failure (6).
Topically, the application of white cohosh can lead to inflammation and skin blistering (6).

Interactions with Herbs & Other Dietary Supplements
None known.

Interactions with Drugs
None known.

Interactions with Foods
None known.

Interactions with Lab Tests
None known.

Interactions with Diseases or Conditions
GASTROINTESTINAL (GI) CONDITIONS: White cohosh can irritate the GI tract. Avoid using in individuals with infectious or inflammatory GI conditions (19).

Dosage and Administration
No typical dosage.

Comments
White cohosh appears to be a substance with no reliable evidence to support its use, yet with documented toxicity. It should not be confused with black cohosh, used for symptoms of menopause, nor with blue cohosh, a substance used as a uterine stimulant and antispasmodic (6). White cohosh is also known as baneberry but it should not be confused with European baneberry.

WHITE DEAD NETTLE FLOWER

Also Known As
Archangel, Bee Nettle, Blind Nettle, Deaf Nettle, Dumb Nettle, Lamii Albi Flos, Stingless Nettle, White Archangel.
CAUTION: See separate listing for Stinging Nettle.

Scientific Names
Lamium album.
Family: Lamiaceae/Labiatae.

People Use This For
Orally, white dead nettle flower is used for mild inflammation of mucous membranes in the upper respiratory tract, and as a sedative.
Topically, white dead nettle flower is used for mild inflammation of the mouth, throat, and skin, and for non-specific vaginal discharge.

Safety
LIKELY SAFE ...when used orally and appropriately (2,18).
There is insufficient reliable information available about the safety of white dead nettle flower for its other uses.
PREGNANCY AND LACTATION: Insufficient reliable information available; avoid using.

Effectiveness
There is insufficient reliable information available about the effectiveness of white dead nettle flower.

Mechanism of Action
White dead nettle flowers contain tannin, mucilage, and saponins (2). These give nettle expectorant and astringent effects.

Adverse Reactions
None reported.

Interactions with Herbs & Other Dietary Supplements
None known.

Interactions with Drugs
None known.

Interactions with Foods
None known.

Interactions with Lab Tests
None known.

Interactions with Diseases or Conditions
None known.

Dosage and Administration
ORAL: The average daily dose is 3 grams (2).
TOPICAL: The typical dosage is 5 grams of the white dead nettle flower is commonly added to a sitz bath (2).

Comments
Avoid confusion with stinging nettle.

WHITE HELLEBORE

Also Known As
European Hellebore, European White Hellebore, Langwort.
CAUTION: See separate listings for Black Hellebore, American Hellebore, and Pheasant's Eye (false hellebore).

Scientific Names
Veratrum album, synonym Veratrum lobelianum.
Family: Melanthiaceae or Liliaceae.

People Use This For
Orally, white hellebore is used to treat cholera, gout, and hypertension.
Topically, white hellebore is used for herpetic lesions.
In manufacturing, white hellebore is used as an insecticide against flies and mosquitoes.

Safety
LIKELY UNSAFE ...when used orally. All plant parts are considered toxic (6). Between 10-20 mg of alkaloids (1-2 grams of rhizome/root) are lethal (6,18). ...when used topically. Toxic alkaloids can be absorbed through intact skin (6,18).
PREGNANCY: LIKELY UNSAFE ...when used orally or topically because it could be teratogenic (6); avoid using.
LACTATION: LIKELY UNSAFE ...when used orally or topically (6); avoid using.

Effectiveness
There is insufficient reliable information available about the effectiveness of white hellebore.

Mechanism of Action
The applicable parts of white hellebore are the rhizome and root. White hellebore contains the toxic ester-alkaloids protoveratirine A and B (13), which are sensory nerve irritants (18). These alkaloids inhibit the inactivation of the sodium ion channels and thus have a paralyzing effect on many excitable cells, including those of the heart (18).

Adverse Reactions
Orally, white hellebore can cause mucous membrane irritation (18), a burning sensation in upper abdomen, salivation, vomiting, gastric erosion, severe hypotension, bradycardia, and shock (6,553). Large doses may cause central respiratory depression, blindness, paralysis, convulsions, cardiac arrhythmias, and death (6).
Topically, it can cause skin irritation (18) and the toxic alkaloids could be absorbed.
By inhalation, the powdered root induces violent sneezing and runny nose (6).

Interactions with Herbs & Other Dietary Supplements
None known.

Interactions with Drugs
None known.

Interactions with Foods
None known.

Interactions with Lab Tests
None known.

Interactions with Diseases or Conditions
None known.

Dosage and Administration
No typical dosage.

Comments
Crude white hellebore is not used therapeutically (13), though it is sometimes used in homeopathic dilutions (18). In Roman times, white hellebore was used as a poison. An extract has been used as an arrow tip poison.

WHITE HOREHOUND

Also Known As
Common Hoarhound, Hoarhound, Horehound, Houndsbane, Marrubii herba, Marrubium, Mastranzo.
CAUTION: See separate listing for Black Horehound.

Scientific Names
Marrubium vulgare.
Family: Lamiaceae/Labiatae.

People Use This For
Orally, white horehound is used for loss of appetite, cough, bronchitis, respiratory tract mucous membrane inflammation, whooping cough, asthma, tuberculosis, indigestion, bloating and flatulence, diarrhea, jaundice, debility, liver and gallbladder complaints, and for painful menstruation. It is also used orally as a laxative, an anthelmintic, as a diuretic, and to induce sweating.
Topically, white horehound is used for skin damage, ulcers, and wounds.
In manufacturing, the extracts of white horehound are used as flavoring in foods and beverages, and as an expectorant in cough syrups and lozenges.

Safety
LIKELY SAFE ...when used orally in amounts commonly found in foods. White horehound has Generally Recognized As Safe (GRAS) status in the US (4912).
POSSIBLY SAFE ...when used orally and appropriately (2,12).
POSSIBLY UNSAFE ...when used orally in excessive amounts; white horehound may have purgative effects (4,12). There is insufficient reliable information available about the safety of the topical use of white horehound.
PREGNANCY: LIKELY UNSAFE ...when used orally; white horehound might have abortifacient effect (19), or stimulate menstrual flow and the uterus (12). There is insufficient reliable information available about the safety of topical use during pregnancy; avoid using.
LACTATION: There is insufficient reliable information available about the safety of oral use during lactation; avoid amounts greater than those commonly found in foods. There is insufficient reliable information available about the safety of topical use during lactation; avoid using.

Effectiveness
There is insufficient reliable information available about the effectiveness of white horehound.

Mechanism of Action
The applicable parts of white horehound are the above ground parts. White horehound contains marrubiin, bitter ingredients, volatile oil, and tannins (515). The constituent, marrubiin does not exist in the fresh plant; it is formed from premarrubiin during processing (515). The volatile oil of white horehound exhibits vasodilation, expectorant (11), and antischistosomal activity (4). Preliminary evidence suggests the hydroxycinnamic derivatives might have weak antioxidant activity (11). Other evidence suggests marrubinic acid may stimulate bile secretion (515). Marrubiin's expectorant effects may result from direct stimulation of bronchial mucosal secretions (512). Marrubiin may act to normalize extrasystolic arrhythmias (4,11), but large amounts might cause arrhythmias (4). An alcoholic extract reduces spasms of gastrointestinal (GI) tract (515). An aqueous extract demonstrates evidence that it can antagonize serotonin (11) and exerts anti-inflammatory activity (4,11).

Adverse Reactions
Orally, large amounts of white horehound can cause purgative effects (4,12).
Topically, skin contact with the plant juice may cause contact dermatitis (4).

Interactions with Herbs & Other Dietary Supplements
None known.

Interactions with Drugs
None known.

Interactions with Foods
None known.

Interactions with Lab Tests
None known.

Interactions with Diseases or Conditions
HEART CONDITIONS: Theoretically, large amounts of white horehound might cause arrhythmias (4).

Dosage and Administration
ORAL: A typical dose is 1-2 grams dried above ground parts or one cup of tea of three times daily before meals to stimulate bile secretion or during the day as an expectorant (8). To make tea, steep 1-2 grams dried above ground parts in 150 mL boiling water 5-10 minutes, and strain (4,8). Up to 4.5 grams dried above ground parts or 2-6 tablespoons of pressed juice (or equivalent preparations) are used per day (2). A typical dose of pressed juice is 30-60 mL daily (18). 1-3 mL of the liquid extract, 1:1 in 25% ethanol, has been used three times daily (4). 1-2 mL of the tincture, 1:10 in 45% alcohol, has been used three times daily (4).
TOPICAL: No typical dosage.

Comments
White horehound derives its name from ancient Greece where it was used for treating mad-dog bites (515).

WHITE LILY

Also Known As
Baurenlilien, Farmer's Lily, Madonna Lily, Meadow Lily, White Pond Lily.

Scientific Names
Lilium candidum.
Family: Liliaceae.

Comments
At the date of publication, there was very little scientific information available about this product. Our staff is continually analyzing the available information on natural medicines and will add data to the online version of *Natural Medicines Comprehensive Database* as it becomes available. See www.naturaldatabase.com.

WHITE MUSTARD

Also Known As
American Yellow Mustard, Mustard, Weibe Senfsamen, Yellow Mustard.
CAUTION: See separate listings for Black Mustard, Clown's Mustard Plant, and Hedge Mustard.

Scientific Names
Sinapis alba, synonym Brassica alba.
Family: Brassicaceae/Cruciferae.

People Use This For
Orally, white mustard is used to clear the voice, for those with a tendency for infection, to induce vomiting, as a diuretic, and as an appetite stimulant.
Topically, white mustard is used for cough and colds, pulmonary congestion, bronchitis, joint and soft tissue inflammation, rheumatism, osteoarthritis, lumbago, inflammation of the mouth and pharynx, hyperemization of the skin, a counterirritant, and a bath to treat paralytic symptoms.
In foods, white mustard is a common flavoring agent in mustard condiments, and is considered a culinary spice.

Safety

LIKELY SAFE ...when used orally in the amounts commonly found in foods. White mustard has Generally Recognized As Safe (GRAS) status in the US (4912).
POSSIBLY SAFE ...when used orally and appropriately for medicinal purposes (12). ...when used topically and appropriately (12,19).
LIKELY UNSAFE ...when used orally as an emetic because mustard is an irritant. Used as an emetic, the esophageal tissue is twice exposed to the corrosive effects of white mustard (19). Ingestion of a large quantity can cause irritant poisoning (12,19). ...when used topically for more than 15-30 minutes because severe burns can occur (12,19). ...when used topically on a regular basis for more than 2 weeks (2,12,19).
CHILDREN: LIKELY UNSAFE ...when used orally in medicinal amounts. ...when used topically in children under 6 years of age (2,12,19).
PREGNANCY: LIKELY UNSAFE ...when used orally in medicianl amounts; white mustard can have abortifacient and menstrual-stimulant properties (19).
LACTATION: Insufficient reliable information available; avoid using.

Effectiveness

There is insufficient reliable information available about the effectiveness of white mustard.

Mechanism of Action

The applicable part of white mustard is the seed. White mustard seeds contain mustard oil glycosides and mustard oils (2). White mustard contains the glucosinolate sinalbin, which on hydrolysis yields p-hydroxybenzyl isothiocyanate, p-hydroxybenzylamine, and other constituents, such as proteins, fatty oil, and sinapine (11,18). These products of hydrolysis possess irritant and bacteriostatic properties (18). White mustard's pungent taste comes from p-hydroxybenzyl isothiocyanate (11). Some evidence suggests the glucosinolate products can have protective effects against carcinogens (11).

Adverse Reactions

Orally, long-term use of white mustard can increase the risk of nerve damage (2,18). Isothiocyanates, such as those in mustard, can cause endemic goiters (6,11).
Topically, white mustard can cause blistering and skin ulceration, as well as nerve damage (2,12,18,19).

Interactions with Herbs & Other Dietary Supplements

None known.

Interactions with Drugs

None known.

Interactions with Foods

None known.

Interactions with Lab Tests

None known.

Interactions with Diseases or Conditions

KIDNEY DISEASE: Irritant poisoning from white mustard can occur in people with kidney disorders (12,19).

Dosage and Administration

ORAL: The average amount of white mustard is 60-150 grams daily (18). To "brighten and clear" the voice, mustard flour, or powdered mustard, is stirred with honey to form balls (18). One or two of these honey balls are taken on an empty stomach (18).
TOPICAL: As a foot bath, 20 to 30 grams of mustard flour is typically mixed in 1 liter of water (18). For a mustard bath, 150 grams of mustard flour in a pouch is commonly placed in the bath (18). For local application, 4 tablespoons (50-70 grams) of the powdered seeds are usually mixed with warm water to form a soft material, which is applied for 10-15 minutes for adults and 5-10 minutes for children older than 6 years of age (2,18). Decrease the application time in individuals with sensitive skin (2). Treatment should not exceed two weeks (2,12,18,19).

Comments

There are approximately 40 different species of mustard plant. Three different types are typically used to make the mustard condiment. Black mustard (Brassica nigra) is the most pungent. White mustard (Brassica alba) is the most mild and is used to make traditional American yellow mustard. Brown mustard (Brassica juncea) is dark yellow, has a pungent taste, and is used to make Dijon mustard.

WHITE SANDALWOOD

Also Known As

Chandana, East Indian Sandalwood, Oil of Sandalwood, Sanderswood, Santal Oil, Santali Lignum Albi, Tan Xiang, White Saunders, Yellow Sandalwood, Yellow Saunders.
CAUTION: See separate listing for Red Sandalwood.

Scientific Names

Santalum album.
Family: Santalaceae

People Use This For

Orally, white sandalwood is used for treating urinary tract infections, common cold, cough, bronchitis, fever, inflammatory conditions of the mouth and pharynx, liver disease, gallbladder complaints, heat stroke, gonorrhea, headache, cardiovascular conditions, and as an anti-aphrodisiac.
In food and beverages, white sandalwood is used as a flavor component.
In manufacturing, white sandalwood oil is used as a fragrance ingredient in soaps, cosmetics, and perfumes.

Safety

LIKELY SAFE ...when used orally in amounts commonly found in foods. White sandalwood oil has Generally Recognized As Safe status (GRAS) for use in foods in the US (4912).
POSSIBLY UNSAFE ...when used orally for longer than 6 weeks. Use for more than 6 weeks is associated with kidney damage (12,19).
There is insufficient reliable information available about the safety of the topical use of white sandalwood in amounts greater than those found in cosmetics.
PREGNANCY: LIKELY UNSAFE ...when used orally in medicinal amounts; sandalwood is reported to have abortifacient effects (19); avoid using.
LACTATION: Insufficient reliable information available; avoid using amounts greater than those found in foods.

Effectiveness

There is insufficient reliable information available about the effectiveness of white sandalwood.

Mechanism of Action

The applicable parts of sandalwood are the oil and wood. White sandalwood oil is reported to have antifungal, antiseptic, diuretic, antibacterial, and spasmolytic activity (2,11). It is considered to be a kidney irritant (19). Although some evidence suggests it is not irritating, sensitizing, or phototoxic when applied to the skin, the constituent, santolol, can cause contact dermatitis (11). The wood is reported to have antibacterial, spasmolytic, and urinary disinfectant activities (2,18).

Adverse Reactions

Orally, white sandalwood can cause itching, nausea, gastrointestinal complaints, and blood in the urine (18). Large doses or use longer than six weeks can cause kidney toxicity (12,18).
Topically, contact dermatitis can occur in sensitive individuals (11).

Interactions with Herbs & Other Dietary Supplements

None known.

Interactions with Drugs

None known.

Interactions with Foods

None known.

Interactions with Lab Tests

None known.

Interactions with Diseases or Conditions

KIDNEY DISEASE: White sandalwood is contraindicated in kidney disease, particularly in individuals with diseases of the kidney parenchyma (2,19).

Dosage and Administration

ORAL: No typical dosage. However, traditionally 1-1.5 grams of oil per day has been used as an enteric-coated product (2). The wood has been used 10-20 grams per day, brewed as a tea or other preparations (2). White sandalwood should not be used for more than a six-week duration (2,12).

Comments
Avoid confusion with red sandalwood (Pterocarpus santalinus).

WHITE SOAPWORT

Also Known As
Gypsophilae radix, Soapwort.
CAUTION: See separate listing for Red Soapwort.

Scientific Names
Gypsophila paniculata.
Family: Caryophyllaceae.

People Use This For
Orally, white soapwort is used for cough, bronchitis, and inflammation of the mucous membranes in the upper and lower respiratory tract.
Topically, white soapwort is used for chronic skin disorders and eczema.

Safety
POSSIBLY SAFE ...when used orally and appropriately (2).
PREGNANCY AND LACTATION: Insufficient reliable information; avoid using.

Effectiveness
There is insufficient reliable information available about the effectiveness of white soapwort.

Mechanism of Action
The applicable part of white soapwort is the root. White soapwort has expectorant, emetic, antibiotic, and insecticidal effects (18). In large amounts, it is cytotoxic (2). The saponin constituents exhibit expectorant effects (2), and they irritate the gastric mucosa to stimulate the bronchial mucous glands via parasympathetic sensory pathways (7). Saponins can cause stomach upset, nausea, and vomiting (7).

Adverse Reactions
Orally, white soapwort can cause stomach irritation (2), nausea, and vomiting (7).

Interactions with Herbs & Other Dietary Supplements
None known.

Interactions with Drugs
None known.

Interactions with Foods
None known.

Interactions with Lab Tests
None known.

Interactions with Diseases or Conditions
GI IRRITATION: Theoretically, the saponin content of white soapwort can exacerbate existing gastrointestinal mucosal irritation (6).

Dosage and Administration
ORAL: The typical dose of white soapwort is 30-150 mg per day of the dried root or 3-15 mg per day of the gysophila saponin or equivalent preparations (2).

Comments
In the Middle Ages, Franciscan and Dominican monks viewed soapwort as a divine gift that was meant to keep them clean (6). Avoid confusion with the red soapwort root.

WILD CARROT

Also Known As

Beesnest Plant, Bird's Nest Root, Daucus, Garijara, Queen Anne's Lace, Shikha-Mula.
CAUTION: See separate listings for Hemlock and Water Hemlock.

Scientific Names

Daucus carota subsp. carota.
Family: Apiaceae/Umbelliferae.

People Use This For

Orally, wild carrot is used for urinary calculus or stones, and high uric acid in urine, cystitis, and gout. The seed oil is used for dysentery, indigestion, uterine pain, heart disease, cancer, kidney problems, as a nerve tonic, a diuretic, an antiflatulent, an aphrodisiac, to induce menstruation, and as an anthelmintic.
In foods, wild carrot oil is used as a flavoring agent in alcoholic and non-alcoholic beverages, frozen dairy desserts, candy, baked goods, gelatins, puddings, meat and meat products, condiments relishes, and soups.
In manufacturing, wild carrot seed oil is used as a fragrance in soaps, detergents, creams, lotions, and perfumes.

Safety

LIKELY SAFE ...when used orally in amounts commonly found in foods. Wild carrot oil has Generally Recognized As Safe (GRAS) status in the US (4912).
POSSIBLY SAFE ...when wild carrot seed oil is used orally and appropriately in medicinal amounts (4,11).
LIKELY UNSAFE ...when an excessive amount of wild carrot seed oil is used orally, it can cause renal irritation (4). Theoretically, high doses of oil could cause neurological effects (6) because the seed contains the psychoactive agent myristicin.
There is insufficient reliable information available about the safety of the oral use of the above ground parts of wild carrot.
PREGNANCY: LIKELY UNSAFE ...when used orally. The seeds, oil, and above ground parts can cause uterine stimulant, abortifacient, and menstrual stimulant effects (19).
LACTATION: POSSIBLY UNSAFE ...when the seed oil is used orally. Wild carrot seed oil has mild estrogenic activity and irritant effects (4). There is insufficient reliable information available about the safety of the oral use of the seeds or above ground parts during lactation.

Effectiveness

There is insufficient reliable information available about the effectiveness of wild carrot.

Mechanism of Action

The applicable parts of wild carrot are the fruit and seed. Wild carrot fruit/seed contains flavones including apigenin, chrysin, luteolin; flavonols including kaempferol and quercetin and various glycosides. The amount and composition of the volatile oil contained in the fruit/seed varies between different cultivars. The furanocoumarins, 8-methoxypsoralen and 5 methoxypsoralen are found in the plant (4). Some evidence suggests that wild carrot might have significant antifertility activity (4,3858). Other evidence suggests that wild carrot has cholinergic-type actions, perhaps due to the choline constituents (4). Wild carrot seed oil shows some evidence of vasodilation, cardiac depressant, and smooth muscle relaxation effects (11). Terpinen-4-ol, a component of the seed oil, is a renal irritant and believed to cause a diuretic effect (4). A tertiary base isolated from wild carrot seed appears to have papaverine-like antispasmodic activity.

Adverse Reactions

Orally, ingesting excessive doses can cause renal irritation or neurological effects. Hypersensitivity reactions and increased sensitivity to UV light and sunburn might occur (4,19).
Wild carrot can cause allergic reactions. People who are sensitive to birch, celery, or mugwort spices are more likely to also be sensitive to wild carrot. This has been called the "celery-carrot-mugwort-spice syndrome" (12192).
Topically, contact with the plant can cause dermatitis (4).

Interactions with Herbs & Other Dietary Supplements

HERBS WITH SEDATIVE PROPERTIES: Theoretically, concomitant use with herbs that have sedative properties might enhance therapeutic and adverse effects. These include California poppy, catnip, German chamomile, hops, Jamaican dogwood, kava, lemon balm, scullcap, valerian, and others.

Interactions with Drugs

ANTIHYPERTENSIVE DRUGS: Theoretically, excessive doses of wild carrot seed oil might interfere with antihypertensive therapy due to cardiotonic effects (4).
ESTROGENS: Theoretically, excessive use of the above ground parts of wild carrot might interfere with hormonal therapy due to estrogenic effects of wild carrot (4).

PHOTOSENSITIZING DRUGS: Theoretically, concomitant use might result in increased photosensitivity (19). Some drugs that cause photosensitivity include amitriptyline (Elavil), quinolones (Ciprofloxacin, others), sulfa drugs (Septra, Bactrim, others), and tetracycline.

Interactions with Foods
None known.

Interactions with Lab Tests
None known.

Interactions with Diseases or Conditions
CROSS-ALLERGENICITY: Wild carrot can cause allergic reactions in patients who are sensitive to other plants and spices including birch, mugwort, and celery (12192). This has been called the "celery-carrot-mugwort-spice syndrome" (12192).
RENAL INFLAMMATION/IRRITATION: Contraindicated due to renal irritant properties (4,19).
UV LIGHT THERAPY: Contraindicated due to photosensitizing effect; avoid excessive periods in the sun (19).

Dosage and Administration
ORAL: No typical dosage. But, the dried above ground parts is 2-4 grams or as tea has been used three times daily. To make tea, steep 2-4 grams of above ground parts in boiling water for 5-10 minutes, strain (4). A liquid extract (1:1 in 25% alcohol) 2-4 mL three times daily has been used (4).

Comments
Carrot seed oil is steam-distilled from the dried root of both the familiar vegetable known as carrot, and the wild carrot. Avoid confusing wild carrot (which has an inedible white tap root) with the common carrot (Daucus carota subspecies sativus) (4).

WILD CHERRY

Also Known As
Black Cherry, Black Choke, Choke Cherry, Rum Cherry Bark, Virginian Prune, Wild Black Cherry.
CAUTION: See separate listing for Cherry Laurel Water.

Scientific Names
Prunus serotina; Prunus virginiana.
Family: Rosaceae.

People Use This For
Orally, wild cherry is used for colds, whooping cough, bronchitis and other lung problems, diarrhea, gout, digestive disorders, pain, and cancer. It is also used in cough syrups because of its sedative, expectorant, astringent, and antitussive effects.
In foods and beverages, wild cherry is used as a flavoring agent.

Safety
LIKELY SAFE ...when used orally in amounts commonly found in foods and beverages. Wild cherry has Generally Recognized As Safe (GRAS) status in the US (4912).
POSSIBLY SAFE ...when used orally and appropriately short-term, in limited amounts (12).
POSSIBLY UNSAFE ...when used orally and long-term or in excessive amounts (12,19). The constituent, prunasin, hydrolyzes to hydrocyanic acid (HCN) (11,12,13,18).
PREGNANCY: LIKELY UNSAFE ...when used orally because prunasin is potentially teratogenic (19).
LACTATION: Insufficient reliable information available; avoid using.

Effectiveness
There is insufficient reliable information available about the effectiveness of wild cherry.

Mechanism of Action
The applicable part of wild cherry is the stem bark. Wild cherry bark has astringent, antitussive, and sedative effects (18). It contains prunasin, a cyanogenic glycoside that is hydrolyzed to toxic hydrocyanic acid (HCN) and benzaldehyde (11). Bark collected in the fall has a higher HCN yield (approximately 0.15%) than bark collected in the spring (approximately 0.05%). Leaves collected in the spring have the highest HCN yield (approximately 0.25%) (11).

Adverse Reactions
Orally, large amounts of wild cherry can lead to fatal poisonings (18).

Interactions with Herbs & Other Dietary Supplements
None known.

Interactions with Drugs
CYTOCHROME P450 3A4 (CYP3A4) SUBSTRATES: There's preliminary evidence that wild cherry can inhibit CYP3A4 enzymes (6450). Theoretically, wild cherry might increase levels of drugs metabolized by CYP3A4. However, so far, this interaction has not been reported in humans. Some drugs metabolized by CYP3A4 include lovastatin (Mevacor), ketoconazole (Nizoral), itraconazole (Sporanox), fexofenadine (Allegra), triazolam (Halcion), and numerous others. Use wild cherry cautiously or avoid in patients taking these drugs.

Interactions with Foods
None known.

Interactions with Lab Tests
None known.

Interactions with Diseases or Conditions
None known.

Dosage and Administration
ORAL: People use 5 to 12 drops of the liquid extract containing wild cherry bark (12-14% by volume) in water two to three times daily (5023).

Comments
Avoid confusion with cherry laurel water. In Chinese medicine, the stem and bark of related species (Prunus armeniaca) may be effective as an antidote for apricot kernel poisoning (18).

WILD DAISY

Also Known As
Bruisewort.

Scientific Names
Bellis perennis.
Family: Asteraceae/Compositae.

Comments
At the date of publication, there was very little scientific information available about this product. Our staff is continually analyzing the available information on natural medicines and will add data to the online version of *Natural Medicines Comprehensive Database* as it becomes available. See www.naturaldatabase.com.

WILD INDIGO

Also Known As
American Indigo, Baptista, False Indigo, Horsefly Weed, Indigo Broom, Rattlebush, Yellow Broom, Yellow Indigo.

Scientific Names
Baptisia tinctoria.
Family: Fabaceae/Leguminosae.

People Use This For
Orally, wild indigo is used for diphtheria, influenza, malaria, septic angina, and typhoid fever with prostration. It is also used orally for upper respiratory tract infections, common head cold, tonsillitis, stomatitis, inflammation of the mouth and throat mucous membranes, fever, lymphadenitis, furunculosis, Crohn's disease, scarlet fever, typhoid, and pharyngitis.
Topically, wild indigo is used for painless ulcers, inflamed nipples, as a douche for leukorrhea, and for cleaning open and inflamed wounds.

Safety
UNSAFE ...when used orally or topically, long-term; contraindicated due to potential toxicity (12,19).
PREGNANCY AND LACTATION: UNSAFE ...when used orally or topically due to its toxic potential (12,19).

Effectiveness
There is insufficient reliable information available about the effectiveness of wild indigo.

Mechanism of Action
The applicable part of wild indigo is the root. Preliminary evidence suggests that glycoprotein constituents might have lymphocyte stimulating activity (393). Quinolizidine alkaloids cause gastrointestinal symptoms with high doses (18).

Adverse Reactions
Orally, large doses of wild indigo can cause vomiting, diarrhea, gastrointestinal complaints, and spasms (12).

Interactions with Herbs & Other Dietary Supplements
None known.

Interactions with Drugs
None known.

Interactions with Foods
None known.

Interactions with Lab Tests
None known.

Interactions with Diseases or Conditions
GASTRIC DISORDERS: Use of wild indigo is contraindicated in patients with inflammatory gastrointestinal conditions, particularly with accompanying capillary congestion (19).

Dosage and Administration
ORAL: One cup of tea is typically taken orally 3 times daily. The tea is prepared by simmering 0.5-1 grams dried root in 150 mL of boiling water for 10-15 minutes and straining (18).
TOPICAL: An ointment is prepared using one part of liquid extract to 8 parts of ointment base and applied to the affected area (18).

WILD LETTUCE

Also Known As
Acrid Lettuce, Bitter Lettuce, German Lactucarium, Green Endive, Lactucarium, Lettuce Opium, Poison Lettuce, Strong-Scented Lettuce.

Scientific Names
Lactuca virosa.
Family: Asteraceae/Compositae.

People Use This For
Orally, wild lettuce is used for whooping cough, mucous inflammations of the bronchial tract, asthma, urinary tract diseases, irritable cough, insomnia, restlessness, excitability in children, priapism, painful menses, nymphomania, muscular or joint pains, for aiding circulation, swollen genitals, and as an opium substitute in cough preparations.
The seed oil is used orally for arteriosclerosis and as a substitute for wheat germ oil.
Topically, wild lettuce latex is used as an antiseptic.
By inhalation, wild lettuce is used for a recreational "high" or hallucinogenic effect.

Safety
POSSIBLY SAFE ...when used orally and appropriately (12,4).
LIKELY UNSAFE ...when used orally in large doses because they can cause stupor, depressed respiration, and death (4).
PREGNANCY AND LACTATION: Insufficient reliable information available; avoid using.

Effectiveness
There is insufficient reliable information available about the effectiveness of wild lettuce.

Mechanism of Action
The applicable parts of wild lettuce are the latex and leaf. Wild lettuce is thought to have mild sedative, analgesic, and hypnotic or tranquilizing effects (4,18). Wild lettuce contains lactucin and lactupicrin (4). The milky latex, known

as lactucarium, can cause mydriasis (4). This effect is theorized to be due to the presence of hyoscyamine (4); however, the dried sap contains no hyoscyamine (4). Wild lettuce has sedative activity (4). Lactucin, lactupicrin, and hyoscyamine have all been proposed responsible for this activity, but the active constituent(s) has not been identified (4). Low concentrations (nanogram amounts) of morphine have been found in Lactuca species and are considered too low to have a pharmacological effect (4).

Adverse Reactions

Orally, large amounts can cause sweating, increased respiration, tachycardia, pupil dilation, dizziness, ringing in the ears, vision disorders, pressure in the head, somnolence, excitatory states (18), respiratory depression, coma, and death (4).

Topically, wild lettuce can cause contact dermatitis (4). It can cause an allergic reaction in individuals sensitive to the Asteraceae/Compositae family. Members of this family include ragweed, chrysanthemums, marigolds, daisies, and many other herbs.

Interactions with Herbs & Other Dietary Supplements

HERBS WITH ANTICOAGULANT/ANTIPLATELET POTENTIAL: Concomitant use of herbs that have antiplatelet/anticoagulant effects could theoretically increase the risk of bleeding in some people. These herbs include clove, danshen, garlic, ginger, ginkgo, ginseng, meadowsweet, poplar, red clover, and others.

HERBS WITH SEDATIVE PROPERTIES: Theoretically, concomitant use with herbs that have sedative properties might enhance therapeutic and adverse effects. These include calamus, California poppy plant, catnip leaves, hops, Jamaican dogwood bark, kava root, passionflower, sage, St. John's wort, sassafras bark, scullcap plant, valerian, and others.

Interactions with Drugs

CNS DEPRESSANTS: Theoretically, concomitant use with drugs with sedative effects might cause additive therapeutic effects and adverse effects (19).

Interactions with Foods

None known.

Interactions with Lab Tests

None known.

Interactions with Diseases or Conditions

BENIGN PROSTATIC HYPERPLASIA (BPH): Contraindicated in prostate enlargement (12). Wild lettuce might contain hyoscyamine (4) which is contraindicated in conditions involving urinary retention, including BPH (15).

CROSS-ALLERGENICITY: Wild lettuce can cause an allergic reaction in individuals sensitive to members of the Asteraceae/Compositae plant family. Members of this family include ragweed, chrysanthemums, marigolds, daisies, and many other herbs.

NARROW-ANGLE GLAUCOMA: Contraindicated (12). Wild lettuce might contain hyoscyamine (4) which can exacerbate narrow-angle (closed-angle) glaucoma (15).

Dosage and Administration

ORAL: A typical dose is 0.5-3 grams dried leaves or as tea three times daily. To make tea, steep 0.5-3 grams dried leaves in 150 mL of boiling water, strain (4). As the liquid extract (1:1 in 25% alcohol), 0.5-3 mL three times daily (4). For the dried latex extract, lactucarium, 0.3-1 grams three times daily (4). Also available as a soft extract, with the usual dose of 0.3-1 grams three times daily (4).

WILD MINT

Also Known As

Hairy Mint, Marsh Mint, Water Mint.

CAUTION: See separate listing for English Horsemint.

Scientific Names

Mentha aquatica, synonym Mentha palustris.

Family: Lamiaceae/Labiatae.

Comments

At the date of publication, this product was not a common ingredient used in brand name supplements marketed to consumers. Details about this product are available in the online version of *Natural Medicines Comprehensive Database.* See www.naturaldatabase.com.

WILD RADISH

Also Known As
Joint-Podded Charlock.

Scientific Names
Raphanus raphanistrum.
Family: Brassicaceae/Cruciferae.

Comments
At the date of publication, this product was not a common ingredient used in brand name supplements marketed to consumers. Details about this product are available in the online version of *Natural Medicines Comprehensive Database*. See www.naturaldatabase.com.

WILD THYME

Also Known As
Mother of Thyme, Serpyllum, Shepherd's Thyme.
CAUTION: See separate listings for Thyme, Spanish Origanum Oil, and Thyme Oil.

Scientific Names
Thymus serpyllum.
Family: Lamiaceae/Labiatae.

People Use This For
Orally, wild thyme is used for cough, bronchitis, inflammation of the respiratory tract, kidney and bladder disorders, to relieve flatulence and colic, as a digestive aid, expectorant, aromatic, and antimicrobial.
Topically, wild thyme is used for arthritis and sprains.

Safety
LIKELY SAFE ...when used in amounts commonly found in foods. Wild thyme has Generally Recognized As Safe (GRAS) status in the US (4912).
POSSIBLY SAFE ...when preparations of the above ground flowering parts are used orally and appropriately (12).
PREGNANCY AND LACTATION: Insufficient reliable information; avoid using in medicinal amounts.

Effectiveness
There is insufficient reliable information available about the effectiveness of wild thyme.

Mechanism of Action
The applicable parts of wild thyme are the above ground, flowering parts. There is insufficient reliable information available about the possible mechanism of action and active ingredients.

Adverse Reactions
None reported.

Interactions with Herbs & Other Dietary Supplements
None known.

Interactions with Drugs
None known.

Interactions with Foods
None known.

Interactions with Lab Tests
None known.

Interactions with Diseases or Conditions
THYROID DISORDERS: Can suppress thyroid function by decreasing hormone production and/or release (19).

Dosage and Administration
ORAL: One cup of tea taken orally before meals. The tea is prepared by steeping 1.5-2 grams dried plant in 150 mL of boiling water for 10 minutes and straining. The daily dose is equivalent to 4-6 grams dried herb (18).

WILD YAM

Also Known As

Atlantic Yam, Barbasco, China Root, Colic Root, Devil's Bones, Dioscorea, Dioscoreae, Mexican Yam, Natural DHEA, Phytoestrogen, Rheumatism Root, Rhizoma Dioscoreae, Wild Mexican Yam, Yam, Yuma.
CAUTION: See separate listings for Pregnenolone and Progesterone.

Scientific Names

Dioscorea composita, synonym Dioscorea tepinapensis; Dioscorea floribunda; Dioscorea mexicana, synonym Dioscorea macrostachya; Dioscorea villosa, synonym Dioscorea hirticaulis.
Family: Dioscoreaceae.

People Use This For

Orally, wild yam is used as a "natural alternative" for estrogen replacement therapy, postmenopausal vaginal dryness, premenstrual syndrome, osteoporosis, increasing energy and libido in men and women, and for breast enlargement. Wild yam is also used orally for treating diverticulosis, gallbladder colic, painful menstruation, cramp, rheumatoid arthritis, and for increasing energy.
Topically, wild yam is used for menopausal vasomotor symptoms such as hot flashes.
In manufacturing, the constituent of wild yam root, diosgenin, is used as a precursor for commercial chemical synthesis of human steroidal hormones.

Safety

POSSIBLY SAFE ...when used orally (12). ...when used topically (10989).
PREGNANCY AND LACTATION: Insufficient reliable information available; avoid using.

Effectiveness

POSSIBLY INEFFECTIVE

Menopausal symptoms. Wild yam applied topically appears to be no better than placebo for relieving vasomotor symptoms such as hot flashes and night sweats in menopausal women using wild yam cream for 3 months. It doesn't appear to cause changes in serum follicle stimulating hormone (FSH), estradiol, or progesterone (10989).

There is insufficient reliable information available about the effectiveness of wild yam for its other uses.

Mechanism of Action

The applicable parts of wild yam are the root and rhizome. The tubers of Dioscorea species contain the glycoside diosgenin, a steroid precursor that was used in the first commercial production of oral contraceptives, topical hormones, systemic corticosteroids, androgens, estrogens, progestogens, and other sex hormones (515). Dioscorea continues to be used as the precursor for manufacturing progesterone contained in some "natural progesterone" cosmetic products. The chemical transformation of diosgenin to estrogen, progesterone, or any other steroidal compound does not occur in the human body (515). Diosgenin prevents estrogen-induced bile flow suppression (5129). It shows some evidence that it might stimulate growth of mammary tissue (5130), and attenuate indomethacin-induced intestinal inflammation (5131). A wild yam extract enhances estradiol binding to estrogen receptors and induces transcription activity in estrogen-responsive cells (6180). Topically applied wild yam doesn't appear to cause changes in serum follicle stimulating hormone (FSH), estradiol, or progesterone (10989).

Adverse Reactions

Orally, ingestion of large amounts of wild yam tincture has caused emesis (12).

Interactions with Herbs & Other Dietary Supplements

None known.

Interactions with Drugs

None known.

Interactions with Foods

None known.

Interactions with Lab Tests

None known.

Interactions with Diseases or Conditions

HORMONE SENSITIVE CANCERS/CONDITIONS: Wild yam has in vitro estrogenic effects, but doesn't appear to affect hormone levels when used topically (6180,10989). Women with hormone sensitive conditions should avoid wild yam until more is known. Some hormone sensitive conditions include breast cancer, uterine cancer, ovarian cancer, endometriosis, and uterine fibroids.

Dosage and Administration

No typical dosage.

Comments

Diosgenin, a component of wild yam, is promoted as a natural precursor to dehydroepiandosterone (DHEA). Some wild yam products are promoted as "natural DHEA." Although diosgenin can be converted to steroidal compounds, including DHEA, in the laboratory, this chemical synthesis does not occur in the human body. So taking wild yam extract will not increase DHEA levels in humans (515,2112). People interested in taking DHEA should avoid wild yam products labeled as "natural DHEA."

WILLARD WATER

Also Known As

Biowater, Carbonaceous Activated Water, Catalyst Altered Water, Williard's Water.

Scientific Names

None.

Comments

At the date of publication, this product was not a common ingredient used in brand name supplements marketed to consumers. Details about this product are available in the online version of *Natural Medicines Comprehensive Database.* See www.naturaldatabase.com.

WILLOW BARK

Also Known As

Basket Willow, Bay Willow, Brittle Willow, Crack Willow, Daphne Willow, Knackweide, Laurel Willow, Lorbeerweide, Osier Rouge, Pupurweide, Purple Osier, Purple Osier Willow, Reifweide, Salicis cortex, Silberweide, Violet Willow, Weidenrinde, White Willow, White Willow Bark.

Scientific Names

Salix alba; Salix daphnoides; Salix fragilis; Salix pentandra; Salix purpurea; other Salix species.
Family: Salicaceae.

People Use This For

Orally, willow bark is used for headache, pain, myalgia, osteoarthritis, dysmenorrhea, gouty arthritis, ankylosing spondylitis, rheumatoid arthritis (RA), and gout. It is also used for fever, common cold, influenza, and weight loss.

Safety

POSSIBLY SAFE ...when used orally and appropriately, short-term (6456,12474,12475,12804,12811). Willow bark has been used safely for up to 12 weeks in one study (12811).
CHILDREN: POSSIBLY UNSAFE ...when used orally for viral infections. Salicylic acid and aspirin are contraindicated in children with viral infections (12801). Although Reye's syndrome has not been reported, the salicin constituent in willow bark is similar to aspirin and might pose the same risk.
PREGNANCY: Insufficient reliable information available; avoid using.
LACTATION: POSSIBLY UNSAFE ...when used orally. Willow bark contains salicylates which are excreted in breast milk and have been linked to adverse effects in breast-fed infants (12802,12803).

Effectiveness

POSSIBLY EFFECTIVE

Back pain. There's some evidence that a willow bark extract providing 120-240 mg of the salicin constituent daily can reduce low back pain in some patients. The higher concentration of 240 mg salicin is more effective than 120 mg of salicin. It can take up to 1 week for significant relief (6456). Some research suggests salicin 240 mg daily is as effective as rofecoxib (Vioxx) for low back pain (12804).

INSUFFICIENT RELIABLE EVIDENCE to RATE

Obesity. Preliminary clinical research suggests that willow bark in combination with ephedra and cola nut might cause modest weight loss in overweight and obese people. Willow bark 600 mg per day (containing 90 mg salicin) in divided doses given for 3 months in combination with CNS stimulants might cause a 2 kg reduction in weight (12811). This combination may not be appropriate due to safety concerns associated with ephedra. Ephedra is banned in the US due to severe adverse effects (10055).

Osteoarthritis. Clinical research on willow bark extract for osteoarthritis is conflicting. Some research suggests it

has a moderate analgesic effect on osteoarthritis, while other research shows it is similar to placebo and inferior to diclofenac (Voltaren, Cataflam) (12474,12475).
Rheumatoid arthritis (RA). Preliminary clinical research suggests that willow bark extract is not effective for rheumatoid arthritis (12475).
More evidence is needed to rate willow bark for these uses.

Mechanism of Action

Willow bark is the bark of salix tree species such as the white willow. Willow bark constituents include flavonoids, tannins, and salicylates. The active constituent of willow bark is thought to be salicin. Salicin is metabolized to salicyl alcohol and then to salicylic acid. From there, metabolism is the same as aspirin (12808).
An ethanolic extract of willow bark seems to inhibit cyclooxygenase (COX)-2 mediated prostaglandin release, but it doesn't seem to directly affect COX-1 or COX-2 activity. Constituents of willow bark other than salicin may have lipoxygenase-inhibiting and antioxidant effects that could contribute to its analgesic effect (6456,12476). They also might prevent prostaglandin and cytokine release (12476). Some research suggests that extended treatment with willow bark may be necessary for a therapeutic effect (12809,12812).
Preliminary research suggests that willow bark extracts have analgesic, anti-inflammatory, and antipyretic effects (12476). Willow bark inhibits platelet aggregation, but to a lesser degree than aspirin (12810).
Willow bark is sometimes included in weight loss supplements. Some evidence suggests that willow bark or aspirin and caffeine might act synergistically with ephedrine for weight loss by inhibiting prostaglandin, which increases norepinephrine release. However aspirin, and theoretically willow bark, have no thermogenic effect when given alone (314,729,10003,12811).
Bioavailability of willow bark may be lower due to manufacturing processes. A dose of 240 mg of salicin is equivalent to 87 mg of aspirin (12808).

Adverse Reactions

Orally, willow bark extract can cause gastrointestinal adverse effects, but these appear to be less frequent than those caused by NSAIDs (12474,12475). Willow bark may cause itching and rash, as well as serious allergic reactions, including anaphylaxis, in people who are allergic to aspirin (10392,12474,12475).
Salicylates can inhibit prostaglandins, which can reduce renal blood flow (12805). Salicin can cause renal papillary necrosis (12806). The risk for toxicity is greater with high acute doses or chronic use (12805).

Interactions with Herbs & Other Dietary Supplements

HERBS WITH ANTICOAGULANT/ANTIPLATELET POTENTIAL: Concomitant use of herbs that have antiplatelet/anticoagulant effects could theoretically increase the risk of bleeding in some people (12810). These herbs include clove, danshen, garlic, ginger, ginkgo, ginseng, meadowsweet, red clover, and others.
SALICYLATE-CONTAINING HERBS: Theoretically, concomitant use may potentiate salicylate effects and adverse effects (12808). Salicylate-containing herbs include aspen bark, black haw, poplar, and meadowsweet.

Interactions with Drugs

ANTICOAGULANT/ANTIPLATELET DRUGS: Concomitant use theoretically might increase the risk of bleeding due to decreased platelet aggregation. Willow bark has antiplatelet effects, but less so than aspirin (12810). Avoid concomitant use with other anticoagulant and antiplatelet drugs. Some of these drugs include aspirin, clopidogrel (Plavix), dalteparin (Fragmin), enoxaparin (Lovenox), heparin, ticlopidine (Ticlid), warfarin (Coumadin), and others.
ASPIRIN: Willow bark contains salicin, a plant salicylate. Theoretically, willow bark might have an additive effect with other salicylate-containing drugs such as aspirin (12808).
CHOLINE MAGNESIUM TRISALICYLATE (Trilisate): Willow bark contains salicin, a plant salicylate. Theoretically, willow bark might have an additive effect with other salicylate-containing drugs such as choline magnesium trisalicylate (12808).
SALSALATE (Disalcid): Willow bark contains salicin, a plant salicylate. Theoretically, willow bark might have an additive effect with other salicylate-containing drugs such as salsalate (12808).

Interactions with Foods

None known.

Interactions with Lab Tests

CREATININE: Theoretically, salicin could cause a rise in serum creatinine without affecting renal function. Salicylates can cause a rise in serum creatine without a change in glomerular filtration rate (GFR). This is thought to be due to changes in plasma protein binding caused by salicylates or competitive inhibition of tubular secretion of creatinine by salicylates (12807).

Interactions with Diseases or Conditions

KIDNEY DYSFUNCTION: Theoretically, salicin might reduce renal blood flow (12805). Chronic use of high doses might contribute to renal failure in predisposed people (12806). Avoid use in people with compromised renal function.
SALICYLATE PRECAUTIONS: Avoid or use cautiously in individuals with aspirin hypersensitivity, asthma,

active peptic ulcer disease, diabetes, gout, hemophilia, hypoprothrombinemia, kidney or liver disease. Willow bark may cause serious allergic reactions, including anaphylaxis, in people who are allergic to aspirin (10392).

Dosage and Administration

ORAL: For back pain, willow bark extract providing 120-240 mg salicin has been used. The higher 240 mg dose might be more effective (6456,12804).

Comments

The composer, Ludwig van Beethoven, is thought to have ingested toxic amounts of salicin, which contributed to his death. His autopsy report is the first recorded case of renal papillary necrosis (12806).

WINE

Also Known As

Alcohol, Ethanol, Wine Extract.
CAUTION: See separate listing for Resveratrol.

Scientific Names

Vitis vinifera.
Family: Vitaceae.

People Use This For

Orally, wine is used for reducing the risk of cardiovascular disease, including coronary heart disease (CHD), atherosclerosis, and myocardial infarction (MI); and for reducing the risk of ischemic stroke and type 2 diabetes. It is also used orally to prevent cognitive decline in later life and to prevent Alzheimer's disease. Wine is also used orally for anxiety, achlorhydria, malabsorption syndromes, and as an appetite stimulant.
Topically, wine is used to stimulate wound healing and improve rheumatoid skin ulcerations.

Safety

LIKELY SAFE ...when used orally, responsibly, and in moderation (11880).
POSSIBLY UNSAFE ...when used orally in excess of 1 to 2 five-ounce glasses of wine per day. Larger amounts can cause minimal to significant adverse effects (11880).
PREGNANCY: LIKELY UNSAFE ...when used orally; alcohol is a teratogen. Use during pregnancy, especially during the first two months after conception, is associated with significant risk of spontaneous abortion, fetal alcohol syndrome, and developmental and behavioral dysfunction in infants and children exposed to alcohol in utero (8100); avoid using.
LACTATION: LIKELY UNSAFE ...when used orally. Alcohol is secreted in breast milk. Chronic use can cause abnormal psychomotor development, and disrupt the infant's sleep wake pattern. Alcohol also seems to reduce milk production (11878); avoid using.

Effectiveness

LIKELY EFFECTIVE

Cardiovascular disease. Consumption of alcoholic drinks, including wine, by otherwise healthy people seems to reduce the risk of developing cardiovascular disease. Moderate alcohol use (one to two drinks per day) reduces the risk of coronary heart disease, atherosclerosis, and myocardial infarction (MI), by approximately 30% to 50% when compared with nondrinkers (2267,2268,2271,6888,6892,8648,8649,10128,11879). Light to moderate alcohol consumption reduces ischemic stroke risk, but there is evidence that consuming any amount of alcohol can increase the risk of hemorrhagic stroke (841,2271,2279,6834,6842,6893). There is some evidence that light to moderate consumption of alcoholic drinks (one to two drinks per day) including wine, can reduce the risk of all-cause mortality in people who are middle-aged or older (2058,6823,6837,6843). Light to moderate consumption of alcohol might also reduce the risk of cardiovascular mortality in otherwise healthy people (2058,2270,6835,6837). Light to moderate alcohol consumption in the year prior to first acute MI is associated with a reduced cardiovascular- and all-cause mortality risk compared with non-drinkers (8650). Consumption of one alcoholic beverage per day or consuming alcohol on at least 3 to 4 days per week is a good rule of thumb for people who drink alcohol. Tell patients not to exceed two drinks per day. More than two drinks daily can increase the risk of cardiovascular and overall mortality (841,2060,2261,6173,6890,8648,11879). In men with established coronary heart disease (CHD), consumption of 1-14 alcoholic drinks per week, including wine, doesn't seem to have any effect on cardiovascular disease or all-cause mortality compared with men who drink less than one drink per week. Consuming three or more drinks per day is associated with increased mortality in men with a history of heart attacks (6173).

POSSIBLY EFFECTIVE

Cognitive function. Elderly men who have a history of consuming up to one alcoholic drink per day seem to maintain better general cognitive function during their late 70's and 80's compared to non-drinkers (6824,6829). However, consumption of more than four drinks per day during middle age seems to be associated with significantly poorer cognitive function in later life (6824).

Diabetes. Light to moderate alcohol consumption from wine and other sources, is associated with a reduced risk of type 2 diabetes in healthy men (6172,6891). Light to moderate alcohol consumption is also associated with a reduced risk of coronary heart disease (CHD) in men and women with type 2 diabetes compared with non-drinkers with type 2 diabetes. The risk reduction of CHD associated with light to moderate alcohol consumption in people with type 2 diabetes is similar to that found in people without diabetes who consume light to moderate amounts of alcohol (8653,8654).

Heart failure. Consuming one to four alcoholic drinks per day is associated with a reduced risk of heart failure in persons aged 65 years or older (8104). Consumption of 1-14 alcoholic drinks per week is associated with reduced all-cause mortality in people with ischemic left ventricular (LV) dysfunction compared with non-drinkers with ischemic LV dysfunction. However, this benefit does not seem to occur for those patients with non-ischemic LV dysfunction (6827).

Helicobacter pylori (H pylori). There is some evidence that moderate to high (more than 75 grams) consumption of alcohol per week from beverages such as beer and wine can reduce the risk of H. pylori infection (8034).

INSUFFICIENT RELIABLE EVIDENCE to RATE

Alzheimer's disease. There is some evidence that 1 to 2 drinks per day can reduce the risk of developing Alzheimer's disease in both men and women compared with non-drinkers (6603).

Anxiety. The effect of alcohol on anxiety is complex, and may be affected by the psychological state of the user. It sometimes reduces anxiety, sometimes increases it, and sometimes has no effect (2266).

Cancer. There is some preliminary evidence that intake of up to 21 alcoholic drinks per week, including wine, might slightly reduce the risk of cancer-related mortality (6823).

Post-menopausal osteoporosis. There is preliminary evidence that moderate alcohol consumption in postmenopausal women is associated with increased bone mineral density in the trochanter, femoral neck, mid-radius, and lumbar spine (6825,6836,8655). Alcohol intake of one-half to one drink per day seems to have the greatest effect on bone mineral density compared with non-drinkers and heavy drinkers of alcohol (8655).

More evidence is needed to rate wine for these uses.

Mechanism of Action

Wine is the natural yeast fermentation product of the juice of sun-ripened grapes, the fruit of Vitis vinifera. Wine normally contains 10% to 14% alcohol, predominantly as ethanol, which is a central nervous system (CNS) depressant (2263).

Several mechanisms have been proposed for the protective effects of alcohol against coronary heart disease (CHD) (2060,2268,2270,6839,6840). One to two alcoholic drinks per day increases high-density lipoprotein (HDL) cholesterol by about 12% (6892) and apolipoprotein A-I by about 2.2% (8649). This increase in HDL cholesterol levels may account for about 50% of the cardioprotective effect of moderate alcohol consumption (2261,6838,6841). Moderate alcohol consumption also decreases low-density lipoprotein (LDL) cholesterol by 5% to 17% (6841,8649), triglycerides by 5% to 10%, and apolipoprotein B levels by 3.7% (8649). There is concern that moderate alcohol consumption can increase systolic blood pressure (6841). However, there is evidence that light to moderate alcohol consumption does not increase the risk of hypertension and may actually decrease the risk (8102). Effects of alcohol on blood clotting include a reduction in clotting potential and enhancement of clot breakdown (2261). Alcohol consumption decreases platelet aggregation, possibly via inhibition of prostaglandin synthesis (6892). Moderate alcohol consumption is also associated with an increase in plasma levels of tissue-type plasminogen activator, an indicator of fibrinolytic capacity (6894). Alcohol also seems to lower fibrinogen and interleukin-1 alpha concentrations (11943). Light to moderate alcohol consumption also seems to produce a reduction in coronary narrowing due to atherosclerosis (2261,6840,8652).

Wine may also have anti-inflammatory effects. It reduces high sensitivity C-reactive protein (hs-CRP) and expression of adhesion molecules, markers of inflammation that seem to be related to early atherosclerosis (11943).

There is also evidence that an increased intake of dietary folate or the use of supplemental folate (400 mcg/day) in moderate alcohol users can lower homocysteine levels compared with nonusers of alcohol (8101). High levels of homocysteine are a risk factor for cardiovascular disease. Homocysteine breakdown and removal requires folate, and alcohol is an antagonist of folate metabolism (8101). The protective effect of alcohol against cardiovascular disease is lost at higher intakes of alcohol (greater than one to two drinks per day). High alcohol consumption can cause increased homocysteine levels, hypertension, hemorrhagic stroke, fatal arrhythmias, and direct damage to heart muscle (alcoholic cardiomyopathy) (2060,2261,2267,2270,8101,8102,8103).

Some alcoholic beverages, in particular red wine, have constituents that may be more protective than others against coronary heart disease, but there is no conclusive evidence of this from clinical studies (2267,2268,6892). Red wine has higher concentrations of polyphenolic compounds than other alcoholic drinks. The antioxidant properties of these polyphenols may contribute to protection against coronary heart disease by reducing oxidation of LDL cholesterol (2268). The polyphenolic compounds in red wine include trans-resveratrol; proanthocyanidins; anthocyanins; and flavonoids such as quercetin, kaempferol, and catechins (1262,2057,8976). However, the polyphenol content of wine is highly dependent on grape type, climate, and practices used to make the wine (2057). Unlike red wines, white wines have very low polyphenol concentrations (2030). The antioxidant potential of plasma and erythrocytes is increased for up to 4.5 hours after red wine consumption (6828). However, there is some evidence that the increase of polyphenols in plasma after red wine consumption is not sufficient to acutely influence lipoprotein oxidation (1262,6826,8976). There is evidence that other foods such as onions and black tea may be better sources of polyphenols than red wine (8976). Additionally, a difference in lifestyle among wine, beer, and other alcohol beverage drinkers, including diet and social class, might also explain why some alcoholic beverages appear to offer more protection than others against CHD (10129).

Several red wine components also have in vitro antiplatelet effects, including trans-resveratrol, quercetin, and catechins (2057). Red wine and white wine seem to have similar activity on platelets (2057,2949). Human data also suggest rebound hypercoagulability can normally occur when acute or chronic alcohol consumption stops, but that red wine attenuates this effect (2060,2061). Red wine might also reduce mutagenic DNA damage and improve endothelial function when added to a high fat diet. Red wine also might have additive vasorelaxing benefits with a low-fat, high plant material diet (2059).

Possible mechanisms by which alcohol could have a protective effect against ischemic stroke include increasing HDL and prostacyclin, decreasing fibrinogen, and inhibiting platelet aggregation (6842). There is evidence that moderate alcohol increases cerebral blood flow (8651). Moderate alcohol consumption is associated with a lower prevalence of white matter changes and brain infarcts on magnetic resonance imaging in adults 65 years of age or older compared to non-drinkers and heavy drinkers (8651).

Moderate alcohol intake may be protective against the development of type 2 diabetes due to an increase in insulin sensitivity (6891). Wine stimulates gastric acid secretion and gastrin release. This may explain why moderate to high alcohol consumption from beverages such as wine seems to prevent Helicobacter pylori infection (8034). Moderate alcohol consumption may be protective against postmenopausal bone loss due to an increase in estrogen levels, increased calcitonin secretion, and reduced parathyroid hormone secretion (6825,6836,8655). However, heavy and chronic alcohol consumption reduces bone mineral density, possibly due to increased calcium and magnesium excretion, increased cortisol secretion, and reduced osteoblast activity (6836,8656). Chronic alcoholics also often have other risk factors for osteoporosis, including poor nutrition, smoking, sedentary lifestyle, and lower body weight (6825,6836).

Adverse Reactions

Orally, wine can cause a variety of side effects due to the alcohol content. The side effects depend on the amount ingested and can vary among individuals. Some common side effects include flushing, confusion, emotional lability, perceptual and sensational disturbances, blackouts, lack of coordination and trouble walking, central nervous system (CNS) depression, drowsiness, respiratory depression, hypothermia, hypoglycemia, nausea, vomiting, diarrhea, abdominal pain, and others. Chronic heavy ethanol ingestion (three or more alcoholic drinks per day) can lead to physical dependence, malnutrition, amnesia, dementia, somnolence, cardiac myopathy, hepatotoxicity, and cirrhosis. Other effects of chronic abuse are pancreatitis, hypomagnesemia, skeletal myopathies, Wernicke's encephalopathy, Korsakoff's psychosis, chronic cerebellar syndrome, mouth cancer, esophageal cancer, pharyngeal cancer, laryngeal cancer, and liver cancer (6843,8972,9004). There is evidence that heavy alcohol consumption is associated with the mutation of the p53 gene in individuals with esophageal carcinoma (9005). There is also some evidence heavy consumption of wine is associated with the highest risk of esophageal cancer compared to heavy consumption of beer and spirits (8972). Chronic intake of three or more drinks per day is associated with an increased risk of all-cause mortality, ischemic stroke, and hypertension (2261,6892,8102). Heavy alcohol consumption (fifteen or more drinks per week) is also associated with a higher percentage of white matter changes and larger ventricular and sulcal size on magnetic resonance imaging of the brain, suggesting heavy alcohol consumption decreases cerebral blood flow and may contribute to brain atrophy (8651). Consumption of any amount of alcohol can increase the risk of hemorrhagic stroke (841,2271).

Daily consumption one or more alcoholic drinks in women might increase the risk of breast cancer by 2% to 15% and increase mortality from breast cancer by as much as 30% (6843,8100,8974). There is also evidence in women who consume alcohol daily that the risk for breast cancer increases when the daily intake of folate is 300 mcg or less (8974).

Some research suggests an association between alcohol consumption and an increased risk for pancreatic cancer, but other studies do not support this association (8038).

Wine is associated with triggering asthmatic reactions in people with a history of asthma, possibly due to salicylates and/or added sulfites contained in wines (6174). People who are allergic to sulfites and/or yeast might react to wine. There is some evidence consumption of more than six beers per week is associated with a larger waist-to-hip ratio than those consuming an equivalent amount of hard liquor or wine. However, an association between moderate alcohol intake equivalent to approximately three beers per week or less and waist-to-hip ratio does not seem to exist (10164,10165). It is also unclear whether waist-to-hip ratios associated with the intake of wine, beer, or other alcoholic beverages have any clinical significance (9007).

Interactions with Herbs & Other Dietary Supplements

HERBS/SUPPLEMENTS WITH SEDATIVE PROPERTIES: Theoretically, concomitant use of wine with herbs that have sedative properties might enhance adverse effects (2262). Some of these supplements include 5-HTP, calamus, California poppy, catnip, hops, Jamaican dogwood, kava, St. John's wort, scullcap, valerian, yerba mansa, and others.

Interactions with Drugs

ASPIRIN: Concomitant use of aspirin with alcohol may increase the risk of gastrointestinal (GI) bleeding (2262).
BARBITURATES: Concomitant consumption of large amounts of alcohol may decrease metabolism of barbiturates (2262). Some of these sedative medications include pentobarbital (Nembutal), phenobarbital (Luminal), secobarbital (Seconal), and others.
BENZODIAZEPINES: Concomitant consumption of large amounts of alcohol may decrease metabolism of benzodiazepines (2262).
CEFAMANDOLE (Mandol): Cefamandole antibiotics can cause a disulfiram-like reaction when taken with alcohol (2262).
CEFOPERAZONE (Cefobid): Cefoperazone can cause a disulfiram-like reaction when taken with alcohol (2262).
CHLORPROPAMIDE (Diabinese): Chlorpropamide can cause a disulfiram-like reaction when taken with alcohol (506).
CISAPRIDE (Propulsid): Concomitant use of cisapride might increase blood alcohol levels and effects, due to the alcohol in wine (2262). Red wine increases plasma cisapride concentrations, possibly by reducing metabolism (1383).
CNS DEPRESSANTS: Concomitant use of antihistamines, barbiturates, benzodiazepines, and tricyclic antidepressants with alcohol may increase sedative and other adverse effects (2262).
CYCLOSPORINE (Neoral, Sandimmune): Red wine reduces plasma cyclosporine concentrations, possibly by reducing cyclosporine absorption. There is evidence the reduction in cyclosporine AUC by red wine is less in Asians (8% to 14%) than Caucasians (35% to 36%) (1384,1387,8977).
DISULFIRAM (Antabuse): The alcohol content of wine can cause a disulfiram reaction when taken within 12 hours of disulfiram (2262). Patients taking disulfiram should not drink any alcoholic beverages including wine.
ERYTHROMYCIN: Concomitant use of erythromycin with alcohol may increase blood alcohol levels and effect (2262).
FELODIPINE (Plendil): Red wine can cause "dose dumping" of extended release felodipine. Red wine taken on an empty stomach with felodipine can alter the pharmacokinetics of extended release felodipine, possibly by changing absorption or metabolism. Red wine can delay the appearance of felodipine in plasma until 4 hours after dosing and can rapidly increase its plasma concentration, producing peak serum levels 3 to 4 times higher than when felodipine is given with water. This can cause an increase in adverse effects 5 hours after dosing (11976).
GRISEOFULVIN (Fulvicin): Griseofulvin can cause a disulfiram-like reaction when taken with alcohol (2262).
H2-BLOCKERS: Concomitant use of cimetidine (Tagamet) and ranitidine (Zantac) with alcohol may increase blood alcohol levels and adverse effects (2262).
HEPATOTOXIC DRUGS: Concomitant use with acetaminophen, isoniazid, and phenylbutazone may increase the risk of hepatotoxicity (2262).
METFORMIN (Glucophage): Concomitant consumption of large amounts of alcohol may increase the risk of lactic acidosis with metformin (2262).
METRONIDAZOLE (Flagyl): Metronidazole can cause a disulfiram-like reaction when taken with alcohol (2262).
MONOAMINE OXIDASE INHIBITORS (MAOIs): Concomitant use of MAOIs with red wine may cause hypertensive crisis due to the tyramine content of wines (506).
NARCOTIC DRUGS: Concomitant consumption of large amounts of alcohol may decrease metabolism of narcotics (2262).
NONSTEROIDAL ANTI-INFLAMMATORY DRUGS (NSAIDs): Concomitant use of nonsteroidal anti-inflammatory drugs with alcohol may increase the risk of gastrointestinal (GI) bleeding (2262).
PHENYTOIN (Dilantin): Concomitant consumption of large amounts of alcohol may induce metabolism, reducing therapeutic effectiveness of phenytoin (2262).
SULFONAMIDE ANTIBIOTICS: Sulfonamide antibiotics can cause a disulfiram-like reaction when taken with alcohol (2262).
TOLBUTAMIDE (Orinase): Tolbutamide can cause a disulfiram-like reaction when taken with alcohol (2262).
WARFARIN (Coumadin): Acute alcohol intoxication can decrease metabolism and increase effects of warfarin (2262). In contrast, chronic intoxication can induce metabolism of warfarin, reducing therapeutic effectiveness (2262).

Drug Influences on Nutrient Levels and Depletion

B VITAMINS: Concomitant chronic use with alcohol might interfere with absorption of B vitamins and other nutrients (2263).

Interactions with Foods

None known.

Interactions with Lab Tests

LIVER FUNCTION TESTS: Chronic alcohol ingestion may increase alkaline phosphatase (Alk phos), alanine aminotransferase (ALT), aspartate aminotransferase (AST), gamma-glutamyltransferase (GGT), and bilirubin test results (2263).
MEAN CORPUSCULAR VOLUME (MCV): Chronic alcohol ingestion may increase MCV (2263).
TRIGLYCERIDES: Chronic alcohol ingestion may increase triglycerides (2263).

Interactions with Diseases or Conditions

ASTHMA: Wine is associated with triggering asthma reactions, possibly due to salicylates and/or added sulfites contained in wines (6174).
GOUT: Alcohol use may exacerbate gout (2263).
HEART CONDITIONS: Alcohol use may exacerbate congestive heart failure (2261,2263,6889) and idiopathic cardiomyopathy (6889).
HIGH BLOOD PRESSURE: Consuming three or more alcoholic drinks a day may increase blood pressure and exacerbate hypertension (2261).
HYPERTRIGLYCERIDEMIA: Alcohol use may exacerbate hypertriglyceridemia (2261,2263,6892).
INSOMNIA: Alcohol use may exacerbate insomnia (2263).
LIVER DISEASE: Alcohol use may exacerbate liver disease (2261).
NEUROLOGICAL CONDITIONS: Alcohol use may exacerbate degenerative neurological conditions (6889).
PANCREATITIS: Alcohol use may exacerbate pancreatitis (2261).
PEPTIC ULCER DISEASE (PUD)/GASTROESOPHAGEAL REFLUX DISEASE (GERD): Alcohol use may exacerbate PUD and GERD (2261,2263).
PORPHYRIA: Alcohol use may exacerbate porphyria (2261).
PSYCHIATRIC DISORDERS: Consuming three or more drinks of alcohol a day may exacerbate psychiatric disorders and increase cognitive impairment (2261).

Dosage and Administration

ORAL: For reducing the risk of cardiovascular disease, ischemic stroke, and all-cause mortality, 1-2 glasses (120-240 mL) per day has been used (2261,2271,6835,6837,6840,6841,6842,6888,6892,6893,8648,8649,8650,10128). Up to four glasses per day has been used to reduce the risk for heart failure (8104). Up to one drink per day has been used to lessen cognitive decline in older men (6824,6829). Between two drinks per week and three or four drinks per day has been used to reduce risk of type 2 diabetes in healthy men (6172,6891). Up to seven drinks per week has been used to reduce the risk of coronary heart disease (CHD) in people with type 2 diabetes (8653,8654). Consumption of more than 75 grams of alcohol from beverages such as wine has been used to reduce the risk of Helicobacter pylori infection (8034).
TOPICAL: No typical dosage.

Comments

One report disputes the "French paradox" and suggests that reduced risk of heart disease in the French population is not due to red wine consumption, but due to the traditional French diet, which is low in animal fat (835).

WINTER CHERRY

Also Known As

Cape Gooseberry, Chinese Lantern, Coqueret, Japanaese Lantern, Strawberry Tomato.
CAUTION: See separate listing for Ashwagandha.

Scientific Names

Physalis alkekengi.
Family: Solanaceae.

Comments

At the date of publication, there was very little scientific information available about this product. Our staff is continually analyzing the available information on natural medicines and will add data to the online version of *Natural Medicines Comprehensive Database* as it becomes available. See www.naturaldatabase.com.

WINTER SAVORY

Also Known As

Mountain Savory Oil, Savory.
CAUTION: See separate listing for Summer Savory.

Scientific Names

Satureja montana; Satureja obovata, synonym Calamintha montana.
Family: Lamiaceae/Labiatae.

People Use This For
Orally, winter savory is used for intestinal disorders including cramps, indigestion, diarrhea, nausea, flatulence, sore throat, as a tonic, expectorant, and to decrease libido.
In manufacturing, the oleoresin of winter savory oil is used as a flavoring agent.

Safety
LIKELY SAFE ...when used orally in amounts commonly found in foods. Summer savory has Generally Recognized As Safe (GRAS) status in the US (4912).
There is insufficient reliable information available about the safety of the medicinal use of winter savory.
PREGNANCY AND LACTATION: Insufficient reliable information available; avoid using.

Effectiveness
There is insufficient reliable information available about the effectiveness of winter savory.

Mechanism of Action
The applicable parts of winter savory are the leaf and stem. Winter savory contains flavonoids (11), ursolic and oleanolic acids, and 1.6% volatile oil. Constituents of the volatile oil include carvacrol, p-cymene, and thymol (6,11). Some evidence suggests the flavonoid, eriodictyol, might have a vasodilator effect (4124). Other information indicates carvacrol, found in both savories, might have diuretic effects (6,11).

Adverse Reactions
None reported.

Interactions with Herbs & Other Dietary Supplements
None known.

Interactions with Drugs
None known.

Interactions with Foods
None known.

Interactions with Lab Tests
None known.

Interactions with Diseases or Conditions
None known.

Dosage and Administration
No typical dosage.

Comments
Although summer savory and winter savory are both used as spices, in the United States summer savory is the most common (6).

WINTER'S BARK

Also Known As
Pepper Bark, Wintera, Wintera Aromatica, Winters Bark, Winter's Cinnamon, Winters Cinnamon.

Scientific Names
Drimys winteri, synonym Drimys chilensis.
Family: Winteraceae.

Comments
At the date of publication, this product was not a common ingredient used in brand name supplements marketed to consumers. Details about this product are available in the online version of *Natural Medicines Comprehensive Database.* See www.naturaldatabase.com.

WINTERGREEN

Also Known As

Boxberry, Canada Tea, Checkerberry, Deerberry, Gaultheria Oil, Ground Berry, Hilberry, Mountain Tea, Oil of Wintergreen, Partridge Berry, Spiceberry, Teaberry, Wax Cluster, Wintergreen leaf, Wintergreen oil.
CAUTION: See separate listing for Periwinkle.

Scientific Names

Gaultheria procumbens.
Family: Ericaceae.

People Use This For

Orally, wintergreen leaf is used for headache, stomachache, flatulence, fever, kidney disorders, asthma, neuralgia (particularly sciatica), pleurisy, ovarian pain, inflammation of the epididymis, inflammation of the diaphragm, gout, arthritis, and dysmenorrhea. Small doses of wintergreen oil have been used to stimulate gastric secretion and aid digestion.
Topically, wintergreen leaf is used as a wash for rheumatism, sore muscles, and lumbago. Wintergreen oil is used topically as a counterirritant, for musculoskeletal pain, and as an antiseptic.
In manufacturing, wintergreen is used as a flavoring agent in food, candies, teas, and in pharmaceutical products.

Safety

LIKELY SAFE ...when used in amounts commonly found in foods. Wintergreen oil has Generally Recognized As Safe status (GRAS) in the US (4912).
POSSIBLY SAFE ...when wintergreen leaf is used orally and appropriately in medicinal amounts (12). ...when wintergreen oil is used topically and appropriately (272).
POSSIBLY UNSAFE ...when wintergreen oil is used orally. Wintergreen oil contains large amounts of methyl salicylate (272).
CHILDREN: LIKELY UNSAFE ...when used orally. Ingesting 4-10 mL of wintergreen oil can be lethal (159). ...when wintergreen oil is used topically in children less than 2 years old (272).
PREGNANCY: Insufficient reliable information; avoid using in amounts greater than those found in foods.
LACTATION: LIKELY UNSAFE ...when used orally or topically. Wintergreen products might be toxic to nursing infants (19).

Effectiveness

There is insufficient reliable information available about the effectiveness of wintergreen.

Mechanism of Action

The applicable parts of wintergreen are the leaf and oil. When freshly harvested, the plant contains galutherin that changes into methyl salicylate as the plant is dried (18). The leaves contain 0.5-0.8% wintergreen oil (6). Wintergreen oil contains 98% methyl salicylate (6). It has antipyretic, anti-inflammatory, and analgesic properties (11), possibly due to its counterirritant effect (6).

Adverse Reactions

Orally, ingestion of wintergreen oil can cause salicylate poisoning (salicylism) including tinnitus, nausea, vomiting, diarrhea, headache, stomach pain, and confusion (272,3805).
Topically, contact dermatitis can occur (18). When applied topically and covered with an occlusive dressing, 12-20% of methyl salicylate is absorbed systemically over 10 hours (272).

Interactions with Herbs & Other Dietary Supplements

None known.

Interactions with Drugs

ASPIRIN: Topical use of wintergreen oil in large amounts, with occlusive dressings, or for prolonged periods of time, can cause additive salicylate toxicity (159, 272).
WARFARIN (Coumadin): Concomitant use of topical wintergreen oil-containing products and warfarin can increase INR and bleeding risk due to systemic absorption of the methyl salicylate contained in wintergreen oil (3811,6181). Topical analgesic gels, lotions, creams, ointments, liniments, and sprays can contain up to 55% methyl salicylate (6181).

Interactions with Foods

None known.

Interactions with Lab Tests

None known.

Interactions with Diseases or Conditions

GASTROINTESTINAL INFLAMMATION: Oral use is contraindicated because it can aggravate inflammation (19).
SALICYLATE ALLERGY/ASTHMA: Individuals with salicylate allergy, asthma, or nasal polyps should use cautiously due to its potential for allergic reaction (272).

Dosage and Administration

ORAL: No typical dosage. However, wintergreen leaf has been used as a tea, 1 teaspoon of the dried leaves in 1 cup boiling water. The tea is taken cold, 1 cup per day (5253,5254).
TOPICAL: Wintergreen is used as a gel, lotion, ointment, or liniment (containing 10-60% methyl salicylate) 3-4 times daily (3). Heat can increase skin absorption; do not apply after strenuous exercise or use a heating pad after application (3).

Comments

Wintergreen oil is obtained by steam distillation of warmed, water-macerated leaves.

WITCH HAZEL

Also Known As

Hamamelis, Hazel, Snapping Tobacco Wood, Spotted Elder, Winter Bloom, Witchazel.

Scientific Names

Hamamelis virginiana.
Family: Hamamelidaceae.

People Use This For

Orally, witch hazel is used for diarrhea, mucus colitis, vomiting blood, coughing up blood, tuberculosis, colds, fevers, tumors and cancer.
Topically, witch hazel is used for itching, skin inflammation, eye inflammation, skin injury, mucous membrane inflammation, varicose veins, hemorrhoids, bruises, insect bites, minor burns, and other skin irritations.
In manufacturing, witch hazel leaf extract, bark extract, and witch hazel water are used as astringents and hemostatics in preparations for insect bites, stings, teething, hemorrhoids, itching, irritations, and minor pain.

Safety

LIKELY SAFE ...when witch hazel water is used topically and appropriately (272).
POSSIBLY SAFE ...when used orally and appropriately (12). In high doses, tannins in witch hazel bark can cause liver damage (8). The volatile oil contains safrole, a known carcinogen, but in amounts too small for concern (4).
PREGNANCY AND LACTATION: Insufficient reliable information available; avoid using.

Effectiveness

POSSIBLY EFFECTIVE

Hemorrhoids. Applying witch hazel water topically may help to temporarily relieve itching, discomfort, irritation, and burning associated with anorectal disorders (272).
Minor bleeding. Applying witch hazel bark, leaf, or water as a styptic seems to reduce minor bleeding (7,8).
Skin irritation. Applying witch hazel cream topically relieve mild skin irritation, but less so than hydrocortisone (11151).

There is insufficient reliable information available about the effectiveness of witch hazel for its other uses.

Mechanism of Action

The applicable parts of witch hazel are the leaf and bark. The active constituents include gallotannins, gallic acid, myricetin, quercetin, kaempferol, and catechol derivatives. Witch hazel leaf and bark possess astringent, styptic, and anti-inflammatory properties (10377). The leaf contains 8-10% tannins (512). The bark contains up to 12% tannins (10377).
Tannins, applied topically to broken skin or mucous membranes induce protein precipitation. They tighten up superficial cell layers and shrink colloidal structures thereby causing capillaries to constrict. The decrease in vascular permeability approximates an anti-inflammatory effect. The astringent activity of tannins also causes an indirect antibacterial effect (7).
Steam distillation used for producing Hamamelis water removes the tannins (13). Thus, the astringent properties of Hamamelis water result from its 14-15% alcohol content (13).

Adverse Reactions

Orally, plants with at least 10% tannins can cause gastrointestinal disturbances, kidney damage, and necrotic conditions of the liver (12). Some evidence suggests that tannins might cause cancer; other evidence shows tannins

may prevent it (12). Regular consumption of herbs with high tannin concentrations correlates with increased incidence of esophageal or nasal cancer (12).
Topically, witch hazel can cause contact dermatitis (6).

Interactions with Herbs & Other Dietary Supplements
None known.

Interactions with Drugs
None known.

Interactions with Foods
None known.

Interactions with Lab Tests
None known.

Interactions with Diseases or Conditions
None known.

Dosage and Administration
ORAL: A typical dose is 2 grams of dried leaves three times daily or as tea. To make tea, steep 2 grams in 150 mL of boiling water for 5-10 minutes, and strain (4). Hamamelis Liquid Extract (1:1 in 45% alcohol), 2-4 mL three times daily, has also been used (4).
TOPICAL: For compresses and irrigations, simmer 5-10 grams leaf and bark per 250 mL of water (2). For poultice, use witch hazel water (Hamamelis water) undiluted or diluted 1:3 with water. Semisolid preparations 20-30% (2). Extracts, semisolid and liquid preparations corresponding to 5-10% leaf and bark (2).
RECTAL: Suppositories, corresponding to 0.1-1 grams leaf and bark applied 1-3 times daily (2). Anorectal disorders, Hamamelis water applied externally up to six times a day or after each bowel movement (272).

Comments
Witch hazel water (Hamamelis water, distilled witch hazel extract) is distilled from dried leaves, bark, and partially dormant twigs of Hamamelis virginiana (11).

WOOD ANEMONE

Also Known As
Crowfoot, Smell Fox, Wind Flower.

Scientific Names
Anemone nemorosa.
Family: Ranunculaceae.

People Use This For
Orally, wood anemone is used orally for stomach pains, delayed menstruation, gout, whooping cough, and asthma.

Safety
LIKELY UNSAFE ...when the fresh plant is used orally. Freshly harvested wood anemone can cause severe irritation to the gastrointestinal tract. Ingesting 30 freshly harvested plants is believed to be fatal (18).
There is insufficient reliable information available about the safety of the dried, cut above ground parts.
PREGNANCY AND LACTATION: LIKELY UNSAFE ...when the fresh plant is used orally or topically (18).
There is insufficient reliable information available about the safety of the oral or topical use of the dried, cut plant during pregnancy and lactation; avoid using.

Effectiveness
There is insufficient reliable information available about the effectiveness of wood anemone.

Mechanism of Action
The applicable parts of wood anemone are the above ground parts. When the fresh plant is crushed or cut into small pieces, the glycoside ranunculin is enzymatically changed into a severely irritating protoanemonin, which, in turn, rapidly degrades into the less toxic anemonin (18). Both protoanemonin and ranunculin are destroyed to an unknown extent during the drying process (2).

Adverse Reactions
Orally, the ingestion of freshly harvested wood anemone can cause colic, diarrhea, and severe irritation to the gastrointestinal tract and the urinary drainage passages (18).
Topically, wood anemone can cause slow-healing blisters and burns after prolonged skin contact (18).

Interactions with Herbs & Other Dietary Supplements
None known.

Interactions with Drugs
None known.

Interactions with Foods
None known.

Interactions with Lab Tests
None known.

Interactions with Diseases or Conditions
None known.

Dosage and Administration
No typical dosage.

Comments
Avoid confusion with the poisonous plant, pasque flower (Pulsatilla pratensis). Although the two plants are from the same botanical family and have similar pharmacological compounds, they are not synonymous (2,18). Wood anemone was traditionally used in Russian folk medicine.

WOOD SAGE

Also Known As
Ambroise, Garlic Sage, Hind Heal, Large-Leaved Germander.
CAUTION: See separate listings for Sage and Tansy.

Scientific Names
Teucrium scorodonia.
Family: Lamiaceae/Labiatae.

Comments
At the date of publication, there was very little scientific information available about this product. Our staff is continually analyzing the available information on natural medicines and will add data to the online version of *Natural Medicines Comprehensive Database* as it becomes available. See www.naturaldatabase.com.

WOOD SORREL

Also Known As
Common Sorrel, Cuckoo Bread, Cuckowes Meat, Fairy Bells, Green Sauce, Hallelujah, Mountain Sorrel, Shamrock, Sour Trefoil, Stickwort, Stubwort, Surelle, Three-Leaved Grass, White Sorrel, Wood Sour.
CAUTION: See separate listing for Sorrel and Yellowdock.

Scientific Names
Oxalis acetosella, synonym Oxalis montana.
Family: Oxalidaceae.

People Use This For
Orally, wood sorrel is used for liver and digestive disorders, scurvy, wounds, and inflammation of the gums.

Safety
POSSIBLY UNSAFE ...when used orally, particularly in large amounts (6,17).
CHILDREN: POSSIBLY UNSAFE ...when used orally. One four-year old child died after consuming rhubarb leaves, which is also a source of oxalic acid (17).

PREGNANCY: LIKELY UNSAFE ...when used orally because it might stimulate menses (19); avoid using.
LACTATION: POSSIBLY UNSAFE ...when used orally (6,17); avoid using.

Effectiveness
There is insufficient reliable information available about the effectiveness of wood sorrel.

Mechanism of Action
The applicable part of wood sorrel is the whole flowering plant. It contains 0.3-1.25% oxalic acid (18). Oxalate content is high in fresh leaves and roots (17,19). Once absorbed, the oxalic acid reacts with calcium in plasma and resulting insoluble calcium oxalate may precipitate in the kidneys, blood vessels, heart, lungs, and liver. This may also cause hypocalcemia (12,17). Oxalate crystals damage mucosal tissue, resulting in severe irritation and possible damage. The systemic absorption of oxalates may result in kidney damage, both in people with pre-existing kidney disease and in healthy kidneys (19).

Adverse Reactions
Orally, consuming excessive amounts of wood sorrel can cause diarrhea, nausea, polyuria (6), dermatitis (4), and gastrointestinal symptoms due to its oxalic acid content. Oxalic acid poisoning affects skin, eyes, respiratory system, and kidneys. Oral symptoms of oxalate irritation include swelling of the mouth, tongue and throat, with difficulty in speaking and suffocation. It has a corrosive effect on the digestive tract. It can lead to oxalic acid crystals in the kidneys, blood vessels, heart, lungs, liver, and/or hypocalcemia (17).

Interactions with Herbs & Other Dietary Supplements
CALCIUM, IRON, ZINC: Concurrent use might decrease mineral absorption. Wood sorrel contains oxalate (7,12), which can bind multivalent metal ions in the gastrointestinal tract and decrease mineral absorption.

Interactions with Drugs
None known.

Interactions with Foods
CALCIUM, IRON, ZINC: Concurrent use might decrease mineral absorption from foods. Wood sorrel contains oxalate (7,12), which can bind multivalent metal ions in the gastrointestinal tract and decrease mineral absorption.

Interactions with Lab Tests
None known.

Interactions with Diseases or Conditions
COAGULATION DISORDERS: Oxalate constituents can alter the calcium concentrations and decrease coagulation time (4,12).
GI CONDITIONS: Theoretically can exacerbate stomach and intestinal ulcers due to mucosal irritant effect (19).
KIDNEY DISEASE: Can damage kidneys with formation of insoluble oxalate; use with caution or avoid in individuals with history of kidney stones or kidney disease (12,19).

Dosage and Administration
No typical dosage.

Comments
Wood sorrel is also called common sorrel, and could be confused with sorrel.

WOODBINE

Also Known As
Clematis, Devil's Darning Needle, Old Man's Beard, Traveler's Joy, Vine Bower, Virgin's Bower.
CAUTION: See separate listings for Clematis, Fringetree, Traveler's Joy, and Usnea.

Scientific Names
Clematis virginiana.
Family: Rananculaceae.

People Use This For
Orally, woodbine is used for skin sores, cuts, itching, venereal disorders, cancer, tumors, itching, fever, nephrosis, ulcers, diuretic, purgative, tuberculosis, and cervical lymphadenitis.

Safety
LIKELY UNSAFE ...when used orally or topically because it is a powerful irritant (6).
PREGNANCY AND LACTATION: LIKELY UNSAFE ...when used orally or topically (6); avoid using.

Effectiveness
There is insufficient reliable information available about the effectiveness of woodbine.

Mechanism of Action
The applicable part of woodbine is the leaf. There is insufficient reliable information available about the possible mechanism of action and active ingredients.

Adverse Reactions
Orally, the juice derived from the woodbine leaf is said to be a powerful local irritant (6).

Interactions with Herbs & Other Dietary Supplements
None known.

Interactions with Drugs
None known.

Interactions with Foods
None known.

Interactions with Lab Tests
None known.

Interactions with Diseases or Conditions
None known.

Dosage and Administration
ORAL: People typically make a liquid preparation of woodbine, combining one heaping teaspoon of leaves and flowers with one cup of water and allowing the mixture to stand for 30 minutes. The dose is one tablespoon 4 to 6 times daily (5263).

Comments
Avoid confusion with American ivy, gelsemium or honeysuckle, which are also known as woodbine.

WORMSEED

Also Known As
Levant, Santonica, Sea Wormwood, Worm Seed.
CAUTION: See separate listings for Chenopodium Oil, Levant Berry, Mugwort. Wormwood, and Wormwood Oil.

Scientific Names
Artemisia cina, synonym Seriphidium cinum.
Family: Asteraceae/Compositae.

People Use This For
Orally, wormseed is used for ascaris and oxyuris infestations.

Safety
UNSAFE ...when used orally due to its highly toxic adverse effects (18).
PREGNANCY AND LACTATION: UNSAFE ...when used orally due to potential for toxicity (18); avoid using.

Effectiveness
There is insufficient reliable information available about the effectiveness of wormseed.

Mechanism of Action
The anthelmintic activity is attributed to the sesquiterpene lactone beta-santonin. When wormseed is used with a laxative, it appears to paralyze the muscles of ascarids and facilitate their elimination from the body. Some data suggest wormseed lowers body temperature when a fever is present (18).

Adverse Reactions
Orally, death has been reported with less than 10 grams of herb. Symptoms of poisoning are possible in amounts used to treat parasitic infestations. Symptoms may include kidney irritation, gastroenteritis, stupor, visual disorders, muscle twitching, and epileptiform spasms (18). It can cause an allergic reaction in individuals sensitive to the Asteraceae/Compositae family. Members of this family include ragweed, chrysanthemums, marigolds, daisies, and many other herbs.

Interactions with Herbs & Other Dietary Supplements
None known.

Interactions with Drugs
None known.

Interactions with Foods
None known.

Interactions with Lab Tests
None known.

Interactions with Diseases or Conditions
CROSS-ALLERGENICITY: Can cause an allergic reaction in individuals sensitive to the Asteraceae/Compositae family. Members of this family include ragweed, chrysanthemums, marigolds, daisies, and many other herbs.

Dosage and Administration
No typical dosage.

Comments
Avoid confusing wormseed with chenopodium oil (or wormseed oil), wormwood oil, or wormwood. Avoid confusing wormseed, also referred to as levant, with levant berry.

WORMWOOD

Also Known As
Absinthe, Absinthii Herba, Absinthites, Ajenjo, Armoise, Artemisia, Artesian Absinthium, Common Wormwood, Green Ginger, Herbe d'Absinthe, Indhana, Lapsent, Vilayati Afsanteen, Wermut, Wermutkraut, Wurmkraut.
CAUTION: See separate listing for Ginger and Mugwort.

Scientific Names
Artemisia absinthium.
Family: Asteraceae/Compositae.

People Use This For
Orally, wormwood is used for loss of appetite, indigestion, biliary dyskinesia, and gastrointestinal complaints such as low acidity gastritis. Wormwood is also used as an anthelmintic, aphrodisiac, tonic, antispasmodic, and to stimulate sweating. It is also used for fever and liver disease. Orally, wormwood oil is used for digestive disorders, as an aphrodisiac, and to stimulate the imagination.
Topically, wormwood is used for healing wounds and insect bites. Wormwood oil is used as a counterirritant.
In foods, wormwood is used as a flavoring agent for products such as alcoholic bitters and vermouth.
In manufacturing, wormwood oil is used as a fragrance component in soaps, cosmetics, and perfumes. It is also used as an insecticide.

Safety
LIKELY SAFE ...when used orally in the amounts commonly found in foods including bitters and vermouth. Wormwood products that are thujone-free have Generally Recognized As Safe status (GRAS) for use in foods in the US (4912).
POSSIBLY UNSAFE ...when products containing thujone are used orally. Thujone is a neurological toxin that is present in the oil contained in wormwood (12617). Seizures, rhabdomyolysis, and acute renal failure can occur when as little as 10 mL of wormwood oil is ingested (662,12817).
There is insufficient reliable information available about the safety of the topical use of wormwood in amounts greater than those found in cosmetics.
PREGNANCY : UNSAFE ...when used orally in amounts greater than those found in foods (662,12817). Some wormwood products contain thujone. Thujone is a CNS stimulant. Theoretically, thujone has potential uterine and menstrual stimulant effects (12617).

There is insufficient reliable information available about the safety of wormwood when used topically in amounts greater than those found in cosmetics. Avoid use.
LACTATION: Insufficient reliable information available; avoid using.

Effectiveness

There is insufficient reliable information available about the effectiveness of wormwood.

Mechanism of Action

The applicable parts of wormwood are the above ground parts. Wormwood is an aromatic bush. It contains up to 1.7% essential oil. It also contains absinthin, anabsinthin, resins, and various organic acids (12814,12815).
Wormwood oil has convulsant effects and insecticidal and vermicidal activity (12817). Other preliminary research suggests it has antiinflammatory, antipyretic, antifertility, antibacterial, antifungal, antimalarial, and anti-amebic activity. An aqueous methanolic extract seems to protect against acetaminophen induced hepatotoxicity, possibly by preventing the breakdown of acetaminophen into reactive metabolites (12818).
The oil in wormwood leaves also contains thujone, which is responsible for its toxicity. Thujone is a CNS stimulant and can cause seizures. Thujone occurs as two isomers, alpha- and beta-thujone. Alpha-thujone is more toxic than beta-thujone (12814,12815). Alpha- and beta- thujone block gamma-aminobutyric acid (GABA) channels, which is likely responsible for their convulsant activity. Alpha-thujone might also increase production of porphyrins, making it potentially more toxic to patients with underlying defects in hepatic heme synthesis (12816).
Thujone is structurally similar to detla-9 tetrahydrocannabinol (THC), the active ingredient in marijuana, but it seems to have low affinity for the cannabinoid receptor (12815).
Preliminary research suggests that thujone is metabolized by the cytochrome P450 enzyme system; the specific human isozyme has not been identified (12816).

Adverse Reactions

Orally, the oil in wormwood leaves can cause nausea, vomiting, diffuse muscle aches, acute renal toxicity, seizures, rhabdomyolysis, and acute renal failure (662). Chronic ingestion of absinthe, an alcoholic beverage that contains wormwood oil, can cause absinthism. Absinthism is characterized by addiction, gastrointestinal adverse effects, insomnia, auditory and visual hallucinations, tremors, paralysis, epilepsy, and brain damage. There is also increased risk of psychiatric disease and suicide (662,12814).
Wormwood can theoretically cause an allergic reaction in people sensitive to the Asteraceae/Compositae family (12815). Members of this family include ragweed, chrysanthemums, marigolds, daisies, and many other herbs.

Interactions with Herbs & Other Dietary Supplements

THUJONE-CONTAINING HERBS: Theoretically, concomitant use might increase the risk of thujone toxicity. Thujone-containing herbs include mugwort, oak moss, oriental arborvitae, sage, savin tops, tansy, thuja (cedar), tree moss, and yarrow (12815); avoid using.

Interactions with Drugs

ANTICONVULSANTS: Theoretically, concomitant use of wormwood might interfere with the effectiveness of anticonvulsant drugs. Thujone, a constituent of wormwood has convulsant effects (12816). Some anticonvulsant drugs include phenobarbital, primidone (Mysoline), valproic acid (Depakene), gabapentin (Neurontin), carbamazepine (Tegretol), phenytoin (Dilantin), and others.

Interactions with Foods

None known.

Interactions with Lab Tests

None known.

Interactions with Diseases or Conditions

CROSS-ALLERGENICITY: Theoretically, wormwood oil can cause an allergic reaction in people sensitive to the Asteraceae/Compositae family (12815). Members of this family include ragweed, chrysanthemums, marigolds, daisies, and many other herbs.
PORPHYRIA: Alpha-thujone, a constituent of wormwood oil, might increase production of porphyrins, making it potentially more toxic to patients with underlying defects in hepatic heme synthesis (12816).
SEIZURE DISORDERS: Theoretically the wormwood constituent, thujone, might lower the seizure threshold (12816).

Dosage and Administration

No typical dosage.

Comments

Absinthe is an emerald-green alcoholic drink that is prepared from wormwood oil. Its use was popularized by famous artists and writers such as Toulouse-Lautrec, Degas, Manet, van Gogh, Picasso, Hemingway, and Oscar

Wilde. It is now banned in many countries, including the US. Traditionally, absinthe is prepared by distilling the essential oil from wormwood. This contains high amounts of the CNS toxin, thujone. Other preparation methods include macerating wormwood in ethanol, which yields a minimal concentration of thujone (12814).

XANTHAN GUM

Also Known As
Bacterial Polysaccharide, Corn Sugar Gum, Xanthan.

Scientific Names
Xanthomonas campestris (Bacterium).

People Use This For
Orally, xanthan gum is used for lowering blood glucose and total plasma cholesterol in people with diabetes. It is also used orally as a laxative.
Topically, xanthan gum is used as a saliva substitute in people with Sjogren's syndrome.
In manufacturing, xanthan gum is used as a thickening, suspending, emulsifying, and stabilizing agent in foods, toothpastes, and pharmaceutical products.

Safety
LIKELY SAFE ...when consumed in amounts found in foods, up to 10 mg/kg per day (4914). It has Generally Recognized As Safe (GRAS) status in the US (4912). ...when used orally for medicinal use in amounts up to 15 grams per day (4914,4916,4917,4918). ...when used topically and appropriately (4914).
PREGNANCY AND LACTATION: Insufficient reliable information is available; avoid using in amounts greater than those found in foods.

Effectiveness
POSSIBLY EFFECTIVE

Constipation. Taking xanthan gum orally as a bulk-forming laxative seems to decrease constipation (4917,4918).
Diabetes. Taking xanthan gum orally seems to lower blood glucose and cholesterol in people with diabetes (4916).
Sjogren's syndrome. Applying xanthan gum topically seems to help as a saliva substitute in people with Sjogren's syndrome (4915).

Mechanism of Action
Xanthan gum is a polysaccharide produced by fermenting carbohydrate with the bacterium Xanthomonas campestris. It is a bulk-forming laxative. In the body, it forms an emollient gel that stimulates peristalsis and passage of intestinal contents (4917). Xanthan gum slows gastric emptying and intestinal absorption of glucose (4916). It mimics saliva as a lubricating and wetting agent in humans (4915), and shows evidence that it might reduce demineralization of tooth enamel (4920).

Adverse Reactions
Orally, xanthan gum can cause flatulence and abdominal distention (4916,4918). Occupational exposure in workers handling xanthan gum powder can cause flu-like symptoms, and nose and throat irritation without acute or chronic loss of pulmonary function (4913).

Interactions with Herbs & Other Dietary Supplements
BULK-FORMING LAXATIVE HERBS AND SUPPLEMENTS: Theoretically, concomitant use may increase likelihood of flatulence and abdominal distention.
HERBS WITH HYPOGLYCEMIC POTENTIAL: Theoretically, concomitant use with pharmacologically active amounts of xanthan gum could result in excessive lowering of blood glucose.

Interactions with Drugs
ANTIDIABETES DRUGS: Xanthan gum seems to lower blood glucose in people with diabetes (4916). Concomitant use of xanthan gum with antidiabetes medication might have additive effects. Monitor blood glucose levels closely. Some antidiabetes drugs include glimepiride (Amaryl), glyburide (DiaBeta, Glynase PresTab, Micronase), insulin, pioglitazone (Actos), rosiglitazone (Avandia), and others.

Interactions with Foods
None known.

Interactions with Lab Tests
BLOOD GLUCOSE: Might lower blood glucose and test results (4916).
CHOLESTEROL: Might lower serum cholesterol and test results (4916).

Interactions with Diseases or Conditions

CONTRAINDICATIONS: Bulk forming laxative are contraindicated in individuals with nausea, vomiting, appendicitis, fecal impaction, intestinal obstruction, or undiagnosed abdominal pain.

Dosage and Administration

ORAL: The World Health Organization (WHO) has set the maximum acceptable intake for xanthan gum as a food additive at 10 mg/kg per day (4914), and as a laxative at 15 grams per day (4918). For safety and effectiveness, bulk laxatives require adequate fluid intake (272). For diabetes a typical dose is 12 grams per day as an ingredient in muffins (4916).
TOPICAL: Saliva substitutes, 0.018% or 0.092% aqueous solutions with added electrolytes and peppermint flavoring (4915).

Comments

Xanthan gum is an ingredient in some sustained release matrix tablets (4914).

XYLITOL

Also Known As

Birch Sugar, E967, Meso-Xylitol, Xylit, Xylite.

Scientific Names

Xylitol; xylo-pentane-1,2,3,4,5-pentol.

People Use This For

Orally, xylitol is used to prevent acute otitis media in young children, and as a sugar substitute for people with diabetes.
Topically, xylitol is used in chewing gums and other oral care products to prevent dental caries and dry mouth.
Intravenously, xylitol is used as an energy source in parenteral nutrition.
In foods, xylitol is used as a sweetener, including sugar-free preparations.

Safety

LIKELY SAFE ...when used orally in amounts commonly found in foods. Xylitol has Generally Recognized As Safe (GRAS) status in the US (4912).
POSSIBLY SAFE ...when used orally and topically, and appropriately in medicinal amounts. Xylitol has been used safely in doses from 20-53 grams per day for up to three years (6815,6819,6821).
POSSIBLY UNSAFE ...when used orally in very high doses, long-term. There is some concern that very high doses for extended periods of use can induce tumor growth (6815,6820). However, this effect has not yet been demonstrated in humans.
CHILDREN: POSSIBLY SAFE ...when used orally and topically, and appropriately in medicinal amounts. Xylitol has been used safely in children in doses up to 20 grams per day for up to three years (6815,6819).
PREGNANCY AND LACTATION: There is insufficient reliable information available about the use of xylitol in medicinal amounts during pregnancy and lactation; avoid using.

Effectiveness

LIKELY EFFECTIVE

Dental caries. Use of xylitol-containing products such as foods, chewing gum, candies, soluble dragees, and toothpaste that provide 1-20 grams of xylitol per day can significantly reduce the rate of cavity formation in both adults and children (6815,6819,6822). Xylitol products appear to be more effective than products containing sorbitol for preventing cavity formation (6822).

POSSIBLY EFFECTIVE

Otitis media. Xylitol 8.4-10 grams per day given orally as a chewing gum, lozenge, or syrup five times a day after meals to preschool children, seems to significantly reduce the number of episodes of acute otitis media and the usage of antibiotics (6816,6817). However, xylitol gum, lozenges, or liquid 8.4-10 grams per day administered at the onset of symptoms of an acute respiratory infection does not seem to prevent acute otitis media (3846).

Mechanism of Action

Xylitol is a polyhydric alcohol (polyol) related to the pentose sugar, xylose (9). Xylitol is found in almost all plant material, including fruits such as raspberries, strawberries, and plums; vegetables; and mushrooms. Commercial preparations are extracted from birch wood (268). In the body, it is produced during metabolism of glucose in the liver (268). Xylitol has several properties that might provide a locally protective effect against dental caries. Xylitol is not fermented by plaque flora to the low pH associated with caries. Xylitol lowers plaque and salivary levels of Streptococcus mutans and lactobacilli, which cause caries. Most children acquire Streptococcus mutans from their mothers after birth. Habitual chewing of xylitol gum by mothers with high bacterial levels beginning three months

after delivery appears to significantly reduce transmission of Streptococcus mutans to their children (6818). Xylitol also reduces bacterial adhesiveness. Xylitol increases salivary flow rates and calcium and phosphate concentrations in saliva, which promote buffering and remineralization of tooth surfaces. Xylitol also stimulates activity of the antimicrobial enzyme lactoperoxidase in saliva (6815,6819).
Due to its five-carbon structure, xylitol is not a substrate for growth of most bacteria, and it may inhibit some bacterial enzymes and interfere with their metabolism of six carbon sugars (6819). In the prevention of acute otitis media, xylitol may work by inhibiting growth of bacteria including Streptococcus pneumoniae, and preventing adhesion of pneumococci and Haemophilus influenzae to nasopharyngeal cells (3846,6819). There is also some preliminary evidence from animal models that suggests xylitol might increase the calcium and phosphorus content of bone and protect against osteoporosis (6819).

Adverse Reactions

Orally, acute administration of large amounts of xylitol (30 to 40 grams) can cause osmotic diarrhea and flatulence. However, if the dose is increased gradually, tolerance to this effect can occur and prevent development of diarrhea and flatulence (9). Intravenous infusion of high doses has been associated with hyperuricemia, changes in liver function tests, and acidosis, including lactic acidosis (6815).

Interactions with Herbs & Other Dietary Supplements

None known.

Interactions with Drugs

None known.

Interactions with Foods

None known.

Interactions with Lab Tests

None known.

Interactions with Diseases or Conditions

None known.

Dosage and Administration

ORAL: For acute otitis media, total daily doses of 8.4 to 10 grams have been used in chewing gum, lozenges, or syrup given in five divided doses, after meals for prevention (3846,6816,6817).
TOPICAL: For prevention of dental caries in adults and children, a wide range of doses has been used. Typically, doses are from 7 to 20 grams per day divided into three to five doses, usually given as candies or chewing gum (6815,6819).
INTRAVENOUS: No typical dosage.

Comments

Xylitol is widely used in other countries as a sugar substitute and in chewing gums, mints, and other candies. Its use in the United States is relatively limited. Sorbitol is the most commonly used sweetener in sugarless gums because it is less expensive than xylitol and easier to formulate into commercial products (8329). Some national brands of chewing gum contain milligram amounts of xylitol, far from the gram doses that seem to prevent tooth decay.

YARROW

Also Known As

Achilee, Achillea, Acuilee, Band Man's Plaything, Bauchweh, Birangasifa, Birangasipha, Biranjasipha, Bloodwort, Carpenter's Weed, Civan Percemi, Common Yarrow, Devil's Nettle, Devil's Plaything, Erba Da Cartentieri, Erba Da Falegname, Gandana, Gemeine Schafgarbe, Green Arrow, Herbe Aux Charpentiers, Katzenkrat, Milefolio, Milfoil, Millefeuille, Millefolii flos, Millefolii herba, Millefolium, Millegoglie, Noble Yarrow, Nosebleed, Old Man's Pepper, Roga Mari, Sanguinary, Soldier's Wound Wort, Staunchweed, Tausendaugbram, Thousand-Leaf, Wound Wort.
CAUTION: See separate listing for Bloodroot.

Scientific Names

Achillea millefolium, synonyms Achillea borealis, Achillea lanulosa, Achillea magna.
Family: Asteraceae/Compositae.

People Use This For

Orally, yarrow is used for fever, common cold, allergic rhinitis, amenorrhea, dysentery, diarrhea, loss of appetite, mild or spastic gastrointestinal (GI) tract discomfort, and to induce sweating. Specifically, yarrow is used orally for thrombotic conditions with hypertension, including cerebral and coronary thromboses.

Orally, the fresh leaves of yarrow are chewed to relieve toothache.
Topically, yarrow is used as a stypticl; for bleeding hemorrhoids; for wounds; and as a sitz bath for painful, lower pelvic, cramp-like conditions of psychosomatic origin in women.
In combination with other herbs, yarrow is used for bloating, flatulence, mild gastrointestinal (GI) cramping, and nervous gastrointestinal complaints.
In foods, the young leaves and flowers of yarrow are used in salads.
In manufacturing, yarrow is also used as a cosmetic cleanser and in snuff. Yarrow oil is used in shampoos.

Safety

LIKELY SAFE ...when used orally in amounts commonly found in foods. Yarrow has Generally Recognized As Safe status (GRAS) for use in foods in the US (4912).
POSSIBLY SAFE ...when used orally and appropriately for medicinal purposes (2,12).
PREGNANCY: LIKELY UNSAFE ...when used orally; yarrow is believed to be an abortifacient and affect the menstrual cycle (12).
LACTATION: Insufficient reliable information available; avoid excessive amounts during lactation (4).

Effectiveness

There is insufficient reliable information available about the effectiveness of yarrow.

Mechanism of Action

The applicable parts of yarrow are the above ground parts. Yarrow has diaphoretic, antipyretic, hypotensive, astringent, diuretic, urinary antiseptic, spasmolytic, and antiflatulent effects (4). Yarrow contains amino acids, fatty acids, ascorbic acid, caffeic acid, folic acid, salicylic acid, succinic acid, alkaloids, flavonoids including rutin, tannins, volatile oil, an unknown cyanogenetic compound, and sugars (4). The volatile oil contains chamazulene, other azulenes (11), and trace amounts of thujone (4,11) The volatile oil content, and especially the azulene content, varies considerably depending on the source (11). Some evidence suggests that achilleine, an alkaloid constituent, might decrease clotting time (4). The alkaloid fraction has shown evidence of antipyretic and hypotensive effects (4). An aqueous extract shows some evidence of anti-inflammatory and diuretic activity (4). Anti-inflammatory and anti-allergy activities may be associated with the constituent chamazulene (6). Not all species contain azulene constituents (6). An ethanolic extract shows moderate antibacterial activity against Staphylococcus aureus, Bacillus subtilis, Mycobacterium smegmatis, Escherichia coli, Shigella sonnei, and Shigella flexneri (4). Some evidence suggests that the volatile oil of yarrow might have CNS depressant activity (4).

Adverse Reactions

Orally, large amounts of yarrow might cause sedative and diuretic effects (4,5).
Topically, yarrow can cause dermatitis (4).
Yarrow may cause an allergic reaction in individuals sensitive to the Asteraceae/Compositae family. Members of this family include ragweed, chrysanthemums, marigolds, daisies, and many other herbs.

Interactions with Herbs & Other Dietary Supplements

THUJONE CONTAINING HERBS: Concomitant use can increase the risk of thujone toxicity.
Thujone-containing herbs include oak moss, oriental arborvitae, sage, tansy, thuja (cedar), tree moss, and wormwood (2,4,11,12); avoid using.

Interactions with Drugs

ANTACIDS: Theoretically, due to reports that yarrow increases stomach acid, yarrow might decrease the effectiveness of antacids (19).
ANTICOAGULANT/ANTIPLATELET DRUGS: Theoretically, concomitant use might cause increased effects and adverse effects (4).
BARBITURATES: Theoretically, concomitant use might prolong barbiturate-induced sleep time (4). Some of these sedative medications include pentobarbital (Nembutal), phenobarbital (Luminal), secobarbital (Seconal), and others.
H2-BLOCKERS: Theoretically, due to reports that yarrow increases stomach acid, yarrow might decrease the effectiveness of H2-blockers (19). The H2 blockers include cimetidine (Tagamet), ranitidine (Zantac), nizatidine (Axid), and famotidine (Pepcid).
PROTON PUMP INHIBITORS (PPIs): Theoretically, due to reports that yarrow increases stomach acid, yarrow might decrease the effectiveness of PPIs (19). PPIs include omeprazole (Prilosec), lansoprazole (Prevacid), rabeprazole (Aciphex), pantoprazole (Protonix), and esomeprazole (Nexium).

Interactions with Foods

None known.

Interactions with Lab Tests

None known.

Interactions with Diseases or Conditions

CROSS-ALLERGENICITY: Yarrow may cause an allergic reaction in individuals sensitive to the Asteraceae/Compositae family. Members of this family include ragweed, chrysanthemums, marigolds, daisies, and many other herbs.

Dosage and Administration

ORAL: No typical dosage.
But, traditionally an oral dose of 2-4 grams of the dried flowerheads or one cup tea three times daily has been used. To make tea, steep 2-4 grams dried flowerhead or 2 grams finely cut above ground parts in 150 mL of boiling water for 10-15 minutes, and strain (4). A daily dose is up to 4.5 grams above ground parts, 3 grams flowerheads, 3 teaspoons pressed juice from fresh plants, or equivalent preparations per day. The liquid extract, 1:1 in 25% alcohol, is typically dosed at 2-4 mL three times daily (4). The tincture, 1:5 in 45% alcohol, is typically dosed at 2-4 mL three times daily (4).
TOPICAL: No typical dosage.
But, traditionally as a sitz bath, 100 grams above ground parts per 20 L of water has been used (2).

YELLOW DOCK

Also Known As

Broad-Leaved Dock, Curled Dock, Curly Dock, Field Sorrel, Narrow Dock, Rumex, Sheep Sorrel, Sour Dock, Yellowdock.
CAUTION: See separate listing for Sorrel

Scientific Names

Rumex crispus; Rumex obtusifolius.
Family: Polygonaceae.

People Use This For

Orally, yellow dock is used for acute and chronic inflammation of nasal passages and the respiratory tract, as an adjunct to antibacterial therapy, a laxative, tonic, and for treating venereal diseases.
Topically, yellow dock is used as a dentifrice.
Historically, yellow dock has been used for chronic skin diseases, dermatitis, rashes, scurvy, obstructive jaundice, and psoriasis with constipation.
For food uses, yellow dock is used in salads.

Safety

POSSIBLY SAFE ...when consumed in amounts commonly found in foods. Young leaves must be boiled to remove the oxalate content; death has occurred after consuming uncooked leaves (6,18). ...when used orally and appropriately for medicinal purposes.
PREGNANCY: POSSIBLY UNSAFE ...when used orally; avoid using. Contains anthraquinone glycosides, and unstandardized laxatives are not desirable during pregnancy (4)
LACTATION: POSSIBLY UNSAFE ...when used orally; avoid using. Anthraquinones are secreted into breast milk (4,5).

Effectiveness

There is insufficient reliable information available about the effectiveness of yellow dock.

Mechanism of Action

The applicable parts of yellow dock are the root and rhizome. Yellow dock contains anthraquinone glycosides (chrysophanic acid, emodin, physcion), oxalates (oxalic acid and calcium oxalate), and tannins (4,5,6,12). Oxalate content is high in the leaves and low in the stalks (17). The anthroquinones (2-4%) have a mild stimulant laxative effect (4,6,12). Anthroid laxative use is not associated with an increased risk of developing colorectal ademoma or carcinoma (6138). The tannins (12-20%) (12,19) are responsible for the astringent effect (5). Yellow dock is reported to stimulate bile production (4). The leaves of yellow dock contain provitamin A (beta-carotene) and iron (19).

Adverse Reactions

Orally, vomiting may occur after ingestion of fresh rhizome (18). Consuming excessive amounts can cause diarrhea, nausea, polyuria (6), or dermatitis (4). Excessive oral use can also cause abdominal cramps, hypokalemia, and intestinal atrophy (4). There is one report of a death, preceded by vomiting, diarrhea, coma, respiratory depression, liver and kidney failure, severe metabolic acidosis, and ventricular fibrillation, after ingestion of 500 grams of yellow dock (17). Oxalic acid reacts with calcium in plasma, forming insoluble calcium oxalate, which can cause hypocalcemia; the crystals may precipitate in the kidneys, blood vessels, heart, lungs, and liver. Individuals with a history of kidney stones should use yellow dock cautiously (12).

Topically, contact with the plant may cause dermatitis in people sensitive to yellow dock (6). Older or uncooked leaves should be avoided (6). Yellow dock can cause allergic reaction in individuals allergic to ragweed (4117).

Interactions with Herbs & Other Dietary Supplements

CALCIUM, IRON, ZINC: Concurrent use might decrease mineral absorption. Yellow dock contains oxalate (7,12), which can bind multivalent metal ions in the gastrointestinal tract and decrease mineral absorption.
CARDIAC-GLYCOSIDE-CONTAINING HERBS: Theoretically, concomitant use may increase the risk of cardiac glycoside toxicity because of the presence of stimulant laxatives in yellow dock, which can decrease serum potassium (19).
STIMULANT LAXATIVE HERBS: Theoretically, concomitant use of yellow dock with other stimulant laxative herbs can increase the risk of potassium depletion. Stimulant laxative herbs include aloe dried leaf sap, blue flag rhizome, alder buckthorn, European buckthorn, butternut bark, cascara bark, castor oil, colocynth fruit pulp, gamboge bark exudate, jalap root, black root, manna bark exudate, podophyllum root, rhubarb root, senna leaves and pods, and wild cucumber fruit (19).

Interactions with Drugs

DIGOXIN (Lanoxin): Toxic effects due to hypokalemia are possible when yellow dock is used chronically or in large amounts (4,19).
DIURETIC DRUGS: Overuse of yellow dock might compound diuretic-induced potassium loss (19). There is some concern that people taking yellow dock along with potassium-depleting diuretics might have an increased risk for hypokalemia. Initiation of potassium supplementation or an increase in potassium supplement dose may be necessary for some patients. Some diuretics that can deplete potassium include chlorothiazide (Diuril), chlorthalidone (Thalitone), furosemide (Lasix), hydrochlorothiazide (HCTZ, Hydrodiuril, Microzide), and others.

Interactions with Foods

CALCIUM, IRON, ZINC: Concurrent use might decrease mineral absorption from foods. Yellow dock contains oxalate (7,12), which can bind multivalent metal ions in the gastrointestinal tract and decrease mineral absorption.

Interactions with Lab Tests

COLORIMETRIC TESTS: Yellow dock might discolor urine (pink, red, purple, orange, rust), interfering with diagnostic tests that depend on a color change, due to its anthraquinone content (12,275).
SERUM POTASSIUM: Excessive use of yellow dock might cause potassium depletion, reducing serum potassium concentrations and test results (4,19).

Interactions with Diseases or Conditions

COAGULATION DISORDERS: Oxalate constituents of yellow dock can alter calcium concentrations and decrease coagulation time (4,12).
GI CONDITIONS: Avoid use in individuals with intestinal obstruction (4). Theoretically, yellow dock can exacerbate stomach and intestinal ulcers due to its mucosal irritant effect (19).
KIDNEY DISEASE: Yellow dock can damage kidneys with formation of insoluble oxalate; use with caution or avoid in individuals with a history of kidney stones (12,19).

Dosage and Administration

ORAL: Typical dose of the dried root is 2-4 grams or as a tea (Simmer 2-4 grams root in 150 mL of boiling water for 5-10 minutes, strain) 3 times daily (4). The liquid extract 2-4 mL (1:1 in 25% alcohol) 3 times daily (4) and a tincture 1-2 mL (1:5 in 45% alcohol) have also been used (4).

YELLOW LUPIN

Also Known As

Hasenklee, Lupin Jaune.

Scientific Names

Lupinus luteus.
Family: Fabaceae/Leguminosae.

People Use This For

Orally, yellow lupin is used for urinary tract disorders, as an anthelmintic for worm infestations, and as a diuretic. Topically, yellow lupin is used for ulcers.

Safety

POSSIBLY UNSAFE ...when the seeds or above ground parts are used orally (18).
There is insufficient reliable information available about the topical safety of yellow lupin.
PREGNANCY AND LACTATION: POSSIBLY UNSAFE ...when used orally (18); avoid using.

Effectiveness

There is insufficient reliable information available about the effectiveness of yellow lupin.

Mechanism of Action

Yellow lupin contains 0.6-1.6% quinolizidine alkaloids in the above ground plant parts, including sparteine, 13-hydroxylupanine, lupinines and p-cumaroyllupinine. The seed contains 0.4-3.3% quinolizidine alkaloids, including lupinines, sparteine, and in some cultivated strains, gramine. At present, we don't know how these components relate to the uses of lupin. Poisoning has been seen in animals, and is known as "lupinosis." It is due to the presence of mycotoxins that are produced by the fugus Phomopsis leptostromiformis, which sometimes lives in lupins (18).

Adverse Reactions

Orally, the symptoms of poisoning following ingestion include salivation, vomiting, dysphagia, cardiac arrhythmias, ascending paralysis and possibly death due to respiratory failure (18).

Interactions with Herbs & Other Dietary Supplements

None known.

Interactions with Drugs

None known.

Interactions with Foods

None known.

Interactions with Lab Tests

None known.

Interactions with Diseases or Conditions

None known.

Dosage and Administration

No typical dosage.

YELLOW TOADFLAX

Also Known As

Brideweed, Butter and Eggs, Buttered Hayhocks, Calves' Snout, Churnstaff, Devil's Head, Devil's Ribbon, Doggies, Dragon-Bushes, Eggs and Bacon, Eggs and Collops, Flaxweed, Fluelli, Gallwort, Larkspur Lion's Mouth, Monkey Flower, Pattens and Clogs, Pedlar's Basket, Pennywort, Rabbits, Ramsted, Toadpipe, Wild Snapdragon, Yellow Rod.

Scientific Names

Linaria vulgaris.
Family: Scrophulariaceae.

Comments

At the date of publication, there was very little scientific information available about this product. Our staff is continually analyzing the available information on natural medicines and will add data to the online version of *Natural Medicines Comprehensive Database* as it becomes available. See www.naturaldatabase.com.

YERBA MANSA

Also Known As

Lizard's Tail, Swamp Root, Yerba Manza.

Scientific Names

Anemopsis californica, synonym Anemia californica.
Family: Saururaceae.

People Use This For
Orally, yerba mansa is used for cancer; catarrh; common cold; cough; gastrointestinal disturbances; orthopedic, skin, and throat ailments; tuberculosis; venereal diseases; and women's ailments. It is also used orally as an analgesic, disinfectant, emetic, laxative, tonic, and to induce sweating.

Safety
There is insufficient reliable information available about the safety of yerba mansa.
Pregnancy and Lactation: Insufficient reliable information is available; avoid using.

Effectiveness
There is insufficient reliable information available about the effectiveness of yerba mansa.

Mechanism of Action
The applicable parts of yerba mansa are the root and rhizome. Yerba mansa is believed to have sedative effects. It is also a urinary irritant (19). In animals, methyleugenol, a constituent of the volatile oil, prolongs the hypnotic effect of barbiturates and CNS depressant effects of chlorpromazine (19).

Adverse Reactions
None reported.

Interactions with Herbs & Other Dietary Supplements
HERBS WITH SEDATIVE PROPERTIES: Theoretically, concomitant use with herbs that have sedative properties might enhance therapeutic and adverse effects. Some of these supplements include 5-HTP, calamus, California poppy, catnip, hops, Jamaican dogwood, kava, St. John's wort, scullcap, valerian, yerba mansa, and others.

Interactions with Drugs
CNS DEPRESSANTS: Theoretically, concomitant use might cause additive or prolonged sedative effects (19).

Interactions with Foods
None known.

Interactions with Lab Tests
None known.

Interactions with Diseases or Conditions
URINARY TRACT INFLAMMATION: Contraindicated due to urinary irritant effects (19).

Dosage and Administration
No typical dosage.

Comments
There is very little scientific information about this product. Our staff is continually analyzing the available information on natural medicines and will add data here as it becomes available.

YERBA SANTA

Also Known As
Bear's Weed, Consumptive's Weed, Eriodictyon, Gum Bush, Gum Plant, Hierba Santa, Holy Herb, Holy Weed, Mountain Balm, Sacred Herb, Tarweed.

Scientific Names
Eriodictyon californicum; Eriodictyon glutinosum; Wigandia californicum.
Family: Hydrophyllaceae.

People Use This For
Orally, yerba santa is used for coughs, colds, tuberculosis, asthma, chronic bronchitis, xerostomia, as an antispasmodic, tonic, an antipyretic, and as an expectorant.
Topically, yerba santa is used as a poultice to treat bruises, sprains, wounds, insect bites, and to relieve rheumatism.
In foods and beverages, a fluid extract of yerba santa is used as a flavoring component.
In manufacturing, yerba santa is used as a pharmaceutical flavoring agent to mask the bitter taste of other drugs.

Safety
LIKELY SAFE ...when consumed in food amounts (11). ...when used orally as a medicinal (6,12).
There is insufficient reliable information about the safety of yerba santa for its other uses.
PREGNANCY AND LACTATION: Insufficient reliable information available.

Effectiveness
There is insufficient reliable information available about the effectiveness of yerba santa.

Mechanism of Action
The applicable part of yerba santa is the leaf. Yerba santa contains several flavonoids including eriodictyonine (6%), eriodictyol (0.5%) (6,11), chrysoeriol, and cirsimaritin (4118); tannins (11); and a trace amount of volatile oil (6,11). Yerba santa may have a mild diuretic effect (18). Eriodictyol is reported to exert an expectorant effect (6,11).

Adverse Reactions
None reported.

Interactions with Herbs & Other Dietary Supplements
None known.

Interactions with Drugs
None known.

Interactions with Foods
None known.

Interactions with Lab Tests
None known.

Interactions with Diseases or Conditions
None known.

Dosage and Administration
ORAL: People typically prepare yerba santa using 1 teaspoon of the leaves added to 1 cup boiling water. The liquid is taken warm, 30 minutes before bedtime or a mouthful taken 3 times a day (5254).

YEW

Also Known As
Chinwood, Common Yew, English Yew, Pacific Yew, Western Yew.

Scientific Names
Taxus brevifolia; Taxus baccata; and other Taxus species.
Family: Taxaceae.

People Use This For
Orally, yew is used for promoting menstruation, inducing abortion, treating diphtheria, tapeworm infestation, tonsillitis, epilepsy, rheumatism, urinary tract conditions, and liver conditions.
Yew is FDA-approved for the treatment of breast and ovarian cancer.

Safety
LIKELY UNSAFE ...when used orally (6,18). All parts of the yew plant are considered poisonous (5604). Ingestion of 50-100 grams of yew needles can cause death (18,5604). Yew can cause severe gastrointestinal irritation and can cause heart rate to slow dangerously (17,159). Many of the reported fatalities have occurred after ingestion of large amounts of plant material, especially yew needles (5603,5604,5605).
CHILDREN: UNSAFE ...when the berries are used orally. One chewed berry is potentially lethal (159).
PREGNANCY AND LACTATION: UNSAFE ...when the needles are used orally. Yew needles have been used as an abortifacient (16,18).

Effectiveness
There is insufficient reliable information available about the effectiveness of yew.

Mechanism of Action
The applicable parts of yew are the bark, branch tip, and needle. The yew bark is reported to have antispasmodic, nerve toxicant, and cardiac metabolism effects (6,18). It contains many alkaloids of which taxine A and B are

considered to be cardiotoxic (5603,5604). Taxine B affects myocardial cells of the heart by inhibiting both calcium and sodium transport across cell membranes (5604). Yew also contains flavonoids (18). Old growth Pacific yew bark contains 0.01% paclitaxel (13,512). Initially, the small yield from the bark limited the amount of drug that could be produced. Efforts to increase the drug without decimating the supply of the Pacific yew resulted in a semi-synthetic process that produces larger yields (512). English yew needles can be used to isolate 10 desacetylbaccatin III which is converted to paclitaxel (13,512). Paclitaxel is available as the prescription drug, Taxol, for treating advanced ovarian cancer, non-small cell lung cancer, metastatic breast cancer, esophageal cancer, bladder cancer, head and neck cancer, and AIDS-related Kaposi's sarcoma (15).

Adverse Reactions

Orally, death has occurred with ingestion of 50-100 grams of yew needles (18,5604). Symptoms of poisoning include queasiness, dry mouth, (18) vomiting, vertigo, severe abdominal pain, weakness (5604), nervousness, trembling, dyspnea, incoordination (5603), tachycardia, bradycardia, arrhythmias, hypotension, unconsciousness, coma (5604), mydriasis, reddening of the lips, pale and cyanotic skin (6,18), and death secondary to cardiac arrest (5604).

Interactions with Herbs & Other Dietary Supplements

None known.

Interactions with Drugs

None known.

Interactions with Foods

None known.

Interactions with Lab Tests

None known.

Interactions with Diseases or Conditions

None known.

Dosage and Administration

No typical dosage.

YIN CHEN

Also Known As

Armoise Capillaire, Capillary Wormwood, Chiu, In Chen, Inchin-Ko-To, Inchinko, Kawara-Yomogi, Kyunchinho, Rumput Roman, Shih Yin Ch'en, Yin Ch'en, Yin Ch'en Hao, Yin Chen Hao.

Scientific Names

Artemisia capillaris; Artemisia scoparia.
Family: Asteraceae/Compositae.

People Use This For

Orally, yin chen is used to treat hepatitis, infectious cholecystitis, and hyperlipidemia. Yin chen is also used to stimulate the bile flow, liver, and gallbladder. It is used orally for newborn kernicterus, for symptoms of intermittent fever and chills, bitter taste in the mouth, chest constriction, flank pain, dizziness, nausea, and loss of appetite. In addition, it is used for headache, constipation, painful urination, fever, itching, tumors, catarrh, rheumatism, painful menses, malaria, and spasms.

In Chinese and Japanese herbal combinations, yin chen is used orally for jaundice with fever, urinary dysfunction, constipation, and abdominal distention.

Yin chen is contained in inchin-ko-to, a Kampo (Chinese/Japanese) medicine used to treat hepatitis C.

Safety

POSSIBLY SAFE ...when the above ground parts are used orally and appropriately (12,4342). However, serious conditions such as hepatitis require medical management by a physician and should not be self-treated.

CHILDREN: POSSIBLY UNSAFE ...when used orally. Children under the age of 12 years should not use except under care of physician (4344).

PREGNANCY AND LACTATION: LIKELY UNSAFE ...when used orally (12); avoid using.

Effectiveness

There is insufficient reliable information available about the effectiveness of yin chen.

Mechanism of Action
The applicable parts of yin chen are the above ground parts which contain varied constituents. Scoparone, chlorogenic acid, and caffeic acid have demonstrated effects in stimulating bile secretion and protecting the liver against carbon tetrachloride injury (4343). The essential oils cause yin chen to have antipyretic (4343) and antifungal properties (4344). Yin chen is also believed to have bactericide, anti-inflammatory, and diuretic properties (4342,4343,4344). Some evidence suggests yin chen can reduce blood pressure, cholesterol levels, and act as an antiasthmatic agent (4342,4343). Inchin-ko-to, a medicine that contains yin chen, shows evidence that it can prevent apoptosis that is believed to be the mechanism of cell death in viral and fulminant hepatitis (4345). Genepin, a metabolite of inchin-ko-to, appears to be responsible for therapeutic effects (4346).

Adverse Reactions
Orally, use of yin chen is associated with nausea, abdominal distention, and dizziness (4343). One study using yin chen and da zao (Fructus Zizyphi Jujubae) orally to treat infectious hepatitis reported that 2 women developed Adams-Stokes syndrome. This syndrome is usually associated with heart block (4342). Yin chen can cause an allergic reaction in individuals sensitive to the Asteraceae/Compositae family. Members of this family include ragweed, chrysanthemums, marigolds, daisies, and many other herbs.

Interactions with Herbs & Other Dietary Supplements
None known.

Interactions with Drugs
None known.

Interactions with Foods
None known.

Interactions with Lab Tests
None known.

Interactions with Diseases or Conditions
None known.

Dosage and Administration
ORAL: A typical dose of yin chen is 9-15 grams. In very serious conditions, up to 30 grams might be used three times daily (4342). Yin chen is most often used in herbal combinations.

Comments
Traditional Chinese medicine nearly always uses herbal combinations. A well accepted motto in herbal medicine translates as "One ruler, two ministers, three aides, and four guides." In this expression, the active principle is the ruler and the other nine are helpers with different degrees of strength (4343).

YLANG YLANG OIL

Also Known As
Ylang Ylang.
CAUTION: See separate listing for Cananga Oil (Cananga odorata macrophylla).

Scientific Names
Cananga odorata forma. genuina, synonym Canangium odoratum forma. genuina.
Family: Annonaceae.

People Use This For
Topically, ylang ylang oil is used as a sedative, antiseptic, hypotensive, and aphrodisiac.
In foods and beverages, ylang ylang oil is used as a flavoring agent.
In manufacturing, it is used as a fragrance for cosmetics (maximum levels 1% in perfumes) and soaps.

Safety
LIKELY SAFE ...when used in amounts commonly found in foods. Ylang ylang has Generally Recognized As Safe (GRAS) status in the US (4912). ...when applied topically in amounts found in cosmetics and soaps (11), it is nonirritating and nonsensitizing to skin, and no phototoxicity is reported (11).
PREGNANCY AND LACTATION: Insufficient reliable information available; avoid using.

Effectiveness
There is insufficient reliable information available about the effectiveness of ylang ylang oil.

Mechanism of Action
There is insufficient reliable information available about the possible mechanism of action and active ingredients.

Adverse Reactions
None reported.

Interactions with Herbs & Other Dietary Supplements
None known.

Interactions with Drugs
None known.

Interactions with Foods
None known.

Interactions with Lab Tests
None known.

Interactions with Diseases or Conditions
None known.

Dosage and Administration
No typical dosage.

Comments
Ylang ylang oil is the distilled oil from freshly harvested Cangana odorata genuina flower.

YOGURT

Also Known As
Acidophilus Milk, Bulgarian Yogurt, Live Culture Yogurt, Probiotics, Yoghurt, Yogourt, Yougurt.
CAUTION: See separate listings for Bifidobacteria, Lactobacillus, and Saccharomyces boulardii.

Scientific Names
None.

People Use This For
Orally, yogurt is used for restoring gastrointestinal normal flora after antibiotic therapy, reducing antibiotic-associated diarrhea, acute diarrhea in children, treating and preventing vaginal candidiasis, bacterial vaginosis, and preventing urinary tract infections. Yogurt is also used orally for lactose intolerance, reducing the risk of colorectal cancer, treating hyperlipidemia, eradicating Helicobacter pylori infection in peptic ulcer disease, and preventing sunburns.
Intravaginally, yogurt is used for treating vaginal candidiasis and bacterial vaginosis in pregnancy.
Yogurt is also eaten as a food and used as an alternative to milk in lactose-intolerant individuals.

Safety
LIKELY SAFE ...when consumed in food amounts. ...when used orally for medicinal purposes (1240,1241,1242,1246,1253,1256,3590,8526).
POSSIBLY SAFE ...when used intravaginally. A small clinical study reported no adverse reactions (1248).
PREGNANCY: LIKELY SAFE ...when consumed in amounts commonly found in foods. POSSIBLY SAFE ...when used intravaginally. A small clinical study in pregnant women reported no adverse reactions (1248).
LACTATION: LIKELY SAFE ...when used in amounts commonly found in foods. There is insufficient reliable information available about the safety of the intravaginal use of yogurt during breast-feeding.

Effectiveness
POSSIBLY EFFECTIVE

Antibiotic-associated diarrhea. There is some clinical evidence that consuming a specific yogurt product fermented with Lactobacillus rhamnosus GG can significantly decrease symptoms of diarrhea, abdominal distress, stomach pain, and flatulence in people taking erythromycin (1255,3589). It's not known if other yogurt products offer the same benefits.

Bacterial vaginosis. Taking yogurt orally seems to help treat bacterial vaginosis (1245,1248).

Diarrhea. Yogurt formula given as a replacement for milk formula in infants and young children seems to relieve persistent diarrhea (1250,1254).

Helicobacter pylori (H pylori). Supplementation with Lactobacillus- and Bifidobacterium-containing yogurt can improve eradication rates of H. pylori by increasing compliance in patients treated for peptic ulcer with standard triple-drug therapy, including lansoprazole (Prevacid), amoxicillin (Amoxil, others), and clarithromycin (Biaxin). It can also restore Bifidobacterium in stools after depletion by triple therapy (8525). However, consuming yogurt without standard triple-drug therapy does not appear to effectively eradicate H. pylori (10053).

Hyperlipidemia. Taking yogurt orally seems to decrease cholesterol in patients with borderline to moderate hyperlipidemia (1240,1241,3590). Fermented milk or yogurt products fermented with specific organisms including Lactobacillus acidophilus and a combination of Enterococcus faecium and Streptococcus thermophilus have been shown to produce mild to moderate reductions in serum cholesterol (1240,1241,3590). In one crossover study, four weeks of treatment with a human strain of Lactobacillus acidophilus resulted in a significant reduction in total serum cholesterol (3.2%) (1240). In another small crossover study, a milk preparation fermented with Lactobacillus acidophilus plus added fructo-oligosaccharides was tested in men. After three weeks of treatment, there was a significant decrease in total cholesterol (4.4%), low-density lipoprotein (LDL) levels (5.4%), and the LDL/high-density lipoprotein (HDL) ratio (5.3%). There were no significant changes in triglyceride or HDL levels (1241). In a larger study, borderline hyperlipidemic men and women taking a specific yogurt fermented with a strain of Enterococcus faecium and two strains of Streptococcus thermophilus (CAUSIDO culture), for an eight week period, had a significant average LDL reduction of 8.4% after adjusting for changes in body mass. Yogurts in this study fermented with a Streptococcus thermophilus/Lactobacillus acidophilus combination and a Streptococcus thermophilus/Lactobacillus rhamnosus combination did not significantly reduce LDL cholesterol (3590).

Lactose intolerance. Continuous consumption of yogurt with live bacterial cultures seems to improve lactose tolerance in children and adults with lactose malabsorption. The presence of actively growing bacteria cultures or the fat content does not seem to influence tolerability (1246,1256,8526,8943,9220).

Vaginal candidiasis. Taking yogurt orally seems to help prevent vaginal candidiasis (1245,1249).

POSSIBLY INEFFECTIVE

Asthma. Taking yogurt orally as an adjunctive treatment doesn't seem to improve asthma (1244,3589).

Malnourishment-related diarrhea. Yogurt formula given as a replacement for milk formula doesn't seem to help acute, noninfectious diarrhea in malnourished infants and children (1242).

INSUFFICIENT RELIABLE EVIDENCE to RATE

Urinary tract infections (UTIs). Preliminary research indicates that consuming a yogurt drink containing Lactobacillus does not seem to prevent recurrent UTIs when used up to 6 months in women with a history of UTIs (8253). More evidence is needed to rate yogurt for this use.

Mechanism of Action

Yogurt is a dairy preparation produced by fermenting milk using one or more of a variety of specific organisms such as Lactobacillus acidophilus, Lactobacillus rhamnosus, Lactobacillus bulgaricus, Enterococcus faecium, Streptococcus thermophilus, and others (1240,1241,3589,3590). The bacteria in yogurt provides the active constituents, peptidoglycans, polysaccharide, and techoic acid, which modulates the immune system, and beta-galactosidase, which improves lactose tolerance (3589,8517). The partial digestion of milk products results in production of solubilized forms of calcium, which are easily absorbed (3589).The medicinal benefit of yogurt is primarily attributed to the live cultures it contains as a source of probiotics. Probiotics are symbiotic micro-organisms similar to the human gastrointestinal normal flora that, when ingested, can pass through the stomach and potentially colonize the lower gastrointestinal tract. It is thought that this colonization might restore the normal flora after antibiotic therapy and maintain the balance of flora to prevent or minimize antibiotic-associated diarrhea (3589). Yogurt is often suggested as a probiotic source, but the two probiotics used in the fermentation of milk to yogurt, Lactobacillus bulgaricus and Streptococcus thermophilus, might not survive transit through the gut to the colon, eliminating their probiotic effects. Other more acid-resistant bacteria such as Lactobacillus acidophilus are sometimes added to yogurt to give it probiotic effects (12778). The lactic acid bacteria found in yogurt seem to suppress growth of pathogenic bacteria such as Salmonella typhimurium (3589). The lactobacillus species in yogurt can also stimulate the production of mucin by intestinal goblet cells, which improves the intestinal environment (8513).

There is preliminary evidence that yogurt might stimulate the immune system (3589). In vitro studies have produced an increase of immune related substances after yogurt consumption or exposure to lactic acid bacteria (3589). Other components of yogurt, such as whey protein, short peptides, and conjugated linoleic acid, may contribute to its proposed immune effects (3589). Yogurt may have an effect on IgE-mediated diseases such as asthma by decreasing IgE production, but human studies have produced conflicting results (3589).

Yogurt may reduce nitrite concentrations in the gastrointestinal tract (3589). Preliminary evidence indicates that nitrites lead to the formation of carcinogenic compounds.

In healthy infants, milk fermented with Lactobacillus casei increases fecal lactobacilli and decreases potentially harmful beta-glucosidase enzyme activity. Beta-glucosidase is a bacterial enzyme that has been associated with enterohepatic circulation of toxins and carcinogens. Beta-glucosidase has been shown to be elevated in diets high in meat (1243).

Lactobacillus is part of the normal vaginal flora. Probiotics, particularly Lactobacillus acidophilus strains, are thought to be beneficial for candidal vaginal infections by helping to restore the normal flora of the vagina. Lactobacillus acidophilus has also been found to inhibit growth of Candida albicans. Presence of lactobacillus species in the rectum has been associated with lactobacillus colonization in the vagina (1245,1249).

For lowering cholesterol in hyperlipidemia, it is thought that certain culture strains found in yogurt might deconjugate bile salts. This action reduces the serum concentrations of low-density lipoprotein (LDL) cholesterol (3590). Other evidence suggests yogurt with live bacterial cultures can increase short-chain fatty acid production, which might improve lipid and glucose metabolism with chronic yogurt consumption (8943).

People with lactase deficiency seem to tolerate and digest pasteurized yogurt or yogurt with live bacterial cultures better than milk. However, lactose absorption seems to be greater with live culture yogurt than pasteurized yogurt. Yogurt seems to have an immediate beneficial effect on lactose digestion and a delayed effect as the intestinal flora adapts to chronic yogurt ingestion (8943). Some evidence suggests yogurt might induce production of endogenous lactase in the intestine, or active bacteria cultures might produce beta-galactosidase and partially replace deficient lactase (1256,8517,8526,8943).

Yogurt, like milk, is rich in B vitamins. However, yogurt might not be a good source of B vitamins because the bioavailability of B vitamins in yogurt might be low. It is likely that some bacteria in yogurt consume B vitamins, especially thiamine (vitamin B1), riboflavin (vitamin B2), and pyridoxine (vitamin B6), making them less available for intestinal absorption (10464). However, some bacteria in yogurt are capable of synthesizing B vitamins such as vitamin B12 and folate (12778).

Adverse Reactions

Orally, yogurt is usually well tolerated (8561). Fatal Lactobacillus rhamnosus septicemia has been reported in an immunocompromised patient consuming yogurt and taking prolonged courses of multiple broad spectrum antibiotics (8561).

Interactions with Herbs & Other Dietary Supplements

None known.

Interactions with Drugs

CIPROFLOXACIN (Cipro): Concomitant administration can significantly reduce absorption of ciprofloxacin (Cipro) (1252).

IMMUNOSUPPRESSANTS: Theoretically, yogurt could cause infection in patients taking medications that suppress the immune system. These include cyclosporine (Neoral, Sandimmune), tacrolimus (Prograf), azathioprine (Imuran), and cancer chemotherapeutic agents like cyclophosphamide (Cytoxan) and cisplatin (Platinol-AQ) (4380,4391,4393,4398).

TETRACYCLINE ANTIBIOTICS: Concomitant administration can reduce the absorption of tetracyclines (15).

Interactions with Foods

None known.

Interactions with Lab Tests

None known.

Interactions with Diseases or Conditions

IMMUNODEFICIENCY: There is some concern that yogurt might cause pathogenic colonization, especially in patients who are immunocompromised. Yogurt and probiotics have caused bacteremia and fungemia in seriously ill, immunocompromised patients, but very rarely. Pathogenic colonization is more likely to occur in severely immunocompromised patients (8561).

Dosage and Administration

ORAL: Yogurt should be labeled with a "Live and Active Cultures" seal from the National Yogurt Association, indicating the product reliably contains at least 100 million active cultures per gram of yogurt (e.g., Dannon, Yoplait). For preventing antibiotic-induced diarrhea, 125 mL (approximately 4 ounces) of yogurt containing Lactobacillus GG taken twice daily throughout the antibiotic treatment course has been used (1255). Some researchers recommend taking 240 mL (8 ounces) of other yogurt preparations twice daily (1736). Separate antibiotic administration and yogurt by at least two hours. For acute diarrhea, 125 grams of yogurt containing Lactobacillus casei twice daily has been used (1253). For reducing cholesterol, several different doses have been tried depending on the preparation. A typical dose of 200 mL of yogurt containing Lactobacillus acidophilus per day has been used (1240). A combination product of 125 mL Lactobacillus acidophilus yogurt with 2.5% fructo-oligosaccharides three times daily has also been used (1241). A dose of 450 mL daily of yogurt containing the CAUSIDO culture has also been used (3590). For preventing vaginal candidiasis and bacterial vaginosis, a typical dose is 150 mL Lactobacillus acidophilus yogurt per day (1245).

INTRAVAGINAL: No typical dosage.

YOHIMBE

Also Known As

Johimbi, Yohimbehe, Yohimbehe cortex, Yohimbine.

Scientific Names

Pausinystalia yohimbe, synonyms Pausinystalia johimbe, Corynanthe johimbi, Corynanthe yohimbi.
Family: Rubiaceae.

People Use This For

Orally, yohimbe is used as an aphrodisiac, for impotence, exhaustion, angina, hypertension, diabetic neuropathy, and postural hypotension. Yohimbe is also used for general sexual dysfunction in men and women, sexual dysfunction caused by selective-serotonin reuptake inhibitors (SSRI), and as an adjunct to conventional antidepressants for refractory depression.

Yohimbe bark is also smoked or snuffed for its hallucinogenic effects.

Safety

POSSIBLY SAFE ...when used orally and appropriately with medical supervision. The primary active constituent, yohimbine has been shown to be safe in several clinical trials lasting up to 10 weeks (3305,3307,3311,3313). However, yohimbe is not appropriate for self-treatment.

LIKELY UNSAFE ...when used orally in excessive doses or without medical supervision. The primary active ingredient, yohimbine, is considered unsafe for unmonitored nonprescription use (515). Large doses can cause significant toxicity including severe hypotension, heart conduction disorders, and death (18).

There is insufficient reliable information available about the safety of inhaling yohimbe bark.

CHILDREN: LIKELY UNSAFE ...when used orally. Children can be extra sensitive to the adverse effects of yohimbe (19).

PREGNANCY AND LACTATION: LIKELY UNSAFE ...when used orally. Yohimbe might have uterine relaxant effects and also cause fetal toxicity (19).

Effectiveness

POSSIBLY EFFECTIVE

Erectile dysfunction (ED). There is evidence suggesting that the primary constituent, yohimbine, can be helpful for impotence. Yohimbine seems to help men with organic, psychogenic, mixed, and unknown vascular erectile dysfunction (3305,3307,3311,3313,10629). Some herbalists suggest that the yohimbe bark actually works better than the isolated yohimbine constituent; however, yohimbe bark has not been evaluated in studies.

Sexual dysfunction. There is evidence from multiple clinical trials that the primary constituent, yohimbine, can improve sexual dysfunction associated with selective-serotonin reuptake inhibitors (SSRIs) (3305,3306,3307,3311,3313,3970,3971,3972,3973). However, this benefit has not been described specifically for the yohimbe bark.

There is insufficient reliable information available about the effectiveness of yohimbe for its other uses.

Mechanism of Action

The applicable part of yohimbe is the bark. The constituent thought to be responsible for yohimbe's effects is the alkaloid yohimbine (10629). Yohimbe bark contains approximately 6% yohimbine. Aphrodisiac activity of yohimbe has been attributed to genital blood vessel dilation, nerve impulse transmission to genital tissue, and increased reflex excitability in the sacral region of the spinal cord (11). The yohimbine constituent readily penetrates the central nervous system (CNS) and works primarily through alpha 2-adrenergic receptor blockade (3305). It also has monoamine oxidase (MOA) inhibiting, calcium channel blocking, and peripheral serotonin receptor blocking effects (11). Yohimbine likely works several ways to affect impotence since it has been effective in men with organic, psychogenic, mixed, and unknown vascular erectile dysfunction (3305,3310,3311,10629). Yohimbine's effect on impotence might be mediated through both increased penile blood flow and increased central sympathetic excitatory impulses to the genital tissue (3305,3309). In women, a nitric oxide-enhanced form of yohimbine (NMI-870) is theorized to improve sexual arousal by increasing vaginal blood flow by dilating vaginal blood vessels (6198).

Adverse Reactions

Orally, yohimbe and the constituent yohimbine in typical doses can cause excitation, tremor, insomnia, anxiety, hypertension, tachycardia, dizziness, gastric intolerance, salivation, sinusitis, irritability, headache, urinary frequency, fluid retention, rash, nausea, and vomiting (3303,3304,3305,3309,3311,3313,10629). Although low doses can stimulate respiration, high doses can cause respiratory depression (11). High doses can also cause other severe toxicities including paralysis, severe hypotension, cardiac conduction disorders, cardiac failure, and death (18). There is also one report of a hypersensitivity reaction including fever; chills; malaise; itchy, scaly skin; progressive renal failure; and lupus-like syndrome associated with ingestion of a one-day dose of yohimbine (6169).

Interactions with Herbs & Other Dietary Supplements

CAFFEINE-CONTAINING HERBS: Theoretically, concomitant use of yohimbe with large amounts of caffeine-containing herbs or products can increase the risk of hypertensive crisis (12). Caffeine-containing herbs include coffee, cola, guarana, mate, and tea.
EPHEDRA: Theoretically, concomitant use of large amounts of ephedra can increase the risk of hypertensive crisis due to ephedrine content (12).
HERBS WITH MONOAMINE OXIDASE INHIBITING (MAOI) ACTIVITY: Theoretically, concomitant use of these herbs with yohimbe can have additive therapeutic and adverse effects (12). Herbs with MAOI activity include California poppy, ginkgo, mace, and St. John's wort (12).

Interactions with Drugs

ANTIHYPERTENSIVE DRUGS: Concomitant use of yohimbe can interfere with blood pressure control and should be used with caution (11).
CLONIDINE (Catapres): Avoid concomitant use; yohimbine antagonizes the effect of clonidine (11,19).
GUANABENZ (Wytensin): Avoid concomitant use; yohimbine antagonizes the effect of guanabenz (11,19).
MONOAMINE OXIDASE INHIBITORS (MAOIs): Concomitant use with yohimbe can result in additive effects (11,12).
NALOXONE (Narcan): Concomitant use can have additive therapeutic and adverse effects (19).
PHENOTHIAZINES: Yohimbe is contraindicated with phenothiazines due to the risk of increased alpha 2-adrenergic antagonism (19).
STIMULANT DRUGS: Yohimbe is contraindicated because concomitant use increases the risk of hypertensive crisis due to yohimbe monoamine oxidase inhibitor MAOI activity (11,12).
TRICYCLIC ANTIDEPRESSANTS (TCAs): Yohimbe is contraindicated due to its potential to increase or decrease blood pressure (19).

Interactions with Foods

TYRAMINE-CONTAINING FOODS: Avoid concomitant consumption of large amounts of tyramine-containing foods, due to the risk of hypertensive crisis (11). Tyramine-containing foods include aged cheeses, fermented meats, red wines, and others (506).
VASOPRESSOR-CONTAINING FOODS: Avoid concomitant consumption of large amounts of vasopressor-containing foods due to the risk of hypertensive crisis (11). Vasopressor-containing foods include overripe fava beans, coffee, tea, colas, and chocolate (506).

Interactions with Lab Tests

None known.

Interactions with Diseases or Conditions

ANGINA, HEART DISEASE: Contraindicated, due to the cardiovascular effects of the yohimbe constituent, yohimbine (515).
ANXIETY: Contraindicated; the yohimbe constituent, yohimbine, might cause anxiety (515).
BENIGN PROSTATIC HYPERPLASIA (BPH): Theoretically, yohimbe might exacerbate symptoms of BPH due to antagonism of alpha-2 receptors and decreased circulation (19).
DEPRESSION: Contraindicated. The constituent yohimbine might elicit manic-like symptoms in individuals with bipolar depression or suicidal tendencies in individuals with endogenous depression (19).
DIABETES: Avoid, due to the monoamine oxidase inhibiting (MAOI) activity of yohimbe (515). Use of MAO inhibitors in patients receiving insulin or oral antidiabetes drugs has been associated with hypoglycemic episodes (15).
HYPERTENSION: Avoid; small amounts of yohimbine can increase blood pressure (19).
HYPOTENSION: Contraindicated; large amounts of yohimbine can cause hypotension (515).
KIDNEY DISEASE: Contraindicated. Theoretically, yohimbine might have antidiuretic effects (19).
LIVER DISEASE: Contraindicated. Theoretically, liver disease might alter metabolism of the constituent yohimbine (19).
POST-TRAUMATIC STRESS DISORDER (PTSD): Avoid; the constituent yohimbine has been associated with triggering acute symptoms in four individuals with PTSD (1294).
SCHIZOPHRENIA: Use with caution; the constituent yohimbine might activate psychoses in patients with schizophrenia (19,515).
YOHIMBE HYPERSENSITIVITY: Contraindicated (19).

Dosage and Administration

ORAL: For sexual dysfunction, including impotence, a typical dose of the constituent yohimbine is 15-30 mg daily (3303,3305,3307,3313,10629). Doses of yohimbine up to 100 mg daily have been used. However, significantly more severe adverse effects would be expected with such a high dose (3312).

Comments

Yohimbe is the name of an evergreen tree that is native to Zaire, Cameroon, and Gabon. The bark of the yohimbe tree contains the alkaloid yohimbine (4201).

YUCCA

Also Known As

Adam's Needle (Yucca filamentosa), Aloe Yucca (Yucca aloifolia), Bear Grass (Yucca filamentosa), Dagger Plant (Yucca aloifolia), Joshua Tree (Yucca brevifolia), Mohave Yucca (Yucca schidigera), Our-Lord's-Candle (Yucca whipplei), Soapweed (Yucca glauca), Spanish Bayonet (Yucca aloifolia).

Scientific Names

Yucca aloifolia; Yucca brevifolia, synonym Yucca arborescens; Yucca filamentosa; Yucca glauca, synonym Yucca angustifolia; Yucca schidigera, synonym Yucca mohavensis; Yucca whipplei; other Yucca species.
Family: Agavaceae.

People Use This For

Orally, yucca is used for osteoarthritis, hypertension, migraine headaches, colitis, hypercholesterolemia, stomach disorders, diabetes, poor circulation, and liver and gallbladder disorders.
Topically, yucca is used for sores, skin diseases, inflammation, bleeding, sprains, broken limbs, joint pain, baldness, and dandruff.
In foods, yucca is fried like potatoes.
In manufacturing, yucca extract is used as a foaming and flavoring agent in carbonated beverages. Many compounds from yucca have been used in the synthesis of new drugs.

Safety

LIKELY SAFE ...when used orally in amounts commonly found in foods. Mojave yucca and Joshua tree have Generally Recognized As Safe status (GRAS) for use in foods in the US (4912).
POSSIBLY SAFE ...when used orally and appropriately, short-term (12).
There is insufficient reliable information available about the safety of yucca used long-term or applied topically.
PREGNANCY AND LACTATION: There is insufficient reliable information about the safety of yucca in medicinal amounts during pregnancy and breast-feeding; avoid using.

Effectiveness

INSUFFICIENT RELIABLE EVIDENCE to RATE

Hypercholesterolemia. Taking yucca orally, in combination with diet and exercise, seems to help lower triglycerides and cholesterol levels (4,6).
Hypertension. Taking yucca orally, in combination with diet and exercise, might help lower blood pressure (4,6).
Osteoarthritis. There is preliminary evidence that a yucca extract might reduce symptoms of osteoarthritis such as pain, swelling, and stiffness (4,6).
More evidence is needed to rate yucca for these uses.

Mechanism of Action

The applicable part of yucca is the root of the non-flowering plant. Yucca contains saponins that are believed responsible for the pharmacologic activity of the plant (4,6,11). However, the mechanism for these effects is unclear because yucca saponins don't seem to be absorbed in the gastrointestinal tract (4). The saponins in yucca are often irritating to mucous membranes and might cause GI irritation (4077). In vitro, saponins have hemolytic activity (11). There is preliminary evidence that yucca has anti-inflammatory, antitumor, and antiviral activity (4,6,11).

Adverse Reactions

Orally, yucca can cause stomach upset, mucous membrane irritation, bitter taste, nausea, and vomiting (7).
Intravenously, yucca administration may result in hemolysis (11).

Interactions with Herbs & Other Dietary Supplements

None known.

Interactions with Drugs

None known.

Interactions with Foods

None known.

Interactions with Lab Tests
None known.

Interactions with Diseases or Conditions
None known.

Dosage and Administration
ORAL: No typical dosage. However, traditionally 380 to 490 mg of the powdered yucca stalk or root has been used two to three times daily. Yucca can be prepared as a decoction by boiling one-fourth ounce of the root in 16 ounces of water for 15 minutes. People have taken 3 to 5 cups of this liquid per day (6006).
TOPICAL: No typical dosage.

ZEDOARY

Also Known As
Cedoaria, Cetoal, E Zhu, E-Zhu, Indian Arrowroot, Kua, Sati, Shati, Temu Kuning, Temu Putih, Turmeric, Zedoaire, Zedoária, Zedoarie rhizoma, Zitwer, Zitwerwirtzelstock.
CAUTION: See separate listings for Turmeric, Goldenseal, and Javanese Turmeric.

Scientific Names
Curcuma zedoaria, synonym Amomum zedoaria.
Family: Zingiberaceae.

People Use This For
Orally, zedoary is used for colic, spasms, stimulating appetite, improving digestion, stimulating bile flow, nervous diseases, and as an anti-inflammatory.
In combination herbal products, zedoary extracts are used for gastrointestinal complaints and stimulating bile flow.

Safety
POSSIBLY SAFE ...when used orally and appropriately (12).
PREGNANCY: LIKELY UNSAFE ...when used orally; avoid using (12) due to potential abortifacient effects (19).
LACTATION: Insufficient reliable information available; avoid using.

Effectiveness
There is insufficient reliable information available about the effectiveness of zedoary.

Mechanism of Action
The applicable part of zedoary is the rhizome. Zedoary contains a volatile oil and curcuminoids (18). Zedoary is thought to stimulate bile production and gallbladder emptying (512). The volatile oil contains sesquiterpene ketones known as turmerones that are believed responsible for increasing bile production (512). The curcuminoid constituents are believed to be responsible for gallbladder emptying effects (512). The isolated sesquiterpene constituent dehydrocurdione shows some evidence of anti-inflammatory activity (4011). Experimental evidence suggests other sesquiterpenes isolated from zedoary might be hepatoprotective (4012). Compounds isolated from zedoary demonstrate some evidence of antifungal (4013) and cytotoxic (4014) activity.

Adverse Reactions
None reported.

Interactions with Herbs & Other Dietary Supplements
None known.

Interactions with Drugs
None known.

Interactions with Foods
None known.

Interactions with Lab Tests
None known.

Interactions with Diseases or Conditions
MENORRHAGIA: Some experts suggest that zedoary should not be used by women who have heavy menstrual periods (12).

Dosage and Administration

ORAL: One cup of tea is typically taken three times daily at meals. To make tea, steep 1-1.5 grams powdered dried rhizome in 150 mL boiling water, 5-10 minutes, and strain (18).

Comments

Traditional methods for preparing zedoary involve prolonged washing with water to remove most of the protein, water-soluble nutrients, and presumably, an unidentified toxic constituent (4015).

ZINC

Also Known As

Zinc Acetate, Zinc Acexamate, Zinc Aspartate, Zinc Citrate, Zinc Gluconate, Zinc Methionine, Zinc Monomethionine, Zinc Oxide, Zinc Picolinate, Zinc Pyrithione, Zinc Sulfate.

Scientific Names

Zinc; Zn; atomic number 30.

People Use This For

Orally, zinc is used for treatment and prevention of zinc deficiency. It is also used orally for treating the common cold, recurrent ear infections, and preventing acute lower respiratory infections. Other oral uses include macular degeneration, night blindness, cataracts, diabetes, hypertension, acquired immunodeficiency syndrome (AIDS), psoriasis, eczema, and acne. It is also used orally for anorexia nervosa, acute diarrhea in children with zinc deficiency, attention deficit-hyperactivity disorder (ADHD), blunted sense of taste (hypogeusia), aphthous ulcers, Crohn's disease, ulcerative colitis, and peptic ulcers. Other oral uses include benign prostatic hyperplasia (BPH); male infertility, male impotence; osteoporosis, rheumatoid arthritis, and muscle cramps in patients with cirrhosis. It is also used orally for sickle cell disease, thalassemia, Alzheimer's disease, Down syndrome, Wilson's disease, Hansen's disease, acrodermatitis enteropathica, necrolytic acral erythema, and delayed wound healing associated with zinc deficiency. Zinc is also used orally for improving athletic performance and strength, improving immune function, improving growth and health in zinc-deficient stunted children, tinnitus, and severe head injuries. It is also used orally and locally for parasitic infections, including prevention and treatment of malaria.

Topically, zinc is used for treating acne, aging skin, herpes simplex infections, resistant trichomonas infection, and speeding wound healing. Zinc citrate is used in toothpaste and mouthwash to prevent dental plaque formation and gingivitis.

Intranasally, zinc is used for treating the common cold.

Ophthalmically, zinc sulfate is used in products for eye irritation.

Intravenously, zinc is used as a component of total parenteral nutrition and for improving outcomes in burn patients.

Safety

LIKELY SAFE ...when used orally or topically and appropriately. Zinc is safe in amounts that do not exceed the tolerable upper intake level (UL) of 40 mg per day (7135).

POSSIBLY SAFE ...when used orally and appropriately in doses higher than the tolerable upper intake level (UL). There is some concern that doses higher than the UL of 40 mg per day might decrease copper absorption and result in anemia. However, there is some evidence doses of elemental zinc as high as 80 mg daily in combination with copper 2 mg can be used safely for approximately six years without significant adverse effects (7303,8622).

POSSIBLY UNSAFE ...when used intranasally. Case reports and animal research suggest that intranasal zinc might cause permanent anosmia (loss of sense of smell) (11155,11156,11703,11704,11705,11706,11707). Until more is known, use intranasal zinc with caution.

LIKELY UNSAFE ...when taken orally in excessive amounts. Chronic intake of 450-1600 mg daily can cause sideroblastic anemia. Ingestion of 10-30 grams of zinc sulfate can be lethal in adults (7135).

CHILDREN: LIKELY SAFE ...when used orally and appropriately (7135). Zinc is safe in amounts that do not exceed the tolerable upper intake level (UL). The UL for children is based on age; 4 mg per day for infants birth to 6 months, 5 mg per day for infants 7 to 12 months, 7 mg per day for children 1 to 3 years, 12 mg per day for children 4 to 8 years, 23 mg per day for children 9 to 13 years, and 34 mg per day for adolescents ages 14 to 18 years (7135). POSSIBLY UNSAFE ...when used orally in high doses. Taking amounts greater than the tolerable upper intake level (UL) can cause sideroblastic anemia and copper deficiency (7135).

PREGNANCY: LIKELY SAFE ...when used orally and appropriately. Zinc is safe in amounts that do not exceed the tolerable upper intake level (UL) of 34 mg per day for pregnant women 14 to 18 years, and 40 mg per day for pregnant women age 19-50 (7135). LIKELY UNSAFE ...when used orally in high doses. Tell pregnant patients not to exceed the tolerable upper intake level (UL) (7135). Taking higher doses during the third trimester can cause premature births and stillbirths (332).

LACTATION: LIKELY SAFE ...when used orally and appropriately. Zinc is safe in amounts that do not exceed the tolerable upper intake level (UL) of 34 mg per day for lactating women age 14 to 18 years, and 40 mg per day for pregnant women age 19-50 (7135). POSSIBLY UNSAFE ...when used orally in high doses. Tell breast-feeding patients not to exceed the tolerable upper intake level (UL). Higher doses can cause zinc-induced copper deficiency in nursing infants (7135).

Effectiveness

EFFECTIVE

Wilson's disease. Taking zinc orally improves symptoms of Wilson's disease (822,823,2693). Zinc blocks copper absorption and increases copper elimination in the stool of people with Wilson's disease (2692).

Zinc deficiency. Taking zinc orally or intravenously prevents and treats zinc deficiency (2619). However, routine zinc supplementation is not recommended (403). Zinc deficiency requiring supplementation may occur in severe diarrhea, malabsorption syndromes, liver cirrhosis and alcoholism, after major surgery, and during long-term administration of total parenteral nutrition (TPN) (3900). Zinc supplementation (136 mg elemental zinc per day) in patients with cirrhosis and zinc deficiency seems to improve liver function and glucose tolerance, possibly by increasing insulin-like growth factor (8624).

LIKELY EFFECTIVE

Diarrhea. Taking zinc orally reduces the duration and severity of acute and persistent diarrhea in malnourished or zinc-deficient children (825,826,827,3455,3456,8633,8638). Zinc supplements lower the probability of continuing diarrhea by approximately 24% in acute diarrhea and lower the rate of treatment failure or mortality by approximately 42% in persistent diarrhea (8633,10248). Zinc also seems to reduce hospital admissions due to acute diarrhea by approximately 23% (10248). Severe zinc deficiency in children is common in developing countries.

POSSIBLY EFFECTIVE

Acne. Taking zinc orally might help treat acne. Research suggests that people with acne might have lower serum and skin zinc levels (2686,6507,6508,6509). Clinical trials have been small, but most suggest that zinc can improve acne (6297,6298,6299,6501,6502,6503,6504). So far, it is not clear how zinc compares to other treatments. Comparative trials with tetracycline have yielded conflicting results (6505,6506). Topically, in combination with erythromycin, zinc also seems to help treat acne (819,820,2687,2688).

Acrodermatitis enteropathica. Taking zinc orally seems to help improve acrodermatitis enteropathica (821,2689,2690,2691). There is one case report of oral zinc sulfate 225 mg twice daily plus interferon alfa-2b for six months resolving all lesions in a woman with necrolytic acral erythema and hepatitis C. Necrolytic acral erythema is categorized in the family of necrolytic erythemas which includes acrodermatitis enteropathica (6192).

Age-related macular degeneration (AMD). Taking zinc orally in combination with antioxidant vitamins might slow the progression of advanced age-related macular degeneration (AMD). Elemental zinc 80 mg plus vitamin C 500 mg, vitamin E 400 IU, and beta-carotene 15 mg daily seems to provide a risk reduction of 27% for visual acuity loss and a risk reduction of 24% for progression of AMD in patients with advanced AMD (7303). Patients with monocular or binocular intermediate AMD or monocular advanced AMD are at high risk for advanced AMD. Theoretically, these patients may also benefit from zinc and antioxidant supplementation (11326). There isn't enough information to determine if zinc plus antioxidants is beneficial for people with less advanced macular disease or for preventing AMD (6583,6584,7303). However, dietary zinc or zinc supplementation alone does not seem to reduce the risk of developing of AMD (6579,6580,6581).

Anorexia nervosa. Taking zinc supplements orally might help increase weight gain and improve depressive symptoms in patients with anorexia nervosa (6905,6906).

Attention deficit-hyperactivity disorder (ADHD). Taking zinc orally in combination with conventional treatment might modestly improve symptoms of hyperactivity, impulsivity, and impaired socialization in some children with ADHD (11350,12060). But zinc might not improve attention deficit (11350). There is some evidence that zinc could be most helpful in children with a high body mass index (BMI), low zinc levels, and low free fatty acid levels (11350). Some research suggests that children with ADHD have lower serum zinc levels than children without ADHD (9965,9966). Other research suggests ADHD patients with lower zinc levels might not respond adequately to stimulant therapy (9967). Studies using zinc for ADHD have taken place in the Middle East where zinc deficiency is relatively common compared to Western countries. It's not known if zinc would have the same potential benefits when used for ADHD in patient populations from Western countries.

Burns. Administering zinc intravenously in combination with other minerals seems to improve the outcomes of burn patients (6520). Supplementation with zinc, copper, and selenium significantly reduced pulmonary infections and shortened intensive care unit stay in patients with serious burns (6520).

Common cold. Using zinc oral lozenges seems to help decrease the duration of the common cold in adults. The majority of studies show a significant decrease in the duration of symptoms of the common cold when adults take zinc gluconate or acetate lozenges providing 9-24 mg elemental zinc per dose. Lozenges should be taken every 2 hours while awake, starting within 48 hours of symptom onset (333,334,335,337,6703,6705). However, not all studies have been positive (333,338,339,6521,6522,6700). The reasons for these different findings are not clear, but might be due to differences in zinc formulations and study methodologies. In some cases, flavoring agents such as citric acid, mannitol, and sorbitol might chelate zinc and decrease zinc ionization. Since zinc ionization is thought to be an important step involved in the effectiveness of zinc, a decrease in zinc ionization could decrease effectiveness (300,340,6522). Some of the positive studies have also been criticized for inadequately blinding the unpleasant, distinctive taste of zinc (6522,6706). Overall, zinc products seem to be beneficial for reducing the duration of symptoms of the common cold in adults. Zinc from supplements taken prophylactically does not seem to prevent the common cold (10780,10784). Research on zinc lozenges in children is conflicting (341,10803).

The role of intranasal zinc to prevent or treat the common cold is controversial. Zinc nasal spray (as a sulfate, gluconate emulsion, or gluconium gel) reduces the severity and duration of cold symptoms according to some research, while other research has found no effect (6471,8628,8629,10247). Zinc nasal spray doesn't seem to prevent experimentally induced colds (8628).

Gingivitis. Using zinc toothpaste or mouthwash alone or in combination with triclosan seems to prevent plaque accumulation, gingivitis, or formation of calculus (6523,6524,6525,6526,6527,6528,6529). Most studies used zinc citrate in combination with triclosan, which is not available in the US (6523).

Herpes simplex virus (HSV). Applying zinc topically seems to help treat herpes simplex infection (6538,6539,6540). Zinc sulfate seems to reduce the severity and duration of symptoms in both orolabial and genital herpes (6538,6539,6540,8623). Zinc oxide (0.3%) in combination with glycine cream applied topically every 2 hours to facial and circumoral herpes seems to reduce symptoms such as blistering, soreness, itching, and tingling. It can also reduce the duration of lesions from 6.5 days to 5 days when treatment is begun within 24 hours of onset of symptoms (8623).

Hypogeusia. Taking zinc orally might be effective for taste dysfunction in some patients with zinc depletion (6542,6546). Zinc also seems to improve hypogeusia conditions unrelated to zinc deficiency, such as gustin/carbonic anhydrase VI deficiency, captopril-induced taste disturbances, hypogeusia secondary to head and neck radiation, and post-traumatic olfactory disorder (6543,6544,6545,6547). In uremic adults, zinc supplementation, orally or via dialysate, might improve taste acuity; but it appears to be ineffective for pediatric dialysis patients (6548,6549,6550).

Leprosy. Taking zinc orally in combination with anti-leprosy drugs seems to help treat leprosy (6534,6535,6536,6537). Zinc levels appear to be reduced in people with leprosy. Early clinical evidence suggests that the addition of zinc to the anti-leprosy drug regimen might allow for lowering or eliminating steroid doses in a severe form of leprosy, erythema nodosum leprosum (6534,6535,6536).

Muscle cramps. Taking zinc orally by people with cirrhosis seems to help treat muscle cramps in zinc-deficient patients (1352).

Peptic ulcers. Taking zinc orally seems to help treat and prevent peptic ulcers (6588,6589,6590,6591). Zinc acexamate (not available in the US) seems to improve peptic ulcers when compared to placebo or H2 receptor antagonist drugs (6589). It is not known if other zinc salts are effective.

Pneumonia. Zinc supplementation seems to reduce the incidence of pneumonia in undernourished children aged six months to three years in developing countries by 25% (8637). However, zinc supplementation does not show any additional benefit, compared with antibiotics and vitamin A alone, when used to reduce the severity of illness in children with both measles and pneumonia (9589). Taking 10 mg of zinc daily for six months seems to help reduce the incidence of acute lower respiratory infection in 45% of children ages 6 to 35 months living in developing countries (8920).

Sickle cell disease. Taking zinc orally seems to help treat sickle cell disease in people with zinc deficiency (6594,6595,6596,8626), and decrease the incidence of sickle-cell crisis and infections (6594,6596). Although zinc might reduce the number of hospitalizations for sickle cell crisis, the severity of a crisis does not appear to be reduced, based on length of hospital stay (6594,6596). In prepubertal children with homozygous sickle cell disease, supplementation with elemental zinc 10 mg per day seems to improve growth, height, and weight gain (8626).

Venous leg ulcers. Taking zinc orally might help treat arterial and venous leg ulcers in people with low zinc levels (6903), and recurrent aphthous ulcers in people with low zinc levels (6593). However, it's not helpful for recurring aphthous ulcers (6592,6593) or arterial and venous leg ulcers (6902) in people with adequate zinc levels. Topical zinc also seems to help treat leg ulcers (2694,6901).

Vitamin A deficiency. Taking zinc orally in combination with vitamin A seems to improve measures of vitamin A adequacy in undernourished children better than vitamin A or zinc alone (8636).

POSSIBLY INEFFECTIVE

AIDS diarrhea-wasting syndrome. Taking zinc orally in combination with vitamins doesn't seem to help treat AIDS diarrhea-wasting syndrome (6564).

Alopecia areata. Although there is preliminary evidence that suggests zinc in combination with biotin might be helpful for alopecia areata (6932), most studies indicate that zinc is not effective for alopecia areata, alopecia totalis, or alopecia universalis (6931,6932).

Atopic dermatitis (eczema). Taking zinc orally doesn't appear to improve the surface area affected and degree of erythema, symptom scores of itch and sleep disturbance, or topical steroid use in children with eczema. Zinc levels appear to be normal in children with eczema (6911).

Cataracts. Taking zinc orally in combination with antioxidant vitamins doesn't seem to help treat or prevent cataracts. Taking elemental zinc 80 mg plus vitamin C 500 mg, vitamin E 400 IU, and beta-carotene 15 mg daily does not seem to have any effect on the development or progression of age-related lens opacities (cataracts) or the need for cataract surgery in well-nourished people 55-80 years of age. However, it is unknown whether earlier intervention and/or a longer period of treatment with supplements would have any effect on cataracts (7304).

Inflammatory bowel disease (IBD). Taking zinc orally doesn't seem to help treat IBD (6913,6915,6916).

Influenza. Supplemental zinc seems to improve cell-mediated immune response in elderly people (824), but it doesn't seem to have a significant effect on antibody response and incidence of flu infection after flu vaccine (6553,6563). Additionally, zinc supplementation in patients on hemodialysis, who have a high risk of zinc deficiency, doesn't seem to improve response to influenza vaccine (10809). Taking zinc supplements orally is unlikely to improve immune function in people without risk factors for zinc deficiency (10789). However, there is preliminary evidence that suggests zinc along with selenium might reduce the incidence of infections in institutionalized older patients (8921).

Malaria. Taking zinc orally doesn't seems to help prevent or treat malaria in undernourished children in developing countries. Zinc supplements don't seem to protect against infection by Plasmodium falciparum (8638). In acute malaria, zinc supplements do not affect fever, parasitemia, or hemoglobin in zinc-deficient children (10246).

Pregnancy-related iron deficiency. Taking zinc orally doesn't seem to help improve iron status in pregnant women taking supplemental iron and folic acid (6104).

Psoriasis. Taking zinc orally doesn't seem to help treat psoriasis (6513,6514,6912). Zinc epidermal levels are reportedly lower in people with psoriasis (6509). However, zinc has no effect on the psoriasis area and severity index (6513,6514).

Psoriatic arthritis. Taking zinc orally, alone or in combination with nonsteroidal anti-inflammatory drugs (NSAIDs), has no effect on the course of psoriatic arthritis (6514,6515).

Rheumatoid arthritis (RA). Taking zinc orally doesn't seem to help treat RA (2823,6516,6517,6518,6519).

Tinnitus. Taking zinc orally doesn't seem to help treat tinnitus (6914,6917,6921).

INSUFFICIENT RELIABLE EVIDENCE to RATE

AIDS-related opportunistic infections. There is some preliminary clinical evidence that taking zinc supplements orally in combination with zidovudine (AZT, Retrovir, a component of Combivir) might reduce opportunistic infections of Pneumocystis carinii and Candida in patients with AIDS (6566). However, zinc supplementation might also adversely affect the overall survival in people with AIDS (6565).

Alzheimer's disease. Preliminary clinical evidence has shown a modest slowing of cognitive decline in patients with Alzheimer's disease who take zinc supplements (2824).

Impotence. Taking zinc orally to treat male impotence secondary to disease or medical treatment has produced varying results (6568,6569,6570,6571,6572,6708).

Neurological trauma. Administering zinc parenterally immediately following post-head trauma seems to improve the rate of neurological recovery (2696).

Wrinkled skin. A topical preparation containing 10% vitamin C as L-ascorbic acid and acetyl tyrosine, zinc sulfate, sodium hyaluronate, and bioflavonoids (Cellex-C High Potency Serum) applied to photo-aged facial skin for 3 months seems to improve fine and coarse wrinkling, yellowing and sallowness, roughness, and skin tone compared to placebo (6155).

More evidence is needed to rate zinc for these uses.

Mechanism of Action

Zinc is a biologically essential trace element and is the second most abundant trace element in the body. The total body content is about 2 grams (8621). It is a cofactor in many biological processes including DNA, RNA, and protein synthesis. About 30% of cellular zinc is found within the nucleus. A large number of proteins that play a role in the regulation of gene expression are thought to contain zinc (8619).

Zinc also plays a role in immune function, wound healing, reproduction, growth and development, behavior and learning, taste and smell, blood clotting, thyroid hormone function, and insulin action (331).

Zinc is found in more than 300 enzymes (8619). Nearly 100 enzymes depend on zinc as a catalyst (7135). Zinc is also required in hepatic synthesis of retinol binding protein, the transport protein of vitamin A (8630). Without adequate zinc, symptoms of vitamin A deficiency can appear, despite vitamin A supplementation (8630).

Meat, seafood, dairy products, nuts, legumes, and whole grains contain relatively high concentrations of zinc (331). Many breakfast cereals are fortified with zinc (7135). Zinc oxide and zinc sulfate are typically used to fortify wheat products (10668). About 15% to 40% of the zinc in foods is absorbed. Bioavailability is influenced by zinc ion status and absorption increases in states of zinc deficiency. Zinc is mostly absorbed in the small intestine, particularly the jejunum (7135).

During lactation, zinc excretion increases via breast milk. The body seems to compensate for this increased demand by increasing zinc absorption and conserving endogenous zinc (8631).

More than 85% of the total zinc in the body is in skeletal muscle and bone; plasma zinc is tightly regulated at a concentration of approximately 10 to 15 micromol/L (7135).

Zinc deficiency is characterized by growth retardation, low insulin levels, reduced levels of insulin-like growth factor (IGF)-1, anorexia, mental lethargy, irritability, low sperm count, generalized hair loss, rough and dry skin, skin lesions, slow wound healing, decreased thyroid function, delayed onset of puberty, poor sense of smell and taste, diarrhea, and nausea (8619). Although zinc deficiency and tri-iodothyronine (T3) have complementary roles in growth and development, growth failure in zinc deficiency does not seem to be the result of impaired T3 function (8619).

Zinc deficiency is not uncommon worldwide, but deficiency is rare in the US; most diets provide more than the recommended dietary allowance (RDA) (8632). Moderate zinc deficiency is associated with malabsorption syndromes, alcoholism, chronic renal disease, and chronic debilitating diseases (8621). Zinc levels also appear to be lower in acute attacks of paranoid schizophrenia (12584).

There is no reliable test in clinical use to determine zinc deficiency. Serum or plasma zinc on its own is neither sensitive nor specific. It seems to be useful to measure zinc status on a population basis, but is an inaccurate measure in individuals, particularly in people with chronic infections or inflammatory conditions (8625). The most reliable method for diagnosing marginal zinc deficiency is a positive response to zinc supplementation and improvement in subtle symptoms such as growth retardation or altered ability to taste or smell (8621).

Zinc plays a key role in the maintenance of vision. It is present in high concentrations in the eye, particularly in the retina and choroid. Zinc deficiency can alter vision, and severe deficiency causes changes in the retina and retinal pigment epithelium (RPE). Zinc interacts with taurine and vitamin A in the retina, modifies plasma membranes in the photoreceptors, regulates the light-rhodopsin reaction within the photoreceptor, modulates synaptic transmission, and serves as an antioxidant in both the RPE and retina. It seems to slow the progression of some degenerative retinal diseases (8621). Topically, zinc sulfate ophthalmic solution acts as a mild astringent, precipitating protein and clearing mucus from the outer surface of the eye (15).

Zinc is responsible for neutrophil, natural killer cell, and T-lymphocyte function (6551). Even mild zinc deficiency might adversely affect T-cell functions (6552). Interestingly, high-dose zinc supplementation, 20 times the RDA, can have a negative effect similar to deficiency on immune function (8625).

For the common cold, zinc doesn't have any effect on interleukin-8 in nasal secretions, suggesting that zinc doesn't affect immune response to colds (10783,10784).

The amount of available ionized zinc might influence the effectiveness of zinc (336). The extent of zinc ionization varies with different lozenge formulations (340). The addition of flavoring agents such as citric acid, mannitol, or sorbitol to zinc gluconate lozenge preparations decreases the extent of zinc ionization, while the addition of glycine to zinc gluconate lozenges does not (300).

Some researchers question the clinical relevance of oral zinc levels since the rhinovirus replicates in the nasal mucosa (8628,8629). Also, zinc inhibits rhinovirus replication in vitro, but there's no evidence this happens in vivo (10783,10784).

Zinc ions might also have effects against other viruses. There's some evidence that zinc ions also have antiviral activity against the herpes virus (6538,6539,6541). Plasma zinc levels are low in people with HIV infection, but this appears to be a marker of disease progression rather than an indication that zinc deficiency. Some evidence suggests that zinc supplementation might increase disease progression and mortality in HIV infected patients, but other evidence suggests that avoiding zinc deficiency might allow normal or improved immune function, particularly T-lymphocyte mediated cellular immunity. It also might inhibit susceptibility of T-lymphocytes to apoptosis (8625). More research is needed to tell if zinc should be avoided or prescribed for zinc deficiency in HIV disease.

People with sickle cell disease (SCD) are commonly zinc deficient. Zinc deficiency in SCD might cause a cell-mediated immune disorder, and increase the risk of infection in SCD. Some researchers think zinc deficiency leads to increased production of tumor necrosis factor (TNF)-alpha and interleukin-1 (IL-1) which might result in vaso-occlusive pain. This may explain the benefit of zinc supplementation in some patients with SCD (8627).

Topical zinc might be effective for treating acne (819,820,2687,2688) due to anti-inflammatory activity resulting from inhibition of polymorphonuclear leukocyte chemotaxis induced by decreased granulocyte zinc levels (2686).

Male fertility appears to be influenced by zinc (6573,6574,6575,6576). Infertile males have lower seminal plasma zinc, with normal or reduced blood zinc (6575,6577). Clinical research suggests that short-term dietary zinc depletion results in reduced serum testosterone concentrations, seminal volume, and total seminal zinc loss per ejaculate (6576). Supplementation with zinc improves sperm parameters in men with reduced sperm mobility (6578); excess zinc might reduce sperm motility (6573). Zinc levels appear to decrease in the prostate tissue and prostatic fluid in men with prostatic carcinoma (6909,6910).

Zinc blocks copper absorption and increases copper elimination in the stool of people with Wilson's disease (2692). In acrodermatitis enteropathica, zinc seems to regulate linoleic acid and serum lipoprotein metabolism (2689). In children with thalassemia major, zinc deficiency is common (6597,6598,6599).

The role of zinc in Alzheimer's disease might be both protective and causative. Laboratory studies suggest that zinc might contribute to aggregation of amyloid beta peptide, but protect against subsequent neurotoxicity as an antioxidant (6510,6511,6512).

Zinc levels appear to be reduced in some people with major depression (6562).

Preliminary research suggests some people with type 2 diabetes might be zinc deficient, possibly as a result of altered zinc metabolism (6531,6532). There's some evidence that zinc can increase glucose transport into cells and potentiate insulin-induced glucose transport, possibly by affecting the insulin intracellular signaling pathway (second messenger system) (8620). In patients with cirrhosis and impaired glucose tolerance, zinc can increase serum levels of insulin-like growth factor (IGF)-1 by 30% and improve glucose tolerance (8624). Whether zinc deficiency is involved in the development of insulin resistance is unknown. In type 1 diabetes with zinc deficiency, zinc supplementation might reduce lipid peroxidation (6533).

In people with osteoporosis, urinary zinc excretion is increased, possibly as a result of bone resorption (6918). Serum zinc levels have been variably reported as normal or decreased in people with osteoporosis (6918,6920). Early clinical evidence suggests that zinc in combination with copper, manganese, and calcium might slow bone loss (1994). However, moderately high dietary zinc intake (53 mg per day) seems to increase magnesium excretion without affecting copper metabolism in postmenopausal women (12424). Supplementation with high doses of zinc, 142 mg/day, also appears to decrease magnesium absorption and magnesium balance in healthy adult males (9624). This might adversely affect bone health. Zinc may compete with magnesium for ion exchange transport in the intestine (12424). More research on the clinical importance of these observations is needed.

For aiding in wound healing, topical zinc might enhance re-epithelialization, decrease inflammation, and inhibit bacterial growth (2699).

Zinc oxide absorption is best in an acidic environment (2809). Zinc acetate is absorbed over a wide pH range and might be a better choice in people with reduced stomach acid (2809). An enteric-coated zinc aspartate preparation (Taurizine) showed no absorption (2740). Zinc uptake in human intestinal epithelial cells is similar for zinc chloride, zinc methionine, and zinc propionate (2739). Most zinc is excreted in the feces, with a small amount eliminated in the urine (7135).

Adverse Reactions

Orally, zinc can cause nausea, vomiting, and a metallic taste in the mouth (2619,11350). There is concern that high daily doses above the tolerable upper intake level (UL) of 40 mg per day might increase the risk of copper deficiency (7135). To prevent copper deficiency, some clinicians give a small dose of copper when zinc is used in high doses, long-term (7303). In overdose, zinc can cause watery diarrhea, irritation and corrosion of the gastrointestinal (GI) tract, acute renal tubular necrosis, and interstitial nephritis (331,1352). Other symptoms of toxicity include flu-like and central nervous system (CNS) symptoms including fever, coughing, nausea, vomiting, diarrhea, epigastric pain, lethargy, fatigue and neuropathy, dehydration, severe vomiting (2663,2681); and zinc-induced copper deficiency with symptoms including sideroblastic anemia, neutropenia, impaired immune function, and an increase in the ratio of low-density-lipoprotein to high-density-lipoprotein (LDL/HDL) cholesterol (2619,2681). However, daily doses of 80 mg elemental zinc in combination with copper 2 mg for five years doesn't seem to cause changes in serum cholesterol or hematocrit (8622). Daily doses of 300 mg of supplemental zinc for six weeks appear to impair immune response (7135). There is preliminary evidence that higher dietary zinc intake might increase the risk for benign prostatic hyperplasia (BPH) (6908). Epidemiological evidence suggests that taking more than 100 mg of supplemental zinc daily or taking supplemental zinc for 10 or more years doubles the risk of developing prostate cancer (10306).
Topically, zinc can cause burning, stinging, itching, and tingling when applied to inflamed tissue (8623). Zinc oxide can be deposited in the submucosal tissue and cause dark discoloration of the skin. This can occur with prolonged topical application to intact skin, application to eroded or ulcerated skin, or penetrating traumatic exposure, and also parenteral administration (8618).

Intranasally, zinc can cause nasal irritation, headache, bad taste, bloody nose, dry nose, loss of sense of smell, dry mouth, and burning and irritation of the throat (8628,8629,11306,11155). There are case reports of complete loss of sense of smell (anosmia) that may be permanent with use of zinc gluconate nasal gel (Zicam). Loss of sense of smell appears to be dose related but has been reported following a single application (11306,11155,11707). Zinc sulfate nasal spray was used unsuccessfully for polio prophylaxis before the polio vaccine was developed. It caused loss of smell and/or taste, which was sometimes permanent (11713). Animal studies suggest that zinc sulfate negatively affects smell, possibly by damaging the olfactory epithelium and neurons (11156,11703,11704,11705,11706). Zinc gluconate nasal spray has not been tested for safety in animals or humans. The clinical studies of intranasal zinc have not described anosmia as an adverse effect, but testing was not done to see if zinc use adversely affected sense of smell (6471,8628,8629,10247).

Occupational inhalation of zinc oxide fumes can cause metal fume fever with symptoms including fatigue, chills, fever, myalgias, cough, dyspnea, leukocytosis, thirst, metallic taste, and salivation (331).

Interactions with Herbs & Other Dietary Supplements

COPPER: Concomitant use with zinc may impair copper absorption (2693).

IP-6 (Phytic Acid): IP-6 in foods can decrease zinc absorption (7135). Theoretically, IP-6 supplements could also interfere with zinc absorption. IP-6 chelates multivalent metal ions in the gastrointestinal tract, preventing absorption (1858).

IRON: Non-heme iron might decrease zinc absorption. Non-heme iron and zinc compete for a common absorption pathway in the gut. However, when iron and zinc are taken concomitantly with food, this interaction is not likely to occur. When taken with food, zinc absorption is facilitated by proteins in food through an alternate pathway that does not compete with iron (7357). Protein-bound heme iron (found in red meats) does not affect zinc absorption (7135).

Interactions with Drugs

AMILORIDE (Midamor): Amiloride reduces urinary zinc excretion and can increase zinc levels (830).

CISPLATIN (Platinol-AQ): Concomitant use with zinc might increase the cytotoxicity of cisplatin when in the presence of the chelate ethylenediaminetetraacetic acid (EDTA), as compared to cisplatin treatment alone (2668).

PENICILLAMINE: Penicillamine chelates zinc and can reduce the effects of supplemental zinc (2678). Separate dose times by at least 2 hours.

POTASSIUM-SPARING DIURETICS: Concomitant use with zinc can lead to zinc accumulation and increase risk of adverse effects (830).

QUINOLONE ANTIBIOTICS: Concomitant use with zinc reduces drug absorption and serum levels of quinolones due to zinc binding (828,2682). Concomitant use can also reduce the effects of zinc supplementation due to reduced zinc absorption.

TETRACYCLINE ANTIBIOTICS: Concomitant use with zinc decreases absorption and serum levels of demeclocycline (Declomycin), minocycline (Minocin), and tetracycline (Achromycin) due to zinc binding. Concomitant use can also reduce the effects of zinc supplementation due to reduced zinc absorption. Doxycycline (Vibramycin) does not interact with zinc (4945).

THIAZIDE DIURETICS: Concomitant use with zinc can interfere with zinc supplementation by increasing urinary zinc elimination (830,831).

Drug Influences on Nutrient Levels and Depletion

SOME DRUGS CAN AFFECT ZINC LEVELS:

CAPTOPRIL (Capoten): Captopril might increase urinary zinc excretion in patients with hypertension. There is no data on other ACE-inhibitors (ACEIs). The clinical consequence of urinary zinc loss in hypertensive patients is unknown (25,26). Patients receiving high doses, greater than 200 mg daily long-term, have developed taste disturbances which resolved in some patients with zinc supplementation (6543).

DEFEROXAMINE (Desferal): Deferoxamine increases urinary zinc elimination (6597,6598).

DIURETICS: Use of loop diuretics and thiazide diuretics can increase urinary zinc loss and reduce serum levels. This is more likely with higher doses or when used in combination with diuretics of another class (4412,4425).

PENICILLAMINE (Cuprimine): Penicillamine can reduce serum zinc levels and might cause zinc depletion in some patients (4453,4531,4534,9630).

QUINOLONES: Treatment with fluoroquinolones can reduce dietary zinc absorption. The clinical significance is yet to be determined, and the need for supplementation has not been adequately studied. Consider zinc supplementation in patients on long-term fluoroquinolone therapy (828,2682).

TETRACYCLINES: Tetracyclines, except doxycycline (Vibramycin), can reduce dietary zinc absorption and serum levels due to zinc binding. The clinical significance is yet to be determined, and the need for supplementation has not been adequately studied. Consider zinc supplementation in patients on long-term tetracycline therapy (4945).

Interactions with Foods

FOODS: Concomitant administration with foods containing bran, phytates, calcium, or phosphorus may decrease supplemental zinc absorption (506).

VEGETARIANISM: Absorption of zinc from vegetarian diets is lower than from non-vegetarian diets most likely due to the higher amount of phytate, calcium, and other inhibitors of zinc absorption (7135). Dietary zinc requirements, particularly in strict vegetarians, may be 50% greater when the major food sources are grains and legumes (7135).

Interactions with Lab Tests

BLOOD ZINC ASSAYS: Avoid using powdered gloves when drawing blood for zinc assays, due to potential for sample contamination (2663).

HEMOGLOBIN A1C (HgbA1c): Supplementation with elemental zinc 50 mg per day has increased HgbA1c in type 1 diabetics (6530).

LIPID PROFILES: Zinc supplementation might reduce high-density lipoprotein (HDL) cholesterol levels and test results (2681). Zinc supplementation might increase the ratio of low-density-lipoprotein to high-density-lipoprotein (LDL/HDL) cholesterol and test results (2681).

Interactions with Diseases or Conditions

ALCOHOLISM: Long-term excessive alcohol consumption is associated with impaired zinc absorption and increased excretion of zinc in the urine (7135).

HUMAN IMMUNODEFICIENCY VIRUS (HIV): Use zinc with caution in people with HIV infection. Some evidence suggests an association between higher intakes of zinc and reduced survival time (6565). However, other researchers have reported no association. Some research suggests that avoiding zinc deficiency in patients with HIV disease might allow normal or improved immune function (8625).

MALABSORPTION SYNDROMES (Sprue, Crohn's disease, short bowel syndrome, etc): People with malabsorption syndromes may be zinc deficient due to decreased zinc absorption and increased urinary zinc losses (7135).

RHEUMATOID ARTHRITIS (RA): Zinc absorption is reduced in people with rheumatoid arthritis (2823).

Dosage and Administration

ORAL: The typical dose for treating the common cold is one zinc gluconate or acetate lozenge, providing 9-24 mg elemental zinc, dissolved in the mouth every two hours while awake when cold symptoms are present (333,335,336).

For acute diarrhea in malnourished or zinc-deficient children, 10-40 mg elemental zinc is given daily (825,826,827,3455,3456,10248).

For preventing pneumonia in babies and children in developing countries, 10 mg per day has been used (8920).

For hypogeusia, 25-100 mg oral zinc has been used in clinical trials (6542). Anorexia nervosa has been treated with 100 mg of zinc gluconate daily (6905).

For treating gastric ulcers, zinc sulfate 200 mg three times daily has been used (6591).

For muscle cramps in zinc deficient patients with cirrhosis, zinc sulfate 220 mg twice daily has been used (1352).

Sickle cell disease has been treated with zinc sulfate 220 mg three times daily (6594).

To increase growth and weight gain in prepubertal children with sickle cell disease, 10 mg elemental zinc per day has been used (8626).

For treating attention deficit-hyperactivity disorder (ADHD) in children, doses of zinc sulfate 55 mg (15 mg elemental zinc) to 150 mg (40 mg elemental zinc) daily has been used (11350,12060).

For treating acne, clinical trials have used 30 to 135 mg elemental zinc daily (6297,6298,6299,6501,6502).

For treating age-related macular degeneration (AMD), elemental zinc 80 mg plus vitamin C 500 mg, vitamin E 400 IU, and beta-carotene 15 mg has been given daily (7303).

For treating advanced cirrhosis, zinc sulfate 200 mg three times daily has been used (8624).

The National Institute of Medicine has established Adequate Intake (AI) levels of zinc for infants birth to 6 months is 2 mg/day (7135). For older infants, children, and adults, Recommended Dietary Allowance (RDA) quantities of zinc have been established: infants and children 7 months to 3 years, 3 mg/day; 4 to 8 years, 5 mg/day; 9 to 13 years, 8 mg/day; girls 14 to 18 years, 9 mg/day; boys and men age 14 and older, 11 mg/day; women 19 and older, 8 mg/day; pregnant women 14 to 18, 13 mg/day; pregnant women 19 and older, 11 mg/day; lactating women 14 to 18, 14 mg/day; lactating women 19 and older, 12 mg/day (7135).

The typical North American male consumes about 13 mg/day of dietary zinc; women consume approximately 9 mg/day (7135).

The Tolerable Upper Intake Levels (UL) of zinc for people who are not receiving zinc under medical supervision: Infants birth to 6 months, 4 mg/day; 7 to 12 months, 5 mg/day; children 1 to 3 years, 7 mg/day; 4 to 8 years, 12 mg/day; 9 to 13 years, 23 mg/day; 14 to 18 years (including pregnancy and lactation), 34 mg/day; adults 19 years and older (including pregnancy and lactation), 40 mg/day (7135).

Different salt forms provide different amounts of elemental zinc. Zinc sulfate contains 23% elemental zinc; 220 mg zinc sulfate contains 50 mg zinc. Zinc gluconate contains 14.3% elemental zinc; 10 mg zinc gluconate contains 1.43 mg zinc (506).

INTRANASAL: For treating or preventing the common cold 2.1 mg of elemental zinc per day has been used (10247).

TOPICAL: For acne vulgaris, zinc acetate 1.2% with erythromycin 4% as a lotion has been applied twice daily (819). For herpes simplex infections, zinc sulfate 0.25% applied 8 to 10 times daily or zinc oxide, 0.3%, with glycine applied every 2 hours while awake has been used (8623). Lower concentrations have shown variable efficacy (6538).

Comments

Zinc acetate (Galzin) is an FDA-approved orphan drug for treating Wilson's disease. Zinc and cadmium are chemically similar and often occur together in nature. Cadmium is not an essential element, and excessive long-term exposure can lead to kidney dysfunction. The concentration of cadmium in zinc-containing supplements can vary as much as 37-fold. Zinc gluconate consistently contains the lowest cadmium concentration (10669).

1 Monographs on the medicinal uses of plant drugs. Exeter, UK: European Scientific Co-op Phytother, 1997.
2 Blumenthal M, ed. The Complete German Commission E Monographs: Therapeutic Guide to Herbal Medicines. Trans. S. Klein. Boston, MA: American Botanical Council, 1998.
3 Tyler VE. Herbs of Choice. Binghamton, NY: Pharmaceutical Products Press, 1994.
4 Newall CA, Anderson LA, Philpson JD. Herbal Medicine: A Guide for Healthcare Professionals. London, UK: The Pharmaceutical Press, 1996.
5 Foster S, Tyler VE. Tyler's Honest Herbal: A Sensible Guide to the Use of Herbs and Related Remedies. 3rd ed., Binghamton, NY: Haworth Herbal Press, 1993.
6 The Review of Natural Products by Facts and Comparisons. St. Louis, MO: Wolters Kluwer Co., 1999.
7 Schulz V, Hansel R, Tyler VE. Rational Phytotherapy: A Physician's Guide to Herbal Medicine. Terry C. Telger, transl. 3rd ed. Berlin, GER: Springer, 1998.
8 Wichtl MW. Herbal Drugs and Phytopharmaceuticals. Ed. N.M. Bisset. Stuttgart: Medpharm GmbH Scientific Publishers, 1994.
9 Martindale W. Martindale the Extra Pharmacopoeia. Pharmaceutical Press, 1999.
10 United States Pharmacopeial Convention, Inc., ed. Drug Information for the Health Care Professional. 19th ed. Englewood, CO: Micromedex Inc., 1999.
11 Leung AY, Foster S. Encyclopedia of Common Natural Ingredients Used in Food, Drugs and Cosmetics. 2nd ed. New York, NY: John Wiley & Sons, 1996.
12 McGuffin M, Hobbs C, Upton R, Goldberg A, eds. American Herbal Products Association's Botanical Safety Handbook. Boca Raton, FL: CRC Press, LLC 1997.
13 Robbers JE, Speedie MK, Tyler VE. Pharmacognosy and Pharmacobiotechnology. Baltimore, MD: Williams & Wilkins, 1996.
15 McKevoy GK, ed. AHFS Drug Information. Bethesda, MD: American Society of Health-System Pharmacists, 1998.
16 Gennaro A. Remington: The Science and Practice of Pharmacy. 19th ed. Lippincott: Williams & Wilkins, 1996.
17 Ellenhorn MJ, et al. Ellenhorn's Medical Toxicology: Diagnoses and Treatment of Human Poisoning. 2nd ed. Baltimore, MD: Williams & Wilkins, 1997.
18 Gruenwald J, Brendler T, Jaenicke C. PDR for Herbal Medicines. 1st ed. Montvale, NJ: Medical Economics Company, Inc., 1998.
19 Brinker F. Herb Contraindications and Drug Interactions. 2nd ed. Sandy, OR: Eclectic Medical Publications, 1998.
21 *Arch Intern Med* 1998;158:2200-11.
22 *Lancet* 1999;354:353.
23 *Pharmacist's Letter/Prescriber's Letter* 1999:15(12);151206.
25 *J Am Coll Nutr* 1998;17:75-8.
26 *Metabolism* 1990;39:665-7.
27 *JAMA* 1991;265:2688-91.
28 *Arch Intern Med* 1995;155:2005-7.
29 *Lancet* 1992;340:9-13.
30 *Am J Hematol* 1995;49:318-22.
31 *Am J Clin Nutr* 1996;64:622-6.
32 *Scand J Clin Lab Invest* 1997;57:521-7.
33 Chevallier A. Encyclopedia of Medicinal Plants. New York, NY: DK Publishing, 1996.
34 *Br Med J (Clin Res Ed)* 1981;282:1823-4.
35 *J Ethnopharmacol* 1986;17:277-82.
36 *Phytother Res* 1993;7:285-9.
37 *Phytomedicine* 1996;294.
38 *Upsala J Med Sci* 1977;82:39-41.
39 *Ann Ottalmol Clin Ocul* 1987;113:1173-7.
40 *Kiln Monastbl Augenheilkd* 1981;178:386-9.
41 *Biol Psychiatry* 1979;14:741-51.
42 *Drug Development Res* 1988;14:213-6.
43 *Altern Med Rev* 1999;4:144-61.
44 *N Engl J Med* 1999;341:1670-9.
45 *J Ethnopharmacol* 1990;30:281-94.
46 *J Ethnopharmacol* 1990;30:295-300.
47 *Townsend Letter for Doctors & Patients* 1998;180:72-84.
48 *J Pharmacol Sci* 1970;59:622-8.
49 *J Herbs Spices Med Plants* 1998;5:95-8.
50 *Lancet* 1997;350:1598-9.
51 *Calcif Tissue Int* 1999;65:285-9.
52 *Arch Intern Med* 1999;159:1750-6.
53 *Calcif Tissue Int* 1996;59:352-6.
54 *J Bone Miner Res* 2000;15:515-21.
55 *Am J Clin Nutr* 2000;71:1031-2.
56 *J Nutr* 1996;126:1187S-91S.
57 *Hematol Oncol Clin North Am* 2000;14:339-53.
58 *Maturitas* 1999;31:161-4.
59 *Lancet* 1998;351:724.
60 *J Bone Joint Surg Br* 1988;70:663-4.
61 *J Bone Joint Surg Br* 1985;60:1268-9.
62 *J Bone Miner Res* 1993;8:1241-5.
63 *Int J Gynaecol Obstet* 1997;56:25-30.
64 *J Nutr* 1996;126:1181S-6S.
65 *Jpn J Pharmacol* 1997;75:135-43.
66 *Gastroenterology* 1977;72:483-7.
68 *JPEN J Parenter Enteral Nutr* 1987;11:447-53.
69 *J Gastroenterol* 2000;35:7-12.
70 *Arch Neurol* 2000;57:956-63.
71 *J Natl Cancer Inst* 1996;88:550-2.
72 *Psychopharmacology (Berl)* 1999;143:358-64.
73 *Intern Med* 1999;38:401-6.
74 *Nutrition* 1999;15:656-60.
75 Institute of Medicine. The role of protein and amino acids in sustaining and enhancing performance. Washington, DC: National Academy Press, 1999. Available at: http://books.nap.edu/books/0309063469/html/309.html#pagetop.
77 *Nutrition* 1996;12:485-90.
78 *Am J Clin Nutr* 1998;68:72-81.
79 *Am J Psychiatry* 1984;141:1212-5.
80 *Med Hypotheses* 1983;12:239-51.
81 *Gastroenterology* 1989;97:1033-42.
82 *JPEN J Parenter Enteral Nutr* 1996;20:159-64.
83 *Arch Ophthalmol* 1993;111:761-72.
84 *Arch Ophthalmol* 1993;111:1462-3.
85 *Arch Ophthalmol* 1993;111:1463;discussion 1463-6.
86 *Arch Ophthalmol* 1993;111:1461-2.
87 *Arch Ophthalmol* 1993;111:1460.
88 *Arch Ophthalmol* 1993;111:1460-1.
89 *J Pediatr* 2000;136:734-8.
90 *Am J Cardiol* 1996;77:545-6.
91 *Ann N Y Acad Sci* 1982;393:361-8.
92 *Am J Pediatr Hematol Oncol* 1979;1:169-73.
93 *JAMA* 1974;230:1300-1.
94 *J Am Coll Cardiol* 2000;36:94-102.
95 *Circulation* 2000;102:191-6.
96 *Eur J Clin Nutr* 2000;54:298-305.
97 *Am J Clin Nutr* 2000;71:1665S-8S.
98 *Am J Clin Nutr* 2000;72:181-9.

99 *Am J Clin Nutr* 1998;67:669-84.
100 *Am J Clin Nutr* 2000;72:202-3.
101 *J Am Acad Dermatol* 1988;18:714-20.
102 *Biol Chem* 1997;378:951-61.
104 *Thromb Res* 1990;57:839-45.
105 *Mycopathologia* 1995;131:107-14.
107 *Urology* 1998;52:1026-9.
108 *Br J Clin Pharmacol* 1998;46:489-97.
109 *Int J Clin Pharmacol Res* 1998;18:145-50.
110 *Circulation* 1998;97:2123-8.
112 *Nephrol Dial Transplant* 1997;12:1437-40.
114 *J Urol* 1997;158:2045-50.
116 *Atherosclerosis* 1997;129:261-9.
117 *J Pharmacol Exp Ther* 1998;286:767-71.
118 *J Virol* 1995;69:4656-7.
119 *Chemotherapy* 1981;27:209-13.
121 *Thorax* 1998;53:172-5.
122 *Liver* 1998;18:27-31.
123 *Am J Clin Nutr* 1983;38:257-63.
126 *Scand J Gastroenterol* 1994;29:178-81.
127 *Biochem J* 1992;288:341-4.
128 *J Lipid Res* 1992;33:385-97.
129 *Br Med J (Clin Res Ed)* 1981;282:1516.
130 *Br Med J (Clin Res Ed)* 1981;283:503.
131 *Proc Natl Acad Sci U S A* 1996;93:3704-9.
132 *Ann Intern Med* 1990;113:82-3.
133 *Br Med J* 1980;281:1682.
134 *Ann Intern Med* 1990;113:483-4.
135 *JCC* 1997;40:146.
136 *JAMA* 1983;289:729-30.
137 *JAMA* 1983;250:729.
139 *Annu Rev Public Health* 1998;19:73-99.
140 *Nutr Rev* 1998;56:9-16.
141 *J Womens Health* 1998;7:525-9.
148 *Epidemiology* 1996;7:472-7.
149 *Prostaglandins Leukot Essent Fatty Acids* 2000;63:119-21.
150 Johnson JA, Lalonde RL. Congestive Heart Failure. Eds. DiPiro JT, et al. Pharmacotherapy, third ed. Stamford: Appleton and Lange, 1997.
151 Sklar S, et al. Drug therapy screening system. Indianapolis, IN: First Data Bank 99.1-99. 2 eds.
152 *Am J Public Health* 1993;83:1155-60.
153 *JAMA* 1996;275:870-5.
155 *Chemotherapy* 1995;41:48-81.
156 *Eur J Clin Nutr* 1995;49:S123-8.
157 Drug Facts and Comparisons. Olin BR, ed. St. Louis, MO: Facts and Comparisons. (updated monthly).
159 Gossel TA, Bricker JD. Principles of Clinical Toxicology. New York, NY:Raven Press, 1994.
160 *Eur J Cancer Prev* 1998;7:S1-83.
161 *Lancet* 1994;344:1046-9.
162 *Gastroenterology* 1992;102:875-8.
164 *Prog Food Nutr Sci* 1987;11:153-74.
165 *Appl Environ Microbiol* 1999;65:4606-10.
166 *Arch Intern Med* 1998;158:2200-11.
167 *Ann Pharmacother* 1998;32:1201-8.
169 *Ann Pharmacother* 1998;32:680-91.
170 *Ann Clin Biochem* 1996;33:162-3.
171 *Cutis* 1993;51:303-5.
172 *Am J Clin Nutr* 1989;49:127-31.
173 *Ann N Y Acad Sci* 1985;447:97-104.
175 *Ann N Y Acad Sci* 1985;447:297-313.
176 *J Pediatr Gastroentereol Nutr* 1998;26:245-50.
178 *Am J Clin Nutr* 1995;61:585-9.
179 *Padiatr Padol* 1993;28:133-6.
180 *Pediatr Med Chir* 1992;14:195-8.
181 *Minerva Med* 1992;83:135-9.
182 *Int J Obes* 1984;8:289-93.
183 *Clin Ter* 1995;146:269-74.
184 *N Engl J Med* 1999;340:814-5.
185 *Nippon Ronen Igakkai Zasshi* 1990;27:555-8.
186 *Oral Surg Oral Med Oral Pathol* 1991;71:288-93.
187 *Otolaryngol Head Neck Surg* 1990;102:326-30.
195 *Am J Ind Med* 1996;29:215-21.
196 *South Med J* 1997;90:1106-9.
197 *Thorax* 1984;39:436-41.
198 *Clin Pharmacokinet* 1988;15:227-44.
199 *Res Commun Chem Pathol Pharmacol* 1983;40:165-8.
200 *Am J Clin Nutr* 2000;72:201-3.
202 *Am J Clin Nutr* 1999;69:156-8.
203 *Pharmacopsychiatry* 1997;30:81-5.
204 *Pharmacopsychiatry* 1997;30:77-80.
205 *Pharmacopsychiatry* 1997;30 Suppl 2:72-6.
206 *Ann Intern Med* 1999;130:510-4.
207 *Am J Psychiatry* 2000;157:836-7.
208 *J Herb Pharmacother* 2001;1:65-9.
209 *Arch Biochem Biophys* 1998;355:43-8.
211 *Neoplasma* 1998;45:266-71.
212 *Pharmacist's Letter/Prescriber's Letter* 1997;13(9):130916.
213 *J Urol* 1996;156:1876-80.
215 Osol and Farar. The Dispensatory of the United States of America. 25th ed. JB Lippincott Co., 1955.
216 Dorland's Illustrated Medical Dictionary, 25th ed. WB Saunders Company, 1974.
218 *Am J Clin Nutr* 1984;40:240-5.
219 *J Am Optom Assoc* 1999;70:39-47.
220 *Am J Clin Nutr* 1997;65:1489-94.
221 *BMJ* 2001;322:73.
222 *BJU Int* 1999;83:269-73.
223 Williamson EM, Evans FJ, eds. Potter's new cyclopaedia of botanical drugs and preparations. Essex, England: CW Daniel Company Ltd., 1998.
224 *Obstet Gynecol* 1999;94:225-8.
225 *J Reprod Med* 1993;38:37-40.
226 *Int J Fertil Womens Med* 1999;44:67-73.
227 *Fertil Steril* 1999;71:614-8.
228 *Obstet Gynecol* 1998;92:982-8.
233 *Ann Allergy* 1993;70(3):237-42.
234 *Immunopharmacology* 1995;30(2):147-55.
235 *Planta Med* 1995;61(1):33-6.
236 *Cancer Lett* 1992;63(1):41-6.
237 *Toxicol Lett* 1998;95(1):23-9.
238 *Anticancer Res* 1998;18(3A):1527-32.
239 *Eur J Cancer Prev* 1999;8:435-40.
240 *Biochem Mol Biol Int* 1999;47(1):153-9.
241 *J Ethnopharmacol* 1996;52:23-6.
242 *Indian J Physiol Pharmacol* 1995;39:59-62.
243 *J Ethnopharmacol* 1991;34:275-8.
245 *J Ethnopharmacol* 1991;31(3):283-9.
246 Medenica RD. Use of Black seed to increase immune function. U.S. Patent 5,482,711, issued January 9, 1996. Obtained from US Patent and Trademark Ofc on April 12, 2000. www.uspto.gov/patft/index.htm.
247 *Am J Clin Nutr* 1997;65:785-9.
248 *Am J Clin Nutr* 1986;43:382-7.
249 *Am J Clin Nutr* 2000;71:458-64.
250 *J Pharm Sci* 1981;70:999-1002.
251 *J Clin Pharmacol* 1981;21:26-30.
252 *J Pharm Sci* 1978;67:1582-6.
253 *J Pharm Sci* 1978 67:1579-82.

REFERENCES

256 *Bioorg Med Chem* 1997;5:501-6.
257 *J Econ Entomol* 1992;85:2353-6.
258 *J Med Chem* 1994;37:1971-6.
259 *Circulation* 1995;91:645-55.
260 *J Anal Toxicol* 1998;22:460-73.
261 *J Forensic Sci* 1995;40:614-8.
266 Facts and Comparisons staff. Drug Facts and Comparisons. St Louis: Wolters Kluwer Company (updated monthly).
267 Chaparral-containing *Herp-Eeze* on the Market. *Pharmacist's Letter/Prescriber's Letter* 1999;15(2):150215.
268 Merck Index, 12th ed. Whitehouse Station: Merck Research Laboratories, 1996.
269 Neal H. Dictionary of Chemical Names and Synonyms. Chelsea: Lewis Publishers, 1992.
270 Parker SP. ed. McGaw Hill Dictionary of Chemistry. New York: McGraw-Hill Book Company 1984.
271 Bruneton J. Pharmacognosy, Phytochemistry, Medicinal Plants. Paris: Lavoisier Publishing, 1995.
272 Covington TR, et al. Handbook of Nonprescription Drugs. 11th ed. Washington, DC: Am Pharmaceutical Assn, 1996.
274 *BMJ* 1994;308:501-3.
275 Young DS. Effects of Drugs on Clinical Laboratory Tests 4th ed. Washington: AACC Press, 1995.
277 *J Hypertension* 1994;12:463-8.
278 *Pharmacotherapy* 1993;13:406-7.
279 *Br J Clin Pract Symp Suppl* 1990;69:3-6.
280 *Fortschr Med* 1995;113:291-2.
281 *Arch Dermatol* 1998;134:1356-60.
282 *Fortschr Med* 1996;114:196-200.
283 *Lancet* 1996;347:292-4.
284 *Vasa* 1992;21:188-92.
285 *Dtsch Med Wochenschr* 1986;111:1321-9.
286 *Prostate* 1992;20:123-31.
287 *Mol Biother* 1991;3:170-8.
289 *Contact Dermatitis* 1981;7:309-10.
291 *Pediatrics* 1996;98(5):944-7.
292 *J Am Vet Med Assoc* 1992;200:817-8.
295 *Eur J Clin Pharmacol* 1997;12:457-61.
296 Agriculture Res Svc. Dr. Duke's phytochemical and ethnobotanical databases. www.ars-grin.gov/duke/ (Accessed 7 July 1999).
297 *Hum Toxicol* 1989;8:501-6.
298 Mann J, Truswell AS, eds. Essentials of Human Nutrition. Oxford: Oxford Univ Press 1998.
300 *J Pharm Sci* 1992;81:128-30.
303 Upton R, ed. Astragalus Root: Analytical, quality control, and therapeutic monograph. Santa Cruz, CA: American Herbal Pharmacopoeia. 1999:1-25.
310 *Ther Drug Monit* 1999;21:304-9.
311 FTC. FTC charges marketer of vitamin O of making false claims. Fed Trade Comm. 1999. Available at: www.ftc.gov/opa/1999/03/rosecreek.htm
313 Mehta DK (Ex Ed). British National Formulary, Number 37. British Medical Association and Royal Pharmaceutical Society of Great Britain: London, England, March 1999.
314 *Int J Obes* 1991;15:359-66.
315 *Thorax* 1999;54:115-8.
316 *J Appl Microbiol* 1999;86:985-90.
317 *J Allergy Clin Immunol* 1999;103:959-60.
319 *J Pediatr* 2000;137:604-7.
320 *Arch Surg* 2000;135:1265-70.
322 *J Rheumatol* 1996;23:1385-91.
323 *Presse Med* 1998;27:1862-5.
324 *Rev Rhum Mal Osteoartic* 1992;59:466-72.
325 *Can J Psychiatry* 1998;43:746-7.
326 *BMJ* 1999;318:1287.
327 *Aust Dent J* 1996;41:294-9.
328 *Natl Med J India* 1998;11:113-6.
329 *Indian J Dent Res* 1997;8:39-45.
330 *Antimicrob Agents Chemother* 1999;43:975-7.
331 *J Toxicol Clin Toxicol* 1999;37:279-92.
332 *Med Lett Drugs Ther* 1997;39:9-10.
333 *Ann Intern Med* 1996;125:81-8.
334 *J Int Med Res* 1992;20:234-6.
335 *J Antimicrob Chemother* 1987;20:893-901.
336 *Antimicrob Agents Chemother* 1984;25:20-4.
337 *Antimicrob Agents Chemother* 1987;31:1183-7.
338 *Antimicrob Agents Chemother* 1989;33:646-8.
339 *Dan Med Bull* 1990;37:279-81.
340 *J Antimicrob Chemother* 1997;40:483-93.
341 *JAMA* 1998;279:1962-7.
345 *Ann N Y Acad Sci* 1993;695:324-6.
347 *Medical Letter* 1999;41:107-8.
348 *Br J Ophthalmol* 2001;85:537-9.
349 *Arch Intern Med* 1999;159:2456-60.
350 *Lancet* 1981;2:122-4.
354 *Nippon Kyobu Shikkan Gakkai Zasshi* 1997;35:1372-7.
355 *Arerugi* 1997;46:1148-55.
356 *Nippon Kyobu Shikkan Gakkai Zasshi* 1997;35:391-5.
357 *Nippon Kyobu Shikkan Gakkai Zasshi* 1992;30:1583-8.
358 *Arerugi* 1995;44:711-4.
359 *Eur Respir J* 1996;9:2691-6.
360 *Nippon Kyobu Shikkan Gakkai Zasshi* 1995;33:1361-6.
361 *Nihon Kokyuki Gakkai Zasshi* 1998;36:776-80.
362 *Microbiol Immunol* 1997;41:835-9.
363 *Gastroenterology* 1999;117:1234-7.
365 FDA. Guide to Inspections of Cosmetic Product Manufacturers: products containing estrogenic hormones, placental extract or vitamins. 2001. Available at: http://www.fda.gov/ora/inspect_ref/igs/cosmet.html
366 *J Assoc Phys India* 1989;37:323-8.
367 *Richters HerbLetter* November 23, 1999.
368 *Klin Padiatr* 1987;199:453-6.
370 *Proc Natl Acad Sci USA* 1999;96:13486-90.
371 *Diabetes* 1994;43:1173-9.
372 *Diabetologia* 1995;38:518-24.
374 *Phytomedicine* 1994;1:177-81.
375 *Gut* 1999;45:840-7.
376 *J Geriatr Psychiatry Neurol* 1994;7 Suppl 1:S12-4.
379 *Wien Med Wochenschr* 1999;149:202-8.
380 *Pharmacy Practice* 1995;11:51-2,54-5.
381 *Lancet* 1981;14:615.
382 *Clin Pharmacol Ther* 1999;66:338-45.
383 *J Assoc Phys India* 1994;42:454-5.
384 *N Engl J Med* 1980;303:355-9.
387 FDA Talk Paper. FDA takes action against firm marketing unapproved drugs. 1999. Available at: www.fda.gov/bbs/topics/ANSWERS/ANS00988.html
388 *J Biol Chem* 1999;274:26617-24.
389 *J Surg Oncol* 1999;72:230-9.
390 *Dtsch Med Wochenschr* 1998;123:1410-4.
391 *Oncology* 1999;13:1003-8.
393 *Planta Med* 1989;55:358-63.
394 *UC Berkeley Wellness Letter* 1997;13:1-2.
395 *Burns* 1998;24:157-61.
396 *Burns* 1996;22:491-3.
397 *Burns* 1994;20:331-3.
398 *Br J Plast Surg* 1993;46:322-3.

399 *Br J Surg* 1991;78:497-8.
401 *Lancet* 1999;354:482-3.
403 Whitney E, Cataldo CB, Rolfes SR, eds. Understanding Normal and Clinical Nutrition. Belmont, CA: Wadsworth, 1998.
405 *Gastroenterology* 1990;98:66-72.
406 Upton R, ed. Hawthorn Leaf with Flower: Analytical, quality control, and therapeutic monograph. Santa Cruz, CA: American Herbal Pharmacopoeia 1999:1-29.
409 *Pediatr Pulmonol* 1994;18:34-8.
410 A Modern Herbal (Mrs.M.Grieve) website. Available at: http://botanical.com/botanical/mgmh/s/squawv85.html (Accessed 25 November 1999).
412 *J Am Coll Cardiol* 1999;34:2002-6.
416 *Allergy* 1997;52:829-35.
417 *Clin Exp Allergy* 1996;26:1401-10.
418 *Singapore Med J* 1995;36(4):387-90.
419 *Cancer Biother* 1994;9(2):153-61.
420 *Mutat Res* 1993;319(1):1-9.
421 *J Urol* 1991;146(2):486-90.
422 *Turk J Pediatr* 2000;42:17-21.
423 *Cancer* 1983;52:70-3.
424 *Lancet* 1999;354:1948-54.
425 *Lancet* 1999;354:1919.
426 *Calcif Tissue Int* 2000;66(1):61-5.
427 *Bone Miner* 1992;19,Suppl 1:S49-56.
428 *Bone Miner* 1992;19,Suppl 1:S43-8.
429 *Am J Phys Med Rehabil* 1999;78(5):457-63.
430 *Horm Res* 1999;51:178-83.
431 *Altern Med Rev* 1999;4:10-22.
432 *Calcif Tissue Int* 1997;61,Suppl 1:S23-7.
433 *Calcif Tissue Int* 1997;61,Suppl 1:S19-22.
434 *Calcif Tissue Int* 1995;56(2):160-5.
441 *Phytother Res* 1999;13:380-7.
442 *FEBS Lett* 1999;444:173-6.
443 *Cancer Lett* 1993;73:161-6.
444 *Planta Med* 1990;56:430-4.
448 *Chem Pharm Bull (Tokyo)* 1995;43(9):1462-5.
449 *Chung Kuo Chung Yao Tsa Chih* 1995;20:36-9, 62-3.
450 *N Engl J Med* 1997;336:1328.
451 *Yao Hsueh Hsueh Pao* 1992;27:358-64.
452 *Chung Kuo Chung Yao Tsa Chih* 1991;16:675-6, 703.
453 *Chung Hsi I Chieh Ho Tsa Chih* 1991;11:390,415-7.
454 *J Clin Oncol* 1998;16:495-500.
455 *Lancet* 1995;346:1104-5.
456 *Diabet Med* 1999;16:312-8.
457 *Mol Aspects Med* 1994;15:s273-80.
461 KeDi High-Tech Ind Co (Xiamen Office). www.eckorea.net/co/kedi/3.asp (Accessed 10 January 2000).
462 Seabuckthorn seed oil. RichNature Inc. www.richnature.com/products/herbal/seaseed.htm (Accessed 10 January 2000).
463 Seabuckthorn berry oil. RichNature Inc. www.richnature.com/products/herbal/seaberry.htm (Accessed 10 January 2000).
466 *Eksp Klin Farmakol* 1998;61:31-5.
467 *Khirurgiia (Sofiia)* 1995;48:30-3.
468 *IARC Sci Publ* 1991;105:568-70.
469 *Chung Kuo Chung Yao Tsa Chih* 1994;19:367-70, 384.
470 *Chung Hua Yu Fang I Hsueh Tsa Chih* 1992;26:227-9.
471 *Chung Kuo Chung Yao Tsa Chih* 1992;17:601, 624-6 (inside back cover).
472 *Hua Hsi I Ko Ta Hsueh Hsueh Pao* 1992;23:98-101.
473 Satietrol press releases. PacificHealth Labs, Inc., Woodbridge, NJ. www.satietrol.com/press.htm and www.satietrol.com/press1.htm (Accessed 01/05/2000).
474 *Blood* 1999;94(8):2735-43.
475 *Circulation* 1996;93(7):1328-30.
476 *J Clin Invest* 1999;103:383-91.
477 *Physiol Behav* 1998;65(3):505-11.
478 *Hippophae* 1993;6:39-41.
479 *Hippophae* 1996;9:40-1.
480 *Hippophae* 1997;10:39-41.
481 *Urology* 1999;54:960-3.
482 *Diabetes Care* 1998;21:2194-5.
483 *Alt Med Rev* 1998;3:140-3.
484 *Br J Cancer* 1999;80:1150-5.
485 *Anticancer Drugs* 1999;10:187-93.
486 *Proc Nutr Soc* 1999;58:139-46.
487 *Eur J Clin Nutr* 1999;53:92-6.
488 Hansten PD, Horn JR. Hansten and Horn's Drug Interactions Analysis and Management. Vancouver, CAN:Appl Therapeut, 1999.
489 *J Steroid Biochem Mol Biol* 1997;63:9-15.
490 *Am Heart J* 1999;138:1082-7.
492 *Biofactors* 1999;9:315-8.
496 *Altern Med Rev* 1998;3:222-3.
498 *Clin Rheumatol* 1988;7:46-9.
499 *Arzneimittelforschung* 1983;33(5):776-9.
500 Brinker F. Herb Contraindications and Drug Interactions. Sandy, OR: Eclectic Medical Publ, 1997.
501 De Smet PAGM, Keller K, Hansel R, Chandler RF, Eds. Adverse Effects of Herbal Drugs 1. Verlag, Berlin: Springer, 1992.
502 De Smet PAGM, Keller K, Hansel R, Chandler RF, Eds. Adverse Effects of Herbal Drugs 2. Verlag, Berlin: Springer, 1993.
504 Holt GA. Food & Possible Interactions with Drugs: Revised and Expanded Ed. Chicago, IL: Precept Press, 1998.
505 Hardman JG, Limbird LL, Molinoff PB, eds. Goodman and Gillman's The Pharmacological Basis of Therapeutics, 9th ed. New York, NY: McGraw-Hill, 1996.
506 Burnham TH, ed. Drug Facts and Comparisons, Updated Monthly. Facts and Comparisons, St. Louis, MO.
509 Dukes, MNG. Meyler's Side Effects of Drugs. 13th ed. Elsevier: Amsterdam, 1997.
510 Meuss AR, transl. Phytotherapy in Paediatrics -- Handbook for Physicians and Pharmacists by H Schilcher. 2nd edition. Stuttgart, Germany: Medpharm GmbH Scientific Publishers, 1997.
511 Spraycar M, ed. Stedman's Medical Dictionary. 26th ed. Baltimore, MD: Williams & Wilkins, 1995.
512 Robbers JE, Tyler VE. Tyler's Herbs of Choice: The Therapeutic Use of Phytomedicinals. New York, NY: The Haworth Herbal Press, 1999.
513 Agri Res Svc: Dr. Duke's phytochemical and ethnobotanical databases. www.ars-grin.gov/duke (Accessed 3 November 1999).
515 Foster S, Tyler VE. Tyler's Honest Herbal, 4th ed., Binghamton, NY: Haworth Herbal Press, 1999.
517 Duke JA, Vasquez R. Amazonian Ethnobotanical Dictionary. Boca Raton, FL: CRC Press, LLC 1994.
518 Schultes RE, Raffauf RF. The Healing Forest, Medicinal and Toxic Plants of the Northwest Amazonia. Portland, OR: Dioscorides Press, 1990.
519 Foster S, Duke JA. Eastern/Central Medicinal Plants. New York, NY: Houghton Mifflin Co., 1990.
522 *J Rheumatol* 1997;24:49-54.
523 *Eur J Clin Pharmacol* 1996;51:189-93.
524 *Clin Pharmacol Ther* 1998;64:286-8.

REFERENCES

525 *Contraception* 1996;53:41-7.
526 *Maturitas* 1994;20:155-63.
527 *Clin Pharmacol Ther* 1998 63:397-402.
528 *Lancet* 1991;337:268-9.
529 *Clin Pharmacol Ther* 1993;54:589-94.
530 *Clin Pharmacol Ther* 1997 61:401-9.
531 *Int J Vitam Nutr Res* 1988;58:414-7.
533 *Eur J Clin Pharmacol* 1984;26:279-81.
535 Swensen JN. Man convicted of driving under the influence of kava. Salt Lake City, UT: Deseret News, 1996.
536 *Ann Intern Med* 1996;125:940-1.
537 *Planta Med* 1987;53:568-9.
538 *Eur J Clin Pharmacol* 1991;41;615-7.
539 *Drug Dev Ind Pharm* 1995;21:1901-6.
540 *Lancet* 1990;35:416.
542 *Am Fam Physician* 1998;57:950,953.
543 *CMAJ* 1996;155:293-5.
553 *Schweiz Med Wochenschr* 1996;126:1085-98.
554 *Ann Pharmacother* 1998;32:428-31.
558 *Lancet* 1993;341:892.
559 *Lancet* 1992;340:1254-6.
560 *N Engl J Med* 1951;244:315-21.
561 *Ann Emerg Med* 1992;21:309-11.
562 *Lancet* 1993;341:370-1.
563 *Aust N Z J Med* 1993;23:268-71.
564 *Nephrol Dial Transplant* 1995;10:157-60.
566 *J Pediatr* 1998;132:550-2.
567 *J Allergy Clin Immunol* 1989;84:353-8.
568 *Aust N Z J Med* 1993;23:526.
569 *JAMA* 1995;273:489-90.
570 *Am J Gastroenterol* 1995;90:831-3.
571 *J Clin Gastroenterol* 1990;12:203-6.
575 *J Pediatr* 1988;112:433-6.
576 *Neurology* 1998;50:1934.
579 *N Engl J Med* 1997;336:1108.
580 *J Allergy Clin Immunol* 1997;100:575-6.
581 *Pneumologie* 1990;44(Suppl 1):337-8.
582 *Chest* 1993;104:1936-7.
583 *Chest* 1993;103:309-11.
584 *Chest* 1992;102:1605-7.
585 *Pediatrics* 1993;91:658-9.
586 *Neurosurg* 1990;26:880-2.
587 *Plast Reconstr Surg* 1995;95:213.
588 *Hosp Pharm* 1996;31:1553-4.
589 *Drugs Exp Clin Res* 1996;22:65-72.
590 *BMJ* 1978;1:1284.
591 *Am J Obstet Gynecol* 1988;159:1121-2.
592 *JAMA* 1983;249:2018.
593 *JAMA* 1990;264:2866.
594 *J Clin Psychopharmacol* 1995;15:447-8.
595 *Neurology* 1995;45:829-30.
596 *Lancet* 1996;313:756.
597 *Eur J Herbal Med* 1997;3:25-8.
598 *Ann Intern Med* 1997;127:169-70.
600 *J Allergy Clin Immunol* 1990;86:562-9.
601 *J Allergy Clin Immunol* 1990;85:785-90.
602 *Am J Gastroenterol* 1992;87:1424-8.
604 *Am J Gastroenterol* 1984;79:319-21.
605 *Eur J Herbal Med* 1997;3:25-8.
606 *Am J Med* 1989;87:89S-91S.
607 *Clin Pharmacol Ther* 1989;45:234-40.
608 *Antimicrob Agents Chemother* 1989;33:474-8.
609 *Biol Psychiatry* 1995;37:348-50.
610 *J Clin Psychiatry* 1988;49:72-3.
611 *J Intern Med* 1997;241:337-9.
612 *Aust N Z J Med* 1995;25:258.
613 *Drug Saf* 1997;17:342-56.
615 *Lancet* 1991;338:706.
616 *Pharm J* 1991;246:722.
617 *J Clin Psychopharmacol* 1985;5:65.
618 *J Clin Psychopharmacol* 1987;7:201-2.
619 *Am J Health Syst Pharm* 1997;54:692-3.
620 *Hautarzt* 1997;48:249-52.
621 *Lancet* 1998;352:1121-2.
622 *Eur J Clin Nutr* 1990;44:301-6.
626 *J Pharm Sci* 1984;73:1056-8.
627 *Lancet* 1979;2:1130.
628 *Pharmacopsychiatry* 1997;30:94-101.
631 *Am J Clin Nutr* 1985;41:1210-3.
636 *Hawaii Med J* 1995;54:669-70.
638 *Med J Aust* 1998;168:170-1.
645 *Lancet* 1992;339:1540.
650 *Ann Intern Med* 1996;124:726-34.
658 *Contact Dermatitis* 1996;35:304-5.
659 *Vet Hum Toxicol* 1995;37:364-5.
661 Berlin R, et al. Wormwood: Oregon Poison Ctr. Portland, OR: Oregon Health Sci Univ 1996.
662 *N Engl J Med* 1997;337:825-7.
665 *N Engl J Med* 1998;339:847-8.
667 *Lancet* 1991;337:914-5.
668 *Am J Clin Nutr* 1992;56:671-7.
669 *Arch Med Res* 1996;27:519-23.
670 *Arch Inst Cardiol Mex* 1995;65:342-8.
671 *Diabetes Care* 1994;17:311-5.
672 *Endocrinol* 1992;131:2909-13.
673 *Nat Med* 1996;2:443-8.
674 *Med Lett Drugs Ther* 1998;40:105-6.
675 *Arch Med Res* 1992;23:163-7.
677 *J Pharm Sci* 1994;83:296-9.
678 *Lancet* 1988;1:1015-8.
679 *Neurology* 1993;43:2466-70.
680 *J Neurol* 1989;236:445-7.
681 *Neurology* 1996;47:1220-6.
682 FDA. FDA warns about products containing gamma butyrolactone or GBL and asks companies to issue a recall. Talk Paper, 21 January 1999.
684 *J Hepatol* 1993;17:308-14.
685 *Gastroenterology* 1985;88:887-95.
686 *Gut* 1986;27:111-5.
687 *Hepatol* 1983;3:475-80.
688 *Liver* 1985;5:282-9.
689 *J Hepatol* 1990;10:291-6.
690 *J Hepatol* 1990;11:92-101.
691 *J Hum Nutr Diet* 1992;5:53-6.
692 *Acta Physiol Scand* 1997;159:41-9.
693 *J Appl Physiol* 1993;74:2711-7.
694 *Am J Physiol* 1994;267:E1010-22.
695 *Int J Obes Relat Metab Disord* 1994;18:99-103.
696 *Int J Obes Relat Metab Disord* 1993;17:S73-7.
698 Cystadane (betaine anhydrous for oral solution) Package insert. Orphan Med. October 1996.
703 *Int J Sport Nutr* 1994;4:104-19.
704 *J Sports Sci* 1991;9:91-116.
705 *Sports Med* 1987 4:9-18.
706 *JAMA* 1990;264:1441-3.
707 *Am J Clin Nutr* 1995;61:621S-4S.
708 *J Lab Clin Med* 1998;132:264-78.
709 *Am J Clin Nutr* 1988;47:186-91.
710 *Am J Clin Nutr* 1983;37:553-6.
711 *J Rheumatol* 1998;25:1986-90.
713 *J Toxicol Clin Toxicol* 1997;35:581-90.

715 *Burns* 1998;24:532-8.
716 *Burns* 1997;23:560-4.
717 *Br J Clin Pract* 1969;23:25-6.
718 *Int Surg* 1972;57:479-82.
719 *Ann Allergy Asthma Immunol* 1997;78:297-300.
720 *J Ethnopharmacol* 1989;26:249-54.
721 *Eur J Obstet Gynecol Reprod Biol* 1991;38:19-24.
722 *Anaesthesia* 1993;48:715-7.
723 *Anaesthesia* 1990;45:669-71.
724 Foster S. Feverfew, Tanacetum parthenium, botanical series #310. Austin, TX: Am Botanical Council, 1996.
726 *HerbalGram* 1997;41:16-7.
728 *JAMA* 1998;280:1596-600.
729 *Am J Clin Nutr* 1987;45:564-9.
730 *Int J Altern Complem Med* 1995;13:9-12.
731 *Arch Intern Med* 1998;158:1189-94.
732 *JAMA* 1998;279:1900-2.
733 *Med Res Rev* 1997;17:327-65.
735 Kingsbury JM. Poison ivy, poison sumac, and other rash-producing plants. York State Coll of Agri, Life Sci, Info Bull #105;1976.
736 *Phytochemistry* 1995;39:1099-101.
737 *Eur J Drug Metab Pharmacokinet* 1995;20:55-60.
738 *Fertil Steril* 1997;68:981-6.
739 *Dermatology* 1996;93:61-2.
740 *Am J Clin Nutr* 1987;46:61-5.
741 *Am J Clin Nutr* 1994;59:763S-9S.
744 *Crit Rev Food Sci Nutr* 1993;33:103-48.
745 *Eur J Clin Nutr* 1995;49:501-7.
746 *Nahrung* 1987;31:427-36.
747 *Br J Nutr* 1996;76:211-21.
748 *Cancer Res* 1997;57:225-8.
749 *Br J Nutr* 1998;80:S209-12.
750 *J Nutr* 1999;129:113-6.
751 *Int J Sport Nutr* 1997;7:318-29.
752 *Clin Ther* 1990;12:263-8.
753 *Endocrinol Jpn* 1980;27:83-6.
754 *Biomed Environ Sci* 1996;9:242-6.
755 *Int J Sport Nutr* 1991;1:170-7.
756 *Indian J Med Res* 1990;92:471-5.
757 *Nippon Sanka Fujinka Gakkai Zasshi* 1982;34:243-51.
758 Upton R, ed. St. John's wort, Hypericum perforatum: Quality control, analytical and therapeutic monograph. Santa Cruz, CA: American Herbal Pharmacopoeia 1997;1-32.
759 *Hosp Pharm* 1997;32:1621-32.
760 *Hosp Pharm* 1997;32:1275-85.
761 *Pharmacopsychiatry* 1998;31:54-9.
762 *Pharmacopsychiatry* 1998;31:7-15.
763 *Pharmacopsychiatry* 1998;31:16-21.
764 *Urology* 1998;51:1003-7.
768 *J Am Acad Dermatol* 1993;28:466-9.
769 *J Clin Endocrinol Metab* 1992;74:108-17.
770 *JAMA* 1996;276:606-7.
772 *Biochem Med Metab Bio* 1990;43:83-92.
773 *Isr J Med Sci* 1995;31:101-5.
774 *Cancer Detect Prev* 1997;21:178-90.
775 *Carcinogenesis* 1986;7:1463-6.
776 *Life Sci* 1994;54:1299-303.
777 *J Antibiot (Tokyo)* 1976;29:950-3.
778 *Eur J Clin Pharmacol* 1980;18:255-61.
779 *Res Commun Chem Pathol Pharmacol* 1976;15:735-42.
780 *Angiology* 1987;38:46-50.
781 *N Engl J Med* 1991;325:1223-7.
782 *HerbalGram* 1997;39:33-44, 46-55.
783 *Allergy* 1996;51:647-9.
785 *Arch Intern Med* 1995;155:2245-8.
787 Foster S. Peppermint, Menta x piperita, botanical series #306. Austin, TX: Am Botanical Council, 1990.
789 *Int J Radiat Oncol Biol Phys* 1993;26:413-6.
790 *Phytomedicine* 1994;1:25-31.
791 *Contact Dermatitis* 1983;9:452-5.
792 *Med J Aust* 1994;160:44.
793 *Urology* 1999;53:590-5.
795 Foster S. Milk Thistle, Silybum marianum, botanical series #305. Austin, TX: Am Botanical Council, 1996.
797 *CMAJ* 1996;155:1237.
798 *Blood* 1998;91:3817-24.
799 *J Nihon Univ Sch Dent* 1994;36:102-11.
800 *J Nihon Univ Sch Dent* 1990;32(1):4-13.
806 *Cancer Res* 1994;54:1004-7.
807 *J Appl Physiol* 1990;69:1651-6.
808 *J Appl Physiol* 1990;68:119-24.
809 *JAMA* 1983;249:2679-80.
812 *Ann N Y Acad Sci* 1998;844:274-92.
813 *Ann N Y Acad Sci* 1998;844:214-26.
816 Germplasm Resources Info. www.ars-grin.gov/npgs (Accessed 3 November 1999).
818 *Ann Otol Rhinol Laryngol* 1983;92:396-7.
819 *Eur J Clin Pharmacol* 1995;49:57-60.
820 *J Am Acad Dermatol* 1980;3:483-91.
821 *Int J Dermatol* 1990;29:134-8.
822 *J Neurol Sci* 1987;77:137-46.
823 *Ann Pharmacother* 1998;32:78-87.
824 *J Am Geriatr Soc* 1998;46:19-26.
825 *Acta Paediatr* 1999;88:154-60.
826 *Arch Dis Child* 1997;77:196-200.
827 *N Engl J Med* 1995;333:839-44.
828 *Clin Ther* 1999;21:3-40.
830 *S Afr Med J* 1983;64:936-41.
831 *Johns Hopkins Med J* 1975;136:137-44.
832 *Circulation* 1992;86:798-802.
833 Blueberry. Eat 5 a day for better health. www.5aday.com/ (Accessed 12 October 2000).
834 *Altern Med Rev* 1999;4:23-8.
835 *BMJ* 1999;318:1471-80.
836 *J Clin Endocrinol Metab* 1999;84:895-8.
837 *Am J Clin Nutr* 1999;69:74-9.
838 *J Nat Prod* 1992;55:999-1003.
840 *Phytochemistry* 2000;53:805-10.
841 *BMJ* 1999;318:1725-9.
842 *Am J Clin Nutr* 1998;68:1375S-9S.
845 *Eur J Clin Nutr* 1995;49(3):169-78.
849 *Int J Dermatol* 1993;32:690.
850 *JAMA* 1992;267:2329.
851 *Arterioscler Thromb Vasc Biol* 1997;17:3392-8.
852 *Rom J Physiol* 1993;30:101-7.
854 *Phytomedicine* 1996;3:231-5.
856 Natural Health Remedies. Health Canada. URL: hc-sc.gc.ca/english/archives/96-97/herbnae.html (Accessed 16 July 1999).
857 *J Dermatol Treatment* 1995;6:31-4.
858 *J Ethnopharmacol* 1997;55(3):179-83.
859 *Planta Med* 1991;57(4):357-60.
860 *J Ethnopharmacol* 1986;17(2):161-9.
865 *J Nutr* 1998;128:865-9.
866 *Biochem Biophys Res Commun* 1998;243:25-9.
868 *Dermatologica* 1982;165:136-40.
869 *Planta Med* 2000;66:35-9.
870 *Fukuoka Igaku Zasshi* 1993;84:257-62.
871 *Basic Life Sci* 1993;61:45-63.
872 *Acta Paediatr Jpn* 1992;34:505-10.

874 *Urol Res* 1992;20:3-6.
876 *Br J Urol* 1991;67:237-40.
877 *Am J Clin Nutr* 1990;52:661-6.
878 *Rev Paul Med* 1989;107:19-24.
879 *Eur J Clin Nutr* 1988;42:857-61.
880 *Br J Urol* 1986;58:592-5.
881 *J Urol* 1984;132:1140-5.
882 *J Urol* 1983;129:1009-11.
884 *Int J Vitam Nutr Res* 1976;46:154-9.
885 *Arch Latinoam Nutr* 1975;25:401-17.
887 *Am Surg* 2001;67:33-5.
888 *Planta Med* 1996;62:212-6.
900 *Biochim Biophys Acta* 2000;1519:117-22.
901 *Altern Med Rev* 1998;3:271-80.
902 *J Rheumatol* 1994;21:2261-5.
903 *Folia Psychiatr Neurol Jpn* 1978;32:223-30.
904 *Arch Gen Psychiatry* 1972;26:234-41.
907 *J Appl Physiol* 1999;86:1817-22.
908 *Brain Res* 2000;866:211-7.
909 *Thromb Res* 1996;84:311-22.
910 *Clin Trials J* 1985;22:149-57.
911 *Planta Med* 1992;58:338-41.
913 *J Int Med Res* 1992;20:182-9.
914 *Am J Clin Nutr* 1992;56:863-7.
915 *J Affect Disord* 1985;8:197-200.
916 *Arch Neurol* 1988;45:1217-22.
917 *Neurology* 1978;28:358-9.
918 *J Amer Geriat Soc* 1977;25:289-98.
919 FDA Talk Paper. Impurities confirmed in dietary supplement 5-hydroxy-L-tryptophan. August 31, 1998. Available at: http://vm.cfsan.fda.gov/~lrd/tp5htp.html
920 *Ann Neurol* 1993;34:169-74.
921 *Ann Neurol* 1994;36:741-6.
922 *Can Assoc Radiol J* 1995;46:386-91.
923 *J Neuropathol Exp Neurol* 1995;54:740-5.
924 *N Engl J Med* 1993;329:745-52.
925 *Biochem Mol Med* 1996;57:125-33.
926 *Postgrad Med J* 1996;72:113-4.
927 *J Inherit Metab Dis* 1995;18:635-7.
929 *Brain Dev* 1992;14:409-12.
930 *Brain Dev* 1992;14:276-7.
931 *Neurochem Res* 1994;19:1073-82.
932 *Agents Actions* 1993;38 Spec No:C139-42.
933 *N Z Med J* 1982;95:803-6.
935 *Ann Rheum Dis* 1985;44:199-201.
936 *N Z Med J* 1984;97:355-7.
937 *Biol Trace Elem Res* 1997;56:273-86.
938 *Minerva Med* 1987;78:1281-9.
939 *Sci Total Environ* 1996;191:283-90.
940 *Am J Clin Nutr* 1995;61:341-5.
941 *Environ Health Perspect* 1994;102:83-5.
942 *Environ Health Perspect* 1994;102(Suppl 7):79-82.
943 *Environ Health Perspect* 1994;102:65-72.
944 *Environ Health Perspect* 1994;102:73-7.
945 Shils M, Olson A, Shike M. Modern Nutrition in Health and Disease. 8th ed. Philadelphia, PA: Lea and Febiger, 1994.
947 *Australas J Dermatol* 1992;33:131-4.
948 *Dermatol Surg Jun* 1998;24(6):641-5.
949 *Cutis* 1998;61:347-50.
950 *Br J Dermatol* 1997;137:934-8.
951 *Arch Dermatol Res* 1996;288:383-90.
952 *Arch Dermatol* 1996;132:631-6.
953 *Dermatol Surg* 1996;22:449-52.
954 *J Am Acad Dermatol* 1996;34:187-95.
955 *Cutis* 1986;37:205-7, 209.
956 *Baillieres Clin Endocrinol Metab* 1998;12:559-79.
957 *Dtsch Zahnarztl Z* 1989;44:830-2.
958 *Biochemistry (Mosc)* 1997;62:1367-74.
959 *Arerugi* 1997;46:1170-3.
960 *Fortschr Med* 1995;113:303-6.
961 *Biokhimiia* 1995;60:118-23.
962 *Cancer Biother* 1995;10:147-52.
963 *Ann Allergy Asthma Immunol* 1998;80:24-30.
964 *Fortschr Med* 1976;94:1579-82.
965 *Fortschr Med* 1995;113:43-8.
966 *Br J Dermatol* 1988;119:535-40.
967 *Ann Allergy* 1985;55:541-3.
968 *MMW Munch Med Wochenschr* 1981;123:745-7.
969 *MMW Munch Med Wochenschr* 1976;118:1253-4.
970 *N Engl J Med* 1999;340:101-7.
971 *N Engl J Med* 1997;337:69-76.
972 *Am J Clin Nutr* 1997;65:652S-60S.
973 *J Obstet Gynaecol Res* 1996;22:425-30.
974 *Ann Epidemiol* 1995;5:96-107.
975 *Int J Artif Organs* 1994;17:37-40.
976 *Am J Hypertens* 1993;6:799-805.
977 *J Clin Endocrinol Metab* 1998;83:3817-25.
978 *Osteoporos Int* 1998;8:255-60.
979 *J Bone Miner Res* 1998;13:168-74.
980 *N Engl J Med* 1997;337:670-6.
981 *Osteoporos Int* 1997;7:23-8.
982 *Aliment Pharmacol Ther* 1996;10:777-86.
984 *Am J Clin Nutr* 1998;68:648-55.
987 *J Bone Miner Res* 1998;13:1045-50.
988 *N Engl J Med* 1997;337:523-8.
990 *Acta Paediatr Jpn* 1996;38:513-9.
994 *J Natl Cancer Inst* 1995;87:1303-7.
995 *J Clin Endocrinol Metab* 1980;51:1359-64.
996 *Nutr Rev* 1994;52:95-7.
997 *South Med J* 1983;76:556-9.
999 *Jpn J Clin Oncol* 1998;28:762-5.
1001 *Thromb Res* 1998;1:105-12.
1002 *Am J Surg* 1990;160:490-5.
1004 *J Am Acad Dermatol* 1998;38:539-47.
1005 *J Clin Periodontol* 1997;24:907-13.
1006 *J Paediatr Child Health* 1997;33:349-51.
1008 *Cancer Lett* 1992;63:189-98.
1010 *Minerva Med* 1987;78(22):1675-81.
1011 *Lipids* 1997;32:535-41.
1012 *J Am Coll Cardiol* 1997;29:1324-31.
1013 *Hepatol* 1997;25:313-6.
1014 *Eur J Clin Nutr* 1996;50:765-71.
1015 *Immunol Invest* 1991;20(7):545-55.
1016 *Lipids* 1992;27:533-8.
1017 *Ann Rheum Dis* 1990;49:76-80.
1018 *Arch Intern Med* 2000;160:1009-13.
1020 *Ann Intern Med* 1995;123:911-8.
1021 *Hepatol* 1995;22:1695-71.
1022 *J Am Coll Cardiol* 1995;25:1492-8.
1023 *Nihon Kyobu Shikkan Gakkai Zasshi* 1995;33:395-402.
1024 *Am J Clin Nutr* 1995;61:831-6.
1025 *Diabetes Res Clin Pract* 1995;28:35-40.
1026 *Br J Obstet Gynaecol* 1995;102:95-100.
1027 *Br J Obstet Gynaecol* 1995;102:123-6.
1028 *Circulation* 1994;90:2248-57.
1029 *Arterioscler Thromb* 1994;14:1425-9.
1030 *J Hypertens* 1994;12:209-13.
1031 *Br J Rheumatol* 1993;32:982-9.
1032 *Lupus* 1993;2:319-23.
1033 *Hypertension* 1993;22:371-9.
1034 *Clin Investig* 1993;71:634-43.

1035 *N Engl J Med* 1993;328:1812-6.
1036 *Am Rev Respir Dis* 1993;147:1138-43.
1037 *Aliment Pharmacol Ther* 1993;7:159-66.
1038 *Eur Heart J* 1992;13:1626-31.
1039 *J Rheumatol* 1992;19:1531-6.
1040 *Gut* 1992;33:922-8.
1041 *Rev Med Chil* 1991;119:267-72.
1042 *Women Health* 1992;19:117-31.
1043 *J Clin Invest* 1996;97:1129-33.
1044 *J Nutr* 1996;126:3032-9.
1045 *Lipids* 1996;31:85-90.
1046 *Ann Intern Med* 1996;125:961-8.
1047 *Cancer Epidemiol Biomarkers Prev* 1997;6:769-74.
1049 *Chronobiol Int* 1998;15:655-6.
1052 *Ann Emerg Med* 1998 32(3 Pt 1):334-40.
1053 *Am J Psychiatry* 1998;155:1119-21.
1054 *Am J Emerg Med* 1998;16:367-70.
1055 *Eur J Clin Nutr* 2000;54:263-7.
1056 *Dev Med Child Neurol* 1998;40:186-92.
1058 *J Pharm Sci* 1997;86:1115-9.
1060 *Gut* 2000;47:646-52.
1061 *JAMA* 1984;251:2348.
1062 *Physiol Behav* 1997;61:795-802.
1063 *Eur J Clin Invest* 1997;27:374-9.
1064 *J Pineal Res* 1996;21:239-42.
1065 *J Am Acad Dermatol* 1986;15:144-9.
1066 *Arch Dermatol Res* 1996;288:522-6.
1067 *Tech Urol* 1997;3:135-9.
1068 *Psychopharmacol (Berl)* 1996;126:179-81.
1069 *Support Care Cancer* 1996;4:313-6.
1070 *J Sleep Res* 1996;5:61-5.
1071 *Clin Exp Rheumatol* 1988;6:261-8.
1072 *Lancet* 1995;346:541-44.
1073 *J Clin Epidemiol* 1988;41:193-205.
1074 *J Rheumatol* 1994;21:105-10.
1075 *Respiration* 1989;56:22-33.
1076 *Clin Endocrinol (Oxf)* 1993;39:193-9.
1077 *Biol Psychiatry* 1993;33:526-30.
1078 *Psychopharmacol (Berl)* 1993;112:490-6.
1079 *Biol Psychiatry* 1992;32:705-11.
1080 *Oncology* 1992;49:336-9.
1082 *J Biol Rhythms* 1991;6:249-61.
1083 *Neuropsychopharmacology* 1990;3:19-23.
1084 *Urol Int* 1991;47:236-9.
1085 *BMJ* 1989;298:705-7.
1086 *J Am Acad Dermatol* 1983;9:770.
1087 *Arch Dis Child Fetal Neonatal Ed* 1998;79:F44-8.
1088 *Nephrol Dial Transplant* 1998;13:2572-7.
1089 *Arch Surg* 1998;133:740-4.
1090 *Nephron* 1998;79:299-305.
1091 *Eur J Haematol* 1998;60:252-9.
1093 *Neuropsychobiology* 1997;35:178-80.
1094 *J Am Acad Dermatol* 1985;13:671-2.
1095 *Lancet* 1996;348:992-6.
1096 *Br J Pharmacol* 1970;40:161P+.
1097 *Am J Cardiol* 1997;79:120-7.
1098 *Cancer Lett* 1997;114:215-6.
1099 *J Intern Med* 1995;238:223-30.
1100 *Am J Clin Nutr* 1999;69:250-5.
1101 *J Trace Elem Med Biol* 1998;12:129-40.
1102 *Biochem Biophys Res Commun* 1998;246:293-8.
1104 *Kobe J Med Sci* 1995;41:1-17.
1105 *Control Clin Trials* 1996;17:60-8.
1106 *Med J Aust* 1990;153:189-92.
1107 *J Med* 1995;26(5-6):193-207.
1108 *Gan To Kagaku Ryoho* 1994;21(13):2323-5.
1109 *Hinyokika Kiyo* 1994;40:119-23.
1110 *Gan To Kagaku Ryoho* 1988;15(4 Pt 2-3):1615-20.
1111 *Gan To Kagaku Ryoho* 1987;14(8):2509-11.
1112 *Gan To Kagaku Ryoho* 1987;14(2):516-22.
1113 *Cancer Detect Prev Suppl* 1987;1:333-49.
1114 *Oral Surg Oral Med Oral Pathol* 1984;58(6):659-66.
1115 *Cutis* 1984;34(4):366-73.
1116 *Arch Dermatol* 1984;120(1):48-51.
1117 *Eur J Clin Nutr* 2000;54:849-55.
1118 *Acta Derm Venereol* 1980;60(1):85-7.
1119 *Dermatologica* 1978;156(5):257-67.
1120 *Dermatologica* 1987;175(4):183-90.
1121 *Am J Kidney Dis* 1996;28:614-7.
1122 *J Nurse Midwifery* 1999;44:205-16.
1123 *Arch Gen Psychiatry* 2000;57:572-9.
1124 *J Am Coll Nutr* 1997;16(1):7-12.
1125 *Anesth Analg* 2000;91:473-9.
1126 *J Clin Pharmacol* 2000;40:781-4.
1127 *Cephalalgia* 1996;16:494-6.
1128 *Lancet* 2000;355:147.
1129 *Lancet* 1999;354:1001-2.
1130 *Calcif Tissue Int* 1998;63(3):183-9.
1131 *Nutr* 1992;8(6):400-5.
1132 *J Biol Rhythms* 1997;12:509-17.
1133 *Arch Gen Psychiatry* 1999;56:171-6.
1134 *Neuropsychobiology* 1997;35:5-10.
1135 *J Physiol (Lond)* 1995;486:789-94.
1136 *Arch Gen Psychiatry* 1994;51:865-74.
1137 *BMJ* 1999;318:999-1003.
1138 *J Behav Med* 1991;14:97-110.
1139 *J Craniomandib Disord* 1991;5:115-20.
1140 *J Am Dent Assoc* 1989;118:457-60.
1141 *J Toxicol Clin Toxicol* 1993;31:603-30.
1142 *Am J Obstet Gynecol* 1986;155:135-9.
1143 *Am J Clin Nutr* 1985;42:366-70.
1144 *Bull Eur Physiopathol Respir* 1983;19:625-9.
1145 *J Psychiatr Res* 1982-83;17:181-6.
1146 *J Nerv Ment Dis* 1979;167:497-9.
1147 *J Gastroenterol* 1998;33:562-5.
1148 *Dermatol* 1998;197:255-7.
1149 *J Allergy Clin Immunol* 1998;101:613-20.
1150 *J Intern Med* 1997;241:85-8.
1151 *Intern Med* 1992;31:1204-6.
1152 *Contact Dermatitis* 1992;27:65-70.
1153 *Contact Dermatitis* 1992;26:228-33.
1154 *Microbes Infect* 2000;2:681-6.
1155 *Yakugaku Zasshi* 1996;116:169-73.
1157 Colloidal minerals in brief. www.colloidal.com.au/ (Accessed 23 July 1999).
1158 Wallach J. Dr. Joel Wallach's colloidal minerals. www.elementsofhealth.com/b1.html (Accessed 23 July 1999).
1159 *Amer J Nat Med* 1997;4:5-10.
1160 *Proc Natl Acad Sci U S A* 1999;96:3358-64.
1161 *Int J of Integrative Med* 1999;1:18-22.
1162 *Avian Dis* 1995;39:631-5.
1167 *Magnes Res* 1998;11:25-42.
1168 *Hum Reprod* 1997;12:63-71.
1170 *J Am Coll Nutr* 1996;15:21-35.
1171 *Diabet Med* 1998;15:503-7.
1172 *Diabetes Care* 1998;21:682-6.
1173 *Eur Respir J* 1997;10:2225-9.
1175 *Immunopharmacol Immunotoxicol* 1989;11:131-42.
1176 *Int J Tissue React* 1986;8(3):239-42.
1177 *Drugs Exp Clin Res* 1985;11(9):665-9.
1178 *Eur J Cancer Clin Oncol* 1987;23(12):1915-9.
1180 *Am J Clin Nutr* 1994;60:129-35.

1181 *Magnes Res* 1994;7:145-53.
1182 *Health Rep* 1994;6:22-7.
1183 *Headache* 1993;33:135-8.
1184 *Headache* 1995;35:597-600.
1185 *Clin Sci (Colch)* 1995;89:633-6.
1186 *Headache* 1991;31:298-301.
1187 *Obstet Gynecol* 1991;78:177-81.
1188 *J Womens Health* 1998;7:1157-65.
1189 *Magnes Res* 1997;10:149-56.
1190 *Lancet* 1997;350:1272-6.
1191 *Am J Cardiol* 1997;79(6):768-72.
1192 *Int J Cardiol* 1996;56:177-83.
1193 *Magnes Res* 1996;9:129-32.
1194 *Am J Obstet Gynecol* 1995;173:175-80.
1195 *Magnes Res* 1994;7:277-83.
1196 *JAMA* 2001;285:1482-8.
1197 *Arch Fam Med* 1994;3:503-8.
1198 *BMJ* 1993;307:585-7.
1199 *Am J Hypertens* 1993;6:41-5.
1201 *Urol Res* 1994;22:161-5.
1202 *Am J Cardiol* 1994;73:1227-9.
1203 *Diabetes* 1999;48:106-11.
1204 *Diabetes* 1999;48:310-20.
1205 *Am J Otolaryngol* 1994;15:26-32.
1206 *Ann Rheum Dis* 1999;58:366-71.
1207 *J Pediatr* 1999;134:384-5.
1208 *Arch Intern Med* 1995;155:496-500.
1211 *Alt Ther Health Med* 1996;2:62-6.
1212 *Biol Pharm Bull* 1994;17:1106-10.
1213 *J Nutr Sci Vitaminol (Tokyo)* 1989;35:91-4.
1214 *J Nutr Sci Vitaminol (Tokyo)* 1987;33:341-6.
1215 *Diabetes Care* 1998;21:1589-95.
1216 *J Reprod Med* 1998;43:568-74.
1217 *Circulation* 1998;97:979-86.
1218 *Clin Exp Obstet Gynecol* 1997;24:228-31.
1219 *Crit Care Med* 1988;16:642-3.
1220 *JAMA* 1995;274:51-7.
1221 *Psychopharmacol (Berl)* 1995;117:424-9.
1223 *J Endocrinol Invest* 1992;15:801-6.
1224 *Br J Clin Pharmacol* 1992;33:293-8.
1225 *Hum Reprod* 1992;7:168-75.
1226 *Maturitas* 1991;13(2):109-15.
1227 *Am J Med* 1998;105:71-2.
1228 *Lancet* 1998;351:1255-6.
1229 *Am J Obstet Gynecol* 1999;180:1504-11.
1230 FDA. www.verity.fda.gov/default.html.
1231 *Lancet* 1998;352:906.
1233 *Lancet* 1987;2:43.
1234 Abul-Ezz SR, Barone GW, Gurley BJ, et al. Effect of herbal supplements on cyclosporine blood levels and associated acute rejection. Am Soc of Nephrol Ann Mtg, Toronto, CAN 2000;Oct. 11-16:abstract A3754.
1236 *J Clin Microbiol* 1999;37:1227-8.
1238 Ascherio A, Zhang SM, Hernan MA, et al. Prospective study of caffeine intake and risk of Parkinson's disease in men and women. Proceedings 125th Ann Mtg Am Neurological Assn. Boston, MA: 2000;Oct 15-18:42 (abstract 53).
1239 *Biol Trace Elem Res* 2001;79:221-33.
1240 *J Am Coll Nutr* 1999;18:43-50.
1241 *Eur J Clin Nutr* 1998;52:436-40.
1242 *J Pediatr* 1998;132:999-1003.
1243 *Am J Clin Nutr* 1998;67:111-7.
1244 *Ann Allergy Asthma Immunol* 1997;79:229-33.
1245 *Arch Fam Med* 1996;5:593-6.
1246 *J Trop Pediatr* 1996;42:133-7.
1247 *Clin Infect Dis* 1999;28:930.
1248 *Acta Obstet Gynecol Scand* 1993;72:17-9.
1249 *Ann Intern Med* 1992;116:353-7.
1250 *Ann Pediatr (Paris)* 1992;39:79-86.
1251 *J Clin Microbiol* 1998;36:2613-7.
1252 *Clin Pharmacol Ther* 1991;50:498-502.
1253 *Pediatrics* 1991;8:90-7.
1254 *J Pediatr Gastroenterol Nutr* 1990;11:509-12.
1255 *Ann Med* 1990;22:57-9.
1256 *Am J Clin Nutr* 1989;49:823-7.
1258 *Arch Ophthalmol* 1999;117(12):1617-22.
1259 *Pharm World Sci* 1999;21:44-6.
1260 *Pharmacol Ther* 1987;33:163-9.
1261 *J R Soc Med* 1999;92:283-5.
1262 *Am J Clin Nutr* 2000;71:67-74.
1263 *AIDS* 1989;3:423-7.
1264 *Thromb Res* 1996;84(5):311-22.
1265 *Ann Pharm Fr* 1996;54(6):280-3.
1266 *J Forensic Sci* 1998;43:1225-7.
1268 *Ophthalmology* 1980;87:222-8.
1269 Magainin Pharmaceuticals announces new research program for anti-angiogenesis agent - Squalamine - at Georgetown Univ Med Ctr. PRNewswire. www.prnewswire.com (Accessed 22 January 2000).
1270 *Arthritis Rheum* 1996;39:349.
1271 *J Toxicol Clin Toxicol* 1999;37:485-9.
1272 *Am J Kidney Dis* 1998;32:153-9.
1273 *Am J Gastroenterol* 1996;91:1436-8.
1274 *J Clin Psychopharmacol* 1997;17:437-9.
1275 *J Neurol Neurosurg Psychiatr* 2000;68:112-3.
1276 *BMJ* 1996;313:756.
1279 Hussain MD, Teixeira MG. Saint John's wort and analgesia: effect of Saint John's wort on morphine induced analgesia. AAPS Ann Mtg & Expo Indianapolis, IN:2000;Oct 29- Nov 2:presentation #3453.
1280 *Klin Wochenschr* 1991;69:722-4.
1281 *J Rheumatol* 2000;27:20-5.
1282 *Clin Infect Dis* 1996;22:200-1.
1283 *J Am Diet Assoc* 1995;95:541-4.
1284 *Am J Med* 1995;98:485-90.
1285 *Int J Vitam Nutr Res* 1994;64:113-8.
1286 *Am J Med* 1991;91:151-5.
1287 *J Ethnopharmacol* 1999;66:11-7.
1290 *Lancet* 2000;355:547-8.
1292 *Lancet* 2000;355:576-7.
1293 *Lancet* 2000;355:548-9.
1294 *Biol Psychiatry* 1999;46:442-4.
1296 *Photochem Photobiol* 1999;69:42S.
1297 *Arch Dermatol* 2000;136:179-84.
1298 *Am J Kidney Dis* 2000;35:310-2.
1299 *Chem Res Toxicol* 1999;12:483-7.
1300 *Electrophoresis* 1997;18:826-33.
1301 Gurley BJ, Barone GW. Herb-drug interaction involving St. John's wort and cyclosporine. AAPS Ann Mtg & Expo Indianapolis, IN:2000;Oct29- Nov2: presentation #3443.
1302 *Forensic Sci Int* 1992;54:9-22.
1303 Gurley BJ, Gardner SF, Hubbard MA. Clinical assessment of potential cytochrome P450-mediated herb-drug interactions. AAPS Ann Mtg & Expo Indianapolis, IN: 2000; Oct 29 - Nov 2:presentation #3460.
1304 *Clin Toxicol* 1981;18:1485-98.
1305 *Leukemia* 1988;2(8):528-33.
1306 *Leukemia* 1992;6(Suppl 3):189S-91S.
1307 *Teratog Carcinog Mutagen* 1994;14:75-81.
1309 *Carcinogenesis* 1991;12(5):939-42.

1310 FDA, CFSAN. FDA approved potassium health claim notification for potassium containing foods. 2000. Available at: www.cfsan.fda.gov/~dms/hclm-k.html.

1311 *Environ Mol Mutagen* 1996;28:121-6.

1312 *Mutagenesis* 1996;11:161-7.

1313 FDA. Center for Food Safety and Applied Nutrition. Letter regarding dietary supplement health claim for omega-3 fatty acids and coronary heart disease. Available at: http://vm.cfsan.fda.gov/~dms/ds-ltr11.html.

1314 *J Nat Prod* 1992;55(9):1241-51.

1315 *Yonsei Med J* 1990;31:225-33.

1316 Foerster KK, Schmid K, Rovati LC. Efficacy of glucosamine sulfate in osteoarthritis of the lumbar spine: a placebo-controlled, randomized, double-blind study. Am Coll Rheumatol 64th Ann Scientific Mtg, Philadelphia, PA: 2000;Oct 29- Nov 2:abstract 1613.

1318 *Ann Emerg Med* 2000;36:S85.

1319 ORCHIC PMG (Protomorphogen). Natural Health Cod. www.nbizz.com/naturalhealthdoc/listings/184.html (Accessed 9 November 2000).

1320 Gambos J. Fooling the bladder cops: the complete drug testing guide. www.csun.edu/~hbcsc096/dt/ftbc.txt (Accessed 9 November 2000).

1321 *J Am Geriatr Soc* 1980; 28(1):46-7.

1322 *Ugeskr Laeger* 1989;151:1753-4.

1323 *Drug Intell Clin Pharm* 1983; 17(10):732-4.

1324 *Gastroenterol Jpn* 1980; 15(1):49-61.

1326 *Ann N Y Acad Sci*, 1993; 691:127-38.

1329 Cardiovascular Benefits Claimed For Cocoa Flavonoids. www.medscape.com/reuters/prof/2000/02/02.21/dd02210b.html (Accessed 21 February 2000).

1330 *West J Med* 2000;172:91-4.

1332 *Phytochemistry* 1990;29:1131-5.

1333 *Acta Virol* 1993;37:241-50.

1334 *Int J Cancer* 1997;71:545-51.

1335 *J Infect Dis* 1991;164:1082-90.

1336 *J Natl Cancer Inst* 1994;86:281-6.

1337 *J Natl Cancer Inst* 1999;91:414-28.

1338 *Int Arch Allergy Immunol* 2000;122:137-42.

1340 *Clin Pharmacol Ther* 2000;68:598-604.

1341 *Scand J Clin Lab Invest* 1994;54:543-7.

1342 *J Rheumatol* 2000;27:205-11.

1343 *Allergy* 2000;55:1005-10.

1344 *Psychiatry Clin Neurosci* 1998;52:311-6.

1345 *Psychiatry Clin Neurosci* 1998;52:483-90.

1346 *Psychiatry Clin Neurosci* 1997;51:275-9.

1347 *Psychiatry Clin Neurosci* 1996;50:203-9.

1348 *Sleep* 1991;14:414-8.

1349 *Neuropsychopharmacology* 1996;15:456-64.

1350 *Med Hypotheses* 1991;36:371-3.

1351 *South Med J* 1999;92:1095-7.

1352 *J Am Coll Nutr* 2000;19:13-5.

1353 *Am J Clin Nutr* 2000;71:480-4.

1354 *Environmental & Nutritional Interactions* 1999;3:115-22.

1355 Dwyer JH, Merz NB, Shirocre AM, et al. Progression of early atherosclerosis and intake of vitamin C and vitamin E from supplements and food. The Los Angeles Atherosclerosis Study. 41st Annual Conference on Cardiovascular Disease Epidemiology and Prevention - Abstract P77. *Circulation* 2001;103:1365d.

1356 Marijuana Use by Middle-Aged Adults Linked to Increased Risk of MI. www.medscape.com/reuters/prof/2000/03/03.03/ep03030b.html (Accessed 3 March 2000).

1357 *Mov Disord* 1996;11:321-3.

1358 *J Allergy Clin Immunol* 2000;104:S340-341 (Abstract 1003).

1359 *J Am Acad Dermatol* 2001;44:425-32.

1360 *Pediatrics* 2000;105:e18.

1362 *J Clin Invest* 1992;90:1248-53.

1363 *J Clin Invest* 1996;97:1989-94.

1364 *Cancer Biother* 1994;9:253-63.

1365 *Med Sci Sports Exerc* 1999;31:1788-92.

1366 *Med J Aust* 1998;169:644-6.

1367 *Med Sci Sports Exerc* 2001;33:183-8.

1368 *Lancet* 1998;352:233-4.

1369 *Clin Cardiol* 1996;19:699-703.

1370 *Arch Dermatol* 2000;136:124-5.

1371 *Arterioscler Thromb Vasc Biol* 2000;20:230-5.

1372 *J Hum Hypertens* 1995;9:345-8.

1373 *Am J Cardiol* 1999;84:370-3.

1374 *Gastroenterol Clin North Am* 1991;20:313-24.

1375 Blue-Green Algae Protein Is a Promising Anti-HIV Microbicide Candidate. www.medscape.com/reuters/prof/2000/03/03.16/dd03160g.html (Accessed 16 March 2000).

1376 *Am J Clin Nutr* 2000;71:472-9.

1377 *Clin Pharmacol Ther* 2000;67:130, abstract PII-64.

1378 *Clin Pharmacol Ther* 2000;67:159, abstract PIII-69.

1380 For Dieter, Nearly the Ultimate Loss. The Washington Post. Available at: www.washingtonpost.com/wp-dyn/articles/A33421-2000Mar17.html (Accessed 19 March 2000).

1381 FDA Takes Aim at Ephedra. The Washington Post. Available at: www.washingtonpost.com/wp-dyn/articles/A33439-2000Mar17.html (Accessed 19 March 2000).

1382 *Clin Pharmacol Ther* 2000;67:156 (abstract PIII-56).

1383 *Clin Pharmacol Ther* 2000;67:110 (abstract PI-83).

1384 *Clin Pharmacol Ther* 2000;67:150 (abstract PIII-35).

1385 *Clin Pharmacol Ther* 2000;67:106 (abstract PI-72).

1386 *Clin Pharmacol Ther* 2000;67:151 (abstract PIII-37).

1387 *Clin Pharmacol Ther* 1998;65:159 (abstract PII-51).

1388 *Clin Pharmacol Ther* 2000;67:107 (abstract PI-71).

1389 *Clin Pharmacol Ther* 2000;67:109 (abstract PI-82).

1390 *Pharm Res* 1999;16:478-85.

1391 *Clin Pharmacol Ther* 1998;65:(abstract PI-60).

1392 *Clin Pharmacol Ther* 1998;65:(abstract PIII-63).

1393 *J Natl Cancer Inst* 1994;86:608-13.

1394 *Clin Pharmacol Ther* 1998;65:(abstract PII-27).

1395 *Thorax* 2000;55:340-2.

1396 *Headache* 2000;40:30-5.

1397 *Cephalalgia* 1994;14:328-9.

1398 *Neurology* 1998;50:466-70.

1401 *Acta Paediatr* 1996;85:943-6.

1402 *Am J Med Genet* 1997;69:89-95.

1403 *N Engl J Med* 1980;303:782-7.

1404 *J Am Acad Dermatol* 1991;25:332-3.

1405 *Am J Clin Nutr* 1999;70:466-73.

1406 *Proc Natl Acad Sci U S A* 1993;90:3304-8.

1409 *Prostaglandins Leukot Essent Fatty Acids* 1993;49:691-4.

1410 *Ann Pharmacother* 1994;28:767-78.

1411 *J Nurse Midwifery* 1999;44:320-4.

1412 *Phytomedicine* 1999;6:1-6.

1413 *Arzneimittelforschung* 1991;41:1076-81.

1414 *Can Pharm J* 1999:512-6.

1416 *Eur J Epidemiol* 1989;5:392-7.

1417 *Int J Cancer* 1988;42:17-22.

1418 *J Neurosci* 1998;18:8047-55.

1419 *J Neurosci* 1999;19:8114-21.

1420 *Clin Immunol Immunopathol* 1989;50:402-6.

1421 *Pharm Ztg* 1995;140:34-7.
1422 *Toxicol Appl Pharmacol* 1997;144:279-86.
1423 *Wien Med Wochenschr* 1973;123:601-5.
1424 *Atherosclerosis* 1977;26:249-53.
1425 *J Pharmacol Exp Therap* 1998;386:1122-8.
1426 *Free Radic Res* 1998;29:247-55.
1427 *Eur J Clin Pharmacol* 1999;55:567-75.
1428 *Dig Dis Sci* 1999;44:462-4.
1430 *MMWR Morb Mortal Wkly Rep* 1999;48:137-40.
1431 *Arch Intern Med* 1999;159:2221-4.
1432 *Oncol Res* 1996;8:121-30.
1433 *J Child Neurol* 1999;14:162-7.
1434 *J Am Coll Cardiol* 1999;34:1618-24.
1435 *J Am Coll Cardiol* 1995;26:1411-6.
1436 *Am J Cardiol* 1997;79:777-80.
1437 *Eur Heart J* 1992;13:251-5.
1438 *J Anal Toxicol* 1996;20:55-8.
1439 *Cardiovasc Drugs Ther* 1991;5 Suppl 1:11-5.
1440 *Circulation* 1999;99:591-5.
1441 *J Am Coll Cardiol* 1998;31:1323-9.
1442 *Arthritis Rheum* 1991;34:1274-81.
1443 *Arch Pediatr Adolesc Med* 1997;151:103-9.
1444 *J Natl Cancer Inst* 1999;91:547-56.
1445 *Clin Immunol Immunopathol* 1987;44:329-34.
1446 *Atherosclerosis* 2000;148:49-56.
1447 *Cancer Res* 1999;59:1225-30.
1448 *J Natl Cancer Inst* 1999;91:2102-6.
1449 *Ann Intern Med* 1999;130:963-70.
1451 *Eur J Epidemiol* 1998;14:669-73.
1452 *J Hypertens* 1999;17:457-63.
1453 *Am J Clin Nutr* 1999;70:1040-5.
1454 *Nat Med* 1999;5:1216.
1455 *Nature* 1999;398:381.
1456 *Bull Cancer* 1999;86:721-4.
1457 *Nutr Cancer* 1998;31:151-9.
1458 *Jpn J Cancer Res* 1993;84:1223-9.
1459 *Natl Cancer Inst Monogr* 1985;69:229-34.
1460 *J Am Diet Assoc* 1995;95:82-3.
1461 *Chin Med J (Engl)* 1989;102:579-83.
1463 *Prev Med* 1992;21:334-50.
1464 *Lancet* 1999;354:203-9.
1465 *Pediatr Infect Dis J* 1999;18:127-33.
1466 *Am J Clin Nutr* 1998;68:187-92.
1467 *Am J Med* 1994;97(6):523-8.
1468 *Nat Med* 1999;5:418-22.
1469 *Arch Intern Med* 1996;156(9):925-35.
1470 *Nutr Rev* 1999;57:201-14.
1471 *Nutr Rev* 1999;57:133-45.
1472 *Arch Otolaryngol Head Neck Surg* 1999;125:1305-10.
1473 *Cancer* 1999;86:1783-92.
1474 *Ann Allergy Asthma Immunol* 1999;82:549-53.
1475 *Am J Vet Res* 1985;46:875-8.
1476 *Clin Immunol Immunopathol* 1978;10:369-80.
1477 *Clin Immunol Immunopathol* 1977;8:238-46.
1478 *Clin Immunol Immunopathol* 1978;10:214-21.
1480 *J Infect Dis* 1990;161:108-12.
1481 *Cancer Res* 1993;53:3172-8.
1482 *Am J Clin Nutr* 1999;69:564-71.
1484 *Am J Clin Nutr* 1999;70:904-10.
1485 *Am J Clin Nutr* 1999;70:911-9.
1486 *Food Chem Toxicol* 1987;25:755-62.
1487 *Carcinogenesis* 1992;13:827-830.
1488 *Gastroenterology* 2001;120:179-89.
1489 *Ann Intern Med* 1997;127:1089-92.
1492 *Am J Epidemiol* 1999;149:421-8.
1493 *Ann N Y Acad Sci* 1993;685:362-8.
1494 *Ann Allergy* 1989;62:170-6.
1495 *Ann Intern Med* 1991;115:294-307.
1496 *Cancer Epidemiol Biomarkers Prev* 1996;5:823-33.
1497 *Am J Clin Nutr* 1997;66:116-22.
1498 *Am J Clin Nutr* 1998;68:1187-95.
1499 USDA. NCC Carotenoid Database for U.S. Foods. 1998. Available at: http://www.nal.usda.gov/fnic/foodcomp/Data/car98/car98.html.
1500 *J Allergy Clin Immunol* 1998;101:S207.
1501 *J Allergy Clin Immunol* 1998;101:281-2.
1502 Medicinal Plants. Springer Verlag: Lavoisier, NY, 1995.
1505 *Indian J Physiol Pharmacol* 1986;30:267-8.
1507 *Annu Rev Pharmacol Toxicol* 1989;29:475-516.
1512 *Bull World Health Organ* 1989;67:613-8.
1514 *JAMA* 1997;278:1327-32.
1515 *Arch Neurol* 1998;55:1409-15.
1516 *J Pak Med Assoc* 1991;41:185-7.
1519 *J Ethnopharmacol* 1998;61:57-65.
1520 *J Rheumatol* 1999;26:2423-30.
1522 *Biol Pharm Bull* 1996;19:1434-9.
1523 *Am J Clin Nutr* 1998;68:1512S-5S.
1524 *Alcohol Clin Exp Res* 1994;18:1443-7.
1525 *Contact Dermatitis* 1993;29:33-5.
1526 *Chem Pharm Bull* 1989;37:3029-32.
1527 *J Ethnopharmacol* 1995;46:101-6.
1528 *Epidemiology* 1994;5:583-90.
1529 *Br J Cancer* 1998;78:1239-43.
1530 *Cancer* 1991;67:536-40.
1531 *Cancer Epidemiol Biomarkers Prev* 1996;5:515-9.
1533 *Am J Chin Med* 1989;17:65-70.
1534 *Arch Immunol Ther Exp* 1991;39:103-8.
1535 *J Ethnopharmacol* 1997;55:141-50.
1536 *Chemotherapy* 1994:40:337-47.
1537 *Planta Med* 1995;61:233-6.
1539 *Eur J Clin Invest* 2000;30:915-29.
1540 *J Pharm Belg* 1996;51:69-71.
1541 *Microbios* 1998;93:43-54.
1543 *Int Arch Allergy Immunol* 1996;111:210-7.
1544 *J Int Med Res* 1979;7:473-83.
1545 *J Int Med Res* 1977;5:217-22.
1546 *Dtsch Med Wochenschr* 1976;101:401-5.
1547 *Altern Med Rev* 1998;3:308-10.
1548 *N Engl J Med* 1979;300:371.
1549 *Crit Care Med* 1986;14:753-4.
1550 *Gen Pharmacol* 1997;29:315-31.
1554 *J Pediatr* 1984;104:65-9.
1555 *Pediatr Res* 1990;27:75-9.
1556 *Neurology* 1998;50:645-51.
1557 *Eur J Pediatr* 1976;122:159-68.
1561 *Free Radic Biol Med* 1997;22:359-78.
1562 *FEBS Lett* 1996;394:9-13.
1563 *Biochem Biophys Res Commun* 1992;189:1709-15.
1571 *Cardiovasc Drugs Ther* 1991;5 Suppl 1:107-11.
1572 *J Cardiovasc Pharmacol* 1992;20:157-64.
1573 *Am J Cardiol* 1994;74:125-30.
1574 *Drugs Exp Clin Res* 1995;21:187-98.
1575 *Cardiovasc Drugs Ther* 1998;12:291-9.
1576 *Drugs Exp Clin Res* 1999;25:29-36.
1577 *J Card Fail* 1997;3:217-24.
1578 *Drugs Aging* 1998;12:243-8; discussion 249-50.
1579 *Cardiovasc Drugs Ther* 1990;4:481-6.
1580 *Cardiovasc Drugs Ther* 1995;9:749-53.
1581 *Eur Heart J* 1996;17:414-20.
1582 *Eur Heart J* 1994;15:1267-73.
1583 *Arzneimittelforschung* 1992;42:1101-4.

1584 *J Am Diet Assoc* 1993;93:910-2.
1586 *Epidemiology* 2003;14:206-12.
1589 *Int J Clin Pharmacol Res* 1990;10:101-7.
1591 *Pharmacol Res* 1991;23:241-6.
1592 *Int J Clin Pharmacol Res* 1990;10:123-8.
1593 *Int J Clin Pharmacol Res* 1995;15:9-15.
1594 *Neurology* 1996;47:705-11.
1595 *Arch Neurol* 1992;49:1137-41.
1596 *Neurology* 1991;41:1726-32.
1597 *Int Psychoger* 1998;10:193-203.
1598 *Neurobiol Aging* 1995;16:1-4.
1599 *Curr Med Res Opin* 1990;11:638-47.
1600 *Life Sci* 1997;60:PL135-40.
1605 FDA. FDA warns against consuming triax metabolic accelerator. Available at: www.fda.gov/bbs/topics/ANSWERS/ANS00984.html.
1607 *Endocrinol Metab Clin North Am* 1998;27(1):187-203.
1608 *J Clin Endocrinol Metab* 1995;80:2033-40.
1609 *J Clin Endocrinol Metab* 1989;69:461-6.
1610 *J Clin Endocrinol Metab* 1992;75:1071-5.
1611 *J Endocrinol Invest* 1988;11:113-8.
1612 *Nuklearmedizin* 1989;28:217-20.
1613 *Prenat Diagn* 1996;16:443-8.
1614 *J Clin Endocrinol Metab* 1999;84:405-10.
1615 *Thyroid* 1997;7:775-8.
1616 *Ann Endocrinol (Paris)* 1995;56:119-26.
1617 *Clin Endocrinol (Oxf)* 1988;28:345-51.
1618 *Clin Endocrinol (Oxf)* 1991;35:123-8.
1620 *Postgrad Med J* 1998;74:121-2.
1621 *Ann Pharmacother* 1992;26:1457-8.
1622 *Lancet* 1986;1:383.
1623 *Ann Med Interne (Paris)* 1982;133:588-9.
1624 *J Toxicol Clin Exp* 1986;6:115-21.
1625 *Acta Clin Belg* 1984;39:285-9.
1627 *Cardiovasc Res* 1981;15:196-205.
1628 *Lancet* 1977;2:221-3.
1629 *Lancet* 1953;2:234.
1630 *Lancet* 1956;1:885-9.
1631 *Acta Endocrinol (Copenh)* 1989;121(5):651-8.
1632 *J Clin Endocrinol Metab* 1997;82:2153-8.
1633 *J Clin Endocrinol Metab* 1992;75(3):901-5.
1634 *J Clin Endocrinol Metab* 1993;77:221-8.
1635 *Gen Pharmacol* 1998;30:1-4.
1636 *J Urol* 1991;145:1082-7.
1637 *Cancer Epidemiol Biomarkers Prev* 1995;4:275-81.
1638 *Res Commun Mol Pathol Pharmacol* 1996;92:140-8.
1639 *In Vivo* 1994;8:241-5.
1640 *Cancer Chemother Pharmacol* 1993;33:171-5.
1641 *Int J Cancer* 1997;70:362-72.
1642 *Cancer Treat Rev* 1984;11:131-55.
1643 *Life Sci* 1997;60:PL383-7.
1644 *Biochem Biophys Res Commun* 1987;148:726-33.
1645 *Chung Kuo Yao Li Hsueh Pao* 1998;19:67-70.
1646 *Gen Pharmacol* 1997;29:269-73.
1647 *Methods Find Exp Clin Pharmacol* 1994;16:723-9.
1648 *Anticancer Res* 1995;15:2907-11.
1649 *Am J Clin Oncol* 1995;18:216-22.
1650 *Anticancer Res* 1997;17:2815-8.
1651 *Lancet* 1994;343:1122-6.
1652 *Cancer Chemother Pharmacol* 1997;40:233-8.
1653 *Cancer Detect Prev* 1997;21:71-7.
1654 *Eur J Cancer* 1996;32A:235-42.
1655 *Cancer Chemother Pharmacol* 1994;33 Suppl:S145-8.
1656 *Cancer* 1992;70:2475-83.
1657 *Dis Colon Rectum* 1992;35:123-30.
1658 *Biotherapy* 1992;4:117-28.
1659 *Biotherapy* 1991;3:287-95.
1660 *Cancer Immunol Immunother* 1990;31:261-8.
1661 *J Int Med Res* 1989;17:141-9.
1662 *Semin Oncol* 1996;23:369-78.
1664 *J Physiol Anthropol Appl Human Sci* 2001;20:81-4.
1665 *Nutr Rev* 2000;58:363-9.
1668 Davies C, Maidment S, Hanley P, et al. Dimethylaminoethanol (DMAE). HSE. Risk assessment document; EH72/2;1997. (TOXLINE).
1669 *Curr Ther Res Clin Exp* 1974;16:1238-42.
1671 *Clin Ther* 1991;13:373-82.
1672 *Aust N Z J Psychiatry* 1981;15:68-71.
1673 *JAMA* 1978;239:1997-8.
1674 *Psychopharmacology (Berl)* 1979;65:219-23.
1675 *Acta Neurol Scand* 1978;58:134-8.
1676 *Neuropsychobiology* 1978;4:140-9.
1677 *Dis Nerv Syst* 1977;38:25-31.
1679 *Clin Pharmacol Ther* 1975;17:534-40.
1680 *Am J Psychiatry* 1981;138:970-2.
1681 *J Am Geriatr Soc* 1977;25:241-4.
1682 *J Gerontol* 1977;32:38-45.
1683 *Mech Ageing Dev* 1988;42:129-38.
1684 *Eur Neurol* 1991;31:423-5.
1685 *Psychopharmacology (Berl)* 1979;62:187-91.
1686 *Med Hypotheses* 1988;26:255-7.
1688 *Oncology* 1991;48:448-50.
1691 FDA. List of orphan designations and approvals. Office of Orphan Products Development. Available at: www.fda.gov/orphan/designat/list.htm.
1692 *Br J Cancer* 1992;66:155-8.
1693 *Cancer* 1994;73:699-701.
1694 *J Pineal Res* 1999;26:169-73.
1695 *Recenti Prog Med* 1996;87:582-5.
1696 *Oncology* 1995;52:360-2.
1697 *Recenti Prog Med* 1995;86:231-3.
1698 *J Nephrol* 1999;12:230-40.
1701 Wallach J. Interpretation of Diagnostic Tests. A synopsis of Laboratory Medicine. Fifth ed; Boston, MA: Little Brown, 1992.
1704 *BMJ* 1997;314:29-34.
1705 *Chest* 1995;107:1437-41.
1706 *J Ethnopharmacol* 1993;38:1139.
1708 *Eur J Med Res* 1998;3:511-4.
1709 *Eur J Med Res* 1997;2:37-43.
1710 *J Natl Cancer Inst* 2000;92:977-86.
1711 *J Toxicol Clin Toxicol* 1997;35:447-51.
1712 *J Hepatol* 1999;30:1081-9.
1713 *J Pharmacol Exp Ther* 1997;22:845-50.
1714 *Arterioscler Thromb Vasc Biol* 1996;16:727-33.
1715 *Medical Update for Psychiatrists* 1997;2:172-6.
1716 *Ann Emerg Med* 1998;31:710-5.
1721 *Ann Emerg Med* 1998;31:699-704.
1722 *J Anal Toxicol* 1999;23:159-67.
1727 *J Clin Pharmacol* 1996;36:647-53.
1729 *Biol Signals Recept* 1999;8:126-31.
1730 Roche, Inc. Xenical package insert. Nutley, NJ. May 1999.
1731 *J Dairy Sci* 1999:82:2308-14.
1733 *Am Heart J* 1999;138:1082-7.
1736 Anon. Yogurt cuts down diarrhea. HealthNews, November 1999.
1738 *Sleep* 1995;18:598-603.
1739 *Clin Endocrinol (Oxf)* 1997;47:463-9.
1740 Pierce A. The American Pharmaceutical Association Practical Guide to Natural Medicines. New York: The Stonesong Press, 1999:19.

1741 *J Clin Endocrinol Metab* 1977;45:768-74.
1742 *J Clin Endocrinol Metab* 1996;81:1882-6.
1743 *Horm Res* 1997;47:97-101.
1744 *Dev Med Child Neurol* 1997;39:319-25.
1745 *Am J Ment Retard* 1999;104:170-86.
1746 *J Pineal Res* 1996;21:193-9.
1747 *Dev Med Child Neurol* 1999;41:123-6.
1749 *Biol Signals Recept* 1999;8:90-5.
1751 *Eur Neuropsychopharmacol* 1997;7:157-60.
1752 *Lancet* 1999;353:294-5.
1753 *Psychopharmacology (Berl)* 1990;100:222-6.
1754 *Lancet* 1995;346:541-4.
1755 *Ann Emerg Med* 1994;23:519-23.
1756 *Proc Natl Acad Sci USA* 1994;91:1824-8.
1757 *Clin Pharmacol Ther* 1995;57:552-8.
1758 *Eur J Pharmacol* 1995;275:213-6.
1759 *Sleep* 1996;19(5):423-31.
1761 *Altern Med Rev* 1998;3:114-27.
1762 *Drug Saf* 2000;22:123-48.
1763 *Respir Med* 1998;92:609-23.
1764 *Am J Psychiatry* 1976;133:1181-1186.
1765 *Cardiologia* 1999;44:633-7.
1766 *J Clin Psychiatry* 1997;58:383-8.
1767 *Int J Biol Markers* 1999;14:268-71.
1768 *Dermatology* 1997;195:248-52.
1769 *Biol Signals Recept* 1999;8:132-5.
1771 *Dev Med Child Neurol* 1999;41:491-500.
1772 *Ann Med* 1998;30:122-30.
1773 *N Engl J Med* 1997;336:186-95.
1774 *BMJ* 1996;312:1242-3.
1775 *Int Clin Psychopharmacol* 1999;14:189-92.
1776 *Biol Signals Recept* 1999;8:111-9.
1777 *Eur J Endocrinol* 1999;141:22-6.
1778 *J Pineal Res* 1998;24:193-200.
1779 *Clin Endocrinol (Oxf)* 1999;51:637-42.
1780 *Eur J Clin Pharmacol* 1999;55:111-5.
1781 *Am J Med* 1999;107:432-6.
1784 *J Am Geriatr Soc* 1989;37:515-20.
1785 *Eur J Clin Pharmacol* 1999;55:349-52.
1786 *J Neuroimaging* 1998;8:197-204.
1787 *Int Clin Psychopharmacol* 1991;6:31-43.
1789 *J Am Geriatr Soc* 1987;35:425-30.
1793 *Angiology* 1995;46:53-8.
1796 *Int Clin Psychopharmacol* 1987;2:325-31.
1797 *Eur J Clin Pharmacol* 1985;28:567-71.
1799 The Natural Pharmacist. Vinpocetine. www.tnp.com/substance.asp?ID=573. (Accessed 16 December 1999).
1800 *Psychopharmacology (Berl)* 1990;101:147-59.
1801 *Eur J Clin Pharmacol* 1992;42:257-9.
1802 *Arzneimittelforschung* 1992;42:914-7.
1803 *Cochrane Database Syst Rev* 2000;2:CD000207.
1804 *Schizophr Res* 1999;39:1-16; discussion 17-18.
1805 *Sb Lek* 2000;101:241-8.
1816 Allen LV. Nutritional Products. In: Covington TR, Ed. Handbook of Nonprescription Drugs. Washington, DC: American Pharmaceutical Association;1996:361-92.
1817 *Bone Marrow Transplant* 1999;23:355-61.
1818 *Ann Intern Med* 1996;124:825-31.
1819 *JAMA* 1996;275:1016-22.
1820 *J Hypertens* 1998;16:1693-9.
1821 *Am J Hypertens* 1999;12:84-92.
1822 *Am J Obstet Gynecol* 1998;179:444-52.
1823 *Psychopharmacol Bull* 1991;27:145-8.
1824 *J Gen Intern Med* 1989;4:183-9.
1825 Lewis CJ. Letter to reiterate certain public health and safety concerns to firms manufacturing or importing dietary supplements that contain specific bovine tissues. FDA. Available at: www.cfsan.fda.gov/~dms/dspltr05.html.
1826 *Gastroenterology* 1994;106:1162-7.
1827 *Nephron* 1998;79:137-41.
1828 *Am J Kidney Dis* 1995;25:879-86.
1829 *Nephron* 1993;65:369-74.
1830 *Calcif Tissue Int* 1999;65:332-6.
1831 *J Rheumatol* 1996;23:995-1000.
1832 *Arthritis Rheum* 1996;39:1791-801.
1833 *Aust N Z J Obstet Gynaecol* 1999;39:12-8.
1834 *Am J Obstet Gynecol* 1999;181:1560-9.
1836 *N Engl J Med* 1992;327:1637-42.
1837 *J Int Med Res* 1999;27:1-14.
1838 *J Clin Pharmacol* 1999;39:1151-4.
1839 *Calcif Tissue Int* 1996;58:226-30.
1840 *Miner Electrolyte Metab* 1995;21:229-31.
1841 *Osteoporos Int* 1999;10:137-42.
1842 *Osteoporos Int* 1999;9:19-23.
1843 *Drugs* 1999;57:855-70.
1844 *Gastroenterology* 1977;72:957-61.
1845 *Dig Dis Sci* 1988;33:409-13.
1846 *J Bone Miner Res* 1999;14:215-20.
1847 *J Endocrinol Invest* 1998;21:263-7.
1848 *Am J Clin Nutr* 1998;68:96-102.
1849 *Am J Clin Nutr* 1992;56:1045-8.
1850 *Am J Clin Nutr* 1998;67:1244-9.
1854 *J Am Diet Assoc* 1996;96:1027-39.
1855 *Free Radic Biol Med* 1990;8:61-69.
1857 *Life Sci* 1997;61:343-54.
1858 *Crit Rev Food Sci Nutr* 1995;35:495-508.
1859 *Anticancer Res* 1999;19:3733-6.
1860 *Anticancer Res* 1999;19:3671-4.
1861 *Carcinogenesis* 1997;18:2023-6.
1862 *Anticancer Res* 1998;18:1479-84.
1863 *Carcinogenesis* 1991;12:2041-5.
1864 *Anticancer Res* 1998;18:4091-6.
1865 *Carcinogenesis* 1995;16:1975-9.
1866 *Carcinogenesis* 1988;9:577-80.
1867 *Anticancer Res* 1999;19:3689-93.
1868 *Anticancer Res* 1999;19:3699-3702.
1869 *Am J Clin Nutr* 1999;70:240-6.
1870 *J Trace Elem Electrolytes Health Dis* 1992;6:99-103.
1871 *J Pharm Pharmacol* 1997;49:908-11.
1873 *Am J Clin Nutr* 1996;64:866-70.
1874 *J Cardiovasc Pharmacol* 1998;31:904-8.
1875 *Nutrition Research* 1987;7:139-49.
1876 *Atherosclerosis* 1999;143:399-404.
1877 *Planta Med* 1994;60:417-20.
1878 *Biol Pharm Bull* 1996;19:305-7.
1879 *Atherosclerosis* 1997;132:37-42.
1880 *Phytomedicine* 1999;6:125-31.
1881 *Nutr Cancer* 1997;27:186-91.
1882 *N Eur J Neurosci* 1998;10:3869-75.
1883 *Toxicology* 1999;132:215-25.
1884 *Cancer Epidemiol Biomarkers Prev* 1994;3:155-60.
1885 *Planta Med* 1999;65:545-8.
1886 *Mayo Clin Proc* 1999;74:1198-206.
1889 *J Neurosci Res* 1999;58:417-25.
1890 *Eur J Dermatol* 1999;9:289-96.
1896 Investigator's Brochure: Ademetionine 1,4-butanedisulfonate. Knoll Pharmaceuticals.
1897 *J Pharmacol Exp Ther* 1979;209:323-6.
1898 *South Med J* 1999;92:866-70.

1899 *Atherosclerosis* 1999;147:317-26.
1900 Lininger SW. The Natural Pharmacy. 1st ed. Rocklin, CA: Prima Publishing; 1998.
1901 *Ann Clin Lab Sci* 1983;13:20-4.
1902 *Semin Nephrol* 1999;19:551-6.
1903 *Psychopharmacology (Berl)* 2000;152:353-361.
1905 *Arch Intern Med* 2000;160:3093-104.
1906 *JAMA* 2000;284:2618-21.
1907 *Drugs Fut* 1999;24:295-320.
1908 *Dermatologica* 1983;167:109-10.
1909 *JPEN J Parenter Enteral Nutr* 2000;24:133-9.
1910 *Dev Med Child Neurol* 1991;33:795-802.
1911 *J Pediatr* 1991;119:799-802.
1912 *Epilepsia* 1993;34:184-7.
1913 *Acta Paediatr* 1995;84:93-5.
1914 *Acta Paediatr* 1996;85:446-9.
1915 *J Child Neurol* 1997;12:461-3.
1916 *Ann Neurol* 1988;24:301.
1917 *Ann Neurol* 1989;26:456.
1918 *J Intern Med* 2000;248:377-86.
1919 *Br J Anaesth* 2000;84:367-71.
1920 *J Am Diet Assoc* 2000;100:257-9.
1921 *Midwifery* 2000;16:224-8.
1922 *Cochrane Database Syst Rev* 2000;2:CD000145.
1923 *Int J Clin Pharmacol Ther* 1999;37:341-6.
1924 *Anaesthesia* 1993;48:1118.
1926 *Phytomedicine* 2000;7(1):1-6.
1927 *Phytomedicine* 2000;7:85-89.
1928 *J Am Coll Nutr* 2000;19:563-9.
1929 *Nutrition* 2000;16:734-9.
1930 *Altern Med Rev* 1998;3(5):345-60.
1931 *Life Sci* 1996;59:1579-99.
1932 *Curr Ther Res* 1993;53:441-3.
1933 *Clin Ther* 1995;17:176-85.
1934 *Diabetes Care* 1994;17:1449-52.
1935 *J Fam Pract* 1998;46:83-6.
1937 *Metabolism* 1987;36:896-9.
1938 *Am J Clin Nutr* 1998;67:1250-5.
1939 *Med Sci Sports Exerc* 1997;29:992-8.
1942 *J Pharm Pharmacol* 1997;49:721-3.
1943 *J Biomed Mater Res* 1997;34:21-28.
1944 *Biomaterials* 1991;12:281-6.
1945 *Biomaterials* 1989;10:598-603.
1946 *Biochem Pharmacol* 1995;49:1403-10.
1947 *Eur J Appl Physiol* 1996;73:434-9.
1948 *Hepatol* 1997;25:148-53.
1949 *J Am Coll Nutr* 2000;19:528S-31S.
1950 *Am J Physiol* 1975;228:1020-3.
1951 *Ann Intern Med* 1997;126:410.
1952 *Nutr Rev* 1998;56:174-7.
1953 *J Am Coll Nutr* 1998;17:548-55.
1954 *J Ethnopharmacol* 2000;72:345-93.
1955 *Angiology* 1973;24:269-87.
1956 *Circulation* 2000;102:1233-8.
1957 *Stroke* 2000;31:2287-94.
1958 *BMJ* 1995;310:1563-6.
1959 *Dermatol Surg* 1998;24:331-4.
1960 *N Engl J Med* 1986;315:708-9.
1961 *Ann Pharmacother* 2000;34:1193-7.
1963 *Adv Exp Med Biol* 1981;135:1-25.
1964 *Am J Med Technol* 1983;49:23-6.
1965 *West J Med* 1980;133:485-92.
1966 *Prog Clin Biol Res* 1982;103:365-73.
1967 *JAMA* 1979;241:908-11.
1968 *J Med Soc N J* 1979;76:765-6.
1969 *Postgrad Med* 1979;66:153-60.
1970 *Osteoarthritis Cartilage* 1998;6:39-46.
1971 *Osteoarthritis Cartilage* 1998;6:25-30.
1972 *Osteoarthritis Cartilage* 1998;6 Suppl A:31-6.
1973 *Altern Med Rev* 1998;3:27-39.
1974 *Am J Ophthalmol* 1987;103:194-7.
1975 *J Nutr* 1998;128:1411-4.
1976 *J Nutr* 1997;127:1435-44.
1977 *Acta Derm Venereol* 1996;76:144-6.
1979 *Prostaglandins Leukot Essent Fatty Acids* 1994;51:311-6.
1980 *Diabet Med* 1994;11:145-9.
1981 *Agents Actions Suppl* 1992;37:120-44.
1982 *J Nutr Sci Vitaminol (Tokyo)* 1991;37:573-9.
1983 *Prostaglandins Leukot Essent Fatty Acids* 1990;40:199-202.
1984 *Diabet Med* 1990;7:319-23.
1985 *Arthritis Rheum* 1990;33:1526-33.
1986 *Biochem Med* 1979;21:78-85.
1987 *Scand J Infect Dis* 1994;26:1-6.
1988 *J Am Coll Nutr* 1995;14:116-23.
1989 *J Clin Epidemiol* 1996;49:1079-84.
1990 *Environ Res* 1998;78:50-8.
1992 *Can J Neurol Sci* 1996;23:95-8.
1994 *J Nutr* 1994;124:1060-4.
1995 *Diabetes* 1999;48:176-81.
1996 *Lik Sprava* 1998;4:122-4.
1997 *Biol Trace Elem Res* 1998;62:135-53.
1998 *J Nutr* 1998;128:593-7.
1999 *Am J Clin Nutr* 1998;67:255-62.
2000 *J Am Coll Nutr* 1991;10:38-43.
2001 *Lancet* 1995;346:270-4.
2002 *J Nutr* 1989;119:1832-8.
2003 *Obstet Gynecol* 1981;58:68S-78S.
2004 *Am J Obstet Gynecol* 1993;168:1417-23.
2005 *J Nutr* 1996;126:2435S-40S.
2006 *J Urol* 1985;133:23.
2007 *J Urol* 1980;124:770–4.
2008 *Nutr Today* 1988;23:13-9.
2009 *Semin Arthritis Rheum* 1974;3:287-321.
2010 *J Biol Response Mod* 1985 Dec;4(6):551-84.
2011 *Lancet* 1989;1:614.
2012 *Ann Intern Med* 1996;125:780-1.
2013 *Am J Health Syst Pharm* 1995;52:1756-60.
2014 Lane IW, Comac L. Sharks don't get cancer. Garden City, NY: Avery Publishing Group; 1992.
2015 *J Clin Oncol* 1998;16:3649-55.
2020 *Int J Fertil* 1985;30(1):85-7.
2021 *Brain Res* 1976;114:105-15.
2023 PKU - Dietary Treatment of the Untreated Adult PKU. National Society for Phenylketonuria (NSPKU). 1996-2001. Available at: web.ukonline.co.uk/nspku/untreatd.htm.
2024 *Lancet* 1998;352:291-2.
2025 *Biol Psychiatry* 1999;45:270-3.
2026 *Isr J Psychiatry Relat Sci* 1995;32:14-21.
2027 *J Affect Disord* 1991;22:165-70.
2028 *N Engl J Med* 1999;340:1314-20.
2030 *Clin Biochem* 1997;30:91-113.
2031 *Am J Obstet Gynecol* 1997;177:937-41.
2032 *Hum Reprod* 1996;11:2085-9.
2033 *Maturitas* 1994;20:191-8.
2034 *Fertil Steril* 1994;62:485-90.
2035 *J Antimicrob Chemother* 2001;48:450-1.
2036 *Int J Impot Res* 1994;6:33-5.
2038 *Urol Int* 1999;63:220-3.
2039 *Br J Dermatol* 1989;121:75-90.

2040 *J Clin Pharmacol* 2001;41:1059-63.
2041 *Am J Obstet Gynecol* 1999;180:42-8.
2044 *Lancet* 1999;354:2048-9.
2045 *Lancet* 1999;354:2025-8.
2047 *Altern Med Rev* 1998;3:432-47.
2048 Nomenclature of Cyclitols. IUPAC Commission on the Nomenclature of Organic Chemistry (CNOC) and IUPAC-IUB Commission on Biochemical Nomenclature (CBN). Available at: http://www.chem.qmw.ac.uk/iupac/cyclitol/ (Accessed 23 January 2004).
2049 *Am J Clin Nutr* 1999;70:817-25.
2052 *Clin Chim Acta* 1983;128:181-98.
2056 *Phytomedicine* 1997;4:369-78.
2057 *J Clin Lab Anal* 1997;11:287-313.
2058 *Arch Intern Med* 1999;159:1865-70.
2059 *Drugs Exp Clin Res* 1999;25:133-41.
2060 *Clin Chim Acta* 1996;246:51-7.
2061 *Clin Chim Acta* 1996;246:77-89.
2063 *Int J Epidemiol* 1998;27:359-64.
2064 *Curr Ther Res* 1996;57:959-68.
2065 *J Infect Dis* 1998;177:955-61.
2067 *J Pediatr Gastroenterol Nutr* 1999;29:452-6.
2068 *J Infect Dis* 1998;177:662-7.
2069 *N Engl J Med* 1988;318:1240-3.
2070 *Am J Trop Med Hyg* 1992;47:276-83.
2071 *J Infect Dis* 1999;180:2056-9.
2072 *J Pediatr Gastroenterol Nutr* 1994;19:228-35.
2074 *Pharmacopsychiatry* 1999;32:235-41.
2075 *Environ Health Perspect* 1999;107:783-9.
2076 GRIN Taxonomy. Available at: http://www.ars-grin.gov/cgi-bin/npgs/html/tax_search.pl? (Accessed 27 February 2000).
2077 *Eur J Clin Nutr* 1988;42:939-44.
2078 *J Pharm Pharmacol* 1993;45:581-4.
2079 *Planta Med* 1997;63:518-24.
2080 *Chung Hua Yu Fang I Hsueh Tsa Chih* 1990;24:132-5.
2081 *Indian J Exp Biol* 1999;37:676-80.
2082 *Ala J Med Sci* 1988;25:306-13.
2083 *Curr Ther Res* 1992;52:478-85.
2084 *Chung Hua I Hsueh Tsa Chih (Taipei)* 1991;71:28, 388-90.
2086 *Fertil Steril* 1999;72:830-6.
2089 *Fertil Steril* 1998;69:96-101.
2091 FDA MedWatch. Summary of safety-related drug labeling changes approved by FDA May 1998. Crinone (progesterone) Gel. May 11, 1998. Available at: http://www.fda.gov/medwatch/safety/1998/may98.htm#crinon.
2092 *Z Allg Med* 1993;69:271–7.
2093 *J Clin Psychopharmacol* 2000;20:84-9.
2094 *Pharmacopsychiatry* 1997;30:1-5.
2095 *Phytomedicine* 1996;3:113-9.
2096 *Fortschr Med* 1991;109:119-22.
2097 *Pharmacopsychiatry* 1994;27:224-30.
2098 *Neuropsychobiology* 1993;27:46-53.
2100 *Med Sci Sports Exerc* 1998;30:73-82.
2101 *J Appl Physiol* 1997;83:2055-63.
2102 *Acta Physiol Scand* 1995;153:207-9.
2103 *Sports Med* 1994;18:268-80.
2104 *J Appl Physiol* 1996;81:232-7.
2105 *Med Sci Sports Exerc* 1995;27:S146.
2106 *Med Sci Sports Exerc* 1996;28:1435-41.
2107 *Molec Aspects Med* 1994;15:S241-8.
2108 *Br Dent J* 1995;178:209-13.
2109 *Acta Physiol Scand* 1997;161:379-84.
2110 *Int J Sport Nutr* 1997;7:197-206.
2111 *Hosp Pract* 1998;33:85-6.
2112 *JAMA* 1996;276:1365-7.
2113 *J Rheumatol* 1998;25:285-9.
2114 *Arth Rheum* 1995;38:1826-31.
2115 *Lancet* 1994;343:1479-81.
2116 *Med Lett Drugs Ther* 1996;38:91-2.
2117 *J Appl Physiol* 1996;80:452-7.
2118 *Lancet* 1998;351:1252-3.
2119 *Med Vet Entomol* 1997;11:355-60.
2120 *Eur J Appl Physiol* 1997;76:566-7.
2121 *Am J Cardiol* 1985;56:247-51.
2122 *Mol Aspects Med* 1994;S265-72.
2123 *Biochem Biophys Res Commun* 1991;176:786-91.
2124 *Biochem Biophys Res Commun* 1988;153:888-96.
2125 *Diabetologia* 1998;41:584-8.
2126 *Mol Aspects Med* 1997;18 Suppl:S307-9.
2127 *Biochem Biophys Acta* 1995;1271:281-6.
2128 *Lancet* 1994;334:1372-3.
2129 *J Agric Food Chem* 2000;48:2576-81.
2130 *J Appl Microbiol* 2000;88:308-16.
2131 *Altern Ther Health Med* 1999;5:42-51.
2133 *Ann N Y Acad Sci* 1995;774:128-42.
2134 *J Clin Pharmacol* 1990;30:596-608.
2136 *Arthritis Rheum* 1994;37:1305-10.
2138 Goodman GA, Rall TW, Nies AS, Taylor P. The Pharmacological Basis of Therapeutics, 9th ed.
2139 *Cancer Res* 1997;57:1098-102.
2140 *Gastroenterology* 1997;112:29-32.
2141 *Int J Cancer* 1997;73:525-30.
2142 *Am J Epidemiol* 1996;144:1005-14.
2143 *J Natl Cancer Inst* 1998;90:57-62.
2144 *Nutr Cancer* 1997;28:52-62.
2145 *Int J Epidemiol* 1991;20:368-74.
2146 *Am J Clin Nutr* 1999;69:99-104.
2147 *J Intern Med* 1995;237:381-8.
2148 *Am J Clin Nutr* 1998;67:858-66.
2149 *Scand J Clin Lab Invest* 1988;48:215-21.
2150 *Oral Surg Oral Med Oral Pathol* 1991;70:565-8.
2151 *J Clin Periodontol* 1987;14:350-6.
2152 *J Clin Periodontol* 1980;7:402-14.
2153 *Acta Derm Venereol* 1997;77:460-2.
2154 *Cutis* 1992;50:39-42.
2155 *Am J Med Genet* 1992;44:676-82.
2156 *Am J Med Genet* 1988;30:393-9.
2157 *Dev Med Child Neurol* 1986;28:624-7.
2158 *Am J Hum Genet* 1985;37:543-52.
2159 *Am J Med Genet* 1986;23:241-62.
2160 *Am J Med Genet* 1986;23:263-71.
2161 *J Natl Cancer Inst* 1996;88:1495-6.
2162 *Ann Intern Med* 1994;121:833-41.
2163 *Arthritis Rheum* 1990;33:9-18.
2164 *J Rheumatol* 1998;25:36-43.
2167 *Int J Sport Nutr Exerc Metab* 2001;11:384-96.
2168 *J Appl Physiol* 1996;81:2095-104.
2169 *Menopause* 1998;5(1):9-15.
2170 *Calcif Tissue Int* 1997;61:142-7.
2171 *Maturitas* 1997;28(1):75-81.
2172 *Osteoporos Int* 1995;5(6):462-6.
2173 *Calcif Tissue Int* 1994;54(5):377-80.
2174 *Int J Gynaecol Obstet* 1995;48(3):283-8.
2175 *Drugs Exp Clin Res* 1989;15(2):97-104.
2176 *Bone Miner* 1992;19 Suppl 1:S35-42.
2177 *Nephron* 1991;58:114-5.
2178 *Br J Pharmacol* 1998;123(4):605-10.
2179 *J Endocrinol Invest* 1992;15(10):755-61.
2184 *Am J Psychiatry* 1995;152:1084-6.
2185 *Am J Psychiatry* 1995;152:792-4.

2186 *Am J Psychiatry* 1996;153:1219-21.
2187 *Eur Neuropsychopharmacol* 1997;7:147-55.
2188 *Eur Neuropsychopharmacol* 1994;4:487-90.
2189 *Prog Neuropsychopharmacol Biol Psychiatry* 1996;20:729-35.
2190 *J Neural Transm* 1997;104:307-10.
2191 *N Engl J Med* 1992;326:1233-9.
2192 *Lung* 1990;168:877-82.
2193 *Acta Neurol Scand* 1983;67:164-72.
2194 *Lancet* 1978;2:1282-4.
2195 *Acta Neurol Scand* 1978;58:241-8.
2197 *Can J Surg* 1993;36:453-60.
2198 *Support Care Cancer* 1998;6:373-7.
2199 *Dermatology* 1997;195(Suppl 2):57-61.
2200 *Acta Derm Venereol* 1996; 76(3):231-5.
2203 *Psychopathology* 1991;24:53-81.
2204 *Headache* 2000;40:451-6.
2208 *J Urol* 1998;160:664-8.
2209 *Urology* 1998;159:1451-5;discussion 1455-6.
2212 *J Pharm Sci* 1978;67:1582-6.
2213 *J Pharm Sci* 1979;68:586-8.
2214 *Thromb Res* 1997;86:183-96.
2215 *J Nutr* 1998;128:1927-32.
2216 *Clin Cardiol* 1988;11:589-94.
2217 *Am J Clin Nutr* 1985;42:207-13.
2219 *JAMA* 1990;263:688-92.
2220 *Am J Epidemiol* 1986;124:903-15.
2221 *Int J Cancer* 1994;58:774-80.
2222 *Cancer Causes Control* 1995;6:545-50.
2223 *J Natl Cancer Inst* 1995;87:110-6.
2224 *Am J Clin Nutr* 1995;61:1368S-73S.
2225 *Am J Clin Nutr* 1992;55:96-9.
2228 *Am J Med* 1989;87:295-300.
2229 *Scand J Rheumatol* 1984;13(2):108-12.
2230 *Lancet* 1981;1:1015-7.
2231 *Curr Ther Res Clin Exp* 1976;20:62-9.
2232 *Am J Med* 1983;74:124-8.
2233 *Eur J Rheumatol Inflamm* 1981;4(2):237-43.
2234 *Anticancer Res* 1996;16(4A):2025-8.
2235 *Acta Oncol* 1987;26:101-4.
2237 *Ann Pharmacother* 2001;35:501-4.
2238 *Transplantation* 1993;55:57-60.
2239 *Transplantation* 1994;57(2):211-7.
2241 *Circulation* 1994;89:1982-91.
2242 *J Pediatr* 1984;105:781-5.
2243 *Am J Cardiol* 1991;67:765-7.
2245 *J Am Coll Cardiol* 1997;29:941-7.
2246 *Eur Heart J* 1988;9:95-100.
2250 *Ann Intern Med* 1998;129:517-24.
2252 *J Natl Cancer Inst* 1983;71:917-20.
2253 *Am J Clin Oncol* 1982;5:657-63.
2254 *Arch Neurol* 1995;52:559-64.
2255 *Dementia* 1994;5:88-98.
2256 *Atherosclerosis* 1996;119:99-106.
2258 *Atherosclerosis* 1996;120:241-4.
2259 *Neurology* 1996;47:1264-8.
2260 *Eur Respir J* 1997;10:1535-41.
2261 *Circulation* 1996;94:3023-5.
2262 *Clin Pharmacokinet* 1997;33:79-90.
2263 Isselbacher KJ, Braunwald E, Wilson JD, et al. Harrison's Principles of Internal Medicine. 13th Ed. New York, NY: McGraw-Hill, 1994.
2264 *Biol Sport* 1998;15:135-44.
2266 *Addict Behav* 1993;18:117-26.
2267 *Stroke* 1998;29:900-7.
2268 *Am J Cardiol* 1997;80:416-20.
2270 *JAMA* 1979;242:1973-4.
2271 *N Engl J Med* 1988;319:267-73.
2273 *Arch Dis Child* 1986;61:1168-72.
2274 *Neurology* 1985;35:237-8.
2275 *Clin Nutr* 1998;17:23-9.
2276 *Intensive Care Med* 1993;19:89-95.
2278 *Br J Surg* 1987;74:701-4.
2279 *Stroke* 1998;29:2467-72.
2280 *Clin Pharmacol Ther* 1992;52:125-33.
2281 *Br J Clin Pharmacol* 1989;28:421-6.
2282 *Br J Clin Pharmacol* 1990;30:573-7.
2284 *Br J Dermatol* 2000;143:680-2.
2286 *Nephron* 1998;79:173-80.
2287 *Clin Nephrol* 1993;40:315-20.
2288 *Miner Electrolyte Metab* 1992;18:203-6.
2290 *Am J Clin Nutr* 1998;68:1466-73.
2291 *Pediatrics* 1993;92:241-7.
2292 *Clin Pediatr (Phila)* 1997;36:135-9.
2293 *Am J Clin Nutr* 1998;68:1385S-9.
2294 *Am J Clin Nutr* 1998;68:1380S-4.
2295 *J Nutr* 1994;124:213-22.
2296 *Menopause* 1999;6:7-13.
2297 *Obstet Gynecol* 1998;91:6-11.
2298 *Cancer Causes Control* 1998;9:553-7.
2299 *Diabetes Care* 2000;23:1407-15.
2300 *Atherosclerosis* 1999;146:361-7.
2301 *Prostaglandins Leukot Essent Fatty Acids* 1999;61:83-7.
2302 *Scand J Clin Lab Invest* 1994;54:273-80.
2303 *J Clin Pharm Ther* 2001;25:369-73.
2307 *Lancet* 1999;354:447-55.
2309 *N Engl J Med* 1995;332:977-82.
2311 *Ann Intern Med* 1999;130:554-62.
2314 *Am J Cardiol* 1996;77:31-6.
2315 *Arterioscler Thromb Vasc Biol* 1997;17:3384-91.
2316 *J Gastroenterol Hepatol* 1990;5:507-13.
2317 *J Nutr* 1996;126:2130-40.
2318 *Am J Clin Nutr* 1997;65:445-50.
2319 *J Natl Med Assoc* 1997;89:673-8.
2320 *Circulation* 1996;94:1553-60.
2321 *Ann Pharmacother* 1995;29:625-7.
2323 *Am J Clin Nutr* 2000;72:714-22.
2324 *Ann Intern Med* 1993;119:545-54.
2326 *Am J Cardiol* 1993;71:759-65.
2327 *Am J Clin Nutr* 1998;67:1286.
2328 *Allergy* 1983;38:363-5.
2329 *Allergy* 1996;51:266-8.
2330 *Ann Allergy* 1994;73:490-2.
2334 *Gastroenterology* 1997;113:1074-81.
2335 *Int J Sport Nutr Exerc Metab* 2000;10:444-51.
2336 *Cancer* 1998;83:1433-9.
2337 *Am J Gastroenterol* 1998;93:972-5.
2338 *J Parenter Enteral Nutr* 1999;23:7-11.
2339 *Invest Urol* 1980;18:155-7.
2340 *Am J Clin Nutr* 1982;35:107-12.
2341 *J Sports Med Phys Fitness* 1998;38:240-4.
2342 *Nutrition* 1997;13:738-42.
2347 *Metabolism* 1976;25(6):655-7.
2350 *J Rheumatol* 1977;4(4):414-9.
2351 *Metabolism* 1976;25(6):655-7.
2352 *Br Med J* 1975;2(5970):530-3.
2353 *Am J Clin Nutr* 1977;30:579-81.
2354 Bigwood EJ, ed. Protein and amino acid functions. Oxford, NY: Pergamon Press, 1972.
2355 Sacher RA, McPherson RA, eds. Widdmann's Clinical Interpretation of Laboratory Tests. 10th ed., Philadelphia, PA: FA Davis Company, 1991.

2360 *Regul Toxicol Pharmacol* 1997;25:211-9.
2361 *Ann Surg* 1995;222:243-54.
2362 *JPEN J Parenter Enteral Nutr* 1995;19:296-302.
2363 *Ann Surg* 1998;227:302-8.
2364 *J Lab Clin Med* 1996;127:223-8.
2365 *Br J Cancer* 1994;70:732-5.
2366 *Ann Intern Med* 1992;116:821-8.
2367 *Am J Clin Nutr* 1982;35:100-6.
2368 *Bone Marrow Transplant* 1998;22:339-44.
2369 *Med Sci Sports Exerc* 1996;28:1193-8.
2370 *Med Sci Sports Exerc* 1990;22:517-22.
2371 *Am J Gastroenterol* 1994;89:566-70.
2372 *Clin Pharm* 1992;11:533-8.
2373 *Dig Dis Sci* 1993;38:2022-7.
2374 DairyEase product information. McNeil-PPC Inc. Fort Washington, PA 19034.
2375 *Am J Gastroenterol* 1988;83:1145-9.
2376 *Arch Intern Med* 1987;147:534-6.
2377 *Ann Intern Med* 1978;89:218-20.
2379 *J Clin Gastroenterol* 1995;21:2-5.
2380 *Lancet* 1995;346:1265-7.
2381 *Lancet* 1995;346:1247-51.
2382 *Lancet* 1994;343:85-6.
2383 *J Paediatr Child Health* 1994;30:539-43.
2385 *Am J Gastroenterol* 1999;94:427-33.
2387 *Am J Surg* 1999;177:307-10.
2388 *Am J Clin Nutr* 1995;62:1448S-61S.
2389 *Exp Eye Res* 1997;65:57-62.
2390 *Am J Clin Nutr* 1998;68:82-9.
2391 *Am J Clin Nutr* 1995;62:604-10.
2392 *J Nutr* 1997;127:1636S-45S.
2393 *Am J Gastroenterol* 1992:87:305-10.
2394 *JAMA* 1994;272:1413-20.
2395 *BMJ* 1992;305:335-9.
2398 *Am J Epidemiol* 1999;149:801-9.
2400 *Am J Epidemiol* 2001:153:157-63.
2401 *Nutr Cancer* 1998;31:199-203.
2403 *J Nutr* 1997;127:1833-7.
2404 *Proc Soc Exp Biol Med* 1998;218(2):125-8.
2405 *Int J Cancer* 1999;80:704-8.
2406 *J Natl Cancer Inst* 1995;87:1767-76.
2407 *J Natl Cancer Inst* 1999;91:317-31.
2409 *Nutr Cancer* 1997;27:65-8.
2410 *Circulation* 1998;98:1848-52.
2411 *Thromb Res* 1997;88:361-4.
2412 *Clin Endocrinol (Oxf)* 1997;47:61-4.
2413 *Arch Intern Med* 1981;141:394-6.
2414 *Anesthesiology* 1994;80:1046-56.
2415 *J Nutr* 1998;128:720-7.
2417 *Int J Sport Nutr* 1992;2:287-91.
2418 *Int J Sport Nutr* 1993;3:290-7.
2424 *Pharmacol Biochem Behav* 2000;67:131-5.
2425 *Exp Gerontol* 2001;36:297-310.
2426 *Circulation* 2000;102:2555-9.
2428 *Breast* 2000;9:271-6.
2429 *Cancer Res* 2000;60:4112-21.
2430 *Cancer Epidemiol Biomarkers Prev* 2000;9:781-6.
2431 *Pharmazie* 2000;55:364-8.
2432 *Circulation* 2001;103:826-30.
2433 Packer L, Midori H, Toshikazu Y, eds. Antioxidant Food Supplements in Human Health. San Diego: Academic Press, 1999.
2434 *Circulation* 1998;97:363-8.
2435 Rice-Evans CA, Packer L, eds. Flavonoids in Health and Disease. Manhattan, NY: Marcel Dekker, Inc., 1998.
2437 *Psychopharmacol Bull* 1992;28:61-6.
2438 *Acta Neurol Scand* 1986;73:136-40.
2439 *Eur Neuropsychopharmacol* 1992;2:149-55.
2440 *Aging (Milano)* 1993;5:123-33.
2441 *Neurology* 1991;41:644-9.
2443 *J Nutr* 1998;128(3):563-9.
2444 *Am J Clin Nutr* 1994;60(3):408-13.
2445 *Metabolism* 1989;38(8 Suppl 1):63-6.
2446 *Ann Surg* 1987;206(5):674-8.
2447 *Stroke* 1978;9:218-22.
2448 *Metabolism* 1995;44(9):1215-22.
2449 *Acta Hepatogastroenterol (Stuttg)* 1977;24(6):434-9.
2450 *Biomedicine* 1979;30:173-7.
2451 *Fitoterapia* 2000;71:236-44.
2452 *Eur J Appl Physiol* 1982;49(3):307-17.
2454 *N Engl J Med* 1967;276:374-9.
2455 *Arzneimittelforschung* 1976;26:577-9.
2456 *Acupunct Electrother Res* 1990;15:121-35.
2457 *Neuropsychopharmacology* 1997;16:136-46.
2458 *Neuropsychopharmacology* 1992;6:241-7.
2459 *Arch Phys Med Rehabil* 1986;67:436-9.
2460 *Phys Ther* 1987;67:203-5.
2461 *Int J Dermatol* 1989;28:545-7.
2462 *Phytomedicine* 2000;7:383-8.
2463 *Dermatology* 1994;88:215-8.
2464 *Z Hautkr* 1987;62:519-23.
2465 *Arch Dermatol Res* 1985;277:126-30.
2466 *J Trop Med Hyg* 1986;89:149-55.
2467 *Pediatr Dermatol* 1989;6:332-5.
2468 *Arch Psychiatr Nervenkr* 1979;227:49-58.
2469 *J Neural Transm* 1984;59:81-7.
2472 *Am J Clin Nutr* 1992;56:630-5.
2473 *Lancet* 1991;338:1020-1.
2474 *Am J Clin Nutr* 1994;59:423-7.
2475 *J Am Diet Assoc* 1999;99:207-12.
2476 *J Appl Physiol* 1991;71:144-9.
2477 *Sports Med* 1998;26:145-67.
2478 *Undersea Hyperb Med* 1993;20:309-20.
2479 *Int J Sports Med* 1996;17:27-33.
2480 *Stroke* 1993;24:1119-24.
2481 *Stroke* 1992;23:967-71.
2482 *Stroke* 1987;18:373-9.
2483 *Lancet* 1987;:405-8.
2484 *Schweiz Med Wochenschr* 1979;109:737-42.
2485 *Int J Obes* 1984;8:129-33.
2486 *Stroke* 1978;9:484-6.
2487 *Am J Clin Nutr* 1994;59:331-7.
2488 *Am J Physiol* 1993;265:H1571-6.
2490 *Adv Exp Med Biol* 1998;443:261-5.
2491 *J Appl Bacteriol* 1992;73:472-9.
2492 *Med Sci Sports Exerc* 1998;30:1263-9.
2493 *Schweizerische Zeitschrift fur GanzheitsMedizin* 1995;3:114-5.
2494 *Aust N Z J Surg* 1998;68(12):856-8.
2495 *Gastrointest Endosc* 1996;43:42-8.
2496 *Am J Kidney Dis* 1997;29:103-5.
2497 *Dig Dis Sci* 1996;41:749-53.
2498 *J Pediatr Surg* 1997;32:1244-6.
2499 *Eur J Appl Physiol* 1996;72:224-30.
2500 *Pharmacopsychiatry* 1998;31:187-92.
2501 *Planta Med* 1997;63:27-30.
2502 *Indian Heart J* 1997;49:507-10.
2503 *J Assoc Physicians India* 1994;42:287-9.
2504 *Int J Cardiol* 1995;49(3):191-9.
2505 *J Ethnopharmacol* 1997;55(3):165-9.
2506 *J Ethnopharmacol* 1996;53(2):57-63.
2507 *Pharmacol Res* 1997;36:315-21.

2508 *Biol Pharm Bull* 1997;20(4):401-4.
2509 *Antiviral Res* 1996;32(2):63-70.
2510 *Nippon Rinsho* 1998;56(1):156-60.
2511 *Southeast Asian J Trop Med Public Health* 1993;24(4):751-5.
2512 *Antiviral Res* 1995;27(1-2):19-37.
2513 *J Ethnopharmacol* 1999 Dec 15;68(1-3):299-306.
2514 *Indian J Med Sci* 1989;43(5):113-7.
2515 *Biol Pharm Bull* 1997;20:1017-9.
2516 *J Ethnopharmacol* 1985;13(3):323-35.
2517 *Int J Cardiol* 1998;67(2):119-214.
2518 *Chem Pharm Bull (Tokyo)* 1995;43(4):641-8.
2519 *Int J Cardiol* 1988;21:167-75.
2520 *Allergy* 1999;54:635-9.
2521 *Ned Tijdschr Geneeskd* 1991;135:478-80.
2522 *Int J Clin Pharmacol Res* 1983;3:363-6.
2523 *Planta Med* 1997;63(3):233-6.
2524 *Eur J Pharmacol* 1995;286(2):115-22.
2525 *Planta Med* 1994;60(2):101-5.
2526 *J Ethnopharmacol* 1989;26:249-54.
2527 *Arch Toxicol Suppl* 1983;6:194-6.
2528 *J Dermatol Sci* 1999;19(2):78-88.
2530 *Immunol Lett* 1999;68:391-5.
2531 *J Pharm Pharmacol* 1999;51:175-80.
2532 *Lancet* 2000;355(9208):967-72.
2533 *JAMA* 2000;283:1469-75.
2534 *JANA* 2000;2:50-8.
2535 *JANA* 2000;2:59-65.
2536 *Phytother Res* 2001;15:219-23.
2537 *Urology* 2000;55:257-61.
2538 *Arzneimittelforschung* 2000;50:109-17.
2539 *Br J Clin Pharmacol* 1999;48:638-40.
2541 *Fitoterapia* 1995;LXVI:291-317.
2542 *CVR&R* 1999;June:326-9.
2543 *Eur Bull Drug Res* 1999;7:5-7.
2544 *Eur Bull Drug Res* 1999;7:8-13.
2545 *Eur Bull Drug Res* 1999;7:14-18.
2546 *J Comput Assist Tomogr* 1999;23:730-5.
2547 *Eur Radiol* 1999;9(2):287-91.
2548 *Chest* 1993;103(3):976-7.
2549 *Oncol Rep* 1999;6(6):1341-4.
2550 *Eur J Biochem* 1997;250:242-8.
2551 *Pharmazie* 1997;52:463-5.
2552 *Ugeskr Laeger* 1991;153:343-6.
2553 *Eur Bull Drug Res* 1999;7:19-25.
2554 *Eur Bull Drug Res* 1999;7:26-9.
2555 *Eur Bull Drug Res* 1999;7:30-2.
2556 *Eur Bull Drug Res* 1999;7:33-6.
2557 *Arch Intern Med* 1992;152:2441-4.
2558 *Cancer Causes Control* 2000;11:679-85.
2559 *Cancer Causes Control* 2000;11:677-8.
2560 *Ann Pharmacother* 2000;34:931-5.
2562 *Phytother Res* 2001;15:58-61.
2563 *Clin Toxicol* 2000;38:671-8.
2564 *Support Care Cancer* 1997;5:126-9.
2565 *J Pineal Res* 2001;30:123-6.
2566 *Nat Immun* 1998;16:27-33.
2567 *Acta Obstet Gynecol Scand* 1981;60:345-7.
2568 *Ann N Y Acad Sci* 2000;917:560-7.
2569 *J Am Coll Nutr* 2000;19:83S-99S.
2570 *J Gerontol A Biol Sci Med Sci* 1999;54:M275-80.
2571 *Postgrad Med* 2000;108:79-82,85-88, 91.
2572 *Am J Clin Nutr* 1998;67:18-24.
2574 *J Neurol Sci* 1997;150:S90.
2575 *Cleve Clin J Med* 2000;67:696-8.
2576 *Bone* 1999;24:279-90.
2577 *Bone* 1997;21:527-33.
2578 *J Am Coll Nutr* 1999;18:406S-412S.
2579 *J Natl Cancer Inst* 2000;92:1881-8.
2580 *Am J Respir Crit Care Med* 1997;156:1447-52.
2581 *J Nutr* 2000;130:2675-82.
2582 *J Natl Cancer Inst* 1996;88:1560-70.
2583 *Antimicrob Agents Chemother* 1988;32:1274-7.
2585 *Prev Med* 2000;31:308-14.
2586 *Am J Clin Nutr* 2000;72:395-400.
2587 *Ann Trop Med Parasitol* 1991;85:417-25.
2588 *Am J Dis Child* 1975;129:866.
2589 *Biol Neonate* 1993;63:201-8.
2590 *J Anal Toxicol* 1993;17:246-7.
2591 *Indian J Med Res* 1969;57:2128-31.
2592 *Am J Clin Nutr* 2000;72:1421-3.
2593 *Am J Clin Nutr* 2000;72:1576-82.
2594 *Am J Clin Nutr* 2000;71:908-13.
2595 *Am J Clin Nutr* 2000;72:990-7.
2596 *Vet Hum Toxicol* 1997 Dec;39(6):373-5.
2597 *Planta Med* 1998;64(5):404-7.
2598 *J Pharm Pharmacol* 1995;47:152-6.
2599 *Lancet* 1999;354:723-9.
2600 *Clin Ther* 1980;3:260-72.
2601 *Ann Pharmacother* 1998;32:580-7.
2602 *Curr Med Res Opin* 1982;8:145-9.
2603 *Curr Med Res Opin* 1980;7:110-4.
2604 *Arzneimittelforschung* 1998;48:469-74.
2605 *Arzneimittelforschung* 1994;44:75-80.
2606 *Eur J Clin Pharmacol* 1996;50:542.
2607 *Arzneimittelforschung* 1993;43:1109-13.
2608 *Ann Pharmacother* 1998;32:574-9.
2609 *Am J Gastroenterol* 1983;78:19-22.
2612 *J Ethnopharmacol* 1986;17:75-83.
2613 *Orv Hetil* 1989;130:2723-7.
2614 *Acta Med Hung* 1988;45:249-56.
2615 *Hum Toxicol* 1983;2:183-95.
2616 *J Hepatol* 1989;9:105-13.
2617 *J Hepatol* 1997;26:871-9.
2618 *Scand J Gastroenterol* 1982;17:517-21.
2619 Hebel SK, ed. Drug Facts and Comparisons. 52nd ed. St. Louis: Facts and Comparisons, 1998.
2620 *J Pharmacol Exp Ther* 1980;213:306-8.
2623 FDA Office of Regulatory Affairs. Sec. 457.100 Pangamic Acid and Pangamic Acid Products Unsafe for Food and Drug Use. (CPG 7121.01). 1995. Available at: www.fda.gov/ora/compliance_ref/cpg/cpgdrg/cpg457-100.html (Accessed 16 July 1999).
2624 *Am J Clin Nutr* 1999;69:231-6.
2628 *Alt Med Rev* 2000;5:530-45.
2629 *Anticancer Res* 1999;19(1A):35-44.
2630 *Prostaglandins Leukot Essent Fatty Acids* 1996;55:441-9.
2631 *Curr Microbiol* 1998;36:24-8.
2632 *Oral Surg Oral Med Oral Pathol* 1990;70:584-6.
2633 *Z Naturforsch [C]* 1988;43:470-2.
2634 *Heart* 2000;84(4):E8.
2635 *Biochem Pharmacol* 1984;33:3933-9.
2636 *Cell Mol Life Sci* 1998;54:1168-72.
2637 *J Cardiovasc Pharmacol* 1998;32:509-15.
2639 *J Am Coll Nutr* 2000;19:220-7.
2640 *J Med Food* 2000;3:1-13.
2641 *Planta Med* 1998;64:324-7.
2642 *N Engl J Med* 1996;334:1150-5.
2644 *Chest* 1994;106:1654-9.
2645 *Med Sci Sports Exerc* 1982;14:424-7.
2646 *N Engl J Med* 1996;334:1145-9.

2648 *J Int Med Res* 1977;5:334-7.
2649 *Ann Chir Gynaecol* 1983;72:62-5.
2650 FDA Talk Paper. FDA Cautions Consumers on "Kombucha Mushroom Tea." Available at: www.vm.cfsan.fda.gov/~lrd/TPMUSHRM.html.
2651 *JAMA* 1998;280:1567-8.
2652 *Crit Path AIDS Proj* 1994;30:31-32 1994-5.
2653 *Sidahora* 1995;90:34-5.
2654 *GMHC Treat Issues* 1995;9:10.
2655 *MMWR Morb Mortal Wkly Rep* 1995;44:892-3,899-900.
2656 *J Gen Intern Med* 1997;12:643-4.
2657 *JAMA* 1996;275:699-703.
2658 *J Natl Cancer Inst* 1993;85:1483-92.
2659 *J Clin Psychiatry* 1999;60:237-40.
2660 *Life Sci* 2000;67:1389-96.
2662 *Analyst* 1998;123:3-6.
2663 *Clin Lab Med* 1998;18:673-85.
2664 *JAMA* 1996;276:1957-63.
2665 *Human Psychopharmacol* 1987;2:159-69.
2666 *Human Psychopharmacol* 1994;9:215-22.
2667 *Br J Urol* 1998;81:730-4.
2668 *In Vitro Cell Dev Biol Anim* 1997;33:218-21.
2669 *Am J Clin Nutr* 2001;74:694-700.
2670 *Am J Clin Nutr* 2001;74:343-7.
2671 *Can J Vet Res* 1986;50:297-306.
2672 *J Lab Clin Med* 1992;119:407-11.
2673 *Epidemiology* 1998;9:9-15.
2675 *Q J Med* 1986;59:569-77.
2676 *J Cardiovasc Risk* 1996;3:42-7.
2677 Shils ME, Olson JA, Shike M, Ross AC, eds. Modern Nutrition in Health and Disease. 9th ed. Baltimore, MD: Williams & Wilkins, 1999.
2678 *J Am Coll Nutr* 1993;12:26-30.
2681 *Am J Clin Nutr* 1990;51:225-7.
2682 *Drug Saf* 1995;12:314-33.
2684 *Arch Intern Med* 1986;146:41-2.
2685 *Arch Intern Med* 1986;146:48-53.
2686 *Acta Derm Venereol* 1992;72:250-2.
2687 *J Am Acad Dermatol* 1990;22:253-60.
2688 *Br J Dermatol* 1989;121:497-502.
2689 *Am J Clin Nutr* 1983;38:512-22.
2690 *Eur J Pediatr* 1985;143:310-4.
2691 *Am J Dermatopathol* 1992;14:304-9.
2692 *Am J Gastroenterol* 1999;94:334-8.
2693 *J Lab Clin Med* 1998;132:264-78.
2694 *Adv Ther* 1996;13:88-94.
2695 *JAMA* 1988;259:3137-41.
2696 *J Neurotrauma* 1996;13:25-34.
2697 *Ann Intern Med* 1990;113:265-9.
2698 *Am J Med* 1991;91:5-14.
2699 *Acta Derm Venereol Suppl (Stockh)* 1990;154:1-36.
2700 *J Ethnopharmacol* 1999;65:1-11.
2702 *Nutrition* 1999;15:860-4.
2703 *JPEN J Parenter Enteral Nutr* 1999;23:309-12.
2704 *Ann Surg* 1998;227:772-8.
2705 *Ann Surg* 1998;227:485-91.
2706 Osol A, Hoover JE, eds. Remington's Pharmaceutical Science, 15th ed. Easton, PA: Mack Publishing Company, 1975.
2708 The National Toxicology Program (NTP). Caffeine. Center for the Evaluation of Risks to Human Reproduction (CERHR). Available at: http://cerhr.niehs.nih.gov/genpub/topics/caffeine-ccae.html.
2709 *N Engl J Med* 1999;341:1639-44.
2710 *N Engl J Med* 1999;341:1688-9.
2711 *Reprod Toxicol* 1998;12:435-44.
2712 *Eur J Epidemiol* 1999;15:181-8.
2713 *Int J Sports Med* 1997;18:40-6.
2714 *J Clin Pharmacol* 1999;39:936-40.
2715 *Cephalalgia* 1999;19:684-91.
2716 *Arch Neurol* 1998;55:210-7.
2717 *Clin Ther* 1999;21:475-91.
2718 *Clin Pharmacol Ther* 1994;56:576-86.
2719 DiPiro JT, Talbert RL, Yee GC, et al; eds. Pharmacotherapy: A pathophysiologic approach. 4th ed. Stamford, CT: Appleton & Lange, 1999.
2720 *Psychopharmacology (Berl)* 1999;145:181-8.
2721 *Am J Med* 1991;91:1-4.
2722 *Eur J Clin Nutr* 1999;53:831-9.
2723 *J Clin Pharmacol* 1999;39:1221-32.
2724 *J Laryngol Otol* 1999;113:341-5.
2725 *Mayo Clin Proc* 1997;72:621-6.
2726 *Can J Anaesth* 1995;42:789-92.
2727 *Reg Anesth Pain Med* 1999;24:51-4.
2728 *Anesth Analg* 1990;70:181-4.
2729 FDA. Proposed rule: dietary supplements containing ephedrine alkaloids. Available at: www.verity.fda.gov (Accessed 25 January 2000).
2730 *Arch Intern Med* 1988;148:1801-5.
2731 *New Engl J Med* 1984;310:1221-5.
2732 *JAMA* 1998;280:1604-9.
2735 *Urology* 1999;53:457-61.
2736 USRF Research. Clinical effects of saw palmetto extract in men with symptomatic BPH webpage: www.usrf.org/spepapers.html (Accessed 23 June 2004).
2737 *JAMA* 1999;282:1539-46.
2738 *Lancet* 1980;1:616-20.
2739 *Biol Trace Elem Res* 1998;61:19-31.
2740 *Pharm Weekbl Sci* 1986;8:85-8.
2743 Dr. Duke's Phytochemical and Ethnobotanical Databases. Ethnobotanical uses: Andrographis paniculata. www.ars-grin.gov/cgi-bin/duke/ethnobot.pl?andrographis%20pnaiculata (Accessed 27 January 2000).
2744 *Phytomedicine* 1999;6:217-23.
2746 Indian Herbs. Andrographis paniculata. www.indianherbs.com (Accessed 23 June 2004).
2748 *J Med Assoc Thai* 1991;74:437-42.
2750 *Indian J Pharm Sci* 1998;60:176-8.
2751 *Pharm Biol* 1998;36:72-4.
2752 *J Environ Sci Health A Tox Hazard Subst Environ Eng.* 1999;34:975-87.
2753 *Indian J Pharm Sci* 1995;57:121-5.
2754 *J Ethnopharmacol* 1991;33:193-6.
2755 *J Ethnopharmacol* 1997;56:97-101.
2756 *J Tongji Med Univ* 1994;14:49-51.
2757 *J Tongji Med Univ* 1996;16:193-7.
2758 *Chin Med J (Engl)* 1991;104:770-5.
2759 *Phytomedicine* 1999;6:27-31.
2760 *Pharmacol Res* 1998;38:413-7.
2761 *Planta Med* 1992;58:146-9.
2762 *J Ethnopharmacol* 1993;40:131-6.
2763 *Arch Pharm Res* 1991;14:93-5.
2764 *J Med Assoc Thai* 1990;73:299-304.
2765 *Proc Soc Exp Biol Med* 1991;197:59-66.
2766 *J Nat Prod* 1993;56:995-9.
2767 *Ind J Physiol Pharmacol* 1975;19;47-9.
2768 *Chem Pharm Bull (Tokyo)* 1994;42:1216-25.
2769 *Indian J Exp Biol* 1990;28:421-6.
2770 *J Ethnopharmacol* 1997;58:219-24.
2771 *Phytomedicine* 1999;6:157-61.
2772 *Phytomedicine* 1997;4:101-4.

2773 *Phytomedicine* 1996;97;3:315-8.
2774 *Phytotherapy Res* 1995;9:559-62.
2776 *Bangladesh Med Res Counc Bull* 1989;15:34-7.
2777 *SAR QSAR Environ Res* 1999;10:47-60.
2778 *Biochem Pharmacol* 1993;46:182-5.
2779 *Int J Pharmacogn* 1993;31:198-204.
2780 *J Ethnopharmacol* 1999;64:249-54.
2781 *Int J Pharmacogn* 1992;30:263-74.
2782 *Chin Med J (Engl)* 1994;107:464-70.
2783 *J Tongji Med Univ* 1993;13:193-8.
2784 *Am J Gastroenterol* 1999;94:3267-73.
2786 *Am J Physiol* 1999;276:G58-G63.
2787 *Antiviral Res* 1994;25:185-92.
2788 *Antiviral Res* 1997;35:91-103.
2790 *Chemotherapy* 1993;39:203-11.
2791 *Antiviral Res* 1993;20:145-54.
2792 *Chemotherapy* 1993;39:212-7.
2793 *Chemotherapy* 1994;40:42-50.
2794 *Antiviral Res* 1993;21:37-45.
2795 *J Pharm Sci* 1979;68:124-6.
2796 *Planta Med* 1989;55:140-3.
2797 *J Nat Prod* 1993;56:899-906.
2798 *Planta Med* 1994;60:541-5.
2799 *J Ethnopharmacol* 1997;58:103-8.
2804 Raintree Nutrition. Sangre de Grado website: www.raintree.com/sangre.htm (Accessed 31 January 2000).
2805 USDA, ARS, National Genetic Resources Program. Germplasm Resources Information Network - (GRIN). Taxon: Croton lechleri mull. Arg website: www.ars-grin.gov/cgi-bin/npgs/html/tax_search.pl?croton+lechleri (Accessed 31 January 2000).
2806 Dicesare D, Dupont HL, Mathewson JJ, et al. A double-blind randomized, placebo-controlled study of SP-303 (Provir) in the symptomatic treatment of acute diarrhea among travelers to Mexico and Jamaica. Infectious Diseases Society of America Annual Meeting, 1998 (abstract).
2807 BioWorld Today. Shaman will sidestep FDA by selling product over internet website. Available at: http://www.bioworld.com. (Accessed 6 January 2000).
2809 *JPEN J Parenter Enteral Nutr* 1995;19:393-7.
2810 *Lipids* 2001;36:669-74.
2811 *J Pediatr* 1999;135:698-702.
2812 *J Urol* 1984;131:1013-6.
2813 *N Engl J Med* 1998;339:1085-6.
2814 *J Urol* 1998;159:559-62.
2815 *Can J Microbiol* 1999;45:691-4.
2816 *J Am Dent Assoc* 1998;129:1719-23.
2819 *Lipids* 2001;36:773-81.
2820 *Nutr Res* 2001;21:955-60.
2821 *Diabetes Care* 2002;25:1516-21.
2823 *J Rheumatol* 1997;24:643-6.
2824 *S Afr Med J* 1997;87:1116-9.
2825 *Int J Sports Med* 1985;6:44-9.
2826 *Cardiovasc Drugs Ther* 1998;12:197-202.
2827 *J Clin Chem Clin Biochem* 1984;22:717-21.
2828 *Int J Sports Med* 1982;3:177-81.
2829 *Int J Sports Med* 1983;4:119-23.
2830 *Med Sci Sports Exerc* 1998;30:1584-91.
2900 *Blood* 1998;92:1191-1198.
2901 *Am J Med* 2001;111:126-9.
2902 *JAMA* 1991;265:94-95.
2909 *Lancet* 1998;352:1721-1722.
2910 *Arch Intern Med* 2000;160:2061-2.
2911 *J Am Geriatr Soc* 1997;45:124-125.
2912 *Nouv Presse Med* 1982; 11(4): 267-9.
2913 *Med Klin* 1981;76(10):291-3.
2915 *Am J Clin Nutr* 1994;60:12-14
2917 *J Assoc Acad Minor Phys* 1998;9(1):9-15.
2918 *Hepatogastroenterology* 1986;33:159-62.
2919 *Am J Clin Nutr* 1994;60:2-11.
2921 *Neurology* 1986;36:1263-4.
2924 *Br J Nutr* 1995;73:433-41.
2925 *Nahrung* 1994;38:373-7.
2927 *Int J Clin Pharmacol Res* 1995;15:159-65.
2928 *Int J Clin Pharmacol Res* 1994;14:27-33.
2929 *Diabetes Care* 1995;18:393-7.
2930 *Int J Clin Pharmacol Ther* 1996;34:134-7.
2931 *Angiology* 1999;50:123-30.
2933 *Int J Tissue React* 1998;20:119-24.
2934 *Br J Nutr* 1997;77:923-32.
2935 *Pharmacol Res* 1996;34:181-5.
2936 *Prostaglandins Leukot Essent Fatty Acids* 1998;58:61-4.
2937 *Pharmacol Res* 1997;36:293-7.
2938 *Int J Clin Pharmacol Res* 1996;16:67-72.
2939 *Biol Res* 1994;27:199-203.
2941 *Int J Clin Pharmacol Ther* 1998;36:469-73.
2943 *Curr Ther Res* 1995;56:819-23.
2944 *Curr Ther Res* 1996;57:691-5.
2948 *Science* 1997;275:218-20.
2949 *Clin Chim Acta* 1996;246:163-82.
2950 *Drugs Exp Clin Res* 1996;22:61-3.
2951 *Clin Chim Acta*, 1995; 235(2): 207-19.
2952 *Drugs Exp Clin Res* 1998; 24(3): 133-8.
2954 *Gen Pharmacol* 1996;27:363-6.
2956 *J Nutr* 2002;132:394-8.
2958 *Carcinogenesis* 1999; 20(2): 237-42.
2959 *Biochem Biophys Res Commun* 1999;254(3):739-43.
2960 *Proc Natl Acad Sci U S A* 1997; 94(25): 14138-43.
2961 *Int J Tissue React* 1995; 17(1): 1-3.
2971 *Plast Reconstr Surg* 1998;102:2088-93; discussion 2094-6.
3001 *Integrative Medicine Consult* 2001;3:17,21.
3005 *Biol Psychiatry* 1994;35:775-80.
3006 *J Clin Endocrinol Metab* 1996;81:1076-82.
3007 *Brain Res* 1993; 615(2): 267-74.
3008 Devlin TM, ed. Textbook of Biochemistry With Clinical Correlations. third ed. New York: Wiley-Liss Inc., 1992.
3011 Klaassen CD, ed. Casarett and Doull's Toxicology: The Basic Science of Poisons. fifth ed. New York: McGraw-Hill, 1996.
3012 *J Am Diet Assoc* 1994;94:891-4.
3013 *Diabetes* 1994;43:9-15.
3014 *Eur J Cancer Prev* 1997;6:58-70.
3016 *Neoplasma* 1994;41:291-6.
3017 *Vet Human Toxicol* 1993;35:495-500.
3018 *Toxicology* 1993;83:115-30.
3019 *Biochem Cell Biol* 1993;71:103-12.
3020 *Mineral Electrolyte Metab* 1998;19:51-6.
3021 *Toxicology* 1991;66:279-87.
3022 Kastrup EK. Drug Facts and Comparisons. 1998 ed. St. Louis, MO: Facts and Comparisons, 1998.
3024 *JAMA* 1991;265:96-97.
3025 *J Nutr* 2000;130:2243-50.
3026 *West J Med* 1984;140:460.
3041 Beers MH, Berkow R. The Merck Manual of Diagnosis and Therapy. 17th ed. West Point, PA: Merck and Co., Inc., 1999.
3042 *JAMA* 1999;281:1415-23.
3046 Hansten PD, Horn JR. Drug Interactions Analysis and Management. Vancouver, WA: Applied Therapeutics Inc., 1997 and updates.

REFERENCES

3047 *J Am Coll Cardiol* 1996;27:517-27.
3051 *Mutat Res* 1994;317:81-8.
3054 *Chem Pharmaceut Bull* 1992;40:174-6.
3055 *Diabetes* 1996;45:659-66.
3056 *J Clin Invest* 1995;95:2501-9.
3057 *Metabolism* 1996;45:1130-5.
3062 *Cancer* 1988;61:1543-9.
3063 *Cancer* 1983;51:269-72.
3066 FDA Talk Paper. Vitamin A and birth defects (T95-56). Food and Drug Administration, U.S.Department of Health and Human Services, Rockville, MD. October 6, 1995.
3070 *Obes Res* 2001;9:129-34.
3072 Tatro DS, ed. Drug Interactions Facts. Facts and Comparisons Inc., St. Louis, MO. 1999.
3073 *Int J Vit Nutr Res* 1997;67:242-7.
3074 *Thromb Res* 1984;35:11-8.
3082 Budavari S, ed. The Merck Index. 12th ed. Whitehouse Station, NJ: Merck & Co., Inc., 1996.
3083 *Geriatr Nephrol Urol* 1998;8:95-100.
3085 *Drugs Aging* 1998; 13(4):263-8.
3086 *J Neural Transm (Budapest)* 1996; 103(10):1187-93.
3088 *J Neural Transm* (Parkinsons Disease & Dementia Section) 1993; 5(2):147-56.
3089 *Acta Neurol Scand Suppl* 1993; 146:32-5.
3090 *Acta Neurol Scand* 1994; 90(5):345-7.
3091 *Biochim Biophys Acta* 1997;1361:59-65.
3092 Fauci AS, Braunwald E, Isselbacher KJ, et al. Harrison's Principles of Internal Medicine, 14th ed. New York, NY: McGraw-Hill, 1998.
3093 *BMJ* 1999;318:1375-81.
3094 *J Am Diet Assoc* 1998;98:699-706.
3095 *Antimicrob Agents Chemother* 1997;41:961-4.
3096 *Clin Diagn Lab Immunol* 1998;5:882-7.
3097 *JAMA* 1999;281:2289-93.
3098 *J Am Coll Nutr* 1999;18:166-70.
3099 *Am J Epidemiol* 1998;147:1162-74.
3100 *J Chromatogr A* 1998;823:331-7.
3101 *Life Sci* 1998;62:687-95.
3102 *Planta Med* 1997;63:409-14.
3103 *Free Radical Biol Med* 1996;21:487-93.
3104 *Cancer Lett* 1996;109:185-91.
3105 *Br J Pharmacol* 1995;116:1985-90.
3106 *Mutagenesis* 1995;10:325-8.
3107 *Gen Pharmacol* 1994;25:575-80.
3109 *Phytother Res* 1999;13;59-64.
3111 *Arthritis Rheum* 1998;41:290-7.
3112 *Arthritis Rheum* 1996;39:623-8.
3113 *Biochem Biophys Res Commun* 1998;243:25-9.
3116 *FASEB J* 1996;10:26-32.
3117 Ghoneum M, Jewett A. Synergistic effect of modified arabinoxylane (MGN-3) and low dose of recombinant IL-2 on human NK cell activity and TNF production [abstract]. American Acadamy of Anti-Aging Medicine Educational Conference, August 15-6, 1998.
3118 *Int J Immunotherapy* 1998;14:89-99.
3119 Ghoneum M, Namatalla G. NK immunomodulatory function in 27 cancer patients by MGN-3, a modified arabinoxylane from rice bran [abstract]. 87th Annual Meeting of the American Association for Cancer Research. April 20-4, 1996.
3120 Ghoneum M. Immunomodulatory and anti-cancer properties of MGN-3, a modified xylose from rice bran, in 5 patients with breast cancer [abstract]. American Association for Cancer Research Special Conference. November 5-8, 1995.
3121 *Planta Med* 2000;66:217-20.
3122 *Cancer Causes Control* 2000;11:565-76.
3123 *Eur J Clin Pharmacol* 2000;56:489-93.
3125 *Arthritis Rheum* 1998;41:191-4.
3126 *Rheum Dis Clin North Am* 1998;24:525-36.
3127 *Aust N Z J Ophthalmol* 1996;24:257-60.
3128 AutoImmune Inc. announces phase III trial results for Colloral. URL http://www.autoimmune.com/clinic/coll.html (Accessed 24 October 1999).
3129 *Chung Kuo Yao Li Hsueh Pao* 1999;20:31-5.
3131 *JAMA* 1997;277:776.
3132 *Chung Kuo Yao Li Hsueh Pao* 1998;19:27-30.
3133 *Chung Kuo Yao Li Hsueh Pao* 1998;19:128-32.
3134 *J Pharmacol Exp Ther* 1999;288:814-9.
3135 *Eur J Pharmacol* 1998;349:137-42.
3136 *Pharmacol Biochem Behav* 1998;60:377-86.
3137 *Fundam Clin Pharmacol* 1997;11:387-94.
3138 *Zhongguo Yao Li Xue Bao* 1995;16:391-5.
3139 *Life Sci* 1994;54:991-7.
3140 *Chung Kuo Yao Li Hsueh Pao* 1991;12:250-2.
3141 *J Neurosci Res* 1989;24:276-85.
3142 Safety Briefs, ISMP Medication Safety Alert, vol.4, #4. Institute for Safe Medication Practices, Warminster, PA. February 24, 1999.
3148 Bupleurum falcatum Bitter & cool. The Australian Naturopath Network web site. Available at: www.comcen.com.au/~sburgess/herbs/Monographs/bupleuru.htm.
3151 *Chung Kuo Chung Yao Tsa Chih* 1996;21:739-41,762.
3152 *J Ethnopharmacol* 1991;34:155-65.
3153 *J Nutr* 2000;130:2943-8.
3154 *Nippon Yakurigaku Zasshi* 1995;106:229-37.
3155 *J Pharm Pharmacol* 1993;45:535-9.
3156 *Nippon Yakurigaku Zasshi* 1991;97:13-21.
3157 *Planta Med* 1998;64:220-4.
3158 *Am J Clin Nutr* 2001;73:807-814.
3159 *Prostaglandins Leukot Essent Fatty Acids* 1991;44:51-6.
3160 *Cell Immunol* 1994;159(1):15-25.
3161 *Int J Immunopharmacol* 1991;13:501-8.
3162 *Int J Infect Dis* 1999;3:197-202.
3163 *Am J Chin Med* 1992;20:257-64.
3164 *Biol Pharm Bull* 1997;20:759-64.
3165 *Planta Med* 1994;60:163-7.
3166 *Planta Med* 1993;59(6):533-6.
3167 *J Nat Prod* 1989;52:267-72.
3168 *Life Sci* 1998;63:1147-56.
3169 *J Med Assoc Thai* 1999;82:S43-S48.
3170 *J Nat Prod* 1994;57:1178-82.
3171 *New Drugs and Clinical Remedies* 1986;5:260-2.
3172 *New Drugs and Clinical Remedies* 1986;5:197-9.
3176 HolisticOnLine website. URL: holisticonline.com/Herbal-Med/_scripts/getHerb_Dir.idc?Herb_Names=365 (Accessed 25 November 1999).
3177 Dharmananda S. PCP prophylaxis with drugs and herbs. Institute for Traditional Medicine Online. URL: www.rdi.gpo.or.th/NetZine/V3N42/pcp.htm (Accessed 25 November 1999).
3180 *Clin Infect Dis* 1999;28:597-601.
3181 *Trends Pharmacol Sci* 1999;20:199-205.
3182 *Med Trop (Mars)* 1998;58:70-2.
3183 *Planta Med* 1994;60:54-7.
3184 *Chung Kuo Chung Yao Tsa Chih* 1993;18:44-48,63-4.
3185 *Chung Kuo Chi Sheng Chung Hsueh Yu Chi Sheng Chung Ping Tsa Chih* 1992;10:290-4.
3190 *Patol Fiziol Eksp Ter* 1997;:22-4.
3191 *Eksp Klin Farmakol* 1997;60:34-6.

3192 *Eksp Klin Farmakol* 1997;60:38-9.
3193 *Eksp Klin Farmakol* 1994;57:61-3.
3194 *Urol Nefrol (Mosk)* 1995;:46-7.
3195 *Bull Eksp Biol Med* 1993;116:175-6.
3196 *Vopr Onkol* 1992;38:1217-22.
3197 *Eksp Onko* 1990;12:55-6.
3198 *Acta Physiol Pharmacol Bulg* 1986;12:3-16.
3219 *Am J Clin Nutr* 1999;70:517-24.
3220 *Am J Clin Nutr* 1999;70:509-16.
3221 *Am J Epidemiol* 1999;149:801-9.
3222 *J Epidemiol Community Health* 1998;52:468-72.
3223 *Acta Ophthalmol Scand* 1997;75:634-40.
3224 *Br J Ophthalmol* 1998;82:907-10.
3225 *Optom Vis Sci* 1997;74:499-504.
3226 *Clin Pharmacol Ther* 1999;65:395-401.
3227 *Clin Pharmacol Ther* 1999;66:118-27.
3228 *Eur J Drug Metab Pharmacokinet* 1998;23:55-9.
3229 Grapefruit-drug interactions. URL: powernetdesign.com/grapefruit (Accessed 26 September 1999).
3230 *Eur J Clin Pharmacol* 1998;54:337-40.
3231 *N Engl J Med* 1999;341:1013-20.
3232 *N Engl J Med* 1999;341:1073-4.
3234 *J Nutr* 2000;130:2662-5.
3235 *N Engl J Med* 1988;318:1720-8.
3236 *Lancet* 1999;354:810-6.
3237 *Am J Clin Nutr* 1999;69:213-9.
3238 *Am J Clin Nutr* 1991;53:1021S-6S.
3239 *Lipids* 1995;30:1179-83.
3240 *Lipids* 1995;30:1171-7.
3241 *Nutr Biochem* 1997;8:290-8.
3242 *Arzneimittelforschung* 1991; 41:768-72.
3243 *Eur J Clin Nutr* 1999;53:379-81.
3244 *Methods Find Exp Clin Pharmacol* 1999;21:357-61.
3246 *N Engl J Med* 1999;341:1158.
3247 *Nippon Rinsho* 1994;52:1817-22.
3248 *J Hepatol* 1994;21:601-9.
3249 *Antiviral Res* 1996;30:171-7.
3250 *Indian J Med Res* 1993;98:69-74.
3251 *J Nutr* 2001;131:1471-8.
3252 *J Endocrinol Invest* 1996;19:624-9.
3253 *J Clin Endocrinol Metab* 1994;78:581-5.
3254 *Clin Pharmacol Ther* 1996;59:62-71.
3255 *J Steroid Biochem Mol Biol* 1994;49:81-5.
3256 *Endocrinol Jpn* 1979;26:661-5.
3257 *Biol Pharm Bull* 1998;21:1277-81.
3259 *Semin Nephrol* 1996;16:567-75.
3260 *J Invest Dermatol* 1996;106:419-27.
3261 *Aliment Pharmacol Ther* 1999;13:1103-8.
3262 *J Rheumatol* 1995;22:953-8.
3263 *Obstet Gynecol* 1999;94:577-82.
3264 *Am J Clin Nutr* 1978; 31:466-9.
3265 *J Biol Chem* 1999;274:22041-7.
3267 *Cardiovasc Drugs Ther* 1994;8:659-64.
3268 *J Dermatol* 1994;21:729-31.
3269 *J Nat Prod* 1987;50:612-7.
3270 *Am J Psychiatry* 1999;156:646-9.
3273 The IOOC's Trade Standard Applying to Olive Oil and Olive Pomace Oil. Available at: sovrana.com/ioocdef.htm (Accessed 23 June 2004).
3274 *Aust Fam Physician* 1999;28:817,828.
3275 *J Am Acad Dermatol* 1999;41:312-5.
3276 *Arch Pediatr Adolesc Med* 1997 Jul;151(7):675-8.
3278 *J Infect Dis* 1985;152:1324-7.
3279 *Hosp Pharm* 1998;33:180-8.
3280 *West J Med* 1999;171:198-200.
3281 *J Fam Pract* 1999;48:628-35.
3282 *Am J Med* 1999;106:138-43.
3283 *Thromb Res* 1999;95:155-61.
3284 *J Pharm Pharmacol* 1999;51:971-4.
3285 *Eur J Clin Nutr* 1989;43 Suppl 2:43-8.
3286 *Am J Clin Nutr* 1992;55:846-50.
3287 *Arterioscler Thromb* 1993;13:1533-42.
3288 *J Intern Med* 1999;246:191-201.
3289 *J Hypertens* 1996;14:1483-90.
3290 *Arterioscler Thromb Vasc Biol* 1999;19:122-30.
3291 *N Engl J Med* 1984;310:483-8.
3292 *Clin Neuropharmacol* 1987;10:527-37.
3293 *Arch Neurol* 1987;44:1003-5.
3294 *Neurology* 1988;38:1245-8.
3300 *Microbiol Immunol* 1997;41:1005-9.
3301 *Braz J Med Biol Res* 1986;19:771-4.
3302 *Indian J Med Res* 1991;93:324-7.
3303 *Eur J Clin Pharmacol* 1987;3:877-82.
3304 *Biol Psychiatry* 1995;38:765-7.
3305 *Urology* 1994;44:732-6.
3306 *J Clin Psychiatry* 1993;54:161-2.
3307 *Arch Sexual Behavior* 1996;25:341-60.
3309 *Urology* 1997;49:441-4.
3310 *BMJ* 1998;316:678-82.
3311 *J Fam Pract* 1998;46:282-3.
3312 *J Urol* 1998;159:122-4.
3313 *Am J Psychiatry* 1994;151:1397.
3314 Anderson PO, Knoben JE, Troutman WG. Handbook of Clinical Drug Data. 9th ed. Stamford, CT: Appleton & Lange, 1999.
3315 *Atherosclerosis* 2000;150:437-8.
3316 *AJG* 2000;95:563-4.
3317 *Contact Dermatitis* 2000;42:108-9.
3318 *JAMA* 2000;284:831.
3319 *Nutrition* 2000;16:236-9.
3320 *Am J Clin Nutr* 2000;72:1047-52.
3321 *Nutrition* 2000;16:787-8.
3322 *Appl Environ Microbiol* 2000;66:2269-73.
3323 *Eur J Clin Nutr* 2000;54:424-8.
3324 *Circulation* 2000;101:2829-32.
3325 US Food and Drug Administration, Center for Food Safety, and Applied Nutrition, Office of Nutritional Products, Labeling, and Dietary Supplements. Letter regarding dietary supplement health claim for folic acid with respect to neural tube defects. 2000. Available at: http://vm.cfsan.fda.gov/~dms/ds-ltr7.html.
3330 *Cardiology* 1998;90:153-5.
3331 *Surgery* 1994;115:205-12.
3332 *Arterioscler Thromb Vasc Biol* 2000;20:2134-9.
3333 *Age Ageing* 2000;29:9-12.
3334 *Home Healthc Nurse* 1997;15:199-202.
3335 *Adv Exp Med Biol* 1996;408:185-6.
3337 *Nutr Rev* 1994;52:168-70.
3338 *Microbios* 1988;55:173-81.
3339 *Nurs Res* 1979;28:287-90.
3340 *Am J Clin Nutr* 2000;72:1095-100.
3341 *Lancet* 2000;356:233-41.
3343 *Cancer Epidemiol Biomarkers Prev* 1998;7:853-6.
3344 *Am J Clin Nutr* 2000;72:1107-10.
3345 *JAMA* 1999;281:2106-12.
3346 *J Clin Gastroenterol* 1997;24:196-8.
3347 *JAMA* 1992;268:3224-7.
3348 *Lancet* 1990;336:677-8.
3349 *Bull N Y Acad Med* 1982;58:323-39.
3350 *Am J Gastroenterol* 2000;95:1008-13.
3351 *J Learn Disabil* 1982;15:258-64.
3353 *JAMA* 1979;241:1614-5.

3354 *Ann Pharmacother* 2000;34:1347-8.
3356 *Med J Aust* 1990;152:613-4.
3357 *Lancet* 2000;356:1213-8.
3358 *Am J Clin Nutr* 2000;72:1142-9.
3359 *Arch Neurol* 2000;57:1503-9.
3360 *Cancer* 2000;89:1205-13.
3361 *Nutr Cancer* 2000;36:90-100.
3362 *J Epidemiol Community Health* 2000;54:756-60.
3364 *Biochem Biophys Res Commun* 1998;248:28-32.
3365 *J Hum Hypertens* 1999;13:203-8.
3366 *Lancet* 2000;356:391-5.
3367 *Clin Pharmacol Ther* 1995;57:62-6.
3368 *Res Commun Chem Pathol Pharmacol* 1977;17:157-64.
3369 *Res Commun Chem Pathol Pharmacol* 1975;12:533-40.
3370 *US Pharm* 2000;28-41.
3371 *Aust N Z J Med* 1990;20:803-5.
3372 *Semin Nephrol* 1990;10:24-30.
3373 *J Clin Endocrinol Metab* 2000;85:2797-800.
3374 *J Nutr* 2000;130:1937-45.
3375 *Atherosclerosis* 2000;152:143-7.
3376 *Pharmacotherapy* 2000;20:981-90.
3378 *J Cancer Res Clin Oncol* 2000;126:448-54.
3380 *Nutr Cancer* 1996;26:289-302.
3381 *Biochem Biophys Res Commun* 1996;223:278-82.
3382 *The Wellness Letter* 2001;17:5.
3383 *Midwifery Today Int Midwife* 1999;52:34-5.
3384 *Am J Hypertens* 1994;7:926-32.
3385 *JAMA* 1997;277:1624-32.
3386 *Ann Epidemiol* 1995;5:85-95.
3387 *Breast Cancer Res Treat* 2000;62:35-49.
3390 *Am J Physiol* 1997;272:H462-8.
3391 *J Nutr* 2001;131:287-90.
3392 *Scand J Plast Reconstr Surg Hand Surg* 2000;34:15-20.
3393 *Proc Soc Exp Biol Med* 1999;221:281-293.
3394 *Curr Med Chem* 2000;7:715-29.
3395 *Int J Cancer* 1997;71:600-4.
3396 *Lancet* 1996;347:1804.
3397 *Biochim Biophys Acta* 1996;1299:175-82.
3398 *Ann Rheum Dis* 1992;51:128-9.
3399 *N Engl J Med* 1989;321:1572-7.
3400 *Pediatrics* 1998;101:148-53.
3401 *N Engl J Med* 1995;333:276-82.
3402 *Arch Intern Med* 1999;159:2070-6.
3403 *J Altern Complement Med* 1998;4:289-303.
3404 *J Altern Complement Med* 1998;4:429-57.
3405 *J Clin Invest* 1995;96:132-40.
3406 *Metabolism* 1998;47:573-7.
3407 *Jpn J Pharmacol* 1999;79:335-41.
3409 *Am J Chin Med* 1998;26:159-70.
3410 *Phytochemistry* 1999;51:891-8.
3411 *Chung Kuo Chung Hsi I Chieh Ho Tsa Chih* 1996;16:733-7.
3412 *J Cell Biochem* 1998;69:483-9.
3414 *Life Sci* 1997;60:2349-59.
3415 *Biol Pharm Bull* 1996;19:294-6.
3416 *Am J Chin Med* 1996;24:111-25.
3417 *Chung Kuo Chung Hsi I Chieh Ho Tsa Chih* 1995;15:476-8.
3418 *Nephrol Dial Transplant* 1995;10:142-3.
3419 *Chung Kuo Chung Hsi I Chieh Ho Tsa Chih* 1994;14:271-3, 259.
3420 *Cancer Invest* 1994;12:611-5.
3421 *Biol Pharm Bull* 1993;16:1291-3.
3424 *Am J Chin Med* 1993;21:257-62.
3425 *Chung Kuo Chung Hsi I Chieh Ho Tsa Chih* 1992;12:267-9, 259.
3427 *Chin Med J (English)* 1992;105:97-101.
3428 *Chung Hua I Hsueh Tsa Chih (Taipei)* 1992;72:27-9, 63.
3429 *Chung Hua I Hsueh Tsa Chih (Taipei)* 1991;71:612-5, 42.
3431 *Chin Med J (English)* 1991;104:4-8.
3432 *Chung Hsi I Chieh Ho Tsa Chih* 1990;10:485-7, 454.
3434 *Biotherapy* 1990;2:199-205.
3435 *Chung Kuo Chung Yao Tsa Chih* 1990;15:53-5, 65.
3436 *Chung Kuo Chung Yao Tsa Chih* 1989;14:616-8, 640.
3437 *Jpn J Exp Med* 1989;59:157-61.
3450 *Arch Intern Med* 1999;159:2170-4.
3451 *J Clin Psychiatry* 1998;59:431-2.
3452 *Anaesth Intensive Care* 1995;23:449-52.
3453 *Anaesthesia* 1998;53:506-10.
3454 *Am J Clin Nutr* 1999;70:1077-82.
3455 *J Pediatr* 1999;135:208-17.
3456 *J Pediatr* 1999;135:689-97.
3457 *J Med Microbiol* 1996;44:70-4.
3458 *Clin Exp Allergy* 2000;30:1604-10.
3460 *J Urol* 1999;161:558-65.
3461 *Arzneimittelforschung* 1999;49:900-4.
3462 *Natural Pharmacy* 1998;2:10.
3463 *J Clin Endocrinol Metab* 1999;84:3988-90.
3464 *J Clin Endocrinol Metab* 1999;84:4541-4.
3465 *J Am Coll Cardiol* 1998;32:1336-44.
3467 *Ann Med* 1999;31:318-26.
3469 *Thorax* 2000;55(2):102-8.
3470 *J Natl Cancer Inst* 2000;92:154-60.
3471 *Atemvegs und Lungenkrankheiten* 1997;23:291-4.
3472 *Lancet* 1999;354(9196):2171.
3473 *Lancet* 1981;1:487-9.
3474 *Am J Gastroenterol* 1982;77:158-61.
3475 *J Pathol* 1989;159:255-64.
3476 *Singapore Med J* 1990;31:463-5.
3477 *Crit Care Clin* 1997;13(4):849-88.
3478 *JAMA* 1979;242:2759-60.
3479 *Ann Emerg Med* 1986;15:470-3.
3480 *South Med J* 1981;74(5):639-40.
3481 *Lancet* 1967;1:437.
3482 *Vet Hum Toxicol* 1982;24:36.
3483 *Med Lett Drugs Ther* 1979;21:29-32.
3484 *Am J Health Syst Pharm* 1999;56:125-38.
3485 *Am J Health Syst Pharm* 2000;57:328,333,335.
3486 *J Pharm Pharmacol* 1999;51:505-12.
3487 *JAMA* 1998;280:1566-7.
3488 *J Toxicol Clin Toxicol* 1995;33(1):83-6.
3490 *Vet Hum Toxicol* 1994;36(3):212-5.
3491 *Monatsschr Kinderheilkd* 1991;139(6):366-7.
3492 *Nat Toxins* 1997;5(5):186-92.
3493 *Biochem Biophys Res Commun* 1995;217:966-71.
3494 *Med Times* 1977;105:63-4.
3495 *Ann Emerg Med* 1985;14(4):350-3.
3496 *JAMA* 1988;259:1943.
3497 *Arch Intern Med* 1997;157:913-9.
3499 *J Fla Med Assoc* 1978;65:188-91.
3501 *Life Sci* 1986;39:263-8.
3502 *Cancer* 1988;62:944-8.
3503 *Arch Surg* 1986;62:1455-9.
3504 *Diabetes* 1998;62:194-7.
3508 *Breast Cancer Res Treat* 1995;35:91-5.
3509 Malloy MJ, Kane JP. Agents used in hyperlipidemia. In: B. Katzung, ed. Basic and Clinical Pharmacology. 4th ed. Norwald, CT: Appleton and Lange, 1989.
3510 *Prev Med* 1996;25:34-7.
3511 *Oncology* 1995;52:265-71.
3513 *Clin Exp Allergy* 1996;26:216-22.

3515 *Experientia* 1995;51:927-35.
3516 *J Gastroenterol Hepatol* 1997;12:495-9.
3521 *Am J Psychiatry* 1993;150:522.
3523 *Br J Psychiatry* 1989;154:48-51.
3524 *J Clin Psychiatry* 1998;59:689.
3525 *Med J Aust* 1999;170:218-9.
3526 *Pharmacotherapy* 1999;19:870-6.
3529 *J Naturopath Med* 1996;6:33-7.
3530 *Alt Med Rev* 1999;4:96-103.
3531 *Bottom Line* 1999;20:1.
3535 Anon. Toxic algae in lake Sammamish. King County, WA. October 28, 1998; URL: splash.metrokc.gov/wlr/waterres/lakes/bloom.htm (Accessed 5 December 1999).
3536 Anon. Health Canada announces results of blue-green algal products testing – only Spirulina found Microcystin-free. Health Canada, September 27, 1999; URL: www.hc-sc.gc.ca/english/archives/releases/99_114e.htm (Accessed 27 October 1999).
3540 *Diabetes Care* 1999;22:1296-301.
3541 *Free Radic Res* 1999;31:171-7.
3542 *Diabetes Care* 1997;20:369-73.
3545 *Diabetes Care* 1999;22:280-7.
3546 *Ann N Y Acad Sci* 1994;738:257-64.
3547 *Skin Pharmacol Appl Skin Physiol* 1999;12:299-304.
3548 *J Nerv Ment Dis* 1999;187:532-9.
3549 *BMJ* 1996;313:253-8.
3550 *Arzneimittelforschung* 1999;49:289-96.
3551 *BMJ* 1999;319:1534-9.
3552 *Arch Intern Med* 2000;160:152-6.
3553 *J Pharmacol Exp Ther* 1999;290:1363-8.
3554 *Lancet* 1999;353:2129.
3555 *Biol Psychiatry* 1999;46:1707-8.
3556 *Ann Pharmacother* 1999;33:502.
3557 *Diabetologia* 1995;38:1425-33.
3558 Huang KC. The Pharmacology of Chinese Herbs. 2nd ed. Boca Raton, FL: CRC Press, LLC 1999:267.
3559 Upton R, ed. Schisandra Berry: Analytical, quality control, and therapeutic monograph. Santa Cruz, CA: American Herbal Pharmacopoeia 1999;1-25.
3561 *Am J Health Syst Pharm* 2000;57:530-4.
3562 *Alternative Medicine Alert* 1999;12:133-5.
3563 Chevallier A. Encyclopedia of Medicinal Plants. New York, NY: DK Publishing 1996;202.
3564 Anon. Lapacho. The Natural Pharmacist 2000. http://www.tnp.com/substance.asp?ID=67 (Accessed 7 April 2000).
3567 Anon. Colostrum. The Natural Pharmacist. Prima Communications, Inc., 2000. http://www.tnp.com/substance.asp?ID=121 (Accessed 5 May 2000).
3568 *J Clin Psychopharmacol* 2000;20:115-7.
3569 *Pharmacotherapy* 2000;20:568-74.
3570 Ereshefsky B, Gewertz N, Lam YMF, et al. Determination of SJW differential metabolism at CYP2D6 and CYP3A4, using dextromethorphan probe methodology. Abstract Poster Presentations, 39th NCDEU Annual Meeting, 1999:Poster 130 128.
3571 Gewertz N, Ereshefsky B, Lam YWF, et al. Determination of the differential effects of St. John's wort on the CYP1A2 and NAT2 metabolic pathways using caffeine probe methodology. Abstract Poster Presentations, 39th NCDEU Annual Meeting, 1999: Poster 131.
3574 Anon. Bee Propolis. MotherNature.com 1999. http://www.mothernature.com/library/books/natmed/bee_propolis.asp (Accessed 28 May 2000).
3577 Anon. PC-SPES. UCSF Cancer Center Communications 2000. Available at: http://cc.ucsf.edu/clinical/uro_pc-spes.html (Accessed 2 June 2000).
3579 *J Agric Food Chem* 1997;45:1638-43.
3580 Anon. OPCs (Oligomeric Proanthocyanidins). The Natural Pharmacist 2000. http://www.tnp.com/substance.asp?ID=181. (Accessed 3 June 2000).
3582 Pizzorno JE, Murray MT, eds. Textbook of Natural Medicine. 2nd ed. New York, NY: Chuchill Livingstone, 1999.
3583 *Fertil Steril* 1996;66:430-4.
3585 *Biol Trace Elem Res* 1996;53:65-83.
3586 *Fertil Steril* 1994;61:929-34.
3589 *Am J Clin Nutr* 2000;71:861-72.
3590 *Eur J Clin Nutr* 2000;54:288-97.
3593 *Am J Cardiol* 1999;15:1488-90.
3595 *Circulation* 1996;93:2135-41.
3596 *J Hypertens* 2000;18:229-34.
3598 *Pharmacist's Letter/Prescriber's Letter* 1999;15(1):150105.
3599 *Life Sci* 2000;66:PL 133-9.
3600 *Drugs Exp Clin Res* 1994;20:169-76.
3601 *Int J Clin Pharmacol Res* 1990;10:75-9.
3602 *Int J Clin Pharmacol Res* 1990;10:355-60.
3603 *Drugs Exp Clin Res* 1990;16:101-6.
3604 *Drugs Exp Clin Res* 1987;13:417-23.
3605 *Clin Immunol* 1999;92:103-10.
3606 *AIDS* 1997;11:185-90.
3607 *Acta Europ Fertil* 1992;23:221-4.
3608 *Hum Reprod Update* 1996;2:87-102.
3609 *Reprod Nutr Develop* 1988;28:1317-27.
3610 *Int J Androl* 1984;7:484-94.
3611 *Fertil Steril* 1977;28:1333-6.
3612 *Int J Fertil* 1977;22:85-91.
3616 Anon. Carnitor (levocarnitine) package insert. Sigma-Tau Pharmaceuticals Inc, Gaithersburg, MD. December 1999.
3617 *J Child Neurol* 1995;10:S40-4.
3618 *Ann Neurol* 1994;35:482-7.
3619 *J Eur Acad Dermatol Venereol* 1999;13:205-9.
3620 *Indian Pediatr* 1992;29:1501-5.
3621 *Pediatr Res* 1984;18:815-9.
3622 *South Med J* 1993;86:1411-2.
3623 *Drugs Exp Clin Res* 1991;17:225-35.
3624 *Int J Clin Pharmacol Ther Toxicol* 1985;23:569-72.
3625 *Am Heart J* 2000;139:S120-3.
3626 *Int J Clin Pharmacol Ther Toxicol* 1988;26:217-20.
3627 *Postgrad Med J* 1996;72:45-50.
3628 *J Am Coll Cardiol* 1995;26:380-7.
3629 *Drugs Exp Clin Res* 1992;18:355-65.
3630 *Neuropsychobiology* 1997;35:16-23.
3631 *Circulation* 1988;77:767-73.
3632 *Proc Assoc Am Physicians* 1997;109:146-53.
3633 *Semin Perinatol* 1999;23:152-61.
3634 *J Pediatr* 1995;126:287-92.
3635 *Biol Neonate* 1990;58:81-8.
3636 *Acta Paediatr Hung* 1986;27:253-8.
3637 *J Pediatr* 1983;102:931-5.
3639 *Sports Med* 1996;22:109-32.
3640 *Clin Chim Acta* 1982;122:369-75.
3641 *Cancer Chemother Pharmacol* 1999;44:170-2.
3642 *Eur J Clin Pharmacol* 1998;54:503-8.
3643 *J Perinat Med* 1995;23:477-85.
3644 *Biol Neonate* 1990;58:89-92.
3645 *J Ren Nutr* 1998;8:118-21.
3646 *Kidney Int* 1999;69:93-106.

3647 *Kidney Int* 1990;38:912-8.
3648 *Drugs Exp Clin Res* 1999;25:167-71.
3649 *Eur J Appl Physiol* 1990;61:486-90.
3650 *Eur J Appl Physiol* 1985;54:131-5.
3651 *J Am Coll Nutr* 1999;18:77-82.
3652 *Diabetes Res Clin Pract* 1991;14:191-5.
3653 *Int J Tissue React* 1990;12:183-6.
3657 *J Affect Disord* 2000;60:121-31.
3658 Anon. W&B Associates Inc. website. URL http://www.wandb.com/cholesterol.6.htm (Accessed 30 March 2000).
3661 *J Lipid Res* 1998;39:1055-61.
3662 *J Lipid Res* 1989;30:1319-30.
3663 *Proc Assoc Am Physicians* 1998;110:32-9.
3667 *Anticancer Res* 1998;18:471-3.
3668 *Anticancer Res* 1996;16:2797-804.
3669 *Int J Immunopharmacol* 1996;18:693-700.
3672 *J Atheroscler Thromb* 1995;2:60-5.
3673 *Metabolism* 1999;48:68-73.
3678 Anon. FDA alert on misuse of consumer products containing GHB, GBL and BD. Food and Drug Administration, Rockville, MD. June 15, 1999. Available at: http://www.fda.gov/cder/graphics/ghb.gif.
3679 Anon. Important message for health professionals: Report serious adverse events associated with dietary supplements containing GBL, GHB or BD. Food and Drug Administration, Rockville, MD. August 25, 1999. Available at: http://vm.cfsan.fda.gov/~dms/mwgblghb.html.
3680 Otto A. Acquaintance rape drug may one day help instead of hurt (news). Pharmacy Today. American Pharmaceutical Association, Washington, DC. April 2000:17.
3681 Hillory J. Farias and Samantha Reid date-rape drug prohibition act of 2000. 106th Congress of the United States of America. HR 2130.
3682 *JAMA* 1991;265:447-8.
3683 *Ann Pharmacother* 1992;26:647-8.
3684 *Lancet* 1998;351:38.
3686 *Lancet* 1989;2:787-9.
3687 *J Am Pharm Assoc* 1999;39:519-25.
3688 *Am J Emerg Med* 1991;9:321-4.
3689 *Sleep* 1990;13:479-90.
3690 *Biol Psychiatry* 1989;26:331-43.
3691 *J Clin Psychiatry* 1985;46:222-5.
3692 *Can J Neurol Sci* 1979;6:1-6.
3693 *Encephale* 1980;6:93-9.
3694 *Eur Arch Psychiatry Clin Neurosci* 1994;244:113-4.
3695 *Neuropsychopharmacology* 1993;9:77-81.
3696 *Alcohol Clin Exp Res* 1992;16:673-6.
3699 *Gen Pharmacol* 1992;23:1027-34.
3700 Goodman LS, Gilman A. The Pharmacological Basis of Therapeutics. 5th ed. New York, NY: Macmillan Publ. Co., Inc., 1975.
3701 *Proc Soc Exp Biol Med* 1998;217(3):369-78.
3702 *Rev Latinoam Microbiol* 1991;33:149-51.
3703 *Int J Food Microbiol* 1991;13(1):81-5.
3704 *Int J Food Microbiol* 1988;6(3):263-8.
3705 *Ann Allergy Asthma Immunol* 1996; 76(5): 416-8.
3706 *Am J Emerg Med* 1997;15:516-20.
3707 *Anticancer Res* 1996 Mar-Apr;16:915-20.
3710 Upton R, ed. Ashwagandha Root (Withania somnifera): Analytical, quality control, and therapuetic monograph. Santa Cruz, CA: American Herbal Pharmacopoeia 2000:1-25.
3711 *Cancer Lett* 2000;148:9-17.
3713 *J Clin Lab Immunol* 1988;25:125-9.
3714 *J Rheumatol* 2001;28:1347-55.
3716 *Ann Allergy Asthma Immunol* 1999;82:194-7.
3717 *Allergol Immunopathol (Madr)* 1998;26:288-90.
3718 *Carcinogenesis* 1998;19:2163-8.
3719 *Int J Obes Relat Metab Disord* 2001;25:316-24.
3720 *Biochem Biophys Res Commun* 1995;208:779-85.
3721 *Gene* 1995;161:151-6.
3722 *Cell Immunol* 1990;126:278-89.
3723 *Cancer Res* 1983;43:5151-5.
3724 *Immunopharmacology* 1987;13:159-71.
3726 *Chung Hua Min Kuo Wei Sheng Wu Chi Mien I Hsueh Tsa Chih* 1992;25:1-11.
3727 *Jpn J Pharmacol* 1992;59:89-96.
3728 *Chem Pharm Bull (Tokyo)* 1997;45:492-4.
3729 *Oncology* 1996;53:382-5.
3730 *Planta Med* 1995;61:527-30.
3731 *Chung Kuo Chung Hsi I Chieh Ho Tsa Chih* 1995;15:284-6.
3732 *Chung Hsi I Chieh Ho Tsa Chih* 1991;11:79-82, 67.
3733 *J Tradit Chin Med* 1989;9:132-4.
3734 *Chung Hsi I Chieh Ho Tsa Chih* 1989;9:270-1, 259-60.
3735 *Chung Hsi I Chieh Ho Tsa Chih* 1989;9:272-3, 260.
3736 *Phytochemistry* 1998;48:1357-60.
3737 *Chem Pharm Bull (Tokyo)* 1996;44:847-9.
3740 *Chem Res Toxicol* 1994;7(6):850-6.
3741 *Ann Intern Med* 1992;117(2):129-32.
3742 *Gastroenterol Clin Biol* 1992;16(1):92-5.
3743 *Therapie* 1997;52(2):97-103.
3744 *Lancet* 1992;340:674.
3745 *Life Sci* 1998;63:1679-84.
3746 *Braz J Med Biol Res* 1996;29:669-75.
3747 *J Ethnopharmacol* 1995;47:129-34.
3748 *Mutagenesis* 1996;11:573-9.
3749 *Proc Natl Acad Sci USA* 1985;82:2478-82.
3750 *Res Commun Chem Pathol Pharmacol* 1994;84:111-8.
3751 *Yao Hsueh Hsueh Pao* 1989;24:366-71.
3752 *Lett Appl Microbiol* 1998;27:207-10.
3753 *Microbios* 1996;86:237-46.
3754 *J Ethnopharmacol* 1994;44:143-6.
3755 *J Ethnopharmacol* 1997;56:233-6.
3756 *Plant Foods Hum Nutr* 1998;52:231-9.
3757 *Indian J Exp Biol* 1998;36:46-50.
3758 *J Ethnopharmacol* 1996;50:167-70.
3759 *Oncology* 1991;48:347-50.
3760 *Cancer Lett* 1993;72:5-9.
3761 *J Ethnopharmacol* 1998;62:15-24.
3762 *Planta Med* 1990;56:426-9.
3763 *Planta Med* 1993;59:408-12.
3764 *J Ethnopharmacol* 1994;44:117-21.
3765 *Pharmacol Res* 1996;33:1-4.
3766 *J Ethnopharmacol* 1986;17:105-38.
3767 *Biol Pharm Bull* 1999;22:265-7.
3768 *J Nat Prod* 1996;59:525-7.
3769 *Pharmacogenetics* 1997;7:391-6.
3771 *Clin Pharmacol Ther* 1998;64:655-60.
3773 *Br J Clin Pharmacol* 1998;45:355-9.
3774 *Clin Pharmacol Ther* 1998;64:477-83.
3775 *Clin Pharmacokinet* 1997;33:103-21.
3800 Tyler VE, Brady LR, Robbers JE. Pharmacognosy. 7th ed. Philadelphia, PA: Lea & Febiger, 1976.
3801 *Cephalalgia* 1994;14:228-34;discussion 182.
3802 *J Gastroenterol* 1997;32:765-8.
3803 *Am J Gastroenterol* 1998;93:1131-5.
3804 *J Adv Nurs* 1997;26:543-9.

3805 United States Pharmacopeial Convention I, editor. Drug Information for the Health Care Professional. 19th ed. Micromedex, 1999.
3807 *J Hosp Infect* 1991;18:301-6.
3808 *Ann Allergy Asthma Immunol* 1996; 76(5):416-8.
3811 *Hum Exp Toxicol* 1996;15:747-50.
3818 *Exp Neurol* 1997;146:518-25.
3822 *Am J Chin Med* 1991;19:223-31.
3823 *J Ethnopharmacol* 1994;44:123-5.
3824 *J Ethnopharmacol* 1988;22:211-21.
3825 *Fund Clin Pharmacol* 1998;12:82-7.
3826 *Am Rev Respir Dis* 1975;111:703-5.
3828 *J Ethnopharmacol* 1987;19:81-4.
3829 *Contact Dermatitis* 1983;9:390-6.
3830 *Phytochemistry* 1996;41:531-6.
3831 *Mol Cell Biochem* 1993;119:143-50.
3832 *J Ethnopharmacol* 1997;57:29-34.
3833 *Int J Food Sci Nutr* 1995;46:47-51.
3834 *J Ethnopharmacol* 1997;58:39-44.
3835 *Derm Beruf Umwelt* 1990;38(6):190-2.
3836 *Experientia* 1978;34(11):1442-3.
3837 *Derm Beruf Umwelt* 1985;33(3):95-8.
3838 *Am J Emerg Med* 1996;14(7):671-4.
3839 *Cutis* 1998;62:139-42.
3841 *Planta Med* 1995;61:307-12.
3842 *Eur J Pharmacol* 1995;273:73-81.
3846 *Pediatrics* 2002;109:E19.
3847 *MMWR Morb Mortal Wkly Rep* 1994;43:525-6.
3850 *Br J Nutr* 1986;55:643-9.
3851 *J Immunol* 1992;148:1519-25.
3852 *J Pharm Sci* 1996;85:518-24.
3853 *Pharm Res* 1995;12:1917-23.
3854 *Lloydia* 1975;38:109-16.
3858 *J Ethnopharmacol* 1997;57:209-12.
3859 *US Pharm* 1999;24:66-76.
3860 *Alt Med Alert* 1999 Dec;138-42.
3861 *JAMA* 2000;283:779-82.
3862 *J Clin Endocrinol Metab* 2000;85(1):55-9.
3863 *Int J Gynaecol Obstet* 1999;67:169-74.
3865 *J Acq Immun Def Synd* 1993;6:459-65.
3866 *AIDS Res Hum Retroviruses* 1992;8:625-31.
3867 *Psychoneuroendocrinology* 1997;22:S11-8.
3868 *Diabet Med* 1999;16:1040-3.
3869 *Hormone Metab Res Suppl* 1980;9:105-7.
3870 *Br J Clin Pharmacol* 1999;48:819-25.
3871 *Free Rad Biol Med* 1995;19:227-50.
3872 *Int J Clin Pharmacol Ther* 1998;36:625-8.
3873 *Diabet Care* 1995;18:1160-7.
3874 *Exp Clin Endocrinol Diabet* 1996;104:284-8.
3875 *Arzneimittelforschung* 1995;45:872-4.
3876 *Free Rad Biol Med* 1999;27:309-14.
3877 *Biochem Mol Biol Int* 1995;37:591-7.
3878 *Diabetes* 1999;48:2045-51.
3879 *Free Rad Biol Med* 1998;24:1023-39.
3880 *Gut* 1982;23:1088-93.
3881 *Hear Res* 1999;128:40-4.
3882 *Biochem Mol Biol Int* 1999;47:815-23.
3883 *Free Rad Biol Med* 1999;27:75-81.
3884 *Neurotoxicol Teratol* 1990;12:619-22.
3885 *Arzneimittelforschung* 1993;43:1359-62.
3886 *Lancet* 2000;355:517-22.
3887 *Lancet* 2000;355:511-2.
3888 *Arterioscler Thromb Vasc Biol* 2000;20:500-6.
3889 *J Pediatr* 1993;122:292-6.
3891 *J Pain Symptom Manage* 2000;19:45-52.
3892 *Biol Psychiatry* 1999;45:1533-41.
3893 *J Clin Endocrinol Metab* 1997;82:2363-7.
3894 Environmental Protection Agency. Cesium. 2002. Available at: www.epa.gov/radiation/radionuclides/cesium.htm.
3896 *N Engl J Med* 2000;342:154-60.
3898 *N Engl J Med* 1993;328:1444-9.
3899 *Circulation* 2001;103:919-25.
3900 Peirce A. The American Pharmaceutical Association Practical Guide to Natural Medicines. New York, NY: William Morrow and Co., 1999.
3901 Tyler VE, Brady LR, Robbers JB. Pharmacognosy. 8th ed. Philadelphia, PA: Lea and Fibiger, 1981.
3902 *Wien Klin Wochenschr* 1990;102:667-73.
3903 *Curr Med Res Opin* 1998;14:127-39.
3904 *Ann Urol (Paris)* 1984;18:193-5.
3905 Whitmore A. FDA warns consumers against dietary supplement products that may contain Digitalis mislabeled as Plantain. Food and Drug Administration, U.S. Department of the Interior, Washington DC, 1997.
3906 *Am J Clin Nutr* 2001;73:219-24.
3907 *Lancet* 2001;357:89-95.
3908 *BMJ* 1994;309:824-825.
3909 *Am J Clin Nutr* 2000;71:386S-392S.
3910 *Lancet* 2001;357:657-63.
3911 *Atherosclerosis* 1990;83(2-3):167-75.
3912 *Dtsch Z Verdau Stoffwechselkr* 1984;44(5):245-51.
3914 *Ann Pharmacother* 2001;35:424-6.
3916 *In Vivo* 1992; 6(2):161-5.
3919 Agricultural Research Service. Dr. Duke's Phytochemical and Ethnobotanical Databases. Available at: www.ars-grin.gov/duke/.
3921 *Braz J Med Biol Res* 1984; 17:313-21. [primary reference in Taylor].
3922 *Endocrinol* 2000;141:980-7.
3924 *N Z Med J* 1994;107:243.
3925 *J Lab Clin Med* 1995; 126:350-2.
3926 *Cancer Lett* 2001;167:175-82.
3927 *J Nat Prod* 1996; 59(2):196-9.
3928 *Indian J Exp Biol* 1995; 33:861-4.
3929 *Onderstepoort Journal Veterinary Res* 1996;63:327-34.
3930 *Clin Immunol Immunopathol* 1979;12:183-90.
3931 *Chung Hsi I Chieh Ho Tsa Chih* 1990;10:85-7.
3932 *Br Med J (Clin Res Ed)* 1981;282:186-7.
3933 *N Engl J Med* 1993;328:1450-6.
3934 *N Engl J Med* 1996;334:1156-62.
3935 *Arch Intern Med* 1998;158:668-75.
3936 *Lancet* 1996;347:781-6.
3937 *Lancet* 1997;349:1715-20.
3938 *Am J Clin Nutr* 1996;64:190-6.
3939 *The Tan Sheet* January 24, 2000;10.
3940 *Anticancer Drugs* 1997;8:265-8.
3941 *Proc Soc Exp Biol Med* 1999;220:271-5.
3942 *Biol Psychiatry* 1998;43:868-72.
3943 *Int Clin Psychopharmacol* 1998;13:147-55.
3944 *J Clin Psychiatry* 1996;57:167-73.
3945 *Am J Psychiatry* 1992;149:391-3.
3946 *Eur Neuropsychopharmacol* 1999;9:475-7.
3947 *Ann Pharmacother* 1999;33:1195-202.
3948 *Am J Psychiatry* 1994;151:925-6.
3949 *N Engl J Med* 1994;330:1029-35.
3951 *Oral Dis* 1998;4:78-83.
3952 *Clin Pharmacol Ther* 1984;35:161-169.
3953 *Cancer Epidemiol Biomarkers Prev* 1999;8:489-93.
3954 *Dis Colon Rectum* 1993;36:227-34.
3955 *N Engl J Med* 1994;331:141-7.
3956 *J Natl Cancer Inst* 1992;84:47-51.

3957 *Cancer Res* 1988;48:4701-5.
3958 *Cancer Epidemiol Biomarkers Prev* 1997;6:769-74.
3959 *J Natl Cancer Inst* 1998;90:440-6.
3960 *Scand J Gastroenterol* 1998;33:294-300.
3961 *Cancer* 1999;86:37-42.
3962 *Am J Clin Nutr* 2000;71:575-82.
3963 *Cancer Causes Control* 1991;2:325-57.
3964 *Cancer Causes Control* 1997;8:575-90.
3965 *J Sex Marital Ther* 1998;24:139-43.
3966 *J Sex Marital Ther* 1999;25:1-2.
3967 *J Clin Psychiatry* 1998;59:199-200.
3969 *J Sex Marital Ther* 1999;25:2-5.
3970 *J Clin Psychiatry* 1992;53:119-22.
3971 *J Clin Psychiatry* 1992;53:207-9.
3972 *Ann Clin Psychiatry* 1995;7:189-201.
3973 *Primary Psychiatry* 1999;6:40-54.
3974 *Lancet* 1999;354:1880.
3975 *Toxicol Appl Pharmacol* 1998;149:210-6.
3976 *Cancer Epidemiol Biomarkers Prev* 2000;9:113-7.
3977 Henkel. FDA. Soy: Health Claims for Soy Protein, Questions About Other Components. May-June 2000. Available at: http://vm.cfsan.fda.gov/~dms/fdsoypr.html#health.
3978 *J Clin Endocrinol Metab* 1998;83:2223-35.
3980 *Am J Clin Nutr* 1998;68:1431S-5S.
3981 *Cancer Epidemiol Biomarkers Prev* 1996;5:785-94.
3982 *J Nutr* 2000;130:654S-5S.
3983 *J Nutr* 2000;130:656S-7S.
3984 *J Endocrinol* 1995;147:295-302.
3985 *J Nutr* 2000;130:658S-9S.
3986 *Menopause* 1997;4:89-94.
3987 *J Nutr* 2000;130:660-1.
3988 *J Clin Endocrinol Metab* 1995;80:1685-90.
3989 *J Clin Endocrinol Metab* 1999;84:3479-84.
3990 *Lancet* 2000;355:163-4.
3991 *J Clin Oncol* 2000;18:1068-74.
3992 *J Nutr* 2000;130:662S-3S.
3993 *Biochem Biophys Res Commun* 1995;212:172-7.
3994 *J Clin Endocrinol Metab* 1999;84:4017-24.
3995 *Biochem Biophys Res Commun* 1994;199:1504-8.
3996 *Med Sci Sports Exerc* 1999;31:1108-10.
3997 *Clin J Sport Med* 1998;8:298-304.
3998 *J Am Pharm Assoc (Wash)* 1999;39:803-10.
3999 *Am J Health Syst Pharm* 1999;56:1608-10.
4001 *Pharmacol Biochem Behav* 1997;58:887-91.
4002 *Eur J Pharmacol* 1994;252:51-9.
4003 *Lancet* 1987;2:453.
4004 *Lancet* 1987;2:274-5.
4005 *Ann Thorac Surg* 1986;41:54-7.
4006 *Pharm Pharmacol Lett* 1996;6:86-9.
4007 *J Herbs Spices Med Plants* 1995;3:71-6.
4008 *Aust Vet J* 1993;70:169-71.
4009 Dukes JA. CRC Handbook of Medicinal Herbs. first ed. Boca Raton, FL: CRC Press, Inc., 1985.
4010 *J Ethnopharmacol* 1985;13:157-63.
4011 *Inflamm Res* 1998;47(12):476-81.
4012 *Bioorg Med Chem Lett* 1998;8:339-44.
4013 *Lloydia* 1976;39:218-22.
4014 *J Nat Prod* 1998;61:1531-4.
4015 *Br J Nutr* 1979;41:57-63.
4016 *Am J Clin Nutr* 1999;70:536-43.
4018 *Clin Pharmacol Ther* 1998;64:144-9.
4019 *Cancer Epidemiol Biomarkers Prev* 1995;4:877-84.
4020 *Planta Med* 1998;64:683-5.
4021 WHO working group. Pyrrolizidine alkaloids. Environmental Health Criteria, 80. WHO: Geneva, 1988.
4022 *J Thorac Cardiovasc Surg* 1985;89:351-7.
4023 *Contact Dermatitis* 1980;6:111-9.
4025 *Thromb Haemost* 1981;46:604-11.
4026 *Clin Sci (Colch)* 1981;61:317-24.
4027 *Australas J Dermatol* 1998;39:244-7.
4028 *J Hosp Infect* 1998;40:175-8.
4029 *Contact Dermatitis* 1997;36:117-8.
4030 *Vet Hum Toxicol* 1995;37:557-8.
4031 *Australas J Dermatol* 1992;33:145-9.
4032 *Hum Psychopharmacol Clin Exp* 2001;16:353-6.
4033 *Contact Dermatitis* 1987;16:84-6.
4034 *Contact Dermatitis* 1988;19:355-7.
4037 *Psychopharmacology (Berl)* 1994;116:469-74.
4038 *Pharmacol Toxicol* 1992;71:120-6.
4039 *Contact Dermatitis* 1982;8:396-400.
4041 *J Ethnopharmacol* 1989;27:285-95.
4042 *Chem Pharm Bull (Tokyo)* 1994;42:1101-5.
4043 *Biol Pharm Bull* 1996;19:1046-8.
4044 *Chem Pharm Bull (Tokyo)* 1990;38:1313-6.
4045 *Planta Med* 1989;55:349-50.
4046 *Chin Med J* 1989;102:327-32.
4047 *Pediatr Neurosurg* 1997;27:45-8.
4048 *J Nat Prod* 1992;55:88-92.
4049 *J Nat Prod* 1992;55:340-6.
4050 *Pharmacol Res* 1995;3:29-32.
4052 *Prostaglandins Leukot Essent Fatty Acids* 1998;59:235-8.
4053 *J Pharm Pharmacol* 1996;48:858-60.
4054 *J Pharm Pharmacol* 1995;47:731-3.
4055 *J Neurol Neurosurg Psychiatry* 1995;58:639-40.
4056 *J Clin Pharmacol* 2000; 40:1150-3.
4058 *Contact Dermatitis* 1990;22:212-7.
4059 *J Hortic Sci* 1992;67:197-202.
4060 *J Food Prot* 1997;60:1262-4.
4062 *J Appl Nutr* 1995;47:96-102.
4063 *Mycopathologia* 1994;128:151-3.
4064 *Bull Tokyo Dent Coll* 1990;31:17-21.
4065 *J Appl Microbiol* 1998;85:211-8.
4066 *J Agric Food Chem* 1998;46:3590-5.
4067 *Food Chem Toxicol* 1994;32:31-6.
4068 *Toxicol Lett* 1984;21:73-81.
4069 *Br Med J* 1978;1:1392-4.
4070 *Chemotherapy* 1996;42:286-93.
4072 *J Am Coll Toxicol* 1987;6:1-22.
4073 *J All Clin Immunol* 1998;101:S31.
4074 *BIBRA Toxicol Int* 1991;6.
4075 *Allergy* 1995;50:269-73.
4077 Tyler VE, Brady LR, Robbers JE. Pharmacognosy. 9th ed. Philadelphia, PA: Lea & Febiger, 1988.
4078 Foster S, Duke JA. The Peterson Field Guide to Medicinal Plants: Eastern and Central North America. Boston, MA: Houghton Mifflin Co., 1990.
4079 *J Allergy Clin Immunol* 1996;98:969-78.
4080 *Allerg Immunol (Paris)* 1988;20:63-6.
4081 *The Herb Companion* 1992;4:32-5.
4084 Drugs in Pregnancy and Lactation. 4th ed. Baltimore, MD: Williams & Wilkens, 1994.
4085 *N Engl J Med* 1999;340:1933-40.
4087 FDA. Center for Science in the Public Interest. A Food Labeling Guide. Available at: http://www.cfsan.fda.gov/~dms/flg-6c.html.
4089 *Semin Urol Oncol* 1999;17:85-90.
4092 *Biochem Biophys Res Commun* 1999;259:157-61.
4096 *Eur J Clin Invest* 1998;28:235-42.
4098 *Food Chem Toxicol* 1995;33:121-8.
4100 *Planta Med* 1989;55(4):379-84.

4101 The Bantam Medical Dictionary. rev ed. New York, NY: Bantam Books, 1990.
4104 *Arch Latinoam Nutr* 1997;47:195-202.
4105 *Cancer Lett* 1991;57:109-14.
4106 *Allergy* 1997;52:633-41.
4107 *Allergy* 1997;52:476-7.
4109 *J Pharm Sci* 1982;71:173-7.
4110 *Experientia* 1975;31:548-9.
4111 *J Allergy Clin Immunol* 1996;97:1416-8.
4112 *Int J Cancer* 1997;Suppl 10:7-9.
4113 *J Ethnopharmacol* 1999;64:91-3.
4114 *J Ethnopharmacol* 1998;62:209-14.
4116 *Indian J Exp Biol* 1997;35:236-9.
4117 *Chung Hua Min Kuo Wei Sheng Wu Chi Mien I Hsueh Tsa Chih* 1985;18:232-9.
4118 *J Nat Prod* 1992;55(3):357-63.
4120 *Leukemia* 1997;11:128-30.
4121 *Biosci Biotechnol Biochem* 1997;61:267-71.
4122 *Mutat Res* 1996;350:153-61.
4123 *Neurosci Lett* 1995;196:85-8.
4124 *Planta Med* 1999;65:234-8.
4125 Lacy CF, Armstrong LL, Ingrim NB, Lance LL. Drug Information Handbook. Hudson, OH: Lexi Comp Inc; 1998-9.
4137 *Cancer Res* 1998;58:2784-92.
4138 *Antimicrob Agents Chemother* 1997;41:1433-8.
4139 *Proc Natl Acad Sci U S A* 1993;90:1354-8.
4140 *Allergy* 1997;52(3):323-30.
4141 *J Chemother* 1996;8(3):207-9.
4142 *J Ethnopharmacol* 1986;15:271-8.
4143 *Int Arch Allergy Immunol* 1997;112:356-64.
4144 *J Allergy Clin Immunol* 1992;89:987-93.
4145 *J Nat Prod* 1979;42(5):483-8.
4146 *Int Arch Allergy Immunol* 1997;114:298-9.
4147 *Ann Trop Paediatr* 1996;16:287-91.
4148 *Am J Contact Dermat* 1996;7:38-40.
4149 *Biochem Biophys Res Commun* 1986;139:780-6.
4150 *Tubercle* 1990;71:293-5.
4151 *Plant J* 1997;12:1251-60.
4152 *Acta Physiol Pharmacol (Bulg)* 1984;10(2):13-20.
4200 *N Engl J Med* 1989;321:1432-7.
4201 Chevallier A. The Encyclopedia of Medicinal Plants. London, UK: Dorling Kindersley, Ltd., 1996.
4202 *Eur J Drug Metab Pharmacokinet* 1982;7:11-6.
4203 *Osteoarthritis Cartilage* 1998;6 Suppl A:14-21.
4205 *Semin Thromb Hemost* 1994;20:281-92.
4208 *Arch Ophthalmol* 2000;118:1556-63.
4211 *Ann Pharmacother* 1999;33:426-8.
4212 *Proc Soc Exp Biol Med* 1999;220:249-54.
4213 *Proc Soc Exp Biol Med* 1999;220:218-24.
4216 *Ann Intern Med* 1998;128:534-40.
4217 *J Cell Biochem Suppl* 1997;27:68-75.
4218 *CMAJ* 1998;158:1033-5.
4221 *Psychopharmacol* 1998;140:116-9.
4222 *Am J Epidemiol* 1999;149:162-7.
4224 *Psychopharmacol* 1998;139:230-8.
4225 *Diabetes Care* 1995;18:1373-5.
4227 *Cancer Lett* 1998;132:219-27.
4230 *J Am Coll Nutr* 1998;17:462-6.
4231 *J Am Diet Assoc* 1997;97:1110-5.
4233 *Biol Psychiatry* 1997;41:311-8.
4236 *Int J Sport Nutr* 1996;6:263-71.
4237 *Mil Med* 1999;164:85-91.
4239 *J Assist Reprod Genet* 1999;16:87-91.
4240 *Fertil Steril* 1999;71:517-22.
4242 *J Clin Endocrinol Metab* 1997;82:3498-505.
4243 *Chung Kuo Chung His I Chieh Ho Tsa Chih* 1995;15:325-7.
4248 *J Clin Pharmacol* 1999;39:327-48.
4249 *Fertil Steril* 1995;63:1027-31.
4250 *Ann N Y Acad Sci* 1995;774:291-3.
4251 *Clin Endocrinol* 1998;49:421-32.
4252 *Am J Obstet Gynecol* 1995;1536-9.
4253 *J Clin Endocrinol Metab* 1998;83:1928-34.
4254 *J Clin Endocrinol Metab* 1998;83:1756-61.
4255 *J Clin Endocrinol Metab* 1999;84:1527-33.
4259 FDA Talk Paper. FDA Warns About GBL-Related Products. 1999. Available at: vm.cfsan.fda.gov/~lrd/tpgbl2.html.
4260 Briggs GB, Freeman RK, Yaffe SJ. Drugs in Pregnancy and Lactation. 5th ed. Philadelphia: Lippincott Williams & Wilkins; 1998.
4261 FDA Talk Paper. FDA Approves Xyrem for Cataplexy Attacks in Patients with Narcolepsy. Issued July 17, 2002. Availbale at: http://www.fda.gov/bbs/topics/ANSWERS/2002/ANS01157.html.
4263 *J AOAC Int* 1995;78:1177-82.
4264 *BMJ* 1998; 17:1341-5.
4265 *Lipids* 1998;33:821-3.
4266 *Arch Pathol Lab Med* 1988;112:1041-4.
4267 *Cancer Causes Control* 1995;6:545-50.
4269 *Biomaterials* 1993;14:39-43.
4270 *Antimicrob Agents Chemother* 1990;34:2019-23.
4274 *N Engl J Med* 1997;337:473-9.
4275 *Vet Med Nauki* 1981;18(4):94-8.
4278 *Biochem Biophys Res Commun* 1999;265:499-502.
4282 National Genetics Resources Program. The Germplasm Resources Information Network. Available at: http://www.ars-grin.gov (Accessed 24 February 2000).
4283 *J Nat Prod* 1999;62:86-8.
4284 Bruneton J. Pharmacognosy Phytochemistry Medicinal Plants. 2nd ed. Paris, FR: Lavoisier, 1999:142.
4289 Protocol Title: A Phase 1B Dose-Range Study to Evaluate the Safety, Pharmacokinetics, and Effects of (+)-calaonlide A on surrogate markers in HIV-positive patients with no previous antiretroviral therapy. Protocol ID numbers: FDA 297A.
4290 Reuters Health. Anti-HIV herbal product shows therapeutic potential in phase I trial. November 1, 1999.
4291 *J Pharm Sci* 1998;87:1077-80.
4292 *Antimicrob Agents Chemother* 1999;43:1827-34.
4293 *J Virol* 1993;67(4):2412-20.
4294 *J Pharmacol Exp Ther* 1996;279:652-61.
4295 *J Pharmacol Exp Ther* 1996;279:645-51.
4299 *Phytother Res* 1999;13(1):75-7.
4300 *Drug Saf* 1998;18:251-72.
4301 *J Urol* 1997;157:2881-7.
4302 *Curr Ther Res* 1995;56:796-817.
4303 *J Clin Periodontol* 1992;19(5):305-10.
4304 Anon. Sida Cordifolia. Metro Marketing, Inc. Available at: http://metromkt.net/viable/1sidacor.shtml. (Accessed 9 March 2000).
4310 Anon. Sida Cordifolia Linn. Available at: http://www.modern-natural.com/sida_cordifolia.htm. (Accessed 9 March 2000).
4314 Anon. Strictly Medicinal Herb Seeds. Available at: http://www.chatlink.com/~herbseed/sida.html. (Accessed 9 March 2000).
4321 Maharishi Ayur-Ved Products Inc. 1998; Ayurvedic Herbs: Bala. http://www.mapi.com/cgi-local/shop.pl/page=herbbala.html/SID=1877132249. (Accessed 9 March 2000).

4322 *Ann Pharmacother* 2002;36:758-63.
4326 *Annu Rev Nutr* 1986;6:273-97.
4330 *Lancet* 1980;1:1134.
4331 *Lancet* 1980;1:1134.
4332 *Appl Microbiol Biotechnol* 1997;48:351-6.
4335 *J Nutr* 1995;125:2483-92.
4336 *Anticancer Res* 1999;19;5223-8.
4337 *Anticancer Res* 1999;19:1849-54.
4338 *Carcinogenesis* 1994;15:15-9.
4339 *Cancer Res* 1995;55:4059-64.
4340 *Carcinogenesis* 1998;19:403-11.
4341 *Immunol Lett* 1999;70:185-9.
4342 Bensky D, Gamble A, Kaptchuk T. Chinese Herbal Medicine Materia Medica. Seattle, WA: Eastland Press, 1996:214-6.
4343 Huang KC. The Pharmacology of Chinese Herbs. 2nd ed. Boca Raton, FL: CRC Press, LLC, 1999:258.
4344 Chevallier A. The Encyclopedia of Medicinal Plants. New York, NY: DK Publishing. 1996:170.
4345 *Hepatol* 1996;23(3):552-9.
4346 *Gastroenterology* 2000;118:380-9.
4347 *Am J Gastroenterol* 2000;95:S16-8.
4348 *Infection and Immun* 1999;67:302-7.
4349 *Intensive Care Med* 1997;23:517-23.
4350 *J Infect* 1998;36:171-4.
4351 *J Infect* 1998;37:307-8.
4352 *JAMA* 1994;271:1913-8.
4353 *Am J Gastroenterol* 1995;90:439-48.
4354 *Am J Gastroenterol* 1989;84:1285-7.
4355 *Gastroenterology* 1989;96:981-8.
4356 *J Pediatr Gastroenterol Nutr* 1993;16:419-25.
4357 *J Pediatr Gastroenterol Nutr* 1995;21:113-5.
4358 *Clin Infect Dis* 1998;27:222-3.
4359 *Eur J Clin Microbiol Infect Dis* 2000;19:16-20.
4360 *Aliment Pharmacol Ther* 1999;13:1663-8.
4361 *Gastroenterology* 1994;106:65-72.
4362 *Z Gastroenterol* 1993;31:73-7.
4363 *Aliment Pharmacol Ther* 1998;12:807-22.
4366 *J Nutr* 2001;131:980S-4S.
4367 *Am J Gastroenterol* 2000;95:S2-S4.
4368 *Am J Gastroenterol* 2000;95:S19-21.
4369 *Am J Clin Nutr* 2000;71:405-11.
4370 *J Pediatr Gastroenterol Nutr* 2000;30:54.
4371 *J Pediatr* 1999;135:564-8.
4372 *Pediatrics* 1999;104:e64.
4373 *J Pediatr* 1999;134:15-20.
4374 *J Travel Med* 1997;4:41-3.
4376 *Food Chem Toxicol* 1998;36:321-6.
4377 *J Pediatr Gastroenterol Nutr* 1997;25:516-9.
4378 *Appl Environ Microbiol* 1997;63:513-8.
4379 *Scand J Immunol* 1996;43:687-9.
4380 *Clin Infect Dis* 1996;22:564-6.
4382 *Nutr Cancer* 1996;25:197-204.
4383 *Med J Aust* 2002;177:440-3.
4387 *Nutr Cancer* 1999;35:153-9.
4388 *Clin Exp Immunol* 1999;116:276-82.
4389 *Int J Food Microbiol* 1998;41:195-204.
4390 *J Clin Microbiol* 1998;36:1781-3.
4391 *J Infect* 1996;32:165-7.
4392 *Am J Gastroenterol* 2000;95:S11-3.
4393 *Br J Nutr* 1998;80:S203-7.
4394 *J Pediatr Gastroenterol Nutr* 1995;21:224-6.
4397 *J Clin Microbiol* 1995;33:1433.
4398 *Clin Infect Dis* 1999;28:1159-60.
4399 *Clin Exp Allergy* 1998;28:1474-9.
4400 *Gastroenterology* 1979;76:603-6.
4404 *Proc Natl Acad Sci USA* 1990;87:8931.
4405 *Mol Aspects Med* 1997;18:S137-44.
4406 *J Clin Pharmacol* 1993;33:226-9.
4407 *Br J Clin Pharmacol* 1996;42:333-7.
4408 *Mol Aspects Med* 1994;15:187-93.
4409 *J Clin Pathol* 1993;46:1055-7.
4410 *Clin Investig* 1993;71:112-5.
4411 *Clin Radiol* 1994;49;874-6.
4412 *J Am Diet Assoc* 1991;91:66-73.
4425 *AFP* 1986;33:165-74.
4426 *J Neurol Sci* 1997;145:109-12.
4427 *Clin Neuropharmacol* 1995;18:165-82.
4428 *Acta Neurol Scan* 1984;69:226-31.
4429 *Eur Neurol* 1983;22:410-6.
4430 *Acta Neurol Scand* 1984;70:77-80.
4431 *Acta Paediatr Scand* 1984;73:325-8.
4434 *J Parenter Enteral Nutr* 1997;21:357-65.
4435 *New Medicines and Clinics* 1986;35:1-3.
4436 *Scand J Infect Dis Suppl* 1986;49:17-30.
4437 *Eur J Cancer Prev* 1997;6:S43-5.
4438 *Clin Invest Med* 1994;17:531-9.
4439 *Am J Gastroenterol* 1994;89:915-23.
4440 *Monatsschr Kinderheilkd* 1990;138:85-7.
4441 *J Antimicrob Chemother* 1988;21:281-300.
4442 *Ann Clin Res* 1985;17:116-9.
4443 *J Antimicrob Chemother* 1984;14:325-30.
4445 *AIDS* 1998;12:1033-7.
4446 *J Antimicrob Chemother* 1998;42:591-5.
4447 *J Nat Prod* 1999;62:665-9.
4448 *J Antimicrob Chemother* 1999;43:427-8.
4449 *Eur Heart J* 1984;5(Suppl A):25-8.
4450 *Antimicrob Agents Chemother* 2000;44:467-9.
4451 *J Antimicrob Chemother* 2000;45:549-50.
4453 *Lancet* 1975;2:711.
4454 *Fed Proc* 1985;44:124-9.
4455 *Gut* 1975;16:93-8.
4456 *S Afr Med J* 1990;77:131-5.
4457 *Arterioscler Thromb Vasc Biol* 1995;15:1057-63.
4458 *Med Toxicol* 1987;2:10-32.
4459 *Clin Ther* 1982;4:423-40.
4460 *Pediatrics* 1980;65:243-50.
4461 *Arch Dis Child* 1996;74:157-60.
4462 *Br J Rheumatol* 1998;37:27-33.
4463 *Br Med J (Clin Res Ed)* 1982;285:330-2.
4464 *Ned Tijdschr Geneeskd* 1998;142:1904-8.
4465 *Br J Rheumatol* 1993;32:11-4.
4466 *Aust N Z J Med* 1986;16:341-6.
4467 *Am J Clin Nutr* 1986;44:287-90.
4468 *Clin Pharmacol Ther* 1968;9:550-60.
4469 *J Pediatr* 2001;138:125-8.
4471 *Ann Pharmacother* 1995;29:726-35.
4472 *J Am Diet Assoc* 1995;95:352-6.
4473 *Epilepsia* 1992;33:712-20.
4475 *Brain Dev* 1994;16:382-5.
4476 *JAMA* 1999;282:233-4; discussion 235.
4477 *J Clin Endocrinol Metab* 1975;41:1125-9.
4478 *JAMA* 1999;282:234; discussion 235.
4480 *JAMA* 1999;282:234; discussion 235.
4481 *Chest* 1985;87:658-61.
4482 *Tubercle* 1980;61:191-6.
4483 *Am J Med* 1998;104:422-30.
4484 *Intern Med* 1996;240:161-4.
4485 *J Am Coll Nutr* 1994;13:584-91.
4486 *Ann Intern Med* 1994;120:211-5.
4487 *J Nutr* 2000;130:2990-5.
4488 *Am J Med Sci* 1951;243-8.

4490 *Diabete Metab* 1976;2:187-90.
4492 *Clin Exp Rheumatol* 1995;13:459-63.
4493 *J Rheumatol* 1998;25:441-6.
4494 *Br J Rheumatol* 1995;34:1172-4.
4495 *Am J Digestive Dis* 1953;19:344-7.
4496 *Am J Dis Child* 1987;141:1210-2.
4498 *Am J Obstet Gynecol* 1976;125:1063-9.
4500 Hocking GM. A dictionary of natural products. 2nd ed. Medford, OR: Plexus Publishing, 1997.
4502 Duke JA. CRC handbook of medicinal herbs. 1st ed. Boca Raton, FL: CRC Press, LLC, 1985.
4504 Weiss RF. Herbal medicine. 5th ed. Beaconsfield, UK: Beaconsfield Publishers Ltd, 1998.
4511 *Acta Med Scand* 1972;191:355-7.
4512 *Acta Med Scand* 1970;187:431-2.
4513 *Int J Clin Pharmacol Ther* 2000;38:500-2.
4515 *Scand J Clin Lab Invest* 1996;56:421-9.
4516 *Gut* 1986;27:868-72.
4517 *Postgrad Med J* 1986;62:307-8.
4518 *Int Clin Psychopharmacol* 2001;16:239-52.
4520 *Phytomedicine* 2000;7:449-53.
4521 *Life Sci* 2001;68:1593-605.
4522 *Int J Vitam Nutr Res* 1988;58:67-72.
4523 *Int J Vitam Nutr Res* 1995;65:211-4.
4524 *J Pediatr* 1986;109:131-4.
4525 *J Pediatr* 1982;101:782-5.
4526 *Am J Dis Child* 1991;145:999-1001.
4527 *Acta Paediatr Hung* 1987;28(2):137-42.
4528 *Epilepsia* 1998;39:1216-25.
4529 *J Child Neurol* 1991;6:7-14.
4530 *Acta Biomed Ateneo Parmense* 1989;60:245-8.
4531 *American Druggist* 1996 Jul;42-8.
4532 Glaxo-Wellcome, Inc. Daraprim package insert. Research Triangle Park, NC; August, 1996.
4533 *N Engl J Med* 1965;273:1182-5.
4534 *J Am Coll Nutr* 1982;1:207-14.
4535 *Diag Microbiol Infect Dis* 1998;30:83-7.
4536 *Drugs* 1985;30:145-55.
4537 *Neth J Med* 1991;38:209-11.
4538 *Phytother Res* 2001;15:367-70.
4539 *Med Toxicol Adverse Drug Exp* 1988;3:430-48.
4540 *Gastroenterol Clin Biol* 1983;7:381-4.
4541 *Scand J Gastroenterol* 1982;17:129-31.
4542 *Arch Dermatol* 2001;137:512-3.
4543 *Am J Med Sci* 1970;259:32-41.
4544 *Gastroenterology* 1969;56:1251.
4545 *N Engl J Med* 1968;279:845-50.
4546 *Arthritis Rheum* 1996;39:723-31.
4547 *Acta Obstet Gynecol Scand* 1985;64:59-63.
4548 *Lancet* 1974;1:836-7.
4549 *J Am Acad Dermatol* 1985;12(2 Pt 1):308-12.
4550 *Br J Clin Pharmacol* 1975;2:94-6.
4556 *Methods Find Exp Clin Pharmacol* 1992;14:315-25.
4558 *Gastroenterology* 1972;62:1232-7.
4559 *Am J Dig Dis* 1972;17:731-4.
4560 *Biochem Pharmacol* 1992;44:1839-42.
4562 *Eur Heart J* 1998;19:617-22.
4563 *Cardiovasc Res* 1995;30:413-8.
4566 *Nat Med* 1999;5:347-50.
4567 *J Neurosci* 1998;18:156-63.
4568 *Exp Neurol* 1999;157:142-9.
4569 *Med Sci Sports Exerc* 2000;32:291-6.
4570 *Int J Sports Med* 2000;21:71-5.
4571 *Acta Physiol Scand* 1998;164:147-55.
4572 *Eur J Appl Physiol* 1999;80:139-44.
4573 *Clin Sci (Colch)* 1996;91:113-8.
4574 *Sports Med* 1999;28:49-60.
4575 *J Am Coll Nutr* 1998;17:216-34.
4576 *Phys Sportsmed* 1999;27:47-50,53-54,56,61,89.
4577 *Eur J Clin Invest* 1999;29:1060-5.
4578 *N Engl J Med* 1981;304:867-70.
4579 *Recent Adv Stud Cardiac Struct Metab* 1975;8:467-81.
4580 *Med Sci Sports Exerc* 1999;31:236-42.
4581 *Scand J Prim Health Care* 1994;12:239-43.
4582 *Acta Physiol Scand* 1995;155:387-95.
4583 *Clin Sci (Colch)* 1992;83:367-74.
4584 *J Am Diet Assoc* 1999;99:593-5.
4587 *Ann Thorac Surg* 1996;61:67-75.
4588 *Eur J Appl Physiol* 1999;80:165-8.
4589 *Am J Physiol* 1996;271:E821-6.
4590 *Am J Clin Nutr* 2000;71:1705S-7S.
4591 *Acta Physiol Scand* 1995;154:303-10.
4592 *Eur J Appl Physiol* 1994;69:268-76.
4593 *Aust J Sci Med Sport* 1995;27:56-61.
4594 *Res Q Exerc Sport* 1997;68:233-40.
4595 *Aust J Sci Med Sport* 1996;28:35-9.
4596 *Can J Appl Physiol* 1997;22:454-67.
4597 *Int J Clin Pharmacol Ther* 1998;36:258-62.
4598 *J Appl Physiol* 1995;78:670-3.
4599 *Med Sci Sports Exerc* 1997;29:216-9.
4600 *J Appl Physiol* 1998;84:1667-73.
4601 *Int J Sport Nutr* 1999;9:251-62.
4602 *J Sports Med Phys Fitness* 1999;39:189-96.
4603 *J Sports Sci* 1999;17:853-9.
4604 *Med Sci Sports Exerc* 1999;31:1763-9.
4605 *Eur J Appl Physiol* 1998;78:236-40.
4606 *J Appl Physiol* 1999;87:2244-52.
4607 *J Sports Sci* 1996;14:175-9.
4608 *South Med J* 2000;93(6):596-8.
4609 *Lancet* 1999;354:2083.
4611 *Pharmacotherapy* 2002;22:1067-9.
4614 *Menopause* 1998;5:250.
4615 *Am J Health Syst Pharm* 1999;56:1400-2.
4616 *Adv Ther* 1998;15:45-53.
4618 *Planta Med* 1999;65:763-4.
4619 *Maturitas* 1996;25:149-53.
4620 *Zentralbl Gynakol* 1988;110:611-8.
4621 *Oral Surg Oral Med Oral Pathol Oral Radiol Endod* 2000;90:651-5.
4623 *J Am Coll Nutr* 1994;15:485-92.
4624 *Zhongguo Yao Li Xue Bao* 1999;20:486-90.
4625 *Mol Pharmacol* 2000;57:409-17.
4626 *Chung Kuo Yao Li Hsueh Pao* 1999;20:601-3.
4627 *Am J Clin Nutr* 1999;69:341-2.
4628 *Photodermatol Photoimmunol Photomed* 2000;16:125-8.
4629 *J Nat Prod* 2001;664:127-30.
4630 *Phytomedicine* 998;6:435-42.
4631 *Antimicrob Agents Chemother* 2001;45:517-24.
4632 *J Ethnopharmacol* 2001;76:49-57.
4634 *J Am Coll Cardiol* 2000;35:277-83.
4635 *N Engl J Med* 1997;336:1216-22.
4636 *Neurology* 2000;54:1265-72.
4637 *Brain Res* 1995;693:88-94.
4638 *Eur J Neurosci* 1999;11:83-90.
4639 *J Neurosci* 1998;18:8047-55.
4640 *Pediatr Nephrol* 2000;14:13-7.
4641 *Free Rad Res* 1999;31:211-6.
4642 *J Med Assoc Thai* 1993;76:146-52.
4644 *Br J Cancer* 1999;80:591-7.
4645 *Cancer Epidemiol Biomarkers Prev* 1999;8:887-92.
4646 *Cancer Epidemiol Biomarkers Prev* 1999;8:893-9.
4647 *Nephrol Dial Transplant* 1997;12:2312-7.

4648 *Pediatrics* 1987;79:61-8.
4649 *Int J Exp Pathol* 2000;81:57-62.
4650 *J Am Coll Cardiol* 1998;32:1672-9.
4651 *Heart* 1998;79:454-8.
4652 *Arch Intern Med* 1999;159:1313-20.
4655 *Pediatrics* 1990;85:578-84.
4656 *Am J Clin Nutr* 1991;53:370S-2S.
4657 *Eur Resp J* 1991;4:188-90.
4658 *N Engl J Med* 1993;329:234-40.
4659 *Cancer Causes Control* 1993;4:29-37.
4660 *Surgery* 1985;97:490-4.
4661 *Surgery* 1990;107:549-51.
4662 *Obstet Gynecol* 1985;65:104-6.
4663 *Ophthalmology* 1998;105:831-6.
4664 *Am J Publ Health* 1994;84:788-92.
4665 *Ann Epidemiol* 1996;6:41-6.
4666 *J Epidemiol Community Health* 1998;52:468-72.
4667 *Acta Ophthalmol Scand* 1998;76:224-9.
4668 *Eur J Cancer Clin Oncol* 1987;23:327-9.
4670 *Epilepsia* 1994;35:368-72.
4671 *Epilepsia* 1989;30:84-9.
4672 *J Clin Oncol* 1999;17:3283-90.
4673 *Br J Radiol* 1998;71:892-4.
4675 *Pediatr Nephrol* 1999;13:649-52.
4676 *Scand J Gastroenterol* 1998;33:294-300.
4677 *Cancer Epidemiol Biomarkers Prev* 1997;6:543-6.
4679 *Cancer Epidemiol Biomarkers Prev* 1994;3:161-6.
4681 *Hautarzt* 1991;42:176-8.
4682 *Int J Vita Nutr Res* 1988;58:184-8.
4683 *J Pediatr* 1986;108:558-561.
4684 *N Engl J Med* 1983;308:1014-7.
4685 *Proc Soc Exp Biol Med* 1999;222:274-82.
4686 *Am J Psychiatry* 1995;152:1771-5.
4687 *JAMA* 1997;277:1380-6.
4688 *Am J Clin Nutr* 2000;71:590-8.
4689 *Am J Clin Nutr* 1999;69:1273-81.
4690 *Can J Physiol Pharmacol* 1998;76:373-80.
4691 *Int J Vita Nutr Res* 1998;68:133-41.
4693 *Fertil Steril* 1995;64:825-31.
4695 *J Androl* 1996;17:530-7.
4696 *Hum Reprod* 1999;14:1028-33.
4697 *J Thorac Cardiovasc Surg* 1994;108:302-10.
4698 *J Thorac Cardiovasc Surg* 1997;113:942-8.
4699 *Ann Thorac Surg* 1995;59:1519-23.
4700 *Am Fam Physician* 1995;52:1794-8.
4701 *ASAIO J* 1992;38:M481-5.
4702 *Arch Intern Med* 1992;152:1877-80.
4703 *Muscle Nerve* 1988;11:1164-8.
4704 *J Intern Med* 1994;235:205-10.
4705 *Circulation* 1997;96:2545-50.
4708 *J Natl Cancer Inst* 1993;85:44-7.
4709 *N Engl J Med* 1993;328:176-83.
4710 *Neurology* 1994;44:1756-9.
4711 *Ann Neurol* 1996;39:37-45.
4712 *Arch Neurol* 1997;54:762-5.
4713 *Br J Dermatol* 1998;139:332-9.
4714 *Dermatology* 1999;198:52-5.
4715 *Free Radic Biol Med* 1998;25:1006-12.
4716 *J Am Acad Dermatol* 1998;38:45-8.
4718 *Br J Obstet Gynaecol* 1997;104:689-96.
4719 *J Reprod Med* 1987;32:400-4.
4720 *J Am Coll Nutr* 1983;2:115-22.
4721 *Dermatol Surg* 1999;25:311-5.
4722 *J Burn Care Rehabil* 1986;7:309-12.
4723 *Ann Rheum Dis* 1997;56:649-55.
4724 *Diabetes Care* 1998;21:1915-8.
4725 *Diabetes Care* 1999;22:1245-51.
4726 *Am J Clin Nutr* 1993;57:650-6.
4727 *Am J Clin Nutr* 1994;59:1291-6.
4730 *Br J Ophthalmol* 1999;83:1277-82.
4732 *Atherosclerosis* 1999;147:193-7.
4733 *Ann Med* 1998;30:542-6.
4735 *Gastroenterology* 1987;93:225-33.
4736 *Ther Drug Monit* 2000;22:131-6.
4737 *Med Lett Drugs Ther* 2000;42:17-8.
4738 *J Nutr* 1998;128:728-32.
4740 *Cancer Res* 1993;53:5815-21.
4741 *Life Sci* 2000;66:1281-91.
4742 *Cancer Res* 1988;48:6257-61.
4743 *Annu Rev Nutr* 1997;17:353-81.
4746 *Calcif Tissue Int* 1997;61:S15-8.
4749 *Int J Gynaecol Obstet* 1998;62:69-75.
4750 *J Nutr* 2000;130:798-801.
4751 *Menopause* 2000;7:105-11.
4752 *Obstet Gynecol* 1999;94:229-31.
4753 *Annu Rev Nutr* 1997;17:353-81.
4755 *Br J Nutr* 1999;82:91-6.
4756 *Arch Gerontol Geriatr* 1994;19:253-63.
4757 *Curr Ther Res* 1991;49:1004-10.
4759 *Invest Ophthalmol Vis Sci* 1995;36:276-88.
4761 *Am J Gastroenterol* 1999;94:1200-2.
4762 *Arch Intern Med* 1999;159:2484-5.
4763 *Am J Gastroenterol* 2000;95:563-4.
4764 *Appl Environ Microbiol* 2000;66:2269-73.
4765 *Am J Gastroenterol* 2000;95:820-1.
4766 *Mycoses* 1996;39:393-5.
4767 *Arzneimittelforschung* 1999;49:544-7.
4768 *Microbes Infect* 1999;1:125-9.
4769 *Planta Med* 1992;58:417-23.
4770 *Am J Epidemiol* 1994;139:1-15.
4771 *Am J Epidemiol* 1996;144:1015-25.
4772 *Epidemiology* 1997;8:658-65.
4773 *Carcinogenesis* 1996;17:477-84.
4774 *Int J Epidemiol* 1998;27:941-4.
4775 *J Natl Cancer Inst* 1989;81:162-4.
4776 *J Epidemiol* 1999;9:297-305.
4777 *Br J Cancer* 1997;76:678-87.
4778 *Cancer Res* 1994;54:6148-53.
4779 *Breast Cancer Res Treat* 1995;33:163-70.
4780 *Planta Med* 2000;66:148-51.
4782 *Arzneimittelforschung* 1992;42:1473-7.
4783 *Am J Med* 1993;94:632-5.
4784 *Arzneimittelforschung* 1990;40:1111-6.
4785 *Arzneimittelforschung* 1992;42:1223-7.
4786 *J R Coll Physicians Lond* 1994;28:39-45.
4787 *Br J Clin Pract Symp Suppl* 1990;69:7-11.
4788 *Ann Intern Med* 1993;119:599-605.
4789 *Am J Clin Nutr* 1997;65:445-50.
4790 *J Natl Med Assoc* 1997;89:673-8.
4791 *Arzneimittelforschung* 1993;43:978-81.
4792 *J Am Coll Cardiol* 2000;35:321-6.
4793 *Atherosclerosis* 1995;113:219-25.
4794 *Arzneimittelforschung* 1986;36:766-8.
4795 *J R Coll Physicians Lond* 1996;30:329-34.
4796 *Arch Pediatr Adolesc Med* 1998;152:1089-94.
4797 *Circulation* 1997;96:2649-55.
4798 *Atherosclerosis* 1999;144:237-49.
4799 *Atherosclerosis* 1981;38:417-21.
4800 Blumenthal M, Goldberg A, Brinckmann J, eds. Herbal Medicine Expanded Commission E Monographs. Newton, MA: Integrative Medicine Communications, 2000.

4801 *Clin Investig* 1993;71:383-6.
4802 *Eur J Clin Pharmacol* 1993;45:333-6.
4803 *Arzneimittelforschung* 1993;43:119-22.
4804 *Prostaglandins Leukot Essent Fatty Acids* 1999;60:43-7.
4805 *Clin Exp Pharmacol Physiol* 1995;22:414-7.
4807 *Atherosclerosis* 1981;39:447-52.
4808 *J Nutr Sci Vitaminol (Tokyo)* 1999;45:785-90.
4809 Jepson RG, Kleijnen J, Leng GC. Garlic for peripheral arterial occlusive disease (Cochrane Review). In: The Cochrane Library, Issue 2, 2000. Oxford: Update Software.
4810 *Lipids* 1996;31:1269-76.
4811 *J Nutr* 1983;113:1746-55.
4812 *Life Sci* 1998;62:71-7.
4813 *Atherosclerosis* 1998;139:333-9.
4814 American Academy Of Pediatrics Policy Statement. Camphor Revisited: Focus on Toxicity (RE9422). Available at: http://www.aap.org/policy/00300.html.
4815 *Carcinogenesis* 1995;16:2649-52.
4816 *J Allergy Clin Immunol* 1997;100:734-8.
4817 *J Am Coll Cardiol* 2000;35:640-6.
4818 *Arch Intern Med* 2000;160:1177-84.
4819 *N Engl J Med* 2000;342:1156-62.
4820 *N Engl J Med* 2000;342:1149-55.
4821 *N Engl J Med* 1999;340:169-76.
4822 *Stroke* 1999;30:1772-9.
4823 *Am J Kidney Dis* 2000;35:227-36.
4824 *Am J Clin Nutr* 2000;71:931-6.
4825 *Cancer Causes Control* 1998;9:559-66.
4826 *Am J Kidney Dis* 2001;38:1105-7.
4828 *Chem Senses* 1995;20:207-9.
4829 *Pediatrics* 1991;88:737-44.
4830 *Pediatr Res* 1993;34:805-8.
4831 *J Hepatol* 2000;33:853-5.
4832 *Contact Dermatitis* 1987;17:265-9.
4833 *Contact Dermatitis* 1991;24:193-6.
4834 *Nephrol Dial Transplant* 2000;15:1473-4.
4835 *Clin Pharmacol Ther* 2001;70:317-26.
4837 *AIDS* 2001;15:420-1.
4838 *Blood* 1994;84:1628-34.
4839 *Cancer Res* 1997;57:2529-37.
4840 *Blood* 1998;91:2536-46.
4841 *Cancer Res* 1999;59:4555-8.
4842 *N Engl J Med* 1985;312:137-41.
4843 *N Engl J Med* 1979;301:687-90.
4844 Food and Nutrition Board, Institute of Medicine. Dietary Reference Intakes for Vitamin C, Vitamin E, Selenium, and Carotenoids. Washington, DC: National Academy Press, 2000. Available at: http://www.nap.edu/books/0309069351/html.
4846 *Int J Clin Pharmacol Ther* 1998;36:506-9.
4847 *J Am Coll Cardiol* 1986;8:1245-55.
4848 *Circulation* 1993;88:2744-53.
4850 *Am J Public Health* 2000;90:727-38.
4851 *Am J Med* 1995;99:378-85.
4852 *J Fam Pract* 1992;34:165-8.
4853 *J Gen Intern Med* 1997;12:591-6.
4854 *Am J Cardiol* 1998;82:74-81;disc. 85U-6U.
4855 *Ann Intern Med* 1994;121:252-8.
4856 *JAMA* 1994;271:672-7.
4857 *Metabolism* 1998;47:1097-104.
4858 *Am J Cardiol* 1998;82:24U-28U;discussion 39U-41U.
4859 *Coron Artery Dis* 1996;7:321-6.
4860 *JAMA* 1990;264:723-6.
4861 *Br J Surg* 2000;87:868-72.
4862 *Chest* 1998;114:1472-4.
4863 *Am J Health Syst Pharm* 1997;54:2815-9.
4864 *Am J Cardiol* 1998;82:35U-38U;discussion 39U-41U.
4865 *J Neurol Neurosurg Psychiatry* 1985;48:628-34.
4866 *Clin Exp Dermatol* 1999;24:167-9.
4867 National Cholesterol Education Program. Cholesterol Lowering in the Patient with Coronary Heart Disease. 1997. Available at: http://www.nhlbi.nih.gov/health/prof/heart/chol/chol_low.pdf.
4868 *Lancet* 1983;2:1439-42.
4869 *J Diarrhoeal Dis Res* 1993;11:97-100.
4870 *Biol Psychiatry* 1997;41:507-13.
4871 *J Cardiovasc Risk* 1997;4:165-71.
4872 *Diabetes Care* 1999;22:B16-20.
4873 *J Pediatr Endocrinol Metab* 1996;9:375-9.
4874 *J Pediatr Endocrinol Metab* 1996;9:501-9.
4875 *Diabetes* 1998;47:980-4.
4876 *Ugeskr Laeger* 1994;156:461-5.
4877 *Eur J Endocrinol* 1997;137:234-9.
4878 *Diabetes Metab Res Rev* 1999;15:181-5.
4879 *Diabetologia* 1995;38:848-52.
4880 *Diabetes Care* 1996;19:1357-63.
4881 *Diabetes* 1996;45:1631-4.
4882 *Acta Diabetol* 1998;35:61-4.
4883 *Inflamm Res* 1996;45:330-4.
4884 *Med Hypotheses* 1999;53:350-60.
4885 *Arch Ophthalmol* 1993;111:1246-53.
4886 *Arch Intern Med* 1994;154:1586-95.
4887 *Am J Cardiol* 1995;76:182-4.
4888 *Arch Intern Med* 1994;154:73-82.
4889 *Am J Cardiol* 1998;82:737-43.
4890 *Am J Kidney Dis* 1995;25:616-22.
4891 *Cephalalgia* 1996;16:257-63.
4892 Richter O. Several countries issue restrictions on St. John's wort. Richter's HerbLetter 7/30/00. Available at: www.richters.com (Accessed 01 March 2002).
4893 *Altern Complement Ther* 2000;6:291.
4894 Neovastat clinical trial abstracts. Presented at the American Association for Cancer Research 92nd annual meeting. March 27, 2001.
4897 *Int Clin Psychopharmacol* 2000;15:61-8.
4898 *Dis Colon Rectum* 1992;35:1085-8.
4899 *Cochrane Database Syst Rev* 2000;2:CD000448.
4900 *Angiology* 1994;45:566-73.
4901 *J Appl Physiol* 1997;83:1144-51.
4903 *Pediatr Infect Dis J* 1998;17:1149-54.
4904 *Acta Paediatr* 1995;84:996-1001.
4905 *J Acquir Immune Defic Syndr Hum Retrovirol* 1996;13:348-54.
4906 *Clin Investig* 1993;71:42-5.
4907 *Clin Investig* 1992;70:588-94.
4908 *AIDS* 1990;4:581-4.
4909 *Acta Paediatr* 1998;87:264-7.
4911 *Gut* 1999;44:653-8.
4912 FDA. Center for Food Safety and Applied Nutrition, Office of Premarket Approval, EAFUS: A food additive database. Available at: vm.cfsan.fda.gov/~dms/eafus.html.
4913 *Occup Med* 1990;32(7):625-30.
4914 Wade A, Weller PJ, eds. Handbook of Pharmaceutical Excipients. 2nd ed. Washington, DC: Am Pharmaceutical Assn, 1994.
4915 *Arthritis Rheum* 1996; 39:57-63.
4916 *Am J Clin Nutr* 1985; 42(4): 597-603.
4917 *Food Addit Contam* 1987;4:17-26.
4918 *Br J Nutr* 1993; 69(3): 897-902.

4919 *Life Sci* 1999;65:337-53.
4920 *Caries Res* 1997;31(3):216-23.
4926 *Clin Invest Med* 1993;16:204-9.
4927 *Ann Allergy* 1992;68:419-24.
4928 *Prev Med* 1993;22:767-74.
4929 *Nutr Sci Vitaminol (Tokyo)* 1997;43:673-8.
4930 *Anticancer Res* 1995;15:2643-9.
4932 *J Am Diet Assoc* 1998;98:460-2.
4933 *Tumor Biol* 1990;11:129-36.
4934 *Infect Immun* 1990;58:2962-5.
4935 *Int Conf AIDS* 1998;12:557 (abstract # 32185).
4936 *Int Conf AIDS* 1991;7:223 (abstract # WB2165).
4937 *Int Conf AIDS* 1994;10:32 (abstract # 421A).
4938 *Arch Dermatol* 2001;137:1149-52.
4939 *J Dairy Res* 1997;64:281-8.
4940 *J Dairy Res* 1995;62:359-68.
4941 *Int Conf AIDS* 1998;12:553 (abstract #32166).
4942 *J Food Prot* 1998;61:1522-4.
4943 *Cancer Lett* 1991;7:91-4.
4944 Semla TP, Beizer JL, Higbee MD. Geriatric Dosage Handbook. 4th ed. Hudson, OH: Lexicomp, 1998.
4945 *Drugs* 1976;11:45-54.
4946 *Phytochemistry* 2003;62:1283-9.
4947 *Am J Clin Nutr* 2004;79:1118-25.
4948 FDA. Center for drug evaluation and research. Generic drug List. 2003. Available at: http://www.fda.gov/cder/ogd/approvals/1stgen0103.htm.
4949 FDA. List of All Orphan Products Designations and Approvals. Levocarnitine. Available at: http://www.fda.gov/orphan/designat/alldes.rtf.
4950 *Menopause* 2004;11:239-41.
4951 *Menopause* 2004;11246-54.
4952 *Menopause* 2004;11:290-98.
4953 FDA Fact Sheet. I. FDA's New Interim Final Rule Prohibiting Use of Certain Cattle Materials that May Carry the Risk of Bovine Spongiform Encephalopathy in Human Foods and Cosmetics. July 9, 2004. Available at: www.www.cfsan.fda.gov/~comm/bsefact2.html.
4954 *Toxicology* 1992;73:179-89.
4956 *Anticancer Res* 1999;19:3237-41.
4959 *Am J Clin Nutr* 1999;70:491-9.
4960 FDA Talk Paper. FDA Allows Whole Oat Foods to make Claim on Reducing the Risk of Heart Disease. 1997. Available at: vm.cfsan.fda.gov/~lrd/tpoats.html.
4961 *Diabetes Care* 1997;20:1774-80.
4962 *Circulation* 1996;94:2720-7.
4963 *Circulation* 1997;95:2701-4.
4964 *JAMA* 1996;275:447-51.
4965 *Am J Clin Nutr* 1995;61:366-72.
4966 *Am J Epidemiol* 1987;126:1093-102.
4967 *Br Med J* 1977;2:1307-14.
4968 *Am J Epidemiol* 1984;119:733-41.
4969 American Dietetic Association Website. Available at: www.eatright.org/adap1097.html (Accessed 16 July 1999).
4970 *Am J Clin Nutr* 1998;68:711-9.
4972 *Pediatrics* 1995;96:1005-9.
4973 *J Am Coll Nutr* 1998;17:601-8.
4974 *Hepatol* 1994;20:1450-7.
4975 *Am J Clin Nutr* 1994;59:66-9.
4976 *Eur J Clin Nutr* 1994;48:465-74.
4977 *JAMA* 1992;267:3317-25.
4979 *N Engl J Med* 1989;320:1148-9.
4980 *J Am Diet Assoc* 1996;96:1254-61.
4981 *Br J Nutr* 1994;72:731-43.
4982 *Diabet Med* 1994;11:312-8.
4983 *Am J Clin Nutr* 1991;53:1425-30.
4984 *Digestion* 1983;28:197-200.
4985 *J Am Geriatr Soc* 1990;38:608.
4986 *J Acquir Immune Defic Syndr* 1991;4:1218-26.
4988 *Calcif Tissue Int* 2000;66:53-5.
4989 *JAMA* 2003;290:2824-30.
5000 *Toxicology* 1996;109:1-13.
5001 *Antiviral Res* 1993;21:317-25.
5002 *JAMA* 1995;273:912-3.
5003 *Planta Med* 1998;64:541-45.
5004 *Contact Dermatitis* 1997;37:70-7.
5005 *Contact Dermatitis* 1993;29:11-5.
5006 *Ann Allergy* 1988;61:53-7.
5007 *Planta Med* 1997;63:472-4.
5011 Lininger S. The Natural Pharmacy. Prima Health. Rocklin, CA: 1998.
5013 Moore M. Herbal Materia Medica fifth edition, Southwest School of Botanical Medicine: Bisbee, AZ 1995.
5019 Manufacturer: Nature's Way. Springville, UT.
5020 Manufacturer: Twinlab. Ronkonkoma, NY.
5023 Manufacturer: Nature's Answer. Hanppange, NY.
5024 Manufacturer: Walgreens. Deerfield, IL.
5028 Personal correspondence. Janna Leppala, jleppala@ucla.edu. March 4, 2000.
5029 *Ann Pharmacother* 2000;34:300-3.
5030 Schardt D. Stevia, A Bittersweet Tale. Nutrition Action Healthletter April 2000- U.S. Edition. Available at: www.cspinet.org/nah/4_00/stevia.html (Accessed 25 June 2004).
5031 *J Ethnopharmacol* 1991;33:257-622.
5032 *Metabolism* 2000;49:208-14.
5033 *J Ethnopharmacol* 1999;67:157-61.
5034 *Drug Chem Toxicol* 1997;20:31-44.
5035 *J Nutr Sci Vitaminol (Tokyo)* 1995;41:105-13.
5036 *Drug Chem Toxicol* 1998;21:207-22.
5037 Stevia: Not Ready For Prime Time. Ctr for Sci in the Public Interest. Available at: www.cspinet.org/additives/stevia (Accessed 28 March 2000).
5038 *Clin Pharmacol Ther* 2000;67:1-6.
5039 *Diabet Med* 1999;16:164-7.
5040 *Ann Intern Med* 1991;115:917-24.
5041 National Collegiate Athletic Association. List of banned drug classes for 2004-2005. Available at: www.ncaa.org.
5043 Magainin Presents Neuroblastoma Data for Squalamine at AACR Meeting. Available at: www.prnewswire.com (Accessed 3 April 2000).
5044 Iron chefs get nutritional boost cooking vegetables. American Chemical Society website. Available at: center.acs.org/applications/news//story.cfm?story=347 (Accessed 6 April 2000).
5047 FDA announces the availability of new Ephedrine and street drug alternative docs. Available at: www.fda.gov (Accessed 6 April 2000).
5049 *J Autism Dev Disord* 1997;27:467-78.
5050 *Neurology* 1971;21:911-9.
5051 *Br J Clin Pharmacol* 2000;49:59-63.
5052 *Br J Dermatol* 2000;142:580-1.
5053 *Am J Clin Nutr* 1994;60:567-72.
5054 *J Allergy Clin Immunol* 2000;105:844.
5055 Mundell EJ. Mussel extract helps arthritic dogs. www.reutershealth.com (Accessed 18 April 2000).
5056 *Nutrition* 2000;16:330-8.
5058 *Nutr Cancer* 2000;38:151-7.

5059 *FASEB J* 2000;14:A750.
5060 *Lancet* 1980;1:1134.
5061 Antioxidant lozenge could help ward off flu. www.reutershealth.com (Accessed 19 April 2000).
5063 *Plant Foods Hum Nutr* 1993;44:63-70.
5064 *J Clin Psychopharmacol* 1997;17:62-3.
5065 *Eur J Clin Pharmacol* 1999;55:405-10.
5066 *Clin Pharmacol Ther* 1999;66:408-14.
5067 *Br J Clin Pharmacol* 1999;48:829-38.
5068 *Clin Pharmacol Ther* 2000:67:201-14.
5069 *Br J Clin Pharmacol* 2000;49:49-58.
5070 *Clin Pharmacokinet* 2000;38:41-57.
5071 Coreg monograph. In: Gillis MC, Ed. Compendium of Pharmaceuticals and Specialities (CPS). 34th ed. Ottawa, Ontario, CAN:Canadian Pharmacists Assn, 1999:395.
5072 *Chem Res Toxicol* 1998;11:252-9.
5073 *Eur J Clin Pharmacol* 1998;54:589-94.
5074 *J Geriatr Psychiatry Neurol* 1999;12:7-10.
5075 *J Clin Psychiatry* 2000;61:575-8.
5076 Fed Trade Comm. Marketers of Vitamin O settles FTC charges of making false health claims. 2000. Available at: www.ftc.gov/opa/2000/05/rosecreek2.htm.
5080 McCrory DC, Matchar DB, Gray RN, et al. Evidence-based guidelines for migraine headache: overview of program description and methodology. US Headache Consortium, April 2000. Available at: www.aan.com/cgi-bin/whatsnewlink.pl?loc=/public/practiceguidelines.
5081 *Ann Intern Med* 2000:132:595.
5082 *JAMA* 1998;279:750.
5084 *J Allergy Clin Immunol* 2000;105:570-6.
5085 *N Engl J Med* 1989;320:1097-1102.
5086 *Am J Epidemiol* 1997;145:432-8.
5087 *Ann Intern Med* 2000;132:738-42.
5089 *Ann Emerg Med* 2000;35:391-3.
5090 *Ann Intern Med* 2000;132:636-40.
5091 *Arch Intern Med* 2000;160:837-42.
5092 *BMJ* 2000;320:1322-4.
5093 *J Urol* 2000;163:1451-6.
5094 *J Urol* 2000;163:1408-12.
5095 *Prostate* 1999;38:208-15.
5096 *JAMA* 2001;285:1978-86.
5097 Harel Z, Gascon G, Riggs S, et al. Fish oil vs olive oil in the management of recurrent headaches in adolescents. Advancing Children's Health 2000. Joint Meeting of Pediatric Academic Soc and Am Acad of Pediatrics; Abstract 30.
5104 *Am J Med* 1999;106:16S-9S.
5105 *Am J Med* 1981;71:193-5.
5106 *N Engl J Med* 1980;302:324-31.
5107 *Eur J Cancer Prev* 1997;6(5):435-41.
5108 *Am J Hosp Pharm* 1978;35:278-87.
5109 Kalant H, Roschlau WHE, Eds. Principles of Med. Pharmacology. New York, NY: Oxford Univ Press, 1998.
5110 Bloom FE, Kupfer DJ. Psychopharmacology: The Fourth Generation of Progress. New York, NY: Raven Press, Ltd., 1995.
5113 *Epilepsy Res* 1994;17:49-53.
5114 *Metabolism* 1982;31:73-7.
5115 *Acta Endocrinol (Copenh)* 1980;93:149-54.
5116 *Psychiatry Res* 1986;19:113-7.
5122 *Urology* 1999;54:319-28.
5129 *Hepatol* 1998;28:129-40.
5130 *Indian J Exp Biol* 1992;30:367-70.
5131 *Am J Physiol* 1997;273:G355-64.
5133 *Clin Pharm* 1993;12:900-8.
5139 Gilman AG, et al, eds. Goodman and Gilman's The Pharmacological Basis of Therapeutics. 8th ed. New York, NY: Pergamon Press, 1990.
5140 *Gastroenterology* 1992;102:1363-70.
5141 *Exerc Sport Sci Rev* 1998;26:287-314.
5142 *Am J Gastroenterol* 1976;65:231-5.
5146 *Am J Psychiatry* 1983;140:1010-2.
5147 *Aust N Z J Med* 1977;7:262-6.
5148 *Eur J Clin Nutr* 1998;52(6):419-24.
5149 *J Gerontol* 1982;37:4-9.
5150 *J Clin Psychopharmacol* 1982;2:281-5.
5151 *J Clin Psychiatry* 1983;44:293-5.
5152 *Neurology* 1981;31:1552-4.
5153 Facts and Comparisons, loose leaf edition. St. Louis, MO: Wolters Kluwer Co., 1999.
5155 *Digestion* 1979;19:251-8.
5156 *BMJ* 1994;308:879-83.
5158 *Clin Biochem* 2000;33:279-84.
5159 *Folia Microbiol (Praha)* 1998;43:505-6.
5160 *Sports Med* 1993;15:90-103.
5161 *Acta Neurol Scand* 1980;62:124-6.
5162 *Neurology* 1980;30:1334-6.
5163 *J Am Diet Assoc* 1997;97:639-46.
5164 *Med Sci Sports Exerc* 1995;27:668-73.
5165 *Indian J Chet Dis Allied Sci* 1997;39:149-56.
5166 *Indian J Chest Dis Allied Sci* 1997;39:107-13.
5170 *Neurobiol Aging* 1980;1:21-5.
5171 *Biol Psychiatry* 1978;13:23-49.
5172 *Am J Psychiatry* 1979;136:1581-4.
5173 *J Neurol Neurosurg Psychiatry* 1980;43:452-4.
5174 *Hepatol* 1995;22:1399-403.
5175 *Magn Reson Med* 1998;39:1005-10.
5177 *Arch Dermatol* 1998;134:1349-52.
5178 *Adv Exp Med Biol* 1997;422:97-107.
5179 *FASEB J* 1999;13:135-42.
5180 *J Am Coll Nutr* 1992;11:473-81.
5184 *Psychiatry Res* 1995;56:295-7.
5188 *J Rheumatol* 1994;21:905-11.
5189 *Acta Neurol Scand Suppl* 1994;154:7-14.
5190 *Acta Neurol Scand Suppl* 1994;154:15-8.
5191 *Pharmacotherapy* 2001;21:509-12.
5192 *Psychother Psychosom* 1993;59:34-40.
5193 *Psychiatry Res* 1992;44:257-62.
5195 *Am J Psychiatry* 1990;147:591-5.
5196 *Acta Psychiatr Scand* 1990;81:432-6.
5197 Heartwire. Antioxidants get a vote of confidence in cardiac transplant patients. Available at: http://www.theheart.org/viewEntityDispatcherAction.do?primaryKey=174806 (Accessed 13 December 2001).
5198 *Drugs* 1990;40:98-110.
5199 *Int J Clin Pharmacol Ther Toxicol* 1989;27:329-33.
5200 *Am J Psychiatry* 1988;145:1110-4.
5201 *Neurosci Biobehav Rev* 1988;12:139-41.
5202 *Am J Med* 1987;83:95-103.
5203 *Am J Med* 1987;83:78-80.
5204 *Am J Med* 1987;83:84-8.
5205 *Am J Med* 1987;83:81-3.
5206 *Am J Med* 1987;83:78-80.
5207 *Am J Med* 1987;83:72-7.
5208 *Am J Med* 1987;83:66-71.
5209 *Am J Med* 1987;83:60-5.
5210 *Am J Hypertens* 2000;13:564-7.
5211 *Am J Med* 1987;83:107-10.
5213 *Am J Med* 1987;83(5A):43-7.
5215 *Int J Clin Pharmacol Res* 1985;5:39-49.
5216 *Am J Psychiatry* 1984;141:448-50.

5217 *Neurology* 1995;45:1678-83.
5218 *J Neurol Neurosurg Psychiatry* 1998;65:23-8.
5219 *Drugs* 1990;40:111-23.
5221 *Scand J Rheumatol* 1997;26:206-11.
5222 *Nephron* 1991;59:100-3.
5223 *Biol Psychiatry* 1985;20:1189-96.
5224 *Liver* 1982;2:77-81.
5225 *Aliment Pharmacol Ther* 1995;9:699-703.
5226 *Hepatogastroenterology* 1998;45:797-804.
5228 *Clin Neuropharmacol* 1993;16:540-9.
5229 *Acta Derm Venereol* 1985;65:19-24.
5231 *Drugs* 1989;38:389-416.
5232 *Drugs* 1994;48:137-52.
5233 *Urol Clin North Am* 1999;26:413-7.
5234 U.S. Department of Agriculture, Agricultural Research Service. USDA Nutrient Database for Standard Reference, Release 14. Nutrient Data Laboratory. Available at: http://www.nal.usda.gov/fnic/foodcomp.
5235 *An Med Interna* 1996;13:9-15.
5236 *Alcohol* 1994;29:597-604.
5238 *Klin Med (Mosk)* 1998;76:45-8.
5239 *Gastroenterology* 1990;99:211-5.
5240 *Hepatogastroenterology* 1990;37:122-5.
5241 *Scand J Rheumatol* 1991;20:294-302.
5244 Botanical Dermatological Database. Annonaceae (Custard apple family). Available at: http://archive.uwcm.ac.uk/uwcm/dm/BoDD/BotDermFolder/BotDermA/ANNO.html. (Accessed 17 August 2001).
5245 *Int J Obes Relat Metab Disord* 2001;25:1095-9.
5246 *Am J Clin Nutr* 1998;67:317-21.
5247 *J Pediatr* 2001;138:649-55.
5248 *Jpn Circ J* 1992;56:95-9.
5249 *J Herb Pharmacother* 2001;1:81-7.
5250 Castleman M. The healing herbs, the ultimate guide to the curative power of nature's medicines. 2nd ed. New York, NY: Bantam Books, 1995.
5251 Reid D. A handbook of Chinese healing herbs. Boston, MA:Shambhala, 1995.
5252 Sifton D, ed. The PDR family guide to natural medicines & healing therapies. New York, NY: Three Rivers Press, 1999.
5253 Hoffman D. The herbal handbook: a user's guide to medical herbalism. rev ed. Rochester, VT:Healing Arts Press, 1998.
5254 Weiner MA, Weiner JA. Herbs that heal: prescription for herbal healing. Mill Valley, CA:Quantum Books, 1999.
5255 Raintree tropical plant database, Amazon plants. www.rain-tree.com/plants.htm (Accessed 30 July 1999).
5260 *J Altern Complement Med* 1995;1:361-9.
5263 Lust J. The herb book. New York, NY: Bantam Books, 1999.
5264 *Ann Rheum Dis* 2001;60:946-9.
5267 Botanical.Com A Modern Herbal. www.botanical.com (Accessed 31 July 1999).
5269 Herbal Monographs. Healthlink. www.healthline.com (Accessed 1 August 1999).
5271 *Clin Cardiol* 1985;8:276-82.
5274 GHS Gold. Gerovital Direct Prod. www:gerivital.co.uk (Accessed 3 August 1999).
5275 *Lancet* 2000;356:1573-4.
5276 Herbal Materia Medica 4.0. website: www.herb.com/materia.htm (Acessed 6 August 1999).
5277 *N Engl J Med* 1993;329(11):745-52.
5278 *Ann Pharmacother* 1995;29:312-3.
5279 Brown D. Encyclopedia of herbs and their uses. New York, NY:Dorland Kindersley Publ., Inc., 1995.
5280 *Adv Pediatr* 1985;32:1-42.
5286 *Eur J Clin Nutr* 1993;47:747-9.
5290 *Prostate* 1998;37(3):187-93.
5292 *Br J Urol* 1990;66(4):398-404.
5293 *Br J Urol* 1993;71:433-8.
5294 *Clin Ther* 1995;17:82-7.
5295 *Urology* 1996;48:12-20.
5296 *Br J Urol* 1989;64:496-9.
5297 *Prostate* 1995;26:133-9.
5298 *Arzneimittelforschung* 1991;41:162-7.
5301 *Arch Intern Med* 1999;159:2090.
5304 *J Psychoactive Drugs* 1983;15:251-9.
5305 *J Ethnopharmacol* 1998;62:167-71.
5306 *Clin Ther* 1983;5:398-408.
5308 *Ann Thorac Surg* 1998;65(3):684-90.
5309 *Lancet* 1990;335(8691):701-3.
5310 *Metabolism* 1995;44(9):1215-22.
5311 *Nephron* 1996;74(2):261-5.
5312 *Lancet* 1995;345(8949):552-3.
5313 *Ann Thorac Surg* 1997;63(6):1625-33.
5314 *Cell Biol Int* 1996;20(5):359-63.
5315 *Fed Proc* 1980;39:2685-90.
5318 Stabilized Oxygen. Portal Market. www.portalmarket.com/earthportals/Portal_Market/eathportals/portal_Ma_/oxygen.htm (Accessed 7 October 1999).
5320 Oxygen caps. Lifeplus vitamins. www.lifeplusvitamins.simpletnet.com/1p27p.html (Accessed 7 October 1999).
5321 How to use Oxy boost. O2oxyboost. www.o2xyboost.com/howto.htm (Accessed 7 October 1999).
5326 *J Lipid Res* 1992;33:945-55.
5327 *Lancet* 1995;345:1529-32.
5328 *Br J Urol* 1997;80:427-32.
5329 *BJU Int* 1999;83:976-83.
5330 *J Pediatr* 1993;122:292-6.
5331 *Dtsch Med Wochenschr* 1976;101:1308-11.
5332 *Atherosclerosis* 1978;30:245-8.
5333 *MMW Munch Med Wochenschr* 1978;120:1575-8.
5334 *Pediatrics* 1992;89:138-42.
5335 *Int J Sports Med* 1999;20:258-62.
5336 *Eur J Clin Nutr* 1998;52:334-43.
5337 *Int J Tubercul Lung Dis* 1997;1:518-22.
5338 *Lancet* 1975;2:721.
5339 *Gastroenterology* 1979;76:1341-6.
5340 *Med Lett Drugs Ther* 1999;41:56-8.
5342 *Altern Med Rev* 1999;4:170-7.
5343 *Obstet Gynecol* 2001;97:577-82.
5344 *Ann Pharmacother* 1995;29:1263-73.
5345 *Am J Epidemiol* 1994;139(5):453-65.
5346 *Am J Obstet Gynecol* 1993;169:1456-61.
5347 *Obstet Gynecol* 1998;92:1012-5.
5348 *Placenta* 1999;20:541-6.
5349 *Free Radic Biol Med* 1999;27:515-20.
5350 *Ann Neurol* 1998;44(3 Suppl 1):S72-84.
5351 *Mov Disord* 1998;(13 Suppl)1:24-34.
5352 *J Neural Transm* 1997;104(6-7):661-77.
5353 *Biochem Pharmacol* 1998;56:645-55.
5354 *Prog Neuropsychopharmacol Biol Psychiatry* 1996;20(7):1159-70.
5357 *Metabolism* 1998;47(8):993-7.
5358 *Diabetes Metab* 1997;23(1):58-60.
5359 *J Nephrol* 1997;10(5):261-5.
5360 *J Am Coll Surg* 1994;179:714-20.
5361 *Gut* 1965;6:472-6.
5362 *Eur J Clin Pharmacol* 1992;43(6):667-9.
5363 *Am J Physiol* 1990;259(4 Pt 1):G530-5.
5364 *Chem Biol Interact* 1991;80(1):89-97.

5367 *J Appl Physiol* 1999;87(1):438-43.
5368 *Thorax* 1993;48(10):985-9.
5369 *Lancet* 1991;338(8761):215-6.
5372 *Am J Respir Crit Care Med* 1997;156(2 Pt 1):425-30.
5373 *Ann Oncol* 1997;8(6):569-73.
5374 *J Clin Oncol* 1995;13(1):26-32.
5375 *Drugs* 1999;57(3):293-308.
5376 *Cancer Chemother Pharmacol* 1992;29(5):385-90.
5377 *Tumori* 1998;84(3):368-71.
5378 *Gynecol Oncol* 1994;55:82-6.
5379 *Tumori* 1993;79(1):37-9.
5380 *Ann Oncol* 1993;4(1):55-61.
5381 *Eur J Cancer* 1995;31A(10):1721.
5382 *Br J Cancer* 1999;79(3-4):491-4.
5383 *J Clin Oncol* 1997;15(11):3313-9.
5384 *Hum Reprod* 1993;8:1657-62.
5386 *Clin Sports Med* 1999;18(3):525-36.
5387 *Chem Biol Interact* 1998;24;111-112:1-14.
5388 *FASEB J* 1999;13(10):1169-83.
5389 *Mol Genet Metab* 1999;67(2):100-5.
5392 *Klin Wochenschr* 1991;69(18):857-62.
5393 *FASEB J* 1997;11(13):1077-89.
5394 *Proc Natl Acad Sci USA* 1997;94(5):1967-72.
5395 *Free Radic Biol Med* 1998;24(5):699-704.
5396 *Brain Res Brain Res Rev* 1997;25:335-58.
5397 *Ital J Gastroenterol Hepatol* 1999;31(5):401-7.
5398 *Med Sci Sports Exerc* 1999;31(7):987-97.
5429 *Metabolism* 1999;48:575-80.
5430 *J Lipid Res* 1999;40(4):593-600.
5431 *Circulation* 1997;96:4226-31.
5432 *Diabetologia* 1994;37(8):773-80.
5433 *J Lipid Res* 1996;37(8):1776-85.
5434 *Am J Cardiol* 1999;145:279-85.
5435 *Am J Clin Nutr* 1999;69(3):403-10.
5436 *Eur J Clin Pharmacol* 1991;40 Suppl 1:S59-63.
5437 *Am J Clin Nutr* 1999;69(6):1144-50.
5438 *J Lipid Res* 1995;36(8):1807-12.
5439 *N Engl J Med* 1995;333(20):1308-12.
5441 *Clin Sci (Colch)* 1994;87:61-7.
5443 *Med Lett Drugs Ther* 1999;41:56-8.
5444 Cowley G. Newsweek July 5, 1999; pp. 46-50.
5446 *Altern Med Rev* 1999;4:73.
5447 *Ann Thorac Surg* 1992;53:391-6.
5448 *Gut* 1999;45:82-8.
5449 *Lancet* 1998;352:772-6.
5450 *Nutrition* 1999;15:108-15.
5451 *JPEN J Parenter Enteral Nutr* 1999;23:117-22.
5452 *Bone Marrow Transplant* 1998;22:281-4.
5453 *Am J Med Sci* 1998;315:4-10.
5454 *Curr Opin Clin Nutr Metab Care* 1999;2:323-7.
5455 *Eur J Appl Physiol* 1998;78:448-53.
5456 *Med Sci Sports Exerc* 1998;30:856-62.
5458 *Eur J Cancer* 1999;35:202-7.
5461 *Am J Gastroenterol* 1998;93:972-5.
5462 *Am J Clin Oncol* 1999;22:258-61.
5464 *Can J Physiol Pharmacol* 1998;76:524-32.
5465 *Can J Appl Physiol* 1999;24:1-14.
5466 *Sports Med* 1998;26:177-91.
5467 *Curr Opin Clin Nutr Metab Care* 1999;2:177-82.
5468 *Ann Pharmacother* 1999;33:348-54.
5469 *Altern Med Rev* 1999;4:239-48.
5470 *Mol Genet Metab* 1999;67:100-5.
5473 Reishi. Mothernature encyclopedia. ww.mothernature.com/ency/herb/reishi.asp. (Accessed 7 November 1999).
5476 *J Tongji Med Univ* 1990;10(4):240-3.
5477 *Crit Rev Immunol* 1999;19:65-96.
5478 *Am J Chin Med* 1990;18:175-9.
5479 *Clin Exp Allergy* 1995;25:440-7.
5480 *Chem Pharm Bull (Tokyo)* 1998;46:1607-12.
5481 *Phytochemistry* 1998;49:1651-7.
5482 *Mol Cells* 1997;7:52-7.
5483 *Int J Cancer* 1997;70:699-705.
5484 *Carcinogenesis* 1999;20:1637-40.
5485 *Am J Chin Med* 1998;26:375-81.
5486 *Chem Pharm Bull (Tokyo)* 1989;37:531-3.
5487 *Planta Med* 1989;55:423-8.
5488 *Chem Pharm Bull (Tokyo)* 1990;38:1359-64.
5489 *Biol Pharm Bull* 1999;22:162-4.
5490 *Arch Pharm Res* 1994;17:438-42.
5491 *J Tradit Chin Med* 1993;13:223-6.
5492 *Transplantation* 1995;60:438-43.
5494 *Int J Biochem Cell Biol* 1996;28:601-7.
5500 *Appl Environ Microbiol* 1999;65:351-4.
5501 Bensky D, Gamble A, Kaptchuk T. Chinese Herbal Medicine Materia Medica. Seattle, WA: Eastland Press. 1996;483-5.
5502 Huang KC. The pharmacology of Chinese herbs. 2nd ed. Boca Raton, FL: CRC Press, LLC 1999;266-7.
5503 *J Ethnopharmacol* 1999;66:41-9.
5504 *Arch Dermatol* 1988;124:768.
5505 Anon. Human clinical trials show significant results for New Zealand deer antler velvet's effect on sports performance. www.prnewswire.com (Accessed 7 March 2000).
5518 *Gen Comp Endocrinol* 1986;3:431-40.
5525 *J Toxicol Clin Toxicol* 1996;34:119-26.
5526 *JAMA* 1995;274:1196-7.
5531 *Surgery* 1992;112:56-67.
5532 *Eur J Surg* 1995;161:115-22.
5533 *Crit Care Med* 1995;23:652-9.
5534 *JPEN J Parenter Enteral Nutr* 1999;23(6):314-20.
5535 *J Trauma* 1997;42(5):793-802.
5536 *Crit Care Med* 1995;23(3):436-49.
5538 *Contact Dermatitis* 1999;41:239.
5539 *Mol Gen Genet* 1998;259:569-76.
5541 Huang KC. The pharmacology of Chinese herbs. 2nd ed. New York, NY: CRC Press LLC. 1999;385-6, 400-1.
5543 *Nutr* 1997;13:470-2.
5544 Bensky D, Gamble A, Kaptchuk T. Chinese Herbal Medicine Materia Medica. Seattle, WA: Eastland Press 1996:107-8.
5545 Huang KC. The Pharmacology of Chinese Herbs. 2nd ed. New York, NY: CRC Press, LLC 1999:113-114, 417.
5546 *Chung Kuo Chung His I Chieh Ho Tsa Chih* 1997;17:666-8.
5547 *Adv Exp Med Biol* 1998;439:191-225.
5548 *N Engl J Med* 1998;339:785-91.
5549 *Eksp Klin Farmakol* 1997;60:49-51.
5550 *Eksp Klin Farmakol* 1997;60:28-30.
5551 *Chung Hsi I Chieh Ho Tsa Chih* 1990;10:278-9, 260.
5552 *Contact Dermatitis* 1999;40:224-5.
5553 *Contact Dermatitis* 1998;38:140-6.
5554 *Allergy* 1998;53:204-9.
5555 *Chung Kuo Chung His I Chieh Ho Tsa Chih* 1993;13:147-9.
5556 *Contact Dermatitis* 1978;4(2):93-102.
5557 *Contact Dermatitis* 1976;2(2):81-8.
5558 Huang KC. The Pharmacology of Chinese Herbs. 2nd ed. New York, NY: CRC Press, LLC 1999:101-102.
5559 Bensky D, Gamble A, Kaptchuk T. Chinese Herbal Medicine Materia Medica. Seattle, WA: Eastland Press, 1996:359-60.

5598 *J Clin Endocrinol Metab* 2000;85:3043-8.
5599 *Ann Nutr Metab* 1998;42:350-9.
5600 *N Engl J Med* 1990;322:338.
5601 *JAMA* 1979;242:2873-4.
5602 *MMWR Morb Mortal Wkly Rep* 1992;41:53-5.
5603 *J Forensic Sci* 1991;36(2):599-601.
5604 *Forensic Sci Int* 1992;56(1):81-7.
5605 *J Toxicol Clin Toxicol* 1998;36(3):219-23.
5606 *J Pediatr* 1978;93:980-2.
5607 *Vet Hum Toxicol* 1981;23:259-60.
5608 *N Engl J Med* 1969;281:51-2.
5609 *Lancet* 1999;353(9164):1623-4.
5610 *J Allergy Clin Immunol* 1996;98:997-8.
5611 *Ann Emerg Med* 1990;19:1177-83.
5612 *J Toxicol Clin Toxicol* 2000;38(1):67-9.
5614 *J Clin Pathol* 1976;29:788-94.
5617 *J Toxicol Clin Toxicol* 1982;19:35-44.
5618 *Pediatrics* 1976;57:419-21.
5619 *Am J Dis Child* 1988;142(6):633-6.
5620 *Am J Forensic Med Pathol* 1988;9:51-3.
5621 *MMWR Morb Mortal Wkly Rep* 1981;30:65-7.
5622 *J Forensic Sci* 1982;27:948-54.
5623 *MMWR Morb Mortal Wkly Rep* 1995;44:41-4.
5624 *J Fla Med Assoc* 1978;65:192-6.
5625 *Am J Psychiatry* 1977;134:312-4.
5626 *South Med J* 1996;89:365-9.
5627 *J Paediatr Child Health* 1999;35:93-5.
5628 Anon. FDA Import Alert #53-03, 1991. Availble at: http://www.fda.gov/ora/fiars/ora_import_ia5303.html.
5629 Pine, D. Cool tips for a hot season. FDA/CFSAN Cosmetics 1992. Available at: http://vm.cfsan.fda.gov/~dms/cos-815.html.
5631 *J Am Acad Dermatol* 1981;4:233.
5632 *J Am Acad Dermatol* 1985;13:660.
5633 *Drug Ther Bull* 1983;21:57.
5634 *Lancet* 1981;1:1419-20.
5635 *JAMA* 1990;264:1141-2.
5636 *Arch Ophthalmol* 1989;107:538-40.
5637 *Am J Clin Nutr* 1991;53:573-4.
5638 *Am Fam Physician* 1988;37:125-6.
5639 *Am J Ophthalmol* 1995;119:801-2.
5640 *Acta Ophthalmol (Copenh)* 1990;68(5):607-11.
5641 *Arch Ophthalmol* 1999;117:412-3.
5642 Anon. Permitted colouring agents for use in medicinal products - E 161 Canthaxanthine. Health and Consumer Protection - The European Commission 1998. Available at: http://europa.eu.int/comm/food/index_en.htm.
5643 *Phytomedicine* 1998;5:1-10.
5644 Anon. Porphyria information for patients and their families. University of Cape Town / Medical Research Council - Liver Research Center 2000. Availble at: http://web.uct.ac.za/depts/porphyria.
5646 *Am J Clin Nutr*. 2001;73:151-152.
5647 *Cancer Epidemiol Biomarkers Prev* 1998;7(8):725-8.
5648 *Cancer Lett* 1992;65(3):209-13.
5649 *Int J Vitam Nutr Res* 1998;68:354-9.
5650 *J Clin Invest* 1958;37:719-35.
5651 *J Thorac Cardiovasc Surg* 1980;80:506-16.
5652 *J Thorac Cardiovasc Surg* 1982;83:390-8.
5653 *Ann Surg* 1984;200(1):1-12.
5654 *Surgery* 1984;96(2):248-55.
5655 *Gastroenterology* 1978;74:900-2.
5656 *J Appl Physiol* 1994;76:1802-9.
5657 *J Appl Physiol* 1995;78(1):146-52.
5658 *J Appl Physiol* 1993;74:2523-8.
5659 *Biochem Soc Trans* 1985;13:885-6.
5660 *J Surg Res* 1989;46:157-62.
5662 *J Nucl Med* 1991;32:193-200.
5663 *J Am Coll Cardiol* 1991;18:1671-81.
5664 *Lancet* 1992;340:507-10.
5665 *J Mol Cell Cardiol* 1998;30:879-87.
5666 *Eur J Med Res* 1998;3:554-8.
5667 Burke ER. D-Ribose What You Need To Know. Garden City Park, NY: Avery Publishing Group 1999;1-43.
5676 *Klin Wochenschr* 1989;67:1205-13.
5677 *Klin Wochenscher* 1986;64:1281-90.
5678 *J Neurol Sci* 1996;136:174-7.
5679 *Ann Nutr Metab* 1991;35:297-302.
5680 *Klin Wochenscher* 1991;69:251-5.
5682 *Ann Intern Med* 1971;74:424-33.
5683 *J Pharm Sci* 1994;83:1081-4.
5684 *J Pharm Sci* 1997;86:396-7.
5685 *Life Sci* 1996;58:1777-84.
5686 *Pharm Biotechnol* 1998;11:575-95.
5687 *J Urol* 1998;160:389-93.
5688 Wessells H, Gralnek DR, Dorr RT, et al. Erectogenic properties of melanotan II in men with organic erectile dysfunction. 1999. Abstract Info-American Urological Association, Inc.
5692 *Urol Clin North Am* 1994;21(1):73-83.
5693 *J Urol* 1997;158:1989-95.
5694 *Urology* 1987;29:17-21.
5695 *Br J Urol* 1987;59(2):142-4.
5696 *Urology* 1981;18(1):21-6.
5697 *Urology* 1978;11(3):215-20.
5698 *Drug Saf* 1995;12(4):245-55.
5699 *Blood Rev* 1990;4(1):41-60.
5701 *Br J Cancer* 1999;81:80-6.
5702 *J Am Coll Cardiol* 2000;35:265-70.
5705 *Am J Clin Nutr* 2000;71:28-35.
5706 *Am J Clin Nutr* 2000;71:232S-7S.
5707 *Am J Clin Nutr* 2000;71:228S-31S.
5708 *Am J Clin Nutr* 2000;71:323S-6S.
5709 *Am J Clin Nutr* 2000;71:339S-42S.
5710 *J Rheumatol* 2000;27:298-303.
5711 *Am J Clin Nutr* 2000;71:327S-30S.
5713 *Arch Gen Psychiatry* 2000;57:716-7.
5714 *Phytomedicine* 1999;6:281-3.
5715 *Invest Ophthalmol Vis Sci* 1999;40:1191-9.
5716 *Curr Opin Pediatr* 2000;12:298-302.
5717 *Phytomedicine* 1998;5:425-34.
5718 *J Altern Complement Med* 2000;6:219-29.
5719 *J Clin Pharmacol* 2000;40:647-54.
5720 *J Am Geriatr Soc* 2000;48:1183-94.
5721 *Arch Phys Med Rehabil* 2000;81:668-78.
5723 *Life Sci* 1998;62:2329-40.
5724 *Endocrinol* 1996;137:5707-18.
5728 *Food Chem Toxicol* 2000;38:99-111.
5729 *Sci Am* 1966;214:40-50.
5730 *Am Fam Physician* 1985;32:137-43.
5731 *J Toxicol Clin Toxicol* 1992;30:493-504.
5732 *Ann Intern Med* 1999;130:7-13.
5733 *Clin Pediatr (Phila)* 1993;32:284-91.
5734 *JAMA* 1967;201:972-4.
5735 *Lancet* 1961;1:310-2.
5736 *Arch Pediatr Adolesc Med* 1998;152:1100-4.
5737 *Ann Pharmacother* 1993;27:1504-9.
5738 *J Cardiovasc Nurs* 1996;10:78-86.
5739 *Altern Med Rev* 1998;3:4-17.
5740 *Am Heart J* 2000;140:139-41.
5741 *J Clin Pharmacol* 1998;38:101-5.
5742 *Circulation* 1997;96:1031-3.

5743 *Altern Ther Health Med* 1995;1:53-7.
5744 *Med Hypotheses* 1999;53:69-70.
5746 *WJM* 1999;171:191-4.
5747 *JAMA* 1975;233:1206-7.
5749 Green S. Chelation therapy: unproven claims and unsound theories. Quackwatch 2000. Available at: http://www.quackwatch.org (Accessed 17 November 2000).
5750 *Am J Cardiol* 1963;11:501-6.
5751 *Med Hypotheses* 1998;27:41-9.
5752 *Am J Surg* 1991;162:122-5.
5753 *J Intern Med* 1992;231:261-7.
5754 *Circulation* 1994;90:1194-9.
5756 Anon. Questions and Answers about chelation therapy. American Heart Association 2000. Available at: www.americanheart.org. (Accessed 17 November 2000).
5757 *Arch Dermatol* 1962;86:95-9.
5758 *Br J Dermatol* 1968;80:184-9.
5759 *Med J Aust* 1969;1:992-1001.
5760 *J Invest Dermatol* 1966;47:235-46.
5761 *Am Heart J* 1967;73:835-7.
5762 *Prog Cardiovasc Dis* 1960;2:432-43.
5763 *Proc Soc Exp Biol Med* 1950;74:415-7.
5764 *FEMS Immunol Med Microbiol* 2000;28:343-6.
5765 *Pharmacotherapy* 1998;18:130-9.
5768 *Am Heart J* 2000;140:4-5.
5769 *Circulation* 1999;99:164-5.
5770 *Altern Ther Health Med* 1995;1:53-6.
5771 Lacy CF, Armstrong LL, Ingrim NB, et al. Drug Information Handbook. 6th ed. Hudson, OH:Lexi-Comp Inc 1998:439-41.
5772 Ellsworth AJ, Witt DM, Dugdale DC, et al. Medical Drug Reference. Saint Louis, MO: Mosby-Year Book Inc 1998:302-3.
5773 *Ophthalmologica* 1975;171:119-22.
5774 Yanoff M, Duker JS. Ophthalmology. Saint Louis, MO: Mosby-Year Book Inc., 1999.
5775 Carey CF, Lee HH, Woeltje KF. The Washington Manual of Medical Therapeutics. Philadelphia, PA: Lippincott-Raven Publishers, 1998.
5784 *Phytomedicine* 2000;7:341-50.
5786 *JAMA* 1991;265:1833-9.
5787 *JAMA* 1992;267:3317-25.
5788 *Am J Clin Nutr* 1999;69:30-42.
5789 *Am J Clin Nutr* 1995;62:1245-51.
5792 *Fed Regist* 1996;61:296-313.
5794 *J Am Diet Assoc* 1986;86:759-64.
5795 *Am J Clin Nutr* 54:678-83.
5796 *Eur J Clin Nutr* 1994;48:465-74.
5797 FDA Talk Paper. FDA Allows Whole Oat Foods To Make Health Claim on Reducing the Risk of Heart Disease. 1997. Available at: http://www.fda.gov/bbs/topics/ANSWERS/ANS00782.html.
5798 *Ann Pharmacother* 2000;34:630-8.
5799 *Epilepsia* 1996;37:687-9.
5800 *Neurosci Biobehav Rev* 1994;18:291-304.
5801 *Prog Neurobiol* 1997;51:337-61.
5802 *Prog Neurobiol* 1996;50:1-7.
5803 *Neurosci Biobehav Rev* 1989;13:187-98.
5804 *J Clin Invest* 1997;100:745-53.
5805 *Med Hypotheses* 1996;47(6):455-9.
5806 *Int Clin Psychopharmacol* 1995;10:245-50.
5807 *J Forensic Sci* 1995;40:501-4.
5808 *Semin Oncol* 1983;10:66-71.
5809 *Lancet* 1977;1:721-4.
5810 *Biol Psychiatry* 1983;18:1023-32.
5811 *Physiol Behav* 1983;30:607-12.
5812 *Neurology* 1980;30:832-8.
5813 *Ann Emerg Med* 1999;33:475-6.
5814 *BMJ* 2000;320:861-4.
5816 *Atherosclerosis* 1987;65:173-9.
5819 *J Autism Dev Disord* 1999;29(3):191-4.
5820 *J Lab Clin Med* 1990;115(4):481-6.
5821 *Ann Pharmacother* 1992;26:935-7.
5822 *Am J Vet Res* 1992;53(5):829-33.
5823 *Epilepsia* 1989;30(1):90-3.
5824 *Pharmacol Biochem Behav* 1985;22(4):641-3.
5825 *J Infect Dis* 1981;143(1):101-5.
5826 *N Engl J Med* 1982;307:1081-2.
5827 *N Engl J Med* 1983;308:527-8.
5828 *Arch Neurol* 1984;41:1129-30.
5829 *Ann Neurol* 1985;17:213.
5830 *Ann Pharmacother* 1994;28:973.
5837 *Proc Natl Acad Sci U S A* 1995;92:6617-9.
5838 *Gastroenterology* 1972;62:642-6.
5839 *Steroids* 2000;65:124-9.
5840 Davidson MH, Weeks C, Lardy H, et al. Clinical Safety and Endocrine Effects of 7-KETO-DHEA. Abstract presented at: Experimental Biology 98, April 19-22, 1998, San Francisco, CA. Abstract obtained from Humanetics Corporation website.
5841 Nelson R, Herron M, Weeks C, Lardy H. Dehydroepiandrosterone and 7-KETO-DHEA augment Interleukin 2 (IL2) Production by Human Lymphocytes In Vitro. Abstract presented at: The 5th Conference on Retroviruses and Opportunistic Infections, February 1-5, 1998, Chicago, IL. Abstract obtained from Humanetics Corporation.
5842 Colker CM, Torina GC, Swain MA, Kalman DS. Double-Blind Study Evaluating the Effects of Exercise Plus 3-Acetyl-7-oxo-dehydroepiandrosterone on Body Composition and the Endocrine System in Overweight Adults. Abstract presented at 2nd ASEP Annual Meeting, October 14-16, 1999, and published in Journal of Exercise Physiology online, Volume 2 Number 4 October 1999.
5847 *Resp Med* 1994;88:555-7.
5848 *J Nutr* 1995;125:2511-5.
5849 *J Nutr* 1997;127:378,380.
5850 *Phytochemistry* 1995;40:1433-7.
5851 *Acta Univ Palacki Olomuc Fac Med* 1982;103:273-9.
5852 *Int J Dermatol* 1984;23:263-8.
5854 *Oncology* 1994;51:344-7.
5855 *Br J Cancer* 1994;69:196-9.
5856 *Mol Cell Endocrinol* 1995;112:169-73.
5857 *Br J Cancer* 1996;74:1466-8.
5862 *J Food Prot* 1998;61:272-5.
5863 *Eisei Shikenjo Hokoku* 1996;:38-42.
5864 *Food Addit Contam* 1995;12(3):347-50.
5865 *Food Addit Contam* 1995;12(3):343-6.
5866 *J Orthomolec Med* 1990;5:155-7.
5867 *Pharmazie* 1999;54(6):452-6.
5868 *Urology* 2000;55:755-8.
5869 *Arterioscler Thromb Vasc Biol* 2000;20:782-92.
5870 *Am J Psychiatry* 1999;156:971.
5871 *J Clin Endocrinol Metab* 2000;85:1834-40.
5872 *J Rheumatol* 1998;25:2352-6.
5873 *Arch Fam Med* 2000;9:241-5.
5874 *Arch Intern Med* 2000;160:2193-8.
5875 *Am J Clin Nutr* 2000;71:530-6.
5876 *Am J Clin Nutr* 2000;71:1181-6.
5877 *Arch Intern Med* 2000;160:931-6.
5878 *Am J Clin Nutr* 2000;72:139-45.

REFERENCES

5879 *Hypertension* 2000;35:936-41.
5880 *Arzneimittelforschung* 2000;50:16-23.
5881 *Arthritis Rheum* 1996;39:648-56.
5882 *Int J Cancer* 2000;86:276-80.
5883 *Int J Clin Pharmacol Ther* 1998;36:403-5.
5884 *Ann Thorac Surg* 1998;66:941-2.
5885 *Allergy* 2000;55:546-50.
5886 *J Agric Food Chem* 2000;48:1340-4
5887 *Nat Med* 2000;6(3):313-9.
5888 *Nat Med* 2000;6:255-6.
5889 *Nature* 2000;404:84-7.
5890 *Phytother Res* 2000;14:167-73.
5891 *Cancer Immunol Immunother* 1985;19:73-8.
5892 *J Ethnopharmacol* 1988;24:135-46.
5893 *Nutr Cancer* 1999;33:188-95.
5894 *Am J Clin Nutr* 1999;69:549-55.
5895 *Anticancer Res* 1998;18:1405-8.
5896 *Arterioscler Thromb Vasc Biol* 1997;17(6):1163-70.
5897 *Nutr Cancer* 1997;27:26-30.
5898 *Rheumatol Int* 1995;14:231-4.
5899 *Br J Nutr* 1993;69:443-53.
5900 *Curr Opin Clin Nutr Metab Care* 1998;1:527-30.
5902 *Int J Cancer* 2000;85:643-8.
5910 Duke J. The Green Pharmacy. Emmaus: Rodale Press, 1997
5911 *Nephron* 1998;80:242-3.
5912 Nutrition Search. Nutrition Almanac, Revised Edition. New York: McGraw-Hill Book Company. 1979.
5914 *Contraception* 2002;65:259-63.
5915 *J Neurooncol* 1994;19:25-35.
5916 *JAMA* 1961;175:187-90.
5919 *Clin Ther* 1982;4:423-40.
5921 *Dig Dis Sci* 1982;27:723-7.
5922 *JAMA* 1994;272:1413-20.
5923 *Am J Vet Res* 1999;60:1558-61.
5924 *Toxicol Sci* 1999;52:107-10.
5925 *Am J Clin Nutr* 1999;70:21-7.
5926 *Anticancer Res* 1999;19:1953-60.
5928 *Am J Physiol* 1998;275:R667-72.
5931 *Nutr Cancer* 1999;33:53-7.
5932 *J Nutr* 128:881-5.
5933 *Am J Clin Nutr* 1998;67:332-7.
5934 *Curr Opin Clin Nutr Metab Care* 1999;2:499-506.
5937 *J Nutr* 2000;130:1695-9.
5939 *Menopause* 2000;7:289-96.
5940 *Int J Dermatol* 1995;34:434-7.
5941 *Dev Med Child Neurol* 2000;42:174-81.
5942 *Lancet* 1995;345:1529-32.
5944 Fleming T, ed. PDR for Herbal Medicines, 2nd ed. Montvale: Medical Economics 2000.
5955 *J Ethnopharmacol* 1996;55:27-33.
5956 *Antiviral Res* 1996;30:75-85.
5957 *J Ethnopharmacol* 1995;48:25-32.
5958 *J Nutr* 1994;124:817-24.
5959 *Arch Invest Med (Mex)* 1991;22:333-6.
5960 *Arch Invest Med (Mex)* 1990;21:99-102.
5961 *Arch Invest Med (Mex)* 1989;20:321-5.
5962 *Arch Invest Med (Mex)* 1989;20:197-201.
5963 *Arch Invest Med (Mex)* 1988;19:143-8.
5964 *Diabetes Care* 1988;11:63-6.
5968 *Am J Chin Med* 1986;14:116-8.
5969 *Gac Med Mex* 1991;127:163-70.
5970 *Gae Med Mex* 1992;128:431-6.
5971 Medical Economic. Physician's Desk Reference. Montvale:Medical Economics, 1999:1289.
5973 McCalla CX. Instantaneous cure of acute frontal cephalalgia. Manufacturer information from High Chemical Company; 1995.
5975 Manufacturer Information. Sarapin. Injection technique in pain control. High Chemical Company. Information not dated.
5979 *Am J Clin Nutr* 1982;36:32-40.
5991 *Ann Allergy Asthma Immunol* 1999;83:377-83.
5993 *Clin Exp Allergy* 1997;27:1203-11.
5994 *Clin Exp Allergy* 1999;29:1256-9.
5995 *Int J Food Sci Nutr* 1998;49:199-203.
5996 *J Investig Allergol Clin Immunol* 1998;8:6-16.
5997 *J Allergy Clin Immunol* 1999;104:889-90.
5998 *Allergy* 1994;49:314-6.
5999 *Epidemiol Infect* 1990;104:389-95.
6000 *JAMA* 1999;281:2020-8.
6001 Roche Laboratories, Inc. Package insert for Xenical. April 1999.
6002 Fetrow CW, Avila JR. Professional's Handbook of Complementary & Alternative Medicines. 1st ed. Springhouse, PA: Springhouse Corp., 1999.
6004 *Diabetes Care* 1983;6:319-27.
6006 Mother Nature Products website: www.mothernature.com (Accessed 23 July 1999).
6007 *Pharmacist's Letter/Prescriber's Letter* 1998;14(12):141212.
6008 *Am J Health Syst Pharm* 2000;57:963-9.
6009 *J Clin Pharmacol* 1997;37:116-22.
6010 *J Clin Endocrinol Metab* 1999;84:2170-6.
6011 *J Clin Endocrinol Metab* 1999;84:3896-902.
6012 *Steroids* 2000;65:98-102.
6013 *Aging (Milano)* 1999;11:30-4.
6014 *J Endocrinol Invest* 1999;22:681-7.
6015 *Nutr Res* 2000;20:505-14.
6016 *Am J Med* 2000;108:518.
6017 *Am J Clin Nutr* 1999;70:951-2.
6018 *Lancet* 1999;354:488.
6019 *J Am Diet Assoc* 1999;99:1249-58.
6020 *Metabolism* 1993;42:463-9.
6022 *JAMA* 2000;283:2674-9.
6023 *South Med J* 2000;93:297-304.
6024 *Diabetes Care* 2000;23:455-9.
6025 *J Am Coll Nutr* 2000;19:256-61.
6026 American Academy of Pediatrics. The transfer of drugs and other chemicals into human milk (RE9403). Available at: www.aap.org/policy/00026.html.
6027 *Am J Clin Nutr* 1999;70:1001-8.
6028 *J Am Coll Cardiol* 2000;35:706-13.
6029 *J Nutr* 1999;129:758S-67S.
6030 *J Am Coll Cardiol* 2000;35:1403-10.
6031 *US Pharm* 2000;May:67-70.
6032 *Eur J Clin Nutr* 2000;54:87-92.
6033 *Am J Clin Nutr* 2000;71:1103-7.
6034 *J Am Pharm Assoc* 200;40:234-42.
6036 *Am J Clin Nutr* 2000;71:352S-6S.
6037 *J Am Coll Cardiol* 1999;33:1549-52.
6038 *Eur Heart J* 1992;13:1528-33.
6039 *Toxicon* 1972;10:377-80.
6040 *Toxicon* 1972;10:581-6.
6041 *Endeavour* 1988;12:60-5.
6042 *FEBS Lett* 1999;448:62-6.
6043 *Allergy* 1999;54:980-4.
6044 *J Rheumatol* 1999;26:2684-90.
6045 *Rheum Dis Clin North Am* 1999;25(4):919-28.
6046 *Am J Emerg Med* 2000;18:22-7.
6047 *Am J Cardiol* 1990;65:521-3.

6048 *Am J Health Syst Pharm* 2000;57:1221-7.
6049 *Thorax* 2000;55:283-8.
6051 *Phytomedicine* 1998;5:253-7.
6052 *Med Sci Sports Exerc* 2000;32:706-17.
6054 *Am J Clin Nutr* 1995;61:625S-30S.
6055 *Am J Respir Crit Care Med* 1998;158:728-33.
6056 *Am J Clin Nutr* 1994;59:110-4.
6057 *Thorax* 2000;55:102-8.
6058 *Am J Respir Crit Care Med* 1995;151:1401-8.
6060 Wobenzym N media kit. Naturally Vitamins (Marlyn Nutraceuticals, Inc.): Scottsdale, AZ.
6061 *Clin Sports Med* 1998;17:283-97.
6062 *J Am Acad Dermatol* 1998;39:611-25.
6064 *Postgrad Med* 1997;102:115-26.
6065 *Arch Dermatol* 2000;136:989-94.
6066 *Int Med* 1998;1:173-6.
6067 *Psychopharmacol Bull* 1998;34:391-7.
6068 Mease PJ, Merrill JT, Lahita RG, et al. GL701 (prasterone, dehydroepiandrosterone) improves systemic lupus erythematosus. 2000 American College of Rheumatology Meeting. Philadelphia, PA. October 29-November 2. Abstract 1230.
6069 *J Ethnopharmacol* 2000;71:83-8.
6070 *Clin Exp Allergy* 1993;23:226-30.
6071 *J Immunol* 1995;154:4027-31.
6072 *N Z Med J* 1986;99:281-3.
6073 *N Engl J Med* 2000;342:1686-92.
6074 Hollister-Stier Laboratories LLC. Instructions and dosing schedule for allergenic extracts hymenoptera venom prodcts. No. 355120-HD1.
6075 *Mayo Clin Proc* 1992;67(2):188-94.
6076 *J Allergy Clin Immunol* 2000;105(2 Pt 1):385-90.
6077 *Allergy* 1987;42:401-13.
6078 *BMJ* 1998;316:1365-8.
6079 Anon. Alpha Hydroxy Acids in Cosmetics. July 31, 1997. FDA. www.fda.gov/opacom/backgrounders/alphabg.html.
6080 Kurtzweil P. Alpha-hydroxy acids for skin care: Smooth sailing or rough seas? FDA 1999. www.fda.gov. (Accessed 18 August 2000).
6081 *Br J Psychiatry* 2000;177:174-8.
6082 *Altern Med Rev* 2000;5:93-108.
6083 *Neurology* 1993;43:2645-7.
6085 *Am J Clin Nutr* 2000;72:30-5.
6086 *J Spinal Cord Med* 2000;23:136-40.
6087 *Gastroenterology* 2000;119:305-9.
6088 *Scand J Infect Dis* 1990;22:43-7.
6089 *FEMS Immunol Med Microbiol* 1993;6:251-64.
6090 *Appl Environ Microbiol* 1996;62:1958-63.
6091 *J Urol* 1987;138:330-5.
6092 *Infect Immun* 1985;47:84-9.
6093 *Infect Immun* 1989;57:2447-51.
6094 *Can J Microbiol* 1988;34:339-43.
6095 *Clin Ther* 1992;14:11-6.
6096 *J Infect Dis* 1998;178:446-50.
6097 Mease PJ, Ginzler EM, Gluck OS, et al. Improvement in bone mineral density in steroid-treated SLE patients during treatment with GL701 (prasterone, dehydroepiandrosterone). 2000 American College of Rheumatology Meeting. Philadelphia, PA. October 29-November 2. abstract 835.
6098 *Rheum Dis Clin North Am* 2000;26:349-62.
6099 *Am J Clin Nutr* 2000;71:1682S-7S.
6101 *Arch Surg* 2000;135:416-23.
6102 *Biol Psychiatry* 1999;45:241-2.
6103 Israel RJ, Sonis ST. Topical dehydroascorbic acid (DHA) reduces moderate to severe mucositis in the hamster acute radiation model. 36th Am Soc Clin Oncol Ann Mtg Prog Proceedings/Abstracts: Abstract 2367.
6104 *Am J Clin Nutr* 2000;71:956-61.
6106 *Eur J Clin Nutr* 2000;54:234-8.
6107 Agrawal A. Potato peel extract holds potential as antiboitic. Reuters Health May 23, 2000. www.medscape.com (Accessed 23 May 2000).
6110 *Arch Ophthalmol* 1995;113:518-23.
6112 *Lancet* May 2000;355:1912.
6114 Miller MJ, Vergnolle N, Wallace JL, et al. Sangre de grado is a potent and unique inhibitor of neurogenic inflammation and promotes healing in experimental necrotizing enterocolitis. Pediatric Academic Soc and Acad Pediatrics Joint Mtg, May 12-6 2000:Abstract 979.
6118 Lewis CJ, Alpert S. Letter to health care professionals -- FDA concerned about botanical products, including dietary supplements, containing aristolochic acid. Office of Nutritional Products, Labeling, Dietary Supplements. Center for Food Safety and Applied Nutrition. May 31, 2000.
6122 *Med Lett Drugs Ther* 2000;42:29-31.
6124 *Ann Pharmacother* 2000;34:622-9.
6126 *Cancer Res* 2000;60:3477-83.
6127 Atkinson C, Compston JE, Robins SP, Bingham SA. The effects of isoflavone phytoestrogens on bone; preliminary results from a large randomized, controlled trial. Endocrine Soc 82nd Ann Mtg, Toronto, CAN 2000;Jun 21-4:abstract 196.
6128 Gerber G, Lowe FC, Spigelman S. The use of a standardized extract of red clover isoflavones for the alleviation of BPH symptoms. Endocrine Soc 82nd Ann Mtg, Toronto, CAN 2000;Jun 21-4:abstract 2359.
6132 Kulkarni PM, Schuman PC, Merlino NS, Kinzie JL. Lactic acidosis and hepatic steatosis in HIV seropositive patients treated with nucleoside analogues. Natl AIDS Treatment Advocacy Project. Dig Disease Week Liver Conf, San Diego,CA. 2000;May 21-4:Rep11.
6133 *Am J Clin Nutr* 2000;71:1187-93.
6134 *Am J Clin Nutr* 2000;71:795-8.
6135 *J Pharm Pharmacol* 1999;51:1391-6.
6136 *N Engl J Med* 1999;341(24):1801-6.
6137 *JAMA* 2000;283:2822-5.
6138 *Gut* 2000;46:651-5.
6140 NCAA prohibits schools from supplying creatine to students. Reuters Health 2000;Jun 13. Available at: www.medscape.com/reuters/prof/ 2000/06/06.13/20000613publ004.html (Accessed 13 June 2000).
6143 *Am J Clin Nutr* 2000;71:1085-94.
6144 *CMAJ* 1999;160:310.
6145 *Br J Dermatol* 1999;141:598-600.
6146 *Contact Dermatitis* 1997;:183.
6147 *Contact Dermatitis* 1992;27:346-7.
6148 *Contact Dermatitis* 1988;18:55-6.
6149 *Contact Dermatitis* 1986;15:303-4.
6150 *Contact Dermatitis* 1980;6:288-9.
6151 *Contact Dermatitis* 1979;5:198-9.
6152 *Am J Clin Nutr* 2000;71:1570-6.
6153 *BMJ* 1999;318:570-5.
6154 *J Nutr* 1998;128:1458-63.
6155 *Arch Otolaryngol Head Neck Surg* 1999;125:1091-8.
6166 Cellex-C product information for professionals. Cellex-C. www.cellex-c.com/pro_side/navigator.html (Accessed 14 June 2000).
6167 *Am J Obstet Gynecol* 1995;173:881-4.

6168 *Obstet Gynecol* 1991;78:33-6.
6169 *Urology* 1993;41(4):343-5.
6170 Wang ZQ, Zhang XH, Baldor LC, et al. Chromium picolinate enhances insulin sensitivity in an animal model for the metabolic syndrome: the obese, insulin resistant JCR:LA-corpulent rat. Am Diabetes Assn's 60th Sci Sessions & Expo, San Antonio, TX 2000;Jun 9-13: abstract 291.
6171 Nelson L, Rao A, Olson P. Unique hydrolyzed whey protein isolates with antihypertensive activity. Institute of Food Tech 2000 Ann Mtg & Food Expo:abstract 38-6. Available at: ift.confex.com/ift/2000/techprogram/paper_5129.htm.
6172 *Arch Intern Med* 2000;160:1025-30.
6173 *Heart* 2000;83:394-9.
6174 *J Allergy Clin Immunol* 2000;105:462-7.
6175 *J Fr Ophthalmol* 1988;11:671-4.
6176 *Clin Ther* 2000;22:209-21.
6177 *Br J Dermatol* 1997;136:973-4.
6178 *Ann Dermatol Venereol* 1993;120:599-603.
6180 Eagon PK, Elm MS, Hunter DS, et al. Medicinal herbs: modulation of estrogen action. Era of Hope Mtg, Dept Defense; Breast Cancer Res Prog, Atlanta, GA 2000;Jun 8-11.
6181 *Ann Pharmacother* 2000;34:729-33.
6182 *Neurology* 2000;54:1848-50.
6183 *Med Sci Sports Exerc* 2000;32:993-6.
6185 *J Nutr* 2000;130(4):767-76.
6186 *Chest* 2000;117:1324-9.
6187 *Pediatrics* 2000;105:E40. Available at: www.pediatrics.org/cgi/content/full/105/3/e40.
6188 *Cereal Chem* 2000:77;297-302.
6190 *Nervenarzt* 1996;67:672-81.
6192 *Arch Dermatol* 2000;136:755-7.
6193 *Am J Clin Nutr* 2000;71:1201-8.
6196 *J Endocrinol Invest* 2003;26:646-50.
6197 *J Allergy Clin Immunol* 1999;103(3 Pt 1):507-13.
6198 Varnell MA. Enhanced herb may help female sexual dysfunction. Reuters Health 2000;Jun 27. www.reutershealth.com/frame/eline.html (Accessed 28 June 2000).
6199 *Ugeskr Laeger* 1998;160:3226-7.
6200 *Med J Aust* 1998;169:583-6.
6201 *Am J Emerg Med* 2000;18:231-2.
6203 *Magnesium* 1986;5:85-94.
6204 *Pharmacist's Letter/Prescriber's Letter* 2000;16(3):160307.
6205 *J Assoc Physicians India* 1992;40:346.
6206 *Phytother Res* 2000;14:30-5.
6208 *Arch Phys Med Rehabil* 2000;81:668-78.
6209 *Clin Sci* 1988;74:595-7.
6210 *Eur Resp J* 1996;9:237-40.
6211 *Am J Med* 2000,108:276-81.
6212 *Chung Kuo Yao Li Hsueh Pao* 1998;19:417-21.
6213 *Vasa* 1998;27:106-10.
6214 *Phytother Res* 1999;13:408-15.
6215 *Int J Clin Pharmacol Res* 1984;4:89-93.
6216 *Curr Med Res Opin* 1991;12:350-5.
6217 *Eur J Clin Pharmacol* 1989;36:239-45.
6218 *Audiol* 1994;33:85-92.
6219 *Presse Med* 1986;15:1562-4.
6220 *Adv Ther* 1998;15:291-304.
6221 *Presse Med* 1986;15:1569-72.
6222 *Arzneimittelforschung* 1994;44:1005-13.
6223 *Br J Clin Pharmacol* 1992;34:352-8.
6224 *Phytomedicine* 2000;6:393-401.
6225 *Pharmacopsychiatry* 1996;29:47-56.
6226 National Institutes of Health. Clinical trials. www.clinicaltrials.gov/ct/gui/c/r (Accessed 15 June 2000).
6227 *Presse Med* 1986;15:1556-8.
6228 *Cochrane Database Syst Rev* 2000;CD001775.
6229 *Rev Fr Gynecol Obstet* 1993;88:447-57.
6230 *Aviat Space Environ Med* 1996;67:445-52.
6231 *Life Sci* 2000;66:141-6.
6232 *Arzneimittelforschung* 2000;50:232-5.
6233 *Life Sci* 1996;58:1315-21.
6234 *Am J Clin Nutr* 2000;71:993-8.
6236 *Clin Sci (Colch)* 1999;96:235-9
6237 *Obstet Gynecol* 2000;95:519-24.
6238 *J Nutr* 1996;126:1992-9.
6239 *Am J Psychiatry* 1997;154:426-8.
6240 *J Am Acad Dermatol* 1994;31:89-97.
6241 *J Am Diet Assoc* 2000;100:88-94.
6242 *J Am Diet Assoc* 1999;99:285.
6243 Food and Nutrition Board, Institute of Medicine. Dietary Reference Intakes for Thiamin, Riboflavin, Niacin, Vitamin B6, Folate, Vitamin B12, Pantothenic Acid, Biotin, and Choline (2000). Washington, DC: National Academy Press, 2000. Available at: http://books.nap.edu/books/0309065542/html.
6245 *Int J Clin Pharmacol Res* 1983;3:239-50.
6246 *Adv Exp Med Biol* 1999;467:85-8.
6247 *J Affect Disord* 1998;50:23-7.
6248 *Pharmacol Biochem Behav* 1982;17:65-71.
6249 *Pharmacopsychiatry* 2000;33:47-53.
6250 *Fundam Clin Pharmacol* 1997;11:127-32.
6251 *J Toxicol Clin Toxicol* 2000;38:63-6.
6252 *Clin Drug Invest* 2000;19:15-23.
6253 *Ann Intern Med* 2000;132:680.
6254 *Drugs Exp Clin Res* 1996;22:323-9.
6255 *Physiol Behav* 1990;48:241-6.
6256 *J Pediatr Gastroenterol Nutr* 2000;30:78-84.
6257 *N Engl J Med* 1996;334:1557-60.
6258 *Dig Dis Sci* 1994;39:2589-94.
6259 *Scand J Gastroenterol* 1996;31:778-85.
6260 *Arch Ophthalmol* 2000;118:401-4.
6261 *Am J Clin Nutr* 2000;71:1433-8.
6262 *Am J Clin Nutr* 1998;67:367-76.
6263 *J Nutr* 1997;127:1973-80.
6264 FDA, Ctr Food Safety, Applied Nutr. FDA allows foods containing psyllium to make health claim on reducing risk of heart disease. Available at: http://vm.cfsan.fda.gov/~lrd/tpsylliu.html.
6265 *Am J Gastroenterol* 2000;95:1244-52.
6266 *N Engl J Med* 2000;342:1392-8.
6269 *Dig Dis Sci* 1993;38:1614-8.
6270 *Gastroenterology* 1997;112:29-32.
6271 *J Cancer Res Clin Oncol* 1993;119:549-54.
6280 *Magnesium* 1988;7:78-83.
6281 *Am J Clin Nutr* 1998;67:919-26.
6282 *Arzneimittelforschung* 2000;50:260-5.
6284 *BJU Int* 1999;84:845-50.
6285 *Prostate* 2000;42:163-71.
6286 *BJU Int* 2000;85:481-5.
6287 *Mol Urol* 1999;3(3):333-6.
6289 *J Clin Pharmacol* 2000;40:457-61.
6290 *Planta Med* 2000;66:91-3.
6291 *Planta Med* 1998;64:571-2.
6292 *J Nat Prod* 1998;61:1413-5.
6293 *Biochim Biophys Acta* 1999;1472:643-50.
6294 *Planta Med* 2000;66:70-1.
6295 *Phytother Res* 2000;14:210-2.

6297 *Acta Derm Venereol* 1978;58:443-8.
6298 *Br J Dermatol* 1977;97:681-4.
6299 *Eur J Dermatol* 2000 May;10:269-73.
6300 *Neurosurg* 1984;14(6):659-63.
6301 *Eur J Clin Pharmacol* 1991;40:113-4.
6302 *Ann N Y Acad Sci* 1983;411:293-308.
6303 *Rheum Dis Clin North Am* 1999;25:899-918.
6304 *Semin Arthritis Rheum* 1985;15:45-60.
6306 *Semin Hematol* 1995;32:60-79.
6307 *Ann Surg* 1996;224:583-9.
6308 *J Am Acad Dermatol* 1983;8:433-6.
6309 *N Z Med J* 1981;94:384-6.
6310 *Br Med J* 1966;2:805-7.
6311 *Br Med J* 1970;4:776-80.
6312 *Scand J Infect Dis* 1981;13:257-62.
6313 *Arthritis Rheum* 1985;28:308-14.
6314 *Rheum Dis Clin North Am* 1990;16:217-41.
6315 *Gut* 1995;37:157-8.
6317 *Pain* 1997;73(2):123-39.
6318 *J Clin Apheresis* 1992;7(3):132-4.
6320 *Anticancer Res* 1998;18:4705-8.
6321 *Intern Med* 1993;32(5):359-64.
6323 *Cancer Nurs* 2000;23:134-40.
6324 *Ann N Y Acad Sci* 1983;411:6-10.
6325 *Clin Biochem* 1983;16(4):261-2.
6326 *Cornell Vet* 1986;76(1):61-90.
6327 *J Clin Oncol* 1984;2(3):227-41.
6328 *Med Hypotheses* 1993;41(6):495-8.
6329 *Neurosci Lett* 1993;150(2):145-8.
6330 *Cryobiology* 1986;23:14-27.
6331 *Cytobios* 1990;63:139-65.
6332 *Br Med J (Clin Res Ed)* 1987;295:1657.
6334 *Clin Toxicol* 1978;12(4):417-26.
6335 *Postgrad Med J* 1987;63(739):363-5.
6337 *Eur J Toxicol Environ Hyg* 1976;9(2):119-25.
6338 *Toxicon* 1999;37(6):841-65.
6339 *J Anim Sci* 1988;66:2407-13.
6340 *Med J Aust* 1995;162:592-3.
6341 *West J Med* 1995;163:573-4.
6344 *NACCT Abstracts* 1996: Abstract #131.
6346 *Neurology* 1975;25(8):730-4.
6347 *Calif Med* 1973;119:78-82.
6348 *J Toxicol Clin Toxicol* 1984;22(2):157-66.
6349 *MMWR Morb Mortal Wkly Rep* 1994;43:229-31.
6350 *JACEP* 1979;8(10):401-3.
6351 *Clin Toxicol* 1979;14(1):87-92.
6353 *West J Med* 1985;142:637-40.
6354 *Can J Public Health* 1976;67:386.
6355 *N Engl J Med* 1969;281:566-7.
6356 *Am J Clin Nutr* 2000;71:999-1002.
6357 *Am J Psychiatry* 2000;157:715-21.
6358 *N Engl J Med* 2000;342:981.
6360 Suzuki Y, Oishi Y, Yamazaki H, et al. How to avoid bone loss in patients with prostatic carcinoma receiving long-term LHRH-analogue. 2000 Abstract Info-Am Urol Assn, Inc.
6362 Minne HW, Pfeifer M, Begerow B, et al. Vitamin D and calcium supplementation reduces falls in elderly women via improvement of body sway and normalization of blood pressure: a prospective, randomized, and double-blind study. Abstracts World Congress on Osteoporosis 2000.
6366 *J Nutr* 2000;130:1584-90.
6367 *Am J Clin Nutr* 2000;71:1448-54.
6368 *Urology* 1999;54:473-8.
6369 *J Forensic Sci* 1970;15:529-36.
6370 *J Sports Med Phys Fitness* 2000;40:71-9.
6371 *Pharmacotherapy* 2000;20:644-52.
6372 Suleman A, Siddiqui NH. Haemodynamic and cardiovascular effects of caffeine. Medicine On Line Int J Medicine 2000. www.priory.com/pharmol/caffeine.htm (Accessed 14 April 2000).
6373 *Neurology* 2000;54(12):2285-92.
6374 *Heart* 2000;83:688-95.
6376 *J Acquir Immune Defic Syndr* 2000;23:246-54.
6377 *Am J Clin Nutr* 2000;71:878-84.
6378 *Ophthalmology* 2000;10:450-6.
6380 *J Natl Cancer Inst* 2000;92:780-1.
6381 *J Natl Cancer Inst* 2000;92:826-32.
6382 *J Natl Cancer Inst* 1996;88:1550-9.
6384 *J Altern Complement Med* 2000;6:327-34.
6385 *Complement Ther Med* 1997;5:40-2.
6386 *Arch Fam Med* 1998;7:541-5.
6387 *Phytomedicine* 1996;3:95-102.
6388 *J Natl Cancer Inst* 1989;81:669-75.
6389 *Infect Immun* 1984;46:845-9.
6390 *Planta Med* 2000;66:241-4.
6391 *Planta Med* 2000;66:54-6.
6392 *Curr Med Res Opin* 1999;15:214-27.
6393 *Nutr Rev* 2000;58:39-53.
6394 *Am J Clin Nutr* 2000;71:914-20.
6395 *Br J Cancer* 1999;81:1238-42.
6396 *Arch Gen Psychiatry* 2000;57:715-6.
6397 *Lancet* 1999;354:2082-3.
6398 *Cancer* 2000;88:1916-28.
6399 *Am J Clin Nutr* 2000;72:389-94.
6400 *Clin Ther* 2000;22:411-9.
6401 Pizzorno JE, Murray MT, eds. Textbook of Natural Medicine. 2nd ed. Edinburgh:Churchill Livingstone, 1999.
6402 *Med J Aust* 1988;148:548-55.
6403 *BMJ* 1995;310:693-6.
6404 *Am J Clin Nutr* 2000;71:1003-7.
6405 *Arterioscler Thromb Vasc Biol* 2001;21:E34-7.
6406 *Lancet* 1985;2:373-7.
6407 *Clin Investig* 1993;71:S134-6.
6408 *J Card Fail* 1995;1:101-7.
6409 *Mol Aspects Med* 1994;15 Suppl:S287-94.
6410 Pizzorno JE, Murray MT, eds. Textbook of Natural Medicine. 2nd ed. New York: Churchill Livingston, 1999.
6412 *Am J Clin Nutr* 2000;71:1077-84.
6413 *Am J Clin Nutr* 2000;71:1462-9.
6414 *Am J Clin Nutr* 2000;71:1166-9.
6415 *J Am Coll Nutr* 2000;19:242-55.
6416 *J Am Coll Nutr* 2000;19:207-9.
6417 *Pharmacotherapy* 2000;20:690-7.
6418 *Am J Health Syst Pharm* 1999;56:121-3.
6420 Anon. Horse Chestnut. The Natural Pharmacist 2000. www.tnp.com/substance.asp?ID=62. (Accessed 24 June 2000).
6423 *J Neurol Neurosurg Psychiatry* 2000;68:679-80.
6424 *Prostate* 1996;29:231-40.
6425 *Clin Pharmacol Ther* 2000;67:451-7.
6426 *Br J Dermatol* 2000;142:979-84.
6427 *Arzneimittelforschung* 1999;49:106-9.
6428 *Ann Intern Med* 2000;132:743-56.
6429 *BJOG* 2000;107:870-6.
6430 Anderson PO, Knoben JE. Handbook of Clinical Drug Data. 8th ed. Stamford, CT: Appleton & Lange, 1997.
6431 *Ann Intern Med* 2000;132:538-46.
6432 *J Am Board Fam Pract* 2000;13:138-40.

REFERENCES

6433 *J Clin Oncol* 1998;16:3918-9.
6434 *BMJ* 2000;321:536-9.
6435 *Ann Pharmacother* 2000;34:1013-6.
6436 *Br J Clin Pharmacol* 2000;49:423-7.
6437 *Int Urol Nephrol* 1988;20:353-9.
6438 *Urol Int* 1986;41:393-6.
6439 *N Engl J Med* 1985;312:953-7.
6440 *Urol Int* 1977;32:348-52.
6441 *J Am Soc Nephrol* 1999;10:840-5.
6442 *J Urol* 1996;155:1847-51.
6443 *Biol Psychiatry* 1989;25:222-8.
6444 *Advances Neurol* 1992;58:303-10.
6445 *Eur J Clin Nutr* 1999;53:771-5.
6446 *Proc Natl Acad Sci U S A* 2000;97:4279-84.
6447 *Lupus* 1999;8:181-7.
6449 *Am J Clin Nutr* 2000;72:844-52.
6450 *Phytomedicine* 2000;7:273-82.
6451 *J Pharm Sci* 1976;65:1218-21.
6453 *Clin Pharmacol Ther* 2000;68:28-34.
6455 *Menopause* 2000;7:236-42.
6456 *Am J Med* 2000;109:9-14.
6457 *Ann Intern Med* 2000;133:420-9.
6458 *Cochrane Database Syst Rev* 2000;2:CD000980.
6459 *JAMA* 2000;284:1425-29.
6460 *JAMA* 2000;284:1432-3.
6461 *Diabetes Care* 2000;23:1221-6.
6462 *J Abnorm Child Psychol* 1987;15:75-90.
6463 *Proc Natl Acad Sci U S A* 2000;97:7500-2.
6464 *Gut* 2000;47:584-5.
6465 Garlic: Effects on cardiovascular risks and disease, protective effects against cancer, and clinical adverse effects. Summary, evidence report/technol assessment: no 20. AHRQ Publ No. 01-E022, 2000;Oct. Agency for Healthcare Res and Quality. Rockville, MD.
6466 *Biochem Pharmacol* 1997;54:1087-96.
6470 *Urol Res* 1992;20:96-7.
6471 *Ear Nose Throat J* 2000;79:778-82.
6472 *Phytomedicine* 2000;7:177-84.
6473 *Arch Intern Med* 2000;160:2548.
6474 *Arch Intern Med* 2000;160:2548.
6475 *J Endocrinol* 2000;166:R11-6.
6477 *Med J Aust* 2000;172:302.
6478 *CMAJ* 2000;163:262-3.
6479 Carey CF, Lee HH, Woeltje KF (eds). Washington Manual of Medical Therapeutics. 29th ed. New York, NY: Lippincott-Raven, 1998.
6480 *Forsch Komplementarmed Klass Naturheilkd* 2000;7:79-84.
6481 *J Aust Coll Midwives* 1999;12:20-5.
6482 *Ann Rheum Dis* 2000;59:631-5.
6483 *J Urol* 2000;164:1229-34.
6484 *J Clin Oncol* 2000;18:3595-603.
6485 *Biol Trace Elem Res* 1997;58:43–53.
6486 *N Engl J Med* 2000;343:1833-8.
6487 *Clin Toxicol* 2000;38:353-4.
6488 *Ther Drug Monit* 2000;22:497.
6490 *Dement Geriatr Cogn Disord* 2000;11:230-7.
6491 *Alzheimer's Dis Assoc Disord* 2000;14:S103-S108.
6492 *Arterioscler Thromb Vasc Biol* 2000;20:e34-e40.
6493 *Med Hypotheses* 2000;54:221-35.
6494 *Eur J Neurosci* 2000;12:1882-90.
6496 *Am J Psychiatry* 1999;156:1392-6.
6497 *Brain Res* 2000;878:98-104.
6498 *Eur J Clin Pharmacol* 2000;56:123-7.
6499 *Arch Gen Psychiatry* 2000 Aug;57:812-3.
6500 Mills S, Bone K. Principles and Practice of Phytotherapy. London: Churchill Livingstone, 2000.
6501 *Arch Dermatol* 1977;113:31-6.
6502 *Acta Derm Venereol* 1989;69:541-3.
6503 *Arch Dermatol* 1978;114:1018-20.
6504 *Acta Derm Venereol* 1977;57:357-60.
6505 *Br J Dermatol* 1979;101:321-5.
6506 *Br J Dermatol* 1977;97:561-6.
6507 *Int J Dermatol* 1982;21:481-4.
6508 *Br J Dermatol* 1977;96:283-6.
6509 *Acta Derm Venereol* 1990;70:304-8.
6510 *J Nutr* 2000;130:1488S-92S.
6511 *J Neurol Sci* 1998;158:47-52.
6512 *Brain Res* 1999;823:88-95.
6513 *Cutis* 1994;54:117-8.
6514 *Isr J Med Sci* 1990;26:306-9.
6515 *Br J Dermatol* 1980;103:411-5.
6516 *Int J Clin Pharmacol Res* 1985;5:25-33.
6517 *Scand J Rheumatol* 1982;11:168-70.
6518 *Clin Rheumatol* 1998;17:378-82.
6519 *Lancet* 1976;2:539-42.
6520 *Am J Clin Nutr* 1998;68:365-71.
6521 *Cochrane Database Syst Rev* 2000;CD001364.
6522 *J Nutr* 2000;130:1512S-5S.
6523 Guide to Clinical Preventive Services. 2nd ed. Natl Institute of Health, 1996. Available at: http://hstat2.nlm.nih.gov/download/409812772438.html.
6524 *J Clin Periodontol* 1996;23:465-70.
6525 *J Periodontol* 1990;61:674-9.
6526 *Scand J Dent Res* 1990;98:301-4.
6527 *Int Dent J* 1993;43:431-9.
6528 *Compend Contin Educ Dent* 1998;19:4-15.
6529 *Med Hypotheses* 1993;40:182-5.
6530 *Metabolism* 1994;43:1558-62.
6531 *J Trace Elem Med Biol* 1997;11:65-70.
6532 *Am J Clin Nutr* 1997;66:639-42.
6533 *Eur J Clin Nutr* 1995;49:282-8.
6534 *Indian J Lepr* 1994;66:51-7.
6535 *Lepr India* 1983;55:547-52.
6536 *Int J Lepr Other Mycobact Dis* 1984;52:331-8.
6537 *Int J Lepr Other Mycobact Dis* 1991;59:20-4.
6538 *Br J Dermatol* 1981;104:191-4.
6539 *Med Hypotheses* 1985;17:157-65.
6540 *Arzneimittelforschung* 1995;45:624-6.
6541 *J Clin Microbiol* 2000;38:1758-62.
6542 *Ann Pharmacother* 1996;30:186-7.
6543 *Am J Hypertens* 1988;1:303S-8S.
6544 *Am J Med Sci* 1999;318:392-405.
6545 *Am J Med Sci* 1999;318:380-91.
6546 *Am J Med Sci* 1976;272:285-99.
6547 *Cancer* 1998;82:1938-45.
6548 *Am J Clin Nutr* 1980;33:1517-21.
6549 *Hum Nutr Clin Nutr* 1983;37:219-25.
6550 *Kidney Int Suppl* 1983;16:S315-8.
6551 *Am J Clin Nutr* 1998;68:447S-63S.
6552 *Mol Cell Biochem* 1998;188:63-9.
6553 *Arch Intern Med* 1999;159:748-54.
6556 *Hum Reprod* 1994;9:1469-70.
6558 *J Am Acad Child Adolesc Psychiatry* 1999;38:357-8.
6562 *J Affect Disord* 1999;56:189-94.
6563 *Age Ageing* 1998;27:715-22.
6564 *AIDS* 1999;13:495-500.
6565 *Am J Epidemiol* 1996;143:1244-56.
6566 *Int J Immunopharmacol* 1995;17:719-27.
6568 *Lancet* 1980;2:618-20.
6569 *J Am Coll Nutr* 1983;2:157-62.

6570 *Cent Afr J Med* 1995;41:312-5.
6571 *Ann Intern Med* 1982;97:357-61.
6572 *Nephrol Dial Transplant* 1989;4:888-92.
6573 *Int Urol Nephrol* 1999;31:401-8.
6574 *Fertil Steril* 1999;71:1138-43.
6575 *J Androl* 2000;21:53-7.
6576 *Am J Clin Nutr* 1992;56:148-57.
6577 *Indian J Pathol Microbiol* 1997;40:451-5.
6578 *Eur J Obstet Gynecol Reprod Biol* 1998;79:179-84.
6579 *Arch Ophthalmol* 1996;114:991-7.
6580 *Ophthalmology* 1999;106:761-77.
6581 *Am J Epidemiol* 1998;148:204-14.
6583 *Arch Ophthalmol* 1988;106:192-8.
6584 *Invest Ophthalmol Vis Sci* 1996;37:1225-35.
6585 *N Engl J Med* 2000;343:1070-7.
6588 *J Rheumatol* 1994;21:927-33.
6589 *Digestion* 1992;51:18-26.
6590 *Rev Esp Enferm Dig* 1996;88:757-62.
6591 *Med J Aust* 1975;2:793-6.
6592 *Oral Surg Oral Med Oral Pathol* 1982;53:469-72.
6593 *South Med J* 1977;70:559-61.
6594 *J Assoc Physicians India* 1995;43:467-9.
6595 *J Pediatr* 1998;132:467-71.
6596 *Am J Hematol* 1999;61:194-202.
6597 *Biol Trace Elem Res* 1999;70:165-72.
6598 *Pediatr Hematol Oncol* 1993;10:257-60.
6599 *Eur J Pediatr* 1995;154:205-8.
6601 Anon. Roasting process to pump up cancer fighting properties of coffee unveiled by oncology sciences corp. PRNewswire 2000; Jun 30. www.prnewswire.com (Accessed 3 July 2000).
6602 *Otolaryngol Pol* 1989;43(3):180-4.
6603 Pennell MM. One to two drinks a day may reduce risk of Alzheimer dementia. Reuters Health. www.medscape.com/reuters/prof/2000/07/07.11/20000711epid005.html (Accessed 11 July 2000).
6604 *Eur J Clin Pharmacol* 1992;43:207-8.
6606 Goldschmidt RH, Dong BJ. Treatment of AIDS and HIV-related conditions: 2000. *J Am Board Fam Pract* 2000;13:274-98. Full text available at www.medscape.com/viewarticle/405799_print.
6607 *J Nutr* 2000;130:1719-23.
6610 Anon. Court backs Food & Drug Administration's check of cholestin. NewsExcite.com. news.excite.com/news/ap/000723/19/cholesterol-dispute (Accessed 25 July 2000).
6611 *N Engl J Med* 2000;343:180-4.
6612 *Addiction* 1997;92(1):89-96.
6613 *Br J Psychiatry* 2000;177:181.
6614 Murray MT. Encyclopedia of Nutritional Supplements. Rocklin, CA: Prima Health, 1996.
6620 Nationwide alert on hallmark labs injectable adrenal cortex extract. FDA. Available at: www.fda.gov/bbs/topics/NEWS/NEW00539.html.
6624 *Cutis* 2000;65:116.
6625 *Pharmaceutical Biology* 2000;38:181-6.
6627 *Minerva Cardioangiol* 1999;47:315-9.
6628 *Minerva Cardioangiol* 1998;46:41-7.
6629 *Minerva Cardioangiol* 1997;45:383-92.
6630 *Minerva Med* 1997;88:537-41.
6631 *Recenti Prog Med* 1995;86:282-9.
6632 *Pediatrics* 2001;108:90.
6633 *Acta Neurol (Napoli)* 1993;15:449-56.
6634 *Int J Dermatol* 1993;32:368-71.
6635 *J Int Med Res* 1993;21:138-46.
6637 *Acta Neurol (Napoli)* 1991;13:255-60.
6638 *Minerva Cardioangiol* 1991;39:395-400.
6639 *Minerva Med* 1991;82:101-5.
6640 *Ann Ital Med Int* 1989;4:378-85.
6641 *Riv Neurol* 1989;59:121-6.
6642 *Int J Tissue React* 1988;10:261-6.
6643 *Angiology* 1987;38:593-600.
6644 *Minerva Med* 1985;76:543-8.
6645 *Minerva Med* 1984;75:1733-8.
6646 *Pharmacol Res Commun* 1984;16:1-8.
6650 *Nippon Yakurigaku Zasshi* 1999;114:233-8.
6652 *JAMA* 1993;269:1635-6.
6653 *Physiol Chem & Physics* 1978;10:449-64.
6654 *West J Med* 2000;173:86-7.
6655 *J Prosthet Dent* 1991;66:361-9.
6656 *Cancer* 1996;77:522-5.
6660 *Crit Rev Biochem Mol Biol* 1989;24(1):1-40.
6661 *Arzneimittelforschung* 1991;41(12):1281-5.
6662 *Lancet* 1991;337(8732):12-3.
6668 Anon. FDA authorizes new coronary heart disease health claim for plant sterol and plant stanol esters. FDA. 2000. Available at: www.fda.gov/bbs/topics/ANSWERS/ANS01033.html.
6669 Anon. FDA takes action against firms marketing unapproved drugs. FDA. 2000. www.fda.gov/bbs/topics/ANSWERS/ANS01032.html.
6672 Anon. Postscript on laetrile. FDA. 1987. Available at: www.fda.gov/bbs/topics/ANSWERS/ANS00309.html.
6673 Anon. Laetrile (Amygdalin, other Names). FDA. 1987. www.fda.gov/ora/fiars/ora_import_ia6201.html.
6675 Anon. FDA warns against consuming dietary supplements containing tiratricol. FDA. 2000. Available at: www.fda.gov/bbs/topics/ANSWERS/ANS01057.html.
6677 *Med Oncol Tumor Pharmacother* 1989;6(1):31-43.
6678 *Clin Immunol Immunopathol* 1984;30(1):11-8.
6679 *Int J Tissue React* 1984;6(3):223-8.
6680 *Thymus* 1988-89;12(2):69-75.
6681 *Respiration* 1997;64:220-3.
6682 *Ann Allergy* 1987;58:379-84.
6683 *J Pediatr Surg* 1986;21:1000-4.
6684 *Immunopharmacol Immunotoxicol* 1993;15:447-59.
6685 *Pediatr Res* 1979;13:797-802.
6686 *Gut* 1984;25:279-83.
6687 *Cancer* 1977;39:575-80.
6688 *J Immunol* 1975;114:1248-54.
6689 *Med Oncol Tumor Pharmacother* 1989;6:5-9.
6690 *FEMS Immunol Med Microbiol* 2000;29:295-301.
6691 *Drugs Exp Clin Res* 1985;11(9):671-4.
6694 *Pediatr Med Chir* 1983;5(5):395-402.
6695 *Ann Allergy* 1989;62:425-8.
6696 *Int J Tissue React* 1989;11(1):21-5.
6697 *Thymus* 1986;8(6):331-9.
6698 *Pediatr Med Chir* 1988;10(6):603-7.
6699 *Pediatr Med Chir* 1990;12(3):229-32.
6700 *Antimicrob Agents Chemother* 1987;31:1263-5.
6703 *Ann Intern Med* 2000;133:245-52.
6705 *Curr Ther Res* 1998;59:595-607.
6706 *Ann Intern Med* 2000;133:302-3.
6708 *Lancet* 1977;2:895-8.
6709 *J Surg Res* 1999;87:108-13.
6711 *Cochrane Database Syst Rev* 2000;3:CD002286.
6712 *Cephalalgia* 1995;15:136-9.
6713 *J Pharm Pharmacol* 1988;40:743-5.
6714 Natl Cancer Institute CancerNet. Cartilage website: www.cancernet.nci.nih.gov/cam/cartilage.htm (Accessed 18 August 2000).

REFERENCES

6716 *Proc Am Soc Clinical Oncol* 1998;17:A240.

6717 *Proc Am Soc Clinical Oncol* 1999;18:A554.

6718 *Proc Am Soc Clinical Oncol* 1999;18:A1938.

6719 *Proc Am Soc Clinical Oncol* 1999;18:A622.

6720 *Proc Am Soc Clinical Oncol* 2000;19:A698.

6721 *Proc Am Soc Clinical Oncol* 1999;18:A698.

6722 *J Natl Cancer Inst* 1993;85:1190-1.

6723 *Mutat Res* 1996;367:204-8.

6724 *Biol Pharm Bull* 1997;20:1151-4.

6725 *Braz J Med Biol* Res 1996;29:643-6.

6726 *Anticancer Res* 1998;18:4435-41.

6727 Anon. AEterna announces the commencement of patient enrollment for the NIH - sponsored phase III clinical trial of AE-941/Neovastat in the treatment of lung cancer. Aeterna 2000 News Release 2000 May 17.

6729 Herb.com. Herbal Materia Medica 4.0 website. Available at: http://herb.com/materia.htm (Accessed 22 August 2000).

6733 Colorado State Univ. Colorado AES project COL00271. 1999-2000 website. www.colostate.edu/depts/aes/projs/271.htm (Accessed 22 August 2000).

6734 Coulombe RA. Improve food safety through discovery and control of natural and induced toxicants and antitoxicants. Fedrip database, Natl Technical Info Svc (Ntis). Fedrip/1999/07801368.

6735 United Plant Savers. United Plant Savers at risk forum website. www.plantsavers.org/endanger2.html (Accessed 5 August 2000).

6736 *J Nat Prod* 1995;58:1047-55.

6738 *Drugs Exp Clin Res* 1991;17:3-7.

6739 *Br J Radiol* 1995;68:841-3.

6740 *Arzneimittelforschung* 1999;49:925-32.

6741 *Arzneimittelforschung* 1996;46:1149-53.

6742 *Phytother Res* 2000;14:20-3.

6743 *Contact Dermatitis* 1995;32:281-4.

6744 *Gut* 1996;39:214-9.

6745 *Nutr Cancer* 1993;19:321-5.

6746 Herb Info Canada. Caraway website. www.herb.plant.org/caraway.htm (Accessed 11 September 2000).

6749 Leicester RJ, Hunt RH. Peppermint oil to reduce colonic spasm during endoscopy. *Lancet* 1982;2:989.

6750 *Br J Clin Pharmacol* 1984;18:461-2.

6751 *Curr Ther Res* 1994;55:776-85.

6752 *Br J Urol* 1986;58:36-40.

6753 *JAMA* 2000;283:1691.

6754 *Eur J Clin Nutr* 2000;54:405-8.

6755 *Phytochemistry* 2000;54:173-81.

6757 *N Engl J Med* 1991;324:1599.

6758 *JAMA* 1994;272:590.

6759 *Can J Urol* 1995;2:98-102.

6760 *J Fam Pract* 1997;45:167-8.

6762 Wilt T, Ishani A, Stark G, et al. Serenoa repens for benign prostatic hyperplasia (Cochrane Review). In: The Cochrane Library, Issue 3, 2000. Oxford: Update Software.

6763 *BJU Int* 2000;86:439-42.

6764 *Urology* 2000;55:533-9.

6765 *Prostate* 1998;37:77-83.

6766 *Eur Urol* 1992;21:309-14.

6767 *Phytother Res* 2000;14:333-8.

6769 *Urol Res* 2000;28:201-9.

6770 *J Urol* 2000;164:876-81.

6771 *Eur Urol* 1994;26:247-52.

6772 *Adv Ther* 1999;16:231-41.

6773 *Prostate* 1999;40:232-41.

6775 *Arch Esp Urol* 1995;48:97-103.

6776 *Arch Esp Urol* 1992; 45:211-3.

6777 *Br J Urol* 1990;66:639-41.

6778 *Clin Drug Invest* 1995; 9:291-7.

6779 *Prostaglandins Leukot Essent Fatty Acids* 1997;57:299-304.

6780 *Gen Pharmacol* 1996;27:171-6.

6781 *J Hum Lact* 1995;11:17-20.

6782 *J Hum Lact* 1995;11:191-4.

6783 *J Hum Lact* 1998;14:231-6.

6784 *Birth* 1993;20:61-4.

6789 *J Am Diet Assoc* 1996;96:46-8.

6790 *Food Chem Toxicol* 1995;33:537-43.

6791 *Anticancer Res* 2000;20:219-24.

6792 *Adv Exp Med Biol* 1999;472:159-68.

6793 *Drug Metabol Drug Interact* 1999;15:215-22.

6796 *Psychoneuroendocrinology* 2000;25:765-71.

6797 *Bone* 1995;17:15-20.

6798 *Ann Intern Med* 1989;111:1001-5.

6799 *Calcif Tissue Int* 2000;66:123-8.

6800 *J Am Coll Nutr* 1993;12:501-4.

6801 *Am J Clin Nutr* 1994;60:122-8.

6802 *Kidney Int* 1995;48:475-80.

6803 *Am J Clin Nutr* 1995;61:62-8.

6804 *Phytother Res* 1990;4:220-31.

6805 *Carcinogenesis* 1996;17:1373-6.

6806 *Atherosclerosis* 1997;132:69-76.

6807 *Atherosclerosis* 1998;136:367-75.

6808 *Am J Clin Nutr* 1999;69:395-402.

6809 *J Allergy Clin Immunol* 1996;98:469-70.

6810 *Arch Intern Med* 2000;160:2546-7.

6811 *Med Hypotheses* 1999;53:383-5.

6812 *Acta Odontol Scand* 1998;56:65-9.

6813 *Alcohol* 1996;13:395-8.

6815 *DICP* 1989;23:691-2.

6816 *BMJ* 1996;313:1180-4.

6817 *Pediatrics* 1998;102:879-84.

6818 *J Dent Res* 2000;79(3):882-7.

6819 *Med Hypotheses* 2000;54:603-13.

6820 *Diabetes Care* 1988;11:174-82.

6821 *J Dent Res* 2000;79:1352-5.

6822 *Ann Pharmacother* 2000;34:98-100.

6823 *Ann Intern Med* 2000;133:411-9.

6824 *Am J Publ Health* 2000;90:1254-9.

6825 *Am J Epidemiol* 2000;151:773-80.

6826 *Am J Clin Nutr* 2000;71:67-74.

6827 *J Am Coll Cardiol* 2000;35:1753-9.

6828 *Curr Med Res Opin* 1999;15:208-13.

6829 *Br J Psychiatry* 2000;177:66-71.

6832 *Lancet* 2000;355:1522.

6833 *J Agri Food Chem* 1999;47:221-30.

6834 *N Engl J Med* 1999;341:1557-64.

6835 *Epidemiology* 1990;1:342-8.

6836 *J Womens Health* 1999;8:65-73.

6837 *Am J Epidemiol* 1986;124:481-9.

6838 *N Engl J Med* 1993;329:1829-34.

6839 *J Intern Med* 1997;242:219-24.

6840 *Clin Chim Acta* 1996;246:59-76.

6841 *Circulation* 1992;85:910-5.

6842 *JAMA* 1999;281:53-60.

6843 *N Engl J Med* 1997;337:1705-14.

6844 *South Med J* 1999;92:1040-7.

6845 *Am J Clin Nutr* 2000;71:921-30.

6846 *J Pain Symptom Manage* 2000;19:35-9.

6847 *J Am Coll Nutrition* 2000;19:3-12.

6848 *Anesthesiology* 1996;84:340-7.

6849 *J Emerg Med* 2000;19:169-71.

6850 *J Reprod Med* 1999;44:601-5.
6851 *Am J Clin Nutr* 2000;72:466-71.
6852 *Am J Clin Nutr* 2000;71:1530-5.
6853 *Am J Clin Nutr* 2000;72:745-50.
6854 *Am J Clin Nutr* 2000;71:1577-81.
6855 *Ann Intern Med* 2000;133:319-20.
6856 *Am J Clin Nutr* 2000;72:690-3.
6857 *Tex Med* 2000;96:64-8.
6858 *Am J Clin Nutr* 1982;35:661-7.
6859 *Metabolism* 1987;36:351-5.
6860 *J Sports Med Phys Fitness* 1995;35:273-80.
6861 *Am J Clin Nutr* 1996;63:954-65.
6862 *Med Sci Sports Exerc* 1996;28:139-44.
6863 *FASEB J* 1995;9:1650-7.
6864 *Curr Ther Res* 1996;57:747-56.
6865 *Am J Clin Nutr* 1997;66:944-9.
6866 *Am J Clin Nutr* 1997;65:890-2.
6867 *Diabetes* 1997;46:1786-91.
6868 *Curr Ther Res* 1998;59:379-88.
6869 *J Nutr* 2000;130:715-8.
6871 Mahan LK, Escott-Stump S. Krause's Food, Nutrition, and Diet Therapy. 9th edition. W.B. Saunders Co., Philadelphia, PA, 1996.
6874 *JAMA* 1988;260:665-70.
6875 *J Am Coll Cardiol* 1992;19:174-85.
6877 *Phytomedicine* 2000;7:365-71.
6878 *Phytother Res* 2000:14:213-4.
6879 Anon. Milk thistle: Effects on liver disease and cirrhosis and clinical adverse effects. Summary, Evidence Report/ Technology Assessment: Number 21, September 2000. Agency for Healthcare Research and Quality, Rockville, MD. Available at: http://www.ahrq.gov/clinic/epcsums/ milktsum.htm.
6880 *Cancer Lett* 2000;154:151-61.
6883 *CMAJ* 2000;163:21-9.
6884 *Kidney Int* 2000;58:851-8.
6885 *BMJ* 1995;311:631.
6887 *Phytomedicine* 2000;7:427-48.
6888 *Ann Intern Med* 1997;126:372-5.
6889 *JAMA* 1994;272:967-8.
6890 *Am J Epidemiol* 1997;146:495-501.
6891 *Br Med J* 1995;310:555-9.
6892 *Circulation* 2001;103:472-5.
6893 *Stroke* 2001;32:77-83.
6894 *JAMA* 1994;272:929-33.
6895 *Am J Gastroenterol* 2000;95:3634-7.
6896 *Eur Heart J* 2001;22:611-2.
6897 *Arch Intern Med* 2001;161:813-24.
6898 *MMWR Morb Mortal Wkly Rep* 1985;34:732-3.
6899 *J Neurol Sci* 2000;176:124-7.
6901 *Br J Dermatol* 1984;111:461-8.
6902 *Cochrane Database Syst Rev* 2000;2:CD001273.
6903 *J Nutr* 1987;117:321-7.
6905 *Int J Eat Disord* 1994;15:251-5.
6906 *J Adolesc Health Care* 1987;8:400-6.
6908 *Urology* 1999;54:284-90.
6909 *Int Urol Nephrol* 1997;29:565-74.
6910 *Int Urol Nephrol* 1996;28:687-94.
6911 *Eur J Clin Nutr* 1991;45:507-10.
6912 *Br J Dermatol* 1990;122:485-9.
6913 *J Gastroenterol Hepatol* 1994;9:472-7.
6914 *J Am Coll Nutr* 1988;7:57-60.
6915 *Aliment Pharmacol Ther* 1993;7:281-6.
6916 *Gut* 1977;18:33-6.
6917 *Scand J Gastroenterol* 1998;33:514-23.
6918 *Age Ageing* 1995;24:303-7.
6920 *J Am Geriatr Soc* 1983;31:790-1.
6921 *Ann Otol Rhinol Laryngol* 1991;100:647-9.
6923 *Am J Clin Nutr* 2000;71:1485-94.
6925 *Int J Sports Med* 2000;21:139-45.
6926 *Med Sci Sports Exerc* 2000;32:379-85.
6927 *J Appl Physiol* 2000;88:1181-91.
6929 *Rheumatology (Oxford)* 2000;39:293-8.
6931 *Br J Dermatol* 1981;104:483-4.
6932 *Pediatr Dermatol* 1999;16:336-8.
6933 *Ann Rheum Dis* 1989;48:547-9.
6935 *Int Med* 1998;1:11-3.
6936 *J Pharm Pharmacol* 1987;39:459-65.
6937 *CMAJ* 1999;160:21-2.
6938 *Phytomedicine* 1996;3:225-30.
6939 *Biochem Pharmacol* 1992;43:2313-20.
6940 Health Canada. Labelling Standard: feverfew leaf. Available at: www.hc-sc.gc.ca/hpd-dgps/therapeut/zfiles/ english/guides/lebel/drug/feverfew_e.html (Accessed 24 July 2000).
6941 *Phytochemistry* 1995;38:267-70.
6942 *Lancet* 1985;1:1071-4.
6943 *Prostaglandins Leukot Med* 1982;8:653-60.
6944 *J Pharm Pharmacol* 1990;42:553-7.
6945 *Folia Haematol Int Mag Klin Morphol Blutforsch* 1988;115:447-9.
6946 *Phytochemistry* 1999;51:417-23.
6947 *J Ethnopharmacol* 1999;68:251-9.
6948 *Lancet* 1991;338:1015.
6950 *J Pharm Pharmacol* 1992;44:737-40.
6951 *Lancet* 1982;2:776.
6953 *Lancet* 1981;2:1054.
6954 *Lancet* 1980;2:922-3.
6957 *Planta Med* 1999;65:126-9.
6958 *Contact Dermatitis* 1996;34:330-5.
6959 *Br Med J (Clin Res Ed)* 1985;291:569-73.
6960 *Lancet* 1988;2:189-92.
6961 *Phytotherapy Res* 1997;11:508-11.
6965 *Cephalalgia* 1998;18:704-8.
6969 *Fitoterapia* 1999;70:586-92.
6971 *Ann Pharm Fr* 1999;57:410-4.
6972 *Int J Dermatol* 1996;35:448-9.
6973 *East Afr Med J* 1992;69:223-6.
6974 *Yakugaku Zasshi* 1996;116:244-50.
6975 *Life Sci* 1995;57:2011-20.
6976 *Biol Pharm Bull* 2000;23:356-8.
6978 *Chin Med J (Engl)* 1989;102:91-3.
6979 *Br Med J* 1985;291:940.
6981 Quackwatch. Unconventional cancer treatments: dietary treatments. www.quackwatch.com/ 01QuackeryRelatedTopics/OTA/ota03.html.
6982 *Br J Rheumatol* 1998;37:274-81.
6983 *Int J Clin Lab Res* 1994;24:171-6.
6984 *Proc Natl Acad Sci USA* 1990;87:8931-4.
6985 *J Clin Pharmacol* 1993;33:226-9.
6986 *Mol Aspects Med* 1997;18:S137-S144.
6987 Georgetown Univ Med Center. Cytochrome P450 interaction table. Available at: www. dml.georgetown. edu/depts/pharmacology.davetab.html.
6988 *Cur Ther Res* 1997;58:964-78.
6990 Am Heart Assn. Am Heart Assn meeting report: Chinese condiment cuts blood cholesterol. www.americanheart. org/Whats_News/AHA_News_Releases/03-25-99- chinese.html (Accessed 2 August 2000).

REFERENCES

6991 Am Heart Assn. Comment: the Am Heart Assn urges caution on cholestin. www.americanheart.org/Whats_News/AHA_News_Releases/03-25-99-comment.htm (Accessed 2 August 2000).

6993 *Chung Hua Nei Ko Tsa Chih* 1997;36:529-31.

6994 US Dept Health, Human Services, FDA. Pharmanex, Inc, administrative proceeding, public docket #97P-0441: final decision. Available at: www.fda.gov/ohrms/dockets/dockets/97p0441/ans0002.pdf.

6995 *Am J Clin Nutr* 1000;69:175-6.

6996 *Am J Clin Nutr* 2000;71:152-7.

6997 *Allergy* 1999;54:1330-1.

6998 *Psychosomatics* 2000;41:58-62.

6999 Federal Trade Commission. FTC Action against Lane Laboratories. Available at: www.ftc.gov/opa/2000/06/lanelabs.htm.

7001 *Eur J Clin Invest* 1988;18:162-5.

7005 *Can Pharm J* 1985;118:517-9.

7006 *Am J Clin Nutr* 1982;35:1452-8.

7007 *Ann Pharmacother* 1993;27:330-6.

7008 *JAMA* 1994;271:751-4.

7010 Brown D. Herbal Prescriptions for Better Health. Rocklin, CA: Prima Publishing, 1996.

7012 *Aust J Med Herb* 1993;5:63-5.

7013 *Qtrly Rev Natural Med* 1994;2:111-21.

7014 *Forschende Komplementarmedizen* 1996;3:329-30.

7015 *Exp Clin Endocrinol* 1994;102:448-54.

7016 *Exp Clin Endocrinol Diabetes* 1996;104:447-53.

7020 *J Alt Comp Med* 1995;1:249-55.

7021 *Lancet* 1990;336:1129.

7022 *J Allergy Clin Immunol* 2000;106:989-90.

7023 *Ann Pharmacother* 2000;34:1419-22.

7024 *BMJ* 2001;322:139.

7025 *Audiol Neurootol* 2000;5:64-8.

7026 *Lancet* 2001;357:251-6.

7027 *Clin Infect Dis* 2002;34:234-8.

7028 *Texas J Rural Health* 1998;26:68-76.

7029 *Clin Pharmacol Ther* 2001;69:14-23.

7030 *Ann Intern Med* 2001;134:344.

7031 *J Fam Pract* 1994;38:601-5.

7032 *Trop Med Int Health* 1999;4:284-7.

7033 *N Engl J Med* 2001;344:632-6.

7035 *Planta Med* 1990;56:44-7.

7038 *Semin Arthr Rheum* 1994;23:41-7.

7039 Natl Cancer Inst. Mistletoe (PDQ). CancerNet. www.cancernet.nci.nih.gov/cam/mistletoe.htm#7 (Accessed 30 March 2001).

7040 *Eur J Cancer* 1999;35:1688-92.

7041 *Br J Cancer* 2001;84:397-9.

7042 *Med Hypotheses* 1999;53:1-5.

7043 *Br J Cancer* 1995;71:854-6.

7044 *CMAJ* 1998;158:1157-9.

7045 *Altern Ther Health Med* 2001;7:57-78.

7046 *Clin Pharmacol Ther* 2001;69:P21.

7047 *Pain* 2000;91:361-5.

7048 *Osteoarth Cartilage* 2000;8:9-12.

7049 Holtmann G, Madisch A, Juergen H, et al. A double-blind, randomized, placebo-controlled trial on the effects of an herbal preparation in patients with functional dyspepsia [Abstract]. Ann Mtg Digestive Disease Week 1999 May.

7050 *Fitoterapia* 2000;71:425-8.

7051 *Der Krankenhaus Arzt* 1983;56:1005-8.

7052 *Pediatrics* 2001;107:e71.

7053 Mulvihill SJ, Debas HT. Regulatory peptides in the gut. In: Greenspan FS, Strewler GJ, Eds. Basic & Clinical Endocrinology. 5th ed. Stamford, CT: Appleton & Lange, 1997:581.

7054 *J Clin Oncol* 2001;19:2739-45.

7055 *Br Med J* 2001;322:134-7.

7056 *Arch Intern Med* 2000;160:3141-3.

7057 *J Am Acad Dermatol* 2001;44:298-9.

7058 *Metabolism* 1997;46:469-73.

7060 *Metabolism* 1992;41:768-71.

7061 *Pharmacist's Letter/Prescriber's Letter* 2000;16(2):160212.

7062 *J Sports Med Phys Fitness* 1978;18:271-8.

7063 *Br J Sports Med* 1982;16:142-5.

7064 *Ann Allergy* 1993;70:147-52.

7065 *Ann Allergy* 1975;35:93-7.

7066 *Pharmacology* 1994;49:392-7.

7067 FDA. Information paper on L-tryptophan and 5-hydroxy-L-tryptophan. Office of Nutritional Products, Labeling, Dietary Supplements. Center for Food Safety and Applied Nutrition. February 2001.

7068 *Ann Intern Med* 2001;135:68

7069 *Fujian Med J* 1988;10:4-6.

7070 *Hunan Med J* 1991;8:259-60.

7071 *Zhingguo Zhong Xi Yi Jie He Za Zhi* 1993;13:278-80.

7072 *Ann Pharmacother* 2001;35:1118-21.

7073 *J Agric Food Chem* 2001;49:4262-6.

7074 *Urology* 2001;57:26-9.

7075 *Pharmacist's Letter/Prescriber's Letter* 2001;17(11):171115.

7076 *Phytomedicine* 1997;4:183-9.

7077 *Forsch Komplementarmed* 1998;5:272-8.

7078 *Arch Gynecol Obstet* 2000;264:150-3.

7079 *J Womens Health Gend Based Med* 2000;9:315-20.

7080 *Pharmacist's Letter/Prescriber's Letter* 2001;17(12):171214.

7081 *J Clin Endocrinol Metab* 2001;86:4727-30.

7082 *Arch Gen Psychiatry* 2001;58:1049-52.

7083 *Eur J Obstet Gynecol Reprod Biol* 1991;42:163-4.

7084 *Arthritis Rheum* 2001;44:2531-38.

7085 *Arthritis Rheum* 2001;44:2461-2.

7086 *Pharmacist's Letter/Prescriber's Letter* 2001;18(1):180115.

7087 *Int J STD AIDS* 2001;12:154-8.

7088 *Science* 2001;292:2083-4.

7089 *Pharmacol Toxicol* 2000;86:250-6.

7090 *Age Ageing* 2001;30:523-5.

7091 *Ann Intern Med* 2002;136:590-5.

7092 Mathijssen RHJ, Verweij J, De Bruijn P, et al. Modulation of irinotecan (CPT-11) metabolism by St. John's wort in cancer patients. American Association for Cancer Research Annual Meeting, San Francisco, April 2002. Abstract 2443.

7093 Health Canada warns public not to use Hua Fo (DIN 02243366). Health Canada Online April 5, 2002. Available at: http://www.hc.sc.gc.ca/english/protestion/warnings/2002/2002_26e.htm (Accessed 5 April 2002).

7095 Mai I, Bauer S, Krueger H, et al. Wechselwirkungen von Johaniskraut mit tacrolismus bei nierentransplantierten patienten. Symposium Phytopharmaka VII. Forschung und Klinische Anwendung, Berlin, October, 2001.

7096 Consultation letter MLX 286: Proposals to prohibit the herbal ingredient Kava-Kava (Piper methysticum) in unlicensed medicines. Medicines Control Agency, United Kingdom, July 19, 2002.

7100 *Postgrad Med* 1980;67:64,69.

7101 *Br J Nutr* 1997;77:59-72.
7102 *J Manipulative Physiol Ther* 1999;22:530-3.
7103 *Eur J Clin Nutr* 2000;54:671-7.
7104 *Eur J Clin Nutr* 1999;53:966-9.
7105 *Eur J Clin Nutr* 2000;54:715-25.
7106 *J Altern Complement Med* 2000;6:305-10.
7107 *Altern Ther Health Med* 1999;5:42-51.
7110 Irikura B, Kennelly E. American Health Consultants. Blue Cohosh: a word of caution. 1999. Available at: www.ahcpub.com/ahc_root_html/hot/archive/atwh1099.html.
7111 *J Antimicrob Chemother* 2000;45:639-43.
7113 *Acta Psychiatr Scand* 1990;81:265-70.
7114 *Prog Clin Biol Res* 1989;317:1235-46.
7115 *Nutrition* 1999;15:778-83.
7116 *Am J Health-Syst Pharm* 1999;56:2038,2043-4.
7117 *Altern Med Rev* 2000;5:402-28.
7118 *Psychopharmacol Bull* 1988;24:130-4.
7119 *Clin Trials J* 1987;24:84-93.
7120 *Clin Trials J* 1987;24:73-83.
7121 *Altern Med Rev* 1996;1:70-84.
7122 Chevallier A. Encyclopedia of Herbal Medicine. 2nd ed. New York, NY: DK Publ, Inc., 2000.
7123 Agricultural Research Service. Dr. Duke's phytochemical and ethnobotanical databases. www.ars-grin.gov/cgi-bin/duke/farmacy2.pl?575 (Accessed 31 January 2001).
7125 *Phytother Res* 2000;14:448-51.
7126 Huang KC. The Pharmacology of Chinese Herbs. 2nd ed. Boca Raton, FL: CRC Press, LLC 1999.
7127 *Phytother Res* 2000;14:15-9.
7128 *Phytother Res* 2000;14:40-2.
7129 *J Allergy Clin Immunol* 2000;106:183-189.
7130 *J Clin Invest* 1993;91:1268.
7131 *Int J Vitam Nutr Res* 1997;67:350-356.
7132 *Metabolism* 1998;47:195-9.
7133 *Proc Nutr Sci* 1997;56:915-37.
7134 *Ann Intern Med* 1998;128:829-832.
7135 Food and Nutrition Board, Institute of Medicine. Dietary Reference Intakes for Vitamin A, Vitamin K, Arsenic, Boron, Chromium, Copper, Iodine, Iron, Manganese, Molybdenum, Nickel, Silicon, Vanadium, and Zinc. Washington, DC: National Academy Press, 2002. Available at: www.nap.edu/books/0309072794/html/.
7136 *J Nutr* 1998;128:73-78.
7137 *Int J Vitam Nutr Res* 2004;74:178-82.
7139 *Am J Clin Nutr* 1999;69:1071-85.
7140 *Fortschr Med* 1989;107:563-6.
7141 *Ann Nutr Metab* 2000;44:263-5.
7142 *Am J Clin Nutr* 1999;69:827-8.
7143 *Am J Clin Nutr* 2000;71:171S-5S.
7144 *Am J Clin Nutr* 2000;71:197S-201S.
7145 *Am J Clin Nutr* 2000;71:251S-5S.
7146 *Br J Nutr* 1998;80:163-7.
7147 *Cancer Epidemiol Biomarkers Prev* 2000;9:335-8.
7148 *Am J Clin Nutr* 1999;70:560S-9S.
7149 *Am J Clin Nutr* 1999;69:872-82.
7150 *Lancet* 1994;343:1454-9.
7151 *Eur J Clin Nutr* 2000;54:865-71.
7152 *BMJ* 1996;313:84-90.
7153 *Am J Clin Nutr* 1999;69:890-7.
7155 *Eur J Clin Nutr* 2000;54:618-25.
7156 *Nutr Metab Cardiovasc Dis* 2000;10:57-61.
7158 *Ann Pharmacother* 2001;35:1199-201.
7161 Chevallier A. Encyclopedia of Herbal Medicine. 2nd ed. New York, NY: DK Publ, Inc., 2000.
7162 Dr. Duke's Phytochemical and Ethnobotanical Databases. www.ars-grin.gov/cgi-bin/duke/farmacy2.pl.
7165 *Eur J Clin Nutr* 1998;52:749-53.
7166 *Atherosclerosis* 1999;142:159-68.
7167 *J Urol* 2000;164:2168-72.
7168 *Eur J Cancer* 2000;36:335-40.
7169 *Osteoarthritis Cartilage* 2000;8:343-50.
7170 Natl Inst Health, Natl Inst Environmental Health Sci. Indole-3-carbinol. Available at: http://ntp-server.niehs.nih.gov.
7171 *Chem Biol Interact* 1998;110:1-5.
7172 *Otolaryngol Head Neck Surg* 1998;118:810-5.
7173 *Gynecol Oncol* 2000;78:123-9.
7174 *J Cell Biochem Suppl* 1997;28-29:111-6.
7175 *Int J Obes Relat Metab Disord* 1998;22:227-9.
7176 *Altern Med Alert* 2000; 3:105-7.
7177 *J Natl Cancer Inst* 1990;82:947-9.
7178 *Proc Soc Exp Biol Med* 1997;216:246-52.
7179 *Carcinogenesis* 1991;12:1571-4.
7180 *Anticancer Res* 1995;15:709-16.
7181 *Cancer Res* 1994;54:1446-9.
7182 *Anticancer Res* 1999;19:1673-80.
7183 *Cancer Res* 1999;59:3991-7.
7184 *Carcinogenesis* 1997;18:377-81.
7185 *J Natl Cancer Inst* 1986;77:269-76.
7186 *IARC Sci Publ* 1991;105:275-80.
7187 *Food Chem Toxicol* 2000;38:15-23.
7188 *Ann N Y Acad Sci* 1999;889:204-13.
7189 *Cancer Lett* 1998;134:91-5.
7190 *J Toxicol Environ Health A* 2000;59:271-9.
7191 *Altern Ther Health Med* 2000;6:77-9.
7192 *Acta Oncol* 1996;35:1021-6.
7193 *J Am Coll Nutr* 1999;18:572-81.
7194 *J Pediatr* 2000;136:503-10.
7195 *Circulation* 2001;103:1177-9.
7196 *J Lipid Res* 2000;41:697-705.
7198 *BJU Int* 2000;85:842-6.
7201 *Acta Med Scand* 1977;210(4):291-7.
7202 *Arch Gen Psychiatry* 1999;56:407-12.
7203 *Neurol India* 1978;26:171-6.
7204 *Pharm World Sci* 1993;15:263-8.
7205 *Int J Food Sci Nutr* 2000;51:279-87.
7206 *Neurol India* 1978;26:179-182.
7207 *Neurol India* 1978;26:177-8.
7208 *J Affect Disord* 1990;19:125-32.
7209 *J Clin Psychiatry* 1988;49:193-5.
7210 *Am J Psychiatry* 1987;144:1071-3.
7211 *Psychopharmacol Bull* 1985;21:146-9.
7212 *Am J Clin Nutr* 2001;73:153-7.
7213 *Cochrane Database Syst Rev* 2000;2:CD001507.
7214 *Am J Clin Nutr* 2001 Feb;73:276-82.
7215 *Aviat Space Environ Med* 1995;66:313-9.
7217 Food and Nutrition Board, Institute of Medicine. The Role of Protein and Amino Acids in Sustaining and Enhancing Performance. Washington, DC: National Academy Press, 1999. Available at: http://www.nap.edu/books/0309063469/html.
7219 *Brain Res* 2000;852:56-61.
7220 *J Ethnopharmacol* 2001;76:233-8.
7221 *J Pak Med Assoc* 1990;40:147-50.
7222 *J Ethnopharmacol* 2001;75:175-80.
7223 *Mov Disord* 1990;5:47-8.
7224 *Anticancer Res* 1998;18:3363-8.
7225 *Free Radic Biol Med* 2000;29:71-78.
7226 *J Pharm Pharmacol* 2000;52:1553-1561.
7227 *J Ethnopharmacol* 1997;57:183-7.

7229 *Altern Med Rev* 2001;6:207-9.
7230 *Int J Clin Pharmacol Ther* 2000;38:430-5.
7231 *Pharm Acta Helv* 1985;60:256-9.
7232 *Pediatrics* 2001;108:972-82.
7233 *Nutrition* 1997;13:748-51.
7234 *Int Conf AIDS* 1996;11:65.
7235 *J Clin Oncol* 2000;18:450-1.
7236 *J Clin Endocrinol Metab* 2000;85:4074-80.
7237 *Immunopharmacology* 1999;42:61-74.
7238 *J Immunol* 1996;156:3418-25.
7239 *J Immunol* 1999;163:3045-52.
7240 *Int J Cancer* 1996;65:377-382.
7241 *Immunopharmacology* 1991;22:139-55.
7242 *Glycobiology* 2000;10:339-46.
7243 *Int J Immunopharmacol* 1987;9:261-7.
7246 *Am Surg* 1997;63:125-31.
7248 *Int J Immunopharmacol* 1998;20:595-614.
7249 *Immunopharmacology* 1999;4:89-107.
7250 *Free Radic Biol Med* 2001;30:393-402.
7251 *Int J Immunopharmacol* 1988;10;405-14.
7252 *Arch Dermatol* 1987;123:751-6.
7255 *Eur Urol* 1997;31:178-81.
7256 *J Rheumatol* 2001;28:173-81.
7258 *Can J Microbiol* 1969;15:1067-76.
7259 *Antimicrob Agents Chemother* 1988;32:1370-4.
7260 *Oncology* 1986;43:131-4.
7261 *Cancer* 1986;58:865-72.
7263 *Acta Otolaryngol Suppl* 1994;511:192-5.
7264 *Gynecol Oncol* 1995;56:412-40.
7265 *Int J Immunopharmacol* 1992;14:535-539.
7266 *Anticancer Res* 1997 Jul-Aug;17:2751-5.
7267 *J Med* 1998;29:305-30.
7268 *Ann Surg* 1990;211:605-12; discussion 612-3.
7269 *Ann Surg* 1994;220:601-9.
7270 *Arch Surg* 1994;129:1204-10.
7271 *Arch Surg* 1999;134:977-83.
7272 *Am J Clin Nutr* 1999;70:208-12.
7273 *Crit Rev Food Sci Nutr* 1999;39:189-202.
7277 *Planta Med* 1985;6:473-7.
7278 *J Cardiovasc Pharmacol* 1990;16(1):93-100.
7279 *Arzneimittelforschung* 1987;37:364-7.
7281 *Clin Pharmacol Ther* 1993;53:76-83.
7282 *S Afr Med J* 1987;71:570-1.
7283 *Arch Ophthalmol* 1987;105:637-41.
7284 *Jpn J Ophthalmol* 30(3):238-44.
7285 *Gut* 2001;48:28-33.
7286 *Abstr Gen Meet Am Soc Microbiol* 1994;94:481.
7288 Robert G. Petit II, Chris French. Phase III Clinical Trial Design Considerations for Oral Treatments of Chemotherapy-Induced Mucositis: AES-14 (Uptake-Facilitated L-Glutamine) Pivotal Studies. 2001 ASCO Annual Meeting. Abstract #2954. Available at: http://www.asco.org/ac/1,1003,_12-002636-00_18-0010-00_19-002954,00.asp.
7289 *Kidney Int* 2001;59:1103-9.
7291 *Am J Psychiatry* 984;141:1302-3.
7292 *J Nutr* 2000;130:1007S-15S.
7293 *J Nutr* 2001;131:2556S-61S.
7294 *J Nutr* 2000;130:1043S-5S.
7295 *Cancer* 1994;74:2879-84.
7296 *JPEN J Parenter Enteral Nutr* 2000;24:61-6.
7297 *Gastroenterology* 1995;108:A766.
7298 *J Am Coll Nutr* 1994;13:251-5.
7299 *Lancet* 1993;341:1363-5.
7300 *JPEN J Parenter Enteral Nutr* 1999;23:S62-6.
7303 *Arch Ophthalmol* 2001;119:1417-36.
7304 *Arch Ophthalmol* 2001;119:1439-52.
7306 *Mayo Clin Proc* 2001;76:883-9.
7307 *Hypertension* 2001;38:166-170.
7308 *Am J Clin Nutr* 1998;68:3-4.
7309 *J Med Assoc Thai* 1998;81:334-43.
7310 *JPEN J Parenter Enteral Nutr* 2000;24:133-9.
7311 *Am J Clin Pathol* 2001;116:403-408.
7312 *Can J Psychiatry* 2001;46:456-457.
7313 *J Mol Evol* 1999;49:290-297.
7314 *Clin Exp Allergy* 1997;27:333-6.
7315 *N Z Med J* 1996;109:325.
7316 *Allergy* 1996;51:440.
7317 *Inflamm Res* 2001;50:442-448.
7318 *Drug Metab Dispos* 2000;28:1270-3.
7319 *Carcinogenesis* 2001;22:1399-403.
7320 *J Pharmacol Exp Ther* 1999;290:1375-83.
7321 *Rev Med Chil* 1992;120:1370-5.
7322 *Gastroenterol Clin Biol* 1989;13:120-4.
7325 *Psychopharmacology (Berl)* 2001;157:277-83.
7326 *Mutat Res* 2000;469:135-45.
7327 *Fertil Steril* 2001;76:241-8.
7328 *Rheumatology (Oxford)* 1999;38:488-95.
7329 *Support Care Cancer* 2000;8:504-5.
7330 *J Nutr* 2001;131:1362S-75S.
7331 *JAMA* 2001;286:807-14.
7332 *Lancet* 1997;350:23-7.
7333 *J Clin Endocrinol Metab* 2001;86:41-7.
7334 *Am J Clin Nutr* 1978;31:2020-5.
7335 *Lancet* 1991;337:1197-200.
7336 *Cancer Epidemiol Biomarkers Prev* 2001;10:483-88.
7337 *Lancet* 1997;350:971-2.
7338 *Am J Epidemiol* 1997;146:294-306.
7339 *Nutr Cancer* 2000;36:14-8.
7340 *Cancer Epidemiol Biomarkers Prev* 2000;9:1051-8.
7341 *Cancer Epidemiol Biomarkers Prev* 2001;10:570.
7342 *Obstet Gynecol* 2001;97:109-15.
7343 *Altern Ther Health Med* 2001;7:S35.
7344 *Mayo Clin Proc* 2000;75:1174-84.
7345 *Am J Clin Nutr* 2001;73:667-8.
7346 *Am J Clin Nutr* 2001;73:728-35.
7347 *J Am Coll Nutr* 2000;19:761-7.
7348 *Altern Ther Health Med* 2001;7:S31-2.
7349 US Department of Justice, Drug Enforcement Agency, Diversion Control Program. Drugs and Chemicals of Concern: Salvia Divinorum, ska Maria Pastora, Salvia (Salvinorin A, Divinorin A). 2002. Available at: http://www.deadiversion.usdoj.gov/drugs_concern/salvia_d/summary.htm.
7350 *J Ethnopharmacol* 1983;7:287-312.
7351 *J Psychoactive Drugs* 1994;26:277-83.
7352 *J Ethnopharmacol* 1994;43:53-6.
7353 *J Clin Microbiol* 2001;39:551-9.
7354 *Biol Pharm Bull* 1994;17:443-5.
7355 *J Hepatol* 1998;28:615-21.
7356 *Int J Clin Pharmacol Ther Toxicol* 1993;31:456-60.
7357 *Am J Clin Nutr* 1998;68:442S-6S.
7358 *Am J Clin Nutr* 1998;68:1413S-7S.
7359 *Lancet* 1989;2:757-61.
7360 *Am J Cardiol* 1995;76:974-7.
7361 *Am J Clin Nutr* 2001;74:50-6.
7362 *Proc Natl Acad Sci U S A* 1994;91:4427-30.
7363 *Circulation* 1999;99:2452-7.
7366 *Am J Clin Nutr* 1998;68:235-41.
7368 *Atherosclerosis* 1998;137:419-27.
7369 *Diabetes Care* 1998;21:717-24.
7372 *Health Rep* 1994;6:22-7.

7373 *JAMA* 2001;285:304-12.
7377 *Clin Drug Invest* 2001;21:175-81.
7378 *Lancet* 2001;357:1764-6.
7380 *Verh K Acad Geneeskd Belg* 1992;54:189-16.
7381 *Am J Clin Nutr* 1997;66:89-96.
7382 *J Am Coll Cardiol* 2000;36:1455-60.
7383 *Nutrition* 2000;16:143-5.
7384 *Nutr Clin Pract* 1993;8:65-72.
7386 *Am J Clin Nutr* 1999;69:261-6.
7387 *Am J Epidemiol* 1999;150:1073-80.
7388 *N Engl J Med* 2001;345:1583-93.
7389 *Prostaglandins Leukot Essent Fatty Acids* 1997;56:379-84.
7390 *Am J Clin Nutr* 2000;72:476-83.
7394 *JAMA* 1999;282:1233-39.
7400 *Acta Otolaryngol* 1998;105:45-9.
7401 *Med Hypotheses* 1989;29:25-8.
7402 *Lancet* 1983;1:958-60.
7403 *Invest Ophthalmol Vis Sci* 1984;25:268-77.
7404 *Arch Women Ment Health* 2000;3:99-101.
7405 *Exp Eye Res* 1984;39(6):745-9.
7406 *Arzneimittelforschung* 1981;31(8):1248-50.
7407 *Arzneimittelforschung* 1983;33(10):1436-41.
7408 *J Cyclic Nucleotide Res* 1981;7(4):201-24.
7409 *Eur J Pharmacol* 1985;111:1-8.
7410 *Vasa* 1995;24:56-61.
7411 *Thromb Haemost* 1989;61:106-10.
7412 *Int J Cancer* 1983;32(6):801-4.
7413 *Cancer* 1990;65(3):446-51.
7501 *Phytochemistry* 1997;46:1349-53.
7502 *Xenobiotica* 1999;29:1241-56.
7503 *Biochem Pharmacol* 1998;55:1369-75.
7504 *Pharm Res* 2000;17:21-6.
7505 *Biochem Pharmacol* 1999;58:431-8.
7506 *Science* 1984;225:1032-4.
7507 *Environ Health Perspect* 1998;106:85-92.
7508 *Arch Pharm Res* 1999;22:309-12.
7509 *Xenobiotica* 1999;29:1227-40.
7510 *Biosci Biotechnol Biochem* 1999;63:1787-90.
7511 *Photochem Photobiol* 1998;67:456-61.
7512 *Proc Natl Acad Sci U S A* 1997;94:6110-5.
7513 *Drug Metab Dispos* 2000;28:1077-82.
7514 *Int J Sport Nutr Exerc Metab* 2000;10:340-59.
7517 World Health Organization. Guidelines for Iodine Prophylaxis following Nuclear Accidents. Available at: www.who.int/environmental_information/Information_resources/on_line_radiation.htm. (Accessed 11 January 2002).
7518 Center for Drug Evaluation and Research. Guidance. Potassium iodide as a thyroid blocking agent in radiation emergencies. Food and Drug Administration December 2001. Available at: http://www.fda.gov/cder/guidance/4825fnl.htm.
7520 *Am J Clin Nutr* 2000;72:1510-5.
7521 *Anticancer Res* 1999;19:3651-7.
7522 *Med Sci Sports Exerc* 1996;28:482-9.
7523 *Zhong Xi Yi Jie He Za Zhi* 1991;11:280-1, 261.
7524 *Zhong Xi Yi Jie He Za Zhi* 1990r;10:155-6, 132.
7525 *J Pharm Sci* 1984;73:270-2.
7526 *Antiviral Res* 2001;50:223-8.
7527 *Zhongguo Zhong Yao Za Zhi* 1994;19:683-5, 703.
7528 *Zhongguo Zhong Yao Za Zhi* 1994;19:746-7, 764.
7529 *Zhongguo Zhong Xi Yi Jie He Za Zhi* 1998;18:472-4.
7530 *Int J Immunopharmacol* 1991;13:549-54.
7531 *J Ethnopharmacol* 1984;10:235-41.
7532 *Alt Ther* 2001;7:S14.
7533 *Am J Clin Nutr* 2001;73:1101-6.
7538 *J Ethnopharmacol* 1998;61:9-16.
7539 *Fertil Steril* 1999;72:686-90.
7540 *Biochem Biophys Res Commun* 1996;219:923-9.
7541 *Planta Med* 2001;67:350-3.
7542 *Proc Natl Acad Sci U S A* 1995;92:8818-22.
7543 *FEBS Lett* 1990;272:12-8.
7555 Food and Nutrition Board, Institute of Medicine. Dietary Reference Intakes for Calcium, Phosphorus, Magnesium, Vitamin D, and Fluoride. Washington, DC: National Academy Press, 1999. Available at: http://books.nap.edu/books/0309063507/html/index.html.
7556 *Lancet* 1991;337:757-60.
7557 *Ann Clin Biochem* 1994;31:459-61.
7558 *Int J Mol Med* 1998;1:143-6.
7559 *J Clin Rheumatol* 1999:5:56-9.
7561 *Arch Intern Med* 1989;149:2501-3.
7562 *Am J Med* 1993 Feb;94(2):197-203.
7563 *Acta Neurol Scand* 1990;82:209-16.
7564 *Acta Neurol Scand* 1999;99:112-6.
7565 *Arch Dis Child* 1996;75:494-7.
7566 *Lancet* 1993;341:1557-60.
7567 *Dermatology* 1996;193:115-20.
7568 *Drugs Exp Clin Res* 1988;14:291-7.
7569 *Br J Dermatol* 1987;117:11-9.
7570 *Drugs Exp Clin Res* 1994;20:77-84.
7571 *Kidney Int* 1993;44:75-86.
7572 *Ann Rheum Dis* 1991;50:463-6.
7573 *Am J Med* 1989;86:158-64.
7574 *Am J Obstet Gynecol* 1996;174:1335-8.
7575 *Nut Res* 2000;20:621-31.
7585 *Lancet* 2000;356:1300-6.
7591 *J Nat Prod* 1986;49:293-7.
7592 *J Nat Prod* 1987;50:1059-64.
7593 *Planta Med* 1986;175-7.
7594 *Eur J Med Res* 2000;5:463-7.
7595 *BMJ* 2002;324:144-6.
7596 *Pharm Acta Helv* 1998;72:378-80.
7597 *Pharm Acta Helv* 1998;72:376-8.
7598 *Drugs Exp Clin Res* 2001;27:17-26.
7599 *J Pediatr* 2001;139:189-96.
7600 *Med Sci Sports Exerc* 1998;30 Suppl:S323.
7601 *Med Sci Sports Exerc* 1998;30 Suppl:S32.
7602 *Alt Ther* 2001;7:S21.
7603 *Neuroepidemiology* 2002;21:107-14.
7604 *J Nutr* 1999 Jul;129(7 Suppl):1471S-3S.
7605 *J Nutr* 1998;128:11-9.
7606 *J Nutr* 2000;130:1197-9.
7607 *Adv Ther* 1998;15:305-14.
7608 *N Engl J Med* 2000;342:1372.
7610 *Neuroepidemiology* 2002;21:105-6.
7611 *Aging (Milano)* 1998;10:385-94.
7612 *Pharmacol Biochem Behav* 1984;21:17-23.
7613 *Pharmacol Biochem Behav* 1984;21:11-3.
7617 *Life Sci* 1996;59:PL147-57.
7619 *Am J Epidemiol* 2001;153:1085-8.
7620 *J Hum Hypertens* 2001;15:549-52.
7621 *Anaesthesia* 1993;48:393-5.
7622 *Prostaglandins Leukot Essent Fatty Acids* 1989;35:183-5.
7623 *ORL J Otorhinolaryngol Relat Spec* 1986;48:282-6.
7624 *Pharmacology* 1991;42:111-20.
7625 *Clin Res Pr Drug Regul Aff* 1988;6:129-36.
7626 *J Gastroenterol Hepatol* 2001;16:115-7.
7627 *Vet Hum Toxicol* 1996;38:280-2.
7628 *Adv Ther* 1998;15:25-44.

R E F E R E N C E S

7629 *Crit Care Med* 1999;27:1409-20.
7630 *Br J Dermatol* 1993;129:95.
7631 *Journal of Planar Chromatography* 1994;7:80-2.
7632 *Br J Dermatol* 1999;140:685-8.
7633 *Br J Dermatol* 2000;143:201.
7634 *J Hypertens* 1992;10:1197-204.
7635 *Biochem Soc Trans* 1997;25:343S.
7636 *BMC Complement Altern Med* 2002;2(1):1.
7637 *Diabetes* 2000;49:926-35.
7638 *J Clin Endocrinol Metab* 2001;86:2099-103.
7639 *Oncol Res* 1995;7:583-90.
7640 *Atherosclerosis* 1990;82:75-83.
7641 *Pol Arch Med Wewn* 1998;100:419-25.
7642 *J Infect Dis* 1991;164:1082-90.
7645 *Am J Gastroenterol* 1999;94:1711.
7646 *Gastroenterology* 1993;31:129-34.
7652 *Mycoses* 1995;38:119-23.
7653 *Am J Epidemiol* 2001;153:790-3.
7654 *J Clin Endocrinol Metab* 1999;84:192-7.
7655 *Arch Intern Med* 2001;161:1161-72.
7656 *Am J Epidemiol* 2001;153:1206-12.
7657 *Biol Pharm Bull* 2001;24:351-6.
7658 *J Clin Oncol* 2002;20:1449-55.
7659 *Menopause* 2001;8:384-92.
7660 *J Clin Endocrinol Metab* 2001;86:5217-21.
7661 *Am J Clin Nutr* 2002;75:126-36.
7662 *Cancer Epidemiol Biomarkers Prev* 2002;11:43-9.
7663 *Br J Cancer* 2000;82:1879-86 .
7664 *Biochem Pharmacol* 2000;60:167-77.
7665 *Cancer Lett* 2000;151:169-79.
7666 *Carcinogenesis* 1998 Sep;19:1631-9.
7667 *Xenobiotica* 1998;28:803-11.
7668 *Biochem Biophys Res Commun* 1996;228:153-8.
7669 *Biochem Pharmacol* 1996;51:1069-76.
7670 *Pharmacol Biochem Behav* 1984;21:7-10.
7671 *Pharmacol Biochem Behav* 1984;21:15-6.
7673 *Allergy* 1991;46:472-4.
7674 *Allergy* 1999;54:287-8.
7685 *Neurosci Lett* 2000;289:189-92.
7686 *Chem Pharm Bull* 1986;34:3053-57.
7687 *Life Sci* 1998;62:1065-8.
7688 *Toxicol Lett* 2000:121:89-96.
7689 *Cancer Lett* 2000;158:119-24.
7690 *Toxicol Lett* 2000;114:155-62.
7691 *Life Sci* 2000;67:2647-53.
7692 *J Ethnopharmacol* 1995;48:53-7.
7693 *Phytother Res* 2002:16:S1-S5.
7694 *Alternative Therapies* 2001;7:S17.
7695 *Life Sci* 1996;58:87-96.
7696 *Free Radic Biol Med* 2001;30:154-60.
7697 *FEBS Lett* 2000:465;93-7.
7698 *FEBS Lett* 1998;431:315-8.
7699 *Biol Pharm Bull* 2000;23:735-7.
7700 *J Ethnopharmacol* 2001;76:139-43.
7701 *Ann Intern Med* 1993;119:867-73.
7702 *Arthritis Rheum* 1996;39:1808-17.
7703 *Bibl Haematol* 1969;33:111-25.
7704 *Semin Arthritis Rheum* 2000;30:87-99.
7706 *Arthritis Rheum* 1998;41:2185-95.
7707 *Clin Exp Immunol* 1993;94:241-6.
7708 *J Allergy Clin Immunol* 1999;103:200-2.
7709 *J Allergy Clin Immunol* 1999;103:321-5.
7710 *J Allergy Clin Immunol* 2001;108:1033-4.
7711 PDR Electronic Library. Montvale, NJ: Medical Economics Company, Inc., 2001.
7712 *JAMA* 2002;287:47-54.
7713 *Ann Intern Med* 1998;129:770-8.
7714 *Clin Investig* 1993;71:3-6.
7715 *Am J Epidemiol* 1994;139:1180-9.
7716 *Arch Intern Med* 1996;156:637-42.
7722 *Nut Res* 2001;21:551-67.
7724 *Am J Epidemiol* 2000;152:149-62.
7725 *J Am Coll Cardiol* 2000;36:758-65.
7726 *Lancet* 1993;342:1007-1011.
7727 *Mov Disord* 2002;17:195-6.
7728 *Lancet* 1990;335:1442-5.
7729 *Nutrition* 1999;15:860-4.
7730 *Clin Nutr* 2001;20:319-23.
7731 *JPEN J Parenter Enteral Nutr* 1990;14:109S-13S.
7732 *Clin Nutr* 2000;19:395-401.
7733 *J Nutr* 2001;131:2505S-8S.
7734 *J Nutr* 2001;131:2515S-22S.
7735 *J Nutr* 2001;131:2543S-9S.
7736 *J Nutr* 2001;131:2552S-5S.
7737 *J Nutr* 2001;131:2562S-8S.
7738 *J Nutr* 2001;131:2578S-84S.
7739 *J Nutr* 2001;131:2539S-42S.
7740 *J Nutr* 2001;131:2585S-9S.
7741 *J Pediatr* 2001;138:361-5.
7742 *Nut Res* 2001;22:65-9.
7743 *J Allergy Clin Immunol* 2002;109:119-21.
7744 *Am J Gastroenterol* 1996;91:1579-85.
7745 *Eur J Pharm Biopharm* 2000;50:389-95.
7746 *Infect Immun* 1997;65:4165-4172.
7747 *Gastroenterology* 1996;111:334-44.
7748 *Int J Food Microbiol* 2000;55:235-8.
7749 *J Infect Dis* 1997;175:218-21.
7750 *J Hepatol* 1997;26:417-24.
7751 *J Pediatr Gastroenterol Nutr* 1997;24:399-404.
7752 *Food Chem Toxicol* 1998;36:1085-94.
7753 *Pediatr Infect Dis J* 1997;16:1103-7.
7754 *Gastroenterology* 1999;116:1107-14.
7755 *Microbial Ecology in Health and Disease* 2000;12:247-85.
7756 *Nutr Res* 2001;21:183-9.
7757 *J Am Coll Nutr* 2001;20:149-56.
7758 *J Am Coll Nutr* 1996;15:408-12.
7759 *Nutr Res* 2002;22:393-403.
7760 *J Syst Bacteriol* 1992;42:487-91.
7771 *Cancer Epidemiol Biomarkers Prev* 2001;10:861-8.
7772 *J Natl Cancer Inst* 2002;94:391-8.
7773 *Cancer Epidemiol Biomarkers Prev* 2001;10:749-56.
7774 *J Urol* 2001;166:613.
7775 *Allergy* 1992;47:380-3.
7776 *Eur J Clin Pharmacol* 2000;56:411-5.
7777 *J Nutr* 2001;131:235-41.
7778 *Life Sci* 1998;62:PL135-42.
7779 *Eur J Clin Pharmacol* 2000;56:693-8.
7780 *Eur J Clin Pharmacol* 2000;56:643-9.
7781 *Clin Pharmacol Ther* 2000;67:690.
7782 *Clin Pharmacol Ther* 2000;68:384-90.
7783 *J Nutr* 2001;131:164S-166S.
7784 *CA Cancer J Clin* 2001;51:199-204.
7785 *Urology* 2001;57:122-6.
7786 *J Altern Complement Med* 2000;6:449-51.
7787 *Urology* 2002;59:444.
7788 *Thymus* 1982;4:335-50.
7789 *Cell Immunol* 1988;115:130-45.
7790 *Vet Immunol Immunopathol* 1992;32:103-21.
7791 *Cell Immunol* 1979;43:192-6.
7792 *Cell Immunol* 1979;47:1-18.
7793 *Mol Med* 2000;6:332-41.

7794 *Am J Med* 1979;67:59-66.
7795 *Ann Neurol* 1979;6:84.
7797 *Proc Soc Exp Biol Med* 1985;178:468-75.
7798 *Lancet* 1980;2:931-4.
7799 *Lancet* 1978;1:851-3.
7800 *Cancer* 1984;54:663-9.
7801 *Menopause* 2001;8:17-26.
7802 *Obstet Gynecol* 2002;99:389-94.
7803 *J Nutr* 2000;130:2590-3.
7804 *J Nutr* 2001;131:1202-6.
7805 *J Clin Endocrinol Metab* 2001;86:3045-52.
7806 *J Clin Nutr* 2002;75:145-53.
7807 *Am J Health Syst Pharm* 2002;59:545-7.
7808 *Phytomedicine* 2001;8:152-60.
7809 *Clin Pharmacol Ther* 2001;71:P25.
7810 *Br J Clin Pharmacol* 2002;53:75-82.
7811 *Can J Psychiatry* 2001;46:77-9.
7812 *Am J Med* 2002;112:507-8.
7813 *Heart* 1999;81:512-7.
7814 *Proc Nutr Soc* 1993;52:387-401.
7815 *J Am Coll Cardiol* 2002;39:37-45.
7816 *Am J Cardiol* 1997;80:331-3.
7817 *Circulation* 2000;101:2160-4.
7818 *Am J Hypertens* 2000;13:547-51.
7819 *Lancet* 2001;358:696-701.
7820 *J Nutr* 2000;130:2626-9.
7821 *J Am Coll Cardiol* 2000;36:410-6.
7822 *Ann Pharmacother* 2001;35:755-64.
7823 *J Natl Cancer Inst* 1993;85:1571-9.
7824 *Prostate* 2001;47:262-8.
7825 *Mutat Res* 2001;475:123-39.
7826 *Urology* 2001;57:90-4.
7827 *Free Radic Biol Med* 1999;26:42-8.
7828 *Life Sci* 2000;68:603-10.
7829 *J Infect Dis* 2000;182 Suppl 1:S69-73.
7830 *Clin Infect Dis* 1996;23:654-6.
7831 *Curr Sci* 2001;81:1215-8.
7832 *Toxicol Appl Pharmacol* 1998;152:309-14.
7833 *J Nutr* 2000;130:2384-9.
7834 *J Nutr* 2000;130:1653-6.
7835 *Arch Dis Child Fetal Neonatal Ed* 1998;78:F225-6.
7836 *J Am Coll Nutr* 2001;20:1-4.
7837 *J Nutr* 2001;131:1355S-8S.
7838 *Acta Paediatr* 1996;85:1143-5.
7839 *Transplant Proc* 2001;33:974-5.
7840 *J Clin Gastroenterol* 2001;32:405-8.
7841 *Cancer Epidemiol Biomarkers Prev* 2001;10:385-90.
7842 *Arch Dermatol Res* 1997;289:404-9.
7843 *J Pediatr* 1982;101:771-4.
7844 *J Am Diet Assoc* 1998;98:49-55.
7845 *Gynecol Obstet Invest* 1997;43:120-4.
7846 *Infect Immun* 1974;9:781-7.
7847 *Lancet* 1993;341:756-7.
7848 *Burns* 1999;25:729-31.
7849 *Br J Surg* 1988;75:679-81.
7850 *Lancet* 1982;1:963.
7851 Lancaster S, Krieder RB, Rasmussen C, et al. Effects of honey on glucose, insulin and endurance cycling performance. Abstract presented 4/4/01 at Experimental Biology 2001, Orlando, FL.
7852 *Arch Surg* 2000;135:1414-7.
7853 *J Allergy Clin Immunol* 1999;104:681-7.
7854 *Lancet* 1999;354:281-6.
7855 *J Ethnopharmacol* 1998;61:81-3.
7856 *Curr Opin Neurol* 1998;11:539-44.
7857 *J Med Chem* 1997;40:2102-6.
7858 *Fitoterapia* 2000;71:183-6.
7859 *J Immunol* 1999;163:6800-9.
7860 *Menopause* 2002;9:145-50.
7861 *Cancer Lett* 2000;158:85-91.
7862 *Cancer Lett* 2001;167:151-6.
7863 *Nutrition Research* 2001;21:747-53.
7864 *Toxicol Lett* 2001;125:83-91.
7865 *Endocrinol* 2000;141:3657-67.
7866 *Antiviral Res* 1999;43:145-55.
7868 *Am J Respir Crit Care Med* 1997;156:1897-901.
7869 *Pharmacotherapy* 2001;21:1331-6.
7870 *Neurology* 2001;57:1515-7.
7871 *Crit Care Med* 1999;27:1100-4.
7872 *Circulation* 1995;92:2855-62.
7873 *Cancer Lett* 1999;147:109-14.
7874 *Transplantation* 2000;69:853-9.
7875 *J Clin Oncol* 1993;11:1216-22.
7876 *Mov Disord* 2002;17:84-90.
7877 *Contraception* 1990;42:573-87.
7878 *Am J Clin Nutr* 2002;75:295-9.
7879 *J Nutr* 2001;131:1479-84.
7880 *Ann N Y Acad Sci* 1985;447: 389-92.
7881 *Arterioscler Thromb Vasc Biol* 1999;19:2918-21.
7882 *Arch Surg* 2002;137:278-82.
7883 *Semin Arthritis Rheum* 2000;30(2 Suppl 1):19-25.
7884 *Semin Arthritis Rheum* 2000;30(2 Suppl 1):11-8.
7885 *J Rheumatol* 1998;25:2203-12.
7886 *Clin Exp Rheumatol* 1998;16:441-9.
7887 *Arch Intern Med* 2002;162:292-8.
7888 *Arch Intern Med* 2002;162:245-7.
7889 *Pharmacist's Letter/Prescriber's Letter* 2002;18(7):180711.
7890 Hyalgan Prescribing Information. Sanofi-Synthelabo, Inc. New York, NY, 2002.
7891 Synvisc Prescribing Information. Wyeth-Ayerst Pharmaceuticals, Philadelphia, PA, 2000.
7892 Gelclair Prescribing Information. Cell Pathways, Inc. Horsham, PA, 2002.
7893 *Can J Ophthalmol* 1994;29:182-6.
7894 *Dermatol Surg* 2002;28:359-60.
7895 *Am J Epidemiol* 2000;151:119-23.
7896 *Am J Clin Nutr* 2000;71:1691S-5S.
7897 *Am J Epidemiol* 1997;146:618-26.
7898 *Allergy* 2000;55:1184-9.
7899 *J Nutr* 2002;132:404-8.
7900 *Clin Pharmacol Ther* 1988;43:381-6.
8000 *Drugs* 1992;43:499-506.
8001 *J Clin Oncol* 1994;12:1126-9.
8002 *J Clin Oncol* 1994;12:1121-5.
8003 *J Clin Oncol* 1994;12:1113-20.
8004 *Cancer* 1987;59:406-10.
8005 *CMAJ* 1998;158:1327-30.
8006 *Prog Neuropsychopharmacol Biol Psychiatry* 2002;26:539-45.
8007 *J Clin Pharm Ther* 2001;26:363-7.
8008 *N Engl J Med* 2001;345:1593-600.
8009 *N Engl J Med* 2001;345:1593-600.
8010 Office of Public Affairs. State health director warns consumers about prescription drugs in herbal products. California Department of Health Services 2002. Available at: http://www.applications.dhs.ca.gov/pressreleases/store/pressreleases/02-03.html (Accessed 8 Feb 2002).
8011 *J Am Acad Dermatol* 1996;35:388-91.
8012 *Planta Med* 2001;67:561-4.
8013 *J Nutr* 1998;128:1411-4.

8014 *J Am Coll Cardiol* 1996;27:1207-13.
8015 *Anesth Analg* 2000;90:840-6.
8016 *Circulation* 1999;99:2113-7.
8017 *Prostaglandins Leukot Essent Fatty Acids* 2000;62:55-73.
8018 *Urol Clin North Am* 2000;27:157-62.
8019 *J Am Acad Dermatol* 2000;43:829-32.
8020 *Cancer Epidemiol Biomarker Prev* 2000;9:719-25.
8021 *J Am Coll Nutr* 2001;20:143-8.
8022 *Cancer Lett* 1991;60:135-42.
8023 *Cancer Lett* 2000;161:47-55.
8024 *Ann N Y Acad Sci* 1990;595:281-90.
8025 *Lancet* 1982;2:1295-9.
8026 *Am J Clin Nutr* 2001;73:1094-100.
8027 *JAMA* 2001;285:41,42.
8028 *Prostaglandins Leukot Med* 1987;27:9-13.
8029 *Thromb Diath Haemorrh* 1967;18:670-3.
8030 *Atherosclerosis* 1977;26:255-60.
8032 *Am J Epidemiol* 2000;152:1034-8.
8033 *Arch Intern Med* 2002;162:657-62.
8034 *BMJ* 1997;315:1489-92.
8035 *Am J Clin Nutr* 2001;73:532-8.
8036 *Am J Epidemiol* 2001:153:353-62.
8037 *Am J Clin Nutr* 2001;73:45-52.
8038 *Cancer Epidemiol Biomarkers Prev* 2001;10:429-37.
8039 *Eur J Cancer Prev* 1998;7:77-82.
8040 *Eur J Cancer Prev* 2000;9:241-56.
8041 *Nutr Cancer* 1998;31:41-8.
8042 Anon. Filtering the news about coffee. University of California, Berkeley Wellness Letter 2001:17:1-2.
8043 *Am J Epidemiol* 1996:144:642-4.
8044 *Am J Clin Nutr* 2002;75:900-7.
8045 *J Nutr* 2001;131:1574-80.
8046 *J Am Coll Nutr* 2001;20:628-36.
8047 *J Clin Endocrinol Metab* 2001;86:3579-94.
8048 *Curr Opin Clin Nutr Metab Care* 2000;3:417-24.
8049 *Arch Intern Med* 1999;159:1143-4.
8050 *JAMA* 1993;269:3108-9.
8051 *Lancet* 1994;344:817-9.
8052 *Arch Intern Med* 1993;153: 2368-73.
8053 *Arch Intern Med* 1996;156:973-9.
8054 *Am J Epidemiol* 1993;138:154-9.
8055 *Ann Hematol* 1998;77:235-8.
8056 *Neurology* 2002;58:130-3.
8057 *Ann Allergy Asthma Immunol* 1995;75:351-9.
8058 *Am J Clin Nutr* 1991;53:1431-5.
8060 *Am J Clin Nutr* 1992;56:93-8.
8061 *Med J Aust* 1994;161:660-4.
8062 *Am J Clin Nutr* 1994;59:1055-9.
8064 *J Am Coll Nutr* 1991;10:364-71.
8065 *Curr Opin Lipidol* 2000;11:49-56.
8066 *JAMA* 1989;261:3419-23.
8067 *Am J Clin Nutr* 1997;65:1524-33.
8068 *Biol Pharm Bull* 1998;21:184-7.
8069 *Am J Clin Nutr* 194;59:395-400.
8070 *J Nutr* 1994;124:78-83.
8071 *Am J Clin Nutr* 1992;55:719-22.
8072 *J Am Coll Nutr* 1993;12:147-54.
8073 *Pediatrics* 1995;96:1005-9.
8074 *J Pediatr* 1993;123:24-9.
8075 *Am J Clin Nutr* 1996;63:96-102.
8076 *J Am Coll Nutr* 1995;14:251-7.
8077 *Dis Colon Rectum* 2000;43:66-9.
8079 *JAMA* 1990;264:2534-6.
8080 *South Med J* 1989;82:1449-50.
8081 *Neurology* 1999;52:670-1.
8082 *J Natl Cancer Inst* 1996;88:857-8.
8083 *Cancer Lett* 1993;75:53-8.
8084 *Lancet* 1992;340:124-5.
8085 *Lancet* 1991;337;1094-5.
8086 *Lancet* 1991;338:66.
8087 *Lancet* 1991;338:641.
8088 *Am Heart J* 1996;132:664-71.
8089 *J Am Coll Nutr* 1997;16:22-31.
8090 *J Am Coll Nutr* 1997;16:4-6.
8091 *Chest* 2000;118:1690-5.
8092 *Am J Hypertens* 2001;14:254-8.
8093 *Am J Obstet Gynecol* 2000;183:717-25.
8094 *Ann Pharmacother* 2002;36:255-60.
8095 *J Emerg Med* 2002;22:185-8.
8096 *JAMA* 1974;230:1302-3.
8097 *J Urol* 1988;139:679-84.
8098 *Hypertension* 1998;31:131-8.
8099 *Am J Clin Nutr* 2002;75:65-71.
8100 *J Nutr* 2001;131:552S-61S.
8101 *Am J Clin Nutr* 2001;73:628-37.
8102 *Arch Intern Med* 2002;162:569-74.
8103 *JAMA* 2001;285:2004-6.
8104 *JAMA* 2001;285:1971-7.
8105 *Clin Immunol Immunopathol* 1981;19:351-9.
8110 *Am J Clin Nutr* 2001;73:607-12.
8111 *N Engl J Med* 1981;305:467.
8112 *Eur J Pharmacol* 2000;390:339-45.
8113 *Arch Dermatol* 2001;137:664.
8114 *Phytomedicine* 2002;9:3-8.
8115 *Altern Comp Ther* 2000;6:296-300.
8116 *Arch Intern Med* 2002;162:1001-6.
8117 *J Clin Oncol* 2001;19:1830-8.
8118 *Life Sci* 2001;68:1207-14.
8119 *Am J Clin Nutr* 2002;75:880-6.
8120 *Circulation* 2002;105:2476-81.
8121 *Am J Epidemiol* 2001;154:495-503.
8122 *Arch Intern Med* 2000;160:3328-9.
8123 *J Nutr* 2001;131:1207-10.
8125 *Atherosclerosis* 1972;16:105-18.
8126 *J Am Geriatr Soc* 1968;16:779-85.
8127 *Urology* 1997;50:173-83.
8128 *JANA* 2000;3:37-44.
8129 *Med J Aust* 1990;153:630-1.
8131 *Int J Epidemiol* 2002;31:474-80.
8132 *Diabetes Care* 2000;23:1472-7.
8133 *Eur J Cancer* 2001;37:402-13.
8134 *Altern Ther* 2001;7:112.
8135 *Cephalalgia* 2002;22:137-41.
8136 Burton TM. Maker of herbal cancer therapy shuts its operations, citing recall. Wall Street Journal. May 2002.
8137 *Cancer* 2002;94:686-9.
8138 *Int J Vitam Nutr Res* 2001;71:293-301.
8139 *Altern Med Rev* 2000;5:164-73.
8140 *Arzneimittelforschung* 1976;26:832-5.
8141 *Arzneimittelforschung* 1976;26:829-32.
8142 *Zhongguo Zhong Yao Za Zhi* 1995;20:173-5, 192.
8143 *Compr Ther* 1998;24:336-9.
8144 *J Womens Health Gend Based Med* 2000;9:381-7.
8145 *Circulation* 2001;103:1961-6.
8146 *J Am Coll Cardiol* 2000;36:2154-9.
8147 *Clin Drug Invest* 2001;21:103–13.
8148 *JAMA* 1995;274:1196-7.
8149 *Cutis* 2000;66:373-4.
8150 *Altern Ther Health Med* 2001;7:120,112-4.
8151 *Alt Ther* 2001;7:S30.
8152 *Curr Ther Res* 1999;60:220-7.

8153 *Planta Med* 1988;54:271-7.
8154 *Indian J Med Res* 1989;90:62-8.
8155 *Ind J Med Res* 1986;84:626-34.
8156 *Life Sci* 1999;65:PL137-41.
8158 *Indian J Med Res* 1977;65:390-5.
8159 *J Neurol* 1998;245:681-5.
8160 *Neurology* 1997;48:1238-43.
8161 *J Neurol Sci* 1998;156:41-6.
8162 *Eur Neurol* 1997;37:212-8.
8163 *J Neurol Sci* 1990;100:70-8.
8165 *Fitoterapia* 2000;71:S117-S23.
8166 *Pharmacol Biochem Behav* 1994;47:1-4.
8167 *Biochem Pharmacol* 1990;40:2227-31.
8168 *Br J Clin Pharmacol* 2001;51:143-6.
8169 *Bioorg Med Chem Lett* 1999;9:869-74.
8170 *Pharm Res* 2001;18:374-9.
8171 *Adv Exp Med Biol* 1998;439:191-225.
8172 *Mutagenesis* 2002;17:45-53.
8175 *Hawaii Med J* 2000;59:420-2.
8176 *BJU Int* 2000;85:836-41.
8177 *Hinyokika Kiyo* 1990;36:495-516.
8178 *Planta Med* 1979;37:115-23.
8179 *J Ethnopharmacol* 2001;76:233-8.
8180 *Phytother Res* 2000;14:592-5.
8181 *Lancet* 1979:1:607.
8182 *Nutrition* 2002;18:130-3.
8183 *Nutrition* 2002;18:123-6.
8184 *Clin Nutr* 2000;19:375-7.
8185 *Gut* 2000;47:199-205.
8186 *Nutrition* 2002;18:127-9.
8187 Secondary Direct Food Additives Permitted in Food for Human Consumption. Safe use of ozone when used as a gas or dissolved in water as an antimicrobial agent on food, including meat and poultry. Federal Register 66 http://www.fda.gov/OHRMS/Dockets/98fr/062601a.htm (Accessed 26 June 2001).
8188 *Diabet Med* 2001;18:1010.
8189 *Chem Pharm Bull (Tokyo)* 1987;35:262-70.
8190 *Ann N Y Acad Sci* 1995;768:243-5.
8191 *Ann N Y Acad Sci* 1997;833:204-7.
8192 *Endocr Relat Cancer* 2001;8:129-34.
8193 *J Altern Complement Med* 2002;8:135-42.
8194 *Alt Ther* 2001;7:S33.
8195 *Ann N Y Acad Sci* 1990;585:321-30.
8196 *N Engl J Med* 1983;309:445-8.
8197 *Dev Med Child Neurol* 1997;39:63-5.
8198 *Ann N Y Acad Sci* 1990;585:250-60.
8199 *Arch Surg* 1989;124:1329-30.
8200 *Ann Neurol* 1984;15:104-7.
8201 *Ann N Y Acad Sci* 1990;585:295-301.
8202 *Am J Clin Nutr* 1979;32:2040-6.
8203 *South Med J* 1989;82:841-2.
8204 *BMJ* 1995;310:1534.
8205 *Am J Nephrol* 1996;16:552-3.
8217 *Prog Clin Biol Res* 1983;125:61-72.
8218 *Int J Cardiol* 1982;2:303-4.
8219 *Acta Med Scand Suppl* 1980;642:79-84.
8220 *Nutr Rev* 1975;33:343-7.
8221 *Adv Exp Med Biol* 1994;359:425-33.
8222 *Prog Clin Biol Res* 1985;179:195-213.
8223 *J Nat Prod* 1996;59:541-3.
8224 *J Ethnopharmacol* 1999;68:3-37.
8225 *Ann Allergy Asthma Immunol* 2002;88:42-51.
8226 *Biochem Pharmacol* 2000;60:155-8.
8227 *Planta Med* 1995;61:510-4.
8228 *Antimicrob Agents Chemother* 2000;44:1708-9.
8229 *Fed Regist* 2002;67:31125-7.
8231 *Pediatrics* 2002;109:325-7.
8232 *Epilepsia* 2001;42:280-1.
8233 *Acta Psychiatr Scand* 1999;100:62-6.
8234 *Pharmacotherapy* 2002;22:551-6.
8235 *J Psychiatry Neurosci* 2001;26:221-8.
8236 *Psychopharmacology (Berl)* 2000;151:416-23.
8238 *Cancer Lett* 2000;151:133-43.
8239 *J Clin Endocrinol Metab* 2000;85:666-70.
8240 *Chronobiol Int* 2000;17:71-6.
8241 *Altern Ther Health Med* 1999;5:49-57.
8242 *Osteoarthritis Cartilage* 2000;8:335-42.
8243 *BMJ* 1989;299:1156-7.
8244 *J Psychosom Res* 2000;48:45-50.
8245 *J Clin Psychiatry* 2000;61:373-7.
8246 *J Clin Endocrinol Metab* 2000;85:2137-44.
8247 *J Clin Endocrinol Metab* 2001;86:129-34.
8248 *Lancet* 1998;351:1254.
8249 *Neurology* 2000;55:1746-8.
8250 *Alternative Therapies* 2001;7:S4.
8251 *Clin Pharmacol Ther* 2000;67:1-6.
8252 *Urology* 2001;57:407-13.
8253 *BMJ* 2001;322:1571.
8254 *J Psychiatr Nurs* 1966;467-70.
8256 *Plant Physiol* 2000;123:327-34.
8257 *Phytochemistry* 2000;54:71-5.
8260 *Geriatr Nephrol Urol* 1998;8:95-100.
8262 *Dev Med Child Neurol* 2000;42:487-91.
8263 *J Clin Endocrinol Metab* 2000;85:2135-6.
8265 *Brain Res* 2000;873:310-7.
8266 *Am Fam Physician* 1999;59:284, 287-8.
8267 *Ann Allergy Asthma Immunol* 1999;82:185-91.
8268 *J Pineal Res* 1997;23:15-9.
8269 *Cochrane Database Syst Rev* 2001;1:CD001520.
8270 *Psychopharmacology (Berl)* 2001;154:403-7.
8271 Briggs, Freeman, Yafee. Update Drugs in Pregnancy and Lactation. Lippincott Williams & Wilkins, 2001.
8272 *Am Heart J* 2001;141:E9.
8273 *Chronobiol Int* 1998;15:655-66.
8274 *Chronobiol Int* 1992;9:380-92.
8275 *J Neural Transm* 2000;107:1475-81.
8277 *Plast Reconstr Surg* 1998;102:2404-7.
8278 *Biosci Biotechnol Biochem* 1999;63:202-5.
8279 *Phytomedicine* 1994;1:17-24.
8280 *Phytomedicine* 2001;8:262-6.
8281 *Am Heart J* 2002;143:910-5.
8282 *Antimicrob Agents Chemother* 2002;46:1614-6.
8283 *Clin Pharmacol Ther* 2002;71:21-9.
8284 *Int J Clin Pharmacol Ther* 2000;38:523-31.
8285 *Eur J Clin Pharmacol* 2002;58:45-53.
8286 *Eur J Clin Pharmacol* 2001;56:799-803.
8287 *Contraception* 1997;55:183-8.
8288 *J Lab Clin Med* 1998;132:32-8.
8289 *Cancer Lett* 1999;135:171-80.
8290 *Contraception* 2000;61:61-7.
8291 *Cancer Lett* 1996;107:37-44.
8292 *Eur J Pharmacol* 1996;313:243-55.
8294 *Life Sci* 1995;57:61-7.
8295 *Invest New Drugs* 1995;13:181-6.
8296 *Planta Med* 1985;2:144-8.
8300 *J Appl Physiol* 1988;65:1821-6.
8301 *Med Sci Sports Exerc* 1986;18(6):674-7.
8302 *Ann Pharmacother* 1997;31(6):683-8.
8303 *Crit Care Med* 1995;23(7):1204-10.
8305 *Am J Med* 2001;110:724-30.
8307 *Phytother Res* 2000;14:472-3.

8308 *J Agric Food Chem* 2002;50:166-71.
8309 *J Nutr* 2001;131:2082-9.
8310 *Atherosclerosis* 2001;158:195-8.
8311 *J Chromatogr* 1988;438:438-42.
8312 *Clin Cancer Res* 1999;5:413-6.
8313 *Artery* 1985;12:234-43.
8314 *Curr Ther Res* 1982;32:380-6.
8315 *Curr Ther Res* 1984;36:314-22.
8316 *Curr Ther Res* 1985;38:719-27.
8317 *Curr Ther Res* 1983;33:1091-7.
8318 *Atherosclerosis* 1984;50:73-83.
8319 *Angiology* 1987;38:241-7.
8320 *Med Hypotheses* 2001;56:314-7.
8321 *Biochim Biophys Acta* 1988;963:389-93.
8322 *Atherosclerosis* 1984;53:255-64.
8323 *Curr Eye Res* 2000;20:17-24.
8324 *Exp Eye Res* 1996;62:11-9.
8325 *Exp Eye Res* 1996;62:75-84.
8329 *Ann Pharmacother* 2000 Jan;34(1):98-100.
8330 *Int Urol Nephrol* 1993;25:565-9.
8407 *J Nutr* 2001;131:989S-93S.
8408 *J Nutr* 2001;131:985S-8S.
8409 *Life Sci* 2000;67:155-63.
8413 *Phytomedicine* 2002;9:41-7.
8414 *J Ethnopharmacol* 1992;37:13-45.
8415 *Life Sci* 2002;70:2581-97.
8417 *CMAJ* 2002;166:777.
8418 *J Allergy Clin Immunol* 1999;103:507-13.
8419 *Gastroenterology* 1993;104:1007-12.
8420 *Nurs Res* 2001;50:203-13.
8421 *Am J Clin Nutr* 2000;72:784-9.
8422 *Scand J Gastroenterol* 1988;23:1237-40.
8423 *Heart Lung* 1991;20:409-13.
8424 *Am J Gastroenterol* 1987;82:333-7.
8425 *Ann Intern Med* 1981;95:53-6.
8426 *Gut* 1987;28:1510-3.
8427 *Gut* 1987;28:150-5.
8428 *Q J Med* 1989:73:931-9.
8429 *Ann Intern Med* 1990;112:386.
8430 *Am J Clin Nutr* 2000;71:401-2.
8431 *Am J Cardiol* 1997;79:34-7.
8432 *Ann Intern Med* 1995;123:493-9.
8433 *Am J Med Sci* 1994;307:269-73.
8434 *JAMA* 1961;175:187-90.
8440 *Planta Med* 2000;66:7-10.
8441 *J Lab Clin Med* 1988;112:458-63.
8442 *Pharmacist's Letter/Prescriber's Letter* 2002;18(6):180614.
8443 *The Tan Sheet* May 13, 2002.
8444 *Clin Cardiol* 2000;23:205-10.
8445 *Contact Dermatitis* 1998;38:44-5.
8446 *Arch Ophthalmol* 1994;112:222-7.
8447 *Nutr Rev* 1996;54:S38-42.
8448 *Metabolism* 1996;45:1547-50.
8449 *Eur J Clin Nutr* 1995;49:S145-52.
8450 *Br J Nutr* 1997;78:215-22.
8451 Abrams SA, Griffin IJ. Calcium absorption is increased in adolescent girls receiveing enriched inulin. World Congress of Pediatric Gastroenterology, Hepatology, & Nutrition, Boston, MA, August 5-9, 2000: Abstract 821.
8452 *Eur J Clin Nutr* 1995;49:346-52.
8453 *Nutr Cancer* 2000;36:59-65.
8454 *Methods Find Exp Clin Pharmacol* 2001;23:79-84.
8455 *Arch Ophthalmol* 1999;117:412-3.
8456 *Nutr Rev* 1999;57:1-10.
8457 *Eur J Clin Nutr* 1996;50:811-5.
8458 *Ann Intern Med* 1993;119:867-73.
8459 *Int Immunopharmacol* 2001;1:2197-9.
8462 *Contraception* 1989;39:579-87.
8463 *Drugs* 1989;38:333-41.
8464 *Mutat Res* 1993;297:293-312.
8466 *J Med* 1991;22:29-44.
8467 Astaxanthin biochemical properties website. URL: http://www.astaxanthin.org. (Accessed 5 June 2002).
8468 *Biomed Pharmacother* 1990;44:511-4.
8469 *Med J Aust* 1976;1:584-5.
8470 *Ann Nutr Metab* 2001;45:47-57.
8472 *J Am Coll Cardiol* 2002;39:1314-22.
8473 *Am J Med* 2000;108:439.
8474 *J Pediatr* 2002;140:425-31.
8475 *J Am Coll Cardiol* 2002;39:1199-203.
8476 *Eur J Clin Nutr* 1998;52:12-6.
8477 *N Engl J Med* 1993;328:603-7.
8478 *J Nutr* 2002;132:1062S-101S.
8479 *Ann Allergy Asthma Immunol* 1999;83:377-83.
8480 *Eur J Clin Nutr* 1998;52:436-40.
8481 *Immunopharmacology* 1986;12:29-35.
8482 *Jpn J Med Sci Biol* 1982;35:75-80.
8483 *J Dairy Res* 2001;68:653-61.
8484 *Br J Nutr* 1992;67:67-75.
8485 *J Ind Microbiol Biotechnol* 2002;28:1-6.
8486 *J Dairy Sci* 1982;65:346-52.
8487 *Lett Appl Microbiol* 2002;35:136-40.
8488 *J Nutr* 2001;131:807-12.
8489 *Jpn J Med Sci Biol* 1983;36:49-53.
8490 *J Dermatol Sci* 1998;16:226-230.
8493 *Acta Otolaryngol Suppl* 1987;442:50-3.
8494 *Acta Ophthalmol (Copenh)* 1990;68:721-7.
8495 *Br J Ophthalmol* 1982;66:714-6.
8496 *Ophthalmic Surg* 1990;21:486-91.
8497 *Surgery* 1991;109:76-84.
8498 *Trans Ophthalmol Soc U K* 1985;104:616-20.
8499 *J Clin Oncol* 2002;20:1436-8.
8501 *Am J Clin Nutr*. 2002;75:179-80.
8502 *Am J Cardiol* 2000;85:1297-301.
8503 *Fertil Steril* 74:3:S25.
8504 *J Am Coll Nutr* 2001;20:398S-402S.
8505 *Nutr Res* 2000;20:1725-33.
8506 *Carcinogenesis* 1999;20:1953-6 .
8507 *J Nutr* 2000;130:1197-9.
8508 *Gastroenterology* 1994;106:A598.
8509 *Am J Clin Nutr* 2001;73:415S-420S.
8511 *BMJ* 2002;324:1361.
8512 *Am J Clin Nutr* 2001;73:444S-450S.
8513 *Am J Clin Nutr* 2001;73:1131S-41S.
8514 *Am J Clin Nutr* 2001;73:437S-443S.
8515 *Lancet* 2001;357:1076-1079.
8516 *Am J Clin Nutr* 2001;73;1124S-1130S.
8517 *Am J Clin Nutr* 2001;73:421S-9S.
8520 *Int Urol Nephrol* 1996;28:49-53.
8521 *J Am Diet Assoc* 2001;101:1319-25.
8522 *Semin Dial* 2002;15:53-9.
8523 *Phytother Res* 2002;16:138-42.
8524 *Med Sci Sports Exerc* 2002;34:1605-13.
8525 *Aliment Pharmacol Ther* 2002;16:1669-75.
8526 *Am J Clin Nutr* 1991;53:1253-8.
8527 *Arterioscler Thromb Vasc Biol* 1997;17:2868-74.
8528 *Am J Clin Nutr* 2002;76:57-64.
8529 *J Nutr* 2002;132:708-14.
8530 *Am J Clin Nutr* 2002;76:78-84.
8531 *Diabetes Care* 2002;25:1709-14.
8532 *J Am Coll Nutr* 2002;21:388-93.

8533 *Heart Lung and Circulation* 2001;10:116-20.
8535 *J Epidemiol Community Health* 2000;54:654-5.
8536 *J Epidemiol Community Health* 2000;54:656-9.
8537 *J Epidemiol Community Health* 2000;54:650-1.
8538 *Arch Intern Med* 2000;160:3393-400.
8539 *BMJ* 1996;313:1362-6.
8540 *Ann Pharmacother* 2002;36:992-5.
8541 *Chem Res Toxicol* 2001;14:1254-8.
8542 *Phytomedicine* 2002;9:442-6.
8543 *Eur Arch Otorhinolaryngol* 2001;258:213-9.
8544 *Hum Psychopharmacol* 2001;16:409-16.
8545 *Am J Cardiol* 2001;87:476-9,A7.
8546 *Am Heart J* 2002;143:514-8.
8547 *Am Heart J* 2000;140:631-6.
8548 *Am J Clin Nutr* 1967;20:393-9.
8549 *Proc Eur Dial Transplant Assoc* 1979;16:727-8.
8550 *Contrib Nephrol* 1987;58:190-2.
8551 *Postgrad Med* 1985;78:38-44, 47-51.
8552 *Ann Allergy* 1975;35:153-8.
8554 *Med Hypotheses* 2000;54:803-7.
8555 *J Womens Health Gend Based Med* 2000;9:131-9.
8556 *J Nutr* 2001;131:1777-86.
8558 *Am J Psychiatry* 2001;158:1511-4.
8559 *Am J Clin Nutr* 2000;71:674-81.
8560 *JAMA* 2002;287:1940-1941.
8561 *Postgrad Med J* 2002;78:366-7.
8562 *Aliment Pharmacol Ther* 2000;14:1625-9.
8563 *Nut Res* 2002;22:71-84.
8564 *J Appl Nutr* 1984;36:125-153.
8565 *BMJ* 2001;322:1327.
8566 *Pediatr Infect Dis J* 2002;21:417-9.
8567 *Pediatr Infect Dis J* 2002;21:411-6.
8568 *Pediatrics* 2002;109:678-84.
8569 *Pharmacotherapy* 2001;21:1574-8.
8570 *Pharmacotherapy* 2002;22:673-5.
8571 *Phytother Res* 2001;15:172-3.
8572 *Int J Obes* 2002;26:870-2.
8573 *Med J Aust* 1990;153:455-8.
8574 *J Altern Complement Med* 2002;8:167-73.
8575 Jacob S, Lawrence RM, Zucker M. The Miracle of MSM: The Natural Solution for Pain. New York: Penguin-Putnam, 1999.
8576 *Patol Fiziol Eksp Ter* 1991;37-9.
8577 *US Pharm* 2000;92-4.
8579 *J Autism Dev Disord* 1993;23:193-9.
8581 *J Herb Pharmacother* 2002;2:57-63.
8582 *Brain Inj* 2002;16:359-67.
8583 *Alt Ther* 2001;7:105.
8584 *J Pharm Pharmacol* 2002;54:661-9.
8586 *JAMA* 2002;288:835-40.
8587 *Hum Psychopharmacol* 2002;17:45-9.
8588 *Hum Psychopharmacol* 2002;17:267-277.
8591 *Hum Psychopharmacol* 2002;17:35-44.
8592 *Am J Health Syst Pharm* 2000;57:2048-50, 2053-4, 2056.
8593 *J Clin Endocrinol Metab* 2002;87:2046-52.
8594 *J Sex Marital Ther* 2002;28:53-60.
8595 *Eur J Obstet Gynecol Reprod Biol* 2001;97:96-7.
8596 *Urol Res* 2001;29:278-81.
8597 *Proc Natl Acad Sci U S A* 2001;98:8145-50.
8598 *HIV Med* 2001;2:136-8.
8599 *Eur J Pharmacol* 2001;419:61-64.
8600 *Herbalgram* 2002;54:34-51.
8601 *Ann Pharmacother* 2002;36:375-9.
8602 *Toxicology* 2002;172:149-56.
8603 *Life Sci* 2001;68:739-49.
8604 *Arch Intern Med* 2000;160:3329.
8605 *Altern Ther* 2001;7:S26.
8608 *Phytomedicine* 2002;9:181-94.
8609 *J Ethnopharmacol* 1984;11:259-74.
8610 *J Ethnopharmacol* 1985;13:193-9.
8611 *Can J Physiol Pharmacol* 1994;72:1532-6.
8612 *Phytomedicine* 2000;6:469-73.
8613 *Ann Rheum Dis* 1981;40:632.
8614 *Planta Med* 1992;58:117-23 .
8615 *Planta Med* 1997;63:171-6.
8616 *Phytomedicine* 2001;8:28-30..
8617 *Can Med Assoc J* 1983;129:249-51.
8618 *J Cutan Pathol* 2002;29:613-5.
8619 *J Nutr* 2001;4:1135-41.
8620 *J Nutr* 2001;131:1414-20.
8621 *J Am Coll Nutr* 2001;20:106-18.
8622 *J Nutr* 2002;132:697-702.
8623 *Altern Ther Health Med* 2001;7:49-56.
8624 *Nut Res* 2000;20:1079-89.
8625 *Nut Res* 2002;22:527-38.
8626 *Am J Clin Nutr* 2002;75:300-7.
8627 *Am J Clin Nutr* 2002;75:181-2.
8628 *Clin Infect Dis* 2001;33:1865-70.
8629 *Am J Med* 2001;111:103-8.
8630 *Am J Clin Nutr* 2001;73:1045-51.
8631 *Am J Clin Nutr* 2002;75:99-103.
8632 *Am J Clin Nutr* 2002;75:2-3.
8633 *Am J Clin Nutr* 2000;72:1516-22.
8636 *Am J Clin Nutr* 2002;75:92-8.
8637 *BMJ* 2002;324:1358.
8638 *BMJ* 2001;322:1567.
8639 Anabolic Steroid Act, Public Law No. 108-358, 2004.
8640 *Int J Obes Relat Metab Disord* 2002;26:589.
8641 *Int J Obes Relat Metab Disord* 2002;26:590-2.
8642 *Mayo Clin Proc* 2002;77:7-9.
8643 *Mayo Clin Proc* 2002;77:12-6.
8644 *Clin Pharmacol Ther* 2002;71:421-32.
8645 *J Altern Complement Med* 2000;6:553-5.
8646 *Med Sci Sports Exerc* 2001;33:1399-403.
8647 *Int J Obes Relat Metab Disord* 2002;26:593-604.
8648 *Arch Intern Med* 2000;160:2605-12.
8649 *Am J Clin Nutr* 2002;75:593-9.
8650 *JAMA* 2001:285:1965-70.
8651 *Stroke* 2001;32:1939-46.
8652 *Atherosclerosis* 2001;156:177-83.
8653 *Circulation* 2000;102:500-5.
8654 *Circulation* 2000;102:494-9.
8655 *Am J Clin Nutr* 2000;72:1206-13.
8656 *Am J Clin Nutr* 2000;72:1073.
8657 *J Clin Pharm Ther* 2001;26:271-8.
8658 *Int J Cardiol* 1995;49:173-7.
8659 *J Intern Med* 2001;250:167-9.
8660 *Proc West Pharmacol Soc* 1998;41:123-4.
8661 *J Rheumatol* 2002;29:678-81.
8662 *Virology* 2000;278:412-22.
8663 *J Altern Complement Med* 2002;8:77-83.
8664 *J Ethnopharmacol* 2002;80:1-7.
8665 *Biosci Biotechnol Biochem* 2000;64:287-93.
8666 *Biosci Biotechnol Biochem* 1995;59:2134-6.
8667 *Exp Toxicol Pathol* 1997;49:329-35.
8668 *Cancer Lett* 1996;105:203-9.
8669 *Cancer Lett* 1998;133:19-26.
8670 *Biosci Biotechnol Biochem* 1998;62:816-7.
8671 *Circulation* 2002;105:1874-5.
8673 *Am J Med* 2002;112:298-304.
8674 *Am J Clin Nutr* 2001;74:603-11.

8676 *Circulation* 2001;103:651-7.
8677 *CMAJ* 2002:166:608-15.
8678 *Am J Clin Nutr* 2001;74:464-73.
8679 *Am J Clin Nutr* 2001;74;415-6.
8680 *Am Heart J* 143:E5.
8681 *Cardiovasc Res* 2002;54:183-90.
8683 *Arterioscler Thromb Vasc Biol* 2000;20:1990-7.
8684 *J Am Soc Nephrol* 2002;13:184-90.
8685 *JANA* 2002;5:46-50.
8686 *J Am Soc Nephrol* 2001;12:791-9.
8687 *Eur Heart J* 2001;22:428-36.
8689 *Urology* 2001;58:283-8.
8690 *Cancer Epidemiol Biomarkers Prev* 2002;11:143-5.
8691 *Cancer Chemother Pharmacol* 2001;47:34-40.
8693 *Nutrition* 2001;17:793-6.
8694 *Nutr Res* 2000;20:1065-77.
8695 *Nutr Res* 2000;20:1091-102.
8696 *Nutr Res* 2001;21:309-41.
8697 *Eur J Clin Nutr* 2000;54:690-4.
8698 *J Am Coll Nutr* 2000;19:745-53.
8699 *Lancet* 1999;353:812-3.
8700 *J Lipid Res* 2001;42:407-18.
8701 *Prostaglandins Leukot Essent Fatty Acids* 2001;64:291-7.
8702 *Eur Neuropsychopharmacol* 2001;11:295-9.
8704 *J Neurochem* 2000;75:2563-73.
8705 *Br J Nutr* 2000;83:337-9.
8706 *Lancet* 1992;339:1003-7.
8707 *Am J Obstet Gynecol* 1993;168:915-22.
8708 *Lancet* 1988;1:378-80.
8709 *Cancer Lett* 2001;163:171-8.
8710 *Aliment Pharmacol Ther* 2001;15:851-5.
8711 *J Am Soc Nephrol* 1999;10:1772-7.
8712 *J Adolesc Health* 2002;31:154-61.
8713 *Cephalalgia* 2001;21:818-22.
8714 *Diabetes Care* 2002;25:17048.
8715 *Neuroscience* 1999;93:237-41.
8716 *Am J Clin Nutr* 2001;73:622-7.
8717 *Clin Nutr* 2000;19:417-23.
8718 *Am J Clin Nutr* 2001;73:539-48.
8720 *Am J Psychiatry* 2002;159:1596-8.
8734 *J Natl Cancer Inst* 1998;90:1219-24.
8735 *Cancer Epidemiol Biomarkers Prev* 2000;9:883-7.
8736 *J Urol* 2001;166:2034-8.
8739 Antony AC. Megaloblastic Anemias. In: Hoffman R, Benz Jr EJ, Shattil SJ, et al. Hematology: Basic Principles and Practice. 3rd ed. New York, NY: Churchill Livingstone 2000: 451-79.
8740 *Planta Med* 1997;63:548-549.
8743 *Drug Metab Dispos* 2002;30:1153-7.
8744 *Eur J Clin Pharmcol* 2002;58:491-4.
8745 *Circulation* 2001;103:2792-8.
8746 *Circulation* 1999;100:1050-5.
8758 *Am J Clin Nutr* 1999;69:504-8.
8800 *Prog Neuropsychopharmacol Biol Psychiatry* 2002;26:233-9.
8801 *J Thromb Thrombolysis* 1998;5:257-61.
8803 *J Pediatr* 1994;125:S39-47.
8805 *Nephron* 2001;88:329-33.
8807 *Diabetes* 2002;51:2377-86.
8808 *J Nutr* 2001;131:717-22.
8809 *Hepatol* 2000;32:386A.
8811 *Fitoterapia* 2001;72:922-6.
8812 *Phytomedicine* 2001 Sep;8(5):382-8.
8813 *J Urol* 2002;168:2070-3.
8814 *Clin Drug Invest* 2001;21:41-5.
8815 *Allergy* 2001;56:462-3.
8816 *Am J Med* 2001;111:452-6.
8817 *Am J Hypertens* 2001;14:206S-12S.
8818 *Osteoporos Int* 2002;13:257-64.
8820 *Nutr Cancer* 2002;43:39-46.
8821 *J Am Coll Nutr* 2002;21:239-44.
8822 *Am J Clin Nutr* 2002;76:419-25.
8823 *J Clin Pharmacol* 2002;42:1251-6.
8824 *J Am Coll Nutr* 2002;21:152S-5S.
8825 *J Am Coll Nutr* 2002;21:146S-51S.
8826 *N Engl J Med* 2002;346:77-84.
8827 *J Clin Endocrinol Metab* 2001;86:4098-103.
8828 *Int J Gynaecol Obstet* 2001;74:17-21.
8830 *J Am Coll Nutr* 2000;19:754-60.
8831 *Nutrition* 2001;17:46-51.
8832 *J Clin Pharmacol* 2000;40:1237-44.
8833 *J Clin Endocrinol Metab* 2000;85:4023-7.
8834 *Diabetes Care* 2000;23:1227-31.
8835 *J Bone Miner Metab* 1999;17:131-6.
8836 *Osteoporos Int* 2000;11:938-43.
8837 *J Am Coll Nutr* 2001;20:198S-207S.
8838 *J Am Coll Nutr* 2001;20:192S-197S.
8839 *J Am Coll Nutr* 2001;20:186S-91S.
8840 *Cancer Lett* 1990;51:103-8.
8841 *J Biol Chem* 1982;257:13263-70.
8842 *Eur J Cancer* 2001;37:23-31.
8843 *Biomed Pharmacother* 1995;49:153-8.
8844 *Cancer Lett* 1995;94:199-205.
8845 *Cancer Lett* 1988;41:307-14.
8846 *Cancer Lett* 1992;66:123-30.
8847 *Cancer Lett* 1989;48:223-7.
8848 *Complement Ther Med* 1998;6:172-7.
8849 *J Biol Chem* 1982;257:13271-7.
8850 *J Clin Gastroenterol* 1992;14:288-92.
8851 *Neuroendocrinology* 1990;52:243-8.
8852 *Eur J Clin Pharmacol* 1992;42:385-8.
8853 *J Neuroimmunol* 1997;75:113-22.
8854 *Neurology* 1993;43:153-63.
8855 *Circulation* 2000;101:841-3.
8856 *J Nutr* 2000 130:2251-5.
8857 *J Biol Chem* 2000;275:35215-23.
8858 *Psychopharmacology (Berl)* 1989;99:316-21.
8859 *Altern Med Rev* 1999;4:249-65.
8860 *J Pediatr* 1983;102:796-8.
8861 *Altern Med Rev* 1998;3:379-81.
8862 *Am J Nephrol* 1991;11:32-6.
8863 *Atherosclerosis* 1987;68:41-9.
8864 *Atherosclerosis* 1985;57:99-106.
8865 *Atherosclerosis* 1982;44:261-73.
8866 *Br J Nutr* 1995;74:417-25.
8867 *Nutr Cancer* 1992;17:153-9.
8868 *J Steroid Biochem Mol Biol* 1992;41:615-9.
8869 *Ann Pharmacother* 1993;27:285-9.
8870 *J Am Coll Nutr* 2001;20:168S-85S.
8871 *Bone* 2000;27:45S.
8872 *Am J Med* 1990;89:380-2.
8873 *Bone* 2000;27:54S.
8874 *J Clin Oncol* 1988;6:1170-6.
8875 *Eur J Clin Nutr* 1992;46:317-27.
8876 *Gastroenterology* 1981;81:1068-71.
8877 Food and Drug Administration Science Background: Safety of Sodium Phosphates Oral Solution. September 17, 2001. Available at: http://www.fda.gov/cder/drug/safety/sodiumphospate.htm.
8880 *Kidney Int* 1997;51:1867-75.
8881 *Chest* 1996;110:42-7.

8882 *Chest* 1992;102:91-5.
8883 *Am Rev Respir Dis* 1990;141:575-9.
8884 *Lancet* 1989;2:45.
8885 *Chest* 1987;91:288-9.
8886 *Chest* 1988;94:763-6.
8887 *Am J Clin Nutr* 1983;37:416-20.
8888 *Br J Gen Pract* 1999;49:729-30.
8889 *Am Rev Respir Dis* 1984;129:329-32.
8890 *Chest* 1986;89:348-51.
8891 *Am Rev Respir Dis* 1990;142:338-42.
8892 *Lancet* 1984;1:51-2.
8893 *Ann Intern Med* 1985;103:68-9.
8894 *Am J Respir Crit Care Med* 1994;149:1359-74.
8900 *Clin Sci* 2000;99:285-92.
8901 *J Urol* 2001;167:374.
8902 *Cell Biol Int* 2001;25:1117-24.
8903 *Int J Cancer* 2001;92:600-4.
8904 *Crit Rev Food Sci Nutr* 2000;40:371-98.
8905 *Arterioscler Thromb Vasc Biol* 2001;21:1084-9.
8906 *Contraception* 1983;27:571-6.
8907 *South Med J* 2001;94:1112-7.
8908 *Br J Pharmacol* 1998;124:1500-6.
8909 *Mol Aspects Med* 1997;18:S159-68.
8910 *JACC* 2000;36:304-5.
8911 *J Sports Med Phys Fitness* 2000;40:51-7.
8912 *Neurology* 2001;56:849-55.
8913 *J Am Coll Nutr* 2001;20:591-8.
8914 *Arterioscler Thromb Vasc Biol* 1997;17:127-33.
8915 *Am Heart J* 2001;142:E2.
8916 *Res Commun Chem Pathol Pharmacol* 1975;11:265-71.
8917 *Res Commun Chem Pathol Pharmacol* 1975;12:111-23.
8918 *Res Commun Chem Pathol Pharmacol* 1976;14:715-9.
8920 *Pediatrics* 2001;108:1280-6.
8921 *Ann Nutr Metab* 1997;41:98-107.
8923 FDA. Center for Devices and Radiological Health. StaarVisc. Sodium Hyaluronate. http://www.fda.gov/cdrh/pdf/P960033c.pdf. (Accessed 11 October 2002).
8924 *J Rheumatol* 2002;29:1708-12.
8925 *Maturitas* 2002;42:187-93.
8926 *Diabetes Care* 1993;16:8-15.
8927 *Am J Clin Nutr* 2002;76:148-55.
8929 *Psychopharmacology (Berl)* 2002;159:432-6.
8930 *Br J Dermatol* 2000;143:1127-8.
8931 *J Clin Anesth* 2000;12:498-9.
8932 *Indian J Exp Biol* 2000;38:36-41.
8933 *Biochem Syst Ecol* 2001;29:659-61.
8934 *Phytochemistry* 2001;56:437-41.
8935 *Int J Pharm* 2001;213:199-208.
8936 *Pharmacopsychiatry* 2001;34:45-9.
8937 *Hand Clin* 1996;12:253-7.
8938 *Arch Neurol* 2002;59:1541-50.
8939 *Neurology* 1998;50:793-5.
8940 *Neurology* 2001;57:397-404.
8941 *J Neurosci* 2002;22:1592-9.
8942 *Arch Intern Med* 2002;162:2113-23.
8943 *Am J Clin Nutr* 2000;72:1474-9.
8944 *J Clin Invest* 2001;108:1341-8.
8945 *Obstet Gynecol* 1982;60:440-3.
8946 *Arzneimittelforschung* 1991;41:1294-8.
8948 *Calcif Tissue Int* 2001;69:252-5.
8949 *Osteoporos Int* 2002;13:158-70.
8950 *J Am Diet Assoc* 2001;101:126-32.
8951 *J Urol* 1959;81:770-2.
8952 *J Am Acad Dermatol* 1982;7:285-312.
8953 *J Invest Dermatol* 1950;399-401.
8954 *Southern Medicine & Surgery* 1942;135-9.
8955 *J Nutr* 2001;131:2837-42.
8956 *J Herb Pharmacother* 2002;2:11-7.
8957 *Am J Gastroenterol* 1998;93:139-43.
8958 *Am J Health-Syst Pharm* 1999;56:519-21.
8959 Kishi T, Makino K, Okamoto T, et al. Inhibition of myocardial respiration by psychotherapeutic drugs and prevention by coenzyme Q. In: Yamamura Y, Folkers K, Ito Y (eds). Biomedical and clinical aspects of coenzyme Q. Amsterdam: Elsevier/North-Holland Biomedical Press 1980;2:139-54.
8961 *Am J Kidney Dis* 2002;39:E13.
8962 *Cancer Res* 1999;59:2324-8.
8963 *J Clin Endocrinol Metab* 2001;86:3053-60.
8964 *Am J Cardiol* 2000;85:1297-301.
8965 *Eur J Obstet Gynecol Reprod Biol* 2002;102:188-94.
8968 *Int J Sport Nutr Exerc Metab* 2001;11:442-50.
8969 *J Ethnopharmacol* 1993 Jan;38(1):63-77.
8970 *J Acquir Immune Defic Syndr Human Retrovirol* 2001;27:56-62.
8971 *Agents Actions* 1981;11:296-305.
8972 *Eur J Clin Nutr* 2000;54:918-20.
8974 *JAMA* 2001;286:2143-51.
8976 *J Nutr* 2001;131:745-8.
8977 *Clin Pharmacol Ther* 2001;70:462-7.
8994 *Med Sci Sports Excerc* 1998;30 Suppl:S278.
8995 *Cochrane Database Syst Rev* 2004;2:CD001322.
8996 *J Am Diet Assoc* 2000;100:1368-80.
8997 *J Am Coll Nutr* 2000 Apr;19:111S-8S.
8998 *Neurosci Lett* 1997;230:37-40.
8999 *Int J Cardiol* 1995;52:95-9.
9000 *Stroke* 1995;26:1183-8.
9001 *Nutr Rev* 1999;57:84-8.
9002 *Circulation* 1998;98:1198-204.
9003 *Stroke* 1998;29:918-23.
9004 *Eur J Clin Nutr* 2000;54:918-20.
9005 *Cancer Lett* 2001;167:65-72.
9006 *JAMA* 2001;286:2143-51.
9007 *Am J Epidemiol* 1995;142:1034-8.
9100 American Dental Association. "ADA Statement on FDA Toothpaste Warning Labels" http://www.ada.org/prof/prac/issues/statements/fluoride.html (Accessed 18 November 2002).
9101 Centers for Disease Control. National Center for Chronic Disease Prevention and Health Promotion. "Dietary Fluoride Supplement Schedule." http://www.cdc.gov/OralHealth/factsheets/fl-supplements.htm (Accessed 18 November 2002).
9102 *BMJ* 2000;321:860-4.
9103 *Arch Intern Med* 2001;161:2325-33.
9104 *Magnes Res* 1993;6:155-63.
9105 *Int Clin Psychopharmacol* 2003;18:61-71.
9106 *J Bone Miner Metab* 2002;20:39-43.
9108 Hardy M, Coulter I, Morton SC, et al. S-Adenosyl-L-Methionine for Treatment of Depression, Osteoarthritis, and Liver Disease. Evidence Report/Technology Assessment Number 64. Agency for Healthcare Research and Quality, US Dept of Health and Human Services; 2002. AHRQ publication 02-E033. Rockville, Md. Available at: http://www.ahrq.gov/clinic/tp/sametp.htm.
9109 *Am J Clin Nutr* 2002;76:1172S-6S.
9110 *Am J Clin Nutr* 2002;76:1151S-7S.
9111 *J Fam Pract* 2002;51:425-30.
9112 *Am J Clin Nutr* 2002;76:1148S-50S.
9113 *Am J Clin Nutr* 2002;76:1158S-61S.
9114 *Am J Clin Nutr* 2002;76:1162S-71S.
9115 *Am J Clin Nutr* 2002;76:1177S-82S.

9116 *Am J Clin Nutr* 2002;76:1183S-17S.
9117 *J Lab Clin Med* 1989;114:213-4.
9118 *Arthritis Rheum* 2004;51:738-45.
9119 Ganu VA, Hu SI, Strassman J, et al. Inhibitors of N-glycosylation Reduce Cytokine-induced Production of Matrix Metalloproteinases, Nitric oxide, and PGE2 from Articular Chondrocytes: A Candidate Mechanism for the Chondroprotective Effects of d-Glucosamine. American College of Rheumatology Meeting; October 25-29, 2002. Abstract 616.
9121 Alvarez-Soria MA, Largo R, Diez-Ortego E, et al. Glucosamine Inhibits IL-1ß-induced NF-kappa B Activation in Human Osteoarthritic chondrocytes. American College of Rheumatology Meeting; October 25-29, 2002. Abstract 118.
9122 Tiku ML, Narla H, Karry SK, et al. Glucosamine Inhibits Advanced Lipoxidation Reaction and Chemical Modification of Lipoproteins by Scavenging Reactive Carbonyl Intermediates. American College of Rheumatology Meeting; October 25-29, 2002. Abstract 11.
9123 *Curr Ther Res* 1989;45:650-63.
9124 *Ann Intern Med* 1998;129:1-8.
9125 *J Clin Endocrinol Metab* 1999;84:3013-20.
9126 *Wound Repair Regen* 1999;7:79-89.
9127 *CMAJ* 2002;167:S1-S34.
9128 *Cochrane Database Syst Rev* 2002;2:CD002280.
9129 *Cochrane Database Syst Rev* 2002;4:CD002825.
9130 *J Rheumatol* 1997;24:2308-13.
9132 *Bone* 2000;27:123-8.
9133 *Osteoporos Int* 1998;8:4-12.
9134 *Eur J Gastroenterol Hepatol* 2000;12:19-24.
9139 *Drugs* 1994;47:536-66.
9140 US Food and Drug Administration. Center for Food Safety & Applied Nutrition. Office of Premarket Approval. Agency Response Letter GRAS Notice No. GRN 00056. DEcember 4, 2000 Available at: http://vm.cfsan.fda.gov/~rdb/opa-g056.html.
9141 Eur *J Intern Med* 2002;13:518-20.
9142 *Am J Clin Nutr* 2002;76:1230-6.
9143 *J Nutr* 2001;131:3204-7.
9144 *J Nutr* 2000;130:792-7.
9145 *J Am Coll Nutr* 2000;19:789-96.
9146 *Ann Nutr Metab* 2001;45:259-64.
9148 *Drugs* 1999;58:211-32.
9149 *J Clin Oncol* 2002;20:371-8.
9150 *JAMA* 1985;253:1444-5.
9151 *J Natl Cancer Inst* 2000;92:321-8.
9152 *Med Pediatr Oncol* 1996;27:165-73.
9153 *J Clin Oncol* 2002;20:362-3.
9154 *Invest New Drugs* 1998;16:81-5.
9155 *JAMA* 1985;253:1427-30.
9156 *Am J Obstet Gynecol* 2002;187:1389-94.
9157 *Anesthesiology* 2002;97:938-42.
9158 *Eur J Clin Pharmacol* 2000;56:49-55.
9159 *Hepatol* 2002;35:421-4.
9160 *J Pharmacol Exp Ther* 2000;294:126-33.
9161 *Caries Res* 1982;16:249-56.
9162 *Osteoporos Int* 2001;12:800.
9163 *J Am Coll Nutr* 2002;21:14-21.
9164 *J Pharm Pharmacol* 1979;31:161-3.
9165 *Am J Psychiatry* 2002;159:1155-9.
9166 *Am J Obstet Gynecol* 2002;187:245-9.
9167 *Neurology* 2003;60:132-5.
9170 *Ann Intern Med* 2003;138. http://www.acponline.org/journals/annals/ephedra.htm (Accessed 02/04/2003).
9171 *Environ Health Perspect* 2000;108:435-9.
9172 *Am J Gastroenterol* 2002;97:3212-13.
9173 *Biochem Pharmacol* 1998;55:1071-6.
9174 *Clin Biochem* 2003;36:79-87.
9175 *J Nutr* 2001;131:1938-41.
9176 *J Allergy Clin Immunol* 1995;96:528-36.
9181 *Cochrane Database Syst Rev* 2002;2:CD001520.
9182 *Ann Allergy Asthma Immunol* 2002;88:272-8.
9183 *Clin Immunol* 2002;104:183-90.
9184 *Allergy* 2001;56:257-8.
9185 *Intern Med* 2001;40:764-8.
9186 *J Nutr* 2001;131:1405-8.
9187 *Cancer Chemother Pharmacol* 2001;47:27-33.
9188 *Eur J Haematol* 2001;66:389-95.
9189 *JAMA* 2002;287:102-4.
9190 *N Engl J Med* 2003;348:287-94.
9191 *N Engl J Med* 2003;348:347-9.
9192 *Bone* 2002;31:685-9.
9193 *Cancer* 2001;92:2318-26.
9194 *Cancer* 2000;88:737-48.
9195 *Am J Respir Crit Care Med* 2001;163:1246-55.
9196 *Am J Clin Nutr* 2001;73:934-40.
9197 *Am J Clin Nutr* 2000;72:1069-70.
9198 *J Cell Biochem Suppl* 1997;28-29:133-9.
9199 *J Natl Cancer Inst* 1983;71:921-5.
9201 *Eur J Obstet Gynecol Reprod Biol* 2001;99:201-6.
9202 *J Ethnopharmacol* 2001;76:229-32.
9203 *J Nutr* 2001;131:1118S-9S.
9204 *Br J Clin Pharmacol* 2002;54:349-56.
9205 *Oncogene* 2002;21:1242-50.
9206 *J Natl Cancer Inst* 2002;94:1247-9.
9208 *J Nutr* 2001;131:1071S-4S.
9209 *Atherosclerosis* 2001;154:213-20.
9219 *J Am Soc Nephrol* 2000;11:1106-16.
9220 *Eur J Clin Nutr* 1992;46:61-7.
9222 *Cancer Causes Control* 1998;9:209-16.
9223 *Jpn J Cancer Res* 1985;76:705-16.
9224 *Life Sci* 2001;70:603-14.
9225 *Jpn J Cancer Res* 1988;79:1067-74.
9226 *Cancer* 1996;77:2449-57.
9227 *Cancer Causes Control* 1991;2:169-74.
9228 *Cancer Epidemiol Biomarkers Prev* 2002;11:713-8.
9229 *Eur J Pharmacol* 2002;434:1-7.
9230 *J Nutr* 2002;132:55-8.
9231 *Eur J Clin Nutr* 2000;54:757-63.
9232 *J Nutr* 2001;131:2248-51.
9233 *Nutr Cancer* 2001;39:176-9.
9234 *Public Health Nutr* 2002;5:419-25.
9235 *Ann Epidemiol* 2002;12:21-6.
9236 *Am J Epidemiol* 2002;155:732-8.
9237 *Eur J Clin Nutr* 2002;56:379-86.
9238 *Lipids* 1984;19:923-8.
9239 *J Ethnopharmacol* 1989;27:91-8.
9241 Upton R, Petrone C, eds. Black Haw Bark, Viburnum prunifolium: Analytical, quality control, and therapeutic monograph. American Herbal Pharmacopoeia and Therapeutic Compendium. Santa Cruz, CA: American Herbal Pharmacopoeia. 2000.
9242 *JANA* 2001;3:35-39.
9243 *J Am Geriatr Soc* 1995;43:261-3.
9244 *J Allergy Clin Immunol* 1991;88:402-8.
9245 *J Allergy Clin Immunol* 1992;89:866-76.
9246 *N Engl J Med* 1990;323:1072-3.
9247 *N Engl J Med* 1990;323:1073.
9248 *Clin Nephrol* 1991;36:309.
9249 *Br J Nutr* 1984;51:371-8.

9250 *Mutation Res* 1996;350:185-97.
9300 *J Nutr* 2001;131:1376S-1382S.
9301 *Am J Clin Nutr* 2002;75:275-82.
9302 *Am J Clin Nutr* 2000;72:1156-63.
9303 *Thromb Res* 2000;100:495-500.
9304 *Am J Clin Nutr* 2001;73:1027-33.
9305 *J Nutr* 2000;130:3090-6.
9306 *Arch Intern Med* 2001;161:774-5.
9307 *Arch Intern Med* 2001;161:695-700.
9308 *Arch Intern Med* 160:3406-12.
9309 *J Nutr* 2001;131:733-9.
9310 *Am J Med* 2002;112:556-65.
9311 *Arch Intern Med* 2000;160:3258-62.
9312 *Circulation* 2001;103:2674-80.
9313 *J Am Coll Cardiol* 2001;37:1858-63.
9314 *Am J Med* 2002;112:535-9.
9315 *J Am Coll Cardiol* 2001;38:1799-805.
9316 *Circulation* 2001:104;1119-23.
9317 *Circulation* 2001;104:1086-8.
9318 *Stroke* 2002;33:1183-8.
9319 *Eur J Clin Pharmacol* 2002;58:1-5.
9320 *Drugs Aging* 2000;16:251-60.
9321 *Nutrition* 2001;17:721-3.
9322 *Circulation* 2000;102:871-5.
9324 *Am J Hematol* 2002;69:239-46.
9325 *Ann Epidemiol* 2001;11:65-72.
9326 *Cancer Epidemiol Biomarkers Prev* 2002;11:227-34.
9327 *Am J Epidemiol* 2001;153:680-7.
9328 *Cancer Res* 2001;61:7136-41.
9329 *J Nutr* 1999;129:25-31.
9330 *Am J Clin Nutr* 2002;75:908-13.
9331 *Am J Clin Nutr* 2002;75:785-6.
9332 *Can Med Assoc J* 1976;115:217-23.
9333 *Appl Neurophysiol* 1979;42:171-83.
9334 *Fertil Steril* 2002;77:491-8.
9335 *J Am Geriatr Soc* 2002;50:1401-4.
9336 *Hepatol* 2002;36:1190-6.
9338 *Pharmacotherapy* 2002;22:188-211.
9339 *Arterioscler Thromb Vasc Biol* 2002;22:1046-50.
9340 *Drug Ther Perspect* 1997;10:11-3.
9341 *Nutr Cancer* 2002;42:158-66.
9342 *J Am Coll Nutr* 2001;20:443S-9S.
9343 *J Nutr* 2000;130:2653-7.
9344 Kokko JP. Fluids and electrolytes. In: Goldman L, Bennett JC. Cecil Textbook of Medicine. 21st ed. Philadelphia, PA: W.B. Saunders Co. 2000:59.
9345 Barshop BA. Homocystiniuria. In: Goldman L, Bennett JC. Cecil Textbook of Medicine. 21st ed. Philadelphia, PA: W.B. Saunders Co. 2000:1115-6.
9346 *Menopause* 2000;7:215-29.
9347 *J Ethnopharmacol* 2001;74(1):45-51.
9348 *J Ethnopharmacol* 1995;46(2):125-9.
9349 *Phytother Res* 1993;7:299-304.
9350 *Chem Pharm Bull (Tokyo)* 1985;33:5568-71.
9351 *J Lab Clin Med* 1984;103:944-8.
9352 *Am J Clin Nutr* 1982;35:73-82.
9353 *New Engl J Med* 1981;305:1513-7.
9354 *Br Med J* 1983;287:577-9.
9355 *Neurology* 1992;42:32-42.
9356 *Ann Pharmacother* 1998;32:802-17.
9357 *Clin Haematol* 1976;5:661-96.
9358 *Proc R Soc Med* 1974;67:68.
9359 *Drugs* 1985;29:570-81.
9360 *Blood* 1971;38:405-16.
9361 *Biochem J* 1992;282:197-202.
9362 *J Neurol* 1993;240:305-8.
9363 *Blood* 1967;29:697-712.
9364 *Gastroenterology* 1986;91:1476-82.
9366 *Diabetes Care* 2000;23:1816-22.
9367 *J Int Med* 1998;244:169-74.
9368 *Scand J Gastroenterol* 1971;6:751-4.
9369 *Cochrane Database Syst Rev* 2000;2:CD000951.
9370 *J Am Med Assoc* 1980;244:633-4.
9371 *Can Med Assoc J* 1982;126:244-7.
9372 *Haematologica* 1979;64:190-5.
9373 *Contraception* 1991;44:277-88.
9374 *Dig Dis Sci* 1980;25:369-73.
9375 *Ann Intern Med* 1970;73:419-24.
9376 *BMJ* 1986;293:1407.
9377 *Arch Intern Med* 1983;143:902-4.
9378 *Clin Pharm* 1985;4:507-16.
9379 *Gastroenterology* 1989;97:255-9.
9380 *J Infect Dis* 1996;173:1294-5.
9381 *Curr Ther Res* 1983;34:436-40.
9382 *Ann Intern Med* 1981;94:780-1.
9383 *Antimicrob Agents Chemother* 1997;41:2466-70.
9384 *Ann Intern Med* 1984;101:565.
9385 *Ann Intern Med* 1985;102:138.
9386 *Ann Intern Med* 1985;102:277.
9387 *J Infect Dis* 1994;170:912-7.
9388 *Gastroenterology* 1970;58:1001.
9389 *Am J Clin Nutr* 1984;39:535-9.
9390 *J Natl Cancer Inst* 1985;74:2638.
9391 *Am J Clin Nutr* 1988;47:484-6.
9392 *Eur J Pediatr* 1992;151:51-3.
9393 *J Nutr* 1995;125:66-72.
9394 *Aust N Z J Med* 1973;3:245-50.
9395 *Q J Med* 1971;40:331-40.
9396 *Tubercle* 1971;52:288-94.
9397 *Arch Intern Med* 1972;130;935-9.
9398 *Scand J Infect Dis* 1988;20:685-6.
9399 *Chest* 1984;86:149-50.
9400 *BMJ* 1998;316:894-8.
9401 *Am J Clin Nutr* 1998;68:1104-10.
9402 *Am J Clin Nutr* 2000;72:324-32.
9403 *Am J Med* 2001;110:536-42.
9404 *Ann Intern Med* 2001;135:133-7.
9405 *Semin Thromb Hemost* 2000;26:341-8.
9406 *J Int Med* 2000;248:223-9.
9407 *Publ Health Rev* 2000;28:117-45.
9408 *Curr Atheroscler Rep* 2001;3:54-63.
9409 *Exp Opin Invest Drugs* 2000;9:2637-51.
9410 *Arterioscler Thromb Vasc Biol* 1998;18:356-61.
9411 *JAMA* 1995;274:1049-57.
9412 *JAMA* 2002;288:973-9.
9413 *J Am Soc Nephrol* 2000;11:1106-16.
9414 *Transplantation* 2000;69:2128-31.
9415 *J Renal Nutr* 2001;11:67-72.
9416 *Kidney Int* 2001;59:s246-s252.
9417 *Clin Nephrol* 1999;51:108-15.
9418 *Rheumatology (Oxford)* 2000;39:1102-9.
9419 *Scand J Rheumatol* 2001;30:129-34.
9420 *Ped Hematol Oncol* 1986;3:241-7.
9421 *Am J Clin Nutr* 1987;46:835-9.
9422 *Heart Lung* 1997;26:229-37.
9423 *J Am Geriatr Soc* 1995;43:666-9.
9424 *Arch Fam Med* 1994;3:955-60.
9425 *J Lipid Res* 1992;33:1183-92.
9426 *J Lipid Res* 1997;38:491-502.
9427 *Radiology* 1995;194:119-23.
9429 *Ann N Y Acad Sci* 1998;854:268-76.
9431 *Phytomedicine* 2002;9:461-7.

9432 *Planta Med* 2000;66:751-3.
9434 *J Nutr Sci Vitaminol (Tokyo)* 1998;44:841-51.
9435 *Breast Cancer Res Treat* 2002;76:1-10.
9436 *Cancer Res* 2002;62:3448-52.
9437 *J Womens Health Gend Based Med* 2002;11:163-74.
9439 *Ann Epidemiol* 1996;6:41-6.
9442 *Eur J Clin Pharmacol* 2000;56:545-53.
9443 *J Nutr* 2000;130:2658-61.
9444 *Am J Clin Nutr* 2001;73:941-8.
9445 *Res Commun Chem Pathol Pharmacol* 1976;13:743-57.
9446 *Res Commun Chem Pathol Pharmacol* 1977;17:165-77.
9447 *Res Commun Chem Pathol Pharmacol* 1981;33:331-44.
9448 *J Occup Environ Med* 1996;38:485-91.
9449 *Proc Natl Acad Sci U S A* 1978;75:3410-2.
9450 *J Neurol* 2002;249:272-80.
9451 *Am J Clin Nutr* 2001;73:759-64.
9452 *Circulation* 2001;103:2788-91.
9453 *Arch Phys Med Rehabil* 1984;65:712-6.
9454 *Am J Epidemiol* 2001;153:688-94.
9455 *J Appl Physiol* 1996;81:1901-7.
9456 *J Appl Physiol* 1997;83:376-82.
9457 *J Ethnopharmacol* 1997;56:179-91.
9458 *Am J Epidemiol* 1968;88:159-77.
9459 *Cardiology* 2001;95:25-30.
9460 *J Pharm Sci* 1991;80:96.
9461 *Pharmacol Biochem Behav* 1981;15:907-9.
9462 *Pharmacol Biochem Behav* 1980;13:403-8.
9465 *Am J Hypertens* 2002;15:691-6.
9466 *Sleep* 1998;21:501-5.
9467 *Am J Clin Nutr* 1991;53:695-7.
9468 *Inflamm Res* 1998;47:334-8.
9469 *Inflamm Res* 1998;47:36-41.
9470 *Phytother Res* 1999;13:258-60.
9472 *Rom J Neurol Psychiatry* 1993;31:55-61.
9473 *N Engl J Med* 2003;348:304-11.
9474 *Br J Dermatol* 2001;144:916-8.
9475 *Nutrition* 2002;18:201-4.
9476 *Psychopharmacology (Berl)* 2002;164:294-300.
9477 *J Nutr* 1997;2:379.
9478 *J Am Coll Nutr* 1993;12:73-6.
9479 *Dermatology* 2000;201:356-60.
9480 *Res Commun Chem Pathol Pharmacol* 1993;79:325-33.
9481 *Anesth Analg* 2001;93:1507-10.
9482 *J Occup Environ Med* 1997;39:949-59.
9483 *Proc Natl Acad Sci U S A* 1982;79:7494-8.
9484 *Forensic Sci Int* 1991;49:57-64.
9492 *N Z Med J* 1996;109:410-1.
9493 *N Z Med J* 1997;110:20-1.
9494 *Ann Intern Med* 2002;137:805-13.
9495 *Clin Pharmacol Ther* 2001;69:365-71.
9496 *Arch Pediatr Adolesc Med* 2000;154:979-83.
9497 *J Intern Med* 2000;247:78-86.
9498 *J Headache Pain* 2000;1:179-86.
9499 *Eur J Neurol* 2000;7:741-4.
9500 *Kidney Int* 2000;58:2462-72.
9502 Goldin BR, Lichtenstein AH, Gorbach SL. Nutritional and metabolic roles of intestinal flora. In: Shils ME, Olson JA, Shike M, eds. Modern Nutrition in Health and Disease, 8th ed. Malvern, PA: Lea & Febiger, 1994.
9503 *Ann N Y Acad Sci* 1990;585:285-94.
9505 *J Reprod Med* 1984;29:547-50.
9507 *Magnes Trace Elem* 1990;9:132-6.
9508 *Clin Rheumatol* 1985;4:143-9.
9509 *Calcif Tissue Int* 1984;36:269-73.
9511 *JAMA* 1974;230:241-2.
9512 *Thromb Res* 2000;100:153-60.
9513 *Ann Pharmacother* 2002;36:812-6.
9514 *Ann Pharmacother* 1992;26:1283-6.
9515 *Aliment Pharmacol Ther* 1994;8:343-6.
9516 *Br J Surg* 1984;71:334-7.
9517 *Clin Sci* 1987;72:135-8.
9518 *Public Health Nutr* 2000;3:125-50.
9519 *Drugs Aging* 1992;2:35-41.
9520 *Br Med J* 1980;280:1214-5.
9521 *Arch Intern Med* 2002;162:484-5.
9522 *Arch Intern Med* 2002;162:2251-2.
9523 *Diabetes Care* 2000;23:1227-31.
9525 *Miner Electrolyte Metab* 1999;25:352-6.
9526 *Am J Gastroenterol* 2001;96:635-43.
9527 *Arch Neurol* 2000;57:380-2.
9528 *Ann Pharmacother* 2003;37:490-3.
9529 *Environ Health Perspect* 1994;102:59-63.
9530 McCormick DB. Riboflavin. In: Shils ME, Olson JA, Shike M, Ross AC, eds. Modern Nutrition in Health and Disease. 9th ed. Baltimore, MD: Williams & Wilkins, 1999. pg.391-9.
9531 *Arch Intern Med* 2003;163:803-8.
9532 *Neurology* 1995;45:1608-10.
9533 *Cancer* 1986;58:1911-4.
9534 *N Z Med J* 1987;100:309-11.
9535 Tanphaichitr V. Thiamin. In: Shils ME, Olson JA, Shike M, Ross AC, Eds. Modern Nutrition in Health and Disease. 9th ed. Baltimore, MD: Williams & Wilkins, 1999. pg.381-9.
9536 *Arch Intern Med* 2003;163:983.
9537 *Ann Intern Med* 1986;104:134-5.
9538 *Clin Pharmacokinet* 1992;22(3):231-7.
9539 *Ann Pharmacother* 1994;28:175-9.
9540 *Am J Clin Nutr* 2001;74:650-6.
9541 *J Am Coll Nutr* 2001;20:477-85.
9542 *Am J Clin Nutr* 2002;76:499-500.
9543 *Am J Clin Nutr* 2002;76:501-3.
9544 *Circulation* 1998;97:1461-6.
9545 *Circulation* 1992;86:803-11.
9546 *Circulation* 1994;89:969-74.
9547 *Circulation* 1993;87:688.
9548 *Am J Cardiol* 1993;72:347-8.
9549 *N Engl J Med* 1994;330:1119-24.
9550 *Circulation* 1999;99:852-4.
9552 *Breast* 2002;11:170-4.
9553 *J Herb Pharmacother* 2002;2:49-72.
9554 *Ann N Y Acad Sci* 1965;130:390-7.
9555 *Arch Dermatol* 1976;112:560.
9556 *J Am Board Fam Pract* 1998;11:478-80.
9557 *Planta Med* 1979;37:367-9.
9558 *J Ethnopharmacol* 2001;78:165-70.
9559 *FASEB J* 1993;7:A690.
9560 *Proc Natl Acad Sci USA* 1998;95:3106-10.
9561 *Atherosclerosis* 1998;140:341-7.
9562 *Stroke* 2002;33(8):2086-93.
9563 *Clin Biochem* 1994;27:245-8.
9564 *Clin Cancer Res* 1996;2:659-67.
9566 *Dig Dis Sci* 1985;30:477-82.
9567 *Clin Pharmacol Ther* 1989;45:220-5.
9568 *Ann Intern Med* 1992;117:1010-3.
9569 *J Nutr* 1998;128:646-50.
9570 *Am J Clin Nutr* 1998;67:593-4.
9571 *Am J Clin Nutr* 1998;67:722-33.
9572 *Am J Clin Nutr* 2001;73:93-8.
9573 *Am J Clin Nutr* 2000;71:1147-60.
9574 Package insert for Paser granules. Jacobus Pharmaceutical Co., Inc. Princeton, NJ. July 1996.

9575 *Am J Dis Child* 1989;143:969-72.
9576 *Ann Rheum Dis* 1990;49:359-62.
9577 *Dis Colon Rectum* 1995;38:1311-21.
9578 *Aliment Pharmacol Ther* 1988;12:83-98.
9579 *Am J Clin Nutr* 1984;40:536-41.
9580 *Am J Clin Nutr* 1989;50:141-4.
9581 *Am J Clin Nutr* 1991;54:152-6.
9582 *Am J Clin Nutr* 1999;69:509-15.
9583 *J Nutr* 2002;132:1860-4.
9584 *Am J Clin Nutr* 1981;34:475-82.
9585 *Lancet* 1970;1:424.
9586 *Nutr Rev* 1997;55:102-10.
9587 *Transplantation* 2002;74:1200-1.
9588 *J Altern Complement Med* 2001;7:133-9.
9589 *Am J Clin Nutr* 2002;76:604-7.
9590 *Oral Surg Oral Med Oral Pathol* 1979;48:416-7.
9591 *J Steroid Biochem Mol Biol* 1994;50:205-12.
9592 *J Steroid Biochem* 1986;25:791-7.
9593 *Nutr Cancer* 1990;13:1-8.
9594 *Circulation* 2003;108:802-7.
9595 *Pharmacotherapy* 2002;22:814-22.
9596 *Arch Surg* 2002;137:316-9.
9597 *Psychopharmacology (Berl)* 2002;164:301-8.
9598 Barrett S. Coral Calcium. June 12, 2003. http://www.quackwatch.org/01QuackeryRelatedTopics/DSH/coral.html (Accessed 26 June 2003).
9599 *J R Coll Phys Lond* 1984;18:190-4.
9601 *J Clin Endocrinol Metab* 2001;86:1968-72.
9602 Research abstract. American Association of Cancer Research. Annual meeting, July 2003.
9603 *Drugs Exp Clin Res* 1993;19:65-8.
9605 Health Canada warns public not to use Vigor-Max. Health Canada Online May 27, 2003. http://www.hc-sc.gc.ca/english/protection/warnings/2003/2003_35.htm (Accessed 28 June 2003).
9606 *Am J Epidemiol* 2003;157:456-66.
9607 *Cochrane Database Syst Rev* 2001;4:CD001112.
9608 *Adv Drug Deliv Rev* 2001;52:105-15.
9609 *Nutrition* 2003;19:137-9.
9610 *Acta Toxicol Ther* 1995;16:199-214.
9612 *Pediatrics* 1998;101:E9 (abstract). Full text at: www.pediatrics.org/cgi/content/full/101/5/e9.
9613 *Am J Med* 1987;82:38-47.
9614 *Am J Med* 1987;82:30-7.
9615 *Surgery* 2002;131:236.
9616 *Dig Dis Sci* 1997;42:858-60.
9617 *Ann Intern Med* 1991;115:665-73.
9618 *DICP* 1990;24:239-40.
9619 *Rev Infect Dis* 1991;13:511-2.
9620 *Transplant Proc* 1997;29:3161-2.
9621 *Magnes Res* 1990;3:197-215.
9622 *Magnesium* 1984;3:248-56.
9623 *FASEB J* 1987;1:394-7.
9624 *J Am Coll Nutr* 1994;13:479-84.
9625 *Miner Electrolyte Metab* 1988;14:114-20.
9626 *Am J Clin Oncol* 1992;15:348-51
9627 *Acta Med Scand* 1972;192:71-6.
9628 *Magnesium* 1986;5:248-72.
9629 *Nephron* 1975;15:261-78.
9630 *Toxicol Appl Pharmacol* 1982;63:344-50.
9631 *Am J Cardiol* 1989;63:39G-42G.
9632 *Lancet* 1984;2:1116-20.
9633 *Lancet* 1985;1:1283-4.
9634 *J Nutr* 1991;121:13-23.
9635 *Scand J Gastroenterol* 1984;19:1031-8.
9636 *J Clin Endocrinol Metab* 1987;65:1301-4.
9637 *Am J Med* 1983;75:973-6.
9638 *Fertil Steril* 1999;71:869-72.
9639 *J Am Coll Nutr* 1993;12:442-58.
9640 *J Am Coll Nutr* 1987;6:313-9.
9641 *Lancet* 1988;1:989.
9671 *Psychopharmacology (Berl)* 2001;157:430-6.
9672 *Ann Pharmacother* 2002;36:1893-6.
9673 *Am J Clin Nutr* 2002;76:588-94.
9674 *J Natl Cancer Inst* 1993;85:1819-27.
9676 *Nutr Cancer* 2002;43:22-30.
9677 *Cancer Epidemiol Biomarkers Prev* 2002;11:1674-7.
9679 *J Nutr* 2001;131:2280-7.
9680 *Neurology* 2002;59:1289-90.
9681 *Fertil Steril* 2001;75:1059-64.
9682 *Nutr Res* 2001;21:1287-98.
9683 *Eur J Clin Nutr* 2003;57:100-6.
9684 *Eur J Clin Nutr* 2003;57:324-7.
9685 *Clin Pharmacol Ther* 2002;71:414-20.
9686 *Curr Med Res Opin* 1999;15:33-7.
9687 *Fertil Steril* 2001;76:1073-4.
9690 *Breast J* 2000;6:14-19.
9691 *Horm Res* 2001;56:134-9.
9692 *Arch Gen Psychiatry* 2003;60:133-41.
9693 *J Clin Pharmacol* 2001;41:1195-205.
9694 *J Clin Endocrinol Metab* 2001;86:4686-92.
9695 *J Child Neurol* 1998;13:501-9.
9696 *Epilepsia* 1995;36:75-8.
9697 *Int J Neurosci* 1992;63:125-35.
9698 *Int J Neurosci* 1992;65:83-90.
9699 *Epilepsia* 2001;42:1208-10.
9700 *Eur Psychiatry* 2001;16:68-70.
9701 *Clin Rheumatol* 2000;19:9-13.
9702 *Headache* 2002;42:787-92.
9703 *Chronobiol Int* 1992;9:124-31.
9704 *Clin Endocrinol (Oxf)* 2000;53:367-72.
9705 *Eur J Clin Invest* 2002;32:831-7.
9706 *Sleep* 2000;23:663-9.
9707 *J Child Neurol* 2001;16:581-4.
9708 *J Child Neurol* 2001;16:86-92.
9709 *J Clin Psychiatry* 2001;62:41-5.
9710 *Biochemistry* 2001;40:14995-5001.
9711 *Eur J Cancer* 2000;36(Suppl 4):117-8.
9712 *Eur J Pharmacol* 2001;426:1-10.
9713 *Clin Endocrinol (Oxf)* 2001;54:339-46.
9714 *J Appl Physiol* 2001;91:1214-22.
9715 *Mayo Clin Proc* 1997;72:1094-5.
9716 *Chem Res Toxicol* 1998;11:234-40.
9717 *Am J Clin Nutr* 1986;44:659-63.
9718 *Br J Nutr* 2001;85:517-47.
9719 *Chem Biol Interact* 1994;91:199-205.
9720 *J Acquir Immune Defic Syndr* 2001;26:360-4.
9721 *Biol Trace Elem Res* 2000;77:273-85.
9722 *Cancer Epidemiol Biomarkers Prev* 2002;11:630-9.
9723 *J Agric Food Chem* 2001;49:2679-83.
9724 *Med Hypotheses* 2002;59:330-3.
9725 *Intensive Care Med* 2001;27:91-100.
9726 *Biol Trace Elem Res* 2001;79:107-14.
9727 *Biol Trace Elem Res* 2001;79:97-105.
9728 *FASEB J* 2001;15:1481-3.
9729 *J Androl* 2001;22:764-72.
9730 *Aliment Pharmacol Ther* 2002;16:1917-22.
9731 *Am J Clin Nutr* 2000;72:5-14.
9732 *Eur J Clin Nutr* 2003;57:243-8.
9733 *Life Sci* 1999;64:53-62.
9734 *Am J Chin Med* 1999;27:331-8.
9735 *Anal Chem* 1999;71:1579-84.

9736 *Pharmacology* 1991;42:223-9.
9737 *Cancer Res* 2001;61:3647-52.
9738 *Invest Ophthalmol Vis Sci* 1997;38:S633.
9739 *Eye* 1998;12:967-9.
9740 *JAMA* 2003;289:1537-45.
9741 *Evid Rep Technol Assess (Summ)* 2003;76:1-4.
9744 *Int J Neurosci* 2001;107:77-85.
9745 *Biol Signals Recept* 1999;8:105-10.
9746 *J Pineal Res* 1997;23:97-105.
9747 *J Neural Transm* 2000;107:271-9.
9748 *Biol Psychol* 2000;53:69-78.
9749 *Fundam Clin Pharmacol* 2000;14:553-60.
9750 *Advances Pineal Res* 1991;5:303-6.
9751 *Bioelectromagnetics* 2001;22:178-84.
9759 *Psychopharmacology (Berl)* 2000;152:353-61.
9760 *Thromb Res* 2002;108:151-60.
9761 *Br J Nutr* 2001;85:157-63.
9762 *Br J Nutr* 1997;77:551-63.
9763 *Scand J Rheumatol* 2001;30:208-12.
9764 *Biol Trace Elem Res* 1998;65:143-51.
9765 *Planta Med* 1995;61:213-6.
9766 *Contact Dermatitis* 1982;8:143.
9767 *Acta Oncol* 1991;30:395-6.
9768 *Contact Dermatitis* 1987;16:50-1.
9769 *Fitoterapia* 2001;72:101-5.
9770 *Complement Ther Med* 2001;9:12-6.
9771 *J Lipid Res* 1995;36:473-84.
9772 *Am J Clin Nutr* 2003;77:565-72.
9773 *Cancer Epidemiol Biomarkers Prev* 2003;12:64-7.
9774 *Am J Clin Nutr* 2003;77:532-43.
9775 *J Clin Endocrinol Metab* 2003;88:1048-54.
9776 *J Nutr* 2003;133:797-800.
9777 *J Urol* 2003;169:507-11.
9780 *J Lipid Res* 2000;41:1901-11.
9781 *Pediatr Int* 1999;41:108-9.
9782 *N Engl J Med* 1999;341:769.
9783 *Plant Foods Hum Nutr* 1999;53:359-65.
9784 *Int J Food Sci Nutr* 2000;51:409-14.
9785 *Int Surg* 1973;58:451-2.
9786 *Angiology* 1990;41:12-8.
9789 *Contact Dermatitis* 1985;13:310-3.
9790 *J Am Soc Nephrol* 2002;13:708-14.
9791 *Fertil Steril* 2002;78:1203-8.
9792 *Prog Neuropsychopharmacol Biol Psychiatry* 2003;27:123-7
9794 *Aust N Z J Surg* 1999;69:492-4.
9796 *J Midwifery Womens Health* 2001;46:51-9.
9797 *J Clin Endocrinol Metab* 2002;87:1687-91.
9798 *Cancer Epidemiol Biomarkers Prev* 2002;11:1285-91.
9800 *J Infect Dis* 2000;182:1084-9.
9801 *AIDS* 2002;16:1935-44.
9802 *Pediatr Hematol Oncol* 2002;19:181-92.
9804 *JAMA* 1971;215:1671.
9805 *JAMA* 1972;219:1479.
9806 *JAMA* 1972;221:1166.
9808 *Life Sci* 2001;68:1751-60.
9809 *CMAJ* 2001;164:353-5.
9810 *J Am Coll Nutr* 1998;17:366-70.
9811 *J Am Diet Assoc* 2002;102:525-9.
9812 *Circ Res* 2000;87:349-54.
9813 *Circulation* 2001;103:1863-8.
9814 *J Am Coll Cardiol* 2001;38:1788-94.
9815 *J Am Coll Cardiol* 2001;38:1795-8.
9816 *Circulation* 2001;104:2182-7.
9817 *Lancet* 2002;360:23-33.
9818 *J Am Coll Cardiol* 2000;35:1616-21.
9819 *J Am Coll Cardiol* 2000;35:1860-6.
9820 *Arterioscler Thromb Vasc Biol* 2000;20:2401-6.
9821 *Hypertension* 2002;40:797-803.
9822 *Hypertension* 2002;40:804-9.
9823 *Ophthalmology* 2002;109:2272-8.
9824 *JAMA* 2002;288:2266-8.
9825 *Am J Gastroenterol* 2001;96:1080-4.
9826 *Cancer Treat Rev* 2002;28:79-91.
9827 *Lancet* 2002;359:1648-54.
9828 *Am J Epidemiol* 2001;154:427-33.
9830 *Eur J Clin Nutr* 2001;55:107-14.
9831 *Int J Sports Med* 1996;17:379-83.
9832 *Med J Aust* 1981;2:411-2.
9833 *Med J Aust* 2001;175:359-62.
9834 *Med Hypotheses* 1999;52:171-8.
9835 *Int J Vitam Nutr Res* 1997;67:329-35.
9836 *Nutrition* 1996;12:804-9.
9837 *Br J Haematol* 2001;112:783-6.
9838 *Cancer Epidemiol Biomarkers Prev* 2001;10:1055-62.
9839 *Am J Epidemiol* 2002;156:1002-10.
9840 FDA Orphan Drug List. http://www.fda.gov/ohrms/dockets/dailys/00/mar00/030100/lst0094.pdf (Accessed 2 May 2003).
9871 *Int J Clin Pharmacol Ther* 2002;40:188-197.
9872 *Phytother Res* 2001;15:34-38.
9873 *Eur J Pharmacol* 2001;433:177-85.
9874 *Prostaglandins Leukot Essent Fatty Acids* 1998;58:257-63.
9875 *Planta Med* 1995;61:356-7.
9876 *J Natl Cancer Inst* 2002;94:1648-51.
9878 *J Intern Med* 1993;233:94.
9880 *Br J Clin Pharmacol* 2003;55:112-3.
9881 *Int J Toxicol* 2001;20:31-9.
9882 The Medicines Control Agency (MCA), Epogam and Efamast (gamolenic acid) - withdrawal of marketing authorizations. http://www.mca.gov.uk/whatsnew/epogam.htm. (Accessed 2 June 2003).
9883 *Ann Allergy Asthma Immunol* 2002;89:91-6.
9885 *Biochem Pharmacol* 2003;65:1483-8.
9890 *Eur J Clin Nutr* 2002;56:1137-42.
9891 *South Med J* 1988;81:1092-4.
9892 *J Am Coll Nutr* 1994;13:6-21.
9893 *Phytother Res* 2002;16:23-7.
9894 *Am Fam Physician* 2003;67:1755-8.
9895 *Pharmacopsychiatry* 1988;21:447-8.
9896 *Phytother Res* 2002;16:650-4.
9898 *J Agric Food Chem* 2002;50:6136-42.
9899 *Psychopharmacology (Berl)* 2001;158:322-8.
9900 *Life Sci* 1974;14:1353-9.
9901 *Eur J Obstet Gynecol Reprod Biol* 1998;80:75-78.
9903 *Rapid Commun Mass Spectrom* 2001;15:1796-801.
9904 *Farmakol Toksikol* 1988;51:57-60.
9905 *Farmakol Toksikol* 1976;39:690-3.
9906 *J Womens Health Gend Based Med* 2002;11:155-62.
9916 *Menopause* 2003;10:147-53.
9917 *J Soc Gynecol Investig* 2002;9:238-42.
9919 *Metabolism* 2002;51:919-24.
9920 *J Ethnopharmacol* 1985;13:307-311.
9921 *J Altern Complement Med* 2002;8:237-263.
9923 *Prog Neuropsychopharmacol Biol Psychiatry* 1998;22:1105-1120.
9924 *J Ethnopharmacol* 1983;7:267-76.
9925 National Academy of Science. Lost Crops of the Incas Little-Known Plants of the Andes with Promise for Worldwide Cultivation (1989). Available at: http://books.nap.edu/books/030904264X/html/57.html.

9926 *Chem Pharm Bull (Tokyo)* 2002;50:988-99.
9927 *J Agric Food Chem* 2002;50:5621-25.
9928 *Andrologia* 2002;34:367-72.
9929 *Economic Botany* 2001;55:255-62.
9930 *Atherosclerosis* 1983;46:321-31.
9931 *Arch Phys Med Rehabil* 2003;84:1258-65.
9932 *Arzneimittelforschung* 2002;52:243-250.
9933 *JAMA* 1998;279:1100-7.
9934 *Pediatrics* 2000;105:1158-70.
9935 *Ann N Y Acad Sci* 2001;931:1-16.
9936 *JAMA* 2001;285:60-6.
9937 *Am J Psychiatry* 1996;153:1138-42.
9938 *Behav Brain Res* 2002;130:97-102.
9939 *Arch Gen Psychiatry* 1999;56:1088-96.
9940 *J Dev Behav Pediatr* 2001;22:60-73.
9941 *Pediatrics* 2001;108:1033-44.
9942 *J Am Acad Child Adolesc Psychiatry* 2002;41:26S-49S.
9943 *Pediatrics* 2003;111:1010-6.
9944 *Am Fam Physician* 2001;64:1355-62.
9945 *Pharmacist's Letter/Prescriber's Letter* 2003;19:190102
9946 *J Dev Behav Pediatr* 2003;24:4-8.
9948 *Psychiatry Res* 1990;33:301-6.
9949 *Biol Psychiatry* 1991;29:15-22.
9950 *Am J Psychiatry* 1987;144:792-4.
9951 *Psychiatry Res* 1985;16:21-6.
9952 *Neuropsychobiology* 1983;10:111-4.
9955 *Clin Pediatr (Phila)* 1987;26:406-11.
9956 *Am J Med Genet* 1999;87:366-8.
9957 *Pediatrics* 1984;74:103-11.
9958 *JAMA* 1978;240:2642-43.
9959 *J Nutr* 1979;109:819-26.
9960 *J Learn Disabil* 1982;15:258-64.
9962 *J Nutr* 2003;133:1468S-72S.
9965 *J Child Psychol Psychiatry* 1996;37:225-7.
9966 *Biol Psychiatry* 1996;40:1308-10.
9967 *Int J Neurosci* 1990;50:103-7.
9969 *Magnes Res* 1997;10:143-8.
9970 Agricultural Research Service- Germplasm Resources Information Network. "Botanicals Generally Recognized As Safe" http://www.ars-grin.gov/duke/syllabus/gras.htm (Accessed 10 July 2003).
9972 *Pharmacotherapy* 2003;23:222-30.
9973 *JAMA* 1995;274:1617-21.
9974 *N Engl J Med* 1994;330:301-7.
9975 *J Consult Clin Psychol* 1986;54:714-8.
9976 *J Pediatr* 1985;106:675-82.
9977 *J Dev Behav Pediatr* 2003;24:155-62.
9978 *Pediatrics* 2003;111:97-109.
9979 *Pediatrics* 2003;111:179-85.
9980 *Eur J Pediatr* 2003;162:554-5.
9981 *Psychopharmacol Bull* 1990;26:249-53.
9984 *J Atten Disord* 2002;6:49-60.
9985 *Phytother Res* 2000;14:195-9.
9986 *Singapore Med J* 2001;42:6-10.
9987 *Obes Res* 2001;9:364-7.
9988 *Arzneimittelforschung* 1993;43:752-6.
9990 *Oncol Rep* 1999;6:1383-7.
9991 *Biol Pharm Bull* 2003;26:10-18.
9993 *J Neurol Neurosurg Psychiatry* 2003;74:863-6.
9994 *Pharmacol Biochem Behav* 2002;72:953-64.
9995 *Phytomedicine* 1999;6:225-30.
9996 *J Steroid Biochem Mol Biol* 2003;84:259-68.
9997 *Menopause* 2003;10:299-313.
9998 *J Agric Food Chem* 2001;49:2472-9.
9999 Davis VL, Jayo MJ, Hardy ML, et al. Effects of black cohosh on mammary tumor development and progression in MMTV-neu transgenic mice. 94th Annual Meeting of the American Association for Cancer Research, Washington, DC. July 11-14, 2003;abstract R910.
10000 Rockwell S, Fajolu O, Liu Y, et al. The herbal medicine black cohosh alters the response of breast cancer cells to some agents used in cancer therapy. Annual Meeting of the American Association for Cancer Research, Washington, DC. July 11-14, 2003;abstract 2721.
10002 *J Am Board Fam Pract* 2002;15:481-4.
10003 *Nutrition* 1989;5:7-9.
10004 *Int J Obes* 2002;26:1363-66.
10005 *Am J Health Syst Pharm* 2003;60:375-7.
10006 *Am J Clin Nutr* 2003;77:319-25.
10007 *Circulation* 2002;106:2747-57.
10008 *J Clin Oncol* 2003;21:129-34.
10009 *Br J Dermatol* 2002;147:1212-7.
10010 *J Toxicol Clin Toxicol* 1994;32:461-4.
10011 *Med J Aust* 1993;159:830-1.
10012 *Med J Aust* 1994;160:236.
10013 *J Toxicol Clin Toxicol* 1995;33:193-4.
10014 *J Antimicrob Chemother* 1995;35:421-4.
10015 *J Am Acad Dermatol* 1994;30:423-7.
10016 *Med J Aust* 1994;160:236.
10017 *Lancet* 1991;337:300.
10018 *Acta Pharmacol Toxicol (Copenh)* 1979;44:7-12.
10019 *Dig Dis* 1996;14:119-28.
10020 *Int J Obes* 2002;26:119-22.
10021 *Adv Drug Deliv Rev* 2001;52:117-26.
10022 *Acta Toxicol Ther* 1996;17:287-302.
10023 *Acta Toxicol Ther* 1996;17:303-320.
10024 *Acta Toxicol Ther* 1995;16:215-29.
10025 *Acta Toxicol Ther* 1996;17:53-70.
10026 *Am J Infect Control* 1996;24:186-9.
10027 *J Hosp Infect* 1998;39:244-5.
10028 *J Appl Microbiol* 2000;88:170-5.
10029 *Trop Med Int Health* 1999;4:630.
10030 *Contact Dermatitis* 1999;41:354-5.
10031 *Contact Dermatitis* 2000;42:309-10.
10032 *Am J Contact Dermat* 2000;11:238-42.
10033 *Australas J Dermatol* 2002;43:175-8.
10034 *Toxicology* 1999;132:147-53.
10035 *Cancer Treat Rep* 1982;66:173-5.
10037 *Chest* 2000;117:591-3.
10038 *Am J Clin Oncol* 1985;8:341-4.
10039 *Med Pediatr Oncol* 1989;17:197-201.
10040 *Acta Neuropathol (Berl)* 1989;79:300-4.
10041 *Clin Nephrol* 1988;30:341-5.
10042 *Am J Kidney Dis* 1993;21:548-52.
10043 *Nephrol Dial Transplant* 1999;14:2464-8.
10044 *Biol Trace Elem Res* 1991;29:267-80.
10045 *Kidney Int* 2000;57:2275-84.
10046 *J Toxicol Environ Health A* 1999;58:289-97.
10047 *Biol Trace Elem Res* 2000;77:193-7.
10048 *Med Hypotheses* 1988;26:207-15.
10049 *Cancer Treat Rep* 1980;64:1051-6.
10050 *Cancer Treat Rep* 1981;65:119-20.
10051 *Mutat Res* 1997;387:141-6.
10052 *J Neurol Sci* 1995;130:220-3.
10053 *Digestion* 2002;65:16-20.
10054 *Am J Chin Med* 1987;15:117-25.
10055 *Fed Regist* 2004;69:6787-6854.
10056 *Am J Chin Med* 1994;22:137-45.
10057 *Gen Pharmacol* 1996;27:713-22.

10058 *Psychopharmacology (Berl)* 2001;156:481-4.
10059 *Indian J Med Res* 1989;90:496-503.
10060 *Fitoterapia* 2001;72:284-5.
10061 *Altern Med Rev* 1999;4(3):144-61.
10062 *Nutrition* 2001;17:558-66.
10063 *Acta Physiol Scand* 1996;158:195-202.
10064 *Med Sci Sports Exerc* 2001;33:814-21.
10065 *J Clin Pharmacol* 2003;43:29-37.
10066 *Biochem Pharmacol* 2000;59:1173-85.
10067 *JAMA* 1985;254:912.
10068 *Angiology* 2000;51:535-44.
10069 *J Altern Complement Med* 2000;6:539-49.
10070 *Drugs Exp Clin Res* 1988;14:277-83.
10071 *Science* 1981;213:909-10.
10072 *Nephron* 1990;54:53-60.
10073 *Nephron* 1992;62:351-6.
10074 *Nephron* 1992;60:436-42.
10075 *Aliment Pharmacol Ther* 2000;14:1671-7.
10076 *BJU Int* 2001;88:63-7.
10077 *Acta Med Scand* 1986;219:341-8.
10080 *J Intern Med* Suppl 1989;225:133-9.
10081 *Life Sci* 1991;48:1401-9.
10082 *Can J Surg* 1986;29:129-31.
10083 *Acta Med Scand* 1983;213:137-44.
10084 *J Rheumatol* 1999;26:2714-7.
10085 *J Am Acad Dermatol* 1996;35:264-6.
10086 *Scand J Gastroenterol* 1991;26:747-50.
10088 *Aliment Pharmacol Ther* 1998;12:491-7.
10089 *Scand J Gastroenterol Suppl* 1987;129:68-72.
10090 *Scand J Clin Lab Invest* 1992;52:697-706.
10091 *Arch Med Res* 1998;29:137-41.
10092 *Mov Disord* 1997;12:946-51.
10094 *J Am Diet Assoc* 1988;88:211-3.
10095 *Arch Intern Med* 1988;148:292-6.
10096 *Gut* 1994;35:1747-52.
10097 *Clin Pharm* 1990;9:206-8.
10098 *Drug Nutr Interact* 1987;5:67-9.
10099 *J Diabetes Complications* 1998;12:273-8.
10101 *Int J Dermatol* 2000;39(10):789-94.
10102 *Int J Dermatol* 2001;40:354-7.
10103 *J Emerg Med* 2002;22(4):353-5.
10104 *J Am Acad Dermatol* 1984;11(5Pt1):867-79.
10105 *J Nutr* 2001;131:839S-40S.
10106 *J Nutr* 2001;131:841S-5S.
10107 *J Nutr* 2001;131:846S-50S.
10108 *J Nutr* 2001;131:856S-60S.
10109 *J Nutr* 2001;131:861S-5S.
10110 *Curr Opin Clin Nutr Metab* 2002;5:63-7.
10111 *Am J Physiol Endocrinol Metab* 2002; 283:E824-35.
10112 *Eur J Biochem* 2002;269:5338-49.
10113 *Am J Physiol Endocrinol Metab* 282:E1092-101.
10114 *J Appl Physiol* 2002;93:1168-80.
10115 *J Nutr* 2001;131:851S-5S.
10116 *J Nutr* 2003;133:261S-7S.
10117 *Br J Psychiatry* 2003;182:210-3.
10118 *Diabetes Care* 2003;26:625-30.
10120 *JAMA* 1993;269:12-13.
10121 Upton R, ed. Chaste Tree Fruit. American Herbal Pharmacopoeia and Therapeutic Compendium. Santa Cruz, CA; American Herbal Pharmacopoeia 2001:1-37.
10122 *Phytomedicine* 2000;7:373-81.
10123 *Acta Haematol* 2000;104:22-4.
10124 *J Nutr* 2001;131:291-3.
10125 *Am J Clin Nutr* 2000;72:762-9.
10126 *J Am Geriatr Soc* 2002;50:146-51.
10127 *Br J Nutr* 1973;30:277-83.
10128 *Circulation* 2002;105:2836-44.
10129 *Circulation* 2002;105:2806-7.
10130 *Am J Epidemiol* 2001;154:145-9.
10131 *Arch Neurol* 2003;60:203-8.
10132 *Nutr Res* 2001;21:797-809.
10133 *Int J Cancer* 94:128-34.
10134 *Am J Clin Nutr* 1997;66:366-72.
10135 *Arch Intern Med* 2001;161:1903-8.
10136 *Nutrition Research* 2001;21:1209-15.
10137 *Best Pract Res Clin Gastroenterol* 2002;16:77-90.
10139 *Lancet* 2001;358:1500-3.
10140 *J Bone Miner Res* 2002;17:709-15.
10141 *Am J Clin Nutr* 2002;75:283-8.
10142 *N Engl J Med* 2001;345:66-7.
10143 *J Clin Endocrinol Metab* 2003;88:4077-9.
10144 *Am J Med* 2003;114:665-74.
10145 *Am J Clin Nutr* 2003;78:221-7.
10146 *Am J Psychiatry* 2003;160:1117-24.
10147 *Nephrol Dial Transplant* 2001;16:1856-62.
10148 *Diabetes Care* 2003;26:770-6.
10149 *Clin Rheumatol* 2002;21:231-43.
10150 Henry-Launois B. Evaluation of the use of financial impact of Chondrosulf 400 in current medical practice. Part of the Proceedings of a Scientific Symposium held at the XIth EULAR Symposium: New approaches in OA: Chondroitin sulfate (CS 4&6) not just a symptomatic treatment. Geneva, 1998.
10151 *Ann Otol Rhinol Laryngol* 2002:111:642-52.
10152 *Mol Cell Biochem* 2003;246:75-82.
10153 *Int J Cancer* 2003;105:113-116.
10154 *Circulation* 2003;108:820-5.
10155 *Br J Nutr* 2003;89:517-22.
10156 *J Clin Pharm Ther* 1998;23:385-89.
10157 *Ann N Y Acad Sci* 2002;957:260-70.
10158 *Am J Med* 2003;114:511-512.
10159 *Clin Pharmacol Ther* 2003;74:121-29 .
10160 *Eur J Clin Nutr* 2003;57:96-9.
10161 *Proc Natl Acad Sci USA* 1998;95:11083-88.
10162 *J Appl Physiol* 2002;92:142-6.
10164 *Eur J Clin Nutr* 2003;57:1250-53.
10165 *Am J Clin Nutr* 2003;78:719-27.
10166 *Am J Clin Nutr* 2003;78:711-18.
10201 *J Neurosci* 2001;21:RC143.
10202 *Am J Clin Nutr* 2001;74:569-70.
10203 *J Appl Physiol* 2000;89:1837-44.
10204 *J Psychosom Res* 2003;54:191-8.
10205 *Eur J Clin Pharmacol* 2000;56:537-44.
10206 *J Am Coll Nutr* 2000;19:591-600.
10207 *Phytomedicine* 2002;9:273-9.
10208 *J Nutr Biochem* 2000;11:491-5.
10209 *Sleep Med* 2000;1:91-9.
10210 *Free Radic Biol Med* 2000;28:1564-1570.
10211 *Biokhimiia* 1987;52:1216-1220.
10212 *Free Radic Biol Med* 2000;28:1249-56.
10213 *Free Radic Biol Med* 2000;28:219-27.
10214 *Nutr Res* 2001;21:1251-60.
10215 *Arch Gen Psychiatry* 2002;59:913-9.
10216 *Ann Med* 1990;22:53-6.
10217 *Biol Trace Elem Res* 2000;77:209-17.
10218 *J Endocrinol* 2003;176:63-168.
10219 *Urology* 2000;55:598-602.
10221 *JANA* 2001;4:25-30.
10222 *Eur J Neurol* 2001;8:81-5.
10223 *Am J Clin Nutr* 2002;75:894-9.
10224 *Mol Carcinog* 2000;28:129-38.
10225 *Nutrition* 2000;16:323-9.

10226 *Aliment Pharmacol Ther* 2000;14:1679-84.
10227 *Angiology* 1997;48:93-8.
10228 *J Clin Endocrinol Metab* 2001;86:3202-6.
10229 *Angiology* 1997;48:77-85.
10230 *Contraception* 1995;51:121-9.
10231 *Chin Med J* 2000;113:159-61.
10232 *Arthritis Rheum* 1993;36:1751-2.
10233 *J Rheumatol* 2003;30:465-7.
10234 *Aliment Pharmacol Ther* 2000;14:1567-79.
10235 *BMJ* 2001;323:13-6.
10237 *Clin Nephrol* 1986;25:70-4.
10238 *Clin Ther* 1986;8:537-45.
10239 *J Immunol* 2000;164:6461-6.
10240 *J Immunol* 2000;165:373-80.
10241 *BMJ* 2001;323:16-21.
10242 *JAMA* 2002;287:1123-31.
10243 *J Nutr* 1998;128:1920-6.
10244 *Eur J Cancer* 2000;36:2115-9.
10245 *Am J Clin Nutr* 2000;71:1555-62.
10246 *Am J Clin Nutr* 2002;76:805-12.
10247 *QJM* 2003;96:35-43.
10248 *BMJ* 2002;325:1059-62.
10249 *Nutr Res* 2000;20:575-84.
10250 *Am J Psychiatry* 1994;151:1234-6.
10251 *Br J Psychiatry* 1996;169:610-7.
10252 *Arch Gen Psychiatry* 1999;56:29-36.
10253 *Am J Psychiatry* 1999;156:145-7.
10254 *Ann Neurol* 1998;44:261-5.
10255 *Pharmatherapeutica* 1985;4:227-30.
10256 *J Pediatr* 1996;129:449-52.
10257 *Biol Psychiatry* 1999;45:668-79.
10258 *Transplantation* 1997;63:1661-7.
10259 *Am J Physiol* 1998;275:F595-604.
10260 *J Pharmacol Exp Ther* 1998;286:1014-9.
10261 *Carcinogenesis* 1999;20:793-8.
10262 *Carcinogenesis* 1999;20:2075-81.
10263 *J Natl Cancer Inst* 2000;92:2018-23.
10264 *Cancer Metastasis Rev* 2002;21:231-55.
10265 *Int J Oncol* 2002;20:631-6.
10266 *Regul Toxicol Pharmacol* 1993;18:419-27.
10267 *J Nutr Sci Vitaminol (Tokyo)* 1994;40:431-41.
10268 *Semin Oncol* 1983;10:56-61.
10269 *Semin Oncol* 1982;9:71-4.
10270 *Cancer Treat Rep* 1986;70:919-20.
10271 *Semin Oncol* 1983;10:72-5.
10272 *Eur J Clin Invest* 2001;31:452-61.
10274 *Ann Nutr Metab* 1999;43:356-64.
10275 *Food Addit Contam* 1988;5:103-9.
10276 *Indian J Exp Biol* 1968;6:181-2.
10277 *Contact Dermatitis* 1993;29:175-9.
10278 *Contact Dermatitis* 1995;33:435-6.
10279 *Optometry* 2000;71:147-64.
10283 *Eur J Clin Nutr* 1988;42:51-4.
10284 *J Assoc Physicians India* 1994;42:33-5.
10285 *Adv Exp Med Biol* 1996;398:373-9.
10286 *J Int Med Res* 1990;18:201-9.
10287 *Eur J Pediatr* 1994;153:344-6.
10288 *Clin Investig* 1994;72:541-9.
10289 *Adv Exp Med Biol* 1999;467:469-80.
10291 *Am J Chin Med* 1997;25:27-35.
10292 *Food Chem Toxicol* 1999;37:1027-38.
10293 *Food Chem Toxicol* 2000;38:599-605.
10294 *Clin Pharmacol Ther* 1985;38:56-9.
10295 *Biophys J* 1980;30:517-21.
10296 *Lancet* 1980;2:1113-4.
10297 *Anticancer Res* 1999;19:3717-22.
10298 *Scand J Urol Nephrol* 1998;32:261-5.
10299 *Lancet* 2003;361:2045-6.
10300 *Drug Metab Dispos* 2002;30:709-15.
10302 *J Ethnopharmacol* 2004;92:291-5.
10303 *N Engl J Med* 1986;314:648-9.
10305 *N Engl J Med* 2003;349:51.
10306 *J Natl Cancer Inst* 2003;95:1004-7.
10307 *Pharmacotherapy* 2001;21:647-51.
10309 *Biol Psychiatry* 2003;53:261-4.
10310 *Arch Intern Med* 2003;163:1514-22.
10311 *Arch Intern Med* 2003;163:1587-90.
10312 *Br J Sports Med* 2003;37:45-9.
10313 *Metabolism* 2001;50:767-70.
10314 *J Am Diet Assoc* 2001;101:655-60.
10315 *Rheumatol Int* 1992;12:81-8.
10316 *Arzneimittelforschung* 2001;51:699-725.
10317 *Diabetes Care* 2003;30:523-8.
10319 *Clin Rheumatol* 2003;22:158-9.
10320 *Eur J Clin Res* 1997;9:261-268.
10321 *Am J Clin Nutr* 2002;76:1007-15.
10322 *Am J Clin Nutr* 2003;78:65-71.
10323 *J Nutr* 2003;133:2210-3.
10324 *Am J Clin Nutr* 2001;73:209-18.
10325 *Clin Nutr* 2001;20:301-5.
10326 *Dig Dis Sci* 2002;47:1697-704.
10327 *J Rheumatol* 2003;30:523-8.
10328 *Diabetes Care* 2002;25:1522-8.
10329 *Nephrol Dial Transplant* 2003;18:819-22.
10332 *BMJ* 2001;323:776-80.
10334 *Pharmacol Biochem Behav* 2003;75:651-9.
10335 *Clin Pharmacol Ther* 2003;74:170-7.
10336 *Int Immunopharmacol* 2002;2:997-1006.
10337 *Clin Exp Allergy* 2003;33:882-6.
10339 *Antimicrob Agents Chemother* 2003;47:2158-60.
10340 *Carcinogenesis* 1996;17:265-9.
10342 *Nutr Cancer* 1995;23:121-30.
10343 *Bioorg Med Chem* 2003;11:1593-6.
10344 *J Agric Food Chem* 2002;508:5197-201.
10345 *Cell Tissue Res* 2003;311:393-9.
10346 *Alt Med Alert* 2001;4:19-22.
10348 *Am J Psychiatry* 2003;160:167-9.
10349 *J Ethnopharmacol* 2001;76:299-304.
10350 *Atherosclerosis* 1999;143:177-83.
10351 *Am J Gastroenterol* 1998;93:697-701.
10352 *Circulation* 2003;108:1059-63.
10353 *Psychopharmacology (Berl)* 2002;159:319-24.
10354 *Hypertension* 2001;37:261-7.
10355 *J Gastroenterol* 2001;36:486-91.
10356 *J Urol* 2003;170:397-401.
10357 *Aliment Pharmacol Ther* 2001;15:677-87.
10358 *J Am Coll Cardiol* 2003;42:246-52.
10359 *Aliment Pharmacol Ther* 2000;14:1303-9.
10360 *J Gastroenterol Hepatol* 2001;16:1206-10.
10361 *BJOG* 2001;108:1181-3.
10362 *Arch Dis Child Fetal Neonatal Ed* 2003;88:F324-8.
10363 *J Clin Oncol* 2003;21:2545-50.
10364 *Am J Clin Nutr* 2003;77:700-6.
10365 *Lancet* 2003;361:2017-23.
10366 *J Clin Oncol* 2003;21:927-31.
10367 *Am J Clin Nutr* 1994;59:1270-4.
10368 *Lancet* 1991;338:212-4.
10369 *Nephrology* 2000;5:1-7.
10370 *Arch Surg* 2003;138:879-83.
10371 *JAMA* 2003;290:765-72.
10372 *J Natl Cancer Inst* 2003;95:1158-64.
10373 *Aliment Pharmacol Ther* 2001;15:1139-45.

10374 *Nutr Res* 2003;23:199-204.
10375 *J Emerg Med* 2001;21:31-3.
10376 *Ann Emerg Med* 2001;38:660-5.
10377 *Phytomedicine* 1994;1:161-71.
10378 *Ophthalmology* 2003;110:359-62.
10379 *Phytomedicine* 2001;8:115-20.
10381 *Arch Dis Child* 2001;85:411-2.
10382 *N Z Med J* 2000;113:315-7.
10383 *Contact Dermatitis* 1980;6:150-1.
10384 *Ann Intern Med* 2000;133:877-80.
10385 *Nutr Cancer* 1981;3:7-12.
10386 *J Altern Complement Med* 2000;6:45-8.
10387 *J Clin Psychopharmacol* 2001;21:335-9.
10388 *CMAJ* 2003;169:111-7.
10389 *J Nat Prod* 2002;65:1194-7.
10390 *Am J Clin Nutr* 2000;72:624S-36S.
10391 *Cochrane Database Syst Rev* 2003;2:CD003158.
10392 *Ann Pharmacother* 2003;37:832-5.
10393 *Clin Neurol Neurosurg* 2003;105:286-7.
10395 *Mol Psychiatry* 2000;5:616-32.
10396 *Mol Cancer Ther* 2002;1:795-802.
10397 *Semin Oncol* 2001;28:620-5.
10398 *Anticancer Res* 2001;21:145-55.
10399 *J Am Acad Dermatol* 2002;47:535-41.
10400 *Drug Metab Dispos* 2003;31:519-22.
10401 *Surgery* 2001;130:947-53.
10403 *Am J Surg* 2003;185:411-5.
10404 *Clin Invest Med* 2000;23:300-10.
10405 *Physiol Res* 2001;50:9-18.
10406 *Arch Intern Med* 2003;163:720-7.
10407 Anon. FDA issue advisory on star anise "teas." FDA News P03-67; September 10, 2003.
10408 *Arthritis Rheum* 2000;43:2853.
10409 *Arthritis Rheum* 2001;44:2943-4.
10410 *J Nutr Biochem* 2001;12:585-94.
10412 *Nutr Res* 1998;18:503-17.
10413 *Eur J Clin Nutr* 1999;53:726-33.
10414 *Gastroenterology* 1995;108:975-82.
10415 *Am J Clin Nutr* 1997;65:1397-402.
10416 *J Sex Marital Ther* 2003;29:207-13.
10417 *J Altern Complement Med* 2001;7:175-85.
10418 *J Nutr* 2003;133:2336-41.
10419 *Am J Gastroenterol* 2000;95:1231-8.
10421 *J Nutr* 2002;132:329-32.
10422 *BMJ* 2002;325:1312-3.
10423 *Fitoterapia* 1999;70:221-8.
10424 *J Clin Psychopharmacol* 2003;23:260-8.
10425 *Am J Med* 2000;109:654-64.
10426 *Cochrane Database Syst Rev* 2002;CD001044.
10427 *Pharmacotherapy* 2003;23:866-70.
10428 *J Am Coll Cardiol* 2002;40:1383-8.
10429 *Respiration* 1999;66:495-500.
10430 *Circulation* 2003;107:992-5.
10431 *Int J Pharm* 2000;209:79-85.
10432 *Eur J Appl Physiol Occup Physiol* 1998;77:486-91.
10433 *Practitioner* 1980;224:208-11.
10434 *Diabet Med* 2001;18:756-60.
10435 *Gastroenterology* 2001;120:387-91.
10436 *Pharmacology* 1980;20 Suppl 1:128-30.
10437 *Forsch Komplementarmed Klass Naturheilkd* 2001;8:373-82.
10438 *Am J Gastroenterol* 2003;98:1563-8.
10439 *J Am Osteopath Assoc* 1984;83:790-1.
10440 *J Intern Med* 2002;252:475-96.
10441 *J Herb Pharmcother* 2003;3:77-92.
10447 *Hum Reprod* 2003;18:2166-8.
10448 *Eur J Pharm Biopharm* 2003;56:231-6.
10450 *Postgrad Med J* 2003;79:531-2.
10451 *Urology* 2002;60:640-4.
10452 *Current Problems in Pharmacovigilance* 2003;29:8.
10453 *Clin Cancer Res* 2001;7:1894-900.
10454 *Prog Clin Biol Res* 1983;125:461-8.
10455 *Am J Dis Child* 1991;145:1401-4.
10456 *Am J Med* 2001;110:616-22.
10457 *J Intern Med* 2001;249:163-6.
10458 *Hypertension* 2001;38:821-6.
10459 *Am J Clin Nutr* 2001;73:225-31.
10460 *Phytomedicine* 2002;9:85-92.
10461 *Anticancer Res* 2000;20:2409-16.
10462 *Nutr Cancer* 2000;38:168-78.
10463 *Nutr Rev* 1998;56:127-30.
10464 *Ann Nutr Metab* 2001;45:13-8.
10465 *Alcohol* 2002;27:151-4.
10466 *Pharmacol Biochem Behav* 1992;43:423-31.
10467 *N Engl J Med* 2002;346:614-6.
10468 *AIDS Patient Care STDS* 2001;15:611-4.
10470 *Am J Clin Nutr* 2002;75:887-93.
10473 *Circulation* 2003;107:947-53.
10501 *Acta Med Scand* 1974;196:525-6.
10502 *Q J Med* 1961;30:231-48.
10503 *J Clin Pathol* 1965;18:593-8.
10504 *J Lab Clin Med* 1973;81:105-15.
10505 *Br J Psychiatry* 1967;113:911-9.
10506 *Am J Med* 1992;93:705-6.
10507 *Am Heart J* 1996;131:1248-50.
10508 *South Med J* 2003;96:114-5.
10509 *J Lab Clin Med* 1999;134:232-7.
10510 *Epilepsy Res* 1993;16:157-63.
10511 *Can J Neurol Sci* 1982;9:37-9.
10512 *Brain Res* 1993;628:179-86.
10513 *J Pharm Sci* 1972;61:798-9.
10514 *J Pharm Sci* 1977;66:1433-5.
10515 *Am J Physiol Cell Physiol* 2000;279:C1782-6.
10516 *J Pharm Sci* 1967;56:1145-9.
10517 *J Pharm Sci* 1970;59:473-7.
10518 *J Clin Invest* 1981;67:1500-6.
10519 *Biochem Pharmacol* 1982;31:3495-9.
10520 *Biochem Pharmacol* 1983;32:2949-53.
10521 *Physiologist* 1985;28:322.
10522 *Lancet* 1985;2:1040-3.
10523 *Am J Clin Nutr* 1975;28:606-15.
10524 *Lancet* 1974;1:1234-5.
10525 *Am J Clin Nutr* 1978;31:247-9.
10526 *Am J Clin Nutr* 1982;35:495-501.
10527 *Am J Clin Nutr* 1980;33:832-8.
10528 *J Nutr Sci Vitaminol* 1991;37:473-7.
10529 *Biochem Pharmacol* 1988;37:1741-4.
10530 *Clin Res* 1983;31;467A.
10531 *N Engl J Med* 1987;317:192-7.
10532 *Eur J Haematol* 1995;55:97-102.
10533 *AIDS* 1990;4:701-2.
10534 *J Biol Chem* 1983;258:5629-33.
10535 *Int J Vit Nutr Res* 1979;49:59-63.
10536 *Int J Vitam Nutr Res* 1979;49:286-90.
10537 *J Nutr Sci Vitaminol* 1976;22:1-2.
10538 *Ann N Y Acad Sci* 1982;378:123-36.
10539 *Am J Clin Nutr* 1990;52:1077-92.
10540 *Ann N Y Acad Sci* 1982;378:137-44.
10541 *Acta Physiol Scand Suppl* 1978;459:1-35.
10542 *Proc Soc Exp Biol Med* 1973;142:1341-4.
10543 *Arzneimittelforschung* 1979;29:97-81.
10544 *Int J Vit Nutr Res* 1976;46:149-53.

10545 *Am J Clin Nutr* 1990;52:183-202.
10546 *Br Med J* 1981;282:19-20.
10547 *Br Med J* 1981;282:568-9.
10548 *J Am Diet Assoc* 1980;76:581-4.
10549 *Lancet* 1991;338:1467.
10550 *Kidney Int* 1991;39:598-601.
10551 *Kidney Int* 1989;35:1413-7.
10552 *Eur J Cancer* 1980;16:1041-5.
10553 *Am J Hematol* 1999;61:155-6.
10554 *Arch Neurol* 1980;37:338-41.
10555 *Contraception* 1975;11:151-4.
10556 *Int J Vit Nutr Res* 1979;49:291-5.
10557 *Annu Rev Pharmacol Toxicol* 1977;17:133-48.
10558 *Am J Clin Nutr* 1974;27:234-53.
10559 *Am J Clin Nutr* 1974;27:774-6.
10560 *Am J Clin Nutr* 1989;49:358-71.
10561 *Am J Clin Nutr* 1983;38:559-66.
10562 *Cutis* 1979;23:600-3, 689-90.
10563 *Clin Chim Acta* 1978;90:71-4.
10564 *Nutr Res* 1981;1:559-64.
10565 *Clin Sci* 1972;42:17P.
10566 *Acta Med Scand* 1976;199:175-80.
10567 *Pediatrics* 1974;54:51-5.
10568 *Metabolism* 1985;34:88-91.
10569 *J Am Med Assoc* 1984;251:351-64.
10570 *JAMA* 1999;281:235-42.
10571 *Lancet* 1998;352:167-73.
10572 *Gastroenterology* 1999;116:813-22.
10573 *Can Pharm J* 1992:399-401.
10574 *Br Med J* 1981;282:1585-6.
10577 *Osteoporos Int* 2000;11(8):637-59.
10578 *Q J Med* 1991;78:113-22.
10580 *Planta Med* 1994;60:197-200.
10582 *Lancet* 1985;1:126-8.
10583 *Nature* 1972;238:277.
10585 *Am J Clin Nutr* 1975;28:550-4.
10586 *J Am Diet Assoc* 1979;75:19-22.
10587 *Eur J Pharmacol* 1998;361:253-9.
10588 *N Engl J Med* 1977;296:1413.
10589 *J Clin Pharmacol* 1980;20:326-31.
10590 *J Clin Pharmacol* 1975;15:36-45.
10591 *Lancet* 1971;1:937-8.
10592 *J Clin Pharmacol* 1978;18:21-8.
10593 *Ann Pharmacother* 1998;32:588-98,601.
10594 *Arch Intern Med* 1986;146:386-8.
10595 *Am J Obstet Gynecol* 1993;168:1265-70.
10596 *Am J Obstet Gynecol* 1994;170:862-9.
10597 *Lancet* 1980;2:650-1.
10598 *Lancet* 1991;338:706.
10599 *Thromb Haemost* 2002;87:182-6.
10600 *Trace Elements Electrolytes* 1994;11:178-81.
10601 Agency for Healthcare Research and Quality. "Evidence Report/Technology Assessment Number 54: Management of Allergic and Nonallergic Rhinitis" http://www.ahrq.gov/clinic/epcsums/rhinsum.pdf (Accessed 4 March 2003).
10602 *J Allergy Clin Immunol* 2001;108:S2-8.
10603 *Chest* 2001;120:1461-1467.
10604 *Am J Med* 2002;113:47S-51S.
10605 *BMJ* 2002;324:144-6.
10607 *J Allergy Clin Immunol* 2000;106:603-614.
10608 *Ear Nose Throat J* 1991;70:54-5.
10609 *Ann Allergy* 1990;65:311-314.
10610 *J Allergy Clin Immunol* 1982;69:484-488.
10611 *J Am Coll Nutr* 1996;15:586-591.
10612 *Prim Care* 2002;29:231-261.
10613 Food and Drug Administration Press Release. "Pacific Biologic Recalls Seven Herbal Products That Contain the Herb Akebia Trifoliata Caulis (Mu Tong) and the Herb Asarum Sieboldii Herba Cum Radix (Xi Xin) Because of a Possible Health Risk." http://www.fda.gov/oc/po/firmrecalls/pacificbio8_01.html (Accessed 10 February 2003).
10614 *Chest* 2001;120:1433-1434.
10615 *J Am Diet Assoc* 2002;102:525-529.
10616 *Antivir Chem Chemother* 1999;10:33-8.
10617 *Cancer Res* 2000;60:5704-9.
10618 *Am J Epidemiol* 2002;156:803-5.
10619 *Postgrad Med J* 2003;79:115-6.
10620 *Am J Epidemiol* 2002;156:842-50.
10621 *BMJ* 2003;326:420.
10622 *Clin J Sport Med* 2002;12:373-8.
10623 *J Allergy Clin Immunol* 1995;96:1004-7.
10624 *BMJ* 1995;311:1472.
10625 *Nature* 1966;209:619-20.
10627 *Clin Pharmacol Ther* 2001;70:518-24.
10628 *Br J Clin Pharmacol* 2003;55:203-11.
10629 *J Urol* 1998;159:433-6.
10630 *Br J Oral Maxillofac Surg* 1984;22:42-9.
10631 *Am J Gastroenterol* 2001;96:2711-7.
10633 *Nutrition* 2002;18:729-33.
10634 *J Agric Food Chem* 2000;48:1150-4.
10635 *WHO Drug Information* 2001;16:15.
10636 *J Am Coll Nutr* 2002;21:422-7.
10637 *Am J Clin Nutr* 2002;76:359-64.
10638 *Atherosclerosis* 2001;156:329-37.
10639 *J Ethnopharmacol* 1988;22:191-203.
10640 *N Engl J Med* 2001;344:87-94.
10641 *Clin J Sport Med* 2001;11:254-9.
10642 *Prostaglandins Leukot Essent Fatty Acids* 1992;46:283-6.
10643 *Australas J Dermatol* 1996;37:159-61.
10644 *Neurosci Lett* 1997;238:135-8.
10645 *Neurosci Lett* 1998;242:105-8.
10646 *Australian Prescriber* 2001;24:6-7.
10647 *Vet Hum Toxicol* 2002;44:291-2.
10648 *Int J Dermatol* 2003;42:549.
10649 *Planta Med* 1989;55:390-1.
10650 *J Am Acad Dermatol* 2001;44:471-8.
10651 *J Clin Psychiatry* 2001;62:933-35.
10653 *Gut* 1989;30:1412-18.
10654 *Neurology* 2003;60:500-2.
10655 *Gut* 2000;47:571-4.
10656 *Ann Emerg Med* 2001;37:147-53.
10657 *J Emerg Med* 2000;19:47-50.
10658 *Acad Emerg Med* 2002;9:730-39.
10659 *Br Med J* 1986;293:1276-7.
10660 *J Clin Psychiatry* 2001;62:936-44.
10661 *Cephalalgia* 1996;16:436-40.
10663 *Headache* 2003;43:601-10.
10664 *Diabetes Care* 2003;26:1147-52.
10665 *Arch Neurol* 2000;57:597-9.
10666 *Neurology* 2003;60:1761-6.
10667 *Pediatr Infect Dis J* 2003;22:706-11.
10668 *Am J Clin Nutr* 2003;78:279-83.
10669 *Int J Food Sci Nutr* 2001;52:379-82.
10670 *Psychiatry Res* 1998;77:57-61.
10671 *Stroke* 2003;34:770-5.
10672 *Int J Cancer* 2003;107:262-7.
10673 *J Nutr* 2003;133:2532-6.
10674 *Semin Arthritis Rheum* 1997;26:713-23.
10675 *Arthritis Rheum* 2002;46:1735-43.

10676 *J Rheumatol* 2001;28:2160-7.
10677 *Pediatr Nephrol* 1994;8:343-4.
10678 *Prostate Cancer Prostatic Dis* 1999;2:S8.
10679 *J Agric Food Chem* 2003;51:3554-9.
10680 *Carcinogenesis* 2003;24:497-503.
10681 *Biochem J* 2002;364:301-7.
10682 *J Biol Chem* 2001;276:32008-15.
10683 *Food Chem Toxicol* 1999;37:271-85.
10684 *J Clin Endocrinol Metab* 1999;84:2249-52.
10685 *J Clin Endocrinol Metab* 2000;85:4912-5.
10686 *Xenobiotica* 2000;30:235-51.
10687 *J Natl Cancer Inst* 2003;95:1477-81.
10688 *J Anal Toxicol* 2003;27:123-4.
10689 *South Med J* 2003;96:718-20.
10690 *J Clin Pharmacol* 2003;43:1283-8.
10691 *Contact Dermatitis* 2001;45:269-72.
10692 *Med J Aust* 2003;179:390-1.
10693 *Arthritis Rheum* 1998;41:81-91.
10694 *Arthritis Rheum* 2002;47:50-8.
10695 *J Rheumatol* 2003;30:1825-34.
10696 *Br J Sports Med* 2003;37:212-8.
10697 *Med Hypotheses* 1987;23:39-42.
10698 *West J Med* 1986;145:245-6.
10699 *West J Med* 1986;145:699.
10700 *Arch Pediatr Adolesc Med* 2004;158:1113-15.
10701 *Nutrition Action Healthletter* 2001;28:3-8.
10702 *Mayo Clin Proc* 2002;77:109-13.
10703 *Am J Public Health* 2002;92:246-9.
10704 *Am Fam Physician* 2000; 61:2131-43.
10705 Guidelines on Overweight and Obesity. National Heart, Lung, and Blood Institute 1998. Available at: http://www.nhlbi.nih.gov/guidelines/obesity (Accessed 11 Feb 2002).
10706 *Pharmacist's Letter/Prescriber's Letter* 2000;12:161202.
10707 *Pharmacist's Letter/Prescriber's Letter* 1998;3:140305.
10708 *Pharmacist's Letter/Prescriber's Letter* 1999;15:150710.
10709 FDA. Information paper on L-tryptophan and 5-hydroxy-L-tryptophan. Feb 2001. Available at: http://vm.cfsan.fda.gov/~dms/ds-tryp1.html.
10710 Health Canada requests recall of certain products containing ephedra/ephedrine. Health Canada Online 2002. www.hc-sc.gc.ca/english/protection/warnings/2002/2002_01e.htm (Accessed 9 January 2002).
10711 *Pharmacist's Letter/Prescriber's Letter* 2002;18:180408.
10728 *J Am Diet Assoc* 1996;96:383-6.
10733 Hoechst Marion Roussel, Inc. Arava (leflunomide) product information. Kansas City, MO: September 1998.
10734 Pavelka K, Gatterova J, Olejarova M, et al. Glucosamine sulfate decreases progression of knee osteoarthritis in a long-term, randomized, placebo-controlled, independent, confirmatory trial. ACR Abstract Concurrent Session. OA-Advances in Management. November 1, 2000. Page S384, Abstract 1908.
10735 Topical Capsaicin NNTs. Bandolier 1996;29-36. www.jr2.ox.ac.uk:80/bandolier.
10736 *Clin Oral Investig* 2000;4:98-105.
10737 *J Biomed Mater Res* 2000;51:117-22.
10738 *Spine* 2002;27:E518-25.
10739 *J Craniofac Surg* 1994;5:213-7.
10741 *Acta Neurochir (Wien)* 1995;133:201-205.
10742 Federal Trade Commission. FTC and FDA Take New Actions in Fight Against Deceptive Marketing. http://www.ftc.gov/opa/2003/06/trudeau.htm (Accessed 28 July 2003).
10743 *Arzneimittelforschung* 2002;52:1-7.
10748 *Invest New Drugs* 1992;10:159-163.
10749 *JAMA* 2002;288:728-37.
10750 *Biol Psychiatry* 1997;41:65-75.
10751 *N Engl J Med* 1999;340:780-8.
10752 *CMAJ* 2003;168:715-22.
10753 *J Am Acad Child Adolesc Psychiatry* 1996;35:264-72.
10754 National Institutes of Health Consensus Development Conference Statement. Phenylketonuria: Screening and Management http://odp.od.nih.gov/consensus/cons/113/113_statement.htm (Accessed 15 August 2003).
10755 *J Clin Pharmacol* 1985;25:276-80.
10756 *Am J Psychiatry* 1973;130:796-8.
10757 *Am J Psychiatry* 1975;132:723-8.
10758 *J Abnorm Child Psychol* 1979;7:145-51.
10759 *Arch Gen Psychiatry* 1978;35:463-73.
10760 *Am J Psychiatry* 1975;132:868-70.
10762 National Institute of Allergy and Infectious Diseases. The Common Cold. http://www.niaid.nih.gov/factsheets/cold.htm (Accessed 28 August 2003).
10763 Gwaltney JM Jr. The Common Cold. In: Principles and Practices of Infectious Diseases, 5th ed. Mandell GL, Bennett JE, Dolin R, eds. New York, NY: Churchill Livingstone; 2000. pgs. 651-6.
10764 National Institute of Allergy and Infectious Diseases. Flu. http://www.niaid.nih.gov/factsheets/flu.htm (Accessed 28 August 2003).
10765 *Paediatr Respir Rev* 2003;4:91-8.
10766 *Lancet* 2003;361:51-9.
10767 Treanor, JJ. Influenza virus. In: Principles and Practices of Infectious Diseases, 5th ed. Mandell GL, Bennett JE, Dolin R, eds. New York, NY: Churchill Livingstone; 2000. pgs. 1823-49.
10768 *N Engl J Med* 1992;326:644-5.
10769 *Ann Epidemiol* 2001;11:225-31.
10770 National Institute of Allergy and Infectious Diseases. Is it a Cold or the Flu? http://www.niaid.nih.gov/publications/cold/sick.pdf (Accessed 29 August 2003).
10771 *N Engl J Med* 1991;325:606-12.
10772 *Epidemiology* 2001;12:345-9.
10773 *MMWR Recomm Rep* 2003:52(RR-8);1-34. Available at: http://www.cdc.gov/mmwr/preview/mmwrhtml/rr5208a1.htm (Accessed 30 August 2003).
10774 FDA News: First Nasal Mist Flu Vaccine Approved. June 17, 2003. http://www.fda.gov/bbs/topics/NEWS/2003/NEW00913.html (Accessed 30 August 2003).
10775 *N Engl J Med* 2000;343:1778-87.
10776 *BMJ* 2003;326:1235.
10777 *J Biol Response Mod* 1983;2:227-37.
10780 *Epidemiology* 2002;13:38-44.
10782 *Cochrane Database Syst Rev* 2000;2:CD000530.
10783 *Antiviral Res* 2001;49:1-14.
10784 *Clin Infect Dis* 2000;31:1202-8.
10785 *J Int Med Res* 1996;24:325-30.
10786 *Am J Clin Nutr* 2003;77:1287-95.
10787 *Adv Ther* 2001;18:189-93.
10788 *JAMA* 2002;288:715-21.
10789 *Br J Nutr* 2003;89:695-703.
10791 *Cochrane Database Syst Rev* 2003;(3):CD002744.
10792 *Cochrane Database Syst Rev* 2003;3:CD001267.
10793 *Ann Intern Med* 1996;125:89-97.
10794 *Cochrane Database Syst Rev* 2001;(3):CD001831.
10795 *Phytomedicine* 2002;9:589-97.
10796 *Eur Cytokine Netw* 2001;12:290-6.
10797 *J Immunother* 2002;25:413-20.
10798 *Food Chem Toxicol* 1985;23:317-9.

10799 *Planta Med* 1994;60:37-40.
10800 *Ann Intern Med* 2002;137:939-46.
10801 *Lancet* 1976;1:256.
10802 *Arzneimittelforschung* 2001;51:563-8.
10803 *Am J Ther* 2002;9:472-5.
10804 *Cochrane Database Syst Rev* 2000;2:CD001957.
10805 *Cochrane Database Syst Rev* 2001;(4):CD001728.
10806 *Chest* 2000;118:1150-7.
10807 *Am J Epidemiol* 2002;155:853-8.
10808 *Eur J Nutr* 2002;41:264-70.
10809 *Int J Artif Organs* 1998;21:274-278.
10810 *J Clin Pharm Ther* 2003;28:53-9.
10811 *Pharmacol Biochem Behav* 2003;75:669-74.
10812 *J Agric Food Chem* 1999;47:2048-54.
10813 *J Agric Food Chem* 2000;48:849-52.
10814 *Am J Epidemiol* 1996;144:501-11.
10815 *BMJ* 1997;314:634-8.
10816 *Circulation* 1995;92:2142-50.
10817 *Am J Clin Nutr* 1980;33:2079-87.
10818 *JAMA* 1995;273:1849-54.
10819 *Am J Clin Nutr* 1995;62:1385S-92S.
10821 *Int J Cancer* 2000;86:122-7.
10822 *J Natl Cancer Inst* 2000;92:1607-12.
10823 *J Natl Cancer Inst* 1996;88:340-8.
10824 *Eur J Cancer* 2000;36:636-46.
10825 *Int J Cancer* 2001;91:563-7.
10826 *Cancer Causes Control* 2000;11:279-83.
10827 *Cochrane Database Syst Rev* 2003;1:CD003119.
10828 *Cochrane Database Syst Rev* 2000;2:CD000480.
10829 *Int J Clin Pharmacol Ther Toxicol* 1990;28:323-8.
10830 *JAMA* 2003;290:1500-4.
10831 *N Engl J Med* 2000;343:1942-50.
10832 *JAMA* 2003;289:3095-105.
10833 *CMAJ* 2002;167:1253-60.
10834 *Am J Psychiatry* 2000;157:1925-32.
10835 *JAMA* 2003;290:215-21.
10841 *Am J Psychiatry* 2001;158:289-94.
10842 *J Nerv Ment Dis* 1999;187:692-5.
10843 *JAMA* 2002;287:1807-14.
10844 *J Am Acad Child Adolesc Psychiatry* 2003;42:908-914.
10845 *Psychosomatics* 2003;44:271-82.
10846 *Am J Obstet Gynecol* 2001;184:191-5.
10847 *Clin Pharmacol Ther* 2002;72:276-87.
10848 *Phytomedicine* 2003;10:334-42.
10849 *Can J Clin Pharmacol* 2003;10:114-118.
10850 *Psychopharmacol Bull* 1995;31:167-75.
10851 *J Neural Transm* 1999;106:795-8.
10852 *Psychopharmacology (Berl)* 2003 Sept 4 [Epub ahead of print].
10853 *Cochrane Database Syst Rev* 2002;1:CD003198.
10854 *Br J Psychiatry* 2001;178:399-405.
10855 *Psychopharmacology (Berl)* 2002;163:42-53.
10856 *Arch Gen Psychiatry* 1976;33:1384-89.
10857 *Biol Psychiatry* 1981;16:291-310.
10858 *J Clin Psychopharmacol* 1987;7:127-37.
10859 *Psychiatry Res* 1999;85:275-91.
10860 *Am J Clin Nutr* 2003;78:40-6.
10861 *CMAJ* 1987;137:722-6.
10862 *J Clin Microbiol* 1987;25:1763-5.
10863 *Clin Infect Dis* 2000;31:136-43.
10864 *Clin Infect Dis* 2001 May 15;32(10):1520.
10865 *Infect Control Hosp Epidemiol* 2000;21:516-9.
10866 *Arch Gen Psychiatry* 2002;59:913-9.
10867 *Arch Gen Psychiatry* 2001;58:512-513.
10868 *Lancet* 1998;351:1213.
10869 *Am J Psychiatry* 2003;160:996-8.
10870 *Arch Gen Psychiatry* 2002;59:592-6.
10871 *Eur Neuropsychopharmacol* 2003;13:267-71.
10872 *Am J Psychiatry* 2002;159:477-9.
10874 *Ann Clin Psychiatry* 1990;2:39-45.
10875 *Gerontology* 1995;41:343-51.
10876 *J Am Geriatr Soc* 1999;47:685-91.
10877 *Am J Geriatr Psychiatry* 1998;6:277-84.
10879 *J Neurol Neurosurg Psychiatry* 2000;69:228-32.
10880 *J Clin Psychopharmacol* 2003;23:309-13.
10881 *Am J Psychiatry* 2002;159:2099-101.
10882 *Psychother Psychosom* 2003;72:80-7.
10883 *J Nutr* 2003;133:3233-6.
10884 *Cochrane Database Syst Rev* 2003;2:CD003390.
10885 *J Affect Disord* 1989;16:103-7.
10886 *Aging (Milano)* 1993;5:63-71.
10887 *Lancet* 1990;336:392-5.
10888 *J Am Coll Nutr* 1992;11:159-63.
10889 *J Affect Disord* 1994;32:197-200.
10892 *J Clin Psychiatry* 2002;63:357-66.
10893 *Hum Psychopharmacol* 2002;17:279-84.
10894 *JAMA* 2003;289:56-64.
10895 *Food Chem Toxicol* 1987;25:807-814.
10896 *Am J Clin Nutr* 1992;56:1056-1060.
10897 *Am J Cardiol* 1988;62:51-55.
10898 *Drugs* 1990;39:917-28.
10899 FDA List of Orphan Designations and Approvals. http://www.fda.gov/orphan/DESIGNAT/list.htm (Accessed 27 October 2003).
10900 *Ann Oncol* 2002;13:1259-63.
10901 *Exp Eye Res* 1997;64:211-8.
10902 *Arch Ophthalmol* 1993;111:104-9.
10903 *Invest Ophthalmol Vis Sci* 1997;38:1795-801.
10904 *J Nutr Med* 1990;1:133-8.
10905 *Bull Wrld Health Org* 1995;73:115-21.
10906 *Am J Epidemiol* 1977;106:17-32.
10907 *Arch Ophthalmol* 1998;116: 219-25.
10908 *Adv Pharmacol* 1997;38:515-36.
10909 *Ophthalmic Res* 1983;15:173-9.
10910 *Am J Clin Nutr* 1997;66:911-6.
10911 *Ophthalmic Epidemiol* 2002;9(1):49-80.
10912 *Nutr Rep Inter* 1987;36:685-92.
10913 *Am J Clin Nutr* 1981;34:861-3.
10914 *Ann Ottalmol Clin Ocul* 1989; 115:109.
10915 *Clin Pharm* 1990;9:446-57.
10916 *Arch Biochem Biophys* 1985;239:491-6.
10917 *Exp Eye Res* 1999;69:109-15.
10918 *Free Radic Res* 1999;30:253-63.
10919 *Arch Ophthalmol* 1987;105:482-5.
10920 Ginkgo may protect against stroke damage. www.medscape.com/reuters/prof/2000/05/05.03/20000503scie003.html (Accessed 3 May 2000).
10921 *J Ocul Pharmacol Ther* 1999;15:233-40.
10922 *Klin Monatsbl Augenheilkd* 1980;177:577-83.
10923 *Curr Opin Ophthalmol* 2000;11:90-3.
10924 *Z Gerontol* 1993;26:243-6.
10925 *Acta Soc Med Upsal* 1964;69:225-32.
10926 *Acta Ophthalmol (Copenh)* 1969;47:685-9.
10927 *Eye Ear Nose Throat Mon* 1967;46:1502-8.
10928 *Arch Ophthalmol* 1998;116:1433-7.
10929 *Am J Epidemiol* 1988;128:700-10.
10930 *Eur J Neurosci* 2001;13:409-12.
10931 *Science* 1975;188:1215-6.
10932 *JAMA* 2001;285:785-95.
10933 *Clin Fam Prac* 2002;4:89-111.

10934 National Osteoporosis Foundation. America's Bone Health: The State of Osteoporosis and Low Bone Mass. Available at: http://www.nof.org/advocacy/prevalence/index.htm (Accessed 11 June 2002).
10935 National Institute of Health Osteoporosis and Related Bone Diseases National Resource Center. "Fast Facts on Osteoporosis." Website: http://www.osteo.org/osteofastfact.html (Accessed 11 June 2002).
10936 National Osteoporosis Foundation. Osteoporosis in Men. Available at: http://www.nof.org/men/strategies_men.htm (Accessed 11 June 2002).
10937 *J R Soc Med* 2001;94:620-3.
10938 *Am J Ther* 1999;6:313-21.
10939 *Phytother Res* 2003;17:227-31.
10940 *Fund App Tox* 1997;35:205-15.
10941 *Bio Trace Elem Res* 2001;82:109-23.
10942 *Magnes Trace Elem* 1990;9:61-9.
10943 *Magnes Res* 1993;6:291-6.
10944 *Menopause* 2000;7:413-6.
10945 *Biol Trace Elem Res* 1995;48:1-11.
10948 *Menopause* 2001;8:259-65.
10949 *J Bone Miner Res* 1995;10:1802-15.
10950 *Osteoporos Int* 1999;9:45-54.
10951 *J Clin Endocrinol Metab* 2002;87:1544-9.
10952 *J Clin Endocrinol Metab* 2002;87:1527-32.
10953 *Cas Lek Cesk* 1996;135:74-8.
10954 *Am J Clin Nutr* 2002;75:609-10.
10955 *Am J Clin Nutr* 2002;75:773-9.
10956 *Am J Clin Nutr* 1999;69:147-52.
10957 *Ann Intern Med* 1998;128(10):801-9.
10958 *JAMA* 2002;288:49-57.
10959 *JAMA* 2002;288:321-33.
10960 *N Engl J Med* 2003;348:1839-54.
10961 *JAMA* 2003;289:2673-84.
10962 *JAMA* 2003;289:2651-62.
10963 *Obstet Gynecol* 2003;101:10S-11S
10964 *JAMA* 2002;287:591-7.
10965 North American Menopause Society. Menopause Core Curriculum Study Guide. 2002. http://www.menopause.org/edumaterials/studyguide/sgtoc.html (Accessed 22 April 2003).
10966 *Lancet* 1999;353:571-80.
10967 *Obstet Gynecol* 2003;101:264-72.
10968 *Obstet Gynecol* 2002;100:1209-18.
10969 *N Engl J Med* 2003;348:1835-7.
10970 *Clin Obstet Gynecol* 2000;43:162-83.
10971 *Obstet Gynecol* 2002;100:18-25.
10972 *Menopause* 2003;10:65-72.
10973 *J Nutr* 2001;131:1826-32.
10975 *Climacteric* 1999;2:85-92.
10976 *Climacteric* 1999;2:79-84.
10977 *J Am Vet Med Assoc* 1998;212:857-9.
10978 *Obstet Gynecol* 2002;100:495-504.
10979 *J Agric Food Chem* 2001;49:2472-9.
10980 *J Agric Food Chem* 2003;51:2193-9.
10981 *Int J Clin Pharmacol Res* 1999;19:89-99.
10982 *Med J Aust* 1981;1:492.
10983 *Br Med J* 1980;281:1110.
10984 *Arch Pharm Res* 2003;26:58-63.
10985 *Eur J Endocrinol* 2001;145:457-61.
10986 *Gynecol Endocrinol* 2000;14:342-63.
10987 *Maturitas* 2003;44:S67-77.
10988 *Menopause* 2003;10:58-64.
10989 *Climacteric* 2001;4:144-50.
10990 *JAMA* 2002;288:2432-40.
10991 *JAMA* 2003;290:207-14.
10992 National Institute of Neurological Disorders and Stroke. Headache: Hope through Research. http://www.ninds.nih.giv/healinfo/DISORDER/Headache/head.htm. Updated 11/19/98.
10993 *Clin Neurosci* 1998;5:24-7.
10994 *Clin Ther* 2001;23:772-88.
10995 Freitag F. What's new in migraine prevention? NHF Headlines 2001 July/Aug No. 121:1-2.
10996 *Pediatr Med Chir* 1993;15:481-8.
10997 *Headache* 1998;38:303-7
10998 *J Eur Acad Dermatol Venereol* 2001;15:484-5.
11000 *N Engl J Med* 1997;337:365-372.
11001 *J Cardiovasc Risk* 1996;3:513-521.
11002 *Epidemiology* 1992;3:194-202.
11003 *Sports Med* 2000;30:105-16.
11004 *Dig Dis Sci* 1995;40:349-56.
11005 *Biochem Pharmacol* 2000;59:1109-16.
11006 *Cancer Lett* 2000;150:41-8.
11007 *Br J Pharmacol* 2000;130:1859-64.
11008 *Allergol Immunopathol (Madr)* 2001;29:272-5.
11009 *Zhonghua Liu Xing Bing Xue Za Zhi* 2002;23:213-7.
11010 *J Nutr* 2002;132:2015-8.
11011 *Int J Antimicrob Agents* 2000;15:235-7.
11012 National Institutes of Health (NIH). Glucosamine/Chondroitin Arthritis Intervention Trial (GAIT) Begins Patient Recruitment. National Center for Complementary and Alternative Medicine, 2000. Available at: http://nccam.nih.gov/news/19972000/121100.
11013 *Methods Find Exp Clin Pharmacol* 1999;21:679-82.
11014 *Nat Genet* 1995;10:111-3.
11016 *East Afr Med J* 1993;70:90-3.
11017 *JAMA* 1979;241:2008.
11018 FDA Talk Paper. FDA Allows Foods Containing Psyllium To Make Health Claim On Reducing Risk Of Heart Disease. 1998. Available at: http://www.fda.gov/bbs/topics/ANSWERS/ANS00850.html.
11019 *Arch Dermatol Res* 1985;278:31-6.
11020 *J Pharm Sci* 1975;64:535-98.
11021 Anon. EPOGAM Capsules. G.D. Searle (South Africa) (Pty) Ltd. January 1990. Available at: http://home.intekom.com/pharm/searle/epogm.html.
11022 *Clin Pharmacol Ther* 1992;51:183.
11023 FDA, HHS. Final Rule Declaring Dietary Supplements Containing Ephedrine Alkaloids Adulterated Because They Present An Unreasonable Risk. 21 CFR Part 119. February 11, 2004. Available at: http://www.fda.gov/OHRMS/DOCKETS/98fr/1995n-0304-nfr0001.pdf.
11024 *BMC Complement Altern Med* 2004;4:12.
11101 *Cochrane Database Syst Rev* 2002;(3):CD000247.
11102 *Pediatrics* 1998;101:163-5.
11103 *Ann Intern Med* 2001;134:479-86.
11104 *Ann Intern Med* 1992;117:37-41.
11105 *J Infect Dis* 1992;166:776-82.
11106 *Am J Rhinol* 2001;15:239-42.
11107 *Pharmacotherapy* 1992;12:331-3.
11108 *Can Fam Physician* 2003;49:168-73.
11109 *Arch Fam Med* 1998;7:39-43.
11110 *J Pharm Pharmacol* 1997;49:1045-9.
11111 *Res Commun Mol Pathol Pharmacol* 1998;100:351-61.
11112 *Prostaglandins Leukot Essent Fatty Acids* 1994;51:101-8.
11113 *Lipids* 1997;32:1129-36.
11114 *Cancer Epidemiol Biomarkers Prev* 1997;6:25-9.
11115 *Chem Biol Interact* 2002;139:1-21.
11116 *Gynecol Oncol* 1997;66:417-24.

11117 *Hepatogastroenterology* 1998;45:727-32.
11118 *J Gastrointest Surg* 2002;6:302-3.
11119 *Acta Chir Scand* 1988;154:395-98.
11120 Food and Nutrition Board, Institute of Medicine. Dietary Reference Intakes for Energy, Carbohydrate, Fiber, Fat, Fatty Acids, Cholesterol, Protein, and Amino Acids (Macronutrients). Washington, DC: National Academy Press, 2002. Available at: http://www.nap.edu/books/0309085373/html.
11121 *MMWR Morb Mortal Wkly Rep* 1992;41:812-4.
11122 *Arch Surg* 2003;138:852-8.
11123 *Phytomedicine* 2001;8:1-7.
11124 *Anticancer Drug Des* 2001;16:261-70.
11125 *Toxicon* 2002;40:1701-8.
11126 *J Ethnopharmacol* 2001;74:89-96.
11127 *Proc Natl Acad Sci U S A* 1995;92:11239-43.
11128 *J Am Acad Dermatol* 1986;15:302.
11129 *J Urol* 1994;152:2089-91.
11130 *Drugs R D* 2003;4:1-18.
11131 *J Androl* 1998;19:479-86.
11132 *Acta Pharmacol Sin* 2003;24:22-30.
11133 *Adv Contracept* 1988;4:307-10.
11134 *J Am Diet Assoc* 1994;94:65-70.
11135 *BMJ* 1988;297:958-60.
11136 *Dtsch Tierarztl Wochenschr* 1995;102:228-32.
11137 *Gastroenterology* 2001;120:636-51.
11138 *Carcinogenesis* 1999;20:445-51.
11139 *Food Chem Toxicol* 2002;40:1091-7.
11140 *Mem Inst Oswaldo Cruz* 2001;96:723-8.
11141 *Mol Cancer Ther* 2003;2:95-103.
11142 *Cell Growth Differ* 1998;9:305-12.
11143 *Biochem Pharmacol* 1999;58:1167-72.
11144 *J Med Assoc Thai* 1989;72:613-20.
11145 *Asia Pac J Clin Nutr* 2002;11:314-8.
11146 *Contact Dermatitis* 1997;36:107-8.
11147 *Immunol Invest* 1999;28:291-303.
11148 *Tumori* 1987;73:29-31.
11149 *Indian J Med Res* 1980;71:632-4.
11150 *Phytother Res* 1999;13:318-22.
11151 *Eur J Clin Pharmacol* 1993;44:315-8.
11152 *Klin Med (Mosk)* 1974;52:142-3.
11153 *J Ethnopharmacol* 2003;84:187-92.
11154 *Lancet Neurol* 2002;1:275.
11155 Jafek BW, Linschoten M, Murrow BW. Zicam Induced Anosmia. American Rhinologic Society 49th Annual Fall Scientific Meeting abstract. Orlando, Florida. September 20, 2003. http://app.american-rhinologic.org/programs/2003ARSFallProgram071503.pdf (Accessed 24 November 2003).
11156 *Physiol Behav* 2001;72:291-6.
11157 *Med Sci Monit* 2002;8:RA210-5.
11158 Society of Surgery of the Alimentary Tract, Inc. Management of ulcerative colitis. SSAT patient care guidelines 2002. Available at: http://www.ssat.com/cgi-bin/colitis.cgi?affiliation.
11159 *Am J Physiol* 1997;273:R710-5.
11160 Product information for infliximab (Remicade). Centocor, Inc. Malvern, PA. April 2003.
11161 *Maturitas* 2002;42:129-35.
11162 *Ann N Y Acad Sci* 2002;962:372-7.
11163 *Lancet Neurol* 2003;2:429-34.
11164 *JAMA* 2002;287:425-7.
11165 *Scand J Gastroenterol* 2002;4:444-9.
11166 *J Pain Symptom Manage* 1995;10:89-97.
11167 *Eur Neurol* 1997;38:44-8.
11168 *Lancet* 2003;362:1517-26.
11215 *Lancet* 2003;361:1359-67.
11216 *Urology* 2003;61:267-73.
11217 *Eur Urol* 2002;42:323-8.
11218 *BJU Int* 2000;85:1037-48.
11219 *Med Clin North Am* 1999;83:1213-29.
11221 *J Urol* 2003;170:530-47.
11222 *Urology* 1999;54:86-9.
11224 *Eur Urol* 2003;44:549-55.
11225 *Clin Pharmacol Ther* 2003;74:536-42.
11226 *Arch Esp Urol* 2003;56:369-78.
11227 *Planta Med* 2000;66:44-7.
11228 *Planta Med* 1997;63:529-32.
11229 *Planta Med* 1997;63:307-10.
11230 *Urologe A* 1985;24:49-51.
11231 *Forsch Komplementarmed Klass Naturheilkd* 2000;7:200-4.
11233 *J Tongji Med Univ* 1994;14:235-8.
11234 *Eur Urol* 2000;37:735-41.
11235 *Oncol Rep* 2003;10:2009-14.
11236 *Methods Find Exp Clin Pharmacol* 2003;25:617-23.
11237 *J Nutr* 2003;133:3356-60.
11238 *Prostate* 1998;34:75-9.
11239 *Prostate* 2003;56:54-64.
11240 *Reprod Fertil Dev* 2001;13:325-9.
11241 *Int Urol Nephrol* 2001; 33: 217-25.
11242 Lee M. Management of benign prostatic hyperplasia. Pharmacotherapy - A Pathophysiological Approach, 5th edition (1999). New, NY: McGraw-Hill Publishing Division.
11243 *Eur Urol* 2002;41:497-506.
11244 *J Agric Food Chem* 1998;46:8-12.
11245 *Int J Immunopharmacol* 1998;20:643-60.
11246 *Arch Pharm Res* 1998;21:147-52.
11247 *J Agric Food Chem* 2004;52:65-70.
11248 *J Am Coll Nutr* 2001;20:327-36.
11249 *Horm Res* 1998;50:177-82.
11250 *JAMA* 2003;289:1837-50.
11251 *Med Lett Drugs Ther* 2000;42:52.
11252 *JAMA* 2003;289:1767-8, 1773.
11253 *N Engl J Med* 2003;348:2082-90.
11254 *N Engl J Med* 2003;348:2074-81.
11255 *Am J Med* 2002;113:30-6.
11256 *JAMA* 2002;287:2414-23.
11257 *Am J Clin Nutr* 2002;76:5-56.
11258 *Am J Clin Nutr* 2002;76:281S-5S.
11259 Ellison S. The good, the bad and the high glycemic. Wall Street Journal. November 24, 2003.
11260 *Am J Med* 2002;113 Suppl 9B:5S-8S.
11261 *Cochrane Database Syst Rev* 2002;2:CD003640.
11262 *Circulation* 2001;104:1869-74.
11263 *J Am Coll Nutr* 2003;22:9-17.
11264 *JAMA* 2003;289:1792-8.
11265 FDA Center for Food Safety and Nutrition. What are some of the questionable weight loss products? http://www.cfsan.fda.gov/~dms/qa-nut4.html. (Accessed December 20, 2003).
11266 *N Engl J Med* 2002;346:591-602.
11267 *J Pharm Biomed Anal* 2002;29:1113-9.
11268 *Curr Ther Res* 1999;60:145-153.
11269 *J Clin Pharmacol* 2002;42:1165-70.
11270 *Clin Pharmacol Ther* 1999;65:237-44.
11271 Food and Drug Administration, Center for Food Safety and Applied Nutrition. Letter to Health Care Professionals on Hazardous Dietary Supplement LipoKinetix. November 19, 2001. Available at: http://www.cfsan.fda.gov/~dms/ds-ltr25.html.

11272 *Nat Toxins* 1996;4:96-102.
11273 *Drug Metab Dispos* 1997;25:1228-33.
11274 *Clin Pharmacol Ther* 1999;66:358-66.
11275 *J Clin Pharmacol* 2003;43:831-9.
11276 *Clin Pharmacol Ther* 2003;73:529-37.
11277 *Clin Pharmacol Ther* 2001;70:311-6.
11278 *Clin Pharmacol Ther* 2002;71:11-20.
11280 *J Clin Pharmacol* 2001;41:435-42.
11282 *Pharmacotherapy* 2003;23:979-87.
11284 Stenson WF, Korzenik J. Inflammatory Bowel Disease. In: Yamada T, ed. Textbook of Gastroenterology. 4th ed. Philadelphia, PA: Lippincott Williams & Wilkins; 2003.
11285 *Br J Nutr* 2000;83:389-99.
11286 *J Am Coll Cardiol* 2001;38:1806-13.
11287 *Drugs Aging* 2002;19:793-805.
11288 *Clin Fam Prac* 2002;4:967-971.
11289 *N Engl J Med* 2003;349:2387-98.
11292 *Chem Senses* 1999;24:387-92.
11293 *Br Med J* 1986;292:591-2.
11294 *Ital J Gastroenterol* 1991;23:421-5.
11295 *J Pediatr* 2000;136:41-5.
11296 *Planta Med* 1996;62:548-51.
11297 *Reprod Toxicol* 2001;15:75-80.
11298 *Reprod Toxicol* 2000;14:507-12.
11299 *Cancer Lett* 1987;36:221-33.
11300 *Pharmacotherapy* 2005;25:165-70.
11301 *Altern Med Rev* 2000;5:334-46.
11302 *Arch Dermatol* 2003;139:451-5.
11303 *JAMA* 2003;290:476-85.
11304 *J Natl Cancer Inst* 2003;95:1563-5.
11305 *J Natl Cancer Inst* 2003;95:1578-86.
11306 Barrett S. Zicam Marketers Sued. United States District Court Western District of Michigan Southern Division, Filed October 14, 2003, Case No. 4:03CV0146.
11307 *Eur J Clin Nutr* 2003;57:721-5.
11308 *Arch Intern Med* 2003;163:1448-53.
11309 *J Urol* 2003;170:773-6.
11310 *Eur J Cancer Prev* 2003;12:383-90.
11311 *Eur J Pharmacol* 1981;72:219-25.
11312 *Gut* 1969;10:299-302.
11313 *Practitioner* 1973;210:820-3.
11314 *BJU Int* 2003;92:267-70.
11315 *Allergy* 2003;58:681-2.
11316 *N Engl J Med* 2002;347:417-29.
11317 *J Nutr* 1993;123:1611-4.
11318 *J Nutr* 2003;133:3228-32.
11320 *Cerebrovasc Dis* 2000;10:49-60.
11321 *Am J Psychiatry* 2000;157:826-8.
11322 *J Clin Psychopharmacol* 1999;19:506-12.
11323 *J Clin Gastroenterol* 2003;36:111-9.
11324 *WHO Drug Inf (Iran)* 2002;16:15-16.
11325 *Clin Experiment Ophthalmol* 2002;30:303-4.
11326 *Arch Ophthalmol* 2003;121:1621-4.
11327 *Eur J Clin Nutr* 2003;57:1268-74.
11328 *Diabetes Care* 2003;26:2695-6.
11330 *Pharmacol Res* 2000;41:255-64.
11331 *Int J Sports Med* 1997;18:369-72.
11332 *Ann Neurol* 2003;53:437-45.
11333 *Arch Ophthalmol* 2003;121:1269-78.
11334 *Neurology* 2003;60:1071-6.
11335 *J Agric Food Chem* 2002;50:2200-6.
11336 *J Herb Pharmacother* 2003;3:5-17.
11337 *J Am Coll Cardiol* 2003;41:2105-13.
11338 *Am J Clin Nutr* 2003;77:1318-23.
11339 *Nutr Cancer* 1995;24:33-45.
11340 *Arthritis Rheum* 2003;49:601-4.
11341 *BMJ* 2003;327:1385.
11342 *BMJ* 2003;327:1358-9.
11343 *Ann Pharmacother* 2004;38:50-2.
11344 *Circulation* 2003;108:1.
11345 *J Am Coll Cardiol* 2003;42:1967-74.
11346 *Am J Obstet Gynecol* 2003;189:1374-7.
11347 *Diabetes Care* 2003;26:3215-8.
11348 *AIDS* 2003;17:2461-9.
11349 *Pharmacist's Letter/Prescriber's Letter* 2003;19(12):191201.
11350 *Prog Neuropsychopharmacol Biol Psychiatry* 2004;28:181-90.
11351 *J Am Geriatr Soc* 2004;52:13-9.
11352 *Diabetes Care* 2004;27:59-65.
11353 *Ann Intern Med* 2004;140:1-8.
11354 *J Urol* 2004;171:284-8.
11355 *JAMA* 2004;291:216-21.
11356 *Neurology* 2004;62:60-5.
11357 *J Am Coll Nutr* 2003;22:36-42.
11358 *Diabetes Care* 2000;23:9-14.
11359 *Diabetes Care* 1999;22:913-9.
11360 *Horm Metab Res* 1983;15:1-3.
11361 *Lancet* 1979;1:987-8.
11362 *Life Sci* 2002;71:1149-60.
11363 *Vasc Med* 2002;7:265-7.
11364 *Eur J Clin Nutr* 2003;57:31-6.
11365 *J Allergy Clin Immunol* 2003;112:805-6.
11366 *Cancer* 2003;97:1442-6.
11367 *Diabetes Care* 2003;26:1277-94.
11368 *Control Clin Trials* 1997;18:286-300.
11369 *Phytomedicine* 2003;10:440-6
11370 *Contact Dermatitis* 2000;42:363-4.
11371 *Phytomedicine* 2003;10:68-73.
11372 *Cochrane Database Syst Rev* 2003;1:CD003383.
11373 *Hum Psychopharmacol* 2003;18:525-33.
11374 *J Nutr* 2003;133:2188-93.
11375 *J Am Coll Cardiol* 2003;41:1744-9.
11376 *Curr Ther Res* 1996;57:445-61.
11377 *Nutr Res* 1999;19:1507-18.
11378 *Scand J Infect Dis* 2003;35:365-7.
11379 *Aliment Pharmacol Ther* 2003;17:895-904.
11380 *Oral Microbiol Immunol* 2002;17:9-15.
11381 *Lancet* 2003;361:1869-71.
11382 *J Antimicrob Chemother* 2003;52:308-11.
11383 *J Allergy Clin Immunol* 1997;99:179-85.
11384 *JAMA* 2004;291:562-3.
11386 *Menopause* 2003;10:352-61.
11387 *JAMA* 2004;291:565-75.
11388 *JAMA* 2004;291:621-2.
11389 *Am J Health Syst Pharm* 2004;61:306-307.
11390 *Arch Neurol* 2004;61:82-8.
11391 *Am J Clin Nutr* 2004;79:282-8.
11392 *N Engl J Med* 2004;350:459-68.
11393 *N Engl J Med* 2004;350:504-6.
11394 *Kidney Int* 2003;64:534-43.
11395 *J Clin Endocrinol Metab* 2002;87:2060-6.
11396 *Calcif Tissue Int* 2001;69:121-9.
11397 *J Bone Miner Res* 2001;16:299-308.
11399 *Am J Med* 1993;95:69S-74S.
11400 *J Clin Endocrinol Metab* 1988;66:1124-31.
11401 *Metabolism* 1999;48:809-16.
11402 *Can Med Assoc J* 1981;125:703-12.
11403 *Isr J Med Sci* 1971;7:393.
11404 *Clin Sci* 1968;34:351-63.
11405 *J Clin Endocrinol Metab* 1966;26:566-72.
11406 *BMJ* 2003;326:1124.

11407 *Int J Obes Relat Metab Disord* 2001;25:1087-94.
11408 *Pharmacopsychiatry* 2001;34:S127-33.
11409 *Neurology* 2003;60:1679-81.
11410 *Neurology* 2003;60:1676-9.
11411 *Neurology* 2003;60:1569-70.
11412 *Mol Genet Metab* 2002;77:21-30.
11413 *Heart* 2002;87:346-9.
11414 *J Neurosci Methods* 2002;115:63-6.
11415 *Neurosci Lett* 2001;306:169-72.
11416 *J Inherit Metab Dis* 2001;24:28-34.
11417 *Altern Med Rev* 2001;6:83-6.
11418 *Lancet* 1999;354:477-9.
11419 *Free Radic Biol Med* 1999;26:1405-17.
11420 *Free Radic Biol Med* 1998;25:480-92.
11421 *Neuropsychobiology* 1997;36:73-82.
11422 *Neurology* 1996;47:583-5.
11423 *Arch Biochem Biophys* 1996;330:395-400.
11424 *Eur J Clin Pharmacol* 1996;51:167-9.
11425 *Lancet* 1992;340:368-9.
11426 *J Neurol Sci* 1989;90:263-71.
11427 *J Neural Transm* 1998;54:301-10.
11428 *Am J Respir Crit Care Med* 2003;168:63-9.
11429 *Phytomedicine* 2002;9:694-9.
11430 *Am Heart J* 2003;146:E23.
11431 *J Agric Food Chem* 2003;51:6452-5.
11432 *J Agric Food Chem* 2003;51:1500-5.
11433 *J Agric Food Chem* 2002;50:3341-5.
11434 *J Agric Food Chem* 2002;50:2125-9.
11435 *Allergy* 2001;56:1020-1.
11436 *Allergy* 2001;56:763-6.
11437 *Allergy* 2001;56:703-4.
11438 *J Agric Food Chem* 2001;49:490-6.
11439 *J Agric Food Chem* 1999;47:4384-7.
11440 *J Am Diet Assoc* 2001;101:586-7.
11441 *Int Immunopharmacol* 2003;3:129-36.
11442 *Indian J Med Res* 1985;81:162-8.
11443 *Ann Allergy Asthma Immunol* 2003;90:355-8.
11444 *Biol Pharm Bull* 2001;24:209-13.
11445 *J Am Diet Assoc* 1999;99:1361.
11446 *J Can Dent Assoc* 1990;56:7-12.
11447 *Eur J Pharmacol* 1979;60:373-7.
11448 *J Toxicol Environ Health* 1987;20:199-208.
11449 *Phytomedicine* 2003;10:363-9.
11450 *J Cardiovasc Pharmacol* 2000;35:700-7.
11451 *J Herb Pharmacother* 2003;3:19-29.
11452 *J Clin Oncol* 2003;21:2372-6.
11453 *J Sports Sci* 2003;21:577-88
11454 *Nutr Res* 2003;23:1619-29.
11455 *Biomed Pharmacother* 1997;51:176-80.
11456 *Phytomedicine* 2003;10:348-57.
11457 *Phytomedicine* 2002;9:681-6.
11458 *Contact Dermatitis* 2002;47:189-98.
11459 *Rheumatology* 2002;41:279-84.
11460 *Planta Med* 2003;69:162-4.
11462 *J Clin Pharmacol* 1977;17:308-18.
11463 *Nutr Res* 2003;23:1631-42.
11464 *Fertil Steril* 2003;80:1495-501.
11465 *World J Urol* 2003;21:346-55.
11466 *Arch Intern Med* 2003;163:983.
11467 *Diabetes* 2003;52:2110-20.
11468 *Curr Opin Pediatr* 2002;14:702-6.
11469 *J Inherit Metab Dis* 2000;23:677-83.
11470 *Amino Acids* 2001;21:139-50.
11472 *Alzheimer Dis Assoc Disord* 2003;17:113-6.
11473 *Anaesthesia* 2001;56:1178-80.
11474 *J Rheumatol Suppl* 1996;46:81-8.
11475 *J Rheumatol Suppl* 1996;46:60-72.
11476 *J Rheumatol Suppl* 1996;46:44-58.
11477 *Mayo Clin Proc* 1994;69:702-4.
11478 *Mayo Clin Proc* 1994;69:620-5.
11479 *Eur J Vasc Endovasc Surg* 2001;22:365-72.
11480 *J Clin Pharm Ther* 2002;27:229-30.
11481 *Bioorg Med Chem Lett* 2000;10:157-60.
11482 *J Natl Cancer Inst* 2002;94:1641-7.
11485 *Planta Med* 2002;68:1024-8.
11486 *Life Sci* 2002;70:3049-58.
11487 *Phytother Res* 2003;17:174-8.
11488 *J Clin Endocrinol Metab* 2002;87:3691-5.
11490 *Phytomedicine* 2001;8:306-9.
11491 *J Ethnopharmacol* 1991;34:61-8.
11492 *J Ethnopharmacol* 1994;41:185-92.
11493 *J Ethnopharmacol* 1989;27:347-52.
11494 *Biochem Pharmacol* 1992;44:180-3.
11501 *J Am Diet Assoc* 1995;95:798-800.
11502 *Cancer* 1992;70:2579-85.
11507 *J Clin Endocrinol Metab* 1987;64:1165-8.
11508 *Arch Dermatol* 1988;124:1802-4.
11509 *Arch Dermatol* 1988;124:1844-8.
11512 *Proc Natl Acad Sci U S A* 1995;92:8171-5.
11513 *Lancet* 1983;1:1215-6.
11514 *Lancet* 1980;1:39-40.
11515 *Indian Pediatr* 2003;40:36-40.
11516 *Ann Intern Med* 1986;105:924-31.
11517 *Pediatr Infect Dis J* 2002;21:1088-90.
11518 *Am J Gastroenterol* 1995;90:1526-8.
11519 *Neth J Med* 2003;61:19-21.
11520 *Ann Pharmacother* 2003;37:510-2.
11521 *Am J Obstet Gynecol* 1993;168:923-8.
11522 *Am J Obstet Gynecol* 1993;168:884-8.
11523 *Eur J Pediatr* 1998;157:663-5.
11524 *JAMA* 1976;235:626-7.
11525 *Drugs* 1995;49:376-87.
11526 *Int J Vitam Nutr Res Suppl* 1982;23:83-90.
11527 *Int J Vitam Nutr Res* 1985;55:197-204.
11528 *Nutr Rep* Int 1977;15:255-64.
11529 *Clin Nephrol* 1986;26:146-9.
11530 *Br J Clin Pract* 1977;31:17-9.
11531 *Digestion* 1990;46:61-4.
11532 *J Lab Clin Med* 1984;104;546-52.
11533 *Clin Pharmacol Ther* 1983;34:529-32.
11534 *J Child Neurol* 1996;11:244-6.
11537 *Arterioscler Thromb Vasc Biol* 2001;21:1320-6.
11538 *Am J Clin Nutr* 1991;54:1193s-7s.
11539 *Practitioner* 1984;228:312-3.
11540 *Ann Intern Med* 1972;77:557-63.
11541 *Pharmacist's Letter* 2003;19(11):191105.
11543 *Circulation* 1998;98:1350-1.
11546 *Altern Med Rev* 2003;8:43-54.
11547 *J Lab Clin Med* 1969;74:789-802.
11548 *Am J Cardiol* 1995;75:348-53.
11555 *Clin Lab Haematol* 1996;18:55-7.
11556 *Urol Int* 1998;61:39-42.
11561 *Tubercle* 1985;66:49-54.
11562 *Clin Endocrinol (Oxf)* 1994;41:831-8.
11563 *J R Soc Med* 1982;75:533-6.
11564 *Tubercle* 1981;62:207-9.
11565 *Clin Pharmacol Ther* 1982;32:525-30.
11566 *Toxicol Appl Pharmacol* 1975;31:544-7.
11567 *Toxicol Appl Pharmacol* 1974;28:53-6.
11571 *Br J Nutr* 2001;85:S181-5.
11574 *Am J Clin Nutr* 1979;32:2269-71.
11575 *Devel Pharmacol Ther* 1989;14:96-101.

11576 *Trop Geog Med* 1985;37:175-7.
11577 *Devel Pharmacol Ther* 1982;5:109-13.
11578 *Pediatr Pharmacol* 1980;1:129-34.
11579 *Am J Clin Nutr* 2004;79:238-43.
11580 *JAMA* 1975;232:19.
11582 *Haematologica* 2002;87:420-6.
11583 *Am J Clin Nutr* 1988;47:700-6.
11584 *Blood* 1989;73:141-9.
11585 *Circulation* 1996;94:2434-40.
11586 *Nutr Rev* 1999;57:306-9.
11587 *Atherosclerosis* 1998;139:179-87.
11588 *Ann Oncol* 1998;9:1331-7.
11589 *J Clin Oncol* 2004;22:517-28.
11595 *J Am Coll Nutr* 1994;13:559-64.
11596 *Clin Nephrol* 1989;31:123-7.
11597 *Am J Physiol* 1985;249:G209-13.
11598 *J Nutr* 1991;121:13-23.
11599 *J Clin Endocrinol Metab* 1987;65:1301-4.
11701 *Biochem Biophys Res Commun* 2000;279:407-11.
11702 *Zhong Yao Cai* 2002;25:651-3.
11703 *Chem Senses* 2003;28:659-70.
11704 *Microsc Res Tech* 1993;24:195-213.
11705 *Eur J Neurosci* 2002;15:1907-17.
11706 *Physiol Behav* 1993;53:587-92.
11707 *Chem Senses* 2000;25:659.
11708 *Am J Cardiol* 2003;91:1510-3, A9.
11709 *J Nutr* 2003;133:1281-5.
11711 *J Agric Food Chem* 2003;51:4213-8.
11712 *Br J Clin Pharmacol* 1989;28:535-44.
11713 *J Ped* 1938;18:60-2.
11714 *Ceska Slov Farm* 1995;44:190-95.
11715 *Eksp Klin Farmakol* 1998;61:69-74.
11716 *JAMA* 1999;281:1998-2004.
11717 *Fed Regist* 1998;63:62977-63015.
11719 *Environ Health Perspect* 2000;108:309-19.
11720 *Phytochemistry* 2002;61:729-36.
11722 *Drug Metab Rev* 2002;34:47-54.
11723 *Drugs* 1980;20:216-24.
11724 *Am J Clin Nutr* 1982;36:950-62.
11725 *Lipids* 1987;22:417-20.
11726 *Arch Int Physiol Biochim* 1980;88:B17-B19.
11727 *South Med J* 1987;80:1290-3.
11728 *Gastroenterology* 1989;97:761-5.
11729 *Am J Perinatol* 1999;16:415-20.
11730 *J Acquir Immune Defic Syndr* 1999;22:253-9.
11731 *JAMA* 2004;291:1213-9.
11732 *JAMA* 2004;291:1199-201.
11733 *Food Addit Contam* 2003;20:1-30.
11734 Food and Nutrition Board, Institute of Medicine. Nutrition during lactation. Washington, DC: National Academy Press, 1991. Available at: http://books.nap.edu/books/0309043913/html.
11735 *Clin Pharmacol Ther* 1995;58:288-98.
11736 *Clin Pharmacol Ther* 1982;31:656-61.
11737 *Eur J Clin Pharmacol* 1985;28:425-8.
11738 *Clin Pharmacol Ther* 1991;50:363-71.
11739 *Pharmacol Exp Ther* 1997;282:1465-72.
11740 *Eur J Clin Pharmacol* 1989;37:279-83.
11741 *Clin Pharmacokinet* 2000;39:127-53.
11742 *Pharmacotherapy* 1995;29:425-7.
11743 *Food Chem Toxicol* 2002;40:1243-55.
11744 *Clin Nephrol* 1985;24:300-4.
11745 *J Periodontol* 1987;58:470-4.
11746 *J Endod* 2002;28:34-5.
11747 *Clin Nucl Med* 2004;29:81-5.
11748 *Eur Urol* 2003;44:519-26.
11749 *J Natl Med Assoc* 2002;94:706-11.
11750 *Oncology* 1998;55:377-81.
11751 *Radiother Oncol* 1994;31:33-40.
11752 *JAMA* 1995;274:420-4.
11753 *Bone* 2001;28:446-53.
11754 *Bone* 1996;18:253-9.
11755 Metastron prescribing information. Medi-Physics, Inc., Amersham Healthcare, Arlington Heights, IL, 1998. http://www.cancerpaintherapy.com/METATECHPAGE.htm. (Accessed 13 March 2004).
11756 *J Can Dent Assoc* 2003;69:221-6.
11757 Drug Enforcement Agency. Peyote and mescaline. http://www.usdoj.gov/dea/concern/peyote.html. (Accessed 14 March 2004).
11758 *S D J Med* 2001;54:27-9.
11759 *Proc West Pharmacol Soc* 2003;46:153-5.
11760 *Lancet* 1982;1:704-5.
11761 *Cancer Res* 2003;63:4786-91.
11762 *J Nutr Biochem* 2001;12:351-56.
11763 *J Natl Cancer Inst* 2002;94:1275-81.
11764 *Ann Pharmacother* 2002;36:921-6.
11765 *Urology* 2001;58:36-8.
11766 *BMJ* 2004;328:797.
11767 *Cancer Chemother Rep* 1975;59:1151-4.
11768 *Pediatrics* 1975;55:814-7.
11769 *Eur J Respir Dis* 1985;66:13-20.
11770 *Cleve Clin J Med* 2002;69:449-50.
11771 *Am J Cardiol* 2004;93:343-6.
11772 *J Nucl Med Technol* 2002;30:123-7.
11773 *Cochrane Database Syst Rev* 2002;3:CD003335.
11774 *CMAJ* 2003;169:1269-73.
11775 *Psychosomatics* 2002;43:508-9.
11776 *Pharm Res* 1994;11:1707-11.
11777 *Br J Clin Pract* 1986;40:292-3.
11778 *Br J Clin Pract* 1984;38:394-98.
11779 *Br Med J* 1979;2:835-6.
11780 *Br J Clin Pharmacol* 1984;18:638-40.
11781 *Clin J Pain* 2002;18:200-2.
11782 *Postgrad Med J* 1987;63:717.
11783 *Clin Pharmacol Ther* 2002;72:247-55.
11784 *J Pharm Sci* 2002;91:77-90.
11785 *Biomed Pap Med Fac Univ Palacky Olomouc Czech Repub* 2001;145:17-26.
11786 Food Standards Agency. Medicines and Healthcare products Regulatory Agency (MHRA). Expert Group on Vitamins and Minerals. Available at: http://www.foodstandards.gov.uk/multimedia/pdfs/vitmin2003.pdf.
11787 *Am J Health Syst Pharm* 1999;56:1950-6.
11788 *Psychosom Med* 2004;66:276-82.
11789 *J Gastroenterol Hepatol* 1988;3:235-8.
11791 *Int J Cancer* 2004;10;109:949-54.
11792 *Arch Biochem Biophys* 2001;389:1-6.
11793 *Clin Dermatol* 1998;16:295-8.
11794 *Med J Aust* 2003;178:451-3.
11795 *Med J Aust* 2003;178:442-3.
11797 *Wien Med Wochenschr* 2002;152:423-6.
11798 *Optometry* 2004;75:216-30.
11799 *Pediatr Emerg Care* 2003;19:169-71.
11800 *Br J Clin Pharmacol* 2002;54:277-82.
11801 *Ann Pharmacother* 2003;37:150.
11802 *J Clin Pharmacol* 2004;44:95-101.
11803 *Pharmacol Res* 1990;22:37-44.
11804 *Life Sci* 2002;70:3077-96.
11805 *Maturitas* 2004;47:1-9.
11806 *Maturitas* 2004;47:11-20.
11807 *J Natl Cancer Inst* 2003;95:906-13.

11808 FDA. Office of Regulatory Affairs. Automatic detention of stevia leaves, extract of stevia leaves, and food containing stevia. http://www.fda.gov/ora/fiars/ora_import_ia4506.html (Accessed 21 April 2004).
11809 *Clin Ther* 2003;25:2797-808.
11810 *Br J Clin Pharmacol* 2000;50:215-20.
11811 *Phytochemistry* 2003;64:913-21.
11812 *Metabolism* 2004;53:73-6.
11813 *Metabolism* 2004;53:101-7.
11814 *J Am Geriatr Soc* 2003;51:1762-7.
11815 *Am J Clin Nutr* 1999;69:842-56.
11816 *Ren Fail* 2003;25:1011-8.
11818 *Endocrinol Metab Clin North Am* 2000;29:591-609.
11819 *Clin Endocrinol (Oxf)* 1995;43:479-90.
11820 *N Engl J Med* 2000;343:1863-75.
11821 *Hepatol* 2001;33:301-7.
11822 *Am J Med* 1999;107:595-605.
11823 *Nephrol Dial Transplant* 2002;17 Suppl 10:6-9.
11824 *Med J Aust* 2004;180:354-9.
11825 *Br J Haematol* 1998;100:516-20.
11826 *Joint Bone Spine* 2001;68:125-9.
11827 *Obstet Gynecol* 2004;103:203-16.
11828 *Acta Obstet Gynecol Scand* 2004;83:103-7.
11829 *Eur J Clin Invest* 1995;25:629-38.
11830 *Ann Allergy Asthma Immunol* 2002;88:67-8.
11831 *Eur J Haematol* 2001;66:195-9.
11832 Institute of Medicine. Caffeine for the Sustainment of Mental Task Performance: Formulations for Military Operations. Washington, DC: National Academy Press, 2001. Available at: http://books.nap.edu/books/0309082587/html/index.html.
11833 *Food Chem Toxicol* 2002;40:1235-42.
11834 *J Am Geriatr Soc* 1991;39:160-4.
11835 *Clin Exp Pharmacol Physiol* 1996;23:559-63.
11836 *Psychopharmacology (Berl)* 1997;129:1-14.
11837 *West J Med* 1992;157:544-53.
11838 *Forensic Sci Int* 2004;139:71-3.
11839 *Food Chem Toxicol* 2002;40:1257-61.
11840 *Clin Pharmacol Ther* 1986;39:265-70.
11842 Youngkin EQ, et al, eds. Pharmacotherapeutics - a primary care clinical guide. Stamford, CT: Appleton & Lange, 1999.
11844 *J Am Pharm Assoc* 2002;42:625-37.
11845 *Med J Aust* 2001;174:520-1.
11847 *J Nat Prod* 1999;62:901-3.
11848 *J Postgrad Med* 1996;42:105-8.
11849 *Teratog Carcinog Mutagen* 2001;21:303-13.
11850 *Phytother Res* 2001;15:307-10.
11851 *J Exp Clin Cancer Res* 2000;19:459-65.
11852 *J Ethnopharmacol* 1999;66:263-9.
11853 *Pharmacol Res* 1998;38:487-92.
11854 *Indian J Exp Biol* 1998;36:371-4.
11855 *Life Sci* 1998;63:1823-34.
11856 *Zhongguo Yao Li Xue Bao* 1992;13:197-200.
11857 *Int Arch Allergy Appl Immunol* 1991;95:128-33.
11858 *J Postgrad Med* 1983;29:89-95.
11859 *Eur J Pharmacol* 2001;433:225-30.
11860 *Free Radic Biol Med* 1990;9:127-31.
11861 *Scand J Urol Nephrol* 1993;27:267-9.
11862 *Eur J Clin Pharmacol* 1993;44:295-8.
11863 *Head Neck* 2003;25:595-601.
11864 *Cancer Epidemiol Biomarkers Prev* 2003;12:508-13.
11865 *J Agric Food Chem* 2004;52:1990-5.
11866 *J Hum Nutr Diet* 2001;14:243-50.
11867 *J Agric Food Chem* 2002;50:4820-6.
11868 *Circulation* 1996;94:2337-40.
11869 *Thorax* 1988;43:93-7.
11872 *Neurology* 2005;64:713-5.
11873 FDA. List of Orphan Designations and Approvals. http://www.fda.gov/orphan/DESIGNAT/list.htm (Accessed 19 June 2004).
11874 Gray J, ed. Therapeutic Choices, second ed. Ottawa: Canadian Pharmacists Association, 1998.
11875 *Am J Clin Nutr* 1973;26:191-6
11876 *Am J Clin Nutr* 1972;25:684-9.
11877 *Atherosclerosis* 2003;168:169-79.
11878 *Alcohol Res Health* 2001;25:230-4.
11879 *N Engl J Med* 2003;348:109-18.
11880 Departments of Health and Human Services and Agriculture. Dietary Guidelines for Americans, 5th edition. Available at: http://www.health.gov/dietaryguidelines/dga2000/document/choose.htm#alcohol.
11881 *Curr Opin Pulm Med* 2000;6:442-7.
11882 *Semin Liver Dis* 2002;22:195-206.
11883 FDA. Pyrrolizidine Alkaloids. Center for Food Safety & Applied Nutrition Foodborne Pathogenic Microorganisms and Natural Toxins Handbook. Available at: http://vm.cfsan.fda.gov/~mow/chap42.html.
11884 *Prostaglandins Leukot Essent Fatty Acids* 2002;67:1-12.
11886 *Br J Clin Pharmacol* 2003;56:683-90.
11887 *Clin Pharmacol Ther* 2003;74:525-35.
11888 *Clin Pharmacol Ther* 2004;76:323-9.
11889 *Drug Metab Dispos* 2004;32:512-8.
11890 *Br J Clin Pharmacol* 2004;57:592-9.
11891 *J Ethnopharmacol* 2001;77:259-64.
11892 *Biochim Biophys Acta* 2004;1660:171-99.
11893 *Endocr Pract* 2003;9:417-70.
11894 *Pharmacotherapy* 2001;21:797-806.
11895 *Mech Ageing Dev* 2004;125:41-6.
11896 *Free Radic Biol Med* 2004;36:1043-57.
11897 *Curr Opin Neurol* 1998;11:193-7.
11898 *JAMA* 2003;289:1681-90.
11899 *Clin Cancer Res* 1996;2:483-91.
11900 *Invest New Drugs* 2001;19:81-3.
11901 *Ann Neurol* 1984;16:723.
11902 *J Cardiovasc Surg (Torino)* 1996;37:229-35.
11903 *Ann Thorac Surg* 1994;58:1427-32.
11904 *Ann Thorac Surg* 1996;61:829-33.
11905 *Thromb Haemost* 2002;87:1075-6.
11906 *Menopause* 2004;11:575-7.
11907 *Diabetes Care* 2004;27:2741-51.
11908 *Diabetes Care* 2004;27:2211-6.
11909 *Med J Aust* 2003;178:411-2.
11910 *Med J Aust* 2004;180:598-600.
11911 *Menopause* 2004;11:281-9.
11912 *Breast Cancer Res Treat* 2004;83:221-31.
11913 *Obstet Gynecol* 2001;97:suppl 1-11.
11915 *Contact Dermatitis* 1999;40:165.
11916 *JAMA* 2004;291:1999-2006.
11917 *J Am Geriatr Soc* 2003;51:1533-8.
11918 *Age Ageing* 2002;31:267-71.
11919 *Am J Clin Nutr* 2002;75:611-5.
11920 *Arch Dermatol* 1976;112:202-3.
11921 *J Bone Miner Res* 2004;19:265-9.
11922 *Osteoporos Int* 2002;13:187-94.
11923 *Arch Intern Med* 2000; 160:1199–203.
11924 *J Bone Miner Res* 2000;15:1113-8.
11925 *J Bone Miner Res* 2002;17:891-7.
11926 *Am J Epidemiol* 1996;143:1129-36.
11927 *J Bone Miner Res* 2002;17:709-15.
11928 *Ann Intern Med* 1996;124:400-6.

11930 *N Engl J Med* 1992;327:1637-42.
11931 *BMJ* 2003;326:469.
11932 *J Am Geriatr Soc* 2004;52:230-6.
11933 *J Am Coll Nutr* 2003;22:142-6.
11935 *Am J Clin Nutr* 2004;79:362-71.
11936 *J Gen Intern Med* 2002;17:733-5.
11937 Arnas LAG, Heaney RP, Hollis BW. Vitamin D2 is much less effective than vitamin D3 in humans (abstract OR22-2). The Endocrine Society 86th Annual Meeting, June 16-19, New Orleans, LA.
11938 *Am J Clin Nutr* 1998;68:854-8.
11939 *J Bone Miner Res* 2003;18:343-51.
11940 *J Am Coll Nutr* 2004;23:303-8.
11941 *Clin Exp Allergy* 2004;34:646-9.
11942 *Ann Allergy Asthma Immunol* 2004;93:56-60.
11943 *Atherosclerosis* 2004;175:117-23.
11944 *Acta Pharmacol Sin* 2002;23:1127-41.
11945 *Br J Pharmacol* 2000;131:1172-8.
11946 *J Pharm Pharmacol* 2000;52:1425-9.
11947 *J Pharm Pharmacol* 2001;53:721-5.
11948 *J Pharm Pharmacol* 2000;52:1017-22.
11949 *Anticancer Drugs* 2003;14:211-7.
11950 *J Pharm Pharmacol* 2003;55:1583-91.
11951 *Am J Chin Med* 2000;28:379-84.
11952 *Biochem Pharmacol* 2000;60:433-40.
11953 *J Nat Prod* 1998;61:808-11.
11954 *J Ethnopharmacol* 2003;87:115-7.
11955 *Biosci Biotechnol Biochem* 1996;60:204-8.
11956 *Planta Med* 2002;68:173-5.
11957 *J Pharmacol Sci* 2003;93:69-73.
11958 *J Ethnopharmacol* 2004;93:391-5.
11959 *J Nutr Sci Vitaminol (Tokyo)* 1999;45:791-5.
11960 *In Vivo* 2004;18:55-62.
11961 *Int J Sports Med*. 2001;22:537-43.
11962 *Int J Obes Relat Metab Disord* 2003;27:522-9.
11963 *Nutr Neurosci* 2001;4:169-78.
11964 *Integr Cancer Ther* 2002;1:110-20.
11965 *Angiogenesis* 2003;6:143-9.
11966 *Pharmacol Biochem Behav* 2002;72:39-43.
11967 Clinicaltrials.gov. Phase I Study of Noni in Cancer Patients. http://www.clinicaltrials.gov/ct/show/NCT00033878?order=1 (Accessed 17 September 2004).
11968 *J Sex Marital Ther* 2003;29:33-44.
11969 *Drugs* 2003;63:1445-57.
11970 *Arch Intern Med* 2004;164:1237-41.
11971 Wiwanikit V, Taungjarwinai W. A case report of suspected ginseng allergy. Medscape General Medicine 6 (3), 2004. http://www.medscape.com/viewarticle/482833 (Accessed 17 September 2004).
11972 *Br J Dermatol* 2004;150:966-9.
11973 *J Pharm Pharmacol* 1999;51:1305-12.
11976 *Clin Pharmacol Ther* 2003;73:529-37.
11977 *Food Chem Toxicol* 2004;42:1513-29.
11978 *Am J Clin Nutr* 2000;71:1325S-33S.
11979 *Cancer* 2004;101:370-8.
11980 *J Spinal Cord Med* 2004;27:35-40.
11981 *Dement Geriatr Cogn Disord* 2004;18:217-26.
11982 *Obstet Gynecol* 1991;78:115-7.
11983 *J Med Food* 2004;7:61-6.
11984 *Aliment Pharmacol Ther* 2004;19:739-47.
11985 *Circulation* 2004;109:966-71.
11986 *J Am Coll Nutr* 2004;23:55-62.
11987 *Ther Drug Monit* 2001;23:698-708.
11988 Food and Drug Administration. FDA Advises Dietary Supplement Manufacturers to Remove Comfrey Products From the Market. July 6, 2001. Available at: http://www.cfsan.fda.gov/~dms/dspltr06.html.
11989 *Circulation* 2002;106:1943-8.
11990 *Public Health Nutr* 2000;3:501-8.
11991 *Am J Med* 1990;89:547-8.
11992 *Fortschr Med Orig* 2002;120:1-9.
11993 *Maturitas* 2004;48:372-80.
11994 *Menopause* 2004;11:400-4.
11995 *J Pharmacol Exp Ther* 2001;299:96-104.
11996 *Neurology* 2004;62:1701-5.
11997 *Am J Clin Nutr* 2004;79:1029-36.
11998 *Arch Dermatol* 1965;92:76-7.
11999 *Am J Clin Nutr* 2004;80:143-8.
12000 *J Altern Complement Med* 2002;8:229.
12001 Health and Human Services. HHS launches crackdown on products containing Andro. March, 2004.
12002 Mangold T. Sampling the Kalahari cactus diet. BBC News; May 30, 2003.
12003 Pfizer returns rights of P57. Phytopharm Press Release; July 30, 2003.
12004 Phytopharm plc successful completion of proof of principle clinical study of P57 for Obesity. Phytopharm Press Release; December 5, 2001.
12005 FDA Warns Distributors of Dietary Supplements Promoted Online for Weight Loss. FDA Press Release; April 1, 2004.
12006 Cohen B, Schardt D. Center for Science in the Public Interest. Letter to Food and Drug Administration. Commissioner Mark McClellan, MD, PhD. March 4, 2004.
12007 FDA Expands Warning About "Green Hornet" To Include All Other Products By Cytotec Solutions, Inc. FDA Press Release, April 9, 2004.
12008 *Curr Ther Res Clin Exp* 2002;63:344-53..
12009 *Clin Radiol* 2003;58:301-5.
12010 *Fertil Steril* 2003;80:459-61.
12011 Neinhuys JW. The True Story of Oscillococcinum. HomeoWatch 2003. http://www.homeowatch.org/history/oscillo.html (Accessed 21 April 2004).
12012 *Nutr Res* 2003;23:1189-98..
12013 *J Nat Prod* 2003;66:1124-7.
12014 *Chem Pharm Bull (Tokyo)* 2003;51:857-9.
12015 *Planta Med* 2002;68:975-9.
12016 *Phytochemistry* 2002;60:541-8.
12017 *Planta Med* 1996;62:471-2.
12018 *Skinmed* 2002;2:117-22.
12019 *Arch Dermatol* 2002;138:1486-93.
12020 *Dermatol Surg* 2004;30:32-6.
12021 *Br J Dermatol* 2003;149:841-9.
12022 *Biochem Biophys Res Commun* 1994;201:665-72.
12023 *Skin Res Technol* 2002;8:164-7.
12024 *JAMA* 2001;285:2486-97.
12026 *Pharmacist's Letter* 2004;20(5):200504.
12027 *Pharmacists's Letter* 2003:18:181202.
12028 *Pharmacist's Letter* 2003;19:191205.
12029 FDA Warning Letter to Hyalogic LLC. May 5, 2004. Available at: http://www.fda.gov/foi/warning_letters/g4681d.htm (Accessed June 30, 2004).
12030 *Ann Pharmacother* 2004;38:812-6.
12031 *J Agric Food Chem* 2004;52:3329-32.
12032 *Ann Intern Med* 2004;141:23-7.
12033 *Arch Intern Med* 2004;164:164:697-705.
12034 *JAMA* 2004;292:65-74.
12035 *Scand J Rheumatol* 1983;12:85-8.

12036 *Ann Rheum Dis* 1988;47:96-104.
12037 *Scand J Rheumatol* 1986;15:103-8.
12038 *Prostaglandins Leukot Med* 1982;8:403-8.
12039 *Psychopharmacology (Berl)* 2001;157:430-6.
12040 *Menopause* 2003;10:196-202.
12041 *Cancer Epidemiol Biomarkers Prev* 2003;12:144-50.
12042 *Circulation* 2004;110:227-39.
12044 *Am J Clin Nutr* 2003;78:593S-609S.
12045 *J Paediatr Child Health* 2004;40:154-5.
12046 *N Engl J Med* 2004;351:56-67.
12047 *N Engl J Med* 2004;351:302-3.
12048 *Pharmacol Biochem Behav* 2003;75:721-9.
12049 *J Nutr* 2002;132:3577-84.
12050 *J Nutr* 2003;133:245S-8S.
12051 *Am J Clin Nutr* 2004;79:907S-12S.
12052 *J Clin Endocrinol Metab* 2004;89:632-7.
12053 *Dig Dis Sci* 1995;40:576-9.
12054 *BMC Musculoskelet Disorders* 2004;5:6.
12055 *Circulation* 2004;110:368-73.
12056 *Acta Neurol Scand* 1993;88:334-8.
12057 *J Neurol* 1992;239:79-81.
12058 *Medical Hypotheses* 1991;34:20-3.
12059 *Clin Neuropharmacol* 1991;14:403-12.
12060 *BMC Psychiatry* 2004;4:9.
12061 *Biochem Biophys Res Commun* 2004;318:1072–8.
12063 *Am J Health-Syst Pharm* 1998;55:1581-3.
12064 *Eur J Endocrinol* 2003;149:351-62.
12069 FDA. U.S. District Judge Issues Permanent Injunction Against Lane Labs-USA, Inc. and Orders Firm to Refund Money to Purchasers of Illegally Marketed Unapproved Drugs. FDA News; July 13, 2004. Available at: www.fda.gov/bbs/topics/news/2004/NEW01086.html (Accessed 3 August 2004).
12070 *Life Sci* 2003;73:1289-98.
12071 *Nutrition* 2003;19:261–4.
12072 *Experientia* 1987;43:1110-1.
12073 *Acta Haematol* 1990;84:139-43.
12074 *Biol Pharm Bull* 1995;18:1387-91.
12075 *Angiology* 2003;54:531-9.
12076 *J Rheumatol* 2004;31:767-74.
12077 *J Neurol Neurosurg Psychiatry* 2004;75:1093-99.
12078 *Pharmacol Rev* 2000;52:673-751.
12079 *Internat J Vit Nutr Res* 1973;43:494-503.
12080 *Internat J Vit Nutr Res* 1977;47:373-82.
12081 *Internat J Vit Nutr Res* 1975;45:51-60.
12082 *J Clin Pharmacol* 1973;13:401-7.
12083 *J Clin Pharmacol* 1973;13:271-5.
12084 *J Agric Food Chem* 2002;50:5837-43.
12085 *Arch Intern Med* 2004;164:1334-40.
12086 *Am J Clin Nutr* 2004;80:391-5.
12087 *J Agric Food Chem* 2004;52:3661-5.
12088 *Rheum Dis Clin North Am* 1995;21:759-77.
12089 *Semin Arthritis Rheum* 1995;25:87-96.
12090 *Biochem Biophys Res Commun* 1993;197:1340-7.
12091 *J Biol Chem* 2001;276:24690-6.
12092 *Federal Practitioner* 2004;April:9-17.
12093 *Eur J Drug Metab Pharmacokinet* 2003;28:179-84.
12094 *JAMA* 2004;292:828-36.
12095 *Int J Sport Nutr Exerc Metab* 2004;14:236-42.
12096 *Trop Med Int Health* 1996;1:505–9.
12097 *Burns* 2003;28:834-6.
12098 *Cancer Nurs* 2002;25:442-51.
12099 *Arch Neurol* 2004;61:889-92.
12100 *Int J Clin Pharmacol Ther Toxicol* 1992;30:331-5.
12101 *J Int Med Res* 1991;19:330-41.
12102 *Ann N Y Acad Sci* 1994;717:253-69.
12103 *Int J Clin Pharmacol Ther Toxicol* 1991;29:103-7.
12104 *J Nat Prod* 2003;66:535-7.
12105 *Fertil Steril* 2004;82:145-8.
12106 *Diabet Med* 2004;21:114-21.
12107 *Osteoarthritis Cartilage* 2004;12:506-11.
12108 *BMJ* 2004;329(7465):548. Epub 2004 Aug 27.
12110 *J Altern Complement Med* 2002;8:493-7.
12111 *J Nutr* 2004;134:1454-8.
12112 *J Agric Food Chem* 2004;52:2879-86.
12113 Pittler MH, Ernst E. Horse chestnut seed extract for chronic venous insufficiency (Cochrane Review). In: The Cochrane Library, Issue 3, 2004. Chichester, UK: John Wiley & Sons, Ltd..
12114 *Blood Coagul Fibrinolysis* 2004;15:303–9.
12115 *Clin Pharmacol Ther* 2004;75:184-90.
12116 *Pharm Res* 2002;19:802-9.
12117 *Am J Clin Nutr* 2004;80:123–30.
12118 *J Natl Cancer Inst* 2003;95:1765-71.
12119 *Nutr Rev* 2004;62:125-31.
12120 *J Natl Cancer Inst* 2004;96:1015-22.
12121 *FASEB J* 2000;14:1132-8.
12122 *Ann Intern Med* 1983;98:800-5.
12124 *J Am Coll Nutr* 2002;21:47-54.
12125 *J Nutr* 2000;130:1734–42.
12126 *Am J Clin Nutr* 2003;77:1448–52.
12127 *J Clin Endocrinol Metab* 2000;85:4635-8.
12128 *Obes Res* 2004;12:582–90.
12129 *Psychopharmacology (Berl)* 1996;127:88-94.
12130 *Arch Neurol* 1996;53:441-8.
12131 Fioravanti M, Yanagi M. Cytidinephosphoholine (CDP choline) for cognitive and behavioural disturbances associated with chronic cerebral disorders in the elderly (Cochrane Review). In: The Cochrane Library, Issue 3, 2004. Chichester, UK: John Wiley & Sons, Ltd.
12132 *Altern Med Rev* 2004;9:17-31.
12133 *J Neurol Sci* 2003;215:105-10.
12134 *J Neurosci Res* 2003;73:308-15.
12135 *Cerebrovasc Dis* 2003;16:199-204.
12136 *Eur J Pharmacol* 2003;468:129-39.
12137 *J Neurosurg* 2003;98:867-73.
12138 *Neuroscience* 2003;118:107-13.
12139 *Stroke* 2002;33:2850-7.
12140 *J Neurosci Res* 2002;70:133-9.
12141 FDA Warning Letter to Mr. Stephen Cheng, Window Rock Enterprises. August 19, 2004. Available at: http://www.fda.gov/foi/warning_letters/g4945d.htm. (Accessed 17 September 2004).
12142 *Circulation* 2004;110:637-41.
12143 *Planta Med* 1987;53:410-4.
12144 *Am J Chin Med* 2002;30:207-14.
12145 *Clin Exp Allergy* 2000;31:779-81.
12146 *Int Immunopharmacol* 2002;2:1183-93.
12147 *Fed Regist* 2004;69:6787-6854.
12148 *Osteoarthritis Cartilage* 2004;12:269-76.
12149 *Neurology* 2004;63:757.
12150 *N Engl J Med* 2004;350:2673-81.
12151 *N Engl J Med* 2004;350:2708-10.
12152 Sauer J, Tabet N, Howard R. Alpha lipoic acid for dementia (Cochrane Review). In: The Cochrane Library, Issue 3, 2004. Chichester, UK: John Wiley & Sons, Ltd.
12153 Pittler MH, Ernst E. Feverfew for preventing migraine (Cochrane Review). In: The Cochrane Library, Issue 3, 2004. Chichester, UK: John Wiley & Sons, Ltd.
12154 *Clin Pharmacol Ther* 2003;73 (Abstract PDII-A-10) P94.
12155 *Clin Pharmacol Ther* 2003;73 (Abstract PDII-A-8):P94.

12156 *Adv Exp Med Biol* 1987;209:183-9.
12158 *Aliment Pharmacol Ther* 2004;19:521-7.
12159 *Oncol Nurs Forum* 2001;28:543-7.
12160 *J Wound Ostomy Continence Nurs* 2003;30:68-71.
12161 *J Burn Care Rehabil* 1988;9:156-9.
12162 *Arch Otolaryngol Head Neck Surg* 1995;121:678-80.
12163 *Int J Radiat Oncol Biol Phys* 1996;36:345-9.
12164 *Br J Gen Pract* 1999;49:823-8.
12165 *Swiss Med Wkly* 2004;134:385.
12166 *Metabolism* 2004;53:1309-14.
12167 *Steroids* 1993;58:40-6.
12168 *Endocrinol* 1981;108:1597-9.
12169 *Fertil Steril* 2004;81:93-8.
12170 *Clin Cardiol* 2004;27:295–9.
12171 *Arch Dermatol* 2004;140:723-7.
12172 *Chem Pharm Bull* 1978;26:2096-7.
12173 *Med Sci Monit* 2003;9:PI24-8.
12174 *Am J Transplant* 2003;3:1608-9.
12175 *Int J Comp Alt Med* 1994;Sept:21-2.
12176 *Clin Ther* 2003;25:178-93
12177 *Cancer Causes Control* 2003;14:319-26.
12178 *Ther Drug Monit* 2003;25:114-6.
12179 *Br J Clin Pharmacol* 2003;57:448-55.
12181 *Ann Pharmacother* 2004;38:1651-4.
12182 *Diabetes Care* 1998;21:494-500.
12183 *Pediatr Emerg Care* 2003;19:206-10.
12184 *Eur J Drug Metab Pharmacokinet* 2004;29:25-9.
12185 *Lancet* 2004;364:1219-28.
12186 *Altern Med Rev* 2004;9:63-9.
12187 *Eur J Drug Metab Pharmacokinet* 1996;21:223-6.
12188 *Hum Psychopharmacol Clin Exp* 2004;19:457–65.
12189 *J Heart Valve Dis* 2004;13:25-6.
12190 *Cur Ther Res* 1997;58:390-401.
12191 *Clin Exp Pharmacol Physiol* 1987;14:543-6.
12192 *Clin Exp Allergy* 1996;26:1161-70.
12193 *Exp Biol Med* 2004;229:698–704.
12194 *Curr Med Res Opin* 2002;18:s14-s17.
12195 *Life Sci* 1995;56:637-60.
12196 *Prog Neuropsychopharmacol Biol Psychiatry* 2003;27:711–17.
12197 *Mutation Res* 2003;523-524:55-62.
12198 *J Pharm Pharmaceut Sci* 2001;4:176-84.
12199 *Int J Cardiol* 2003;88:101-2.
12200 *Phytochemistry* 2003;64:903-6.
12206 *Arthritis Rheum* 2004;50:72-7.
12207 *Hum Psychopharmacol Clin Exp* 2003;18:191–195.
12208 *Aliment Pharmacol Ther* 2003;18:1099–105.
12209 *Ann Intern Med* 2002;137:E-76
12210 *J Allergy Clin Immunol* 2004;114:459-60.
12211 Brackett RE. Letter Responding to Health Claim Petition dated August 28, 2003: Monounsaturated Fatty Acids from Olive Oil and Coronary Heart Disease. CFSAN/Office of Nutritional Products, Labeling and Dietary Supplements. 2004 Nov 1; Docket No 2003Q-0559. Available at: http://www.fda.gov/ohrms/dockets/dailys/04/nov04/110404/03q-0559-ans0001-01-vol9.pdf.
12212 *Ann Intern Med* 2005;142:60520-53.
12213 *J Alt Comp Med* 2004;431-7.
12214 *J Pharm Pharmaceut Sci* 2004;7:265-73.
12215 *JAMA* 2004;292:2243-8.
12216 *Altern Ther Health Med* 2003;9:74-8.
12217 *Biol Pharm Bull* 2002;25:809-12.
12218 *Biol Pharm Bull* 2002;25:260-3.
12219 *J Ethnopharmacol* 2003;89:67-71.
12220 *Emerg Med J* 2004;21:742-4.
12223 FDA warning letter to Berkeley Premium Nutraceuticals. October 14, 2004. Available at: http://www.fda.gov/foi/warning_letters/g5013d.htm.
12226 Buscemi N, Vandermeer B, Pandya R, et al. Melatonin for treatment of sleep disorders. Summary, Evidence Report/Technology Assessment #108. (Prepared by the Univ of Alberta Evidence-based Practice Center, under Contract#290-02-0023.) AHRQ Publ #05-E002-2. Rockville, MD: Agency for Healthcare Research & Quality. November 2004.
12227 *Br Med J* 2004;329:1375-6.
12228 *Br Med J* 2004;329:1376.
12229 *Proc Soc Exp Biol Med* 1972;140:457-61.
12230 *Int J Toxicol* 2001;20:41-56.
12231 *Pharmacotherapy* 2004;24:1501-7.
12232 *J Neurol Neurosurg Psychiatry* 2004;75:1672-77.
12234 *Circulation* 2004;110:2837-42.
12235 *J Int Med Res* 2004;32:132-40.
12236 *Indian J Exp Biol* 2003;41:1329-33.
12237 *Indian J Exp Biol* 2002;40:1151-60.
12238 *Indian J Exp Biol* 2002;40:1079-82.
12239 *Indian J Exp Biol* 1999 37:1136-8.
12240 *Indian J Exp Biol* 1998;36:1028-31.
12241 *Indian J Exp Biol* 1997;35:380-3.
12242 *Int J Clin Pharmacol Ther* 1996;34:406-9.
12243 *Indian J Exp Biol* 1981;19:975-6.
12244 *Indian J Exp Biol* 1972;10:23-5.
12245 *Cochrane Database Syst Rev* 2004;1:CD001957.
12246 *J Ethnopharmacol* 1987;21:153-63.
12247 *J Ethnopharmacol* 2002;80:15-20.
12248 *J Ethnopharmacol* 2003;88:293-6.
12249 *J Ethnopharmacol* 2003;84:105-8.
12250 *J Ethnopharmacol* 2002;79:95-100.
12251 *JAMA* 1998;280:1397-98.
12252 Anon. Dermatologists can help consumers find the best products to rejuvenate their skin. American Academy of Dermatology, 1999. Available at: http://www.aad.org/PressReleases/rejuvenate.html.
12253 Anon. Skin trauma: A tan is an early warning sign. American Academy of Dermatology, 1996. Available at: www.aad.org.PressReleases/PHOTOAGE.html.
12254 Drake LA, Dinehart SM, Farmer ER, et al. Guidelines of care for photoaging/photodamage. American Academy of Dermatology, 2000. Available at: www.aad.org/Guidelines/Photoagingdamage.html.
12255 Young LY, Koda-Kimble MA, eds. Photosensitivity and Burns. Applied Therapeutics: The Clinical Use of Drugs. 6th ed. Vancouver, WA: Applied Thera Inc., 1995.
12256 *Drug Topics* 1997;17:92-101.
12257 McEvoy GK, ed. AHFS Drug Information. Bethesda, MD: American Society of Health-system Pharmacists, 2000.
12258 Anon. Cosmetic dermatology handbook. American Academy of Dermatology, 2000. Available at: www.aad.org/ss00/cosmetic.html.
12259 *Ann Pharmacother* 1998;32:1365-67.
12261 Anon. Adding vitamins to the mix: Skin care products that can benefit the skin. American Academy of Dermatology, 2000. Available at: www.aad.org/PressReleases/skincare.html.
12262 Anon. All dried out. American Academy of Dermatology, 2000. Available at: www.aad.org/ss98driedou.html.
12263 Anon. Mature skin. American Academy of Dermatology, 2000. Available at: www.aad.org/pamphlets/mature.html.
12264 Anon. Skin tips. American Academy of Dermatology, 1999. Available at: www.aad.org/ss99/stips.html.

12265 *J Cell Biochem Suppl* 1997;27:59-67.
12276 *Trends Pharmacol Sci* 1989;Suppl:85-8.
12277 *Neurosurg* 1984;15:514-8.
12278 *J Neurosurg* 1989;71:481-6.
12279 *Arch Neurol* 1997;54:465-73.
12283 *Prog Neurobiol* 1999;57:301-23.
12284 *Brain Pathol* 1999;9:133-46.
12285 *Free Radic Biol Med* 1999;26:1346-55.
12286 *J Neural Transm Suppl* 1998;54:211-9.
12287 *J Am Geriatr Soc* 1997;45:718-24.
12288 *Int J Geriatr Psychiatry* 1998;13:235-9.
12289 *Arch Neurol* 1998;55:1449-55.
12290 *Age Ageing* 1998;27:485-91.
12291 *Nutr Health* 1998;12:215-26.
12292 *Dev Neurosci* 1996;18:6-21.
12293 *Recent Prog Horm Res* 1997;52:1-32.
12294 *Life Sci* 1996;59:1651-7.
12295 *Ann N Y Acad Sci* 1995;774:111-20.
12296 *Lancet* 1989;2:570.
12297 *Biol Psychiatry* 1991;30:684-90.
12299 *Lancet* 1992;340:1136-9.
12300 *Ther Hung* 1985;33:13-21.
12301 *Journal of Naturopathic Medicine* 1998;8:26-41.
12304 *Neurology* 1998;50:A231-32.
12305 *Int J Geriatr Psychiatry* 1998;13:611-6.
12308 European Commission. Scientific Committee on food. Opinion on stevioside as a sweetener. Adopted on June 17, 1999. Available at: http://europa.eu.int/comm/food/fs/sc/scf/out34_en.pdf.
12310 *Am J Med* 2002;113:17S-24S.
12311 *Diabetes Care* 2000;23:S43-6.
12312 Jermain DM. Sleep disorders. In: DiPiro JT, Talbert RL, Yee GC, et al (eds). Pharmacotherapy: A Pathophysiologic Approach. 4th edition. Stamford, CT: Appleton & Lange, 1999.
12313 Wincor MZ, Cyr M. Sleep disorders. In: Herfindal ET, Gourley DR (eds). Textbook of Therapeutics: Drug and Disease Management. 6th edition. Baltimore, MD: Williams & Wilkins, 1996.
12314 Arana GW, Hyman SE. Handbook of Psychiatric Drug Therapy. 2nd edition. Boston, MA: Little, Brown & Company, 1991.
12315 Rostler S. More studies should target health effects of sleep herbs. Reuters Health, June 15, 2000.
12316 Sonnenblick E. Detecting and treating heart failure: An update on strategies. www.ConsultantLive.com (Accessed 24 January 2001).
12317 *Pharmacotherapy* 2000;20:787-804.
12318 Pharmacotherapy Self-Assessment Program. Module 1: Cardiology. 3rd Ed. Kansas City, MO: American College of Clinical Pharmacy, 1998.
12319 *Pharmacotherapy* 2000;20:495-522.
12320 *Prescriber's Letter* 2000;170104.
12321 *N Engl J Med* 1999;341:709-17.
12322 *N Engl J Med* 2004;351:526-8.
12323 *Mol Cell Biochem* 2000;213:37-41.
12324 *J Natl Cancer Inst* 2000;92:1740-52.
12325 Alternative Medicine Alert, October 2000, p 120.
12326 *Gut* 1998;43:578-85.
12327 *Gastroenterology* 1996;111:445-54.
12328 *N Engl J Med* 2000;342:1946-52.
12329 *Lancet* 1971;I:95-100.
12330 *Scand J Gastroenterol Suppl* 1997;222:76-82.
12331 *Carcinogenesis* 1983;4:45-8.
12332 *Dis Colon Rectum* 1999;42:1300-5.
12333 *Ann Intern Med* 2001;134:89-95.
12334 *JAMA* 1998;280:1074-9.
12335 *Am Fam Physician* 2000;62:1575-82, 1587.
12336 *Arthritis Rheum* 1998;41:778-99.
12337 *Pharmacist's Letter/Prescriber's Letter* 2000;16(8):160803.
12338 *Am J Med* 1992;92:363-7.
12339 *Arthritis Rheum* 1994;37:1593-601.
12341 *Arthritis Rheum* 1992;35:550-6.
12342 *Pharmacist's Letter* 2005;21:210103.
12343 *Journal of Musculoskeletal Pain* 1998;6(Suppl 2):147.
12344 *Arthritis Rheum* 1986;29:1371-7.
12345 *J Rheumatol* 1985;12:980-3.
12346 *JAMA* 2004;292:2388-95.
12347 *Pharmacist's Letter* 2000:16(12):67.
12348 *Am J Med* 1998;104:227-31.
12349 The American College of Obstetricians and Gynecologists. Clinical management guidelines for premenstrual syndrome. ACOG Practice Bulletin. No. 15. April 2000.
12350 *US Pharmacist CE*. September 2004.
12351 *Toxicol Lett* 2001;123:169-77.
12352 *Fertil Steril* 2004;81:1578-84.
12353 *Urology* 2004;63:641-6.
12354 *Clin Infect Dis* 2004;38:1367-71.
12355 *J Clin Pharm Ther* 2004;29:75-83.
12356 *Br J Dermatol* 1993;128:301-5.
12357 *J Agric Food Chem* 2002;50:1581-6.
12358 *Br J Nutr* 2001;85:583-9.
12359 *J Allergy Clin Immunol* 1999;103:1180-5.
12360 *Allergy* 2003;58:825-6.
12361 *Am J Clin Nutr* 1985;42:190-7.
12362 *J Nutr* 2004;134:410-5.
12363 *J Nutr* 2003;133:3422-7.
12366 *Clin Exp Pharmacol Physiol* 2003;30:38-43.
12367 *Singapore Med J* 2002;43:617-21.
12368 *J Ethnopharmacol* 2002;80:203-6.
12369 *J Agric Food Chem* 2004;52:2541-5.
12370 *J Pharm Pharmacol* 2001;53:1139-43.
12371 *Mol Cell Biochem* 2003;243:23-8.
12372 *J Nutr Biochem* 2003;14:452-8.
12373 *J Ethnopharmacol* 2004;90:145-50.
12374 *Diabetes Care* 2004;27:2047-8.
12375 *Am J Clin Nutr* 2004;80:22-8.
12376 *Naunyn Schmiedebergs Arch Pharmacol* 2001;364:21-6.
12377 *Neurosci Lett* 1996;214:107-10.
12378 *Experientia* 1979;35:1283-4.
12379 *Neurochem Res* 1993;18:1179-82.
12380 *J Clin Pharm Ther* 2004;29:37-45.
12381 *Phytother Res* 2004;18:47-53.
12382 *Phytomedicine* 2003;10:271-85.
12383 *Public Health Nutr* 2000;3:509-14.
12384 *Cephalalgia* 2002;22:523-32.
12385 Geohas J, Finch M, Juturu V, et al. Improvement in Fasting Blood Glucose with the Combination of Chromium Picolinate and Biotin in Type 2 Diabetes Mellitus. American Diabetes Association 64th Annual Meeting, June 2004, Orlando, Florida, abstract 191-OR.
12386 *Headache* 2003;43:76-8.
12387 *Eur J Neurol* 2004;11:475-7.
12388 *Headache* 2002;42:114-9.
12389 *Headache* 2004;44:885-90.
12390 Albarracin C, Fuqua B, Finch M, et al. Glycemic Control Is Improved by the Combination of Chromium Picolinate and Biotin in Type 2 Diabetes Mellitus. American Diabetes Association 64th Annual Meeting, June 2004, Orlando, Florida, abstract 2483-PO.

12391 *Prostaglandins Leukot Essent Fatty Acids* 2003;69:61-6.
12392 *J Toxicol Clin Toxicol* 1999;37:731-51.
12393 *Ann Emerg Med* 2002;39:273-86.
12394 *J Toxicol Clin Toxicol* 2004;42:133-43.
12395 *Am J Gastroenterol* 1981;75:192-6.
12396 *Am J Gastroenterol* 1999;94:208-12.
12397 *Eur J Clin Pharmacol* 1989;37:225-30.
12398 *J Clin Pharmacol* 1988;28:416-9.
12399 *Neth J Med* 1988;33:209-16.
12400 *J Toxicol Clin Toxicol* 2002;40:59-67.
12401 *BMJ* 2004;328:991.
12402 *J Ethnopharmacol* 1996;52:61-70.
12403 *Am J Gastroenterol* 2003;98:1214-5.
12404 *Food Chem Toxicol* 1996;34:313-6.
12405 *Eur J Drug Metab Pharmacokinet* 1995;20:173-8.
12406 *Eur J Pharmacol* 1991;202:129-31.
12407 *Thromb Res* 1984;36:497-507.
12408 *Ann Emerg Med* 1995;25:713-5.
12409 *Ophthalmology* 2000;107:2186-9.
12410 *Aliment Pharmacol Ther* 2002;16:1075-82.
12411 *Br J Clin Pharmacol* 1995;40:423-9.
12412 *J Clin Pharmacol* 1995;39:271-6.
12413 *Am J Respir Crit Care Med* 1994;150:374-80.
12414 *Ann Allergy* 1990;65:322-3.
12415 *Lancet* 1999:13;353:536-40.
12416 *Ann Emerg Med* 1994;23:1116-8.
12417 *J Chromatogr Sci* 2002;40:441-6.
12418 *Am J Gastroenterol* 1994;89:1577-8.
12420 *Clin Pharmacol Ther* 1971;12:491-5.
12421 *Contraception* 2000;62:253-7.
12422 FDA Import Alert #IA2111. Detention Without Physical Examination Of Ackees (All Types) Due To Contamination By Natural Toxins. Issued on 7/3/00. Available at: http://www.fda.gov/ora/fiars/ora_import_ia2111.html.
12423 *J Neurosci Nurs* 2000;32:229-32.
12424 *Eur J Clin Nutr* 2004;58:703-10.
12425 *J Bone Miner Res* 2004;19:297-307.
12426 *Analyst* 2004;129:87-91.
12427 *J Ethnopharmacol* 2000;73:429-36.
12428 *J Antimicrob Chemother* 1999;43:667-74.
12429 *Planta Med* 1995;61:45-9.
12430 *Yakugaku Zasshi* 1989;109:672-6.
12431 *Fitoterapia* 2001;72:221-9.
12432 *Phytomedicine* 2003;10:3-7.
12433 *Z Rheumatol* 1998;57:11-6.
12434 *Phytomedicine* 1996;3:91-4..
12435 *Carcinogenesis* 2002;23:2087-93.
12436 *Z Gastroenterol* 2001;39:11-17.
12437 *Arzneimittelforschung* 1998;48:668-74.
12438 *Planta Med* 2001;67:391-5.
12439 *Indian J Exp Biol* 2003;41:1460-2.
12440 *Transplant Proc* 2001;33:539-41.
12441 *Phytomedicine* 2004;11:255-60.
12442 *Contact Dermatitis* 2004;51:91-2.
12443 *Phytochemistry* 2003;62:537-41.
12444 *J Pharmacol Exp Ther* 2004;310:528-35.
12445 *Chem Pharm Bull (Tokyo)* 2003;51:1106-8.
12446 *Chem Pharm Bull (Tokyo)* 2003;51:673-8.
12447 *Chem Pharm Bull (Tokyo)* 2003;51:152-7.
12448 *J Ethnopharmacol* 2003;84:51-5.
12449 *Chem Pharm Bull (Tokyo)* 1986;34:3854-60.
12450 *J Ethnopharmacol* 1990;29:341-4.
12451 *J Pharm Pharmacol* 2003;55:1275-82.
12452 *Biol Pharm Bull* 2004;27:324-7.
12453 *Planta Med* 1998;64:714-9.
12454 *Planta Med* 2001;67:437-42.
12455 *Planta Med* 2001;67:428-31.
12456 *Phytother Res* 2001;15:481-6.
12457 *Planta Med* 2002;68:204-8.
12458 *J Altern Complement Med* 2000;6:557-9.
12459 *J Trad Chinese Med* 1999;19:3-9.
12460 *Eur J Clin Nutr* 2003;57:138-42.
12461 *Menopause* 2004;11:138-43.
12462 *Am J Med* 2004;117:643-9.
12463 *Arthritis Rheum* 2004;51:738-45.
12464 *Rheum Dis Clin North Am* 2003;29:789-801.
12465 *Cochrane Database Syst Rev* 2001;1:CD002946.
12466 *Ann Rheum Dis* 2004 Nov 4 [Epub ahead of print].
12467 *J Rheumatol* 2004;31:826.
12468 *Ann N Y Acad Sci* 2004;1012:115-28.
12469 *Clin Drug Invest* 2004;24:353-63.
12470 *J Clin Immunol* 2002;22:83-91.
12471 *J Biol Chem* 2000;275:721-4.
12472 *Osteoarthritis Cartilage* 2003;11:783-9.
12473 *In Vitro Cell Dev Biol Anim* 2004;40:95-101.
12474 *Phytother Res* 2001;15:344-50.
12475 *J Rheumatol* 2004;31:2121-30.
12476 *Phytomedicine* 2004;11:135-8.
12477 *BMC Complement Altern Med* 2004;4:13.
12478 *J Pharmacol Sci* 2003;93:367-71.
12479 *Rapid Commun Mass Spectrom* 2004;18:2273-81.
12480 *J Ethnopharmacol* 2003;85:61-7.
12481 ClinicalTrials.gov. Treating Rheumatoid Arthritis with Tripterygium Wilfordi Hook F or Sulfasalazine. Available at: http://www.clinicaltrials.gov/ct/show/NCT00062465?order=1.
12482 *Oncogene* 2004 Oct 18 [Epub ahead of print].
12483 *Biochem Biophys Res Commun* 1996;226:810-8.
12484 *Bioorg Med Chem* 2004;12:5571-8.
12485 *Free Radic Biol Med* 2002;33:1097-105.
12486 *J Nutr* 2002;132:341-6.
12487 *Proc Natl Acad Sci U S A* 1999;96:4524-9.
12488 *J Ethnopharmacol* 1999;66:227-33.
12489 *J Nutr* 2004;134:552-7
12490 *J R Soc Med* 2000;93:305-9.
12491 Baker K, Zhang YQ, Goggins J, et al. Hypovitaminosis D and its association with muscle strength, pain, and physical function in knee osteoarthritis (OA). American College of Rheumatology Meeting; San Antonio, Texas, October 16-21, 2004. Abstract 1755.
12492 *Arch Intern Med* 2004;164:1552-6.
12493 *J Gen Intern Med* 2004;19:380-9.
12494 *Am J Clin Nutr* 2001;74:714-22.
12495 *Clin Chim Acta* 2004;339:11-25.
12496 *J Nutr* 2003;133:3137-40.
12497 *Metabolism* 2004;53:236-40.
12498 *Am J Clin Nutr* 2004;80:1194-200.
12499 *Eur J Intern Med* 2004;15:97-107.
12500 *J Nutr* 2004;134:79-85.
12501 *Am J Clin Nutr* 1999;69:727-36.
12502 *J Nutr* 1995;125:1229-37.
12503 *Am J Clin Nutr* 1997;65:1831-9.
12504 *Gynecol Endocrinol* 1994;8:55-8.
12505 *J Am Coll Nutr* 2000;19:715-37.
12506 *J Reprod Med* 1990;35:503-7.
12507 *J Bone Miner Res* 1998;13:749-58.
12508 FDA. Dietary Supplement Enforcement Report July 2003. Available at: http://www.fda.gov/oc/whitepapers/chbn_summary.html.
12509 *Curr Opin Nephrol Hypertens* 2002;11:403-10.
12510 *Heart* 2003;89:411-6.

12511 *J Nutr* 2003;133:2879-82.
12513 *Gastroenterol Clin North Am* 2003;32:659-83.
12514 *N Engl J Med* 2003;349:1360-8.
12515 *Allergy* 2002;57:1215.
12516 *Eur J Clin Nutr* 2003;57:163-9.
12517 *Am J Clin Nutr* 2003;78:790-5.
12518 *Arch Intern Med* 2004 26;164:1534-40.
12519 *Diabetes Care* 2003;26:1714-8.
12520 *Arch Dermatol* 2001;137:42-3.
12521 *Diabetes Res Clin Pract* 2004;65:227-34.
12522 *J Agric Food Chem* 2002;50:6929-34.
12523 *Mutat Res* 2002;512:37-65.
12524 *J Agric Food Chem* 2003;51:7495-503.
12525 *Biol Pharm Bull* 2003;26:739-42.
12526 *Int J Obes Relat Metab Disord* 1999;23:98-105.
12527 *J Nutr* 2001;131:2848-52.
12528 *Biol Pharm Bull* 1995;18:683-6.
12529 *Planta Med* 2003;69:1091-5.
12530 *Bangladesh Med Res Counc Bull* 1999;25:11-3.
12531 *Planta Med* 1969;17:14-8.
12532 *J Ethnopharmacol* 2003;88:73-7.
12533 *Food Chem Toxicol* 2004;42:1769-75
12534 *J Assoc Physicians India* 2001;49:1057-61.
12535 *J Hum Lact* 2002;18:274-9.
12536 *J Am Coll Nutr* 2004;23:248-58.
12537 *J Clin Endocrinol Metab* 2004;89:3510-5.
12538 *Pharmacol Res* 2003;48:511-3.
12539 *Tohoku J Exp Med* 1983;141:677-81.
12540 *Dig Dis Sci* 2003;48:1221-9.
12541 *Am J Clin Nutr* 1993;58:513-8.
12542 *Diabet Med* 1996;13:358-64.
12543 *J Formos Med Assoc* 1992;91:15-9.
12544 *Diabet Med* 1990;7:242-5.
12545 *Am J Clin Nutr* 1988;48:98-103.
12546 *Clin Pharmacokinet* 1996;30:359-71.
12547 *Am J Prev Med* 1999;17:18-23.
12548 *J Am Diet Assoc* 1998;98:912-4.
12549 *J Endocrinol* 1999;163:207-12.
12550 *N Engl J Med* 1989;320:1148-9.
12551 *Diabetes Care* 2003;26:2470-1.
12552 *Eur J Clin Nutr* 2002;56:830-42.
12553 *Acta Med Scand* 1982;212:237-9.
12554 *Gastroenterology* 1985;88:901-7.
12555 *J Nutr* 2004;134:1874-80.
12556 *Eur J Clin Nutr* 2003;57:1292-4.
12557 *J Clin Endocrinol Metab* 1995;80:3311-20.
12558 *J Clin Endocrinol Metab* 2001;86:1410-7.
12559 *Eur J Endocrinol* 2004;151:1-14.
12560 *Mol Cell Endocrinol* 2004;218:57-64.
12561 *Arthritis Rheum* 2004;50:2858-68.
12562 *J Clin Endocrinol Metab* 2002;87:4935-41.
12563 *Chin Med J (Engl)* 2002;115:402-4.
12564 *Clin Endocrinol (Oxf)* 2000;53:561-8.
12565 *Fertil Steril* 2004;81:595-604.
12566 *Int J Cancer* 2003;105:321-5.
12568 *Endocrinol Metab Clin North Am* 1999;28:265-93.
12569 *JAMA* 1998;280:1565.
12570 *J AOAC Int* 2000;83:847-57.
12571 *Gynecol Obstet Invest* 2003;55:135-8.
12572 *Planta Med* 2002;68:748-9.
12573 Genelabs Technologies, Inc. Prestara Background. Available at: http://www.genelabs.com/development/prestaraBackground.html (Accessed 10 December 2004).
12574 *Arthritis Rheum* 2002;46:1820-9.
12575 *Gastroenterology* 2001;121:554-60.
12576 *Am Fam Physician* 2003;67:2517-24.
12577 Federal Register April 17,2003. Anti-Diarrheal Products for over-the-counter human use; final monograph. Available at: http://www.fda.gov/OHRMS/DOCKETS/98fr/03-9380.pdf (Accessed 27 December, 2004).
12578 *Diabetes Res Clin Pract* 1998;39:19-22.
12579 *J Nat Prod* 2001;64:993-6.
12580 *Allergy* 1995;50:514-6.
12581 *Contact Dermatitis* 1984;11:21-5.
12583 *Curr Med Res Opin* 2004;20:63-71.
12584 *J Am Coll Nutr* 2004;23:549S-51S.
12595 *J Clin Pharmacol* 2002;42:605-12.
12596 *Eur J Pharmacol* 2004;485:69-79.
12597 *J Chromatogr B Analyt Technol Biomed Life Sci* 2003;789:43-57.
12598 *J Nutr* 2003;133:1060-3.
12599 *Arch Intern Med* 2000;160:1154-8.
12600 *Allergy* 2005;60:130-1.
12601 *Ann Allergy Asthma Immunol* 2000;85:385-6.
12602 *J Allergy Clin Immunol* 1997;99:502-7.
12603 *J Am Acad Dermatol* 1996;35:482-4.
12604 *Fitoterapia* 2000;71:713-5.
12605 *Int Immunopharmacol* 2005;5:209-17.
12606 *Clin Chim Acta* 2003;330:165-71.
12607 *Chem Pharm Bull (Tokyo)* 2003;51:333-5.
12608 *Phytochemistry* 2000;54:795-9.
12609 *Antiviral Res* 1995;27:367-74.
12610 *Prostaglandins Leukot Essent Fatty Acids* 1992;45:307-12.
12611 *Cutis* 1993;51:424.
12612 *Natl Med J India* 1993;6:199-201.
12613 *Arch Dis Child* 1993;68:468-71.
12614 *J Herb Pharmcother* 2003;2:35-40.
12615 *J Pharm Pharmacol* 2003;55:1275-82.
12616 *Clin Cancer Res* 2003;9:3115-23.
12617 *Inflammation* 2003;27:129-35.
12618 *Phytochemistry* 2001;56:815-8.
12619 *Chem Pharm Bull (Tokyo)* 1992;40:1196-8.
12620 *J Clin Pharmacol* 2002;42:30-6.
12621 *J Ethnopharmacol* 1997;56:103-8.
12622 *Immunopharmacol Immunotoxicol* 1999;21:705-15.
12623 *Biol Pharm Bull* 2000;23:599-601.
12624 *Zhongguo Zhong Yao Za Zhi* 1993;18:598-600, 638.
12625 *Biomed Chromatogr* 2002;16:229-33.
12626 *Life Sci* 2004;74:935-68.
12627 *Lancet* 1992;340:13-17.
12628 *Br J Dermatol* 1992;126:179-84.
12629 *Cochrane Database Syst Rev* 2004;4:CD002291.
12630 *Int J Dermatol* 1999;38:387-92 .
12631 *Lancet* 1993;342:1175-6.
12632 *J Pharmacobiodyn* 1984;7:836-48.
12633 *J Cardiovasc Pharmacol* 2005;45:74-80.
12634 *Prostaglandins Leukot Essent Fatty Acids* 2002;67:475-8.
12635 *Contact Dermatitis* 1996;35:157-62.
12636 *J Pharm Pharmacol* 2004;56:101-5.
12637 *Ann Intern Med* 2002;137:1001-2.
12638 *Arch Intern Med* 2003;163:699-704.
12639 *Phytomedicine* 2003;10:66-86.
12640 *Biochem Pharmacol* 2004;67:167-74.
12641 *Planta Med* 2002;68:875-80.
12642 *Nat Cell Biol* 1999;1:60-7.
12643 *Biotechnol Appl Biochem* 2004;39:123-8.
12644 *Phytomedicine* 2002;9:419-24.
12645 *J Nat Prod* 2001;64:1297-300.
12646 *Phytochemistry* 2004;65:3261-8.

12647 *Phytochemistry Reviews* 2002;1:333-44.
12648 *J Nat Prod* 2002;65:537-41.
12649 *Chem Pharm Bull (Tokyo)* 1998;46:655-62.
12650 *J Ethnopharmacol* 2000;72:443-50.
12651 *J Agric Food Chem* 2001;49:5880-2.
12652 *J Agric Food Chem* 2003;51:4291-5.
12653 *J Am Soc Nephrol* 2004;15:3225-32.
12654 *J Antimicrob Chemother* 2004;54:577-8.
12656 *Biol Pharm Bull* 2000;23:365-7.
12657 *Biol Pharm Bull* 1997;20:861-4.
12658 *J Nat Prod* 1998;61:377-9.
12659 *J Biomed Sci* 2002;9:401-9.
12660 *Int J Dermatol* 2003;42:472-3.
12661 *Int J Biol Macromol* 2003;33:135-40.
12662 *J Toxicol Clin Toxicol* 1984-85;22:581-4.
12663 *Am J Chin Med* 1996;24:127-37.
12664 *Cancer Lett* 2000;155:79-88.
12665 *Chem Pharm Bull (Tokyo)* 2003;51:378-84.
12666 *Mem Inst Oswaldo Cruz* 2002;97:1027-31.
12667 *Contact Dermatitis* 1995;33:134-5.
12668 *BMJ* 2003;327:1454.
12669 *J Am Diet Assoc* 2001;101:1406-8.
12670 *J Clin Pathol* 2001;54:553-5.
12671 *N Engl J Med* 1990;322:849-50.
12672 *J Clin Endocrinol Metab* 2003;88:2384-92.
12673 *Life Sci* 2003;73:2963-71.
12674 *Reprod Fertil Dev* 1992;4:135-44.
12675 *J Ethnopharmacol* 2005;96:127-32.
12676 *Fitoterapia* 2003;74:583-91.
12677 *Life Sci* 2002;71:1385-96.
12678 *J Ethnopharmacol* 2002;83:153-9.
12679 *Zhong Yao Cai* 2002;25:420-2.
12680 *Phytomedicine* 2002;9:753-6.
12681 *J Ethnopharmacol* 2003;85:257-60.
12682 *Curr Med Res Opin* 2004;20:1377-84.
12683 *BJU Int* 2002;89:895-900.
12684 *Drugs Exp Clin Res* 1993;19:213-7.
12685 *Pharmacol Res* 1995;31:67-72.
12686 *Horm Metab Res* 1990;22:622-6.
12687 *Neuroendocrinology* 1993;57:985-90.
12688 *Ann N Y Acad Sci* 2004;1033:117-31.
12689 *Photodermatol* 1985;2:119-20.
12690 *Cutis* 2002;69:339-40.
12691 *Planta Med* 1991;57:212-6.
12692 *Phytother Res* 2001;15:377-81.
12693 *Br Med J* 1980;280:1044.
12694 *Planta Med* 1993;59:330-2.
12696 *Indian J Clin Biochem* 2003;18:54-63.
12697 *Biochem J* 1993;292:267-70.
12698 *Indian J Pharmacol* 2004;36:249-250.
12699 *J Ethnopharmacol* 2003;84:163-8.
12700 *J Nutr Biochem* 2003;14:173-9.
12701 *Mutat Res* 1998;402:111-20.
12702 *J Ethnopharmacol* 1995;49:101-10.
12703 *J Ethnopharmacol* 2002;82:117-25.
12704 *J Chromatogr Sci* 2004;42:196-9.
12705 *J Nat Prod* 1997;60:1210-3.
12706 *Ann Allergy* 1985;55:678-9.
12707 *J Agric Food Chem* 2004;52:7532-40.
12708 *Medicina (Kaunas)* 2004;40:787-94.
12709 *Cancer Chemother Pharmacol* 1998;42:111-7.
12710 *Mutagenesis* 2001;16:329-32.
12711 *Immunopharmacol Immunotoxicol* 2003;25:285-94.
12712 *Hum Exp Toxicol* 2000;19:457-66.
12713 *Appl Microbiol Biotechnol* 2003;61:269-77.
12714 *J Nutr* 1999;129:775S-778S.
12715 *J Am Acad Dermatol* 2002;47:709-14.
12716 *Contact Dermatitis* 2003;49:108-9.
12717 *Toxicology* 2002;170:75-88.
12718 *Drug Metab Dispos* 2002;30:602-7.
12719 *Drug Metab Pharmacokinet* 2003;18:261-6.
12720 *Anesth Analg* 2004;98:353-8.
12721 *J Pediatr Gastroenterol Nutr* 1993;17:407-13.
12722 *Lancet* 1991;338:1153.
12723 *Am J Gastroenterol* 2000;95:1932-8.
12724 *Digestion* 2004;69:45-52.
12725 *Biochem Pharmacol* 2000;59:1387-94.
12726 *J Pharmacol Sci* 2003;92:50-5.
12727 *Phytomedicine* 2003;10:657-64.
12728 *J Agric Food Chem* 2004;52:6956-61.
12729 *J Agric Food Chem* 2005;53:191-6.
12730 *Biol Pharm Bull* 2002;25:256-9.
12731 *Hum Exp Toxicol* 2004;23:21-8.
12732 *Urology* 2004;64:394-8.
12733 *Biol Pharm Bull* 2001;24:92-5.
12734 *J Pharm Pharmacol* 2001;53:1323-9.
12735 *Planta Med* 1992;58:338-41.
12736 *J Ethnopharmacol* 2004;94:143-8.
12738 *J Agric Food Chem* 2002;50:1168-71.
12739 *Fitoterapia* 2000;71:46-9.
12740 *J Ethnopharmacol* 1999;66:187-92.
12741 *Phytother Res* 2002;16:751-3.
12742 *Contact Dermatitis* 1991;24:382-3.
12743 *Drugs R D* 2002;3:223-31.
12744 *Ann N Y Acad Sci* 2004;1033:30-41.
12745 *AIDS* 2004;18:1549-60.
12746 *J Diabetes Complications* 1999;13:251-3.
12747 *J Peripher Nerv Syst* 1997;2:250-2.
12748 *Ann N Y Acad Sci* 2004;1033:42-51.
12749 *JAMA* 2002;288:2579-88.
12750 *Diabetes* 2002;51:2619-28.
12751 *Diabetes Res Clin Pract* 2002;56:173-80.
12752 *Neurosci Res* 1999;33:207-13.
12753 *Diabetologia* 1995;38:123..
12754 *Ann N Y Acad Sci* 2004;1033:99-107.
12755 *Clin Cancer Res* 2003;9:5756-67.
12756 *Clin Pharmacokinet* 2003;42:941-67.
12758 *J Child Neurol* 1998;13:546-9.
12759 *Pharmacol Rev* 2002;54:589-98.
12760 *J Pharmacol Exp Ther* 1999;290:1482-92.
12761 *Ann N Y Acad Sci* 2004;1033:158-67.
12762 *Ann Allergy Asthma Immunol* 2004;93:S33-7.
12763 *Am J Gastroenterol* 2002;97:2744-9.
12764 *Eur J Gastroenterol Hepatol* 2001;13:25–9.
12765 *J Antimicrob Chemother* 2001;47:709-10.
12766 *Digestion* 2002;65:16-20.
12767 *Gut* 2002;51:405-9.
12768 *Best Pract Res Clin Gastroenterol* 2003;17:821-31.
12769 *Gut* 2004;53:108-14.
12770 *Dig Dis Sci* 2002;47:2615-20.
12771 *Dig Liver Dis* 2000;32:294-301.
12772 *J Intern Med* 2005;257:78-92.
12773 *J Allergy Clin Immunol* 2003;111:389-95.
12774 *J Nutr* 2004;134:2022S-2026S.
12775 *J Am Coll Nutr* 2003;22:56-63.
12776 *Clin Infect Dis* 2003;36:775-80.
12777 *J Clin Gastroenterol* 2004;38:S67-9.
12778 *Am J Clin Nutr* 2004;80:245-56.
12779 *J Pharmacol Exp Ther* 1999;289:695-702.
12780 *Ann Intern Med* 2000;133:911-3.
12782 *Mutagenesis* 2002;17:265-77.
12783 *Nephrol Dial Transplant* 2002;17:524-5.

12784 *Am J Nephrol* 2001;21:441-8.
12785 *Lancet* 2001;358:1515-6.
12786 *Lancet* 1999;354:481-2.
12787 *Toxicology* 2002;181-182:577-80.
12788 *Exp Biol Med (Maywood)* 2004;229:473-8.
12789 *Environ Res* 1999;80:S175-S182.
12790 *BMC Complement Altern Med* 2004;4:10.
12791 *Rev Esp Fisiol* 1984;40:227-30.
12792 *J Nat Prod* 1993;56:478-88.
12793 *J Agric Food Chem* 2002;50:840-5.
12794 *Antimicrob Agents Chemother* 1988;32:1742-5.
12795 *J Biol Chem* 1993;268:21770-6.
12796 *Biol Pharm Bull* 2004;27:266-70.
12797 *Thromb Res* 1997;85:479-91.
12798 *Biochem Pharmacol* 2003;65:173-9.
12799 *J Cosmet Sci* 2002;53:1-9.
12800 *Nephrol Dial Transplant* 1998;13:526-7.
12801 Food and Drug Administration, HHS. Labeling for oral and rectal over-the-counter drug products containing aspirin and nonaspirin salicylates; Reye's Syndrome warning. Final rule. *Fed Regist* 2003;68:18861-9. Available at: http://fr.cos.com/cgi-bin/getRec?id=20030417a147.
12802 *Ann Rheum Dis* 1987;46:638-9.
12803 *Clin Pediatr (Phila)* 1981;20:53-4.
12804 *Rheumatology (Oxford)* 2001;40:1388-93.
12805 *Am J Kidney Dis* 1996;28:S24-9.
12806 *Am J Kidney Dis* 1993;21:643-52.
12807 *J Intern Med* 1999;246:247-52.
12808 *Eur J Clin Pharmacol* 2001;57:387-91.
12809 *Clin Pharmacol Ther* 2003;73:272-4.
12810 *Planta Med* 2001;67:209-12.
12811 *Int J Obes Relat Metab Disord* 2004;28:1411-9.
12812 *Clin Pharmacol Ther* 2003;74:96.
12813 *Toxicol Lett* 2004;150:97-110.
12814 *Forensic Sci Int* 2002;130:183-6.
12815 *J Toxicol Sci* 2003;28:471-8.
12816 *Chem Res Toxicol* 2001;14:589-95.
12817 *Proc Natl Acad Sci U S A* 2000;97:4417-8.
12818 *Gen Pharmacol* 1995;26:309-15.
12819 *J Trauma* 2002;53:761-3.
12820 *J Am Board Fam Pract* 2000;13:134-7.
12821 *Am J Sports Med* 2000;28:112-6.
12822 *Life Sci* 2004;75:2867-78.
12823 *Curr Sci* 2002;82:1336-45.
12824 *J Ethnopharmacol* 2004;90:99-103.
12825 *Int J Immunopharmacol* 1992;14:1187-93.
12826 *Indian J Exp Biol* 1999;37:1251-4.
12827 *J Ethnopharmacol* 1998;60:235-46.
12828 *Contraception* 2003;68:225-9.
12829 *Indian J Exp Biol* 2003;41:636-40.
12830 *Oral Dis* 2003;9:95-8.
12831 *Indian J Exp Biol* 1992;30:738-40.
12832 *Indian J Physiol Pharmacol* 2000;44:64-8.
12833 *J Ethnopharmacol* 1992;35:267-73.
12834 *J Ethnopharmacol* 1994;42:71-2.
12835 *J Ethnopharmacol* 2004;94:25-41.
12836 Environmental Protection Agency. Azadirachtin (121701) Clarified Hydrophobic Extract of Neem Oil (025007) Fact Sheet. Available at: http://www.epa.gov/pesticides/biopesticides/ingredients/factsheets/factsheet_025007.htm.(Accessed 2005 March 9).
12837 *N Engl J Med* 1990;322:850.
12838 *Fitoterapia* 2001;72:695-7.
12839 *Phytother Res* 1999;13:188-91.
12840 *Eur Neurol* 2004;51:89-97.
12841 *J Hepatol* 2003;39:437-46.
12842 *Pharmazie* 1995;50:83-98.
12847 *Immunopharmacology* 2000;49:295-306.
12848 *Anesth Analg* 2003;97:1724-9.
12849 *J Surg Res* 2004;119:138-42 .
12850 *Ann Nutr Metab* 2004;48:151-5.
12851 *J Ethnopharmacol* 2003;85:25-32.
12853 *Arch Pharm (Weinheim)* 2002;335:262-6.
12854 *Phytother Res* 2000;14:575-7.
12855 *J Biochem Biophys Methods* 2002;53:45-9.
12856 *Clin Exp Pharmacol Physiol* 2005;32:47-53.
12857 *Clin Pharmacol Ther* 2004;75:259-73.
12858 *Am J Med Sci* 1993;306:317-9.
12859 *Masui* 1997;46:823-6.
12860 *Toxicol Lett* 2005;155:411-20.
12865 *J Toxicol Environ Health* 1983;12:633-40.
12866 *J Ethnopharmacol* 2003;89:277-83.
12867 *Fitoterapia* 2002;73:269-75.
12868 *J Neurol* 1999;246:667-70.
12869 *Australas J Dermatol* 1998;39:265-7.
12870 *Lett Appl Microbiol* 2004;39:60-4.
12871 *J Nutr* 1998;128:2319-23.
12872 *BJU Int* 2004;93:1139-50.
12873 *Cancer Epidemiol Biomarkers Prev* 2004;13:378-82.
12874 *Cancer Epidemiol Biomarkers Prev* 2003;12:518-26.
12875 *Mol Cancer Ther* 2003;2:797-803.
12876 *Prostate* 2001;46:33-8.
12877 *Cancer Causes Control* 2000;11:617-26.
12878 *Cancer Epidemiol Biomarkers Prev* 2004;13:340-5.
12879 *J Agric Food Chem* 2005;53:2897-2900.
12880 *Ann Pharmacother* 2004;38:257-60.
12881 *Br J Clin Pharmacol* 2005;59:425-32.
12882 *Prostaglandins Leukot Essent Fatty Acids* 2004;71:25-31.
12883 *Urol Clin North Am* 2002;29:83-93.
12884 *Cancer Sci* 2004;95:238-42.
12885 *Eur Urol* 2004;45:245-51.
12886 *Cancer Epidemiol Biomarkers Prev* 2004;13:2277-9.
12887 *J Natl Cancer Inst* 1998;90:1637-47.
12888 *Cancer Epidemiol Biomarkers Prev* 2004;13:644-8.
12889 *Gen Pharmacol* 1996;27:629-33.
12890 *J Ethnopharmacol* 2003;87:241-6.
12891 *J Ethnopharmacol* 1997;55:107-11.
12892 *Pharmacol Biochem Behav* 2003;74:739-45.
12894 *J Ethnopharmacol* 2005;96:295-301.
12895 *Exp Biol Med (Maywood)* 2003;228:967-71.
12896 *J Pharm Pharmacol* 2003;55:1267-73.
12897 *Oral Surg Oral Med Oral Pathol* 1992;73:555-8.
12898 *Arch Intern Med* 1997;157:2007-9.
12899 *J Am Acad Dermatol* 2002;47:774-5.
12900 *N C Med J* 1992;53:98-9.
12901 *Mol Cell Biochem* 2003;250:27-40.
12902 *Regul Toxicol Pharmacol* 2001;33:117-37.
12903 *Clin Infect Dis* 2002;35:S210-24.
12904 *Sex Transm Infect* 2003;79:270-5.
12912 Wilde-Mathews A, Schaefer-Munoz S. Judge overturns ban on ephedra, roils FDA policy. Wall Street Journal, April 15, 2005.
12913 Anon. High-dose ephedra pills still illegal, FDA says. Reuters, April 15, 2005.
12914 *Prev Cardiol* 2003;6:136-46.
12915 *Evid Rep Technol Assess (Summ)* 2004 Mar;(94):1-8.
12916 *Arch Intern Med* 2005;165:725-30.
12917 *Cochrane Database Syst Rev* 2004;(4):CD003177.
12918 *Am J Clin Nutr* 2003;77:783-95.
12919 *Am J Clin Nutr* 2005;81:50-4.

12920 *Am J Clin Nutr* 2005;81:416-20.
12921 Balk E, Chung M, Lichtenstein A, et al. Effects of omega-3 fatty acids on cardiovascular risk factors and intermediate markers of cardiovascular disease. Evidence report/technology assessment no. 93. AHRQ publication no. 04-E010-2. Rockville (MD): Agency for Healthcare Research and Quality; 2004. Available at http://www.ahrq.gov/clinic/o3cvrinv.htm.
12922 *Am J Clin Nutr* 1997;65:1645S-54S.
12923 *Arch Intern Med* 2005;165:200-6.
12924 *J Clin Epidemiol* 1995;48:1379-90.
12925 Agency for Healthcare Research and Quality. Effects of Omega-3 Fatty Acids on Lipids and Glycemic Control in Type II Diabetes and the Metabolic Syndrome and on Inflammatory Bowel Disease, Rheumatoid Arthritis, Renal Disease, Systemic Lupus Erythematosus, and Osteoporosis. AHRQ Publication No. 04-E012-1; 2004. Available at: http://www.ahcpr.gov/clinic/epcsums/o3lipidsum.htm.
12926 National Osteoporosis Foundation. Physician's Guide to Prevention and Treatment of Osteoporosis. Universal Recommendations for All Patients. Available at: http://www.nof.org/physguide/univeral_recommendations.htm#adequate. (Accessed May 14, 2005).
12928 *Crit Care Med* 2004;32:S146-54.
12929 *BMJ* 2005;330:1003.
12930 *J Bone Miner Res* 2004;19:370-8.
12931 *Lancet* 2005;365:1599-600.
12933 *JAMA* 2005;293:2257-64.
12934 *Osteoporos Int* 2005;16:239-54.
12935 *Am J Ther* 1995;2:546-52.
12936 *Eur J Drug Metab Pharmacokinet* 1996;21:351-7.
12937 *Cleve Clin J Med* 2001;68:945-51.
12938 *J Am Acad Dermatol* 1997;37:929-34.
12939 *J Am Coll Nutr* 2000;19:119s-136s.
12940 *Postgrad Med J* 1999;75:554-6.
12942 *Lancet* 1978;1:638-9.
12943 *Kidney Int* 2004;65:1914-26.
12944 *Kidney Int Suppl* 2004;90:S25-32.
12945 *Cochrane Database Syst Rev* 2000(2):CD000952.
12946 *J Accid Emerg Med* 2000;17:188-91.
12947 *Acad Emerg Med* 2000;7:1089-96.
12948 *Ann N Y Acad Sci* 2005;1040:53-8.
12949 *Am J Clin Nutr* 2005;81:1147-54.
12950 *Cochrane Database Syst Rev* 2004;(1):CD003548.
12951 *Thorax* 1998;53:425-9.
12952 *Endocr Rev* 2002;23:560-9.
12953 *J Rheumatol* 2004;31:1551-6.
12954 *Cochrane Database Syst Rev* 2002; (2):CD001283.
12955 *Am J Epidemiol* 2005;161:948-59.
12956 *Am J Clin Nutr* 2005;81:934-8.
12958 *Int J Cancer* 2004;112:1-7.
12959 *Am J Epidemiol* 2005;161:462-71.
12960 *Cancer Epidemiol Biomarkers Prev.* 2005;14:835-41.
12961 *Am J Clin Nutr* 2004;80:204-16.
12962 *Am J Clin Nutr* 2004;79:935-45.
12963 *J Allergy Clin Immunol* 2004;114:807-13.
12964 *J Am Diet Assoc* 2005;105:350-1.
12965 *Ann Intern Med* 2004;141:977-80.
12966 *Environ Health Perspect* 2005;113:552-6.
12967 US Food and Drug Administration, Center for Food Safety and Applied Nutrition, Office of Seafood. Mercury levels in seafood species. Available at: http://www.cfsan.fda.gov/~frf/sea-mehg.html.
12968 US Environmental Protection Agency. Fish Advisories web page. Available at: http://www.epa.gov/waterscience/fish.
12969 *Clin Exp Allergy* 2004;34:1237-42.
12970 *Lipids* 2004;39:195-206.
12971 *J Allergy Clin Immunol* 2003;112:1178-84.
12972 *BJOG* 2000;107:382-95.
12973 *Environ Res* 2005;98:133-42.
12975 *Cleve Clin J Med* 2004;71:208-10, 212, 215-8 passim.
12976 *Circulation* 2003;107:1372-7.
12977 *Am J Epidemiol* 2004;160:1005-10.
12978 *J Nutr* 2004;134:919-22.
12979 *J Ethnopharmacol* 1995;46:63-9.
12980 *Contact Dermatitis* 2001;44:101-2.
12981 *Chem Res Toxicol* 2004;17:55-62.
12982 Reliant Pharmaceuticals. Omacor package insert. Liberty Corner, NJ; December, 2004.
12983 *Chemosphere* 1998;37:1241-52.
12984 *J Am Coll Cardiol* 2005;45:1723-8.
12986 *JAMA* 2005;293:2884-91.
12987 *Pharmacol Ther* 2003;98:355-77.
12988 *J Am Coll Cardiol* 2005;45:1716-22.
12989 *Circulation* 2005;111:157-64.
12990 *Circulation* 2005;111:2921-6.
12991 *Hypertension* 2005;45:368-73.
12992 *Lancet* 2001;357:4-6.
12993 *J Am Acad Dermatol* 2003;49:1204-6.
12994 *Cancer Res* 2005; 65:5470-9.
12995 *J Nutr* 2005;135:332-7.
12996 *J Clin Endocrinol Metab* 2005;90:3215-24.
12997 *J Nutr* 2005;135:317-22.
12998 *Aviat Space Environ Med* 2005;76:569-75.
12999 *J Cell Biochem* 2003;88:296-307.
13000 *Photochem Photobiol* 2005 Nov 1; [Epub ahead of print].
13001 *Therapiewoche* 1986;36:3352-8.
13002 *Br J Plast Surg* 2005;58:100-1.
13003 *Neurology* 2004;63:2240-4.
13004 *Bioorg Med Chem Lett* 2004;14:1329-32.
13005 Federal Trade Commission, Plaintiff, v. Enforma Natural Products, Inc. and Andrew Grey, Defendants, and Twenty-Four Seven LLC, Michael Ehrman and Donna DiFerdinando, Respondents, United States District Court, Central District of California. Civil Action No.: CV 00-04376-SVW (CWx).
13006 *Psychosomatics* 2004;45:536-7.
13007 *Diabetes Care* 2005;28:89-94.
13008 *Pediatrics* 2005;115:178-81.
13009 *Arch Pathol Lab Med* 2005;129:74-7.
13010 *J Med Food* 2003;6:309-16.
13011 *Cochrane Database Syst Rev* 2001;3:CD003205.
13012 *Arch Pathol Lab Med* 2003;127:1603-5.
13013 *Am J Clin Nutr* 1997;65:1874-81.
13014 *Drug Metab Dispos* 2004;32:1333-6.
13015 *Hum Psychopharmacol* 2004;19:275-6.
13016 *Planta Med* 2004;70:293-8.
13017 *Pharmazie* 2004;59:643-5.
13018 *Phytochemistry* 2001;58:641-4.
13019 *Planta Med* 2001;67:282-4.
13020 *J Nat Prod* 2000;63:485-8.
13021 *BMJ* 2005;330:503.
13022 *J Med Food* 2004;7:305-8.
13023 *Clin Nutr* 2004;23:423-33.
13024 *J Agric Food Chem* 2000;48:4581-9.

13025 Aviram M. Polyphenolic flavonoids content and antioxidant activities of various juices: a comparative study. Proceedings of the 11th Biennial Meeting of the Society for Free Radical Research International, 2002 Feb:1-9.
13026 *Diabetologia* 2004;47:1016-9.
13027 *Breast Cancer Res* 2004;6:R170-R179.
13028 *Altern Med Rev* 2001;6:293-302.
13029 *Ann Pharmacother* 2004;38:1222-5.
13030 *J Womens Health (Larchmt)* 2004;13:830-3.
13031 *Circulation* 2005;835:835-8.
13032 *J Am Diet Assoc* 2005;105:65-71.
13033 *Life Sci* 2004;75:1735-46.
13034 *Chem Pharm Bull (Tokyo)* 1999;47:1725-9.
13035 *J Ethnopharmacol* 1997;56:145-52.
13036 *JAMA* 2005;293:1338-47.
13037 *Ann Intern Med* 2005;142:477-8.
13038 Lau WC, Carville DGM, Guyer KE, et al. St. John's Wort Enhances the Platelet Inhibitory Effect of Clopidogrel in Clopidogrel "Resistant" Healthy Volunteers. American College of Cardiology Annual Meeting, Orlando, FL 2005: Presentation 1043-129.
13039 *Mayo Clin Proc* 2004;79:1059-62.
13040 *Circulation* 2005;111:465-71.
13041 *Carcinogenesis* 2004;25:2115-23.
13042 *Br J Haematol* 2002;117:577-87.
13043 *J Natl Cancer Inst* 2005;97:396-9.
13044 *Am J Hypertens* 2004;17(11 Pt 1):1056-8.
13045 *J Dairy Sci* 1998;81:2850-7.
13046 *Br J Nutr* 2000;84:S111-7.
13047 *Ann Allergy Asthma Immunol* 2002;89:3-10.
13048 *FEBS Lett* 2002;531:369-74.
13049 *Am J Physiol Gastrointest Liver Physiol* 2002;283:G521-8.
13050 *Exp Biol Med (Maywood)* 2001;226:1031-6.
13051 *Allergy* 2001;56:35-8.
13052 *Biopolymers* 1997;43:129-34.
13053 *Diabetes Care* 2005;28:712-3.
13054 *Gastroenterology* 2005;128:541-51.
13055 *J Natl Cancer Inst* 2005;97:481-8.
13056 *J Ethnopharmacol* 1990;28:143-50.
13057 *Ann Intern Med* 2004;141:650-1.
13058 *Pediatrics* 2004;114:e653-6.
13059 *Fitoterapia* 2004;75:612-4.
13060 *N Engl J Med* 2005;352:2379-88.
13062 FDA. Warning Letter for Weight Loss Product "Dream Shape." FDA Warning Letter. 2004 March 26. Available at: http://www.cfsan.fda.gov/~dms/wl-ltr2.html.
13063 Centers for Disease Control and Prevention. Telebriefing Transcript CDC Adopts New Repellent Guidelines for Upcoming Mosquito Season. Available at: http://www.cdc.gov/od/oc/media/transcripts/t050428.htm. (Accessed 28 April 2005).
13064 *Fitoterapia* 2002;73:261-2.
13065 *Phytother Res* 2003;17:202-5.
13066 *J Rheumatol* 2002;29:2585-91.
13067 *Phytomedicine* 2005;12:247-8.
13068 *Arch Neurol* 2005;62:641-5.
13069 *Prog Lipid Res* 2004;43:553-87.
13070 *Pediatr Infect Dis J* 2005;24:278-80.
13071 *Obstet Gynecol* 2005;105:849-56.
13072 *Exp Clin Endocrinol Diabetes* 2003;111:341-3.
13073 *Lancet* 2005;365:1621-8.
13074 *J Med Entomol* 2002;39:895-9.
13075 US Environmental Protection Agency. p-Menthane-3,8-diol (011550) Biopesticide Registration Eligibility Document. Available at: http://www.epa.gov/oppbppd1/biopesticides/ ingredients/tech_docs/tech_011550.htm#BIBLIOGRAPHY (Accessed 18 May 2005).
13076 *J Am Mosq Control Assoc* 2002;18:107-10.
13077 *N Engl J Med* 2002;347:13-8.
13078 *Eur J Clin Nutr* 2002;56:368-77.
13080 *Obstet Gynecol* 2004;103:639-45.
13081 *Med Vet Entomol* 2000;14:441-4.
13083 Public Health Agency of Canada. Canadian Recommendations for the Prevention and Treatment of Malaria Among International Travellers. Available at: http://www.phac-aspc.gc.ca/publicat/ccdr-rmtc/04vol30/30s1/page2_e.html (Accessed 24 May 2005).
13084 Public Health Agency of Canada. Safety Tips on Using Personal Insect Repellents Available at: http://www.phac-aspc.gc.ca/wn-no/repellents-insectifuge_e.html. (Accessed 24 May 2005).
13085 *Alcohol Clin Exp Res* 2005;29:756-62.
13086 *Cancer* 2005:published online May 23, 2005;doi:10.1002/cncr.21107.
13087 *J Agric Food Chem* 2004;52:1539-45.
13088 *Magn Reson Imaging* 2004;22:389-93.
13089 *Aliment Pharmacol Ther* 2004;20:1279-87.
13090 *Int J Obes Relat Metab Disord* 2000;24:1419-25.
13091 *Mayo Clin Proc* 2005;80:541-5.
13092 *Diabetes Care* 2004;27:3019-20.
13093 *Life Sci* 2003;74:593-602.
13094 *Arch Intern Med* 2005;165:1246-52.
13095 Vanderperren B, Rizzo M, Angenot L, et al. Acute liver failure with renal impairment related to the abuse of senna anthraquinone glycosides. *Ann Pharmacother* 2005 Jun 14; (July/August) [Epub ahead of print] DOI 10.1345/aph.1E670.
13097 Health Canada Press Release. Health Canada warns consumers not to use human growth hormone drug called GHR-15. June 7, 2005. Available at: http://www.hc-sc.gc.ca/english/protection/warnings/2005/2005_55.html (Accessed 17 June 2005).
13099 *Contraception* 2005;71:402-8
13100 *J Am Geriatr Soc* 2005;53:824-8.
13101 *Breast Cancer Res Treat* 2005;90:233-9.
13102 *Arch Intern Med* 2005;165:1161-6.
13103 *Phytother Res* 2005;19:148-51.
13104 *J Strength Cond Res* 2005;19:475-80.
13105 *J Strength Cond Res* 2005;19:115-21.
13106 *Arch Intern Med* 2005;165:1167-72.
13107 *Eur J Gastroenterol Hepatol* 2005;17:445-7.
13108 *Pharmacogenetics* 2004;14:841-50.
13109 *Int J Sport Nutr Exerc Metab* 2004;14:298-307.
13111 *Contact Dermatitis* 2003;48:348-9.
13112 *Gut* 2005 May 24; [Epub ahead of print].
13113 *J Nutr* 2005;135:1120-3.
13114 *Dent Update* 1995;22:36-7.
13115 *J Med Entomol* 2004;41:1064-7.
13116 *J Med Entomol* 2002;39:736-41.
13117 *Phytother Res* 1996;10:313-16.
13118 *Phytother Res* 1993;7:17-20.
13119 *Food Chem Toxicol* 2003;41:867-74.
13120 *J Asthma* 2004;41:825-32.
13121 *Headache* 2005;45:196-203.
13122 *Food Chem Toxicol* 1991;29:765-70.
13123 *Vascul Pharmacol* 2004;40:279-84.
13124 *Bioorg Med Chem Lett* 2001;11:1839-42.
13125 *Planta Med* 1988;54:413-4.

13126 *J Nat Prod* 1992;55:696-8.
13127 *J Ethnopharmacol* 2000;73:199-207.
13128 *J Nat Prod* 1993;56:1805-10.
13129 *Life Sci* 2004;74:2467-78.
13131 *JAMA* 2005;294:56-65.
13132 *Ann N Y Acad Sci* 2004;1031:435-8.
13138 *J Clin Endocrinol Metab* 2005;90:3824-9.
13143 *Obstet Gynecol* 2005;105:1074-83.
13144 *Dig Dis Sci* 2005;50:538-9.
13145 *Phytomedicine* 2005;12:178-82.
13159 *Am J Clin Nutr* 2002;76:549-55.
13251 *J Ethnopharmacol* 2001;78:139-43.
13252 *Fitoterapia* 2001;72:669-70.
13253 *J Ethnopharmacol* 2000;72:29-34.
13254 *J Ethnopharmacol* 1999;65:13-9.
13255 *Int J Sport Nutr Exerc Metab* 2000;10:208-15.
13256 *Breast Cancer Res Treat* 2003;79:301-12.
13257 *J Natl Cancer Inst* 2004;96:696-703.
13258 *J Natl Cancer Inst* 2004;96:645-7.
13259 *BJU Int* 2003;91:608-12.
13276 Dawson-Hughes B, Heaney RP, Holick MF, et al. Estimates of optimal vitamin D status. *Osteoporos Int* 2005 Mar 18; [Epub ahead of print].
13277 *Zhong Yao Cai* 2004;27:77-8.
13278 *Zhongguo Zhong Xi Yi Jie He Za Zhi* 2001;21:31-3 .
13279 *Zhong Xi Yi Jie He Za Zhi* 1990;10:82-4,68.
13280 *Zhongguo Zhong Xi Yi Jie He Za Zhi* 1997;17:339-41.
13281 *J Pharmacol Sci* 2004;96:420-7.
13282 *Zhongguo Zhong Yao Za Zhi* 1995;20:619-21,640.
13283 *Zhongguo Yao Li Xue Bao* 1994;15:180-2.
13284 *Zhongguo Zhong Yao Za Zhi* 2003;28:853-6.
13285 *Arch Pharm Res* 2000;23:461-6.
13286 *Zhong Yao Cai* 2002;25:273-5.
13287 *Zhongguo Zhong Xi Yi Jie He Za Zhi* 1998;18:282-4.
13288 *Life Sci* 2000;67:2997-3006
13289 *Alcohol Clin Exp Res* 1996;20:1083-7.
13290 *J Med Food* 2004;7:168-79.
13291 *Zhong Yao Cai* 1997;20:468-9.
13292 *J Nat Prod* 2003;66:788-92.
13293 *Pharmacol Biochem Behav* 2003;75:619-25.
13294 *Clin Chim Acta* 2004;347:121-8.
13295 *J Steroid Biochem Mol Biol* 2005;94:375-81.
13296 *Toxicol Appl Pharmacol* 2005 Jun 2; [Epub ahead of print].
13297 *Fitoterapia* 2000;71:S38-42
13298 *Beijing Da Xue Xue Bao* 2004;36:45-6.
13299 *Curr Atheroscler Rep* 1999;1:204-9.
13300 *Diabetes Care* 2004;27:2777-83.
13301 *Circulation* 2004;109:1609-14.
13302 *Respir Med* 2003;97:250-6.
13303 *J Paediatr Child Health* 1994;30:190-1.
13304 *Clin Toxicol (Phila)* 2005;43:23-30.
13305 *Pediatr Dermatol* 1997;14:423-5.
13306 *Am J Cardiol* 2004;93:21A-22A.
13307 *J Clin Psychiatry* 2004;65:92-6.
13308 *J Nutr* 2003;133:3540-5.
13309 Food and Drug Administration. A Catalog of FDA Approved Drug Products. Available at: http://www.accessdata.fda.gov/scripts/cder/drugsatfda/ (Accessed 28 June 2005).
13310 *J Nutr* 2005;135:1585S-90S.
13398 *Digestion* 2004;70:257-64.
13776 *J Clin Endocrinol Metab* 1995;80:2227-32.
13777 *Psychosomatics* 1985;26:597-601.
13778 *Gynecol Obstet Invest* 1991;31:146-52.
13779 *N Engl J Med* 1995;332:1529-34.
13780 *J Clin Psychiatry* 1997;58:4-14.

Some Brand Name Natural Products - What they Contain

www.NaturalDatabase.com contains MANY more listings than appear here.
Editor's Notes are located on pages 2155-2163.

#FPMS Female Premenses Syndrome - Systemic Formulas
Vitamin B6 • Cystine • Vitamin A • Magnesium Sulfate • Vitamin E • L-Thionine • Muirapuama • Blue Malva • Pata de Vaca • RNA/DNA Pituitary Factors • L-Methionine • RNA/DNA Duodenal Factors • Choline • Motherwort • Angelica • Cyani Blossoms • Niacin • Inositol • Histidine • Superoxidedismutase • Dong Quai • Zinc Chelate • Vitamin B12 • Octacosanol.
See Editor's Note No. 31.

@zit.gone - Pacific BioLogic
Kochia fruit • Licorice root • Phellodendron bark • Coptis rhizome • Chrysanthemum flower • Forsythia fruit • Ophiopogonis tuber • Rehmannia root (fresh) • Trichosanthis root • Scrophularia root.

1-AD - ErgoPharm/Proviant Technologies
Each capsule contains: 1-Androstene-3beta, 17beta-diol 100 mg. Other Ingredients: Gelatin, Microcrystalline Cellulose, Modified Cornstarch, Magnesium Stearate, Silica.

1-Testabolin - BSN Inc.
Each capsule contains: 17-Hydroxy-5-Alpha-Androst-1-ene-3-one-ECMM (ether carbon molecular modification) 75 mg • Clomitrophin-Q (cissus quadragularis) 150 mg • Kre-Alkalyn 334 mg. Other Ingredients: Magnesium Stearate, Magnesium Silicate, Gelatine, Syloid, White Rice.

1-TU - Nutrex, Inc.
Each liqui-cap contains: 1-TU Proprietary Blend 50 mg: 5-Androst-1-Ene-3-One-17-8-Undecanoate, Oleic Acid. Other Ingredients: Sesame Oil, Gelatin.

2:1 Ratio Calcitron Magnesium/Calcium - Nature's Plus
Two tablets contain: Vitamin D (as ergocalciferol) 50 IU • Calcium (as citrate, aspartate, amino acid complex) 400 mg • Magnesium (as citrate, aspartate, amino acid complex) 800 mg • Horsetail root (from equisetum arvense) 400 mg. Other Ingredients: Microcrystalline Cellulose, Stearic Acid, Di-calcium Phosphate, Magnesium Stearate, Silica, Pharmaceutical Glaze.

2AEP Complex (Ca+Mg+K) - Atrium Biotechnologies
Each cap contains: Calcium (elemental) 25 mg • Magnesium (elemental) 60 mg • Potassium (elemental) 21.5 mg • 2-AEP Complex (2-aminoethylphosphate) 750 mg • Magnesium Stearate • Gelatin.

2DaySlimDown – Momentum
Vitamin C • Vitamin B6 • Vitamin B12 • Vitamin B3 (niacin) • Chromium Polynicotinate • Aloe Vera gel • Garcinia Cambogia • Ginseng tea • Burdock root tea • Licorice root tea • Fennel seed tea • Sumac tea • Pau d'Arco tea • Ginkgo Biloba tea • Peppermint tea.

2nd Wind - Resource Wellness
Two capsules contain: Proprietary Blend 698 mg: Flammulina Velutipes, Eleutherococcus Senticosus (siberian ginseng root extract), Citrus Reticulata (peel extract), Ganoderma lucidum, Panax Ginseng (root extract) • Cordyceps sinensis. Other Ingredients: Gelatin, Maltodextrin, Magnesium Stearate, Silicon Dioxide, Sodium Lauryl Sulfate, Polysorbate 80.

2nd Wind - The Sports Nutrition Source, Inc.
Each scoop contains: Vitamin C 180 mg • Caffeine 20 mg • Ginseng powdered root 10 mg • Chromium Picolinate 200 mcg.

3A Calcium – LaneLabs
Three capsules contain: Calcium (as calcium hydroxide, calcium oxide, combined with algae amino acid extract) 450 mg. Other Ingredients: Gelatin, Water, Glycerin.

3-Daily - The Vitamin Shoppe
Three capsules contain: Vitamin A Activity 25000 IU • Vitamin E 400 IU • Green Tea extract 50 mg • L-Glutathione 10 mg • Vitamin D 400 IU • Vitamin C 500 mg • CoQ10 100 mcg • Selenium 50 mcg • Pycnogenol 100 mcg • N-Acetyl Cysteine 15 mg • Molybdenum 50 mcg • Vitamin B1 50 mg • Vitamin B2 50 mg • Niacinamide 50 mg • Vitamin B6 50 mg • Vitamin B12 500 mcg • Folic Acid 800 mcg • Inositol 50 mg • Choline 50 mg • PABA 50 mg • Vitamin K 30 mcg • Biotin 50 mcg • Pantothenic Acid 50 mg • Calcium 100 mg • Magnesium 50 mg • Zinc 15 mg • Iron 10 mg • Iodine 150 mcg • Potassium 50 mg • Manganese 5 mg • Chromium 100 mcg • Boron 3 mg • Apple Pectin 50 mg • Betaine HCl 25 mg • Glutamic Acid 25 mg • Papain 25 mg • Pepsin 25 mg • Amylase 10 mcg • Lipase 10 mcg • Chlorophyll 10 mg • Spirulina 45 mg • Chlorella 45 mg • Barley Grass 45 mg • Alfalfa concentrate 45 mg • Bee Pollen 45 mg • Rutin 50 mg • Bioflavonoids 50 mg • Shark Cartilage 50 mg • Siberian Ginseng 45 mg • Royal Jelly 15 mg • Echinacea/Golden Seal 50 mg • Shiitake/Reishi Mushrooms 45 mg • RNA/DNA 45 mg. A concentrated blend of: broccoli, tomato, garlic, onions, cauliflower, brussel sprouts, carrots, parsley, watercress, and pure dry cold-pressed borage.

3-Tree Oil - Forest Herbs Research
Tea Tree oil (melalucca alternifolia essential oil) • Pine oil (pinus sylvestris essential oil) • Eucalyptus oil (eucalyptus globulus essential oil) • White Thyme oil (thymus vulgaris/zygis essential oil).

3-Way Calcium Complex - Life Enhancement Products, Inc.
Four capsules contain: Vitamin A (as beta-carotene) 3 mg • Vitamin C (as calcium ascorbate) 221 mg • Vitamin D (as cholecalciferol) 800 IU • Calcium (as tricalcium phosphate, calcium citrate, and calcium ascorbate) 1000 mg • Boron (as calcium borate) 4 mg.

4-Diol 250 - AST Sports Science
Each capsule contains: 4-Androstenediol 250 mg.
See Editor's Note No. 54.

4-in-1 Body Slim - Pro Health
Three capsules contain: Chromium (50% picolinate, 50% polynicotinate) 150 mcg • Psyllium husk fiber 600 mg • Konjak Glucomannan 450 mg • Guar Gum 300 mg • Oat Bran fiber 300 mg • Chitosan (93% deacetylate) 300 mg • Apple Pectin 300 mg • Gymnema Sylvestre extract (2.5% gymnemic acids) 75 mg • L-Carnitine (tartrate) 30 mg. Other Ingredients: Gelatin, Dicalcium Phosphate Anhydrous, Silica, Magnesium Stearate.

4 Sight - Ortho Molecular Products
Two capsules contain: Zinc (as Chelazome brand amino acid chelate) 15 mg • Taurine 400 mg • N-Acetyl Cysteine USP 200 mg • Bilberry fruit extract (standardized to contain 25% anthocyanodins) 150 mg • Liopoic Acid 150 mg • Quercetin 100 mg • Ginkgo Biloba leaf extract (standardized to contain 24% gingko flavonglycosides and 6% terpene lactones) 60 mg • Lutein 30 mg • Lycopene 6 mg. Other Ingredients: Natural Vegetable Capsules, Ascorbyl Palmitate, Microcrystalline Cellulose, Silicon Dioxide.

5-Diol 250 - AST Sports Science
Each capsule contains: 5-Androstenediol 250 mg.
See Editor's Note No. 54.

5-HTP - BioGenesis Nutraceuticals
Each veggie capsule contains: 5-Hydroxy L-Tryptophan 50 mg.

5-HTP - DaVinci Laboratories
Each capsule contains: Vitamin B6 5 mg • 5-Hydroxytryptophan 50 mg. Other Ingredients: Cellulose, Silicon Dioxide, Gelatin.

Some Brand Name Natural Products - What they Contain

www.NaturalDatabase.com contains MANY more listings than appear here.
Editor's Notes are located on pages 2155-2163.

BRAND NAMES

5-HTP Plus Formula **-** Douglas Laboratories/AMNI
Each vegetarian capsule contains: L-5-Hydroxytryptophan 75 mg • Pyridoxal-5-Phosphate 7.5 mg • Proprietary Blend 50 mg: L-Tyrosine, L-Glutamine.

5-HTP **-** J. R. Carlson Laboratories, Inc.
Each tablet contains: Vitamin B6 2 mg • 5-Hydroxytryptophan 50 mg.

5-HTP 50 mg **-** Jarrow Formulas
Each capsule contains: 5-HTP (5-hydroxytryptophan) 50 mg. Other Ingredients: Rice Powder, Magnesium Stearate, Silicon Dioxide, Gelatin.

5-HTP 100 mg **-** Jarrow Formulas
Each capsule contains: 5-HTP (5-hydroxytryptophan) 100 mg. Other Ingredients: Rice Powder, Magnesium Stearate, Silicon Dioxide, Gelatin.

5-HTP (50 mg) **-** Life Enhancement Products, Inc.
Each capsule contains: 5-HTP (5-hydroxytryptophan) 50 mg.

5-HTP (100 mg) **-** Life Enhancement Products, Inc.
Each capsule contains: 5-HTP (5-hydroxytryptophan) 100 mg.

5-HTP SeroTonic II capsules **-** Life Enhancement Products, Inc.
Each capsule contains: Thiamine (vitamin B1 as thiamine mononitrate) 2 mg • Niacin (vitamin B3 as inositol hexaniacinate) 45 mg • Vitamin B6 (as pyridoxal-5-phosphate) 10 mg • Calcium (as calcium citrate) 75 mg • Magnesium (as magnesium hydroxide) 50 mg • 5-Hydroxytryptophan 50 mg • Hyperforin 300 mcg.

5-HTP SeroTonic II powder **-** Life Enhancement Products, Inc.
Each heaping teaspoon (3.75 g) contains: Thiamine (vitamin B1 as thiamine mononitrate) 2 mg • Niacin (vitamin B3 as inositol hexaniacinate) 45 mg • Vitamin B6 (as pyridoxal-5-phosphate) 10 mg • Calcium (as calcium citrate) 75 mg • Magnesium (as magnesium hydroxide) 50 mg • 5-Hydroxytryptophan 50 mg • Hyperforin 300 mcg.

5-HTP **-** Metabolic Response Modifiers
Each capsule contains: 5-HTP (5-hydroxytryptophan) 100 mg.

5-HTP **-** Natural Balance
Each capsule contains: Vitamin B6 (as pyridoxine hydrochloride) 10 mg • 5-HTP (5-hydroxytryptophan from griffonia simplicifolia seed extract) 50 mg. Other Ingredients: Cellulose, Gelatin, Magnesium Stearate.

5 HTP Plus **-** Olympian Labs
Each capsule contains: 5-HTP (L-5 hydroxytryptophan) 100 mg • Vitamin B-6 10 mg • Magnesium Citrate 40 mg • Valerian powder 100 mg • Hops 50 mg • Calcium Citrate 80 mg.

5 HTP **-** Ortho Molecular Products
Each capsule contains: 5-HTP 100 mg. Other Ingredients: Natural Vegetable Capsules, Magnesium Stearate, Microcrystalline Cellulose.

5 HTP 50mg **-** Ortho Molecular Products
Each capsule contains: 5-HTP 50 mg. Other Ingredients: Natural Vegetable Capsules, Magnesium Stearate, Microcrystalline Cellulose.

5-HTP 50 MG **-** Pain & Stress Center
Each capsule contains: 5-Hydroxytryptophan (5-HTP) 50 mg • Glycine 220 mg. Other Ingredients: Gelatin Capsule.

5 HTP **-** Physician Formulas
Each capsule contains: 5-HTP 50 mg • Vitamin C 30 mg • Vitamin E 10 IU.

5 HTP 50 mg Capsules **-** Pro Health
Each capsule contains: 5HTP (5-hydroxy-l-tryptophan, from griffonia seed) 50 mg. Other Ingredients: Rice Flour, Gelatin, Water.

5 HTP 200 mg Xtra Strength Capsules **-** Pro Health
Each capsule contains: 5 HTP (5-hydroxy-L-tryptophan) 200 mg. Other Ingredients: Gelatin, Rice Flour, Magnesium Trisillicate, Magnesium Stearate.

5-HTP (5-Hydroxytryptophan) 50 mg **-** Pure Encapsulations
Each vegetable capsule contains: 5-Hydroxytryptophan (griffonia simplicifolia) 50 mg.

5-HTP (5-Hydroxytryptophan) 100 mg **-** Pure Encapsulations
Each vegetable capsule contains: 5-Hydroxytryptophan (griffonia simplicifolia) 100 mg.

5-HTP **-** Swanson Health Products
Each capsule contains: L-5 HTP (L-5 hydroxytryptophan) 50 mg.

5HTP 50 mg **-** Vital Nutrients
Each capsule contains: 5HTP 50 mg • Pyridoxine HCl 5 mg • Pyridoxal-5-Phosphate 2 mg.

5HTP 100mg **-** Vital Nutrients
Each vegetarian capsule contains: 5-HTP 100 mg • Pyridoxine HCl 10 mg • Pyridoxal-5-Phosphate 4 mg.

5-Hydroxy L-Tryptophan **-** Progressive Labs
Each capsule contains: 5-Hydroxy L-Tryptophan 100 mg.

6-OXO **-** ErgoPharm/Proviant Technologies
Three capsules contain: 6-OXO (3;6;17-androstenetrione) 300 mg. Other Ingredients: Microcrystalline Cellulose.

7 Day Smoke Away Aromatherapy Formula **-** The Quit Smoking Co.
Active Ingredients: Ylang Ylang • Rosemary • Peppermint • Eucalyptus • Virgin Olive Oil • Alcohol.
See Editor's Note No. 1.

7 Day Smoke Away Calming Dietary Supplement **-** The Quit Smoking Co.
Each capsule contains: Avena Sativa (Oats) 10:1 Concentration • Lobelia Inflata (lobelia leaf) 1% lobeline • Capsicum Annuum (cayenne fruit) • Glycyrrhiza Glabra (deglycerized licorice root) • Zingiber Officinale (ginger root) 5% • Piper Methysticum (kava kava leaf) 30% kavalactones • Myristica Fragrans (nutmeg fruit).

7 day Smoke Away Cleanse and Calm Formula **-** The Quit Smoking Co.
Each capsule contains: Proprietary Blend 575 mg: Avena Sativa (Oats) 10:1 Concentration, Lobelia Inflata (lobelia leaf) 1% lobeline, Capsicum Annuum (cayenne fruit), Glycyrrhiza Glabra (deglycerized licorice root), Zingiber Officinale (ginger root) 5%, Piper Methysticum (kava kava leaf) 30% kavalactones, Myristica Fragrans (nutmeg fruit).

7 Day Smoke Away Craving Control Formula **-** The Quit Smoking Co.
Each tablet contains: Plantain major 3X • Caladium seguinum 6X • Daphne indica 6X.
See Editor's Note No. 14.

Some Brand Name Natural Products - What they Contain

www.NaturalDatabase.com contains MANY more listings than appear here.
Editor's Notes are located on pages 2155-2163.

7 Day Smoke Away Lung Saver - The Quit Smoking Co.
Each capsule contains: Vitamin C • Vitamin B6 • Picrorhiza Kurroa • Boswellia Serrata • Piper Longum extract • Lobelia • Adhtoda Vasica • Licorice • Ginger • Piper Nigrum fruit • Tylophora Asmatica • N-Acetyl-Cysteine (NAC) • Marshmallow (Althea Officinalis).

7 Day Souper Cabbage Diet System - Puritan's Pride
Three caplets contain: Souper Cabbage Diet (standardized concentrations) 1500 mg: 3 Green Onions (organo-sulfers), 1 Green Pepper (flavonoids), 1 small stalk of Celery (polyacetylenes), 1 whole Tomato (lycopene), 2 large Carrots (carotenoids), 1 Zucchini Squash (sulforaphane), 1 small head of Cabbage (indole-3-carbinole (I-3-C)). Other Ingredients: Dicalcium Phosphate, Cellulose (plant origin), Croscarmellose, Cellulose Coating, Vegetable Magnesium Stearate.

7 Herb Formula - Daniel Chapter One
Cat's Claw (Una de Gato) • Sheep Sorrel • Siberian Ginseng • Slippery Elm • Burdock root • Turkey Rhubarb • Watercress.

7-Keto - Enzymatic Therapy
Each capsule contains: 7-Keto brand 7-Keto DHEA Acetate 25 mg. Other Ingredients: Cellulose, Gelatin, Magnesium Stearate, Titanium Dioxide.

7-Keto DHEA – PhysioLogics
Each softgel contains: 7-Keto Dehydroepiandrosterone Acetate 25 mg. Other Ingredients: Soybean Oil, Gelatin, Lecithin, Beeswax / Soybean Oil Mixture, Glycerin, Titanium Dioxide Color.

7 Keto DHEA - Pro Health
Each capsule contains: 7-Keto DHEA (3-acetyl-7-oxo-dehydroepiandrosterone, synthetic) 25 mg. Other Ingredients: Rice Flour, Gelatin, Water.

7-KETO DHEA 25 mg - Pure Encapsulations
Each vegetable capsule contains: DHEA-Acetate-7-one 25 mg.

7-KETO DHEA 50 mg - Pure Encapsulations
Each vegetable capsule contains: DHEA-Acetate-7-one 50 mg.

7-KETO DHEA 100 mg - Pure Encapsulations
Each vegetable capsule contains: DHEA-Acetate-7-one 100 mg.

7-Keto Fuel – TwinLab
Each capsule contains: 7-Keto DHEA (3-Acetyl-7-Oxo-Dehydroepiandrosterone) 50 mg.

7-Keto Lean – PhytoPharmica
Each capsule contains: Iodine (potassium iodide) 100 mcg • Copper (gluconate) 500 mcg • Manganese (Krebs cycle chelate) 500 mcg • 7 KETO DHEA 100 mg • L-Tyrosine 100 mg • Asparagus root/ rhizome extract (asparagus officinalis, standardized to contain 4.0%-8.0% asparagosides) 100 mg • Choline Bitartrate 50 mg • Inositol (rice) 50 mg.

7-Keto Naturalean - Enzymatic Therapy
Each capsule contains: 7-Keto DHEA 100 mg • L-Tyrosine 100 mg • Asparagus root extract (asparagus officinalis standardized to contain minimum 4% asparagosides) 100 mg • Choline Bitartrate 50 mg • Inositol 50 mg • Copper (as copper gluconate) 500 mcg • Manganese (krebs cycle chelate) 500 mcg • Iodine (potassium iodine) 100 mcg. Other Ingredients: Magnesium Stearate, Silicon Dioxide, Gelatin, Titanium Dioxide.

7 Vitamin Treatment Cream – Orjene
Vitamin A • Vitamin B5 • Vitamin C • Vitamin D • Vitamin E • Vitamin F • Vitamin H • Antioxidants. Fortified with Beta Carotene.

8 Billion Acidophilus & Bifidus - NOW Foods
Each capsule contains: A guaranteed potency of: Lactobacillus Acidophilus 4 billion • Bifidobacterium Bifidum 3.2 billion • Bifidobacterium Longum 0.8 billion.

8% Plus Antioxidant Cuticle Cream – Jason
Vitamin A • Vitamin C • Vitamin E.

10 Mushroom Combination - Olympia Nutrition
Contains: Cordyceps, Reishi, Maitake, Shitake, Poria, Polyporus, Coriolus, Tremella, Hericium, and Wood Ear mushrooms.

10% Plus Nighttime Cream – Jason
Alpha Hydroxy Acids.

#12 B Brain - Systemic Formulas
RNA/DNA Brain Factors • Italian Pimiento • L-Alanine • Stevia • Tayuya • Vitamin B2 • Rutin • Niacin • Vitamin B6 • L-Glutamic Acid • Hydroxyproline • L-Proline • RNA/DNA Pituitary Factors • RNA/DNA Thalamus Factors.
See Editor's Note No. 31.

12-1/2% Plus with SPF 12-1/2 Protective Moisturizer – Jason
Antioxidant Ester-C • Vitamin E.

#14 Colon - Systemic Formulas
Psyllium Husks • Cascara Sagrada • Licorice Root • Peach Bark • Stillingia • Dolomite • Calcium Carbonate • Citric Acid • Potassium Bicarbonate.

#17 D Digestive - Systemic Formulas
Pancrelipase Enzyme • Golden Seal • RNA/DNA Oxbile Factors • Aspartic Acid • Betaine HCl • L-Glutamic Acid • Echinacea • Lipase • Amylase • Protease • Pepsin • Ammonium Chloride.
See Editor's Note No. 14.

#18 DS Digestive Stabilizer - Systemic Formulas
Kola Nut • Pancrelipase Enzyme • RNA/DNA Oxbile Factors • Betaine HCl • Echinacea • Glutamic Acid • Spearmint • RNA/DNA Liver Factors • Calcium • Papaya leaves • Golden Seal • Aspartic Acid • Ammonium Chloride • Pancreatin Enzyme • Gentian root • Guava powder • Bromelain • Pepsin 1/3000.
See Editor's Note No. 14.

19-Nor-3-Andro - AST Sports Science
Each capsule contains: 19-Norandrostenedione 100 mg • Androstenediol 100 mg • Androstenedione 100 mg.
See Editor's Note No. 47 and 54.

19-Nor 250 - AST Sports Science
Each capsule contains: 19-Norandrostenedione 250 mg.

19-Nor Andro 100 - Metabolic Response Modifiers
Each capsule contains: 19-norandrostenedione (19-nor-4-androstene-3, 17-dione) 100 mg.

19-Nor Xtreme - Metabolic Response Modifiers
Two capsules contain: 19-norandrostenedione 100 mg • 19-nor-4-androstene-3, 17-diol 100 mg • 5-androstenediol 50 mg.
See Editor's Note No. 54.

21 Grain Lecithin – Schiff
Each softgel contains: Lecithin Proprietary Blend 1.36 g: Choline Phosphatides, Inositol Phosphatides, Cephalin, Linoleic Acid. Other Ingredients: Gelatin, Glycerin.

Some Brand Name Natural Products - What they Contain

www.NaturalDatabase.com contains MANY more listings than appear here.
Editor's Notes are located on pages 2155-2163.

#22 F+ Female Plus - Systemic Formulas
Sarsaparilla • Blue Cohosh • Dong Quai • Tayuya • False Unicorn • Cana do Brejo • Carrapichinho • Pfaffia • Motherwort • Balm Mint • Agoniada.

24/7 Instant Relief - Mosaic Nutraceuticals Corp
Celadrin brand Cetylated Fatty Acids • Bowellian extract.

30 Day Beauty Secret - Futurebiotics LLC
Formula I - Two tablets contain: Royal Jelly (freeze dried) 50 mg • Horsetail (extract equivalent to) 300 mg • Dong Quai (extract equivalent to) 100 mg • Polygonum Multiflorum (extract equivalent to) 140 mg • Peony root (extract equivalent to) 120 mg • Betaine HCl 75 mg • Selenium (amino acid chelate) 50 mcg • Iodine (kelp) 175 mcg • Iron (amino acid chelate) 8 mg • Magnesium (oxide, amino acid chelate) 150 mg • Manganese (amino acid chelate) 10 mg • Boron 3 mg • Zinc (gluconate) 15 mg • Calcium (carbonate, phosphate, casein) 300 mg • Phosphorus (calcium phosphate) 150 mg • Collagen 100 mg • Ribonucleic Acid (RNA) 50 mg • Sodium Phosphate 1 mg • Gelatin 200 mg • Papain 25 mg • Keratin 30 mg. Formula II - Each caplet contains: Beta Carotene 10,000 IU • Vitamin C 150 mg • Vitamin B1 (thiamin) 10 mg • Vitamin B2 (riboflavin) 10 mg • Niacinamide 60 mg • Vitamin D (fish liver oil) 200 IU • Vitamin E (natural mixed tocopherols) 30 IU • Vitamin B6 (pyridoxine) 10 mg • Vitamin B12 (cyanocobalamin) 16 mcg • Folic Acid 400 mcg • Biotin 300 mcg • Pantothenic Acid 30 mg • Inositol 50 mg • Para Amino Benzoic Acid (PABA) 50 mg • Choline (bitartrate) 150 mg.

#31 GA Adrenal - Systemic Formulas
RNA/DNA Adrenal Factors • Echinacea • Vitamin C • D-Calcium Pantothenate • Inositol • Ma Huang • Sete Sangrias • RNA/DNA Spleen Factors • Zinc Chelate • Selenium Aspartate.
See Editor's Note No. 14 and 30.

#32 GB Pituitary - Systemic Formulas
RNA/DNA Brain Factors • Whey Protein • RNA/DNA Pituitary Factors • Peach Bark • Jaborandi • RNA/DNA Orchic Factors • L-Methionine • Vitamin B6 • Superoxidedismutase.
See Editor's Note No. 31.

#39 GF Thyroid - Systemic Formulas
Irish Moss • Thyroid-6x dilution • Pata de Vaca • Abutua Kelp • Cucurbita Pepo • RNA/DNA Lung Factors • RNA/DNA Thymus Factors.
See Editor's Note No. 14.

#41 GT Thymus - Systemic Formulas
Vitamin C • Sweet Basil • Golden Seal • RNA/DNA Thymus Factors • Poke Root • Pau d'Arco • RNA/DNA Liver Factors and Lung Factors • Calcium Carbonate • Zinc Aspartate • RNA/DNA Spleen Factors • Magnesium Chloride • Bitter Root • Beta Carotene • Thymol Iodide • RNA/DNA Stomach Factors • Selenium Yeast • Chromium Chelate • Vitamin B2 • Inositol • Niacinamide • PABA • Vitamin B1 • Calcium Pantothenate • Vitamin B6 • Niacin • Vitamin B12 • Folic Acid • Biotin.
See Editor's Note No. 14.

#44 H Heart - Systemic Formulas
RNA/DNA Heart Factors • Lecithin • Chromium Chelate • Phenylalanine • Sete Sangrias • Tayuya • RNA/DNA Thymus Factors • Woodruff • RNA/DNA Spleen Factors • Tyrosine • Vitamin B2 • Carnitine • Vitamin B1 • Niacin • Vitamin B6 • Calcium (from Pantothenate) • Folic Acid • Biotin.
See Editor's Note No. 14.

#45 HCV Heart Cardio Vascular - Systemic Formulas
Sete Sangrias • RNA/DNA Heart Factors • Pimiento • Cassia Bark • Stevia • Hawthorne berries • Potassium Bitartrate.

#46 HN Heart Nerve - Systemic Formulas
RNA/DNA Brain and Spleen Factors • Hesperidin • RNA/DNA Lung Factors • Calcium Pantothenate • Niacin • Tayuya • Vitamin B2 • L-Threonine • RNA/DNA Aorta Factors • L-Methionine • Selenium Chelate • RNA/DNA Heart Factors • Beta Carotene • Chromium Chelate.
See Editor's Note No. 31.

50+ - Futurebiotics LLC
Three capsules contain: Beta-carotene 10,000 IU • Vitamin C (buffered ascorbate) 300 mg • Vitamin E (natural) 100 IU • Vitamin D (as Vitamin D3) 400 IU • Vitamin B1 25 mg • Vitamin B2 25 mg • Vitamin B3 (niacinamide) 25 mg • Vitamin B6 25 mg • Vitamin B12 100 mcg • Pantothenic Acid 25 mg • Biotin 300 mcg • Folic Acid 400 mcg • PABA 25 mg • Choline Bitartrate 50 mg • Inositol 25 mg • Calcium (ascorbate, carbonate, chelate) 200 mg • Magnesium (oxide, chelate) 3 mg • Potassium (chloride, iodide) 20 mg • Zinc (gluconate) 15 mg • Copper (gluconate) 2 mg • Manganese (amino acid chelate) 3 mg • Iodine (potassium iodide) 150 mcg • Selenium (amino acid chelate) 150 mcg • Chromium (amino acid chelate) 200 mcg • Molybdenum (amino acid chelate) 50 mcg • Siberian Ginseng 50 mg • Ginkgo Biloba 25 mg • Turmeric 25 mg • Garlic (Pure-Gar 1500 deodorized concentrate) 200 mg • Cayenne 25 mg • Gotu Kola 100 mg • Alfalfa 50 mg.

#50 I Eyes - Systemic Formulas
Rue Herb • Eye Bright • Vitamin A • Vitamin E • Chap'u de Couro • Proline • Cystine • RNA/DNA Eye Factors • Vitamin B6 • Valine • Niacin • RNA/DNA Brain Factors.
See Editor's Note No. 31.

#58 Ks Kidney Stabilizer - Systemic Formulas
Rose Hips • Gelatin • RNA/DNA Kidney Factors • Magnesium Sulfate • Juniper Berries • Vitamin C • Sete Sangrias • Spearmint Herb • Calcium Carbonate, Hesperidin Complex • Serine • Phenylalanine • RNA/DNA Adrenal and Thalamus Factors • Tyrosine • Vitamin A • Sodium Copper Chlorophyll.
See Editor's Note No. 31.

#60 L Liver - Systemic Formulas
RNA/DNA Liver Factors • Mountain Mahogany • Spearmint Leaves • Vitamin A • Vitamin D • Ragweed • Golden Seal • Quince Seed • Boldo • Vitamin C • Vitamin E.
See Editor's Note No. 14.

#61 LB Liver Normalizer - Systemic Formulas
Red Beet • Betaine HCl • Choline Bitartrate • Lipase 24.

#62 LS Liver Stimulant - Systemic Formulas
Rose Hips • Vitamin C • Chromium Chelate • Magnesium Chelate • Red Beet • Sete Sangrias • Chde Bugre • Potassium Chelate • RNA/DNA Adrenal Factors • Choline Bitartrate • Iron Chelate • RNA/DNA Thymus Factors • Vitamin A • RNA/DNA Pituitary and Liver Factors.
See Editor's Note No. 31.

#70 M+ Male Endocrine - Systemic Formulas
RNA/DNA Orchic Factors • Hops • Boldo (from Chile) • Cipó Caboclo • Abacateiro • Agoniada • Chinese Bamboo • Cipó Cravo • RNA/DNA Prostate Factors • African Yohimbe • Eucalyptus • Catuaba • Muirapuama.
See Editor's Note No. 14.

#72 Mpc Prostata Corrector - Systemic Formulas
Cucurbita Pepo Oil • Pau D'Arco • RNA/DNA Prostate Factors • Ginkgo leaf • Pau D'Alho • RNA/DNA Orchic, Thymus, Pituitary & Hypothalamus Factors • Golden Seal • Echinacea Purpurea • Thyme.
See Editor's Note No. 31.

#73 Mpr Prostata Ovatum - Systemic Formulas
Cucurbita Pepo Oil.

#75 N3 Anti-Tensive - Systemic Formulas
Tayuya • Blue Vervain • Valerian Root Extract • Senna Leaves • L-Methionine • Passion Flower Extract • Calcium Chelate • Saw Palmetto • Sete Sangrias • Mandrake Root • Ephedra • Tyrosine.
See Editor's Note No. 30.

#77 NC Calm - Systemic Formulas
Calcium Carbonate • Dulse • Passion Flowers • Muirapuama • RNA/DNA Brain Factors • Tayuya • Boldo • Selenium Chelate • RNA/DNA Spleen and Lung Factors • Valerian • Niacin • Vitamin B12 • Vitamin B2 • Vitamin B1.
See Editor's Note No. 31.

#78 P Pancreas - Systemic Formulas
RNA/DNA Pancreas Factors • Catuaba • Cynita Cactus • Japecanga • Pata de Vaca • Pedra Hume Ca • Zinc Oxide.
See Editor's Note No. 14.

#79 Ps Pancreas Stabilizer - Systemic Formulas
RNA/DNA Pancreas Factors • Catuaba • Cynita Cactus • Japecanga • Pata de Vaca • Pedra Hume Ca • Zinc Oxide.
See Editor's Note No. 14.

#80 R Lung - Systemic Formulas
Golden Seal • RNA/DNA Lung Factors • Pancreatin 4x • RNA/DNA Thymus Factors • L-Lysine • Aspartic Acid • Allantoin • Tayuya • Aloe Vera.
See Editor's Note No. 14.

#82 S Spleen - Systemic Formulas
RNA/DNA Spleen Factors • Pedra Hume Ca • Nettle • Sweet Gum Tree • RNA/DNA Liver Factors and Pancreas Factors • Lysine • L-Methionine • Leucine • Isoleucine.
See Editor's Note No. 14.

90% Protein Powder - Puritan's Pride
Two tablespoons (20 g) contain: L-Isoleucine 850 mg • L-Leucine 1122 mg • L-Lysine 1092 mg • L-Methionine 225 mg • L-Threonine 659 mg • L-Phenylalanine 902 mg • L-Valine 867 mg • L-Histidine 451 mg • L-Arginine 1318 mg • L-Aspartic Acid 2012 mg • L-Cysteine 225 mg • L-Serine 902 mg • L-Glutamic Acid 3312 mg • L-Tryptophan 225 mg • L-Proline 884 mg • L-Glycine 728 mg • L-Alanine 746 mg • L-Tyrosine 659 mg.

99% Aloe Vera Gel - Vitamin World
Aloe Vera • Carbomer • Triethanolamine • Vitamin E Acetate • Polysorbate 20 • Trisodium EDTA • Sodium Benzoate • Potassium Sorbate • Diazolidinyl Urea • Methylchloroisothiazolinone • Methylisothiazolinone.

#100 ABC Acidophilus/Bifidum Complex - Systemic Formulas
Each capsule contains: "A minimum of one billion Lactobacillus acidophilus (NAS strain) and one billion Bifidobacterium bifidum (Malyoth strain) uniquely suspended in an anaerobic, sunflower oil matrix containing vitamin E as a natural antioxidant."

100% ANY WHEY Protein - Optimum Nutrition
Each scoop (20.5 g) contains: Protein Blend: Whey Protein Isolate, Whey Protein Concentrate, Whey Protein Hydrosylate • Natural Flavor.

100% Egg Protein - Healthy 'N Fit Nutritionals
100% pure extracted egg albumen (with a protein efficiency ratio of 3.9 or greater), enzymatic digest of egg albumia containing naturally occurring amino acids, vanilla flavoring, bromelain and papain.

100% Egg Protein - Optimum Nutrition
Each scoop (29.4 g) contains: Egg Albumen • Cocoa • Artificial Flavor • Lecithin • Sucralose.

100% Natural Vitamin E – GNC
Each capsule contains: Vitamin E (as d-alpha Tocopheryl Acetate) 400 IU. Other Ingredients: Soybean oil, Gelatin, Glycerin.

100% Natural Whey Protein - Optimum Nutrition
Each scoop (31.4 g) contains: Stevia leaf extract (stevia rebaudiana, standardized to 90% steviosides) 70 mg • Enzyme Blend 10 mg: Aminogen, Lactase (standardized to 100,000 FCC units/g) • Protein Blend: Whey Protein Isolate, Whey Protein Concentrate, Whey Peptides • Cocoa • Fructose • Lecithin • Natural Flavor.

100% Whey Protein - Optimum Nutrition
Each scoop (28.4 g) contains: Enzyme Blend 10 mg: Aminogen, Lactase (standardized to 100,000 FCC units/g) • Protein Blend: Whey Protein Concentrate, Whey Protein Isolate, Whey Peptides • Natural and Artificial Flavor, Lecithin, Acesulfame Potassium • Salt.

#101 ACP Vitamin ACP - Systemic Formulas
Rose Hips • Orange peel • Bone Meal • Vitamin C • RNA/DNA Liver Factors • Lemon Bioflavonoid • Vitamin E • RNA/DNA Thymus Factors • Pedra Hume Ca • Acacia Gum flower • Vitamin A.
See Editor's Note No. 14.

#102 ACX Vitamin Detox - Systemic Formulas
Rose Hips • Vitamin C • RNA/DNA Liver Factors • Lemon Bioflavonoid • Pimiento • Vitamin E • Damiana • Pedra Hume Ca • RNA/DNA Thymus Factors • Vitamin A • Acacia Gum Flower • Hesperidin • RNA/DNA Spleen Factors • Peach Bark • Sun Dew.
See Editor's Note No. 14.

#111 AZV Multi-Vitamin and Mineral Supplement - Systemic Formulas
RNA/DNA Liver Factors • Rose Hips • Kelp • Linseed Oil • Vitamin A • Vitamin D • Vitamin E • Vitamin C • Calcium • Niacin • Phosphorus • Iron • Vitamin B1 (Thiamine) • Vitamin B2 (Riboflavin) • Magnesium • Vitamin B6 (Pyridoxine HCl) • Pantothenic Acid • Potassium • Zinc • Manganese • Vitamin B12 (Cyanocobalamin) • Lemon Bioflavonoid • Autolyzed RNA/DNA Yeast.
See Editor's Note No. 14.

#115 BSV Vitamin B Stress Complex - Systemic Formulas
Abuta • Centuary • Red Bone Marrow • Nettle • Poke Root • Spearmint • RNA/DNA Liver Factors and Parotid Factors • Guarana • Vitamin B2 • Fringe Tree • Choline Bitartrate • Inositol • Niacinamide • PABA • Vitamin B1 • Calcium Pantothenate • Vitamin B6 • Niacin • Vitamin B12 • Folic Acid • Biotin.
See Editor's Note No. 14.

#120 CAL Calcium Plus - Systemic Formulas
Calcium (from Citrate, Lactate, Hydroxide, Bone Meal, Bone Ash, Carbonate, Oyster Shell, Lysinate, Methionate, and Aspartate) • Lecithin • Magnesium Oxide • Vitamin C • Vitamin E • Trace Minerals • Iron Chelate • Copper Carbonate • Vitamin D • Betaine HCl • Boron Chelate.

#126 CTV Vitamin C Therapeutic - Systemic Formulas
Ascorbic Acid • Sodium Ascorbate • Beta-carotene (source of Vit. A) • Sago Palm • Calcium Ascorbate • Calcium Carbonate • Bioflavonoids • Potassium Bitartrate • Hesperidin • Rose Hips • Thymol Iodide.

#130 EZV 200 IU Vitamin E - Systemic Formulas
Lactose • Fructose • Vitamin E • Honey Bake.

Some Brand Name Natural Products - What they Contain

www.NaturalDatabase.com contains MANY more listings than appear here.
Editor's Notes are located on pages 2155-2163.

#132 FLX Vegetable Omega-3 Flaxseed Oil **- Systemic Formulas**
Superunsaturate; Alphalinolenic Acid, Omega-3 • Polyunsaturate; Linoleic Acid, Omega-6 • Monounsaturate; Oleic Acid • Saturated Fatty Acid • Beta Carotene • Vitamin E • Phytosterols • Lecithin and Traces of Fiber.

#134 LEV Lecithin **- Systemic Formulas**
Lecithin • Inositol • Choline • Phospholipids.

#140 Min Multi-Mineral Plus **- Systemic Formulas**
Great Salt Lake Water • Calcium Carbonate • Horse Tail • Magnesium Oxide • Calcium Lactate • Calcium Citrate • Irish Moss • Magnesium Chloride • Red Root • Zinc Chelate • Kelp • Manganese Chelate • Iron Chelate • Vitamin C • Iron Aspartate • Potassium Bitartrate • Copper Chelate • Manganese Picolinate • Zinc Picolinate • Molybdenum Chelate • Vanadium Chelate • Chromium Chelate • Selenium Chelate.

#150 PRO Nutro Protein **- Systemic Formulas**
Whey Protein • Pasteurized Saccharomyces Cerevisiae • Rice Protein • Green Lipped Mussel • RNA/DNA Trachea Factors • Dolomite • Dulse • Pimiento • Choline • Papain • Horse Tail (source of silica) • Niacin • Pancreatin Enzyme • Vitamin C • Tyrosine • Valine • Aspartic Acid • Cystine • Methionine • Vitamin B6 • Vitamin E • RNA/DNA Thalamus Factors.
See Editor's Note No. 31.

#155 PTM Potassium Stabilizer **- Systemic Formulas**
Potassium Bitartrate • Potassium Chloride • Magnesium Oxide • Boldo • Pfaffia • Kelp • Maracuja • Chamomile.

200 mg of Zen **- Allergy Research Group**
Two capsules contain: GABA (gamma-aminobutyric acid) 550 mg • L-Theanine 200 mg. Other Ingredients: Silicon Dioxide, Carbowax.

#400 APHA pH Control **- Systemic Formulas**
Rhubarb Root • Spearmint • Calcium Carbonate • Nettle • Seaweed • Hyssop • Shave Grass • RNA/DNA Adrenal Factors • Potassium Bitartrate.
See Editor's Note No. 14.

#402 ARTA Arthro Support **- Systemic Formulas**
Chapu de Couro • Spearmint Leaves • Pomegranate • Vitamin B2 • RNA/DNA Adrenal Factors • Potassium Bitartrate • Magnesium Sulfate • Vitamin B6 • Niacin • Chaparral • Mistletoe • Yucca • Tayuya • Burdock Seed • Lysine • Isoleucine • Methionine • Magnesium Chelate • RNA/DNA Pituitary Factors • Zinc Chelate • Chromium Chelate.
See Editor's Note No. 31.

#403 ATAK Shield Rejuvenator **- Systemic Formulas**
Pau d'Arco • Yarrow • Stevia • Calcium Carbonate • Betaine HCl • Tayuya • Gravel Root • Pimpinella Root • Yellow Dock • Echinacea • Rose Hips.

#405 BLDB Blood Builder **- Systemic Formulas**
RNA/DNA Blood Factors • Burdock • RNA/DNA Liver Factors • Wahoo • RNA/DNA Spleen Factors • L-Cystine • L-Leucine • Chlorophyll.
See Editor's Note No. 14.

#408 CLNZ Toxin Chelator **- Systemic Formulas**
Dandelion root • Pfaffia • Cinquefoil • Milk Thistle • Mountain Mahogany • Yucca • Vitamin E • Wahoo • RNA/DNA Liver Factors • L-Methionine.
See Editor's Note No. 14.

#425 DIJS Stomach Antacid **- Systemic Formulas**
Oregon Grape • Golden Seal • Spearmint • Sodium Bicarbonate • Potassium Bitartrate • Sodium Chloride • Spearmint Oil • Anise Oil • Potassium Bicarbonate • Sodium Citrate • Malt Diastase • Chlorophyll.

#428 DSIR Digestant Internal Regenerator **- Systemic Formulas**
RNA/DNA Stomach and Duodenal Factors • Echinacea • Rose Hips • Ma Huang • Stevia • Allantoin • RNA/DNA Thymus Factors • Hesperidin • Vitamin C • L-Methionine • Senna Pod • L-Glutamic Acid • Vitamin A • Pau d'Arco • Vitamin B6 • Spearmint Oil • Aloe Vera • Sodium Copper Chlorophyll.
See Editor's Note No. 14 and 30.

#435 Gold Shield Plus **- Systemic Formulas**
Golden Seal • Niacin • Vitamin B6 • Rose Hips • Vitamin C • Fenugreek • Garlic • Vitamin B1 • Elder Berry • Spearmint Oil • Lomatium Dissecutim.

#450 KDIR Diuretic **- Systemic Formulas**
Manganese Chelate • Ch de Bugre • Juniper berry • Peach bark • Saw Palmetto • Zinc Aminoate • Magnesium Sulfate • Peach leaves • Uva Ursi.

#460 KYRO Muscle/Ligament/Tissue Strengthener **- Systemic Formulas**
Orange peel • Beta Carotene • Collagen • Bone Meal • Pfaffia • Vitamin C • Manganese Chelate • Slippery Elm • RNA/DNA Liver Factors • Vitamin B12 • Sete Sangrias • Vitamin E • Lemon Bioflavonoid • Pimiento • RNA/DNA Heart Factors • Hesperidin • Stevia • Cassia bark • Potassium Bitartrate • Vitamin A • Hawthorne berry.

#481 OXAA Cell Organizer **- Systemic Formulas**
Centaury herb • Red Clover blossom • Peach bark • Stillingia • Buckthorn bark • Oregon Grape • Cascara Sagrada • Prickly Ash bark • Cinquefoil • Saw Palmetto • Burdock root.

#482 OXCC Cell Cleanser **- Systemic Formulas**
Choke Cherry • Irish Moss • Pimiento • Blessed Thistle • Peach Bark • Oregon Grape • Fringe Tree • Red Clover • Burdock root.

#483 OXOX Cell Activator **- Systemic Formulas**
Fenugreek • Cyani Petals • Pulsatilla • Mandrake • Myrrh Gum • Gentian Root • Primrose • Pfaffia • Bugleweed • Barberry • Prickly Ash • Golden Seal • Blue Vervain • Catnip • Allantoin • Comfrey Root.

#486 SENG Red Ginseng Plus **- Systemic Formulas**
Red Ginseng • Pasteurized Saccharomyces Cerevisiae • Potassium Phosphate • Yucca • Chaparral.

#488 VIVI Anti Viro **- Systemic Formulas**
Pau D'Arco • Lomatium Dissecutim Oil • Vitamin E.

#491 VRM1 Large Pathogens **- Systemic Formulas**
Pau d'Arco • Rose Hips • Garlic • Valerian Root • Hops • Bromelain • Zapilopatle Beans • Hojas de Jalapa • Dolomite • Worm Seed Oil.

#492 VRM2 Small Pathogens **- Systemic Formulas**
Black Walnut Husks • Wormseed Herb • Kamala • Quassia Chips • Bromelain Enzyme • Bethyl Nut.

#493 VRM3 Micro Pathogens **- Systemic Formulas**
Black Walnut Husks • Carrapichinho • Erva Tostao • Aniz Estrelado • Bromelain Enzyme • Worm Seed Oil • Yerba Santa.

Some Brand Name Natural Products - What they Contain

www.NaturalDatabase.com contains MANY more listings than appear here.
Editor's Notes are located on pages 2155-2163.

#494 VRM4 Cellular Pathogens - Systemic Formulas
Kamala • Guarana • Carrapichinho • Maracuj • Wormseed Herb • Papain • Alfazema.

500-C Methoxyflavone – Metagenics
Each tablet contains: Vitamin C (as ascorbic acid) 500 mg • Citrus Bioflavonoid Complex (standardized to 45% full spectrum bioflavonoids) 500 mg.

707 Wei Yao Gastropathy Capsules - Zhengjiang Chinese Medicine Works
Yuan Hu • Wu Zei Gu • Qing Ma Ziang • Zhen Hu Mu • Ming Fan • Fen Huang Yi.
See Editor's Note No. 46.

714X - CERBE Distribution Inc.
Each 6.5 mL vial contains: Camphor or a nitrogenated derivative 0.09 mg/mL • NaCl 8.2 mg/mL • Aluminum <0.5 ppm • Antimony <1.0 ppm • Arsenic <1.0 ppm • Barium 0.7 ppm • Bore <0.05 ppm • Cadmium <0.05 ppm • Calcium 0.5 ppm • Chromium <0.1 ppm • Cobalt <1.0 ppm • Copper 0.01 ppm • Iron <0.1 ppm • Lead <1.0 ppm • Magnesium 6.5 ppm • Mercury <1.0 ppm • Molybdenum <1.0 ppm • Nickel <0.1 ppm • Phosphorus <5.0 ppm • Zinc 2.0 ppm.

911 Caps - Global Health Trax
Each capsule contains: Chitosan 600 mg • Garcinia (whole plant) 375 mg • Gymnema Sylvestre root 250 mg • Kidney Bean (phaseolus vulgaris) 250 mg. Other Ingredients: Methylcellulose, Gelatin.

1000-K Alternative Formula - Douglas Laboratories/AMNI
Each caplet contains: Proprietary Blend 1000 mg: Alpha-Carotene, Beta-Carotene, Bioflavonoids, Burdock, Astragalus, Echinacea Angustifolia, Echinacea Purpurea, Evening Primrose oil (dry), Ellagic Acid (cherries), GLA (borage seed oil, dry), Genistein (isoflavone), Ginger root, L-Glutathione, Grape seed extract, Green Tea extract, Glycyrrhetinic Acid, Lignans, Ligusticum, Lutein, Lycopene, Maitake, Shitake, and Reishi Mushrooms, Quercetin, Pectin (apple), Nucleic acids (RNA and DNA), Cartilage powder (bovine and shark), Sesame seed powder, Cruciferous Vegetables (broccoli, cabbage, cauliflower, kale), Solanaceous Foods (tomatoes, peppers, eggplant), Umbelliferous Vegetables (carrots, celery, parsnips).
See Editor's Note No. 14.

1000 mg MSM, Bones and Joints - CVS Pharmacy
Each tablet contains: MSM 1000 mg. Other Ingredients: Cellulose, Stearic Acid, Magnesium Stearate, Silicon Dioxide.

25,000 IU Natural Vitamin A & Beta Carotene - Progressive Labs
Each softgel capsule contains: Vitamin A (as beta carotene) 15,000 IU • Vitamin A (from fish liver oil) 10,000 IU • Alfalfa 5 mg • Cranberry juice concentrate 5 mg • Carrot oil 6 mg • Lecithin 5 mg. Other Ingredients: Gelatin.

A & D Natural Capsules - Progressive Labs
Each softgel contains: Vitamin A (from fish liver oil, Skip Jack liver oil) 10,000 IU • Vitamin D (from fish liver oil, Skip Jack liver oil) 400 IU.

A & D Vitamins - Puritan's Pride
Each softgel contains: Vitamin A 5000 IU • Vitamin D 400 IU.

A & E Mulsion - Aspen Group, Inc.
Each drop contains: Emulsified Vitamin A (palmitate) 5000 IU • Vitamin E (dl-alpha tocopheryl acetate) 10 IU.

A Bonanza of B Vitamins - Swanson Health Products
Each capsule contains: Thiamin (as thiamin HCl, vitamin B1) 100 mg • Riboflavin (vitamin B2) 100 mg • Niacinamide USP 100 mg • Vitamin B6 USP (as pyridoxine HCl) 100 mg • Folic Acid 400 mcg • Vitamin B12 (as cyanocobalamin) 100 mcg • Biotin USP 100 mcg • Pantothenic Acid (as D-calcium pantothenate) 100 mg • Choline (as choline bitartrate) 100 mg • Inositol 100 mg • PABA (para-aminobenzoic acid) 100 mg.

A Kid's Companion High Potency Chewable Multi-Vitamin Mineral Formula - Natrol, Inc.
Two wafers contain: Vitamins/Minerals: Vitamin A Activity (Palmitate) 2500 IU • Vitamin A (Beta Carotene) 2500 IU • Vitamin D (Calciferol) 400 IU • Vitamin E (d-Alpha Tocopheryl Succinate) 30 IU • Vitamin C (Ascorbic Acid) 60 mg • Vitamin B1 (Thiamine HCl) 2.5 mg • Vitamin B2 (Riboflavin) 2.5 mg • Vitamin B6 (Pyridoxine HCl) 2.5 mg • Vitamin B12 (Cyanocobalamin) 10 mcg • Niacinamide 20 mg • Calcium (Carbonate) 200 mg • Iron (Gluconate) 5 mg • Folic Acid 400 mcg • Biotin 150 mcg • Pantothenic Acid (Calcium d-Pantothenate) 12.5 mg • Choline (Bitartrate) 10 mg • Inositol 10 mg • PABA (Para Amino Benzoic Acid) 5 mg • Iodine (Kelp) 150 mcg • Magnesium (Oxide) 50 mg • Zinc (Gluconate) 2.5 mg • Copper (Gluconate) 200 mcg • Vitamin K 25 mcg • Selenium, organically bound concentrate 5 mcg • Chromium (ChromeMate) 10 mcg • Manganese (Gluconate) 1 mg • Potassium (Chloride) 1 mg • Silica from standardized Horsetail extract 1.5 mg • Glycine 200 mg • Lemon Bioflavonoids 25 mg • Bee Pollen 25 mg • Acerola 25 mg • Black Currant 25 mg. Other Ingredients: Lemon Fruit Extract, Orange Fruit Extract, Natural Flavors (butterscotch, vanilla), Fructose.

A Perfect You Booster Drink (cherry flavor) - Advocare International
Two wafers contain: Caffeine 100 mg • L-Carnitine 30 mg • Taurine 300 mg • L-Glutamine 100 mg • Shisandra fruit extract (schisandra chinensis) 50 mg • Golden root extract (rhodiola rosea) 50 mg. Other Ingredients: Citric Acid, Potassium Bicarbonate, Natural Flavors, Modified Cellulose, Silica, Polysorbate, Stearic Acid, Sucralose, Carmine, Magnesium Stearate.

A Perfect You Energy Drink - Advocare International
Each packet contains: Vitamin A (as beta-carotene and vitamin A palmitate) 2500 IU • Vitamin C (as ascorbic acid) 180 mg • Vitamin E (as alpha tocopheryl acetate) 30 IU •Thiamine (as HCl) 3 mg • Riboflavin 3.4 mg • Niacin (as niacinamide and niacin) 60 mg • Pyridoxine (as HCl) 15 mg • Vitamin B12 (as cyanocobalamin) 45 mcg • Pantothenic Acid (as calcium pantothenate) 50 mg • Zinc (as monomethionine - OptiZinc) 3 mg • Copper (as amino acid chelate) 200 mcg • Chromium (as polynicotinate - ChromeMate) 24 mcg • L-Carnitine (as HCl) 10 mg • Taurine 200 mg • Gamma Aminobutyric Acid (GABA) 100 mg • L-Glycine 100 mg • L-Phenylalanine 500 mg • Ribonucleic Acid 2 mg • Ubiquinone (coenzyme Q-10) 100 mcg • Choline (as citrate and bitartrate) 450 mg • Caffeine 100 mg • Green Orange extract (pericarp - citrus aurantium) 125 mg. Other Ingredients: Maltodextrin, Natural Flavor, Citric Acid, Xanthan Gum, Sucralose.
See Editor's Note No. 40.

A Perfect You Gold - Advocare International
Each 4-packet strip (two white packets and two gold packets) contains: Vitamin A (as palmitate) 2500 IU • Vitamin A (as beta-carotene) 12,500 IU • Vitamin C (as ascorbic acid and mineral ascorbates) 600 mg • Vitamin D (as cholecalciferol) 400 IU • Vitamin E (as D-alpha tocopheryl succinate) 150 IU • Thiamine 9 mg • Riboflavin 10.2 mg • Niacin (as niacin and niacinamide) 120 mg • Vitamin B6 (as pyridoxine HCl) 12 mg • Folic Acid 800 mcg • Vitamin B12 (as cyanocobalamin) 36 mcg • Biotin 300 mcg • Pantothenic Acid 40 mg • Calcium (as amino acid chelate) 150 mg • Phosphorus (as amino acid chelate) 100 mg • Iodine (from kelp) 150 mcg • Magnesium (as amino acid chelate and phosphate) 200 mg • Zinc (as zinc monomethionine) 15 mg • Selenium (L-selenomethionine) 80 mcg • Copper (as amino acid chelate) 2 mg • Manganese (as amino acid chelate) 4 mg • Chromium (as chromium polynicotinate) 100 mcg • Molybdenum (as amino acid chelate) 50 mcg • Potassium (as amino acid chelate and phosphate) 100 mg • Inositol 6 mg • Choline (as bitartrate) 60 mg • Boron (as amino acid

chelate) 300 mcg • Vanadium (as bis-glycinate-oxovanadium) 50 mcg • Silicon (as amino acid chelate) 500 mcg • Coenzyme Q-10 150 mcg • Octacosanol 2 mg • Ribonucleic Acid (RNA) 2 mg • Garlic bulb powder (allium sativum) 50 mg • L-Glutathione 5 mg • Gamma-oryzanol 5 mg • Citrus flavonoids 100 mg • Grape seed (vitis vinifera) 5 mg • Milk Thistle extract (silybum marianum) 5 mg • Ginkgo seed extract (ginkgo biloba) 10 mg • Eicosapentaenoic Acid (from marine lipids) 360 mg • Docosahexaenoic Acid (from marine lipids) 240 mg • D-Limonene powder 300 mg • Grapefruit juice powder 200 mg • 5-Hydroxytryptophan (as griffonia simplicifolia seed) 25 mg • Garcinia fruit extract (garcinia cambogia) 2000 mg • Tulsi leaf extract (ocimum sanctum) 50 mg • Taurine 50 mg • Beta-sitosterol 25 mg • L-Carnitine (as tartrate) 25 mg • Gymnema leaf extract (gymnena sylvestre) 10 mg • Oolong Tea leaf extract (camellia sinensis) 200 mg • Guarana seed extract (paullinia cupana) 550 mg • Eleuthero root extract (eleutherococcus senticosus) 50 mg • Green Tea leaf extract (camellia sinensis) 20 mg • Green Orange pericarp extract (citrus aurantium) 1000 mg • Lactobacillus Acidophilus 50 mg • Bifidobacterium Bifidum 50 mg • Fructooligosaccharides 250 mg • Moomiyo 25 mg • Aloe Vera rind powder 50 mg. Other Ingredients: Dicalcium Phosphate, Silicon Dioxide, Cellulose, Stearic Acid, Magnesium Stearate, Peppermint Extract, Vanillin, Beet Root Powder (for color), Gelatin, Glycerin, Water.
See Editor's Note No. 40.

***A Perfect You Meal Replacement Shake (Chocolate)* -** Advocare International
APY Protein Concentrate: Whey Protein concentrate, Calcium Caseinate, Sodium Caseinate, Milk Protein Isolate, Soy Protein Isolate, L-Glutamine, L-Lysine Hydrochloride, L-Leucine, L-Isoleucine, L-Valine • Fructose • Maltodextrin • Cocoa (processed with alkali) • Vitamin/Mineral Mix: Calcium Phosphate, Magnesium Oxide, Potassium Citrate, Potassium Chloride, Ascorbic Acid, Ferrous Fumarate, Vitamin E Acetate, Choline Bitartrate, Inositol, Niacinamide, Zinc Oxide, Manganese Sulfate, Calcium Pantothenate, Copper Sulfate, Vitamin A Palmitate, Pyridoxine Hydrochloride, Riboflavin, Thiamine Mononitrate, Chromium Chloride, Folic Acid, Sodium Molybdate, Biotin, Potassium Iodide, Sodium Selenite, Phytonadione, Cholecalciferol, Cyanocobalamin • Natural and Artificial Flavors • Gum Acacia • Guar Gum • Medium-Chain Triglycerides • Apple powder • Soy Fiber • Oat Fiber • Cellulose • Soy Lecithin • Rice Syrup solids • Corn Syrup solids • Lactobacillus Acidophilus • Bifidobacterium Bifidum • Sucralose • Bromelain • Papain.

***A Perfect You Nutritional Supplements* -** Advocare International
Two white packets contain: Vitamin A (as palmitate) 2500 IU • Vitamin A (as beta-carotene) 12,500 IU • Vitamin C (as ascorbic acid/mineral ascorbates) 600 mg • Vitamin D (as ergocalciferol) 400 IU • Vitamin E (as d-alpha tocopheryl succinate) 150 IU • Thiamine 9 mg • Riboflavin 10.2 mg • Niacin / Niacinamide 120 mg • Vitamin B6 12 mg • Folic Acid 800 mcg • Vitamin B12 (as cyanocobalamin) 36 mcg • Biotin 300 mcg • Pantothenic Acid 40 mg • Calcium (as amino acid chelate) 150 mg • Phosphorus (as amino acid chelate) 100 mg • Iodine (from kelp) 150 mcg • Magnesium (as amino acid chelate) 200 mg • Zinc (as monomethionine - Opti Zinc) 15 mg • Selenium (as selenomethionine) 80 mcg • Copper (as amino acid chelate) 2 mg • Manganese (as amino acid chelate) 4 mg • Chromium (as polynicotinate - ChromeMate) 100 mcg • Molybdenum (as amino acid chelate) 50 mcg • Potassium (as amino acid chelate/phosphate) 100 mg • Boron (as amino acid chelate) 300 • Vanadium (as bis-maltolato-oxovanadium) 50 mcg • Silicon (as amino acid chelate) 500 mg • Inositol 6 mg • Choline (as bitartrate) 60 mg • Coenzyme Q-10 150 mcg • Octacosanol 2000 mcg • Ribonucleic Acid (RNA) 2000 mcg • Odorless Garlic (bulb powder - allium sativum) 50 mg • L-Glutathione 5 mg • Gamma-Oryzanol 5 mg • Citrus Bioflavonoids 100 mg • Red Wine Polyphenols 5 mg • Milk Thistle extract (fruit - silybum marianum) 5 mg • Ginkgo extract (leaf - ginkgo biloba) 10 mg • L-Methionine 100 mg • Eicosapentaenoic Acid (from marine lipids) 360 mg • Docosahexaenoic Acid (from marine lipids) 240 mg • 5-Hydroxytryptophan (seed - griffonia simplicifolia) 25 mg • D-Limonene powder 300 mg • Grapefruit juice powder 200 mg. Two silver packets contain: Garcinia extract (fruit - garcinia cambogia) 2000 mg • Tulsi extract (leaf - ocimum sanctum) 50 mg • Taurine 50 mg • L-Carnitine 25 mg • Beta-Sitosterol 25 mg • Gymnema extract (leaf - gymnema sylvestre) 10 mg • Green Orange extract (pericarp - citrus aurantium) 1000 mg • Guarana extract (seed - paullinia cupana) 550 mg • Green Tea extract (leaf - camellia sinensis) 20 mg • Oolong Tea extract (leaf - camellia sinensis) 200 mg • Siberian Ginseng extract (root - eleutherococcus senticosus) 50 mg • Lactobacillus Acidophilus 0.5 billion • Bifidobacterium Bifidus 0.5 billion • Fructooligosaccharides 250 mg • Moomiyo 25 mg • Aloe Vera powder 50 mg. Other Ingredients: Dicalcium Phosphate, Silicon Dioxide, Cellulose, Stearic Acid, Magnesium Stearate, Vanillin, Gelatin, Water, Beet Root Powder (for color).
See Editor's Note No. 40.

***A Perfect You Platinum Multinutrient Dietary Supplements* -** Advocare International
Each 4-packet strip (two white packets and two gold packets) contains: Vitamin A (as palmitate) 2500 IU • Vitamin A (as beta-carotene) 12,500 IU • Vitamin C (as ascorbic acid and mineral ascorbates) 600 mg • Vitamin D (as cholecalciferol) 400 IU • Vitamin E (as D-alpha tocopheryl succinate) 150 IU • Thiamine 9 mg • Riboflavin 10.2 mg • Niacin (as niacin and niacinamide) 120 mg • Vitamin B6 (as pyridoxine HCl) 12 mg • Folic Acid 800 mcg • Vitamin B12 (as cyanocobalamin) 36 mcg • Biotin 300 mcg • Pantothenic Acid 40 mg • Calcium (as amino acid chelate) 150 mg • Phosphorus (as amino acid chelate) 100 mg • Iodine (from kelp) 150 mcg • Magnesium (as amino acid chelate and phosphate) 200 mg • Zinc (as zinc monomethionine) 15 mg • Selenium (L-selenomethionine) 80 mcg • Copper (as amino acid chelate) 2 mg • Manganese (as amino acid chelate) 4 mg • Chromium (as chromium polynicotinate) 100 mcg • Molybdenum (as amino acid chelate) 50 mcg • Potassium (as amino acid chelate and phosphate) 100 mg • Inositol 6 mg • Choline (as bitartrate) 60 mg • Boron (as amino acid chelate) 300 mcg • Vanadium (as bis-glycinate-oxovanadium) 50 mcg • Silicon (as amino acid chelate) 500 mcg • Coenzyme Q-10 150 mcg • Octacosanol 2 mg • Ribonucleic Acid (RNA) 2 mg • Garlic bulb powder (allium sativum) 50 mg • L-Glutathione 5 mg • Gamma-oryzanol 5 mg • Citrus flavonoids 100 mg • Grape seed (vitis vinifera) 5 mg • Milk Thistle extract (silybum marianum) 5 mg • Ginkgo seed extract (ginkgo biloba) 10 mg • Eicosapentaenoic Acid (from marine lipids) 360 mg • Docosahexaenoic Acid (from marine lipids) 240 mg • Garcinia fruit extract (garcinia cambogia) 2000 mg • Tulsi leaf extract (ocimum sanctum) 50 mg • Taurine 50 mg • Beta-sitosterol 25 mg • L-Carnitine (as tartrate) 25 mg • Gymnema leaf extract (gymnena sylvestre) 10 mg • Oolong Tea leaf extract (camellia sinensis) 800 mg • Kola Nut extract (cola acuminata) 500 mg • Guarana seed extract (paullinia cupana) 150 mg • Coleus Forskolii root extract 30 mg • Resveratrol (from polygonum cuspidatum) 25 mg • Eleuthero root extract (eleutherococcus senticosus) 50 mg • White Willow bark extract (salix alba) 50 mg • L-Tyrosine 800 mg • L-Glutamine 1600 mg • Green Tea leaf extract (camellia sinensis) 20 mg • Green Orange pericarp extract (citrus aurantium) 1000 mg • Lactobacillus Acidophilus 50 mg • Bifidobacterium Bifidum 50 mg • Fructooligosaccharides 250 mg • Moomiyo 25 mg • Aloe Vera rind powder 50 mg. Other Ingredients: Dicalcium Phosphate, Silicon Dioxide, Cellulose, Stearic Acid, Magnesium Stearate, Peppermint Extract, Vanillin, Beet Root Powder (for color), Gelatin, Glycerin, Water.
See Editor's Note No. 40.

***A thru Z Advantage tablets* -** Walgreens
Each tablet contains: Vitamin A (20% as beta carotene) • Vitamin C 120 mg • Vitamin D • Vitamin E • Vitamin K 25 mcg • Thiamin 4.5 mg • Riboflavin 5.1 mg • Niacin 40.0 mg • Vitamin B6 6 mg • Folic Acid 400 mcg • Vitamin B12 18 mcg • Biotin 40 mcg • Pantothenic Acid 10 mg • Calcium 100 mg • Iron 18 mg • Phosphorus 48 mg • Iodine 150 mcg • Magnesium 40 mg • Zinc 15 mg • Selenium 70 mcg • Copper 2 mg • Manganese 4 mg • Chromium 120 mcg •

Molybdenum 75 mcg • Chloride 72 mg • Potassium 80 mg • Panax Ginseng root standardized extract 50 mg • Ginkgo Biloba leaf standardized extract 60 mg • Boron 60 mcg • Nickel 5 mcg • Silicon 4 mg • Tin 10 mcg • Vanadium 10 mcg.

A.C. Formula - Pure Encapsulations
Two vegetable capsules contain: Barberry 6:1 extract (berberis vulgaris) 100 mg • Grapefruit seed extract 40 mg • Calcium (calcium undecylenate) 15 mg • Lavender extract (standardized to contain 15% essential oil) 266 mg • Tea Tree oil extract (standardized to contain 15% essential oil) 266 mg • Red Thyme extract (standardized to contain 15% essential oil 133 mg.

A.C.E. - Golden Glow Natural Health Products
Each capsule contains: Vitamin C (ascorbic acid) 500 mg • D-Alpha-Tocopherol 250 IU • Beta Carotene 25 mg • Lecithin 20 mg.

A.D.P. - Biotics Research Corporation
Each tablet contains: Oregano standardized extract (in emulsified form, incorporated into a sustained release mechanism) 50 mg.

A.H.C.C. (AHCC) - Quality of Life Labs
Two capsules contain: Proprietary Blend 500 mg: Mushroom Mycelia extract, Candelilla Wax, Cyclodextrin, Microcrystalline Cellulose. Other Ingredients: Silica, Gelatin, Glycerin.

A.I Enzymes - Pure Encapsulations
Each vegetale capsule contains: Bromelain (2400 gdu/gram) 120 mg • Papain (50,000 USP units/mg) 120 mg • Amylase (10,000 DU) 100 mg • Protease (30,000 HUT) 50 mg • Lipase (1000 LU) 60 mg • Rutin 60 mg.

A.I. Formula - Pure Encapsulations
Each vegetable capsule contains; Quercetin 250 mg • Turmeric extract (curcuma longa, standardized to contain 97% curcuminoids) 150 mg • Bromelain (2400 gdu/gram) 200 mg • Ginger extract (zingiber officinale, standardized to contain 5% gingerols) 100 mg • Vitamin C (as ascorbyl palmitate) 14 mg.

A.M.P. - Molo-Cure Research, Inc.
Each capsule contains: Freeze-dried Aloe Vera 125 mg • Soy Lecithin 375 mg.

A.M.P. MoloCure - Molo-Cure Research, Inc.
Each capsule contains: Proprietary blend 500 mg: Stabilized Aloe Mucilaginous Polysaccharide molecules • L-Glutamine powder.

A.P. Formula - Pure Encapsulations
Each vegetable capsule contains: Berberine sulfate 125 mg • Gentian 5:1 extract (gentiana lutea) 50 mg • Garlic 100:1 extract (odorless) 25 mg • Ginger extract (zingiber officinale, standardized to contain 5% gingerols) 50 mg • Quassia 5:1 extract 50 mg • Vitamin C (as ascorbyl palmitate) 9 mg.

A.S.A.P. - The Herbalist
Black Cohosh root • Passionflower herb • Scullcap herb • Valerian root • Lobelia leaf • Prickly Ash bark.

A-25 Plex - Progressive Labs
Each softgel contains: Vitamin A (beta carotene) 15,000 IU • Vitamin A (from fish liver oil) 10,000 IU • Alfalfa 5 mg • Cranberry juice concentrate 5 mg • Carrot oil 6 mg • Lecithin 5 mg.

A-25,000 IU Fish Oil - Rexall - Sundown
Each softgel contains: Vitamin A (from fish liver oil) 25,000 IU. Other Ingredients: Soybean Oil, Gelatin, Glycerin.

AARP Pharmacy Service Formula 502 (Seniors Vitamins) - Retired Persons Services, Inc.
Each caplet contains: Vitamin A (as vitamin A acetate and 3% as beta carotene) 5200 IU • Vitamin C (as ascorbic acid) 60 mg • Vitamin D (as cholecalciferol) 200 IU • Vitamin E (as dL-alpha tocopheryl acetate) 15 IU • Thiamin (vitamin B1 as thiamine mononitrate) 1.2 mg • Riboflavin 1.4 mg • Niacin (as niacinamide) 16 mg • Vitamin B6 (as pyridoxine hydrochloride) 2.2 mg • Folic Acid (folate) 400 mcg • Vitamin B12 (as cyanocobalamin) 3 mcg • Pantothenic Acid (as D-calcium pantothenate) 10 mg • Calcium (as dicalcium phosphate and calcium carbonate) 100 mg • Iron (as ferrous fumarate) 10 mg • Phosphorous (as dicalcium phosphate) 77 mg • Iodine (as potassium iodide) 150 mcg • Magnesium (as magnesium oxide) 30 mg • Zinc (as zinc oxide) 15 mg • Copper (as cupric sulfate) 2 mg • Manganese (as manganese sulfate) 1 mg • Potassium (as potassium sulfate) 5 mg.

Abana - The Himalaya Drug Company
Each tablet contains: Arjuna (terminalia arjuna) 30 mg • Ashvagandha (withania somnifera) 20 mg • Badranj Boya (nepeta hindostana) 20 mg • Dashamoola 20 mg: Aegle Marmelos root, Gmelina Arborea root, Oroxylum Indicum root, Clerodendrum Phlomidis root, Stereospermum Chelonoides root, Desmodium Gangeticum root, Uraria Picta root, Solanum Indicum root, Solanum Surattense root, Tribulus Terrestris root • Guduchi (tinospora cordifolia) 10 mg • Amalaki (emblica officinalis) 10 mg • Haritaki (terminalia chebula) 10 mg • Bhringaraja (eclipta alba syn. e. prostrata) 10 mg • Yashti-Madhu (glycyrrhiza glabra) 10 mg • Shatavari (asparagus racemosus) 10 mg • Punarnava (boerhaavia diffusa) 10 mg • Guggulu (balsamodendron mukul syn. commiphora wightii, purified) 30 mg • Shilajeet (mineral pitch, purified) 20 mg • Mandukaparni (centella asiatica) 10 mg • Shankhapushpi (convolvulus pluricaulis syn. c.microphyllus) 10 mg • Vishnu Priya (ocimum sanctum syn. o.tenuiflorum) 10 mg • Jatamansi (nardostachys jatamansi) 10 mg • Pippali (piper longum) 10 mg • Yawani (carum copticum syn. trachyspermum ammi) 10 mg • Sunthi (zingiber officinale) 10 mg • Nagapashana Bhasma (calx serpentine, magnesium silicate) 10 mg • Shankh Bhasma (conch shell/ash) 10 mg • Makardwaj (sulphide of mercury) 10 mg • Musta (cyperus rotundus) 5 mg • Vacha (acorus calamus) 5 mg • Vidanga (embelia ribes) 5 mg • Lavanga (syzygium aromaticum) 5 mg • Jyotishmati (celastrus paniculatus) 5 mg • Chandana (santalum album) 5 mg • Ela (elettaria cardamomum) 5 mg • Shatapuspha (foeniculum vulgare) 5 mg • Satapatrika (rosa damascena syn. r.centifolia) 5 mg • Tvak Patra (cinnamomum cassia) 5 mg • Abhrak Bhasma (powdered talc, biotite calx) 5 mg • Mukta Pishti (processed pearl) 5 mg • Akik Pishti (processed agate) 5 mg • Yeshab Pishti (processed vyomashma) 5 mg • Yakut Pishti (processed manikya) 5 mg • Praval Pishti (processed coral) 5 mg • Kumkuma (crocus sativus) 2 mg.

ABC Dophilus - Solgar
Each 1/2 tsp serving contains: ABC Dophilus powder complex (supplying 1 billion live microorganisms) 1 g: B. Bifidum 350 million viable organisms, S. Thermophilus 350 million viable microorganisms, B. Infantis 350 million viable microorganisms. Other Ingredients: Maltodextrin, Silica, Casein (a milk derivative).

ABC Plus SENIOR - Vitamin World
Each tablet contains: Vitamin A (as vitamin A acetate and beta carotene) 3500 IU • Vitamin C (as ascorbic acid) 60 mg • Vitamin D (as cholecalciferol) 400 IU • Vitamin E (as dL-alpha tocopheryl acetate) 45 IU • Vitamin K (as phytonadione) 10 mcg • Thiamin (vitamin B1, as thiamin mononitrate) 1.5 mg • Riboflavin (vitamin B2) 1.7 mg • Niacin (as niacinamide) 20 mg • Vitamin B6 (as pyridoxine hydrochloride) 3 mg • Folic Acid 400 mcg • Vitamin B12 (as cyanocobalamin) 25 mcg • Biotin (as D-biotin) 30 mcg • Pantothenic Acid (as D-calcium pantothenate) 10 mg • Calcium (as calcium carbonate and dicalcium phosphate) 200 mg • Phosphorus (as dicalcium phosphate) 48 mg • Iodine (as potassium iodide) 150 mcg • Magnesium (as magnesium oxide) 100 mg • Zinc (as zinc oxide) 15 mg • Selenium (as sodium selenate) 20 mcg • Copper (as cupric oxide) 2 mg • Manganese (as manganese sulfate) 2 mg • Chromium (as chromium chloride) 150 mcg • Molybdenum (as sodium molybdate) 75 mcg • Chloride (as potassium chloride) 72 mg • Potassium (as potassium chloride) 80 mg • Boron (as sodium borate) 150 mcg • Nickel (as nickel sulfate) 5 mcg • Silica (as silicon dioxide) 2 mg • Vanadium (as sodium metavanadate) 10 mcg • Lycopene (from tomato extract) 300 mcg • Lutein (from marigold extract) 250 mcg. Other Ingredients: Cellulose, Croscarmellose,

Vegetable Stearic Acid, Vegetable Magnesium Stearate, Mannitol, Cellulose Coating, Starch, FD&C Blue No. 2 Lake, Titanium Dioxide Color, FD&C Yellow No. 6 Lake, FD&C Red No. 40 Lake.

ABC Plus SENIOR **- Puritan's Pride**

Each tablet contains: Vitamin A (as vitamin A acetate and beta carotene) 3500 IU • Vitamin C (as ascorbic acid) 60 mg • Vitamin D (as cholecalciferol) 400 IU • Vitamin E (as dL-alpha tocopheryl acetate) 45 IU • Vitamin K (as phytonadione) 10 mcg • Thiamin (vitamin B1 as thiamin mononitrate) 1.5 mg • Riboflavin (vitamin B2) 1.7 mg • Niacin (as niacinamide) 20 mg • Vitamin B6 (as pyridoxine hydrochloride) 3 mg • Folic Acid 400 mcg • Vitamin B12 (as cyanocobalamin) 25 mcg • Biotin (as D-biotin) 30 mcg • Pantothenic Acid (as D-calcium pantothenate) 10 mg • Calcium (as calcium carbonate and dicalcium phosphate) 200 mg • Phosphorus (as dicalcium phosphate) 48 mg • Iodine (as potassium iodide) 150 mcg • Magnesium (as magnesium oxide) 100 mg • Zinc (as zinc oxide) 15 mg • Selenium (as sodium selenate) 20 mcg • Copper (as cupric oxide) 2 mg • Manganese (as manganese sulfate) 2 mg • Chromium (as chromium chloride) 150 mcg • Molybdenum (as sodium molybdate) 75 mcg • Chloride (as potassium chloride) 72 mg • Potassium (as potassium chloride) 80 mg • Boron (as sodium borate) 150 mcg • Nickel (as nickel sulfate) 5 mcg • Silica (as silicon dioxide) 2 mg • Vanadium (as sodium metavanadate) 10 mcg • Lycopene (from tomato fruit extract) 300 mcg • Lutein (from marigold flower extract) 250 mcg. Other Ingredients: Cellulose (plant origin), Croscarmellose, Vegetable Stearic Acid, Vegetable Magnesium Stearate, Mannitol, Cellulose Coating, Starch, FD&C Blue No. 2 Lake, Titanium Dioxide Color, FD&C Yellow No. 6 Lake, FD&C Red No. 40 Lake.

ABC Plus Tablets **- Vitamin World**

Each tablet contains: Vitamin A (as retinyl acetate and beta carotene) 3500 IU • Vitamin C (as ascorbic acid) 60 mg • Vitamin D (as cholecalciferol) 400 IU • Vitamin E (as dL-alpha tocopheryl acetate) 30 IU • Vitamin K (as phytonadione) 25 mcg • Thiamin (vitamin B1, as thiamin mononitrate) 1.5 mg • Riboflavin (vitamin B2) 1.7 mg • Niacin (as niacinamide) 20 mg • Vitamin B6 (as pyridoxine hydrochloride) 2 mg • Folic Acid 400 mcg • Vitamin B12 (as cyanocobalamin) 6 mcg • Biotin (as D-biotin) 30 mcg • Pantothenic Acid (as D-calcium pantothenate) 10 mg • Calcium (as dicalcium phosphate and calcium carbonate) 162 mg • Iron (as ferrous fumarate) 18 mg • Phosphorus (as dicalcium phosphate) 109 mg • Iodine (as potassium iodide) 150 mcg • Magnesium (as magnesium oxide) 100 mg • Zinc (as zinc oxide) 15 mg • Selenium (as sodium selenate) 20 mcg • Copper (as cupric oxide) 2 mg • Manganese (as manganese sulfate) 2 mg • Chromium (as chromium chloride) 120 mcg • Molybdenum (as sodium molybdate) 75 mcg • Chloride (as potassium chloride) 72 mg • Potassium (as potassium chloride) 80 mg • Boron (as sodium borate) 150 mcg • Nickel (as nickel sulfate) 5 mcg • Silica (as silicon dioxide) 2 mg • Tin (as tin chloride) 10 mcg • Vanadium (as sodium metavanadate) 10 mcg • Lutein (from marigold extract) 250 mcg • Lycopene (from tomato extract) 300 mcg. Other Ingredients: Cellulose, Croscarmellose, Vegetable Stearic Acid, Vegetable Magnesium Stearate, Mannitol, Cellulose Coating, Starch, FD&C Yellow No. 6 Lake, Titanium Dioxide Color.

ABC Plus with Lutein & Lycopene **- Puritan's Pride**

Each tablet contains: Vitamin A (as retinyl acetate and beta carotene) 3500 IU • Vitamin C (as ascorbic acid) 60 mg • Vitamin D (as cholecalciferol) 400 IU • Vitamin E (as dL-alpha tocopheryl acetate) 30 IU • Vitamin K (as phytonadione) 25 mcg • Thiamin (vitamin B1, as thiamin mononitrate) 1.5 mg • Riboflavin (vitamin B2) 1.7 mg • Niacin (as niacinamide) 20 mg • Vitamin B6 (as pyridoxine hydrochloride) 2 mg • Folic Acid 400 mcg • Vitamin B12 (as cyanocobalamin) 6 mcg • Biotin (as D-biotin) 30 mcg • Pantothenic Acid (as D-calcium pantothenate) 10 mg • Calcium (as dicalcium phosphate and calcium carbonate) 162 mg • Iron (as ferrous fumarate) 18 mg • Phosphorus (as dicalcium phosphate) 109 mg • Iodine (as potassium iodide) 150 mcg • Magnesium (as magnesium oxide) 100 mg • Zinc (as zinc oxide) 15 mg • Selenium (as sodium selenite) 20 mcg • Copper (as cupric oxide) 2 mg • Manganese (as manganese sulfate) 2 mg • Chromium (as chromium chloride) 120 mcg • Molybdenum (as sodium molybdate) 75 mcg • Chloride (as potassium chloride) 72 mg • Potassium (as potassium chloride) 80 mg • Boron (as sodium borate) 150 mcg • Nickel (as nickel sulfate) 5 mcg • Silica (as silicon dioxide) 2 mg • Tin (as tin chloride) 10 mcg • Vanadium (as sodium metavanadate) 10 mcg • Lutein (from marigold flower extract) 250 mcg • Lycopene (from tomato fruit extract) 300 mcg. Other Ingredients: Cellulose (plant origin), Croscarmellose, Vegetable Stearic Acid, Vegetable Magnesium Stearate, Mannitol, Cellulose Coating, Starch, FD&C Yellow No. 6 Lake, Titanium Dioxide Color.

AB-Fem Glandular **- American Biologics**

Each tablet contains: Ovarian tissue 40 mg • Thymus tissue 20 mg • Spleen tissue 20 mg • Adrenal concentrate 20 mg • Superoxide Dismutase 20 mcg • Catalase (of bovine origin) 20 mcg. Other Ingredients: Dicalcium Phosphate, Cellulose, Magnesium Stearate. See Editor's Note No. 14.

AbGone **- Albion Medical**

Two capsules contain: Vitamin C (ascorbic acid) 175 mg • Zinc (zinc citrate) 7.5 mg • Chromium 100 mcg • Dandelion root/leaf powder 150 mg • AbGone Proprietary Blend 820 mg: Phosphatidylserine, CLA, L-Leucine, L-Isoleucine, L-Valine. Other Ingredients: Soybean Oil, Beeswax, Kosher Gelatin, Glycerin, Titanium Dioxide, Purified Water, FD&C Red #40, FD&C Blue #1, FD&C Blue #6.

Able Eyes **- J. R. Carlson Laboratories, Inc.**

Each softgel contains: Vitamin A (from fish liver oil) 500 IU • Vitamin C (as ascorbic acid) 180 mg • Vitamin E (as D-alpha tocopherol) 200 IU • Magnesium (as magnesium oxide) 80 mg • Zinc (as zinc citrate) 7 mg • Selenium (as L-selenomethionine) 70 mcg • Chromium 120 mcg • Quercetin Bioflavonoid 50 mg • Zeaxanthin 264 mg • Silymarin seeds 50 mg • Bilberry (vaccinium myrtillus, 25% anthocyanosides) 50 mg • Lutein (FloraGlo brand, from marigolds) 6 mg • NAC (N-Acetyl cysteine) 20 mg • Citrus Bioflavonoids complex 50 mg • DHA (docosahexaenoic acid) 100 mg • L-Taurine 25 mg.

Ablene **- Progressive Health Nutraceuticals**

Vitamin A 10,000 IU • Vitamin C 75 mg • Vitamin D (D3) 200 IU • Vitamin E 100 IU • Vitamin B1 12.5 mg • Vitamin B2 12.5 mg • Vitamin B3 50 mg • Vitamin B6 12.5 mg • Folic Acid 400 mcg • Vitamin B12 200 mcg • Biotin 10 mcg • Vitamin B5 25 mg • Iron 25.01 mg • Iodine 65 mcg • Magnesium 2.601 mg • Zinc 20 mg • Copper 0.13 mg • Manganese 3 mg • Para-Aminobenzoic Acid 12 mg • Citrus Bioflavonoids 12.5 mg • Rutin 12.5 mg • Betaine HCl 12.5 mg • Hesperidin 2.5 mg • Huperzine A extract 0.5 mg • Choline 0.08 mg • Inositol 0.13 mg • L-Glutamine 1000 mg • Cat's Claw 200 mg • Licorice 100 mg • Olive extract 50 mg.

AB-Male Glandular **- American Biologics**

Each tablet contains: Orchic tissue 40 mg • Thymus tissue 20 mg • Spleen tissue 20 mg • Adrenal concentrate 20 mg • Superoxide Dismutase 20 mcg • Catalase (of bovine origin) 20 mcg. Other Ingredients: Dicalcium Phosphate, Cellulose, Magnesium Stearate. See Editor's Note No. 14.

Absorbable Calcium **- PhysioLogics**

Two softgels contain: Vitamin D (as cholecalciferol) 100 IU • Calcium (as calcium carbonate) 1000 mg. Other Ingredients: Soybean Oil, Gelatin, Glycerin, Lecithin, Titanium Dioxide Color.

Absorbable Calcium with Vitamin D **- Puritan's Pride**

Two softgels contain: Vitamin D (as cholecalciferol) 100 IU • Calcium (as calcium carbonate) 1000 mg. Other Ingredients: Soybean Oil, Gelatin, Glycerin, Lecithin, Titanium Dioxide Color.

Absorbable Calcium with Vitamin D **- Nature's Bounty**

Two softgels contain: Vitamin D (as Cholecalciferol) 100 IU • Calcium (as Calcium Carbonate) 1000 mg. Other Ingredients: Soybean Oil, Gelatin, Glycerin, Lecithin, Titanium Dioxide Color.

Some Brand Name Natural Products - What they Contain

www.NaturalDatabase.com contains MANY more listings than appear here.
Editor's Notes are located on pages 2155-2163.

Absorbable Iron with Hematinic Factors - The Vitamin Shoppe
Each tablet contains: Iron 50 mg • Heme Iron 25 mg • Vitamin C 75 mg • Copper 1 mg • Folic Acid 200 mcg • Vitamin B12 12.5 mcg.

AbsorbAid - Nature's Sources
Two capsules contain: Lipase 1145 LU • Amylase 8316 SKBU • Protease (from Bromelain) 36 GDU • Cellulase 299 CU • Lactase 900 LacU.

Absorbitol Fat Binder - Natrol, Inc.
Two capsules contain: Chitosan Complex 900 mg. Other Ingredients: Magnesium Stearate, Gelatin.

Abundance of Greens - Abundance Marketing
Each scoop contains: Soy Lecithin (97% phosphatides) 1000 mg • Enzyme-Active brand 10:1 concentrate 1600 mg: Alfalfa, Barley greens, Buckwheat, Kamut, Red Beet, Wheat Grass • Hawaiian Spirulina Pacifica 1600 mg • Multi-Algae blend 400 mg • Non-dairy four-culture Probiotic blend (provides 2.5 billion organisms) with patented Dahlulin PB Inulin and FOS from Dahlia, Chicory and Jerusalem Artichoke 500 mg • Five-Fibre blend 100 0mg • Milk Thistle 30:1 extract 60 mg • Sprouted Multi-Grains 400 mg • Whole Brown Rice powder 250 mg • Acerola berry 4:1 extract 125 mg • Ginkgo Biloba 2000:1 standardized extract 30 mg • Royal Jelly (from lyophilized 3.5:1 concentrate) 150 mg • Multi-flora wildflower Bee Pollen 150 mg • Astragalus root 60 mg • Grape seed extract (50% proanthocyanidins) 9 mg • European Bilberry 50:1 standardized extract (25% anthocyanosides) 10 mg • Siberian Ginseng root standardized extract (0.5% eleutherosides) 75 mg • Licorice root standardized extract (15% glycyrrhizin) 125 mg • Stevia leaf extract 20 mg • Tomato powder (10:1 concentrate) 100 mg. Other Ingredients: Natural Flavors, BeFlora Plus brand (50% fructooligosaccharides, 47.5% soy extract, and 2.5% potato starch), Silica.

A-C Carbamide - Standard Process, Inc.
Each capsule contains: Proprietary Blend: 2675 mg: Carbamide, Arrowroot flour • Vitamin A 825 IU • Vitamin C 6 mg. Other Ingredients: Gelatin, Water, Colors.

Acai - Life Dynamics
Two capsules contain: Acai 4:1 extract (euterpe oleracea) 1000 mg.

Acai Lite - Life Dynamics
Two capsules contain: Acai 1:1 extract (euterpe oleracea) 800 mg • Acerola extract - 15% (malpighiaceae) 200 mg.

Accel Dietary Supplement - Atkins Nutritionals, Inc.
Each capsule contains: Niacin (B3) 15 mg • Chromium (as chromium polynicotinate) 100 mcg • Glucomannan (konjac flour) 350 mg • Green Tea leaf extract (providing caffeine 50 mg, epigallocatechin gallate 90 mg) 350 mg. Other Ingredients: Gelatin, Magnesium Stearate.

Acceleration - PhytoPharmica
Each capsule contains: Cola Nut extract (cola nitida) 250 mg (contains 35 mg of caffeine) • Green Tea extract (Camellia sinensis) 250 mg (contains 15 mg of caffeine) • Ma Huang extract (Ephedra sinensis) 250 mg (contains 15 mg of ephedrine).
See Editor's Note No. 21 and No. 30.

Acceleration (Ephedra Free!) - PhytoPharmica
Each capsule contains: Bitter Orange fruit extract (citrus x aurantium, standardized to contain 6% synephrine) 250 mg • Cola nut extract (cola nitida, standardized to contain 35 mg caffeine) 250 mg • Green Tea leaf extract (camellia sinensis, containing 15 mg caffeine) 110 mg. Other Ingredients: Gelatin, Cellulose, Magnesium Stearate, Silicon Dioxide, Titanium Dioxide Color.
See Editor's Note No. 40.

Accu-Mind & Memory - Leiner Health Products
Each caplet contains: Ginkgo Biloba extract (Ginkgo biloba) leaf 60 mg • Vinpocetine 5 mg. Other Ingredients: Dicalcium Phosphate, Cellulose, Silicon Dioxide, Croscarmellose Sodium, Stearic Acid, Dextrin, Crospovidone, Magnesium Stearate, Dextrose, Lecithin, Sodium Carboxymethylcellulose, Sodium Citrate.

Accunatural - Skinutrients, LLC
Three tablets contain: Vitamin A (acetate) 5000 IU • Vitamin E (tocopherol succinate) 400 IU • Vitamin B6 50 mg • Pantothenic Acid 500 mg • Zinc 50 mg • Selenium 200 mcg • Chromium 200 mcg. Other Ingredients: Stearic Acid, Magnesium Stearate, Croscarmellose Sodium, Microcrystalline Cellulose, Silicon Dioxide, Dicalcium.

ACE Antioxidant Complex - Nature's Life
Each tablet contains: Beta Carotene (Vitamin A equivalent to 5000 IU) 3 mg • Vitamin C 500 mg • Vitamin E (d-Alpha Tocopheryl Succinate) 200 IU • Selenium (Selenomax Selenomethionine) 25 mcg. In a natural base of Rose Hips powder & Nature's Life Greens (A proprietary blend of 24 vegetables & herbs, microalgae, sea vegetables & sprouts).

ACE Ultimate Antioxidant Plus - Nature's Life
Two capsules contain: Antioxidant Nutrients: Beta Carotene (vitamin A equivalent to 25,000 IU) 15 mg • Vitamin C 1000 mg • Vitamin E (D-alpha tocopheryl succinate) 300 IU • Vitamin B2 (riboflavin, riboflavin-5-phosphate) 10 mg • Selenium (selenite, methionine) 200 mcg • Glutathione (glutamine/cysteine / glycine tripeptide) 100 mg • Superoxide Dismutase - inducing Minerals: Zinc (citrate, picolinate) 10 mg • Manganese (citrate) 10 mg • Copper (citrate, gluconate) 1 mg • Antioxidant Flavonoids: Lemon Bioflavonoids Complex (TESTLAB 50% total bioflavonoids as flavanones, hesperidin, naringenin & eriocitrin = 50%) 25 mg • Quercetin (dimorphandra pod) 25 mg • Rutin (saphora japonica) 25 mg • Hesperidin (citrus) 25 mg • Pine bark Proanthocyanidins (pinus maritima extract) 5 mg • Epigallocatechin Gallate (camellia sinensis (green tea) extract) 5 mg.

Acerola Chewable C 120 mg - Source Naturals
Each tablet contains: Vitamin C (as ascorbic acid & sodium ascorbate) 120 mg • Bioflavonoids 20 mg • Rutin 20 mg • Acerola Cherry 5 mg • Rosehips 4 mg.

Acerola Chewable C 500 mg - Source Naturals
Each tablet contains: Vitamin C (as ascorbic acid & sodium ascorbate) 500 mg • Bioflavonoids 20 mg • Rutin 20 mg • Acerola Cherry 5 mg • Rosehips 4 mg.

Acerola Plus - Pure Encapsulations
Each vegetable capsule contains: Acerola extract (malpighia glabra L., providing 17% vitamin C) 150 mg • Vitamin C (as ascorbyl palmitate, providing 43% vitamin C) 13 mg • Ascorbic Acid (providing 100% vitamin C) 200 mg • Hesperidine Methyl Chalcone (98% pure) 150 gm • Naringin (98% pure) 150 mg.

ACES - J. R. Carlson Laboratories, Inc.
Two softgels contain: Vitamin A (as beta carotene) 10,000 IU • Vitamin C (as calcium ascorbate) 1000 mg • Vitamin E (as D-alpha tocopherol) 400 IU • Calcium (as calcium ascorbate) 100 mg • Selenium (as L-selenomethionine) 100 mcg.

ACES + Zn - J. R. Carlson Laboratories, Inc.
Two softgels contain: Vitamin A (as beta carotene) 10,000 IU • Vitamin C (as calcium ascorbate) 500 mg • Vitamin E (as D-alpha tocopherol) 400 IU • Calcium (as calcium ascorbate) 50 mg • Zinc (as zinc citrate) 15 mg • Selenium (as L-selenomethionine) 100 mcg.

ACES Gold - J. R. Carlson Laboratories, Inc.
Two tablets contain: Vitamin A (as beta carotene) 10,000 IU • Vitamin C (as calcium ascorbate) 1000 IU • Vitamin E (as D-alpha tocopheryl sucinate) 400 IU • Calcium (as calcium ascorbate) 100 mg • Zinc (as zinc glycinate chelate) 7 mg • Selenium (as L-selenomethionine) 100 mcg • Copper (as copper glycinate chelate) 1 mg • Manganese (as manganese glycinate chelate) 2 mg • Lutein 1 mg • Quercetin Bioflavonoid 30 mg • Alpha Lipoic 6 mg • Citrus Bioflavonoids Complex 100 mg • Co-Q10 (coenzyme Q10) 15 mg • Garlic bulb (allium sativum, odorless) 100 mg • Glutathione 3 mg • Grape seed extract 10 mg • Green Tea 3 mg • L-Cysteine (N-acetyl) 50 mg.

Some Brand Name Natural Products - What they Contain

www.NaturalDatabase.com contains MANY more listings than appear here.
Editor's Notes are located on pages 2155-2163.

BRAND NAMES

Acetabolan **-** MuscleTech
Six capsules contain: Acetyl-L-Carnitine 1000 mg • Glutamine 2000 mg • L-Leucine 1000 mg • L-Valine 250 mg • L-Isoleucine 250 mg • OKG 100 mg • Zinc 60 mg • Taurine 1000 mg.

Acetabolan II **-** MuscleTech
Six capsules contain: NAC (as N-acetyl-cysteine hydrochloride) 400 mg • Acetyl-L-Carnitine • Tribulus Terrestris • ZincTech brand blend: Chelated Zinc, Magnesium, Vitamin B6.

Acetyl Glucosamine **-** Life Enhancement Products, Inc.
Each capsule contains: Acetyl Glucosamine 500 mg. Other Ingredients: Silicon Dioxide, Gelatin Capsule.

Acetyl L Carnitine **-** Physician Formulas
Each capsule contains: Acetyl-L-Carnitine 300 mg • Alpha Lipoic Acid 10 mg.

Acetyl L-Carnitine **-** Source Naturals
Each tablet contains: Acetyl-l-Carnitine 500 mg.

Acetyl L-Carnitine **-** NSI - Nutraceutical Sciences Institute
Each tablet contains: Acetyl L-Carnitine 500 mg.

Acetyl L-Carnitine **-** PhysioLogics
Each capsule contains: Acetyl L-Carnitine (as acetyl l-carnitine hydrochloride) 250 mg. Other Ingredients: Dicalcium Phosphate, Gelatin, Vegetable Magnesium Stearate.

Acetyl L-Carnitine **-** Optimum Nutrition
Each capsule contains: Acetyl L-Carnitine 1000 mg. Other Ingredients: Gelatin, Magnesium Stearate.

Acetyl L-Carnitine **-** Life Enhancement Products, Inc.
Each capsule contains: Acetyl L-Carnitine (as acetyl l-carnitine hydrochloride) 500 mg.

Acetyl L-Carnitine **-** Ortho Molecular Products
Each capsule contains: N-Acetyl L-Carnitine HCl 500 mg. Other Ingredients: Natural Vegetable Capsules, Ascorbyl Palmitate, Microcrystalline Cellulose, Silicon Dioxide.

Acetyl L-Carnitine **-** Pro Health
Each capsule contains: Acetyl L-Carnitine 500 mg. Other Ingredients: Rice Flour, Gelatin, Magnesium Stearate.

Acetyl L-Carnitine 167mg **-** N.V. Perricone M.D. Cosmeceuticals
Each capsule contains: Acetyl L-Carnitine (as 260 mg galactarate) 167 mg. Other Ingredients: Gelatin, Calcium Sulfate, Croscarmellose Sodium, Magnesium Stearate, Silica.

Acetyl L-Carnitine 250 **-** Jarrow Formulas
Each capsule contains: Acetyl-L-Carnitine 250 mg. Other Ingredients: Cellulose, Magnesium Stearate, Silicon Dioxide, Gelatin.

Acetyl L-Carnitine 250 mg **-** Vitamin World
Each capsule contains: Acetyl L-Carnitine (as acetyl L-carnitine hydrochloride) 250 mg. Other Ingredients: Dicalcium Phosphate, Gelatin, Vegetable Magnesium Stearate.

Acetyl L-Carnitine 500 **-** Jarrow Formulas
Each capsule contains: Acetyl-L-Carnitine 500 mg. Other Ingredients: Cellulose, Magnesium Stearate, Silicon Dioxide, Gelatin.

Acetyl L-Carnitine 500 mg with Alpha Lipoic Acid 200 mg **-** Vitamin World
Each capsule contains: Acetyl L-Carnitine 500 mg • Alpha Lipoic Acid 200 mg. Other Ingredients: Gelatin, Marnesium Silicate, Vegetable Magnesium Stearate.

Acetyl L-Carnitine Powder **-** Vital Nutrients
Each 1/4 teaspoon contains: Acetyl-L-Carnitine HCl 1500 mg.

Acetyl-L-Carnitine **-** Douglas Laboratories/AMNI
Each capsule contains: Acetyl-L-Carnitine 500 mg.

Acetyl-L-Carnitine (250 mg) **-** Allergy Research Group
Each capsule contains: Acetyl-L-Carnitine 250 mg. Other Ingredients: Cellulose, Silicon Dioxide, Stearic Acid.

Acetyl-L-Carnitine (500 mg) **-** Allergy Research Group
Each capsule contains: Acetyl-L-Carnitine 500 mg. Other Ingredients: Cellulose, Silicon Dioxide, Stearic Acid.

Acetyl-L-Carnitine 250 mg **-** Solgar
Each capsule contains: Calcium (as dicalcium phosphate) 60 mg • Acetyl-L-Carnitine (as acetyl-L-carnitine chloride) 250 mg. Other Ingredients: Dicalcium Phosphate, Vegetable Cellulose, Microcrystalline Cellulose, Vegetable Magnesium Stearate, Silica, Water, Vegetable Glycerin.

Acetyl-l-Carnitine 250 mg **-** Pure Encapsulations
Each vegetable capsule contains: Acetyl-L-Carnitine (free-form) 250 mg • Vitamin C (as ascorbyl palmitate) 4 mg.

Acetyl-L-Carnitine 500 **-** GNC
Each capsule contains: Acetyl-L-Carnitine Hydrochloride 500 mg. Other Ingredients: Gelatin, Cellulose.

Acetyl-l-Carnitine 500 mg **-** Pure Encapsulations
Each vegetable capsule contains: Acetyl-L-Carnitine (free-form) 500 mg • Vitamin C (as ascorbyl palmitate) 8 mg.

ACF 223 **-** Gero Vita International
Each capsule contains: Vitamin A (as beta-carotene) 900 IU • Vitamin B3 (as niacinamide) 60 mg • Zinc (as gluconate) 7.6 mg • Selenium 13.6 mcg • Copper (as copper gluconate) 0.6 mg • Manganese 0.136 mg • Chromium 28 mcg • Molybdenum 15.2 mcg • L-Carnitine Fumarate 100 mg • MultiMins 78 mg • Uncaria Tomentosa bark extract 50 mg • Tocotrienols 30 mg • CoQ10 10 mg. Other Ingredients: Silica, Magnesium Stearate, Gelatin, Cellulose, Dicalcium Phosphate.

Acid Defense Nature's Acid Relief Formula **-** Garden of Life, Inc.
Each tablespoon (12 g) contains: Mineral Matrix from Goat's Milk Whey 10,060 mg • Potassium 411 mg • Calcium 146 mg • Chloride 130 gm • Phosphorus 116 mg • Sodium 88 mg • Zinc 370 mcg • Iron 240 mcg • Molybdenum 29 mcg • Chromium 5.5 mcg • Selenium 1 mcg • Copper 8 mcg • Manganese 0.7 mcg • Beet juice concentrate (33:1) 600 mg • Carrot juice concentrate (33:1) 600 mg • Barley Grass juice concentrate (33:1) 600 mg • Stomach Soothe Enzyme Blend 150 mg: Amylase 9000 DU, Glucoamylase 20 AGU, Lipase 400 LU, Alpha Galactosidase 150 GalU, Malt Diastase 950 DP, Cellulose 800 CU, Sucrose 675 SU, Lactose 650 ALU.

Acid Redux **-** NOW Foods
Each lozenge contains: Vitamin C (as ascorbic acid) 12 mg • Vitamin D (as cholecalciferol) 150 IU • Calcium (as calcium carbonate) 116 mg • Magnesium (from magnesium hydroxide) 11 mg • Potassium (from potassium hydroxide) 4 mg • Acid Redux 373 mg: Calcium Carbonate, Magnesium Hydroxide, Potassium Hydroxide • Stevia Rebaudiana leaf extract (enzyme-treated, min. 80% glycosylsteviosides). Other Ingredients: Fructose, Maltodextrin, Sorbitol, Stearic Acid, Natural Peppermint Flavor, Gum Acacia (food grade).

Acid-A-Cal **-** Enzymatic Therapy
Two capsules contain: Calcium (from calcium chloride and calcium phosphate) 108 mg • Magnesium (glycerophosphate) 11 mg • Vitamin C 100 mg • Vitamin B6 (pyridoxine HCl) 50 mg • Betaine HCl 192 mg • Ammonium Chloride 192 mg • Kidney extract (freeze-dried) 60 mg • Citrus Bioflavonoids 60 mg. Other Ingredients: Gelatin, Cellulose, Silicon Dioxide, Magnesium Stearate, Titanium Dioxide. See Editor's Note No. 14.

Acida-Zyme **-** Progressive Labs
Each capsule contains: Betaine HCl 200 mg • Glutamic Acid HCl 100 mg • Ammonium Chloride 35 mg • Pepsin USP/NF 25 mg • Protease (from plant enzymes) 150 Units.

Some Brand Name Natural Products - What they Contain

www.NaturalDatabase.com contains MANY more listings than appear here.
Editor's Notes are located on pages 2155-2163.

Acid-Ease - Enzymatic Therapy
Two capsules contain: Slippery Elm bark (ulma rubra) 200 mg • Marshmallow root extract (althaea officinalis) 200 mg • Gamma-Oryzanol (from rice bran) 150 mg • Pure Plant Enzymes Blend 109 mg: Amylase, Lipase II, Cellulase I. Other Ingredients: Gelatin, Microcrystalline Cellulose, Ascorbyl Palmitate.

AcidFree - Performance Labs
Each tablet contains: Calcium (precipitated calcium, carbonated) 200 mg • FOS (fructooligosaccharides) 40 mg • Proprietary Digestive Enzyme Blend 15 mg: Amylase, Neutral Protease, Lactase, Lipase, Cellulase. Other Ingredients: Sorbitol, Sucrose, Mannitol, Pregelatinized Starch, Cellulose Gum, Natural Flavor, Sodium Potassium Polyphosphate, Stearic Acid, Magnesium Stearate.

Acidophilase - Wakunaga of America
Each caspule contains: Lactobacillus acidophilus 1 billion live cells • Food Enzyme complex 155 mg: Protease, Amylase, & Lactase in a vegetable starch complex.

Acidophilus - Trophic
Each capsule contains: 6 Billion Active Cells: L. Acidophilus 50% • Bifidobacteria Bifidus 34% • S. Faecium 16%.

Acidophilus - Nature Made
Each tablet contains: L. Acidophilus cells 500 million.

Acidophilus - Cell Tech
Two capsules contain: Vitamin K 6.8 mcg • Proprietary Blend 410 mg: Lactobacillus Acidophilus, Blue-Green Algae (aph. flos-aquae) 170 mg. Other Ingredients: Maltodextrin, Plant Cellulose, Gelatin Capsule.

Acidophilus - PhytoPharmica
Each capsule contains: Proprietary blend of active cultures 4 billion. Contains a specific mixture of Lactobacillus acidophilus, Lactobacillus rhamnosus, Bifidobacteria longum, Bifidobacteria breve.
See Editor's Note No. 21.

Acidophilus - PhysioLogics
Each softgel contains: Lactobacillus Acidophilus (contains over 100 million active lactobacillus acidophilus, including naturally occurring metabolic product produced by lactobacilli, at time of manufacture) 10 mg. Other Ingredients: Soybean Oil, Gelatin, Glycerin, Beeswax / Soybean Oil Mixture, Lecithin, Titanium Dioxide Color.

Acidophilus E.C. - Progressive Labs
Each high potency capsule contains 2.8 billion live organisms from specially selected strains of lactobacillus acidophilus and lactobacillus casei subsp. Rhamnosus in a base of maltodextrin.

Acidophilus Pearls - Enzymatic Therapy
Each pearl capsule contains: Proprietary Probiotic Blend 1 Billion CFU: Lactobacillus Acidophilus, Bifidobacterium Longum. Other Ingredients: Palm Oil, Gelatin, Glycerin, Lecithin, Pectin.

Acidophilus Plus 1 billion cells - Nature's Own
Each tablet contains: 1 billion viable cells comprising of: Lactobacillus Acidophilus 500 million cells • Bifidobacterium Lactis 500 million.

Acidophilus XTRA - Rexall - Sundown
Two caplets contain: Proprietary Blend (40,000 CFU) 40 mg: Lactobacillus Acidophilus • Lactobacillus Bulgaricus • Streptococcus Thermophilus • Bifidobacterium Bifidum. Other Ingredients: Rice Maltodextrin, Cellulose, Croscarmellose Sodium, Magnesium Stearate, Silica, Stearic Acid.

Acidophilus, Milk Free - Schiff
Each tablet contains: Calcium (as dicalcium phosphate anhydrous) 47 mg • Lactobacillus Acidophilus 1,000,000,000 CFU. Other Ingredients: Cellulose, Silicon Dioxide, Modified Cellulose Gum, Magnesium Stearate.

Acidophilus/Bifidobacter/FOS - Vital Nutrients
Each capsule contains: Lactobacillus Acidophilus 2 billion • Bifidobacter Lactis 2 billion • FOS (fructooligosaccharides) 150 mg.

Acidophilus-Lactobacillus - Jamieson
Each capsule contains: Minimum two billion active cells of Lactobacillus acidophilus and probiotic cultures.

Acidophilus-Super Strain - Jamieson
Each capsule contains: Lactobacillus Acidophilus 10% • Lactobacillus Rhamnosus 50% • Streptococcus Thermophilus 20% • Bifidobacterium Longum 10% • Bifidobacterium Bifidum 10%.

Ack-Nee with MAT - Olympian Labs
Two capsules contain: Vitamin A 10000 IU • Beta Carotene (pro-vitamin A) 500 IU • Vitamin E (d-a-tocopheryl acetate) 120 IU • L-Carnitine Fumarate 200 mg • Vitamin C 60 mg • Pantothenic Acid 20 mg • Vitamin B-6 (pyridoxine HCl) 5 mg • Chromium (picolinate, Cromax) 100 mcg • Selenium (l-selenomethionine) 70 mcg • Proprietary Blend 500 mg: Goldenseal, Curcumin extract, Enzyme blend (protease, lipase, amylase), MAT.

Acktiva 100% Pure Coral Calcium - Progressive Health Nutraceuticals
Two capsules contain: Coral Calcium 2000 mg: Yielding Calcium 480 mg, Magnesium 240 mg • Vitamin D 800 IU. Other Ingredients: Rice Powder, Gelatin.

Acne - Nature's Sunshine
Echinacea Angustifolia (cone flower) 4X • Kali Bromatum (potassium bromide) 4X • Mezereon (spurge olive) 4X • Belladonna (nightshade) 6X • Ledum Palustre (wild rosemary) 6X • Graphite 10X • Carbo Vegetabilis (vegetable carbon) 12X • Hepar Sulfuris Calcareum (calcium sulfide) 12X. Other Ingredients: Purified Water, 20% USP Alcohol.
See Editor's Note No. 1.

Acne Formula - HERBALmax
Dandelion • Baical Skullcap root • Red Sage root • Red Peony root • Yedoens violet.

Acti-Flex - FreeLife International
Six caplets contain: Proprietary Blend 1350 mg: Bromelain (80 GDU), Ashwagandha root (withania somnifera), Yucca root extract (yucca schidigera, standardized 10% saponins) • Glucosamine Hydrochloride 1200 mg • Turmeric Rhizome standardized extract (curcuma longa, 92% curcuminoids) 1200 mg • Ginger root standardized (zingiber officinale, 0.8% essential oils, 0.4% amino acids) 1200 mg • Feverfew herb standardized extract (chrysanthemum parthenium, 0.4% parthenolide) 600 mg • Pregnenolone (pharmeceutical-grade) 50 mg • Boron (chelated) 1 mg.

ActiFolate - Metagenics
Each tablet contains: Proprietary blend 800 mcg: Folic Acid, L-5-methyl Tetrahydrofolate, 5-formyl Tetrahydrofolate.

Actilife Super Antioxidant - Crystal Springs
Two tablets contain: Red Grape extract seeds 100 mg • Polygonum cuspidatum extract root 100 mg • Trans-Resveratrol 20 mg • Total Resveratrols 24 mg • Emodin 10 mg • Zinc 30 mg.

Actimine - Progressive Health Nutraceuticals
Vitamin A 5000 IU • Selenium 50 mcg • Vitamin E 200 IU • Zinc 10 mg • Methylsulfonyl Methane 1500 mg • Gum Guggul extract 50 mg.

Actisyn - SportPharma
Each packet contains: Actipro Protein Substrate: Ion Exchanged Whey Protein Isolate, Whey Protein Concentrate, Enzymatically Hydrolyzed Whey Protein, Pepti-Lean Select Micro-Peptides • Actiplex: Specific Ratios of L-Glutamine, Taurine, L-Leucine, & N-Acetyl-L-Cysteine • Anticell Vitamins & Minerals: Ascorbic Acid, DL-Alpha Tocopheryl Acetate, Vitamin A Palmitate, Potassium Chloride, Magnesium Aspartate, Magnesium Fumerate, Magnesium Oxide, Pyridoxine HCl, Niacinamide, Calcium Phosphate, Magnesium Orotate, Sodium Chloride, Alpha Lipoic Acid, Calcium

BRAND NAMES

Alpha-Ketoglutarate, Zinc Gluconate, L-Selenomethionine • Maltodextrin • Actigen: Tri-Methyl Glycine, Specific Nucleotides including: Purine and Pyrimidine Isolates, RNA Hydrolysates • Natural & Artificial Vanilla & Cream Flavors • CMC Gum • Aspartame • Sunett Brand Sweetener (Acesulfame K).

Activ Essentials **-** Xymogen
Two packets contain: Four ActivNutrients capsules: Vitamin A (as mixed carotenoids and cis-retinol palmitate) 7500 IU • Vitamin C (as potassium ascorbate, zinc ascorbate, calcium ascorbate and sodium ascorbate) 250 mg • Calcium (as dicalcium malate) 100 mg • Vitamin D (D3, as cholecalciferol) 200 IU • Vitamin E (as D-alpha tocopheryl succinate) 200 IU • Vitamin B1 (as thiamine mononitrate) 20 mg • Vitamin B2 (as riboflavin 5'-phosphate) 20 mg • Vitamin B3 (as niacinamide and niacin) 63 mg • Vitamin B6 (as pyridoxal 5'-phosphate) 20 mg • Folate (as folic acid and 5-formyl tetrahydrofolate) 400 mcg • Vitamin B12 (as methylcobalamin) 500 mcg • Biotin 1000 mcg • Pantothenic Acid (as D-calcium pantothenate) 200 mg • Iodine (as potassium iodide) 100 mcg • Magnesium (as dimagnesium malate) 100 mg • Zinc (as zinc bis-glycinate) 13 mg • Selenium (as selenium glycinate) 100 mcg • Copper (as copper bis-glycinate chelate) 1 mg • Manganese (as manganese bis-glycinate) 500 mcg • Chromium (as chromium nicotinate glycinate) 500 mcg • Molybdenum (as molybdenum glycinate) 50 mcg • Potassium (as potassium glycinate and potassium ascorbate) 99 mg • Inositol 36 mg • Choline (as choline dihydrogen citrate) 36 mg • PABA 13 mg • Vanadium (as vanadium niacinate glycinate) 750 mcg. Other Ingredients: Cellulose, Magnesium Stearate.
Two Oraxinol capsules: Oraxinol Proprietary Blend 1000 mg: RosemarinX brand Rosemary extract and Berr-X brand Berry extract (standardized to provide 6000 trolox equivalents). Other Ingredients: Cellulose, Magnesium Stearate.
Two OmegaPure 300EC softgels: Vitamin E 20 IU • EPA (eicosapentaenoic acid) 360 mg • DHA (docosahexaenoic acid) 240 mg. Other Ingredients: Gelatin, Glycerin, Purified Water, Enteric Coating, Vanillin.

Activ Essentials WOMEN **-** Xymogen
Two packets contain: Four ActivNutrients capsules: Vitamin A (as mixed carotenoids and cis-retinol palmitate) 7500 IU • Vitamin C (as potassium ascorbate, zinc ascorbate, calcium ascorbate and sodium ascorbate) 250 mg • Calcium (as dicalcium malate) 100 mg • Iron 5 mg • Vitamin D (D3, as cholecalciferol) 200 IU • Vitamin E (as D-alpha tocopheryl succinate) 200 IU • Vitamin B1 (as thiamine mononitrate) 50 mg • Vitamin B2 (as riboflavin 5'-phosphate) 13 mg • Vitamin B3 (as niacinamide and niacin) 63 mg • Vitamin B6 (as pyridoxal 5'-phosphate) 13 mg • Folate (as folic acid and 5-formyl tetrahydrofolate) 400 mcg • Vitamin B12 (as methylcobalamin) 500 mcg • Biotin 1000 mcg • Pantothenic Acid (as D-calcium pantothenate) 125 mg • Iodine (as potassium iodide) 100 mcg • Magnesium (as dimagnesium malate) 100 mg • Zinc (as zinc bis-glycinate) 13 mg • Selenium (as selenium glycinate) 100 mcg • Copper (as copper bis-glycinate chelate) 1 mg • Manganese (as manganese bis-glycinate) 500 mcg • Chromium (as chromium nicotinate glycinate) 1000 mcg • Molybdenum (as molybdenum glycinate) 50 mcg • Potassium (as potassium glycinate and potassium ascorbate) 50 mg • Inositol 36 mg • Choline (as choline dihydrogen citrate) 36 mg • PABA 13 mg • Vanadium (as vanadium niacinate glycinate) 750 mcg. Other Ingredients: Cellulose, Magnesium Stearate.
Two Oraxinol capsules: Oraxinol Proprietary blend 1000 mg: RosemarinX brand Rosemary extract and Berr-X brand Berry extract (standardized to provide 6000 trolox equivalents). Other Ingredients: Cellulose, Magnesium Stearate.
Two OmegaPure 300EC softgels: Vitamin E 20 IU • EPA (eicosapentaenoic acid) 360 mg • DHA (docosahexaenoic acid) 240 mg. Other Ingredients: Gelatin, Glycerin, Purified Water, Enteric Coating, Vanillin.
Two Ossopan capsules: Calcium 700 mg. Other Ingredients: HPMC, Magnesium Stearate, Stearic Acid.

Activated Charcoal **-** Nature's Sunshine
Eight capsules contain: Charcoal powder 2080 mg. Other Ingredients: Kosher Gelatin, Water.

Activated Coral Calcium Capsules **-** Nature's Plus
Three capsules contain: Vitamin A (as beta carotene) 2917 IU • Vitamin C (as ascorbic acid) 70 mg • Vitamin D (as ergocalciferol) 816 IU • Vitamin E (as D-alpha tocopheryl succinate) 35 IU • Phytavail Complex Proprietary Blend: Soluble plant based minerals, Aminoate, rare earth elements, Fructooligosaccharides from Dahlia inulin and Chicory root • Calcium (from coral calcium, AquaMin, Phytavail complex proprietary blend) 345 mg • Iodine (from kelp) 150 mcg • Magnesium (from coral calcium) 183 mg • Zinc (Phytavail complex proprietary blend) 16 mg • Selenium (Phytavail complex proprietary blend) 30 mcg • Copper (Phytavail complex proprietary blend) 2.4 mg • Manganese (Phytavail complex proprietary blend) 1.44 mg • Chromium (Phytavail complex proprietary blend) 86 mcg • Coral Calcium 1000 mg • Aquamin brand Lithothamnium Corallioides 305 mg • Bioperine brand Black Pepper extract (from piper nigrum fruit, standardized to 95% 1-piperoylpiperidine) 1 mg • Boron (Phytavail complex proprietary blend) 1 mg. Other Ingredients: Microcrystalline Cellulose, Silica, Magnesium Stearate, Vegetable Cellulose, Purified Water.

Activated Quercetin **-** Source Naturals
Three tablets contain: Quercetin 1000 mg • Vitamin C (magnesium ascorbate) 600 mg • Magnesium (magnesium ascorbate) 47 mg • Bromelain (2000 GDU per g) 300 mg.

Activated Selenium **-** Jarrow Formulas
Each capsule contains: Vitamin E (D-alpha tocopheryl succinate) 30 IU • Vitamin B2 (riboflavin) 2 mg • Selenium (as methylselenocysteine) 200 mcg • Broccoli 150 mg. Other Ingredients: Cellulose, Magnesium Stearate, Silicon Dioxide, Gelatin.

Active A **-** Source Naturals
Each tablet contains: Beta Carotene (pro-vitamin A) 15,000 IU • Vitamin A (palmitate) 10,000 IU.

Active Aloe brand **-** Aloecorp
Aloe Vera.
See Editor's Note No. 44.

Active B-50 **-** The Vitamin Shoppe
Each capsule contains: Vitamin B1 (Thiamin) 50 mg • Vitamin B2 (Riboflavin) 50 mg • Vitamin B6 (Pyridoxine HCl) 50 mg • Vitamin B12 (Cobalamin Concentrate) 50 mcg • Niacinamide 50 mg • Folic Acid 400 mcg • Pantothenic Acid (d-Calcium Pantothenate) 50 mg • Biotin 50 mcg • Choline 50 mg • Inositol 50 mg • PABA (Para Amino Benzoic Acid) 50 mg. In a base of Alfalfa, Watercress, Parsley, Lecithin, and Rice Concentrate.

Active Booster Compound **-** Starlight International
Each caplet contains: Potassium (as Potassium Gluconate) 8.3 mg • Uva Ursi extract, 4:1 (Arctostaphylos uva ursi, leaf) 300 mg • Corn Silk Pistils extract, 4:1 (Zea mays, flower) 300 mg • Citric Acid 200 mg • Parsley leaf extract (Petroselinum crispum, leaf) 50 mg. Other Ingredients: Dicalcium Phosphate, Microcystalline Cellulose, Stearic Acid, Sodium Starch Glycolate, Croscarmellose Sodium, Magnesium Stearate, Silicon Dioxide, Pharmaceutical Shellac, Hydroxypropylmethylcellulose, Carbowax Powder, Calcium Carbonate, Mono & Diglycerides, Gum Acacia.

Active Calcium **-** USANA Health Sciences
Four tablets contain: Calcium (as Citrate and Carbonate) 800 mg • Magnesium (as Citrate, Amino Acid Chelate and Oxide) 400 mg • Vitamin K (as Phylloquinone) 60 mcg • Vitamin D (Vitamin D3 as Cholecalciferol) 400 IU • Boron (as Citrate) 1.32 mg • Silicon (as Amino Acid Complex) 9 mg. Other Ingredients: Microcrystalline Cellulose, Pregelatinized Starch, Ascorbyl Palmitate, Dextrin, Croscarmellose Sodium, Dextrose.

Active Calcium Chewable - USANA Health Sciences
Each tablent contains: Vitamin D (vitamin D3 as cholecalciferol) 100 IU • Calcium (as citrate and carbonate) 200 mg • Magnesium (as oxide and citrate) 100 mg • Boron (as amino acid complex) 0.33 mg • Silicon (as amino acid complex) 2 mg. Other Ingredients: Xylitol, Maltodextrin, Dextrose, Lecithin, Vegetable-Derived Stearic Acid, Natural Flavor Blend, Natural Flavors, Citric Acid, Guar Gum, Malic Acid, Natural Carmine Color.

Active Enzymes - Global Health Trax
Each capsule contains: Digeseb Plus Proprietary Blend 450 mg: Protease, Carbohydrases, Lipase • Cellulase 75 mg • Proprietary Enzyme Blend 75 mg: Xylanase, Beta-Glucanases, Phytase, Hemicellulases • Probiotic Blend 75 mg: Lactobacillus Biffidum, Lactobacillus Longum.

Active Joints - Health Smart Vitamins
Each caplet contains: Vitamin C (ascorbic acid) 60 mg • Manganese (as manganese glycinate) 2 mg • Glucosamine Sulfate 500 mg • Sea Cucumber 100 mg • Chondroitin Sulfate 400 mg.
See Editor's Note No. 15.

Active Joints with MicroLactin - Vitamin World
Two caplets contain: MicroLactin brand Milk Protein Concentrate 2000 mg. Other Ingredients: Dextrose, Crospovidone, Cellulose, Lactose, Cellulose Coating, Titanium Dioxide (color), Silica, Vegetable Magnesium Stearate, Triacetin, Vegetable Stearic Acid.

Active One Senior Multivitamin - Rainbow Light
Each tablet contains: Vitamin A (50% beta-carotene, 50% palmitate) 5000 IU • Vitamin C (ascorbic acid) 120 mg • Vitamin D (D3, cholecalciferol) 400 IU • Vitamin E (D-alpha tocopheryl succinate) 100 IU • Thiamin (vitamin B1) 10 mg • Riboflavin (vitamin B2) 10 mg • Niacinamide (vitamin B3) 30 mg • Pyridoxine (vitamin B6) 15 mg • Folic Acid 800 mcg • Cyanocobalamin (vitamin B12) 200 mcg • Biotin 150 mcg • Pantothenic Acid (vitamin B5) 20 mg • Calcium (carbonate) 200 mg • Magnesium (oxide) 100 mg • Zinc (citrate) 15 mg • Selenium (amino acid chelate, selenomethionine) 15 mg • Copper (amino acid chelate) 1.5 mg • Manganese (citrate) 2 mg • Chromium (amino nicotinate) 200 mcg • Molybdenum (amino acid chelate) 100 mcg • Potassium (citrate) 10 mg • Plant-Source Enzymes: Protease 664 HUT, Amylase 226 DU, Lipase 3 LU, Cellulase 2 CU • Citrus Bioflavonoids 25 mg • Betaine HCl 20 mg • Choline (bitartrate) 30 mg • Inositol 10 mg • Boron (glycinate) 1 mg • Lutein (esters) 1 mg • Lycopene (from tomato extract) 500 mcg • Green Foods/Superfoods: Spirulina 20 mg, 4:1 Organic Vegetable Juice Extract 50 mg: Alfalfa, Kamut, Barley grass, Oat grass, Stinging Nettle leaf, Kale, Broccoli, Cabbage, Parsley • Rosemary leaf essential oil 2 mg. Other Ingredients: Cellulose, Modified Cellulose Gum, Stearic Acid (vegetable), Silica, Magnesium Stearate, Vegetable Food Glaze.

Active Slim Meal - Nature's Plus
Active Slim Meal Tri-Protein Blend: Whey Protein concentrate and isolate, Rice Protein concentrate, Partially Hydrolyzed Rice Protein, Milk Protein • MultiCarb/MultiFiber: Fibersol-2 brand Maltodextrin Fiber, Xylitol, Rice Starch, Stabilized Rice Bran, Rice Bran Solubles • Fructose • Cocoa powder • Cellulose gel • Cellulose gum • Multi-Vitamin/Mineral Blend: Potassium Chloride, Dicalcium Phosphate, Magnesium Oxide, Ascorbic Acid, Ferric Orthophosphate, D-Alpha Tocopheryl Acetate, Niacinamide, Zinc Oxide, Copper Gluconate, Vitamin A Palmitate, D-Calcium Pantothenate, Manganese Sulfate, Pyridoxine Hydrochloride, Riboflavin, Thiamin Mononitrate, Chromium Picolinate, Vitamin D (D3), Folic Acid, Biotin, Potassium Iodide, Sodium Molybdate, Vitamin K, Sodium Selenate, Cyanocobalamin • Lo Han Kuo • Natural Chocolate flavors • Carrageenan • Lecithin.

ActiveCal Caramel Chews - GNC
Each chew contains: Vitamin D 100 IU • Vitamin K 40 mcg • Calcium 500 mg. Ingredients: Corn syrup, Calcium Carbonate, Sugar, Sweetened Condensed Skim Milk, Partially Hydrogenated Soybean oil, Whey, Mono & Diglycerides, Soy Lecithin, Artificial Flavor, Vitamin D, Vitamin K.

ActiveCal Chocolate Chews - GNC
Each chew contains: Vitamin D 100 IU • Vitamin K 40 mcg • Calcium 500 mg. Ingredients: Corn syrup, Calcium Carbonate, Sugar, Sweetened Condensed Skim Milk, Partially Hydrogenated Soybean oil, Whey, Cocoa (processed with alkali), Mono & Diglycerides, Soy Lecithin, Artificial Flavor, Vitamin D, Vitamin K.

Activin 50 Mg Grape Seed Extract - Natrol, Inc.
Each tablet contains: ActiVin brand Grape seed extract 50 mg. Other Ingredients: Dicalcium Phosphate, Microcrystalline Cellulose, Mono & Di-Glycerides, Stearic Acid, Silicon Dioxide, Magnesium Stearate.

ActivNutrients - Xymogen
Four capsules contain: Vitamin A (as mixed carotenoids and cis-retinol palmitate) 7500 IU • Vitamin C (as potassium ascorbate, zinc ascorbate, calcium ascorbate and sodium ascorbate) 250 mg • Calcium (as dicalcium malate) 100 mg • Iron 5 mg • Vitamin D (D3, as cholecalciferol) 200 IU • Vitamin E (as D-alpha tocopheryl succinate) 200 IU • Vitamin B1 (as thiamine mononitrate) 20 mg • Vitamin B2 (as riboflavin 5'-phosphate) 20 mg • Vitamin B3 (as niacinamide and niacin) 63 mg • Vitamin B6 (as pyridoxal 5'-phosphate) 20 mg • Folate (as folic acid and 5-formyl tetrahydrofolate) 400 mcg • Vitamin B12 (as methylcobalamin) 500 mcg • Biotin 1000 mcg • Pantothenic Acid (as D-calcium pantothenate) 200 mg • Iodine (as potassium iodide) 100 mcg • Magnesium (as dimagnesium malate) 100 mg • Zinc (as zinc bis-glycinate) 13 mg • Selenium (as selenium glycinate) 100 mcg • Copper (as copper bis-glycinate chelate) 1 mg • Manganese (as manganese bis-glycinate) 500 mcg • Chromium (as chromium nicotinate glycinate) 500 mcg • Molybdenum (as molybdenum glycinate) 50 mcg • Potassium (as potassium glycinate and potassium ascorbate) 99 mg • Inositol 36 mg • Choline (as choline dihydrogen citrate) 36 mg • PABA 13 mg • Vanadium (as vanadium niacinate glycinate) 750 mcg. Other Ingredients: Cellulose, Magnesium Stearate.

ActivNutrients without Iron - Xymogen
Four capsules contain: Vitamin A (as mixed carotenoids and cis-retinol palmitate) 7500 IU • Vitamin C (as potassium ascorbate, zinc ascorbate, calcium ascorbate and sodium ascorbate) 250 mg • Calcium (as dicalcium malate) 100 mg • Vitamin D (D3, as cholecalciferol) 200 IU • Vitamin E (as D-alpha tocopheryl succinate) 200 IU • Vitamin B1 (as thiamine mononitrate) 20 mg • Vitamin B2 (as riboflavin 5'-phosphate) 20 mg • Vitamin B3 (as niacinamide and niacin) 63 mg • Vitamin B6 (as pyridoxal 5'-phosphate) 20 mg • Folate (as folic acid and 5-formyl tetrahydrofolate) 400 mcg • Vitamin B12 (as methylcobalamin) 500 mcg • Biotin 1000 mcg • Pantothenic Acid (as D-calcium pantothenate) 200 mg • Iodine (as potassium iodide) 100 mcg • Magnesium (as dimagnesium malate) 100 mg • Zinc (as zinc bis-glycinate) 13 mg • Selenium (as selenium glycinate) 100 mcg • Copper (as copper bis-glycinate chelate) 1 mg • Manganese (as manganese bis-glycinate) 500 mcg • Chromium (as chromium nicotinate glycinate) 500 mcg • Molybdenum (as molybdenum glycinate) 50 mcg • Potassium (as potassium glycinate and potassium ascorbate) 99 mg • Inositol 36 mg • Choline (as choline dihydrogen citrate) 36 mg • PABA 13 mg • Vanadium (as vanadium niacinate glycinate) 750 mcg. Other Ingredients: Cellulose, Magnesium Stearate.

Acti-Zyme - Nature's Plus
Two capsules contain: Live Food Enzymes: Aminogen (Aspergillus niger & Aspergillus oryzae proteolytic enzyme complex) 100 mg • Lugamase (Saccharamyces cerevisae & Aspergillus oryzae oligosaccharide enzyme complex) 100 mg • Amylase (30000 units/gram) 50 mg • Lactase (1000 units/gram) 50 mg • Lipase (5000 units/gram) 50 mg • Cellulase (5000 units/gram) 50 mg • Protease (100000 units/gram) 50 mg • Oxidase (5000 units/gram) 50 mg • Bromelain (2000 GDU/gram) 50 mg • Diastase (1000 units/gram) 5 mg • Maltase (1000 units/gram) 5 mg. Lactic Flora and Growth Accelerants: FOS (Fructooligosaccharides), lactic flora growth accelerant 100 mg • Lactospor, micro-encapsulated pure culture of B. Coagulans, provides 300 million viable cells 50 mg. Bioavailability

Enhancing Phytonutrient: Bioperine brand Black Pepper extract (from piper nigrum fruit, standardized to 95% 1-piperoylpiperidine) 5 mg.

ActoTherm - Advocare International
Each caplet contains: Niacin 20 mg • Vitamin A (as beta-carotene) 1000 IU • Magnesium (as phosphate) 50 mg • Potassium (as phosphate) 100 mg • Guarana seed extract (paullinia cupana) 200 mg • Green Tea leaf extract (camellia sinensis) 10 mg • Capsicum fruit extract (capsicum annuum) 16 mg • Proprietary Blend Thermogen-HC 112 mg: Gotu Kola extract, Cinnamon Ramulus extract, Peppermint extract, Lemon Verbana extract, Chamomile extract, Ginger extract, Chinese Licorice root extract, Sweet Citrus peel extract, Chicory extract. Other Ingredients: Calcium Sulfate, Dicalcium Phosphate, Silicon Dioxide, Cellulose, Stearic Acid, Magnesium Stearate.

ACTRA-Rx (Yilishen) - Body Basics
Some ingredients include: Proline • Histidine • Glutamic Acid • Arginine • Aspartic Acid • Tyrosine • Phenylalanine • Lycium fruit • Epimedium • Cistanche • Enzymes • Vitamin B1 • Vitamin B2 • Vitamin B12 • Vitamin E • Calcium • Iron • Magnesium • Phosphorus • Zinc • Selenium • Iodine • Copper.
See Editor's Note No. 58.

Actrim Plus - Arden Healthcare
Two tablets contain: Pineapple extract 150 mg • Fig extract 140 mg • Papaya extract 70 mg • Grapefruit extract 90 mg • L-Carnitine L-Tartrate 100 mg • Chromium Tri-Picolinate 0.100 mg. Other Ingredients: Cellulose Fibre, Sorbitol, Stearic Acid, Vanilline, Tricalcium Phosphate.

Actrim2 - Arden Healthcare
Two tablets contain: Pineapple extract 395 mg • Fig extract 235 mg • Papaya extract 330 mg • Grapefruit extract 328 mg • Spirulina 60 mg. Other Ingredients: Sorbitol, Cellulose Fibre, Stearic Acid, Vanilline, Tricalcium Phosphate.

Acutrim Natural A.M. - Heritage Consumer Products
Two tablets contain: Orange extract (4% synephrine) 100 mg • Niacin 100 mg • Guarana seed extract 300 mg • Polygonum cuspidatum root extract 25 mg • L-Arginine 450 mg • Guar Gum 200 mg • Citrus Pectin 50 mg.
See Editor's Note No. 40.

Acutrim Natural P.M. - Heritage Consumer Products
Two tablets contain: Niacin 180 mg • L-Arginine 450 mg • Polygonum cuspidatum 30 mg • Inositol Hexanicotinate 100 mg • L-Glutamine 40 mg • Guar Gum 250 mg • Citrus Pectin 50 mg.

Adagin - Dazzle, Inc.
Each tablet contains: Calcium (as calcium carbonate) 36 mg • Proprietary Blend 520 mg: L-Arginine, Mucuna Pruriens 15% L-dopa, Ashwaganda, Alpha GPC, Tribulis Terrestris Extract 40%, Cordyceps Sinensis Extract, Optizine. Other Ingredients: Silicon Dioxide, Magnesium, Gelatin.

Adam's Equalizer - Zeller
Purified Water • Natural Glycerin • Stearal Konium Chloride • D-Alpha Tocopherol (vitamin E) • Avocado oil • Jojoba oil • Saw Palmetto • Pygeum Africanum • Ginseng • Uva-Ursi • Pumpkin seed extract • Sarsaparilla • Natural Progesterone • Vitamin C (acerola) • OptiZinc Zinc • Rosemary extract • Carrot oil • Lemon Grass oil.

Adapt - InterPlexus
Each capsule contains: Vitamin B6 (as pyridoxine HCl) 25 mg • Biotin 1000 mcg • Pantothenic Acid (as calcium pantothenate) 250 mg • Zinc (as malate) 5 mg • Copper (as citrate) 5 mg • Proprietary Blend 320 mg: Rosemary extract, Ashwaganda extract, Hesperidin Methyl Chalcone. Other Ingredients: Cellulose.

Adaptagen Green Tea PhytoSerum - Abra Therapeutics
Apple juice • ABRA6 brand PhytoSerum Complex: Green Tea extract, Grape seed extract, Sage leaf extract, Schisandra berry extract, Siberian Ginseng extract • Limnanthes oil • Green Tea Phytoliposomes (standardized polyphenols from green tea) • Phospholipids • Sea Algae Complex • Clover Honey • Sorbitol • Tocopherol (vitamin E) • Xanthan gum • Sweet Orange oil • Grapefruit oil • Lavender oil • Peppermint oil • Glucose • Glucose Oxidase • Lactose Peroxidase • Acetic Acid • Lactic Acid • Methylparaben • Propylparaben.

AdaptaMax - Nature's Sunshine
Two capsules contain: Chromium (amino acid chelate) 40 mcg • Proprietary Blend 770 mg: Korean Ginseng root extract (panax ginseng), Rhodiola root extract (rhodiola rosea), Eleuthero root (eleutherococcus senticosus), Gynostemma whole plant extract (gynostemma pentaphyllum), Ashwagandha root (withania somnifera), Schizandra fruit (schisandra chinensis), Suma bark (pfaffia paniculata), Alfalfa aerial parts (medicago sativa), Astragalus root (astragalus membranaceus), Kelp leaf and stem (ascophyllum nodosum and laminaria digitata), Reishi mushroom (ganoderma lucidum), Rosemary leaf extract (rosmarinus officinalis), Ginkgo leaf concentrate (ginkgo biloba). Other Ingredients: Broccoli, Carrot, Red Beet, Tomato, Turmeric, Cabbage, Chinese Cabbage, Grapefruit Bioflavonoid, Hesperidin, Orange Bioflavonoid, Gelatin, Water.

AdaptaPhase I - Vitamin Research Products
Each full dropper (1 mL) contains: Proprietary Blend 1000 mg: Eleutherococcus senticosus root, Manchurian Thorn Tree (Aralia manchuria) root, Hawthorn (Crataegus oxyacantha) fruit extract, Echinopanax Elatum root, Schisandra (Schisandra chinensis) seed. Other Ingredients: Vegetable Glycerin, Deionized Water.

AdaptaPhase II - Vitamin Research Products
Each capsule contains: Adjuga Turkistanica root (2% turkesterone) 100 mg • Aralia Mundshurica root extract (20% aralosides) 100 mg • Rhaponticum Carthamoids extract (5% ecdysterone) 100 mg • Rhodiola (rhodiola rosea) root extract (5% rosavin & 1% salidrosides) 30 mg • Myricetin 30 mg.

Adaptrin - Pacific BioLogic
Each capsule contains: Proprietary Blend 500 mg: Iceland Moss • Red Sandalwood • Hardy Orange • Vetiver • Margosa • Spiral Flag • White Sandalwood • Cloves • Columbine • Wild Lettuce • Marigold • Knotgrass • Licorice • Valerian • Camphor bark • Gypsum • Cardamom • Jamaican Pepper • Ribwort (plantain) • Heartleaved Sida Cordifolia • Myrobalan • Blackthorn • Golden Cinquefoil • Gingerlily • Homeopathic Monkshood.
See Editor's Note No. 39.

ADE Cream - J. R. Carlson Laboratories, Inc.
Each gram contains: Vitamin A (as palmitate) 5000 IU • Vitamin D 200 IU • Vitamin E (as D-alpha tocopheryl acetate) 100 IU.

ADE Ointment - J. R. Carlson Laboratories, Inc.
Each gram contains: Vitamin A (as palmitate) 10,000 IU • Vitamin D 200 IU • Vitamin E (as D-alpha tocopheryl acetate) 100 IU.

Adenergy - Optimum Nutrition
Each caplet contains: Calcium 20 mg • Adenosine 5'-Triphosphate Disodium (peak ATP) 125 mg • Proprietary Adenergizing Blend 406 mg: ATP, Caffeine, Theophylline, Polyphenols (including EGCG). Other Ingredients: Enteric Coating (enteric polymer (methacrylic acid/methlmethacrylate), titanium dioxide, triethyl citrate, talc), Calcium Citrate, Microcystalline Cellulose, Dicalcium Phosphate, Solutab, Stearic Acid, Magnesium Stearate, Silica.

AD-FX - CV Technologies Inc.
Each capsule contains: American Ginseng (standardized extract HT-1001containing >15% ginsenosides) 125 mg • Ginkgo biloba standardized extract 29 mg (containing >4% terpenelactones).

Adipo Rx PM Formula - Athletic Technologies Inc.
Two capsules contain: Legume Protein • Phaseolus Vulgaris • Chitosan • Garcinia Cambogia • Gymnema Sylvestre • Cider Vinegar • Aloe Vera.

Some Brand Name Natural Products - What they Contain

www.NaturalDatabase.com contains MANY more listings than appear here.
Editor's Notes are located on pages 2155-2163.

Adipokinetix - Syntrax Innovations
Each capsule or tablet contains: Caffeine 100 mg • Phenylpropanolamine (PPA) 25 mg • Yohimbine HCl 3 mg.

Adipoxil - I Force
Three capsules contain: Vitamin B5 (D-cal pantothenate) 50 mg • Green Tea extract 500 mg • Guarana extract (22% caffeine) 450 mg • Citrus Aurantium (6.9% synephrine) 400 mg • Lecithin (phosphatidyl choline 105 mg) 300 mg • L-Carnitine L-Tartrate 300 mg • White Willow bark extract (15% salicin) 105 mg • 2,3-Aminomutase 100 mg • 5-Methyl-7-Methoxy-Isoflavone 60 mg • 7-Isopropoxyisoflavone 55 mg • Coleus Forskohlii (95% forskolin) 50 mg • Ginger root powder 50 mg. Other Ingredients: Gelatin, Microcrystalline Cellulose, Magnesium Stearate, Silica.
See Editor's Note No. 40.

ADR Complex - Professional Botanicals
Each caplet contains: Vitamin C 100 mg • Vitamin B6 25 mg • Pantothenic Acid 250 mg • Adrenal 150 mg • Pituitary 30 mg • Barberry 150 mg • Blessed Thistle 100 mg.

ADR Formula - Pure Encapsulations
Each vegetable capsule contains: Panax Ginseng extract (standardized to contain 27-30% total ginsenosides) 200 mg • Eleutherococcus Senticosus extract (standardized to contain 0.8% eleutheroside E & B) 100 mg • Licorice (standardized to contain 12% glycyrrhizic acid) 100 mg • Whole Adrenal (bovine) 150 mg • Adrenal Cortex (bovine) 75 mg • Calcium Pantothenate (B5) 100 mg • Vitamin C (as ascorbyl palmitate) 15 mg.

Adrenal - Pure Encapsulations
Each vegetable capsule contains: Whole Adrenal (bovine) 150 mg • Adrenal Cortex (bovine) 80 mg.

Adrenal 100 - Professional Botanicals
Each tablet contains: Raw Adrenal substance (freeze-dried) 100 mg. Base: Thymus, Lymph, Duodenal Substance.

Adrenal Chelate - Atrium Biotechnologies
Each tablet contains: Raw Adrenal concentrate (not an extract) 80 mg • L-Leucine 10 mg • L-Isoleucine 20 mg • D-Calcium Pantothenate 60 mg • Sodium Ascorbate 120 mg • Potassium Aspartate 30 mg • Hesperidin Complex 150 mg • Bioflavonoid Complex 75 mg • Chlorophyll 10 mg. In a base of Alfalfa, Celery & Parsley.
See Editor's Note No. 14.

Adrenal Cortex 75 - Professional Botanicals
Each tablet contains: Raw Adrenal Cortex substance (freeze-dried) 75 mg. Base: Thymus, Lymph, Duodenal Substances.

Adrenal Energy - Pro Health
Two capsules contain: Vitamin C (as ascorbic acid) 250 mg • Pantothenic Acid 50 mg • Licorice root (glycyrrhiza glabra) 250 mg • L-Tyrosine 250 mg • Eleuthero root (eleutherococcus senticosus) 200 mg • Pregnenolone 50 mg • CoQ10 30 mg • DHEA 10 mg. Other Ingredients: Gelatin (capsule shell), Silica, Rice Flour, Magnesium Stearate.

Adrenal Essence - Xymogen
Each capsule contains: Cordyceps Sinensis (standardized 8% cordyceptic acid and 0.25% adenosine) 400 mg • Panax Ginseng (standardized 27-30% ginsenosides) 200 mg • Rhodiola Rosea (standardized 1% salidroside) 100 mg • Pantothenic Acid (as D-calcium pantothenate) 50 mg • Vitamin B6 (as pyridoxine hydrochloride) 25 mg • PABA 25 mg.

Adrenal Glandular - American Biologics
Each tablet contains: Raw Adrenal Concentrate 160 mg. Other Ingredients: Dicalcium Phosphate, Magnesium Stearate.
See Editor's Note No. 14.

Adrenal Health - Enzymes, Inc.
Two capsules contain: n-zimes Proprietary Enzyme Blend 65 mg: pHysioProtease (177,600 pHysio-U), CereCalase Plus • Panax Ginseng root extract (standardized to contain 8% ginsenosides) 160 mg • Bupleurum root extract (equivalent to 400 mg raw herb) 100 mg • Rice Bran 65 mg • Siberian Ginseng root extract (standardized to contain 0.8% eleutherosides) 40 mg. Other Ingredients: Plant Cellulose, Water.

Adrenal Plus - Futurebiotics LLC
Raw Adrenal concentrate 80 mg • Vitamin C (Ascorbic Acid) 150 mg • Pantothenic Acid 60 mg • Zinc (Gluconate) 5 mg • Manganese (Amino Acid Chelate) 1 mg • Schizandra (6:1) 20 mg • Chinese Licorice (10:1) 12 mg • Niacinamide 80 mg.
See Editor's Note No. 14.

Adrenal Power + - EnerGreens, Inc.
Each capsule contains: 10-HDA Royal Jelly 700 mg • Pantothenic Acid 25 mg. Other Ingredients: Gelatin.

Adrenal Support - Nature's Sunshine
Each capsule contains: Vitamin C (as ascorbic acid) 25 mg • Vitamin B1 (as thiamine mononitrate) 10 mg • Riboflavin Phosphates (including riboflavin-5-phosphate, as vitamin B2) 5 mg • Vitamin B6 (as pyridoxal-5-phosphate) 5 mg • Pantothenic Acid (as D-calcium pantothenate) 45 mg • Magnesium (as citrate) 10 mg • Zinc (as citrate) 5 mg • Potassium (as citrate) 5 mg • Proprietary Blend 240 mg: Adrenal Substance, Schizandra fruit (schisandra chinensis), Borage oil (borago officinalis), Licorice root (glycyrrhiza glabra), Protease Blend. Other Ingredients: Cellulose, Gelatin, Water.

Adrenal Support - Vital Nutrients
Two capsules contain: Adrenal (whole, bovine) 300 mg • Adrenal (cortex, bovine) 150 mg • Eleuthero extract (eleutherococcus senticosus, 28:1) 200 mg • Ashwagandha extract (5:1) 200 mg • Cordyceps Sinensis extract (4:1) 100 mg • Pantothenic Acid 100 mg.
See Editor's Note No. 14.

Adrenal Support - PhytoPharmica
Two capsules contain: Vitamin C (ascorbic acid/rose hip fruit) 125 mg • Vitamin B6 (pyridoxine HCl) 25 mg • Pantothenic Acid (calcium D-pantothenate) 125 mg • L-Tyrosine 250 mg • Betaine 125 mg • Pituitary extract 60 mg • Adrenal extract (predigested soluble concentrate) 50 mg • Ginger root and rhizome 6.5:1 extract (zingiber officinale) 50 mg • Adrenal cortex extract 17 mg.
See Editor's Note No. 21 and No. 31.

Adrenal Support Plus - BioGenesis Nutraceuticals
Two capsules contain: Vitamin C (ascorbic acid & ascorbyl palmitate) 100 mg • Vitamin B1 (thiamine) 50 mg • Vitamin B2 (riboflavin) 50 mg • Vitamin B3 (niacinamide & nicotinic acid) 50 mg • Vitamin B6 (pyridoxine HCl & pyridoxine 5' phosphate) 50 mg • Folic Acid 400 mcg • Vitamin B12 (hydroxycobalamine) 100 mcg • Biotin 1500 mcg • Pantothenic Acid (calcium) 200 mg • Zinc (malate) 1 mg • Copper (citrate) 50 mcg • PABA 100 mg • Bioflavonoid complex 100 mg • Choline (bitartrate) 50 mg • Inositol 50 mg • Siberian Ginseng extract (0.8% eleutheros) 50 mg • Rosemary 4:1 extract 36 mg • Naringen 36 mg • Hesperidin Methyl Chalcone 36 mg • Rutin 10 mg • DHEA 6.7 mg • Pregnenolone 6.7 mg.

Adrenal Trophic - Progressive Labs
Each capsule contains: Pantothenic Acid (as d-calcium panothenate) 50 mg • Raw Porcine Adrenal concentrate 80 mg. Other Ingredients: Rice Flour, Magnesium Stearate.

Adrenal, Desiccated - Standard Process, Inc.
Two tablets contain: Proprietary Blend 444 mg: Bovine Adrenal, Carrot root. Other Ingredients: Calcium Lactate, Honey, Arabic Gum, Calcium Stearate.
See Editor's Note No. 14.

Adrenal, Organic Glandular - Allergy Research Group
Each capsule contains: Adrenal tissue (bovine) 300 mg. Other Ingredients: Cellulose, Silicon Dioxide, Stearic Acid.
See Editor's Note No. 14.

Adrenal-Cortex Complex **-** Enzymatic Therapy
Each capsule contains: Adrenal Cortex extract 250 mg • Multi-Glandular Complex 100 mg: Liver, Lung, Pancreas, Heart, Kidney, Spleen. Other Ingredients: Gelatin, Cellulose, Magnesium Stearate, Titanium Dioxide Color.
See Editor's Note No. 14.

Adrenal-Cortex Fractions **-** PhytoPharmica
Each capsule contains: Adrenal-Cortex Complex 250 mg • Multi-Glandular Complex 100 mg: Raw Liver, Raw Lung, Raw Pancreas, Raw Heart, Raw Kidney, Raw Spleen, Raw Brain. All organs & glands derived from bovine sources except raw pancreas (porcine).
See Editor's Note No. 31.

AdrenaLyze Vegetarian **-** DaVinci Laboratories
Each capsule contains: Vitamin C (as ascorbic acid and ascorbate) 100 mg • Thiamin 25 mg • Riboflavin 25 mg • Niacin (as niacinamide) 25 mg • Vitamin B6 (as pyridoxal-5-phosphate) 25 mg • Folic Acid 100 mcg • Vitamin B12 (methylcobalamin) 20 mcg • Biotin 75 mcg • Pantethine 50 mg • Eleutherococcus Sinensis root extract (siberian ginseng) 150 mg • Ashwaganda extract (yielding withanolides 3.75 mg) 150 mg • Phosphatidylserine 50 mg • Panax Ginseng extract 50 mg • Licorice (deglyzhirized) 10 mg. Other Ingredients: Rice Flour, Vegetable Cellulose, Vegetable Stearate.

Adren-Comp **-** Enzymatic Therapy
Each capsule contains: Bupleurum root extract 150 mg • Panax Ginseng root extract 100 mg • Eleuthero root extract (eleutherococcus senticosus) 100 mg • Wild Yam root extract (dioscorea villosa) 100 mg • Licorice root, rhizome extract (glycyrrhiza glabra) 50 mg • Turmeric rhizome extract (curcuma longa) 15 mg. Other Ingredients: Gelatin, Magnesium Stearate, Titanium Dioxide, Silicon Dioxide.

Adrenerlin **-** Bodyonics, Ltd.
Two capsules contain: Maca Pure brand Lepidium Meyenii (standardized to contain 0.6% macamides and macaenes) 450 mg • Jeevani Botanical Complex 150 mg: Tricopus Zylanicus, Ashwanga (withania somnifera), Piper Longum, Vishnukranthi (Evolvus alsinoies) • Peptide GPX 250 mg • D-Ribose 10 mg • Acetyl-L-Carnitine 10 mg • Bitter Orange (standardized 4% synephrine) 83.3 mg • Yerba Mate and Guarana Extract (standardized) 200 mg Methylxanthines/ Caffeine 910 mg • Mucuna Pruriens (standardized 15% L-Dopa) 33.3 mg • Calcium Pyruvate 10 mg. Other Ingredients: Magnesium Stearate, Gelatin.
See Editor's Note No. 40.

Adreno Chelate **-** Progressive Labs
Each capsule contains: Calcium (Proteinate) 27 mg • Chloride (Proteinate) 50 mg • Sodium (Proteinate) 20 mg • Potassium (Proteinate) 20 mg • Raw Bovine Adrenal concentrate 40 mg • L-Isoleucine 10 mg • L-Leucine 10 mg.
See Editor's Note No. 14.

Adreno Trophic **-** Progressive Labs
Each capsule contains: Pantothenic Acid (calcium pantothenate) 50 mg • Raw Bovine Adrenal concentrate 80 mg.
See Editor's Note No. 14.

Adreno-Cortex **-** Atrium Biotechnologies
Each tablet contains: Adrenal Cortex • Pituitary Anterior 20 mg • Pineal, bovine source 10 mg • Vitamin C (calcium ascorbate) 25 mg.
See Editor's Note No. 14.

Adrenogen **-** Metagenics
Each tablet contains: Raw Adrenal Concentrate (bovine) 80 mg • Pantothenic Acid (as D-calcium pantothenate) 50 mg • Vitamin B6 (as pyridoxine hydrochloride) 25 mg • Para-Aminobenzoic Acid (PABA) 25 mg • Riboflavin 10 mg.

Adreno-Medulla Plus **-** Atrium Biotechnologies
Each tablet contains: Adrenal Medulla 100 mg • Hypothalamus 15 mg • Pituitary Posterior Bovine Source 10 mg • Vitamin C (calcium ascorbate) 25 mg.
See Editor's Note No. 14.

Adren-Plus **-** PhytoPharmica
Each capsule contains: Bupleurum Chinense root 150 mg • Eleuthero root extract (eleutherococcus senticosus, standardized to contain a minimum of 0.5% eleutheroside E) 100 mg • Licorice root and rhizome extract (glycyrrhiza glabra, standardized to contain 5% glycyrrhizic acid) 50 mg • Panax Ginseng root extract (standardized to contain minimum of 7% ginsenosides) 100 mg • Tumeric rhizome extract (curcuma longa, standardized to contain 85-100% curcumin) 15 mg • Wild Yam root extract (dioscorea villosa, standardized to contain 10% diosgenin) 100 mg.

Adreset **-** Metagenics
Each capsule contains: Cordyceps Mycelium extract (paecilomyces hepiali) 400 mg • Asian Ginseng root extract (panax ginseng, standardized to 8% ginsenosides) 200 mg • Rhodiola root extract (rhodiola rosea, standardized to 1% salidroside) 50 mg.

Adult Echinacea+C+Zinc (cherry flavor) **-** LiFizz Effervescent Vitamins
Each tablet contains: Vitamin C (Ascorbic Acid) 1500 mg • Zinc 15 mg • Echinacea extract (Echinacea purpurea) 100 mg. Other Ingredients: Citric Acid, Sodium Bicarbonate, Sorbitol, Mannitol, Polyethylene Glycol 6000, Cherry Flavor, Povidone, Aspartame, Acesulfame Potassium, Magnesium Stearate, Silicon Dioxide, Simethicone.

Adult Echinacea+C+Zinc (lemon/lime flavor) **-** LiFizz Effervescent Vitamins
Each tablet contains: Vitamin C (Ascorbic Acid) 1500 mg • Zinc 15 mg • Echinacea extract (Echinacea purpurea) 100 mg. Other Ingredients: Citric Acid, Sodium Bicarbonate, Sorbitol, Mannitol, Polyethylene Glycol 6000, Lemon Flavor, Povidone, Aspartame, Acesulfame Potassium, Lemon/Lime Flavor, Magnesium Stearate, Silicon Dioxide, Simethicone.

Adult Multi-Vitamin (orange flavor) **-** LiFizz Effervescent Vitamins
Each tablet contains: Vitamin A (Palmitate and Beta Carotene) 5000 IU • Vitamin C 60 mg • Vitamin D 400 IU • Vitamin E 15 IU • Thiamin 1.5 mg • Riboflavin 1.7 mg • Niacinamide 20 mg • Vitamin B6 2 mg • Folic Acid 400 mcg • Vitamin B12 6 mcg • Biotin 300 mcg • Pantothenic Acid 10 mg • Calcium 200 mg • Iron 6 mg • Magnesium 80 mg • Zinc 5 mg.

Adult Multi-Vitamin and Mineral **-** Golden Glow Natural Health Products
Each tablet contains: Ascorbic Acid (vitamin C) 75 mg • Calcium Pantothenate (vitamin B5) 8 mg • Cholecalciferol (vitamin D3 10 mcg) 400 IU • Cyanocobalamin (vitamin B12) 2 mcg • DL-Alpha Tocopheryl Acetate (vitamin E 10 mg) 10 IU • Nicotinamide (vitamin B3) 25 mg • Pyridoxine Hydrochloride (vitamin B6) 2 mg • Retinyl Acetate (vitamin A) 1250 IU • Riboflavin (vitamin B2) 10 mg • Thiamine Nitrate (vitamin B1) 10 mg • Calcium Hydrogen Phosphate 43 mg: Calcium 10 mg • Copper (as cupric sulfate anhydrous) 1 mg • Iodine (as potassium iodide) 145 mcg • Iron (as ferrous fumarate) 5 mg • Magnesium (as magnesium oxide) 36 mg • Manganese (as manganese sulphate monohydrate) 1 mg • Potassium (as potassium sulphate) 5 mg • Zinc (as zinc oxide) 1.5 mg. Other Ingredients: Glucose, Sucrose.

Adult Multivitamin Chewable **-** Nature Made
Two tablets contain: Vitamin A (2% as beta carotene) 5000 IU • Vitamin C 250 mg • Vitamin D 400 IU • Vitamin E 30 IU • Thiamin 1.5 mg • Riboflavin 1.7 mg • Niacin 20 mg • Vitamin B6 2 mg • Folic Acid 400 mcg • Vitamin B12 6 mcg • Biotin 40 mcg • Pantothenic Acid 10 mg • Calcium 200 mg • Phosphorus 100 mg • Iodine 150 mcg • Magnesium 20 mg • Zinc 15 mg • Copper 2 mg • Sodium 15 mg. Other Ingredients: Dibasic Calcium Phosphate, Sorbitol, Fructose, Xylitol, Stearic Acid, Mono and Diglycerides of Fatty Acids, Carrageenan, Gelatin, Aspartame, Yellow 6 Lake, Corn Starch,

Silicon Dioxide, Magnesium Stearate, Natural and Artificial Flavors, Modified Food Starch, Red 40 Lake.
See Editor's Note No. 45.

Adult-C-Vitamin (pink grapefruit flavor) - LiFizz Effervescent Vitamins
Each tablet contains: Vitamin C (Ascorbic Acid) 500 mg. Other Ingredients: Citric Acid, Sorbitol, Potassium Bicarbonate, Sodium Bicarbonate, Mannitol, Grapefruit Flavor, Polyethylene Glycol 6000, Orange Flavor, Aspartame, Acesulfame Potassium, Wild Berry Powder, Silicon Dioxide, Lemon/Lime flavor, Magnesium Stearate.

Adult-C-Vitamin (raspberry flavor) - LiFizz Effervescent Vitamins
Each tablet contains: Vitamin C (Ascorbic Acid) 500 mg. Other Ingredients: Citric Acid, Sodium Bicarbonate, Potassium Bicarbonate, Sorbitol, Mannitol, Polyethylen Glycol 6000, Red Beet Powder, Raspberry Flavor, Aspartame, Acesulfame Potassium, Magnesium Stearate.

Adults 50 + Vita-Vim - Jamieson
Each caplet contains: Vitamin A (Acetate) 3000 IU • Beta Carotene 3000 IU • Vitamin D 400 IU • Vitamin C 90 mg • Vitamin E 75 IU • Vitamin B1 2.25 mg • Vitamin B2 3.2 mg • Vitamin B3 (No Flush Niacinamide) 40 mg • Vitamin B5 10 mg • Vitamin B6 8 mg • Vitamin B12 25 mcg • Folic Acid 600 mcg • Biotin 45 mcg • Calcium 200 mg • Copper (from Oxide) 2 mg • Iodine 0.15 mg • Magnesium 50 mg • Zinc (from Zinc Oxide) 15 mg • Potassium (Non Citrate form) 80 mg • Manganese (Sulfate Source) 5 mg • Chromium (Non Chelated) 100 mcg • Selenium (Non Chelated) 25 mcg • Vanadium 10 mcg • Molybdenum 1 mcg • Nickel 5 mcg • Tin 10 mcg • Phosphorus 125 mcg • Silicon 10 mcg • Ginkgo Biloba 250 mg • Lutein 300 mcg • Lycopene 300 mcg • Digestive Enzyme Absorption Factors: derived from Peppermint, Bromelain, Papain, Amylase, Lipase, Cellulose 2000 mcg.

Adult's Chewable - Nature's Plus
Each tablet contains: Vitamin A (as beta carotene) 5000 IU • Vitamin C (as ascorbic acid) 150 mg • Vitamin D (as ergocalciferol) 400 IU • Vitamin E (as D-alpha tocopheryl succinate) 100 IU • Thiamin (vitamin B1, as thiamine HCl) 15 mg • Riboflavin (vitamin B2) 15 mg • Niacin (as niacinamide) 25 mg • Vitamin B6 (as pyridoxine HCl) 15 mg • Folate (as folic acid) 100 mcg • Vitamin B12 (as cyanocobalamin) 15 mcg • Biotin 20 mcg • Pantothenic Acid (as calcium pantothenate) 20 mg • Calcium (as gluconate) 10 mg • Iron (as gluconate) 5 mg • Iodine (as potassium iodide) 100 mcg • Magnesium (as gluconate) 0.145 mg • Zinc (as gluconate) 0.325 mg • Copper (as gluconate) 0.05 mg • Manganese (as gluconate) 0.017 mg • Lecithin (from soy) 25 mg • Choline (as bitartrate) 5 mg • Hesperidin (from citrus limon exocarp) 5 mg • Betaine HCl (from beet molasses) 5 mg • Rutin (from saphora japonica leaf) 2.5 mg • Citrus Bioflavonoids (from citrus limon exocarp) 2.5 mg • PABA (para-aminobenzoic acid) 2.5 mg • Inositol 2.5 mg. Other Ingredients: Fructose, Stearic Acid, Silica, Microcrystalline Cellulose, Rice Bran, Rose Hips (rosa canina fruit).

AdvaCal - LaneLabs
Three capsules contain: Elemental Calcium (as calcium hydroxide, calcium oxide, combined with algae amino acid extract) 450 mg. Other Ingredients: Citric Acid, Gelatin, Water, Glycerine.

AdvaClear - Metagenics
Two capsules contain: Vitamin A (33% as retinyl palmitate and 67% as beta-carotene) 2,500 IU • Vitamin C (as magnesium ascorbate) 133 mg • Vitamin D (as cholecalciferol) 33 IU • Vitamin E (as D-alpha tocopheryl acetate and mixed tocopherols) 66 IU • Thiamin (as thiamin mononitrate) 10 mg • Riboflavin 5 mg • Niacin (as niacinamide and niacin) 23 mg • Vitamin B6 (as pyridoxine hydrochloride) 17 mg • Folate (as L-5-methyl tetrahydrofolate and 5-formyl tetrahydrofolate) 267 mcg • Vitamin B12 (as cyanocobalamin) 33 mcg • Biotin 66 mcg • Pantothenic Acid (as D-calcium pantothenate) 33 mg • Magnesium (as magnesium ascorbate) 19 mg • Zinc (as zinc citrate) 6.5 mg • Selenium (as selenomethionine) 50 mcg • Copper (as copper citrate) 0.65 mg • Manganese (as manganese citrate) 1.65 mg • Molybdenum (as molybdenum amino acid chelate) 66 mcg • N-Acetylcysteine 66 mg • Sodium Sulfate 100 mg • Taurine 117 mg • Choline (as choline bitartrate) 66 mg • Silymarin (as silybin, silychristin, silydianin) 50 mg • Catechins 34 mg • Epigallocatechin Gallate (EGCG, from decaffeinated green tea leaf, camellia sinensis) 22 mg • Artichoke leaf extract (cynara scolymus) 166 mg • Watercress whole plant 4:1 extract (nasturtium officinale) 134 mg • Ellagic Acid (from pomegranate rind extract, punica granatum) 33 mg.

AdvaLean - Optalife Nutrition
Four capsules contain: Proprietary Blend (Metabolism) 1050 mg: Green Tea extract, Alpha Lipoic Acid, L-Carnitine • Proprietary Blend (Energy) 750 mg: Ginseng, Yerba Mate extract • Proprietary Blend (Thyroid Support) 550 mg: Bladderwrack, Bovine • Proprietary Blend (Appetite Control) 900 mg: Garcinia Cambogia, Hoodia Gordonii extract • Proprietary Blend (Fat & Carb Block) 910 mg: Chitosan, Vitamin C, Chromium Polynicotinate, Phaseolus Vulgaris • 5-Hydroxytryptophan 100 mg • Vitamin B6 75 mg • Vitamin B12 150 mcg. Other Ingredients: Rice Flour, Gelatin.
See Editor's Note No. 14.

Advanced Aminos - American Biologics
Three capsules contain: Proprietary Blend 677 mg: L-Lysine HCl, L-Isoleucine, L-Glutamine, L-Tyrosine, L-Threonine, L-Alanine, L-Leucine, L-Histidine, L-Arginine HCl, L-Aspartic Acid, L-Valine, Ornithine Alpha Ketoglutarate, L-Methionine, L-Cystine, L-Glutamic Acid, Glycine, L-Phenylalanine, Alpha Lipoic Acid, N-Acetyl-L-Tyrosine, L-Serine, Taurine, L-Proline. Other Ingredients: Microcrystalline Cellulose, Magnesium Stearate.

Advanced Antioxidant Formula - Waiora
Each capsule contains: Proprietary U.W. Blend 600 mg: Grape seed extract (phenolic components 95%), Green Tea extract (camellia sinensis - 40% EGCG), Wild Blueberry concentrate, Wild Bilberry concentrate, Cranberry concentrate, Tart Cherry concentrate, Prune concentrate, Raspberry concentrate, Strawberry concentrate, Resveratrol, Quercetin. Other Ingredients: Gelatin, Rice Flour, Silicon Dioxide, Magnesium Stearate.

Advanced B Heart Health Formula - Nature Made
Each tablet contains: Vitamin B6 (pyridoxine hydrochloride) 10 mg • Natural Folate (Metafolin, L-methylfolate) 400 mcg • Vitamin B12 (cyanocobalamin) 200 mcg • Phytonutrient Blend 100 mg: Green Tea extract, Grape seed extract, Blueberry, Strawberry, Blackberry, Raspberry, Cranberry, Sour Cherry fruit, Blueberry extract. Other Ingredients: Cellulose Gel, Dibasic Calcium Phosphate, Talc, Gelatin, Silicon Dioxide, Croscarmellose Sodium, Magnesium Stearate, Hydroxypropyl Methylcellulose, Polyethylene Glycol.

Advanced Calcium Complex - Solgar
Four tablets contain: Vitamin D (as cholecalciferol) 600 IU • Vitamin K (as phytonadione) 65 mcg • Calcium (as calcium carbonate, citrate, malate, glycinate) 800 mg • Iron 3 mg • Magnesium (as magnesium glycinate, citrate, oxide) 500 mg • Zinc (as zinc glycinate) 5 mg • Copper (as copper lysinate) 0.5 mg • Manganese (as manganese glycinate) 2 mg • Sodium 60 mg • Silica (from red algae-Lithothamnium corallioides) 15 mg • Boron (as boron glycinate complex) 2 mg. Other Ingredients: Microcrystalline Cellulose, Vegetable Cellulose, Titanium Dioxide, Vegetable Magnesium Stearate, Silica, Vegetable Glycerin, Carnauba Wax.

Advanced Chromium HCA - Health Smart Vitamins
Each capsule contains: Calcium (as calcium salt of hydroxy citric acid) 79 mg • Chromium (as chromium picolinate) 100 mcg • Garcinia cambogia fruit (50% (-) hydroxycitric acid [HCA], 250 mg) 500 mg.

Advanced C-Jointin - Puritan's Pride
Three softgels contain: Vitamin C (as Ascorbic Acid) 60 mg • Vitamin E (as d-Alpha-Tocopherol) 10 IU • Manganese (as Manganese Aspartate) 1 mg • Boron (as Boron Citrate) 1.5 mg • Evening

Primrose Oil 250 mg • MSM (Methylsulfonylmethane) 750 mg • Chondroitin Sulfate 200 mg • Glucosamine Sulfate 1,000 mg. See Editor's Note No. 15.

Advanced C-Jointin - Vitamin World
Three softgels contain: Vitamin C (as ascorbic acid) 60 mg • Vitamin E (as d-alpha tocopherol) 10 IU • Manganese (as manganese aspartate) 1 mg • Glucosamine Sulfate (2KCl) 1000 mg • MSM (methylsulfonylmethane) 750 mg • Chondroitin Sulfate 200 mg • Evening Primrose Oil 250 mg • Boron (as boron citrate) 1.5 mg. Other Ingredients: Soybean Oil, Gelatin, Glycerin, Beeswax / Soybean Oil Mixture, Lecithin, Caramel Color. See Editor's Note No. 15.

Advanced Colloidal Chromium/Vanadium - Futurebiotics LLC
Each 1 tsp serving contains: Chromium 0.18 ppm • Vanadium 0.18 ppm. Other Ingredients: Deionized Water.

Advanced CoQ10 - Goldshield Elite
Each capsule contains: Coenzyme Q10 50 mg.

Advanced E + Grape Seed Extract - Leiner Health Products
Each softgel contains: Vitamin E (DL-alpha tocopherol) 400 IU • Grape seed extract 20 mg. Other Ingredients: Gelatin, Vegetable Oil, Glycerin, Yellow Beeswax, Unbleached Lecithin, Titanium Dioxide, Carmine.

Advanced E with Alpha Lipoic Acid - Leiner Health Products
Each softgel contains: Vitamin C (Ascorbic Acid) 20 mg • Vitamin E (dl-Alpha Tocopherol, d-Alpha Tocopherol) 400 IU • Alpha Lipoic Acid 30 mg • Rice Bran oil 5 mg. Other Ingredients: Gelatin, Glycerin, Yellow Beeswax, Soybean Oil, Lecithin, Titanium Dioxide, Turmeric.

Advanced Formula - Biotech Corp.
Each tablet contains: Folate 400 mg • Pantothenic Acid 100 mg • Biotin 700 mcg • Iodine 75 mcg • Zinc 75 mg • Shen Min 225 mg • Shen Min root powder (he shou wu) 435 mg • Isoflavones 10 mg • Saw Palmetto berries standardized extract 160 mg • Silica 20 mg • Black Pepper extract 2.5 mg.

Advanced Formula AntioxidEnz - Enzymes, Inc.
Each capsule contains: Vitamin A (from dualiella algae) 3000 IU • Vitamin C (from acerola cherries extract) 50 mg • Vitamin E (from D-alpha tocopheryl acid succinate) 100 IU • Zinc (from zinc citrate) 7.5 mg • Selenium (from kelp) 30 mcg • n-zimes Proprietary Blend 166 mg: pHysioprotease brand, Catalase • Proprietary Blend 130 mg: Turmeric root extract, Quercetin, Green Tea leaf extract, Lycopenes, Grape seed extract, Bilberry fruit extract, Alpha-Lipoic Acid, Lutein. Other Ingredients: Cellulose, Water.

Advanced Formula CarbohydrEnz - Enzymes, Inc.
Each capsule contains: n-zimes Proprietary Blend 512 mg: Amylase, Protease blend, alpha-Galactosidase, CereCalase Plus, Glucoamylase, Malt Diatase, Lipase, Pectinase, Invertase, Cellulase, Lactase, Xylanase • Proprietary Blend 190 mg: Ginger root extract, Fennel seed extract. Other Ingredients: Cellulose, Water.

Advanced Formula DairyEnz - Enzymes, Inc.
Each capsule contains: n-zimes Proprietary Blend 213 mg: Lactase, Proteases, Invertase, Lipase. Other Ingredients: Gelatin, Water.

Advanced Formula DigestEnz - Enzymes, Inc.
Each capsule contains: n-zimes Proprietary Blend 652 mg: Proteases, Amylase, Lipase, CereCalase Plus, Glucoamylase, Malt Diastase, alpha-Galactosidase, Invertase, Lactase, Pectinase, Cellulase. Other Ingredients: Cellulose, Water.

Advanced Formula FlorEnz - Enzymes, Inc.
Each capsule contains: Proprietary Blend 473 mg: Bifidobacterium longum, Lactobacillus plantarum, Lactobacillus salivarius, Lactobacillus acidophilus, Lactobacillus rhamnosis. Other Ingredients: Cellulose, Water.

Advanced Formula GastrEnz - Enzymes, Inc.
Each capsule contains: Proprietary Blend 450 mg: Marshmallow extract, Green Papaya concentrate, Deglycyrrhizinized Licorice root extract, Licorice root extract • n-zimes Proprietary Blend 251 mg: Lipase, Amylase, Peptidase, Catalase, CereCalase Plus, Glucoamylase, Papain, Malt Diastase, Cellulase, Pectinase, alpha-Galactosidase, Ivertase, Lactase. Other Ingredients: Cellulose, Water.

Advanced Formula ImmunEnz - Enzymes, Inc.
Each capsule contains: Proprietary Blend 375 mg: Echinacea purpurea root extract, Ginkgo biloba leaf extract, Garlic concentrate, Thyme extract, Reishi Mushroom extract, Mullein leaf extract, Eucalyptus leaf extract, Wild Indigo root extract • pHysioProtease 322 mg. Other Ingredients: Cellulose, Water.

Advanced Formula InflammEnz - Enzymes, Inc.
Each capsule contains: Vitamin C (from calcium and potassium ascorbates) 150 mg • Calcium (from ascorbate and citrate) 30 mg • Potassium (from potassium ascorbate) 10 mg • n-zimes Proprietary Blend 442 mg: pHysioProtease brand, Bromelain • Proprietary Blend 90 mg: Rutin, Grape seed extract. Other Ingredients: Cellulose, Water.

Advanced Formula LipidEnz - Enzymes, Inc.
Each capsule contains: Chromium (50% from Chromium Polynicotinate and 50% from Chromium Picolinate) 100 mcg • Proprietary Blend 500 mg: Garcinia fruit rind extract, Garlic concentrate, Guggulipids extract, Globe Artichoke leaf extract • n-zimes Proprietary Blend 181 mg: Lipase, pHysioProtease. Other Ingredients: Cellulose, Water.

Advanced Formula ProactEnz - Enzymes, Inc.
Each capsule contains: Calcium (from Calcium Citrate) 32 mg • n-zimes pHysioProtease 607 mg. Other Ingredients: Cellulose, Water.

Advanced Formula ProtEnz 375 - Enzymes, Inc.
Each capsule contains: n-zimes Protease Blend 625 mg. Other Ingredients: Cellulose, Water.

Advanced Formula Shen Min For Men - Biotech Corp.
Two tablets contain: Folate (as folic acid) 800 mcg • Pantothenic Acid (as dicalcium pantothenate) 200 mg • Biotin 1400 mcg • Iodine (from kelp) 150 mcg • Zinc (as zinc monomethionine) 15 mg • Shen Min Herb Blend 1320 mg: He Shou Wu (12:1 extract, standardized for chrysophanics and resveratrol), He Shou Wu root powder (polygonum multiflorum) • Shen Min Botanical Blend 450 mg: Saw Palmetto berries (sabal serrulata), Beta Sitosterol, Isoflavones (from pueraria lobata root and soybeans) • Silica (from colloidals) 40 gm • Bioperine brand Black Pepper extract (piper nigrum standardized extract 5 mg). Other Ingredients: Microcrystalline Cellulose, Croscarmellose Sodium, Stearic Acid, Magnesium Stearate, Pharmaceutical Glaze.

Advanced Formula Shen Min For Women - Biotech Corp.
Two tablets contain: Vitamin A (as retinyl palmitate) 5000 IU • Vitamin B6 (pyridoxine HCl) 10 mg • Niacin (as nicotinic acid) 20 mg • Pantothenic Acid 200 mg • Biotin 1400 mcg • Shen Min (polygonum multiflorum, 12:1 standardized extract) 450 mg • He Shou Wu root powder 870 mg • Soy Isoflavones (glycine max, from 50 mg 40% standardized soybean extract) 20 mg • Black Cohosh root (cimicifuga racemosa, 2.5% sesquiterpene lactones) 40 mg • Horse Chestnut standardized extract (20% escin) 50 mg • Hydrolyzed Collagen 250 mg • Silica (from plant sources) 100 mg • Ginkgo Biloba leaf 100 mg • Uva Ursi root standardized extract (10% arbutin) 50 mg • Burdock root (4:1 extract) 25 mg • Cayenne pepper (80,000 scoville heat units) 25 mg • Bioperine brand Black Pepper extract (piper nigrum standardized extract) 2 mg. Other Ingredients: Microcrystalline Cellulose, Croscarmellose Sodium, Stearic Acid, Magnesium Stearate, Dicalcium Phosphate, Pharmaceutical Glaze.

Advanced Geri-Max - Puritan's Pride
Each tablet contains: Vitamin A 10,000 IU • Vitamin C 250 mg • Vitamin D 400 IU • Vitamin E 150 IU • Thiamin 50 mg • Riboflavin 50 mg • Niacin 100 mg • Vitamin B6 50 mg • Folic Acid 400 mcg • Vitamin B12 50 mcg • Biotin 300 mcg • Pantothenic Acid 100 mg •

Calcium 10 mg • Iron 1 mg • Iodine 150 mcg • Magnesium 1.54 mg • Zinc 1.15 mg • Copper 0.25 mg • Manganese 0.61 mg • Potassium 1 mg • PABA 50 mg • Inositol 250 mg • Choline Bitartrate 250 mg • Rutin 25 mg • Citrus Bioflavonoid complex 25 mg • Hesperidin complex 25 mg • Betaine Hydrochloride 25 mg • L-Glutamic Acid 25 mg • Omega-3 EPA / DHA 50 mg. In a natural base of Alfalfa, Watercress, Parsley, Lecithin, and Rice Polishings.

Advanced Herbals Ginkgo Biloba Phytosome - Golden Glow Natural Health Products
Each capsule contains: Ginkgo Biloba leaf 2700 mg: Ginkgo Flavonglycosides 12 mg, Ginkgolide A 3.5 mg, Bilobalide 3.5 mg.

Advanced Joint Support - Futurebiotics LLC
Four capsules contain: Glucosamine Sulfate 1000 mg • Vitamin C (Buffered Ascorbate) 750 mg • Vitamin E (natural) 400 IU • Calcium (Ascorbate) 185 mg • Selenium (Amino Acid Chelate) 100 mcg • Zinc (Amino Acid Chelate) 15 mg • Bovine Cartilage 200 mg • Pancreatin 4X (Quadruple Strength) 100 mg containing: (Lipase 1600 USP units, Amylase 10000 USP units, Protease 10000 USP units) • Papain 60 mg • Bromelain 50 mg • Turmeric (standardized Curcumin) 250 mg • Cayenne powder 15 mg • Ginger powder 100 mg • Boswellin (standardized for 65% Boswellic Acid) 100 mg • Devil's Claw 50 mg • Rutin 50 mg.
See Editor's Note No. 14.

Advanced Prostate Formula - Rx Vitamins
Three capsules contain: Saw Palmetto fruit 320 mg • Stinging Nettle root 100 mg • African Pygeum bark 50 mg • Zinc 50 mg • Glycine 50 mg • Alanine 50 mg • Glutamic Acid 50 mg • Vitamin B6 50 mg • Vitamin E 100 IU in Borage seed oil.

Advanced Strength Ginkgo Biloba - Leiner Health Products
Each caplet contains: Ginkgo Biloba extract (Ginkgo biloba) leaf 75 mg • Lecithin 15 mg. Other Ingredients: Dicalcium phosphate, Cellulose, Silicon Dioxide, Stearic Acid, Croscarmellose Sodium, Dextrin, Magnesium Stearate, Dextrose, Sodium Carboxymethylcellulose, Sodium Citrate.

Advanced Strength Kava Kava - Leiner Health Products
Each caplet contains: Kava Kava extract (Piper methysticum) root 400 mg. Other Ingredients: Dicalcium Phosphate, Cellulose, Talc, Stearic Acid, Croscarmellose Sodium, Silicon Dioxide, Magnesium Stearate, Crospovidone, Hydroxypropyl Methylcellulose, Hydroxypropyl Cellulose, Polysorbate 80, Polyethylene Glycol 3350.

Advanish cream - Gero Vita International
Active Ingredient: Hydroquinone 2.0%. Inactive Ingredients: Deionized Water, Glycolic Acid, Triethanolamine, Glycerin, Petrolatum, Cetyl Alcohol, Glyceryl Stearate, Stearic Acid, DEA-Cetyl Phosphate, Octyl Methoxycinnamate, Sodium Bisulfite, Kojic Dipalmitate, Mulberry extract, Licorice root extract, Ascorbic acid, Tocopheryl Acetate, Dimethicone, Sodium Lauroyl Oat Amino Acids, Phenoxyethanol, Disodium EDTA, Xanthan Gum, Fragrance, Methylparaben, Propylparaben.

Advantage - Metabolic Nutrition, Inc.
Each packet (62 g) contains: Vitamin A • Vitamin B6 • Vitamin B12 • Vitamin C • Vitamin D • Vitamin E • Biotin • Calcium • Copper • Folic Acid • Iodine • Iron • Magnesium • Niacin • Pantothenic Acid • Phosphorus • Riboflavin • Thiamine • Zinc • Enzyme Additives: Betaine HCl, Pancreatin, Pepsin, Papain, Amylase.

Advantage Shake (cafe au lait flavor) - Atkins Nutritionals, Inc.
Water • Calcium Caseinate • Soybean oil • Whey Protein Concentrate • Coffee powder • Cellulose gel • Cellulose gum • Natural and Artificial flavor • Soy Lecithin • Sucralose (a non-nutritive sweetener) • Carrageenan • Magnesium Chloride • Magnesium Phosphate • Potassium Phosphate • Tricalcium Phosphate • D-Biotin • D-Calcium Pantothenate • Folic Acid • Niacinamide • Pyridoxine Hydrochloride • Sodium Ascorbate • Thiamin Mononitrate • Vitamin A Palmitate • Vitamin B12 • Riboflavin • Vitamin E Acetate • Vitamin K (K1) • Chromium Chloride • Copper Sulfate • Ferrous Sulfate • Manganese Sulfate • Potassium Chloride • Potassium Citrate • Potassium Iodide • Sodium Citrate • Sodium Molybdate • Sodium Selenite • Zinc Sulfate • Maltodextrin.

Advantage Shake (chocolate delight flavor) - Atkins Nutritionals, Inc.
Water • Calcium Caseinate • Soybean oil • Whey Protein Concentrate • Cocoa (processed with alkali) • Cellulose gel • Potassium Phosphate • Cellulose gum • Soy Lecithin • Natural and Artificial flavor • Carrageenan • Sucralose (a non-nutritive sweetener) • Magnesium Chloride • Magnesium Phosphate • Tricalcium Phosphate • D-Biotin • D-Calcium Pantothenate • Folic Acid • Niacinamide • Pyridoxine Hydrochloride • Sodium Ascorbate • Thiamin Mononitrate • Vitamin A Palmitate • Vitamin B12 • Riboflavin • Vitamin E Acetate • Vitamin K (K1) • Chromium Chloride • Copper Sulfate • Ferrous Sulfate • Manganese Sulfate • Potassium Chloride • Potassium Citrate • Potassium Iodide • Sodium Citrate • Sodium Molybdate • Sodium Selenite • Zinc Sulfate • Maltodextrin.

Advantage Shake (chocolate royale flavor) - Atkins Nutritionals, Inc.
Water • Calcium Caseinate • Soybean oil • Cocoa (processed with alkali) • Whey Protein Concentrate • Cellulose gel • Natural and Artificial flavor • Cellulose gum • Soy Lecithin • Carrageenan • Sucralose (a non-nutritive sweetener) • Magnesium Chloride • Magnesium Phosphate • Potassium Phosphate • Tricalcium Phosphate • D-Biotin • D-Calcium Pantothenate • Folic Acid • Niacinamide • Pyridoxine Hydrochloride • Sodium Ascorbate • Thiamin Mononitrate • Vitamin A Palmitate • Vitamin B12 • Riboflavin • Vitamin E Acetate • Vitamin K (K1) • Chromium Chloride • Copper Sulfate • Ferrous Sulfate • Manganese Sulfate • Potassium Chloride • Potassium Citrate • Potassium Iodide • Sodium Citrate • Sodium Molybdate • Sodium Selenite • Zinc Sulfate • Maltodextrin.

Advantage Shake (strawberry flavor) - Atkins Nutritionals, Inc.
Water • Calcium Caseinate • Soybean oil • Whey Protein Concentrate • Cellulose gel • Natural and Artificial flavor • Potassium Phosphate • Cellulose gum • Soy Lecithin • Carrageenan • Sucralose (a non-nutritive sweetener) • Cochineal extract • Magnesium Chloride • Magnesium Phosphate • Tricalcium Phosphate • D-Biotin • D-Calcium Pantothenate • Folic Acid • Niacinamide • Pyridoxine Hydrochloride • Sodium Ascorbate • Thiamin Mononitrate • Vitamin A Palmitate • Vitamin B12 • Riboflavin • Vitamin E Acetate • Vitamin K (K1) • Chromium Chloride • Copper Sulfate • Ferrous Sulfate • Manganese Sulfate • Potassium Chloride • Potassium Citrate • Potassium Iodide • Sodium Citrate • Sodium Molybdate • Sodium Selenite • Zinc Sulfate • Maltodextrin.

AdvantaSoy brand - Cargill Health & Food Technologies
Soy.
See Editor's Note No. 44.

Advantin - Advocare International
Each capsule contains: Ginger root extract (zingiber officinale) 200 mg • Boswellia gum resin extract (boswellia serrata) 150 mg • Curcumin root powder (curcuma longa) 100 mg • Whole Papaya fruit powder (carica papaya) 50 mg • Papain 50 mg • Bromelain 50 mg. Other Ingredients: Silicon Dioxide, Magnesium Stearate, Gelatin.

Advantra Z (Advantra-Z, AdvantraZ) brand - Nutratech
Citrus Aurantium.
See Editor's Note No. 40 and No. 44.

AdvoKids Spark - Advocare International
Each pouch contains: Vitamin A (as beta-carotene from D. satina mixed carotenoids) 2500 IU • Vitamin C (as ascorbic acid) 180 mg • Vitamin E (as D-alpha-tocopheryl acetate) 30 IU • Thiamine 3 mg • Riboflavin 3.4 mg • Niacin (as niacin and niacinamide) 60 mg • Vitamin B6 (as pyridoxine HCl) 6 mg • Vitamin B12 (as cyanocobalamin) 45 mcg • Pantothenic Acid (as calcium

pantothenate) 30 mg • Zinc (as OptiZinc brand monomethionine) 3 mg • Copper (as glycinate) 200 mcg • Chromium (as ChromeMate brand polynicotinate) 60 mcg • Sodium (as phosphate) 20 mg • L-Tyrosine 500 mg • Choline (as citrate and bitartrate) 400 mg • Taurine 200 mg • Glycine 100 mg • Gamma-Aminobutyric Acid 100 mg • Caffeine 60 mg • L-Carnitine (as tartrate) 10 mg • Coenzyme Q-10 100 mcg. Other Ingredients: Maltodextrin, Citric Acid, Natural Flavor, Artificial Flavor, Sodium Phosphate, Sucralose, Silicon Dioxide.

A-F Betafood - Standard Process, Inc.
Two tablets contain: Proprietary Blend 590 mg: Carrot root, Dried Beet leaf juice, Beet root, Oat Flour, Calcium Lactate, Defatted Wheat Germ, Magnesium Citrate, Bovine Prostate, Nutritional Yeast, Bovine Liver, Bovine Kidney, Alfalfa Flour, Bovine Orchic extract, Bovine Liver fat extract, Flaxseed oil extract, Mixed Tocopherols, Soybean Lecithin • Vitamin A 3000 IU • Vitamin B6 0.3 mg • Iodine 40 mcg • Potassium 10 mg. Other Ingredients: Honey, Arabic Gum, Gelatin.
See Editor's Note No. 14.

Aflexa - McNeil Consumer Healthcare
Each tablet contains: Glucosamine 340 mg (Glucosamine Sulfate, Glucosamine Hydrochloride). Other Ingredients: Cellulose, Hydroxypropyl, Methylcellulose, Polyethylene Glycol, Silicon Dioxide, Propylene Glycol, Crospovidone, Hydroxypropyl Cellulose, Titanium Dioxide, Magnesium Stearate, Polysorbate 80, Povidone.

After Max - Optimum Nutrition
Three scoops (97 g) contain: Proprietary Protein Blend: Whey Protein Concentrate, Glutamine Peptides, Whey Protein Isolate, Hydrolyzed Whey Peptides • Maltodextrin • Cocoa • Natural and Artificial Flavors • Salt • Acesulfame Potassium • Vitamin/Mineral Blend: Ascorbic Acid, D-Alpha Tocopheryl Succinate, Maltoxextrin, Niacinamide, D-Calcium Pantothenate, Pyridoxine Hydrochloride, Chromium Polynicotinate, Riboflavin, Vitamin A Palmitate, Biotin, Folic Acid, Cholecalciferol, Cyanocobalamin • Sucralose.

AfterFX Bar (Bavarian mint flavor) - Nutripeak
Each bar contains: Protein 34 g • Vitamin A (Retinyl Palmitate) 5000 IU • Vitamin C (Ascorbic Acid) 120 mg • Vitamin D (Cholecalciferol) 400 IU • Vitamin E (dl-Alpha Tocopheryl Acetate) 60 IU • Thiamin Mononitrate (Vitamin B1) 1.5 mg • Riboflavin (Vitamin B2) 1.7 mg • Niacin (Niacinamide) 20 mg • Vitamin B6 (Pyridoxine Hydrochloride) 2 mg • Folic Acid 400 mcg • Vitamin B12 (Cyanocobalamin) 6 mcg • Biotin 300 mcg • Pantothenic Acid (Calcium D-Pantothenate) 10 mg • Calcium (Tricalcium Phosphate and Monocalcium Phosphate) 500 mg • Iron (Ferrous Fumarate) 18 mg • Phosphorus 300 mg • Iodine (Potassium Iodide) 150 mcg • Magnesium Oxide 100 mg • Zinc Amino Acid Chelate 15 mg • Copper Gluconate 2 mg • Sodium 75 mg • Potassium 250 mg • HMB (as calcium-b-hydroxy-b-methylbutyrate) 585 mg • L-Glutamine 3 mg. Other Ingredients: Metamyosyn Protein Blend: Bovine Hydrolyzed Collagen, Calcium Caseinate, Milk Protein Concentrate, Whey Protein Isolate, Whey Protein Concentrate, Dried Egg Albumen; Coating: Maltitol, Salatrim, Cocoa (processed with alkali), Butter Oil, Soy Lecithin, Acesulfame K, Vanilla; Glycerin; Water; Natural and Artificial Flavors; Brown Rice Syrup; Medium Chain Triglycerides; Cocoa (processed with alkali); Cocoa extract; Polydextrose; Potassium Sorbate (preservative); Salt; Sucralose; Partially Hydrogenated Soybean Oil; Partially Hydrogenated Cottonseed Oil. May contain traces of peanuts and/or other nuts.

Age Resistance Cream - Abra Therapeutics
Green Tea extract • Apricot kernel oil • Vegetable Emulsifying Wax • Beta Glucan (from oat) • Sea Algae extract • Shea Butter • Squalane (from olives) • Glycerin • Borage seed oil • Wheat Germ oil • Bulgarian Rosewater • Aloe Vera gel • Calophyllum Inophyllum berry (foraha) • Milk Thistle extract • White Willow bark extract • Neroli oil • Chamomile • Daucus Carota subsp. carota • Lavender • Vitamin A • Vitamin C • Vitamin E • Superoxide Dismutase • Methylparaben • Propylparaben.

Age Right Formula - Nature's Way
Four capsules contain: Acetylcarnitine 50 mcg • Acetylcysteine 50 mcg • Betaine Anhydrous 50 mg • Biotin (Biotin Triurate) 500 mcg • Boron (Amino Acid Chelate) 500 mcg • Calcium 43 mg • Calcium Pantethonate 175 mg • Caromix (Mixed Carotenoids) 2000 IU • Chromium Picolinate 100 mcg • Citrus Bioflavonoids 250 mg • Coenzyme Q10 (Ubiquinone) 15 mg • Copper (Amino Acid Chelate) 500 mcg • Fizyme Enzyme Formula 65 mg • Folic Acid (Folate) 250 mcg • Grape seed dried extract 15 mg • Green Tea (Polyphenol Catechin extract) 75 mg • Inositol 15 mg • Kelp (whole Thallus) 25 mcg • Manganese (Amino Acid Chelate) 2.5 mg • Molybdenum Triturate 25 mcg • Niacinamide 47.5 mg • Potassium (Aspartate, Chloride) 25 mg • Riboflavin (Vitamin B2) 25 mg • Selenium (l-Selenomethione) 25 mcg • Thiamine (Vitamin B1) 25 mg • Vitamin A (Retinol Palmitate) 2530 IU • Vitamin B12 (Cyanocobalamin) 250 mcg • Vitamin B6 (Pyridoxine HCL) 25 mg • Vitamin C (Ascorbic Acid) 250 mg • Vitamin D (as Vitamin D3) (Cholecalciferol) 200 IU • Vitamin E (d-Alpha Tocopheryl) 200 IU • Vitamin K (Phytonadione) 30 mcg • Zinc (Amino Acid Chelate) 5 mg. Other Ingredients: Gelatin, Magnesium Stearate, Millet.

AgeErasers SAMe - Bodyonics, Ltd.
Each tablet contains: Vitamin B12 50 mcg • Folic Acid 100 mcg • SAMe 200 mg. Other Ingredients: Calcium Phosphate, Stearic Acid, Croscarmellose, Magnesium Strearate.

Ageless - Oasis Wellness Network
Four capsules contain: Vitamin B3 (as niacin, niacinamide) 35 mg • Vitamin B6 (as pyridoxal-5-phosphate) 8 mg • Serenix Corn extract 1000 mg • Energetix 3-Ginseng Complex 750 mg: Panax Ginseng extract, Rhodiola extract, Eleuthero extract • Green Tea extract (70% polyphenols/25% EGCG, 5% theanine) 440 mg • Ornithine Ketoglutarate 300 mg • Protectin Proprietary Blend 300 mg: Catechu bark, Scullcap root • MaxCell Proprietary Blend 30 mg: Zisyphus Jujube, Piper Nigrum, Aloe Vera, Glycyrrhiza Glabra. Other Ingredients: Magnesium Stearate, Cellulose.

AGEless - Life Enhancement Products, Inc.
Four capsules contain: Vitamin C (as ascorbyl palmitate) 17 mg • Thiamine (vitamin B1 as thiamine hydrochloride) 20 mg • Vitamin B6 (as pyridoxine hydrochloride) 25 mg • Chromium (as chromium aspartate and chromium nicotinate) 200 mcg • American Ginseng (panax quinquefolius, 5%) 2 g • Diosmin 300 mg • Nutmeg, fresh ground powder 150 mg • Allspice, fresh ground powder 104 mg • Clove powder 100 mg • Kola nut 67 mg • Hesperidin, 98+% 33 mg • Cinnamon powder 10 mg.

AHA (Alpha Hydroxy Acids) 2oz - Derma E
Purified Water • Glycolic Acid • Glycerin • Caprylic Triglyceride • Jojoba Oil • Cetearyl Alcohol • Ceteарate 20 • Stearic Acid • Glyceryl Stearate • Peg 100 Stearate • Cetyl Alcohol • Xanthan Gum • Green Tea extract • Lemon extract • Passion Fruit extract • Dimethicone • Methylparaben • Sodium Hydroxide • I. Urea.

AHCC - Source Naturals
Two capsules contain: AHCC Proprietary Blend 1 g: Mushroom mycelia extract, Candelilla wax, Cyclodextrin, Microcrystalline Cellulose • Bioperine brand Black Pepper extract 6 mg. Other Ingredients: Gelatin, Magnesium Stearate.

Air Power - Enzymatic Therapy
Each tablet contains: Glycerol Guaiacolate 200 mg • Fenugreek seed 4:1 extract (trigonella foenum-graecum) 350 mg • Marshmallow root 3.5:1 extract (althaea officinalis) 125 mg • PABA (para-aminobenzoic acid) 50 mg • Mullein leaf (verbascum nigrum) 50 mg. Other Ingredients: Carnauba Wax, Cellulose, Lecithin, Magnesium Stearate, Modified Cellulose, Modified Cellulose Gum.

Airborne Effervescent Health Formula Lemon-Lime - Knight-McDowell Labs
Each tablet contains: Vitamin A (100% acetate) 5000 IU • Vitamin C 1000 mg • Vitamin E 30 IU • Magnesium (sulfate) 40 mg • Zinc (sulfate) 8 mg • Selenium (sodium selinite) 15 mcg • Manganese

(gluconate) 3 mg • Potassium (bicarbonate) 75 mg • Organic Herbal Extracts 350 mg: Lonicera, Forsythia, Schizonepeta, Ginger, Chinese Vitex, Isatis root, Echinacea • Amino Acids 50 mg: Glutamine, Lysine. Other Ingredients: Citric Acid, Sorbitol, Sodium Bicarbonate, Natural Lemon-Lime Flavor, Polyethylene Glycol, Sucralose, Mineral Oil.

Airborne Effervescent Health Formula Original - Knight-McDowell Labs
Each tablet contains: Vitamin A (100% acetate) 5000 IU • Vitamin C 1000 mg • Vitamin E 30 IU • Magnesium (sulfate) 40 mg • Zinc (sulfate) 8 mg • Selenium (sodium selinite) 15 mcg • Manganese (gluconate) 3 mg • Potassium (bicarbonate) 75 mg • Organic Herbal Extracts 350 mg: Lonicera, Forsythia, Schizonepeta, Ginger, Chinese Vitex, Isatis root, Echinacea • Amino Acids 50 mg: Glutamine, Lysine. Other Ingredients: Citric Acid, Sorbitol, Sodium Bicarbonate, Natural Orange Flavor, Mineral Oil, Sucralose, Acesulfame Potassium.

Airborne Health Formula Lemon-Lime - Knight-McDowell Labs
Each tablet contains: Vitamin A (100% acetate) 5000 IU • Vitamin C 1000 mg • Vitamin E 30 IU • Magnesium (sulfate) 40 mg • Zinc (sulfate) 8 mg • Selenium (sodium selinite) 15 mcg • Manganese (gluconate) 3 mg • Potassium (bicarbonate) 75 mg • Organic Herbal Extracts 350 mg: Lonicera, Forsythia, Schizonepeta, Ginger, Chinese Vitex, Isatis root, Echinacea • Amino Acids 50 mg: Glutamine, Lysine. Other Ingredients: Citric Acid, Sorbitol, Sodium Bicarbonate, Natural Lemon-Lime Flavor, Polyethylene Glycol, Sucralose, Mineral Oil.

Airborne Health Formula Original - Knight-McDowell Labs
Each tablet contains: Vitamin A (100% acetate) 5000 IU • Vitamin C 1000 mg • Vitamin E 30 IU • Magnesium (sulfate) 40 mg • Zinc (sulfate) 8 mg • Selenium (sodium selinite) 15 mcg • Manganese (gluconate) 3 mg • Potassium (bicarbonate) 75 mg • Organic Herbal Extracts 350 mg: Lonicera, Forsythia, Schizonepeta, Ginger, Chinese Vitex, Isatis root, Echinacea • Amino Acids 50 mg: Glutamine, Lysine. Other Ingredients: Citric Acid, Sorbitol, Sodium Bicarbonate, Natural Orange Flavor, Mineral Oil, Sucralose, Acesulfame Potassium.

Airborne Jr - Knight-McDowell Labs
Each tablet contains: Vitamin A (100% acetate) 500 IU • Vitamin C 500 mg • Vitamin E 15 IU • Magnesium (sulfate) 20 mg • Zinc (sulfate) 4 mg • Selenium (sodium selinite) 8 mcg • Manganese (gluconate) 1.5 mg • Potassium (bicarbonate) 38 mg • Herbal Extracts 200 mg: Lonicera, Forsythia, Schizonepeta, Ginger, Chinese Vitex, Isatis root, Echinacea • Amino Acids 25 mg: Glutamine, Lysine. Other Ingredients: Citric Acid, Sorbitol, Sodium Bicarbonate, Natural Grape Flavors, Polyethylene Glycol, Sucralose, Mineral Oil.

Airborne Sore Throat Gummi Lozenges - Knight-McDowell Labs
Each lozenge contains: Vitamin C 7.5 mg • Vitamin E 1.25 IU • Thiamin 0.175 mg • Riboflavin 0.2 mg • Niacin 2.25 mg • Vitamin B6 0.25 mg • Folic Acid 25 mcg • Vitamin B12 0.125 mcg • Biotin 18.75 mcg • Pantothenic Acid 0.75 mg • Magnesium (lactate) 1 mg • Zinc (citrate) 1 mg • Organic Herbal Extract 22 mg: Lonicera, Forsythia, Schizonepeta, Ginger, Chinese Vitex, Isatis root, Echinacea. Other Ingredients: Sugar, Gum Arabic, Corn Syrup, Citric Acid, Licorice, Honey, Natural Fruit Flavors, Natural and Naturally Processed Colors.

Airborne Sore Throat Lozenges - Knight-McDowell Labs
Each lozenge contains: Vitamin C 7.5 mg • Vitamin E 1.25 IU • Thiamin 0.175 mg • Riboflavin 0.2 mg • Niacin 2.25 mg • Vitamin B6 0.25 mg • Folic Acid 25 mcg • Vitamin B12 0.125 mcg • Biotin 18.75 mcg • Pantothenic Acid 0.75 mg • Magnesium (lactate) 1 mg • Zinc (citrate) 1 mg • Organic Herbal Extract 22 mg: Lonicera, Forsythia, Schizonepeta, Ginger, Chinese Vitex, Isatis root, Echinacea. Other Ingredients: Sugar, Gum Arabic, Corn Syrup, Citric Acid, Licorice, Honey, Natural Fruit Flavors, Natural and Naturally Processed Colors.

AirDefense - NaturalCare
Active Ingredients: Pink Root (spigelia anthelmia) 3X • Origanum Vulgare (oregano) 3X, 6X • Luffa Operculata (luffa fruit) 6X • Hydrastis Canadensis (golden seal) 3X, 6X, 12X • Echinacea Angustifolia (cone flower) 3X, 6X, 12X • Zinc Gluconate (zincum gluconicum) 2X, 6X • Euphorbium Officinarum 4X, 6X, 12X • Silver (argentum metallicum) 8X • Potassium Sulfate (kali sulphuricum) 3X, 6X, 12X • Allium Cepa (red onion) 6X • Ragweed (ambrosia artemisiaefolia) 6X • Calcium Sulfide (hepar sulphuris calcareum) 8X • Potassium Dichromate (kali bichromicum) 6X, 10X • Sanguinaria Canadensis (blood root) 6X • Lemna Minor (duckweed) 3X • Pulsatilla (windflower) 3X • Sabadilla (cevadilla seed) 6X • Silicea (silicon dioxide) 8X. Other Ingredients: Aloe Vera Extract, Bitter Melon Fruit Extract (momordica charantia), Colloidal Silver, D-Mannose (natural saccharide), Grapefruit Seed Extract, Green Tea Extract, Licorice Extract (root), Tea Tree Oil.
See Editor's Note No. 1.

Airzene - Progressive Health Nutraceuticals
Vitamin C 250 mg • Zinc 20 mg • N-Acetyl L-Cysteine 750 mg • Licorice root 100 mg • Cordyceps 500 mg • Astragalus 200 mg • Echinacea Purpurea 50 mg • Citrus Aurantium 150 mg.
See Editor's Note No. 40.

AKG Fuel - TwinLab
Three capsules contain: Alpha-Ketoglutaric Acid (from Magnesium Alpha-Ketoglutarate) 1250 mg • Magnesium (from Magnesium Alpha-Ketoglutarate) 210 mg • L-Glutamine 1000 mg.

AKN Skin Care - Nature's Way
Two capsules contain: Proprietary Blend 930 mg: Burdock root, Capsicum root, Dandelion root, Echinacea Purpurea root, Kelp (whole thallus), Licorice root, Plantain root, Sarsaparilla root, Yellow Dock root. Other Ingredients: Gelatin.

ALA 300 (Alpha-Lipoic Acid) - America's Finest
Each capsule contains: Alpha-Lipoic Acid 300 mg. Other Ingredients: Di-Calcium Phosphate, Cellulose, Magnesium Stearate, Silica.

ALA Eye Area Therapy - N.V. Perricone M.D. Cosmeceuticals
Water • Cetearyl Alcohol • Ceteareth-20 • Glycerin • Isopropyl Palmitate • Butylene Glycol • Glycosaminoglycans • Sodium Chondroitin Sulfate • Sodium Carboxymethyl Betaglucan • C12-C15 Alkyl Benzoate • Lipoic Acid • Petrolatum • Cyclomethicone • Dimethyl MEA (DMAE) • Glyceryl Stearate • PEG-100 Stearate • Squalane • Tocopheryl Acetate • Tyrosine • Dimethicone • Urea • Propylene Glycol • Camellia Oleifera extract (green tea) • Citric Acid • Diazolidinyl Urea • Allantoin • Bisabolol • Zinc Sulfate • Methylparaben • Pyridoxine HCl • Pantethine • Propylparaben • Disodium EDTA • BHT • Sodium Hyaluronate.

Alapars - Metagenics
Each tablet contains: Niacin (as niacinamide) 500 mg • N-Acetylcysteine 200 mg • Vitamin C (as ascorbic acid) 100 mg.

Al-Assist - FreeLife International
Each caplet contains: Respiratory Support Blend 500 mg: Stinging Nettle leaf extract (urtica dioica), Chinese Skullcap root (scutellaria baicalensis), Feverfew leaf (tanacetum parthenium), Purple Butterbur root and rhizome standardized extract (petasites hybridus), Citrus Bioflavonoids, Tylophora leaf standardized extract (tylophora asthmatica), Boswellia Serrata gum resin, Licorice root (glycyrrhiza glabra), Quercetin Dihydrate, Wild Cherry bark (prunus serotina), Cayenne fruit (capsicum annuum), Fenugreek seed (trigonella foenum-graecum), Bromelain, Curcumin, Horseradish root (armoracia rusticana), Lungwort (pulmonaria officinalis), Black Seed (nigella sativa), Yerba Santa leaf (eriodictyon californicum). Other

BRAND NAMES

Ingredients: Calcium Hydrogen Phosphate, Cellulose, Cellulose Gum, Vegetable Stearic Acid, Vegetable Magnesium Stearate, Silica, Vita-Coat brand (modified vegetable cellulose, alpha-lipoic acid).

Albaplex **-** Standard Process, Inc.
Two capsules contain: Proprietary Blend 940 mg: Choline Bitartrate, Dried Kidney bean juice, Oat Flour, Betaine Hydrochloride, Bovine Liver PMG extract, Carrot root, Tillandsia Usneoides, Inositol, Calcium Glycerophosphate, Bovine Adrenal, Bovine Kidney PMG extract, Nutritional Yeast, Bovine Thymus Cytosol extract, Soy bean, Dried Pea vine juice, Bovine Liver, Dried Buckwheat leaf juice, Buckwheat seed, Dried Alfalfa juice, Mushroom, Bovine Bone, Bovine Kidney, Defatted Wheat germ, Dried Beet leaf juice, Veal Bone meal, Enzymatically Processed Tillandsia Usneoides and Beet root, Peanut bran, Mixed Tocopherols, Soybean Lecithin • Vitamin A 2160 IU • Vitamin C 12 mg • Niacin 10 mg • Vitamin B6 2 mg • Sodium 10 mg • Potassium 30 mg. Other Ingredients: Gelatin, Water, Colors.
See Editor's Note No. 14.

ALC arginate **-** Pure Encapsulations
Each vegetable capsule contains: Acetyl-L-Carnitine Arginate Dihydrochloride 500 mg.

ALC Fuel **-** TwinLab
Each capsule contains: Acetyl-L-Carnitine (ALC) 1000 mg.

Alcodol **-** Unicus Health
Two capsules contain: Vitamin A 213 IU • Vitamin C 1.8 mg • Vitamin D 320 IU • Vitamin E 0.1 IU • Thiamin (B1) 12 mcg • Riboflavin (B2) 18 mcg • Vitamin B12 3 mcg • Bitoin 3 mcg • Pantothenic Acid 28 mcg • Phosphorus 1.5 mg • Magnesium 50 mcg.

Alcohol Free Astragalus Root **-** Vitamin World
Each 1 mL serving contains: Astragalus root (astragalus membranaceus) 500 mg. Other Ingredients: Vegetable Glycerin, Water, Caramel Color.

Alcohol-Free Melissa Supreme **-** Gaia Herbs
Fifteen drops contain: Proprietary Blend 120 mg: Lemon Balm (melissa off.), German Chamomile flowers (matricaria recutita), Passionflower vine (passiflora incarnata), Fresh Skullcap herb (scutellaria lateriflora), Fresh Wild Oats milky seed (avena sativa), Gotu Kola concentrated glycerite (centella asiatica), Mineral Salts extracted from Kelp, 50-60% Pure Vegetable Glycerine.

Alcohol-Free Recovery Supreme **-** Gaia Herbs
Forty drops contain: Proprietary Blend 120 mg: Schizandra berry (schizandra chinensis), Milk Thistle seed (silybum marianum), Wild Oats milky seed (avena sativa), Kudzu root (pueraria lobata), Indian Gooseberry (emblica officinalis), Passionflower (passiflora incarnata), Licorice root (glycyrrhiza glabra), Peppermint leaf (mentha piperita), Ginger root juice (zingiber officinale), Spring Water, 45-55% Pure Vegetable Glycerin.

Alcohol-Free Valerian Poppy Supreme **-** Gaia Herbs
Forty drops contain: Proprietary Blend 90 mg: Valerian root (valeriana officinalis), Fresh Skullcap herb (scutellaria lateriflora), California Poppy herb (eschscholzia california), Kava Kava rhizome and root (piper methysticum), Passionflower vine (passiflora incarnata), German Chamomile flowers (matricaria recutita), Mugwort herb (artemisia vulgaris), 60% Pure Vegetable Glycerine, Spring Water.

Aler-Key **-** J. R. Carlson Laboratories, Inc.
Two capsules contain: Vitamin C (as calcium ascorbate) 800 mg • Riboflavin (vitamin B2) 10 mg • Vitamin B6 (as pyridoxine hydrochloride) 10 mg • Pantothenic Acid (as di-calcium pantothenate) 200 mg • Calcium (as calcium ascorbate and di-calcium pantothenate) 116 mg • Quercetin bioflavonoid 300 mg.

Alert **-** PhytoPharmica
Each capsule contains: Cola Nut extract (Cola nitida; contains 35 mg caffeine) 250 mg • Green Tea extract (Camellia sinensis; contains 15 mg caffeine) 250 mg • Oat Straw extract 10:1 (Avena sativa) 50 mg • Schisandra extract (standardized to contain 9% schizandrin) 50 mg • Siberian Ginseng extract (Eleutherococcus senticosus; (standardized to contain greater than 1% eleutheroside E) 50 mg • Ginger root extract 6.5:1 (Zingiber officinale) 25 mg • Korean Ginseng root extract (Panax ginseng; standardized to contain 7% saponis calculated as ginsenoside Rg1) 10 mg • Chromium (Polynicotinate) 100 mcg.

Alert Vitalizing Formula **-** Starlight International
Two capsules contain: Potassium (as potassium glycerophosphate) 35 mg • Schisandra extract 4:1 (schisandra chinensis, berry) 250 mg • Oriental Ginseng (panax ginseng, root) 300 mg • Guarana extract 6:1 (paulina cupana, seed) 600 mg • Caffeine 132 mg • Adrenal Substance 150 mg • Coenzyme Q10 5.0 mg • Siberian Ginseng (eicutherococcus senticosus, root) 1.0 mg • Spirulina 1.0 mg. Other Ingredients: Dicalcium Phosphate, Magnesium Stearate, Silicon Dioxide, Gelatin.
See Editor's Note No. 14.

Aletris Compound **-** The Herbalist
False Unicorn root • Squaw Vine herb • Cramp bark • Blue Cohosh root • Ginger root.

Alfalfa **-** Nature's Sunshine
Two capsules contain: Alfalfa aerial parts (medicago sativa) 680 mg. Other Ingredients: Kosher Gelatin, Water.

Alfalfa **-** Puritan's Pride
Three tablets contain: Alfalfa leaf (Medicago sativa) 1,500 mg. Other Ingredients: Dicalcium Phosphate, Vegetable Stearic Acid, Vegetable Magnesium Stearate, Croscarmellose.

Alfalfa **-** Quest
Each tablet contains: Organic Alfalfa 650 mg. Other Ingredients: Terra Alba, Silica, Magnesium Stearate (vegetable source).

Alfalfa Compleet **-** J. R. Carlson Laboratories, Inc.
Three tablets contain: Vitamin C (as ascorbic acid) 30 mg • Alfalfa (from leaves, seeds & juice concentrate) 1554 mg.

Alfalfa Complex **-** Shaklee
Ten tablets contain: Calcium 300 mg • Iron 0.36 mg • Phosphorus 150 mg • Magnesium 10 mg • Sodium 10 mg • Alfalfa powder (Medicago sativa) leaf 2.85 g. Other Ingredients: Dicalcium Phosphate, Maltodextrin, Fructose, Tricalcium Phosphate, Spearmint Oil (Mentha spicata) Leaf.

Alfalfa Concentrate **-** Marlyn
Each tablet contains: Vegetarian Organically Grown Alfalfa 648 mg.

Alfalfa Leaves **-** Nature's Way
Three capsules contain: Alfalfa leaf 1.22 g • Vitamin C 1.46 mg.

Alfalfa-Devil's Claw Formula **-** Quest
Each caplet contains: Alfalfa leaf powder (medicago sativa) 70 mg • Alfalfa seed powder 70 mg • Burdock root powder (arctium lappa) 70 mg • Celery seed powder (apium graveolens) 70 mg • Devil's Claw root powder (herpagophytum procumbens) 70 mg • Cayenne powder (capsicum) 35 mg • Kelp powder (fucus versiculosis) 35 mg • Queen of the Meadow root powder (filipendula ulmaria) 5 mg • Sarsaparilla root powder (smilax officinalis) 5 mg. Other Ingredients: Calcium Phosphate, Microcrystalline Cellulose, Vegetable Stearin, Croscarmellose Sodium, Magnesium Stearate (vegetable source).

Alfa-Max **-** Nature's Way
Each capsule contains: Alfalfa leaf 420 mg.

Algin **-** Nature's Sunshine
Two capsules contain: Algin (sodium alginate, from brown seaweed) 950 mg. Other Ingredients: Gelatin, Water.

Algosan **-** Xymogen
Deionized Water • Aloe Vera gel • Caprylic/Capric Triglycerides • Shea Butter • Sunflower seed oil • Cis-9-Cetylmyristoleate •

Vegetable Glycerin • Artichoke extract • Sarsaparilla extract • Isopropyl Palmitate • Cetearyl Alcohol • Ceteareth-20 • Stearic Acid • Carbomer • MSM • DL Panthenol • Hydroxypropyl Cellulose • Nutmeg oil • Rosemary oil • Menthol • Camphor • Boswellin • Glucosamine HCl • Disodium EDTA • Allantoin • Methyl Paraben • Propyl Paraben • Diazolidinyl Urea • TEA • Capsicum • Oleoresin.

Alive! Whole Food Energizer (Iron Free) Veggie Cap - Nature's Way
Six capsules contain: Amino Acids Blend 225 mg: Glutamine, Asparagine, Leucine, Alanine, Arginine, Lysine, Threonine, Valine, Glycine, Isoleucine, Serine, Proline, Phenylalanine, Tyrosine, Histidine, Methionine, Tryptophan, Cysteine • Biotin Triurate 300 mcg • Boron Amino Acid Chelate 1 mg • Calcium (citrate, carbonate) 250 mg • Chlorophyll (from spirulina) 4 mg • Choline Bitartrate 30 mg • Chromium Polynicotinate 120 mcg • Citrus Bioflavonoid Complex 60 mg: Eriocitrin 600 mcg, Naringin/Narirutin/other Flavonones 1.8 mg, Flavonols 600 mcg, Flavones/related Phenolic compounds 600 mcg • Copper Amino Acid Chelate 2 mg • Digestive Enzyme Blend 100 mg: Protease I, Protease II, Peptizyme SP, Amylase, Lactase, Invertase, Lipase, Cellulase, Alpha Galactosidase, Betaine HCl, Bromelain (from pineapple), Papain (from papaya) • DNA (from spirulina, chlorella) 4 mg • Eleuthero root 50 mg • Folic Acid (folate) 400 mcg • Garden Veggies Juice Powder Blend 500 mg: Parsley, Kale, Spinach, Wheat Grass, Brussels Sprouts, Asparagus, Broccoli, Cauliflower, Beet, Carrot, Cabbage, Garlic • Green Food/Spirulina Blend 500 mg: Spirulina (microalgae), Alfalfa (leaf, stem), Barley Grass, Dandelion (leaf), Wheat Grass, Spinach (leaf), Lemon Grass, Nettle (leaf), Blessed Thistle (stem, leaf, flower), Chlorella (broken-cell microalgae), Chickweed (stem, leaf, flower), Blue Green Algae (microalgae), Cilantro (leaf) • Hesperidin 2 mg • Inositol 50 mg • Iodine 150 mcg • Lutein (from marigold) 200 mcg • Magnesium (as citrate, oxide) 125 mg • Manganese Amino Acid Chelate 4 mg • Molybdenum Triurate 75 mcg • MycoDefense Mushroom Blend 100 mg: Cordyceps, Reishi, Shiitake, Hiratake, Maitake, Ymabushitake, Mimembatsutake, Kawaratake, Chaga, Zhu Ling, Agarikon, Mesima • Niacinamide 125 mg • Omega Fatty Acid Seed Blend 100 mg: Flax seed powder, Sunflower seed powder, providing: Alpha-Linoleic Acid, Oleic Acid, Linoleic Acid, Palmitic Acid, Stearic Acid, Behenic Acid, Gadoleic Acid, Palmitoleic Acid, Eicosanoic Acid, Lignoceric Acid • Orchard Fruits Juice Powder blend 100 mg: Plum, Cranberry, Blueberry, Strawberry, Blackberry, Bilberry, Cherry, Apricot, Papaya, Orange, Grape, Pineapple • PABA (para aminobenzoic acid) 25 mg • Pantothenic Acid 125 mg • Potassium Amino Acid Chelate 50 mg • Riboflavin (vitamin B2) 25 mg • RNA (from spirulina, chlorella) 14 mg • Rutin 25 mg • Selenium Monomethionine 70 mcg • Sodium 15 mg • Thiamine (vitamin B1) 25 mg • Vitamin A (retinol, palmitate) 15,000 IU • Vitamin B12 (cyanocobalamin) 200 mcg • Vitamin B6 (pyridoxine HCl) 50 mg • Vitamin C (ascorbic acid) 1 g • Vitamin D (D3, cholecalciferol) 400 IU • Vitamin E (d-alpha tocopheryl succinate) 200 IU • Vitamin K (phytonadione) 80 mcg • Zinc Amino Acid Chelate 15 mg. Other Ingredients: Plant-Derived Cellulose, Vegetable Magnesium Stearate.

Alive! Whole Food Energizer (Iron-free) - Nature's Way
Three tablets contain: Amino Acids Blend 225 mg: Glutamine, Asparagine, Leucine, Alanine, Arginine, Lysine, Threonine, Valine, Glycine, Isoleucine, Serine, Proline, Phenylalanine, Tyrosine, Histidine, Methionine, Tryptophan, Cysteine • Beta Carotene 10,000 IU • Biotin Triurate 300 mcg • Boron Amino Acid Chelate 1 mg • Calcium (citrate, carbonate) 250 mg • Chlorophyll (from spirulina) 4 mg • Choline Bitartrate 30 mg • Chromium Polynicotinate 120 mcg • Citrus Bioflavonoid Complex 60 mg: Eriocitrin 600 mcg, Naringin/Narirutin/other Flavonones 1.8 mg, Flavonols 600 mcg, Flavones/related Phenolic compounds 600 mcg • Copper Amino Acid Chelate 2 mg • Digestive Enzyme Blend 100 mg: Protease I, Protease II, Peptizyme SP, Amylase, Lactase, Invertase, Lipase, Cellulase, Alpha Galactosidase, Betaine HCl, Bromelain (from pineapple), Papain (from papaya) • DNA (from spirulina, chlorella) 4 mg • Eleuthero root 50 mg • Folic Acid (folate) 400 mcg • Garden Veggies Juice Powder Blend 500 mg: Parsley, Kale, Spinach, Wheat Grass, Brussels Sprouts, Asparagus, Broccoli, Cauliflower, Beet, Carrot, Cabbage, Garlic • Green Food/Spirulina Blend 500 mg: Spirulina (microalgae), Alfalfa (leaf, stem), Barley Grass, Dandelion (leaf), Wheat Grass, Spinach (leaf), Lemon Grass, Nettle (leaf), Blessed Thistle (stem, leaf, flower), Chlorella (broken-cell microalgae), Chickweed (stem, leaf, flower), Blue Green Algae (microalgae), Cilantro (leaf) • Hesperidin 2 mg • Inositol 50 mg • Iodine 150 mcg • Lutein (from marigold) 200 mcg • Magnesium (as citrate, oxide) 125 mg • Manganese Amino Acid Chelate 4 mg • Molybdenum Triurate 75 mcg • MycoDefense Mushroom Blend 100 mg: Cordyceps, Reishi, Shiitake, Hiratake, Maitake, Ymabushitake, Mimembatsutake, Kawaratake, Chaga, Zhu Ling, Agarikon, Mesima • Niacinamide 125 mg • Omega Fatty Acid Seed Blend 100 mg: Flax seed powder, Sunflower seed powder, providing: Alpha-Linoleic Acid, Oleic Acid, Linoleic Acid, Palmitic Acid, Stearic Acid, Behenic Acid, Gadoleic Acid, Palmitoleic Acid, Eicosanoic Acid, Lignoceric Acid • Orchard Fruits Juice Powder Blend 100 mg: Plum, Cranberry, Blueberry, Strawberry, Blackberry, Bilberry, Cherry, Apricot, Papaya, Orange, Grape, Pineapple • PABA (para aminobenzoic acid) 25 mg • Pantothenic Acid 125 mg • Potassium Amino Acid Chelate 50 mg • Riboflavin (vitamin B2) 25 mg • RNA (from spirulina, chlorella) 14 mg • Rutin 25 mg • Selenium Monomethionine 70 mcg • Sodium 15 mg • Thiamine (vitamin B1) 25 mg • Vitamin A (retinol, palmitate) 5000 IU • Vitamin B12 (cyanocobalamin) 200 mcg • Vitamin B6 (pyridoxine HCl) 50 mg • Vitamin C (ascorbic acid) 1 g • Vitamin D (D3, cholecalciferol) 400 IU • Vitamin E (d-alpha tocopheryl succinate) 200 IU • Vitamin K (phytonadione) 80 mcg • Zinc Amino Acid Chelate 15 mg. Other Ingredients: Glycerin, Vegetable Magnesium Stearate, Vegetable Modified Cellulose, Vegetable Modified Cellulose Gum, Vegetable Stearic Acid.

Alive! Whole Food Energizer (with Iron) - Nature's Way
Three tablets contain: Amino Acids blend 225 mg: Glutamine, Asparagine, Leucine, Alanine, Arginine, Lysine, Threonine, Valine, Glycine, Isoleucine, Serine, Proline, Phenylalanine, Tyrosine, Histidine, Methionine, Tryptophan, Cysteine • Beta Carotene 10,000 IU • Biotin Triurate 300 mcg • Boron Amino Acid Chelate 1 mg • Calcium (citrate, carbonate) 250 mg • Chlorophyll (from spirulina) 4 mg • Choline Bitartrate 30 mg • Chromium Polynicotinate 120 mcg • Citrus Bioflavonoid Complex 60 mg: Eriocitrin 600 mcg, Naringin/Narirutin/other Flavonones 1.8 mg, Flavonols 600 mcg, Flavones/related Phenolic compounds 600 mcg • Copper Amino Acid Chelate 2 mg • Digestive Enzyme blend 100 mg: Protease I, Protease II, Peptizyme SP, Amylase, Lactase, Invertase, Lipase, Cellulase, Alpha Galactosidase, Betaine HCl, Bromelain (from pineapple), Papain (from papaya) • DNA (from spirulina, chlorella) 4 mg • Eleuthero root 50 mg • Folic Acid (folate) 400 mcg • Garden Veggies Juice Powder Blend 500 mg: Parsley, Kale, Spinach, Wheat Grass, Brussels Sprouts, Asparagus, Broccoli, Cauliflower, Beet, Carrot, Cabbage, Garlic • Green Food/Spirulina Blend 500 mg: Spirulina (microalgae), Alfalfa (leaf, stem), Barley Grass, Dandelion (leaf), Wheat Grass, Spinach (leaf), Lemon Grass, Nettle (leaf), Blessed Thistle (stem, leaf, flower), Chlorella (broken-cell microalgae), Chickweed (stem, leaf, flower), Blue Green Algae (microalgae), Cilantro (leaf) • Hesperidin 2 mg • Inositol 50 mg • Iodine 150 mcg • Iron Amino Acid Chelate 18 mg • Lutein (from marigold) 200 mcg • Magnesium (as citrate, oxide) 125 mg • Manganese Amino Acid Chelate 4 mg • Molybdenum Triurate 75 mcg • MycoDefense Mushroom Blend 100 mg: Cordyceps, Reishi, Shiitake, Hiratake, Maitake, Ymabushitake, Mimembatsutake, Kawaratake, Chaga, Zhu Ling, Agarikon, Mesima • Niacinamide 125 mg • Omega Fatty Acid Seed Blend 100 mg: Flax seed powder, Sunflower seed powder, providing: Alpha-Linoleic Acid, Oleic Acid, Linoleic Acid, Palmitic Acid, Stearic Acid, Behenic Acid, Gadoleic Acid, Palmitoleic Acid, Eicosanoic Acid, Lignoceric Acid • Orchard Fruits Juice Powder Blend 100 mg: Plum, Cranberry, Blueberry, Strawberry, Blackberry, Bilberry, Cherry, Apricot, Papaya, Orange, Grape, Pineapple • PABA (para aminobenzoic acid) 25 mg • Pantothenic Acid 125 mg • Potassium Amino Acid Chelate 50 mg • Riboflavin (vitamin B2) 25 mg • RNA (from spirulina, chlorella) 14 mg • Rutin 25 mg • Selenium Monomethionine 70 mcg • Sodium 15 mg • Thiamine (vitamin B1) 25 mg • Vitamin A (retinol, palmitate)

5000 IU • Vitamin B12 (cyanocobalamin) 200 mcg • Vitamin B6 (pyridoxine HCl) 50 mg • Vitamin C (ascorbic acid) 1 g • Vitamin D (D3, cholecalciferol) 400 IU • Vitamin E (d-alpha tocopheryl succinate) 200 IU • Vitamin K (phytonadione) 80 mcg • Zinc Amino Acid Chelate 15 mg. Other Ingredients: Glycerin, Vegetable Magnesium Stearate, Vegetable Modified Cellulose, Vegetable Modified Cellulose Gum, Vegetable Stearic Acid.

Alive! Whole Food Energizer (with Iron) Veggie Cap **-** Nature's Way
Six capsules contain: Amino Acids blend 225 mg: Glutamine, Asparagine, Leucine, Alanine, Arginine, Lysine, Threonine, Valine, Glycine, Isoleucine, Serine, Proline, Phenylalanine, Tyrosine, Histidine, Methionine, Tryptophan, Cysteine • Biotin Triurate 300 mcg • Boron Amino Acid Chelate 1 mg • Calcium (citrate, carbonate) 250 mg • Chlorophyll (from spirulina) 4 mg • Choline Bitartrate 30 mg • Chromium Polynicotinate 120 mcg • Citrus Bioflavonoid Complex 60 mg: Eriocitrin 600 mcg, Naringin/Narirutin/other Flavonones 1.8 mg, Flavonols 600 mcg, Flavones/related Phenolic compounds 600 mcg • Copper Amino Acid Chelate 2 mg • Digestive Enzyme Blend 100 mg: Protease I, Protease II, Peptizyme SP, Amylase, Lactase, Invertase, Lipase, Cellulase, Alpha Galactosidase, Betaine HCl, Bromelain (from pineapple), Papain (from papaya) • DNA (from spirulina, chlorella) 4 mg • Eleuthero root 50 mg • Folic Acid (folate) 400 mcg • Garden Veggies Juice Powder Blend 500 mg: Parsley, Kale, Spinach, Wheat Grass, Brussels Sprouts, Asparagus, Broccoli, Cauliflower, Beet, Carrot, Cabbage, Garlic • Green Food/ Spirulina Blend 500 mg: Spirulina (microalgae), Alfalfa (leaf, stem), Barley Grass, Dandelion (leaf), Wheat Grass, Spinach (leaf), Lemon Grass, Nettle (leaf), Blessed Thistle (stem, leaf, flower), Chlorella (broken-cell microalgae), Chickweed (stem, leaf, flower), Blue Green Algae (microalgae), Cilantro (leaf) • Hesperidin 2 mg • Inositol 50 mg • Iodine 150 mcg • Iron Amino Acid Chelate 18 mg • Lutein (from marigold) 200 mcg • Magnesium (as citrate, oxide) 125 mg • Manganese Amino Acid Chelate 4 mg • Molybdenum Triurate 75 mcg • MycoDefense Mushroom Blend 100 mg: Cordyceps, Reishi, Shiitake, Hiratake, Maitake, Ymabushitake, Mimembatsutake, Kawaratake, Chaga, Zhu Ling, Agarikon, Mesima • Niacinamide 125 mg • Omega Fatty Acid Seed Blend 100 mg: Flax seed powder, Sunflower seed powder, providing: Alpha-Linoleic Acid, Oleic Acid, Linoleic Acid, Palmitic Acid, Stearic Acid, Behenic Acid, Gadoleic Acid, Palmitoleic Acid, Eicosanoic Acid, Lignoceric Acid • Orchard Fruits Juice Powder Blend 100 mg: Plum, Cranberry, Blueberry, Strawberry, Blackberry, Bilberry, Cherry, Apricot, Papaya, Orange, Grape, Pineapple • PABA (para aminobenzoic acid) 25 mg • Pantothenic Acid 125 mg • Potassium Amino Acid Chelate 50 mg • Riboflavin (vitamin B2) 25 mg • RNA (from spirulina, chlorella) 14 mg • Rutin 25 mg • Selenium Monomethionine 70 mcg • Sodium 15 mg • Thiamine (vitamin B1) 25 mg • Vitamin A (retinol, palmitate) 15,000 IU • Vitamin B12 (cyanocobalamin) 200 mcg • Vitamin B6 (pyridoxine HCl) 50 mg • Vitamin C (ascorbic acid) 1 g • Vitamin D (D3, cholecalciferol) 400 IU • Vitamin E (d-alpha tocopheryl succinate) 200 IU • Vitamin K (phytonadione) 80 mcg • Zinc Amino Acid Chelate 15 mg. Other Ingredients: Plant-Derived Cellulose, Vegetable Magnesium Stearate.

ALJ Capsules **-** Nature's Sunshine
Four capsules contain: Proprietary Blend 1760 mg: Boneset aerial parts (eupatorium perfoliatum), Horseradish root (armoracia rusticana), Mullein leaf (verbascum thapsus), Fennel seed (foeniculum vulgare), Fenugreek seed (trigonella foenum-graecum). Other Ingredients: Kosher Gelatin, Water.

ALJ Liquid **-** Nature's Sunshine
Boneset aerial parts (eupatorium perfoliatum) • Fenugreek seed (trigonella foenum-graecum) • Horseradish root (armoracia rusticana) • Mullein leaf (verbascum thapsus) • Fennel seed (foeniculum vulgare). Base: 80% Glycerin, 20% Water.

ALJ Vegitabs **-** Nature's Sunshine
Four tablets contain: Proprietary Blend 1920 mg: Boneset aerial parts (eupatorium perfoliatum), Horseradish root (armoracia rusticana), Mullein leaf (verbascum thapsus), Fennel seed (foeniculum vulgare), Fenugreek seed (trigonella foenum-graecum). Other Ingredients: Cellulose, Sorbitol, Stearic Acid, Maltodextrin, Silicon Dioxide, Guar Gum (cyam-opsis tetragonolobus).

AlkaSlim (Alka-Slim, Alka Slim, AlkaSlim) **-** Dr. M.T. Morter
Barley malt • Soy Protein complex • Fiber Complex: Psyllium, Guar, Apple Pectin • Alkalizing Complex: Bee Pollen, Barley grass, Alfalfa juice concentrate, Spinach, Parsley, Celery, Spirulina • Barley grass juice • Natural Fruit and Vanilla Flavors • Lecithin • Bromelain (pineapple enzyme) • Methionine • RNA - DNA complex • Schizandra • Siberian Ginseng • Foti • Bioflavonoid - Hesperidin complex • Beta Sitosterol plant lipid complex • Gamma Oryzanol (brown rice extract) • Octacosonal.

All Capsule Health Pak Iron Free **-** Jarrow Formulas
Each packet contains: Mineral Balance (three clear white capsules): Vitamin A (from fish liver oil) 2500 IU • Vitamin D (D3, cholecalciferol, from fish liver oil) 200 IU • Calcium (as microcrystalline hydroxyapatite) 500 mg • Magnesium (as oxide) 300 mg • Potassium (as chloride) 50 mg • Zinc (as monomethionate) 7.5 mg • Manganese (as citrate) 0.5 mg • Copper (as gluconate) 1 mg • Iodine (from potassium iodine) 113 mcg • Selenium (as L-selenomethionine) 50 mcg • Chromium 100 mcg • Molybdenum (trivalent sodium molybdate) 100 mcg.
Marine Beta Carotene (dunaliella salinas, small oval brown softgel): Vitamin A (10,000 IU equivalent, pre-formed vitamin A from fish liver oil) 6 mg • Natural Vitamin E (golden softgel, D-alpha tocopherol acetate) 400 IU.
Odorless B-RIGHT Complex (smaller white capsule): Vitamin B1 (thiamin mononitrate) 25 mg • Vitamin B2 (riboflavin) 25 mg • Niacin 25 mg • Niacinamide 25 mg • Vitamin B5 (D-calcium pantothenate) 100 mg • Pantethine 25 mg • Vitamin B6 (pyridoxine HCl) 25 mg • Pyridoxal-5-Phosphate 10 mg • Vitamin B12 (methylcobalamin) 100 mcg • Folic Acid (folate) 400 mcg • Biotin 300 mcg • PABA (para-aminobenzoic acid) 30 mg • Choline Bitartrate 50 mg • Inositol 50 mg.
Vitamin C (off-white two-peice capsules): Vitamin C (ascorbic acid) 1000 mg • Rosemary extract antioxidant 50 mg. Other Ingredients: Magnesium Stearate, Rice Powder, Silicon Dioxide, Titanium Dioxide, Gelatin, Soybean Oil, Natural Annatto Extract, Lecithin, Gelatin, Glycerin, Water.

All Cell Detox **-** Nature's Sunshine
Two capsules contain: Proprietary blend 950 mg: Gentian root (gentiana lutea), Irish Moss plant (chondrus crispus), Cascara Sagrada bark (rhamnus purshiana), Fenugreek seed (trigonella foenum-graecum), Goldenseal root and rhizome (hydrastis canadensis), Slippery Elm bark (ulmus fulva), Safflower flower (carthamus tinctorius), Black Walnut hulls (juglans nigra), Myrrh gum (commiphora molmol), Parthenium root (parthenium integrifolium), Yellow Dock root (rumex crispus), Dandelion root (taraxacum officinale), Oregon Grape root and rhizome (berberis aquifolium), Uva Ursi leaf (arctostaphylos uva ursi), Chickweed aerial parts (stellaria media), Catnip leaf (nepeta cataria), Cyani flower (centaurea cyanus). Other Ingredients: Gelatin, Water.

All Purpose Multivitamin/Mineral **-** Leiner Health Products
Each tablet contains: Vitamin E (dl-Alpha Tocopheryl Acetate) 15 IU • Magnesium Oxide 100 mg • Calcium 160 mg • Phosphorus 125 mg • Folate (Folic Acid) 400 mcg • Iodine 150 mcg • Iron (Ferrous Fumarate) 18 mg • Niacin (Niacinamide) 20 mg • Riboflavin (Vitamin B2) 1.7 mg • Thiamin Mononitrate (Vitamin B1) 1.5 mg • Vitamin A Palmitate 5000 • Vitamin B12 (Cyanocobalamin - USP Method 2) 6 mcg • Vitamin B6 (Pyridoxine Hydrochloride) 2 mg • Vitamin C (Ascorbic Acid) 60 mg • Vitamin D (Ergocalciferol) 400 IU. Other Ingredients: Dicalcium Phosphate, Gelatin, Hydroxypropyl Methylcellulose, Croscarmellose Sodium, Sodium Starch Glycolate, Niacinamide, dl-Alpha Tocopheryl Acetate, Cellulose, Tricalcium Phosphate, Silicon Dioxide, Titanium Dioxide, Starch, Polyethylene Glycol 3350, Hydroxypropyl Cellulose, Magnesium Stearate, Yeast,

Pyridoxine Hydrochloride, Polysorbate 80, Pharmaceutical Glaze, Resin, Povidone, Potassium Iodide.

All Purpose Skin Therapy - All Terrain Company
Calendula flower extract • Rosemary extract • Lavender extract. Base: Canola Oil, Caster Oil, Beeswax, Corn Starch.

All You Can Eat - Vitalabs, Inc
Two 2-piece capsules contain: Proprietary Blend 1300 mg: Legume Protein concentrate, Chitosan, Garcinia Cambogia, Gymnema Sylvestre, Cider Vinegar, Cascara Sagrada, Aloe Vera.

All-Day Complete - Swanson Health Products
Each rounded scoop (15 g) contains: Vitamin A (as palmitate) 8000 IU • Vitamin A (as beta-carotene) 1000 IU • Vitamin C (as ascorbic acid) 1 g • Vitamin D (as cholecalciferol) 500 IU • Vitamin E (as d-alpha tocopheryl acetate) 400 IU • Vitamin K 5 mcg • Thiamin (as thiamin HCl; vitamin B-1) 25 mg • Riboflavin (vitamin B-2) 25 mg • Niacin (as niacinamide) 100 mg • Vitamin B-6 (as pyridoxine HCl) 25 mg • Folic Acid 400 mcg • Vitamin B-12 (as cyanocobalamin) 25mcg • Biotin 300 mcg • Pantothenic Acid (as d-calcium pantothenate) 100 mg • Calcium (from calcium carbonate and dicalcium phosphate) 500 mg • Iron (as ferrous gluconate) 18 mg • Phosphorus (from d-calcium phosphate) 200 mg • Iodine (from potassium iodide) 150 mcg • Magnesium (from magnesium oxide) 200 mg • Zinc (from zinc oxide) 15 mg • Selenium (as proteinate) 50 mcg • Copper (from copper gluconate) 1 mg • Manganese (from manganese sulfate) 4 mg • Chromium (as chromium proteinate complex) 50 mcg • Molybdenum (as amino acid chelate) 50 mcg • Potassium (as potassium citrate) 99 mg • Lecithin 750 mg • Lemon Bioflavonoid complex 400 mg • Hesperidin complex 25 mg • PABA (para-aminobenzoic acid) 25 mg • Rutin (from buckwheat) 25 mg • Choline (from lecithin) 20 mg • Inositol (from lecithin) 15 mg • Betaine HCl 2 mg • Papain (from papaya) 2 mg • Kelp 1.5 mg.

All-Day Complete (for Seniors) - Swanson Health Products
Each rounded scoop (15 g) contains: Vitamin A (as palmitate) 8000 IU • Vitamin A (as beta-carotene) 1000 IU • Vitamin C (as ascorbic acid) 1 g • Vitamin D (as cholecalciferol) 500 IU • Vitamin E (as d-alpha tocopheryl acetate) 400 IU • Vitamin K 5 mcg • Thiamin (as thiamin HCl; vitamin B-1) 25 mg • Riboflavin (vitamin B-2) 25 mg • Niacin (as niacinamide) 100 mg • Vitamin B-6 (as pyridoxine HCl) 25 mg • Folic Acid 400 mcg • Vitamin B-12 (as cyanocobalamin) 25 mcg • Biotin 300 mcg • Pantothenic Acid (as d-calcium pantothenate) 100 mg • Calcium (from calcium carbonate and dicalcium phosphate) 500 mg • Iron (as ferrous gluconate) 18 mg • Phosphorus (from d-calcium phosphate) 200 mg • Iodine (from potassium iodide) 150 mcg • Magnesium (from magnesium oxide) 200 mg • Zinc (from zinc oxide) 15 mg • Selenium (as proteinate) 50 mcg • Copper (from copper gluconate) 1 mg • Manganese (from manganese sulfate) 4 mg • Chromium (as chromium proteinate complex) 50 mcg • Molybdenum (as amino acid chelate) 50 mcg • Potassium (as potassium citrate) 99 mg • Lecithin 1.4 g • Fructooligosaccharides (FOS) 1 g •Lemon Bioflavonoid complex 400 mg • Inositol (from inositol and lecithin) 100 mg • Choline (from lecithin) 50 mg • Ginkgo Biloba powder 25 mg • Hesperidin complex 25 mg • PABA (para-aminobenzoic acid) 25 mg •Rutin (from buckwheat) Coenzyme Q10 20 mg • Reishi Mushroom extract 5 mg • Betaine HCl 2 mg • Papain (from papaya) 2 mg • Kelp 1.5 mg.

Aller Ease - Nutritional Therapeutics, Inc.
Three tablets contain: Vitamin C (as calcium ascorbate) 750 mg • Vitamin B6 (as pyridoxine HCl) 15 mg • Vitamin A (as natural beta-carotene, mixed carotenioids, acetate) 7500 IU • Vitamin E (as D-alpha, mixed tocopherols) 15 IU • Folic Acid 120 mcg • Calcium 240 mg • Magnesium 39 mg • Phosphorus 60 mg • Arginine HCl 107 mg • Bromelain 40 mg • Garlic (as odorless) 78 mg • N-Acetyl-D-Glucosamine 84 mg • NT Factor (as tablet base) 600 mg • Pantethine (as coenyme A precursor) 75 mg • Papain 40 mg • Phosphoglycolipids 117 mg • Quercetin 150 mg. Other Ingredients: Calcium Phosphate, Croscarmellose Sodium, Food Glaze, Vegetable Magnesium Stearate, Silica.

Aller-7 Formula - Natural Factors
Each capsule contains: Aller-7 Herbal Extract Proprietary Blend 330 mg: Amla fruit powdered extract (phyllanthus emblica), Chebulic Myrobalan fruit powdered extract (terminalia chebula), Belleric Myrobalan fruit powdered extract (terminalia bellerica), Indian Walnut bark powdered extract (albizia lebeck), Ginger root powdered extract (zingiber officinale), Long Pepper fruit powdered extract (piper longum), Black Pepper fruit powdered extract (piper nigrum); providing standardized levels of Polyphenols, Glycosides, Piperine, Gallic Acid and Gingerols • Licorice root powdered extract (glycyrrhiza glabra) 25 mg • Glycyrrhizin 3 mg • Grape seed 100:1 powdered extract 20 mg • Polyphenols 19 mg • Proanthocyanidins 16 mg • Wild Cherry powdered bark (prunus serotina) 25 mg • Quercetin 25 mg. Other Ingredients: Gelatin Capsule (gelatin, purified water), Rice Powder, Magnesium Stearate (vegetable grade), Silica.

Aller-7 Rx-Respiration - Nature's Plus
Each capsule contains: Zinc (as OptiZinc brand monomethionine) 7.5 mg • Aller-7 brand herbal extract 330 mg: Phyllanthus Emblica fruit extract, Terminalia Chebula fruit extract, Terminalia Bellerica fruit extract, Albizia Lebbeck bark extract, Zingiber Officinale root extract, Piper Longum fruit extract, Piper Nigrum fruit extract providing Polyphenols 81 mg, Chebulic Acid 26 mg, Gallic Acid 15 mg, Glycosides as Corilagin and Tri-Galloyl Glucose 7 mg, Ellagic Acid 1.2 mg, Piperine 0.25 mg, Gingerols 0.05 mg • Georgian Blueberry leaf (vaccinium myrtillus) 12.5 mg supplying Chlorogenic Acid (standardized 20%) 2.5 mg • Lemon Bioflavonoids (from citrus limon exocarp) 12.5 mg supplying Active Flavones (standardized 24%) 3 mg • Active Flavonols and Flavones (standardized 20%) 2.5 mg. Other Ingredients: Microcrystalline Cellulose, Silica, Gelatin, Natural Color, Purified Water.

Aller-7 Support - Health Unlimited Ministries
Three caplets contain: Vitamin C 100 mg • Proprietary Herbal Blend 660 mg: Phyllanthus Emblica fruit extract, Terminalia Chebula fruit extract, Terminalia Bellerica fruit extract, Albizia Lebbeck bark extract, Zingiber Officinale root extract, Piper Longum fruit extract • Quercetin 500 mg • MSM 1300 mg • Stinging Nettles freeze dried leaf (urtica dioica) 200 mg • Bromelain (protease enzyme) 2400 GDUs/g • Proprietary Berry Blend 25 mg: Wild Blueberry, Strawberry, Cranberry, Wild Bilberry, Elderberry, Raspberry • Feverfew leaf (tanacetum parthenium) 25 mg • Tumeric rhizome (curcuma longa) 50 mg • Ginger rhizome (zingiber officinale) 25 mg.

Aller-B - Progressive Labs
Each capsule contains: Thiamin (Vitamin B1) 50 mg • Riboflavin (Vitamin B2) 50 mg • Niacinamide 50 mg • Vitamin B6 50 mg • Folate (Folic Acid) 400 mcg • Vitamin B12 60 mcg • Biotin 50 mcg • Pantothenic Acid 100 mg • Choline Bitartrate 50 mg • Inositol 25 mg • PABA (Para Aminobenzioc Acid) 50 mg.

Aller-C - Vital Nutrients
Each capsule contains: Vitamin C (pure ascorbic acid) 450 mg • Quercetin 250 mg • Citrus Bioflavonoids (60%) 150 mg • Bromelain (2400 gdu, pure uncut) 50 mg.

Aller-C Support Formula - The Vitamin Factory
Each tablet contains: Vitamin C (Calcium Ascorbate) 500 mg • Calcium (Ascorbate, Citrate, Pantothenate) 100 mg • Vitamin B5 (Calcium Pantothenate) 50 mg • Pycnogenol (Maritime Pine bark extract) 15 mg.

Aller-Cal - Atrium Biotechnologies
Each tablet contains: Adrenal 80 mg • Pituitary 10 mg • Liver Substance 6 mg • Parathyroid 5 mg • Calcium 20.4 mg • Pantothenic Acid 26 mg • Folic Acid 130 mcg • Ammonium Chloride 30 mg • Choline Bitartrate 25 mg • Methionine 14 mg • Inositol 12 mg • Glutamic Acid HCl 12 mg • Betaine HCl 3.6 mg • Hydrolized Amino Acids 150 mg • Dulse 50 mg • Persic oil 36 mg • Linseed oil 12 mg. See Editor's Note No. 14.

Some Brand Name Natural Products - What they Contain

www.NaturalDatabase.com contains MANY more listings than appear here.
Editor's Notes are located on pages 2155-2163.

Allercetin Allergy & Sinus - Source Naturals
Each tablet contains: Ambrosia Artemisiaefolia (ragweed) 30X • Hydrochloricum (histamine hydrochloride) 12X • Quercetin 12X • Succinicum Acidum (succinic acid) 12X • Euphrasia Officinalis (eyebright) 6X • Kali Iodatum (potassium iodide) 6X • Sabadilla (cevadilla seed) 6X • Sticta Pulmonaria (lungwort) 6X. Other Ingredients: Lactose, Magnesium Stearate.
See Editor's Note No. 1.

AllerClear - Enzymatic Therapy
Active Ingredient: Ephedra Sinensis (providing pseudophedrine HCl 60 mg). Other Ingredients: Vitamin E (DL-alpha tocopherol) 75 IU • Vitamin C (ascorbic acid) 150 mg • Pantothenic Acid (D-calcium pantothenate) 150 mg • Choline (bitartrate) 150 mg • Macrocystis Pyrifera 150 mg • Lung extract 90 mg • Adrenal extract 80 mg • Methionine 75 mg • Pancreatic Enzymes (3X) 65 mg • Ammonium Chloride 50 mg • Calcium Chloride 50 mg • Glutamic Acid HCl 50 mg • Betaine HCl 50 mg • Pepsin (1:10000) 49 mg • Magnesium Glycerophosphate 30 mg • Spleen extract 25 mg • Pancreas extract 15 mg • Thymus extract 15 mg • Niacinamide 10 mg • Liver Fractions 10 mg • Vitamin B6 (Pyridoxine HCl) 5 mg.
See Editor's Note No. 14, No. 21 and No. 30.

Aller-G Formula 25 - Olympian Labs
Two capsules contain: Vitamin C 200 mg • Histidine 60 mg • Citrus Aurantium extract 200 mg • Bee Pollen 75 mg • Propolis 25 mg • Pantothenic Acid 75 mg • Citrus Bioflavonoid Complex 30 mg • Niacin 20 mg • Goldenseal 25 mg • Echinacea 50 mg • Garlic 25 mg • Yerba Santa 50 mg • Nettle 80 mg • Mullein 40 mg • White Willow Bark 6 mg.
See Editor's Note No. 40.

Allergia - HerbaSway
Bitter Orange • Ginger • Panax Ginseng • Blackberry • Kudzu • HerbaSwee (Cucurbitaceae fruit).
See Editor's Note No. 40.

Allergies- Molds, Yeast & Dust - Nature's Sunshine
Adrenalinum (adrenalin) 6X • Lycopodium Clavatum (club moss) 6X • Natrum Sulfuricum (sodium sulfate) 6X • Silicea (silica) 6X • Phosphorus 8X • Histaminum (histamine hydrochloride) 12X • Mixed Mold/Yeast/Dust Allersodes: Aspergillus Flavus, A. Fumigatus, A. Glaucus, A. Nidulans, A. Niger, Candida Albicans, Curvularia Spicifera, Farinae (mite), Fusarium Moniliforme, Geotrichum Candidum, House Dust, Mucor Plumbeus, Penicillinum Camemberti, P. Chrysogenum, P. Digitatum, P. Notatum, P. Roqueforti, Pullularia Pullulans, Rhizopus Nigricans, Saccharomyces Boulardii (baker's and brewer's yeast), Trichophyton Mentagrophytes, all at 12X. Other Ingredients: Purified Water, 20% USP Alcohol.
See Editor's Note No. 1.

Allergies-Hayfever/Pollen - Nature's Sunshine
Adrenalinum (adrenalin) 6X • Allium Cepa (red onion) 6X • Eyebright (euphrasia) 6X • Lycopodium Clavatum (club moss) 6X • Sabadilla (cevadilla) 6X • Silicea (silica) 6X • Histaminum (histamine hydrochloride) 12X • Mixed Pollen Allersodes: Amaranthus, Chenopodium, Cocklebur, Daisy, Dandelion, Goldenrod, Honeysuckle, Marsh Elder, Mugwort, Ragweed, Timothy Grass, all at 12X. Other ingredients: Purified Water, 20% USP Alcohol.
See Editor's Note No. 1.

Allergy - Nature's Sunshine
Arnica Montana (mountain arnica) 6X • Eyebright (euphrasia officinalis) 6X • Ignatius Bean (ignatia amara) 6X • Lycopodium Clavatum (club moss) 6X • Skunk Cabbage (pothos foetidus) 6X • Thuja Occidentalis (tree of life) 6X • Antimonium Crudum (antimonious sulfide) 10X • Histaminum (histamine hydrochloride) 12X. Other Ingredients: Purified Water, 20% USP Alcohol.
See Editor's Note No. 1.

allergy & hayfever - Nelson Bach
Active Ingredients: Allium Cepa 30C HPUS • Euphrasia 30C HPUS • Sabadilla 30C HPUS. Inactive Ingredients: Lactose, Sucrose.
See Editor's Note No. 1.

Allergy Essentials - Swanson Health Products
Three capsules contain: Vitamin C (as calcium ascorbate) 100 mg • Zinc (from zinc chelate and zinc gluconate) 15 mg • Ma Huang extract (6% ephedra) 250 mg • Bromelain (2400 GDU) 100 mg • Licorice root extract (1% glycyrrhizic acid) 100 mg • N-Acetyl-Cysteine 100 mg • Nettle extract (5:1) 100 mg • Quercetin 100 mg • White Willow Bark 100 mg • Cayenne pepper 100,000 HU 50 mg • Echinacea root extract (4% echinacosides) 50 mg • Goldenseal root 50 mg • Grapeseed extract (95% proanthocyanidins) 30 mg.
See Editor's Note No. 30.

Allergy Eye Drops - Natural Ophthalmics
Active Ingredients: Apis HPUS 6x • Sabadilla HPUS 6x • Allium Cepa HPUS 6x • Eyebright (euphrasia) HPUS 4x. Inactive Ingredients: Sterile Water, Sodium Chloride, Sodium Citrate, Citrate, Polysorbate 80.

Allergy MD - Long Life, Inc.
Amylase • Cellulase • Fenugreek • Licorice • Methionine • Lipase • Mullein • Niacinamide • Pantothenic Acid • Protease • Sida Cordifolia extract • Vitamin A • Vitamin C • Yerba Santa.
See Editor's Note No. 39.

Allergy Multi Caps - TwinLab
Six hard gel capsules contain: Buffered Vitamin C (sago palm) 1000 mg • Dry Vitamin A Acetate (non-fish source) 10,000 IU • Dry Beta-Carotene 15,000 IU • Total Vitamin A activity 25,000 IU • Dry Vitamin D (D3, non-fish source) 400 IU • Dry Vitamin E (non-soybean source) 400 IU • Vitamin B1 25 mg • Vitamin B2 25 mg • Vitamin B3 (niacinamide) 100 mg • Vitamin B6 50 mg • Vitamin B12 100 mcg • Pantothenic Acid 50 mg • Biotin 150 mcg • Folic Acid 400 mcg • PABA 25 mg • Choline 25 mg • Inositol 25 mg • Calcium (from calcium carbonate) 1000 mg • Magnesium (from magnesium oxide (magnesium aspartate) 500 mg • Potassium (from potassium chloride & potassium aspartate) 99 mg • Zinc (from zinc picolinate) 30 mg • Manganese (from manganese asparate) 10 mg • Copper (from copper aspartate) 2 mg • Iron (from iron aspartate) 10 mg • Selenium (from yeast free selenomethionine & selenate) 200 mcg • Chromium (from yeast free GTF chromium) 200 mcg • Molybdenum (from molybdate) 500 mcg.

Allergy Relief - Futurebiotics LLC
Three capsules contain: Vitamin A (as beta-carotene) 5000 IU • Vitamin C 1000 mg • Pantothenic Acid 100 mg • Zinc (as OptiZinc zinc monomethionine) 15 mg • MSM (methyl-sulfonyl-methane) 500 mg • Citrus Bioflavonoids 100 mg • Quercetin 25 mg • Rutin 25 mg • Bitter Orange (Citrus aurantium) peel powder extract (standardized for 4% synephrine, 4 mg) 100 mg • Grape Seed extract powder (standardized for 95% polyphenols, 29 mg) 30 mg • Stinging Nettle extract powder (leaf) (standardized for 2% plant silica, 2 mg) 100 mg • N-Acetyl-Cysteine (NAC) 100 mg • L-Histidine 200 mg. Other Ingredients: Gelatin, Cellulose, Magnesium stearate, Water.
See Editor's Note No. 40.

Allergy Shield - NSI - Nutraceutical Sciences Institute
Four capsules contain: MSM 1.5 g • Bioflavoniod as Quercetin 500 mg • Bioflavonoid as Rutin 150 mg • Bioflavonoid as Hesperidin 350 mg • Protease 50,000 HUT • Vitamin C (as magnesium ascorbate, Ester C) 1 g.

Allergy Support - Olympia Nutrition
Quercetin • Nettle • Licorice • Vitamin C.

AllergyCare - Nature's Way
Each capsule contains: Pseudoephedrine HCl 60 mg. Other Ingredients: Brigham Tea Herb, Elder Flowers, Eyebright (stem, leaf, flower), Ginger, Golden Rod Herb, Licorice Root.

Aller-Leaf - Gaia Herbs
Two capsules contain: Turmeric root and leaf (curcuma longa) 132 mg • Eyebright herb (euphrasia officinalis) 132 mg • Nettle leaf (urtica dioica) 106 mg • Bayberry bark (myrica cerifera) 100 mg • Chinese Skullcap root (scutellaria baicalensis) 36 mg • Goldenseal rhizome (hydrastis canadensis) 16 mg • Yarrow flower (achillea millefolium) 14 mg • Calamus rhizome (acorus calamus) 8 mg. Other Ingredients: Vegetable Glycerin, Vegetable Cellulose (capsule).

Allerplex - Standard Process, Inc.
Three capsules contain: Proprietary Blend 860 mg: Tillandsia Usneoides, Fenugreek seed, Betaine Hydrochloride, Soy bean, Bovine Lung PMG extract, Carbamide, Carrot root, Oat flour, Bovine Adrenal PMG extract, Bovine Liver fat extract (yakriton), Alfalfa flour, Dried Alfalfa juice, Bovine Bone, Dried Buckwheat leaf juice, Defatted Wheat germ, Bovine Kidney, Veal Bone meal, Soybean Lecithin, Peanut bran, Mixed Tocopherols, Carrot oil • Vitamin A 525 IU • Vitamin C 4 mg • Calcium 20 mg • Magnesium 12 mg. Other Ingredients: Gelatin, Water, Colors.
See Editor's Note No. 14.

AllerPlus - PhytoPharmica
Two capsules contain: Pseudoephedrine HCl (from Ephedra sinensis) 60 mg • Vitamin E (DL-Alpha Tocopherol) 75 IU • Vitamin C (Ascorbic Acid) 150 mg • Pantothenic Acid (D-Calcium Pantothenate) 150 mg • Choline (Bitartrate) 150 mg • Macrocystis Pyrifera 150 mg • Lung extract 90 mg • Adrenal extract 80 mg • Methionine 75 mg • Pancreatic Enzymes (3X) 65 mg (Treated for enteric activity) • Ammonium Chloride 50 mg • Calcium Chloride 50 mg • Glutamic Acid HCl 50 mg • Betaine HCl 50 mg • Pepsin (1:10000) 49 mg • Magnesium Glycerophosphate 30 mg • Spleen extract 25 mg • Pancreas extract 15 mg • Thymus extract 15 mg • Niacinamide 10 mg • Liver Fractions 10 mg • Vitamin B6 (Pyridoxine HCl) 5 mg.
See Editor's Note No. 14, No. 21 and No. 30.

Aller-Response - Source Naturals
Three tablets contain: Quercetin 600 mg • Vitamin C (ascorbic acid and zinc ascorbate) 500 mg • Bitter orange standardized extract 500 mg • Bromelain (2000 GDU per g) 300 mg • Nettle root extract 100 mg • Ginkgo Biloba standardized leaf extract 75 mg • Licorice root extract 50 mg • Magnesium (amino acid chelate) 50 mg • Vitamin A (palmitate) 2500 IU • Vitamin B-6 (pyridoxine HCl) 5 mg • Vitamin B-12 (cyanocobalamin) 12 mcg • Zinc (ascorbate) 10 mg.
See Editor's Note No. 40.

Aller-Sin Caps - Douglas Laboratories/AMNI
Each capsule contains: Proprietary Blend 440 mg: Boneset herb, Fenugreek seeds, Horseradish root, Mullein leaves, Fennel seeds.

Aller-SP - Benepure, Inc
Each tablet contains: Vitamin C (as calcium ascorbate) 250 mg • Quercetin Chalcone 250 mg • Bromelain (600 GDU) 250 mg • Grape seed extract (yielding proanthocyanidins 142.5 mg) 150 mg • N,N-Dimethylglycine HCl 100 mg • Perilla seed extract (perilla frutescens) 75 mg: Polyphenols 2.5 mg, Rosemarinic Acid 1.13 mg, Luteolin 80 mcg. Other Ingredients: Stearic Acid, Vegetable Stearate, Croscarmellose Sodium, Silicon Dioxide, Microcrystalline Cellulose, Hydroxy Propyl Methyl Cellulose.

AllerZinc - Quantum, Inc.
Each drop contains: Zinc 9 mg • Ephedrine from Ephedra Extract 2 mg • Quercetin 80 mg • Lobelia 15 mg • Licorice 15 mg. Other Ingredients: Sugar, Corn Syrup, Natural Flavor.
See Editor's Note No. 21 and No. 30.

Allicin Rich Garlic Powder 1,500 mg - Jamieson
Each caplet contains: Allicin Garlic (equivalent to 2 cloves of garlic) 1500 mg.

Allicin Rich Garlic Powder 300 mg - Jamieson
Each caplet contains: Garlic bulb powder (containing 750 mcg Allicon and 5000 mcg Alliin) 300 mg.

Allisyn Garlic Cinnamon Oil - Genestra - Seroyal
Each capsule contains: Garlic extract (yielding allicin, no less than 5 mg) 500 mg • Cinnamon bark oil (yielding cinnamaldehyde, no less than 40 mg) 200 mg.

Allorganic Trace Minerals-B12 - Standard Process, Inc.
Each tablet contains: Proprietary Blend 173 mg: Kelp, Alfalfa, Magnesium Citrate, Dried Pea (vine) juice, Bovine Orchic extract, Bovine Bone, Dried Buckwheat (leaf) juice, Buckwheat (seed), Defatted Wheat (germ), Oat Flour, Dicalcium Phosphate, Carrot (root), Peanut (bran) • Manganese Lactate 16 mg • Potassium Para-Aminobenzoate 10 mg • Honey • Iron Liver Chelate 1.4 mg • Calcium Stearate • Prolamine Iodine (zein) 145 mcg • Cyanocobalamin 5 mcg.

Alluna - SmithKline Beecham
Two tablets contain: Valerian root extract 500 mg • Hops extract 120 mg. Other Ingredients: Microcrystalline Cellulose, Soy Polysaccharide, Hydrogenated Castor oil, Hydroxypropyl Methylcellulose, Titanium Dioxide (less than 20%), Propylene Glycol, Magnesium Stearate, Silica, Polyethylene Glycol (400, 6000, 20000), Blue 2 Lake, Artificial flavoring.

Allurex Female - Westport Group Inc.
Each 300 mg capsule contains: Avena Sativa 1X • Sabal Serrulata 2X.
See Editor's Note No. 1.

Allurex Male - Westport Group Inc.
Each 300 mg capsule contains: Avena Sativa 1X.
See Editor's Note No. 1.

Aloe & Chamomile Skin Soothing Moisturizer 4oz - Derma E
Purified Water • Stearic Acid • Jojoba oil • Cetyl Alcohol • Stearyl Alcohol • Aloe Vera Gel • Glyceryl Stearate SE • Caprylic Triglyceride • Glycerin • Almond oil • Chamomile extract • Tocopheryl Acetate (vitamin E) • Retinyl Palmitate (vitamin A) • Ergocalciferol (vitamin D) • Allantoin • Panthenol • Methylparaben • TEA • I. Urea • Fragrant Oils.

Aloe & Chamomile Skin Toner 8oz - Derma E
Purified Water • Herbal Extracts Blend: Aloe Vera, Chamomile, Cucumber, Lavender, Rose Hips, Rosemary • NAPCA • Sodium Citrate • DL-Panthenol • Polysorbate 20 • Natural Color • Methylparaben • I. Urea • Fragrant Oils.

Aloe & E Moisturizing Lotion 10.1oz - Derma E
Purified Water • Aloe Vera Gel • Safflower oil • Cetyl Alcohol • Glyceryl Stearate • PEG 100 Stearate • Stearic Acid • Glycerin • Tocopheryl Acetate (vitamin E) • Retinyl Palmitate (vitamin A) • Ergocalciferol (vitamin D) • Allantoin • Panthenol • Methylparaben • TEA • I. Urea • Fragrant Oils.

Aloe & E with Allantoin - Derma E
Aloe Vera gel • Vitamin E.

Aloe Gel Skin Repair - All Terrain Company
Aloe Vera Gel (10% polysaccharides) • Glycerin • Bisabolol • Allantoin • Chamomile • Comfrey • Sweet Clover leaf • Sea Algae • Sodium Carbomor • Bladderwrack • Cucumber • Ginseng • Ginkgo Biloba • Sodium PCA • Polysorbate 20 • Methylparaben • Propylparaben • Lavender oil.

Aloe Gold - Oasis Wellness Network
Each ounce (30 mL) contains: FOS (fructo-oligosaccharide) 1.7 g • Active Aloe (200:1) 280 mg • Carragel 95 mg • Pine Needle leaf extract 28 mg • Citric Acid 11 mg • Green Tea root extract 2.8 mg • MaxCell Proprietary Blend 25 mg: Jujube fruit extract, Black Pepper extract, Aloe Vera (dried gel), Chinese Licorice root. Other Ingredients: Sodium Benzoate, Potassium Sorbate.

Aloe Immune 150 mg - 4R Health Products
Each capsule contains: Aloe Vera gel 150 mg. Other Ingredients: Rice Flower.

Aloe Immune 500 mg - 4R Health Products
Each capsule contains: Aloe Vera gel 500 mg. Other Ingredients: Magnesium Stearate.

Aloe Isolate - Progressive Labs
Each capsule contains: Aloe Vera Mucilaginous Polysaccharide (freeze-dried) 30 mg.

Aloe Seltzer C - Nutraceutics Corp.
Each tablet contains: Vitamin C (as l-ascorbic acid) 1000 mg • Lyopilized whole Aloe Vera gel (betamannin) 50 mg • Other Ingredients: Sodium Bicarbonate, Citric Acid, Glucose, Orange Flavor, Magnesium Carbonate, Polyethylene Glycol, Calcium Carbonate, Sodium Carbonate.

Aloe Vera - Leiner Health Products
Each softgel contains: Aloe Vera gel 25 mg. Other Ingredients: Vegetable Oil, Gelatin, Hydrogenated Soybean and Cottonseed Oil, White Beeswax.

Aloe Vera - Puritan's Pride
Each capsule contains: Aloe Vera (Aloe barbadensis, leaf) 470 mg. Other Ingredients: Gelatin, Silica, Vegetable Magnesium Stearate.

Aloe Vera - 4 Life
100% Pure Aloe Vera 10:1 concentrate.

Aloe Vera (Aloe barbadensis) - Solgar
Each capsule contains: Aloe Vera leaf 200:1 extract 1.2 mg • Raw Aloe Vera leaf powder 308 mg. Other Ingredients: Vegetable Cellulose, Microcrystalline Cellulose, Vegetable Magnesium Stearate, Vegetable Stearic Acid, Water, Vegetable Glycerin.

Aloe Vera 200 - New Chapter, Inc.
Two tablets contain: Freeze dried Aloe Vera juice concentrate (200:1) 300 mg.

Aloe Vera Deep Skin Moisturizer Vitamin D Cell Refining Cream - Orjene
85% pure Aloe Vera • Bee Pollen • Vitamin F Complex • PABA-free sunblock.

Aloe Vera Gel - Jamieson
Contains: Purified Water • Carrageenan (gelling agent from red seaweed) • 100% Aloe Vera Concentrate.

Aloe Vera Gel - Puritan's Pride
Each softgel contains: Premium Concentrated Aloe Vera Gel 200:1 (Equivalent to 5000 mg or approximately one teaspoonful of 100% pure aloe vera inner leaf gel) 25 mg.

Aloe Vera Gel - Nature's Bounty
Each softgel contains: Aloe Vera Gel (200:1 extract: Equivalent to 5,000 mg or approximately one teaspoonful of 100% pure aloe vera inner leaf gel) 25 mg. Other Ingredients: Beeswax/Soybean Oil Mixture, Gelatin, Glycerin, Cottonseed Oil.

Aloe Vera Gel - Nature's Sunshine
Aloe Vera gel (aloe barbadensis, from aloe vera concentrate and purified water) • Xanthan Gum • Citric Acid • Potassium Sorbate • Sodium Benzoate • Carrageenan extract.

Aloe Vera Gel - J. R. Carlson Laboratories, Inc.
Each softgel contains: Aloe Vera concentrate (200:1) 25 mg.

Aloe Vera Jelly - Golden Glow Natural Health Products
Aloe Barbadensis leaf juice 970 mg/g. Other Ingredients: Hydroxybenzoates 0.11%, Diazolidinylurea 0.3%.

Aloe Vera Juice - Nature's Sunshine
Aloe Vera gel concentrate • Purified Water • Citric Acid • Potassium Sorbate • Sodium Benzoate.

Aloe Vera Juice - Progressive Labs
Aloe Vera gel (98.94% pure, naturally processed, cold stabilized) • Fructose • Citric Acid • Ascorbic Acid.

Aloe Vera Moisture Cream - Jamieson
Contains: 200 Biologically Active Compounds of Aloe Vera Concentrate • Almond Oil • Avocado Oil • Cactus • Yucca.

Aloe Vera Moisturizing Gel 8oz - Derma E
Aloe Vera Gel • Purified Water • Glycerine • Carbomer • Potassium Sorbate • Triethanolamine • Polysorbate 20 • Methylparaben • Fragrant Oils • Plant Extracts.

Aloe Vera Soothing Moisturizing Gel - Jamieson
Contains: Aloe Vera Concentrate • Cactus • Yucca.

Aloe Vital - Source Naturals
Each tablet contains: Organic whole leaf aloe vera powder (200:1 concentrate) 200 mg.

Alozone-M - T-Up Biosystems
Each teaspoon (5mL) contains: Proprietary Blend 670 mg: Aloe Vera • Iron • Boron • Lithium • Fluoride • Copper • Zinc • Selenium • Chromium • Valadium • Cobalt • Nickel • All Natural Ultra-Wide Mineral System.

Alpha Base Capsules w/o Iron - Ortho Molecular Products
Four capsules contain: Vitamin A (as Betatene brand natural mixed carotenoids, palmitate) 7500 IU • Vitamin C (as ascorbic acid USP, ascorbate) 500 mg • Vitamin D (D3, as cholecalciferol) 400 IU • Vitamin E (as D-alpha-tocopherol succinate) 100 IU • Vitamin K (as phytonadione) 50 mcg • Thiamine (B1 from thiamine HCl USP) 25 mg • Riboflavin (vitamin B2 USP) 25 mg • Niacin (as niacin USP, niacinamide) 25 mg • Vitamin B6 (as pyridoxine HCl USP) 38 mg • Folic Acid 400 mcg • Vitamin B12 (as methylcobalamin) 500 mcg • Biotin 200 mc g • Pantothenic Acid (as D-calcium pantothenate) 150 mg • Calcium (as Citrimal brand, malate) 100 mg • Iodine (from kelp) 113 mcg • Magnesium (as buffered amino acid chelate, malate, ascorbate) 20 mg • Zinc (as Chelazome brand amino acid chelate) 10 mg • Selenium (as amino acid complex) 100 mcg • Copper (as lysinate) 1 mg • Manganese (as Chelazome brand) 2500 mcg • Chromium (as ChromeMate brand) 200 mcg • Molybdenum (as amino acid chelate) 25 mc g • Potassium (as citrate) 50 mg • Choline Bitartrate 50 mg • Inositol 50 mg • Mixed Tocopherols 50 mg • Lipoic Acid 25 mg • Trace Minerals 74 (Montmorillonite) 25 mg • N-Acetyl Cysteine USP 25 mg • Rutin 25 mg • Lutein 3 mg • Boron (as proteinate) 1500 mcg • Lycopene 1 mg • Vanadyl Sulfate 1 mg. Other Ingredients: Natural Vegetable Capsules, Ascorbyl Palmitate, Magnesium Stearate, Microcrystalline Cellulose, Silicon Dioxide.

Alpha Base Capsules with Iron - Ortho Molecular Products
Four capsules contain: Vitamin A (as Betatene brand natural mixed carotenoids, palmitate) 7500 IU • Vitamin C (as ascorbic acid USP, ascorbate) 500 mg • Vitamin D (D3, as cholecalciferol) 400 IU • Vitamin E (as D-alpha-tocopherol succinate) 100 IU • Vitamin K (as phytonadione) 50 mcg • Thiamine (B1 from thiamine HCl USP) 25 mg • Riboflavin (vitamin B2 USP) 25 mg • Niacin (as niacin USP, niacinamide) 25 mg • Vitamin B6 (as pyridoxine HCl USP) 38 mg • Folic Acid 400 mcg • Vitamin B12 (as methylcobalamin) 500 mcg • Biotin 200 mc g • Pantothenic Acid (as D-calcium pantothenate) 150 mg • Calcium (as Citrimal brand, malate) 100 mg • Iron (as Ferrochel brand) 15 mg • Iodine (from kelp) 113 mcg • Magnesium (as buffered amino acid chelate, malate, ascorbate) 20 mg • Zinc (as Chelazome brand amino acid chelate) 10 mg • Selenium (as amino acid complex) 100 mcg • Copper (as lysinate) 1 mg • Manganese (as Chelazome brand) 2500 mcg • Chromium (as ChromeMate brand) 200 mcg • Molybdenum (as amino acid chelate) 25 mc g • Potassium (as citrate) 50 mg • Choline Bitartrate 50 mg • Inositol 50 mg • Mixed Tocopherols 50 mg • Lipoic Acid 25 mg • Trace Minerals 74 (Montmorillonite) 25 mg • N-Acetyl Cysteine USP 25 mg • Rutin 25 mg • Lutein 3 mg • Boron (as proteinate) 1500 mcg • Lycopene 1 mg • Vanadyl Sulfate 1 mg. Other Ingredients: Natural Vegetable Capsules, Ascorbyl Palmitate, Magnesium Stearate, Microcrystalline Cellulose, Silicon Dioxide.

Alpha Base Foundation Pak - Ortho Molecular Products
Two packets contain: Vitamin A (as Betatene brand natural mixed carotenoids, palmitate) 15,000 IU • Vitamin C (as ascorbic acid USP) 1000 mg • Vitamin D (D3, as cholecalciferol) 400 IU • Vitamin E (as D-alpha tocopherol) 400 IU • Vitamin K (as phytonadione) 100 mcg • Thiamine (B1 from thiamine HCl USP) 50 mg • Riboflavin (vitamin B2 USP) 50 mg • Niacin (as niacin USP, niacinamide) 50 mg • Vitamnin B6 (as pyridoxine HCl USP) 75 mg • Folic Acid 800 mcg • Vitamin B12 (as methylcobalamin) 950 mcg • Biotin 400 mcg • Pantothenic Acid (as D-calcium pantothenate) 400 mg • Calcium (as Citrimal brand, malate) 350 mg • Iodine (from kelp) 225 mcg • Magnesium (as buffered amino acid chelate, malate) 350 mg • Zinc (as Chelazome brand amino acid chelate) 20 mg • Selenium (as amino acid complex) 200 mcg • Copper (as lysinate) 2 mg • Manganese (as Chelazome brand) 5 mg • Chromium (as ChromeMate brand) 5 mg • Molybdenum (as amino acid chelate) 50 mcg • Potassium (as citrate) 100 mg • EPA 840 mg • DHA 600 mg • Total non-Alpha Tocopherol forms 200 mg • Gamma Tocopherols 146 mg • Delta Tocopherols 33 mg • Lipoic Acid 100 mg • N-Acetyl Cysteine USP 100 mg • Choline Bitartrate 50 mg • Inositol 50 mg • Trace Minerals 74 (montmorillonite) 50 mg • Rutin 50 mg • Lutein 6 mg • Boron (as proteinate) 3 mg • Lycopene 2 mg • Vanadyl Sulfate 2 mg.

Alpha Base Tablets - Ortho Molecular Products
Three tablets contain: Vitamin A (as Betatene brand natural mixed carotenoids, palmitate) 7500 IU • Vitamin C (as ascorbic acid USP, ascorbate) 500 mg • Vitamin D (D3, cholecalciferol) 400 IU • Vitamin E (as D-alpha tocopherol succinate) 100 IU • Vitamin K (as phytonadione) 50 mcg • Thiamine (B1 from thiamine HCl USP) 25 mg • Riboflavin (vitamin B2 USP) 25 mg • Niacin (as niacin USP, niacinamide) 25 mg • Vitamin B6 (as pyridoxine HCl USP) 38 mg • Folic Acid 400 mcg • Vitamin B12 (as methylcobalamin) 500 mcg • Biotin 200 mcg • Pantothenic Acid (as D-calcium pantothenate) 150 mg • Calcium (as Citrimal brand, malate) 100 mg • Iodine (from kelp) 113 mcg • Magnesium (as buffered amino acid chelate, malate, ascorbate) 200 mg • Zinc (as Chelazome brand amino acid chelate) 10 mg • Selenium (as amino acid complex) 100 mcg • Copper (as lysinate) 1 mg • Manganese (as Chealzome brand) 2500 mg • Chromium (as ChromeMate) 200 mcg • Molybdenum (as amino acid chelate) 25 mcg • Potassium (as citrate) 50 mg • Choline Bitartrate 50 mg • Inositol 50 mg • Mixed Tocopherols 50 mg • Lipoic ACid 25 mg • Trace Minerals 74 (montmorillonite) 25 mg • N-Acetyl Cysteine USP 25 mg • Rutin 25 mg • Lutein 3 mg • Boron (as proteinate) 1500 mcg • Lycopene 1 mg • Vanadyl Sulfate 1 mg.

Alpha Base Tablets w/o Iron - Ortho Molecular Products
Six tablets contain: Vitamin A (from fish liver oil and 40% as beta carotene) 25,000 IU • Vitamin C (as ascorbic acid, ascorbate, Ca ascorbate, Mg ascorbate) 570 mg • VItamin D (D3, as cholecalciferol) 100 IU • Vitamin E (as D-alpha tocopherol acid succinate) 200 IU • Thiamine (B1 as thiamine HCl) 75 mg • Vitamin B2 (as riboflavin 5 phosphate) 87 mg • Niacin (67% as niacinamide) 75 mg • Vitamin B6 (as pyridoxine HCl, pyridoxal 5 phosphate) 150 mg • Folic Acid 800 mcg • Vitamin B12 (as cyanocobalamin) 150 mcg • Biotin 75 mcg • Pantothenic Acid (as D-calcium pantothenate) 100 mg • Calcium (as hydroxyapatite, calcium ascorbate) 250 mg • Iodine (from kelp) 225 mcg • Magnesium (as buffered amino acid chelate, ascorbate, citrate, aspartate) 500 mg • Zinc (as picolinate) 20 mg • Selenium (as amino acid complex0 200 mcg • Copper (Chelazome brand) 2 mg • Manganese (as aspartate) 5 mg • Chromium (as aspartate) 200 mcg • Molybdenum (as amino acid chelate) 50 mcg • Potassium (as citrate) 99 mg • PABA (as para aminobenzoic acid) 150 mg • Inositol 100 mg • Choline Bitartrate 100 mg • Lemon Bioflavonoids 100 mg • L-Glutathione (99% reduced) 25 mcg • Vanadium (Chelavite brand) 50 mcg • Montmorillonite 50 mg. Other Ingredients: Hydroxypropyl Cellulose, Croscarmellose Sodium, Stearic Acid, PEG, Silica, Magnesium Stearate, Sodium Copper Chlorophyllin.

Alpha Base Ultimate Pak - Ortho Molecular Products
Two packets contain: Vitamin A (as Betatene brand natural mixed carotenoids, palmitate) 15,000 IU • Vitamin C (as ascorbic acid USP) 1000 mg • Vitamin D (D3, as cholecalciferol) 400 IU • Vitamin E (as D-alpha tocopherol) 400 IU • Vitamin K (as phytonadione) 100 mcg • Thiamine (B1 from thiamine HCl USP) 50 mg • Riboflavin (vitamin B2 USP) 50 mg • Niacin (as niacin USP, niacinamide) 50 mg • Vitamin B6 (as pyridoxine HCl USP) 75 mg • Folic Acid 800 mcg • Vitamin B12 (as methylcobalamin) 950 mcg • Biotin 400 mcg • Pantothenic Acid (as D-calcium pantothenate) 400 mg • Calcium (as Citrial, malate) 350 mg • Iodine (from kelp) 225 mg • Magnesium (as buffered amino acid chelate, malate) 350 mg • Zinc (as Chelazome brand amino acid chelate) 20 mg • Selenium (as amino acid complex) 200 mcg • Copper (as lysinate) 2 mg • Manganese (as Chelazome brand) 5 mg • Chromium (as ChromeMate brand) 400 mcg • Molybdenum (as amino acid chelate) 50 mcg • Potassium (as citrate) 100 mg • Proprietary Blend 4200 mg: Greens Blend 738 mg: Alfalfa grass juice powder, Spirulina, Barley juice powder, Wheat grass juice powder; Foods Blend 3198 mg: Apple, Carrot, Raspberry, Spinach, Strawberry, Blueberry, Tomato, Kale, Lecithin; ORAC Blend 264 mg: Acacia, Blueberry fruit extract, Grapeseed extract, Cranberry, Prune, Cherry, Raspberry seed extract, Bilberry fruit extract • EPA 840 mg • DHA 600 mg • Total Non-Alpha Tocopherol forms 200 mg • Gamma Tocopherols 146 mg • Delta Tocopherols 33 mg • Green Tea extract (standardized to contain 60% polyphenopls and 40% EGCG) 150 mg • Broccoli powder extract 100 mg • Lipoic Acid 100 mg • Milk Thistle seed extract (standardized to contain 60% 80% silymarin) 100 mg • N-Acetyl Cysteine USP 100 mg • Red Wine concentrate 75 mg • Turmeric root extract (standardized to contain 95% curcumin) 75 mg • Choline Bitartrate 50 mg • Inositol 50 mg • Trace Minerals 74 (montmorillonite) 50 mg • Rutin 50 mg • Ginkgo Biloba leaf extract (standardized to contain 24% ginkgo flavonglycosides and 6% terpene lactones) 40 mg • Lutein 6 mg • Boron (as proteinate) 3 mg • Lycopene 2 mg • Vanadyl Sulfate 2 mg.

Alpha betic - Abkit
Each caplet contains: Vitamin A 5000 IU • Vitamin C (ascorbic acid) 120 mg • Vitamin D (as cholecalciferol) 400 IU • Vitamin E (as D-alpha tocopheryl succinate) 60 IU • Thiamin (vitamin B1) 1.5 mg • Riboflavin (vitamin B2) 1.7 mg • Niacin 20 mg • Vitamin B6 (as pyridoxine hydrochloride) 2 mg • Folic Acid 400 mcg • Vitamin B12 (as cyanocobalamin) 6 mcg • Biotin 150 mcg • Pantothenic Acid (as D-calcium pantothenate) 10 mg • Calcium (as calcium sulfate) 200 mg • Iodine (as sodium iodide) 150 mcg • Magnesium (as magnesium oxide) 200 mg • Zinc (as zinc citrate) 15 mg • Selenium (as selenomethionine) 50 mcg • Manganese (as manganese sulfate) 5 mg • Chromium (as chromium picolinate) 200 mcg • Potassium (as potassium chloride) 100 mg • Vanadium (as vanadium sulfate) 100 mcg • Lutein (as lutein ester) 500 mcg • Alpha Lipoic Acid 60 mg. Other Ingredients: Stearic Acid, Cellulose, Magnesium Stearate, Beta Carotene.

Alpha CF Liquid 1 oz - Boericke & Tafel
Aconitum Napellus 4X • Bryonia Alba 3X • Eupatorium Perfoliatum 2X • Gelsemium Sempervirens 4X • Ipecacuanha 3X • Phosphorus 5X • Eucalyptus Globulus 1X.
See Editor's Note No. 1.

Alpha Enzyme Peel - Abra Therapeutics
Apple juice • Raw Cane Sugar • Lemon juice • Apple Pectin • Nonfat Dry Milk • Vitamin E • Vitamin C • Xanthan Gum • Salicylic Acid • Glucose • Glucose Oxidase (from corn sugar) • Lactose Peroxidase (from milk whey) • Grape seed oil • Lactic Acid (from milk whey) • Acetic Acid (from apple cider) • Lavender oil.

Alpha GPC - Source Naturals
Two capsules contain: L-Alpha-Glycerylphosphorylcholine 600 mg. Other Ingredients: Gelatin, Magnesium Stearate.

Alpha GPC 300 - Jarrow Formulas
Each vegetarian capsule contains: Alpha GPC (L-alphaglycerylphosphorylcholine) 300 mg. Other Ingredients: Cellulose, Dicalcium Phosphate, Silicon Dioxide.

Alpha KG - Pain & Stress Center
Each capsule contains: Vitamin C (as ascorbyl palmitate) 10 mg • Vitamin B6 (as pyridoxine HCl) 10 mg • Potassium (as potassium

citrate and aspartate) 60 mg • Magnesium (as magnesium citrate and magnesium aspartate) 40 mg • Alpha-Ketoglutaric Acid 300 mg • Aspartic Acid 50 mg. Other Ingredients: Gelatin Capsule.

Alpha Lipoderm & Green Tea Extract 2oz - Derma E
Purified Water • Green Tea extract • Stearic Acid • Alpha Lipoic Acid • Allantoin • Pantehnol • Caprylic Triglyceride • Jojoba Oil • Cetyl Alcohol • Polysorbate 20 • Glyceryl Stearate • PEG 100 Stearate • Tocopheryl Acetate (vitamin E) • Ascorbyl Palmitate (vitamin C) • Dimethicone • Allantoin • TEA • Retinyl Palmitate (vitamin A) • Ergocalciferol (vitamin D) • Methylparaben • Citricidal • Phenoxyethanol.

Alpha Lipoic 100 mg - J. R. Carlson Laboratories, Inc.
Each tablet contains: Alpha Lipoic 100 mg.

Alpha Lipoic 300 mg - J. R. Carlson Laboratories, Inc.
Each tablet contains: Alpha Lipoic 300 mg.

Alpha Lipoic Acid - Pain & Stress Center
Each capsule contains: Vitamin C (ascorbic acid & ascorbyl palmitate) 80 mg • Alpha Lipoic Aicd (thioctic acid) 300 mg. Other Ingredients: Gelatin Capsule.

Alpha Lipoic Acid - Optimum Nutrition
Each capsule contains: Alpha Lipoic Acid 100 mg. Other Ingredients: Microcrystalline Cellulose, Gelatin, Magnesium Stearate.

Alpha Lipoic Acid - Olympian Labs
Each capsule contains: Crystalline Alpha Lipoic Acid 100 mg.

Alpha Lipoic Acid - Life Extension
Each capsule contains: Alpha Lipoic Acid (100% pharmaceutically pure) 100 mg.

Alpha Lipoic Acid - Progressive Labs
Each capsule contains: Alpha Lipoic Acid 100 mg • Bioperine brand Black Pepper extract (piper nigrum) 5 mg. Other Ingredients: Rice Flour, Gelatin.

Alpha Lipoic Acid - NSI - Nutraceutical Sciences Institute
Each capsule contains: Alpha Lipoic Acid 300 mg.

Alpha Lipoic Acid - Swanson Health Products
Each capsule contains: Alpha Lipoic Acid 50 mg.

Alpha Lipoic Acid - NOW Foods
Each Vcap contains: Vitamin C (as ascorbic acid) 250 mg • Vitamin E (as d-alpha tocopheryl succinate) 30 IU • Alpha Lipoic Acid 100 mg. Other Ingredients: Rice Flour, Cellulose (capsule).

Alpha Lipoic Acid - Leiner Health Products
Each tablet contains: Alpha Lipoic Acid 50 mg. Other Ingredients: Cellulose, Calcium Carbonate, Croscarmellose Sodium, Stearic Acid, Magnesium Stearate, Silicon Dioxide, Hydroxypropyl Methylcellulose, Polyethylene Glycol, Hydroxypropyl Cellulose.

Alpha Lipoic Acid - Metabolic Response Modifiers
Each capsule contains: Alpha Lipoic acid 100 mg.

Alpha Lipoic Acid 100 MG - PhysioLogics
Each capsule contains: Alpha Lipoic Acid 100 mg. Other Ingredients: Dicalcium Phosphate, Gelatin, Silica, Vegetable Magnesium Stearate.

Alpha Lipoic Acid 100 - GNC
Each capsule contains: Alpha Lipoic Acid 100 mg. Other Ingredients: Soybean oil, Gelatin, Glycerin, Corob extract, Titanium Dioxide.

Alpha Lipoic Acid 100 mg - Vitamin World
Each capsule contains: Alpha Lipoic Acid 100 mg. Other Ingredients: Rice Powder, Gelatin, Silica, Vegetable Magnesium Stearate.

Alpha Lipoic Acid 100 mg - Pro Health
Each tablet contains: Alpha Lipoic Acid 100 mg. Other Ingredients: Cellulose, Stearic Acid, Silica, Magnesium Stearate.

Alpha Lipoic Acid 100 mg - Puritan's Pride
Each capsule contains: Alpha Lipoic Acid 100 mg.

Alpha Lipoic Acid 100 mg - Pure Encapsulations
Each vegetable capsule contains: Alpha Lipoic Acid (thioctic acid) 100 mg • Vitamin C (as ascorbyl palmitate) 8 mg.

Alpha Lipoic Acid 200 - Xymogen
Each capsule contains: Alpha-Lipoic Acid 200 mg. Other Ingredients: Cellulose, Silicone Dioxide, Magnesium Stearate.

Alpha Lipoic Acid 200 MG - PhysioLogics
Each capsule contains: Alpha Lipoic Acid 200 mg. Other Ingredients: Cellulose (plant origin), Dicalcium Phosphate, Gelatin, Vegetable Magnesium Stearate, Silica.

Alpha Lipoic Acid 200 mg - Pure Encapsulations
Each vegetable capsule contains: Alpha Lipoic Acid (thioctic acid) 200 mg • Vitamin C (as ascorbyl palmitate) 16 mg.

Alpha Lipoic Acid 200 mg - Vitamin World
Each capsule contains: Alpha Lipoic Acid 200 mg. Other Ingredients: Rice Powder, Gelatin, Silica, Vegetable Magnesium Stearate.

Alpha Lipoic Acid 200 mg - Puritan's Pride
Each capsule contains: Alpha Lipoic Acid 200 mg.

Alpha Lipoic Acid 30 mg - Puritan's Pride
Each capsule contains: Alpha Lipoic Acid 30 mg.

Alpha Lipoic Acid 30 mg - Vitamin World
Each capsule contains: Alpha Lipoic Acid 30 mg. Other Ingredients: Dicalcium Phosphate, Gelatin, Silica, Vegetable Magnesium Stearate.

Alpha Lipoic Acid 300 mg - Pro Health
Each tablet contains: Alpha Lipoic Acid 300 mg. Other Ingredients: Calcium Phosphate, Stearic Acid, Magnesium Stearate, Silicon Dioxide, Vanilla, Natural Food Glaze.

Alpha Lipoic Acid 300 mg - Vitamin World
Each capsule contains: Alpha Lipoic Acid 300 mg. Other Ingredients: Soybean Oil, Soy Lecithin, Gelatin, Glycerin, Caramel Color.

Alpha Lipoic Acid 400 - Pure Encapsulations
Each vegetarian capsule contains: Alpha Lipoic Acid (thioctic acid) 400 mg • Vitamin C (as ascorbyl palmitate) 16 mg. Inactive Ingredients: Hypo-allergenic Plant Fiber, Vegetable Capsule.

Alpha Lipoic Acid 400 mg - Pure Encapsulations
Each vegetable capsule contains: Alpha Lipoic Acid (thioctic acid) 400 mg • Vitamin C (as ascorbyl palmitate) 16 mg.

Alpha Lipoic Acid 50 - GNC
Each capsule contains: Alpha Lipoic Acid 50 mg. Other Ingredients: Soybean oil, Gelatin, Glycerin, Carob extract, Titanium Dioxide.

Alpha Lipoic Acid 600 mg - Pure Encapsulations
Each vegetable capsule contains: Alpha Lipoic Acid (thioctic acid) 600 mg • Vitamin C (as ascorbyl palmitate) 30 mg.

Alpha Lipoic Acid capsules - Jarrow Formulas
Each capsule contains: Biotin 333 mcg • Alpha Lipoic Acid (thioctic acid) 100 mg. Other Ingredients: Rice Powder, Magnesium Stearate, Gelatin, Glycerin, Water.

Alpha Lipoic Acid Extra Strength with MAT - Olympian Labs
Each capsule contains: Crystalline Alpha Lipoic Acid 200 mg. Other Ingredients: MAT (a proprietary blend of nutritional ingredients).

Alpha Lipoic Acid tablets - Jarrow Formulas
Each tablet contains: Biotin 333 mcg • Alpha Lipoic Acid (thioctic acid) 100 mg. Other Ingredients: Cellulose, Calcium Phosphate, Magnesium Stearate, Silicon Dioxide, Vanilla.

BRAND NAMES

Alpha Lipoic Sustain 300 - Jarrow Formulas
Each tablet contains: Biotin 333 mcg • Alpha Lipoic Acid 300 mg. Other Ingredients: Polyacrylate, Calcium Phosphate, Cellulose, Stearic Acid, Magnesium Stearate, Silicon Dioxide, Vanilla.

Alpha Male Plus+ - Albert M. O'Connor, M.D.
Each capsule contains: Thiamin 1 mg • Riboflavin 1 mg • Niacin 1 mg • Vitamin B6 1 mg • Folic Acid 1 mg • Vitamin B12 1 mcg • Biotin 1 mg • Pantothenic Acid 1 mg • Zinc 15 mg • Elk Velvet Antler 250 mg • Nettle root powder 100 mg • Oriental Ginseng 80 mg • Oligomeric Proanthocyanidins 50 mg • Cnidium Monnier 25 mg • Saw Palmetto extract 25 mg • Inositol 1 mg • Choline (bitartrate) 1 mg • PABA 1 mg.

Alpha Night Therapy - Abra Therapeutics
Purified Water • Sugarcane extract • Citrus extract • Apple extract • Green Tea extract • Vegetable Emulsifying Wax • Apricot Kernel oil • Squalane (from olives) • Beta Glucan from Oat • Borage oil • White Willowbark extract • Bulgarian Rosewater • Shea Butter • Wheat Germ oil • Calophyllum Inophyllum berry (foraha) • Aloe Vera gel • Sea Algae extract • Vegetable Glycerin • Phospholipid Complex: Retinyl Palmitate, Tocopheryl Acetate, Ascorbyl Palmitate • High Oleic Safflower oil • Nettle extract • Rosebud extract • Soy Lecithin • Neroli oil • Roman Chamomile • French Lavender • Vitamin A • Vitamin C • Vitamin E • Xanthan Gum • Methylparaben • Propylparaben.

Alpha R-Lipoic Acid - BioGenesis Nutraceuticals
Each veggie capsule contains: Alpha R-Lipoic Acid 50 mg.

Alpha Sun Capsules - Cell Tech
Four capsules contain: Vitamin K 40 mcg • Blue-Green Algae (aph. flos-aquae) 1 g. Other Ingredients: Plant Fiber, Water.

Alpha Sun Tablets - Cell Tech
Four tablets contain: Vitamin K 40 mcg • Blue-Green Algae (aph. flos-aquae) 1 g. Other Ingredients: Croscarmellose Sodium, Stearic Acid, Maltodextrin, Calcium Carbonate.

Alpha-GPC - Pure Encapsulations
Each vegetable capsule contains: Stabilized Alpha-GPC (L-alpha-glycerophosphatidylcholine, providing 50% L-alpha-glycerophosphatidylcholine) 400 mg • Vitamin C (as ascorbyl palmitate) 20 mg. Other Ingredients: Calcium Phosphate, Silicon Dioxide.

Alpha-Lipoic Acid - Source Naturals
Each tablet contains: Alpha-Lipoic acid 50 mg.

Alpha-Lipoic Acid - Rexall - Sundown
Each caplet contains: Alpha-Lipoic Acid 50 mg. Other Ingredients: Maltodextrin, Microcrystalline Cellulose, Crospovidone, Hydrogenated Cottonseed Oil, Silica, Turmeric, Natural & Artificial Flavors, Magnesium Stearate.

Alpha-Lipoic Acid 100 mg - Trophic
Each capsule contains: Alpha-Lipoic Acid 100 mg.

Alphastat Rx-Prostate - Nature's Plus
Each softgel contains: Zinc 15 mg • Alphastat complex 200 mg: Serenoa Repens fruit extract and Haematococcus pluvialis algae extract providing free fatty acids and astaxanthin.

Alternecal-Rx - Alternecare Health Products
Each tablet contains: Tri- Calcium Phosphate 1000 mg • Magnesium 500 mg • Zinc 10 mg • Copper 3 mg • Oat Straw 25 mg • Boron 3 mg • Vitamin C 30 mg • Vitamin D 400 IU • Ashwagandha 25 mg • Silica 25 mg.

Alticort - PhytoPharmica
Contains: 1.8% Salicylic Acid. Other Ingredients: Purified Water • Organic Fatty Acid Complex (C11-C18), Glyceryl Stearate, Chamomile extract (0.5% Flavonoid Content) • 18-Beta-Glycyrrhetinic Acid (from Licorice root extract) • Allantoin 2.0% from Comfrey root extract • Dimethicone, Vitamin E (Antioxidant). Hypoallergenic Fragrance.

Altovis - Berkeley Premium Nutraceuticals
Each caplet contains: Altovis Proprietary Blend 906 mg: Green Tea leaf extract (provides caffeine 100 mg), Cordyceps extract (mycelium), Eleutherococcus Senticosus root standardized extract, Panax Ginseng root standardized extract, Vinpocetine (from vocanga tree seeds), Octacosanol. Other Ingredients: Dicalcium Phosphate, Microcrystalline Cellulose, Croscarmellose Sodium, Stearic Acid, Silica, Magnesium Stearate, Film Coat (hypromellose, hydroxypropyl cellulose, polyethylene glycol, propylene glycol, titanium dioxide, FD&C yellow #6 lake, riboflavin, FD&C blue #2 lake).

Alzare - Alzare LLC
Each tablet contains: Zinc 50 mg • Yohimbe 400 mg • Maca 125 mg • I-arginine 100 mg • Bioperine brand Black Pepper extract 10 mg • DHEA 50 mg • Saw Palmetto 50 mg • Ginseng Blend 50 mg • Proprietary Blend 250 mg: Oat Straw, Catuaba, Muira Puama, Nettle leaf, Tribulus, Sarsaparilla, Astragalus, Pumpkin seed, Licorice, Boron, Damiana.

AM Herbal Cleansing Program Replenishing Formula - Herbalife International of America, Inc.
Two tablets contain: Calcium (as calcium carbonate) 340 mg • Exclusive Blend 1110 mg: Beet root, Fructooligosaccharides, Apple Pectin, Lemon Pectin, Lactobacillus Sporogenes, German Chamomile flower, Hesperidin fruit, Valerian root, Horsetail stem, Uncaria Tormentosa bark, Grapefuit Bioflavonoids, Carrot root, Dandelion leaf, Echinacea root, Quercetin, Lactobacillus Acidophilus. Other Ingredients: Corn Starch, Stearic Acid, Croscarmellose Sodium, Silicon Dioxide, Magnesium Stearate, Shellac, Glycerine, Carnauba Wax.

AM Herbal Maximizer - Slimlife
Three caplets contain: Chromium (as picolinate) 200 mcg • Bladderwrack powder 5 mg • Goldenrod leaf powder 5 mg • Corn Silk pistils powder 5 mg • Hawthorn berries powder 20 mg • Licorice root powder 20 mg • Marshmallow root powder 25 mg • Guarana extract 25 mg • Kola nut extract 30 mg • Cayenne Pepper powder • Chitosan 180 mg • Garcinia Cambogia powder 50 mg. Other Ingredients: Dicalcium Phosphate, Cellulose, Stearic Acid, Magnesium Stearate, Silicone Dioxide, Croscarmellose Sodium, Pharmaceutical Glaze, Talc USP.

AM Menopause Formula - PhytoPharmica
Each tablet contains: Green Tea (Camellia sinesis) leaf extract (standardized to contain 14% caffeine) 250 mg • Panax Ginseng root phytosome (bound to phosphatidylcholine under patent) 50 mg •Black Cohosh (Cimicifuga racemosa) root and rhizome extract 20 mg.

AM Plus (Brain 111 Formula) AM Super Capsule - Alpha Zebra
Two capsules contain: Beta Carotene 25 IU • Thiamine HCl (vitamin B1) 50 mg • Riboflavin (vitamin B2) 50 mg • Niacin (vitamin B3) 20 mg • Pantothenic Acid (vitamin B5) 75 mg • Pyridoxine HCl (vitamin B6) 50 mg • Cyanocobalamin concentrate (vitamin B12/ Sorbitol) 500 mcg • Vitamin C 55 mg • Bioflavonoids with Rose Hips 45 mg • Vitamin E (dry, DL-alpha tocopherol) 25 IU • Biotin 300 mcg • Choline Bitartrate (phosphatidyl) 75 mg • Soy Lecithin (phospholipids) 50 mg • Folic Acid 500 mcg • Inositol 50 mg • Inosine 40 mg • Para-Aminobenzioc Acid (PABA) 30 mg • Calcium Phosphate (chelated) 40 mg • Chromium Picolinate (chelated) 200 mcg • Copper (oxide, chelated) 1 mg • Magnesium (oxide, chelated) 25 mg • Manganese (oxide, chelated) 45 mg • Phosphorus (oxide, chelated)12 mg • Potassium (oxide, chelated) 50 mg • Zinc (oxide, chelated) 50 mg • Boron (chelated) 1 mg • Molybdenum (oxide, chelated) 100 mcg • Selenium (oxide, chelated) 200 mcg • Silicon 400 mcg • L-Aspartic Acid 25 mg • L-Cysteine 15 mg • L-Glutamine 115 mg • L-Glycine 15 mg • L-Leucine 50 mg • L-Lysine 15 mg • L-Methionine 70 mg • L-Tyrosine 70 mg • L-Phenylalanine 100 mg • L-Serine 25 mg • A-Ketoglutaric Acid 15 mg • Raw Adrenal freeze dried concentrate 25 mg • Gamma Aminobutyric Acid - GABA 25 mg • Glutamic Acid 5 mg • RNA/DNA (complex) 25 mg • Beta

BRAND NAMES

Hydrochloride 5 mg • Bromelain 3 mg • Pancreatin 10 mg • Papain 10 mg • Pepsin 10 mg • Protease Enzyme 3 mg • Bee Pollen 40 mg • Royal Jelly 35 mg • Ginkgo Biloba (50:1, contains 24% ginkgolides heterosides) 50 mg • Ginkgo Biloba (8:1, contains 24% ginkgolides) 160 mg • Gotu Kola 128 mg • Panax Korean Ginseng 88 mg • Ginger root 80 mg • Mexican Yam 80 mg • Echinacea Angustifolia 76 mg • Spirulina Algae 75 mg • Fo-Ti 60 mg • Oat Straw 60 mg • Siberian Ginseng 60 mg • Beet root powder 60 mg • Alfalfa 50 mg • Peppermint leaves 60 mg • Eyebright (euphrasia herb) 60 mg • Licorice root (de-glycyrrhiznated) 56 mg • Passionflower 48 mg • Capsicum 40 mg • Dandelion root 40 mg • Hawthorn berry 40 mg • Mexican Damiana leaves 32 mg • Kelp 28 mg • Aloe Vera 28 mg • Fennel 28 mg • Sarsaparilla 28 mg • Cabbage seed 24 mg • Sea Plant concentrate 20 mg • Saw Palmetto berry 20 mg • Burdock root 20 mg • Chamomile 20 mg • Slippery Elm 20 mg • Kava Kava 16 mg • Horseradish 16 mg • Suma 12 mg.

AM Plus (Brain 111 Formula) Energizer Formula **-** Alpha Zebra

Each capsule contains: Niacinamide (vitamin B3) 40 mg • Pyridoxine HCl (vitamin B6) 25 mg • Cyanocobalamin concentrate (vitamin B12, sorbitol) 500 mcg • Bioflavonoids (including rose hips) 30 mg • L-Glutamine 50 mg • L-Phenylalanine 50 mg • L-Methionine 30 mg • L-Tyrosine 25 mg • L-Aspartic Acid 10 mg • L-Taurine 10 mg • L-Asparigne 10 mg • L-Alanine 10 mg • L-Glycine 10 mg • Pancreatin 20 mg • Gamma Aminobutyric Acid (GABA) 10 mg • Soy Lecithin (phospholipids) 10 mg • Royal Jelly 25 mg • Beet root powder 80 mg • Cantaloupe 80 mg • Yucca 60 mg • American Cenuary 60 mg • Mexican Yam 60 mg • Bissy Nut 60 mg • Kava Kava root 56 mg • Fo-Ti 48 mg • Oat Straw 48 mg • Capsicum / Cayenne 44 mg • Bee Pollen 40 mg • Dandelion root 40 mg • Brigham Tea 40 mg • Artichoke 40 mg • Wild Lettuce 40 mg • Rosemary leaves 40 mg • Yerba Mate 32 mg • Peppermint leaves 32 mg • Sarsaparilla 25 mg • Ginger root 24 mg • Suma 24 mg • Hawthorn berry 16 mg • American Ginseng 16 mg • Cabbage seed 16 mg • Parsley 16 mg • Fenugreek 16 mg • Gotu Kola 16 mg • Muira Puama 12 mg • Spirulina Algae 12 mg.

AM/PM Menopause Formula **-** Enzymatic Therapy

AM Formula: Each white tablet contains: Green Tea leaf extract (camellia sinensis, standardized to contain 35 mg caffeine) 250 mg • Panax Ginseng root phytosome (one part panax ginseng extract, standardized to contain 37.5% ginsenosides, bound to two parts phosphatidylcholine) 50 mg • Black Cohosh root and rhizome extract (standardized to contain 2.5% triterpene glycosides calculated as 27-deoxyactein) 20 mg. Other Ingredients: Cellulose, Modified Cellulose, Modified Cellulose Gum, Titanium Dioxide Color, Magnesium Stearate, Lecithin, Carnauba Wax.

PM Formula: Each red tablet contains: Valerian root extract (valeriana officinalis, standardized to contain a minimum of 0.8% valerenic acids) 200 mg • Hops flower 6.6:1 extract (humulus lupulus) 100 mg • L-Theanine 50 mg • Black Cohosh root and rhizome extract (standardized to contain 2.5% triterpene glycosides calculated as 27-deoxyactein) 20 mg. Other Ingredients: Cellulose, Modified Cellulose, Modified Cellulose Gum, Magnesium Stearate, Carrot and Paprika Extract Color, Lecithin, Carnauba Wax.

AM/PM Menopause Formula **-** PhytoPharmica

AM Formula: Each yellow tablet contains: Green Tea leaf extract (camellia sinensis, standardized to contain 35 mg caffeine) 250 mg • Panax Ginseng root phytosome (one part panax ginseng extract, standardized to contain 37.5% ginsenosides, bound to two parts phosphatidylcholine) 50 mg • Black Cohosh root and rhizome extract (standardized to contain 2.5% triterpene glycosides calculated as 27-deoxyactein) 20 mg. Other Ingredients: Cellulose, Modified Cellulose, Modified Cellulose Gum, Titanium Dioxide Color, Magnesium Stearate, Lecithin, Carnauba Wax.

PM Formula: Each purple tablet contains: Valerian root extract (valeriana officinalis, standardized to contain a minimum of 0.8% valerenic acids) 200 mg • Hops flower 6.6:1 extract (humulus lupulus) 100 mg • L-Theanine 50 mg • Black Cohosh root and rhizome extract (standardized to contain 2.5% triterpene glycosides calculated as 27-deoxyactein) 20 mg. Other Ingredients: Cellulose, Modified Cellulose, Modified Cellulose Gum, Magnesium Stearate, Carrot and Paprika Extract Color, Lecithin, Carnauba Wax.

AM/PM PeriMenopause Formula **-** Enzymatic Therapy

AM Formula: Each yellow tablet contains: Green Tea leaf extract (camellia sinensis, standardized to contain 35 mg caffeine) 250 mg • Rhodiola root extract (rhodiola rosea, standardized to contain 3% rosavins and 1% salidroside) 205 mg • Chaste Tree berry extract (vitex agnus-castus, standardized to contain 0.5% agnusides) 40 mg • Black Cohosh root and rhizome extract (standardized to contain 2.5% triterpene glycosides calculated as 27-deoxyactein) 20 mg. Other Ingredients: Cellulose, Modified Cellulose, Modified Cellulose Gum, Titanium Dioxide Color, Magnesium Stearate, Lecithin, Carnauba Wax.

PM Formula: Each purple tablet contains: Valerian root extract (valeriana officinalis, standardized to contain a minimum of 0.8% valerenic acids) 200 mg • Hops flower 6.6:1 extract (humulus lupulus) 100 mg • L-Theanine 50 mg • Black Cohosh root and rhizome extract (standardized to contain 2.5% triterpene glycosides calculated as 27-deoxyactein) 20 mg. Other Ingredients: Cellulose, Modified Cellulose, Modified Cellulose Gum, Magnesium Stearate, Carrot and Paprika Extract Color, Lecithin, Carnauba Wax.

AM/PM PeriMenopause Formula **-** PhytoPharmica

AM Formula: Each yellow tablet contains: Green Tea leaf extract (camellia sinensis, standardized to contain 35 mg caffeine) 250 mg • Rhodiola root extract (rhodiola rosea, standardized to contain 3% rosavins and 1% salidroside) 205 mg • Chaste Tree berry extract (vitex agnus-castus, standardized to contain 0.5% agnusides) 40 mg • Black Cohosh root and rhizome extract (standardized to contain 2.5% triterpene glycosides calculated as 27-deoxyactein) 20 mg. Other Ingredients: Cellulose, Modified Cellulose, Modified Cellulose Gum, Titanium Dioxide Color, Magnesium Stearate, Lecithin, Carnauba Wax.

PM Formula: Each purple tablet contains: Valerian root extract (valeriana officinalis, standardized to contain a minimum of 0.8% valerenic acids) 200 mg • Hops flower 6.6:1 extract (humulus lupulus) 100 mg • L-Theanine 50 mg • Black Cohosh root and rhizome extract (standardized to contain 2.5% triterpene glycosides calculated as 27-deoxyactein) 20 mg. Other Ingredients: Cellulose, Modified Cellulose, Modified Cellulose Gum, Magnesium Stearate, Carrot and Paprika Extract Color, Lecithin, Carnauba Wax.

Amazing Herbs Black Seed & Green Tea Blend **-** TNC International, Inc.

Thirty grams (1.06 ounces) contain: Proprietary Blend: Black Cumin Seed powder, Green Tea leaves.

Amazing Herbs Black Seed & Peppermint Tea **-** TNC International, Inc.

Thirty grams (1.06 ounces) contain: Proprietary Blend: Black Cumin Seed powder, Peppermint leaves.

Amazing Herbs Black Seed Female Energy Tea **-** TNC International, Inc.

Thirty grams (1.06 ounces) contain: Proprietary Blend: Black Cohosh, Ginseng, Ginkgo, Black Cumin Seed, St. John's Wort, Gotu Kola, Green Tea, Red Raspberry leaf, Rose Hips.

Amazing Herbs Black Seed Ground Herb **-** TNC International, Inc.

Three ounces contain: Black Cumin Seed herb (100% pure, non-irradiated, untreated, unwashed, finely ground).

Amazing Herbs Black Seed Herbal Honey: Energizing Blend **-** TNC International, Inc.

Sixteen ounces contain: Proprietary Blend: Black Seed oil (100% pure), Ginger, Ginseng, Ginkgo Biloba, Raw Natural Honey.

Some Brand Name Natural Products - What they Contain

www.NaturalDatabase.com contains MANY more listings than appear here.
Editor's Notes are located on pages 2155-2163.

Amazing Herbs Black Seed Herbal Honey: Immune Boost - TNC International, Inc.
Sixteen ounces contain: Proprietary Blend: Black Seed oil (100% pure), Echinacea, Elderberry, Garlic, Raw Natural Honey.

Amazing Herbs Black Seed Herbal Honey: Soothing Blend - TNC International, Inc.
Sixteen ounces contain: Proprietary Blend: Black Seed oil (100% pure), Hyssop, Chamomile, Thyme, Raw Natural Honey.

Amazing Herbs Black Seed Male Energy Tea - TNC International, Inc.
Thirty grams (1.06 ounces) contain: Proprietary Blend: Ginseng, Ginkgo, Yohimbe, Saw Palmetto, Green Tea, Black Cumin Seed, Echinacea, Mint, Rose Hips.

Amazing Herbs Black Seed Original Plain - TNC International, Inc.
Each capsule contains: Pure Black Seed herb (black cumin, nigella sativa) 500 mg.

Amazing Herbs Black Seed Relaxing Blend - TNC International, Inc.
Thirty grams (1.06 ounces) contain: Proprietary Blend: Black Cumin Seed powder, Hops, Valerian, Passion Flower, Mint, Orange peel, Chamomile, Stevia.

Amazing Herbs Black Seed Rooibos Tea Blend - TNC International, Inc.
Thirty grams (1.06 ounces) contain: Proprietary Blend: Black Cumin Seed powder, South African Rooibos.

Amazing Herbs Black Seed Whole Herb - TNC International, Inc.
Four ounces contain: Black Cumin Seed herb (100% pure, non-irradiated, untreated, unwashed).

Amazing Herbs GlyMordica Bitter Melon - TNC International, Inc.
Bitter Melon (Momordica Charantia).

Amazon A-F - Raintree Nutrition, Inc.
Each capsule contains: Proprietary Blend 650 mg: Jatoba, Fedegoso, Brazilian Peppertree, Pau d'Arco, Clavillia, Anamu.

Amazon A-P - Raintree Nutrition, Inc.
Each capsule contains: Proprietary Blend 650 mg: Epazote, Graviola, Fedegoso, Anama, Simarouba, Carqueja, Guaco, Amargo, Erva Tostao, Cat's Claw.

Amazon Athletic Support - Raintree Nutrition, Inc.
Each capsule contains: Proprietary Blend 650 mg: Suma, Sarsaparilla, Maca, Chuchuhuasi, Muria Puama, Yerba Mate, Tayuya, Iporuru.

Amazon A-V - Raintree Nutrition, Inc.
Each capsule contains: Proprietary Blend 600 mg: Bitter Melon, Clavillia, Mullaca, Macela, Vassourinha, Chanca Piedra, Jergon Sacha, Corqueja.

Amazon Blood Support - Raintree Nutrition, Inc.
Each capsule contains: Proprietary Blend 600 mg: Artichoke, Suma, Cat's Claw, Bitter Melon, Yerba Mate, Sarsaparilla, Vassourinha, Maca.

Amazon Bowel Support - Raintree Nutrition, Inc.
Each capsule contains: Proprietary Blend 650 mg: Cat's Claw, Macela, Boldo, Jurubeba, Simarouba, Tayuya, Anamu.

Amazon Calm Support - Raintree Nutrition, Inc.
Each capsule contains: Proprietary Blend 650 mg: Graviola, Manaca, Mulungu, Passionflower, Catuaba, Muira Puama, Damiana, Chamomile.

Amazon C-F - Raintree Nutrition, Inc.
Each capsule contains: Proprietary Blend 650 mg: Picao Preto, Fedegoso, Amor Seco, Bitter Melon, Clavillia, Mullaca, Gervao, Cat's Claw, Simarouba, Brazillian Peppertree.

Amazon CNS Support - Raintree Nutrition, Inc.
Each capsule contains: Proprietary Blend 650 mg: Iporuru, Tayuya, Manaca, Pau d'Arco, Amor Seco, Mulungu.

Amazon Detox Support - Raintree Nutrition, Inc.
Each capsule contains: Proprietary Blend 600 mg: Boldo, Amor Seco, Artichoke, Sarsaparilla, Cat's Claw, Carqueja, Nettles.

Amazon Digestion Support - Raintree Nutrition, Inc.
Each capsule contains: Proprietary Blend 650 mg: Boldo, Carqueja, Espinheira Santa, Picao Preto, Jurubeba, Gervao, Cat's Claw.

Amazon Energy Support - Raintree Nutrition, Inc.
Each capsule contains: Proprietary Blend 650 mg: Jatoba, Guarana, Yerba Mate, Maca, Suma.

Amazon F-Tonic Support - Raintree Nutrition, Inc.
Each capsule contains: Proprietary Blend 650 mg: Abuta, Suma, Simarouba, Sarsaparilla, Chuchuhuasi, Damiana, Pau d'Arco.

Amazon Gallbladder Support - Raintree Nutrition, Inc.
Each capsule contains: Proprietary Blend 600 mg: Chanca Piedra, Boldo, Artichoke, Erva Tostao, Carqueja, Jurubeba.

Amazon Hair Support - Raintree Nutrition, Inc.
Each capsule contains: Proprietary Blend 650 mg: Nettles, Mutamba, Muira Puama, Sarsaparilla, Avenco, Gervao, Catuaba, Chuchuhuasi.

Amazon Heart Support - Raintree Nutrition, Inc.
Each capsule contains: Proprietary Blend 650 mg: Abuta, Hawthorn, Chanca Piedra, Picao Preto, Stevia, Brazilian Peppertree, Erva Tostao.

Amazon Hypertension Support - Raintree Nutrition, Inc.
Each capsule contains: Abuta • Artichoke • Bitter Melon • Chanca Piedra • Graviola • Jurubeba • Mullaca • Suma • Periwinkle • Stevia • Pedra hume caa.

Amazon Immune Support - Raintree Nutrition, Inc.
Each capsule contains: Proprietary Blend 650 mg: Cat's Claw, Mullaca, Erva Tostao, Sarsaparilla, Anamu, Fedegoso.

Amazon Joint-Muscle Support - Raintree Nutrition, Inc.
Each capsule contains: Proprietary Blend 650 mg: Amor Seco, Cat's Claw, Chuchuhuasi, Tayuya, Iporuru, Picao Preto, Guaco, Sarsaparilla.

Amazon Kidney Support - Raintree Nutrition, Inc.
Each capsule contains: Proprietary Blend 650 mg: Chanca Piedra, Boldo, Cipo Cabeludo, Erva Tostao, Abuta.

Amazon Liver Support - Raintree Nutrition, Inc.
Each capsule contains: Proprietary Blend 600 mg: Carqueja, Picao Preto, Erva Tostao, Artichoke, Boldo, Chanca Piedra, Guaco.

Amazon Lung Support - Raintree Nutrition, Inc.
Each capsule contains: Proprietary Blend 650 mg: Amor Seco, Embauba, Samambaia, Mullaca, Mutamba, Jatoba, Avenca.

Amazon Menopause Support - Raintree Nutrition, Inc.
Each capsule contains: Proprietary Blend 650 mg: Muira Puama, Suma, Damiana, Maca, Dong Quai, Black Cohosh, Sarsaparilla, Passionflower.

Amazon Menstrual Support - Raintree Nutrition, Inc.
Each capsule contains: Proprietary Blend 650 mg: Abuta, Chuchuhuasi, Tayuya, Iporuru, Cramp Bark, Periwinkle, Erva Tostao.

Amazon Mood Support - Raintree Nutrition, Inc.
Each capsule contains: Proprietary Blend 650 mg: Tayuya, Damiana, Muira Puama, Passion Flower, Chamomile, Graviola, Mulungu.

Some Brand Name Natural Products - What they Contain

www.NaturalDatabase.com contains MANY more listings than appear here.

Editor's Notes are located on pages 2155-2163.

Amazon M-Tonic Support **-** Raintree Nutrition, Inc.
Each capsule contains: Proprietary Blend 650 mg: Muira Puama, Catuaba, Chuchuhuasi, Suma, Maca, Nettles, Sarsaparilla, Jatoba.

Amazon Prostate Support **-** Raintree Nutrition, Inc.
Each capsule contains: Proprietary Blend 650 mg: Mutamba, Brazilian Peppertree, Jatoba, Nettles, Pau d'Arco, Graviola, Cipo Cabeludo.

Amazon Sinus Support **-** Raintree Nutrition, Inc.
Each capsule contains: Proprietary Blend 650 mg: Nettles, Yerba Mate, Jatoba, Gervao, Pau d'Arco, Picao Preto, Carqueja.

Amazon Skin-A Support **-** Raintree Nutrition, Inc.
Each capsule contains: Proprietary Blend 650 mg: Abuta, Bitter Melon, Chuchuhuasi, Espinheira Santa, Fedegoso, Sarsaparilla, Tayuya.

Amazon Skin-P Support **-** Raintree Nutrition, Inc.
Each capsule contains: Proprietary Blend 650 mg: Samambaia, Cat's Claw, Suma, Sarsaparilla, Fedegoso, Boldo, Pau d'Arco.

Amazon Urinary Support **-** Raintree Nutrition, Inc.
Each capsules contains: Proprietary Blend 650 mg: Chanca Piedra, Anamu, Jatoba, Brazilian Peppertree, Pau d'Arco, Erva Tostao.

Amazon Weight Loss Support **-** Raintree Nutrition, Inc.
Each capsule contains: Proprietary Blend 650 mg: Cha de Bugre, Carqueja, Guarana, Jurubeba, Picao Preto, Yerba Mate, Annatto.

AmbroDerm Lotion **-** Mannatech
Water • Emu Oil • Glycereth-26 • Sorbitol • Glycerin • Germaben II (propylene glycol, diazolidinyl urea, methylparaben, propylparaben) • Polysorbate 80 • Tocopherol Acetate • Ambrotose Complex (patent pending; naturally occurring plant saccharides, including freeze-dried Aloe Vera gel extract - manapol powder) • Carbomer • Aminomethyl Propanol • Retinyl Palmitate • Fragrance • Allantoin.

AmbroStart Drink Mix, Orange **-** Mannatech
Each 1 tbsp serving contains: Vitamin A (100% as beta-carotene) 400 IU • Proprietary Blend Energy Complex 5.9 g: Fructose, Citric Acid, Medium Chain Triglycerides, Calcium Citrate, Magnesium Aspartate, Magnesium Succinate, Potassium Aspartate, Potassium Succinate, Choline Bitartrate, Lecithin • Mannatech 2001 brand Arabinogalactan Fiber 3 g • Ambrotose Complex (patent pending) 697 mg: Arabinogalactan gum (larix decidua), Manapol brand Aloe Vera gel extract (inner leaf gel), Gum Ghatti, Gum Tragacanth • Stevia leaf extract. Other Ingredients: Silicon Dioxide, Natural Flavors, Calcium Pyruvate.

Ambrotose AO **-** Mannatech
Each capsule contains: Vitamin E (as mixed D-alpha-, D-beta-, D-delta-, and D-gamma-tocopherols) 18 IU • Proprietary Blend MTech AO 113 mg: Quercetin Dihydrate, Grape skin extract (fruit), Green Tea extract (leaves), Australian Bush Plum (terminalia ferdinandiana fruit) • Ambrotose Phyto Formula 333 mg: Gum Arabic, Xanthan Gum, Gum Tragacanth, Gum Ghatti, Aloe Vera gel extract (inner leaf gel - manapol powder) • Phyt•Aloe Complex: Broccoli, Brussels Sprout, Cabbage, Carrot, Cauliflower, Garlic, Kale, Onion, Tomato, Turnip, Papaya, Pineapple. Other Ingredients: Vegetable-Based Cellulose Capsules.

Ambrotose Complex capsules **-** Mannatech
Each capsule contains: Proprietary Blend Ambrotose Complex (patent pending) 150 mg: Arabinogalactan (larix decidua gum), Manapol Aloe Vera gel extract (inner leaf gel), Gum Ghatti, Gum Tragacanth. Other Ingredients: Brown Rice Flour, Silicon Dioxide, Magnesium Stearate.

Ambrotose Complex powder **-** Mannatech
Each 1/4 tsp serving contains: Proprietary Blend Ambrotose Complex (patent pending) 0.44 g: Arabinogalactan (larix decidua gum), Rice Starch, Manapol Aloe Vera gel extract (inner leaf gel), Gum Ghatti, Glucosamine HCl, Gum Tragacanth.

Ambrotose with Lecithin **-** Mannatech
Each capsule contains: Calcium 70 mg • Proprietary Blend Ambrotose Complex (patent pending) 150 mg: Arabinogalactan gum (larix decidua), Manapol brand Aloe Vera gel extract (inner leaf gel), Gum Ghatti, Gum Tragacanth • Lecithin powder 50 mg. Other Ingredients: Calcium Carbonate, Dibasic Calcium Phosphate, Gelatin, Brown Rice Flour, Cellulose, Silicon Dioxide, Magnesium Stearate.

Ameal S **-** Calpis Co, Ltd
Three tablets contain: Lactotripeptide (derived from milk protein) 6 mg. Other Ingredients: Whey Powder, Sorbitol, Corn Starch, Maltodextrin, Natural & Artificial Flavors, Cellulose, Polyglycerol Esters of Fatty Acids, Anhydride Citric Acid, Aspartame, Calcium Triphosphate.

American Ginseng **-** Nature's Way
Two capsules contain: American Ginseng root 1.1 g. Other Ingredients: Gelatin, Magnesium stearate.

American Ginseng 500 mg **-** Vitamin World
Each capsule contains: American Ginseng root extract (panax quinquefolius) 500 mg. Other Ingredients: Gelatin.

American Ginseng 500 mg **-** Vital Nutrients
Each capsule contains: Panax Quinquefolius (american ginseng, minimum 4% ginsenosides) 500 mg.

American Ginzing **-** Traditional Medicinals
Contains: American Ginseng root • Licorice root • Ginger rhizome • Cinnamon bark • Sarsaparilla root • Dong Quai root.

American Wild Ginseng and Tian Qi capsules **-** Eu Yan Sang
American Wild Ginseng • Tian Qi.

Amino 1000 **-** Puritan's Pride
Three tablets contain: Vitamin C (as ascorbyl palmitate) 30 mg • Hydrolyzed Protein 3000 mg • L-Alanine 210 mg • L-Arginine 189 mg • L-Aspartic Acid 114 mg • L-Cysteine 9.9 mg • L-Glutamic Acid 114 mg • L-Glycine 588 mg • L-Histidine 23.4 mg • L-Hydroxyproline 378 mg • L-Isoleucine 40.8 mg • L-Leucine 66.6 mg • L-Lysine 99 mg • L-Methionine 22.8 mg • L-Phenylalanine 45 mg • L-Proline 303 mg • L-Serine 106.8 mg • L-Threonine 38.4 mg • L-Tyrosine 17.1 mg • L-Valine 57.3 mg.

Amino 1500 **-** Puritan's Pride
Six tablets contain: L-Ornithine HCl 161.1 mg • L-Lysine 836.2 mg • L-Histidine 198.6 mg • L-Arginine 329.2 mg • L-Aspartic Acid 861.3 mg • L-Threonine 376.3 mg • L-Serine 629.2 mg • L-Glutamic Acid 1259.7 mg • L-Proline 635.6 mg • L-Glycine 162.0 mg • L-Alanine 388.8 mg • L-Cystine 250.9 mg • L-Valine 445.3 mg • L-Methionine 203.8 mg • L-Isoleucine 543.5 mg • L-Leucine 977.4 mg • L-Tyrosine 339.7 mg • L-Phenylalanine 376.3 mg.

Amino 2000 **-** Puritan's Pride
Each tablet contains: L-Lysine 282.4 mg • L-Histidine 61.6 mg • L-Arginine 84.6 mg • L-Aspartic Acid 326.0 mg • L-Threonine 211.8 mg • L-Serine 164.6 mg • L-Proline 190.4 mg • L-Alanine 127.2 mg • L-Glycine 59.2 mg • L-Glutamic Acid 275.4 mg • L-Cysteine 80.4 mg • L-Valine 173.6 mg • L-Methionine 64.2 mg • L-Isoleucine 187.6 mg • L-Leucine 321.8 mg • L-Tyrosine 90.4 mg • L-Phenylalanine 97.6 mg • L-Tryptophan 52.2 mg • L-Carnitine 10.0 mg.

Amino 21 **-** DaVinci Laboratories
Each capsule contains: Glutamic Acid 225 mg • L-Glutamine 75 mg • L-Taurine 75 mg • L-Aspartic Acid 45 mg • L-Glycine 45 mg • L-Lysine 30 mg • DL-Phenylalanine 30 mg • L-Tyrosine 30 mg • L-Arginine 22.5 mg • L-Cystine 22.5 mg • L-Leucine 22.5 mg • L-Methionine 22.5 mg • L-Alanine 15 mg • L-Serine 15 mg • L-Threonine 15 mg • L-Citrulline 15 mg • L-Valine 15 mg • L-Histidine 7.5 mg • L-Isoleucine 7.5 mg • L-Ornithine 7.5 mg • L-Proline 7.5 mg. Other Ingredients: Gelatin.

Some Brand Name Natural Products - What they Contain

www.NaturalDatabase.com contains MANY more listings than appear here.
Editor's Notes are located on pages 2155-2163.

Amino 2222 Capsules **-** Optimum Nutrition
Two capsules contain: Pharmaceutical Grade 3Amino Acids2 (derived from Predigested Lactalbumen, Soy Protein Isolate & Whey Protein concentrate) 2222 mg • L-Ornithine • L-Carnitine.

Amino Acid 1000 mg **-** Nature's Life
Ten capsules contain: Casein Hydrolysate • Glycine • L-Proline • L-Arginine • L-Alanine • Pyridoxine HCl • L-Ornithine • L-Serine • L-Cystine • Whole Egg powder. Providing, based on a typical analysis: L-Alanine 663 mg • L-Arginine 665 mg • L-Aspartic Acid 447 mg • L-Cystine 4 mg • L-Glutamic Acid 1222 mg • Glycine 1806 mg • L-Histidine 157 mg • L-Isoleucine (esssential amino acid) 313 mg • L-Leucine (essential amino acid) 512 mg • L-Ornithine 250 mg • L-Lysine (essential amino acid) 471 mg • L-Methionine (essential amino acid) 166 mg • L-Phenylalanine (essential amino acid) 313 mg • L-Proline 1640 mg • L-Serine 505 mg • L-Threonine (essential amino acid) 262 mg • L-Tryptophan (essential amino acid) 70 mg • L-Tyrosine 200 mg • L-Valine (essential amino acid) 408 mg.

Amino acid chelated Magnesium 500mg **-** Nature's Own
Each tablet contains: Magnesium Chelate 500 mg: Elemental Magnesium 100 mg.

Amino acid chelated Potassium 495mg **-** Nature's Own
Each tablet contains: Potassium Amino Acid Chelate 495 mg: Elemental Potassium 100 mg.

Amino acid chelated Zinc 220mg **-** Nature's Own
Each tablet contains: Zinc Amino Acid Chelate 220 mg: Elemental Zinc 22 mg.

Amino acid chelates Calcium plus Magnesium **-** Nature's Own
Each tablet contains: Calcium Amino Acid Chelate 500 mg: Elemental Calcium 100 mg • Calcium Carbonate 375 mg: Elemental Calcium 150 mg • Magnesium Amino Acid Chelate 125 mg: Elemental Magnesium 25 mg • Magnesium Oxide 42.96 mg: Elemental Magnesium 25 mg • Vitamin D (as D3) 200 IU: Cholecalciferol 5 mcg.

Amino Acid Complex **-** Pro Health
Each tablet contains: Vitamin C (as ascorbic acid) 15 mg • Vitamin B6 (as pyridoxine HCl) 5 mg • Proprietary Blend 1 g: L-Lysine, L-Glutamic Acid base, L-Leucine, L-Tyrosine, L-Aspartic Acid, L-Alanine, L-Glutamine, Glycine, L-Methionine, L-Threonine, L-Serine, L-Valine, L-Proline, L-Phenylalanine, L-Ornithine, L-Isoleucine, L-Arginine base, L-Histidine, L-Cysteine HCl, L-Cystine base, Taurine, L-Carnitine, L-Tartrate, L-Citruline. Other Ingredients: Stearic Acid, Dibasic Calcium Phosphate, Colloidal Silicon Dioxide, Modified Cellulose Gum, Magnesium Stearate, Calcium Ascorbate.

Amino Acids from Whey Protein **-** Rexall - Sundown
Two tablets contain: Calcium 178 mg • Whey Protein concentrate 200 mg • Glutamic Acid 12.3 mg • Aspartic Acid 7.6 mg • Leucine 7.3 mg • Lysine 6.5 mg • Threonine 4.6 mg • Proline 4.2 mg • Isoleucine 3.9 mg • Serine 3.9 mg • Valine 3.9 mg • Alanine 3.4 mg • Phenylalanine 2.3 mg • Cystine 2.1 mg • Arginine 1.7 mg • Histidine 1.5 mg • Glycine 1.4 mg • Tyrosine 1.3 mg • Methionine 1.2 mg • Tryptophan 1.1 mg. Other Ingredients: Dicalcium Phosphate, Microcrystalline Cellulose, Croscarmellose Sodium, Silica, Magnesium Stearate.

Amino Athlete **-** Source Naturals
Each tablet contains: Vitamin B6 5 mg • Vitamin C (ascorbic acid) 15 mg.

Amino Blend **-** Progressive Labs
Three capsules contain: L-Alanine 147 mg • L-Arginine 138 mg • L-Cysteine 23 mg • L-Cystine 26 mg • L-Glutamine 28 mg • Glycine 95 mg • L-Histidine 73 mg • L-Isoleucine 71 mg • L-Leucine 203 mg • L-Lysine 203 mg • L-Methionine 55 mg • L-Ornithine 23 mg • L-Proline 77 mg • L-Serine 95 mg • L-Threonine 91 mg • L-Tyrosine 77 mg • L-Valine 120 mg • Taurine 48 mg • L-Aspartic Acid 206 mg • L-Phenylalanine 102 mg • L-Glutamic Acid 349 mg.

Amino Complex **-** Puritan's Pride
Each tablet contains: L-Arginine 50 mg • L-Cysteine 50 mg • L-Histidine 50 mg • L-Isoleucine 50 mg • L-Leucine 50 mg • L-Lysine Hydrochloride 50 mg • L-Methionine 50 mg • L-Ornithine Hydrochloride 50 mg • L-Phenylalanine 50 mg • L-Threonine 50 mg • L-Tyrosine 50 mg • L-Valine 50 mg.

Amino Day **-** Source Naturals
Each tablet contains: Vitamin B6 5 mg • Vitamin C (ascorbic acdi) 15 mg.

Amino Fuel (Anabolic Amino Acid Drink) **-** TwinLab
Peptide Bonded & Free Amino Acids (derived from the natural Pancreatic digests of Whey Protein & Egg White Protein) 20 g • Protein-sparing Carbohydrates (predominantly from Glucose Polymers) 50 g. Other Ingredients: L-Carnitine, Branched Chain Amino Acids (L-Leucine, L-Isoleucine & L-Valine), Essential Vitamins & Minerals, Zinc Picolinate, Boron, GTF Chromium, Chromium Picolinate & Chromium Polynicotinate.

Amino Fuel (Mega Anabolic Chewable Wafers) 7500 mg **-** TwinLab
Two wafers contain: Peptide Bonded & Free Amino Acids 7500 mg (7.5 g). Each wafer contains: L-Carnitine • Branched Chain Amino Acids (L-Leucine, L-Isoleucine & L-Valine) • Pharmaceutical Grade Peptide Bonded & Free Amino Acids derived from the natural Pancreatic digests of Whey Protein (Lactalbumin) & Egg White (Albumin).

Amino Fuel (Peptide Bonded Amino Acid Liquid Concentrate) **-** TwinLab
L-Carnitine • Branched Chain Amino Acids (L-Leucine, L-Isoleucine & L-Valine) • Pharmaceutical Grade, Peptide Bonded & Free Amino Acids • Stress B Complex Vitamins • Lipotropic Factors: Choline & Inositol • Complex Carbohydrates (Glucose Polymers) • Pure Crystalline Fructose. Each serving contains: Peptide Bonded & Free Amino Acids [derived from the natural Pancreatic digests of Whey Protein (Lactalbumin), Egg Protein (Albumin), Liver Protein & other Animal Proteins] 15 g.

Amino Fuel (Peptide Bonded Amino Acid Tablets) **-** TwinLab
L-Carnitine • Branched Chain Amino Acids (L-Leucine, L-Isoleucine & L-Valine) • Peptide Bonded Amino Acids [derived from Pharmaceutical Grade Pancreatic (Enzymatic) digests of Whey Protein (Lactalbumin) & Egg White Protein (Albumin)].

Amino Fuel 1000 Tabs **-** TwinLab
L-Carnitine • Branched Chain Amino Acids (L-Leucine, L-Isoleucine & L-Valine) • Peptide Bonded Amino Acids [derived from Pharmaceutical Grade Pancreatic (Enzymatic) digests of Whey Protein (Albumin)].

Amino Fuel 1500 Tablets **-** TwinLab
Each tablet contains: Peptide Bonded Amino Acids & Branched Chain Amino Acids [derived from Pharmaceutical Grade Pancreatic digests of Whey Protein (Lactalbumin) & Egg White Protein (Albumin)] 1500 mg. No lower quality amino acid sources are present, such as soy or casein.

Amino Fuel 2000 (Extra Strength Amino Acid Tablets) **-** TwinLab
Each tablet contains: Protein (as Peptide Bonded Amino Acids) derived from Pharmaceutical Grade Pancreatic digests of Whey Protein (Lactalbumin) & Egg White Protein 2000 mg.

Amino Fuel Stack **-** TwinLab
Six capsules contain: HMB (B-Hydroxy B-Methylbutyrate Monohydrate) 3000 mg • L-Glutamine 2000 mg • Acetyl-L-Carnitine 1000 mg • Taurine 200 mg • N-Acetyl-Cysteine (NAC) 200 mg.

Amino Mass **-** Source Naturals
Four tablets contain: L-Arginine Pyroglutamate 1,000 mg • L-Lysine HCl 1,000 mg • ChromeMate Chromium GTF (Chromium Polynicotinate) 100 mcg.

Some Brand Name Natural Products - What they Contain

www.NaturalDatabase.com contains MANY more listings than appear here.
Editor's Notes are located on pages 2155-2163.

BRAND NAMES

Amino Night - Source Naturals
Four tablets contain: Arginine Pyroglutamate 816 mg • L-Lysine HCl 816 mg • L-Ornithine (from 469 mg of L-ornithine HCl) 368 mg.

Amino Strength - Source Naturals
Each tablet contains: Arginine Pyroglutamate 330 mg • l-Ornithine (from 382 mg of L-Ornithine HCl) 300 mg.

Amino Surge - Jarrow Formulas
Each tablet contains: Vitamin C 20 mg • Vitamin B1 (thiamin) 2 mg • Vitamin B2 (riboflavin) 2 mg • Vitamin B3 (niacin) 2 mg • Vitamin B5 (pantothenic acid) 5 mg • Vitamin B6 (pyridoxine) 2 mg • Essential Amino Acids 487 mg: Isoleucine 60 mg, Leucine 104 mg, Lysine 89 mg, Methionine 19 mg, Phenylalanine / Tyrosine 63 mg, Threonine 69 mg, Tryptophan 24 mg, Valine 50 mg • Non-Essential Amino Acids 552 mg: Alanine 47 mg, Arginine 26 mg, Aspartic Acid 110 mg, Cysteine / Cystine 23 mg, Glutamic Acid 182 mg, Glycine 20 mg, Histidine 21 mg, Proline 69 mg, Serine 54 mg. Other Ingredients: Dicalcium Phosphate, Modified Cellulose Gum, Magnesium Stearate (vegetable source), Cellulose, Silicon Dioxide.

Amino Ty - Genestra - Seroyal
Each capsule contains: L-Tyrosine 403 mg • Amino Acids 100 mg.

Amino Vital Fast-Charge - Ajinomoto USA
Each packet contains: Vitamin A (as retinyl palmitate) 600 IU • Vitamin C (as ascorbic acid) 125 mg • Vitamin D (as cholecalciferol) 8 IU • Vitamin E (as D-alpha tocopherol) 41 IU • Vitamin B1 (as thiamin mononitrate) 0.3 mg • Vitamin B2 (as riboflavin) 0.4 mg • Niacin (as nicotinic acid) 4.7 mg • Vitamin B6 (as pyridoxine hydrochloride) 0.5 mg • Vitamin B12 (as cyanocobalamin) 0.5 mg • Pantothenic Acid (as calcium pantothenate) 1.8 mg • Amino Acids 2400 mg: L-Glutamine 590 mg, L-Leucine 500 mg, L-Isoleucine 400 mg, L-Valine 340 mg, L-Arginine 570 mg.

Amino Vital Mix-and-Shake - Ajinomoto USA
Each 1 tbsp serving contains: Vitamin C (ascorbic acid) 70 mg • Calcium 55 mg • Phosphorus 30 mg • Chloride 20 mg • Amino Acids 960 mg: L-Arginine 230 mg, L-Glutamine 230 mg, L-Leucine 200 mg, L-Isoleucine 160 mg, L-Valine 140 mg.

Amino Vital Pro - Ajinomoto USA
Each 8 fl oz serving (250 mL) contains: Calcium 20 mg • Sodium 10 mg • Potassium 35 mg • Amino Acids 1440 mg: L-Leucine 400 mg, L-Isoleucine 325 mg, L-Valine 265 mg, L-Arginine 450 mg.

Amino Vital Ready-to-Drink - Ajinomoto USA
Each 8 fl oz serving (250 mL) contains: Calcium 20 mg • Chloride 25 mg • Sodium 10 mg • Potassium 35 mg • Amino Acids 740 mg: L-Leucine 205 mg, L-Isoleucine 165 mg, L-Valine 135 mg, L-Arginine 235 mg.

Amino-BC - ANS - Applied Nutrition Sciences
Branched Chain Amino Acids.

AminoBuild (chocolate flavor) - Pharmanex
Three scoops (45 g) contain: Vitamin A (as Vitamin A Palmitate) 1000 IU • Vitamin C (as Ascorbic Acid) 60 mg • Vitamin D (as Vitamin D3) (as Cholecalciferol) 40 IU • Vitamin E (as d-Alpha Tocopheryl Acetate) 30 IU • Thiamin (as Thiamin Mononitrate) 0.3 mg • Riboflavin (as Riboflavin) 0.34 mg • Niacin (as Niacinamide) 4 mg • Vitamin B6 (as Pyridoxine Hydrochloride) 0.4 mg • Folate (as Folic Acid) 80 mcg • Vitamin B12 (as Cyanocobalamin) 1.2 mcg • Biotin (as Biotin) 60 mcg • Pantothenic Acid (as d-Calcium Pantothenate) 2 mg • Calcium (as Dicalcium Phosphate) 540 mg • Phosphorus (as Dicalcium Phosphate) 400 mg • Iodine (as Calcium Iodate) 15 mcg • Magnesium (as Magnesium Citrate) 80 mg • Zinc (as Zinc Gluconate) 3 mg • Selenium (as Sodium Selenate) 14 mcg • Copper (as Copper Gluconate) 0.2 mg • Manganese (as Manganese Gluconate) 0.4 mg • Chromium (as Chromium Polynicotinate 24 mcg • Molybdenum (as Sodium Molybdate) 15 mcg • Sodium (as Sodium Chloride, Soy Protein Isolate) 250 mg • Potassium (from Soy Protein Isolate) 360 mg • Stevia (Stevia Rebaudiana) (Leaves) 50 mg. Other Ingredients: Protein Blend (Supro7 Soy Protein Isolate, Cross Flow Microfiltration Whey Protein Isolate, Whey Protein Hydrolysate), Crystalline Fructose, Natural Flavors, Alkalized Cocoa Powder, Magnesium Citrate, Sodium Chloride, Dicalcium Phosphate, Ascorbic Acid, dl-Alpha Tocopheryl Acetate, Stevia, Medium Chain Triglycerides, Zinc Gluconate, Chromium Polynicotinate, Biotin, Vitamin A Palmitate, Niacinamide, Manganese Gluconate, Copper Gluconate, d-Calcium Pantothenate, Pyridoxine Hydrochloride, Cholecalciferol, Riboflavin, Thiamin Mononitrate, Cyanocobalamin, Folic Acid, Calcium Iodate, Sodium Molybdate, Sodium Selenate.

AminoBuild (vanilla flavor) - Pharmanex
Three scoops (45 g) contain: Vitamin A (as Vitamin A Palmitate) 1000 IU • Vitamin C (as Ascorbic Acid) 60 mg • Vitamin D3 (as Cholecalciferol) 40 IU • Vitamin E (as d-Alpha Tocopheryl Acetate) 30 IU • Thiamin (as Thiamin Mononitrate) 0.3 mg • Riboflavin (as Riboflavin) 0.34 mg • Niacin (as Niacinamide) 4 mg • Vitamin B6 (as Pyridoxine Hydrochloride) 0.4 mg • Folate (as Folic Acid) 80 mcg • Vitamin B12 (as Cyanocobalamin) 1.2 mcg • Biotin (as Biotin) 60 mcg • Pantothenic Acid (as d-Calcium Pantothenate) 2 mg • Calcium (as Dicalcium Phosphate) 540 mg • Phosphorus (as Dicalcium Phosphate) 400 mg • Iodine (as Calcium Iodate) 15 mcg • Magnesium (as Magnesium Citrate) 80 mg • Zinc (as Zinc Gluconate) 3 mg • Selenium (as Sodium Selenate) 14 mcg • Copper (as Copper Gluconate) 0.2 mg • Manganese (as Manganese Gluconate) 0.4 mg • Chromium (as Chromium Polynicotinate 24 mcg • Molybdenum (as Sodium Molybdate) 15 mcg • Sodium (as Sodium Chloride, Soy Protein Isolate) 250 mg • Potassium (from Soy Protein Isolate) 360 mg • Stevia (Stevia Rebaudiana) (Leaves) 50 mg. Other Ingredients: Protein Blend (Supro7 Soy Protein Isolate, Cross Flow Microfiltration Whey Protein Isolate, Whey Protein Hydrolysate), Crystalline Fructose, Natural Vanilla Flavors, Magnesium Citrate, Sodium Chloride, Dicalcium Phosphate, Ascorbic Acid, Stevia, Medium Chain Triglycerides, dl-Alpha Tocopheryl Acetate, Zinc Gluconate, Chromium Polynicotinate, Biotin, Vitamin A Palmitate, Niacinamide, Manganese Gluconate, Copper Gluconate, d-Calcium Pantothenate, Pyridoxine Hydrochloride, Cholecalciferol, Riboflavin, Thiamin Mononitrate, Cyanocobalamin, Folic Acid, Calcium Iodate, Sodium Molybdate, Sodium Selenate.

Amino-Cartilage - Nutri-Quest Rx
Six tablets contain: Natural Hydrolyzed Protein 6000 mg. Typically Providing: Isoleucine 66 mg • Leucine 174 mg • Lysine 216 mg • Methionine 30 mg • Phenylalanine 126 mg • Threonine 120 mg • Valine 168 mg • Arginine 468 mg • Histidine 36 mg • Alanine 546 mg • Tyrosine 24 mg • Serine 198 mg • Aspartic Acid 336 mg • Glutamic Acid 582 mg • Glycine 1362 mg • Hydroxlysine 60 mg • Hydroxyproline 654 mg • Proline 834 mg.

Amino-Gram Forte - Douglas Laboratories/AMNI
Each tablet contains: L-Lysine 148 mg • L-Histidine 30 mg • L-Arginine 39 mg • L-Aspartic 74 mg • L-Threonine 41 mg • L-Serine 53 mg • L-Glutamic Acid 230 mg • L-Proline 110 mg • L-Alanine 34 mg • L-Cystine 9.4 mg • L-Valine 71.5 mg • L-Methionine 32 mg • L-Isoleucine 59 mg • L-Tyrosine 16 mg • L-Leucine 102.1 mg • L-Phenylalanine 22 mg • L-Tryptophan (naturally occurring) 13 mg • L-Cysteine 10 mg • L-Glutamine 15.3 mg • Taurine 10.7 mg. In a base of Carnitine.

Aminologic - PhysioLogics
Three capsules contain: L-Glutamine 185 mg • L-Aspartic Acid 107 mg • L-Tyrosine 103 mg • L-Leucine 97 mg • L-Valine 97 mg • Taurine 90 mg • L-Phenylalanine 88 mg • L-Proline 82 mg • L-Lysine 77 mg • L-Isoleucine 71 mg • L-Serine 71 mg • L-Alanine 60 mg • L-Threonine 59 mg • L-Methionine 55 mg • L-Arginine 54 mg • Papain NF 50 mg • Bromelain 50 mg • Glycine 48 mg • L-Histidine 41 mg • Pancreatin 4X 25 mg • L-Cystine 23 mg.
See Editor's Note No. 14.

Amino-Plex tablets - Golden Glow Natural Health Products
Each tablet contains: Cysteine Hydrochloride 10 mg • Pyridoxine Hydrochloride (vitamin B6) 5 mg • Riboflavin (vitamin B2) 2.3 mg •

Glycine 50 mg • Ascorbic Acid (vitamin C) 5 mg • Isoleucine 28 mg • Leucine 52 mg • Lysine Hydrochloride 47 mg • Phenylalanine 25 mg • Threonine 22 mg • Tryptophan 5 mg • Valine 36 mg • Methionine 17 mg • Cysteine 5 mg • Alanine 100 mg • Arginine 57 mg • Aspartic Acid 38 mg • Glutamic Acid 115 mg • Histidine 22.5 mg • Proline 92 mg • Serine 29 mg • Tyrosine 28 mg • Ornithine Monohydrochloride 25 mg • Zinc Amino Acid Chelate (equivalent to 500 mcg zinc) 5 mg • Magnesium Amino Acid Chelate (equivalent to 1 mg magnesium) 5 mg.

Amino-VIL - J. R. Carlson Laboratories, Inc.
Each 1 tbsp serving contains: Isoleucine 2000 mg • L-Valine 1600 mg • Leucine 3000 mg.

AminoZyme - Nature's Plus
Each capsule contains: AMINOGEN (Aspergillus niger & Aspergillus oryzae proteolytic complex) 250 mg • Vitamin B6 (Pyridoxine HCL) 10 mg • CoQ10 (Ubiquinone) 2.5 mg • Chromium (Polynicotinate) 25 mcg • Vanadium (Sulfate) 10 mcg.

Amla Kalp - R-U Ved U.S.A.
Indian Gooseberry standardized extract (AMLA) • Dried Catkins • Indian Gallnut • Long Pepper • Indian Pennywort • Cardamom • Nutmeg • Cinnamon • Bamboo Mana • Sandalwood • Asparagus • Bael fruit • Tribulus • Terminalia Chebula • Adhatoda Vesica • Leptadenia Reticulata • Aquilaria Agallocha • Kuch • Ashwagandha • Cyperus • Butterfly pea • Thatch grass • Turmeric • Indian Trumpet flower • Calotropis • Gymnema Auraniticum • Speading Hogweed • Kudju • Uraria Picta • Cashmere bark • Arni • Phaseolus Triobus • Desmodium Gangeticum • Castor oil root • Indian Nightshade • Clarified Butter • Dehydrated Sugar cane • Honey.

AmlaPaste - InterPlexus
Amla fruit (Indian gooseberry, cooked in herbal extract of 31 plants) • Pippali • Indian Gallnut • Ashwaganda • Sesame oil • Clarified Butter • Honey • Bamboo Manna • Dehydrated Cane juice • Cardamom • Haritaki • Satawari • Nutmeg • Sandalwood oil • Pennywort • Cinnamon • Cloves • Saffron.

Amore Plus-Rx - H Enterprise
Vitamin E • Calcium • Arginine • Saw Palmetto • Damiana • Celery • Chinese Cinnamon • Pygeum Africanum bark • Gotu Kola • Rice flour • Magnesium Stearate • Silica.

Amoryn - BioNeurix Corporation
Each capsule contains: Hyperforin from 450 mg Hypericum Perforatum extract (St. John's wort aerial portion, standardized to 5% hyperforin, 0.3% hypericin) 22.5 mg • 5-HTP (5-hydroxytryptophan, from griffonia simplicifolia extract) 25 mg • Vitamin B6 20 mg • Vitamin B12 30 mcg • Folate 200 mcg • Selenium 100 mcg • Vitamin D (D3, cholecalciferol) 250 IU. Other Ingredients: Gelatin, Rice Powder, Magnesium Stearate.

Amp Energy Drink - PepsiCo, Inc
Carbonated Water • High Fructose Corn Syrup and/or Sugar • Citric Acid • Orange juice from concentrate • Natural Flavors • Guarana • Sodium Benzoate • Sodium Polyphosphates • Maltodextrin • Caffeine • Gum Arabic • Erythoric Acid • Taurine • Panax Ginseng • Calcium Disodium EDTA • Potassium Benzoate • Brominated Vegetable oil • Yellow 5.

Amplifico (Nero Amplifico) - Caesars Empire
Zinc Oxide • Yohimbe • Maca (lepidium meyenii) • L-Arginine • Oat Straw • Deer Antler • Muira Puama • Oyster meat • Orchic substance • Tribulus Terrestris • Boron Citrate • Nettle leaf • Cayenne • Pumpkin • Licorice • Astragalus • Ginseng Blend: Korean Ginseng, American Ginseng, Siberian Ginseng.

Amplify - NDS Nutrition
Each level scoop contains: Proprietary Blend 908 g: Cold-Filtered Whey Protein concentrate, Whey Protein isolate, Hydrolyzed Whey Protein (producing di, tri-oligo and poly-peptides from speically filtered and ion-exchanged whey protein concentrate (comprising B-lactoglobulin [approx. 46%], A-lactobumin [approx. 24%], immunoglobin [approx. 10%], lactoferrin)), Natural Flavors.

AmyNex-I - Global Life Laboratory Corp.
Each capsule contains: Turmeric (Curcuma longa) 200 mg • Ginger (Zingiber officinale) 190 mg • Ginkgo (Ginkgo biloba) 120 mg. Other Ingredients: Gelatin, Magnesium.

An Fu Le capsules - Eu Yan Sang
Spina Gleditsiae • Flos Lonicerae • Radix Trichosanthis • Myrrha • Olibanum • Radix Angelicae Dahuricae • Radix Paeonia Rubra • Bulbus Fritillariae Thunbergii • Radix Glycyrrhizae • Radix Angelicae Sinensis • Pericarpium Citri Reticulatae • Radix Lebedouriellae.

An Ji Le capsules - Eu Yan Sang
Pericarpium Acecae • Radix Angelicae Dahuricae • Folium Perillae • Poria • Rhizoma Pinelliae • Rhizoma Atractylodis Macroephalae • Pericarpium Citri Reticulatae • Radix Platycodi • Herba Pogostemonis • Radix Glycyrrhizae • Rhizoma Zingiberis Recens • Fructus Ziziphi Jujubae.

Anabolic Complex - The Kutting Edge
Two capsules contain: 10-Norandrosenedione 100 mg • 5-Andro-3B-17B Diol 100 mg • Androstenedione 100 mg • Phosphatidylserine 100 mg • Tribulus 150 mg • Chrysin 50 mg.
See Editor's Note No. 47.

Anabolic Fuel - TwinLab
Four capsules contain: L-Leucine 2000 mg • L-Valine 500 mg • L-Isoleucine 500 mg.

Anamu - Nature's Sunshine
Each capsule contains: Anamu leaf (petiveria alliacea) 400 mg. Other Ingredients: Gelatin, Water.

Anatrin - Progressive Health Nutraceuticals
Vitamin B1 25 mg • Magnesium 400 mg • Malic Acid 300 mg • Creatine Monohydrate 500 mg • Cordyceps 500 mg • Astragalus 300 mg • 5-Methyl-7-Methyloxflavone 10 mg • Turmeric 2 mg.

Andro Infusion - Mass Quantities, Inc.
Each capsule contains: 4-Androstenediol 100 mg • 5-Androstenediol 50 mg • Silymarin 20 mg • Niacin 10 mg • Zinc 5 mg.
See Editor's Note No. 54.

Andro Surge - MRM
Each capsule contains: Androstenedione 100 mg.
See Editor's Note No. 47.

Andro Surge - Country Life Vitamins
Each capsule contains: Tribulus Terrestris 100 mg • Moomiyo 50 mg • Dehydroepiandrosterone 50 mg • Vitamin E 25 IU.

Andro-6 - EAS, Inc.
Four tablets contain: DHEA 50 mg • Androstenedione 100 mg • Tribulus terrestris 250 mg • Chrysin 150 mg • Saw Palmetto extract 180 mg • Indole-3-Carbinol 50 mg • Zinc Glycinate 8 mg.
See Editor's Note No. 47.

Androbolic - ProLab
Two tablets contain: 19-Norandrostenedione 100 mg • 4-Androstene-3,17 Diol 100 mg • 5-Androstene-3,17 Diol 50 mg • Tribulus Terrestris 250 mg • Saw Palmetto 180 mg • Chrysin 150 mg • Indole 3 Carbinol 50 mg.

Andro-Diol - New Hope Health Products
Each capsule contains: 4-androstene-3, 17-diol 100 mg.

Androdiol Select 300 - ErgoPharm/Proviant Technologies
Each capsule contains: 4-Androstenediol (androdiol) 300 mg. Other Ingredients: Corn Starch.
See Editor's Note No. 54.

Some Brand Name Natural Products - What they Contain

www.NaturalDatabase.com contains MANY more listings than appear here.
Editor's Notes are located on pages 2155-2163.

BRAND NAMES

Androdyne - Cytodyne LLC
Three capsules contain: 19-Norandrostenedione 100 mg • 5-Androstene-3B, 17b-Diol 50 mg • 4-Androstene-3,17-dione 50 mg • AA-t3 Anti-Aromatase Complex 100 mg: Chrysin, Indole 3-Carbinol, 7-IsoPropoxyIsoflavone • Zinc Gluconate 20 mg • B3 Nicotinic Acid 50 mg.
See Editor's Note No. 47.

Andro-Edge - Aarisse Health Care
Each 1.75 oz pump contains: 4-Androstene-3, 17-Dione Androstenediol • Tribulus Terrestris • Chrysin • Damiana extract • Vitamin E • Zinc.
See Editor's Note No. 54.

Andrographis Plus - Metagenics
Two tablets contain: Andrographis leaf extract (andrographis paniculata, standardized to 2.5% andrographolides) 400 mg • Amla fruit 4:1 extract (emblica officinalis, containing a minimum of 30% tannins) 200 mg • Proprietary 5:1 Herbal Extract 400 mg: Adenophora root (adenophora tetraphylla), Apricot seed (prunus armeniaca), White Mulberry leaf (morus alba), Gardenia fruit (gardenia jasminoides), Soybean (glycine max), Zhejiang Fritillaria bulb (fritillaria thunbergii), Pear fruit (pyrus pyri).

Androplex - Ortho Molecular Products
Each capsule contains: Muira Puama root 4:1 extract 400 mg • Panax Ginseng root extract (standardized to contain 10% ginsenosides) 100 mg • Ginkgo Biloba leaf extract (standardized to contain 24% ginkgo flavonglycosides and 6% terpene lactones) 60 mg. Other Ingredients: Natural Vegetable Capsules, Magnesium Stearate, Microcrystalline Cellulose.

Andro-Plex - Unknown
Each tablet contains: Vitamin A (fish liver oil) 2500 IU • Vitamin C 100 mg • Vitamin E (D-alpha tocopherol) 50 IU • Calcium (amino acid chelate) 50 mg • Magnesium (amino acid chelate) 25 mg • Zinc (amino acid chelate) 15 mg • Orchic (testicle substance) 100 mg • Raw Adrenal Tissue 10 mg • Raw Pituitary Tissue 5 mg • Raw Prostate Tissue 100 mg • Proprietary Blend 123.5 mg: Saw Palmetto (serenoa repens), Damiana leaf (turmera aphrodesiaca), Licorice root (glycyrrhiza glabra), Sarsparilla (smilax medica), Ginseng (panax ginseng), Hibisucs, DNA, RNA.
See Editor's Note No. 14.

AndroPlex 700 - AST Sports Science
Two capsules contain: Tribulus Terrestris 500 mg • Androstenedione 100 mg • DHEA 100 mg.
See Editor's Note No. 47.

Andro-Stack 850 - Optimum Nutrition
Two capsules contain: pharmaceutical grade Androstenedione (Delta-4-androstene-3-17-dione) 100 mg • pharmaceutical grade DHEA (Dehydroepiandrosterone) 100 mg • Tribulus terrestris 650 mg.
See Editor's Note No. 47.

AndrosteDERM - MedLean
2 ml contain: 4-Androstenediol (Androdiol from Pat Arnold's LPJ Research) 90 mg • Androstenedione 30 mg.
See Editor's Note No. 47 and No. 54.

Androstene Power - Olympian Labs
Each capsule contains: 4-Androstene 3, 17-dione 50 mg.

Androstenediol 300 - Higher Power
Each capsule contains: Androstenediol (4-Androstene,17-diol) 300 mg.
See Editor's Note No. 54.

Androstenedione with Yohimbe - Puritan's Pride
Each capsule contains: Androstenedione 100 mg • Yohimbe bark extract (standardized for 8 mg Yohimbine) 400 mg.
See Editor's Note No. 47.

Androstenetrione Powder - ErgoPharm/Proviant Technologies
Each 1/4 tsp serving contains: Androstenetrione 440 mg.

Andro-Surge - Metabolic Response Modifiers
Each capsule contains: Androstenedione (4-androstene-3, 17-dione) 100 mg.
See Editor's Note No. 47.

Andro-Surge - New Hope Health Products
Each capsule contains: Androstenedione (4-androstene-3, 17-dione) 100 mg.
See Editor's Note No. 47.

Andro-Xtreme - Metabolic Response Modifiers
Two capsules contain: Dehydroepiandrosterone (DHEA) 100 mg • Androstenedione (4-androstene-3, 17-dione) 100 mg • 5-androstenediol (5-androstene 3, 17- diol) 50 mg • Tribulus terrestris 500 mg • Chrysin 250 mg.
See Editor's Note No. 47 and No. 54.

ANDRO-Xtreme - New Hope Health Products
Each capsule contains: Dehydroepiandrosterone (DHEA) 100 mg • Androstenedione (4-androstene-3, 17-dione) 100 mg • 5-androstenediol (5-androstene-3, 17-diol) 50 mg • Tribulus terrestris 500 mg • Chrysin 250 mg.
See Editor's Note No. 47 and No. 54.

Androzyme - Progressive Labs
Each capsule contains: Vitamin E (d-alpha tocopheryl succinate) 50 IU • Zinc (as zinc aspartate) 15 mg • Raw Orchic concentrate (bovine) 100 mg • Siberian Ginseng (Eleutherococcus senticosus) 100 mg • L-Carnitine 30 mg.
See Editor's Note No. 14.

Angel Hair - Physicians Laboratories
Two ounces contain: Certified Isoflavone 15 mg. Other Ingredients: Soy Protein Isolate, Niacin, Iron (ferrous sulfate), Thiamin Mononitrate, Riboflavin, Folic Acid.

Animal Chews - Puritan's Pride
Two tablets contain: Vitamin A (as retinyl palmitate & beta carotene) 5,000 IU • Vitamin C (as calcium ascorbate) 120 mg • Vitamin D (as cholecalciferol) 400 IU • Vitamin E (as d-alpha tocopheryl acid succinate) 30 IU • Vitamin K (as phytonadione) 2 mcg • Thiamin (Vitamin B1; as thiamine mononitrate) 1.5 mg • Riboflavin (Vitamin B2) 1.7 mg • Niacin (as niacinamide) 20 mg • Vitamin B6 (as pyridoxine hydrochloride) 2 mg • Folic Acid 400 mcg • Vitamin B12 (as cyanocovalamin) 6 mcg • Biotin (as d-biotin) 300 mcg • Pantothenic Acid (as d-calcium pantothenate) 10 mg • Calcium (as calcium carbonate, calcium citrate, and calcium ascorbate) 250 mg • Iron (as ferrous fumarate) 4 mg • Iodine (as potassium iodide and kelp) 75 mcg • Magnesium (as magnesium ascorbate and magnesium oxide) 100 mg • Zinc (as zinc amino acid chelate) 7.5 mg • Selenium (as L-Selenomethionine) 15 mcg • Copper (as cupric gluconate) 1 mg • Manganese (as manganese gluconate) 1 mg • Chromium (as chromium polynicotinate) 15 mcg • Molybdenum (as sodium molybdate) 10 mcg • Boron (sodium borate) 10 mcg • Vanadium (as vanadyl sulfate) 5 mcg • Nickel (as nickelous sulfate) 2 mcg • Tin (as stannous chloride) 2 mcg • Choline Phosphatides (as lecithin) 2 mg • Inositol Phosphatides (as lecithin) 5 mg • Rutin 5 mg • Green Barley juice powder 3 mg • Chlorella powder 3 mg • Spirulina powder 5 mg • Alfalfa juice powder 5 mg • Rice Bran powder 10 mg • Carrot juice powder 5 mg • Natural Licorice root 4 mg.

Animal Chews with Calcium - Puritan's Pride
Two tablets contain: Vitamin A (50% as retinyl palmitate and 50% as beta-carotene) 5,000 IU • Vitamin C (as calcium ascorbate) 120 mg • Vitamin D (as cholecalciferol) 400 IU • Vitamin E (as d-alpha tocopheryl acid succinate) 30 IU • Thiamin (as thiamine mononitrate) 1.5 mg • Riboflavin 1.7 mg • Niacin (as niacinamide) 20 mg • Vitamin B6 (as pyridoxine hydrochloride) 2 mg • Folic Acid 0.4 mg • Vitamin B12 (as cyanocobalamin) 6 mcg • Biotin 100 mcg •

Pantothenic Acid (as d-calcium pantothenate) 10 mg • Calcium (as calcium carbonate, calcium citrate, and calcium ascorbate) 250 mg. In a base containing Raspberry Juice Concentrate, Rose Hips, Acerola, Black Currant Juice, Fructose, Fruit Juice Solids, Dried Dates, Dried Apricots, and Dried Peaches.

Animal Cuts Free **-** Universal Nutrition
Each pack contains: Niacin (as niacinamide) 15 mg • Vitamin B6 (as pyridoxine HCl) 2 mg • Thermogenic Complex 575 mg: Synephrine, Octopamine, Tyramine, EGCG (epigallocatechin gallate), L-Theanine, PEA (phenylethylamine) • Lipotropic Complex 75 mg: Choline Citrate, Betaine HCl, Inositol Monophosphate • Metabolic Complex 900 mg: Guarana (22% caffeine), L-Carnitine • Diuretic Complex 750 mg: Dandelion extract (taraxol, taraxerol), Uva Ursi extract (arbutin, methyl-arbutin) • Thyroid Complex 175 mg: Guggul (2.5% guggulsterones), Soy Isoflavones • Insulin Potentiators 100 mg: Alpha Lipoic Acid, Chromium Polynicotinate, Chromium Picolinate • Nucleotide Regulators 300 mg: Phospate, Inosine, Phosphatidylcholine • Neurotransmitter Regulators 250 mg: St. John's Wort (0.3% hypericin), L-Tyrosine • Animal Cuts Complex 812 mg: Citriline Hydroxycitric Acid, Grapefruit extract (naringin, naringenin), White Willow bark, Phenylalanine (as L-phenylalanine), Ginger root extract (gingerols, shoagols). Other Ingredients: Bitter Orange Extract, Green Tea Extract, Cocoa Extract, Potassium Phosphate, Magnesium Phosphate, Magnesium Stearate, Gelatin, Stearic Acid.
See Editor's Note No. 40.

Animal Mix **-** Professional Complementary Health Formulas
Adrenal 3X, 4X • ACTH 6X, 30X • Histamine 12X • Liver 6X, 12X • Camel, Cat (short and long haired), Chicken, Cow, Dog (short and long haired), Duck, Fish Scale (fresh and salt water), Goat (angora/mohair), Goose, Guinea Pig Hog, Horse, Llama, Mouse, Pheasant, Quail, Rabbit, Rat, Sheep (wool), Turkey 6X, 12X, 60X, 100X • Purified Water • 20% USP Alcohol.
See Editor's Note No. 1.

Animal Pak **-** Universal Nutrition
Two paks (22 tablets) contain: Vitamin A (as acetate & 66% as beta-carotene) 9900 IU • Vitamin C (as ascorbic acid) 1 g • Vitamin D (as ergocalciferol) 680 IU • Vitamin E (as D-A-tocopheryl acetate) 300 IU • Thiamin (as thiamin HCl) 76 mg • Riboflavin 76 mg • Niacin (as niacinamide) 82 mg • Vitamin B6 (as pyridoxine HCl) 72 mg • Folic Acid 400 mcg • Vitamin B12 (as cyanocobalamin) 6 mcg • Biotin 300 mcg • Pantothenic Acid (as calcium pantothenate) 76 mg • Calcium (as citrate, carbonate) 2 g • Phosphorus (as calcium phosphate) 228 mg • Iodine (from kelp) 150 mcg • Magnesium (as oxide) 133 mg • Zinc (as oxide) 30 mg • Selenium (as selenite) 50 mcg • Copper (as sulfate) 600 mcg • Manganese (as sulfate) 11 mg • Chromium (as picolinate) 6 mcg • Potassium (as sulfate) 200 mg • Amino Acid Blend: Lysine (from lactalbumin) 300 mg, Methionine (from lactalbumin) 500 mg, Leucine (from lactalbumin) 100 mg, Valine (from lactalbumin) 760 mg, Threonine (from lactalbumin) 48 mg, Glutamic Acid (from lactalbumin) 700 mg, Phenylalanine (from lactalbumin) 560 mg, Arginine (as L-arginine) • Performance Optimizers: Siberian Ginseng root 2 g, Oriental Ginseng root 250 mg, Smilax Officinalis root 500 mg, Protogen A (as thioctic acid) 200 mg, Inosine (as hypoxanthine riboside) 500 mg, Pyridoxine A-Ketoglutarate (PAK) 200 mg, Carnitine (as L-carnitine) 25 mg, Chromium Picolinate 50 mcg, Coenzyme A 20 mg, Coenzyme B12 10 mg, Phosphatidylcholine 200 mg, Para-Aminobenzoic Acid (PABA) 400 mg, Colostrum (bovine) 25 mg, Argentine Liver (bovine) 3.9 g, Shark Cartilage 1 g, Choline Complex 1.2 g, Citrus Bioflavonoids 1 g • Essential Fatty Acid Complex: Linoleic Acid 200 mg, Oleic Acid 100 mg • Digestive Enzymes: Betaine HCl 200 mg, Pepsin 64 mg, Papain 64 mg, Ox Bile (bovine) 120 mg, Pancreatin 700 mg, Mycozyme 64 mg. Other Ingredients: Maltodextrin, Calcium Sulfate, Choline Citrate, Magnesium Stearate, Stearic Acid, Parsley, Goldenseal, Dong Quai, Burdock, Alfalfa, Watercress, Rice Bran, Cellulose, Rose Hips.
See Editor's Note No. 14.

Animal Parade Children's Chewable Calcium **-** Nature's Plus
Two chewable tablets contain: Calcium (as amino acid/chelate complex) 250 mg • Magnesium (as aminoate complex) 50 mg. Other Ingredients: Fructose, Natural Vanilla, Spinach Leaf Extract (spinacia oleracea), Broccoli Floret extract (brassica oleracea), Fig Concentrate (ficus carica), Date Concentrate (phoenix dactylifera), Stearic Acid, Magnesium Stearate.

Animal Stak **-** Universal Nutrition
Each pak contains: Vitamin C (as ascorbic acid) 50 mg • Vitamin B6 (as pyridoxine HCl) 10 mg • Calcium (as sulfate, phosphate) 200 mg • Zinc (as picolinate) 15 mg • Chromium (as picolinate) 100 mcg • Prohormone Complex: 19-Nor-5-Androstenedione 100 mg, 5-Androxydiol 100 mg, Dehydroepiandrosterone 50 mg • LH Boosters: Tribulus extract (standardized to 20-29% steroidal saponins) 250 mg, Acetyl-L-Carnitine 250 mg, L-Carnitine 100 mg • Growth Hormone Secretagogues: L-Arginine Pyroglutamate 2.5 g, L-Ornithine Alpha-Ketoglutarate 1.3 g, L-Taurine 750 mg, Colostrum (bovine) 250 mg • Anti-Aromatase Inhibitors: Chrysin 250 mg, Kudzu extract (isoflavones) 150 mg • DHT Blockers: Beta Sitosterol 250 mg, Saw Palmetto fruit 200 mg, Pygeum Africanum Hook f. bark 50 mg • Thermogenic Factors: Guarana extract (standardized for 20-29% steroidal saponins) 570 mg, Bitter Orange extract (standardized for 4% synephrine) 500 mg, Coleus Forskohlii extract (standardized for 20% forskohlin) 50 mg • Liver Detoxifiers: Lysolphosphatidylcholine 100 mg, Milk Thistle seed 75 mg.
See Editor's Note No. 40.

Animi-3 **-** PBM Pharmaceuticals, Inc.
Each capsule contains: Folic Acid 1 mg • Vitamin B6 12.5 mg • Vitamin B12 500 mcg • Omega-3 Acids 500 mg: Docosahexaenoic Acid (DHA) 350 mg and Eicosapentaenoic Acid (EPA) 35 mg. Other Ingredients: Yellow Beeswax, Sunflower Oil, Bleached Lecithin, Ascorbic Acid, Glycerin, Titanium Dioxide, FD&C Red 40, Purified Water.

Anise Star Galaxy **-** RedSafari
100% Pure Anise Star essential oil.

Anistil **-** Progressive Health Nutraceuticals
Vitamin B1 10 mg • Vitamin B2 4 mg • Vitamin B3 20 mg • Vitamin B6 10 mg • Methylcobalamin 500 mcg • Folic Acid 400 mcg • Magnesium 250 mg • Zinc 10 mg • N-Acetyl L-Carnitine HCl 50 mg • N-Acetyl Cysteine HCl 75 mg • Alpha Lipoic Acid 75 mg • CoEnzyme Q10 1 mg • Butcher's Broom 300 mg • Ginkgo Biloba extract 100 mg • Larch Arabinogalactan 150 mg • Resveratrol 5 mg.

Anorex **-** Klein-Becker
Two capsules contain: Calcium (amino acid chelate) 264 mg • Vitamin B6 25 mg • Anorex (Leptoprin) Proprietary Blend 989 mg: Acetylsalicylic Acid 324 mg, Caffeine (34 mg from standardized kola nut) (280 mg) 200 mg, Green Tea leaf extract (standardized for polyphenols/catechins content), L-Tyrosine, Kelp (0.155 Iodine [100 mg]), Ephedrine Alkaloids from Ma Huang (10% extract from whole plant 200 mg), Cayenne (fruit).
See Editor's Note No. 30 and No. 51.

Anorex-SF **-** Klein-Becker
Two capsules contain: Calcium (amino acid chelate) 132 mg • Anorex (Leptoprin S-F) Proprietary Blend 1493.5 mg: Calcium Phosphate, Commiphora Mukul extract, Garcinia Cambogia (HCA 125 mg), L-Tyrosine, Acetylsalicylic Acid (162.5 mg), Dipotassium Phosphate, Sodium Phosphate, Disodium Phosphate, Phosphatidyl Choline, Scutellaria root, Bupleurum root, Epimedium herb. Other Ingredients: Rice Flour.
See Editor's Note No. 22.

Anotesten **-** MuscleTech
Six capsules contain: 4-Androstenediol 150 mg • Androstenedione 250 mg • DHEA 100 mg • Tribulus Terrestris 1000 mg • Chrysin

150 mg • Indole-3-Carbinol (I3C) 50 mg • Saw Palmetto (standardized for 25% fatty acids) 320 mg.
See Editor's Note No. 47 and No. 54.

Antacid - Progressive Labs
Each tablet contains: Calcium Carbonate 500 mg which supplies: Calcium (from calcium carbonate) 200 mg. Other Ingredients: Dextrose, Mannitol, Cellulose, Magnesium Stearate, Glycine and Spearmint oil. Free of Sodium & Aluminum.

Anthocyan - PhytoPharmica
Two capsules contain: Vitamin A (beta-carotene) 10,000 IU • Vitamin C (ascorbic acid) 200 mg • Riboflavin (vitamin B2) 10 mg • Bilberry (Vaccinium myrtillus fruit berry) extract (standardized to contain 25% anthocyanosides [40 mg per 2 capsules] calculated as anthocyanidins) 160 mg.
See Editor's Note No. 21.

AnthoMax - Pure Encapsulations
Each vegetable capsule contains: Bilberry fruit extract (vacinium myrtillus, standardized to contain 18% anthocyans) 100 mg • Bilberry fruit extract (vaccinium myrtillus, standardized to contain 50% antohocyanosides) 50 mg • Vitamin C (as ascorbyl palmitate) 2 mg.

Anti - Grandma's Herbs
Each capsule contains: Proprietary Blend 0.451 g: Garlic herb, Goldenseal root, Echinacea Angustifolia root, Myrrh gum, Plantain leaves, Propolis herb. Other Ingredients: Gelatin.

Anti Oxidant - Nutritional Therapeutics, Inc.
Two tablets contain: Vitamin B2 (as riboflavin/ribose-5-phosphate) 50 mg • Vitamin B6 (as pyridoxine HCl/P-5-P) 40 mg • Vitamin E (as D-alpha, mixed tocopherols) 200 IU • Vitamin c (as calcium ascorbate) 160 mg • Vitamin A (as natural beta-carotene, mixed carotenoids, acetate) 10,000 IU • Zinc (as monomethionine) 30 mg • Selenium (as selenomethionine) 100 mcg • Folic ACid 80 mcg • Calcium (as calcium ascorbate) 25 mg • Garlic (as odorless) 8 mg • Grape seed (as Activin brand) 10 mg • Green Tea extract 100 mg • L-Arginine 20 mg • L-Glycine 17 mg • N-Acetyl-L-Cysteine 50 mg • NT Factor (as tablet base) 380 mg • Pantethine (as coenzyme A precursor) 11 mg • Phosphoglycolipids 11 mg. Other Ingredients: Microcrystalline Cellulose, Croscarmellose Sodium Food Glaze, Silica, Vegetable Magnesium Stearate.

Anti-Age/Energy Formula - Body Language Vitamin Co.
Each capsule contains: Alpha Lipoic Acid 150 mg • Acetyl L-Carnitine 150 mg • Coenzyme Q10 60 mg • Glutathione 30 mg.

Anti-Aging - Vidafit
Each serving contains: Biotin 30 mcg • Folate 400 mcg • Niacin 20 mg • Pantothenic Acid 10 mg • Riboflavin 1.7 mg • Thiamine 1.5 mg • Vitamin A 3300 IU • Vitamin B12 6 mcg • Vitamin B6 10 mg • Vitamin C 120 mg • Vitamin D 400 IU • Vitamin E 30 IU • Boron 1 mg • Calcium 500 mg • Magnesium 250 mg • Phosphorus 500 mg • Selenium 70 mcg • Zinc 15 mg • Acetyl-L-Carnitine 50 mg • Coenzyme Q10 20 mg • Quercetin 20 mg • Bilberry 50 mg • Ginkgo extract 50 mg • Grape seed extract 50 mg • Soy Protein 2 g.

Anti-Anxiety - PhytoPharmica
Twenty drops contain: Cicuta Virosa 4X • Gaultheria 4X • Ignatia 4X • Staphysagria 4X • Asa Foetida 3X • Corydalis Formosa 3X • Hyoscyamus 3X • Sumbulus 3X • Valeriana Officianalis 3X • Avena sativa 1X. In a base of 40% USP alcohol by volume.
See Editor's Note No. 1 and No. 21.

Anti-Arthritis Glucosamine Chondroitin - Crystal Springs
Each tablet contains: Glucosamine (Sulfate) 600 mg • Chondroitin Sulfate 400 mg.
See Editor's Note No. 15.

AntiBetic Pancreas Tonic - Gero Vita International
Each capsule contains: Pterocarpus Marsupium (Indian kino tree, fabaceae family) 195 mg • Gymnema Sylvestre (gymnema) 175 mg • Momordica Charantia (bitter melon) 40 mg • Azadirachta Indica (neem) 20 mg • Tinospora Cordifolia (heart leaved moonseed) 30 mg • Aegle Marmelos (bael) 40 mg • Syzygium Cumini (jambolan) 50 mg • Cinnamonum Tamala (cinnamon leaf) 20 mg • Trigonella Foenum-Graecum (fenugreek) 65 mg • Ficus Racemosa (cluster fig) 15 mg.

AntiBio 1 - Dial Herbs
Echinacea • Goldenseal • Poke root • Cayenne.

AntiBio 2 - Dial Herbs
Echinacea • Myrrh • Poke root • Cayenne.

Anti-Catabolic Fuel - TwinLab
Four capsules contain: L-Leucine 1000 mg • L-Valine 225 mg • L-Isoleucine 225 mg • Ketoisocaproate (KIC) 100 mg • L-Ornithine, Alpha-Ketoglutarate 1000 mg • L-Glutamine 250 mg.

Anti-Cholesterol Formula - Body Language Vitamin Co.
Three tablets contain: Artichoke (Cynara scolymnus, 15% caffeoylquinic/chlorogenic acids) 100 mg • Chitosan 300 mg • Garlic 300 mg • Chinese Red Yeast Rice 500 mg • Garcinia fruit 100 mg • Myristica fragrans 100 mg • Grapefruit Pectin 400 mg • Gugulipid 200 mg • Beta-sitosterol 200 mg • Hyaluronic Acid 200 mg • EDTA 200 mg • Milk Thistle 250 mg • Policosanol 10 mg • Vitamin B12 mcg • Folate 400 mcg.

Anti-Depressant Formula With St. John's Wort - Life Extension
Each capsule contains: Standardized Herbal Blend 0.450 mg: St. John's Wort (standardized for 0.3% hypericin), Kava Kava, Ginkgo Biloba.

Anti-Fatigue - PhytoPharmica
Twenty drops contain: Zincum Muriaticum 8X • Gelsemium Sempervirens 6X • Picricum Acidum 6X • Acidum Phosphoricum 3X • Valeriana Officinalis 1X. In a base of 45% USP alcohol by volume.
See Editor's Note No. 1 and No. 21.

Anti-Fungal - The Herbalist
Thuja leaf • Usnea lichen • Spilanthes herb • Pau D'Arco inner bark • Echinacea root • Calendula flower • Cayenne pepper.

Anti-Fungal Salve - Blessed Herbs
Jewelweed • Black Walnut hulls • Pau d'Arco bark • Usnea lichen • Calendula flowers • Spilanthes • Echinacea Angustifolia root • Goldenseal root • Myrrh Gum • Organic Cold-Pressed Olive oil • Beeswax • Essential oils of Tea Tree & Thyme linalol.

Anti-Gas - Nature's Sunshine
Two capsules contain: Proprietary Blend 982 mg: Papaya fruit (carica papaya), Ginger rhizome (zingiber officinale), Peppermint leaf (mentha piperita), Wild Yam root (dioscorea villosa), Fennel seed (foeniculum vulgare), Dong Quai root (angelica sinensis), Lobelia aerial parts (lobelia inflata), Spearmint leaf and flower (mentha spicata), Catnip aerial parts (nepeta cataria). Other Ingredients: Gelatin, Water.

Anti-HangOver - Jamieson
Each capsule contains: Botanical Complex AK280 243 mg: Perilla Frutescens, Agastache Rugosa • Taurine 37 mg.

Anti-Insom - Dial Herbs
Hops • Lobelia • Valerian • Cayenne.

Anti-Nausea Ginger Gum - Sea-Band LTD
Each piece contains: Ginger oil (equivalent to 8 g fresh ginger root) 25 mg.

Anti-Ox: Herbal Antioxidant - The Herbalist
Pau D'Arco inner bark • Astragalus root • Ginkgo leaf • Milk Thistle seed • Licorice root • Cayenne pepper.

Antioxidant - Oasis Wellness Network
Each tablet contains: Vitamin C (as ascorbic acid) 125 mg • Vitamin E (as D-alpha-tocopheryl acetate) 50 IU • Niacin (as niacinamide

ascorbate) 25 mg • Folate (as folic acid) 100 mcg • Calcium (as calcium sulfate) 15 mg • MaxCell Proprietary Blend 125 mg: Zisyphus Jujube, Aloe Vera gel, Piper Nigrum, Glycyrrhiza Glabra • L-Cysteine (base) 50 mg • Bioflavonoid Complex 25 mg • Green Tea leaf extract 25 mg • Rosemary leaf extract 25 mg • Turmeric rhizome extract 25 mg • Carotenoid mixture 10 mg • Grape seed extract 10 mg. Other Ingredients: Calcium Sulfate, Stearic Acid, Cellulose, Silica, Magnesium Stearate.

Antioxidant - Enzymes, Inc.
Three capsules contain: Vitamin A (as beta-carotene from dunaliella algae) 7500 IU • Vitamin C (from acerola cherry) 45 mg • Vitamin E (from D-alpha tocopheryl acid succinate) 90 IU • Zinc (from zinc citrate) 9 mg • Selenium (from selenium citrate) 45 mcg • Copper (from copper citrate) 0.75 mg • Manganese (from manganese citrate) 3 mg • n-zimes brand Proprietary Enzyme Blend 36 mg: pHysioProtease (88,800 pHysio-U), CereCalase Plus • Proprietary Herbal Blend 159 mg: Quercetin, Rutin, Hesperidin extract, Citrus Bioflavonoids, Rice Bran, Green Tea leaf extract, Lutein extract, Lycopenes extract, Grape seed extract, Lipoic Acid, Milk Thistle seed extract, Ginkgo Biloba leaf extract, Bilberry fruit extract, conc. of Brococoli, Cabbage, Brussel sprouts, Cauliflower, Kale, Watercress. Other Ingredients: Plant Cellulose, Water.

AntiOxidant - HealthMinded
Each tablet contains: Vitamin C (ascorbic acid and calcium ascorbate) 300 mg • Selenium (L-selenomethionine) 100 mcg • Antioxidant Proprietary Blend 44 mg: Alpha Lipoic Acid, Lutein, Lycopene, Zeaxanthin, Alpha Carotene, Pycnogenol, CoQ10. Other Ingredients: Di Calcium Phosphate, Stearic Acid, Croscarmellose Sodium, Magnesium Stearate, Micro Crystalline Cellulose, Silicon Dioxide.

Anti-oxidant - Douglas Laboratories/AMNI
Three capsules contain: Vitamin C (as ascorbic acid/ascorbyl palmitate complex) 200 mg • Bioflavonoids 200 mg • L-Cysteine 200 mg • Choline Bitartrate 200 mg • Inositol 200 mg • Vitamin E 150 IU • L-Methionine 20 mg • Vitamin A (as beta carotene) 12,500 IU • Vitamin B1 40 mg • Vitamin B2 20 mg • Niacinamide 20 mg • Pantothenic Acid 20 mg • Vitamin B6 (as pyridoxal-5-phosphate) 20 mg • DMG (dimethylglycine) 20 mg • Glutathione 15 mg • Selenium (as selenium Krebs) 50 mcg.

Antioxidant & Multivitamin Formula - Weil Lifestyle, LLC
Each Daily Antioxidant capsule contains: Vitamin A as Beta Carotene 15,000 IU • Vitamin D 400 IU • Selenium 200 mcg • Alpha-Carotene 1 mg • Astaxanthin 750 mcg • Coenzyme Q10 (CoQ10) 30 mg • Gamma Carotene 132 mcg • Lutein 5 mg • Lycopene 10 mg • Phytoene 800 mcg • Phytofluene 800 mcg • Zeaxanthin 300 mcg • Natural Mixed Tocopherols 159 mg • Palm Tocotrienols Complex 17 mg: D-Alpha Tocotrienols 5 mg, D-Gamma Tocotrienols 10 mg, D-Delta Tocotrienols 2 mg.
Each Daily Mulitvitamin Tablet contains: Vitamin C 125 mg • Thiamin (vitamin B1) 25 mg • Riboflavin (vitamin B2) 25 mg • Niacin (vitamin B3) 25 mg • Vitamin B6 25 mg • Folate, Folic Acid, Folacin 200 mcg • Vitamin B12 50 mcg • Biotin 50 mcg • Pantothenic Acid 25 mg • Calcium 30 mg • Iodine 75 mcg • Magnesium 15 mg • Zinc 7.5 mg • Copper 0.75 mg • Manganese 0.5 mg • Chromium 100 mcg • Molybdenum 37.5 mcg • Potassium 0.5 mg • Choline 25 mg • Inositol 25 mg • PABA 25 mg • Citrus Bioflavonoid Complex 20 mg • Rutin 20 mg • Flavones 9.8 mg • Sulphur 2.5 mg • Silicon 1 mg • Flavonols 0.2 mg • Vanadium 5 mcg.

Antioxidant 4000 Vitamins & Mineral - Nature's Bounty
Two softgels contain: Vitamin A (as Beta Carotene) 20000 IU • Vitamin C (as Ascorbic Acid) 400 mg • Vitamin E (as dl-Alpha Tocopheryl Acetate) 250 IU • Selenium (as Selenium Yeast) 50 mcg • Proprietary Blend: Carrot powder, Broccoli powder, Spinach powder 6 mg. Other Ingredients: Gelatin, Soy Lecithin, Glycerin, Vegetable Oil.

Antioxidant Booster - Advocare International
Two caplets contain: Vitamin E (as D-alpha tocopheryl succinate) 250 IU • Vitamin C (as ascorbic acid & ascorbyl palmitate) 1000 mg • Beta-Carotene 15,000 IU • Selenium (as selenomethionine) 35 mcg • Zinc (as OptiZinc brand monomethionine) 5 mg • Manganese (as amino acid chelate) 1 mg • Green Tea leaf extract (camellia sinensis) 50 mg • Milk Thistle fruit extract (silybum marianum) 50 mg • ActiVin brand Grape seed and skin extract (vitis vinifera) 100 mg. Other Ingredients: Dicalcium Phosphate, Silicon Dioxide, Cellulose, Stearic Acid, Magnesium Stearate.

Antioxidant Caps - NOW Foods
Two capsules contain: Vitamin A (from 15 mg Beta-Carotene) 25000 IU • Vitamin C (from Calcium Ascorbate) 500 mg • Vitamin E (natural d-Alpha Succinate) 300 IU • Calcium (Ascorbate) 50 mg • Zinc (Picolinate) 5 mg • Selenium (L-Selenomethionine) 25 mcg • N-Acetyl-Cysteine 100 mg • L-Glutathione 25 mg • Alfalfa juice concentrate (Green Superfood) 250 mg • Wheat Sprout concentrate (Enzyme active) 100 mg.

Anti-Oxidant Caps - Vital Nutrients
Each capsule contains: Natural Mixed Carotenes 10,000 IU • Vitamin C (ascorbic acid 100%) 250 mg • Vitamin E (natural source) 200 IU • Selenium (selenomethionine) 50 mcg • Selenium (sodium selenite) 50 mcg • N-Acetyl-Cysteine 100 mg • Ginkgo extract (50:1, 24%/6%) 25 mg • Green Tea extract (80% catechins) 25 mg.

Antioxidant Cocktail Custom Paks - The Vitamin Shoppe
Each packet contains: Vitamin A (as 100% beta-carotene) 15 mg (25000 IU) • Vitamin C (as ascorbic acid) 2000 mg • Vitamin E (as d-alpha, d-gamma, d-beta, d-delta tocopherol) 400 IU • Selenium (as selenomethionine) 200 mcg • Alpha-carotene 1 mg (833 IU) • Lycopene (LYC-O-MATO) 5 mg • Lutein 5 mg • Zeaxanthin 0.24 mg • Phytoene 0.055 mg • Phytofluene 0.026 mg • Citrus Bioflavonoids 1000 mg • Hesperidin 100 mg • Rutin 100 mg • Rose Hips (Rosa canina) fruit 160 mg • Acerola 20 mg.

Antioxidant Cocktail II - The Vitamin Shoppe
Two capsules contain: Pine bark extract (pycnogenol) 30 mg • ActiVin brand Grape seed extract (vitis vinifera) 50 mg • Alpha Lipoic Acid 50 mg • Green Tea leaf (camellia sinensis, standardized to 75% polyphenols) 50 mg.

Antioxidant Formula - Nature's Way
Two capsules contain: Beta Carotene 25,000 IU • Coenzyme Q10 (ubiquinone) 5 mg • Copper amino acid chelate 2 mg • Green Tea, polyphenol catechin extract 10 mg • L-Cysteine 100 mg • Quercetin (eucalyptus) 100 mg • Selenium (l-selenomethione) 200 mcg • Vitamin C 500 mg • Vitamin E (d-alpha tocopheryl) 400 IU • Zinc amino acid chelate 15 mg. Other Ingredients: Gelatin, Magnesium stearate, Maltodextrin, Silica.

Antioxidant Formula - Body Language Vitamin Co.
Two tablets contain: N-Acetyl-L-Cysteine 100 mg • Vitamin E (D-alpha) 400 IU • Beta Carotene 12,000 IU • Vitamin C 800 mg • L-Glutathione 60 mg • Chromium Picolinate 120 mcg • Niacinamide 100 mg • Selenium (methionate) 200 mcg • Vitamin B12 100 mcg • Folic Acid 800 mcg • Manganese (glycinate) 5 mg • Zinc (monomethionate) 30 mg • Ginkgo Biloba (24% ginkgo flavoglycosides) 60 mg • Korean Ginseng (25% ginsenosides) 25 mg • Grape seed extract 45 mg • Green Tea extract 25 mg • Alpha Lipoic Acid 25 mg • Coenzyme Q10 10 mg • Citrus Bioflavonoids 100 mg • Lutein 5 mg • DL-Methionine 60 mg.

Antioxidant Formula - America's Finest
Each tablet contains: Vitamin A (as beta carotene) 8000 IU • Vitamin E (as alpha tocopheryl acetate) 200 IU • Selenium (selenomethionine) 100 mcg • CurcuminC3 Complex from Turmeric root extract (95% curcuminoids) 250 mg • Bioperine Black Pepper fruit extract 5 mg. Other Ingredients: Cellulose, Magnesium Stearate, Pharmaceutical Glaze.

Some Brand Name Natural Products - What they Contain

www.NaturalDatabase.com contains MANY more listings than appear here.

Editor's Notes are located on pages 2155-2163.

BRAND NAMES

AntiOxidant Formula **-** Pure Encapsulations
Each vegetable capsule contains: N-Acetyl-L-Cysteine (NAC) 100 mg • Milk Thistle extract (silybum marianum, standardized to contain 80% silymarin) 100 mg • Vitamin C (as ascorbyl palmitate) 100 gm • Mixed Carotenoids (Betatene brand) 10,000 IU: Beta Carotene 5712 mcg, Alpha Carotene 180 mcg, Zeaxanthin 36 mcg, Cryptoxanthin 44 mcg, Lutein 28 mcg • D-Alpha Tocopherol Succinate (natural vitamin E) 100 IU • Selenium (selenomethionine) 100 mcg • Riboflavin (B2) 25 mg • Zinc (picolinate) 5 mg.

Anti-Oxidant Formula #1 **-** Olympian Labs
Two capsules contain: Cat's Claw (uncaria tomentosa) 500 mg • Ginkgo Biloba extract 60 mg • Crystalline CoQ10 30 mg • Grape seed extract 50 mg.

Antioxidant Fuel **-** TwinLab
Three capsules contain: Beta-Carotene (pro-Vitamin A) 25000 IU • Vitamin C 1000 mg • Natural Vitamin E (Succinate) 800 IU • CoQ10 (Coenzyme Q10) 30 mg • N-Acetyl Cysteine (NAC) 200 mg • L-Glutathione 100 mg • Selenium (from Selenomethionine & Selenate 50/50 mixture) 100 mcg • Alpha-Lipoic Acid (reduced) 100 mcg.

Antioxidant Optimizer **-** Jarrow Formulas
Three tablets contain: Vitamin C (ascorbic acid) 250 mg • Gamma Tocopherol 100 mg • Lutein 5 mg • Lyc-O-Mato brand Lycopene 2 mg • LeucoSelect brand Grape seed OPCs 50 mg • Grape skin extract (30% polyphenols) 150 mg • Silymarin 80% (milk thistle seed 30:1 concentrate) 80 mg • Olive fruit polyphenols (OleaSelect brand) 30 mg • Green Tea 5:1 concentrate (45% polyphenols) 250 mg • Curcumin root 18:1 concentrate 300 mg • Freeze dried Ginger 6:1 200 mg. Other Ingredients: Cellulose, Calcium Phosphate, Modified Cellulose Gum, Stearic Acid, Vegetable Magnesium Stearate, Silicon Dioxide.

Anti-Oxidant Supreme **-** Gaia Herbs
Two capsules contain: Hawthorn berry, solid extract (crataegus spp.) 100 mg • Green Tea leaf, decaffeinated (camellia sinensis) 100 mg • Bilberry berry (vaccinium myrtillus) 50 mg • Ginkgo leaf (ginkgo biloba) 20 mg • Rosemary leaf, supercritical CO2 extract (rosmarinus off.) 8 mg • Prickly Ash bark (xanthoxylum clava-herculis) 8 mg • Astaxanthin 2 mg. Other Ingredients: Vegetable Glycerin, Vegetable Cellulose (capsule).

Antioxidant Tablet **-** Leiner Health Products
Each tablet contains: Vitamin E (d-Alpha Tocopherol Acid Succinate and dl-Alpha Tocopheryl Acetate) 200 IU • Vitamin C (Ascorbic Acid) 250 mg • Selenium 70 mcg • Lutein 0.5 mg • Pine bark extract (Pycnogenol brand) 1 mg. Other Ingredients: Calcium Carbonate, Gelatin, Cellulose, Maltodextrin, Crospovidone, Croscarmellose Sodium, Silicon Dioxide, Spinach, Magnesium Stearate, Tricalcium Phosphate, Starch, Dicalcium Phosphate, Hydroxypropyl Methylcellulose, Pharmaceutical Glaze, Vegetable Oil, Ethylcellulose, Hydroxypropyl Cellulose, Sorbitol, Polysorbate 80, Ascorbyl Palmitate, Sodium Selenate, Polyethylene Glycol, Tocopherols, Zeaxanthin.

AntiSpasmodic **-** Dial Herbs
Scullcap • Skunk Cabbage • Black Cohosh • Myrrh • Lobelia • Cayenne

Anti-Stress **-** Oasis Wellness Network
Each tablet contains: Ashwagandha root extract 150 mg • MaxCell Proprietary Blend 125 mg: Zisyphus Jujube, Aloe Vera gel, Piper Nigrum, Glycyrrhiza Glabra • Gotu Kola extract (whole plant) 100 mg • Taurine 100 mg • Jujube seed extract (zisyphus spinosa) 100 mg • Kava Kava root extract 50 mg. Other Ingredients: Calcium Sulfate, Stearic Acid, Cellulose, Silica, Magnesium Stearate.

Anti-Stress Support **-** Weil Lifestyle, LLC
Each B-50 Complex tablet contains: Thiamin (vitamin B1) 50 mg • Riboflavin (vitamin B2) 50 mg • Niacin (vitamin B3) 50 mg • Vitamin B6 50 mg • Folate, Folic Acid, Folacin 400 mcg • Vitamin B12 50 mcg • Biotin 50 mcg • Pantothenic Acid 50 mg • Choline 50 mcg • Inositol 50 mcg • PABA 50 mg.

Antronex **-** Standard Process, Inc.
Each tablet contains: Calcium 40 mg • Bovine Liver Fat extract (yakriton) 15 mg. Other Ingredients: Arabic Gum, Mixed Tocopherols.
See Editor's Note No. 14.

Anxietol 7 **-** MedaBiotics
Two capsules contain: Vitamin C (as ascorbic acid) 80 mg • Vitamin B6 (as pyridoxine HCl) 3 mg • Vitamin B12 (as cyanocobalamin) 500 mg • Folic Acid (vitamin B9) 200 mg • Serotain brand Griffonia Simplicifolia 250 mg • 5-Hyonaytratophan 45 mg • GABA 200 mg • SunTheanine brand L-Theanine 120 mg • Sensoril 100 mg • Panax Ginseng 100 mg • L-Tyrosine 60 mg • Vinpocetine 10 mg. Other Ingredients: Gelatin, Cellulose, Magnesium Stearate.

Anxiety Control **-** Pain & Stress Center
Two capsules contain: Magnesium (as magnesium oxide) 100 mg • Vitamin B6 (as pyridoxine HCl) 10 mg • Gamma Amino Butyric Acid (GABA) 400 mg • Glycine 100 mg • Glutamine 140 mg • Passion Flower 150 mg • Primula Officinalis herb powder 150 mg. Other Ingredients: Gelatin Capsule.

Anxiety-X **-** Olympian Labs
Two capsules contain: GABA (gamma aminobutyric acid) 150 mg • Niacinamide 150 mg • L-Tyrosine 40 mg • Glycine 40 mg • L-Glutamine 40 mg • Inositol 150 mg • Kava Kava 20 mg • Motherwort 20 mg • Wintergreen 30 mg.

AO Elite **-** VitaCube Systems (V3S)
Two tablets contain: L-Arginine HCl 625 mg • L-Ornithine HCl 375 mg • VitaCube Activating System Proprietary Blend 50 mg: Orange Bioflavonoid Complex, Grapefruit Bioflavonoid Complex, Alfalfa leaf, Ginkgo Biloba leaf, Spirulina algae, Cayenne, Apple Pectin, Odorless Garlic, 7-Isopropoxy Isoflavone, L-Glutathione, Lemon Bioflavonoid Complex, Lycopene 1%, Dimethylglycine, Potassium Glycerophosphate, Rutin, Bromelain, Lutein 5% • Hawthorne berries 10 mg • Capsicum fruit (cayenne pepper herb) 5 mg. Other Ingredients: Cellulose, Stearic Acid, Croscarmellose Sodium, Silicon Dioxide, Magneisum Stearate, White Cellulose Film Coat containing Titanium Dioxide.

Aorta-Glycan **-** Enzymatic Therapy
Each capsule contains: Glycosaminoglycans (GAGs) 50 mg: Dermatan Sulfate, Heparan Sulfate, Hyaluronic Acid, Chondroitin Sulfate, Hexosaminoglycans. Other Ingredients: Gelatin, Magnesium Stearate, Silicon Dioxide, Titanium Dioxide color.
See Editor's Note No. 15.

Aphrodesia **-** Life Extension
Each tablet contains: Yohimbine 25 mg • Kelp 10 mg • Zinc Orotate 120 mg • Niacin 20 mg • Selenium 200 mcg • Siberian Ginseng 60 mg • Damiana leaf 20 mg • Bee Pollen 75 mg • Lecithin 25 mg • L-Lysine 20 mg • Calcium Gluconate 90 mg • Pituitary Gland extract 35 mg.
See Editor's Note No. 31.

Apis-Homaccord **-** Heel/BHI, Inc.
Antimonium Tartaricum 2X, 10X, 30X, 200X • Apisinum 6X, 30X • Scilla Martima 3X, 10X, 30X • Apis Mellifera 2X, 10X, 30X, 200X, 1000X • Ethyl Alcohol 35% by volume.
See Editor's Note No. 1.

APM 60 double-shot (chocolate flavor) **-** Nutripeak
Each packet contains: Protein 60 g • Vitamin A (Retinyl Palmitate and Beta Carotene) 4500 IU • Vitamin C (Ascorbic Acid) 60 mg • Vitamin D (Cholecalciferol) 240 IU • Vitamin E (dl-Tocopheryl Acetate) 45 IU • Vitamin K (Phytonadione) 40 mcg • Thiamin (Vitamin B1) 0.9 mcg • Riboflavin (Vitamin B2) 1 mg • Niacin (Niacinamide) 20 mg • Vitamin B-6 (Pyridoxine Hydrochloride) 1 mg

• Folic Acid 400 mcg • Vitamin B-12 (Cyanocobalamin) 3 mcg • Biotin 180 mcg • Pantothenic Acid (Calcium D-Pantothenate) 4 mg • Calcium Lactate 2 g • Iron (Ferrous Fumarate) 7.2 mg • Phosphorus (Tricalcium Phosphate and Dicalcium Phosphate) 1.3 mg • Iodine (Potassium Iodide) 52 mg • Magnesium (Trimagnesium Phosphate and Magnesium Oxide) 440 mg • Zinc Oxide 5.2 mg • Selenium (Sodium Molybdate) 31 mcg • Copper (Cupric Sulfate) 0.7 mg • Manganese Sulfate 1 mg • Chromium 48 mcg • Molybdenum (Sodium Molybdate) 60 mcg • Sodium 340 mcg • Potassium Chloride and Citrate 1 g • ARS Proprietary Blend: L-Glutamine, Potassium Bicarbonate, Monosodium Orthophosphate, Sodium Citrate Dihydrate, L-Carnosine, Trans-Ferulic Acid 1.6 g •TNA Proprietary Blend: DL-Phenylalanine, L-Tyrosine, Taurine 800 mg • Proulin Proprietary Blend: Myo-Inositol, Alpha-Lipoic Acid, Vanadium, Chromium 201 mg. Other Ingredients: Metamyosyn Protein Blend: Milk Protein Concentrate, Calcium Sodium Caseinate, Whey Protein Concentrate, Dried Egg Albumen, Whey Protein Isolate, Bovine lactoferrin; Cocoa (processed with alkali); Xanthan Gum; Sodium Carboxymethylcellulose; Maltodextrin; Sucralose; Acesulfame Potassium; Natural and Artificial Flavors.

Appeal French Delight - Pharmanex
Each packet contains: Vitamin A (62% as beta-carotene) 2000 IU • Vitamin C 30 mg • Calcium 350 mg • Iron 2.7 mg • Vitamin D 200 IU • Vitamin E 9 mg • Thiamin 0.45 mg • Riboflavin 0.76 mg • Niacin 5 mg • Vitamin B6 0.6 mg • Folate 120 mcg • Vitamin B12 2.7 mcg • Biotin 75 mcg • Pantothenic Acid 3.5 mg • Phosphorus 300 mg • Iodine 52.5 mg • Magnesium 60 mg • Zinc 5.25 mg • Selenium 20 mcg • Copper 0.3 mg • Manganese 560 mcg • Chromium 20 mcg • Molybdenum 50 mcg. Other Ingredients: Gelatin, Silicon Dioxide, Microcrystalline Cellulose, Magnesium Stearate.

Appeal Swiss Truffle - Pharmanex
Nonfat Milk • Crystalline Fructose • Milk Protein • Maltodextin • Canola Oil • Cocoa powder • Soy Fiber • Custard Flavor • Soy Lecithin • Oat Fiber • Magnesium Chelate • Gelatin • Sodium Chloride • Liquid Molasses • Calcium Chelate • Potassium Citrate • Barley Malt • Rice Syrup Solids • Potassium Chloride • Gum Arabic • Microcrystalline and Carboxymethyl Cellulose • Potassium Iodide • Zinc Chelate • L-Carnitine • Molybdenum Yeast Concentrate • Locust Bean Gum • Xanthan Gum • Citrus Pectin • Selenium Yeast Concentrate • Rose Hips • Ascorbic Acid • Copper Chelate • Beta-Carotene • Bee Pollen • D-Alpha Tocopheryl Acetate • Ferric Orthophosphate • Peppermint stick flavor • Manganese Chelate • Iron Chelate • Chromium Chelate • Folic Acid • Citrus Bioflavonoid • Lemon Bioflavonoid • Bromelain • Papain • L-Isoleucine • L-Valine • L-Leucine • L-Cysteine • L-Methionine • L-Aspartate • Magnesium • Vitamin A Palmitate • Niacinamide • D-Calcium Pantothenate • Dicalcium Phosphate • Calcium Lactate • Pyridoxine Hydrochloride • Riboflavin • Thiamine Mononitrate • Cyanocobalamin • Cholecalciferol • Biotin.

Appetite Control - Nature's Sunshine
Antimonium Crudum (antimonious sulfide) 6X • Fucus Vesiculosus (kelp) 6X • Graphite 6X • Iodine (iodium) 6X • Pulsatilla (wind flower) 6X • Aurum Metallicum (gold) 12X • Sulfur 12X. Other ingredients: Purified Water, 20% USP Alcohol.
See Editor's Note No. 1.

Appetite Control - The Council On Natural Health
Two tablets contain: Vitamin C (as ascorbic acid) 50 mg • Chromium (as patented chromium dinicotinate glycinate) 200 mcg • Garcinia Cambogia fruit extract (50% [-] hydroxycitric acid) 250 mg • Chitosan 500 mg • 5-HTP (from griffonia simplicifolia seed extract) 12.5 mg • Capsicum (cayenne) Pepper 30 mg • Ginger root 15 mg. Other Ingredients: Dicalcium Phosphate, Microcrystalline Cellulose, Croscarmellose Sodium, Stearic Acid, Magnesium Stearate, Silica, Pharmaceutical Glaze.

Appetite Suppressant with Carb Blocker - EnerGreens, Inc.
Each capsule contains: Proprietary Blend 650 mg: Green Tea standardized extract (minimum 25%), White Kidney bean SE, Garcinia Cambogia SE, Citrus Aurantium SE, Phosphatidyl Serine SE. Other Ingredients: Gelatin.
See Editor's Note No. 40.

Apple Cider Vinegar - Natural Brand
Two tablets contain: Apple Cider Vinegar 600 mg • Cayenne Pepper fruit powder (capsicum frutescens) 100 mg • Ginger root powder (zingiberis officinale) 100 mg • Garcinia Cambogia fruit extract (50% hydroxycitric acid 50 mg) 100 mg. Other Ingredients: Cellulose, Dicalcium Phosphate.

Apple Cider Vinegar - American Health
Two tablets contain: Apple Cider Vinegar (equivalent to pure cider vinegar 1 tsp) 600 mg. Other Ingredients: Dicalcium Phosphate, Cellulose (plant origin), Vegetable Stearic Acid, Croscarmellose, Silica, Vegetable Magnesium Stearate.

Apple Cider Vinegar - Source Naturals
Each tablet contains: Apple Cider Vinegar (concentrated to 35% acetic acid) 500 mg. Other Ingredients: Sorbitol, Stearic Acid, Modified Cellulose Gum, Colloidal Silicon Dioxide, Magnesium Stearate.

Apple Cider Vinegar - Only Natural, Inc.
Each capsule contains: Apple Cider Vinegar 500 mg.

Apple Cider Vinegar 500 mg - Natural Factors
Each caplet contains: Apple Cider Vinegar 500 mg. Other Ingredients: Gelatin Capsule (gelatin, purified water), Maltodextrin, Food Starch, Magnesium Stearate (vegetable grade).

Apple Cider Vinegar Plus - Only Natural, Inc.
Each capsule contains: Apple Cider Vinegar 500 mg • Cayenne Pepper 100 mg • Grapefruit rind 100 mg.

Apple Cinnamon Celebration - Physicians Laboratories
Each bar contains: Certified Isoflavone 160 mg. Other Ingredients: Soy Protein Isolate, Rice Flour, Malt, Salt, Corn Syrup, Sugar, Corn Starch, Water, Gelatin, Artificial Flavoring, Dried Apples, Glycerin, Sunflower Oil, Natural Flavors, Soy Lecithin, Ground Cinnamon.

Appleheart Chondroitin Sulfate - Appleheart
Each capsule contains: Chondroitin Sulfate 300 mg. Other Ingredients: Cellulose, Gelatin, Vegetable Stearate.
See Editor's Note No. 15.

Appleheart Echinacea - Appleheart
Each capsule contains: standarized Echinacea Angustifolia and Echinacea Purpurea 250 mg • Rice Protein • Gelatin • Cellulose • Vegetable Stearate.

Appleheart Glucosamine Sulfate - Appleheart
Each capsule contains: Glucosamine Sulfate (from Glucosamine Sulfate Potassium) 500 mg • Potassium 65 mg. Other Ingredients: Gelatin, Cellulose, Vegetable Stearate.

Appleheart Melatonin - Appleheart
Each capsule contains: Melatonin 3mg.
See Editor's Note No. 16 and No. 21.

Appleheart Saw Palmetto - Appleheart
Each capsule contains: Saw Palmetto berry 160 mg • Olive Oil • Water • Gelatin.

Appleheart St. John's Wort - Appleheart
Each capsule contains: standardized St. John's Wort 250 mg • Gelatin • Rice Protein • Cellulose • Magnesium Stearate (Vegetable Source).

Apple-Honey Lactobacillus Acidophilus - Nature's Life
Unfiltered Apple juice • Purified Water • Pasteurized Honey • Soy Protein Isolate • Lactobacillus Acidophilus Culture.

AppSignal - Pharmanex
Two wafers contain: Sucrose • Cocoa Powder • Microcrystalline Cellulose • Protein Complex (Hydrolyzed Soy Protein, Soy Protein Isolate, Egg Albumin) • L-Tyrosine • AbsorbaLean Fiber Complex:

BRAND NAMES

Apple Pectin, Fructooligosaccharides, Locust Bean Gum, Carrageenan, Microcrystalline Cellulose • Stearic Acid • Lecithin Powder • Natural and Artificial Flavors • Sorbitol • L-Histidine Hydrochloride • Pyridoxine Hydrochloride • Magnesium Stearate • Folic Acid.

APS-II - Nature's Sunshine
Two capsules contain: Proprietary Blend 700 mg: White Willow bark (salix alba), Lettuce leaf (lactuca virosa), Valerian root (valeriana officinalis), Capsicum fruit (capsicum annuum). Other Ingredients: Gelatin, Water.

Aqua Ban - Thompson Medical Co.
Each tablet contains: Active Ingredient: Pamabrom 50 mg (Diuretic). Other Ingredients: Carnauba Wax • Croscarmellose Sodium • FD&C Blue No. 1 Aluminum Lake • Hydroxypropyl Methylcellulose • Lactose • Magnesium Stearate • Microcrystalline Cellulose • Polyethylene Glycol • Polysorbate 80 • Starch • Titanium Dioxide.

Aqua Gem-E 400 IU - J. R. Carlson Laboratories, Inc.
Each softgel contains: Vitamin E (as D-alpha tocopherol) 400 IU.

Aqua Greens - Futurebiotics LLC
Twelve tablets contain: Chlorella 1000 mg • Spirulina 2500 mg • Klamath Blue/Green Algae 500 mg • Kelp 250 mg • D. Salina 100 mg.

AquaActin - Nature's Plus
Two capsules contain: Chinese Green Tea [(Camellia sinensis leaf) decaffeinated, standardized 50% Polyphenols] 250 mg • Horsetail [(Equisetum arvense stem) standardized 10% Silicic Acid, 7% Silica] 150 mg • Uva Ursi [(Arctostaphylos uva-ursi leaf) standardized 20-25% Arbutin] 100 mg • Vitamin B6 (Pyridoxine HCl) 75 mg • Goldenseal [(Hydrastis canadensis root & rhizome) standardized 10% Alkaloids, 5% Hydrastine] 50 mg • Artichoke [(Cynara scolymus flower) standardized 2.5-5% Caffeylquinic Acids] 50 mg.

Aqua-Action - Nature's Plus
Each capsule contains: Buchu leaves 125 mg • Couchgrass 100 mg • Juniper berries 100 mg • Parsley leaves 100 mg • Corn Silk 75 mg • Uva Ursi leaves 50 mg • Celery seed 50 mg.

Aqua-Flow - Enzymatic Therapy
Two capsules contain: Potassium Citrate 70 mg • Magnesium Oxide 50 mg • Vitamin B6 (pyridoxine HCl) 25 mg • Uva Ursi leaf extract (standardized to contain 20% arbutin) 200 mg • Boldo leaf 2:1 extract (peumus boldus) 100 mg • Dandelion root 4:1 extract (taraxacum officinale) 100 mg • Early Goldenrod aerial part extract (solidago serotina standardized to contain 5% flavonoids) 100 mg. Other Ingredients: Gelatin, Magnesium Stearate, Titanium Dioxide Color, Silicon Dioxide.

Aqua-Lim - Aspen Group, Inc.
Each tablet contains: Buchu leaves 70 mg • Couch Grass 70 mg • Hydrangea root 35 mg • Corn Silk 35 mg • Uva Ursi 10 mg • Hypothalamus 30 mg • Raw Kidney concentrate 30 mg • Vitamin B6 16 mg • Bladder Wrack 100 mg • Magnesium: Protein Chelated 50 mg.
See Editor's Note No. 31.

AquaSport SPF 15 - All Terrain Company
Active Ingredients: Zinc Oxide • Octyl Methoxycinnamate. Other Ingredients: Water, Aloe Vera Gel, Starch, Octyl Palmitate, Glycerin, Isopropyl Palmitate, Shea Butter, Cetearyl Glucoside, Glyceryl Stearate, PEG-100 Stearate, Tricontanyl PVP, Beeswax, Magnesium Aluminum Silicate, Rose Hip Seed Oil, Xantham Gum, Arginine, Squalane, Glycereth-26, Tocopheryl Acetate (Vitamin E Acetate), Retinyl Palmitate (Vitamin A Palmitate), Cholecalciferol (Vitamin D3), Capryl Glycine, Methylparaben, Propylparaben.

AquaSport SPF 30 - All Terrain Company
Active Ingredients: Titanium Dioxide • Octyl Methoxycinnamate. Other Ingredients: Water, Aloe Vera Gel, Starch, Octyl Palmitate, Glycerin, Isopropyl Palmitate, Shea Butter, Cetearyl Glucoside, Glyceryl Stearate, PEG-100 Stearate, Tricontanyl PVP, Beeswax, Magnesium Aluminum Silicate, Rose Hip Seed Oil, Xantham Gum, Arginine, Squalane, Glycereth-26, Tocopheryl Acetate (Vitamin E Acetate), Retinyl Palmitate (Vitamin A Palmitate), Cholecalciferol (Vitamin D3), Capryl Glycine, Methylparaben, Propylparaben.

Aquatone - PharmAssure
Two tablets contain: Vitamin B6 (as Pyridoxine Hydrochloride) 15 mg • Magnesium (as Magnesium Gluconate) 25 mg • Potassium (as Potassium Gluconate) 99 mg • Uva Ursi Extract (Arctostaphylos uva ursi;20% Arbutin=150 mg) 750 mg. Other Ingredients: Cellulose, Calcium Carbonate.

Arabinogalactan - Pure Encapsulations
Each vegetable capsule contains: Arabinogalactan extract (larix spp.) 500 mg • Vitamin C (as ascorbyl palmitate) 50 mg.

Arabinogalactan Powder - Vital Nutrients
Each 1 slightly rounded tsp serving contains: Arabinogalactan powder (from larix occidentalis) 2000 mg.

Arbu-Tone - PhytoPharmica
Two capsules contain: Boldo leaf 2:1 extract (peumus boldus) 100 mg • Dandelion root 4:1 extract (taraxacum officinale) 100 mg • Early Goldenrold aerial part extract (solidago serotina, standardized to contain 5% flavonoids) 100 mg • Magnesium (as magnesium oxide) 50 mg • Potassium (as potassium citrate) 70 mg • Uva-Ursi leaf extract (arctostaphylos uva-ursi, standardized to contain 20% arbutin) 200 mg • Vitamin B6 (as pyridoxine HCl) 25 mg.

Arctic Cod Liver Oil (peach, orange, or unflavored) - Nordic Naturals
Each 1 tsp serving contains: Vitamin A 875-1950 IU • Vitamin D 5-40 IU • Natural Vitamin E 8 IU • DHA 700 mg • EPA 450 mg • Other Omega-3 Fatty Acids 250 mg.

Arctic Cod Liver Oil Capsules (peach) - Nordic Naturals
Two softgels contain: Vitamin A 350-780 IU • Vitamin D 2-16 IU • Natural Vitamin E 33 IU • DHA 280 mg • EPA 180 mg • Other Omega-3 Fatty Acids 100 mg.

Arctic Cod Liver Oil Singles (orange) - Nordic Naturals
Each packet (1 tsp, or 5 mL) contains: Vitamin A 875-1950 IU • Vitamin D 5-40 IU • Natural Vitamin E 8 IU • DHA 700 mg • EPA 450 mg • Other Omega-3 250 mg.

Arctic Omega (lemon or unflavored) - Nordic Naturals
Two softgels contain: Vitamin E (mixed tocopherols) 28 IU • Omega-3 Fatty Acids 700 mg (EPA 360 mg, DHA 240 mg, Other Omega-3 100 mg).

Arctic Omega Liquid (lemon) - Nordic Naturals
Each 1/2 tsp (2.5 mL) serving contains: Vitamin E (mixed tocopherols) 35 IU • Omega-3 Fatty Acids 875 mg (EPA 450 mg, DHA 300 mg, Other Omega-3 125 mg).

Arctic Root - Swedish Herbal Institute
Each tablet contains: Rhodiola Rosea extract SHI-Rr5 180 mg.

A-Retic - Douglas Laboratories/AMNI
Each tablet contains: Proprietary Blend 480 mg: Juniper berry dried powder, Buchu leaves, Uva-Ursi, Cubeb, Asparagus.

Arginex - Standard Process, Inc.
Each tablet contians: Proprietary Blend 362 mg: Dried Buckwheat juice, Buckwheat seed, Dried Pea vine juice, Oat Flour, Bovine Liver, Beet root, Rhizopus Oryzae extract, Tillandsia Usneoides, Beet root, Dried Beet leaf juice, Ascorbic Acid • Vitamin A 990 IU. Other Ingredients: Honey, Calcium Stearate, Gelatin.
See Editor's Note No. 14.

Arginine - Vital Nutrients
Each capsule contains: Arginine (l-form, from pure 100% l-arginine base) 750 mg.

Some Brand Name Natural Products - What they Contain

www.NaturalDatabase.com contains MANY more listings than appear here.
Editor's Notes are located on pages 2155-2163.

Arginine & Ornithine - Olympian Labs
Each capsule contains: L-Arginine 500 mg • L-Ornithine 250 mg.

Arginine + Ornithine - Jarrow Formulas
Each capsule contains: L-Arginine (from 602 mg L-arginine hydrochloride) 500 mg • L-Ornithine (from 319 mg of L-ornithine hydrochloride) 250 mg. Other Ingredients: Cellulose, Magnesium Stearate, Gelatin.

Arginine 1000 - Jarrow Formulas
Each tablet contains: L-Arginine (from 1024 mg of L-arginine hydrochloride) 1000 mg. Other Ingredients: Calcium Phosphate, Cellulose, Stearic Acid, Modified Cellulose, Modified Cellulose Gum, Magnesium Stearate, Silicon Dioxide.

Arginine 1000 - GNC
Each tablet contains: L-Arginine 1000 mg. Other Ingredients: Cellulose.

Arginine 500 MG - Pain & Stress Center
Each capsule contains: Vitamin C (ascorbyl palmitate) 5 mg • L-Arginine 500 mg. Other Ingredients: Gelatin Capsule.

Arginine Plus with ActiFolate - Metagenics
Two tablets contain: ActiFolate brand Folate (as folic acid, L-5-methyl tetrahydrofolate, 5-formyl tetrahydrofolate) 400 mcg • L-Arginine 1500 mg • L-Glycine 10 mg.

Arginine Pyroglutamate/Lysine - Ultimate Nutrition
Each capsule contains: L-Arginine Pyroglutamate 500 mg • L-Lysine 250 mg.

Arginine Ultra - FreeLife International
Two caplets contain: Calcium as Calcium carbonate and Calcium hydrogen phosphate 100 mg • L-Arginine Hydrochloride 1500 mg. Other Ingredients: Galactomannan, Cellulose, Fractionated Vegetable oil, Fruit Pectin, Vita-Coat: vegetable resin, alpha-lipoic acid.

Arginine-Ornithine 1500 - Puritan's Pride
Two capsules contain: L-Arginine 1000 mg • L-Ornithine 500 mg • Chromium picolinate 6.2 mcg.

ArginMax for Female Sexual Fitness - The Daily Wellness Company
Six tablets contain: Vitamin A (as palmitate) 5000 IU • Vitamin C (as ascorbic acid) 60 mg • Vitamin E (as d-alpha-tocopherol) 30 IU • Thaimin (B1, as thiamin mononitrate) 1.7 mg • Riboflavin (B2) 1.7 mg • Niacin (B3, as niacinamide) 20 mg • Vitamin B6 (as pyridoxine hydrochloride) 2 mg • Folate, Folic Acid, Folacin (as folic acid) 400 mcg • Vitamin B12 (as cyanocobalamin) 6 mcg • Biotin 300 mcg • Pantothenic Acid (as calcium d-pantothenate) 10 mg • Calcium (as carbonate) 500 mg • Iron (as gluconate) 9 mg • Zinc (as gluconate) 7.5 mg • Proprietary Blend: L-Arginine 2500 mg, Korean Ginseng root extract (panax ginseng, root/aerial parts) 100 mg, Ginkgo Biloba leaf extract 50 mg • Damiana leaf (turnera aphrodisiaca) leaf 50 mg. Other Ingredients: Microcrystalline Cellulose, Hydroxypropyl Methylcellulose, Pharmaceutical Glaze, Silica, Titanium Dioxide (color), Magnesium Stearate, PEG, Polysorbate 80.

ArginMax for Men - The Daily Wellness Company
Six capsules contain: L-Arginine 3000 mg • American Ginseng 100 mg • Korean Ginseng 100 mg • Ginkgo Biloba 50 mg • Vitamin A 5000 IU • Vitamin C 60 mg • Vitamin E 30 IU • Thiamin 1.5 mg • Riboflavin 1.7 mg • Niacin 20 mg • Vitamin B6 2 mg • Folate 400 mcg • Vitamin B12 6 mcg • Biotin 300 mcg • Pantothenic Acid 10 mg • Calcium 500 mg • Iron 9 mg • Zinc 7.5 mg.

Arizona Odourless Garlic 1000 - Golden Glow Natural Health Products
Each tablet contains: Allium Sativum bulb powder (equivalent to garlic bulb 1000 mg).

Arko-Lesterol - Arkopharma
Each capsule contains: Gugulon (commiphora mukul) 170 mg • Chrysanthellum (chrysanthellum americanum) 170 mg.

Armovita - Aboca USA, Inc
Two capsules contain: St. John's Wort WPC (whole phytocomplex concentrate; hypericum perforatum, standardized to 0.16% total hypericin) 384 mg • Lemon Balm leaf WPC (melissa officinalis, standardized to 4% rosmarinic acid) 160 mg • Passiflo 2-LMF brand Passionflower leaf (multifration freeze-dried extract, passiflora incarnata, standardized to 8% total flavonoids) 96 mg. Other Ingredients: Gelatin.

Arnica Gel - Jamieson
Contains: Arnica Montana Flowers Tincture 1.5% w/w (European Arnica Equivalent to 7.5% of a 20% NFXI).

Arnica Oil - Blessed Herbs
Arnica flower & leaf • Organic Cold-Pressed Olive oil.

ArnicAid - Hyland's
Three tablets contain: Arnica Montana 30X • Hypericum Perfoliatum 6X • Ruta Graveolens 6X • Ledum Palustre 6X • Bellis Perennis 6X. Base: Lactose N.F.

See Editor's Note No. 1.

ArniSport - Hyland's
Three tablets contain: Arnica Montana 30X • Hypericum Perfoliatum 6X • Ruta Graveolens 6X • Ledum Palustre 6X • Bellis Perennis 6X • Hyland's Bioplasma: Calcarea Fluorica 6X, Calcarea Phosphorica 3X, Calcarea Sulphurica 3X, Ferrum Phosphoricum 3X, Kali Muriaticum 3X, Kali Phosphoricum 3X, Kali Sulphuricum 3X, Magnesia Phosphorica 3X, Natrum Nuriaticum 6X, Natrum Phosphoricum 3X, Natrum Sulphuricum 3X, Silicea 6X. Base: Lactose N.F.

See Editor's Note No. 1.

Aroma Baby Lavender Massage Oil - Golden Glow Natural Health Products
Sweet Almond oil • Jojoba oil • Natural Vitamin E oil • Lavender oil.

Aromadex - VPX Sports
Each 8 cc serving contains: 3;6; 17-Androstenetrione 100 mg • 4-Androsten-4-ol-3Beta-dione 50 mg. Other Ingredients: Lipoject Technologies Proprietary Liposomal Matrix, Vegetable Gum, Sucralose, Potassium Sorbate, Artificial Flavors, Natural Colors.

Aromasaurus Rex Aromatherapy Bath - Abra Therapeutics
Sodium Borate • Sodium Carbonate • Sodium Sesquicarbonate • Sodium Laurel Sulfoacetate • Sweet Almond oil • Wheat Germ oil • Hops flower extract • Valerian root extract • Sweet Orange oil • Tangerine oil • Lime oil • Lavender oil • Cedarwood oil.

ArteClear - Pacific BioLogic
Rhubarb rhizome • Salvia root • Sea Weed • Polygonum root • Polygonatum rhizome • Cassia seeds • Aucklandia root • Hawthorn fruit • Pseudoginseng root.

Artemisia - Pure Encapsulations
Each vegetable capsule contains: Artemisia whole plant extract (artemisia annua L., standardized to contain 5% artemisinin) 400 mg • Vitamin C (as ascorbyl palmitate) 10 mg.

Artemisia Combination - Nature's Sunshine
Two capsules contain: Proprietary Blend 780 mg: Elecampane root (inula helenium), Mugwort aerial parts (artemisia vulgaris), Clove flower bud (eugenia caryophyllata), Garlic bulb (allium sativum), Ginger rhizome (zingiber officinale), Spearmint leaf & flower (mentha spicata), Turmeric root (curcuma longa), Olive leaf extract (olea europa), Wormwood aerial parts (artemisia annua). Other Ingredients: Cellulose, Magnesium Stearate, Silicon Dioxide, Gelatin, Water.

Artemisinin - EcoNugenics
Each capsule contains: Artemisinin 100 mg. Other Ingredients: Gelatin, Maltodextrin, Magnesium Stearate.

Arth Rx - Symmetry
Each packet contains: Glucosamine • Chondroitin Sulfate • Hydrolyzed gelatin • Boswellia • Curcumin • Bilberry • Grape seed extract • Grape skin extract • Tumeric extract.
See Editor's Note No. 15.

Arth-9 - Rx Vitamins
Four capsules contain: Glucosamine Sulfate (Aminomonosaccharide) 1000 mg • Vitamin C (Ascorbic Acid) 250 mg • Bromelain 250 mg • Calcium (Citrate) 250 mg • Boswellin 250 mg • Curcumin 100 mg • Zinc (L-Monomethionine) 30 mg • Chondroitin Sulfate A (CSA) 25 mg • Copper (Glycinate) 2 mg.
See Editor's Note No. 15.

Arthenol - Health Logics
Four capsules contain: BioCell Collagen II 2000 mg: Type II Collagen 1400 mg, Chondroitin Sulfate (from chicken collagen) 40 mg, Hyaluronic Acid 200 mg. Other Ingredients: Kosher Gelatin, Rice Powder, Magnesium Stearate.

Artho-Health Formula - Youngevity
Cosamin (Glucosamine Sulfate 200 mg, Chondroitin Sulfate 160 mg) • Vitamin C 15 mg • Manganese 500 mcg • Vilcabamba Mineral Essence: Potassium, Calcium, Magnesium, Zinc, Chromium, Selenium, Iron, Copper, Molybdenum, Vanadium, Iodine, Cobalt, Manganese.
See Editor's Note No. 15.

Artho-Therapy - PhytoPharmica
Each tablet contains: Capsaicin 0.025%. Other Ingredients: Purified water, Alcohol, Glycerin, Triethanolamine, Escin (Horse chestnut extract), Glory Lily, Methylparaben, Lavender essential oil.
See Editor's Note No. 21.

Arthred brand - Degussa Food Ingredients/BL BioActives
Hydrolyzed Collagen.

ArthRed capsules - Pure Encapsulations
Each vegetable capsule contains: Hydrolyzed Collagen Peptides (bovine) 500 mg.

ArthRed powder - Pure Encapsulations
Each scoop contains: Hydrolyzed Collagen Peptides (bovine, enzymatically hydrolyzed from bovine collagen) 8 g.

Arth-Rid Us - The Herbalist
Devil's Claw root bark • Yucca root • Yerba Mansa root • Black Cohosh root • Wild Yam root.

Arthri-Gesic Liquid Glucosamine - Quantum, Inc.
Each 10 mL serving contains: Glucosamine HCl 500 mg • White Willow Bark extract 50 mg • Devil's Claw extract 25 mg • Curcumin extract 500 mcg. Other Ingredients: Glycerin, Water, Potassium Sorbate, Stevia, Natural Beet Color, Tangerine Oil.

Arthrimin Effervescent Drink Crystals Complex - Jamieson
Each pouch contains: Glucosamine Complex (Derived from Sulfate and HCl) 1500 mg • Hyaluronic Acid (Derived from Glucosamine Complex) 300 mg • Chondroitin Sulfate 1200 mg • MSM (Methylsulfonylmethane) 1000 mg.
See Editor's Note No. 15.

Arthrimin Glucosamine Sulfate - Jamieson
Each capsule contains: Glucosamine Sulfate (from Potassium Chloride Complex) 500 mg.

Arthrimin GS Glucosamine Sulfate 500 mg - Jamieson
Each capsule contains: Glucosamine Sulfate (from Potassium Chloride Complex) 500 mg. Other Ingredients: Peppermint Leaf, and Betaine Hydrochloride.

Arthrimin GS Zinaxin Ev.Ext 77 - Jamieson
Each capsule contains: Ginger Extract (Zinaxin Ev. Ext 77 standardized equivalent to 3500 dried ginger) 255 mg.

Arthrimin Joints + Bones Glucosamine Chondroitin Complex - Jamieson
Each capsule contains: Glucosamine HCl 250 mg • Chondroitin Sulfate 200 mg.
See Editor's Note No. 15.

Arthrimin Joints + Bones Glucosamine MSM Complex - Jamieson
Each capsule contains: Glucosamine HCl 333 mg • MSM (Methylsulfonylmethane) 250 mg • Turmeric Extract 25 mg.

Arthrimin Joints + Bones MSM 1000 mg - Jamieson
Each caplet contains: MSM (methylsulfonylmethane) 1000 mg.

Arthrin - BotanicLab
Glycyrrhiza Glabra L. (licorice; gan-cao) • Epimedium Brevicornum Maxim (epimedium; yin-yang-huo) • Ostrea Gigas Thunberg (oyster shell; mu-li) • Ganoderma Lucidum Karst (lucid ganoderma; ling-zhi) • Isatis Indigotica Fort (isatidis; ta-ching-yeh) • Corydalis Bulbosa (corydalis; yen-hu-suo).

Arthrit-Eze - Xtend-Life Nutraceuticals Inc.
Three tablets contain: Boron Citrate 1.5 mg • Copper Gluconate 1. 5mg • Manganese Citrate 5 mg • Potassium Monophosphate 10 mg • Selenium (as sodium selenite) 0.1 mg • Sodium Metasilicate 2.5 mg • Strontium Chloride 5 mg • MSM (methylsulfonylmethane) 200 mg • Zinc (as zinc citrate) 15 mg • Vitamin B3 (niacinamide) 20 mg • Vitamin D (D3, as cholecalciferol) 150 IU • Vitamin E (succinate) 15 mg • L-Proline 50 mg • Proprietary Blend 102.5 mg: Bromelain, Lysozyme SC, Papain, Protease • Chondroitin Sulphate 200 mg • CMO (cerasomal-cis-9-cetylmyristoleate) 100 mg • Glucosamine Sulfate 250 mg • D-Glucosamine Hydrochloride 100 mg • Green Lipped Mussel lipids 50 mg • Ipriflavone (7-IPF from soy) 50 mg • Poly-N-Acetyl-Glucosamine 150 mg • Rutin 100 mg • SAMe (S-adenosylmethionine) 150 mg • Boswellia Serrata extract 100 mg • Celery seed extract 75 mg • Chasteberry extract (vitex agnus-castus) 25 mg • Ginger extract (zingiber officinale) 100 mg • Phellodendron Amurense bark extract 100 mg • Piperine 25 mg • Turmeric root extract (95% curcumin) 300 mg. Other Ingredients: Magnesium Stearate, Silicon Dioxide, Microcrystalline Cellulose, Maltodextrin, Calcium Phosphate, Enteric Coating.

ArthritiCare - Aarisse Health Care
CMO (cis-9-cetylmyristoleate) • Shea Butter • Speedwell • Glucosamine sulfate • Chondroitin sulfate • MSM (methyl-sulfonyl-methane) • Pregnenolone • Comfrey • Ginger • Primrose Oil • Dong Quai • Citric Acid • Vitamin A • Vitamin E • Panthenol (vitamin B5) • Glycerine • Allantoin.
See Editor's Note No. 15.

Arthritis - Nature's Sunshine
Bryonia (white bryony) 4X • Cimicifuga Racemosa (black cohosh) 4X • Rhus Toxicodendron (poison ivy) 4X • Apis Mellifera (honeybee) 6X • Arnica Montana (mountain arnica) 6X • Berberis Vulgaris (barberry) 8X • Causticum (Hahnemann's causticum) 8X • Calcium Carbonate (calcarea carbonica) 9X. Other Ingredients: Purified Water, 20% USP Alcohol.
See Editor's Note No. 1.

Arthritis & Joint Relief Cream - DermaTechRx
Purified Water • Linoleic Acid • Glyceryl Monostearate • Chondroitin Sulfate • D-Glucosamine Hydrochloride • MSM (methyl sulfonylmethane) • Cetyl Alcohol • Steryl Alcohol • Pregnenolone.

Arthritis Pain - Nelson Bach
Active Ingredients: Berberis Vulgaris 30C HPUS • Calc Fluor 30C HPUS • Causticum 30C HPUS • Dulcamara 30C HPUS • Rhus Toxicodendron 30C HPUS • Bryonia 30C HPUS • Rhododendron 30C HPUS • Nux Vomica 30C HPUS • Actaea 30C HPUS • Pulsatilla 30C HPUS. Other Ingredients: Lactose, Sucrose.
See Editor's Note No. 1.

BRAND NAMES

Arthritis Pain Formula **-** Hyland's
Two tablets contain: Arnica Montana 6X • Cimicifuga Racemosa 3X • Guaiacum 3X • Bryonia 3X • Rhus Toxicodendron 6X. Base: Lactose USP.
See Editor's Note No. 1.

Arthritis Relief **-** Dr. Mike's Vitamins
Four vegetarian capsules contain: Glucosamine Sulfate Potassium (from shellfish) 1500 mg • Methylsulfonylmethane (MSM, natural organic sulfur compound) 750 mg • Shark Cartilage 150 mg • Ginger root 120 mg • Curcumin (turmeric root extract) 115 mg. Other Ingredients: Cellulose (plant derivative), Magnesium Stearate (vegetable oil derivative).

Arthritis Remedy **-** PhytoPharmica
Each tablespoon contains: Aurum Muriaticum Natronatum 8X • Mercurius Corrosivus 6X • Silicea 6X • Sulphur 4X • Bryonia 3X • Colchicum 3X • Natrum Salicylicum 3X • Viscum Album 3X • Dulcamara 2X • Kalium Iodatum 2X • Betula 1X • Rubia Tinctorum 1X. Base: 20% USP Alcohol by volume.
See Editor's Note No. 1 and No. 21.

Arthro Enzyme **-** Nutri-Health
Each tablet contains: Serratiopeptidase 330 mg. Other Ingredients: Microcrystalline Cellulose, Hydroxypropylethylcellulose, Magnesium Stearate, Hydroxypropylmethylcellulosephthalate.

Arthro Herbal-Rx **-** Alternecare Health Products
Two capsules contain: Chondroitin Sulfate (bovine cartilage) 150 mg • Glucosamine Sulfate 350 mg • Cat's Claw 25 mg • Quercetin 50 mg • Bromelain 50 mg • Alfalfa 25 mg • Devil's Claw 10 mg • Yucca 20 mg • Pycnogenol 5 mg • Grape seed 5 mg • Suma 25 mg • Siberian Ginseng 25 mg • Lipoic Acid 25 mg.
See Editor's Note No. 15.

Arthro-7 **-** Gero Vita International
Each capsule contains: Chicken Collagen type II 400 mg • Methylsulfonylmethane (MSM) 50 mg • Cetyl Myristoleate (CMO) 50 mg • Bromelain (2400 GDU) 15 mg • Curcuma Longa Extract (root, 95% Curcumin) • Vitamin C (as Ascorbic Acid) 70 mg • Lipase (30 USP units) 50 mg.
See Editor's Note No. 14.

Arthro-7 Topical Gel **-** Gero Vita International
Active Ingredient: 1.26% Menthol. Other Ingredients: Purified Water, Methylsulfonylmethane (MSM), Glycerine, Hyaluronic Acid, Carbomer, Ginger root extract (10% total gingerols), Cetyl Myristoleate (CMO), Triethanolamine, Polysorbate 20, Methylparaben, FD&C Blue #1.

ArthroColl brand **-** Cyvex Nutrition, Inc.
Chicken Collagen Type II.

ArthroGenx **-** MK Supplements
Four capsules contain: Vitamin B3 (niacinamide) 600 mg • Glucosamine Sulfate 1500 mg • MSM (methyl sulfonyl methane) 500 mg • Chondroitin 4-Sulfate 250 mg • Boswellia Serrata extract (60% boswellic acid) 100 mg • Ginger extract (5% Gingerols) • Rosemary • Turmeric extract • Cetyl Myristoleate.
See Editor's Note No. 15.

ArthroGenx **-** BioGenesis Nutraceuticals
Four capsules contain: Vitamin B3 (niacinamide) 600 mg • Glucosamine Sulfate (KCl, stabilized) 1500 mg • MSM (methyl sulfonyl methane) 500 mg • Chondroitin-4-Sulfate 250 mg • Boswellia Serrata extract (60% boswellic acid) 100 mg • Ginger extract (5% gingerols) 50 mg • Rosemary 50 mg • Turmeric extract (95% curcuminoids) 50 mg • Cetyl Myristoleate 30 mg.

Arthro-Glucosamine **-** Nutri-Quest Rx
Each tablet contains: Glucosamine Sulfate 100 mg • N-Acetyl Glucosamine 50 mg • L-Glutathione 2 mg • N-Acetyl Cysteine 5 mg • L-Cysteine 50 mg • L-Glutamic Acid 50 mg • L-Glycine 50 mg • L-Taurine 25 mg • Vitamin C 50 mg • Vitamin E (Succinate) 25 IU • Pantothenic Acid 50 mg • Soluble Trachea (16% Chondroitin Sulfate-A) 25 mg • Silymarin 5 mg • Milk Thistle 100 mg • Green Lipped Mussel 25 mg (natural source of Mucopolysaccharides & Superoxide Dismutase).
See Editor's Note No. 15.

ArthroPlex **-** Aidan Products, LLC
Each capsule contains: Methylsulfonylmethane 250 mg • Glucosamine Sulfate 325 mg • Chondroitin Sulfate 300 mg • Bromelain (600 GDU) 25 mg. Other Ingredients: Gelatin (capsule), Maltodextrin.
See Editor's Note No. 15.

ArthroPro System **-** Life Extension
Four capsules contain: Nettle leaf extract (super-concentrate) 1125 mg • Chondroitin Sulfate 2450 mg • N-Acetyl-D-Glucosamine 500 mg • Glucosamine Sulfate (from shellfish) 500 mg • Nexrutine 750 mg • Ginger (powdered extract, 5% gingerols) 60 mg • Chondroitin Sulfate 1650 mg. Other Ingredients: Gelatin, Water.
See Editor's Note No. 15.

Arthro-SYN **-** Douglas Laboratories/AMNI
Four capsules contain: Vitamin A 2500 IU • Vitamin B1 (thiamin) 40 mg • Vitamin B2 (riboflavin) 20 mg • Niacin / Niacinamide 100 mg • Vitamin B5 (pantothenic acid) 50 mg • Vitamin B6 50 mg • Vitamin C 500 mg • Hesperidin Complex 25 mg • Rutin 25 mg • Bioflavonoids 150 mg • Folic Acid 200 mcg • Vitamin E 100 IU • Choline Bitartrate 20 mg • Inositol 20 mg • PABA (para-aminobenzoic acid) 10 mg • Calcium (citrate complex) 125 mg • Magnesium (aspartate complex) 125 mg • Manganese (sulfate) 100 mg • Zinc (amino acid chelate) 25 mg • Potassium (aspartate complex) 25 mg • Selenomethionine 50 mcg • Copper (sebacate complex) 2 mg • Chromium (GTF) 100 mcg • L-Cystine 75 mg • L-Histidine 25 mg • DL-Phenylalanine 100 mg • Omega-3 Fatty Acids (DHA/EPA) 100 mg • Trypsin 25 mg • Chymotrypsin 25 mcg • Bromelain 150 mcu • Bovine Tracheal Cartilage (BTC) 100 mg • Papain 25 mg • Raw Veal Bone 25 mg • Yucca extract 100 mg.
See Editor's Note No. 14.

Arthrovedic **-** Gero Vita International
Two capsules contain: Herbal Proprietary Blend 830 mg: Commiphora Mukul gum extract (24% lipids), Withania Somnifera root extract (0.5% alkaloids), Boswellia Serrate gum extract (basalic acid 4.5%), Cyperus Rotundus tuber extract (0.45% alkaloids), Paederia Foetida leaf extract (0.45% alkaloids), Vitex Negundo leaf extract (0.10% alkaloids), Holarrhena Antidysenterica bark extract (0.10% alkaloids), Smilax China root extract (60% water-soluble extractive), Boerhoavia Diffusa root extract (0.8% alkaloids), Tribulus Terrestris root extract (7% saponins), Apium Graveolens seed extract (60% water-soluble extractive), Sida Cordifolia root extract (50% water-soluble extractive), Trachyspermum Ammi fruit extract (60% water-soluble extractive), Trigonella Foenum-Graecum seed extract (10% saponins) • Proprietary Phytominerals Blend 200 mg. Other Ingredients: Dicalcium Phosphate, Silicon Dioxide, Vegetable Magnesium Stearate, Gelatin, ACF 223.
See Editor's Note No. 39.

Arthryx **-** Herbal Research International
Three capsules contain: Proprietary Blend: Citrus Reticulata, Ligusticum Sinense, Forsythia Suspensa, Sinapis Alba, Codonopsis Pilosula, Pubescent Angelica, Eucommia Ulmoides, Bupleurum Chinensis, Saposhnikovia Divaricata, Foeniculum Vulgare, Alpinia Officinarum, Taraxacum Mongolicum, Loranthus Parasiticus, Gleditsia Sinensis, Rehmannia Glutinosa, Phellodendron Chinense, Leonurus Sibiricus, Glycyrrhiza Glabra, Zingiber Officinale, Scutellaria Baicalensis, Picrasma Excelsa, Polygonum Multiflorum, Achyranthes Bidentata, Prunus Mume, Rheum Palmatum, Coptis Teeta, Wolfiporia Cocos, Paenoia Lactiflora, Angelica Sinensis, Laminaria Japonica, Berberis Vulgaris, Actaehera Cleifolia, Cinnamomum Aromaticum, Gentiana Macrophylla, Prunus

Armeniaca, Isatis Indigotica, Lycium Chinense, Sophora Flavescens, Gentiana Triflora, Artemisia Annua, Tabebuia Impetiginosa. Other Ingredients: Vegetable Gelatin.

Arth-Support Formula **- Douglas Laboratories/AMNI**
Four tablets contain: Proprietary Blend 500 mg: Turmeric (curcuma longa), Pancreatin 8X (providing protease, amylase, lipase activity), Licorice (glycyrrhiza glabra), Quercetin, Betaine HCl / Glutamic Acid HCl, Shark Cartilage powder, Glucosamine Sulfate, Pepsin, Bromelain (minimum 2000 m.c.u.), SOD / Glutathione Peroxidase (young wheat sprouts), Feverfew, Devil's Claw, Proanthocyanidins (red wine grapes), Ginseng (panax), Skullcap, N-Acetyl-L-Cysteine / L-Cysteine HCl, L-Methionine • Beta-Carotene (vitamin A activity) 15,000 IU • Vitamin A (palmitate, water dispersible) 5000 IU • Vitamin D (D3) 50 IU • Vitamin E (succinate) 200 IU • Vitamin C (ascorbic acid) 1000 mg • Vitamin B1 (thiamine HCl) 50 mg • Vitamin B2 (riboflavin) 25 mg • Niacin 20 mg • Niacinamide 100 mg • Pantothenic Acid (as d-calcium pantothenate) 150 mg • Vitamin B6 (as pyridoxine HCl/pyridoxal-5-phosphate complex) 25 mg • Vitamin B12 100 mcg • Folic Acid 800 mcg • Biotin 300 mcg • Choline (from choline citrate/bitartrate) 20 mg • Inositol 25 mg • Citrus Bioflavonoid Complex 100 mg • PABA (para-aminobenzoic acid) 300 mg • Calcium (citrate/ascorbate complex) 300 mg • Magnesium (aspartate/ascorbate complex) 300 mg • Potassium (aspartate complex) 75 mg • Zinc (aspartate complex) 50 mg • Copper (amino acid chelate) 2 mg • Manganese (aspartate complex) 15 mg • Chromium GTF (organically bound with GTF activity-low allergenicity) 200 mcg • Selenium (organic selenium in Krebs Cycle (citrate, fumarate, malate, glutarate, succinate complex) and kelp) 300 mcg • Molybdenum (Krebs) 50 mcg • Vanadium (Krebs) 25 mcg • Boron (aspartate/citrate complex) 1 mg • Trace Elements (sea vegetation) 100 mg.

Arthur Children's Chewable Multivitamins **- Jamieson**
Each tablet contains: Vitamin A 5000 IU • Vitamin D (as Vitamin D3) 3 400 IU • Vitamin E 10 IU • Vitamin C 40 mg • Vitamin B1 1.5 mg • Vitamin B2 1.7 mg • Niacinamide 20 mg • Pantothenic Acid 10 mg • Vitamin B6 2 mg • Vitamin B12 4 mcg • Folic Acid 0.1 mg • Biotin 30 mcg • Calcium 162 mg • Phosphorus 125 mg • Copper 1 mg • Iodine 0.15. Blended in a base of concentrated fruits and vegetables derived from: Tomato, Broccoli, Carrot, Orange Fiber, Cranberry, and Lemon Bioflavonoids.

Artichoke **- Arkopharma**
Each capsule contains: Artichoke (cynara scolymus) 400 mg.

Artichoke 350 mg **- Vitamin World**
Each capsule contains: Artichoke leaf extract (cynara scolymus, standardized to contain 2.2% Cynarin) 350 mg. Other Ingredients: Gelatin, Rice Powder, Vegetable Magnesium Stearate, Silica.

Artichoke 500 **- Jarrow Formulas**
Each capsule contains: Artichoke leaf extract (cynara scolymus, 15% cholorogenic acid, 5% cynarin) 500 mg. Other Ingredients: Cellulose, Magnesium Stearate, Silicon Dioxide, Gelatin.

Artichoke Extract **- Enzymatic Therapy**
Two capsules contain: Artichoke leaf extract (cynara scolymus standardized to contain 13-18% caffeylquinic acids calculated as chlorogenic acid) 320 mg. Other Ingredients: Gelatin, Magnesium Stearate, Silicon Dioxide, Titanium Dioxide Color.

Artichoke Extract **- Nature's Way**
Two capsules contain: Artichoke dried extract 600 mg • Milk Thistle seed 300 mg. Other Ingredients: Gelatin, Magnesium stearate, Maltodextrin, Silica.

Artichoke Extract **- PhytoPharmica**
Two capsules contain: Artichoke (Cynara scolymus leaf extract 5:1) 320 mg.

Artichoke Leaf **- Aboca USA, Inc**
Two capsules contain: Artichoke leaf WPC (whole phytocomplex concentrate, cynara scolymus, standardized to 3% caffeoylquinic acids, yielding 7 mg per capsule) 468 mg. Other Ingredients: Gelatin.

Artichoke leaf extract **- Pure Encapsulations**
Each vegetable capsule contains: Artichoke leaf extract (cynara scolymus L.) 400 mg • Vitamin C (as ascorbyl palmitate) 5 mg.

AS With Gymnema **- Nature's Sunshine**
Two capsules contain: Proprietary Blend 880 mg: Garcinia fruit (garcinia indica), Gymnema leaf (gymnema sylvestre), Marshmallow root (althaea officinalis), Psyllium hull (plantago ovata). Other Ingredients: Gelatin, Water.

Ascend'n See **- Life Enhancement Products, Inc.**
Each rounded tablespoon (14.5 g) contains: Vitamin A (as beta-carotene) 2500 IU • Vitamin C (as ascorbic acid and niacinamide ascorbate) 325 mg • Vitamin E (as D,L-alpha-tocopheryl acetate) 30 IU • Thiamine (vitamin B1 as thiamine hydrochloride) 1.5 mg • Riboflavin (vitamin B2) 3 mg • Niacin (vitamin B3 as niacinamide ascorbate) 75 mg • Vitamin B6 (as pyridoxine hydrochloride) 16 mg • Folic Acid 100 mcg • Vitamin B12 (cyanocobalamin) 20 mcg • Pantothenic Acid (vitamin B5 as calcium pantothenate) 18 mg • Zinc (as zinc gluconate) 3 mg • Copper (as copper gluconate) 420 mcg • Chromium (as chromium aspartate) 25 mcg • L-Phenylalanine 600 mg • Taurine 200 mg • Glycine 150 mg • Caffeine 42 mg • Tea Polyphenols 280 mg.

As-Comp **- Enzymatic Therapy**
Each capsule contains: Ephedrine from Ma Huang extract (ephedra sinensis) 200 mg 12 mg. Other Ingredients: Ginger root extract 6.5:1 (Zingiber officinale) 65 mg • Licorice root extract (Glycyrrhiza glabra) standardized to contain 5% Glycyrrhizic acid) 50 mg • Marshmallow root extract 4:1 (Althaea officinalis) (Mucilage content 30-40%) 50 mg • Sundew Herb extract 4:1 (Drosera rotundifolia) 40 mg • Euphorbia Herb extract 4:1 (Euphorbia hirta) 40 mg • Senega root extract 4:1 (Polygala senega) 40 mg • Goldenseal root extract (Hydrastis canadensis) standardized to contain 5% total Alkaloids including Berberine, Hydrastine & Canadine 20 mg.
See Editor's Note No. 21 and No. 30.

Ascorbate-C **- Atrium Biotechnologies**
Each teaspoon (5 gm) contains: Vitamin C (Calcium Ascorbate) 2000 mg • Rose Hips 1450 mg • Acerola 1000 mg • Lemon Bioflavonoids 500 mg • Rutin 25 mg • Hesperidin 25 mg • Calcium (from Calcium Ascorbate) 230 mg.

Ascorbplex 1,000 (Buffered) **- Douglas Laboratories/AMNI**
Each tablet contains: Vitamin C (ascorbates) 1000 mg • Calcium 90 mg • Magnesium 125 mcg • Potassium 60 mg • Pectin 100 mg • Bioflavonoid complex 100 mg.

Ascorbyl Palmitate **- Pure Encapsulations**
Each vegetable capsule contains: Ascorbyl Palmitate 500 mg.

Ascorbyl Palmitate (500 mg) **- NOW Foods**
Each capsule contains: Vitamin C (from ascorbyl palmitate) 200 mg • Ascorbyl Palmitate 500 mg. Other Ingredients: Cellulose (vegetable source), Magnesium Stearate (vegetable source), Silica.

AShwagandha **- Pure Encapsulations**
Each vegetable capsule contains: Ashwagandha extract (withania somnifera, standardized to contain 5% withanolides) 500 mg.

Ashwagandha 300 mg **- Vitamin World**
Each tablet contains: Ashwagandha root extract (withania somnifera, standardized to contain 1.5% Withanolides) 300 mg. Other Ingredients: Cellulose, Dicalcium Phosphate, Acacia Gum, Croscarmellose, Vegetable Stearic Acid, Silica, Vegetable Magnesium Stearate, Cellulose Coating.

Ashwagandha Root Extract **- America's Finest**
Each capsule contains: Ashwagandha root (withania somnifera, 1.5% withanolides, 1% alkaloids) 300 mg. Other Ingredients: Gelatin, Water, Cellulose, Magnesium Stearate, Silica.

Asian Ginseng Root - Aboca USA, Inc
Each capsule contains: Asian Ginseng root WPC (whole phytocomplex concentrate, panax ginseng, standardized to 3.6% ginsenosides, yielding 10 mg per capsule) 280 mg. Other Ingredients: Gelatin.

Asotas Plus for HER - Unknown
Two tablets contain: Niacin (as niacinamide) 10 mg • Dong Quai (1% extract) 200 mg • Avena Sativa (4:1 extract) 200 mg •Yohimbe (2% extract) 100 mg • Sarsaparilla (root) 600 mg • Siberian Ginseng (8% extract) 300 mg • Panax Ginseng (10% extract) 300 mg • Maca (herb powder) 100 mg • Damiana (4:1 extract) 100 mg • Black Cohosh (2.5% extract) 40 mg • False Unicorn (root) 40 mg • Asparagus 60 mg • Artichoke 40 mg • Wild Yam (6% extract) 50 mg.
Other Ingredients: Magnesium Stearate, Stearic Acid, Microcrystalline Cellulose.

Asotas Plus for HIM - Unknown
Two tablets contain: Niacin (as niacinamide) 10 mg • Yohimbe bark (as 2% extract) 250 mg • Avena Sativa (as 10:1 extract) 150 mg • Androstenedione 100 mg • Saw Palmetto (as 4:1 extract) 100 mg • Guarana (as 22% extract) 300 mg • Taurine (as l-taurine HCl) 200 mg • Siberian Ginseng (as 40% extract) 30 mg • Panax Ginseng (as 40% extract) 30 mg • Tribulus Terrestris (as 40% extract) 50 mg • Rhodiola Rosea (as extract) 10 mg • Wild Yam (as 10:1 extract) 250 mg • Maca (as powder) 100 mg • Arginine (as l-arginine HCl) 100 mg. Other Ingredients: Di-calcium Phosphate, Magnesium Stearate, Stearic Acid.
See Editor's Note No. 47.

Asparagus Extract - Enzymatic Therapy/PhytoPharmica
Each capsule contains: Asparagus rhizome extract (asparagus officinalis standardized to contain 4-8% asparagosides) 170 mg. Other Ingredients: Cellulose, Gelatin, Magnesium Stearate, Titanium Dioxide Color.

AspirActin - Nature's Plus
Three capsules contain: White Willow bark [(Salix alba) standardized 7-9% Salicin] 500 mg • Kava Kava [(Piper methysticum root) standardized 29-31% Kavalactones] 50 mg • Inositol Hexanicotinate (Flush-Free Niacin) 50 mg • Cayenne [(Capsicum frutescens fruit) standardized 100000 STU] 25 mg • Ginkgo Biloba leaf (standardized 24% Ginkgo Flavone-Glycosides, 6% Terpene Lactones) 10 mg.

Aspitive - Progressive Health Nutraceuticals
Vitamin B12 1 mg • Folic Acid 400 mcg • Magnesium 100 mg • Schizandra extract 100 mg • Siberian Ginseng 500 mg • Bee Pollen 250 mg • Bee Propolis 50 mg • Royal Jelly 8 mg • Coenzyme Q10 5 mg • Korean Ginseng 25 mg • Rhodiola extract 100 mg • DHEA 25 mg • Cordyceps 100 mg.

Astaxanthin - Pure Encapsulations
Each softgel capsule contains: Astaxanthin (naturally derived from haematococcus pluvialis microalgae) 4 mg • Lutein 40 mcg • Vitamin A (as beta carotene) 40 mcg • Vitamin E (D-alpha tocopherol) 65 IU. Other Ingredients: Rosemary Liquid Extract, High Oleic Safflower Oil, Gelatin.

Astaxanthin 4 mg - NOW Foods
Each softgel contains: Vitamin A (100% as natural beta-carotene) 105 IU • Vitamin E (as natural D-alpha tocopherol) 50 IU • BioAstin Natural Astaxanthin (from haematococcus pluvialis extract) 4 mg • Lutein 40 mcg. Other Ingredients: Safflower Oil, Gelatin, Glycerin, Water, Carob Extract (natural color).

Astaxanthin Complex - Solgar
Each softgel contains: Proprietary Blend 4 mg: Astaxanthin (from h. pluvialis, 3.4 mg), Lutein, Beta Carotene, Canthaxanthin, Other Carotenoids. Inactive Ingredients: Safflower oil, Gelatin, Glycerin, Yellow Beeswax, Lecithin, Caramel.

AstaZANTHIN - La Haye Labs
Astaxanthin.
See Editor's Note No. 44.

AstaZanthin - Source Naturals
Marine Algae (Haematococcus pluvialis) 10 mg. Natural concentrate (AstaZanthin) yielding Astaxanthin complex 1 mg.

Astazanthin & Pycnogenol Age Protection Creme 2oz - Derma E
Purified Water • Glycerin • Caprylic Triglyceride • Stearic Acid • Jojoba oil • Glyceryl Stearate • Cetyl Alcohol • Stearyl Alcohol • Astazanthin Astaxanthin (1%) • Pycnogenol (1%) • Tocopheryl Acetate (vitamin E) • Ergocalciferol (vitamin D) • Retinyl Palmitate (vitamin A) • TEA • Polysorbate 20 • Titanium Dioxide • Methylparaben • Ethylparaben • I. Urea • Fragrant Oils.

Asthma - Nature's Sunshine
Zingiber Officinale (ginger) 3X • Aralia Racemosa (spikenard) 6X • Eucalyptus Globulus (eucalyptus) 6X • Grindelia (gum plant) 6X • Hypericum Perforatum (St. John's wort) 6X • Lobelia Inflata (Indian tobacco) 6X • Sanguinaria Canadensis (blood root) 6X • Cinchona Officinalis (Peruvian bark) 12X. Other Ingredients: Purified Water, 20% USP Alcohol.
See Editor's Note No. 1.

Asthma & Allergy Remedy - PhytoPharmica
Twenty to fifty drops contain: Adrenalinum 6X • Stramonium 6X • Belladonna 4X • Ephedra Vulgaris 4X • Ipecacuanha 4X • Lobelia 3X • Solidago Virgaurea 3X • Yerba Santa 3X • Sambucus 1X. In a base of 40% USP alcohol by volume.
See Editor's Note No. 1 and No. 21.

Asthma-X5 - Olympian Labs
Each capsule contains 500 mg: Proprietary Blend: Schisandra Berries, Green Tea, Mormon Tea, Coleus Forskohlii, Lobelia, Feverfew, Skullcap, Licorice root, Ginger.

Astragalus - Nature's Sunshine
Two capsules contain: Astragalus root (astragalus membranaceus) 840 mg. Other Ingredients: Gelatin, Water.

Astragalus - NOW Foods
Two capsules contain: Total Carbohydrate 0.7 g • Dietary Fiber 0.5 g • Astragalus root powder (a. membranaceus) 1.0 g. Other Ingredients: Stearic Acid.

Astragalus - Pharmanex
Each capsule contains: Astragalus root extract (Astragalus membranaceus) (10:1) 250 mg. Other Ingredients: Rice Flour, Gelatin, Magnesium Stearate, Silicon Dioxide.

Astragalus - Jamieson
Each caplet contains: Astragalus Root Formula (T-Cell 7) 3000 mg.

Astragalus - Nature's Way
Three capsules contain: Astragalus root 1.41 g. Other Ingredients: Gelatin, Magnesium stearate.

Astragalus - Pro Health
Each capsule contains: Astragalus root powder (A. membranaceus) 500 mg. Other Ingredients: Stearic Acid.

Astragalus Jade Screen - Planetary Formulas
Two tablets contain: Proprietary Blend 1.7 g: Astragalus root, Atractylodes root, Siler root. Other Ingredients: Dibasic Calcium Phosphate, Sorbitol, Stearic Acid, Modified Cellulose Gum, Acacia Gum, Colloidal Silicon Dioxide, Magnesium Stearate.

Astragalus Plus - The Herbalist
Astragalus root • Echinacea root • Lomatium root • Myrrh Gum • Poke root • Wild Indigo root • Yarrow flower • Cayenne pepper.

Astragalus Root - Solgar
Each capsule contains: Iron 1 mg • Astragalus root 2:1 extract 2:1 90 mg • Raw Astragalus root powder 350 mg. Other Ingredients: Vegetable Cellulose, Vegetable Magnesium Stearate, Microcrystalline Cellulose, Water, Vegetable Glycerin.

Some Brand Name Natural Products - What they Contain

www.NaturalDatabase.com contains MANY more listings than appear here.
Editor's Notes are located on pages 2155-2163.

BRAND NAMES

Astragalus Root - Aboca USA, Inc
Two capsules contain: Astragalus root WPC (whole phytocomplex concentrate, astragalus membranaceus, standardized to 0.0086% astragaloside IV, yielding 0.025 mg per capsule) 580 mg. Other Ingredients: Gelatin.

Astragalus Root Extract - Vital Nutrients
Each capsule contains: Astragalus Membranaceus root 15:1 extract 300 mg.

Astragalus Supreme - Gaia Herbs
Thirty drops contain: Proprietary Blend 125 mg: Chinese Astragalus root (astragalus membranaceus), Chinese Schizandra berry (schizandra chinensis), Chinese Ligustrum berry (ligustrum lucidum), 30-40% Pure Grain Alcohol, Spring Water.

Astragalus Supreme capsules - Gaia Herbs
Two capsules contain: Astragalus root (astragalus membranaceus) 380 mg • Schizandra berry (schizandra chinensis) 370 mg • Ligustrum berry (ligustrum lucidum) 120 mg. Other Ingredients: Lecithin, Vegetable Cellulose (capsule).

Astragalus-Shitake Virtue - Blessed Herbs
Astragalus root • Echinacea angustifolia root • Licorice root • Shitake mycelium • Grain alcohol & Distilled Water.

A-Supreme - Advocare International
Each 1 fl oz serving contains: Riboflavin 3.4 mg • Niacin (as niacinamide) 40 mg • Vitamin B6 (as pyridoxine HCl) 4 mg • Folic Acid 800 mcg • Vitamin B12 (as cyanocobalamin) 500 mcg • Pantothenic Acid (as calcium pantothenate) 20 mg • Betaine 100 mg • Proprietary Blend 2 g: Eleutherococcus Senticosus (leaf, stem, root), Schisandra Chinensis seed, Aralia Mondshurica flower, Crataegus Oxyacantha leaf, Viburnum Sargenti (leaf, berry), Glycyrrhiza Uralensis root, Rhaponticum Carthamoides root, Rhodiola Rosea flower, Sorbus Aucuparia (whole plant), Iconotus Obliquus root.

A-Team: Adrenal Support - The Herbalist
Siberian Ginseng fresh-dried root (Eleuthero sent) • Oats fresh milky seed (Avena sativa) • Licorice fresh-dried root (Glycyrrhiza glabra) • Gotu Kola fresh herb (Hydrocotyle asiatica) • Cayenne fresh-dried pepper (Capsicum anuum).

Athero Chelates - PhytoPharmica
Twelve tablets contain: Ammonium Chloride 291 mg • Betaine HCl 300 mg • Bromelain (1800 MCU/g) 150 mg • Calcium (as monocalcium phosphate) 150 mg • Copper (as copper gluconate) 113 mcg • Iodine (from kelp) 600 mcg • L-Methionine 600 mcg • Magnesium (as magnesium orotate and magnesium ascorbate) 146 mg • Manganese (as manganese ascorbate) 6 mg • Mucopolysaccharide (soluble) 300 mg • Niacin (as niacinamide and niacin) 630 mg • Potassium (as potassium orotate, potassium aspartate, potassium chloride, and potassium phosphate) 75 mg • Proprietary Phytosterol Blend 450 mg: Beta Sitosterol, Campesterol, Stigmasterol, other Plant Sterols • Selenium (as selenium ascorbate) 300 mcg • Taurine 300 mg • Vitamin B6 (as pyridoxine HCl) 150 mg • Vitamin C (ascorbic acid) 1.5 g • Zinc (as zinc ascorbate) 9 mg.

Athero-Plus - Atrium Biotechnologies
Two film coated tablets contain: Vitamin A Palmitate 3334 IU • Vitamin D (as Vitamin D3) (Fish oil) 67 IU • Vitamin B1 (Thiamine Mononitrate) 34 mg • Vitamin B2 (Riboflavin) 17 mg • Vitamin B6 (Pyridoxine HCL) 34 mg • Vitamin B12 (Cyanocobalamin) 34 mcg • Vitamin C (Ascorbic Acid, Sago Palm) 400 mg • Vitamin E Succinate 134 IU • Beta Carotene 5000 IU • Biotin 100 mcg • Niacin/ Niacinamide 67 mg • D-Calcium Pantothenate 167 mg • Folic Acid 267 mcg • Calcium Orotate 170 mg • Chromium Aspartate 67 mcg • Copper Gluconate 0.67 mg • Iodine (Kelp) 40 mcg • Iron (Ferrous Fumerate) 6.67 mg • Magnesium Orotate 170 mg • Magnesium Aspartate 6.67 mg • Molybdenum (Kelp) 34 mcg • Potassium Orotate 34 mg • Selenium Aspartate 67 mcg • Zinc Orotate 6.67 mg • Bromelain 50 mg • Choline Bitartrate 34 mg • L-Methionine 20 mg • PABA 17 mg • Rutin 17 mg.

Athle-Peak - The Herbalist
Jamaican Sarsaparilla root • Siberian Ginseng root • American Ginseng root • Licorice root • Wild Yam root • Cinnamon bark • Cayenne pepper.

Athlete's Nutra-Pack - Nature's Plus
Each pack contains: Vitamin A (as beta carotene) 30,000 IU • Vitamin C (as mineral ascorbate, ascorbic acid) 1250 mg • Vitamin D (as ergocalciferol) 1000 IU • Vitamin E (as D-alpha tocopheryl succinate) 500 IU • Thiamin (as thiamine hydrochloride, vitamin B1) 100 mg • Riboflavin (vitamin B2) 100 mg • Niacin (as niacinamide) 125 mg • Vitamin B6 (pyridoxine HCl) 125 mg • Folate (as folic acid) 400 mcg • Vitamin B12 (as cyanocobalamin) 500 mcg • Biotin 125 mcg • Pantothenic Acid (as calcium pantothenate) 125 mg • Calcium (as amino acid chelate/complex) 550 mg • Iron (as amino acid chelate/ complex) 39 mg • Phosphorus (as amino acid complex) 100 mg • Iodine (from kelp) 262.5 mcg • Magnesium (as amino acid chelate/ complex, ascorbate) 275 mg • Zinc (as amino acid chelate/complex, ascorbate) 50 mg • Selenium (as amino acid complex) 200 mcg • Manganese (as amino acid chelate/complex) 15 mg • Chromium (as amino acid chelate) 300 mcg • Molybdenum (as amino acid complex) 50 mcg • Potassium (as amino acid complex) 64.5 mg • Bromelain (from pineapple fruit) 250 mg • PABA (para-aminobenzoic acid) 100 mg • Raw Adrenal Concentrate (bovine) 80 mg • Choline (as bitartrate) 75 mg • Inositol 75 mg • Citrus Bioflavonoids (from citrus limon exocarp) 50 mg • Rutin (from saphora japonica leaf) 50 mg • L-Methionine (free form amino acid) 50 mg • L-Glutamic Acid (free form amino acid) 25 mg • Betaine HCl (from beet molasses) 25 mg • Hesperidin (from citrus limon exocarp) 10 mg. Other Ingredients: Di-calcium Phosphate, Microcrystalline Cellulose, Stearic Acid, Magnesium Stearate, RNA, DNA, Brewer's Yeast, Lecithin, Silica, Hydroxypropyl Methylcellulose, Isolated Soy Protein, Rose Hips (rosa canina fruit), Spinach, Carrot, Broccoli, Bee Pollen, Wheat Germ.
See Editor's Note No. 14.

Athletic Performance - Vidafit
Each serving contains: Niacin 6 mg • Pantothenic Acid 4 mg • Riboflavin 1.3 mg • Thiamine 1.2 mg • Vitamin B12 2.4 mcg • Vitamin B6 1.3 mg • Vitamin C 75 mg • Vitamin E 10 IU • Complex Carbohydrates 12 g • Soy Protein 4 g • Whey Protein 8 g.

Athletic Performance Plus - Vidafit
Each serving contains: Niacin 6 mg • Pantothenic Acid 4 mg • Riboflavin 1.2 mg • Thiamine 1.1 mg • Vitamin B12 2.4 mcg • Vitamin B6 1.5 mg • Vitamin C 75 mg • Vitamin E 10 IU • Complex Carbohydrates 15 g • Creatine Monohydrate 1000 mg • Siberian Ginseng 150 mg • Guarana Extract 100 mg • Soy Protein 5 g • Whey Protein 10 g.

Athletic Recovery - Vidafit
Each serving contains: Vitamin C 75 mg • Vitamin E 10 IU • Calcium 100 mg • Copper 0.5 mg • Magnesium 120 mg • Phosphorus 100 mg • Potassium 700 mg • Zinc 5 mg • Complex Carbohydrates 15 g • Soy Protein 3 g • Whey Protein 7 g.

Athletic Strength - Vidafit
Each serving contains: Niacin 10 mg • Riboflavin 1.3 mg • Thiamine 1.2 mg • Vitamin B12 2.4 mcg • Vitamin B6 1.3 mg • Vitamin C 75 mg • Vitamin E 10 IU • Chondroitin Sulfate 250 mg • Glucosamine 500 mg • Siberian Ginseng 150 mg • Soy Protein 7 g • Whey Protein 18 g.
See Editor's Note No. 15.

Athletica - HerbaSway
Bitter Orange • Kudzu • Panax Ginseng • Siberian Ginseng • Astragalus • Schisandra • Ginger • Knotweed • Blackberry • Licorice • HerbaSwee (Cucurbitaceae fruit).
See Editor's Note No. 40.

Atkins Allergy - Atkins Nutritionals, Inc.
Six tablets contain: Pantethine (co-enzyme A precursor) 360 mg • Bioperine brand Black Pepper extract (piperine) 5 mg • Citrus

Bioflavonoids 1000 mg • Grape seed extract (Activin) 60 mg • Vitamin B12 (cyanocobalamin) 1000 mcg • Vitamin B6 (pyridoxine) 50 mg • Vitamin C (buffered) 2000 mg • Vitamin A (Acetate) 10000 IU • Quercetin (flavonoid) 840 mg • Calcium (3-phosphate, ascorbate) 700 mg • Magnesium (carbonate) 200 mg.

Atkins Basic #3 **- Atkins Nutritionals, Inc.**
Each tablet contains: Magnesium Oxide 8 mg • Copper Sulfate 200 mcg • Vitamin E (d Alpha Tocopherol) 20 IU • Cyanocobalamin (Vitamin B12) 30 mcg • Biotin 75 mcg • Folic Acid 100 mcg • Pyridoxine (HCL) (Vitamin B6) 20 mg • Pyridoxal 5-Phosphate 2 mg • Calcium Pantothenate (Vitamin B5) 25 mg • Pantethine (80%) 25 mg • Niacinamide 5 mg • Niacin (Vitamin B3) 2 mg • Vitamin C (Calcium Ascorbate) 120 mg • Riboflavin (Vitamin B2) 4 mg • Thiamine (HCL) (Vitamin B1) 5 mg • Vitamin D (as Vitamin D2) 15 IU • Beta Carotene 500 IU • Vitamin A 200 IU • L-Glutathione (reduced) 5 mg • N-Acetyl-L-Cysteine 20 mg • Octacosanol 150 mcg • Selenium 40 mcg • Vanadyl Sulfate 15 mcg • Molybdenum (Sodium) 10 mcg • Chromium (Polynicotinate) 50 mcg • Zinc (Chelate) 10 mg • Manganese (Chelate) 4 mg • PABA 100 mg • Inositol 80 mg • Choline Bitartrate 100 mg.

Atkins Blood Pressure **- Atkins Nutritionals, Inc.**
Six tablets contain: Taurine 1500 mg • Bioperine brand Black Pepper extract (piperine) 5 mg • Hawthorn (1.5% vitexin conc.) 300 mg • Calcium (from ascorbate) 75 mg • Magnesium (carbonate, glycinate) 600 mg • Vitamin C (buffered) 600 mg • Pantethine (co-enzyme A precursor) 35 mg • L-Arginine base 100 mg • Inositol 600 mg • N-Acetyl-L-Cysteine 150 mg • Chromium (picolinate) 200 mcg • Garlic 600 mg • Vitamin B6 (pyridoxine) 150 mg • Potassium (citrate) 99 mg.

Atkins Blood Sugar Tablets **- Atkins Nutritionals, Inc.**
Six tablets contain: Chromium (picolinate) 500 mcg • Bioperine brand Black Pepper extract (piperine) 5 mg • Folic Acid (folate) 800 mcg • Vitamin E natural 150 IU • Manganese (glycinate) 30 mg • Selenium (selenomethionine) 120 mcg • Inositol 900 mg • Niacinamide 300 mg • Vitamin C (buffered) 1200 mg • Bis-Glycinato Oxovanadium Complex (BGOV) 15 mg • Biotin 4 mg • Taurine 600 mg • Alpha-Lipoic Acid 240 mg • Magnesium (glycinate, carbonate) 600 mg • Zinc (monomethionine) 50 mg.

Atkins Cold & Flu **- Atkins Nutritionals, Inc.**
Four tablets contain: natural Beta-Carotene 20000 IU • Bioperine brand Black Pepper (piperine) 5 mg • Copper (chelate) 4 mg • Vitamin B6 (pyridoxine) 16 mg • Vitamin B3 (niacinamide) 60 mg • Vitamin B2 (riboflavin) 8 mg • Dimethylglycine (DMG) 80 mg • Folic Acid (folate) 800 mcg • Garlic 640 mg • Magnesium (ascorbate) 60 mg • Selenium (selenate) 120 mcg • Citrus Bioflavonoids 320 mg • Calcium Pantothenate (vitamin B5) 320 mg • Vitamin C buffered 2000 mg • Zinc (monomethionine) 100 mg • Quercetin (flavonoid) 320 mg • Vitamin A (acetate) 13333 IU.

Atkins Dieters Advantage **- Atkins Nutritionals, Inc.**
Four tablets contain: Citrin (55% Hydroxycitric Acid) 450 mg • Chromium (Polynicotinate) 200 mcg • Soy extract (containing active Saponins) 1500 mg • Methionine 250 mg • L-Carnitine Peptide Complex 500 mg • Vitamin B6 (pyridoxine) 20 mg • Pantethine (co-enzyme A precursor) 20 mg • Asparagus concentrate 50 mg • Parsley concentrate 50 mg • Kelp 20 mg • Spirulina 50 mg • Potassium (citrate) 99 mg • Magnesium (citrate/carbonate) 60 mg • L-Glutamine 75 mg • DL-Phenylalanine 150 mg • L-Tyrosine 75 mg • Bioperine brand Black Pepper extract (piperine) 5 mg.

Atkins Essential Oils **- Atkins Nutritionals, Inc.**
Each capsule contains: Flaxseed oil 400 mg • Vitamin E 5 IU • Fish oil (50% Omega-3 potency) 400 mg • Borage seed oil 400 mg.

Atkins Heart Care **- Atkins Nutritionals, Inc.**
Eight tablets contain: Magnesium (glycinate, carbonate) 400 mg • Bioperine brand Black Pepper extract (piperine) 5 mg • Cayenne 500 mg • Bromelain (proteolytic enzyme) 500 mg • Vitamin B6 (pyridoxine) 10 mg • Folic Acid (folate) 800 mcg • Selenium (methionate) 150 mcg • Hawthorn (1.5% vitexin conc.) 100 mg • Ginkgo Biloba (6% terpene conc.) 60 mg • Natural Beta-Carotene (dunaliella salina) 12000 IU • Chromium (picolinate) 200 mcg • Vitamin C (buffered) 1000 mg • Natural Vitamin E 400 IU • Taurine 500 mg • Calcium (3-phosphate) 500 mg.

Atkins Memory **- Atkins Nutritionals, Inc.**
Eight tablets contain: Phosphatidylserine (PS) 160 mg • Bioperine brand Black Pepper extract (piperine) 5 mg • Folic Acid (folate) 800 mcg • Vitamin B12 (cyanocobalamin) 1000 mcg • Vitamin B1 (thiamine) 100 mg • N-Acetyl-L-Cysteine 1000 mg • Octacosanol 6 mg • Ginkgo Biloba (6% terpene lactone conc.) 60 mg.

Atkins Menopause **- Atkins Nutritionals, Inc.**
Four tablets contain: Black Cohosh (cimicifuga rademosal, 2.5% triterpenes) 25 mg • Vitamin E (D-alpha-tocopheryl) 200 IU • Bioperine brand Black Pepper extract (piperine) 5 mg • Vitamin K 50 mg • Folic Acid 800 mcg • Mixed Tocotrienols 3 mg • Boron (boroglutamate) 3 mg • Alpha Lipoic Acid 10 mg • Pantethine (co-enzyme A precursor) 25 mg • Vitamin B6 (pyridoxine) 50 mg • Calcium (sulfate) 65 mg • Magnesium (sulfate) 70 mg • Beta-Sitosterol 50 mg • Gamma Oryzanol 150 mg • PurGar brand Garlic 250 mg • Soy Phosphatidylcholine 400 mg • PABA (para amino benzoic acid) 500 mg • Soy Isoflavones concentrate (23.6% Genistein/Genistin; 3.8% Daidzin/Daldzein) 100 mg.

Atkins Shake Mix (cappuccino flavor) **- Atkins Nutritionals, Inc.**
Cappuccino shake mix contains: Lipo-Pro Blend (special formulation containing: Calcium Caseinate, Milk Protein concentrate, Egg Whites, Glutamine Peptides, Hydrolyzed Whey Protein concentrate & Whey Protein Isolate) • High Oleic Sunflower oil • Lecithin • Enzyme Modified Soy Protein • Carmel Color • Guar Gum • Vitamins & Minerals • Natural & Artificial Flavors • Acesulfame Potassium • Beta-Carotene.

Atkins Shake Mix (chocolate flavor) **- Atkins Nutritionals, Inc.**
Chocolate shake mix contains: Lipo-Pro Blend (special formulation containing: Calcium Caseinate, Milk Protein concentrate, Egg Whites, Glutamine Peptides, Hydrolyzed Whey Protein concentrate & Whey Protein Isolate) • Dutch Cocoa • High Oleic Sunflower oil • Polydextrose • Lecithin • Guar Gum • Vitamins & Minerals • Vanillin • Acesulfame Potassium • Beta-Carotene.

Atkins Shake Mix (vanilla flavor) **- Atkins Nutritionals, Inc.**
Vanilla Shake Mix contains: Lipo-Pro Blend (special formulation containing: Calcium Caseinate, Milk Protein concentrate, Egg Whites, Glutamine Peptides, Hydrolyed Whey Protein concentrate & Whey Protein Isolate) • High Oleic Sunflower oil • Lecithin • Guar Gum • Vitamins & Minerals • Natural & Artificial Flavors • Acesulfame Potassium • Beta-Carotene.

Atkins Vita-Chol **- Atkins Nutritionals, Inc.**
Three tablets contain: Calcium 200 mg • Phosphorus 100 mg • Inositol Hexanicotinate 1.6 g • Guggul Lipids 100 mg • Phytosterols 225 mg • Garlic 300 mg • Pantethine 100 mg • L-Arginine 100 mg. AbsorbBest base 345 mg: Lecithin extracts, Garlic, Arginine, Licorice, Bromelain, Spirulina, Pantethine, Inulin, Lactoferrin, Bioperine brand Black Pepper extract, Acidophilus.
This product was formerly known as Enhanced Cholesterol.

Atomic X Energy Drink **- Atomic X**
Water • High Fructose Corn Syrup • Glucose • Natural and Artificial Flavors • Taurine • Citric Acid • Malic Acid • Gluconolactone • Ascorbic Acid • Inositol • Choline • Caffeine • Niacin (vitamin B3) • Pantothenic Acid (vitamin B5) • FD&C Yellow #5 and #6 • Pyridoxine (vitamin B6) • Cyanocobalamin (vitamin B12).

ATP Fuel **- TwinLab**
Three capsules contain: Creatine Monohydrate & Creatine Pyruvate 3000 mg • Potassium Phosphate 300 mg • ATP (adenosine triphosphate) 60 mg.

BRAND NAMES

ATP Plus - Progressive Labs
Six tablets contain: Magnesium (as magnesium hydroxide) 300 mg • Malic Acid 1200 mg.

Atri A.S.F - Atrium Biotechnologies
Each tablet contains: Raw Tissue concentrates (not extracts) of Bovine source of the following 200 mg: Thymus 80 mg • Partoid 80 mg • Adrenal 20 mg • Spleen 20 mg.
See Editor's Note No. 14.

Atri CU- Chelate - Atrium Biotechnologies
Each tablet contains: Spleen 28.5 mg • Brain 7.5 mg • Liver 5 mg • Heart 3.5 mg • Kidney 3.5 mg • Thymus 2 mg • Adrenal 2 mg • Pituitary 1 mg • Pancreas 1 mg • Duodenum 1 mg • Copper (Protein Chelated) 2 mg.
See Editor's Note No. 31.

Atri E-Derm - Atrium Biotechnologies
Each gram contains: Natural Vitamin E (d-Alpha Tocopheryl Acetate) 30 IU. In an absorbent base containing unsaturated fatty acids from Flax & Beet Lipids, Natural Vitamin A & Lecithin.

Atri Flexile - Atrium Biotechnologies
Each capsule contains: Glucosamine Sulfate 500 mg • Uncaria tomentosa 200 mg • Curcumin 50 mg • Bromelain 25 mg.

Atri Free Amino - Atrium Biotechnologies
Each capsule contains: Free Form Amino Acids: L- Alanine • L-Arginine • L-Aspartic Acid • L-Citruline • L-Cystine • L-Glutamic Acid • L-Glutamine • L-Glysine • L-Histidine HCl • L-Hydroxproline • L-Isoleucine • L-Leucine • L-Lysine • L-Methionine • L-Phenylalanine • L-Proline • L-Serine • L-Threonine • L-Tyrosine • L-Valine • L-Taurine.

Atri K-Chelate - Atrium Biotechnologies
Each tablet contains: As chelated proteinates (Amino Acid Chelated Minerals): Potassium 100 mg • Raw Tissue concentrate 55 mg: Spleen 28.5 mg, Brain 7.5 mg, Liver 5 mg, Heart 3.5 mg, Kidney 3.5 mg, Thymus 2 mg, Adrenal 2 mg, Pituitary 1 mg, Pancreas 1 mg, Duodenum 1 mg.
See Editor's Note No. 31.

Atri Multi-Hypo - Atrium Biotechnologies
Three tablets contain: Vitamin A (from Fish Liver oil) 10000 IU • Vitamin D (as Vitamin D3) 400 IU • Vitamin B 10 mg • Vitamin B2 10 mg • Vitamin B6 10 mg • Vitamin B12 50 mcg • Niacinamide 100 mg • Pantothenic Acid 50 mg • Folic Acid 400 mcg • Vitamin C 120 mg • Vitamin E (d-Alpha Tocopherol Succinate) 15 mg • Biotin 30 mcg • Calcium 97 mg • Magnesium 72 mg • Manganese 15 mg • Potassium 53 mg • Zinc 15 mg • Iron (from Iron Sulfate) 18 mg • Iodine (from Kelp) 150 mcg • Choline Bitartrate 30 mg • Inositol 30 mg • PABA (Para Amino Benzoic Acid) 30 mg • Citrus Bioflavonoids 100 mg • Hesperidin 25 mg • Rutin 20 mg • Glutamic Acid 18 mg • L-Lysine (Monohydrochloride) 30 mg • L-Methionine 30 mg.

Atri Zinc Plus - Atrium Biotechnologies
Each tablet contains: Ascorbic Acid & Sodium Ascorbate 125 mg • Zinc Gluconate 25 mg • Rutin 25 mg.

Atri-770 - Atrium Biotechnologies
Each capsule contains: Cold Pressed concentrated Wheat Germ oil 770 mg.

Atri-A + E Mulsion High concentrate - Atrium Biotechnologies
Each drop contains: Emulsified Vitamin A Palmitate 15000 IU • Vitamin E (d-Alpha Tocopheryl Acetate) 10 IU.

Atri-A + E Mulsion Regular concentrate - Atrium Biotechnologies
Each drop contains: Emulsified Vitamin A Palmitate 5000 IU • Vitamin E (d-Alpha Tocopheryl Acetate) 10 IU.

Atri-Acidic - Atrium Biotechnologies
Each tablet contains: Raw Stomach concentrate (Bovine) 50 mg • Raw Duodenum concentrate (Bovine) 50 mg • Betaine HCl 460 mg • Glutamic Acid HCl 200 mg • Pepsin 1:20000 25 mg • Potassium Chloride 25 mg.
See Editor's Note No. 14.

Atri-Aloe-Lax - Atrium Biotechnologies
Each capsule contains: Aloe 450 mg.

Atri-Aloe-V - Atrium Biotechnologies
Each capsule contains: Aloe ferox (Aloe Vera resin) 430 mg • Aloe barbadensis (Aloe Vera leaf) 100 mg.

Atri-Amino - Atrium Biotechnologies
Six tablets contain: Isoleucine 90 mg • Leucine 216 mg • Lysine 270 mg • Methionine 54 mg • Phenylalanine 132 mg • Threonine 132 mg • Valine 156 mg • Arginine 528 mg • Histidine 48 mg • Alanine 660 mg • Tyrosine 18 mg • Serine 252 mg • Aspartic Acid 402 mg • Cystine 18 mg • Glutamic Acid 684 mg • Glycine 1650 mg • Hydroxylysine 54 mg • Hydroxyproline 846 mg • Proline 984 mg.

Atri-Arthritis Spray - Atrium Biotechnologies
Four fluid ounces contains: Oil of Wintergreen (Methyl Salicylate) 15% • Menthol 6% • IPA Alcohol. In a specially formulated, non-greasy base.

Atri-Bio-C - Atrium Biotechnologies
Each tablet contains: Calcium Ascorbate 500 mg • Bioflavonoids 500 mg • Acerola 10 mg • Hesperidin 10 mg • Rutin 10 mg.

Atri-BLP - Atrium Biotechnologies
Each capsule contains: Cayenne 200 mg • Parsley 90 mg • Ginger root 50 mg • Goldenseal root 40 mg • Garlic 35 mg • Siberian Ginseng 30 mg.

Atri-Cal Chelate - Atrium Biotechnologies
Three tablets contain: As Chelated Proteinates (Amino Acid Chelated Minerals) Calcium 450 mg • Raw Tissue concentrate 135 mg: Spleen 74.1 mg, Brain 19.5 mg, Liver 13 mg, Heart 9.1 mg, Kidney 9.1 mg, Thymus 2 mg, Adrenal 2 mg, Pituitary 1 mg, Pancreas 2.6 mg, Duodenum 2.6 mg.
See Editor's Note No. 31.

Atri-C-Flu - Atrium Biotechnologies
Each capsule contains: Garlic 300 mg • Parsley 60 mg • Rose Hips 60 mg • Rosemary 25 mg • Watercress 20 mg.

Atri-Daily Essentials - Atrium Biotechnologies
Three tablets contain: Vitamin E (D-alpha) 200 IU • Beta Carotene 5000 IU • Vitamin D 400 IU • Folic Acid 400 mcg • Thiamine 1.5 mg • Riboflavin 1.7 mg • Niacin 20 mg • Vitamin B6 2 mg • Vitamin B12 6 mcg • Biotin 300 mcg • Pantothenic Acid 10 mg • Calcium Citrate 600 mg • Phosphorous 450 mg • Iodine (Kelp) 150 mcg • Magnesium (carbonate) 200 mg • Copper (gluconate) 2 mg • Zinc (gluconate) 15 mg • Vitamin K 100 mcg • Selenium (yeast) 75 mcg • Manganese (gluconate) 5 mg • Chromium (aspartate) 200 mcg • Molybdenum 150 mcg • Nickel 15 mcg • Tin 15 mcg • Vanadium 5 mg • Boron (citrate) 2 mg • Potassium (gluconate) 100 mg • Grape seed extract 10 mg • CoQ10 10 mg.

Atri-Detox - Atrium Biotechnologies
Each capsule contains: Red Clover Blossoms 150 mg • Chaparral 80 mg • Licorice root 50 mg • Peach bark 50 mg • Oregon Grape root 40 mg • Stillingia 35 mg • Cascara Sagrada bark 30 mg • Sarsaparilla root 30 mg • Burdock root 15 mg • Buckthorn bark 10 mg.

Atri-Disco - Atrium Biotechnologies
Each tablet contains: First Phase (in Stomach) Manganese Sulfate 200 mg • Calcium Ascorbate 100 mg • Magnesium Aspartate 50 mg. Second Phase (in Duodenum) Alpha-Chymotrypsin 4 mg • Papain 100 mg • Bromelain 100 mg • Pancreatin 5x 50 mg.
See Editor's Note No. 14.

Some Brand Name Natural Products - What they Contain

www.NaturalDatabase.com contains MANY more listings than appear here.
Editor's Notes are located on pages 2155-2163.

Atri-DMG Plus - Atrium Biotechnologies
Each tablet contains: NN Dimethyl Glycine 19.3 mg • Calcium Gluconate 30.7 mg • Glycine 25 mg • Lysine 25 mg.

Atri-EPA Plus - Atrium Biotechnologies
Each capsule contains: Salmon oil [containing EPA (eicosapentaenoic acid) 180 mg & DHA (docosahexaenoic acid) 120 mg] 1000 mg • Vitamin A (fish oil) 100 IU • Vitamin E (fish oil) 5 IU.

Atri-F - Atrium Biotechnologies
Each capsule contains: Cold Processed Persic oil (yielding the following Lipid Acids referred to as Vitamin F factors: Oleic 192 mg, Linoleic 109 mg, Palmitic 18 mg, Stearic 4 mg, Linolenic 701 mcg, Heptodecanoic 400 mcg, Arachadic 330 mcg, Arachidonic 111 mcg) 370 mg • Potassium 113 mcg • Sodium 14 mcg • Magnesium 7 mcg • Phosphorus 4 mg • Calcium 4 mcg • "trace amounts of: Manganese, Chromium, Zinc, Iron, Copper, Boron & Barium" • Palmitoleic 5 mg.

Atri-Fem-Reg - Atrium Biotechnologies
Each capsule contains: Goldenseal root 120 mg • Blessed Thistle 100 mg • Cramp bark 80 mg • Uva Ursi leaves 70 mg • False Unicorn 50 mg • Raspberry leaves 30 mg • Squaw Vine 20 mg • Ginger root 10 mg.

Atri-Flav-1000 - Atrium Biotechnologies
Three tablets contain: Vitamin C 1000 mg • Citrus Bioflavonoids 1000 mg • Rutin 100 mg. Other Ingredients: Rose Hips & Acerola, in a base containing Raw Spleen concentrate 4 mg.
See Editor's Note No. 14.

Atri-FM-H - Atrium Biotechnologies
Each capsule contains: Black Cohosh 200 mg • Sarsaparilla root 150 mg • Siberian Ginseng 40 mg • Licorice root 35 mg • False Unicorn 30 mg • Blessed Thistle 25 mg • Squaw Vine 20 mg.

Atri-Gastro Atrium Biotechnologies
Each capsule contains: Colloidal Silica 200 mg • Irish Moss 50 mg • Beef Duodenum 20 mg • Pepsin 20 mg • Stomach Mucosa 10 mg • Di-Sodium Phosphate 10 mg.
See Editor's Note No. 14.

Atri-GE-132 - Atrium Biotechnologies
Each capsule contains: Germanium Sesquioxide 150 mg.

Atri-GE-132 Sub - Atrium Biotechnologies
Each tablet contains: Germanium Sesquioxide 25 mg.

Atri-Gesic - Atrium Biotechnologies
Three ounces contain: Lanolin • Menthol • Methyl Salicylate • Oil of Cassia • Stearic Acid • Spermwax • GMS • Tea • Methyl Gluceth E 10 • Camphor • Methyl Nicotinate • Propyl Parasept • Deionized Water.

Atri-Glucomannan - Atrium Biotechnologies
Each capsule contains: Glucomannan Dietary Fiber (Konjac root source) 500 mg.

Atri-Greens Plus - Atrium Biotechnologies
Each tablet contains: Vitamin A (Palmitate) 5000 IU • Vitamin C (Ascorbic Acid) 240 mg • Vitamin E (Acetate) 45 mg • Beta Carotene 150 mg • Selenium (Yeast) 50 mcg • Spirulina 25 mg • Chlorophyll 2 mg. In a base of cruciferous vegetables: Broccoli, Brussels Sprouts, Cabbage, Carrot, Cauliflower, Kale, Mustard Greens, Pumpkin, Spinach & Turnip Greens.

Atri-Herb-CLS - Atrium Biotechnologies
Each capsule contains: Gentian root 50 mg • Valerian root 50 mg • Catnip 40 mg • Goldenseal root 40 mg • Barberry bark 30 mg • Cascara Sagrada 30 mg • Irish Moss 30 mg • Fenugreek seed 30 mg • Bugleweed 25 mg • Yellow Dock root 25 mg • St. John's Wort 25 mg • Brigham Tea 25 mg • Red Clover Blossoms 25 mg • Chickweed 25 mg.

Atri-IBC - Atrium Biotechnologies
Each capsule contains: Eyebright 100 mg • Goldenseal root • Barberry bark 100 mg • Red Raspberry leaves 100 mg • Cayenne 100 mg.

Atri-INF - Atrium Biotechnologies
Each capsule contains: Plantain 200 mg • Black Walnut leaves 100 mg • Goldenseal root 60 mg • Marshmallow root 50 mg • Bugleweed 40 mg.

Atri-Kid-Uri - Atrium Biotechnologies
Each capsule contains: Juniper berries 200 mg • Parsley 120 mg • Uva Ursi leaves 50 mg • Marshmallow root 45 mg • Ginger root 40 mg • Goldenseal root 20 mg.

Atri-Lacto - Atrium Biotechnologies
Each capsule contains: Lactobacillus Acidophilus & Bulgaras culture 400 mg. Contains a minimum two million total bacteria count.

Atri-Lax - Atrium Biotechnologies
Each capsule contains: Psyllium husks 100 mg • Cascara Sagrada bark 100 mg • Prune concentrate 100 mg • Senna leaves 100 mg • Licorice root 45 mg • Chlorophyll 10 mg.

Atri-LB-CLS - Atrium Biotechnologies
Each capsule contains: Cascara Sagrada 150 mg • Bayberry root bark 75 mg • Cayenne 75 mg • Ginger root 50 mg • Goldenseal root 50 mg • Lobelia 30 mg • Red Raspberry leaves 30 mg • Turkey Rhubarb root 30 mg • Fennel seed 20 mg.

Atri-Lipotropic - Atrium Biotechnologies
Three capsules contain: Choline Bitartrate 1000 mg • Inositol 1000 mg • Methionine 300 mg.

Atri-Liv-GLB - Atrium Biotechnologies
Each capsule contains: Barberry root bark 120 mg • Wild Yam 80 mg • Cramp bark 60 mg • Fennel seed 50 mg • Yellow Dock 40 mg • Ginger root 35 mg • Catnip 30 mg • Peppermint leaves 30 mg.

Atri-Ly Poll - Atrium Biotechnologies
Each tablet contains: Raw Bovine Tissue concentrate (not extracts) 20 mg: Pituitary 5 mg, Adrenal 15 mg • Bee Pollen 250 mg • L-Lysine 400 mg.
See Editor's Note No. 14.

Atri-Lym-Inf - Atrium Biotechnologies
Each capsule contains: Cayenne 150 mg • Echinacea 120 mg • Myrrh Gum 100 mg • Hawthorn berries 100 mg • Licorice root 30 mg.

Atri-Mag Chelate Plus - Atrium Biotechnologies
Each tablet contains: Amino Acid Chelated Minerals as: Magnesium 300 mg • Raw Tissue concentrates (bovine source): Spleen 29 mg • Brain 8 mg • Liver 5 mg • Heart 4 mg • Kidney 4 mg • Thymus 2 mg • Adrenal 2 mg • Pituitary 1 mg • Duodenum 1 mg • Pancreas 1 mg.
See Editor's Note No. 31.

Atri-Medicated Psoriasis Shampoo - Atrium Biotechnologies
Eight fluid ounces contain: Active Ingredients: Coal Tar solution USP 5% • Colloidal Sulfur 2% • Salicylic Acid 2%. In a special base of Surface Active Cleansers, Wetting Agents & Lanolin.

Atri-Mega Plus - Atrium Biotechnologies
Four tablets contain: Vitamin A Acetate 25000 IU • Vitamin D (as Vitamin D3) Cholecalciferol 1000 IU • Vitamin E Acetate 100 IU • Vitamin C (with Rose Hips) 500 mg • Folic Acid 0.1 mg • Thiamine (Vitamin B1) 50 mg • Riboflavin (Vitamin B2) 50 mg • Niacin 100 mg • Vitamin B6 50 mg • Vitamin B12 50 mcg • Biotin 50 mcg • Pantothenic Acid 50 mg • Choline Bitartrate 50 mg • Calcium (as Oyster Shell & Calcium Carbonate) 700 mg • Iodine (Kelp) 225 mcg • Iron (Ferrous Fumerate) 30 mg • Magnesium (as Oxide) 200 mg • Zinc (as Sulfate) 36 mg • Manganese (as Carbonate) 3 mg • Potassium (Chloride & Kelp) 99 mg • Chromium (as Chelate) 20 mcg • Selenium (Yeast) 60 mcg • Betaine HCl 50 mg • Papain 200 mg • Para Aminobenzoic Acid 50 mg • Citrus Bioflavonoids 50 mg • Inositol 50 mg • Ribonucleic Acid (Yeast extract) 200 mg.

Atri-Mega-Lacto - Atrium Biotechnologies
Each capsule contains: Lactobacillus Acidophilus with Bifidus Four Billion CFU (Colony Forming Units).

Some Brand Name Natural Products - What they Contain

www.NaturalDatabase.com contains MANY more listings than appear here.
Editor's Notes are located on pages 2155-2163.

BRAND NAMES

Atri-Min 74 - Atrium Biotechnologies
Each tablet contains: Sea Bed Montmorillonite (also known as Mineral 74100 mg Volcanic Montmorillonite) 900 mg.

Atri-Multi - Atrium Biotechnologies
Each tablet contains: Vitamin A (from Fish Liver oil) 3333 IU • Vitamin D (as Vitamin D3) 133 IU • Vitamin B1 4 mg • Vitamin B2 3 mg • Vitamin B6 3 mg • Vitamin B12 11 mcg • Niacinamide 34 mg • Pantothenic Acid 17 mg • Folic Acid 134 mcg • Vitamin C 40 mg • Vitamin E (d-Alpha Tocopherol) 5 mg • Biotin 10 mcg • Calcium 32 mg • Magnesium 24 mg • Manganese 5 mg • Potassium 18 mg • Zinc 5 mg • Iron (from Sulfate) 6 mg • Iodine (from Kelp) 50 mcg • Choline Bitartrate 10 mg • PABA 9 mg • Citrus Bioflavonoids 100 mg • Hesperidin 9 mg • Rutin 7 mg • Glutamic Acid 6 mg • L-Lysine 10 mg • L-Methionine 10 mg • RNA (from Yeast) 15 mg. In a base of Watercress, Kelp, Alfalfa, Parsley.

Atri-Nerv - Atrium Biotechnologies
Each capsule contains: Black Cohosh 100 mg • Cayenne 100 mg • Hops Flowers 80 mg • Scullcap 70 mg • Wood Betony 50 mg • Passiflora 40 mg • Valerian root 20 mg • Lady's Slipper 10 mg.

Atri-Neuro - Atrium Biotechnologies
Each tablet contains: Choline (Choline Bitartrate) 200 mg • L-Histidine 50 mg • L-Phenylalanine 50 mg • GABA (Amino Buteric Acid) 50 mg • L-Tyrosine 50 mg • Raw Brain concentrate 25 mg • Niacin 15 mg • Pyridoxine HCl 50 mg.
See Editor's Note No. 31.

Atri-NTL-CA - Atrium Biotechnologies
Each capsule contains: Horsetail grass 300 mg • Oat Straw 100 mg.

Atri-Ortho-Phos - Atrium Biotechnologies
Each drop contains: Ortho Phosphoric Acid 13 mg • Inositol 0.57 mg • Choline Bitartrate 0.27 mg. Thirty drops contain: Ortho Phosphoic Acid 390 mg • Inositol 17 mg • Choline Bitartrate 8 mg.

Atri-Oxy - Atrium Biotechnologies
Two tablets contain: Vitamin A (beta carotene) 25000 IU • Vitamin E (D-alpha tocopherol) 400 IU • Vitamin C 1000 mg • Bioflavonoid Complex 150 mg • Superoxide Dismutase 100 mg • Selenium 100 mcg • Zinc 25 mg • Copper 2 mg • Astragalus 50 mg • Rosemary 50 mg • Milk Thistle (silymarin) 50 mg • Spirulina 100 mg • Chromium Picolinate 25 mcg • Grape seed extract 50 mg • CoEnzyme Q-10 10 mg • L-Glutathione 10 mg • L-Cysteine 100 mg • Reishi Mushroom 50 mg • Curcumin 50 mg.

Atri-PMS - Atrium Biotechnologies
Three tablets contain: Vitamin A Acetate 5000 IU • Vitamin B6 (pyridoxine HCl) 100 mg • Adrenal concentrate 50 mg • Hypothalamus concentrate 10 mg • Ovary concentrate 50 mg • Pituitary concentrate 10 mg • Passion Flower 75 mg • Dong Quai 50 mg • Cramp bark 50 mg • Chionanthus 50 mg • Valerian 75 mg • Magnesium (Oxide) 200 mg • Iron (Peptonate) 20 mg • Red Raspberry 50 mg.
See Editor's Note No. 31.

Atri-Pros - Atrium Biotechnologies
Each capsule contains: Cayenne 160 mg • Uva Ursi leaves 70 mg • Parsley 60 mg • Goldenseal root 50 mg • Gravel root 50 mg • Juniper berries 30 mg • Marshmallow root 25 mg • Ginger root 20 mg • Siberian Ginseng 15 mg.

Atri-Psoriasis Ointment - Atrium Biotechnologies
Four ounces contains: Sulfur ppt 1.5% • Salicylic Acid 1.5% • Coal Tar Solution USP 2%.

Atri-Res - Atrium Biotechnologies
Each capsule contains: Marshmallow root 200 mg • Mullein 120 mg • Comfrey leaves 100 mg • Chickweed 50 mg. Professional Formula.

Atri-RNA/DNA - Atrium Biotechnologies
Each tablet contains: RiboNucleic Acid (RNA) 180 mg • DeoxyNucleic Acid (DNA) 40 mg.

Atri-SDT - Atrium Biotechnologies
Each tablet contains: Trypsin 4 mg • Chymotrypsin 2 mg • Pancreatin 2 mg • Bromelain 3 mg • Papayotin 4 mg • Thymus concentrate (Bovine) 2 mg • Mannitol 13 mg. In a specially prepared natural spearmint flavored slow dissolving tablet base.
See Editor's Note No. 14.

Atri-Selenium+E - Atrium Biotechnologies
Each tablet contains: Vitamin C (Ascorbic Acid) 250 mg • Vitamin E (d-Alpha Tocopherol) 200 IU • Vitamin B1 (Thiamine HCL) 4 mg • Vitamin B2 (Riboflavin) 4 mg • Vitamin B6 (Pyridoxine HCL) 4 mg • Niacin 10 mg • Pantothenic Acid 50 mg • Selenium (Selenium Yeast) 50 mcg • Raw Heart concentrate 10 mg. In a base of Bone Meal.
See Editor's Note No. 14.

Atri-S-G-V - Atrium Biotechnologies
Each tablet contains: Selenium 50 mcg • Germanium 225 mcg • Vanadium 225 mcg, as Protein Chelates.

Atri-Statin - Atrium Biotechnologies
Each tablet contains: Caprylic Acid 110 mg.

Atri-Stress-B+C - Atrium Biotechnologies
Two tablets contain: Vitamin C (Ascorbic Acid) 500 mg • Vitamin B1 (Thiamine HCl) 100 mg • Vitamin B2 (Riboflavin) 100 mg • Vitamin B6 (Pyridoxine HCl) 100 mg • Vitamin B12 (Cyanocobalamin) 500 mcg • Niacinamide 100 mg • Pantothenic Acid 100 mg • Folic Acid 400 mcg • Biotin 100 mcg • Lemon Bioflavonoids 250 mg • Choline (Choline Bitartrate) 100 mg • Inositol 100 mg • PABA 50 mg.

Atri-Thy-Kelp - Atrium Biotechnologies
Each capsule contains: Mullein 140 mg • Parsley 90 mg • Watercress 80 mg • Kelp (Norwegian) 70 mg • Irish Moss 60 mg • Iceland Moss 40 mg.

Atri-Trace - Atrium Biotechnologies
Three tablets contain: Calcium (Egg & Oyster Shells) 250 mg • Magnesium (Gluconate) 50 mg • Manganese (Gluconate) 10 mg • Potassium (Gluconate) 50 mg • Zinc (Gluconate)15 mg • Vitamin D (as Vitamin D3) 133 IU • Vitamin B6 50 mg • Glutamic Acid HCL 325 mg.

Atri-V&M+Complete - Atrium Biotechnologies
Six tablets contain: Vitamin A (Fish oil) 10000 IU • Vitamin D (Fish oil) 400 IU • Vitamin C (Calcium Ascorbate, Acerola, Rose Hips) 400 mg • Vitamin E 60 IU • Vitamin B1 • Vitamin B2 10 mg • Vitamin B6 10 mg • Vitamin B12 25 mcg • Niacin 60 mg • Calcium (Bone Meal & Calcium Carbonate) 750 mg • Magnesium (Oxide) 375 mg • Phosphorus (Bone Meal) 700 mg • Iron (Amino Acid Chelate) 20 mg • Iodine (Kelp) 150 mcg • Potassium (Proteinate) 20 mg • Zinc (Amino Acid Chelate) 20 mg • Manganese (Amino Acid Chelate) 15 mg • Choline (Bitartrate) 50 mg • Inositol 500 mg • Lecithin 50 mg • Pantothenic Acid 50 mg • Folic Acid 400 mcg • PABA 30 mg • RNA-DNA 15 mg • Betaine HCL 25 mg • Biotin 100 mcg. In a base of Alfalfa, Kelp, Rose Hips, Acerola, Fish Liver oils, Bone Meal, Citrus Bioflavonoids, Papaya, Bromelain Enzymes & Essential Amino Acids.

Atri-Vana - Atrium Biotechnologies
Each capsule contains: Vanadyl Sulfate 25 mg.

Atri-Verm - Atrium Biotechnologies
Each capsule contains: Pumpkin seed 100 mg • Culver's root 70 mg • Violet leaves 60 mg • Cascara Sagrada bark 50 mg • Slippery Elm bark 45 mg • Witch Hazel bark 40 mg • Mullein 30 mg • Echinacea 20 mg.

Atri-Yeast - Atrium Biotechnologies
Four tablets contain: Protein from a Special Yeast 1200 mg • Niacin 66 mg • Pantothenic Acid 13 mg • Vitamin B1 13 mg • Vitamin B2 13 mg • Vitamin B6 3 mg • Chromium 25 mcg • Selenium 7.5 mcg.

Atri-Zinc Chelate Plus - Atrium Biotechnologies
Each tablet contains: Amino Acid Chelated Minerals: Zinc 29 mg. Raw Tissue concentrates (bovine source) from: Spleen 29 mg • Brain

8 mg • Liver 5 mg • Heart 4 mg • Kidney 4 mg • Thymus 2 mg • Adrenal 2 mg • Pituitary 1 mg • Duodenum 1 mg.
See Editor's Note No. 31.

Attend - Vaxa International
Each capsule contains: Proprietary Blend 715 mg: L-Isoleucine, L-Leucine, L-Valine, L-Tyrosine, L-Cysteine, L-Cystine, DL-Methionine, DLPA, L-Glutamic Acid, GABA, L-Glycine, L-Glutathione, Catechol, Pregnenolone, Trifolium Pratense (trans-cis-cloramide), Flax Seed powder, Pyridoxine, Calcium Pantothenate, Magnesium Aspartate, OptiZinc brand Zinc, Niacinamide, Radix Heraclei, Gotu Kola, Ginkgo Biloba, ChromeMate GTF brand Chromium, DMAE, Pycnogenol, Pine Bark extract, NADH, Sodium Bicarbonate, Phosphatidylcholine, Phosphatidylethanolamine, Phosphatidylserine, Phosphatidylinositol, Medium Chain Triglycerides, Caprylic Acid, Lauric Acid, Myristic Acid, Palmitic Acid, Stearic Acid, Oleic Acid, Linoleic Acid, Linolenic Acid, Arachidic Acid, EPA (eicosapentaenoic acid), Ecicosatrienoic Acid, Arachidonic Acid, Gamma Linolenic Acid, DHA (docosahexaenoic acid), Agaricus Muscarius, Argentum Nitricum, Avena Sativa, Caffeinum, Cimicifuga Racemosa, Fluoricum Acidum, Humulus Lupulis, Hyoscyamus Niger, Ignatia Amara, Iodum, Kali Bromatum, Kali Phosphoricum, Lithium Bromatum, Lithium Carbonicum, Natrum Muriaticum, Hypothalamus, Corticohypothalmic Axis, Diopside, Parasympathetic Ganglia, Rhodonite.
See Editor's Note No. 31.

Attention! - Olympia Nutrition
Contains DHA 250 mg • Phosphatidylserine 20 mg • DMAE 100 mg • Choline 100 mg • TMG.

Attentive Child - Source Naturals
Two chewable wafers contain: Magnesium (from magnesium aspartate) 109 mg • Zinc (as zinc picolinate) 2 mg • L-Aspartate (from magnesium aspartate) 310 mg • DMAE (as DMAE bitartrate) 100 mg • Standardized Soybean Lecithin (yielding 40% phosphatidylserine, 20 mg) 50 mg • Phosphatidylcholine 6 mg • Phosphatidylethanolamine 3.5 mg • Phosphatidylinositol 1.5 mg • DHA (docosahexaenoic acid, Neuromins brand) 15 mg • Grape seed extract 15 mg. Other Ingredients: Xylitol, Crystalline Fructose, Citric Acid, Stearic Acid, Magnesium Stearate, Colloidal Silicon Dioxide, Natural Peach, Cherry, and Chocolate Flavors.

Avacor nutricap DHT Blocker - Global Vision
Active Ingredients: Maidenhair Tree • Vaccinium Myrtillus • Equisetum • Sabal Serrulata.

Avadio - Progressive Health Nutraceuticals
Vitamin B6 10 mg • Vitamin B12 200 mcg • Vitamin E 45 IU • Selenium 50 mcg • Potassium 99 mg • Magnesium 400 mg • Coenzyme Q10 20 mg • L-Arginine base 25 mg • Hawthorne berry 25 mg • Garlic 25 mg.

Avatrol - Progressive Health Nutraceuticals
Horse Chestnut 100 mg • Arginine 100 mg • Oat Straw 75 mg • Cascara Sagrada 60 mg • Bilberry 50 mg • Butcher's Broom 40 mg • Mullein 25 mg • Cayenne 15 mg • Zinc 5 mg.

Avena Sativa Complex - Puritan's Pride
Each capsule contains: Avena Sativa 300 mg • Siberian Ginseng 150 mg • Nettle 50 mg.

Avlimil - Berkeley Premium Nutraceuticals
Each tablet contains: Avlimil Proprietary Blend 756 mg: Salvia Officinalis (sage leaf), Rubus Idaeus (red raspbery leaf), Isoflavones [from pueraria montana (kudzu) root extract/ trifolium pratense (red clover) extract], Capsicum Annuum (capsicum pepper), Glycyrrhiza Glabra (licorice root), Morella Cerifera (bayberry fruit), Turnera Diffusa (damiana leaf), Valeriana Officinalis (valeriana root), Zingiber Officinale (ginger root), Actaea Caremosa (black cohosh root). Other Ingredients: Dicalcium Phosphate, Microcrystalline Cellulose, Croscarmellose Sodium, Stearic Acid, Magnesium Stearate, Silica, Hypromellose, Titanium Dioxide, Propylene Glycol, FD&C Blue #1 Lake, FD&C Red #3.

Avocado & E Dry Skin Relief Creme 4oz - Derma E
Purified Water • Safflower oil • Stearic Acid • Cetyl Alcohol • Glyceryl Stearate • Avocado oil • Glycerin • Tocopheryl Acetate (vitamin E) • Retinyl Palmitate (vitamin A) • Ergocalciferol (vitamin D) • Panthenol • Sunflower oil • Wheat Germ oil • Allantoin • Methylparaben • TEA • I. Urea • Natural Plant extract • Fragrant oils.

Avosoy ASU - Supplement Testing Institute, Inc.
Each tablet contains: Vitamin C (ascorbic acid) 60 mg • Vitamin E (D-alpha tocopheryl, mixed tocopherols) 30 IU • Manganese (manganese sulfate) 2 mg • ASU Avocado - Soybean Unsaponifiables standardized to greater-than-or-equal-to 30% Phytosterols 300 mg. Other Ingredients: Cellulose, Dicalcium Phosphate, Sodium Croscarmellose, Silicon Dioxide, Gum Acacia, Stearic Acid, Film Coating (hydroxypropyl methylcellulose, polyethylene glycol, hydroxypropyl cellulose, carnauba wax), Magnesium Stearate.

Avosoy Complete - Supplement Testing Institute, Inc.
Three tablets contain: Vitamin C (ascorbic acid) 60 mg • Vitamin E (D-alpha tocopheryl acetate, D-alpha tocopherol, mixed tocopherols) 30 IU • Calcium (calcium phosphate) 35 mg • Manganese (manganese sulfate) 2 mg • Glucosamine HCl (vegetarian, shellfish-free) 1500 mg • Chondroitin Sulfate (porcine) 800 mg • ASU Avocado - Soy Unsaponifiables, standardized to greater-than-or-equal-to 30% Phytosterols. Other Ingredients: Cellulose, Dicalcium Phosphate, Gum Arabic, Silicon Dioxide, Stearic Acid, Film Coating (hydroxypropyl methyl cellulose, polyethylene glycol, hydroxypropyl cellulose, carnauba wax), Magnesium Stearate.

Avosoy Plus - Supplement Testing Institute, Inc.
Two tablets contain: Vitamin C (ascorbic acid) 60 mg • Vitamin E (D-alpha tocopheryl acetate, D-alpha tocopherol, mixed tocopherols) 30 IU • Manganese (manganese sulfate) 2 mg • Glucosamine HCl (vegetarian, shellfish-free) 1500 mg • ASU Avocado - Soybean Unsaponifiables, standardized to greater-than-or-equal-to 30% Phytosterols 300 mg. Other Ingredients: Dicalcium Phosphate, Stearic Acid, Silicon Dioxide, Cellulose, Film Coating (hydroxypropyl methylcellulose, polyethylene glycol, hydroxypropyl cellulose, carnauba wax), Magnesium Stearate.

Avotone - Meliorra LLC
Acetyl Hexapeptide-3 (10%) • Avocado oil • Propylene Glycol • Acrylamide Copolymer • Natural Fragrance • Ethylparaben • Methylparaben • Propylparaben.
This product used to be called "Avotox."

Ayurceutics Ashwagandha (formerly Pegasus) - Renaissance Herbs
Each capsule contains: Ashwagandha root extract (withania somnifera) 500 mg: 5% Withanolides 25 mg. Other Ingredients: Vegetarian Capsules, Rice Flour, Maltodextrin, Silicon Dioxide.

Ayurceutics Boswellia (formerly BosWell) - Renaissance Herbs
Each tablet contains: Boswellia Serrata tree resin extract 500 mg: 85% Boswellic Acids 425 mg. Other Ingredients: Cellulose, Silicon Dioxide, Stearic Acid, Croscarmellose Sodium, Magnesium Stearate, Vegetable Glaze.

Ayurceutics Gymnema (formerly Gymulin) - Renaissance Herbs
Each capsule contains: Gymnema leaf extract (gymnema sylvestre) 300 mg: 75% Gymnemic Acids 225 mg, 35% Gymnemogenin 105 mg. Other Ingredients: Vegetarian Capsules, Rice Flour, Silicon Dioxide.

Ayurceutics Shatavari - Renaissance Herbs
Each capsule contains: Shatavari root extract (asparagus racemosus) 500 mg: 40% Saponins 200 mg. Other Ingredients: Vegetarian Capsules, Rice Flour, Silicon Dioxide.

Ayurceutics Tribulus (formerly TriBull) - Renaissance Herbs
Each capsule contains: Tribulus Terrestris whole plant extract 500 mg: 60% saponins 300 mg. Other Ingredients: Vegetarian Capsules, Rice Flour, Silicon Dioxide.

Ayurceutics Triphala - Renaissance Herbs
Each tablet contains: Triphala 750 mg: Terminalia Bellerica fruit extract, Terminalia Chebula fruit extract, Phyllanthus Emblica fruit extract (in equal parts): 50% Tannins 375 mg. Other Ingredients: Cellulose, Silicon Dioxide, Stearic Acid, Croscarmellose Sodium, Magnesium Stearate, Vegetable Glaze, Organic Peppermint Oil.

Ayurvedic Blood Sugar Formula - Nature's Sunshine
Two capsules contain: Proprietary Blend 1140 mg: Gymnema Sylvestre leaf, Momordica Charantia fruit bark, Pterocarpus Marsupium gum, Aegle Marmelos leaf, Enicostemma Littorale herb, Andrographis Paniculata herb, Curcuma Longa rhizome, Syzygium Cumini seed, Azadirachta Indica leaf, Picrorhiza Kurroa root, Trigonella Foenum-Graecum seed, Cyperus Rotundus tuber. Other Ingredients: Gelatin, Water.

Ayurvedic Bronchial Formula - Nature's Sunshine
Two capsules contain: Proprietary Blend 1042 mg: Verbascum Thapsus leaf, Adhatoda Vasica leaf extract, Glycyrrhiza Glabra root extract, Alpinia Galanga rhizome extract, Clerodendrum Indicum root, Inula Racemosa root extract, Myrica Nagi bark extract, Phyllanthus Emblica fruit, Hedychium Spicatum root, Picrorhiza Kurroa root extract, Pimpinella Anisum fruit, Pistacia Integerrima gall, Zingiber Officinale rhizome, Ocimum Sanctum leaf extract, Tylophora Asthmatica leaf, Abies Webbina leaf, Elettaria Cardamomum seed, Ferula Assa-Foetida gum. Other Ingredients: Gelatin, Water.

Ayurvedic Joint Health - Nature's Sunshine
Two capsules contain: Proprietary Blend 820 mg: Withania Somnifera root, Commiphora Mukul gum extract, Smilax China root, Boswellia Serrata gum, Holarrhena Antidysenterica bark, Paederia Foetida leaf extract, Vitex Negundo leaf extract, Tinospora Cordifolia stem, Cyperus Rotundus tuber, Apium Graveolens seed, Boerhaavia Diffusa root, Trachyspermum Ammi fruit, Tribulus Terrestris fruit, Trigonella Foenum-Graecum seed. Other Ingredients: Magnesium Stearate, Gelatin, Water.

Ayurvedic Skin Detox - Nature's Sunshine
Two capsules contain: Proprietary Blend 1040 mg: Taraxacum Officinale root, Acacia Catechu bark extract, Azadirachta Indica bark extract, Smilax China root, Picrorhiza Kurroa root, Hemidesmus Indicus root, Holarrhena Antidysenterica bark, Rubia Cordifolia Root, Swertia Chirata whole plant extract, Caesalpinia Crista seed extract, Fumaria Parviflora whole plant, Alstonia Scholaris bark extract, Tinospora Cordifolia stem, Curcuma Longa rhizome, Phyllanthus Emblica fruit, Terminalia Belerica fruit, Terminalia Chebula fruit. Other Ingredients: Gelatin, Water.

Azeo-Pangen - Metagenics
Three tablets contain: Raw porcine pancreas concentrate: Protease 156,000 USP • Amylase 156,000 USP • Lipase 24,960 USP.

Azeo-Pangen Extra Strength - Metagenics
Each tablet contains: Raw porcine pancreas concentrate: Protease 104,000 USP • Amylase 104,000 USP • Lipase 16,640 USP.

Azulene Eye Elixir - Abra Therapeutics
Deionized Water • Eyebright extract • Vegetable Glycerin • Sea Algae extract • German Blue Chamomile Azulene • Vitamin Liposome Complex: D-Alpha-Tocopherol (vitamin E), Retinyl Palmitate (vitamin A), Panthenol (pro-vitamin B5), Sodium PCA • Herbal Liposome Complex: Green Tea, Ginkgo Biloba, Grape seed, Locust Bean gum, Fruit Sorbitol • Soy Protein • Chamomile oil • Olibanum oil • Xanthan gum • Methylparaben • Propylparaben.

B Complex - Benepure, Inc
Each tablet contains: Thiamine 55 mg • Riboflavin 55 mg • Niacin (as niacinamide) 55 mg • Vitamin B6 55 mg • Folic Acid 200 mcg • Vitamin B12 12 mcg • Biotin 100 mcg • Pantothenic Acid 55 mg • PABA (para-aminobenzoic acid) 55 mg • Choline 55 mg • Inositol 55 mg. Other Ingredients: Calcium Carbonate, Cellulose, Xanthan Gum, Stearic Acid, Vegetable Stearate.

B Complex - Shaklee
Two capsules contain: Thiamin (as Thiamin mononitrate) 20.25 mg • Riboflavin 22.95 mg • Niacin (as Niacinamide) 270 mg • Vitamin B6 (as Pyridoxine hydrochloride) 27 mg • Folate (as Folic acid) 400 mcg • Vitamin B12 (as Cyanocobalamin) 81 mcg • Biotin (as D-Biotin) 300 mcg • Pantothenic acid (as D-Calcium pantothenate) 135 mg. Other Ingredients: Microcrystalline Cellulose, Torula Yeast, Brewer's Yeast, Hydroxypropyl Methylcellulose, Croscarmellose Sodium, Hydroxylated Soy Lecithin.

B Complex 100 with Iron - Schiff
Each tablet contains: Vitamin B1 (as thiamin mononitrate) 100 mg •Vitamin B2 (as riboflavin) 100 mg • Vitamin B3 (as niacinamide) 100 mg • Vitamin B6 (as pyridoxine hydrochloride) 100 mg • Folate (as folic acid) 200 mcg • Vitamin B12 (as cyanocobalamin) 100 mcg • Biotin 100 mcg • Pantothenic Acid (as d-calcium pantothenate) 100 mg • Calcium (as calcium carbonate and dicalcium phosphate) 145 mg • Iron (as ferrous fumarate) 18 mg • Proprietary Blend 5 mg: Alfalfa Herb powder, Lecithin powder, Parsley leaf powder, Watercress leaf extract, Whole Brown Rice concentrate • Choline Bitartrate 100 mcg • Inositol 100 mcg • PABA (para-aminobenzoic acid) 100 mcg. Other Ingredients: Cellulose, Stearic Acid, Cellulose Gum, Silicon Dioxide, Magnesium Stearate, Coating (hydroxypropyl methylcellulose, polyethylene glycol).

B Complex 100% RDA - Rexall - Sundown
Each tablet contains: Thiamin (vitamin B1, from thiamin mononitrate) 1.5 mg • Riboflavin (vitamin B2) 1.7 mg • Niacin (as niacinamide) 20 mg • Vitamin B6 (as pyridoxine HCl) 2 mg • Folic Acid 400 mcg • Vitamin B12 (as cyanocobalamin) 6 mcg • Calcium 35 mg. Other Ingredients: Dicalcium Phosphate, Microcrystalline Cellulose, Croscarmellose Sodium, Hydroxypropyl Methylcellulose, Magnesium Stearate, Thiethyl Citrate.

B Complex Capsules - Nature's Sunshine
Each capsule contains: Vitamin B1 (thiamine) 33 mg • Vitamin B2 (riboflavin) 33 mg • Niacinamide 33 mg • Vitamin B6 (pyridoxine HCl) 33 mg • Folic Acid 133 mcg • Vitamin B12 (cyanocobalamin) 33 mcg • Biotin 100 mcg • Pantothenic Acid (D-calcium pantothenate) 33 mg • Choline (bitartrate) 33 mg • Inositol 33 mg.

B Complex Forte - Nature's Own
Each tablet contains: Vitamin B1 (thiamine nitrate) 15 mg • Vitamin B2 (riboflavin) 15 mg • Vitamin B3 (nicotinamide) 30 mg • Vitamin B5 (calcium pantothenate) 8 mg • Vitamin B6 (pyridoxine hydrochloride) 5 mg • Vitamin B12 (cyanocobalamin) 10 mcg • Folic Acid 150 mcg.

B Complex Maxi - Rexall - Sundown
Two softgels contain: Thiamin (vitamin B1, as thiamin mononitrate) 15 mg • Riboflavin (vitamin B2) 17 mg • Niacin (as niacinamide) 200 mg • Vitamin B6 (as pyridoxine HCl) 20 mg • Folic Acid 400 mcg • Vitamin B12 (as cyanocobalamin) 60 mcg • Pantothenic Acid (as calcium D-pantothenate) 100 mg • B Complex Base Blend 600 mcg: Choline Bitartrate, Inositol, Para-Aminobenzoic Acid (PABA). Other Ingredients: Soybean Oil, Gelatin, Glycerin, Soy Lecithin, Silica, Caramel, Magnesium Stearate, Dicalcium Phosphate, Titanium Dioxide, D-alpha-tocopherol.

B Complex Vitamins - Nature's Bounty
Each tablet contains: Thiamin (vitamin B1, as thiamin hydrochloride) 5 mg • Riboflavin (as vitamin B2) 5 mg • Niacin (as niacinamide) 40 mg • Vitamin B6 (as pyridoxine hydrochloride) 1 mg • Vitamin B12 (as cyanocobalamin) 1 mcg • Pantothenic Acid (as D-calcium pantothenate) 4.6 mg • Inositol 10 mg • Choline Bitartate 20 mg • Desiccated Liver powder 100 mg • Brewer's Yeast 50 mg. Other Ingredients: Dicalcium Phosphate, Cellulose (plant origin), Vegetable

Stearic Acid, Croscarmellose, Cellulose Coating, Silica, Vegetable Magnesium Stearate, Mannitol.
See Editor's Note No. 14.

B Complex Vitamins plus B-12 - Nature's Bounty
Each tablet contains: Thiamin (vitamin B1, as thiamin hydrochloride and brewer's yeast) 7 mg • Riboflavin (vitamin B2, as riboflavin and brewer's yeast) 14 mg • Niacin (as niacin and brewer's yeast) 4.5 mg • Vitamin B12 (as cyanocobalamin and brewer's yeast) 25 mcg • Protease (as papain powder) 10 mg. Other Ingredients: Dicalcium Phosphate, Cellulose (plant origin), Vegetable Stearic Acid, Croscarmellose, Silica, Mannitol, Vegetable Magnesium Stearate.

B Complex Vitamins plus Iron - Nature's Bounty
Each tablet contains: Thiamin (vitamin B1, as thiamin hydrochloride) 5 mg • Riboflavin (vitamin B2) 5 mg • Niacin (as niacinamide) 50 mg • Vitamin B6 (as pyridoxine hydrochloride) 1 mg • Vitamin B12 (as cyanocobalamin) 1 mcg • Pantothenic Acid (as D-calcium pantothenate) 4.6 mg • Iron (as ferrous sulfate) 10 mg • Choline Bitartrate 20 mg • Inositol 10 mg • Dessicated Liver 100 mg • Brewer's Yeast 50 mg. Other Ingredients: Cellulose (plant origin), Dicalcium Phosphate, Vegetable Stearic Acid, Silica, Croscarmellose, Cellulose Coating, Vegetable Magnesium Stearate, Mannitol.
See Editor's Note No. 14.

B Complex with Rice Bran - Nature's Plus
Each tablet contains: Thiamin (vitamin B1, as thiamine hydrochloride) 10 mg • Riboflavin (vitamin B2) 10 mg • Niacin (as niacinamide) 50 mg • Vitamin B6 (as pyridoxine HCl) 10 mg • Folate (as folic acid) 100 mcg • Vitamin B12 (as cyanocobalamin) 10 mcg • Biotin 20 mcg • Pantothenic Acid (as calcium pantothenate) 15 mg • Choline (as bitartrate) 50 mg • Inositol 50 mg • PABA (as para-aminobenzoic acid) 10 mg. Other Ingredients: Microcrystalline Cellulose, Stearic Acid, Rice Bran, Magnesium Stearate, Pharmaceutical Glaze, Silica.

B Complex with Vitamin C - Jamieson
Each tablet contains: Vitamin B1 5 mg • Vitamin B2 5 mg • Niacinamide 50 mg • Vitamin B6 5 mg • Vitamin B12 10 mcg • Biotin 10 mcg • Pantothenic Acid 25 mg • Folic Acid 0.05 mg • Vitamin C 250 mg • Lipotropic Factors: Choline Bitartrate 50 mg • Inositol 50 mg. Also contains Para-Aminobenzoic Acid.

B Healthy - iVillage Inc.
Each tablet contains: Thiamin 16.67 mg • Riboflavin 16.67 mg • Niacin 16.67 mg • Vitamin B6 16.67 mg • Folic Acid 133.33 mcg • Vitamin B12 16.67 mcg • Biotin 100 mcg • Pantothenic Acid 16.67 mg • Calcium 110 mg • iVillage Blend 5 mg: Spinach leaf, Acerola fruit extract (malpighia glabra), Broccoli floweret. Other Ingredients: Microcrystalline Cellulose, Maltodextrin, Acacia, Magnesium Stearate, Sodium Carboxymethylcellulose, Hydroxypropyl Methylcellulose, Glycerin.

B-1 100 mg - Puritan's Pride
Each tablet contains: Vitamin B1 (thiamine hydrochloride) 100 mg.

B-1 250 mg - Puritan's Pride
Each tablet contains: Vitamin B1 (thiamine hydrochloride) 250 mg.

B100 Complex - Natrol, Inc.
Each tablet contains: Vitamin B1 (Thiamine) 100 mg • Vitamin B2 (Riboflavin) 100 mg • Vitamin B6 (Pyroxidoxine) 100 mg • Vitamin B12 (Cobalamin) 100 mcg • Niacinamide 100 mg • Folic Acid 400 mcg • Biotin 100 mcg • Pantothenic Acid 100 mg • Choline 100 mg • Inositol 100 mg • PABA 100 mg • ULTRAGREEN 150 mg. Other Ingredients: Microcrystalline Cellulose, Calcium Carbonate, Croscarmellose Sodium, Stearic Acid, Silicon Dioxide, Magnesium Stearate.

B-100 Complex - Vitamin World
Each capsule contains: Thiamin (vitamin B1, as thiamin mononitrate) 100 mg • Riboflavin (vitamin B2) 100 mg • Niacin (as niacinamide) 100 mg • Vitamin B6 (as pyridoxine hydrochloride) 100 mg • Folic Acid 400 mcg • Vitamin B12 (as cyanocobalamin) 100 mcg • Biotin 100 mcg • Pantothenic Acid (as D-calcium pantothenate) 100 mg • Choline Bitartrate 100 mg • PABA (para-aminobenzoic acid) 100 mg • Inositol 100 mg • Proprietary Blend 7.5 mg: Alfalfa, Watercress, Parsley, Lecithin, Rice Bran. Other Ingredients: Gelatin, Vegetable Magnesium Stearate, Silica.

B-100 Complex - Rexall - Sundown
Each tablet contains: Thiamin (vitamin B1, as thiamin HCl) 1.5 mg • Riboflavin (vitamin B2) 1.7 mg • Niacin (as niacinamide) 20 mg • Vitamin B6 (as pyridoxine HCl) 2 mg • Folic Acid 400 mcg • Vitamin B12 (as cyanocobalamin) 6 mcg • Pantothenic Acid (as calcium d-pantothenate) 10 mg • Calcium 120 mg • Vitamin Co-Factor Blend 1 mg: Choline Bitartrate, Para-Aminobenzoic Acid (PABA), Inositol. Other Ingredients: Dicalcium Phosphate, Microcrystalline Cellulose, Croscarmellose Sodium, Magnesium Stearate.

B100 Complex Timed Release - Jamieson
Each caplet contains: Vitamin B1 100 mg • Vitamin B2 100 mg • Vitamin B3 100 mg • Vitamin B6 100 mg • Vitamin B12 100 mcg • Biotin 100 mcg • Pantothenic Acid 100 mg • Folic Acid 0.4 mg • Lipotropic Factors: Choline Bitartrate 100 mg, Inositol 100 mg. Also contains Para-Aminobenzoic Acid.

B-100 Complex Yeast Free - Rexall - Sundown
Each caplet contains: Thiamin (vitamin B1, as thiamin mononitrate) 100 mg • Riboflavin (vitamin B2) 100 mg • Niacin (as niacinamide) 100 mg • Vitamin B6 (as pyridoxine HCl) 100 mg • Folic Acid 400 mcg • Vitamin B12 (as cyanocobalamin) 100 mcg • Biotin 100 mg • Pantothenic Acid (as calcium D-pantothenate) 100 mg • Calcium 60 mg • B-Factor Blend 3.4 mg: Alfalfa (aerial parts), Choline Bitartrate, Para-Aminobenzoic Acid (PABA), Inositol, Parsley (aerial parts), Rice Bran, Watercress (aerial parts). Other Ingredients: Microcrystalline Cellulose, Dicalcium Phosphate, Croscarmellose Sodium, Stearic Acid, Soy Polysaccharides, Hydroxypropyl Methylcellulose, Silica, Magnesium Stearate, Hydroxypropyl Cellulose, PEG.

B-100 Mg Complex Timed - Rexall - Sundown
Each caplet contains: Thiamin (vitamin B1, as thiamin mononitrate) 100 mg • Riboflavin (vitamin B2) 100 mg • Niacin (as niacinamide) 100 mg • Vitamin B6 (as pyridoxine HCl) 100 mg • Folic Acid 400 mcg • Vitamin B12 (as cyanocobalamin) 100 mcg • Biotin 100 mcg • Pantothenic Acid (as calcium D-pantothenate) 100 mg • Calcium 90 mg • Base Complex Blend 4.4 mg: Alfalfa (leaves), Choline Bitartrate, Para-Aminobenzoic Acid (PABA), Soy Lecithin, Inositol, Parsley (aerial parts), Rice Bran, Watercress (aerial parts). Other Ingredients: Dicalcium Phosphate, Cellulose, Methylcellulose, Hydrogenated Vegetable Oil, Stearic Acid, Hydroxypropyl Methylcellulose, Silica, Magnesium Stearate, Hydroxypropyl Cellulose, PEG.

B-100 Ultra B-Complex - Puritan's Pride
Each tablet contains: Thiamin (Vitamin B1; as thiamine mononitrate) 100 mg • Riboflavin (Vitamin B2) 100 mg • Niacin (as niacinamide) 100 mg • Vitamin B6 (as pyridoxine hydrochloride) 100 mg • Folic Acid 400 mcg • Vitamin B12 (as cyanocobalamin) 100 mcg • Biotin (as d-biotin) 100 mcg • Pantothenic Acid (as d-calcium pantothenate) 100 mg • Inositol 100 mg • PABA (para-aminobenzoic acid) 100 mg • Choline Bitartrate 100 mg • Proprietary Blend: Parsley leaves powder, Rice Bran defatted powder, Watercress leaves powder, Alfalfa leaves powder, Lecithin granules 5 mg.

B12 - Wild Rose
Each tablet contains: Vitamin B12 (cyanocobalamin) 1000 mcg • Folic Acid 0.1 mg. Other ingredients: Mannitol, Sorbitol, Microcrystalline Cellulose, Silicon Dioxide, Magnesium Stearate (vegetable source), Natural Pineapple Flavor.

B-12 100 mcg - Puritan's Pride
Each tablet contains: Vitamin B-12 (Cyanocobalamin) 100 mcg.

B-12 1000 mcg - Puritan's Pride
Each tablet contains: Vitamin B-12(Cyanocobalamin) 1000 mcg.

B-12 1000 mcg - Arrowroot
Each tablet contains: Vitamin B12 1000 mcg.

B-12 1000 mcg - Rexall - Sundown
Each tablet contains: Vitamin B12 (as cyanocobalamin) 1 mg • Calcium 26 mg. Other Ingredients: Dextrose Direct Compression, Dicalcium Phosphate, Croscarmellose Sodium, Magnesium Stearate.

B-12 1500 mcg - Puritan's Pride
Each tablet contains: Vitamin B-12 (Cobalamin concentrate) 1500 mcg.

B-12 1500 mcg - Rexall - Sundown
Each caplet contains: Vitamin B12 (as cyanocobalamin) 1.5 mg • Calcium 150 mg. Other Ingredients: Dicalcium Phosphate, Calcium Sulfate, Hydroxypropyl Methylcellulose, Hydrogenated Cottonseed Oil, Stearic Acid, Silica, Magnesium Stearate.

B-12 250 mcg - Puritan's Pride
Each tablet contains: Vitamin B-12 (Cyanocobalamin) 250 mcg.

B-12 500 mcg - Puritan's Pride
Each tablet contains: Vitamin B-12 (Cyanocobalamin) 500 mcg.

B-12 500 mcg - Arrowroot
Eact tablet contains: Vitamin B12 500 mcg.

B-12 500 mcg - Rexall - Sundown
Each caplet contains: Vitamin B12 (as cyanocobalamin) 500 mcg • Calcium 50 mg. Other Ingredients: Dicalcium Phosphate, Croscarmellose Sodium, Magnesium Stearate.

B12 Active Form - Benepure, Inc
Each tablet contains: Vitamin B12 (methylcobalamin) 1000 mcg • Folic Acid 100 mcg. Other Ingredients: Mannitol, Sorbitol, Natural Cherry Flavor, Cellulose, Vegetable Stearate, Silica.

B12 Folic - Pure Encapsulations
Each vegetable capsule contains: Methylcobalamin (B12) 800 mcg • Folic Acid 800 mcg • Vitamin C (as ascorbyl palmitate) 2 mg.

B12 Herbal Lozenges - Nature's Plus
Each lozenge contains: Vitamin B12 (as cyanocobalamin) 1000 mcg • Dandelion root 25 mg • Sarsaparilla root 25 mg • Raspberry leaf (rubus idaeus) 25 mg • Beet root (beta vulgarist) 25 mg. Other Ingredients: Fructose, Acacia Gum, Guar Gum, Di-Calcium Phosphate, Stearic Acid, Natural Flavor, Silica.

B-12 Lingual - Progressive Labs
Each tablet contains: Vitamin B12 1000 mcg • Folate (folic acid) 400 mcg, in a base of Mannitol and Natural Cherry flavor.

B-12 Neurobolic - Pharmalogic
Four sprays contain: Vitamin B12 500 mcg • Dibencozide (coenzyme B12) 500 mcg • ATP (adenosine triphosphate) 10,000 mcg • Alpha-glycerylphosphorylcholine 10,000 mcg. Other Ingredients: Purified Water, Sodium Benzoate, Potassium Sorbate, Glycerin, Citric Acid, Sodium Citrate (to adjust the pH to approximately 6.2).

B-12 Time - J. R. Carlson Laboratories, Inc.
Each tablet contains: Vitamin B12 (cyanocobalamin) 1000 mcg.

B-12/Folate - Vital Nutrients
Each capsule contains: Vitamin B12 (as hydroxocobalamin powder) 1000 mcg • Folic Acid powder 800 mcg.

B12-Active - PhytoPharmica
Each tablet contains: Vitamin B12 (methylcobalamin) 1,000 mcg.

B-12-SL - J. R. Carlson Laboratories, Inc.
Each tablet contains: Vitamin B12 (cyanocobalamin) 1000 mcg.

B-150 - Puritan's Pride
Each tablet contains: Thiamin (Vitamin B1; as thiamine mononitrate) 150 mg • Riboflavin (Vitamin B2) 150 mg • Niacin (as niacinamide) 150 mg • Vitamin B6 (as pyridoxine hydrochloride) 150 mg • Folic Acid 150 mcg • Vitamin B12 (as cyanocobalamin) 150 mcg • Biotin (as d-biotin) 150 mcg • Pantothenic Acid (as d-calcium pantothenate) 150 mg • Choline Bitartrate 150 mg • PABA (para-aminobenzoic acid) 150 mg • Inositol 150 mg • Proprietary Blend 7.5 mg: Alfalfa, Watercress, Parsley, Lecithin, Rice Bran.

B-2 - Puritan's Pride
Each tablet contains: Vitamin B-2 (Riboflavin) 100 mg.

B-2 (100 mg) - Marlyn
Each tablet contains: Riboflavin (vitamin B2) 100 mg.

B4 Skin Formula - Life Extension
Each tablet contains: Polysaccharides (marine protein fractions) 50 mg • L- Ascorbic Acid 30 mg • Silicon Dioxide 7 mg • L-Cysteine 5 mg • Zinc Gluconate 2 mg • Calcium Gluconate 1.8 mg • Selenomethionine 50 mcg • Vitamin A 2600 IU • D-Alpha Acetate 6 IU.

B-50 B-Complex Vitamin - Puritan's Pride
Each tablet contains: Thiamin (vitamin B1, as thiamin mononitrate) 50 mg • Riboflavin (vitamin B2) 50 mg • Niacin (as niacinamide) 50 mg • Vitamin B6 (as pyridoxine hydrochloride) 50 mg • Folic Acid 400 mcg • Vitamin B12 (as cyanocobalamin) 50 mcg • Biotin (as D-biotin) 50 mcg • Pantothenic Acid (as D-calcium pantothenate) 50 mg • PABA (para-aminobenzoic acid) 50 mg • Inositol 50 mg • Choline Bitartrate 50 mg • Proprietary Blend 2.5 mg: Alfalfa, Watercress, Parsley, Lecithin, Rice Bran. Other Ingredients: Cellulose (plant origin), Dicalcium Phosphate, Vegetable Stearic Acid, Croscarmellose, Cellulose Coating, Silica, Mannitol, Vegetable Magnesium Stearate.

B-50 Caps With C - NOW Foods
Each capsule contains: Vitamin B1 (Thiamine) 50 mg • Vitamin B2 (Riboflavin) 50 mg • Vitamin B3 (Niacinamide) 50 mg • Vitamin B6 (Pyridoxine) 50 mg • Vitamin B12 100 mcg • Biotin 100 mcg • Folic Acid 400 mcg • Pantothenic Acid 100 mg • Vitamin C (Ascorbic Acid) 250 mg • PABA 50 mg • Choline (Bitartrate) 50 mg • Inositol 50 mg.

B50 Complex - Jamieson
Each caplet contains: Vitamin B1 50 mg • Vitamin B2 50 mg • Vitamin B3 50 mg • Vitamin B6 50 mg • Vitamin B12 mcg • Biotin 50 mcg • Pantothenic Acid 50 mg • Folic Acid 0.4 mg. Lipotropic Factors: Choline Bitartrate 50 mg, Inositol 50 mg. Also contains Para-Aminobenzoic Acid.

B-50 Complex - NOW Foods
Each capsule contains: Vitamin B1 (Thiamine HCl) 50 mg • Vitamin B2 (Riboflavin) 50 mg • Vitamin B3 (Niacinamide) 50 mg • Vitamin B5 Pantothenic Acid 50 mg • Vitamin B6 (Pyridoxine HCl) 50 mg • Vitamin B12 (Cyanocobalamin) 50 mcg • Biotin 50 mcg • Folic Acid 400 mcg • PABA 50 mg • Choline (Bitartrate) 50 mg • Inositol 50 mg.

B-50 Complex - Rexall - Sundown
Each caplet contains: Thiamin (vitamin B1, as thiamin mononitrate) 50 mg • Riboflavin (vitamin B2) 50 mg • Niacin (as niacinamide) 50 mg • Vitamin B6 (as pyridoxine HCl) 50 mg • Folic Acid 400 mcg • Vitamin B12 (as cyanocobalamin) 50 mg • Biotin 50 mg • Pantothenic Acid (as calcium D-pantothenate) 50 mg • Calcium 36 mg • PABA (para-aminobenzoic acid) 50 mg • Choline Bitartrate 50 mg • Inositol 5 mg • Alfalfa Base Complex 222 mcg: Alfalfa leaves, Parsley (aerial parts), Watercress (aerial parts), Rice Bran. Other Ingredients: Dicalcium Phosphate, Microcrystalline Cellulose, Croscarmellose Sodium, Hydrogenated Vegetable Oil, Hydroxypropyl Methylcellulose, Silica, Magnesium Stearate, Titanium Dioxide.

B-50 Gel - J. R. Carlson Laboratories, Inc.
Each softgel contains: Thiamin (vitamin B1, as thiamin hydrochloride) 50 mg • Riboflavin (vitamin B2) 50 mg • Niacin (vitamin B3, as niacinamide) 50 mg • Vitamin B6 (as pyridoxine hydrochloride) 50 mg • Folate (folic acid) 400 mcg • Vitamin B12 (cyanocobalamin) 50 mcg • Biotin 50 mcg • Pantothenic Acid (as di-calcium pantothenate) 50 mg • Phosphatidyl Choline 50 mg.

B-50 Vitamin B-Complex - Puritan's Pride
Each capsule contains: Thiamin (Vitamin B1; as thiamine mononitrate) 50 mg • Riboflavin (Vitamin B-2) 50 mg • Niacin (as niacinamide) 50 mg • Vitamin B6 (as pyridoxine hydrochloride) 50 mg • Folic Acid 100 mcg • Vitamin B12 (as cyanocobalamin) 50 mcg • Biotin (as d-biotin) 50 mcg • Pantothenic Acid (as d-calcium pantothenate) 50 mg • PABA (as para-aminobenzoic acid) 50 mg • Inositol 50 mg • Choline Bitartrate 50 mg • Proprietary Blend 2.5 mg: Alfalfa, Watercress, Parsley, Lecithin, Rice Bran.

B-6 - Arrowroot
Each tablet contains: Vitamin B6 100 mg.

B-6 100 mg - Puritan's Pride
Each tablet contains: Vitamin B-6 (Pyridoxine Hydrochloride) 100 mg.

B-6 100 mg - Progressive Labs
Each capsule contains: Vitamin B6 (pyridoxine HCl) 100 mg. Other Ingredients: Rice Flour, Magnesium Stearate, Gelatin.

B-6 100 mg - Rexall - Sundown
Each tablet contains: Vitamin B6 (as pyridoxine HCl) 100 mg • Calcium 38 mg. Other Ingredients: Dicalcium Phosphate, Croscarmellose Sodium, Magnesium Stearate.

B-6 200 mg - Puritan's Pride
Each tablet contains: Vitamin B-6 (Pyridoxine Hydrochloride) 200 mg.

B-6 50 mg - Puritan's Pride
Each tablet contains: Vitamin B-6 (Pyridoxine Hydrochloride) 50 mg.

B6 Complex - Pure Encapsulations
Each vegetable capsule contains: Pyridoxine HCl (B6) 250 mg • Pyridoxal 5' Phosphate (activated B6) 10 mg • Thiamine HCl (B1) 100 mg • Riboflavin (B2) 5 mg • Riboflavin 5' Phosphate (activated B2) 10 mg • Niacinamide 100 mg • Inositol Hexaniacinate (no-flush niacin) 10 mg • Pantothenic Acid (calcium pantothenate, B5) 100 mg • Methylcobalamin (B12) 400 mcg • Folic Acid 400 mcg • Biotin 400 mcg • Vitamin C (as ascorbyl palmitate) 15 mg.

B6 Min - Atrium Biotechnologies
Each capsule contains: Vitamin B6 (Pyridoxine HCL) 200 mg • Magnesium Gluconate 120 mg • Potassium Gluconate 120 mg.

B6 Niacinamide - Standard Process, Inc.
Each tablet contains: Proprietary Blend 247 mg: Nutritional Yeast, Bovine Liver, Mushroom, Ascorbic Acid • Niacin 10 mg • Vitamin B6 50 mg. Other Ingredients: Honey, Calcium Stearate, Arabic Gum. See Editor's Note No. 14.

B-6 Timed Release - Source Naturals
Each tablet contains: Vitamin B6 (as pyridoxine HCl, from vegetables) 100 mg • Calcium 31 mg. Other Ingredients: Dibasic Calcium Phosphate, Microcrystalline Cellulose, Stearic Acid, Modified Cellulose Gum, Colloidal Silicon Dioxide, Magnesium Stearate.

B6+B Complex - Vital Nutrients
Each capsule contains: Thiamine HCl (vitamin B1) 50 mg • Riboflavin (vitamin B2) 20 mg • Riboflavin 5' Phosphate 5 mg • Niacinamide (vitamin B3) 100 mg • Pyridoxine HCl (vitamin B6) 250 mg • Pyridoxal 5 Phosphate 15 mg • Folic Acid 400 mcg • Hydrocobalamin (vitamin B12) 200 mcg • Biotin 200 mcg • Calcium Pantothenate (vitamin B5) 75 mg.

B75 Complex - Jamieson
Each tablet contains: Vitamin B1 75 mg • Vitamin B2 75 mg • Niacinamide 75 mg • Vitamin B6 75 mg • Vitamin B12 75 mcg • Biotin 75 mcg • Pantothenic Acid 75 mg • Folic Acid 0.6 mg. Lipotropic Factors: Choline Bitartrate 75 mg, Inositol 75 mg. Also contains Para-Aminobenzoic Acid.

Ba Wei Di Huang Wan (Rehmannia Eight Formula) - Qualiherb
Six honey-pills contain: Poria Cocos Rx. (fu ling) 39 mg • Moutan Radicis Cx. (mu dan pi) 39 mg • Alismatis Rz. (ze xie) 39 mg • Rehmanniae Rx. Prep. (shou di huang) 104 mg • Corni Fr. (shan zhu yu) 52 mg • Dioscoreae Rz. (shan yao) 52 mg • Fu Zi B. 13 mg • Cinnamomi Cx. (rou gui) 13 mg • Honey 249 mg.

Ba Zhen Tang Plus - Secara
Organic Licorice root (gan cao) 356 mg • Asian Ginseng root 5:1 extract (ren shen) 285 mg • Atractylodes rhizome 5:1 extract (bai zhu) 238 mg • Chinese Peony root 5:1 extract (bai shao) 238 mg • Dong Quai root 5:1 extract 238 mg • Ligusticum Wallichii rhizome 5:1 extract (chuan xiong) 238 mg • Poria Sclerotium 5:1 extract (fu ling) 238 mg • Rehmannia cured root tuber 5:1 extract (shu di huang) 238 mg • Gynostemma leaves & stems 5:1 extract 181 mg.

Baby & Me Daily Foods - MegaFood
Six tablets contain: Vitamin A 3000 IU • Vitamin C 100 mg • Vitamin D (vitamin D3) 400 IU • Vitamin E 75 IU • Vitamin K (vitamin K1) 65 mcg • Thiamine (vitamin B1) 2 mg • Riboflavin (vitamin B2) 2 mg • Niacinamide 20 mg • Vitamin B6 10 mg • Folic Acid 800 mcg • Vitamin B12 50 mcg • Biotin 300 mcg • Pantothenic Acid 10 mg • Calcium 200 mg • Iron 18 mg • Iodine 150 mcg • Magnesium 75 mg • Zinc 15 mg • Selenium 50 mcg • Copper 500 mcg • Manganese 5 mg • Chromium (GTF) 50 mcg • Molybdenum 50 mcg • Beta Carotene 3000 IU • Bioflavonoids (from vitamin C) 250 mg • Choline 25 mg • Inositol 25 mg • Potassium 10 mg • PABA 5 mg • Alfalfa 450 mg • Barley grass/juice concentrate 100 mg • Wild Blueberry fruit (6:1) 50 mg • Cranberry (25:1) 25 mg • Red Raspberry leaf (4:1) 75 mg • Chamomile flower (4:1) 30 mg • Dandelion leaf (4:1) 23 mg • Dandelion root (4:1) 22 mg. Other Ingredients: Vegetable Lubricant, Food Glaze.

Baby and Me Daily Foods - MegaFood
Six tablets contain: Vitamin A 3000 IU • Vitamin C 100 mg • Vitamin D (vitamin D3) 400 IU • Vitamin E 75 IU • Vitamin K (vitamin K1) 65 mcg • Thiamine (vitamin B1) 2 mg • Riboflavin (vitamin B2) 2 mg • Niacinamide 20 mg • Vitamin B6 10 mg • Folic Acid 800 mcg • Vitamin B12 50 mcg • Biotin 300 mcg • Pantothenic Acid 10 mg • Calcium 200 mg • Iron 18 mg • Iodine 150 mcg • Magnesium 75 mg • Zinc 15 mg • Selenium 50 mcg • Copper 500 mcg • Manganese 5 mg • Chromium (GTF) 50 mcg • Molybdenum 50 mcg • Beta Carotene 3000 IU • Bioflavonoids (from vitamin C) 250 mg • Choline 25 mg • Inositol 25 mg • Potassium 10 mg • PABA 5 mg • Alfalfa 450 mg • Barley grass/juice concentrate 100 mg • Wild Blueberry fruit (6:1) 50 mg • Cranberry (25:1) 25 mg • Red Raspberry leaf (4:1) 75 mg • Chamomile flower (4:1) 30 mg • Dandelion leaf (4:1) 23 mg • Dandelion root (4:1) 22 mg. Other Ingredients: Vegetable Lubricant, Food Glaze.

Baby-Cal Syrup - Hadas Natural Products
Natural Citrus flavored Fructose-Glucose syrup • Fennel 200 mg • Chamomile 200 mg • Caraway 200 mg.

Baby's Bliss Gripe Water - MOM Enterprises, Inc.
Ingredients: Ginger • Fennel • Sodium Bicarbonate • Fructose • Deionized Water.

Baby's Jarro-Dophilus - Jarrow Formulas
Each 1/4 tsp serving contains: Probiotic Bacteria 3 billion organisms: Bifidobacterium Breve M-16v 750 million, Bifidobacterium Infantis Bi-07 450 million, Bifidobacterium Longum BB536 (morinaga) 450 million, Bifidobacterium Bifidum Bb-02 450 million, Lactobacillus Casei Lc-11 450 million, Lactobacillus Rhamnosus Lr-32 450 million • Vitamin C 4 mg • Inulin (source of FOS) 973 mg.

BackAche with Arnica - Hyland's
Two tablets contain: Benzoicum Acidum 3X • Colchicum Autumnale 3X • Sulphur 3X • Arnica Montana 6X • Rhus Toxicodendron 6X. Base: Lactose N.F.
See Editor's Note No. 1.

BRAND NAMES

Some Brand Name Natural Products - What they Contain

www.NaturalDatabase.com contains MANY more listings than appear here.
Editor's Notes are located on pages 2155-2163.

BRAND NAMES

Back-Relief - Futurebiotics LLC
Four capsules contain: Magnesium (as magnesium amino acid chelate) 300 mg • Alfalfa whole juice 225 mg • Yucca root powder 200 mg • Cayenne fruit powder extract 25 mg • Valerian root powder extract 12 mg • Pancreatin 4X quadruple strength (supplying 1600 USP units lipase, 10000 USP units amylase, 1000 USP protease) 125 mg • DL-Phenylalanine 250 mg. Other Ingredients: Magnesium stearate, Gelatin, Water.
See Editor's Note No. 14.

Bacopa monniera - Pure Encapsulations
Each vegetable capsule contains: Bacopa Monniera leaf extract (standardized to contain 20% bacosides A & B) 200 mg • Vitamin C (as ascorbyl palmitate) 5 mg.

Bacopa Vitality - Life Enhancement Products, Inc.
Each capsule contains: Bacopa Monniera 100 mg. Other Ingredients: Rice Flour, Gelatin Capsule.

Bacopin - America's Finest
Each capsule contains: Bacopin brand Bacopa Monniera extract 120 mg. Other Ingredients: Dicalcium Phosphate, Cellulose, Magnesium Stearate, Silica.

Bakol Basikol - Arkopharma
Each capsule contains: Non-esterfied Phytosterols 200 mg • Vitamin E 2.5 mg.

Balance - Ortho Molecular Products
Each capsule contains: Paeonia Lactiflora root powder 400 mg • Licorice root extract (standardized to contain 12% glycyrrhizin) 200 mg • Chaste Berry 10:1 extract 20 mg. Other Ingredients: Natural Vegetable Capsules, Magnesium Stearate, Microcrystalline Cellulose.

Balance Meal Neutralizer - Legacy for Life
Two capsules contain: Betasanne Chitosan, Betaine HCl complex 450 mg.

BALANCE Shake (cafe mocha) - Legacy for Life
Protein blend: Whey Protein Isolate, Whey Protein Concentrate, Soy Protein Isolate, Egg Powder with immune components • Inulin • Decaffeinated Coffee • Natural and Artificial flavors • Cocoa (processed with alkali) • L-Taurine • Glucomannan • Cellulose Gum • Potassium Citrate • Calcium Carbonate • Dipotassium Phosphate • Soy Lecithin • Magnesium Oxide • Psyllium • Maltodextrin • Enzyme Blend: Proteases, Amylase, Lactase, Cellulase • Acesulfame Potassium • Sucralose.

BALANCE Shake (Dutch chocolate) - Legacy for Life
Protein blend: Whey Protein Isolate, Whey Protein Concentrate, Soy Protein Isolate, Egg Powder with immune components • Cocoa (processed with alkali) • Inulin • Natural and Artificial flavors • L-Taurine • Glucomannan • Cellulose Gum • Potassium Citrate • Calcium Carbonate • Dipotassium Phosphate • Soy Lecithin • Magnesium Oxide • Psyllium • Maltodextrin • Enzyme Blend: Proteases, Amylase, Lactase, Cellulase • Acesulfame Potassium • Sucralose.

BALANCE Shake (vanilla creme) - Legacy for Life
Protein Blend: Whey Protein Isolate, Whey Protein Concentrate, Soy Protein Isolate, Egg powder with immune components • Inulin • Natural and Artificial flavors • Potassium Citrate • L-Taurine • Glucomannan • Cellulose Gum • Calcium Carbonate • Dipotassium Phosphate • Soy Lecithin • Magnesium Oxide • Psyllium • Maltodextrin • Enzyme Blend: Proteases, Amylase, Lactase, Cellulase • Acesulfame Potassium • Sucralose.

Balanced B Complex Tablets - Nature's Sunshine
Each tablet contains: Vitamin B1 (thiamine) 5 mg • Vitamin B2 (riboflavin) 6 mg • Niacin (niacinamide) 50 mg • Vitamin B6 (pyridoxine HCl) 9 mg • Folic Acid 400 mcg • Vitamin B12 (cyanocobalamin) 50 mcg • Biotin 100 mcg • Pantothenic Acid (D-calcium pantothenate) 45 mg • Calcium (di-calcium phosphate) 120 mg • Phosphorus (di-calcium phosphate) 90 mg. Other Ingredients: Cellulose, Wheat Germ, Stearic Acid, Choline, Para-Amino Benzoic Acid (PABA), Magnesium Stearate, Wild Lettuce Leaf (lactuca virosa), Watercress Leaf (nasturtium officinale), Cabbage Leaf (brassica oleracea), Rice Bran Polish.

Balanced B-100 Capsules - Arrowroot
Each capsule contains: Vitamin B1 100 mg • Vitamin B2 100 mg • Vitamin B6 100 mg • Vitamin B12 100 mcg • PABA 50 mg • Niacinamide 100 mg • Choline 100 mg • Biotin 100 mcg • Inositol 100 mg • Folic Acid 400 mcg • Pantothenic Acid 100 mg.

Balanced B-100 Tablets - Arrowroot
Each tablet contains: Vitamin B1 100 mg • Vitamin B2 100 mg • Vitamin B6 100 mg • Vitamin B12 100 mcg • PABA 50 mg • Niacinamide 100 mg • Choline 100 mg • Biotin 100 mcg • Inositol 100 mg • Folic Acid 400 mcg • Pantothenic Acid 100 mg.

Balanced B-100 Timed Release - Nature Made
Each tablet contains: Thiamin (thiamin mononitrate) 100 mg • Riboflavin 100 mg • Niacin (niacinamide) 100 mg • Vitamin B6 (pyridoxine hydrochloride) 100 mg • Folic Acid 400 mcg • Vitamin B12 (cyanocobalamin) 100 mcg • Biotin 100 mcg • Pantothenic Acid (D-calcium pantothenate) 100 mg. Other Ingredients: Dibasic Calcium Phosphate, Cellulose, Hydroxypropyl Methylcellulose, Stearic Acid, Silicon Dioxide, Magnesium Stearate, Croscarmellose Sodium, Polyethylene Glycol, Carnauba Wax.

Balanced B-125 PR Tablets - Arrowroot
Each prolonged-release tablet contains: Vitamin B1 125 mg • Vitamin B2 125 mg • Vitamin B6 125 mg • Vitamin B12 125 mcg • PABA 125 mg • Choline 125 mg • Niacinamide 125 mg • Inositol 125 mg • Biotin 125 mcg • Folic Acid 400 mcg • Pantothenic Acid 125 mg.

Balanced B-50 Capsules - Arrowroot
Each capsule contains: Vitamin B1 50 mg • Vitamin B2 50 mg • Vitamin B6 50 mg • Vitamin B12 50 mcg • Choline 50 mg • Niacinamide 50 mg • Inositol 50 mg • Biotin 50 mcg • Folic Acid 400 mcg • Pantothenic Acid 50 mg • PABA 50 mg.

Balanced B-50 softgels - Golden Glow Natural Health Products
Each capsule contains: Thiamine Nitrate 50 mg: Thiamine (vitamin B1) 40.7 mg • Riboflavin (vitamin B2) 50 mg • Nicotinamide (vitamin B3) 50 mg • Calcium Pantothenate 50 mg: Pantothenic Acid (vitamin B5) 46 mg • Pyridoxine Hydrochloride (vitamin B6) 50 mg • Cyanocobalamin (vitamin B12) 50 mcg • Folic Acid 100 mcg • Biotin (vitamin H) 50 mcg • Choline Bitartrate 50 mg • Inositol 50 mg.

Balanced B-50 tablets - Golden Glow Natural Health Products
Each tablet contains: Thiamine Nitrate (vitamin B1) 50 mg • Riboflavin (vitamin B2) 50 mg • Nicotinamide (vitamin B3) 50 mg • Calcium Pantothenate 50 mg: Pantothenic Acid (vitamin B5) 45.8 mg • Pyridoxine Hydrochloride (vitamin B6) 50 mg • Cyanocobalamin (vitamin B12) 50 mcg • Folic Acid 100 mcg • Biotin (vitamin H) 50 mcg • Choline Bitartrate 50 mg • Inositol 50 mg.

Balanced B-50 Tablets - Arrowroot
Each tablet contains: Vitamin B1 50 mg • Vitamin B2 50 mg • Vitamin B6 50 mg • Vitamin B12 50 mcg • Choline 50 mg • Niacinamide 50 mg • Inositol 50 mg • Biotin 50 mcg • Folic Acid 400 mcg • Pantothenic Acid 50 mg • PABA 50 mg.

Balanced B-50 Timed Release - Nature Made
Each tablet contains: Thiamin (thiamin mononitrate) 50 mg • Riboflavin 50 mg • Niacin (niacinamide) 50 mg • Vitamin B6 (pyridoxine hydrochloride) 50 mg • Folic Acid 400 mcg • Vitamin B12 (cyanocobalamin) 50 mcg • Biotin 50 mcg • Pantothenic Acid (D-calcium pantothenate) 50 mg. Other Ingredients: Dibasic Calcium Phosphate, Cellulose, Hydroxypropyl Methylcellulose, Stearic Acid, Silicon Dioxide, Magnesium Stearate, Polyethylene Glycol, Carnauba Wax.

Some Brand Name Natural Products - What they Contain

www.NaturalDatabase.com contains MANY more listings than appear here.
Editor's Notes are located on pages 2155-2163.

Balanced EPA-DHA Liquid - Metagenics
Each 1 tsp (5 mL) serving contains: EPA (eicosapentaenoic acid) 630 mg • DHA (docosahexaenoic acid) 630 mg • Other Omega-3 Fatty Acids 240 mg. Other Ingredients: Natural Lemon Flavor, Rosemary, Ascorbyl Palmitate, Citric Acid, Mixed Tocopherols.

Balanced Omega Combination (lemon) - Nordic Naturals
Two softgels contain: Vitamin E (mixed tocopherols) 30 IU (EPA 36 mg, DHA 24 mg) • Evening Primrose oil 800 mg (GLA 76 mg).

Balanced Vitamin B-50 - Nature's Valley
Each tablet contains: Thiamine (vitamin B1) 50 mg • Riboflavin (vitamin B2) 50 mg • Niacin 50 mg • Vitamin B6 50 mg • Vitamin B12 50 mcg • Biotin 50 mcg • Pantothenic Acid 50 mg • Folic Acid 100 mcg. Other Ingredients: Calcium Carbonate, Cellulose, Maltodextrin, Croscarmellose Sodium, Sodium Starch Glycolate, Polyethylene Glycol, Tricalcium Phosphate, Hydroxypropyl Methylcellulose, Resin, Dicalcium Phosphate, Silicon Dioxide, Magnesium Stearate, Pharmaceutical Glaze, Hydroxypropyl Cellulose, Mannitol, Starch, Rice Bran, Yeast, Polysorbate 80, Alfalfa, Lecithin, Para-Aminobenzoic Acid, Parsley, Watercress. See Editor's Note No. 45.

Bao He Wan Plus - Secara
Three tablets contain: Chinese Hawthorn fruit 5:1 extract (shan zha) 516 mg • Organic Artichoke leaf 354 mg • Ban Xia 5:1 extract (pinellia rhizome) 231 mg • Hoelen Sclerotium 5:1 extract (fu ling) 231 mg • Organic Gentian root (qin jiao) 192 mg • Massa Fermentata 5:1 extract (shen qu) 192 mg • Tangerine peel 4:1 extract (chen pi) 153 mg • Papain 135 mg • Radish seed 5:1 extract (lai fu zi) 96 mg • Forsythia fruit 5:1 extract (lian qiao) 93 mg • Bromelain 2400 GDU/gram 45 mg • Lactase 12 mg.

Barlean's Flax Oil - The Vitamin Shoppe
Each 1 tsp serving provides: Omega-3 7.7 g • Omega-6 2.3 g • Omega 9 2.2 g • VitaLox [a natural protectant blend of Ascorbic Acid and Rosemary extracts] 30 mg.

Barlean's Flax Oil High Lignin Formula - The Vitamin Shoppe
Each 1 tbsp serving contains: Omega-3 6.1 g • Omega-6 1.8 g • Omega 9 1.7 g • Flaxseed Particles 2.6 g • VitaLox brand ascorbic acid and rosemary extract 30 mg.

Barlean's Vita-Flax - The Vitamin Shoppe
Certified Organic Flax Seed Powder containing: Protein (NX6.25) 34.7% • Fat 14.7% • Energy 435 Kcal/100 g. Vitamin E 0.01% • Dietary Fiber 34.2%. Total Fiber: Soluble Fiber 38%, Insoluble Fiber 62%.

Barley Juice Powder - Nature's Sunshine
Eight capsules contain: Barley plant juice powder extract (hordeum vulgare) 3840 mg. Other Ingredients: Gelatin, Water.

BarleyGreen Premium - The AIM Companies
Ten caplets contain: Vitamin A (as beta-carotene) 1000 IU • Vitamin C 9 mg • Calcium 35 mg • Iron 0.5 mg • Sodium 50 mg • Magnesium 12 mg • Potassium 240 mg • Iodine 20 mcg • Chlorophyll 13 mg. Ingredients: Organic Young Barley Grass Juice, Organic Maltodextrin, Organic Brown Rice, Kelp (Kombu), Magnesium Stearate.

BarleyLife - The AIM Companies
Each 1 tbsp serving contains: Vitamin A (beta-carotene) 1370 IU • Vitamin B1 (thiamin) 0.04 mg • Vitamin B2 (riboflavin) 0.0895 mg • Vitamin B6 0.0635 mg • Vitamin B12 0.0385 mg • Folic Acid 5.3 mg • Niacin 0.4295 mg • Pantothenic Acid 0.11 mg • Vitamin C 1.39 mg • Vitamin E 0.505 IU • Vitamin K 121.5 mcg • Calcium 45.25 mg • Chromium 1.1 mcg • Copper 0.0255 mg • Iodine 22 mcg • Iron 0.745 mg • Magnesium 11 mg • Manganese 0.1595 mg • Molybdenum 0.0015 mg • Phosphorous 20.7 mg • Zinc 0.1135 mg. Other Ingredients: Green Barley Juice, Maltodextrin, Brown Rice, Kelp.

Basic Antioxidant - GNC
Each capsule contains: Vitamin A (as Natural beta-Carotene) 5000 IU •Vitamin C (as Ascorbic Acid) 300 mg • Vitamin E (as d-alpha Tocopherol) 200 IU • Selenium (as Selenium Yeast) 200 mcg. Other Ingredients: Soybean Oil, Gelatin, Glycerin, Caramel Color, Titanium Dioxide.

Basic Elemental Minerals - American Biologics
Each capsule contains: Lithium 10 mcg • Rubidium 15 mcg • Vanadium 5 mcg • Germanium 30 mcg • Selenium 5 mcg • Molybdenum 10 mcg • Chromium 25 mcg • Superoxide Dismutase (plant source) 5 mcg • Catalase (plant source) 5 mg. Other Ingredients: Magnesium Stearate.

Basic Mindell Plus - FreeLife International
Eight caplets contain: Vitamin A (100% from Betatene brand mixed carotenoids: beta-carotene, alpha-carotene, cryptoxanthin, zeaxanthin, lutein) 20,000 IU • Vitamin C (as buffered ascorbic acid) 600 mg • Vitamin D (as cholecalciferol) 400 IU • Vitamin E (from E-Plex brand D-alpha tocopheryl succinate with mixed tocopherols and tocotrienols) 400 IU • Vitamin K (as phytonadione) 80 mcg • Thiamin (vitamin B1 as food-bound thiamin HCl with cocarboxylase coenzyme) 50 mg • Riboflavin (vitamin B2 food-bound with riboflavin-5-phosphate coenzyme) 50 mg • Niacin (as food-bound vitamin B3, 50% as niacinamide) 50 mg • Vitamin B6 (as food-bound pyridoxine HCl with pyridoxal-5-phosphate coenzyme) 50 mg • Folate (as food-bound folic acid) 800 mcg • Vitamin B12 (as food-bound cyanocobalamin with cobamamide coenzyme) 100 mcg • Biotin (as food-bound D-biotin) 300 mcg • Pantothenic Acid (vitamin B5 as food-bound D-calcium pantothenate with pantethine coenzyme) 50 mg • Calcium (as hydroxyapatite and glycinated purified calcite) 1000 mg • Phosphorus (as hydroxyapatite) 320 mg • Iodine (from kelp) 150 mcg • Magnesium (as glycinated purified magnesite) 400 mg • Zinc (as glycinated zinc citrate) 15 mg • Selenium (as selenomethionine) 200 mcg • Copper (as glycinated copper gluconate) 2 mg • Manganese (as glycinated manganese gluconate) 2.5 mg • Chromium (as Chelavite brand chromium dinicotinate glycinate) 200 mcg • Molybdenum (as glycinated molybdenum amino acid chelate) 75 mcg • Potassium (as glycinated potassium citrate) 99 mg • Alpha-Lipoic Acid 100 mg • L-Carnosine (beta-alanyl-L-histidine dipeptide) 50 mg • Betatene brand Mixed Carotenoids from Dunaliella Salina Sea Algae 175 mg: Beta-Carotene 12,500 mcg, Alpha-Carotene 394 mcg, Cryptoxanthin 92 mcg, Zeaxanthin 79 mcg, Lutein 59 mcg • Plant Enzymes 37,000 units: Alpha-Amylase, Beta-Amylase, Cellulase, Lactase, Papain, Bromelain, Dual-Action Protease (acid and alkaline), Lipase • Essential lipid complex 630 mg: Vegetable Oil Free Fatty Acids and Esters, Soy Activation Complex (purified soy phosphatides), Flaxseed oil, Borage seed oil, Rice Bran • Probiotics with Growth Factors 1,000 mg: Lactospore brand 100 million microencapsulated active Lactobacillus cells, Growth Factor Blend: Vegetable Cellulose, Dahlulin PB brand Chicory and Dahlia Inulin fructans, Mannan-oligosaccharides, Beta-Glucan soluble fiber • Antioxidant Support Complex 825 mg: Soygenol 100 brand Soy Phosphatidebonded Grape seed OPCs, Green Tea leaf standardized extract, Citrus Bioflavonoids, Jamaican Ginger root, N-Acetylcysteine, Grape skin extract, Quercetin (from rutin), Turmeric rhizome, Bilberry fruit extract • Fruit and Vegetable extract Complex 500 mg: Allium Vegetables (deodorized garlic and aged garlic concentrate), Cruciferous Vegetables: Cabbage, Broccoli, Brussels Sprouts, Kale, Cauliflower, Ellagic Fruits: Strawberry, Cherry, Grape, Anthocyanin fruits: Bilberry, Grape seed, Cranberry, Umbelliferous Vegetables: Carrot, Celery, Parsnip, Soy Isoflavones: Genistein, Daidzein, Sea vegetables: Nori, Sea Kelp, Wakame, Kombu, Carotenoid Vegetables: Cayenne, Tomato, Mustard Greens, Turmeric, Vegetable fiber, Citrus Bioflavonoids • Herbal Extract Complex 500 mg: Aloe Vera leaf, Ashwagandha root, Astragalus root, Burdock root, Butcher's Broom, Cinnamon bark, Dandelion root, Dong Quai root, Fo Ti root, Hawthorn berry, Ligusticum root, Milk Thistle seed, Schizandra fruit, Wild Yam root, Vegetable fiber • SuperFoods complex 500 mg: Alfalfa sprouts, Barley grass, Bee Pollen, Blackstrap Molasses, Green

Tea, Reishi Mushroom, Shiitake Mushroom • Nutrient co-factors 275 mg: Inositol, RNA and DNA concentrates, Choline Bitartrate, PABA • Trace mineral factors 165 mg: Glycinated Boron Chelate, Colloidal Silica, Glycinated Vanadium Amino Acid Chelate • UltraSoy Complex III Proprietary blend 200 mg: Standardized Soy Kernel Concentrate, Soybean sprout Concentrate, Pine Bark extract, Grape seed extract, Glutathione, Red Cabbage, Green Tea, Carrots, Broccoli, Celery, Brussels Sprouts, Kale, Cauliflower, Green Onion, Yams • UltraSoy brand 10,000 IU: Soy Polysaccharides, Plant Enzymes. Other ingredients: Vita-Coat brand (modified vegetable cellulose, alpha-lipoic acid).

Basic Multivitamin - Arrowroot
Each tablet contains: Vitamin A 8000 IU • Biotin 30 mcg • Beta Carotene 2,000 IU • Folic Acid 400 mcg • Vitamin D (D3) 400 IU • Copper 1 mg • Vitamin E 30 IU • Phosphorus 50 mg • Vitamin C 100 mg • Iron 18 mg • Vitamin B1 10 mg • Iodine 150 mcg • Vitamin B2 10 mg • Manganese 1 mg • Vitamin B3 20 mg • Magnesium 50 mg • Vitamin B6 10 mg • Zinc 15 mg • Vitamin B12 15 mcg • Calcium 100 mg • Pantothenic Acid 20 mg • Selenium 25 mcg • Molybdenum 5 mcg • Chromium 25 mcg.

Basic Vita-Vim Level 1 Potency Multivitamin - Jamieson
Each caplet contains: Vitamin A (Acetate) 2000 IU • Beta Carotene 3000 IU • Vitamin D 400 IU • Vitamin C 90 mg • Vitamin E 25 IU • Vitamin B1 2.25 mg • Vitamin B2 3.2 mg • Vitamin B3 (No Flush Niacinamide) 40 mg • Vitamin B5 10 mg • Vitamin B6 3 mg • Vitamin B12 14 mcg • Folic Acid 400 mcg • Biotin 45 mcg • Calcium 175 mg • Iron (from Fumarate) 10 mg • Copper 2 mg • Iodine 0.15 mg • Magnesium 50 mg • Phosphorus 125 mg • Lutein 300 mcg.

B-Assure - The Vitamin Shoppe
Each capsule contains: 100 mg Champignon (Agaricus bisporus) stem and cap.

Bayberry - Nature's Sunshine
Each capsule contains: Bayberry root bark (myrica cerifera) 440 mg. Other Ingredients: Gelatin, Water.

B-Basic - PhysioLogics
Each capsule contains: Vitamin B6 (as pyridoxine hydrochloride) 25 mg • Folic Acid 800 mcg • Vitamin B12 (as cyanocobalamin) 100 mcg • Betaine Hydrochloride 50 mg. Other Ingredients: Rice Powder, Gelatin, Vegetable Magnesium Stearate, Silica.

BCAA - Pain & Stress Center
Each capsule contains: Vitamin B6 (as 5 mg pyridoxal 5'phosphate) 3 mg • Chromium (as chromium nicotinate) 50 mcg • L-Leucine 225 mg • L-Valine 175 mg • L-Isoleucine 100 mg. Other Ingredients: Gelatin Capsule.

BCAA 1000 Caps - Optimum Nutrition
Two capsules contain: L-Leucine 500 mg • L-Isoleucine 250 mg • L-Valine 250 mg. Other Ingredients: Gelatin, Magnesium Stearate.

BCAA 5000 Powder - Optimum Nutrition
Each 1 tsp (5 g) serving contains: L-Valine 1250 mg • L-Leucine 2500 mg • L-Isoleucine 1250 mg.

BCAA capsules - Pure Encapsulations
Each vegetable capsule contains: Branched Chain Amino Acids (free-form) 600 mg: L-Leucine 300 mg, L-Isoleucine 150 mg, L-Valine 150 mg.

BCAA Plus - Solgar
Two capsules contain: Vitamin B6 (as pyridoxine HCl) 20 mg • L-Leucine 540 mg • L-Isoleucine 360 mg • L-Valine 300 mg. Other Ingredients: Vegetable Cellulose, Vegetable Magnesium Stearate, Microcrystalline Cellulose, Vegetable Stearic Acid, Water, Vegetable Glycerin.

BCAA powder - Pure Encapsulations
Each scoop contains: Branched Chain Amino Acids (free-form) 3000 mg: L-Leucine 1500 mg, L-Isoleucine 750 mg, L-Valine 750 mg.

B-Com - Professional Botanicals
Each capsule contains: Thiamin (vitamin B1) 50 mg • Riboflavin (vitamin B2) 50 mg • Niacin (as niacinamide) 50 mg • Vitamin B6 50 mg • Folate (folic acid) 100 mcg • Vitamin B12 50 mcg • Pantothenic Acid 100 mg • D-Biotin 50 mcg • Choline Bitartrate 50 mg • Inositol 50 mg • PABA (para amino benzoic acid) 50 mg. Other Ingredients: Alfalfa, Watercress, Parsley, Lecithin, Rice Bran, EDS Enzymes/Cofactors.

B-Compleet - J. R. Carlson Laboratories, Inc.
Two tablets contain: Vitamin C (as ascorbic acid & from rose hips) 500 mg • Thiamin (vitamin B1, as thiamin hydrochloride) 10 mg • Riboflavin (vitamin B2) 10 mg • Niacin (vitamin B3, as niacinamide) 100 mg • Vitamin B6 (as pyridoxine hydrochloride) 10 mg • Folate (folic acid) 800 mcg • Biotin 300 mcg • Pantothenic Acid (as di-calcium pantothenate) 200 mg • PABA (para-aminobenzoic acid) 30 mg • Vitamin B12 (as cobalamin concentrate) 30 mcg • Choline (as choline bitartrate) 100 mg • Inositol 100 mg.

B-Compleet-100 - J. R. Carlson Laboratories, Inc.
Each tablet contains: Thiamin (vitamin B1, as thiamin hydrochloride) 100 mg • Riboflavin (vitamin B2) 100 mg • Niacin (vitamin B3, as niacinamide) 100 mg • Vitamin B6 (as pyridoxine hydrochloride) 100 mg • Folate (folic acid) 400 mcg • Vitamin B12 (cyanocobalamin) 100 mcg • Biotin 100 mcg • Pantothenic Acid (as di-calcium pantothenate) 100 mg • PABA (para-aminobenzoic acid) 100 mg • Choline (as choline bitartrate) 100 mg • Inositol 100 mg.

B-Compleet-50 - J. R. Carlson Laboratories, Inc.
Each tablet contains: Thiamin (vitamin B1, as thiamin hydrochloride) 50 mg • Riboflavin (vitamin B2) 50 mg • Niacin (vitamin B3, as niacinamide) 100 mg • Vitamin B6 (as pyridoxine hydrochloride) 50 mg • Folate (folic acid) 400 mcg • Vitamin B12 (cyanocobalamin) 50 mcg • Biotin 50 mcg • Pantothenic Acid (as di-calcium pantothenate) 200 mg • PABA (para-aminobenzoic acid) 50 mg • Choline (as choline bitartrate) 50 mg • Inositol 50 mg.

B-Complex - Nutri-Quest Rx
Two tablets contain: Vitamin B1 100 mg • Vitamin B2 100 mg • Vitamin B6 50 mg • Niacinamide 100 mg • Pantothenic Acid 100 mg • Vitamin B12 100 mcg • Folic Acid 300 mcg • Biotin 100 mcg • Choline Bitartrate 100 mg • Inositol 100 mg • PABA 50 mg.

B-Complex - Health Smart Vitamins
Each caplet contains: Thiamin (as thiamin mononitrate) 100 mg • Riboflavin 100 mg • Niacin (as niacinamide) 100 mg • Vitamin B6 (as pyridoxine hydrochloride) 100 mg • Folate (folic acid) 400 mcg • Vitamin B12 (as cyanocobalamin) 100 mcg • Biotin 300 mcg • Pantothenic acid (as calcium pantothenate) 100 mg • Calcium (as dicalcium phosphate, calcium pantothenate, calcium stearate) 100 mg • Phosphorus (as dicalcium phosphate) 70 mg • Choline (as choline bitartrate) 100 mg • Inositol 100 mg • Para-aminobenzoic acid 100 mg.

B-Complex - Vital Nutrients
Each capsule contains: Thiamine HCl (vitamin B1) 100 mg • Riboflavin (vitamin B2) 25 mg • Riboflavin 5' Phosphate (activated vitamin B2) 10 mg • Pyridoxine HCl (vitamin B6) 25 mg • Pyridoxal 5' Phosphate (activated vitamin B6) 15 mg • Calcium Pantothenate (vitamin B5) 200 mg • Hydroxocobalamin (vitamin B12, pure powder) 500 mcg • Inositol Hexaniacinate (no-flush niacin) 25 mg • Niacinamide 75 mg • Folic Acid (pure powder) 800 mcg • Biotin (pure powder) 400 mcg.

B-Complex "100" Tablets - Solgar
Each tablet contains: Thiamin (as thiamin mononitrate) 100 mg • Riboflavin 100 mg • Niacin (as niacinamide) 100 mg • Vitamin B6 (as pyridoxine HCl) 100 mg • Folic Acid 400 mcg • Vitamin B12 (as cobalamin) 100 mcg • Biotin (as D-biotin) 100 mcg • Pantothenic Acid (from D-calcium pantothenate) 100 mg • Inositol 100 mg • Choline (as choline bitartrate) 41 mg. Other Ingredients: Microcrystalline Cellulose, Silica, Vegetable Cellulose, Vegetable

Magnesium Stearate, Titanium Dioxide, Vegetable Glycerin, Natural Powdered Base: Alfalfa, Acerola, Kelp, Parsley, Rose Hips, Watercress, Carnauba Wax.

B-Complex "100" Vegetable Capsules - Solgar
Each capsule contains: Thiamin (as thiamin mononitrate) 100 mg • Riboflavin 100 mg • Niacin (as niacinamide) 100 mg • Vitamin B6 (as pyridoxine HCl) 100 mg • Folic Acid 400 mcg • Vitamin B12 (as cobalamin) 100 mcg • Biotin (as D-biotin) 100 mcg • Pantothenic Acid (from D-calcium pantothenate) 100 mg • Inositol 100 mg • Choline (as choline bitartrate) 41 mg. Other Ingredients: Vegetable Cellulose, Silica, Vegetable Magnesium Stearate, Water, Vegetable Glycerin.

B-Complex "50" - Solgar
Each capsule contains: Thiamin (as thiamin mononitrate) 50 mg • Riboflavin 50 mg • Niacin (as niacinamide) 50 mg • Vitamin B6 (as pyridoxine HCl) 50 mg • Folic Acid 400 mcg • Vitamin B12 (as cobalamin) 50 mcg • Biotin (as D-biotin) 50 mcg • Pantothenic Acid (from D-calcium pantothenate) 50 mg • Inositol 50 mg • Choline (as choline bitartrate) 21 mg • Natural Powder Blend 3.5 mg: Acerola berry 4:1 extract, Alfalfa whole plant, Kelp whole plant, Parsley aerial parts, Rose Hips fruit, Watercress whole plant. Other Ingredients: Vegetable Cellulose, Vegetable Magnesium Stearate, Silica, Microcrystalline Cellulose, Citric Acid, Water.

B-Complex & B-12 - Puritan's Pride
Each tablet contains: Thiamin (Vitamin B1; as Thiamine Hydrochloride and Brewer's Yeast) 7 mg • Riboflavin (Vitamin B2) (as Riboflavin and Brewer's Yeast) 14 mg • Niacin (as Niacin and Brewer's Yeast) 4.5 mg • Vitamin B12 (as Cyanocobalamin and Brewer's Yeast) 25 mcg • Protease (as Papain Powder) 10 mg.

B-Complex 100 - The Vitamin Shoppe
Each capsule contains: Vitamin B1 100 mg • Vitamin B2 100 mg • Vitamin B6 100 mg • Vitamin B12 100 mcg • Niacinamide 100 mg • Folic Acid 400 mcg • Pantothenic Acid 100 mg • D-Biotin 100 mcg • Choline Bitartrate 100 mg • Inositol 100 mg • PABA 100 mg.

B-Complex 125 - GNC
Each tablet contains: Vitamin C (as Ascorbic Acid) 125 mg • Thiamin (as Thiamin Mononitrate) 125 mg • Riboflavin 125 mg • Niacin (as Niacinamide) 125 mg • Vitamin B6 (Pyridoxine Hydrochloride) 125 mg • Folate, Folic Acid, Folacin 400 mcg • Vitamin B12 (as Cyanocobalamin) 125 mcg • Biotin 125 mcg • Pantothenic Acid (as Calcium d-Pantothenate) 125 mg • Choline Bitartrate 125 mg • Inositol 125 mcg • Para-aminobenzoic Acid (PABA) 75 mg. Other Ingredients: Cellulose, Dicalcium Phosphate, Vegetable Acetoglycerides, Rose Hips powder (Rosina canina), Brewer's Yeast, Lecithin, Alfalfa leaf powder (Medicago sativa), Watercress herb powder (Nasturtium officinale), Parsley herb powder (Petroselinum sativum), Whole Brown Rice (Oryza sativa).

B-Complex 50 - GNC
Each capsule contains: Thiamin (as Thiamin Mononitrate) 50 mg • Riboflavin (vitamin B2) 50 mg • Niacin (as Niacinamide) 50 mg • Vitamin B6 (as Pyridoxine Hydrochloride) 50 mg • Folate, Folic Acid, Folacin 400 mcg • Vitamin B12 (as Cyanocobalamin) 50 mcg • Biotin 50 mcg • Pantothenic acid (as Calcium d-Pantothenate) 50 mg • Choline Bitartrate 50 mg • Inositol 50 mg • Para-aminobenzoic Acid (PABA) 50 mg. Other Ingredients: Gelatin, Mono- & Diglycerides, Whole Brown rice powder (Oryza sativa), Brewer's Yeast, Lecithin, Alfalfa leaf powder (Medicago sativa), Watercress herb powder (Nasturtium officinale), Parsley herb powder (Petroselinum sativum).

B-Complex 50 mg - Nature's Life
Each tablet contains: Vitamin B1 (Thiamine HCl) 50 mg • Vitamin B2 (Riboflavin) 50 mg • Vitamin B6 (Pyridoxine HCl) 50 mg • Vitamin B12 (Cobalamin concentrate) 50 mcg • Niacinamide 50 mg • Pantothenic Acid (d-Calcium Pantothenate) 50 mg • Choline (Bitartrate) 50 mg • Inositol 50 mg • Biotin 50 mcg • Folic Acid 400 mcg • PABA (Para Aminobenzioc Acid) 50 mg • Lecithin 8 mg. In a natural base of Alfalfa, Parsley, Rice Bran & Watercress.

B-Complex 75 Complete - GNC
Two tablets contain: Vitamin A (50% as beta-Carotene and 50% as Retinyl Acetate) 10,000 IU • Vitamin C (as Ascorbic Acid) 500 mg • Vitamin D (as Cholecalciferol) 400 IU • Vitamin E (as d-alpha tocopheryl succinate) 100 IU • Thiamin (as Thiamin Mononitrate) 75 mg • Riboflavin 75 mg •Niacin (as Niacinamide and Niacin) 75 mg • Vitamin B6 (as Pyridoxine Hydrochloride) 75 mg • Folate, Folic Acid, Folacin 400 mcg • Vitamin B12 (as Cyanocobalamin) 250 mcg • Biotin 75 mcg • Pantothenic acid (as Calcium d-Pantothenate) 100 mg • Iron (as Ferrous Fumarate) 18 mg • Selenium (as Hydrolyzed Rice Protien Chelate) 50 mcg • Copper (as Copper Gluconate) 2 mg • Chromium (as Hydrolyzed Rice Protien chelate) 25 mcg • Citrus Bioflavonoid Complex 100 mg • Bee Pollen 50 mg • Valerian root powder (Valeriana officinalis) 25 mg • Licorice root powder (Glycyrrhiza glabra) 25 mg • Goldenseal herb powder (Hydrastis Canadensis) 50 mg • Korean Ginseng root powder (Panax Ginseng) 50 mg • Guarana seed extract (Paullinia cupana) 50 mg. Other Ingredients: Dicalcium Phosphate, Cellulose, Food Glaze.

B-Complex Forte - Golden Glow Natural Health Products
Each tablet contains: Thiamine Nitrate (vitamin B1) 15 mg • Riboflavin (vitamin B2) 15 mg • Nicotinamide (vitamin B3) 30 mg • Calcium Pantothenate (vitamin B5) 8 mg • Pyridoxine Hydrochloride (vitamin B6) 5 mg • Cyanocobalamin (vitamin B12) 10 mcg • Folic Acid 150 mcg.

B-Complex Plus - Pure Encapsulations
Each vegetable capsule contains: Thiamine HCl (B1) 100 mg • Riboflavin HCl (B2) 5 mg • Riboflavin 5' Phosphate (activated B2) 10 mg • Niacinamide 100 gm • Inositol Hexaniacinate (no-flush niacin) 10 mg • Pyridoxine HCl (B6) 10 mg • Pyridoxal 5' Phosphate (activated B6) 10 mg • Pantothenic Acid (calcium pantothenate, B5) 100 mg • Methylcobalamin (B12) 400 mcg • Folic Acid 400 mcg • Biotin 400 mcg • Vitamin C (as ascorbyl palmitate) 16 mg.

B-Complex Sublingual Liquid - Puritan's Pride
Each 1 dropper serving (1.0 cc) contains: Vitamin C (as Ascorbic Acid) 60 mg • Riboflavin (Vitamin B2; as Riboflavin 5-Phosphate Sodium) 1.7 mg • Niacin (as Niacinamide) 20 mg • Vitamin B6 (as Pyridoxine Hydrochloride) 2 mg • Vitamin B12 (as Cyanocobalamin) 1,200 mcg • Pantothenic Acid (as Dexpanthenol) 30 mg.

B-Complex Sublingual Liquid - Vitamin World
Each dropperful (1 mL) contains: Riboflavin (vitamin B2, as riboflavin 5-phosphate sodium) 1.7 mg • Niacin (as niacinamide) 20 mg • Vitamin B6 (as pyridoxine hydrochloride) 2 mg • Vitamin B12 (as cyanocobalamin) 1200 mcg • Pantothenic Acid (as dexpanthenol) 30 mg. Other Ingredients: Purified Water, Sorbitol, Glycerin, Citric Acid, Potassium Sorbate, Natural Flavors.

B-Complex Supplement - Leiner Health Products
Each tablet contains: Thiamin Mononitrate (Vitamin B1) 10 mg • Riboflavin (Vitamin B2) 10 mg • Vitamin B6 (Pyridoxine Hydrochloride) 10 mg • Niacin (Niacinamide) 10 mg • Biotin (USP Method 2) 10 mcg • Folate (Folic Acid) 100 mcg • Vitamin B12 (Cyanocobalamin - USP Method 2) 10 mcg • Pantothenic Acid 10 mg. Other Ingredients: Calcium Carbonate, Maltodextrin, Hydroxypropyl Methycellulose, d-Calcium Pantothenate, Cellulose, Starch, Para-Aminobenzoic Acid, Croscarmellose Sodium, Sodium Starch Glycolate, Silicon Dioxide, Hydroxypropyl Cellulose, Red 40 Lake, Polyethylene Glycol 3350, Magnesium Stearate, Resin, Dicalcium Phosphate, Polysorbate 80, Titanium Dioxide, Povidone, Pharmaceutical Glaze.

B-Complex with B-12 Sublingual Liquid - Nature's Bounty
Each dropperful (1 mL) contains: Riboflavin (vitamin B2, as riboflavin 5'-phosphate sodium) 1.7 mg • Niacin (as niacinamide) 20 mg • Vitamin B6 (as pyridoxine hydrochloride) 2 mg • Vitamin B12 (as cyanocobalamin) 1200 mcg • Pantothenic Acid (as dexpanthenol) 30 mg. Other Ingredients: Purified Water, Sorbitol, Glycerin, Citric Acid, Potassium Sorbate, Natural Flavors.

Some Brand Name Natural Products - What they Contain

www.NaturalDatabase.com contains MANY more listings than appear here.
Editor's Notes are located on pages 2155-2163.

BRAND NAMES

B-Complex with Folic Acid - Nutritional Therapeutics, Inc.
Two tablets contain: Vitamin B12 (as cyanocobalamin) 200 mcg • Vitamin B2 (as riboflavin) 50 mg • Vitamin B1 (as thiamin HCl) 40 mg • Vitamin B6 (as pyridoxine HCl/P-5-P) 40 mg • Pantothenic Acid (as D-calcium pantothenate) 90 mg • Vitamin B3 (as niacinamide) 100 mg • Folic Acid 800 mcg • Biotin 200 mcg • Calcium 100 mg • Vitamin E (as D-alpha, mixed tocopherols) 1.5 IU • Choline Bitartrate 250 mg • Inositol 100 mg • NT Factor (as tablet base) 190 mg • PABA (as para amino benzoate) 50 mg • Pantethine (as coenxyme A precursor) 27 mg. Other Ingredients: Microcrystalline Cellulose, Croscarmellose Sodium, Food Glaze, Vegetable Magnesium Stearate, Silica.

B-Complex with Vitamin C - Nature Made
Each caplet contains: Vitamin C (from ascorbic acid) 300 mg • Thiamin (from thiamin mononitrate) 15 mg • Riboflavin 10.2 mg • Niacin (from niacinamide ascorbate) 50 mg • Vitamin B6 (from pyridoxine hydrochloride) 5 mg • Pantothenic Acid (from D-calcium pantothenate) 10 mg. Other Ingredients: Dibasic Calcium Phosphate, Cellulose Gel, Croscarmellose Sodium, Hydroxypropyl Methylcellulose, Magnesium Stearate, Polyethylene Glycol.
See Editor's Note No. 45.

B-Complex With Vitamin C Stress Formula - Solgar
Two tablets contain: Vitamin C (as L-ascorbic acid) 500 mg • Thiamin (as thiamin mononitrate) 10 mg • Riboflavin 10 mg • Niacin (as niacinamide) 100 mg • Vitamin B6 (as pyridoxine HCl) 10 mg • Folic Acid 100 mcg • Vitamin B12 (as cobalamin) 25 mcg • Biotin (as D-biotin) 25 mcg • Pantothenic Acid (as D-calcium pantothenate) 100 mg • Inositol 100 mg • Choline (as choline bitartrate) 41 mg. Other Ingredients: Microcrystalline Cellulose, Vegetable Cellulose, Silica, Vegetable Magnesium Stearate, Vegetable Stearic Acid, Titanium Dioxide, Vegetable Glycerin, Carnauba Wax, Natural Powdered Base: Alfalfa, Acerola, Kelp, Parsley, Rose Hips, Watercress.

BCQ - Vital Nutrients
Each capsule contains: Boswellia Serrata (65% boswellic acids) 200 mg • Bromelain (2400 gdu/2600 mcu) 100 mg • Curcuma Longa (curcumin 95%) 200 mg • Quercetin 100 mg.

Be Sure - Wakunaga of America
Two caplets contain: Aspergillus Enzyme Complex 300 mg. Other Ingredients: Cellulose, Silica, Magnesium Stearate (vegetable source).

Bean & Vegi Formula - Enzymatic Therapy
Two capsules contain: Pure Plant Enzymes Blend 235 mg: Alpha-Galactosidase (FCC IV [pH5.5]) 900 GalU, Amylase (USP XXI [pH6.8]) 16,500 USP (FCC IV [pH4.8]) 7140 DU, Cellulase I, II (FCC IV [Ph4.5]) 332 CU, Protease I,II,III (USP XXIII [Ph7.5]) 6550 USP (FCC IV [Ph7.0] 10,500 PC. FCC IV [Ph4.7] 11,900 HUT, Lipase II (FCC III [Ph6.5]) 54 LU. Other Ingredients: Gelatin, Microcrystalline Cellulose, Ascorbyl Palmitate.

Bean Pods - Arkopharma
Each capsule contains: White Kidney Bean pods (phaseolus vulgaris) 320 mg.

Bearberry Leaf - Aboca USA, Inc
Two capsules contain: Bearberry leaf WPC (whole phytocomplex concentrate, arctostaphylos uva-ursi, standardized to contain 9.84% arbutin, yielding 30 mg per capsule) 610 mg. Other Ingredients: Gelatin.

beCalm'd - Neurogenesis Inc.
Each capsule contains: D / L-Phenylalanine 300 mg • L-Glutamine 150 mg • 5-HTP 5 mg • Vitamin B6 (pyridoxine HCl) 1 mg • Calcium (chelate, citrate) 50 mg • Magnesium (chelate, oxide) 25 mg • Folic Acid 0.01 mg.

Bedwetting Tablets - Hyland's
Each tablet contains: Equisetum hyemale as Scouring Rush 3X HPUS • Rhus aromatica (Fragrant Sumac) 3X HPUS • Belladonna 3X HPUS (0.0003% Allkaloids). In a base of Lactose NF (Milk Sugar).
See Editor's Note No. 1.

Bee Complete - Futurebiotics LLC
Two tablets contain: Bee Pollen 1,000 mg • Royal Jelly 25 mg • Bee Propolis 500 mg.

Bee Pollen - Nature's Sunshine
Two capsules contain: Bee Pollen 900 mg. Other Ingredients: Gelatin, Water.

Bee Pollen - Source Naturals
Each tablet contains: Whole nugget Bee Pollen 500 mg.

Bee Pollen Chewable - Atrium Biotechnologies
Each tablet contains: Bee Pollen 300 mg.

Bee Pollen Complex - Puritan's Pride
Each tablet contains: Bee Pollen 1000 mg • Bee Propolis 10 mg • Royal Jelly 10 mg.

Beef Liver 1500 mg - Nature's Life
Six tablets contain: Argentine Beef Liver (defatted, desicated, pesticide free) 9000 mg • Vitamin B12 (cobalamin concentrate) 1000 mcg • Vitamin B2 457 mcg • Vitamin B6 224 mcg • Vitamin B12 1 mg • Niacin 2.2 mg • Choline 94 mg • Calcium 2.7 mg • Copper 90 mcg • Iron 6.3 mg • Manganese 90 mcg • Potassium 94 mg • Sodium 28 mg • Zinc 1.3 mg • Amino Acids (naturally occurring): Alanine 747 mg • Arginine 297 mg • Aspartic Acid 99 mg • Cysteine 351 mg • Cystine 103 mg • Glutamic Acid 108 mg • Glysine 792 mg • Histidine (essential amino acid) 198 mg • Isoleucine (essential amino acid) 207 mg • Leucine (essential amino acid) 198 mg • Lysine (essential amino acid) 558 mg • Methionine (essential amino acid) 315 mg • Phenylalanine (essential amino acid) 369 mg • Proline 99 mg • Serine 441 mg • Threonine (essential amino acid) 306 mg • Tyrosine 396 mg • Tryptophan (essential amino acid) 36 mg • Valine (essential amino acid) 90 mg.
See Editor's Note No. 14.

Bee-Happy Plus - Bee-Alive Inc.
Each capsule contains: Rhodiola Rosea root extract (standardized to 1% rosavins 0.5 mg) 50 mg • St. John's Wort flowering tops extract (standardized to 0.3% hypericin 0.45 mg) 150 mg • Siberian Ginseng root (eleutherococcus senticosus) 25 mg • Honey (dried) 25 mg. Other Ingredients: Microcrystalline Cellulose, Stearic Acid, Magnesium Stearate, Calcium Silicate, Gelatin (capsule shell).

Beelith - Beach Pharmaceuticals
Each tablet contains: Magnesium Oxide (equivalent to 362 mg of magnesium) 600 mg • Pyridoxine Hydrochloride (equivalent of Vitamin B6) 20 mg.

Beer Neutralizer - EGOceutical
Two capsules contain: Calcium (as carbonate) 150 mg • Vitamin B2 6 mg • Chromium (as picolinate) 120 mcg • Vitamin B12 9 mcg • White Kidney Bean powder (phaseolus vulgaris) 1000 mg • Vegetable Carbon 300 mg • Kudzu root (supplying isoflavones) 100 mg • Vanadium Chelate 1% 400 mcg • CoEnzyme Q10 100 mcg. Other Ingredients: Maltodextrin, Kosher, NF, Gelatin Capsule.

beeSatisfied Fruit Bar (Blueberry) - Bee-Alive Inc.
Each bar (35 g) contains: Apples • Honey • Blueberries • Natural Flavor • Ascorbic Acid • Non-Freeze Dried Royal Jelly.

beeSatisfied Fruit Bar (Raspberry) - Bee-Alive Inc.
Each bar (35 g) contains: Apples • Honey • Raspberries • Natural Flavor • Ascorbic Acid • Non-Freeze Dried Royal Jelly.

beeSatisfied Fruit Bar (Strawberry) - Bee-Alive Inc.
Each bar (35 g) contains: Apples • Honey • Strawberries • Natural Flavor • Ascorbic Acid • Non-Freeze Dried Royal Jelly.

Some Brand Name Natural Products - What they Contain

www.NaturalDatabase.com contains MANY more listings than appear here.
Editor's Notes are located on pages 2155-2163.

Before & AfterGlow **-** Life Enhancement Products, Inc.
Two capsules contain: Pantothenic Acid (from vitamin B5 from calcium pantothenate) 22 mg • L-Arginine 1000 mg • Ginkgo Biloba leaf extract 80 mg • Choline (from choline citrate) 67 mg • DHEA (dehydroepiandrosterone) 8 mg. Other Ingredients: Silicon Dioxide, Gelatin Capsule.

Bend & Flex **-** Gero Vita International
Two capsules contain: Glucosamine Sulfate 500 mg • Turmeric rhizome extract (95% curcumin) 400 mg • Nexrutine (phellodendron bark extract) 250 mg • Exclzyme (proprietary blend of enzymes) 200 mg • Black Pepper fruit extract (10% volatile oil) 20 mg • Piper Longum fruit extract (2.5% piperine) 20 mg • Ginger rhizome extract (5% volatile oils) 20 mg. Other Ingredients: Gelatin, Silicon Dioxide, Magnesium Stearate.

BeneCardia **-** Natrol, Inc.
Each tablet contains: Niacin (as inositol hexa-nicotinate) 600 mg • Bovine Protein Hydrolysate 25 mg • Policosanol (from rice bran, carnauba and candelilla wax) 5 mg. Other Ingredients: Cellulose, Stearic Acid, Silica, Cellulose Gum, Magnesium Stearate, Methylcellulose, Glycerin.

Benecol Light Spread **-** McNeil Consumer Healthcare
Liquid Canola oil • Water • Partially Hydrogenated Soybean oil • Liquid Soybean oil • Plant Stanol Esters • Salt • Emulsifiers (vegetable mono- and diglycerides, soy lecithin, polyglycerol esters of fatty acids) • Potassium Sorbate • Citric Acid • Calcium Disodium EDTA • Artificial Flavor • DL-Alpha Tocopheryl Acetate • Vitamin A Palmitate • Beta Carotene.

Benecol Regular Spread **-** McNeil Consumer Healthcare
Liquid Canola oil • Water • Partially Hydrogenated Soybean oil • Liquid Soybean oil • Plant Stanol Esters • Salt • Emulsifiers (vegetable mono- and diglycerides, soy lecithin, polyglycerol esters of fatty acids) • Potassium Sorbate • Citric Acid • Calcium Disodium EDTA • Artificial Flavor • DL-Alpha Tocopheryl Acetate • Vitamin A Palmitate • Beta Carotene.

Benecol Smart Chews **-** McNeil Consumer Healthcare
Each chew contains: Plant Stanol Esters 0.85 g.

Benecol softgels **-** McNeil Consumer Healthcare
Three softgels contain: Plant Stanol Esters 1.5 g. Other Ingredients: Gelatin, Glycerin, Sunflower Oil, Titanium Dioxide, Soybean Oil, Annatto Extract, Red 40, Yellow 8, Blue 1, Yellow 5.

Benefiber **-** Novartis
Partially hydrolyzed Guar Gum.

BeneFin Caplets **-** LaneLabs
Four caplets contain: BeneFin Organically Processed Whole Shark Cartilage 750 mg • Calcium 591 mg • Phosphorous 315 mg • Magnesium 8 mg • Zinc 135 mcg • Sodium 18 mg • Potassium 1 mg. Other Ingredients: Carnauba Wax, Hypromellose, Magnesium Stearate, Microcrystalline Cellulose, Tragacanth Gum.
See Editor's Note No. 9 and No. 21.

Benejoint **-** LaneLabs
Menthol (1.25%) • Aloe Vera • Apricot kernal oil • BeneFin Shark Cartilage (providing glucosamine, collagen, chondroitin sulfate) • Capsaicin • Carbomer • Cetyl Esters Wax • Citrus seed extract • Imidazolidinyl Urea • Jojoba oil • Lanolin Anhydrous • Lavender oil • Lemon • Methylhydroxybenzoate • Polawax GP200 • Propylhydroxybenzoate • Soft White Parafin • Water.

BenfoMax **-** Pure Encapsulations
Each vegetable capsule contains: Benfotiamine (S-benzoylthiamine-O-Monophosphate) 200 mg • Vitamin C (ascorbyl palmitate) 5 mg.

Bentonite **-** Ortho Molecular Products
Each scoop contains: Bentonite 1.46 g.

Benzo Berries **-** Unknown
Two tablets contain: 5-HTP extract 10X • Phenepropaloxamine • Valerian root extract 10X • Wild Berry extract 10X • Kava Kava extract 10X • Bioperine brand Black Pepper extract.

Berberine Complex **-** PhytoPharmica
Two capsules contain: Berberis Vulgaris bark of root 6:1 extract (barberry) 400 mg • Oregon Grape root 6:1 extract (berberis aquifolium) 400 mg • Goldenseal root and rhizome 4:1 extract (hydrastis canadensis, standardized to contain 5% total alkaloids including berberine, hydrastine, and canadine) 100 mg.

Berberis Formula **-** Genestra - Seroyal
Each capsule contains: Barberry extract 4:1 (equivalent to 800 mg) 200 mg • Oregon Grape extract 4:1 (equivalent to 800 mg) 200 mg • Goldenseal extract (standardized 5%) 50 mg • Barberry 25 mg • Oregon Grape 25 mg. Contains no less than 4,500 mcg Hydrastine and Berberine.

Bergamot Essential Oil **-** Golden Glow Natural Health Products
Citrus Aurantium var. Bergamia fruit peel essential oil.

Bergamot Pure Essential Oil **-** Nature's Sunshine
Pure Organic Citrus Bergamia oil.

BerrX brand **-** Xymogen
Proprietary Berry extract blend.
See Editor's Note No. 44.

Berry Barley Essence **-** Green Foods Corp.
Each 5.3 oz jar contains: Proprietary Blend 150 g: Young Barley Grass powdered juice, Maltodextrin, Raspberry, Strawberry, Other Natural Flavors, Chicory root extract (contains FOS), Brown rice, Stevia Extract.

Berry Healthy Drink Mix **-** Nature's Sunshine
Each scoop (9.2 g) contains: Vitamin C (ascorbic acid) 60 mg • Proprietary Blend 9180 mg: Chokeberry fruit (aronia melanocarpa), Blueberry fruit (vaccinium corymbosum), Raspberry fruit (rubus idaeus), Malic Acid, Citric Acid, Blackberry fruit (rubus fruticosus), Dried Cranberry fruit juice (vaccinium macrocarpon), Stevia extract (stevia rebaudiana).

Berry High **-** Jarrow Formulas
Each scoop contains: Bilberry 325 mg • Blueberry powder 1575 mg • Red Raspberry powder 750 mg • Blackberry powder 750 mg • Peach powder 750 mg • Apple fiber powder 1000 mg • Apple powder 525 mg • Cranberry powder 500 mg • Strawberry powder 480 mg • Apricot powder 750 mg • Cherry powder 325 mg • Elderberry powder 380 mg.

Berry StandardBar **-** Standard Process, Inc.
Brown Rice Syrup • Whey Protein • Almond Butter • Pure Wildflower Honey • Cherry • Soybean Lecithin • Cranberry • Apple juice concentrate • Blueberry • Glycerin • Sesame seed • Cranberry Puree • Extra Virgin Olive oil • Black Currant seed oil • Blueberry Puree • Calcium Lactate • Oat fiber • Apple fiber • Magnesium Citrate.

BerryVida brand **-** Cyvex Nutrition, Inc.
High ORAC Berries with Polyphenols, Anthocyanin and Ellagic Acid.

BerryVin brand **-** Cyvex Nutrition, Inc.
Berry Blend: Strawberries, Blueberries, Blackberries, Cranberries, Grape, Pomegranate.
See Editor's Note No. 44.

Best Defense High-Potency Herbal Defense Complex **-** Pro Health
Three tablets contain: Vitamin A (as palmitate 4000 IU, beta carotene 1000 IU) 5000 IU • Vitamin C (from ascorbic acid, zinc, calcium, magnesium ascorbates) 1278 mg • Calcium 47 mg • Zinc (as zinc ascorbate) 23 mg • Selenium (as sodium selenate) 25 mcg • Copper

(as copper sebacate) 300 mcg • Garlic Clove 360 mg • Propolis 324 mg • Boneset leaf 238 mg • Polygonum Odoratum rhizome 200 mg • Echinacea root 196 mg • Echinacea extract 164 mg • Isatis root/leaf 159 mg • Horehound stems 150 mg • Propolis extract 126 mg • Bioflavonoids 120 mg • Astragalus root 90 mg • Angelica root 87 mg • Mullein leaf 80 mg • Goldenseal root 75 mg • Eleutherococcus Senticosus root 65 mg • Hawthorn berry 55 mg • Oregon Grape root 55 mg • Eleutherococcus Senticosus root extract 54 mg • Pau D'Arco bark extract 36 mg • Cayenne fruit 30 mg. Other Ingredients: Modified Cellulose Gum, Stearic Acid, Colloidal Silicon Dioxide, Magnesium Ascorbate, Magnesium Stearate.

Best Friends **- Goldshield Elite**
Each tablet contains: Vitamin A (as Alpha- and Beta-Carotene with mixed Carotenoids from D. Salina algae) 5000 IU • Vitamin C (as Ascorbic Acid with Sodium and Calcium Ascorbates) 100 mg • Vitamin D (as Cholecalciferol) 400 IU • Vitamin E (as mixed natural D-Alpha and DL-Alpha-Tocopherol Acetate) 80 IU • Thiamin (as Thiamin HCl) 1.5 mg • Riboflavin 1.7 mg • Niacin (as Niacinamide) 2 mg • Vitamin B6 (as Pyridoxine HCl) 2 mg • Folate (as Folic Acid) 400 mcg • Vitamin B12 (as Cyanocobalamin) 12 mcg • Biotin 75 mcg • Pantothenic Acid (as D-Calcium Pantothenate) 10 mg • Calcium (as Calcium Carbonate and Citrate) 125 mg • Iron (as Ferrous Fumarate) 5 mg • Iodine (as Potassium Iodide) 75 mcg • Magnesium (as Magnesium Oxide, Glycinate, and Citrate) 40 mg • Zinc (as Zinc Citrate and Glycinate) 5 mg • Selenium (as Selenomethionine) 25 mcg • Copper (as Copper Oxide, Citrate, Gluconate, and Glycinate) 2 mg • Manganese (as Manganese Sulfate, Citrate, Gluconate, and Glycinate) 1 mg • Chromium (as Chromium Dinicotinate Glycinate) 50 mcg • Molybdenum (as natural Molybdic Acid) 50 mcg • Fruit and vegetable phytonutrient concentrates 1500 mg: Dunaliela salina algae, Parsley, Tomato, Spinach, Kale, Yellow Squash, Turmeric, Orange, Cranberry, Lemon, Tangerine, Grapefruit, Red Grape, Strawberry, Cherry, Peach, Raspberry, Onion, Garlic, Leek, Broccoli, Cauliflower, Mustard Greens, Cabbage. Other Ingredients: Fructose, Sorbitol, Natural and Artificial flavors, Microcrystalline Cellulose, Stearic Acid, Carrageenan, Glycine, Maltodextrin, Citric Acid, Magnesium Stearate, Silica, Fractionated vegetable oil, Salt, and Carmine red.

Beta 1,3 Glucan **- PhysioLogics**
Each tablet contains: Beta 1,3 Glucan (saccharomyces cerevisiae, from cell wall concentrate). Other Ingredients: Cellulose (plant origin), Dicalcium Phosphate, Acacia Gum, Vegetable Stearic Acid, Croscarmellose, Silica, Cellulose Coating, Vegetable Magnesium Stearate.

Beta 1,3 Glucans **- Solgar**
Each tablet contains: Beta 1,3 Glucans (from yeast cell wall concentrate Saccaromyces cerevisiae) 200 mg. Other Ingredients: Microcrystalline Cellulose, Vegetable Cellulose, Vegetable Stearic Acid, Titanium Dioxide, Vegetable Glycerin, Silica, Vegetable Magnesium Stearate, Caramel.

Beta Carotene **- Puritan's Pride**
Each softgel contains: Beta Carotene (25,000 IU) 15 mg.

Beta Carotene **- Pure Encapsulations**
Each softgel capsule contains: Mixed Carotenoids (Betatene brand, naturally derived from D. salina) 25,000 IU: Beta Carotene 14,280 mcg, Alpha Carotene 450 mcg, Zeaxanthin 90 mcg, Cryptoxanthin 110 mcg, Lutein 70 mcg.

Beta Carotene **- American Biologics**
Each softgel contains: Beta Carotene 25,000 IU. Other Ingredients: Gelatin, Water, Carrot Oil.

Beta Carotene **- Olympian Labs**
Each softgel contains: Beta Carotene 25000 IU.

Beta Carotene 10,000 IU **- Jamieson**
Each caplet contains: Beta Carotene 10,000 IU.

Beta Carotene 11,000 IU **- Solgar**
Each softgel contains: Vitamin A (as 100% beta carotene from carrot oil) 11,000 IU. Other Ingredients: Gelatin, Glycerin, Beeswax, Caramel, Safflower Oil.

Beta Carotene 25,000 IU **- Sunmark**
Each softgel contains: Beta Carotene 25,000 IU. Other Ingredients: Soybean Oil, Gelatin, Corn Oil, Glycerin, Yellow Beeswax, Purified Water, Silica, Lecithin.
See Editor's Note No. 45.

Beta Carotene 25,000 IU **- Jamieson**
Each caplet contains: Beta Carotene (pro-vitamin A) 25,000 IU.

Beta Carotene 25,000 IU **- Rexall - Sundown**
Each softgel contains: Vitamin A (100% as beta-carotene) 25,000 IU. Other Ingredients: Soybean Oil, Gelatin, Glycerin, Water.

Beta Carotene 25,000 IU **- Solgar**
Each softgel contains: Vitamin A (100% as natural beta carotene from D. salina) 25,000 IU • Alpha Carotene (from D. salina) 500 mcg • Cryptoxanthin (from D. salina) 130 mcg • Zeaxanthin (from D. salina) 100 mcg • Lutein (from D. salina) 86 mcg. Other Ingredients: Soybean Oil, Gelatin, Glycerin, Safflower Oil, Beeswax, Water.

Beta Carotene 25,000 IU **- Nature Made**
Each softgel contains: Vitamin A as Beta Carotene 25,000 IU. Other Ingredients: Soybean Oil, Gelatin, Glycerin, Partially Hydrogenated Cottonseed Oil, Soybean Oil, Water.
See Editor's Note No. 45.

Beta Carotene 25,000 IU **- Nature's Valley**
Each softgel contains: Beta Carotene 25,000 IU. Other Ingredients: Soybean Oil, Gelatin, Glycerin, Vegetable Oil, Yellow Beeswax, Beta Carotene, Carrot Oil.
See Editor's Note No. 45.

Beta Carotene 25,000 IU with Vitamin C & E **- Jamieson**
Each caplet contains: Beta Carotene 25,000 IU (15 mg) • Vitamin C (Ascorbic Acid) 250 mg • Vitamin E (Succinate) 100 IU.

Beta Carotene 5000 IU Chewable **- Jamieson**
Each tablet contains: Beta Carotene (Pro-Vitamin A) 5000 IU (3 mg).

Beta Carotene 6 **- GNC**
Each capsule contains: Vitamin A (as beta-Carotene 6 mg) 10,000 IU. Other Ingredients: Soybean oil, Gelatin, Glycerin, Partially Hydrogenated Corn oil.

Beta Carotene Provitamin A **- Puritan's Pride**
Each softgel contains: Beta Carotene (10000 IU) 6 mg.

Beta Carotene Provitamin A **- Nature's Bounty**
Each softgel contains: Vitamin A (as 100% Beta Carotene) 10000 IU. Other Ingredients: Soybean Oil, Gelatin, Beeswax, Glycerin, Lecithin.

Beta Carotene Pro-Vitamin A **- Westcoast Naturals**
Each softgel contains: Beta Carotene 25,000 IU.

Beta Carotene with Vitamin D **- Puritan's Pride**
Each softgel contains: Beta Carotene (25,000 IU) 15 mg • Vitamin D 400 IU.

Beta Fast GXR **- Informulab**
Each tablet contains: Gymnema Sylvestre (25% standardized extract) 400 mg.

Beta Glucan **- Source Naturals**
Each capsule contains: Purified beta-1, 3-glucan (derived from baker's yeast cell wall) 7.5 mg.

Beta Glucan **- Life Source Basics**
Each capsule contains: Beta-1-6,1,3-Beta-Glucan (micronized and naturall derived from baker's yeast cell wall, saccharomyces cerevisiae) 75 mg. Other Ingredients: Chitin, Manno-Protein, Microcrystalline Cellulose, Magnesium Stearate, Gelatin, Water.

Some Brand Name Natural Products - What they Contain

www.NaturalDatabase.com contains MANY more listings than appear here.
Editor's Notes are located on pages 2155-2163.

Beta Glucan 500 mg - Pro Health
Each capsule contains: Saccharomyces Cerevisiae Glucan-A extract (cell wall, providing 70-75% polysacharrides as beta 1-3-glucans 350-375 mg) 500 mg. Other Ingredients: Gelatin, Magnesium Stearate, Water.

Beta Glucans - Natrol, Inc.
Two capsules contain: Oat Bran extract Seed (Avena sativa) 1500 mg, supplying Beta Glucan 185 mg. Other Ingredients: Oat Bran powder, Magnesium Stearate, Gelatin.

Beta Sitosterol - Source Naturals
Three tablets contain: Soybean Hull 750 mg (yielding total sterols 660 mg, 324 mg as beta-sitosterol). Other Ingredients: Microcrystalline Cellulose, Dibasic Calcium, Phosphate, Sorbitol, Stearic Acid, Colloidal Silicon Dioxide, Magnesium Stearate, Modified Cellulose Gum.

Beta1, 3 Glucan - America's Finest
Each capsule contains: Beta 1,3 Glucans (saccharomyces cerevisiae) 500 mg. Other Ingredients: Dicalcium Phosphate, Cellulose, Magnesium Stearate, Silica.

BETA-C - Pharmagel
Beta Hydroxy Acid • Stabilized Vitamin C.

Beta-Carotene - Benepure, Inc
Each capsule contains: Vitamin A (100% as beta-carotene) 25,000 IU. Other Ingredients: Gelatin, Carrot Oil.

Beta-Carotene 15 - GNC
Each capsule contains: Vitamin A (100% as beta-Carotene 15mg) 25,000 IU. Other Ingredients: Soybean Oil, Gelatin, Partially Hydrogenated Corn Oil, Glycerin.

Beta-Carotene 25 - GNC
Each tablet contains: Vitamin A (as beta-Carotene) 41,666 IU. Other Ingredients: Dicalcium Phosphate, Cellulose.

Beta-Carotene 25,000 IU - Trophic
Each softgel contains: Beta-Carotene 25,000 IU.

Beta-Carotene 25,000 IU - Schiff
Each softgel contains: Vitamin A as Beta Carotene 25,000 IU. Other Ingredients: Carrot Oil, Soybean Oil, Gelatin, Glycerin), Purified Water.

Beta-Carotene 6mg - Nature's Own
Each tablet contains: Beta Carotene 6 mg.

Betacol - Standard Process, Inc.
Each capsule contains: Proprietary Blend 293 mg: Tillandsia Usneoides, Soy bean, Bovine Liver PMG extract, Betaine Hydrochloride, Calcium Lactate, Defatted Wheat germ, Potassium Bicarbonate, Choline Bitartrate, Inositol, Disodium Phosphate, Bovine Adrenal Cytosol extract, Oat flour, Ascorbic Acid • Niacin 10 mg • Vitamin B6 2 mg.

Betafood - Standard Process, Inc.
Each tablet contains: Proprietary Blend 316 mg: Beet root, Beet leaf, Oat flour, Dried Beet root juice. Other Ingredients: Honey, Calcium Stearate.

BetaGen - EAS, Inc.
Each 6.6 gram serving contains: Ca HMB Monohydrate 1000 mg • Creatine Monohydrate 2000 mg • Potassium Phosphate 50 mg • L-Glutamine 400 mg • Taurine 200 mg. Ingredients: Dextrose, Phosphagen (HPCE pure Creatine Monohydrate) • Calcium b-Hydroxy b-Methylbutyrate Monohydrate • Citric Acid • L-Glutamine • Natural Flavors • Taurine • Potassium Phosphate • Aspartame • Beta-Carotene for color. Contains Phenylalanine.

Beta-glucan - Pure Encapsulations
Each vegetable capsule contains: Beta-Glucan (providing 60% beta-1,3/1,6-glucan min.) 425 mg.

Betaine & Pepsin - Ortho Molecular Products
Two capsules contain: Betaine HCl USP 1040 mg • Pepsin 1:3000 208 mg. Other Ingredients: Natural Vegetable Capsules, Magnesium Stearate, Microcrystalline Cellulose.

Betaine HCl Pepsin - Pure Encapsulations
Each vegetable capsule contains: Betaine HCl 520 mg • Pure Pepsin (1:15,000 potency, lactose free, porcine) 21 mg • Vitamin C (as ascorbyl palmitate) 10 mg.

Betaine HCl/Pepsin & Gentian - Vital Nutrients
Each capsule contains: Betaine HCl 520 mg • Pepsin (1:15,000, pure un-cut pepsin, lactose free) 21 mg • Gentian root extract (5:1, equivalent to gentian root powder 250 mg) 50 mg.

Betaine Hydrochloride - Standard Process, Inc.
Two tablets contain: Proprietary Blend 605 mg: Betaine Hydrochloride, Ammonium Chloride, Calcium Lactate, Pepsin (1:10,000), Magnesium Citrate. Other Ingredients: Cellulose, Lactose, Calcium Stearate.

BetaLean Ephedra Free - EAS, Inc.
Two tablets contain: Calcium (from calcium carbonate) 360 mg • Chromium (from chromium polynicotinate) 150 mcg • Green Tea leaf extract (50% polyphenols, 150 mg; 35% catechins, 105 mg; 9% epigallocatechin gallate, EGCG, 27 mg) 300 mg • Bitter Orange fruit (6% synephrine, 18 mg) 300 mg • Proprietary Blend 225 mg: L-Tyrosine, Potassium Phosphate, White Willow bark, L-Carnitine (tartate) • Caffeine (from caffeine anhydrous, green tea leaf) 200 mg • Naringin (from grapefruit) 75 mg. Other Ingredients: Stearic Acid, Microcrystalline Cellulose, Magnesium Stearate, Silicon dioxide, Coating.
See Editor's Note No. 40.

Betalin-7-EC - BSN Inc.
Two capsules contain: 20-Hydroxy-Beta-Ecdysterone (96% extract from rhaponticum carthamoides) 100 mg • 7-Hydroxy-ECMM (5-methyl-7-hydroxy isoflavone ethyl carbonate molecular modification) 267 mg • 4-Hydroxyisoleucine (extracted from fenugreek) 50 mg. Other Ingredients: Cellulose, Magnesium Stearate, Gelatin.

Beta-mannan - Alotek Supplement Company
Two capsules contain: Vitamin E (as d-alpha-tocopherol) 100 IU • Proprietary blend of freeze-dried Aloe vera gel concentrates and extracts containing beta-mannans and beta-glucans 600 mg • IP6 (inositol hexaphosphate, derived from grains) 184 mg. Other Ingredients: defatted rice bran flour.

Beta-Sea 10,000 IU - Holista
Each capsule contains: Beta Carotene (from Dunaliella salina algae) 10000 IU. Other Ingredients: Carotenoids.

Beta-Sea 25,000 IU - Holista
Each capsule contains: Beta Carotene (from Dunaliella salina algae) 25000 IU. Other Ingredients: Carotenoids.

Beta-sitosterol - Pure Encapsulations
Each vegetable capsule contains: Beta-Sitosterol (from 150 mg of a phytosterol complex) 68 mg • Vitamin c (as ascorbyl palmitate) 20 mg.

Better BodyEnergy for Life - HealthWatchers System
Ma Huang • Chromium Picolinate • Brindel Berry • White Willow Bark • Ginger Root • Hawthorn Berry • Licorice Root • Gotu Kola • Passion Flower • Siberian Ginseng • Guarana • Rhemannia Root • Bladderwrack • Reishi Mushroom • Astragalus.
See Editor's Note No. 30.

Better Living Multi Vitamins - Health Center for Better Living
Each tablet contains: Vitamin A (Natural Fish Liver Oil) 10,000 IU• Beta Carotene (6 mg) 10000 mg • Vitamin B1 (Thiamine HCL) 75 mg • Vitamin B2 (Riboflavin) 75 mg • Vitamin B3 (Niacinamide) 75 mg • Vitamin B5 (Pantothenic) 75 mg • Vitamin B6 (as pyridoxine

HCl) 75 mg • Vitamin B12 (as cyanocobalamin) 100 mcg • Biotin 100 mcg• Folic Acid 400 mcg • Vitamin C (Ascorbic Acid) 250 mg • Vitamin D (Natural FLO) 400 IU • Vitamin E (100% Natural d-alpha) 150 IU • Calcium (Ostershell) 100 mg • Magnesium (Oxide, amino acid chelate) 60 mg • Zinc (Amino acid chelate) 1 mg • Iodine (Kelp) 150 mcg • Iron (Amino acid chelate) • Chromium (Yeast Free GFT) 50 mcg • Boron (Amino acid chelate) 500 mcg • Molybdenum (Amino acid chelate) 50 mcg • Nucleic 50 mg.

BetterMan **- Interceuticals**
Each capsule contains: Proprietary Blend: Radix Ginseng, Rhizoma Dioscoreae, Radix Paeonia Alba, Herba Epimedii, Cornu Cervi Pantotrichum, Radix Astragali, Poria Cocos, Radix Morindae Officinalis, Fructus Corni, Cortex Eucommiae, Radix Angelicae Sinensis, Fructus Lycii, Radix Rehmanniae, Rhizoma Chuanxiong, Fructus Schisandrae, Acanthopanax Senticosus, Cynomorium Songaricum Rupr, Cortex Cinnamomi.

BetterWOMAN **- Interceuticals**
Each capsule contains: Proprietary Blend 400 mg: Asian Ginseng root, Chinese Yam rhizome, Chinese Peony root, Deer Antler velvet, Astragalus root, Poria Sclerotium, Morinda root, Asiatic Dogwood fruit, Eucommia stem, Dong Quai root, Bupleurum root, Lycium fruit, Rehmannia root, Epimedium leaf, Szechuan Lovage root, Schisandra fruit, Eleuthero root, Cynomorium stem, Cassia bark, Palm-leaf Raspberry fruit. Other Ingredients: Gelatin, Microcrystalline Celluose, Water, Magnesium Stearate, Silicon Dioxide.

Beyond Basics **- Metabolic Response Modifiers**
Three tablets contain: Vitamin A (as beta-carotene palmitate) 15,000 IU • Vitamin C (as ascorbic acid) 500 mg • Vitamin E (as D-alpha tocopherol acetate) 200 IU • Vitamin B1 (as thiamine HCl) 20 mg • Vitamin B2 (as riboflavin) 30 mg • Vitamin D (as cholecalciferol) 400 IU • Vitamin K (K1, as phylloquinine) 60 mcg • Niacin (niacinamide 1:1) 30 mg • Pantothenic Acid (as calcium D-pantothenate) 25 mg • Vitamin B6 (as pyridoxine HCl) 20 mg • Vitamin B12 (as cyanocobalamin) 200 mcg • Biotin 75 mcg • Folic Acid 400 mcg • Calcium (as calcium carbonate citrate 4:1) 200 mg • Magnesium (as oxide glycinate 4:1) 125 mg • Zinc (as zinc citrate) 10 mg • Copper (as copper citrate) 2 mg • Potassium (as potassium citrate) 75 mg • Molybdenum (as molybdate) 100 mcg • Iodine (as kelp) 150 mcg • Selenium (as L-selenomethionine) 50 mcg • Chromium (as chromium chelate) 200 mcg • Boron (as potassium borate) 3 mg • Silica (as colloidal silica) 10 mg • Organic Horsetail 275 mg • Vanadium (as vanadyl sulfate) 50 mcg • Choline (as choline bitartrate) 25 mg • Inositol 30 mg.

Beyond Echinacea **- Flora Inc.**
Echinacea • Balsam root • Peruvian Cat's Claw bark.

BF & SC **- MMS Pro**
Each capsule contains: Calendula flowers • White Oak bark • Marshmallow root • Mullein leaves • Black Walnut hulls • Gravel root • Slippery Elm bark • Wormwood • Scullcap.

B-Fruitful **- TriLight Herbs**
False Unicorn • Vitex • Squaw Vine • True Unicorn root • Black Haw • Ginger.

BGSE Mint Mouthwash Treatment **- FreeLife International**
Purified Water • Vegetable Glycerin • Xylitol • Aloe Vera gel • Peppermint oil • Spearmint oil • Anise oil • Wintergreen oil • Sodium Benzoate • BioEnhanced Grapefruit seed extract (BGSE) • Stevia • Licorice extract • Willowherb extract • Harmonic Essence • Xanthan Gum.

BGSE Mint Toothpaste **- FreeLife International**
Glycerin • Purified Water • Silica • Sorbitol (fruit base) • Silicone Dioxide • Lauryl Polyglucoside: Coconut oil & Glucose • Peppermint oil • Spearmint oil • Anise oil • Wintergreen oil • Xylitol • Sodium Benzoate • Xanthan Gum • Dicalcium Phosphate Dihydrate • BioEnhanced Grapefruit seed extract (BGSE) • Peelu bark • Methylsulfonylmethane (MSM) • Natural Orange • Stevia • Licorice extract • Cranberry extract • Willowherb extract • Grape seed oil.

BHI Alertness **- Heel/BHI, Inc.**
Phosphoricum Acidum 4X, 10X • Anacardium Orientale 6X • Arsenicum Iodatum 6X • Kali Phosphoricum 6X • Staphysagria 6X • Lycopodium Clavatum 8X • Calcarea Phosphorica 10X • Ignatia Amara 10X • Silicea 10X • Selenium Metallicum 12X • Nux Vomica 30X.
See Editor's Note No. 1.

BHI Allergy oral vials **- Heel/BHI, Inc.**
Each vial contains: Arnica Montana, radix 6X • Ignatia Amara 6X • Lycopodium Clavatum 6X • Thuja Occidentalis 6X • Lappa Major 8X • Arsenicum Album 8X • Formicum Acidum 8X • Histaminum 8X, 12X, 30X • Ledum Palustre 8X • Antimonium Crudum 10X • Graphites 10X • Pix Liquida 10X • Tellurium Metallicum 10X • Selenium Metallicum 12X• Sulphur 12X• Sulphuricum Acidum 30X.
See Editor's Note No. 1.

BHI Allergy tablets **- Heel/BHI, Inc.**
Each tablet contains: Arnica Montana, radix 6X • Ignatia Amara 6X • Lycopodium Clavatum 6X • Thuja Occidentalis 6X • Lappa Major 8X • Arsenicum Album 8X • Formicum Acidum 8X • Histaminum 8X, 12X, 30X, 200X • Ledum Palustre 8X • Antimonium Crudum 10X • Graphites 10X • Pix Liquida 10X • Tellurium Metallicum 10X • Selenium Metallicum 12X • Sulphur 12X • Sulphuricum Acidum 30X.
See Editor's Note No. 1.

BHI Arnica ointment **- Heel/BHI, Inc.**
Arnica Montana, radix 3X.
See Editor's Note No. 1.

BHI Arnica PC **- Heel/BHI, Inc.**
Arnica Montana, radix 6X, 12X, 30X, 200X.
See Editor's Note No. 1.

BHI Arthritis **- Heel/BHI, Inc.**
Each tablet contains: Bryonia Alba 4X, 8X, 12X, 30X • Rhus Toxicodendron 4X, 8X, 12X, 30X • Colocynthis 5X • Arnica Montana radix 6X • Colchicum Autumnale 6X • Dulcamara 6X • Ledum Palustre 6X • Ranunculus Bulbosus 6X • Berberis Vulgaris 8X • Causticum 8X • Rhododendron Chrysanthemum 8X • Lycopodium Clavatum 10X • Sulphur 10X • Ferrum Phosphoricum 12X.
See Editor's Note No. 1.

BHI Asthma **- Heel/BHI, Inc.**
Each tablet contains: Arsenicum Album 12X • Carbo Vegetabilis 12X • Sulphur 12X.
See Editor's Note No. 1.

BHI Back **- Heel/BHI, Inc.**
Each tablet contains: Colocynthis 5X • Gnaphalium Polycephalum 5X • Ammonium Muriaticum 6X • Gelsemium Sempervirens 6X • Rhus Toxicodendron 8X • Arsenicum Album 10X • Chamomilla 10X.
See Editor's Note No. 1.

BHI Bleeding **- Heel/BHI, Inc.**
Each tablet contains: Rhlaspi Bursa Pastoris 4X • Aceticum Acidum 6X • Crocus Sativus 6X • Ipecacuanha 6X • Arnica Montana, radix 8X • Erigeron Canadensis 8X • Hammamelis Virginiana 8X • Millefolium 8X • Bovista 12X • Phosphorus 12X • Crotalus Horridus 15X.
See Editor's Note No. 1.

BHI Body Pure **- Heel/BHI, Inc.**
Each tablet contains: Alpha-Lipoicum Acidum 3X, 6X, 8X • Avena Sativa 3X • Ricinus Communis 3X • Solidago Virgaurea 4X • Viola Tricolor 4X • Berberis Vulgaris 6X • Caffeinum 6X • Juglans Regia 6X • Rhamnus Purshiana 6X • Urita Urens 6X • Cholesterinum 10X •

Influenzinum 12X • Petroleum 12X • Tabacum 12X • X-Ray 12X • Nux Vomica 30X.
See Editor's Note No. 1.

BHI Bone **- Heel/BHI, Inc.**
Each tablet contains: Asafoetida 6X • Kalmia Latifolia 8X • Aurum Metallicum 12X • Hekla Lava 12X • Mercurius Praecipitatus Ruber 12X • Natrum Sulphuricum 12X • Aranea Diadema 15X • Lycopodium Clavatum 30X.
See Editor's Note No. 1.

BHI Bronchitis **- Heel/BHI, Inc.**
Each tablet contains: Lobelia Inflata 4X • Hyoscymus Niger 5X • Sticta Pulmonaria 5X • Antimonium Tartaricum 5X • Belladonna 6X • Bryonia Alba 6X • Hepatic Triloba 6X • Ipecacuanha 6X • Kreosotum 6X • Pertussinum 30X.
See Editor's Note No. 1.

BHI Calendula ointment **- Heel/BHI, Inc.**
Calendula Officinalis 1X.
See Editor's Note No. 1.

BHI Calming **- Heel/BHI, Inc.**
Each tablet contains: Chamomilla 2X • Humulus Lupulus 2X • Passiflora Incarnata 2X • Valeriana Officinalis 2X • Veratrum Album 4X • Ignatia Amara 8X • Coffea Cruda 10X • Moschus 10X • Sulphur 12X • Nux Vomica 30X.
See Editor's Note No. 1.

BHI Chamomilla Complex **- Heel/BHI, Inc.**
Each tablet contains: Chamomilla 4X • Plantago Major 4X • Pulsatilla 4X • Aconitum Napellus 5X • Capsicum Annuum 6X • Kali Chloricum 6X • Ferrum Phosphoricum 10X • Hepar Sulphuris Calcareum 10X.
See Editor's Note No. 1.

BHI Chelidonium Complex **- Heel/BHI, Inc.**
Each tablet contains: Belladonna 8X • Chelidonium Majus 8X • Cinchona Officinalis 8X • Veratrum Album 8X • Calcarea Carbonica 10X • Cholesterinum 10X • Lycopodium Clavatum 10X.
See Editor's Note No. 1.

BHI Chest **- Heel/BHI, Inc.**
Each tablet contains: Bryonia Alba 4X • Ranunculus Bulbosus 4X • Asclepias Tuberosa 6X • Kali Carbonicum 6X • Natrum Sulphuricum 6X • Sticta Pulmonaria 6X • Arsenicum Iodatum 8X • Dulcamara 8X • Colocynthis 10X • Sulphur 30X.
See Editor's Note No. 1.

BHI Cold **- Heel/BHI, Inc.**
Each tablet contains: Pulsatilla 6X • Sulphur 8X.
See Editor's Note No. 1.

BHI Constipation **- Heel/BHI, Inc.**
Each tablet contains: Dioscorea Villosa 4X • Nux Vomica 8X • Natrum Muriaticum 200X.
See Editor's Note No. 1.

BHI Cough **- Heel/BHI, Inc.**
Each tablet contains: Illicium Anisatum 4X • Ipecacuanha 4X • Stachys Betonica 4X • Hepatica Triloba 5X • Lobelia Inflata 5X • Arsenicum Iodatum 6X • Belladonna 6X • Naphthalinum 6X • Natrum Sulphuricum 6X • Quebracho 6X • Antimonium Tartaricum 6X • Blatta Orientalis 8X • Bryonia Alba 8X.
See Editor's Note No. 1.

BHI Diarrhea **- Heel/BHI, Inc.**
Each tablet contains: Aloe Socotrina 4X • Tormentilla 4X • Veratrum Album 5X • Arsenicum Album 6X • Colocynthis 6X • Cuprum Aceticum 6X • Mercurius Corrosivus 6X • Podophyllum Peltatum 6X • Ferrum Phosphoricum 10X • Carbo Vegetabilis 12X.
See Editor's Note No. 1.

BHI Echinacea P.C. **- Heel/BHI, Inc.**
Each tablet contains: Echinacea Angustifolia 6X, 12X, 30X, 200X • Echinacea Purpurea 6X, 12X, 30X, 200X.
See Editor's Note No. 1.

BHI Eczema **- Heel/BHI, Inc.**
Each tablet contains: Berberis Vulgaris 6X • Rhus Toxicodendron 8X • Arsenicum Album 10X • Graphites 10X • Hydrofluoricum Acidum 10X • Kreosotum 10X • Petroleum 10X • Sepia 10X • Lycopodium Clavatum 12X • Sulphur 12X.
See Editor's Note No. 1.

BHI Enzyme **- Heel/BHI, Inc.**
Each tablet contains: Nicotine Acid Amide 4X • Vitamin B1 4X • Vitamin B2 4X • Vitamin B6 4X • Vitamin B12 6X • Cysteinum 6X • Magnesia Phosphorica 6X • Natrum Oxalaceticum 6X • Alpha-Lipoicum Acidum 8X • Cerium Oxalicum 8X • Cis-Aconitate 8X • Citricum Acidum 8X • Coenzyme A 8X • Fumaricum Acidum 8X • Alpha-Ketoglutaricum Acidum 8X • Malonicum Acidum 8X • Natrum Pyruvicum 8X • Succinicum Acidum 8X • Pulsatilla 8X • Baryta Oxalsuccinicum 10X • ATP (adenosine-triphosphate) 10X • Manganum Gluconicum 10X • Nadidum 10X • Hepar Sulphuris Calcareum 10X • Sulphur 30X.
See Editor's Note No. 1.

BHI Exhaustion **- Heel/BHI, Inc.**
Each tablet contains: Cinchona Officinalis 4X • Cocculus Indicus 5X • Aletris Farinosa 6X • Citricum Acidum 6X • Kali Phosphoricum 6X • Phosphorus 6X • Picricum Acidum 6X • Muriaticum Acidum 8X • Sepia 12X.
See Editor's Note No. 1.

BHI Eye **- Heel/BHI, Inc.**
Each tablet contains: Euphrasia Officinalis 6X • Kalmia Latifolia 8X • Rhus Toxicodendron 8X • Staphysagria 8X • Aethiops Mercurialis-Mineralis 10X • Apis Mellifica 12X • Graphites 12X • Belladonna 30X.
See Editor's Note No. 1.

BHI Feminine **- Heel/BHI, Inc.**
Each tablet contains: Pulsatilla 4X • Sanguinaria Canadensis 4X • Lilium Tigrinum 5X • Apis Mellifica 6X • Cocculus Indicus 6X • Palladium Metallicum 10X • Sepia 10X • Sulphur 10X • Lachesis Mutus 12X • Oophorinum 12X.
See Editor's Note No. 1.

BHI FluPlus **- Heel/BHI, Inc.**
Each tablet contains: Zincum Gluconicum 3X • Zincum Metallicum 3X • Aconitum Napellus 4X • Bryonia Alba 4X • Eupatorium Perfoliatum 4X • Ipecacuanha 6X • Pulsatilla 6X • Mercurius Corrosivus 8X • Phosphorus 8X • Sulphur 8X • Influenzinum 12X • Lachesis Mutus 12X • Anas Barbariae, Hepatis et Cordis extractum 200 CK.
See Editor's Note No. 1.

BHI Gastro-Cleanse **- Heel/BHI, Inc.**
Each tablet contains: Cinchona Officinalis 4X • Leptandra Virginica 6X • Cynara Scolymus 8X • Fel Tauri • Galium Aparine 8X • Lycopodium Clavatum 8X • Phosphorus 10X • Sulphur 10X • Niccolum Metallicum 12X.
See Editor's Note No. 1.

BHI Ginkgo Complex **- Heel/BHI, Inc.**
Each tablet contains: Ginkgo Biloba 2X • Baryta Carbonica 8X.
See Editor's Note No. 1.

BHI Hair & Skin **- Heel/BHI, Inc.**
Each tablet contains: Galium Aparin 6X • Ignatia Amara 6X • Lycopodium Clavatum 6X • Thuja Occidentalis 6X • Urtica Urens 6X • Phosphoricum Acidum 8X • Arsenicum Album 10X • Natrum Muriaticum 12X • Selenium Metallicum 12X.
See Editor's Note No. 1.

BHI Hayfever nasal spray - Heel/BHI, Inc.
Galphimia Glauca 4X, 12X, 30X • Luffa Operculata 4X, 12X, 30X • Histaminum 12X, 30X, 200X • Sulphur 12X, 30X, 200X.
See Editor's Note No. 1.

BHI Headache - Heel/BHI, Inc.
Each tablet contains: Cimicifuga Racemosa 4X • Gelsemium Sempervirens 4X • Rhus Toxicodendron 4X.
See Editor's Note No. 1.

BHI Headache II - Heel/BHI, Inc.
Each tablet contains: Cinchona Officinalis 4X • Condurango 4X • Pulsatilla 4X • Aceticum Acidum 6X • Arsenicum Album 6X • Asafoetida 6X • Lycopodium Clavatum 6X • Natrum Sulphuricum 6X • Phosphoricum Acidum 6X • Secale Cornutum 6X • Aranea Diadema 8X • Kalmia Latifolia 8X • Strychninum Nitricum 8X • Calcarea Phosphorica 10X • Carbo Vegetabilis 10X • Curare 10X • Mercurius Praecipitatus Ruber 10X • Silicea 10X • Uranium Nitricum 12X • Bryonia Alba 30X.
See Editor's Note No. 1.

BHI Hemorrhoid Relief - Heel/BHI, Inc.
Paeonia Officinalis 1X.
See Editor's Note No. 1.

BHI Hemorrhoid suppositories - Heel/BHI, Inc.
Each suppository contains: Aesculus Hippocastanum 4X • Aloe Socotrina 4X • Collinsonia Canadensis 4X • Nux Vomica 5X • Leptandra Virginica 6X • Muriaticum Acidum 6X • Paeonia Officinalis 6X • Sulphur 10X.
See Editor's Note No. 1.

BHI Hemorrhoid tablets - Heel/BHI, Inc.
Each tablet contains: Aesculus Hippocastanum 4X • Aloe Socotrina 4X • Collinsonia Canadensis 4X • Nux Vomica 5X • Leptandra Virginica 6X • Muriaticum Acidum 6X • Paeonia Officinalis 6X • Sulphur 10X.
See Editor's Note No. 1.

BHI Infection - Heel/BHI, Inc.
Each tablet contains: Echinacea Angustifolia 3X • Echinacea Purpurea 3X • Mercurius Solubilis 8X • Hepar Sulphuris Calcareum 10X.
See Editor's Note No. 1.

BHI Inflammation - Heel/BHI, Inc.
Each tablet contains: Echinacea Purpurea 2X • Belladonna 4X • Bryonia Alba 5X • Arnica Montana radix 6X • Dulcamara 6X • Phytolacca Decandra 6X • Pulsatilla 6X • Rhus Toxicodendron 6X • Thuja Occidentalis 6X • Argentum Nitricum 8X • Arsenicum Album 10X • Hepar Sulphuris Calcareum 10X • Mercurius Solubilis 10X • Lachesis Mutus 12X • Pyrogenium 12X • Staphylococcinum 12X • Streptococcinum 12X • Influenzinum 15X.
See Editor's Note No. 1.

BHI Injury - Heel/BHI, Inc.
Each tablet contains: Aconitum Napellus 4X • Arnica Montana radix 4X • Calendula Officinalis 4X • Chamomilla 4X • Echinacea Angustifolia 4X • Echinacea Purpurea 4X • Hamamelis Virginiana 4X • Hypericum Perforatum 4X • Symphytum Officinale 5X • Aristolochia Clematitis 6X • Belladonna 6X • Bellis Perennis 6X • Millefolium 6X • Rhus Toxicodendron 6X • Hepar Sulphuris Calcareum 10X • Veratrum Album 10X • Carbo Vegetabilis 12X • Mercurius Solubilis 12X • Arsenicum Album 15X • Sulphur 30X.
See Editor's Note No. 1.

BHI Intestine - Heel/BHI, Inc.
Each tablet contains: Bryonia Alba 5X • Colocynthis 5X • Lycopodium Clavatum 5X • Nux Vomica 5X • Mercurius Corrosivus 6X • Sulphur 10X.
See Editor's Note No. 1.

BHI Lightheaded - Heel/BHI, Inc.
Each tablet contains: Conium Maculatum 5X • Cocculus Indicum 6X • Phosphorus 5X • Petroleum 8X • Ambra Grisea 12X.
See Editor's Note No. 1.

BHI Masculine - Heel/BHI, Inc.
Each tablet contains: Agnus Castus 4X • Cinchona Officinalis 4X • Lycopodium Clavatum 4X • Petroselinum Sativum 4X • Picricum Acidum 6X • Orchitinum 8X • Sepia 10X.
See Editor's Note No. 1.

BHI Menstrual - Heel/BHI, Inc.
Each tablet contains: Aceticum Acidum 4X • Pulsatilla 4X • Caulophyllum Thalictroides 6X • Hydrastis Canadensis 6X • Lilium Tigrinum 6X • Kreosotum 8X • Asterias Rubens 10X • Mercurius Iodatus Flavus 10X • Thuja Occidentalis 12X.
See Editor's Note No. 1.

BHI Nausea - Heel/BHI, Inc.
Each tablet contains: Anacardium Orientale 6X • Ipecacuanha 6X • Argentum Nitricum 8X • Rovinia Pseudoacacia 10X • Carbo Vegetabilis 12X • Iodium 12X • Sepia 30X.
See Editor's Note No. 1.

BHI Neuralgia - Heel/BHI, Inc.
Each tablet contains: Spigelia Anthelmia 8X • Gelsemium Sempervirens 10X • Kali Bichromium 10X • Thuja Occidentalis 10X • Silicea 12X • Stannum Metallicum 12X • Theridion 12X • Belladonna 30X.
See Editor's Note No. 1.

BHI Pancreas - Heel/BHI, Inc.
Each tablet contains: Leptandra Virginica 6X • Momordica Balsamina 6X • Ceanothus Americanus 8X • Podophyllum Peltatum 8X • Carbo Vegetabilis 10X • Lycopodium Clavatum 10X • Mercurius Iodatus Flavus 10X • Pancreatinum 10X • Lachesis Mutus 12X.
See Editor's Note No. 1.

BHI Perspiration - Heel/BHI, Inc.
Each tablet contains: Salvia Officinalis 4X • Sambucus Nigra 4X • Pilocarpus 5X • Cedron 6X • Nitricum Acidum 6X • Petroleum 6X • Sanguinaria Canadensis 6X • Thuja Occidentalis 6X • Salicylicum Acidum 8X • Sulphuricum Acidum 8X • Calcarea Carbonica 10X • Sepia 10X.
See Editor's Note No. 1.

BHI PMS-Mulimen - Heel/BHI, Inc.
Each tablet contains: Agnus Castus 3X • Hypericum Perforatum 3X • Urtica Urens 3X • Ambra Grisea 4X • Cimicifuga Racemosa 4X • Gelsemium Sempervirens 4X • Kali Carbonicum 4X • Calcarea Carbonica 8X • Sepia 8X.
See Editor's Note No. 1.

BHI Pure Eye Drops - Heel/BHI, Inc.
Active Ingredients: Cochlearia officinalis 5X • Echinacea angustifolia 5X • Euphrasia officinalis 5X • Pilocarpus 5X. Other Ingredient: Saline Solution.
See Editor's Note No. 1.

BHI Recuperation - Heel/BHI, Inc.
Each tablet contains: Causticum 8X • Gelsemium Sempervirens 8X • Plumbum Metallicum 30X.
See Editor's Note No. 1.

BHI Rendimax - Heel/BHI, Inc.
Each tablet contains: Ilex Aquifolium 2X • Oleander 5X • Arnica Montana radix 7X • Orchitinum 10X • Sarcolacticum Acidum 11X.
See Editor's Note No. 1.

BHI Rhus tox P.C. - Heel/BHI, Inc.
Each tablet contains: Rhus Toxicodendron 6X, 12X, 30X, 200X.
See Editor's Note No. 1.

BRAND NAMES

BHI Saw Palmetto Complex **-** Heel/BHI, Inc.
Each tablet contains: Petroselinum Sativum 4X • Populus Termuloides 4X • Sabal Serrulata 4X • Chimaphila Umbellata 5X • Kreosotum 6X • Succinum Acidum 8X • Hepar Sulphuris Calcareum 10X • Conium Maculatum 30X.
See Editor's Note No. 1.

BHI Sinus **-** Heel/BHI, Inc.
Each tablet contains: Pulsatilla 4X • Euphorbium Officinarum 6X • Hydrastis Canadensis 6X • Kali Bichromicum 6X • Thuja Occidentalis 6X • Kali Iodatum 8X • Phosphorus 8X • Mercurius Sulphuratus Ruber 10X • Influenzinum 10X.
See Editor's Note No. 1.

BHI Skin **-** Heel/BHI, Inc.
Each tablet contains: Berberis Vulgaris 6X • Rhus Toxicodendron 8X • Arsenicum Album 10X • Graphites 10X • Hydrofluoricum Acidum 10X • Kreosotum 10X • Petroleum 10X • Sepia 10X • Lycopodium Clavatum 12X • Sulphur 12X.
See Editor's Note No. 1.

BHI Spasm-Pain **-** Heel/BHI, Inc.
Each tablet contains: Aconitum Napellus 4X • Bryonia Alba 4X • Colocynthis 4X • Atropinum Sulphuricum 6X • Cuprum Sulphuricum 6X.
See Editor's Note No. 1.

BHI Stomach **-** Heel/BHI, Inc.
Each tablet contains: Nux Vomica 4X • Pulsatilla 4X • Argentum Nitricum 6X • Arsenicum Album 6X • Natrum Phosphoricum 6X • Antimonium Crudum 10X • Carbo Vegetabilis 10X.
See Editor's Note No. 1.

BHI Stramonium Complex **-** Heel/BHI, Inc.
Each tablet contains: Kali Phosphoricum 6X • Rauwolfia Serpentina 6X • Arnica Montana radix 8X • Plumbum Metallicum 8X • Aurum Iodatum 10X • Lycopodium Clavatum 10X • Stramonium 10X • Baryta Iodata 12X • Conium Maculatum 12X • Sulphur 12X.
See Editor's Note No. 1.

BHI Throat **-** Heel/BHI, Inc.
Arum Triphyllum 4X • Paris Quadrifolia 5X • Argentum Nitricum 6X • Causticum 6X • Hyoscyamus Niger 6X • Arnica Montana radix 8X • Verbascum Thapsus 8X • Carbo Vegetabilis 10X • Phosphorus 10X • Calcarea Carbonica 30X.
See Editor's Note No. 1.

BHI Uri-Cleanse **-** Heel/BHI, Inc.
Each tablet contains: Solidago Virgaurea 4X • Ammi Visnaga 6X • Berberis Vulgaris 6X • Citricum Acidum 6X • Pareira Brava 6X • Cantharis 8X • Hepar Sulphuris Calcareum 8X • Nitricum Acidum 8X • Mercurius Solubilis 10X • Arsenicum Album 30X.
See Editor's Note No. 1.

BHI Uri-Control **-** Heel/BHI, Inc.
Each tablet contains: Belladonna 4X • Apis Mellifica 6X • Argentum Nitricum 6X • Cantharis 6X • Equisetum Hyemale 6X • Pulsatilla 6X • Sarsaparilla 6X • Causticum 8X • Petroselinum Sativum 8X • Terebinthina 8X.
See Editor's Note No. 1.

BHI Varicose **-** Heel/BHI, Inc.
Each tablet contains: Hamamelis Virginiana 4X • Pulsatilla 4X • Aesculus Hippocastanum 6X • Carduus Marianus 6X • Lycopodium Clavatum 6X • Picricum Acidum 6X • Secale Cornutum 6X • Carbo Vegetabilis 10X • Mercurius Praecipitatus Ruber 10X • Apis Mellifica 12X.
See Editor's Note No. 1.

BHI Varicose Relief ointment **-** Heel/BHI, Inc.
Hamamelis Virginiana 1X.
See Editor's Note No. 1.

BHT Plus **-** Life Enhancement Products, Inc.
Each capsule contains: BHT 100 mg • Ascorbyl Palmitate 80 mg. Other Ingredients: Gelatin.

Bicreatol XS **-** BSN Inc.
Two scoops contain: Calcium 310 mg • Magnesium 400 mg • Phosphorus 200 mg • Folic Acid 800 mcg • Vitamin B12 (cyanocobalamin) 500 mcg • Vitamin B6 (pyridoxine HCl) 50 mg • Bicreaplex 11 g: Micronized Creatine - Magnesium Hydrate, Glycovol Glycocyamine, Betapure Trimethylglycine • L-Glutamine & Glutamine Peptides 5 mg • Phosphoplexx 600 mg: Di-Potassium Phosphate, Sodium Bi-Phosphate, Calcium Phosphate • Nitrolen-4 300 mg: 4-Hydroxyisoleucine from Fenugreek and Vanadyl Sulfate. Other Ingredients: Micro-Filtered Whey Protein Concentrate, Rice Protein Concentrate, Maltodextrin, Canola Oil, MCT Oil, Natural & Artificial Flavors, Corn Syrup Solids, Sucralose, Sodium Caseinate, Mono and Diglycerides, Sodium Alginate, Lecithin.

Bifidophilus Chewables **-** American Biologics
Each tablet contains: Bifidobacterium Bifidum 1 billion • Lactobacillus Acidophilus 1 billion. Other Ingredients: Silicon Dioxide, Vegetable Magnesium Stearate, Vegetable Stearic Acid, Ascorbic Acid, Natural Raspberry Flavoring.

Bifidophilus Flora Force **-** Nature's Sunshine
Two capsules contain: Lactobacillus Rhamnosus 2.5 billion • Lactobacillus Casei 2 billion • Lactobacillus Acidophilus 2.5 billion • Bifidobacterium Longum 1 billion. Other Ingredients: FOS (short and long chain), Kosher Gelatin, Water.

Bifidus - Super Blue Green **-** Cell Tech
Two capsules contain: Vitamin K 6.8 mcg • Proprietary Blend 470 mg: Bifidobacterium Bifidum, Blue-Green Algae (aphanizomenon flos-aquae) 170 mg. Other Ingredients: Maltodextrin, rice bran, gelatin capsule (gelatin, water), vegetable magnesium stearate (encapsuling aid).

Bifidus Balance + FOS **-** Jarrow Formulas
Each capsule contains: FOS (fructooligosaccharides) 210 mg • Bifidobacterium Breve R070 40% 800 million • Bifidobacterium Longum R023 40% 800 million • Bifidobacterium Bifidum R071 15% 300 million • Bifidobacterium Infantis R033 5% 100 million. Other Ingredients: Maltodextrin, Magnesium Stearate, Ascorbic Acid, Gelatin.

Bifoviden **-** Metagenics
Each capsule contains: Proprietary Blend 15 billion live organisms: Bifidobacterium Lactis BI-07, Bifidobacterium Lactis BI-01, Streptococcus Thermophilus St-21.

Big 100 **-** GNC
Each tablet contains: Thiamin (as Thiamin Mononitrate) 100 mg • Riboflavin 100 mg • Niacin (as Niacinamide) 100 mg • Vitamin B6 (as Pyridoxine Hydrochloride) 100 mg • Folate, Folic Acid, Folacin 400 mcg • Vitamin B12 (as Cyanocobalamin) 100 mcg • Biotin 100 mcg • Pantothenic Acid (as Calcium d-Pantothenate) 100 mg • Choline Bitartrate 100 mg • Inositol 100 mcg • Para-Aminobenzoic Acid (PABA) 30 mg. Other Ingredients: Cellulose, Dicalcium Phosphate, Vegetable Acetoglycerides.

Big 150 **-** GNC
Each tablet contains: Thiamin (as Thiamin Mononitrate) 150 mg •Riboflavin 150 mg •Niacin (as Niacinamide) 150 mg • Vitamin B6 (as Pyridoxine Hydrochloride) 150 mg • Folate, Folic Acid, Folacin 400 mcg • Vitamin B12 (as Cyanocobalamin) 150 mcg •Biotin 150 mcg •Pantothenic acid (as Calcium d-Pantothenate) 150 mg • Choline Bitartrate 150 mg •Inositol 150 mcg • Para-aminobenzoic Acid (PABA) 150 mg. Other Ingredients: Dicalcium Phosphate, Cellulose, Whole Brown Rice Powder (oryza sativa).

Big 50 Timed Release **-** GNC
Each tablet contains: Thiamin (as thiamin mononitrate) 50 mg • Riboflavin 50 mg • Niacin (as niacinamide) 50 mg • Vitamin B6 (as

pyridoxine hydrochloride) 50 mg • Folate, Folic Acid, Folacin 400 mcg • Vitamin B12 (as cyanocobalamin) 50 mcg • Biotin 50 mcg • Pantothenic Acid (as calcium d-pantothenate) 50 mg • Choline Bitartrate 50 mg •Inosotil 50 mg •Para Amino Benzoic Acid (PABA) 30 mg. Other Ingredients: Dicalcium Phosphate, Cellulose, Brewer's Yeast, Lecithin, Alfalfa leaf powder (medicago sativa), Watercress herb powder (nasurtium officinale), Parsley herb powder (petroselinium sativum), Whole Brown Rice (oryza powder), Vegetable Acetoglycerides.

Big Daddy - The Sports Nutrition Source, Inc.
Each 225 gram serving contains: Sodium 50 mg • Potassium 145 mg • Protein 40 g.

Bilberry - Jamieson
Each capsule contains: Bilberry fruit 2500 mg.

Bilberry - GNC
Each capsule contains: Bilberry fruits powder (Vaccinium myrtillus) 500 mg. Other Ingredients: Gelatin, Cellulose.

Bilberry - Progressive Labs
Each all-vegetable capsule contains: Bilberry leaf powder (Vaccinum myrtillus) 370 mg • Bilberry extract (Vaccinum myrtillus) 80 mg • Anthocyanids (from above) 25 mg.

Bilberry - Leiner Health Products
Each caplet contains: Bilberry extract (Vaccinium myrtillus) berry 80 mg. Other Ingredients: Calcium Carbonate, Cellulose, Maltodextrin, Hydroxypropyl Methylcellulose, Silicon Dioxide, Polyethylene Glycol 3350, Croscarmellose Sodium, Hydroxypropyl Cellulose, Pharmaceutical Glaze, Yellow 5 Lake, Blue 1 Lake, Crospovidone, Magnesium Stearate, Polysorbate 80, Titanium Dioxide.

Bilberry - Rexall - Sundown
Two capsules contain: Bilberry Extract 4:1 (fruit) 80 mg. Other Ingredients: Gelatin, Natural Vegetable Fiber.

Bilberry (Vaccinium myrtillus) - Solgar
Each capsule contains: Bilberry extract (vaccinium myrtillus, standardized to anthocyanosides 15 mg) 60 mg • Blueberry powder (vaccinium angustilolium) 100 mg • Ginkgo Biloba leaf powder 322 mg. Other Ingredients: Vegetable Cellulose, Vegetable Magnesium Stearate, Water, Vegetable Glycerin.

Bilberry + Grapeskin Polyphenols - Jarrow Formulas
Each capsule contains: Swedish Bilberry 100:1 extract (vaccinium myrtillus, 25% anthocyanosides) 80 mg • Grapeskin extract (vitis vinifera, 30% polyphenols) 200 mg. Other Ingredients: Cellulose, Magnesium Stearate, Silicon Dioxide, Gelatin.

Bilberry 1000 mg, Concentrated - GNC
Each capsule contains: Bilberry Fruits (vaccinum myrtillus; from 10 mg bilberry fruit extract 100:1) 1000 mg. Other Ingredients: Soybean Oil, Gelatin, Glycerin, Caramel Color, Titanium Dioxide (natural mineral whitener).

Bilberry 160 mg - Pure Encapsulations
Each vegetable capsule contains: Bilberry extract (vaccinium myrtillus, standardized to contains 25% anthocyanosides) 160 mg • Vitamin C (as ascorbyl palmitate) 6 mg.

Bilberry 5000 - Golden Glow Natural Health Products
Each capsule contains: Vaccinium Myrtillus fruit extract (bilberry) 5000 mg: Anthocyanosides 12.5 mg. Other Ingredients: Lactose.

Bilberry 80 mg - Pure Encapsulations
Each vegetable capsule contains: Bilberry extract (vaccinium myrtillus, standardized to contains 25% anthocyanosides) 80 mg • Vitamin C (as ascorbyl palmitate) 3 mg.

Bilberry Complex w/Lutein - Pro Health
Each capsule contains: Vitamin A (as beta carotene) 10,000 IU • Riboflavin (vitamin B2) 10 mg • Bilberry extract (vaccinium myrtillus, standardized for 25% anthocyanidins 20 mg) 80 mg • Carrot root powder (daucus carota sativa) 300 mg • Citrus Bioflavonoid complex (35% hesperidin 40 mg) 114 mg • Floraglo Lutein extract (from marigold flowers, standardized for 5% lutein 3 mg, 0.22% zeaxanthin 132 mcg) 60 mg. Other Ingredients: Rice Flour, Gelatin, Maltodextrin, Water.

Bilberry Extract - Source Naturals
Each tablet contains: Bilberry (Vaccinium myrtillus, standardized extract, yielding 18.5 mg Anthocyanosides) 50 mg.

Bilberry Extract - NSI - Nutraceutical Sciences Institute
Each capsule contains: Bilberry extract (standardized to 25% anthocyanosides) 160 mg.

Bilberry Extract - Nature's Way
Each capsule contains: Bilberry fruit (dried extract 25% anthocyanins) 80 mg • Elderberry 125 mg • Other Ingredients: Gelatin, Millet.

Bilberry Extract - Enzymatic Therapy
Two capsules contain: Bilberry fruit extract (vaccinium myrtillus) 160 mg. Other Ingredients: Cellulose, Gelatin, Magnesium Stearate, Titanium Dioxide.

Bilberry Extract - PhytoPharmica
Two capsules contain: Bilberry berry extract (vaccinium myrtillus fructus, standardized to contain 25% anthocyanosides [40 mg] calculated as anthocyanidins) 160 mg.

Bilberry Extract - Swanson Health Products
Each capsule contains: Bilberry extract (25% anthocyanidins) 60 mg • Bilberry powder 360 mg • Citrus Bioflavonoids 50 mg.

Bilberry Formula - Quest
Each caplet contains: Bilberry (Vaccinium myrtillus) (provided by 50 mg P.E. 1:100 standardized to contain 25% anthocyanosides) 5000 mg • Citrus Bioflavonoids (providing Hesperidin 50 mg) 200 mg • Carrot powder (Daucus carota) 100 mg. Other Ingredients: Calcium Phosphate, Microcrystalline Cellulose, Vegetable Stearin, Croscarmellose Sodium, Magnesium Stearate (vegetable source).

Bilberry Fruit - Nature's Sunshine
Two tablets contain: Calcium (di-calcium phosphate) 200 mg • Phosphorus (di-calcium phosphate) 160 mg • Bilberry fruit concentrate (vaccinium myrtillus, standardized to 25% anthocyanidins) 80 mg. Other Ingredients: Cellulose, Stearic Acid, Magnesium Stearate, Silicon Dioxide.

Bilberry Fruit - PhysioLogics
Each capsule contains: Bilberry fruit extract (vaccinium myrtillus, standardized to contain 25% anthocyanosides 15 mg) 60 mg. Other Ingredients: Cellulose (plant origin), Beet Root Concentrate, Gelatin, Dicalcium Phosphate, Vegetable Magnesium Stearate, Silica.

Bilberry i sight - Nature's Life
Two capsules contain: Vitamin A (100% as beta carotene from dunaliella salina algae) 15,000 IU • Vitamin E (as d-alpha tocopheryl succinate) 400 IU • Vitamin C (from calcium ascorbate) 300 mg • Riboflavin (vitamin B2) 3 mg • Niacin 40 mg • Calcium (from calcium ascorbate) 30 mg • Bilberry fruit extract (vaccinium myrtillus, standardized to 25% anthocyanosides) 360 mg • Alpha Carotene (from D. salina algae) 288 mcg • Cryptoxanthin (from D. salina algae) 70 mcg • Zeaxanthin (from D. salina algae) 58 mcg • Lutein (from D. salina algae) 45 mcg. Other Ingredients: Cellulose, Vegetarian Magnesium Stearate.

Bilberry Plus - J. R. Carlson Laboratories, Inc.
Each softgel contains: Vitamin A (as palmitate) 2000 IU • Vitamin E (as D-alpha tocopheryl) 100 IU • Bilberry (vaccinium myrtillus, 25% anthocyanosides) 25 mg.

Bilberry-Go! - Wakunaga of America
Each caplet contains: Bilberry standardized extract (fruit) 120 mg. Other Ingredients: Cellulose, Starch, Magnesium Stearate (vegetable source), Silica.

Some Brand Name Natural Products - What they Contain

www.NaturalDatabase.com contains MANY more listings than appear here.
Editor's Notes are located on pages 2155-2163.

Bile Acid Factors - Jarrow Formulas
Three tablets contain: Total Bile Acids (from 1530 bovine/ovine bile concentrate) 1000 mg • Conjugated Bile Acid (as glycocholic acid, taurocholic acid, glycodeoxycholic acid, taurodeoxycholic acid, glycochenodeoxycholic acid, taurochenodeoxycholic acid) 945 mg • Unconjugated Bile Acid (as cholic acid and deoxycholic acid) 53 mg. Other Ingredients: Magnesium Stearate, Natural Vanilla Flavor, Gelatin.

Bile-Gest - Atrium Biotechnologies
Each tablet contains: Ox Bile concentrate 195 mg • Collinsonia root 310 mg • Glycine 50 mg • Pepsin 30 mg • Raw Liver concentrate 30 mg.
See Editor's Note No. 14.

Biliherb - Wild Rose
Each tablet contains: Black Radish root 109 mg • Barberry root bark 72.7 mg • Wood Betony herb 36.4 mg • Dandelion root 36.4 mg • Ginger root 36.4 mg • Parsley root 36.4 mg • Marshmallow root 36.4 mg • Cramp Bark 36.4 mg.

Binge Breaker - Enforma Natural Products
Two capsules contain: St. John's Wort (.2 -.3 hypericin) • Kava Kava (70% kavalactones) • Vitamin C (ascorbic acid) • Vitamin B1 (thiamine) • Vitamin B2 (riboflavin) • Vitamin B6 (pyridoxine) • Vitamin B3 (niacin).
See Editor's Note No. 65.

Bio Alkalizer - BioGenesis Nutraceuticals
Each 5 gm serving contains: Vitamin C (magnesium ascorbate, potassium asorbate, sodium ascorbate, calcium ascorbate) 250 mg • Zinc (glycinate) 10 mg • Selenium (selenomethionine) 25 mcg • Rubidium (carbonate) 25 mg • Magnesium (ascorbate, carbonate) 100 mg • Potassium (ascorbate, bicarbonate) 99 mg • Cesium (carbonate) 25 mg • Rye grass 1000 mg • Barley grass 1000 mg • Blue Green Algae 1300 mg • Sea Kelp powder 100 mg • Bee Pollen powder 500 mg. Other Ingredients: Silicon Dioxide.

Bio Alkalizer - BioGenesis Nutraceuticals
Each 5 g serving contains: Vitamin C (magnesium ascorbate, potassium ascorbate, sodium ascorbate, calcium ascorbate) 250 mg • Zinc (glycinate) 10 mg • Selenium (selenomethionine) 25 mcg • Rubidium (carbonate) 25 mg • Magnesium (ascorbate & carbonate) 100 mg • Potassium (ascorbate & bicarbonate) 99 mg • Cesium (carbonate) 25 mg • Rye grass 1000 mg • Barley grass 1000 mg • Blue Green algae 1300 mg • Sea Kelp powder 100 mg • Bee Pollen powder 500 mg. Other Ingredients: Silicon Dioxide.

Bio Berry Grape Seed Extract Plus - Flora Inc.
Grape Seed Extract 50 mg • Bilberry 10 mg. In a base of Cranberry powder.

Bio Block Sport Sun & Insect Repellent lotion - HOMS LLC
Soybean oil • Coconut oil • Purified Water • Cyclomethicone • Glycerin • Geranium oil • Aloe • Citric Acid • Lecithin • Vanillin • Zinc Oxide.

Bio C-Complex 1000 - The Vitamin Shoppe
Each capsule contains: Pure Crystalline Vitamin C (fortified with Rose Hips) 1000 mg • Citrus Bioflavonoids Complex 100 mg.

Bio C-Complex 500 - The Vitamin Shoppe
Vitamin C (fortified with Rose Hips Conc.) 500 mg • Citrus Bioflavonoids Complex 250 mg.

Bio Q-Gel Mega 100 - Solanova
Each softsule contains: Vitamin E (d-alpha tocopherol concentrate) 150 IU • Coenzyme Q10 (Ubidecarenone USP) 100 mg. Other Ingredients: Gelatin, Sorbitol, Glycerin, Purified Water, Hydroxylated Lecithin, Medium Chain Triglycerides, Annato Seed Extract, Soybean Oil.

Bio Rejuvenate - Windspirit Productions, Inc.
Two softgets contain: Astaxanthin 5 mg. Other Ingredients: Algal Meal extract (haematococcus pluvialis), Rice Bean oil, Gelatin, Vegetable Glycerin Water, Beta-carotene, Lutein.

Bio Selenium - America's Finest
Each tablet contains: Selenium (as selenomethionine) 50 mcg • Proprietary Blend 20 mg: Kelp, Ginger root, Bioperine brand Black Pepper fruit extract (98% piperine). Other Ingredients: Di-Calcium Phosphate, Calcium Sulfate Monohydrate, Magnesium Stearate, Pharmaceutical Glaze.

Bio St. John's - Pharmanex
Each capsule contains: Cordyceps Sinensis (CordyMax Cs-4, standardized to adenosine & mannitol content) 375 mg • St. John's Wort (hypericum extract, standardized to 0.3% hypericin) 225 mg.

Bio Trim - Dial Herbs
Ma Huang • Kola Nut • Ginger • White Willow • Ginkgo Biloba • Bladderwrack • Fo-Ti • Hawthorn berries • Saw Palmetto • Beet Powder • Chromium Proteinate • Zinc Picolinate • Boron Proteinate • Chromium Picolinate • Kola Nut extract.
See Editor's Note No. 30.

Bioactive B12 - Enzymatic Therapy
Each tablet contains: Vitamin B12 (as methylcobalamin) 1 mg. Other Ingredients: Fructose, Mannitol, Stearic Acid, Cellulose, Natural Cherry Flavor, Magnesium Stearate, Silicon Dioxide.

BioAdaptogen - MK Supplements
Two capsules contain: Eleutherococcus 300 mg • Panax Ginseng 300 mg • Ashwagandha 300 mg • Licorice root 40 mg.

BioAdaptogen - BioGenesis Nutraceuticals
Two capsules contain: Calcium 210 mg • Siberian Ginseng root extract (0.8% eleutherosides) 300 mg • Panax Ginseng extract (20% ginsenosides) 300 mg • Ashwaganda extract (1.5% withanolides) 300 mg • Licorice root (glycyrrhiza glabra) 40 mg.

BioAdreno - BioGenesis Nutraceuticals
Each capsule contains: Vitamin C (ascorbic acid) 100 mg • Pantothenic Acid (vitamin B5) 250 mg • Adrenal cortex (freeze dried, New Zealand bovine) 300 mg.
See Editor's Note No. 14.

BioAllergy - BioGenesis Nutraceuticals
Two capsules contain: Vitamin C (ascorbyl palmitate) 13 mg • Citrus Bioflavonoids 250 mg • Bromelain (3200 mcu/gm) 100 mg • Uritca Dioica (nettle root) 300 mg • Protease 2500 HUT • Lipase 50 LU • Amylase 3500 DU • Cellulase 200 CU • Rice Bran 100 mg • Curcuma Longa (tumeric rhizome) 100 mg • Glycyrrhiza Glabra (licorice) 100 mg • Zingiber Officianle (ginger) 100 mg • Tanacetum Parthenium (feverfew) 100 mg.

BioAstin Brand - Nutrex, Inc.
Natural Astaxanthin from Microalgae.

Bio-Balanced Calcium Magnesium - Pro Health
Each tablet contains: Calcium (amino acid chelate, from oyster shells) 250 mg • Magnesium (amino acid chelate) 125 mg • Vitamin D (cholecalciferol) 200 IU. Other Ingredients: Calcium Phosphate Dibasic, Stearic Acid, Hydroxypropyl Cellulose, Croscarmellose Sodium, Magnesium Stearate, Silicon Dioxide, Sodium Lauryl Sulfate.

BioBeads - Natrol, Inc.
Each bead contains: Proprietary Blend 1 Billion: Lactobacillus Acidophilus, Bifidobacterium Bifidum, Bifidobacterium Longum, Lactobacillus Rhamnosus. Other Ingredients: Vegetable Oil, Gelatin, Glycerine, Lecithin, Pectin.

Bio-Bifidus Complex Powder - American Biologics
Each 1 tbsp serving contains: Bifidobacterium Bifidum 800 million • Lactobacillus Acidophilus 200 million. Other Ingredients: Lactose, Whey, Herbal Stabilizers.

Some Brand Name Natural Products - What they Contain

www.NaturalDatabase.com contains MANY more listings than appear here.
Editor's Notes are located on pages 2155-2163.

BRAND NAMES

BioBuilde - BodyHealth
L-Isoleucine • L-Leucine • L-Valine • L-Lysine • L-Methionine • L-Phenylalanine • L-Threonine • L-Tryptophan.

BioBurn Extreme - For Youthful Health
Two capsules contain: Chromium 200 mcg • Citrus Aurantium fruit 500 mg • BioBurn Complex 200 mg: Garcinia Cambogia fruit (standardized to 50% hydroxycitric acid), Guggulipids (commiphora mukul/gum resin standardized to 2.5% guggulsterones), Metabromine-G brand Cocoa / Guarana extract, N-Acetyl L-Tyrosine, L-Tyrosine • BioBurn Tea Blend 200 mg: Caffeine Anhydrous USP, Green Tea powder (camellia sinensis leaf), Green Tea extract (camellia sinensis leaf standardized to 40% catechins).
See Editor's Note No. 40.

BIO-C 1 gram - Golden Glow Natural Health Products
Each tablet contains: Ascorbic Acid (vitamin C from calcium ascorbate 302.24 mg and sodium ascorbate 844.09 mg) 1000 mg • Rosehips extract (rosa canina) 50 mg • Rutin 50 mg • Citrus Bioflavonoid extract 50 mg • Hesperidin 50 mg. Other Ingredients: Gluten (from maltodextrin, derived from wheat).

Bio-C Caps - Arrowroot
Each tablet contains: Vitamin C 1000 mg • Bioflavonoids 500 mg.

BioCalth Bone and Joint - BioCalth International
Three caplets contain: Calcium L-Threonate 775 mg • Calcium (elemental) 100 mg. Other Ingredients: Microcrystalline Cellulose, Maltodextrin, Carboxymethylcellulose, Magnesium Silicate, Magnesium Stearate.

BioCalth Caplets - Nature's Solution
Three caplets contain: Calcium L-Threonate 2325 mg • Calcium (element) 300 mg. Other Ingredients: Microcrystalline Cellulose, Carboxymenthylcellulose, Magnesium Silicate, Magnesium Stearate, Maltodextrin.

BioCalth Kids - Nature's Solution
Each piece of gum contains: Vitamin A (as vitamin A palmitate) 2500 IU • Vitamin C (as calcium ascorbate) 30 mg • Vitamin D (as cholecalciferol) 200 • Vitamin E (as d-alpha tocopheryl acetate) 19 IU • Vitamin K (as phytonadione) 40 mcg • Thiamin (as thiamine mononitrate) 0.75 mg • Riboflavin 0.85 mg • Niacin (as niacinamide) 10 mg • Vitamin B6 (as pyridoxine hydrochloride) 1 mg • Folic Acid 200 mcg • Vitamin B12 (as cyanocobalamin) 3 mcg • Biotin 25 mcg • Pantothenic Acid (as d-calcium) 5 mg • Calcium D-Threonate (BioCalth) 200 mg. Other Ingredients: Pharmagums, Tutti-Frutti (natural), Natural Color, Citric Acid, Sucralose, Magnesium Stearate.

BioCalth Powder - Nature's Solution
Two packets contain: Calcium L-Threonate 2320 mg • Calcium (element) 300 mg.

BioCell Collagen II brand - Biocell Technology LLC
Hydrolyzed Chicken Collagen Type II.
See Editor's Note No. 44.

Biochem Aller-Max - Country Life Vitamins
Two capsules contain: Quercetin 250 mg • N-Acetyl Cysteine 200 mg • Bromelain 100 mg • L-Histidine 200 mg • Vitamin A (Palmitate) 2500 IU • Vitamin C (Calcium Ascorbate) 250 mg • Pantothenic Acid 200 mg • Zinc 10 mg • Grape seed extract 5 mg • Stinging Nettle 100 mg • Cayenne 20 mg.

BioChem Anabolic Max - Country Life Vitamins
Four tablets contain: L-Glutamine 1000 mg • L-Arginine (pyroglutamate) 900 mg • Creatine Monohydrate 500 mg • L-Citrulline 300 mg • Taurine 300 mg • Betaine HCl 300 mg • Cinnamon extract 250 mg • Green Tea extract 100 mg • DHA (docosahexaenoic acid) 100 mg • Ginseng (panax ginseng) 50 mg • PAK (pyridoxine, alpha-ketoglutarate) 25 mg • Niacin 25 mg • Pantothenic Acid / Pantethine 90/10 25 mg.

Biochem Chrom-Adyl Surge - Country Life Vitamins
Each capsule contains: Chromium 500 mcg • BMOV (Bis-Maltol OXO Vandium) 5 mg • Vanadyl Sulfate 5 mg.

Biochem Prosta-Max for Men - Country Life Vitamins
Two tablets contain: Glycine 250 mg • L-Glutamic Acid 250 mg • Bromelain 100 mg • Vitamin A (beta carotene) 10,000 IU • Vitamin E 200 IU • Vitamin C 250 mg • Vitamin B1 (thiamin) 25 mg • Vitamin B2 (riboflavin) 20 mg • Vitamin B6 (pyridoxine) 20 mg • Zinc 50 mg • Saw Palmetto 100 mg • Pygeum 100 mg • Parsley 75 mg.

Biochem Ultimate Athlete's Pain Formula - Country Life Vitamins
Three softgel capsules contain: Boswellia Serrata extract 500 mg • Omega-3 Fish oil concentrate 400 mg • Glucosamine HCl 250 mg • Glucosamine Sulfate 250 mg • Chondroitin Sulfate 200 mg • Poly-NAG (N-acetyl glucosamine) 50 mg • Vitamin C (ascorbyl palmitate) 50 mg • Green Lipped Mussel extract 50 mg • CMO (cetyl myristoleate) 50 mg • Gamma-Linolenic Acid (borage seed oil) 50 mg • Vitamin E (d-alpha tocopheryl acetate) 25 IU • Manganese (sulfate) 5 mg • Boron (borogluconate) 1.5 mg.
See Editor's Note No. 15.

Biochem Ultimate Fat Metabolizer - Country Life Vitamins
Three tablets contain: Choline Bitartrate 500 mg • Inositol 500 mg • L-Carnitine 500 mg • L-Methionine 500 mg • Taurine 500 mg • Phosphatidyl Choline 200 mg • Betaine HCl 200 mg • Dandelion 100 mg • Milk Thistle 100 mg • Barberry 100 mg • Artichoke extract 50 mg • Vitamin B6 (Pyridoxine/Alpha-Ketoglutarate/Pyridoxal-5-Phosphate) 10 mg • Chromium 400 mcg.

Biochem Ultimate Sports Multiple - Country Life Vitamins
Four tablets contain: Vitamin A (carotene complex) 5000 IU • Vitamin D (ergocalciferol) 200 IU • Vitamin E (D-alpha tocopheryl succinate) 400 IU • Vitamin C (ascorbic acid) 1000 mg • Grape seed extract / Grape skin 100 mg • Vitamin B1 (thiamine HCl/thiamine cocarboxylase) 100 mg • Vitamin B2 (riboflavin/riboflavin 5 phosphate) 100 mg • Vitamin B3 (niacin/niacinamide) 200 mg • Vitamin B5 (D-calcium pantothenate/pantethine) 200 mg • Vitamin B6 (pyridoxine HCl/pyridoxal 5 Phosphate) 100 mg • Folic Acid 400 mcg • Vitamin B12 (cyanocobalamine/dibencozide) 200 mcg • D-Biotin 300 mcg • PABA 200 mcg • Selenium 100 mcg • Molybdenum 10 mcg • Choline Bitartrate 200 mg • Inositol 100 mg • Bromelain 100 mg • Betaine HCl 200 mg • L-Methionine 50 mg • Taurine 50 mg.

BioChoice Immune Support (chocolate flavor) - Legacy for Life
Each packet (27 g) contains: Sodium 160 mg • Potassium 55 mg • Protein 7 g • Vitamin A 5000 IU • Vitamin C 60 mg • Vitamin D (as Vitamin D3) 400 IU • Vitamin E 30 IU • Niacin 20 mg • Folic Acid 0.4 mg • Pantothenic Acid 10 mg • Vitamin B6 2 mg • Vitamin B2 (Riboflavin) 1.7 mg •Vitamin B1 (Thiamin) 1.5 mg • Vitamin B12 6 mcg • Biotin 0.3 mg • Calcium 100 mg • Copper 0.6 mg • Iodine 45 mcg • Iron 5.4 mg • Magnesium 10 mg • Phosphorus 120 mg • Zinc 4.5 mg • Vitamin K (as Vitamin K1) 80 mcg • Manganese 0.6 mg • Chromium 36 mcg. Other Ingredients: Protein blend (Egcel [egg powder], soy protein isolate, milk protein), Maltodextrin, Oat fiber, Cocoa, Natural Chocolate and Vanilla flavor, Soy lecithin, Guar Gum, Xanthan Gum.

BioChoice Immune Support (strawberry flavor) - Legacy for Life
Each packet (24 g) contains: Sodium 160 mg • Potassium 55 mg • Protein 7 g • Vitamin A 5000 IU • Vitamin C 60 mg • Vitamin D (as Vitamin D3) 400 IU • Vitamin E 30 IU • Niacin 20 mg • Folic Acid 0.4 mg • Pantothenic Acid 10 mg • Vitamin B6 2 mg • Vitamin B2 (Riboflavin) 1.7 mg • Vitamin B1 (Thiamin) 1.5 mg • Vitamin B12 6 mcg • Biotin 0.3 mg • Calcium 100 mg • Copper 0.6 mg • Iodine 45 mcg • Iron 5.4 mg • Magnesium 10 mg • Phosphorus 120 mg • Zinc 4.5 mg • Vitamin K (as Vitamin K1) 80 mcg • Manganese 0.6 mg • Chromium 36 mcg. Other Ingredients: Protein Blend (Egcel

[egg powder], Soy protein isolate, milk protein), Maltodextrin, Oat fiber, artificial Strawberry flavor, Beet extract, Soy lecithin, Guar Gum, Xanthan Gum.

BioChoice Immune Support (vanilla flavor) - Legacy for Life
Each packet (24 g) contains: Vitamin A 5000 IU • Vitamin C 60 mg • Vitamin D (Vitamin D3) 400 IU • Vitamin E 30 IU • Niacin 20 mg • Folic Acid 0.4 mg • Pantothenic Acid 10 mg • Vitamin B6 2 mg • Vitamin B2 (Riboflavin) 1.7 mg • Vitamin B1 (Thiamin) 1.5 mg • Vitamin B12 6 mcg • Biotin 0.3 mg • Calcium 100 mg • Copper 0.6 mg • Iodine 45 mcg • Iron 5.4 mg • Magnesium 10 mg • Phosphorus 120 mg • Zinc 4.5 mg • Vitamin K (as Vitamin K1) 80 mcg • Manganese 0.6 mg • Chromium 36 mcg. Other Ingredients: Protein blend (Egcel [egg powder], soy protein isolate, milk protein), Maltodextrin, Oat fiber, Natural Vanilla flavor, Soy lecithin, Guar Gum, Xanthan Gum.

BioChoice Immune Support Drink Mix (chocolate) - Legacy for Life
Each 27 g serving contains: Vitamin A 5000 IU • Vitamin C 60 mg • Vitamin D (D3) 400 IU • Vitamin E 30 IU • Niacin 20 mg • Folic Acid 0.4 mg • Pantothenic Acid 10 mg • Vitamin B6 2 mg • Vitamin B2 (riboflavin) 1.7 mg • Vitamin B1 (thiamin) 1.5 mg • Vitamin B12 6 mcg • Biotin 0.3 mg • Calcium 100 mg • Copper 0.6 mg • Iodine 45 mcg • Iron 5.4 mg • Magnesium 10 mg • Phosphorus 120 mg • Zinc 4.5 mg • Vitamin K (K1) 80 mcg • Manganese 0.6 mg • Chromium 26 mcg. Other Ingredients: Protein Blend (Egcel egg powder, soy protein isolate, milk protein), Maltodextrin, Oat Fiber, Cocoa, Natural Chocolate and Vanilla Flavor, Soy Lecithin, Guar Gum Xanthan Gum.

BioChoice Immune Support Drink Mix (strawberry) - Legacy for Life
Each 24 g serving contains: Vitamin A 5000 IU • Vitamin C 60 mg • Vitamin D (D3) 400 IU • Vitamin E 30 IU • Niacin 20 mg • Folic Acid 0.4 mg • Pantothenic Acid 10 mg • Vitamin B6 2 mg • Vitamin B2 (riboflavin) 1.7 mg • Vitamin B1 (thiamin) 1.5 mg • Vitamin B12 6 mcg • Biotin 0.3 mg • Calcium 100 mg • Copper 0.6 mg • Iodine 45 mcg • Iron 5.4 mg • Magnesium 10 mg • Phosphorus 120 mg • Zinc 4.5 mg • Vitamin K (K1) 80 mcg • Manganese 0.6 mg • Chromium 26 mcg. Other Ingredients: Protein Blend (Egcel egg powder, soy protein isolate, milk protein), Maltodextrin, Oat Fiber, Artificial Strawberry Flavor, Beet Extract, Soy Lecithin, Guar Gum Xanthan Gum.

BioChoice Immune Support Drink Mix (vanilla) - Legacy for Life
Each 24 g serving contains: Vitamin A 5000 IU • Vitamin C 60 mg • Vitamin D (D3) 400 IU • Vitamin E 30 IU • Niacin 20 mg • Folic Acid 0.4 mg • Pantothenic Acid 10 mg • Vitamin B6 2 mg • Vitamin B2 (riboflavin) 1.7 mg • Vitamin B1 (thiamin) 1.5 mg • Vitamin B12 6 mcg • Biotin 0.3 mg • Calcium 100 mg • Copper 0.6 mg • Iodine 45 mcg • Iron 5.4 mg • Magnesium 10 mg • Phosphorus 120 mg • Zinc 4.5 mg • Vitamin K (K1) 80 mcg • Manganese 0.6 mg • Chromium 26 mcg. Other Ingredients: Protein Blend (Egcel egg powder, soy protein isolate, milk protein), Maltodextrin, Oat Fiber, Cocoa, Natural Vanilla Flavor, Soy Lecithin, Guar Gum Xanthan Gum.

BioChoice Immune26 capsules - Legacy for Life
Each capsule contains: Hyperimmune Egg powder (Egcel).

BioChoice Immune26 packets - Legacy for Life
Each 4.5 g packet contains: Hyperimmune Egg powder (Egcel).

BioChoice Immune26 powder - Legacy for Life
Each 4.5 g scoop contains: Hyperimmune Egg powder (Egcel).

Biochol - Ketopharm USA
Each capsule contains: Fenugreek seed 305 mg • Garlic bulb 55 mg • Cloves 55 mg • Cinnamon bark 55 mg • Ginger root 55 mg • Costus root 55 mg.

BioCleanse Powder - BioGenesis Nutraceuticals
Two scoops (45.5 g) contain: Vitamin A (as Betatene brand mixed carotenoids and palmitate) 5000 IU • Vitamin D (D3, cholecalciferol) 80 IU • Vitamin C (sodium ascorbate) 300 mg • Vitamin E (D-alpha tocopherol) 80 IU • Vitamin B1 (thiamin hydrochloride) 2 mg • Vitamin B2 (riboflavin 5'phosphate) 2 mg • Vitamin B3 (niacinamide) 7 mg • Pantothenic Acid (calcium pantothenate) 36 mg • Vitamin B6 (pyridoxal 5'phosphate) 3.4 mg • Vitamin B12 (cyanocobalamin) 3.6 mg • Biotin 135 mg • Folate (folic acid) 80 mcg • Sodium 120 mg • Potassium (dipotassium phosphate and rice protein) 120 mg • Calcium (citrate and rice protein) 225 mg • Magnesium (glycinate) 200 mg • Iron (glycinate and rice protein) 4.6 mg • Phosphorus (rice protein and dipotassium phosphate) 235 mg • Iodine (potassium iodide) 53 mcg • Zinc (glycinate) 10 mg • Copper (glycinate) 1 mg • Manganese (glycinate) 1 mg • Chromium (nicotinate) 50 mcg • Selenium (selenomethionine) 40 mcg • L-Glycine 1500 mg • L-Lysine 540 mg • L-Threonine 540 mg • N-Acetyl Cysteine (NAC) 50 mg • L-Cysteine 10 mg • Taurine 150 mg • Sodium Sulfate 75 mg • MSM (methylsulfonylmethane) 100 mg • Calcium D-Glucarate) 200 mg • Silymarin (milk thistle) 200 mg.

BioCosanol brand - Cyvex Nutrition, Inc.
Policosanol.
See Editor's Note No. 44.

Biodelivery Nutritional Systems C 1000 mg with Mixed Bioflavonoids - Nutritional Therapeutics, Inc.
Vitamin C (as calcium ascorbate/niascorbate) 3000 mg • Vitamin B3 (as niacinamide) 150 mg • Calcium (as calcium ascorbate) 100 mg • Citrus Bioflavonoids 75 mg • Bioflavonoids - Quercetin 75 mg • Bioflavonoids - Rosehips 75 mg • Bioflavonoids - Rutin 75 mg • NT Factor (as tablet base) 240 mg • Pantethine (as coenzyme A precursor) 15 mg. Other Ingredients: Microcrystalline Cellulose, Croscarmellose Sodium, Food Glaze, Vegetable Magnesium Stearate, Silica.

Biodelivery Nutritional Systems Calcium Magnesium with Vitamin D - Nutritional Therapeutics, Inc.
Magnesium (as glycinate) 250 mg • Calcium (as citrate) 500 mg • Vitamin D (D3) 75 IU • NT Factor (as tablet base) 420 mg • Pantethine (as coenzyme A precursor) 18 mg. Other Ingredients: Croscarmellose Sodium, Food Glaze, Vegetable Magnesium Stearate, Silica.

Biodelivery Nutritional Systems Choless - Nutritional Therapeutics, Inc.
Pantothenic Acid (as D-calcium pantothenate) 200 mg • Vitamin E (as D-alpha tocopherol, mixed tocopherols) 40 IU • Gugulipids 100 mg • Inositol Hexanicotinate 400 mg • NT Factor (as tablet base) 600 mg • Pantethine (as coenzyme A precursor) 200 mg. Other Ingredients: Microcrystalline Cellulose, Croscarmellose Sodium, Food Glaze, Vegetable Magnesium Stearate, Silica.

Biodelivery Nutritional Systems Circulatory Assist - Nutritional Therapeutics, Inc.
Vitamin B6 (as pyridoxine HCl) 90 mg • Magnesium (as carbonate, glycinate) 375 mg • Potassium (as citrate) 99 mg • Garlic (as odorless) 750 mg • Hawthorn extract 150 mg • NT Factor (as tablet base) 570 mg • Pantethine (as coenzyme A precursor) 18 mg • Phosphoglycolipids 17 mg. Other Ingredients: Microcrytsalline Cellulose, Croscarmellose Sodium, Food Glaze, Vegetable Magnesium Stearate, Silica.

Biodelivery Nutritional Systems Clean Energy - Nutritional Therapeutics, Inc.
Vitamin B6 HCl 60 mg • Vitamin E (as D-alpha tocopherol, mixed tocopherols) 5 IU • Alpha-Keto Glutarate 250 mg • Co Q-10 3 mg • Creatine Monohydrate 175 mg • Creatine Phosphate 45 mg • L-Tyrosine 125 mg • NT Factor (as tablet base) 300 mg • Pantethine (as coenzyme A precursor) 90 mg. Other Ingredients: Croscarmellose Sodium, Food Glaze, Vegetable Magnesium Stearate, Silica.

Some Brand Name Natural Products - What they Contain

www.NaturalDatabase.com contains MANY more listings than appear here.
Editor's Notes are located on pages 2155-2163.

BRAND NAMES

Biodelivery Nutritional Systems Daily Complete - Nutritional Therapeutics, Inc.
Biotin 300 mcg • Chromium (as nicotinate) 120 mcg • Copper (as glycinate) 2 mg • Folic Acid 400 mcg • Iodine (as kelp) 150 mcg • Magnesium (as carbonate) 400 mg • Manganese (as glycinate) 2 mg • Molybdenum (as glycinate) 75 mcg • Pantothenic Acid (as D-calcium pantothenate) 10 mg • Selenium (as selenomethionate) 70 mcg • Vitamin A (50% as natural beta-carotene) 5000 IU • Vitamin B1 (as thiamin) 1.5 mg • Vitamin B12 6 mcg • Vitamin B2 (as riboflavin/ riboflavin phosphate) 1.7 mg • Vitamin B3 (as niacinamide) 20 mg • Vitamin B6 (as pyridoxine HCl) 2 mg • Vitamin C 60 mg • Vitamin D 400 IU • Vitamin E (as D-alpha, mixed tocopherols) 30 IU • Zinc (as monomethionine) 15 mg • Calcium (as phosphate) 500 mg • Phosphorus 109 mg • Potassium (as citrate) 80 mg • NT Factor (as tablet base) 200 mg • Pantethine (as coenzyme A precursor) 3 mg. Other Ingredients: Calcium Phosphate, Microcrystalline Cellulose, Croscarmellose Sodium, Food Glaze, Vegetable Magnesium Stearate, Silica.

Biodelivery Nutritional Systems EatLite - Nutritional Therapeutics, Inc.
Chromium (as nicotinate) 200 mcg • Iodine (as kelp) 100 mcg • 5-HTP 50 mg • Citrin brand Garcina Cambogia extract 1000 mg • NT Factor (as tablet base) 760 mg • Pantethine (as coenzyme A precursor) 24 mg • Phosphoglycolipids 23 mg. Other Ingredients: Microcrystalline Cellulose, Croscarmellose Sodium, Food Glaze, Vegetable Magnesium Stearate.

Biodelivery Nutritional Systems Essential Fatty Acids - Nutritional Therapeutics, Inc.
ALA (as alpha-linolenic acid, as omega-3) 699 mg • Borage oil 1200 mg • DHA (as docosahexaenoic acid, as omega-3) 138 mg • EPA (as eicosapentaenoic acid, as omega-3) 216 mg • Flax oil (as certified organic) 1200 mg • GLA (as gamma-linolenic acid, as omega-6) 288 mg • LA (as cis-linolenic acid, as omega-6) 652 mg • Northern deep-sea, cold-water, Fish oil (as salmon, halibut, cod, pilchard) 1200 mg. Other Ingredients: Gelatin, Glycerin, Purified Water.

Biodelivery Nutritional Systems HomoCysteine Reducing Formula - Nutritional Therapeutics, Inc.
Vitamin B12 (as cyanocobalamin) 250 mcg • Vitamin B6 (as pyridoxine HCl) 50 mg • Folic Acid 800 mcg • Vitamin E (as D-alpha, mixed tocopherols) 24 IU • NT Factor (as tablet base) 135 mg • Pantethine (as coenyzme A precursor) 4 mg • Phosphoglycolipids 5 mg. Other Ingredients: Microcrystalline Cellulose, Croscarmellose Sodium, Food Glaze, Vegetable Magnesium Stearate, Silica.

Biodelivery Nutritional Systems Menstrual Relief - Nutritional Therapeutics, Inc.
Vitamin B6 (as pyridoxine HCl) 80 mg • Vitamin B12 (as cyanocobalamin) 50 mcg • Vitamin B2 (as riboflavin) 10 mg • Vitamin B1 (as thiamin HCl) 8 mg • Folic Acid 400 mcg • Pantothenic Acid (as D-calcium pantothenate) 10 mg • Vitamin E (as D-alpha, mixed tocopherols) 24 IU • Vitamin B3 (as niacinamide) 10 mg • Biotin 100 mcg • Magnesium 35 mg • Calcium 65 mg • Potassium (as glycerol phosphate) 50 mg • Bromelain 40 mg • Cramp bark 40 mg • DGL as deglycyrrhizinated Licorice 45 mg • Fennel 40 mg • Garlic (as odorless) 130 mg • Inositol 10 mg • Lactoferrin 2 mg • Lipoic Acid 5 mg • NT Factor (as tablet base) 1120 mg • Pantethine (as coenzyme A precursor) 20 mg • Peppermint 40 mg • Phosphoglycolipids 195 mg. Other Ingredients: Microcrystalline Cellulose, Croscarmellose Sodium, Food Glaze, Vegetable Magnesium Stearate, Silica.

Biodelivery Nutritional Systems Mood Right - Nutritional Therapeutics, Inc.
Folic Acid 270 mg • DL-Phenylalanine 500 mg • L-Glutamine 250 mg • L-Glutamine 250 mg • L-Glycine 330 mg • L-Tyrosine 250 mg • NT Factor (as tablet base) 200 mg • Pantethine (as coenzyme A precursor) 6 mg. Other Ingredients: Microcrystalline Cellulose, Croscarmellose Sodium, Food Glaze, Vegetable Magnesium Stearate, Silica.

Biodelivery Nutritional Systems Multi Vitamin - Nutritional Therapeutics, Inc.
Vitamin B1 (as thiamin/thiamin pyrophosphate) 25 mg • Vitamin B12 (as cyanocobalamin) 100 mcg • Vitamin B2 (as riboflavin/ ribose-5-phosphate) 25 mg • Vitamin B6 (as pyridoxine HCl/P-5-P) 25 mg • Vitamin B5 (as pantothenic acid) 100 mg • Vitamin C (as buffered) 500 mg • Vitamin E (as D-alpha, mixed tocopherols) 150 IU • Vitamin A (as natural beta-carotene) 12,500 IU • Vitamin B3 (as niacinamide, inositol hexanicotinate) 50 mg • Folic Acid (as folate) 800 mcg • Biotin 100 mcg • Vitamin D (D3) 100 IU • Vitamin K 10 mcg • Catechin complex as Gambir 50 mg • Choline (as phosphoglycolipid complex) 100 mg • Citrus Bioflavonoids 200 mg • Inositol Hexanicotinate 100 mg • NT Factor (as tablet base) 640 mg • PABA (para amino benzoate) 100 mg • Pantethine (as coenzyme A precursor) 30 mg • Phosphoglycolipids 4 mg • Quercetin (as bioflavonoid) 50 mg. Other Ingredients: Croscarmellose Sodium, Food Glaze, Vegetable Magnesium Stearate, Silica.

Biodelivery Nutritional Systems Multi-Mineral - Nutritional Therapeutics, Inc.
Manganese (as glycinate) 10 mg • Chromium (as nicotinate) 200 mcg • Selenium (as selenomethionine) 100 mcg • Magnesium (as glycinate, carbonate) 500 mg • Molybdenum (as glycinate) 80 mcg • Calcium (as phosphate, citrate) 700 mg • Zinc (as monomethionine) 10 mg • Iodine (as kelp) 75 mcg • Phosphorus 350 mg • Vitamin D (as vitamin D3) 100 IU • Copper (as tyrosinate) 300 mcg • Vitamin E (as D-alpha succinate, mixed tocopherols) 1.5 IU • Potassium (as glycerol phosphate) 50 mg • Boron (as calcium borogluconate) 1 mg • Horsetail (as silica) 50 mg • NT Factor (as tablet base) 200 mg • Pantethine (as coenzyme A precursor) 25 mg • Phosphoglycolipids 128 mg. Other Ingredients: Dicalcium Phosphate, Croscarmellose Sodium, Food Glaze, Vegetable Magnesium Stearate, Sililca.

Biodelivery Nutritional Systems Nursing Support - Nutritional Therapeutics, Inc.
Calcium 200 mg • Brewers Yeast 400 mg • NT Factor (as tablet base) 800 mg • Pantethine (as coenzyme A precursor) 20 mg. Other Ingredients: Citrate Phosphate Protein Complex from Milk, Croscarmellose Sodium, Food Glaze, Vegetable Magnesium Stearate, Silica.

Biodelivery Nutritional Systems Odorless Garlic - Nutritional Therapeutics, Inc.
Garlic (as odorless) 1000 mg • Lactoferrin 2 mg • NT Factor (as tablet base) 150 mg • Pantethine (as coenzyme A precursor) 20 mg. Other Ingredients: Microcrytsalline Cellulose, Croscarmellose Sodium, Food Glaze, Vegetable Magnesium Stearate.

Biodelivery Nutritional Systems Phytoestrogen Complete - Nutritional Therapeutics, Inc.
Vitamin B6 (as pyridoxine HCl) 16 mg • Vitamin E (as D-alpha, mixed tocopherols) 145 IU • Folic Acid 600 mcg • Vitamin K 60 mcg • Selenium 11 mcg • Calcium 55 mg • Phosphorus 19 mg • Betaine HCl 60 mg • Betasitosterol 75 mg • Black Cohosh 30 mg • Boron 2 mg • Bromelain 75 mg • DGL as deglycyrrhizinated Licorice 75 mg • Dong Quai 30 mg • Gamma Oryzanol 75 mg • Isoflavones as Genistein, Daidzein 15 mg • Lactoferrin 6 mg • Lipoic Acid 8 mg • N-Acetyl-D-Glucosamine 60 mg • NT Factor (as tablet base) 540 mg • Pancreatin 75 mg • Pantethine (as coenzyme A precursor) 30 mg • Papain 75 mg • Phosphoglycolipids 320 mg. Other Ingredients: Dicalcium Phosphate, Croscarmellose Sodium, Food Glaze, Silica, Vegetable Magnesium Stearate.

Biodelivery Nutritional Systems Probiotics Plus - Nutritional Therapeutics, Inc.
Magnesium 18 mg • Calcium 35 mg • Beet root fiber 300 mg • Garlic (as odorless) 75 mg • Lactoferrin 3 mg • NT Factor (as capsule base) 1065 mg • Pantethine (as coenzyme A precursor) 24 mg • Phosphoglycolipids 58 mg. Other Ingredients: Gelatin, Vegetable Magnesium Stearate, Silica.

Some Brand Name Natural Products - What they Contain

www.NaturalDatabase.com contains MANY more listings than appear here.
Editor's Notes are located on pages 2155-2163.

Biodelivery Nutritional Systems Pros Health - Nutritional Therapeutics, Inc.
Manganese (as chelate) 30 mg • Vitamin B6 22 mg • Zinc (as monomethionine) 30 mg • Folic Acid 600 mcg • Vitamin E (as D-alpha, mixed tocopherols) 30 IU • African Pygeum extract 150 mg • Betasitosterol 60 mg • Bioperine brand Black Pepper extract 4 mg • Lactoferrin 3 mg • L-Alanine 188 mg • L-Glutamic Acid 450 mg • L-Glycine 300 mg • NT Factor (as tablet base) 630 mg • Pantethine (as coenzyme A precursor) 40 mg • Phosphoglycolipids 240 mg. Other Ingredients: Microcrystalline Cellulose, Croscarmellose Sodium, Food Glaze, Vegetable Magnesium Stearate, Silica.

Biodelivery Nutritional Systems Relief-Joint Support - Nutritional Therapeutics, Inc.
Vitamin C (as calcium ascorbate) 500 mg • Manganese (as manganese glycinate) 10 mg • Zinc (as monomethionine) 12 mg • Bromelain 200 mg • Glucosamine Sulfate 1500 mg • NT Factor (as tablet base) 940 mg • Pantethine (as coenzyme A precursor) 24 mg • Phosphoglycolipids 58 mg. Other Ingredients: Microcrystalline Cellulose, Croscarmellose Sodium, Food Glaze, Vegetable Magnesium Stearate, Silica.

Biodelivery Nutritional Systems Vitamin E Complete - Nutritional Therapeutics, Inc.
Vitamin E (as D-alpha, mixed tocopherols) 400 IU • Calcium (as phosphate) 450 gm • Selenium (as selenomethionate) 25 mcg • Folic Acid 40 mcg • Magnesium 10 mg • NT Factor (as tablet base) 95 mg • Pantethine (as coenzyme A precursor) 50 mg. Other Ingredients: Microcrystalline Cellulose, Silica, Croscarmellose Sodium, Food Glaze, Vegetable Magnesium Stearate.

Bio-Dent - Standard Process, Inc.
Five tablets contain: Proprietary Blend 695 mg: Defatted Wheat germ, Carrot root, Bovine Adrenal, Bovine Spleen, Licorice root, Peanut bran • Calcium 100 mg • Phosphorus 50 mg • Manganese 7 mg • Potassium 5 mg. Other Ingredients: Bovine Bone, Honey, Cellulose, Veal Bone Meal, Arabic Gum.
See Editor's Note No. 14.

Bio-Directed Antioxidant - Nikken Inc.
Two capsules contain: Vitamin A (as d. salina, beta carotene, spirulina pacifica, chlorella vulgaris) 10,000 IU • Vitamin C (as ascorbic acid, calcium ascorbate, acerola cherry) 300 mg • Vitamin E (as D-alpha tocopheryl succinate, D-alpha tocopheryl acetate, alpha, beta, gamma, delta tocopherols) 150 IU • Zinc (as zinc citrate) 15 mg • Selenium (L-selenomethionine) 140 mcg • Green Tea polyphenol extract (camellia sinensis) 500 mg • Alpha Lipoic Acid 50 mg • N-Acetyl L-Cysteine 50 mg • Grape Seed extract (vitis vinifera l.) 25 mg • Glutathione (reduced) 20 mg • Lycopenes 2 mg. Other Ingredients: Gelatin, Maltodextrin, Magnesium Stearate, Silicon Dioxide.

Bio-Directed Digestion - Nikken Inc.
Three capsules contain: Protease (from papaya) 450 mg • Fructooligosaccharides (100% fiber) 375 mg • Amylase 150 mg • Cellulase 75 mg • Lactase 75 mg • Broccoli sprout powder 45 mg • Tomato fruit powder 45 mg • Wheat Grass powder 45 mg • Lactobacillus Sporogenes 45 mg • Papaya fruit powder 45 mg • Fiber 375 mg. Other Ingredients: Gelatin, Magnesium Stearate.

Bio-Directed Fat Metabolism - Nikken Inc.
Two tablets contain: Vitamin C (as ascorbic acid) 30 mg • Vitamin B1 (as thiamine mononitrate) 1.5 mg • Vitamin B2 (as riboflavin) 1.7 mg • Vitamin B6 (as pyridoxine hydrochloride) 2 mg • Folate (as folic acid) 200 mcg • Vitamin B12 (as cyanocobalamin) 6 mcg • Chromium (as chromium picolinate, chromium chelate) 180 mcg • Garcinia Cambogia fruit 500 mg • L-Carnitine (as l-carnitine tartrate) 250 mg • Inositol (as myo-inositol) 25 mg • Bioperine brand Black Pepper extract 2.5 mg. Other Ingredients: Croscarmellose Sodium, Cellulose, Stearic Acid, Calcium Carbonate, Silicon Dioxide, Magnesium Stearate, Dextrin, Dextrose, Lecithin, Sodium Carboxymethylcellulose, Sodium Citrate.

Bio-Directed For Men - Nikken Inc.
Two tablets contain: Vitamin C (as ascorbic acid) 120 mg • Vitamin E (as D-alpha tocopheryl succinate, alpha, beta, gamma, delta tocopherols) 120 IU • Vitamin B6 (as pyridoxine hydrochloride) 5 mg • Folate (as folic acid) 400 mcg • Vitamin B12 (as cyanocobalamin) 30 mcg • Calcium (as calcium carbonate) 300 mg • Zinc (as zinc citrate) 15 mg • Selenium (as L-selenomethionine) 140 mcg • Saw Palmetto fruit extract (serenoa repens, 25% phytosterols) 250 mg • Echinacea Purpurea leaf 50 mg • Taurine 50 mg • Ginkgo Biloba leaf extract (standardized to 24% ginkgoflavoneglycosides, 6% terpene lactones) 30 mg • Curcumin root extract complex (curcuma longa) 25 mg • Garlic bulb (allium sativum) 25 mg • Green Tea polyphenol extract (camellia sinensis) 25 mg • Glycine 25 mg • L-Glutamine 25 mg • Pygeum Africanum root extract 25 mg • Glutathione (reduced) 10 mg • Alpha Lipoic Acid 5 mg • Lycopenes 0.25 mg. Other Ingredients: Dextrose, Cellulose, Dicalcium Phosphate, Croscarmellose Sodium, Stearic Acid, Silicon Dioxide, Dextrin, Magnesium Stearate, Lecithin, Sodium Carboxymethylcellulose, Sodium Citrate.

Bio-Directed For Women - Nikken Inc.
Four tablets contain: Vitamin C (as ascorbic acid, ascorbyl palmitate) 250 mg • Vitamin D (as cholecalciferol) 200 IU • Vitamin E (as D-alpha tocopheryl succinate, alpha, beta, gamma tocopherols) 30 IU • Vitamin B6 (as pyridoxine hydrochloride, pyridoxal 5 phosphate) 10 mg • Folate (as folic acid) 210 mcg • Vitamin B12 (as cyanocobalamin) 12 mcg • Calcium (as calcium carbonate, calcium citrate) 750 mg • Iron (as iron amino acid chelate) 18 mg • Magnesium (magnesium oxide, magnesium citrate) 100 mg • Cranberry fruit powder 250 mg • IsoflavonePlus complex 210 mg: Fenugreek whole plant, N-Acetyl L-Cysteine, Dong Quai root, Soy Isoflavones, Black Cohosh root • Grape Seed extract (vitis vinifera l.) 25 mg • Lutein 1.5 mg • Melatonin 0.1 mg. Other Ingredients: Cellulose, Dextrose, Croscarmellose Sodium, Stearic Acid, Silicon Dioxide, Magnesium Stearate, Dextrin, Lecithin, Sodium Carboxymethylcellulose, Sodium Citrate.

Bio-Directed Immunity - Nikken Inc.
Each capsule contains: Proprietary Blend 500 mg: Cordyceps Sinensis, Agaricus Blazei, Maitake (grifolia frondosa), Reishi (ganoderma lucidum), Trametes Versicolor, Shiitake (lentinula edodes), Hericium Erinaceus, Tremella Mesenterica, Phellinus Linteus, Pleurotus Tuber-Regium, Oyster (pleurotus ostreatus), Chaga (inonotus obliques), Lepiota Prorera, Enoki (flammulina velutipes). Other Ingredients: Magnesium Stearate, Hydroxypropyl Methylcellulose (vegetarian capsule).

Bio-Directed Joint - Nikken Inc.
Three softgels contain: Glucosamine Hydrochloride 300 mg • Methylsulfonylmethane (MSM) 150 mg • High Potency CM Complex 1125 mg: Cetyl Myristoleate complex 900 mg, EPA (eicosapentaenoic acid) 135 mg, DHA (docosahexaenoic acid) 90 mg. Other Ingredients: Gelatin, Glycerin,Titanium Dioxide, Chlorophyll.

Bio-Directed Liver Support - Nikken Inc.
Three capsules contain: Maximum Purifying Blend 1260 mg: Artichoke leaf extract (cynara floridanum), Sarsaparilla root extract (smilax aristolochaiefolii). Other Ingredients: Gelatin, Cellulose, Magnesium Stearate.

Bio-Directed Mental Clarity - Nikken Inc.
Two capsules contain: Vitamin C (as ascorbic acid, ascorbyl palmitate) 150 mg • Vitamin E (as D-alpha tocopheryl succinate, D-alpha tocopheryl acetate, alpha, beta, gamma, delta tocopherols) 100 IU • Green Tea polyphenol extract (camellia sinensis) 500 mg • L-Glutamine 250 mg • L-Tyrosine 250 mg • Cordyceps Sinensis 200 mg • Ginkgo Biloba leaf extract (standardized to 24% ginkgoflavoneglycosides, 6% terpene lactones) 60 mg • Alpha Lipoic Acid 50 mg • N-Acetyl L-Cysteine 25 mg • Grape Seed extract (vitis vinifera l.) 20 mg • Glutathione (reduced) 10 mg. Other Ingredients: Gelatin, Silicon Dioxide, Magnesium Stearate.

Some Brand Name Natural Products - What they Contain

www.NaturalDatabase.com contains MANY more listings than appear here.
Editor's Notes are located on pages 2155-2163.

Bio-Directed Multi-Vitamin/Mineral - Nikken Inc.
Four tablets contain: Vitamin A Palmitate (100% as beta carotene, d. salina) 12,500 IU • Vitamin C (as ascorbic acid, calcium ascorbate, ascorbyl palmitate) 500 mg • Vitamin D (as cholecalciferol) 200 IU • Vitamin E (as d-alpha tocopheryl succinate, alpha, beta, gamma tocopherols) 180 IU • Vitamin K (as phytonadione) 20 mcg • Thiamin (vitamin B1) 4.5 mg • Riboflavin (vitamin B2) 5.1 mg • Niacin (as niacinamide) 60 mg • Vitamin B6 (as pyridoxine hydrochloride, pyridoxal 5 phosphate) 10 mg • Folate (as folic acid) 400 mcg • Vitamin B12 (as cyanocobalamin) 18 mcg • Biotin 300 mcg • Pantothenic Acid (as d-calcium pantothenate) 30 mg • Iodine (as potassium iodide) 150 mcg • Magnesium (as magnesium oxide, magnesium citrate) 100 mg • Zinc (as zinc citrate) 15 mg • Selenium (as yeast, sodium selenate) 70 mcg • Copper (as copper citrate) 2 mg • Manganese (as manganese citrate) 2 mg • Chromium (as chromium picolinate, yeast) 120 mcg • Potassium (as chloride) 50 mg • Nikkomannan Glucomannan root (amorphophallus konjac, 100% fiber) 250 mg • Taurine 250 mg • L-Glutamine 100 mg • Deep Sea Mineral Complex Trace Minerals 100 mg • L-Tyrosine 100 mg • Bromelain 50 mg • N-Acetyl-L-Cysteine 50 mg • Alpha Lipoic Acid 10 mg • Choline (choline bitartrate, choline dihydrogen citrate) 200 mg. Other Ingredients: Cellulose, Dextrose, Starch, Stearic Acid, Silicon Dioxide, Magnesium Stearate, Dextrin, Lecithin, Sodium Carboxymethylcellulose, Sodium Citrate, Chromium Picolinate.

Bio-Directed Restful Night - Nikken Inc.
Two tablets contain: Ascorbic Acid (vitamin C) 28.9 mg • Ascorbyl Palmitate (equivalent to vitamin C 1.1 mg) 2.62 mg • Calcium (as carbonate) 249 mg • Calcium (as citrate hydrate) 1 mg • Cholecalciferol (equiv vit DC 100 IU) 2.5 mcg • D-alpha-Tocopheryl Acid Succinate (vitamin E 14 IU) 11.6 mg • Mixed Tocopherols concentrate (high alpha type) 840 mcg • Phytomenadione (vitamin K) 20 mcg • Magnesium (as oxide) 99 mg • Magnesium (as citrate) 1 mg • Manganese (as gluconate) 1 mg • Alpha Lipoic Acid 5 mg • Matricaria Recutita herb powder (chamomile) 5 mg • Humulus Lupulus flower powder (hops) 5 mg • Valeriana Officinalis root powder 5 mg • Vitis Vinifera extract (grape seed, standardized to procyanidins 4.75 mg) 450 mg.

Bio-Dophilus Complex - American Biologics
Each capsule contains: Bifidobacterium Bifidum 1.25 billion • Lactobacillus Acidophilus 1.25 billion.

Bio-EFA Borage Oil 90 - Health From The Sun
Each capsule contains: Cis- Linoleic Acid (Omega-6) 190 mg • Gamma Linolenic Acid (GLA) (Omega-6) 90 mg • Oleic Acids (Omega-9) 75 mg. Ingredients: 100% Pure Borage oil 500 mg.

BioEFA with CLA - 4 Life
Two softgels contain: Vitamin E (as D-alpha, beta, delta and gamma tocopherols) 15 IU • Alpha Linolenic Acid (ALA, from organic flax seed oil, linum usitatissimum seed) 275 mg • Conjugated Linoleic Acid (CLA, from sunflower seed, helianthus annuus seed) 244 mg • Gamma Linolenic Acid (from borage seed oil, boraga officinalis seed) 69 mg • Eicosapentaenoic Acid (EPA, from fish oil) 66 mg • Docosahexaenoic Acid (DHA, from fish oil) 44 mg. Other Ingredients: Gelatin, Glycerin, Purified Water.

Bio-Energy - Oasis Wellness Network
Each tablet contains: Magnesium (as potassium magnesium aspartate) 100 mg • Chromium (as chromium polynicotinate) 100 mcg • Alpha-Ketoglutaric Acid 100 mg • MaxCell Proprietary Blend 83 mg: Zisyphus Jujube, Piper Nigrum, Aloe Vera gel, Glycyrrhiza Glabra • Siberian Ginseng root extract 67 mg • Panax Ginseng root extract 17 mg • Coenzyme Q10 6 mg. Other Ingredients: Calcium Sulfate, Stearic Acid, Cellulose, Silica, Magnesium Stearate.

BioEnhance - Life Enhancement Products, Inc.
Three caps contain: Vitamin A (as 2500 IU beta-carotene and 2000 IU vitamin A palmitate) 500 mg • Vitamin C 500 mg • Vitamin D (as cholecalciferol) 50 IU • Vitamin E (as D, L-alpha-tocopheryl acetate) 100 mg • Vitamin K (as phytonadione) 22.5 mcg • Thiamine (vitamin B1 as thiamine hydrochloride) 7.5 mg • Riboflavin (vitamin B2) 5 mg • Niacin (vitamin B3) 70 mg • Vitamin B6 (as pyridoxine hydrochloride) 9 mg • Folic Acid 200 mcg • Vitamin B12 (cyanocobalamin) 150 mcg • Biotin 188 mcg • Pantothenic Acid (vitamin B5 as calcium pantothenate) 62.5 mg • Calcium 100 mg • Iodine (as potassium iodide) 25 mcg • Magnesium (as magnesium oxide, magnesium aspartate, and magnesium citrate) 113 mg • Zinc (as zinc gluconate) 5 mg • Selenium (as sodium selenate) 50 mcg • Copper (as copper gluconate) 625 mcg • Manganese (as manganese gluconate) 2 mg • Chromium (as chromium aspartate, chromium nicotinate, and chromium picolinate) 50 mcg • Molybdenum (as molybdenum gluconate) 20 mcg • Taurine 188 mg • PABA (para-aminobenzoic acid) 60 mg • Hesperidin 60 mg • Choline (as choline bitartrate) 50 mg • Inositol 50 mg • Cysteine (anhydrous) 50 mg • Betaine (as betaine hydrochloride) 25 mg • N-Acetylcysteine 25 mg • Quercetin 25 mg • Lipoic Acid 25 mg • DMAE (as dimethylaminoethanol bitartrate) 10 mg • Coenzyme Q10 8 mg • Boron (as calcium borate) 750 mcg • Vanadium (as vanadyl sulfate) 5 mcg.

BioEnhance with DNAble - Life Enhancement Products, Inc.
Four caps contain: Vitamin A (as 2500 IU beta-carotene and 2000 IU vitamin A palmitate) 500 mg • Vitamin C 871 mg • Vitamin D (as cholecalciferol) 50 IU • Vitamin E (as D, L-alpha-tocopheryl acetate) 200 mg • Vitamin K (as phytonadione) 22.5 mcg • Thiamine (vitamin B1 as thiamine hydrochloride) 7.5 mg • Riboflavin (vitamin B2) 5 mg • Niacin (vitamin B3) 550 mg • Vitamin B6 (as pyridoxine hydrochloride) 9 mg • Folic Acid 200 mcg • Vitamin B12 (cyanocobalamin) 150 mcg • Biotin 188 mcg • Pantothenic Acid (vitamin B5 as calcium pantothenate) 62.5 mg • Calcium 224 mg • Phosphorus 235 mg • Iodine (as potassium iodide) 25 mcg • Magnesium (as magnesium oxide, magnesium aspartate, and magnesium citrate) 113 mg • Zinc (as zinc gluconate) 5 mg • Selenium (as sodium selenate) 50 mcg • Copper (as copper gluconate) 625 mcg • Manganese (as manganese gluconate) 2 mg • Chromium (as chromium aspartate, chromium nicotinate, and chromium picolinate) 50 mcg • Molybdenum (as molybdenum gluconate) 20 mcg • Taurine 188 mg • PABA (para-aminobenzoic acid) 60 mg • Hesperidin 60 mg • Choline (as choline bitartrate) 50 mg • Inositol 50 mg • Cysteine (anhydrous) 50 mg • Betaine (as betaine hydrochloride) 25 mg • N-Acetylcysteine 25 mg • Quercetin 25 mg • Lipoic Acid 25 mg • DMAE (as dimethylaminoethanol bitartrate) 10 mg • Coenzyme Q10 8 mg • Resveratrol 2 mg • Boron (as calcium borate) 750 mcg • Vanadium (as vanadyl sulfate) 5 mcg.

BioFem HRT - MK Supplements
Two capsules contain: Red Clover 230 mg • Black Cohosh 200 mg • Wild Yam 200 mg • Dong Quai 100 mg • Pregnenolone 10 mg • Ferulic Acid 25 mg.

BioFem PMS - MK Supplements
Two capsules contain: Vitamin C 250 mg • Vitamin E 100 IU • Vitamin B6 50 mg • Calcium D-Glucarate 200 mg • Magnesium 400 mg • Curcuma Longa 250 mg • Dioscorea Villosa 250 mg • Cimicifuga Racemosa 250 mg • Vitex Agnus-Castus 250 mg • Viburnum Opulus 250 mg • Caulophyllum Thalictroides 250 mg • Angelica Sinensis 250 mg • Zingiber Officinale 150 mg • Peony root 150 mg • Rutin 600 mg • Taurine 300 mg • Choline (citrate) 300 mg.

Bioflavonex - Pure Encapsulations
Each vegetable capsule contains: Grape seed extract (vitis vinifera, standardized to cotnain 92% oligomeric proanthocyanidins) 50 mg • Green Tea extract (standardized to contain a minimum of 65% total tea catechins, providing epigallocatechin gallate [EGCG] 23 mg, caffeine 7 mg) 100 mg • Milk Thistle extract (silybum marianum, standardized to contain 80% silymarin) 100 mg • Resveratrol extract (polygonum cuspidatum, standardized to contain 20% total resveratrol and 10% emodin) 100 mg • Vitamin C (as ascorbyl palmitate) 6 mg.

Bioflavonoid Tablets - Arrowroot
Each tablet contains: Bioflavonoids (from lemon) 500 mg.

Some Brand Name Natural Products - What they Contain

www.NaturalDatabase.com contains MANY more listings than appear here.
Editor's Notes are located on pages 2155-2163.

Bioflavonoids - J. R. Carlson Laboratories, Inc.
Each tablet contains: Rose Hips fruit powder (rosa L. spp) 5 mg • Citrus Bioflavonoids complex 500 mg.

Bioflavonoids 1000 mg - Nature's Plus
Each tablet contains: Bioflavonoids from Citrus Limon exocarp (supplying 24% active flavonones & 20% active flavonols and flavones) 1000 mg. Other Ingredients: Microcrystalline Cellulose, Dicalcium Phosphate, Stearic Acid, Magnesium Stearate, Silica, Pharmaceutical Glaze.

Bioflavonoids 500 mg - Nature's Plus
Each tablet contains: Bioflavonoids from Citrus Limon exocarp (supplying 24% active flavonones & 20% active flavonols and flavones) 500 mg. Other Ingredients: Microcrystalline Cellulose, Stearic Acid, Magnesium Stearate, Pharmaceutical Glaze.

Bioflora - PhysioLogics
Each caplet contains: Fructooligosaccharides (FOS) 500 mg • Lactobacillus Acidophilus (providing 1.02 billion active cells) 255 mg • Lactobacillus Bifidus (providing 0.12 billion active cells) 30 mg • Lactobacillus Bulgaricus (providing 0.12 billion active cells) 30 mg • Turmeric root (curcurma longa) 10.8 mg. Other Ingredients: Cellulose (plant origin), Vegetable Stearic Acid, Croscarmellose, Silica, Vegetable Magnesium Stearate, Cellulose Coating.

BioGenistein Plus - 4 Life
Each capsule contains: Proprietary Blend 400 mg: Soy isoflavone extract (contains 35 mg of genistein and genistin and 40 mg of total isoflavones, Glycine max., seeds), Broccoli sprouts powder extract (brassica oleracea, contains highly concentrated sulforaphane compounds), Quercitin, Curcumin (from turmeric, curcuma longa L.), Dietary indoles, including Indole-3-Carbinol. Other Ingredients: Gelatin Capsule, Peppermint Leaf, and Vegetable Oil.

BioGinkgo 27/7 - Pharmanex
Each tablet contains: Ginkgo leaf extract (ginkgo biloba, 50:1) 60 mg. Other Ingredients: Lactose Anhydrous, Microcrystaline Cellulose, Corn Starch, Sodium Starch Glycolate, Opadry Colors (containing yellow lake 5, blue lake 1), Colloidal Silicon Dioxide, Magnesium Stearate.

Biogra - Olympian Labs
Each capsule contains: DHEA 10 mg • Thymus Gland 20 mg • Octacosanol 600 mg • Raw Orchic 20 mg • L-Tyrosine 250 mg • Vitamin C 30 mg • Vitamin B-6 10 mg • Damiana 80 mg • Wild Yam 20 mg • Yohimbe Bark 20 mg • Gotu Kola 20 mg • Siberian Ginseng 20 mg • Licorice root powder 20 mg • Jamaican Ginger 20 mg • Dong Quai 20 mg • Sarsaparilla 20 mg • Zinc Gluconate 20 mg.
See Editor's Note No. 14.

Biogra for Women - Olympian Labs
Each capsule contains: Proprietary Blend: Damiana, Wild Yam, Gotu Kola, Sarsaparilla, Saw Palmetto, Siberian Ginseng, Dong Quai, Kelp, L-Tyrosine, L-Phenylalanine, Fo-Ti, Para-Aminobenzoic Acid, Bee Propolis 685 mg.

BioGreens - The Vitamin Shoppe
Three teaspoons contain: Organically grown wheatgrass, alfalfa 1923 mg • Soy Lecithin (99% oil-free, 97% phosphatides) 1862 mg • Royal Jelly, Bee Pollen, Honey Extract 1070 mg • Spirulina, Chlorella 700 mg • Vegetable Concentrate (carrot, spinach, bean sprout, celery, tomato, daikon) 700 mg • High Pectin Fruit Fibers (apple, banana, pineapple, papaya) 500 mg • Fructooligosaccharides from Chicory root 400 mg • Dairy-Free Probiotic Cultures (Lactobacillus acidophilus, L. bifidus, L. plantarum, L. rhamnosus, S. thermopilus) 360 mg • Wheat Germ Extract 350 mg • Vitamin E 120 IU • Acerola Berry Powder 120 mg • Licorice Root Extract 120 mg • Brown Rice 112 mg • Red Beet Extract 90 mg • Lipase 0.5 units • Amylase 0.5 skb units • Protease 10 hut • Aloe Vera 50 mg • Green Tea extract 30 mg • Reishi Mushroom 30 mg • Cat's Claw Extract 30 mg • Yucca Root Extract 30 mg • Ginger Root 30 mg • Ginkgo Biloba 20 mg • Bilberry Extract (25% anthocyanidins) 20 mg • Garcinia Extract 20 mg • Konjac Yam extract 20 mg • Maltodextrin 900 mg. Plus 60 mg of the following herbal extracts: Milk Thistle, Siberian Ginseng, Echinacea, American Ginseng.

Bio-Guard - Progressive Labs
Each 2 mL serving contains: Vitamin A 10000 IU • Beta Carotene 2500 IU • Vitamin C 50 mg • Vitamin E 100 IU • Selenium (as selenomethionine) 50 mcg.

BioIsoflavone - MK Supplements
Each capsule contains: NovaSoy brand Soy Isoflavones 50 mg.

BioLax - Body Wise International, Inc.
Two caplets contain: Aloe Vera leaf extract 200:1 500 mg • Senna leaf 400 mg • Prune fruit 250 mg • Fig fruit 200 mg • Psyllium whole husks 100 mg • Celery seed 100 mg • Green Barley Grass 100 mg • Cruciferous Vegetables 100 mg • Lactobacillus Acidophilus 100 mg • Anise Seed 20 mg.

BioLean - Wellness International Network, Ltd.
Each AM serving of 2 tablets and 1 capsule contains: Calcium (as calcium carbonate, dicalcium phosphate anhydrous) 317 mg • Proprietary Blend 1300 mg: Ephedra Alkaloids (25 mg, as ma huang), Caffeine (12 mg, as green tea leaf), Schisandrae berry, Rehmannia root, Hawthorne berry, Jujube seed, Alisma root, Angelicae Dahuricae root, Epimedium, Poria Cocos, Rhizoma Rhei, Stephania root, Angelicae Sinensis root, Codonopsis root, Euconium bark, Panax Notoginseng root • L-Phenylalanine 196 mg • L-Tyrosine 196 mg • L-Carnitine 9.42 mg. Other Ingredients: Cellulose, Stearic Acid, Starch, Sodium Lauryl Sulfate, Hydroxypropyl Cellulose, Magnesium Stearate, Croscarmelose Sodium, Silicon Dioxide.
See Editor's Note No. 30.

BioLean Accelerator - Wellness International Network, Ltd.
Each caplet contains: Proprietary Blend 250 mg: Microcrystalline Cellulose, Black Sesame seed, Raw Chinese Foxglove root, Chinese Wolfberry root, Achyranthes root, Cornelian Cherry fruit, Chinese Yam, Eclipta herb, Rose Hips, Privet fruit, Mulberry fruit spike, Polygonat rhizome, Cooked Chinese Foxglove root, Poria Cocos, Cuscuta seed, Foxnut seed, Alisma rhizome, Moutan bark, Phellodendron bark, Anemarrhena rhizome, Schisandra berry, Royal Jelly • L-Phenylalanine 200 mg • L-Tyrosine 200 mg. Other Ingredients: Calcium Carbonate, Calcium Phosphate Dibasic, Partially Hydrogenated Vegetable Oil, Hydroxypropyl Cellulose, Croscarmellose Sodium, Magnesium Stearate, Silicon Dioxide, Sodium Lauryl Sulfate.

BioLean Free - Wellness International Network, Ltd.
Four caplets contain: Niacin (as niacinamide) 40 mg • Vitamin B6 (as pyridoxine HCl) 16 mg • Chromium (as chromium Chelavite, dinicotinate glycinate) 400 mcg • Potassium (as potassium citrate) 100 mg • Standardized Botanical Extracts 2972 mg: Green Tea leaf extract (10% methylxanthines), Yerba Mate leaf extract (10% methylxanthines), Korean Ginseng root extract (4% ginsenosides), Uva Ursi leaf (20% arbutin), Guarana seed (22% methylxanthines), Quebracho bark extract (10% quebrachine) • Non-Irradiated Pure Herbs and Thermogenic Spices 1440 mg: Gotu Kola leaf (centella asiatica), Ceylon Cinnamon bark, Chinese Horseradish root, Jamaican Ginger root, Tumeric rhizome, Nigerian Cayenne Pepper (fruit), English Mustard seed, Ho Shou Wu root, Ginkgo Biloba leaf (24% ginkgoflavoneglycosides and 6% bilobalides) • L-Tyrosine 500 mg • DL-Methionine 100 mg • Vanadium (as BMOV) 400 mcg. Other Ingredients: Dicalcium Phosphate, Cellulose, Cellulose Gum, Vegetable Stearic Acid, Silica, Vegetable Magnesium Stearate, Vegetable Resin Glaze.

BioLean LipoTrim - Wellness International Network, Ltd.
Each capsule contains: Chromium (as ChromeMate brand chromium polynicotinate) 100 mcg • Garcinia Cambogia fruit (as CitriMax brand hydroxycitrate) 500 mg. Other Ingredients: Gelatin, Calcium Sulfate, Talc, Magnesium Stearate, Silicon Dioxide.

BioMax Limited Adrenal Cortex Extract - Progressive Labs
Each dropper (0.166 ml) contains: Adrenal Cortex extract (bovine) 66.66 mcg. Other Ingredients: Glycerin, Alcohol, Stevia.

BiOmega-3 - USANA Health Sciences
Each capsule contains: Natural Mixed Tocopherols 1 mg • EPA (as fish oil) 180 mg • DHA (as fish oil) 120 mg • Total Omega-3 (as fish oil) 330 mg. Other Ingredients: Gelatin, Glycerin.

Biomune OSF Express - Matol Botanical International Ltd
Silica • Silver Nitrate • Belladonna extract. Inactive Ingredients: Filtered Water, Ai/E[10] Colostrum and Whey extract, 2 Deoxy-D-Glucose, Eucalyptus Oil, Benzalkonium Chloride, Disodium EDTA, Sodium Hydroxide.

Bionate SE - Johnston-Keay Laboratories, Inc
Each tablet contains: Protease (from pancreatin) 60,000 USP units 300 mg • Papain 60,000 USP units 180 mg • Bromelain 324 GDU 135 mg • Trypsin 5400 USP units 72 mg • Chymotrypsin 75 USP units 3 mg • Rutin 150 mg • Boswellia extract (20% boswellic acid) 150 mg • White Willow extract 150 mg. Other Ingredients: Calcium Carbonate, Microcrystalline Cellulose, Starch Ethylcellulose, Hydroxypropyl Methyl Cellulose, Silicon Dioxide, Magnesium Stearate, Fractionated Coconut Oil, Oleic Acid, Triethyl Citrate.

Bio-Organics Breathe-Eze - Mayne Group Ltd
Each capsule contains: Inula helenium (Elecampane) root & rhiz dry 500 mg • Grindelia robusta (Grindelia) herb fl. dry 400 mg • Thymus vulgaris (Thyme) herb fl. dry 300 mg • Glycyrrhiza glabra (Licorice) root & stolon dry 250 mg • Euphorbia hirta (Euphorbia) herb dry 40 mg.

BioPectin - Flora Inc.
Modified citrus pectin.

Bioperine - Source Naturals
Each tablet contains: Bioperine brand Black Pepper extract (95% pure piperine) 10 mg.

Bioperine - America's Finest
Each tablet contains: Bioperine brand Black Pepper fruit extract (98% piperine) 5 mg. Other Ingredients: Dicalcium Phosphate, Emocell Emcompress, Calcium Sulfate Monohydrate, Magnesium Stearate, Pharmaceutical Glaze.

Bioperine brand - Sabinsa Corporation
Black Pepper extract.
See Editor's Note No. 44.

Bio-Phoria - Olympian Labs
Two capsules contain: Proprietary Blend 700 mg: St. John's Wort extract, Phosphatidyl Serine, Acetyl L-Carnitine, Gotu Kola.

BioPro - PhytoPharmica
Two capsules contain: Vitamin A (fish liver oil) 3,000 IU • Vitamin B6 (pyridoxine HCl) 20 mg • Zinc (chelate) 40 mg • Essential fatty acids (unrefined vegetable lipids) 1,260 mg • Amino acid complex 300 mg • Prostate extract (freeze-dried) 300 mg • Saw Palmetto berry extract (4:1) 200 mg.
See Editor's Note No. 21.

BioProstate - MK Supplements
Two capsules contain: Zinc (aspartate) 10 mg • Copper (glycinate) 1 mg • Saw Palmetto extract 350 mg • Nettle leaf powder 150 mg • Pygeum Africanum extract 125 mg • Pumpkin seed 80 mg • Beta-Sitosterol 15 mg • Lycopene 200 mg.

Biopure E 400 - Dial Herbs
Natural Vitamin E (soy-free d-alpha tocopherol) • Medium Chain Triglycerides (coconut) • Oleic Acid (canola oil). Capsule Shell: Gelatin, Vegetable Glycerine, Water.

BioPure Protein - Metagenics
Two scoops (20 g) contain: Immunoglobulins 1.5 g • Calcium 60 mg • Phosphorus 60 mg • Magnesium 10 mg • Sodium 40 mg • Potassium 120 mg • L-Alanine 333 mg • L-Arginine 410 mg • L-Aspartic Acid 1960 mg • L-Cysteine 380 mg • L-Glutamic Acid 2860 mg • L-Glutamine 1240 mg • Glycine 1090 mg • L-Histidine 310 mg • L-Isoleucine (BCAA) 970 mg • L-Leucine (BCAA) 1760 mg • L-Lysine 1590 mg • L-Methionine 280 mg • L-Phenylalanine 520 mg • L-Proline 1090 mg • L-Serine 960 mg • L-Threonine 1290 mg • L-Tryptophan 280 mg • L-Tyrosine 550 mg • L-Valine (BCAA) 920 mg.

Bio-Q10 - America's Finest
Each softgel contains: CoQ10 enzyme (ubiquinone) 30 mg • Selenium (selenomethionine) 100 mcg • CurcuminC3 complex from Turmeric root extract (95% curcuminoids) 250 mg • Bioperine brand Black Pepper fruit extract (98% piperine) 5 mg. Other Ingredients: Gelatin, Glycerine, Medium Chain Triglycerides, Water, Natural Colors, Natural Vitamin E, Polysorbate, Sorbitan Monooleate, Propylene Glycol.

Bio-Rizin - American Biologics
Glycyrrhizic Acid Sodium Salt 8.3 mg/ml. Other Ingredients: Distilled Water.

Biorutin - Nature's Plus
Each tablet contains: Rutin (from saphora japonica leaf) 500 mg • Bioflavonoids from Citrus Limon exocarp 500 mg. Other Ingredients: Microcrystalline Cellulose, Stearic Acid, Magnesium Stearate, Pharmaceutical Glaze, Silica.

Bios Life 2 - Unicity International, Inc.
Each packet contains: Vitamin A (from beta-carotene) 1000 IU • Vitamin C 60 mg • Vitamin E 30 IU • Thiamin (B1) 2.7 mg • Riboflavin (B2) 3.06 mg • Niacinamide (B3) 36 mg • Pyridoxine (B6) 3.6 mg • Biotin (B7) 30 mcg • Folic Acid (B9) 120 mcg • Cyanocobalamin (B12) 10.8 mcg • Calcium 100 mg • Chromium (as polynicotinate) 45 mcg • Selenium 5.5 mcg • Zinc 0.9 mg. Ingredients: Guar Gum, Gum Arabic, Locust Bean Gum, Pectin, Oat Fiber, Calcium Carbonate, Natural Orange Flavor, Ascorbic Acid, Stevia, Niacinamide, dl-Alpha-Tocopheryl Acetate, Natural Cream Flavor, Maltodextrin, Zinc Gluconate, Pyridoxine HCl, Riboflavin, Thiamin HCl, Beta-Carotene, Chromium Polynicotinate (ChromeMate), Folic Acid, Biotin, Sodium Selenite, Cyanocobalamin.

BioSculpt - For Youthful Health
Each 1 oz serving (30 mL) contains: Vitamin B5 60 mg • Vitamin B6 4 mg • Hydrolyzed Collagen 3000 mg • BioSculpt Complex 8500 mg: Aloe Vera gel, Garcinia Cambogia fruit (standardized to 50% hydroxycitric acid), Potassium Pyruvate, CLA, L-Carnitine • Proprietary Blend 1000 mg: L-Alanine, L-Lysine, L-Proline, L-Glutamine, L-Leucine, Hydroxyproline, Dimethyl Glycine.

BioSculpt Extreme - For Youthful Health
Each 1.5 ounce serving contains: Vitamin B5 (as calcium pantothenate) 60 mg • Vitamin B6 (as pyridoxine HCl) 4 mg • Collagen (porcine) 10,000 mg • BioSculpt Extreme Blend 10,000 mg: Aloe Vera gel, Potassium Pyruvate, Ornithine Alpha Ketoglutarate (OKG), Conjugated Linoleic Acid (CLA), Acetyl L-Carnitine, L-Alpha-Glycerylphosphorylcholine (Alpha GPC).

BioSET Antioxidant - Enzymes, Inc.
Each capsule contains: Vitamin A (100% as Beta-Carotene from Dunaliella) 5000 IU • Vitamin C (100% from Acerola Cherries) 47 mg • Vitamin E (100% from d-Alpha Tocopheryl Succinate) 100 IU • Zinc (100% from Zinc Citrate) 5 mg • Selenium (100% from SeaSel Kelp) 15 mcg • Manganese (100% from Manganese Citrate) 3 mg • Proprietary Enzyme Blend 81 mg: pHysioProtease, Catalase • Proprietary Herbal Blend 81 mg: Turmeric root extract, Green Tea leaf extract, Quercetin, Lutein extract, Bilberry fruit extract, Grape seed extract, Alpha-Lipoic Acid. Other Ingredients: Plant Cellulose, Water.

BioSET Blood Sugar - Enzymes, Inc.
Each capsule contains: Vitamin E (100% from d-Alpha Tocopheryl Acid Succinate) 30 mg • Zinc (100% from Zinc Citrate) 5 mg •

Manganese (100% from Manganese Citrate) 1 mg • Chromium (50% from Chromium Picolinate, 50% from Chromium GTF Polynicotinate) 1 mg • Proprietary Herbal Blend 415 mg: Gymnema leaf extract, Bitter Melon extract, Jambolan seed extract, Garlic bulb conc., Green Tea leaf extract, Black Currant seed extract • Lipase 25 mg. Other Ingredients: Plant Cellulose, Water.

BioSET Bone - Enzymes, Inc.
Two capsules contain: Calcium (100% from Calcium Citrate) 114 mg • Magnesium (100% from Magnesium Aspartate) 76 mg • Manganese (100% from Manganese Citrate) 2 mg • Proprietary Herbal Blend 125 mg: Horsetail herb extract, Oat straw extract, Soy Isoflavones • Proprietary Enzyme Blend 73 mg: pHysioProtease, Phytase • Boron Citrate 10 mg. Other Ingredients: Plant Cellulose, Water.

BioSET Digestion - Enzymes, Inc.
Each capsule contains: Proprietary Enzyme Blend 460 mg: Amylase, Protease, Lipase, CereCalase, Invertase, Glucoamylase, alpha-Galactosidase, Malt Diastase, Lactase, Pectinase, Cellulase, Peptidase. Other Ingredients: Plant Cellulose, Water.

BioSET Female Balance - Enzymes, Inc.
Each capsule contains: Vitamin E (100% from d-Alpha Tocopheryl Acid Succinate) 30 IU • Proprietary Herbal Blend 408 mg: Black Cohosh root extract, Chaste Tree berry extract, Ginkgo Biloba leaf extract, Oat straw extract, Soy Isoflavones • pHysioProtease 40 mg. Other Ingredients: Plant Cellulose, Water.

BioSET Immune - Enzymes, Inc.
Each capsule contains: Proprietary Herbal Blend 375 mg: Astragalus root extract, Goldenseal root extract, Echinacea Angustifolia root extract, Echinacea Purpurea root extract, Reishi Mushroom extract, Shiitake Mushroom extract • pHysioProtease 150 mg. Other Ingredients: Plant Cellulose, Water.

BioShape - Royal BodyCare
Four caplets contain: Vitamin C (from ascorbyl palmitate) 40 mg • Calcium (from Super CitriMax Full Strength brand) 200 mg • Chromium (polynicotinate) 160 mcg • Potassium (From Super CitriMax Full Strength brand) 290 mg • Garcinia Cambogia fruit extract (Super CitriMax brand, providing (-) hydroxycitric acid 1120 mg) 1867 mg • Gymnema Sylvestre leaves extract (providing gymnemic acids 40 mg) 160 mg • Proprietary Amino Acid Blend 2000 mg: Isoleucine (as L-isoleucine), L-Lysine (as L-lysine HCl), Phenylalanine (as L-phenylalanine), Arginine (as L-arginine HCl), Glutamine (as L-glutamine), Leucine (as L-leucine), Methionine (as L-methionine), Threonine (as L-threonine), Valine (as L-valine), Histidine (as L-histidine HCl), L-5 Hydroxytryptophan. Other Ingredients: Microcrystalline Cellulose, Stearic Acid, Cellulose Gum, Silicon Dioxide.

BioSil capsules - Jarrow Formulas
Each capsule contains: Silicon (as stabilized orthosilicic acid) 5 mg.

BioSil liquid - Jarrow Formulas
2% elemental Silicon (Si, as stabilized, concentrated orthosilicic acid [Si(OH)4]) • 47% Choline Chloride • 33% Glycerol (vegetable) • 18% Distilled Water.

Biosol Liquid Calcium - Nature's Own
Each tablet contains: Calcium Carbonate 875 mg: Elemental Calcium 350 mg • Vitamin D (D2, as ergocalciferol 2.5 mcg) 100 IU.

BioSom (BioSom) - Metagenics
Each spray contains: Dehydroepiandrosterone (DHEA) 5 mg • Stevia leaf extract (stevia rebaudiana) 7 mg • Grapefruit seed extract (citricidal spp.) 330 mcg.

Biosorb Silymarin - Metabolic Response Modifiers
Each capsule contains: Biosorb Silymarin (yielding 80 mg silymarin) 250 mg.

Biospec Muscle Builder - BioTherapies, Inc.
Two rounded tablespoons (28.4 g) contain: Riboflavin 0.136 mg • Niacin 0.8 mg • Calcium 200 mg • Phosphorus 150 mg • Iron 1.44 mg. Typical Amino Acid Profile: Alanine 1000 mg, Arginine 1490 mg, Aspartic Acid 2390 mg, Cystine 360 mg, Glycine 840 mg, Histidine 700 mg, Isoleucine 1490 mg, Leucine 2400 mg, Lysine 1900 mg, Methionine 590 mg, Phenylalanine 1370 mg, Proline 2160 mg, Serine 1420 mg, Threonine 1080 mg, Tryptophan 380 mg, Tyrosine 1260 mg, Valine 1000 mg.

Biost - Standard Process, Inc.
Each tablet contains: Proprietary Blend 258 mg: Veal Bone PMG extract, Calcium Lactate, Magnesium Citrate • Manganese 6 mg • Sodium 10 mg. Other Ingredients: Honey, Cellulose.

Biotic Buddies - Advocare International
Each packet contains: Lactobacillus Acidophilus 1 billion • Bifidobacterium Bifidus 1 billion • Fructooligosaccharides 500 mg. Other Ingredients: Dextrose, Maltodextrin, Inulin, Natural Strawberry Flavor, Silicon Dioxide.

Biotin - Source Naturals
Each tablet contains: Biotin 600 mcg.

Biotin - J. R. Carlson Laboratories, Inc.
Each tablet contains: Biotin 1000 mcg.

Biotin - Jamieson
Each tablet contains: Biotin 250 mcg.

Biotin - GNC
Each tablet contains: Biotin 600 mcg. Other Ingredients: Dicalcium Phosphate, Cellulose, Magnesium Stearate.

Biotin - Pure Encapsulations
Each vegetable capsule contains: Biotin 8 mg.

Biotin - Nature's Bounty
Each tablet contains: Biotin 300 mcg. Other Ingredients: Dicalcium Phosphate, Cellulose, Vegetable Stearic Acid, Vegetable Magnesium Stearate.

Biotin & Folic Acid Sustained Release Tablets - Nature's Plus
Each tablet contains: Folic Acid 800 mcg • Biotin 2000 mcg. Other Ingredients: Microcrystalline Cellulose, Di-calcium Phosphate, Hydroxypropyl Methylcellulose, Stearic Acid, Magnesium Stearate, Rice Bran, Riboflavin, Pharmaceutical Glaze, Silica.

Biotin 1000 mcg Vegetarian Formula - Vitamin World
Each tablet contains: Biotin (D-biotin) 1000 mcg. Other Ingredients: Dicalcium Phosphate, Cellulose (plant origin), Vegetable Stearic Acid, Croscarmellose, Cellulose Coating, Silica, Vegetable Magnesium Stearate.

Biotin 300 - GNC
Each tablet contains: Biotin 300 mg. Other Ingredients: Dicalcium Phosphate, Cellulose, Whole Brown Rice powder (Oryza sativa).

Biotin 300 mcg - Vitamin World
Each tablet contains: Biotin 300 mcg. Other Ingredients: Dicalcium Phosphate, Cellulose (plant origin), Vegetable Stearic Acid, Croscarmellose, Silica, Vegetable Magnesium Stearate.

Biotin 300mcg - Nature's Own
Each tablet contains: Biotin 300 mcg.

Biotin 5 mg - Jarrow Formulas
Each capsule contains: D-Biotin 5 mg. Other Ingredients: Rice Powder, Magnesium Stearate, Silicon Dioxide, Gelatin.

Biotin 500 mcg - Arrowroot
Each capsule contains: Biotin 500 mcg.

Biotin 600 - GNC
Each tablet contains: Biotin 600 mcg. Other Ingredients: Dicalcium Phosphate, Cellulose.

Some Brand Name Natural Products - What they Contain

www.NaturalDatabase.com contains MANY more listings than appear here.

Editor's Notes are located on pages 2155-2163.

Biotin 800 mcg **-** Rexall - Sundown
Each tablet contains: Biotin 800 mcg • Calcium 20 mg. Other Ingredients: Dextrose, Dicalcium Phosphate, Croscarmellose Sodium, Magnesium Stearate.

Biovigora **-** Oasis Biotech
Each capsule contains: Proprietary Blend 400 mg: Aframomum, Kola Nitida, Digestive Enzymes. Other Ingredients: Gelatin Capsule.

BioVin brand **-** Cyvex Nutrition, Inc.
Grape extract.

BioVin Plus brand **-** Cyvex Nutrition, Inc.
Grape seed extract.

BioVinca brand **-** Cyvex Nutrition, Inc.
Vinpocetine.

Biovital Plus **-** Enzymatic Therapy
Vitamin A (Beta Carotene) non-toxic form of Vitamin A 40,000 IU • Vitamin A Fish Liver oil 25,000 IU • Vitamin E (D-Tocopherol Succinate) 800 IU • Vitamin D Fish Liver oil 600 IU • Vitamin C (Ascorbic Acid/Rose Hips) 3000 mg • Calcium (Carbonate, Citrate, Aspartate, Gluconate) 625 mg • Potassium Aspartate 375 mg • Magnesium Aspartate 375 mg • Pantothenic Acid (D-Calcium Pantothenate) 250 mg • Thiamine HCl (Vitamin B1) 250 mg • Niacin/Niacinamide 250 mg • Manganese (Aspartate) 186 mg • Vitamin B6 (Pyridoxine HCl) 150 mg • Riboflavin (Vitamin B2/ Liver) 100 mg • Zinc (Aspartate) 92 mg • Iron (Aspartate) 60 mg • Copper (Aspartate) 2 mg • Biotin 1 mg • Folic Acid 800 mcg • Chromium Aspartate 428 mcg • Iodine (Kelp) 225 mcg • Selenium (Aspartate) 120 mcg • Vitamin B12 /Liver (Cyanocobalamin) 100 mcg • Other ingredients: Choline Bitartrate /Liver 750 mg • Bromelain (600 MCU) 400 mg • Pancreatic Enzymes (10X) 400 mg • PABA (Para Aminobenzoic Acid) 250 mg • Citrus Bioflavonoids 250 mg • Lipase 200 mg • L-Methionine 200 mg • Trace Mineral Complex "Containing 72 trace minerals" 200 mg • Alfalfa juice concentrate 200 mg • Liver concentrate (20X) 200 mg • Multi-Glandular concentrate 200 mg • Adrenal extract freeze-dried 200 mg • Thymus extract freeze-dried 200 mg • Saw Palmetto Berry extract 4:1 (Serenoa repens) 125 mg • Ma Huang extract (Ephedra sinensis) standardized to contain 6% Ephedrine 125 mg • Sarsaparilla root 4:1 (Smilax officinalis) 125 mg • Inositol 100 mg.
See Editor's Note No. 14, No. 21, and No. 30.

Bio-Zyme **-** PhytoPharmica
Two tablets contain: Amylase 10 mg • Bromelain (1200 MCU/g) 50 mg • Chymotrypsin 2 mg • Lipase 10 mg • Lysozyme 10 mg • Pancreatic Enzymes 10X 325 mg • Papain 50 mg • Trypsin 75 mg.

Bite Blocker lotion **-** HOMS LLC
Soybean oil • Coconut oil • Purified Water • Glcyerin • Geranium oil • Cetearyl Alcohol • Citric Acid • Lecithin • Vanillin.

Bite Blocker spray **-** HOMS LLC
Soybean oil • Purified Water • Coconut oil • Glycerin • Geranium oil • Citric Acid • Lecithin • Soidum Bicarbonate • Vanillin.

Biting Insect Mix **-** Professional Complementary Health Formulas
Adrenal 3X, 4X • ACTH 6X, 30X • Histamine 12X • Liver 6X, 12X • Ant (black/fire/red), Bedbug, Bee (five types), Chigger, Cockroach, Deerfly, Flea, Horsefly, House Fly, Lice (head and body), Mosquito, Moth, Spider (five types), Tick, Wasp 6X, 12X, 60X, 100X • Purified Water • 20% USP Alcohol.
See Editor's Note No. 1.

Bitter Melon Complex **-** Susan Ambrosino's Herb Club, Inc.
Bitter Melon concentrate • Fenugreek seed powder • White Panax Ginseng powder.

Bitters Virtue **-** Blessed Herbs
Aloe • Myrrh Gum • Senna • Camphor • Turkey Rhubarb root • Zedoary root • Manna • Carline Thistle • Angelica root • Licorice root • Fennel seed • Anise seed • Pomeranz peel • Gentian root • Galangal root & Peach brandy.

Black Cohosh **-** Leiner Health Products
Each caplet contains: Black Cohosh extract powder (Cimicifuga racemosa) root 40 mg • Lecithin 25 mg. Other Ingredients: Calcium Carbonate, Dicalcium Phosphate, Cellulose, Maltodextrin, Stearic Acid, Croscarmellose Sodium, Silicon Dioxide, Magnesium Stearate, Dextrin, Hydroxypropyl Methylcellulose, Polyethylene Glycol 3350.

Black Cohosh **-** Enzymatic Therapy
Each tablet contains: Black Cohosh root/rhizome extract (cimicifuga racemosa, standardized to contain 2.5% triterpene glycosides calculated as 27-deoxyactein) 20 mg. Other ingredients: Cellulose, Modified Cellulose, Magnesium Stearate, Lecithin, Peppermint Leaf, Carnauba Wax.

Black Cohosh **-** Ortho Molecular Products
Two capsules contain: Black Cohosh root extract (standardized to contain 2.5% triterpene glycosides) 160 mg. Other Ingredients: Natural Vegetable Capsules, Magnesium Stearate, Microcrystalline Cellulose.

Black Cohosh **-** Jarrow Formulas
Each tablet contains: Black Cohosh 2.5% extract (cimicifuga racemosa) 40 mg. Other Ingredients: Cellulose, Modified Cellulose, Modified Cellulose Gum, Silicon Dioxide, Magnesium Stearate.

Black Cohosh **-** Source Naturals
Each tablet contains: Black Cohosh standardized extract 2.5% (Cimicifuga racemosa roots and rhizome) (yielding 2 mg of Triterpene Glycosides) (containing 27-deoxyactein) 80 mg.

Black Cohosh **-** PhysioLogics
Two softgels contain: Black Cohosh root/rhizome extract (cimicifuga racemosa, standardized to contain 2.5% triterpene glycosides conatining 27-deoxyactein, 2 mg) 80 mg. Other Ingredients: Soybean Oil, Gelatin, Glycerin, Beeswax / Soybean Oil Mixture, Lecithin, Caramel Color, Titanium Dioxide Color.

Black Cohosh **-** Nature's Way
Each capsule contains: Black Cohosh root 515 mg. Other Ingredients: Gelatin, Magnesium stearate, Millet.

Black Cohosh **-** Nature's Sunshine
Each capsule contains: Black Cohosh root (cimicifuga racemosa) 525 mg. Other Ingredients: Magnesium Stearate, Silicon Dioxide, Kosher Gelatin, Water.

Black Cohosh **-** Jamieson
Each caplet contains: Black Cohosh Root 40 mg.

Black Cohosh 1000 mg, Concentrated **-** GNC
Each capsule contains: Black Cohosh Root (cimicifuga racemosa; from 250 mg black cohosh root extract 4:1) 1000 mg. Other Ingredients: Soybean Oil, Gelatin, Glycerin, Partially Hydrogenated Soybean Oil, Caramel Color, Titanium Dioxide (natural mineral whitener).

Black Cohosh 2.5 **-** Pure Encapsulations
Each vegetable capsule contains: Black Cohosh extract (cimicifuga racemosa, standardized to provide 2.5% triterpene glycosides) 250 mg.

Black Cohosh 500 mg **-** Nature's Own
Each tablet contains: Black Cohosh rhizome extract (cimicifuga racemosa) 500 mg.

Black Cohosh Extract **-** Nature's Way
Each tablet contains: Black Cohosh dried extract 40 mg. Other Ingredients: Cellulose, Maltodextrin, Modified Cellulose Gum, Silica, Stearic Acid.

Some Brand Name Natural Products - What they Contain

www.NaturalDatabase.com contains MANY more listings than appear here.
Editor's Notes are located on pages 2155-2163.

Black Cohosh Plus - Metagenics
Each tablet contains: Black Cohosh root and rhizome extract (actaea racemosa, standardized to 2.5% triterpene glycosides expressed as 27-deoxyactein) 80 mg • Motherwort aerial parts 6.5:1 extract (leonurus cardiaca) 100 mg • Lemon Balm leaf 5:1 extract (melissa officinalis) 50 mg.

Black Cohosh Root - NOW Foods
Two capsules contain: Black Cohosh (Cimicifuga Racemosa) root 1100 mg. Other Ingredients: Gelatin (capsule), Stearic Acid.

Black Cohosh Root - Aboca USA, Inc
Each capsule contains: Black Cohosh root WPC (whole phytocomplex concentrate, cimicifuga racemosa, standardized to contain 0.7% actein and 27-deoxyactein, yielding 2 mg per capsule) 290 mg. Other Ingredients: Gelatin.

Black Cohosh Standardized Extract - NOW Foods
Two capsules contain: Black Cohosh root & rhizome 160 mg • Cimicfuga racemosa (standardized to contain 2.5% total triterpene Glycosides, calculated as 27-Deoxyactein) 4 mg • Licorice root 250 mg • Dong Quai root (Angelica sinensis) 250 mg.

Black Cohosh Whole Herb - Rexall - Sundown
Each capsule contains: Black Cohosh (root) 540 mg. Other Ingredients: Gelatin.

Black Cohosh-Blue Cohosh Virtue - Blessed Herbs
Black Cohosh root • Blue Cohosh root • Ginger root • Beth root • Grain alcohol & Distilled Water.

Black Currant - Wild Rose
Each capsule contains: Black Currant oil 1000 mg • Alpha-Linolenic Acid (omega-3) 128 mg • Cis-Linoleic Acid (omega-6) 433 mg • Gamma-Linolenic Acid (omega-6) 170 mg • Oleic Acid (omega-9) 87 mg • Stearidonic Acid 25 mg.

Black Currant 1000 - Health From The Sun
Each capsule contains: Alpha-Linolenic Acid (ALA) (Omega-3) 130 mg • Gamma Linolenic Acid (Omega-6) 170 mg • Linoleic Acid (Omega-6) 430 mg • Oleic Acid (Omega-9) 90 mg • Stearidonic Acid (Omega -3) 25 mg. Ingredients: Black Currant seed oil, Gelatin, Glycerine, Water.

Black Currant 500 - Health From The Sun
Each capsule contains: Alpha-Linolenic Acid (ALA)(Omega-3) 65 mg • Gamma Linolenic Acid (GLA)(Omega-6) 85 mg • Linoleic Acid (Omega-6) 215 mg • Oleic Acid (Omega-9) 45 mg • Stearidonic Acid (Omega-3) 12 mg. Ingredients: Black Currant seed oil, Gelatin, Glycerine, Water.

Black Currant Oil - Puritan's Pride
Each softgel contains: Black Currant oil 460 mg.

Black Currant Oil - Nature's Sunshine
Each capsule contains: Black Currant oil (Providing 12% gamma-linolenic acid) 250 mg. Other Ingredients: Gelatin, Glycerin, Water.

Black Currant Seed Oil - Pure Encapsulations
Each softgel capsule contains: Black Currant Seed Oil (typical fatty acid composition: 16:0 palmitic, 18:0 stearic, 18:1 oleic, 18:2 linoleic, 18:3 gamma linolenic [GLA] 18:3 linolenic, other fatty acids 10 mg) 500 mg • Vitamin E (D-alpha-tocopherol) 10 IU.

Black Currant Seed Oil - Vital Nutrients
Each capsule contains: Black Currant seed oil 460 mg: Gamma Linolenic Acid 70 mg.

Black Currant Seed Oil - Standard Process, Inc.
Each perle contains: Black Currant seed oil 320 mg • Gamma-Linolenic Acid 47 mg. Other Ingredients: Gelatin, Glycerin, Water, Carob.

Black Currant seed oil - Nutri-Quest Rx
Each capsule contains: Black Currant seed oil 250 mg • Fatty Acid composition: Gamma Linolenic acid 16.9% • Linoleic 45.2% • Oleic 12.7% • Alpha Linolenic 11.7% • Palmitic 7.4% • Stearidonic 2.9% • Stearic 1.6% • Eicosenoic Acid 1.1%. Other Ingredients: Myristic, Arachidic, Behenic, Lignoceric, Palmitoleic Acids with natural Vitamin E 5 IU.

Black Elderberry - Gaia Herbs
Two capsules contain: Black Elderberries (sambucus nigra) 200 mg. Other Ingredients: Vegetable Glycerin, Vegetable Cellulose (capsule).

Black Ointment - Nature's Sunshine
Chaparral herb • Lobelia herb • Comfrey herb • Red Clover herb • Plantain root • Golden Seal root • Myrrh gum • Marshmallow root • Mullein herb • Chickweed herb. Base: Olive Oil, Beeswax, Pine Tar, Vitamin E Oil.

Black Walnut - Nature's Sunshine
Two capsules contain: Black Walnut hull (juglans nigra) 1000 mg. Other Ingredients: Magnesium Stearate, Silicon Dioxide, Kosher Gelatin, Water.

Blackcurrant C 500mg - Nature's Own
Each tablet contains: Vitamin C 500 mg (from ascorbic acid 200 mg and sodium ascorbate 337.5 mg).

Blackstrap Molasses with Iron - Swanson Health Products
Each tablet contains: Blackstrap Molasses with 29 mg of Iron.

Bladderwrack-Dandelion Virtue - Blessed Herbs
Ma Huang • Guarana seed • Dandelion blend of flower, leaf & root • Bladderwrack • Grain alcohol & Distilled Water.
See Editor's Note No. 30.

BLAST - Life Enhancement Products, Inc.
Each rounded tablespoon (13.6 g) contains: Vitamin A (as beta-carotene) 2500 IU • Vitamin C (as ascorbic acid and niacinamide ascorbate) 325 mg • Vitamin E (as D,L-alpha-tocopheryl acetate) 30 IU • Thiamine (vitamin B1 as thiamine hydrochloride) 1.5 mg • Riboflavin (vitamin B2) 3 mg • Niacin (vitamin B3 as niacinamide ascorbate) 75 mg • Vitamin B6 (as pyridoxine hydrochloride) 16 mg • Folic Acid 100 mcg • Vitamin B12 (cyanocobalamin) 20 mcg • Pantothenic Acid (vitamin B5 as calcium pantothenate) 18 mg • Zinc (as zinc gluconate) 3 mg • Copper (as copper gluconate) 420 mcg • Chromium (as chromium aspartate) 25 mcg • L-Phenylalanine 600 mg • Taurine 200 mg • Glycine 150 mg • Caffeine 80 mg • Tea Polyphenols 50 mg.

BLAST Caps - Life Enhancement Products, Inc.
Two capsules contain: Vitamin A (as beta-carotene) 2500 IU • Vitamin C (as ascorbic acid and niacinamide ascorbate) 325 mg • Vitamin E (as D,L-alpha-tocopheryl acetate) 30 IU • Thiamine (vitamin B1 as thiamine hydrochloride) 1.5 mg • Riboflavin (vitamin B2) 3 mg • Niacin (vitamin B3 as niacinamide ascorbate) 75 mg • Vitamin B6 (as pyridoxine hydrochloride) 16 mg • Folic Acid 100 mcg • Vitamin B12 (cyanocobalamin) 20 mcg • Pantothenic Acid (vitamin B5 as calcium pantothenate) 18 mg • Zinc (as zinc gluconate) 3 mg • Copper (as copper gluconate) 420 mcg • Chromium (as chromium aspartate) 25 mcg • L-Phenylalanine 600 mg • Taurine 200 mg • Glycine 150 mg • Caffeine 80 mg.

Blast of Grass - Green Foods Corp.
Active Ingredient: Barley Grass Essence.

Blessed Thistle - Nature's Sunshine
Two capsules contain: Blessed Thistle aerial parts (cnicus benedictus) 650 mg. Other Ingredients: Kosher Gelatin, Water.

BLF # Breathe Easy Without Stimulants - Health Center for Better Living
Two tablets contain: Siberian Ginseng root extract (0.8% eleutherosides) 250 mg • American Ginseng root 250 mg • Ginger root standardized extract (5% gingerols) • Peppermint leaf 75 mg •

Chickweed herb (aerial parts) 50 mg • Myrrh resin 50 mg • Mullein leaf 50 mg • Yerba Mate leaf (20% alkaloids) • MSM (methyisulforaimethan, 36% organic sulfur) 1,000 mg.

BLF #1 Clear Complexion - Health Center for Better Living
Each capsule contains: Burdock root 84 mg • Dandelion root 84 mg • Red Clover tops 84 mg • Echinacea root 56 mg • Yellow Dock root 56 mg • Capsicum 28 mg • Alfalfa leaf 28 mg • Valerian root 28 mg.

BLF #12 Cholest-A Ingredients - Health Center for Better Living
Each capsule contains: Hawthorn Berry 113 mg • Fenugreek Seed 75 mg • Capsicum 75 mg • Plantain Herb 75 mg • Red Clover Blossom 75 mg • Black Cohosh Root 38 mg.

BLF #125 Woman's Balance Health Center for Better Living
Each capsule contains: Dong Quai Root 102 mg • Damiana Leaf 61 mg • Kelp Atlantic 61 mg • Sarsaparilla Root 61 mg • Saw Palmetto Berry 41 mg • Chickweed Herb 41 mg • Capsicum 41 mg • Black Cohosh Root 41 mg.

BLF #13 Body Circulation - Health Center for Better Living
Each capsule contains: Capsicum 84 mg • Bayberry Bark 34 mg • Hyssop Leaf 17 mg • Skullcap 17 mg • Witch Hazel Bark 17 mg.

BLF #16 Colon Helper - Health Center for Better Living
Each capsule contains: Slippery Elm Bark 145 mg • Aloe 145 mg • White Oak Bark 73 mg • Blue Vervain Herb 73 mg • Gentain Root 36 mg • Goldenseal Herb 15 mg.

BLF #17 Regularity Ingredients - Health Center for Better Living
Each capsule contains: Buckthorn Bark 113 mg • Cascara Sagrada Bark 113 mg • Chickweed Herb 75 mg • Elder Flower 75 mg • Oregon Grape Root 38 mg • Mandrake Root 38 mg.

BLF #2 Allergy First Aid - Health Center for Better Living
Each caplet contains: Allergy Herbal Blend 200 mg: Hyssop whole plant, Mullein leaves, Thyme whole plant, Chrysanthemum flower, Magnolia flower, Angelica root, Vitex fruit, Atractylodes Rhizome, Bellflower root, Field Mint, Immature Tangerine peel, Ledebouriella root, Moutan bark, Perilla leaf and Schizonepeta stem • Boswellia Gum resin (40% boswellic acid) 100 mg • Yerba Mate leaf (20% alkaloids) 50 mg • Meadowsweet 4:1 extract 50 mg • Eucalyptus leaf extract 25 mg • Fennel seed 25 mg.

BLF #21 Endless Energy - Health Center for Better Living
Each capsule contains: Ginseng Root 75 mg • Foti Root • Bee Pollen Granules 75 mg • Damiana Leaf 75 mg • Capsicum 50 mg • Kola Nut 50 mg • Echinacea Root 25 mg • Licorice Root 25 mg.

BLF #225 Man's Rejuvenator - Health Center for Better Living
Each capsule contains: Saw Palmetto Berry 75 mg • Cornsilk 75 mg • Gota Kola Herb 75 mg • Damiana Leaf 75 mg • Juniper Berry 38 mg • Kelp Atlantic 38 mg • Parsley Leaf 38 mg • Uva Ursi Leaf 38 mg.

BLF #23 Vision Booster - Health Center for Better Living
Vitamin A [as retinyl palmitate and 75% as beta-carotene with natural mixed carotenoids (alpha-carotene, beta-carotene, cryptoxanthin, zeaxanthin and lutein)] 10,000 IU • Vitamin C (as ascorbic acid) 250 mg • Vitamin E (as d-alpha-tocopheryl succinate and 50% as dl-alpha-tocopheryl acetate) 100 IU • Selenium (as selenomethionine) 100 mcg • Bilberry Herb blend [Bilberry leaf and Bilberry fruit standardized extract (25% anthocyanins)] 75 mg • Eyebright herb blend [Eyebright herb and eyebright herb 4:1 extract (whole plant)] 75 mg • Lutein (from marigold flower) 5 mg • L-Glutathione 5 mg • Taurine 5 mg • Quercetin dihydrate 75 mg • Lycium berry 5:1 extract 50 mg.

BLF #24 Fresh Start - Health Center for Better Living
Alfalfa • Hyssop • Chamomile • Cornsilk • "Vitamins and minerals with antioxidant and diuretic qualities."

BLF #3 Love Formula - Health Center for Better Living
Two caplets contain: Tribulus terrestris extract (20% furanosterois) fruit and root 400 mg • Damiana leaf 125 mg • Fo-ti root 125 mg • Gota Kola leaf extract (10% total asiaticosides) 50 mg • Saw Palmetto berry extract (85-95% sterols and fatty acid) 150 mg • Korean Ginseng root extract (10% ginsenosides) 200 mg.

BLF #30 Head-X - Health Center for Better Living
Each capsule contains: Fenugreek seed 107 mg • Feverfew herb 107 mg • Passion Flower herb 43 mg • Rosemary leaf 43 mg • Peppermint leaf 43 mg • Thyme leaf 21 mg • Marjoram leaf 21 mg • Blue Violet leaf 21 mg • Wood Betony herb 21 mg • Lobelia herb 21 mg.

BLF #31 Healthy Heart - Health Center for Better Living
Each capsule contains: Angelica root 45 mg • Blue Cohosh root 45 mg • Borage herb 45 mg • Capsicum 45 mg • Blue Vervain herb 45 mg • Peppermint leaf 45 mg • Wood Betony herb 45 mg • Sheep Sorrel herb 23 mg • Garlic Bulb 23 mg • Barberry Bark 23 mg • Goldenseal root 23 mg • Motherwort herb 23 mg • Scullcap herb 23 mg.

BLF #35 Sleep Like a Baby - Health Center for Better Living
Each capsule contains: Hops flower 113 mg • Passion flower 113 mg • Scullcap herb 75 mg • Catnip leaf 38 mg • Peppermint leaf 38 mg • Rosemary leaf 38 mg • Mullein leaf 38 mg.

BLF #38 Kidney Flush - Health Center for Better Living
Each caplet contains: Vitamin B6 (as pyridoxine HCl) 5 mg • Magnesium (as magnesium oxide) • Potassium (as potassium citrate) • Uva Ursi Leaf standardized extract (20% arbutin) 100 mg • Chokeberry fruit standardized extract (35% quinic acid) 100 mg • Cranberry juice 10:1 concentrate 50 mg • Dandelion root standardized extract (20% taraxasterol) 50 mg • Aloe Vera 200x gel 25 mg • Herbal Blend 200 mg: Couchgrass (whole plant), Buchu leaf, Uva Ursi leaf, Juniper berry, Hydrangea root, Cornsilk stylus.

BLF #41 Liver De-Tox - Health Center for Better Living
Each capsule contains: Fennel seed 107 mg • Chicory root 107 mg • Angelica root 54 mg • Cleavers herb 54 mg • Dandelion root 27 mg • Gentian root 27 mg • Hops flower 27 mg • Elder flower 27 mg • Wormwood herb 11 mg • Lobelia herb 11 mg.

BLF #42 Prime Lung - Health Center for Better Living
Each capsule contains: Mullein leaf 101 mg • Coltsfoot herb 101 mg • Chickweed herb 67 mg • Fenugreek seed 34 mg • Pennyroyal leaf 34 mg • Myrrh Gum 34 mg • Yarrow flower 34 mg • Nettle leaf 34 mg • Lobelia herb 13 mg.

BLF #43 Bone & Nail Builder - Health Center for Better Living
Each capsule contains: Bee Pollen Granules 87 mg • Horsetail 43 mg • Oatstraw 43 mg • Kelp Atlantic 43 mg • Ginseng root 43 mg • Foti root 43 mg • Chamomile flower 43 mg • Rose hips 43 mg • Red Clover blossom 43 mg • Lobelia Herb 17 mg.

BLF #44 Woman's Change - Health Center for Better Living
Two tablets contain: Black Cohosh root extract (2.5% triterpene glycosides) 160 mg • Dong Quai root extract (1% lingustilide) 200 mg • Chaste Tree berry extract (5% vitexi capcin) 100 mg • Licorice root extract (13% glycyrrhizin) 100 mg • Soybean and Kudzu root extract (20% total isoflavones) 150 mg • Damiana leaf 100 mg • Wild Yam root extract (5% diosgenin) 150 mg • Red Clover flowers 100 mg.

BLF #47 Rest Ease - Health Center for Better Living
Each capsule contains: Valerian root 101 mg • Wintergreen leaf 67 mg • Peppermint leaf 67 mg • Spearmint leaf 67 mg • Sassafras root bark 34 mg • Capsicum 34 mg • Burdock root 34 mg • Buckthorn bark 34 mg • Lobelia herb 13 mg.

Some Brand Name Natural Products - What they Contain

www.NaturalDatabase.com contains MANY more listings than appear here.
Editor's Notes are located on pages 2155-2163.

BLF #48 Anti-Stress - Health Center for Better Living
Each capsule contains: Hops flower 99 mg • Valerian root 99 mg • Scullcap herb 66 mg • Catnip leaf 66 mg • Passion Flower herb 66 mg • Red Clover herb 33 mg • Black Cohosh root 20 mg.

BLF #49 Stable Sugar - Health Center for Better Living
Each capsule contains: Juniper berry 94 mg • Uva Ursi leaf 94 mg • Garlic bulb 94 mg • Dandelion root 47 mg • Capsicum 47 mg • Mullein leaf 47 mg • Licorice root 28 mg.

BLF #52 Fatigue Fighter - Health Center for Better Living
Prime Ingredients: Capsicum • Ginseng.

BLF #53 Male Vigor - Health Center for Better Living
Two caplets contain: Yohimbe bark extract (2% yohimbe, 4% total alkaiods) 500 mg • Tribulus terrestris extract (20% furanosterols) fruit and root • Korean Ginseng root extract (10% ginsenosides) 200 mg • Yerba Mate leaf extract (20% total alkaloids) 125 mg • Saw Palmetto berry extract (85-95% sterols and fatty acid) 160 mg • Male support blend of Damiana leaf, Fo-ti root, Gota Kola leaf, and Pumpkin Seed concentrate 250 mg.

BLF #54 Sinus & Hayfever Ingredients - Health Center for Better Living
Each capsule contains: Myrrh Gum 148 mg • Echinacea Root 74 mg • Bayberry Bark 74 mg • Plantain Herb 74 mg • Saw Palmetto Berry 22 mg • Licorice Root 22 mg • Goldenseal Herb.

BLF #55 Pro Skin Enhancer - Health Center for Better Living
Each capsule contains: Red Clover blossom 115 mg • Spikenard root 115 mg • Dandelion root 58 mg • Chickweed herb 29 mg • Plantain herb 29 mg • Blue Vervain herb 29 mg • Sarsaparilla root 29 mg • Buckthorn bark 29 mg • Goldenseal root 17 mg.

BLF #57 Vein Vanish - Health Center for Better Living
Each capsule contains: White Oak bark 87 mg • Witch Hazel bark 87 mg • Bayberry bark 87 mg • Capsicum 87 mg • Kelp Atlantic 43 mg • Goldenseal root 43 mg • Lobelia herb 17 mg.

BLF #59 Weight Loss - Health Center for Better Living
Each capsule contains: Nettle leaf 139 mg • Chickweed herb 93 mg • Seawrack 93 mg • Kelp Atlantic 35 mg • Fennel seed 23 mg • Hawthorn berry 23 mg • Dandelion root 12 mg • Echinacea root 12 mg • Burdock root 12 mg • Licorice root 5 mg • Chia seed 5 mg.

BLF #6 Healthy Joints - Health Center for Better Living
Burdock • Alfalfa • Kelp • Vitamin C • Vitamin E • Vitamin B6.

BLF #61 P.M.S. Stop - Health Center for Better Living
Each capsule contains: Black Cohosh Root 82 mg • Dong Quai Root 82 mg • Red Raspberry Leaf 82 mg • Chaste Tree Berry 57 mg • Ginger Root 49 mg • Dandelion Root 41 mg • Motherwort Herb 33 mg • Valerian Root 25 mg.

BLF #75 Prostate Support - Health Center for Better Living
Two tablets contain: Zinc (as zinc glycinate) 15 mg • Saw Palmetto berry extract (85-95% sterols and fatty acid) 320 mg • Pygeum bark 4:1 extract 100 mg • Pumpkin seed 10:1 concentrate 100 mg • Tomato lycopene concentrate (10,000 lycopene) 100 mg • Urinary tract support blend [Chokeberry extract (35% quinic acid), Cranberry juice 10:1 concentrate, Uva-Ursi leaf extract (20% arbutin)].

BLF #9: 120 Over 80 - Health Center for Better Living
Two tablets contain: Calcium (as calcium carbonate and calcium citratemalate-glycinate) 500 mg • Magnesium (as magnesium oxide and magnesium amino acid chelate) 200 mg • Potassium (as postassium citrate) • Ginger root extract (5% gingerols) 100 mg • Odor-controlled Garlic extract (10,000 ppm allicin) 300 mg • Hawthorn berry extract (5% flavonoid glycosides) 250 mg • Capsicum pepper 50 mg • Panax Ginseng root extract (10% ginsenosides) 100 mg • Onion bulb 50 mg • Parsley leaf 50 mg.

Block It - PotentHerbs
Two capsules contain: Proprietary Blend 1000 mg: Chromium Polynicotinate 200 mcg, Phaseolus Vulgaris L (Phase 2), Chitosan (Quik-o-san), Gymnema Sylvestre. Other Ingredients: Certified Kosher Gel Caps.
See Editor's Note No. 37.

Blood Nutrients - J. R. Carlson Laboratories, Inc.
Each capsule contains: Vitamin A (from fish liver oil) 5000 IU • Vitamin C (as ascorbic acid) 120 mg • Vitamin E (as D-alpha tocopheryl succinate) 30 IU • Thiamin (vitamin B1, as thiamin hydrochloride) 10 mg • Riboflavin (vitamin B2) 10 mg • Niacin (vitamin B3, as niacinamide) 20 mg • Vitamin B6 (as pyridoxine hydrochloride) 10 mg • Folate (folic acid) 400 mcg • Vitamin B12 (cyanocobalamin) 300 mcg • Pantothenic Acid (as di-calcium pantothenate) 10 mg • Iron (as iron glycinate chelate) 28 mg • Copper (as copper glycinate chelate) 2 mg • Molybdenum (as molybdenum glycinate chelate) 200 mcg • Edible Hemoglobin 25 mg • Stomach substance 10 mg • Liver concentrate 100 mg.

Blood Pressure - Nutrivention
Three tablets contain: Vitamin B6 100 mg • Calcium 50 mg • Potassium 45 mg • Magnesium 30 mg • Manganese 15 mg • Vitamin D 50 IU • Hawthorne berries 500 mg • Apple Pectin 500 mg • Garlic powder concentrate 500 mg • Cayenne pepper 500 mg • Black Cohosh 300 mg • Valerian root (Star root) 200 mg • Hops 200 mg • L-Taurine 100 mg.

Blood Pressure - Grandma's Herbs
Each capsule contains: Proprietary Blend 0.477 g: Cayenne Pepper fruit, Garlic clove, Black Cohosh root, Mistletoe leaf, Sassafras root, Ginko leaf, Valerian root, Wild Yam root, Nettle leaf, Horsetail grass, Bladderwrack leaf, Hyssop herb, Ginseng root, Bladder Pod herb, Dong Quai root, Bayberry bark. Other Ingredients: Gelatin.

Blood Pressure Control - TwinLab
Two tablets contain: C-12 Peptide (enzymatically hydrolyzed casein) 100 mg. Other Ingredients: Maltodextrin, Cellulose, Vegetable Stearic Acid, Calcium Phosphate, Croscarmellose Sodium, Silica, Magnesium Stearate, Polyethylene Glycol, Carrageenan, Water.

Blood Pressure Formula - HERBALmax
Gouteng branches • Ju flowers • Xiakucao flowers • Juming seeds.

Blood Pressurex - Nature's Sunshine
Each capsule contains: Vitamin E 30 IU • Proprietary Blend 385 mg: L-Arginine, Olive leaf extract (olea europaea), Goldenrod aerial parts (solidago virgaurea), Coleus root extract (coleus forskohlii), Hawthorn berry extract (crataegus oxyacanthoides), Grape seed extract (vitis vinifera). Other Ingredients: Magnesium Stearate, Silicon Dioxide, Gelatin, Water.

Blood Sugar Blues - The Herbalist
Devil's Club root bark • Blueberry leaf • Dandelion root • Oregon Grape root • Uva Ursi leaf • Juniper berry • Licorice root • Elecampane root.

Blood Sugar Essentials - Swanson Health Products
Each tablet contains: Vitamin C (as calcium ascorbate) 100 mg • Vitamin E (as d-alpha tocopheryl succinate) 133.3 IU • Magnesium (from magnesium oxide) 66.7 mg • Biotin 333.3 mcg • Zinc (OptiZinc) 5 mg • Chromium (from Chromax chromium picolinate) 66.7 mcg • Gymnema Sylvestre powder 134 mg • Momordica Charantia (2.5%) 100 mg • Fenugreek seed powder 67 mg • Inositol 50 mg • Vanadyl Sulfate 4 mg.

Blood Sugar Formula - Nature's Way
Three capsules contain: Bilberry leaf 255 mg • Bitter Melon dried extract 150 mg • Caromix (Mixed Carotenoids) 30 mg • Chromium Polynicotinate 300 mcg • Fenugreek dried extract 210 mg • Gymnema sylvestre dried extract 66 mg • Prickly Pear leaf pad 420 mg. Other Ingredients: Gelatin, Magnesium Stearate, Millet.

Some Brand Name Natural Products - What they Contain

www.NaturalDatabase.com contains MANY more listings than appear here.
Editor's Notes are located on pages 2155-2163.

BRAND NAMES

Bloodroot Celandine Supreme **-** Gaia Herbs
Fifteen drops contain: Proprietary Blend 20 mg: Bloodroot (sanguinaria canadensis), Celandine tops and roots (chelidonium majus), Prickly Ash bark (xanthoxylum clava-herculis), Spring Water, 55-65% Pure Grain Alcohol USP.

Bloussant **-** WellQuest International, Inc.
Each tablet contains: Saw Palmetto extract (serenoa repens) leaf 150 mg • Fennel seed (foeniculum vulgare) fruit 50 mg • Dong Quai leaf 50 mg • Damiana (tumera diffusa) leaf 100 mg • Blessed Thistle (cnicus benedictus) leaf 40 mg • Dandelion (taraxaci herba) root 40 mg • Watercress (nasturtium officinale) leaf 40 mg • Black Cohosh (cimicifuga racemosa) root 50 mg • Wild Yam (dioscorea villosa) root 40 mg. Other Ingredients: Silicon Dioxide, Magnesium Stearate, Titanium Dioxide, Gelatin, and Water.

Blubberwack **-** The Herbalist
Bladderwrack • Gotu Kola herb • Kelp • Echinacea root • Kola Nut • Licorice root.

Blue Cohosh **-** Nature's Sunshine
Each capsule contains: Blue Cohosh root (caulophyllum thalictroides) 450 mg. Other Ingredients: Gelatin, Water.

Blue Green Algae **-** PhysioLogics
Each capsule contains: Klamath Lake Blue Green Algae (aphanizomenon flos-aquae) 500 mg. Other Ingredients: Gelatin, Vegetable Magnesium Stearate, Silica.

Blue Green Algae **-** Rexall - Sundown
Two capsules contain: Blue Green Algae Blend: Spirulina Blue-Green Algae (spirulina platensis), Watercress (aerial parts), Klamath Blue-Green Algae (aphanizomenon flos-aquae) 750 mg. Other Ingredients: Gelatin.

Blue Green Algae from Upper Klamath Lake **-** Futurebiotics LLC
Blue-Green algae 500 mg.

Blue Green Micro Algae **-** Olympian Labs
Each capsule contains: Blue Green Micro Algae 380 mg.

Blue Joint Soother **-** Home Health Products, Inc.
Aloe Vera Gel • Emu Oil • SD-Alcohol 40-B • Glucosamine Sulfate (from shellfish) • Dimethyl Sulfone (MSM) • Oleoresin of Capsicum • Arnica extract • Sorbitol • Chondroitin Sulfate • Menthol • White Nettle extract • Witch Hazel • Coriander Oil • Kava Kava extract • Willow bark extract • Propylene Glycol • Methylparaben • Propylparaben • Diazolidinyl Urea • Carbomer • Chamomile • Marigold extract • Triethanolamine • Ascorbyl Palmitate (vitamin C) • Tocopherol Acetate (vitamin E) • Fragrance • FD&C Blue #1.
See Editor's Note No. 15.

Blue Vervain Liquid **-** Nature's Sunshine
Blue Vervain herb extract (verbena officinalis) • Vegetable Glycerin.

Blue-Green Connection **-** HealthWatchers System
Spirulina • Chlorella • Klamath Lake Algae • Ginkgo Biloba • CoQ10 • Wheatgrass • Alfalfa • Chlorophyll.

Blue-Green Stuff **-** Blue Stuff, Inc.
Each gel cap contains: Organic Wheatgrass juice powder • Barley Grass juice powder • organic Oatgrass juice powder • organic Spirulina.

B-Nase **-** Nutraceutics Corp.
Four sprays contain: Vitamin B12 500 mcg • Dibencozide (coenzyme B12) 500 mcg • ATP (adenosine triphosphate) 10,000 mcg • Alpha Glycerylphosphorylcholine 10,000 mcg. Other Ingredients: Purified Water, Sodium Benzoate, Potassium Sorbate, Glycerin, Citric Acid, Sodium Citrate.

Body Answers Grapefruit Diet **-** GNC
Each capsule contains: CitraSens Grapefruit extract 500 mg. Other Ingredients: Gelatin, Cellulose.

Body Balance **-** Life Force International
Each 30 mL contains: Proprietary Blend: Aloe Vera juice, Black Cherry, Raw Honey, Pure Water, Fucus Gardneri, Ulva Latuca, Alaria Valida, Nerecocystis Leutkeana, Laminaria, Ulva Linza, Gigartina, Costaria Costata, Phodymenia Pertusa.

Body Booster with Power **-** Aspen Group, Inc.
Each tablet contains: Raw bovine testicular concentrate 300 mg • Multiple Glans Raw Gland concentrate 225 mg: Porcine Liver, Porcine Duodenum, Porcine Pancreas, Bovine Heart, Bovine Pituitary, Bovine Kidney, Bovine Spleen, Bovine Thymus, Bovine Adrenal concentrate • Cayenne 25 mg • Gotu Kola 25 mg • Fo-Ti 25 mg • Damiana 32 mg • Guarana 50 mg.
See Editor's Note No. 31.

Body Contouring Cream **-** Herbalife International of America, Inc.
Water • Cetyl Esters • Isopropyl Myristate • Stearyl Alcohol •Hydrogenated Coco-glycerides • Steareth-20 • Caffeine • Propylene Glycol • Lecithin • Aminophylline • Imidazolidinyl • Urea •Methylparaben • Carbomer • Propylparaben • Triethanolamine • Algae • Magnolia Bark extract • Fragrance • Horsetail extract • Rose Hips extract • Mate.

Body Detox **-** BodyHealth
Oligopolysaccharides • Glycoproteins • Phospholipids • Colloidal sea minerals • Micro-cluster Structured Water • Microactivated Enzymes • Microactivated Mercury-free Chlorella • Lipoic Acid • NAC • Glutathione • Vitamin C • Hyaluronic Acid • Fulvic Acid • Ferulic Acid • Protease Inhibitors.

Body Fortress Hardcore Formula Creatine Powder **-** U.S. Nutrition
Each scoop (5 g) contains: HPLC Pure Creatine Monohydrate 5000 mg.

Body Guard **-** Jamieson
Chlorhexidine Gluconate • Glycerin • Nonoxynol-9 • Witch Hazel Herbal Extract.

Body Octane **-** MAN
Each level 1 tsp (8 grams) serving contains: Citruline Malate 3500 mg • L-Carnitine L-Tartrate 1500 mg • Beta-Alanine 1000 mg • Histidine 500 mg. Other Ingredients: Maltodextrin, Citric Acid, Natural Orange Flavor, Natural Vanilla, Sucralose, Sodium Chloride.

Body Rewards Daily Multiple **-** Enzymatic Therapy
Each tablet contains: Vitamin A (50% as beta carotene and as retinyl acetate) 5000 IU • Vitamin C (ascorbic acid) 200 mg • Vitamin D (as cholecalciferol) 400 IU • Vitamin E (as d-alpha tocopheryl acid succinate) 100 IU • Vitamin K (as phytonadione) 80 mcg • Thiamin (as thiamin HCl, vitamin B1) 15 mg • Riboflavin (vitamin B2) 17 mg • Niacin (as niacin and niacinamide) 20 mg • Vitamin B6 (as pyridoxine HCl) 20 mg • Folic Acid 800 mcg • Vitamin B12 (as cyanocobalamin) 60 mcg • Biotin 300 mcg • Pantothenic Acid (as calcium D-pantothenate) 10 mg • Calcium (from tricalcium phosphate) 200 mg • Phosphorus (as tricalcium phosphate) 100 mg • Iodine (as potassium iodide) 150 mcg • Magnesium (as magnesium oxide and magnesium aspartate) 1000 mg • Zinc (as zinc ascorbate) 15 mg • Selenium (as L-selenomethionine) 70 mcg • Manganese (as manganese citrate) 2 mg • Chromium (as chromium picolinate) 120 mcg • Molybdenum (as sodium molybdate) 75 mcg • Green Tea leaf extract (camellia sinensis, standardized to contain 4.2 mg caffeine) 30 mg • Boron (as sodium borate) 1 mg • Vanadium (as vanadyl sulfate) 16 mcg. Other Ingredients: Cellulose, Modified Cellulose, Modified Cellulose Gum, Magnesium Stearate, Lecithin, Riboflavin Color, Carnauba Wax.

Body Rewards Digestion Formula **-** Enzymatic Therapy
Each capsule contains: Proprietary Plant Enzyme Blend 156 mg: Protease, Amylase, Lipase, Lactase, Phytase, Cellulase, Sucrase, Maltase. Other Ingredients: Gelatin, Cellulose, Titanium Dioxide Color.

Body Rewards Fruit & Veggie 5 - Enzymatic Therapy
Eight capsules contain: Vitamin A (as beta carotene) 11,822 IU • Vitamin C (ascorbic acid) 480 mg • Psyllium husk (plantago ovata) 2665 mg • Pectin (from citrus fruits) 16 mg • Proprietary PhytoRedoxin Blend 19 mg: Lutein 5% (from calendula officinalis), Lycopene, Quercetin. Other Ingredients: Cellulose, Gelatin, Titanium Dioxide Color, Magnesium Stearate, Silicon Dioxide.

Body Rewards Healthy Skin - Enzymatic Therapy
Three softgels contain: Proprietary Essential Oils Blend 2402 mg: Fish oil, Borage seed oil (borago officinalis), Flax seed oil (linum usitatissimum). Other Ingredients: Gelatin, Glycerin, Mixed Tocopherols (preservative).

Body Rox - USANA Health Sciences
Each tablet contains: Vitamin A (as Beta Carotene) 3000 IU • Vitamin C (as Calcium Ascorbate) 167 mg • Vitamin D (Vitamin D3 as Cholecalciferol) 133 IU • Vitamin E (as D-Alpha Tocopheryl Succinate) 66.7 IU • Vitamin K (as Phylloquinone) 12 mcg • Thiamine (as Thiamine HCl) 3 mg • Riboflavin 3 mg • Niacin (as Niacin and Niacinamide) 5 mg • Vitamin B6 (as Pyridoxine HCl) 3 mg • Folate (as Folic Acid) 267 mcg • Vitamin B12 (as Cyanocobalamin) 20 mcg • Biotin 100 mcg • Pantothenic Acid (as D-Calcium Pantothenate) 10 mg • Calcium (as Ascorbate and Citrate) 50 mg • Iodine (as Potassium Iodide) 50 mcg • Magnesium (as Amino Acid Chelate) 25 mg • Zinc (as Citrate) 4 mg • Selenium (as Amino Acid Complex) 40 mcg • Copper (as Gluconate) 0.33 mg • Manganese (as Amino Acid Chelate) 1 mg • Chromium (as Amino Acid Chelate) 50 mcg • Molybdenum (as Amino Acid Chelate) 10 mcg • Bioflavonoid Complex 30 mg: Rutin, Hesperidin (Citrus SPP. L. fruit), Green Tea Extract Decaffeinated (Camellia Sinensis Hunt leaf) • Inositol 10 mg • Choline Bitartrate 15 mg • Cruciferous Extract (Brassica Oleracea L.) 25 mg • N-Acetyl-L-Cysteine 10 mg • Boron (as Amino Acid Complex) 0.33 mg. Other Ingredients: Microcrystalline Cellulouse, Croscarmellose Sodium, Maltodextrin, Ascorbyl Palmitate, Sodium Citrate, Collodial Silicon Dioxide, Lecithin.

Body Shape - Hydroderm
Organic Kukui nut oil • Organic Caffeine • Organic Lecithin (liposomes). Other Ingredients: Water, Potassium Sorbate, Peg 8 Stearate, Cetyl Alcohol, Stearic Acid, Polysorbate 80, Decamethyltetrasiloxane, Silicone Resin Dimethicone, Green Tea Extract, Carbomer, Triethanolamine, Silicone Glycol Copolymer, Propylene Glycol, Sodium Chloride, Tocopheryl Acetate Dl-a, Disodium EDTA, Glycolic Acid, Fragrance Tropical, Propylparaben, Methylparaben.

Body Solutions Evening Formula - Mark Nutritionals, Inc.
Each tablespoon contains: Chromium (as chromium picolinate, chromium polynicotinate, and chromium cruciferate) 15 mcg • Proprietary Blend of Aloe Vera Gel, Collmark, Fosmark, Leanmark, Conjugated Linoleic Acid, Stevia 6 mL. Other Ingredients: Purified Water, Glycerin, Natural Kiwi Flavor, Natural Strawberry Flavor, Xanthan Gum, Sodium benzoate, Potassium sorbate.

Body Stuff - Blue Stuff, Inc.
Each 8 oz bottle contains: Whole leaf Aloe Vera concentrate • Purified Water • Squalene • Emu oil • Glyceryl Stearate • Lanolin Alcohol • Propylene Glycol • Sorbitan Sesquioleate • Stearic Acid • Dimethicone • PEG-75 Lanolin • Allantoin • Polysorbate-60 • Apricot Kernel oil • Sesame Seed oil • Jojoba oil • Carbomer-940 • Treithanolamine • Methylparaben • Fragrance • Imidazolidinyl Urea • Proylparaben.

BodyLean Bars - Advocare International
Maltitol Syrup • BodyLean Protein Blend (whey protein isolate, calcium caseinate, soy protein isolate, milk protein isolate) • Dark Chocolate flavored coating (sugar, fractionated palm kernel oil, cocoa [processed with alkali], lactose, dextrose, soy lecithin, natural flavor) • High Fructose Corn Syrup • Rice Syrup • Partially Defatted Peanut Flour • Crisp Grain (soy protein isolate, rice flour, malt, salt) • Ground Peanuts • Natural Flavor • Honey • Salt • Magnesium Oxide • Glycerin • Potassium Chloride • L-Leucine • Sucralose • Ascorbic Acid • L-Valine • L-Isoleucine • Maltodextrin • Niacinamide • Calcium Pantothenate • Bromelain • Papain • Manganese Sulfate • Pyridoxine HCl • Riboflavin • Thiamine Mononitrate • Biotin • Cyanocobalamin.

BodyLean Shake, Vanilla - Advocare International
Metabolically Balanced Protein Isolate (containing total milk protein, calcium, sodium caseinate, whey protein concentrate, soy protein concentrate, branched chain amino acids [L-leucine, L-isoleucine, L-valine]) • Fructose • Natural Flavors • Artificial Flavors • Magnesium Oxide • Ascorbic Acid • Acesulfame Potassium • Pyridoxine Hydrochloride • Calcium Pantothenate • Niacin • Manganese Sulfate • Papain • Bromelain • Thiamine Hydrochloride • Riboflavin • Biotin • Cyanocobalamin.

BodyQUICK - BrainQUICKEN LLC Research and Technologies
Four capsules contain: Niacinamide 20 mg • Vitamin B6 (pyridoxine HCl) 25 mg • Folic Acid 400 mcg • Vitamin B12 (cobalamin) 1000 mcg • Pantothenic Acid (calcium pantothenate) 40 mg • Proprietary Cognamine Complex 1610 mg: Cordyceps Sinensis, Choline Bitartrate, L-Glutamine, L-Tyrosine, Salix Alba, Phosphatidylserine, Ciwujia, 2-Dimethylaminoethanol, Salisburia Adiantifolia, Vinpocetine, Huperzine A • Paullinia Cupana 810 mg • Alpha-Lipoic Acid 30 mg. Other Ingredients: Gelatin, Magnesium Stearate, Silica. This product is also known as BrainQUICKEN.

Body-Spirit-Mind Enhancer - Alacer
Each tablet contains: Vitamin C (as calcium amgnesium ascorbate) 80 mg • Ginkgo Biloba 50 mg • Siberian Ginseng 100 mg • Flower Pollen extract 25 mg • Magnesium Aspartate 25 mg.

BodySynergy Anti-Craving Formula - Rexall - Sundown
Two tablets contain: Vitamin B-6 (from pyridoxine HCl and pyridoxal-5-phophate) 12 mg • Calcium 125 mg • Chromium (from chromium polynicotinate) 133 mcg • Sodium 10 mg • BodySynergy proprietary blend 1237 mg: DL-Phenylalanine, L-Tyrosine, Stinging Nettle leaf, L-Glutamine, L-Carnitine. Other Ingredients: Dicalcium Phosphate, Cellulose, Croscarmellose Sodium, Silica, Stearic Acid, Calcium Citrate, Hydroxypropyl Methylcellulose, Magnesium Stearate, PEG.

BodySynergy Meal Replacement Drink Mix (chocolate flavor) - Rexall - Sundown
Each packet contains: Sodium 100 mg • Protein 18 g • Vitamin A (Retinyl Palmitate) 1250 IU • Vitamin C (Ascorbic Acid) 15 mg • Calcium 500 mg • Electrolytic Iron 4.5 mg • Vitamin D (Cholecalciferol) 100 IU • Vitamin E (dl-Alpha Tocopheryl Acetate) 7.5 IU • Thiamin Mononitrate 0.375 mg • Riboflavin 0.425 mg • Niacin (Niacinamide) 5 mg • Vitamin B6 (Pyridoxine Hydrochloride) 0.5 mg • Folate (Folic Acid) 100 mcg • Vitamin B12 (Cyanocobalamin) 1.5 mg • Biotin 75 mcg • Pantothenic Acid (Calicum D-Pantothenate) 2.5 mg • Phosphorous (Dicalcium Phosphate) 700 mg • Iodine (Potassium Iodide) 37.5 mcg • Magnesium 8 mg • Zinc Oxide 3.75 mg • Copper Gluconate 0.5 mg. Other Ingredients: Fructose, Maltodextrin, Soy Protein isolate, Whey Protein isolate, Whey Protein concentrate, Cocoa Processed with Alkali, Dicalcium Phosphate, Natural and Artificial Chocolate flavor, Carrageenan, Dipotassium Phosphate, Natural Cream flavor, Xanthan Gum, Stevia extract.

BodySynergy Meal Replacement Drink Mix (vanilla flavor) - Rexall - Sundown
Each packet contains: Sodium 100 mg • Protein 18 g • Potassium 340 mg • Vitamin A (Retinyl Palmitate) 1250 IU • Vitamin C (Ascorbic Acid) 15 g • Calcium 500 mg • Electrolytic Iron 4.5 mg • Vitamin D (Cholecalciferol) 100 IU • Vitamin E (dl-Alpha Tocopheryl Acetate) 7.5 IU • Thiamin Mononitrate 0.375 mg • Riboflavin 0.425 mg • Niacin (Niacinamide) 5 mg • Vitamin B6 (Pyridoxine Hydrochloride) 0.5 mg • Folate (Folic Acid) 100 mcg • Vitamin B12

BRAND NAM

Cyanocobalamin) 1.5 mcg • Biotin 75 mcg • Pantothenic Acid (Calcium D-Pantothenate) 2.5 mg • Phosphorus (Dicalcium Phosphate) 700 mg • Iodine (Potassium Iodide) 37.5 mcg • Magnesium 8 mg • Zinc Oxide 3.75 mg • Copper Gluconate 0.5 mg. Other Ingredients: Fructose, Maltodextrin, Soy Protein isolate, Whey Protein isolate, Whey Protein concentrate, Cocoa Processed with Alkali, Natural and Artificial Chocolate Flavor, Carrageenan, Dipotassium Phosphate, Natural Cream Flavor, Xanthan Gum, Stevia extract.

Bodyworx Nutri-Genics Complete - Bodyworx Nutri-Genics
Each 2 tbsp serving contains: Vitamin A (palmitate) 5000 IU • Vitamin C (Ester C brand) 300 mg • Vitamin D (cholecalciferol) 400 IU • Vitamin E (D-alpha tocopherol) 150 IU • Vitamin K (phytonadione) 30 mcg • Vitamin B1 (thiamine HCl) 500 mcg • Vitamin B2 (ribo-5-phosphate) 1700 mcg • Vitamin B3 (niacinamide) 20 mcg • Vitamin B5 (D-panthenol) 10 mg • Vitamin B6 (pyridoxine HCl) 2 mg • Vitamin B12 (cyanocobalamin) 50 mcg • Acetyl Carnitine 500 mg • Folic Acid 400 mcg • Biotin (D-biotin) 300 mcg • Choline (choline chloride) 20 mg • Myoinositol (inositol) 20 mg • Cat's Claw (uncaria tomentosa) 10 mg • Coenzyme Q10 200 mg • Tumeric Flavonoids 200 mg • Bioflavonoid from Grape seed extract (OPC) 50 mg • Calcium 1000 mg • Chloride (calcium/chromium) 15.33 mg • D-Mannose 1000 mg • Ginkgo Biloba 60 mg • Magnesium (magnesium sulfate) 400 mg • Milk Thistle (silymarin) 60 mg • Potassium (phosphate/iodide) 50 mg • Sodium (sodium benzoate) 4.8 mg • Sulfur (magnesium/zinc/manganese/iron/copper) 31 mg • Boron (boric acid) 2 mg • Chromium (chromium chloride) 200 mcg • Copper (copper sulfate) 2 mg • Germanium (sesquioxide) 55 mcg • Iodine (potassium iodide) 150 mcg • Iron (ferrous sulfate) 10 mg • Manganese (manganese sulfate) 3 mg • Molybdenum (molybenum glycinate) 200 mcg • Protein (whey) 10 mg • Selenium (sodium selenite) 200 mcg • Zinc (zinc sulfate) 15 mg • Amino Acids from Whey Protein 10 mg/oz: Alanine, Arginine, Aspartic Acid, Cystine, Glutamic Acid, Histadine, Hydroxyproline, Isoleucine, Leucine, Lysine, Methionine, Phenylalanine, Proline, Serine, Threonine, Tryptophan, Tyrosine, Valine • Trace Minerals 900 mg: Antimony, Barium, Beryllium, Bismuth, Bromine, Carbon, Cerium, Cesium, Cobalt, Dysprosium, Erbium, Europium, Fluorine, Gadolinium, Gallium, Gold, Hafnium, Holmium, Hydrogen, Indium, Iridium, Lanthanum, Lithium, Lutetium, Nickel, Niobium, Nitrogen, Osmium, Oxygen, Palladium, Platinum, Praseodymium, Rhenium, Rhodium, Rubidium, Ruthenium, Samarium, Scandium, Silicon, Silver, Strontium, Tantalum, Tellurium, Terbium, Thallium, Thorium, Thulium, Tin, Titanium, Tungsten, Vanadium, Ytterbium, Yttrium, Zirconium • Fatty Acids: Olive oil, Omega 3 Fatty Acids (linolenic acid), Omega 6 Fatty Acids (linoleic acid), Omega 9 Fatty Acids (oleic acid). Other Ingredients: Purified Water, Fructose, Sorbitol, Sodium Benzoate, Natural Flavoring.

Bold BBQ Soynuts - Physicians Laboratories
Each 1/6 cup contains: Certified Isoflavone 10 mg. Other Ingredients: Soy Protein (whole roasted soybeans), Soybean Oil, Salt, Dextroxe, Spices, Malto Dextrin, Smoke Flavor, Paprika, Extractives of Spice and Paprika.

Bone & Joint Care - Natrol, Inc.
Three capsules contain: Vitamin D (as cholecalciferol) 20 IU • Vitamin K (as Phytonadione) 10 mcg • Calcium (as calcium carbonate & calcium citrate) 250 mg • Magnesium (as Magnesium oxide) 125 mg • Zinc (as zinc citrate) 5 mg • Copper (as copper gluconate) 100 mcg • Glucosamine Sulfate 250 mg • MSM (Methyl Sulfonyl Methane) 250 mg • Ipriflavone 100 mg • Sea Cucumber • 100 mg Mucopolysaccarides (26%) 26 mg • Horsetail grass 100 mg • Silica (8%) 8 mg • Bamboo 100 mg • Salicylic Acid 10 mg • Boron 2 mg. Other Ingredients: Silicon Dioxide, Magnesium Stearate, Gelatin.

Bone & Joint Defense System - Puritan's Pride
Each tablet contains: Vitamin A 208.34 IU • Vitamin C 8.33 mg • Vitamin D 66.67 IU • Vitamin E 8.33 IU • Vitamin K 8.33 mcg • Vitamin B6 1.33 mg • Folic Acid 100 mcg • Vitamin B12 8.33 mcg • Pantothenic Acid 8.33 mg • Calcium 333.33 mg • Magnesium 83.33 mg • Zinc 6 mg • Selenium 2 mcg • Copper 1 mg • Manganese 3.67 mg • Molybdenum 83.33 mcg • Potassium 33 mg • Silica 667 mcg • Boron 1.33 mg • Vanadium 66.67 mcg • Glucosamine Sulfate 41.67 mg • N-Acetyl Cysteine 4.3 mg • Pycnogenol Pine bark extract 80 mcg • Coenzyme Q-10 84 mcg • DL-Phenylalanine 4.33 mg • L-Proline 4.33 mg • Glycine 16.67 mg • S.O.D. 8.33 mcg • Mucopolysaccharide complex 21 mg • Hydrolyzed Collagen Protein 21 mg • Herbal Support Complex 36.67 mg. Other Ingredients: Milk Thistle, Alfalfa, Garlic, Young Barley Grass, Spirulina, Kelp, Devil's Claw, Hydrangea Root, Irish Moss, Yucca Root, White Willow Bark, Slippery Elm Bark.

Bone & Joint Formula - Oasis Wellness Network
Two tablets contain: Vitamin C 100 mg • Vitamin D (D3) 100 IU • Calcium (as aspartate, phosphate) 95 mg • Magnesium (as citrate) 24 mg • Manganese (as amino acid chelate) 2.5 mg • Glucosamine Sulfate 250 mg • Microcrystalline Hydroxyapatite (MCHC) 200 mg • Chondroitin Sulfate 150 mg • Horsetail stems/leaf extract (4:1) 10 mg • MaxCell Proprietary Blend 50 mg: Zisyphus Jujube, Aloe Vera gel, Piper Nigrum, Glycyrrhiza Glabra • Boron (as citrate) 1.5 mg. Other Ingredients: Stearic Acid, Cellulose, Magnesium Stearate, Silica. See Editor's Note No. 15.

Bone 350 Plus - Atrium Biotechnologies
Each tablet contains: Raw Calf Bone concentrate 350 mg • Equisetum (Horsetail Rush) 150 mg.
See Editor's Note No. 14.

Bone Assure - Life Extension
Six capsules contain: Calcium (from bis-glycinate, supplying elemental calcium) 1000 mg • Magnesium Oxide (supplying elemental magnesium) 320 mg • Zinc Citrate (supplying elemental zinc 12 mg) 35 mg • Manganese Citrate (supplying elemental manganese 3 mg) 10 mg • Boron (from amino acid chelate) 2 mg • Copper Sulfate (supplying elemental copper 1.5 mg) 3.7 mg • Oat Straw (10:1 silica source) 40 mg • Vitamin D (D3) 400 IU • Folic Acid 200 mcg • TMG (trimethylglycine/betaine) 100 mg • Vitamin B6 15 mg.

Bone Balance - Source Naturals
Each tablet contains: Vitamin C (as magnesium & calcium ascorbates, ascorbic acid & manganese ascorbate) 72 mg • Vitamin D (as cholecalciferol) 50 IU • Vitamin B6 (as pyridoxine HCl) 5 mg • Folate (as folic acid) 150 mg • Calcium (as calcium citrate, carbonate, malate, fumarate, ethanolamine phosphate & ascorbate) 150 mg • Magnesium (as magnesium oxide, citrate, fumarate, malate, & ascorbate) 150 mg • Zinc (as zinc chelate) 2 mg • Copper (as copper sebacate) 250 mg • Manganese (as manganese ascorbate) 2 mg • Genistein-Rich Soy concentrate (SoyLife brand, yielding 6.4 mg total isoflavones) 208 mg • L-Lysine (HCl) 15 mg • Silica (from horsetail) 3 mg • Boron (as amino acid chelate) 750 mcg.

Bone Builder - Schiff
Three tablets contain: Calcium (carbonate, chelate, citrate-malate) 1000 mg • Magnesium (oxide, chelate) 400 mg • Vitamin D (as vitamin D3, cholecalciferol) 400 IU • Vitamin C (ascorbic acid) 150 mg • Vitamin K (phytonadione) 25 mcg • Vitamin B6 (pyridoxine, coenzyme pyridoxal-5-phosphate) 10 mg • Vitamin B12 (cyanocobalamin, coenzyme dibencozide) 25 mcg • Folic Acid (folic acid, coenzyme tetrahydrafolate) 200 mcg • Boron (chelate) 1 mg • Zinc (Optizinc) 7.5 mg • Copper (lysinate) 1 mg • Manganese (glycinate) 10 mg • Molybdenum (chelate) 50 mcg • Silica (magnesium trisillicate) 25mg • Strontium (chloride) 100 mcg • Vanadium (vanadyl sulfate) 50 mcg • Sulphur (vanadyl sulfate) 30 mcg • Betaine HCl 50 mg • Glucose Polymers (maltodextrin) 50 mcg • Citrus Bioflavonoids Complex 250 mg • Fennel (4:1 extract) 100 mg • Black Cohosh (4:1 extract) 100 mg • Blessed Thistle (4:1 extract) 100 mg. Natural base: Cellulose, Vegetable Sterates, Silica.

Some Brand Name Natural Products - What they Contain

www.NaturalDatabase.com contains MANY more listings than appear here.
Editor's Notes are located on pages 2155-2163.

Bone Building Hair Teeth & Nails Formula - Youngevity
Calcium 250 mg • Magnesium 100 mg • Manganese 0.5 mg • Boron 240 mg • Vitamin D (as Vitamin D3) 150 IU • Horsetail grass 25 mg • Rose Hips 25 mg • Vilcabamba Mineral Essence: Potassium, Calcium, Magnesium, Zinc, Chromium, Selenium, Iron, Copper, Molybdenum, Vanadium, Iodine, Cobalt, Manganese.

Bone Calcium - NOW Foods
Four tablets contain: Calcium (from 4000 mg Microcrystalline Hydroxyapatite) 1000 mg • Magnesium (from 835 mg Magnesium Oxide) 500 mg • Phosphorus (Hydroxyapatite) 500 mg • Zinc (Amino Acid Chelate) 15 mg • Copper (Amino Acid Chelate) 2 mg • Vitamin D (Cholecalciferol) 200 IU • Manganese (Amino Acid Chelate) 7 mg • Boron (Amino Acid Chelate) 3 mg.

Bone Care - Puritan's Pride
Two tablets contain: Vitamin D (as Cholecalciferol) 800 IU • Vitamin K (as Phytonadione) 100 mcg • Calcium (as Calcium Carbonate and Calcium Gluconate) 1,200 mg • Magnesium (as Magnesium Oxide and Magnesium Gluconate) 300 mg. Other Ingredients: Cellulose (Plant Origin), Croscarmellose, Cellulose Coating, Vegetable Magnesium Stearate, Mannitol.

Bone Enrich with Ostivone - Pro Health
Two caplets contain: Vitamin D (cholecalciferol) 200 IU • Calcium (citrate, carbonate) 600 mg • Ostivone Ipriflavone (7-isopropoxyisoflavone) 300 mg • SoyLife Soy extract (3% isoflavones) 100 mg • Boron (citrate, glycinate, aspartate) 1.5 mg. Other Ingredients: Microcrystalline Cellulose (plant fiber), Stearic Acid, Magnesium Stearate, Croscarmellose Sodium, Glaze.

Bone Essentials - Swanson Health Products
Two capsules contain: Vitamin D (as cholecalciferol) 400 IU • Vitamin K (as phytonadione) 100 mcg • Calcium (from citrate/citrate maleate) 350 mg • Magnesium (from glycinate/oxide) 174 mg • Zinc (from zinc oxide) 30 mg • Copper (from copper gluconate) 2 mg • Manganese (from manganese gluconate) 3.6 mg • SoyLife Soy extract (3% soy isoflavones) 50 mg • Lactose 5 mg • L-Arginine 5 mg • L-Lysine (HCl) 5 mg • Silica (horsetail herb) 5 mg • Boron (from gluconate) 3 mg • Strontium Chloride 20 mcg.

Bone Formula - Pharmanex
Two capsules contain: Vitamin C (as Ester C brand calcium ascorbate complex) 60 mg • Vitamin D (as Vitamin D3, cholecalciferol) 50 IU • Vitamin K (as vitamin K1, phytonadione) 20 mcg • Calcium (as calcium carbonate, calcium propionate) 250 mg • Magnesium (as magnesium asparate, magnesium oxide) 125 mg • Isoflavones from Soy extract 12.5 mg • Silicon (as sodium metasilicate) 5 mg • Boron (as boron citrate) 1.5 mg. Other Ingredients: Magnesium Stearate, Sodium Carboxymethylcellulose.

Bone Health - Enzymes, Inc.
Two capsules contain: Manganese (from Manganese Citrate) 1.5 mg • Boron (from Boron Citrate) 2 mg • Proprietary Enzyme Blend 84 mg: Protease Blend (alkaline, neutral and acid proteases), CereCalase Plus • Proprietary Herbal Blend 310 mg: Chlorella Algae (cracked-wall), Red Clover flower extract (equivalent to 300 mg raw herb), Almond concentrate, Horsetail herb extract (equivalent to 160 mg raw herb), Oat straw extract (equivalent to 400 mg raw herb), Rice Bran. Other Ingredients: Plant Cellulose, Water.

Bone Maximizer - Metabolic Response Modifiers
Six capsules contain: Hydroxyapatite (MCHC) 4,000 mg • Calcium (from MCHC) 1,000 mg • Protein (from MCHC) 1,000 mg • Phosphorus (from MCHC) 500 mg • Magnesium oxide glycinate 300 mg • Zinc (citrate) 18 mg • Boron (citrate) 2 mg • Vitamin D (as Vitamin D3 cholecalciferol) 480 IU • Vitamin K (as Vitamin K1, phylloquinone) 120 mcg • Vitamin C (ascorbic acid) 72 mg • MSM (methyl-sulfonyl-methane) 120 mg • Glucosamine (HCl) 120 mg • Horsetail extract (silica) 25 mg • Pregnenolone 10 mg.

Bone Maximizer II - Metabolic Response Modifiers
Six capsules contain: Hydroxyapatite (MCHC) 4,000 mg • Calcium (from MCHC) 1,000 mg • Protein (from MCHC) 1,000 mg • Phosphorus (from MCHC) 500 mg • Magnesium Glycinate 200 mg • Zinc (citrate) 18 mg • Boron (citrate) 2 mg • Vitamin D (as Vitamin D3 cholecalciferol) 480 IU • Vitamin K1 (phylloquinone) 120 mcg • Vitamin C (ascorbic acid) 72 mg • MSM (methyl-sulfonyl-methane) 120 mg • Glucosamine (HCl) 120 mg • Horsetail extract (silica) 25 mg.

Bone Meal Powder - Solgar
Each 1 tsp (5 g) serving contains: Vitamin B12 (as cobalamin) 25 mcg • Calcium (as calcium oxide, from bone meal) 1000 mg • Phosphorus (as phosphorus oxide, from bone meal) 600 mg • Sodium 35 mg • Bone Meal powder (as tricalcium phosphate) 5000 mg.

Bone Meal with Natural Vitamin D - Puritan's Pride
Four tablets contain: Vitamin D (as Cholecalciferol) 400 IU • Calcium (as Bone Meal) 880 mg • Iron (as Ferrous Sulfate) 1.8 mg • Phosphorus (as Bone Meal) 400 mg • Magnesium (as Magnesium Gluconate) 3.7 mg • Zinc (as Zinc Gluconate) 0.080 mg • Copper (as Copper Gluconate) 0.013 mg • Manganese (as Manganese Gluconate) 0.011 mg • Red Beef Bone Marrow 15 mg.

Bone Power - Nature's Plus
Four softgels contain: Vitamin A (as beta carotene) 1000 IU • Vitamin C (as ascorbic acid) 200 mg • Vitamin D (as ergocalciferol) 200 IU • Vitamin B6 (as pyridoxine HCl) 20 mg • Vitamin B12 (as cyanocobalamin) 120 mcg • Calcium (as amino acid chelate, aspartate, carbonate) 1000 mg • Phosphorus (as amino acid complex) 100 mg • Magnesium (as amino acid chelate, aspartate, oxide) 200 mg • Zinc (as picolinate, amino acid chelate) 10 mg • Boron (as citrate, glycinate, aspartate) 3 mg. Other Ingredients: Soy Oil, Gelatin, Glycerin, Purified Water.

Bone Protector with Ostivone - Natrol, Inc.
Six capsules contain: Calcium (as calcium citrate) 1200 mg • 7-Isopropoxy-Isoflavone 600 mg. Other Ingredients: Rice powder, Magnesium Stearate, Gelatin.

Bone Reinforcer with Hydroxyapatite - Puritan's Pride
Four tablets contain: Vitamin C 60 mg • Vitamin D 400 IU • Calcium 1200 mg • Magnesium 400 mg • Zinc 15 mg • Copper 2 mg • Manganese 2.5 mg • Boron 3 mg • Silica 20 mg • Betaine Hydrochloride 100 mg.

Bone Renew with Ostivone - Source Naturals
Four tablets contain: Calcium (as Calcium Citrate, Ethanolamine Phosphate and Malate) 800 mg • Ipriflavone (Ostivone) 600 mg.

Bone Support - Zone Labs
Three softgels contain: Vitamin D (cholecalciferol) 200 IU • Vitamin K (phytonadione) 10 mcg • Calcium (as carbonate, citrate, gluconate, aspartate, malate, micronized hydroxyapatite) 750 mg • Magnesium (as oxide, aspartate, citrate) 400 mg • Boron (as calcium borogluconate) 1 mg • Horsetail extract (equisetum arvense) 25 mg. Other Ingredients: Gelatin, High Oleic Safflower Oil, Glycerin, Purified Water, Titanium Dioxide, Lecithin, Silicon Dioxide.

Bone Support - Eidon Inc.
Each 1 tbsp serving contains: Boron 27 mcg • Calcium 2250 mcg • Copper 18 mcg • Magnesium 2250 mcg • Manganese 45 mcg • Silica 131250 mcg • Sulfur 7500 mcg • Zinc 135 mcg. Other Ingredients: Purified Water.

Bone Support - TwinLab
Four tablets contain: Vitamin D (from Cholecalciferol) 800 IU • Calcium (from Calcium Citrate & Carbonate) 1500 mg • Magnesium (from Magnesium Aspartate & Oxide) 750 mg • Ostivone brand Ipriflavone (7-Isopropoxy Isoflavone) 600 mg • Novasoy Phytoestrogen extract (containing 40 mg of Soy Isoflavones) 100 mg • Boron (from Boron Citrate, Glycinate & Aspartate) 3 mg. Other Ingredients: Pharmaceutical Glaze, Cellulose, Stearic Acid Sodium Lauryl Sulfate, Magnesium Stearate, Colloidal Silicon Dioxide.

Some Brand Name Natural Products - What they Contain

www.NaturalDatabase.com contains MANY more listings than appear here.

Editor's Notes are located on pages 2155-2163.

BRAND NAMES

Bone Support Formula with Vitamin D - Health Smart Vitamins
Four caplets contain: Vitamin A (as beta-carotene) 25,000 IU • Vitamin D (cholecalciferol) 4 mg • Vitamin K (phytonadione) 0.08 mg • Calcium (as 50% calcium carbonate, 25% calcium citrate, 25% calcium glycinate) 1000 mg • Magnesium (as 75% magnesium oxide, 25% magnesium glycinate) 400 mg • Zinc (as zinc citrate) 15 mg • Copper (as copper asparate) 1.50 mg • Boron (as sodium borate) 1.50 mg.

Bone Support Plus D & K (female) - Weil Lifestyle, LLC
Each Cal-Mag Citrate Complex tablet contains: Calcium 250 mg • Magnesium 125 mg.
Each Dr. Weil Bone Support tablet contains: Vitamin D 200 IU • Vitamin K (phytonadione) 50 mcg • Calcium 125 mg • Magnesium 62.5 mg.

Bone Support Plus D & K (male) - Weil Lifestyle, LLC
Each Cal-Mag Citrate Complex tablet contains: Calcium 250 mg • Magnesium 125 mg.
Each Dr. Weil Bone Support tablet contains: Vitamin D 200 IU • Vitamin K (phytonadione) 50 mcg • Calcium 125 mg • Magnesium 62.5 mg.

Bones & Joints Body Benefits Pak - Leiner Health Products
Each packet contains: Magnesium 233 mg • Calcium Carbonate 498 mg • Iron 8 mg • Manganese 7.5 mg • Riboflavin (vitamin B2) 5.1 mg • Thiamin (vitamin B1) 4.5 mg • Vitamin B12 18 mcg • Vitamin B6 6 mg • Selenium 200 mcg • Molybdenum 208 mcg • Niacin 40 mg • Biotin 60 mcg • Chloride 72 mg • Potassium 80 mg • Copper 3.5 mg • Chromium 200 mcg • Vitamin E 460 IU • Vitamin A 7500 IU • Zinc 20 mg • Phosphorus 130 mg • Vitamin C 620 mg • Folate 400 mcg • Iodine 150 mcg • Pantothenic Acid 10 mg • Vitamin D 400 IU • Vitamin K 80 mcg • Boron 200 mcg • Citrus Bioflavonoids complex 10 mg • Ginkgo Biloba leaf 25 mg • Grape seed extract (vitis vinefera) seed 1 mg • Hesperidin complex 5 mg • Kelp powder (macrocystis pyrifera) frond 5 mg • Lecithin 10 mg • Mixed Carotenoids complex 10 mg • Nickel 6.5 mcg • Siberian Ginseng powder (eleutherococcus senticosus) root 25 mg • Silicon Dioxide 2 mg • Tin 13 mcg • Tocotrienol complex 5 mg • Trace Mineral complex 10 mg • Vanadium 13 mcg. Other Ingredients: Glucosamine Sulfate, Glucosamine Hydrochloride, Cellulose, Methylcellulose, Maltodextrin, Hydroxypropyl Methylcellulose, Polyethylene Glycol 3350, Propylene Glycol, Starch, Crospovidone, Croscarmellose Sodium, Acacia.

BoneSeltzer Fizz - Abundance Marketing
Vitamin C (as ascorbic acid) 60 mg • Vitamin D (cholecalciferol) 400IU • Folate (as folic acid) 400 mcg • Calcium (as carbonate, citrate) 1000 mg • Magnesium (as oxide, citrate) 400 mg • Zinc (as citrate) 15 mg • Potassium 330 mg • Hydrolyzed Gelatin 250 mg • Herbal Formula 100 mg: Glucosamine HCl, Grape seed extract (95% polyphenols), Grape skin extract (15% phenolics), Turmeric. Other Ingredients: Malic Acid, Citric Acid, Natural Flavors, Beet Juice Powder, Silica.

Bone-Up - Jarrow Formulas
Six capsules contain: Vitamin C (ascorbic acid) 200 mg • Vitamin D (D3, cholecalciferol) 500 IU • Vitamin K (K1, phylloquinone) 100 mcg • MK-7 (vitamin K2 as menaquinone-7) 10 mcg • Folic Acid 400 mcg • Methylcobalamin (methyl B12) 100 mcg • Microcrystalline Hydroxyapatite (MCHS) 4762 mg: Calcium (from MCHA) 1000 mg, Phosphorus (from MCHA) 510 mg, Protein (from MCHA) 1514 mg • Magnesium (as oxide) 600 mg • Zinc (as monomethionate) 10 mg • Copper (as gluconate) 1 mg • Manganese (as citrate) 1 mg • Glucosamine HCl 300 mg • Boron (from citrate) 3 mg. Other Ingredients: Magnesium Stearate, Silicon Dioxide, Gelatin.

Bone-Up (vegetarian) - Jarrow Formulas
Six tablets contain: Vitamin C (ascorbic acid) 200 mg • Vitamin D (D2, ergocalciferol) 500 IU • Vitamin K (K1, phylloquinone) 100 mcg • MK-7 (vitamin K2 as megaquinone-7) 10 mcg • Vitamin B1 (thiamin HCl) 5 mg • Folic Acid 400 mcg • Methylcobalamin (methyl B12) 100 mcg • Calcium (as calcium citrate) 1000 mg • Magnesium (as oxide) 500 mg • Zinc (as citrate) 10 mg • Copper (as gluconate) 1 mg • Manganese (as citrate) 1 mg • Boron (as borate) 3 mg • Glucosamine HCl 300 mg. Other Ingredients: Microcrystalline Cellulose, Modified Cellulose Gum, Modified Cellulose, Stearic Acid, Magnesium Stearate.

Bong Water (chronic tonic flavor) - Real Things Distributing Co.
Carbonated Water • High Fructose Corn Syrup and/or Sugar • Natural and Artificial Flavors • Citric Acid • Caffeine • Sodium Benzoate • Potassium Sorbate • Thiamine.

Bong Water (cottonmouth quencher flavor) - Real Things Distributing Co.
Carbonated Water • High Fructose Corn Syrup and/or Sugar • Citrus Oils • Natural and Artificial Flavors • Vanillin • Citric Acid • Caffeine • Vitamin C • Vitamin B3 • Vitamin B5 • Vitamin B6 • Vitamin B2 • Vitamin B1 • Vitamin B9 • Vitamin B12 • Sodium Benzoate.

Bong Water (green dreams flavor) - Real Things Distributing Co.
Carbonated Water • High Fructose Corn Syrup and/or Sugar • Citrus Oils • Natural and Artificial Flavors • FD&C Yellow #5 • FD&C Blue #1 • Citric Acid • Caffeine • Vitamin C • Vitamin B3 • Vitamin B5 • Vitamin B6 • Vitamin B2 • Vitamin B1 • Vitamin B9 • Vitamin B12 • Sodium Benzoate.

Bong Water (purple haze flavor) - Real Things Distributing Co.
Carbonated Water • High Fructose Corn Syrup and/or Sugar • Gum Arabic • Natural and Artificial Flavors • FD&C Red #40 • FD&C Blue #1 • Citric Acid • Caffeine • Vitamin C • Vitamin B3 • Vitamin B5 • Vitamin B6 • Vitamin B2 • Vitamin B1 • Vitamin B9 • Vitamin B12 • Sodium Benzoate.

Bonnisan drops - The Himalaya Drug Company
Each 1 mL serving contains: Dill oil (anethum sowa) 0.00162 mL • Guduchi (tinospora cordifolia) 0.45 mg • Himsra (caparis spinosa) 0.45 mg • Pippali (piper longum) 0.45 mg • Amalaki (emblica officinalis) 0.45 mg • Kasani (cichorium intybus) 0.45 mg • Kasamarda (cassia occidentalis) 0.45 mg • Haritaki (terminalia chebula) 0.45 mg • Ela (elattaria cardamomum) 0.45 mg • Biranjasipha (achillea millefolium) 0.45 mg • Jhavuka (tamarix gallica) 0.45 mg • Gokshura (tribulus terrestris) 0.45 mg • Punarnava (boerhaavia diffusa) 0.45 mg.

Bonnisan liquid - The Himalaya Drug Company
Each 1 tsp serving contains: Dill oil (anethum sowa) 0.0018 mL • Guduchi (tinospora cordifolia) 0.5 mg • Himsra (capparis spinosa) 0.5 mg • Pippali (piper longum) 0.5 mg • Amalaki (emblica officinalis) 0.5 mg • Kasani (cichorium intybus) 0.5 mg • Kasamarda (cassia occidentalis) 0.5 mg • Haritaki (terminalia chebula) 0.5 mg • Ela (elattaria cardamomum) 0.5 mg • Biranjasipha (achillea millefolium) 0.5 mg • Jhavuka (tamarix gallica) 0.5 mg • Gokshura (triblus terrestris) 0.5 mg • Punarnava (boerhaavia diffusa) 0.5 mg.

Borage CP-240 - Xymogen
Each softgel contains: Vitamin E (as D-alpha tocopherol acetate) 10 IU • Borage seed oil (borago officinalis) 1000 mg • Gamma-Linolenic Acid (GLA) 240 mg. Other Ingredients: Gelatin, Glycerin, Purified Water.

Borage GLA-125 - Jarrow Formulas
Each softgel contains: Borage oil (yielding 125 mg of gammalinolenic acid (GLA)) 550 mg. Other Ingredients: Gelatin, Glycerine, Water.

Borage GLA-240 - Jarrow Formulas
Each softgel contains: Borage oil (yielding 240 mg of GLA) 1000 mg • Gamma Tocopherol 10 mg. Other Ingredients: Gelatin, Glycerin, Water.

Some Brand Name Natural Products - What they Contain

www.NaturalDatabase.com contains MANY more listings than appear here.

Editor's Notes are located on pages 2155-2163.

Borage Oil - Rexall - Sundown
Each two softgels contain: Vitamin E (as d-alpha-tocopherol) 30 IU • Borage (seed oil) 1 g • Gamma Linolenic Acid (GLA) 200 mg. Other Ingredients: Gelatin, Glycerin, Water.

Borage Oil - Vital Nutrients
Each capsule contains: Borage oil (extracted without chemicals, contains gamma linolenic acid 240 mg) 1000 mg.

Borage Oil - Pure Encapsulations
Each softgel capsule contains: Borage Oil (provides GLA 240 mg, typical fatty acid composition: 16:0 palmitic, 18:0 stearic, 18:1 oleic, 20:1 eicosenoic, 18:2 linoleic, 18:3 gamma linolenic [GLA], other fatty acids 69 mg) 1045 mg • Vitamin E (D-alpha-tocopherol) 10 IU.

Borage Oil - PhysioLogics
Each softgel contains: Borage (borago officinalis seed oil) 1000 mg containing: Gamma Linolenic Acid (GLA) 240 mg, Linoleic Acid (LA) 360 mg. Other Ingredients: Gelatin, Glycerin.

Borage Oil - Ortho Molecular Products
Each soft gel capsule contains: Pure Borage seed oil providing 200 mg Gamma-Linolenic Acid 1000 mg. Other Ingredients: Gelatin, Glycerin, Water.

Borage Oil 1000 mg - Arrowroot
Each capsule contains: Borage seed oil 1000 mg.

Borage Oil 1000mg - N.V. Perricone M.D. Cosmeceuticals
Each softgel contains: Borage oil (borage officinalis, which contains: gamma-linolenic acid (GLA) 200 mg, palmitic acid 100 mg, stearic acid 30 mg, oleic acid 150 mg, linoleic acid 450 mg) 1000 mg. Other Ingredients: Gelatin, Glycerin, Purified Water, Mixed Tocopherols Concentrate.

Borage Oil 1300 mg - Nature's Plus
Each softgel contains: Borage seed oil (borago officinalis standardized 24% gamma-linolenic acid) 1300 mg. Other Ingredients: Gelatin, Glycerin, Purified Water.

Borage Oil 240 - Health From The Sun
Each capsule contains: Gamma Linolenic Acid (GLA) (Omega-6) 240 mg • Linoleic Acid (Omega-6) 370 mg • Oleic Acid (Omega-9) 15 mg. Other Ingredients: Borage seed oil, Gelatin, Glycerine, Water.

Borage Oil 300 - Health From The Sun
Each capsule contains: Gamma Linolenic Acid (GLA) (Omega-6) 300 mg • Linoleic Acid (Omega-6) 480 mg • Oleic Acid (Omega-9) 190 mg. Ingredients: Borage seed oil, Gelatin, Glycerine, Water.

Borage-Licorice Virtue - Blessed Herbs
Borage • Astragalus root • Licorice root • Siberian Ginseng root • Wild American Ginseng root • Suma root • Reishi mycelium • Ginger root • Grain alcohol & Distilled water.

Born Again Meno-Herbs - At Last Naturals, Inc.
Wild Yam • Black Cohosh • Red Clover • Dong Quai • Raspberry leaf • Chaste Tree berry • Siberian Ginseng • Squaw Vine • Nettles.

Born Again Vaginal Gel - At Last Naturals, Inc.
Water • Wild Yam extract • Glycerin • Sodium Alginate • Tocopheryl Acetate • Methylparaben • Citric Acid.

Born Again Wild Yam Cream - At Last Naturals, Inc.
Wild Yam extract • Aloe Vera gel • Soybean Oil • Stearic Acid • Cetyl Alcohol • Triethanolamine • Tocopheryl Acetate • Glycerin • Methylparaben • Propylparaben.

Born Again Wild Yam Extra Strength Gel - At Last Naturals, Inc.
Wild Yam extract • Aloe Vera gel • Glycerin • Oleth-20 • Carbomer • Triethanolamine • Methylparaben.

Boron - Nature's Way
Each capsule contains: Boron amino acid chelate 3 mg. Other Ingredients: Cellulose, Gelatin, Maltodextrin, Millet.

Boron (glycinate) - Pure Encapsulations
Each vegetable capsule contains: Boron (glycinate) 2 mg.

Boron Complex Plus - The Vitamin Shoppe
Four capsules contain: Boron 3 mg • Calcium 1000 mg • Magnesium 500 mg • Vitamin D (as Vitamin D3) 400 IU • Zinc 15 mg • Manganese 5 mg • Copper 500 mcg • Betaine HCl 324 mg.

Boswell Relief - Life Enhancement Products, Inc.
Each capsule contains: Boswellia extract 300 mg • Curcuma extract 65 mg. Other Ingredients: Ascorbyl Palmitate, Gelatin Capsule.

Boswellia - Pure Encapsulations
Each vegetable capsule contains: Boswellic Acids (from 429 mg of a standardized extract of boswellia serrata gum resin containing 70% boswellic acids) 300 mg • Vitamin C (as ascorbyl palmitate) 10 mg.

Boswellia Extract - Source Naturals
Three tablets contain: Boswellia serrata extract (yielding 788 mg of Boswellic Acids) 1,125 mg.

Boswellia Extract - Vital Nutrients
Each veg capsule contains: Boswellia Serrata extract (65% boswellic acids as organic acids, true boswellic acids 30%-40% by HPLC, alpha and beta boswellic acids, 3-acetyl-beta boswellic acid, 3-acetyl alpha boswellic acid, 11-keto-beta-boswellic acid, 3-acetyl-11-ketone-beta boswellic acid) 400 mg.

Boswellin - NOW Foods
Each capule contains: Boswellin (Boswellia serrata; extract of gum resins standardized to contain 65% [162 mg] Boswellic Acids) 250 mg • Curcumin extract (Curcuma longa; min 90% standardized extract of turmeric root powder) 100 mg • Turmeric root powder 150 mg. Other Ingredients: Rice Flour, Magnesium Stearate, Silica.

Boswellis & Curcuminoids - America's Finest
Each tablet contains: Boswellin brand Boswellia Serrata gum extract (65% boswellic acids) 200 mg • Turmeric root extract (95% curcuminoids) 200 mg. Other Ingredients: Cellulose, Stearic Acid, Magnesium Silicate, Magnesium Stearate, Pharmaceutical Glaze.

Botanaflor - Pharmanex
Each capsule contains: Jerusalem Artichoke with Fructooligosaccharides 100 mg • Cellulose Powder 100 mg • Citrus Pectin 98 mg • Apple Pectin Fiber 66 mg • Konjac Root (Glucomannan) 59 mg • Date Fiber 52 mg • Prune Fiber 48 mg • Soybean Fiber 43 mg • Papaya Powder with Papain 30 mg • Pineapple Powder with Bromelain 30 mg • Bifidobacterium Bifidum 30 mg • Lactobacillus Acidophilus.

Botaname - Pharmanex
Two capsules contain: Garcinia Cambogia 500 mg • Peppermint powder 104 mg • Brewer's Yeast 100 mg • Cinnamon Ramulus powder 86 mg • Lemon Verbena powder 86 mg • Chamomile flower powder 69 mg • Ginger root powder 69 mg • Chinese Licorice root extract 35 mg • Sweet Citrus Peel 35 mg • Chicory powder 16 mg.

Botanelle - Matol Botanical International Ltd
Deionized Water • Wild Yam extract • Liposome Complex • Aloe Vera • Glycerine • Stearic Acid • Safflower oil • Almond oil • Triethanolamine • Vitamin E oil (as D-tocopheryl acetate) • Jojoba oil • Avocado oil • Burdock root extract • Black Cohosh root extract • Siberian Ginseng extract • Chamomile extract • Isopropyl Myristate • PEG-100 Stearate • Methylparaben • Diazolidinyl Urea • Carbomer • Dimethicone • Disodium EDTA • Propylparaben.

Botanic Choice #739 Colon Cleanse Formula - Indiana Botanic Gardens
Two capsules contain: Psyllium husk hulls powder 660 mg • Karaya dried gum 200 mg • Slippery Elm bark powder 140 mg. Other Ingredients: Gelatin, Water.

Botanic Choice 5-HTP 50 mg Capsules - Indiana Botanic Gardens
Each capsule contains: L-5 Hydroxytryptophan 50 mg. Other Ingredients: Rice Flour, Gelatin, Water.

Botanic Choice 7X Herbal Weight Loss - Indiana Botanic Gardens
Two capsules contain: Calcium (as calcium pyruvate) 25 mg • Chromium (as Chromax brand chromium picolinate) 50 mcg • Calcium Pyruvate (80% pyruvic ion) 150 mg • Bromelain (2400 GDU, from pineapple) 300 mg • Guarana seed extract (standardized to 22% alkaloids as caffeine) 455 mg • Cayenne fruit powder 25 mg • Green Tea leaf extract (standardized to 20% polyphenols) 50 mg • Chitosan (90% deacetylated chitlin) 150 mg. Other Ingredients: Gelatin, Rice Flour, Water, Magnesium Stearate.

Botanic Choice Accu Hear Tablets - Indiana Botanic Gardens
Each tablet contains: Folate (as folic acid) 2000 mcg • Vitamin B12 (as cyanocobalamin) 2000 mcg. Other Ingredients: Dicalcium Phosphate, Microcrystalline Cellulose, Stearic Acid, Magnesium Stearate, Purified Water, Methylcellulose, Polyethylene Glycol.

Botanic Choice Acidophilus 1 mg Capsules - Indiana Botanic Gardens
Each capsule contains: Lactobacillus Acidophilus (supplying 100 million organisms) 1 mg • Apple Pectin 100 mg. Other Ingredients: Maltodextrin, Rice Flour, Gelatin, Water, Magnesium Stearate.

Botanic Choice Age Spot Reducing Cream - Indiana Botanic Gardens
Purified Water • Grapeseed oil • Stearic Acid • Natural Beeswax • Triethanolamine • Cetyl Alcohol • Sweet Almond oil • Masil VV Silicone • Glyceryl Stearate SE • Fragrance • Aloe Vera juice concentrate • Pure Pearl powder • Methylparaben.

Botanic Choice Aloe Vera 500 mg Capsules - Indiana Botanic Gardens
Each capsule contains: Aloe Vera leaf powder 500 mg. Other Ingredients: Gelatin, Water.

Botanic Choice Aloe Vera Gel - Indiana Botanic Gardens
Aloe Vera concentrate • Purified Water • SD Alcohol 40 • Triethanolamine • Propylene Glycol • Glycerin • Carbopol 940 • Imidazolidinyl Urea Menthol • Artificial Coloring.

Botanic Choice Aloe Vera Juice Concentrate - Indiana Botanic Gardens
Each 3 tbsp serving contains: Sodium 27 mg • Calcium 47.7 g • Aloe Vera juice 45 g.

Botanic Choice Aloe Vera Moisturizing Cream - Indiana Botanic Gardens
Purified Water • Mineral oil • Vegetable Glycerin • Safflower oil • Stearic Acid • Aloe Vera juice concentrate • Cucumber extract • Glyceryl Stearate SE • Cetyl Alcohol • Triethanolamine • Natural Beeswax • Fragrance • Methylparaben.

Botanic Choice Alpha Lipoic Acid 50 mg Tablets - Indiana Botanic Gardens
Each tablet contains: Alpha Lipoic Acid 50 mg. Other Ingredients: Dicalcium Phosphate, Microcrystalline Cellulose, Stearic Acid, Croscarmellose Sodium, Magnesium Stearate, Pharmaceutical Glaze.

Botanic Choice Andrographis Extract 300 mg Tablets - Indiana Botanic Gardens
Each tablet contains: Andrographis Paniculata leaf extract (standardized to 10% andrographolide) 300 mg. Other Ingredients: Dicalcium Phosphate, Microcrystalline Cellulose, Stearic Acid, Magnesium Stearate, Croscarmellose Sodium, Silicon Dioxide, Pharmaceutical Glaze.

Botanic Choice Apple Cider Vinegar 500 mg Tablets - Indiana Botanic Gardens
Each tablet contains: Apple Cider Vinegar powder (25% acetic acid) 500 mg. Other Ingredients: Microcrystalline Cellulose, Dicalcium Phosphate, Stearic Acid, Magnesium Stearate, Croscarmellose Sodium, Pharmaceutical Glaze.

Botanic Choice Apple Cider Vinegar Plus - Indiana Botanic Gardens
Two capsules contain: Apple Cider Vinegar powder (25% acetic acid) 600 mg • Cayenne fruit powder 100 mg • Ginger root powder 100 mg • Bromelain (from pineapple, supplying 600 gelatin digestive units per gram) 100 mg • Citrin 1 brand Garcinia Cambogia extract (50% (-) hydroxycitric acid) 100 mg. Other Ingredients: Gelatin, Rice Flour, Water, Magnesium Stearate.

Botanic Choice Arnica Plus Cream - Indiana Botanic Gardens
Purified Water • Refined Avocado oil • Propylene Glycol • Arnica oil • Stearic Acid • Triethanolamine • Natural Lanolin (anhydrous) • Aloe Vera juice concentrate • Soluble Collagen • Hydrolyzed Soy Protein • Cetyl Alcohol • Natural Beeswax • Glyceryl Stearate SE • Imidazolidinyl Urea • Arnica Solid extract • Natural Vitamin E.

Botanic Choice Astaxanthin 1 mg Tablets - Indiana Botanic Gardens
Each tablet contains: Astaxanthin 1 mg. Other Ingredients: Dicalcium Phosphate, Microcrystalline Cellulose, Stearic Acid, Magnesium Stearate, Croscarmellose Sodium, Silicon Dioxide, Hydrolyzed Gelatin, Vegetable Oil, Oleoresin, Sucrose, Ascorbyl Palmitate, Natural Mixed Tocopherols, Modified Corn Starch, Water, Pharmaceutical Glaze.

Botanic Choice Back Formula Tablets - Indiana Botanic Gardens
Two tablets contain: Vitamin C (as ascorbic acid) 200 mg • Vitamin D (as cholecalciferol) 60 IU • Vitamin B6 (as pyridoxine HCl) 20 mg • Calcium (as calcium carbonate) 200 mg • Magnesium (as magnesium oxide) 100 mg • Zinc (as zinc oxide) 10 mg • Manganese (as manganese sulfate) 6 mg • Potassium (as potassium citrate) 12 mg • Citrus Pectin (fruit and peel) 26 mg • Pepsin 1:3000 (porcine) 10 mg • Horsetail herb extract (standardized for 7% silic acid, 700 mcg) 10 mg • Bovine Cartilage Trachea powder (45% mucopolysaccharides, 4.50 mg) 10 mg. Other Ingredients: Dicalcium Phosphate, Microrystalline Cellulose, Stearic Acid, Magnesium Stearate, Croscarmellose Sodium, Silicon Dioxide, Pharmaceutical Glaze.
See Editor's Note No. 14.

Botanic Choice Bay Rum Aftershave - Indiana Botanic Gardens
Alcohol 39-B • Purified Water • Bay oil • Orange oil • Sucrose Octa Acetate • Lemon oil • Pimento oil • Talc.

Botanic Choice Bee Pollen 500 mg - Indiana Botanic Gardens
Two tablets contain: Bee Pollen powder 1 g. Other Ingredients: Dicalcium Phosphate, Stearic Acid, Magnesium Stearate, Silicon Dioxide, Pharmaceutical Glaze.

Botanic Choice Bee Pollen 580 mg - Indiana Botanic Gardens
Two capsules contain: Bee Pollen powder 1.16 g. Other Ingredients: Gelatin, Water.

Botanic Choice Bend Free Spray - Indiana Botanic Gardens
Alcohol 398 • Menthol • Lemon oil • Peppermint oil • Nutmeg oil • Cassia oil • Lemongrass oil • Masil VV Silicone • Lavender oil • Clove oil.

Botanic Choice Beta Carotene 25,000 IU Softgels - Indiana Botanic Gardens
Each softgel contains: Beta Carotene 25,000 IU.

Botanic Choice Bilberry 60 mg Tablets - Indiana Botanic Gardens
Each tablet contains: Bilberry extract (standardized to 10% anthocyanidins) 60 mg. Other Ingredients: Dicalcium Phosphate, Microcrystalline Cellulose, Stearic Acid, Magnesium Stearate, Silicon Dioxide, Pharmaceutical Glaze.

Botanic Choice Bilberry Plus Tablets - Indiana Botanic Gardens
Two tablets contain: Vitamin A (as acetate) 5000 IU • Riboflavin (vitamin B2) 20 mg • Citrus Bioflavonoid complex (50% total bioflavonoids) 200 mg: Hesperidin 70 mg, Naringin, Naringenin 7-beta-rutinoside and others 28 mg, Flavonols, Flavones and related Phenolic compounds 2 mg • Carrot root powder 100 mg • Bilberry extract (standardized to 25% anthocyanidins). Other Ingredients: Dicalcium Phosphate, Microcrystalline Cellulose, Stearic Acid, Magnesium Stearate, Croscarmellose Sodium, Silicon Dioxide, Pharmaceutical Glaze.

Botanic Choice Biotin 1000 mcg Tablets - Indiana Botanic Gardens
Each tablet contains: Biotin 1000 mcg. Other Ingredients: Dicalcium Phosphate, Microcrystaline Cellulose, Stearic Acid, Magnesium Stearate, Croscarmellose Sodium, Silicon Dioxide, Pharmaceutical Glaze.

Botanic Choice Prostate 9 Complex - Indiana Botanic Gardens
Each tablet contains: Iodine (from kelp) 150 mcg • Zinc (as zinc oxide) 15 mg • Lycopene (from tomatoes, as Lycobeads brand) 500 mcg • Pumpkin seed powder 50 mg • Pygeum Africanum bark powder 50 mg • Saw Palmetto berry powder 100 mg • Parsley leaf powder 100 mg • Cornsilk styles and stigmas powder 25 mg • Buchu leaf powder 25 mg. Other Ingredients: Dicalcium Phosphate, Microcrystalline Cellulose, Croscarmellose Sodium, Hydrolyzed Gelatin, Vegetable Oil, Vegetalbe Oleoresin, Sucrose, Corn Starch, Water, Ascorbyl Palmitate, Natural Tocopherol, Pharmaceutical Glaze.

Botanical Chi - Naturally Safe Technologies
Lycium berry • Cassia bark • Aloe Vera barbadensis • Schisandra berry • Dandelion root • Passion flower • Chinese Wild Yam • Kudzu root • Rosemary • American Ginseng • Rhodiola crenulata • Fo-Ti • Astragalus • Rosehips • Bee Pollen • Lemon Balm • Grapefruit seed extract • Phytonutrients.

Botopical the Botanical Instant Wrinkle Eraser Eye Repair - pH Beauty Labs LLC
Water (aqua) • Stearic Acid • Ethylene/Acrylic Acid Copolymer • Glyceryl Stearate • PEG-100 Stearate • Caprylic/Capric Triglyceride • Sodium Polystyrene Sulfonate • Propylene Glycol • Phytonadione (vitamin K1) • Green Coffee extract • Cucumis Sativus fruit extract (cucumber) • Algae extract • Artemisia Vulgaris extract • Polyquaternium-10 • Hyaluronic Acid • Aloe Barbadensis leaf juice • Glycerin • Propylene Glycol • Diazolidinyl Urea • Methylparaben • Propylparaben • Cyclopentasiloxane • C30-45 Alkyl Dimethicone/Polycyclohexane Oxide • Crosspolymer • Acrylates/Acrylamide Copolymer • Mineral oil • Polysorbate 85 • Carbomer • Triethanolamine • Trisodium EDTA • Propylparaben • Methylparaben • Fragrance (parfum).

Botopical the Botanical Instant Wrinkle Eraser Forehead Smoother - pH Beauty Labs LLC
Water (aqua) • Stearic Acid • Ethylene/Acrylic Acid Copolymer • Glyceryl Stearate • PEG-100 Stearate • Caprylic/Capric Triglyceride • Sodium Polystyrene Sulfonate • Propylene Glycol • Camellia Sinensis seed extract (green tea) • Saccharomyces-Copper-Ferment • Glycerin • Carbomer • Propylene Glycol • Diazolidinyl Urea • Methylparaben • Propylparaben • Aloe Barbadensis leaf juice • Chamomilla Recutita flower extract (matricaria) • Algae extract • Artemisia Vulgaris extract • Cyclopentasiloxane • C30-45 Alkyl Dimethicone/Polycyclohexane Oxide • Triethanolamine • Crosspolymer • Trisodium EDTA • Propylparaben • Methylparaben • Fragrance (parfum).

Botopical the Botanical Instant Wrinkle Eraser Lip Treatment - pH Beauty Labs LLC
Water (aqua) • Stearic Acid • Ethylene/Acrylic Acid Copolymer • Glyceryl Stearate • PEG-100 Stearate • Caprylic/Capric Triglyceride • Sodium Polystyrene Sulfonate • Propylene Glycol • Olea Europaea extract (olive) • Glycerin • Carbomer • Aloe Barbadensis leaf juice • Algae extract • Artemisia Vulgaris extract • Cyclopentasiloxane • C30-45 Alkyl Dimethicone/Polycyclohexane Oxide • Propylene Glycol • Diazolidinyl Urea • Methylparaben • Propylparaben • Crosspolymer • Triethanolamine • Trisodium EDTA • Propylparaben • Methylparaben • Fragrance (parfum).

Bountiful Harvest - 4 Life
Each packet contains: Vitamin A (as beta carotene) 5000 IU • Vitamin C (as ascorbic acid) 60 mg • Vitamin D 200 IU • Thiamin (as thiamine mononitrate) 2 mg • Riboflavin 2 mg • Niacin (as niacinamide) 15 mg • Vitamin B6 (as pyridoxine) 4 mg Folic Acid 500 mcg • Calcium 250 mg • Magnesium 100 mg • Zinc (as zinc gluconate) 5 mg • Onion 300 mg • Apple 250 mg • Sweet Potato 225 mg • Cabbage 200 mg • Paprika 200 mg • Celery 200 mg • Citrus Bioflavonoids (lemon, orange, grapefruit) 130 mg • Tomato 110 mg • Garlic 100 mg • Carrot 100 mg • Broccoli 100 mg • Parsley 100 mg • Spinach 100 mg • Capsicum 100 mg • Beet 75 mg • Cranberry 70 mg • Pineapple 50 mg • Cauliflower 50 mg • Chinese Cabbage 50 mg • Papaya 30 mg • Boron 2 mg • NDS Proprietary Blend 210 mg: Fungal Protease, Fungal Amylase, Fungal Lipase, Cellulase, Pectinase.

Bounty Bears Plus Extra C - Nature's Bounty
Each tablet contains: Vitamin A (as Retinyl Acetate and Beta Carotene) 2500 IU • Vitamin C (as Ascorbic Acid and Sodium Ascorbate) 250 mg • Vitamin D (as Cholecalciferol) 400 IU • Vitamin E (as d-Alpha Tocopheryl Acetate) 15 IU • Thiamin (as Thiamine Mononitrate) 1.05 mg • Riboflavin (Vitamin B-2) 1.2 mg • Niacin (as Niacinamide) 13.5 mg • Vitamin B-6 (as Pyridoxine Hydrochloride) 1.05 mg • Folic Acid 300 mg • Vitamin B-12 (as Cyanocobalamin) 4.5 mcg. Other Ingredients: Sugar, Vegetable Stearic Acid, Natural Orange Flavor, Vegetable Magnesium Stearate, Silica, Mannitol, FD&C Red No. 40, FD&C Yellow No. 6, FD&C Blue No. 2.

Bovine Cartilage - Pure Encapsulations
Each vegetable capsule contains: Bovine Cartilage (hormone-free) 500 mg: Glycosaminoglycans (mucopolysaccharides, including chondroitin-4-sulfate and dermatan sulfate) 225 mg • Vitamin C (as ascorbyl palmitate) 10 mg.

Bovine Cartilage Plus - Atrium Biotechnologies
Each capsule contains: Freeze Dried Bovine Cartilage 600 mg • Freeze Dried Soluble Trachea Substance 150 mg.
See Editor's Note No. 14.

Bowel & Intestinal Cleanser - Nature's Own
Each tablet contains: Fenugreek seed extract (trigonella foenum-graecum) 400 mg • Ginger root extract (zingiber officinale) 125 mg • Psyllium seed powder (plantago afra) 100 mg • Inulin 400 mg.

Bowel Detox - Nature's Sunshine
Three capsules contain: Vitamin A (beta-carotene) 800 IU • Vitamin C 30 mg • Vitamin E (D-alpha tocopherol) 6 IU • Zinc (gluconate) 3 mg • Selenium (amino acid chelate) 16 mcg • Betaine HCl 24 mg • Bile Salts 24 mg • Pancreatin 108 mg • Pepsin 24 mg. Base: Psyllium hull (plantago ovata), Algin (from brown seaweed), Cascara Sagrada bark (rhamnus purshiana), Bentonite Clay, Apple Pectin, Marshmallow root (althaea officinalis), Parthenium root (parthenium integrifolium), Charcoal, Ginger root (zingiber officinale), Sodium, Copper, Chlorophyllin. Other Ingredients: Silicon Dioxide, Gelatin, Water.

Bowel EZ - Pro Health
Two capsules contian: Peppermint oil 300 mg • Evening Primrose oil 200 mg • Psyllium 200 mg • Licorice 200 mg • Colostrum 200 mg • Grapefruit seed extract 200 mg • Ginger 100 mg. Other Ingredients: Gelatin, Silica, Magnesium Stearate, Microcrystalline Cellulose.

BRAND NAMES

Some Brand Name Natural Products - What they Contain

www.NaturalDatabase.com contains MANY more listings than appear here.
Editor's Notes are located on pages 2155-2163.

BowelSoothe - Vita Pharmica - formerly Neopharmica
Each packet contains: Herbal Concentrate 10 g: White Peony Root, Atractylodes Rhizome, Cardamon Seed, Paederia Scandens stem, Sonchus Brachyotus, Chinese Licorice root.

B-Plex Plus C - Wild Rose
Each tablet contains: Vitamin B1 (thiamine mononitrate) 12.5 mg • Vitamin B2 (riboflavin) 6.5 mg • Vitamin B3 (niacin) 60 mg • Vitamin B5 (pantothenic acid) 50 mg • Vitamin B6 (pyroxidine HCl) 17 mg • Vitamin B12 (cyanocobalamin) 22.5 mg • Vitamin B15 (calcium pangamate) 5 mg • Folic Acid 0.4 mg • Biotin 32 mcg • Vitamin C (ascorbic acid) 250 mg • Choline (choline bitartrate) 50 mg • Inositol 2.5 mg • Para-Aminobenzoic Acid (PABA) 12 mg. Base: Alfalfa, Rose Hips, Rice Bran, Passion Flower.

BP-X - Nature's Sunshine
Two capsules contain: Proprietary Blend 890 mg: Burdock root (arctium lappa), Pau d'Arco bark (tabebuia heptaphylla), Red Clover tops (trifolium pratense), Dandelion root (taraxacum officinale), Sarsaparilla root (smilax officinalis), Yellow Dock root (rumex crispus), Buckthorn bark (rhamnus frangula), Cascara Sagrada bark (rhamnus purshiana), Yarrow flower (achillea millefolium), Oregon Grape root (berberis aquifolium), Prickly Ash bark (zanthoxylum clava-herculis). Other Ingredients: Gelatin, Water.

Brain - Enzymes, Inc.
Each capsule contains: Proprietary Herbal Blend 460 mg: Ginkgo Biloba leaf extract, Ginseng root extract, Gotu Kola extract, Rice Bran, Bacopin, Schizandra extract, Grape seed extract, Lecithin • pHysioProtease 40 mg. Other Ingredients: Plant Cellulose, Water.

Brain & Eye Nutritional Fertilizer - Life Extension
Each softgel contains: DHA (docosahexaenoic acid, from microalgae) 200 mg • EPA (eicosapentanoic acid) 180 mg • Lecithin 800 mg • Vitamin E 5 IU. Other Ingredients: Soybean Oil, Purified Water, Glycerin.

Brain Actives - VitaStore
Six tablets contain: Ginkgo Biloba (24% flavoneglycosides, 6% terpene lactones) 100 mg • Phosphatidylserine 300 mg • L-Methionine 300 mg • OPC Complex (pine bark and grapeseed extracts) 100 mg • Vitamin B1 (thiamine) 1.5 mg • Vitamin B2 (riboflavin) 1.5 mg • Vitamin B3 (niacin) 20 mg • Vitamin B5 (pantothenic acid) 10 mg • Vitamin B6 (pyridoxine) 2 mg • Vitamin B12 6 mcg • Lecithin 1000 mcg • Acetyl L-Carnitine 500 mg • L-Glutamine 250 mg • Manganese 35 mg.

Brain Alert - Nutrapathic
Two tablets contain: Vitamin B1 10 mg • Vitamin B6 20 mg • Vitamin B12 40 mcg • Niacin 10 mg • Niacinamide 10 mg • Biotin 30 mcg • Choline Bitartrate 20 mg • Inositol 10 mg • PABA 20 mg • Vitamin F 4 mg • Calcium 20 mg • Chloride 4 mg • Copper 4 mg • Magnesium 10 mg • Manganese 6 mg • Phosphorus 10 mg • Potassium 10 mg • Selenium 10 mcg • Silica 4 mg • Zinc 20 mg. Other Ingredients: Brain, Egg Lecithin, Rye Green, Red Clover, Peppermint leaves, L-Tyrosine, L-Arginine, Lecithin granules, Barley Green, Bee Pollen, Gotu Kola, Ginkgo, Glutamic Acid, L-Phenylalanine, L-Glutamine, DNA, RNA, Hypothalamus, Pineal, Pituitary, Valerian, Ginseng, Spirulina, Wood Betony, Bupleurum root, Chondroitin Sulfate, CoQ10.
See Editor's Note No. 14 and No. 31.

Brain Booster - Optimum Nutrition
Each capsule contains: Ginkgo Biloba Extract (standardized for 24% flavone glycosides and 6% terpene lactones) 60 mg • Siberian Ginseng Extract (standardized for Eleutheroside B 400 mcg and D 300 mcg) 150 mg • Gotu Kola 250 mg. In a base of Bee Pollen and Ginkgo biloba leaf powders.
See Editor's Note No. 21.

Brain Care - Quantum, Inc.
Two tablets contain: Vitamin E (d-Alpha Tocopherol) 100 IU • Phosphatidylserine complex 100 mg • Phosphatidyl Choline 95 mg • Ginkgo leaf (Ginkgo Biloba) (24% Ginkgo Flavone Glycosides) 60 mg • Alpha-Linolenic Acid (Borage Oil) 50 mg • Coenzyme Q10 30 mg • DHA (Docosahexaenoic Acid) 10 mg • EPA (Eicosahexaenoic Acid) 10 mg. Other Ingredients: Stearic Acid, Guar Gum, Magnesium Stearate.

Brain E - Life Enhancement Products, Inc.
Two capsules contain: Vitamin E (dL-alpha-tocopheryl acetate) 1000 IU. Other Ingredients: Gelatin, Ascorbyl Palmitate.

Brain Essentials - Swanson Health Products
Each capsule contains: Vitamin E (as d-alpha tocopheryl succinate) 100 IU • Vitamin B-6 (as pyridoxine HCl) 25 mg • Vitamin B-12 (as cyanocobalamin) 250 mcg • Pantothenic Acid (as d-calcium pantothenate) 25 mg • Gotu Kola extract (10% asiaticosides) 150 mg • L-Glutamine 100 mg • L-Tyrosine 100 mg • Phosphatidylcholine (from lecithin) 100 mg • Ginkgo Biloba leaf extract (24% flavone glycosides, 6% terpene lactones) 60 mg • DHA (docosahexaenoic acid) 30 mg • Alpha Lipoic Acid 25 mg • DMAE Bitartrate 2 mg • Phosphatidylserine 1 mg.

Brain Essentials - PhytoPharmica
Three tablets contain: Vitamin C (Ascorbic Acid) 300 mg • Magnesium Aspartate 100 mg • Potassium Aspartate 100 mg • Zinc Aspartate 30 mg • Manganese (Chelate) 15 mg • Folic Acid 800 mcg • Vitamin B12 (Cyanocobalamin) 500 mcg • L-Glutamine 300 mg • L-Phenylalanine 300 mg • Brain extract freeze-dried 300 mg • Choline (Bitartrate) 200 mg • Gamma-Aminobutyric Acid (GABA) 100 mg • Alpha-Ketoglutaric Acid 100 mg • Glycine 100 mg • L-Tyrosine 100 mg • Pituitary extract freeze-dried 65 mg • L-Methionine 50 mg • RNA/DNA Complex 50 mg • L-Cysteine 50 mg • Pyridoxal Phosphate 15 mg.
See Editor's Note No. 21 and No. 31.

Brain Fuel - Futurebiotics LLC
Three tablets contain: Ginkgo Biloba (24% standardized extract) 45 mg • Korean Ginseng (7% ginsenoside extract) 15 mg • American Ginseng (7% ginsenoside extract) 10 mg • Gotu Kola extract (4:1 extract equivalent to) 150 mg • Ginkgo Biloba leaves 200 mg • Gotu Kola leaves 250 mg • Chinese Licorice extract (glycyrrhiza) 150 mg • Tyrosine 150 mg • Glutamine 275 mg • Phosphatidyl Choline (55% strength) 250 mg • Vitamin C 60 mg • Vitamin E (natural succinate) 5 IU • Vitamin B6 25 mg • Folic Acid 400 mcg • Vitamin B12 25 mcg • Vitamin B5 35 mg • Potassium 200 mg • Betaine HCl 50 mg • Bromelain 50 mg • Para Amino Benzoic Acid (PABA) 75 mg • L-Methionine 75 mg • Ribonucleic Acid (RNA) 50 mg.

Brain Fuel II - Futurebiotics LLC
Two capsules contain: Vitamin E (as d-alpha tocopheryl acetate) 100 IU • Vitamin B6 (as pyridoxine hydrochloride) 25 mg • Vitamin B12 (as Cyanocobalamin) 25 mcg • Pantothenic acid (as calcium pantothenate) 25 mg • DHA (decosahexaenoic acid) 100 mg • Phosphatidylcholine (supplying 55% (110 g) choline) 200 mg • Alpha Lipoic Acid 100 mg • Ginkgo biloba leaf powder extract [standardized for 24% (11 g) ginkgo heterosides] 45 mg • Korean ginseng root powder extract [standardized for 7% (1 mg) ginsenosides] 15 mg • Gotu Kola leaf 4:1 powder extract 38 mg. Other Ingredients: Gelatin, Water.

Brain Glandular - American Biologics
Each tablet contains: Raw Brain Concentrate (bovine origin) 360 mg. Other Ingredients: Dicalcium Phosphate, Magnesium Stearate.
See Editor's Note No. 31.

Brain Lightning - Novus Research
Three capsules contain: Vitamin E 100 IU • Vitamin B-1 (Thiamin) 25 mg • Vitamin B-3 (Niacin, non-flushing, as niacinamide) 10 mg • Vitamin B-5 (Pantothenic Acid) 25 mg • Vitamin B-6 (Pyridoxine 5-Phosphate) 25 mg • Vitamin B-12 (as Cyanocobalamin) 250 mcg • Magnesium 50 mg • Zinc (as Amino Acid Chelate) 10 mg • Manganese (as Manganese Chelate) 5 mg • Selenium (as Amino Acid Chelate) 200 mcg • Proprietary Synergistic Blend: [DMAE (dimethylaminoethanol), Pregnenolone, Trimethylglycine (TMG), L-

BRAND NAMES

Tyrosine, Huperzine A (pure molecular alkaloid), Vinpocetine, DL Phenylalanine (DLPA), GABA (gamma aminobutyric acid), Ginkgo Biloba] 1490 mg. Other Ingredients: Magnesium Silicate, Calcium Carbonate, Silicon Dioxide, Cellulose (non-reactive mixing agents).

Brain Link Complex - Pain & Stress Center
Six scoops contain: Vitamin A (as palmitate and beta carotene) 4035 IU • Vitamin C (as ascorbic acid) 500 mg • Vitamin D (as cholecalciferol) 160 IU • Vitamin E (as D-alpha tocopheryl succinate) 50 IU • Thiamine (as thiamine mononitrate) 0.3 mg • Riboflavin 0.3 mg • Niacin 8 mg •Vitamin B6 (as pyridoxine HCl) 5 mg • Folate (as folic acid) 242 mcg • Vitamin B12 (as cyanocobalamin) 40 mcg • Biotin 120 mcg • Pantothenic acid (as clacium pantothenate) 50 mg • Calcium (from calcium citrate & calcium carbonate) 240 mg • Iron (as iron citrate) 2 mg • Phosphorus (from dipotassium phosphate and whey protein) 60 mg • Iodine (from potassium iodide) 30 mcg • Magnesium (from magnesium oxide and magnesium chloride) 100 mg • Zinc (from zinc citrate) 6 mg • Selenium (from sodium selenite) 20 mcg • Copper (from copper citrate) 0.4 mg • Manganese (from manganese citrate) 0.1 mg • Chromium (from chromium nicotinate) 100 mcg • Molybdenum (from sodium molybdate) 20 mcg • Potassium (from dipotassium phosphate and whey protein) 125 mg • Barin Link Amino Acid Profile 9675 mg: L-Glutamine 3100 mg, L-Glycine 2105 mg, L-Taurine 1600 mg, GABA (gamma amino butyric acid) 1500 mg, L-Tyrosine 858 mg, L-Leucine 723 mg, Glutamic Acid 621 mg, Aspartic Acid, L-Isoleucine, L-Valine, L-Lysine, L-Phenylalanine, L-Threonine, Proline, Serine, L-Alanine, L-Arginine, L-Methionine, L-Cystine / L-Cysteine, Histidine, Tryptophan (from natural milk and egg proteins) 82 mg, 5-HTP (5-hydroxytryptophan) 25 mg. Other Ingredients: Food Starch, Fructose, Whey Protein Isolate, Maltodextrin, Egg Albumin Powder, Lecithin Powder, Natural Flavors (vanilla and banana), Medium Chain Triglycerides.

Brain Nutrition - Enzymatic Therapy
Three tablets contain: Vitamin C (ascorbic acid) 300 mg • Magnesium Aspartate 100 mg • Potassium Aspartate 100 mg • Zinc Aspartate 30 mg • Manganese (chelate) 15 mg • Folic Acid 800 mcg • Vitamin B12 (cyanocobalamin) 500 mcg • L-Glutamine 300 mg • L-Phenylalanine 300 mg • Brain extract (freeze-dried) 300 mg • Choline (bitatrate) 200 mg • Gamma-Aminobutyric Acid (GABA) 100 mg • Alpha-Ketoglutaric Acid 100 mg • Glycine 100 mg • L-Tyrosine 100 mg • Pituitary extract (freeze-dried) 65 mg • L-Methionine 50 mg • RNA-DNA Complex 50 mg • L-Cysteine 50 mg • Pyridoxal Phosphate 15 mg.
See Editor's Note No. 21 and No. 31.

Brain Pep - Pep Products, Inc.
Each capsule contains: Ginkgo Biloba • Kola Nut • Gotu Kola • Siberian Ginseng • Schizandra • Ginger • L-Glutamine 130 mg.

Brain Plus - Progressive Labs
Each capsule contains: Raw Porcine Brain concentrate 100 mg • Choline (bitartrate) 100 mg • Inositol 100 mg. This product contains naturally occuring RNA/DNA qualitatively from the brain concentrate.
See Editor's Note No. 14.

Brain Protex with Huperzine A - Nature's Sunshine
Two capsules contain: Proprietary Blend 321 mg: Soybean Lecithin Complex: Phosphatidyl Serine, Phosphatidyl Choline, Ethanolamine and Inositol, Ginkgo Biloba leaf, Lycopene, Alpha Lipoic Acid, Rhododendron Caucasicum root extract, Chinese Club Moss (huperzia serrata) • Huperzine A 50 mcg. Other Ingredients: Maltodextrin, Magnesium Stearate, Cellulose, Gelatin, Water.

Brainpower - Gero Vita International
Each capsule contains: Vitamin C (as ascorbic acid) 60 mg • Vitamin E (as dl-alpha-tocopheryl acetate) 30 IU • Thiamin (as thiamin mononitrate) 3 mg • Riboflavin 1.7 mg • Niacin 15 mg • Vitamin B6 (as pyridoxine hydrochloride) 1.2 mg • Folic Acid 200 mcg • Vitamin B12 (as cyanocobalamin) 7.5 mcg • Pantothenic Acid (as calcium pantothenate) 15 mg • Pyroglutamic Acid 125 mg • L-Tyrosine 75 mg • Choline (as choline bitartrate) 37.5 mg • Acetyl-L-Carnitine 32 mg • Cola seed extract 32 mg • L-Glutamine 18 mg • Ginkgo leaf extract (ginkgo biloba, 24% ginkgo flavoneglycosides, 6% terpene lactones) 15 mg • Vinpocetine 10 mg • L-Phenylalanine 3 mg • L-Cysteine 3 mg. Other Ingredients: Silicon Dioxide, Magnesium Stearate, Purified Talc, Gelatin.

BrainQUICKEN (Cognamine) - BrainQUICKEN LLC Research and Technologies
Two capsules contain: Niacinamide 10 mg • Vitamin B6 (pyridoxine HCl) 12.5 mg • Folic Acid 200 mcg • Vitamin B12 (cobalamin) 500 mcg • Pantothenic Acid (calcium pantothenate) 20 mg • Proprietary Cognamine Complex 805 mg: Cordyceps Sinensis, Choline Bitartrate, L-Glutamine, L-Tyrosine, Salix Alba, Phosphatidylserine, Ciwujia, 2-Dimethylaminoethanol, Salisburia Adantifolia, Vinpocetine, Huperzine A • Paullinia Cupana 405 mg • Alpha-Lipoic Acid 15 mg. Other Ingredients: Gelatin, Magnesium Stearate, Silica.

Brainwash Shampoo - Evergreen Research
Active Ingredients: Ginkgo Biloba • Grape seed extract. Other Ingredients: Peppermint Oil, Calendula Oil, Arnica.

BrainWave Plus - Allergy Research Group
Each capsule contains: Acetyl-L-Carnitine 100 mg • L-Glutamine 80 mg • Choline Bitartrate 40 mg • Phosphatidylserine 30 mg • Ginkgo Biloba extract (standardized to 24% ginkgo flavonglycosides and 6% terpene lactones) 24 mg • Siberian Ginseng extract (15:1) 20 mg • Panax Ginseng extract (standardized to 7% ginsenosides) 20 mg • Ashwaganda extract 20 mg • Gotu Kola, powdered 10 mg • Royal Jelly 20 mg • Bacopa Monniera extract (standardized to 30% bacosides) 20 mg • Vinpocetine 2 mg • CDP-Choline 50 mg • Huperzine A 20 mcg • Thymus 20 mg • DMAE (dimethylaminoethanol) 20 mg. Other Ingredients: Cellulose, Magnesium Stearate, Silicon Dioxide.

Branch Chain Amino Acid Complex - Jarrow Formulas
Two capsules contain: Vitamin B6 (pyridoxine hydrochloride) 5 mg • L-Leucine 300 mg • L-Isoleucine 150 mg • L-Valine 150 mg • L-Glutamine 500 mg. Other Ingredients: Rice Powder, Magnesium Stearate, Gelatin.

Brave Hart Deer Velvet Capsules - Hart Products
Deer Velvet 300 mg.

Breakfast Blend - Physicians Laboratories
Eight fluid ounces contain: Certified Isoflavone 15 mg. Other Ingredients: Whole Roasted Soybeans, Natural and Artificial Flavors.

Breast Assured - Nature's Sunshine
Three capsules contain: Proprietary Blend 1485 mg: Calcium Glucarate, Ellagic Acid (from pomegranate), Maitake mushroom (grifola frondosa), Kudzu extract (pueraria omeiensis), Flax meal (linum usitatissimum), Lutein (from marigold). Other Ingredients: Magnesium Stearate, Gelatin, Water.

Breast Care System-3 - Natrol, Inc.
Calcium 24 mg • Calcium D-Glucarate 200 mg. Breast Care Formula: Selenium 50 mcg • Green Tea Extract 50 mg • Garlic 50 mg • Grape Seed Extract 20 mg. Ultra Green Breast Care Ingredients: Rice Powder, Silica, Magnesium Stearate, Gelatin.
See Editor's Note No. 21.

Breast Enhance - Nature's Sunshine
Each capsule contains: Proprietary Blend 482 mg: Kudzu root extract (pueraria omeiensis), Alfalfa herb (medicago sativa), Dong Quai root extract (angelica sinensis), Saw Palmetto fruit extract (serenoa repens). Other Ingredients: Magnesium Stearate, Silicon Dioxide, Gelatin, Water.

Breast Enhance - NewLibido
Each six tablets contain: Saw Palmetto extract (30% sterols) 300 mg • Kava Kava (10% kava lactones) 300 mg • Dandelion (4:1 extract) 150 mg • Dong Quai extract (.08% ligustilide) 150 mg • Wild Yam extract 10:1 (4%-7% std) 150 mg • Chasteberry extract (4:1) 150 mg

BRAND NAMES

• Oat Bran 300 mg • Motherwort 500 mg • Blessed Thistle 500 mg • Folic Acid (as folate) 300 mcg • Biotin 300 mcg • Zinc (as amino acid chelate) 12 mg • Selenium (as amino acid chelate) 120 mcg. Other Ingredients: Di-calcium Phosphate, Magnesium Stearate, Stearic Acid.

Breast Essentials - Swanson Health Products
Two capsules contain: Calcium (from calcium d-glucarate) 24 mg • Selenium (as selenomethionine) 100 mcg • SoyLife Soy extract (3% soy isoflavones) 400 mg • Calcium D-Glucarate 200 mg • Green Tea extract (48% polyphenols) 200 mg • Rosemary leaf extract (6% rosemaric acid) 200 mg • Citrus Bioflavonoids (Citrus aurantium; 25% bioflavonoids) 100 mg • Boron (from boron aspartate) 3 mg. See Editor's Note No. 40.

Breast Gain Plus - Ultra Herbal, LLC
Two tablets contain: Vitamin E (as D-alpha tocopheryl succinate) 60 IU • Fenugreek seed (trigonella foenum-graecum) 400 mg • Fennel seed (foeniculum vulgare) 350 mg • Dong Quai root (angelica chinensis) 250 mg • Blessed Thistle root (cnicus benedictus) 125 mg • Dandelion root (taraxacum officinale) 125 mg • Kelp (ascophyllum nodosum) 50 mg • Watercress leaf (nasturtium officinale) 50 mg • L-Tyrosine 50 mg. Other Ingredients: Calcium Carbonate, Dibasic Calcium Phosphate, Tribasic Calcium Phosphate, Microcrystalline Cellulose, Croscarmellose Sodium, Stearic Acid, Magnesium Stearate, Silicon Dioxide, Modified Cellulose, Maltodextrin, Hydroxopropyl Methylcellulose, Hydroxopropyl Cellulose, Pharmaceutical Glaze, Water.

Breast Health - Schiff
Two capsules contain: Calcium (as calcium d-gluconate and calcium borogluconate) 37 mg • Selenium (as selenium yeast) 100 mcg • Calcium D-Gluconate 200 mg • Green Tea leaf extract (carnellia sinensis) 200 mg • Polyphenols 100 mg • Rosemary leaf extract (rosmarinus officinalis) 155 mg • Rosmarinic Acid 14 mg • Soy Isoflavones concentrate 31 mg • Isoflavones 12 mg • Citrus Bioflavonoids 25 mg • Boron (as calcium boroglucarate) 3 mg. Other Ingredients: Maltodextrin, Gelatin, Silicon Dioxide, Magnesium Stearate.

Breast Health Formula - Great American Nutrition
Two capsules contain: Calcium (as calcium d-glucarate) 24 mg • Selenium (as selenomethionine, from SelenoMax) 100 mcg • Calcium D-Glucarate 200 mg • Green Tea leaf extract (Ccellia sinensis, standardized to 48% polyphenols) 200 mg • Rosemary folia extract (rosemarinus officialis, standardized to 6% rosemaric acid) 200 mg • Soy extract (standardized to 3% isoflavones) 400 mg • Citrus peel bioflavonoids (citrus aurantium, standardized to 25% bioflavonoids) 100 mg • Boron Aspartate 3 mg. Other Ingredients: White Rice powder.
See Editor's Note No. 40.

BreastSuccess - EyeFive, Inc.
Three capsules contain: Fenugreek seed 219 mg • Fennel Seed 162 mg • L-Tyrosine 135 mg • Mexican Wild Yam root 96 mg • Pacific Kelp 90 mg • Damiana leaf 51 mg • Dong Quai root 48 mg • Mother's Wort herb 48 mg • Black Cohosh root extract 45 mg • Oat grass 42 mg • Blessed Thistle herb 39 mg • Hops flower 30 mg.

Breath Aid - D & E Pharmaceuticals
Each tablet contains: Ephedrine 12.5 mg • Guaifenesin 100 mg.

Breathe Easy - Traditional Medicinals
Each brewed cup contains: Pseudoephedrine (ephedra sinisa, naturally occurring in whole ma huang herb) 0.5 mg Other Ingredients: Peppermint leaf, Licorice root, Fennel seed, Eucalyptus leaf, Pleurisy root, Calendula flower, Ginger rhizome.
See Editor's Note No. 30.

Breathe Easy Tea - Traditional Medicinals
Each brewed cup contains: Manganese 0.04 mg • Licorice root 300 mg • Eucalyptus leaf 285 mg • Bitter Fennel seed 255 mg • Proprietary Blend 255 mg: Peppermint leaf, Calendula flower, Pleurisy root, Ginger rhizome.

Breathe Free Oil - Nature's Sunshine
Geranium oil • Rosemary oil • Peppermint oil • Niauli oil.

Breathe Well - Gero Vita International
Each capsule contains: Vitamin E (as dl-alpha-tocopheryl acetate) 50 IU • Proprietary Herbal Blend 390 mg: Adhatoda Vasika leaf extract, Glycyrrhiza Globra root extract (25% glycyrrhizine), Alpinia Golango root extract (30% ASE 90), Inula Racemosa root extract (30% ASE 90), Phyllanthus Emblica fruit extract (5% tannins), Myrica Nagi bark extract, Sida Cordifolia root extract, Clerodendrum Indicum root extract (0.5% active principle), Hedychium Spicatum root extract (0.5% volatile oil), Pistacia Integerrima gall extract (0.5% tannins), Picrorhiza Kurroa root extract (1% bitter), Zingiber Officinale rhizome extract (0.5% volatile oil), Ocimum Sanctum leaf extract, Abies Webbiana leaf extract • Quercetin 75 mg • PhytoSel 30 mg. Other Ingredients: Gelatin, Magnesium Stearate, Silica, Rice Flour. See Editor's Note No. 39.

Breathe-Aid Formula - Nature's Way
Two capsules contain: Proprietary Formula: Chickweed leaf & stem • Ephedra HCL • Guafinesin • Lobelia herb • Marshmallow root • Mullein leaf. Other Ingredients: Gelatin, Magnesium Stearate, Millet. See Editor's Note No. 30.

BreatheSmart - Health Smart Vitamins
Each capsule contains: Vitamin C (ascorbic acid) 150 mg • Piper Longum fruit (1.5% piperine, 1.5 mg) 100 mg • Picrorhiza Kurroa root (4%-5% kutkin, 2 mg - 2.5 mg) 50 mg • Quercetin 50 mg • Ginkgo leaf (24% ginkgo flavonglycosides, 9.6 mg; 6% terpene lactones, 2.4 mg) 40 mg • Tylophora asthmatica leaf (0.1%- 0.25% tylophorine alkaloids, 0.03 mg - 0.075 mg) 30 mg • Serratiopeptidase 7.5 mg.

Breath-EZ - Indiana Botanic Gardens
Two capsules contain: Breath EZ Herbal Blend 900 mg: Licorice root powder, Echinacea Purpurea powder, Saw Palmetto berry powder, Bayberry root bark powder, Myrrh gum powder, Plantain herb powder, Goldenseal root powder. Other Ingredients: Gelatin, Rice Flour, Water.

Brevail - Lignan Research
Each capsule contains: Vitamin D (as vitamin D3) 400 IU • Lignan extract from Flaxseed (Brevail) 200 mg • Secoisolariciresinol Diglycoside (from Brevail) 50 mg. Other Ingredients: Rice Powder, Maltodextrin, Magnesium Stearate, Silica, Gelatin, Titanium Dioxide, Vanilla Extract.

Brewers Yeast - J. R. Carlson Laboratories, Inc.
Twelve tablets contain: Thiamin (vitamin B1) 720 mcg • Riboflavin (vitamin B2) 240 mg • Niacin (vitamin B3) 1800 mg.

Brewer's Yeast - Nature's Life
Twelve tablets contain: Vitamin B1 1 mg • Vitamin B2 1 mg • Vitamin B6 240 mg • Choline 23 mg • Folic Acid 120 mcg • Niacin 3 mg • Inositol 23 mg • Pantothenic Acid 600 mcg • Calcium 360 mcg • Chromium 9 mcg • Copper 300 mcg • Iodine 18 mcg • Iron 2 mg • Magnesium 6 mg • Manganese 30 mcg • Phosphorus 8 mg • Potassium 10 mg • Selenium 12 mcg • Sodium 460 mcg • Zinc 600 mcg • Protein Profile 2.9 g: Alanine 216 mg, Arginine 155mg, Aspartic Acid 302 mg, Cysteine 72 mg, Glycine 148 mg, Glutamic Acid 402 mg, Histidine (essential amino acid) 78 mg, Isoleucine (essential amino acid) 140 mg, Leucine (essential amino acid) 222 mg, Lysine (essential amino acid) 234 mg, Methionine (essential amino acid) 43 mg, Phenylalanine (essential amino acid) 135 mg, Proline 140 mg, Serine 150 mg, Threonine (essential amino acid) 143 mg, Tryptophan (essential amino acid) 50 mg, Tyrosine 81 mg, Valine (essential amino acid) 179 mg.

Brewer's Yeast - The Vitamin Shoppe
Six tablets contain: Vitamin B1 48 mg • Vitamin B2 16 mg • Niacin 1.6 mg • Folic Acid 13 mcg • Vitamin B6 160 mcg • Choline 15 mg • Pantothenic Acid 200 mcg • Biotin 20 mcg • Inositol 15 mg.

Some Brand Name Natural Products - What they Contain

www.NaturalDatabase.com contains MANY more listings than appear here.
Editor's Notes are located on pages 2155-2163.

Brewer's Yeast 500 - GNC
Eight tablets contain: Thiamin .4 mg •Riboflavin .1 mg •Niacin 1.2 mg. Ingredients: Dry Debittered Brewer's Yeast.

Brewer's Yeast Powdered - GNC
Two tablespoons contain: Thiamin 1.05 mg • Riboflavin 1.36 mg •Niacin 9 mg • Vitamin B6 0.7 • Folate, Folic Acid, Folacin 40 mcg •Vitamin B12 0.12 mcg • Biotin 12 mcg •Pantothenic Acid 0.6 mg •Iron 1.8 mg •Phosphorus 20 mg •Magnesium 32 mg • Zinc 3 mg • Copper 1 mg. Ingredients: Brewer's Yeast.

Brigham Tea - Nature's Way
Two capsules contain: Brigham Tea herb 830 mg. Other Ingredients: Gelatin, Magnesium stearate, Millet.

B-Right - Jarrow Formulas
Each capsule contains: Vitamin B1 (thiamin mononitrate) 25 mg • Vitamin B2 (riboflavin) 25 mg • Vitamin B3 (niacin) 25 mg • Vitamin B5 (D-calcium pantothenate) 100 mg • Pantethine (vitamin B5 derivative) 25 mg • Vitamin B6 (pyridoxine HCl) 25 mg • Vitamin B6 (pyridoxal-5-phosphate) 10 mg • Vitamin B12 (as methylcobalamin) 100 mcg • Folic Acid (folate) 400 mcg • Biotin 300 mcg • PABA (para-aminobenzoic acid) 30 mg • Choline Bitartrate 50 mg • Inositol 50 mg. Other Ingredients: Cellulose, Silicon Dioxide, Magnesium Stearate, Gelatin, Titanium Dioxide.

Bright Eyes - Grandma's Herbs
Each capsule contains: Proprietary Blend 0.450 g: Eyebright herb, Fennel seed, Rue herb, Chamomile flower, Goldenseal root, Red Raspberry leaf/seed, Blue Vervain herb, Bayberry bark, Cayenne Pepper (40,000 HU).

Brighten-Up - Goldshield Elite
Two caplets contain: St. John's Wort standardized extract aerial parts (0.3% hypericin) 300 mg • Panax Ginseng root standardized extract (4% ginsenosides) 200 mg • Ashwagandha root (Withania somnifera) 200 mg • Green Tea leaf standardized extract (20% methylxanthines) 150 mg • Kava Kava root standardized extract (30% kavalactones) 50 mg • Siberian Ginseng root standardized extract (0.8% eleutherosides) 50 mg • Schizandra berry standardized extract (9% schizandrins) 50 mg. Other Ingredients: Dicalcium Phosphate, Vegetable Cellulose, Fractionated vegetable oil, Soy polysaccharides, Silica, and Vegetable resin glaze.

Bright-Eyes - Futurebiotics LLC
Three tablets contain: Bilberry extract (standardized for 25% anthocyanidins) 10 mg • Eyebright (extract equivalent to) 500 mg • Chamomile (extract equivalent to) 250 mg • Rosemary (extract equivalent to) 200 mg • Beta Carotene 20,000 IU • Vitamin A 5000 IU • Quercetin 100 mg • Citrus bioflavonoids 100 mg • Vitamin C 1000 mg • Natural Vitamin E (d-alpha succinate) 200 IU • Vitamin B2 (riboflavin) 40 mg • Rutin 100 mg • Selenium (from selenomethionine) 100 mcg • Zinc (monomethionine) 15 mg • Vitamin B6 5 mg • Niacinamide 10 mg • Pantothenic Acid (B5) 40 mg • Chromium (GTF) 200 mcg • L-Cysteine 100 mg • L-Glutamine 75 mg. In a base of: Alfalfa, Carrot, Parsley & Dandelion.

BRIO Adult Multivitamin - Functional Products
Each wafer contains: Vitamin A (Retinol Palmitate) 2667 IU • Vitamin C (Ascorbic Acid) 60 mg • Vitamin D (Calciferol D3) 0.005 mg • Vitamin E (dl-alpha tocopherol) 10 mg • Vitamin B1 (Thiamine) 1.4 mg • Vitamin B2 (Riboflavin) 1.6 mg • Niacin 18 mg • Vitamin B6 (Pyridoxine) 2 mg • Folic Acid 0.2 mg • Vitamin B12 (Cyanocobalamin) 0.001 mg • Biotin 0.15 mg • Pantothenic Acid 6 mg • Calcium (Calcium Carbonate) 1200 mg • Magnesium (Magnesium Oxide) 45 mg • Zinc (Zinc Sulfate) 3 mg. Ingredients: Citric Acid, Sodium Carbonate, Potassium Carbonate, Corn Starch, Natural Orange Flavor, Mannitol, Potassium Chloride, Beet Root Color, Aspartame, Acesulfame K, Maltodextrin.

BRIO Children's Multivitamin - Functional Products
Each wafer contains: Vitamin A (Retinol Palmitate) 1333 IU • Vitamin C (Ascorbic Acid) 30 mg • Vitamin D (Calciferol D3) 0.0025 mg • Vitamin E (dl-Alpha Tocopherol) 5 mg • Vitamin B1 (Thiamine) 0.7 mg • Vitamin B2 (Riboflavin) 0.8 mg • Niacin 9 mg • Vitamin B6 (Pyridoxine) 1 mg • Folic Acid 0.1 mg • Vitamin B12 (Cyanocobalamin) 0.0005 mg • Biotin 0.075 mg • Pantothenic Acid 3 mg • Calcium (Calcium Carbonate) 250 mg. Ingredients: Citric Acid, Sodium Carbonate, Potassium Hydrogen Carbonate, Beet Root Color, Maltodextrin, Rice Starch, Artificial Strawberry Flavor, Potassium Chloride, Aspartame, Acesulfame K.

BRIO Echinacea - Functional Products
Each wafer contains: Vitamin C (Ascorbic Acid) 200 mg • Echinacea (Dried Juice) 200 mg. Ingredients: Citric Acid, Sodium Hydrogen Carbonate, Potato Starch, Aspartame, Acesulfame K, Natural Lemon Flavor.

Brite-Life - Advocare International
Each caplet contains: Pyridoxine (as HCl) 100 mg • St. John's Wort leaf/flower extract (hypericum perforatum) 450 mg • L-Tyrosine 300 mg. Other Ingredients: Dicalcium Phosphate, Silicon Dioxide, Cellulose, Stearic Acid, Magnesium Stearate.

BroccoPhane brand - Cyvex Nutrition, Inc.
Standardized Broccoli sprout powder.

BroccoSinolate brand - Cyvex Nutrition, Inc.
Broccoli extract.

Bromelain - Source Naturals
Each tablet contains: Bromelain (2000 GDU per g) 500 mg.

Bromelain 1000 - Jarrow Formulas
Each tablet contains: Bromelain 1000 GDU 500 mg. Other Ingredients: Calcium Phosphate, Cellulose, Stearic Acid, Modified Cellulose Gum, Magnesium Stearate, Modified Cellulose.

Bromelain 2400 - Vitaline Formulas
Each capsule contains: Bromelain (2400 mcu/gm) 500 mg.

Bromelain 2400 250 mg - Pure Encapsulations
Each vegetable capsule contains: Bromelain (2400 gdu/gram) 150 mg • Vitamin C (ascorbyl palmitate) 3 mg.

Bromelain 2400 500 mg - Pure Encapsulations
Each vegetable capsule contains: Bromelain (2400 gdu/gram) 500 mg • Vitamin C (ascorbyl palmitate) 6 mg.

Bromelain 2400 gdu - Vital Nutrients
Each capsule contains: Bromelain (2400 gdu/3600 mcu per gram) 375 mg.

Bromelain Complex - PhytoPharmica
Two capsules contain: Vitamin C (calcium ascorbate) 225 mg • Pantothenic Acid (calcium D-pantothenate) 125 mg • Bromelain (1800 MCU/g, enzymes derived from pineapple stems) 750 mg.

Bromelain Forte - Ortho Molecular Products
Each capsule contains: Bromelain (2400 GDU/g) 500 mg • Papain (6000 USP/mg) 30 mg. Other Ingredients: Other Ingredients: Natural Vegetable Capsules, Ascorbyl Palmitate, Microcrystalline Cellulose, Silicon Dioxide.

Bromelain Joint-Ease - Nature's Life
Four capsules contain: Bromelain [an enzyme from Pineapple fruit (Ananassa sativa) activity of 1500 mg = 3000 GDU (4500 MCU)] 1500 mg • Quercetin (Dimorphandra pod) 400 mg • Vitamin C (Ascorbic Acid) 750 mg • Zinc (Picolinate, Gluconate, Citrate) 15 mg • Copper (Gluconate, Citrate) 1 mg • Manganese (Citrate, Aspartate) 3 mg.

Bromelain Plus - Enzymatic Therapy
Each tablet contains: Vitamin C (Calcium Ascorbate) 225 mg • Pantothenic Acid (D-Calcium Pantothenate) 125 mg. Other Ingredients: Bromelain (1800 MCU) pineapple enzyme 750 mg.

Editor's Notes are located on pages 2155-2163.

Bromezyme - Progressive Labs
Each capsule contains: Bromelain 50 mg • Papain 20 mg • Raw Spleen concentrate 20 mg • Raw Calf Thymus 10 mg.
See Editor's Note No. 14.

Bronchitis Remedy - PhytoPharmica
Twenty drops contain: Antimonium tartaricum 4x • Ipecacuanha 4x • Pimpinella saxifraga 2x • Cetraria islandica 1x • Eucalyptus globulus 1x. In a base of 45% USP alcohol by volume.
See Editor's Note No. 1 and No. 21.

Bronchoril - PhytoPharmica
Each tablet contains: Glycerol Guaiacolate 200 mg • Fenugreek seed powder 4:1 (trigonella foenum-graecum) 350 mg • Marshmallow 4:1 extract (althaea officinalis, mucilage content 30%-40%) 125 mg • PABA (para-aminobenzoic acid) 50 mg • Mullein leaf (verbascum nigrum) 50 mg.

Bronchostem - American Biologics
Each drop contains: Spongia 4X • Causticum 6X • Lachesis 5X • Hepar. Sulph 5X • Thyme 3X • Tartar Emt. 6X • Aconite 6X • Drosera 4X. Other Ingredients: 20% Alcohol, Distilled Water.
See Editor's Note No. 1.

BryantLabs Select Olivine - Bryant Nutrients
Two tablets contain: 15% Olivine brand standardized Olive leaf extract (150 mg standardized oleuropein) 1000 mg. Other Ingredients: Spirulina, Stearic Acid.

BryantLabs Select Prosta-Max Pro 320 - Bryant Nutrients
Each softgel contains: Saw Palmetto extract (serenoa repens, standardized to 85%-95% fatty acids and active sterols) 160 mg. Other Ingredients: Pumpkin Seed Oil, Gelatin, Glycerin.

BryantLabs Select Virucept - Bryant Nutrients
Two tablets contain: Red Marine Algae concentrate 600 mg. Other Ingredients: Di-Calcium Phosphate, Dextrose, Stearic Acid, Magnesium Stearate.

BryantLabs Select Virucept Pro - Bryant Nutrients
Two tablets contain: Proprietary Blend 1000 mg: Red Marine Algae concentrate, Olive leaf extract, Astragalus extract. Other Ingredients: Di-Calcium Phosphate, Dextrose, Stearic Acid, Magnesium Stearate.

B-Stress with Siberian Ginseng and Coenzymes - Nature's Way
Two capsules contain: Biotin (biotin triurate) 300 mcg • Calcium Pantethonate 150 mg • Choline Bitartrate 50 mg • Chromium Picolinate 200 mcg • Folic Acid (folate) 400 mcg • Inositol 100 mg • Niacin (Vitamin B3) 25 mg • Niacinamide 100 mg • PABA (para aminobenzoic acid) 50 mg • Pyridoxine HCl 100 mg • Riboflavin (Vitamin B2) 40 mg • Siberian Ginseng root 250 mg • Thiamine (Vitamin B1) 50 mg • Vitamin B12 (Cyanacobalamin) 100 mcg • Vitamin C (Ascorbic Acid) 500 mg.

B-to-the-E - Anheuser-Busch
Beer • Caffeine • Guarana • Ginseng.

B'Tweens - 4 Life
Each chew contains: Niacin 0.59 mg • Vitamin B6 0.79 mg • Folic Acid 137 mcg • Vitamin B12 2.4 mcg • Sodium 20 mg • Proprietary Blend 215 mg: Maca, Cocoa - Almond extract, Opuntia Ficus-Indica leaf, Quercetin, L-Tyrosine, 5-Hydroxytryptophan, Bromelain, Schisandra Chinensis fruit. Other ingredients: Corn Syrup, Sugar, Condensed Whole Milk, Palm Kernel Oil, Chocolate, Mono- & Diglycerides, Salt, Soya Lecithin, Natural Flavors.

Bu Zhong Yi Qi Tang Plus - Secara
Three tablets contain: Organic Ginger rhizome (gan jiang) 405 mg • Organic Gentian root (qin jiao) 300 mg • Astragalus root 5:1 extract (huang qi) 300 mg • Shiitake fruit body [20% polysaccharides (40 mg)] 201 mg • Atractylodes root 5:1 extract (bai zhu) 198 mg • Dong Quai root 5:1 extract (dang gui) 198 mg • Asian Ginseng root [ren shen, 5% ginsenosides (10 mg)] 198 mg • Tangerine peel 4:1 extract (chen pi) 141 mg • Bupleurum root 5:1 extract (chai hu) 120 mg • Licorice root 5:1 extract (gan cao) 99 mg • Chinese Cimicifuga rhizome 5:1 extract (sheng ma) 60 mg.

Buckley's Mixture Cough Suppresant - W.K. Buckley Limited
Each teaspoon (5 mL) contains: Dextromethorphan Hydrobromide 12.5 mg • Ammonium Carbonate • Camphor • Canada Balsam • Carrageenan • Glycerine • Menthol • Pine Needle Oil • Sodium Butylparaben • Sodium Propylparaben • Sodium Saccharin • Tincture of Capsicum • Water.

Buffalo Liver - J. R. Carlson Laboratories, Inc.
Six capsules contain: Riboflavin (vitamin B2) 300 mcg • Niacin (vitamin B3) 2 mg • Vitamin B12 (cyanocobalamin) 2 mcg • Iron (as iron glycinate chelate) 5 mg • Copper 300 mcg • Buffalo Liver concentrate 3000 mg.

Buffered Vitamin C - Life Enhancement Products, Inc.
Each capsule contains: Vitamin C (from calcium ascorbate) 500 mg • Calcium (from calcium ascorbate) 65 mg. Other Ingredients: Gelatin.

Buffered Ascorbic Acid capsules - Pure Encapsulations
Each vegetable capsule contains: Buffered Ascorbic Acid (providing vitamin C equivalent of 511 mg from calcium ascorbate 520 mg, magnesium ascorbate 340 mg, potassium ascorbate 140 mg) 1000 mg • Vitamin C (as ascorbyl palmitate) 20 mg.

Buffered Ascorbic Acid powder - Pure Encapsulations
Each heaping teaspoon (4.4 g) contains: Buffered Ascorbic Acid (providing vitamin C equivalent of 2200 mg from calcium ascorbate 2288 mg, magnesium ascorbate 1496 mg, potassium ascorbate 616 mg) 4400 mg.

Buffered C 1000 mg - Arrowroot
Each tablet contains: Vitamin C (ascorbic acid, calcium ascorbate) 1000 mg • Manganese (manganous carbonate) 0.1 mg • Calcium (calcium ascorbate) 40 mg • Potassium (potassium citrate, aspartate) 30 mg • Magnesium (magnesium hydroxide, aspartate) 40 mg • Bioflavonoids (from lemon) 50 mg • Zinc (zinc oxide) 2 mg.

Buffered C 500 mg - Vital Nutrients
Each capsule contains: Buffered Vitamin C (from calcium ascorbate 367 mg) 300 mg • Buffered Vitamin C (from magnesium ascorbate 145 mg) 100 mg • Buffered Vitamin C (from potassium ascorbate 112 mg) 100 mg • Calcium (ascorbate) 34 mg • Magnesium (ascorbate) 7 mg • Potassium (ascorbate) 22 mg.

Buffered C Capsules - Ortho Molecular Products
Two capsules contain: Vitamin C (as ascorbic acid USP) 700 mg • Calcium (as carbonate USP) 100 mg • Magnesium (as carbonate USP) 100 mg • Potassium (as gluconate USP) 20 mg. Other Ingredients: Natural Vegetable Capsules, Ascorbyl Palmitate, Magnesium Stearate, Microcrystalline Cellulose, Silicon Dioxide.

Buffered C Powder - Ortho Molecular Products
Each heaping teaspoon contains: Vitamin C (as ascorbic acid USP) 2350 mg • Calcium (as ascorbate) 350 mg • Magnesium (as ascorbate) 350 mg • Potassium (as gluconate) 99 mg. Other Ingredients: Ascorbic Acid, Calcium Carbonate, Magnesium Carbonate.

Buffered C Powder 2000 mg - The Vitamin Shoppe
Each teaspoon contains: Vitamin C (calcium ascorbate) 2000 mg • Rose Hips 1450 mg • Acerola 1000 mg • Lemon Bioflavonoids 500 mg • Rutin 25 mg • Hesperidin 25 mg • Calcium (ascorbate) 230 mg.

Buffered Lemon C-Powder - Ortho Molecular Products
Each heaping teaspoon contains: Vitamin C (as ascorbic acid USP) 2350 mg • Calcium (as ascorbate) 350 mg • Magnesium (as ascorbate) 350 mg • Potassium (as gluconate) 99 mg. Other Ingredients: Ascorbic Acid, Calcium Carbonate, Magnesium Carbonate, Natural Lemon Flavor.

Some Brand Name Natural Products - What they Contain

www.NaturalDatabase.com contains MANY more listings than appear here.
Editor's Notes are located on pages 2155-2163.

Buffered TLC - Jarrow Formulas
Each 2 1/2 level tsp contains: Vitamin C (ascorbic acid, calcium and magnesium asocrbates) 4500 mg • L-Lysine 750 mg • L-Proline 750 mg • L-Taurine 250 mg • Magnesium (carbonate, ascorbate) 375 mg • Potassium (bicarbonate) 99 mg • Calcium (carbonate, ascorbate) 676 mg • Bromelain 1200 GDU. Other Ingredients: Silicon Dioxide, Lime Oil.

Buffered Vitamin C - Bee-Alive Inc.
Each capsule contains: Vitamin C (from calcium ascorbate, magnesium ascorbate, potassium ascorbate, zinc and rose hips fruit) 500 mg • Calcium 45 mg • Proprietary Blend 200 mg: Citrus Bioflavonoid complex, Rose Hips fruit, Hesperidin, Rutin, Acerola fruit. Other Ingredients: Cellulose, Calcium Phosphate, Gelatin, Vegetable Stearate, Silica.

Buffered Vitamin C 500 with Rose Hips - Schiff
Each tablet contains: Vitamin C (as calcium ascorbate) 500 mg • Calcium (as calcium ascorbate) 31 mg • Rose Hips fruit (rosa canina) 25 mg. Other Ingredients: Cellulose, Hydroxypropyl Methylcellulose, Maltodextrin, Polyethylene Glycol, Magnesium Stearate.

Bug Off! Kids Biting Insect Repelling Wrist Band - Kaz, Inc.
Active Ingredients: Citronella Oil • Geraniol Oil • Lemongrass Oil (15.75%). Inactive Ingredient: Polyethylene (84.25%).

Bugleweed Motherwort Supreme - Gaia Herbs
Thirty drops contain: Proprietary Blend 30 mg: Bugleweed herb (lycopus virginicus), Motherwort flowering tops (leonurus cardiaca), Lemon Balm leaf (melissa officinalis), Spring Water, 45-55% Pure Grain Alcohol USP.

Bulk & Muscle Formula (chocolate flavor) - Herbalife International of America, Inc.
Soy Protein Isolate • Calcium Caseinate • Maltodextirn • Whey Protein Concentrate • Dextrose • Fructose • Dutch processed Cocoa powder • Artificial Flavor • Tricalcium Phosphate • Dipotassium Phosphate • Medium Chain Triglycerides • Magnesium Oxide • Honey powder • Soy Lecithin • Bacterially-Derived Patented Proteases (from Aminogen) • Choline Bitartrate • Potassium Citrate • Aspartame • Egg Albumin solids powder • L-Carnitine Hydrochloride • L-Glutamine • Beta Carotene • Ascorbic Acid • DL-Alpha Tocopheryl Acetate • Molybdenum Amino Acid Chelate • Potassium Glycerophosphate • Ornithine Alpha Ketoglutarate • Biotin • Selenium Amino Acid Chelate • Ferrous Fumarate • Niacin • Manganese Amino Acid Chelate • Zinc Oxide • D-Calcium Pantothenate • Potassium Iodide • Vitamin A Palmitate • Vitamin K • Copper Sulfate • Eleuthero powder • Astragalus root powder • Pyridoxine Hydrochloride • Riboflavin • Thiamin Hydrochloride • Chromium Nicotinate • Cyanocobalamin • Vitamin D (D2) • Folic Acid.

Bulk & Muscle Formula (vanilla flavor) - Herbalife International of America, Inc.
Soy Protein Isolate • Calcium Caseinate • Maltodextirn • Whey Protein Concentrate • Dextrose • Fructose • Natural and Artificial Flavors • Tricalcium Phosphate • Dipotassium Phosphate • Medium Chain Triglycerides • Magnesium Oxide • Honey powder • Soy Lecithin • Bacterially-Derived Patented Proteases (from Aminogen) • Choline Bitartrate • Potassium Citrate • Aspartame • Egg Albumin solids powder • L-Carnitine Hydrochloride • L-Glutamine • Beta Carotene • Ascorbic Acid • DL-Alpha Tocopheryl Acetate • Molybdenum Amino Acid Chelate • Potassium Glycerophosphate • Ornithine Alpha Ketoglutarate • Biotin • Selenium Amino Acid Chelate • Ferrous Fumarate • Niacin • Manganese Amino Acid Chelate • Zinc Oxide • D-Calcium Pantothenate • Potassium Iodide • Vitamin A Palmitate • Vitamin K • Copper Sulfate • Eleuthero powder • Astragalus root powder • Pyridoxine Hydrochloride • Riboflavin • Thiamin Hydrochloride • Chromium Nicotinate • Cyanocobalamin • Vitamin D (D2) • Folic Acid.

Burdock - Nature's Sunshine
Two capsules contain: Burdock root (arctium lappa) 720 mg. Other Ingredients: Magnesium Stearate, Silicon Dioxide, Gelatin, Water.

Burdock - Nature's Way
Two capsules contain: Burdock root 1.08 g. Other Ingredients: Gelatin, Magnesium stearate.

Burdock Root - Aboca USA, Inc
Two capsules contain: Burdock root WPC (whole phytocomplex concentrate, arctium lappa, standardized to 1.9% caffeoylquinic acids, yielding 5 mg per capsule) 524 mg. Other Ingredients: Gelatin.

Burdock-Dandelion Formula - Quest
Each caplet contains: Burdock root powder (Arctium lappa) 90 mg • Dandelion root powder (Taraxacum officinale) 90 mg • Oregon Grape root powder (Mahonia aquifolium) 90 mg • Red Clover blossoms powder (Trifolium praetense) 90 mg • Echinacea angustifolia root powder (Echinacea angustifolia) 30 mg • Yellow Dock root powder (Rhumex) 30 mg • Cayenne powder (Capsicum) 20 mg • Kelp powder (Fucus vesiculosis) 20 mg • Licorice root powder (Glycirrhiza glabra) 5 mg. Other Ingredients: Calcium Phosphate, Microcrystalline Cellulose, Vegetable Stearin, Croscarmellose Sodium, Magnesium Stearate (vegetable source).

Burn Bar - Metagenics
Each bar contains: Vitamin A (as retinyl acetate) 1250 IU • Vitamin D (as cholecalciferol) 100 IU • Riboflavin (vitamin B2) 425 mcg • Thiamin (as thiamin mononitrate) 750 mcg • Folate (as folic acid) 200 mcg • Vitamin B12 (as cyanocobalamin) 3 mcg • Vitamin B6 (as pyridoxine HCI) 1 mg • Niacin 5 mg • Biotin 75 mcg • Pantothenic Acid (as calcium D-pantothenate) 2.5 mg • Vitamin C (as ascorbic acid) 60 mg • Vitamin E (as D-alpha tocopheryl acetate) 7.5 IU • Vitamin K 20 mcg • Calcium (as calcium phosphate, calcium gluconate, and calcium citrate) 150 mg • Magnesium (as magnesium oxide) 80 mg • Phosphorus 100 mg • Zinc (as zinc arginate) 3.75 mg • Copper (as copper gluconate) 120 mcg • Iron (as ferrous sulfate) 1mg • Chromium (as chromium dinicotinate glycinate) 120 mcg • Selenium (as sodium selenite) 17.5 mcg • Molybdenum (as sodium molybdate) 7.5 mcg • Manganese (as manganese sulfate) 200 mcg. Other Ingredients: High Fructose Corn Syrup, Protein Blend (whey protein isolate, calcium caseinate), Coating (sugar, fractionated palm kernel oil, cocoa powder, whey powder, nonfat milk powder, lecithin, natural vanilla flavor), Natural Peanut Butter (peanuts), Fibersol 2 brand Maltodextrin with soluble fiber, Natural Peanut Flavor, Glycerin, Salt, Mono- and Diglycerides, Lecithin Emulsifiers.

Burn Gel - Nature's Way
Calendula Officinalis (marigold) 1X • Cantharis (cantharides) 3X • Sulphur (sulfur) 6X • Urtica Dioica (stinging nettle) 1X.
See Editor's Note No. 1.

Burn It - ANS - Applied Nutrition Sciences
Chromium Picolinate • Vitamin E • Selenium • Zinc.

BustPrep - HealthMinded
Four capsules contain: BustPrep Proprietary Blend 1960 mg: Saw Palmetto berry, Wild Yam root & rhizome dried extract, Damiana leaf, Black Cohosh root dried extract, Dong Quai root dried extract, Fennel seed, Blessed Thistle herb, Dandelion root, Watercress leaf. Other Ingredients: Gelatin, Stearic Acid, Magnesium Stearate.

BustPro - HealthMinded
Four capsules contain: BustPro Proprietary Blend 2000 mg: Saw Palmetto berry, Wild Yam extract, Damiana, Dong Quai extract, Fennel seed, Black Cohosh extract, Dandelion root, Blessed Thistle, Watercress leaf. Other Ingredients: Stearic Acid, Magnesium Stearate.

Butcher's Broom - Nature's Way
Two capsules contain: Butchers Broom root 940 mg. Other Ingredients: Gelatin, Magnesium stearate.

Butcher's Broom - NOW Foods
Two capsules contain: Butchers Broom 5:1 extract (rascus aculeatus) (root) 200 mg. Other Ingredients: Rice Flour.

BRAND NAMES

Butcher's Broom **- Source Naturals**
Each tablet contains: Butcher's Broom 500 mg.

Butcher's Broom **- Nature's Sunshine**
Two capsules contain: Butcher's Broom root (ruscus aculeatus) 800 mg. Other Ingredients: Kosher Gelatin, Water.

Butchers Broom (Ruscus aculeatus) **- Solgar**
Each capsule contains: Iron 1 mg • Butcher's Broom root 5:1 extract 50 mg • Raw Butcher's Broom root powder 283 mg. Other Ingredients: Vegetable Cellulose, Vegetable Magnesium Stearate, Rosemary Oil Powder, Water, Vegetable Glycerin.

BUTTitOUT **- Paradise**
Each capsule contains: Lobelia Inflata leaf 130 mg. In Base of Organic Brown Rice Flour.

Buzz Away Lotion With Sunblock SPF 15 **- Quantum**
Padimate-0 (octo-dimethyl paba) • Benzophenone-3 • Purified Water • Aloe Vera gel • Hybrid Safflower oil • Octyl Palmitate Glycerine • Coconut oil • Sesame oil • Jojoba oil • Avocado oil • Stearic Acid • PVP-Eicosene Copolymer • Glyceryl Stearate • Cetyl Alcohol • Citronella oil • Dimethicone • Allantoin • Panthenol • Tocopherol (vitamin E) • Cocoa butter • Lecithin • TEA-Carbomer-040 • Methylparaben • Propylparaben • Cedarwood oil • Eucalyptus oil • Lemongrass oil • Peppermint oil • Diazolidinyl Urea • Polysorbate 80.

Buzz Away Spray **- Quantum**
Citronella oil • Cedarwood oil • Eucalyptus oil • Lemongrass oil • Peppermint oil • Water • Denatured Ethyl Alcohol • Modified Castor oil.

Buzz Away Towelettes **- Quantum**
Water • Denatured Ethyl Alcohol • Modified Castor oil • Citronella oil • Cedarwood oil • Eucalyptus oil • Lemongrass • Peppermint oil.

Bye Mygrain **- DreamPharm**
Two capsules contain: Bay (laurus nobilis) 60 mg • Feverfew (tanacetum parthenium) 80 mg • Evening Primrose herb (oenothera biennis) 60 mg • Willow bark (salix species) 50 mg • Ligusticum Chuan Xiang root 100 mg • Angelica Dahurica root 100 mg • Gastrodia Elata rhizome 50 mg.

Bye-Lori **- Life Enhancement Products, Inc.**
Four capsules contain: Mastic Gum 1000 mg.

Bye-Lori II **- Life Enhancement Products, Inc.**
Four capsules contain: Mastic gum 1000 mg • Thyme extract 8.75 mg • Hyperforin 4 mg • Cinnamon extract 2.5 mg.

C + Herbs **- Jarrow Formulas**
Each tablet contains: Silymarin (Silybum marianum) 30:1 Concentrate (standardized to 80% silybin) 75 mg • PicroLiv (3.5- 4% Kutkin from Picrorrhiza kurroa) 50 mg • Astragalus Root 6:1 Concentrate 150 mg • Schisandra 5:1 Concentrate 75 mg • Scutelluria root (Skullcap) 4:1 concentrate 150 mg • Vitamin C (Ascorbic Acid) 500 mg. Other Ingredients: Magnesium Stearate.

C All Inclusive 1000 mg **- Rexall - Sundown**
Each tablet contains: Vitamin C 600 mg • Calcium 74 mg • Bioflavonoid Complex 48 mg: Rose Hips & Seeds, Citrus Bioflavonoids, Rutin, Hesperidin, Acerola Fruit Extract 4:1. Other Ingredients: Ascorbic Acid, Calcium Sulfate, Microcrystalline Cellulose, Croscarmellose Sodium, Magnesium Stearate, Hydroxypropyl Methylcellulose, Sweet Orange (peel and fruit), Bitter Orange (fruit), PEG.
See Editor's Note No. 40.

C Aspa Scorb **- Progressive Labs**
Each teaspoon (5100 mg) supplies: Vitamin C 4000 mg • Magnesium (from magnesium ascorbate and magnesium aspartate) 250 mg • Zinc (from zinc ascorbate) 30 mg • Selenium (from selenium ascorbate) 50 mcg • Manganese (from manganese ascorbate) 4.2 mg • Potassium (from potassium ascorbate and potassium aspartate) 96 mg.

C Complex 500mg with rosehips and bioflavonoids **- Nature's Own**
Each tablet contains: Vitamin C (ascorbic acid) 500 mg • Bioflavonoids 100 mg • Hesperidin complex 50 mg • Rosehips (rosa canina) extract 50 mg • Rutin 25 mg.

C Every Day **- Hadas Natural Products**
Each 5 mL serving contains: Orange flavored Sorbitol syrup • Rose Hip extract with Vitamin C 300 mg.

C Herbaplex 500 **- Wild Rose**
Each tablet contains: Vitamin C (ascorbic acid) 500 mg • Lemon Bioflavanoids (10%) 250 mg • Rutin 50 mg • Hesperidin Complex (15%) 50 mg • Rose Hips 250 mg • Parsley leaf 8.5 mg • Red Raspberry leaf 8.5 mg • Mullein leaf 2 mg.

C&E **- Nature's Bounty**
Each softgel contains: Vitamin C (as ascorbic acid and rose hips) 500 mg • Vitamin E (as D-alpha tocopherol plus D-beta, D-gamma and D-delta tocopherols) 400 IU. Other Ingredients: Gelatin, Glycerin, Soybean Oil, Soy Lecithin, Caramel Color, Yellow Beeswax.

C&F Formula **- Dial Herbs**
Vinegar • Glycerine • Honey • the Tinctures of Garlic, Comfrey, Wormwood, Marshmallow, White Oak bark, Black Walnut, Mullein, Scullcap, Uva Ursi, Lobelia.

C-1000 **- PhysioLogics**
Each capsule contains: Vitamin C (as ascorbic acid) 1000 mg • Citrus Bioflavonoids (citrus spp., fruit) 30 mg. Other Ingredients: Gelatin, Vegetable Magnesium Stearate, Titanium Dioxide Color.

C-1000 **- Source Naturals**
Each tablet contains: Vitamin C (as ascorbic acid) 1000 mg. Other Ingredients: Microcrystalline Cellulose, Stearic Acid, Hydroxypropyl Cellulose, Modified Gum, Magnesium Stearate, Colloidal Silicon Dioxide.

C-1000 **- Nutritional Therapeutics, Inc.**
Each tablet contains: Vitamin C (Calcium Ascorbate-Niascorbate) 1000 mg • Bioflavonoids 100 mg • Pantethine 5 mg • NT Factor tablet base 50 mg.

C-1000 **- Ortho Molecular Products**
Each tablet contains: Vitamin C (as ascorbic acid) 1000 mg • Rose Hips 25 mg. Other Ingredients: Cellulose, Stearic Acid, Magnesium Stearate, Dicalcium Phosphate, Vegetable Coating.

C-1000 mg Ascorbic Acid **- Rexall - Sundown**
Each caplet contains: Vitamin C (as ascorbic acid) 1 g. Other Ingredients: Cornstarch, Crospovidone, Magnesium Stearate, Hydroxypropyl Methylcellulose, PEG.

C-1000 mg Rosehip Timed **- Rexall - Sundown**
Each caplet contains: Vitamin C 1 g • Calcium 35 mg • Bioflavonoid Complex 19 mg: Rose Hips & Seeds, Citrus Bioflavonoids, Rutin, Acerola Fruit Extract 4:1. Other Ingredients: Hydrogenated Cottonseed Oil, Dicalcium Phosphate, Hydroxypropyl Methylcellulose, Silica, Magnesium Stearate, Orange (fruit), Bitter Orange (fruit).
See Editor's Note No. 40.

C-1000 with Rosehips **- Rexall - Sundown**
Each caplet contains: Vitamin C 1 g • Bioflavonoid Complex 17 mg: Rose Hips & Seeds, Citrus Bioflavonoids, Rutin, Acerola Fruit Extract 4:1. Other Ingredients: Microcrystalline Cellulose, Stearic Acid, Silica, Croscarmellose Sodium, Magnesium Stearate, Orange (fruit), Bitter Orange (fruit).
See Editor's Note No. 40.

C-1000-TR **- Atrium Biotechnologies**
Each tablet contains: Vitamin C 1000 mg • Naturally Associated Bioflavonoid Complex 100 mg.

C-250 mg Ascorbic Acid - Rexall - Sundown
Each tablet contains: Vitamin C (as ascorbic acid) 250 mg. Other Ingredients: Dicalcium Phosphate, Microcrystalline Cellulose, Stearic Acid, Croscarmellose Sodium, Magnesium Stearate.

C-500 - Nutritional Therapeutics, Inc.
Each tablet contains: Vitamin C (Calcium Ascorbate-Niascorbate) 500 mg • Bioflavonoids 100 mg • Pantethine 5 mg • NT Factor tablet base 50 mg.

C-500 mg Ascorbic Acid - Rexall - Sundown
Each tablet contains: Vitamin C (as ascorbic acid) 500 mg. Other Ingredients: Cornstarch, Crospovidone, Magnesium Stearate.

C-500 mg Chew w/Rosehips - Rexall - Sundown
Each tablet contains: Vitamin C (as sodium ascorbate, ascorbic acid & rose hips with seeds) 500 mg • Sodium 40 mg. Other Ingredients: Compressible Sugar, Hydrogenated Cottonseed Oil, Stearic Acid, Natural Orange Flavor (with other natural flavors), Magnesium Stearate, Yellow 6 Lake.

C-500 mg Time Release - Rexall - Sundown
Each capsule contains: Vitamin C (as ascorbic acid) 500 mg. Other Ingredients: Gelatin, Pharmaceutical Glaze, Sucrose, Starch, Talc, Titanium Dioxide, Yellow 5 (tartrazine), Yellow 6, Red 40.

C-500 mg with Mixed Bioflavonoids - Nutritional Therapeutics, Inc.
Three tablets contain: Vitamin C (as calcium ascorbate/niascorbate) 1500 mg • Vitamin B3 (as niacinamide) 75 gm • Calcium (as calcium ascorbate) 90 mg • Citrus Bioflavonoids 75 mg • Quercetin 75 mg • Rosehips 75 mg • Rutin 75 mg • NT Factor (as tablet base) 250 mg • Pantethine (as coenzyme A precursor) 15 mg. Other Ingredients: Microcrystalline Cellulose, Croscarmellose Sodium, Food Glaze, Vegetable Magnesium Stearate, Silica.

C-500 Timed Colorfree - Rexall - Sundown
Each capsule contains: Vitamin C (as ascorbic acid) 500 mg. Other Ingredients: Gelatin, Pharmaceutical Glaze, Sucrose, Talc, Food Starch.

C-500 with Rosehips - Rexall - Sundown
Each caplet contains: Vitamin C 500 mg • Bioflavonoid Complex 9 mg: Rose Hips & Seeds, Citrus Bioflavonoids, Rutin, Acerola Fruit Extract 4:1. Other Ingredients: Microcrystalline Cellulose, Stearic Acid, Silica, Croscarmellose Sodium, Magnesium Stearate, Orange (fruit), Bitter Orange (fruit).
See Editor's Note No. 40.

C-500 XTRA - Rexall - Sundown
Each tablet contains: Vitamin C 500 mg • Zinc (as zinc oxide) 5 mg • Selenium (as selenium yeast chelate) 33 mcg • Orange Peel Extract 100 mg • Citrus Bioflavonoids 25 mg • Rutin 50 mg • XTRA Premium Blend 5.25 mg: Alfalfa (leaf), Rose Hips & Seeds, Parsley (aerial parts), Acerola Fruit Extract 1:4. Other Ingredients: Ascorbic Acid, Dicalcium Phosphate, Croscarmellose Sodium, Hydroxypropyl Methylcellulose, Magnesium Stearate, PEG.

Caballo Negro Energy Drink - Distribuidores De La Energia Inc.
Carbonated Water • High Fructose Corn Syrup • Sucrose • Citric Acid • Sodium Citrate • Taurine • Gluconolactone • Potassium Benzoate (as a preservative) • Caramel Color • Natural & Artificial Flavors • Caffeine • Inositol • Niacin • D-Panthenol • Pyridoxine HCl • Cyanocobalamin (vitamin B12) • Guarana extract • Ginseng extract • Epimedium extract • Cat's Claw extract.

CAC Tabs - Dial Herbs
Cascara Sagrada • Buckthorn • Burdock • Chaparral • Dandelion • Licorice root • Barberry • Red Clover.

Cacao - Nature's Way
Two capsules contain: Cacao (whole fruit) 1.1 g. Other Ingredients: Cellulose, Gelatin.

Cactus (Nopal) - Natural Dynamics
Each capsule contains: Nopal 650 mg.

Cactus Diet - Cactu-Life
Each capsule contains: Opuntia Streptacantha 500 mg.

Caffeine Detox - Nature's Sunshine
Chamomilla (chamomile) 3X • Coffee (coffea cruda) 6X • Gratiola Officinalis (hedge-hyssop) 6X • Ignatius Bean (ignatia amara) 6X • Nux Vomica (quaker button) 6X • Thuja Occidentalis (tree of life) 6X. Other ingredients: Purified Water, Glycerin, Citric Acid, Potassium Benzoate.
See Editor's Note No. 1.

Caffeine Mix - Professional Complementary Health Formulas
Adrenal 3X, 4X • ACTH 6X, 30X • Histamine 12X • Liver 6X, 12X • Methylxanthine-bearing foods: Caffeine, Chocolate (milk, dark, white), Coffee (five types), Decaffeinated Coffee, Cola, Espresso, Tea 6X, 12X, 60X, 100X • Purified Water • 20% USP Alcohol.
See Editor's Note No. 1.

CAL (+ CAL +) - Pure Encapsulations
Seven vegetable capsules contain: Calcium (citrate/malate) 900 mg • Ipriflavone 500 mg • Horsetail 5:1 extract (equisetum arvense) 300 mg • Magnesium (aspartate) 115 mg • Manganese (aspartate) 10 mg • Zinc (picolinate) 30 mg • Copper (glycinate) 2.5 mg • Boron (glycinate) 2 mg • Vitamin C (as ascorbyl palmitate) 102 mg • Vitamin D (D3) 400 IU • Vitamin K (K1) 500 mcg.

Cal Apatite - Metagenics
Three tablets contain: Microcrystalline Hydroxyapatite Concentrate (MCHC) 1500 mg • Calcium (as MCHC and dicalcium phosphate) 626 mg • Phosphorus (as MCHC and dicalcium phosphate) 398 mg.

Cal Apatite 1000 - Metagenics
Three tablets contain: Microcrystalline Hydroxyapatite Concentrate (MCHC) 3000 mg • Calcium (as MCHC and dicalcium phosphate) 1011 mg • Phosphorus (as MCHC and dicalcium phosphate) 609 mg.

Cal Apatite Chewable - Metagenics
Three tablets contain: Microcrystalline Hydroxyapatite Concentrate (MCHC) 750 mg • Calcium (as MCHC and dicalcium phosphate) 300 mg • Phosphorus (as MCHC and dicalcium phosphate) 189 mg • Vitamin D (as cholecalciferol) 75 IU • Magnesium (as magnesium bis-glycinate) 75 mg • Zinc (as zinc glycinate) 6 mg • Copper (as copper glycinate) 750 mcg • Manganese (as manganese glycinate) 750 mcg.

Cal Apatite Forte Capsules - Metagenics
Three capsules contain: MCHC 3036 mg • Calcium (as MCHC) 684 mg • Phosphorus (as MCHC) 357 mg • Vitamin D (as cholecalciferol) 600 IU.

Cal Apatite Plus - Metagenics
Three tablets contain: Microcrystalline Hydroxyapatite concentrate (MCHC) 1500 mg • Vitamin D (as cholecalciferol) 600 IU • Calcium (as MCHC and dicalcium phosphate) 660 mg • Phosphorus (as MCHC and dicalcium phosphate) 423 mg • Ipriflavone 150 mg.

Cal Apatite with Boron - Metagenics
Three tablets contain: Microcrystalline Hydroxyapatite Concentrate (MCHC) 1500 mg • Calcium (as MCHC and dicalcium phosphate) 626 mg • Phosphorus (as MCHC and dicalcium phosphate) 398 mg • Boron (as boron citrate) 300 mcg.

Cal Apatite with Magnesium - Metagenics
Three tablets contain: Microcrystalline Hydroxyapatite Concentrate (MCHC) 1500 mg • Calcium (as MCHC and dicalcium phosphate) 600 mg • Phosphorus (as MCHC and dicalcium phosphate) 378 mg • Magnesium (as magnesium citrate, aspartate, and bis-glycinate) 300 mg.

Cal Mag + D - Wild Rose
Each tablet contains: Calcium (citrate) 150 mg • Magnesium (oxide) 75 mg • Vitamin D (as D3) 100 IU • Bromelain (1:10) 20 mg • Pacific Kelp 50 mg • Parsley leaf 10 mg.

Cal Mag Liquid - Genestra - Seroyal
Each tablespoon contains: Calcium Carbonate 600 mg • Magnesium Oxide 300 mg • Vitamin D (as vitamin D3) 100 IU. Other Ingredients: Natural Spearmint Flavor.

Cal Mag with D - Benepure, Inc
Two tablets contain: Vitamin D (D3) 50 IU • Calcium 500 mg • Magnesium 200 mg. Other Ingredients: Calcium Amino Acid Chelate, Magnesium Amino Acid Chelate, Microcrystalline Cellulose, Vegetable Stearate, Stearic Acid, Silica.

Cal Matrix - Metagenics
Six tablets contain: Microcrystalline Hydroxyapatite Concentrate (MCHC) 2688 mg • Calcium (as MCHC and dicalcium phosphate) 1224 mg • Phosphorus (as MCHC and dicalcium phosphate) 774 mg • Glucosamine Sulfate (as D-glucosamine sulfate KCl) 500 mg • Vitamin C (as ultra potent-C) 500 mg • Niacin (as niacinamide ascorbate) 18 mg • Manganese (as manganese glycinate) 1 mg • Vitamin D (as cholecalciferol) 400 IU • Magnesium (as magnesium bis-glycinate) 220 mg • Zinc (as zinc glycinate) 15 mg • Copper (as copper glycinate) 2 mg • Boron (as boron citrate) 390 mcg • Chromium (as chromium nicotinate glycinate) 240 mcg • Horsetail aerial parts (equisetum arvense) 600 mg.

Cal/Mag 500/250 mg - Nature's Plus
Each tablet contains: Calcium (as amino acid chelate/complex) 500 mg • Magnesium (as amino acid chelate/complex) 250 mg. Other Ingredients: Stearic Acid, Microcrystalline Cellulose, Di-calcium Phosphate, Magnesium Stearate, Isolated Soy Protein, Silica, Pharmaceutical Glaze.

Cal/Mag Balance - Nutri-Quest Rx
Each tablet contains: Calcium Aspartate 175 mg • Calcium Citrate 175 mg • Magnesium Aspartate 175 mg • Magnesium Glycinate 175 mg • Vitamin C 25 IU • Vitamin D 20 mg of HCL.

Cal/Mag Caps 500/250 mg - Nature's Plus
Two capsules contain: Calcium (as amino acid chelate/complex) 500 mg • Magnesium (as amino acid chelate/complex) 250 mg. Other Ingredients: Isolated Soy Protein, Silica, Vegetable Cellulose, Purified Water.

Cal/Mag Citrate - Nature's Plus
Three capsules contain: Calcium (as citrate) 500 mg • Magnesium (as citrate) 250 mg • Boron (as citrate) 3 mg. Other Ingredients: Microcrystalline Cellulose, Magnesium Stearate, Vegetable Cellulose, Purified Water.

Cal/Mag Citrate with Vitamin D - Country Life Vitamins
Each four softgels contain: Calcium (citrate, carbonate) 400 mg • Magnesium (carbonate, citrate) 400 mg • Vitamin D (cholecalciferol) 100 IU. Inactive Ingredients: Soybean Oil, Lecithin, Gelatin, Glycerin, Purified Water, Titanium Dioxide.

Cal/Mag Complex - Country Life Vitamins
Each tablet contains: Calcium (as calcium hydroxyapatite, citrate, asparate, alpha-ketoglutartate, lysinate) 1000 mg • Phosphorous (from calcium hydroxyapatite) 500 mg • Magnesium (as magnesium oxide, citrate, taurinate, alpha-ketoglutarate, magnesium aspartate) 500 mg.

Cal/Mag/Zinc 1000/500/75 mg - Nature's Plus
Four tablets contain: Calcium (as amino acid chelate/complex) 1000 mg • Magnesium (as amino acid chelate/complex) 500 mg • Zinc (as amino acid chelate/complex) 75 mg. Other Ingredients: Di-calcium Phosphate, Microcrystalline Cellulose, Stearic Acid, Isolated Soy Protein, Silica, Pharmaceutical Glaze.

Cal-1000 Complete - Puritan's Pride
Two tablets contain: Vitamin A (as Retinyl Acetate) 5,000 IU • Vitamin C (as Ascorbic Acid) 60 mg • Vitamin C (as Cholecalciferol) 400 IU • Vitamin E (as dl-Alpha Tocopheryl Acetate) 30 IU • Thiamin (Vitamin B-1; as Thiamine Mononitrate) 1.5 mg • Riboflavin (Vitamin B-2) 1.7 mg • Niacin (as Niacinamide) 20 mg • Vitamin B-6 (as Pyridoxine Hydrochloride) 2 mg • Folic Acid 400 mcg • Vitamin B-12 (as Cyanocobalamin) 6 mcg • Biotin (as d-Biotin) 300 mcg • Pantothenic Acid (as d-Calcium Pantothenate) 10 mg • Calcium (as Calcium Carbonate) 1,000 mg • Iron (as Ferrous Fumarate) 18 mg.

Cal-Acid Complex - Atrium Biotechnologies
Four tablets contain: Calcium (from oyster shell, oyster shell-citrus juice complex, & calcium caseinate) 750 mg • Magnesium (from magnesium citrus juice complex & oxide) 210 mg • Manganese (manganese-citrus carbonate juice complex) 5 mg • Copper (as gluconate) 0.1 mg • Vitamin D (fish oil) 400 USP IU • Vitamin C with Rose Hips 40 mg • Vitamin E 10 IU • Betaine HCl & Glutamic Acid HCl sufficient to provide dilute HCL10 min • Amino Acids, Peptides, & Polypeptides from Hydrolized Soy Protein with Lecithin & Alfalfa juice concentrate.

Cal-Acid Maxi - Atrium Biotechnologies
Four tablets contain: Calcium (Calcium Citrate, Calcium Caseinate & Oyster Shell) 1500 mg • Magnesium (Magnesium Citrus Juice Complex & Oxide) 500 mg • Manganese (Manganese Citrus Carbonate Juice) 10 mg • Vitamin D (Fish oil) 500 IU • Vitamin C with Rose Hips 100 mg • Vitamin E (d-Alpha Tocopherol) 20 IU • Horsetail (Silica) 250 mg • Boron (Citrate) 3 mg. Betaine HCL & Glutamic Acid HCL sufficient to provide dilute HCL. Amino acids, peptids & polypeptids from hydrolyzed soy protein with Lecithin & Alfalfa juice concentrate.

Calamacin - MMS Pro
Each capsule contains: Scullcap herb • Wood Betony • Black Cohosh root • Hops flowers • Valerian root • Cayenne.

Cal-Amo - Standard Process, Inc.
Each tablet contains: Calcium 30 mg • Magnesium 6 mg • Chloride 100 mg • Betaine Hydrochloride.

Calcet Triple Calcium - Mission Pharmacal
Two tablets contain: Vitamin D (Vitamin D3; as cholecalciferol) 200 IU • Calcium (as calcium carbonate, calcium gluconate, calcium lactate) 300 mg. Other Ingredients: Polyethylene Glycol, HPMC, Croscarmellose Sodium, Color, Magnesium Stearate, FD & C Yellow 5 Lake, Magnesium Silicate, Carnauba Wax.

Cal-Chew Calcium 350 mg - Jamieson
Each tablet contains: Calcium (as Calcium Carbonate, Calcium Citrate, Calcium Malate, Calcium Succinate, Calcium Aspartate, Calcium Glutamate, Calcium Fumarate) 350 mg • Iron 0.4 mg.

Calcifood - Standard Process, Inc.
Two wafers contain: Proprietary Blend 800 mg: Defatted Wheat germ, Carrot root, Date fruit, Veal Bone meal, Rice bran extract, Peanut bran • Calcium 200 mg. Other Ingredients: Bovine Bone, Cellulose, Honey, Dicalcium Phosphate, Calcium Stearate, Arabic Gum.

Calcifood Powder - Standard Process, Inc.
Each 1 tbsp (9 g) serving contains: Proprietary Blend 5.15 g: Defatted Wheat germ, Carrot root, Oat flour, Date powder, Peanut bran • Calcium 600 mg • Sodium 8 mg • Potassium 3.5 mg. Other Ingredients: Bovine Bone Meal, Veal Bone Meal.

Calci-Lean - Gero Vita International
Two capsules contain: Vitamin C (as magnesium ascorbate) 77 mg • Calcium (as calcium gluconate) 19 mg • Magnesium (as magnesium ascorbate) 10 mg • Proprietary Herbal Blend 890 mg: Guggul gum extract (24% lipids), Nut Grass tuber extract (0.15% alkaloids), Plumbago Zeylanica root extract (0.01% alkaloids), Embelia Ribes fruit extract, Operculina Turpenthurn root extract (2.5% resins), Picorhiza Kurroa root extract (1% bitter), Emblic fruit extract (5% tannins), Tropical Almond fruit extract (7.5% tannins), Belleric Myrobalan fruit extract (5% tannins), Piper Longum fruit extract (0.5% volatile oil), Black Pepper fruit extract (1% volatile oil), Ginger rhizome extract (0.5% volatile oils) • Proprietary Enzyme Blend 100 mg: Bromelain, Amylase, HermiSeb, Peptizyme SP, Catalase, Lipase, Amla. Other Ingredients: Gelatin, Silicon Dioxide, Magnesium Stearate.

Calcimate - GNC
Two tablets contain: Vitamin D (as cholecalciferol) 200 IU • Calcium (as calcium citrate malate) 500 mg • Magnesium (as magnesium oxide) 125 mg • Zinc (as zinc oxide) 8 mg • Copper (as cupric oxide) 1 mg • Boron (as boron citrate) 1 mg. Other Ingredients: Cellulose.

Calcimate 400 - GNC
Three tablets contain: Vitamin D (as Cholecalciferol) 200 IU • Calcium (as Calcium Citrate Malate) 400 mg. Other Ingredients: Cellulose.

Calcimate Plus 800 - GNC
Four tablets contain: Vitamin D (as Cholecalciferol) 200 IU • Calcium (as Calcium Citrate Malate) 800 mg • Magnesium (as Magnesium Oxide) 100 mg • Potassium (as Potassium Chloride) 99 mg. Other Ingredients: Cellulose, Titanium Dioxide, Vegetable Acetoglycerides.

Calcium - Vital Nutrients
Each capsule contains: Calcium (citrate/malate) 150 mg.

Calcium - Natrol, Inc.
Three tablets contain: Calcium 500 mg • Magnesium 200 mg • Fruitbase 640 mg. Other Ingredients: Mono- and Di-Glycerides, Croscarmellose Sodium, Silicon Dioxide, Stearic Acid, Magnesium Stearate.

Calcium - GNC
Each tablet contains: Calcium (as Calcium Carbonate) 600 mg. Other Ingredients: Gelatin, Cellulose, Soy Fiber, Titanium Dioxide, Vegetable Acetoglycerides, Magnesium Stearate.

Calcium - PhytoPharmica
Each tablet contains: Calcium (from tricalcium phosphate and calcium citrate) 333 mg • Magnesium (as magnesium oxide and magnesium aspartate) 133 mg • Phosphorus (from tricalcium phosphate) 150 mg • Sodium 5 mg • Vitamin D (as cholecalciferol) 133 IU.

Calcium & Magnesium - NSI - Nutraceutical Sciences Institute
Each four capsules contain: Calcium (from 2,227 mg calcium citrate malate) 500 mg • Magnesium (from 1,190 mg magnesium citrate) 250 mg.

Calcium & Magnesium - Nature's Way
Three capsules contain: Calcium (citrate, carbonate, malate) 500 mg • Magnesium (oxide, aspartate) 250 mg •Sodium 5 mg. Other Ingredients: Cellulose, Gelatin, Magnesium Stearate.

Calcium & Magnesium - Matol Botanical International Ltd
Each 2 tbsp (30 mL) serving contains: Vitamin D (as cholecalciferol) 200 IU • Calcium (as carbonate, lactate, and citrate) 600 mg • Magnesium (as oxide and citrate) 270 mg • Zinc (as citrate) 9 mg. Other Ingredients: Purified Water, Sorbitol, Glycerin, Xanthan Gum, Natural Flavor, Methylparaben, Propylparaben.

Calcium & Magnesium - Source Naturals
Each tablet contains: Calcium (from 1,250 mg of Amino Acid Chelate) 250 mg • Magnesium (from 625 mg of Amino Acid Chelate) 125 mg • Vitamin D (Cholecalciferol) 500 IU.

Calcium & Magnesium Complex - Health Smart Vitamins
Three caplets contain: Calcium (as 80% calcium citrate, 19% calcium carbonate, 1% calcium stearate) 503 mg • Magnesium (as 50% magnesium citrate, 50% magnesium glycinate) 250 mg.

Calcium & Magnesium Complex - Nature's Way
Three capsules contain: Calcium (citrate, carbonate, malate) 500 mg • Magnesium (oxide, aspartate) 250 mg • Sodium 5 mg. Other Ingredients: Cellulose, Gelatin, Magnesium-Stearate.

Calcium (aspartate) - Pure Encapsulations
Each vegetable capsule contains: Calcium (aspartate) 140 mg • Vitamin C (as ascorbyl palmitate) 11 mg.

Calcium (citrate) - Pure Encapsulations
Each vegetable capsule contains: Calcium (citrate) 150 mg • Vitamin C (as ascorbyl palmitate) 16 mg.

Calcium (citrate/malate) - Pure Encapsulations
Each vegetable capsule contains: Calcium (citrate/malate) 150 mg • Vitamin C (as ascorbyl palmitate) 8 mg.

Calcium (microcrystalline hydroxyapatite) - Pure Encapsulations
Each vegetable capsule contains: Calcium (microcrystalline hydroxyapatite, bovine) 150 mg.

Calcium + D, Natural Source - Leiner Health Products
Each tablet contains: Calcium Carbonate 600 mg • Vitamin D (Cholecalciferol) 200 IU. Other Ingredients: Maltodextrin, Hydroxypropyl Methylcellulose, Talc, Croscarmellose Sodium, Acacia, Hydroxypropyl Cellulose, Titanium Dioxide, Silicon Dioxide, Starch, Magnesium Stearate, Polysorbate 80, Polyethylene Glycol 3350, Sodium Citrate, Yellow 6 Lake.

Calcium +D - Rexall - Sundown
Three tablets contain: Vitamin D (as cholecalciferol) 400 IU • Calcium (from oyster shell) 1 g. Other Ingredients: Maltodextrin, Cellulose, Mineral Oil, Croscarmellose Sodium, Hydroxypropyl Methylcellulose, Carboxymethylcellulose Sodium, PEG, Carnauba Wax, Crospovidone, Magnesium Stearate, Stearic Acid.

Calcium +D 500 mg - Rexall - Sundown
Each caplet contains: Vitamin D (as cholecalciferol) 200 IU • Calcium (from oyster shell) 500 mg. Other Ingredients: Maltodextrin, Microcrystalline Cellulose, Mineral Oil, Hydroxypropyl Methylcellulose, Soy Poly-Saccharides, Titanium Dioxide, PEG, Polysorbate 80, Yellow 5 Lake (tartrazine), Blue 1 Lake, Carnauba Wax, Stearic Acid, Magnesium Stearate, Crospovidone.

Calcium 1000 Magnesium 400 - GNC
Three tablets contain: Calcium (as Calcium Carbonate) 1000 mg •Magnesium (as Magnesium Oxide) 400 mg •Zinc (as Zinc Oxide) 15 mg •Copper (as Cupric Oxide) 1 mg. Other Ingredients: Cellulose.

Calcium 1200 with D - Rexall - Sundown
Two softgels contain: Vitamin D (as cholecalciferol) 200 IU • Calcium (as calcium carbonate) 1.2 g. Other Ingredients: Soybean Oil, Gelatin, Glycerin, Soy Lecithin, Water, Titanium Dioxide (color).

Calcium 500 mg - Nature Made
Each tablet contains: Calcium (from calcium carbonate) 500 mg. Other Ingredients: Maltodextrin, Cellulose, Hydroxypropyl Methylcellulose, Soy Polysaccharides, Polyethylene Glcyol. See Editor's Note No. 45.

Calcium 500 mg - Rexall - Sundown
Each caplet contains: Calcium (from oyster shell) 500 mg. Other Ingredients: Maltodextrin, Cellulose, Hydroxypropyl Methylcellulose, Mineral Oil, Titanium Dioxide (color), PEG, Yellow 5 Lake, Polysorbate 80, Blue 1 Lake, Stearic Acid, Magnesium Stearate, Crospovidone.

Calcium 500 mg - Sunmark
Each tablet contains: Calcium (calcium carbonate from oyster shell) 500 mg. Other Ingredients: Maltodextrin, Cellulose, Hypromellose, Mineral Oil, Titanium Dioxide, Polyethylene Glycol, Triethyl Citrate, FD&C Yellow No. 5 Lake, Carnauba Wax, FD&C Blue No. 1 lake, Stearic Acid, Magnesium Stearate, Crospovidone. See Editor's Note No. 45.

Calcium 500 mg Plus D - Nature's Valley
Each tablet contains: Vitamin D 200 IU • Calcium (from oyster shell) 500 mg. Other Ingredients: Maltodextrin, Cellulose, Hydroxypropyl Methylcellulose, Carboxymethylcellulose Sodium, Croscarmellose Sodium, Starch, Mineral Oil, Titanium Dioxide, Gelatin, Yellow 5 Lake, Blue 1 Lake, Polyethylene Glycol 3350, Polysorbate 80, Acacia, Crospovidone, Magnesium Stearate, Stearic Acid. See Editor's Note No. 45.

Some Brand Name Natural Products - What they Contain

www.NaturalDatabase.com contains MANY more listings than appear here.
Editor's Notes are located on pages 2155-2163.

BRAND NAMES

Calcium 600 **- Solgar**
Two tablets contain: Vitamin D (as cholecalciferol) 600 IU • Calcium (as calcium carbonate from oyster shell) 1200 mg • Iron 1 mg • Sodium 15 mg. Other Ingredients: Microcrystalline Cellulose, Vegetable Cellulose, Vegetable Magnesium Stearate, Vegetable Glycerin.

Calcium 600 **- Walgreens**
Each tablet contains: Calcium (as calcium carbonate) 600 mg. Other Ingredients: Croscarmellose Sodium, Hydroxypropyl Methylcellulose, Sodium Lauryl Sulfate, Titanium Dioxide, Magnesium Stearate, Polyethylene Glycol, Carnauba Wax.

Calcium 600 **- Pro Health**
Each tablet contains: Vitamin D (as cholecalciferol) 400 IU • Calcium (as carbonate, citrate, mined from earth deposits) 600 mg. Other Ingredients: Stearic Acid, Microcrystalline Cellulose, Croscarmellose Sodium, Magnesium Stearate, Pharmaceutical Glaze.

Calcium 600 / Magnesium 300 **- GNC**
Three capsules contain: Vitamin D (as cholecalciferol) 100 IU • Calcium (as calcium carbonate) 600 mg • Magnesium (as magnesium oxide) 300 mg. Other Ingredients: Gelatin, Cellulose.

Calcium 600 + Vitamin D **- AIE Pharmaceuticals**
Two tablets contain: Vitamin D (as cholecalciferol) 250 IU • Calcium (from calcium carbonate) 1200 mg. Other Ingredients: Cellulose, Croscarmellose Sodium, Guar Gum, Magnesium Stearate, Ethylcellulose.

Calcium 600 +D **- Rexall - Sundown**
Each caplet contains: Vitamin D (as cholecalciferol) 200 IU • Calcium (as calcium carbonate) 600 mg. Other Ingredients: Maltodextrin, Cellulose, Hydroxypropyl Methylcellulose, Titanium Dioxide (color), Mineral Oil, PEG, Polysorbate 80, Stearic Acid, Magnesium Stearate, Crospovidone.

Calcium 600 mg **- Nature's Plus**
Each tablet contains: Calcium (as amino acid chelate) 600 mg. Other Ingredients: Magnesium Stearate, Pharmaceutical Glaze, Silica.

Calcium 600 mg **- Sunmark**
Each tablet contains: Calcium (carbonate) 600 mg. Other Ingredients: Maltodextrin, Powdered Cellulose, Hypromellose, Mineral Oil, Titanium Dioxide, Polysorbate 80, Sodium Lauryl Sulfate, Carnauba Wax, Stearic Acid, Magnesium Stearate, Crospovidone, Gluten.
See Editor's Note No. 45.

Calcium 600 mg **- Nature Made**
Each tablet contains: Vitamin D 200 IU • Calcium 600 mg. Other Ingredients: Maltodexrin, Cellulose, Hydroxypropyl Methylcellulose, Soy Polysacchardies, Polyethylene Glycol.
See Editor's Note No. 45.

Calcium 600 mg Plus with Vitamin D & Minerals **- Sunmark**
Each tablet contains: Vitamin D 200 IU • Calcium 600 mg • Magnesium 40 mg • Zinc 7.5 mg • Copper 1 mg • Manganese 0.60 mg • Boron 250 mcg. Other Ingredients: Maltodextrin, Powered Cellulose, Hydroxypropyl Methylcellulose, Mineral Oil, Soy Polysaccharides, Titanium Dioxide, Polysorbate 80, Polyethylene Glycol, Carnauba Wax, FD&C Red No. 40 Lake, FD&C Yellow No. 6 Lake, FD&C Blue No. 1 Lake, Magnesium Stearate, Stearic Acid, Crospovidone, Gluten.
See Editor's Note No. 45.

Calcium 600 mg With D **- Sunmark**
Each tablet contains: Vitamin D 200 IU • Calcium (carbonate) 600 mg. Other Ingredients: Maltodextrin, Powdered Cellulose, Hyprocellulose, Mineral Oil, Titanium Dioxide, Polysorbate 80, Polyethlene Glycol, Carnauba Wax, FD&C Yellow No. 6 Lake, Stearic Acid, Magnesium Stearate, Crospovidone, Gluten.
See Editor's Note No. 45.

Calcium 600 Plus Soy **- Walgreens**
Each tablet contains: Vitamin D (as cholecalciferol) 200 IU • Calcium (as calcium carbonate) 600 mg • Soy Isoflavones (from Novasoy brand soybean extract) 25 mg. Other Ingredients: Crospovidone, Powdered Cellulose, Stearic Acid, Magnesium Stearate, Hydroxypropyl Methylcellulose, Carnauba Wax, Polyethylene Glycol.

Calcium 600+D **- Walgreens**
Each tablet contains: Vitamin D (as cholecalciferol) • Calcium (as calcium carbonate) 600 mg. Other Ingredients: Croscarmellose Sodium, Hydroxypropyl Methylcellulose, Sodium Lauryl Sulfate, Titanium Dioxide, Magnesium Stearate, Polyethylene Glycol, Carnauba Wax, FD&C Yellow No. 6 Lake.

Calcium A.E.P. **- American Biologics**
Five capsules contain: Calcium Hydroxide 740 mg • Phosphorus 1150 mg. Other Ingredients: Magnesium Stearate.

Calcium and Magnesium Chelate **- Golden Glow Natural Health Products**
Each tablet contains: Calcium Amino Acid Chelate 500 mg: Calcium 100 mg • Magnesium Amino Acid Chelate 250 mg: Magnesium 50 mg.

Calcium and Magnesium with Zinc **- Nature Made**
Each tablet contains: Calcium (from calcium carbonate) 333 mg • Magnesium (from magnesium oxide) 133 mg • Zinc (from zinc sulfate) 5 mg. Other Ingredients: Maltodextrin, Croscarmellose Sodium, Silicon Dioxide, Magnesium Stearate, Hydroxypropyl Methylcellulose, Cellulose, Polyethylene Glycol.
See Editor's Note No. 45.

Calcium Ascorbate **- Atrium Biotechnologies**
Each tablet contains: Vitamin C (Ascorbic Acid) 1000 mg.

Calcium Ascorbate **- Source Naturals**
Each half-rounded teaspoon contains: Vitamin C (as calcium ascorbate) 2150 mg • Calcium (as calcium ascorbate) 245 mg.

Calcium Ascorbate 1000mg **- Nature's Own**
Each tablet contains: Calcium Ascorbate 1000 mg • Bioflavonoids 100 mg • Rutin 50 mg • Hesperidin 25 mg.

Calcium Ascorbate Buffered Vitamin C **- Jarrow Formulas**
Each tablet contains: Vitamin C (from calcium ascorbate) 820 mg • Calcium (as ascorbate) 100 mg. Other Ingredients: Cellulose, Calcium Phosphate, Stearic Acid, Magnesium Stearate (vegetable source), Silicon Dioxide.

Calcium Ascorbate C-Complex 1000 mg **- The Vitamin Shoppe**
Each 1000 mg capsule contains: Vitamin C as calcium ascorbate 750 mg • Citrus Bioflavonoids 100 mg • Hesperidin 50 mg • Rutin 25 mg • Calcium 75 mg.

Calcium Ascorbate Crystals **- Nature's Life**
Each teaspoon contains: Vitamin C (Calcium Ascorbate) 3240 mg • Calcium (Calcium Ascorbate) 360 mg.

Calcium Ascorbate powder **- Nature's Own**
Each 1 tsp serving contains: Calcium Ascorbate 4000 mg.

Calcium Ascorbate powder **- Golden Glow Natural Health Products**
Each level 5 mL metric spoonful (4.12 g) contains: Ascorbic Acid (vitamin C, from Calcium Ascorbate 4.12 g) 3.41 g.

Calcium Aspartate **- American Biologics**
Each tablet contains: Elemental Calcium 100 mg. Other Ingredients: Dicalcium Phosphate, Cellulose, Magnesium Stearate.

Calcium Citrate - Walgreens
Two tablets contain: Calcium (as calcium citrate) 400 mg. Other Ingredients: Microcrystalline Cellulose, Stearic Acid, Silicon Dioxide, Magnesium Stearate, Hydroxypropyl Methylcellulose, Polyethylene Glycol, Carnauba Wax.

Calcium Citrate + with Vitamin D - Sunmark
Two caplets contain: Calcium 630 mg • Vitamin D 400 IU. Other Ingredients: Microcrystalline Cellulose, Acacia, Modified Cellulose Gum, Stearic Acid, Magnesium Stearate, Hydroxypropyl Methylcellulose, Hydroxypropyl Cellulose, Artificial Color (Titanium Dioxide), Polyethylene Glycol, Sodium Lauryl Sulfate, Gelatin, Starch, Sodium Citrate, Gluten.
See Editor's Note No. 45.

Calcium Citrate 1000 - GNC
Four tablets contain: Calcium (as calcium citrate) 1000 mg. Other Ingredients: Cellulose.

Calcium Citrate 250 mg - Pro Health
Each tablet contains: Calcium (as calcium citrate) 250 mg. Other Ingredients: L-Glutamic Acid, Cellulose, Modified Cellulose Gum, Stearic Acid, Silica, Magnesium Stearate.

Calcium Citrate Capsules - Optimum Nutrition
Two capsules contain: Vitamin D (as cholecalciferol) 200 IU • Calcium (as calcium citrate) 300 mg • Magnesium (as magnesium oxide, aspartate) 150 mg. Other Ingredients: Gelatin, Magnesium Stearate.

Calcium Citrate Malate - Rexall - Sundown
Two caplets contain: Vitamin D (as cholecalciferol) 200 IU • Calcium (as calcium citrate malate) 500 mg. Other Ingredients: Microcrystalline Cellulose, Stearic Acid, Titanium Dioxide (color), Dextrose, Silica, Magnesium Stearate, Hydroxypropyl Methylcellulose, PEG, Sodium Carboxymethylcellulose, Carnauba Wax, Mineral Oil, Sodium Citrate, Polysorbate 80, Dextrin.

Calcium Citrate Plus - GNC
Four tablets contain: Vitamin D (as cholecalciferol) 100 IU • Calcium (as calcium citrate) 800 mg • Magnesium (as magnesium oxide) 400 mg • Casein Phosphopeptide 75 mg. Other Ingredients: Cellulose, Titanium Dioxide, Vegetable Acetoglycerides.

Calcium Citrate Plus Vitamin D - Progressive Labs
Four tablets contain: Calcium (as calcium citrate) 3240 mg • Calcium (Calcium Ascorbate) 360 mg.

Calcium Citrate Plus with Magnesium - Walgreens
Two caplets contain: Vitamin D (as cholecalciferol) • Vitamin B6 (as pyridoxine hydrochloride) 10 mg • Calcium (as calcium citrate) 500 mg • Magnesium (as magnesium oxide) 80 mg • Zinc (as zinc oxide) 10 mg • Copper (as copper gluconate) 1 mg • Manganese (as manganese gluconate) 1 mg • Boron (as sodium borate) 1 mg. Other Ingredients: Microcrystalline Cellulose, Croscarmellose Sodium, Hydroxypropyl Methylcellulose, Titanium Dioxide, Magnesium Stearate, Polyethylene Glycol, Carnauba Wax.

Calcium Citrate with Vitamin D - Solgar
Four tablets contain: Vitamin D (as ergocalciferol) 600 IU • Calcium (as calcium citrate) 1000 mg. Other Ingredients: Microcrystalline Cellulose, Vegetable Cellulose, Vegetable Magnesium Stearate, Silica, Vegetable Glycerin, Carnauba Wax.

Calcium Citrate with Vitamin D - Nature Made
Three tablets contain: Vitamin D 300 IU • Calcium (from calcium citrate) 750 mg. Other Ingredients: Cellulose Gel, Stearic Acid, Hydroxypropyl Methylcellulose, Croscarmellose Sodium, Titanium Dioxide Artificial Color, Magnesium Stearate, Polyethylene Glycol, Triethyl Citrate, Polysorbate 80, Sodium Citrate, Corn Starch.
See Editor's Note No. 45.

Calcium Citrate with Vitamin D - Walgreens
Two tablets contain: Vitamin D (as cholecalciferol) • Calcium (as calcium citrate) 630 mg. Other Ingredients: Croscarmellose Sodium, Magnesium Stearate, Hydroxypropyl Methylcellulose, Polyethylene Glycol, Carnauba Wax.

Calcium Citrate with Zinc & Magnesium - NOW Foods
Two tablets contain: Vitamin D (Fish oil) 100 IU • Calcium (Citrate) 600 mg • Magnesium (Oxide, Aspartate) 300 mg • Zinc (Amino Acid Chelate) 15 mg • Manganese (Amino Acid Chelate) 5 mg • Copper (Amino Acid Chelate) 1 mg.

Calcium Citrate/Malate Complex - Nature's Way
Two capsules contain: Calcium (citrate, carbonate, malate) 500 mg. Other Ingredients: Cellulose, Gelatin, Magnesium Stearate, Silica.

Calcium Complete Capsules - GNC
Two capsules contain: Calcium (as Cacium Carbonate) 600 mg • Magnesium (as Magnesium Oxide) 300 mg. Other Ingredients: Soybean Oil, Gelatin, Glycerin, Titanium Dioxide.

Calcium Complete Tablets - GNC
Three tablets contain: Vitamin C (as ascorbic acid) 300 mg • Calcium (as calcium carbonate) 1200 mg • Magnesium (as magnesium oxide) 600 mg • Betaine hydrochloride 50 mg. Other Ingredients: Cellulose, Soy fiber, Titanium Dioxide, Rose Hips powder (rosina canina).

Calcium Complex 750 - Optimum Nutrition
Each tablet contains: Vitamin D (as cholecalciferol) 200 IU • Calcium (as calcium carbonate, citrate) 500 mg • Magnesium (as magnesium oxide, aspartate) 250 mg. Other Ingredients: Pharmaceutical Glaze, Stearic Acid, Magnesium Stearate, Croscarmellose Sodium (disintegrant), Silica.

Calcium Complex Bone Formula - Nature's Way
Three capsules contain: Boron Amino Acid Chelate 1.5 mg • Calcium (citrate, carbonate, malate) 500 mg • Copper Amino Acid Chelate 500 mcg • Folic Acid (folate) 100 mcg • Horsetail Grass 12.6 mg • Magnesium (oxide, aspartate) 2.5 mg • Manganese Aspartate 2.5 mg • Vitamin B6 (as pyridoxine HCl) 12.5 mg • Vitamin D (D3, cholecalciferol) 100 IU • Vitamin K (phytonadione) 37.5 mcg • Zinc Amino Acid Chelate 5 mg. Other Ingredients: Cellulose, Gelatin, Magnesium-Stearate.

Calcium D-Glucarate - Source Naturals
Each two tablets contain: Calcium from 1000 mg Calcium d-Glucarate 1230 mg.

Calcium D-Glucarate - Tyler Encapsulations
Three capsules contain: Calcium (as calcium d-glucarate) 180 mg • Calcium D-Glucarate USP 1.5 g. Other Ingredients: Microcrystalline Cellulose, Gelatin, Water.

Calcium Effervescent - Progressive Labs
Two tablets contain: Calcium (from calcium carbonate) 1000 mg • Vitamin D (as cholecaciferol) 400 IU. Ingredients: Citric Acid, Calcium Carbonate, Sorbitol, Sodium Bicarbonate, Sodium Carbonate, Magnesium Carbonate, Aspartame, Mineral oil, Natural Orange flavor, Cholecalciferol. Contains Phenylalanine.

Calcium Gluconate - Solgar
Six tablets contain: Calcium (as calcium gluconate) 360 mg. Other Ingredients: Microcrystalline Cellulose, Vegetable Cellulose, Silica, Vegetable Stearic Acid, Vegetable Magnesium Stearate.

Calcium Lactate - Solgar
Nine tablets contain: Calcium (as calcium lactate) 760 mg • Sodium 10 mg. Other Ingredients: Microcrystalline Cellulose, Vegetable Cellulose, Silica, Vegetable Magnesium Stearate, Vegetable Glycerin, Carnauba Wax.

Calcium Lactate - Standard Process, Inc.
Six tablets contain: Calcium 250 mg • Magnesium 50 mg. Other Ingredients: Arabic Gum.

Some Brand Name Natural Products - What they Contain

www.NaturalDatabase.com contains MANY more listings than appear here.

Editor's Notes are located on pages 2155-2163.

BRAND NAMES

Calcium Lactate - Puritan's Pride
Three tablets contain: Calcium (as calcium lactate trihydrate) 250 mg.

Calcium Lactate Powder - Standard Process, Inc.
Each 1 tbsp (10 g) serving contains: Calcium (from calcium lactate) 800 mg • Magnesium (from magnesium citrate) 160 mg.

Calcium Magnesium - Solgar
Three tablets contain: Calcium (as calcium carbonate, calcium citrate, calcium gluconate) 1000 mg • Magnesium (as magnesium oxide, magnesium citrate, magnesium gluconate) 400 mg. Other Ingredients: Microcrystalline Cellulose, Titanium Dioxide, Vegetable Cellulose, Citric Acid, Vegetable Magnesium Stearate, Vegetable Stearic Acid, Vegetable Glycerin, Carnauba Wax.

Calcium Magnesium - Pro Health
Each tablet contains: Calcium (amino acid chelate) 250 mg • Magnesium (amino acid chelate) 125 mg • Vitamin D (cholecalciferol) 200 IU. Other Ingredients: Calcium Phosphate Dibasic, Stearic Acid, Hydroxypropyl Cellulose, Croscarmellose Sodium, Magnesium Stearate, Silicon Dioxide.

Calcium Magnesium (aspartate) - Pure Encapsulations
Each vegetable capsule contains: Calcium (aspartate) 80 mg • Magnesium (aspartate) 80 mg • Vitamin C (as ascorbyl palmitate) 10 mg.

Calcium Magnesium (citrate) - Pure Encapsulations
Each vegetable capsule contains: Calcium (citrate) 80 mg • Magnesium (citrate) 80 mg • Vitamin C (as ascorbyl palmitate) 10 mg.

Calcium Magnesium (citrate/malate) - Pure Encapsulations
Each vegetable capsule contains: Calcium (citrate/malate) 75 mg • Magnesium (citrate/malate) 75 mg • Vitamin C (as ascorbyl palmitate) 10 mg.

Calcium Magnesium Ascorbate - Alacer
Two tablets contain: Vitamin C (as mineral ascorbates) 1860 mg • Lemon and Orange Bioflavonoids 200 mg • Calcium (as mineral ascorbate) 100 mg • 100 mg • Magnesium Citrate 72 mg • Magnesium (as mineral ascorbate) 40 mg • Vitamin B6 (pyridoxine HCl) 10 mg • Melatonin 100 mcg. Other Ingredients: Cellulose, Chlorophyll, Citric Acid, Guar Gum, Hydroxypropylcellulose, Magnesium Stearate, Methyl- and Ethylcellulose, Polyethylene Glycol, Psyllium Husk Powder, Shellac, Titanium Dioxide, Vegetable Stearic Acid.
See Editor's Note No. 26.

Calcium Magnesium Citrate - Solgar
Five tablets contain: Calcium (as calcium citrate) 1000 mg • Iron 0.6 mg • Magnesium (as magnesium oxide, citrate) 500 mg. Other Ingredients: Microcrystalline Cellulose, Vegetable Cellulose, Silica, Vegetable Stearic Acid, Vegetable Magnesium Stearate, Vegetable Glycerin, Carnauba Wax.

Calcium Magnesium Phosphorus Superabsorbeze - Nature's Life
Each tablespoon contains: Calcium (Calcium Phosphate) 600 mg • Magnesium (Hydroxide, Carbonate) 300 mg • Vitamin D (as Vitamin D3) (Cholecalciferol) 200 IU. In a natural base of Purified Water, Citric Acid, Sorbital, natural Orange flavor & Cellulose.

Calcium Magnesium Plus Boron - Solgar
Three tablets contain: Calcium (as calcium carbonate, calcium citrate, calcium gluconate) 1000 mg • Magnesium (as magnesium oxide, magnesium citrate, magnesium gluconate) 400 mg • Boron (as boron citrate) 3 mg. Other Ingredients: Microcrystalline Cellulose, Vegetable Cellulose, Citric Acid, Vegetable Magnesium Stearate, Vegetable Stearic Acid, Vegetable Glycerin, Carnauba Wax.

Calcium Magnesium Superabsorbeze - Nature's Life
Each tablespoon contains: Calcium (Citrate, Lactate/ Gluconate) 600 mg • Phosphorus (Calcium Phosphate) 600 mg • Magnesium (Hydroxide, Carbonate) 300 mg • Vitamin D (as Vitamin D3) (Cholecalciferol) 200 IU. In a natural base of Purified Water, Citric Acid, Fructose, natural Orange flavor, Cellulose & Ascorbic Acid.

Calcium Magnesium Zinc - Nature's Life
Three tablets contain: Calcium (carbonate, citrate/malate) 1000 mg • Magnesium (oxide, citrate) 600 mg • Zinc (picolinate, citrate) 15 mg • Copper (gluconate, citrate) 1 mg • Silicon (dioxide) 20 mg • Boron (citrate) 100 mcg • Glutamic Acid HCl 100 mg. Base: Springtime Horsetail Herb (equisetum arvense).

Calcium Mineral Supplement - Eidon Inc.
Each 1 tbsp serving contains: Calcium (providing approx. 590 ppm calcium) 3 mg. Other Ingredients: Purified Water.

Calcium Night - Source Naturals
Four tablets contain: Calcium (citrate, malate, carbonate, fumarate and ascorbate) 600 mg • Magnesium (oxide, malate, citrate, fumarate and ascorbate) 600 mg • Vitamin C (magnesium and calcium ascorbate, ascorbic acid, and manganese ascorbate) 275 mg • Vitamin B6 (pyridoxine HCl) 20 mg • Vitamin D (D3, cholecalciferol) 200 IU • Folic Acid 200 mcg • Silica (horsetail silica extract) 9 mg • Manganese (ascorbate) 6 mg • Boron (amino acid chelate) 3 mg • Copper Sebacate 1 mg.

Calcium Oyster Shell 1000 mg - Rexall - Sundown
Three tablets contain: Vitamin D (as cholecalciferol) 400 IU • Calcium (from oyster shell) 1 g. Other Ingredients: Maltodextrin, Cellulose, Mineral Oil, Croscarmellose Sodium, Hydroxypropyl Methylcellulose, Carboxymethylcellulose Sodium, PEG, Carnauba Wax, Crospovidone, Magnesium Stearate, Stearic Acid.

Calcium Pantothenate - Golden Glow Natural Health Products
Each tablet contains: Calcium Pantothenate 275 mg: Pantothenic Acid (vitamin B5) 250 mg.

Calcium Plus 1000 - GNC
Three tablets contain: Vitamin A (as retinyl palmitate) 4000 IU • Vitamin C (as ascorbic acid) 100 mg • Vitamin D (as cholecalciferol) 400 IU • Calcium (as calcium carbonate) 1000 mg • Iron (as ferrous gluconate) 10 mg • Magnesium (as magnesium oxide) 500 mg. Other Ingredients: Cellulose, Rose Hips Powder (rosina canina).

Calcium Plus Soy - Rexall - Sundown
Each tablet contains: Vitamin D 200 IU • Calcium 600 mg • Magnesium 50 mg • Soy Isoflavones 25 mg • Trans-Resveratrol 2 mg. Other Ingredients: Calcium Carbonate, Magnesium Oxide, Soybean Extract, Microcrystalline Cellulose, Lactose, Hydroxypropyl Methylcellulose, Magnesium Stearate, Titanium Dioxide (color), Silica, Croscarmellose Sodium, Tricetin, Polygonum Cuspidatum Siebold & Zucc. Extract (root), Stearic Acid, Cholecalciferol.

Calcium Plus Vitamin D - Nature's Sunshine
Each tablet contains: Vitamin D 120 IU • Calcium (amino acid chelate, calcium citrate, bone meal, di-calcium phosphate) 250 mg • Phosphorus (bone meal, di-calcium phosphate) 110 mg • Magnesium (amino acid chelate, magnesium oxide, magnesium stearate) 125 mg. Other Ingredients: Sorbitol, Cellulose, Magnesium Stearate, Alfalfa Herb (medicago sativa), Wheat Germ Flour.

Calcium Plus Vitamin D & Minerals - Leiner Health Products
Each tablet contains: Manganese Sulfate 1.8 mg • Calcium Carbonate 600 mg • Copper (Cupric Oxide) 1 mg • Vitamin D (Cholecalciferol) 200 IU • Zinc Oxide 7.5 mg • Magnesium Oxide 40 mg • Boron 250 mcg. Other Ingredients: Maltodextrin, Hydroxypropyl Methylcellulose, Titanium Dioxide, Magnesium Stearate, Sodium Borate, Red 40 Lake, Yellow 6 Lake, Blue 1 Lake, and may contain less than 2% of Cellulose, Talc, Starch, Mineral Oil, Croscarmellose Sodium, Hydroxypropyl Cellulose, Silicon Dioxide, Polyethylene Glycol 8000, Polysorbate 80, Sodium Lauryl Sulfate, Polyethylene Glycol 3350, Crospovidone, Gelatin, Stearic Acid.

Calcium Plus Vitamins D3 & K1, Magnesium - Nature's Own
Each tablet contains: Calcium Carbonate 1500 mg: Calcium 600 mg • Magnesium Oxide 54.08 mg: Magnesium 30 mg • Vitamin D (D3, as cholecalciferol 5 mcg) 200 IU • Vitamin K (K1, as phytomenadione) 40 mcg.

Calcium Pyruvate - Natrol, Inc.
Each capsule contains: Calcium (as calcium pyruvate) 122 mg • Pyruvate (as calcium pyruvate) 528 mg • Cayenne Pepper 50 mg. Other Ingredients: Magnesium Stearate, Silica, Gelatin.

Calcium Pyruvate - Allergy Research Group
Each capsule contains: Calcium (as calcium pyruvate) 110 mg • Pyruvate 530 mg. Other Ingredients: Stearic Acid.

Calcium Rich Antacid Relief - Walgreens
Active Ingredients: Calcium Carbonate 550 mg • Magnesium Hydroxide 110 mg. Other Ingredients: FD&C Yellow No. 10, FD&C Blue No. 1, FD&C Yellow No. 6, Flavors, Magnesium Stearate, Starch, Stearic Acid, Sugar.

Calcium Support A (female) - Weil Lifestyle, LLC
Each Cal-Mag Citrate Complex tablet contains: Calcium 250 mg • Magnesium 125 mg.

Calcium Support A (male) - Weil Lifestyle, LLC
Each Cal-Mag Citrate Complex tablet contains: Calcium 250 mg • Magnesium 125 mg.

Calcium with Vitamin D 500 mg - Nature Made
Each tablet contains: Vitamin D 200 IU • Calcium (from calcium carbonate) 500 mg. Other Ingredients: Maltodextrin, Cellulose Gel, Soy Polysaccharides, Hydroxypropyl Methylcellulose, Corn Starch, Polyethylene Glycol.
See Editor's Note No. 45.

Calcium with Vitamin D 600 mg - Nature Made
Each tablet contains: Vitamin D 200 IU • Calcium (from calcium carbonate) 600 mg. Other Ingredients: Maltodextrin, Cellulose, Hydroxypropyl Methylcellulose, Soy Polysaccharides, Polyethylene Glycol.
See Editor's Note No. 45.

Calcium with Vitamin D3 - Pure Encapsulations
Six vegetable capsules contain: Calcium (citrate/malate) 900 mg • Vitamin D (D3) 800 IU • Vitamin C (as ascorbyl palmitate) 48 mg.

Calcium Xtra - Puritan's Pride
Three tablets contain: Vitamin A (as Retinyl Acetate) 4,000 IU • Vitamin C (as Ascorbic Acid) 100 mg • Vitamin D (as Cholecalciferol) 400 IU • Calcium (as Calcium Carbonate) 1,000 mg • Iron (as Ferrous Gluconate) 10 mg • Magnesium (as Magnesium Oxide) 500 mg.

Calcium, Magnesium & Phosphorus Plus Vitamin D (vanilla flavor) - Westcoast Naturals
Each 1 tbsp serving contains: Calcium 600 mg • Magnesium 300 mg • Phosphorus 300 mg • Vitamin D (as D3) 400 IU. Other Ingredients: Citric Acid, Sorbitol, Flavor, Purified Water, Sorbic Acid, Sodium Benzoate, Potassium Sorbate.

Calcium, Magnesium & Vitamin D - Nature's Way
Three capsules contain: Calcium (citrate, carbonate, malate) 500 mg • Magnesium (oxide, aspartate) 250 mg • Vitamin D (D3, cholecalciferol) 400 IU. Other Ingredients: Cellulose, Gelatin, Magnesium-Stearate.

Calcium, Magnesium & Zinc Plus Vitamin D - Westcoast Naturals
Each tablet contains: Calcium (HVP chelate from calcium carbonate) 500 mg • Magnesium (HVP chelate from magnesium oxide) 250 mg • Zinc (HVP chelate from magnesium oxide) 25 mg • Vitamin D (as D3, from natural source) 200 IU. • Glutamic Acid Hydrochloride 50 mg • Betaine Hydrochloride 50 mg.

Calcium, Magnesium and Zinc - Sunmark
Each caplet contains: Calcium 1000 mg • Magnesium 400 mg • Zinc 15 mg. Other Ingredients: Maltodextrin, Talc, Soy Polysaccharide, Citric Acid, Hypromellose, Cellulose, Mineral Oil, Titanium Dioxide, Magnesium Stearate, Polysorbate 80, Sodium Lauryl Sulfate, Carnauba Wax, Crospovidone, Stearic Acid, Gluten.
See Editor's Note No. 45.

Calcium/Magnesium - Vital Nutrients
Each capsule contains: Calcium (50% succinate and carbonate) 200 mg • Magnesium (40% citrate and 60% oxide) 100 mg.

Calcium/Magnesium (Citrate) - Vital Nutrients
Each capsule contains: Calcium (citrate/malate) 90 mg • Magnesium (citrate) 90 mg.

Calcium/Magnesium with Vitamin D - Jamieson
Each caplet contains: Vitamin D (as Cholecalciferol) 133 IU • Calcium (as Calcium Carbonate, Calcium Citrate, Calcium Succinate, Calcium Asparate, Calcium Glutamate, Calcium Furmarate) 333 mg • Magnesium (as Magnesium Oxide, Magnesium Citrate, Magnesium Malate, Magnesium Succiante, Magnesium Asparate, Magnesium Glutamate, Magnesium Fumarate) 167 mg.

Calcium+Minerals - Walgreens
Each tablet contains: Vitamin D (as cholecalciferol) • Calcium (as calcium carbonate) 600 mg • Magnesium (as magnesium oxide) 40 mg • Zinc (as zinc oxide) 7.5 mg • Copper (as cupric oxide) 1 mg • Manganese (as manganese sulfate) 1.8 mg • Boron (as sodium borate) 250 mcg. Other Ingredients: Microcrystalline Cellulose, Crospovidone, Hydroxypropyl Methylcellulose, Titanium Dioxide, Sodium Lauryl Sulfate, Magnesium Stearate, Triacetin, Polysorbate 80, FD&C Red No. 40 Lake, FD&C Yellow No. 6 Lake, FD&C Blue No. 1 Lake.

Calcium-d-Glucarate - Pure Encapsulations
Each vegetable capsule contains: Calcium-D-Glucarate 500 mg.

Calcium-Magnesium - Nutritional Therapeutics, Inc.
Each tablet contains: Calcium (Citrate) 250 mg • Magnesium (Oxide) 250 mg • NT Factor tablet base 200 mg.

Calcium-Magnesium Complex - The Vitamin Shoppe
Four tablets contain: Calcium 1500 mg • Magnesium 420 mg • Vitamin D 1000 IU • Vitamin E 20 IU • Vitamin C 80 mg • Manganese 10 mg. Plus Betaine HCl and Glutamic Acid HCl. In a base containing: Hydrolyzed Soy Protein, Lecithin, and Alfalfa Powder.

Calcium-Magnesium for Children - The Vitamin Shoppe
Each tablet contains: Calcium 200 mg • Magnesium 100 mg.

Calcium-Magnesium with Vitamin D - Schiff
Two softgels contain: Vitamin D (from fish liver oil and as cholecalciferol) 100 IU • Calcium (as calcium carbonate) 600 mg • Magnesium (as magnesium oxide) 300 mg. Other Ingredients: Vegetable Oil, Lecithin, Gelatin, Glycerin, Titanium Dioxide, Silicon Dioxide.

Calcium-Magnesium-Zinc - The Vitamin Shoppe
Three tablets contain: Elemental Calcium 1500 mg • Elemental Magnesium 750 mg • Elemental Zinc 45 mg.

CalciWise - Resource Wellness
Each chew contains: Vitamin A 1,000 IU • Vitamin D 200 IU • Vitamin K 40 mcg • Riboflavin 0.8 mg • Calcium 600 mg • Sodium 10 mg. Other Ingredients: Corn Syrup, High Fructose Corn Syrup, Sweetened Condensed Skim Milk, Sugar, Chocolate Liqueur, High Oleic Sunflower Oil, Cocoa (Processed with Alkali), Glycerol Monostearate, Salt, Artificial Flavor, Maltodexrin, Soy Lecithin.

Calendula Oil - Blessed Herbs
Calendula flower & Organic Cold-Pressed Olive oil.

BRAND NAMES

BRAND NAMES

Calendula Salve - Dial Herbs
Calendula • Chamomile • Mullein. In a base of Beeswax, Glycerine & Cold Pressed Olive oil.

Calgest - PhytoPharmica
Two capsules contain: Vitamin C (ascorbic acid/rose hips) 100 mg • Vitamin B6 (pyridoxine HCl) 50 mg • Calcium chloride 192 mg •Calcium phosphate 180 mg • Magnesium glycerophosphate 104 mg • Betaine HCl 192 mg • Ammonium chloride 192 mg • Kidney extract (freeze-dried) 60 mg • Mixed Bioflavonoids (citrus) 60 mg.
See Editor's Note No. 21 and No. 53.

California Poppy Flowering Top - Aboca USA, Inc
Each capsule contains: California Poppy flowering top WPC (whole phytocomplex concentrate, eschscholzia californica, standardized to 0.045% protopine, yielding 0.1 mg per capsule) 220 mg. Other Ingredients: Gelatin.

Calm (Stress Relief) Herbal Transdermal 1/4oz - Derma E
Jojoba oil • Sweet Almond oil • Tocopheryl Acetate (vitamin E) • Champaca Absolute • Jonquil.

Calm Aid Formula - Nature's Way
Two capsules contain: Blue Vervain stem, leaf, flower, fruit 150 mg • Chamomile flower 75 mg • Kava (dried extract 30% Kavalactones) 350 mg • L-5 Hydroxytryptophan (Griffonia bean extract) 5 mg • Niacin (Vitamin B3) 6.66 mg • Passion flower stem, leaf, flower, fruit 75 mg • Riboflavin (Vitamin B2) 568 mcg • Scullcap herb 60 mg • Thiamine (Vitamin B1) 500 mcg • Vitamin B12 (Cyanocobalamin) 2 mcg • Vitamin B6 (Pyridoxine HCL) 660 mcg • Wood Betony stem, leaf, flower 100 mg. Other Ingredients: Gelatin, Magnesium Stearate, Millet.

Calm Colon - Samra Health and Beauty
Each capsule contains: Proprietary Blend 500 mg: Yin Chen, Atractylodes root, Schisandra fruit, Job's Tears seed, Codonopsis, Huo Xiang, Chinese Thoroughwax root, Raxinus Chinensis bark, Polyporus, Asian Psyllium seed, Phellodendron bark, Licorice root, Ginger root, Magnolia bark, Fang Feng root, Tangerine peel, White Peony root, Costus root, Chinese Goldthread root, Fragrant Angelica root. Other Ingredients: Gelatin, Silicon Dioxide, Magnesium Stearate.

Calm Thoughts - Source Naturals
Three tablets contain: Kava root extract (Piper methysticum) (Standardized to 30% kavalactones yielding 105 mg of kavalactones) 350 mg • Siberian Ginseng root 200 mg • Bacopa Monniera leaf extract (Standardized to 20% bacosides yielding 20 mg of bacosides) 100 mg • Lemon Balm herb 100 mg • St. John's Wort extract (hypericum perforatum) (50 mg standardized to 0.3% hypericin and 50 mg 4:1 extract) 100 mg • Valerian root 60 mg • Ashwagandha root 50 mg • Ginger root 50 mg • Licorice root 4:1 extract 50 mg • Ginkgo Biloba leaf 50:1 extract (standardized to 24% ginkgo flavone glycosides and 6% terpene lactones) 30 mg • Schizandra fruit 30 mg • Vitamin C (as ascorbic acid) 100 mg • Vitamin B1 (thiamin) 25 mg • Vitamin B2 (riboflavin) 25 mg • Niacinamide 25 mg • Vitamin B6 (Pyridoxine HCl) 25 mg • Vitamin B12 (cyanocobalamin) 25 mcg • Vitamin B5 (pantothenic acid) 50 mg • Calcium (as calcium citrate) 100 mg • Magnesium (magnesium oxide 275 mg, magnesium taurinate 25 mg) 300 mg • Zinc (as zinc citrate) 15 mg • Manganese (as manganese citrate) 3 mg • GABA (gamma amino butyric acid) 500 mg • Taurine (as magnesium taurinate) 300 mg • L-Tyrosine (L-tyrosine 200 mg, N-acetyl L-tyrosine 50 mg) 250 mg.

Calm Thoughts Kava - Source Naturals
Three tablets contain: Kava root extract (Piper methysticum) standardized to 30% Kavalactones, Yielding 105 mg to Kavalactones 350 mg • Siberian Ginseng root 200 mg • Bacopa monniera leaf extract, standardized to 20% Bacosides, Yielding 20 mg of Bacosides 100 mg • Lemon Balm herb 100 mg • St. John's wort extract (Hypericum perforatum) 50 mg standardized to 0.3 % Hypericin and 50 mg 4:1 extract 100 mg • Valerian root 60 mg • Ashwagandha root 50 mg • Ginger root 50 mg • Licorice root extract (4:1) 50 mg • Ginkgo Biloba leaf extract (50:1) standardized to 24% Ginkgo Flavone Glycosides and 6% Terpene Lactones 30 mg • Schizandra fruit 30 mg • Vitamin C (as Ascrobic Acid) 100 mg • Vitamin B1 (Thiamin) 25 mg • Vitamin B2 (Riboflavin) 25 mg • Niacinamide 25 mg • Vitamin B6 (Pyridoxine HCl) 25 mg • Vitamin B12 (Cyanocobalamin) 25 mcg • Vitamin B5 (Pantothenic Acid) 50 mg • Calcium (as Calcium Citrate) 100 mg • Magnesium (275 mg Magnesium Oxide and 25 mg Magnesium Taurinate) 300 mg • Zinc (as Zinc Citrate) 15 mg • Manganese (as Manganese Citrate) 3 mg • GABA (Gamma Amino Butyric Acid) 500 mg • Taurine (as Magnesium Taurinate) 300 mg • L-Tyrosine (200 mg as L-Tyrosine and 50 mg N-Acetyl-l-Tyrosine) 250 mg.

Cal-Ma Plus - Standard Process, Inc.
Three tablets contain: Calcium (from calcium lactate, calcium chloride, and calcium stearate) 170 mg • Bovine Parathyroid 2.3 mg. Other Ingredients: Honey, Magnesium Citrate.
See Editor's Note No. 14.

CALMadvantage CM-01 - Advanced Nutritional Innovations
Each capsule contains: L-Theanine (Suntheanine brand) 100 mg • 5-Hydroxytryptophan (5-HTP) 50 mg • Methylsulfonylmethane (MSM) 50 mg. Other Ingredients: Gelatin, Titanium Dioxide, FD&C Blue #1, Red #3.

CAL-MAG - The Vitamin Shoppe
Each tablet contains: Calcium 500 mg • Magnesium 250 mg.

Cal-Mag Boron - Puritan's Pride
Three tablets contain: Calcium (as Calcium Carbonate, Calcium Citrate and Calcium Gluconate) 1,000 mg • Magnesium (as Magnesium Oxide, Magnesium Citrate, and Magnesium Gluconate) 400 mg • Boron (as Boron Citrate) 3 mg.

Cal-Mag Caps - Arrowroot
Three capsules contain: Calcium (calcium carbonate) 1000 mg • Magnesium (magnesium oxide) 500 mg.

Cal-Mag Chelate - Arrowroot
Three tablets contain: Calcium (carbonate, amino acid chelate) 100 mg • Magnesium (oxide, amino acid chelate) 500 mg • Betaine HCl 10 mg.

Cal-Mag Chewable - Quest
Each tablet contains: Elemental Calcium (Citrate, Phosphate) 300 mg •Elemental Magnesium (Citrate, Oxide) 150 mg • Vitamin D (as Vitamin D3) 100 IU. Other Ingredients: Sorbitol, Silicon Dioxide, Magnesium Stearate, Sucralose and Spearmint Flavor.

Cal-Mag Citrate - Puritan's Pride
Four tablets contain: Calcium (as Calcium Carbonate, Calcium Aspartate) 1,000 mg • Magnesium (as Magnesium Oxide and Magnesium Citrate) 500 mg.

Cal-Mag Citrate - Arrowroot
Four tablets contain: Calcium (citrate, hydroxyapatite complex, ascorbate, aspartate)1000 mg • Magnesium (oxide, citrate) 500 mg. Other Ingredients: Phosphorus, Magnesium, Zinc, Potassium, Manganese, Fluorine, Silicon, Proteins, Matrix materials, Mucopolysaccharide Compounds.

CalMag Citrates 2:1 - Jarrow Formulas
Three tablets contain: Vitamin D (D2, ergocalciferol) 200 IU • Calcium (as calcium citrate) 500 mg • Magnesium (as magnesium citrate) 250 mg. Other Ingredients: Cellulose, Stearic Acid, Magnesium Stearate, Modified Cellulose Gum.

Cal-Mag Fizz - Baywood International
Each scoop contains: Vitamin D 200 IU • Vitamin B1 (Thiamin HCL) 750 mcg • Vitamin B2 (Riboflavin) 850 mcg • Vitamin B3 (Niacinamide) 10 mg • Vitamin B6 (Pyridoxine HCL) 1 mg • Vitamin B12 (Cyanocobalamin) 3 mcg • Vitamin B5 (Pantothenic Acid) 5 mg • Calcium 500 mg • Magnesium 200 mg • Proprietary Blend 12 mg: Selenium, Potassium, Boron.

Some Brand Name Natural Products - What they Contain

www.NaturalDatabase.com contains MANY more listings than appear here.
Editor's Notes are located on pages 2155-2163.

Cal-Mag Liquid - Cardiovascular Research
Each 1 tbsp serving contains: Calcium (carbonate) 240 mg • Vitamin D (D3) 100 IU • Magnesium (hydroxide) 180 mg. Other Ingredients: Purified Water, Glycerine, Celulose, Spearmint Oil, Peppermint Oil.

Cal-Mag Potassium - Puritan's Pride
Two tablets contain: Calcium (carbonate, citrate, asparate) 500 mg • Magnesium (oxide, citrate, aspartate) 500 mg • Potassium (gluconate, aspartate, citrate) 99 mg.

CAL-MAG w/Zinc and Vitamin D - Dial Herbs
Vitamin D • Calcium from Gluconate & Lactate • Magnesium • Zinc • Aqueous Extracts from: Hibiscus, Chamomile, Fennel, Spinach • Fructose • Mango Juice • Orange Juice • Natural Flavor • Locust Seed Flour.

Cal-Mag-Zinc - Schiff
Two tablets contain: Vitamin D (as cholecalciferol) 100 IU • Calcium (as calcium carbonate) 500 mg • Magnesium (as magnesium oxide) 250 mg • Zinc (as zinc citrate) 25 mg • Proprietary Blend 56 mg: Citrates, Fumarates, Succinates, Gluconates, Aspartates, Ascorbates, Amino Acid Chelates, Ketoglutarates. Other Ingredients: Cellulose, Stearic Acid, Croscarmellose Sodium, Methylcellulose Titanium Dioxide, Polyethylene Glycol, Magnesium Stearate.

Cal-Mag-Zinc - Puritan's Pride
Three tablets contain: Calcium (as Calcium Carbonate and Calcium Gluconate) 1,000 mg • Magnesium (as Magnesium Oxide and Magnesium Gluconate) 400 mg • Zinc (as Zinc Gluconate and Zinc Citrate) 25 mg.

Cal-Mag-Zinc - Arrowroot
Two tablets contain: Calcium 1000 mg • Magnesium 500 mg • Zinc 25 mg • Vitamin D 200 IU • Glutamic Acid HCl 80 mg • Betaine HCl 100 mg.

Cal-Mag-Zinc Liquid - Metabolic Response Modifiers
Each tablespoon contains: Vitamin D (as Vitamin D3 cholecalciferol) 400 IU • Calcium (tri-calcium phosphate citrate, gluconate, lactate) 600 mg • Magnesium (hydroxide, carbonate) 300 mg • Phosphate (tri-calcium phosphate) 300 mg • Zinc (citrate) 22.5 mg • Potassium (citrate) 50 mg.

Calmatrol - Ortho Molecular Products
Each capsule contains: Valerian root extract (standardized to contain 0.8% valerenic acids) 200 mg • German Chamomile flower 100 mg • Hops strobile 50 mg • Passionflower aerial portion 50 mg. Other Ingredients: Natural Vegetable Capsules, Magnesium Stearate, Microcrystalline Cellulose, Silicon Dioxide.

CalmEz - Allergy Research Group
Three tablets contain: Proprietary Blend 1800 mg: Ramulus Uncariae hook extract, Ziziphus Spinosa seed extract, Albisia Julibrissin bark extract. Other Ingredients: Rice Starch.

Cal-Min - Progressive Labs
Each tablet contains: Calcium (as calcium proteinate) 300 mg. In a base of mixed vegetable concentrate from: Cultured Peas, Lentils, Buckwheat, Millet, and Chlorophyll, carefully dried to preserve their natural trace nutrient and enzyme content.

CalmingBlend - Rexall - Sundown
Each capsule contains: Ashwaganda root extract (standardized to 1.5% withanolides, 3 mg; standardized to 1% alkaloids, 2 mg) 200 mg • Valerian root extract (standardized to 0.8% valerenic acid, 0.5 mg) 67 mg • Proprietary Blend: Kava Kava root, German Chamomile flower head, Hops (strobiles) 133 mg. Other Ingredients: Gelatin.

Calms Forte - Hyland's
Each tablet contains: Passiflora 1X • Avena Sativa 1X • Chamomilla 2X • Calcarea Phosphorica 2X HPUS • Ferrum Phosphoricum 3X HPUS • Kali Phosphoricum 3X HPUS • Natrum Phosphoricum 3X HPUS • Magnesia Phosphoricum 3X HPUS.

CalmTabs - Puritan's Pride
Four tablets contain: Valerian root 258 mg • Passiflora flower 258 mg • Celery seed 258 mg • Catnip leaf 258 mg • Hops flower 129 mg • Dried Orange Peel 129 mg.

Calorad - Essentially Yours Industries, Inc. (EYI)
Demineralized Water • Collagen Hydrolysat • Aloe Vera • Vegetal Glycerin • Potassium Sorbate • Citrus Extracts • Natural Peach Flavor.

Calotren - Formula Master Botanicals
Each 500 mL bottle contains: Purified Water • Collagen Hydrolysate • Aloe Vera • Glycerin • Potassium Sorbate • Natural Flavoring • Methyl Paraben.

Cal-Para - Atrium Biotechnologies
Each tablet contains: Alkalinizing Calcium Lactate 325 mg • Calcium Aspartate (supplying Elemental Calcium 52) 80 mg • Magnesium Aspartate 75 mg • Magnesium Citrate (supplying Elemental Magnesium 21 mg) 70 mg.

Calsol - Standard Process, Inc.
Five tablets contain: Calcium (from calcium glycerophosphate, calcium lactate, calcium stearate, and calcium acid phosphate) 225 mg • Phosphorus 170 mg • Carbamide 165 mg. Other Ingredients: Magnesium Citrate.

Calsorb - PhysioLogics
Three caplets contain: Calcium (as 80% calcium citrate, 19% calcium carbonate, 1% calcium stearate) 500 mg • Magnesium (as 50% magnesium citrate, 50% magnesium glycinate) 250 mg. Other Ingredients: Microcrystalline Cellulose, Stearic Acid, Croscarmellose Sodium, Hydroxypropyl Methylcellulose, Silicon Dioxide, Magnesium Silicate, Polyethylene Glycol.

Calsure - Rexall - Sundown
Each tablet contains: Calcium 250 mg. Other Ingredients: Stearic Acid, Titanium Dioxide, Silica, Magnesium Stearate, Hydroxypropyl Methylcellulose, Microcrystalline Cellulose.

Cal-Sym - Atrium Biotechnologies
Each tablet contains: Acidifying Calcium Phosphate 100 mg • Calcium Ascorbate 50 mg • Calcium Aspartate (supplies Elemental Calcium 34 mg compounded to insure acidic pH) 35 mg • Ammonium Chloride 100 mg • Betaine HCL 12 mg • Glutamic Acid HCL120 mg.

Caltrate 600 + Soy - Wyeth
Each two tablets contain: Soy Isoflavones 50 mg • Calcium 1200 mg • Vitamin D 400 IU.

Caltrate Plus - Wyeth
Each tablet contains: Vitamin D 200 IU • Calcium 600 mg • Magnesium 40 mg • Zinc 7.5 mg • Copper 1 mg • Manganese 1.8 mg • Boron 250 mcg. Other Ingredients: Maltodextrin, Cellulose, Mineral Oil, Hydroxypropyl Methylcellulose, Titanium Dioxide, Sodium Lauryl Sulfate, Cupric Oxide, FD&C Red No. 40, FD&C Yellow No. 6, FD&C Blue No. 1, Gelatin, Crospovidone, Stearic Acid, Magnesium Stearate.

CamoCare Bamboo Gentle Face Scrub - Abkit
Bamboo extract • German Chamomile extract. Base: Purified Water, PEG-6 Stearate, Ceteth-20, Glyceryl Stearate, Stearate 20, Shea Butter, Isostearyl Isostearate, Glycerin, Cetyl Alcohol, Dimethicone, Lactic Acid, Phenonip.

CamoCare Cleansing Therapy - Abkit
German Chamomile extract. Base: Deionized Water, Safflower Oil, Sorbitol, Dimethicone, Glyceryl Stearate, Cetearyl Alcohol, Ceteareth-20, PEG-8, Distearate, Allantoin, Carbomer 934, Methylparaben, Imidazolidinyl Urea, Triethanolamine, Xanthan Gum.

CamoCare Clear Solution - Abkit
German Chamomile extract • Alpha Lipoic Acid. Other Ingredients: Camillosan Camomile, Alpha Lipotene Antioxidant, Levomenol, Flavonoids, Essential Oils.

Some Brand Name Natural Products - What they Contain

www.NaturalDatabase.com contains MANY more listings than appear here.
Editor's Notes are located on pages 2155-2163.

BRAND NAMES

CamoCare Conditioner - Abkit
Purified Water • Cetearyl Alcohol • PEG 40 • Castor oil • Stearalkonium Chloride • Aloe Vera gel • Glycerin • Propylene Glycol • Retinyl Palmitate (vitamin A) • Ascorbyl Palmitate (vitamin C), Tocopherol Acetate (Vitamin E) • Soy Protein • Hydrolyzed Silk Protein • Hydolyzed Wheat Protein • German Chamomile extract • DL Panthenol (vitamin B5) • Methylparaben • Imidazolidinyl Urea • Herbal Fragrance.

CamoCare C-Spot - Abkit
German Chamomile extract (chamomile recutita) • Mulberry root extract (morus alba) • Licorice root extract (glycyrrhea glabra) • Ester-C extract. Base: Deionized Water, Glycerin, Dioctyl Sebacate, Dimenthicone, Caprylic/capric Triglycerides, Lactic Acid, Sorbitol, Glyceryl Stearate, Polyacrylamide, Calcium Ascorbate, C13-14 Isoparaffin, Laureth-7, Imdazoudnyl Urea, Methylparaben, Propylparaben, Allantoin, Panthenol, Mica, Titanium Dioxide.

CamoCare Day Skin Firmer - Abkit
German Chamomile extract. Base: Deionized Water, Glycerin Ascorbate, Sorbitol Ascorbate, Calcium Ascorbate (ester-C), Dioctyl Sebacate, Caprylic/Capric Triglycerides, Glyceryl Stearate, Cetyl Alcohol, Cetearyl Alcohol, Ceteareth20 brand, Tocopheryl Acetate (vitamin E), Dimethicone, Bilberry Extract, Sugar Cane Extract, Tocopherol (vitamin E), Sugar Maple Extract, Orange Extract, Lemon Extract, Polyacrylamide, C13-14 Isoparaffin, Laureth-7, Sodium Citrate, Methylparaben, Propylparaben, Imidazolidinyl Urea.

CamoCare EPF With SPF 15 - Abkit
Octyl Methoxycinnamate • Zinc Oxide • Benzophenone • Deionized Water • Caprylic/Capric Triglycerides • Glycerin • Glyceryl Stearate • PEG-100 Stearte • Cetearyl Alcohol • Ceteareth-20 • Polyacrylamide • C13/14 Isoparaffin • Laureth-7 • German Chamomile extract • Diazolidnyl Urea, Methylparaben • Propylparaben.

CamoCare Eye Lifting Moisture Cream - Abkit
German Chamomile extract. Base: Purified Water, Caprylic/Capric Triglycerides, Cetearyl Alcohol, Polyglucose, Octyl Palmitate, Glycerine, Sodium Cetearyl Sulfate, Panthenol, Tocopherol (vitamin E), Allantoin, Disodium EDTA, Methylparaben, Cornflower Extract, Yeast Extract, Tocopherol Acetate, Alpha Lipoic Acid, Ceramide III, Imidazolidinyl Urea.

CamoCare Face Lifting 12% Liquid - Abkit
Chamomile extract. Base: Deionized Water, Sugar Cane Extract, Citrus Extract, Apple Extract, Green Tea Extract, PEG-400, Willow Bark Extract, Peppermint Extract, Rosemary Extract, Lavender Extract, Orange Fruit Extract, Lemon Extract, Lemon Grass Extract, Angelica Extract, Sodium Citrate, Witch Hazel Extract, Cucumber Extract, Nettle Extract, Calendula Extract, Comfrey Extract, Grapefruit Extract, Germaben II.

CamoCare Face Lifting 12% Refining Cream - Abkit
Chamomile extract. Base: Deionized Water, Sugar Cane Extract, Citrus Extract, Apple Extract, Green Tea Extract, Dicapryl Ether, Glyceryl Stearate, PEG-100 Stearate, Stearic Acid, Shea Butter, Cyclomethicone, Cetearyl Alcohol, Ceteareth-20, Dimethicone, Squalane, Polyacrylamide, C13-14 Isoparaffin, Laureth-7, Alpha Lipoic Acid, Sodium Citrate, Willow Bark Extract, Ginger Extract, Grapefruit Extract, Orange Fruit Extract, Xanthan Gum, Methylparaben, Imidazolidinyl Urea.

CamoCare Face Lifting 8% Liquid - Abkit
Chamomile extract. Base: Deionized Water, Sugar Cane Extract, Citrus Extract, Apple Extract, Green Tea Extract, Peg-4, Willow Bark Extract, Alpha Lipoic Acid, Peppermint Extract, Rosemary Extract, Lavender Extract, Orange Fruit Extract, Lemon Extract, Lemon Grass Extract, Angelica Extract, Sodium Citrate, Witch Hazel Extract, Cucumber Extract, Nettle Extract, Calendula Extract, Comfrey Extract, Grapefruit Extract, Propylene Glycol, Diazolidinyl Urea, Methylparaben, Propylparaben.

CamoCare Face Lifting 8% Refining Cream - Abkit
Chamomile extract. Base: Deionized Water, Sugar Cane Extract, Citrus Extract, Apple Extract, Green Tea Extract, Dicapryl Ether, Glyceryl Stearate, PEG-100 Stearate, Stearic Acid, Shea Butter, Cyclomethicone, Cetearyl Alcohol, Ceteareth-20, Dimethicone, Squalene, Polyacrylamide, C13-14 Isoparaffin, Laureth-7, Alpha Lipoic Acid, Sodium Citrate, Willow Bark Extract, Ginger Extract, Grape Fruit Extract, Orange Fruit Extract, Xanthan Gum, Methylparaben, Imidazolidinyl Urea.

CamoCare Facial Therapy - Abkit
Chamomile extract. Base: Deionized Water, Sorbitol, Propylene Glycol Dicaprylate/Dicaprate, Glyceryl Stearate, Safflower Oil, Lanoline Oil, Squalane, Stearic Acid, Dimethicone, Cetyl Alcohol, Cetearyl Alcohol, Ceteareth-20, Alpha Lipoic Acid, Tocopheryl Acetate, Retinyl Pamlitate, Carbomer, Allantoin, Methylparaben, Xanthan Gum, Triethanolamine, Imidazolidinyl Urea, Titanium Dioxide.

CamoCare Hand & Body Lotion - Abkit
Purified Water • Canola oil • Stearic Acid • Glycerol Stearate • Propylene Glycol • Glycerin • Cetyl Alcohol • Lecithin • Aloe Vera gel • Squalane (vegetable) • Avocado oil • Vitamin E • Vitamin A • Vitamin D • D-Panthenol • Allantoin • Chamomile extract • Herbal Fragrance • Propylparaben • Methylparaben • Triethanolamine.

CamoCare Intense Facial Therapy - Abkit
Chamomile extract. Base: Deionized Water, Sorbitol, Caprylic/Capric Triglycerides, Glyceryl Stearate, Safflower Oil, Sqalane, Sericin, Stearic Acid, Dimethicone, Cetyl Alcohol, Cetearyl Alcohol, Ceteareth-20, Vitamin E, Allantoin, Vitamin A, Vitamin C, Vitamin B5, Lecithin, Carbomer, Methylparaben, Xanthum Gum, Triethanolamine, Imidazolidinyl Urea, Disodium EDTA.

CamoCare Light Facial Therapy - Abkit
Chamomile extract • Camillosan Camomile • Levomenol • Flavonoids • Essential Oils. Base: Deionized Water, Sorbitol, Propylene Glycol Dicaprylate/Dicaprate, Glyceryl Stearate, Safflower Oil, Stearic Acid, Dimethicone, Lanolin Oil, Squalane (vegetable), Cetyl Alcohol, Cetearyl Alcohol, Ceteareth-20, Tocopheryl Acetate, Allantoin, Alpha Lipoic Acid, Panthenol, Retinyl Palmitate, Carbomer, Methylparaben, Xanthan Gum, Triethanolamine, Disodium Edta, Imidazolidinyl Urea.

CamoCare Light Foaming Cleanser - Abkit
Chamomile extract. Base: Deionized Water, Lauryl Glucoside, Sodium Laureth Sulfate, Lauramide DEA, PEG-7 Glyceryl Cocoate, Sea Salt, Xanthan Gum, Glycol Stearate, Stearamide AMP, Comphrey Extract, Calendula Extract, Rosemary Extract, Lavender Extract, Witch Hazel Extract, Elder Flower Extract, Propylene Glycol, Diazolidinyl UREA, Methylparaben, Propylparaben.

CamoCare Moisturizing Cleanser - Abkit
Chamomile extract. Base: Deionized Water, Safflower Oil, Sorbitol, Dimethicone, Glyceryl Stearate, Cetearyl Alcohol, Ceteareth-20, Allantoin, Stearyl Alcohol, PEG-8 Distearate, Xanthan Gum, Carbomer, Methylparaben, Imidazolidinyl Urea, Triethanolamine, Alpha Lipotene Antioxidant.

Camocare Night Skin Firmer - Abkit
Chamomile extract. Base: Deionized Water, Glycerin, Sorbitol, Calcium Ascorbate (ester-C), Caprylic/Capric Triglycerides, Cetearyl Alcohol, Cetearyl Polyglucose, Octyl Palmitate, Sunflower Oil, Jojoba Oil, Tocopheryl Acetate (vitamin E), Sodium Cetearyl Sulfate, Tocopherol (vitamin E), Allantoin, Panthenol (vitamin B5), Methylparaben, Imidazolidinyl Urea. Ester-C (14% vitamin concentrate), Camillosan Camomile.

CamoCare Oil Free Toner - Abkit
Chamomile extract. Base: Deionized Water, Willow Bark Extract, PPG-7 Glyceryl Cocoate, Polysorbate-20, Lipoic Acid, Comfrey Extract, Calendula Extract, Rosemary Extract, Lavender Extract, Witch Hazel Extract, Elder Flower Extract, Propylene Glycol,

Diazolidinyl Urea, Methylparaben, Propylparaben. Alpha Lipotene Antioxidant, Camillosan Camomile, Levomenol, Flavonoids, Essential Oils.

CamoCare Revitalizing Mask **- Abkit**
Chamomile extract. Base: Glacial Clay, Glycerine, Diazolidinyl Urea, Methylparaben.

CamoCare Shampoo **- Abkit**
Purified Water • Sodium Myreth Sulfate • Lauramide MEA • Cocamidopropyl Betaine • Aloe Vera gel • D-calcium pantothenate (vitamin B5) • Chamomile extract • Tocopherol (vitamin E) • Herbal Fragrance • Linoleic Acid • Linolenic Acid (vitamin F) • Horse Chestnut oil • Biotin (vitamin H) • Retinol (vitamin A) • Henna extract • Methylparaben • Propylparaben • Polysorbate-20, Citric Acid • Imidazolidinyl Urea.

CamoCare Soothing Cream **- Abkit**
Water • Cetearyl Alcohol • Lanolin • Hydrogenated Peanut oil • Glyceryl Stearate • Sodium Cetearyl Sulfate • Isopropyl Myristate • Glycerin • Chamomile extract • Methylparaben • Propylparaben.

CamoCare Stimulating Toner **- Abkit**
Chamomile extract. Base: Deionized Water, Polysorbate-20, Propylene Glycol, Rosemary Extract, Lavender Extract, Alpha Lipoic Acid, Allantoin, Sodium Hydroxymethylglycinate, Sodium Citrate, Citric Acid, Disodium EDTA, Sodium Benzoate, Imidazolidinyl Urea, Camillosan Camomile, Levomenol, Flavonoids, Essential Oils, Alpha Lipotene Antioxidant.

CamoCare Toning Therapy **- Abkit**
Chamomile extract. Base: Deionized Water, Polysorbate-20, Ppropylene Glycol, Allantoin, Sodium Hydroxyglycinate, Sodium Citrate, Citric Acid, Disodium EDTA, Sodium Benzoate, Imidazolidinyl Urea.

CamoCare Ultimate Body Therapy **- Abkit**
Chamomile extract • Deionized Water • Sorbitol • Sunflower oil • Caprylic/Capric Triglycerides • Cetearyl Alcohol • Ceteareth-20 • Dimethicone • Squalane (vegetable) • Lecithin (vegetable) • Cornflower extract • Tocopherol (vitamin E) • Tocopheryl Acetate (Vitamin E) • Retinyl Palmitate (Vitamin A) • Ascorbyl Palmitate (Vitamin C) • Alantoin • Stearic Acid • Methylparaben • Imidazolidinyl Urea • Carbomer • Xanthan Gum • Lavender oil • Tangerine oil • Blackcurrant oil • Disodium EDTA • Triethanolamine.

CamoCare Under Eye Therapy **- Abkit**
Chamomile extract. Base: Deionized Water, PEG-40, Sorbitol, Xanthan Gum, Sodium PCA, Lemon Extract, Witch Hazel Extract, Cornflower Extract, Hyaluronic Acid, Citric Acid, Disodium EDTA, Propylene Glycol, Diazolidinyl Urea, Methylparaben, Propylparaben.

cAMP-Coleus Forskohlii Supreme **- Gaia Herbs**
Thirty drops contain: Proprietary Blend 65 mg: Coleus Forskohlii (coleus forskohlii), Bupleurum root (bupleurum falcatum), Feverfew herb (chrysanthemum parthenium), Chinese Skullcap root (scutellaria baicalensis), Jujube dates (ziziphus jujube), Licorice root (glycyrrhiza glabra), Ginger rhizome (zingiber officinalis), Spring Water, 50-60% Pure Grain Alcohol USP.

Canadian Ginseng **- Jamieson**
Each capsule contains: Canadian Ginseng whole root (Panax quinquefolium, containing a minimum of 5% Ginsenosides) 250 mg.

Candex **- Pure Essence Labs**
Two capsules contain: Cellulase 74,000 CU • Hemicellulase 30,000 HCU • Amylase 4000 DU • Invertase 1000 SU • Malt Diastase 200 DP • Glucoamylase 100 AGU. Other Ingredients: Cellulose, Rice Bran, Water, Soya Lecithin Oil.

Candibactin-AR **- Metagenics**
Each softgel contains: Red Thyme oil (thymus vulgaris, providing 30%-50% thymol) 0.2 ml • Oregano oil (origanum vulgare, providing 55% to 75% carvacrol) 0.1 ml • Sage leaf 5.5:1 extract (salvia officinalis) 75 mg • Lemon Balm leaf 5:1 extract (melissa officinalis) 50 mg.

Candibactin-BR **- Metagenics**
Two tablets contain: Coptis root and rhizome extract (coptis chinensis, containing berberine) 30 mg • Indian Barberry root extract (berberis aristata, containing berberine) 70 mg • Berberine Sulfate 400 mg • Proprietary 4:1 Extract 300 mg: Coptis root and rhizome (coptis chinensis), Chinese Skullcap root (scutellaria baicalensis), Phellodendron bark (phellodendron chinense), Ginger rhizome (zingiber officinale), Chinese Licorice root (glycyrrhiza uralensis), Chinese Rhubarb root and rhizome (rheum officinale).

Candicid Forte **- Ortho Molecular Products**
Two capsules contain: Biotin 300 mcg • Sodium Caprylate 200 mg • Oregano leaf 10:1 extract 180 mg • Pau d'Arco inner bark 5:1 extract 180 mg • Berberine sulfate 100 mg • Cinnamon bark 5:1 extract 100 mg • Ginger root 100 mg • Goldenseal root extract (standardized to contain 4.8% hydrastine) 100 mg • Grapefruit seed extract (Citricidal brand) 100 mg • German Chamomile flower 50 mg. Other Ingredients: Natural Vegetable Capsules, Magnesium Stearate, Microcrystaline Cellulose, Silicon Dioxide.

Candicid IT **- Ortho Molecular Products**
Extra Virgin Olive oil • Modified Coconut oil.

Candicidal **- Source Naturals**
Each capsule contains: Brevibacterium linens 2 billion cells • Vitamin B-6 (pyridoxine HCl) 10 mg • Methionine 200 mg.

Candicin **- Genestra - Seroyal**
Each capsule contains: Oregano oil • Clove oil • Wormwood extract • Ginger extract • Evening Primrose oil.

Candid Care **- Natrol, Inc.**
Two capsules contain: Zinc 9 mg • FOS 500 mg • Garlic 100 mg • Undecylenic Acid (as Zinc undecylenate acid) 50 mg • Citrus extract, dried powder from grapefruit Seed 25 mg. Other Ingredients: Microcrystalline Cellulose, Silicon Dioxide, Magnesium Stearate, Gelatin.

Candida **- Nature's Sunshine**
Baptisia Tinctoria (wild indigo) 4X • Bryonia (white bryony) 4X • Echinacea Angustifolia (cone flower) 4X • Eupatorium Perfoliatum (boneset) 4X • Hydrastis Canadensis (goldenseal) 4X • Thuja Occidentalis (tree of life) 4X • Viscum Album (mistletoe) 6X • Candida Albicans (candida yeast extract) 12X. Other ingredients: Purified Water, 20% USP Alcohol.
See Editor's Note No. 1.

Candida **- Aspen Group, Inc.**
Each capsule contains: Pau D'Arco 4:1 extract 100 mg • Calcium Caprylate 100 mg • Goldenseal root extract 100 mg • Garlic extract (odorless) 50 mg • Licorice root extract 50 mg • Caprilic Acid 25 mg • Oregano 25 mg • Tea Tree oil 5 mg.

Candida Albicans **- American Biologics**
Each drop contains: Candida Albicans 6X-12X-30X-60X-100X-200X-500X. Other Ingredients: 20% Alcohol, Distilled Water.
See Editor's Note No. 1.

Candida Formula **- Enzymatic Therapy**
Each capsule contains: Oregano oil extract (Origanum vulgare) 0.1 ml • Thyme oil extract (Thymus vulgaris) 0.05 ml • Peppermint oil extract (Mentha piperta) 0.05 ml • Goldenseal root (Hydrastis canadensis) standardized to contain 5% total Alkaloids including: Berberine, Hydrastine, & Canadine 50 mg.

Candida Forte **- Nature's Plus**
Two softgels contain: Safflower oil 1000 mg • Vitamin C (ascorbate) 500 mg • L-Cysteine free-form amino acid 100 mg • Zinc (ascorbate) 50 mg • Pau D'Arco 50 mg • Vitamin B6 (pyridoxine HCl) 50 mg • Acidophilus (lactobacillus) supplying 80 million viable cells 20 mg • Vitamin A (fish liver oil) 10,000 IU • Beta Carotene (supplying 15,000 IU Vitamin A activity) 9 mg • Garlic (equivalent to 500 mg of fresh garlic) 1 mg • Biotin 100 mcg • Free-Form Amino Acid Complex 198.08 mg: L-Glutamine 40.8 mg, L-Lysine 25 mg,

L-Leucine 20.2 mg, L-Proline 16.2 mg, L-Valine 14 mg, L-Serine 12.6 mg, L-Isoleucine 11 mg, L-Phenylalanine 9.32 mg, L-Threonine 8.64 mg, L-Arginine 7.3 mg, L-Alanine 6.28 mg, L-Aspartic Acid 7 mg, L-Methionine 6.08 mg, L-Histidine 5.74 mg, L-Glycine 3.52 mg, L-Tyrosine 3 mg, L-Cysteine 1.4 mg. In a Base of Black Walnut.

candida/yeast - Nelson Bach
Active Ingredients: Candida alb 30c HPUS • Kreosotum 30c HPUS • Thuja occ 30c HPUS. Inactive Ingredients: Lactose, Sucrose.
See Editor's Note No. 1.

Candidase - Enzymedica
Each capsule contains: Protease Thera-Blend 100,000 HUT • Cellulase Thera-Blend 30,000 CU.

CandiGONE - Renew Life Formulas, Inc.
Part I: Two capsules contain: Uva Ursi (arctostaphylos uva-ursi) • Garlic bulb • Magnesium Caprylate (caprylic acid) • Citricidal extract from Grapefruit seed and rind • Pau d'Arco root bark 4:1 extract • Calcium Undecylenate (undecylenic acid) • Barberry root alkaloids (berberis vulgaris) • Neem leaf (azadirachta indica) • Olive leaf (olea europa 18% oleuropein) • Berberine Sulphate. Other Ingredients: Vegetable Cellulose, Hypromellose, Water.
Part II: 20 drops contain: Oregano leaf (origanum vulgare) • Orange peel (citrus sinensis) • Oregon Grape root (mahonia auquifolium) • Pau d'Arco root bark (tabebuia heptaphylla) • Cinnamon bark (cinnamomum casia) • Clove bud (syzgium aromaticum) • Peppermint leaf (mentha piperita). Other Ingredients: Filtered Water, Ethyl Alcohol 45-55%.

Candistatin - PhysioLogics
Two capsules contain: Calcium (as calcium caprylate) 58 mg • Magnesium (as magnesium caprylate) 46 mg • Caprylic Acid 800 mg • Goldthread root (coptis groenlandica, standardized to contain 10% alkaloids) 100 mg • Pau D'Arco herb (tabebuia impetiginosa) 60 mg. Other Ingredients: Gelatin, Vegetable Magnesium Stearate, Silica.

Candistroy - Nature's Secret
Two tablets contain: Zinc tannates • Barberry root extract • Goldenseal root • Pau d'Arco bark • Oregon Grape root • Peppermint oil • Orange peel • Licorice root • Cinnamon bark • Clove buds • Thyme leaf • Allicin.

CandiZYME - Renew Life Formulas, Inc.
Three capsules contain: Ultrazyme Blend 1860 mg: Protease 300,000 HUT • Cellulase 112,500 CU • Hemicellulase 45,000 HCU • Lysozyme 22,500 mcg • Amylase 18,000 DU • Invertase 1050 Sumner = 345 INVU • Lactase 750 ALU • Malt Diastase 375 DP • Lipase 300 FCCFIP = 1500 LU • Glucoamylase 150 AG.

Canelim - Xi'an Zheng Da Pharmaceutical
Each capsule contains: Proprietary Blend: Radix Curcumae 23.5%, Fructus Aurantii 45.5%, Faeces Trogopterori 18%, Herba Agrimoniae 13%.

Cang Er Zi San Plus - Secara
Magnolia flower 5:1 extract (xin yi) 792 mg • Xanthium fruit 5:1 extract (cang er zi) 396 mg • Organic Eyebright herb 285 mg • Organic Peppermint leaf 240 mg • Fragrant Angelica root 5:1 extract (bai zhi) 198 mg • Eucalyptus leaf 5:1 extract 150 mg • Reishi fruit body (ling zhi, 10% polysaccharides (16 mg) 159 mg • Organic Peppermint oil 21 mg.

Cankermelts-GX - Orahealth
Each disc contains: Proprietary Blend 30 mg: Glycyrrhiza extract (includes 1.4 mg glycyrrhizin), Hydrophilic Gums, Potassium.

Canserfx170 - Kangniling (KNL) Pharmaceutical Company
Renshen • Reishi • Dangshen • San Qi • Ciwujia.
See Editor's Note No. 57.

Capisette - Progressive Health Nutraceuticals
Magnesium 150 mg • Potassium 99 mg • Uva Ursi extract 40 mg • Dandelion extract 200 mg • Ginkgo Biloba 5 mg • Horse Chestnut 50 mg • Buchu extract 25 mg.

Cappuccino Comfort Fructose - Physicians Laboratories
Each packet contains: Certified Isoflavone 160 mg. Other Ingredients: Soy Protein Isolate, Fructose, Sucrose, Real Coffee Powder, Natural and Artificial Flavor, Dutch Processed Cocoa, Soy Lecithin, Calcium Phosphate, Potassium Chloride, Sodium Chloride, Xanthan Gum, Carboxymethylcellulose, Undegraded Carrageenan.

Cappuccino Comfort Splenda - Physicians Laboratories
Each packet contains: Certified Isoflavone 160 mg. Ingredients: Soy Protein Isolate, Cocoa, Maltodextrin, Caclium Phosphate, Soy Lecithin, Salt, Potassium Chloride, Artificial Flavor, Carrageenan, Carboxymethylcellulose, Xanthan Gum, Sucralose.

Cappuccino Comfort Unsweetened - Physicians Laboratories
Each packet contains: Certified Isoflavone 160 mg. Other Ingredients: Soy Protein Isolate, Real Coffee Powder, Natural and Artificial Flavor, Dutch Processed Cocoa, Soy Lecithin, Calcium Phosphate, Potassium Chloride, Sodium Chloride, Xanthan Gum, Carboxymethylcellulose, Undegraded Carrageenan.

Caprylate Complex - Progressive Labs
Three capsules contain: Caprylic Acid (as caprylate) 1290 mg • Calcium (as caprylate) 100 mg • Magnesium (as caprylate) 50 mg • Zinc (as caprylate) 5 mg.

Caprylic Acid Combination - Nature's Sunshine
Two capsules contain: Caprylic Acid 600 mg • Proprietary Blend 200 mg: Black Walnut hull (juglans nigra), Elecampane root (inula helenium), Red Raspberry leaf (rubus idaeus). Other Ingredients: Gelatin, Water.

Caprylic Acid Complex - Jamieson
Each capsule contains: Caprylic Acid (from calcium and magnesium caprilate) 200 mg • Garlic (odour controlled allicin-rich) 150 mg • Thyme 100 mg • Black Walnut Hulls 50 mg • Borage Oil 50 mg.

Caprylimune - Nature's Sunshine
Two tablets contain: Vitamin A 3666 IU • Vitamin C (ascorbic acid) 333 mg • Vitamin E (D-alpha tocopherol) 100 IU • Biotin 133 mcg • Pantothenic Acid (D-calcium pantothenate) 120 mg • Calcium (di-calcium phosphate) 185 mg • Phosphorus (di-calcium phosphate) 144 mg • Zinc (gluconate) 13 mg • Selenium (amino acid chelate) 133 mcg • Caprylic Acid 100 mg. Base: Pau d'Arco bark (tabebuia heptaphylla), Garlic bulb (allium sativum), Goldenseal root (hydrastis canadensis), Yucca root (yucca baccata), Lemongrass herb (cymbopogon citratus), Rose Hips concentrate (rosa canina), Lemon Bioflavonoid, Hesperidin, Rutin. Other Ingredients: Cellulose, Maltodextrin, Silicon Dioxide, Magnesium Stearate, Stearic Acid, Guar Gum (cyamopsis tetragonolobus), Gelatin.

CapsiCool Cayenne - Nature's Way
Two capsules contain: Proprietary Formula: Cayenne pepper fruit • Ginger • Glucomannan root. Other ingredients: Gelatin.

Capsicum - Nature's Sunshine
Each capsule contains: Capsicum fruit (capsicum annuum) 520 mg. Other Ingredients: Kosher Gelatin, Water.

Capsicum & Garlic with Parsley - Nature's Sunshine
Two capsules contain: Proprietary Blend 1000 mg: Garlic bulb (allium sativum), Capsicum fruit (capsicum annuum), Parsley herb (petroselinum crispum). Other Ingredients: Gelatin, Water.

Capsicum Extract - Nature's Sunshine
Capsicum fruit (capsicum annuum) • Water • Alcohol 15-20%.

Caramel Corn - Physicians Laboratories
Eight fluid ounces contain: Certified Isoflavone 15 mg. Ingredients: Roasted Whole Soybeans, Natural and Artificial Flavors.

Cararthron - Chalmers Dale
Each tablet contains: Extract Blend: Trichosanthes Kirilowii root (Chinese snakegourd) 4 g • Clematis Siinensis root (wellingxian) 2 g • Prunella Vulgaris flower (self heal) 2 g.
Available in Australia.

Some Brand Name Natural Products - What they Contain

www.NaturalDatabase.com contains MANY more listings than appear here.
Editor's Notes are located on pages 2155-2163.

Caratomax **- Shaklee**
Each capsule contains: Vitamin A 5000 IU • Lycopene 5 mg • Lutein 5 mg • Zeaxanthin 200 mcg • Alpha Carotene 1.5 mg • CaratoMax Proprietary Blend 70 mg: Quercitin, Grapeseed extract (Vitis vinifera) seed/skin, Broccoli Sprouts extract (Brassica oleracea italica) whole sprout. Other Ingredients: Soybean Oil, Beeswax, Palm Oil, Soy Lecithin, Gelatin, Glycerine, Water, Annatto.

Carb BLX Type 1 **- 4 Life**
Each capsule contains: Proprietary Blend 490 mg: White Kidney bean extract, Wheat Grass extract, Green Tea extract (polyphenols 90%, catechins 70%), Jaborandi extract, Arabinose. Other Ingredients: Gelatin.

Carb BLX Type 2 **- 4 Life**
Each capsule contains: Proprietary Blend 490 mg: Cassia Nomame extract, White Kidney bean extract, Cocoa - Almond extract, Green Tea extract (polyphenols 90%, catechins 70%), Jaborandi extract, Arabinose. Other Ingredients: Gelatin.

Carb Cutter with Phase 2 Starch Neutralizer **- Health and Nutrition Systems**
Each tablet contains: Phase 2 brand Starch Neutralizer from White Kidney Bean extract (phaseolus vulgaris) 500 mg • Proprietary Carb Free Blend 50 mg: Gymnema Sylvestre leaf, Fenugreek seed, Garcinia Cambogia fruit extract (50% hydroxycitric acid), Vanadium (as vanadyl sulfate). Other Ingredients: Dicalcium Phosphate, Microcrystalline Cellulose, Croscarmellose Sodium, Stearic Acid, Magnesium Stearate, Silica, Pharmaceutical Glaze.

Carb Defense **- Dynamic Nutritional Products**
Each vegetarian tablet contains: Chromium (as chromium polynicotinate) 100 mcg • Vanadium (as vanadyl sulfate) 100 mcg • Northern White Kidney Bean extract (phaseolus vulgaris) 750 mg. Other Ingredients: Cellulose, Calcium Phosphate, Stearic Acid, Vegetable Magnesium Stearate, Modified Cellulose Gum, Silicon Dioxide.

Carb Explosion (orange flavor) **- Rexall - Sundown**
Each scoop contains: Vitamin A 3000 IU • Vitamin C (Ascorbic Acid) 6 mg •Vitamin D (Cholecalciferol) 40 IU •Vitamin E (dl-Alpha Tocopheryl Acetate) 3 IU • Thiamin Mononitrate (Vitamin B-1) 0.15 mg • Riboflavin (Vitamin B-2) 0.17 mg • Niacin (Niacinamide) 2 mg • Vitamin B-6 (Pyridoxine HCl) 0.2 mg • Folic Acid 40 mcg • Vitamin B-12 (Cyanocobalamin) 0.6 mcg • Biotin 30 mcg • Pantothenic Acid (Calcium D-Pantothenate) 1 mg • Electrolytic Iron 1.8 mg • Phosphorus 50 mg • Iodine 0.15 mg •Magnesium Phosphate Dibasic 40 mg • Zinc Oxide 1.5 mg •Copper Gluconate 0.2 mg • Chromium Polynicotinate 90 mcg •Sodium Chloride 100 mg • Potassium Chloride 75 mg • Carb Explosion Enzyme Blend: Glucoamylase, Malt Diastase, Amylase, Phytase,Hemicellulase,Beta-Glucanase 250 mg. Other Ingredients: Crystalline Fructose, Maltodextrin, Dextrose, Natural and Artificial Orange Flavor, Citric Acid, Malic Acid, Dicalcium Phosphate, Beta-Carotene, Potassium Iodide.

Carb Intercept with Phase 2 Starch Neutralizer **- Natrol, Inc.**
Two capsules contain: White Kidney Bean extract (phaseolamin vugaris) 1 g. Other Ingredients: Gelatin, Silica, Magnesium Stearate.
See Editor's Note No. 37.

Carb Zapper **- New Sun**
Two tablets contain: Magnesium (as oxide) 50 mg • Phaseolin EX Phaseolus Vulgaris extract 750 mg • Gymnemalin Gymnema Sylvestre extract 100 mg • Alpha Lipoic Acid 25 mg • Chromium Picolinate 150 mcg • Chromium Polynicotinate 50 mcg • Vanadium (as BMOV) 100 mcg. Other Ingredients: Magnesium Stearate, Stearic Acid.
See Editor's Note No. 37.

Carba-E-A-C **- Atrium Biotechnologies**
Each rounded teaspoon contains approximately: Vitamin A Acetate 4000 IU • Vitamin C from Ascorbic Acid 100 mg • Vitamin E 33 IU. In a carrier of Carbamide (food grade).

Carbo **- Enzymedica**
Each capsule contains: Amylase Thera-Blend 22,000 DU • Glucoamylase 30 AG • Alpha-Galactosidase 1000 GAL • Protease Thera-Blend 15,000 HUT • Lipase Thera-Blend 150 FCCLU • Cellulase Thera-Blend 400 CU • Lactase 400 ALU • Maltase 300 DP • Pectinase with Phytase 20 endo-PGU.

Carbo Fuel (Complex Carbohydrate Peak Performance Energy Drink) **- TwinLab**
Each serving contains: Carbohydrates (from Glucose Polymers & Crystalline Pure Fructose) (no high fructose corn syrups are present) 80 grams. Other Ingredients: Vitamin B1, Vitamin B2, Vitamin B3, Vitamin B6, Pantothenic Acid, Biotin, Potassium, Magnesium, Yeast-Free GTF Chromium, Inosine, L-Carnitine, CoQ10, Lipoic Acid, Pantetheine, Pyridoxine-Alpha-Ketoglutarate, Soluble Potassium (Phosphate & Succinates), Citrates, Aspartates, Fumarates, Malates, Alpha-Ketoglutarates.

Carbo Grabbers **- Nature's Sunshine**
Two capsules contain: White Kidney Bean extract (phaseolus vulgaris) 600 mg. Other Ingredients: Cellulose, Magnesium Sterate, Silicon Dioxide, Gelatin, Water.

Carboburn **- United Healthcare Labs**
Three capsules contain: Proprietary Blend 3000 mg: Phaseolus Vulgaris, Critzine, Magnolia bark extract (magnolia officinalis, 1.5% honokiol), Beta-Sitosterol, L-Theanine, L-Phenylalanine, Niacinamide, Chromium Picolinate, Citrus Aurantium extract, Guarana.
See Editor's Note No. 40.

Carbolin **- Phytobase, Inc.**
Two vegetable capsules contain: Magnesium (citrate) 14 mg • Chromium (polynicotinate) 42 mcg • Proprietary Blend 1180 mg: Phaseolamine complex (phaseolamine, phaseolamine 2250), Citrin HCA, American Ginseng, Cassia Nomame 10:1 extract, Green Tea 50% extract, Vanadyl Sulfate.

Carbo-Meta **- Atrium Biotechnologies**
Each tablet contains: Pyridoxal-5-Phosphate 20 mg • Pyridoxine HCL 50 mg • Chromium Aspartate 500 mcg • Magnesium 50 mg • Manganese 5 mg • Zinc Aspartate 15 mg.

Carbonyl Iron 25 mg **- Rexall - Sundown**
Two tablets contain: Calcium 117 mg • Iron (as carbonyl iron) 50 mg. Other Ingredients: Dicalcium Phosphate, Maltodextrins, Corn Syrup Solids, Croscarmellose Sodium, Magnesium Stearate.

CarboTame **- Jarrow Formulas**
Each capsule contains: Chromium GTF (from saccharomyces cerevisiae) 50 mcg • Phase 2 brand Starch Neutralizer, Phaseolus Vulgaris 500 mg • Green Tea (camellia sinensis, 45% polyphenols) 150 mg. Other Ingredients: Magnesium Stearte, Silicon Dioxide.

CarbOut 255 **- Unknown**
Each tablet contains: Phaseolus Vulgaris extract (kidney bean) 500 mg. Other Ingredients: Gelatin, Glycerin, Water, Cellulose, Magnesium Stearate, Vegetable Stearin, Silica.

Carbs Away **- FreeLife International**
Each caplet contains: Chromium (as patented Chelavite chromium dinicotinate glycinate) 200 mcg • Carbohydrate Reducing Blend 125 mg: Phaseolus Vulgaris seed (2500 units/gm), Gymnema Sylvestre leaf standardized extract (25% gymnemic acid), Banaba leaf standardized extract (lagerstoemia speciosa, 1% corosolic acid), Momordica Charantia fruit (2.5% bitter principles) • Proprietary Blend 25 mg: Purified Methylsulfonylmethane, Piper Nigrum fruit standardized extract (95% piperine) • Vanadium (from glycinate chelate) 100 mcg. Other Ingredients: Calcium Hydrogen Phosphate, Cellulose, Cellulose Gum, Fractionated Vegetable Oil, Colloidal Silica, Vita-Coat (vegetable resin, alpha-lipoic acid).

Carbs Away Plus **- FreeLife International**
Each caplet contains: Vitamin B6 (as pyridoxine hydrochloride) 2 mg • Chromium (as Chelavite brand chromium dinicotinate glycinate)

200 mcg • Carbitol brand Herbal Complex 125 mg: Amylase inhibitor factor from Phaseolus vulgaris seed, Gymnema sylvestre leaf extract, Banaba leaf (lagerstroemia speciosa), Momordica charantia fruit • Lipitol brand Complex 610 mg: Green Tea leaf extract, Cinnamon twig extract, Galangal root extract • Appitol brand Complex 275 mg: Purified Vegetable Cellulose, Griffonia Simplicifolia seed extract, 5-Hydroxytryptophan • Absorption Enhancement Complex 25 mg: MSM brand purified Methylsulfonylmethane, Bioperine brand Black Pepper extract (from piper nigrum fruit) • Vanadium (from glycinated chelate) 100 mcg. Other Ingredients: Calcium Hydrogen Phosphate, Cellulose Gum, Fractionated Vegetable Oil, Silica, Vita-Coat brand (modified cellulose, alpha-lipoic acid).

Carbs Away Shake - FreeLife International
Whey Protein Isolate • Calcium Carbonate • Safflower Essential Fatty Acids Complex: Non-Hydrogenated Safflower Oil, Dextrose, Sodium Caseinate, Dipotassium Phosphate, Mono- and Diglycerides, Lecithin, Mixed Tocopherols, Natural Flavor, Silicon Dioxide • Potassium Phosphate • Natural Flavors • Vegetable Gum Blend: Xanthan Gum, Cellulose Gum, Irish Moss extract • Potassium Citrate • Magnesium Phosphate • Lecithin • Magnesium Oxide • Salt • Silica • Oat Bran • Choline Bitartrate • Sodium Ascorbate • Sucralose • Sodium Molybdate • Niacinamide • D-Alpha-Tocopheryl Succinate • Kelp • Manganese Gluconate • Copper Gluconate • Calcium Pantothenate • Phylloquinone • Sodium Selenite • Cholecalciferol • Retinyl Palmitate • Pyridoxine Hydrochloride • Thiamin Mononitrate • Cyanocobalamin • Chromium Chloride • Folic Acid.

CarbWatchers Lean Body Meal Replacement Shake - Labrada Bodybuilding Nutrition
Lean Pro blend: Milk Protein Isolate, Whey Protein Concentrate, Whey Protein Isolate, Hydrolyzed Whey Protein Isolate peptides, Calcium Caseinate, L-Glutamine, Taurine • Maltodextrin • Vitamin and Mineral Blend: Potassium Chloride, Calcium Phosphate, Magnesium Oxide, Alpha Tocopherol Acetate, Ascorbic Acid, Ferrous Fumarate, Niacinamide, Zinc Oxide, Manganese Sulfate, Calcium Pantothenate, Vitamin A Palmitate, Vitamin K (K1), Zinc Picolinate, Copper Sulfate, Vitamin D (D3), Pyridoxine Hydrochloride, Chromium Polynicotinate, Riboflavin, Thiamin Hydrochloride, Vitamin B12, Folic Acid, Sodium Molybdate, Chromium Chloride, Biotin, Potassium Iodide, Sodium Selenite • Polydextrose • Natural and Artificial flavor • Soy Lecithin • Xanthan gum • Sucralose • Cellulose fiber • Beta Carotene (color).

Carctol - IvyComm Systems
Each capsule contains: Hemidesmus Indicus 20 mg • Tribulus Terrestris 20 mg • Piper Cubeba Linn 120 mg • Ammani Vesicatoria 20 mg • Lepidium Sativum Linn 20 mg • Blepharis Edulis 200 mg • Smilax China Linn 80 mg • Rheumemodi Wall 20 mg.

Cardimax - Ortho Molecular Products
Four capsules contain: Hawthorne leaf & flower extract (standardized to contain 1.8% vitex-2"O-rhamnosides) 320 mg • L-Carnitine (as L-tartrate) 250 mg • Taurine 1000 mg • Berberine sulfate 1200 mg • Quercetin 400 mg. Other Ingredients: Natural Vegetable Capsules, Magnesium Stearate, Microcrystalline Cellulose, Silicon Dioxide, Ascorbyl Palmitate.

Cardio 150 - Atrium Biotechnologies
Each tablet contains: Raw Heart concentrate (not an extract) of Bovine source 150 mg.
See Editor's Note No. 14.

Cardio 20 - Futurebiotics LLC
Six capsules contain: Beta-carotene 25,000 IU • Vitamin C (buffered ascorbate)1000 mg • Vitamin E (natural) 400 IU • Niacin (timed release, flush-free) 250 mg • Choline Bitartrate 150 mg • Inositol 75 mg • Calcium (ascorbate) 250 mg • Magnesium (oxide, chelate) 400 mg • Potassium (gluconate) 99 mg • Coenzyme Q10 15 mg • L-Carnitine 100 mg • Taurine 100 mg • Procyanidol 35 mg • Hawthorn berries (4:1 extract) 250 mg • Soy Isoflavone extract 100 mg • Cholestatin Beta-sitosterol complex 250 mg • Garlic (pure-gar 1500 deodorized concentrate) 400 mg • Cayenne 100 mg • Ginger 50 mg • Chlorella 250 mg.

Cardio ACES - J. R. Carlson Laboratories, Inc.
Two softgels contain: Vitamin A (as beta carotene) 5000 IU • Vitamin C (as calcium ascorbate) 500 mg • Vitamin E (as D-alpha tocopheryl acetate) 400 IU • Calcium (as calcium ascorbate) 50 mg • Magnesium (as magnesium oxide and magnesium glycinate) 200 mg • Selenium (as L-selenomethionine) 100 mcg • Potassium (as potassium citrate) 49 mg • DHA (docosahexaenoic acid) 160 mg • EPA (eicosapentaenoic acid) 240 mg • Co-Q10 (coenzyme Q10) 30 mg • Fish Oil concentrate 800 mg • Garlic bulb (allium sativum, odorless) 50 mg.

Cardio Assurance - Nature's Sunshine
Each capsule contains: Vitamin B6 (as pyridoxine HCl) 4 mg • Vitamin B12 (as cyanocobalamin) 50 mcg • Folic Acid 300 mcg • Proprietary Blend 432 mg: Hawthorn berry extract (crataegus oxyacanthoides), Red Clover flower extract (trifolium pratense), Ginkgo Biloba leaf concentrate, Capsicum fruit (capsicum annuum), Choline (bitartrate), Taurine. Other Ingredients: Magnesium Stearate, Silicon Dioxide, Gelatin, Water.

Cardio B - Ortho Molecular Products
Each capsule contains: Vitamin B6 (as pyridoxine HCl USP) 50 mg • Folic Acid 5 mg • Vitamin B12 (as methylcobalamin) 1 mg • Trimethyl Glycine 500 mg. Other Ingredients: Natural Vegetable Capsules, Ascorbyl Palmitate, Magnesium Stearate, Microcrystalline Cellulose, Silicon Dioxide.

Cardio Care - Vidafit
Each serving contains: Biotin 30 mcg • Folate 400 mcg • Niacin 16 mg • Pantothenic Acid 5 mg • Riboflavin 1.3 mg • Thiamine 1.2 mg • Vitamin A 3300 IU • Vitamin B12 2.4 mcg • Vitamin B6 1.7 mg • Vitamin C 100 mg • Vitamin D 200 IU • Vitamin E 10 IU • Calcium 500 mg • Chromium 50 mcg • Copper 2 mg • Iodine 70 mcg • Magnesium 320 mg • Phosphorus 500 mg • Potassium 700 mg • Zinc 15 mg • Coenzyme Q10 25 mg • Bilberry 50 mg • Garlic 10 mg • Ginkgo extract 100 mg • Grape Seed extract 50 mg • Soy Protein 5 grams.

Cardio Chelate - Nutri-Quest Rx
Six tablets contain: Vitamin A (palmitate) 3000 IU • Beta Carotene 7500 IU • Vitamin D (as D3) 100 IU • Vitamin C 300 mg • Vitamin B1 30 mg • Vitamin B2 30 mg • Vitamin B6 75 mg • Vitamin B12 500 mcg • Biotin 200 mcg • Niacin 60 mg • D-Calcium Pantothenate (pantothenic acid) 150 mg • Folic Acid 300 mcg • Vitamin E (succinate) 300 IU • Iodine (kelp) 100 mcg • PABA 100 mg • Lecithin 120 mg • Choline Bitartrate 250 mg • Cysteine HCl 250 mg • L-Methionine 75 mg • L-Lysine 100 mg • Bromelaine 30 mg • Lemon Bioflavonoid 900 mg • Rutin 30 mg • Inositol 75 mg • Garlic 120 mg • Cayenne 30 mg • Hawthorne berry 100 mg • Pancreatin 6X 25 mg • Thymus 30 mg • Spleen 30 mg • Heart 30 mg • Adrenal (nutritrophic) 30 mg • Whole Pituitary 30 mg • Papain 30 mg • L-Glycine 75 mg • Calcium Gluconate 37 mg • Manganese Chelate 2.5 mg • Copper Gluconate 7.8 mcg • Molybdenum Chelate 12 mcg • Chromium Chelate 102 mcg • Selenium Chelate 30 mcg • Calcium Ascorbate 100 mg • Calcium Aspartate 100 mg • Potassium Aspartate 25 mg • Magnesium Ascorbate 75 mg • Magnesium Aspartate 75 mg • Ferrous Gluconate 15 mg • Zinc Aspartate 15 mg. Base: Calcium Phosphate, Magnesium Phosphate, Calcium Flouride, Ferric Phosphate, Kali Phosphate, Silica, Chiorinum, Peppermint Leaf, Black Cohosh, Scullcap, Licorice Root, Watercress, Siberian Ginseng, Red Beet Root, Parsley.
See Editor's Note No. 31.

Cardio Cholestamax - Biotech Corp.
Two tablets contain: Shen Min (he shou wu, 12:1 extract standardized to 10% chrysophanics and 1.9% resveratrol) 100 mg • Natural Vitamin E (dl-alpha tocopherol succinate) 400 IU • Folic Acid 800 mcg • Selenium (as organic selenomethionine) 150 mcg • Chromium (as patented dinicotinate glycinate) 200 mcg • Potassium

(citrate) 50 mg • Aged Garlic (5:1 extract, equivalent to one clove of fresh garlic) 360 mg • Guggulipid Commiphora Mukul standardized extract 100 mg • Inula root (inula racemose, standardized to 2% analactones) 100 mg • Cholestatin purified Plant Phytosterols 100 mg • Tomato concentrate (a source of lycopene) 100 mg • Hawthorne berry (crutageous oxycantha, standardized to 5% vitexin-2' rhamnoside) 100 mg. Other Ingredients: Dicalcium Phosphate, Microcrystalline Cellulose, Croscarmellose Sodium, Stearic Acid, Magnesium Stearate, Pharmaceutical Glaze.

Cardio Complex - Leiner Health Products
Each softgel contains: Vitamin E (dl-Alpha Tocopherol and d-Alpha Tocopherol) 400 IU • Folate (Folic Acid) 400 mcg • Vitamin B12 (Cyanocobalamin) 6 mcg • Vitamin B6 (Pyridoxine Hydrochloride) 2 mg. Other Ingredients: Gelatin, Vegetable Oil, Glycerin, Yellow Beeswax, Unbleached Lecithin, Titanium Dioxide, Dicalcium Phosphate, Red 40.

Cardio EDTA Chelate - Olympia Nutrition
EDTA 400 mg • MSM 100 mg • NAC 50 mg • Vitamin C 100 mg.

Cardio Essentials - Royal Numico
Six capsules contain: Coenzyme Q10 100 mg • Proprietary Blend 3.5 g: L-Carnitine, L-Taurine, Hawthorn berry (standardized to 1.8% vitexin). Other Ingredients: Gelatin (capsules), Stearic Acid, Calcium Silicate, Silicon Dioxide.

Cardio Flow - Progressive Labs
Six capsules contain: Vitamin A (retinyl palmitate) 10,000 IU • Vitamin C (ascorbic acid and zinc ascorbate) 640 mg • Elemental Potassium (from Potassium Aspartate 684 mg, from Potassium Orotate 300 mg) 210 mg • Elemental Magnesium (from Magnesium Aspartate 1400 mg, from Magnesium Orotate 714 mg) 330 mg • Elemental Zinc (from Zinc Ascorbate 168 mg) 25 mg • Elemental Selenium (Selenium Ascorbate 70 mg) 70 mcg • Sodium 28 mg • EDTA (Ethylenediamine tetra-acetic acid) 800 mg • Disodium EDTA 200 mg • L-Glutathione, reduced 20 mg • Bromelain (2000 GDU) 300 mg • Papain (525 TU/mg) 30 mg • Cilantro (coriander) 500 mg • Butcher's Broom 150 mg • Cardio Flow 600 mg: a proprietary blend of the following extracts: [Inula racemosa (root), Saussurea lappa (root), Terminalia arjuna (root), Desmodium gingatic (leaves), Commiphora mukul (resin), Bacopa monniera (leaves), Convolvulous pluricaulis (leaves)]. Other Ingredients: Rice flour, Magnesium Stearate.

Cardio Formula - Pharmanex
Three capsules contain: Vitamin E (D-alpha tocopherol) 100 IU • Vitamin B6 (as pyridoxine hydrochloride) 20 mg • Folate (as folic acid) 400 mcg • Vitamin B12 (as cyanocobalamin) 60 mcg • Marine Fish Oil (providing omega-3 fatty acids) 2000 mg • EPA 360 mg • DHA 240 mg • Garlic powder (allium sativum) 325 mg • White Willow bark (salix alba) 250 mg • Rosemary leaf extract (rosarinus officinalis) 12 mg • Policosanol (beeswax extract) 10 mg.

Cardio Plus - Atrium Biotechnologies
Three tablets contain: Vitamin E Acetate 300 IU • Vitamin C (with Rose Hips) 60 mg • Thiamine Mononitrate 15 mg • Vitamin B2 Riboflavin 2 mg • Niacin 100 mg • Vitamin B6 15 mg • Vitamin B12 2 mcg • Magnesium (as Citrus Juice Complex & Oxide) 100 mg • Zinc (as Gluconate) 5 mg • Potassium (as Citrus Juice Complex & Chloride) 99 mg • Chromium (amino acid complex) 10 mcg • Selenium (in yeast) 48 mcg • Choline Bitartrate 66 mg. In a base containing Lecithin 80 mg, Para Aminobenzoic Acid 30 mg, Inositol 4 mg, Cold Processed Heart Protein 90 mg.
See Editor's Note No. 14.

Cardio ProtoChol - Inverness Medical Innovations, Inc.
Each capsule contains: Vitamin E (as D-Alpha Tocopheryl Acid Succinate) 10 IU • Niacin Powder 3 mg • Soybean Isoflavones extract (Novasoy brand, isoflavones 13 mg) 33 mg • Garlic bulb extract (allicin 333 mcg) 33 mg • Guggulipids extract (guggulsterones 0.8 mg) 33 mg • Red Rice Yeast Extract (lovastatin 134 mcg) 33 mg • Lemon Bioflavonoids Complex 10 mg • Chitosan Powder 50 mg. Other Ingredients: Calcium Carbonate, Hydroxymethyl Propylcellulose, Magnesium Stearate, Silicon Dioxide.

Cardio Q10 - PhysioLogics
Each capsule contains: Vitamin E (as d-Alpha Tocopherol) 200 IU • Calcium (as Dicalcium Phosphate) 2 mg • Selenium (as Selenomethionine) 25 mcg • Coenzyme Q10 30 mg.

Cardio Q10 - Health Smart Vitamins
Two capsules contain: Vitamin E (as d-alpha tocopheryl acetate) 542 IU • Calcium (as dicalcium phosphate) 3 mg • Selenium (as selenonmethionine) 50 mcg • Coenzyme Q10 60 mg.

Cardio Results - Goldshield Elite
Two caplets contain: Vitamin B6 (as Pyridoxine HCl) 15 mg • Folate (as Folic acid) 400 mcg • Vitamin B12 (as Cyanocobalamin) 250 mcg • Red Yeast rice (from fermentation of Monascus pupureus Went) 600 mg • Purified Soy phytosterols (45-55% Beta-Sitosterol) 50 mg. Other Ingredients: Dicalcium phosphate, Vegetable cellulose, Fractionated vegetable oil, Soy polysaccharides, Silica, and Vita-Lok vegetable resin glaze.

Cardio Stack - Maruda Nutrition
Three capsules contain: Vitamin B6 10 mg • Folate 400 mcg • Vitamin B12 50 mcg • Carnitine blend 1000 mg • Rhodiola Rosea 200 mg • Green Tea / Guarana (200 mg total active caffeine) 500 mg • Lipotropic Blend 100 mg: DL-Methionine, Choline Bitartrate, Inositol • Electrolyte Replenishing Blend 100 mg: Calcium Citrate, Magnesium Oxide, Potassium Gluconate • Krebs Cycle blend 100 mg.

Cardio Support Formula - The Vitamin Factory
Each tablet contains: Vitamin E (d-Alpha Tocopheryl-Succinate) 100 IU • Folic Acid 100 mcg • White Willow bark extract 4:1 100 mg • Hawthorne berry extract 50 mg • Coenzyme Q10 30 mg • Oat Beta Glucan powder (min 18%) 25 mg • Pycnogenol (Maritime Pine bark extract) 15 mg.

Cardio Support with Q-Gel - Zone Labs
Each softgel contains: Natural Vitamin E (D-alpha tocopheryl acetate) 22 IU • Natural Coenzyme Q-10 (ubidecarenone) 15 mg. Other Ingredients: Gelatin, Sorbitol, Glycerin, Purified Water, Polysorbate 80, Hydroxylated Lecithin, Medium Chain Triglycerides, Annatto Seed Extract.

Cardio ToconOx - Herbalife International of America, Inc.
Each capsule contains: Vitamin E (from Tocomins) 6 IU • Natural Mixed Tocotrienols (from Tocomins) 20 mg • Dried Olive leaf extract (olea europaea) 20 mg • Coenzyme Q10 4 mg. Other Ingredients: Rice Bran Oil, Gelatin, Glycerin, Lecithin, Beeswax, Olive Oil, Water, Natural Vanilla Flavor.

Cardio Tonic - Puritan's Pride
Three caplets contain: Coenzyme Q10 20 mg • Vitamin E 100 IU • Vitamin C 300 mg • Folic Acid 400 mcg • Niacin (Vitamin B3) 20 mg • Vitamin B6 (pyridoxine) 50 mg • Calcium 100 mg • Magnesium 100 mg • Potassium 99 mg • Selenium Proteinate 150 mcg • L-Carnitine 50 mg • L-Taurine 300 mg • Garlic 100 mg • Hawthorn berry 5:1 50 mg • Lecithin 50 mg • Ginger 25 mg.

Cardioace - Vitabiotics
Two capsules contain: Omega-3 Fish oil 800 mg • Vitamin D 5 mcg • Vitamin E 80 mg • Vitamin C 60 mg • Vitamin B1 (thiamin) 10 mg • Vitamin B2 (riboflavin) 1.6 mg • Vitamin B6 (pyridoxine HCl) 10 mg • Folic Acid 500 mcg • Vitamin B12 (cyanocobalamin) 20 mcg • Zinc 10 mg • Manganese 3 mg • Copper 2 mg • Chromium 100 mcg • Selenium 160 mcg • Natural Mixed Carotenoids 4 mg • Garlic 200 mg • Lecithin 40 mg.

CardioAntioxidant - Advocare International
Four capsules contain: Vitamin A (as beta-carotene from D. salina mixed carotenoids) 10,000 IU • Vitamin C (as magnesium ascorbate) 600 mg • Vitamin E (as d-alpha-tocopheryl succinate) 400 IU •

Thiamine 1.5 mg • Niacin (as inositol hexanicotinate) 60 mg • Vitamin B6 (as pyridoxine HCl) 20 mg • Folic Acid 1000 mg • Vitamin B12 (as cyanocobalamin) 60 mcg • Zinc (as monomethionine OptiZinc) 5 mg • Selenium (as selenomethionine) 35 mcg • Manganese (as gluconate) 0.5 mg • Taurine 600 mg • Coenzyme Q-10 100 mg • Golden Root extract (root - rhodiola rosea) 50 mg • Green Tea extract (leaf - camellia sinensis Sinensa) 50 mg • Lipoic Acid 50 mg • L-Carnitine 50 mg • Ascorbyl Palmitate 15 mg. Other Ingredients: Silicon Dioxide, Magnesium Stearate, Gelatin.

CardioBALANCE - Mannatech
Each capsule contains: Vitamin C (as ascorbic acid, acerola [fruit], camu-camu [fruit]) 60 mg • Vitamin E (as d-alpha tocopheryl acetate, mixed d-alpha-, d-beta-, d-delta-, and d-gamma-tocopherols and mixed tocotrienols) 15 IU • Folate (as folic acid) 200 mcg • Vitamin B6 (as pyridoxine hydrochloride and pyridoxal 5-phosphate) 2 mg • Vitamin B12 (as cyanocobalamin) 16.7 mcg • Magnesium (as magnesium oxide, magnesium citrate and magnesium glycinate) 34 mg • L-Arginine 333.3 mg • Proprietary Herbal Blend 88 mg: Garlic extract (root), Grape extract (seed & skin), Hawthorn extract (crataegus pinnatifida fruit), Carambola (fruit) • Taurine 100 mg • Trimethylglycine 83.3 mg • Alpha-Lipoic Acid 20 mg • N-Acetyl-L-Cysteine 16.7 mg • Ambrocosanol Complex 8.3 mg: Ambrotose Complex (patent pending) [arabinogalactan (larix decidua gum), Aloe Vera gel extract (inner leaf gel), Manapol powder, Gum Ghatti, Gum Tragacanth], Octacosanol, Triacontanol, Hexacosanol, Tetracosanol, Heptacosanol • Coenzyme Q10 1.67 mg. Other Ingredients: Gelatin, Magnesium Stearate.

Cardio-Basics - Rexall - Sundown
Each two tablets contain: Vitamin A (100% as beta-carotene) 2500 IU • Vitamin C (as ascorbyl palmitate and ascorbic acid) 300 mg • Vitamin D (as cholecalciferol) 200 IU • Vitamin E (as d-alpha-tocopheryl acid succinate) 200 IU • Thiamin (as thiamin mononitrate) 10 mg • Riboflavin (Vitamin B-2) 10 mg • Niacin (as niacinamide and niacin) 65 mg • Vitamin B-6 (as pyridoxine HCl) 15 mg • Folic Acid 130 mcg • Vitamin B-12 (as cyanocobalamin) 30 mcg • Biotin 100 mcg • Pantothenic Acid (as calcium d-pantothenate) 60 mg • Calcium 50 mg • Phosphorus 20 mg • Magnesium (as magnesium oxide) 60 mg • Zinc (as zinc oxide) 10 mg • Selenium (as sodium selenate) 30 mcg • Copper (as cupric oxide) 0.5 mg • Manganese (as manganese sulfate) 2 mg • Chromium (as chromium amino acid chelate) 15 mcg • Molybdenum (as molybdenum yeast chelate) 6 mcg • Sodium 5 mg • Potassium (as potassium chloride) 30 mg • L-Proline 150 mg • L-Lysine HCl 150 mg • L-Arginine HCl 50 mg • L-Carnitine Tartrate 50 mg • L-Cysteine HCl 50 mg • Inositol 50 mg • Coenzyme Q-10 10 mg • Pycnogenol Pine Bark extract 10 mg. Inactive Ingredients: Cellulose, Tricalcium Phosphate, Croscarmellose Sodium, Stearic Acid, Povidone, Dicalcium Phosphate, Silica, Pharmaceutical Glaze, Magnesium Stearate, Hydroxypropyl Methylcellulose, Hydroxypropyl Cellulose, PEG.

CardioBran - Pure Encapsulations
Two vegetable capsules contain: Oat bran concentrate (standardized to contain 54% oat beta glucan) 1400 mg.

Cardio-Chelate - Metabolic Response Modifiers
Each capsule contains: EDTA (Ethylenediamine-Tetra-Acetic acid) 400 mg • MSM (Methyl-Sulfonyl-Methane) 100 mg • NAC (N-Acetyl-Cysteine) 50 mg • Vitamin C (ascorbic acid) 100 mg.

Cardiogarl - Olympian Labs
Three capsules contain: Ginkgo Biloba leaf extract 120 mg • Garlic extract 600 mg • Bilberry extract 150 mg • Coenzyme Q10 60 mg • Hawthorn Berry extract 210 mg.

Cardiogenics - Metagenics
Three tablets contain: L-Taurine 600 mg • Magnesium (as amino acid chelate and magnesium aspartate) 320 mg • Potassium (as potassium chloride, aspartate) 310 mg • Calcium (as amino acid chelate and calcium aspartate) 160 mg • Raw Heart concentrate (bovine) 150 mg • Selenium (as selenium aspartate) 99 mcg • Chromium (as chromium aspartate) 99 mcg • Hawthorn berry (crataegus oxyacantha) 50 mg • Gentian root (gentiana lutea) 50 mg • Green Pea (pisum sativum) 50 mg.

Cardiogenics Intensive Care - Metagenics
Three tablets contain: Calcium (as calcium aspartate) 100 mg • Magnesium (as magnesium citrate) 200 mg • Selenium (as selenium aspartate) 50 mcg • Potassium (as potassium aspartate) 100 mg • L-Taurine 600 mg • Hawthorn leaf and flower 5.5:1 extract (crataegus oxyacantha) 400 mg • Arjuna bark 8:1 extract (terminalia arjuna) 200 mg.

Cardio-Glycan - PhytoPharmica
Each capsule contains: Glycosaminoglycans (GAGs) 50 mg. See Editor's Note No. 14.

Cardio-Health - Aspen Group, Inc.
Each caplet contains: Vitamin E (d-alpha tocopheryl acetate) 200 IU • Vitamin C 50 mg • Garlic extract (allium sativum) 300 mg • Hawthorn extract of leaf & flower (crategus laevigata) 50 mg • Co-Enzyme Q10 (ubiquinone) 5 mg.

CardioLogics with Policosanol - PhysioLogics
Two softgels contain: Vitamin E (as d-alpha tocopherol) 200 IU • Vitamin B6 (as pyridoxine hydrochloride) 20 mg • Folic Acid 400 mcg • Vitamin B12 (as cyanocobalamin) 50 mcg • Fish Oil 1000 mg (containing EPA (eicosapentaenoic acid) 180 mg, DHA (docosahexaenoic acid) 120 mg) • Policosanol (oryza sp., from rice wax) 10 mg • Co-Enzyme Q-10 30 mg. Other Ingredients: Gelatin, Glycerin, Yellow Beeswax, Lecithin, Caramel Color, Mannitol.

CardioMate - FreeLife International
Each softgel conains: Natural Vitamin E (from mixed tocopherols) 60 IU • Coenzyme Q10 60 mg • Hawthorne flower and leaf standardized extract (1.8-2.2% vitexin) 200 mg • Aged Garlic (from standardized 70:1 exract) 200 mg • Capsicum standardized extract (2500 SHU) 5 mg • Parsley seed oil (2000:1 concentrate) 7 mg. Other Ingredients: Rice Bran Oil, Gelatin, Glycerin, Water, Yellow Beeswax, Annatto, Carob, Other Natrual Coloring Agents.

Cardio-Natto - Gero Vita International
Each capsule contains: Nattokinase (fermented soybean extract) 150 mg. Other Ingredients: Gelatin, Silicon Dioxide, Magnesium Stearate.

Cardio-Plus - Standard Process, Inc.
Two tablets contain: Proprietary Blend: 626 mg Bovine Heart PMG extract, Bovine Liver, Choline Bitartrate, Calcium Lactate, Porcine Stomach, Bovine Orchic extract, Tillandsia Usneoides powder, Defatted Wheat germ, Nutritional Yeast, Allantoin, Inositol, Bovine Spleen, Ovine Spleen, Bovine Adrenal Cytosol extract, Porcine Brain, Oat flour • Vitamin C 14.5 mg • Vitamin E 2 IU • Riboflavin 1.6 mg • Niacin 14 mg • Vitamin B6 0.5 mg • Selenium 2.8 mcg • Potassium 5 mg. Other Ingredients: Honey, Selenium Yeast, Niacinamide, Ascorbic Acid, Mixed Tocopherols, Potassium Para-Aminobenzoate, Calcium Stearate, Arabic Gum, Glycerin, Riboflavin 5'-Phosphate, Pyridoxal 5'-Phosphate.
See Editor's Note No. 14.

CardiOptima - Advocare International
Each pouch contains: Vitamin C (as potassium/calcium ascorbates) 1000 mg • Vitamin E (as d-alpha tocopheryl acetate) 150 IU • Niacin (as inositol hexanicotinate) 70 mg • Vitamin B6 (as pyridoxine HCl) 20 mg • Folic Acid 400 mcg • Vitamin B12 (as cyanocobalamin) 60 mcg • Calcium (as ascorbate and citrate) 100 mg • Magnesium (as citrate) 60 mg • Sodium 10 mg • Potassium (as ascorbate) 170 mg • L-Lysine (as HCl) 800 mg • L-Proline 200 mg • Taurine 500 mg • L-Carnitine 100 mg • Coenzyme Q-10 5 mg • Turmeric extract 50 mg • Grape extract (seed/skin, vitis vinifera, Activin brand) 100 mg • Proprietary Blend 375 mg: Hawthorn leaf and flower extract, Hibiscus flower extract, Hawthorn Berry extract, Gotu Kola extract, Golden Root extract. Other Ingredients: Fructose, Maltodextrin, Citric Acid, Gum Arabic, Natural Flavors, Artificial Flavors, Beet Root Powder, Sucralose, Silicon Dioxide.

Some Brand Name Natural Products - What they Contain

www.NaturalDatabase.com contains MANY more listings than appear here.

Editor's Notes are located on pages 2155-2163.

Cardio-SP **-** Benepure, Inc
Each tablet contains: Vitamin B6 (pyridoxal 5-phosphate) 25 mg • Folic Acid 150 mg • Vitamin B12 (methylcobalamin) 240 mcg • Magnesium (as magnesium citrate) 50 mg • Potassium (as potassium citrate) 65 mg • Dimethylglycine HCl 200 mg • Acetyl-L-Carnitine 100 mg • Betaine HCl 100 mg • Coenzyme Q10 50 mg. Other Ingredients: Microcrystalline Cellulose, Stearic Acid, Vegetable Stearate, Silicon Dioxide, Croscarmellose Sodium, Hydroxypropyl Methylcellulose.

CardioSupport **-** Aidan Products, LLC
Each tablet contains: Vitamin A (25% palmitate/75% carotenoids) 4000 IU • Vitamin C (ascorbic acid) 250 mg • Vitamin D (D3) 50 IU • Vitamin E (d-alpha tocopheryl succinate) 65 IU • Thiamine (mononitrate, vitamin B1) 20 mg • Riboflavin (vitamin B2) 20 mg • Niacin (vitamin B3) 35 mg • Pyridoxine (hydrochloride, vitamin B6) 20 mg • Folic Acid 40 mcg • Cyanocobalamin (vitmain B12) 20 mcg • D-Biotin 30 mcg • Pantothenic Acid (CA salt) 20 mg • Calcium (carbonate) 50 mg • Iodine (kelp) 15 mcg • Magnesium (oxide, granular) 40 mg • Zinc (monomethionine) 3 mg • Selenium (amino acid chelate) 25 mcg • Copper (gluconate) 20 mcg • Manganese (gluconate) 0.5 mg • Chromium (picolinate, Nutrition 21) 30 mcg • Potassium (amino acid chelate, 20%) 10 mg • Choline (bitartrate) 72 mg • Inositol 4 mg • L-Carnitine 20 mg • DL-Methionine 20 mg • Citric Acid 15 mg • Para Aminobenzoic Acid 20 mg • Bioflavonoids (lemon) 150 mg • Bromelain (1200 MCU/GM) 10 mg • Coenzyme Q-10 (ubiquinone) 5 mg • EDTA (disodium salt) 15 mg. Other Ingredients: Silicon Dioxide, Hydrogenated Vegetable Oil, Magnesium Stearate (vegetable source).

Cardiotonic Pill **-** Tasly Pharmaceutical Group Co. Ltd.
Each 25 mg pill contains: Salviae Miltiorrhizae • Radix Notoginseng • Cinnamomum Camphora extract.

Cardiotrate **-** Progressive Labs
Each capsule contains: Raw Bovine heart concentrate 140 mg prepared by a special process which does not exceed physiological temperature (37º C). Guaranteed to be free of chemical pesticides and synthetic hormones.
See Editor's Note No. 14.

Cardiotrophin PMG **-** Standard Process, Inc.
Each tablet contains: Proprietary Blend 185 mg: Bovine Heart PMG extract, Magnesium Citrate • Calcium (from calcium lactate and calcium stearate) 20 mg. Other Ingredients: Cellulose.
See Editor's Note No. 14.

Cardiovascular Health **-** Enzymes, Inc.
Two capsules contain: Vitamin E (from d-Alpha Tocopheryl Acid Succinate) 50 IU • Coenzyme Q10 (Ubiquinone) 25 mg • n-zimes Proprietary Enzyme Blend 72 mg: pHysioProtease (177,600 pHysio-U), CereCalase Plus • Proprietary Herbal Blend 300 mg: Hawthorne leaf and flower extract (standardized to contain 1.8% vitexin), Garlic bulb concentrate, Grape seed extract (standardized to contain 95% proanthocyanidins), Rice Bran. Other Ingredients: Plant Cellulose, Water.

Cardio-Vite **-** Atrium Biotechnologies
Each tablet contains: Vitamin B1 2.2 mg • Vitamin B2 2.2 mg • Vitamin B6 50 mg • Pantothenic Acid 50 mg • Niacinamide 15 mg • Magnesium 50 mg • Potassium 50 mg.

CardioZyme **-** VP Nutrition
Each capsule contains: Nattokinase NSK-SD 700 FU • Amylase 2525 DU • Protease 11,000 HUT • Minerals 40 mg • Glucoamylase 30 AGU • Lipase 450 FCCFIP • Cellulase 700 SU.

Cardiphenol Plus **-** Gero Vita International
Each capsule contains: Morinda Citrifolia fruit extract (4:1) 100 mg • Red Wine extract (30% polyphenols) 100 mg • Prune extract (60% polyphenols) • Blueberry extract (16% chlorogenic acid) 50 mg • Pomegranate extract (40% ellagic acid, 60% polyphenols) 50 mg • Apple extract (60% polyphenols, 5% chlorogenic acid) 50 mg • Proprietary Enzyme Blend 30 mg: Amylase, Cellulase, Hemicellulase, Protease, Xylanase, Beta-Glucanase. Other Ingredients: Gelatin, Silicon Dioxide, Magnesium Stearate, Rice Flour Powder.

Cardi-Rite **-** J. R. Carlson Laboratories, Inc.
Six tablets contain: Vitamin A (as beta carotene) 8000 IU • Vitamin C (as calcium ascorbate) 1000 mg • Vitamin D (D3, cholecalciferol) 600 IU • Vitamin E (as D-alpha tocopheryl succinate) 600 IU • Thiamin (vitamin B1, as thiamin mononitrate) 40 mg • Riboflavin (vitamin B2) 40 mg • Niacin (vitamin B3, as niacin and niacinamide) 200 mg • Vitamin B6 (as pyridoxine hydrochloride) 50 mg • Folate (folic acid) 400 mcg • Vitamin B12 (cyanocobalamin) 100 mcg • Biotin 300 mcg • Pantothenic Acid (as di-calcium pantothenate) 200 mg • Calcium (carbonate and ascorbate) 1000 mg • Magnesium (as mangesium glycinate chelate) 200 mg • Zinc (as zinc glycinate chelate) 30 mg • Selenium 105 mcg • Copper (as copper glycinate chelate) 2 mg • Manganese (as citrate) 2 mg • Chromium (as an amino acid and kelp) 180 mcg • Molybdenum (as molybdenum glycinate chelate) 20 mcg • Potassium (as potassium chloride) 99 mg • Lutein (FloraGlo brand from marigolds) 600 mcg • Co-Q 10 12 mcg • Lecithin 60 mcg • L-Carnitine 150 mg • L-Lysine (as L-lysine monohydrohcloride) 500 mg • L-Proline 500 mg.

Careseng **-** Blossom Portfolio
Active Ingredient: Wild American Ginseng 50 mL. Inactive Ingredient: Normal Saline 250 mL.

Careseng #1 Solution of Ginseng Extract (Ginsenoside Rh2 and Aglycon Sapogenins) **-** EcoNugenics
Each bottle contains: Ginseng extract (Ginsenosides, Sapogenins) 600 mg.

Caribbean Tanning Secret **-** Futurebiotics LLC
Each tablet contains: Vitamin C 13 mg • Vitamin B 625 mg • Copper Gluconate 0.7 mg • Para Amino Benzoic Acid (PABA) 13 mg. In a base containing: L-tyrosine, Aloe Vera, Carrot powder, & Yucca powder.

Carmidas **-** Hadas Natural Products
Each 5 mL serving contains: Natural Citrus flavored Sucrose syrup • Fennel 200 mg • Chamomile 200 mg • Caraway 200 mg.

Carni Fuel **-** TwinLab
Each capsule contains: Carni Fuel L-Carnitine Magnesium Citrate 500 mg • L-Carnitine 200 mg • Magnesium 30 mg.

Carni Fuel (L-Carnitine Liquid Concentrate) **-** TwinLab
Each tablespoonful (15 ml) contains: L-Carnitine 1000 mg.

Carni Lean **-** The Sports Nutrition Source, Inc.
Each capsule contains: L-Carnitine 1000 mg.

CarniteX **-** Xymogen
Each capsule contains: Free form L-Carnitine (from 500 mg of L-carnitine) 340 mg. Other Ingredients: Cellulose, Magnesium Stearate.

Carnitine **-** Pain & Stress Center
Each capsule contains: Vitamin C (ascorbyl palmitate) 4 mg • L-Carnitine (as 373 mg of L-carnitine tartrate) 250 mg • Silicon (as silicon dioxide) 5 mg. Other Ingredients: Gelatin Capsule.

Carnitine + Co-Q10 **-** Jarrow Formulas
Each capsule contains: Pantothenic Acid (D-calcium pantothenate, vitamin B5) 10 mg • L-Carnitine (from 431 mg L-carnitine fumarate) 250 mg • Co-Q10 (ubiquinone) 30 mg • Lecithin (35% phosphatidylcholine) 50 mg. Other Ingredients: Cellulose, Rice Powder, Silicon Dioxide, Magnesium Stearate, Gelatin.

Carnitine 500 mg **-** Vital Nutrients
Each capsule contains: L-Carnitine (from carnitine tartrate 752 mg) 500 mg.

BRAND NAMES

Some Brand Name Natural Products - What they Contain

www.NaturalDatabase.com contains MANY more listings than appear here.
Editor's Notes are located on pages 2155-2163.

Carnitine with Chromium Pic - Pain & Stress Center
Each capsule contains: Vitamin C (as ascorbic acid and ascorbyl palmitate) 125 mg • Chromium (as chromium picolinate) 200 mcg • L-Carnitine (as 375 mg of L-carnitine) 250 mg. Other Ingredients: Guar Gum, Gelatin Capsule.

Carnosine Extreme - America's Finest
Each capsule contains: Carnosine 500 mg. Other Ingredients: Dicalcium Phosphate, Magnesium Stearate, Gelatin, Water.

Caro-Plete 19.5mg-25 - J. R. Carlson Laboratories, Inc.
Two softgels contain: Vitamin A (as alpha carotene) 6 mg • Vitamin A (as beta carotene) 19,500 IU • Vitamin E (as D-alpha tocopherol) 1 IU • Other Carotenoids 1 mg • Zeaxanthin 44 mcg • Lutein (FloraGlo brand, from marigolds) 1 mg.

Caro-Plete 78 mg-100 - J. R. Carlson Laboratories, Inc.
Each softgel contains: Vitamin A (as alpha carotene) 26 mg • Vitamin A (as beta carotene) 78,000 IU • Vitamin E (as D-alpha tocopherol) 1 IU • Lutein 1 mg • Other Carotenoids 4 mg • Zeaxanthin 44 mcg.

Carotenoid Blend - Nature's Sunshine
Each capsule contains: Vitamin A (as beta-carotene) 4000 IU • Proprietary Blend 375 mg: Alpha Carotene, Beta-Carotene, Lycopene, Lutein, Zeaxanthin, Cryptoxanthin, Astaxanthin, Phytoene, Phytofluene, Hibiscus flower (hibiscus sabdariffa). Other Ingredients: Maltodextrin, Gelatin, Water.

Carotenoid Complex - The Vitamin Shoppe
Each softgel contains: Phytofluene 0.033 mg • Lycopene (LYC-O-MATO) 5 mg • Lutein 5 mg • Beta-carotene (6251 IU Vitamin A) 3.75 mg • Alpha-carotene (1042 IU Vitamin A) 1.25 mg • Zeaxanthin 0.26 mg • Phytoene 0.098 mg. In a base of tomato and carrot concentrate.

Carpal-X - Olympian Labs
Two capsules contain: Vitamin C 120 mg • Vitamin B6 (pyridoxine HCl) 100 mg • Vitamin B2 (riboflavin) 10 mg • Zinc 5 mg • Copper 500 mcg • Proprietary Blend 795 mg: Grape Seed extract, CoQ10, White Willow Bark extract, Horse Chestnut extract, Cayenne Pepper, Enzyme blend (protease, lipase, amylase), Sea Cucumber, Yucca, Devil's Claw, Boswellia Serrata extract, Curcumin extract.

Carrot Essence - Green Foods Corp.
Each 6.8 oz jar contains: Proprietary Blend 192 g: Powdered Carrot juice, Maltodextrin, Acerola.

Carrot-Tein Energy Shake - Nature's Plus
Each scoop (33 g) contains: Vitamin A 25,000 IU • Vitamin C 60 mg • Calcium 300 mg • Iron 4.5 mg • Vitamin D 400 IU • Vitamin E 30 IU • Thiamin 1.5 mg • Riboflavin 1.7 mg • Niacin 20 mg • Vitamin B6 2 mg • Folic Acid 400 mcg • Vitamin B12 6 mcg • Biotin 300 mcg • Pantothenic Acid 10 mg • Phosphorus 200 mg • Iodine 150 mcg • Magnesium 80 mg • Zinc 15 mg • Selenium 21 mcg • Manganese 5 mg • Chromium 18 mcg • Molybdenum 20 mcg • Inositol 50 mg • Choline (as bitartrate) 21 mg. Other Ingredients: Non-GMO Isolated Soy Protein, Fructose, Carrot, Natural Carrot Flavor, Guar Gum, Psyllium, Oat Bran, Microcrystalline Cellulose, Spirulina, Apple Pectin, Bee Pollen, Lecithin, Lemon Bioflavonoids, Papaya, Bromelain, Chlorophyll.

Carry On - TriLight Herbs
Black Haw • Wild Yam • False Unicorn.

Cartilade - BioTherapies, Inc.
Shark Cartilage.

Cartilage Care - PhysioLogics
Each capsule contains: Vitamin C (as ascorbic acid) 60 mg • Manganese (as manganese glycinate) 2 mg • Sodium (from chondroitin sulfate) 10 mg • Glucosamine Sulfate KCl 200 mg • Chondroitin Sulfate 100 mg • Glucosamine Hydrochloride 100 mg • Sea Cucumber 100 mg. Other Ingredients: Rice Powder, Gelatin, Vegetable Magnesium Stearate, Silica.
See Editor's Note No. 15.

Cartilage Companion - PhysioLogics
Each capsule contains: Glucosamine Sulfate 200 mg • Chondroitin Sulfate 67 mg • Methylsulfonylmethane (MSM) 333 mg.
See Editor's Note No. 15.

Cartilage Companion HP - PhysioLogics
Three tablets contain: Glucosamine Sulfate 2KCl 1500 mg • Chondroitin Sulfate 1200 mg • Methylsulfonylmethane (msm) 500 mg. Other Ingredients: Cellulose (plant origin), Cellulose Coating, Vegetable Magnesium Stearate, Silica, Titanium Dioxide Color.
See Editor's Note No. 15.

Cartilage Companion With MSM - PhysioLogics
Each capsule contains: Methylsulfonylmethane (msm) 333 mg • Glucosamine Sulfate (2KCl) 200 mg • Chondroitin Sulfate 67 mg. Other Ingredients: Rice Powder, Gelatin, Silica, Vegetable Magnesium Stearate.
See Editor's Note No. 15.

Cartilage Factors - Pure Encapsulations
Each vegetable capsule contains: Shark Cartilage concentrate 200 mg: Glycosaminoglycans (mucopolysaccharides, including chondroitin-4-sulfate and dermatan sulfate) 42 mg, Protein 54 mg • Bovine Cartilage (hormone-free) 200 mg: Glycosaminoglycans (mycopolysaccharides, including chondroitin-4-sulfate and dermatan sulfate) 90 mg, Protein 90 mg • Purified Chondroitin Sulfate (bovine, 95%, from 210 mg of chondroitin sulfate) 200 mg • Vitamin C (as ascorbyl palmitate) 12 mg • Manganese (ascorbate) 4 mg.

Cartilage Formula - Pharmanex
Two capsules contain: Vitamin C (Ascorbic Acid) 100 mg • Vitamin E (d-Alpha Tocopheryl Succinate, Beta, Delta, Gamma Tocopherols) 50 IU • Zinc (Zinc Propionate) 7.5 mg • Boron (Boron Citrate) 3 mg • Glucosamine (Glucosamine Sulfate, Glucosamine Hydrochloride) 750 mg • Boswellia Serrata extract (Min. 95% Boswellic Acids) 150 mg • Tumeric extract (Min. 95% Curcumin) 100 mg • Quercetin 25 mg • Rutin 25 mg. Other Ingredients: Silicon Dioxide, Magnesium Stearate.

Cascara Sagrada - Nature's Way
Two capsules contain: Cascara Sagrada bark 850 mg. Other Ingredients: Plant-derived Cellulose.

Cascara Sagrada Capsules - Nature's Sunshine
Two capsules contain: Cascara Sagrada bark (rhamnus purshiana) 780 mg. Other Ingredients: Kosher Gelatin, Water.

Cascara Sagrada Vegitabs - Nature's Sunshine
Two tablets contain: Cascara Sagrada bark (rhamnus purshiana) 820 mg. Other Ingredients: Cellulose, Maltodextrin, Stearic Acid, Silicon Dioxide, Magnesium Stearate.

Castor Oil - Home Health Products, Inc.
Castor Oil.

Cata-Comp - Enzymatic Therapy
Two capsules contain: Vitamin A (Beta Carotene) non-toxic form of Vitamin A 10000 IU • Vitamin E (D-Alpha Tocopherol Succinate) 75 IU • Vitamin C (Ascorbic Acid) 500 mg • Zinc (Picolinate) 10 mg • Manganese (Picolinate) 2 mg • Riboflavin (Vitamin B2) 2 mg • Selenium selenomethionine 75 mcg • Other Ingredients: Hachimijiogan Herbal Complex 200 mg • Curcuma root extract (curcuma longa, standardized to contain 97% Curcumin) 100 mg • L-Cysteine 50 mg • L-Glutamine 50 mg • L-Glycine 50 mg.

Catalyn - Standard Process, Inc.
Three tablets contain: Proprietary Blend 832 mg: Defatted Wheat (germ), Carrot (root), Calcium Lactate, Nutritional Yeast, Bovine Adrenal, Bovine Liver, Bovine Spleen, Bovine Kidney, Dried Pea (vine) juice, Dried Alfalfa juice, Ganoderma Lucidum (mushroom), Lentinula Edodes (mushroom) Oat Flour, Soy Bean Lecithin, Rice Bran extract • Honey • Magnesium Citrate • Glycerine • Arabic Gum • Ascorbic Acid 4 mg • Pyridoxine Hydrochloride 1 mg • Vitamin A

Palmitate 1200 IU • Gelatin • Cocarboxylase • Riboflavin 0.2 mg • Cholecalciferol 312 IU.
See Editor's Note No. 14.

Catalyn (Chewable) - Standard Process, Inc.
Three tablets contain: Proprietary Blend 468 mg: Cherry powder, defatted Wheat (germ), Carrot (root), Calcium Lactate, nutritional Yeast, Bovine Adrenal, Bovine Liver, Magnesium Citrate, Bovine Spleen, Bovine Kidney, Ganoderma Lucidum, Lentinula Edodes, dried Alfalfa juice, Soy Bean Lecithin, Rice Bran extract. Other Ingredients: Dried Cane Juice, Maltodextrine, Honey, Calcium Stearate, Natural Cherry Flavor, Glycerine, Arabic Gum, Ascorbic Acid, Pyridoxine Hydrochloride, Vitamin A Palmitate, Gelatin, Cocarboxylase, Riboflavin, Cholecalciferol.
See Editor's Note No. 14.

Catalyst - Advocare International
Three capsules contain: L-Glutamine 1200 mg • L-Leucine 450 mg • L-Isoleucine 225 mg • L-Valine 225 mg. Other Ingredients: Silicon Dioxide, Magnesium Stearate, Gelatin.

Catalyst Plus - 4 Life
Each capsule contains: Chromium 120 mcg • Proprietary Blend 410 mg: Gymnema Sylvestre powder, Gymnema Sylvestre extract, Momordica Charantia, Lagerstroemia Speciosa leaf extract, Vanadium (bis-glycinate oxo vanadium), Alpha-Lipoic Acid.

Cataplex A - Standard Process, Inc.
Two tablets contain: Proprietary Blend 584 mg: Carrot root, Calcium Lactate, Defatted Wheat germ, Bovine Kidney, Oat flour, nutritional Yeast, Rice Bran extract, Magnesium Citrate, Alfalfa flour, Mixed Tocopherols, Ascorbic Acid, Carrot oil, Soybean Lecithin • Vitamin A 3000 IU. Other Ingredients: Honey, Arabic Gum, Gelatin.

Cataplex A-C - Standard Process, Inc.
Two tablets contain: Proprietary Blend 514 mg: Carrot root, Echinacea root, Calcium Lactate, Bovine Adrenal, Bovine Kidney, Nutritional Yeast, Magnesium Citrate, Alfalfa flour, Dried Alfalfa juice, Mushroom, Dried Buckwheat leaf juice, Buckwheat seed, Bovine Bone, Defatted Wheat germ, Oat flour, Soybean Lecithin, Veal Bone meal, Mixed Tocopherols, Peanut bran, Carrot oil • Vitamin A 1500 IU • Vitamin C 11 mg. Other Ingredients: Honey, Ascorbic Acid, Arabic Gum, Gelatin.

Cataplex A-C-P - Standard Process, Inc.
Three tablets contain: Proprietary Blend 852 mg: Dried Buckwheat juice, Buckwheat seed, Carrot root, Calcium Lactate, Nutritional Yeast, Bovine Adrenal, Bovine Kidney, Alfalfa flour, Dried Alfalfa juice, Magnesium Citrate, Mushroom, Bovine Bone, Echinacea root, Defatted Wheat germ, Oat flour, Soybean Lecithin, Veal Bone meal, Calcium Phosphate, Mixed Tocopherols, Peanut bran, Carrot oil • Vitamin A 2250 IU • Vitamin C 17 mg. Other Ingredients: Honey, Arabic Gum, Gelatin.

Cataplex B - Standard Process, Inc.
Two tablets contain: Proprietary Blend 60 mg: Bovine Liver, Nutritional Yeast, Porcine Duodenum, Beet root, Carrot root, Dried Beet root juice, Choline Bitartrate, Rice bran extract, Defatted Wheat germ, Bovine Adrenal, Oat flour, Soybean Lecithin, Mixed Tocopherols, Ascorbic Acid, Manganese Lactate, Inositol, Riboflavin • Thiamine 1 mg • Niacin 20 mg • Vitamin B6 1 mg • Potassium 10 mg. Other Ingredients: Honey, Potassium Para-Aminobenzoate, Arabic Gum, Cocarboxylase.

Cataplex B12 - Standard Process, Inc.
Each tablet contains: Proprietary Blend 363 mg: Carrot root, Bovine Liver, Calcium Lactate, Porcine Stomach Parenchyma, Bovine Spleen, Ovine Spleen, Bovine Adrenal Cytosol extract, Dicalcium Phosphate, Oat flour, Ascorbic Acid • Vitamin B12 6 mcg. Other Ingredients: Cellulose, Honey.
See Editor's Note No. 14.

Cataplex C - Standard Process, Inc.
Three tablets contain: Proprietary Blend 643 mg: Veal Bone PMG extract, Bovine Adrenal, Dried Buckwheat leaf juice, Buckwheat seed, Nutritional Yeast, Dried Alfalfa juice, Alfalfa flour, Mushroom, Magnesium Citrate, Bovine Bone, Defatted Wheat germ, Calcium Phosphate, Echinacea root, Carrot root, Veal Bone meal, Soybean Lecithin, Mixed Tocopherols, Rice bran extract, Peanut bran • Vitamin C 17 mg • Calcium 30 mg • Sodium 25 mg. Other Ingredients: Honey, Arabic Gum.

Cataplex D - Standard Process, Inc.
Each tablet contains: Vitamin A (from palmitate) 1000 IU • Vitamin D (cholecalciferol) 400 IU • Calcium (from calcium lactate, milk powder, and calcium stearate) 10 mg. Other Ingredients: Potassium Citrate, Glycerin, Arabic Gum, Ascorbic Acid.

Cataplex E - Standard Process, Inc.
Each two tablets contain: Proprietary Blend 523 mg: Bovine Orchic extract, Inositol, Dried Pea (vine) juice, Ribonucleic Acid, Oat Flour, Bovine Adrenal, Beet (root), Bovine Spleen, Ovine Spleen, Beet (root) juice, Bovine Liver, Manganese Lactate, Ascorbic Acid • Honey • Selenium Yeast 11 mcg • Potassium Para-Aminobenzoate • Mixed Tocopherols 5 IU • Arabic Gum.

Cataplex E2 - Standard Process, Inc.
Two tablets contain: Proprietary Blend 492 mg: Bovine Orchic extract, Calcium Lactate, Tillandsia Usneoides, Bovine Spleen, Ovine Spleen, Inositol, Bovine Adrenal Cytosol extract, Oat flour, Ascorbic Acid • Vitamin E 4 IU • Selenium 9 mcg. Other Ingredients: Honey, Arabic Gum, Mixed Tocopherols, Calcium Stearate.
See Editor's Note No. 14.

Cataplex F perles - Standard Process, Inc.
Each perle contains: Proprietary Blend 348 mg: Flaxseed oil, Bovine Liver fat extract, Flaxseed oil extract, Bovine Orchic extract • Vitamin B6. Other Ingredients: Gelatin, Glycerin, Beeswax, Water, Pyridoxine Hydrochloride, Carob.
See Editor's Note No. 14.

Cataplex F tablets - Standard Process, Inc.
Each tablet contains: Proprietary Blend: 285 mg Calcium Lactate, Defatted Wheat germ, Carrot root, Bovine Prostate, Bovine Liver, Magnesium Citrate, Oat flour, Bovine Orchic extract, Bovine Liver fat extract, Flaxseed oil extract, Potassium Para-Aminobenzoate, Mixed Tocopherols, Ascorbic Acid, Soybean Lecithin • Vitamin B6 0.8 mg • Iodine 95 mcg. Other Ingredients: Honey, Glycerin, Arabic Gum, Calcium Stearate, Pyridoxal 5'-phosphate.
See Editor's Note No. 14.

Cataplex G - Standard Process, Inc.
Each tablet contains: Proprietary Blend 225 mg: Bovine Liver, Porcine Stomach, Choline Bitartrate, Calcium Lactate, Nutritional Yeast, Defatted Wheat germ, Potassium Para-Aminobenzoate, Allantoin, Porcine Brain • Vitamin C 6.5 mg • Riboflavin 1.3 mg • Niacin 12 mg • Vitamin B6 0.3 mg. Other Ingredients: Honey, Niacinamide, Ascorbic Acid, Glycerin, Riboflavin 5'-phosphate, Arabic Gum, Calcium Stearate, Pyridoxal 5'-phosphate.

Cataplex GTF - Standard Process, Inc.
Each tablet contains: Proprietary Blend 330 mg: Bovine Liver, Nutritional Yeast, Dried Buckwheat juice, Buckwheat seed, Bovine Pancreas Cytosol extract, Inositol, L-Cysteine Hydrochloride, Bovine Adrenal Cytosol extract, Oat flour • Vitamin A 500 IU • Vitamin C 1.6 mg • Niacin 9.5 mg • Chromium 48 mcg • Potassium 5 mg. Other Ingredients: Honey, Calcium Stearate.

Catnip - Nature's Sunshine
Two capsules contain: Catnip aerial parts (nepeta cataria) 600 mg. Other Ingredients: Kosher Gelatin, Water.

Catnip - Nature's Way
Two capsules contain: Catnip (stem, leaf, flower) 760 mg. Other Ingredients: Gelatin.

Some Brand Name Natural Products - What they Contain

www.NaturalDatabase.com contains MANY more listings than appear here.
Editor's Notes are located on pages 2155-2163.

Catnip & Fennel Extract **- Nature's Sunshine**
Catnip (nepeta cataria) leaf extract • Fennel oil (foeniculum vulgare). Other Ingredients: Vegetable Glycerin (80% glycerin, 20% water).

Catnip and Fennel **- Dial Herbs**
Catnip • Peppermint • Fennel • Lobelia.

Catnip and Peppermint **- Dial Herbs**
Catnip • Peppermint • Lobelia.

Cat's Claw **- Pure Encapsulations**
Each vegetable capsule contains: Cat's Claw extract (uncaria tomentosa, standardized to contain 3% oxindole alkaloids and 15% polyphenols) 500 mg • Vitamin C (as ascorbyl palmitate) 10 mg.

Cat's Claw **- Nature's Way**
Three capsules contain: Cat's Claw bark 1.45 g. Other Ingredients: Gelatin, Magnesium stearate, Millet.

Cat's Claw **- Olympian Labs**
Each capsule contains: Cat's Claw (uncaria tomentosa) 500 mg.

Cat's Claw **- NutraMedix**
Two capsules contain: Cat's Claw bark (uncaria tomentosa) 1 g. Other Ingredients: Gelatin Capsule, Magnesium Stearate.

Cat's Claw **- Jarrow Formulas**
Each capsule contains: Cat's Claw 6:1 extract (from inner bark) 500 mg. Other Ingredients: Rice Powder, Magnesium Stearate, Gelatin.

Cat's Claw 1000 **- Golden Glow Natural Health Products**
Each tablet contains: Uncaria Tomentosa bark (cat's claw) 1 g: Oxindole Alkaloids (as mitraphylline) 7.5 mg.

Cat's Claw 1000mg **- Nature's Own**
Each tablet contains: Cat's Claw stem and bark extract (uncaria tomentosa) 1000 mg.

Cat's Claw 5000 **- NOW Foods**
Each capsule contains: Cat's Claw (Uncaria tomentosa) (Inner bark) 15:1 standardized extract equivalent 333 mg. Other Ingredients: Stearic Acid.

Cat's Claw Caplet **- Leiner Health Products**
Each caplet contains: Cat's Claw extract (Uncaria tomentosa) 250 mg. Other Ingredients: Calcium Carbonate, Cellulose, Maltodextrin, Hydroxypropyl Methylcellulose, Silicon Dioxide, Polyethylene Glycol 3350, Croscarmellose Sodium, Hyroxypropyl Cellulose, Pharmaceutical Glaze, Crospovidone, Magnesium Stearate, Yellow 5 Lake, Blue 1 Lake, Polysorbate 80, Titanium Dioxide.

Cat's Claw Defense Complex **- Source Naturals**
Four tablets contain: Cat's Claw inner bark (Uncaria Tomentosa) 2000 mg • Whole-Leaf Aloe Vera powder (200:1 Concentrate) 200 mg • Proanthodyn (from Grape Seed extract) 60 mg • Quercetin 400 mg • Green Tea extract 40 mg • Turmeric root extract (Yielding 95% Curcumin) 400 mg • Silymarin (Milk Thistle seed extract) 50 mg • Reishi Mycelia biomass 200 mg • Shiitake Mycelia biomass 200 mg • Maitake Mycelia biomass 150 mg • Astragalus root 200 mg • St. John's Wort herb extract 100 mg • St. John's Wort herb powder 100 mg • Siberian Ginseng root 100 mg • Siberian Ginseng root extract 100 mg • Schizandra berries 200 mg • Pau d'Arco bark 100 mg • Pau d'Arco bark extract 100 mg • Isatis leaf 150 mg • Vitamin A (Beta Carotene) 10000 IU • Vitamin C (Ascorbic Acid, Magnesium and Zinc Ascorbates) 350 mg • Magnesium (Ascorbate) 10 mg • Zinc (Ascorbate) 12 mg • N-Acetyl Cysteine 600 mg.

Cat's Claw Super 547 **- Susan Ambrosino's Herb Club, Inc.**
Each capsule contains: Cat's Claw inner bark full-spectrum powder (una de gato) 500 mg • Cat's Claw extract 3% 47 mg.

Cayenne **- NOW Foods**
Each capsule contains: Cayenne Pepper (Capsium Frutescens) 500 mg.

Cayenne **- Nature's Way**
Each capsule contains: Cayenne pepper fruit 450 mg. Other Ingredients: Gelatin.

Cayenne **- Pharmanex**
Each capsule contains: Cayenne (Capisicum Annum, Pepper, 40000 Heat Units) 450 mg. Other Ingredients: Gelatin, Magnesium Stearate, Silicon Dioxide.

Cayenne **- Leiner Health Products**
Each softgel contains: Oleoresin Capsicum extract (Oleoresin capsicum) fruit 25 mg. Other Ingredients: Soybean Oil, Gelatin, Glycerin, Beeswax, Lecithin, Caramel, Titanium Dioxide, Red 40, Yellow 6, Blue 1.

Cayenne 500 **- Golden Glow Natural Health Products**
Each tablet contains: Capsicum Annuum fruit powder (cayenne) 100 mg • Capsicum Annuum extract 400 mg.

Cayenne Extra Hot **- Nature's Way**
Each capsule contains: Proprietary Formula: Cayenne pepper fruit • Ginger • Hawthorne berry. Other Ingredients: Gelatin.

Cayenne Garlic **- Nature's Way**
Two capsules contain: Proprietary Blend 1.06 g: Cayenne pepper fruit, Garlic bulb. Other Ingredients: Gelatin.

Cayenne Goldenseal (formerly B/P) **- Nature's Way**
Two capsules contain: Proprietary Blend 1000 mg: Cayenne pepper fruit, Eleuthero root, Garlic bulb, Ginger, Goldenseal stem/leaf/flower, Parsley herb. Other Ingredients: Gelatin.

Cayenne Hawthorn with Vitamin E **- Nature's Way**
Two capsules contain: Proprietary Blend 1040 mg: Cayenne pepper fruit, Hawthorn berry, Lecithin, Vitamin E (d-alpha tocopheryl). Other Ingredients: Gelatin.

Cayenne Herbal Pain Relieving Ointment **- Nature's Way**
Primary Ingredients: Capsaicin • Menthol. Other Ingredients: Beeswax, Eucalyptus, Olive oil, Vitamin E (d-alpha tocopheryl).

Cayenne Pepper **- Standard Process, Inc.**
Each capsule contains: Cayenne Pepper (capsicum annuum) 35,000 Scoville Units 350 mg. Other Ingredients: Cellulose, Water, Calcium Stearate.

Cayenne, Super **- Swanson Health Products**
Two capsules contain: Cayenne pepper (100,000 heating units) 450 mg • Ginger root powder 200 mg • Hawthorn berry powder 200 mg • Lecithin granules 50 mg.

C-Blast Lemon Lime **- GNC**
Each packet contains: Vitamin C (ascorbic acid) 1000 mg • Thiamin HCl 0.38 mg • Riboflavin 0.43 mg • Niacin (niacinamide) 5 mg • Vitamin B6 (pyridoxine HCl) 10 mg • Folate, Folic Acid, Folacin 12.5 mcg • Vitamin B12 (cyanocobalamin) 25 mcg • Pantothenic Acid 2.5 mg • Calcium (ascorbate) 50 mg • Magnesium (ascorbate) 60 mg • Zinc (ascorbate) 2 mg • Manganese (ascorbate) 1 mg • Chromium (ascorbate) 10 mcg. Other Ingredients: Fructose, Natural Lemon Lime Flavors, Potassium Bicarbonate, Citric Acid, Tartaric Acid, Malic Acid, Sodium Bicarbonate, Aspartic Acid, Quercetin, Calcium Pantothenate.

C-Blast Tangerine **- GNC**
Each packet contains: Vitamin C (ascorbic acid) 1000 mg • Thiamin HCl 0.38 mg • Riboflavin 0.43 mg • Niacin (niacinamide) 5 mg • Vitamin B6 (pyridoxine HCl) 10 mg • Folate, Folic Acid, Folacin 12.5 mcg • Vitamin B12 (cyanocobalamin) 25 mcg • Pantothenic Acid 2.5 mg • Calcium (ascorbate) 50 mg • Magnesium (ascorbate) 60 mg • Zinc (ascorbate) 2 mg • Manganese (ascorbate) 1 mg • Chromium (ascorbate) 10 mcg. Other Ingredients: Fructose, Natural Tangerine Flavors, Potassium Bicarbonate, Citric Acid, Tartaric Acid, Malic Acid, Sodium Bicarbonate, Aspartic Acid, Quercetin, Calcium Pantothenate.

CBlock **-** Absolute Nutrition
Two caplets contain: Chromium (as chormium dinicotinate glycinate) 200 mcg • Vanadium (as BMOV) 100 mg • Trim Plex brand Phaseolus Vulgaris (as white kidney bean extract) 700 mg. Other Ingredients: Dicalcium Phosphate, Cellulose, Cellulose Gum, Vegetable Stearic Acid, Silica, Vegetable Magnesium Stearate, Vegetable Resin Gum.

C-B-R **-** Source Naturals
Each tablet contains: Vitamin C (as ascorbic acid) 500 mg • Citrus Bioflavonoid Complex 500 mg • Rutin 52 mg • Hesperidin Complex 50 mg • Acerola Cherry fruit 1 mg.

CC-A **-** Nature's Sunshine
Two capsules contain: Proprietary Blend 800 mg: Rose Hips (rosa canina), Chamomile flower (matricaria recutita), Slippery Elm bark (ulmus fulva), Yarrow flower (achillea millefolium), Capsicum fruit (capsicum annuum), Goldenseal root (hydrastis canadensis), Myrrh gum (commiphora molmol), Peppermint leaf (mentha piperita), Sage leaf (salvia officinalis), Lemongrass herb (cymbopogon citratus). Other Ingredients: Gelatin, Water.

CC-A with Yerba Santa **-** Nature's Sunshine
Rose Hips fruit (rosa canina) • Chamomile flowers (matricaria recutita) • Mullein leaf (verbascum thapsus) • Yarrow flower (achillea millefolium) • Yerba Santa leaf (eriodictyon californicum) • Goldenseal rhizome (hydrastis canadensis) • Myrrh gum (commiphora molmol) • Peppermint leaf (mentha piperita) • Sage leaf (salvia officinalis) • Astragalus root (astragalus membranaceus) • Slippery Elm bark (ulmus fulva) • Lemongrass aerial parts (cymbopogon citratus) • Capsicum fruit (capsicum annuum). Other Ingredients: Water, Alcohol.

CCM Calcium **-** Source Naturals
Each tablet contains: Calcium (from Calcium Citrate and Calcium Malate) 300 mg.

C-Complex 1000 **-** Puritan's Pride
Each tablet contains: Vitamin C (as Ascorbic Acid and Rose Hips) 1000 mg • Citrus Bioflavonoids 100 mg • Rutin 50 mg • Hesperidin complex 25 mg • Acerola powder 1 mg • Alfalfa leaf powder 1 mg • Barley grass powder 1 mg.

C-Complex 500 **-** Puritan's Pride
Each tablet contains: Vitamin C (with rose hips and other natural sources) 500 mg • Citrus Bioflavonoids 100 mg • Rutin (buckwheat) 50 mg • Hesperidin complex 25 mg • Acerola 1.0 mg • Alfalfa leaf 1 mg •Barley grass 1 mg. Other Ingredients: Vegetable Stearic Acid, Cellulose Coating, Silica, Vegetable Magnesium Stearate.

C-Complex Sustained Release **-** Golden Glow Natural Health Products
Each tablet provides: Total Ascorbic Acid 1 g (from calcium ascorbate 608.6 mg and ascorbic acid 500 mg) • Hesperidin 50 mg • Citrus Bioflavonoids 50 mg • Rutin 50 mg • Rosehips extract (rosa canina) 50 mg.

C-Complex/ Bioflavonoids/ Rutin **-** Nature's Life
Each tablet contains: Vitamin C 500 mg • Lemon Bioflavonoids Complex (natural whole unaltered TESTLAB concentrate containing Hesperidin, Eriocitrin, Flavonols, & Flavones derived from freshly dejuiced Lemons) 500 mg • Acerola (Malpighia glabra) 50 mg • Hesperidin 50 mg • Rutin (Saphora japonica) 50 mg • Calcium (naturally buffering Calcium Carbonate) 12 mg. In a natural base of Bell Peppers & Rose Hips powder.

C-Crystals **-** Arrowroot
Each 1 tsp serving contains: Vitamin C 5000 mg.

CDC Chondro Forte **-** Genestra - Seroyal
Each tablet contains: Vitamin C (ascorbic acid) 150 mg • Chondroitin Sulfate (collagen, 8:1) 100 mg • Glucosamine Sulfate 100 mg • Manganese Citrate 65 mg • Marine Mucopolysaccharides 50 mg • Papain 25 mg • Wild Yam (10:1, equivalent to 250 mg) 25 mg • L-Proline 25 mg • L-Glutamic Acid 20 mg • L-Cysteine 15 mg • Zinc (aspartate acid chelate) 10 mg • Non-citrus Bioflavonoids 15 mg • Hesperidin 15 mg.
See Editor's Note No. 15.

CDG EstroDIM **-** Ortho Molecular Products
Two capsules contain: Vitamin E (as D-alpha tocopherol succinate) 100 IU • Folic Acid 3 mg • Calcium (as D-glucorate) 120 mg • Calcium D-Glucorate 1000 mg • I3C (indole 3 carbinol) 200 mg • DIM (diindolylmethane) 100 mg. Other Ingredients: Natural Vegetable Capsules, Ascorbyl Palmitate, Microcrystaline Cellulose, Silicon Dioxide.

CDP Choline **-** Jarrow Formulas
Each capsule contains: Citicoline (from stabilized cytidine 5'diphosphocholine) 250 mg. Other Ingredients: Rice Powder, Magnesium Stearate, Gelatin.

CDP Choline Caps 250 MG **-** Life Extension
Each capsule contains: CDP-Choline (cytidine-5-diphosphocholine, elemental choline 51.25 per capsule) 250 mg. Other Ingredients: Rice Flour, Magnesium Stearate, Silica, Gelatin, Water.

CDP-Choline **-** Life Enhancement Products, Inc.
Each capsule contains: Citicoline 250 mg. Other Ingredients: Silicon Dioxide, Gelatin Capsule.

CDP-Choline Caps **-** Prolongevity
Each capsule contains: Cytidine 5-diphosphocholine 250 mg. Other Ingredients: Rice Flour, Magnesium Stearate, Silica, Gelatin, Water.

CDT CoQ10 **-** Olympian Labs
Each capsule contains: Crystalline Coenzyme Q10 60 mg.

CE **-** EAS, Inc.
Two capsules contain: Green Tea (catechins 200 mg, epigallocatechin gallate 135 mg) 225 mg • Phosphatidylserine 150 mg • Ashwaganda Sensoril (oligosaccharides 40 mg, withanolides 10 mg) 125 mg • Theanine 100 mg • Beta Sitosterol 50 mg • Choline 50 mg • Inositol 50 mg. Other Ingredients: Microcrystalline Cellulose, Magnesium Stearate (vegetable source), Silicon Dioxide.

Celadrin **-** Doctor's Best, Inc.
Each capsule contains: Celadrin brand proprietary blend 500 mg: Esterified Fatty Acid Carbons (EFAC) of Myristate, Myristoleate, Laurate, Oleate, Palmitate, Palmitoleate with Tapioca. Other Ingredients: Gelatin.

Celadrin brand **-** Proprietary Nutritionals, Inc.
Cetylated Fatty Acids.
See Editor's Note No. 44.

Celadrin Complex with Glucosamine **-** Doctor's Best, Inc.
Each tablet contains: Glucosamine Sulfate KCl 500 mg • Celadrin brand proprietary blend 500 mg: Esterified Fatty Acid Carboms of Myristate, Myristoleate, Laurate, Oleate, Palmitate, Palmitoleate with Tapioca. Other Ingredients: Cellulose, Croscarmellose Sodium, Silicon Dioxide.

Celadrin Creme **-** Abundance Marketing
Active Ingredients: Menthol (1.25%). Inactive Ingredients: Benzyl Alcohol, Butylparaben, Carbomer, Celadrin brand Esterified Fatty Acid Carrbons proprietary blend, Ethylparaben, Glycerin, Glyceryl Stearate, Isobutylparaben, Lecithin, Methylparaben, Olea Europaea fruit oil (olive), PEG-100 Stearate, Peppermint oil, Phenoxyethanol, Potassium Hydroxide, Propylparaben, Tocopheryl Acetate, Water.

Celadrin Joint Health **-** Natural Factors
Three softgels contain: Celadrin Proprietary Blend 1050 mg: Esterified Fatty Acid Carbons including CMO. Other Ingredients: Softgel Capsule (gelatin, glycerin, carob), Soy Oil, Salmon Oil.

Some Brand Name Natural Products - What they Contain

www.NaturalDatabase.com contains MANY more listings than appear here.
Editor's Notes are located on pages 2155-2163.

Celadrin tablets - Abundance Marketing
Each tablet contains: Celadrin brand EFAC (esterified fatty acid carbons) proprietary blend 500 mg. Other Ingredients: Dicalcium Phosphate, Microcrystalline Cellulose, Croscarmellose Sodium, Stearic Acid, Magnesium Stearate, Silica, Pharmaceutical Glaze.

Celadrin Topical Analgesic Pain Cream - NSI - Nutraceutical Sciences Institute
Purified Water • Glyceryl Stearate • PEG 100 Stearate • Glycerin • Celadrin brand proprietary blend: Esterified Fatty Acid Carbons of Myristate, Myristoleate, Laurate, Oleate, Palmitate, Palmitoleate with Tapioca • Lecithin • Tocopheryl Acetate (vitamin E) • Phenylcarbinol • Phenoxyethanol • Menthol • Carbomer 940 • Potassium Hydroxide • Methylparaben.

Celapro - Metagenics
Each softgel contains: Green Tea leaf extract (camellia sinensis, providing 47.5%-52.5% total polyphenols (catechins), 1%-3% L-theanine, 5%-10% caffeine, 0.3%-1.2% theobromine) 200 mg • D-Limonene (from citrus sinensis peel oil) 500 mg • Lycopene 2.5 mg • Turmeric rhizome extract (curcuma longa, standardized to 95% curcuminoids) 50 mg.

Celasine - Aidan Products, LLC
Water • Aloe Barbadensis leaf juice • Cyclomethicone • Propylene Glycol • Arachidyl Propionate • Stearyl Alcohol • Glyceryl Stearate • PEG-100 Stearate • Glycine Soja (soybean) oil • Glycerin • Cetyl Alcohol • Cetearyl Alcohol • Ceteareth-20 • Tetrahexadecyl Ascorbate • L-Carnosine • Sodium Hyaluronate • Tocopheryl Acetate • Carbomer • Acrylates/C10-30 Alkyl Acrylate Crosspolymer • Triethanolamine • Dimethicone Copolyol • Tetrasodium EDTA • Methylparaben • Propylparaben • Imidazolidinyl Urea • DMDM Hydantoin.

Celebrity Diet Quickstart Peach Mango Juice - Celebrity Products Direct, Inc.
Purified Water • Juice Concentrates: Pear, Grape, Mango, Peach, Kiwi, Plum • Natural Flavoring • Potassium Citrate • Ascorbic Acid (vitamin C), D-Alpha-Tocopheryl Acetate (vitamin E) • Niacinamide (vitamin B3) • Calcium Pantothenate (vitamin B5) • Vitamin A Palmitate • Pyridoxine Hydrochloride (vitamin B6) • Riboflavin -5' Phosphate (vitamin B2) • Thiamine Mononitrate (vitamin B1) • Bilberry extract • Green Tea extract • Ginkgo Biloba extract • Grape Seed extract • Biotin • Cyanocobalamin (vitamin B12).

Celebrity Diet Quickstart Wild Berry Juice - Celebrity Products Direct, Inc.
Purified Water • Juice Concentrates: Pear, Cherry, Strawberry, Raspberry, Blueberry, Kiwi, Cranberry, Blackberry • Natural Flavoring • Potassium Citrate • Ascorbic Acid (vitamin C), D-Alpha-Tocopheryl Acetate (vitamin E) • Niacinamide (vitamin B3) • Calcium Pantothenate (vitamin B5) • Vitamin A Palmitate • Pyridoxine Hydrochloride (vitamin B6) • Riboflavin -5' Phosphate (vitamin B2) • Thiamine Mononitrate (vitamin B1) • Bilberry extract • Green Tea extract • Ginkgo Biloba extract • Grape Seed extract • Biotin • Cyanocobalamin (vitamin B12).

Celery 750mg & Juniper 500mg - Nature's Own
Each tablet contains: Celery seed extract (apium graveolens) 750 mg • Juniper berry extract (juniperus communis) 500 mg.

Celery 750mg & Juniper Berries 500mg - Golden Glow Natural Health Products
Each tablet contains: Apium Graveolens seed extract (celery) 750 mg • Juniperus Communis berry (juniper) 500 mg.

Celery Seed 250mg - Nature's Own
Each tablet contains: Wild Celery seed extract (apium graveolens) 250 mg.

Celite Complex 75 - Jamieson
Two capsules contain: Concentrated Citrus Bioflavonoids (Vitamin P) 100 mg • Ginkgo Biloba extract flavoglycoside-rich JGB24 250 mg • Bilberry extract anthocyanoside-rich JMF25 750 mg • Oil of Madagascar Cinnamon 20 mg • South Pacific Sea Kelp extract 25 mg • Bromelain Enzyme (from Pineapple) 100 mg • Kola Nut extract 250 mg. Other Ingredients: Soybean Oil, Vegetable Oil, Gelatin, Glycerin, Lecithin, Purified Water.

Celite Complex 75 Firming Gel - Jamieson
Water • Glycerin • Butylene Glycol • Kola Nut (Cola acuminata) extract • Coneflower (Echinacea purpurea) extract • Propylene Glycol • Butylene Glycol • Camellia oleifera extract • Arnica montana extract • Dimethylsilanol Hyaluronate • Jojoba Esters • Butcher's Broom (Rucus aculeatus) extract • Kelp (Macrocystis pyrifera) extract • Imidazolidinyl Urea • Triethanolamine • Carbomer • Methyl Paraben • Ethyl Paraben • Fragrance.

Celite Complex 75 Smoothing & Firming Gel - Jamieson
Contains: Jojoba Esters (toning beads) • Kola Nut Extract • Echinacea Extract • Camellia Oleifera Extract • Arnica Montana Extract • Butcherbroom Extract • Kelp Extract.

Cell Boost with IP-6 - Ultimate Nutrition
Two capsules contain: Calcium 101 mg • Phosphorous 195 mg • Calcium Magnesium Phytate (Inositol Hexaphosphate) 1000 mg.

Cell Forte Max 3 Maitake - Enzymatic Therapy
Two capsules contain: Ip-6 (inositol hexaphosphate) 800 mg • Inositol 220 mg • Maitake Mushroom extract (grifola frondosa, standardized to contain pure d-fraction 9 mg) 30 mg • Poa Cat's Claw root extract (uncaria tomentosa, pentacyclic chemotype, standardized to contain a minimum of 1.3% pentacyclic oxindole alkaloids) 10 mg. Other Ingredients: Gelatin, Magnesium Stearate, Titanium Dioxide Color, Silicon Dioxide.

Cell Forte with IP-6 - Enzymatic Therapy
Each capsule contains: IP-6 (inositol hexaphosphate, from rice) 400 mg • Inositol (from rice) 110 mg.

Cell Guard - Source Naturals
Three tablets contain: Vitamin A (beta carotene 15000 IU and palmitate 10000 IU) 25000 IU • Vitamin B-1 (thiamin) 10 mg • Vitamin B-2 (riboflavin) 10 mg • Niacin 30 mg • Vitamin B-5 (calcium D-Pantothenate) 50 mg • Vitamin B-6 (pyridoxine HCl) 30 mg • Vitamin B-12 (cyanocobalamin) 100 mcg • Vitamin C (ascorbic acid, magnesium and calcium ascorbates) 2000 mg • Vitamin E D-alpha Tocopheryl (natural) 400 IU • Folic acid 800 mcg • Calcium (ascorbate) 30 mg • Copper (sebacate) 1 mg • Magnesium (ascorbate, citrate, succinate and oxide) 120 mg • Selenium (from high-selenium yeast and sodium selenite) 200 mcg • Zinc (OptiZinc zinc monomethionine) 30 mg. Other Ingredients: N-Acetyl Cysteine 300 mg, N,N-Dimethyl Glycine HCl 150 mg, Coenzyme Q10 (ubiquinone) 30 mg, Herbal blend (unique) 600 mg.

Cell Strength - Source Naturals
Each tablet contains: Calcium ethanolamine phosphate 600 mg.

Cell Strength - Source Naturals
Four tablets contain: Phosphorus 460 mg • Calcium 300 mg.

Cell U Less - Olympian Labs
Each capsule contains: Grape Seed extract 50 mg • Bladderwrack extract 100 mg • Gotu Kola extract 300 mg • Horse Chestnut extract 100 mg.

Cell Well - Gaia Herbs
Two capsules contain: Coleus root (coleus forskohlii) 114 mg • Chinese Skullcap (scutellaria baicalensis) 88 mg • Bupleurum root (bupleurum chinense) 70 mg • Feverfew flowering herb (tanacetum parthenium) 60 mg • Jujube date seed (zizyphus jujuba) 32 mg • Licorice root (glycyrrhiza glabra) 20 mg • Ginger rhizome, supercritical CO2 extract (zingiber off.) 8 mg. Other Ingredients: Vegetable Glycerin, Lecithin, Vegetable Cellulose (capsule).

Cella Free - Bodyonics, Ltd.
Six tablets contain: Herbal BioModulators 1000 mg: Evening primrose Oil (contains Gamma Linolenic Acid (GLA), Borage Seed Oil, Bladderwrack extract, dried Fucus Vesiculosus extract, Fish Oil

BRAND NAMES

(containing the Omega-3 polyunsaturated fatty acids EPA (eicosapentaenoic acid) and DHA (docosahexaenoic acid)), Grape Seed extract, Bioflavonoids, Soy Lecithin, Fatty Acids, dried Sweet Red Clover extract (Mellotus Officinals,Tri Folium pratense, standardized to 1% biochanina), dried Ginkgo Biloba extract (standardized to contain flavonglycosides) • Protein/Fiber BioModulators 1750 mg: A mixture of Bioactive Oligopeptides prepared from food grade proteins by means of enzymatic hydrolysis of Bovine Globin Proteins, Casein and Wheat Protein; Chitosan (Fibrabind) • Therma/ Fluid Balance BioModulators 1000 mg: Uva Ursi (standardized to contain 120 mg of yydroxyquinone), Yerba Mate (standardized to contain 300 mg methyl xanthines). Other Ingredients: Calcium Carbonate, Stearic Acid, Croscarmellose, Magnesium Stearate.
See Editor's Note No. 14.

Cellasene - Thompson Nutritional Products
Three softgels contain: Iodine 720 mcg • Cellasene Lipovascolen 702 mg • Cellasene support blend 1230 g. Other Ingredients: Bladderwrack extract, Grape seed extract, Sweet Clover extract, Ginko Biloba, Borage, Fish oil, Soya Lecithin.

Cellex-C Betaplex Clear Complexion Mask - Cellex-C International Inc.
Kaolin • Glycolic Acid • Echinacea • Peppermint • Rosemary • Olive leaf extract • Green Tea extract.
See Editor's Note No. 17.

Cellex-C Betaplex Facial Firming Water - Cellex-C International Inc.
Witch Hazel • Glycolic Acid • Malic Acid • Willow Bark extract • Clover extract • Pomegranate extract.
See Editor's Note No. 17.

Cellex-C Betaplex Fresh Complexion Mist - Cellex-C International Inc.
Witch Hazel • Rice Wine • Lactic Acid • Malic Acid • Willow bark extract • Cucumber extract • Horsetail extract • Lavender oil • Peppermint oil • Thyme oil.
See Editor's Note No. 17.

Cellex-C Betaplex Gentle Cleansing Milk - Cellex-C International Inc.
Sunflower seed oil • Lactic Acid • Willow Bark extract • Aloe Barbadensis gel • Vitamin E • Allantoin • Sassafras extract • Chamomile extract • Ginseng extract • Milfoil extract • Lemongrass extract.
See Editor's Note No. 17.

Cellex-C Betaplex Gentle Foaming Cleanser - Cellex-C International Inc.
Aloe Barbadensis gel • Lactic Acid • Willow Bark extract • Cucumber extract • Clover extract.
See Editor's Note No. 17.

Cellex-C Betaplex Line Smoother - Cellex-C International Inc.
Lactic Acid • Glycolic Acid • Malic Acid • Sodium Hyaluronate • Willow Bark extract.
See Editor's Note No. 17.

Cellex-C Betaplex New Complexion Cream - Cellex-C International Inc.
Lactic Acid • Glycolic Acid • Malic Acid • Glycerin • Willow Bark extract • Aloe Barbadensis gel • Vitamin E • Allantoin • Evening Primrose Oil • Chamomile extract.
See Editor's Note No. 17.

Cellex-C Betaplex Smooth Skin Complex - Cellex-C International Inc.
Lactic Acid • Glycolic Acid • Malic Acid • Vitamin E • Willow Bark extract • Aloe Barbadensis gel • Lecithin • Allantoin.
See Editor's Note No. 17.

Cellex-C Bio-Botanical - Cellex-C International Inc.
Aloe Vera gel • Primrose oil • Sodium Hyaluronate • Phospholipids • Vitamin E • Chamomile extract • Allantoin • Lavandula Vera.
See Editor's Note No. 17.

Cellex-C Bio-Tan - Cellex-C International Inc.
DHA • Tyrosine • Melanin • Erythrulose • Walnut extract • Phospholipids.
See Editor's Note No. 17.

Cellex-C Body Smoothing Lotion - Cellex-C International Inc.
Ascorbic Acid • Vitamin E • Tomato extract • Evening Primrose oil • Tyrosine • Zinc • Hyaluronic Acid • Aloe Vera extract • Chamomile extract • Allantoin • Bioflavonoids.
See Editor's Note No. 17.

Cellex-C Eye Contour Cream Plus - Cellex-C International Inc.
Ascorbic Acid • Tyrosine • Zinc • Bioflavonoids • Vitamin E • Sodium Hyaluronate • Evening Primrose Oil • Tomato oil • Aloe Barbadensis gel • Chamomile extract • Allantoin.
See Editor's Note No. 17.

Cellex-C Eye Contour Gel - Cellex-C International Inc.
Ascorbic Acid • Tyrosine • Zinc • Bioflavonoids • Sodium Hyaluronate.
See Editor's Note No. 17.

Cellex-C Fade Away Gel For Sun & Age Spots - Cellex-C International Inc.
Glucosamine • Ascorbic Acid • Tyrosine • Zinc • Green Tea extract • Sodium Hyaluronate • Cucumber extract • Thyme extract.
See Editor's Note No. 17.

Cellex-C G.L.A. - Cellex-C International Inc.
Gamma Linolenic Acid • Evening Primrose Oil • Vitamin A Palmitate • Vitamin E • Wheat Germ Oil • Witch Hazel • Liposomes • Milk Thistle seed extract • Lemon oil flavonoids.
See Editor's Note No. 17.

Cellex-C G.L.A. Extra Moist - Cellex-C International Inc.
Glycophospholipids • Evening Primrose Oil • Witch Hazel extract • Wheat Germ oil • Retinyl Palmitate • Vitamin E • Allantoin • Milk Thistle seed extract • Chamomile extract.
See Editor's Note No. 17.

Cellex-C G.L.A. Eye Balm - Cellex-C International Inc.
Gamma Linolenic Acid • Evening Primrose Oil • Vitamin A Palmitate • Vitamin E • Wheat Germ oil • Witch Hazel • Liposomes • Milk Thistle seed extract • Lemon oil flavonoids.
See Editor's Note No. 17.

Cellex-C High-Potency Serum - Cellex-C International Inc.
10% L-Ascorbic Acid • Tyrosine • Zinc • Sodium Hyaluronate • Bioflavonoids.
See Editor's Note No. 17.

Cellex-C Hydra 5 B-Complex - Cellex-C International Inc.
Hyaluronic Acid • Pantothenic Acid.
See Editor's Note No. 17.

Some Brand Name Natural Products - What they Contain

www.NaturalDatabase.com contains MANY more listings than appear here.
Editor's Notes are located on pages 2155-2163.

Cellex-C Hydra Hand Cream SPF 15 - Cellex-C International Inc.
Kukui nut oil • Vitamin E • Lecithin • Shea Butter • Horse Chestnut extract • Hyaluronic Acid • Glycerin • Allantoin • Chamomile.
See Editor's Note No. 17.

Cellex-C Sea Silk Oil-Free Moisturizer - Cellex-C International Inc.
Jojoba esters • Sodium Hyaluronate • Seasilk • Plankton extract • Sea Buckthorn extract • Watercress extract • Marine Algae extract • Seaweed extract.
See Editor's Note No. 17.

Cellex-C Seline-E - Cellex-C International Inc.
Vitamin E • Bioflavonoids • Herbal essence.
See Editor's Note No. 17.

Cellex-C Serum For Sensitive Skin - Cellex-C International Inc.
Ascorbic Acid • Tyrosine • Zinc • Sodium Hyaluronate • Pine Bark extract.
See Editor's Note No. 17.

Cellex-C Skin Firming Cream Plus - Cellex-C International Inc.
Ascorbic Acid • Tyrosine • Vitamin E • Zinc • Bioflavonoids • Sodium Hyaluronate • Evening Primrose Oil • Tomato extract • Aloe Barbadensis gel • Chamomile extract • Allantoin.
See Editor's Note No. 17.

Cellex-C Skin Firming Hand Cream - Cellex-C International Inc.
L- Ascorbic Acid • Tyrosine • Zinc • Chamomile.
See Editor's Note No. 17.

Cellex-C Skin Perfecting Pen - Cellex-C International Inc.
Olive leaf • Rosemary • Lavender • Thyme • Eucalyptus extract • Peppermint extract • Zinc • Hyaluronic Acid.
See Editor's Note No. 17.

Cellex-C Speed Peel & Polish Gel - Cellex-C International Inc.
Ficin Enzyme • Melon extract • Natural Bamboo extract (providing micro-cylinders of silica) • Jojoba oil • Hyaluronic Acid.
See Editor's Note No. 17.

Cellex-C Sun Care SPF 15 - Cellex-C International Inc.
Octinoxate 7% • Octisalate 4% • Zinc Oxide 2% • Titanium Dioxide 2% • Total Hydroxy-Benzoates 0.17%.
See Editor's Note No. 17.

Cellex-C Sun Care SPF 30+ - Cellex-C International Inc.
Octinoxate 7.5% • Octisalate 5% • Zinc Oxide 3% • Titanium Dioxide 2% • Total Hydroxybanzoates 0.17%.
See Editor's Note No. 17.

Cellex-C Sun Rescue Gel - Cellex-C International Inc.
L- Ascorbic Acid • Tyrosine • Zinc • Green Tea extract • Glycine • Peppermint.
See Editor's Note No. 17.

Cellex-C Under-Eye Toning Gel - Cellex-C International Inc.
Azulene • Cornflower • Nicotinic Acid • Beta 1,3 glucans • Witch Hazel • Glycosaminoglycans • Plant Tannins • Cucumber extract • Kigelia extract.
See Editor's Note No. 17.

Cell-FX - CV Technologies Inc.
Each capsule contains: Shark Cartilage extract 200 mg.

Cell-FX (Bulk Powder) - CV Technologies Inc.
Water-soluble concentrated Shark Cartilage 227 mg.

Cell-FX 500 mg - CV Technologies Inc.
Each capsule contains: Shark Cartilage extract 500 mg.

CellMend IP-6 - Nature's Way
Three tablets contain: C-Med-100 patented Cat's Claw extract 300 mg • Inositol 150 mg • IP-6 (inositol hexaphosphate from rice) 1.6 g • Ribose (as d-ribose) 90 mg.

CellSparc 360 - The AIM Companies
Each softgel contains: Coenzyme Q10 60 mg • Tocotrienols 100 mg • Fish Oil 240 mg.

CELL-Tech - MuscleTech
Each serving contains: Creatine Monohydrate 10 g • Insulin-releasing Dextrose 75 g • Insulin-potentiating Lipoic Acid 200 mg • Chromium Picolinate 300 mcg • Potassium 150 mg • Phosphates 100 mg • Taurine • Magnesium.

Celltrex Skin Hydrating Fluid (original) - Nu Skin Enterprises
Water • Aloe Vera gel • Propylene Glycol • Hydroxypropyl Methylcellulose • Avian Collagen • Hyaluronic Acid • Linoleic Acid • Linolenic Acid • Oleic Acid • Tocopherol • Citric Acid • Arachidonic Acid • Triethanolamine • Disodium EDTA • Methylparaben • Propylparaben.

Celltrex Ultra Recovery Fluid - Nu Skin Enterprises
Water • Glycerin • Guar Hydroxypropyl-Trimonium Chloride • Ethoxydigylcol • Olea Europaea oil (olive fruit) • PEG-60 Hydrogenated Castor oil • Tocopheryl Acetate • Retinyl Palmitate • Citrus Aurantium var. Dulcis oil (orange) • Lavandula Angustifolia oil (lavender) • Anthemis Nobilis flower oil • Isoceteth-20 • Oleth-10 • Sodium Hydroxide • Citric Acid • Sodium Chloride • Disodium EDTA • Methylparaben • Ethylparaben • Propylparaben.

Cellular Build - Nature's Sunshine
Each capsule contains: Proprietary Blend 295 mg: Nucleotides (nucleoside monophosphate), Fructooligosaccharides (FOS), Astragalus root (astragalus membranaceus), Milk Thistle fruit and seed extract (silybum marianum). Other Ingredients: Cellulose, Magnesium Stearate, Silicon Dioxide, Gelatin, Water.

Cellular Detox Bath - Abra Therapeutics
Sodium Borate • Sodium Sulfate • Sodium Chloride • Sodium Sesquicarbonate • Olive Oil • Essential Oils Blend: Grapefruit oil, Juniper oil, Lavender oil, Lemongrass oil, Cedar leaf oil, Fir oil, Peru Balsam oil • Herbal Extracts Blend: Dandelion root, Burdock root • Vitamin A • Vitamin C • Vitamin E • Chromium Oxide • Trace Mineral Salts.

Cellular Detox Lotion - Abra Therapeutics
Purified Water • Aloe Vera • Coconut oil • Stearic Acid • Glycerin • Glyceral Stearate • Cetyl Alcohol • Olive oil • Burdock extract • Dandelion extract • Comfrey extract • Ginseng extract • Vitamin A • Vitamin D • Vitamin E • Grapefruit oil • Juniper oil • Sodium PCA • TEA • Allantoin • Lecithin • Methylparaben • Propylparaben.

Cellular Detox Salt Scrub - Abra Therapeutics
20% Volcanic ash • Natural Mineral Blend: Sodium Borate, Sodium Sulfate, Sodium Chloride • Organic Oils Blend: Almond oil, Olive oil, Sunflower oil, Jojoba oil, Grapefruit oil, Tea Tree oil, Juniper oil, Lime oil • Organic Comfrey • Dandelion • Burdock root • Natural Trace Minerals • Natural Vitamin E.

Cellular Energy - Nature's Sunshine
Each capsule contains: Vitamin E 10 IU • Vitamin B1 (thiamine mononitrate) 5 mg • Vitamin B2 (riboflavin) 5 mg • Niacin (as niacinamide) 2.5 mg • Pantothenic Acid 5 mg • Magnesium (as citrate) 5 mg • Zinc (as citrate) 2.5 mg • Manganese (as amino acid chelate) 5 mg • Proprietary Blend 85 mg: L-Carnitine, Alpha Ketoglutaric Acid, Coenzyme Q10, Alpha Lipoic Acid, Dimethyl Glycine HCl, Ferulic Acid. Other Ingredients: Cellulose, Di-Calcium Phosphate, Magnesium Stearate, Silicon Dioxide, Gelatin, Water.

Cellular Firming Mask - Abra Therapeutics
Deionized Water • Kaolin (china clay) • Vegetable Glycerin • Sorbitol • Titanium Dioxide • Colloidal Oats (avena) • Almond Glycerides • Angelica extract • Chamomile extract • Calendula extract • Elder flower extract • Thyme extract • Sodium PCA • Sea Algae extract • Panthenol (pro-vitamin B5) • Allantoin • Ascorbyl Palmitate (vitamin C) • Tocopherol (vitamin E) • Retinyl Palmitate (vitamin A) • Ylang Ylang oil • Rosemary oil • Methylparaben • Propylparaben.

Cellular Fort MAX3 - PhytoPharmica
Two capsules contain: Calcium (from calcium magnesium phytate) 130 mg • Inositol 220 mg • IP-6 (inositol hexaphosphate, from calcium magnesium phytate) 800 mg • Magnesium (from calcium magnesium phytate) 40 mg • Maitake mushroom extract (grifola frondosa, standardized to contain 9 mg of pure D-fraction) 30 mg • Phosphorus (from calcium magnesium phytate) 190 mg • POA Cat's Claw root extract (uncaria tomentosa, pentacyclic chemotype, Saventaro brand, standardized to contain a minimum of 1.3% pentacyclic oxindole alkaloids (POAs) and to be free of tetracyclic oxindole alkaloids (TOAs)) 10 mg.

Cellular Forte with IP-6 and Inositol capsules - PhytoPharmica
Two capsules contain: Calcium (from calcium magneisum phytate) 130 mg • Inositol 220 mg • IP-6 (inositol hexaphosphate) 800 mg • Magnesium (from calcium magnesium phytate) 40 mg • Phosphorus (from calcium mangeisum phytate) 190 mg.

Cellular Forte with IP-6 and Inositol Powder - PhytoPharmica
Each heaping scoop contains: Calcium (from calcium magnesium phytate) 520 mg • Inositol 880 mg • IP-6 (inositol hexaphosphate, from calcium magnesium phytate) 3.2 g • Magnesium (from calcium magnesium phytate) 160 mg • Phosphorus (from calcium magnesium phytate) 760 mg • Stevia leaf 12:1 extract (stevia rebaudiana) 60 mg.

Cellular Gold Calendula PhytoSerum - Abra Therapeutics
Calendula extract • Chamomile extract • Rose bud extract • Elder flower extract • Jojoba oil • Camellia oil • Kukui nut oil • Evening Primrose oil • Rose Hip oil • Foraha berry oil • Italian Neroli oil • D-Alpha-Tocopheryl (vitamin E).

Cellular Lift Marine Plasma SeaSerum - Abra Therapeutics
Aonori extract • Sea Palm extract • Laminaria extract • Irish Moss extract • Wakame extract • Ulva extract • Dulse extract • Aloe Vera juice • Vegetable Glycerin • Blue Green Algae • Microburst Seaweed oil • Glycosaminoglycans • Sea Buckthorn extract • Grapefruit oil • Lavender oil • Clary Sage oil • Tea Tree oil • Geranium oil • Methylparaben • Propylparaben.

Cellular Support Advanced (No Iron) - Pro Health
Two tablets contain: Vitamin A (as beta carotene 7500 IU, palmitate 5000 IU) 12,500 IU • Vitamin C (as ascorbic acid, ascorbyl palmitate) 500 mg • Vitamin D (D3, as cholecalciferol) 200 IU • Vitamin E (as natural d-alpha tocopheryl) 200 IU • Thiamin (vitamin B1) 50 mg • Riboflavin (vitamin B2) 50 mg • Niacinamide 35 mg • Niacin 15 mg • Vitamin B6 (as pyridoxine HCl) 50 mg • Folate (as folic acid) 400 mcg • Vitamin B12 (as cyanocobalamin) 100 mcg • Biotin 150 mcg • Pantothenic Acid (as calcium d-pantothenate) 50 mg • Calcium (as calcium chelate, citrate, malate) 100 mg • Iodine (from kelp) 100 mcg • Magnesium (as magnesium chelate, citrate, oxide) 100 mg • Zinc (as zinc citrate, monomethionine) 15 mg • Selenium (as l-selenomethionine, sodium selenite) 100 mcg • Copper (as copper sebacate) 1 mg • Manganese (as manganese citrate) 3 mg • Chromium (as chromium polynicotinate) 100 mcg • Molybdenum (as molybdenum chelate) 100 mcg • Potassium (as potassium citrate) 50 mg • N-Acetyl Cysteine 100 mg • Hawthorn berry 75 mg • Milk Thistle seed extract (yielding silymarin 60 mg) 72 mg • L-Tyrosine 50 mg • Choline (as bitartrate) 50 mg • Inositol 50 mg • DMAE (as bitartrate) 30 mg • Alpha-Lipoic Acid 25 mg • MSM (methylsulfonylmethane) 25 mg • Grape Seed extract 25 mg • Coenzyme Q-10 20 mg • Ginkgo Biloba leaf 24% (50:1 extract) 20 mg • Turmeric rhizome extract (95%) 15 mg • Bilberry standardized extract 10 mg • Pepper fruit extract 3 mg • Boron Amino Acid Chelate 2 mg. Other Ingredients: Stearic Acid, Acacia Gum, Modified Cellulose Gum, Colloidal Silicon Dioxide, Magnesium Stearate.

Cellular Support Advanced (With Iron) - Pro Health
Two tablets contain: Vitamin A (as beta carotene 7500 IU, palmitate 5000 IU) 12,500 IU • Vitamin C (as ascorbic acid, ascorbyl palmitate) 500 mg • Vitamin D (D3, as cholecalciferol) 200 IU • Vitamin E (as natural d-alpha tocopheryl) 200 IU • Thiamin (vitamin B1) 50 mg • Riboflavin (vitamin B2) 50 mg • Niacinamide 35 mg • Niacin 15 mg • Vitamin B6 (as pyridoxine HCl) 50 mg • Folate (as folic acid) 400 mcg • Vitamin B12 (as cyanocobalamin) 100 mcg • Biotin 150 mcg • Pantothenic Acid (as calcium d-pantothenate) 50 mg • Calcium (as calcium chelate, citrate, malate) 100 mg • Iron (as iron fumarate) 6 mg • Iodine (from kelp) 100 mcg • Magnesium (as magnesium chelate, citrate, oxide) 100 mg • Zinc (as zinc citrate, monomethionine) 15 mg • Selenium (as l-selenomethionine, sodium selenite) 100 mcg • Copper (as copper sebacate) 1 mg • Manganese (as manganese citrate) 3 mg • Chromium (as chromium polynicotinate) 100 mcg • Molybdenum (as molybdenum chelate) 100 mcg • Potassium (as potassium citrate) 50 mg • N-Acetyl Cysteine 100 mg • Hawthorn berry 75 mg • Milk Thistle seed extract (yielding silymarin 60 mg) 72 mg • L-Tyrosine 50 mg • Choline (as bitartrate) 50 mg • Inositol 50 mg • DMAE (as bitartrate) 30 mg • Alpha-Lipoic Acid 25 mg • MSM (methylsulfonylmethane) 25 mg • Grape Seed extract 25 mg • Coenzyme Q-10 20 mg • Ginkgo Biloba leaf 24% (50:1 extract) 20 mg • Turmeric rhizome extract (95%) 15 mg • Bilberry standardized extract 10 mg • Pepper fruit extract 3 mg • Boron Amino Acid Chelate 2 mg. Other Ingredients: Stearic Acid, Acacia Gum, Modified Cellulose Gum, Colloidal Silicon Dioxide, Magnesium Stearate.

CelluPhase - Pure Encapsulations
Each vegetable capsule contains: Broccoli sprout concentrate 20:1 (brassica oleracea italica, standardized to contain a minimum of 2000 mcg sulforaphane) 500 mg • Broccoli extract (brassica oleracea italica/alba, standardized to contain 4% glucosinolates) 100 mg.

CelluPlex - Jamieson
Each capsule contains: Bilberry extract 750 mg • Kola Nut extract 250 mg • Ginkgo Biloba extract 250 mg • Concentrated Citrus Bioflavonoids PF 100 (vitamin P) 100 mg • Active PSP Bromelain Enzyme (from fresh pineapple) 100 mg • Mineral-Rich Pacific Sea Kelp Extract 25 mg • Oil of Madagascar Cinnamon Leaf 20 mg.

Cellu-Rid - Biotech Corp.
Two tablets contain: Vitamin C (ascorbic acid) 80 mg • Iron (as ferrous fumarate) 9 mg • HerbaCell! Proprietary Herb Blend 200 mg: Senna leaves (cassia angustifolia), Cascara Sagrada bark, Apple rind extract, Milk Thistle root extract (silybum marianum), Bioperine brand Black Pepper extract, Cinnamon root extract (cinnamomum verum) • White Willow bark (salix alba) 100 mg • Kelp 33 mg • Apple Cider Vinegar 33 mg • Guarana seed (paullinia cupana) 20 mg • Soy Lecithin 16 mg • Rose Hips 10 mg • Buchu leaves (betulina bosma) 5 mg • Couch Grass (cynodon dactylon) 5 mg • Hydrangea Arborescens root 5 mg • Uva Ursi (arctostaphylos uva-ursi) 5 mg • Juniper berries (juniperus vulgaris) 5 mg. Other Ingredients: Gelatin, Silica, Potassium (as potassium chloride).

Cellu-Smooth with Coleus - Nature's Sunshine
Each capsule contains: Proprietary Blend 405 mg: Coleus Forskohlii root extract, Bladderwrack plant (fucus vesiculosus), Milk Thistle fruit concentrate (silybum marianum), Ginkgo leaf concentrate (ginkgo biloba), Rhodiola root extract (rhodiola rosea), Rhododendron root (rhododendron caucasicum). Other Ingredients: Cellulose, Gelatin, Water.

Cellu-Tone Essential Oil - Nature's Sunshine
Geranium oil • Pink Grapefruit oil • Rosemary oil • Thyme Linalol • Cypress oil • Juniper oil • Vetiver • Niauli oil.

Some Brand Name Natural Products - What they Contain

www.NaturalDatabase.com contains MANY more listings than appear here.
Editor's Notes are located on pages 2155-2163.

BRAND NAMES

Cellu-Trim **-** Enforma Natural Products
Two capsules contain: White Willow bark • Vitamin C (ascorbic acid) • Hydragia root • Sida Cordifolia • Uva Ursi • Tinospora Cordifolia • Potassium Chloride.
See Editor's Note No. 39 and No. 65.

Cellu-Var Capsules **-** Enzymatic Therapy/PhytoPharmica
Each capsule contains: Butchers Broom extract (Ruscus aculeatus) standardized to contain 10% Saponins calculated as Ruscogenin 100 mg • Gotu Kola extract (Centella asiatica) standardized to contain 70% of selected Triterpenic Acids: Asiaticoside, Asiatic Acid, & Madecassic Acid from Centella 30 mg • Escin extract (Aesculus hippocastanum) 10 mg.
See Editor's Note No. 21.

Cellu-Var Cream **-** Enzymatic Therapy
Deionized Water • Horse Chestnut (Escin) extract • Sea Ware extract • Cola vera extract • Rosemary extract in a base of Cholestanol (Dihydrocholesterol), a natural emulsifying agent.

Cenitol **-** Metagenics
Two scoops (7.4 g) contain: Inositol (as myo-inositol) 4 g • Magnesium (as magnesium bis-glycinate) 200 mg • Citric Acid 800 mg.

Censor **-** NDS Nutrition
Each capsule contains: Proprietary Blend 1000 mg: CLA (conjugated linoleic acid), GLA (gamma linoleic acid), ALA (alpha linoleic acid), EPA (eicosapentaenoic acid), DHA (docosahexaenoic acid), Omega 3-6-9 Blend.

Central-Vite Select Formula Plus **-** Leiner Health Products
Each tablet contains: Folate (Folic Acid) 200 mcg • Iron (Ferrous Fumarate) 9 mg • Phosphorus 48 mg • Vitamin B12 (Cyanocobalamin, USP Method 2) 25 mcg • Magnesium Oxide 100 mg • Molybdenum 160 mcg • Calcium Carbonate 200 mg • Chloride 72 mg • Potassium Chloride and Iodide 80 mg • Manganese Sulfate 3.5 mg • Vitamin A (Acetate) 7500 IU • Vitamin B6 (Pyridoxine Hydrochloride) 3 mg • Vitamin C (Ascorbic Acid) 90 mg • Vitamin E (dl-Alpha Tocopheryl Acetate) 45 IU • Zinc Oxide 22.5 mg • Vitamin K (Phytonadione) 10 mcg • Chromium Chloride 130 mcg • Copper Oxide 2 mg • Iodine 150 mcg • Niacin (Niacinamide) 20 mg • Pantothenic Acid 10 mg • Riboflavin (Vitamin B2) 1.7 mg • Selenium 70 mcg • Thiamin Mononitrate (Vitamin B1) 1.5 mg • Vitamin D 400 IU • Biotin (USP Method 2) 30 mcg • Boron 150 mcg • Nickel (Nickelous Sulfate) 5 mcg • Silicon Dioxide 10 mcg • Vanadium 10 mcg. Other Ingredients: Dicalcium Phosphate, Gelatin, Cellulose, Starch, Croscarmellose Sodium, Sodium Starch Glycolate, Hydroxypropyl Methylcellulose, Polyethylene Glycol 3350, Tricalcium Phosphate, Magnesium Stearate, Hydroxypropyl Cellulose, Resin, Beta Carotene, Polysorbate 80, Pharmaceutical Glaze, Sodium Metasilicate.

Centrum **-** Wyeth
Each tablet contains: Nickel (Nickelous Sulfate) 5 mcg • Vitamin A Acetate 5000 IU • Tin (Stannous Chloride) 10 mcg • Vitamin C (Ascorbic Acid) 60 mg • Vitamin D 400 IU • Vanadium (Sodium Metavanadate) 10 mcg • Silicon Dioxide 2 mg • Vitamin E (dl-Alpha Tocopheryl Acetate) 30 IU • Boron (Potassium Borate) 150 mcg • Vitamin K (Phytonadione) 25 mcg • Thiamin Mononitrate (Vitamin B1) 1.5 mg • Riboflavin (Vitamin B2) 1.7 mg • Niacin (Vitamin B3, Niacinamide) 20 mg • Vitamin B6 (Pyridoxine Hydrochloride) 2 mg • Folate (Folic Acid) 400 mcg • Vitamin B12 (Cyanocobalamin) 6 mcg • Biotin 30 mcg • Pantothenic Acid (Calcium Pantothenate) 10 mg • Calcium Carbonate 162 mg • Iron (Ferrous Fumarate) 18 mg • Phosphorus (Calcium Carbonate) 109 mg • Iodine 150 mcg • Magnesium Oxide 100 mg • Zinc Oxide 15 mg • Selenium (Sodium Selenate) 20 mcg • Copper (Cupric Acid) 2 mg • Manganese Sulfate 3.5 mg • Chromium 65 mcg • Molybdenum 160 mg • Chloride 72 mg • Potassium Chloride 80 mg. Other Ingredients: Microcrystalline Cellulose, Gelatin, Crospovidone, Hydroxypropyl Methylcellulose, Titanium Dioxide, Magnesium Stearate, Stearic Acid, Triethyl Citrate, Polysorbate 80, FD&C Yellow #6.

Centrum Carb Assist **-** Wyeth
Each tablet contains: Vitamin A (29% as beta carotene) 3500 IU • Vitamin C 120 mg • Vitamin D 400 IU • Vitamin E 60 IU • Vitamin K 25 mcg • Thiamin 4.5 mg • Riboflavin 5.1 mg • Niacin 40 mg • Vitamin B6 6 mg • Folic Acid 400 mcg • Vitamin B12 18 mcg • Biotin 40 mcg • Pantothenic Acid 10 mg • Calcium 100 mg • Iron 18 mg • Phosphorus 48 mg • Iodine 150 mcg • Magnesium 40 mg • Zinc 15 mg • Selenium 70 mcg • Copper 2 mg • Manganese 4 mg • Chromium 120 mcg • Molybdenum 75 mcg • Chloride 72 mg • Potassium 80 mg • Ginseng root standardized extract (panax ginseng) 50 mg • Ginkgo Biloba leaf standardized extract (ginkgo biloba) 60 mg • Boron 60 mcg • Nickel 5 mcg • Silicon 4 mg • Tin 10 mcg • Vanadium 10 mcg. Other Ingredients: Dibasic Calcium Phosphate, Microcrystalline Cellulose, Gelatin, Crospovidone, Starch, Acacia Senegal Gum, BHT, FD&C Red #40 Aluminum Lake, FD&C Yellow #6 Aluminum Lake, Glucose, Hypromellose, Lactose Monohydrate, Magnesium Stearate, Polyethylene Glycol, Polysorbate 80, Purified Water, Sucrose, Titanium Dioxide, Tribasic Calcium Phosphate, Maltodextrin.

Centrum Chewables **-** Wyeth
Each tablet contains: Vitamin A (29% as beta carotene) 3500 IU • Vitamin C 60 mg • Vitamin D 400 IU • Vitamin E 30 IU • Vitamin K 10 mcg • Thiamin 1.5 mg • Riboflavin 1.7 mg • Niacin 20 mg • Vitamin B6 2 mg • Folic Acid 400 mcg • Vitamin B12 6 mcg • Biotin 45 mcg • Pantothenic Acid 10 mg • Calcium 108 mg • Iron 18 mg • Phosphorus 50 mg • Iodine 150 mcg • Magnesium 40 mg • Zinc 15 mg • Copper 2 mg • Manganese 1 mg • Chromium 20 mcg • Molybdenum 20 mcg. Other Ingredients: Sucrose, Dibasic Calcium Phosphate, Mannitol, Stearic ACid, Pregelatinzed Starch, Microcrystalline Cellulose, Acacia, Aspartame, BHT, Carrageenan, Dextrose, FD&C Yellow #6 Aluminum Lake, Gelatin, Glucose, Guar Gum, Lactose, Magnesium Stearate, Malic Acid, Mono- and Di-glycerides, Natural and Artificial Flavors, Purified Water, Sorbic Acid, Starch, Tribasic Calcium Phosphate, Vanillin, Fructose, Maltodextrin.

Centrum Focused Formula Stress **-** Wyeth
Each tablet contains: Vitamin C 150 mg • Vitamin E 22.5 IU • Thiamin (B1) 15 mg • Riboflavin (B2) 4.8 mg • Niacin (B3) 50 mg • Vitamin B6 5 mg • Folate, Folic Acid, Folacin 200 mcg • Vitamin B12 12.5 mcg • Biotin 15 mcg • Pantothenic Acid 12.5 mg • Zinc 7.5 mg • Copper 1 mg • Ginseng standardized root extract (Panax ginseng) 62.5 mg.
See Editor's Note No. 21.

Centrum Focused Formulas Bone Health **-** Wyeth
Each two tablets contain: Supplement facts: Vitamin D 200 IU • Calcium (Citrate) 500 mg • Magnesium 40 mg • Zinc 7.5 mg • Copper 1 mg • Manganese 1.8 mg • Boron 250 mcg • Lycopene 1.5 mg • Saw Palmetto (Standardized lipophilic fruit extract, Serenoa repens) 160 mg. Ingredients: Calcium Citrate, Magnesium Oxide, Talc, Hydroxypropyl Methylcellulose, Sodium Starch Glycolate, Titanium Dioxide, Magnesium Stearate, Zinc Oxide, Mineral Oil, Manganese Sulfate Monohydrate, Vitamin D (Cholecalciferol), Polysorbate 80, Sodium Borate, Polyethlene Glycol, Cupric Oxide, Gelatin, Sucrose, Starch, Carnauba Wax, Vegetable Oil, DL-Alpha-Tocopherol.
See Editor's Note No. 21.

Centrum Focused Formulas Energy **-** Wyeth
Each tablet contains: Supplement facts: Thiamin (Vitamin B1) 3 mg • Riboflavin (Vitamin B2) 0.85 mg • Niacin (Vitamin B3) 10 mg • Vitamin B6 1 mg •Vitamin B12 3 mcg • Biotin 15 mcg • Pantothenic Acid 5 mg • Taurine 100 mg • Panax Ginseng standardized extract (root) 62.5 mg. Ingredients: Dibasic Calcium Phosphate, Taurine, Ginseng standardized root extract (Panax Ginseng), Microcrystalline Cellulose, Crospovidone, Maltodextrin, Hydroxypropyl Methylcellulose, Niacinamide, Calcium Pantothenate, Magnesium Stearate, Titanium Dioxide, Polyethylene Glycol, Thiamin Mononitrate, Polysorbate 80, FD&C Yellow #6 Aluminum Lake,

Pyridoxine Hydrochloride, Riboflavin, Starch, Biotin, Citric Acid, Sodium Citrate, Silicon Dioxide, Cyanocobalamin, Sodium Benzoate, Sorbic Acid.
See Editor's Note No. 21.

Centrum Focused Formulas Heart **- Wyeth**
Each tablet contains: Supplement facts: Vitamin E 200 IU • Vitamin B6 5 mg • Folate, Folic Acid, Folacin 200 mcg • Vitamin B12 200 mcg • Selenium 25 mcg • Manganese 1 mg • Garlic Powder (bulb) (Allium sativum) 300 mg • Taurine 33 mg • Coenzyme Q10 4 mg. Ingredients: DL-Alpha Tocopherol Acetate, Garlic powder (Bulb, Alium sativum), Microcrystalline Cellulose, Dibasic Calcium Phosphate, Calcium Silicate, Taurine, Croscarmellose sodium, Sodium Selenate, Gelatin, Hydroxypropyl methylcellulose, Silicon Doxide, Magnesium Stearate, Pyridoxine Hydrochloride, Ubidecarenone, Titanium Dioxide, Polyethylene Glycol, Polysorbate 80, Magnesium Sulfate Monohydrate, FD&C Red #40 Aluminum Lake, FD&C Blue #2 Aluminum Lake, Folic Acid, Cyanocobalamin, Citric Acid, Starch, Sodium Citrate, Sodium Benzoate, Sorbic Acid.
See Editor's Note No. 21.

Centrum Focused Formulas Mental Clarity **- Wyeth**
Each tablet contains: Supplement Facts: Vitamin E 20 IU • Thiamin (B1) 0.55 mg • Riboflavin (B2) 0.85 mg • Niacin (B3) 10 mg • Vitamin B6 1 mg • Folate, Folic Acid, Folacin 200 mcg • Vitamin B12 3 mcg • Biotin 5 mcg • Pantothenic Acid 7.5 mg • Ginkgo Biloba standardized leaf extract 60 mg • Choline 8 mg. Ingredients: Dibasic Calcium Phosphate, Microcrystalline Cellulose, Ginkgo Biloba standardized extract, Dl-alpha Tocopheryl Acetate, Choline Bitartrate, Hydroxypropyl methylcellulose, Crospovidone, maltodextrin, Niacinamide, Zinc Oxide, Calcium Pantothenate, Calcium Silicate, Magnesium Stearate, Titanium Dioxide, Gelatin, Polyethylene Glycol, Polysorbate 80, Silicon Dioxide, FD&C Blue #2 Aluminum Lake, FD&C Red #40 Aluminum Lake, FD&C Yellow #6 Aluminum Lake, Pyridoxine Hydrochloride, Riboflavin, Thiamine Mononitrate, Folic Acid, Starch, Citric Acid, Sodium Citrate, Cyanocobalamin, Sodium Benzoate, Sorbic Acid.
See Editor's Note No. 21.

Centrum Focused Formulas Prostate **- Wyeth**
Each softgel contains: Vitamin A as Beta-carotene 5000 IU • Lycopene 1.5 mg • Saw Palmetto standardized Lipophilic fruit extract (Serenoa repens) 160 mg.
See Editor's Note No. 21.

Centrum Herbals Echinacea **- Wyeth**
Each capsule contains: Echinacea extract flower and root (Echinacea purpurea) 100 mg. Standardized to contain (based on extract weight): Total Phenols (marker) 3.0%, Cichoric Acid (natural active), Isobutyl Alkylamides (natural active), Activity Measure 15-lipoxygenase enzymatic assay. Other Ingredients: Dibasic Calcium Phosphate, Cellulose, Lactose Monohydrate, Hydroxypropyl Cellulose, Ethylcellulose, Castor Oil, Gelatin, Silicon Dioxide, Sodium Lauryl Sulfate, Propylene Glycol, Titanium Dioxide.
See Editor's Note No. 21.

Centrum Herbals Garlic **- Wyeth**
Each capsule contains: Garlic powder (bulb) Allium sativum 300 mg • Allin (marker) allicin potential 45% 1300 mcg. Standardized to contain: Gamma Glytamyl-S allyl-cysteine (natural active) • Gamma Glytamyl-S-trans-1-propenyl-cysteine (natural active) • Gamma glutamyl-phenylalanine (natural active) • Activity Measure Angiotensin converting enzyme assay.
See Editor's Note No. 21.

Centrum Herbals Ginkgo Biloba **- Wyeth**
Each capsule contains: Ginkgo Biloba leaf extract 60 mg. Standardized to contain (based on extract weight): Ginkgo Flavone glycosides (marker) 24%, Terpene Lactones (marker) 6%, ginkgolide A (natural active), Ginkgolide B (natural active), Amentoflavone (natural active). Activity measure: GABA Central binding assay. Other Ingredients: Sucrose, Cellulose, Lactose, Monohydrate, Dibasic Calcium Phosphate, Hydroxypropyl Cellulose, Ethylcellulose, Castor Oil, Flavor Extractives of St. John's Bread, Glucose, Caramel color, Silicon Dioxide, Sodium Lauryl Sulfate, Propylene Glycol, Titanium Dioxide.
See Editor's Note No. 21.

Centrum Herbals Ginseng **- Wyeth**
Each capsule contains: Ginseng root extract 100 mg. Standardized to contain (based on extract weight): Total Ginenosides (marker) 7.0%, Ginsenoside Rb1 (natural active), Ginsenoside Rg1 (natural active). Activity measure: Phospholipase A2 enzymatic assay. Other Ingredients: Dibasic Calcium Phosphate, Cellulose, Lactose, Monohydrate, Hydroxypropyl Cellulose, Ethylcellulose, Castor Oil, Gelatin, Silicon Dioxide, Sodium Lauryl Sulfate, Propylene Glycol, Titanium Dioxide.
See Editor's Note No. 21.

Centrum Herbals Saw Palmetto **- Wyeth**
Each softgel contains: Saw Palmetto berry extract (Serenoa repens) 160 mg. Total Fatty Acids (marker) 80% (Standardized to contain-based on extract weight): Linolenic Acid (natural active) • Lauric Acid, Ethyl Ester (natural active) • Linoleic Acid, Ethyl Ester (natural active) • Activity measure: Adrenergic alpha 1B binding assay. Inactive Ingredients: Corn Oil, Yellow Wax, Gelatin, Propylene Glycol, Hydroxypropyl Methylcellulose, Titanium Dioxide, Carmine.
See Editor's Note No. 21.

Centrum Herbals St. John's Wort **- Wyeth**
Each capsule contains: St. John's Wort (Hypericum perforatum) flower and leaves 300 mg. Standardized to contain (based on extract weight): Total Hypericin compounds (marker) 0.3%, Hyperforin (marker), Quercetin (natural active), Amentoflavone (natural active), Gaba & Proline (natural actives). Activity measure: Muscarinic M1 binding assay. Other Ingredients: Dibasic Calcium Phosphate, Maltodextrin, Cellulose, Lactose Monohydrate, Silicon Dioxide, Hydroxypropyl Cellulose, Ethycellulose, Castor Oil, Gelatin, Sodium Lauryl Sulfate, Propylene Glycol, Titanium Dioxide.
See Editor's Note No. 21.

Centrum Kids **- Wyeth**
Each tablet contains: Vitamin A Acetate 5000 IU • Sodium 14 mg • Vitamin C (Ascorbic Acid and Sodium Ascorbate) 250 mg • Vitamin D 400 IU • Vitamin E (dl-Alpha Tocopheryl Acetate) 15 IU • Thiamin Mononitrate (Vitamin B1) 1.5 mg • Riboflavin (Vitamin B2) 1.7 mg • Niacin (Niacinamide, Vitamin B3) 13.5 mg • Vitamin B6 (Pyridoxine Hydrochloride) 1 mg • Folate (Folic Acid) 300 mcg • Vitamin B12 (Cyanocobalamin) 5 mcg • Calcium Carbonate 108 mg • Phosphorus (Calicum Phosphate) 50 mg • Zinc Oxide 4 mg • Copper (Cupric Oxide) 0.5 mg. Other Ingredients: Sugar, Mannitol, Mono- and Diglycerides, Microcrystalline Cellulose, Modified Food Starch, Gelatin, Stearic Acid, FD&C Yellow #6 Lake, Food Starch, Aspartame, Carrageenan, Magnesium Stearate, Natural and Artificial Flavors, Guar Gum, FD&C Red #40 Lake, FD&C Blue #2 Lake, Silicon Dioxide, Partially Hydrogenated Coconut Oil, Dextrose, Beta Carotene, Lactose, Acacia.

Centrum Kids Jimmy Neutron Complete **- Wyeth**
Each tablet contains: Vitamin A (20% as beta carotene) 5000 IU • Vitamin C 60 mg • Vitamin D 400 IU • Vitamin E 30 IU • Vitamin K 10 mcg • Thiamin 1.5 mg • Riboflavin 1.7 mg • Niacin 20 mg • Vitamin B6 2 mg • Folic Acid 400 mcg • Vitamin B12 6 mcg • Bitoin 45 mcg • Pantothenic Acid 10 mg • Calcium 108 mg • Iron 18 mg • Phosphorus 50 mg • Iodine 150 mg • Magnesium 40 mg • Zinc 15 mg • Copper 2 mg • Manganese 1 mg • Chromium 20 mcg. Other Ingredients: Sucrose, Dibasic Calcium Phosphate, Mannitol, Calcium Carbonate, Stearic Acid, Microcrystalline Cellulose, Pregelatinized Starch, Gelatin, Acacia, Aspartame, Butylate Hydroxytoluene, Carrageenan, FD&C Blue 2 Aluminum Lake, FD&C Red 40 Aluminum Lake, FD&C Yellow 6 Aluminum Lake, Glucose, Guar Gum, Lactose, Magnesium Stearate, Malic ACid, Maltodextrin, Mono- and Diglycerides, Natural and Artificial Flavors, Purified Water, Starch, Tribasic Calcium Phosphate, Vanillin, Fructose.

Some Brand Name Natural Products - What they Contain

www.NaturalDatabase.com contains MANY more listings than appear here.
Editor's Notes are located on pages 2155-2163.

B R A N D N A M E S

Centrum Kids Jimmy Neutron Extra C - Wyeth
Each tablet contains: Vitamin A (20% as beta carotene) 5000 IU • Vitamin C 250 mg • Vitamin D 400 IU • Vitamin E 15 IU • Thiamin 1.5 mg • Riboflavin 1.7 mg • Niacin 13.5 mg • Vitamin B6 1 mg • Folic Acid 300 mcg • Vitamin B12 5 mcg • Calcium 108 mg • Phosphorus 50 mg • Zinc 4 mg • Copper 0.5 mg • Sodium 16 mg. Other Ingredients: Sucrose, Dibasic Calcium Phosphate, Mannitol, Stearic Acid, Microcrystalline Cellulose, Pregelatinized Starch, Starch, Aspartame, Butylated Hydroxytoluene, Carrageenan, Citric Acid, FD&C Blue 2 Aluminum Lake, FD&C Red 40 Aluminum Lake, FD&C Yellow 6 Aluminum Lake, Gelatin, Guar Gum, Lactose, Magnesium Stearate, Maltodextrin, Mono- and Diglycerides, Natural and Artificial Flavors, Purified Water, Tribasic Calcium Phosphate, Vanillin, Dextrose, Fructose.

Centrum Kids Rugrats Complete - Wyeth
Each tablet contains: Vitamin A (20% as beta carotene) 5000 IU • Vitamin C 60 mg • Vitamin D 400 IU • Vitamin E 30 IU • Vitamin K 10 mcg • Thiamin 1.5 mg • Riboflavin 1.7 mg • Niacin 20 mg • Vitamin B6 2 mg • Folic Acid 400 mcg • Vitamin B12 6 mcg • Bitoin 45 mcg • Pantothenic Acid 10 mg • Calcium 108 mg • Iron 18 mg • Phosphorus 50 mg • Iodine 150 mg • Magnesium 40 mg • Zinc 15 mg • Copper 2 mg • Manganese 1 mg • Chromium 20 mcg. Other Ingredients: Sucrose, Dibasic Calcium Phosphate, Mannitol, Calcium Carbonate, Stearic Acid, Microcrystalline Cellulose, Pregelatinized Starch, Gelatin, Acacia, Aspartame, Butylate Hydroxytoluene, Carrageenan, FD&C Blue 2 Aluminum Lake, FD&C Red 40 Aluminum Lake, FD&C Yellow 6 Aluminum Lake, Glucose, Guar Gum, Lactose, Magnesium Stearate, Malic Acid, Maltodextrin, Mono- and Diglycerides, Natural and Artificial Flavors, Purified Water, Starch, Tribasic Calcium Phosphate, Vanillin, Fructose.

Centrum Kids Rugrats Extra C - Wyeth
Each tablet contains: Vitamin A (20% as beta carotene) 5000 IU • Vitamin C 250 mg • Vitamin D 400 IU • Vitamin E 15 IU • Thiamin 1.5 mg • Riboflavin 1.7 mg • Niacin 13.5 mg • Vitamin B6 1 mg • Folic Acid 300 mcg • Vitamin B12 5 mcg • Calcium 108 mg • Phosphorus 50 mg • Zinc 4 mg • Copper 0.5 mg • Sodium 16 mg. Other Ingredients: Sucrose, Dibasic Calcium Phosphate, Mannitol, Stearic Acid, Microcrystalline Cellulose, Pregelatinized Starch, Starch, Aspartame, Butylated Hydroxytoluene, Carrageenan, Citric Acid, FD&C Blue 2 Aluminum Lake, FD&C Red 40 Aluminum Lake, FD&C Yellow 6 Aluminum Lake, Gelatin, Guar Gum, Lactose, Magnesium Stearate, Maltodextrin, Mono- and Diglycerides, Natural and Artificial Flavors, Purified Water, Tribasic Calcium Phosphate, Vanillin, Dextrose, Fructose.

Centrum Kids Rugrats Extra Calcium - Wyeth
Each tablet contains: Vitamin A (20% as beta carotene) 5000 IU • Vitamin C 60 mg • Vitamin D 400 IU • Vitamin E 15 IU • Thiamin 1.5 mg • Riboflavin 1.7 mg • Niacin 13.5 mg • Vitamin B6 1 mg • Folic Acid 300 mcg • Vitamin B12 5 mcg • Calcium 200 mg • Phosphorus 50 mg • Zinc 4 mg • Copper 0.5 mg. Other Ingredients: Sucrose, Dibasic Calcium Phosphate, Mannitol, Stearic Acid, Microcrystalline Cellulose, Cellulose, Pregelatinized Starch, Starch, Aspartame, Butylated Hydroxytoluene, Carrageenan, Citric Acid, FD&C Blue 2 Aluminum Lake, FD&C Red 40 Aluminum Lake, FD&C Yellow 6 Aluminum Lake, Gelatin, Guar Gum, Lactose, Magnesium Stearate, Malic Acid, Maltodextrin, Mono- and Diglycerides, Natural and Artificial Flavors, Purified Water, Sorbic Acid, Tribasic Calcium Phosphate, Vanillin, Dextrose, Fructose.

Centrum Liquid - Wyeth
Each 1 tbsp serving (15 mL) contains: Vitamin A Palmitate 2500 IU • Vitamin C (Ascorbic Acid) 60 mg • Vitamin D (as Vitamin D3) 400 IU • Vitamin E (dl-Alpha Tocopheryl Acetate) 30 IU • Thiamin Hydrochloride (Vitamin B1) 1.5 mg • Riboflavin 5-Phosphate Sodium (Vitamin B2) 1.7 mg • Niacin (Vitamin B3, Niacinamide) 20 mg • Vitamin B6 (Pyridoxine Hydrochloride) 2 mg • Vitamin B12 (Cyanocobalamin) 6 mcg • Biotin 300 mcg • Pantothenic Acid (D-Panthenol) 10 mg • Iron (Ferrous Gluconate) 9 mg • Iodine (Potassium Iodide) 150 mcg • Zinc Gluconate 3 mg • Manganese Chloride 2 mg • Chromium Chloride 25 mcg • Molybdenum (Sodium Molybdate) 25 mg. Other Ingredients: Water, Sucrose, Ethyl Aclohol 5.4% w/v, Glycerin, Polysorbate 80, Citric Acid, Sodium Benzoate, D-Panthenol, BHA, Natural and Artificial Flavor, Food Starch, Edetic Acid.

Centrum Multivitamin/Multimineral - Wyeth
Each tablet contains: Vitamin A (29% as beta carotene) 3500 IU • Vitamin C 60 mg • Vitamin D 400 IU • Vitamin E 30 IU • Vitamin K 25 mcg • Thiamin (B1) 1.5 mg • Riboflavin (B2) 1.7 mg • Niacin (B3) 20 mg • Vitamin B6 2 mg • Folate, Folic Acid, Folacin 400 mcg • Vitamin B12 6 mcg • Biotin 30 mcg • Pantothenic Acid 10 mg • Calcium 162 mg • Iron 18 mg • Phosphorus 109 mg • Iodine 150 mcg • Magnesium 100 mg • Zinc 15 mg • Selenium 20 mcg • Copper 2 mg • Manganese 2 mg • Chromium 120 mcg • Molybdenum 75 mcg • Chloride 72 mg • Potassium 80 mg • Nickel 5 mcg • Tin 10 mcg • Silicon 2 mg • Vanadium 10 mcg • Boron 150 mcg • Lutein 250 mcg • Lycopene 300 mcg. Other Ingredients: Dibasic Calcium Phosphate, Magnesium Oxide, Potassium Chloride, Microcrystalline Cellulose, Gelatin, Acacia Senegal Gum, Butylated Hydroxytoluene, Crospovidone, FD&C Yellow 6, FD&C Yellow 6 Aluminum Lake, Hypromellose, Magnesium-Stearate, Polysorbate 80, Pregelatinized Starch, Purified Water, Starch, Sucrose, Titanium Dioxide, Calcium Stearate, Glucose, Lactose Monohydrate.

Centrum Performance - Wyeth
Each tablet contains: Ginseng root extract 50 mg • Vitamin A 5000 IU • Ginkgo root extract 60 mg • Vitamin C 120 mg • Vitamin D 400 IU • Boron 60 mg • Vitamin E 60 IU • Nickel 5 mcg • Silicon 4 mg • Vitamin K 25 mcg • Tin 10 mg • Thiamin (B1) 4.5 mg • Vanadium 10 mcg • Riboflavin (B2) 5.1 mg • Niacin (B3) 40 mg • Vitamin B6 6 mg • Folate (Folic Acid) 400 mcg • Vitamin B12 18 mcg • Biotin 40 mcg • Pantothenic Acid 10 mg • Calcium 100 mg • Iron 18 mg • Phosphorus 48 mg • Iodine 150 mcg • Magnesium 40 mg • Zinc 15 mg • Selenium 70 mcg • Copper 2 mg • Manganese 4 mg • Chromium 120 mcg • Molybdenum 75 mg • Chloride 72 mg • Potassium 80 mg.

Centrum Silver - Wyeth
Each tablet contains: Nickel (Nickelous Sulfate) 5 mcg • Vitamin A Acetate 5000 IU • Silicon Dioxide 2 mg • Vitamin C (Ascorbic Acid) 60 mg • Vitamin D 400 IU • Vanadium (Sodium Metavanadate) 10 mcg • Boron (Borates) 150 mcg • Vitamin E (dl-Alpha Tocopheryl Acetate) 45 IU • Vitamin K (Phytonadione)10 mcg • Thiamin Mononitrate (Vitamin B1) 1.5 mg • Riboflavin (Vitamin B2) 1.7 mg • Niacin (Niacinamide, Vitamin B3) 20 mg • Vitamin B6 (Pyridoxine Hydrochloride) 3 mg • Folate (Folic Acid) 400 mcg • Vitamin B12 (Cyanocobalamin) 25 mcg • Biotin 30 mcg • Pantothenic Acid (Calcium Pantothenate) 10 mg • Calcium Carbonate 200 mg • Phosphorus 48 mg • Iodine (Potassium Iodide) 150 mcg • Magnesium Oxide 100 mg • Zinc Oxide 15 mg • Selenium (Sodium Selenate) 20 mcg • Copper (Cupric Oxide) 2 mg • Manganese Sulfate 2 mg • Chromium Chloride 150 mcg • Molybdenum (Sodium Molybdate) 75 mg • Chloride 72 mg • Potassium Chloride 80 mg. Other Ingredients: Microcrystalline Cellulose, Gelatin, Starch, Crospovidone, Hydroxypropyl Methylcellulose, Titanium Dioxide, Sucrose, Magnesium Stearate, Triethyl Citrate, Lactose, Polysorbate 80, Beta Carotene, Lutein, Glucose, FD&C Yellow No. 6 Lake, FD&C Blue No. 2 Lake, FD&C Red No. 40 Lake.

Centrum with Lutein - Wyeth
Each tablet contains: Boron (Borates) 120 mcg • Vitamin A Acetate 5000 IU • Nickel (Nickelous Sulfate) 5 mcg • Vitamin C (Ascorbic Acid) 60 mg • Silicon Dioxide 2 mcg • Vitamin D 400 IU • Vitamin E (dl-Alpha Tocopheryl Acetate) 30 IU • Tin (Stannous Chloride) 10 mcg • Vanadium (Sodium Metavanadate) 10 mcg • Vitamin K (Phytonadione) 25 mcg • Lutein 250.0 mcg • Thiamin Mononitrate (Vitamin B1) 1.5 mg • Riboflavin (Vitamin B2) 1.7 mg • Niacin (Vitamin B3, Niacinamide) 20 mg • Vitamin B6 (Pyridoxine HCl) 2 mg • Folate (Folic Acid) 400 mcg • Vitamin B12 (Cyanocobalamin) 6 mcg • Biotin 30 mcg • Pantothenic Acid (Calcium Pantothenate) 10 mg • Calcium Carbonate 162 mg • Iron (Ferrous Fumarate) 18 mg

• Phosphorus 109 mg • Iodine (Potassium Iodide) 150 mcg • Magnesium Oxide 100 mg • Zinc Oxide 15 mg • Selenium (Sodium Selenate) 20 mcg • Copper (Cupric Oxide) 2 mg • Manganese Sulfate 2 mg • Chromium Chloride 120 mcg • Molybdenum (Sodium Molybdate) 75 mg • Potassium Chloride 80 mg. Other Ingredients: Calcium Phosphate, Microcrystalline Cellulose, Gelatin, Crospovidone, Hydroxypropyl Methylcellulose, Starch, Titanium Dioxide, Sucrose, Magnesium Stearate, Triethyl Citrate, Lactose, Polysorbate 80, Beta Carotene, Glucose, FD&C Yellow #6 Lake.

Century Formula **-** Swanson Health Products
Each tablet contains: Vitamin A (as acetate) 5000 IU • Vitamin C USP (as ascorbic acid) 90 mg • Vitamin D USP (as cholecalciferol) 400 IU • Vitamin E (as d-alpha tocopheryl acetate) 30 IU • Vitamin K (as phytonadione) 25 mcg • Thiamin USP (as thiamin mononitrate; vitamin B-1) 2.25 mg • Riboflavin USP (vitamin B-2) 2.6 mg • Niacinamide 20 mg • Vitamin B-6 (pyridoxine HCl) 3 mg • Folic Acid 400 mcg • Vitamin B-12 (as cyanocobalamin) 9 mcg • Biotin 25 mcg • Pantothenic Acid (as d-calcium pantothenate) 10 mg • Calcium (from dicalcium phosphate) 162 mg • Iron (as ferrous fumarate) 27 mg • Iodine (as potassium iodide) 150 mcg • Magnesium (from magnesium oxide) 100 mg • Zinc (from zinc fultate) 15 mg • Selenium (as sodium selenate) 25 mcg • Copper (from copper gluconate) 2 mg • Manganese (from manganese sulfate) 5 mg • Chromium (as chromium chloride) 25 mcg • Molybdenum (sodium molybdate) 25 mcg • Potassium (as potassium chloride) 57.2 mg.

Ceralin **-** Metagenics
Each tablet contains: Vitamin A (as mixed carotenoids) 2500 IU • Thiamin (as thiamin hydrochloride) 25 mg • Riboflavin 25 mg • Niacin (as niacinamide) 250 mg • Vitamin B6 (as pyridoxine hydrochloride) 12.5 mg • Folate (as 5-formyl tetrahydofolate) 200 mcg • Vitamin B12 (as methylcobalamin and cyanocobalamin) 100 mcg • Lutein (from tagetes erecta flower) 1.5 mg • Resveratrol (from polyganum cuspidatum root extract) 1 mg • Acetyl-L-Carnitine 200 mg • N-Acetylcysteine 300 mg • Ginkgo leaf extract (ginkgo biloba, standardized to 24% ginkgoflavonglycosides and 6% terpene lactones) 30 mg.

Cerebra **-** Natrapharm, Inc.
Each tablet contains: Huperzine A (Chinese club moss) 50 mcg • Vitamin E.

Cerebrex **-** Gero Vita International
Each capsule contains: Vitamin B6 (as pyridoxol-5-phosphate) 6.7 mg • Folic Acid 300 mcg • Citrus Bioflavonoids (13% bioflavonoids) 300 mg • Phosphatidylserine 150 mg • Ginkgo Biloba leaf extract (24% ginkgo flavoneglycosides/6% terpene lactones) 50 mg • Mixed Tocopherols 20 IU • Methylcobalamin 100 mcg. Other Ingredients: Rice Flour, Silicon Dioxide, Magnesium Stearate, Gelatin Capsule, ACF 223.

CerebroPlex **-** Life Enhancement Products, Inc.
Three capsules contain: Pantothenic Acid (vitamin B5 as calcium pantothenate) 75 mg • Ginkgo Biloba extract 360 mg • Citicoline (as cytidine 5'-diphosphocholine sodium salt) 250 mg • DHA (docosahexaenoic acid) 200 mg • Choline (as choline dihydrogen citrate) 150 mg • DMAE (as dimethylaminoethanol bitartrate) 150 mg • Phosphatidylserine 50 mg • Pregnenolone 25 mg • Vinpocetine 15 mg.

CerebroPlex (without pregnenolone) **-** Life Enhancement Products, Inc.
Three capsules contain: Pantothenic Acid (vitamin B5 as calcium pantothenate) 75 mg • Ginkgo Biloba extract 360 mg • Citicoline (as cytidine 5'-diphosphocholine sodium salt) 250 mg • DHA (docosahexaenoic acid) 200 mg • Choline (as choline dihydrogen citrate) 150 mg • DMAE (as dimethylaminoethanol bitartrate) 150 mg • Phosphatidylserine 50 mg • Vinpocetine 15 mg. Other Ingredients: Silicon Dioxide, Gelatin Capsule.

Cerebrovascular Support **-** Weil Lifestyle, LLC
Each Magnesium Glycinate tablet contains: Magnesium Glycinate 200 mg.

Cernilton Flower Pollen **-** Cernitin America
Two tablets contain: Rye Grass Pollen (Cernitin Flower Pollen) Extract Water-Soluble Pollen Extract (T60) 120 mg • Cernitin Flower Pollen Extract Fat-Soluble Pollen Concentrate (GBX) 6 mg. Other Ingredients: Cellulose (plant fiber), Magnesium Stearate (vegetable source).

Cernilton T.S. Flower Pollen Triple Strength **-** Cernitin America
Two capsules contain: Rye Grass Pollen (Cernitin Flower Pollen) Extract Water-Soluble Pollen concentrate (T60) 360 mg • Cernitin Flower Pollen extract fat-soluble pollen concentrate (GBX) 18 mg. Other Ingredients: Cellulose (plant fiber), Magnesium Stearate (vegetable source).

Certain Sleep **-** Gero Vita International
Two capsules contain: Vitamin B6 (as pyridoxine hydrochloride) 0.5 mg • Magnesium (as magnesium aspartate) 18.74 mg • Zinc (as zinc monomethionine, aspartate) 1.26 mg • Proprietary Blend 900 mg: Jujube seed extract, Schisandra fruit extract (10% schisandrin), Polygala root extract, Anemorrhena rhizome extract (1% sarsosapogenin), Chinese Thoroughwax root extract, Uncaria Rhynchophylla stem extract • 5-Hydroxytryptophan 100 mg. Other Ingredients: Silicon Dioxide, Magnesium Stearate, Gelatin.

Cetyl Myristoleate Complex **-** PhysioLogics
Each capsule contains: Cetyl Myristoleate Complex 550 mg. Other Ingredients: Gelatin, Vegetable Magnesium Stearate, Silica.

CetylPure **-** Natrol, Inc.
Two capsules contain: Cetyl Myristoleate proprietary blend (CetylPure) 1100 mg. Other Ingredients: Silica, Magnesium Stearate, Gelatin.

C-Flav **-** Ortho Molecular Products
Each capsule contains: Vitamin C (as ascorbic acid USP, acerola fruit extract) 400 mg • Acerola fruit extract (standardized to contain 17% vitamin C) 100 mg • Quercetin 70 mg • Hesperidin complex 50 mg • Hibiscus flowers 50 mg • Rutin 50 mg. Other Ingredients: Other Ingredients: Natural Vegetable Capsules, Ascorbyl Palmitate, Microcrystalline Cellulose, Silicon Dioxide.

CFS Supreme **-** Gaia Herbs
Thirty drops contain: Proprietary Blend 100 mg: Astragalus root (astragalus membranaceus), Eleuthero root (eleutherococcus senticosus), Gotu Kola leaf and root (centella asiatica), Ginkgo leaf (ginkgo biloba), Chinese Skullcap root (scutellaria baicalensis), Reishi mushroom (ganoderma lucidum), Wild Oats milky seed (avena sativa), Licorice root (glycyrrhiza glabra), Prickly Ash bark (xanthoxylum clava-herculis), Spring Water, 45% Pure Grain Alcohol USP.

C-Gel **-** J. R. Carlson Laboratories, Inc.
Each softgel contains: Vitamin C (as ascorbic acid) 1000 mg.

CGP **-** Metabolic Nutrition, Inc.
Each scoop (2 tsp) contains: Creatine - Glycerol - Phosphate 10 g • Potassium 720 mg • Alpha-Lipoic Acid 100 mg • Magnesium 75 mg • Calcium 50 mg • Sodium 30 mg.

C-Grams **-** Advocare International
Two caplets contain: Vitamin C (as potassium/magnesium/calcium ascorbates and ascorbic acid) 1000 mg • L-Lysine 300 mg • Mixed Citrus Flavonoids 100 mg • Alpha-Ketoglutaric Acid 50 mg. Other Ingredients: Dicalcium Phosphate, Silicon Dioxide, Cellulose, Stearic Acid, Magnesium Stearate.

CGT10 **-** Optimum Nutrition
Each 2 tsp (20 g) serving contains: Creatine Monohydrate 5 g • L-Glutamine 3 g • Taurine 2 g. Other Ingredients: Dextrose, Citric Acid, Beet Color, Artificial Flavor, Acesulfame Potassium.

Chai Hu Shu Gan San Plus **-** Secara
Bupleurum root 5:1 extract (chai hu) 316 mg • Tangerine peel 5:1 extract (chen pi) 316 mg • Organic Licorice root (gan cao) 269 mg •

BRAND NAMES

Bitter Orange young fruit 5:1 extract (zhi ke) 236 mg • Chinese Peony root 5:1 extract (bai shao) 236 mg • Cyperus rhizome 5:1 extract (xiang fu) 236 mg • Ligusticum Wallichii rhizome 5:1 extract (chuan xiong) 236 mg • Organic Cardamom seed 158 mg • Organic Caraway seed 113 mg • Organic Fennel seed 113 mg • Organic Fennel oil 78 mg • Caraway oil 7 mg • Bitter Orange oil 7 mg.
See Editor's Note No. 40.

Chamomile **-** Nature's Sunshine
Each capsule contains: Chamomile flower (matricaria recutita) 250 mg. Other Ingredients: Kosher Gelatin, Water.

Chamomile **-** Nature's Way
Two capsules contain: Chamomile flower 700 mg. Other Ingredients: Gelatin.

Chamomile & Ylang Ylang Body Lotion 8oz **-** Derma E
Purified Water • Jojoba Oil • Safflower oil • Glycerin • Octylpalmitate • Glyceryl Stearate • PEG 100 Stearate • Cetyl Alcohol • Tocopheryl Acetate (vitamin E) • Lavender oil • Geranium oil • Panthenol • Allantoin • Retinyl Palmitate (vitamin A) • Ergocalciferol (vitamin D) • Methylparaben • I. Urea • Fragrant Oils.

Chamomile Calm **-** Botanical Laboratories
Each 1 mL serving contains: Skullcap herb • Chamomile flowers • Fennel seed • Hops strobiles • Catnip herb. Other Ingredients: Kosher Coconut and/or Palm Kernal Glycerine, Purified Water, Citric Acid.

Chanca-Piedra **-** Jarrow Formulas
Each capsule contains: Phyllanthus Niruri 10:1 500 mg. Other Ingredients: Microcrystalline Cellulose.

Change of Life Menopause Relief **-** Abundance Marketing
Isoflavones (from kudzu root and soy green extracts) • Black Cohosh root extract • Licorice root extract • Chaste Tree berry extract • Raspberry leaf • Ginkgo Biloba leaf extract • Elderberry fruit extract.

Change-O-Life 7 Herb Blend Formula **-** Nature's Way
Three capsules contain: Proprietary Blend 1320 mg: Black Cohosh root, Blessed Thistle, Eleuthero root, False Unicorn root, Licorice root, Sarsaparilla root, Squaw Vine (vine, leaf, fruit). Other Ingredients: Gelatin, Magnesium Stearate.

Changes Now **-** Goldshield Elite
Two capsules contain: Vitamin C (Ascorbic acid) 50 mg • Lipase 300 LU • Calcium sulfate 100 mg • Multi-Source Fiber Complex 650 mg: Chitosan (Deacylated cellulose biopolymer), Glucomannan, Citrus Pectin, and Oat fiber. Other Ingredients: Gelatin, Magnesium stearate, and Silica.

Changes Relief **-** Goldshield Elite
Three caplets contain: Vitamin C (as Ascorbic Acid) 100 mg • Calcium (as Calcium Monohydrogen Phosphate) 300 mg • Phosphorus (as Calcium Monohydrogen Phosphate) 225 mg • Zinc (as Zinc Monomethionine) 13.75 mg • Copper (as Copper Gluconate) 500 mcg • Manganese (as Manganese Sulfate) 5 mg • Glucosamine Hydrochloride/Glucosamine Sulfate/N-Acetyl Glucosamine blend (with Chondroitin precursors) 750 mg • Turmeric rhizome standardized extract (12x) 300 mg • Boswellia serrata gum-resin 300 mg • Devil's Claw root standardized extract (5% harpagosides) 125 mg • Bromelain (80 GDU/g) 125 mg • White Willow bark 4:1 extract 150 mg • Ginger root standardized extract (5% gingerols) 125 mg • Alpine Snow Rose leaf (50% active polyphenolic proanthocyanidins) 213 mg. Other Ingredients: Vegetable cellulose, Fractionated vegetable oil, Soy polysaccharides, Silica, and Vegetable resin glaze.
See Editor's Note No. 15.

Changing Times **-** Nature's Plus
Two tablets contain: Wild Brazilian SUMA [Pfaffia paniculata (Martius) Kuntze] 300 mg • Calcium amino acid chelate/complex 200 mg • Magnesium amino acid chelate/complex 100 mg • Vitamin B6 (Pyridoxine HCL) 100 mg • Pantothenic Acid 100 mg • Phosphatidylcholine 100 mg • Siberian Ginseng (Eleutherococcus senticosus) 100 mg • Niacinamide 25 mg • Vitamin E natural 200 IU • Vitamin B12 from Cobalamin 200 mcg • Selenium yeast free, amino acid complex 50 mcg. Yeast free. Sugar & starch free.

Chaparral and Red Clover **-** Dial Herbs
Chaparral • Red Clover • Echinacea • Buchu leaves • Blood root.

Charcoal **-** Nature's Way
Two capsules contain: Activated Charcoal 560 mg. Other Ingredients: Gelatin.

Charcoal **-** Source Naturals
Each capsule contains: Charcoal 260 mg.

Charcoal **-** Country Life Vitamins
Each capsule contains: Activated Charcoal 520 mg.

Charco-Zyme **-** Atrium Biotechnologies
Each capsule contains: Papaya leaf 65 mg • Papain 32.5 mg • Mycozyme 32.5 mg • Rennin NF 3.75 mg • Activated Charcoal 130 mg. In a base of Alfalfa & Peppermint.

Chase Kolic Gripe Water **-** Stella Pharmaceutical Canada, Inc.
Each 5 mL contains: Alcohol Anhydrous 0.1945 mL • Ginger 0.05 mL • Dill Oil 0.002 mL • Sodium Bicarbonate 50 mg.

Chase Kolik Alcohol Free Gripe Water **-** Stella Pharmaceutical Canada, Inc.
Each 150 mL contains: Fennel Oil 0.05% • Sodium Bicarbonate 1%.

Chaser **-** Living Essentials
Each two capsules contain: Activated Calcium Carbonate 618 mg • Vegetable Carbon 332 mg.

Chaser Wine **-** Living Essentials
Each two caplets contains: Activated Calcium Carbonate 650 mg • Vegetable Carbon 350 mg • Vitamin B2 1 mg. Other Ingredients: Croscarmellose Sodium, Sucrose, Cellulose, Stearic Acid, Magnesium Citrate.

Chaste Tree-Siberian Ginseng Virtue **-** Blessed Herbs
Chaste Tree berry • Siberian Ginseng root • Hawthorn berry, leaf & flower • Lavender flower • Wild Yam root • Licorice root • Grain alcohol & Distilled Water.

Chasteberry Extract **-** Enzymatic Therapy
Each capsule contains: Chaste Tree berry extract (vitex agnus-castus, standardized to contain 0.5% agnusides) 225 mg. Other Ingredients: Gelatin, Cellulose, Magnesium Stearate, Silicon Dioxide, Titanium Dioxide Color.

Chasteberry Plus **-** Metagenics
Each tablet contains: Chasteberry fruit 10:1 extract (vitex agnus-castus) 100 mg • Black Cohosh root and rhizome extract (actaea racemosa, containing triterpene glycosides) 40 mg • Ashwagandha root extract (withania somnifera, standardized to 2% withanolides) 60 mg.

Cheat Tabs **-** Fizogen Precision Technologies Inc.
Three tablets contain: Enzytrox (calorie intercepting agent) 2000 mg: Glucomannan, Phaseolus Vulgaris extract, Platycodi radix extract, Garcinia Cambogia extract, Pandalidus Biopolymer extract • Neurotrol (appetite controlling blend) 130 mg: Hoodia Gordonii cactus extract, Caralluma cactus extract, Simthin Jojoba seed extract, Griffonia Simplicifolia seed extract • Digestol (hyper digestive fusion) 75 mg: Terminalia Chebula fruit extract, Terminlais Belerica fruit extract, Emblica Officinalis fruit extract. Other Ingredients: Di Calcium Phosphate, Magnesium Stearate, Stearic Histrene, Maltodextrin, Plasdone, Acesulfame-K.

Chelated Calcium **-** J. R. Carlson Laboratories, Inc.
Each tablet contains: Calcium (as calcium glycinate chelate) 250 mg.

Chelated Calcium **-** Puritan's Pride
Six tablets contain: Calcium (as Calcium Amino Acid Chelate) 900 mg.

Chelated Calcium Magnesium **-** Nature's Bounty
Two tablets contain: Calcium (as calcium carbonate, oyster shell, and calcium gluconate) 1000 mg • Magnesium (as magnesium oxide and magnesium gluconate) 500 mg. Other Ingredients: Cellulose (plant origin), Croscarmellose, Titanium Dioxide Color, Cellulose Coating, Vegetable Magnesium Stearate.

Chelated Calcium Magnesium 1:1 **-** Solgar
Four tablets contain: Calcium (as glycinate, carbonate, citrate) 500 mg • Magnesium (as glycinate, oxide, citrate) 500 mg • Iron 0.6 mg • Sodium 10 mg. Other Ingredients: Microcrystalline Cellulose, Vegetable Cellulose, Citric Acid, Maltodextrin, Silica, Titanium Dioxide, Vegetable Magnesium Stearate, Vegetable Glycerin, Carnauba Wax.

Chelated Calcium Magnesium Zinc **-** Nature's Bounty
Three tablets contain: Calcium (as Calcium Carbonate and Calcium Gluconate) 1000 mg • Magnesium (as Magnesium Oxide and Magnesium Gluconate) 400 mg • Zinc (as Zinc Gluconate and Zinc Citrate) 25 mg. Other Ingredients: Cellulose, Croscarmellose, Acacia Gum, Maltodextrin, Titanium Dioxide Color, Cellulose Coating, Vegetable Magnesium Stearate.

Chelated Calcium-Magnesium **-** Schiff
Six tablets contain: Calcium (as calcium glycinate from rice protein chelate) 780 mg • Magnesium (as magnesium glycinate from rice protein chelate) 468 mg. Other Ingredients: Citric Acid, Cellulose, Croscarmellose Sodium, Magnesium Stearate.

Chelated Cal-Mag **-** J. R. Carlson Laboratories, Inc.
Two tablets contain: Calcium (as calcium glycinate chelate) 400 mg • Magnesium (as magnesium glycinate chelate) 200 mg.

Chelated CAL-MAG **-** Puritan's Pride
Each tablet contains: Calcium 500 mg • Magnesium 250 mg.

Chelated Chromium **-** J. R. Carlson Laboratories, Inc.
Each tablet contains: Niacin (vitamin B3) 0 mg • Chromium (as chromium glycinate chelate) 200 mg.

Chelated Copper **-** J. R. Carlson Laboratories, Inc.
Each tablet contains: Copper (as copper glycinate chelate) 5 mg.

Chelated Iron **-** J. R. Carlson Laboratories, Inc.
Each tablet contains: Iron (as iron glycinate chelate) 27 mg.

Chelated Iron **-** Solgar
Each tablet contains: Calcium (as dicalcium phosphate) 45 mg • Iron (as iron bisglycinate) 25 mg. Other Ingredients: Dicalcium Phosphate, Microcrystalline Cellulose, Vegetable Cellulose, Vegetable Stearic Acid, Vegetable Magnesium Stearate, Vegetable Glycerin, Carnauba Wax.

Chelated Magnesium **-** J. R. Carlson Laboratories, Inc.
Two tablets contain: Magnesium (as magnesium glycinate chelate) 400 mg.

Chelated Magnesium **-** Solgar
Four tablets contain: Calcium (as dicalcium phosphate) 135 mg • Iron 0.7 mg • Magnesium (as magnesium glycinate amino acid chelate) 400 mg • Sodium 10 mg. Other Ingredients: Microcrystalline Cellulose, Dicalcium Phosphate, Vegetable Cellulose, Vegetable Stearic Acid, Vegetable Glycerin.

Chelated Magnesium Calcium 2:1 **-** Solgar
Three tablets contain: Magnesium (as citrate, oxide, glycinate) 600 mg • Calcium (as carbonate, glycinate, citrate) 300 mg • Iron 0.7 mg • Sodium 10 mg. Other Ingredients: Microcrystalline Cellulose, Vegetable Cellulose, Titanium Dioxide, Vegetable Magnesium Stearate, Vegetable Stearic Acid, Vegetable Glycerin, Silica, Carnauba Wax.

Chelated Manganese **-** J. R. Carlson Laboratories, Inc.
Each tablet contains: Manganese (as manganese glycinate chelate) 20 mg.

Chelated Manganese **-** Solgar
Each tablet contains: Calcium (as dicalcium phosphate) 50 mg • Manganese (as manganese glycinate amino acid chelate) 8 mg. Other Ingredients: Dicalcium Phosphate, Microcrystalline Cellulose, Vegetable Cellulose, Vegetable Magnesium Stearate.

Chelated Mineral Compleet **-** J. R. Carlson Laboratories, Inc.
Three tablets contain: Calcium (as calcium glycinate chelate) 300 mg • Iron (as iron glycinate chelate) 18 mg • Iodine (from kelp) 100 mcg • Magnesium (as magnesium glycinate chelate) 150 mg • Zinc (as zinc glycinate chelate) 15 mg • Selenium (from kelp) 77 mcg • Copper (as copper glycinate chelate) 1 mg • Manganese (as manganese glycinate chelate) 7 mg • Chromium (from kelp) 75 mcg • Potassium (as potassium glycinate complex) 60 mg.

Chelated Minerals **-** Arrowroot
Three tablets contain: Calcium 100 mg • Magnesium 500 mg • Manganese 30 mg • Zinc 30 mg • Potassium 14 mg • Iron 10 mg • Copper 1 mg • Iodine 150 mcg • Chromium 15 mcg • Selenium 15 mcg.

Chelated Molybdenum **-** Solgar
Each tablet contains: Calcium (as dicalcium phosphate) 85 mg • Molybdenum (as molybdenum amino acid chelate) 150 mcg. Other Ingredients: Dicalcium Phosphate, Vegetable Stearic Acid, Vegetable Cellulose, Casein, Vegetable Magnesium Stearate.

Chelated Zinc **-** J. R. Carlson Laboratories, Inc.
Each tablet contains: Zinc (as zinc glycinate chelate) 30 mg.

Chelated Zinc 100 mg **-** Puritan's Pride
Each tablet contains: Zinc (from Zinc Gluconate) 100 mg.

Chelated Zinc 25 mg **-** Puritan's Pride
Each tablet contains: Zinc (from Zinc Gluconate) 25 mg.

Chelated Zinc 50 mg **-** Puritan's Pride
Each tablet contains: Zinc (from Zinc Gluconate) 50 mg.

CheleX **-** Xymogen
Four capsules contain: DMSA 100 mg • EDTA 300 mg • Cilantro (coriandrum sativum) 300 mg • Chlorella 300 mg • Garlic (organic high-allicin) 600 mg • Humifulvate 160 mg • N-Acetyl-L-Cysteine 200 mg • Alpha-Lipoic Acid 100 mg.

Chem-Defense **-** Source Naturals
Each tablet contains: Molybdenum (aspartate, citrate) 120 mcg • Glutathione 50 mg • Coenzymated Vitamin B-2 (flavin mononucleotide) 2.25 mg.

Chem-Ex **-** Enzymatic Therapy
Two capsules contain: Pantothenic Acid (D-Calcium Pantothenate) 80 mg • Zinc (Chelate) 40 mg • L-Cysteine 300 mg • L-Methionine 200 mg • Alpha-Ketoglutarate 60 mg • Taurine 50 mg • Glycine 40 mg. This exclusive formula also contains Licorice root extracts (Glycyrrhiza glabra).

Chemotain **-** Ortho Molecular Products
Four capsules contain: Red root 4:1 extract 800 mg • Aloe Vera leaf exudate concentrate 200:1 extract 500 mg • Eclipta Alba leaf, root 10:1 extract 500 mg • Lipoic Acid 400 mg • Ginger root 300 mg • Rabdosia Rubescens 5:1 extract 200 mg • Ashwagandha root extract (standardized to contain 1.5% withanolides) 100 mg. Other Ingredients: Natural Vegetable Capsules, Magnesium Stearate, Microcrystalline Cellulose.

Cherry Fruit Extract **-** Enzymatic Therapy/PhytoPharmica
Two capsules contain: Sweet Cherry fruit 10:1 extract (prunus avium) 1000 mg.

Chew Chew Vites Multiple **-** Nature's Life
Two tablets contain: Vitamin A (Fish Liver oil) 5000 IU • Vitamin D (as Vitamin D3) (Cholecalciferol) 400 IU • Vitamin E (d-Alpha Tocopheryl with Beta, Gamma, & Delta Tocopherols) 30 IU • Vitamin B1 (Thiamine HCl) 5 mg • Vitamin B2 (Riboflavin) 5 mg • Vitamin

B6 Pyridoxine HCl) 5 mg • Vitamin B12 (Cyanocobalamin) 10 mcg • Niacinamide 10 mg • Pantothenic Acid (d-Calcium Pantothenate) 10 mg • Folic Acid 0.1 mg • Choline (Bitartrate) 25 mcg • Inositol 25 mcg • PABA (Para Aminobenzoic Acid) 300 mcg • Biotin 75 mcg • Vitamin C (with Rose Hips) 150 mg • Calcium (Carbonate, Gluconate, Citrate) 28 mg • Chromium (Picolinate Nutrition 21) 50 mcg • Copper (Full ranged Amino Acid Chelate) 0.1 mg • Iodine (Kelp) 0.1 mg • Iron (Full ranged Amino Acid Chelate) 5 mg • Magnesium (Full ranged Amino Acid Chelate)15 mg • Manganese (Full ranged Amino Acid Chelate) 0.3 mg • Phosphorus (Proteinate) 4 mg • Potassium (Proteinate) 11.5 mg • Silicon (Dioxide) 5 mg • Zinc (Picolinate) 2 mcg • Essential Fatty Acids 5 mg • Hawaiian Spirulina 10 mg • Chlorophyll, Alfalfa 10 mg • Chlorella algae 10 mg. In a natural base of low Glycemic pure Crystalline Fructose, pasteurized Honey powder, natural Lemon flavor, Vegetarian Acidophilus powder, natural Pineapple flavor, Rose Hips powder, Lecithin, Lemon Bioflavonoids, Barley Grass, Sunflower Seed powder, Rice Bran, Wheat Germ, Alfalfa leaf, Watercress & Parsley.

***Chewable Acerola C Complex 500 mg* - The Vitamin Shoppe**
Each wafer contains: Vitamin C (fortified with Acerola extract & Rose Hips Concentrate) 500 mg • Bioflavonoid complex 50 mg. Sweetened exclusively with fructose, a naturally occurring sweetener found in fruit, and all-natural Acerola cherry flavoring.

***Chewable C 500 (cherry flavor)* - GNC**
Each tablet contains: Vitamin A (100% as beta-carotene) 1000 IU •Vitamin C (as ascorbic acid and sodium ascorbate) 500 mg • Vitamin E (as dl-alpha tocopheryl acetate) 5 mg • Citrus Bioflavonoids Complex 5 mg. Other Ingredients: Sorbitol, Cellulose, Artificial and Natural Flavors, Stevia leaves powder.

***Chewable C 500 (fruit flavor)* - GNC**
Each tablet contains: Vitamin C (as ascorbic acid) 500 mg • Citrus Bioflavonoids Complex 5 mg. Other Ingredients: Dextrose, Turbinado Sugar, Cellulose, Artificial Flavor, Rose Hips powder (Rosina Canina), Acerola, Black Currant powder, Green Pepper powder, Hesperidin Complex, Rutin powder, Citrus Pectin, Potassium Chloride, Magnesium Oxide.

***Chewable C 500 (orange flavor)* - GNC**
Each tablet contains: Vitamin C (as ascorbic acid and sodium ascorbate with other natural sources of Vitamin C) 500 mg • Vitamin E (as dl-alpha tocopheryl acetate) 5 IU • Citrus Bioflavonoids Complex (from 12.5 mg of citrus bioflavonids complex 4X) 50 mg. Other Ingredients: Sorbitol, Natural Color (annatto), Natural Flavors, Magnesium Stearate, Cellulose, Acrola, Black Currant, Green Pepper.

***Chewable C 500 mg* - Sunmark**
Each chewable tablet contains: Vitamin C 500 mg. Other Ingredients: Sugar, Sodium Ascorbate, Stearic Acid, Microcrystalline Cellulose, Starch, FD&C Yellow No. 6 Lake, Artificial Flavor, Magnesium Stearate, Lactose, Gluten.
See Editor's Note No. 45.

***Chewable C 500 mg (tropical fruit flavor)* - Sunmark**
Each chewable tablet contains: Vitamin C 500 mg. Other Ingredients: Sorbitol, Sugar, Sodium Ascorbate, Natural and Artificial Flavors, Magnesium Stearate, Aspartame, Lactose, FD&C Yellow No. 5 Lake, FD&C Yellow No. 6 Lake, FD&C Blue No. 1 Lake, FD&C Red No. 40 Lake, Gluten.
See Editor's Note No. 45.

***Chewable C-500 mg with Rose Hips* - Puritan's Pride**
Each tablet contains: Vitamin C with Rose Hips 500 mg.

***Chewable Cal Mag Plus* - Shaklee**
Four tablets contain: Vitamin D (as Cholecalciferol) 200 IU • Calcium (as Calcium carbonate and Calcium citrate) • 1000 mg • Magnesium (as Magnesium oxide) 100 mg • Zinc (as Zinc gluconate) 1.5 mg • Copper (as Copper gluconate) 0.2 mg • Manganese (as Manganese gluconate) 0.2 mg • Boron (as Boron protein hydrolysate) 1.0 mg. Other Ingredients: Dextrose, Mannitol, Sorbitol, Acacia Gum, Natural Berry, Other Flavors, Citric Acid.

***Chewable Calcium* - Rexall - Sundown**
Each tablet contains: Vitamin D (as cholecalciferol) 100 IU • Calcium (as calcium carbonate) 600 mg. Other Ingredients: Dicalcium Phosphate, Microcrystalline Cellulose, Hydroxypropyl Merthylcellulose, Hydrogenated Cottonseed Oil, Magnesium Stearate, PEG.

***Chewable Calcium + D* - Leiner Health Products**
Each tablet contains: Calcium Carbonate 300 mg • Vitamin D (Ergocalciferol) 100 IU • Calories 5. Other Ingredients: Sorbitol, Stearic Acid, Cocoa, Magnesium Stearate, Maltodextrin, Silicon Dioixde, Natural Vanilla, Maltol, Gelatin.

***Chewable Calcium 500 mg* - Solgar**
Two wafers contain: Calcium (as calcium carbonate) 1000 mg • Iron 0.6 mg. Other Ingredients: Natural Sweetener (granulated cane juice), Natural Coconut Flavor With Other Natural Flavors, Vegetable Magnesium Stearate, Silica.

***Chewable Calcium 600 (cherry flavor)* - GNC**
Each tablet contains: Vitamin D (as cholecalciferol) 200 IU • Calcium (as calcium carbonate, tricalcium phosphate and calcium citrate) 600 mg • Boron (as boron gluconate) 1 mg. Other Ingredients: Sorbitol, Mannitol, Natural Flavor.

***Chewable Calcium for Women (caramel flavor)* - Walgreens**
Each chew contains: Vitamin D • Vitamin K 40 mcg • Calcium 500 mg • Sodium 10 mg. Other Ingredients: Corn Syrup, Sugar, Sweetened Condensed Milk, Cocoa Butter, Glycerin, Caramel Color, Artificial Cream Caramel Flavor, Soy Lecithin, Glyceryl Monostearate, Salt, Artificial Toffee Milk Flavor, Vanillin, Carrageenan.

***Chewable Calcium for Women (milk chocolate flavor)* - Walgreens**
Each chew contains: Vitamin D • Vitamin K 40 mcg • Calcium 500 mg • Sodium 10 mg. Other Ingredients: Corn Syrup, Sugar, Chocolate, Nonfat Milk, Cocoa Butter, Glycerin, Caramel Color, Salt, Soy Lecithin, Natural and Artificial Chocolate Flavor, Glyceryl Monostearate, Carrageenan.

***Chewable Calcium Malted Milk Balls* - Nature's Plus**
Four chewable tablets contain: Vitamin D (as ergocalciferol) 400 IU • Calcium (as lactate, aspartate, gluconate, carbonate) 1000 mg. Other Ingredients: Fructose, Acacia Gum, Microcrystalline Cellulose, Stearic Acid, Silica, Malted Milk, Nonfat Milk, Vanilla, Whey.

***Chewable Calcium with Vitamin D* - Nature's Bounty**
Four wafers contain: Vitamin D (as Ergocalciferol) 400 IU • Calcium (as Calcium Carbonate and Dicalcium Phosphate) 560 mg • Phosphorus (as Dicalcium Phosphate) 100 mg • Buckwheat (Fagopyrum esculentum) seed 10.4 mg • Corn Bran (Zea mays) seed 10.4 mg. Other Ingredients: Sucrose, Dextrose, Cellulose, Acacia Gum, Cottonseed Oil, Artificial Flavor, Silica, Vegetable Magnesium Stearate, Sodium Chloride.

***Chewable Cellular Forte with IP-6 and Inositol* - PhytoPharmica**
Each tablet contains: Calcium (from calcium magnesium phytate) 130 mg • Inositol 220 mg • IP-6 (inositol hexaphosphate from calcium magnesium phytate) 800 mg • Magnesium (from calcium magnesium phytate) 40 mg • Phosphorus (from calcium magnesium phytate) 190 mg.

***Chewable Digestion* - Enzymes, Inc.**
Each chewable tablet contains: Proprietary Enzyme Blend 209 mg: Amylase, Invertase, Glucoamylase, Protease, Lipase, Malt Diastase, Lactase, Cellulase, Pectinase, CereCalase, alpha-Galactosidase, Peptidase. Other Ingredients: Dextrose (Corn Sugar), Fructose (Fruit Sugar), Natural Raspberry Flavor, Silica (Mineral), Plant Cellulose, Citric Acid, Veg. Magnesium Stearate, Proprietary Plant-derived Sweetener.

Chewable E - Country Life Vitamins
Each wafer contains: Vitamin E (D-alpha tocopheryl succinate) 450 IU.

Chewable E 400 - GNC
Each tablet contains: Vitamin E (as d-alpha Tocopheryl Succinate) 400 IU. Other Ingredients: Dextron, Sorbitol, Fructose, Cellulose, Natural Flavors.

Chewable Echinacea - Leiner Health Products
Two tablets contain: Vitamin C (Ascorbic Acid) 60 mg • Total Carbohydrates 2 g • Echinacea Purpurea root powder 25 mg. Other Ingredients: Dextrose, Natural Raspberry Flavor, Magnesium Stearate, Silicon Dioxide, Carmine.

Chewable Ester-C 300 - GNC
Each tablet contains: Vitamin C (as Ester-C Calcium Ascorbate) 300 mg. Other Ingredients: Sorbitol, Sucrose, Dextrose, Fructose, Carrageenan, Citric Acid, Natural Wildberry Flavor, Sucralose.

Chewable Iron w/Vitamin C & Herbs - Nature's Plus
Each chewable tablet contains: Vitamin C (as ascorbic acid) 100 mg • Iron (as amino acid chelate) 27 mg. Other Ingredients: Fructose, Rose Hips (rosa canina), Beet Root (beta vulgaris), Raspberry Leaf (rubus idaeus), Stearic Acid, Silica.

Chewable Orange Juice C 500 mg - The Vitamin Shoppe
Each chewable tablet contains: 500 mg Vitamin C, blend of natural Orange Juice concentrate, Orange Juice pulp, Orange peels, and natural fruit sugar.

Chewable Q-60 + Creatine - Jarrow Formulas
Each tablet contains: Coenzyme Q10 (USP grade) 60 mg • Creatine 500 mg. Other Ingredients: Xylitol, Fibersol-2 Brand Maltodextrin, Magnesium Stearate (vegetable source), Lo Han Kuo (m. grosvenorii), Microcrystalline Cellulose, Silicon Dioxide, Stearic Acid (vegetable source), Natural Orange Cream Flavor.

Chewable Vita C - Shaklee
Each tablet contains: Vitamin C (as Ascorbic acid) 100 mg. Other Ingredients: Sorbitol, Rosehips Powder, Natural Lemon Flavor, Lemon Bioflavonoid, Hesperidin Complex, Orange Bioflavonoid, Grapefruit Bioflavonoid, Grapefruit Oil.

Chewable Vitamin C - GNC
Each tablet contains: Vitamin C (as Ascorbic Acid and other natural sources of Vitamin C) 100 mg • Citrus Bioflavonoids Complex 5 mg. Other Ingredients: Dextrose, Turbinado Sugar, Stearic Acid, Magnesium Stearate, Artificial Flavor, Rose hips, Acerola, Black Currant, Green Pepper, Hesperidin, Rutin, Citrus pectin, Potassium Chloride, Magnesium Oxide.

Chewable Vitamin C - Ortho Molecular Products
Each chewable tablet contains: Vitamin C (as ascorbic acid, sodium ascorbate) 600 mg • Acerola fruit juice powder (18% vitamin C) 75 mg • Quercetin Dihydrate 30 mg • Hesperidin complex 25 mg • Rosehips 25 mg • Rutin 15 mg. Other Ingredients: Natural Oragne Flavor, Natural Cane Sugar.

Chewable Vitamin C - Nature's Sunshine
Two tablets contain: Vitamin C (ascorbic acid) 500 mg. Other Ingredients: Fructose, Sorbitol, Freeze-Dried Orange Juice, Stearic Acid, Xylitol, Rose Hips Fruit (rosa canina), Magnesium Stearate, Silicon Dioxide, Natural Orange Flavor, Natural Lemon-Lime Flavor.

Chewable Vitamin C 500 mg - Walgreens
Each tablet contains: Vitamin C (ascorbic acid) 500 mg. Other Ingredients: Sorbitol, Sodium Ascorbate, Natural Orange Juice Powder, Natural Flavors, Artificial Flavors, Magnesium Stearate, Sucrose, Sucralose Non-Nutritive Sweetener, FD&C Yellow No. 6 Lake.

Chewable Vitamin C 500 mg - Nature Made
Each tablet contains: Vitamin C (from sodium ascorbate, ascorbic acid, lemon bioflavonoids) 500 mg. Other Ingredients: Sugar, Fructose, Stearic Acid, Dextrose, Maltodextrin, Corn Starch, Magnesium Stearate, Natural Orange Flavors with Other Natural Flavors, Silica Gel.
See Editor's Note No. 45.

Chewable Vitamin C with Acerola - Leiner Health Products
Each wafer contains: Vitamin C 500 mg • Other Ingredients: Sugar, Ascorbic Acid, Stearic Acid, Cellulose, Silicon Dioxide, Artificial Flavor, Acerola, Magnesium Stearate, Starch, Rose Hips, Lemon Bioflavonoids Complex, Hesperidin Complex, Buckwheat, Caramel, Rutin, Green Pepper Extract, Black Currant Extract.

Chew-Iron - J. R. Carlson Laboratories, Inc.
Each tablet contains: Iron (as iron glycinate chelate) 27 mg.

Chewy C 500 Orange - GNC
Each chew contains: Vitamin C 500 mg. Ingredients: Corn syrup, Sugar, Partially Hydrogenated Soybean oil, Ascorbic Acid, Mono & Diglycerides, Soy Lecithin, Salt, Natural Flavor, FD&C Yellow #6.

Chezyn - Standard Process, Inc.
Each tablet contains: Proprietary Blend 153 mg: Bovine Liver, Beet root, Dried Beet root juice, Oat flour • Iron 5 mg • Zinc 10 mg • Copper 0.2 mg. Other Ingredients: Honey, Arabic Gum, Calcium Stearate.

CHI Chinese Herbal Bar - Nature's Plus
Each bar contains: Vitamin A 1000 IU • Vitamin C 12 mg • Calcium 200 mg • Iron 3.6 mg • Vitamin D 80 IU • Vitamin E 6 IU • Thiamin 0.3 mg • Riboflavin 0.34 mg • Niacin 4 mg • Vitamin B6 0.4 mg • Folic Acid 80 mcg • Vitamin B12 1.2 mcg • Biotin 60 mcg • Pantothenic Acid 2 mg • Iodine 30 mcg • Magnesium 80 mg • Zinc 3 mg • Selenium 5 mcg • Copper 0.4 mg • Manganese 1 mg • Chromium 5 mcg • Molybdenum 5 mcg • Huang Qi (astragalus root) 312 mg • Dang Shen (relative root) 228 mg • Ling Zhi (reishi mushroom) 192 mg • Bai Zhu (atractylodes root) 144 mg • Ji Xue Teng (millettia stem) 144 mg • Tu Si Zi (dodder seed) 144 mg • Shan Yao (Chinese yam root) 144 mg • Nu Zhen Zi (privet fruit) 144 mg • Di Huang (rehmannia root) 138 mg • Bei Sha Shen (sand root) 136 mg • Wu Wei Zi (schisandra fruit) 114 mg • Jiang (ginger root) 114 mg • Suan Zao Ren (jujube seed) 114 mg • Chieh Keng (balloon flower root) 114 mg • Gan Cao (licorice root) 108 mg • Peony root (bai shoa) 72 mg • Ju Luo (tangerine peel) 72 mg.

Chickweed - Nature's Sunshine
Two capsules contain: Chickweed aerial parts (stellaria media) 750 mg. Other Ingredients: Kosher Gelatin, Water.

Chickweed Formula - Quest
Each caplet contains: Chickweed powder (Stellaria media) 120 mg • Fennel seed powder (Foeniculum vulgare) 80 mg • Burdock root powder (Actium lappa) 80 mg • Chia seeds powder (Salvia columbariae) 70 mg • Bladderwrack powder (Fucus Vesiculosis) 30 mg • Kelp powder (Fucus Vesiculosis) 30 mg. Other Ingredients: Calcium Phosphate, Microcrystalline Cellulose, Vegetable Stearin, Croscarmellose Sodium, Magnesium Stearate (vegetable source).

Child Lax - Dial Herbs
Senna • Fennel • Rhubarb.

Children Immu-C - Nutri-Quest Rx
Each tablet contains: Vitamin C (Sago Palm) 125 mg • Biotin 20 mcg • Folic Acid 10 mcg • Vitamin A (Palmitate) 1500 IU • Rutin 7.5 mg • Lemon Bioflavonoids 10 mg • Hesperidin Complex 7.5 mg • Propolis 1 mg • Lymph 1 mg • Thymus 1 mg • Spleen 1 mg. In a base of Fructose & Maltodextrin, with pleasant tasting Tropical Fruit Flavoring.
See Editor's Note No. 14.

Children's Calming - Nature's Sunshine
Gelsemium Sempervirens (yellow jessamine) 4X • Henbane (hyoscyamus niger) 6X • Saccharum Officinale (cane sugar) 6X • Hepar Sulfuris Calcareum (calcium sulfide) 8X • Lycopodium Clavatum

BRAND NAMES

(club moss) 8X • Ambra Grisea (ambergris) 10X. Other Ingredients: Purified Water, Glycerin, Potassium Benzoate. See Editor's Note No. 1.

Children's Chewable Multivitamin - Arrowroot
Each tablet contains: Vitamin A 2500 IU • Biotin 50 mcg • Beta Carotene 2500 IU • Folic Acid 10 mcg • Vitamin D 400 IU • Copper 0.01 mg • Vitamin E 25 IU • PABA 0.4 mg • Vitamin C 75 mg • Iron 5 mg • Vitamin B1 5 mg • Iodine 0.1 mg • Vitamin B2 5 mg • Manganese 3 mcg • Vitamin B6 5 mg • Magnesium 6 mcg • Vitamin B12 10 mcg • Zinc 20 mcg • Niacinamide 10 mg • Calcium 10 mg • Pantothenic Acid 10 mg.

Children's Chewable Vita-Bear - The Vitamin Shoppe
Each tablet contains: Vitamin C 200 mg • Citrus Bioflavonoid Complex 20 mg.

Children's Chewable Vitamin C - Health Smart Vitamins
Each tablet contains: Vitamin C (as ascorbic acid) 250 mg.

Children's Chewable Vitamins with Minerals - Schiff
Each tablet contains: Vitamin A (as palmitate) 5000 IU • Vitamin C (as ascorbic acid) 60 mg • Vitamin D (as cholecalciferol) 400 IU • Vitamin E (as D-alpha tocopheryl succinate) 30 IU • Thiamin (as mononitrate) 1.5 mg • Riboflavin 1.7 mg • Niacin (as niacinamide) 20 mg • Vitamin B6 (as pyridoxine hydrochloride) 2 mg • Folic Acid 400 mcg • Vitamin B12 (as cyanocobalamin) 6 mcg • Calcium (as calcium phosphate) 41 mg • Iron (as ferrous fumarate) 18 mg • Phosphorus (as calcium phosphate) 31 mg • Magnesium (as oxide) 6 mg • Zinc (as oxide) 2 mg. Other Ingredients: Fructose, Cellulose, Sorbitol, Stearic Acid, Natural Flavor, Silica, Magnesium Stearate, Citric Acid.

Children's Chewables - Swanson Health Products
Each tablet contains: Vitamin A (as acetate, beta-carotene) 2500 IU • Vitamin C USP (as ascorbic acid) 60 mg • Vitamin D (as cholecalciferol) 400 IU • Vitamin E (as d-alpha tocopheryl acetate) 15 IU • Thiamin USP (as thiamin HCl; vitamin B-1) 1.05 mg • Riboflavin USP (vitamin B-2) 1.2 mg • Niacinamide 13.5 mg • Vitamin B-6 (pyridoxine HCl) 1.05 mg • Folic Acid 300 mcg • Vitamin B-12 (cyanocobalamin) 4.5 mcg.

Children's Echinacea+C+Zinc (raspberry flavor) - LiFizz Effervescent Vitamins
Each tablet contains: Vitamin C 400 mg • Zinc (Zinc Oxide, Zinc Sulfate) 10 mg • Echinacea extract (Echinacea purpurea) 67 mg. Other Ingredients: Citric Acid, Sodium Bicarbonate, Sorbitol, Mannitol, Red Beet Powder, Raspberry Flavor, Polyethylene Glycol 6000, Aspartame, Acesulfame Potassium, Wild Berry Powder, Magnesium Stearate, Silicon Dioxide.

Children's Imu-A liquid extract - Ortho Molecular Products
Proprietary Blend 13 mg: Coriander seed extract, Echinacea Purpurea whole plant extract, Pau d'Arco bark extract, Cinnamon bark extract, Echinacea Angustifolia root extract, Goldenseal root extract.

Children's Multi Chewables - Benepure, Inc
Each wafter contains: Vitamin A (1250 IU as fish liver oil and 1250 IU as beta-carotene) 2500 IU • Vitamin C 50 mg • Vitamin D 40 IU • Vitamin E (as D-alpha tocopheryl succinate) 11 IU • Thiamin 1.2 mg • Riboflavin 1.4 mg • Niacin 16 mg • Vitamin B6 1.6 mg • Folic Acid 200 mcg • Vitamin B12 3 mcg • Biotin 65 mcg • Pantothenic Acid 4 mg • Calcium 40 mg • Iron 2 mg • Iodine (from kelp) 40 mcg • Magnesium 20 mg • Zinc 0.5 mg • Selenium 5 mcg • Copper 0.002 mg • Magnanese 0.25 mg • Chromium 5 mcg • Molybdenum 2.5 mcg • Potassium 10 mg • Lecithin 10 mg • Choline 2 mg • Inositol 2 mg • PABA (para-aminobenzoic acid) 2 mg • Mixed Citrus Bioflavonoids 5 mg • Hesperidin 2.5 mg • Pectin 2.5 mg. Other Ingredients: Fructose, Honey, Fruit Juice Powder, Natural Grape and Strawberry Flavors, Calcium Carbonate, Magnesium Oxide, Vegetable Stearate, Potassium Gluconate, Stearic Acid, Calcium Pantothenate, Ferrous Fumarate, Zinc Gluconate, Magnesium Gluconate, Amino Acid Chelates (selenium, chromium, molybdenum), Cupric Gluconate.

Children's Multi Vitamins - Jamieson
Each tablet contains: Vitamin A 5000 IU • Vitamin D (as Vitamin D3) 400 IU • Vitamin C 100 mg • Vitamin E 5 IU • Vitamin B1 1.5 mg • Vitamin B2 1.2 mg • Vitamin B6 1 mg • Vitamin B12 6 mcg • Pantothenic Acid 10 mg • Niacinamide 10 mg • Iron 5 mg.

Children's Multivitamin Liquid - Schiff
Two teaspoons (10 ml) contain: Vitamin A (as vitamin A acetate) 2500 IU • Vitamin C (as ascorbic acid) 40 mg • Vitamin D (as cholecalciferol) 400 IU • Vitamin E (as alpha tocopheryl acetate) 10 IU • Thiamin (as thiamin hydrochloride) 0.7 mg • Riboflavin (as riboflavin-5-phosphate) 0.8 mg • Niacin (as niacinamide) 9 mg • Vitamin B6 (as pyridoxine hydrochloride) 0.7 mg • Folate (as folic acid) 200 mcg • Vitamin B12 (as cyanocobalamin) 3 mcg • Biotin 150 mcg • Pantothenic Acid (as D-calcium pantothenate) 5 mg • Iron (as ferrous sulfate) 10 mg • Zinc (as zinc sulfate) 8 mg. Other Ingredients: Mannitol, Water, Glycerin, Propylene Glycol, Natural Flavor, Carrageenan, Citric Acid.

Children's Multivitamins - AIE Pharmaceuticals
Each chew contains: Vitamin A (as retinylacetate) • Vitamin C (as ascorbic acid) • Vitamin D (as cholecalciferol) • Vitamin E (as D-alpha tocopheryl acetate) • Thiamin (as thiamin mononitrate) • Riboflavin • Niacin (as niacinamide) • Vitamin B6 (as pyridoxine hydrochloride) • Folic Acid • Vitamin B12 (as cyanocobalamin).

Children's Multi-Vitamins - LiFizz Effervescent Vitamins
Each tablet contains: Vitamin A 2500 IU • Vitamin C 60 mg • Vitamin D 200 IU • Vitamin E 9 IU • Thiamin 1.05 mg • Riboflavin 1.19 mg • Niacinamide 14 mg • Vitamin B6 1.4 mg • Folic Acid 280 mcg • Vitamin B12 4.2 mcg • Biotin 210 mcg • Pantothenic Acid 7.9 mg • Calcium 200 mg. Available in Grape, Bubblegum, Orange, and Fruit Punch flavors.

Children's Vita-Gels - Nature's Plus
Each softgel contains: Vitamin A (as beta carotene) 5000 IU • Vitamin C (as ascorbic acid) 50 mg • Vitamin D (as ergocalciferol) 200 IU • Vitamin E (as d-alpha tocopheryl acetate) 25 IU • Vitamin B1 (as thiamine HCl) 5 mg • Vitamin B2 (as riboflavin) 5 mg • Niacin (as niacinamide) 10 mg • Vitamin B6 (as pyridoxine HCl) 5 mg • Folate (as folic acid) 10 mcg • Vitamin B12 (as cyanocobalamin) 10 mcg • Biotin 50 mcg • Pantothenic Acid (as calcium pantothenate) 10 mg • Calcium (as gluconate) 10 mg • Iron (as gluconate) 5 mg • Iodine (from kelp) 100 mcg • Magnesium (as gluconate) 0.25 mg • Zinc (as gluconate) 0.25 mg • Manganese (as gluconate) 0.05 mg • Potassium (as gluconate) 1 mg • Choline (as bitartrate) 2 mg • Inositol 1 mg • PABA (para-aminobenzoic acid) 0.6 mg.

Child's Chewable Vitamins + Iron - Penwel
Each tablet contains: Vitamin A (Acetate & Beta Carotene) 2500 IU • Vitamin D (Ergocalciferol) 400 IU • Vitamin E (dl-Alpha tocopheryl Acetate) 15 IU • Vitamin C (Ascorbic Acid & Sodium Ascorbate) 60 mg • Folic Acid 0.3 mcg • Thiamine Mononitrate (Vitamin B1) 1.05 mg • Riboflavin (Vitamin B2) 1.2 mg • Niacin (Niacinamide) 13.5 mg • Vitamin B6 (Pyridoxine HCl) 1.05 mg • Vitamin B12 (Cyanocobalamin) 4.5 mcg • Iron (Ferrous Fumarate) 15 mg. Other Ingredients: Sugar, Corn Syrup Solids, Partially Hydrogenated Vegetable Oil, Stearic Acid, Maltodextrin, Natural and Artificial Flavorings, Starch, Tartaric Acid, Artificial Colors (Red #40, Blue #2, Yellow #6), Magnesium Stearate, and Gelatin.

Chill Out - Pacific BioLogic
Gotu Kola • Peony root • Polygoni vine • Valerian root • Passion flower • Skullcap • Lemon Balm • Sweetflag rhizome • Polygala root • Citrus peel (unripened) • Salvia root • Schizandra fruit.

Chill Pill - Futurebiotics LLC
Three tablets contain: Vitamin B1 (thiamin) 5 mg • Vitamin B2 (riboflavin) 5 mg • Niacinamide 200 mg • Calcium (carbonate, phosphate, amino acid chelate) 150 mg • Vitamin B6 5 mg. In a balanced formula of Herbal extracts & powders: Valerian root, Chamomile, Avena Sativa, Kava Kava, Hops, Skullcap, Spearmint, Nettles, Hawthorn, Fennel, Horsetail, Peppermint, Motherwort.

Some Brand Name Natural Products - What they Contain

www.NaturalDatabase.com contains MANY more listings than appear here.
Editor's Notes are located on pages 2155-2163.

China Balsem - Districare
Lignum Sappan • Herba Linderniae Angustifoliae • Perucarpium Zanthoxyli • Folium Artemissiae Argyi • Radix Angelica Pubescentis • Cortex Acanthopanacis Radicis • Herba Veronicae Pergrinae • Herba Lycopodi • Rhizoma Seu Radix Notopterygi • Radix Angelica Sinensis • Olibanum • Myrrha • Resina Draconis • Eupolyphaga Seu Steleophaga • Metholum • Rhizoma Spargami • Rhizoma Zedoariae • Camphora.
See Editor's Note No. 1.

China Chlorella 200 Mg - Natrol, Inc.
Fifteen tablets contain: Protein 2 mg • Vitamin A 1665 mg • Vitamin C 500 mg • Thiamine (B1) 45 mcg • Riboflavin (B2) 140 mcg • Niacin 714 mcg • Calcium 6.2 mg • Iron 5 mg • Vitamin E 0.03 IU • Vitamin B6 51 mcg • Folic Acid 0.8 mcg • Vitamin B12 4 mcg • Phosphorus 30 mg • Iodine 18 mcg • Potassium 27.3 mg • Magnesium 10 mg • Zinc 2.2 mg • Copper 3 mcg • Biotin 6 mcg • Pantothenic Acid 40 mcg • Chlorophyll 90.1 mg • RNA 89.1 mg • DNA 8.5 mg • Germanium 76 ppm.

Chinac Digestive Health Formula - Metabolife International, Inc.
Each caplet contains: Amomum longiligulare (Chinese Amomum) • Oryza sativa (Rice) • Artemisia annua (Sweet Wormwood) • Crataegus cuneata (Chinese Hawthorn) • Armeniaca amarum (Apricot) • Xanthium sibiricum (Xanthium) • Wolfiporia cocos (Poria) • Coix Lacryma-jobi (Job's Tears).

Chinac Joint Health Formula - Metabolife International, Inc.
Each caplet contains: Achryanthes bidentata (achyranthes) • Wenyujin concisa (wen curcuma) • Erythrina variegata (coral tree) • Atractylodes Macrocephala (bai-zhu atractylodes) • Notopterygium Incisum (notopterygium) • Angelica Pubescens (pubescent angelica).

Chinac Menstrual Health Formula - Metabolife International, Inc.
Each caplet contains: Lindera Aggregata (lindera) • Leonurus Japonicus (Chinese motherwort) • Angelica Sinensis (dong quai) • Cyperus Rotundus (cyperus) • Corydalis Yanhusuo (corydalis).

Chinac Stress and Tension Formula - Metabolife International, Inc.
Each caplet contains: Corydalis yanhusuo (Corydalis) • Angelica dahurica (Fragrant Angelica) • Ligusticum sinense (Sichuan Lovage) • Saposhnikovia divaricata (Siler) • Arctium lappa (Burdock).

Chinese Anti-Gas - Nature's Sunshine
Three capsules contain: Proprietary Blend 1605 mg: Agastache tops (agastache rugosa), Crataegus Pinnatifida fruit, Poria Cocos (hoelen sclerotium), Magnolia bark (magnolia liliflora and officinalis), Oryza Sativa, Shen-Chu whole plant (xanthium stramonium), Citrus Aurantium peel, Gastrodia rhizome (gastrodia elata), Panax Ginseng root, Typhonium rhizome (typhonium flagelliforme), Atractylodes rhizome (atractylodes lancea), Cardamon fruit (amomum villosum), Platycodon root (platycodon grandiflorum), Ginger rhizome (zingiber officinale), Licorice root (glycyrrhiza uralensis). Other Ingredients: Gelatin, Water.
See Editor's Note No. 40.

Chinese Blood Build - Nature's Sunshine
Three capsules contain: Proprietary Blend 1410 mg: Dong Quai root (angelica sinensis), Ganoderma Lucidum plant, Lycium fruit (lycium chinense), Peony root (paeonia officinalis and lactiflora), Bupleurum root (bupleurum chinense), Cornus fruit (cornus officinalis), Curcuma root (curcuma longa), Salvia root (salvia sclarea), Achyranthes root (achyranthes aspera), Alisma rhizome (alisma plantago-aquatica), Astragalus root (astragalus membranaceus), Atractylodes rhizome (atractylodes lancea), Ho Shou Wu root (polygonum multiflorum), Ligustrum Lucidum rhizome, Cnidium Japonicum, Ligusticum Wallchii, Rehmannia root (rehmannia glutinosa), Cyperus rhizome (cyperus rotundus), Panax Ginseng root. Other Ingredients: Gelatin, Water.

Chinese Green Tea 400 mg - Nature's Plus
Each capsule contains: Chinese Green Tea leaf (camellia sinensis, decaffeinated and standardized to 50% polyphenols) 400 mg. Other Ingredients: Di-calcium Phosphate, Silica, Vegetable Cellulose, Purified Water.

Chinese Herbal Formula - Futurebiotics LLC
Four tablets contain: Proprietary Blend of extracts and powders equivalent to a minumum of 7000 mg: Siberian Ginseng, Foti, Astragalus, Schizandra, LEM, Shiitake - Ganoderma Mushroom Complex, Chinese Licorice, Codonopsis, Echinacea • Beta Carotene 10,000 IU • Vitamin E (mixed tocopherols) 100 IU • Vitamin C 1000 mg • Selenium 100 mcg.

Chinese Red Ginseng 550 mg - Vitamin World
Each capsule contains: Chinese Red Ginseng root (Panax ginseng) 550 mg. Other Ingredients: Gelatin, Vegetable Magnesium Stearate, Silica.

Chisukit Syrup - Hadas Natural Products
Each 5 mL serving contains: Fructose-Glucose syrup with Sorbitol • Echinacea Angustifolia & Purpurea standardized organic extract 250 mg • Propolis standardized extract 250 mg • Rose Hip extract with Vitamin C 300 mg.

Chito Block 2000 Plus C - Tiffin International, Inc.
Three capsules contain: Chitosan 990 mg • Iron 0.5 mg • Vitamin C 60 mg. Other Ingredients: Microcrystalline Cellulose, Gelatin, Sodium Lauryl Sulfate, Colloidal Silicon Dioxide, Purified Water, Stearic Acid, Hydrogenated Vegetable Oil.
See Editor's Note No. 37.

Chitodrene - Sterling-Grant Laboratories
Two tables contain: Vitamin C (as ascorbic acid) 100 mg • Chitosan (marine fiber concentrate) 1000 mg • Calcium 200 mg • Vegetable Cellulose 200 mg. Other Ingredients: Gelatin, Dicalcium Phosphate, Magnesium Stearate, Silica.

ChitoLite - 4 Life
Each capsule contains: Proprietary Blend 340 mg: Chitosan, L-Ascorbic Acid, Erythorbic Acid, Aloe Vera. Other Ingredients: Gelatin.

Chitoplex - Gero Vita International
Each teaspoon contains: Vitamin B6 (as pyridoxine hydrochloride) 10 mg • Chromium (as chromium polynicotinate) 500 mcg • Vitamin C (from acerola) 30 mg • Chitosan (15%) 3000 mg. Other Ingredients: Purified Water, Glycerine, Fructose, Natural Flavor, Citric Acid, Potassium Sorbate, Grapefruit Seed Extract.

Chitorex - Selmedica Healthcare
Pure 100% Chitosan liquid.

Chitosan - Puritan's Pride
Two tablets contain: Chitosan 1000 mg.

Chitosan - Swanson Health Products
Two capsules contain: LipoSan Ultra Chitosan (90%-93% deacetylated) 1 g.

Chitosan - The Vitamin Shoppe
Each capsule contains: Chitosan, minimum 90% Deacetylated Chitin 250 mg • Aloe Vera 50 mg.

Chitosan - Leiner Health Products
Two tablets contain: Chromium (Chromium picolinate) 100 mcg • Vitamin C 120 mg • Chitosan 1000 mg. Other Ingredients: Calcium Carbonate, Cellulose, Sodium Ascorbate, Maltodextrin, Acacia, Stearic Acid, Hydroxypropyl Methylcellulose, Magnesium Stearate, Hydroxypropyl Cellulose, Starch, Polysorbate 80, Polyethylene Glycol 3350.

Chitosan - Pro Health
Two capsules contain: Chitosan 1000 mg. Other Ingredients: Gelatin.

Some Brand Name Natural Products - What they Contain

www.NaturalDatabase.com contains MANY more listings than appear here.
Editor's Notes are located on pages 2155-2163.

BRAND NAMES

Chitosan **-** Olympian Labs
Two capsules contain: Chitosan 1000 mg.

Chitosan **-** PhysioLogics
Two tablets contain: Chitosan 1000 mg. Other Ingredients: Dicalcium Phosphate, Cellulose (plant origin), Vegetable Stearic Acid, Croscarmellose, Silica, Cellulose Coating, Vegetable Magnesium Stearate.

Chitosan 500 mg **-** Natrol, Inc.
Two capsules contain: Chitosan (95% deacetylated) 1000 mg. See Editor's Note No. 37.

Chitosan 750mg **-** Nature's Own
Each tablet contains: Chitosan 750 mg.

Chitosan Diet Formula **-** Optimum Nutrition
Two capsules contain: Vitamin C (ascorbic acid) 200 mg • Chitosan (fiber, 90-95% deacetylated) 1 g. Other Ingredients: Gelatin, Microcrystalline Cellulose, Magnesium Stearate.

Chitosan LipoSan Ultra **-** Pure Encapsulations
Each vegetable capsule contains: Chitosan (90% pure, shellfish) 435 mg. Other Ingredients: Succinic Acid.

Chitosan Plus **-** Progressive Labs
Each capsule contains: Chitosan (marine fiber concentrate) 250 mg • Citric Acid 75 mg • Lipase (3000 units) 25 mg.

Chit-O-Slim Plus **-** Aspen Group, Inc.
Each capsule contains: Chitosan 500 mg • Chromium (picolinate) 50 mcg.

Chitosol **-** Sheldon Marketing
Four capsules contain: Chitosan 2000 mg • Vitamin C 400 mg.

Chizukit Forte For Adults **-** Hadas Natural Products
Each tablet contains: Echinacea Angustifolia & Purpurea standardized extract 500 mg • Propolis standardized extract 500 mg • Astragalus standardized extract 100 mg • Cat's Claw standardized extract 100 mg • Vitamin C 15 mg • Vitamin E 1 mg • Beta-Carotene 0.8 mg.

Chizukit Gold **-** Hadas Natural Products
Each tablet contains: Echinacea Angustifolia & Purpurea standardized extract 500 mg • Propolis standardized extract 330 mg • Astragalus standardized extract 150 mg • Cat's Claw standardized extract 150 mg • Panax Ginseng standardized extract 20 mg • Green Tea standardized extract 12.5 mg • Vitamin C 30 mg • Vitamin E 4 mg • Beta Carotene 0.4 mg.

Chizukit Syrup **-** Hadas Natural Products
Each 5 mL serving contains: Echinacea Angustifolia/Purpurea extract 250 mg • Propolis standardized extract 250 mg • Vitamin C 30 mg • Rose Hip extract 30 mg. Other Ingredients: Fructose-Glucose Syrup.

Chlorella **-** Earthrise Nutritionals, LLC.
Fifteen tablets contain: Sodium 3 mg • Vitamin A (100% Beta Carotene) 1500 IU • Calcium 4 mg • Iron 2 mg • Niacin 0.75 mg • Riboflavin 0.15 mg • Protein 1.8 g • Total Carb. 0.4 g • Potassium 35 mg • Vitamin C 4 mg • Vitamin E 0.7 IU • Magnesium 8.0 mg • Thiamin 0.05 mg • Vitamin B6 0.05 mg • Vitamin B12 0.12 mcg • Chlorophyll 80 mg • Mixed Carotenoids 8 mg.

Chlorella **-** Pro Health
Three tablets contain: Vitamin A (100% as beta carotene) 3000 IU • Vitamin B12 3 mcg • Iron 3 mg • Zinc 2 mg • Chlorella 3000 mg • Chlorophyll 60 mg • RNA 89 mg • DNA 8.3 mg. Other Ingredients: Cellulose, Croscarmellose Sodium, Magnesium Stearate.

Chlorella **-** Nature's Way
Three capsules contain: Chlorella Microalgae 1.23 g. Other Ingredients: Gelatin.

Chlorella **-** Source Naturals
Six tablets contain: Vitamin A (Beta Carotene) 1,665 IU • Vitamin B1 (Thiamin) 45 mcg • Vitamin B2 (Riboflavin) 140 mcg • Vitamin B3 (Niacin) 710 mcg • Vitamin B6 (Pyridoxine) 50 mcg • Vitamin B12 (Cyanocobalamin) 3.75 mcg • Biotin 5.7 mcg • Vitamin C (Ascorbic Acid) 460 mcg • Calcium 6 mg • Iodine 18 mcg • Iron 5 mg • Magnesium 9.45 mg • Phosphorus 29 mg • Zinc 2.1 mg • Chlorella Growth Factor (CGF) 60 mg • Chlorophyll 60 mg.

Chlorella Regularis **-** New Chapter, Inc.
Six capsules contain: Chlorella regularis 2340 mg.

Chlorofresh Liquid **-** Nature's Way
Each tablespoon conatins: Chlorophyll Copper complex 50 mg. Other Ingredients: Glycerin, Oil Of Mint, Water.

Chlorofresh Softgels **-** Nature's Way
Each softgel contains: Chlorophyll Copper complex 50 mg. Other Ingredients: Oil Of Mint.

Chlorophyll Complex **-** Standard Process, Inc.
Each two perles contain: Proprietary Blend 754 mg: Fat Soluble Extract from Sesame seed, Alfalfa, Tillandsia Usneoides, Buckwheat, Pea (vine), & Carrot; Soy Bean Lecithin. Inactive Ingredients: Gelatin, Glycerine, Water, Carob.

Chlorophyll Complex Ointment **-** Standard Process, Inc.
Soybean Lecithin • Crude Chlorophyll extract: Alfalfa, Pea vine, Buckwheat, Tillandsia Usneoides, Lard, Lanolin, Beeswax, Flaxseed oil, Bovine Orchic glandular extract.

Chlorophyll Concentrate **-** Puritan's Pride
Each softgel contains: Chlorophyllin Copper 50 mg.

Chlorophyll Liquid **-** Dial Herbs
Chlorophyllin Copper complex • Water • Oil of Mint • Glycerine, vegetable derived.

Chlorophyll Softgels **-** Dial Herbs
Chlorophyllin Copper complex • Water • Oil of Mint • Glycerine, vegetable derived.

Chloroplex **-** Progressive Labs
Each softgel contains: Chlorophyllin 50 mg.

Chloroplus **-** Atrium Biotechnologies
Each capsule contains: Vitamin A 11000 IU • Vitamin D (as Vitamin D3) 250 IU • Chlorophyll (oil soluble) 10 mg • Vitamin E (d-Alpha Tocopherol) 3 IU • Lecithin (Raw Unbleached) 210 mg • Pumpkin seed oil 45 mg • Sesame seed oil 22 mg • Halibut Liver oil • Skip Jack Liver oil.

Chlorotene **-** Metagenics
Each softgel contains: Vitamin A (as beta-carotene from dunaliella salina algae) 12,500 IU • Chlorophyll oil 8 mg • Vitamin E (as D-alpha tocopherol) 2 IU.

Chocolate Daydream Fructose **-** Physicians Laboratories
Each packet contains: Certified Isoflavone 160 mg. Other ingredients: Soy Protein Isolate, Fructose, Sucrose, Cocoa, Calcium Phosphate, Maltodextrin, Soy Lecithin, Salt, Potassium Chloride, Artificial Flavor, Carrageenan, Carboxymethylcellulose, Xanthan Gum.

Chocolate Daydream Splenda **-** Physicians Laboratories
Each packet contains: Certified Isoflavone 160 mg. Other Ingredients: Soy Protein Isolate, Cocoa, Maltodextrin, Calcium Phosphate, Soy Lecithin, Salt, Potassium Chloride, Artificial Flavor, Carrageenan, Carboxymethylcellulose, Xanthan Gum, Sucralose.

Chocolate Daydream Unsweetened **-** Physicians Laboratories
Each packet contains: Certified Isoflavone 160 mg. Other Ingredients: Soy Protein Isolate, Cocoa, Maltodextrin, Calcium Phosphate, Soy Lecithin, Salt, Potassium Chloride, Artificial Flavor, Carrageenan, Carboxymethylcellulose, Xanthan Gum.

Some Brand Name Natural Products - What they Contain

www.NaturalDatabase.com contains MANY more listings than appear here.
Editor's Notes are located on pages 2155-2163.

Chocolate Temptation - Physicians Laboratories
Each bar contains: Certified Isoflavone 160 mg. Other Ingredients: Corn syrup, Corn starch, Water, Gelatin, Soy Protein Isolate, Rice flour, Malt, Salt, Glycerin, Chocolate Liquor, Cocoa butter and dextrose, Soy Lecithin, Sunflower oil, Natural and Artificial Flavors, Cocoa powder.

Chocolate-covered Soynuts - Physicians Laboratories
Each 1/6 cup contains: Certified Isoflavone 10 mg. Other Ingredients: Milk Chocolate (sugar, whole milk powder, cocoa butter, chocolate liquor, lecithin), Soy Protein (whole roasted soybeans), Vanillin, Corn Syrup, Starch Gum, Soybean Oil, Confectioner's Glaze.

Choice 50 - 4 Life
Each capsule contains: Vitamin C (as ascorbic acid) 75 mg • Vitamin E (as D-alpha tocopheryl acetate) 30 IU • Grapeseed extract (vitis vinifera) 50 mg • Proprietary Blend 365 mg: Fo-Ti (polygonum multiflorum), Citrus Bioflavonoids, Rutin, Milk Thistle (80% silybum marianum seed), Quercitin, Bilberry (25% vaccinium myrtillus fruit), Curcumin (from tumeric root), Trans-Resveratrol (polygonum cuspidatum root). Other Ingredients: Vegetable Oil, Gelatin.

Choice Prime - 4 Life
Maritime Pine bark extract • Proprietary Enzyme Blend: Peptidase • Pectinase • Amylase • Lipase • Hemicellulase • Protease • Cellulase • Synergistic Herbal Blend: Citrus Bioflavonoids, Spirulina Platensis, Acerola, Arctic Root, Schisandra Chinensis, Green Tea extract.

Cholacol - Standard Process, Inc.
Two tablets contain: Proprietary Blend 721 mg: Collinsonia root, Purified Bovine bile salts • Iron 0.2 mg. Other Ingredients: Honey, Calcium Stearate.

Cholacol II - Standard Process, Inc.
Four tablets contain: Proprietary Blend 1954 mg: Bentonite (montmorillonite), Collinsonia root, Purified Bovine bile salts • Iron 3 mg • Sodium 20 mg. Other Ingredients: Honey, Calcium Stearate.

Cholaplex - Standard Process, Inc.
Each capsule contains: Proprietary Blend 476 mg: Collinsonia root, Choline Bitartrate, Defatted Wheat germ, Bovine Liver, Calcium Lactate, Dried Buckwheat leaf juice, Buckwheat seed, Porcine Stomach, Tillandsia Usneoides, Purified Bovine Bile salts, Bovine Orchic Cytosol extract, Soy bean, Inositol, Soybean Lecithin, Bovine Spleen, Ovine Spleen, Betaine Hydrochloride, Carrot root, Manganese Glycerophosphate, Bovine Prostate, Porcine Brain, Allantoin, Bovine Adrenal Cytosol extract, Bovine Orchic extract, Oat flour, Ascorbic Acid • Riboflavin 0.3 mg • Niacin 22 mg • Vitamin B6 4 mg • Iodine 130 mcg. Other Ingredients: Gelatin, Water, Potassium Bicarbonate, Potassium Para-Aminobenzoate, Colors.

Cholarest SC - Metagenics
Each tablet contains: Policosanol from sugar cane wax (saccharum officinarum) 10 mg.

CholeRx - Xymogen
Each capsule contains: Policosanol (from sugar cane wax) 10 mg • Magnesium (as magnesium glycinate/lysinate and magnesium malate) 100 mg. Other Ingredients: Cellulose, Ascorbyl Palmitate, Magnesium Stearate.

CholesFiber - Source Naturals
Three heaping scoops contain: Dietary Fiber 15 g • Soluble Fiber 15 g • Protein 15 g • Soy Isoflavones 60 mg. Other Ingredients: Soy Protein, Apple Pectin, Grapefruit Pectin, Mixed Gums: Guar Gum, Arabic Gum, Xanthan Gum.

Choles-Response - Source Naturals
Three tablets contain: Vitamin C (as ascorbic acid) 600 mg • Vitamin E (as succinate) 200 IU • Niacin (as inositol hexanicotinate) 500 mg • Iodine (from kelp) 150 mcg • Chromium (as chromium picolinate & ChromeMate brand) 100 mcg • Phytosterols Complex 40% (yielding beta sitosterol 300 mg) 750 mg • Inositol (as inositol hexanicotinate) 640 mg • Garlic powder extract (standardized to 8000 ppm allicin) 600 mg • Turmeric extract (95% curcumin) 526 mg • Artichoke extract (standardized to 2.5% cynarins) 250 mg • Methylmethioninesulfonium Chloride (vitamin U) 200 mg • Green Tea extract 95% 100 mg • Soy Bean concentrate (yielding 40 mg total isoflavones) 100 mg • Guggul Gum resin extract 100 mg • Ginkgo Biloba leaf 50:1 extract, 24% 60 mg • Dandelion root 4:1 extract 50 mg • Hawthorn berry 4:1 extract 50 mg • Myricetin 30 mg. Other Ingredients: Sorbitol, Stearic Acid, Colloidal Silicon dioxide, Modified Cellulose Gum, Magnesium Stearate.

Cholesta Balance - PhysioLogics
Each softgel contains: Pantethine (80% purity, 307 mg) 384 mg • Gamma Oryzanol (from Rice Bran) 100 mg.

CholestaCare - Your Vitamins
Each capsule contains: CholestaCare Proprietary Sterol Blend 400 mg. Other Ingredients: Gelatin Capsule, Vegetable Magnesium Stearate, Vegetable Stearine, Silicon Dioxide.

Cholestaid - Omni Nutraceuticals
Two tablets contain: Esterin extract of Alfalfa 900 mg • Citric Acid 100 mg. Other Ingredients: Microcrystalline, Croscarmellose Sodium, Stearic Acid, Silica.

Cholesta-Lo - Futurebiotics LLC
Three tablets contain: Cholestatin 600 mg • Niacin (flush free) 200 mg • Chromium (polynicotinate) 100 mcg • Garlic (odorless) concentrate (2:1) 350 mg • Siberian Ginseng extract (10:1) 75 mg • Parsley 250 mg • Chickweed 200 mg • Hawthorn 150 mg • Ginger 200 mg • Cayenne 200 mg. ("75 mg of 10:1 Siberian Ginseng extract is equal to 750 mg of raw Siberian Ginseng. 350 mg of 2:1 Garlic is equal to 875 mg of raw Garlic.")

CholesTame - Jarrow Formulas
Four tablets contain: Red Yeast Rice Extract (Monascus purpureus) (Xie Zhi Kang) 4% Statins 2400 mg • Coenzyme Q10 (Ubiquinone) 30 mg • Artichoke Leaf Extract (Cynara scolymus) 2% cynarine 400 mg • Guggul (Commiphora mukul) 4% guggulsterones 500 mg • Alpha Lipoic Acid 100 mg • Grape Seed Extract (Vitis vinifera) 95% polyphenols 50 mg • Pantethine 200 mg • Lutein 10 mg • Taurine 250 mg.

CholesTame (New Formula with Sytrinol!) - Jarrow Formulas
Four tablets contain: Sytrinol (polymethoxylated flavonoid-tocotrienol complex) 300 mg • Plant Sterols (phytosterols) 2000 mg • Coenzyme Q10 (ubiquinone) 30 mg • Artichoke leaf extract (cynara scolymus, 2.5% cynarine) 400 mg • Alpha Lipoic Acid 100 mg • Grape seed extract (vitus vinifera, 95% polyphenols) 50 mg • Pantethine (coenzyme vitamin B5) 200 mg • Lutein (tagetes erecta, from 20 mg lutein esters) 10 mg • Taurine 250 mg • Lecithin (35% phosphatidylcholine) 200 mg. Other Ingredients: Dicalcium Phosphate, Silicon Dioxide, Modified Cellulose Gum, Stearic Acid, Magnesium Stearate, Modified Cellulose.

Cholestatin - Futurebiotics LLC
Each tablet contains: Beta Sitosterol 200 mg • Campesterol 100 mg • Stigmasterol 80 mg. Other Ingredients: Dicalcium phosphate, Cellulose, Magnesium Stearate, Silica.

Cholestatin brand - Degussa Food Ingredients/BL BioActives
Phytosterols complex.
See Editor's Note No. 44.

CholestePure - Pure Encapsulations
Each vegetable capsule contains: Phytosterol Complex (derived from soybean oil, typically providing: total phytosterols 450 mg, beta-sitosterol 230 mg, campesterol 135 mg, stigmasterol 82 mg, brassicasterol 1.5 mg, sitostanol 1.5 mg) 500 mg • Vitamin C (as ascorbyl palmitate) 50 mg.

Some Brand Name Natural Products - What they Contain

www.NaturalDatabase.com contains MANY more listings than appear here.
Editor's Notes are located on pages 2155-2163.

Cholesterol Essentials - Swanson Health Products
Two tablets contain: Vitamin C (ascorbic acid) 500 mg • Thiamin (as thiamin HCl; vitamin B-1) 7 mg • Riboflavin (vitamin B-2) 7 mg • Niacin (100 mg as flush-free inositol hexanicotinate and 7 mg as niacinamide) 107 mg • Vitamin B-6 (as pyridoxine HCl) 7 mg • Folic Acid 200 mcg • Vitamin B-12 (as cyanocobalamin) 200 mcg • Biotin 6.24 mcg • Pantothenic Acid (as d-calcium pantothenate) 6.24 mg • Chromium (from Chromax® chromium picolinate) 200 mcg • Gugulipid® (Commiphora mukul, 2.5% guggulsterones) 500 mg • Lecithin 300 mg • Oat Bran fiber 300 mg • Phosphatidylcholine (from lecithin and phosphatidylcholine) 200 mg • Odor-Controlled Garlic bulb (PureGar® 10,000 ppm allicin potential) 150 mg • Beta Sitosterol 50 mg • Citrus Bioflavonoids 50 mg • Choline Bitartrate 6.4 mg • Inositol 6.4 mg • PABA (para-aminobenzoic acid) 6.4 mg.

Cholesterol Formula - HERBALmax
Shanzha fruits • Taoren seeds • Ezhu rhizoma • Zexie rhizoma • DAnshen radi • Danggui radix.

Cholesterol Metabolism - Nutrivention
Six tablets contain: Choline 500 mg • Inositol 500 mg • Niacinamide 200 mg Unsaturated Fatty Acids (7% GAMA Linolenic Acid • 64% Linoleic Acid) 500 mg • Pantothenic Acid 200 mg • Magnesium 200 mg • Vitamin B6 100 mg • Vitamin D 600 IU • Lecithin 600 mg • Hawthorne berries 400 mg • Garlic powder concentrate 400 mg • Apple Pectin 360 mg • L-Methionine 340 mg • Capsicum 200 mg • Ginger root 200 mg • Butcher's Broom 100 mg • Betaine HCL 100 mg.

Cholesterol Regulation Complex - Shaklee
Six tablets contain: Protein 2 g • Sodium 60 mg • Hydrolyzed Soy Protein Blend 3000 mg: Phytopeptides with bound phospholipids • N-acetylcysteine 200 mg. Other Ingredients: Dicalcium Phosphate, Croscarmellose Sodium.

Cholesterol Success - TwinLab
Each two tablets contain: Phytosterols (Reducol) 900 mg.

Cholesterol Support - Zone Labs
Three capsules contain: Garlic (odor reduced, 10,000 ppm allicin) 500 mg • Policosanol 10 mg • Phytosterols Complex (a source of plant sterols including beta sitosterol, capesterol and stigmasterol) 900 mg • Citrus Pectin 5 mg • Apple Pectin 5 mg • Ginger extract 5 mg. Other Ingredients: Gelatin, Microcrystalline Cellulose, Magnesium Stearate, Silica, Sodium Lauryl Sulfate.

Cholesterol Support II - Weil Lifestyle, LLC
Each Dr. Weil Heart Health tablet contains: Coenzyme Q10 (CoQ10) 30 mg • EPA Omega 3 335 mg • DHA Omega 3 167.5 mg.

Cholesterol Vital Maintenance - Gaia Herbs
Two capsules contain: Pantethine 200 mg • Artichoke leaf (cynara scolymus) 200 mg • Coleus root (coleus forskholii) 160 mg • Guggulu resin (commiphora mukul) 150 mg • Arjuna bark (terminalia arjuna) 100 mg • Wild Yam rhizome (dioscorea villosa) 8 mg • Policosanol 8 mg • Greater Celandine tops and roots (chelidonium majus) 8 mg. Other Ingredients: Vegetable Glycerin, Vegetable Cellulose (capsule).

Cholester-Reg II - Nature's Sunshine
Each capsule contains: Proprietary Blend 500 mg: Artichoke leaf (cynara scolymus), Phytosterol (contains beta-sitosterol, campesterol, and stigmasterol), Inositol Nicotinate, Resveratrol (Japanese knotweed root), Policosanol. Other Ingredients: Gelatin, Water.

CholesteSoy - FreeLife International
Two caplets contain: Niacin (from flush-free inositol hexanicotinate 250 mg) 200 mg • Vitamin B6 (as pyridoxine HCl) 10 mg • Folate (as folic acid) 200 mcg • Vitamin B12 (as cyanocobalamin) 100 mcg • Red Yeast Rice (from fermentation of monascus purpureus went) 1200 mg • Proprietary Blend 100 mg: Octadecanoic Acid, Magnesium Octadecanoate (from vegetable oil), Soy Phytosterols (beta-sitosterol, campesterol, stigamasterol), 2.5% Guggulsterone extract (commiphora mukul). Other Ingredients: Calcium Hydrogen Phosphate, Cellulose, Cellulose Gum, Silica, Vita-Coat (vegetable resin, alpha-lipoic acid).

Cholestin - Pharmanex
Each capsule contains: Policosanol (Beeswax extract 5:1) 15 mg. Other Ingredients: Soybean Oil, Lecithin, Gelatin, Glycerin, Purified Water, Carmine (for color).

Cholestinol Red - MedaBiotics
Three capsules contain: Red Yeast Rice (from traditional fermentation) 1080 mg. Other Ingredients: Gelatin, Cellulose, Magnesium Stearate.

Cholest-Off - Nature Made
Each tablet contains: Proprietary Blend 450 mg: Plant Sterols, Plant Stanols, Cellulose Gel, Gum Acacia, Magnesium Silicate, Croscarmellose Sodium, Silica Gel, Hydroxypropyl Methylcellulose, Titanium Dioxide (artificial color), Magnesium Stearate, Polyethylene Glycol, Triethyl Citrate, Polysorbate 80, Sodium Citrate.

Cholestoril - Enzymatic Therapy
Each tablet contains: Pantethine 300 mg.

Cholestoril Plus - Enzymatic Therapy
Each tablet contains: Proprietary Phytosterol Blend 400 mg: Beta Sitosterol, Campesterol, Stigmasterol, Brassicasterol, Other Plant Sterols • Pantethine 200 mg. Other Ingredients: Cellulose, Modified Cellulose Gum, Modified Cellulose, Silicon Dioxide, Magnesium Stearate, Lecithin, Carnauba Wax.

CholestOut II - Life Enhancement Products, Inc.
Four capsules contain: Niacin (vitamin B3 as inositol hexanicotinate) 1.2 g • Green Tea extract (total polyphenols 337 mg; catechins 150 mg, theaflavins 75 mg) 375 mg • Policosanol 20 mg • Coenzyme Q10 30 mg.

Cholestra - HerbaSway
Soy • Hawthorn berry • Green Tea • He Shou Wu • Cassia tora • Blackberry • HerbaSwee (Cucurbitaceae fruit).

Cholest-Response - Source Naturals
Three tablets contain: Vitamin C (as ascorbic acid) 600 mg • Vitamin E (from gamma-vitamin E complex) 16 IU • Niacin (as inositol hexanicotinate) 500 mg • Iodine (from kelp) 150 mcg • SelenoPure brand Selenium (as l-selenomethionine and sodium selenite) 100 mcg • ChromeMate brand Chromium (as chromium polynicotinate and chromium picolinate) 100 mcg • Phytosterol Complex 40% (yielding 300 mg beta-sitosterol) 750 mg • Garlic powder extract (standardized to 8000 ppm allicin) 600 mg • Turmeric extract (yielding 500 mg curcumin) 526 mg • Gamma-Vitamin E complex 500 mg • Inositol (as inositol and inositol hexanicotinate) 350 mg • Red Yeast Rice (yielding 1.5% mevinolinic acid monacolins) 350 mg • Artichoke extract (standardized to 2.5% cynarins) 250 mg • L-Arginine (as L-arginine HCl) 240 mg • Methylmethioninesulfonium Chloride (vitamin U) 200 mg • Green Tea extract (yielding 100 mg polyphenols, 36 mg EGCG) 105 mg • Sytrinol brand Proprietary Blend of Citrus Polymethoxylated Flavones and palm tocotrienols 100 mg • Soy bean concentrate (yielding 40 mg total isoflavones) 60 mg • Ginkgo leaf 50:1 extract 60 mg • Guggul extract (10% guggulsterones) 50 mg • Dandelion root 4:1 extract 50 mg • Hawthorne berry 4:1 extract 50 mg • Myricetin 30 mg • Policosanol 10 mg • Coenzyme Q10 5 mg. Other Ingredients: Stearic Acid, Acacia Gum, Modified Cellulose Gum, Colloidal Silicon Dioxide.

Cholestrex - Source Naturals
Nine tablets contain: Niacin 480 mg • Vitamin C (Calcium Ascorbate, Ascorbic Acid and Zinc Ascorbate) 900 mg • Vitamin E (D-Alpha Tocopheryl) (Natural) 100 IU • Calcium (Calcium Ascorbate) 100 mg • Zinc (Zinc Ascorbate) 6 mg • Copper (Copper Sevacate) 2 mg • Chromium (ChromeMate GTF Chromium Polynicotinate) 300 mcg • Oats (bran and fiber) 2500 mg • Grapefruit Pectin 1400 mg • Psyllium seed husk 1100 mg • Lecithin (with 24% Phosphatidyl Choline) 900 mg • Alfalfa seed 600 mg • Beta Sitosterol 300 mg • L-Arginine 300 mg.

BRAND NAMES

Cholest-Rite - Nu-Creations
Each capsule contains: Niacin 20 mg • Red Yeast 600 mg. Other Ingredients: Hawthorn extract, Artichoke extract, Gelatin, Magnesium Stearate.

Cholest-SP - Benepure, Inc
Three capsules contain: Chromium (as chromium polynicotinate) 200 mcg • Red Yeast Rice 600 mg • Policosanol (from sugar cane) 20 mg • Phytosterols Complex (from soy) 600 mg • Coenzyme Q10 20 mg • Guggul lipids 200 mg • Artichoke leaf extract 100 mg • Eicosapentaenoic Acid (EPA) 180 mg. Other Ingredients: Rice Flour, Vegetable Cellulose, Vegetable Stearate.

Choline - Nature's Bounty
Each tablet contains: Choline Bitartrate 650 mg. Other Ingredients: Cellulose, Vegetable Stearic Acid, Food Glaze, Silica, Vegetable Magnesium Stearate, Magnesium Silicate, Croscarmellose.

Choline - Puritan's Pride
Each tablet contains: Choline (from Choline Bitartrate) 650 mg.

Choline - Standard Process, Inc.
Each tablet contains: Choline 180 mg. Other Ingredients: Honey, Calcium Stearate.

Choline & Inositol - Puritan's Pride
Each tablet contains: Choline Bitartrate 250 mg • Inositol 250 mg.

Choline & Inositol 250 mg & 250 mg - Nature's Way
Two capsules contain: Choline Bitartrate 500 mg • Inositol 500 mg. Other Ingredients: Cellulose, Magnesium Stearate, Silica.

Choline & Inositol 500 mg - Nature's Plus
Each tablet contains: Choline (as bitartrate) 500 mg • Inositol 500 mg. Other Ingredients: Stearic Acid, Rice Bran, Microcrystalline Cellulose, Di-calcium Phosphate, Silica, Magnesium Stearate, Pharmaceutical Glaze.

Choline 600 mg Sustained Release Tablets - Nature's Plus
Each tablet contains: Choline (as bitartrate) 600 mg. Other Ingredients: Microcrystalline Cellulose, Hydroxypropyl Methylcellulose, Stearic Acid, Magnesium Stearate, Rice Bran, Silica, Pharmaceutical Glaze.

Choline Bitartrate 500mg - Nature's Own
Each tablet contains: Choline Bitartrate 500 mg.

Choline/Inositol 250/250 - Solgar
Each capsule contains: Choline (as choline bitartrate) 250 mg • Inositol 250 mg. Other Ingredients: Vegetable Cellulose, Silica, Vegetable Magnesium Stearate, Water, Vegetable Glycerin.

Choline/Inositol Tablets - Solgar
Each tablet contains: Calcium (as dicalcium phosphate) 25 mg • Choline (as choline bitartrate) 103 mg • Inositol 250 mg. Other Ingredients: Microcrystalline Cellulose, Dicalcium Phosphate, Vegetable Cellulose, Silica, Titanium Dioxide, Vegetable Stearic Acid, Vegetable Magnesium Stearate, Vegetable Glycerin.

Cholinex (Niuhuang Jiedu Pian) - Shanghai Chinese Herbal Co. Ltd.
Each tablet contains: Proprietary Blend 500 mg: Rhubarb root (radix et rhizoma rhei), Scutellaria root (radix scutellariae), Lonicera flower (lonicera japonica), Coptis rhizome (coptis chinensis), Gardenia fruit (gardenia jasminoides), Angelica root (angelica sinensis), Mentha herb (mentha hapocalyx), Ligusticum rhizome (ligusticum sinensis).

ChondroCare - Metagenics
Six tablets contain: D-Glucosamine Sulfate 1500 mg • Chondroitin Sulfate 1200 mg • MSM (methyl-sulfonyl-methane) 1000 mg • Zinc (as zinc glycinate) 15 mg • Selenium (as selenium amino acid complex) 300 mcg • Copper (as copper lysinate) 1.5 mg • Manganese (as manganese ascorbate) 1.5 mg.

Chondro-Flx - Ortho Molecular Products
Three capsules contain: Vitamin C (as ascorbic acid USP) 60 mg • Glucosamine Sulfate 1500 mg • Chondroitin Sulfate 900 mg • Bromelain (2400 GDU/g) 45 mg. Other Ingredients: Natural Gelatin Capsules, Ascorbyl Palmitate, Magnesium Stearate, Microcrystalline Cellulose, Silicon Dioxide.

Chondroitin 400 - Jarrow Formulas
Each capsule contains: Chondroitin Sulfate (from 420 mg chondroitin sulfate calcium) 400 mg. Other Ingredients: Rice Powder, Magnesium Stearate.

Chondroitin Complex - Puritan's Pride
Each capsule contains: Glucosamine Sulfate (2KCl) 250 mg • Chondroitin Sulfate 200 mg • Vitamin C (Ascorbic Acid) 100 mg • Manganese 1 mg.
See Editor's Note No. 15.

Chondroitin Plus - Atrium Biotechnologies
Two capsules contain: Calcium Ascorbate 60 mg • Magnesium Ascorbate 60 mg • Vitamin C Content 100 mg • Thiamine HCL 25 mg • Pyridoxine HCL 10 mg • Niacinamide 60 mg • Manganese (Sulfate) 65 mg • Potassium (Citrate) 25 mg • Zinc (Citrate) 25 mg • Chondroitin Sulfates 125 mg • Mocopoly Saccharides 65 mg • Bioflavonoid Complex 50 mg • Betaine HCL 15 mg • Rutin 10 g • Black Cohosh 75 mg • Passiflora 75 mg • Valerian root 75 mg • Equestium 65 mg.
See Editor's Note No. 15.

Chondroitin Sulfate - Jamieson
Each caplet contains: Chondroitin Sulfate (Equivalent to 400 mg Sodium Chondroitin Sulfate) 360 mg.
See Editor's Note No. 15.

Chondroitin Sulfate - Swanson Health Products
Each capsule contains: Chondroitin Sulfate 500 mg.
See Editor's Note No. 15.

Chondroitin Sulfate - Leiner Health Products
Each tablet contains: Chondroitin Sulfate 600 mg. Other Ingredients: Cellulose, Dicalcium Phosphate, Stearic Acid, Croscarmellose Sodium, Magnesium Stearate, Silicon Dioxide, Titanium Dioxide, Hydroxypropyl Methylcellulose, Talc, Polyethylene Glycol 3350, Wax, Polysorbate 80.
See Editor's Note No. 15.

Chondroitin Sulfate - PhysioLogics
Each capsule contains: Chondroitin Sulfate 250 mg. Other Ingredients: Rice Powder, Gelatin.
See Editor's Note No. 15.

Chondroitin Sulfate - Olympian Labs
Each capsule contains: Chondroitin Sulfate 400 mg.
See Editor's Note No. 15.

Chondroitin Sulfate (bovine) - Pure Encapsulations
Each vegetable capsule contains: Chondroitin Sulfate (bovine, from 444 mg of bovine chondroitin sulfate) 400 mg • Vitamin C (as ascorbyl palmitate) 5 mg.
See Editor's Note No. 15.

Chondroitin Sulfate (marine) - Pure Encapsulations
Each vegetable capsule contains: Chondroitin Sulfate (marine, from 416 mg of marine chondroitin sulfate) 400 mg • Vitamin C (as ascorbyl palmitate) 5 mg.

Chondroitin Sulfate 250 MG - Puritan's Pride
Each capsule contains: Chondroitin Sulfate 250 mg. Other Ingredients: Cellulose (plant origin), Gelatin, Dicalcium Phosphate, Vegetable Stearic Acid, Vegetable Magnesium Stearate.
See Editor's Note No. 15.

Some Brand Name Natural Products - What they Contain

www.NaturalDatabase.com contains MANY more listings than appear here.
Editor's Notes are located on pages 2155-2163.

BRAND NAMES

Chondroitin Sulfate 400 - GNC
Each capsule contains: Chondroitin Sulfate Sodium 400 mg. Other Ingredients: Cellulose, Gelatin, Calcium Carbonate.
See Editor's Note No. 15.

Chondroitin Sulfate 90% - Vital Nutrients
Each capsule conatins: Chondroitin Sulfate 400 mg.
See Editor's Note No. 15.

Chondroitin Sulfate, Joint Support, 600 mg - NOW Foods
Two capsules contain: Sodium 110 mg • Sodium Chondroitin Sulfate (from bovine cartilage) 1200 mg. Other Ingredients: Rice, Flour, Gelatin (capsule), Magnesium Stearate.
See Editor's Note No. 15.

Chondroitin Sulfate/Glucosamine Sulfate - Metabolic Response Modifiers
Each capsule contains: Glucosamine sulfate KCl 500 mg • Chondroitin sulfate 400 mg.
See Editor's Note No. 15.

Chondroytamine HCl - Olympian Labs
Each capsule contains: Chondroitin Sulfate 200 mg •Glucosamine HCl 250 mg.
See Editor's Note No. 15.

Chondroytamine HCl (Double Strength) - Olympian Labs
Each capsule contains: Chondroitin Sulfate 400 mg • Glucosamine HCl 500 mg • Cat's Claw 30 mg • White Willow Bark 30 mg.
See Editor's Note No. 15.

Christopher's Complete Tissue Formula - Dr. Christopher's
Each capsule contains: White Oak bark • Lungwort • Slippery Elm bark • Marshmallow root • Mullein leaf • Black Walnut leaf • Wormwood • Lobelia • Scullcap • Plantain • Gravel root • Aloe Vera gel 100:1 extract.

Christopher's Joint Formula - Dr. Christopher's
Each capsule contains: Proprietary Blend 450 mg: Hydrangea root, Brigham Tea herb, Yucca root, Chaparral leaves, Black Walnut leaves, Lobelia herb, Burdock root, Sarsaparilla root, Wild Lettuce leaves, Valerian root, Wormwood herb, Cayenne Pepper, Black Cohosh root. Other Ingredients: 100% Vegetable Base Capsule.

Chroma Slim Apple Cider Vinegar - Richardson Labs
Two caplets contain: Vitamin B6 (as pyridoxine HCl) 20 mg • Calcium 70 mg • Chromium (as chromium polynicotinate) 120 mcg • Apple Cider Vinegar Complex 600 mg • Grapefruit powder 400 mg • Premium Herbal Blend 300 mg: Buchu leaf extract, Parsley leaf/stem, Juniper berry, Uva-Ursi leaf, Dandelion root • Soy Lecithin 100 mg. Other Ingredients: Microcrystalline Cellulose, Maltodextrin, Dicalcium Phosphate, Crospovidone, Modified Food Starch, Hydroxypropyl Methylcellulose, Calcium Silicate, Silica, Magnesium Stearate, PEG.

Chromax brand - Nutrition 21
Chromium Picolinate.
See Editor's Note No. 44.

Chromax II - Nature's Plus
Each tablet contains: Chromium (as picolinate) 200 mcg. Other Ingredients: Microcrystalline Cellulose, Di-calcium Phosphate, Stearic Acid, Magnesium Stearate, Natural Color, Pharmaceutical Glaze, Silica.

Chromemate - Natrol, Inc.
Each capsule contains: Chromium (polynicotinate) 200 mcg • L-Arginine 50 mg • L-Lysine 50 mg • Vitamin B6 (pyridoxine) 10 mg. Other Ingredients: Microcrystalline Cellulose, Magnesium Stearate, Gelatin.

ChromeMate GTF 200 - Pure Encapsulations
Each vegetable capsule contains: Chromium (from chromium polynicotinate) 200 mcg • Niacin (from chromium polynicotinate) 1.1.-1.2 mg.

ChromeMate GTF 200 - Pure Encapsulations
Each vegetarian capsule contains: Chromium (from chromium polynicotinate) 200 mg • Niacin (from chromium polynicotinate) 1.1-1.2 mg.

ChromeMate GTF 600 - Pure Encapsulations
Each vegetable capsule contains: Chromium (from chromium polynicotinate) 600 mcg • Niacin (from chromium polynicotinate) 3.3-3.6 mg.

Chromic Fuel (Chromium Picolinate) - TwinLab
Pure Crystalline Chromium Picolinate (supplying of Trivalent Chromium 200 mcg) 1.67 mg.

Chromium - GNC
Each capsule contains: Chromium (as Chromium Picolinate) 200 mcg. Other Ingredients: Soybean oil, Gelatin, Glycerin, Magnesium Stearate, Caramel color, Titanium Dioxide.

Chromium - Source Naturals
Each tablet contains: Chromium (amino acid chelate) 200 mcg.

Chromium (picolinate) 200 mcg - Pure Encapsulations
Each vegetable capsule contains: Chromium (picolinate) 200 mcg.

Chromium (picolinate) 500 mcg - Pure Encapsulations
Each vegetable capsule contains: Chromium (picolinate) 500 mcg.

Chromium (polynicotinate) 200 mcg - Vital Nutrients
Each capsule contains: Chromium (polynicotinate) 200 mcg.

Chromium Chelated 200 mcg - Jamieson
Each tablet contains: Chromium (vegetable protein chelate) 200 mcg.

Chromium GTF - Jarrow Formulas
Each capsule contains: Chromium (in food matrix of 100 mg of saccharomyces cerevisiae nutritional yeast) 200 mcg. Other Ingredients: Rice Powder, Magnesium Stearate, Gelatin.

Chromium GTF - Nature's Sunshine
Each tablet contains: Calcium (di-calcium phosphate) 80 mg • Phosphorus (dicalcium phosphate) 61 mg • Chromium (chromium amino acid chelate, chromium nicotinate) 500 mcg • Proprietary Blend 60 mg: Horsetail (equisetum arvense), Red Clover tops (trifolium pratense), Yarrow flower (achillea millefolium).

Chromium GTF - Source Naturals
Each tablet contains: Chromium GTF (polynicotinate) 200 mcg • Niacin (polynicotinate) 1.8 mg.

Chromium GTF - Pro Health
Two tablets contain: Chromium GTF (as polynicotinate, from chromate [niacin bound to chromium]) 400 mcg. Other Ingredients: Dicalcium Phosphate, Dextrose, Magnesium Stearate, Stearic Acid.

Chromium GTF - Quest
Each capsule contains: Chromium (HVP Chelate) 200 mcg. Other Ingredients: Microcrystalline Cellulose, Magnesium Stearate (vegetable source).

Chromium HCA - PhysioLogics
Each capsule contains: Calcium (as Calcium Salt of Hydroxy Citric Acid) 79 mg • Chromium (as Chromium Picolinate) 100 mcg • Garcinia cambogia [50% (-)- Hydroxy Citric Acid (HCA) 250 mg] 500 mg.

Chromium Nicotinate Complex - Progressive Labs
Each capsule contains: Niacin (as polynicotinate) 1300 mcg • Chromium (as polynicotinate) 200 mcg • Glutathione 250 mcg • Glycine 50 mcg • Cysteine 100 mcg • Aspartic Acid 100 mcg.

Chromium Picolinate - PhytoPharmica
Each capsule contains: Chromium (picolinate) 200 mcg.

Chromium Picolinate - PhysioLogics
Each tablet contains: Chromium (as chromium picolinate) 200 mcg. Other Ingredients: Dicalcium Phosphate, Cellulose (plant origin), Vegetable Stearic Acid, Croscarmellose, Silica, Vegetable Magnesium Stearate.

Chromium Picolinate - Olympian Labs
Each capsule contains: Chromium (picolinate) 200 mcg.

Chromium Picolinate - Metabolic Response Modifiers
Each capsule contains: Chromium (picolinate) 200 mcg.

Chromium Picolinate - Great American Nutrition
Each tablet contains: Chromium (picolinate) 200 mcg. Other Ingredients: Calcium Carbonate, Cellulose, Magnesium Stearate.

Chromium Picolinate - Metagenics
Three tablets contain: Chromium (as chromium picolinate) 600 mcg.

Chromium Picolinate - Pro Health
Each capsule contains: Chromium (as chromax chromium picolinate, from white rice) 200 mcg. Other Ingredients: Rice Flour, Gelatin, Water.

Chromium Picolinate - Swanson Health Products
Each capsule contains: Chromium (from chromax chromium picolinate) 200 mcg.

Chromium Picolinate - Optimum Nutrition
Each capsule contains: Chromium (as chromium picolinate) 200 mcg. Other Ingredients: Gelatin, Microcrystalline Cellulose, Magnesium Stearate, Silica.

Chromium Picolinate - Source Naturals
Each tablet contains: Trivalent Chromium (from Chromax brand of yeast-free Chromium Picolinate) 200 mcg.

Chromium Picolinate - Nature's Way
Each capsule contains: Chromium Picolinate 200 mcg. Other Ingredients: Cellulose, Maltodextrin, Millet.

Chromium Picolinate - The Vitamin Shoppe
Each softgel contains: Chromium Picolinate (compound of yeast-free trivalent chromium and picolinic acid) 200 mcg.

Chromium Picolinate - GNC
Each tablet contains: Chromium (as Chromium Picolinate) 400 mcg. Other Ingredients: Dicalcium Phosphate, Cellulose, Stearic Acid, Silica, Magnesium Stearate.

Chromium Picolinate 200 Capsules - GNC
Each capsule contains: Chromium (as chromax chromium picolinate) 200 mcg. Other Ingredients: Soybean oil, Gelatin, Glycerin, Titanium Dioxide.

Chromium Picolinate 200 mcg - Puritan's Pride
Each tablet contains: Chromium (as chromium picolinate) 200 mcg. Other Ingredients: Dicalcium Phosphate, Cellulose (plant origin), Vegetable Stearic Acid, Silica, Vegetable Magnesium Stearate.

Chromium Picolinate 200 mcg - Kroger
Each tablet contains: Chromium (as chromium picolinate) 200 mcg. Other Ingredients: Calcium Carbonate, Maltodextrin, Cellulose, Croscarmellose Sodium, Silicon Dioxide, Magnesium Stearate, Dextrin, Dextrose, Lecithin, Sodium Carboxymethylcellulose, Sodium Citrate.

Chromium Picolinate 200 mcg - Nature Made
Each tablet contains: Chromium 200 mcg. Other Ingredients: Dibasic Calcium Phosphate, Cellulose, Magnesium Stearate.
See Editor's Note No. 45.

Chromium Picolinate 200 mcg - Rexall - Sundown
Each tablet contains: Calcium 120 mg • Chromium (as chromium picolinate) 200 mcg. Other Ingredients: Dicalcium Phosphate, Microcrystalline Cellulose, Croscarmellose Sodium, Magnesium Stearate.

Chromium Picolinate 200 mcg - Sunmark
Each tablet contains: Chromium Picolinate 200 mcg. Other Ingredients: Microcrystalline Cellulose, Silicon Dioxide, Magnesium Stearate.
See Editor's Note No. 45.

Chromium Picolinate 200 Tablets - GNC
Each tablet contains: Chromium (as chromax chromium picolinate) 200 mcg. Other Ingredients: Dicalcium Phosphate, Cellulose.

Chromium Picolinate 400 mcg XTRA - Rexall - Sundown
Each tablet contains: Calcium 128 mg • Chromium (as chromium picolinate) 400 mcg • Grapefruit Extract (fruit) 1 mg • Weight Loss Complement Blend 76 mg: Inositol, Soy Lecithin, Choline Bitartrate. Other Ingredients: Dicalcium Phosphate, Microcrystalline Cellulose, Croscarmellose Sodium, Silica, Magnesium Stearate.

Chromium Picolinate 400mcg - Nature's Own
Each tablet contains: Chromium Picolinate 400 mcg: Elemental Chromium 50 mcg.

Chromium Picolinate 500 - GNC
Each tablet contains: Chromium (as chromium picolinate) 500 mcg. Other Ingredients: Cellulose, Dicalcium Phosphate, Red Beet juice powder.

Chromium Picolinate GTF - Atrium Biotechnologies
Each capsule contains: Chromium (Chromium Picolinate) 200 mcg.

Chromium Picolinate High Potency - Optimum Nutrition
Each tablet contains: Chromium (as Chromium Picolinate) 200 mcg. Other Ingredients: Gelatin, Microcrystalline Cellulose, Magnesium Stearate, Silica.

Chromium Picolinate Plus - Progressive Labs
Each capsule contains: Chromium 200 mcg (from chromium picolinate 1640 mg) • Gamma Oryzanol 15 mg • Boron (as boron aspartate) 2 mg.

Chromium Picolinate Plus - Life Extension
Each capsule contains: Chromium Picolinate 300 mcg • Lipase 20 mg (blended in natural herb base).

Chromium Plus Vanadium - Trophic
Each capsule contains: Chromium (amino acid/niacin chelate) 200 mcg • Vanadium (from 400 mcg vanadyl sulphate) 75 mcg • Vitamin C 200 mg • Niacinamide 40 mg • Niacin 20 mg • Vitamin B6 (HCl) 20 mg.

Chromium Plus with Oxidative Factors - The Vitamin Shoppe
Each tablet contains: Zinc 30 mg • Chromium 100 mcg • Selenium 100 mcg.

ChronFS-X - Olympian Labs
Each capsule contains: Raw Adrenal 50 mg • Licorice Rhizome 150 mg • Shitake Mushrooms 30 mg • Maitake Mushrooms 30 mg • Malic Acid 200 mg • Magnesium Glycinate 50 mg • Manganese Glycinate 10 mg • Potassium Gluconate 30 mg • Zinc Gluconate 20 mg.
See Editor's Note No. 14.

Chronic Red Eye Drops - Natural Ophthalmics
Active Ingredients: Argentum Nitricum HPUS 10x • Hepar Sulphur HPUS 10x • Eyebright (euphrasia) HPUS 6x • Pulsatilla HPUS 6x • Rhus Toxicodendron HPUS 12x. Inactive Ingredients: Sterile Water, Sodium Chloride, Sodium Citrate, Citrate, Polysorbate 80.

BRAND NAMES

Some Brand Name Natural Products - What they Contain

www.NaturalDatabase.com contains MANY more listings than appear here.
Editor's Notes are located on pages 2155-2163.

Chrysin - ProLab
Each capsule contains: Chrysin (5,7-Dihydroxyflanone) 250 mg.

Chrysin - Metabolic Response Modifiers
Each capsule contains: Chrysin (5,7-dihydroxyflavone) 500 mg.

Chrysin - America's Finest
Each capsule contains: 100% pure Chrysin (5.7 dihydroxyflavone) 250 mg. Other Ingredients: Rice Powder, Magnesium Stearate, Silica.

Chrysin 500 Flavone X - Jarrow Formulas
Each capsule contains: Chrysin (5,7-dihydroxyflavone) 500 mg. Other Ingredients: Cellulose, Magnesium Stearate, Gelatin.

Chrysin Deluxe - Mass Quantities, Inc.
Each capsule contains: Chrysin 250 mg • Daidzein 25 mg.

Cider Source - Nature's Health Connection
Six caplets contain: Apple Cider Vinegar 60,000 mg • Calcium 144 mg • Magnesium 54 mg.

Cider Vinegar - Naturally Vitamins
Each tablet contains: Apple Cider Vinegar (equivalent to apple cider vinegar 5 ml) 100 mg. Other Ingredients: Dicalcium Phosphate, Colloidal Silica, Modified Cellulose Gum, Cholesterol Free Magnesium Stearate, Stearic Acid.

Cider Vinegar Diet Formula - NOW Foods
Each capsule contains: Vitamin B6 (pyridoxine HCl) 3.5 mg • Chromium (as amino acid chelate) 100 mcg • Apple Cider Vinegar powder 250 mg • Lecithin 100 mg • Glucomannan tuber fiber (amorphophallus rivieri) 50 mg • Kelp algae (ascophyllum nodosum) 37 mg • Grapefruit fiber 15 mg. Other Ingredients: Gelatin (capsule), Silica, Magnesium Stearate.

CigNo - M.E. Cody Products, Inc.
Plantain (plantago major) 1X, Alchohol 18-22%.
See Editor's Note No. 1.

Cimi-Fem - Source Naturals
Each table contains: Black Cohosh root (Cimi-Pure, standardized extract 2.5% yielding 2 mg triterpene glycosides, containing 27-deoxyactein) 80 mg.

Cineraria Eye Drops - Natural Ophthalmics
Active Ingredients: Cineraria Maritima 5x • Eyebright (euphrasia) 5x. Inactive Ingredients: Sterile Water, Sodium, Citrates, Polysorbate 80.

CinnaBeticII - Hero Nutritionals
Two capsules contain: Cinnulin PF water extract of Cassia Cinnamon 250 mg. Other Ingredients: Gelatin (capsules), Magnesium Stearate.

Cinnamon Quills 1:2 - Standard Process, Inc.
Each 5 mL serving contains: Cinnamon quills stem bark 1:2 extract (from cinnamomum zeylanicum 2.5 g) 5 mL. Other Ingredients: Purified Water, 70% Alcohol.

Cinnamon-Ginger - Susan Ambrosino's Herb Club, Inc.
Chinese Cinnamon • Ginger root.

Cinnulin PF - Pure Encapsulations
Each vegetable capsule contains: Cinnamon bark 20:1 extract (cinnamomi cassia) 125 mg • Vitamin C (as ascorbyl palmitate) 5 mg.

Cinnulor - Dr. Mark's
Each capsule contains: Cinnulin PF Cinnamomum Mairei extract 250 mg.

Circulate Dietary Supplement Tablets - HealthWatchers System
Vitamin B6 • Vitamin B2 • Vitamin B12 • Vitamin B15 • Vitamin D • OrthoPhosphoric Acid • EDTA • Fenugreek Seed • Superoxide Dismutase • Rutin • Catalase • Beet Leaf • Phosphatidyl Choline • Alfalfa • Spanish Moss • Urea • Orchick Hyaluridase • Beta Carotene • Protomorphagens Pituitary • Heart • Liver • Kidney • Brain.
See Editor's Note No. 31.

Circulatone - TriLight Herbs
Bilberry • Rosehips • Cleavers herb • Ginkgo.

Circuleg - Puritan's Pride
Each tablet contains: Horse Chestnut Seed extract (aesculus hippocastanum: Standardized to 20% Aescin) 300 mg • Proprietary Herbal Blend 200 mg: Butcher's Broom (Ruscus aculeatus) root, Bilberry (Vaccinium myrtillus) fruit, Cayenne (Capsicum annum) fruit, Ginger (Zingiber officinale) fruit, Ginkgo leaf extract (Ginkgo biloba).

Circulite Oil - The Herbalist
Oils of Sweet Almond, Eucalyptus, Camphor, St. John's Wort flower, Calendula flower, French Lavender, Peppermint, Sage & Extracts of Prickly Ash bark, Ginger root, Lobelia leaf.

Circuplex - Futurebiotics LLC
Two tablets contain: Vitamin C 100 mg • Vitamin B1 (thiamin) 8 mg • Niacinamide 414 mg • Vitamin B2 (riboflavin) 8 mg • Niacin 20 mg • Vitamin B6 20 mg • Vitamin B12 10 mcg • Zinc (gluconate) 5 mg • Manganese (amino acid chelate) 5 mg. In a tablet base of: Betaine HCl 20 mg, Citrus Bioflavonoids 50 mg, Alfalfa seed meal 200 mg, Oyster Shell Calcium 50 mg, Cayenne 10 mg, Ginger 200 mg, Prickly Ash bark 200 mg, Peppermint 100 mg.

Circuplex - Standard Process, Inc.
Each capsule contains: Proprietary Blend 425 mg: Ribonucleic Acid, Arrowroot flour, Dried Buckwheat leaf juice, Buckwheat seed, Bovine Liver, Phosphoric Acid, Porcine Stomach, Bovine Spleen, Bvine Spleen, Soy bean, Calcium Lactate, Defatted Wheat germ, Bovine Adrenal Cytosol extract, Inositol, Porcine Brain, Ascorbic Acid, Magnesium Citrate • Niacin 30 mg • Vitamin B6 4.7 mg • Potassium 5 mg. Other Ingredients: Gelatin, Water, Calcium Stearate, Natural Colors.
See Editor's Note No. 14.

Circusome - Jamieson
Horse Chestnut 5% • Arnica Flower 5% • Calendula 5% • Witch Hazel 4% • Butcher's Broom 2.5% • Peppermint Oil • Aloe Vera.

Circutone - The Herbalist
Prickly Ash bark • Hawthorn berry, leaf & flower • Bayberry root bark • Ginger root • Yarrow flower • Cayenne pepper.

Citicoline - QualiCeutix
Each capsule contains: Citicoline 500 mg. Other Ingredients: Gelatin, Microcrystalline Cellulose, Magnesium Stearate, Silicon Dioxide.

Citra Garcinia Cambogia - Olympian Labs
Each capsule contains: Garcinia (hydroxycitrate) 500 mg.

Citracal Calcium Citrate 250 mg + D - Mission Pharmacal
Two tablets contain: Vitamin D (as vitamin D3; as cholecalciferol) 125 IU • Calcium (as Ultradense calcium citrate) 500 mg. Other Ingredients: Polyethylene Glycol, Citric Acid, Microcrystalline Cellulose, HPMC, Croscarmellose Sodium, Color, Magnesium Silicate, Magnesium Stearate.

Citracal Calcium Citrate caplets - Mission Pharmacal
Two caplets contain: Vitamin D (D3, as cholecalciferol) 400 IU • Calcium (as Ultradense calcium citrate) 630 mg. Other Ingredients: Polyethylene Glycol, Croscarmellose Sodium, HPMC, Color Added, Magnesium Silicate, Magnesium Stearate.

Citracal Calcium Citrate Caplets + D - Mission Pharmacal
Two caplets contain: Vitamin D (as Vitamin D3; as cholecalciferol) 400 IU • Calcium (as Ultradense calcium citrate) 630 mg. Other Ingredients: Polyethylene Glycol, Croscarmellose Sodium, HPMC, Color, Magnesium Silicate, Magnesium Stearate.

Citracal Calcium Citrate Liquitab - Mission Pharmacal
Each dissolved tablet contains: Calcium (as calcium citrate) 500 mg. Other Ingredients: Citric Acid, Adipic Acid, Saccharin Sodium, Orange Flavor, Cellulose Gum, Aspartame. This Product contains Nutrasweet. Phenylketonurics: contains 6 mg Phenylalanine per tablet.

Citracal Calcium Citrate tablets - Mission Pharmacal
Two tablets contain: Calcium (as Ultradense calcium citrate) 400 mg. Other Ingredients: Polyethylene Glycol, Croscarmellose Sodium, HPMC, Color, Magnesium Silicate, Magnesium Stearate.

Citracal Plus - Mission Pharmacal
Two tablets contain: Vitamin D (as vitamin D3; as cholecalciferol) 250 IU • Vitamin B6 (as pyridoxine hydrochloride) 10 mg • Calcium (as Ultradense calcium citrate) 500 mg • Magnesium (as magnesium oxide) 80 mg • Zinc (as zinc oxide) 10 mg • Copper (as copper gluconate) 1 mg • Manganese (as manganese gluconate) 1 mg • Boron (as sodium borate) 1 mg. Other Ingredients: Polyethylene Glycol, Povidone, Croscarmellose Sodium, HPMS, Color, Magnesium Stearate, Magnesium Silicate, Maltodextrin, Carnauba Wax.

Citracal Prenatal Rx - Mission Pharmacal
Each tablet contains: Vitamin A (Vitamin A palmitate) 2700 IU • Vitamin C (Ascorbic acid) 120 mg • Calcium (Calcium citrate) 125 mg • Iron (Carbonyl iron, Ferrous gluconate) 27 mg • Vitamin D (as Vitamin D3) (Cholecalciferol) 400 IU • Vitamin E (dl Alpha Tocopheryl acetate) 30 IU • Thiamin (Vitamin B1) 3 mg • Riboflavin (Vitamin B2) 3.4 mg • Niacinamide (Vitamin B3) 20 mg • Vitamin B6 (Pyridoxine HCl) 20 mg • Folic Acid 1 mg • Iodine (Potassium iodide) 150 mcg • Zinc (Zinc oxide) 25 mg • Copper (Cupric oxide) 2 mg • Docusate Sodium 50 mg.

Citramannan - The Vitamin Shoppe
Each capsule contains: Citrimax brand Hydroxy Citric Acid 400 mg • Glucomannan root (konjac) 400 mg.

Citratherm - MetPro
Citrus aurantium • Chromium Picolinate • Vitamin C • Niacin • St. John's Wort.
See Editor's Note No. 40.

Citri-Caps - Progressive Labs
Each capsule contains: Malibar Tamarind [Garcinia cambogia, standardized to contain 50% (-) hydroxycitric acid] 333 mg • Atractylodes (Atractylodes lancea) 50 mg • Seville Orange flower (Citrus aurantii) 50 mg • Chromium (as chromium picolinate) 50 mcg • Chromium (as chromium arginate) 15 mcg.
See Editor's Note No. 40.

Citri-Caps Plus - Progressive Labs
Each capsule contains: Malibar Tamarind [Garcinia cambogia, standardized to contain 50% (-) hydroxycitric acid] 333 mg • Ma Huang Extract (Ephedra sinica) 200 mg • Yerba Mate 75 mg • Atractylodes (Atractylodes lancea) 50 mg • Seville Orange flower (Citrus Aurantii) 50 mg • Chromium (as chromium picolinate) 50 mcg • Chromium (as chromium arginate) 15 mcg.
See Editor's Note No. 30 and No 40.

CitriChrome - Swanson Health Products
Each capsule contains: Chromium (from Chromax brand chromium picolinate) • CitriMax brand Garcinia Cambogia fruit extract, (-) hydroxycitric acid 250 mg) 500 mg.

CitriGenics - Roex
Six tablets contain: Citrimax Garcinia Cambogia 1500 mg • L-Carnitine 300 mg • Choline Bitartrate 100 mg • Inositol 100 mg • Betaine HCl 50 mg • Chromium 200 mcg • Green Tea extract 150 mg • Kola Nut extract 150 mg • Yerba Mate 100 mg • Ginger 100 mg • Spirulina 100 mg • Kelp with Trace Minerals 100 mg • Vitamin C 100 mg • Vitamin E 30 IU • Potassium 25 mg • Biotin 300 mcg • Niacinamide 50 mg • Vitamin A 5000 IU • Vitamin B6 20 mg • Vitamin B2 20 mg • Vitamin B12 6 mcg • Folic Acid 400 mcg • Iodine 150 mcg • Selenium 50 mcg.

CitriLean - Enzymatic Therapy
Each capsule contains: Garcinia cambogia extract (CitriMax) standardized to contain 50% (-) hydroxycitrate (125 mg/capsule) 250 mg • Ginger root extract 6.5:1 (Zingiber officinale) 50 mg • Fenugreek seed extract 4:1 (Trigonella foenum-graecum) 50 mg • Curcuma root extract (Curcuma longa) standardized to contain 4% curcumin 50 mg • Chromium Polynicotinate (ChromeMate) 25 mcg.

CiTrim - E'OLA
Each tablet contains: Garcinia Cambogia (CitriMax) 500 mg • Proprietary Blend 97 mg: Triphala, Cayenne Pepper, Piper Longum, Vanadyl Sulfate. Other Ingredients: DiCalcium Phosphate, Microcrystalline Cellulose, Calcium Stearate, Vegetable Stearine, Cros Carmellose Sodium.

CiTrim 250 - E'OLA
0.75 ml (Approx. 15 drops) contains: Chromium 50 mcg • CitriMax Garcinia Cambogia 543 mg • L-Carnitine 125 mg • DMAE Bitartrate 20 mg. Other Ingredients: Purified Water, Sodium Benzoate.

Citrimate - Nature's Plus
Two tablets contain: Chromium (as polynicotinate) 200 mcg • Garcinia Cambogia fruit (standardized to 50% {-} hydroxycitrate extract) 1000 mg. Other Ingredients: Di-Calcium Phosphate, Microcrystalline Cellulose, Stearic Acid, Silica, Magnesium Stearate, Pharmaceutical Glaze.

CitriMax - JBN (Just Be Natural)
Two capsules contain: Hydroxycitric Acid (CitriMax brand) 1500 mg.

Citrimax - Trophic Canada
Each caplet contains: Garcinia Cambogia (CitriMax brand, supplying HCA 300 mg) 600 mg. Base: Ginkgo Biloba Leaves, Black Currant Extract.

CitriMax (-)Hydroxycitric Acid (HCA) 750 mg - Vitamin World
Two tablets contain: (-) Hydroxycitric Acid (HCA, provided by 1 500 mg of CitriMax brand from garcinia cambogia) 750 mg. Other Ingredients: Cellulose (plant origin), Dicalcium Phosphate, Cellulose Coating, Vegetable Stearic Acid, Silica, Vegetable Magnesium Stearate.

Citrimax 1000 mg - Nature's Plus
Each tablet contains: Calcium (as hydroxycitrate) 150 mg • Garcinia Cambogia fruit (standardized to 50% {-} hydroxycitrate extract) 1000 mg. Other Ingredients: Di-Calcium Phosphate, Stearic Acid, Microcrystalline Cellulose, Silica, Magnesium Stearate, Pharmaceutical Glaze.

CitriMax Balance with GlucoSupport Factors - Natrol, Inc.
Two tablets contain: Vitamin B6 (as pyridoxine HCl) 6.5 mg • Magnesium (as magnesium amino acid chelate) 86 mg • Chromium (as ChromeMate brand chromium polynicotinate) 100 mcg • Vanadium (as vanadyl sulfate) 340 mg • (-) HydroxyCitric Acid extract (HCA, from garcinia cambogia fruit, CitriMax brand) 500 mg • Green Tea leaf extract 400 mg • Gymnema Sylvestre leaf extract 400 mg • Bitter Orange rind extract (from citrus aurantium) 100 mg. Other Ingredients: Cellulose, Stearic Acid, Cellulose Gum, Silica, Magnesium Stearate, Methylcellulose, Glycerine.
See Editor's Note No. 40.

CitriMax brand - InterHealth Nutraceuticals
Hydroxycitric Acid (HCA, extracted from garcinia cambogia fruit).
See Editor's Note No. 44.

Citrimax Fat Burners - Optimum Nutrition
Citrimax brand H.C.A.

Citrimax Forte - Ortho Molecular Products
Each capsule contains: Vitamin B6 (as pyridoxine HCl USP) 15 mg • Folic Acid 200 mcg • Vitamin B12 (as methylcobalamin) 50 mcg • Manganese (as Chelazome brand) 2.5 mg • Chromium (as ChromeMate brand) 50 mcg • CitriMax brand Garcinia Cambogia fruit extract (standardized to contain 60% hydroxycitric acid) 900 mg • Vanadyl Sulfate 1 mg. Other Ingredients: Natural Vegetable Capsules, Magnesium STearate, Microcrystalline Cellulose.

CitriMax plus ChromeMate - Pure Encapsulations
Each vegetable capsule contains: Garcinia Cambogia extract (CitriMax brand of standardized garcinia cambogia extract, standardized to contain 60^ (-)hydroxycitric acid) 500 mg •

BRAND NAMES

Some Brand Name Natural Products - What they Contain

www.NaturalDatabase.com contains MANY more listings than appear here.
Editor's Notes are located on pages 2155-2163.

Chromium (polynicotinate, ChromeMate brand of niacin-bound chromium) 100 mcg • Vitamin C (as ascorbyl palmitate) 10 mg.

Citrimax Plus ChromeMate - Pro Health
Each capsule contains: Calcium (from citrimax) 83 mg • Iodine (from kelp) 150 mcg • ChromeMate Chromium (from chromium polynicotinate) 100 mcg • Potassium 120 mg • Super Citrimax Garcinia Cambogia fruit extract (containing (-) hydroxycitric acid 450 mg) 750 mg • Panax Ginseng powder 100 mg. Other Ingredients: Gelatin (capsule), Cellulose, Magnesium Stearate, Silica.

CitriMax Plus with ChromeMate - Natrol, Inc.
Each capsule contains: Calcium [from (-)hydroxycitric acid] 75 mg • Chromium (as chromium polynicotinate) 100 mcg • (-) HydroxyCitric Acid (HCA, from 500 mg garcinia cambogia fruit, CitriMax brand) 250 mg • Uva Ursi leaf 100 mg • Cascara Sagrada bark 75 mg. Other Ingredients: Gelatin, Magnesium Stearate.

CitrimaxPlus with ChromeMate - Natrol, Inc.
Each capsule contains: Chromium (Polynicotinate) 100 mcg • (-) Hydroxycitric Acid 250 mg • Uva Ursi 100 mg • Cascara Sagrada 75 mg. Other Ingredients: Gelatin, Magnesium Stearate.

Citrin + Chromium - Olympia Nutrition
Hydroxycitrate (-) HCA • Chromium Picolinate.

Citrin Forte - America's Finest
Each tablet contains: Citrin brand Garcinia Cambogia fruit extract [50% (-) HCA] 1000 mg • Bioperine brand Black Pepper fruit extract (98% piperine) 5 mg. Other Ingredients: Cellulose, Magnesium Stearate, Pharmaceutical Glaze.

CitriSate - Advocare International
Each caplet contains: D-Limonene powder 300 mg • Grapefruit juice powder 200 mg • 5-Hydroxytryptophan (seed - griffonia simplicifolia) 25 mg. Other Ingredients: Dicalcium Phosphate, Silicon Dioxide, Cellulose, Stearic Acid, Magnesium Stearate.

Citri-Shape - 4 Life
Each capsule contains: Thiamin (as thiamine mononitrate) 750 mcg • Riboflavin 850 mcg • Niacin (niacinamide) 10 mg • Vitamin B6 (as pyridoxine hydrochloride, pyridoxal 5-phosphate) 1 mg • Folate (folic acid) 200 mcg • Vitamin B12 (as cyanocobalamin) 3 mcg • Biotin 150 mcg • Pantothenic Acid (as D-calcium pantothenate) 5 mg • Manganese (as amino acid chelate) 2 mg • Chromium (as chromium chelate) 200 mcg • Garcinia Cambogia fruit extract (minimun 50% hydroxycitric acid 250 mg) 500 mg. Other Ingredients: Gelatin, Rice Flour, Magnesium Stearate, Silicon Dioxide.

CitriThin - PhytoPharmica
Two capsules contain: Garcinia Cambogia extract (CitriMax) 500 mg standardized to contain 50% (-)hydroxycitrate (125 mg per capsule) • Ginger root extract 6.5:1 (Zingiber officinale) 100 mg • Fenugreek seed extract 4:1 (Trigonella foenum-graecum) 100 mg • Curcuma root extract (Curcuma longa) 100 mg standardized to contain 4% curcumin • Chromium Polynicotinate (ChromeMate) 50 mcg.

Citrucel caplets - GlaxoSmithKline (GSK)
Each caplet contains: Methylcellulose 500 mg. Other Ingredients: Crospovidone, Dibasic Calcium Phosphate, FD&C Yellow No. 6 Aluminum Lake, Magnesium Stearate, Maltodextrin, Povidone, Sodium Lauryl Sulfate.

Citrucel Clear-Mix - GlaxoSmithKline (GSK)
Each 11.5 g serving contains: Methylcellulose 2 g. Other Ingredients: Maltodextrin, Flavors (natural and artificial), Potassium Citrate, Riboflavin, Sucrose, Malic Acid.

Citrucel Orange Mix - GlaxoSmithKline (GSK)
Each 19 g serving contains: Methylcellulose 2 g. Other Ingredients: Citric Acid, FD&C Yellow #6, Orange Flavors (natural and artificial), Potassium Citrate, Riboflavin, Sucrose.

Citrucel Sugar Free Orange Mix - GlaxoSmithKline (GSK)
Each 10.2 g serving contains: Methylcellulose 2 g containing Phenylalanine 52 mg. Other Ingredients: Aspartame, Dibasic Calcium Phosphate, FD&C Yellow #6, Malic Acid, Maltodextrin, Orange Flavors (natural and artificial), Potassium Citrate, Riboflavin.

Citrus Balm (Royal Image Cosmetics) - InterPlexus
Aloe Barbadensis gel • Olive extract • Olive Squalane • Glucose Stearate • Shea Butter • Rose Hip oil • Olive oil • Coconut oil • Glycerin • Extracts Blend: Arnica, Comfrey, Ginkgo, Ginseng, Bioflavonoids • Hyaluronic Acid • Allantoin • Natural Gums • Natural Essences • Tocopherol (vitamin E) • Retinyl Palmitate (vitamin A) • Cholecalciferol (vitamin D3) • Citric Acid.

Citrus Bioflavonoids - Nature's Sunshine
Two tablets contain: Vitamin C (ascorbic acid) 1000 mg • Calcium (di-calcium phosphate) 180 mg • Phosphorus (di-calcium phosphate) 140 mg • Proprietary Blend 525 mg: Citrus Bioflavonoids: Grapefruit, Lemon, Orange, Hesperidin, Rutin • Rose Hips (rosa canina). Other Ingredients: Magnesium Stearate, Cellulose, Stearic Acid.

Citrus Bioflavonoids Complex 1000 - GNC
Each tablet contains: Citrus Bioflavonoids 1000 mg. Other Ingredients: Dicalcium Phosphate, Povidine.

Citrus Slender - Nature's Way
Each 14 g scoop contains: Arabinogalactan 2 g • Chromium Polynicotinate 100 mcg • Citrin 1.5 g • L-Carnitine L-Tartrate 800 mg. Other Ingredients: Citric Acid, Fructose, Lemon Crystals, Lemon/Lime Crystals, Lime Crystals, Sodium Chloride, Sorbitol, Stevia, dried extract.

C-Jointin With Glucosamine, MSM, Chondroitin And Other Joint Nutrition Factors - Puritan's Pride
Three softgels contain: Vitamin C (as ascorbic acid) 60 mg • Vitamin E (as d-alpha tocopherol) 10 IU • Manganese (as manganese aspartate) 1 mg • Glucosamine Sulfate (2KCl) 1000 mg • MSM (methylsulfonylmethane) 750 mg • Chondroitin Sulfate 200 mg • Evening Primrose Oil 250 mg • Boron (as boron citrate) 1.5 mg. Other Ingredients: Soybean Oil, Gelatin, Glycerin, Lecithin, Yellow Beeswax, Caramel Color.
See Editor's Note No. 15.

CL Herbal Extract - Wild Rose
20 drops contain: Licorice root • Yarrow • Burdock • Uva Ursi (bearberry) • Juniper berry • Corn Silk.

CLA - NOW Foods
Three softgels contain: Safflower oil (high linoleic acid) 3 g • Conjugated Linoleic Acid (CLA) 2.25 g • Cis-9, Trans-11 Isomer 1.05 g • Trans-10, Cis-12 Isomer 1.08 g • Other Isomers 120 mg. Other Ingredients: Gelatin, Glycerin, Water, Natural Color.

CLA - Nature's Sunshine
Each capsule contains: CLA (conjugated linoleic acid) 750 mg. Other Ingredients: Safflower Oil, Gelatin, Glycerin, Natural Caramel Color, Water.

CLA - Wild Rose
Each capsule contains: Sunflower oil 1000 mg: Alpha-Linolenic Acid (omega-3) 550 mg, Cis-Linoleic Acid (omega-6) 140 mg, Oleic Acid (omega-9) 145 mg.

CLA - EAS, Inc.
Each capsule contains: Vegetable Oil 1000 mg: 60% Conjugated Linoleic Acid (CLA), 40% other Monounsaturated & Saturated Fatty Acid. Other Ingredients: 0.02% TBHQ.

CLA (1000 mg) - Pro Health
Each softgel contains: Sunflower Oil, Safflower Oil (high linoleic acid) 1000 mg • Conjugated Linoleic Acid (CLA) 700 mg • Cis-9 Trans-11 Isomer 330 mg • Trans-10 Cis-12 Isomer 330 mg. Other Ingredients: Gelatin, Glycerin, Water, Carob.

CLA (conjugated linoleic acid) 1,000 mg - Pure Encapsulations
Each softgel capsule contains: Conjugated Linoleic Acid [from

safflower oil, providing pure conjugated linoleic acid (CLA) 770 mg, palmitic acid 44 mg, stearic acid 21 mg, oleic acid 120 mg, linoleic acid 13 mg] 1000 mg.

CLA (conjugated linoleic acid) 500 mg - Pure Encapsulations
Each softgel capsule contains: Conjugated Linoleic Acid [from safflower oil, providing pure conjugated linoleic acid (CLA) 385 mg, palmitic acid 22 mg, stearic acid 10.5 mg, oleic acid 60 mg, linoleic acid 6.5 mg] 500 mg.

CLA 1000 - Human Development Technologies (HDT)
Each softgel capsule contains: Tonalin 1000 mg yielding Conjugated Linoleic Acid 700 mg.

CLA 1000 - AST Sports Science
Each two softgels contain: Conjugated Linoleic Acid 80% 800 mg.

CLA 1000 mg - Vitamin World
Two softgels contain: Tonalin CLA (from safflower oil, 74-82% conjugated linoleic acid) 2000 mg. Other Ingredients: Gelatin, Glycerin, Caramel Color, Titanium Dioxide Color.

CLA 1000mg - Vital Nutrients
Each softgel contains: Safflower oil 1000 mg: CLA (conjugated linoleic acid) 700 mg.

CLA 750 - Jarrow Formulas
Each softgel contains: Conjugated Linoleic Acid 750 mg • Safflower oil base 250 mg. Other Ingredients: Gelatin, Glycerin, Water, Natural Caramel.

CLA One brand - Pharmanutrients
Conjugated Linoleic Acid.

CLA Softgels - Optimum Nutrition
Each softgel contains: CLA One 1000 mg • CLA (conjugated linoleic acid) 750 mg. Other Ingredients: Gelatin, Glycerin, Water, Natural Caramel Color, Titanium Dioxide.

Clarifying Facial Cleanser - FreeLife International
Purified Water • Ahnfeltia Concinna • Himanthalia Elongata • Gigartina Stellata • Porphyra Umbilicalis (nori) • Spirulina Maxima (spirulina) • Crithmum Maritmum (sea fennel) • Palmaria Palmata (dulse) • BioEnhanced Grapefruit seed extract (BGSE) • Chrysanthellum Indicum extract • Arnica Montana • Aloe Barbadensis gel • Plant-Based Decyl Glucoside • Vegetable Glycerin • Glyceryl Stearate • Olive Squalane • Stearic Acid • Shea Butter • Sodium Stearoyl Lactylate • Tocopheryl Acetate (vitamin E) • Sodium Lactate • Sodium PCA • Proline • Sorbitol • Potassium Sorbate • Chlorphenesin • Vegetable Xanthan Gum • Essential Lavender oil, Essential Geranium oil, Essential Neroli oil, Essential Rose oil.

Clarina Cream - The Himalaya Drug Company
Kumari (aloe barbadensis syn. a.vera) 200 mg • Badama (prunus amygdalus) 10 mg • Matsyakshi (alternathera sessilis) 10 mg • Manjishtha (rubia cordifolia) 5 mg • Tankana (sodium biborate) 12.5 mg • Yashad Bhasma (zinc calx) 12.5 mg • Base q.s. ad. 750 mg.

Classic Perfor-Max - Goldshield Elite
Each capsule contains: Proanthocyanidin Blend (85% Proanthocyanidins) Grape seed extract and Pine Bark 4:1 extract 50 mg • Turmeric rhizome extract 25 mg. Other Ingredients: Maltodextrin, Calcium Sulfate, Gelatin, Cellulose, Magnesium Stearate, Silica, and Riboflavin color.

Classic Thermo-Lift (Classic ThermoLift) - Goldshield Elite
Each capsule contains: Chromium (as Chromium picolinate) 200 mcg • MaHuang extract (aerial parts) (Standardized for 25 mg Ephedrine alkaloids) 310 mg • Proprietary herbal blend 260 mg: Guarana seed extract (39 mg Caffeine), White Willow bark, Siberian Ginseng root, Astragalus root, Bee Pollen, Bladderwrack kelp (Fucus vesiculosus), Ginger root, Gotu Kola leaf, Licorice root, Rehmannia root, and Reishi mushroom (fruiting body). Other Ingredients: Gelatin, Maltodextrin, Magnesium stearate, Wheat Germ, Silica, and Turmeric extract.
See Editor's Note No. 30.

Clay Pack - Nu Skin Enterprises
Water (aqua) • Aloe Barbadensis • Kaolin • Butylene Glycol • Glycerin • Bentonite • Sodium PCA • RNA • Tocopheryl Acetate • Retinyl Palmitate • Royal Jelly • Honey (mel) • Hypnea Musciformis extract • Gelidiela Acerosa extract • Sargassum Filipendula extract • Sorbitol • Carbomer • Cellulose Gum • Triethanolamine • Methylparaben • Propylparaben • Disodium EDTA.

Cleansaherb - Wild Rose
Each tablet contains: Red Clover 130 mg • Burdock root 65 mg • Echinacea Angustifolia herb 65 mg • Mullein leaf 65 mg • Uva Ursi leaf 65 mg • Parsley leaf 65 mg • Marshmallow root 65 mg.

Cleanse Maintenance - Gaia Herbs
Two capsules contain: Corydalis tubers (dicentra canadensis) 40 mg • Yellow Dock root (rumex crispus) 36 mg • Black Alder bark (alnus serrulata) 36 mg • Mayapple rhizome (podophyllum peltatum) 32 mg • Figwort herb (scrophylaria nodosa) 32 mg. Other Ingredients: Vegetable Glycerin, Vegetable Cellulose (capsule).

CleanseMORE - Renew Life Formulas, Inc.
Two capsules contain: Magnesium (as magnesium hydroxide) • Cape Aloe gel (aloe ferox) • Rhubarb root (rheum officinalis) • Slippery Elm bark (ulmus rubra) • Marshmallow root (althaea officinalis) • Triphala blend: Indian Gooseberry fruit, Belleric Myrobalan fruit, Tropical Almond fruit. Other Ingredients: Hypromellose, Water.

CleanseSMART - Renew Life Formulas, Inc.
Part I: Two capsules contain: Artichoke leaf (cynara scolymus) • Ashwaganda root (withania somnifera) • Beet leaf (beta vulgaris) • Bupleurum root (bupleurum chinense) • Burdock root (arctium lappa) • Celandine leaf (chelidonium majus) • Chlorella (cracked shell) • Corn Silk (zea mays) • Dandelion root (taraxacum officinale) • Hawthorne berry (crataegus laevigata) • Larch Arabinogalactan gum (larex occidentalis) • Milk Thistle seed (silybum marianum) • Silymarin • Mullein leaf (verbascum thapsus) • Red Clover leaf and stem (trifolium pratense) • Turmeric root (curcuma Longa). Other Ingredients: Hypromellose, Water.
Part II: Two capsules contain: Magnesium (as magnesium hydroxide) • Cape Aloe gel (aloes ferox) • Rhubarb root (rheum officinalis) • Slippery Elm bark (ulmas fulva) • Marshmallow root (althaea officinalis) • Fennel seed (foeniculum vulgare) • Ginger root (zingiber officinale) • Triphala blend: Indian Gooseberry fruit (phyllanthus emblica), Belleric Myrobalan fruit (terminalia bellerica), and Tropical Almond fruit (terminalia chebula). Other Ingredients: Hypromellose, Water.

Cleansing Herbs - Youngevity
Vitamin B2 • Cascara sagrada • Fennel • Peppermint • Yucca root • Pau d'Arco • Yellow Dock root • Vilcabamba Mineral Essence: Potassium, Calcium, Magnesium, Zinc, Chromium, Selenium, Iron, Copper, Molybdenum, Vanadium, Iodine, Cobalt, Manganese.

Cleansing Laxative - Zand
Each tablet contains: Cascara Sagrada bark 150 mg. Other Ingredients: Chinese Rhubarb Root, Frangula Bark, Gentian Root, Goldenseal Root, Fennel Seed, Kaolin Clay, Anise Seed, Oregon Grape Root.

Clear Energy Mind and Muscle Power - Garden of Life, Inc.
Three caplets contain: Poten-Zyme Adaptogen Blend 2700 mg: Eleutherococcus Senticosus, American Ginseng (panax quinquefolium), Cordyceps Sinensis, Reishi (ganoderma lucidum), Codonopsis root, Astragalus root, Polygonum Multiflorum, Schizandra berry, Lycium fruit, Licorice root, Aralia Racemosa, Black Diamond truffle, Maca extract • Rhodiola Rosea extract (3% rosavin) 300 mg • 5% Ecdysterone (from rhaponticum carthamoides) 100 mg. Other Ingredients: Cellulose, Stearates (vegetable source).

Clear Headache - Clear Products, Inc.
Each capsule contains: Aconitum Napellus 3X • Belladonna 6X • Bryonia 6X • Gelsemium 3X • Hypericum 3X • Kali Phosphoricum 3X • Natrum Muriaticum 6X. Other Ingredients: Angelica Dahuricae

Root, Chrysanthemum Flower, Ligustici Root, Notopterygium Root, Pueraria Root, Vitex Fruit, Mint Herb, Ginger Root, Sesame Seed, Tangarine Peel, Licorice Root.
See Editor's Note No. 1.

Clear Migraine **-** Clear Products, Inc.
Three capsules contain: Aconitum Napellus 3X • Belladonna 6X • Bryonia 6X • Cimicifuga Racemose 3X • Hypericum 3X • Iris Versicolor 6X • Kali Bichromicum 3X • Natrum Muriaticum 6X • Sanguinaria 3X • Spigellia 6X. Other Ingredients: Corydalis Tuber, Angelica Sinensis Root, Ligustici Root, Peony Root, Pueraria Root, Angelica Dahurica Root, Chrysanthemum Flower, Gastrodia Tuber, Rehmannia Root, Siler Root, Ginger, Root, Lycium Fruit, Tangerine Peel, Licorice Root.
See Editor's Note No. 1.

Clear Sinus & Ear **-** Clear Products, Inc.
Each capsule contains: Herbal Blend: Pueraria root, Angelica root, Peony root, Magnolia flower, Platycodon root, Coix seed, Ginger root, Perilla leaf, Silver root, Scutellaria root, Cinnamon bark, Licorice root. Other Ingredients: Magnesium Stearate, Gelatin, Silacone Dioxide.
See Editor's Note No. 1.

Clear Skin **-** PhytoPharmica
Twenty drops contain: Cantharis 8x • Croton tiglium 8x •Arsenicum album 6x • Mercurius currosivus 6x • Pulsatilla 4x •Cistus canadensis 3x •Natrum phosphoricum 2x • Echinacea 1x • Juglans 1x • Viola tricolor 1x. In a base of 45% USP alcohol by volume.
See Editor's Note No. 1.

Clear Skin 1 Problem Skin Cleanser 6oz **-** Derma E
Purified Water • Tea Tree oil • Glycerin • Glyceryl Stearate • PEG 100 Stearate • Stearic Acid • Caprylic Triglyceride • Willow bark • Cetyl Alcohol • Cocobetaine • Lavender oil • Rosewood oil • Chamomile • Polysorbate-20 • Methylparaben • Ethylparaben • I. Urea.

Clear Skin 2 Spot Blemish Treatment 1/2oz **-** Derma E
Purified Water • Glycerin • Tea Tree oil • Willow bark • Xanthan Gum • Chamomile • Rosewood oil • Lavender oil • Methylparaben • Ethylparaben • I. Urea.

Clear Skin 3 Problem Skin Moisturizer 2oz **-** Derma E
Purified Water • Tea Tree oil • Lavender oil • Rosewood oil • Chamomile • Stearic Acid • Glyceryl Stearate • PEG 100 Stearate • Xanthan Gum • Glycerin • Caprylic Triglyceride • Willow bark • Cetyl Alcohol • Methylparaben • Ethylparaben • I. Urea.

Clear Thoughts **-** Rexall - Sundown
Two capsules contain: Vitamin E (as dl-alpha-tocopheryl acetate and d-alpha-tocopheryl succinate) 30 IU • Niacin (as niacinamide) 20 mg • Folic Acid 400 mcg • Vitamin B-12 (as cyanocobalamin) 60 mcg • Zinc (as zinc amino acid chelate) 15 mg • Ginkgo Biloba extract (standardized to 24% ginkgo flavonol glycosides, 14.4 mg; standardized to 6% terpene lactones, 3.6 mg) 60 mg • Gotu Kola aerial parts 150 mg • L-Glutamine 200 mg • L-Tyrosine 100 mg • Choline (as choline bitartrate) 50 mg • Phosphatidylserine complex (standardized to 30% phosphatidylserine, 15 mg) 50 mg • Damiana leaf 50 mg. Other Ingredients: Gelatin, Maltodextrin, Silica, Talc, Magnesium Stearate.

Clear Tinnitus **-** Clear Products, Inc.
Each capsule contains: Calcarea Carbonica 6X • Cinchona Officinalis 3X • Chininum Sulphuricum 3X • Graphites 3X • Kali Carbonicum 6X • Lycopodium 3X • Salicylicium Acidum 3X • Proprietary Herbal Extracts Blend 500 mg: Pueraria root (ge gen), Platycodon root (jie geng), Angelica root (bai zhi), Coix seed (yi yi ren), Ginger root (sheng jiang), Ligustici root (chuan xiong), Peony root (bai shao), Perillia leaf (zi su ye), Magnolia flower (zin yi hua), Asarum leaf (xi xin), Cinnamon bark (gui zhi), Huang Qin (scutallaria root), Licorice root (gan cao). Other Ingredients: Magnesium Stearate, Gelatin, Silicon Dioxide.
See Editor's Note No. 1.

Clear Vein Creme/Spider Vein & Bruise Solution 2oz **-** Derma E
Purified Water • Horse Chestnut extract • Witch Hazel extract • Grape skin extract • White Oak extract • Glycerin • Stearic Acid • Jojoba oil • Green Tea extract • Caprylic Triglyceride • Polysorbate 20 • Dimethicone • Glyceryl Stearate • PEG 100 Stearate • Pycnogenol • Cetyl Alcohol • Stearyl Alcohol • Tocopheryl Acetate (vitamin E) • Methylparaben • I. Urea.

ClearAc **-** Hyland's
Two tablets contain: Echinacea Angustifolia 6X • Berberis Vulgaris 6X • Sulphur Lod. 6X • Hepar Sulph. 6X. Base: Lactose.
See Editor's Note No. 1.

ClearDetox (chocolate flavor) **-** Pure Encapsulations
Each scoop contains: Calcium (naturally occurring) 58 mg • Phosphorus (nturally occurring) 190 mg • Magnesium (naturall occurring) 58 mg • Potassium (naturally occurring) 211 mg • Vitamin C (as ascorbyl palmitate) 12 mg • L-Glutathione (reduced, free-form) 200 mg • N-Acetyl-L-Cysteine (free-form) 100 mg • Methylsulfonylmethane (MSM) 100 mg • Alpha Lipoic Acid (thioctic acid) 50 mg • Milk Thistle extract (silybum marianum, standardized to contain 80% silymarin) 100 mg • Artichoke extract (cynara scolymus, standardized to 3% carreolyquinic acids) 150 mg • turmeric extract (curcuma longa, standardized to contain 97% curcuminoids) 150 mg • Greater Celandine 4;1 extract (chelindonium majus) 100 mg • Barberry 6:1 extract (berberis vulgaris) 75 mg • Stevia 30 mg. Other Ingredients: Rice Protein Concentrate, Natural Flavors, Lo Han (momordica grosvenori fruit extract), Cocoa, Xylitol.

ClearDetox (pineapple coconut flavor) **-** Pure Encapsulations
Each scoop contains: Calcium (naturally occurring) 50 mg • Phosphorus (naturally occurring) 150 mg • Magnesium (naturally occurring) 30 mg • Potassium (naturally occurring) 36 mg • Vitamin C (as ascorbyl palmitate) 12 mg • L-Glutathione (reduced, free-form) 200 mg • N-Acetyl-L-Cysteine (free-form) 100 mg • Methylsulfonylmethane (MSM) 100 mg • Alpha Lipoic Acid (thioctic acid) 50 mg • Milk Thistle extract (silybum marianum, standardized to contain 80% silymarin) 100 mg • Artichoke extract (cynara scolymus, standardized to 3% carreolyquinic acids) 150 mg • turmeric extract (curcuma longa, standardized to contain 97% curcuminoids) 150 mg • Greater Celandine 4:1 extract (chelindonium majus) 100 mg • Barberry 6:1 extract (berberis vulgaris) 75 mg • Stevia 10 mg. Other Ingredients: Rice Protein Concentrate, Natural Flavors, Lo Han (momordica grosvenori fruit extract).

ClearDetox (strawberry banana creme flavor) **-** Pure Encapsulations
Each scoop contains: Calcium (naturally occurring) 50 mg • Phosphorus (naturally occurring) 150 mg • Magnesium (naturally occurring) 30 mg • Potassium (naturally occurring) 36 mg • Vitamin C (as ascorbyl palmitate) 12 mg • L-Glutathione (reduced, free-form) 200 mg • N-Acetyl-L-Cysteine (free-form) 100 mg • Methylsulfonylmethane (MSM) 100 mg • Alpha Lipoic Acid (thioctic acid) 50 mg • Milk Thistle extract (silybum marianum, standardized to contain 80% silymarin) 100 mg • Artichoke extract (cynara scolymus, standardized to 3% carreolyquinic acids) 150 mg • turmeric extract (curcuma longa, standardized to contain 97% curcuminoids) 150 mg • Greater Celandine 4:1 extract (chelindonium majus) 100 mg • Barberry 6:1 extract (berberis vulgaris) 75 mg • Stevia 10 mg. Other Ingredients: Rice Protein Concentrate, Natural Flavors, Lo Han (momordica grosvenori fruit extract).

CLENbutical **-** NutraBolics
Two capsules contain: Coleus Forskohlii 175 mg • Guarana extract (22% caffeine) 300 mg • White Kidney bean extract 400 mg • Green Tea extract (50% polyphenols) 200 mg • Citrus Aurantium (6% synephrine) 200 mg • Cayenne 100 mg • Ginger root 100 mg.
See Editor's Note No. 40.

Clensa-Herb **-** Dial Herbs
Red Clover • Burdock • Echinacea • Chaparral • Mullein • Uva Ursi • Parsley • Marshmallow • Cascara Sagrada.

Clif BAR Apricot - Clif Bar Inc
Brown Rice Syrup • Rolled Oats • Evaporated Cane Juice • Soy Protein Isolate • Rice Flour • Oat Flour • Soy Flour • Soybean • Dried Apricots (sulfured) • Apple Fiber • Oat Fiber • Milled Flaxseed • Soy Fiber • Chicory Extract • Lemon Fiber • Psyllium • Dried Apples • Prunes • Brown Rice • Malt Extract • Natural Flavor • Citric Acid • Sea Salt • Baking Soda • Decaffeinated Green Tea Extract.

Clif BAR Carrot Cake - Clif Bar Inc
Brown Rice Syrup • Rolled Oats • Evaporated Cane Juice • Soy Protein Isolate • Rice Flour • Oat Flour • Soy Flour • Soybean • Dried Apples • Apple Fiber • Oat Fiber • Milled Flaxseed • Soy Fiber • Chicory Extract • Lemon Fiber • Psyllium • Cocoa Butter • Soy Milk • Soy Lecithin • Dried Carrots • Brown Rice • Malt Extract • Soy Butter • Raisins • Coconut • Sea Salt • Natural Flavors • Spices • Baking Soda • Decaffeinated Green Tea Extract.

Clif BAR Chocolate Almond Fudge - Clif Bar Inc
Brown Rice Syrup • Rolled Oats • Soy Protein Isolate • Rice Flour • Oat Flour • Soy Flour • Soybean • Evaporated Cane Juice • Soy Butter • Unsweetened Chocolate • Cocoa Butter • Soy Lecithin • Fig Paste • Almonds • Apple Fiber • Oat Fiber • Milled Flaxseed • Soy Fiber • Chicory Extract • Lemon Fiber • Psyllium • Natural Flavors • Sea Salt • Baking Soda • Decaffeinated Green Tea Extract.

Clif BAR Chocolate Brownie - Clif Bar Inc
Brown Rice Syrup • Rolled Oats • Soy Protein Isolate • Rice Flour • Oat Flour • Soy Flour • Soybean • Evaporated Cane Juice • Unsweetened Chocolate • Cocoa Butter • Soy Lecithin • Fig Paste • Soy Butter • Dutch Process Cocoa • Apple Fiber • Oat Fiber • Milled Flaxseed • Soy Fiber • Chicory Extract • Lemon Fiber • Psyllium • Natural Flavors • Sea Salt • Baking Soda • Decaffeinated Green Tea Extract.

Clif BAR Chocolate Chip - Clif Bar Inc
Brown Rice Syrup • Rolled Oats • Soy Protein Isolate • Rice Flour • Oat Flour • Soy Flour • Soybean • Evaporated Cane Juice • Unsweetened Chocolate • Cocoa Butter • Soy Lecithin • Soy Butter • Apple Fiber • Oat Fiber • Milled Flaxseed • Soy Fiber • Chicory Extract • Lemon Fiber • Psyllium • Fig Paste • Raisins • Brown Rice • Malt Extract • Natural Flavors • Sea Salt • Baking Soda • Cinnamon • Decaffeinated Green Tea Extract.

Clif BAR Chocolate Chip Peanut Crunch - Clif Bar Inc
Unsweetened Chocolate • Cocoa Butter • Soy Lecithin • Peanut Butter • Peanut Flour • Apple Fiber • Oat Fiber • Milled Flaxseed • Soy Fiber • Chicory Extract • Lemon Fiber • Psyllium • Fig Paste • Peanuts • Natural Flavors • Sea Salt • Baking Soda • Decaffeinated Green Tea Extract.

Clif BAR Cookies 'N Cream - Clif Bar Inc
Brown Rice Syrup • Rolled Oats • Soy Protein Isolate • Rice Flour • Oat Flour • Soy Flour • Soybean • Evaporated Cane Juice • Dutch Cocoa • Cocoa Butter • Chocolate Liquor • Oat Flour • Gum Arabic • Brown Rice • Malt Extract • Apple Fiber • Oat Fiber • Milled Flaxseed • Soy Fiber • Chicory Extract • Lemon Fiber • Psyllium • Soy Milk • Soy Lecithin • Almond Butter • Fig Paste • Natural Flavors • Cocoa • Sea Salt • Baking Soda • Decaffeinated Green Tea Extract.

Clif BAR Crunchy Peanut Butter - Clif Bar Inc
Brown Rice Syrup • Rolled Oats • Soy Protein Isolate • Rice Flour • Oat Flour • Soy Flour • Soybean • Evaporated Cane Juice • Peanut Butter • Peanut Flour • Apple Fiber • Oat Fiber • Milled Flaxseed • Soy Fiber • Chicory Extract • Lemon Fiber • Psyllium • Fig Paste • Peanuts • Natural Flavor • Sea Salt • Baking Soda • Decaffeinated Green Tea Extract.

Clif BAR GingerSnap - Clif Bar Inc
Brown Rice Syrup • Rolled Oats • Soy Protein Isolate • Rice Flour • Oat Flour • Soy Flour • Soybean • Evaporated Cane Juice • Ginger in cane syrup • Apple Fiber • Oat Fiber • Milled Flaxseed • Soy Fiber • Chicory Extract • Lemon Fiber • Psyllium • Soy Butter • Molasses • Fig Paste • Brown Rice • Malt Extract • Natural Flavors • Ground Ginger • Sea Salt • Baking Soda • Decaffeinated Green Tea Extract.

Clif SHOT Mmm...CHOCOLATE - Clif Bar Inc
Brown Rice Syrup • Cocoa Powder • Chocolate Liquor • Natural Flavors • Sea Salt • Potassium Citrate • Magnesium Oxide.

Clif SHOT Mocha Mocha with Caffeine - Clif Bar Inc
Brown Rice Syrup • Natural Flavors • Cocoa Powder • Kola Nut Extract (contains caffeine) • Sea Salt • Potassium Citrate • Magnesium Oxide.

Clif SHOT Razz Sorbet - Clif Bar Inc
Brown Rice Syrup • Raspberry Puree • Sea Salt • Potassium Citrate • Magnesium Oxide.

Clif SHOT Sonic Strawberry with Caffeine - Clif Bar Inc
Brown Rice Syrup • Strawberry Puree • Natural Flavor • Kola Nut Extract (contains caffeine) • Sea Salt • Potassium Citrate • Magnesium Oxide.

Clif SHOT Viva Vanilla - Clif Bar Inc
Brown Rice Syrup • Natural Flavors • Sea Salt • Potassium Citrate • Magnesium Oxide.

Clinical Nutrients Antioxidant - PhytoPharmica
Three capsules contain: Vitamin A (beta-carotene) 10,000 IU • Vitamin C (ascorbic acid) 500 mg • Vitamin E (D-alpha tocopheryl succinate) 200 IU • Riboflavin (vitamin B2) 6 mg • Zinc (picolinate) 15 mg • Selenium (L-selenomethionine) 200 mcg • Manganese (gluconate) 2 mg • N-Acetylcysteine 100 mg • Red Cabbage (brassica oleracea) leaf extract 4:1 100 mg • Garlic (Allium sativum) bulb extract (deodorized) 100 mg • Ginger root/rhizome extract (zingiber officinale) 100 mg • Green Tea leaf extract (camellia sinensis) 100 mg • Blue-Green Algae 100 mg • Turmeric root extract (curcuma longa, standardized to contain 85%-100% curcumin) 50 mg • Grape seed extract [vitis vinifera, PCO, standardized to contain 95% procyanidolic oligomers (PCOs)] 10 mg.

Clinical Nutrients Eye Formula - PhytoPharmica
Three tablets contain: Bilberry fruit extract (vaccinium myrtillus, standardized to contain 25% anthocyanosides calculated as anthocyanidins) 160 mg • Copper (as copper gluconate) 1 mg • Grape seed extract (vitis vinifera, standardized to contain 95% procyanidolic oligomers (PCOs)) 50 mg • Hachimijiogan Herbal Complex 400 mg: Rehmannia root (rehmannia glutinosa), Poria whole plant (wolfiporia cocos), Chinese Yam root (dioscorea oppositafolia), Asiatic Dogwood aerial part (cornus officinalis), Barrenwort aerial part (epimedium grandiflorum), Water Plantain aerial part (alisma plantago-aquatica), Astragalus root (astragalus membranaceus), Cassia bark (cinnamomum aromaticum) • Lutein 5% (from calendula officinalis) 2 mg • Riboflavin (vitamin B2) 1.5 mg • Selenium (as L-selenomethionine) 50 mcg • Turmeric rhizome extract (curcuma longa, standardized to contain 85-100% curcumin) 50 mg • Vitamin A (50% as beta carotene and as retinyl acetate) 5000 IU • Vitamin C (ascorbic acid) 600 mg • Vitamin E (as D-alpha tocopheryl acid succinate) 60 IU • Zinc (as zinc picolinate) 9 mg.

Clinical Nutrients Flax Oil - PhytoPharmica
Each 1 tbsp serving (14 mL) contains: Flaxseed Oil 11 mL • Pumpkin Seed oil 2 mL • Borage seed oil 1 mL.

Clinical Nutrients Flax Oil Capsules - PhytoPharmica
Seven softgels contain: Flaxseed oil 5250 mg • Pumpkin seed oil 1050 mg • Borage seed oil 700 mg.

Clinical Nutrients for 45-Plus Women - PhytoPharmica
Six tablets contain: Betain HCl 25 mg • Bilberry fruit 4:1 extract (vaccinium myrtillus) 10 mg • Biotin 600 mcg • Black Tea leaf 5:1 extract (camellia sinensis) 50 mg • Boron (as sodium borate) 3 mg • Calcium (as calcium carbonate, tricalcium phosphate, and calcium citrate) 800 mg • Choline Bitartrate 215 mg • Chromium (as chromium picolinate) 200 mcg • Copper (as copper gluconate) 2 mg • Cranberry fruit extract (vaccinium macrocarpon, standardized to contain 5% anthocyanidins and 30% organic acids (quinic, malic, and citric acid) 25 mg • Folic Acid 800 mcg • Ginger rhizome extract

(zingiber officinale) 60 mg • Grape seed 4:1 extract (vitis vinifera) 20 mg • Green Tea leaf 3:1 extract (camellia sinensis) 30 mg • Inositol 30 mg • Iodine (as potassium iodide) 450 mcg • Lipase 5 mg • Lutein (from calendula officinalis) 1.5 mg • Magnesium (as magnesium aspartate and magnesium oxide) 300 mg • Manganese (as manganese citrate) 2 mg • Molybdenum (as sodium molybdate) 75 mcg • Niacin (as niacinamide and niacin) 90 mg • Pantothenic Acid (as calcium D-pantothenate) 50 mg • Papain 15 mg • Pepsin (acid-stable protease) 5 mg • Phosphorus (from tricalcium phosphate) 180 mg • Potassium (as potassium aspartate) 100 mg • Riboflavin (vitamin B2) 60 mg • Selenium (as L-selenomethionine) 200 mcg • Silicon (as magnesium trisilicate) 1 mg • Sour Cherry fruit 10:1 extract (prunus cerasus) 50 mg • Soy (glycine max) 30 mg • Thiamin (as thiamin HCl, vitamin B1) 60 mg • Vanadium (as vanadyl sulfate) 100 mcg • Vitamin A (75% as beta carotene and as retinyl acetate) 10,000 IU • Vitamin B12 (as cyanocobalamin) 800 mcg • Vitamin B6 (as pyridoxine HCl) 60 mg • Vitamin C (ascorbic acid) 300 mg • Vitamin D (as cholecalciferol) 400 IU • Vitamin E (as D-alpha tocopheryl acid succinate) 200 IU • Vitamin K (as phytonadione) 120 mcg • Zeaxanthin (from calendula officinalis) 60 mcg • Zinc (as zinc gluconate) 15 mg.
This product was formerly known as Clinical Nutrients for Senior Women.

Clinical Nutrients for 50-Plus Men **-** PhytoPharmica
Four tablets contain: Betaine HCl 25 mg • Bilberry fruit 4:1 extract (vaccinium myrtillus) 10 mg • Biotin 600 mcg • Black Tea leaf 5:1 extract (camellia sinensis) 50 mg • Boron (as sodium borate) 3 mg • Bromelain (1200 MCU/g) 15 mg • Calcium (as calcium carbonate and calcium citrate) 400 mg • Choline Bitartrate 275 mg • Chromium (as chromium picolinate) 200 mcg • Copper (as copper gluconate) 2 mg • Folic Acid 800 mcg • Ginger rhizome extract (zingiber officinale) 40 mg • Grape seed 4:1 extract (vitis vinifera) 20 mg • Green Tea leaf 3:1 extract (camellia sinensis) 30 mg • Inositol 30 mg • Lipase 5 mg • Lutein (from calendula officinalis) 1.5 mg • Lycopene 2 mg • Magnesium (as magnesium aspartate and magnesium oxide) 250 mg • Manganese (as manganese citrate) 2 mg • Molybdenum (as sodium molybdate) 75 mcg • Niacin (as niacinamide and niacin) 120 mg • Panax Ginseng root extract (standardized to contain a minimum of 7% ginsenosides) 15 mg • Pantothenic Acid (as calcium D-pantothenate) 100 mg • Papain 15 mg • Pepsin (acid-stable protease) 5 mg • Potassium (as potassium aspartate) 100 mg • Riboflavin (vitamin B2) 60 mg • Saw Palmetto berry 4:1 extract (serenoa repens) 80 mg • Selenium (as L-selenomethionine) 200 mcg • Sodium 15 mg • Sour Cherry fruit 10:1 extract (prunus cerasus) 50 mg • Thiamin (as thiamin HCl, vitamin B1) 60 mg • Vanadium (as vanadyl sulfate) 100 mcg • Vitamin A (75% as beta carotene and as retinyl acetate) 10,000 IU • Vitamin B12 (as cyanocobalamin) 800 mcg • Vitamin B6 (as pyridoxine HCl) 60 mg • Vitamin C (ascorbic acid) 300 mg • Vitamin D (as cholecalciferol) 400 IU • Vitamin E (as D-alpha tocopheryl acid succinate) 200 IU • Vitamin K (as phytonadione) 120 mcg • Zeaxanthin (from calendula officinalis) 60 mcg • Zinc (as zinc gluconate) 30 mg.

Clinical Nutrients for Bone Health **-** PhytoPharmica
Three tablets contain: Vitamin C (ascorbic acid) 100 mg • Vitamin D (fish liver oil) 300 IU • Vitamin K (phytonadione) 300 mcg • Folic Acid 800 mcg • Vitamin B12 (cyanocobalamin) 800 mcg • Calcium (Krebs cycle chlelate/carbonate) 600 mg • Magnesium (Krebs cycle chelate) 150 mg • Zinc (picolinate) 15 mg • Copper (picolinate) 1 mg • Sodium 5 mg • Mixed flavonoids (citrus) 100 mg • Betaine HCl 30 mg • Soy (Glycine Max.) bean extract 20 mg • Boron (sodium tetrahydroborate) 3 mg • Silicon (sodium metasilicate) 1 mg • Strontium (chloride) 500 mcg.

Clinical Nutrients for Glucose Regulation **-** PhytoPharmica
2 tablets contain: Bilberry (vaccinium myrtillus extract standardized to contain 25% anthocyanosides calculated as anthocyanidins) 40 mg • Biotin 1 mg • Bitter Melon 2:1 extract (momordica charantia) 200 mg • Chromium (as chromium picolinate) 200 mcg • Copper (as copper gluconate) 0.5 mg • Fenugreek seed 4:1 extract (trigonella foenum-graceum) 100 mg • Folic Acid 400 mcg • Gymnema leaf extract (gymnema sylvestre, standardized to contain 25% gymnemic acids) 200 mg • Magnesium (as magnesium Krebs cycle chelates) 100 mg • Manganese (as manganese Krebs cycle chelates) 3.5 mg • Mixed Citrus Bioflavonoids 50% (from citrus fruits) 25 mg • Selenium (as L-selenomethionine) 50 mcg • Sodium 20 mg • Vanadium (as vanadyl sulfate) 1.6 mg • Vitamin B12 (as cyanocobalamin) 400 mcg • Vitamin B6 (as pyridoxine HCl) 10 mg • Vitamin C 300 mg • Vitamin E (as mixed tocopherols) 100 IU • Zinc (as zinc picolinate) 7.5 mg.
This product was formerly known as Clinical Nutrients for Diabetics.

Clinical Nutrients for Heart Health **-** PhytoPharmica
Two tablets contain: Vitamin C (ascorbic acid) 100 mg • Vitamin E (D-alpha tocopheryl acetate) 100 IU • Niacin 100 mg • Vitamin B6 (pyridoxine HCl) 10 mg • Folic Acid 200 mcg • Vitamin B12 (cyanocobalamin) 200 mcg • Calcium pangamate 20 mg • Magnesium (oxide) 150 mg • Potassium (chloride) 75 mg • Hawthorn (Crataegus oxyacantha) leaf and flower extract (standardized to contain 1.8% vitexin-2-rhamnoside) 150 mg • Super seven complex mixture of herbs: Hydrangea (Hydrangea arborescens) root, Black Cohosh (Cimicifuga racemosa) root, (Rhizome) extract, Buchu (Barosma crenata) leaf extract, Couch Grass (Elytrigia repens) rhizome extract, Cornsilk (Zea mays) extract, Dandelion (Taraxacum officinale) leaf, Ginger (Zingiber officinale) root] 150 mg • Khella (ammi visnaga) fruit extract (standardized to contain a minimum of 10% pyrones calculated as khellin) 100 mg • L-Cysteine 100 mg • Carbamide 100 mg.

Clinical Nutrients for Joint Health capsules **-** PhytoPharmica
Four capsules contain: Vitamin C (ascorbic acid) 100 mg • Niacin/ Niacinamide 330 mg • Vitamin B6 (pyridoxine HCl) 20 mg • Pantothenic Acid (calcium D-pantothenate) 100 mg • Magnesium (oxide) 100 mg • Zinc (picolinate) 3 mg • Copper (gluconate) 200 mcg • Manganese (chelate) 10 mg •Chloride (from glucosamine sulfate) 78 mg • Sodium 60 mg • Stabilized Glucosamine Sulfate 500 mg •Boswellia Serrata (gum resin) standardized to contain 65% boswellic acids 400 mg • Bio-Min T.R. 8 (a source of trace minerals) 100 mg • Chlorophyll 10 mg • Boron (sodium borate) 3 mg.

Clinical Nutrients for Joint Health tablets **-** PhytoPharmica
Two tablets contain: Vitamin C (ascorbic acid) 100 mg • Niacin/ Niacinamide 330 mg • Vitamin B6 (pyridoxine HCl) 20 mg • Pantothenic Acid (calcium D-pantothenate) 100 mg • Magnesium (oxide) 100 mg • Zinc (picolinate) 3 mg • Copper (gluconate) 200 mcg • Manganese (chelate) 10 mg • Chloride (from glucosamine sulfate) 78 mg • Stabilized Glucosamine Sulfate 500 mg • Boswellia Serrata (gum resin) standardized to contain 65% boswellic acids 400 mg • Bio-Min T.R. 8 (a source of trace minerals) 100 mg • Chlorophyll 10 mg • Boron (sodium borate) 3 mg.

Clinical Nutrients for Male Teens **-** PhytoPharmica
Four tablets contain: Vitamin A (86% beta-carotene and 14% retinol) 17,500 IU • Vitamin C (ascorbic acid) 300 mg • Vitamin D (cholecalciferol) 100 IU • Vitamin E (D-alpha tocoptheryl succinate) 200 IU • Vitamin K (phytonadione) 60 mcg • Thiamin (thiamin HCl; vitamin B1) 30 mg • Riboflavin (vitamin B2) 30 mg • Niacin/ Niacinamide 45 mg • Vitamin B6 (pyridoxine HCl) 30 mg • Folic Acid 800 mcg • Vitamin B12 (cyanocobalamin) 800 mcg • Biotin 300 mcg • Pantothenic Acid (calcium D-pantothenate) 30 mg • Calcium (citrate, carbonate) 400 mg • Iodine (kelp) 300 mcg • Magnesium (aspartate) 200 mg • Zinc (picolinate) 30 mg • Selenium (L-selenomethionine) 100 mcg • Copper (gluconate) 1.5 mg • Manganese (citrate) 15 mg • Chromium (polynicotinate) 200 mcg • Molybdenum (sodium molybdate) 25 mcg • Sodium 30 mg • Potassium (aspartate) 99 mg • Mixed flavonoids (citrus) 100 mg • Alfalfa leaf and stem juice concentrate (medicago sativa) 60 mg • Dandelion root 4:1 extract (taraxacum officinale) 60 mg • Ginger root/rhizome extract (zingiber officinale) 60 mg • Sarsaparilla root 4:1 extract (smilax officinalis) 60 mg • Choline Bitartrate 30 mg • Inositol 30 mg • Boron (sodium tetraborate decahydrate) 2 mg • Vanadium (sulfate) 50 mcg.

Some Brand Name Natural Products - What they Contain

www.NaturalDatabase.com contains MANY more listings than appear here.
Editor's Notes are located on pages 2155-2163.

Clinical Nutrients for Men - PhytoPharmica
Three tablets contain: Bilberry fruit 4:1 extract (vaccinium myrtillus) 10 mg • Biotin 600 mcg • Black Tea leaf 5:1 extract 50 mg • Boron (as sodium borate) 2 mg • Calcium (as calcium carbonate and calcium citrate) 300 mg • Choline Bitartrate 215 mg • Chromium (as chromium picolinate) 200 mcg • Copper (as copper gluconate) 2 mg • Folic Acid 800 mcg • Ginger rhizome extract (zingiber officinale) 30 gm • Grape seed 4:1 extract (vitis vinifera) 20 mg • Green Tea leaf 3:1 extract (camellia sinensis) 30 mg • Inositol 30 mg • Iodine (as potassium iodide) 300 mcg • Lutein (from calendula officinalis) 1.5 mg • Lycopene 2 mg • Magnesium (as magnesium aspartate and magnesium oxide) 250 mg • Manganese (as manganese citrate) 2 mg • Molybdenum (as sodium molybdate) 75 mcg • Muira Puama root 6:1 extract (ptychopetalum olacoides) 30 mg • Niacin (as niacinamide and niacin) 90 mg • Panax Ginseng root extract (standardized to contain a minimum of 7% ginsenosides) 15 mg • Pantothenic Acid (as calcium D-pantothenate) 60 mg • Potassium (as potassium aspartate) 100 mg • Riboflavin (vitamin B2) 60 mg • Selenium (as L-selenomethionine) 200 mcg • Sodium 15 mg • Sour Cherry fruit 10:1 extract (prunus cerasus) 50 mg • Thiamin (as thiamin HCl, vitamin B1) 60 mg • Vanadium (as vanadyl sulfate) 100 mcg • Vitamin A (75% as beta carotene and as retinyl acetate) 10,000 IU • Vitamin B12 (as cyanocobalamin) 500 mcg • Vitamin B6 (as pyridoxine HCl) 60 mg • Vitamin C (ascorbic acid) 300 mg • Vitamin D (as cholecalciferol) 400 IU • Vitamin E (as D-alpha tocopheryl acid succinate) 200 IU • Vitamin K (as phytonadione) 80 mcg • Zeaxanthin (from calendula officinalis) 60 mcg • Zinc (as zinc gluconate) 30 mg.

Clinical Nutrients for Teens: Female Formula - PhytoPharmica
Four tablets contain: Vitamin A (88% beta-carotene and 12% retinol) 17,000 IU • Vitamin C (ascorbic acid) 300 mg • Vitamin D (ergocalciferol) 100 IU • Vitamin E (d-alpha tocopheryl succinate) 200 IU • Vitamin K (phytonadione) 60 mcg • Thiamin (thiamin HCl; vitamin B1) 30 mg • Riboflavin (vitamin B2) 30 mg • Niacin/ Niacinamide 45 mg •Vitamin B6 (pyridoxine HCl) 90 mg • Folic Acid 800 mcg • Vitamin B12 (cyanocobalamin) 800 mcg • Biotin 300 mcg • Pantothenic Acid (calcium D-pantothenate) 30 mg • Calcium (citrate, carbonate) 500 mg • Iron (ferrous succinate) 30 mg • Iodine (kelp) 300 mcg • Magnesium (aspartate) 200 mg • Zinc (picolinate) 20 mg • Selenium (L-selenomethionine) 100 mcg • Copper (gluconate) 1.5 mg • Manganese (citrate) 15 mg • Chromium (polynicotinate) 200 mcg • Molybdenum (sodium molybdate) 25 mcg • Sodium 30 mg • Potassium (aspartate) 99 mg • Mixed flavonoids (citrus) 100 mg • Alfalfa (Medicago sativa) leaf and stem juice concentrate 60 mg • Choline Bitartrate 60 mg • Inositol 60 mg • Ginger (Zingiber officinale) root (rhizome) extract 60 mg • Dandelion (Taraxacum officinale) root extract 4:1 60 mg • Licorice (Glycyrrhiza glabra) root extract (standardized to contain 5% glycyrrhizic acid) 30 mg • Boron (sodium tetraborate decahydrate) 2 mg • Silica (sodium metasilicate) 1 mg • Vanadium (sulfate) 50 mcg.

Clinical Nutrients for Women - PhytoPharmica
Three tablets contain: Bilberry fruit 4:1 extract (vaccinium myrtillus) 10 mg • Biotin 600 mcg • Black Tea leaf 5:1 extract (camellia sinensis) 50 mg • Boron (as sodium borate) 3 mg • Calcium (as calcium carbonate, tricalcium phosphate, and calcium citrate) 500 mg • Chaste Tree berry extract (vitex agnus-castus, standadized to contain 0.5% agnusides) 20 mg • Choline Bitartrate 215 mg • Chromium (as chromium picolinate) 200 mcg • Copper (as copper gluconate) 2 mg • Cranberry fruit extract (vaccinium macrocarpon, standardized to contain 5% anthocyanidins and 30% organic acids (quinic, malic, and citric acid) 25 mg • Folic Acid 800 mcg • Ginger rhizome extract (zingiber officinale) 30 mg • Grape seed 4:1 extract (vitis vinifera) 20 mg • Green Tea leaf 3:1 extract (camellia sinensis) 30 mg • Inositol 30 mg • Iodine (as potassium iodide) 300 mcg • Iron (as ferrous succinate) 18 mg • Lutein (from calendula officinalis) 1.5 mg • Magnesium (as magnesium aspartate and magnesium oxide) 300 mg • Manganese (as manganese citrate) 2 mg • Molybdenum (as sodium molybdate) 75 mcg • Niacin (as niacinamide and niacin) 90 mg • Pantothenic Acid (as calcium D-pantothenate) 30 mg • Phosphorus (from tricalcium phosphate) 113 mg • Potassium (as potassium aspartate) 100 mg • Riboflavin (vitamin B2) 60 mg • Selenium (as L-selenomethionine) 200 mcg • Silicon (as magnesium trisilicate) 1 mg • Sour Cherry fruit 10:1 extract (prunus cerasus) 50 mg • Thiamin (as thiamin HCl, vitamin B1) 60 mg • Vanadium (as vanadyl sulfate) 100 mcg • Vitamin A (75% as beta carotene and as retinyl acetate) 10,000 IU • Vitamin B12 (as cyanocobalamin) 800 mcg • Vitamin B6 (as pyridoxine HCl) 95 mg • Vitamin C (ascorbic acid) 300 mg • Vitamin D (as cholecalciferol) 400 IU • Vitamin E (as D-alpha tocopheryl acid succinate) 200 IU • Vitamin K (as phytonadione) 90 mcg • Zeaxanthin (from calendula officinalis) 60 mcg • Zinc (as zinc gluconate) 20 mg.

Clinical Nutrients Prenatal Formula - PhytoPharmica
Four tablets contain: Biotin 600 mcg • Boron (as sodium borate) 1 mg • Calcium (as calcium carbonate, tricalcium phosphate, and calcium citrate) 1 g • Choline Bitartrate 90 mg • Chromium (as chromium polynicotinate) 200 mcg • Copper (as copper gluconate) 1.5 mg • Dandelion root 4:1 extract (taraxacum officinale) 60 mg • Folic Acid 800 mcg • Inositol 90 mg • Iodine (as potassium iodide) 300 mcg • Iron (as ferrous succinate) 30 mg • Magnesium (as magnesium citrate and magnesium oxide) 400 mg • Manganese (as manganese citrate) 2 mg • Mixed Citrus Bioflavonoids 50% (from citrus fruits) 90 mg • Molybdenum (as sodium molybdate) 25 mcg • Niacin (as niacin and niacinamide) 45 mg • Pantothenic Acid (as calcium D-pantothenate) 100 mg • Phosphorus (from tricalcium phosphate) 225 mg • Potassium (as potassium aspartate) 100 mg • Riboflavin (vitamin B2) 60 mg • Selenium (as L-selenomethionine) 100 mcg • Silicon (as magnesium trisilicate) 1 mg • Thiamin (as thiamin HCl, vitamin B1) 60 mg • Vanadium (as vanadyl sulfate) 50 mcg • Vitamin A (as beta carotene) 10,000 IU • Vitamin B12 (as cyanocobalamin) 800 mcg • Vitamin B6 (as pyridoxine HCl) 100 mg • Vitamin C (ascorbic acid) 300 mg • Vitamin D (as cholecalciferol) 200 IU • Vitamin E (as D-alpha tocopheryl acid succinate) 200 IU • Vitamin K (as phytonadione) 500 mcg • Zinc (as zinc picolinate) 30 mg.

Clinical Nutrients to Retain Healthy Cholesterol Levels - PhytoPharmica
Each capsule contains: Red Yeast (Monascus purpureus) rice 475 mg • Artichoke (Cynara scolymus) leaf extract (standardized to contain 13%-18% caffeylquinic acids calculated as chlorogenic acid) 50 mg • Ginger (Zingiber officinale) root (rhizome) extract 50 mg • Coenzyme Q10 (CoQ10) 8 mg.
See Editor's Note No. 21.

Clinician's Choice Arthritis Guardian - American Health Sciences, Inc.
Three tablets contain: Shark Cartilage 1500 mg • Glucosamine Sulfate 450 mg • Linoleic Acid, Gamma Linolenic Acid (sunflower oil, borage oil) 150 mg • Boswellia 30 mg • Cayenne Fruit 30 mg • Glycosaminoglycan 30 mg • White Willow Bark 30 mg • Proprietary blend: Carrot Powder, Citrus Bioflavonoids Complex, Grape Powder 9 mg.

Clinician's Choice Cardio Guardian - American Health Sciences, Inc.
Three tablets contain: Vitamin C (ascorbic acid) 180 mg • Vitamin E (dl-alpha tocopheryl acetate) 400 IU • Niacin (niacinamide) 300 mg • Niacin 100 mg • Vitamin B6 (pyridoxine hydrochloride) 23 mg • Folate (folic acid) 600 mcg • Vitamin B12 (cyanocobalmin) 150 mcg • Magnesium (glycinate) 15 mg • Zinc (gluconate) 15 mg • Selenium (aspartate) 120 mcg • RoseOx (patented, standardized process for an extract of Rosemary) 150 mg • Hawthorn 4:1 Extract 150 mg • Triphala Extract (Sstd. 40% tannin) 90 mg • White Willow Bark 60 mg • Motherwort 4:1 Extract 30 mg • L-Carnitine 30 mg • Seacol 30 mg • Linoleic Acid, Gamma Linolenic Acid (sunflower oil, borage oil) 30 mg • Proprietary blend 45 mg: Grape Powder, Cayenne Fruit, Coenzyme Q10.

Clinician's Choice Energy Reserve - American Health Sciences, Inc.
Two tablets contain: Thiamin (mononitrate) 20 mg • Riboflavin 20 mg • Vitamin B12 (cyanocobalamin) 20 mcg • Siberian Ginseng Root 400 mg • Panax Ginseng Leaves 400 mg • Brazilian Guarana Seeds 200 mg • Green Tea Leaves 200 mg • Wild American Ginseng Root 100 mg • Red Chinese Ginseng Root 100 mg • Tienchi Ginseng Root 100 mg • Cayenne Fruit 20 mg • Proprietary Blend 6 mg: Bee Pollen, Citrus Bioflavonoids, Soy Isoflavones.

Clinician's Choice Immune Guardian - American Health Sciences, Inc.
Three tablets contain: Vitamin C (ascorbic acid, calcium ascorbate) 150 mg • Vitamin E (dl-alpha tocopheryl acetate) 90 IU • Zinc (amino acid chelate) 90 IU • Selenium (selenomethionine) 150 mcg • Echinacea Angustifolia 450 mg • Echinacea Purpurea root 300 mg • Golden Seal root 150 mg • Kudzu root 150 mg • Odor Modified Garlic Bulb 150 mg • Bee Pollen 150 mg • RoseOx (patented, standardized process for an extract of Rosemary) 90 mg • Ascorbyl Palmitate 75 mg • Schizandra fruit 75 mg • Proprietary Blend 15 mg: Beta-Carotene, Reishi Mushroom, Shiitake Mushroom, Cinnamon bark, Grape powder.

Clinician's Choice Macular Guardian - American Health Sciences, Inc.
Two tablets contain: Vitamin A (as retinyl acetate) 2000 IU • Vitamin C (as ascorbic acid) 120 mg • Vitamin E (as dl-alpha tocopheryl acetate) 200 IU • Riboflavin 6 mg • Selenium (as selenomethionine) 40 mcg • Manganese (as amino acid chelate) 10 mg • Eyebright Herb 200 mg • RoseOx (patented, standardized process for an extract of Rosemary) 100 mg • Ascorbyl Palmitate 20 mg • L-Lysine HCl 20 mg • Lutein 12 mg • L-Glutathione 10 mg • Lycopene 10 mg • Beta-Carotene 6 mg • Proprietary blend 8 mg: Cruciferex, Carrot Powder, Citrus Bioflavonoid Complex, Bilberry, Zeaxanthin.

Clinician's Choice Men's AM Multi - American Health Sciences, Inc.
Two tablets contain: Vitamin A (retinyl acetate & 26% as beta-carotene) 3900 IU • Vitamin C (ascorbic acid) 250 mg • Vitamin D (cholecalciferol) 400 IU • Vitamin E (dl-alpha tocopheryl acetate) 150 IU • Thiamin (mononitrate) 1 mg • Riboflavin 1 mg • Niacin (niacinamide) 10 mg • Vitamin B6 (pyridoxine hydrochloride) 1 mg • Folate (folic acid) 200 mcg • Vitamin B12 (cyanocobalamin) 4 mcg • Biotin 210 mcg • Pantothenic Acid (d-calcium pantothenate) 5 mg • Iodine (potassium iodide) 76 mcg • Calcium (amino acid chelate) 4 mg • Magnesium (oxide, amnio acid chelate) 9 mg • Potassium (chloride, amino acid chelate) 12 mg • Zinc (amino acid chelate, gluconate) 2 mg • Selenium (selenomethionine) 100 mcg • Copper (amino acid chelate) 1 mg • Manganese (amino acid chelate) 3 mg • Chromium (nicotinate, amino acid chelate, chelavite, picolinate) 40 mcg • Molybdenum (amino acid chelate) 4 mcg • RoseOx (patented, standardized process for an extract of Rosemary) 50 mg • Citrus Bioflavonoid Complex 10 mg • Saw Palmetto Berries 10 mg • Whole Oats 10 mg • Panax Ginseng Extract 4 mg • Proprietary Blend 12 mg: Gingko Biloba Leaf, Echinacea Angustifolia, Panax Ginseng Root, Bee Pollen, Cruciferex, Grape Powder.

Clinician's Choice Men's PM Multi - American Health Sciences, Inc.
Two tablets contain: Vitamin A (retinyl acetate & 20% as beta-carotene) 1250 IU • Vitamin C (ascorbic acid) 450 mg • Vitamin D (cholecalciferol) 60 IU • Vitamin E (dl-alpha tocopheryl acetate) 150 IU • Thiamin (mononitrate) 0.5 mg • Riboflavin 0.7 mg • Niacin (niacinamide) 10 mg • Vitamin B6 (pyridoxine hydrochloride) 1 mg • Folate (folic acid) 200 mcg • Vitamin B12 (cyanocobalamin) 2 mcg • Biotin 90 mcg • Pantothenic Acid (d-calcium pantothenate) 5 mg • Calcium (carbonate, amino acid chelate) 84 mg • Iodine (potassium iodide) 74 mcg • Magnesium (oxide, amino acid chelate) 20 mg • Potassium (chloride, amino acid chelate) 16 mg • Zinc (oxide, amino acid chelate, gluconate) 32 mg • Selenium (selenomethionine) 100 mcg • Copper (amino acid chelate) 1 mg • Manganese (amino acid chelate) 1 mg • Chromium (nicotinate, picolinate, chelavite, amino acid chelate) 10 mcg • Molybdenum (amino acid chelate) 2 mcg • RoseOx (patented, standardized process for an extract of Rosemary) 50 mg • Citrus Bioflavonoid Complex 10 mg • Chamomile Flowers 10 mg • Passion Flower 10 mg • Valerian Root 10 mg • Mint Leaves 10 mg • Saw Palmetto Berries 10 mg • Whole Oats 10 mg • Hesperidin Complex 4 mg • Proprietary Blend 8 mg: Reishi Mushroom, Shiitake Mushroom, Cruciferex, Grape Powder.

Clinician's Choice Mood Enhancer - American Health Sciences, Inc.
Three tablets contain: Valerian root 300 mg • St. John's Wort extract (std. 0.3% hypericin) 300 mg • Chamomile flowers 300 mg • L-Tyrosine 30 mg • Proprietary Blend 15 mg: Passion Flower, Sage leaves, Isoflavones, Grape powder, Acetyl-L-Carnitine.

Clinician's Choice Neuro Guardian - American Health Sciences, Inc.
Two tablets contain: Vitamin E (as dl-alpha tocopheryl acetate) 200 IU • Thiamin (as mononitrate) 10 mg • Riboflavin 10 mg • Niacin (as niacinamide) 50 mg • Pantothenic Acid (d-calcium pantothenate) 10 mg • Zinc (as amino acid chelate) 10 mg • Selenium (selenomethionine) 50 mcg • Chromium (as nicotinate, chelavite, picolinate) 100 mcg • Ginkgo Biloba Leaf Extract 4:1 150 mg • Lecithin 100 mg • Natural Beta Carotene 40 mg • Acetyl-L-Carnitine 30 mg • RoseOx (patented, standardized process for an extract of Rosemary) 30 mg • Lecithin (standardized to 30% phosphatidyl serine) 30 mg • Aminogen 20 mg • Cayenne Fruit Powder 200 mg • Choline (as choline bitartrate) 20 mg • L-Tyrosine 20 mg • Proprietary Blend 8 mg: Astragalus, Carrot Powder, Pacific Kelp, Piper Longum Fruit Powder.

Clinician's Choice Osteo Guard - American Health Sciences, Inc.
Four tablets contain: Vitamin C (ascorbic acid) 120 mg • Vitamin D (cholecalciferol) 400 IU • Calcium (carbonate, glycinate, gluconate, citrate, succinate, amino acid chelate, aspartate) 1000 mg • Magnesium (oxide, carbonate, citrate, amino acid chelate) 480 mg • Zinc (amino acid chelate) 10 mg • Manganese (amino acid chelate) 1 mg • L-Glutamic Acid 20 mg • Betaine Hydrochloride 20 mg • Proprietary Blend 20 mg: Piper Longum Fruit, Pacific Kelp, Carrot Powder, Astragalus Membranaceus, Silica (horsetail herb), Boron (boron aspartate).

Clinician's Choice Pediatric Chewable - American Health Sciences, Inc.
One tablet contains: Vitamin A (as retinyl acetate & 50% as betacarotene) 2500 IU • Vitamin C (as ascorbic acid & sodium ascorbate) 60 mg • Vitamin D (as cholecalciferol) 200 IU • Vitamin E (as dl-alpha tocopheryl acetate) 15 IU • Thiamin (as mononitrate) 0.75 mg • Riboflavin 0.9 mg • Niacin (as niacinamide) 10 mg • Vitamin B6 (as pyridoxine hydrochloride) 1 mg • Folate (as folic acid) 200 mcg • Vitamin B12 (as cyanocobalamin) 3 mcg • Biotin 30 mcg • Pantothenic Acid (as d-calcium pantothenate) 5 mg • Calcium (as carbonate & gluconate) 85 mg • Iodine (as potassium Iodide) 75 mcg • Magnesium (as oxide) 15 mg • Zinc (as oxide) 7.5 mg • Copper (as cupric oxide) 1 mg • Manganese (as citrate) 0.5 mg • Chromium (as nicotinate) 10 mcg • Molybdenum (sodium molybdate) 5 mcg • Proprietary blend 6 mg: Acerola powdered extract 4:1 • Carrot Powder, Spinach Powder.

Clinician's Choice Prostate Guardian - American Health Sciences, Inc.
Three tablets contain: Vitamin E (dl-alpha tocopheryl acetate) 150 IU • Zinc (glycinate) 15 mg • Niacin (niacinamide) 15 mg • Pygeum Bark Powder 30 mg • Saw Palmetto Berries 450 mg • Kudzu Root 450 mg • Pumpkin Seeds 360 mg • Panax Ginseng Root 150 mg • Siberian Ginseng Root 150 mg • Oat Straw Extract (10:1) 150 mg • Horny Goat Weed 90 mg • RoseOx (patented, standardized process for an extract of Rosemary) 75 mg • Cayenne Fruit • Proprietary blend 12 mg: Lycopene 1%, Citrus Bioflavonoid Complex, Horsetail Herb, Isoflavones.

Clinician's Choice Super Antioxidant Tablets - American Health Sciences, Inc.
Two tablets contain: Vitamin C (as ascorbic acid) 120 mg • Vitamin E (as dl-alpha tocopheryl acetate) 200 IU • Zinc (as amino acid chelate) 4 mg • Selenium (selenomethionine) 100 mcg • RoseOx Rosemary extract 200 mg • Schizandra Fruit Powder 100 mg • Grape Powder 60 mg • Ascorbyl Palmitate 20 mg • Proprietary Blend 10 mg: Astragalus, Beta Carotene, Carrot Powder, Coenzyme Q10, Cruciferex, Pycnogenol.

Clinician's Choice Women's AM Multi - American Health Sciences, Inc.
Two tablets contain: Vitamin A (retinyl acetate & 26% as beta-carotene) 3900 IU • Vitamin C (ascorbic acid) 250 mg • Vitamin D (cholecalciferol) 400 IU • Vitamin E (dl-alpha tocopheryl acetate) 150 IU • Thiamin (mononitrate) 1 mg • Riboflavin 1 mg • Niacin (nianicamide) 10 mg • Vitamin B6 (pyridoxine hydrochloride) 2 mg • Folate (folic acid) 250 mg • Vitamin B12 (cyanocobalamin) 4 mcg • Biotin 200 mcg • Pantothenic Acid (d-calcium pantothenate) 5 mg • Calcium (carbonate, amino acid chelate, ascorbate, aspartate, citrate, gluconate) 220 mg • Iron (amino acid chelate) 12 mg • Iodine (potassium iodide) 76 mcg • Magnesium (oxide, amino acid chelate) 9 mg • Zinc (oxide, amino acid chelate, gluconate) 8 mg • Selenium (selenomethionine) 100 mcg • Copper (amino acid chelate) 1 mg • Manganese (amino acid chelate) 3 mg • Potassium (chloride, amino acid chelate) 12 mg • Chromium (nicotrate, picolinate, chelavite, amino acid chelate) 40 mcg • Molybdenum (amino acid chelate) 4 mcg • RoseOx (patented, standardized process for an extract of Rosemary) 60 mg • Citrus Bioflavonoid Complex 10 mg • Dong Quai 10 mg • Wild Yam 10 mg • Black Currant 10 mg • Red Raspberry Leaf 10 mg • Proprietary Blend 12 mg: Panax Ginseng Extract, Schizandra Fruit, Echinacea Angustifolia, Grape Powder, Bee Pollen, Cruciferex.

Clinician's Choice Women's Guardian - American Health Sciences, Inc.
Two tablets contain: Vitamin B6 (pyridoxine HCl) 2 mg • Pantothenic Acid (calcium pantothenate) 50 mg • Beta-Sitosterol 300 mg • Dong Quai Herb 200 mg • Red Raspberry Leaf 160 mg • Kudzu Root 100 mg • Wild Yam 100 mg • Squaw Vine 50 mg • L-Isoleucine 40 mg • L-Leucine 40 mg • L-Valine 40 mg • Aminogen 20 mg • Black Cohosh Root 20 mg • Evening Primrose 20 mg • Lycopene (1%) 20 mg • Proprietary Blend 12 mg: Lutein (5%), Chamomile Flowers, Passion Flower, Sage Leaves, Isoflavones, Grape Powder.

Clinician's Choice Women's PM Multi - American Health Sciences, Inc.
Two tablets contain: Vitamin A (retinyl acetate & 20% as beta-carotene) 1250 IU • Vitamin C (ascorbic acid) 250 mg • Vitamin D (cholecalciferol) 60 IU • Vitamin E (dl-alpha tocopheryl acetate) 150 IU • Thiamin (mononitrate) 0.5 mg • Riboflavin 0.7 mg • Niacin (niacinamide) 10 mg • Folate (folic acid) 200 mcg • Vitamin B12 (cyanocobalamin) 2 mcg • Biotin 150 mcg • Pantothenic Acid (d-calcium pantothenate) 5 mg • Calcium (amino acid chelate, aspartate, citrate, gluconate) 16 mg • Iron (glycinate) 6 mg • Iodine (potassium iodide) 76 mcg • Magnesium (oxide, amino acid chelate) 20 mg • Potassium (chloride, amino acid chelate, gluconate) 16 mg • Zinc (oxide, amino acid chelate, gluconate) 12 mg • Selenium (selenomethionine) 100 mcg • Copper (amino acid chelate) 1 mg • Manganese (amino acid chelate) 1 mg • Chromium (nicotinate, picolinate, chelavite, amino acid chelate) 10 mcg • Molybdenum (amino acid chelate) 2 mcg • RoseOx (patented, standardized process for an extract of Rosemary) 50 mg • Citrus Bioflavonoid Complex 10 mg • Chamomile Flower 10 mg • Passion Flower 10 mg • Valerian Root 10 mg • Mint Leaves 10 mg • Dong Quai 10 mg • Wild Yam 10 mg • Black Currant 10 mg • Red Raspberry Leaf 10 mg • Hesperidin 4 mg • Proprietary Blend 10 mg: Isoflavones, Echinacea, Milk Thistle Fruit, Cruciferex, Grape Powder.

CM Complex - Source Naturals
Three 500 mg softgels contain: Cetyl Myristoleate 180 mg • Cetyl Oleate (base of mixed fatty acid esters, olive oil and vitamin E) 375mg.

CM Source - NOW Foods
Each 500 mg capsule contains: Cetyl Myristoleate 100 mg.

CM Super - 4 Life
Three tablets contain: Vitamin C (as ascorbic acid) 20 mg • Vitamin D (as cholecalciferol) 400 IU • Vitamin K (as phytonadione) 80 mcg • Vitamin B6 (as pyridoxine hydrochloride) 1 mg • Calcium (as carbonate, citrate, amino acid chelate, di-calcium phosphate) 632 mg • Magnesium (as oxide, citrate, amino acid chelate) 270 mg • Zinc (as amino acid chelate) 2 mg • Copper (as amino acid chelate) 1 mg • Manganese (as glycinate) 1mg • L-Lysine (as L-Lysine monohydrochloride) 20 mg • Soy Lecithin 20 mg • Horsetail (equisetum arvense) 10 mg • Boron (as amino acid chelate) 3 mg • Strontium (as strontium chloride) 15 mcg. Other Ingredients: Croscarmellose Sodium, Magnesium Stearate, Stearic Acid, Silicon Dioxide, Microcystaline Cellulose.

CM+ - Metabolic Response Modifiers
Each softgel contains: Cetylmyristoleate (CMO) complex (Yielding 100 mg CMO) 500 mg.

CMG - Natrol, Inc.
Two capsules contain: Cetyl Myristoleate Proprietary Blend (CetylPure) 500 mg • MSM (Methyl Sulfonyl Methane) 500 mg • Glucosamine Sulfate 500 mg • Sea Cucumber 25 mg. Other Ingredients: Silica, Magnesium stearate, Gelatin.

C-M-K Citrate - Progressive Labs
Each capsule contains: Calcium (as calcium citrate) 100 mg • Magnesium (as magnesium citrate) 100 mg • Potassium (as potassium citrate) 25 mg.

CMO - Health Logics
Two capsules contain: Cetyl Myristoleate extract 760 mg. Other Ingredients: Kosher Gelatin, Calcium Phosphate, Silica.

CNM-FO (Flossing Oil) - CNM Co.
Origanum Vulgare • Melaleuca Alternifolia • Azadirachta Siamenesis • Virgin Olive oil.

Co Enzyme Q10 - Jamieson
Each capsule contains: Co-Enzyme Q10 30 mg.

Co Q10 - Pharmanex
Each softgel contains: Vitamin E (from Mixed Tocopherols) 30 IU • Coenzyme Q10 (Ubiquinone) 30 mg. Other Ingredients: Rice Bran Oil, Gelatin, Glycerin, Yellow Beeswax, Annatto Extract, Titanium Dioxide.

Cobra Powerful Men's Performance Enhancer - Natural Balance
Two capsules contain: Proprietary Blend 986 mg: Kola nut seed extract (contains caffeine), Yohimbe bark extract/powder, Oatstraw aerial portion extract, Nettles leaf extract, Eleuthero root, Horny Goat Weed aerial portion (epimedium), Catuaba bark, Muira Puama root, Korean Ginseng root/rhizome, Damiana leaf, Saw Palmetto fruit. Other Ingredients: Gelatin, Magnesium Stearate.

Cocoa Butter & E Replenishing Creme 4oz - Derma E
Purified Water • Safflower oil • Stearic Acid • Cetyl Alcohol • Glyceryl Stearate • PEG 100 Stearate • Cocoa butter • Glycerin • Tea • Tocopheryl Acetate (vitamin E) • Retinyl Palmitate (vitamin A) • Ergocalciferol (vitamin D) • Panthenol • Sunflower oil • Wheat Germ oil • Allantoin • Methylparaben • I. Urea • Annatto • Fragrant oils.

Cocoa Cherry StandardBar - Standard Process, Inc.
Protein blend: Whey Protein concentrate, Calcium Caseinate, Whole Egg powder • Maltitol Syrup • Almond Butter • Glycerin • Brown Rice syrup • Whey crisps • Natural Chocolate flavoring • Cherries • Grape seed oil • Cocoa powder • Soybean Lecithin • Vanilla extract • Natural Cherry flavor.

Cocoa Crisp StandardBar - Standard Process, Inc.
Protein Blend: Whey protein concentrate, Egg whites, Rice protein • Maltitol syrup • Almond Butter • Glycerin • Brown Rice syrup • Cocoa powder • Whey crisps (whey protein and rice flour) • Natural Flavors • Almond • Grape seed oil • Soybean Lecithin oil.

Cocoon GH Liquid Spray - Cocoon Nutrition
Each 1 oz dropper contains: Growth Hormone 600 ng. Other Ingredients: Purified Water, Sodium Citrate.

Cod Liver Oil - Puritan's Pride
Each softgel contains: Natural Vitamin A 2,664 IU • Natural Vitamin D (from 1,000 mg of Cod Liver Oil) 200 IU. Provides a rich source of Omega 3 fatty acids, EPA and DHA.

Cod Liver Oil - Jamieson
Each capsule contains: Vitamin A (Retinol) 1250 IU • Vitamin D 100 IU (Natural Vitamin A & D from North Atlantic Cod Liver Oils).

Cod Liver Oil - Nature's Way
Each softgel contains: Cod Liver Oil 1000 mg • Vitamin A (from cod liver oil) 1250 IU • Vitamin D (from cod liver oil) 135 IU. Other Ingredients: Gelatin, Glycerin, Water.

Cod Liver Oil - GNC
Each capsule contains: Vitamin A (as cod liver oil) 1250 IU • Vitamin D (as cod liver oil) 135 IU. Other Ingredients: Gelatin, Soybean oil, Glycerin.

Cod Liver Oil - Sunmark
Each softgel contains: Vitamin A as Cod Liver Oil 1250 IU • Vitamin D 135 IU. Other Ingredients: Soybean Oil, Gelatin, Glycerin. See Editor's Note No. 45.

Cod Liver Oil - J. R. Carlson Laboratories, Inc.
Three softgels contain: Vitamin A 3750 IU • Vitamin D (D3) 400 IU • Other Omega-3 Fatty Acids 60 mg • Omega-3 Fatty Acids (from cod liver oil) 300 mg • DHA (docosahexaenoic acid) 135 mg • EPA (eicosapentaenoic acid) 105 mg.

Cod Liver Oil & Evening Primrose Oil - Puritan's Pride
Each softgel contains: Natural Vitamin A 2,664 IU • Natural Vitamin D (from 500 mg of Cod Liver Oil) 200 IU • Evening Primrose Oil 500 mg. Provides a rich source of Omega-3 fatty acids, EPA and DHA.

Cod Liver Oil (A-2500, D-270) - Rexall - Sundown
Each softgel contains: Vitamin A (from cod liver oil) 2500 IU • Vitamin D (from cod liver oil) 270 IU • Cod Liver Oil 650 mg • Docosahexaenoic Acid (DHA) 52 mg • Eicosapentaenoic Acid (EPA) 52 mg. Other Ingredients: Gelatin, Glycerin, Water.

Cod Liver Oil Lemon Flavor - J. R. Carlson Laboratories, Inc.
Each 1 tsp serving contains: Vitamin A 1100 IU • Vitamin D 400 IU • Vitamin E (as D-alpha tocopherol) 10 IU • ALA (alpha-linolenic acid) 45 mg • DHA (docosahexaenoic acid) 500 mg • EPA (eicosapentaenoic acid) 460 mg.

Cod Liver Oil Regular Flavor - J. R. Carlson Laboratories, Inc.
Each 1 tsp serving contains: Vitamin A 1100 IU • Vitamin D 400 IU • Vitamin E (as D-alpha tocopherol) 10 IU • ALA (alpha-linolenic acid) 45 mg • DHA (docosahexaenoic acid) 500 mg • EPA (eicosapentaenoic acid) 460 mg.

Cod Liver Oil with Low Vitamin A - J. R. Carlson Laboratories, Inc.
Each softgel contains: Omega-3 Fatty Acids (from cod liver oil) 270 mg • DHA (docosahexaenoic acid) 110 mg • EPA (eicosapentaenoic acid) 110 mg.

Cod Liver Oil with Omega-3 Fatty Acids - GNC
Each capsule contains: Vitamin A (as cod liver oil) 1250 IU • Vitamin D (as cod liver oil) 135 IU • Vitamin E (as d-alpha Tocopherol) 1 IU • EPA (Eicosapentaenoic Acid) 50 mg • DHA (Docosahexaenoic Acid) 40 mg. Other Ingredients: Gelatin, Soybean oil, Glycerin, Peppermint oil.

CodPure Plus - Xymogen
Each 1 tsp serving contains: Vitamin A (from cod liver oil) 1500 IU • Vitamin D (as cholecalciferol) 100 IU • Vitamin E (as mixed tocopherols) 10 IU • EPA (eicosapentaenoic acid) 363 mg • DHA (docosahexaenoic acid) 545 mg.

CoenZest - Holista
Each capsule contains: CoEnzyme Q10 (ubiquinone) 30 mg. Other Ingredients: Organic Flax Seed Oil.

Coenzymated B-1 - Source Naturals
Each tablet contains: Coenzyme Vitamin B1 (Cocarboxylase) (Yielding 16.25 mg of activated Vitamin B1) 25 mg. In a base of Mannitol, Sorbitol, Natural Peppermint, and Sodium Citrate.

Coenzyme Q10 - Optimum Nutrition
Each capsule contains: Coenzyme Q10 100 mg. Other Ingredients: Microcrystalline Cellulose, Gelatin, Magnesium Stearate.

Coenzyme Q10 - DreamPharm
Each capsule contains: Coenzyme Q10 30 mg • Radix Salviae Miltiorrhizae 170 mg • Angelica Sinensis 100 mg • Cinnamomi Ramulus 100 mg • Sclerotium Poriae Cocos 100 mg.

Coenzyme Q10 - American Biologics
Each capsule contains: Co-Enzyme Q-10 50 mg. Other Ingredients: Magnesium Stearate.

Coenzyme Q10 - Source Naturals
Each sublingual tablet contains: Coenzyme Q10 30 mg.

Coenzyme Q10 - Solanova
Each softsule contains: Vitamin E (d-alpha tocopherol concentrate) 150 IU • Coenzyme Q-10 (ubidecarenone Hydrosoluble) 60 mg. Other Ingredients: Gelatin, Glycerin, Purified Water, Titanium Dioxide, Annato seed extract, plus a proprietary Bio-Solv base (polysorbate 80, lecithin, sorbitan monoleate, medium chain triglycerides).

Coenzyme Q10 - Benepure, Inc
Each capsule contains: Coenzyme Q10 (ubiquinone) 30 mg. Other Ingredients: Maltodextrin, Gelatin, Cellulose, Vegetable Stearate, Silicon Dioxide.

Coenzyme Q10 - CVS Pharmacy
Each softgel contains: Coenzyme Q10 100 mg. Other Ingredients: Soybean Oil, Gelatin, Glycerin, Yellow Beeswax, Lecithin, Titanium Dioxide, Annatto, D-Alpha Tocopheryl, Turmeric.

Coenzyme Q-10 - Natrol, Inc.
Each capsule contains: CoEnzyme Q10 30 mg. Other Ingredients: Rice Powder, Magnesium Stearate, Gelatin.

Coenzyme Q-10 - GNC
Each capsule contains: Coenzyme Q-10 30 mg. Other Ingredients: Dicalcium Phosphate, Cellulose, Gelatin, Stearic Acid.

Coenzyme Q-10 - Puritan's Pride
Each softgel contains: Coenzyme Q-10 10 mg. Other Ingredients: Ricebran Oil, Gelatin, Glycerin, Yellow Beeswax.

Coenzyme Q-10 - The Vitamin Shoppe
Each capsule contains: Co-Enzyme Q10 75 mg. Other Ingredients: Cellulose, Magnesium Stearate, Water.

Coenzyme Q10 50 mg Softgels - Pro Health
Each softgel contains: Vitamin E (D-alpha tocopherol acetate) 30 IU • Selenium (L-selenomethionine) 70 mcg • Coenzyme Q10 (from soy) 50 mg. Other Ingredients: Rice Bran Oil, Beeswax, Lecithin, Gelatin, Glycerine, Water, Annatto (natural color).

Coenzyme Q10 & L-Carnitine - PhysioLogics
Each softgel contains: Vitamin C (as ascorbyl palmitate) 12 mg • Vitamin E (as d-alpha tocopherol) 75 IU • Gamma Tocopherol 10 mg • L-Carnitine (as l-carnitine fumarate) 250 mg • Coenzyme Q10 30 mg. Other Ingredients: Polysorbate 80, Gelatin, Glycerin, Lecithin, Oleyl Lactylic Acid, Titanium Dioxide Color, Beeswax (yellow), Annato Color.

Coenzyme Q10 (100 mg) - Life Enhancement Products, Inc.
Each capsule contains: Coenzyme Q10 100 mg.

Coenzyme Q10 100 mg - PhysioLogics
Each capsule contains: Coenzyme Q10 100 mg. Other Ingredients: Rice Powder, Gelatin, Vegetable Magnesium Stearate.

Coenzyme Q10 100 mg - Leiner Health Products
Each capsule contains: Coenzyme Q10 100 mg. Other Ingredients: Maltodextrin, Gelatin, Magnesium Stearate.

Coenzyme Q10 100 mg - Pro Health
Each capsule contains: Coenzyme Q10 100 mg. Other Ingredients: Microcrystalline Cellulose, Gelatin, Magnesium Stearate, Silicon Dioxide.

Coenzyme Q10 100 mg - DaVinci Laboratories
Each tablet contains: Coenzyme Q10 (ubiquinone) 100 mg. Other Ingredients: Xylitol, Calcium Carbonate, Fibrosol, Silicon Dioxide, Magnesium Stearate.

CoEnzyme Q10 100 mg - Vital Nutrients
Each capsule contains: Coenzyme Q10 100 mg.

Coenzyme Q10 100 mg with Vitamin E - Pro Health
Each softgel contains: Vitamin A (beta carotene from D. salina) 2000 IU • Vitamin E (D-alpha-tocopherol with mixed tocopherols) 100 IU • Coenzyme Q10 (from soy) 100 mg • Betatene brand Beta Carotene 1.18 mg. Other Ingredients: Rice Bran Oil, Yellow Beeswax, Gelatin, Glycerin, Water, Annatto Extract, Titanium Dioxide.

Coenzyme Q-10 100MG - Nature Made
Each softgel contains: Coenzyme Q-10 100 mg.

CoEnzyme Q10 200 mg - Vital Nutrients
Each capsule contains: Coenzyme Q10 200 mg.

Coenzyme Q-10 200mg - Nature Made
Each softgel contains: Coenzyme Q-10 200 mg.

Coenzyme Q10 30 mg - Pro Health
Each Vcap contains: Coenzyme Q10 (from vegetable/plant lipids) 30 mg. Other Ingredients: White Rice Powder, Cellulose.

Coenzyme Q10 30 mg - PhysioLogics
Each capsule contains: Coenzyme Q10 30 mg. Other Ingredients: Rice Powder, Gelatin, Silica, Vegetable Magnesium Stearate.

CoEnzyme Q10 30 mg - Life Enhancement Products, Inc.
Each capsule contains: Coenzyme Q10 30 mg.

CoEnzyme Q10 30 mg - Vital Nutrients
Each capsule contains: Coenzyme Q10 30 mg.

Coenzyme Q10 30 mg - Leiner Health Products
Each softgel contains: Coenzyme Q10 30 mg. Other Ingredients: Hydrogenated Vegetable Oil, Refined Soybean Oil, Gelatin, Glycerin, Lecithin, Titanium Dioxide, Red 40 Lake, d-Alpha Tocopherol, Yellow 6 Lake, Blue 1 Lake.

Coenzyme Q-10 30MG - Nature Made
Each softgel contains: Coenzyme Q-10 30 mg.

Coenzyme Q10 400 mg - Pro Health
Each softgel contains: Vitamin E (d-alpha-tocopherol) 30 IU • Coenzyme Q10 400 mg • Soy Lecithin 50 mg. Other Ingredients: Rice Bran Oil, Gelatin, Glycerine (vegetable source), Lecithin, Purified Water, Beeswax, Annatto Extract (natural colorant).

Coenzyme Q10 50 mg Capsules - Pro Health
Two capsules contain: Coenzyme Q10 50 mg. Other Ingredients: Microcrystalline Cellulose, Gelatin, Magnesium Stearate, Silicon Dioxide.

Coenzyme Q10 50 mg Sublingual Tablets - Pro Health
Each tablet contains: Coenzyme Q10 50 mg. Other Ingredients: Sorbitol, Mannitol, Partially Hydrogenated Vegetable Oil, Artificial Flavor, Microcrystalline Cellulose, Silicon Dioxide, Magnesium Stearate, Croscarmelose Sodium, Gelatin.

Co-Enzyme Q10 50mg - Nature's Own
Each tablet contains: Co-Enzyme Q10 (ubidecarenone) 50 mg.

CoEnzyme Q10 60 mg - Vital Nutrients
Each capsule contains: Coenzyme Q10 60 mg.

Coenzyme Q10 Lozenges 200 mg - Pro Health
Each lozenge contains: Vitamin E (as d-alpha tocopheryl succinate) 100 IU • CoQ10 (coenzyme Q10 as ubidecarenone, from plant lipids) 200 mg • Non-GE Soy Lecithin 50 mg. Other Ingredients: Fructose, Cellulose, Sorbitol, Stearic Acid (vegetable source), Silica, Citric Acid, Natural Orange Flavor, Magnesium Stearate (vegetable source).

CoEnzyme Q10 Powder - Vital Nutrients
Each 1/4 tsp serving contains: Coenzyme Q10 300 mg.

Coenzyme Q10 Q-Sorb 120 MG - PhysioLogics
Each softgel contains: Q-Sorb Coenzyme Q10 120 mg. Other Ingredients: Rice Bran Oil, Gelatin, Glycerin, Lecithin, Beeswax / Soybean Oil Mixture, Titanium Dioxide Color.

Coenzyme Q10 Q-Sorb 200 MG - PhysioLogics
Each softgel contains: Q-Sorb Coenzyme Q10 200 mg. Other Ingredients: Rice Bran Oil, Gelatin, Glycerin, Lecithin, Titanium Dioxide Color, Beeswax / Soybean Oil Mixture.

Coenzyme Q10 Q-Sorb 75 MG - PhysioLogics
Each softgel contains: Coenzyme Q10 75 mg. Other Ingredients: Rice Bran oil, Gelatin, Glycerin, Lecithin, Beeswax / Soybean Oil Mixture, Titanium Dioxide Color.

Coffeccino - Advocare International
Each packet contains: Garcinia Cambogia extract 500 mg • Caffeine 120 mg • L-Tyrosine 800 mg. Other Ingredients: Fructose, Sugar, Polydextrose, Canola Oil, Corn Syrup Solids, Modified Casein, Coffee Powder, L-Tyrosine, Garcinia Cambogia Extract, Cocoa Powder, Caffeine, Natural Flavors, Artificial Flavors, Xanthan Gum, Ascorbic Acid, Calcium Pantothenate, Pyridoxine Hydrochloride, Chromium Polynicotinate (ChromeMate), Folic Acid.

CoFlu - AIE Pharmaceuticals
Echinacea Purpurea root • Vitamin C (as ascorbic acid) • Zinc (as zinc oxide) • Dyer's Woad root • Japanese Honeysuckle flower • Forsythia fruit • Balloon Flower root • Baikal Skullcap root • Apricot seed • Magnolia flower • Chinese Licorice root • Tangerine rind.

Cognicine - Pacific BioLogic
DMAE • Bacopin • Ashwagandha extract • Bioperine brand Black Pepper extract.

Cogni-Flex - Jarrow Formulas
Two capsules contain: Phosphatidylserine (from 250 mg of mixed phospholipids) 100 mg • Ginkgo Biloba 50:1 (minimum 6% terpene lactones; minimum 24% ginkgoflavonglycosides) 40 mg • Phospholipids (from lecithin) 150 mg • Gamma Tocopherol 19 mg. Other Ingredients: Cellulose, Magnesium Stearate, Silicon Dioxide, Gelatin.

Cognimax IQ - For Youthful Health
Two softgels contain: Phosphatidylserine Complex 500 mg: Phosphatidylserine 100 mg, Phosphatidylcholine 45 mg, Phosphatidylethanolamine 10 mg, Phosphatidylinositol 5 mg • DMAE (as bitartrate) 74 mg • DHA 13 mg • Vinpocetine 10 mg • Bioperine brand Black Pepper extract 5 mg • Dibencozide (coenzyme

of B12) 250 mcg • Huperzine A (huperzia serrata) 25 mcg. Other Ingredients: Soybean Oil, Gelatin, Glycerine, Water, Carob, Titanium Dioxide.

Cognita (Preventive Nutrition) - GNC
Three capsules contain: Vitamin E (as natural D-alpha tocopheryl acetate) 272 IU • Thiamin (B1, as thiamin mononitrate) 100 mg • Folate, Folic Acid, Folacin 200 mcg • Vitamin B12 (as cyanocobalamin) 25 mcg • Phosphatidyl Choline (as soy lecithin) 250 mg • Ginkgo Biloba leaf extract 120 mg • EPA (eicosapentaenoic acid, as fish body oil) 75 mg • DHA (docosahexaenoic acid, as fish body oil) 50 mg • Coenzyme Q10 10 mg • Huperzine A 100 mg. Other Ingredients: Soybean Oil, Gelatin, Glycerin, Caramel Color, Titanium Dioxide (natural mineral whitener).

Cognitive Aminos - Pure Encapsulations
Two vegetable capsules contain: DL-Phenylalanine (free-form) 250 mg • Taurine (free-form) 250 mg • L-Tyrosine (free-form) 250 mg • Acetyl-L-Carnitine (HCl) 295 mg • Vitamin C (as ascorbyl palmitate) 10 mg.

Cognitive Factors - Pure Encapsulations
Each vegetable capsule contains: Vinpocetine 20 mg • Ginkgo Biloba 50:1 extract (standardized to contain 24% ginkgoheterosides and 6% terpene lactones; terpene lactones typically provide ginkgolide A 1.2%, ginkgolide B 0.8%, ginkgolide C 1.0%, bilobalides 2.5%) 80 mg.

Cognizin 250 mg - Pure Encapsulations
Each vegetable capsule contains: Citicoline (cytidine 5' diphosphocholine) 250 mg.

Cognizin brand - Kyowa Hakko U.S.A., Inc.
Citicoline.

CognoBlend - Unicity International, Inc.
Two capsules contain: Bacopa monniera leaf extract (standardized to 20% bacosides A&B, 30 mg) 150 mg • Ginkgo Biloba leaf extract (standardized to 24% ginkgo flavone glycosides, 14.4 mg; standardized to 6% terpene lactones, 3.6 mg) 60 mg • Cognitive Proprietary Blend 600 mg: Cat's Claw bark PTI-00703 (uncaria tomentosa), Gotu Kola leaf, Rosemary leaf. Other Ingredients: Gelatin.

Cold & Flu (Cold and Flu) Capsules - Quantum, Inc.
Three capsules contain: Vitamin C 25 mg • Echinacea angustifolia standardized to 4% phenolic compounds 100 mg • Elderberry (10:1 extract) 100 mg • Goldenseal root (3:1 extract) 25 mg. Other Ingredients: Vegetable Sterine, Magnesium stearate, Micro Crystalline Cellulose.

Cold & Flu (Cold and Flu) Liquid Extract - Quantum, Inc.
Each two ounces contain: Fresh undried Echinacea purpurea whole plant 30% • Goldenseal root 20% • Elderberry 40% • Echinacea angustifolia 10%. In a base of Alcohol (approximately 20%), Distilled Water.

Cold & Flu Bath - Abra Therapeutics
Sodium Borate • Sodium Sulfate • Sodium Chloride • Sodium Sesquicarbonate • Olive Oil • Essential Oils Blend: Eucalyptus oil, Peppermint oil, Rosemary oil, Tea Tree oil • Herbal Extracts Blend: Echinacea, Sage leaves, Melissa, Dandelion, Berberry, Pepperwood • Chromium Oxide • Trace Mineral Salts.

Cold & Flu Remedy - PhytoPharmica
Twenty-five drops contain: Gelsemium sempervirens 6x • Aconitum napellus 4x •Arnica montana 4x • Belladonna 4x • Cinchona officinalis 4x • Bryonia 3x • Drosera rotundifolia 3x • Eupatorium 3x • Senega officinalis 3x • Eucalyptus globulus 1x. In a base of 50% USP alcohol by volume.
See Editor's Note No. 1.

Cold & Flu Remedy - Metagenics
Each drop contains: Aconitum Napellus 30X • Bryonia 12X • Eucalyptus Globulus 6X • Eupatorium Perfoliatum 6X • Ipecacuanha 12X • Gelsemium Sempervirens 12X • Phosphorus 6X • Pulsatilla 12X.
This product was formerly known as HP2. See Editor's Note No. 1.

Cold and Flu Formula - Body Language Vitamin Co.
Each capsule contains: Vitamin C (ascorbic acid) 333 mg • Zinc 12 mg • Proprietary Blend 425 mg: Echinacea purpurea, Echinacea pallida, Goldenseal, Astragalus, Elder Flower, Linden Flower, Meadowsweet, L-Arginine, Quercetin, Bioflavonoids.

Cold Care P.M. - Traditional Medicinals
Active Ingredient: Menthol: 5 mg per cup as it naturally occurs in the Peppermint leaf (Mentha x piperia) present in the blend. Other Herbal Ingredients: Licorice root, Chamomile flower, Tilla Starflower, Yarrow flower, Passion flower herb, Eucalyptus leaf, Elder flower.

Cold Cayenne - Olympian Labs
Each capsule contains: Cayenne (40000 h.u.) 500 mg.

Cold Chews - Westcoast Naturals
Each chewable tablet contains: Vitamin C (from Ester-C CG brand calcium ascorbate) 250 mg • Zinc (zinc citrate) 5 mg • Echinacea powder 4:1 extract (from echinacea angustifolia and echinacea purpurea) 50 mg.

Cold Fusion NO2 - Legal Gear
Each 1 tsp serving contains: Arginine Complex: Arginine AKG 2:1 / Diarginine Malate 3500 mg, Taurine 1000 mg, Ornithine 250 mg, Acetyl-L-Carnitine 250 mg. Other Ingredients: Filtered Water, Glycerine, Sugar, Citric Acid, Natural and Artificial Flavors, Red no 40, Blue no 1, Sodium Saccharin, Sodium Benzoate.

Cold FX - CV Technologies Inc.
Each capsule contains: Concentrated North American Ginseng extract (panax quinquefolium) 200 mg.

Cold Pressed Flax Oil - Golden Glow Natural Health Products
100% pure cold pressed Flax oil (linseed).

Cold Relief - Jamieson
Each capsule contains: Ephedra (Ma Huang) 63.75 mg • Grindelia 2 mg • Andrographis 10 mg • Echinacea Purpurea 8.33 mg • Picrorrhiza 2.5 mg.
See Editor's Note No. 30.

Cold Season Formula - Nature's Way
Three capsules contain: Echinacea purpurea (stem, leaf, flower) 450 mg • Ester-C (patented form of Vitamin C) 200 mg • Isatis 150 mg • Ligustrum fruits 70 mg • Sambucol (patented Black Elderberry extract) 100 mg • Siberian Ginseng root 150 mg • Usnea Barbata 100 mg • Vitamin A (retinol palmitate) 6,722 IU • Zinc amino acid chelate 25 mg. Other Ingredients: Cellulose, Gelatin, Magnesium stearate.

Cold Season Nutrition Booster - Advocare International
Each capsule contains: Echinacea root extract (echinacea purpurea) 200 mg • Astragalus root extract (astragalus membranaceus) 50 mg • Goldenseal root extract (hydrastis canadensis) 25 mg • Shiitake mushroom mycelium extract (lentinus edodes) 100 mg • Elderberry flower/fruit extract (sambucus canedensis) 10 mg • Quercetin 50 mg. Other Ingredients: Silicon Dioxide, Magnesium Stearate, Gelatin.

Cold Season Plus+ Zinc Lozenges - Quantum, Inc.
Each lozenge contains: Zinc acetate 14 mg • Vitamin A acetate 500 IU • Slippery Elm bark (Ulmus fulva) 20 mg • Propolis 5 mg. In a base of Goldenseal, Sugar, Dextrose, Fructose.

Cold Sore Relief - Golden Glow Natural Health Products
Each tablet contains: Lysine Hydrochloride 500 mg.

Some Brand Name Natural Products - What they Contain

www.NaturalDatabase.com contains MANY more listings than appear here.
Editor's Notes are located on pages 2155-2163.

***Cold Sore Relief* - PhytoPharmica**
Allantoin (1%), Lemon Balm leaf 65-75:1 extract (melissa officinalis), White Soft Paraffin, Benzyl Alcohol.
This product was formerly known as Herpalieve.

***Cold Sores therapeutic formula* - Nature's Own**
Each tablet contains: L-Lysine Hydrochloride 500 mg • Vitamin C (ascorbic acid) 500 mg • Zinc Sulfate 52.77 mg: Elemental Zinc 12 mg • Aloe Vera leaf extract (aloe barbadensis) 1000 mg • Black Walnut leaf powder (juglans nigra) 10 mg • Lemon Bioflavonoids 50 mg • Eucalyptus oil 2 mg.

***Cold-Eeze* - Quigley Co.**
Each lozenge contains: Zinc Gluconate 11.5 mg. Other Ingredients: Glycine, corn syrup, sucrose, and natural flavors.

***Cold-Eezer Plus* - Quigley Co.**
Each lozenge contains: Zinc Gluconate 14.5 mg. Other Ingredients: Glycerine, corn syrup, sucrose, and natural flavors.

***Coldflua* - HerbaSway**
Bitter Orange • Kudzu • Ginger • Echinacea • Astragalus • Knotweed • Schisandra • Blackberry • Licorice • Skullcap • Cayenne pepper • HerbaSwee (Cucurbitaceae fruit).
See Editor's Note No. 40.

***ColdFX* - CV Technologies Inc.**
Each capsule contains: Concentrated North American Ginseng extract (panax quinquefolium) 200 mg.

***Cold-FX* - CV Technologies Inc.**
Each capsule contains: Concentrated North American Ginseng (Panax quinquefolium) extract 200 mg.

***Colds & Flu* - Nature's Own**
Each tablet contains: Potassium Chloride 35 mg: Potassium 18.3 mg • Iron Phosphate 20 mg: Iron 3.2 mg.

***colds & flu* - Nelson Bach**
Active Ingredients: Anas barbariae 30C HPUS • Arsenicum Iod 30C HPUS • Gelsemium 30C HPUS • Eupatorium perf 30C HPUS.
Inactive Ingredients: Lactose, Sucrose.
See Editor's Note No. 1.

***Cold-X10* - Olympian Labs**
Three capsules contain: Ester C 180 mg • Zinc Gluconate 15 mg • Garlic 500 mg • Cat's Claw 250 mg • Echinacea 500 mg • Gotu Kola 100 mg • Proteolytic Enzymes 100 mg.

***Colest-Oil* - Aboca USA, Inc**
Three capsules contain: Fish Oil 720 mg (eicosapentaenoic acid 150 mg, docosahexaenoic acid 370 mg) • Guggul Olec-Gum-Resin extract in Flaxseed oil (1:10) 330 mg • Garlic bulb extract in Flaxseed oil (1:10) 110 mg. Other Ingredients: Gelatin (capsule), Essential Oil Of Rosemary.

***Coleus Forskohlii* - America's Finest**
Each capsule contains: Forslean brand Coleus Forskohlii 10% extract 100 mg. Other Ingredients: Dicalcium Phosphate, Cellulose, Magnesium Stearate, Silica.

***Coleus forskohlii* - Vital Nutrients**
Each capsule contains: Coleus Forskohlii extract (standardized to 10% forskolin) 90 mg.

***Coleus Forskohlii extract* - Enzymatic Therapy**
Each capsule contains: Coleus Forskohlii extract standardized to contain 18% Forskolin (9 mg per capsule) 50 mg.

***Colic Tablets* - Hyland's**
Each tablet contains: Dioscorea as Wild Yam 2X HPUS • Chamomilla as Chamomile 3X HPUS • Colocynth as Bitter Apple 3X HPUS. In a base of Lactose NF (Milk Sugar).
See Editor's Note No. 1.

***Colic-Ease Gripe Water* - Colic-Ease, Inc.**
Active Ingredients: Dill Oil • Caraway Oil • Cinnamon bark oil • Clove oil (clove bud) • Cardamon Oil. Inactive Ingredients: Deionized Water, Fructose.

***Collagen 15 PhytoShield* - Abra Therapeutics**
Active Ingredient: Titanium Dioxide. Other Ingredients: Aloe Vera Gel, Vegetable Emulsifying Wax, Lemon Juice, Vegetable Glycerine, Orange Wax, Shea Butter, Sesame Oil, Squalane (from olives), Kukui Nut Oil, Rose Water, Grape Seed Extract, Algae Extract, Foraha Berry Oil, Extracts of Green Tea, Comfrey, Red Clover and Horsetail; Ascorbic Acid and Ascorbyl Palmitate (vitamin C), Glucose and Glucose Oxidase, Lactose Peroxidase, Rose Geranium Oils, Lavender, Neroli, Palmarosa Balsam, Peru Balsam, Tocopherol (vitamin E), Citric Acid, Lecithin, Chamomile CO2, Hyaluronic Acid, Cellulose Gum, Methylparaben, Propylparaben.

***Collagen 30 PhytoShield* - Abra Therapeutics**
Active Ingredients: Octyl Methoxycinnamate, Octyl Salicylate, Benzophenone-3, Avobenzone. Other Ingredients: Aloe Vera Gel, Vegetable Emulsifying Wax, Lemon Juice, Vegetable Glycerine, Orange Wax, Shea Butter, Sesame Oil, Squalane (from olives), Kukui Nut Oil, Rose Water, Grape Seed Extract, Algae Extract, Foraha Berry Oil, Extracts of Green Tea, Comfrey, Red Clover and Horsetail; Ascorbic Acid and Ascorbyl Palmitate (vitamin C), Glucose and Glucose Oxidase, Lactose Peroxidase, Rose Geranium Oils, Lavender, Neroli, Palmarosa Balsam, Peru Balsam, Tocopherol (vitamin E), Citric Acid, Lecithin, Chamomile CO2, Hyaluronic Acid, Cellulose Gum, Methylparaben, Propylparaben.

***Collagen C* - Standard Process, Inc.**
Each tablet contains: Proprietary Blend 246 mg: Echinacea root, Rose Hips, Veal Bone meal, Defatted Wheat germ, Bovine Adrenal, Dried Buckwheat leaf juice, Buckwheat seed, Acerola berry, Mushroom • Vitamin C 100 mg. Other Ingredients: Honey, Calcium Stearate.
See Editor's Note No. 14.

***Collagen Support Cream* - Abra Therapeutics**
Deionized Water • Hamamelis Water • Sweet Almond oil • Jojoba oil • Macadamia nut oil • Vegetable Glycerin • Stearic Acid • Shea Butter • Rose Hip seed oil • Glucosamine • Methylsulfonylmethane (MSM) • Quercitin Bioflavonoids • Evening Primrose Oil • N-Acetyl Cysteine • L-Proline • L-Lysine • Pyridoxine HCl (vitamin B6) • D-Alpha-Tocopheryl (vitamin E) • Retinyl Palmitate (vitamin A) • Ascorbyl Palmitate (vitamin C) • Neroli oil • Lavender oil • Sweet Orange oil • Boswellia • Methylparaben • Propylparaben.

***Collagen Type II* - Swanson Health Products**
Six capsules contain: Hydrolyzed Type II Collagen (certified 100% chicken sternal cartilage) 3 g.
See Editor's Note No. 14.

***Collagenics* - Metagenics**
Two tablets contain: MSM (methylsulfonylmethane) 100 mg • Vitamin C (as ascorbic acid) 100 mg • L-Proline 100 mg • L-Lysine (as L-lysine hydrochloride) 100 mg • L-Cysteine 100 mg • Glycine 100 mg • Manganese (as manganese sulfate) 3.3 mg • Magnesium (as magnesium bis-glycinate) 50 mg • L-Glutamine 50 mg • D-Xylose 50 mg • L-Taurine 20 mg • Vitamin B6 (as pyridoxine hydrochloride) 20 mg • Pantothenic Acid (as D-calcium pantothenate) 20 mg • Alpha-Ketoglutaric Acid 10 mg • Zinc (as zinc glycinate) 10 mg • Iron (as iron glycinate) 4 mg • Copper (as copper lysinate) 2 mg • Horsetail aerial parts (equisetum arvense, natural source of silica) 50 mg.

***Collagenics Intensive Care* - Metagenics**
Each tablet contains: Glucosamine Sulfate (as D-glucosamine sulfate KCl) 250 mg • Niacin (as niacinamide ascorbate) 15 mg • Ultra Potent-C brand Vitamin C 200 mg • Vitamin E (as D-alpha tocopheryl succinate) 33 IU • SOD Precursor Blend: Zinc (as zinc glycinate) 3 mg, Manganese (as manganese glycinate) 1 mg, Copper (as copper glycinate) 0.3 mg • Grape seed extract (vitis vinifera) 4 mg.

Some Brand Name Natural Products - What they Contain

www.NaturalDatabase.com contains MANY more listings than appear here.
Editor's Notes are located on pages 2155-2163.

Collagenisis - Sterling-Grant Laboratories
Oxygenated Water • Collagen Hydrolysate (bovine source) • Aloe Vera • Vegetable Glycerin • Natural/Artifical Flavoring from Raspberries • Potassium Sorbate • Methylparaben.
See Editor's Note No. 14.

Collinsonia Root - Standard Process, Inc.
Two capsules contain: Collinsonia root • Gelatin • Water • Calcium Stearate • Colors.

Colloidal Magnesium Plus - Progressive Labs
Each capsule contains: Colloidal Calcium 25 mg • Colloidal Magnesium 50 mg • Colloidal Zinc 1.5 mg • Colloidal Copper 1 mg • Colloidal Manganese 0.1 mg • Colloidal Chromium 0.03 mg • Colloidal Molybdenum 0.012 mg.

Colloidal Minerals - Progressive Labs
Each 1/2 oz serving contains: Calcium 109 mg • Iron 0.24 mg • Phosphorus 109 mg • Iodine 180 mcg • Magnesium 56.9 mg • Zinc 16.3 mg • Selenium 0.09 mcg • Copper 1.24 mg • Manganese 2.8 mg • Chromium 0.4 mcg • Molybdenum 0.01 mcg • Chloride 0.1 mg • Sodium 0.74 mg • Potassium 171 mg • Sulfur 0.08 mg • Aluminum 2.15 mg • Silicon 0.4 mg • Lanthanum 0.1 mg • Thallium 0.02 mg • Cesium 0.4 mcg • Strontium 5.8 mcg • Vanadium 5.4 mcg • Boron 4.62 mcg • Nickel 4.45 mcg • Scandium 3.3 mcg • Ruthenium 3.13 mcg • Lithium 2.15 mcg • Titanium 1.57 mcg • Neodynium 0.15 mcg • Antimony 1.3 mcg • Cobalt 1.06 mcg • Flouride 0.94 mcg • Bismuth 0.33 mcg • Thallium 0.28 mcg • Zirconium 0.23 mcg • Beryllium 0.2 mcg • Cerium 0.2 mcg • Erbium 0.2 mcg • Bromine 0.16 mcg • Indium 0.13 mcg • Rubidium 0.13 mcg • Silver 0.1 mcg • Tin 0.1 mcg • Yttrium 0.1 mcg • Gallium 0.08 mcg • Tellurium 0.07 mcg • Praseodymium 0.05 mcg • Samarium 0.05 mcg • Barium 0.02 mcg • Cadmium 0.02 mcg • Dysprosium 0.02 mcg • Germanium 0.01 mcg • Gold < 0.01 mcg • Europium < 0.01 mcg • Niobium < 0.01 mcg • Palladium < 0.01 mcg • Ytterbium < 0.01 mcg • Hafnium < 0.01 mcg • Iridium < 0.01 mcg • Rhodium < 0.01 mcg • Terbium < 0.01 mcg • Holmium < 0.01 mcg • Lutetium < 0.01 mcg • Rhenium < 0.01 mcg • Tantalum < 0.01 mcg • Thorium < 0.01 mcg • Tungsten < 0.01 mcg • Plantium < 0.01 mcg • Carbon 7.8%. Other Ingredients: Water, Glycerine, Natural Flavor, Grapefruit seed extract, Stevia.

Colloidal Silver - Nature's Sunshine
Each 1 tsp (5 mL) serving contains: Colloidal Silver 70 mcg. Other Ingredients: Deionized Water.

Colloidal Silver - Goldshield Elite
Four droppers (4 mL) contain: Colloidal Silver 20 mcg. Other Ingredients: Demineralized water.

Colloidal Trace Minerals - Source Naturals
Two droppers (approximately 2.5 ml) contain: Boron, Calcium, Chromium, Copper, Iodine, Iridium, Iron, Lithium, Magnesium, Manganese, Molybdenum, Phosphorus, Potassium, Rhodium, Selenium, Silica, Silver, Sulfur, Vanadium, Zinc, Electrolyte complex (from colloidally suspended minerals, desalinated seawater, methylparaben).

Colloidal Vitamins - Progressive Labs
Each 1/2 oz serving contains: Vitamin A (as beta carotene) 5000 IU • Vitamin C (ascorbic acid) 300 mg • Vitamin D 400 IU • Vitamin E 60 IU • Vitamin K 300 mcg • Thiamin (Vitamin B1) 3 mg • Riboflavin (Vitamin B2) 3.4 mg • Niacin (as niacinamide) 40 mg • Vitamin B6 4 mg • Folate (folic acid) 400 mcg • Vitamin B12 3 mcg • Biotin 300 mcg • Pantothenic Acid 20 mg • Choline Bitartrate 50 mg • Myonositol (inositol) 50 mg • Essential Fatty Acid complex 10 mg • Amino Acid complex 10 mg • Aloe powder 3 mg. Other Ingredients: Water, Glycerine, Natural Flavor, Grapefruit seed extract, Stevia.

Coloklysis - PhysioLogics
Each scoop (12 g) contains: Dietary Fiber 9 g • Calcium (as tricalcium phosphate) 25 mg • Sodium 10 mg • Potassium 10 mg • Psyllium seed husk (plantago ovata) 9.1 g • Oat fiber (avena sativa) 1 g • Rice Bran 500 mg • Fructooligosaccharides 250 mg • Stevia leaf extract (stevia rebaudiana) 72 mg • Alfalfa (medicago sativa) 38 mg • Barley leaf (hordium vulgare) 38 mg • Apple Pectin (malus sylvestris) 38 mg • Buckthorn bark (frangula alnus) 38 mg • Papain (from carica papaya) 38 mg • Cascara Sagrada (rhamnus purshiana) 38 mg • Goldenseal (hydrastis canadensis) 38 mg • Triphala Blend 30 mg: Belleric Myrobalan fruit (terminalia bellerica), Emblic Myrobalan fruit (emblica officinalis), Tropical Almond fruit (terminalia chebula). Other Ingredients: Natural Flavors, Maltodextrin, Potato Starch, Acacia Gum.

Coloklysis Daily - PhysioLogics
Each scoop (13 g) contains: Dietary Fiber 10 mg • Calcium (as tricalcium phosphate) 30 mg • Sodium 10 mg • Psyllium seed husk (plantago ovata) 3.4 g • Oat fiber (avena sativa) 2.5 g • Guar Gum seed (cyamopsis tetragonolobus) 2.5 g • Acacia Gum 1.2 g • Apple Pectin 1 g • Rice Bran 500 mg • Fructooligosaccharides (FOS) 250 mg • L-Glutamine 100 mg • Aloe Vera leaf (aloe barbadensis) 100 mg • Licorice root extract (glycyrrhiza glabra) 100 mg • Ginger root (zingiber officinale) 100 mg • Stevia leaf extract (stevia rebaudiana) 59 mg. Other Ingredients: Maltodextrin, Natural Flavors, Acesulfame Potassium, Annatto, Riboflavin, Cornstarch.

Colon Cleanse - American Biologics
Each tablet contains: Calcium 267 mg • Proprietary Blend 835 mcg: Psyllium seed, Fennel seed, Cascara Sagrada, Buckthorn bark, Licorice root, Rhubarb root, Ginger, Goldenseal. Other Ingredients: Calcium Carbonate, Gum Acacia, Silicon Dioxide, Stearic Acid, Magnesium Stearate, Croscarmellose Sodium, Modified Cellulose.

Colon Cleanse - Nature's Rx
Each capsule contains: Bentonita Clay • Micro-Crystalline Cellulose • Psyllium Seed • Senna Leaf • Citrus Pectin • Oat Bran • Nutra Flora FOS • Acidophilus Blend • Barley Grass • Golden Seal • Prune Concentrate • Slippery Elm Bark • Aloe Vera Leaf Extract • Bio-Perine • Cascara Sagrada.

Colon Cleanser Daily - Health Smart Vitamins
Each scoop contains: Dietary Fiber 11 g • Blonde Psyllium (seed husks) 3 g • Oat Fiber 3 g • Guar Gum 3 g • Acacia Gum 1 mg • Apple Pectin 1 g • Rice Bran 500 mg • Fructooligosaccharides (FOS; from chicory root) 250 mg • Aloe Vera leaf 100 mg • Ginger root 100 mg • L-Glutamine 100 mg • Licorice root 100 mg • Stevia leaf 10 mg.

Colon Clear - Metabolic Response Modifiers
Each capsule contains: AG (Arabinogalactan) 200 mg • Cascara Sagrada bark 100 mg • Fennel seed 75 mg • Licorice root 50 mg • Ginger root 50 mg • Senna leaf 50 mg • Peppermint leaf 25 mg • Celery seed 25 mg • Triphala (Anala, Behada, Harada) 25 mg.

Colon Green - Futurebiotics LLC
Six capsules contain: Psyllium seed husk powder 2490 mg • Alfalfa leaf powder 600 mg • Alfalfa juice powder 180 mg • Lactobacillus acidophilus (supplying 12 billion cells) 60 mg • Pau D'Arco bark powder 120 mg • Echinacea leaf powder extract 120 mg • Black Walnut hull powder extract 120 mg • Fenugreek seed powder 120 mg • Watercress powder 120 mg • Parsley leaf powder 120 mg • Rosemary leaf powder 120 mg • Clove flower powder 120 mg • Bayberry bark powder 120 mg • Cayenne fruit powder 120 mg • Lipase 114 LU* • Protease 1380 HUT* • Amylase 114 DU*. Other Ingredients: LU are Lipase Units, HUT are Hemoglobin Units-Tyrosine basis, DU are Alpha-Amylase Dextrinizing Units.

Colostrum - Ortho Molecular Products
Each capsule contains: Colostrum (bovine) 500 mg. Other Ingredients: Natural Vegetable Capsules, Magnesium Stearate, Microcrystalline Cellulose.

Colostrum - Olympian Labs
Two capsules contain: Colostrum 1000 mg.

Colostrum - Abundance Marketing
Each capsule contains: 100% Bovine Colostrum (minimum 30% immunoglobulins) 500 mg.

Colostrum **-** PhysioLogics
Each tablet contains: Colostrum (standardized to contain 30% (195 mg) of naturally occurring immunoglobins) 650 mg. Other Ingredients: Cellulose (plant origin), Povidone, Croscarmellose, Silica, Cellulose Coating, Vegetable Magnesium Stearate.

Colostrum **-** Jamieson
Each capsule contains: Concentrated Colostrum 250 mg.

Colostrum **-** DaVinci Laboratories
Each capsule contains: Bovine Colostrum (yielding Ig [immunoglobulins] 180 mg) 600 mg. Other Ingredients: Gelatin.

Colostrum **-** Pro Health
Two capsules contain: Colostrum (20% IGG, bovine source) 800 mg. Other Ingredients: Cellulose, Magnesium Stearate, Silicon Dioxide.

Colostrum 30% IgG **-** Pure Encapsulations
Each vegetable capsule contains: Bovine Colostrum (standardized to contain 30% IgG) 600 mg.

Colostrum 40% IgG **-** Pure Encapsulations
Each vegetable capsule contains: Bovine Colostrum (standardized to contain 40% IgG) 450 mg.

Colostrum 80/40 **-** Proper Nutrition - PNI
Three capsules contain: Immunoglobulin G 600 mg. Other Ingredients: Gelatin.

Colostrum FM Capsules **-** Global Health Trax
Four capsules contain: Vitamin A 873 IU • Vitamin C 10 mg • Calcium 59 mg • Bovine Colostrum 2000 mg. Other Ingredients: Gelatin Capsules.

Colostrum Lozenges **-** Olympian Labs
Two lozenges contain: Colostrum 1000 mg.

Colostrum Prime Life **-** Jarrow Formulas
Each capsule contains: Colostrum 500 mg. Other Ingredients: Cellulose, Magnesium Stearate, Silicon Dioxide, Gelatin.

Colostrum Specific **-** Jarrow Formulas
Each capsule contains: Freeze Dried Colostrum 500 mg. Other Ingredients: Cellulose, Magnesium Stearate, Silicon Dioxide, Hydroxypropyl-Methyl Cellulose, Ethyl Cellulose, Gelatin.

Colpermin **-** Pharmacia Corp.
Active Ingredient: Peppermint oil BP 0.2. Other Ingredients: Gelatin, Colloidal Silica, Titanium Dioxide (E171), Indigotine (E132), Eudragit S100, Endragit L30 D55, Triethyl Citrate, Ammonia Solution 10%, Monostearin, Polyethylene Glycol 4000, Talc, Purified Water, Beeswax, Refined Arachis oil (peanut).

Comfrey and Fenugreek **-** Dial Herbs
Comfrey • Fenugreek.

Comfrey Ointment **-** Nature's Way
Beeswax • Comfrey leaves • Olive oil • Soybean oil • Tallow.

Comfrey/Aloe Capsules **-** Aloe Farms
Comfrey powder 100 mg • Aloe Vera powder 50 mg.

Commando 2000 **-** Nature's Plus
Two tablets contain: Vitamin A (as beta carotene) 10,000 IU • Vitamin C (as ascorbic acid) 1000 mg • Vitamin E (as D-alpha tocopheryl succinate) 200 IU • Zinc (as monomethionine) 20 mg • Selenium (as selenomethionine) 100 mcg • Echinacea Purpurea root and rhizome 250 mg • Citrus Bioflavonoids (from citrus limon exocarp) 200 mg • Astragalus root (astragalus membranaceus) 150 mg • Garlic clove (allium sativum, odorless) 70 mg • NAC (N-acetyl-cysteine) 20 mg • L-Methionine (free form amino acid) 15 mg • L-Glutathione 10 mg • Ginkgo Biloba leaf (standardized to 24% ginkgo flavone-glycosides and 6% terpene lactones) 5 mg. Other Ingredients: Microcrystalline Cellulose, Di-Calcium Phosphate, Silica, Stearic Acid, Magnesium Stearate, Carrot, Dunaliella Salina, Pycnogenol (pine bark extract), Plant Enzymes (catalase, glucose oxidase, peroxidase), Broccoli, Green Cabbage, Cauliflower, Tomato, Pharmaceutical Glaze.

Compete **-** Mission Pharmacal
Each tablet contains: Vitamin A 5,000 IU • Vitamin C 90 mg • Vitamin D (as Vitamin D3) 400 IU • Vitamin E 43 IU • Thiamine 2 mg • Riboflavin 2.6 mg • Niacin 30 mg • Vitamin B6 20 mg • Folate 0.4 mg • Vitamin B12 9 mcg • Iron 27 mg • Zinc 25 mg. Other Ingredients: Microcrystalline Cellulose, Sugar, Calcium Carbonate, Color, Croscarmellose Sodium, Povidone, Food Glaze, Cyanocobalamin, Magnesium Stearate, Yellow 6 Lake, Carnauba Wax, White Beeswax, Sodium Benzoate.

Complete Amino **-** Arrowroot
Each tablet contains: L-isoleucine 60 mg • L-leucine 104 mg • L-lysine 127 mg • L-methionine 32 mg • L-phenylalanine 53 mg • L-threonine 50 mg • L-tryptophan 14 mg • L-valine 79 mg • L-alanine 37 mg • L-arginine 38 mg • L-aspartic acid 86 mg • L-cysteine 7 mg • L-glutamic acid 235 mg • L-histidine 30 mg • L-proline 117 mg • L-serine 66 mg • L-tyrosine 39 mg.

Complete B **-** Puritan's Pride
Two tablets contain: Thiamin (Vitamin B1: as thiamine mononitrate) 10 mg • Riboflavin (Vitamin B2) 15 mg • Niacin (as niacinamide) 25 mg • Vitamin B6 (as pyridoxine hydrochloride) 10 mg • Folic Acid 400 mcg • Vitamin B12 (as cyanocobalamin) 25 mcg • Biotin (as d-biotin) 100 mcg • Pantothenic Acid (as d-calcium pantothenate) 100 mg • PABA (para-aminobenzoic acid) 50 mg • Choline Bitartrate 250 mg • Inositol 250 mg.

Complete Calcium plus Boron **-** Golden Glow Natural Health Products
Each tablet contains: Calcium (as calcium citrate 714.29 mg and calcium hydroxyapatite 434.78 mg) 250 mg • Phosphorus (from hydroxyapatite) 43.5 mg • Magnesium (as oxide) 125 mg • Zinc (as amino acid chelate) 2 mg • Vitamin D (D3, as cholecalciferol 2.5 mcg) 100 IU • Boron (from boric acid) 750 mcg • Horsetail herb extract (equisetum arvense) 100 mg.

Complete Cleanse **-** PhysioLogics
Two caplets contain: Calcium (from di-calcium phosphate) 260 mg • Phosphorous (from di-calcium phosphate) 200 mg • Enzyme-Activated Herbal Digestive Extract Blend 500 mg: Cellulose, Beet fiber root, Fenugreek seed, Licorice root, Fennel seed, Lipase (from Aspergullus cryzae), Date fruit, Fig fruit, Ginger root, Prune fruit • Herbal Detox Extract Blend 250 mg: Green Tea leaf, Grapefruit seed, Burdock root, Chickweed aerial parts, Gentian root, Milk Thistle seed, Red Clover blossom, Dandelion root, Marshmallow root, Rosemary leaf, Yarrow flower, Yellow Dock root • Enzyme-Activated Cleansing Fiber and Herb Blend 250 mg: Butternut bark, Beet fiber root, Licorice root, Flax seed, Peppermint Oil • Probiotic Flora Replenishment Complex 75 million cells: Fructooligosaccharides, Inulides (from dahlia tuber and chicory root), Lactic Culture of B. Coagulins • Intestinal Tract Immune Complex 250 mg: Black Walnut leaf, Methylsulfonylmethane (MSM), Garlic bulb. Inactive Ingredients: Stearic Acid, Vegetable Stearine, Silica, Croscarmellose Sodium, Magnesium Stearate, Spirulina, Lac-Resin.

Complete Cleanse Fiber Formula **-** PhysioLogics
Each tablet contains: Proprietary Blend 588 mg: Cascara Sagrada bark (rhamnus purshiana), Fennel seed (foeniculum vulgare), Psyllium seed husk (plantago ovata), Ginger root (zingiber officinale), Acacia Gum sap (acacia senegal), Apple Pectin (malus sylvestris), Apple Powder (malus sylvestris), Alfalfa leaf (medicago sativa), Barley Rice seed (hardeum vulgare), Beet root (beta vulgaris), Glucomannan root (amorphophallus riviori), Karaya Gum sap (sterculia urens), Lemon Fiber (citrus limon), Peppermint leaf (mentha piperita), Oat Bran seed (avena sativa), Red Raspberry leaf (rubus idaeus), Slippery Elm bark (ulmus fulva), Chlorella Algae plant (chlorella pyrenoidosa), Lactobacillus Acidophilus, Guar Gum

seed (cyamopsis tetragonolobus). Other Ingredients: Calcium Carbonate, Cellulose (plant origin), Vegetable Stearic Acid, Croscarmellose, Silica, Cellulose Coating.

Complete Cleanse Herb Formula **-** PhysioLogics
Each tablet contains: Proprietary Blend 588 mg: Ginger root (zingiber officinale), Dandelion root (taraxacum officinale), Fenugreek seed (trigonella foenum-graecum), Alfalfa leaf (medicago sativa), Fennel seed (foeniculum vulgare), Yarrow flower (achillea millefolium), Hawthorn berry (crataegus laevigata), Horsetail (equisetum arvense, aerial parts), Marshmallow root (althaea officinalis), Licorice root (glycyrrhiza glabra), Peppermint leaf (mentha piperita), Skullcap (scutellaria baicalensis, aerial parts), Red Clover flower (trifolium pratense), Safflower seed oil (carthamus tinctorius), Red Raspberry leaf (rubus idaeus), Chickweed (stellaria media, aerial parts), Papaya leaf (carica papaya), Mullein leaf (lychnis coronaria), Burdock root (arctium lappa), Cayenne Pepper fruit (capsicum annuum), Irish Moss (chondrus crispus), Black Cohsosh root (cimicufuga racemosa), Kelp (macrocystis pyrifera), Milk Thistle seed (silybum marianum), Slippery Elm bark (ulmus rubra), Ginkgo Biloba leaf (ginkgo biloba), Echinacea (echinacea angustifolia, aerial parts), Plantain seed (plantago lanceolata), Yellow Dock root (rumex crispus). Other Ingredients: Calcium Carbonate, Cellulose (plant origin), Vegetable Stearic Acid, Acacia Gum, Croscarmellose, Silica, Cellulose Coating.

Complete Diet Boost **-** Optimum Nutrition
Two capsules contain: Vitamin A (as mixed carotenoids) 1000 IU • Vitamin C (as ascorbic acid) 30 mg • Vitamin E (as D-alpha tocopheryl succinate) 30 IU • Vitamin B6 (as pyridoxine hydrochloride) 2 mg • Folic Acid 400 mcg • Vitamin B12 (as cyanocobalamin) 6 mcg • Pantothenic Acid (as D-calcium pantothenate) 10 mg • Magnesium (as magnesium aspartate) 5 mg • Chromium (as chromium GTF polynicotinate) 120 mcg • Proprietary Diet Boost Blend 1418 mg: Guarana seed extract (paullinia cupana, 30% caffeine), Green Tea leaf extract (camellia sinensis L., 40% EGCG/22% caffeine), Phase 2 - Brand Bean fruit extract (phaseolus vulgaris), Yerba Mate leaf (ilex paraguayensis, 20% caffeine), Kola Nut fruit extract (cola acuminata, 20% caffeine), Advantra-Z Citrus Aurantium fruit (citrus aurantium L., 30% synephrine), Metabromine-G (cocoa/guarana extract, 5% caffeine/5% theobromine), Ginger root powder, Cayenne fruit powder, DL-Methionine, Dandelion root powder, White Willow bark powder, DL-Phenylalanine, DMAE (2-dimethylaminoethanol), L-Tyrosine, Grape Seed extract (vitis vinifera L., 95% polyphenols), Acetyl-L-Tyrosine. Other Ingredients: Gelatin, Dicalcium Phosphate, Microcrystalline Cellulose, Magnesium Stearate, Stearic Acid, Silica. See Editor's Note No. 40.

Complete Energy **-** Rexall - Sundown
Each caplet contains: Vitamin A (25% [1250 IU] as beta-carotene) 5000 IU • Vitamin C (as ascorbic acid) 120 mg • Vitamin D (as cholecalciferol) 400 IU • Vitamin E (as dl-alpha-tocopheryl acetate) 60 IU • Vitamin K (as phytonadione) 25 mcg • Thiamin (as thiamin mononitrate) 4.5 mg • Riboflavin (vitamin BC) 5.1 mg • Niacin (as niacinamide) 35 mg • Vitamin B6 (as pyridoxine HCl) 6 mg • Folic Acid 400 mcg • Pantothenic Acid (as calcium d-pantothanate) 10 mg • Calcium (as dicalcium phosphate and calcium carbonate) 100 mg • Iron (as carbonyl iron) 18 mg • Phosphorus 48 mg • Iodine (as potassium iodide) 150 mcg • Magnesium (as magnesium oxide) 40 mg • Zinc (as zinc oxide) 15 mg • Selenium (as sodium selenate) 70 mcg • Copper (as cupric oxide) 2 mg • Manganese (as manganese sulfate) 4 mg • Chromium (chromium chloride) 120 mcg • Molybdenum (as sodium molybdate) 75 mcg • Chloride 75 mg • Potassium (as potassium chloride) 80 mg • Lutein 250 mcg • Ginkgo Biloba Extract (leaf) 60 mg • Citrus Bioflavonoids 25 mg • Guarana Extract (seed) 45 mg • American Ginseng (root) 50 mg • Nickel (as nickel sulfate) 5 mcg • Tin 10 mcg • Silicon 4 mg • Vanadium 10 mcg • Boron 150 mcg. Other Ingredients: Microcrystalline Cellulose, Croscarmellose Sodium, Hydroxypropyl Methylcellulose, Magnesium Stearate, Yellow 6 Lake, Caffeine, Corn Starch, PEG, Titanium Dioxide (color), Retinyl Acetate, Red 40 Lake, Polysorbate 80.

Complete Enzyme **-** Benepure, Inc
Each tablet contains: Calcium 50 mg • Pepsin 50 mg • Bromelain 50 mg • Ox Bile 30 mg • Pancreas Substance 200 mg • Papain 50 mg • Protease enzymes 100 mg • Amylase enzymes 100 mg • Lipase enzymes 25 mg • Cellulase enzymes 10 mg • Betaine Hydrochloride 100 mg. Other Ingredients: Calcium Carbonate, Cellulose, Magnesium Stearate.

Complete Essential Fatty Acids **-** Source Naturals
Three softgels contain: Vitamin E (as mixed tocopherols) 30 IU • Alpha-Linolenic Acid (ALA, omega-3) 636 mg • Linoleic Acid (omega-6) 522 mg • Oleic Acid (omega-9) 402 mg • Eicosapentaenoic Acid (EPA, omega-3) 360 mg • Docosahexaenoic Acid (DHA, omega-3) 240 mg • Gamma-Linolenic Acid (GLA, omega-6) 228 mg. Other Ingredients: Borage Seed Oil (non-GMO), Fish Oil (non-GMO), Flaxseed Oil (non-GMO), Gelatin, Glycerin, Purified Water.

Complete Flu Care **-** Hyland's
Eupatorium Perfoliatum 3X HPUS • Bryonia Alba 3X HPUS • Gelsemium Sempervirens 3X HPUS • Euphrasia Officinalis 3X HPUS • Anas Barbariae hepatis et cordis extractum 200C HPUS • Kali iodatum 3X HPUS.
See Editor's Note No. 1.

Complete La Femme Capsules **-** Baywood International
Four capsules contain: 2272 mg Proprietary Blend: Saw Palmetto berry, Pueraria Mirifica leaf, Dong Quai root, Damiana leaf, Hops flower, Fenugreek seed, Blessed Thistle leaf, Wild Yam root. Other Ingredients: Gelatin.

Complete La Femme Liquid **-** Baywood International
Each two mL serving contains: Proprietary Blend 565 mg: Saw Palmetto berry, Pueraria Mirifica leaf, Dong Quai root, Damiana leaf, Hops flower, Fenugreek seed, Blessed Thistle leaf, Wild Yam root. Other Ingredients: Distilled Water, Glycerin.

Complete Multi 50+ **-** Rexall - Sundown
Each caplet contains: Vitamin A (25% [1500 IU] as beta-carotene) 6000 IU • Vitamin C (as ascorbic acid) 120 mg • Vitamin D (as cholecalciferol) 400 IU • Vitamin E (as dl-alpha-tocopherol acetate) 60 IU • Vitamin K (as phytonadione) 10 mcg • Thiamin (as thiamin mononitrate) 1.5 mg • Riboflavin (vitamin B2) 1.7 mg • Niacin (as niacinamide) 20 mg • Vitamin B6 (as pyridoxine HCl) 3 mg • Folic Acid 400 mg • Vitamin B12 (as cyanocobalamin) 30 mcg • Biotin 30 mcg • Pantothenic Acid (as calcium d-pantothenate) 15 mg • Calcium (as calcium carbonate and dicalcium phosphate) 200 mg • Phosphorus 48 mg • Iodine (as potassium iodide) 150 mcg • Magnesium (as magnesium oxide) 100 mg • Zinc (as zinc oxide) 22.5 mg • Selenium (as sodium selenate) 95 mcg • Copper (as cupric oxide) 2 mg • Manganese (as manganese sulfate) 4 mg • Chromium (chromium chloride) 120 mcg • Molybdenum (as sodium molybdate) 75 mcg • Chloride 75 mg • Potassium (as potassium chloride) 8 mg • Lutein 300 mcg • Citrus Bioflavonoids (from orange peel extract) 25 mg • Billberry (fruit) 10 mg • Blueberry (fruit) 10 mg • Elderberry (fruit) 10 mg • Nickel (as nickel sulfate) 5 mcg • Tin (as stannous chloride) 10 mcg • Silicon (as silica) 2mg • Vanadium (as sodium metavanadate) 10 mcg • Boron (as sodium borate and potassium borate) 150 mcg. Other Ingredients: Microcrystalline Cellulose, Croscarmellose Sodium, Hydroxypropyl Methylcellulose, Titanium Dioxide (color), Magnesium Stearate, Corn Starch, PEG, Retinyl Acetate, Blue 2 Lake, Polysorbate 80, Red 40 Lake, Yellow 6 Lake.

Complete Multi Daily **-** Rexall - Sundown
Each caplet contains: Vitamin A (40% [2000 IU] as beta-Carotene) 5000 IU • Vitamin C (as ascorbic acid) 120 mg • Vitamin D (as cholecalciferol) 400 IU • Vitamin E (as dl-alpha-tocopherol acetate) 45 IU • Vitamin K (as phytonadione) 25 mcg • Thiamin (as thiamin mononitrate) 1.9 mg • Riboflavin (vitamin B2) 2.1 mg • Niacin (as niacinamide) 25 mg • Vitamin B6 (as pyridoxine HCl) 2.5 mg • Folic Acid 400 mcg • Vitamin B12 (as cyanocobalamin) 7.5 mcg • Biotin 37.5 mcg • Pantothenic Acid (as calcium d-pantothenate) 12.5 mg •

Calcium (as dicalcium phosphate and calcium carbonate) 162 mg • Iron (as carbonyl iron) 18 mg • Phosphorus 77 mg • Iodine (as potassium iodide) 150 mcg • Magnesium (as magnesium oxide) 100 mg • Zinc (as zinc oxide) 15 mg • Selenium (as sodium selenate) 70 mcg • Copper (as cupric oxide) 2 mg • Manganese (as manganese sulfate) 2.5 mg • Chromium (chromium chloride) 120 mcg • Molybdenum (as sodium molybdate) 75 mcg • Chloride 75 mg • Potassium (as potassium chloride) 80 mg • Lutein 300 mcg • Citrus Bioflavonoids (from orange peel extract) 25 mg • Nickel (as nickel sulfate) 5 mcg • Tin (as stannous chloride) 10 mcg • Silicon (as silica) 2 mg • Vanadium (as sodium metavanadate) 10 mcg • Boron (as sodium borate and potassium borate) 150 mcg. Other Ingredients: Microcrystalline Cellulose, Croscarmellose Sodium, Hydroxypropyl Methylcellulose, Titanium Dioxide (color), Magnesium Stearate, Corn Starch, PEG, Retinyl Acetate, Polysorbate 80, Yellow 5 Lake, Yellow 6 lake, Blue 2 lake.

Complete Multi Vitamin/Mineral **-** Benepure, Inc
Each tablet contains: Vitamin A (4000 IU as vitamin A palmitate and 10,000 IU as beta-carotene) 14,000 IU • Vitamin C 300 mg • Vitamin D 400 IU • Vitamin E (as D-alpha tocopheryl succinate) 120 IU • Thiamine 60 mg • Riboflavin 60 mg • Niacin (as niacinamide) 60 mg • Vitamin B6 60 mg • Folic Acid 400 mcg • Vitamin B12 60 mcg • Biotin 150 mcg • Pantothenic Acid 60 mg • Calcium 100 mg • Iron 10 mg • Phosphorus 45 mg • Iodine (from kelp) 25 mcg • Magnesium 50 mg • Zinc 10 mg • Selenium 20 mcg • Copper 0.25 mg • Manganese 2 mg • Chromium 20 mcg • Molybdenum 10 mcg • Sodium 5 mg • Potassium 20 mg • Boron 1 mg • Choline 40 mg • Inositol 40 mg • PABA (para-aminobenzoic acid) 60 mg • Mixed Citrus Bioflavonoids 50 mg • Hesperidin 10 mg • Pectin 25 mg • Betaine Hydrochloride 30 mg • Alfalfa leaf 5 mg • Chamomile 5 mg • Rose Hips 5 mg • Red Raspberry 5 mg • Parsley leaf 5 mg.

Complete Multi Women **-** Rexall - Sundown
Each caplet contains: Vitamin A (25% [1250 IU] as beta-carotene) 5000 IU • Vitamin C (as ascorbic acid) 120 mg • Vitamin D (as cholecalciferol) 400 IU • Vitamin E (as dl-alpha-tocopherol acetate) 45 IU • Vitamin K (as phytonadione) 80 mg • Thiamin (as thiamin mononitrate) 1.9 mg • Riboflavin (vitamin B2) 2.1 mg • Niacin (as niacinamide) 25 mg • Vitamin B6 (as pyridoxine HCl) 2.5 mg • Folic Acid 400 mcg • Vitamin B12 (as cyanocobalamin) 7.5 mcg • Biotin 37.5 mcg • Pantothenic Acid (as calcium d-pantothenate) 12.5 mg • Calcium (as dicalcium phosphate and calcium carbonate) 250 mg • Iron (as carbonyl iron) 27 mg • Phosphorus 77 mg • Iodine (as potassium iodide) 150 mcg • Magnesium (as magnesium oxide) 100 mg • Zinc (as zinc oxide) 15 mg • Selenium (as sodium selenate) 70 mcg • Copper (as cupric oxide) 2 mg • Manganese (as manganese sulfate) 2 mg • Chromium (chromium chloride) 120 mcg • Molybdenium (as sodium molybdate) 75 mcg • Chloride 37 mg • Potassium (as potassium chloride) 40 mg • Lutein 300 mcg • Citrus Bioflavonoids (from orange peel extract) 25 mg • Soy Isoflavones (from soybean extract) 10 mg • Blueberry (fruit) 10 mg • Cranberry (fruit) 10 mg • Elderberry (fruit) 10 mg • Nickel (as nickel sulfate) 5 mcg • Tin (as stannous chloride) 10 mcg • Vanadium (as sodium metavanadate) 10 mcg • Boron (as sodium borate and potassium borate) 150 mcg. Other Ingredients: Microcrystalline Cellulose, Croscarmellose Sodium, Hydroxypropyl Methylcellulose, Titanium Dioxide (color), Magnesium Stearate, Corn Starch, Triacetin, Retinyl Acetate, Yellow 6 Lake.

Complete Nutrition Center Ultra Choice Premium for Women **-** Walgreens
Two tablets contain: Vitamin A (50% as beta-carotene and 50% as retinyl acetate) • Vitamin C (as ascorbic acid) 200 mg • Vitamin D (D3, as cholecalciferol) • Vitamin E (as D-alpha tocopheryl acetate) • Vitamin K (as phytonadione) 75 mcg • Thiamin (vitamin B1, as thiamin mononitrate) 80 mg • Riboflavin (vitamin B2) 80 mg • Niacin (as niacinamide) 80 mg • Vitamin B6 (as pyridoxine hydrochloride) 80 mg • Folic Acid 400 mcg • Vitamin B12 (as cyanocobalamin) 80 mcg • Biotin 80 mcg • Pantothenic Acid (as calcium D-pantothenate) 80 mg • Calcium (as calcium carbonate) 500 mg • Iodine (as kelp) 150 mcg • Magnesium (as magnesium oxide) 200 mg • Zinc (as zinc oxide) 15 mg • Selenium (as hydrolyzed protein chelate) 100 mcg • Copper (as hydrolyzed protein chelate) 2 mg • Manganese (as hydrolyzed protein chelate) 5 mg • Chromium (as hydrolyzed protein chelate) 100 mcg • Molybdenum (as hydrolyzed protein chelate) 50 mcg • Boron (as hydrolyzed protein chelate) 2 mcg • Silica (as hydrolyzed protein chelate) 2 mg • Choline (as choline bitartrate) 10 mg • Inositol 10 mg • Para-Aminobenzoic Acid 10 mg • Citrus Bioflavonoid Complex 25 mg • Royal Jelly 5 mg • Bee Pollen powder 25 mg • Dong Quai root powder (angelica sinensis) 50 mg • Yarrow flower (achillea millefolium) 2.0 mg • Garlic (allium sativum) 2.0 mg • Red Raspberry leaf (rubus idaeus) 2.0 mg. Other Ingredients: Stearic Acid, Magnesium Stearate, Maltodextrin, Acacia, Hydroxypropylmethylcellulose, Microcrystalline Cellulose, Titanium Dioxide, Magnesium Silicate, Gelatin, Sucrose, Mannitol, Triacetin, Mineral Oil, FD&C Blue No. 1 Lake, FD&C Yellow No. 6 Lake, Glycine, Methocel, Polyvinylpyrolidone.

Complete Protein Diet **-** Optimum Nutrition
Each serving contains: Vanilla flavor Ingredients: Proprietary Protein Blend of Calcium Caseinate, Whey Protein Concentrate, Egg Albumen, Hydrolyzed Whey Peptides, Whey Protein Isolate, L-Glutamine • Canola oil • Artificial Flavor • Complete Vitamin Mineral Blend: di-Potassium Phosphate, Magnesium Oxide, Potassium Chloride, Ascorbic Acid, dl-Alpha Tocopherol Acetate, Niacinamide, Vitamin A Palmitate, Zinc Oxide, Potassium Iodide, Vitamin K, D-Calcium Pantothenate, Copper Sulfate, Manganese Sulfate, Vitamin D (as Vitamin D3), Pyridoxine Hydrochloride, Thiamine Mononitrate, Riboflavin, Selenium Glycinate, Molybdenum Glycinate, Chromium Picolinate, Folic Acid, Biotin, Cyanocobalamin • Lecithin • Cellulose Gum • Xanthan Gum • Aspartame • Acesulfame Potassium • Salt • FD&C Yellow #5 • FD&C Yellow #6.

Complete Protein Diet Bars **-** Optimum Nutrition
Each bar (50 g) contains: Protein Blend: Calcium Caseinate, Whey Protein Isolate, Soy Protein Isolate • Glycerine • Maltitol • Coating: Maltitol, Palm Kernal Oil, Non Fat Dry Milk Solids, Cocoa, Whole Milk Solids, Lecithin, Salt, Natural Flavor • Filtered Water • Natural and Artificial Flavor • Peanut Flour • Lecithin • Gum Arabic • Salt • Sucralose.

Complete Senior Formula **-** Sunmark
Each tablet contains: Vitamin A (29% as beta carotene) 3500 IU • Vitamin B6 3 mg • Vitamin B12 25 mcg • Vitamin C 60 mg • Vitamin D 400 IU • Vitamin E 45 IU • Vitamin K 10 mcg • Thiamin 1.5 mg • Riboflavin 1.7 mg • Niacin 20 mg • Folic Acid 400 mcg • Iodine 150 mcg • Magnesium 100 mg • Zinc 15 mg • Selenium 20 mcg • Copper 2 mg • Manganese 2 mg • Chromium 150 mcg • Molybdenum 75 mcg • Chloride 72 mg • Potassium 80 mg • Biotin 30 mcg • Pantothenic Acid 10 mg • Calcium 200 mg • Phosphorus 48 mg • Boron 150 mcg • Silicon 2 mg • Vanadium 10 mcg • Lutein 250 mcg • Lycopene 300 mcg. Other Ingredients: Microcrystalline Cellulose, Gelatin, Acacia, Modified Cellulose Gum, Stearic Acid, Dextrin, Titanium Dioxide, Crospovidone, Calcium Silicate, Hypromellose, Magnesium Stearate, Silicon Dioxide, Polyethylene Glycol, FD&C Blue No. 2 Lake, Lactose, FD&C Red No. 40 Lake, Sodium Molybdate, Gluten, FD&C Yellow No. 6 Lake.
See Editor's Note No. 45.

Complete Ultra **-** Rexall - Sundown
Each caplet contains: Vitamin A (as beta carotene) 5000 IU • Vitamin C (as ascorbic acid) 200 mg • Vitamin D (as cholecalciferol) 400 IU • Vitamin E (as dl-alpha tocopheryl acetate) 150 IU • Vitamin K (as phytonadione) 40 mcg • Thiamin (as thiamin mononitrate) 50 mg • Riboflavin (vitamin B2) 50 mg • Niacin (as niacinamide) 35 mg • Vitamin B6 (as pyridoxine HCl) 50 mg • Folic Acid 400 mcg • Vitamin B12 (as cyanocobalamin) 50 mcg • Biotin 50 mcg • Pantothenic Acid (as calcium d-pantothenate) 50 mg • Calcium (as dicalcium carbonate and calcium carbonate) 100 mg • Iron (as carbonyl iron) 9 mg • Phosphorous 35 mcg • Iodine (as potassium iodide) 150 mcg • Magnesium (as magnesium oxide) 25 mg • Zinc

BRAND NAMES

(as zinc oxide) 15 mg • Selenium (as sodium selenate) 70 mcg • Copper (as cupric acid) 2 mg • Manganese (as manganese sulfate) 2 mg • Chromium (as chromium chloride) 120 mcg • Molybdenum (as sodium molybdate) 75 mcg • Chloride 38 mg • Potassium (as potassium chloride) 40 mg • Bilberry extract (4:1, fruit) 15 mg • Blueberry (fruit) 15 mg • Citrus Bioflavonoids (from orange peel extract) 25 mg • Nickel (as nickel sulfate) 5 mcg • Tin (as stannous chloride) 10 mcg • Vanadium (as sodium metavanadate) 10 mcg • Boron (as sodium borate and potassium borate) 150 mcg. Other Ingredients: Microcrystalline Cellulose, Croscarmellose Sodium, Silica, Dextrin, Hydroxypropyl Methylcellulose, Titanium Dioxide, Corn Starch, Magnesium Stearate, PEG, Blue 1 Lake, Dextrose, Soy Lecithin, Retinyl Acetate.

CompleteGest **-** PhytoPharmica
Each capsule contains: Proprietary Plant Enzyme Blend 305 mg: Amylase, Protease, Lipase, Lactase, Phytase, Cellulase, Sucrase, Maltase. Other Ingredients: Modified Cellulose, Cellulose, Titanium Dioxide Color.

Completia Diabetic Multivitamin **-** Nature's Way
Two tablets contain: Alpha Lipoic Acid 50 mg • Beta Carotene 1000 IU • Betaine HCl 25 mg • Biotin, Biotin Triurate 300 mcg • Boron Amino Acid Chelate 1 mg • Calcium (calcium ascorbate, d-calcium pantothenate) 45 mg • Choline Bitartrate 50 mg • Chromium Polynicotinate 300 mcg • Cinnamon bark 300 mg • Citrus Bioflavonoid complex 25 mg • Copper Amino Acid Chelate 1 mg • Fenugreek seed 50 mg • Folic Acid (folate) 400 mcg • Hesperidin 1 mg • Inositol 100 mg • Iodine 10 mcg • L-Carnitine L-Tartrate 20 mg • Lutein (from marigold) 200 mcg • Magnesium (as citrate, oxide) 300 mg • Manganese Amino Acid Chelate 5 mg • Molybdenum Triturate 50 mcg • Neem leaf 50 mg • Niacinamide 20 mg • PABA (para aminobenzoic acid) 25 mg • Pantothenic Acid 100 mg • Potassium Amino Acid Chelate 10 mg • Quercetin, Eucalyptus 50 mg • Riboflavin (vitamin B2) 100 mg • Rutin 25 mg • Selenium Monomethionine 200 mcg • Taurine 100 mg • Thiamine (vitamin B1) 100 mg • Vanadium Triturate 10 mcg • Vitamin A (retinol palmitate) 5000 IU • Vitamin B12 (cyanocobalamin) 100 mcg • Vitamin B6 (as pyridoxine HCl) 100 mg • Vitamin C (ascorbic acid, calcium ascorbate) 500 mg • Vitamin D (D3, cholecalciferol) 400 IU • Vitamin E (d-alpha tocopheryl) 200 IU • Zinc Amino Acid Chelate 15 mg. Other Ingredients: Silica, Vegetable Magnesium Stearate, Vegetable Modified Cellulose, Vegetable Modified Cellulose Gum, Vegetable Stearic Acid, Vegetarian Glycerin.

Completia Healthy Heart Multi (Iron free) **-** Nature's Way
Each tablet contains: Beta Carotene 10,000 IU • Betaine HCl 25 mg • Biotin Triurate 75 mcg • Boron Amino Acid Chelate 500 mcg • Calcium (citrate, carbonate) 20 mg • Choline Bitartrate 25 mg • Chromium Polynicotinate 25 mcg • Citrus Bioflavonoid complex 25 mg • Copper Amino Acid Chelate 500 mcg • Folic Acid (folate) 800 mcg • Heart Herbal Blend 100 mg • Hesperidin 1 mg • Inositol 25 mg • Iodine 150 mcg • Lutein (from marigold) 100 mcg • Magnesium (as citrate, oxide) 10 mg • Manganese Amino Acid Chelate 1 mg • Molybdenum Triurate 25 mcg • Niacinamide 100 mg • PABA (para amionbenzoic acid) 25 mg • Pantothenic Acid 50 mg • Potassium Amino Acid Chelate 2 mg • Riboflavin (vitamin B2) 25 mg • Selenium Monomethionine 200 mcg • Sodium 10 mg • Thiamine (vitamin B1) 25 mg • Vitamin A (retinol, palmitate) 5000 IU • Vitamin B12 (cyanocobalamin) 400 mcg • Vitamin B6 (as pyridoxine HCl) 25 mg • Vitamin C (ascorbic acid) 150 mg • Vitamin D (D3, cholecalciferol) 400 IU • Vitamin E (d-alpha tocopheryl) 150 IU • Zinc Amino Acid Chelate 15 mg. Other Ingredients: Silica, Vegetable Magnesium Stearate, Vegetable Modified Cellulose, Vegetable Modified Cellulose Gum, Vegetable Stearic Acid, Vegetarian Glycerin.

Completia Prenatal Multivitamin **-** Nature's Way
Two tablets contain: Beta Carotene 8000 IU • Biotin Triurate 300 mcg • Calcium (citrate, carbonate) 600 mg • Choline Bitartrate 4 mg • Chromium Polynicotinate 50 mcg • Copper Amino Acid Chelate 2 mg • Dandelion root 50 mg • DHA (docosahexaenoic acid) 100 mg • Diatomaceous plant 10 mg • Folic Acid (folate) 800 mcg • Inositol 10 mg • Iodine 150 mcg • Iron Gluconate 45 mg • Magnesium (citrate, oxide) 300 mg • Manganese Amino Acid Chelate 2 mg • Nettle herb 50 mg • Niacinamide 20 mg • PABA (para aminobenzoic acid) 2 mg • Pantothenic Acid 10 mg • Peppermint leaves 50 mg • Peppermint oil 86 mg • Potassium Amino Acid Chelate 50 mg • Red Raspberry leaves 50 mg • Riboflavin (vitamin B2) 2 mg • Selenium Monomethionine 25 mcg • Sodium 10 mg • Thiamine (vitamin B1) 1.7 mg • Vitamin B12 (cyanocobalamin) 8 mcg • Vitamin B6 (pyridoxine HCl) 2.5 mg • Vitamin C (calcium ascorbate) 120 mg • Vitamin D (D3, cholecalciferol) 400 IU • Vitamin E (d-alpha tocopheryl) 30 IU • Vitamin K (phytonadione) 90 mcg • Zinc Amino Acid Chelate. Other Ingredients: Silica, Vegetable Cellulose, Vegetable Magnesium Stearate, Vegetable Modified Cellulose, Vegetable Modified Cellulose Gum, Vegetable Stearic Acid, Vegetarian Glycerin.

Completia Ultra Energy Multi (Iron-free) **-** Nature's Way
Each tablet contains: Beta Carotene 10,000 IU • Betaine HCl 25 mg • Biotin Triurate 75 mcg • Boron Amino Acid Chelate 500 mcg • Calcium (citrate, carbonate) 20 mg • Choline Bitartrate 31 mg • Chromium Polynicotinate 25 mcg • Citrus Bioflavonoid complex 25 mg • Copper Amino Acid Chelate 1 mg • Energizing Herbal Blend 100 mg • Folic Acid (folate) 400 mcg • Hesperidin 1 mg • Inositol 25 mg • Iodine 150 mcg • Magnesium (as citrate, oxide) 10 mg • Manganese Amino Acid Chelate 2 mg • Molybdenum Amino Acid Chelate 25 mcg • Niacinamide 100 mg • PABA (para aminobenzoic acid) 25 mg • Pantothenic Acid 100 mg • Potassium Amino Acid Chelate 1.8 mg • Riboflavin (vitamin B2) 100 mg • Rutin 25 mg • Selenium Monomethionine 25 mcg • Thiamine (vitamin B1) 100 mg • Vitamin A (retinol palmitate) 5000 IU • Vitamin B12 (cyanocobalamin) 100 mcg • Vitamin B6 (as pyridoxine HCl) 100 mg • Vitamin C (ascorbic acid) 150 mg • Vitamin D (D3, cholecalciferol) 400 IU • Vitamin E (d-alpha tocopheryl) 100 IU • Zinc Amino Acid Chelate 10 mg. Other Ingredients: Silica, Vegetable Magnesium Stearate, Vegetable Modified Cellulose, Vegetable Modified Cellulose Gum, Vegetable Stearic Acid, Vegetable Glycerin.

Complex SPP **-** VitaCube Systems (V3S)
Each softgel contains: Zinc 10 mg • Selenium 50 mcg • Saw Palmetto berries 160 mg • Soybean oil 90 mg • Pumpkin seed oil 25 mg • VitaCube Activating System 30 mg: Orange Bioflavonoid Complex, Grapefruit Bioflavonoid Complex, Alfalfa leaf, Ginkgo Biloba, Cayenne, Apple Pectin, Odorless Garlic, L-Glutathione, Lemon Bioflavonoid, Potassium, Rutin, Bromelain, Lutein 5% • Soy Lecithin 15 mg • Epimedium Grandiflorum herb 5 mg • Pygeum Africanum bark extract 5 mg. Other Ingredients: Gelatin, Glycerin, Silicon Dioxide.

Complexed Potassium **-** J. R. Carlson Laboratories, Inc.
Each tablet contains: Potassium (as potassium glycinate complex) 99 mg.

Complexion Clarifier **-** Abra Therapeutics
Apple juice • Raw Cane Sugar • ABRA5 PhytoSerum Complex: Echinacea extract, White Willow bark extract, Usnea extract, Horsetail extract • Salicylic Acid • Lemon juice • Apple Pectin • Nonfat Dry Milk • Zinc Sulfate • Retinyl Palmitate (vitamin A) • Tocopheryl Acetate (vitamin E) • Ascorbyl Palmitate (vitamin C) • Tea Tree oil • Lavender oil • Geranium oil • Xanthan gum • Glucose • Glucose Oxidase • Lactose Peroxidase • Jojoba oil • Lactic Acid • Acetic Acid • Methylparaben • Propylparaben.

Complexion Perfect **-** Aspen Group, Inc.
Four tablets contain: Vitamin A 5000 IU • Beta Carotene 5000 IU • Vitamin B1 (thiamine) 25 mg • Vitamin B2 (riboflavin) 25 mg • Vitamin B3 (niacin) 50 mg • Vitamin B5 (pantothenic acid) 25 mg • Vitamin B6 (pyridoxine HCl) 50 mg • Biotin 300 mcg • Vitamin C (calcium ascorbate) 500 mg • Vitamin E (succinate) 400 IU • Magnesium Oxide 200 mg • Zinc (gluconate) 12 mg • Burdock root 600 mg • L-Lysine HCl 500 mg • L-Proline 500 mg •

Yellow Dock 500 mg • Silica (derived from horsetail extract) 400 mg • Grape seed extract (proanthodyn) 50 mg • Selenomethionine 200 mcg • Chromium Picolinate 50 mcg • GTF Chromium 25 mcg.

Composition 1 - Dial Herbs
Bayberry • White Pine bark • Clove • Cinnamon • Ginger • Cayenne.

Concentrate - Enzymatic Therapy
Two capsules contain: DMAE (as 2-dimethylaminoethanol bitartrate) 100 mg • Phosphatidylserine (from soy) 60 mg • Taurine 25 mg • N-Acetylcysteine 25 mg • L-Theanine 25 mg. Other Ingredients: Gelatin, Cellulose, Magnesium Stearate.

Concentrated Broccoli - Jamieson
Each caplet contains: Concentrated Broccoli florets (Equivalent to 25000 mg fresh Broccoli) 450 mg • Concentrated Kale leaf and Radish root (Standardized to Active Isothiocyanates 450 mcg) 10 mg.

Concentrated Garlic - Leiner Health Products
Two tablets contain: Garlic (Allium sativum) clove powder 300 mg. Other Ingredients: Dicalcium Phosphate, Cellulose, Starch, Silicon Dioxide, Vanilla Flavor, Magnesium Stearate, Ethylcellulose, may contain less than 2% of Croscarmellose Sodium.

Concentrated Lung-Tan-Xie-Gan pills - China Beijing Tong-Ren Tang
Unknown.
See Editor's Note No. 46.

Concentrated Saw Palmetto - GNC
Each capsule contains: Saw Palmetto berries (serenoa repens) (from 38.5 mg of saw palmetto berries extract 26:1) 1000 mg. Other Ingredients: Soybean Oil, Gelatin, Glycerin, Caramel Color, Titanium Dioxide.

Concentrated Ultra Prostagen - Metagenics
Each tablet contains: Vitamin A (as retinyl palmitate) 2500 IU • Vitamin B6 (as pyridoxine hydrochloride) 10 mg • Zinc (as zinc glycinate) 7.5 mg • Glycine 50 mg • L-Alanine 50 mg • L-Glutamine 50 mg • Saw Palmetto berry extract (serenoa repens, standardized to 45% fatty acids and sterols) 320 mg • Nettle root 10:1 extract (urtica dioica) 100 mg.

ConceptionXR - Theralogix
Four tablets contain: Vitamin C 500 mg • Vitamin E 400 IU • Folic Acid 1000 mcg • Zinc 20 mg • Selenium 200 mcg • L-Carnitine 1000 mg • Lycopene 10 mg.

Confido (Speman forte) - The Himalaya Drug Company
Each tablet contains: Salabmisri (orchis mascula) 78 mg • Kokilaksha (astercantha longifolia syn. hygophila auriculata) 38 mg • Vanya Kahu (lactuca scariola syn. l.serriola) 20 mg • Kapikachchhu (mucuna pruriens) 20 mg • Suvarnavang (mosaic gold, unsublimed tin preparation) 20 mg • Sarpagandha (rauwolfia serpentina, standardised to contain 1.5 mg of the total alkaloids) • Vriddadaru (argyreia speciosa syn. a.nervosa) 38 mg • Gokshura (tribulus terrestris) 38 mg • Jeevanti (leptadenia reticulata) 38 mg • Shaileyam (parmelia perlata) 20 mg.

Congaplex - Standard Process, Inc.
Three capsules contain: Proprietary Blend 673 mg: Bovine Thymus Cytosol extract, Carrot root, Ribonucleic Acid, Bovine Bone, Nutritional Yeast, Defatted Wheat germ, Bovine Adrenal, Dried Alfalfa juice, Oat flour, Alfalfa flour, Bovine Kidney, Veal Bone Meal, Veal Bone PMG extract, Reishi / Shiitake Mushroom blend, Dried Buckwheat leaf juice, Buckwheat seed, Peanut bran, Soy bean Lecithin, Mixed Tocopherols, Carrot oil. Other Ingredients: Calcium Lactate, Gelatin, Magnesium Citrate, Water, Ascorbic Acid, Colors, Calcium Stearate, Vitamin A Palmitate.

Congaplex (Chewable) - Standard Process, Inc.
Three tablets contain: Proprietary Blend 320 mg: Raspberry powder, Bovine Thymus Cytosol extract, Carrot root, Ribonucleic Acid, Bovine Bone, Defatted Wheat germ, Bovine Adrenal, Dried Alfalfa juice, Nutritional Yeast, Oat flour, Alfalfa flour, Bovine Kidney, Veal Bone meal, Veal Bone PMG extract, Reishi / Shiitake Mushroom blend, Dried Buckwheat leaf juice, Buckwheat seed, Peanut bran, Soy Bean Lecithin, Carrot oil, Mixed Tocopherols. Other Ingredients: Dehydrated Cane Juice, Cellulose, Maltodextrine, Calcium Lactate, Magnesium Citrate, Natural Flavor, Calcium Stearate, Ascorbic Acid, Vitamin A Palmitate.

Congest-Away - Rainbow Light
Two tablets contain: Vitamin A (from beta-carotene, palmitate 1:1) 5000 IU • Vitamin C (ascorbic acid) 1000 mg • Zinc (citrate) 5 mg • Copper (amino acid chelate) 500 mcg • Spirulina 100 mg • Herbal Extract Blend (equivalent to 4824 mg of herbal powder) 1200 mg: Magnolia flower 4:1 extract (magnolia liliflorae), Yerba Santa leaves 4:1 extract, HoreHound herb 4:1 extract, Mullein herb 4:1 extract, Iceland Moss lichen 4:1 extract, Chinese Goldthread rhizome 4:1 extract, Ligusticum root 4:1 extract, Pinellia Ternata rhizome 4:1 extract, Platycodon 4:1 extract (platycodi grandiflorum), Chinese Licorice root 4:1 extract, Tangerine peel 5:1 extract (standardized to 3% synephrine). Other Ingredients: Stearic Acid (vegetable), Modified Cellulose Gum, Silica, Magnesium Stearate, Vegetable Food Glaze.
See Editor's Note No. 40.

Conjugated Linoleic Acid - PhysioLogics
Two softgels contain: Tonalin CLA (from safflower oil, contains 74-82% conjugated linoleic acid) 2000 mg. Other Ingredients: Gelatin, Glycerin, Caramel Color, Titanium Dioxide Color.

Conjugated Linoleic Acid (CLA) - EcoNugenics
Each softgel contains: Conjugated Linoleic Acid 700 mg. Other Ingredients: Safflower Oil, Gelatin, Glycerin, Carob, Water, Titanium Dioxide, Tenox 20A Antioxidant.

Conjugated Linoleic Acid (CLA) 500MG - Nature Made
Two softgels contain: Vitamin E 2 IU • Conjugated Linoleic Acid 500 mg.

Conjugated Linoleic Acid 1000 mg 70% - NOW Foods
Each softgel contains: Sunflower/Safflower Oil (high linoleic acid) 1000 mg • Conjugated Linoleic Acid (CLA) 700 mg • Cis, Trans-11 Isomer 330 mg • Trans-10, Cis-12 Isomer 330 mg. Other Ingredients: Gelatin, Glycerin, Water, Carob.

ConjuLean 1000 - Xymogen
Each softgel contains: Conjugated Linoleic Acid (CLA) Blend 1000 mg: Pure Conjugated Linoleic Acid 780 mg • Palmitic Acid 57 mg • Stearic Acid 24 mg • Oleic Acid 125 mg • Linoleic Acid 20 mg. Other Ingredients: Gelatin, Glycerin, Purified Water.

Connect-All - Nature's Plus
Two tablets contain: Glucosamine Sulfate (Aminomonosaccharide) 300 mg • Bromelain, proteolytic enzyme 600 GDU/gram, 200 mg • Calcium (Aminoate) 200 mg • Vitamin C corn free 60 mg • Aloe Vera leaf naturally rich in Mucopolysaccharide 50 mg • Chondroitin Sulfate A (CSA) 50 mg • Zinc (Monomethionine) 15 mg • Chinese Sea Cucumber (Microchele nobilis) 10 mg • Copper (Aminoate) 1 mg. In a highly active base of Alfalfa, Chlorella, Spirulina & low temperature dried Barley Grass juice, supplying naturally occuring chlorophyll & trace minerals.
See Editor's Note No. 15.

Contract Ease - TriLight Herbs
Crampbark • Wild Yam • Black Haw • Scullcap • Valerian root • Hops • Chamomile • Fennel • Catnip.

Control C/P - Pure Encapsulations
Two vegetable capsules contain: Flower Pollwn extract (secale cereale L., containing water and fat soluble fractions in a 20:1 ration) 537 mg • Lipid-Free Pumpkin seed 20:1 extract (curcurbita pepo L., standardized to contain a minimum of 2% phenolic derivatives) 525 mg.

Some Brand Name Natural Products - What they Contain

www.NaturalDatabase.com contains MANY more listings than appear here.

Editor's Notes are located on pages 2155-2163.

BRAND NAMES

Controlled-Release Melatonin - Douglas Laboratories/AMNI
Each tablet contains: Melatonin 2 mg.
See Editor's Note No. 16.

Control-X - Gero Vita International
Each capsule contains: Asian Ginseng root extract (20% ginsenosides) 100 mg • Astragalus root extract (1% isoflavones, 10% amino acids) 100 mg • Psoralea fruit extract (8:1) 100 mg • Sharp-leaf Galongal fruit extract (8:1) 100 mg • Palm-leaf Raspberry fruit extract (12% organic acids) 100 mg • Cherokee Rose fruit extract (8:1) 100 mg • Cassia bark extract (5% cinnamaldehdyde) 50 mg • Chinese Cimicifuga rhizome extract (5% ferulic acid) 25 mg • Ginger rhizome extract (5% gingerols) 25 mg • Vinpocetine 5 mg. Other Ingredients: Gelatin, Dicalcium Phosphate, Magnesium Stearate, Silicon Dioxide.

Copper - GNC
Each tablet contains: Copper (as copper gluconate) 2mg. Other Ingredients: Dicalcium Phosphate, Cellulose.

Copper (citrate) - Pure Encapsulations
Each vegetable capsule contains: Copper (citrate) 2 mg.

Copper (glycinate) - Pure Encapsulations
Each vegetable capsule contains: Copper (glycinate) 2 mg.

Copper 3 mg Tablets - Nature's Plus
Each tablet contains: Copper (as amino acid chelate) 3 mg. Other Ingredients: Di-calcium Phosphate, Microcrystalline Cellulose, Stearic Acid, Magnesium Stearate, Pharmaceutical Glaze, Silica.

Copper Liver Chelate - Standard Process, Inc.
Each tablet contains: Proprietary Blend 339 mg: Bovine Liver, Dried Beet root juice, Carrot root, Oat flour • Iron 0.4 mg • Copper 2 mg. Other Ingredients: Honey, Cellulose, Calcium Stearate.
See Editor's Note No. 14.

Copper Mineral Supplement - Eidon Inc.
Each 1 tsp serving contains: Copper 0.2 mg. Other Ingredients: Purified Water.

Copper Sebacate - Source Naturals
Each tablet contains: Copper sebacate 22 mg.

CoQ Absorb 60 mg - Pro Health
Each softgel contains: Vitamin A (as beta carotene from D. salina) 1630 IU • Natural Vitamin E (D-alpha tocopherol with mixed tocopherols) 60 IU • CoQsol brand Coenzyme Q10 60 mg. Other Ingredients: Rice Bran Oil, Gelatin, Glycerin, Water, Beeswax, Annatto Extract, Titanium Oxide.

CoQ Heart - Shaklee
Each capsule contains: Coenzyme Q10 30 mg • Mixed tocopherols 5 mg • Resveratrol (Polygonum cuspidatum) root 640 mcg. Other Ingredients: Soybean Oil, Glyceryl Palmitostearate, Polyglyceryl Dioleate, Gelatin, Glycerine, Water, Annatto, Titanium Dioxide.

CoQ10 - Nature's Way
Each capsule or softgel contains: Coenzyme Q10 (ubiquinone) 60 mg. Other Ingredients: Gelatin, Millet, Turmeric Root.

CoQ10 - NOW Foods
Each capsule contains: Coenzyme Q10 30 mg. Other Ingredients: White Rice Powder.

CoQ10 - Xymogen
Each softgel contains: Coenzyme Q10 (ubiquinone) 200 mg.

CoQ10 - Enzymatic Therapy
Each softgel contains: Coenzyme Q10 (CoQ10, ubiquinone 10) 50 mg. Other Ingredients: Soybean Oil, Gelatin, Beeswax, Lecithin.

Co-Q10 - J. R. Carlson Laboratories, Inc.
Each softgel contains: Vitamin E (as D-alpha tocopherol) 1 IU • Co-Q10 (as coenzyme Q10) 50 mg.

CoQ-10 - Ortho Molecular Products
Each softgel contains: Vitamin E (as mixed tocopherols) 100 IU • Coenzyme Q10 100 mg. Other Ingredients: Rice Bran Oil, Gelatin, Glycerin, Yellow Beeswax, Beta Carotene, Titanium Dioxide, Annatto Extract, Water.

CoQ-10 - Solgar
Each capsule contains: CoEnzyme Q-10 (ubiquinone) 30 mg. Other Ingredients: Microcrystalline Cellulose, Gelatin, Vegetable Cellulose, Silica, Vegetable Magnesium Stearate, Water.

CoQ-10 - Metabolic Response Modifiers
Each capsule contains: Ubiquinone (Coenzyme Q-10) 30 mg.

CoQ-10 - Schiff
Each capsule contains: Coenzyme Q-10 30 mg. Other Ingredients: Rice Powder, Silica.

Co-Q10 (100 mg) - Jarrow Formulas
Each capsule contains: CoEnzyme Q-10 100 mg. Other Ingredients: Cellulose, Magnesium Stearate.

Co-Q10 (200 mg) - Jarrow Formulas
Each capsule contains: CoEnzyme Q-10 200 mg. Other Ingredients: Cellulose, Magnesium Stearate.

Co-Q10 (30 mg) - Jarrow Formulas
Each capsule contains: CoEnzyme Q-10 30 mg. Other Ingredients: Cellulose, Magnesium Stearate.

Co-Q10 (60 mg) - Jarrow Formulas
Each capsule contains: CoEnzyme Q-10 60 mg. Other Ingredients: Cellulose, Magnesium Stearate.

Co-Q-10 10 mg - J. R. Carlson Laboratories, Inc.
Each softgel contains: Vitamin E (as D-alpha tocopherol) 1 IU • Co-Q10 (coenzyme Q10) 10 mg.

CoQ10 100 mg - PhytoPharmica
Each capsule contains: Coenzyme Q10 (CoQ10) verified by HPLC 100 mg.

CoQ10 100 mg - Nature's Way
Each capsule contains: Coenzyme Q10 (ubiquinone) 100 mg • Vitamin E (d-alpha tocopheryl) 5 IU. Other Ingredients: Annatto Oil, Gelatin, Glycerin, Rice Bran Oil, Titanium Dioxide, Water.

Co-Q-10 100 mg - J. R. Carlson Laboratories, Inc.
Each softgel contains: Vitamin E (as D-alpha tocopherol) 1 IU • Co-Q10 (coenzyme Q10) 100 mg.

COQ10 100 mg PLUS E - Progressive Labs
Each capsule contains: Co-Enzyme Q10 100 mg • Vitamin E (dl-alpha tocopheryl acetate) 100 IU.

CoQ-10 100mg - Sundown
Each softgel contains: Vitamin E (as D-alpha tocopherol) 5 IU • Coenzyme Q-10 100 mg. Other Ingredients: Soybean Oil, Gelatin, Glycerin, Water, Yellow Beeswax, Titanium Dioxide, Yellow 6 Lake, Red 40 Lake, Blue 1 Lake.

CoQ10 120 mg - Pure Encapsulations
Each vegetable capsule contains: Coenzyme Q10 120 mg.

Co-Q-10 200 mg - J. R. Carlson Laboratories, Inc.
Each softgel contains: Vitamin E (as D-alpha tocopherol) 1 IU • Co-Q10 (coenzyme Q10) 200 mg.

CoQ10 250 mg - Pure Encapsulations
Each vegetable capsule contains: Coenzyme Q10 250 mg.

CoQ10 30 mg - Swanson Health Products
Each capsule contains: Coenzyme Q10 30 mg.

CoQ10 30 mg - PhytoPharmica
Each capsule contains: Coenzyme Q10 (CoQ10) verified by HPLC 30 mg.

CoQ10 30 mg **-** Nature's Plus
Each softgel contains: Coenzyme Q10 30 mg. Other Ingredients: Soy Oil, Gelatin, Glycerin, Natural Annatto Color, Purified Water.

CoQ10 30 mg **-** Pure Encapsulations
Each vegetable capsule contains: Coenzyme Q10 30 mg.

Co-Q-10 30 mg **-** J. R. Carlson Laboratories, Inc.
Each softgel contains: Vitamin E (as D-alpha tocopherol) 1 IU • Co-Q10 (coenzyme Q10) 30 mg.

CoQ-10 30 mg **-** Rexall - Sundown
Each softgel contains: Vitamin E (as d-alpha-tocopherol) 5 IU • Coenzyme Q-10 30 mg. Other Ingredients: Soybean Oil, Gelatin, Glycerin, Water, Titanium Dioxide, Yellow 6 Lake, Yellow Beeswax, Red 40 Lake, Blue 1 Lake.

Co-Q-10 300 mg **-** J. R. Carlson Laboratories, Inc.
Each softgel contains: Vitamin E (as D-alpha tocopherol) 3 IU • Co-Q10 (coenzyme Q10) 300 mg.

CoQ10 50 mg **-** PhytoPharmica
Each capsule contains: Coenzyme Q10 (CoQ10) verified by HPLC 50 mg.

CoQ-10 50 mg **-** Rexall - Sundown
Each softgel contains: Vitamin E (as d-alpha-tocopherol) 5 IU • Coenzyme Q10 50 mg. Other Ingredients: Soybean Oil, Gelatin, Glycerin, Water, Yellow Beeswax, Titanium Dioxide, Yellow 6 Lake, Red 40 Lake, Blue 1 Lake.

CoQ10 500 mg **-** Pure Encapsulations
Each vegetable capsule contains: Coenzyme Q10 500 mg.

CoQ10 60 mg **-** Pure Encapsulations
Each vegetable capsule contains: Coenzyme Q10 60 mg.

Co-Q10 75 **-** Nature's Sunshine
Each capsule contains: Co-Enzyme Q10 75 mg. Other Ingredients: Soybean Oil, Beeswax, Lecithin, Beta-Carotene, Gelatin, Glycerin, Water.

CoQ-10 75 mg **-** Rexall - Sundown
Each softgel contains: Vitamin E (as d-alpha-tocopherol) 5 IU • Coenzyme Q-10 75 mg. Other Ingredients: Soybean Oil, Gelatin, Glycerin, Water, Yellow Beeswax, Titanium Dioxide, Yellow 6 Lake, Red 40 Lake, Blue 1 Lake.

CoQ10 Extra Strength **-** Olympian Labs
Each capsule contains: Crystalline Coenzyme Q10 150 mg.

CoQ10 l-Carnitine fumarate **-** Pure Encapsulations
Each vegetable capsule contains: L-Carnitine (from 586 mg L-carnitine fumarate) 340 mg • Coenzyme Q10 60 mg • Vitamin C (as ascorbyl palmitate) 13 mg.

CoQ10 Spray **-** Nature's Plus
Each spray contains: Vitamin E 1 IU • CoQ10 (pharmaceutical grade ubiquinone) 30 mg. Other Ingredients: Purified Water, Capric/Caprylic Triglyceride, Fructose, Polysorbate 80, Lecithin, Natural Flavors, Potassium Sorbate, N-Acetyl-Glucosamine, Citrus Sinensis Seed Extract, Vegetable Glycerin.

CoQ-10 ST **-** Metagenics
Each softgel contains: Coenzyme Q10 (ubiquinone) 30 mg • Vitamin E (as D-alpha tocopherol) 30 IU.

CoQ10 ST-100 **-** Metagenics
Each softgel contains: Coenzyme Q10 (ubiquinone) 100 mg • Vitamin E (as mixed tocopherols) 100 IU • Vitamin A (100% as beta-carotene) 2334 IU.

CoQsol brand **-** Soft Gel Technologies, Inc.
CoQ10.
See Editor's Note No. 44.

CoQuinone 30 **-** USANA Health Sciences
Each capsule contains: Coenzyme Q10 30 mg • Alpha Lipoic Acid 12.5 mg. Inactive Ingredients: Medium Chain Triglycerides, Gelatin, Glycerin Monooleate, Lecithin, Glycerin, Purified Water, Annatto seed extract, Titanium Dioxide.

Coral Calcium **-** Sojourn Health
Three capsules contain: Coral Calcium 1500 mg yielding Calcium 260 mg, Magnesium 180 mg • Vitamin D 400 IU. Other Ingredients: Rice Powder, Magnesium Stearate, Gelatin.

Coral Calcium **-** GNC
Two capsules contain: Vitamin D (as Cholecalciferol) 200 IU • Calcium (as Coral calcium 1100 mg) 400 mg • Magnesium (as Magnesium oxide) 200 mg. Other Ingredients: Gelatin, Polyalditol, Titanium Dioxide.

Coral Calcium **-** Pure Source
Two capsules contain: Vitamin A (as beta-carotene) 1945 IU • Vitamin C (as ascorbic acid) 47 mg • Vitamin D (as cholecalciferol) 544 IU • Vitamin E (as dl-alpha tocopheryl) 23 IU • Calcium (from coral calcium) 167 mg • Iodine (kelp) 100 mcg • Magnesium (from coral calcium) 83 mg • Magnesium (as magnesium citrate) 39 mg • Zinc (as amino acid chelate)10.9 mg • Selenium (as amino acid chelate) 20 mcg • Copper (as amino acid chelate) 1.6 mg • Manganese (as amino acid chelate) 0.96 mg • Chromium (as amino acid chelate) 57 mcg • Coral Calcium (70+ trace minerals with natural variability) 667 mg • Cesium 2 mg • Strontium (from coral calcium) 1.9 mg • Boron (as amino acid chelate) 43 mcg. Other Ingredients: Gelatin.

Coral Calcium **-** NSI - Nutraceutical Sciences Institute
Three capsules contain: Beta Carotene 2500 IU • Vitamin C (as Magnesium ascorbate) 86 mg • Vitamin D (D3, as Cholecalciferol) 869 IU • Vitamin E (as D-alpha tocopherol succinate) 50 IU • Vitamin K (as Phytonadione) 18 mcg • Thiamine (as Vitamin B1) 1.5 mg • Riboflavin (as Vitamin B2) 1.7 mg • Niacinamide (as Vitamin B3) 20 mg • Pyridoxine HCl (as Vitamin B6) 2 mg • Folic Acid 400 mcg • Methylcobalamin (Vitamin B12) 6 mcg • Pantothenic Acid (Vitamin B5) 10 mg • Calcium (from Coral mineral powder) 400 mg • Iodine (from Kelp) 100 mcg • Magnesium (from Coral mineral powder) 24 mg • Magnesium (as Ascorbate) 5 mg • Magnesium (as Oxide) 169 mg • Zinc 8 mg • Selenium (as Selenomethionine) 70 mcg • Manganese (as Citrate) 2 mg • Chromium (as Polynicotinate) 100 mcg • L-Lysine (as HCl) 100 mg • Boron (as Citrate) 1.5 mg • Horsetail extract (standardized to 7% Silica) 29 mg. Other Ingredients: Magnesium Searate, Cellulose, Gelatin.

Coral Calcium **-** PhysioLogics
Two capsules contain: Calcium (from coral calcium 1000 mg) 370 mg. Other Ingredients: Gelatin, Rice Powder, Silica, Vegetable Magnesium Stearate.

Coral Calcium **-** Source Naturals
Two capsules contain: Vitamin D (D3, as Cholecalciferol) 400 IU • Calcium 420 mg • Magnesium 8 mg • Coral Calcium 1.2 g. Other Ingredients: Gelatin, Dibasic Calcium Phosphate, Colloidal Silicon.

Coral Calcium **-** For Youthful Health
Two capsules contain: Vitamin D (as cholecalciferol) 400 IU • Coral Calcium (naturally occurring coral minerals, Calcium 240 mg, Magnesium 120 mg) 1200 mg.

Coral Calcium **-** DreamPharm
Three capsules contain: Vitamin A (as palmitate) 300 IU • Vitamin C (as ascorbic acid) 80 mg • Vitamin D (vitamin D3) 820 IU • Vitamin E (d-alpha tocopheryl succinate) 60 IU • Calcium (from 1475 mg of coral calcium) 530 mg • Magnesium (from 1475 coral calcium & magnesium oxide) 265 mg • Zinc (as zinc oxide) 15 mg • Copper (as copper oxide) 3 mg • Coral Calcium (in proprietary base) 1475 mg. Other Ingredients: Cellulose, Silicon Dioxide, Magnesium Stearate.

Some Brand Name Natural Products - What they Contain

www.NaturalDatabase.com contains MANY more listings than appear here.
Editor's Notes are located on pages 2155-2163.

BRAND NAMES

Coral Calcium - Bob Barefoot's Best
Three caplets contain: Vitamin A (as Beta carotene) 5000 IU • Vitamin C (as Ascorbic acid) 60 mg • Vitamin D (as Cholecalciferol) 2000 IU • Vitamin E (as D-alpha-tocopherol) 30 IU • Thiamin (as Thiamin HCl) 1.5 mg • Riboflavin 1.7 mg • Niacin (as Niacinamide) 20 mg • Vitamin B6 (as Pyridoxine HCl) 2 mg • Folic acid 800 mcg • Vitamin B12 (as Cyanocobalamin) 6 mcg • Pantothenic Acid (as Calcium pantothenate) 10 mg • Calcium (from Coral calcium) 500 mg • Calcium 95 mg • Iron (as Amino acid chelate) 18 mg • Iodine (from Kelp) 108 mcg • Magnesium (from Coral calcium) 250 mg • Magnesium (from Citrate) 42 mg • Magnesium 7 mg • Zinc (as Amino acid chelate) 15 mg • Selenium (as Amino acid chelate) 30 mcg • Copper (as Amino acid chelate) 2 mg • Manganese (as Amino acid chelate) 1.44 mg • Chromium (as Amino acid chelate) 120 mcg • Coral Calcium 2000 mg • Cesium (as Chloride) 3 mg • Boron (as Amino acid chelate) 1000 mcg • Strontium (from Coral calcium) 3200 mcg. Other Ingredients: Cellulose, Croscarmellose Sodium, Maltodextrin, Microcrystalline Cellulose, Magnesium Stearate, Silica, Stearic Acid.
See Editor's Note No. 28.

Coral Calcium - Pro Health
Two Vcaps contain: Vitamin D (as ergocalciferol) 400 IU • Calcium (from fossilized coral calcium 35%) 500 mg • Magnesium (from magnesium oxide, citrate, aspartate 17%) 250 mg • Fossilized Coral Calcium (gross weight) 1430 mg. Other Ingredients: Cellulose, Maltodextrin, Mixed Tocopherols.

Coral Calcium - Natrol, Inc.
Three capsules contain: Vitamin D (as Cholecalciferol) 400 IU • Calcium (as Coral Calcium) 400 mg • Magnesium (from Coral and Amino Acid Chelate) 200 mg. Other Ingredients: Rice Powder, Gelatin, Silica, Magnesium Stearate.

Coral Calcium - Elation Therapy, Inc.
Two capsules contain: Coral Calcium 1000 mg • Calcium 240 mg • Magnesium 120 mg • Vitamin D 400 IU.

Coral Calcium 1 - PhysioLogics
Two capsules contain: Proprietary Blend of Coral Calcium 1000 mg: Calcium (from coral calcium) 240 mg, Magnesium (from coral calcium magnesium citrate) 120 mg, Vitamin D3 (as cholecalciferol) 800 IU • Trace Minerals. Other Ingredients: Cellulose, Modified Cellulose, Stearic Acid.

Coral Calcium 1000 mg Plus - Nature's Bounty
Two capsules contain: Vitamin C 5 mg • Vitamin D 400 IU • Calcium 370 mg • Magnesium 56 mg. Other Ingredients: Rice Powder, Gelatin, Vegetable Magnesium Stearate, Silica.

Coral Calcium 500 mg - Puritan's Pride
Two capsules contain: Calcium (from 1000 mg of coral calcium) 370 mg. Other Ingredients: Rice Powder, Gelatin, Silica, Vegetable Magnesium Stearate.

Coral Calcium Complex - PhysioLogics
Two capsules contain: Vitamin C (as ascorbic acid) 5 mg • Vitamin D (as cholecalciferol) 400 IU • Calcium (from coral calcium 1000 mg) 370 mg • Magnesium (as magnesium oxide, magnesium citrate) 56 mg. Other Ingredients: Rice Powder, Gelatin, Vegetable Magnesium Stearate, Silica.

Coral Calcium Factor - Coral Calcium Factor
Three capsules contain: Okinawa Marine Coral Calcium 1500 mg • Calcium (from coral) 360 mg • Magnesium (from coral) 180 mg • Vitamin D 800 mg. Also contains 75 other trace minerals and nutrients. Other Ingredients: Gelatin, Rice Powder.

Coral Calcium Factor Plus - Nature's Solution
Two capsules contain: Vitamin D 400 IU • Calcium 240 mg • Magnesium 120 mg • Coral Calcium 1000 mg. Other Ingredients: Silicon Dioxide, Cellulose, Magnesium Stearate, Gelatin.

Coral Calcium Mineral Complex - Nature's Rx
Each capsule contains: Coral Calcium 600 mg • Calcium (from coral) 230 mg • Vitamin D (D3, as cholecalciferol) 50 IU • Magnesium (from coral & 50 mg gluconate) 9 mg • Boron (chelate) 1 mg.

Coral Calcium plus - DaVinci Laboratories
Three capsules contain: Beta Carotene 2900 IU • Vitamin C (ascorbic acid) 70 mg • Vitamin D (D3, cholecalciferol) 400 IU • Calcium (from coral) 800 mg • Magnesium (168 mg from coral and 232 mg from magnesium oxide) 400 mg • Copper 2 mg • Manganese 2000 mcg • Boron (as boron amino acid chelate) 2 mg. Other Ingredients: Coral Powder, Vegetable Stearate, Vegetable Cellulose.

Coral Calcium with Magnesium - Source Naturals
Three tablets contain: Sodium 5 mg • Vitamin D (D3,as Cholecalciferol) 400 IU • Calcium (from Coral) 1200 mg • Magnesium (as Magnesium oxide, Chelate, Citrate from Coral) 600 mg • Coral Calcium 3.4 g. Other Ingredients: Stearic Acid, Acacia Gum, Magnesium Stearate, Modified Cellulose, Colloidal Silicon Dioxide.

Coral Calcium, Magnesium & Phosphorus Plus Vitamin D (strawberry and chocolate flavors) - Westcoast Naturals
Each 1 tbsp serving contains: Coral Calcium 600 mg • Magnesium 300 mg • Phosphorus 300 mg • Vitamin D (as D3) 400 IU. Other Ingredients: Sorbitol, Flavor, Purified Water, Sorbic Acid, Sodium Benzoate, Potassium Sorbate.

Coral Complete - Global Health Trax
Two capsules contain: Vitamin C (as ascorbic acid) 10 mg • Vitamin D (as cholecalciferol) 800 IU • Calcium (from coral) 460 mg • Magnesium (from coral) 116 mg • Proprietary Blend 30 mg: Trace Minerals From Coral, Malic Acid, Betaine HCl. Other Ingredients: Gelatin, Magnesium Stearate (from vegetable source), Silica, Cellulose (from rice bran).

CORALadvantage Coral Calcium - Advanced Nutritional Innovations
Three capsules contain: Vitamin A (as beta carotene) 2500 IU • Vitamin C (as ascorbic acid) 86 mg • Vitamin D (D3) 869 IU • Vitamin E (as d-alpha tocopherol) 43 IU • Vitamin K (as phytonadione) 18 mcg • Thiamin (B1) 960 mcg • Riboflavin (B2) 1.09 mg • Niacinamide (B3) 12.8 mg • Vitamin B6 (as pyridoxine HCl) 4 mg • Folic Acid 256 mcg • Vitamin B12 (as cyanocobalamin) 3.84 mcg • Pantothenic Acid (B5) 6.4 mg • Calcium (from marine coral) 230 mg • Calcium (from calcium citrate) 136 mg • Iodine (from kelp) 96 mcg • Magnesium (from marine coral) 110 mg • Magnesium (from magnesium citrate) 88 mg • Zinc (amino acid chelate) 8 mg • Selenium (amino acid chelate) 70 mcg • Copper (amino acid chelate) 1 mg • Manganese (citrate) 2 mg • Chromium (amino acid chelate) 77 mcg • Lysine HCl 100 mg • Red Algae powder (Lithothamnium coralloides, yeilding 2 cups of elemental silicon) 29 mg • Malic Acid 15 mg • Boron (citrate) 1.5 mg • Strontium 1.6 mg • Cesium 1 mg. Other Ingredients: Plant Cellulose Capsules, Titanium Dioxide, At least 49 Trace Elements from Marine Coral and Red Algae.

CoralCalcium 1 - Vision Enterprises
Two capsules contain: Proprietary Blend 1000 mg: Coral Calcium, Calcium (from coral calcium) 240 mg, Magnesium (from coral calcium magnesium citrate) 120 mg, Vitamin D (D3, as cholecalciferol) 800 IU. Other Ingredients: Cellulose, Modified Cellulose, Stearic Acid.

CoraLife brand - BI Nutraceuticals
Sea Coral Calcium.

CoralPrep - HealthMinded
Three capsules contain: Vitamin D (as cholecalciferol) 200 IU • Calcium (from coral calcium 1600 mg) 400 mg • Magnesium (from coral calcium) 200 mg. Other Ingredients: Gelatin, Stearic Acid, Magnesium Stearate.

Coratain - Metagenics
Each tablet contains: Proprietary Blend 1100 mg: Asian Ginseng root (panax ginseng), Schisandra fruit (schisandra chinensis), Ophiopogon root (ophiopogon japonicus).

Cordephrine XC - HealthDesigns International
Each vegicap contains: Cordyceps Mycelia (Cordyceps sinensis) 450 mg. Other Ingredients: Pure plant cellulose (vegicaps). Does not contain ephedra or ephedrine.

Cordyceps - Metabolic Response Modifiers
Each capsule contains: Cordyceps mycelia (Cordyceps sinensis) 750 mg.

Cordyceps (Caterpillar Fungus) - Olympia Nutrition
Caterpillar fungus 500 mg.

Cordyceps Power 800 mg - Planetary Formulas
Two capsules contain: Cordyceps Proprietary Blend 1600 mg. Other Ingredients: Dibasic Calcium Phosphate, Colloidal Silicon Dioxide, Magnesium Stearate, Modified Cellulose Gum, Stearic Acid.

Cordyceps with Siberian Ginseng - Natrol, Inc.
Each capsule contains: Cordyceps 300 mg • Siberian Ginseng 50 mg. Other Ingredients: Rice powder, silica, & gelatin.

CordyMax Cs-4 - Pharmanex
Two capsules contain: Cordyceps Cs-4 Mushroom Mycelia (cordyceps sinensis [berk.] sacc.) 1050 mg. Other Ingredients: Gelatin.

CorEnergy - Shaklee
Three capsules contain: Cordyceps 4:1 extract (Cordyceps sinensis) mushroom 750 mg • Ginseng root extract (Panax ginseng standardized to contain 10% ginsenosides) 200 mg • Green Tea extract (Camellia sinensis standardized to contain 50% polyphenols) leaf 200 mg. Other Ingredients: Microcrystalline Cellulose, Gelatin, Water, Titanium Dioxide.

Coreplex - Flora Inc.
Hawthorn blossoms & leaves • Passion Flower Herb • Hibiscus flowers • Hawthorn berry extract (1:4).

CorePlex - Advocare International
Three caplets contain: Vitamin A (as palmitate) 2500 IU • Vitamin A (as beta-carotene) 12,500 IU • Vitamin C (as ascorbic acid) 600 mg • Vitamin D (as ergocalciferol) 400 IU • Vitamin E (as d-alpha tocopheryl succinate) 150 IU • Thiamine 9 mg • Riboflavin 10.2 mg • Niacin/Niacinamide 120 mg • Pantothenic Acid 40 mg • Vitamin B6 (pyridoxine HCl) 12 mg • Vitamin B12 (as cyanocobalamin) 36 mcg • Folic Acid 800 mcg • Biotin 300 mcg • Inositol 6 mg • Choline (as bitartrate) 60 mg • Calcium (as amino acid chelate) 150 mg • Magnesium (as amino acid chelate) 200 mg • Zinc (as monomethionine - OptiZinc) 15 mg • Iodine (from kelp) 150 mcg • Selenium (as selenomethionine) 80 mcg • Manganese (as amino acid chelate) 4 mg • Chromium (as polynicotinate - ChromeMate) 100 mcg • Molybdenum (as amino acid chelate) 50 mcg • Copper (as amino acid chelate) 2 mg • Potassium (as amino acid chelate) 100 mg • Boron (as amino acid chelate) 300 mcg • Vanadium (as bis-maltolato-oxovanadium) 50 mcg • Phosphorus (as amino acid chelate) 100 mg • Silicon (as amino acid chelate) 500 mcg • Coenzyme Q-10 150 mcg • Octacosanol 2 mg • Ribonucleic Acid (RNA) 2 mg • Odorless Garlic bulb powder (allium sativum) 50 mg • L-Glutathione 5 mg • Gamma-Oryzanol 5 mg • Citrus Flavonoids 100 mg • Red Wine Polyphenols 5 mg • Milk Thistle fruit extract (silybum marianum) 5 mg • Ginkgo Biloba leaf extract (ginkgo biloba) 10 mg • L-Methionine 100 mg. Other Ingredients: Dicalcium Phosphate, Silicon Dioxide, Cellulose, Stearic Acid, Magnesium Stearate, Peppermint Extract.

Coromega (orange flavor) - European Reference Botanical Laboratories, Inc.
Each packet contains: Vitamin C 45 mg • Vitamin E 7 IU • Folic Acid 100 mcg • Omega-3 fatty acids (EPA 350 mg, DHA 230 mg) 650 mg • Stevia Leaf extract 5 mg. Other Ingredients: Water, Egg Yolk, Natural Orange Flavor, Citric Acid, Sodium Benzoate, Vanillin, Beta Carotene, Potassium Sorbate, Menthol, Folic Acid.

CoroWise Sterol Esters - Cargill Health & Food Technologies
Two capsules contain: Phytosterol esters (from vegetable oil) 1300 mg. Other Ingredients: Gelatin.

Cort-Bloc - Muscle-Link
Two capsules contain: Phosphatidylserine 200 mg • Glutamine peptide 800 mg. Other Ingredients: Gelatin, Magnesium Stearate.

Cortiblock - Heaven Sent Naturals
Each tablet contains: Vitamin C 50 mg • Vitamin B1 1.25 mg • Vitamin B2 1.25 mg • Vitamin B6 2.5 mg • Vitamin B12 3 mcg • Folic Acid 200 mcg • Calcium (carbonate) 75 mg • Chromium (polynicotinate) 25 mcg • Biotin 75 mcg • Ridicort Blend 157.5 mg: Magnolia bark extract (1.5% honokiol), Beta-Sitosterol, Phosphatidylserine (20% extract), Valerian root, Rhodiola rosea, Suntheanine brand 100% L-Theanine • Synocet Blend 127.5 mg: Green Tea 50% extract (camellia sinensis), Bitter Orange peel 5% extract (citrus aurantium) • BAVA-K Blend 19.5 mg: Banaba leaf (lagerstromia speciosa, 1%), Vanadyl Sulfate (providing 2.5 mcg vanadium). Other Ingredients: Cellulose, Stearic Acid, Silica, Magnesium Stearate.
See Editor's Note No. 40.

CortiBurn (adrenalzide) - MedaBiotics
Two capsules contain: Vitamin B6 (as pyridoxine HCl) 3 mg • Vitamin B12 (as cyanocobalamin) 250 mcg • Folic Acid (vitamin B9) 200 mcg • Advantra Z brand Citrus Aurantium 5% extract (contains 17.5 mg of synephrine) 350 mg • Green Tea leaf extract (50% catechins and 35% polyphenols) 300 mg • Guggulsterones 200 mg • Caffeine 150 mg • Phosphatidylserine 100 mg. Other Ingredients: Gelatin, Cellulose, Magnesium Stearate.
See Editor's Note No. 40.

CortiCarb3000 (Phasisol) - Dynamic Nutritional Research
Two capsules contain: Chromium 100 mcg • Selenium 500 mcg • White Kidney bean extract 600 mg • Guggul 2.5% 300 mg • Green Tea extract 50% 250 mg • L-Tyrosine 150 mg • Citrus Aurantium extract 6% 85 mg • Alpha Lipoic Acid 60 mg • Valerian root powder 50 mg • St. John's Wort powder 50 mg. Other Ingredients: Gelatin, Dicalcium Phosphate, Magnesium Stearate, Silica.
See Editor's Note No. 40.

CortiCept Rx - Nature's Rx
Each capsule contains: Vitamin C (as calcium ascorbate) 100 mg • Calcium (as calcium carbonate, calcium ascorbate) 100 mg • Magnesium (as magnesium chelate) 50 mg • Chromium (as chromium polynicotinate) 50 mg • Proprietary Blend 155 mg: Magnolia bark extract (magnolia officinalis, 1.5% honokiol), Beta-Sitosterol, Suntheanine brand 100% L-Theanine • Proprietary Blend 125 mg: Green Tea leaf extract (camellia sinensis, 50% EGCG), Bitter Orange peel extract (citrus aurantium, providing 5% synephrine) • Proprietary Blend 16.5 mg: Banaba leaf extract (lagerstroemia speicosa, 1% corosolic acid), Vanadyl Sulfate (providing 5 mcg vanadium).
See Editor's Note No. 40.

Cortico-B5B6 - Metagenics
Each tablet contains: Pantothenic Acid (as D-calcium pantothenate) 500 mg • Vitamin C (as ascorbic acid) 240 mg • Citrus Bioflavonoid complex (standardized to 45% full spectrum bioflavonoids) 100 mg • Vitamin B6 (as pyridoxine hydrochloride) 100 mg • Magnesium (as magnesium oxide) 75 mg.

Corti-Cut - Olympian Labs
Each capsule contains: Vitamin C (as ascorbyl palmitate) 60 mg • Chromium (as chromium polynicotinate) 50 mcg • L-Theanine 100 mg • Soy Phospholipids 100 mg: Phosphatidylserine 20-22%, Phosphatidylcholine 14-18%, Phosphatidylethanolamine 10-12%, Phosphatidylinositol 7-10% • Essential Fatty Acid Blend 20 mg:

BRAND NAMES

Caprylic Acid, Linoleic Acid, Capric Acid, Oleic Acid, Palmitic Acid, Linolenic Acid, Stearic Acid • Magnolia fresh flower 4:1 extract 100 mg • Proprietary Herbal Blend 200 mg: Rhodiola Rosea root (4% rosavins), Green Tea leaf extract (camellia sinensis, 50% polyphenols), Citrus Aurantium fruit (6% synephrine). Other Ingredients: Gelatin, Rice Flour, Microcrystalline Cellulose (plant fiber), Magnesium Stearate, Silica.
See Editor's Note No. 40.

Corti-Cut PM - Olympian Labs
Two capsules contain: L-Tyrosine 300 mg • L-Arginine Pyroglutamate 300 mg • L-Carnitine Fumarate 150 mg • L-Theanine 100 mg • Soy Phospholipids 100 mg: Phosphatidylserine, Phosphatidylcholine, Phosphatidylethanolamine, Phosphatidylinositol • Proprietary Herbal Blend 200 mg: Holy Basil leaves (ocimum sanctum, 2.5% ursolic acid), Rhodiola Rosea root (4% rosavins), GABA, Inositol. Other Ingredients: Gelatin, Rice Flour, Microcrystalline Cellulose (plant fiber), Magnesium Stearate, Silica.

CortiDrene (Vitopril) - Wellspring Laboratories
Two capsules contain: Niacin (niacinamide, B3) 20 mg • Green Tea extract PE (40% (EGCG & polyphenols) 150 mg • Epimedium 100 mg • L-Theanine 66.7 mg • Citrus Aurantium 4% extract (synephrine) 55 mg • Beta Sitosterol complex 40 mg • Phosphatidylserine (20% extract) 8.3 mg • Grape seed extract 95% 30 mg • Chromium (picolinate) 50 mcg • St. John's Wort (powder) 50 mg • Valerian root (powder) 20 mg. Other Ingredients: Gelatin, Dicalcium Phosphate, Magnesium Stearate, Silica.
See Editor's Note No. 40.

CortiFast - AmerMed
Each capsule contains: Vitamin C (as calcium ascorbate) 120 mg • Coral Calcium 240 mg • Calcium (from coral calcium and calcium ascorbate) 100 mg • Chromium (as chromium polynicotinate) 50 mcg • Magnolia bark (magnolia officinalis, equivalent from 200 mg of 4:1 extract) 800 mg • Beta-Sitosterol 30 mg • Green Tea extract (camellia sinensis, 50% polyphenols) 175 mg • Hoodia cactus (equivalent from 25 mg of 4:1 extract) 100 mg • Banaba leaf extract (lagerstroemia speciosa, 1% corosolic acid) 25 mg • Vanadium (as amino acid chelate) 10 mcg. Other Ingredients: Gelatin Capsule, Maltodextrin.

Cortigen - Genetix Nutraceuticals
Two capsules contain: Vitamin B6 3 mg • Vitamin B12 500 mcg • Folic Acid 200 mcg • Vitamin C 80 mg • Calcium 100 mg • Chromium 100 mcg • Vanadium 60 mcg • Cortiol Proprietary Blend 530 mg: Green Tea extract, Magnolia bark extract, L-Theanine, Phosphatidylserine, Beta-Sitosterol.

CortiLess - Diet a Day, Inc.
Each capsule contains: Vitamin C (as calcium ascorbate) 100 mg • Calcium (as calcium carbonate and calcium ascorbate) 150 mg • Chromium (as ChromeMate brand chromium polynicotinate) 50 mcg • Blend 1 155 mg: Magnolia bark extract, Beta-Sitosterol, Suntheanine brand 100% L-Theanine • Blend 2 125 mg: Green Tea leaf extract (50% EGCG), Cocoa bean extract (12% theobromine) 125 mg • Blend 3 16.5 mg: Banaba leaf extract (1% corosolic acid), Vanadyl Sulfate (with 50 mcg vanadium). Other Ingredients: Gelatin, Cellulose, Magnesium Stearate, Silica.

Cortiloss - Delmar Labs
Each capsule contains: Vitamin C (as calcium ascorbate) 100 mg • Calcium (as calcium carbonate, calcium ascorbate) 150 mg • Chromium (as chromium polynicotinate) 50 mcg • Proprietary Blend 155 mg: Magnolia bark extract (magnolia officinalis, 1.5% honokiol), Beta-Sitosterol, Suntheanine brand 100% L-Theanine • Proprietary Blend 125 mg: Green Tea leaf extract (camellia sinensis, 50% EGCG), Bitter Orange peel extract (citrus aurantium, 5% synephrine) • Proprietary Blend 16.5 mg: Banaba leaf extract (lagerstroemia speciosa, 1% corosolic acid), Vanadyl Sulfate (providing 5 mcg vanadium). Other Ingredients: Gelatin, Magnesium Stearate.
See Editor's Note No. 40.

Cortimin - Pure Encapsulations
Each vegetable capsule contains: Milk Protein Hydrosylate (standardized to contain 2.5 mga-s1 casein peptide) 150 mg. Other Ingredients: Sodium Caseinate.

Cortipren - Window Rock Health Laboratories
Each capsule contains: Proprietary Blend 155 mg: Magnolia bark (honokiol), Beta-Sitosterol, Suntheanine brand 100% L-Theanine • Proprietary Blend 125 mg: Green Tea extract (EGCG), Bitter Orange peel extract (synephrine) • Proprietary Blend 16.5 mg: Banaba leaf extract (corosolic acid), Vanadyl Sulfate • Vitamin C (as calcium ascorbate) 100 mg • Calcium (as calcium carbonate, calcium ascorbate) 150 mg • Chromium (as chromium polynicotinate) 50 mcg. Other Ingredients: Gelatin, Magnesium Stearate.
See Editor's Note No. 40.

CortiPrep - HealthMinded
Each capsule contains: Vitamin C (as calcium ascorbate) 100 mg • Calcium (as calcium carbonate, calcium ascorbate) 150 mg • Chromium (as chromium polynicotinate) 50 mg • CortiPrep Proprietary Blend 296.5 mg: Magnolia bark extract (magnolia officinalis, 1.5% honokiol), Beta-Sitosterol, Suntheanine brand 100% L-Theanine, Green Tea leaf extract (camellia sinensis, 50% EGCG), Bitter Orange peel extract (citrus aurantium, 5% synephrine), Banaba leaf extract (lagerstroemia speciosa, 1% corosolic acid), Vanadyl Sulfate (providing 5 mcg vanadium). Other Ingredients: Gelatin, Stearic Acid, Magnesium Stearate.
See Editor's Note No. 40.

CortiShed - Higher Power
Each capsule contains: Vitamin C 100 mg • Calcium Citrate 150 mg • Chromium 125 mcg • Vitamin E 25 IU • Green Tea extract 100 mg • Citrus Aurantium 100 mg • Phosphatidylserine 100 mg • Alpha Lipoic Acid 50 mg • Acetyl L-Carnitine 50 mg • Phenylalanine 50 mg • Vanadyl Sulfate 10 mg. Other Ingredients: Magnesium Stearate, Silica.
See Editor's Note No. 40.

CortiSlim - Window Rock Health Laboratories
Each capsule contains: Vitamin C (as calcium ascorbate) 100 mg • Calcium (as calcium carbonate, calcium ascorbate) 150 mg • Chromium (as chromium polynicotinate) 50 mg • Cortiplex Proprietary Blend 155 mg: Magnolia bark extract (magnolia officinalis, 1.5% honokiol), Beta-Sitosterol, L-Theanine (Suntheanine) • Leptiplex Proprietary Blend 125 mg: Green Tea leaf extract (camellia sinensis, 50% EGCG), Bitter Orange peel extract (citrus aurantium, 5% synephrine) • Insutrol Proprietary Blend 16.5 mg: Banaba leaf extract (lagerstroemia speciosa, 1% corosolic acid), Vanadyl Sulfate (providing 5 mcg vanadium). Other Ingredients: Gelatin, Microcrystalline Cellulose, Water, Silicon Dioxide, Magnesium Stearate (vegetable derived).
See Editor's Note No. 33 and No. 40.

Cortisol Appetite Control - Irwin Naturals
Two caps contain: Green Tea extract 200 mg • Beta-Sitosterol (as 100% L-theanine) 200 mg • Magnolia bark extract 500 mg • Epimedium 200 mg • Bioperine brand Black Pepper extract complex 8 mg.

Cortisol X - ANSI - Advanced Nutrient Science International
Each capsule contains: Vitamin B6 5 mg • Vitamin C 60 mg • Calcium 150 mg • Chromium 50 mcg • Magnesium 20 mg • Proprietary Leanplex Blend 520 mg: Phosphatidyl Serine, Green Tea leaf, CLA, Bitter Orange extract, Magnolia bark extract, L-Theonine, Apple Cider Vinegar, Beta Sitosterol, Hoodia Gordonii cactus, Banaba leaf extract, Alpha Lipoic Acid. Other Ingredients: Gelatin, Microcrystalline Cellulose, Magnesium Stearate, Water, Silicon Dioxide.
See Editor's Note No. 40.

BRAND NAMES

Some Brand Name Natural Products - What they Contain

www.NaturalDatabase.com contains MANY more listings than appear here.

Editor's Notes are located on pages 2155-2163.

Cortistat-PS - Champion Nutrition
Four capsules contain: Phosphatidylserine 100 mg • Phosphatidylcholine 105 mg • Phosphatidylethanolamine 70 mg • Phosphatidylinositol 30 mg • Arginine Aspartate 576 mg • Potassium Succinate 576 mg • Quercetin 100 mg • Feverfew 100 mg.

Cortitrol - Pharmanex
Each capsule contains: Magnolia 4:1 extract (magnolia officinalis) 133 mg • Epimedium water 6:1 extract (epimedium koreanum) 100 mg • L-Theanine 70:1 extract (from camillia sinensis) 66.7 mg • Beta-Sitosterol 40 mg • Phosphatidylserine 8.3 mg.

CortiZide - MedaBiotics
Two capsules contain: Calcium (chelate) 100 mg • Vitamin C (as ascorbic acid) 80 mg • Vitamin B6 (as pyridoxine HCl) 3 mg • Vitamin B12 (as cyanocobalamin) 500 mcg • Folic Acid (vitamin B9) 200 mcg • Chromium (as chromium dinicotinate glycinate) 100 mcg • Green Tea leaf extract (50% catechins and 35% polyphenols) 300 mg • Magnolia Officinalis bark 4:1 extract 70 mg • Suntheanine brand L-Theanine (100%) 60 mg • Phosphatidylserine 100 mg • Beta-Sitosterol 40 mg • Vanadium 60 mcg. Other Ingredients: Gelatin, Cellulose, Magnesium Stearate.

CORvalen - Bioenergy, Inc.
Each scoop contains: D-Ribose 5 g.

Coryza Forte - Progressive Labs
Each capsule contains: Vitamin A (as retinol & beta carotene) 4000 IU • Vitamin C (ascorbic acid) 300 mg • Vitamin B6 (pyridoxine HCl) 15 mg • Pantothenic Acid (as d-calcium pantothenate) 25 mg • Calcium (as calcium carbonate) 40 mg • Zinc (as zinc picolinate) 5 mg • Echinacea 50 mg • Citrus Bioflavonoid 5X complex (as undiluted hesperidin, naringin and rutin) 150 mg. Other Ingredients: Pollen, Raw Bovine Trachea, Raw Bovine Thymus, Raw Bovine Adrenal, Raw Bovine Lymph, Raw Bovine Spleen, RNA, Rose Hips, Whey, Cellulose, Magnesium Stearate, Gelatin.
See Editor's Note No. 14.

Coryza-Comp - Atrium Biotechnologies
Each tablet contains: Vitamin A (Fish oil) 2000 IU • Vitamin C Ascorbic Acid 300 mg • Vitamin B6 Pyridoxine HCL 15 mg • Pantothenic Acid 25 mg • Calcium (Aspartate) 10 mg • Magnesium (Aspartate) 10 mg • Zinc (Aspartate) 2 mg • Citrus Bioflavonoids 150 mg • High RNA Yeast 50 mg • Bee Pollen 10 mg • Raw Spleen concentrate (Bovine) 10 mg • Raw Thymus concentrate (Bovine) 10 mg • Raw Adrenal concentrate 5 mg • Raw Lymph concentrate (Bovine) 5 mg. In a base of Alfalfa & Rose Hips.
See Editor's Note No. 14.

Cosamin - Nutramax Laboratories, Inc.
Each capsule contains: Glucosamine HCl (99%) 250 mg • Sodium Chondroitin Sulfate (95%) with Mixed Glycosaminoglycans (5%) 200 mg • Ascorbate (as manganese ascorbate) 33 mg • Manganese (as manganese ascorbate) 5 mg.
See Editor's Note No. 4.

Cosamin DS Double Strength Capsules - Nutramax Laboratories, Inc.
Each tablet contains: Vitamin C (as manganese ascorbate) 16 mg • Manganese (as manganese ascorbate) 3 mg • High Purity FCHG-49 Glucosamine HCl 99% 500 mg • Low Molecular Weight TRH122 Sodium Chondroitin Sulfate 95% 400 mg.

Cosamin DS Double Strength Tablets - Nutramax Laboratories, Inc.
Each tablet contains: Vitamin C (as manganese ascorbate) 16 mg • Manganese (as manganese ascorbate) 3 mg • High Purity FCHG-49 Glucosamine HCl 99% 500 mg • Low Molecular Weight TRH122 Sodium Chondroitin Sulfate 95% 400 mg. Other Ingredients: Microcrystalline Cellulose, Croscarmellose Sodium, Magnesium Stearate.

Cosamin ProTek - Nutramax Laboratories, Inc.
Each capsule contains: Sodium 30 mg • Vitamin C 359 mg • Vitamin D3 400 IU • Vitamin E (d-alpha tocopherol) 35 IU • Manganese 1 mg • Glucosamine HCl 200 mg • Sodium Chondroitin Sulfate 95% and Mixed Glycosaminoglycans 5% 400 mg.
See Editor's Note No. 4.

Cosamin ProTek Women's Formula - Nutramax Laboratories, Inc.
Each capsule contains: Sodium 30 mg • Vitamin C 9 mg • Vitamin D3 400 IU • Calcium 115 mg • Manganese 1 mg • Glucosamine HCl 200 mg • Sodium Chondroitin Sulfate 95% and Mixed Glycosaminoglycans 5% 400 mg.
See Editor's Note No. 4.

CosaminDS (Cosamin DS) - Nutramax Laboratories, Inc.
Each capsule contains: Glucosamine HCl (99%) 500 mg • Sodium Chondroitin Sulfate (95%) with Mixed Glycosaminoglycans (5%) 400 mg • Ascorbate (as manganese ascorbate) 16 mg • Manganese (as manganese ascorbate) 3 mg.
See Editor's Note No. 15.

Cosamine 500 mg - Kripps Pharmacy
Each capsule contains: Chondroitin Sulfate & Glucosamine powder (1:1 ratio) 500 mg.
See Editor's Note No. 15.

Cositin - Life Extension
Each capsule contains: Glucosamine HCL 99+% 250 mg • Sodium Chondroitin Sulfate 95%/Mixed Glycosaminoglycans 5% 200 mg • Ascorbate (manganese ascorbate) 33 mg • Selenium (seleniomethionine) 25 mg • Bromelain 25 mg • Manganese (ascorbate) 5 mg.

CosMedix - Ortho Molecular Products
Three capsules contain: Vitamin A (as palmitate USP) 5000 IU • Vitamin D (D3, as cholecalciferol) 50 IU • Folic ACid 400 mcg • Vitamin B12 (as methylcobalamin) 100 mcg • Biotin 500 mcg • Selenium (as amino acid complex) 25 mcg • Methylsulfonylmethane 400 mg • Stinging Nettles leaf 315 mg • Saw Palmetto fruit extract (standardized to contain 50% fatty acids) 300 mg • Horsetail grass (aerial portion) 250 mg • Fo-Ti root 200 mg • PABA USP 150 mg • Betaine HCl USP 100 mg. Other Ingredients: Natural Vegetable Capsules, Magnesium Stearate, Microcrystalline Cellulose.

Cosmopolitan Nutrition - Vitabiotics
Each capsule contains: Vitamin D (as vitamin D3 200 IU) 5 mcg • Vitamin E (natural source) 20 mg • Vitamin C 60 mg • Thiamin (vitamin B1) 10 mg • Riboflavin (vitamin B2) 5 mg • Niacin (vitamin B3) 18 mg • Pyridoxine Hydrochloride (vitamin B6) 25 mg • Folacin (as folic acid) 400 mcg • Cyanocobalamin (vitamin B12) 15 mcg • Biotin 0.15 mg • Pantothenic Acid 6 mg • Iron 14 mg • Magnesium 50 mg • Zinc 12 mg • Iodine 120 mcg • Manganese 2 mg • Copper 1.5 mg • Chromium (chelated) 100 mcg • Selenium 100 mcg • L-Carnitine 50 mg • Taurine 10 mg • Tyrosine 10 mg • Green tea extract (60% polyphenols) 40 mg • Cranberry extract 100 mg • Wheatgerm oil 200 mg • Natural Mixed Carotenoids 2 mg • Lecithin 15 mg.

Cough Syrup - Progressive Labs
Each 10 ml contains: Dextromethorphan Hydrobromide 10 mg • Guaifenesin 100 mg • Potassium Citrate 85 mg • Citric Acid 35 mg.

Cough Syrup with Honey - Hyland's
Ipecacuanha as Ipecac 6X HPUS • Aconitum napellus as Aconite 6X HPUS • Spongia tosta as Sponge 6X HPUS • Antimonium tartaricum as Potassium antimonium tartrate 6X HPUS. In simple syrup with Honey.
See Editor's Note No. 1.

Cough-Eze Syrup - The Herbalist
Herbs of Marshmallow root, Slippery Elm bark, Elecampane root, Wild Cherry bark, Mullein leaf, Horehound leaf, Licorice root, Cubeb berry, Orange peel, Cinnamon bark & Ginger root, Extracts of Skunk Cabbage root & Lobelia leaf, Honey, Vegetable Glycerine & Peppermint Oil.

CoughFree - Heel/BHI, Inc.
Each 1 tsp (5 mL) serving contains: Drosera Rotundifolia 4X • Ipecacuanha 4X • Rumex Crispus 4X • Antimonium Tartaricum 6X • Cuprum Sulphuricum 6X • Spongia Tosta 8X.
See Editor's Note No. 1.

Covitol brand - Cognis
Vitamin E.
See Editor's Note No. 44.

COX2 Tame - Jarrow Formulas
Three softgels contain: Sardine oil (source of omega 3 fatty acids, providing 113 mg of EPA & 25 mg DHA) 293 mg • GLA (gamma linoleic acid, from 200 mg of borage seed oil 24% extract) 50 mg • Resveratrol (polygonum cuspidatum, derived from 160 mg resveratrol 10% extract) 16 mg • Curcumin (curcuma longa, 95% curcuminoids) 300 mg • Ginger rhizome (zingiber officinale, 5% gingerols and shogaols) 250 mg • Green Tea (camellia sinensis, 45% polyphenols) 150 mg • Devil's Claw (phytum procumbens, 5% iridoid glycosides) 250 mg • White Willow bark (salicis cortex, 15% salicin) 200 mg • Quercetin 250 mg. Other Ingredients: Soybean Oil, Gelatin, Glycerin, Purified Water, Carob, Beeswax, Lecithin.

C-Plus Cold Tablets - Hyland's
Each tablet contains: Eupatorium perforliatum as Boneset 3X HPUS • Euphrasia officinalis as Eyebright 2X HPUS • Gelsemium sempervirens as Yellow Jasmine 3X HPUS • Kali iodatum as Potassium Iodide 3X HPUS. In a base of Lactose NF (Milk Sugar).
See Editor's Note No. 1.

C-Plus-Citrus - Atrium Biotechnologies
Each level teaspoon (3300 mg approx. wt.) contains: Vitamin C from: (Ascorbic Acid 900 mg & Sodium Ascorbate 625 mg) 1500 mg • Mannitol 1395 mg • Lemon Bioflavonoids 150 mg • Rose Hips 100 mg • Hesperidin Complex 50 mg • Rutin 30 mg. Contains natural Orange Juice flavor.

Cracked Skin Relief Creme 2oz - Derma E
Purified Water • Aloe Vera gel • Arnica extract • Bay leaf oil • Glycerin • Clove oil • Cetyl Alcohol • Caprylic Triglyceride • Glyceryl Stearate • PEG 100 Stearate • Stearic Acid • Allantoin • Panthenol • Jojoba oil • Dimethicone • Polysorbate 20 • Tocopheryl Acetate (vitamin E) • Retinyl Palmitate (vitamin A) • Methylparaben • Ethylparaben • Silica 3X • TEA • I. Urea.

Cramp Bark-Catnip Virtue - Blessed Herbs
Cramp bark • Catnip flower & herb • Motherwort • Scullcap • Yarrow flower & herb • Grain alcohol & Distilled Water.

Cramp Free - Health Center for Better Living
Calcium • Magnesium • Potassium • Other Herbs.

Cran Clearance - Jarrow Formulas
Two capsules contain: Vitamin C 60 mg • Cranberry 10:1 1300 mg. Other Ingredients: Magnesium Stearate, Silicon Dioxide, Gelatin.

Cran Support - Natrol, Inc.
Each capsule contains: Guaranteed Potency Cranberry extract supplying 90% solids 30-40% organic acids 400 mg • Uva Ursi leaves 115 mg • Vitamin C (Ascorbic Acid) 100 mg • FOS (Fruiti-Vin FructoOligoSaccharides) 100 mg • Cat's Claw root 50 mg • Corn Silk 30 mg • Kava Kava root 8.5 mg. Other Ingredients: Silica, Magnesium Stearate, Annatto, Gelatin.

Cran-Aid - Traditional Medicinals
Roselle Hibiscus flower • Cranberry Fruit concentrate • German Chamomile flower • Rose Hip • Uva Ursi leaf • Cleavers herb • Althea root • Peppermint leaf • Stevia leaf.

Cranberry - Leiner Health Products
Two caplets contain: Cranberry extract (Vaccinium macrocarpon) berry 600 mg. Other Ingredients: Calcium Carbonate, Cellulose, Maltodextrin, Croscarmellose Sodium, Talc, Silicon Dioxide, Polyethylene Glycol 3350, Crospovidone, Hyroxypropyl Methylcellulose, Magnesium Stearate, Hydroxypropyl Cellulose, Polysorbate 80.

Cranberry - GNC
Each capsule contains: Cranberry fruit powder (Vaccinium Macrocarpon) 500 mg. Other Ingredients: Gelatin, Cellulose, Magnesium Stearate.

Cranberry - Aspen Group, Inc.
Each tablet contains: Cranberry extract (25:1 extract) 250 mg • Vitamin C 60 mg • Echinacea (4:1 extract) 30 mg • Buchu (4:1 extract) 15 mg • Juniper berry (4:1 extract) 15 mg • Uva Ursi (4:1 extract) 15 mg.

Cranberry - Pharmanex
Each capsule contains: Cranberry fruit (15:1) concentrate (Vaccinium macrocarpon) 500 mg. Other Ingredients: Gelatin and Titanium Dioxide.

Cranberry + - PhysioLogics
Each softgel contains: Vitamin C (as ascorbic acid) 100 mg • Vitamin E (as d-alpha tocopherol acetate) 3 IU • Cranberry concentrate powder (vaccinium macrocarpon, from 12:1 concentrate, equivalent to fresh cranberries 1680 mg) 140 mg. Other Ingredients: Soybean Oil, Gelatin, Lecithin, Glycerin, Beeswax / Soybean Oil Mixture.

Cranberry 1000 mg, Concentrated - GNC
Each capsule contains: Cranberry Juice (vaccinium macrocarpon; from 58.5 mg of cranberry juice concentrate 19:1) 1000 mg. Other Ingredients: Soybean Oil, Gelatin, Glycerin, Caramel Color, Titanium Dioxide (natural mineral whitener).

Cranberry 5000 - Nature's Own
Each tablet contains: Cranberry extract (vaccinium macrocarpon) 5000 mg.

Cranberry Apple Cherry - Clif Bar Inc
Brown Rice Syrup • Rolled Oats • Soy Protein Isolate • Rice Flour • Oat Flour • Soy Flour • Soybean • Evaporated Cane Juice • Dried Apples • Cranberries • Apple Juice • Prunes • Apple Fiber • Oat Fiber • Milled Flaxseed • Soy Fiber • Chicory Extract • Lemon Fiber • Psyllium • Brown Rice • Malt Extract • Dried Cherries • Natural Flavor • Sea Salt • Baking Soda • Decaffeinated Green Tea Extract.

Cranberry Concentrate - J. R. Carlson Laboratories, Inc.
Four softgels contain: Vitamin C (as ascorbic acid) 40 mg • Cranberry (juice concentrate) 4000 mg.

Cranberry Concentrate - NOW Foods
Two capsules contain: Vitamin C (as ascorbic acid) 20 mg • Cranberry concentrate fruit (1400 mg of 8:1 concentrate) 1.4 g. Other Ingredients: Magnesium Stearate.

Cranberry Concentrate - Pro Health
Two capsules contain: Vitamin C (as ascorbic acid) 20 mg • Cranberry 8:1 concentrate 1.4 g. Other Ingredients: Magnesium Stearate.

Cranberry Concentrate - Schiff
Two softgels contain: Vitamin C (as ascorbic acid) 10 mg • Cranberry fruit (vaccinium macrocarpon) 1 g. Other Ingredients: Soybean Oil, Softgel (gelatin, glycerin, water, caramel color), Lecithin, Silicon Dioxide.

Cranberry Juice Concentrate 1000 mg - Jamieson
Each capsule contains: Vitamin C (as Ascorbic Acid) 10 mg • Cranberry juice concentrate 1000 mg.

Cranberry Juice Maximum Concentrate - Jamieson
Each capsule contains: Cranberry Juice Concentrate 1:34 500 mg.

Some Brand Name Natural Products - What they Contain

www.NaturalDatabase.com contains MANY more listings than appear here.
Editor's Notes are located on pages 2155-2163.

Cranberry NS - Pure Encapsulations
Each vegetable capsule contains: Cranberry juice extract 500 mg.

Cranberry Plus - Futurebiotics LLC
Cranberry Extract (25:1 extract) 250 mg • Vitamin C 50 mg • Echinacea (4:1 extract equivalent to) 25 mg • Buchu (4:1 extract equivalent to) 12.5 mg • Juniper Berry (4:1 extract equivalent to) 12.5 mg • Uva Ursi (4:1 extract equivalent to) 12.5 mg.

Cranberry/d-Mannose - Pure Encapsulations
Each vegetable capsule contains: Cranberry fruit juice extract 100 mg • D-Mannose 450 mg • Vitamin C (as ascorbyl palmitate) 11 mg.

Cran-C - Holista
Each capsule contains: Vitamin C 100 mg • Concentrated Cranberries (Vaccinum macrocarpon) of 25:1 extract (equivalent to 1132 mg of fresh cranberry juice) 45.3 mg.

Cran-Caps - Progressive Labs
Three softgels contain: Vitamin C 30 mg • Cranberry juice concentrate 3000 mg • Phosphatide complex 90 mg. Free of sugar and artificial sweeteners.

CranExtra - Enzymatic Therapy
Each capsule contains: Vitamin C (Ascorbic Acid) 1000 mg. Other Ingredients: Cranberry extract (Vaccinium macrocarpon) standardized to contain 5% Anthocyanidins & 30% Organic Acids: Quinic, Malic, Citric & Hippuric Acid 100 mg • Uva Ursi (Arctostaphylos uva ursi) standardized to contain 20% Arbutin 100 mg.

CranGuard - PhytoPharmica
Two capsules contain: Vitamin C (ascorbic acid) 200 mg • Cranberry extract[(vaccinium macrocarpon, standardized to contain 5% anthocyanidins & 30% organic acids (quinic, malic, citric & hippuric acid)] 200 mg • Uva Ursi (arctostaphylos uva ursi, standardized to contain 20% arbutin) 200 mg.

Cravex Capsules - Natrol, Inc.
Two capsules contain: Calcium (from garcinia cambogia) 180 mg • Chromium (as chromium picolinate) 120 mcg • Garcinia Cambogia extract 1000 mg: Hydroxycitric Acid (HCA) 600 mg • Green Tea extract (25% polyphenols) 300 mg: Polyphenols 75 mg, Caffeine 60 mg. Other Ingredients: Gelatin Capsules, Silica, Magnesium Stearate.

Cravex Tablets - Natrol, Inc.
Two tablets contain: Calcium 230 mg • Iodine (as Potassium Iodine) 150 mcg • Chromium (as Chromium Picolinate) 200 mcg • Gymnema Sylvestre powdered extract leaves 300 mg • Licorice root 250 mg Deglycyrrhizinated Licorice • powdered extract Glycerinic Acid (1%) 2.5 mg • L-Glutamine 250 mg • DL-Phenylalanine 250 mg • 5-Hydroxytryptophan (5-HTP) 10 mg. Other Ingredients: Calcium Sulfate Dihydrate, Mono & Di-Glycerides, Microcrystalline Cellulose, Croscarmellose Sodium, Stearic Acid, Silicon Dioxide, Magnesium Stearate.

CreActiv - Metabolic Response Modifiers
Two scoops (95.5 g) contains: Creatine monohydrate 12 g • L-Glutamine 5 g • BCAA blend 2 g • Alpha Lipoic Acid 300 mg • Dextrose 70 g • L-Taurine 1 g • L-Arginine 500 mg • Vitamin C 250 mg • Calcium 21 mg • Potassium 101 mg • Sodium 85 mg • Magnesium 100 mg • Phosphorus 160 mg • Chloride 122 mg • RNA 200 mg.

Creagen - ANS - Applied Nutrition Sciences
Creatine Monohydrate.

Creagen Plus - ANS - Applied Nutrition Sciences
Creatine Monohydrate • Dextrose • Taurine.

Cream of Youth - Life Extension
Biologically Active Placenta Enzymes, Apricot kernal oil, Collagen, Elastin, Vitamin E, NaPCA, Aloe, Emollients, Fragrances.

Creamy Cleansing Lotion (normal to dry skin) - Nu Skin Enterprises
Water (aqua) • Caprylic/Capric Triglycerides • Butylene Glycol • Isodecyl Neopentanoate • Glyceryl Stearate • PEG-100 Stearate • Disodium Cocoamphodiacetate • Limnanthes Alba seed oil (meadowfoam) • Glycine Soja lipds (soybean) • Dipotassium Glycyrrhizate • Artemisia Vulgaris extract (mugwort) • Laminaria Digitata extract (algae) • Glycerin • Carbomer • Stearyl Alcohol • Triethanolamine • Tetrasodium EDTA • Fragrance (parfum) • Phenoxyethanol • Chlorphenesin • Methylparaben • Benzoic Acid.

Creamy Hydrating Masque - Nu Skin Enterprises
Water (aqua) • Isocetyl Stearate • Glycerin • Butylene Glycol • Decyl Oleate • Stearic Acid • Saccharide Isomerate • Cetearyl Ethylhexanoate • Cetyl Alcohol • Opuntia Tuna extract (cactus) • Pinus Strobus cone extract • PVM/MA Copolymer • Sodium Polyacrylate • Polyacrylamide • C13-14 Isoparaffin • Carbomer • Oleth-10 • Laureth-7 • Triethanolamine • Anthemis Nobilis flower oil • Lavandula Angustifolia oil (lavender) • Salvia Officinalis oil (sage) • Camellia Sinensis leaf extract • Disodium EDTA • Chlorphenesin • Ethylparaben • Methylparaben • Phenoxy-Ethanol • Propylparaben • Titanium Dioxide.

Creapure brand - Degussa Food Ingredients/BL BioActives
Creatine Monohydrate.

Creatine - Source Naturals
Each tablet contains: Creatine Monohydrate 1,000 mg.

Creatine - Life Extension
Each teaspoon contains: Creatine Monohydrate (99% pure, crystallized) 5000 mg.

Creatine - J. R. Carlson Laboratories, Inc.
Each 1 tsp serving contains: Creatine Monohydrate 2800 mg.

Creatine 1000 - Higher Power
Each 1 tsp (5 g) serving contains: 100% Pure Creatine Monohydrate 5 g.

Creatine 2500 Caps - Optimum Nutrition
Two capsules contain: Creatine Monohydrate 2.5 g. Other Ingredients: Gelatin, Magnesium Stearate.

Creatine 6000-ES - MuscleTech
Each teaspoon contains: Creatine Monohydrate 6000 mg • Proprietary blend 500 mg: Creatine Monohydrate, L-Methionine, L-Arginine, L-Glycine.

Creatine 750 Caps - Optimum Nutrition
Each capsule contains: Creatine Monohydrate 750 mg. Other Ingredients: Gelatin, Calcium Phosphate, Magnesium Stearate, Silica.

Creatine Blast - Pharmanex
Each scoop (42 g) contains: Phosphorus (as Dimagnesium Phosphate) 60 mg • Magnesium (as Dimagnesium Phosphate) 50 mg • Creatine Monohydrate 4 g • Taurine 1000 mg. Other Ingredients: Dextrose, Citric Acid, Natural Grape Flavor, Grape Skin Extract (color).

Creatine Caps 800 - Jarrow Formulas
Each capsule contains: Pure Creatine Monohydrate 800 mg. Other Ingredients: Rice Powder, Magnesium Stearate, Gelatin.

Creatine Fuel - TwinLab
Each capsule contains: Creatine Monohydrate 700 mg. Each teaspoonful of powder contains: Creatine Monohydrate 5 g (5000 mg).

Creatine Fuel Loading Drink - TwinLab
HPLC Pure Creatine Monohydrate with added Dextrose (a high glycemic carbohydrate) • Chromium • Taurine • Magnesium • Alpha Lipoic Acid. Other Ingredients: L-Glutamine 2 g.

Some Brand Name Natural Products - What they Contain

www.NaturalDatabase.com contains MANY more listings than appear here.
Editor's Notes are located on pages 2155-2163.

BRAND NAMES

Creatine Fuel Plus - TwinLab
Creatine (Creatine Monohydrate) 7 g. It also contains muscle cell volumizers, insulin potentiators & anti-catabolic, lean body mass stimulators. Fat free.

Creatine Fuel Stack - TwinLab
Six capsules contain: Creatine Monohydrate 5000 mg • L-Glutamine 2000 mg • Taurine 200 mg.

Creatine Fuelchews - TwinLab
Each chew contains: Pure Creatine Monohydrate 1 g • Dextrose 3 g. No sucrose or fructose is present.

Creatine Monohydrate - Pro Health
Five tablets contain: Creatine Monohydrate (from sarcosine [n,n dimethylglycine]) 5000 mg. Other Ingredients: Stearic Acid, Dibasic Calcium Phosphate, Fiber (vegetable), Modified Cellulose Gum, Colloidal Silicon Dioxide, Magnesium Stearate.

Creatine Monohydrate - Jarrow Formulas
Each scoop contains: Creatine Monohydrate 6 g.

Creatine Monohydrate Powder - ProLab
Each teaspoon contains: Creatine Monohydrate 5 g.

Creatine Now (wild cherry flavor) - Rexall - Sundown
Each packet contains: Vitamin C (Ascorbic Acid) 1000 mg • Thiamin Hydrochloride (Vitamin B-1) 15 mg • Riboflavin USP (Vitamin B-2) 20 mg • Niacin (Niacinamide) 50 mg • Vitamin B-6 (Pyridoxine Hydrochloride) 8.3 mg • Vitamin B-12 (Cyanocobalamin) 10 mcg • Biotin 150 mcg • Pantothenic Acid (Calcium D-Pantothenate) 25 mg • Calcium Citrate 175 mg • Sodium Bicarbonate 200 mg • Potassium Bicarbonate 180 mg • Creatine Citrate 5 g • Stevia extract 26 mg. Other Ingredients: Dextrose, Citric Acid, Natural and Artificial Cherry flavor, Cochineal extract.

Creatine Plus - Life Extension
Two capsules contain: Pure Creatine Monohydrate 1500 mg • Sodium Phosphate (dibasic) 50 mg • Potassium Bicarbonate 50 mg.

Creatine Powder - Olympian Labs
Each teaspoon contains: Creatine Monohydrate 5000 mg.

Creatine Powder - Optimum Nutrition
Each 5 g serving (1 rounded tsp) contains: Creatine Monohydrate 5 g.

Creatine powder - Pure Encapsulations
Each scoop contains: Creatine Monohydrate 4 g.

Creatine pyruvate capsules - Pure Encapsulations
Each vegetable capsule contains: Creatine Pyruvate (providing pyruvic acid 40%, creatine monohydrate 68%; total assay exceeds 100% due to conversion of creatine monohydrate to anhydrous in creatine pyruvate) 800 mg • Vitamin C (as ascorbyl palmitate) 16 mg.

Creatine pyruvate powder - Pure Encapsulations
Each scoop contains: Creatine Pyruvate (providing pyruvic acid 40%, creatine monohydrate 68%; total assay exceeds 100% due to conversion of creatine monohydrate to anhydrous in creatine pyruvate) 3 g.

Creatine Sport Gel - Metabolic Response Modifiers
Contains: Creatine monohydrate 6,000 mg • L-Glutamine 1,000 mg • L-Taurine 500 mg • Dextrose 25 g.

Creatine Surge - Jarrow Formulas
Each scoop contains: Pure Creatine Monohydrate (HPLC tested) 6 g • L-Glutamine (USP/FCC) 2 g • Ribose 1 g • Taurine 1 g • Vitamin C 500 mg • Alpha Lipoic Acid 25 mg. Other Ingredients: Dextrose (glucose), Xanthan Gum, Natural Flavors, Beet Extract.

Creative Creatine - Life Enhancement Products, Inc.
Three rounded tablespoons (22 g) contain: Riboflavin (vitamin B2) 3 mg • Phosphorus (as potassium phosphate and sodium phosphate) 170 mg • Sodium (as sodium phosphate) 116 mg • Potassium (as potassium phosphate) 113 mg • Creatine Monohydrate 5 g • Taurine 1 g

CreaVATE - ProLab
Each capsule contains: Creatine Pyruvate 750 mg.

Creavescent - GEN - Genetic Evolutionary Nutrition
Each serving contains: L-Glutamine 2 g • TCT (Total Creatine Transport) Proprietary Blend 5 g: Creatine Monohydrate. Ingredients: Creatine Monohydrate • Fructose • L-Glutamine • Mono Poly-Saccharide • 2-Hydroxy-1, 2, 3-Propanetricarboxylic Acid • Sodium Hydrogen Carbonate • Orange Solids • Calcium Phosphate • Vitamin A • Vitamin D • Riboflavin.

CreaVol ATP - SportPharma
Each 41 g serving contains: 99% pure microfine Crystalline Creatine 5 g • Adenine Mucleotides including ATP • Vanadyl Sulfate • Taurine • Disodium & Potassium Phosphate • Dextrose (about 35 g per serving).

Critical Keto-Nutrients - Nature's Plus
Three tablets contain: Vitamin A (as beta carotene) 10,000 IU • Vitamin C (as ascorbic acid) 500 mg • Vitamin D (as ergocalciferol) 200 IU • Vitamin E (as D-alpha tocopheryl succinate) 200 IU • Vitamin K 5 mcg • Thiamin (vitamin B1, as thiamine HCl) 25 mg • Riboflavin (vitamin B2) 25 mg • Niacin (as niacinamide) 25 mg • Vitamin B6 (as pyridoxine HCl) 25 mg • Folate (as folic acid) 800 mcg • Vitamin B12 (as cyanocobalamin) 1000 mcg • Biotin 300 mcg • Pantothenic acid (as calcium pantothenate) 60 mg • Calcium (as amino acid chelate/complex) 300 mg • Iron (as amino acid chelate/complex) 4.5 mg • Phosphorus (as amino acid complex) 200 mg • Iodine (from kelp) 150 mcg • Magnesium (as amino acid chelate/complex) 150 mg • Zinc (as amino acid chelate/complex) 25 mg • Selenium (as amino acid chelate) 100 mcg • Copper (as aminoate) 2 mg • Manganese (as amino acid chelate/complex) 5 mg • Chromium (as polynicotinate) 300 mcg • Molybdenum (as amino acid chelate/aminoate) 30 mcg • Potassium (as amino acid complex) 99 mg • Critical Metabolism 150 mg: Super CitriMax brand Garcinia Cambogia extract, Carnitine, Taurine, Apple Cider Vinegar • Critical Green Whole Food Blend 100 mg: Phenalgin, Spirulina, Chlorella, Red Kelp, Brown Kelp, Ulva, Red Seaweed, Dulse, Alfalfa sprout, Barley grass juice, Parsley, Broccoli floret, Olive leaf, Spinach, beet greens, Irish Moss, Green Oats, Kale leaf, Chicory, Artichoke flower, Collards, Parsnips, Green Zucchini, Dandelion greens, Turnip greens, Peas, Mustard greens, Green Tea, Cabbage leaf, Cayenne, Onion bulb, Shiitake mushroom, Celery seed, Carrot root, Garlic clove, Reishi mushroom, Apple, Apricot, Banana, Black Currant, Camu-Camu, Cranberry, Orange, Peach, Red Raspberry, Strawberry, Tomato, Papaya, Pineapple, Red Wine Grape • Bioflavonoids (from citrus limon exocarp) 100 mg • Critical Enzyme 50 mg: Bromelain, Papain, Protease • Inositol 50 mg • PABA (para-aminobenzoic acid) 50 mg • Choline (as bitartrate) 21 mg • Critical Flora 50 million cells: Lactobacillus Acidophilus, Bifidobacterium Longum, B. Bifidum. Other Ingredients: Di-calcium Phosphate, Microcrystalline Cellulose, Spirulina, Stearic Acid, Magnesium Stearate, Silica, Chlorophyll, Red Yeast Rice, Lecithin, Hawthorn, Gugulipid, Pharmaceutical Glaze.

Cruciferous Complete - Standard Process, Inc.
Each capsule contains: Vitamin K 10 mcg • Potassium 10 mcg • Kale 300 mg • Brussels sprouts 300 mg. Other Ingredients: Gelatin, Water, Calcium Stearate, Colors.

C-Statin - Aidan Products, LLC
Each capsule contains: Convolvulus Arvensis leaves extract 250 mg. Other Ingredients: Gelatin Capsule, Maltodextrin.

C-Statin II - Aidan Products, LLC
Each capsule contains: Resveratrol 300 mg • Bromelain 125 mg • Curcumin 125 mg • Baikal Skullcap 50 mg • Quercetin 40 mg • Vitamin E (succinate) 30 IU. Other Ingredients: Gelatin Capsule, Maltodextrin.

C-Time 1000 with Rose Hips - Puritan's Pride
Each tablet contains: Vitamin C with Rose Hips 1000 mg.

C-Time 1500 with Rose Hips - Puritan's Pride
Each tablet contains: Vitamin C with Rose Hips 1500 mg.

C-Time 500 with Rose Hips - Puritan's Pride
Each tablet contains: Vitamin C with Rose Hips 500 mg.

CTR Support - PhysioLogics
Three capsules contain: Turmeric root (curcuma longa, standardized to contain 95% curcuminoids, 713 mg) 750 mg • Boswellia Serrate gum resin (frankincense, standardized to contain 60% boswellic acids, 300 mg) 500 mg • Bromelain (pineapple, from 600 [GDU] per gram) 250 mg • Ginger root (zingiber officinale, standardized to contain 5% gingerols, 5 mg) 100 mg • Devil's Claw root (harpagophytum procumbens, standardized to contain 2% harpagosides, 0.9 mg) 50 mg • Quercetin root (dimorphandra gardina) 50 mg • Yucca plant (yucca schidigera, standardized to contain 14% saponins, 7 mg) 50 mg. Other Ingredients: Gelatin, Rice Powder, Silica, Vegetable Magnesium Stearate.

C-Ultratabs - Metagenics
Each tablet contains: Vitamin C (as mineral ascorbates) 1031 mg • Calcium (as calcium ascorbate) 65 mg • Magnesium (as magnesium ascorbate) 35 mg • Sodium (as sodium ascorbate) 30 mg • Potassium (as potassium ascorbate) 15 mg.

Culturelle with Lactobacillus GG - Klaire Laboratories
Each capsule contains: Lactobacillus GG 10 billion cells. Other Ingredients: Gelatin, Inulin (plant carbohydrate).

Curazyme - Enzymatic Therapy
Each capsule contains: Vitamin C (Ascorbic Acid) 50 mg • Pantothenic Acid (D-Calcium Pantothenate) 25 mg • Magnesium (Oxide) 25 mg • Curcuma root extract (Curcuma longa) standardized to contain 97% Curcumin 200 mg • Bromelain (2000 MCU) 200 mg • Butchers Broom extract (Ruscus aculeatus) standardized to contain 10% Saponins calculated as Ruscogenin 100 mg • Pancreatic Enzymes (10X) 50 mg • L-Cysteine 25 mg.
See Editor's Note No. 14.

Curb Your Cravings Plus patch - Curb Your Cravings LLC
Fucus Vesiculosus • Guarana • 5-HTP • Zinc Pyruvate • DHEA • Yerba Mate • Lecithin • Flaxseed oil • L-Carnitine • Zinc Citrate.

CurcuMax - PhytoPharmica
Each capsule contains: Bromelain (2000 MCU/g) 200 mg • Butcher's Broom root and rhizome extract (ruscus aculeatus, standardized to contain 9-11% saponins calculated as ruscogenins) 100 mg • L-Cysteine (as L-cysteine HCl) 25 mg • Magnesium (as magnesium oxide) 50 mg • Pancreatic Enzymes (10X) 25 mg • Turmeric rhizome extract (curcuma longa, standardized to contain 85-100% curcumin) 200 mg • Vitamin C (ascorbic acid) 50 mg.
See Editor's Note No. 14.

Curcumin - Physician Formulas
Each capsule contains: Curcumin (95% curcuminoids) 400 mg • Turmeric 100 mg.

Curcumin 95 - Jarrow Formulas
Each capsule contains: Curcumin (from turmeric root) 380 mg • Demethoxycurcumin 90 mg • Bisdemethoxycurcumin 15 mg • Other Turmeric substances 15 mg. Other Ingredients: Cellulose, Magnesium Stearate, Silicon Dioxide, Gelatin.

Curcumin 97 - Pure Encapsulations
Each vegetable capsule contains: Turmeric extract (curcuma longa, standardized to contain 97% cucuminoids) 250 mg.

Curcumin Extract 500 mg - Vital Nutrients
Each vegetarian capsule contains: Curcumin extract (curcuma longa, total curcuminoids minimum 90% by HPLC) 500 mg • Bioperine brand Black Pepper extract (95%) 2.5 mg.

Curcuminoids - America's Finest
Each capsule contains: Curcuminoids from Turmeric root extract (95%) 500 mg. Other Ingredients: Gelatin, Water, Mineral Oil, Magnesium Stearate.

Curves For Her - Athletic Technologies Inc.
Each tablet contains: Ma Huang 150 mg • Guarana 190 mg • Vitamin E 6 IU • Magnesium Chelate 75 mg • Zinc Chelate 5 mg • Chromium Picolinate 75 mcg • Gymnema Sylvestre 100 mg • Garcinia Cambogia 50 mg • Proprietary Blend: Bee Pollen, Ginseng root, Ginger root, Lecithin, Bovine complex, Damiana herb, Sarsaparilla, Golden Seal root, Nettle leaf, Gotu Kola, Spirulina, Royal Jelly.
See Editor's Note No. 30.

CV Forte - Pure Encapsulations
Each vegetable capsule contains: Hawthorn extract (crataegus oxycantha, standardized to contain 2% vitexins) 200 mg • Ginger extract (zingiber officinale, standardized to cotnain 5% gingerols) 100 mg • Motherwort 4:1 extract (leonurus cardiaca) 200 mg • Magnesium (citrate) 50 mg • Tuarine 100 mg • Vitamin C (as ascorbyl palmitate) 19 mg.

CV-10 (Cardiovascular Nutritional Support) - Rx Vitamins
Six capsules contain: L-Taurine 500 mg • L-Carnitine 500 mg • Magnesium (Taurate) 400 mg • Hawthorne berry 100 mg • Potassium (Citrate) 99 mg • CoQ10 30 mg • Vitamin B3 (Niacin) 25 mg • Vitamin B6 (Pyridoxine) 25 mg • Folic Acid 400 mcg • Vitamin E 200 IU.

CVS Echinacea - CVS Pharmacy
Three capsules contain: Echinacea 1140 mg. Other Ingredients: Echinacea Purpurea Herb powder, Gelatin, Maltodextrin, Cellulose, Calcium Carbonate, Magnesium Stearate, Silicon Dioxide, Dicalcium Phosphate, Microcrystalline Cellulose, Stearic Acid, Croscarmellose Sodium, Hydroxypropyl Methylcellulose, Hydroxypropyl Cellulose, Polyethylene Glycol.

CVS Saw Palmetto - CVS Pharmacy
Two capsules contain: Maltodextrin • Cellulose • Gelatin • Saw Palmetto extract • Calcium carbonate • Magnesium stearate • Silicon Dioxide.

CVS Saw Palmetto Softgels - CVS Pharmacy
Each softgel contains: Saw Palmetto extract (serenoa repens) fruit 160 mg. Other Ingredients: Olive Oil, Gelatin, Purified Water, Glycerin, FD&C Red #40, FD&C Yellow #6.

Cycla-Action - Nature's Plus
Each capsule contains: Blue Cohosh root 150 mg • Black Currant seed 125 mg • Mustard seed 75 mg • Red Raspberry leaves 75 mg • Cramp bark 75 mg • Squaw Vine 50 mg • False Unicorn 50 mg.

Cycl-A-Vites - Nature's Plus
Two tablets contain: whole Black Currant seeds naturally supplying GLA 300 mg • Magnesium amino acid chelate/complex 250 mg • Vitamin B6 (Pyridoxine HCL) 200 mg • Bromelain natural pineapple 150 mg • Calcium amino acid chelate/complex 125 mg • Iron amino acid chelate/complex 18 mg. In a natural base of Red Raspberry leaves, Strawberry Leaves, Dong Quai, Uva Ursi, & Peppermint. Yeast free. Sugar & starch free.

Cyclo 3 Fort - Unknown
Each capsule contains: Ruscus aculeatus root extract 150 mg • Trimethylhesperidin-chalcon 150 mg • Ascorbic acid 100 mg.

CycloDiol-4 (Sports One Cycloplex Pro-Hormone) - Sports One
Each lozenge contains: 4-Androstenediol Cycloplex (cyclodextrin complex) 25 mg.
See Editor's Note No. 54.

CycloDiol-5 (Sports One Cycloplex Pro-Hormone) - Sports One
Each lozenge contains: 5-Androstenediol Cycloplex (cyclodextrin complex) 25 mg.
See Editor's Note No. 54.

Some Brand Name Natural Products - What they Contain

www.NaturalDatabase.com contains MANY more listings than appear here.
Editor's Notes are located on pages 2155-2163.

BRAND NAMES

CycloDiol-XS (Sports One Cycloplex Pro-Hormone) - Sports One
Each lozenge contains: Nor-4-Androstenediol Cycloplex (cyclodextrin complex) 10 mg • 4-Androstenediol Cycloplex (cyclodextrin complex) 15 mg.
See Editor's Note No. 54.

Cyclovar - Warner Laboratories
Proprietary Blend 250 mg: L-Arginine, Cnidium Monnier extract, Xanthoparmelia extract, ZMA, Gamma Amino Butyric acid, Narigen, Quebracho extract, Microcrystalline Cellulose, Lactose Solutab, Magnesium Stearate.

Cynara-SL Artichoke - Lichtwer Pharma
Each capsule contains: Artichoke extract (Dried leaf extract) 320 mg. Other Ingredients: Gelatin, Magnesium Stearate, Silicon Dioxide, Talc, Titanium Dioxide, Sodium Lauryl Sulphate, FD&C Blue No. 1, FD&C Yellow No. 5.

Cyntol - Progressive Health Nutraceuticals
Iodine 250 mg • Zinc 10 mg • Acetyl L-Carnitine HCl 250 mg • Methylcobalamin 1 mg • Phosphatidylserine 10 mg • Choline 25 mg • Ginkgo Biloba 15 mg • Bacopa extract 5 mg • Korean Ginseng extract 20 mg • Vinpocetine 50 mcg • Huperzine A extract 50 mcg • Lecithin 50 mg.

Cyrofood - Standard Process, Inc.
Four tablets contain: Proprietary Blend 700 mg: Carrot root, Nutritional Yeast, Defatted Wheat germ, Date fruit, Oat flour, Bovine Bone, Bovine Adrenal, Peanut bran, Veal Bone meal, Bovine Spleen, Ovine Spleen, Bovine Kidney, Bovine Liver, Mushroom, Dried Alfalfa juice, Dried Pea vine juice, Soybean Lecithin, Rice bran, Ascorbic Acid, Pyridoxine Hydrochloride, Vitamin A Palmitate, Riboflavin, Cocarboxylase, Cholecalciferol • Calcium 20 mg • Potassium 10 mg. Other Ingredients: Honey, Calcium Lactate, Magnesium Citrate, Arabic gum, Glycerin.
See Editor's Note No. 14.

Cyrofood Powder - Standard Process, Inc.
Each 1 tbsp serving contains: Proprietary Blend 5.55 g: Defatted Wheat germ, Oat flour, Peanut bran, Date powder, Honey, Nutritional Yeast, Bovine Adrenal, Bovine Liver, Magnesium Citrate, Glycerin, Bovine Spleen, Ovine Spleen, Bovine Kidney, Pea (whole plant), Mushroom, Alfalfa powder, Lecithin, Arabic gum, Rice bran, Pyridoxine Hydrochloride, Cholecalciferol, Cocarboxylase, Riboflavin • Vitamin A 100 IU • Calcium 200 mg • Iron 1 mg. Other Ingredients: Bovine Bone meal, Veal Bone meal.
See Editor's Note No. 14.

Cyro-Yeast - Standard Process, Inc.
Each wafer contains: Proprietary Blend 1094 mg: Nutritional Yeast, Whey, Malt Syrup, Defatted Wheat germ, Carrot root, Bovine Liver, Bovine Adrenal, Bovine Kidney, Bovine Spleen, Ovine Spleen, Dried Alfalfa juice, Rice bran, Mushroom, Soybean Lecithin, Ascorbic Acid • Vitamin A 400 IU • Vitamin D 100 IU • Thiamine 0.1 mg • Riboflavin 0.1 mg • Vitamin B6 0.12 mg. Other Ingredients: Honey, Arabic gum, Calcium Stearate, Cocarboxylase.
See Editor's Note No. 14.

Cyruta - Standard Process, Inc.
Each tablet contains: Proprietary Blend 350 mg: Dried Buckwheat leaf juice, Buckwheat seed, Inositol, Bovine Adrenal Cytosol extract, Oat flour • Vitamin C 3 mg. Other Ingredients: Honey, Calcium Stearate.

Cyruta Plus - Standard Process, Inc.
Each tablet contains: Proprietary Blend 322 mg: Dried Buckwheat leaf juice, Buckwheat seed, Bovine Adrenal Cytosol extract, Oat flour • Vitamin C 3 mg • Potassium 10 mg. Other Ingredients: Honey, Calcium Stearate.

Cystistatin - Ortho Molecular Products
Each capsule contains: Uva Ursi leaf extract (standardized to contain 20% arbutin) 325 mg • Goldenseal root extract (standardized to contain 4.8% hydrastin) 250 mg • Berberine Sulfate 50 mg • Bromelain (2400 GDU/g) 50 mg • Marshmallow root 50 mg • Buchu leaf 4:1 extract 40 mg • Bladderwrack leaf 40 mg. Other Ingredients: Natural Vegetable Capsules, Magnesium Stearate, Microcrystalline Cellulose.

Cystone - The Himalaya Drug Company
Each tablet contains: Shilapuspha (didymocarpus pedicellata) 130 mg • Pasanabheda (saxifraga ligulata syn. bergenia ligulata/ciliata) 98 mg • Manjishtha (rubia cordifolia) 32 mg • Nagarmusta (cyperus scariosus) 32 mg • Apamarga (achyranthes aspera) 32 mg • Gojiha (onosma bracteatum) 32 mg • Sahadevi (vernonia cinerea) 32 mg • Shilajeet (mineral pitch, purified) 26 mg • Hajrul Yahood Bhasma (lime silicate calx) 32 mg.

Cytodrene - Weightlosscontrol
Each capsule contains: Proprietary Blend 700 mg: Sida cordifolia extract, Kola Nut extract, Green Tea extract, Yohimbe bark extract, White Willow bark, Chromium picolinate, Guggulsterones.
See Editor's Note No. 39.

Cytodyne - Cytodyne LLC
Six capsules contain: Acetyl L-Carnitine 1100 mg • Phosphatidylserine 175 mg • L-Alanine 200 mg • Alpha Ketoglutaric Acid 150 mg • L-Glutamine 2150 mg • Taurine 1050 mg • Ketoisocaporate 50 mg • Inositol 50 mg.

Cytomax - Champion Nutrition
Each 25 gram serving contains: Apple: Alpha-L-Polyactate • Energy 90 Kcal • Total Fat 0g • Sodium 100 mg • Potassium 120 mg • Total Carbohydrate 22 g • Sugars 10 g • Protein 0 g. Citrus: Energy 90 Kcal • Total Fat 0g • Sodium 100 mg • Potassium 120 mg • Total Carbohydrate 22 g • Sugars 10 g • Protein 0 g. Tangy-Orange: Energy 90 Kcal •Total Fat 0g • Sodium 100 mg • Potassium 120 mg • Total Carbohydrate 21 g • Sugars 11 g • Protein 0. Tropical: Energy 90 Kcal • Total Fat 0g • Sodium 100 mg • Potassium 100 mg • Total Carbohydrate 22 g • Sugars 11 g • Protein 0. Ingredients: Fructose • Alpha-L-Polyactate: our non-acidic patented L-Lactate formula combined with Sodium L-Lactate & Potassium L-Lactate •Metacarb (Champion Nutrition's original complex carbohydrate blend including Amylopectin Starches & Maltodextrins from Corn Hybrids) • Glucose • Citric Acid •Succinate ETF Our Exclusive Succinate Compound containing: Potassium Succinate, L-Glutamic Acid, Inosine, Magnesium Succinate, Calcium Succinate • Natural Flavoring • Malic Acid • L-Alanine • L-Glutamine • Ascorbic Acid • Natural Caramel Coloring • Potassium Citrate • Xanthan Gum • Sunett (Acesulfame-K) • Chromium Polynicotinate (Chromemate - GTF).

CytoPro - Cytodyne LLC
Each rounded scoop contains: Cross Flow Micro/Ultra Filtered 100% pure Whey Protein Isolate (beta lactoglobulin 19,100 MW/50% alpha lactoalbumin 14,700 MW/20%, glycomacropeptides 16,200 MW/20%, glutamine peptides 6700 MW/5%, immunoglobulin 95,000 MW/3%, bovine serum albumin 65,000 MW/2%, protease peptone). CytoPro WPI (typical amino acid profile) 23.976 mg: L-Alanine 1071 mg, L-Arginine 538 mg, L-Aspartic Acid 2303 mg, L-Cysteine 276 mg, L-Glutamic Acid 3870 mg, L-Glutamine 548 mg, L-Glycine 522 mg, L-Histidine 393 mg, L-Isoleucine 1433 mg, L-Leucine 2341 mg, L-Lysine 1999 mg, L-Methionine 409 mg, L-Phenylalanine 768 mg, L-Proline 1553 mg, L-Serine 1184 mg, L-Taurine 1000 mg, L-Threonine 1409 mg, L-Tryptophan 464 mg, L-Tyrosine 567 mg, L-Valine 1328 mg.

CytoVol - EAS, Inc.
Each 15 gram serving contains: L-Glutamine 2500 mg • Taurine 2000 mg • Manganese 50 mcg • Calcium AKG 1500 mg • Inositol 500 mg • Glycine 500 mg • RNA 250 mg • L-Alanine 2000 mg. Ingredients: Dextrose • L-Glutamine • Taurine • L-Alanine • Calcium

Alpha-Ketoglutarate (AKG) • Citric Acid • Natural Flavors • Inositol • Glycine • Sodium Ribonucleic Acid (RNA) • Sodium Phosphate • Turmeric mixed with Maltodextrin for color • Aspartame • Manganese Glycinate. Contains Phenylalanine.

Cytozyme-AD - Biotics Research Corporation
Each tablet contains: Neonatal Adrenal complex (bovine) 80 mg • Superoxide Dismutase (from vegetable culture) 20 mcg • Catalase (from vegetable culture) 20 mcg.
See Editor's Note No. 14.

D.A. #34 - J. R. Carlson Laboratories, Inc.
Each tablet contains: Ox Bile 30 mg • Pancreatin concentrate 330 mg.

D-400 IU - Rexall - Sundown
Each softgel contains: Vitamin A (from fish liver oil) 700 IU • Vitamin D (from fish liver oil) 400 IU. Other Ingredients: Soybean Oil, Gelatin, Glycerin, Water.

Daily 3 Complete - The Vitamin Shoppe
Each tablet contains: Vitamin D 400 IU • Vitamin A Activity 25000 IU • Vitamin C 500 mg • Vitamin E 400 IU • Vitamin B1 50 mg • Vitamin B2 50 mg • Vitamin B6 50 mg • Vitamin B12 500 mcg • Niacinamide 50 mg • PABA 50 mg • Pantothenic Acid 50 mg • Choline Bitartrate 50 mg • Inositol 50 mg • Biotin 50 mcg • Folic Acid 800 mcg • Vitamin K 30 mcg • Selenium 50 mcg • Green Tea extract 50 mg • CoQ10 100 mcg • L-Glutathione 10 mg • Pycnogenol 100 mcg • N-Acetyl Cysteine 15 mg • Molybdenum 50 mcg • Calcium 100 mg • Magnesium 50 mg • Potassium 50 mg • Zinc 15 mg • Iodine 150 mcg • Iron 10 mg • Manganese 5 mg • Chromium 100 mcg • Boron 3 mg • Apple pectin 50 mg • Papain 25 mg • Lipase 10 mcg • Probiotics 10 mg • Betaine HCl 25 mg • Pepsin 25 mg • Protease 10 mcg • Glutamic Acid 25 mg • Amylase 10 mcg • Chlorophyll 10 mg • Spirulina 45 mg • Bee Pollen 45 mg • Echinacea / Golden Seal 50 mg • Shiitake / Reishi mushrooms 45 mg • Barley grass 45 mg • Royal Jelly 15 mg • Alfalfa concentrate 45 mg • Siberian Ginseng 45 mg • Chlorella 45 mg • RNA/DNA 45 mg. A concentrated blend of: broccoli, tomato, garlic, onions, cauliflower, brussel sprouts, carrots, parsley, watercress. Pure dry, cold-pressed borage, flaxseed, safflower oils providing the essential fatty acids, Omega 3-6-9.

Daily 3 with Antioxidant Factors - Puritan's Pride
Three capsules contain: Vitamin A (as Beta-Carotene) 25,000 IU • Vitamin C (as Calcium Ascorbate) 500 mg • Vitamin D (as Cholecalcifeol) 400 IU • Vitamin E (as d-Alpha Tocopherol Succinate) 400 IU • Vitamin K (as Phytonadione) 30 mcg • Thiamin (Vitamin B-1; as Thiamine Hydrochloride) 50 mg • Riboflavin (Vitamin B-2) 50 mg • Niacin (as Niacinamide) 50 mg • Vitamin B-6 (as Pyridoxine Hydrochloride) 50 mg • Folic Acid 800 mcg • Vitamin B-12 (as Coenzyme B-12) 500 mcg • Biotin 50 mcg • Pantothenic Acid (as d-Calcium Pantothenate) 50 mg • Calcium (as Calcium Carbonate) 100 mg • Iron (as Carbonyl Iron) 10 mg • Iodine (as Kelp) 150 mcg • Magnesium (as Magnesium Oxide) 50 mg • Zinc (as Zinc Picolinate) 15 mg • Selenium (as Selenomethionate) 50 mcg • Manganese (as Manganese Carbonate) 5 mg • Chromium (as GTF Chromium Yeast) 100 mcg • Potassium (as Potassium Chloride) 50 mg • Green Tea (Camellia sinensis) leaf 50 mg • N-Acetyl Cysteine 15 mg • L-Glutathione 10 mg • Coenzyme Q10 100 mcg • Pine bark extract (Pycnogenol) 100 mcg • Choline Bitartrate 50 mg • Inositol 50 mg • PABA (Para-Aminobenzoic Acid) 50 mg • Boron (as Boron Citrate) 3 mg • Spirulina (Spirulina plantensis) plant 20 mg • Chinese Chlorella (Chlorella pyrenoidosa) 20 mg • Barley Grass (plant) 20 mg • Alfalfa juice concentrate 20 mg • Octacosanol 100 mcg • Siberian Ginseng (Eleutherococcus senticosus) root 20 mg • Bee Pollen 20 mg • Citrus Bioflavonoids 20 mg • Rutin 20 mg • Echinacea / Goldenseal (Echinacea purpurea / Hydrastis canadensis) root 20 mg • Royal Jelly 15 mg • Reishi Mushroom (Ganoderma lucidum) aerial 15 mg • Shiitake Mushroom (Lentinus edodes) aerial 15 mg • Shark Cartilage 45 mg • Apple Pectin 20 mg • Betaine Hydrochloride 20 mg • L-Glutamic Acid 20 mg • Papain (Papaya) 20 mg • Pepsin Enzyme 20 mg • Lipase 10 mg • Amylase 10 mg • Chlorophyll (as Sodium Copper Chlorophyllin) 10 mg • Proprietary Blend: Broccoli, Tomato, Orange, Lemon, Blueberry, Cranberry, Garlic, Onion, Cauliflower, and Brussels Sprout Concentrates 20 mg.

Daily Antioxidant Packs - Puritan's Pride
Each pack (2 softgels, 3 tablets) contains: Beta Carotene 25,000 IU • Multi-Vitamin: Providing Vitamin A (as beta carotene), Vitamin D, and B-Complex Vitamins • Vitamin E 400 IU • Vitamin C with Rose Hips 500 mg • Multi-Mineral: A full accompaniment of major and trace minerals including Chromium, Calcium, Zinc, and the antioxidant Selenium.

Daily Balance Energy Vitalizer - Doctor's Preferred, Inc.
Each four capsules contains: L-Carnitine 200 mg • L-Tyrosine 500 mg • Coenzyme Q10 30 mg • Ginkgo Biloba 80 mg • Chromium Picolinate 100 mg • Sodium Bicarbonate 350 mg • Vitamin C 500 mg • Vitamin B 120 mg • Vitamin B2 25 mg • Vitamin B3 40 mg • Vitamin B5 250 mg • Vitamin B6 25 mg • Folic Acid 200 mcg • Vitamin B12 25 mg • Biotin 200 mcg • Choline 25 mg • Inositol 25 mg • PABA 25 mg • Calcium 100 mg • Magnesium 200 mg • Iodine 25 mcg • Zinc 7.5 mg • Selenium 70 mcg • Potassium 50 mg.

Daily Balance Hot Flash - Doctor's Preferred, Inc.
Each softgel contains: Vitamin E (as d-alpha tocopheryl) 200 mg • Soy Germ extract (providing 10% soy isoflavones 25 mg) 250 mg • Gamma Oryzan (from rice bran oil) 150 mg • Black Cohosh extract (providing 2.5% triterpine glycosides) 2 mg.

Daily Balance Iron - Doctor's Preferred, Inc.
Each capsule contains: Vitamin C (as ascorbic acid) 30 mg • Iron (as bisglynate) 25 mg.

Daily Balance Menorrhagia - Doctor's Preferred, Inc.
Each two capsules contain: Vitamin C (as ascorbic acid magnesium and calcium ascorbates) 350 mg • Vitamin E (as d-alpha tocopheryl succinate) 100 mg • Calcium (as ascorbate) 3 mg • Bromelain (from pineapples) 250 mg • Lemon Bioflavonoid complex 175 mg • Rutin (from buckwheat) 150 mg • Chaste Tree extract (from berry, providing 0.3% casticin 0.34 mg and 0.15% agnuside 0.17 mg) 112.5 mg • Chaste Tree powder (from berry) 25 mg • Quercetin (as dihydrate) 25 mg.

Daily Balance PMS - Doctor's Preferred, Inc.
Each two softgels contains: Vitamin E (as d-alpha tocopheryl) 100 mg • Calcium (as carbonate) 200 mg • Magnesium (as oxide, ascorbate) 112.5 mg • Chaste Tree extract (from berry, providing 0.3% casticin 0.34 mg and 0.15% agnuside 0.17 mg) 112.5 mg • GLA (from borage oil) 75 mg • Cramp Bark 30 mg • Grapeseed extract 25 mg.

Daily Balance Women's Multinutrient - Doctor's Preferred, Inc.
Each packet contains: Multinutrient (6 capsules): Vitamin A (as palmitate) 1000 IU • Vitamin C (as ascorbic crystals, mineral ascorbates) 600 mg • Vitamin D3 (as cholecalciferol) 400 IU • Vitamin K (as phytonadione) 30 mcg • Thiamine (as mononitrate) 40 mg • Riboflavin (vitamin B2) 40 mg • Niacin (as niacinamide, niacin) 50 mg • Vitamin B6 (as pyridoxine HCl) 100 mg • Folic Acid 400 mcg • Vitamin B12 (as cyanocabalamin) 100 mcg • Biotin 300 mcg • Pantothenic Acid (as calcium pantothenate) 150 mg • Calcium (as carbonate, malate, citrate, ascorbate) 700 mg • Magnesium (as oxide, ascorbate) 350 mg • Zinc (as chelate) 15 mg • Selenium (as methionine) 200 mcg • Copper (as gluconate) 2 mg • Manganese (as ascorbate) 5 mg • Chromium (as chelate) 200 mcg • Molybdenum (as ascorbate) 100 mcg • Potassium (as citrate) 100 mg • Lemon Bioflavonoid Complex 500 mg • Rutin (from buckwheat) 200 mg • Choline (as bitartrate) 50 mg • Para-Aminobenzoic Acid (PABA) 25 mg • Boron (from chelate) 2 mg • Inositol 25 mg. Essential Fatty Acids (2 softgels): Docosahexaenoic Acid (DHA) 300 mg • Eicosapentaenoic Acid (EPA) 200 mg • Other Omega-3 Fatty Acids 100 mg • Gamma-linolenic Acid (as borage oil) 50 mg • Proprietary Antioxidant B (ascorbyl palmitate, rosemary leaf extract, mixed tocopheryls) 6 mg. Antioxidant (2 softgels): Vitamin A (as

beta-carotene) 10,000 IU • Vitamin C (as ascorbyl palmitate) 26 mg • Vitamin E (as d-alpha-tocopheryl acetate) 600 IU • Alpha Lipoic Acid 30 mg • Mixed Tocopherols 10 mg • Tocotrienols (from rice bran oil) 10 mg • Lycopene (from tomatoes) 5 mg • Lutein (from marigold extract) 4 mg.

Daily Basics Original **-** Rexall - Sundown
Each packet contains: Vitamin A (100% as Beta-Carotene) 1,000 IU • Vitamin C (Ascorbic Acid) 60 mg • Vitamin E (dl-Alpha Tocopheryl Acetate) 30 IU • Niacin (Niacinamide) 36 mg • Vitamin B12 (Cyanocobalamin) 10.8 mcg • Selenium Chelate (Sodium Selenite) 4 mcg • Calcium Carbonate 100 mg • Thiamin HCl 2.7 mg •Vitamin B6 (Pyridoxine HCl) 3.6 mg • Biotin 29 mcg • Chromium Polynicotinate (ChromeMate) 52 mcg • Riboflavin 3 mg • Folate (Folic Acid) 120 mcg • Zinc Gluconate 0.9 mg. Other Ingredients: Guar Gum, Locust Bean Gum, Pectins, Oat Fiber, Maltodextrin, Gum Arabic, Natural and Artifical Orange Flavor, Aspartame, Artifical Vanilla Flavor.

Daily Detox **-** M.D. Labs
Sarsaparilla • Milk Thistle • Red Clover • Dandelion • Yellow Dock • Burdock • Hibiscus • Echinacea • Fenugreek • Ginger • Cascara Sagrada. Other Ingredients: All Natural Fruit & Spice extracts.

Daily Enzyme Complex **-** Futurebiotics LLC
Pancreas* 235 mg • Ox bile 35 mg • Duodenum 20 mg • Papaya enzyme 125 mg • Betaine 20 mg • Liver 20 mg • Vitamin B1 (thiamin) 3 mg • Bromelain 50 mg • Niacinamide 10 mg • Vitamin B2 (riboflavin) 3 mg • Peppermint 25 mg • Anise 25 mg • Chamomile 25 mg. *Whole dried pancreas, a source of Pancreatin, Trypsin, Amylase, Lipase, Lisotozyme, Diatase & Chymosin.
See Editor's Note No. 14.

Daily Essentials **-** Aspen Group, Inc.
Each three tablets contain: Vitamin E (d-alpha) 200 IU • Vitamin A 5000 IU • Beta Carotene 5000 IU • Vitamin D 400 IU • Vitamin C 400 mg • Folic Acid 400 mcg • Thiamine 1.5 mg • Riboflavin 1.7 mg • Niacin 20 mg • Vitamin B6 2 mg • Vitamin B12 6 mcg • Biotin 300 mcg • Pantothenic Acid 10 mg • Calcium (citrate) 600 mg • Phosphorus 450 mg • Iodine (kelp) 150 mcg • Magnesium (carbonate) 200 mg • Copper (gluconate) 2 mg • Zinc (gluconate) 15 mg • Vitamin K 100 mcg • Selenium (yeast) 75 mcg • Manganese (gluconate) 5 mg • Chromium (aspartate) 200 mcg • Molybdenum 150 mcg • Nickel 15 mcg • Tin 15 mcg • Vanadium 5 mg • Boron (citrate) 2 mg • Potassium (gluconate) 100 mg • Grape seed extract 10 mg • Co Q10 10 mg.

Daily Essentials **-** Aspen Group, Inc.
Three tablets contain: Vitamin E (d-alpha) 200 IU • Vitamin A 5000 IU • Beta Carotene 5000 IU • Vitamin D 400 IU • Vitamin C 400 mg • Folic Acid 400 mcg • Thiamine 1.5 mg • Riboflavin 1.7 mg • Niacin 20 mg • Vitamin B6 2 mg • Vitamin B12 6 mcg • Biotin 300 mcg • Pantothenic Acid 10 mg • Calcium (citrate) 600 mg • Phosphorus 450 mg • Iodine (kelp) 150 mcg • Magnesium (carbonate) 200 mg • Copper (gluconate) 2 mg • Zinc (gluconate) 15 mg • Vitamin K 100 mcg • Selenium (yeast) 75 mcg • Manganese (gluconate) 5 mg • Chromium (aspartate) 200 mcg • Molybdenum 150 mcg • Nickel 15 mcg • Tin 15 mcg • Vanadium 5 mg • Boron (citrate) 2 mg • Potassium (gluconate) 100 mg • Grape seed extract 10 mg • CoQ10 10 mg.

Daily Essentials for Men **-** Health Smart Vitamins
Two caplets contain: Vitamin A (as 83% beta-carotene, 17% palmitate) 15,000 IU • Vitamin C (ascorbic acid) 250 mg • Vitamin D (as cholecalciferol) 400 IU • Vitamin E (as d-alpha tocopheryl) 200 IU • Vitamin K (as phytonadione) 25 mcg • Thiamin (as thiamin mononitrate) 25 mg • Riboflavin 25 mg • Niacin (as 50% nicotinic acid, 50% niacinamide) 50 mg • Vitamin B6 (as pyridoxine HCl) 25 mg • Folate (folic acid) 400 mcg • Vitamin B12 (as cyanocobalamin) 50 mcg • Biotin 300 mcg • Pantothenic acid (as calcium pantothenate) 25 mg • Calcium (as 87% calcium carbonate, 13% mixed calcium complexes) 258 mg • Iron (as iron sulfate) 6 mg • Iodine (as potassium iodide) 150 mcg • Magnesium (as 80% magnesium oxide, 10% magnesium citrate, 10% mangesium glycinate) 125 mg • Zinc (as zinc ascorbate) 30 mg • Selenium (as selenomethionine) 75 mcg • Copper (as copper citrate) 3 mg • Manganese (as manganese gluconate) 2 mg • Chromium (as chromium polynicotinate) 100 mcg • Molybdenum (as molybdenum amino acid chelate) 50 mcg • Oriental Ginseng root (Panax ginseng) 75 mg • Pumpkin seed 75 mg • Saw Palmetto berry 75 mg • Betaine HCl 25 mg • Citrus bioflavonoids 25 mg • Choline (as bitartrate) 25 mg • Insitol 25 mg • Lecithin (from soybean) 25 mg • Bromelain (from pineapple 6,000 PU/g, 120 PU) 20 mg • Lipase (from fermentation of Aspergillus niger) 10 mg • Papain (from latex of fruit) 10 mg • Para-aminobenzoic acid (PABA) 10 mg • Boron (as boron aspartate) 2 mg • Silicon (as silicon dioxide) 2 mg • Vanadium (as vanadium amino acid chelate) 10 mcg.

Daily Essentials for Women **-** Health Smart Vitamins
Two caplets contain: Vitamin A (as 83% beta-carotene, 17% palmitate) 15000 IU • Vitamin C (ascorbic acid) 250 mg • Vitamin D (as cholecalciferol) 400 IU • Vitamin E (as d-alpha-tocopherol) 200 IU • Vitamin K (as phytonadione) 25 mcg • Thiamin (as thiamin mononitrate) 25 mg • Riboflavin 25 mg • Niacin 50 mg • Vitamin B-6 (as pyridoxine HCl) 25 mg • Folate (folic acid) 400 mcg • Vitamin B-12 (cyanocobalamin) 100 mcg • Biotin 300 mcg • Pantothenic Acid (as calcium pantothenate) 25 mg • Calcium 507 mg • Iron (as iron glycinate) 18 mg • Magnesium 200 mg • Iodine (as potassium iodide) 150 mcg • Zinc (as zinc ascorbate) 15 mg • Selenium (as selenomethionine) 75 mcg • Copper (as copper citrate) 2 mg • Manganese (as manganese gluconate) 2 mg • Chromium (as chromium polynicotinate) 100 mcg • Molybdenum 50 mcg • Dong Quai root 50 mg • Royal Jelly from bees 50 mg • Betaine HCl 25 mg • Bioflavonoids (from citrus) 25 mg • Choline (as choline bitartrate) 25 mg • Inositol 25 mg • Lecithin (from soybean) 25 mg • Bromelain 20 mg • Lipase 10 mg • Papain 10 mg • PABA (Para-Amino Benzoic Acid) 10 mg • Rutin 5 mg • Boron (as boron aspartate) 2 mg • Silicon (as silicon dioxide) 2 mg • Vanadium 10 mcg.

Daily Heart Basics **-** Waiora
Each sotfgel contains: Vitamin E (as D-alpha tocopherol) 1 IU • Fish Oil (containing omega-3 fatty acids: EPA [eicosapentaenoic acid] 180 mg, DHA [docosahexaenoic acid] 120 mg). Other Ingredients: Gelatin, Glycerin, Purified Water.

Daily Heart Essentials **-** Waiora
Two tablets contain: Vitamin C (as Beyond C brand ascorbic acid, ascorbyl palmitate, sodium ascorbate) 500 mg • Vitamin E (as a mix of tocopherols) 500 IU • Vitamin B6 (as pyridoxine hydrochloride) 10 mg • Folate (as folic acid) 400 mcg • Vitamin B12 (as cyanocobalamin) 100 mcg • Magnesium (as magnesium oxide) 200 mg • Selenium (as selenomethionine) 200 mcg • L-Arginine 500 mg • Taurine 350 mg • L-Proline 250 mg • Hawthorne berry fruit 160 mg • Alpha Lipoic Acid 100 mg • Coenzyme Q10 (CoQ10) 30 mg. Other Ingredients: Microcrystalline Cellulose, Croscarmellose Sodium, Stearic Acid, Silicon Dioxide, Magnesium Stearate.

Daily Multi Essentials **-** Nature's Own
Each tablet contains: Beta Carotene 1.5 mg • Vitamin B1 (thiamine nitrate) 15 mg • Vitamin B2 (riboflavin) 15 mg • Vitamin B3 (nicotinamide) 15 mg • Vitamin B5 (calcium pantothenate) 20 mg • Vitamin B6 (pyridoxine hydrochloride) 25 mg • Vitamin B12 (cyanocobalamin) 25 mcg • Folic Acid 250 mcg • Vitamin C (ascorbic acid) 100 mg • Citrus Bioflavonoid extract 25 mg • Vitamin D (cholecalciferol 5 mcg) 200 IU • Vitamin E (D-alpha-tocopherol 33.6 mg) 50 IU • Calcium Carbonate 300 mg: Elemental Calcium 120 mg • Magnesium Oxide 99.6 mg: Elemental Magnesium 60 mg • Ferrous Fumarate 15.7 mg: Elemental Iron 5 mg • Zinc Oxide 6.2 mg: Elemental Zinc 5 mg • Kelp powder (fucus vesiculosus) 3.3 mg • Iodine 10 mcg • Winter Cherry root extract (withania somnifera) 200 mg.

Daily Multi Peak Performance **-** Nature's Own
Each tablet contains: Vitamin A 2500 IU • Vitamin B1 (thiamine nitrate) 35 mg • Vitamin B2 (riboflavin) 35 mg • Vitamin B3 (nicotinamide) 50 mg • Vitamin B5 (calcium pantothenate) 35 mg • Vitamin B6 (pyridoxine hydrochloride) 40 mg • Vitamin B12 (cyanocobalamin) 50 mcg • Vitamin C (from calcium ascorbate dihydrate 303 mg) 250 mg • Vitamin E (D-alpha-tocopheryl acid succinate 61.9 mg) 75 IU • Vitamin K (K1, as phytomenadione) 5 mcg • Vitamin D (D3, as cholecalciferol 5 mcg) 200 IU • Folic Acid 95 mcg • Citrus Bioflavonoid extract 50 mg • Hesperidin 20 mg • Rutin 25 mg • Biotin 50 mcg • Choline Bitartrate 30 mg • Inositol 30 mg • Boron (from boric acid) 1.5 mg • Calcium (from calcium hydrogen phosphate) 46.6 mg • Chromium (from chromium picolinate) 50 mcg • Copper (from cupric sulfate anhydrous) 200 mcg • Iodine (from potassium iodide) 50 mcg • Iron (from ferrous fumarate) 5 mg • Magnesium (from magnesium oxide) 10 mg • Manganese (from manganese sulfate monohydrate) 10 mg • Selenium (from selenomethionine) 26 mcg • Zinc (from zinc sulfate monohydrate) 7.5 mg • L-Lysine 50 mg • L-Tyrosine 50 mg • L-Glutamine 50 mg • Lutein (from tagetes erecta standardized extract, equivalent to dry flower 12.5 mg) 125 mcg.

Daily Multi-Vitamin & Mineral **-** Swanson Health Products
Each capsule contains: Vitamin A (from fish liver oil) 10000 IU • Vitamin C (Ester-C®, as calcium ascorbate) 200 mg • Vitamin D (from fish liver oil) 400 IU • Vitamin E (as d-alpha tocopheryl succinate) 15 IU • Thiamin (as thiamin mononitrate; vitamin B-1) 10 mg • Riboflavin USP (vitamin B-2) 10 mg • Niacinamide 100 mg • Vitamin B-6 (as pyridoxine HCl) 5 mg • Folic Acid 400 mcg • Vitamin B-12 (as cyanocobalamin) 5 mcg • Pantothenic Acid (as d-calcium pantothenate) 20 mg • Calcium (from bone meal and dolomite) 125 mg • Iron (from ferrous sulfate) 12 mg • Iodine (from kelp) 150 mcg • Magnesium (from magnesium oxide) 32.5 mg • Zinc (from zinc sulfate) 15 mg • Copper (from copper sulfate) 2 mg • Manganese (from manganese sulfate) 1 mg.

Daily Nutrition Pack **-** All Terrain Company
Each packet contains: Vitamin A (as acetate and 34% beta carotene) 4950 IU • Vitamin C (as ascorbic acid) 500 mg • Vitamin D 340 IU • Vitamin E (as D-alpha tocopherol) 300 IU • Thiamin (as thiamin HCl) 38 mg • Riboflavin 38 mg • Niacin (as niacinamide) 41 mg • Vitamin B6 (as pyridoxine HCl) 36 mg • Folic Acid 200 mcg • Vitamin B12 (as cyanocobalamin) 3 mcg • Biotin 150 mcg • Pantothenic Acid (as calcium aantothenate) 38 mg • Calcium (as calcium phosphate, citrate) 100 mg • Iodine (from kelp) 100 mcg • Magnesium (as magnesium citrate) 51 mg • Zinc (as zinc picolinate) 7.5 mg • Selenium (from selenium yeast) 25 mcg • Copper (as copper picolinate) 3 mg • Manganese (as maganese sulfate) 15 mg • Chromium (as chromium picolinate) 3.6 mcg • Potassium (as potassium citrate) 99 mg • Choline (as choline bitartrate) 200 mg • Inositol (as inositol monophosphate) 200 mg • Para Aminobenzoic Acid (PABA) 200 mg. Other Ingredients: Whey Protein, Magnesium Stearate, Stearic Acid, Trace Mineral Complex (Ruthenium, Tantalum, Hafnuim, Berylium, Thallium, Rhenium, Iridium, Bromine, Tin, Gallium, Antimony, Tellerium, Platinum, Holmium, Bismuth, Thorium, Rhodium, Lanthanum, Cadmium, Palladium, Uranium, Barium, Terbium, Terbium, Sulfur, Boron, Thulium, Rubidium, Lithium, Titanium, Samarium, Chlorine, Scandium, Silver, Nickel, Fluorine, Zirconium, Praseodymium, Cerium, Tungsten, Molybdenum, Dysprosium, Ytterbium, Sodium, Niobium, Gadolinium, Luteium, Cesium, Silicon, Neodymium, Erbium, Yttrium, Strontium, Osmium).

Daily One Caps With Iron **-** TwinLab
Each capsule contains: Beta-Carotene (pro-vitamin A) 4000 IU • Vitamin A 6000 IU • Vitamin D (from natural form vitamin D3) 400 IU • Vitamin C 150 mg • Natural Vitamin E (succiante) 100 IU • Vitamin B1 (thiamine) 25 mg • Vitamin B2 (riboflavin) 25 mg • Vitamin B6 (pyridoxine) 25 mg • Vitamin B12 (cobalamin concentrate) 100 mcg • Niacinamide 100 mg • Pantothenic Acid 50 mg • Biotin 300 mcg • Folic Acid 400 mcg • Flora Glo brand Lutein 500 mcg • Choline 25 mg • Inositol 25 mg • Calcium (from calcium citrate & calcium carbonate) 25 mg • Magnesium (from magnesium aspartate & magnesium oxide) 7.2 mg • Zinc (from zinc picolinate) 15 mg • Copper (from copper gluconate) 2 mg • Iron (from ferronyl carbonyl) 10 mg • Manganese (from manganese gluconate) 5 mg • Iodine (from potassium iodide) 150 mcg • Selenium (from selenomethionine & selenate-50/50 mixture) 200 mcg • Chromium (GTF) 200 mcg • Molybdenum (natural molybdate) 150 mcg.

Daily One Without Iron **-** TwinLab
Each capsule contains: Beta-Carotene (pro-vitamin A) 4000 IU • Vitamin A 6000 IU • Vitamin D (from natural form vitamin D3) 400 IU • Vitamin C 150 mg • Natural Vitamin E (succinate) 100 IU • Vitamin B1 (thiamine) 25 mg • Vitamin B2 (riboflavin) 25 mg • Vitamin B6 (pyridoxine) 25 mg • Vitamin B12 (cobalamin concentrate) 100 mcg • Niacinamide 100 mg • Pantothenic Acid 50 mg • Biotin 300 mcg • Folic Acid 400 mcg • Flora Glo brand Lutein 500 mcg • Choline 25 mg • Inositol 25 mg • Calcium (from calcium citrate & calcium carbonate) 25 mg • Magnesium (from magnesium aspartate & magnesium oxide) 7.2 mg • Zinc (from zinc picolinate) 15 mg • Copper (from copper gluconate) 2 mg • Manganese (from manganese gluconate) 5 mg • Iodine (from potassium iodide) 150 mcg • Selenium (from selenomethionine & selenate-50/50 mixture) 200 mcg • Chromium (GTF) 200 mcg • Molybdenum (natural molybdate) 150 mcg.

Daily Rx Multi-Vitamin **-** Athletic Technologies Inc.
Each capsule contains: Vitamin A 10,000 IU • Vitamin C 150 mg • Vitamin D 200 IU • Vitamin E 150 IU • Vitamin B1 25 mg • Vitamin B2 25 mg • Niacin 25 mg • Vitamin B6 25 mg • Folic Acid 25 mcg • Biotin 25 mcg • Pantothenic Acid 25 mg • Calcium 25 mg • Iron 7.5 mg • Iodine 75 mcg • Magnesium 5 mg • Zinc 7.5 mg • Selenium 12.5 mcg • Copper 1 mg • Manganese 5 mg • Chromium 1.5 mcg • Potassium 15 mg • Boron 500 mcg • Rutin 5 mg • Citrus Bioflavonoids 15 mg • Royal Jelly 2.5 mg • Garlic oil 68 mg • Choline 25 mg • Inositol 25 mg • PABA 25 mg • Lecithin 40 mg • Octacosanol 5 mcg • RNA 1 mg • DNA 1 mg • CoQ10 50 mcg.

Daily Therapy 7-Vitamin Foaming Cleansing Gel **-** Orjene
Mistletoe extract • Ginseng extract • Purified Water • Sodium Laureth Sulfate • Chamomile extract • Sea Algae Polypeptides • Methyl Gluceth-20 • Panthenol (vitamin B5) • Tocopheryl Acetate (vitamin E) • Retinyl Palmitate (vitamin A) • Ascorbyl Palmitate (vitamin C) • Bisabolol • Cholecalciferol (vitamin D) • Vitamin F (essential fatty acid) • Biotin (vitamin H) • Polyquaternium-10 • Butylene Glycol • Triethanolamine • Carbomer • Chamomile Essential oil • Geranium Essential oil • Methylparaben • Propylparaben.

Daily Vita Plus **-** Global Health Trax
Each tablespoon (0.5 fl oz) contains: Vitamin A (as palmitate, natural carotenese) 5000 IU • Vitamin C (as ascorbic acid) 300 mg • Vitamin D (as cholecalciferol) 400 IU • Vitamin E (as d-alpha tocopherol) 60 IU • Vitamin K (K1, as phyto-menadione) 300 mcg • Thiamin (as thiamine HCl) 3 mg • Riboflavin (as riboflavin) 3.4 mg • Niacin (as niacinamide, niacin) 35 mg • Vitamin B6 (as pyridoxine HCl) 4 mg • Folic Acid 400 mcg • Vitamin B12 (as cyanocobalamin) 6 mcg • Biotin 300 mcg • Pantothenic Acid (as D-calcium pantothenate) 20 mg • Gluconodeltalactone 1 g • Choline Bitartrate 50 mg • Inositol 50 mg • Glucosamine Sulfate 30 mg • Essential Fatty Acid Complex 25 mg • Amino Acid Complex 25 mg • CMO (as cetyl myristoleate, cetyl oleate) 25 mg • Methylsulfonylmethane (MSM) 20 mg • PABA 20 mg • Coenzyme Q10 10 mg • Aloe Vera powder 10 mg. Other Ingredients: Purified Water, Glycerin, Citric Acid, Malic Acid, Pepper Extract (piper nigris), Natural Flavorings, Potassium Sorbate, Sodium Benzoate, Stevia.

Daily Vita Plus, Vegetarian **-** Global Health Trax
Each tablespoon (0.5 fl oz) contains: Vitamin A (as palmitate, natural carotenese) 5000 IU • Vitamin C (as ascorbic acid) 300 mg • Vitamin D (as cholecalciferol) 400 IU • Vitamin E (as d-alpha tocopherol) 60 IU • Thiamin (as thiamine HCl) 3 mg • Riboflavin (as riboflavin) 3.4 mg • Niacin (as niacinamide, niacin) 35 mg • Vitamin B6 (as

pyridoxine HCl) 4 mg • Folic Acid 400 mcg • Vitamin B12 (as cyanocobalamin) 6 mcg • Biotin 300 mcg • Pantothenic Acid (as D-calcium pantothenate) 20 mg • Gluconodeltalactone 1 g • Choline Bitartrate 50 mg • Inositol 50 mg • Astragalus (as astragalus membranaceus) 30 mg • Boswellin (as boswellia serrata) 30 mg • Milk Thistle (as silybum marianum) 30 mg • Essential Fatty Acid Complex 25 mg • Amino Acid Complex 25 mg • Methylsulfonylmethane (MSM) 20 mg • PABA 20 mg • Coenzyme Q10 10 mg • Aloe Vera powder 10 mg. Other Ingredients: Purified Water, Glycerin, Citric Acid, Malic Acid, Pepper Extract (piper nigris), Natural Flavorings, Potassium Sorbate, Sodium Benzoate, Stevia.

Daily Vits One-A-Day Multiple **-** NOW Foods
Each tablet contains: Vitamin A (100% as Beta Carotene) 5000 IU • Vitamin B1 (Thiamine HCL) 1.5 mg • Vitamin B2 (Riboflavin) 1.7 mg • Vitamin B3 (Niacinamide) 20 mg • Vitamin B5 (Pantothenic Acid) 10 mg • Vitamin B6 (Pyridoxine HCL) 3 mg • Vitamin B12 (Cyanocobalamin) 9 mcg • Biotin 300 mcg • Folic Acid 400 mcg • Vitamin C (Ascorbic Acid) 90 mg • Vitamin D (Calciferol) 400 IU • Vitamin E (natural d-Alpha Tocopherol) 30 IU • Calcium (Carbonate, Phosphate) 100 mg • Magnesium (Oxide) 80 mg • Zinc (Amino Acid Chelate) 15 mg • Iron (Ferrochel Bisglycinate) 9 mg • Copper (Amino Acid Chelate) 1 mg • Iodine (Kelp) 150 mcg • Potassium (Chloride) 50 mg • Manganese (Amino Acid Chelate) 2 mg • Selenium (Amino Acid Chelate) 70 mcg • Chromium (Chelavite Chelate) 120 mcg • Molybdenum (Amino Acid Chelate) 50 mcg • Choline (Bitartrate) 10 mg • Inositol 10 mg • PABA 10 mg • Boron (Amino Acid Chelate) 500 mcg • Vanadium (Amino Acid Chelate) 50 mcg • Panax ginseng (5% Ginsenosides) 100 mg.

Daily VM Caps **-** The Vitamin Shoppe
Each capsule contains: Vitamin A 10000 IU • Vitamin D 400 IU • Vitamin C 250 mg • Thiamin 8 mg • Riboflavin 8 mg • Niacin 25 mg • Vitamin B6 10 mg • Vitamin B12 25 mcg • Vitamin E 100 IU • Pantothenic Acid 25 mg • Biotin 300 mcg • Folate 400 mcg • Calcium 100 mg • Magnesium 50 mg • Iron 10 mg • Manganese 2 mg • Zinc 7 mg • Selenium 70 mcg • Chromium 50 mcg • Iodine 125 mcg • Citrus Bioflavonoids 25 mg • Para Aminobenzoic Acid 10 mg • Choline 10 mg • Inositol 10 mg • Potassium 10 mg • Betaine HCl 10 mg • Pepsin 10 mg • Papain 10 mg • Pancreatin 10 mg.
See Editor's Note No. 14.

Dairy Digest **-** Enzymes, Inc.
Each capsule contains: n-zimes Proprietary Enzyme Blend 112 mg: Lactase, Invertase, Amylase, Glucoamylase, Malt Diastase, Lipase, Protease (alkaline, neutral and acid proteases plus peptidase), CereCalase, Cellulase, Xylanase, Pectinase • Proprietary Herbal Blend 385 mg: Ginger root extract (5% gingerols) plus whole root, Caraway seed, Blackberry leaf. Other Ingredients: Plant Cellulose, Water, Lecithin, Rice Bran.

Dairy Enzyme Formula **-** Enzymatic Therapy
Two capsules contain: Pure Plant Enzymes Blend 183 mg: Protease I, II, III, IV (USP XXIII [pH7.5]) 29,250 USP (FCC IV [pH7.0]) 46,650 PC.. (FCC IV [pH4.7]) 36,200 HUT, Lactase I,II (FCC III [pH4.5]) 3350 LacU, Amylase (USP XXI [pH6.8]) 5500 USP (FCC IV [pH4.8]) 2350 DU., Lipase II (FCC IV [pH6.5]) 54 LU.

Dairy Mix **-** Professional Complementary Health Formulas
Adrenal 3X, 4X • ACTH 6X, 30X • Histamine 12X • Liver 6X, 12X • Cheeses: American, Cheddar, Camembert, Cream, Brie, Swiss, Blue, Cottage, Parmesan, Ricotta, Edam • Milks: Cow, Goat, Human 6X, 12X, 60X, 100X • Purified Water • 20% USP Alcohol.
See Editor's Note No. 1.

Dairyzimes **-** Pure Encapsulations
Each vegetable capsule contains: Proprietary Blend 105 mg: Lactase, Proteases (providing 1000 ALU [acid lactase units], 630 BLGU [beta-lactoglobulin units]).

d-Alpha-Gems **-** J. R. Carlson Laboratories, Inc.
Each softgel contains: Vitamin E (as D-alpha tocopheryl acetate) 400 IU.

Damiana Leaf **-** Aboca USA, Inc
Each capsule contains: Damiana leaf WPC (whole phytocomplex concentrate, turnera aphrodisiaca, standardized to 2% arbutin, yielding 4 mg per capsule) 198 mg. Other Ingredients: Gelatin.

Damiana Leaf 1000 mg, Concentrated **-** GNC
Each capsule contains: Damiana Leaves (turnera aphrodisiaca; from 250 mg of damiana leaf extract 4:1) 1000 mg. Other Ingredients: Cellulose, Calcium Carbonate, Gelatin.

Damiana/Ginseng Formula **-** Nature's Way
Two capsules contain: Proprietary Formula: Damiana leaves • Fo-Ti root • Gotu Kola stem, leaf • Licorice root • Sarsaparilla root • Saw Palmetto berry • Siberian Ginseng root • Wild Yam root • Other Ingredients: Gelatin.

Damiana-Sarsaparilla Formula **-** Quest
Each caplet contains: Damiana leaf powder (Tunera aphrodisiaca) 120 mg • Sarsaparilla root powder (Smilax officinalis) 90 mg • Saw Palmetto berry powder (Serenoa serrulata) 90 mg • Siberian Ginseng root powder (Eleutherococcus senticosus) 90 mg • Licorice root powder (Glycyrrhiza glabra) 60 mg • Kelp powder (Fucus versiculosis) 50 mg. Other Ingredients: Calcium Phosphate, Microcrystalline Cellulose, Vegetable Stearin, Croscarmellose Sodium, Magnesium Stearate (vegetable source).

Dandelion **-** Nature's Way
Three capsules contain: Dandelion root 1.62 g. Other Ingredients: Gelatin.

Dandelion 1000mg **-** Nature's Own
Each tablet contains: Dandelion extract (taraxacum officinale), equivalent to whole dry plant 1000 mg.

Dandelion Root **-** NOW Foods
Two capsules contain: Total Carbohydrate 0.7 g • Dandelion root (Taraxacom Officinale) 1.0 g. Other Ingredients: Magnesium Stearate.

Dandelion Root **-** Aboca USA, Inc
Two capsules contain: Dandelion root WPC (whole phytocomplex concentrate, taraxacum officinale, standardized to 0.3% caffeic acid derivatives, yielding 0.96 mg per capsule) 640 mg. Other Ingredients: Gelatin.

Dandelion Root (Taraxacum officinale) **-** Solgar
Each capsule contains: Iron 1 mg • Dandelion root, rhizome 4:1 extract 52 mg • Raw Dandelion root powder 328 mg. Other Ingredients: Vegetable Cellulose, Vegetable Magnesium Stearate, Water, Vegetable Glycerin.

Dandelion-Milk Thistle Virtue **-** Blessed Herbs
Dandelion blend of flower, leaf & root • Milk Thistle seed • Bladderwrack • Reishi mycelium • Scullcap • Licorice root • Prickly Ash bark • Grain alcohol & Distilled Water.

Dasimix Shiulit Herbal Extracts Syrup **-** Hadas Natural Products
Herb Extract Blend: Thyme, Echinacea, Elderberry, Sage, Anise.

DayBreak Instant Beverage **-** Starlight International
Each scoop contains: Vitamin A •Calcium • Vitamin D • Thiamin • Niacin • Folate • Biotin • Phosphorus • Selenium • Zinc • Chromium • Vitamin C • Iron •Vitamin E • Riboflavin • Vitamin B6 • Vitamin B12 • Pantothenic Acid • Iodine • Magnesium • Copper.

Daytime Defense Cream **-** Abra Therapeutics
Green Tea extract • Aloe Vera gel • Coconut oil • Apricot Kernel oil • Camellia oil • Vegetable Emulsifying Wax • Vegetable Glycerin • Burdock extract • Comfrey extract • Dandelion extract • Ginkgo extract • Rose Hips extract • Vitamin A (retinyl palmitate) • Vitamin C (ascorbyl palmitate) • Vitamin E (alpha tocopherol acetate) • Grapefruit oil • Lemongrass oil • Juniper oil • Boswellia oil • Sodium PCA • Allantoin • Soy Lecithin • Chlorophyllin (from alfalfa) • Methylparaben • Propylparaben.

Decaffeinated Green Tea Extract - Pain & Stress Center
Each capsule contains: Green Tea leaf powdered decaffeinated extract 500 mg: Epigallocatechin Gallate (EGCG) 200 mg, Other Polyphenols 275 mg, Total Tea Polyphenols 475 mg. Other Ingredients: Gelatin Capsule.

Deep Pore Cleanser - Jason
Vitamin C Complex • Alpha Lipoic Acid.

Deep Sea Fish Oil - Golden Glow Natural Health Products
Each capsule contains: Deep Sea Fish Oil 1000 mg: Omega-3 Marine Triglycerides 300 mg, Eicosapentaenoic Acid 180 mg, and Docosahexaenoic Acid 120 mg.

Deep Sea Kelp 1000mg - Nature's Own
Each tablet contains: Kelp (fucus vesiculosus) extract (equivalent to dry blade 1000 mg • Iodine 240 mcg.

Deeper Greens capsules - Ortho Molecular Products
Each capsule contains: Greens Blend 123 mg: Alfalfa grass juice powder, Spirulina, Barley juice powder, Wheat grass juice powder • Foods Blend 533 mg: Apple, Carrot, Raspberry, Spinach, Strawberry, Blueberry, Tomato, Kale, Lecithin • ORAC Blend 44 mg: Acacia, Blueberry fruit extract, Grapeseed extract, Cranberry, Prune, Cherry, Raspberry seed extract, Bilberry fruit extract. Other Ingredients: Natural Vegetable Capsules, Ascorbyl Palmitate, Microcrystalline Cellulose, Silicon Dioxide.

Deeper Greens powder - Ortho Molecular Products
Each scoop contains: Greens Blend 2.5 g: Alfalfa grass juice powder, Spirulina, Barley grass jiuce, Wheat grass juice powder • Foods Blend 11.2 g: Apple, Carrot, Raspberry.

Deer Antler Plus - Ultra Herbal, LLC
Two tablets contain: Thiamin 1 mg • Riboflavin 1 mg • Niacin (niacinamide) 1 mg • Vitamin B6 (as pyridoxine HCl) 1 mg • Folic Acid 1 mg • Vitamin B12 (as cyanocobalamin) 1 mcg • Biotin 1 mg • Pantothenic Acid (as calcium pantothenate) 1 mg • Zinc 15 mg • Elk Velvet Antler 250 mg • Nettle root powder 110 mg • Oriental Ginseng root 70 mg • Oligomeric Proanthocyanidins 50 mg • Cnidium Monnier 25 mg • Saw Palmetto extract 25 mg • Inositol 1 mg • Choline (bitartrate) 1 mg • PABA 1 mg. Other Ingredients: Gelatin, Whey, Magnesium Stearate, Stearic Acid.

Defend & Resist Complex - Shaklee
Six tablets contain: Zinc (as Zinc gluconate) 15 mg • Echinacea extract (Echinacea purpurea) herb & root 168 mg • Larch tree extract (Larix sp.) heartwood 300 mg • Defend & Resist Proprietary Blend 480 mg: Elderberry extract & Juice concentrate (Sambucus nigra) fruit, Stevia (Stevia rebaudiana) leaf. Other Ingredients: Maltose, Microcrystalline Cellulose.

Defender - Health Factor
Each tablet contains: Beta Carotene 5000 IU • Vitamin C (Ascorbic Acid) 60 mg • Vitamin E (d-Alpha Tocopheryl) 30 IU • Zinc (Amino Acid Chelate) 20 mg • Copper (Citrate) 2 mg • Selenium (Amino Acid Chelate) 100 mcg • Manganese (Citrate) 2 mg • Chromium (Nicotinate) 100 mcg • Boron (Citrate) 100 mcg • Vanadium (Citrate) 50 mcg • Molybdenum (Citrate) 50 mcg • Silicon (Citrate) 20 mcg • Grape seed (95% Polyphenols) 20 mg • Bilberry (25% Anthocyanidins) 5 mg.

Defender BVM - PhysioLogics
Two caplets contain: Vitamin A (as Beta Carotene) 5000 IU • Vitamin C (as Ascorbic Acid) 100 mg • Vitamin E (as d-Alpha Tocopherol Succinate) 240 IU • Selenium (as Selenomethionine) 400 mcg • Manganese (as Manganese Glycinate) 1.75 mg • Tea Green leaf (50% Polyphenols, 75 mg) 150 mg • N-Acetyl L-Cysteine 50 mg • Resveratrol (8% Resveratrol, 4 mg) 50 mg • Alpha Lipoic Acid 25 mg.

Defender FX - PhysioLogics
Three capsules contain: Vitamin A (as beta carotene) 25,000 IU • Vitamin C (as ester-c calcium ascorbate) 500 mg • Vitamin E (as d-alpha tocopherol acetate) 400 IU • Calcium (as ester-c calcium ascorbate) 65.7 mg • Selenium (as l-selenomethionine) 50 mcg • Coenzyme Q10 3000 mcg • Pycnogenol 3000 mg • Citrus Bioflavonoid complex (citrus sinensis) 50 mg • Quercetin fruit (from dimorphandra mollis) 30 mg • L-Glutathione 1000 mcg • N-Acetyl-Cysteine 100 mg • Green Tea leaf extract (camellia sinensis, standardized to contain 50% polyphenols, 1.5 mg) 3 mg • Bilberry fruit (vaccinium myrtillus) 30 mg. Other Ingredients: Gelatin, Cellulose (plant origin), Silica, Vegetable Magnesium Stearate.

Defense Formula - Bee-Alive Inc.
Two half-droppers (2 mL) contain: Echinacea root extract (echinacea angustifolia) 0.8 ml • Goldenseal root extract 0.06 mgl • Royal Jelly (non-freeze dried) 50 mg. Other Ingredients: Vegetable Glycerin, Clover Honey, Deionized Water, Almond Extract.

Deferol - GeoDist, LLC
Each capsule contains: Pyridoxine HCl 50 mg • Folic Acid 0.4 mg • Proprietary Blend: Passiflora Coerulea leaf extract, Griffonia seed extract, Pyridoxyl 5-phosphate 125 mg. Other Ingredients: Magnesium Stearate, Rice Powder, Gelatin.

Definite Difference Body Lotion - Advocare International
Purified Water • Caprylic/Capric Triglyceride • Cetyl Esters • QutiPlex-DD brand Proprietary Blend: Alkoxylated Diester, Hydrolyzed Algin, Chlorella Vulgaris extract, Seawater, Glycerin, Butylene Glycol, Carbomer, Polysorbate 20, Palmitoyl Pentapeptide-3, Glucosamine HCl, Laminaria Digitata extract, Saccharomyces Cerevisiae extract, Urea • Cetyl Alcohol • Sorbitan Stearate • Aloe Barbadensis leaf gel • Camellia Sinensis leaf extract • Tocopherol • Ascorbyl Palmitate • Squalane • Cyclopentasiloxane • Glyceryl Stearate • PEG-40 Stearate • Polyacrylamide • C13-14 Isoparaffin • Xanthan Gum • Laureth-7 • Dimethicone/Vinyl Dimethicone Crosspolymer • Alpha Lipoic Acid • Imidazolidinyl Urea • Phenoxyethanol • Methylparaben • Propylparaben • Fragrance.

Definite Difference Daily Protective Moisturizer - Advocare International
Purified Water • Octinoxate • QutiPlex-DD brand Proprietary Blend: Alkoxylated Diester, Hydrolyzed Algin, Chlorella Vulgaris extract, Seawater, Glycerin, Butylene Glycol, Carbomer, Polysorbate 20, Palmitoyl Pentapeptide-3, Glucosamine HCl, Laminaria Digitata extract, Saccharomyces Cerevisiae extract, Urea • Avobenzone • Cyclomethicone • Dimethicone • Oxybenzone • C12-15 Alkyl Benzoate • Octisalate • Cetyl Alcohol • C14-22 Alkyl Alcohol • Glyceryl Stearate • PEG-100 Stearate • Phenoxyethanol • Myristyl Alcohol • Solanum Tuberosum starch (modified) • C12-20 Alkyl Glucoside • Imidazolidinyl Urea • Allantoin • Methylparaben • Myristyl Glucoside • Triethanolamine • Acrylates/C10-30 Alkyl Acrylate Crosspolymer • Propylparaben • Fragrance • Disodium EDTA • Retinyl Palmitate • Tocopherol • Panthenol.

Definite Difference Eye Repair Creme - Advocare International
Purified Water • QutiPlex-DD brand Proprietary Blend: Alkoxylated Diester, Hydrolyzed Algin, Chlorella Vulgaris extract, Seawater, Glycerin, Butylene Glycol, Carbomer, Polysorbate 20, Palmitoyl Pentapeptide-3, Glucosamine HCl, Laminaria Digitata extract, Saccharomyces Cerevisiae extract, Urea • Cyclopentasiloxane • Cetyl Esters • Cyclomethicone • Cetyl Alcohol • Dimethicone • Glyceryl Stearate • PEG-100 Stearate • Sorbitan Stearate • Caprylic/Capric/Myristic/Stearic Triglycerides • Phenoxyethanol • Dimethicone/Vinyl Dimethicone Crosspolymer • Imidazolidinyl Urea • Sodium Metabisulfite • Methylparaben • Panthenol • Potassium Hydroxide • Propylparaben • Tocopherol.

Definite Difference Foaming Cleanser - Advocare International
Purified Water • Sodium Methyl Cocoyl Taurate • Lauramidopropyl Betaine • Sodium PCA Dimethicone Copolyol • Quillaja Saponaria extract • Butylene Glycol • Saponaria Officinalis extract • Yucca

Schidigera extract • Benzoic Acid • Trisodium EDTA • Carica Papaya extract • Phenoxyethanol • Hydroxypropyl Methylcellulose • Methylparaben • Citric Acid • Chlorphenesin • Benzyl Alcohol • Fragrance.

Definite Difference Gentle Cleansing Creme **-** Advocare International
Purified Water • Cocamidopropyl Betaine • Butylene Glycol • Glycereth-26 • Cetearyl Alcohol • Coco-Glucoside • Stearic Acid • Sodium Methyl Cocoyl Taurate • Sodium Cocoyl Isethionate • Phenoxyethanol • Coconut Alcohol • Glyceryl Stearate • PEG-100 Stearate • Hydroxyethylcellulose • Cetrimonium Laureth-12 Succinate PEG-7 Dimethicone • Imidazolidinyl Urea • Methylparaben • Potassium Hydroxide • Propylparaben • Disodium EDTA • Fragrance • Tocopherol • QutiPlex-DD brand Proprietary Blend: Alkoxylated Diester, Hydrolyzed Algin, Chlorella Vulgaris extract, Seawater, Glycerin, Butylene Glycol, Carbomer, Polysorbate 20, Palmitoyl Pentapeptide-3, Glucosamine HCl, Laminaria Digitata extract, Saccharomyces Cerevisiae extract, Urea.

Definite Difference Hand Creme **-** Advocare International
Purified Water • Caprylic/Capric Triglyceride • Cetyl Esters • Glycerin • Cetyl Alcohol • QutiPlex-DD brand Proprietary Blend: Alkoxylated Diester, Hydrolyzed Algin, Chlorella Vulgaris extract, Seawater, Glycerin, Butylene Glycol, Carbomer, Polysorbate 20, Palmitoyl Pentapeptide-3, Glucosamine HCl, Laminaria Digitata extract, Saccharomyces Cerevisiae extract, Urea • Sorbitan Stearate • Cyclopentasiloxane • PEG-40 Stearate • Aloe Barbadensis gel • Camellia Sinensis extract • Tocopherol • Ascorbyl Palmitate • Squalane • Glyceryl Stearate • Sodium PCA • Alpha Lipoic Acid • Polyacrylamide • C13-14 Isoparaffin • Laureth-7 • Dimethicone/Vinyl Dimethicone Crosspolymer • Xanthan Gum • Fragrance • Phenoxyethanol • Imidazolidinyl Urea • Methylparaben • Propylparaben.

Definite Difference Night Recovery Ceme **-** Advocare International
Purified Water • Cetyl Alcohol • Squalane • QutiPlex-DD brand Proprietary Blend: Alkoxylated Diester, Hydrolyzed Algin, Chlorella Vulgaris extract, Seawater, Glycerin, Butylene Glycol, Carbomer, Polysorbate 20, Palmitoyl Pentapeptide-3, Glucosamine HCl, Laminaria Digitata extract, Saccharomyces Cerevisiae extract, Urea • Cyclopentasiloxane • Butylene Glycol • Glyceryl Stearate • PEG-100 Stearate • Glycerin • Dimethicone • Phenoxyethanol • Sodium Hyaluronate • Imidazolidinyl Urea • Allantoin • Panthenol • Methylparaben • Dimethicone/Vinyl Dimethicone Crosspolymer • Disodium EDTA • Hydrogenated Lecithin • Propylparaben • Tocopheryl Acetate • Retinyl Palmitate • Fragrance • Chamomile extract (anthemis nobilis) • Acanthopanax Senticosus extract • Piper Methysticum extract • Lavandula Angustifolia extract • Rosmarinus Officinalis extract.

Definite Difference Renewing Exfoliant Scrub **-** Advocare International
Purified Water • Cocamidopropyl Betaine • Butylene Glycol • Glyceryl Stearate • Cetyl Alcohol • Polyethylene • Sodium Methyl Cocoyl Taurate • Sodium Cocoyl Isethionate • PEG-150 Pentaerythrityl Tetrastearate • Sorbitan Stearate • QutiPlex-DD brand Proprietary Blend: Alkoxylated Diester, Hydrolyzed Algin, Chlorella Vulgaris extract, Seawater, Glycerin, Butylene Glycol, Carbomer, Polysorbate 20, Palmitoyl Pentapeptide-3, Glucosamine HCl, Laminaria Digitata extract, Saccharomyces Cerevisiae extract, Urea • Tocopherol • PEG-100 Stearate • Guar Hydroxypropyltrimonium Chloride • Hydroxyethylcellulose • Methylchlorisothiazolinone • Methylisothiazolinone • Fragrance • Disodium EDTA.

Definite Difference Second Look **-** Advocare International
Two capsules contain: Zinc (as monomethionine) 2 mg • Manganese (as amino acid chelate) 3 mg • Silicon (as silicic acid) 20 mg • Shave Grass herb extract (equisetum arvense) 100 mg • MariPlex PG Proprietary Blend 725 mg: Chondroitin Sulfate, Shark Cartilage concentrate, L-Pyroglutamic Acid, N-Acetyl Glucosamine, Ribonucleic Acid. Other Ingredients: Silicon Dioxide, Magnesium Stearate, Gelatin.
See Editor's Note No. 15.

Definite Difference Vitamin C Reparative **-** Advocare International
Purified Water • Safflower oil • Butylene Glycol • Cyclomethicone • Cyclopentasiloxane • PEG-40 Stearate • Urea • Aluminum Starch Octenylsuccinate • Ascorbyl Palmitate • Cetyl Alcohol • Stearyl Alcohol • PEG-100 Stearate • Phenoxyethanol • Sodium Hyaluronate • Tocopherol • Imidazolidinyl Urea • Methyparaben • Sodium Metabisulfite • Dimethicone/Vinyl Dimethicone Crosspolymer • Dimethylaminoethanol Bitartrate • Disodium EDTA • Panthenol • Propyl Gallate • Propylparaben • Pyridoxine HCl • Xanthan Gum • Fragrance • Caramel • QutiPlex-DD brand: Alkoxylated Diester, Hydrolyzed Algin, Chlorella Vulgaris extract, Seawater, Glycerin, Butylene Glycol, Carbomer, Polysorbate 20, Palmitoyl Pentapeptide-3, Glucosamine HCl, Laminaria Digitata extract, Saccharomyces Cerevisiae extract, Urea • Hydrogenated Lecithin.

Defy Your Age **-** Pharmagel
10% Alpha Hydroxy Acids • Stabilized Oxygen.

Denta Shield **-** Jarrow Formulas
Each chewable tablet contains: Calcium (as citrate) 100 mg • Coenzyme Q10 30 mg • Lactoferrin (freeze dried) 50 mg • Green Tea 5:1 extract (camellia sinensis, 45% polyphenols) 25 mg • Metabolin 100 mg • Cranberry (vaccinium macrocarpon) 300 mg • Gamma Tocopherol 4 mg • Xylitol 1000 mg. Other Ingredients: Lo Han Kuo (momordica grosvenorii), Dicalcium Phosphate, Celluose, Croscarmellose Sodium, Stearic Acid, Magnesium Stearate, Silicon Dioxide.

Dental-Aid **-** Futurebiotics LLC
Three capsules contain: Vitamin C (as ascorbic acid) 1000 mg • Calcium (as calcium citrate) 250 mg • MSM (methyl-sulfonyl methane) 200 mg • Citrus Bioflavonoids 110 mg • Hesperidin 55 mg • Rutin 55 mg • Quercetin 50 mg • CoEnzyme Q-10 15 mg • Ginger root powder 110 mg • Chamomile flower powder 35 mg • Prickly Ash bark powder 50 mg • Barberry fruit powder 35 mg • Cloves 17 mg • Lemon Grass 15 mg • Sage 12 mg • Angelica root 12 mg. Other Ingredients: Magnesium stearate, Gelatin, Water.

Dentalgel **-** NutriBiotic
Contains 0.4% Grapefruit extract.

Dentaplex **-** MediNiche, Inc.
Each tablet contains: Vitamin A (20% [1000 IU] as Beta Carotene, 80% [4000 IU] as Vitamin A Acetate) 5000 IU • Vitamin C (as Ascorbic Acid) 300 mg • Vitamin D 200 IU • Vitamin E (as dl-Alpha Tocopheryl Acetate) 30 IU • Thiamin (Vitamin B1) 7.5 mg • Riboflavin (Vitamin B2) 8.5 mg • Vitamin B6 (as Pyridoxine Hydrochloride) 10 mg • Folic Acid 400 mcg • Vitamin B12 (as Cyanocobalamin) 30 mcg • Calcium (as Calcium Carbonate) 333 mg • Magnesium (as Magnesium Oxide) 40 mg • Zinc (as Zinc Oxide) 20 mg • Selenium (as Sodium Selenate) 15 mcg • Copper (as Cupric Oxide) 2 mg • Molybdenum (as Sodium Molybdate) 25 mcg • Vanadium (as Sodium Metavanadate) 10 mcg.

Depeze **-** FreeLife International
Each caplet contains: Calcium (as calcium hydrogen phosphate) 100 mg • St. John's Wort dual-standardized extract (hypericum perforatum with 0.3% hypericin, 3.0% hyperforin) 300 mg • Jujube seed standardized extract (ziziphus jujuba var. spinosa with 2% saponins) 150 mg. Other Ingredients: Cellulose, Cellulose Gum, Vegetable Stearic Acid, Magnesium Stearate, Silica, VitaCoat brand Proprietary Blend: Modified Vegetable Cellulose, Spirulina Blue-Green Algae, Alpha-Lipoic Acid.

Depremin - FreeLife International
Each tablet contains: St. John's Wort extract (hypericum perforatum EV.EXT 119) 300 mg. Other Ingredients: Calcium Hydrogen Phosphate, Potato Starch, Hydrous Magnesium Silicate, Silica Dioxide, Microcrystalline Cellulose, Magnesium Stearate.

Depress-X - Olympian Labs
Each capsule contains: 5-HTP 10 mg • Ginkgo Biloba extract 40 mg • Vitamin B-6 50 mg • Magnesium 120 mg • Vitamin B-3 (niacinamide) 20 mg.

Derma Beauty HA dietary supplement - Health Logics
Two capsules contain: Vitamin C (as calcium ascorbate) 120 mg • Vitamin E (as natural D-alpha tocopherol) 30 IU • Calcium (as calcium ascorbate) 20 mg • Hyaluronic Acid (from BioCell Collagen II) 100 mg • Bio-Optimized Proprietary Blend 1160 mg: BioCell Collagen II brand: Patented Collagen Type II, Hyaluronic Acid, Chondroitin Sulfate (from chicken collagen); Citrus Bioflavonoids (fruit), Rosemary Antioxidant extract, Peppermint oil extract, Green Tea leaf extract (standardized for antioxidant epigallocatechin gallate, polyphenols), L-Leucine, Grape Seed extract (standardized for antioxidant oligomeric proanthocyanidins), Ascorbyl Palmitate, Alpha Lipoic Acid, DMAE Bitartrate. Other Ingredients: Kosher Gelatin.

Derma Beauty HA Gold Dramatic Effects Serum - Health Logics
Purified Water • Glycerin • BioCell Collagen II brand Type II Collagen, Hyaluronic Acid, Chondroitin Sulfate (from chicken collagen) • Cunninghami A (sneezeweed) • Broussonetia Kazinoki (paper mulberry) • Arcostaphylos • Camellia Sinensis extract (green tea) • Uva Ursi (bearberry) • Grape seed extract (vinis vinifera) • 1,3 Butylene Glycol • Hydroxyethyl Cellulose • Panthenol • Disodium Edetate • Co-Enzyme Q10 • Imiduria • Methylparaben • Propylparaben • Fragrance.

Derma Beauty HA topical serum - Health Logics
Purified Water • Glycerin • BioCell Collagen brand Type II Collagen, Hyaluronic Acid, Chondroitin Sulfate (from chicken collagen) • Butylene Glycol • Hydroxyethyl Cellulose • Triethanolamine • Methylparaben • Propylparaben • Imiduria • Fragrance.

Derma Care - PhytoPharmica
Two softgel capsules contain: Biotin 1 mg • Choline Bitartrate 100 mg • Folic Acid 100 mcg • Inositol 66 mg • Lecithin (from soy) 400 mg • Niacin (as niacinamide and niacin) 66 mg • Pantothenic Acid (as calcium D-pantothenate) 17 mg • Proprietary Omega Blend 700 mg: Wheat germ oil, Safflower seed oil • Riboflavin (vitamin B2) 3.4 mg • Vitamin A (from fish liver oil) 3332 IU • Vitamin B6 (as pyridoxine HCl) 20 mg • Vitamin C (ascorbic acid) 200 mg • Vitamin D (as cholecalciferol) 666 IU • Vitamin E (as D-alpha tocopherol) 66 IU • Zinc (as zinc chelate) 10 mg.

Derma Cleanse - Raging Creations, Ltd.
Each capsule contains: Flos Lonicerae (Jin yin hua) 70 mg • Fructus Forsythia (Lian Qiao) 70 mg • Yellow Dock (Radiz Rumicis) 84 mg • Fructus Gardenia Jasminoidis (Zhi zi) 56 mg • Radix Paeoniae Rubra (Chi shao yao) 56 mg • Cortex Moutan Radicis (Mu dan pi) 56 mg • Burdock Root seed (Fructus arttii) 84 mg • Chastetree Berry (Fructus Viticis angi-casti) 91 mg • Herba Schizsizonepetae (Jing jie) 42 mg • Dandelion root (Radix taraxici) 56 mg • Chamomile (Flos Anthemis seu Matricariae) 35 mg.

Derma Klear Healthy Skin - Enzymatic Therapy
Two capsules contain: Vitamin A (as retinyl acetate) 10,000 IU • Vitamin C (ascorbic acid) 200 mg • Niacin 10 mg • Vitamin B6 (as pyridoxine HCl) 8 mg • Vitamin B12 (as cyanocobalamin) 3 mcg • Pantothenic Acid (as calcium D-pantothenate) 10 mg • Calcium (as calcium lactate) 11 mg • Magnesium (as magnesium oxide) 72 mg • Zinc (as zinc chelate) 30 mg • Potassium (as potassium chloride) 200 mg • Sulfur (sublimed) 200 mg • Bromelain (1200 M.C.U./g) 200 mg • Thymus extract 25 mg • Ribonucleic Acid (RNA) 20 mg • Burdock root 4:1 extract (arctium lappa) 10 mg. Other Ingredients: Gelatin, Silicon Dioxide, Titanium Dioxide Color, Magnesium Stearate.
See Editor's Note No. 14.

Derma Q-Gel - Tishcon-GelTec
Active Ingredients: Coenzyme Q10 • Vitamin E • Vitamin C • Vitamin A (Retinyl palmitate) • Alpha-Lipoic Acid (Thioctic Acid) • Vitamin K (as Vitamin K1) • Vitamin D • Biotin • Panthenol • Grape Seed extract • Green Tea extract • Chamomile extract • GLA from Borage Oil, Evening Primrose Oil • Aloe Vera gel • Squalane • Kikui Nut oil • Jojoba oil • Sweet Almond oil • Wheat Germ oil • Avocado oil.

Derma Teen - Futurebiotics LLC
MSM, combination of vitamins, minerals, and horsetail.

Derma-Glo Dietary Supplement - N.V. Perricone M.D. Cosmeceuticals
Each softgel contains: Vitamin C (as ascorbyl palmitate) 20 mg • DMAE (as DMAE bitartrate) 75 mg • Grape seed extract (90% polyphenols) 25 mg • Pycnogenol brand Maritime Pine bark extract 5 mg • Ascorbyl Palmitate 50 mg. Other Ingredients: Flaxseed Oil, Gelatin, Glycerin, Borage Oil, Soy Lecithin, Beeswax, Caramel Color, Titanium Dioxide.

Derma-Klear Akne Treatment Cream - Enzymatic Therapy
Sulfur 2.5%. Other Ingredients: Purified Water, Zinc, Sage extract, Silymarin phytosome, Hawthorne extract, Chamomile extract, 18-Beta-Glycyrrhetinic Acid, essential oil of Rosemary, Urea, Vitamin E (tocopherol). Fragrance is natural & hypoallergenic. Contains no Benzoyl Peroxide.

DermaKlear Akne-Zyme - Enzymatic Therapy
Two capsules contain: Vitamin A (as retinyl acetate) 10,000 IU • Vitamin C (ascorbic acid) 200 mg • Niacin 10 mg • Vitamin B6 (as pyridoxine HCl) 8 mg • Vitamin B12 (as cyanocobalamin) 3 mcg • Pantothenic Acid (as calcium d-pantothenate) 10 mg • Calcium (from calcium lactate 60 mg) 11 mg • Magnesium (from magnesium oxide 120 mg) 72 mg • Zinc (as zinc chelate) 30 mg • Potassium (from potassium chloride 200 mg) 105 mg • Sulfur (sublimed) 200 mg • Bromelain (1200 M.C.U./G) 200 mg • Thymus extract 25 mg • Ribonucleic Acid (rna) 20 mg • Burdock root extract (acrtium lappa, 4:1) 10 mg. Other Ingredients: Gelatin, Silicon dioxide, Titanium Dioxide Color, Magnesium Stearate.
See Editor's Note No. 14.

Dermalin-APg - Klein-Becker
Lecithin • Octyl Palmitate • Water • Aminophylline • Isopropylparaben • Isobutylparaben • Butylparaben • Fragrance.

DermaSlim TD - Alvin Last
Abies Canadensis • Ammonium Bromatum • Ammonium Carbonicum • Antimonium Crudem • Argentum Metallicum • Argentum Nitircum • Calcarea Carbonica • Capsicum Annuum • Cinchona Officinalis • Fucus Vesiculosus • Graphites • Kali Bichromicum • Kali Carbonicum • Kali Phosphoricum • Lycopodium Clavatum • Natrum Muriaticum • Phosphorus • Pulsatilla • Silicea • Spongia Tosta • Staphsagria • Sulphur • Thyroidunum • Veratrum Album.

Dermatin - Progressive Health Nutraceuticals
Selenium 100 mcg • Zinc 10 mg • Omega-3 Fatty Acids 20 mg • Artichoke 100 mg • Grape seed extract 100 mg • Milk Thistle 100 mg • Olive leaf extract 100 mg • Gamma Linolenic Acid 20 gm • BioCell brand Type II Collagen 500 mg • Hyaluronic Acid 50 mg • Chondroitin Sulfate 100 mg.
See Editor's Note No. 15.

Dermatrophin PMG - Standard Process, Inc.
Each tablet contains: Proprietary Blend 132 mg: Bovine Epithelial PMG extract, Magnesium Citrate • Calcium 20 mg • Sodium 10 mg. Other Ingredients: Cellulose.

DermaVite Dietary Supplement - Stiefel Laboratories
Each tablet contains: Vitamin A (29% as beta carotene) 3500 IU • Vitamin C 120 mg • Vitamin E 60 IU • Riboflavin 8.5 mg • Vitamin B-6 10 mg • Folate 400 mcg • Biotin 600 mcg • Calcium 270 mg • Zinc 45 mg • Selenium 50 mcg • Copper 2 mg • Manganese 5 mg • Chromium 200 mcg • Lycopene 5 mg • Silicon 20 mg.

Some Brand Name Natural Products - What they Contain

www.NaturalDatabase.com contains MANY more listings than appear here.
Editor's Notes are located on pages 2155-2163.

BRAND NAMES

Desert Balm (Royal Image Cosmetics) - InterPlexus
Aloe Barbadensis gel • Olive extract • Olive Squalane • Shea Butter • Rose Hip oil • Olive oil • Coconut oil • Glycerin • Extracts blend: Arnica, Comfrey, Gingko, Ginseng, Bioflavonoids • Hyaluronic Acid • Myrrh extract • Spikenard • Myrtle • Gurjum Balsam • Rosewood • Lemongrass • Natural Essences • Natural Gums • Glucose Stearate • Allantoin • Menthol • Tocopherol (vitamin E) • Retinyl Palmitate (vitamin A) • Cholecalciferol (vitamin D3) • Citric Acid.

Desert Burn - Desert Burn Industries, LLC
Two capsules contain: Hoodia Gordonii powder 150 mg. Other Ingredients: Gelatin, Magnesium Stearate, Stearic Acid.

Desiccated Liver Tablets with B-12 and B-Complex - Puritan's Pride
Each tablet contains: Thiamin (Vitamin B-1; Thiamine Hydrochloride) 1 mg • Vitamin B-12 (as Cyanocobalamin) 1 mcg • Desiccated Liver 680 mg.

Designer Whey Protein powder (chocolate flavor) - Next Nutrition
Each level scoop contains: Designer Whey full spectrum Whey Peptides: Modified molecular weight and partially pre-digested Whey Protein concentrate, PDUF Whey Protein isolate, Whey Glutamine Peptides (including natural glutamine peptides), Taurine, L-Leucine, L-Phenylalanine • Cocoa (treated with alkali) • Whey Mineral complex • Lecithin • Natural and Artificial Chocolate flavor • Glutasynth: L-Glutamine, Oligofructose, Glutamine Peptides • Natural and Artificial Flavor Zinmag-6: Magnesium Oxide, Magnesium Aspartate, Zinc Aspartate, Pyridoxine • Artificial Peanut butter flavor • Salt • Cellulose gum • Dried Cream extract • Xanthan gum • Sodium Alginate • Artificial Caramel flavor • Acesulfame Potassium • Sucralose • Vanillin • Natural Vitamin E (as mixed tocopherols) • Lactoperoxidase.

Dessert Avert - Enforma Natural Products
Each lozenge contains: Gymnema Sylvestre • Clove oil (or Clove powder) • Fructose.
See Editor's Note No. 65.

Detox - The Herbalist
Oregon Grape root • Yellow Dock root • Dandelion root • Burdock root • Fennel seed.

Detox Complexion Wash - Abra Therapeutics
Apple juice • Mineral Water • Vegetable Polyglucose • Lemon juice • Soapbark extract • Soapwort extract • Yucca extract • Methyl Glucose Dioleate (from grape sugar) • Raw Cane Sugar • Guar Gum • Acacia Gum • Xanthan Gum • Corn Glucose • Vitamin E (tocopherol) • Lactic Acid (from milk whey) • Acetic Acid (from apple cider) • Grapefruit oil • Lavender oil.

Detox Formula - Gary Null & Associates (GNA)
Each capsule contains: Apple Pectin 25 mg • Buckthorn bark 25 mg • Burdock root 25 mg • Cascara Sagrada bark 25 mg • Chrysanthemum 25 mg • Dandelion root 25 mg • Fennel seed 25 mg • Fiber 75 mg • Garlic 25 mg • Ginger root 25 mg • Goldenseal root 50 mg • Hibiscus 25 mg • Kelp 25 mg • Licorice root 25 mg • Marshmallow 25 mg • Orange peel 25 mg • Oregon Grape root 25 mg • Peppermint 25 mg • Prickly Ash bark 25 mg • Psyllium 50 mg • Red Clover 25 mg • Rose Hips 25 mg • Sarsaparilla root 25 mg • Stillingia 25 mg • Yellow Dock 25 mg.

DeTox Formula - Vital Nutrients
Two capsules contain: Glutamine 250 mg • Glycine 250 mg • Taurine 250 mg • Milk Thistle extract (80%) 80 mg • Silybin A & B extract (80%) 20 mg • Curcumin extract (90%) 100 mg • N-Acetyl-Cysteine 100 mg • Alpha Lipoic Acid 100 mg • Grape seed extract (60:1) 50 mg • MSM 50 mg • Broccoli sprout extract 50 mg • Yellow Dock extract (4:1) 50 mg • Schisandra extract (30:1) 50 mg • Green Tea extract (80% catechins) 25 mg • Glutathione (reduced) 20 mg.

Detox Formula - Pharmanex
Each capsule contains: Vitamin C (as calcium ascorbate) 150 mg • N-Acetyl-L-Cysteine 125 mg • Calcium D-Glucarate 125 mg • Silymarin (as milk thistle fruit extract 30:1 (silybum marianum L.)) 70 mg. Other Ingredients: Gelatin, Calcium Carbonate, Stearic Acid, Silicon Dioxide.

Detox Support - NOW Foods
Each capsule contains: Milk Thistle • Sodium Alginate • Chlorella • MSM as central ingredients.

Detoxagen Milk Thistle PhytoSerum - Abra Therapeutics
Grapefruit juice • ABRA9 PhytoSerum Complex: Milk Thistle extract, Echinacea extract, Agrimony extract, Burdock root extract, Dandelion root extract, Thyme extract • Limnanthes oil, Time Release Milk Thistle Phytoliposomes (standardized silymarin flavonoids from milk thistle seed) • Phospholipids • Sea Algae Complex • Clover Honey • Sorbitol • Tocopherol (vitamin E) • Ascorbic Acid (vitamin C) • Xanthan Gum • Grapefruit oil • Lavender oil • Clary Sage oil • Tea Tree oil • Glucose • Glucose Oxidase • Lactose Peroxidase • Acetic Acid • Lactic Acid • Methylparaben • Propylparaben.

Detoxene - Health Smart Vitamins
Two capsules contain: Vitamin C (as ascorbic acid) 50 mg • Vitamin E (as d-alpha tocopheryl acetate) 10 IU • Pectin (from citrus) 120 mg • Chlorella 60 mg • Algin (as alginic acid) 50 mg • Burdock root 50 mg • Red Clover flower 50 mg • Sarsaparilla root 50 mg • Cornsilk style and stigma 30 mg • Bromelain (from pineapple) 20 mg • Garlic bulb 20 mg • Goldenseal (whole herb) 20 mg • Juniper berry 20 mg • Kelp 20 mg • Turmeric root (95% curcumin; 19 mg) 20 mg • Dandelion root 10 mg • Milk Thistle seed (80% silymarin; 8 mg) 10 mg.

Detoxication Factors - Tyler Encapsulations
Two capsules contain: Vitamin A (as natural beta-carotene with mixed carotenoids, palmitate) 6665 IU • Vitamin C (as magnesium ascorbate) 167 mg • Vitamin E (as d-alpha tocopheryl succinate) 83 IU • Thiamine (as thiamine HCl, thiamine pyrophosphate) 8.3 mg • Riboflavin (as riboflavin-5'-phosphate) 8.3 mg • Niacin 10 mg • Vitamin B6 (as pyridoxal-5'-phosphate) 10 mg • Folic Acid 200 mcg • Vitamin B12 (as cyanocobalamin, adenosylcobalamin) 41.6 mcg • Biotin 66.7 mcg • Pantothenic Acid (as calcium pantothenate) 33.3 mg • Magnesium (as magnesium citrate, ascorbate, malate) 78 mg • Zinc (as zinc picolinate) 10 mg • Selenium (as l-selenomethionine) 66.7 mcg • Copper (as copper sebicate) 66.7 mcg • Manganese (as manganese glycinate) 3.3 mg • Molybdenum (as molybdenum citrate) 50 mcg • Calcium d-Glucarate 66.7 mg • L-Methionine 66.7 mg • Glycine 66.7 mg • L-Glutamic Acid HCl 66.7 mg • Taurine 66.7 mg • L-Glutamine 66.7 mg • Choline (as choline bitartrate) 66.7 mg • NAC (n-acetyl cysteine) 66.7 mg • Quercetin 66.7 mg • Inositol 33.3 mg • L-Ornithine-L-Aspartate 33.3 mg • Broccoli aerial parts extract (Brassica oleracea, 0.7% total sulfur) 33.3 mg • Milk Thistle seed extract (Silybum marianium, 80% silymarin) 16.7 mg • L-Glutathione reduced 16.7 mg • L-Serine 16.7 mg • L-Histidine 16.7 mg • L-Carnitine (as l-carnitine tartrate) 16.7 mg • Coenzyme Q10 (ubiquinone) 8.3 mg • Proanthocyanidins (from grape seed extract, vinis vinifera) 3.3 mg • Superoxide Dismutase 33.3 mcg • Catalase 16.7 mcg. Other Ingredients: Microcrystalline Cellulose, Silicon Dioxide, Gelatin, Water.

Detoxil - Vitabiotics
Two tablets contain: Vitamin A (1333 IU) 400 mcg • Vitamin D (as D3 200 IU) 5 mcg • Vitamin E (natural source) 30 mg • Vitamin C 120 mg • Vitamin B1 (thiamin) 12 mg • Vitamin B2 (riboflavin) 5 mg • Vitamin B3 (niacin) 27 mg • Vitamin B6 (pyridoxine HCl) 30 mg • Folacin (as folic acid) 400 mcg • Vitamin B12 (cyanocobalamin) 20 mcg • Biotin 0.03 mg • Pantothenic Acid 50 mg • Iron 5 mg • Magnesium 50 mg • Zinc 15 mg • Manganese 8 mg • Copper 2 mg • Iodine 200 mcg • Selenium 120 mcg • Natural Mixed Carotenoids 2 mg • N-Acetyl Cysteine 30 mg • Methionine 40 mg • Phosphatidylcholine 10 mg • Artichoke concentrate extract 50 mg • Grapefruit concentrate extract 50 mg • Dandelion root extract 50 mg.

Detoxinal **-** PhysioLogics
Two capsules contain: Vitamin C (as ascorbic acid) 200 mg • Chlorella 200 mg • Garlic bulb (allium sativum) 100 mg • Milk Thistle seed (silybum marianum, 80% silymarin, 80 mg) 100 mg • Sodium Alginate 50 mg • Bromelain (from 600 gelatin digestive units, GDU, per gram) 50 mg • Burdock root (arctium lappa) 50 mg • Cascara Sagrada bark (rhamnus purshiana) 50 mg • Dandelion root (taraxacum officinale) 50 mg • Citrus Pectin (citrus spp.) 50 mg • Red Clover (trifolium pratense) 50 mg. Other Ingredients: Gelatin, Rice Flower Powder, Silica, Vegetable Magnesium Stearate.

Detox-Kit **-** Heel/BHI, Inc.
Berberis-Homaccord: Each 100 mL serving contains: Colocynthis 3X 3 mL • Berberis Vulgaris 4X, 10X, 30X, 200X 0.4 mL • Veratrum Album 3X, 10X, 30X, 200X 0.3 mL • Colocynthis 10X, 30X, 200X 0.3 mL. Other Ingredients: Ethyl Alcohol 35% by volume.
Nux vomica-Homaccord: Each 100 mL serving contains: Colocynthis 3X, 10X, 30X, 200X 0.3 mL • Lycopodium Clavatum 3X, 10X, 30X, 200X, 1000X 0.3 mL • Bryonia Alba 3X, 6X, 10X, 15X, 30X, 200X, 1000X 0.2 mL • Nux Vomica 3X, 10X, 15X, 30X, 200X, 1000X 0.2 mL. Other Ingredients: Ethyl Alcohol 35% by volume.
Lymphomyosot: Each 100 mL serving contains: Geranium Rovertianum 4X 10 mL • Nasturtium Aquaticum 4X 10 mL • Ferrum Iodatum 12X 10 mL • Juglan Rgia 3X 5 mL • Myosotis Arvensis 3X 5 mL • Scrophularia Nodosa 3X 5 mL • Teucrium Scorodonia 3X 5 mL • Veronica Officinalis 3X 5 mL • Equisetum Hyemale 4X 5 mL • Fumaria Officinalis 4X 5 mL • Natrum Sulphuricum 4X 5mL • Pinus Sylvestrus 4X 5 mL • Gentiana Lutea 5X 5 mL • Aranea Diadema 6X • Sarsaparilla 6X 5 mL • Calcarea Phosphorica 12X 5 mL • Levothyroxine 12X 5 mL. Other Ingredients: Ethyl Alcohol 35% by volume.
See Editor's Note No. 1.

Detoxygen **-** Nature's Plus
Two tablets contain: Hibiscus (Hibiscus sabdariffa) 250 mg • Red Clover (Trifolium pratense) 200 mg • Dandelion (Taraxacum officinale) 200 mg • Shiitake Mushroom (Lentinus edodes) 150 mg • Reishi Mushroom (Ganoderma lucidum) 50 mg • Echinacea (Echinacea purpurea) 100 mg • Cayenne (Capsicum frutescens) 75 mg • Yellow Dock (Rumex crispus) 50 mg • Milk Thistle (standardized 80% Silymarin) 50 mg • Celery Seed (Apium graveolens) 25 mg • Ginger root (Zingiber officinale) 25 mg • Juniper berries (Juniperus communis) 20 mg • Creatine Monohydrate Energy Precursor 100 mg • Co-Enzyme Q10 (Ubiquinone) 10 mg • Vitamin B12 (Cobalamin concentrate) 250 mcg.

Devil's Claw **-** Jarrow Formulas
Each capsule contains: Devil's Claw 5:1 extract (harpagophytum procumbens, containing 5% iridoid glycosides) 500 mg. Other Ingredients: Rice Powder, Magnesium Stearate.

Devil's Claw Chaparral Supreme **-** Gaia Herbs
Thirty drops contain: Proprietary Blend 80 mg: Devil's Claw root (harpagophytum procumbens), Chaparral leaf (larrea tridentata), Echinacea Supreme (echinacea angustifolia roots and echinacea purpurea roots, seeds, & flowers), Burdock root and seed (arctium lappa), Black Cohosh root (cimicifuga racemosa), Licorice root (glycyrrhiza glabra), Prickly Ash bark (xanthoxylum clava-herculis), 45-55% Pure Grain Alcohol USP, Spring Water.

Devil's Claw Complex **-** PhytoPharmica
Two capsules contain: Devil's Claw (Harpagophytum procumbens) root extract (standardized to contain 1.8%-2.2% harpagoside) 500 mg • Nettle leaf (Urticae dioica) leaf extract (standardized to contain 1% silicic acid) 500 mg • Ginger (Zingiber officinale) root extract (standardized to contain a minimum of 4.5% pungent compounds) 200 mg.
See Editor's Note No. 21.

Devil's Claw Root **-** Aboca USA, Inc
Two capsules contain: Devil's Claw root WPC (whole phytocomplex concentrate, harpagophytum procumbens, standardized to 1.53% harpagoside, yielding 4 mg per capsule) 524 mg. Other Ingredients: Gelatin.

Devil's Club Supreme **-** Gaia Herbs
Thirty drops contain: Proprietary Blend 40 mg: Devil's Club root bark (oplopanax horridum), Indian Jambul seed (syzygium jambolanum), Dandelion leaf and root (taraxacum officinalis), Uva Ursi leaf (arctostaphylos uva ursi), Turmeric rhizome (curcuma longa), Spring Water, 45-55% Pure Grain Alcohol USP.

Devil's Club-Bilberry Virtue **-** Blessed Herbs
Devil's Club Root bark • Bilberry leaf • Reishi mycelium • Siberian Ginseng root • Grain alcohol & Distilled Water.

Dexatrim **-** Chattem, Inc.
Each gelcap contains: Phenylpropanolamine HCl 75 mg. Other Ingredients: Carnauba wax, FD&C Yellow No. 10 Aluminum Lake, FD&C Yellow No. 6 Aluminum Lake, Hydroxypropyl Methylcellulose, Iron Oxide, Magnesium Stearate, Microcrystalline Cellulose, Polyethylene Glycol, Polysorbate 80, Povidone, Silicon Dioxide, Stearic Acid, Titanium Dioxide.
See Editor's Note No. 21.

Dexatrim Natural Ephedrine-Free Formula **-** Chattem, Inc.
Each caplet contains: Calcium 23 mg • Chromium (as Chromium Dinicotinate Glycinate) 83 mcg • Bitter Orange Peel powder extract 120 mg • Proprietary Blend: Siberian Ginseng extract, Green Tea leaf with added Caffeine, Fenugreek seed extract, Guarana seed extract with added Caffeine, Kola Nut extract with added Caffeine, Ginger root, Licorice root, and Vanadium amino acid chelate 340 mg. Other Ingredients: Microcrystalline Cellulose, Maltodextrin, Dicalcium Phosphate, Croscarmellose Sodium, Stearic Acid, Silicon Dioxide, Hydroxypropyl Methylcellulose, Polyethylene Glycol.
See Editor's Note No. 40.

Dexatrim Natural Green Tea Formula **-** Chattem, Inc.
Each caplet contains: Iodine (from kelp) 30 mcg • Chromium (as chromium dinicotinate glycinate) 250 mcg • Vanadium (as vanadium amino acid chelate) 100 mcg • Green Tea leaf standardized extract (40 mg caffeine) 200 mg • Heartleaf standardized extract (12 mg ephedrine alkaloids) 120 mg • Herbal Blend 150 mg: Panax Ginseng root standardized extract, Licorice root, Cinnamon bark, Ginger root, Sarsaparilla root, Kelp. Other Ingredients: Dicalcium Phosphate, Microcrystalline Cellulose, Croscarmellose Sodium, Stearic Acid, Silica, Magnesium Stearate, Hydroxypropyl Methylcellulose, Hydroxypropyl Cellulose, Polyethylene Glycol, Titanium Dioxide, Riboflavin, Caramel.
See Editor's Note No. 39.

Dexatrim Natural No Caffeine Formula **-** Chattem, Inc.
Each caplet contains: Chromium (as chromium dinicotinate glycinate) 250 mcg • Vanadium (as vanadium amino acid chelate) 100 mcg • Heartleaf standardized extract (12 mg naturally ocurring ephedrine) 120 mg • Thermonutrient Blend 100 mg: Steatite, Atractylodes rhizome, Baikal Skullcap root, Balloon-Flower root, Licorice root, Terra Alba, Da Huang root, Mirabilite, Dong Quai root, Field Mint leaf, Forsythia fruit, Gardenia fruit, Ginger root, Lovage root, Schizonepeta stem, Siler root, White Peony root. Other Ingredients: Dicalcium Phosphate, Microcrystalline Cellulose, Croscarmellose Sodium, Stearic Acid, Hydroxypropyl Cellulose, Polyethylene Glycol.
See Editor's Note No. 39.

Dexatrim No Caffeine **-** Chattem, Inc.
Each gelcap contains: Phenylpropanolamine HCl 75 mg. Other Ingredients: Carnauba wax, FD&C Yellow No. 10 Aluminum Lake, Edetate Disodium, FD&C Blue No. 1, FD&C Red No. 40 Aluminum Lake, FD&C Yellow No. 6 Aluminum Lake, Gelatin, Glycerin, Hydroxypropyl Methylcellulose, Magnesium Stearate, Microcrystalline Cellulose, Pharmaceutical Glaze, Polyethylene Glycol, Polysorbate 80, Povidone, Propylene Glycol, Silicon Dioxide, Stearic Acid, Titanium Dioxide.

Dexatrim Results **-** Chattem, Inc.
Each caplet contains: Proprietary Blend 185 mg: Ephedra stem, Yohimbe bark, Siberian Ginseng root, Licorice root, Rutin, Kelp, Fenugreek seed, Hesperidin complex • Proprietary Blend 130 mg:

Cocogen, Caffeine, Green Tea extract • Vitamin C 10 mg • Vitamin E 5 IU • Vitamin B6 2 mg • Pantothenic Acid 5 mg • Calcium 97 mg • Iron 54 mcg • Phosphorus 70 mg • Magnesium 6.7 mg • Chromium 40 mcg.
See Editor's Note No. 21 and No. 30.

Dexatrim Results Ephedrine Free Formula - Chattem, Inc.
Each caplet contains: Vitamin C (as ascorbic acid) 10 mg • Vitamin E (as d-alpha tocopheryl succinate) 5 IU • Vitamin B6 (as pyridoxine Hydrochloride) 2 mg • Pantothenic Acid (as d-calcium pantothenate) 5 mg • Calcium (as dicalcium phosphate) 90 mg • Phosphorus (as dicalcium phosphate) 70 mg • Magnesium (as magnesium oxide) 6.7 mg • Zinc (as zinc oxide) 2.5 mg • Manganese (as amino acid chelate) 0.67 mg • Chromium (as amino acid chelate) 40 mcg • Proprietary Herbal Blend #1 202 mg: Bitter Orange peel extract, Yohimbe bark, Eleuthero root, Licorice root, Rutin, Kelp, Fenugreek seed, Hesperidin complex • Proprietary Blend #2 130 mg: Cocoa extract, Caffeine, Green Tea leaf extract. Other Ingredients: Gelatin, Microcrystalline Cellulose, Croscarmellose Sodium, Stearic Acid, Silicon Dioxide, Pharmaceutical Glaze, Carnauba Wax.
See Editor's Note No. 40.

DGC - AST Sports Science
Four level teaspoons (46 g) contain: Pure Dextrorotatory Glucose Crystals.

DGL - Enzymatic Therapy
Each chewable tablet contains: Licorice root extract 4:1 Deglycyrrhizinated (Glycyrrhiza glabra) 380 mg • Glycine (Amino Acid) 50 mg. In a base of Fructose.

DGL - Ortho Molecular Products
Each tablet contains: L-Glutamine USP 750 mg • Deglycrrhized Licorice root extract 500 mg.

DGL Chewable Licorice - Puritan's Pride
Each tablet contains: Deglycyrrihizinated Licorice root (Glycyrrihiza glabra) extract (4:1) 380 mg • Glycine (Amino Acid) 50 mg.

DGL Plus - Pure Encapsulations
Each vegetable capsule contains: Deglycyrrhizinated Licorice 300 mg • Unripe Plantain banana (musa paradisiaca) 150 mg • Slippery Elm (ulmus fulva) 100 mg • Marshmallow root 8:1 extract (althaea officinalis) 200 mg • Vitamin C (as ascorbyl palmitate) 15 mg.

DGL Plus - Progressive Labs
Two capsules contain: Licorice root (Glycyrrhiza glabra): Deglycyrrhizinated Licorice extract 400 mg • NAG (N-Acetyl Glucosamine) 60 mg • Parotid Gland 10 mg • Gamma Oryzanol 50 mg • Glycine 50 mg.

DGL Plus Ginger - America's Finest
Each wafer contains: Sucrose 1440 mg • Deglycyrrhizinated Licorice (<3% glycyrrhizinic acid) 380 mg • Proprietary Blend 140 mg: Glycine, Carob powder, Ginger root extract, Prosweet (flavor enhancer). Other Ingredients: Stertex, Magnesium Stearate, Aerosil.

DGL Powder - Vital Nutrients
Each level 1/8 teaspoon contains: Deglycyrrhinzinated Licorice (DGL) powder 300 mg.

DHA - Nordic Naturals
Two softgels contain: Vitamin E (mixed tocopherols) 12 IU • Omega-3 Fatty Acids 740 mg • DHA (docosahexaenoic acid) 500 mg • EPA (eicosapentaenoic acid) 150 mg • Other Omega-3 90 mg. Other Ingredients: Purified Deep Sea Fish Oil, Softgel Capsule (gelatin, water, glycerine, strawberry essence), Antioxidant Blend (lecithin, ascorbyl palmitate).

DHA - PhysioLogics
Each softgel contains: DHA (docosahexaenoic acid, as algal oil) 100 mg. Other Ingredients: Sunflower oil, Gelatin, Glycerin.

DHA Brain Support Complex - Leiner Health Products
Each softgel contains: DHA (Docosahexaenoic Acid) 100 mg. Other Ingredients: High Oleic Sunflower Oil, Algal Oil, Gelatin, Glycerin, Vanillin, Ascorbyl Pamitate, Mixed Natural Tocopherols.

DHA Enhance - Pure Encapsulations
Each softgel contains: Fish oil concentrate (typically providing DHA [docosahexaenoic acid] 100 mg, DPA [eicosapentaenoic acid] 50 mg) 600 mg. Other Ingredients: Natural Lemon Flavor, Proprietary Antioxidant Blend (rosemary extract, ascorbyl palmitate, natural tocopherols), Gelatin.

DHA Gold brand - OmegaTech
Docosahexaenoic Acid.

DHA Junior (strawberry) - Nordic Naturals
Four soft gels contain: Vitamin A 175-390 IU • Vitamin D 1-8 IU • Natural Vitamin E 2 IU • Omega-3 Fatty Acids 280 mg (DHA 140 mg, EPA 90 mg, Other Omega-3 50 mg).

DHA LemonGels - Metagenics
Each softgel contains: DHA (docosahexaenoic acid) 100 mg • EPA (eicosapentaenoic acid) 55 mg • Other Omega-3 Fatty Acids 25 mg.

DHA Neuromins - Source Naturals
Each softgel contains: Docosahexaenoic acid 100 mg.

DHA Omega - Life Enhancement Products, Inc.
Each capsule contains: DHA (docosahexaenoic acid) 200 mg. Other Ingredients: Silicon Dioxide, Magnesium Stearate, Gelatin Capsule.

DHEA - Schiff
Each tablet contains: Calcium (as calcium carbonate) 137 mg • DHEA (dehydroepiandrosterone) 25 mg • Trans-Ferolic Acid 1 mg. Other Ingredients: Cellulose, Magnesium Stearate, Croscarmellose Sodium.

DHEA - Olympian Labs
Each capsule contains: DHEA (dehydroepiandrosterone) 25 mg.

DHEA - NewLibido
Each capsule contains: DHEA 100 mg. Other Ingredients: Gelatin, Dicalcium Phosphate, Magnesium Stearate, Stearic Acid, Microcrystalline Cellulose.

DHEA - AIE Pharmaceuticals
Each tablet contains: DHEA (dehydroepiandrosterone) 25 mg.

DHEA - GNC
Each capsule contains: Dehydroepiandrosterone (DHEA) 25 mg. Other Ingredients: Cellulose, Calcium Carbonate, Gelatin, Magnesium Stearate.

DHEA - Optimum Nutrition
Each tablet contains: Calcium 110 mg • Phosphorus 85 mg • Dehydroepiandrosterone (DHEA) 50 mg. Other Ingredients: Dicalcium Phosphate, Stearic Acid, Microcrystalline Cellulose, Magnesium Stearate, Silica, Croscarmellose Sodium (disintegrant).

DHEA - Leiner Health Products
Each tablet contains: DHEA (dehydroepiandrosterone) 25 mg. Other Ingredients: Dicalcium Phosphate, Cellulose, Stearic Acid, Silicon Dioxide, Magnesium Stearate, Polyethylene Glycol 3350, Crospovidone, Croscarmellose Sodium, Hydroxypropyl Methylcellulose, Hydroxypropyl Cellulose, Polysorbate 80.

DHEA - Life Extension
Each capsule contains: Dehydroepiandrosterone (DHEA, 100% pharmaceutical grade) 50 mg.

DHEA - Swanson Health Products
Each capsule contains: DHEA (dehydroepiandrosterone) 25 mg.

DHEA - Body Wise International, Inc.
Each capsule contains: DHEA (dehydroepiandrosterone) 25 mg • Calcium (from dicalcium phosphate) 6 mg.

DHEA **- DreamPharm**
Each capsule contains: DHEA 30 mg • Korean Ginseng (Panax ginseng) 200 mg • Chinese Yam (dioscorea opposite) 200 mg • Poria Cocos 70 mg.

DHEA (50 mg) **- Olympian Labs**
Each capsule contains: DHEA (dehydroepiandrosterone) 50 mg.

DHEA 10 mg **- Vital Nutrients**
Each capsule contains: DHEA (dehydroepiandrosterone) 10 mg.

DHEA 10 mg **- Pro Health**
Each capsule contains: DHEA (dehydroepiandrosterone) 10 mg. Other Ingredients: Cellulose, Gelatin, Water, Magnesium Stearate.

DHEA 10 mg **- Pure Encapsulations**
Each vegetable capsule contains: DHEA (dehydroepiandrosterone, C19-H28-O2, micronized) 10 mg.

DHEA 25 **- GNC**
Each capsule contains: DHEA (dehydroepiandrosterone) 25 mg. Other Ingredients: Cellulose, Calcium Carbonate, Gelatin.

DHEA 25 mg **- Pure Encapsulations**
Each vegetable capsule contains: DHEA (dehydroepiandrosterone, C19-H28-O2, micronized) 25 mg • Vitamin C (as ascorbyl palmitate) 3 mg.

DHEA 25 mg **- Pro Health**
Each capsule contains: DHEA (dehydroepiandrosterone) 25 mg. Other Ingredients: Cellulose, Gelatin, Water, Magnesium Stearate.

DHEA 25 mg **- Nature's Bounty**
Each tablet contains: DHEA (dehydroepiandrosterone) 25 mg. Other Ingredients: Cellulose (plant origin), Dicalcium Phosphate, Croscarmellose, Vegetable Stearic Acid, Vegetable Magnesium Stearate, Silica.

DHEA 25 mg **- Vital Nutrients**
Each capsule contains: DHEA (dehydroepiandrosterone) 10 mg.

DHEA 25 Timed Release **- GNC**
Each tablet contains: DHEA (dehydroepiandrosterone) 25g. Other Ingredients: Dicalcium Phosphate, Cellulose, Vegetable Acetoglycerides.

DHEA 25mg **- Ortho Molecular Products**
Each capsule contains: DHEA 25 mg. Other Ingredients: Natural Gelatin Capsules, Magnesium Stearate, Microcrystalline Cellulose.

DHEA 5 mg **- Pure Encapsulations**
Each vegetable capsule contains: DHEA (dehydroepiandrosterone, C19-H28-O2, micronized) 5 mg.

DHEA 50 mg **- Pure Encapsulations**
Each vegetable capsule contains: DHEA (dehydroepiandrosterone, C19-H28-O2, micronized) 50 mg • Vitamin C (as ascorbyl palmitate) 3 mg.

DHEA 50 mg **- Pro Health**
Each capsule contains: DHEA (dehydroepiandrosterone) 50 mg. Other Ingredients: Cellulose, Gelatin, Water, Magnesium Stearate.

DHEA 5mg **- Ortho Molecular Products**
Each tablet contains: Dehydroepiandrosterone 1.2 mg.

DHEA Creme With Antioxidants **- At Last Naturals, Inc.**
Aloe Vera gel • Soybean Oil • Stearic Acid • Cetyl Alcohol • Triethanolamine • Glycerin • DHEA • Tocopheryl Acetate (vitamin E) • Wild Yam extract • Grape seed extract • Ascorbic Acid (vitamin C) • Retinyl Palmitate (vitamin A) • Methylparaben.

DHEA Eye Lift Serum **- At Last Naturals, Inc.**
Aloe Vera Gel • Carageenan extract (Irish Moss) • Jojoba oil • Glyceryl Stearate with PEG-100 Stearate • Kojic Acid • DHEA • Chamomile extract • Elder flower extract • Corn flower extract • Green Tea extract • Methylparaben • Propylparaben.

DHEA Fuel **- TwinLab**
Each hard gelatin capsule contains: Pharmaceutical Grade DHEA (dehydroepiandrosterone) 25 mg. Other Ingredients: Potato Starch, Cellulose, Gelatin, Purified Water, Magnesium Stearate, MCT.

DHEA Lipoceutical Spray **- Nature's Plus**
Each spray contains: Vitamin E 1 IU • DHEA (micronized dehydroepiandrosterone) 12 mg • Proprietary NADH Complex 2.5 mg: Nicotinamide Adenine Dinucleotide Hydrate, Phosphatidylcholine. Other Ingredients: Purified Water, Fructose, Caprylic/Capric Triglyceride, Natural Flavor, Vegetable Glycerin, Polysorbate-60, Glyceryl Stearate, Citric Acid, Lecithin, Potassium Sorbate.

DHEA MAX **- Nutraceutics Corp.**
Each caplet contains: DHEA (dehydroepiandrosterone) 25 mg. Other Ingredients: Microcrystalline Cellulose, Non-Pariel Beads, Magnesium Stearate, Stearic Acid, Pharmaceutical Glaze, Lactose, FD&C Lake Blue Lake #1, FD&C Yellow Lake #6.

DHEA Original (10 mg) **- Life Enhancement Products, Inc.**
Each capsule contains: Vitamin C (as ascorbyl palmitate) 10 mg • DHEA (dehydroepiandrosterone) 10 mg.

DHEA Original (100 mg) **- Life Enhancement Products, Inc.**
Each capsule contains: Vitamin C (as ascorbyl palmitate) 10 mg • DHEA (dehydroepiandrosterone) 100 mg.

DHEA Original (25 mg) **- Life Enhancement Products, Inc.**
Each capsule contains: Vitamin C (as ascorbyl palmitate) 10 mg • DHEA (dehydroepiandrosterone) 25 mg.

DHEA Original (50 mg) **- Life Enhancement Products, Inc.**
Each capsule contains: Vitamin C (as ascorbyl palmitate) 10 mg • DHEA (dehydroepiandrosterone) 50 mg.

DHEA PLUS **- Nutraceutics Corp.**
Two caplets contain: Vitamin C (as ascorbic acid) 25 mg • Vitamin B6 (as pyridoxine hydrochloride) 6 mg • Pantothenic Acid (as calcium pantothenate) 25 mg • Proprietary Blend 1350 mg: Pentasterone, Smilex Aristolochiafolii (dried root), Beta sitosterol, Adrenal Cortex.

DHEA Plus **- Xymogen**
Deionized Water • Aloe Vera gel • Caprylic/Capri Triglycerides • Shea Butter • Sunflower seed oil • Stearic Acid • Natural DHEA • Glyceryl Stearate • PEG-100-Stearate • Beeswax • Isopropyl Palmitate • MSM • Evening Primrose oil (oenothera biennis) • Burdock root extract • Chamomile extract • Ginseng extract • Lavender extract • Lecithin • Vegetable Glycerin • Stearyl Alcohol or Cetyl Alcohol • Carbomer • Triethanolamine • Xanthan Gum • Hydroxypropylmethylcellulose • Allantoin • Disodium EDTA • Potassium Sorbate • Grape seed extract.

DHEA SL **- Nutraceutics Corp.**
Each caplet contains: DHEA (dehydroepiandrosterone) 25 mg. Other Ingredients: Magnesium Stearate.

DHEA Ultra **- FreeLife International**
Each tablet contains: DHEA (dehydroepiandrosterone) 25 mg • Proprietary Metabolic Activation Factor Blend 10 mg: Thiamin (as thiamin mononitrate) 0.15 mg, Riboflavin (as riboflavin-5-phosphate) 0.17 mg, Niacin (as nicotinamide) 8.5 mg, Vitamin B6 (as pyridoxal-5-phosphate) 0.2 mg, Pantothenic Acid 1 mg • Bioperine brand Black Pepper extract (standardized 95% piperoylpiperidine) 2.5 mg • Trikatu Herbal Blend 10 mg: Black Pepper fruit, Long Pepper fruit, Ginger root. Other ingredients: Calcium Hydrogen Phosphate, Cellulose, Cellulose Gum, Vegetable Stearic Acid, Silica, Vegetable Magnesium Stearate, Vita-Coat brand (vegetable resin, alpha-lipoic acid).

DHEA X-TRA **- Progressive Labs**
Each capsule contains: DHEA (dehydroepiandrosterone) 50 mg • Herbal Base 250 mg: Green Tea leaf extract (Camellia sinensis) 35% polyphelols, Schizandra berry (Schizandra chinensis), Soybean

extract (Glycine max) 1% isoflavones (hypoallergenic), Ginkgo Biloba leaf extract (24% ginkgoflavonglycosides), Grape seed extract (Vitis vinifera) 40% proanthocyanidins.

DHEA-10 - Nature's Plus
Each capsule contains: DHEA (dehydroepiandrosterone) 10 mg • Bioperine brand Black Pepper extract (from piper nigrum fruit, standardized to 95% 1-piperoylpiperidine) 5 mg. Other Ingredients: Silica, Gelatin, Purified Water.

DHEA-25 - Nature's Plus
Each capsule contains: DHEA (dehydroepiandrosterone) 25 mg • Bioperine brand Black Pepper extract (from piper nigrum fruit, standardized to 95% 1-piperoylpiperidine) 5 mg. Other Ingredients: Silica, Gelatin, Purified Water.

DHEA-25 - PhytoPharmica
Each capsule contains: DHEA (Dehydroepiandrosterone) pharmaceutical grade 25 mg.

DHEA-25-X-TRA - Progressive Labs
Each capsule contains: DHEA (dehydroepiandrosterone) 25 mg • Herbal Base 250 mg: Green Tea leaf extract (Camellia sinensis) 35% polyphenols, Schizandra berry (Schizandra chinensis), Soybean extract (Glycine max) 1% isoflavones (hypoallergenic), Ginkgo Biloba leaf extract (24% ginkgoflavonglycosides), Grape seed extract (Vitis vinifera) 40% proanthocyanidins.

DHEA-5 - PhytoPharmica
Each capsule contains: DHEA 5 mg.

DHEAX - HealthWatchers System
Dioscorea Villosa • Alpha Ketoglutaric Acid • Phosphatidyl Serine • Pantothenic Acid • Gotu Kola Powder • Ginkgo Biloba Powder • Siberian Ginseng Powder • L-Glutamine • L-Tyrosine • L-Glycine • L-Arginine-HCl • L-Ornithine • L-Lysine • Pantethine • Beta Sitosterol.

Diabecon - The Himalaya Drug Company
Each tablet contains: Meshashringi (gymnema sylvestre) 30 mg • Pitasara (pterocarpus marsupium) 20 mg • Yashti-Madhu (glycyrrhiza glabra) 20 mg • Saptarangi (casearia esculenta) 20 mg • Jambu (eugenia jambolana syn. syzygium cumini) 20 mg • Shatavari (asparagus racemosus) 20 mg • Punarnava (boerhaavia diffusa) 20 mg • Mundatika (sphaeranthus indicus) 10 mg • Guduchi (tinospora cordifolia) 10 mg • Kairata (swertia chirata syn. s.chirayita) 10 mg • Gokshura (tribulus terrestris) 10 mg • Bhumyaamlaki (phyllanthus amarus) 10 mg • Gumbhari (gmelina arborea) 10 mg • Karpasa (gossypium herbaceum) 10 mg • Daru Haridra (berberis aristata) 5 mg • Kumari (aloe vera syn. a.barbadensis) 5 mg • Triphala 3 mg: Emblica Officinalis, Terminalia Chebula, Terminalia Bellirica • Guggul (commiphora wightii, purified) 30 mg • Shilajeet (mineral pitch, purified) 30 mg • Sushavi (momordica charantia) 20 mg • Maricha (piper nigrum) 10 mg • Vishnu Priya (ocimum sanctum syn. o.tenuiflorum) 10 mg • Atibala (abutilon indicum) 10 mg • Haridra (curcuma longa) 10 mg • Jungli Palak (rumex maritimus) 5 mg • Vidangadi Lauham 27 mg: Embelia Ribes, Cyperus Rotundus, Terminalia Chebula, Terminalia Bellirica, Emblica Officinalis, Cedrus Deodara, Piper Longum, Piper Chaba, Plumbago Zeylanica, Zingiber Officinalis, Piper Nigrum, Iron Calx • Vang Bhasma (tin calx) 5 mg • Abhrak Bhasma (powdered talc, biotite calx) 10 mg • Praval Bhasma (coral calx) 10 mg • Akik Pishti (processed agate) 5 mg • Shingraf (cinnabar) 5 mg • Yashad Bhasma (zinc calx) 5 mg • Trikatu 5 mg: Piper Nigrum, Piper Longum, Zingiber Officinale.

Diabest - PhysioLogics
Three tablets contain: Vitamin A (palmitate) 2500 IU • Vitamin E (d-alpha tocopherol) 300 IU • Vitamin C (ascorbic acid) 300 mg • Magnesium (glycinate) 300 mg • Niacin 150 mg • Zinc (glycinate) 23 mg • Vitamin B6 (pyridoxine HCl) 15 mg • Copper (glycinate) 3 mg • Biotin 900 mcg • Chromium (niacin/glycine chelate) 200 mcg • Selenium (as selenomethionine) 50 mcg • Quercetin 150 mg • Ginkgo leaf (24% ginkgo flavonglycosides 75 mg, 6% terpene lactones 4.5 mg) 75 mg • Vanadyl Sulfate 750 mcg. Other Ingredients: Cellulose (plant origin), Croscarmellose, Vegetable Stearic Acid, Silica, Vegetable Magnesium Stearate, Cellulose Coating.

Diabest 2 - PhysioLogics
Each capsule contains: Chromium (as 67% chromium amino acid chelate, 33% chromium picolinate) 300 mcg • Gymnema Sylvestre leaf (standardized to contain 25% gymnemic acid, 50 mg) 200 mg • Bitter Melon fruit (momordica charantia, standardized to contain 7% bitter principles, 7 mg) 100 mg • Bis-Glycinate-Oxovanadium (BGOV) 10 mg • Vanadyl Sulfate 10 mg. Other Ingredients: Gelatin, Dicalcium phosphate, Cellulose (plant origin), Silica, Vegetable Magnesium Stearate.

Diabetic Support Formula - Puritan's Pride
Each tablet contains: Vitamin C (as Ascorbic Acid) 100 mg • Vitamin E (as dl-Alpha Tocopheryl Acetate) 30 IU • Biotin 350 mcg • Calcium (as Dicalcium Phosphate) 85 mg • Magnesium (as Magnesium Oxide) 250 mg • Zinc (as Zinc Oxide) 7.5 mg • Selenium (as Sodium Selenate) 70 mcg • Manganese (as Manganese Sulfate) 2 mg • Chromium (as Chromium Picolinate) 500 mcg • Lipoic Acid 30 mg • Vanadyl Sulfate 10 mg • Ginkgo Biloba (24% flavone glycosides) 20 mg • Coenzyme Q-10 5 mg • Taurine 50 mg • L-Carnitine 125 mg.

Diabetica Tea - HerbaSway
Panax Ginseng • Siberian Ginseng • Astragalus • Kudzu • Blackberry • Licorice • HerbaSwee (Cucurbitaceae fruit).

Diabeticine - Techmedica Health Inc.
Each capsule contains: Vitamin C (ascorbic acid) 50 mg • Vitamin E (D-alpha tocopheryl acetate) 15 IU • Magnesium (oxide) 125 mg • Biotin 300 mcg • Zinc (oxide) 7.5 mg • Magnanese (amino acid chelate) 1 mg • Chromium (amino acid chelate) 200 mcg • Banaba (1% extract) 25 mg • Guggle 50 mg • Bitter Melon extract 50 mg • Licorice extract 50 mg • Cinnamon herb powder 50 mg • Gymnema Sylvestre herb powder 50 mg • Yarrow herb powder 25 mg • Cayenne herb powder 25 mg • Juniper berries herb powder 25 mg • Huckleberry herb powder 25 mg • Vanadyl Sulfate 3 mg • Alpha Lipoic Acid 30 mg • L-Taurine 25 mg • L-Carnitine 25 mg. Other Ingredients: Gelatin, Magnesium Stearate, Stearic Acid, Microcrystalline Cellulose.

Diabinil - Thorne Research Inc.
Two capsules contain: Chromium (Ultachrome) 100 mcg • Vanadyl sulfate 3 mg • Gymnena sylvestre extract leaf (25% Gymnemic acid) 200 mg • Bilberry extract fruit (Vaccinium myritillus) (25% Anthocyanocides) 80 mg • Bitter Melon extract fruit (mormordica charantia) (0.5% Charantin) 80 mg • Quercetin Chalcone 400 mg • Alpha Lipoic Acid 100 mg.

Diablo - NutraBolics
Each (4 cc) serving contains: L-Citruline Malate 3000 g • Designer Cell-Oxidizing Complex 1000 g: DiArginine Malate, Bis-Carboxyethyl Germanium Sesquioxide, Trimethyl-Aminoethanol, Nicotinamide Adenine Dinucleotide.

Dia-B-Tea - Raintree Nutrition, Inc.
Each rounded teaspoon contains: Pata de Vaca • Pedra Hume Caa • Bitter Melon • Chanca Piedra • Stevia.

Diachrome - Nutrition 21
Each tablet contains: Biotin 150 mcg • Chromium (as Chromax brand chromium picolinate) 300 mcg. Other Ingredients: Dicalcium Phosphate Anhydrous, Stearic Acid, Magnesium Trisilicate, Magnesium Stearate.

Di-Acid Dim - Atrium Biotechnologies
Each tablet contains: First Phase (in Stomach): Glycine 32 mg • Pepsin 100 mg • Papain 50 mg. Second Phase (in Duodenum): Pancreatin 100 mg • Pancrelipase 50 mg • Amylase 30 mg • Bromelain 30 mg • Ox Bile extract 65 mg.
See Editor's Note No. 14.

BRAND NAMES

Some Brand Name Natural Products - What they Contain

www.NaturalDatabase.com contains MANY more listings than appear here.
Editor's Notes are located on pages 2155-2163.

Di-Acid Stim - Atrium Biotechnologies
Each tablet contains: First Phase (in Stomach): Betaine HCL 100 mg • Glutamic Acid HCL 110 mg • Pepsin 100 mg • Papain 50 mg. Second Phase (in Duodenum): Pancreatin 100 mg • Pancrelipase 50 mg. Amylase 30 mg • Bromelain 40 mg • Ox Bile extract 60 mg. See Editor's Note No. 14.

Dia-Comp - Enzymatic Therapy
Two capsules contain: Vitamin E (Mixed Tocopherols) 50 IU • Magnesium (Chelate) 100 mg • Vitamin C (Ascorbic Acid) 100 mg • Vitamin B6 (Pyridoxine HCL) 10 mg • Manganese (Chelate) 10 mg • Zinc (Picolinate) 5 mg • Biotin 1000 mcg • Vitamin B12 (Cyanocobalamin) 250 mcg • Chromium (Picolinate) 50 mcg • Selenium (Aspartate) 40 mcg • Other Ingredients: Blueberry extract 4:1 (Vaccinium myrtillus fructus) 300 mg • Gymnema sylvestre extract standardized to contain 24% Gymnemic Acid 150 mg • Bitter Melon extract (Momordica charanita) 100 mg • Fenugreek seed extract (4:1) (Trigonella foenum-Ggaecum) 100 mg.

Diakof - The Himalaya Drug Company
Each 1 tsp (5 mL) serving contains: Guggulu (balsamodendron mukul syn. commiphora wightii, purified) 35 mg • Draksha (vitis vinifera) 35 mg • Bishnupriya (ocimum sanctum syn. o.tenuiflorum) 25 mg • Jufa (hyssopus officinalis) 25 mg • Guduchi (tinospora cordifolia) 20 mg • Vasaka (adhatoda vasica syn. a.zeylanica) 15 mg • Jaatipatree (myristica fragrans, mace) 15 mg • Yashti-Madhu (glycyrrhiza glabra) 15 mg • Gojihva (onosma bracteatum) 10 mg • Neelapuspha (viola odorata) 10 mg • Triphala 9 mg: Emblica Officinalis, Terminalia Chebula, Terminalia Bellirica • Trikatu 9 mg: Piper Nigrum, Piper Longum, Zingiber Officinale • Vidanga (embelia ribes) 8 mg • Kantakari (solanum xanthocarpum syn. s.surattense) 8 mg • Taja (cinnamomum cassia) 8 mg • Navasagara (ammonii chloridum) 3 mg.

Diaper Ointment - Hyland's
Calendula flowers extract (calendula officinalis) 1X HPUS. Base: Petrolatum USP, 5% Lanolin USP.
See Editor's Note No. 1.

Diaplex - Standard Process, Inc.
Two capsules contain: Proprietary Blend 966 mg: Betaine Hydrochloride, Bovine Pancreas PMG extract, Alfalfa, Calcium Lactate, Buckwheat juice, Buckwheat seed, Pea vine juice, Carrot root, Oat flour, Beet leaf juice, Bovine Pancreas Cytosol extract, Bovine Liver, Bovine Spleen Cytosol extract, Ammonium Chloride, Defatted Soy bean, Pancreatin 3X, Beet root, Pepsin 1:10,000, Bovine Pituitary PMG extract, Bovine Kidney, Bovine Prostate, Inositol, Enzymatically processed Tillandsia Usneoides, Beet root, Bovine Orchic extract, L-Cysteine Hydrochloride, Bovine Adrenal Cytosol extract, Bovine Liver fat extract, Flaxseed oil extract • Vitamin A 2400 IU • Vitamin C 1 mg • Niacin 1 mg • Vitamin B6 0.2 mg • Iodine 10 mcg • Magnesium 8 mg • Chromium 55 mcg. Other Ingredients: Gelatin, Water, Lactose, Cellulose, Potassium Bicarbonate, Fatty Acids, Colors.
See Editor's Note No. 14.

Diarex - The Himalaya Drug Company
Each tablet contains: Kutaja (holarrhena antidysenterica) 245 mg • Guduchi (tinospora cordifolia) 16 mg • Bilva (aegle marmelos) 245 mg • Dadima (punica granatum) 82 mg • Shankh Bhasma (conch shell calx, conch shell ash) 61 mg • Musta (cyperus rotundus) 51 mg.

Diaxinol - Ortho Molecular Products
Two capsules contain: Biotin 3000 mcg • Chromium (ChromeMate brand chromium polynicotinate) 800 mcg • Gymnema leaf extract (standardized to contain 25% gymnemic acids) 400 mg • Lipoic Acid 300 mg • Vanadyl Sulfate 50 mg. Other Ingredients: Natural Vegetable Capsules, Ascorbyl Palmitate, Microcrystalline Cellulose, Silicon Dioxide.

Dibencozide - Source Naturals
Each tablet contains: Dibencozide (Coenzyme Vitamin B12) 10,000 mcg.

Diene-O-Lean - Pharmanex
Two capsules contain: Sunflower oil 2000 mg • Conjugated Linoleic Acid 1200 mg • Capsaicin 100 mg.

Diet Chitosan - Source Naturals
Each capsule contains: Chitosan (minimum 80% Deacetylated Chitin) 250 mg.

Diet Chrome-Care - Bluebonnet
Three capsules contain: Vitamin B6 (pyridoxine HCl) 35 mg • Magnesium (citrate) 50 mg • Potassium (citrate) 50 mg • Chromium (picolinate) 200 mcg • Super CitriMax brand Garcinia Cambogia extract 1500 mg • HCA (hydroxycitric acid) 900 mg • L-Carnitine (L-carnitine tartrate) 500 mg • L-Methionine 50 mg • Choline (bitartrate) 50 mg • Inositol 50 mg. Other Ingredients: 100% Kosher Vegetable Capsules, Silica, Magnesium Stearate.

Diet CitriMax - Source Naturals
Each tablet contains: Garcinia cambogia extract [yielding 500 mg of (-) Hydroxycitric Acid as Calcium Hydroxycitrate] 1,000 mg • Chromium (60 mcg ChromeMate Chromium Polynicotinate and 60 mcg of Chromium Picolinate) 120 mcg.

Diet CitriMax Complex - Source Naturals
Three tablets contain: Garcinia cambogia extract [yielding 1,000 mg of (-) Hydroxycitric Acid as Calcium Hydroxycitrate] 2,000 mg • L-Phenylalanine 200 mg • Chromium (200 mcg ChromeMate Chromium Polynicotinate and 200 mcg Chromium Picolinate) 400 mcg.

Diet Clear Cleanse Fiber Re:Fresh - Source Naturals
Each scoop (3.75 g) contains: Proprietary Concentrate 3300 mg: Psyllium Husk Powder, Rice Bran Fiber, Oat Bran Powder, Grapefruit Pectin, Flax Seed, Barley Bran, and Acacia Gum • Lipase 100 mg • Stevia rebaudiana 100 mg • NutraFlora FOS (Fructooligosaccharides) 74 mg • Ginger Root 74 mg • Lactobacillus Acidophilus (providing 3 billion cells at packaging) 30 mg • Green Citrus Peel 25 mg • Anise Seed 20 mg.

Diet Clear Cleanse Herbal Re:Store - Source Naturals
Three tablets contain: L-Glutamine 300 mg • Oregon Grape root 225 mg • Blessed Thistle root 180 mg • Plantain herb 180 mg • Red Clover blossom 180 mg • Cloves fruit 180 mg • Artemesia herb 150 mg • Black Walnut hull extract (4:1) 150 mg • Bupleurum root 150 mg • Burdock root 150 mg • Ginger root 150 mg • Grapefruit Seed extract (80:1) 150 mg • Licorice root 150 mg • Quercetin 150 mg • Slippery Elm bark 150 mg • Vitamin C (as ascorbic acid) 150 mg • Yellow Dock root 150 mg • Dandelion root 120 mg • Cat's Claw bark 100 mg • Dandelion root extract (4:1) 100 mg • Milk Thistle seed extract (standardized to 83% silymarin) 90 mg • Bioflavonoid Complex 75 mg • Garlic clove 75 g • Sarsaparilla root 75 mg • Turmeric root 75 mg.

Diet Esteem Plus - Esteem Products, Ltd.
Two capsules contain: Super CitriMax brand Garcinia Cambogia 200 mg • L-Carnitine 25 mg • Bromelain 100 mg • GTF ChromeMate brand Chromium 100 mcg • Siberian Ginseng (25x1) 500 mg • Gymnema Sylvestre 100 mg • Choline 200 mg • Lecithin 100 mg • Lipase 125 mg • Inositol 35 mg • Biotin 200 mcg • Pacific Kelp 150 mcg • Pyridoxine (B-6) 25 mg • Cayenne 30 mg.

Diet Fuel - TwinLab
Three capsules contain: Chromium 200 mcg • Citrimax: Garcinia cambogia, Hydroxycitrate extract 500 mg • Guarana extract 909 mg • L-Carnitine 100 mg • Ma Huang extract 334 mg • Potassium & Magnesium Phosphate 100 mg.
See Editor's Note No. 30.

Diet Fuel Ephedra Free - TwinLab
Two capsules contain: Guarana Seed Extract (22% caffeine) 800 mg • Proprietary Blend 685 mg: Citrus Aurantium Fruit Extract (standardized for 19.5 mg synephrine alkaloids), St. John's Wort Extract (aerial parts; standardized for 0.9 mg hypericin),

L-Phenylalanine, Green Tea Leaf Extract (standardized for epigallocatechin gallate), Quercetin, Citrus Bioflavonoid Complex (containing naringin), Ginger Root, Cayenne Fruit. Other Ingredients: Gelatin, Purified Water, MCT, Magnesium Stearate, Silica.
See Editor's Note No. 40.

Diet Fuel With Chitosan Formula **-** TwinLab
Two capsules contain: Chitosan (fiber) 1000 mg. Other Ingredients: Cellulose, Gelatin, Purified Water, Magnesium Stearate, MCT.

Diet Lean Carb Blocker **-** Naturade
Two tablets contain: Calcium (as dibasic calcium phosphate) 200 mg • Phase2 Phaseolus Vulgaris bean extract 1000 mg. Other Ingredients: Croscarmellose Sodium, Vegetable Stearic Acid, Magnesium Stearate, Silicon Dioxide, Hydroxypropyl Methylcellulose, Water.

Diet Lean Low Carb Dieter's Shake (chocolate flavor) **-** Naturade
Protein Blend: Soy Protein Isolate, Whey Protein Isolate, Whey Protein Concentrate • Tricalcium Phosphate • Ferric Orthophosphate • Zinc Oxide • Potassium Iodide • Copper Gluconate • Sodium Selenite • Manganese Sulfate • Chromium Chloride • Sodium Molybdate • Cocoa • Natural Flavors • Sunflower oil • Polydextrose • Guar Gum • Xanthan Gum • Sodium Caseinate • Sodium Chloride • Lecithin • Vitamin A Palmitate • D-Alpha-Tocopheryl Succinate • Ergocalciferol • Folic Acid • Ascorbic Acid • Niacinamide • Calcium Pantothenate • Pyridoxine Hydrochloride • Riboflavin • Thiamine Mononitrate • Biotin • Cyanocobalamin • Mono- and Diglycerides • Sucralose.

Diet Lean Low Carb Dieter's Shake (vanilla flavor) **-** Naturade
Protein Blend: Soy Protein Isolate, Whey Protein Isolate, Whey Protein Concentrate • Tricalcium Phosphate • Ferric Orthophosphate • Zinc Oxide • Potassium Iodide • Copper Gluconate • Sodium Selenite • Manganese Sulfate • Chromium Chloride • Sodium Molybdate • Natural Flavors • Sunflower oil • Polydextrose • Carrageenan • Xanthan Gum • Sodium Caseinate • Sodium Chloride • Lecithin • Vitamin A Palmitate • D-Alpha-Tocopheryl Succinate • Ergocalciferol • Folic Acid • Ascorbic Acid • Niacinamide • Calcium Pantothenate • Pyridoxine Hydrochloride • Riboflavin • Thiamine Mononitrate • Biotin • Cyanocobalamin • Mono- and Diglycerides • Sucralose.

Diet Metabo-7 **-** Source Naturals
Each tablet contains: Vitamin C (as ascorbic acid) 80 mg • Niacinamide 30 mg • Vitamin B6 (as pyridoxine HCl) 30 mg • Pantothenic Acid (as calcium-d-pantothenate) 80 mg • Chromium (as picolinate & polynicotinate) 400 mcg • Potassium (as potassium citrate) 20 mg • Iodine (from kelp) 100 mcg • GABA (gamma-aminobutyric acid) 500 mg • Phenylalanine (as l-& dl-phenylalanine) 500 mg • Sida cordifolia extract (6% yielding 30 mg ephedrine alkaloids) 500 mg • Gymnema sylvestre extract (GS4) 400 mg • Green Tea leaf extract (20% yielding 60 mg of caffeine) 300 mg • Glutamine 200 mg • Yogaraj Guggul Gum Resin 200 mg • Kola Nut extract (20% yielding 30 mg of caffeine) 150 mg • Yerba Mate extract (8% yielding 10 mg of caffeine) 125 mg • Dandelion leaf 100 mg • Bupleurum root 100 mg • L-Tryosine 100 mg • Horse Chestnut extract (yielding 14 mg Aescin) 70 mg • Dandelion root extract (4:1) 50 mg • Bladderwrack extract 30 mg • Ginkgo Biloba leaf extract (50:1) 30 mg • Ginger root 30 mg • N-Acetyl-Cysteine 30 mg • Bioperine brand Black Pepper extract 3 mg.
See Editor's Note No. 39.

Diet Pyruva-Nectar **-** Source Naturals
Two scoops (32 g) contain: Calcium Pyruvate Monohydrate 5 g. Other Ingredients: Fructose, Natural Flavorings, Gum Arabic, Red Beet Root (natural color), and Citric Acid.

Diet Pyruvate 500 mg **-** Source Naturals
Each capsule contains: Calcium Pyruvate Monohydrate 500 mg.

Diet Pyruvate 750 mg **-** Source Naturals
Each capsule contains: Calcium Pyruvate Monohydrate 750 mg.

Diet Rockstar Energy Drink **-** Rockstar, Inc.
Carbonated Water • Citric Acid • Taurine • Sodium Citrate • Maltodextrin • Natural and Artificial Flavors • Guarana seed extract • Ascorbic Acid • Caramel Color • Caffeine • Poatssium Sorbate • Sodium Benzoate • Acesulfame Potassium • Sucralose • L-Carnitine • Inositol • Milk Thistle extract • Ginkgo Biloba leaf extract • Niacinamide • Calcium Pantothenate • Siberian Ginseng root extract • Riboflavin • Pyridoxine Hydrochloride • Cyanocobalamin.

Diet Slim **-** Gaia Herbs
Three capsules contain: Garcinia fruit (garcinia cambogia) 300 mg • Green Tea leaf (camellia sinensis) 150 mg • Coleus root (coleus forskholii) 138 mg • Turmeric rhizome (curcuma longa) 90 mg • Elderberry (sambucus canadensis) 90 mg • Bitter Orange peel (citrus aurantium) 57 mg • Gymnema leaf (gymnema sylvestre) 51 mg • Yohimbe bark (coryanthe yohimbe) 36 mg • Bladderwrack fronds (fucus vesiculosus) 18 mg • Ginger rhizome, supercritical CO2 extract (zingiber off.) 12 mg. Other Ingredients: Vegetable Glycerin, Lecithin, Vegetable Cellulose (capsule).
See Editor's Note No. 40.

Diet Support Formula **-** NOW Foods
Two capsules contain: Vitamin B6 (pyridoxine HCL) 10 mg • Chromium (chelavite chelate) 300 mcg • Iodine (kelp extract) 300 mcg • Bitter Orange extract (Citrus aurantium) containing 6% synepherine 350 mg • L-Carnitine (from 365 mg l-carnitine tartrate) 250 mg • Super Citrimax as Garcinia cambogia extract containing 225 mg (-)hydroxycitric acid 375 mg • Uva Ursi (Uvae ursi folium) 4:1 extract 50 mg • Green Tea extract (Carmellia sinenis) 30% calechins 200 mg.
See Editor's Note No. 40.

Diet System 6 **-** Applied Nutrition
Six capsules contain: Super Citrimax: Garcinia extract 1500 mg. Energizing Herbs (Thermogenic Herbs): Kola nut extract 550 mg, Guarana extract 100 mg, Ginger 100 mg. Three Lipotropics including: Choline Bitartrate 100 mg, Inositol 100 mg, Betaine HCL 25 mg. Chromium (Chromium Picolinate 150 mcg, ChromeMate 150 mcg). L-Carnitine (L-Carnitine Complex) 300 mg. Vitamins & Minerals: "72 Trace Mineral Complex" 100 mg: Vitamin B3 20 mg, Vitamin B6 2 mg, Vitamin B12 6 mcg, Vitamin B2 1.7 mg, Vitamin E 15 IU, Folic Acid 400 mcg, Selenium 50 mcg , Vitamin C 60 mg, Potassium 25 mg, Iodine 150 mcg.

Diet Tonalin **-** Source Naturals
Three softgels contain: Conjugated Linoleic Acid 1800 mg. Other Ingredients: Gelatin (capsule), Glycerin, Purified Water, Caramel, Carob, Titanium Dioxide.

Diet Ultra III **-** The Vitamin Shoppe
Three tablets contain: Vitamin A (as acetate, beta-carotene) 10000 IU • Vitamin C (as ascorbic acid) 100 mg • Vitamin D (cholecalciferol) 400 IU • Vitamin E (as d-alpha tocopherol) 50 IU • Vitamin B1 (as thiamin hydrochloride) 25 mg • Vitamin B2 (as riboflavin) 25 mg • Vitamin B12 (as cobalamin) 25 mcg • Niacin (as nicotinic acid) 25 mg • Folic Acid 100 mcg • Biotin 100 mcg • Pantothenic Acid (as d-calcium pantothenate) 20 mg • Iron (as chelate) 10 mg • Calcium (as citrate) 100 mg • Iodine (from kelp) 150 mcg • Magnesium (as citrate) 50 mg • Zinc (as chelate) 15 mg • Selenium (as chelate) 25 mcg • Chromium (as chelate) 300 mcg • Gotu Kola (Centella asiatica) 50 mg • Siberian Ginseng (Eleutherococcus senticosus) root 50 mg • L-Carnitine 50 mg • Choline 150 mg • Inositol 150 mg • Omega-3 (fish) 15 mg.

Dietary Fat Metaboliser **-** Nature's Own
Each tablet contains: Inositol 300 mg • Choline Bitartrate 300 mg • Dandelion extract (taraxacum officinale) equivalent to dry whole plant 100 mg • Chelidonium Majus extract, equivalent to dry herb 30 mg • Levocarnitine (from levocarnitine tartrate 36.6 mg) 25 mg • Vitamin B6 (pyridoxine hydrochloride) 25 mg • Biotin 50 mcg • Vitamin B12 (cyanocobalamin) 50 mcg • Chromium (from chromium picolinate 200 mcg) 24.8 mcg.

BRAND NAMES

Dieter's Green Tea - Triple Leaves Brand
Malva verticillata • Loquat leaf.

DietMaxx - MK Supplements
Hoodia Gordonii 500 mg • Vitamin B6 2 mg • Glucomannan 200 mg • Chromium (chelate) 100 mcg • Vanadium (chelate) 150 mcg.

DIETMAXXX - MKSupplements
Hoodia Gordonii 500 mg • Vitamin B6 2 mg • Glucomannan 200 mg • Chromium Chelate 100 mcg • Vanadium Chelate 150 mcg.

Diet-Phen - Source Naturals
Three tablets contain: St. John's Wort standardized extract (hypericum perforatum, 0.3%, yielding hypericin 2.7 mg) 900 mg • Vitamin B3 (niacinamide) 25 mg • Vitamin B6 (pyridoxine hydrochloride) 25 mg • Chromium (100 mcg chromium polynicotinate, 100 mcg chromium picolinate) 200 mcg • Acetyl L-Carnitine 50 mg • L-Phenylalanine 500 mg • Green Tea leaf extract (yielding 33 mg caffeine) 300 mg • Ginger root 50 mg • Bitter Orange peel extract (8%, yielding 24 mg synephrine) 300 mg. Other Ingredients: Sorbitol, Stearic Acid, Colloidal Silicon Dioxide, Magnesium Stearate.
See Editor's Note No. 40.

Diet-Phen Ephedra Free - Source Naturals
Three tablets contain: St. John's Wort extract (hypericum perforatum standardized extract 0.3% yielding 2.7 mg of hypericin) 900 mg • L-Phenylalanine 750 mg • Green Tea 300 mg • Cayenne 100 mg • Mustard seed 100 mg • Ginger root 100 mg • Piper Nigrum 100 mg • Acetyl L-Carnitine 50 mg • Niacinamide 25 mg • Vitamin B6 (pyridoxine HCl) 25 mg • ChromeMate brand Chromium (100 mcg chromium polynicotinate, 100 mcg chromium picolinate) 200 mcg.

Diet-Phen Ephedra Free (New Formula) - Source Naturals
Three tablets contain: Niacinamide 25 mg • Calcium 135 mg • Vitamin B6 (as pyridoxine HCl) 25 mg • Chromium (as chromium picolinate 100 mcg and polynicotinate 100 mcg) 200 mcg • St. John's Wort leaf/flower standardized extract (0.3%, yielding 2.7 mg hypericin) 900 mg • L-Phenylalanine 750 mg • Green Tea leaf extract 165 mg • Cayenne fruit 100 mg • Mustard seed 100 mg • Ginger root 100 mg • Piper Nigrum seed 100 mg • Acetyl L-Carnitine 50 mg. Other Ingredients: Dibasic Calcium Phosphate, Stearic Acid, Colloidal Silicon Dioxide, Modified Cellulose Gum, Magnesium Stearate.

Diet-Phen for Men - Source Naturals
Two tablets contain: Niacinamide 17 mg • Vitamin B6 (as pyridoxine HCl) 17 mg • Chromium (as ChromeMate chromium polynicotinate and picolinate) 270 mcg • St. John's Wort leaf/flower extract (yielding 1.8 mg hypericum) 600 mg • Bitter Orange peel extract (yielding 16 mg synephrine) 400 mg • L-Phenylalanine 333 mg • Creatine Monohydrate 330 mg • L-Glutamine 133 mg • Panax Ginseng root extract (standardized to 8% ginsenosides) 67 mg • L-Carnitine L-Tartrate 33 mg. Other Ingredients: Dibasic Calcium Phosphate, Stearic Acid, Modified Cellulose Gum, Colloidal Silicon Dioxide, Magnesium Stearate.
See Editor's Note No. 40.

Dietrine Carb Blocker - Ultra Herbal, LLC
Two capsules contain: Chelavite brand Chromium Dinicotinate Glycinate 200 mcg • Phase 2 brand White Kidney Bean extract (phaseolus vulgaris) 1000 mg • Vanadium (as vanadium amino acid chelate) 100 mg. Other Ingredients: Gelatin, Water, Cellulose, Magnesium Stearate.

Diet-Tech - MuscleTech
Four capsules contain: Chromium (as chromium polynicotinate) 300 mcg • GLUCO-TECH 2.2 g: Glucomannan (amorphophallus konjac), Xanthan gum • METABO-TECH 843 mg: Green Tea leaf extract (standardized for 95% polyphenols [70% catechins, 45% epigallocatechins gallate - 300 mg EGCG]), Caffeine (as caffeine anhydrous), Guarana seed extract, Yerba Mate leaf (ilex paraguariensis, standardized for 200 mg of caffeine), Alpha Lipoic Acid. Other Ingredients: Gelatin, Magnesium Stearate, Silica, Cellulose.

Digest - Enzymedica
Each capsule contains: Amylase Thera-Blend 12,000 DU • Protease Thera-Blend 42,000 HUT • Invertase 1.75 INVU • Alpha-Galactosidase 75 GALU • Lactase 850 ALU • Pectinase with Phytase 50 endo Pgu • Maltese 200 DP • Cellulase Thera-Blend 200 CU • Lipase Thera-Blend 500 FCCFIP • Lactobacillus Acidophilus 100 Million CFU • Bifidobacterium Longum 25 Million CFU.

Di-Gest - Wild Rose
Each capsule contains: L-Glutamic Acid HCl 100 mg • Pancreatin NF 360 mg • Betaine HCl 100 mg • Calcium Ascorbate 50 mg • Bromelain (1:10) 80 mg • Papain NF 75 mg.

Digest Gold - Enzymedica
Each capsule contains: Amylase Thera-Blend 23,000 DU • Protease Thera-Blend 80,000 HUT • Maltase 200 DP • Glucoamylase 50 AG • Alpha-Galactosidase 450 GALU • Lipase Thera-Blend 3500 FCCFIP • Cellulase Thera-Blend 3000 CU • Lactase 900 ALU • Beta Glucanase 25 BGU • Xylanase 550 XU • Pectinase with Phytase 45 endo-PGU • Hemicellulase 30 HCU • Invertase 79 INVU • L. Acidophilus 250 million CFU.

Digest RC - Life Extension Foundation
Each two capsules contain: Black Radish extract 75 • Linden bark charcoal 75 mg • Artichoke extract 47 mg • Calcium Phosphate 45 mg • Cholic Acid 40 mg • Peppermint 15 mg. Inactive Ingredients: Beet Sugar, Talcum, Vegetable Starch, Magnesium Stearate, Arabic Gum, Gelatin, Silicon Dioxide.

Digest Support - Natrol, Inc.
Two capsules contain: Proteolytic Enzymes: Protease I (20000 HUT) 200 mg • Protease II (16600 FCC) 8 mg • Amylolytic Enzymes: Amylase (10200 DU) 408 mg • Cellulase (410 CMC) 100 mg • Lactase (200 LAC) 20 mg • Lipolytic Enzymes: Lipase (300 LU) 100 mg • Maltase (90 DU) 90 mg • Sucrase (200 SU) 20 mg • Anti Gas Factor: Alpha Galactosidase (54 GAL) 54 mg. Other Ingredients: TriCalcium Phosphate, Silica, Magnesium Stearate, Gelatin.

Digestabs - Puritan's Pride
Two tablets contain: Pancreatin 600 mg • Amylase 260 mg • Pepsin 130 mg • Papain 130 mg • Ox Bile 130 mg • Betaine HCl 130 mg • Duodenal substance 60 mg.
See Editor's Note No. 14.

DigestActiv - Source Naturals
Two capsules contain: Vegetal Analong of Pancreatin 286 mg (28625 FCC) • Acid-Stable Protease 12 mg (785 FCC) • Lipase 125 mg (785 FCC) • Alpha-Amylase 52 mg (630 FCC) • Amyloglucosidase 12 mg (2 FCC) • Cellulase 5 mg (100 FCC) • Hemicellulase 3 mg (325 FCC) • Lactase 5 mg (40 FCC) • Bromelain 50 gm • Papain 50 mg • Gentian root 50 mg • Ginger root 25 mg • Peppermint 25 mg • Bioperine brand Black Pepper extract 6 mg • Quassia 4:1 extract 50 mg • Betaine HCl 200 mg. Other Ingredients: Gelatin (capsule), Magnesium Stearate, Colloidal Silicon Dioxide.

Digest-Aid (Bile Salts) - Trophic
Each tablet contains: Bile Salts (derived from ox bile extract) 100 mg • Lipase 10 mg • Bromelain 10 mg • Trypsin 10 mg • Chamomile 10 mg • Charcoal 10 mg • Goldenseal 10 mg.

DigestEase - Pacific BioLogic
Ginger • Rhubarb • Elecampane • Gentian • Long Pepper • Tropical Almond • Emblic Myrobalan • Beleric Myrobalan • Glauber's Salt • Kaolin.

Di-Gest-Eze - Nutri-Quest Rx
Each two-phase tablet contains: Phase One (Stomach): Betaine HCl 155 mg • L-Glutamic Acid HCl 100 mg • Pepsin 105 mg • Papain 50 mg. Phase Two (Duodenum): Pancreatin 100 mg •

BRAND NAMES

Pancrelipase 50 mg • Amylase 30 mg • Bromelain 30 mg • Ox Bile 65 mg • Parotid 2 mg.
See Editor's Note No. 14.

DigestiMax **-** FreeLife International
Each capsule contains: Proprietary DigestiMax Pure Plant Enzyme Blend 425 mg: Alpha-Amylase, Beta-Glucosidase, Cellobiase, Glucoamylase, Cellulase, Hemicellulase, Xylanase, Pectinase, High-Activity Lipase (fatty acid esterase), Acid Protease, Aminopeptidase, Bromelain, Carboxypeptidase, Neutral Protease, Papain • Base: Pure Microencapsulated Peppermint oil. Other ingredients: Gelatin, Glucose Polymers, Vegetable Magnesium Stearate, Silica.

Digestion Formula **-** Nature's Way
Two capsules contain: Angelica root 90 mg • Barberry bark 135 mg • Beet root 100 mg • Cayenne pepper fruit 25 mg • Dandelion root 315 mg • Fizyme enzyme formula 100 mg • Gentian root 135 mg. Other Ingredients: Gelatin, Magnesium stearate, Millet.

Digestion Formula **-** Nature's Way
Two capsules contain: Angelica root 90 mg • Barberry bark 135 mg • Beet root 100 mg • Cayenne pepper fruit 25 mg • Dandelion root 315 mg • Fizyme Enzyme Formula 100 mg • Gentian root 135 mg. Other Ingredients: Gelatin, Magnesium Stearate, Millet.

Digestive Advantage IBD **-** Ganeden Biotech
Each tablet contains: Lactobacillus cultures • Saccharomyces Boulardii • Maltodextrose • Microcrystalline Cellulose • L-Lysine • Vitamin A • Vitamin C • Vitamin D • Vitamin E • Vitamin K • Vitamin B12 • Folic Acid • Selenium.

Digestive Advantage IBS **-** Ganeden Biotech
Each tablet contains: Cellulose • Lactobacillus cultures • L-Lysine • Hydroxypropyl Methylcellulose • Maltodextrin • Magnesium Stearate • Flavor • FD&C Blue Lake • Red Sucrose Specs.

Digestive Advantage LI **-** Ganeden Biotech
Each caplet contains: Lactase Enzyme 3000 FCC units • Lactobacillus cultures (total ingredient weight per caplet 200 mg) 400 million. Other Ingredients: Cellulose, Stearic Acid, Hydroxypropylmethylcellulose, Polyethylene Glycol, Maltodextrin, FD&C Blue #1 Lake.

Digestive Cleanser **-** Nature's Own
Each tablet contains: Olive leaf extract (olea europaea) 1000 mg • Chinese Wormwood herb extract (artemisia annua) 400 mg • Chamomile flowering herb extract (matricaria recutita) 250 mg • Black Walnut fruit hull extrct (juglans nigra) 200 mg • Barberry root bark extract (berberis vulgaris) 200 mg • Peppermint leaf extrat (mentha piperita) 200 mg.

Digestive Enzymes **-** Jamieson
Each caplet contains: Papain 50 mg • Bromelain 30 mg • Lipase 30 mg • Amylase 50 mg • Lactase 30 mg • Cellulase 15 mg • Calcium Gluconate • Peppermint Leaf • Fennel Complex.

Digestive Enzymes **-** Always Young
Each vegetarian capsule contains: N-Zymes brand Proprietary Plant Enzyme Blend 275 mg: Amylase 3500 DU • Glucoamylase 5.25 AGU • Lipase 350 FCCLU • Protease I pH 3.0 15 SAPU • Protease II pH 4.5 20,000 HUT • Protease III pH 6.0 35,000 HUT • Cellulase 200 CU • CereCalase 250 MU • Alpha Galactosidase 75 GalU • Lactase 150 ALU • Invertase 150 SU • Malt Diastase 325 DP • Peptidase 2500 HUT • Bromelain 650,000 FCCPU • Papain 250,000 FCCPU. Other Ingredients: Rice Bran, Vegetable Cellulose, Water.

Digestive Enzymes and Probiotics **-** 4 Life
Each caplet contains: Vitamin C (as calcium ascorbate) 60 mg • Proprietary Enzyme Blend 221 mg: Amylase, Invertase, Glucoamylase, Protease, Cellulase, Peptidase FP, Alpha-Galactosidase, Lipase • Proprietary Probiotic Blend 250 million CFU: Lactobacillus Acidophilus, Lactobacillus Casei, Bifidobacterium Bifidum, Bifidobacterium Longum, Lactobacillus Plantarum, Lactobacillus Reuteri • Proprietary Digestive Blend 150 mg: Fructooligosaccharides (FOS), Jerusalem Artichoke. Other Ingredients: Microcrystalline Cellulose, Maltodextrin, Croscarmellose Sodium, Glucose Polymers, Magnesium Stearate, Silica, Stearic Acid.

Digestive Formula **-** 4 Life
Each capsule contains: Ginger root 180 mg • Turmeric root 65 mg • Digestive Proprietary Blend 45 mg: Milk Thistle leaf extract, Artichoke root extract, Dandelion root extract, Gentian root extract, Ginger root extract, Turmeric root extract • Milk Thistle seed 30 mg • Dandelion root 30 mg • Artichoke leaf 30 mg • Gentian leaf 20 mg. Other Ingredients: Gelatin, Rice Bran, Silicon Dioxide, Magnesium Stearate.

Digestive Formula **-** Pharmanex
Each capsule contains: Ginger root 5:1 extract (zingiber officinale) 200 mg • Proprietary Enzyme Blend 145 mg: Amylase, Protease, Bromelain, acid stable Protease, Lipase, Cellulase, Lactase • Artichoke leaf 5:1 extract (cynara scolymus) 135 mg. Other Ingredients: Gelatin, Stearic Acid, Corn Starch.

DigestMORE **-** Renew Life Formulas, Inc.
Each capsule contains: Protease • Amylase • Lipase • Lactase • Cellulase • Invertase (sucrase) • Malt Diatase • Pectinase with Phytase • L-Glutamine • Ginger root (zingiber officinale) • Marshmallow root (althaea officinalis) • Papaya fruit (cariaca papaya) • Bromelain • N-Acetyl D-Glucosamine • Gamma Oryzanol. Other Ingredients: Gelatin, Water.

DigestMORE ULTRA **-** Renew Life Formulas, Inc.
Each capsule contains: Protease • Amylase • Lipase • Lactase • Cellulase • Invertase • Glucoamylase • Alpha Galactosidase • Beta Glucanase • Xylanase • Hemicellulase • Pectinase • Phytase • Papain. Other Ingredients: Gelatin, Water.

DIM Bioavailable Diindolylmethane **-** PhysioLogics
Each capsule contains: Diindolylmethane 100 mg. Other Ingredients: Rice Powder, Gelatin, Silica, Vegetable Magnesium Stearate.

Dinomins **-** Herbalife International of America, Inc.
Each tablet contains: Vitamin A (as 50% retinyl acetate and 50% beta-carotene) 2500 IU • Vitamin C (as ascorbic acid) 30 mg • Vitamin D (as cholecalciferol) 200 IU • Vitamin E (as dL-alpha tocopheryl acetate) 15 IU • Thiamin (as monoitrate) 0.75 mg • Riboflavin 0.9 mg • Niacin (as niacinamide) 10 mg • Vitamin B6 (as pyridoxine hydrochloride) 1 mg • Folate (as folic acid) 100 mcg • Vitamin B12 (as cyanocobalamin) 3 mcg • Biotin 30 mcg • Pantothenic Acid (as D-calcium pantothenate) 5 mg • Calcium (as carbonate and gluconate) 85 mg • Iron (as ferrous fumarate) 5 mg • Iodine (as potassium iodide) 50 mcg • Magnesium (as magnesium oxide) 15 mg • Zinc (as zinc oxide) 5 mg • Copper (as cupric oxide) 0.5 mg • Manganese (as manganese citrate) 0.5 mg • Chromium (as chromium nicotinate) 10 mcg • Molybdenum (as sodium molybdate) 5 mcg. Other Ingredients: Dextrose, Hydrogenated Vegetable Oil, Stearic Acid, Citric Acid, Magnesium Stearate, Trusil Natural and Artificial Fruit Flavor, Artificial Strawberry Flavor, Orange-Vanilla Flavor, Guar Gum, Blue 2, Red 40, Sucralose, Carrot Powder, Spinach Powder, Licorice Sweetener Powder.

DinoPals **-** FreeLife International
Two chewable tablets contain: Vitamin A (as alpha and beta carotene with dunaliella salina algae) 5000 IU • Vitamin C (as ascorbic acid) 60 mg • Vitamin D (as cholecalciferol) 400 IU • Vitamin E (natural D-alpha tocopheryl succinate) 30 IU • Vitamin K (as phylloquinone) 25 mcg • Vitamin B1 (as thiamin mononitrate) 1.5 mg • Vitamin B2 (as riboflavin) 1.7 mg • Niacin (as niacinamide) 20 mg • Vitamin B6 (as pyridoxine HCl) 2 mg • Folate (as folic acid) 400 mcg • Vitamin B12 (cyanocobalamin) 6 mcg • Biotin 300 mcg • Pantothenic Acid (as D-calcium pantothenate) 10 mg • Calcium (as calcium carbonate/glycine complex) 100 mg • Iodine (as potassium iodide) 150 mcg • Magnesium (as magnesium oxide/glycine complex) 25 mg • Zinc (as zinc citrate/glycine complex) 15 mg • Selenium (as selenomethionine) 20 mcg • Copper (as copper oxide/glycine

complex) 2 mg • Manganese (as manganese sulfate/glycine complex) 2 mg • Chromium (as chromium dinicotinate glycinate) 50 mcg • Molybdenum (molybdenum/glycine complex) 75 mcg • Vanadium (vanadyl sulfate) 25 mcg • Boron (as boron citrate/glycine complex) 1 mg • DinoPals 10:1 Fruit Complex 500 mg: Strawberry, Banana, Raspberry, Melon, Cranberry, Pineapple, Black Currant, Apricot, Cherry, Tangerine, Kiwi, Grape, Apple, Tomato, Peach, Papaya, Guava, Mango • DinoPals 10:1 Vegetable Complex 500 mg: Broccoli, Carrot, Spinach, Beet Greens, Asparagus, Onion, Garlic, Alfalfa, Barley Grass, Artichoke, Peas, Summer Squash • DinoPals Phytoplankton Complex 300 mg: Spirulina, Klamath Blue/Green Algae, Chlorella, Kombu, Cystoseira Brown Algae • DinoPals Friendly Flora Blend 250 million cells: Lactobacillus Acidophilus, L. plantarum, L. salivarius, L. bulgaricus, L. casei, Bifidobacterium infantis, B. bifidum. Other Ingredients: Crystalline Fructose (natural fruit sugar), Sorbitol, Microcrystalline Cellulose, Fruit Flavors, Dried Canola Oil, Vegetable Stearic Acid, Irish Moss Extract, Maltodextrin, Citric Acid, Silica, Vegetable Stearine, Vegetable Magnesium, Natural Color.

Dioxychlor DC3 - American Biologics
2% NaCl • Combined Oxygen. Other Ingredients: Distilled Water.

Dioxychlor OXY-C2 - American Biologics
2% NaCl • Combined Oxygen. Other Ingredients: Water, Carbomer 940.

Disc/Joint - Enzymes, Inc.
Two capsules contain: Vitamin C (100% from Acerola Cherries) 8 mg • Copper (100% as Copper Gluconate) 0.2 mg • Manganese (100% as Manganese Citrate) 5 mg • Proprietary Herbal Blend 750 mg: Methylsulfonylmethane (MSM), Devil's Claw root extract, Boswellia Gum extract, Yucca root extract, Tumeric root extract, Celery seed extract, Grape seed extract • Proprietary Enzyme Blend 221 mg: pHysioProtease, Bromelain, Peptidase • Boron Citrate 10 mg. Other Ingredients: Plant Cellulose, Water.

Disodium Phosphate - Standard Process, Inc.
Three capsules contain: Disodium Phosphate: Phosphorus 580 mg • Sodium 150 mg. Other Ingredients: Gelatin, Calcium Stearate, Water, Colors.

Ditox - Ditox Limited
Each 5 mL bottle contains: Vitamin B1 0.4 mg • Vitamin B6 0.4 mg. Other Ingredients: Alcohol 18%.

Diurex Long Acting Water Capsules - Alva-Amco Pharmacal Cos., Inc.
Each capsule contains: Active Ingredients: Caffeine Anhydrous • Acetaminophen • Potassium Salicylate. Other Ingredients: Non-Pariell seeds, Magnesium Oxide, Titanium Dioxide, plus other coloring & coating ingredients.

Diurex Water Caplets - Alva-Amco Pharmacal Cos., Inc.
Each caplet contains: Active Ingredient: Pamabrom 50 mg. Other Ingredients: Dicalcium Phosphate, FD&C Blue #1, Hydroxypropyl Methylcellulose, Magnesium Stearate, Polyethylene Glycol, Potassium Gluconate, Riboflavin, Stearic Acid, Titanium Dioxide. May also contain: Calcium Sulfate, Croscarmellose Sodium, Microcrystalline Cellulose, Mineral Oil, Polysorbate, Silicon Dioxide, Sodium Lauryl Sulfate.

Diurex Water Pills - Alva-Amco Pharmacal Cos., Inc.
Each pill contains: Active Ingredients: Potassium Salicylate • Caffeine Anhydrous • Salicylamide. Other Ingredients: Calcium Sulfate, Dicalcium Phosphate, Magnesium Trisilicate, Microcrystalline Cellulose, Starch, Magnesium Stearate, Stearic Acid, plus other fillers, coloring & coating ingredients.

Diutrate - Atrium Biotechnologies
Each tablet contains: Buchu leaves 70 mg • Couch grass 70 mg • Hydrangea root 35 mg • Corn Silk 35 mg • Uva Ursi 10 mg • Hypothalamus 30 mg • Raw Kidney concentrate 60 mg • Vitamin B6 16 mg • Magnesium (protein chelated) 50 mg.
See Editor's Note No. 31.

DL-Alpha Vitamin E - GNC
Each capsule contains: Vitamin E (as dl-alpha Tocopheryl Acetate) 400 IU. Other Ingredients: Gelatin, Glycerin.

DLPA - American Biologics
Each capsule contains: DL-Phenylalanine 750 mg. Other Ingredients: Gelatin, Water, Silica, Calcium Sulfate.

DLPA (DL-Phenylalanine) - J. R. Carlson Laboratories, Inc.
Each capsule contains: DL-Phenylalanine 500 mg.

DLPA (DL-phenylalanine) 500 mg - Solgar
Each capsule contains: DLPA (as DL-phenylalanine) 500 mg. Other Ingredients: Vegetable Cellulose, Vegetable Magnesium Stearate, Water, Vegetable Glycerin.

DLPA 750 mg - Pain & Stress Center
Each capsule contains: Vitamin C (as ascorbyl palmitate) 10 mg • Vitamin B6 (as pyridoxine HCl) 15 mg • DL-Phenylalanine 750 mg. Other Ingredients: Gelatin Capsule.

DLPA Factors - Ortho Molecular Products
Two capsules contain: Vitamin B6 (as pyridoxine HCl USP) 40 mg • Folic Acid 800 mcg • DL Phenylalanine 550 mg • L-Methionine USP 225 mg • L-Carnitine Tartrate 100 mg • L-Leucine 40 mg • Valine 25 mg • L-Isoleucine 20 mg. Other Ingredients: Natural Vegetable Capsules, Magnesium Stearate, Microcrystalline Cellulose.

DL-Phenylalanine - J. R. Carlson Laboratories, Inc.
Each 1 tsp serving contains: DL-Phenylalanine 1700 mg.

dl-Phenylalanine - Pure Encapsulations
Each vegetable capsule contains: DL-Phenylalanine (free-form) 500 mg • Vitamin C (as ascorbyl palmitate) 10 mg.

DMAE - Source Naturals
Each tablet contains: DMAE Bitartrate 351 mg. Other Ingredients: Stearic Acid, Dibasic Calcium Phosphate, Magneisum Stearate, Colloidal Silicon Dioxide, Modified Cellulose Gum.

DMAE - PhysioLogics
Each capsule contains: DMAE (as dimethylaminoethanol bitartrate) 100 mg. Other Ingredients: Cellulose (plant origin), Gelatin, Silica, Vegetable Magnesium Stearate.

DMAE - Life Enhancement Products, Inc.
Each capsule contains: DMAE (as dimethyaminoethanol bitartrate) 125 mg.

DMAE 75 mg - N.V. Perricone M.D. Cosmeceuticals
Each softgel contains: DMAE (as 225 mg bitartrate) 75 mg • Nutriene brand Tocotrienols and Tocopherols complex 5 mg. Other Ingredients: Gelatin, Glycerin, Purified Water.

DMAE Firming Fluid - Reviva Labs
Demineralized spring water • DMAE Bitartrate • Glycerin (veg.) • Polysorbate 20 • Sodium Chloride • Simethicone • Hydroxytethylcellulose • Methyl Paraben • Propyl Paraben.

d-Mannose - Pure Encapsulations
Each 1/2 tsp serving contains: D-Mannose 0.9 g.

D-Mannose Powder Plus - Nutrifactor
Each level teaspoon (4.7 g) contains: D-Mannose 1500 mg • Cranberry (vaccinium macrocarpon) 800 mg • Vitamin C (as ascorbic acid) 60 mg. Other Ingredients: Natural Mixed Berry Flavor, Xylitol, Citric Acid, Sucralose.

D-Mannose U-Tract X-Tra - Progressive Labs
Four capsules contain: D-Mannose 2000 mg • Cratavin bark standardized extract (crataeva nurbula) 40 mg • White Willow bark standardized extract (salix alba) 60 mg • Salicin (from white willow bark extract) 9 mg • Swedish Pollen extract (cernitin 63) 20 mg. Other Ingredients: Gelatin, Magnesium Stearate.

Some Brand Name Natural Products - What they Contain

www.NaturalDatabase.com contains MANY more listings than appear here.
Editor's Notes are located on pages 2155-2163.

DMG dimethylglycine - Pure Encapsulations
Each vegetable capsule contains: N,N-Dimethylglycine (free-form, DMG) 125 mg • Vitamin C (as ascorbyl palmitate) 5 mg.

DMG-B15-Plus - Enzymatic Therapy
Each capsule contains: Potassium Aspartate 125 mg • Magnesium Aspartate 125 mg • Calcium Gluconate 31 mg • Other Ingredients: Trimethylglycine (TMG) 100 mg • N,N-Dimethylglycine 100 mg • Glycine 25 mg.

D-MNS - Dial Herbs
Mistletoe • Blessed Thistle • Witch Hazel • Nettle • Shepherd's Purse • Red Raspberry • Cayenne.

DMSA 100 mg - Vital Nutrients
Each capsule contains: DMSA (meso-2, 3-dimercaptosuccinic acid) 100 mg.

DMSA 250 mg - Vital Nutrients
Each capsule contains: DMSA (meso-2, 3-dimercaptosuccinic acid) 250 mg.

DN-24 Hydracreme - Pharmagel
Vitamin Retinyl-A 25000 IU.

DNAble - Life Enhancement Products, Inc.
Three capsules contain: Vitamin C (from niacinamide ascorbate) 500 mg • Vitamin E (from dL-alpha-tocopheryl acetate) 267 IU • Niacin (vitamin B3, as niacinamide and niacinamide ascorbate) 667 mg • Calcium (from tricalcium phosphate) 127 mg • Phosphorus (tricalcium phosphate) 65 mg • N-Acetylcysteine 333 mg • Taurine 33 mg • Resveratrol 8 mg. Other Ingredients: Gelatin, Silicon Dioxide.

DNE Ephedrana 12.5 - D & E Pharmaceuticals
Each tablet contains: Ephedrine HCL 12.5 mg. In a proprietary herbal base of Ephedra, Guarana, Chromium.
See Editor's Note No. 30.

Doctor's A-Z Advanced Ginkgo 24% - Great American Health Products
Each softgel contains: Ginkgo Biloba leaf extract (24% flavone glycosides, 6% terpene lactones) 60 mg.

Doctor's A-Z Advanced Lutein & Bilberry - Great American Health Products
Each softgel contains: Bilberry extract (25% anthocyanidins) 20 mg • FloraGLO Lutein extract (from marigold) 6 mg.

Doctor's A-Z Prostate Health - Great American Health Products
Each capsule contains: Zinc (as zinc picolinate) 15 mg • Saw Palmetto extract (20% fatty acids) 160 mg • Stinging Nettle concentrate 120 mg • Korean Ginseng root 50 mg • Pygeum extract (3% sterols) 50 mg • Pumpkin Seed concentrate 40 mg • Glycine 25 mg • L-Alanine 25 mg • L-Glutamic Acid 25 mg • Beta Sitosterol 20 mg.

Doctor's Choice Antioxidant - Enzymatic Therapy
Three capsules contain: Vitamin A (Beta Carotene) non-toxic form of Vitamin A 10000 IU • Vitamin E (D-Alpha Tocopherol) 200 IU • Vitamin C (Ascorbic Acid) 500 mg • Zinc (Picolinate) 15 mg • Manganese (Gluconate) 15 mg • Riboflavin (Vitamin B2) 6 mg • Selenium (L-Selenomethionine) 200 mcg • N-Acetylcysteine 100 mg • Cabbage extract (Brassica oleracea) 100 mg • Garlic extract, deodorized 100 mg • Ginger root extract 6.5:1 (Zingiber officinale) 100 mg • Green Tea extract (Camellia sinensis) 100 mg • Klamath Blue-Green Algae 100 mg • Curcuma root extract (Curcuma longa) standardized to contain 97% Curcumin 50 mg • Grape seed (PCO) extract (Procyanidolic oligomers (PCO) from grape seed extract) 10 mg. Other Ingredients: Cellulose, Calcium Silicate, Silicon Dioxide, & Gelatin Capsule.

Doctor's Choice Eye Formula - Enzymatic Therapy
Three tablets contain: Vitamin A (Fish Liver oil) 2500 IU • Vitamin A (Beta Carotene) non-toxic form of Vitamin A 2500 IU • Vitamin C (Ascorbic Acid) 600 mg • Vitamin E (D-Alpha Tocopheryl Acetate) 60 IU • Vitamin B2 (Riboflavin) 1.5 mg • Zinc (Picolinate) 9 mg • Selenium (L Selenomethionine) 50 mcg • Copper (Picolinate) 1 mg • Hachimijiogan Herbal Complex 400 mg • Bilberry (Vaccinium myrtillus fructus) Berry extract standardized to contain 25% Anthocyanosides (calculated as Anthocyanidins) 160 mg • Curcuma (Curcuma Longa) root extract standardized to contain 85-97% Curcumin) 50 mg • Grape (Vitis vinifera) seed (PCO) extract standardized to contain 95% Procyanidolic Oligomers (PCOs) 50 mg • Lutein (Marigold flower extract) 2 mg. Other Ingredients: Cellulose, Calcium Carbonate, Cellulose Gum, Stearic Acid, Silicon Dioxide & Magnesium Stearate.

Doctor's Choice Flax Oil - Enzymatic Therapy
Seven softgels contain: Flaxseed Oil 1050 mg • Pumpkin seed oil 1050 mg • Borage seed oil (borago officinalis) 700 mg • Omega-3 (ALA) 2625 mg • Omega-6 (LA) 1313 mg • Omega-9 (oleic acid) 1300 mg • Gamma Linolenic Acid (GLA) 163 mg. Other Ingredients: Gelatin Capsule, Rosemary Leaf Antioxidant (rasemarinus officinalis) S-327.

Doctor's Choice Flax Oil fortified with Borage & Pumpkin - Enzymatic Therapy
Flaxseed oil • Pumpkin seed oil • Borage seed oil • Rosemary Antioxidant S-327 • Average analysis per tablespoon: Omega-3 (LNA) 5250 mg • Omega-6 (LA) 2625 mg • Omega-9 (Oleic) 2600 mg • Gamma-Linolenic Acid (GLA) 325 mg.

Doctor's Choice for 45-Plus Women - Enzymatic Therapy
Six tablets contain: Vitamin A (Beta Carotene) 15000 IU • Vitamin A (Retinol) 2500 IU • Vitamin D 400 IU • Vitamin E (D-Alpha Tocopherol Succinate) 200 IU • Vitamin D 400 IU • Calcium (Citrate, Carbonate) 600 mg • Vitamin C (Ascorbic Acid) 300 mg • Magnesium (Aspartate) 300 mg • Potassium (Aspartate) 99 mg • Vitamin B6 (Pyridoxine HCL) 60 mg • Thiamine HCL (Vitamin B1) 60 mg • Riboflavin (Vitamin B2) 60 mg • Pantothenic Acid (D-Calcium Pantothenate) 50 mg • Niacin/Niacinamide 45 mg • Zinc (Picolinate) 15 mg • Manganese (Citrate) 15 mg • Copper (Gluconate) 1.5 mg • Folic Acid 800 mcg • Vitamin B12 (Cyanocobalamin) 800 mcg • Biotin 600 mcg • Vitamin K (Phytonadione) 60 mcg • Iodine (Kelp) 300 mcg • Chromium (Polynicotinate) 200 mcg • Selenium (L-Selenomet hionine) 100 mcg • Molybdenum (Sodium Molybdate) 25 mcg • Flavonoids mixed 100 mg • Alfalfa juice concentrate 100 mg • Dong Quai extract 4:1 (Angelica sinensis) 90 mg • Ginger root extract 6.5:1 (Zingiber officinale) 15 mg • Green Tea extract (Camellia sinensis) 30 mg • Choline Bitartrate 30 mg • Fennel seed extract 6:1 (Foeniculum vulgare) 30 mg • Inositol 30 mg • PABA (Para-Aminobenzoic Acid) 30 mg • Betaine HCL 25 mg • Glutamic Acid HCL 25 mg • Bromelain 15 mg • Papain 15 mg • Protease acid stable 5 mg • Lipase 5 mg • Boron (Sodium Tetraborate Decahydrate 3 mg • Silica (Sodium Metasilicate) 1 mg • Vanadium (Sulfate) 50 mcg. Other Ingredients: Cellulose, Cellulose Gum, Stearic Acid, Silicon Dioxide & Magnesium Stearate.

Doctor's Choice for 50-Plus Men - Enzymatic Therapy
Four tablets contain: Vitamin A (Beta Carotene) 15000 IU • Vitamin A (Retinol) 2500 IU • Vitamin E (d-Alpha Tocopherol Succinate) 200 IU • Vitamin D (Ergocalciferol) 100 IU • Vitamin C (Ascorbic Acid) 300 mg • Magnesium (Aspartate) 250 mg • Calcium (Citrate Carbonate) 250 mg • Niacin/Niacinamide 120 mg • Pantothenic Acid (D-Calcium Pantothenate) 100 mg • Potassium (Aspartate) 99 mg • Thiamine HCL (Vitamin B1) 60 mg • Riboflavin (Vitamin B2) 60 mg • Vitamin B6 (Pyridoxine HCL) 60 mg • Zinc (Picolinate) 30 mg • Manganese (Citrate) 15 mg • Copper (Gluconate) 1.5 mg • Folic Acid 800 mcg • Vitamin B12 (Cyanocobalamin) 800 mcg • Biotin 600 mcg • Iodine (Kelp) 300 mcg • Chromium (Polynicotinate) 200 mcg • Selenium (L-Selenomethionine) 100 mcg • Vitamin K (Phytonadione)

BRAND NAMES

60 mcg • Molybdenum (Sodium Molybdate) 25 mcg • Mixed Flavonoids citrus 100 mg • Saw Palmetto Berry extract 4:1 (Serenoa repens) 80 mg • Ginger root extract 6.5:1 (Zingiber officinale) 60 mg • Alfalfa juice concentrate 60 mg • Choline Bitartrate 30 mg • Inositol 30 mg • PABA (Para-Aminobenzoic Acid) 30 mg • Green Tea extract (Camellia sinensis) 30 mg • Betaine HCL 25 mg • Glutamic Acid HCL 25 mg • Korean Ginseng root extract (Panax ginseng) standardized to contain 7% Saponins (calculated as Rg1) 15 mg • Bromelain 15 mg • Papain 15 mg • Protease acid stable 5 mg • Lipase 5 mg • Boron (Sodium Tetraborate Decahydrate) 2 mg • Vanadium (Sulfate) 50 mcg. Other Ingredients: Cellulose, Stearic Acid, Cellulose Gum, Silicon Dioxide, & Magnesium Stearate.

Doctor's Choice for Arthritics - Enzymatic Therapy
Two tablets contain: Niacin/Niacinamide 330 mg • Pantothenic Acid (D-Calcium Pantothenate) 100 mg • Magnesium (Oxide) 100 mg • Calcium Chloride 32 mg • Vitamin C (Ascorbic Acid) 30 mg • Zinc (Picolinate) 3 mg • Manganese (Chelate) 3 mg • Glucosamine Sulfate 500 mg • PABA (Para-Aminobenzoic Acid) 400 mg • Bio-Min TR8 a source of trace minerals 100 mg • Glutamic Acid HCL 40 mg • Ammonium Chloride 32 mg • Betaine HCL 20 mg • Chlorophyll 10 mg • Boron (Sodium Tetraborate Decahydrate) 3 mg. Other Ingredients: Cellulose, Cellulose Gum, Stearic Acid, Silicon Dioxide, Magnesium Stearate, Alfalfa (Medicago sativa) leaves & stems juice concentrate, Black Cohosh (Cimicituga racemosa) root, Licorice (Glycyrrhiza glabra) root extract & Scullcap (Scutellaria baicalensis) whole plant.

Doctor's Choice for Bone Health - Enzymatic Therapy
Three tablets contain: Vitamin C (Ascorbic Acid) 100 mg • Vitamin D (Fish Liver oil) 300 IU • Vitamin K (Phytonadione) 300 mcg • Folic Acid 800 mcg • Vitamin B12 (Cyanocobalamin) 800 mcg • Calcium (Krebs Cycle Chelate) 600 mg • Magnesium (Krebs Cycle Chelate) 150 mg • Vitamin C (Ascorbic Acid) 100 mg • Zinc (Picolinate) 15 mg • Sodium 6 mg • Copper (Picolinate) 1 mg • Mixed Flavonoids (Citrus) 100 mg • Betaine HCL 30 mg • Soy Bean extract standardized to contain 25% Saponins & 13-17% Isoflavones calculated as Genistein 20 mg • Boron (Sodium Tetrahydroborate) 3 mg • Silicon (Sodium Metasilicate) 1 mg • Strontium (Chloride) 500 mcg. Other Ingredients: Cellulose, Cellulose Gum, Stearic Acid, Silicon Dioxide, Magnesium Stearate.

Doctor's Choice for Diabetics - Enzymatic Therapy
Two tablets contain: Vitamin E (Mixed Tocopherols) 100 IU • Vitamin C (Ascorbic Acid) 300 mg • Magnesium (Krebs Cycle Chelate) 100 mg • Vitamin B6 (Pyridoxine HCL) 10 mg • Manganese (Krebs Cycle Chelate) 7.5 mg • Zinc (Picolinate) 7.5 mg • Copper (Picolinate) 0.5 mg • Biotin 1000 mcg • Folic Acid 400 mcg • Vitamin B12 (Cyanocobalamin) 400 mcg • Chromium (Picolinate) 200 mcg • Selenium (Aspartate) 50 mcg • Gymnema sylvestre leaves extract standardized to contain 25% Gymnemic Acid 200 mg • Bitter Melon extract (Momordica charantia) 200 mg • Fenugreek seed extract (4:1) (Trigonella foenum-graecum) 100 mg • Bilberry extract (Vaccinium myrtillus fructus) standardized to contain 25% Anthocyanosides calculated as Anthocyanidins) 40 mg • Mixed Bioflavonoids (Citrus) 25 mg • Vanadyl Sulfate 5 mg. Other Ingredients: Calcium Carbonate, Cellulose, Cellulose Gum, Silicon Dioxide, Dicalcium Phosphate, Magnesium Stearate & Calcium Silicate.

Doctor's Choice for Female Teens - Enzymatic Therapy
Four tablets contain: Vitamin A (Beta Carotene) 15000 IU • Vitamin A (Retinol) 2500 IU • Vitamin E (D-Alpha Tocopherol Succinate) 200 IU • Vitamin D (Ergocalciferol) 100 IU • Calcium (Citrate, Carbonate) 500 mg • Vitamin C (Ascorbic Acid) 300 mg • Magnesium (Aspartate) 200 mg • Potassium (Aspartate) 99 mg • Vitamin B6 (Pyridoxine HCL) 90 mg • Niacin/Niacinamide 45 mg • Iron (Ferrous Succinate) 30 mg • Pantothenic Acid (D-Calcium Pantothenate) 30 mg • Thiamine HCL (Vitamin B1) 30 mg • Riboflavin (Vitamin B2) 30 mg • Zinc (Picolinate) 20 mg • Manganese (Citrate) 15 mg • Copper (Gluconate) 1.5 mg • Folic Acid 800 mcg • Vitamin B12 (Cyanocobalamin) 800 mcg • Biotin 300 mcg • Iodine (Kelp) 300 mcg • Chromium (Polynicotinate) 200 mcg • Selenium (L-Selenomethionine) 100 mcg • Vitamin K (Phytonadione) 60 mcg • Molybdenum (Sodium molybdate) 25 mcg • Mixed Flavonoids (Citrus) 100 mg • Alfalfa juice concentrate 60 mg • Choline Bitartrate 60 mg • Inositol 60 mg • Ginger root extract 6.5:1 (Zingiber officinale) 60 mg • 8 Dandelion root extract 4:1 (Taraxacum officinale) 60 mg • Licorice root extract (Glycyrrhiza glabra) standardized to contain 5% Glycyrrhizic Acid 30 mg • Boron (Sodium Tetraborate Decahydrate) 2 mg • Silica (Sodium Metasilicate) 1 mg • Vanadium (Sulfate) 50 mcg. Other Ingredients: Cellulose, Cellulose Gum, Stearic Acid, Magnesium Stearate & Silicon Dioxide.

Doctor's Choice for Healthy Cholesterol Levels - Enzymatic Therapy
Each capsule contains: Red Yeast Rice (Standardized to contain 1% Mevinolin) 475 mg • Artichoke (Cynara scolymus) leaf extract 50 mg • Ginger (Zingiber officinale) root extract 50 mg • Coenzyme Q10 (CoQ10) 8 mg. Other Ingredients: Soybean oil, Vegetable oil, Beeswax, Lecithin, and Gelatin capsule.

Doctor's Choice for Heart Health - Enzymatic Therapy
Two tablets contain: Vitamin E (D-Alpha Tocopherol) 100 IU • Magnesium (Oxide) 150 mg • Niacin 100 mg • Vitamin C (Ascorbic Acid) 100 mg • Potassium (Chloride) 75 mg • Calcium Pangamate 20 mg • Vitamin B6 (Pyridoxine HCL) 10 mg • Sodium 6 mg • Folic Acid 200 mcg • Vitamin B12 (Cyanocobalamin) 200 mcg • Hawthorne berry extract (Crataegus oxyacantha) standardized to contain 1.8% Vitexin-2'-Rhamnoside 150 mg • Super Seven Complex Mixture of Herbs: Hydrangea, Black Cohosh (Cimicifuga racemosa), Buchu leaves, Couch Grass, Corn Silk, Dandelion leaf (Taraxacum officinale) & Ginger root (Zingiber officinale) 150 mg • Khella extract (Ammi visnaga) standardized to contain a minimum of 10% Pyrones calculated as Khellin 100 mg • L-Cysteine 100 mg • Carbamide 100 mg. Other Ingredients: Cellulose, Cellulose Gum, Stearic Acid, Sodium Starch, Glycolate, Silicon Dioxide, Magnesium Stearate & Vanillin.

Doctor's Choice for Joint Health Capsules - Enzymatic Therapy
Four capsules contain: Vitamin C (ascorbic acid) 100 mg • Niacin (as niacinamide, niacin) 330 mg • Vitamin B6 (as pyridoxine HCl) 20 mg • Pantothenic Acid (as calcium d-pantothenate) 100 mg • Magnesium (as magnesium oxide) 100 mg • Zinc (as zinc picolinate) 3 mg • Copper (as copper gluconate) 200 mcg • Manganese (as manganese chelate) 2.5 mg • Chloride (from glucosamine sulfate) 78 mg • Sodium 55 mg • Glucosamine Sulfate (stabilized) 500 mg • Boswellia Serrata gum resin extract (standardized to contain 65% boswellic acids) 400 mg • Proprietary Trace Mineral Blend 24 mg: Selenium (as selenium yeast), Silicon (as magnesium trisilicate), Boron (as sodium borate), Nickel (as nickel chelate), Tin (as tin chelate), Molybdenum (as sodium molybdate), Vanadium (as vanadyl sulfate) • Boron (as sodium borate) 3 mg. Other Ingredients: Cellulose, Gelatin, Magnesium Stearate, Titanium Dioxide Color, Silicon Dioxide, Alfalfa Aerial Part Extract 10:1, Black Cohosh Root Extract 4:1, Licorice Root/Rhizome Extract, Chinese Skullcap Root Extract 4:1.

Doctor's Choice for Joint Health Tablets - Enzymatic Therapy
Two tablets contain: Vitamin C (ascorbic acid) 100 mg • Niacin (as niacinamide, niacin) 330 mg • Vitamin B6 (as pyridoxine HCl) 20 mg • Pantothenic Acid (as calcium d-pantothenate) 100 mg • Magnesium (as magnesium oxide) 100 mg • Zinc (as zinc picolinate) 3 mg • Copper (as copper gluconate) 200 mcg • Manganese (as manganese chelate) 2.5 mg • Chloride (from glucosamine sulfate) 78 mg • Sodium 60 mg • Glucosamine Sulfate (stabilized) 500 mg • Boswellia Serrata gum resin extract (standardized to contain 65% boswellic acids) 400 mg • Proprietary Trace Mineral Blend 24 mg: Selenium (as selenium yeast), Silicon (as magnesium trisilicate), Boron (as sodium borate), Nickel (as nickel chelate), Tin (as tin chelate), Molybdenum (as sodium molybdate), Vanadium (as vanadyl sulfate) • Boron (as

sodium borate) 3 mg. Other Ingredients: Cellulose, Modified Cellulose, Modified Cellulose Gum, Magnesium Stearate, Titanium Dioxide Color, Lecithin, Alfalfa Aerial Part Extract 10:1, Black Cohosh Root Extract 4:1, Licorice Root/Rhizome Extract, Chinese Skullcap Root Extract 4:1, Carnauba Wax.

Doctor's Choice for Male Teens - Enzymatic Therapy
Four tablets contain: Vitamin A (Beta Carotene) 15000 IU • Vitamin A (Retinol) 2500 IU • Vitamin E (D-Alpha Tocopherol Succinate) 200 IU • Vitamin D (Ergocalciferol) 100 IU • Calcium (Citrate, Carbonate) 400 mg • Vitamin C (Ascorbic Acid) 300 mg • Magnesium (Aspartate) 200 mg • Potassium (Aspartate) 99 mg • Niacin/Niacinamide 45 mg • Pantothenic Acid (D-CalciumPantothenate) 30 mg • Vitamin B6 (Pyridoxine HCL) 30 mg • Thiamine HCL (Vitamin B1) 30 mg • Riboflavin (Vitamin B2) 30 mg • Zinc (Picolinate) 30 mg • Manganese (Citrate) 15 mg • Copper (Gluconate) 1.5 mg • Folic Acid 800 mcg • Vitamin B12 (Cyanocobalamin) 800 mcg • Iodine (Kelp) 300 mcg • Chromium (Polynicotinate) 200 mcg • Selenium (L-Selenomethionine) 100 mcg • Vitamin K (Phytonadione) 60 mcg • Molybdenum (sodium Molybdate) 25 mcg • Biotin 300 mcg • Mixed Flavonoids (Citrus) 100 mg • Alfalfa juice concentrate 60 mg • Dandelion root extract 4:1 (Taraxacum officinale) 60 mg • Ginger root extract 6.5:1 (Zingiber officinale) 60 mg • Sarsaparilla root extract 4:1 (Simlax officinalis) 60 mg • Choline Bitartrate 30 mg • Inositol 30 mg • Boron (Sodium Tetraborate Decahydrate) 2 mg • Vanadium (Sulfate) 50 mcg.

Doctor's Choice for Men - Enzymatic Therapy
Three tablets contain: Vitamin A (Beta Carotene) non-toxic form of Vitamin A 15000 IU • Vitamin A (Retinol) 2500 IU • Vitamin E (D-Alpha Tocopherol Succinate) 200 IU • Vitamin D 100 IU • Magnesium (Aspartate, Chloride) 400 mg • Vitamin C (Ascorbic Acid) 300 mg • Calcium (Citrate, Carbonate) 200 mg • Potassium (Aspartate) 99 mg • Niacin 90 mg • Thiamine HCL (Vitamin B1) 60 mg • Riboflavin (Vitamin B2) 60 mg • Vitamin B6 (Pyridoxine HCL) 60 mg • Pantothenic Acid (D-Calcium Pantothenate) 60 mg • Zinc (Picolinate) 30 mg • Manganese (Citrate) 5 mg • Copper (Gluconate) 1 mg • Folic Acid 800 mcg • Vitamin B12 (Cyanocobalamin) 800 mcg • Biotin 600 mcg • Iodine (Kelp) 300 mcg • Chromium (Polynicotinate) 200 mcg • Selenium (Selenomethionine) 200 mcg • Vitamin K (Phytonadione) 60 mcg • Molybdenum (Sodium Molybdate) 25 mcg • Flavonoids mixed 50 mg • Alfalfa juice concentrate 50 mg • Choline Bitartrate 30 mg • Inositol 30 mg • Ginger root extract 6.5:1 (Zingiber officinale) 30 mg • Green Tea extract (Camellia sinensis) standardized to contain 70% Polyphenols 30 mg • Muira Puama extract 6:1 (Ptychopetalum olacoides) 30 mg • PABA (Para-Aminobenzoic Acid) 30 mg • Saw Palmetto Berry extract 4:1 (Serenoa repens) 30 mg • Korean Ginseng root extract (Panax ginseng) standardized to contain 7% Saponins (calculated as Ginsenoside Rg1) 15 mg • Carotenes from natural sources 5 mg • Boron (Sodium Tetraborate Decahydrate) 2 mg • Vanadium (Sulfate) 50 mcg. Other Ingredients: Cellulose, Cellulose Gum, Stearic Acid, Silicon Dioxide & Magnesium Stearate.

Doctor's Choice for Women - Enzymatic Therapy
Four tablets contain: Vitamin A (Beta Carotene) non-toxic form of Vitamin A 15000 IU • Vitamin A (Retinol) 2500 IU • Vitamin E (D-Alpha Tocopherol Succinate) 200 IU • Vitamin D 100 IU • Calcium (Citrate, Carbonate) 400 mg • Vitamin C (Ascorbic Acid) 300 mg • Magnesium (Aspartate, Chloride) 300 mg • Potassium (Aspartate) 99 mg • Vitamin B6 (Pyridoxine HCL) 90 mg • Niacin/Niacinamide 90 mg • Thiamine HCL (Vitamin B1) 60 mg • Riboflavin (Vitamin B2) 60 mg • Pantothenic Acid (D-Calcium Pantothenate) 30 mg • Zinc (Picolinate) 20 mg • Iron (Ferrous Succinate) 18 mg • Manganese (Citrate) 5 mg • Vitamin B6 (Pyridoxal-5-Phosphate) 5 mg • Copper (Gluconate) 1 mg • Folic Acid 800 mcg • Vitamin B12 (Cyanocobalamin) 800 mcg • Biotin 600 mcg • Iodine (Kelp) 300 mcg • Chromium (Polynicotinate) 200 mcg • Selenium (Selenomethionine) 200 mcg • Vitamin K (Phytonadione) 60 mcg • Molybdenum (Sodium molybdate) 25 mcg • Flavonoids, mixed 50 mg • Alfalfa juice concentrate 50 mg • Choline Bitartrate 30 mg • Inositol 30 mg • Dong Quai extract 4:1 (Angelica sinensis) 30 mg • Ginger root extract (6.5:1) (Zingiber officinale) 30 mg • Licorice root extract (Glycyrrhiza glabra) standardized to contain 5% Glycyrrhizic Acid 30 mg • PABA (Para-Aminobenzoic Acid) 30 mg • Chaste Tree Berry extract 5:1 (Vitex agnus-castus) 15 mg • Fennel seed extract 6:1 (Foeniculum vulgare) 15 mg • Carotenes from natural sources 5 mg • Boron (Sodium Tetraborate Decahydrate) 3 mg • Silica (Sodium Metasilicate) 1 mg • Vanadium (Sulfate) 50 mcg. Other Ingredients: Cellulose, Cellulose Gum, Magnesium Stearate, Stearic Acid, & Silicon Dioxide.

Doctor's Choice Prenatal Supplement - Enzymatic Therapy
Four tablets contain: Vitamin A (Beta Carotene) 15000 IU • Vitamin E (D-Alpha Tocopherol Succinate) 200 IU • Vitamin D (Ergocalciferol) 100 IU • Calcium (Citrate, Carbonate) 800 mg • Magnesium (Citrate) 400 mg • Vitamin C (Ascorbic Acid) 300 mg • Vitamin B6 (Pyridoxine HCL) 120 mg • Pantothenic Acid (D-Calcium Pantothenate) 100 mg • Potassium (Aspartate) 99 mg • Thiamine HCL (Vitamin B1) 60 mg • Riboflavin (Vitamin B2) 60 mg • Niacin/Niacinamide 45 mg • Iron (Ferrous succinate) 30 mg • Zinc (Picolinate) 30 mg • Manganese (Citrate) 15 mg • Copper (Gluconate) 1.5 mg • Folic Acid 800 mcg • Vitamin B12 (Cyanocobalamin) 800 mcg • Biotin 600 mcg • Vitamin K (Phytonadione) 500 mcg • Iodine (Kelp) 300 mcg • Chromium (Polynicotinate) 200 mcg • Selenium (L-Selenomethionine) 100 mcg • Molybdenum (Sodium Molybdate) 25 mcg • Ginger root extract 6.5:1 (Zingiber officinale) 150 mg • Mixed Flavonoids (Citrus) 90 mg • Choline Bitartrate 90 mg • Inositol 90 mg • Dandelion root extract 4:1 (Taraxacum officinale) 60 mg • Red Raspberry leaves 60 mg • Boron (Sodium Tetraborate Decahydrate) 1 mg • Silica (Sodium Metasilicate) 1 mg • Vanadium (Sulfate) 50 mcg. Other Ingredients: Cellulose, Cellulose Gum, Stearic Acid, Silicon Dioxide & Magnesium Stearate.

Dolicare Cold & Flu - Dolisos
Each tablet contains: Aconitum Napellus 3C • Belladonna 3C • Echinacea Angustifolia 3C • Eupatorium Perfoliatum 3C • Ferrum Phosphoricum 3C • Gelsemium Sempervirens 3C • Anas Barbariae Hepatis et Cordis Extractum 200C. Other Ingredients: Dextrose, Magnesium Stearate.
See Editor's Note No. 1.

Dolicare Fatigue - Dolisos
Each tablet contains: Ignatia 4C • Phosphoric Acid 4C • Rhus Toxicodendron 4C • Selenium 4C. Other Ingredients: Dextrose, Magnesium Stearate.
See Editor's Note No. 1.

Dolicare Hayfever & Allergy - Dolisos
Each tablet contains: Allium Cepa 3C • Amrosia Artemisaefolia 3C • Euphrasia Officinalis 3C • Sabadilla 3C • Sticta Pulmonatira 3C • Apis Mellifica 5C. Other Ingredients: Dextrose, Magnesium Stearate.
See Editor's Note No. 1.

Dolicare Heartburn - Dolisos
Each tablet contains: Solidago Virgaurea 3X • Abies Nigra 3C • Argentum Nitricum 3C • Bryonia Alba 3C • Condurango 3C • Nux Vomica 3C • Robinia Pseudoacacia 3C. Other Ingredients: Dextrose, Magnesium Stearate.
See Editor's Note No. 1.

Dolicare Leg Cramps - Dolisos
Each tablet contains: Arnica Montana 4C • Colocynthis 4C • Cuprum Metallicum 4C • Magnesia Phosphorica 4C • Nux Vomica 4C.
See Editor's Note No. 1.

Dolicare Motion Sickness - Dolisos
Each tablet contains: Conium Maculatum 4C • Tabacum 4C • Calcarea Carbonica 5C • Cocculus Indicus 5C • Ignatia Amara 5C • Petroleum 5C. Other Ingredients: Dextrose, Magnesium Stearate.
See Editor's Note No. 1.

Some Brand Name Natural Products - What they Contain

www.NaturalDatabase.com contains MANY more listings than appear here.
Editor's Notes are located on pages 2155-2163.

Dolicare Nasal Decongestant - Dolisos
Each tablet contains: Belladonna 3C • Euphorbium Officinarum 3C • Sanquinaria Canadensis 3C • Hydrastis Canadensis 4C • Sticta Pulmonaria 4C • Corallium Rubrum 4C • Kali Bichromicum 5C. Other Ingredients: Dextrose, Magnesium Stearate.
See Editor's Note No. 1.

Dolicare Night-Time Sleep-Aid - Dolisos
Two tablets contain: Coffea Cruda 4C • Ignatia Amara 4C • Passiflora Incarnata 3X • Phosphoricum Acidum 7C. Other Ingredients: Dextrose, Magnesium Stearate.
See Editor's Note No. 1.

Dolicare Stop Smokin - Dolisos
Each tablet contains: Lobelia Inflata 4C • Antimonium Crudum 5C • Argentumnitricum 5C • Gelsemium Sempervirens 5C • Nux Vomica 5C • Staphysagria 5C. Other Ingredients: Dextrose, Magnesium Stearate.
See Editor's Note No. 1.

Dolicare Weight Control - Dolisos
Each tablet contains: Anacardium Orientale 4C • Antimonium Crudum 4C • Calcarea Carbonica 4C • Graphites 4C • Iodium 4C • Nux Vomica 4C. Other Ingredients: Dextrose, Magnesium Stearate.
See Editor's Note No. 1.

Dolichild Calm (grape flavor) - Dolisos
Active Ingredients: Passiflora Incarnata 3X • Chamomilla 5C • Cina 5C • Correa Cruda 7C • Tarentula Hispanica 7C • Zincum Valerianicum 7C. Base: Ascorbic Acid, Citric ACid, Glycerin, Natural Grape Flavoring, Purified Water, < 0.3% Ethanol USP.
See Editor's Note No. 1.

Dolichild Colic - Dolisos
Twenty drops contain: Colocynthis 3C • Chamomilla 3C • Bryonia 5C • Magnesia Phosphorica 5C • Nux Vomica 5C • Veratrum Album 5C • Cuprum Metallicum 6C. Base: Ascorbic Acid, Citric Acid, Glycerin, Natural Peach Flavoring, Purified Water, < 0.3% Ethanol USP.
See Editor's Note No. 1.

Dolichild Cough (cherry flavor) - Dolisos
Solidago Virgaurea 1C • Arnica Montana 3C • Belladonna 3C • Cina 3C • Coccus Cacti 3C • Drosera Rotundifolia 3C • Ipecacuanha 3C • Corallium Rubrum 5C • Ferrum Phosphoricum 5C • Cuprum Metallicum 6C. Base: Ascorbic Acid, Citric Acid, Glycerin, Natural Cherry Flavoring, Purified Water, < 0.3% Ethanol USP.
See Editor's Note No. 1.

Dolichild Earache (banana flavor) - Dolisos
Twenty drops contain: Plantago Major 3X • Arsenicum Album 5C • Belladonna 5C • Capsicum Annuum 5C • Chamomilla 5C • Ferrum Phosphoricum 5C. Base: Ascorbic Acid, Citric Acid, Glycerin, Natural Banana Flavoring, Purified Water, < 0.4% Ethanol USP.
See Editor's Note No. 1.

Dolichild Teething (raspberry flavor) - Dolisos
Twenty drops contain: Plantago Major 3X • Belladonna 3C • Coffea Cruda 3C • Chamomilla 3C • Rheum Officinale 3C • Borax 5C • Calcarea Phosphorica 5C. Base: Ascorbic Acid, Citric Acid, Glycerin, Natural Raspberry Flavoring, Purified Water, < 0.1% Ethanol USP.
See Editor's Note No. 1.

Dolicoccil Flu Solution - Dolisos
Each single dose tube contains: Anas Barbariae Hepatis Et Cordis Extractum (HPUS) 9C • Cuprum Gluconicum 3C • Echinacea Angustifolia (HPUS) 3C. Other Ingredients: Lactose, Sucrose.
See Editor's Note No. 1.

Dolicough Solution - Dolisos
Solidago Virga Aurea 1C • Arnica Montana 3C • Belladonna 3C • Cina 3C • Coccus Cacti 3C • Drosera Rotundifolia 3C • Ipecacuanha 3C • Corallium Rubrum 5C • Ferrum Phosphoricum 5C • Ascorbic Acid • Citric Acid • Ethanol (1.25%) • Glycerin • Honey • Natural Lemon Flavor • Purified Water.
See Editor's Note No. 1.

Dolivaxil - Dolisos
Each tube contains: Influenzium (HPUS) 9C. Inactive Ingredients: Sucrose, Lactose.
See Editor's Note No. 1.

Dolomite - Nature's Plus
Four tablets contain: Calcium (from dolomite) 633 mg • Magnesium (from dolomite) 360 mg • Dolomite (44 grains) 2850 mg. Other Ingredients: Microcrystalline Cellulose, Stearic Acid, Magnesium Stearate, Silica, Pharmaceutical Glaze.

Dolomite - The Vitamin Shoppe
Four tablets contain: Calcium 520 mg • Magnesium 312 mg.

Dolomite - Puritan's Pride
One tablet contains: Calcium (as Dolomite) 130 mg • Magnesium (as Dolomite) 78 mg.

Dolomite 1g - Golden Glow Natural Health Products
Each tablet contains: Dolomite 1 g: Calcium 215 mg, Magnesium 130 mg. Other Ingredients: Sucrose, Gluten.

DONA Crystalline Glucosamine Sulfate - Rotta Pharmaceuticals
Each packet contains: Sodium 150 mg • Crystalline Glucosamine Sulfate 1884 mg • Glucosamine Sulfate 1500 mg.

Dona Glucosamine Sulfate - Rotta Pharmaceuticals
Each packet contains: Crystalline Glucosamine Sulfate 1500 mg.

Dong Quai - Leiner Health Products
Each caplet contains: Dong Quai extract (Angelica sinensis) root 200 mg • Ligustilides (Dong Quai extract) 2 mg. Other Ingredients: Cellulose, Calcium Carbonate, Stearic Acid, Croscarmellose Sodium, Silicon Dioxide, Magnesium Stearate.

Dong Quai - Nature's Way
Two capsules contain: Dong Quai root 1110 mg. Other Ingredients: Gelatin, Magnesium stearate.

Dong Quai - Olympian Labs
Each capsule contains: Dong Quai 500 mg.

Dong Quai & Royal Jelly - Puritan's Pride
Each capsule contains: Dong Quai root powder 200 mg • Royal Jelly powder (from Royal Jelly 2:1 150 mg) 300 mg.

Dong Quai (Angelica sinensis) - Solgar
Each capsule contains: Iron 1 mg • Dong Quai root 2:1 extract 50 mg • Raw Dong Quai root Powder 200 mg. Other Ingredients: Vegetable Cellulose, Microcrystalline Cellulose, Vegetable Magnesium Stearate, Silica, Water, Vegetable Glycerin.

Dong Quai and Royal Jelly - GNC
Each capsule contains: Dong Quai 300 mg • Agnus Castus berry 50 mg • Royal Jelly 50 mg • Wild Yam root 50 mg.

Dong Quai Extract - Montana Naturals, Inc.
Each capsule contains: Dong Quai 200 mg.

Dong Quai Extract in Vegetable Glycerin - Nature's Herbs
Each drop contains: Dong Quai 565 mg.

Dong Quai Root - GNC
Each capsule contains: Dong Quai 250 mg.

Dong Quai Supreme - Gaia Herbs
Thirty drops contain: Proprietary Blend 100 mg: Dried Chinese Dong Quai root (angelica sinensis), Helonias root (chamaelirium luteum), Black Cohosh root (cimicifuga racemosa), Partridgeberry (mitchella repens), Saw Palmetto berry (serenoa repens), Dried Licorice root (glycyrrhiza glabra and glycyrrhiza uralensis), Fresh Ginger rhizome (zingiber officinale), 30-40% Pure Grain Alcohol USP, Spring Water.

Double C - Life Enhancement Products, Inc.
Each capsule contains: Vitamin C (from calcium ascorbate and ascorbyl palmitate) 608 mg • Calcium (from calcium ascorbate) 61 mg. Other Ingredients: Gelatin Capsule.

Double Deers Formula Cardioflex - Kingsway Trading Inc
Unknown.
See Editor's Note No. 55.

Double Deers Formula Expellin Extract - Kingsway Trading Inc
Unknown.
See Editor's Note No. 55.

Double G SuperPower - DreamPharm
Each capsule contains: Panax Ginseng 250 mg • Ginkgo Biloba leaf extract (standardized to 20%) 80 mg • Ligusticum Chuan Xiang root 100 mg • Angelica Sinensis root 70 mg.

Double Strength Glucosamine 500 MG Chondroitin 400 MG - Puritan's Pride
Three tablets contain: Glucosamine Hydrochloride 1500 mg • Chondroitin Sulfate 1200 mg. Other Ingredients: Povidone, Beet Juice Color, Vegetable Magnesium Stearate, Silica, Cellulose (plant origin).
See Editor's Note No. 15.

Double Strength Pro Energy - Pro Health
Three capsules contain: Thiamin (vitamin B1 as thiamine HCl) 51 mg • Vitamin B6 (as pyridoxine HCl) 51 mg • Magnesium (as magnesium glycinate) 52.6 mg • Malic Acid from Apple 1200 mg • L-Tyrosine 75 mg. Other Ingredients: Rice Flour, Gelatin, Microcrystalline Cellulose, Magnesium Stearate, Water.

Double Strength Ultra ATP+ - Pro Health
Three tablets contain: Magnesium (from magnesium oxide) 125 mg • Malic Acid 1200 mg. Other Ingredients: Dicalcium Phosphate, Microcrystalline Cellulose, Stearic Acid, Magnesium Stearate, Silicon Dioxide, Pharmaceutical Glaze.

Down Size - Dial Herbs
Purified Water • Hydrolyzed Collagen • Glycerine • Natural Flavors • Aloe concentrate • Acesulfame Potassium • Citric Acid • Potassium Sorbate • Sodium Benzoate • Potassium Iodide.

DP-Transdermal Cream - Life Enhancement Products, Inc.
Aloe Vera gel • Distilled Water • C10-C18 Triglycerides • Tocopherol • Polyethylene Glycol esters • Octyl Palmitate • Glyceryl Stearate • Isopropyl Alcohol • Cetyl Alcohol • Emulsifying wax NF • Avocado oil • Glycerine • Pregnenolone • Dehydroepiandrosterone • Panthenol • Hydrolyzed Protein • Hyaluronic Acid • Lemon oil • Carbomer 940 • Methylparaben • Proplyparaben.

Dr. Art Ulene's Glucosamine Plus Dietary Supplement - Nature's Bounty
Two tablets contain: Niacin (B3) 100 mg • Curcumin 100 mg • Glucosamine Hydrochloride 730 mg • Frankincense Extract (boswellia serrata, roxb. excolabr, gum resin) 300 mg • Glucosamine Sulfate 50 mg • Quercetin 100 mg • Turmeric (Curcuma longa, rhizome powder) 100 mg.

Dr. Bob Martin's Ring Stop - NaturalCare
Active Ingredients: Calcarea Carbonica (calcium carbonate) 8X, 30X • Cimicufuga Racemose (black snake root) 3X, 6X, 12X, 30X • Carbo Vegetabilis (vegetable charcoal) 8X, 12X, 30X • Cinchona Officinalis (peruvian bark) 3X, 6X, 30X • Chininum Sulphuricum (sulphite of quinine) 12X, 30X • Coffea Cruda (unroasted coffee) 3X, 12X • Graphites (plumbago) 8X, 12X, 30X • Kali Carbonicum (potassium carbonate) 12X, 30X • Lycopodium (club moss) 6X, 12X, 30X • Natrum Salicylicum (sodium salicylate) 6X • Salicylicum Acidum (salicyclic acid) 6X. Inactive Ingredients: Alpha Lipoic Acid, Butcher's Broom leaf extract, Chinese herbs: Black Sesame seed (hei zhi ma), Cassia bark (gui zhi), Peony root (chi shao), Pueraria (ge gen)(root), Jobs Tears seed (yi yi ten), Ligusticum Wallichii root (chuan xiong) • CoEnzyme Q10, Cyanocobalamin, Folic Acid, Garlic bulb extract (odor-controlled), Ginger (root), Ginkgo Biloba leaf extract 24/6%, Inositol Hexaniacinate, Kelp Extract, L-Arginine Hydrochloride, Magnesium Amino Acid Chelate, Methyl Cobalamin, N-Acetyl-Carnitine HCl, N-Acetylcystine, Pyridoxine HCl, Riboflavin, Thiamine Mononitrate, Vinpocetine, Vitamin A Acetate, Zinc Amino Acid Chelate.
See Editor's Note No. 1.

Dr. Earl Mindell's 4-SIGHT - FreeLife International
Two caplets contain: Vitamin A as Beta-Carotene 5000 IU • Vitamin C (from Citri-C brand complex) 60 mg • Vitamin E (as natural D-alpha tocopheryl succinate) 30 IU • Selenium (as selenomethionine) 50 mcg • Taurine 400 mg • Bilberry fruit standardized extract (25% anthocyanosides) 160 mg • Citri-C brand complex 100 mg: Ascorbic Acid, Iso-Ascorbic Acid, Citrus Glycosyl Flavones • Vision Support Herbal Blend 100 mg: Eyebright aerial parts, Ginkgo Biloba leaf extract, Green Tea leaf extract, Grape seed extract • N-Acetylcysteine 50 mg • Quercetin Dihydrate 25 mg • Lutein (as mixed xanthophylls from marigold flower) 6 mg. Other ingredients: Calcium Hydrogen Phosphate, Cellulose, Cellulose Gum, Vegetable Stearic Acid, Colloidal Silica, Vegetable Magnesium Stearate, Vita-Coat brand: Vegetable Resin, Alpha-Lipoic Acid.

Dr. Earl Mindell's Okinawan Coral Calcium - FreeLife International
Two caplets contain: Coral Calcium (Okinawa marine grade) 1500 mg • Vitamin D (as cholecalciferol) 200 IU • Calcium (from coral calcium) 360 mg • Magnesium (from coral calcium) 180 mg • MSM brand purified Methylsulfonylmethane 200 mg • Aquamin brand Trace Minerals (from phymatolithon calcareum sea algae) 50 mg • Soyatab brand (caplet disintegration accelerant from soy polysaccharides) 60 mg. Other Ingredients: Cellulose, Cellulose Gum, Vegetable Stearic Acid, Silica, Vegetable Magnesium Stearate, Vita-Coat brand (modified vegetable cellulose, alpha-lipoic acid).

Dr. Earl Mindell's Russian Gold - FreeLife International
Each 1 mL serving contains: Proprietary Adaptogenic Formula 665 mg: Eleuthero root • Ashwagandha root • Schizandra seed • Korean Ginseng root • Rhodiola root • Pantocrene • American Ginseng root • Milky Oats seed • Cordyceps Mushroom • Reishi Mushroom • Elderberry • Green Tea • Hawthorn leaf, flower, berry • Licorice root • Grape seed • Grape skin • Ginger root • Stevia extract. Other Ingredients: Deionized Water, Vegetable Glycerin, Pure Grain Alcohol (20% by volume), Honey, Luo Han Guo, Natural Flavors.

Dr. Harris' Original Snore - Baywood International
Each caplet contains: Calcium (as dicalcium phosphate) 105 mg • Phosphorus (as dicalcium phosphate) 65 mg • Proprietary Blend 415 mg: Protease, Amylase, Lipase, Cellulase, Acerola concentrate fruit, Cayenne fruit, Echinacea root & aerial parts, Rose Hips fruit, Fenugreek seed, Slippery Elm bark, Red Clover aerial part, Yarrow flower, Eucalyptus leaf, Elderberry flower, fruit, Yellow Dock. Other Ingredients: Microcrystalline Cellulose, Silica, Maltodetrin, Croscarmellose Sodium, Magnesium Stearate.

Dr. Morrow's Blood Formula - Nutrition Dynamics, Inc.
Ten drops contain: Hamamelis virginica 3C • Pulsatilla nigricans 3C • Echinacea angustifolia 3C • Acidum hydrofluoricum 3C • Viburnum prunifolium 3C • Tussilago farfara 3C • Aesculus hippocastanum 3X.
See Editor's Note No. 1.

Dr. Morrow's Body Ache Formula - Nutrition Dynamics, Inc.
Ten drops contain: Aconite 3C • Bryonia alba 3C • Eupatorium perfoliatum 3C • Ferrum Phosphate 6C • Apis mellifica 3C • Mercurius dulcis 6C • Arnica 3C.
See Editor's Note No. 1.

Dr. Morrow's Digestion Formula - Nutrition Dynamics, Inc.
Ten drops contain: Nux vomica 3C • Bryonia alba 3C • Argentum nitricum 3C • Condurango 3C • Abies nigra 3C • Robinia pseudacacia 3C • Solidago 3X.
See Editor's Note No. 1.

Some Brand Name Natural Products - What they Contain

www.NaturalDatabase.com contains MANY more listings than appear here.
Editor's Notes are located on pages 2155-2163.

Dr. Morrow's Hives, Allergies, Poison Ivy, Poison Oak Formula - Nutrition Dynamics, Inc.
Ten drops contain: Ammonium carbonate 12X • Apis mellifica 30X • Arsinucum album 30X • Gridelia robusta 30X • Echinacea 6X • Crotalus horridus 20X.
See Editor's Note No. 1.

Dr. Morrow's Insomnia Formula - Nutrition Dynamics, Inc.
Ten drops contain: Passiflora 3X • Ignatia 4C • Coffee cruda 5C • Tellurium 6C • Acid phosphorica 7C • Palladium 6C • Magnesia phosphorica 6C.
See Editor's Note No. 1.

Dr. Morrow's Liver Formula - Nutrition Dynamics, Inc.
Ten drops contain: Chelidonium 3X • Taraxacum 3X • Carduus marianus 3X • Solidago 3X • Hydrastis 3C • Magnesia muriatica 3C • Cinchona 3C.
See Editor's Note No. 1.

Dr. Morrow's Motion Sickness Formula - Nutrition Dynamics, Inc.
Ten drops contain: Tabacum 3C • Cocculus indicus 3C • Arnica montana 3C • Petroleum 3C • Belladonna 3C • Ipecac 3C • Ignatia 3C.
See Editor's Note No. 1.

Dr. Morrow's Overexertion Formula - Nutrition Dynamics, Inc.
Ten drops contain: Phosphoric Acid 3C • Kali phosphoricum 6C • Anacardium 3C • Arnica 3C • Gelsemium 3C • Selenium 6C • Argentum nitricum 3C • Avena sativa 3X.
See Editor's Note No. 1.

Dr. Morrow's Pile Formula - Nutrition Dynamics, Inc.
Ten drops contain: Aesculus hippocastanum 10X • Hamamelis canadensis 10X • Hydrastis canadensis 10X • Viburnum prunifolium 10X.
See Editor's Note No. 1.

Dr. Morrow's Runny Nose Formula - Nutrition Dynamics, Inc.
Ten drops contain: Allium cepa 3C • Belladonna 3C • Euphrasia 3C • Mercurius dulcis 6C • Hydrastis 3C • Kali bichromicum 3C • Sambucus nigra 3C.
See Editor's Note No. 1.

Dr. Morrow's Skin Formula - Nutrition Dynamics, Inc.
Ten drops contain: Saponaria officinalis 3X • Fumaria officinalis 3X • Sarsaparilla 3X • Hydrocotyle asiatica 3X • Viola tricolor 3X • Rhus venenata 3C • Lappa major 3C • Berberis vulgaris 3C.
See Editor's Note No. 1.

Dr. Morrow's Sore Muscle Formula - Nutrition Dynamics, Inc.
Ten drops contain: Rhus toxicodendron 3C • Urtica urens 3C • Benzoic Acid 3C • Formic Acid 3C • Berberis vulgaris 3C • Ranunculus bulbosus 3C • Lithium carbonate 3C.
See Editor's Note No. 1.

Dr. Morrow's Stop Cough Formula - Nutrition Dynamics, Inc.
Ten drops contain: Drosera 3C • Arnica 3C • Belladonna 3C • Cina 3C • Coccus cacti 3C • Corallium rubrum 6C • Cuprum metallicum 6C •Ferrum Phosphate 6C • Ipecac 3C • Solidago 1C.
See Editor's Note No. 1.

Dr. Nanba's Maitake Beta Factor 4 fl oz - Planetary Formulas
Twenty-seven drops (approximately 1.25 ml) contain: Vitamin C (as ascorbic acid) 37.5 mg • Maitake (beta-glucan) Fraction++ 12.5 mg. Other Ingredients: Distilled Water, Vegetable Glycerin.

Dr. Nanba's Maitake Beta-Factor 163 mg - Planetary Formulas
Two tablets contain: Vitamin C (as ascorbic acid) 20 mg • Calcium 326 mg • Maitake (beta-glucan) Fraction 6 mg • Maitake Blend 320 mg: Maitake Fruiting Body, Maitake Mycelia Biomass. Other Ingredients: Dibasic Calcium Phosphate, Stearic Acid, Colloidal Silicon Dioxide, Modified Cellulose Gum, Magnesium Stearate.

Dr. Nanba's Maitake-Pro - Planetary Formulas
Two tablets contain: Dietary Fiber 1 g • Protein 1 g • Vitamin C (as ascorbic acid) 20 mg • Calcium 32 mg • Maitake (beta-glucan) Fraction++ 12.5 mg • Maitake Blend 2.07 g: Maitake Fruiting Body, Maitake Mycelia Biomass. Other Ingredients: Acacia Gum, Stearic Acid, Dibasic Calcium Phosphate, Colloidal Silicon Dioxide, Modified Cellulose Gum, Magnesium Stearate.

Dr. Powers Liquid Colloidal Mineral Source with Trace Minerals - Puritan's Pride
Each 1 fl oz (30 mL) contains: Vitamin B12 1100 mcg • Biotin 200 mcg • Calcium 25 mg • Magnesium 100 mg • Zinc 10 mg • Selenium 50 mcg • Manganese 5 mg • Chromium 50 mcg • Potassium 10 mg • Silica 1000 mcg.

Dream Cream - Sensaquest
Deionized Water • L-Arginine Monohydrochloride • Dimethicone Copolyolmethyl Ether (edicol 421) • Squalene (fitoderm) • Ethoxydiglycol (polawax a) • Acrylate/Aminoacrylates/C10-30 Alkyl PEG20 Itaconate Copolymer (structure plus 3802) • Glycerin / Glyceryl Monostearate • Silwet-7087 (emulsifying wax) • Cremaphor RH40 (hydrogenated castor oil) • Carbopol 940 • Methyl Paraben • Imidazolidinyl Urea (germall 115) • Propyl Paraben.

Dream Shape - Ecommerce Transactions, LLC
Each cap contains: Gamma-AminoButyric Acid (GABA) 665 mg.
See Editor's Note No. 62.

Dream Sleep - The Herbalist
Hops blossom • Passionflower herb • Skullcap herb • Valerian root.

Dream Time - Health Smart Vitamins
Two capsules contain: Calcium (as calcium stearate) 1 mg • Valerian root (0.8% valernic acids, 3 mg) 380 mg • German Chamomile flowers 180 mg • Peppermint leaf 180 mg • Bee Propolis extract 90 mg • Passionflower aerial parts 90 mg • American Ginseng root 80 mg.

Drenamin - Standard Process, Inc.
Three tablets contain: Proprietary Blend 717 mg: Defatted Wheat germ, Nutritional Yeast, Bovine Liver, Bovine Adrenal, Porcine Stomach, Bovine Adrenal PMG extract, Choline Bitartrate, Oat flour, Dried Buckwheat leaf juice, Buckwheat seed, Alfalfa flour, Magnesium Citrate, Mushroom, Bovine Bone, Allantoin, Porcine Brain, Carrot root, Soybean Lecithin, Veal Bone meal, Peanut bran, Mixed Tocopherols • Vitamin C 9 mg • Riboflavin 1 mg • Niacin 12 mg • Vitamin B6 0.3 mg. Other Ingredients: Honey, Calcium Lactate, Cellulose, Water, Potassium Para-Aminobenzoate, Calcium Stearate.
See Editor's Note No. 14.

Drenatrophin PMG - Standard Process, Inc.
Each tablet contains: Proprietary Blend 134 mg: Bovine Adrenal PMG extract, Magnesium Citrate • Calcium 20 mg • Sodium 10 mg. Other Ingredients: Calcium Lactate, Cellulose, Calcium Stearate.

Drink Ease - Global Source
Each tablet contains: Avena Sativa (oats) 30C • Capsicum Annuum (pepper) 30C • Nux Vomica 30C • Veratrum Album (white hellebore) 30C • Zinc Metallicum (zinc metal) 30C. Other Ingredients: Sorbitol, Sterilized Talc E 553b, Magnesium Stearate E 470b.
See Editor's Note No. 1.

Some Brand Name Natural Products - What they Contain

www.NaturalDatabase.com contains MANY more listings than appear here.
Editor's Notes are located on pages 2155-2163.

BRAND NAMES

Drinkables Hawaiian Noni - Remington Health Products, LLC
Each 1 fl oz serving contains: Vitamin C (ascorbic acid) 60 mg • Noni juice (morinda citrifolia) 10 mL. Other Ingredients: Purified Water, Fructose, Aloe Vera gel, Natural Citrus Flavor, Citric Acid, Potassium Sorbate, Sodium Benzoate.

Drinkables Liquid Calcium 3 - Remington Health Products, LLC
Each 1 fl oz serving contains: Vitamin K 80 mcg • Calcium 1200 mg: Calcium Malate 600 mg, Calcium Citrate 200 mg, Tricalcium Phosphate 400 mg • Magnesium (as magnesium citrate) 600 mg • Zinc (as zinc gluconate) 4 mg • Manganese (as manganese gluconate) 2 mg • Vitamin D (as D3) 400 IU • Sodium Borate 5 mg.

Drinkables Liquid Colloidal Minerals - Remington Health Products, LLC
Each 1 fl oz serving contains: Vitamin C (ascorbic acid) 60 mg • Purified Water • Crystalline Fructose • Trace Minerals • Natural Flavors • Honey • Aloe Vera gel • Citric Acid • OPC Grape extract • Plant-derived Mineral Blend • Seawater-derived Minerals • Sodium Benzoate • Potassium Sorbate • Potassium Citrate • Natural Color • Xanthan Gum.

Drinkables Liquid Coral Calcium - Remington Health Products, LLC
Each 1/2 fl oz serving contains: Vitamin D (D3, as cholecalciferol) 200 IU • Calcium (from coral calcium) 360 mg • Coral Calcium 1000 mg • Purified Water • Artifical Flavor • Propylene Glycol • Maltodextrin • Titanium Dioxide • Potassium Citrate • Citric Acid • Potassium Sorbate • Sodium Benzoate • Cellulose Gel • Xanthan Gum • Sucralose • Methylparaben • Propylparaben.

Drinkables Liquid Joint Care - Remington Health Products, LLC
Each 1 fl oz serving contains: Vitamin C (ascorbic acid) 60 mg • Glucosamine HCl 2 g • Chondroitin Sulfate 1.2 g • Methylsulfonylmethane 500 mg • Collagen 50 mg.

Drinkables Liquid Joint Relief - Remington Health Products, LLC
Each 1/2 fl oz serving contains: Vitamin C (ascorbic acid) 30 mg • Glucosamine HCl 1000 mg • Methylsulfonylmethane 250 mg • Purified Water • Natural Flavors • Citric Acid • Potassium Benzoate • Potassium Sorbate • Potassium Citrate • Xanthan Gum • Sucralose • FD&C Red 40.

Drinkables Liquid Multi Vitamins for Seniors - Remington Health Products, LLC
Each 1 fl oz serving contains: Vitamin A (palmitate) 5000 IU • Vitamin C (ascorbic acid) 78 mg • Vitamin D (cholecalciferol) 400 IU • Vitamin E (alpha tocopherol acetate) 30 IU • Vitamin K (phytonadione) 80 mcg • Thiamine 1.5 mg • Riboflavin 1.7 mg • Niacin 20 mg • Vitamin B6 (pyridoxine HCl) 2.7 mg • Folic Acid 400 mcg • Vitamin B12 (cyanocobalamin) 5 mcg • Biotin 300 mcg • Pantothenic Acid (calcium pantothenate) 10 mg • Manganese (gluconate) 2 mg • Chromium 120 mcg • Lutein 1 mg • Choline (bitartrate) 3 mg • Inositol 3 mg • PABA 3 mg.

Drinkables Ultimate Liquid Coral Calcium - Remington Health Products, LLC
Each 1 fl oz serving contains: Vitamin D (D3, as cholecalciferol) 400 IU • Calcium (from coral calcium) 760 mg • Coral Calcium 2000 mg • Purified Water • Artificial Flavor • Propylene Glycol • Maltodextrin • Titanium Dioxide • Potassium Citrate • Citric Acid • Potassium Sorbate • Potassium Benzoate • Cellulose Gel • Xanthan Gum • Sucralose • Methylparaben • Propylparaben.

Drinkables Ultimate Liquid Joint Care - Remington Health Products, LLC
Each 1 fl oz serving contains: Vitamin C (ascorbic acid) 60 mg • Glucosamine HCl 2000 mg • Chondroitin Sulfate 1200 mg • Methylsulfonylmethane 500 mg • Collagen 50 mg.

Drinkables Ultimate Multi Vitamins - Remington Health Products, LLC
Each 1 fl oz serving contains: Vitamin A (palmitate) 5000 IU • Vitamin C (ascorbic acid) 73 mg • Vitamin D (cholecalciferol) 400 IU • Vitamin E (alpha tocopherol acetate) 30 IU • Vitamin K (phytonadione) 50 mcg • Thiamin 1.5 mg • Riboflavin 1.7 mg • Niacin 20 mg • Vitamin B6 (pyridoxine hydrochloride) 2.7 mg • Folic Acid 400 mcg • Vitamin B12 (cyanocobalamin) 5 mcg • Biotin 300 mcg • Pantothenic Acid (calcium pantothenate) 10 mg • Manganese (gluconate) 2 mg • Chromium (chromium chloride) 120 mcg • Lutein 250 mcg • Lycopene 300 mg • Choline (bitartrate) 3 mg • Inositol 3 mg.

Drinkers Champion - Unknown
Potassium (as potassium glycerophosphate) • Schisandra berry extract (schisandra chinensis) • Oriental Ginseng root (panax ginseng) • Coenzyme Q 10 • Siberian Ginseng root (eleutherococcus senticosus) • Spirulina • Unknown Proprietary Blend.

Dromias - Berkeley Premium Nutraceuticals
Each tablet contains: Magnesium (as magnesium oxide) 50 mg • Valerian root standardized extract 200 mg • Wild Jujube seed standardized extract 75 mg. Other Ingredients: Guar Gum, Dicalcium Phosphate, Microcrystalline Cellulose, Calcium Carbonate, Vegetable Stearin, Vanillin, Stearic Acid, Magnesium Stearate, Silica, Citrus Pectin, Sugar Coat Ingredients (to be determined).

Dry Beta Carotene 10,000 IU - Solgar
Each tablet contains: Vitamin A (as 100% natural beta carotene) 10,000 IU • Carotenoid Mix 114 mcg: Alpha Carotene, Lutein, Zeaxanthin, Cryptoxanthin. Other Ingredients: Microcrystalline Cellulose, Vegetable Cellulose, Vegetable Stearic Acid, Silica, Vegetable Magnesium Stearate, Annatto, Titanium Dioxide, Vegetable Glycerin, Caramel, Carnauba Wax.

Dry E-400 - Jarrow Formulas
Each capsule contains: Vitamin E (as a natural D-alpha tocopheryl succinate) 400 IU. Other Ingredients: Cellulose, Calcium Stearate, Magnesium Stearate, Silicon Dioxide, Stearic Acid, Gelatin.

Dry Eyes - Natural Ophthalmics
Active Ingredients: Alumina • Arsenicum Album • Eyebright (euphrasia) 8x • Nux Moschata • Zincum Metalicum. Inactive Ingredients: Sterile Water, Sodium Chloride, Citrates, Polysorbate 80.

Dry Mouth Citrus Lozenges - Thayers Natural Pharmaceuticals
Each lozenge contains: Sorbitol (natural sugar-free sweetener derived from cherries, berries, pears, and plums) • Apple Pectin • Vitamin C (ascorbic acid) • Natural Lemonade Flavor • Potassium Chloride • Stearic Acid • Calcium Stearate.

Dry Mouth Spray, Citrus - Thayers Natural Pharmaceuticals
Glycerin • Tris Amino • Potassium Chloride • Natural Lemon Flavor • Natural Lime Flavor • Purified Water.

Dry Mouth Spray, Menthol - Thayers Natural Pharmaceuticals
Vegetable Glycerin • Tris Amino • Potassium Chloride • Natural Peppermint Flavor • Purified Water.

Dry Vitamin D - Nature's Way
Each capsule contains: Vitamin D (as Vitamin D3) cholecalciferol 400 IU. Other Ingredients: Cellulose, Gelatin, Maltodextrin, Millet.

D-Snore - WellQuest International, Inc.
Sweet Almond Oil • Sesame Oil • Sunflower Oil • Olive Oil • Grape Seed Oil • Lecithin • Orange Seed Extract in a base of glycerin • Purified de-ionized Water • Natural Peppermint extract.

Du Huo Ji Shen Tang Plus - Secara
Organic Licorice root (gan cao) 291 mg • Boswellia gum resin (60% boswellic acids) 288 mg • Organic Cinnamon bark (rou gui) 276 mg • Pubescent Angelica root 5:1 extract (du huo) 153 mg • Eucommia

bark 5:1 extract (du zhong) 132 mg • Siler root 5:1 extract (du zhong) 132 mg • Large Leaf Gentian root 5:1 extract (qin jiao) 114 mg • Achyranthes root 5:1 extract (niu xi) 96 mg • Asian Ginseng root (ren shen, 5% ginsenosides (5 mg)) 96 mg • Chinese Peony root 5:1 extract (bai shao) 96 mg • Dong Quai root 5:1 extract (dang gui) 96 mg • Hoelen sclerotium 5:1 extract (fu ling) 96 mg • Ligusticum Wallichii rhizome 5:1 extract (chaun xiong) 96 mg • Loranthus twig 5:1 extract (sang ji sheng) 96 mg • Rehmannia tuber 5:1 extract (shu di huang) 96 mg • Sichuan Teasel root 5:1 extract (xu duan) 96 mg.

Dymetadrine 25 - AST Sports Science
Each tablet contains: Ephedrine HCL 25 mg • Guaifenesin 200 mg.

Dymetadrine Xtreme - AST Sports Science
Each capsule contains: Vitamin B6 5 mg • Vitamin C 30 mg • Magnesium (as magnesium salicylate) 50 mg • Ephedra extract (standardized for 24 mg ephedrine alkaloids) 300 mg • L-Phenylalanine 150 mg • L-Tyrosine 150 mg • Caffeine (as anhydrous caffeine) 100 mg • Yohimbine HCl 2 mg.
See Editor's Note No. 21 and No. 30.

Dymetadrine Xtreme (Ephedra Free) - AST Sports Science
Two capsules contain: Magnesium (as magnesium salicylate) 60 mg • Vitamin C 44 mg • Vitamin B6 18 mg • NGRX Green Tea leaf extract (standardized for epigallocatechin gallate EGCG, l-phenylalanine, l-tyrosine, caffeine as caffeine anhydrous, norsynephrine HCl, theobromine HCl and yohimbine HCl) 1393 mg.

DynaTrim - America's Finest
Each capsule contains: Citrin brand Garcinia Cambogia fruit extract (50% [-] HCA) 500 mg • Chromium (from chromium polynicotinate) 100 mcg • Gugulipid brand 2.5% Guggulsterones 400 mg • Forslean brand Coleus Forskohlii extract 10% 70 mg • Biopoerine brand Black Pepper extract 25 mg.

Dyno-Vites Sustained Release Tablet - Nature's Plus
Two tablets contain: Vitamin A (as beta carotene) 25,000 IU • Vitamin C (as mineral ascorbate) 1000 mg • Vitamin D (as ergocalciferol) 1000 IU • Vitamin E (as D-alpha tocopheryl succinate) 200 IU • Thiamin (vitamin B1, as thiamine HCl) 100 mg • Riboflavin (vitamin B2) 100 mg • Vitamin B6 (as pyridoxine HCl) 125 mg • Folate (as folic acid) 400 mcg • Vitamin B12 (as cyanocobalamin) 500 mcg • Biotin 125 mcg • Calcium (as ascorbate) 50 mg • Pantothenic Acid (as calcium pantothenate) 125 mg • Iron (as amino acid chelate/complex) 25 mg • Iodine (from kelp) 150 mcg • Magnesium (as ascorbate) 25 mg • Zinc (as ascorbate) 25 mg • Selenium (as amino acid complex) 100 mcg • Manganese (as amino acid chelate/complex) 10 mg • Chromium (as amino acid chelate) 200 mcg • Molybdenum (as amino acid complex) 50 mcg • Potassium (as citrate) 15 mg • PABA (para-aminobenzoic acid) 100 mg • Inositol 75 mg • Choline (as bitartrate) 75 mg • L-Methionine (free form amino acid) 50 mg • Citrus Bioflavonoids (from citrus limon exocarp) 50 mg • Rutin (from saphora japonica leaf) 25 mg • Betaine HCl (from beet molasses) 25 mg • L-Glutamine (free form amino acid) 25 mg • Hesperidin (from citrus limon exocarp) 10 mg. Other Ingredients: Microcrystalline Cellulose, Stearic Acid, Di-Calcium Phosphate, Magnesium Stearate, Hydroxypropyl Methylcellulose, Silica, Bee Pollen, Wheat Germ, RNA, DNA, Brewer's Yeast, Lecithin, Pharmaceutical Glaze.

E 400 I.U. - Nature's Bounty
Each softgel contains: Vitamin E (as dL-alpha tocopheryl acetate and D-alpha tocopherol plus D-beta, D-gamma and D-delta tocopherol) 400 IU. Other Ingredients: Gelatin, Glycerin, Soybean Oil.

E Complex 1:1 - Metagenics
Two capsules contain: Vitamin E (D-alpha tocopherol) 400 IU • Gamma-Tocopherol 270 mg • Delta-Tocopherol 98 mg • Beta-Tocopherol 6 mg.

E Force - VitaCube Systems (V3S)
Each pouch (160 g) contains: Corn Syrup Solids • Citric Acid • Fructose • Maltodextrin • Malic Acid • Natural Flavors • Inulin • Sodium Citrate • Guar Gum • Ribose • Gum Arabic • Sodium Chloride • Magnesium Phosphate • Sucralose • Calcium Citrate • Dipotassium Phosphate • Elderberry concentrate • Potassium Chloride • D-Alpha-Tocopheryl Acetate.

E Succinate 400 IU - Vital Nutrients
Each vegetarian capsule contains: Vitamin E (D-alpha tocopheryl succinate) 400 IU.

E.P.O. evening primrose oil - Pure Encapsulations
Each softgel capsule contains: Evening Primrose oil (provides GLA 50 mg; typical fatty acid composition: 16:0 palmitic, 18:1 oleic, 18:2 linoleic, 18:3 gamma linolenic [GLA], other fatty acids 13 mg) 530 mg

E.T.- Essiac Tonic - The Herbalist
Burdock root • Sheep Sorrel leaf • Slippery Elm bark • Turkey Rhubarb root.

E-1000 Mixed - Rexall - Sundown
Each softgel contains: Vitamin E (as dl-alpha-tocopheryl acetate and d-alpha-tocopherol) 1000 IU. Other Ingredients: Gelatin, Glycerin, Water.

E-1000 Natural - Rexall - Sundown
Each softgel contains: Vitamin E (as d-alpha-tocopherol) 1000 IU. Other Ingredients: Gelatin, Glycerin, Water.

E-12 Super Enzymes - Cell Tech
Each capsule contains: Proprietary Blend 500 mg: Plant-Based Enzyme Blend 193 mg: Blue-Green Algae (aphanizomenon flos-aquae) 25 mg, Fennel seed, Ginger root, Cayenne Pepper fruit • Amylase 5750 DU • Glucoamylase 13.5 AG • Invertase 0.2 IAU • Lactase 1000 ALU • Pectinase (with phytase) 15 endo-PGU • Cellulase 100 CU • Lipase 150 LU • Protease (I) 13,500 HUT • Protease (II) 3000 HUT • Acid-Stable Protease 5.35 SAPU • Bromelain 25,600 FCC PU • Papain 50,000 FCC PU. Other Ingredients: Rice Bran, Gelatin Capsule (gelatin, water).

E-200 Mixed - Rexall - Sundown
Each softgel contains: Vitamin E (as dl-alpha-tocopheryl acetate and d-alpha-tocopherol) 200 IU. Other Ingredients: Gelatin, Glycerin, Water.

E-200 Natural - Rexall - Sundown
Each softgel contains: Vitamin E (as d-alpha-tocopherol) 200 IU. Other Ingredients: Soybean Oil, Gelatin, Glycerin, Water.

E-400 - Jarrow Formulas
Each softgel contains: Vitamin E as 100% natural D-Alpha Tocopherol 400 IU. Other Ingredients: Soybean Oil, Gelatin, Glycerin, Water.

E-400 Caps - TwinLab
Each capsule contains: Vitamin E 400 IU. Other Ingredients: Cellulose, Magnesium, Silicate, Croscarmellose, Sodium, Gelatin, Crospovidone, Purified Water, Silica, Magnesium Stearate, MCT.

E-400 D-Alpha Water Soluble - Rexall - Sundown
Each softgel contains: Vitamin E (as dl-alpha-tocopheryl acetate) 400 IU. Other Ingredients: Gelatin, Polysorbate 80, Glycerin, Water.

E-400 Mixed - Rexall - Sundown
Each softgel contains: Vitamin E (as dl-alpha-tocopheryl acetate and d-alpha-tocopherol) 400 IU. Other Ingredients: Gelatin, Glycerin, Water.

E-400 Natural - Rexall - Sundown
Each softgel contains: Vitamin E (as d-alpha-tocopherol) 400 IU. Inactive Ingredients: Gelatin, Glycerin, Water.

E-400 Plus Selenium - The Vitamin Shoppe
Each softgel contains: Vitamin E (d-alpha, d-beta, d-delta tocopheryls) 400 IU • Selenium (Selenomethionine) 50 mcg.

E-400 Selenium - Metagenics
Each tablet contains: Vitamin E (as D-alpha tocopheryl succinate) 400 IU • Selenium (as selenium L-aspartate) 50 mcg.

E-400 Sesame **-** Progressive Labs
Each softgel capsule contains: Vitamin E (d-alpha tocopherol) 400 IU • Sesame oil 200 mg. With Natural, Unesterified Mixed Tocopherols.

E-400 with Folic Acid **-** Rexall - Sundown
Each softgel contains: Vitamin E (as dl-alpha-tocopheryl acetate and d-alpha-tocopherol) 400 IU • Vitamin B6 (as pyridoxine HCl) 2 mg • Folic Acid 400 mcg • Vitamin B12 (as cyanocobalamin) 6 mcg. Inactive Ingredients: Gelatin, Glycerin, Soybean Oil, Water, Yellow Beeswax, Soy Lecithin, Polysorbate 80.

E-600 **-** Jarrow Formulas
Each softgel contains: Vitamin E as 100% natural D-Alpha Tocopherol 600 IU. Other Ingredients: Soybean Oil, Gelatin, Glycerin, Water.

Ear Drops **-** NutriBiotic
Contains 0.1% grapefruit extract in a base of tea tree oil and vegetable glycerin.

Ear Oil **-** Blessed Herbs
Calendula flower • St. John's Wort flower • Mullein flower • Garlic & Organic Cold-Pressed Olive oil.

Earache Remedy (formerly HP 15) **-** Metagenics
Each tablet contains: Kali Muriaticum 3X • Mercurius Dulcis 6X • Lac Caninum 30X • Belladonna 30X • Ferrum Phosphoricum 12X • Pulsatilla 12X.
See Editor's Note No. 1.

Earache Tablets **-** Hyland's
Each tablet contains: Pulsatilla as Passion Flower 30C HPUS • Chamomilla as Chamomile 30C HPUS • Sulphur 30C HPUS • Calcarea carbonica as Carbonate of Lime 30C HPUS • Belladonna 30C HPUS (3x10-60% Alkaloids) • Lycopodium as Club Moss 30C HPUS. In a base of Lactose NF (Milk Sugar).
See Editor's Note No. 1.

Earthmends Breast Health Program **-** Cancer Wellness Institute
Each packet (containing one softgel and four capsules) contains: Vitamin A (as natural beta-carotene and mixed carotenes from natural antioxidant blend) 9000 IU • Vitamin E (as natural vitamin E succiante and d-alpha tocopherol) 200 IU • Selenium (from selenium yeast) 150 mcg. Energizing Complex - Yellow: Glutamine (as L-glutamine polypeptides) 100 mg • Propolis 75 mg • Bee Pollen 75 mg • Ginger extract (root) (3.75 mg gingerols/shoagols) 75 mg • Turmeric extract (root) (71.25 mg curcumins) 75 mg • Oriental Ginseng extract (root) (3.5 mg ginsenosides) 50 mg • Garlic concentrate (bulb) 50 mg. Mushroom Complex - Speckled: Chinese Skullcap (aerial) 75 mg • Maitake Mushroom (aerial) 50 mg • Reishi Mushroom (mycelia) 50 mg • Shitake Mushroom (aerial) 50 mg • Agaricus Mushroom (aerial) 50 mg • Panax Pseudoginseng Wal. (root) 50 mg • Rabdosia Rubescens (Hemsl.) Hara. (aerial) 35 mg • Dyer's Woad (aerial) 35 mg • Licorice (root) 25 mg • Chrysanthemum (flower) 25 mg • Agaricus Mushroom extract (aerial) 25 mg • Maitaki Mushroom extract (6.25 mg polysaccharides) 25 mg • Shitake Mushroom Lenode extract mycelia (aerial) (0.375 mg) 25 mg • Reishi Mushroom extract (aerial) (3.125 mg polysaccharides) 25 mg. Antioxidant Complex - Burgundy: Broccoli concentrate (with natural sulforophanes) (aerial) 200 mg • Colostrum 200 mg • Green Tea extract (leaf) (50 mg polyphenols) 100 mg • Grape seed extract (45 mg gallic acid equivalent) (40 mg polyphenols) 100 mg • Quercetin (flavonoid) 50 mg • Indole-3-Carbinol 40 mg. Red Clover Complex - Brown: Red Clover extract (flower) (20 mg isoflavones) 200 mg • Black Cohosh extract (root) (2.83 mg triterpeneglycosides) 113 mg • Dong Quai extract (root) (0.042 mg ferulic acids) 83 mg • Tocotrienols 43 mg. Flax Seed Oil Complex - Red: Flax Oil (seed) 200 mg • Natural Antioxidant Blend 100 mg from Carrot oil (root), Palm (fruit), Marigold (flower), Tomato (fruit), supplying Lutein, Lycopene, Phytoene, Phytofluene, Tocotrienols/Tocopherols, Zeaxanthin • Beta Sitosterol Complex (90 mg free sterols) 100 mg • Natural Lycopene (from Tomato fruit) 5 mg • Astaxanthin 2 mg. Other Ingredients: Gelatin, Soybean Oil, Lecithin, Glycerin, Rice Flour, Magnesium Stearate, Silicon Dioxide, Natural Beeswax.

Earthmends Prostate Health Program **-** Cancer Wellness Institute
Each packet (containing two softgels and three capsules) contains: Vitamin A (as natural beta-carotene and mixed carotenes from natural antioxidant blend) 9000 IU • Vitamin E (as natural vitamin E succinate and d-alpha-tocopherol) 200 IU • Zinc (as zinc amino acid chelate) 15 mg • Selenium (from selenium yeast) 150 mcg. Energizing Complex - Yellow: Glutamine (as L-glutamine polypeptides) 100 mg • Propolis 75 mg • Bee Pollen 75 mg • Ginger extract (root) (3.75 mg gingerols/shoagols) 75 mg • Turmeric extract (root) (71.25 mg curcumins) 75 mg • Oriental Ginseng extract (root) (3.5 mg ginsenosides) 50 mg • Garlic concentrate (bulb) 50 mg. Mushroom Complex - Speckled: Chinese Skullcap (aerial) 75 mg • Maitake Mushroom (aerial) 50 mg • Reishi Mushroom (mycelia) 50 mg • Shitake Mushroom (aerial) 50 mg • Agaricus Mushroom (aerial) 50 mg • Panax Pseudoginseng Wall. (root) 50 mg • Rabdosia Rubescens (Hemsl.) Hara. (aerial) 50 mg • Dyer's Woad (aerial) 35 mg • Licorice (root) 25 mg • Chrysanthemum (flower) 25 mg • Agaricus Mushroom extract (aerial) 25 mg • Maitake Mushroom extract (6.25 mg polysaccharides) 25 mg • Shitake Mushroom Lenode extract mycelia (aerial) (0.375 mg) 25 mg • Reishi Mushroom extract (aerial) (3.125 mg polysaccharides) 25 mg. Antioxidant Complex - Burgundy: Broccoli concentrate (with natural sulforophanes) (aerial) 200 mg • Colostrum 200 mg • Green Tea extract (leaf) (50 mg polyphenols) 100 mg • Grape Seed extract (45 mg gallic acid equivalent) (40 mg polyphenols) 100 mg • Quercetin (flavonoid) 50 mg • Indole-3-Carbinol 40 mg. Saw Palmetto Complex - Brown: Red Clover (flower) 200 mg • Saw Palmetto berry extract (seed) (136 mg free fatty acids) 160 mg • Stinging Nettle extract (root) (0.96 mg beta sitosterol) 120 mg • Pygeum extract (Pygeum africanum bark) (6.5 mg sterols) 50 mg • Beta Sitosterol complex (45 mg free sterols) 50 mg. Flax Seed Complex - Red: Flax Oil (seed) 200 mg • Natural Antioxidant Blend 150 mg: Carrot oil (root), Palm (fruit), Marigold (flower), Tomato (fruit), supplying Lutein, Lycopene, Phytoene, Phytofluene, Tocotrienols/Tocopherols, Zeaxanthin • Beta Sitosterol Complex (90 mg free sterols) 100 mg • Natural Lycopene (from Tomato fruit) 5 mg • Astaxanthin 2 mg. Other Ingredients: Gelatin, Soybean Oil, Lecithin, Glycerin, Magnesium Stearate, Silicon Dioxide, Natural Beeswax.

Earthmends Total Health Program **-** Cancer Wellness Institute
Five capsules contain: Fruit extract blend 900 mg: Banana (fruit), New Jersey Tomato (fruit), Delicious Apple (fruit), Strawberry (fruit), Kiwi (fruit), Peach (fruit), Whole Red Wine Grape (fruit), Wild Blueberry (fruit), Mango (fruit), Cantaloupe Melon (fruit), Hawaiian Pineapple (fruit), Cranberry (fruit), Bing Cherry (fruit), Plum (fruit), Elderberry (fruit), Apricot (fruit), Red Raspberry (fruit), Red Pepper (fruit), Eggplant (fruit) • Root Vegetable Extract Blend 450 mg: Carrot (root), Ginger (root), Beet (root), Onion (bulb), Sweet Potato (root), Potato (root) • Cruciferous Vegetable Extract Blend 375 mg: Broccoli (aerial), Spinach (leaf), Kale (leaf), Brussel Sprout (bud), Cabbage (leaf) • Citrus Fruit Extract Blend 350 mg: Orange (fruit), Grapefruit (fruit), Lemon (fruit), Lime (fruit) • Micro-Algae Blend 250 mg: Spirulina (Spirulina planatensis whole cell), Broken Cell Wall Chlorella (Chlorella spp. broken cells) • Soy isolate protein extract (Soybeans)(seed) 250 mg • Whole Cereal Grains and Grass Extract Blend 100 mg: Alfalfa (aerial), Barley (whole plant), Wheat (whole plant), Rye (whole plant) • Vegetable Extract Blend 75 mg: Cauliflower (florets), Corn (seed). Other Ingredients: Malarin, Collagen, Silicon Dioxide, Magnesium Stearate.

Earth's Promise (elderberry flavor) **-** Enzymatic Therapy
Each packet or 2 rounded tbsp serving contains: Fiber Blend 4 g: Inulin (from chicory root) 3 g, Guar Gum seed extract 1 g • Greens Blend 3.73 g: Barley grass 950 mg, Alfalfa sprouts 810 mg, Broccoli sprouts 810 mg, Radish sprouts 786 mg, Oat grass 250 mg, Wheat

grass 100 mg, Alfalfa juice concentrate 25 mg • European Elderberry 4:1 extract 462 mg • Vegetable Blend 446 mg: Broccoli flower 66 mg, Cabbage leaf 66 mg, Carrot root 66 mg, Collard greens 66 mg, Tomato fruit 66 mg, Mustard greens 50 mg, Kale leaf 33 mg, Spinach leaf 33 mg • Green Tea leaf extract 200 mg • Seaweed Blend 125 mg: Dulse 60 mg, Blue-Green Algae 60 mg, Kelp leaf and stem 5 mg • Stevia leaf extract 80 mg. Other Ingredients: Natural Flavors, Malic Acid, Raspberry Powder, Silicon Dioxide.

Earth's Promise (peppermint-tea flavor) **-** Enzymatic Therapy
Each packet or 4 tsp serving contains: Fiber Blend 4 g: Inulin (from chicory root) 3 g, Guar Gum seed extract 1 g • Greens Blend 3.73 g: Barley grass 950 mg, Alfalfa sprouts 810 mg, Broccoli sprouts 810 mg, Radish sprouts 786 mg, Oat grass 250 mg, Wheat grass 100 mg, Alfalfa juice concentrate 25 mg • Peppermint leaf (mentha piperita) 1.54 g • Vegetable Blend 446 mg: Broccoli flower 66 mg, Cabbage leaf 66 mg, Carrot root 66 mg, Collard greens 66 mg, Tomato fruit 66 mg, Mustard greens 50 mg, Kale leaf 33 mg, Spinach leaf 33 mg • Green Tea leaf extract 200 mg • Seaweed Blend 125 mg: Dulse 60 mg, Blue-Green Algae 60 mg, Kelp leaf and stem 5 mg • Stevia leaf extract 120 mg. Other Ingredients: Silicon Dioxide.

Earth's Promise (strawberry kiwi flavor) **-** Enzymatic Therapy
Each packet or 5 tsp serving contains: Fiber Blend 4 g: Inulin (from chicory root) 3 g, Guar Gum seed extract 1 g • Greens Blend 3.73 g: Barley grass 950 mg, Alfalfa sprouts 810 mg, Broccoli sprouts 810 mg, Radish sprouts 786 mg, Oat grass 250 mg, Wheat grass 100 mg, Alfalfa juice concentrate 25 mg • Fruit Blend 2.4 g: Mango fruit 1.2 g, Kiwi fruit 625 mg, Strawberry fruit 525 mg • Vegetable Blend 446 mg: Broccoli flower 66 mg, Cabbage leaf 66 mg, Carrot root 66 mg, Collard greens 66 mg, Tomato fruit 66 mg, Mustard greens 50 mg, Kale leaf 33 mg, Spinach leaf 33 mg • Green Tea leaf extract 200 mg • Seaweed Blend 125 mg: Dulse 60 mg, Blue-Green Algae 60 mg, Kelp leaf and stem 5 mg • Stevia leaf extract 110 mg. Other Ingredients: Natural Flavors, Natural Kiwi Flavor, Malic Acid, Citric Acid, Silicon Dioxide.

Easy Iron **-** Puritan's Pride
Each capsule contains: Iron (as Ferrous Bis-Glycinate) 28 mg • Vitamin C (as Ascorbic Acid) 60 mg • Folate (as Folic Acid) 400 mcg • Vitamin B12 (as Cyanocobalamin) 8 mcg.

Easy Now **-** Traditional Medicinals
Peppermint leaf • Spearmint leaf • Passion flower herb • Valerian root • Licorice root • Catnip leaf • Chamomile flower • Rosemary leaf • Lavender flower • Natural flavors.

Easy Soy **-** J. R. Carlson Laboratories, Inc.
Each capsule contains: Soy Isoflavone concentrate 500 mg.

Easy Soy Powder **-** J. R. Carlson Laboratories, Inc.
Each 100 g serving contains: Soy Isoflavone concentrate 2500 mg.

Easylax **-** R-U Ved U.S.A.
Terminalia chebula • Fennel • Trychospermum • Senna extract (8% sennodides).

Eat Ease **-** Life Enhancement Products, Inc.
Each capsule contains: Betaine Hydrochloride 324 mg • Pepsin 65 mg.

Eater's Digest **-** Traditional Medicinals
Peppermint leaf • Ginger rhizome • Fennel seed • Rose Hip • Papaya leaf • Alfalfa Herb • Cinnamon bark.

EB Capsules **-** Jarrow Formulas
Three capsules contain: Alpha Linoleic Acid (omega-3) 880 mg • Linoleic Acid (omega-6) 880 mg • Oleic Acid (omega-9) 730 mg • Lignans 0.5 mg. Other Ingredients: Unrefined Oils (flax, pumpkin, high oleic sunflower), Gelatin, Glycerine, Purified Water, Carob, Flax Seed Particulate.

EB5 Age Spot Formula **-** Pharmacist Heldfond's eb5 Formulas for Younger Looking Skin
Hydroquinone 2% • Deionized Water • Mineral Oil • Cetearyl Alcohol • Cetearyl Phosphate • Glycerin • Petroleum • Steareth-2 • Stearyl Alcohol • Steareth-10 • Bilberry Extract • Sugar Cane Extract • Sugar Maple Extract • Orange Extract • Lemon Extract • Octyl Methoxcinnamate • Benzophenone-3 • Sodium Sulfite • Sodium Meta Bisulfite • Citric Acid • Propylene Glycol • Diazolidinyl Urea • Methylparaben • Propylparaben.

EB5 Body Formula **-** Pharmacist Heldfond's eb5 Formulas for Younger Looking Skin
Purified Water • Methylsilanol Mannuronate • Mate Extract • Gotu Kola Extract • Thea Sinensis Extract • Butylene Glycol • Glyeryl Stearate • Stearic Acid • Cyclomehticome • Octyl Palmitate • Myristy Myristate • Dimethicone • Sunflower Oil • Isopropyl Lanolate • Soy Serol • Cetareth 20 • Tocopheryl Acetate • Choleth-24 • Ceteth 24 • Panthenol • Ivy Extract • Horsetail Extract • Kelp Extract • Algae Extract • Ginkgo Extract • Arnica Extract • Triethanolamine • Carbomer • Hydroxykpropyl • Methylcellulose • Disodium EDTA • Methylparaben • Propylparaben • Imadazolidinyl Urea • Fragrance.

EB5 Body Lotion **-** Pharmacist Heldfond's eb5 Formulas for Younger Looking Skin
Water • Tocopheryl Acetate • Stearic Acid • Propylene Glycol • Dicaprylate/Dicaprate • Mineral Oil • Butylene glycol • Clyeryl Stearate SE • Sorbitan Stearate • Polysorbate-60 • Squalane • Soy Sterol • Panthenol • Oat Flour • Lanolin Alcohol • Retinyl Palmitate • Ergocalciferol • Dimenthicone • Imidazolidinyl Urea • Disodium EDTA • Carbomer-940 • Polyamino Sugar • Condensate • Urea • Methylparaben • Propylparaben • Triethanolamine • Fragrance.

EB5 Cleansing Formula **-** Pharmacist Heldfond's eb5 Formulas for Younger Looking Skin
Purified Water • Cycerin • Caprylic/Capric Triglyceride • Stearic Acid • Peg 8 • Glycol Distearate • Cetyl Alcohol • Triethanolamine • Tocopheryl Acetate • Lactic Acid • Polyquatemium-7 • Panthenol • Peg-10 • Soya Sterol • Oat Flour • Cetearyl Alcohol • Peg-40 Castor Oil • Sodium Cetearyl Sulfate • Cocamide DEA • Carbomer • Disodium • EDTA • BHA • Methylparaben • Propylparaben • Quantemium-15 • Fragrance.

EB5 Facial Creme **-** Pharmacist Heldfond's eb5 Formulas for Younger Looking Skin
Water • Propylene Glycol • Tocopheryl Acetate • Stearic Acid • Mineral Oil • Cetyl Alcohol • Oat Flour • Retinyl Palmitate • Ergocalciferol • Propylparaben • Triethanolamine • Methylparaben • Potassium Sorbate • Allantoin • Imidazolidinyl • Urea • Panthenol • Cobomer-940 • Soluble Animal Collagen.

EB5 Footcare Formula **-** Pharmacist Heldfond's eb5 Formulas for Younger Looking Skin
Deionized Water • Mineral oil • Propylene Glycol • Stearic Acid • Microcystalline Wax • Cetyl Alcohol • PEG-100 Stearate • Vitamin E Acetate • Oat Protein • Triethanolamine • Menthol • Eucalyptus oil • Fragrance • DL Panthenol • Allantoin • Imidazolidiny Urea • Methylparaben • Propylparaben • Potassium Sorbate • Chamomile • Comfrey • Tea Tree oil • White Lily extract • Corn flower extract • Sandalwood extract • Sunflower extract • Basil extract • Sage extract • Jasmine extract • Sugar Cane extract • Maple extract • Citrus extract • Apple extract • Vitamin A • Vitamin D (as vitamin D3) • Dipotassium • Glycyrrhzinate • Soluble Collagen • FD&C Blue #1 • FD&C Yellow #5.

EB5 Men's Facial Formula **-** Pharmacist Heldfond's eb5 Formulas for Younger Looking Skin
Water • Propylene Glycol • Tocopheryl Acetate • Stearic Acid • Mineral Oil • Cetyl Alcohol • Oat Flour • Sodium PCA • Retinyl Palmiate • Ergocalciferol • Allantoin • Panthenol • Soluble Animal Collagen • Propylparaben • Triethanolamine • Methylparaben • Potassium Sorbate • Imidazolidinyl Urea • Carbomer-940 • Fragrance • FD&C Blue No. 1 • FD&C Red No. 33.

Some Brand Name Natural Products - What they Contain

www.NaturalDatabase.com contains MANY more listings than appear here.
Editor's Notes are located on pages 2155-2163.

BRAND NAMES

EB5 Toning Formula - Pharmacist Heldfond's eb5 Formulas for Younger Looking Skin
Purified Water • Hydrolyzed Wheat Protein • Arnica Extract • Barley Extract • Triethanolamine • Lactic Acid • Polysorbate 20 • Sodium PCA • Vitamin E Acetate • Allantoin • Panthenol • Witch Hazel Distillate • Sage Extract • Birch Leaf Extract • Comfrey Extract • Sambucus Extract • Blackberry Extract • Horsetail Extract • Tetrasodium EDTA • Methylparaben • Imidazolidinyl Uera • Quantemium-15 • Fragrance.

E'balance - E'OLA
Two capsules contain: Proprietary Blend 665 mg: Soy Isoflavones, Black Cohosh (root) (Cimicifuga Racemosa), St. John's Wort (herb), Dong Quai (herb), Licorice (root), Chaste Tree (berry), Fennel (seed). Other Ingredients: Rice Flour, Gelatin, Magnesium Stearate.

EB-C - MMS Pro
Each capsule contains: Eyebright • Golden Seal root • Bayberry root bark • Red Raspberry • Cayenne.

ECA Stack - Nutra Sport
Two capsules contain: Ephedrine alkaloids (from whole ma huang plant extract) 20 mg • Caffeine (32.2 mg from bissey nut) 200 mg • Acetylsalicylic Acid 324 mg. Other Ingredients: Rice flour.
See Editor's Note No. 30.

EchinaCare Capsules - PhytoPharmica
Each capsule contains: Echinacea purpurea (aerial part) concentrate 50:1 50 mg.

EchinaCare Liquid - PhytoPharmica
Forty to sixty drops contain: Echinacea purpurea (fresh-pressed juice from stems, leaves, and flowers) 1.5 ml.
See Editor's Note No. 21.

Echinacea - Pharmanex
Each capsule contains: Echinacea purpurea root 6:1 extract 225 mg. Other Ingredients: Rice Flour, Gelatin.

Echinacea - Nature's Way
Three capsules contain: Echinacea Purpurea stem, leaf, flower 1.20 g. Other Ingredients: Gelatin.

Echinacea - Nature's Bounty
Each capsule contains: Echinacea (Echinacea purpurea) root 400 mg. Other Ingredients: Gelatin, Vegetable Stearic Acid.

Echinacea - Benepure, Inc
Each capsule contains: Echinacea Angustifolia root and rhizome extract (yielding echinacosides 10 mg) 250 mg. Other Ingredients: Rice Powder, Gelatin, Vegetable Stearate, Vegetable Cellulose.

Echinacea - Puritan's Pride
Each capsule contains: Echinacea (Echinacea purpurea) root 400 mg. Other Ingredients: Gelatin, Vegetable Stearic Acid.

Echinacea - Solgar
Each capsule contains: Vitamin A 135 IU • Echinacea root 4:1 extract 65 mg • Raw Echinacea powder 265 mg. Other Ingredients: Vegetable Cellulose, Vegetable Magnesium Stearate, Water, Vegetable Glycerin.

Echinacea - DreamPharm
Each capsule contains: Echinacea herb 400 mg • Glycyrrhizae radix (licorice root) 100 mg.

Echinacea - NOW Foods
Two capsules contain: Total Carbohydrate 620 mg • Echinacea purpurea powder root 800 mg. Other Ingredients: Stearic Acid.

Echinacea - Leiner Health Products
Each caplet contains: Echinacea extract (Echinacea angustifolia & Echinacea purpurea) root 125 mg. Other Ingredients: Calcium Carbonate, Cellulose, Maltodextrin, Hydroxypropyl Methylcellulose, Silicon Dioxide, Polyethylene Glycol 3350, Croscarmellose Sodium, Hydroxypropyl Cellulose, Red 40 Lake, Blue 2 Lake, Pharmaceutical Glaze, Crospovidone, Magnesium Stearate, Polysorbate 80, Titanium Dioxide.

Echinacea - Gaia Herbs
Echinacea standardized for 1% isobutylamides and 4% phenolic compounds. Standardized Full Spectrum 90 mg of extract per capsule. Guaranteed Potency 45 mg of extract per capsule.

Echinacea - Elderberry Syrup - Planetary Formulas
Each 1/2 tsp serving contains: Proprietary Blend 2.5 mL: Elderberry, Echinacea purpurea root, Isatis root, Honeysuckle flower, Forsythia flower, Boneset leaf, Platycodon root, Licorice root, Apricot seed, Gastrodia Tuber. Inactive Ingredients: Vegetable Glycerine, Purified Water, Honey, 1/10th of 1% Potassium Sorbate added as a preservative.

Echinacea & Elderberry - Leiner Health Products
Each softgel contains: Zinc Gluconate 8 mg • Echinacea extract (Echinacea angustifolia, Echinacea purpurea) root and aerial parts 150 mg • Elderberry extract (Sambucus nigra) fruit 100 mg • Golden Seal extract (Hydrastis canadensis) root 100 mg. Other Ingredients: Flaxseed Oil, Gelatin, Lecithin, Wax, Yellow Turmeric, Caramel Powder, Titanium Dioxide.

Echinacea & Golden Seal Combo - Optimum Nutrition
Each capsule contains: Horse Chestnut extract (Aesculus hippocastanum) root 250 mg • Butcher's Broom powdered root 145 mg • Ginger powdered root 145 mg. Other Ingredients: Gelatin, Magnesium Stearate.

Echinacea & Goldenseal - Leiner Health Products
Each caplet contains: Echinacea extract (Echinacea angustifolia & Echinacea purpurea) root 75 mg • Golden Seal extract (Hydrastis canadensis) root 100 mg • Hesperidin 40 mg • Quercetin 20 mg • Rutin 40 mg. Other Ingredients: Calcium Carbonate, Cellulose, Maltodextrin, Hydroxypropyl Methylcellulose, Stearic Acid, Silicon Dioxide, Polyethylene Glycol 3350, Croscarmellose Sodium, Talc, Magnesium Stearate, Hydroxypropyl Cellulose, Pharmaceutical Glaze, Crospovidone, Yellow 5 Lake, Red 40 Lake, Blue 2 Lake, Titanium Dioxide, Polysorbate 80.

Echinacea & Goldenseal 1000 mg, Concentrated - GNC
Each capsule contains: Echinacea Root (echinacea angustifolia; from 72 mg of echinacea root extract 7:1) 500 mg • Goldenseal Root (hydrastis canadensis; from 72 mg of goldenseal root extract 7:1) 500 mg. Other Ingredients: Soybean Oil, Gelatin, Glycerin, Caramel Color, Titanium Dioxide (natural mineral whitener).

Echinacea & Goldenseal Combo - Atrium Biotechnologies
Two fluid ounces contains: Echinacea • Goldenseal. In a synergistic base of Red Clover, Burdock, Parsley, Fennel, Ginger, Chamomile, Barberry & Cayenne. Contains 16-18% Grain Alcohol.

Echinacea & Goldenseal Root - NOW Foods
Two capsules contain: Echinacea Purpurea root powder 450 mg • Goldenseal root powder (hydrastis canadensis) 450 mg.

Echinacea & Goldenseal, Peppermint - GNC
Each dropperful (1mL) contains: Echinacea Extract (echinacea angustifolia, root; standardized to contain 4% echinacosides = 6 mg) 150 mg • Goldenseal Dried Root Extract (hydrastis canadesis) 0.025 mg • Stevia Extract (stevia rebaudiana, leaf) 3 mg. Other Ingredients: Deionized Water, USP Alcohol, Fructose, Glycerin, Natural Peppermint Flavor, Natural Vanilla Flavor, Methylparaben (a preservative), Natural Wintergreen Flavor, Propylparaben (a preservative).

Echinacea 1000 mg - Jamieson
Each capsule contains: Echinacea root 1000 mg.

Echinacea 150 mg - Jamieson
Each capsule contains: Echinacea (Echinacea purpurea, powdered extract 1:3) 150 mg • Panax Ginseng (Standardized to 4% ginsenosides) 250 mg.

Echinacea 150 mg with Ginseng 250 mg - Jamieson
Each capsule contains: Echinacea Purpurea (powdered extract 1:3) 150 mg • Panax Ginseng 250 mg.

Echinacea 2500 - Golden Glow Natural Health Products
Each capsule contains: Echinacea Purpurea herb juice 45:1 powder 2500 mg.

Echinacea 2500mg - Nature's Own
Each tablet contains: Echinacea dry herb juice (echinacea purpurea), equivalent to fresh herb 2500 mg.

Echinacea 300 mg - Jamieson
Each capsule contains: Echinacea herb (Echinacea Purpurea, powdered 1:3) 300 mg • Allicin Rich Garlic bulb powder 300 mg • Ginger root (Zingiber Officinale, powdered Extract 1:6) 300 mg.

Echinacea 300 mg with Garlic and Ginger - Jamieson
Each capsule contains: Echinacea Purpurea (powdered extract 1:3) 300 mg • Allicin Rich Garlic Bulb Powder 300 mg • Ginger Root (Zingiber officinale, powdered extract 1:6) 300 mg.

Echinacea 350 mg - Jamieson
Each capsule contains: Echinacea Purpurea (1:3 powdered extract) 350 mg.

Echinacea 400 mg - Puritan's Pride
Each capsule contains: Echinacea (echinacea purpurea, aerial) 400 mg. Other Ingredients: Gelatin.

Echinacea 5000 Complex - Golden Glow Natural Health Products
Each capsule contains: Echinacea Purpurea juice powder 3.5 g: Beta-1, 2-D-Oligofructofuranocides 1.87 mg • Echinacea Purpurea extract 1.5 g • Ascorbic Acid (vitamin C) 125 mg • Calcium Ascorbate 125 mg • Magnesium 13.8 mg • Zinc (as sulfate monohydrate) 5 mg • Manganese (as sulfate monohydrate) 1 mg • Bioflavonoids 50 mg.

Echinacea 5000 softgels - Golden Glow Natural Health Products
Each capsule contains: Echinacea Purpurea extract (equivalent to herb juice 5000 mg).

Echinacea and Golden Seal - Optimum Nutrition
Echinacea Angustifolia extract • Goldenseal powder.

Echinacea and Goldenseal - Dial Herbs
Echinacea • Goldenseal • Cayenne.

Echinacea and Goldenseal - Jamieson
Each capsule contains: Echinacea Root 740 mg • Goldenseal Root 90 mg.

Echinacea and Goldenseal Tincture - Jamieson
Each 15 drops (1 ml) contains: Echinacea Purpurea 375 mg • Echinacea Angustifolia 100 mg • Goldenseal Root 25 mg.

Echinacea Angustifolia - Optimum Nutrition
Each capsule contains: Echinacea Angustifolia root extract (standardized to 4% echinacosides) 125 mg • Echinacea Angustifola root, powdered 225 mg • Echinacea Purpurea aerial 10 mg. Other Ingredients: Gelatin, Magnesium Stearate.

Echinacea Angustifolia - NOW Foods
Each 1 1/2 droppersful contains: Echinacea Angustifolia root extract 1.2 ml. Other Ingredients: Grain Alcohol, Water.

Echinacea Angustifolia, Extract - Nature's Way
Each capsule contains: Echinacea Angustifolia, dried extract 250 mg • Echinacea Purpurea stem, leaf, flower 190 mg. Other Ingredients: Gelatin, Millet.

Echinacea Balance - HerbaSway
Echinacea • Green Tea • Ginger • Blackberry • HerbaSwee (Cucurbitaceae fruit).

Echinacea Complete Care - Celestial Seasonings
Two capsules contain: Vitamin C (as ascorbic acid) 180 mg • Zinc (as gluconate) 15 mg • Proprietary Blend 1000 mg: Echinacea (root, stem, leaf, flower), Echinacea (standardized extract), Arabinogalactan. Other Ingredients: Dicalcium phosphate, gelatin, rice flour, stearic acid, magnesium stearate and silicon dioxide.

Echinacea Extract - Ortho Molecular Products
Each capsule contains: Echinacea Angustifolia extract 200 mg • Echinacea Purpurea 200 mg.

Echinacea Extract - Jamieson
Each capsule contains: Echinacea herb (Echinacea purpurea 1:3 powdered extract) 350 mg. Other Ingredients: Dicalcium Phosphate, Micorcrystalline Cellulose, Magnesium Stearate, Silicon Dioxide.

Echinacea Extract - Progressive Labs
Each capsule contains: Echinacea 250 mg • Polysaccharides (from Echinacea) 37.5 mg • Phenolic compounds (from Echinacea) 10 mg.

Echinacea Extract 4% 500 mg - Vital Nutrients
Each capsule contains: Echinacea Purpurea extract (4% phenolics) 500 mg.

Echinacea Goldenseal - Jamieson
Each capsule contains: Calcium (as Calcium Sulfate) 30 mg • Echinacea root extract 4:1 (Echinacea purpurea Moench.) (4% Phenolic Compounds) 185 mg • Goldenseal root extract 2:1 (Hydrastis canadensis L.) (5% Alkaloids and Hydrastine Compounds) 45 mg.

Echinacea Goldenseal - Gaia Herbs
Three capsules contain: Echinacea Purpurea root 66 mg • Echinacea Pupurea flowering top 66 mg • St. John's Wort flower buds (hypericum perforatum) 60 mg • Goldenseal root (hydrastis canadensis) 60 mg • Echinacea Angustifolia root 54 mg • Barberry root (berberis vulgaris) 45 mg • Oregon Grape root (berberis aquifolium) 45 mg • Echinacea Purpurea seed 12 mg. Other Ingredients: Vegetable Glycerin, Vegetable Cellulose (capsule).

Echinacea Plus - Aboca USA, Inc
Each capsule contains: Echinacea Purpurea flowering top whole phytocomplex concentrate (WPC, standardized to 2% total polyphenols, yielding 2.48 mg per capsule) 124 mg • Echinacea Pallida root WPC (standardized to 1.1% echinacoside, yielding 1.36 mg per capsule) 124 mg • Echinacea Angustifolia root WPC (standardized to 0.9% echinacoside, yielding 0.38 mg per capsule) 42 mg. Other Ingredients: Gelatin (capsule).

Echinacea Plus - Traditional Medicinals
Echinacea purpurea herb • Lemongrass leaf • Spearmint leaf • Echinacea angustifolia herb • concentrated extract of E. Purpurea root.

Echinacea Red Root Supreme - Gaia Herbs
Thirty drops contain: Proprietary Blend 60 mg: Echinacea Angustifolia root, Echinacea Pupurea root, flowerhead and seed, Red Root (ceanothus americanus), Wild Indigo root (baptisia tinctoria), Thuja leaf (thuja occidentalis), Blue Flag root (iris versicolor), Stillingia root (stillingia sylvatica), Prickly Ash bark (xanthoxylum clava-herculis), 50-60% Pure Grain Alcohol USP, Spring Water.

Echinacea Root - GNC
Each dropperful (1 mL) Contains: Echinacea extract (echinacea angustifolia, root, standardized to contain 4% echinacosides = 6 mg) 150 mg • Stevia extract (as steavia rebaudiana, leaf) 3 mg. Other

BRAND NAMES

Ingredients: Deionized Water, USP Alcohol, Fructose, Glycerin, Natural Peppermint flavor, Natural Vanilla flavor, Methylparaben, Natural Wintergreen flavor, Propylparaben (a preservative).

Echinacea Root 1000 mg, Concentrated - GNC
Each capsule contains: Echinacea Root Extract (echinacea angustifolia; from 142.9 mg of echinacea root extract 7:1) 1000 mg. Other Ingredients: Gelatin, Soybean Oil, Glycerin, Caramel Color, Titanium Dioxide (natural mineral whitener).

Echinacea Root Complex - Nature's Way
Two capsules contain: Echinacea Angustifolia root • Echinacea Purpurea stem, leaf, flower • Proprietary Blend 900 mg. Other Ingredients: Gelatin, Magnesium Stearate.

Echinacea Supreme - Gaia Herbs
Two capsules contain: Echinacea Pupurea flowering top 120 mg • Echinacea Purpurea root 72 mg • Echinacea Angustifolia root 72 mg • Echinacea Pupurea seed 2 mg. Other Ingredients: Vegetable Glycerin, Lecithin, Vegetable Cellulose (capsule).

Echinacea Synergy - Metagenics
Each tablet contains: Ultra Potent-C brand Vitamin C 100 mg • Niacin (as niacinamide ascorbate) 7 mg • Echinacea Purpurea root 4:1 extract (containing polyphenols) 300 mg • Perilla seed extract (perilla frutescens, containing rosmarinic acid and luteolin) 25 mg • Ginger rhizome extract (zingiber officinale, containing gingerols and shogoals) 25 mg • Licorice root extract (glycyrrhiza glabra, containing glycyrrhizic acid) 50 mg.

Echinacea Syrup - Pure Encapsulations
Each 1 tsp serving contains: Echinacea syrup (providing 50% echinacea purpurea fresh pressed juice) 5 mL. Base: Maltitol Syrup (consisting of the sugar alcohol maltitol and hydrated oligosaccharides).

Echinacea Tincture - Jamieson
Each 2 mL (40 drops) contains: Echinacea angustifolia (1:2 pure tincture in 45% Ethanol) Derived from alcohol maceration of fresh plants (aerial parts) 1000 mg.

Echinacea Whole Herb, 350 mg - Nature Made
Each capsule contains: Echinacea Purpurea aerial part 350 mg: Cichoric Acid 2.5 mg.

Echinacea with Goldenseal Liquid Extract - Quantum, Inc.
Two ounces contain: Fresh undried Echinacea purpurea whole plant 70% • Echinacea angustifolia 10% • Goldenseal root 20% • Alcohol 50%.
See Editor's Note No. 21.

Echinacea with Vitamin C - J. R. Carlson Laboratories, Inc.
Each capsule contains: Vitamin C (as ascorbic acid) 500 mg • Echinacea (4% phenolics) 250 mg.

Echinacea with Zinc - Aspen Group, Inc.
Each capsule contains: Echinacea Purpurea 380 mg • Zinc (citrate) 3 mg.

Echinacea, Propolis & Ester C - Futurebiotics LLC
Two capsules contain: Vitamin C (as Ester-C ascorbate) 500 mg • Calcium (as calcium ascorbate) 59 mg • Echinacea angustifolia leaf powder extract [standardized for 4% (5 mg) echinacosides] 125 mg • Echinacea angustifolia leaf powder 150 mg • Echinacea purpurea leaf powder 150 mg • Citrus bioflavonoid peel powder 250 mg • Bee Propolis powder 100 mg • Acerola berry (Rose Hips) powder 50 mg. Other Ingredients: Magnesium stearate, Gelatin, Water.

Echinacea/Astragalus/Reishi Formula - Nature's Way
Three capsules contain: Proprietary Formula: Astragalus root • Echinacea Purpurea stem, leaf, flower • Reishi (dried extract 10% Polysaccharides). Other Ingredients: Gelatin.

Echinacea/Ester-C Formula - Nature's Way
Two capsules contain: Calcium 27 mg • Echinacea Purpurea stem, leaf, flower 722 mg • Ester-C (Patented form of Vitamin C) 207 mg. Other Ingredients: Gelatin.

Echinacea/Ginseng Formula - Nature's Way
Two capsules contain: Proprietary Formula: Echinacea Angustifolia root • Echinacea Purpurea stem, leaf, flower • Siberian Ginseng root . Other Ingredients: Gelatin, Magnesium Stearate, Millet.

Echinacea/Goldenseal - Gaia Herbs
Echinacea and Goldenseal standardized for 1% isobutylamides and 15% total alkaloids. Standardized Full Spectrum 100 mg of extract per capsule. Guaranteed Potency 50 mg of extract per capsule.

Echinacea/Goldenseal/Cats Claw Complex - Solgar
Two capsules contain: Echinacea root extract 4:1 (echinacea angustifolia) 50 mg • Echinacea root 4:1 extract (echinacea purpurea) 50 mg • Raw Echinacea powder (echinacea purpurea) 200 mg • Goldenseal root 4:1 extract (hydrastis canadensis) 100 mg • Raw Goldenseal root powder (hydrastis canadensis) 200 mg • Peruvian Cat's Claw bark 3:1 extract (uncaria tomentosa) 300 mg. Other Ingredients: Vegetable Cellulose, Vegetable Magnesium Stearate, Water, Vegetable Glycerin.

Echinacea/GSR Formula - Nature's Way
Three capsules contain: Proprietary Formula: Burdock root • Cayenne pepper fruit • Echinacea Angustifolia root • Echinacea Purpurea stem, leaf, flower • Gentain root • Goldenseal stem, leaf, flower • Wood Betony stem, leaf, flower. Other Ingredients: Gelatin.

Echinacea-C - Standard Process, Inc.
Each tablet contains: Proprietary Blend 400 mg: Acerola berry, Rose Hips, Dried Buckwheat juice, Buckwheat seed • Vitamin C 5.4 mg • Echinacea root 135 mg. Other Ingredients: Honey, Calcium Stearate.

Echinacea-C 2500 - Nature's Own
Each tablet contains: Echinacea dry herb juice (echinacea purpurea) equivalent to fresh herb 2500 mg • Vitamin C (from ascorbic acid 270 mg and sodium ascorbate 260 mg) 500 mg • Acerola extract (malpighia punicifolia), equivalent to dry fruit 60 mg.

Echinacea-Go! - Wakunaga of America
Each capsule contains: Echinacea standardized extract (angustifolia & purpurea blend) leaf/root, standardized to 4% phenolic compounds. Other Ingredients: Cellulose, Colloidal Silica, Magnesium Stearate (vegetable source).

Echinacea-Goldenseal Formula - Quest
Each caplet contains: Echinacea angustifolia powder (provided by 100 mg P.E. 1:7 standardized to contain 4% echinacosides) 700 mg • Goldenseal root powder (Hydrastis canadensis) (provided by 50 mg P.E. 1:6 standardized to contain 5% hydrastine) 300 mg • Echinacea purpurea powder (Provided by 50 mg P.E. 1:5 standardized to contain 0.7% flavonoids) 250 mg • Astragalus root powder (Astragalus membranaceus) 100 mg. Other Ingredients: Calcium Phosphate, Microcrystalline Cellulose, Vegetable Stearin, Croscarmellose Sodium, Magnesium Stearate (vegetable source).

Echinacea-Reishi Virtue - Blessed Herbs
Astragalus root • Echinacea Angustifolia root • Pau d'Arco bark • Suma root • Siberian Ginseng root • Reishi mycelium • Licorice root • German Chamomile flower • Calendula flower • Grain alcohol & Distilled Water.

Echinaforce - Bioforce AG
Two tablets contain: Echinacea purpurea extract (95% herb and 5% roots) 538 mg • Lactose 250 mg.

EchinaFresh - Enzymatic Therapy
Each capsule contains: Echinacea purpurea 50:1 concentration of powder from the fresh-pressed juice of stems, leaves, & flowers of organically grown Echinacea purpurea 50 mg.

BRAND NAMES

EchinaGold - Pure Encapsulations
Each vegetable capsule contains: Echinacea Angustifolia extract (standardized to contain 4% echinacosides) 200 mg • Goldenseal extract (standardized to contain 8% berberine and hydrastine) 250 mg • Vitamin C (as ascorbyl palmitate) 9 mg.

EchinaGuard - Nature's Way
Each capsule contains: Echinacea purpurea (stem, leaf, flower) 250 mg • EchinaGuard (Echinacea purpurea dried extract) 85 mg. Other Ingredients: Gelatin, Silica.

EchinaGuard Flexitabs - Nature's Way
Each flexitab contains: EchinaGuard (Echinacea Purpurea dried extract) 88 mg. Other Ingredients: Cherry Flavor, Citric Acid, Corn Starch, Fructose, Gelatin, Glycerol, Guar Gum, Lecithin.

Echinamax - Progena
Each capsule contains: Echinacea purpurea herb (standardized to a minumum level of 4% phenolics, 0.1% alkylamides, and 15% minimum polysaccharides) 100 mg • Echinacea purpurea herb (standardized to a minimum level of 1.5% cichoric acid) 400 mg.

Echinex - Chattem, Inc.
Each tablet contains: Standardized extract of Echinacea purpurea root & herb (4% total phenolic compounds) 250 mg • Standardized extract of Siberian Ginseng root (0.8% eleutherosides) 100 mg • Standardized extract of Ginger root (5% gingerols) 100 mg. Other Ingredients: Cellulose, Croscarmellose Sodium, Stearic Acid, Magnesium Stearate, Silicon Dioxide, Hydroxypropyl Methylcellulose (aqueous film coating).

EchinKids - Health Smart Vitamins
Two drops contains: Zinc (as zinc glycinate) 4 mg • Copper (as copper glycinate) 0.50 mg • Echinacea (root, aerial parts) 150 mg.

EchinSeal - Health Smart Vitamins
Two capsules contain: Goldenseal root 800 mg • Echinacea purpurea aerial parts 400 mg.

EchinZinC lozenge - Nature's Own
Each lozenge contains: Echinacea dried herb juice (echinacea purpurea), equivalent to fresh herb juice 751.5 mg • Sodium Ascorbate 66.27 mg, equivalent to Ascorbic Acid 59 mg • Zinc Gluconate 10.2 mg equivalent to elemental Zinc 1.46 mg.

EcoGen Fermented Soy Drink - EcoNugenics
Each bottle (8 oz) contains: Soy Isoflavones 150 mg • Providing: Genistein 70%, Daidzein 23%, Glycitein 7% • Protein 5.7 g • Calcium 32 mg • Iron 1 mg.

EcoGen Soybean Isoflavone Concentrate Powder - EcoNugenics
Five teaspoons (10 g) contain: EcoGen Soy Isoflavone Concentrate 10 g • Soy Isoflavones 191 mg: Glyciteins 92 mg, Genisteins 31 mg, Daidzeins 68 mg • Protein 4 g • Iron 1 mg.

EcoGen Soybean Isoflavone Concentrate Tablets - EcoNugenics
Four tablets contain: EcoGen Soy Isoflavone Concentrate 3 g • Soy Isoflavones 77 mg: Glyciteins 27 mg, Genisteins 10 mg, Daidzeins 40 mg • Protein 1 g • Iron 0.3 g. Other Ingredients: Calcium Sulfate, Stearic Acid, Silica, Magnesium Sulfate, Cellulose.

Eco-Green Multi - NOW Foods
Two tablets contain: Vitamin A (Beta Carotene) (15 mg) 25000 IU • Vitamin B1 (Thiamine HCl) 50 mg • Vitamin B2 (Riboflavin) 50 mg • Vitamin B3 (Niacinamide) 50 mg • Vitamin B5 (Pantothenic Acid) 50 mg • Vitamin B6 (Pyridoxine HCl) 50 mg • Vitamin B12 (Cyanocobalamin) 200 mcg • Biotin 100 mcg • Folic Acid 800 mcg • Vitamin C (Calcium Ascorbate) 500 mg • Vitamin D (Calciferol) 200 IU • Vitamin E (d-Alpha Succinate) 200 IU • Vitamin K (from green foods) 70 mcg • Calcium (Ascorbate, Citrate, Carbonate) 100 mg • Magnesium (50% Citrate, 50% Oxide) 100 mg • Zinc (Picolinate) 15 mg • Copper (Amino Acid Chelate) 500 mcg • Iodine (Kelp) 150 mcg • Potassium (Chloride) 25 mg • Manganese (Amino Acid Chelate) 5 mg • Selenium (L-Selenomethionine) 50 mcg • Chromium (Picolinate) 100 mcg • Molybdenum (Amino Acid Chelate) 50 mcg • Spirulina US grown 250 mg • Barley grass organically grown 250 mg • Chlorella (broken cell wall) 100 mg • Wheat grass organically grown 100 mg • Alfalfa juice concentrate 100 mg • Green Tea extract (40% Catechins) 50 mg • Choline (Bitartrate) 50 mg • Inositol 50 mg • PABA 30 mg • Trace Mineral concentrate 100 mg • Boron (Amino Acid Chelate) 1 mg • Vanadium (Amino Acid Chelate) 50 mcg • Panax ginseng (5% Ginsenosides) 100 mg • Bioflavonoids (40%) 50 mg • Rutin 25 mg • Bromelain (2000 GDU from pineapple) 50 mg • Papain (140 MCU from papaya) 25 mg • Pepsin Enzymes (NF 1:10000) 25 mg • Lipase (3400 Usp Units) 25 mg • Amylase (20000 USP Units) 10 mg • Chlorophyll from green foods 8 mg • Amino Acids from green foods 350 mg. Vegetarian formula base ingredients contain: Di-Calcium Phosphate, Cellulose, Stearic Acid, Magnesium Stearate & Silica.

E-Complete 400 - GNC
Each capsule contains: Vitamin E (as d-alpha Tocopherol) 400 IU • Tocotrienols 40 mg. Other Ingredients: Gelatin, Glycerin.

Edemex - Gero Vita International
Each capsule contains: Alisma rhizome extract (alisma orientale) 70 mg • Zhu Ling sclerotium extract (polyporus umbellatus) 70 mg • White Mulberry root extract (morus alba) 70 mg • Betel nut palm seed extract (areca catechu) 70 mg • Winter Melon fruit rind extract (benincasa hispidum) 50 mg • Bai-Zhu Atractylodes rhizome extract (atractylodes macrocephala) 50 mg • Cassia bark extract (cinnamomum cassia) 50 mg • Corn style extract (zea mays) 50 mg • Ginger rhizome extract (zingiber officinale) 35 mg. Other Ingredients: Silica, Magnesium Stearate, Gelatin.

EDTA Chelator Complex - Life Enhancement Products, Inc.
Each capsule contains: Malic Acid 500 mg • EDTA (as calcium disodium ethylenediaminetetraacetate) 100 mg • Garlic, deodorized (1500 ppm of allicin) 115 mg.

EDTA Chelator Complex Original - Life Enhancement Products, Inc.
Each capsule contains: Garlic powder 400 mg • EDTA (as calcium disodium ethylenediaminetetraacetate) 100 mg.

EFA Attention Formula - Health From The Sun
Each capsule contains: Vitamin E (as d-Alpha Tocopherol) 5 IU • Magnesium from Magnesium Oxide 55 mg • Zinc from Zinc Sulfate 0.5 mg • High DHA Fish oil (70 mg Omega-3 DHA) 175 mg • Arachidonic Acid (from Fish oil) 3 mg • Borage oil (16 mg Omega-6 GLA) 80 mg • Lecithin 50 mg • Ashwagandha root extract 25 mg • Bacopa Monnieri Whole Plant extract 25 mg. Other Ingredients: Gelatin, Glycerine, Beeswax (emulsifier), Water, Carob powder.

EFA Complex - PhysioLogics
Two softgels contain: Vitamin E (as d-Alpha Tocopherol) 20 IU • Eicosapentaenoic Acid (from Marine Lipids) 120 mg • Docosahexaenoic Acid (from Marine Lipids) 80 mg • Gamma-linolenic Acid (from Borage oil) 30 mg.

EFA Complex - New Improved Formula - PhysioLogics
Each softgel contains: Vitamin E (as d-alpha tocopherol) 5 IU • Flaxseed oil 400 mg • Borage seed oil 400 mg • Fish oil (50% omega-3) 400 mg • Fatty Acid Profile: Oleic Acid 152 mg, Linoleic Acid 180 mg, Gamma Linolenic Acid (GLA) 96 mg, Alpha Linolenic Acid 220 mg, Eicosapentaenoic Acid (EPA) 120 mg, Docosahexaenoic Acid (DHA) 80 mg. Other Ingredients: Gelatin, Glycerin.

EFA Derma-Skin Formula - Health From The Sun
Each capsule contains: Vitamin A from Palmitate 3000 IU • Vitamin C from Ascorbic Acid 60 mg • Vitamin D as Cholecalciferol 100 IU • Vitamin E as d-Alpha Tocopherol 40 IU • Zinc from Zinc Sulfate 10 mg • Organic Flax seed oil (450 mg Omega-3 ALA) 800 mg • Borage seed oil (120 mg Omega-6 GLA) 600 mg • Burdock root extract 4:1 50 mg • Yellow Dock root extract 4:1 50 mg. Other Ingredients: Gelatin, Glycerine, Beeswax (emulsifier), Water, Carob powder, Lecithin.

EFA gelcaps **-** Matol Botanical International Ltd
Each capsule contains: Flaxseed oil • Borage oil • Marine oil • Flaxseed Particulate • Mixed Carotenoids • Rosemary.

EFA Heart Formula **-** Health From The Sun
Three capsules contain: Borage oil (180 mg GLA) 900 mg • Fish oil (18% EPA, 12% DHA) 1200 mg • Flax seed oil, organic 300 mg • Folic Acid 300 mcg • Garlic extract (0.8% Allicin) 300 mg • Gugulipid (10% Gugulsterone) 300 mg • Hawthorne extract (2% Vitexin) 105 mg • Tocopherols, mixed 3.9 mg • Tocotrienols 11 mg • Vitamin B6 from Pyridoxine Hydrochloride 1.2 mg.

EFA Joint Formula **-** Health From The Sun
Three capsules contain: Protein 1 g • Vitamin C as Ascorbic Acid 75 mg • Vitamin D (as Vitamin D3) as Cholecalciferol 100 IU • Vitamin E as d-Alpha Tocopherol 30 IU • Zinc from Zinc Sulfate 15 mg • Manganese from Manganese Gluconate 330 mcg • Borage seed oil 300 mg • GLA 1500 mg • Glucosamine Sulfate 1200 mg • Organic Flax seed oil (250 mg ALA) 450 mg • Boswellic Acid from Boswellia Resin extract 100 mg. Ingredients: Gelatin, Glycerine, Beeswax (emulsifer), Water, Carob powder, Soy Lecithin.

EFA liquid **-** Matol Botanical International Ltd
Each 1 tbsp serving contains: Flaxseed oil • Flaxseed Particulate • Borage oil • Marine oil • Soybean oil • Canola oil • Mixed Carotenoids • Ascorbic Acid • Rosemary.

Efalex **-** Efamol Ltd.
Two capsules contain: Efamol brand Evening Primrose oil 280 mg • DHA 120 mg • GLA 24 mg • Arachidonic Acid 10.5 mg • Thyme oil 2 mg • Vitamin E 15 IU. Other Ingredients: Tuna Oil, Gelatin, Glycerin.

Efalex Liquid **-** Efamol Ltd.
Each 4 tsp serving contain: Efamol brand Evening Primrose oil 1200 mg • DHA 480 mg • GLA 96 mg • Arachidonic Acid 42 mg • Thyme oil 8 mg • Vitamin E 15 IU. Other Ingredients: Sunflower Oil, Tuna Oil, Lemon Oil, Lime Oil.

Efamol Fortify **-** Efamol Ltd.
Two capsules contain: Efamol Pure Evening Primrose Oil 800 mg • EPA 14 mg • GLA 64 mg • Vitamin E 30 IU • Calcium 200 mg. Other Ingredients: Calcium Carbonate, Gelatin, Glycerin, Marine Fish Oil, Glyceryl Monostearate, Titanium Dioxide Color.
See Editor's Note No. 21.

Efamol PMS Control **-** Efamol Ltd.
Two capsules contain: Efamol Pure Evening Primrose Oil 500 mg • GLA 40 mg • Vitamin C 60 mg • Vitamin E 30 IU • Niacin 12 mg • Vitamin B6 40 mg • Biotin 80 mcg • Magnesium 40 mg • Zinc 4 mg. Other Ingredients: Gelatin, Sorbitol Syrup, Glyceryl Monostearate, Glycerin, Ascorbic Acid, Heavy Magnesium Oxide, Pyridoxine HCl, Lecithin, Nicotinamide, Zinc Sulphate Monohydrate, d-Biotin.

Efamol Pure Evening Primrose Oil **-** Efamol Ltd.
Two capsules contain: Efamol Pure Evening Primrose Oil 1000 mg • Linoleic Acid 330 mg • Gamma Linolenic Acid 80 mg. Other Ingredients: Gelatin, Glycerin.

Efanatal **-** Efamol Ltd.
Two capsules contain: Efamol Pure Evening Primrose Oil 500 mg • DHA (Docosahexaenoic Acid) 107 mg • Arachidonic Acid 9.4 mg • GLA 40 mg • Vitamin E 15 IU. Inactive Ingredients: Fish Oil, Gelatin, Glycerol, Carmine Color, Titanium Dioxide Color, Ammonium Phosphatide, Ascorbyl Palmitate.

Effect **-** Salitos Beverages
Each 100 mL serving cotnains: Water • Sucrose • Glucose • Citric Acid • Taurine 400 mg • Inositol (0.2%) • Carbonic Acid • Glucuronolactone 240 mg • Sodiumbenzoate • Flavours • Caffeine 32 mg • Niacin • Pantothenic Acid • Vitamin B2 • Vitamin B6 • Vitamin B12 • E150B Colouring.

Effervescent Glucosamine / Chondroitin **-** GNC
Fructose • Glucosamine HCl • Chondroitin Sulfate • Sodium Bicarbonate • Methyl Sulfonyl Methane (MSM) • Ascorbic Acid • Ascorbic Acid • Potassium Bicarbonate • Natural Pineapple flavor • Artificial Pineapple flavor • Calcium Pantothenate • Pyridoxine HCl • Cyanocobalamin.
See Editor's Note No. 15.

Effisoy **-** FermaHealth
Each capsule contains: AglyMax standardized fermented Soy germ extract (includes 40 mg of the isoflavone aglycones, daidzein, glycitein and genistein). Other Ingredients: Gelatin, Soybean Oil, Glycerin, Dextrin, Carob, D-Alpha Tocopherol, Lecithin, Titanium Dioxide.

E-Gem Cream **-** J. R. Carlson Laboratories, Inc.
Each gram contains: Vitamin A (as palmitate) 5000 IU • Vitamin D 200 IU • Vitamin E (as D-alpha tocopheryl acetate) 100 IU.

E-Gem Lip Care **-** J. R. Carlson Laboratories, Inc.
Vitamin E (as D-alpha tocopheryl acetate) 1 IU.

E-Gem Oil Drops **-** J. R. Carlson Laboratories, Inc.
Vitamin E (as D-alpha tocopheryl acetate) 100 IU.

E-Gem Skin-Care Soap **-** J. R. Carlson Laboratories, Inc.
Vitamin A 1000 IU • Vitamin E (as D-alpha tocopheryl acetate) 1000 IU.

E-Gems 100 IU **-** J. R. Carlson Laboratories, Inc.
Each softgel contains: Vitamin E (as D-alpha tocopheryl acetate) 100 IU.

E-Gems 1000 IU **-** J. R. Carlson Laboratories, Inc.
Each softgel contains: Vitamin E (as D-alpha tocopheryl acetate) 100 IU.

E-Gems 1200 IU **-** J. R. Carlson Laboratories, Inc.
Each softgel contains: Vitamin E (as D-alpha tocopheryl acetate) 1200 IU.

E-Gems 30 IU **-** J. R. Carlson Laboratories, Inc.
Each softgel contains: Vitamin E (as D-alpha tocopheryl acetate) 30 IU.

E-Gems 400 IU **-** J. R. Carlson Laboratories, Inc.
Each softgel contains: Vitamin E (as d-alpha tocopheryl acetate) 400 IU.

E-Gems 600 IU **-** J. R. Carlson Laboratories, Inc.
Each softgel contains: Vitamin E (as D-alpha tocopheryl acetate) 600 IU.

E-Gems 800 IU **-** J. R. Carlson Laboratories, Inc.
Each softgel contains: Vitamin E (as D-alpha tocopheryl acetate) 800 IU.

E-Gems Elite **-** J. R. Carlson Laboratories, Inc.
Each capsule contains: Vitamin E (as D-alpha tocopherol) 400 IU • D-Gamma Tocopherol 100 mg • D-Alpha, D-Beta, D-Delta Tocotrienols 20 mg • D-Beta and D-Delta Tocopherol 40 mg.

E-Gems Plus 200 IU **-** J. R. Carlson Laboratories, Inc.
Each softgel contains: Vitamin E (as D-alpha tocopherol) 200 IU • Mixed Tocopherols 67 mg.

E-Gems Plus 400 IU **-** J. R. Carlson Laboratories, Inc.
Each softgel contains: Vitamin E (as D-alpha tocopherol) 400 IU • Mixed Tocopherols 67 mg.

E-Gems Plus 800 IU **-** J. R. Carlson Laboratories, Inc.
Each softgel contains: Vitamin E (as D-alpha tocopherol) 800 IU • Mixed Tocopherols 134 mg.

E-Gems with C **-** J. R. Carlson Laboratories, Inc.
Two softgels contain: Vitamin C (as ascorbic acid) 1000 mg • Vitamin E (as D-alpha tocopheryl acetate) 400 IU.

Some Brand Name Natural Products - What they Contain

www.NaturalDatabase.com contains MANY more listings than appear here.
Editor's Notes are located on pages 2155-2163.

Egg Fuel - TwinLab
Each serving contains: Pure egg white protein.

EgSENTIALS - Bio Tech Pharmacal
Each capsule contains: Vitamin B6 (pyridoxal 5'-phosphate) 9 mg • Proprietary Blend 670 mg: Alpha Ketoglutaric Acid, L-Leucine, L-Valine, L-Lysine, L-Isoleucine, L-Phenylalanine, L-Threonine, L-Methionine, L-Tryptophan.

El Toro Loco Lemon-Lime Loco - Unknown
Purified Water • Crystalline Fructose • Corn Syrup Solids • Natural and Artificial Flavors • Ascorbic Acid • Pyridoxine Hydrochloride • Taurine • Caffeine • Potassium Gluconate • Sodium Chloride • Sodium Gluconate • Acesulfame Potassium • FD&C Yellow No. 5 • FD&C Blue No. 1 • Xanthan Gum • Sodium Benzoate • Potassium Sorbate (as preservatives).

El Toro Loco Orange Stomp - Unknown
Purified Water • Crystalline Fructose • Corn Syrup Solids • Natural and Artificial Flavors • Ascorbic Acid • Pyridoxine Hydrochloride • Taurine • Caffeine • Potassium Gluconate • Sodium Chloride • Sodium Gluconate • Acesulfame Potassium • FD&C Yellow No. 5 • FD&C Blue No. 1 • Xanthan Gum • Sodium Benzoate • Potassium Sorbate (as preservatives).

Elan Vital Multiple - Source Naturals
Six tablets contain: Pro-Vitamin A (beta carotene) 25000 IU • Vitamin A (palmitate) 10000 IU • Total Vitamin A activity 35000 IU • Vitamin B-1 (thiamin nitrate) 100 mg • Vitamin B-2 (riboflavin) 100 mg • Inositol Hexanicotinate, Niacinamide and Niacin 200 mg • Vitamin B-5 (calcium D-pantothenate) 100 mg • Vitamin B-6 (pyridoxine HCl) 100 mg • Vitamin B-12 (cyanocobalamin) 200 mcg • Biotin 500 mcg • Folic acid 800 mcg • Vitamin C (magnesium, manganese and zinc ascorbates) 1800 mg • Fat-Soluble Vitamin C (from 476 mg of ascorbyl palmitate) 200 mg • Total Vitamin C activity 2000 mg • Vitamin D (as Vitamin D-3, cholecalciferol) 400 IU • Vitamin E D-alpha Tocopheryl (natural) 600 IU • Boron (amino acid chelate) 2 mg • Calcium (succinate, carbonate, malate) 200 mg • Chromium (ChromeMate yeast-free polynicotinate 150 mcg and yeast-free picolinate 150 mcg) 300 mcg • Copper (sebacate) 1 mg • Iodine (from kelp) 150 mcg • Magnesium (ascorbate, oxide, succinate) 300 mg • Manganese (ascorbate) 10 mg • Molybdenum (amino acid chelate) 300 mcg • Potassium (succinate, alpha-ketoglutarate) 99 mg • Selenium (L-selenomethionine and sodium selenite) 250 mcg • Zinc (OptiZinc zinc monomethionine and ascorbate) 30 mg. Other Ingredients: N-Acetyl Cysteine 600 mg, Succinic Acid (free form) 300 mg, Choline (bitartrate) 100 mg, Inositol (hexanicotinate and inositol) 100 mg, N-A-G (N-acetyl glucosamine) 200 mg, DMAE (bitartrate) 40 mg, N-Acetyl L-Tyrosine 80 mg, Coenzyme Q10 (ubiquinone) 40 mg, alpha-Lipoic acid (thioctic acid) 40 mg, Quercetin 300 mg, Silymarin (milk thistle seed extract) 200 mg, Proanthodyn (from grape seed extract) 100 mg, Ginkgo Biloba 24% (50:1 extract) 40 mg, Bilberry extract (37% anthocyanosides) 20 mg.

Elations Cranberry Apple Twist - Proctor & Gamble
Each 4 oz bottle contains: Glucosamine HCl 1500 • Calcium 300 mg • Vitamin C 60 mg. Ingredients: Water, fructose, 2% or less juices from concentrate (apple, pear, cranberry), Citric Acid, Malic Acid, Calcium Hydroxide, Ascorbic Acid (vitamin C), Calcium Disodium EDTA, Red 40, Blue 1, Natural and Artificial Flavors.

Elations Ruby Red Grapefruit Lift - Proctor & Gamble
Each 4 oz bottle contains: Glucosamine HCl 1500 • Calcium 300 mg • Vitamin C 60 mg. Ingredients: Water, fructose, 2% or less juices from concentrate (cranberry, apple, grapefruit), Citric Acid, Malic Acid, Calcium Hydroxide, Ascorbic Acid (vitamin C), Calcium Disodium EDTA, Red 40, Blue 1, Natural and Artificial flavors.

Ela-Vites L-Phenylalanine Complex - Nature's Plus
Two tablets contain: L-Phenylalanine free form amino acid 600 mg • Vitamin C with Rose Hips 400 mg • L-Tyrosine free form amino acid 200 mg • Vitamin B6 (Pyridoxine HCl) 100 mg. In a natural herbal base containing Ginseng, Gotu Kola & Fo-Ti.

Elderberry - Pure Encapsulations
Each vegetable capsule contains: Elderberry extract (standardized to contain 28% anthocyanins) 700 mg.

Elderberry - Natrol, Inc.
Each lozenge contains: Vitamin C (as Calcium Ascorbate) 50 mg • Zinc (as Zinc Gluconate) 7.5 mg • Echinacea angustfolia entire plant 10 mg • Bee Propolis 10 mg • Slippery Elm Bark 10 mg • Elderberry 10 mg • Bee Pollen 10 mg. Other Ingredients: Hydrogenated Starch, Hydrolysate, natural Elderberry flavor, Grape skin for color.

Elderberry - Extra Strength - Jamieson
Each capsule contains: Elderberry fruit (Sambucus Nigra L. 40 mg powdered extract 1:50) 2000 mg.

Elderberry Lozenges - Quantum, Inc.
Each lozenge contains: Elderberry extract standardized to 5% total flavonoids (Sambucus nigra) 200 mg • Vitamin C (ascorbic acid) 100 mg • Marshmallow Althea powder 50 mg • Echinacea angustifolia standardized powder extract 4% phenolic compounds 25 mg • Mullein powder 10 mg. Other Ingredients: Menthol Crystals, Eucalyptus Oil, Peppermint Oil, Stevia Leaves and Stevioside, Sorbitol, Raspberry Flavoring.

Elderberry Syrup - Planetary Formulas
Each 1 tsp serving contains: Proprietary Blend 1.5 mL: Elderberry (4:1). Other Ingredients: Honey, Grain Alcohol (20-25%), Purified Water.

Elder-Zinc Lozenges - NOW Foods
Two lozenges contain: Vitamin C (Ascorbic Acid • Sodium Ascorbate) 300 mg • Zinc (as Zinc Gluconate) 24 mg • Elderberry (Sambucus nigra) 10:1 extract 200 mg • Echinacea purpurea root 50 mg • Bee Propolis 50 mg • Slippery Elm bark (Ulmus fulva) 50 mg.

Electro MIX - Alacer
Each packet contains: Potassium 100 mg • Calcium 25 mg • Magnesium 30 mg • Manganese 0.5 mg • Chromium 5 mcg. Other Ingredients: Citric Acid, Potassium Bicarbonate, Calcium, Magnesium Carbonates, Potassium Carbonates, Malic Acid, Magnesium Hydroxide, Manganese Gluconate, Chromium Aspartate, Natural Flavors.

Electrolyte Balance - The Vitamin Shoppe
Two tablets contain: Potassium 99 mg • Magnesium 500 mg • Calcium 250 mg • Boron 3 mg • Vitamin D 100 IU.

Elemax - Naturodoc
Each capsule contains: L-Glycine 200 mg • L-Tyrosine 150 mg • St. John's Wort (hypericum perforatum extract, 0.3% hypericin) 150 mg • Niacin (niacinol) 100 mg • 5-HTP (5-hydroxytryptophan) 25 mg • Siberian Ginseng (eleutherococcus senticosus, 1.2% eleutherosides) 25 mg • Ginkgo Biloba Extract (24% ginkgo extract) 25 mg • Colecus Forskohlii Extract (5-10% forskolin) 25 mg • Coenzyme B6 (pyridoxal-5-phosphate) 5 mg • Folic Acid 500 mcg.

Eleotin tea - Eastwood Bio Medical Research Inc.
Morning Formula: Balloon flower extract • Schizandra fruit extract • Solomon's Seal extract • Mulberry leaf lextract • Licorice root extract • Abyssinian Myrrh extract • Chinese Motherwort extract.
Afternoon Formula: Schizandra fruit extract • Solomon's Seal extract • Balloon flower extract • Chicory extract • Wild Yam root • Chinese Motherwort extract.
Night Formula: Lycium fruit extract • Jujube fruit extract • Wild Yam • Balloon flower extract • Schizandra fruit extract • Abyssinian Myrrh extract • Licorice root extract.

Eleuthero 0.8% E & B - Pure Encapsulations
Each vegetable capsule contains: Eleutherococcus Senticosus extract (standardized to contain 0.8% eleutheroside E & B) 250 mg.

Eleuthero 500 mg - Pro Health
Two capsules contain: Eleutherococcus Senticosus 500 mg. Other Ingredients: Magnesium Stearate.

Eleuthero Extract - PhytoPharmica
Each capsule contains: Siberian Ginseng root extract (eleutherococcus senticosus, standardized to contain a minimum of 0.5% eleutheroside E) 200 mg.
This product was formerly known as Siberian Ginseng Formula.

Eleuthero Root - Gaia Herbs
Two capsules contain: Eleuthero root (eleutherococcus senticosus) 400 mg. Other Ingredients: Vegetable Glycerin, Vegetable Cellulose (capsule).

Elim Slim Supreme - Gaia Herbs
Forty drops contain: Proprietary Blend 450 mg: Green Tea leaf (camellia sinensis), Garcinia Malabar tamarind (garcinia cambogia), Coleus root (coleus forskohlii), Elderberry (sambucus canadensis), Gymnema leaf (gymnema sylvestre), Bladderwrack fronds (fucus vesiculosus), Licorice root (glycyrrhiza glabra), Jujube date seed (ziziphus jujuba), Turmeric root (curcuma longa), Ginger root (zingiber officinale), 40-50% Pure Grain Alcohol USP, Spring Water.

Elo-Plex - Progressive Labs
Each capsule contains: Vitamin C 100 mg • Vitamin B6 10 mg • Pantothenic Acid 50 mg • Zinc (as zinc proteinate) 3.3 mg • Copper (as copper proteinate) 0.3 mg • L-Tyrosine 150 mg • DL-Phenylalanine 80 mg • Adrenal 10 mg • Hypothalamus 15 mg.
See Editor's Note No. 31.

EluHair - Dolisos
Two softgels contain: Vitamin E (as D-alpha tocopherol) 16 IU • Zinc (as zinc sulfate) 15 mg • Pantothenic Acid (as calcium pantothenate) 6 mg • Vitamin B6 (as pyridoxine hydrochloride) 2 mg • Biotin 150 mcg • Wheat Germ oil providing Linoleic Acid and Gammalinolenic Acid 200 mg • L-Cysteine 160 mg • L-Methionine 160 mg • Watercress extract (nasturtium officinale) 30 mg • Bilberry extract (vaccinium myrtillus L., standardized to 25% anthocyanins) 5 mg. Other Ingredients: Sunflower Oil, Soy Lecithin, Yellow Beeswax, Gelatin, Caramel Color, Colloidal Silica, Maltodextrin.

Elusan Prostate - Plantes & Medecines Inc.
Each capsule contains: Serenoa Repens Lipidosterolic extract 160 mg.

EluSlim - Dolisos
Each tablet contains: Calcium 67 mg • Iodine (from kelp extract) 150 mcg • Chromium (chromium as chromium polynicotinate) 100 mcg • Kelp extract (ascophyllum nodosum) 100 mg • Garcinia extract (garcinia cambogia, standardized to 50% (-) hydroxycitric acid, HCA) 100 mg • Green Tea extract (camellia sinensis, standardized to 3% caffeine) 80 mg • Guarana extract (paulinia cupana, standardized to 10% caffeine) 60 mg • Bitter Orange extract (citrus aurantium L., standardized to 6% synephrine) 60 mg • Hieracium Pilosella (hawkweed extract, standardized to 6% ombelliferones) 60 mg • Hibiscus extract (hibiscus sabdariffa, standardized to 30% (-)hydroxycitric acid, HCA) 50 mg. Other Ingredients: Dicalcium Phosphate Dihydrate, Microcrystalline Cellulose, Maltodextrin, Croscarmellose Sodium, Magnesium Stearate (vegetable source), Hydroxypropyl Methylcellulose, Glycerin, Silica.
See Editor's Note No. 40.

EluSun - Dolisos
Two softgels contain: Borage oil (borago officinalis, standardized to 20% gamma linolenic acid) 20 mg • Tocotrienols 1 mg. Other Ingredients: Sunflower Oil, Gelatin (vegetable), Carrot Oil Macerate, Glycerin, Yellow Beeswax, Soy Bean Oil, Cornstarch, Soy Lecithin.

EluSun - Plantes & Medecines Inc.
Two capsules contain: Vitamin C (ascorbic acid) 30 mg • Vitamin E (alpha tocopherol acetate) 5 IU • Natural Carotenes 20 mg • Borage Oil 20 mg. Ingredients: Carrot Oil Macerate, Sunflower Oil, Soy Bean Oil, Lecithin, Gelatin, Glycerin, Purified Water.

EM PACT Drink Mix, Citrus (EMPACT, EM-PACT, EMPACT) - Mannatech
Each tablespoon contains: Calcium 40 mg • Proprietary Blend Energy/Endurance Complex 16.1 g: Fructose, Medium Chain Triglycerides, Creatine Monohydrate, Calcium Citrate, Magnesium Aspartate, Magnesium Succinate, Choline Bitartrate, L-Carnitine, Lecithin • Ambrotose Complex (patent pending) 25 mg: Arabinogalactan (larix decidua gum), Manapol Aloe Vera gel extract (inner leaf gel), Gum Ghatti, Gum Tragacanth. Other Ingredients: Citric Acid, Silicon Dioxide, Natural Flavors.

E-Manganese - Standard Process, Inc.
Each tablet contains: Proprietary Blend 204 mg: Bovine Anterior Pituitary, Magnesium Citrate, Ascorbic Acid • Vitamin E 7.7 IU • Calcium 30 mg • Manganese 8 mg. Other Ingredients: Honey, Mixed Tocopherols.
See Editor's Note No. 31.

E-mergen-C - Alacer
Each packet contains: Vitamin C 1000 mg • Vitamin B1 (thiamine HCl) 0.38 mg • Vitamin B2 (riboflavin) 0.43 mg • Special Niacin complexes 5 mg • Vitamin B6 (pyridoxine HCl) 10 mg • Folic Acid 12.5 mcg • Vitamin B12 (cyanocobalamin) 25 mcg • Pantothenic Acid 2.5 mg • Calcium 50 mg • Magnesium 20 mg • Zinc 2 mg • Sodium 60 mg • Potassium 200 mg • Manganese 1.5 mg • Chromium (ascorbate) 10 mg. In a base of Citric, Tartaric, Aspartic, & Malic (apple) Acids.

Emer'gen-C Fizzing Drink Mix (assorted flavors) - Alacer
Each packet contains: Vitamin C (as ascorbates) 1000 mg • Vitamin B1 (as thiamine HCl) 0.38 mg • Vitamin B2 (as riboflavin) 0.43 mg • Vitamin B3 (as niacin complexes) 5 mg • Vitamin B6 (as pyridoxine HCl) 10 mg • Folic Acid 12.5 mg • Vitamin B12 (as cyanocobalamin) 25 mcg • Pantothenic Acid (as calcium pantothenate) 2.5 mg • Potassium 200 mg • Magnesium 60 mg • Calcium 50 mg • Zinc 2 mg • Manganese 1 mg • Chromium 10 mcg • Alpha Lipoic Acid 1000 mg. Other Ingredients: Sweetened with Fructose, Ascorbic Acid, Carbonates of Potassium, Sodium, Magnesium and Calcium, Citric, Malic, Aspartic, Tartaric Acids, Sodium, Potassium and Calcium Phosphates, Tapioca Starch, Glycine, Magnesium Hydroxide, Quercetin, Manganese Gluconate, Naturally Flavored with one or more of the following, depending on flavor: Cranberry Powder 1000 mg • Instant Coffee (decaffeinated) 2400 mg • Raspberry Powder 1000 mg • Orange Juice Super Concentrate 1250 mg.

Emer'gen-C Fizzing Drink Mix (Lite, Lite Triple Power and Lite with MSM) - Alacer
Each packet contains: Vitamin C (as ascorbates) 1000 mg • Vitamin B3 (as niacin complexes) 10 mg • Folic Acid 25 mcg • Vitamin B12 (as cyanocobalamin) 25 mcg • Potassium • 200 mg • Magnesium 60 mg • Calcium 50 mg • Zinc 2 mg • Manganese 1 mg • Chromium 10 mcg • Alpha-Lipoic Acid 1 mg. Triple Power flavor also contains: Glucosamine Sulfate (12% potassium) 500 mg • Chondroitin Sulfate (5% sodium) 400 mg. Lite with MSM also contains: MSM (methyl sulfonyl methane) 1000 mg. Other Ingredients: Ascorbic Acid, Carbonates of Potassium, Sodium, Magnesium and Calcium, Citric, Malis, Aspartic, and Tartaric Acids, Sodium, Potassium and Calcium Phosphates, Tapioca Starch, Glycine, Magnesium Hydroxide, Quercetin, Manganese Gluconate, Naturally Flavored.

Emer'gen-C Fizzing Drink Mix Multivitamin (strawberry flavor) - Alacer
Each packet contains: Vitamin A 1500 IU • Vitamin B1 (as thiamine HCl) 0.75 mg • Vitamin B2 (as riboflavin) 0.85 mg • Vitamin B3 (as niacin complexes) 5 mg • Vitamin B6 (as pyridoxine HCl) 1 mg • Vitamin B12 (as cyanocobalamin) 3 mcg • Folic Acid 200 mcg • Pantothenic Acid (as calcium pantothenate) 5 mg • Iodine 75 mcg • Biotin 150 mcg • Vitamin C (as ascorbates) 1000 mg • Vitamin D 200 IU • Vitamin E (as mixed tocopherols) 15 IU • Vitamin K 40 mcg • Potassium 200 mg • Calcium 50 mg • Phosphorus 28 mg • Magnesium 60 mg • Zinc 2 mg • Manganese 1 mg • Chromium

10 mcg • Strawberry Powder 1000 mg. Other Ingredients: Sweetened with Fructose, Ascorbic Acid, Carbonates of Potassium, Sodium, Magnesium and Calcium, Citric, Malic, Aspartic, and Tartaric Acids, Sodium, Potassium, and Calcium Phospahtes, Tapioca Starch, Glycine, Magnesium Hydroxide, Quercetin, Manganese Gluconate, Natural Flavors.

Emer'gen-C Fizzing Drink Mix Power for Joints - Alacer
Each packet contains: Vitamin C (as ascorbates) 1000 mg • Vitamin B3 (as niacin complexes) 10 mg • Folic Acid 25 mcg • Vitamin B12 (as cyanocobalamin) 25 mcg • Potassium • 200 mg • Magnesium 60 mg • Calcium 50 mg • Zinc 2 mg • Manganese 1 mg • Chromium 10 mcg • Alpha-Lipoic Acid 1 mg • Glucosamine Sulfate (12% potassium) 500 mg • Chondroitin Sulfate (5% sodium) 400 mg. Other Ingredients: Ascorbic Acid, Carbonates of Potassium, Sodium, Magnesium and Calcium, Citric, Malis, Aspartic, and Tartaric Acids, Sodium, Potassium and Calcium Phosphates, Tapioca Starch, Glycine, Magnesium Hydroxide, Quercetin, Manganese Gluconate, Naturally Flavored.

Emer'gen-C Jr. Fizzing Drink Mix Multivitamin for Kids (strawberry flavor) - Alacer
Each packet contains: Vitamin A 2500 IU • Vitamin B1 (as thiamine HCl) 0.7 mg • Vitamin B2 (as riboflavin) 0.8 mg • Vitamin B3 (as niacin complexes) 5 mg • Vitamin B6 (as pyridoxine HCl) 0.7 mg • Vitamin B12 (as cyanocobalamin) 3 mcg • Folic Acid 200 mcg • Pantothenic Acid (as calcium pantothenate) 5 mg • Iodine 70 mcg • Biotin 150 mcg • Vitamin C (as ascorbates) 500 mg • Vitamin D 400 IU • Vitamin E (as mixed tocopherols) 10 IU • Vitamin K 0.3 mcg • Potassium 111 mg • Calcium 25 mg • Phosphorus 14 mg • Magnesium 31 mg • Zinc 2 mg • Manganese 1 mg • Chromium 5 mcg • Strawberry Powder 1000 mg. Other Ingredients: Sweetened with Fructose, Ascorbic Acid, Carbonates of Potassium, Sodium, Magnesium and Calcium, Citric, Malic, Aspartic, and Tartaric Acids, Sodium, Potassium, and Calcium Phospahtes, Tapioca Starch, Glycine, Magnesium Hydroxide, Quercetin, Manganese Gluconate, Natural Flavors.

Emerita - Transitions for Health, Inc.
Aloe Vera gel • Distilled Water • D-Alpha Tocopherol • Mixed Tocopherols • Cetyl Alcohol • Almond oil • Octyl Palmitate • Panthenol • Peg 8 Stearate • Glycerine • Progesterone • Polysorbate 60 • Hyaluronic Acid, Oil of Lemon, Keratin, Carbomer 940 • Grapefruit seed extract.

Emerita Hot Flash Formula - Transitions for Health, Inc.
Each capsule contains: Vitamin C (sodium ascorbate) 400 mg • Vitamin E (as d-alpha tocopheryl succinate) 100 mg • Bioflavonoids (as citrus bioflavonoid complex) 200 mg • Para-aminobenzoic acid 20 mg • Pantothenic acid (as calcium pantothenate) 20 mg • Adrenal Complex 5 mg. Other Ingredients: Rice Bran, Gelatin, Water, and Glycerin.

Emerita Libido Formula - Transitions for Health, Inc.
Each caplet contains: Calcium (from dicalciumphosphate) 86 mg • Muira Puama extract (4:1, equivalent to 700 mg, providing ptychopetalum olacoides) 175 mg • Ginkgo Biloba extract (standardized 24% ginko flavone glycosides, 6% terpene lactones) 120 mg • Motherwort (leonurus cardiaca) 100 mg • Damiana extract (turnera diffusa, 6.5:1, equivalent to 200 mg) 31 mg • Panax Ginseng root extract (50:1, equivalent to 300 mg) 6 mg. Other Ingredients: Vegetable Sterols, Cellulose, Magnesium Stearate.

Emerita Menopause Plus Formula - Transitions for Health, Inc.
Two caplets contain: Red Clover extract (standardized 8% isoflavonoids, trifolium pratense flowering tops) 500 mg • Siberian Ginseng root (eleutherococcus senticosus) 100 mg • Dandelion (taraxacum officinale) 100 mg • Alfalfa leaf (medicago sativa) 100 mg • Black Cohosh extract (standardized 2.5% triterpene glycosides, cimicifuga racemosa root) 80 mg. Other Ingredients: Dicalcium Phosphate, Vegetable Sterols, Cellulose, Magnesium Stearate.

Emerita Natural Lubricant - Transitions for Health, Inc.
Deionized Water • Sorbitol • Glycerin • Tocopheryl Acetate • Xylitol • Cinnamon oil (cinnamomum cassia) • Allantoin • Isopropyl Myristate • Sucrose Laurate • Hydroxypropyl Methylcellulose • Caromer • Potassium Sorbate • Vanillin • Polysorbate 20 • Methylparaben • Triethanolamine.

Emerita Personal Lubricant - Transitions for Health, Inc.
Deionized Water • Glycerin • Carbomer • Aloe Vera Gel • Butylene Glycol • Hydroxpropyl Methylcellulose • Calendula Extract • Black Walnut Leaf Extract • Imidazolidinyl Urea • Methylparaben • Allantoin • Citric Acid • Tocopheryl Acetate • Retinyl Palmitate • Squalene.

Emerita Phytoestrogen Body Cream - Transitions for Health, Inc.
Deionized Water • Carbomer • Jojoba Oil • Caprylic / Capric Triglycerides • Cetyl Ester • Glyceryl Stearate • Ginseng Extract • Glycerin • Peg-100 Stearate • Stearic Acid • Aloe Vera Gel • Hydrolyzed Glycosaminoglycans • Black Walnut Leaf Extract • Black Cohosh Extract • Licorice Root Extract • Chaste Tree Berry Extract • Evening Primrose Oil • Tocopheryl Acetate • Triethanolamine • Imidazolidinyl Urea • Methylparaben • Xanthan Gum • Grape Seed Extract • Red Clover Blossom Extract • Propylparaben • Butylene Glycol • Orange Oil.

Emerita Pro-Gest Body Cream - Transitions for Health, Inc.
Distilled Water • Aloe Barbadensis gel • Tocopheryl Acetate • Cetyl Alcohol • Octyl Palmitate • Sweet Almond oil (prunus amygdalus dulcis) • Panthenol • PEG-8 Stearate • Stearic Acid • Glycerin • USP Progesterone • Polysorbate 65 • Propylene Glycol • Lemon oil (citrus medica limonum) • Carbomer • Methylparaben • Propylparaben • Triethanolamine • Phenoxyethanol.

Emerita Response Cream - Transitions for Health, Inc.
Water • Glycerine • L-Arginine • L-Phenylalanine • L-Tyrosine • Sorbitol • Sucrose Stearate • Ginger extract (zingiber officinale) • Rosemary oil (rosemarinus officinalis) • Niacin • L-Histidine • Ginseng extract (panax ginseng) • Natural L-Menthol • Cinnamon oil (cinnamomum cassia) • Bergamot (citrus bergamia) • Cetosteryl alcohol • Ascorbyl Palmitate • Isopropyl Myristate • Octyl Palmitate • Carbomer • Triethanolamine.

Emerita Sleep Formula - Transitions for Health, Inc.
Each capsule contains: Valerian root 100 mg • Scullcap leaf and flower 100 mg • Wild Lettuce leaves 50 mg • Lavender flowers 50 mg • Oat Straw tops 50 mg • Lady's Mantle leaves 50 mg. Other Ingredients: Rice Bran, Gelatin, Water, and Glycerin.

Em-Pact - Mannatech
Energy Complex: Fructose, Medium chain triglycerides, Creatine monohydrate, Calcium citrate, Magnesium aspartate, Magnesium succinate, Potassium aspartate, Potassium succinate, Choline bitartrate, L-carnitine, Lecithin • Ambrotose Complex: naturally occurring plant polysaccharides including freeze-dried Aloe Vera inner leaf gel extract - Manapol powder. Other Ingredients: Citric Acid, Natural Flavors.
See Editor's Note No. 17.

Emphaplex - Standard Process, Inc.
Two capsules contain: Proprietary Blend 1180 mg: Fenugreek seed, Defatted Wheat germ, Oat flour, Bovine Bone, Soy bean, Bovine Adrenal, Carrot root, Bovine Lung PMG extract, Choline Bitartrate, Buckwheat seed, Arrowroot flour, Nutritional Yeast, Okra, Bovine Liver, Bovine Adrenal PMG extract, Porcine Stomach, Veal Bone meal, Dried Alfalfa juice, Ribonucleic Acid, Calcium Lactate, Phosphoric Acid, Mushroom, DL-Methionine, Bovine Spleen, Ovine Spleen, L-Lysine Mono-Hydrochloride, Glutamic Acid, Mixed Tocopherols, Peanut bran, Allantoin, Soybean Lecithin, Porcine Brain, Inositol, Rice bran • Vitamin A 3925 IU • Vitamin C 5.6 mg • Vitamin D 102 IU • Thiamine 0.1 mg • Riboflavin 0.5 mg • Niacin 4.2 mg • Vitamin B6 0.3 mg. Other Ingredients: Gelatin, Water, Colors, Cocarboxylase.
See Editor's Note No. 14.

Empower Plus - Truehope
Three capsules contain: Vitamin A (as retinyl palmitate) 1067 IU • Vitamin C (as ascorbic acid) 111 mg • Vitamin D (as cholecalciferol) 267 IU • Vitamin E (as d-alpha tocopheryl succinate) 67 IU • Vitamin B1 (as thiamine mononitrate) 3.33 mg • Vitamin B2 (as riboflavin) 2.5 mg • Vitamin B3 (as niacinamide) 16.7 mg • Vitamin B5 (as d-calcium pantothenate) 4 mg • Vitamin B6 (as pyridoxine hydrochloride) 6.7 mg • Vitamin B9 (as folic acid) 267 mcg • Vitamin B12 (as cyanocobalamin) 167 mcg • Vitamin H (as biotin) 20 mcg • Calcium 244 mg • Phosphorous 155 mg • Magnesium 111 mg • Potassium 44 mg • Iodine (from Pacific kelp) 33 mcg • Zinc 9 mg • Selenium 44 mcg • Copper 1.33 mg • Manganese 1.77 mg • Chromium 110 mcg • Molybdenum 29 mcg • Iron 2.66 mg • CNS Proprietary Blend 414.45 mg: DL-Phenylalanine, Glutamine, Citrus Bioflavonoids, Grape Seed, Choline Bitartrate, Inositol, Ginkgo Biloba, Methionine, Germanium Sesquioxide, Boron, Vanadium, Nickel. Other Ingredients: Gelatin.

Emprizone Gel - Mannatech
Water • Polyglyceryl Methacrylate/Propylene Glycol • Glycerin • Sorbitol • Glycereth-26 • Polysorbate 80 • Carbomer • Germaben II (propylene glycol, diazolidinyl urea, methylparaben, propylparaben) • Aminomethyl Propanol • Ambrotose Complex (patent pending): Arabinogalacan, Manapol Aloe Vera gel extract, Gum Ghatti, Gum Tragacanth • Benzethonium Chloride • Sodium Hyaluronate • Retinyll Palmitate • Allantoin • Tocopheryl Acetate.

Emulsified A Complex - Nature's Life
Each capsule contains: Vitamin A (Fish Liver oil) 7500 IU • Beta Carotene (Vitamin A equivalent to 7500 IU) 4.5 mg.

Emulsified Vitamin A Complex with Vitamin D - Puritan's Pride
Each softgel contains: Vitamin A 10,000 IU • Vitamin D 400 IU • Apple Pectin.

ENADA NADA 2.5 mg - Prof. Birkmayer Health Products USA
Each tablet contains: NADH (reduced B-nicotinamide adenine dinucleotide) 2.5 mg. Other Ingredients: D-Mannitol, Sodium Bicarbonate, Microcrystalline Cellulose, Magnesium Stearate, Sodium Ascorbate, Enteric Coating (methacrylic acid copolymer).

ENADA NADH - Life Extension
Each tablet contains: NADH (reduced B-nicotinamide adenine dinucleotide) 5 mg. Other Ingredients: D-mannitol, Sodium Bicarbonate, Sodium Ascorbate, Microcrystalline Cellulose, Magnesium Stearate, Enteric Coating.

ENADA NADH 5 mg - Prof. Birkmayer Health Products USA
Each tablet contains: NADH (reduced B-nicotinamide adenine dinucleotide) 5 mg. Other Ingredients: D-Mannitol, Microcrystalline Cellulose, Magnesium Stearate, Sodium Ascorbate, Enteric Coating (methacrylic acid copolymer).

ENADAlert - Pro Health
Each tablet contains: NADH (reduced 6-beta-nicotinamide adenine dinudeotide) 10 mg. Other Ingredients: D-Mannitol, Sodium Bicarbonate, Microcrystalline Cellulose, Natural Flavoring, Magnesium Stearate.

ENADAlert - Prof. Birkmayer Health Products USA
Each tablet contains: NADH (reduced B-nicotinamide adenine dinucleotide) 10 mg. Other Ingredients: D-Mannitol, Sodium Bicarbonate, Microcrystalline Cellulose, Natural Flavoring, Magnesium Stearate.

ENADAlert 10 mg - Source Naturals
Each tablet contains: NADH (reduced B-nicotinamide adenine dinucleotide) 10 mg. Other Ingredients: D-Mannitol, Sodium Bicarbonate, Microcrystalline Cellulose, Magnesium Stearate, Vitamin C (as sodium ascorbate).

ENADAlert 2.5 mg - Source Naturals
Each tablet contains: NADH (reduced B-nicotinamide adenine dinucleotide) 2.5 mg. Other Ingredients: D-Mannitol, Sodium Bicarbonate, Microcrystalline Cellulose, Magnesium Stearate, Vitamin C (as sodium ascorbate).

ENADAlert 5 mg - Source Naturals
Each tablet contains: NADH (reduced B-nicotinamide adenine dinucleotide) 5 mg. Other Ingredients: D-Mannitol, Sodium Bicarbonate, Microcrystalline Cellulose, Magnesium Stearate, Vitamin C (as sodium ascorbate).

EnadaNADH 2.5 Mg - Natrol, Inc.
Each micro tab contains: NADH (reduced 5-nicotinamide adenine dinucleotide) 2.5 mg • Baking Soda (Sodium Bicarbonate) 0.3 mg • Vitamin C (Sodium Ascorbate) 0.3 mg. Other Ingredients: D-Mannitol, Microcrystalline Cellulose, Magnesium Stearate.

EnadaNADH 5 Mg - Natrol, Inc.
Each microtab contains: NADH (reduced 5-nicotinamide adenine dinucleotide) 5 mg • Baking Soda (Sodium Bicarbonate) 0.3 mg • Vitamin C (Sodium Ascorbate) 0.3 mg. Other Ingredients: D-Mannitol, Microcrystalline Cellulose, Magnesium Stearate.

End Fatigue Adrenal Stress-End - PhytoPharmica
Two capsules contain: Adrenal cortex extract 33 mg • Adrenal Polypeptide Fractions 400 mg • Betaine 250 mg • Licorice root and rhizome extract (glycyrrhiza glabra standardized to contain 5% glycyrrhizic acid) • L-Tyrosine 250 mg • Pantothenic Acid (calcium D-pantothenate) 100 mg • Vitamin B6 (pyridoxine HCl) 50 mg • Vitamin C (ascorbic acid/rose hip fruit) 150 mg.
This product was formerly known as Adrenal Soluble. See Editor's Note No. 14.

End Fatigue Daily Energy B Complex - PhytoPharmica
Each capsule contains: Choline Bitartrate 100 mg • Folic Acid 800 mcg • Niacin (as niacinamide) 50 mg • Pantothenic Acid (as calcium D-pantothenate) 50 mg • Riboflavin (vitamin B2) 75 mg • Thiamin (vitamin B1, as thiamin HCl) 75 mg • Vitamin B12 (as cyanocobalamin) 500 mcg • Vitamin B6 (as pyridoxine HCl) 85 mg. Other Ingredients: Gelatin, Cellulose, Modified Cellulose Gum, Magnesium Stearate, and Titanium Dioxide Color.

End Fatigue Energy Revitalization System - PhytoPharmica
Each rounded scoop contains: Betaine 750 mg • Biotin 200 mcg • Boron (as sodium borate) 2 mg • Chromium (as chromium picolinate) 200 mcg • Copper (as copper gluconate) 500 mcg • Glycine 390 mg • Hesperidin 50% (from citrus fruits) 500 mg • Inositol 750 mg • Inulin (from chicory root) 750 mg • Iodine (as potassium iodide) 150 mcg • L-Serine 240 mg • L-Tyrosine 377 mg • Magnesium (as magnesium glycinate) 200 mg • Malic Acid 900 mg • Manganese (as manganese citrate) 4 mg • Molybdenum (as sodium molybdate) 250 mcg • N-Acetylcysteine (NAC) 250 mg • Potassium (from whey protein, guar gum, potassium citrate, and potassium iodide) 50 mg • Selenium (as L-selenomethionine) 200 mcg • Stevia leaf 15:1 extract (stevia rebaudiana) 150 mg • Taurine 500 mg • Vitamin A (as 50% beta carotene and as retinyl acetate) 7000 IU • Vitamin C (ascorbic acid) 750 mg • Vitamin D (as cholecalciferol) 600 IU • Vitamin E (as D-alpha tocopheryl acetate) 100 IU • Whey Protein 7 g • Zinc (as zinc sulfate) 15 mg. Other Ingredients: Guar Gum, Natural Flavors.

End Fatigue Revitalizing Sleep Formula - PhytoPharmica
Each capsule contains: Hops flower 6.6:1 extract (humulus lupulus) • Jamaica Dogwood root extract (piscidia piscipula) 12 mg • L-Theanine (Suntheanine brand) 50 mg • Passionflower leaf and flower 4:1 extract (passiflora incarnata) 90 mg • Valerian root extract (valeriana officinalis, standardized to contain a minimum of 0.8% valerenic acids) 200 mg • Wild Lettuce leaf extract (lactuca virosa) 18 mg • Wild Lettuce leaf (lactuca virosa) 10 mg. Other Ingredients: Gelatin, Magnesium Stearate, Titanium Dioxide Color, and Silicon Dioxide.

Some Brand Name Natural Products - What they Contain

www.NaturalDatabase.com contains MANY more listings than appear here.
Editor's Notes are located on pages 2155-2163.

Endefen - Metagenics
Each 2 tbsp serving contains: Vitamin C (as calcium ascorbate) 300 mg • Calcium (as calcium ascorbate) 34 mg • Sodium 12 mg • Potassium 130 mg • Arabinogalactan 1500 mg • Soy Lecithin 1000 mg • Phosphatides 970 mg • Astaxanthin 1 mg • D-Mannose 250 mg • D-Xylitol 950 mg • Green Tea leaf extract (camellia sinensis, standardized to 40% epigallocatechingallate) 250 mg • Cinnamon bark (cinnamomum burmanii) 700 mg • Plantain fruit (musa paradisiaca) 2000 mg • Apple fruit powder 2000 mg.

EndoKinase - Longevity Plus
Each VegeCap (vegetarian) capsule contains: Nattokinase (1000 fibrin units of activity per capsul, active enzyme at 20,000 FU/gram) 50 mg.

Endorphin+ - PhysioLogics
Each capsule contains: DL-Phenylalanine 450 mg • White Willow bark (7.5% Salicin, 1.9 mg) 25 mg • Feverfew flower, leaf (1.2% Parthenolide, 0.3 mg) 25 mg • Ginger root (5% Gingerols, 1.25 mg) 25 mg.

Endura - Metagenics
Two scoops (35 g) contain: Vitamin E (as D-alpha tocopheryl acetate) 28 IU • Citric Acid 1000 mg • Malic Acid 500 mg • Taurine 500 mg • Potassium (as potassium phosphate) 176 mg • Magnesium (as magnesium bis-glycinate) 174 mg • Chloride (as sodium chloride) 148 mg • Vitamin C (as ascorbic acid) 120 mg • Sodium (as sodium chloride) 96 mg • Phosphorus (as dipotassium phosphate) 69 mg • Calcium (as calcium citrate) 60 mg • Pantothenic Acid (as D-calcium pantothenate) 28 mg • L-Carnosine 20 mg • Niacin (as niacinamide) 10 mg • Vitamin B6 (as pyridoxine hydrochloride) 5 mg • Riboflavin 5 mg • Thiamin (as thiamin mononitrate) 2 mg • Chromium (as chromium nicotinate glycinate) 83 mcg.

Endura Optimizer - Metagenics
Two scoops (78 g) contain: Vitamin A (50% from retinyl palmitate and 50% from beta carotene and Betatene brand mixed carotenoids) 2500 IU • Vitamin C 15 mg • Vitamin D 100 IU • Vitamin E 15 IU • Thiamin 0.75 mg • Riboflavin 1 mg • Niacin 5 mg • Vitamin B6 26 mg • Folic Acid 0.2 mg • Vitamin B12 3 mcg • Biotin 0.15 mg • Pantothenic Acid 25 mg • Calcium 230 mg • Iron 2.5 mg • Phosphorus 104 mg • Magnesium 145 mg • Zinc 2.7 mg • Selenium 13 mcg • Copper 0.38 mg • Manganese 1 mg • Chromium 100 mcg • Molybdenum 5 mcg • Sodium 190 mg • Potassium 310 mg • Betaine 50 mg • Inositol 50 mg • Alpha Ketoglutarate 21 mg • Boron 245 mcg • Alpha Lipoic Acid 100 mcg.

Endurabolic - Metagenics
Each tablet contains: Thiamin (as thiamin mononitrate) 25 mg • Riboflavin 10 mg • Niacin (as niacinamide) 25 mg • Magnesium (as magnesium citrate) 70 mg • Zinc (as zinc taurinate) 5 mg • Chromium (as chromium nicotinate glycinate) 200 mcg • Vanadium (as vanadyl sulfate) 5 mg.

Endurance Armor - All Terrain Company
Each capsule contains: Niacin 10 mg • Vitamin B6 3.5 mg • Zinc 10 mg • 5-methyl-7-methoxyisoflavone 100 mg • 7-isopropooxyisoflavone 100 mg • 5,7 dihydroxyflavone 25 mg • Isoflavonol 150 mg • Triboxybol 200 mg • Lysophosphatidylcholine 10 mg. Other Ingredients: Tribulus Terrestris Extract, Pueraria Jobata, Zinc Aspartate, Niacinamide, Pyridoxine HCl, Gelatin, Magnesium Stearate, Stearic Acid.

Endurance Formula - Gaia Herbs
Thirty drops contain: Proprietary Extract Blend 300 mg: Eleuthero root (eleutherococcus senticosus), Schizandra berries (schizandra chinensis), Rose Hips solid extract (rosa canina), Fresh Royal Jelly, Yellow Dock root (rumex crispus), Prickly Ash bark (xanthoxylum clava-herculis), Gentian root (gentiana lutea), Chlorella Algae, Blend of Sea Vegetation and Marine Algae, 18-25% Grain Alcohol USP, Spring Water.

Endurox - PacificHealth Laboratories, Inc.
Two caplets contain: Ciwujia root extract 800 mg • Calcium (sulfate) 130 mg. Other Ingredients: Microcrystalline Cellulose, Stearic Acid, Hydroxypropyl Cellulose, Magnesium Stearate, Titanium Dioxide, P.E.G., Caramel Color, Beet juice powder & Annatto extract.

Endurox Excel - PacificHealth Laboratories, Inc.
Each two caplets contain: Endurox (standardized root extract of the herb ciwujia) 1200 mg • Vitamin E 60 IU.

Endurox R4 - PacificHealth Laboratories, Inc.
Two scoops contain: Vitamin C 470 mg • Vitamin E 400 IU • Calcium 100 mg • Iron 1.8 mg • Magnesium 250 mg • Chloride 270 mg • Ciwujia (Endurox) 600 mg • L-Glutamine 420 mg • L-Arginine 1420 mg. Other Ingredients: Glucose, Whey Protein Concentrate, Crystalline Fructose, L-Arginine, Vitamin E Acetate, Ciwujia, Ascorbic Acid, Sodium Chloride, Citric Acid, L-Glutamine, Magnesium Oxide, Artificial Flavor, Potassium Phosphate, FD&C Red #40.

Endurox R4 Performance/Recovery Drink - PacificHealth Laboratories, Inc.
Each two rounded scoops (74.08 g) contains: Vitamin C 470 mg • Vitamin E 400 IU • Calcium 100 mg • Magnesium 250 mg • Sodium 220 mg • Potassium 120 mg • L-Glutamine 2560 mg • Branched Chain Amino Acids 2719 mg • L-Arginine 1247 mg.

Enedyn - Progressive Health Nutraceuticals
Folic Acid 400 mcg • Magnesium 90 mg • Schizandra extract 100 mg • Siberian Ginseng 500 mg • Bee Pollen 250 mg • Bee Propolis 50 mg • Coenzyme Q10 1 mg • L-Carnitine HCl 10 mg • Ashwagandha 300 mg • Royal Jelly 8 mg • Korean Ginseng 60 mg • Rhodiola extract 100 mg • Astragalus 50 mg • Cordyceps 100 mg.

Enerblast - Nature's Plus
Each tablet contains: Potassium Glycero-Phosphate 250 mg • Pyridoxal Alpha Ketoglutarate (PAK) 50 mg • Trimethylglycine (TMG) 25 mg • Inosine (HXR-Hypoxanthine Riboside) 25 mg • Creatine Phosphate 50 mcg.

Ener-G One Per Day - Vitol
Each tablet contains: Dibencozide (coenzyme B12) 3000 mcg • Boron (chelate, citrate, aspartate) 1000 mcg • Chromium (picolinate-yeast free gtf) 100 mcg • Vitamin C (calcium ascorbate/rose hips) 300 mg • Vitamin E (d-alpha tocopherol) 200 IU • Vitamin A (as beta carotene) 15,000 IU • Vitamin A (as palmitate) 10,000 IU • Vitamin D (cholecalciferol) 1000 IU • Vitamin B1 (thiamine) 75 mg • Vitamin B2 (riboflavin) 75 mg • Vitamin B6 (pyridoxine HCl) 75 mg • Vitamin B12 (cobalamin) 75 mcg • Vitamin B3 (niacinamide, niacin) 75 mg • Choline Bitartrate 30 mg • Inositol 30 mg • Para Aminobenzoic Acid 30 mg • Pantothenic Acid 30 mg • Biotin 75 mcg • Folic Acid 400 mcg • Rutin 10 mg • Citrus Bioflavonoids, Hesperidin Complex 20 mg • Quercetin (saphora japonica) 20 mg • Betaine HCl (beet molasses) 10 mg • Papain, Bromelain, Amylase, Protease, Lipase 30 mg • Glutamic Acid 10 mg • Iodine (kelp) 150 mcg • Calcium Chelate, Citrate 60 mg • Potassium Chelate, Citrate 10 mg • Iron Chelate, Citrate 10 mg • Magnesium Chelate, Citrate 20 mg • Manganese Chelate, Aspartate 3 mg • Molybdenum Chelate, Aspartate 75 mcg • Vanadium (amino acid chelate) 50 mcg • Strontium (amino acid chelate) 10 mcg • Sulfur (amino acid chelate) 5 mg • Silicon (amino acid chelate) 10 mcg • Zinc Chelate, Picolinate 20 mg • Copper Chelate, Aspartate 5 mg • Selenium (l-selenomethionine) 10 mcg • 74 Minerals, Trace Minerals 50 mg • L-Glutathione 5 mg • Free Form Amino Acids 60 mg: L-Lysine, L-Histidine, L-Isoleucine, L-Leucine, L-Phenylalanine, L-Threonine, L-Carnitine, L-Valine, L-Methionine, L-Arginine, L-Glycine, L-Taurine (5 mg each) • Dong Quai 20 mg • Echinacea Purpurea 20 mg • Suma 20 mg • Siberian Ginseng 20 mg • Gotu Kola 10 mg • Golden Seal root 10 mg.

Energel Ephedra Free **-** GNC
Two capsules contain: Iodine (as kelp) 37.5 mcg • Ginger Root Extract 4:1 (zingiber officinale) 25 mg • Mustard Seed Powder (sinapsis alba) 75 mg • Meadowsweet Powder (filipendula ulmaria) 100 mg • Guarana Seed Extract (paullinia cupana; 36% caffeine = 90 mg) 250 mg • Schisandra Extract 6:1 (schisandra chinensis) 8.3 mg • Indian Turmeric Extract 10:1 (curcuma longa) 4 mg • Siberian Ginseng Powder (eleutherococcus senticosus) 25 mg. Other Ingredients: Soybean Oil, Gelatin, Glycerin, Caramel Color, Titanium Dioxide (natural mineral whitener).

Energenics **-** Metagenics
Each tablet contains: L-Tyrosine 200 mg • Raw Liver powder (bovine) 80 mg • Riboflavin 15 mg • Niacin (as niacinamide) 15 mg • Zinc (as zinc glycinate) 5 mg • Copper (as copper tyrosinate) 500 mcg • Iodine (as potassium iodide) 50 mcg • Chromium (as nicotinate glycinate) 50 mcg.
See Editor's Note No. 14.

EnerGFX Energy Booster **-** EnerGreens, Inc.
Each scoop contains: Vitamin C 180 mg • Vitamin E 30 IU • Beta Carotene 3333 IU • Vitamin B1 3 mg • Vitamin B2 3.5 mg • Niacinamide 40 mg • Pantothenic Acid 50 mg • Vitamin B6 15 mg • Vitamin B12 50 mcg • Chromium Picolinate 25 mcg • Zinc 3 mg • Choline Bitartrate 500 mg • L-Taurine 200 mg • L-Tyrosine 100 mg • L-Glycine 100 mg • L-Phenylalanine 250 mg • L-Carnitine 10 mg • GABA 50 mg • Guarana extract 100 mg • Caffeine 100 mg • Siberian Ginseng extract 50 mg. Other Ingredients: Maltodextrin, Citric Acid, Beet Juice Powder, Sucralose, Natural Flavors.

EnerGFX Energy Builder **-** EnerGreens, Inc.
Each 1 ounce serving contains: Vitamin A (as beta carotene) 500 IU • Vitamin C (ascorbic acid) 60 mg • Proprietary Blend 10 mL: Aloe vera gel juice (from concentrate), Aloe leaf gel (from concentrate), Aloe Vera gel fillet, Activin brand Grape skin extract, Cat's Claw bark, Hawaiian Spirulina, Russian Adaptagenic herbs, Aulterra powder, Ascorbic Acid, Colloidal Minerals, Pine bark extract, Cat's Claw bark tea, Echinacea leaf tea, Spirulina Tea (from whole plant), Ginkgo leaf tea, Pau d'Arco bark tea, Siberian Ginseng leaf tea, Suma leaf tea. Other Ingredients: Purified Water, Crystalline Fructose, Natural Flavor Blend (Mango, Lemon, Passion Fruit, Orange), Citric Acid, Xanthan Gum, Sodium Benzoate, Potassium Sorbate.

EnerGFX O2 **-** EnerGreens, Inc.
Ten drops contain: Chloride 41 mg • Sodium 2.6 mg • Chromium 0.04 mcg • Iodine 0.05 mcg • Trace amounts of: Carbon, Calcium, Copper, Lithium, Iron, Magnesium, Potassium, Phosphorus, Selenium, Sulfur, Silicon, Coablt, Zinc.

Energiza **-** HerbaSway
Bitter Orange • Panax Ginseng • Siberian Ginseng • Schisandra • Astragalus • Ginger • Kudzu • Blackberry • Licorice • HerbaSwee (Cucurbitaceae fruit).
See Editor's Note No. 40.

Energizer Formula **-** Nature's Way
Two capsules contain: Proprietary Formula: Bee Pollen • Cayenne pepper fruit • Coenzyme Q10 (Ubiquinone) • Magnesium Stearate • Siberian Ginseng root • Spirulina • Thiamine (Vitamin B1) • Vitamin B12 (Cyanocobalamin). Other Ingredients: Gelatin, Millet.

Energizer Purifying Gel **-** FreeLife International
Purified Water • Neroli Hydrolate (orange blossom water) • Aloe Barbadensis gel • Anafeltia • Himanthalia Elongata • Gigartina Stellata • Palmaria Palmata • Porphyra Umbilicalis • Arnica Montana • Spirulina Maxima • Willowherb • BioEnhanced Grapefruit seed extract (BGSE) • Vegetable Glycerin • Methylsulfonylmethane (MSM) • Lonicera Japonica (Japanese honeysuckle) • Chrysanthellum extract • Beta 1,3 Glucans in Sorbitol • Orange fruit extract (vitamin C) • Hesperidin • Other Bioflavonoids • Tocopherol (vitamin E) • Xanthan • Astragalus gum • Rosa Canina fruit oil • Sweet Orange oil (essential) • Peppermint oil (essential) • Sodium Lactate • Sodium PCA • Proline • Chlorphenesin • Potassium Sorbate • Annatto extract.

Energizing Soy Protein (creamy cocoa flavor) **-** Shaklee
Three tablespoons (28 g) contain: Sugars (as fructose) 8 g • Soy protein isolate 14 g • Thiamin (as thiamin mononitrate) 2 mg • Riboflavin 2 mg • Niacin (as niacinamide) 10 mg • Vitamin B6 (as pyridoxine hydrochloride) 0.5 mg • Pantothenic acid (as calcium pantothenate) 2 mg • Calcium (as tricalcium phosphate and calcium carbonate) 500 mg • Iron 2 mg • Phosphorus (as tricalcium phosphate) 250 mg • Sodium 160 mg • Histidine 340 mg • Isoleucine 540 mg • Leucine 1160 mg • Lysine 900 mg • Methionine 180 mg • Phenylalanine 730 mg • Threonine 530 mg • Tryptophan 190 mg • Valine 690 mg. Other Ingredients: Cocoa Processed With Alkali, Natural Cocoa Flavor, Soy Lecithin, Guar Gum, Potassium Chloride.

Energizing Soy Protein (natural vanilla flavor) **-** Shaklee
Three tablespoons (28 g) contain: Sugars (as fructose and dextrose) 9 g • Soy protein isolate 14 g • Thiamin (as thiamin mononitrate) 2 mg • Riboflavin 2 mg • Niacin (as niacinamide) 10 mg • Vitamin B6 (as pyridoxine hydrochloride) 0.5 mg • Pantothenic acid (as calcium pantothenate) 2 mg • Calcium (as tricalcium phosphate and calcium carbonate) 500 mg • Iron 2 mg • Phosphorus (as tricalcium phosphate) 250 mg • Sodium 170 mg • Histidine 340 mg • Isoleucine 630 mg • Leucine 1160 mg • Lysine 890 mg • Methionine 180 mg • Phenylalanine 720 mg • Threonine 520 mg • Tryptophan 180 mg • Valine 650 mg. Other Ingredients: Soy Lecithin, Natural Vanilla Flavor, Guar Gum.

EnerGreens Capsules **-** EnerGreens, Inc.
Two capsules contain: Vitamin A 430 IU • Proprietary Blend 2g: Barley grass, Kamut grass, Wheat Grass, Lemon Grass, Shave grass, Strawberry leaf, Alfalfa leaf, Blackberry leaf, Dandelion leaf, Bilberry leaf, Black Walnut leaf, Goldenseal leaf, Red Raspberry leaf, Blueberry leaf, Boldo leaf, Plantain leaf, Papaya leaf, Slippery Elm bark, Cornsilk, White Willow leaf, Lecithin, Marshmallow root, Rosemary, Pau d'Arco, Betatene, Soy sprout concentrate, Meadowsweet, Oat, Dog Grass, Rose Hip, Oat grass, Echinacea Purpurea tops, Aloe leaf gel, Watercress, Parsley leaf, Kale, Cabbage, Broccoli, Celery, Okra, Spinach, Alfalfa juice concentrate, Tomato, Turmeric, Sage, Wintergreen leaf, Rosemary leaf, Thyme, Peppermint leaf, Spearmint leaf, High Frequency Mineral Complex.

EnerGreens Powder **-** EnerGreens, Inc.
Each 1 tsp serving contains: Vitamin A 430 IU • Proprietary Blend 2g: Barley grass, Kamut grass, Wheat Grass, Lemon Grass, Shave Grass, Strawberry leaf, Alfalfa leaf, Blackberry leaf, Dandelion leaf, Bilberry leaf, Black Walnut leaf, Goldenseal leaf, Red Raspberry leaf, Blueberry leaf, Boldo leaf, Plantain leaf, Papaya leaf, Slippery Elm bark, Cornsilk, White Willow leaf, Lecithin, Marshmallow root, Rosemary, Pau d'Arco, Betatene, Soy sprout concentrate, Meadowsweet, Oat, Dog Grass, Rose Hip, Oat grass, Echinacea Purpurea tops, Aloe leaf gel, Watercress, Parsley leaf, Kale, Cabbage, Broccoli, Celery, Okra, Spinach, Alfalfa juice concentrate, Tomato, Turmeric, Sage, Wintergreen leaf, Rosemary leaf, Thyme, Peppermint leaf, Spearmint leaf, High Frequency Mineral Complex.

Energ-V **-** Nature's Sunshine
Two capsules contain: Proprietary Blend 900 mg: Bee Pollen, Gotu Kola aerial parts (hydrocotyle asiatica), Kelp leaf and stem (ascophylum nodosum and laminaria digitata), Licorice root (glycyrrhiza glabra), Eleuthero root (eleutherococcus senticosus), Yellow Dock root (rumex crispus), Barley grass aerial parts (hordeum vulgare), Rose Hips (rosa canina), Schizandra fruit (schisandra chinensis), Capsicum fruit (capsicum annuum). Other Ingredients: Silicon Dioxide, Gelatin, Water.

Energy **-** Nutrivention
Each tablet contains: Pantothenic Acid 100 mg • Vitamin B12 300 mcg • Folic Acid 200 mcg • Aspartic Acid 100 mg • Gotu Kola 100 mg • Licorice root 100 mg • Siberian Ginseng 100 mg.

Energy **-** NOW Foods
Two capsules contain: Vitamin E (as d-alpha tocopheryl succinate) 15 IU • Vitamin B1 (from Thiamine HCL) 10 mg • Riboflavin (Vitamin B2) 10 mg • Niacin (Vitamin B3) 25 mg • Vitamin B6 (from

Pyridoxine HCL) 10 mg • Vitamin B12 (as Cyanocobalamin) 100 mg • Vitamin B5 (from Calcium Pantothenate) 10 mg • Iodine (from Kelp) 225 mg • Chromium (as Chromium Chelavite) 200 mg • Potassium (from Potassium Aspartate) 55 mg • Guarana standardized extract (Paullinia Cupane, seed extract contains 42 mg caffeine) 280 mg • Green Tea extract (Camellia Sinensis, leaf extract contains 8 mg caffeine) 200 mg • Bitter Orange extract (Citrus Aurantium) fruit (min. 3% Synephrine) 150 mg • Panax Ginseng (5% Ginsenosides) root 150 mg • Siberian Ginseng (Eleutherococcus Senticosus) root 150 mg • Licorice (Glycyrrhiza Glabra) root 100 mg • Gotu Kola (Centella Asiatica) whole plant 100 mg • Cayenne (Capsicum annuum: 40,000 SHU) fruit 50 mg • Alpha Lipoic Acid 25 mg • COQ10 10 mg • Octacosanol (Spinach) 30 mcg. Other Ingredients: Gelatin (capsule), Magnesium Stearate.
See Editor's Note No. 40.

Energy Body Benefits Pak - Leiner Health Products
Each packet contains: Thiamin Mononitrate (Vitamin B1) 100 mg • Riboflavin (Vitamin B2) 100 mg • Vitamin B6 (Pyridoxine Hydrochloride) 100 mg • Niacin (Niacinamide) 100 mg • Biotin 100 mcg • Vitamin B12 100 mcg • Pantothenic Acid (d-Calcium Pantothenate)100 mg • Folate 400 mcg • American Ginseng extract (Panax quinquefolius) root 70 mg • Chinese Panax Ginseng extract (Panax ginseng) root 60 mg • Damiana (Turnera diffusa) leaf 2 mg • Fo-Ti (Polygonum multiflorum) root 2 mg • Gotu Kola (Centella asiatica) leaf 78 mg • Green Tea extract (Camellia sinensis) leaf (50% catechins) 2 mg • Guarana extract (Paullinia cupana) seed 78 mg • Jamaican Ginger (Zingiber officinalis) rhizome 2 mg • Korean Ginseng extract (Panax ginseng) root 70 mg • Siberian Ginseng (Eleutherococcus senticosus) root 500 mg • Yerba Mate extract (Ilex paraguariensis) leaf 575 mg. Other Ingredients: Dicalcium Phosphate, Calcium Carbonate, Croscarmellose Sodium, Hydrogenated Vegetable Oil, Cellulose.

Energy Cycle II - Life Enhancement Products, Inc.
Each 1 1/2 tbsp (22.5 g) serving contains: Vitamin A (from beta carotene, 0.75 mg) 1250 IU • Vitamin C (from ascorbic acid and niacinamide ascorbate) 200 mg • Vitamin E (from DL-alpha-tocopherol acetate) 45 IU • Thiamine (vitamin B1 thiamine hydrchloride) 1.5 mg • Riboflavin (vitamin B2) 11 mg • Niacin (vitamin B3 from niacinamide ascorbate) 40 mg • Vitamin B6 (from pyridoxine hydrochloride) 6 mg • Folic Acid 100 mcg • Vitamin B12 (from cyanocobalamin) 18 mcg • Pantothenic Acid (vitamin B5 from calcium pantothenate) 100 mg • Zinc (from zinc gluconate) 5.25 mg • Selenium (from sodium selenite) 25 mcg • Copper (from copper gluconate) 750 mcg • Chromium (from chromium asparate) 50 mcg • Potassium (from potassium citrate) 150 mg • Choline (from choline dihydrogen citrate) 200 mg • Glycine 200 mg • Taurine 200 mg • Quercetin 20 mg • Hesperidin 18 mg.

Energy Elixir - Nature's Plus
Each tube contains: Royal Jelly (lyophilized 3X-4.2% (10.5 mg) 10-HDA) 250 mg • Guarana seed 125 mg • Spanish Bee Pollen 125 mg • Korean Ginseng 50 mg • Eleuthero 50 mg • American Ginseng 12.5 mg. Base: Purified Water, Wild Clover Honey, Citric Acid, Potassium Sorbate.

Energy Endurance Formula - Hansen's
Each can (246 mL) contains: Vitamin C 60 mg • Vitamin B2 1.7 mg • Niacin 20 mg • Vitamin B6 2 mg • Vitamin B12 6 mcg • Sodium 210 mg • Taurine 100 mg • L-Carnitine 300 mg • Panax Ginseng 200 mg. Ingredients: Carbonated Water, Sucrose, Glucose, Citric Acid, Taurine, Natural Flavors, Sodium Citrate, L-Carnitine, Natural Color, Panax Ginseng, Ascorbic Acid, Caffeine, Sodium Chloride, Niacinamide, Riboflavin, Inositol, Glucatronalactone, Pyridoxine Hydrochloride, Guarana, Cyanocobalamin.

Energy Formula - Weil Lifestyle, LLC
Each Dr. Weil Energy Factor tablet contians: Siberian Ginseng 200 mg • Cordyceps powder 150 mg • Ashwagandha extract 50 mg.

Energy Formula - Pharmanex
Each capsule contains: Ginseng, Panax root 4:1 extract (Panax ginseng c.a. meyer) 300 mg • Schisandra berry 10:1 extract (schisandra chinensis) 100 mg • Rhodiola root (sedum rosium) 100 mg.

Energy Plus - Vital Nutrients
Each capsule contains: American Ginseng root powder (minimum 4% ginsenosides) 250 mg • Schisandra Chinensis 20:1 extract 150 mg • Polygonum Multiflorum 12:1 extract 150 mg • Astragalus Membranaceus 15:1 extract 100 mg • Atractylodes 15:1 extract 100 mg • Licorice root extract (glycyrrhiza glabra) 50 mg.

Energy Plus - Ortho Molecular Products
Each capsule contains: Vitamin B12 (as methylcobalamin) 150 mcg • Pantothenic Acid (as D-calcium pantothenate USP) 50 mg • Chromium (as ChromeMate brand) 100 mcg • Wheat grass 200 mg • Eleuthero root extract (siberian ginseng, standardized to contain 0.8% eleutherosides) 150 mg • Royal Jelly 100 mg • Licorice root extract (standardized to contain 12% glycyrrhizin) 50 mg • ActiVin brand Grape seed extract 8 mg • Cayenne pepper 50 mg • Ginkgo Bilpba leaf extract (standardized to contain 24% ginkgo flavonglycosides & 6% terpene lactones) 20 mg • Bromelain (2400 GDU/g) 80 mg. Other Ingredients: Natural Vegetable Capsules, Magnesium Stearate, Microcrystalline Cellulose.

Energy Plus B-12 Sublingual 1000 mcg - Pro Health
Each lozenge contains: Folic Acid 100 mcg • Vitamin B12 (as cyanocobalamin) 1 mg. Other Ingredients: Cellulose, Sorbitol, Mannitol, Fructose, Croscarmellose Sodium, Magnesium Stearate (vegetable source), Natural Cherry Flavor.

Energy Rush Ephedra Free - GNC
Two capsules contain: Cocoa Seed Extract (theobroma cacao) 750 mg • Guarana Seed Extract (paullinia cupana; 22% caffeine = 82.5 mg) 375 mg • Citrus Aurantium Fruit Exchange (4% synephrine = 4 mg). Other Ingredients: Cellulose, Gelatin.
See Editor's Note No. 40.

Energy Tonic Bath - Abra Therapeutics
Sodium Borate • Sodium Sulfate • Sodium Chloride • Sodium Sesquicarbonate • Olive Oil • Essential Oils Blend: Rosemary, Peppermint oil, Lemon, Lime, Nutmeg, Fir, Peru Balsam • Herbal Extracts Blend: Ginseng root, Ginkgo leaves, St. John's Wort flower • Chromium Oxide • Trace Mineral Salts.

Energy Vitality - Gaia Herbs
Two capsules contain: Green Tea leaf (camellia sinensis) 90 mg • Eleuthero root (eleutherococcus senticosus) 90 mg • Schizandra berry (schizandra chinensis) 75 mg • Korean Ginseng root (panax ginseng) 51 mg • Cola nut (cola nitida) 42 mg • Ginkgo leaf (ginkgo biloba) 36 mg • Licorice root (glycyrrhiza glabra) 30 mg • Nettle seed (urtica diocia) 6 mg • Prickly Ash bark (xanthoxylum clava-herculis) 6 mg. Other Ingredients: Vegetable Glycerin, Vegetable Cellulose (capsule).

EnergyPrep - HealthMinded
Each tablet contains: EnergyPrep Proprietary Blend 906 mg: Green Tea leaf extract, Cordyceps mycelium extract, Eleutherococcus Senticosus root standardized extract, Panax Ginseng root standardized extract, Vinpocetine (from vocanga tree seeds), Octacosanol. Other Ingredients: Di Calcium Phosphate, Microcrystalline Cellulose, Croscarmellose Sodium, Stearic Acid, Magnesium Stearate, Silicon Dioxide.

Ener-Jazz - Wild Rose
Each capsule contains: Siberian Ginseng root 100 mg • Astragalus root 25 mg • American Ginseng root 25 mg • Reishi mushroom 25 mg • Licorice root 200 mg • Codonopsis root 25 mg • Fo-Ti root 50 mg.

EnerKids Chewable - EnerGreens, Inc.
Two chewable tablets contain: Beta Carotene 3000 IU • Vitamin C (from ascorbic acid) 125 mg • Vitamin D (D3, as cholecalciferol) 100 IU • Vitamin E (D-alpha tocopherol) 60 IU • Vitamin B1

(cocarboxylase) 3.5 mg • Vitamin B2 1.5 mg • Niacinamide 25 mg • Vitamin B6 2 mg • Folic Acid 400 mcg • Vitamin B12 6 mcg • Biotin 75 mcg • Pantothenic Acid 50 mg • Calcium (from citrate and ascorbate) 50 mg • Magnesium (from aspartate and ascorbate) 50 mg • Iodine 70 mcg • Zinc (as aspartate) 5 mg • Selenium (as selenomethionine) 30 mcg • Copper (as chelate) 500 mcg • Manganese (as chelate) 2.5 mg • Chromium (GTF) 50 mcg • Molybdenum (from chelate) 25 mcg • Potassium (from aspartate) 10 mg • Citrus Bioflavonoids 15 mg • Bilberry 4:1 extract 100 mg. Other Ingredients: Dicalcium Phosphate, Fructose, Stevia, Natural Flavors (raspberry, cherry), Silicon Dioxide.

Ener-T **-** Atrium Biotechnologies
Each tablet contains: Primary Yeast 705 mg. Specially grown & formulated because of its content of an accessory factor known as Termitin, Complex-T or Vitamin T. This yeast also typically contains 50% Protein, trace amounts of many B-Complex Vitamins & Inositol as well as trace amounts of many minerals.

EnerX **-** WellQuest International, Inc.
Niacin • Zinc • Yohimbe • Tribulus Terrestris • Panax Ginseng • Guarana • Ashwagandha • Arginine • Damiana • Muira Puama • Potent Herbal Blend.

Engystol **-** Heel/BHI, Inc.
Asclepias Vincetoxicum 6X, 10X, 30X • Sulphur 4X, 10X.
See Editor's Note No. 1.

Enhancer Skin Conditioning Gel **-** Nu Skin Enterprises
Water (aqua) • Aloe Barbadensis leaf juice • Propylene Glycol • Glycerin • Polysorbate 20 • Hyaluronic Acid • Sodium PCA • Zinc Amino Acid Chelate • Algae extract • Sorbitol • Allantoin • Panthenol • Royal Jelly • RNA • Octyl Methoxycinnamate • Carbomer • Fragrance (parfum) • Triethanolamine • Diaxolidinyl Urea • Methylparaben • Propylparaben • Chlorophyllin - Copper complex.

Enhance-Rx **-** Body Wise International, Inc.
Each three capsules contain: Niacin 20 mg • Muira Puama root extract (4:1) 450 mg • L-Arginine 250 mg • Ashwagandha root extract (1% alkaloids) 150 mg • Ginkgo Biloba leaf extract (8:1) 150 mg • Oat Straw concentrate (5:1) 150 mg • Damiana leaf extract (4:1) 100 mg • Mucuna Pruriens seed extract (10% L-DOPA) 100 mg • Nettle root extract (0.8% beta sitosterols) 100 mg • Tribulus Terrestris fruit extract (45% saponins) 100 mg • Korean Ginseng root extract (5% ginsenosides) 75 mg • Horny Goat Weed aerial parts 75 mg • Catuaba bark 60 mg • Siberian Ginseng root extract (5:1) 15 mg. Inactive Ingredients: Gelatin, Cellulose, Magnesium Stearate, Silicon Dioxide.

Enlargo **-** Unknown
Two tablets contain: Zinc (oxide) 10 mg • Proprietary Blend 1300 mg: Jujube dates (ziziphus jujuba), L-Arginine HCl, Oat straw powder, Muira Puama bark powder, Nettles leaf powder, Cayenne powder (40 mhu), Korean Ginseng powder, Siberian Ginseng root powder, Boron Citrate, Licorice root powder, Pumpkin seed powder, Sarsaparilla root powder, Maca root powder, Oyster meat extract (4:1).

Enlast **-** Ultra Herbal, LLC
Water • Glycerin • Glycereth-7 Trimethyl Ether • Saccharide Isomerate • Flavor • Ptychopetalum Olacoides (muria puama) • Jatropha Macrantha (huanarpo macho) • Arginine • Sodium Saccharin • Acrylamidopropyltrimonium Chloride • Arcylamide Copolymer • Phenoxyethanol • Methylparaben • Ethylparaben • Butylparaben.

Enova Oil **-** ADM Kao
Dicylglycerol Oil (made from Soybean Oil and Canola Oil) • Vitamin E • Vitamin C • Polyglycerol Esters of Fatty Acids.

EnraX **-** Herbal Technologies, LLC
Two capsules contain: Proprietary Blend 800 mg: Epimedium Sagittatum (horny goat weed), Damiana leaves, Muira Puama, Oat Straw extract, Panax Ginseng root, Ginkgo Biloba leaves, Soy Protein, Oyster Meat, Stinging Nettle leaves, Saw Palmetto berries, Cayenne fruit powder, Tribulus Terrestris fruit, Inosine, Velvet Deer Antler. Other Ingredients: Gelatin, Magnesium Stearate.

Ensorb E **-** Golden Glow Natural Health Products
Each capsule contains: D-Alpha-Tocopherol 335.6 mg: Natural Vitamin E 500 IU.

Enterosin **-** Ortho Molecular Products
Twelve capsules contain: Vitamin C (as ascorbic acid USP 800 mg • Bee Propolis extract 2x 3000 mg • Calcium / Magnesium Inositol Hexaphosphate 2000 mg • Quercetin Dihydrate 1300 mg • Berberine Sulfate 500 mg • Tumeric root extract (standardized to contain 95% curcumin) 400 mg • Burdock root 4:1 extract 50 mg. Other Ingredients: Natural Vegetable Capsules, Magnesium Stearate, Microcrystalline Cellulose.

Entrox **-** Baywood International
Each softgel contains: Vitamin E 0.6 IU • Perilia Oil 500 mg • Omega 3-alpha linolenic acid (ALA) 270 mg • Omega 6-linoleic acid (LA) 70 mg • Omega 9-oleic acid (OA) 65 mg.

EnurAid **-** Hyland's
Two tablets contain: Belladonna 6X • Cantharis 6X • Apris Mell 6X • Arnica Mont 6X • Allium Cepa 6X • Rhus Arom 6X • Equisetum Hyem 6X. Base: Lactose.
See Editor's Note No. 1.

EnVigor **-** Resource Wellness
Each caplet contains: Vitamin C 60 mg • Vitamin E 30 IU • Thiamin 1.5 mg • Riboflavin 1.7 mg • Niacin 20 mg • Vitamin B6 2 mg • Vitamin B12 6 mcg • Biotin 300 mcg • Pantothenic Acid 10 mg • Calcium 260 mg • Standardized Ginkgo Biloba extract leaves 120 mg • Standardized Panax Ginseng extract root 200 mg. Other Ingredients: Dicalcium Phosphate, Microcrystalline Cellulose, Croscarmellose Sodium, Calcium Silicate, Stearic Acid, Magnesium Stearate, Methylcellulose, Hydroxypropyl Cellulose, Polyethylene Glycol.

Enviro-Gard **-** Aspen Group, Inc.
Four tablets contain: Vitamin A Palmitate 8000 IU • Beta Carotene 16,000 IU • Vitamin C 800 mg • Vitamin E 320 IU • Quercetin 160 mg • Zinc (gluconate) 12 mg • Copper Gluconate 0.1 mg • Yellow Dock 364 mg • Bupleurum 192 mg • Poria Cocos 192 mg • Gentian root 192 mg • Goldenseal 192 mg • Myrrh Gum 192 mg • Echinacea extract 192 mg • Milk Thistle extract (83% silymarin) 192 mg • N-Acetyl Cysteine 160 mg • Rosemary extract 160 mg • Hawthorn Berry extract 80 mg • Wild Yam root 80 mg • Wild Yam extract 77 mg • Marshmallow root 58 mg • Magnesium Ascorbate 24 mg • Grape seed extract 20 mg • Ginkgo Biloba 4 mg • Manganese Ascorbate 4 mg • Selenomethionine 80 mcg.

Enviromend **-** American Biologics
Each drop contains: Alumina 30X, 60X • Argentum Met. 30X, 60X • Aurum Met. 30X, 60X • Beryllium 30X, 60X • Cadmium 30X, 60X • Cuprum Met. 30X, 60X • Hepar Sulf. 12X • Merc. Sol 30X, 60X • Plantago 4X • Platina 30X, 60X • Plumbum Met. 30X, 60X • Pulsatilla 6X • Selenium 30X, 60X • Stannum Met. 30X, 60X. Other Ingredients: 20% Alcohol, Distilled Water.
See Editor's Note No. 1.

ENZOGENOL **-** Pharmacy Express Ltd.
Each tablet contains: Enzogenol (Pinus radiata bark extract) 50 mg • Citrus Bioflavonoids 100 mg • Beta carotene (ProVitA) 5 mg • Natural Vitamin E (80 IU) 66.7 mg • Ester C 250 mg • Selenium (from selenomethionine) 75 ug • Zinc (from OptiZinc) 7.5 mg • Pyridoxine Hydrochloride (Vitamin B6) 25 mg • Cysteine 50 mg • Methionine 50 mg • Folic Acid 100 ug.

Enzolen **-** Enzo Nutraceuticals Ltd.
Each capsule contains: Shiitake mushroom extract 250 mg • Vitamin C 120 mg.

Enzy-Derm - Atrium Biotechnologies
Each gram contains: Pancreatin 12 mg • Papayotin 7 mg • Bromelain 6 mg • Trypsin 4 mg • Lipase 1.5 mg • Amylase 1.5 mg • Chymotrypsin 0.15 mg. In a base containing Vitamin A & Vitamin E.
See Editor's Note No. 14.

Enzygen - Rexall - Sundown
Each tablet contains: Calcium 100 mg • Enzyme Blend 200 mg: Lipase 2400 LU, Cellulase 250 CAU, Amylase 750 SKBU, Lactose 350 LacU, Protease 100 SAPU. Other Ingredients: Dicalcium Phosphate, Croscarmellose Sodium, Magnesium Stearate.

Enzymall - Schiff
Each tablet contains: Calcium (as dicalcium phosphate, calcium carbonate) 115 mg • Phosphorous (as dicalcium phosphate) 44 mg • Pancreatic Enzymes 50 mg • Cellulase 30 mg • Papain (from papaya) 15 mg • Amylase 10 mg. Other Ingredients: Cellulose, Stearic Acid, Acacia Powder, Whey Powder, Cellulose Gum, Silicon Dioxide, Vegetable Oil Powder, Magnesium Stearate, Annatto Seed Powder, Curcumin Powder.

Enzyme Aid Digestive Support - Nature's Life
Each tablet contains: Pancreatin (concentrate 4X NF) containing: (Protease activity 50000 USP IU; Amylase activity 50000 USP IU, Lipase activity 4000 USP IU) 500 mg • Glutamic Acid Hydrochloride 200 mg • Ox Bile extract 200 mg • Pepsin (NF 10000X) 200 mg • Lipase (activity 425 USP IU) 50 mg • Cellulase (activity 10 CMC-ASE IU) 10 mg.
See Editor's Note No. 14.

Enzyme Digestant - Natural Brand
Each tablet contains: Pancreatin 400 mg • Alpha Amylase 130 mg • Betaine hydrochloride 65 mg • Pepsin 65 mg • Papain 65 mg • Ox Bile Extract (8:1) 8.1 mg. Other Ingredients: Dicalcium Phosphate, Cellulose, Food Glaze.
See Editor's Note No. 14.

Enzymes - Nutrivention
Each capsule contains: Pancreatin 100 mg • Papain 60 mg • Anise (Pimpinella anisum) 50 mg • Fennel (Foeniculum vulgare) 50 mg • Rutin 50 mg • Bromelain (natural Pineapple Enzyme) 45 mg • Trypsin 24 mg • Amylase 10 mg • Lipase 10 mg • L-Chymotrypsin 1 mg.
See Editor's Note No. 14.

Enzymes - Matol Botanical International Ltd
Two capsules contain: nº zimes blend 132 mg: Amylase 3000 DU, Protease 14,000 HUT, Glucoamylase 10 AGU, Invertase 0.4 IAU, Acid Stable Protease 15 SAPU, Pepsidase FP 2400 HUT, Lipase 100 FCCLU, Lactase 240 ALU, Cellulase 70 CU, Malt Diastase 40 DP, Hemicellulase 70 HCU • Probiotic Blend 50 mg: Bifidobacterium Bifidum 200,000,000 c.f.u., Lactobacillus Brevis 200,000,000 mil c.f.u., Lactobacillus Acidophilus 1,200,000,000 mil c.f.u., Lactobacillus Rhamnosus 200,000,000 mil c.f.u., Bifidobacterium Longum 200,000,000 mil c.f.u. • Herb Blend 125 mg: Mentha Piperita leaf, Soy sprouts, Taraxacum Officinale root, Fructo-Oligosaccharides (FOS) 600 mg. Other Ingredients: Rice Bran, Gelatin, Water.

Enzy-Rite - 4 Life
Each capsule contains: Vitamin C (as ascorbic acid) 60 mg • Proprietary NDS Enzyme Blend 210 mg: Fungal Protease (aspergillus oryzae), Fungal Amylase (aspergillus oryzae), Fungal Lipase (rhizopus oryzae), Cellulase (aspergillus niger), Pectinase (aspergillus niger) • Citrus Bioflavonoids (from lemon, orange, and grapefruit peel) 130 mg.

Enzyte - Berkeley Premium Nutraceuticals
Each tablet contains: Niacin 30 mg • Zinc (as zinc oxide) 15 mg • Enzyte Proprietary Blend 1494 mg: Tribulus Terrestris extract (aerial), L-Arginine Base, Korean Ginseng, Maca root (lepidium meyenii), Orhcic Substance, Epimedium Sagitatum extract (aerial), Yohimbe bark (pausinystalia yohimba) extract, Muira Puama (aerial), Avena Sativa extract (aerial), Ginkgo Biloba leaf extract, Saw Palmetto berries (serenoa repens), Copper Gluconate, Octacosonal, Thymus Gland. Other Ingredients: Dicalcium Phosphate, Micro-Crystalline Cellulose, Croscarmellose Sodium, Stearic Acid, Magnesium Stearate, Silica, Hypromellose, Hydroxypropyl Cellulose, Polyethylene Glycol, Titanium Dioxide, Propylene Glycol, FD&C Blue #2 Lake.
See Editor's Note No. 59.

E'OLA Pak - E'OLA
Seven capsules contain: Vitamin A (as Palmitate) 12500 IU • Vitamin C (as Ascorbic Acid) 1000 mg • Calcium (as Calcium Carbonate) 1000 mg • Iron (as Ferrous Fumarate) 10 mg • Vitamin D (as Cholecalciferol) 667 IU • Vitamin E (as dl-Alpha Tocopheryl Succinate) 400 IU • Vitamin K (as Phytonadione) 50 mcg • Thiamin (Vitamin B1) 75 mg • Riboflavin (Vitamin B2) 75 mg • Niacin (80% as Niacinamide) 150 mg • Vitamin B6 (as Pyridoxine HCl) 75 mg • Folic Acid 800 mcg • Vitamin B12 (as Cyanocobalamin) 1000 mcg • Biotin 200 mcg • Pantothenic Acid (as D-Calcium Pantothenate) 150 mg • Phosphorus (as Phosphorus Protienate) 30 mg • Iodine (as Potassium Iodide) 100 mcg • Magnesium (as Magnesium Oxide) 500 mg • Zinc (as Amino Acid Chelate) 10 mg • Selenium (as Amino Acid Chelate) 100 mcg • Copper (as Amino Acid Chelate) 1 mg • Manganese (as Amino Acid Chelate) 2 mg • Chromium (as Amino Acid Chelate) 100 mcg • Molybdenum (as Amino Acid Chelate) 10 mcg • Boron 2 mg • Pine bark extract 5 mg • Grape (Seed) Extract 40 mg • Green Tea Extract 100 mg • Alpha-Lipoic Acid 35 mg • E'OLA Mineral Blend 10 mg. Other Ingredients: Potassium Chloride, Silica, Magnesium Stearate.

EPA - Nordic Naturals
Two softgels contain: Vitamin E (mixed tocopherols) 22 IU • Omega-3 Fatty Acids 1200 mg • EPA (eicosapentaenoic acid) 900 mg • DHA (docosahexaenoic acid) 200 mg • Other Omega-3 100 mg. Other Ingredients: Purified Deep Sea Fish Oil, Softgel Capsule (gelatin, water, glycerin, natural lemon oil), Antioxidant Blend (lecithin, ascorbyl palmitate), Rosemary Extract.

EPA Complex - AIE Pharmaceuticals
Eicosapentaenoic Acid (EPA) • Docosahexaenoic Acid (DHA) • Vitamin E.

EPA Gems - J. R. Carlson Laboratories, Inc.
Each softgel contains: Vitamin E (as D-alpha tocopherol) 10 IU • Other Omega-3 Fatty Acids 80 mg • Omega-3 Fatty Acids (from fish oil) 580 mg • DHA (docosahexaenoic acid) 100 mg • EPA (eicosapentaenoic acid) 400 mg.

EPA Natural Fish Oil - Puritan's Pride
Each softgel contains: EPA (Eicosapentaenoic Acid) 180 mg • DHA (Docosahexaenoic Acid) 120 mg.

EPA with Garlic - Puritan's Pride
Each softgel contains: Marine Lipid Concentrate 1000 mg • EPA (Eicosapentaenoic Acid) 180 mg • DHA (Docosahexaenoic Acid) 120 mg • Odorless Garlic powder 50 mg • Vitamin E (d-Alpha Tocopherol) 10 IU.

EPA/DHA Essentials - Pure Encapsulations
Each softgel capsule contains: Fish Oil concentrate (providing EPA [eicosapentaenoic acid] 300 mg, DHA [docosahexaenoic acid] 200 mg) 1000 mg • Vitamin E (D-alpha-tocopherol) 10 IU.

EPA/DHA Liquid - Pure Encapsulations
Each 1 tsp serving contains: Fish Oil concentrate (typically providing EPA [eicosapentaeonic acid] 740-825 mg, DHA [docosahexaenoic acid] 460-550 mg) 4600 mg. Other Ingredients: Natural Lemon Flavor, Proprieatary Antioxidant Blend (rosemary extract, ascorbyl palmitate, natural tocopherols).

EPA/DHA with lemon - Pure Encapsulations
Each softgel capsule contains: Fish Oil concentrate (providing EPA [eicosapentaenoic acid] 300 mg, DHA [docosahexaenoic acid] 200 mg) 900 mg. Other Ingredients: Natural Lemon Flavor, Proprietary Antioxidant Blend (rosemary extract, ascorbyl palmitate, natural tocopherols), Gelatin.

EPA-1000 - PhysioLogics
Each softgel contains: Vitamin E (d-Alpha Tocopherol) 10 IU • Marine Lipid concentrate (18% EPA, 12% DHA) 1000 mg.

EPA-DHA 6:1 Enteric-Coated - Metagenics
Each softgel contains: Natural Marine Lipid Concentrate 1 g • EPA (eicosapentaenoic acid) 500 mg • Vitamin E (mixed tocopherols) 5 IU. Other Ingredients: Rosemary, Ascorbyl Palmitate, Citric Acid.

EPA-DHA 6:1 TG - Metagenics
Each softgel contains: Natural Marine Lipid Concentrate 1 g • EPA (eicosapentaenoic acid) 500 mg • Vitamin E (as mixed tocopherols) 10 IU. Other Ingredients: Rosemary, Ascorbyl Palmitate, Citric Acid.

EPA-DHA 720 - Metagenics
Two softgels contain: Natural Marine Lipid Concentrate 2.4 g • EPA (eicosapentaenoic acid) 840 mg • DHA (docosahexaenoic acid) 600 mg • Vitamin E (mixed tocopherols) 20 IU. Other Ingredients: Rosemary, Ascorbyl Palmitate, Citric Acid.

EPA-DHA Complex - Metagenics
Each softgel contains: Natural Marine Lipid Concentrate 1 g • EPA (eicosapentaenoic acid) 180 mg • DHA (docosahexaenoic acid) 120 mg • Vitamin E (as mixed tocopherols) 9 IU.

EPA-DHA Extra Strength EE - Metagenics
Two softgels contain: Natural Marine Lipid Concentrate 2 g • EPA (eicosapentaenoic acid) 600 mg • DHA (docosahexaenoic acid) 400 mg • Vitamin E (as D-alpha tocopherol and mixed tocopherols) 10 IU.

EPA-DHA Extra Strength EE Enteric Coated - Metagenics
Two softgels contains: Natural Marine Lipid Concentrate 2 g • EPA (eicosapentaenoic acid) 600 mg • DHA (docosahexaenoic acid) 400 mg • Vitamin E (as D-alpha-tocopherol and mixed tocopherols) 10 IU.

EPA-DHA Extra Strength Lemon Flavored - Metagenics
Two softgels contain: EPA (eicosapentaenoic acid) 600 mg • DHA (docosahexaenoic acid) 400 mg • Vitamin E (as D-alpha tocopherol and mixed tocopherols) 10 IU. Other Ingredients: Lemon Extract, Rosemary, Ascorbyl Palmitate, Citric Acid.

EPA-DHA Extra Strength TG Enteric Coated - Metagenics
Two softgels contain: Natural Marine Lipid Concentrate 2 g • EPA (eicosapentaenoic acid) 600 mg • DHA (docosahexaenoic acid) 400 mg • Vitamin E (as D-alpha tocopherol and mixed tocopherols) 20 IU. Other Ingredients: Rosemary, Ascorbyl Palmitate, Citric Acid.

EPA-DHA High Concentrate Liquid - Metagenics
Each 1 tsp serving contains: Omega-3 Fatty Acids 2800 mg: EPA (eicosapentaenoic acid) 1400 mg, DHA (docosahexaenoic acid) 925 mg, Other Omega-3 Fatty Acids 475 mg. Other Ingredients: Natural Lemon Flavor, Rosemary Extract, Ascorbyl Palmitate, Natural Tocopherols.

EPA-DHA Lemon Softgels - Metagenics
Two softgels contain: Natural Marine Lipid Concentrate 2.5 g • EPA (eicosapentaenoic acid) 720 mg • DHA (docosahexaenoic acid) 560 mg. Other Ingredients: Natural Lemon Flavor, Rosemary, Ascorbyl Palmitate, Citric Acid, Mixed Tocopherols.

EPAForte - Nature's Plus
Each softgel contains: Marine Lipid concentrate 900 mg supplying: Eicosapentaenoic Acid (EPA) 162 mg, Docosahexaenoic Acid (DHA) 108 mg, total Omega-3 Fatty Acids 270 mg • Magnesium Aspartate equivalent to 60 mg of elemental Magnesium 300 mg • Vitamin E natural 50 IU • Vitamin B6 (Pyridoxine HCL) 10 mg • Garlic equivalent to 500 mg of fresh garlic 1 mg • Selenium, Biotron yeast-free amino acid complex 25 mcg.

EPH-833 - AST Sports Science
Each capsule contains: standardized 8% Ephedra extract 750 mg.
See Editor's Note No. 30.

EPH-833 (ephedra free) - AST Sports Science
Two capsules contain: Magnesium (as magnesium salicylate) 60 mg • TX-6 1460 mg: Green Tea leaf extract (standardized for epigallocatechin gallate EGCG), L-Phenylalanine, Caffeine (as caffeine anhydrous), Norsynephrine HCl, Theobromine HCl.

Ephedra Plus - PhytoPharmica
Each capsule contains: Ephedrine from 200 mg of Ma Huang extract (Ephedra sinensis) 12 mg • Ginger root extract 6.5:1 (Zingiber officinale) 65 mg • Licorice root extract (Glycyrrhiza glabra) standardized to contain 5% glycyrrhizic acid 50 mg • Marshmallow root extract 4:1 (Althaea officinalis; Mucilage content of 30-40%) 50 mg • Sundew Herb extract 4:1 (Drosera rotundifolia) 40 mg • Euphorbia Herb extract 4:1 (Euphorbia hirta) 40 mg • Senega root extract 4:1 (Polygala senega) 40 mg • Goldenseal root extract (Hydrastis canadensis) standardized to contain 5% total alkaloids, including berberine, hydrastine, & canadine 20 mg.
See Editor's Note No. 21 and No. 30.

Ephedra Super Cap - D & E Pharmaceuticals
Each capsule contains: 883 mg of pure Ephedra extract.
See Editor's Note No. 30.

Ephedra-Free - GNC
Two tablets contain: Proprietary Blend 1350 mg: Guarana Seed Extract (paullinia cupana), Black Tea Leaves Extract (camellia sinensis), Grape Skin Extract (vitis vinifera), Ginger Root Extract (zingiber officinale), Grape Seed Extract (vitis vinifera), Dill Weed Extract (anethum graveolens). Other Ingredients: Dextrose, Cellulose, Starch Caramel Color, Titanium Dioxide, Ethyl Vanillin.

Epidril Cutting Gel (100% Solution) - Nutra Sport
Lecithin • Octyl-Palmitate • Water • Aminophylline • Isopropylparaben • Isobutylparaben • Butylparaben • Fragrance.

Episilk hand & body lotion - Hyalogic LLC
De-Ionized Water • Emulsifying wax • Vitis Vinifera Grapeseed oil • Caprylic/Capric Glycerides • Soy wax • Hyaluronic Acid • Persea Gratissima (avocado oil) • Simmondsia Chinensis (jojoba seed oil) • Aloe Barbadensis leaf juice • Stearyl Alcohol • Limnanthes Alba (meadowfoam) seed oil • Glucose • Glucose Oxidase • Lactoperoxidase • Butyrospermum Parkii (shea butter) • Vegetable Glycerine • Sorbitol • Tocopherol (vitamin E) • Bees wax • Methyl Cellulose • Cyamopsis Tetragonoloba (guar) gum • Allantoin.

Episilk premium facial cream - Hyalogic LLC
De-Ionized Water • Emulsifying Wax • Grapeseed oil • Caprylic/Capric Glycerides • Soy Wax • Stearyl Alcohol • Avocado oil • Jojoba oil • Aloe Vera • Meadowfoam seed oil • Hyaluronic Acid • Shea Butter • Vegetable Glycerine • Sorbitol • Vitamin E • Bees Wax • Methyl Cellulose • Guar Gum • Lactoperoxidase • Glucose Oxidase • Allantoin.

Epoch Rare Earth Mineral Infusions Firming - Nu Skin Enterprises
Copper Gluconate • Diospyros Virginiana leaf powder (persimmon).

Epoch Rare Earths Mineral Infusions Clarifying - Nu Skin Enterprises
Calcium Carbonate • Citrus Aurantium Amara powder (bitter orange).

Epoch Rare Earths Mineral Infusions DeStressing - Nu Skin Enterprises
Mother of Pearl Powder • Cucumis Sativus fruit powder (cucumber).

Epogam - Pharmacia Corp.
Each capsule contains: Gamolenic Acid (GLA) 40 mg • Vitamin E (d-alpha tocopheryl acetate) 10 mg.
See Editor's Note No. 27.

e-Poise - Standard Process, Inc.
Two capsules contain: Proprietary Blend 820 mg: Defatted Wheat germ, Carrot root, Bovine Adrenal, Nutritional Yeast, Tillandsia Usneoides extract, Magnesium Citrate, Bovine Liver, Bovine Spleen, Ovine Spleen, Bovine Kidney, Mushroom, Dried Alfalfa juice, Bovine Bone, Carbamide, Oat flour, Bovine Spleen PMG extract, Soybean Lecithin, Porcine Duodenum, Rice bran, Choline Bitartrate, Veal Bone meal, Citric Acid, Porcine Stomach Parenchyma, Peanut bran, Licorice root, Dicalcium Phosphate, Mixed Tocopherols, Bovine Liver fat extract, Flaxseed oil extract • Vitamin A 1400 IU • Vitamin C 10.8 mg • Vitamin D 300 IU • Thiamine 0.2 mg • Riboflavin 0.3 mg • Vitamin B6 1.2 mg • Vitamin B12 0.4 mcg • Calcium 27 mg • Iron 2 mg. Other Ingredients: Gelatin, Water, Colors, Cocarboxylase, Potassium Para-Aminobenzoate.
See Editor's Note No. 14.

Epresat Multivitamin - Flora Inc.
Each tablet contains: Vitamin A • Vitamin B1 • Vitamin B2 • Vitamin B6 • Vitamin C • Vitamin D • Vitamin E • Niacinamide

E-Prime - USANA Health Sciences
Each capsule contains: Vitamin E (as d-alpha tocopherol) 200 IU • D-Gamma Tocotrienol 7 mg • Mixed Tocopherols 3.4 mg. Other Ingredients: Medium Chain Glycerides, Gelatin, Purified Water, Lecithin.

Epsom Salt (1 lb and 4 lb) - All Terrain Company
Active Ingredient: Magnesium Sulfate (Heplahydrate) • Saline Laxative.

EQ-10 - E'OLA
Ten drops contain: Proprietary Blend 149 mg: DMAE Bitartrate, Aloe Vera Juice, Ginseng Root, Co-Enzyme Q-10, Chromium Chelavite, Kelp, Licorice Root, Royal Jelly, White Willow Bark, L-Arginine, L-Tyrosine, Manganese Chelazome, Cyanocobalamin. Other Ingredients: Water, Glycerin, Sodium Benzoate.

Equal Ratio CAL-MAG - Quest
Each tablet contains: Calcium (HVP Chelate) 100 mg • Magnesium (HVP Chelate) 100 mg • Vitamin D (as Vitamin D3) 200 IU. Other Ingredients: Croscarmellose Sodium, Magnesium Stearate (vegetable source), Microcrystalline Cellulose, Vegetable Stearin.

Equaline B Complex with C - Leiner Health Products
Vitamin C 300 mg • Thiamine (vitamin B1) 15 mg • Riboflavin (vitamin B2) 10.2 mg • Niacin 50 mg • Vitamin B6 5 mg • Folic Acid 400 mcg • Vitamin B12 6 mcg • Pantothenic Acid 10 mg. Other Ingredients: Dextrose, Cellulose, Croscarmellose Sodium, Hydroxypropyl Methylcellulose, Starch Oligosaccharides, Starch, Dextrin, Magnesium Stearate, Silicon Dioxide, Resin, Sodium Carboxymethylcellulose, Sodium Citrate.
See Editor's Note No. 45.

Equaline Beta Carotene Softgels - Leiner Health Products
Each softgel contains: Vitamin A from Beta Carotene 25,000 IU. Other Ingredients: Soybean Oil, Gelatin, Glycerin, Vegetable Oil (partially hydrogenated cottonseed and soybean oils), Yellow Beeswax, Carrot Oil.
See Editor's Note No. 45.

Equaline Calcium Citrate Plus D tablets - Leiner Health Products
Two tablets contain: Vitamin D (as cholecalciferol) 400 IU • Calcium (as calcium citrate) 630 mg. Other Ingredients: Cellulose, Talc, Sodium Starch Glycolate, Croscarmellose Sodium, Stearic Acid, Titanium Dioxide, Dextrose, Hydroxypropyl Methylcellulose, Magnesium Stearate, Magnesium Oxide, Silicon Dioxide, Polyethylene Glycol, Sodium Carboxymethylcellulose, Gelatin, Mineral Oil, Sodium Citrate, Micro Fine Wax, Polysorbate 80, Carnauba Wax, Destrin.
See Editor's Note No. 45.

Equaline Central Vite Select tablets - Leiner Health Products
Each tablet contains: Vitamin A 5000 IU • Vitamin C 60 mg • Vitamin D 400 IU • Vitamin E 45 IU • Vitamin K 10 mcg • Thiamin (vitamin B1) 1.5 mg • Riboflavin (vitamin B2) 1.7 mg • Niacin 20 mg • Vitamin B6 3 mg • Folate 400 mcg • Vitamin B12 25 mcg • Biotin 30 mcg • Pantothenic Acid 10 mg • Calcium 200 mg • Phosphorus 48 mg • Iodine 150 mcg • Magnesium 100 mg • Zinc 15 mg • Selenium 20 mcg • Copper 2 mg • Manganese 2 mg • Chromium 150 mcg • Molybdenum 75 mcg • Chloride 72 mg • Potassium 80 mg • Boron 150 mcg • Nickel 5 mcg • Silicon 2 mg • Vanadium 10 mcg • Lutein 250 mcg. Other Ingredients: Cellulose, Gelatin, Maltodextrin, Starch, Croscarmellose, Sodium, Crospovidone, Magnesium Stearate, Dextrin, Titanium Dioxide, Hydroxypropyl Methylcellulose, Polyethylene Glycol, Resin, Vegetable Oil and Oleoresins, Mannitol, Sucrose, Blue 2 Lake, Sodium Molybdate, Red 40 Lake, Sodium Metasilicate, Yellow 6 Lake, Sodium.
See Editor's Note No. 45.

Equaline Central Vite tablets - Leiner Health Products
Each tablet contains: Vitamin A 5000 IU • Vitamin C 60 mg • Vitamin D 400 IU • Vitamin K 25 mcg • Thiamin 1.5 mg • Riboflavin 1.7 mg • Niacin 20 mg • Vitamin B6 2 mg • Vitamin B12 6 mcg • Biotin 30 mcg • Pantothenic Acid 10 mg • Calcium 162 mg • Iron 18 mg • Phosphorus 109 mg • Iodine 150 mcg • Magnesium 100 mg • Zinc 15 mg • Selenium 20 mcg • Copper 2 mg • Manganese 3.5 mg • Chromium 120 mcg • Molybdenum 75 mcg • Chloride 72 mg • Potassium 80 mg • Nickel 5 mcg • Tin 10 mcg • Silicon 2 mg • Vanadium 10 mcg • Boron 150 mcg • Vitamin E 30 IU • Folic Acid 400 mcg. Other Ingredients: Cellulose, Gelatin, Croscarmellose Sodium, Crospovidone, Magnesium Stearate, Dextrin, Titantium Dioxide, Hydroxypropyl Methylcellulose, Silicon Dioxide, Starch, Maltodextrin, Polyethylene Glycol, Mannitol, Vegetable Oil and Oleoresins, Sucrose, Yellow 6 Lake, Sodium Metasilicate.
See Editor's Note No. 45.

Equaline Children's Multivitamin Complete Chewable - Leiner Health Products
Each chewable tablet contains: Vitamin A 5000 IU • Vitamin C 60 mg • Vitamin D 400 IU • Vitamin E 30 IU • Thiamin (vitamin B1) 1.5 mg • Riboflavin (vitamin B2) 1.7 mg • Niacin 20 mg • Vitamin B6 2 mg • Vitamin B12 6 mcg • Biotin 40 mcg • Pantothenic Acid 10 mg • Calcium 100 mg • Iron 18 mg • Phosphorus 100 mg • Iodine 150 mcg • Magnesium 20 mg • Zinc 15 mg • Folic Acid 400 mcg • Copper 2 mg • Sodium 10 mg. Other Ingredients: Sorbitol, Fructose, Stearic Acid, Mono- and Diglycerides, Xylitol, Natural and Artificial Flavors, Gelatin, Sodium Ascorbate, Carrageenan, Aspartame, Red 40 Lake, Yellow 6 Lake, Starch, Magnesium Stearate, Blue 2 Lake, Hydroxypropyl Methylcellulose, Mononitrate, Resin, Hydroxypropyl Cellulose, Lactose, Polyvinyl Pyrrolidone. Phenylketonurics: Contains Phenylanine.
See Editor's Note No. 45.

Equaline Children's Multivitamin Plus Iron Chewable - Leiner Health Products
Each chewable tablet contains: Vitamin A 2500 IU • Vitamin C 60 mg • Vitamin D 400 IU • Vitamin E 15 IU • Thiamin 1.05 mg • Riboflavin 1.2 mg • Niacin 13.5 mg • Vitamin B6 1.05 mg • Vitamin B12 4.5 mcg • Iron 15 mg • Folic Acid 300 mcg. Other Ingredients: Sucrose, Sodium Ascorbate, Mono- and Diglycerides, Gelatin, Mannitol, Maltodextrin, Stearic Acid, Natural and Artificial Flavors, Magnesium Stearate, Yellow 6 Lake, Red 40 Lake, Blue 2 Lake, Starch, Mono Ammonium Glycyrrhizinate, Resin, Lactose, Ethylmaltol.
See Editor's Note No. 45.

Equaline Chromium Picolinate - Leiner Health Products
Each tablet contains: Chromium 400 mcg. Other Ingredients: Calcium Carbonate, Maltodextrin, Cellulose, Croscarmellose Sodium, Silicon Dioxide, Magnesium Stearate, Dextrin, Dextrose, Lecithin, Sodium Carboxymethylcellulose, Sodium Citrate.
See Editor's Note No. 45.

Equaline Ester C with Bioflavonoids tablets **-** Leiner Health Products
Each tablet contains: Ester-C brand Vitamin C 500 mg • Citrus Bioflavonoid Complex 200 mg. Other Ingredients: Calcium Carbonate, Cellulose, Croscarmellose Sodium, Crospovidone, Silicon Dioxide, Maltodextrin, Polyethylene Glycol 3350, Talc, Magnesium Stearate, Hydroxypropyl Methylcellulose, Hydroxypropyl Cellulose, Polysorbate 80.
See Editor's Note No. 45.

Equaline L-Lysine 500 mg tablets **-** Leiner Health Products
Each tablet contains: L-Lysine 500 mg. Other Ingredients: Monohydrochloride, Cellulose, Polyethylene Glycol 3350, Croscarmellose Sodium, Silicon Dioxide, Magnesium Stearate.
See Editor's Note No. 45.

Equaline One Daily Multivitamin & Mineral tablets **-** Leiner Health Products
Each tablet contains: Vitamin A 5000 IU • Vitamin C 60 mg • Vitamin D 400 IU • Vitamin E 30 IU • Thiamin 1.5 mg • Riboflavin 1.7 mg • Niacin 20 mg • Folate 400 mcg • Vitamin B12 6 mcg • Biotin 30 mcg • Pantothenic Acid 10 mg • Calcium 162 mg • Iron 18 mg • Phosphorus 109 mg • Iodine 150 mcg • Magnesium 100 mg • Zinc 15 mg • Selenium 20 mcg • Copper 2 mg • Manganese 3.5 mg • Chromium 65 mcg • Molybdenum 160 mcg • Chloride 72 mg • Potassium 80 mg • Vitamin K 25 mcg • Vitamin B6 2 mg • Nickel 5 mcg • Tin 10 mcg • Silicon 2 mg • Vanadium 10 mcg • Boron 150 mcg. Other Ingredients: Cellulose, Gelatin, Croscarmellose Sodium, Dextrin, Magnesium Stearate, Crospovidone, Hydroxypropyl Methylcellulose, Red 40 Lake, Maltodextrin, Starch, Polyethylene Glycol, Dextrose, Mannitol, Titanium Dioxide, Resin, Sodium Molybdate, Blue 2 Lake, Sodium Carboxymethylcellulose, Sodium Metasilicate.
See Editor's Note No. 45.

Equaline One Daily Women's tablets **-** Leiner Health Products
Each tablet contains: Vitamin A 2500 IU • Vitamin C 60 mg • Vitamin D 400 IU • Vitamin E 30 IU • Thiamine (vitamin B1) 1.5 mg • Riboflavin (vitamin B2) 1.7 mg • Folic Acid 400 mcg • Niacin 10 mg • Vitamin B6 2 mg • Vitamin B12 6 mcg • Pantothenic Acid 5 mg • Calcium 450 mg • Iron 18 mg • Magnesium 50 mg • Zinc 15 mg. Other Ingredients: Acacia, Cellulose, Croscarmellose Sodium, Magnesium Stearate, Titanium Dioxide, Dextrin, Hydroxypropyl Methylcellulose, Gelatin, Starch, Polyethylene Glycol, Silicon Dioxide, Dextrose, Yellow 5 Lake, Yellow 6 Lake, Blue 2 Lake.
See Editor's Note No. 45.

Equaline Prenatal Formula **-** Leiner Health Products
Each tablet contains: Vitamin A 4000 IU • Vitamin C 100 mg • Vitamin D 400 IU • Vitamin E 11 IU • Thiamin (vitamin B1) 1.84 mg • Riboflavin (vitamin B2) 1.7 mg • Niacin 18 mg • Vitamin B6 2.6 mg • Folic Acid 800 mcg • Vitamin B12 4 mcg • Calcium 200 mg • Iron 27 mg • Zinc 25 mg. Other Ingredients: Cellulose, Maltodextrin, Corn Starch, Croscarmellose Sodium, Sodium Starch Glycolate, Gelatin, Dextrin, Tricalcium Phosphate, Hydroxypropyl Methylcellulose, Magnesium Stearate, Polyethylene Glycol, Titanium Dioxide, Red 40 Lake, Yellow 6 Lake, Dextrose, Blue 2 Lake, Ergocalciferol.
See Editor's Note No. 45.

Equaline Selenium 200 mcg **-** Leiner Health Products
Each tablet contains: Selenium 200 mcg. Other Ingredients: Calcium Carbonate, Maltodextrin, Cellulose, Croscarmellose Sodium, Tricalcium Phosphate, Crospovidone, Polyethelene Glycol 3350, Silicon Dioxide, Magnesium Stearate, Hydroxypropyl Methylcellulose, Hydroxypropyl Cellulose, Polysorbate 80.
See Editor's Note No. 45.

Equaline Stress Formula with Iron **-** Leiner Health Products
Each tablet contains: Vitamin C 500 mg • Vitamin E 30 IU • Thiamin (vitamin B1) 10 mg • Riboflavin (vitamin B2) 10 mg • Niacin 100 mg • Vitamin B6 5 mg • Folate 400 mcg • Vitamin B12 12 mcg • Biotin 45 mcg • Pantothenic Acid 20 mg • Iron 18 mg. Other Ingredients: Starch, Hydroxypropyl Methylcellulose, Gelatin, Cellulose, Croscarmellose Sodium, Sodium Starch Glycolate, Maltodextrin, Hydroxypropyl Cellulose, Polyethylene Glycol 3350, Magnesium Stearate, Yellow 6 Lake, Phamaceutical Glaze, Crospovidone, Titanium Dioxide, Polysorbate 80, Red 40 Lake, Mannitol.
See Editor's Note No. 45.

Equaline Stress Formula with Zinc **-** Leiner Health Products
Each tablet contains: Vitamin C 500 mg • Vitamin E 30 IU • Niacin 100 mg • Vitamin B6 5 mg • Vitamin B12 12 mcg • Biotin 45 mcg • Pantothenic Acid 20 mg • Zinc 23.9 mg • Copper 3 mg • Thiamin 10 mg • Riboflavin 10 mg. Other Ingredients: Sodium Starch Glycolate, Starch, Hydroxypropyl Methylcellulose, Gelatin, Cellulose, Croscarmellose Sodium, Maltodextrin, Silicon Dioxide, Pharmaceutical Glaze, Hydroxypropyl Cellulose, Polyethylene Glycol 3350, Titanium Dioxide, Magnesium Stearate, Crospovidone, Polysorbate 80, Resin, Povidone, Yellow 6 Lake.
See Editor's Note No. 45.

Equaline Vitamin B1 100 mg **-** Leiner Health Products
Each tablet contains: Thiamin 100 mg. Other Ingredients: Dicalcium Phosphate, Stearic Acid, Hydrogenated Vegetable Oil, Croscarmellose Sodium, Cellulose, Magnesium Stearate, Sillicon Dioxide.
See Editor's Note No. 45.

Equaline Vitamin B12 500 mcg tablets **-** Leiner Health Products
Each tablet contains: Vitamin B12 500 mcg. Other Ingredients: Lactose, Dicalcium Phosphate, Starch, Magnesium Stearate, Red 40 Lake.
See Editor's Note No. 45.

Equaline Vitamin B6 100 mg tablets **-** Leiner Health Products
Each tablet contains: Vitamin B6 (as pyridoxine hydrochloride) 100 mg. Other Ingredients: Dicalcium Phosphate, Cellulose, Starch, Crocarmellose Sodium, Polyethylene Glycol 3350, Silicon Dioxide, Magnesium Stearate.
See Editor's Note No. 45.

Equaline Vitamin C 1000 mg **-** Leiner Health Products
Each tablet contains: Vitamin C 1000 mg. Other Ingredients: Starch, Crospovidone, Cellulose, Magnesium Stearate, Stearic Acid, Silicon Dioxide.
See Editor's Note No. 45.

Equaline Vitamin C 500 mg **-** Leiner Health Products
Each tablet contains: Vitamin C 500 mg. Other Ingredients: Starch, Cellulose, Crospovidone, Silicon Dioxide, Stearic Acid, Magnesium Stearate, Hydroxypropyl Cellulose, Croscarmellose Sodium.
See Editor's Note No. 45.

Equaline Vitamin C 500 mg Chewable Orange Tablets **-** Leiner Health Products
Each chewable tablet contains: Vitamin C 500 mg. Other Ingredients: Sucrose, Sodium Ascorbate, Natural Flavor, Sorbitol, Starch, Cellulose, Crospovidone, Silicon Dioxide, Stearic Acid, Magnesium Stearate, Yellow 6 Lake, Lactose, Ethylmaltol.
See Editor's Note No. 45.

Equaline Vitamin C 500 mg Chewable Wafers with Acerola **-** Leiner Health Products
Each chewable wafer contains: Vitamin C 500 mg. Other Ingredients: Sugar, Stearic Acid, Cellulose, Silicon Dioxide, Artificial Flavor, Acerola, Magnesium Stearate, Starch, Rose Hips, Lemon Bioflavonoids Complex, Hesperidin Complex, Buckwheat, Caramel, Rutin, Green Pepper Extract, Black Currant Extract.
See Editor's Note No. 45.

BRAND NAMES

Some Brand Name Natural Products - What they Contain

www.NaturalDatabase.com contains MANY more listings than appear here.
Editor's Notes are located on pages 2155-2163.

Equaline Vitamin C 500 mg with Rose Hips - Leiner Health Products
Each tablet contains: Vitamin C 500 mg. Other Ingredients: Starch, Cellulose, Hydroxypropyl Methylcellulose, Crospovidone, Stearic Acid, Rose Hips, Magnesium Stearate, Silicon Dioxide, Hydroxypropyl Cellulose, Croscarmellose Sodium.
See Editor's Note No. 45.

Equaline Vitamin E 400 IU softgels - Leiner Health Products
Each softgel contains: Vitamin E 400 IU. Other Ingredients: Gelatin, Glycerin, Vegetable Oil.
See Editor's Note No. 45.

Equigest Natural Progesterone Cream - At Last Naturals, Inc.
Water • Isopropyl • Palmitate • Progesterone (from wild yam) • Glyceryl Stearate (vegetable derived) • Stearic Acid (vegetable derived) • Glycerin (vegetable derived) • PEG-100 Stearate • Cetyl Alcohol • Aloe Vera gel • Tocopheryl Acetate (vitamin E) • Citrus Aurantium • Citrus Grandis extract • Maritime Pine bark extract (pycnogenol) • Zea Mays oil • Retinyl Palmitate (vitamin A) • Cholecalciferol (vitamin D3) • Carbomer • Triethanolamine.

Er Chen Tang Plus - Secara
Pinellia ternata rhizome 5:1 extract (ban xia) 547 mg • Tangerine peel 5:1 extract (chen pi) 547 mg • Organic Licorice root (gan cao) 502 mg • Poria sclerotium 5:1 extract (fu ling) 328 mg • Organic Elecampane 315 mg • Tangerine oil 11 mg.

Ericsson's Alka-Mine Coral Calcium - KingsWay, Inc.
Coral Calcium • Magnesium • Ascorbic Acid • Silver.

Erotikava - Pacific Sensuals
Each 1 oz. serving contains: Vanuatu Kava Kava • Honey • Ginger • Lycium • Epimedium • Polygala • Liquid Amber • Saigon Cinnamon bark • Licorice • Vegetable Glycerine • Cnidium seed.

Esberitox - Enzymatic Therapy/PhytoPharmica
Three tablets contain: Echinacea Purpurea and Pallida root 1:1 (coneflower root) 22.5 mg • Thuja leaf (thuja occidentalis/white cedar leaf) 6 mg • Wild Indigo root (baptisia tinctoria) 30 mg.

Escalation - Enzymatic Therapy
Each capsule contains: Cola Nut extract (Cola nitida) (contains Caffeine 35 mg) 250 mg • Green Tea extract (Camellia sinensis) (contains Caffeine 15 mg) 250 mg • Ma Huang extract (Ephedra sinensis) (contains Ephedrine 15 mg) 250 mg.
See Editor's Note No. 21 and No. 30.

Escalation (Ephedra-FREE!) - Enzymatic Therapy
Each capsule contains: Bitter Orange fruit extract (citrus x aurantium, standardized to contain 6% synephrine) 250 mg • Cola nut extract (cola nitida, standardized to contain 35 mg caffeine) 250 mg • Green Tea leaf extract (camellia sinensis, containing 15 mg caffeine) 110 mg. Other Ingredients: Gelatin, Cellulose, Magnesium Stearate, Silicon Dioxide, Titanium Dioxide Color.
See Editor's Note No. 40.

Escalert - Enzymatic Therapy
Two capsules contain: Cola Nut extract (cola nitida, contains caffeine 35 mg) 250 mg • Green Tea extract (camellia sinensis, contains Caffeine 15 mg) 250 mg • Oat Straw extract 10:1 (avena sativa) 50 mg • Schisandra extract (standardized to contain 9% schizandrin) 50 mg • Siberian Ginseng extract (eleutherococcus senticosus, standardized to contain greater than 1% eleutherosides E) 50 mg • Ginger root extract 6.5:1 (zingiber officinale) 25 mg • Korean Ginseng root extract (panax ginseng, standardized to contain 7% saponins calculated as ginsenoside Rg1) 10 mg • Chromium (polynicotinate) 100 mcg.

E-Sel - J. R. Carlson Laboratories, Inc.
Each softgel contains: Vitamin E (as D-alpha tocopherol) 400 IU • Selenium (as L-selenomethionine) 100 mcg.

Esiak Caps - NOW Foods
Each capsule contains: 450 mg Proprietary Blend: Burdock (Articum Lappa) root (4:1 extract) • Sheep Sorrel (Rumex Acetosella) leaf (4:1 extract) • Slippery Elm bark (Ulmus fulva) bark (4:1 extract) • Turkey Rhubarb (Rheum palmatum) root (4:1 extract). Other Ingredients: Maltodextrin, Magnesium Stearate.

Eskimo-3 - Enzymatic Therapy
Each softgel contains: Omega-3 Fatty Acids (provides EPA [eicosapentaenoic acid] 260 mg, DHA [docosahexaenoic acid] 165 mg) 600 mg. Other Ingredients: Gelatin, Glycerin, Mixed Tocopherols, Lemon Oil, Rosemary, Lecithin, Ascorbyl Palmitate.

Eskimo-3 - PhytoPharmica
Three softgel capsules contain: Eskimo-3 brand Fish Oil containing Omega-3 Fatty Acids including 210-270 mg EPA (eicosapentaenoic acid) and 125-175 mg DHA (docosahexaenoic acid) 1.5 g. Other Ingredients: Gelatin, Glycerin, Mixed Tocopherols, Natural Lime Flavor, Natural Rosemary Flavor, Lecithin, Ascorbyl Palmitate.

Eskimo-3 capsules - Tyler Encapsulations
Three capsules contain: Vitamin E (mixed tocopherols) 6.7 IU • Omega-3 Fatty Acids 600 mg • EPA (eicosapentaenoic acid) 260 mg • DHA (docosahexaenoic acid) 166 mg. Ingredients: Fish Oil, Gelatin, Glycerin, Mixed Tocopherols, Lemon Oil, Rosemary, Lecithin, Ascorbyl Palmitate.

Eskimo-3 liquid - Tyler Encapsulations
Each teaspoon (5 mL) contains: Vitamin E (as mixed tocopherols) 20 IU • Omega-3 Fatty Acids 1.8 g • EPA (eicosapentaenoic acid) 750 mg • DHA (docosahexaenoic acid) 500 mg. Ingredients: Fish Oil, Mixed Tocopherols, Lemon Oil, Rosemary, Lecithin, Ascorbyl Palmitate.

Esotyne - Progressive Health Nutraceuticals
Vitamin C 500 mg • Bromelain 20 mg • Quercetin 200 mg • Bee Pollen 500 mg • Bee Propolis 50 mg • Royal Jelly 10 mg • Golden Seal 40 mg.

Especially for MEN - The Vitamin Shoppe
Two capsules contain: Vitamin A 5000 IU • Vitamin C 30 mg • Vitamin D 200 IU • Vitamin E 100 IU • Vitamin K 75 mcg • Niacin 30 mg • Vitamin B1 30 mg • Vitamin B2 30 mg • Vitamin B6 30 mg • Folic Acid 400 mcg • Vitamin B12 30 mcg • Biotin 250 mcg • Pantothenic Acid 30 mg • Calcium 200 mg • Iodine 150 mcg • Magnesium 100 mg • Zinc 25 mg • Selenium 100 mcg • Copper 2 mg • Manganese 5 mg • Chromium 50 mcg • Chloride 28 mg • Beta-carotene 3 mg • Potassium 30 mg • Silica 10 mcg • Choline 10 mg • Inositol 10 mg • PABA 10 mg • Citrus Bioflavonoids 25 mg • Korean Ginseng 70 mg • Damiana leaf 70 mg • Oat Straw 50 mg • Garlic 50 mg • Oyster extract 50 mg • Prostate Glandular 50 mg • Saw Palmetto 50 mg • L-Cysteine 50 mg • Nettles leaf 30 mg • Pumpkin seed 30 mg • L-Methionine 10 mg • Alpha Lipoic Acid 5 mg • Lycopene 1 mg.

Especially for Women - The Vitamin Shoppe
Three capsules contain: Vitamin A Activity 10000 IU • Vitamin E 200 IU • Vitamin D 200 IU • Vitamin C 250 mg • Selenium 50 mcg • Vitamin B1 25 mg • Vitamin B2 25 mg • Niacinamide 25 mg • Vitamin B6 25 mg • Vitamin B12 250 mcg • Pantothenic Acid 25 mg • Citrus Bioflavonoids 100 mg • Biotin 100 mcg • Folic Acid 400 mcg • Choline Bitartrate 25 mg • Inositol 25 mg • PABA 25 mg • Calcium 200 mg • Magnesium 100 mg • Potassium 25 mg • Phosphorus 50 mg • Manganese 15 mg • Zinc 15 mg • Iron 18 mg • Chromium 50 mcg • Iodine 225 mcg • Boron 3 mg • Silica 5 mg • Black Currant 100 mg • Dong Quai 50 mg • Royal Jelly 100 mg.

Especially Yours Bar - Nature's Plus
High Fructose Complex (from fruit concentrate, corn and/or malt) • Rolled Oats • Fructose • Rice Flour • Non-GMO Isolated Soy Protein • Wild Clover Honey • Fractionated Vegetable oil (soy, safflower and/or palm kernel) • Calcium Carbonate • Di-Calcium Phosphate • Barley Malt syrup • Cocoa • Natural Flavors • Dry Roasted Almond • Soybean Lecithin oil • Oat Bran • Malt extract • Rice Bran •

BRAND NAMES

Magnesium Oxide • Canola oil • Distilled Monoglycerides • Ascorbic Acid • Ferric Orthophosphate • D-Alpha Tocopheryl Acetate • Sodium Chloride • Calcium Citrate • Niacinamide • Calcium Pantothenate • Zinc Gluconate/Oxide • Copper Gluconate • Vitamin A Palmitate • Pyridoxine HCl • Thiamine Mononitrate • Riboflavin • Folic Acid • Biotin • Sodium Selenite • Potassium Iodide • Cyanocobalamin.

Especially Yours Tablets **-** Nature's Plus
Three tablets contain: Vitamin A (as beta carotene) 10,000 IU • Vitamin C (as ascorbic acid) 300 mg • Vitamin D (as ergocalciferol) 400 IU • Vitamin E (as D-alpha tocopheryl succinate) 400 IU • Vitamin B1 (as thiamine HCl) 10 mg • Vitamin B2 (as riboflavin) 10 mg • Niacin 10 mg • Vitamin B6 (as pyridoxine HCl) 100 mg • Folate (as folic acid) 800 mcg • Vitamin B12 (as cyanocobalamin) 100 mcg • Biotin 200 mcg • Pantothenic Acid (as calcium pantothenate) 50 mg • Calcium (as aminoate) 150 mg • Iron (aspartate) 40 mg • Iodine (from kelp) 225 mcg • Magnesium (as aminoate) 300 mg • Zinc (picolinate) 20 mg • Selenium (as aminoate) 10 mcg • Manganese (ascorbate) 6.1 mg • Chromium (as aminoate) 15 mcg • Potassium (citrate) 15 mg • Flax seed 100 mg • Lemon Bioflavonoid Complex (from citrus limon exocarp; active flavonols, flavonones, flavones, and naringen 44%) 50 mg • Suma root (pfaffia paniculata) 50 mg • Damiana (whole herb) 50 mg • Dong Quai root 50 mg • Inositol 25 mg • Rutin (from saphora japonica) 25 mg • Amylase 25 mg • Lipase 25 mg • Black Currant seed 25 mg • Buchu leaf 25 mg • Protease 15 mg • PABA (para-aminobenzoic acid) 10 mg • Choline (as bitartrate) 11 mg. Other Ingredients: Di-Calcium Phosphate, Microcrystalline Cellulose, Stearic Acid, Silica, Magnesium Stearate, Pharmaceutical Glaze.

Essential 50+ **-** Nature Made
Each tablet contains: Vitamin A (vitamin A acetate) 5000 IU • Vitamin C (ascorbic acid) 120 mg • Vitamin D 400 IU • Vitamin E (DL-alpha tocopherol acetate) 60 IU • Vitamin K (phylloquinone) 10 mcg • Thiamin (B1, thiamin mononitrate) 3 mg • Riboflavin (B2) 3.4 mg • Niacin (B3, niacinamide ascorbate) 20 mg • Vitamin B6 (pyridoxine hydrochloride) 4 mg • Folate, Folic Acid, Folacin 400 mcg • Vitamin B12 (cyanocobalamin) 25 mcg • Biotin 30 mcg • Pantothenic Acid (D-calcium pantothenate) 10 mg • Calcium (calcium carbonate) 200 mg • Phosphorus 48 mg • Iodine (potassium iodide, kelp) 150 mcg • Magnesium (magnesium oxide) 100 mg • Zinc (zinc oxide) 15 mg • Selenium (sodium selenate) 50 mcg • Copper (copper oxide) 2 mg • Manganese (manganese sulfate) 2 mg • Chromium (chromium chloride) 120 mcg • Molybdenum (sodium molybdate) 25 mcg • Chloride 72 mg • Potassium (potassium chloride) 80 mcg • Nickel (nickelous sulfate) 5 mcg • Silicon (sodium metasilicate) 2 mg • Boron (sodium borates) 150 mcg • Vanadium (sodium metavanadate) 10 mcg • Lutein 250 mcg. Other Ingredients: Dibasic Calcium Phosphate, Cellulose Gel, Crospovidone, Gelatin, Acacia, Hydroxypropyl Methylcellulose, Silicon Dioxide, Corn Starch, Magnesium Stearate, Corn Oil, Modified Food Starch, Polyethylene Glycol.
See Editor's Note No. 45.

Essential Amino Complex **-** Solgar
Each capsule contains: L-Histidine 75 mg • L-Isoleucine 75 mg • L-Leucine 75 mg • L-Lysine (as L-lysine HCl) 75 mg • L-Methionine 75 mg • L-Phenylalanine 75 mg • L-Threonine 75 mg • L-Valine 75 mg. Other Ingredients: Vegetable Cellulose, Microcrystalline Cellulose, Vegetable Magnesium Stearate, Water, Vegetable Glycerin.

Essential Aminos capsules **-** Pure Encapsulations
Each vegetable capsule contains: L-Histidine (free-form) 56 mg • L-Isoleucin (free-form) 88 mg • L-Leucine (free-form) 153 mg • L-Lysine (HCl) 167 mg • L-Methionine (free-form) 86 mg • L-Phenylalanine (free-form) 64 mg • L-Threonine (free-form) 76 mg • L-Valine (free-form) 83 mg • Vitamin C (as ascorbyl palmitate) 9 mg.

Essential Aminos powder **-** Pure Encapsulations
Each scoop contains: L-Histidine (free-form) 198 mg • L-Isoleucine (free-form) 311 mg • L-Leucine (free-form) 540 mg • L-Lysine (HCl) 590 mg • L-Methionine (free-form) 304 mg • L-Phenylalanine (free-form) 226 mg • L-Threonine (free-form) 268 mg • L-Valine (free-form) 293 mg.

Essential B Complete **-** Rexall - Sundown
Each tablet contains: Thiamin (as thiamin mononitrate) 1.5 mg • Riboflavin (Vitamin B-2) 1.7 mg • Niacin (as niacinamide) 20 mg • Vitamin B-6 (as pyridoxine HCl) 2 mg • Folic Acid 400 mcg • Vitamin B-12 (as cyanocobalamin) 6 mcg • Calcium 35 mg. Other Ingredients: Dicalcium Phosphate, Cellulose, Croscarmellose Sodium, Hydroxypropyl Methylcellulose, Magnesium Stearate, Triethyl Citrate.

Essential Balance **-** Nature Made
Each tablet contains: Vitamin A (vitamin A acetate) 5000 IU • Vitamin C (ascorbic acid) 120 mg • Vitamin D (vitamin D3) 400 IU • Vitamin E (DL-alpha tocopherol acetate) 50 IU • Vitamin K (phylloquinone) 25 mcg • Thiamin (B1, thiamin mononitrate) 1.5 mg • Riboflavin (B2) 1.7 mg • Niacin (B3, niacinamide ascorbate) 20 mg • Vitamin B6 (pyridoxine hydrochloride) 2 mg • Folate, Folic Acid, Folacin 400 mcg • Vitamin B12 (cyanocobalamin) 6 mcg • Biotin 20 mcg • Pantothenic Acid (D-calcium pantothenate) 10 mg • Calcium (dibasic calcium phosphate) 100 mg • Iron (ferrous fumarate) 9 mg • Phosphorus 77 mg • Iodine (potassium iodide) 150 mcg • Magnesium (magnesium oxide) 100 mg • Zinc (zinc oxide) 15 mg • Selenium (sodium selenate) 25 mcg • Copper (copper oxide) 2 mg • Manganese (manganese sulfate) 2 mg • Chromium (chromium chloride) 120 mcg • Molybdenum (sodium molybdate) 25 mcg • Chloride 36 mg • Potassium (potassium chloride) 40 mg • Nickel (nickelous sulfate) 5 mcg • Tin (stannous chloride) 10 mcg • Silicon (sodium metasilicate) 2 mg • Vanadium (sodium metavanadate) 10 mcg • Boron (sodium borate) 150 mcg • Lutein 250 mcg. Other Ingredients: Cellulose Gel, Croscarmellose Sodium, Stearic Acid, Gelatin, Magnesium Stearate, Silicon Dioxdie, Corn Starch, Hydroxypropyl Methylcellulose, Polyethylene Glycol.
See Editor's Note No. 45.

Essential Balance oil **-** Jarrow Formulas
Each 1 tbsp serving contains: Organic unrefined Flax seed oil • Organic Pumpkin seed oil • Organic Flax seed particulate • Organic high oleic Sunflower seed oil.

Essential Balance, Jr. oil **-** Jarrow Formulas
Each 1 tsp serving contains: Unrefined, virgin, organic Flax seed oil • Sunflower oil • Sesame oil • Pumpkin oil • Borage oil • Natural Butterscotch flavoring.

Essential Bodyguard **-** Rexall - Sundown
Two tablets contain: Vitamin A (from retinyl acetate and 25% as beta-carotene) 4000 IU • Vitamin C 600 mg • Vitamin D (from cholecalciferol) 160 IU • Vitamin E (from dl-alpha-tocopheryl acetate and d-alpha-tocopheryl acid succinate) 120 IU • Thiamin (from thiamin HCl) 4 mg • Riboflavin (Vitamin B2) 8 mg • Niacin (as niacinamide) 4 mg • Vitamin B-6 (from pyridoxine HCl) 40 mg • Folic Acid 160 mcg • Vitamin B-12 (as cyanocobalamin) 100 mcg • Biotin 100 mcg • Pantothenic Acid (from calcium d-pantothenate) 40 mg • Calcium 20 mg • Iron (from ferrous fumarate) 4 mg • Magnesium (from magnesium oxide) 80 mg • Zinc (from zinc gluconate) 20 mg • Selenium (from selenium amino acid chelate) 80 mcg • Copper (from copper gluconate) 0.8 mg • Manganese (from manganese gluconate) 2 mg • Sodium 5 mg • Whey Protein Concentrate 200 mg • Echinacea Purpurea root 120 mg • Rutin 30 mg • Choline Bitartrate 40 mg • Goldenseal aerial parts 24 mg • Garlic extract 15:1 bulb 8 mg. Other Ingredients: Croscarmellose Sodium, Cellulose, Stearic Acid, Sodium Starch Glycolate, Magnesium Stearate, Silica, Hydroxypropyl Methylcellulose, Hydroxypropyl Cellulose, PEG.

BRAND NAMES

Essential Daily - Nature Made
Each tablet contains: Vitamin A (vitamin A acetate) 5000 IU • Vitamin C (ascorbic acid) 60 mg • Vitamin D 400 IU • Vitamin E (DL-alpha tocopherol acetate) 30 IU • Thiamin (B1, thiamine mononitrate) 1.5 mg • Riboflavin (B2) 1.7 mg • Niacin (B3, niacinamide ascorbate) 20 mg • Vitamin B6 (pyridoxine hydrochloride) 2 mg • Folate, Folic Acid, Folacin 400 mcg • Vitamin B12 (cyanocobalamin) 6 mcg • Pantothenic Acid (D-calcium pantothenate) 10 mg • Calcium (calcium carbonate) 450 mg • Iron (ferrous fumarate) 18 mg • Zinc (zinc oxide) 15 mg. Other Ingredients: Cellulose Gel, Croscarmellose Sodium, Glycerides of Fatty Acids, Acacia, Maltodextrin, Hydroxypropyl Methylcellulose, Magnesium Stearate, Corn Starch, Modified Food Starch, Polyethylene Glycol.
See Editor's Note No. 45.

Essential Defense (formerly TCB 16) - Metagenics
Two tablets contain: 5:1 Proprietary Blend 1000 mg: Forsythia fruit (forsythia suspensa), Lonicera flower (lonicera japonica), Platycodon root (platycodon grandiflorum), Great Burdock fruit (actrium lappa), Chinese Mint leaf (mentha haplocalyx), Chinese Licorice root (glycyrrhiza uralensis), Fermented Soybean (glycine max), Schizonepeta herb (schizonepeta multifida), Laphaterium leaf (lophaterum gracile), Dyer's Woad root (isatis tinctoria), Ginger rhizome (zingiber officinale).

Essential E - PhysioLogics
Each softgel contains: Vitamin E (as d-alpha tocopheryl acetate) 400 IU. Other Ingredients: Gelatin, Soybean Oil, Glycerin.

Essential Enzymes - Source Naturals
Each capsule contains: Vegetal analog of Pancreatin with acid-stable Protease (28652 FCC) 298 mg • Lipase (375 FCC) 125 mg • Alpha Amylase (630 FCC) 52 mg • Amyloglucosidase (2 FCC) 12.5 mg • Cellulase (100 FCC) 5 mg • Hemicellulase (650 FCC) 3 mg • Lactase (40 FCC) 5 mg.
See Editor's Note No. 14.

Essential Fatty Acid Complex - Health Smart Vitamins
Three softgels contain: Vitamin E (as d-alpha tocopherol) 30 IU • Eicosapentaenoic Acid (EPA: from marine lipids) 180 mg • Docosahexaenoic Acid (DHA: from marine lipids) 120 mg • Gamma Linolenic Acid (GLA: from borage oil) 45 mg.

Essential Fatty Acids - Nutri-Quest Rx
Each capsule contains: Cod Liver 500 mg • Flaxseed oil 135 mg • Extra Virgin Olive oil 135 mg • Vitamin A 1190 IU • Vitamin D 124 IU. Also contains: Oleic, Linoleic, Palmitic, Arachidic & Linolenic, Eicosapentaenoic, & Docosahexaenoic.

Essential Fish Oil Concentrate - Rexall - Sundown
Three softgels contain: Vitamin E (as dl-alpha-tocopheryl acetate) 300 IU • Fish Oil (Eicosapentaenoic Acid 540 mg, Docosahexaenoic Acid 360 mg) 3 g. Other Ingredients: Gelatin, Glycerin, Water.

Essential Man - Nature Made
Each tablet contains: Vitamin C 120 mg • Vitamin K 25 mcg • Thiamin 1.5 mg • Riboflavin 1.7 mg • Niacin 20 mg • Vitamin B6 2 mg • Folic Acid 400 mcg • Vitamin B12 6 mcg • Biotin 30 mcg • Pantothenic Acid 10 mg • Calcium 100 mg • Phosphorus 77 mg • Iodine 150 mcg • Magnesium 100 mg • Zinc 15 mg • Selenium 25 mcg • Copper 2 mg • Manganese 2 mg • Chromium 120 mcg • Molybdenum 25 mcg • Chloride 36 mg • Potassium 40 mg • Boron 150 mcg • Nickel 5 mcg • Silicon 2 mg • Tin 10 mcg • Lutein 250 mcg • Vanadium 10 mcg • Lycopene 2 mg. Other Ingredients: Dibasic Calcium Phosphate, Cellulose Gel, Croscarmellose Sodium, Gelatin, Sugar, Corn Starch, Magnesium Stearate, Hydroxypropyl Methylcellulose, Modified Food Starch, Polyethylene Glycol.
See Editor's Note No. 45.

Essential Man 50+ - Nature Made
Each tablet contains: Vitamin C 120 mg • Vitamin K 10 mcg • Thiamin 2 mg • Riboflavin 3.4 mg • Niacin 20 mg • Vitamin B6 4 mg • Folic Acid 400 mcg • Vitamin B12 25 mcg • Biotin 30 mcg • Pantothenic Acid 10 mg • Calcium 2000 mg • Phosphorus 48 mg • Iodine 150 mcg • Magnesium 100 mg • Zinc 15 mg • Selenium 100 mcg • Copper 2 mg • Manganese 2 mg • Chromium 120 mcg • Molybdenum 25 mcg • Chloride 72 mg • Potassium 80 mg • Boron 150 mcg • Nickel 5 mg • Silicon 2 mg • Vanadium 10 mcg • Lutein 250 mcg • Lycopene 2 mg • Vitamin A 5000 IU • Vitamin D 400 IU • Vitamin E 60 IU. Other Ingredients: Dibasic Calcium Phosphate, Cellulose Gel, Croscarmellose Sodium, Gelatin, Sugar, Corn Starch, Acacia, Magnesium Stearate, Hydroxypropyl Methylcellulose, Modified Food Starch, Polyethylene Glycol.
See Editor's Note No. 45.

Essential Meal - Gary Null & Associates (GNA)
Fortified with branched chain amino acids.

Essential Minerals - Futurebiotics LLC
Four tablets contain: Calcium (carbonate, aspartate, citrate) 1000 mg • Magnesium (oxide, aspartate, citrate) 800 mg • Vitamin D 200 IU • Boron (citrate) 3 mg • Iron (gluconate) 9 mg • Manganese (amino acid chelate) 5 mg • Copper (gluconate) 1.5 mg • Zinc (gluconate) 15 mg • Betaine HCl 250 mg • Potassium (chloride, proteinate) 75 mg.

Essential Nutrients - Progressive Labs
Six capsules contain: Vitamin A (retinyl palmitate) 10,000 IU • Vitamin A (beta carotene) 15,000 IU • Vitamin C (ascorbic acid) 1000 mg • Vitamin D (cholecalciferol) 80 IU • Vitamin E (d-alpha tocopheryl succinate) 400 IU • Thiamin (Vitamin B1) 50 mg • Riboflavin-5-Phosphate (Vitamin B2) 20 mg • Niacin 25 mg • Niacinamide 125 mg • Vitamin B6 (pyridoxine HCl with pyridoxal-5'-phosphate) 20 mg • Folate (folic acid) 800 mcg • Vitamin B12 (cyanocobalamin with adenosylocobalamin) 500 mcg • Biotin 800 mcg • Pantothenic Acid (d-calcium pantothenate) 500 mg • Calcium (aspartate & carbonate) 500 mg • Iodine (potassium iodide) 225 mcg • Magnesium (aspartate and oxide) 500 mg • Zinc (picolinate) 25 mg • Selenium (selenomethionine) 200 mcg • Copper (glycinate & oxide) 2 mg • Manganese (aspartate & sulfate) 20 mg • Chromium (as chromium picolinate) 200 mcg • Molybdenum (sodium molybdate) 100 mcg • Potassium (aspartate and chloride) 99 mg • Boron (chelate) 3 mg • Vanadium (vanadyl sulfate) 100 mcg • Choline Citrate 250 mg.

Essential Oils - Puritan's Pride
Each softgel contains: Flaxseed oil 400 mg • Borage oil 400 mg • Super EPA 400 mg • Oleic Acid (Omega 9) 152 mg • Linoleic Acid (Omega 6) 180 mg • Gamma/Alpha Linolenic Acid (Omega 3) 260 mg • Eicosapentaenoic Acid (EPA) 120 mg • Docosahexaenoic Acid (DHA) 80 mg • Vitamin E (d-alpha tocopherol) 5 IU.

Essential Omega-3 Complex - Shaklee
Three capsules contain: Vitamin E 9 IU • EPA (Eicosapentaenoic acid) 545 mg • DHA (Docosahexaenoic acid) 235 mg • Omega-3 fatty acid blend 195 mg. Other Ingredients: Natural Marine Lipid Concentrate, Mixed Tocopherols Concentrate, Gelatin, Glycerin, Water.

Essential Stuff Gel Caps 1000 mg - Blue Stuff, Inc.
Each gel cap contains: Proprietary Blend 1000 mg: Pure Emu oil • Gelatin • Vitamin E.

Essential Stuff Gel Caps 750 mg - Blue Stuff, Inc.
Each gel cap contains: Proprietary Blend 750 mg: Pure Emu oil • Gelatin • Vitamin E.

Essential Stuff Liquid - Blue Stuff, Inc.
Each 16 oz bottle contains: Emu oil • Safflower oil • Natura & Artificial Flavor • Aloe Vera oil • Stevia • Tocopherol.

Essential Woman - Nature Made
Each tablet contains: Vitamin A 3000 IU • Vitamin C 120 mg • Vitamin D 400 IU • Vitamin E 50 IU • Vitamin K 100 mcg • Thiamin 1.5 mg • Riboflavin 1.7 mg • Niacin 20 mg • Vitamin B6 2 mg • Folic Acid 400 mcg • Vitamin B12 6 mcg • Biotin 30 mcg • Pantothenic Acid 10 mg • Calcium 250 mg • Iron 18 mg • Phosphorus 77 mg • Iodine 150 mcg • Magnesium 100 mg • Zinc 15 mg • Selenium 25 mcg • Copper 2 mg • Manganese 2 mg • Chromium 120 mcg • Molybdenum 25 mcg • Chloride 36 mg • Potassium 40 mg • Boron 150 mcg • Nickel 5 mcg • Silicon 2 mg • Tin 10 mcg • Vanadium 10 mcg • Lutein 250 mcg.
See Editor's Note No. 45.

Essential Woman 50+ - Nature Made
Each tablet contains: Vitamin A 3000 IU • Vitamin C 120 mg • Vitamin D 400 IU • Vitamin E 60 IU • Vitamin K 50 mcg • Thiamin 3 mg • Riboflavin 3.4 mg • Niacin 20 mg • Vitamin B6 4 mg • Folic Acid 400 mcg • Vitamin B12 25 mcg • Biotin 30 mcg • Pantothenic Acid 10 mg • Calcium 250 mg • Phosphorus 48 mg • Iodine 150 mcg • Magnesium 120 mg • Zinc 22 mg • Selenium 50 mcg • Copper 2 mg • Manganese 2 mg • Chromium 120 mcg • Molybdenum 25 mcg • Chloride 72 mg • Potassium 80 mg • Boron 150 mcg • Nickel 5 mcg • Silicon 2 mg • Tin 10 mcg • Vanadium 10 mcg • Lutein 250 mcg. Other Ingredients: Dibasic Calcium Phosphate, Cellulose Gel, Crospovidone, Gelatin, Acacia, Maltodextrin, Magnesium Stearate, Hydroxypropyl Methylcellulose, Corn Starch, Corn Oil, Modified Food Starch, Polyethylene Glycol.
See Editor's Note No. 45.

Essentially All - Alacer
Three tablets contain: Vitamin A (beta carotene) 10,000 IU • Vitamin B1 (thiamin HCl) 20 mg • Vitamin B2 (riboflavin) 20 mg • Vitamin C (mineral ascorbates) 750 mg • Vitamin D (cholecalciferol) 100 IU • Vitamin E (acetate) 100 IU • Niacin 30 mg • Vitamin B6 (pyridoxine HCl) 20 mg • Folic Acid 400 mcg • Vitamin B12 (cyanocobalamin) 200 mcg • D-Biotin 100 mcg • Pantothenic Acid (D-calcium pantothenate) 40 mg • Calcium (citrate, ascorbate) 100 mg • Iron (ferrous, gluconate) 9 mg • Iodine (kelp) 75 mcg • Magnesium (citrate, ascorbate) 40 mg • Zinc (ascorbate) 5 mg • Potassium (citrate-ascorbate) 60 mg • Copper (gluconate) 500 mcg • PABA (P-Aminobenzoic acid) 20 mg • Inositol 25 mg • Chromium (ascorbate-aspartate) 20 mcg • Manganese (ascorbate) 500 mcg • Molybdenum (ascorbate) 200 mcg • Selenium (L-selenomethionine) 50 mcg • Vanadium (proteinate, ascorbate) 50 mcg • Lecithin 50 mg.

Essentials - Chelated Mineral - USANA Health Sciences
Three tablets contain: Calcium (as Calcium Citrate) 270 mg • Magnesium (as Magnesium Citrate, Amino Acid Chelate, and Oxide) 300 mg • Iodine (as Potassium Iodide) 225 mcg • Zinc (as Zinc Citrate) 20 mg • Selenium (as L-Selenomethionine and Amino Acid Complex) 200 mcg • Copper (as Copper Gluconate) 3 mg • Manganese (as Manganese Gluconate) 5.1 mg • Chromium (as Chromium Picolinate and Polynicotinate) 300 mcg • Molybdenum (as Molybdenum Citrate) 50 mcg • Boron (as Boron Citrate) 3 mg • Silicon (as Amino Acid Complex) 3 mg • Vanadium (as Vanadyl Sulfate) 30 mcg • Ultra Trace Minerals 3 mg. Other Ingredients: Microcrystalline Cellulose, Pregelatinized Starch, Croscarmellose Sodium, Collodial Silicon Dioxide, Ascorbyl Palmitate, Dextrin, Dextrose.

Essentials - Mega Antioxidant - USANA Health Sciences
Three tablets contain: Vitamin A (as Beta Carotene) 15000 IU • Vitamin C (as Calcium, Potassium, Magnesium, Zinc Ascorbates) 1300 mg • Vitamin D 450 IU • Vitamin E (as D-Alpha Tocopheryl Succinate) 450 IU • Vitamin K (as Phylloquinone) 60 mcg • Vitamin B1 (as Thiamine HCl) 27 mg • Riboflavin 27 mg • Niacin (as Niacin and Niacinamide) 40 mg • Vitamin B6 (as Pyridoxine HCl) 27 mg • Folate (as Folic Acid) 1000 mcg • Vitamin B12 (as Cyanocobalamin) 60 mcg • Biotin 300 mcg • Pantothenic Acid (as D-Calcium Pantothenate) 90 mg • Olive Extract (Olea Europaea L., fruit) 30 mg • Bioflavonoid Complex: Rutin, Quercetin, Hesperidin (Citrus Spp. L., fruit), Green Tea Extract - Decaffeinated (Camillia Sinensis Hunt, leaves), Bilberry Extract (Vaccinium Myrtillus L., fruit) 193 mg • Inositol 150 mg • Choline Bitartrate 100 mg • N-Acetyl L-Cysteine 65 mg • Bromelain 50 mg • Alpha Lipoic Acid 15 mg • Coenzyme Q10 12 mg • Glutathione 10 mg • Curcumin Extract (Curcuma Longa L., Root) 15 mg • Lutein (Tagetes Erecta L., flower) 600 mcg • Lycopene 1 mg • Broccoli Concentrate (Brassica Oleracea V. Botrytis L.) Flower 15 mg. Other Ingredients: Microcrystalline Cellulose, Pregelatinized Starch, Croscarmellose Sodium, Ascorbyl Palmitate, Dextrin, Collodial Silicon Dioxide, Dextrose.

Essentum - Vital Living, Inc.
Two packets contain: Vitamin A (as palmitate) 2500 IU • Vitamin C (as ascorbic acid) 30 mg • Calcium (amino acid chelate, aac) 50 mg • Vitamin D (as cholecalciferol) 200 IU • Vitamin E (as d-alpha tocopherol) 20 IU • Vitamin B1 (as thiamin mononitrate) 750 mcg • Vitamin B2 (as riboflavin) 850 mcg • D-Biotin 0.15 mg • Vitamin B5 (as calcium d-pantothenate) 5 mg • Phosphorous (as di-calcium phosphate) 48 mg • Iodine (as potassium iodide) 750 mcg • Magnesium (aac) 50 mg • Zinc (aac) 7.5 mg • Selenium (aac) 35 mcg • Copper (aac) 1 mg • Manganese (aac) 1 mg • Chromium (as chromium picolinate) 0.06 mg • Molybdenum (aac) 37.5 mcg • Potassium (as potassium chloride) 80 mg • Vitamin B Homocysteine Blend: Vitamin B6 (as pyridoxine HCl) 12.5 mg, Vitamin B9 (as folic acid/folate) 400 mcg, Vitamin B12 (as cyanocobalamin) 500 mcg • Plant Sterols Proprietary Blend 900 mg • Omega 3 Fatty Acids (as ethyl esters) Proprietary Blend 550 mg • Vitamin B3 (as niacin) 250 mg.

Essiac - Dial Herbs
Burdock • Sheep Sorrel • Rhubarb • Slippery Elm.

Ester C - Derma E
Each tablet contains: Vitamin C • Vitamin E • Antioxidants and Skin Rejuvenators.

Ester C - EnerGreens, Inc.
Each capsule contains: Vitamin C (from ester C) 1000 mg • Pepsin (1:10,000) 20 mg • Betaine Hydrochloride 50 mg. Other Ingredients: Gelatin.

Ester C - Westcoast Naturals
Each vegetarian capsule contains: Vitamin C (from Ester-C brand calcium ascorbate) 600 mg • Citrus Bioflavonoids 150 mg.

Ester C 1000 mg - The Vitamin Shoppe
Each tablet contains: Vitamin C (Calcium Ascorbate) 1000 mg • Calcium (as Ascorbate, Threonate) 125 mg.

Ester C 1000 mg with Bioflavonoids - The Vitamin Shoppe
Each tablet contains: Vitamin C (Calcium Ascorbate) (from 1250 mg Ester C) 1000 mg, plus Bioflavonoids Complex.

Ester C 500 mg - The Vitamin Shoppe
Each tablet contains: Vitamin C (Calcium Ascorbate) 500 mg • Calcium (as Ascorbate, Threonate) 60 mg.

Ester C 500 mg with Bioflavonoids - The Vitamin Shoppe
Each tablet contains: Vitamin C (Calcium Ascorbate) (from 625 mg Ester C) 500 mg, plus Bioflavonoids Complex.

Ester C Caps - Progressive Labs
Each capsule contains: Vitamin C (as calcium polyascorbate) 500 mg • Calcium (as calcium polyascorbate) 50 mg.

Ester C Chewable - Natrol, Inc.
Each soft chew contains: Vitamin C (from Ester C brand calcium ascorbate, sodium ascorbate) 250 mg • Calcium (from Ester C brand calcium ascorbate) 12 mg • Sodium (from sodium ascorbate and salt) 25 mg. Other Ingredients: Sugar, Corn Syrup, Palm Kernal Oil, Mono- and Diglycerides, Natural Orange Flavor, Citric Acid, Soy Lecithin, Yellow 6.

Ester C Plus Bioflavonoids and Pycnogenol 500 mg - The Vitamin Shoppe
Each capsule contains: Vitamin C (Calcium Ascorbate) (from 625 mg Ester C) 500 mg • Calcium (Calcium Ascorbate) 60 mg • Quercetin 25 mg • Pycnogenol 2.5 mg • Citrus Bioflavonoid Complex with Hesperidin and Rutin 200 mg.

Ester C Powder 2000 mg with Bioflavonoids - The Vitamin Shoppe
Each teaspoon contains: Vitamin C (Calcium Ascorbate) 2000 mg, plus Bioflavonoids Complex.

Ester C Vitamin C 500 mg - Jamieson
Each caplet contains: Vitamin C (Ester C) 500 mg • Grape Seed 1200 mg.

Ester C with Bioflavonoids, Vitamin C - Leiner Health Products
Each tablet contains: Vitamin C 500 mg • Citrus Bioflavonoids complex 200 mg. Other Ingredients: Ester-C Calcium Ascorbate, Calcium Carbonate, Cellulose, Croscarmellose Sodium, Crospovidone, Silicon Dioxide, Maltodextrin, Polyethylene Glycol 3350, Talc, Magnesium Stearate, Hydroxypropyl Methylcellulose, Hydroxypropyl Cellulose, Polysorbate 80.

Ester-C - PhysioLogics
Each capsule contains: Vitamin C (as ester-c calcium ascorbate) 500 mg • Calcium (as ester-c calcium ascorbate) • Citrus Bioflavonoid (citrus spp.) 100 mg • Rutin fruit (dimorphandra mollis) 5 mg • Hesperidin fruit complex (as citrus aurantium, citrus spp.) 5 mg. Other Ingredients: Gelatin, Cellulose (plant origin), Silica, Vegetable Magnesium Stearate.
See Editor's Note No. 40.

Ester-C 1000 Mg with Bioflavonoids - Natrol, Inc.
Each tablet contains: Vitamin C (as calcium ascorbate) 1000 mg • Calcium (as calcium ascorbate) 100 mg • Lemon Bioflavonoid Complex consisting of extracts from lemon 200 mg. Other Ingredients: Mono & Di-Glycerides, Stearic Acid, Croscarmellose Sodium, Silicon Dioxide, Magnesium Stearate.

Ester-C 250 Mg with Bioflavonoids - Natrol, Inc.
Each tablet contains: Vitamin C (as calcium ascorbate) 250 mg • Calcium (as calcium ascorbate) 25 mg • Lemon Bioflavonoid Complex consisting of extracts from lemon 100 mg. Other Ingredients: Microcrystalline Cellulose, Stearic Acid, Croscarmellose Sodium, Silicon Dioxide, Magnesium Stearate.

Ester-C 500 Mg with Bioflavonoids - Natrol, Inc.
Each tablet contains: Vitamin C (as calcium ascorbate) 500 mg • Calcium (as calcium ascorbate) 50 mg • Lemon Bioflavonoid Complex consisting of extracts from lemon 200 mg. Other Ingredients: Mono & Di-Glycerides, Stearic Acid, Croscarmellose Sodium, Silicon Dioxide, Magnesium Stearate.

Ester-C 1000 - GNC
Each tablet contains: Vitamin C (as calcium ascorbic) 1000 mg • Calcium (as calcium ascorbic) 94 mg • Citrus Bioflavonoids Complex (from 50 mg of cirtus bioflavoniods complex 4X) 200 mg. Other Ingredients: Cellulose, Calcium Carbonate.

Ester-C 1000 - NOW Foods
Each tablet contains: Vitamin C 1000 mg • Citrus Bioflavonoids (40%) 200 mg • Acerola powder 25 mg • Rose Hips powder 25 mg • Rutin 20 mg • Calcium 125 mg.

Ester-C 1000 mg tablets - Source Naturals
Each tablet contains: Vitamin C (as calcium ascorbate [Ester-C]) 500 mg • Calcium (as bioflavonoids & calcium ascorbate [Ester-C]) 90 mg • Bioflavonoid Complex 130 mg • Rutin 36 mg • Hesperidin Complex 35 mg.

Ester-C 1000 Timed Release - GNC
Each tablet contains: Vitamin C (as calcium ascorbate) 1000 mg •Calcium (as calcium ascorbate) 94 mg •Citrus Bioflavonoids Complex (from 50 mg of citrus biofalvonoids complex 4X) 200 mg. Other Ingredients: Cellulose, Food Glaze.

Ester-C 250 Mg - Natrol, Inc.
Each tablet contains: Vitamin C (as calcium ascorbate) 250 mg • Calcium (as calcium ascorbate) 25 mg. Other Ingredients: Microcrystalline Cellulose, Stearic Acid, Mono & Di-Glycerides, Croscarmellose Sodium, Magnesium Stearate.

Ester-C 250 Mg Chewable - Natrol, Inc.
Each wafer contains: Vitamin C (as calcium ascorbate) 250 mg • Calcium (as calcium ascorbate) 25 mg. Other Ingredients: Fructose, Glycine, Mono & Di-Glycerides, Stearic Acid, natural Orange flavor, Citric Acid, Silicon Dioxide, Microcrystalline Cellulose, Gum Acacia, Magnesium Stearate.

Ester-C 500 Mg capsules - Natrol, Inc.
Each capsule contains: Vitamin C (as calcium ascorbate) 500 mg • Calcium (as calcium ascorbate) 50 mg. Other Ingredients: Magnesium Stearate, Microcrystalline Cellulose, Gelatin.

Ester-C 500 Mg tablets - Natrol, Inc.
Each tablet contains: Vitamin C (as calcium ascorbate) 500 mg • Calcium (as calcium ascorbate) 50 mg. Other Ingredients: Microcrystalline Cellulose, Stearic Acid, Croscarmellose Sodium, Magnesium Stearate, Silicon Dioxide.

Ester-C 500 mg tablets - Puritan's Pride
Each tablet contains: Vitamin C (as Ester-C calcium ascorbate) 500 mg • Calcium (as Ester-C calcium ascorbate) 55 mg • Citrus Bioflavonoid fruit complex (citrus spp.) 200 mg • Rutin fruit (dimorphandra mollis) 10 mg • Hesperidin fruit complex (citrus spp.) 10 mg. Other Ingredients: Cellulose (plant origin), Vegetable Stearic Acid, Croscarmellose, Silica, Cellulose Coating, Vegetable Magnesium Stearate.

Ester-C 500 mg With Bioflavonoids - Nature's Valley
Each tablet contains: Vitamin C (as Ester-C brand calcium ascorbate) 500 mg • Citrus Bioflavonoid Complex 200 mg. Other Ingredients: Calcium Carbonate, Cellulose, Croscarmellose Sodium, Crospovidone, Silicon Dioxide, Maltodextrin, Polyethylene Glycol 3350, Talc, Magnesium Stearate, Hydroxypropyl Methylcellulose, Hydroxpropyl Cellulose, Polysorbate 80.
See Editor's Note No. 45.

Ester-C 500 mg With Bioflavonoids capsules - Puritan's Pride
Each capsule contains: Vitamin C (as Ester-C calcium ascorbate) 500 mg • Calcium (as Ester-C calcium ascorbate) 55 mg • Citrus Bioflavonoid fruit (citrus sinensis) 100 mg • Rutin fruit (dimorphandra mollis) 5 mg • Hesperidin fruit complex (citrus spp.) 5 mg. Other Ingredients: Gelatin, Cellulose (plant origin), Silica, Vegetable Magnesium Stearate.

Ester-C 500 Mg with Bioflavonoids Vegetarian capsules - Natrol, Inc.
Each capsule contains: Vitamin C (as calcium ascorbate) 500 mg • Calcium (as calcium ascorbate) 50 mg • Citrus Bioflavonoid Complex consisting of extracts from: lemon, orange, grapefruit, lime, & tangerine 200 mg. Other Ingredients: Magnesium Stearate, Silicon Dioxide, Vegetable Carbohydrate Gum, Glycerine.

Ester-C 500 Mg with Echinacea - Natrol, Inc.
Each tablet contains: Vitamin C (as calcium ascorbate) 500 mg • Calcium (as calcium ascorbate) 50 mg • Echinacea extract (Phenolic compounds 4%) 50 mg • Echinacea (angustifolia) leaf powder 80 mg • Echinacea (Purpurea) leaf powder 80 mg • Echinacea (angustifolia) root powder 20 mg • Echinacea (Purpurea) root powder 20 mg. Other Ingredients: Calcium Carbonate, Mono & Di-Glycerides, Croscarmellose Sodium, Stearic Acid, Silicon Dioxide, Magnesium Stearate.

Ester-C 500 Mg with Pycnogenol & Proanthocyanidins capsules **- Natrol, Inc.**
Each capsule contains: Vitamin C (as calcium ascorbate) 500 mg • Calcium (as calcium ascorbate) 50 mg • Grape skin powder 50 mg • Rutin 50 mg • Hesperidin Complex 50 mg • Quercetin 25 mg • Pycnogenol (pine bark extract) 5 mg. Other Ingredients: Silicon Dioxide, Magnesium Stearate, Gelatin.

Ester-C 500 Mg with Pycnogenol & Proanthocyanidins tablets **- Natrol, Inc.**
Each tablet contains: Vitamin C (as calcium ascorbate) 500 mg • Calcium (as calcium ascorbate-carbonate) 70 mg • Grape skin powder 50 mg • Rutin 50 mg • Hesperidin 50 mg • Quercetin 25 mg • Pycnogenol (pine bark extract) 5 mg. Other Ingredients: Mono & Di-Glycerides, Calcium Carbonate, Croscarmellose Sodium, Silicon Dioxide, Stearic Acid & Magnesium Stearate.

Ester-C 500 with Citrus Bioflavonoids **- GNC**
Each tablet contains: Vitamin C (as calcium ascorbate) 500 mg •Calcium (as calcium ascorbate and dicalcium phosphate) 110 mg •Citrus Bioflavonoids Complex (from 50 mg of Citrus Bioflavonoids Complex 4X) 200 mg. Other Ingredients: Cellulose Calcium Carbonate.

Ester-C 500mg **- Nature's Bounty**
Each tablet contains: Vitamin C (as Ester-C calcium ascorbate) 500 mg • Calcium (as Ester-C calcium ascorbate) 55 mg • Citrus Bioflavonoid fruit complex (citrus spp.) 200 mg • Rutin fruit (dimorphandra mollis) 10 mg • Hesperidin fruit complex (citrus spp.) 10 mg. Other Ingredients: Cellulose (plant origin), Vegetable Stearic Acid, Croscarmellose, Silica, Cellulose Coating, Vegetable Magnesium Stearate.

Ester-C Antioxidant **- Natrol, Inc.**
Two tablets contain: Vitamin A (as d-Salina beta carotene) 5000 IU • Vitamin C (as calcium ascorbate) 500 mg • Vitamin E (as d-alpha tocopheryl succinate with mixed tocopherols) 200 IU • Calcium (as ascorbate) 50 mg • Lemon Bioflavonoid Complex consisting of extracts from lemon 25 mg • a-Lipoic Acid 25 mg. Other Ingredients: TriCalcium Phosphate, Microcrystalline Cellulose, Stearic Acid, Silicon Dioxide, Croscarmellose Sodium, Magnesium Stearate.

Ester-C brand **- Zila Nutraceuticals**
Vitamin C.
See Editor's Note No. 44.

Ester-C Cold Season **- Natrol, Inc.**
Two capsules contain: Vitamin C (as calcium ascorbate) 500 mg • Calcium (as calcium ascorbate) 50 mg • Zinc (chelate) 10 mg • Reishi/Shiitake/ Maitake Blend, powdered extract (mushrooms) 150 mg • Echinacea 50:50 (purpurea & angustifolia), powdered extract supplying Phenolic compounds (4%) 75 mg • Citrus Bioflavonoid Complex extracts of: lemon, orange, grapefruit, lime & tangerine 50 mg • Black Elderberry extract, powdered 30 mg • Garlic, powdered extract bulb 30 mg • Licorice root extract supplying 25 % Glycerenic Acid 25 mg • Astragalus 25 mg • Cayenne supplying 40000 SCU 10 mg • Beta Glucans, oats 5 mg. Other Ingredients: Silica, Magnesium Stearate, Rice powder, Gelatin.

Ester-C Complex **- Olympian Labs**
Each capsule contains: Vitamin C (Ester C) 500 mg • Citrus Bioflavonoid Complex 200 mg.

Ester-C Complex 1370 mg **- Pro Health**
Each tablet contains: Vitamin C (from Ester-C brand calcium ascorbate) 1000 mg • Calcium (from Ester-C brand calcium ascorbate) 125 mg • Citrus Bioflavonoid Complex 200 mg • Acerola extract 25 mg • Rose Hip seed powder (rosae pseudofructus) 25 mg • Rutin 25 mg. Other Ingredients: Stearic Acid, Microcrystalline Cellulose, Magnesium Stearate, Croscarmellose Sodium, Pharmaceutical Glaze.

Ester-C Complex Extra Strength **- Olympian Labs**
Each tablet contains: Ester C (Vitamin C) 1000 mg • Calcium (from Ester-C) 80 mg • Citrus Bioflavonoid Complex 50 mg • Grape Skin extract 50 mg • Rose Hips 50 mg.

Ester-C Complex Plus Calcium **- Olympian Labs**
Each capsule contains: Ester C (Vitamin C) 500 mg • Calcium (from Ester-C) 40 mg • Citrus Bioflavonoid Complex 200 mg.

Ester-C For Kids **- Natrol, Inc.**
Each wafer contains: Vitamin C (as calcium ascorbate) 100 mg • Calcium (as calcium ascorbate) 10 mg • Citrus Bioflavonoids consisting of extracts from lemon 25 mg. Other Ingredients: Fructose, Mono & Di-Glycerides, Glycine, Cellulose, natural Tropical fruit flavor, Stearic Acid, Silica, Magnesium Stearate, Guar Gum, Citric Acid.

Ester-C Nightime Formula **- Natrol, Inc.**
Each tablet contains: Vitamin C (as calcium ascrobate) 500 mg • Calcium (as calcium ascorbate) 50 mg • Kava Kava root supplying 30% Kavalactones 100 mg • Valerian root supplying 0.8% Valerenic Acid 100 mg • Melatonin 1 mg. Other Ingredients: TriCalcium Phosphate, Cellulose, Stearic Acid, Silica, Magnesium Stearate.
See Editor's Note No. 26.

Ester-C Powder **- Natrol, Inc.**
Each teaspoon contains: Vitamin C (as calcium ascorbate) 3200 mg • Calcium (as calcium ascorbate) 320 mg.

Ester-C Powder with Bioflavonoids **- Natrol, Inc.**
Each teaspoon contains: Vitamin C (as calcium ascorbate) 3000 mg • Calcium (as calcium ascorbate) 300 mg • Citrus Bioflavonoid Complex consisting of extracts from: lemon, orange, grapefruit, lime, & tangerine 300 mg.

Ester-C with Bioflavonoids **- Natrol, Inc.**
Each capsule contains: Vitamin C (as calcium ascorbate) 500 mg • Calcium (as calcium ascorbate) 50 mg • Citrus Bioflavonoid Complex consisting of extracts from: lemon, orange, grapefruit, lime & tangerine 200 mg. Other Ingredients: Magnesium Stearate, Gelatin.

Ester-C with Bioflavonoids 500 mg Vitamin C **- Longs**
Each tablet contains: Vitamin C (Ester-C brand calcium ascorbate) 500 mg • Citrus Bioflavonoids complex (standardized to 25% total bioflavonoids) 20 mg. Other Ingredients: Cellulose, Stearic Acid, Croscarmellose Sodium, Crospovidone, Calcium Carbonate, Magnesium Stearate, Dextrin, Silicon Dioxide, Dextrose, Lecithin, Acacia, Sodium Carboxymethylcellulose, Sodium Citrate.

Ester-C with Echinacea **- Natrol, Inc.**
Each capsule contains: Vitamin C (as calcium ascorbate) 500 mg • Calcium (as calcium ascorbate) 50 mg Echinacea extract (Phenolic compounds 4%) 50 mg • Echinacea (angustifolia) leaf powder 80 mg • Echinacea (Purpurea) leaf powder 80 mg • Echinacea (angustifolia) root powder 20 mg • Echinacea (Purpurea) root powder 20 mg. Other Ingredients: Silicon Dioxide, Magnesium Stearate, Gelatin.

Ester-C with Echinacea & Goldenseal Root **- Puritan's Pride**
Each capsule contains: Ester C (Polysascorbate) 500 mg • Echinacea (Eachinacea angustifolia) 100 mg • Goldenseal root (Hydrastis canadensis) 50 mg.

Ester-C Zinc Lozenges **- Natrol, Inc.**
Each lozenge contains: Vitamin C (as calcium ascorbate) 150 mg • Calcium (as calcium ascorbate) 15 mg • Citrus Bioflavonoids consisting of extracts from lemon 25 mg • Zinc (Gluconate) 4.5 mg. Other Ingredients: Fructose, Mono & Di-Glycerides, Glycine, Cellulose, Natural Fruit Flavors, Stearic Acid, Silica, Magnesium Stearate, Guar Gum, Citric Acid.

Ester-E brand **- Zila Nutraceuticals**
Vitamin E.
See Editor's Note No. 44.

Some Brand Name Natural Products - What they Contain

www.NaturalDatabase.com contains MANY more listings than appear here.
Editor's Notes are located on pages 2155-2163.

EstrAttune **-** Health Smart Vitamins
Each capsule contains: Vitamin E (as d-alpha tocopheryl acetate) 50 IU • Vitamin B6 (as pyridoxine HCl) 25 mg • Folate (folic acid) 200 mcg • Magnesium (as magnesium oxide) 100 mg • Zinc (as zinc amino acid chelate) 3.75 mg • Copper (as copper amino acid chelate) 0.5 mg • Black Cohosh root 100 mg • Chastetree berry (5% flavonoids) 100 mg • Dong Quai root (>= 0.8% ligustilides, >= 0.8 mg) 100 mg • Soy bean (5% isoflavones, 2.5 mg) 50 mg • Kava Kava root (30% kavalactones, 7.5 mg) 25 mg.

Estrin D **-** Klein-Becker
Two capsules contain: Vitamin B6 25 mg • Magnesium (as oxide) 100 mg • Estrin D Proprietary Blend 1323 mg: Yerba Mate leaf SE (standardized extract), Caffeine, Guarana seed SE, Damiana leaf/stem SE, Green Tea leaf SE, Ginger root, Kola nut SE, DHEA, Schisandra fruit, Scutellaria root SE, Tibetan Ginseng root SE, Cocoa nut SE, Jujube fruit, Thea Sinensis leaf complex SE.

Estrium (formerly EstroBalance) **-** Metagenics
Two scoops (45 g) contain: Vitamin A (as retinyl palmitate) 1250 IU • Vitamin A (as mixed carotenoids) 2500 IU • Vitamin C (as Ultra Potent-C brand) 60 mg • Vitamin D (as cholecalciferol) 200 IU • Vitamin E (as D-alpha tocopheryl succinate) 300 IU • Vitamin K 40 mcg • Thiamin (as thiamin hydrochloride) 0.75 mg • Riboflavin 0.85 mg • Niacin (as niacinamide) 10 mg • Vitamin B6 (as pyridoxine hydrochloride) 50 mg • Folate (as folic acid) 500 mcg • Vitamin B12 (as cyanocobalamin, methylcobalamin) 30 mcg • Biotin 150 mcg • Pantothenic Acid (as D-calcium pantothenate) 5 mg • Calcium (as calcium citrate) 350 mg • Iron (as ferrochel amino acid chelate) 9 mg • Phosphorus 260 mg • Iodine (as potassium iodide) 75 mcg • Magnesium (as magnesium bis-glycinate, citrate) 240 mg • Zinc (as zinc citrate) 7.5 mg • Selenium (as amino acid complex) 35 mcg • Copper (as copper citrate) 1 mg • Manganese 1 mg • Chromium (as chromium polynicotinate) 100 mcg • Molybdenum (as amino acid chelate) 37.5 mcg • Potassium (as potassium phosphate) 350 mg • L-Lysine 17.5 mg • L-Threonine 17.5 mg • Isoflavones (from kudzu) 25 mg • Defatted Flaxseed meal 1 g • Choline (as choline bitartrate) 250 mg • Turmeric rhizome extract (curcuma longa, standardized to 95% [200 mg] curcuminoids) 210 mg • Trimethylglycine 200 mg • N-Acetylcysteine 100 mg. Other Ingredients: Rice Protein Concentrate, Rice Syrup Solids, Fructose, Olive Oil, Natural Flavors, Xanthan, Carrageenan, Cellulose Gum, Pueraria Root Extract, Xylitol.

Estro 2 OZ **-** Young Living Essential Oils
Black Cohosh Extract • Blue Cohosh Extract • Royal Jelly • Fennel Oil (Foeniculum Vulgare) • Lavender Oil (Lavandula Angustifolia • Clary Sage Oil (Salvia Sclarea).

Estro Balance **-** Puritan's Pride
Each tablet contains: Vitamin E 30 IU • Thiamin (Vitamin B1) 2 mg • Riboflavin (Vitamin B2) 2 mg • Niacin 20 mg • Vitamin B6 10 mg • Calcium 150 mg • Selenium 150 mg • Boron 1.5 mg • Soy Isoflavones 50 mg • Kava Kava root extract (30% kavalactones) 100 mg • Black Cohosh root (cimicifuga racemosa) 40 mg.

Estro Suppress **-** SciFit
Each capsule contains: 5,7-Chrysin (dihydroxy-flavone) 200 mg • 3,6,17-Androstenetrione 100 mg. Other Ingredients: Magnesium Stearate, Gelatin.

EstroCare **-** Xymogen
Deionized Water • Aloe Vera gel • Caprylic/Capri Triglycerides • Shea Butter • Sunflower seed oil • Stearic Acid • Glyceryl Stearate • PEG-100-Stearate • Beeswax • Isopropyl Palmitate • Y-Oryzanol • MSM • Red Clover tops extract • Chasteberry extract • Borage oil • Black Cohosh extract • Dong Quai root extract • Fo-ti Tieng root extract • Saw Palmetto extract • Damiana extract • Vanilla Planifolia fruit extract • Lavender extract • Tocotrienols • Lecithin • Vegetable Glycerin • Stearyl Alcohol or Cetyl Alcohol • Flavonoids (extracts of artichoke and sarsaparilla) • Carbomer • Triethanolamine • Xanthan Gum • Hydroxypropylmethylcellulose • Allantoin • Disodium EDTA • Potassium Sorbate • Grape seed extract.

EstroFactors **-** Metagenics
Three tablets contain: Vitamin A (50% as Betatene mixed carotenoids and 50% retinyl palmitate) 2500 IU • Vitamin D (as cholecalciferol) 200 IU • Vitamin E (as d-alpha tocopheryl acetate) 200 IU • Vitamin K 40 mcg • Vitamin B6 (pyridoxine HCl) 50 mg • Folate [Metafolin (as l-5-methyl tetrahydrofolate), folic acid, and 5-formyl tetrahydrofolate] 800 mcg • Vitamin B12 (as methylcobalamin and cyanocobalamin) 30 mg • Proprietary Blend of Isoflavones 100 mg: Red Clover flowering top extract (Trifolium pratense), Kudzu root extract (Pueraria lobata) • Turmeric rhizome extract (Curcuma longa, standardized to 95% curcuminoids) 210 mg • Rosemary leaf extract (Rosmarinus officinalis, contains 5.1%-7.6% carnosic acid/carnosol) 200 mg • Resveratrol (from Polygonum cuspudatum root extract) 2 mg • Trimethylglycine 200 mg • Chrysin 90 mg.

Estrogen Balance IF **-** Vital Nutrients
Two capsules contain: Indole 3 Carbinol 150 mg • Flax Lignan powder (20% secoisolariciresinol diglycoside flax lignan) 150 mg • Curcumin 90% extract 100 mg • Trimethylglycine 100 mg • Green Tea extract (80% catechins) 50 mg • Rosemary extract 50 mg • Red Clover Isoflavones 25 mg • Piper Nigrum (95% piperine) 2.5 mg • 5 Methyl Tetrahydro Folate (activated folic acid) 100 mcg • Folic Acid 300 mcg.

EstroGentle **-** Bodyonics, Ltd.
Black Cohosh • Soy germ • Red Clover leaf extract • Licorice root • Wild Yam • Chaste Tree berry • Other botanicals.

Estrolean Fat Burner Supreme **-** Bodyonics, Ltd.
Two capsules contain: Apple Extract (standardized for 5% phloridzin) 100 mg • Pomegranate Extract (standardized for 2% estrone) 100 mg • Sea Vegetable Extract (standardized for 5% phloroglucinols and 150 mcg iodine) 150 mg • Plant Based Enzymes: Lipase 1000 FIP, Protease 50,000 HUT, Amylase 5000 SKB • Herbal Metabogenics 300 mg: Guarana Extract, Green Tea Extract, Yerba Mate Extract (standardized for 66.6 mg caffeine) • Proprietary Blend 100 mg: Ginger Root Extract (zingiber officinale), Black Pepper Extract (piper nigrum), Licorice (glycyrrhiza glabra) • Citrus Aurantium (bitter orange; standardized for 4% synephrine) 66.6 mg • Rhodiola Rosea Extract (standardized for 3% rosavins) 50 mg • Rhododendron Caucasicum Extract (standardized for 3% taxifolian) 50 mg • Herbal Modulators 200 mg: Chromium Polynicotinate, L-Carnitine Tartrate, Garcinia Cambogia Extract, Grapefruit Extract, Cinnamon Twig Bar, Dong Quai Extract, Barberry Extract, Chaste Berry Extract. Other Ingredients: Cellulose, Talc, Magnesium Stearate, Gelatin.
See Editor's Note No. 40.

EstroSense **-** Preferred Nutrition
Two capsules contain: Calcium D-Glucarate 150 mg • Indole-3-Carbinol 150 mg • Green Tea extract (caffeine free, 60% polyphenols) 100 mg • Turmeric (95% curcumin) 50 mg • Milk Thistle extract (standardized to 80% silymarin) 50 mg • Rosemary extract (6% carnosic acid) 25 mg • Lycopene 5% (Lyc-O-Mato brand) 5 mg • Sulphoraphane (broccoli sprout extract) 200 mcg.

EstroSoy **-** Nature's Way
Two capsules contain: Fermented Soy extract 890 mg • Red Clover blossoms 100 mg.

EstroSoy Plus **-** Nature's Way
Two capsules contain: Black Cohosh dried extract 40 mg • Fermented Soy extract 890 mg • Red Clover Blossoms 100 mg.

Estrotone **-** New Chapter, Inc.
Two softgels contain: Dong Quai (Angelica sinensis) root, extract (1% lingustilide- .80 mg) 80 mg • Schizandra (wu-wei-zi) berry extract (2% schizandrins- 1.6 mg) 80 mg • Ginger rhizome, certified organic, extract (minimum 20% pungent compounds- 10 mg, 5% ziniberene- 2.5 mg) 50 mg • Black Cohosh root and rhizome, extract (8% triterpene glycoside- 3.2 mg) 40 mg • Chaste Tree berry, extract (0.6% aucubin- 2.4mg, % 0.5 agnuside- 20 mg) 40 mg • Rosemary leaf and essential oil, extract (23% total phenolic anitoxidants- 2.3 mg) 10 mg. Other Ingredients: Evening primrose oil, Olive Oil, Yellow Beeswax, Gelatin, Vegetable glycerin, Purified Water, Carob.

Estroven Calci-Fresh Calcium Gum - Amerifit Nutrition
Two pieces contain: Vitamin C (as sodium ascorbate) 30 mg • Vitamin D (as cholecalciferol) 200 IU • Vitamin K (as phytonadione) 40 mcg • Calcium (as calcium carbonate and citrate) 333 mg. Other Ingredients: Sorbitol, Gum Base, Xylitol, Malitol Syrup, Natural and Artificial Flavors, Sucralose, Carnauba Wax, Resinous Glaze, FD&C Blue #1, Yellow #5.

Estroven Calcium Advantage - Amerifit Nutrition
Each caplet contains: Vitamin D (as cholecalciferol) 200 IU • Vitamin K (as phytonadione) 25 mcg • Calcium (as calcium carbonate) 600 mg • Magnesium (as magnesium oxide) 40 mg • Citrus Bioflavonoid Complex 25 mg • Isoflavones (from GMO-free soybeans and pueraria lobata root extract) 25 mg. Other Ingredients: Microcrystalline Cellulose, Croscarmellose Sodium, Vegetable Stearic Acid, Silica, Vegetable Magnesium Stearate, Citrus Oil, Titanium Dioxide, Natural Coating.

Estroven caplets/gelcaps - Amerifit Nutrition
Each gelcap/caplet contains: Vitamin E (as natural D-alpha tocopherol succinate) 30 IU • Thiamin (as thiamin mononitrate) 2 mg • Riboflavin 2 mg • Niacin (niacinamide) 20 mg • Vitamin B6 (as pyridoxine HCl) 10 mg • Vitamin B12 (as cyanocobalamin) 6 mcg • Folate (as folic acid) 400 mcg • Calcium (from calcium carbonate) 150 mg • Selenium (from L-selenomethionine) 70 mcg • Boron (chelate) 1.5 mg • Purified Isoflavones from Soybean & Other Plants 55 mg • Estroven Calming Herbal Blend 150 mg: Date seed extract (zizyphus spinosa), Magnolia bark extract • Black Cohosh root 40 mg. Other Ingredients: Pueraria Lobata Root Extract, Cellulose, Croscarmellose Sodium, Silica, Vegetable Magnesium Stearate, Titanium Dioxide (natural mineral source), Vanilla, Caramel Color.

Estroven Extra Strength - Amerifit Nutrition
Two caplets contain: Vitamin E (as natural D-alpha tocopherol succinate) 30 IU • Thiamin (as thiamin mononitrate) 5 mg • Riboflavin 5 mg • Niacin (as niacinamide) 20 mg • Vitamin B6 (as pyridoxine HCl) 25 mg • Folate (as folic acid) 400 mcg • Vitamin B12 (as cyanocobalamin) 25 mcg • Calcium 200 mg • Selenium (as L-selenomethionine) 70 mcg • Chromium (as chromium dinicotinate glycinate) 120 mcg • Cranberry juice (from 12:1 extract) 300 mg • Estroven Balancing Herbal Blend 200 mg: Green Tea extract, Date seed extract, Cinnamon twig extract, Galangal root extract, Magnolia bark extract • Isoflavones (from GMO-free soybeans and pueraria lobata root extract, with Isolase enzymes) 80 mg • Black Cohosh root standardized extract 40 mg • Boron (as boron chelate) 1.5 mg. Other Ingredients: Microcrystalline Cellulose, Croscarmellose Sodium, Vegetable Stearic Acid, Vegetable Magnesium Stearate, Silica, Cellulose, Titanium Dioxide, Sodium Citrate.

Estroven Feminine Moisturizer & Lubricant - Amerifit Nutrition
Purified Water • Glycerin • Polysorbate 60 • Sorbitol • Soy extract • Hydroxyethylcellulose • Aloe Barbadensis leaf juice • Vitamin E (as tocopheryl acetate) • Methylparaben • Propylparaben.

Estroven Healthy Heart - Amerifit Nutrition
Each caplet contains: Vitamin E (as natural D-alpha tocopheryl succinate) 200 IU • Vitamin B6 (as pyridoxine HCl) 10 mg • Folate (as folic acid) 400 mcg • Vitamin B12 (as cyanocobalamin) 25 mcg • Niacin (as flush-free inositol hexanicotinate) 100 mg • Selenium (as L-selenomethionine) 70 mcg • Coenzyme Q10 30 mg • Policosanol 10 mg • Proprietary Blend 125 mg: Green Tea leaf standardized extract, Red Wine Grape extract (resveratrol 2 mg), Garlic bulb, Blueberry fruit extract, Hawthorn berry extract • Isoflavones (from pueraria lobata root and GMO-free soy) 10 mg. Other Ingredients: Dicalcium Phosphate, Microcrystalline Cellulose, Croscarmellose Sodium, Vegetable Stearic Acid, Vegetable Magnesium Stearate, Silica, Vegetable Coating.

Estroven Joint & Bone - Amerifit Nutrition
Four caplets contain: Vitamin C (as ascorbic acid) 100 mg • Vitamin D (as cholecalciferol) 400 IU • Vitamin K (as phytonadione) 80 mcg • Folate (as folic acid) 400 mcg • Calcium (as calcium carbonate) 600 mg • Glucosamine HCl 1500 mg • Chondroitin Sulfate 1200 mg • Isoflavones (from pueraria lobata root and non-GMO soybeans) 25 mg. Other Ingredients: Microcrystalline Cellulose, Vegetable Stearic Acid, Silica, Vegetable Coating.
See Editor's Note No. 48.

Estroven Memory - Amerifit Nutrition
Each tablet contains: Zinc 7.5 mg • Ginkgo Biloba leaf standardized extract 60 mg • Panax Ginseng root standardized extract 125 mg • Green Tea leaf standardized extract 250 mg • Isoflavones 10 mg • Grape skin standardized extract 75 mg.
See Editor's Note No. 21.

Estroven Multi-Vitamin - Amerifit Nutrition
Two caplets contain: Vitamin A (100% as beta-carotene with natural mixed carotenoids) 5000 IU • Vitamin C (as non-acidic Ester-C brand) 150 mg • Vitamin D (as cholecalciferol) 400 IU • Vitamin E (as natural D-alpha tocopheryl succinate with tocotretinols) 100 IU • Vitamin B1 (as thiamin hydrochloride) 10 mg • Vitamin B2 (riboflavin) 10 mg • Niacin (as flush-free inositol hexaniacinate) 50 mg • Vitamin B6 (as pyridoxine hydrochloride) 10 mg • Folate (as folic acid) 400 mcg • Vitamin B12 (as cyanocobalamin) 25 mcg • Biotin 300 mcg • Pantothenic Acid (as D-calcium pantothenate) 20 mg • Calcium (as calcium carbonate and Citrimal brand calcium citrate malate glycinate) 200 mg • Iron (as carbonyl iron) 8 mg • Iodine (as potassium iodide) 150 mcg • Magnesium (as magnesium oxide and magnesium chelate) 100 mg • Zinc (as zinc citrate) 15 mg • Selenium (as amino acid chelate) 200 mcg • Copper (as copper bisglycinate chelate) 2 mg • Manganese (as manganese citrate chelate) 5 mg • Chromium (as Chelavite brand chromium dinicotinate glycinate) 200 mcg • Molybdenum (as molybdenum amino acid chelate) 75 mcg • Panax Ginseng root standardized extract 100 mg • Purified Isoflavones (from pueraria lobata root extract and GMO-free soybeans) 15 mg • Cranberry juice 12:1 extract 300 mg • Lutein 1000 mcg • Boron (as boron chelate) 0.5 mg. Other Ingredients: Dicalcium Phosphate, Microcrystalline Cellulose, Croscarmellose Sodium, Vegetable Stearic Acid, Vegetale Magnesium Stearate, Silica.

Estroven PMS - Amerifit Nutrition
Two tablets contain: Thiamin (as thiamin mononitrate) 1.5 mg • Riboflavin 1.7 mg • Niacin (as niacinamide) 20 mg • Vitamin B6 (as pyridoxine HCl) 25 mg • Folate (as folic acid) 200 mcg • Vitamin B12 (as cyanocobalamin) 6 mcg • Pantothenic Acid (as D-calcium pantothenate) 10 mg • Calcium (as calcium carbonate) 200 mg • Magnesium (as magnesium oxide) 50 mg • Anti-bloating Herbal Diuretic Blend 300 mg: Couch Grass plant (agropyron repens), Buchu leaf (agathosma betulina), Arctostaphylos Uva Ursi leaf, Juniper berry (juniperus communis), Hydrangea Arborescens root, Cornsilk stylus (zea mays) • Feverfew standardized extract (aerial parts, tanacetum parthenium) 125 mg • Estroven Calming Herbal Blend 200 mg: Date seed extract (zizyphus spinosa), Magnolia bark extract • Chaste Berry standardized extract (vitex agnus castus) 60 mg • Ginger root (zingiber officinalis) 50 mg • Cramp bark (viburnum opulus) 20 mg • Isoflavones (from pureria lobata root and non-GMO soybeans) 10 mg. Other Ingredients: Cellulose, Cellulose Gum, Fractionated Vegetable Oil, Silica, Natural Glaze, Titanium Dioxide, Vanilla.

E-TOCO 400 - Progressive Labs
Each softgel contains: Vitamin E (mixed tocopherols) 400 IU • Sesame seed oil 200 mg • Nutriene 100 mg.

Eucalyptus Salve - Dial Herbs
Eucalyptus • Camphor • Mint. In a base of Beeswax, Glycerine & Cold Pressed Olive Oil.

Euphorbium Sinus Relief - Heel/BHI, Inc.
Each 100 mL serving contains: Pulsatilla 2X • Luffa Operculata 2X • Euphorbium Officinarum 4X • Mercurius Iodatus Ruber 8X • Mucosa Nasalis Suis 8X • Argentum Nitricum 10X • Hepar Sulphuris Calcareum 10X • Sinusitisinum 13X. Other Ingredients: Benzalkonium Chloride 0.01%.
See Editor's Note No. 1.

European Grape Seed Extract 50 mg - Jamieson
Each caplet contains: Calcium 30 mg • Grape Seed 60:1 extract (Vitis vinifera) (Standardized to 95% Oligomeric Procyanidins) 50 mg.

Evecare Capsules - The Himalaya Drug Company
Each capsule contains: Ashoka (saraca indica syn. s.asoca) 85 mg • Dashamoola 35 mg: Aegle Marmelos root, Gmelina Arborea root, Oroxylum Indicum root, Clerodendrum Phlomidis root, Stereospermum Chelonoides root, Desmodium Gangeticum root, Uraria Picta root, Solanum Indicum root, Solanum Surattense root, Tribulus Terrestris root • Lodhra (symplocos racemosa) 35 mg • Guduchi (tinospora cordifolia) 35 mg • Kakamachi (solanum nigrum) 35 mg • Punarnava (boerhaavia diffusa) 35 mg • Shatavari (asparagus racemosus) 35 mg • Kumari (aloe vera) 25 mg • Chandana (santalum album) 25 mg • Musta (cyperus rotundus) 25 mg • Vasaka (adhatoda vasica syn. a.zeylanica) 20 mg • Triphala 20 mg: Emblica Officinalis, Terminalia Chebula, Terminalia Bellirica • Trikatu 20 mg: Piper Nigrum, Piper Longum, Zingiber Officinale • Shalmali (bombax malabaricum syn. b.ceiba) 15 mg • Kasisa Godanti Bhasma (ferrous sulphate, gypsum calx) 35 mg • Yashada Bhasma (zinc calx) 35 mg.

Evecare Syrup - The Himalaya Drug Company
Each 1 tsp (5 mL) serving contains: Gandapushpa (saraca indica syn. s.asoca) 50 mg • Dashamoola 33 mg: Aegle Marmelos root, Gmelina Arborea root, Oroxylum Indicum root, Clerodendrum Phlomidis root, Stereospermum Chelonoides root, Desmodium Gangeticum root, Uraria Picta root, Solanum Indicum root, Solanum Surattense root, Tribulus Terrestris root • Lodhra (symplocos racemosa) 33 mg • Guduchi (tinospora cordifolia) 33 mg • Kakamachi (solanum nigrum) 33 mg • Punarnava (boerhaavia diffusa) 32 mg • Shatavari (asparagus racemosus) 32 mg • Narikela (cocos nucifera) 32 mg • Kumari (aloe barbadensis) 25 mg • Chandana (santalum album) 25 mg • Vabbula (acacia arabica syn. a.nilotica) 25 mg • Musta (cyperus rotundus) 25 mg • Anantamul (hemidesmus indicus) 25 mg • Triphala 20 mg: Emblica Officinalis, Terminalia Chebula, Terminalia Bellirica • Vasaka (adhatoda vasica syn. a.zeylanica) 20 mg • Manjishtha (rubia cordifolia) 20 mg • Trikatu 20 mg: Piper Nigrum, Piper Longum, Zingiber Officinalis • Shalmali (bombax malabaricum syn. b.ceiba) 12 mg • Shilajeet (mineral pitch, purified) 5 mg.

Evening Primrose 1300 - Jarrow Formulas
Each softgel contains: Oil of Evening Primrose 1300 mg: GLA (gammalinolenic acid) 117 mg. Other Ingredients: Gelatin, Glycerine, Water.

Evening Primrose Deluxe - Health From The Sun
Each capsule contains: Gamma Linolenic Acid (GLA) (Omega-6) 130 mg • Linoleic Acid (Omega-6) 950 mg • Oleic Acid (Omega-9) 80 mg. Other Ingredients: Evening Primrose seed oil, Gelatin, Glycerine, Water.

Evening Primrose Oil - PhysioLogics
Each softgel contains: Evening Primrose Oil 500 mg • Cis-Linoleic Acid (LA) 365 mg • Gamma-Linolenic Acid (GLA) 45 mg. Other Ingredients: Gelatin, Glycerin.

Evening Primrose Oil - Ortho Molecular Products
Each soft gel contains: Evening Primrose seed oil Providine 117 mg Gamma-Linolenic Acid 1300 mg. Other Ingredients: Gelatin, Glycerin, Water.

Evening Primrose Oil - Olympian Labs
Each softgel contains: Evening Primrose Oil 500 mg.

Evening Primrose Oil - Health From The Sun
Two capsules contain: Gamma-Linolenic Acid (GLA) (Omega-6) 100 mg • Linoleic Acid (Omega-6) 730 mg • Oleic Acid (Omega-9) 60 mg. Other Ingredients: Evening Primrose seed oil, Gelatin, Glycerine, Water.

Evening Primrose Oil - Trophic
Each softgel contains: Evening Primrose oil 500 mg • Vitamin E Acetate (as D-alpha tocopherol) 15 IU.

Evening Primrose Oil - Leiner Health Products
Each softgel contains: Evening Primrose Oil (Oenothera biennis) seed 500 mg. Other Ingredients: Gelatin, Glycerin, Purified Water.

Evening Primrose Oil - Pro Health
Three softgels contain: Evening Primrose Oil 1.5 g • Gamma Linolenic Acid (gla) 135 mg • Cis-Linoleic Acid (omega-6) 1.08 g • Cis-Oleic Acid (omega-9) 120 mg. Other Ingredients: Gelatin, Glycerin, Water.

Evening Primrose Oil - Jamieson
Each capsule contains: Vitamin E (as D-Alpha Tocopheryl Acetate) 13.6 IU • Gamma Linolenic Acid (GLA) 50 mg.

Evening Primrose Oil - Optimum Nutrition
Each softgel contains: Evening Primrose Oil 500 mg • Cis-Linoleic Acid 350 mg • Gamma-Linolenic Acid (GLA) 45 mg. Other Ingredients: Gelatin, Glycerin.

Evening Primrose Oil 1.3g softgel - Golden Glow Natural Health Products
Each softgel contains: Evening Primrose oil 1.3 g: Gamma-Linolenic Acid (GLA) 117 mg.

Evening Primrose Oil 1000mg vegicap - Golden Glow Natural Health Products
Each vegicap contains: Evening Primrose oil 1 g: Gamma-Linolenic Acid (GLA) 100 mg.

Evening Primrose Oil 1300 mg - Nature's Way
Each capsule contains: Evening Primrose oil, cold pressed 1.3 g • Vitamin E d-alpha tocopheryl 6 IU. Other Ingredients: Gelatin, Glycerin, Water.

Evening Primrose Oil 500 mg - Nature's Bounty
Each softgel contains: Evening Primrose Oil 500 mg: Cis-Linoleic Acid (LA) 365 mg, Gamma-Linolenic Acid (GLA) 45 mg. Other Ingredients: Gelatin, Glycerin.

Evening Primrose Oil 500 mg - Arrowroot
Each capsule contains: Evening Primrose oil 500 mg.

Evening Primrose Oil 500 mg - Puritan's Pride
Each softgel contains: Evening Primrose Oil 500 mg: Cis-Linoleic Acid (LA) 365 mg, Gamma-Linolenic Acid (GLA) 45 mg. Other Ingredients: Gelatin, Glycerin.

Evening Primrose Oil 500 mg - Nature's Way
Each softgel contains: Evening Primrose Oil (cold pressed) 500 mg • Vitamin E (d-alpha tocopheryl) 6 IU. Other Ingredients: Gelatin, Glycerin, Water.

Evening Primrose Oil 500 mg - Vital Nutrients
Each softgel contains: Evening Primrose oil (providing 45 mg of gamma linolenic acid [GLA]) 500 mg.

Evening Primrose Oil 500 mg - Jamieson
Each capsule contains: Evening Primrose Oil 500 mg • Vitamin E Natural d-Alpha Tocopheryl Acetate 13.6 IU.

Evening Primrose Oil Extra Strength - Olympian Labs
Each softgel contains: Evening Primrose Oil 1300 mg.

Evening Primrose Oil, 500mg - Ortho Molecular Products
Each soft gel capsule contains: Evening Primrose seed oil providing 45 mg Gamma-Linolenic Acid 500 mg. Other Ingredients: Gelatin, Glycerin, Water.

Evening Primrose Oil, 500mg - Nature Made
Two softgels contain: Vitamin E 30 IU • Evening Primrose seed oil 1 g: Cis-Linoleic Acid 720 mg, Gamma-Linolenic Acid 90 mg.

Ever Thin - Dynamic Nutritional Products
Two tablets contain: Vitamin B6 (as pyridoxine HCl) 50 mg • Chromium (as chromium polynicotinate) 200 mcg • L-Carnitine (as l-carnitine fumarate) 250 mg • Alpha Lipoic Acid (thioctic acid) 25 mg

• Kelp powder 200 mg • Ever Thin Proprietary Thermogenic Blend 600 mg: Natural Cocoa extract (theobroma cacao), Theobromine, Citrus Aurantium (6% synephrine), Green Tea extract (98% polyphenols, 70% catechins, 40% EGCG, 6% caffeine).
See Editor's Note No. 40.

EverCLR - Halo Supply Co.
Each capsule contains: Burdock root • Ashwaganda root • Echinacea Angustifolia root • Echinacea Purpurea root • Hydrangea root.

EverFlex - Nature's Sunshine
Two tablets contain: Proprietary Blend 1900 mg: Glucosamine Hydrochloride, Methylsulfonylmethane (MSM), Chondroitin Sulfate, Devil's Claw root (harpagophytum procumbens). Other Ingredients: Cellulose, Stearic Acid, Silicon Dioxide, Magnesium Stearate.

Everyday Detox - Traditional Medicinals
Sweet Tea Vine herb (Gynostemma pentaphyllum) • Schisandra fruit dried aqueous extract • Licorice root • Ginger rhizome • Star Anise fruit • Lycium fruit dried aqueous extract • Schisandra fruit • Kukicha twig (Camellia sinensis).

Everyday Essentials - iVillage Inc.
Each tablet contains: Vitamin A (20% as beta carotene) 5000 IU • Vitamin C 90 mg • Vitamin D 400 IU • Vitamin E 30 IU • Vitamin K 80 mcg • Thiamin 2.3 mg • Riboflavin 2.6 mg • Niacin 20 mg • Vitamin B6 2 mg • Folic Acid 400 mcg • Vitamin B12 9 mcg • Biotin 300 mcg • Pantothenic Acid 10 mg • Calcium 200 mg • Iron 6 mg • Phosphorus 45 mg • Iodine 150 mcg • Magnesium 100 mg • Zinc 15 mg • Selenium 70 mcg • Copper 2 mg • Manganese 2 mg • Chromium 120 mcg • Molybdenum 75 mcg. Other Ingredients: Microcrystalline Cellulose, Corn Starch, Sodium Carboxymethylcellulose, Sucrose, Acacia, Maltodextrin, Magnesium Stearate, Hydroxypropyl Methylcellulose, Glycerin.

Evolution 2 - Element I - Viogenix Corp.
Each spray contains: Proprietary Blend 200 mg: Alpha GPC (alpha glycerlphosphoryl choline), GABA (gamma amino butyric acid), Mucuna Pruriens (l-dopa bean extract), Moomiyo extract (Russian Mumie) • Proprietary Blend 300 mg: Ornithine Alpha Ketoglutarate, L-Glutamine, L-Arginine, L-Lysine, L-Valine, L-Isoleucine, L-Tyrosine, Glycine. Inactive Ingredients: Deionized Water, Lecithin Phospholipids, Sodium Citrate, Citric Acid, Potassium Sorbate, Maltodextrin, Methyl-Paraben, Propylparaben, Natural & Artificial Flavors.

Evolution 2 - Element II - Viogenix Corp.
Each scoop (12 g) contains: Calcium (lactate) 25 mg • Magnesium (oxide) 7.2 mg • Zinc (oxide) 15 mg • Copper (gluconate) 2 mg • Manganese (gluconate) 5 mg • Chromium (amino nicotinate) 200 mcg • Iodine (postassium iodide) 150 mcg • Selenium (sodium) 200 mcg • Molybdenum (sodium molybdate) 150 mcg • Vitamin A (acetate) 10,000 IU • Vitamin E (d-alpha-tocopheryl acetate) 100 IU • Vitamin D (vitamin D3, cholecalciferol) 400 IU • Vitamin C (ascorbic acid) 500 mg • Vitamin B1 (thiamine HCl) 25 mg • Vitamin B2 (riboflavin) 25 mg • Vitamin B3 (niacin) 50 mg • Vitamin B3 (niacinamide) 50 mg • Vitamin B5 (calcium pantothenate) 50 mg • Vitamin B6 (pyridoxine HCl) 25 mg • Vitamin B12 (cyanocobalamin) 100 mcg • Folic Acid 400 mcg • Biotin 300 mcg • PABA (para amino benzoic acid) 25 mg • Choline Bitartrate 25 mg • Inositol 25 mg • N-Acetyl L-Cysteine 175 mg • Enzyme Premix 50 mg. Inactive Ingredients: Fructose, Natural Orange Powder, Potassium Bicarbonate, Citric Acid, Natural Orange Flavor, Digestive Enzymes (blend containing amylase, papain, lipase, bromelain, lactase, cellulase, maltase, sucrase), Stevia, Cholecalciferol, Silicon Dioxide.

Evolution 2 - Element III - Viogenix Corp.
Each spray contains: Phosphatidylserine 75 mg • Vinpocetine 5 mg • Carnitine Fumerate 100 mg • Ginko Biloba 5 mg • L-Theanine 2 mg • 5-HTP 1 mg • Choline Bitartrate 5 mg. Other Ingredients: Deionized Water, Lecithin Phospholipids, Citric Acid, Sodium Citrate, Potassium Sorbate, Sodium Benzoate, Maltodextrin, Glycine, Natural & Artificial Flavors.

Evolution 2 - Element IV - Viogenix Corp.
Each spray contains: N-Acetyl L-Cysteine 50 mg • Ellagic Acid 50 mg • Calcium D-Glucarate 15 mg • Acetyl L-Carnitine 10 mg • Carnosine 10 mg • Alpha Lipoic Acid 5 mg • Magnesium Citrate 5 mg • Coenzyme Q10 2 mg • Proprietary Blend (IMMONOSEB) 2 mg: Bromelain, Peptizine, Lactoperoxidase, Catalase, Lysozyme, Lactoferrin. Other Ingredients: Deionized Water, Lecithin Phospholipids, Polysorbate 60, Glycine, Citric Acid, Sodium Citrate, Potassium Sorbate, Sodium Benzoate, Methylparaben, Natural & Artificial Flavors.

Evolution 2 - Element V - Viogenix Corp.
Each spray contains: Vitamin A 2500 IU • Vitamin E 15 IU • Green Tea extract 10 mg • Grape Seed extract 10 mg • Pine Bark extract 10 mg • Bilberry extract 5 mg • Citrus Bioflavonoids 5 mg • Glutathione 1 mg • Selenium Citrate 50 mcg. Inactive Ingredients: Deionized Water, Lecithin Phospholipids, Polysorbate 60, Stevia extract, Glycine, Citric Acid, Sodium Citrate, Potassium Sorbate, Sodium Benzoate, Methylparaben, Natural & Artificial Flavors.

Exandra Lean - The Kutting Edge
Two capsules contain: Citrus Aurantium 125 mg • Nor-Ephedrine 23 mg • L-Phenylalanine 300 mg • Citri Max 500 mg • Acetyl L-Carnitine 100 mg • L-Tyrosine 80 mg • Ginger Root 50 mg • Vitamin B5 40 mg.
See Editor's Note No. 40.

Exec-U-Stress - Nature's Plus
Three tablets contain: Vitamin C with Rose Hips 600 mg • Niacinamide (Vitamin B3) 300 mg • Pantothenic Acid (Vitamin B5) 300 mg • L-Cysteine free form amino acid 200 mg • L-Glycine free form amino acid 200 mg • Vitamin B1 (Thiamine) 200 mg • Vitamin E natural 200 IU • Vitamin B6 (Pyridoxine HCl) 100 mg • Inositol 100 mg • PABA (Para-aminobenzoic acid) 75 mg • Zinc amino acid chelate/complex 50 mg • Vitamin B2 (Riboflavin) 50 mg • Choline (Bitartrate) 32 mg • Beta Carotene supplying 15000 IU Vitamin A activity 9 mg • Folic Acid 400 mcg • Vitamin B12 from Cobalamin 200 mcg • Selenium amino acid complex 100 mcg • Biotin 100 mcg.

Exercise In A Bottle - Enforma Natural Products
Two capsules contain: Calcium Pyruvate 300 mg • CitriMax brand Garcinia Cambogia extract (providing 40 mg of (-)hydroxycitric acid) 60 mg • Chromium Picolinate 25 mcg • Ginkgo Biloba 10 mg.
See Editor's Note No. 65.

Exfoliant Scrub - Nu Skin Enterprises
Water • Aloe Barbadensis • Stearic Acid • Diatomaceous Earth • Propylene Glycol Stearate SE • Cetyl Alcohol • Glycerin • Allantoin • Tocopheryl Acetate • Retinyl Palmitate • Dioctyl Adipate • Octyl Stearate • Octyl Palmitate • Triethanolamine • Diazolidinyl Urea • Fragrance • Methylparaben • Propylparaben • Disodium EDTA.

Exhilarin - Metagenics
Two tablets contain: Proprietary Blend 615 mg: Holy Basil leaf 10:1 extract (ocimum sanctum, containing urosolic acid), Ashwagandha root 5:1 extract (withania somnifera, containing withanolides), Amla fruit 3:1 extract (emblica officinalis, containing tannins), Bacopa leaf 4:1 extract (bacopa monnieri, containing bacosides A & B).

Exitor - Progressive Health Nutraceuticals
Citrus Aurantium extract 120 mg • Guarana extract 460 mg • Vitamin B6 10 mg • Caffeine Anhydrous 99 mg • Green Tea extract 200 mg • Theobromine Cocoa complex 200 mg • DMAE 50 mg • N-Acetyl L-Tyrosine 100 mg • L-Tyrosine 350 mg • Dandelion 50 mg • Gum Guggul extract 8 mg • Garcinia Cambogia 25 mg • Ginger 1 mg • Gotu Kola 8 mg • Horse Chestnut 9 mg.
See Editor's Note No. 40.

EXO - Agel
Each packet contains: Vitamin C 6 mg • Proprietary Blend 20 g: Dark Grape puree, Cranberry puree, Bilberry puree, Aronia juice from concentrate (aronia melanocarpa), Blueberry puree, Pomegranate juice from concentrate, Aloe Vera juice from concentrate, Para Guava

puree (psidium acutangulum), Noni puree, Acerola puree, Wolfberry juice from concentrate, Acai puree, Ashwagandha, Rooibos. Other Ingredients: Water, Proprietary Sweetening Blend (inulin, xylitol, neotame, acesulfame-K, lactobacillus acidophilus), Fructose, Natural Flavoring, Guar Gum, Grapefruit Seed Extract, Xanthan Gum, Sodium Benzoate.

Exomine - Progressive Health Nutraceuticals
Chondroitin Sulfate 400 mg • Hyaluronic Acid 200 mg • Glucosamine HCl 1500 mg • BioCell brand Type II Collagen 2000 mg • Methylsulfonyl Methane (MSM) 800 mg • Vitamin B 3 10 mg • Vitamin C 250 mg • Boron 1 mg • Boswellia Serrata extract 100 mg • Ginger 100 mg • Cat's Claw 25 mg • Tumeric 10 mg • Grape seed extract 25 mg.
See Editor's Note No. 15.

Exomine RH - Progressive Health Nutraceuticals
Chondroitin Sulfate 400 mg • Hyaluronic Acid 200 mg • BioCell brand Type II Collagen 2000 mg • Vitamin B5 25 mg • Vitamin C 250 mg • Vitamin E 30 IU • Selenium 100 mcg • Copper 1 mg • Zinc 15 mg • Methylsulfonyl Methane (MSM) 250 mg • Omega 3 Fatty Acids 25 mg • Gamma Linolenic Acid 10 mg • Boswellia Serrata extract 10 mg • Cat's Claw 35 mg • Tumeric 5 mg.
See Editor's Note No. 15.

Expectorant - Dial Herbs
Garlic • Bayberry • Mullein • Blood root • Cayenne • Lobelia.

Ex-Stress Formula - Nature's Way
Two capsules contain: Proprietary Formula: Black Cohosh root • Cayenne pepper fruit • Hops flower • Scullcap herb • Valerian root • Wood Betony stem, leaf, flower. Other Ingredients: Gelatin.

Extend Libido Booster for Men - Rbhealth
Each capsule contains: Zinc 50 mg • Orchic substance 75 mg • Yohimbe powder 500 mg • Oyster Shell powder 75 mg • L-Arginine Hydrochloride 250 mg • Cayenne pepper 50 mg • Maca powder 250 mg • Tribulus Terrestris powder 50 mg • Oat Straw powder 150 mg • Astragalus powder 25 mg • Ginseng blend powder 125 mg • Sarsaparilla powder 25 mg • Catuaba powder 100 mg • Licorice root powder 20 mg • Muira Puama stem powder 75 mg • Pumpkin seed powder 20 mg • Nettle leaf powder 75 mg • Boron 2 mg. Other Ingredients: Magnesium Stearate, Silicon Dioxide, Gelatin, Titanium Dioxide.

Ex-Tox - Progressive Labs
Three capsules contain: Vitamin C 600 mg • Bentonite 300 mg • L-Lysine 60 mg • DL-Methionine 600 mg • Sodium Alginate 450 mg • Chlorophyll 60 mg • Fruit pectin 150 mg • Garlic powder 30 mg.

Extra Strength Glucosamine & Chondroitin, Joint Support Factors - NOW Foods
Three capsules contain: Vitamin B3 (niacinamide) 100 mg • Vitamin B5 (pantothenic acid) 100 mg • Vitamin B6 (pyridoxine HCl) 50 mg • Vitamin C (ascorbic acid) 100 mg • Magnesium (oxide) 200 mg • Zinc (picolinate) 15 mg • Manganese (amino acid chelate) 7 mg • Copper (amino acid chelate) 3 mg • Glucosamine HCl 1000 mg • Boswellin (boswellia serrata standardized extract) 300 mg • Sea Cucumber 150 mg • Bromelain (2000 GDU activity from pineapple) 150 mg • PABA (para-aminobenzoic acid) 100 mg • Alfalfa juice concentrate 100 mg.

Extra Strength Glucosamine Chondroitin - Source Naturals
Two tablets contain: Glucosamine (as glucosamine sulfate) 1.5 g • Chondroitin (as chondroitin sulfate) 1.2 g.
See Editor's Note No. 15.

Extra Strength Joint Maintenance - Puritan's Pride
Three tablets contain: Vitamin C (as ascorbic acid) 500 mg • Manganese (as manganese glycinate) 5 mg • Glucosamine Sulfate 1500 mg • Chondroitin Sulfate 1200 mg. Other Ingredients: Cellulose (plant origin), Crospovidone, Vegetable Stearic Acid, Titanium Dioxide Color, Cellulose Coating, Vegetable Magnesium Stearate, Silica.
See Editor's Note No. 15.

Extra Strength Joint Maintenance Gels - Puritan's Pride
Three softgels contain: Glucosamine Sulfate 1500 mg • Chondroitin Sulfate 1200 mg • Citrus Bioflavonoids 45 mg • Manganese (as manganese aspartate) 1.02 mg.
See Editor's Note No. 15.

Extra Strength Joint Maintenance Gels - Vitamin World
Three softgels contain: Manganese (as manganese aspartate) 1 mg • Glucosamine Sulfate (2KCl) 1500 mg • Chondroitin Sulfate 1200 mg • Citrus Bioflavonoids 45 mg. Other Ingredients: Soybean Oil, Gelatin, Glycerin, Lecithin, St. John's Bread extract, Beeswax & Soybean Oil Mixture.
See Editor's Note No. 15.

Extra Strength Joint Maintenance tablets - Vitamin World
Three tablets contain: Vitamin C (as ascorbic acid) 500 mg • Manganese (as manganese glycinate) 5 mg • Glucosamine Sulfate (KCl) 1500 mg • Chondroitin Sulfate 1200 mg. Other Ingredients: Cellulose, Crospovidone, Vegetable Stearic Acid, Titanium Dioxide Color, Cellulose Coating, Vegetable Magnesium Stearate, Silica.
See Editor's Note No. 15.

Extra Strength Prosta-Metto - Puritan's Pride
Each softgel contains: Saw Palmetto extract (Serenoa repens: standardized to contain 85-95% fatty acids and biologically active sterol compounds) 160 mg • Pumpkin Seed oil extract (Cucurbita pepo) 40 mg • Pygeum Africanum extract 10 mg • Bearberry extract (Uva Ursi) 5 mg • Zinc (as Zinc Gluconate) 15 mg • Vitamin B6 5 mg.

Extra Strength Shen Min - Biotech Corp.
Two tablets contain: Shen Min Proprietary Blend 1755 mg: 12:1 He Shou Wu root (fo ti) standardized extract, He Shou Wu root powder • Herbal Purification Blend 600 mg: Eclipta Prostrata root, Radix Rehmannia root, Discorea Villosa root, Pocos Cocos aerial parts, Frucus Mori Albae root and stems, Frucus Ligusti Lucidi whole plant • Bioperine brand Black Pepper extract (piper nigrum) 3 mg. Other Ingredients: Dicalcium Phosphate, Microcrystalline Cellulose, Croscarmellose Sodium, Stearic Acid, Magnesium Stearate, Pharmaceutical Glaze.

Extra Strength Water Pill - Puritan's Pride
Each tablet contains: Potassium (as Potassium Gluconate) 40 mg • Buchu (Barosma betulina) leaf (25 mg of 4:1 extract) 100 mg • Uva Ursi (Arctostaphylos uva-ursi) leaf (33.3 mg of 3:1 extract) 100 mg • Juniper (Juniperus communis) berry 20 mg • Parsley (Petroselinum crispum) leaf 100 mg.

Extract Alpha - Gero Vita International
Three capsules contain: Proprietary Herbal Blend 2070 mg: CLA, Momordica Charantia extract (10% bitter principle), Green Tea extract (50% polyphenols), Choline Bitartrate, Wheat extract alpha (50%), L-Methionine, Inositol. Other Ingredients: Gelatin, Silicon Dioxide, Magnesium Stearate.

Extra-Time - Unknown
Each tablet contains: Salabmisri 78 mg • Kokilaksha 38 mg • Vanya Kahu 20 mg • Kapikachchhu 20 mg • Suvarnavang 20 mg • Vriddadaru extract 38 mg • Gokshura extract 38 mg • Jeevanti extract 38 mg • Shaileyam extract 20 mg.

Extreme Power Plus - Dutch International Products
Green Tea • Kola Nut • 72 Trace Mineral Complex • Siberian Ginseng • Royal Jelly • White Willow bark • Ginger • Fo-Ti • Hawthorn berries • Saw Palmetto • Beet root powder • Chromium Picolinate • Guarana • Ma Huang • Zi Chi • Kelp • CitriMax brand Garcinia Cambogia extract • Calcium Carbonate • Magnesium Carbonate • Korean Ginseng • American Ginseng • Yerba Mate • Vitamin B12 • Bee Pollen.
See Editor's Note No. 30.

Exulin - Progressive Health Nutraceuticals
L-Phenylalanine 150 mg • Rhodiola Rosea extract 250 mg • Vitamin B6 20 mg • Folic Acid 400 mcg • Methylcobalamin 1 mg • St. John's Wort extract 300 mg • Ginkgo Biloba extract 10 mg.

BRAND NAMES

Eye Beaute Pads - Pharmagel
Chamomile • Cucumber • Cornflower • Rosemary • Yarrow • Birch leaf • Sage • Nettle • Clover blossom.

Eye Care Complex - Leiner Health Products
Each tablet contains: Selenium 40 mcg • Vitamin A (Acetate) 2500 IU • Vitamin C (Ascorbic Acid) 30 mg • Bilberry 30 mg • Lutein 8 mg • Spinach 70 mg • Zeaxanthin 640 mcg. Other Ingredients: Calcium Carbonate, Gelatin, Glycerol, Starch, Cellulose, Maltodextrin Hydroxypropyl Methylcellulose, Croscarmellose Sodium, Crospovidone, Silicon Dioxide, Ascorbyl Palmitate, Dicalcium Phosphate, Polyethylene Glycol 3350, Tocopherols, Hydroxypropyl Cellulose, Magnesium Stearate, Pharmaceutical Glaze, Riboflavin, Blue 1 Lake, Titanium Dioxide, Polysorbate 80, Sodium Selenate.

Eye Complex II with Lutein - Hillestad
Each tablet contains: Vitamin A (as beta carotene) 5000 IU • Vitamin C (as ascorbic acid) 60 mg • Zinc (as zinc gluconate) 15 mg • Selenium (as selenium chelate) 100 mcg • Lutein 10 mg • Taurine 20 mg • L-Glutathione 20 mg • Eyebright herb 50 mg • Bilberry fruit 50 mg. Other Ingredients: Oyster Shell, Stearic Acid, Magnesium Stearate, Croscarmellose Sodium.

Eye D'Clare - Life Enhancement Products, Inc.
Glycerin • Carboxymethylcellulose Sodium • Sterile Water (opthalmic-grade isotonic solution, pH 6.3 to 6.5) • N-Acetylcarnosine • Vitamin A • Vitamin E • Borates • Potassium Bicarbonate • Purified Benzyl Alcohol.

Eye Defense - Nature Made
Two tablets contain: Vitamin A (100% as beta carotene) 5000 IU • Vitamin C (as ascorbic acid) 350 mg • Vitamin E (as dL-alpha tocopheryl acetate) 100 IU • Zinc (as zinc oxide) 15 mg • Copper (as copper oxide) 0.4 mg • Lutein 5 mg • Zeaxanthin 1 mg. Other Ingredients: Cellulose Gel, Talc, Gelatin, Sugar, Hydroxypropyl Methylcellulose, Corn Starch, Croscarmellose Sodium, Titanium Dioxide Artificial Color, Silica Gel, Magnesium Stearate, Polyethylene Glycol, Triethyl Citrate, Polysorbate 80, Sodium Citrate.

Eye Firming Gel - Pharmagel
Ginseng and plant extracts.

Eye Formula - Pharmanex
Each capsule contains: Beta-Carotene (Dunaliella Salina) 2500 IU • Vitamin C (Calcium Ascorbate, Ascorbic Acid) 150 mg • Vitamin E (d-Alpha Tocopheryl Succinate, Beta, Delta, Gamma Tocopherols) 75 IU • Zinc (Zinc Propionate) 2.5 mg • Selenium (L-Selenomethionine) 35 mcg • N-Acetyl-L-Cysteine 100 mg • Taurine 100 mg • Tumeric extract (Min. 95% Curcumin) 50 mg • Ginkgo Biloba extract (Min. 95% Flavonglycosides, Min. 6% Terpene Lactones) 30 mg • Alpha-Lipoic Acid 10 mg • Lutein (from Marigold flower extract) 2.5 mg. Other Ingredients: Calcium Carbonate, Sodium Carboxymethylcellulose, Magnesium Stearate, Talc.

Eye Guard Plus - Puritan's Pride
Four capsules contain: Beta Carotene (pro-vitamin A) 40,000 IU • Natural Vitamin E (succinate) 400 IU • Vitamin C 1,500 mg • Citrus Bioflavonoids Complex 250 mg • Quercetin (bioflavonoid) 100 mg • Bilberry extract (standardized 25%) 10 mg • Rutin 100 mg • Zinc (picolinate) 25 mg • Selenium (selenomethionine) 100 mcg • Taurine 200 mg • N-Acetyl-Cysteine 200 mg • L-Glutathione 10 mg • Vitamin B2 (Riboflavin) 50 mg • Chromium (GTF) 200 mcg • Lutein 20 mg.

Eye Support - NOW Foods
Three capsules contain: Vitamin A (natural Beta Carotene • D. salina) 15 mg/25 000 IU • Vitamin C (as Ascorbic Acid) 300 mg • Vitamin E (as d-Alpha-Tocopheryl Succinate) 200 IU • Riboflavin (Vitamin B2) 20 mg • Zinc (as L-OptiZinc) 25 mg • Selenium 100 mcg • Bilberry standardized extract (Vaccinum myrtillus) (25% Anthocyanidins) 100 mg • Lutein 10 mg • Green Tea extract (Camellia sinensis) (40% Catechins) 150 mg • N-Acetyl-Cysteine (NAC) 100 mg • Rutin 100 mg.

Eye Support - Alacer
Each tablet contains: Vitamin A (Betatene brand carotenoid complex) 5000 IU • Bilberry extract 100 mg • Vitamin C (as calcium magnesium ascorbate) 80 mg • Ginkgo Biloba 40 mg • Quercetin Bioflavonoid 25 mg • Siberian Ginseng 25 mg • Vitamin B3 (magnesium niacinate) 10 mg • 8 Mixed Bioflavonoids 25 mg • Grape seed extract 15 mg • Lutein 6 mg • Zinc Niacinate 1.5 mg • Magnesium Aspartate 25 mg.

Eye Treatment - Jason
Complete Vitamin C Complex • Vitamin E • Aloe Vera gel • Rose Hips.

Eyebright (Euphrasia officinalis) - Solgar
Each capsule contains: Eyebright flower 4:1 extract 57 mg • Raw Eyebright leaf powder 295 mg. Other Ingredients: Vegetable Cellulose, Vegetable Magnesium Stearate, Water, Vegetable Glycerin.

Eyebright Formula - Nature's Way
Two capsules contain: Proprietary Formula: Bayberry bark • Cayenne pepper fruit • Eyebright stem, leaf, flower • Goldenseal root • Red Raspberry leaves. Other Ingredients: Gelatin.

Eyebright Herb - NOW Foods
Two capsules contain: Total Carbohydrate 650 mg • Eyebright herb (Euphrasia Officinalis) leaves and stems 940 mg. Other Ingredients: Stearic Acid.

Eye-Rite - J. R. Carlson Laboratories, Inc.
Two capsules contain: Vitamin C (as ascorbic acid) 240 mg • Vitamin E (as D-alpha tocopheryl succinate) 30 IU • Zinc (as zinc glycinate chelate) 7 mg • Chromium (as chromium glycinate chelate) 100 mcg • Soy Isoflavone concentrate 100 mg • Bilberry (vaccinium myrtillus, 25% anthocyanosides) 240 mg • Lutein (FloraGlo brand, from marigolds) 6 mg • Citrus Bioflavonoids complex 90 mg • Cranberry extract (vaccinium macrocarpon) 185 mg • Grape seed extract 10 mg • Quercetin 60 mg • Alpha Lipoic 30 mg.

Eye-Vites - Nature's Bounty
Each tablet contains: Vitamin A (as Beta Carotene) 5000 IU • Vitamin C (as Ascorbic Acid) 60 mg • Vitamin E (as dl-Alpha Tocopheryl Acetate) 30 IU • Zinc (as Zinc Oxide) 40 mg • Selenium (as Sodium Selenate) 40 mcg • Copper (as Cupric Oxide) 2 mg. Other Ingredients: Whey, Calcium Carbonate, Cellulose, Gelatin, Dicalcium Phosphate, Vegetable Stearic Acid, Croscarmellose, Cellulose Coating, Crospovidone, Vegetable Magnesium Stearate.

EZ Flex - Metagenics
Each tablet contains: Niacin (as niacinamide) 250 mg • Magnesium (as magnesium bis-glycinate) 50 mg • Vitamin B6 (as pyridoxine hydrochloride) 50 mg • Riboflavin 36 mg • Folate (as folic acid, L-5-methyl tetrahydrofolate, 5-formyl tetrahydrofolate) 400 mcg • Vitamin B12 (as cyanocobalamin) 200 mcg • Turmeric rhizome (curcuma longa) 100 mg.

EZ Lung - E-Z QUIT, INC.
Two tablets contain: Vitamin A (as retinyl palmitate, 10% as beta-carotene) 5000 IU • Vitamin C (as ascorbic acid) 150 mg • Vitamin D (as cholecalciferol) 200 IU • Vitamin E (as d-alpha-tocopheryl acetate) 30 IU • Thiamin (as thiamin HCl) 5 mg • Riboflavin 5 mg • Niacin (as niacinamide) 20 mg • Vitamin B6 (as pyridoxine HCl) 5 mg • Folate (as folic acid) 400 mcg • Vitamin B12 (as cyanocobalamin) 10 mcg • Pantothenic Acid (as d-calcium pantothenate) 10 mg • Calcium (as calcium carbonate) 300 mg • Iodine (from kelp) 150 mcg • Magnesium (as magnesium oxide) 100 mg • Zinc (as zinc citrate) 20 mg • Selenium (as selenium l-methionine) 200 mcg • Copper (as copper sulfate) 2 mg • Manganese (as manganese citrate) 2.5 mg • Chromium (as chromium dinicotinate glycinate) 120 mcg • Molybdenum (as sodium molybdate) 75 mcg • Stress Fighting Complex 150 mg: Korean Ginseng root extract (4% ginsenosides), Chamomile (flowering tops), Eleuthero root extract (0.8% total eleutherosides), Hops (strobile), Passion flower (whole plant) • Stress Fighting Complex 100 mg: Orange Bioflavonoids

(30-40% total flavanones, flavonols, flavones, calculated as hesperidin), MSM (methylsulfonylmethane), Green Tea leaf extract, Ginger root standardized extract (5% gingerols), Calcium D-Glucarate, Bilberry fruit standardized extract. Other Ingredients: Microcrystalline Cellulose, Croscarmellose Sodium, Stearic Acid, Magnesium Stearate, Silica, Pharmaceutical Glaze.

EZ QUIT Cleanser - E-Z QUIT, INC.
Six tablets contain: Iodine (from kelp) 200 mcg • Crave Control Blend 2500 mg: Alfalfa leaf, Eleuthero root, Licorice root, Echinacea Purpurea (aerial parts), Ginger root, Peppermint leaf, Lobelia (whole plant), Safflower seed oil, Bioperine brand Black Pepper extract (standardized to 95-97% piperine) • Cleansing Blend 1200 mg: Dandelion root, Cayenne Pepper, Sarsaparilla root, Buckhorn bark, Cascara Sagrada bark, Hyssop (aerial parts), Oregon Grape root, Barley grass, Bayberry fruit, Golden Seal (aerial parts) Lemon Verbena leaf, Oxbile extract, Elderberry fruit 10:1 extract. Other Ingredients: Dicalcium Phosphate, Microcrystalline Cellulose, Croscarmellose Sodium, Stearic Acid, Magnesium Stearate, Silica, Pharmaceutical Glaze.

E-Z Vite Multiple - Nature's Life
Two tablets contain: Vitamin A (Fish Liver oil) 10000 IU • Vitamin D (as Vitamin D3, Cholecalciferol) 400 IU • Vitamin B1 (Thiamine HCl) 10 mg • Vitamin B2 (Riboflavin) 10 mg • Vitamin B6 Pyridoxine HCl) 10 mg • Vitamin B12 (Cobalamin) 100 mcg • Niacin 30 mg • Pantothenic Acid (d-Calcium Pantothenate) 20 mg • Folic Acid 400 mcg • PABA (Para Aminobenzoic Acid) 30 mg • Biotin (d-Biotin) 3.5 mcg • Choline (Choline Bitartrate) 3 mg • Inositol 50 mg • Vitamin E (d-Alpha tocopherol, with Beta, Gamma & Delta Tocopherols) 10 IU • Vitamin C 100 mg • Lemon Bioflavonoids (TESTLAB) 30 mg • Rutin (Saphora japonica) 20 mg • Hesperidin Complex 5 mg • Calcium (Bone Meal) 40 mg • Copper (Gluconate) 100 mcg • Phosphorus (Bone Meal) 25 mg • Iodine (Icelandic Kelp) 100 mcg • Iron (Ferrous Fumarate) 10 mg • Magnesium (Oxide) 10 mg • Zinc (Gluconate) 2 mg • Potassium (Chloride) 10 mg • Manganese (Gluconate) 2 mg • Betaine HCl 25 mg • Liver (Defatted & Desiccated) 100 mg • RNA powder (Torula Yeast) 25 mg • Pancreatin (4 X N.F.) 25 mg. In a natural base of Raw Pancreas, Sodium Alginate, Torula B Yeast, Rose Hips & Acerola berries. See Editor's Note No. 14.

EZ-Breather Lung System - Susan Ambrosino's Herb Club, Inc.
Each capsule contains: Proprietary Blend 50 mg: Jatoba, Licorice root, Schizandra berry, Catnip, Marshmallow root, Fenugreek seed, Wild Cherry bark, Mullein.

EZ-Go - Doctor's Choice, Naturally
Two capsules contain: Proprietary Blend 1430 mg: Cape Aloe gel (aloe ferox), Slippery Elm bark (ulmus rubra), Marshmallow root (althaea officinalis), Triphala: Indian Gooseberry fruit, Belleric Myrobalan fruit, and Tropical Almond fruit, Magnesium (as magnesium hydroxide), Rhubarb root (rheum officinalis). Other Ingredients: Hypromellose, Water.

EZorb Capsules - Elixir Industry
Each capsule contains: Calcium Aspartate Anhydrous (CalAA) 560 mg.

EZorb Powder - Elixir Industry
Calcium Aspartate Anhydrous (CalAA) powder.

Face & Body Soap - Omega Nutrition
Spring Water • Food grade Coconut oil • Potassium Hydroxide • Unrefined & certified organic Almond • Unrefined & certified organic Brazilnut or Hazelnut oil • Virgin Olive oil.

Face Lift Activator (original formula) - Nu Skin Enterprises
Water • Aloe Barbadensis • Bladderwrack extract (fucus vesiculosus) • Allantoin • Panthenol • Sodium PCA • RNA • Benzalkonium Chloride • Butylene Glycol • Methylparaben • Phenoxyethanol • Disodium EDTA.

Face Lift Activator (sensitive formula) - Nu Skin Enterprises
Water • Aloe Vera gel (aloe barbadensis) • Hydrolyzed Wheat Protein • Allantoin • Panthenol • Sodium PCA • Citric Acid • Methylparaben • Phenoxyethanol • Tetrasodium EDTA • Methylchloroisothiazolinone • Methylisothiazolinone.

Face Lift Powder (original formula) - Nu Skin Enterprises
Albumin • Corn starch (zea mays) • Aloe Barbadensis • Silica • Hydrolyzed Elastin • Allantoin • Panthenol • Methylparaben.

Face Lift Powder (sensitive formula) - Nu Skin Enterprises
Acacia powder • Corn starch • Aloe • Allantoin • Panthenol • Ascorbic Acid • Methylparaben.

Facial Cleansing Bar - Nu Skin Enterprises
Sodium Cocoyl Isethionate • Maltodextrin • Stearic Acid • Cetyl Alcohol • Water • Nu Skin Cleansing Lotion: Water, Aloe Vera gel, Stearic Acid, Glyceryl Stearate SE, Dioctyl Adipate, Octyl Stearate, Octyl Palmitate, Propylene Glycol, Sodium PCA, Allantoin, RNA, Fragrance, Bladderwrack extract, Retinyl Palmitate, Ergocalciferol, Royal Jelly, Caramel, Cetearyl Alcohol, Ceteareth-20, Triethanolamine, Disodium EDTA, Butylparaben, Isobutylparaben, Isopropylparaben, Methylparaben, Phenoxyethanol • Sodium Isosteroyl Lactylate • Methyl Gluceth-20 • Sodium Lactate • Lactic Acid • Glycerin • Tocopheryl Acetate • Jojoba oil • Polyacrylamide • Titanium Dioxide • Fragrance.

Facial Scrub - Nu Skin Enterprises
Water • Aloe Barbadensis • Stearic Acid • Walnut shell powder (juglans regina) • Propylene Glycol Stearate SE • Cetyl Alcohol • Glycerin • Allantoin • Tocopheryl Acetate • Retinyl Palmitate • Dioctyl Adipate • Octyl Stearate • Octyl Palmitate • Triethanolamine • Quaternium-15 • Diazolidinyl Urea • Fragrance • Methylparaben • Propylparaben.

Fade-Out Creme - Pharmagel
Vitamin C • Licorice Extract • PABA-free sunblock.

Fallodox - Progressive Health Nutraceuticals
Black Cohosh 100 mg • Saw Palmetto extract 70 mg • Saw Palmetto 285 mg • Blessed Thistle 20 mg • Red Raspberry 20 mg • Fennel extract 50 mg • Wild Yam 25 mg • Dandelion 100 mg • Dong Quai 75 mg • Oat straw 50 mg • Fenugreek 50 mg • Chasteberry 25 mg • Red Clover 15 mg • Olive extract 25 mg • Cat's Claw 35 mg.

False Unicorn-Squaw Vine Virtue - Blessed Herbs
False Unicorn root • Squaw vine • Black Haw bark • Grain alcohol & Distilled Water.

familE - Jarrow Formulas
Each softgel contains: Vitamin E (D-alpha tocopherol) 41 mg • D-Beta Tocopherol 6.3 mg • D-Gamma Tocopherol 250 mg • D-Delta Tocopherol 84 mg • Palm fruit distillate 100 mg: D-Beta Tocotrienol 1.5 mg, D-Gamma Tocotrienol 22 mg, D-Delta Tocotrienol 5 mg, D-Alpha Tocotrienol 2 mg, Squalene 10 mg, Phytosterols 3.5 mg • Lutein (from 20 mg esters, tagetes erecta, marigold petal extract) 10 mg • Zeaxanthin (as esters, tagetes erecta, marigold petal extract) 0.5 mg • Pantethine 100 mg. Other Ingredients: Soybean Oil, Gelatin, Glycerin, Water, Carob.

Fast Balance-G.I. - FoodScience of Vermont
Each capsule contains: Mannon Oligosaccharides (MOS) 450 mg • Proprietary Probiotic Blend 50 mg: Lactobacillus Acidophilus, Lactobacillus Rhamnosus, Bifidobacterium Tongum (300 million CFU).

Fast Food - The Sports Nutrition Source, Inc.
Two scoops contain: Sodium 300 mg • Potassium 600 mg • Protein 38 g • Vitamin A 2500 IU • Vitamin C 30 mg • Calcium 500 mg • Iron 9 mg • Vitamin D 200 IU • Vitamin E 15 IU • Vitamin K 35 mcg • Vitamin B-1 75 mg • Vitamin B-2 85 mg • Vitamin B-3 10 mg • Vitamin B-6 1 mg • Vitamin B-12 3 mcg • Biotin 125 mcg • Zinc 7.5 mcg • Copper 1 mg.

Fast-Acting Zinaxin - FreeLife International
Each softgel contains: Patented Extract EV.EXT 77 [highly standardized extracts of rhizomes of Ginger (Zungiber officinale and Alpinia galanga)] 255 mg. Other Ingredients: Sunflower Seed oil, Gelatin, Beeswax, Lecithin, Vegetable Glycerin, Purified Water, Natural Chlorophyll Complex, Titanium Dioxide (natural mineral color).

FastBLAST - Life Enhancement Products, Inc.
Each rounded tablespoon (14.5 g) contains: Vitamin A (as beta-carotene) 2500 IU • Vitamin C (as ascorbic acid and niacinamide ascorbate) 325 mg • Vitamin E (as D,L-alpha-tocopheryl acetate) 30 IU • Thiamine (vitamin B1 as thiamine hydrochloride) 1.5 mg • Riboflavin (vitamin B2) 3 mg • Niacin (vitamin B3 as niacinamide ascorbate) 75 mg • Vitamin B6 (as pyridoxine hydrochloride) 16 mg • Folic Acid 100 mcg • Vitamin B12 (cyanocobalamin) 20 mcg • Pantothenic Acid (vitamin B5 as calcium pantothenate) 18 mg • Zinc (as zinc gluconate) 3 mg • Copper (as copper gluconate) 420 mcg • Chromium (as chromium aspartate) 25 mcg • L-Phenylalanine 800 mg • Citric Acid 50 mg • Malic Acid 200 mg • Taurine 200 mg • Glycine 150 mg • Fumaric Acid 30 mg • Caffeine 80 mg.

Fat & Sugar Block - E'OLA
Two tablets contain: Vitamin C (as Ascorbic Acid) 75 mg • Proprietary Blend 1050 mg: Chitosan, Gymnema Sylvestre, Garcinia Cambogia. Other Ingredients: Dicalcium Phosphate, Microcrystalline Cellulose, Croscarmellose Sodium, Stearic Acid, Silicon Dioxide.

Fat Binding Diet System 6 - Applied Nutrition
Two capsules contain: Vitamin C (ascorbic acid) 14 mg • Vitamin E (dl-alpha tocopheryl acetate) 4 IU • Riboflavin 0.5 mg • Niacin (niacinamide) 5 mg • Vitamin B6 (pyridoxine hydrochloride) 0.54 mg • Folic Acid 107 mcg • Vitamin B12 (cyanocobalamin) 2 mcg • Iodine (potassium iodine) 40 mcg • Selenium (sodium selenite) 14 mcg • Chromium (picolinate & 50% as polynicotinate) ChromeMate 80 mcg • Potassium (chloride) 6 mg • Garcinia Cambogia fruit (Super CitriMax, 60% Hydroxycitric acid extract) 460 mg • Chitosan (82% Deacetylated) 190 mg • Kola nut seed kernel extract (10% caffeine) 146 mg • Guarana seed extract (15% guaranine) 26 mg • Choline (bitartrate) 26 mg • Inositol 26 mg • Carnitine (L-Carnitine fumarate) 20 mg • Betaine (hydrochloride) 7 mg • Proprietary blend: [Ginger root, "72 Trace Minerals", Bioperine brand Black Pepper extract (piper nigrum extract, standardized to 95% piperine) 60 mg. Other Ingredients: Gelatin, montnirollinite, silica & magnesium stearate.

Fat Bloc Chitosan 1000 - Ultimate Nutrition
Each capsule contains: Vitamin C 50 mg • Chitosan 1000 mg. Other Ingredients: Cellulose, Dicalcium Phosphate, Gelatin, Magnesium Stearate.

Fat Bloc Chitosan 500 - Ultimate Nutrition
Each capsule contains: Vitamin C 40 mg • Chitosan 500 mg. Other Ingredients: Cellulose, Dicalcium Phosphate, Gelatin, Magnesium Stearate.

Fat Burner - Swanson Health Products
Three tablets contain: Vitamin B-6 (as pyridoxine HCl) 50 mg • Chromium (from Chromax brand chromium picolinate) 200 mcg • CitriMax brand Garcinia Cambogia fruit extract 1 g • Hydroxycitric Acid 500 mg • Choline Bitartrate 500 mg • Inositol 250 mg • L-Methionine 200 mg • Cider Vinegar powder 100 mg • Grapefruit powder 100 mg • Lecithin 100 mg • Taurine 100 mg.

Fat Burner Non-Ephedra - Natrol, Inc.
Three capsules contain: Chromium (as chromium picolinate) 100 mcg • Mucuna Prurient extract (l-dopa root)15 mg • Bitter Orange rind extract 20 mg • Synephrine 1.2 mg • Caffeine 100 mg. Other Ingredients: Rice Powder, Gelatin Capsule, Silica, Magnesium Stearate.
See Editor's Note No. 40.

Fat Burner with CLA - EnerGreens, Inc.
Each capsule contains: CLA 400 mg • Basil 200 mg • Phosphatidyl Serine 100 mg. Other Ingredients: Gelatin.

Fat Burners - Amerifit Nutrition
Two caplets contain: Vitamin B6 (as pyridoxine HCl) 10 mg • Iron (as ferrous fumarate) 4 mg • Chromium (chromium picolinate) 50 mcg • Choline Complex 1000 mg: Choline Citrate, Buchu leaves, Uva Ursi root & fiber • Inositol 250 mg • L-Carnitine (as carnitine tartrate, carnitine HCl) 50 mg • L-Lysine 100 mg • Methionine 200 mg • Lecithin (from glycine max) 100 mg • Betaine HCl 200 mg • Essential Fatty Acids: (Linoleic, Oleic) 100 mg. Other Ingredients: Dicalcium Phosphate, Microcrystalline Cellulose, Magnesium Stearate, Croscarmellose Sodium • Stearic Acid & Vegetable glaze.
See Editor's Note No. 21.

Fat Busters Shake - Nature's Plus
Each scoop (34 g) contains: Vitamin A 5000 IU • Vitamin C 60 mg • Calcium 300 mg • Iron 4.5 mg • Vitamin D 400 IU • Vitamin E 30 IU • Thiamin 1.5 mg • Riboflavin 1.7 mg • Niacin 20 mg • Vitamin B6 2 mg • Folic Acid 400 mcg • Vitamin B12 6 mcg • Biotin 300 mcg • Pantothenic Acid 10 mg • Phosphorus 200 mg • Iodine 150 mcg • Magnesium 80 mg • Zinc 15 mg • Selenium 21 mcg • Manganese 5 mg • Chromium 18 mcg • Molybdenum 18.75 mcg • Clarinol brand Conjugated Linoleic Acid (CLA) isomers 1500 mg • ForsLean brand Coleus Forskohlii extract (standardized 10% forskolin) 250 mg • Lipase (fat-digesting enzyme) 50 mg • Gugulipid brand Commiphora Mukul Gum resin (standardized 2.5% guggulsterones) 50 mg • Inositol 50 mg • Rhodiola Rosea root (standardized 2.8% salidroside, 2.3% rosavin, 1.44% rosin, 1.24% rosarin, 70% total polyphenols) 25 mg • Choline (bitartrate) 21 mg • Non-GMO Isolated Soy Protein • Fructose • Vanilla Flavor • Maltodextrin • Cinnamon powder • Guar Gum • Psyllium • Oat Bran • Microcrystalline Cellulose • Spirulina • Bee Pollen • Lemon Bioflavonoids • Papaya • Bromelain • Chlorophyll.

Fat Busters Tablets - Nature's Plus
Each tablet contains: Calcium (as aminoate) 120 mg • Chromium (as polynicotinate) 120 mcg • Coleus Forskohlii extract (standardized to 10% forskolin) 250 mg • Green Tea (camellia sinensis leaf, decaffeinated, standardized to 50% polyphenols) 200 mg • Green Orange (from fructus immaturus Citrus aurantium exocarp, standardized to 4% synephrine) 125 mg • Korean Ginseng (Panax ginseng root, standardized to 15% ginsenosides) 100 mg • Ginger (zingiber officinale root, standardized to 4% volatile oils) 100 mg. Other Ingredients: Di-Calcium Phosphate, Hydroxypropyl Methylcellulose, Stearic Acid, Magnesium Stearate, Silica, Pharmaceutical Glaze.
See Editor's Note No. 40.

Fat Defense - Country Life Vitamins
Two tablets contain: Chromium (as chromium polynicotinate) 200 mcg • Brindall berry rind extract (Super CitriMax brand, providing 60% hydroxycitric acid (HCA), equal to 500.4 mg) 834 mg • Gymnema Sylvestre leaf 40:1 extract 5 mg • Vanadium (from 2 mg vanadyl sulfate) 620 mcg. Other Ingredients: Cellulose, Stearic Acid, Magnesium Stearate, Cellulose, Glycerin, Silica.

Fat Digestion - Enzymes, Inc.
Each capsule contains: Proprietary Enzyme Blend 381 mg: Amylase, Lipase, Protease, Glucoamylase, Peptidase, alpha-Galactosidase, Cellulase. Other Ingredients: Plant Cellulose, Water.

Fat Enzyme Formula - Enzymatic Therapy
Two capsules contain: Pure Plant Enzymes Blend 221 mg: Lipase I/II (FIP (pH7.0)) 1500 LU, (FCC III (pH6.5)) 1400 LU, Protease I/II/III/IV, (USP XXIII (pH7.5)) 16,350 USP, (FCC IV (pH7.0)) 26,100 PC.. (FCC IV (pH4.7)) 22,350 HUT, Amylase (USP XXI (pH6.8)) 16,500 USP, (FCC IV (pH4.8)) 7140 DU, Cellulase I (FCC IV (pH4.5)) 47.5 CU.

Fat Fighter Forte - Nature's Own
Each tablet contains: Brindleberry extract (garcinia quaesita), equivalent to dry fruit 4000 mg • Milk Thistle extract (silybum marianum), equivalent to dry fruit 500 mg • Bitter Orange extract (citrus aurantium), equivalent to dry fruit 500 mg • Siberian Ginseng

extract (eleutherococcus senticosus), equivalent to dry root 300 mg • Gymnema extract (gymnema sylvestre), equivalent to dry leaf 250 mg • L-Carnitine 100 mg • Chromium (from chromium picolinate 125 mcg) 15.5 mcg • Choline Bitartrate 50 mg • Inositol 50 mg • Vitamin B1 (thiamine nitrate) 25 mg • Vitamin B2 (riboflavin) 25 mg • Vitamin B3 (nicotinamide) 25 mg • Vitamin B5 (pantothenic acid, from calcium pantothenate) 25 mg • Vitamin B6 (pyridoxine hydrochloride) 25 mg • Vitamin B12 (cyanocobalamin) 15 mcg.
See Editor's Note No. 40.

Fat Free Gainers Fuel 1000 - TwinLab
Each serving contains: Chromium (from Chromic Fuel Chromium Picolinate) 400 mcg. Other Ingredients: Branched Chain Amino Acids (L-Leucine, L-Isoleucine, L-Valine), Milk & Egg White Proteins, L-Carnitine & Kreb's Cycle Mineral Complexes (including Citrates, Aspartates, Succinates & Alpha-Ketoglutarates).

Fat Free Gainers Fuel 2500 - TwinLab
Chromium (from patented Chromic Fuel Chromium Picolinate) 400 mcg • Kreb's Cycle Mineral Complexes (including Citrates, Aspartates, Succinates & Alpha-Ketoglutarates) •Milk & Egg White Proteins • Branched Chain Amino Acids (L-Leucine, L-Isoleucine & L-Valine), L-Carnitine.

Fat Grabbers - Nature's Sunshine
Four capsules contain: Proprietary Blend 2100 mg: Guar Gum (cyamopsis tetragonolobus), Psyllium hulls (plantago ovata), Lecithin, Chickweed herb (stellaria media). Other Ingredients: Silicon Dioxide, Kosher Gelatin, Water.

Fat Metabolism Factors - Michael's Naturopathic Programs
Three tablets contain: Vitamin B6 (as pyridoxine) 100 mg • Iodine (from kelp) 225 mcg • Chromium (as chromium polynicotinate) 200 mcg • Potassium (as potassium amino acid complex) 210 mg • Proprietary Blend: Lecithin (from soy), Choline (as choline bitartrate), Inositol, Chickweed leaf (stellaria media), Fucus Vesiculosus leaf (sea wrack), Guggul gum (from commiphora mukul, 2.5% guggulsterones, 2.5 mg), Methionine (as L-methionine hydrochloride), Phenylalanine (as L-phenylalanine), White Ash bark (fraxinus americana), Bitter Orange fruit (citrus aurantium). Other Ingredients: Dicalcium Phosphate, Maltodextrin, Stearic Acid, Magnesium Stearate.
See Editor's Note No. 40.

Fat Metabolizer 2000 - Youngevity
Cat's Claw • Siberian Ginseng • Bee Pollen • Kelp • Ephedra Sinica herb • White Willow bark • Licorice root • Hops flowers • Valerian root • Pantothenic Acid • Chromium Chelavite • Manganese Chelazome • Vilcabamba Mineral Essence: Potassium, Calcium, Magnesium, Zinc, Chromium, Selenium, Iron, Copper, Molybdenum, Vanadium, Iodine, Cobalt, Manganese.
See Editor's Note No. 21 and No. 30.

Fat Metabolizer 2001+ - Youngevity
Cat's Claw • Ephedra Sinica herb • White Willow bark • Caffeine • Kelp • Pantothenic Acid • Chromium Chelavite • Manganese Chelazome • Vilcabamba Mineral Essence: Potassium, Calcium, Magnesium, Zinc, Chromium, Selenium, Iron, Copper, Molybdenum, Vanadium, Iodine, Cobalt, Manganese.
See Editor's Note No. 21 and No. 30.

Fat Predator - Predator Industries Nutritional
Each capsule contains: Ephedra extract • Cola Nut extract • White Willow bark
See Editor's Note No. 21 and No. 30.

Fat Predator Diet Capsules (no ephedra) - Predator Industries Nutritional
Two capsules contain: Pantothenic Acid (as d-calcium pantothenate) 40 mg • Citrus Aurantium 255 mg • Guarana 910 mg • White Willow bark 101 mg • Proprietary Blend 355 mg: L-Tyrosine, Acetyl L-Carnitine, Bitter Orange, Green Tea extract, Grape seed extract.
See Editor's Note No. 40.

Fat Snatcher - Youngevity
Chitosan • Aloe Vera leaf • Citric Acid • Iso-Ascorbic Acid (Vitamin C).

Fat Stopper Formula - Health Tech Industries (Dr. Bussan's)
Two capsules contain: Chitosan 250 mg • TAT Metabolite (a proprietary process of Dews Research Laboratories) 100 mg • Bile Salts Extract NF 50 mg • Vitamin C (polyascorbic acid) 50 mg • Acetyl Pyruvate Bile 12 mg • Niacin 5 mg • Chromium Picolinate 25 mcg. Other Ingredients: Magnesium trisilicate, Magnesium stearate, trace FD& C Yellow #5 and natural Gelatin capsules.

Fat Trap - The Sports Nutrition Source, Inc.
Each capsule contains: Chitosan shellfish 500 mg • Fiber 500 mg.

Fat Trapper - Enforma Natural Products
Two capsules contain: Psyllium seed husk 420 mg • Chitin 80 mg.
See Editor's Note No. 65.

Fat Trapper Plus - Enforma Natural Products
Two capsules contain: Psyllium seed husk 420 mg • Chitin 80 mg. Other Ingredients: Gelatin, Magnesium Stearate, Vegetable Stearine, Glycerin.
See Editor's Note No. 65.

Fat-B-Gone - Biotech Corp.
Two tablets contain: Natural Vitamin E (d-alpha tocopherol succinate) 10 IU • Vitamin C (ascorbic acid) 500 mg • Chitosan 500 mg • Explosive Proprietary Tablet Dissolution 120 mg: Croscarmellose Sodium, Soy Fibers. Other Ingredients: Dicalcium Phosphate, Microcrystalline Cellulose, Stearic Acid, Silica, Magnesium Stearate, Pharmaceutical Glaze.

FatBlast - E.V.A. Pharmaceutics
Three capsules contain: Chitosan (HD) 554 mg • Psyllium husk 150 mg • Malic Acid 28 mg • Lipase (vegetarian) 14 mg • Aloe Vera leaf (concentrate 1200) 14 mg. Other Ingredients: Rice Flour, Partially Hydrogenated Cottonseed Oil Kosher, NF, Gelatin Capsule.

FatFree - Starlight International
Each two tablets contain: Maitake Mushroom extract, 4:1 (grifola frondosa, plant) 50 mg • Platycodon grandiflorum extract 5:1 (root) 140 mg • Glucomannan (amorphophalius konjac, root) 1000 mg • Gymnema sylvestre leaf 100 mg. Inactive Ingredients: Dicalcium Phosphate, Microcrystalline Cellulose, Stearic Acid Croscarmellose Sodium, Magnesium Stearate, Silicon Dioxide, Food Glaze, Ethylcellulose, Dextrin, Dextrose, Lecithin, Sodium Citrate.

Fatigue-Aid - Futurebiotics LLC
Two capsules contain: Vitamin C (as buffered calcium ascorbate) 120 mg • Thiamin (as thiamin HCl) 25 mg • Riboflavin 25 mg • Niacin (as niacinamide) 25 mg • Vitamin B6 (as pyridoxine hydrochloride) 25 mg • Vitamin B12 (as cyanocobalamin) 250 mcg • Folic Acid 400 mcg • Pantothenic Acid 25 mg • Selenium (as amino acid chelate) 100 mcg • Citrus Bioflavonoids 250 mg • MSM (methyl-sulfonyl-methane) 200 mg • St. John's Wort powder extract (standardized for 0.3% (0.75 mg) hypericin) 250 mg • Astragalus root powder 200 mg • Pancreatin 4x (quadruple strength) (supplying 1600 USP units Lipase, 10000 USP units Amylase, 10000 USP units Protease) 125 mg • Spirulina 100 mg • Blackstrap Molasses powder 25 mg • Red Beet powder 25 mg • Licorice root powder 25 mg • Siberian Ginseng (50:1) root powder 25 mg. Other Ingredients: Gelatin, Water.
See Editor's Note No. 14.

Fatigued to Fantastic! Daily Energy B Complex - Enzymatic Therapy
Each capsule contains: Thiamin (as thiamin HCl, vitamin B1) 75 mg • Riboflavin (vitamin B2) 75 mg • Niacin (as niacinamide) 50 mg • Vitamin B6 (as pyridoxine HCl) 85 mg • Folic Acid 800 mcg • Vitamin B12 (as cyanocobalamin) 500 mcg • Pantothenic Acid (as calcium D-pantothenate) 50 mg • Choline Bitartrate 100 mg. Other Ingredients: Gelatin, Cellulose, Modified Cellulose Gum, Magnesium Stearate, Titanium Dioxide Color.

Some Brand Name Natural Products - What they Contain

www.NaturalDatabase.com contains MANY more listings than appear here.
Editor's Notes are located on pages 2155-2163.

Fatigued to Fantastic! Daily Energy Enfusion **-** Enzymatic Therapy
Each level scoop (17 g) contains: Vitamin A (as 50% beta carotene and as retinyl acetate) 3500 IU • Vitamin C (ascorbic acid) 750 mg • Vitamin D (as cholecalciferol) 600 IU • Vitamin E (as d-alpha tocopheryl acetate) 100 IU • Biotin 200 mcg • Iodine (as potassium iodide) 150 mcg • Magnesium (as magnesium glycinate) 200 mg • Zinc (as zinc oxide) 15 mg • Selenium (as L-selenomethionine) 200 mcg • Copper (as copper gluconate) 500 mcg • Manganese (as manganese citrate) 4 mg • Chromium (as chromium picolinate) 200 mcg • Molybdenum (as sodium molybdate) 250 mcg • Sodium 20 mg • Potassium (as potassium citrate) 50 mg • Whey Protein 7 g • Malic Acid 900 mg • Inositol 750 mg • Inulin (from chicory root) 750 mg • Hesperidin (50% from citrus fruits) 500 mg • Taurine 500 mg • Glycine 390 mg • L-Tyrosine 377 mg • N-Acetylcysteine (NAC) 250 mg • L-Serine 240 mg • Boron (as sodium borate 2 mg). Other Ingredients: Guar Gum, Natural Flavors, Stevia Leaf.

Fatigued to Fantastic! Revitalizing Sleep Formula **-** Enzymatic Therapy
Each capsule contains: Valerian (valeriana officinalis; root extract standardized to contain a minimum of 0.8% valerenic acids) 200 mg • Passionflower (passiflora incarnata; leaf and flower extract 4:1) 90 mg • L-Theanine (suntheanine brand) 50 mg • Hops (humulus lupulus; flower extract 6.6:1) 30 mg • Wild Lettuce (lactuca virosa; leaf extract) 18 mg • Jamaica Dogwood (piscidia piscipula; root extract) 12 mg. Other Ingredients: Gelatin, Magnesium Stearate, Titanium Dioxide Color, Silicon Dioxide.

FATmelt with Gymnema Sylvestre **-** Slimming and Nutrition Consultancy
Each capsule contains: L-Carnitine • Gymnema Sylvestre • Chromium Picolinate • Forskolii 4:1 extract • Bioperine brand Black Pepper extract. Base: Maltodextrin, Magnesium Stearate base.

FBL101 **-** FBL Sciences LLC
Three capsules contain: Proprietary Blend 1379 mg: Soy, Dong Quai root, Black Cohosh root, Licorice root, Gamma Oryzanol, Red Clover blossoms powder.

FBlock Chitosan Caps **-** Absolute Nutrition
Two capsules contain: Vitamin C (as ascorbic acid) 100 mg • Chitosan (marine fiber concentrate) 1000 mg • Lipase 300 LU • Calcium Sulfate 150 mg • Vegetable Cellulose 100 mg. Other Ingredients: Gelatin, Vegetable Magnesium Stearate, Silica. See Editor's Note No. 37.

FBlock Xtra **-** Absolute Nutrition
Two capsules contain: Vitamin C (as ascorbic acid) 100 mg • Chitosan (marine fiber concentrate) 1000 mg • Lipase 300 LU • Calcium Sulfate 150 mg • Vegetable Cellulose 100 mg. Other Ingredients: Gelatin, Vegetable Magnesium Stearate, Silica.

Feel Good Formula **-** Bee-Alive Inc.
Each capsule contains: Royal Jelly (non-freeze dried) 150 mg.

Feelfine **-** Feelfine
Active Ingredients: Fructose • Glucose • Sodium Bicarbonate • Vitamin C • Potassium Citricity • L-Cysteine • Magnesium Oxide • L-Glutamine • Kolin • Vitamin B1 (thiamine) • Vitamin B6 (pyridoxine) • Tricalciumphosphate. Other Ingredients: Passion Fruit flavor.

Feeling Buzzed Formula **-** Sojourn Health
Six capsules contain: Vitamin B1 (thiamin HCl) 75 mg • Vitamin B2 (riboflavin) 75 mg • Vitamin B3 (niacinamide) 75 mg • Vitamin B6 (pyridoxine HCl) 75 mg • Folic Acid 400 mcg • Vitamin B12 75 mg • Biotin 200 mcg • Vitamin B5 (pantothenic acid) 75 mg • Magnesium (aspartate) 400 mg • Zinc (AA chelate) 15 mg • Chromium (AA chelate) 150 mcg • Proprietary Base 3975 mg: Lecithin, Dandelion, Milk Thistle, Artichoke extract (cynara floridanum), L-Carnitine, Vitamin B10 (PABA), Choline (bitartrate), Inositol.

Feeling Young **-** FreeLife International
Four capsules contain: Vitamin A as Beta-Carotene 5000 IU • Vitamin C (as buffered calcium ascorbate) 100 mg • Vitamin D (as cholecalciferol) 400 IU • Vitamin E (as natural D-alpha tocopheryl succinate) 100 IU • Vitamin K (as phytonadione) 50 mcg • Thiamin (as food-bound thiamin HCl with cocarboxylase coenzyme) 50 mg • Riboflavin (food-bound with riboflavin-5-phosphate coenzyme) 50 mg • Niacin (as food-bound vitamin B3, 50% as niacinamide) 50 mg • Vitamin B6 (as food-bound pyridoxine HCl with pyridoxal-5-phosphate coenzyme) 50 mg • Folate (as food-bound folic acid) 400 mcg • Vitamin B12 (as food-bound cyanocobalamin with cobamamide coenzyme) 100 mcg • Biotin (as food-bound D-biotin) 300 mcg • Pantothenic Acid (as food-bound D-calcium pantothenate with pantethine coenzyme) 50 mg • Calcium (as glycinated purified calcite) 250 mg • Iodine (from kelp) 150 mcg • Magnesium (as glycinated purified magnesite) 100 mg • Zinc (as glycinated zinc citrate) 15 mg • Selenium (as selenomethionine) 100 mcg • Copper (as glycinated copper gluconate) 2 mg • Manganese (as glycinated manganese gluconate) 2.5 mg • Chromium (as patented Chelavite brand chromium dinicotinate glycinate) 200 mcg • Molybdenum (as glycinated molybdenum amino acid chelate) 50 mcg • Potassium (as glycinated potassium citrate) 99 mg • Plant Enzyme Proprietary blend 40,500 units: Alpha-Amylase, Beta-Glucosidase, Cellobiase, Glucoamylase, Cellulase, Hemicellulase, Xylanase, Pectinase, High-Activity Lipase (fatty acid esterase), Acid Protease, Aminopeptidase, Carboxypeptidase, Neutral Protease, Papain, Bromelain • Essential Lipid Complex 460 mg: Fatty Acids and Esters, Soy Activation Complex (purified soy phosphatides), Microencapsulated Flaxseed Oil (source of omega 3 fatty acids), Borage Seed Oil (source of gamma-linolenic acid), Octacosanool (from rice bran) 1000 mcg • Probiotics with growth factors 500 mg: Lactospore brand 100 million microencapsulated active lactobacillus cells • Growth Factor Blend: Vegetable Cellulose, Dahlulin PB brand Chicory, Dahlia Inulin Fructans, Mannanoligosaccharides, Beta-Glucan Soluble Fiber • Fruit and Vegetable Extract Complex 500 mg: Vegetable Fiber, Multi-Fruit and Vegetable extract, Deodorized/Aged Garlic Concentrate, Cabbage, Broccoli, Brussels Sprouts, Kale, Cauliflower, Citrus Bioflavonoids, Strawberry, Cherry, Grape fruit, Bilberry, Grape seed, Cranberry, Carrot, Celery, Parsnip, Soy Isoflavones, Nori, Sea Kelp, Wakame, Kombu, Capsaicin (from cayenne), Lycopene (from tomato), Lutein (from mustard greens), Curcumin (from turmeric) • Herbal Extract Complex 500 mg: Aloe Vera leaf, Ashwagandha root, Astragalus root, Burdock root, Butcher's Broom, Cinnamon bark, Dandelion root, Dong Quai root, Fo Ti root, Ginger root, Hawthorn berry, Ligusticum root, Milk Thistle seed, Schizandra fruit, Wild Yam root • SuperFoods brand Complex 500 mg: Alfalfa sprouts, Barley Grass, Bee Pollen, Blackstrap Molasses, Green Tea, Reishi Mushroom, Shiitake Mushroom • Nutrient Co-factors 275 mg: Inositol, RNA and DNA concentrates, Choline, PABA • Trace Mineral factors 165 mg: Glycinated Boron Chelate, Colloidal Silica, Glycinated Vanadium Amino Acid Chelate • UltraSoy brand 2,500 IU: Soy Polysaccharides, Plant Enzymes. Other Ingredients: Vita-Coat brand (vegetable resin, alpha-lipoic acid).

Fem Balance **-** The Vitamin Shoppe
Each capsule contains: Black Cohosh 20 mg.

Fem Essentials **-** Metagenics
Six tablets contain: Vitamin A (25% [5000 IU] as retinyl acetate and 75% [15,000 IU] as beta carotene) 20,000 IU • Vitamin E (as D-alpha tocopheryl succinate) 100 IU • Vitamin D (as cholecalciferol) 20 IU • Vitamin C (as ascorbic acid) 1200 mg • Niacin (as niacinamide and niacin) 420 mg • Betaine Hydrochloride 325 mg • Choline (as choline bitartrate) 200 mg • Inositol 188 mg • Pantothenic Acid (as D-calcium pantothenate) 200 mg • Bioflavonid Complex 100 mg • Para-Aminobenzoic Acid (PABA) 50 mg • Vitamin B6 (as pyridoxine hydrochloride) 40 mg • Riboflavin 34 mg • Thiamin (as thiamin mononitrate) 30 mg • Folate (as folic acid) 800 mcg • Biotin 300 mcg • Vitamin B12 (as cyanocobalamin) 200 mcg • Calcium (as calcium citrate) 500 mg • Magnesium (as magnesium bis-glycinate, citrate) 250 mg • Potassium (as potassium aspartate) 99 mg • Iron (as iron

BRAND NAME

glycinate) 10 mg • Zinc (as zinc aspartate) 20 mg • Manganese (as manganese aspartate) 1 mg • Copper (as copper lysinate) 2 mg • Chromium (as chromium dinicotinate glycinate) 200 mcg • Selenium (as selenium aspartate) 200 mcg • Iodine (as potassium iodide) 150 mcg • Molybdenum 100 mcg • Vanadium (as vanadyl sulfate) 39 mcg • Quercetin (as quercetin dihydrate) 25 mg • Alpha-Carotene 132 mcg • Cryptoxanthin 32 mcg • Zeaxanthin 28 mcg • Lutein 20 mcg.

Fem Estro **- Metagenics**
Three tablets contain: Vitamin E (as D-alpha tocopheryl succinate) 500 IU • Citrus Bioflavonoid Complex (standardized to 45% full spectrum bioflavonoids) 500 mg • Pantothenic Acid (as D-calcium pantothenate) 300 mg • Para-Aminobenzoic Acid (PABA) 300 mg • Vitamin C (as ascorbic acid) 250 mg • Raw Adrenal Concentrate (bovine) 125 mg • White Korean Ginseng root (panax ginseng) 1000 mg.
See Editor's Note No. 1 and No.14.

Fem Estro HP (formerly HP 3) **- Metagenics**
Each drop contains: Sepia Officinalis 12X • Sanguinaria Canadensis 12X • Sulphuric Acdi 6X • Pulsatilla Pratensis 12X • Lachesis Mutus 12X • Lycopodium Clavatum 6X.

Fem EstroPlex **- Metagenics**
Three tablets contain: Rutin 800 mg • Vitamin C (as ascorbic acid) 300 mg • Pantothenic Acid (as d-calcium pantothenate) 300 mg • Vitamin B6 (as pyridoxine hydrochloride) 50 mg • Vitamin E (as d-alpha tocopheryl succinate) 100 IU • Proprietary Herbal Extract Blend 1050 mg: Dandelion root (taraxacum officinale, 4.5:1 extract), Chasteberry fruit (vitex agnus-castus), Valerian root (valeriana officinalis), Motherwort aerial parts (leonurus cardiaca, 6.5:1 extract), Nettle root (urtica dioica, 10:1 extract).

Fem Fit **- The Sports Nutrition Source, Inc.**
Two scoops contain: Sodium 200 mg • Potassium 400 mg • Protein 26 g • Vitamin A 1675 IU • Vitamin C 20 mg • Calcium 335 mg • Iron 6 mg • Vitamin D 134 IU • Vitamin E 10 IU • Vitamin K 23 mcg • Vitamin B-1 50 mg • Vitamin B-2 57 mg • Vitamin B-3 6.7 mg • Vitamin B-6 670 mcg • Vitamin B-12 3 mcg • Biotin 64 mcg • Zinc 5 mcg • Copper 670 mcg.

Fem Osteo HRT **- Metagenics**
Six tablets contain: Microcrystalline Hydroxyapatite Concentrate (MCHC) 3361 mg • Calcium (as MCHC and dicalcium phosphate) 1515 mg • Phosphorus (as MCHC and dicalcium phosphate) 975 mg • Vitamin A (100% as beta-carotene) 25,000 IU • Vitamin E (as D-alpha tocopheryl succinate) 400 IU • Vitamin D (as cholecalciferol) 400 IU • Ultra Potent-C brand Vitamin C 300 mg • Magnesium (as magnesium bis-glycinate) 200 mg • Niacin (as niacinamide and niacinamide ascorbate) 200 mg • Pantothenic Acid (as D-calcium pantothenate) 150 mg • Vitamin B6 (as pyridoxine hydrochloride) 50 mg • Riboflavin 17 mg • Thiamin (as thiamin mononitrate) 15 mg • Zinc (as zinc glycinate) 15 mg • Copper (as copper glycinate) 2 mg • Manganese (as manganese glycinate) 250 mcg • Folate (as folic acid) 800 mcg • Quercetin (as quercetin dihydrate) 42 mg • Alpha-Carotene 270 mcg • Cryptoxanthin 77 mcg • Zeaxanthin 39 mcg • Lutein 39 mcg.

Fem Premenstrual **- Metagenics**
Six tablets contain: Taurine 300 mg • Vitamin C (as ascorbic acid) 200 mg • Magnesium (as magnesium citrate, bis-glycinate) 200 mg • Choline (as choline bitartrate) 150 mg • Pantothenic Acid (as D-calcium pantothenate) 75 mg • Vitamin B6 (as pyridoxine hydrochloride) 75 mg • Proprietary Herbal Blend 5:1 extract 2000 mg: Bupleurum root (bupleurum chinense), Chinese Peony root (paeonia lactiflora), Dong Quai root (angelica sinensis), Bai-Zhu Atractylodes root (atractylodes macrocephala), Poria Cocos (poria sclerotium), Ginger rhizome (zingiber officinale), Chinese Licorice root (glycyrrhiza uralensis), Chinese Mint leaf (mentha haplocalyx).

Fem Prenatal **- Metagenics**
Each packet contains: Vitamin A (50% as retinyl acetate and 50% as beta-carotene) 8000 IU • Vitamin E (as D-alpha tocopheryl succinate) 30 IU • Vitamin K 65 mcg • Vitamin C (as niacinamide ascorbate) 120 mg • Thiamin (as thiamin mononitrate) 3.4 mg • Riboflavin 3.4 mg • Niacin (as niacinamide ascorbate) 40 mg • Pantothenic Acid (as D-calcium pantothenate) 20 mg • Vitamin B6 (as pyridoxine hydrochloride) 10 mg • Biotin 300 mcg • Folate (as folic acid, L-5-methyl tetrahydrofolate, 5-formyl tetrahydrofolate) 800 mcg • Vitamin B12 (as cyanocobalamin) 12 mcg • Iron (as iron glycinate) 30 mg • Zinc (as zinc glycinate) 25 mg • Copper (as copper lysinate) 2 mg • Manganese (as manganese glycinate) 1.2 mg • Iodine (as potassium iodide) 175 mcg • Selenium (as selenium aspartate) 13 mcg • Molybdenum (as molybdenum aspartate) 25 mcg • Chromium (as chromium dinicotinate glycinate) 25 mcg • Inositol 50 mg • Quercetin (as quercetin dihydrate) 6 mg • Magnesium (as magnesium citrate, bis-glycinate) 250 mg • Calcium (as calcium citrate, dicalcium phosphate, microcrystalline hydroxyapatite concentrate) 520 mg • Phosphorus 160 mg • Vitamin D (as cholcalciferol) 400 IU.

FemActin **- Nature's Plus**
Three capsules contain: Dong Quai (angelica sinensis root, standardized to 0.9% ligustilide) 100 mg • Evening Primrose (oenothera biennis seed, standardized 4% gamma-linolenic acid) 100 mg • Uva Ursi (arctostaphylos uva-ursi leaf, standardized to 20-25% arbutin) 75 mg • Suma (pfaffia paniculata root, standardized to 5% beta-ecdysterone) 50 mg • Butcher's Broom (ruscus aculeatus L. rhizome, standardized to 10% saponin glycosides) 50 mg • Nettle (urtica dioica leaf, standardized 1-2% plant silica) 50 mg • Goldenseal (hydrastis canadensis root & rhizome, standardized to 10% alkaloids, 5% Hydrastine) 50 mg • Chasteberry (vitex agnus-castus fruit, standardized to 0.5% agnuside, 0.6% Aucubin) 50 mg • Vitamin B6 (pyridoxine HCl) 25 mg • Iron (amino acid chelate) 12 mg.

Femaherb **- Wild Rose**
Each tablet contains: Dong Quai root 172 mg • Black Cohosh root 57 mg • Blue Cohosh root 57 mg • Blessed Thistle herb 57 mg • Cramp Bark 57 mg.

Femal **- Natumin Pharma**
Each tablet contains: PI 82 Pollen Pistil extract 120 mg • GC FEM Pollen extract 36 mg • Royal Jelly (freeze dried) 6 mg • Vitamin E (50%) 20 mg. Other Ingredients: Microcrystalline Cellulose 87 mg, Dicalcium Phosphate 87 mg, Magnesium Stearate 4 mg.

Female Advantage **- Body Wise International, Inc.**
Each three capsules contain: Magnesium 15 mg • Zinc 10 mg • Soy Protein Concentrate 516 mg • Valerian root 300 mg • Kava Kava root 250 mg • Alpha-Ketoglutaric Acid 50 mg • Dong Quai root 200 mg • Mexican Yam root 100 mg • Flaxseed 100 mg • Korean Ginseng root 75 mg • Siberian Ginseng root 75 mg • Indole-3-Carbinol 50 mg • L-Arginine HCL 50 mg • L-Lysine HCL 50 mg • Black Cohosh root 50 mg • Evening Primrose seed oil 50 mg • Passion Flower whole plant 50 mg • Suma root 50 mg • Gotu Kola whole plant 50 mg • Bromelain 50 mg • Goldenseal root 50 mg • Echinacea Purpurea root 20 mg • Licorice root 10 mg. Inactive Ingredients: Gelatin, Magnesium Stearate NF, Cellulose.

Female Balance **- Olympia Nutrition**
Borage Oil powder • Wild Yam root • Dong Quai • Vitex Agnus • Vitamin B6.

Female Balance **- Enzymatic Therapy**
Three capsules contain: Vitamin A (Beta Carotene) (Non-toxic form of Vitamin A) 16665 IU • Vitamin E (D-Alpha Tocopherol Succinate) 200 IU • Vitamin C (Ascorbic Acid) 200 mg • Magnesium L-Aspartate 150 mg • Pantothenic Acid (D-Calcium Pantothenate) 100 mg • Thiamine HCL (Vitamin B1) 50 mg • Riboflavin (Vitamin B2) 50 mg • Calcium Citrate 50 mg • Iron (Ferrous Succinate) 18 mg • Zinc (Gluconate) 15 mg • Chromium (Polynicotinate) 250 mcg • Folic Acid 100 mcg • Vitamin B12 (Cyanocobalamin concentrate)

50 mcg • Selenium (L-Selenomethionine) 50 mcg • Dong Quai extract (4:1) (Angelica sinensis) 75 mg • Licorice root extract (Glycyrrhiza glabra) standardized to contain 5% Glycyrrhizic acid) 60 mg • Milk Thistle extract (Silybum Marianum) standardized to contain 70% Silymarin calculated as Silybin) 50 mg • Black Cohosh extract (4:1) (Cimicifuga racemosa) 30 mg • Chaste Berry extract (5:1) (Vitex agnus-castus) 20 mg • Pyridoxal-5'-Phosphate 10 mg.

Female Balance **-** Pro Health
Three capsules contain: Vitamin B6 (as pyridoxine HCl) 50 mg • Folic Acid 400 mcg • Borage oil powder (45 mg GLA) 325 mg • Wild Yam root extract (dioscorea villosa with 6% diosgenin) 225 mg • Dong Quai root 5:1 extract (angelica sinensis) 150 mg • Vitex Agnus Castus extract (0.5% agnusides) 150 mg. Other Ingredients: Rice Flour, Gelatin, Cramp Bark, Silica, Magnesium Stearate.

Female Balance **-** NOW Foods
Three capsules contain: Vitamin B6 50 mg • Folic Acid 400 mcg • Borage oil powder (45 mg GLA) 325 mg • Wild Yam root extract (6% Diosgenin) 225 mg • Dong Quai root extract 5:1 150 mg • Vitex Agnus castus extract 10:1 150 mg.

Female Cycle **-** Enzymes, Inc.
Two capsules contain: Vitamin E (100% from d-alpha Tocopheryl Acid Succinate) 100 IU • Proprietary Herbal Blend 850 mg: Chaste Tree berry extract, Dong Quai Rhizome extract, Cramp bark extract, Black Currant seed extract, Damiana leaf extract, Dandelion leaf extract, Soy Isoflavones • pHysioProtease 80 mg. Other Ingredients: Cellulose, Water.

Female Formula **-** Oasis Wellness Network
Each tablet contains: Vitamin D (as cholecalciferol) 100 IU • Calcium (as citrate/malate/carbonate) 100 mg • Iron (as glyco amino acid chelate) 15 mg • Dong Quai root extract 100 mg • Rehmannia Glutinosa root extract 100 mg • MaxCell Proprietary Blend 100 mg: Zisyphus Jujube, Aloe Vera gel, Piper Nigrum, Glycyrrhiza Glabra • Jujube fruit extract 100 mg • Soy Isoflavone extract. Other Ingredients: Stearic Acid, Cellulose, Magnesium Stearate, Silica, Modified Food Starch.

Female Formula **-** 4 Life
Each capsule contains: Fenugreek seed 85 mg • Black Cohosh root 68 mg • Dong Quai root 68 mg • Ginger root 68 mg • Female Proprietary Extract Blend 45 mg: Black Cohosh root extract, Red Raspberry leaf extract, Dong Quai root extract, Valerian root extract, Fenugreek seed extract, Ginger seed extract, Licorice root extract, Black Hawk bark extract • Red Raspberry leaf extract 33 mg • Licorice root 33 mg. Other Ingredients: Gelatin Capsule, Rice Bran, Magnesium Stearate.

Female Multi Vitamin **-** Health Center for Better Living
Each tablet contains: Vitamin A (as retinyl palmitate and 50% from beta-carotene) 3000 IU • Vitamin C (as ascorbic acid) 100 mg • Vitamin D (as cholecalciferol) 200 IU • Vitamin E (as dl-alpha-tocopheryl acetate) 25 IU • Thiamin (as thiamin HCl) 7 mg • Riboflavin 7 mg • Niacin (as niacinamide) 25 mg • Vitamin B6 (as pyridoxine HCl) 25 mg • Folate (as folic acid) 200 mcg • Vitamin B12 (as cyanocobalamin) 50 mcg • Biotin 35 mcg • Pantothenic Acid (as D-calcium patothenate) 25 mg • Calcium (as dicalcium phosphate) 75 mg • Iron (as ferrous fumarate) 18 mg • Iodine (from Kelp) 25 mcg • Magnesium (as magnesium oxide) 75 mg • Zinc (as zinc citrate) 5 mg • Copper (as copper gluconate) 250 mcg • Manganese (as manganese gluconate) 1 mg • Chromium (as chromium dinicotinate glycinate) 50 mcg • Inositol 10 mg • Choline bitartrate 10 mg • Bioflavonoids Complex: Citrus Bioflavonoids, Hesperidin, Rutin, and Quercetin trace.

Female Sage **-** Traditional Medicinals
Each cup brewed tea contains: Calcium 10 mg • Magnesium 4 mg • Manganese 0.04 mg • Potassium 25 mg • Essential Oil (of sage leaf) 750 mg • Chaste Tree Fruit 75 mg • Chaste Tree Fruit Dry Extract (10:1) 75 mg • Proprietary Blend 600 mg: Blue Vervain Herb, Organic Oatstraw Herb, Organic Lemongrass Leaf, Organic Bitter Fennel Seed, Rosemary Leaf, Organic Blessed Thistle Herb, Organic Stevia Leaf.

Female Support **-** Nutripeak
Fifteen drops contains: Oophorinum Sarcode (Ovary Gland) 8X. Other Ingredients: Purified Water, 20% USP Alcohol.
See Editor's Note No. 1.

Female Toner **-** Traditional Medicinals
Spearmint leaf • Rose Hip • Red Raspberry leaf • Licorice root • Strawberry Leaf • Lemongrass leaf • Lemon Verbena leaf • Nettle leaf • Ginger rhizome • Chamomile flower • Angelica root • Blessed Thistle herb • Cramp bark.

Femaprin **-** Nature's Way
Each capsule contains: Vitamin B6 (as pyridoxine HCl) 100 mg • Vitex Agnus Castus (fruit) 100 mg • Vitex Agnus Castus dried extract (fruit, 0.6% agnusides) 225 mg. Other Ingredients: Gelatin, Magnesium Stearate, Millet.

Femarelle **-** Se-Cure Pharmaceuticals/Ventiv Health
Each capsule contains: Tofu (powder form - DT56a) 322 mg • Flaxseed 108 mg. Other Ingredients: Kosher Gelatin.

Femarin **-** Ortho Molecular Products
Two capsules contain: Gamma Oryzanol 300 mg • Black Cohosh root extract (standardized to congain 2.5% triterpene glycosides) 160 mg • Dong Quai root extract (standardized to contian 1% ligustilide) 75 mg • Licorice root extract (standardized to contain 12% glycyrrhizin) 75 mg • Protykin root 200:1 extract (polygonum cuspidatum) 8 mg. Other Ingredients: Natural Vegetable Capsules, Magnesium Stearate, Microcrystalline Cellulose.

Femarin Classic **-** Ortho Molecular Products
Each capsule contains: Dong Quai root extract (standardized to contain 1% ligustilide) 350 mg • Licorice root extract (standardized to contain 12% glycyrrhizin) 100 mg • Chaste Berry 10:1 extract (standardized to contain 0.5% agnuside) 75 mg • Black Cohosh root 4:1 extract 50 mg • St. John's Wort extract (standardized to contain 0.3% hypericin and 3% hyperforin) 50 mg. Other Ingredients: Natural Vegetable Capsules, Magnesium Stearate, Microcrystalline Cellulose.

Femarone 17 **-** Unknown
Purified Water • Wild Yam extract • Polyacrymide/Isoparrafin/ Laureth-7 • Emulsifying Wax • C 12-15 Alkyl Benzoate • Glyceryl Stearate/PEG-100 Stearate • Progesterone (from wild yam) • Chaste Tree berry extract (vitex) • Glycerin / Alcohol • Jojoba oil • Swalane • Allantoin • Water/Phospholipids • Retinyl Palmitate • Ascorbyl Palmitate • A-Alpha Tocopherol • Liposomes of Vitamin A, C & E • Dong Quai extract • Licorice extract • Black Cohosh extract • Grapefruit seed extract • Sorbic Acid.

Fematril **-** Optimal Therapeutics
Three capsules contain: Clovevine powder 500 mg • Damiana leaf 4:1 extract 480 mg • Muira Puama 4:1 extract 260 mg • Di-Arginine Malate 250 mg • Avena Sativa 10:1 extract (oat straw) 150 mg • Catuaba bark 4:1 extract 150 mg • Cnidium Monnier 25 mg • Bioperine brand Piperine extract 3 mg. Other Ingredients: Gelatin, Cellulose, Magnesium Stearate.

Femdiol **-** PhytoPharmica
Each capsule contains: Vitamin E (D-Alpha Tocopherol) 150 IU • Barlean's Flaxseed oil 300 mg • Gamma-Oryzanol 100 mg • Pumpkin seed oil (Curcurbita pepo) 50 mg • Soy extract 20 mg.

FemEssence **-** Advocare International
Three capsules contain: Niacin 20 mg • Vitamin B6 30 mg • Iron (as ferrous glycinate Ferrochel) 13.5 mg • Glucosamine (as HCl) 500 mg • Moomiyo 100 mg • Wild Yam extract (root - Dioscorea floribunda) 100 mg • Saw Palmetto extract (fruit - serenoa repens) 60 mg • Ginkgo extract (leaf - ginkgo biloba) 75 mg • Cranberry extract (fruit - vaccinium macrocarpon) 200 mg • Raspberry extract

BRAND NAMES

(leaf - rubus idaeus) 50 mg • Resveratrol (from polygonum cuspidatum) 5 mg • Lactobacillus Acidophilus 200 MM. Other Ingredients: Silicon Dioxide, Magnesium Stearate, Gelatin.

FemFactor - HealthMinded
Each capsule contains: Proprietary Blend 550 mg: Sage leaf, Red Raspberry leaf, Pueraria root, Red Clover, Cayenne pepper, Licorice root, Bayberry fruit, Damiana leaf, Valerian root, Ginger root, Black Cohosh root.

FEMFOCUS - Solgar
Three tablets contain: Protein 1 g • Vitamin A (as palmitate 5000 IU, 75% as natural beta-carotene from D.salina) 20000 IU • Vitamin C (as L-ascorbic acid) 400 mg • Vitamin D (as cholecalciferol) 400 IU • Vitamin E (as D-alpha tocopheryl succinate) 400 IU • Vitamin K (as phytonadione) 20 mcg • Thiamin (as thiamin mononitrate) 50 mg • Riboflavin 50 mg • Niacin (as niacinamide) 60 mg • Vitamin B-6 (as pyridoxine HCl) 50 mg • Folic Acid 800 mcg • Vitamin B-12 (as cobalamin) 200 mcg • Biotin (as D-biotin) 300 mcg • Pantothenic Acid (as D-ca pantothenate) 80 mg • Calcium (as calcium carbonate, glycinate, citrate) 400 mg • Iron (as iron bisglycinate) 18 mg • Iodine (as kelp) 150 mcg • Magnesium (as magnesium oxide, glycinate, citrate) 400 mg • Zinc (as zinc glycinate, histidinate) 30 mg • Selenium (as L-selenomethionine) 200 mcg • Copper (as copper glycinate) 1.5 mg • Manganese (as manganese glycinate) 2 mg • Chromium (as chromium nicotinoglycinate) 200 mcg • Molybdenum (as molybdenum glycinate) 50 mcg • Sodium 25 mg • Potassium (as potassium glycinate complex) 99 mg • Citrus Bioflavonoids 100 mg • Choline (as choline bitartrate) 100 mg • Inositol 100 mg • Pantethine 7 mg • Cocarboxylase 6 mg • Pyridoxal-5-Phosphate 6 mg • Riboflavin-5-Phosphate 6 mg • Dibencozide 21 mcg • Boron (as boron glycinate complex) 500 mcg • Dong Quai extract root (angelica sinensis) 25 mg • Uva Ursi extract leaf (arcostaphylos uva ursi) 25 mg • Chaste berry extract (vitex agnus-castus) 25 mg • American Ginseng extract root 25 mg • Milk Thistle extract aerial (silybum marianum) 25 mg • Black Cohosh extract root (cimicifuga racemosa) 25 mg • Soy Isoflavone extract seed 25 mg • Carotenoid Mix (alpha carotene, lutein, zeaxanthin, cryptoxanthin) 172 mcg. Other Ingredients: Microcrystalline Cellulose, Vegetable Cellulose, Vegetable Stearic Acid, Red Beet Powder, Titanium Dioxide, Vegetable Glycerin, Silica, Vegetable Magnesium Stearate.

FEMFOCUS Black Cohosh - Solgar
Each vegicap contains: Black Cohosh extract root (triterpine glycosides 5 mg as 27-deoxyactein) 200 mg •Raw Black Cohosh powder root 200 mg • Soy Isoflavone concentrate seed (isoflavone 6 mg) 200 mg. Other Ingredients: Microcrystalline Cellulose; Vegetable Cellulose; Vegetable Magnesium Stearate; Vegetable Glycerin; Phyt02X Blend: Vitamin E, Beta Carotene and other Carotenoids, Rosemary extract aerial, Vitamin C (L-Ascorbic Acid), Water.

FEMFOCUS Bone Support - Solgar
Four tablets contain: Vitamin D (as cholecalciferol) 600 IU •Vitamin K (as phytonadione) 80 mcg •Calcium (as calcium carbonate, glycinate, citrate) 800 mg •Iron 0.7 mg •Magnesium (as magnesium glycinate, citrate, oxide) 400 mg •Zinc (as zinc glycinate, histidinate) 10 mg •Copper (as copper lysinate) 0.5 mg •Sodium 20 mg •Ipriflavone (as 7-isopropoxyisoflavone) 600 mg •Soy Isoflavone Concentrate seed 400 mg •Boron (as boron glycinate complex) 1.5 mg. Other Ingredients: Microcrystalline Cellulose; Vegetable Cellulose; Methacrylic Acid; Vegetable Magnesium Stearate; Vegetable Stearic Acid; Glyceryl Triacetate; Vegetable Glycerin; PhytO2X Blend: Vitamin E, Beta-Carotene and other Carotenoids, Rosemary extract aerial, Vitamin C (L-Ascorbic Acid), Annatto, Grapeskin.

FEMFOCUS Calcium Citrate - Solgar
Four tablets contain: Vitamin D (as cholecalciferol) 600 IU •Calcium (as calcium citrate) 1000 mg. Other Ingredients: Microcrystalline Cellulose, Silica, Vegetable Magnesium Stearate, Titanium Dioxide, Vegetable Cellulose, Vegetable Glycerin.

FEMFOCUS Cranberry Berry Extract - Solgar
Each vegicap contains: Cranberry extract berry (organic acids 30 mg) 100 mg •Cranberry concentrate powder berry 300 mg. Other Ingredients: Vegetable Cellulose; Microcrystalline Cellulose; Silica; Vegetable Magnesium Stearate; Vegetable Glycerin; PhytO2X Blend: Vitamin E, Beta-Carotene and other Carotenoids, Rosemary extract aerial, Vitamin C, Water.

FEMFOCUS Cranberry Extract with Vitamin C - Solgar
Each vegicap contains: Vitamin C (as L-ascorbic acid) 60 mg •Cranberry extract berry 400 mg. Other Ingredients: Vegetable Cellulose, Silica, Vegetable Magnesium Stearate, Vegetable Glycerin, Water.

FEMFOCUS Dong Quai - Solgar
Each vegicap contains: Dong Quai extract root 150 mg •Raw Dong Quai powder root 300 mg. Other Ingredients: Microcrystalline Cellulose; Vegetable Cellulose; Vegetable Magnesium Stearate; Vegetable Glycerin; Phyt02X Blend: Vitamin E, Beta Carotene and other Carotenoids, Rosemary extract aerial, Vitamin C (L-Ascorbic Acid), Water.

FEMFOCUS Ester-C Plus - Solgar
Each vegicaps contain: Vitamin C (as Ester-C calcium ascorbate) 500 mg •Calcium (as calcium ascorbate) 62 mg •Citrus Bioflavonoids 25 mg •Acerola 10 mg •Rose Hips fruit 10 mg •Rutin 5 mg. Other Ingredients: Vegetable Cellulose, Vegetable Magnesium Stearate, Silica, L-Threonic Acid, Vegetable Glycerin, Water.

FEMFOCUS Evening Primrose Oil - Solgar
Each softgel contains: Vitamin E (as D-alpha tocopheryl acetate) 14 IU • Linoleic Acid 360 mg •Gamma-Linolenic Acid 50 mg • Oleic Acid 50 mg •Other Fatty Acids 40 mg. Other Ingredients: Evening Primrose Oil, Gelatin, Glycerin, Water.

FEMFOCUS Flaxseed Oil - Solgar
Two softgels contain: Linolenic Acid 1425 mg •Oleic Acid 450 mg •Linoleic Acid 400 mg •Palmitic Acid 150 mg •Stearic Acid 75 mg. Other Ingredients: Flaxseed Oil, Gelatin, Glycerin, Carob Flavor, Water.

FEMFOCUS Folic Acid - Solgar
Each tablet contains: Folic Acid 400 mcg • Calcium (as dicalcium phosphate) 70 mg. Other Ingredients: Vegetable Stearic Acid, Silica, Vegetable Cellulose.

FEMFOCUS Gentle Iron - Solgar
Each vegicap contains: Iron (as iron bisglycinate) 25 mg. Other Ingredients: Microcrystalline Cellulose, Vegetable Cellulose, Vegetable Magnesium Stearate, Vegetable Glycerin, Water.

FEMFOCUS Herbal Female Complex - Solgar
Each vegicap contains: Iron 1 mg • Standardized Chaste berry extract 75 mg • Dong Quai extract root 75 mg •Soy Isoflavone extract seed 100 mg • Milk Thistle extract aerial, seed (silymarin 40 mg) 50 mg •Black Cohosh extract root 100 mg •Motherwort extract aerial 75 mg •Raw Astragalus powder root 75 mg •Raw Korean Ginseng powder root 50 mg •Raw Dong Quai powder root 50 mg. Other Ingredients: Microcrystalline Cellulose; Vegetable Cellulose; Vegetable Stearic Acid; Vegetable Magnesium Stearate; Vegetable Glycerin; Phyt02X Blend: Vitamin E, Beta-Carotene and other Carotenoids, Rosemary extract aerial, Vitamin C (L-Ascorbic Acid), Water.

FEMFOCUS Ipriflavone - Solgar
Each vegicap contains: Ipriflavone (as 7-isopropoxyisoflavone) 200 mg. Other Ingredients: Microcrystalline Cellulose, Vegetable Cellulose, Vegetable Magnesium Stearate, Vegetable Glycerin, Water.

FEMFOCUS Non-GMO Isoflavones - Solgar
Each tablet contains: Total Soy Isoflavones seed (from soy isoflavone extract) 38 mg. Other Ingredients: Microcrystalline Cellulose, Vegetable Cellulose, Silica, Vegetable Magnesium Stearate, Caramel, Titanium Dioxide, Vegetable Glycerin.

Some Brand Name Natural Products - What they Contain

www.NaturalDatabase.com contains MANY more listings than appear here.
Editor's Notes are located on pages 2155-2163.

FEMFOCUS Oceanic Silica **-** Solgar
Each vegicap contains: Calcium 30 mg •Silica (from red algae powder, 25 mg elemental silicon) 54 mg. Other Ingredients: Vegetable Cellulose, Microcrystalline Cellulose, Vegetable Magnesium Stearate, Vegetable Glycerin, Water.

FEMFOCUS Prenatal Tablets **-** Solgar
Four tablets contain: Vitamin A (as palmitate 3000 IU, 63% as natural beta-carotene from d. salina) 8000 IU • Vitamin C (as l-ascorbic acid) 100 mg • Vitamin D (as cholecalciferol) 400 IU • Vitamin E (as d-alpha tocopheryl succinate) 30 IU • Thiamin (as thiamin mononitrate) 1.7 mg • Riboflavin 2 mg • Niacin (as niacinamide) 20 mg • Vitamin B6 (as pyridoxine HCl) 2.5 mg • Folic Acid 800 mcg • Vitamin B12 (as cobalamin) 8 mcg • Biotin 300 mcg • Pantothenic Acid (as d-ca pantothenate) 10 mg • Calcium (as calcium carbonate, calcium citrate) 1300 mg • Iron (as iron bisglycinate) 27 mg • Iodine (as kelp) 150 mcg • Magnesium (as magnesium oxide, magnesium citrate) 450 mg • Zinc (as zinc chelate, zinc oxide) 15 mg • Copper (as copper chelate, copper gluconate) 2 mg • Selenium (as l-selenomethionine) 25 mcg • Manganese (as manganese chelate, manganese gluconate) 2 mg • Chromium (as chromium picolinate) 25 mcg • Potassium (from potassium amino acid complex, potassium gluconate) 50 mg • Inositol 10 mg • Choline (as choline bitartrate) 4 mg • PABA (as para aminobenzoic acid) 2 mg • Alpha Carotene 114 mcg • Cryptoxanthin 28 mcg • Zeaxanthin 23 mcg • Lutein 18 mcg • Soy Protein Isolate/Amino Acid Blend 160 mg: L-Glutamic Acid, L-Aspartic Acid, L-Leucine, L-Arginine, L-Lysine, L-Phenylalanine, L-Serine, L-Proline, L-Valine, L-Isoleucine, L-Alanine, Glycine, L-Threonine, L-Tyrosine, L-Histidine, L-Cysteine, L-Methionine, L-Ornithine, Taurine. Other Ingredients: Microcrystalline Cellulose, Vegetable Cellulose, Vegetable Stearic Acid, Grape skin, Titanium Dioxide, Silica, Vegetable Magnesium Stearate, Vegetable Glycerin.

FEMFOCUS Red Clover **-** Solgar
Each vegicap contains: Standardized Red Clover extract leaf (biochanin A 3 mg) 250 mg •Raw Red Clover powder leaf 225 mg. Other Ingredients: Vegetable Cellulose; Vegetable Magnesium Stearate; Vegetable Glycerin; PhytO2X Blend: Vitamin E, Beta-Carotene and other Carotenoids, Rosemary extract aerial, Vitamin C (L-absorbic acid), Water.

FEMFOCUS Super GLA **-** Solgar
Each softgel contains: Linoleic Acid 498 mg •Gamma-Linolenic Acid 300 mg •Other Fatty Acids 296 mg •Oleic Acid 206 mg • Borage Oil 1300 mg. Other Ingredients: Gelatin, Glycerin, Water.

FEMFOCUS Vitamin B12 **-** Solgar
Each nugget contains: Vitamin B-12 (as cobalamin) 1000 mcg. Other Ingredients: Mannitol, Vegetable Magnesium Stearate, Vegetable Stearic Acid, Natural Cherry Flavor.

FEMFOCUS Vitamin B-6 **-** Solgar
Each tablet contains: Vitamin B-6 (as pyridoxine HCl) 50 mg • Calcium (as dicalcium phosphate) 50 mg. Other Ingredients: Dicalcium Phosphate, Vegetable Stearic Acid, Vegetable Magnesium Stearate, Vegetable Cellulose.

FEMFOCUS Vitamin K **-** Solgar
Each tablet contains: Calcium (as dicalcium phosphate) 90 mg •Vitamin K (as phytonadione) 100 mcg. Other Ingredients: Vegetable Cellulose, Vegetable Stearic Acid, Vegetable Magnesium Stearate.

Fem-Gest **-** Progressive Labs
Ingredients: Stabilized Aloe Vera gel • Mexican Yam extract • Chamomile extract • Chaste Tree berry • Tocopheryl Acetate • Lavender extract • Jojoba oil • Safflower oil • Progesterone 950 mg • Carbomer 940 • Glyceryl Stearate (and) PEG-100 Stearate • C12-15 Alkyl Benzoate • Stearic Acid • Octyl Palmitate • Triethanolamine •Cetyl Alcohol • Methylparaben • Tetrasodium EDTA • Dimethicone • Propylparaben • Diazolidyl Urea.

FemGest Cream **-** Home Health Products, Inc.
Water • Vitamin E Acetate • Stearic Acid • Cetyl Alcohol • Glyceryl Stearate • Grapefruit Extract • Octyl Palmitate • Cetyl Esters • Progesterone • Aloe Vera Gel • Glycerin • Keratin • Propylene Glycol • Polysorbate 80 • Diazolidinylurea • Carbomer • Sweet Almond Oil • Triethanolamine • Methylparaben • Panthenol • Sodium Hyaluronate • Propylparaben.

FEM-H **-** MMS Pro
Each capsule contains: Black Cohosh root • Sarsaparilla root • Siberian Ginseng root • Licorice root • Blessed Thistle herb • Squaw Vine • False Unicorn root.

Feminene Female Support Formula **-** Market America, Inc.
Two tablets contain: Thiamin HCl (vitamin B1) 20 mg • Riboflavin (vitamin B2) 20 mg • Niacin (vitamin B3) 20 mg • D-Calcium Pantothenate (vitamin B5) 11.8 mg • Pyridoxine HCl (vitamin B6) 10 mg • Folic Acid 400 mcg • Cyanocobalamin (vitamin B12) 200 mcg • D-Alpha-Tocopherol (vitamin E) 50 IU • Soy extract (soy isoflavones, 3%) 200 mg • Dong Quai root 1% extract 200 mg • Evening Primrose oil 200 mg • Wild Yam 180 mg • Black Cohosh root 2.5% extract 160 mg • Chaste berry extract (vitex agnus-castus) 150 mg • Horsetail 150 mg • Red Clover 140 mg • Passiflora 120 mg • Valerian root 120 mg • Sage 100 mg • St. John's Wort 70 mg. Other Ingredients: Dicalcium Phosphate, Microcrystalline Cellulose, Stearic Acid, Magnesium Stearate, Croscarmellose Sodium, Silicon Dioxide.

FeminEstra **-** Pacific BioLogic
Poria Plant Fungus (hoelen) • Polygonum root (thin) • Moutan Root bark • Chinese Yam • Cherry (cornelian asiatic) • Rehmannia root (fresh) • Rehmannia root (cooked in wine) • Curculigo rhizome • Alisma (water plantain rhizome) • Pearl No Concentration.

FeminiCare **-** DreamPharm
Two capsules contain: Proprietary Blend: Astragalus radix, Ginseng radix, Atractylodes rhizoma, Sclerotium Poriae Cocos, Ziziphi semen, Longanae Arillus, Angelica Sinensis radix, Polygala radix, Glycyrrhiza radix, Saussurea radix, Zingiberis radix, Zizyphi fructus.

FeminiMate **-** DreamPharm
Two capsules contain: Proprietary Blend: Myrrha, Forsythiae Suspensae fructus, Glycyrrhizae radix, Coisis semen, Gardeniae fructus, Talcum, Scirpi rhizoma, Mantidis Vagina Oyorum, Phellodentri cortex, Sargentodoxa Cuneata, Patrinia Scabiosaefolia, Bullrush pollen, Dandelion, Ailanthus Altissima.

Feminine Balance **-** Advocare International
Two capsules contain: Pantothenic Acid 30 mg • Pyridoxine (as HCl) 12 mg • Vitamin E (as d-alpha tocopheryl succinate) 10 IU • Red Clover extract (flower/leaf - trifolium pratense) 500 mg • Black Cohosh extract (root - cimicifuga racemosa) 75 mg • Dong Quai extract (root - angelica plymorpha) 50 mg • Chaste Tree extract (berry - vitex agnus-castus) 200 mg. Other Ingredients: Silicon Dioxide, Magnesium Stearate, Gelatin.

Femme Advantage Creatine Serum **-** Muscle Marketing USA
Each serving contains: Creatine Monohydrate • Vitamin B12 • Ginseng • Royal Jelly • Vitamin B5 • Soluable Bioflavonoids • Ginkgo extract • Wild Yam extract • Papain extract.

Femme Alzare **-** Alpha Male Nutrition
Each tablet contains: Yohimbe bark extract (15:1) 400 mg • Maca extract (6:1) 250 mg • Arginine Alpha Ketoglutarate 190 mg • Arginine Ketoisocaproate 10 mg • 4-Androstenediol 2 mg • Bioperine brand Black Pepper extract 10 mg • Deer Antler 100 mg • Proprietary Blend 45 mg: Korean Ginseng powder, Siberian Ginseng powder, Tribulus Terrestris powder, Dong Quai powder, White Peony root powder, Lycium powder, Wild Yam powder, Sarsaparilla powder, Black Cohosh powder, Damiana powder. Other Ingredients: Gelatin, Magnesium Stearate, Stearic Acid, Microcrystalline Cellulose.
See Editor's Note No. 54.

Some Brand Name Natural Products - What they Contain

www.NaturalDatabase.com contains MANY more listings than appear here.
Editor's Notes are located on pages 2155-2163.

Fem-Mend Formula - Nature's Way
Two capsules contain: Proprietary Formula: Blessed Thistle • Cayenne pepper fruit • Cramp bark • False Unicorn root • Ginger • Goldenseal stem, leaf, flower • Red Raspberry leaves • Squaw Vine vine, leaf, fruit • Uva Ursi leaves. Other Ingredients: Gelatin.

FemPrep - HealthMinded
Each capsule contains: FemPrep Proprietary Blend 550 mg: Sage leaf dried extract, Red Raspberry leaf dried extract, Kudzue root dried extract, Red Clover flowers dried extract, Bayberry root bark, Cayenne Pepper fruit, Damiana leaf dried extract, Licorice root, Valerian root, Black Cohosh root, Ginger root. Other Ingredients: Gelatin, Stearic Acid, Magnesium Stearate.

FemRatio - Life Enhancement Products, Inc.
Four capsules contain: Vitamin C (as ascorbic acid and ascorbigen) 110 mg • Vitamin B12 (cyanocobalamin) 400 mcg • Iodine (as potassium iodide) 100 mcg • Selenium (as sodium selenite) 250 mcg • Vitex Agnus-Castus extract 1000 mg • Indole-3-Carbinol 200 mg • Diindolylmethane 80 mg • DHEA (dehydroepiandrosterone) 10 mg.

Fem-Restore - Gaia Herbs
Two capsules contain: Fraxinu bark (fraxinum americana) 60 mg • Red Root (ceanothus americanus) 40 mg • Mayapple rhizome (podophyllum peltatum) 30 mg • True Unicorn root (aletris farinosa) 20 mg • Black Haw root (viburnum prunifolium) 20 mg • Goldenseal rhizome (hydrastis canadensis) 20 mg • Corydalis root (corydalis yanhusuo) 16 mg • Butterbur root (petasites hybridus) 16 mg • Ginger rhizome (zingiber officinale) 14 mg • Lobelia herb and seed (lobelia inflata) 10 mg. Other Ingredients: Vegetable Glycerin, Vegetable Cellulose (capsule).

Fem-Restore Supreme - Gaia Herbs
Thirty drops contain: Proprietary Blend 35 mg: Fraxinus bark (fraxinus americana), Red Root (ceanothus americanus), Mayapple rhizome (podophyllum peltatum), True Unicorn root (aletris farinosa), Black Haw root (viburnum prunifolium), Goldenseal rhizome (hydrastis canadensis), Corydalis root (corydalis yanhusuo), Butterbur root (petasites frigida), Ginger rhizome (zingiber officinale), Lobelia herb/seed (lobelia inflata), 45-55% Pure Grain Alcohol USP, Spring Water.

FemRite - 4 Life
Purified Water • Wild Yam concentrate (dioscorea villosa) • Glyceryl Stearate • Cetyl Alcohol • Glycerin • Sodium Behenoyl Lactylate • USP Natural Progesterone (from soy) • Aloe Barbadensis gel • Cucumber extract (cucumis sativus) • Jojoba oil (buxus chinensis) • Hydrid Sunflower oil (helianthus annus) • Avocado extract (persea gratissima) • NaPCA • Sodium Hyaluronate • Hydrolyzed Glycosaminoglycans • Sodium Lactate • Sorbitol • Proline • D-Tocopheryl Acetate • Disodium EDTA • Propylene Glycol • Diazolidinyl Urea • Methylparaben • Propylparaben.

FemTone - PhytoPharmica
Two capsules contain: Black Cohosh root 4:1 extract (cimicifuga racemosa) 50 mg • Chaste Tree berry extract (vitex agnus-castus, standardized to contain 0.5% agnusides) 50 mg • Dong Quai root 3.2:1 extract (angelica sinensis) 250 mg • False Unicorn root 3:1 extract (chamaelirium luteum) 50 mg • Fennel seed 3.9:1 extract (foeniculum vulgare) 25 mg • Hesperidin 50% (from citrus fruits) 200 mg • Licorice root and rhizome extract (glycyrrhiza glabra, standardized to contin 5% glycyrrhizic acid) 50 mg • Vitamin C (ascorbic acid) 100 mg.

Femtrol - Enzymatic Therapy
Two capsules contain: Vitamin C (Ascorbic Acid) 100 mg. Other Ingredients: Dong Quai extract 4:1 (Angelica sinensis) 250 mg • Hesperidin Complex standardized to contain 50% Bioflavonoids 200 mg • Licorice root extract (Glycyrrhiza glabra) standardized to contain 5% Glycyrrhizic Acid 50 mg • Chaste Tree Berry extract 5:1 (Vitex agnus-castus) 50 mg • Black Cohosh root extract 4:1 (Cimicifuga racemosa) 50 mg • False Unicorn root extract 4:1 (Helonias opulus) 50 mg • Fennel seed extract 6:1 (Foeniculum vulgare) 25 mg.

Fen-Cho - Standard Process, Inc.
Two capsules contain: Proprietary Blend 700 mg: Collinsonia root, Fenugreek seed, Okra, Purified Bovine Bile Salts • Sodium 100 mg • Potassium 5 mg. Other Ingredients: Gelatin, Exsiccated Disodium Phosphate, Water, Colors, Calcium Stearate.

Fen-Gre - Standard Process, Inc.
Three capsules contain: Proprietary Blend 1268 mg: Fenugreek seed, Okra, Rice bran. Other Ingredients: Gelatin, Water, Calcium Stearate, Colors.

Fennel Wild Yam Supreme - Gaia Herbs
Thirty drops contain: Proprietary Blend 50 mg: Fennel seed (foeniculum vulgare), Wild Yam root (dioscorea villosa), Mayapple root (pdophyllum peltatum), Dandelion leaf and root (taraxacum officinalis), Fresh Celandine roots and tops (chelidonium major), Fresh California Poppy (eschscholzia californica), Peppermint oil (mentha piperita), 40-50% Pure Grain Alcohol USP, Spring Water.

Fennel-Yam - Atrium Biotechnologies
Each capsule contains: Fennel 250 mg •Wild Yam 250 mg.

Fen-Tastic - The Vitamin Shoppe
Two tablets contain: St. John's Wort root standardized for 3% hypericin 400 mg • Citrus Aurantium fruit 600 mg • 5-HTP 150 mg • Yerba Santa • Mate leaves standardized 20% methylzanthine 250 mg • White Willow bark 400 mg.
See Editor's Note No. 40.

Fenucin - Ortho Molecular Products
Each rounded scoop contains: FenuLife brand Fenugreek extract (contains 75% soluble fiber) 2000 mg • Cinnamon bark 1000 mg • Cinnulin brand Cinnamon bark extract 200 mg. Other Ingredients: Apple Fruit Extract, Stevia Leaf Extract.

Fenugreek - Nature's Way
Two capsules contain: Fenugreek seed 1.22 g. Other Ingredients: Gelatin.

Fenugreek & Thyme - Nature's Sunshine
Two capsules contain: Proprietary Blend 950 mg: Fenugreek seed (trigonella foenum-graecum), Thyme herb (thymus vulgaris). Other Ingredients: Kosher Gelatin, Water.

Fenugreek (Trigonella foenum-graecum) - Solgar
Each capsule contains: Fenugreek seed 4:1 extract 150 mg • Raw Fenugreek seed powder 370 mg. Other Ingredients: Vegetable Cellulose, Water, Vegetable Glycerin.

Fenugreek 1000mg - Nature's Own
Each tablet contains: Fenugreek dry seed powder (trigonella foenum-graecum) 1000 mg.

Fenugreek 85 - Pure Encapsulations
Each vegetable capsule contains: Fenugreek extract (trigonella foenum-graecum L., standardized to contain 85% total dietary fiber, typically providing 70% soluble fiber) 750 mg • Vitamin C (as ascorbyl palmitate) 15 mg.

Fenugreek Plus - Metagenics
Two capsules contain: Fenugreek seed 6.5:1 extract (trigonella foenum-graecum, containing a minimum of 70% [700 mg] soluble fiber) 1000 mg • Bitter Gourd fruit 10:1 extract (momordica charantia, standardized to 2.5% [3.8 mg] bitter principles) 152 mg • Gymnema leaf 10:1 extract (gymnema sylvestra, standardzied to 24% [24 mg] gymnemic acids) 100 mg.

Fenugreek Seed - Motherlove Herbal Co.
Each 2 oz bottle contains: Fenugreek seed. Base: Certified Kosher Alcohol, Glycerin.

Fenu-Thyme Formula - Nature's Way
Two capsules contain: Proprietary Formula: Fenugreek seed • Thyme leaf. Other Ingredients: Gelatin.

Feosol **-** SmithKline Beecham
Each tablet contains: Iron 65 mg. Inactive Ingredients: Calcium Sulfate, Starch, Glucose, Hydroxypropyl Methylcellulose, Talc, Stearic Acid, Polyethylene Glycol, Sodium Lauryl Sulfate, Mineral Oil, Titanium Dioxide, FD&C Yellow #10, FD&C Blue #2.

Fermalac Vaginal **-** Rougier Pharma
Each capsule contains: Over 2 billion fully viable bacilli (lyophilized cultures): Lactobacillus acidophilus, Lactobacillus bulgaricus, Streptococcus lactic (var. thermophilus).

Fermented Soy Essence **-** Jarrow Formulas
Organic Soy Milk Yogurt fermented with Lactobacillus Acidophilus, Lactobacillus Bulgaricus, Lactobacillus Casie, Lactobacillus Plantarum, S. Thermophilus, Apple Pectin, L-Selenomethionine, Folic Acid, L-Methionine • Fibersol-2 brand indigestible Starch • Magnesium Citrate • Bromelain • Papain • Lecithin (non-GMO) • Natural Vanilla flavor • Natural Lo Han Kuo extract (momordica grosvenorii).

Feroglobin B12 Capsules **-** Vitabiotics
Each capsule contains: Iron 24 mg • Zinc 12 mg • Copper 2 mg • Folic Acid 500 mcg • Vitamin B12 10 mcg • Vitamin B6 5 mg.

Feroglobin B12 Liquid **-** Vitabiotics
Five milliliters contain: Vitamin B1 4 mg • Vitamin B2 1 mg • Vitamin B6 2 mg • Vitamin B12 5 mcg • Vitamin C 10 mg • Folic Acid 150 mcg • Pantothenic Acid 2 mg • Calcium Glycerophosphate 10 mg • Niacin (vitamin B3) 8 mg • Iron 7 mg • Zinc 5 mg • Copper 0.25 mg • Manganese 0.25 mg • Lysine 40 mg • Iodine 40 mcg • Honey 100 mg • Malt 500 mg.

FerroComp **-** PhytoPharmica
Each capsule contains: Vitamin C (Ascorbic Acid) 60 mg • Iron (Ferrous Succinate) 25 mg • Folic Acid 200 mcg • Vitamin B12 (Cyanocobalamin) 100 mcg • Liquid Liver Fractions (predigested soluble concentrate) 250 mg • Chlorophyll (Fat-Soluble) 5 mg. See Editor's Note No. 14.

Ferrofood **-** Standard Process, Inc.
Each capsule contains: Proprietary Blend 405 mg: Bovine Liver, Bovine Bone, Carbamide, Defatted Wheat germ, Porcine Duodenum, Bovine Spleen PMG extract, Bovine Adrenal, Carrot root, Oat flour, Veal Bone meal, Choline Bitartrate, Bovine Spleen, Ovine Spleen, Citric Acid, Porcine Stomach Parenchyma, Dried Alfalfa juice, Mushroom, Tillandsia Usneoides, Peanut bran, Dicalcium Phosphate, Licorice root, Potassium Para-Aminobenzoate, Magnesium Citrate, Flaxseed oil extract, Bovine Liver fat extract, Mixed Tocopherols • Vitamin C 30 mg • Vitamin B12 1.7 mcg • Iron 10 mg • Sodium 10 mg. Other Ingredients: Gelatin, Water, Colors. See Editor's Note No. 14.

Ferro-Sequels **-** Inverness Medical Innovations, Inc.
Each tablet contains: Iron 50 mg. Inactive Ingredients: Lactose, Ferrous Fumarate (equivalent to 50 mg of Elemental Iron), Microcrystalline Cellulose, Hydroxypropyl Methylcellulose, Docusate Sodium, Magnesium Stearate, Sodium Benzoate, Silicon Dioxide, Sodium Triethyl Citrate, Titanium Dioxide, Yellow #10, Blue #1, Sodium Lauryl Sulfate.

Ferrous Gluconate **-** Puritan's Pride
Each tablet contains: Iron (from 246 mg of ferrous gluconate) 28 mg. Other Ingredients: Cellulose (plant origin), Dicalcium Phosphate, Vegetable Stearic Acid, Cellulose Coating, Croscarmellose, Vegetable Magnesium Stearate.

Ferrous Gluconate **-** Walgreens
Each tablet contains: Iron (ferrous sulfate 240 mg) 27 mg. Other Ingredients: Dicalcium Phosphate, Microcrystalline Cellulose, Modified Cellulose Gum, Hydroxypropyl Methylcellulose, Crospovidone, Stearic Acid, Titanium Dioxide, FD&C Yellow No. 5 Lake Tartrazine, FD&C Blue No. 1 Lake, Propylene Glycol, Magnesium Stearate, Polyethylene Glycol, Silicon Dioxide, Sodium Lauryl Sulfate.

Ferrous Gluconate 28 mg Iron **-** Nature's Bounty
Each tablet contains: Iron (from 246 mg of ferrous gluconate) 28 mg. Other Ingredients: Cellulose (plant origin), Dicalcium Phosphate, Vegetable Stearic Acid, Cellulose Coating, Croscarmellose, Vegetable Magnesium Stearate.

Ferrous Sulfate **-** Nature's Bounty
Each tablet contains: Iron (as Ferrous Sulfate, anhydrous) 28 mg. Inactive Ingredients: Dicalcium Phosphate, Calcium Carbonate, Cellulose (Plant Origin), Croscarmellose, Vegetable Stearic Acid, Vegetable Magnesium Stearate, Cellulose Coating.

Fertil Male **-** LaneLabs
Each capsule contains: Lepidium Meyenii g. root 500 mg • HAI (heated algal ingredient) Amino Acid extract (from sea algae) 1.2 mg. Other Ingredients: Gelatin, Magneisum Stearate, Cellulose.

Fertility Blend for Men **-** The Daily Wellness Company
Two capsules contain: Vitamin C as ascorbic acid 120 mg • Vitamin E as d-alpha tocopherol 150 mg • Vitamin B6 as pyridoxine hydrochloride 2 mg • Vitamin B12 as cyanocobalamin 6 mcg • Folate as folic acid 400 mcg • Zinc as gluconate 15 mg • Selenium as sodium selenate 70 mcg • Proprietary Blend 610 mg: L-Carnitine as tartrate, Dong Quai (standardized to .1% ferulic acid), Coenzyme Q10. Inactive Ingredients: Rice Flour Powder, Magnesium Stearate, Silica.

Fertility Blend for Women **-** The Daily Wellness Company
Three capsules contain: Vitamin E (as d-alpha tocopherol) 150 mg • Vitamin B6 (as pyridoxine hydrochloride) 6 mg • Vitamin B12 (as cyanocobalamin) 12 mcg • Folate (as folic acid) 400 mcg • Iron (as gluconate) 18 mg • Magnesium (as oxide) 400 mg • Zinc (as gluconate) • Selenium (as sodium selenate) 70 mcg • Proprietary Blend 1080 mg: Chasteberry (Vitex agnus castus standardized to .5% agnusides), Green Tea (Camellia sinensis standardized to 50% phenols), L-arginine. Inactive Ingredients: Rice Flour Powder, Magnesium Stearate, Silica.

Fevera **-** HerbaSway
Cassia tora • Kudzu • Skullcap • Knotweed • Licorice • Blackberry • HerbaSwee (Cucurbitaceae fruit).

Feverfew **-** PhytoPharmica
Each capsule contains: Feverfew flower and leaf (tanacetum parthenium, standardized to contain 600 mcg of parthenolide) 100 mg. Other Ingredients: Gelatin, Cellulose, Modified Cellulose Gum, Magnesium Stearate, Titanium Dioxide Color. This product was formerly known as MygraFree.

Feverfew **-** Leiner Health Products
Each caplet contains: Feverfew extract (Tanacetum parhenium) leaf 100 mg • Feverfew leaf (Tanacetum parthenium) 20 mg. Other Ingredients: Calcium Carbonate, Cellulose, Maltodextrin, Mannitol, Hydroxypropyl Methylcellulose, Silicon Dioxide, Polyethylene Glycol 3350, Croscarmellose Sodium, Titanium Dioxide, Hydroxypropyl Cellulose, Pharmaceutical Glaze, Crospovidone, Magnesium Stearate, Polysorbate 80, Blue 1 Lake, Yellow 6 Lake.

Feverfew **-** Pharmanex
Each capsule contains: Feverfew leaves and flowers (12:1) extract (Tanacetum parthenium) 125 mg. Other Ingredients: Rice Flour, Gelatin.

Feverfew **-** Source Naturals
Each tablet contains: Feverfew extract 200 mg • Feverfew whole herb 50 mg • Magnesium (Oxide) 70 mg • Calcium (Carbonate) 35 mg • Vitamin C (Ascorbic Acid) 10 mg.

Feverfew **-** NOW Foods
Each capsule contains: Feverfew 0.9% 400 mg.

Some Brand Name Natural Products - What they Contain

www.NaturalDatabase.com contains MANY more listings than appear here.
Editor's Notes are located on pages 2155-2163.

Feverfew (Nomigraine) Caplets - Life Brand
Each caplet contains: Dried Feverfew leaf (Tanacetum parthenium) 125 mg. This product is guaranteed to contain a minimum of 0.2% Parthenolide. Other Ingredients: Dicalcium Phosphate, Microcrystalline Cellulose, Silicon Dioxide, Magnesium Stearate (plant source), Stearic Acid (plant source).

Feverfew 0.7% 120 mg - Vital Nutrients
Each capsule contains: Feverfew (tanacetum parthenium, standardized to 0.7% parthenolide) 120 mg.

Feverfew 1.2 - Pure Encapsulations
Each vegetable capsule contains: Feverfew extract (standardized to contain 1.2% parthenolide, hypo-allergenic plant fiber added to complete capsule volume requirement) 80 mg.

Feverfew 400mg and Willowbark 200mg - Nature's Own
Each tablet contains: Feverfew extract (tanacetum parthenium), equivalent to dry herb 400 mg • Willowbark extract (salix purpurea MIS), equivalent to dry stem bark 200 mg.

Feverfew Jamaican Dogwood Supreme - Gaia Herbs
Forty drops contain: Proprietary Blend 45 mg: Feverfew herb (tanacetum parthenium), Jamaican Dogwood (piscidia erythrina), Black Haw bark (viburnum prunifolium), St. John's Wort flower buds (hypericum perforatum), Butterbur root (petasites frigida), Meadowsweet herb (filipendula ulmaria), Willow bark (salix nigra), Ginger root (zingiber officinalis), 50-60% Pure Grain Alcohol USP, Spring Water.

Fiber 10 - Advocare International
Each pouch (0.7 oz/20 g) contains: Fiber Blend: Psyllium husk, Oat fiber, Carboxymethylcellulose, Guar Gum, Citrus Pectin, Butternut bark powder • Fructose • Maltodextrin • Citric Acid • Natural Flavors • Artificial Flavors • Acesulfame Potassium • Papaya fruit powder • Prune powder • Rhubarb root extract • Black Walnut hull extract • Licorice root powder • Lactobacillus Acidophilus • Bifidobacterium Bifidum • Digestive Enzyme Complex: Lipase, Cellulase, Protease.

Fiber Clense - Nutri-Quest Rx
Three tablets contain: Vitamin C 300 mg • Apple Pectin 150 mg • Garlic 150 mg • Rice Bran 600 mg • Sodium Alginate 300 mg • L-Cysteine 200 mg • DL-Methionine 100 mg • L-Lysine 30 mg • Chlorophyll 10 mg • Oat Bran 600 mg • Red Beet root 100 mg.

Fiber Delights (chocolate flavor) - PhytoPharmica
Two chewable tablets contain: Proprietary Fiber Blend 4.4 g: Enriched Inulin Fiber with Fructooligosaccharides (FOS) from Chicory root, Oat Bran Fiber (avena sativa). Other Ingredients: Fructose, Cocoa Powder, Stearic Acid, Natural Flavors, Lecithin

Fiber Delights (vanilla flavor) - PhytoPharmica
Two chewable tablets contain: Proprietary Fiber Blend 4.4 g: Enriched Inulin Fiber with Fructooligosaccharides (FOS) from Chicory root, Oat Bran fiber (avena sativa). Other Ingredients: Fructose, Stearic Acid, Lecithin, Natural Flavor.

Fiber Digestion - Enzymes, Inc.
Each capsule contains: Proprietary Enzyme Blend 488 mg: Amylase, CereCalase, Protease, Glucoamylase, alpha-Galactosidase, Malt Diastase, Pectinase, Cellulase, Lipase, Peptidase. Other Ingredients: Plant Cellulose, Water.

Fiber Formula - PhytoPharmica
Eight capsules contain: Proprietary Fiber Blend 3455 mg: Psyllium husk (plantago ovata), Oat Bran (avena sativa), Guar Gum seed extract (cyamopsis tetragonoloba), Pectin (from citrus fruit), Marshmallow roo 3.5:1 extract (althaea officinalis). Other Ingredients: Cellulose, Gelatin, Magnesium Stearate, Silicon Dioxide.

Fiber Fusion Drink Mix (incrediberry flavor) - Enzymatic Therapy
Each well-rounded teaspoon (6 g) contains: Psyllium husk (plantago ovata) 4 g • Stevia leaf 15:1 extract (stevia rebaudiana) 55 mg. Other Ingredients: Raspberry Powder, Citric Acid, Natural Flavor, Silicon Dioxide, Malic Acid.

Fiber Fusion Drink Mix (unflavored) - Enzymatic Therapy
Each slightly rounded teaspoon (5.15 g) contains: Psyllium husk (plantago ovata) 4 g. Other Ingredients: Silicon Dioxide.

Fiber Max - FreeLife International
Four caplets contain: Calcium (as calcium hydrogen phosphate) 400 mg • Lactospore brand microencapsulated active Lactobacillus cells 300 million CFU • Lipase enzyme 500 units • Triphala standardized extract 25 mg: Emblica officinalis, Terminalia chebula, Terminalia bellirica • Aloe Vera whole leaf 50 mg • Butternut bark 750 mg • Multi-fiber/Green Food Cleansing Blend 915 mg: Vegetable Cellulose, Oat fiber, Alfalfa, Golden Pea fiber, Scandinavian Beet fiber, Barley greens, Slippery Elm bark, Oat greens • Glyco-Nutrient Blend 500 mg: Fructo-Oligosaccharides from Chicory and Jerusalem Artichoke, Larch Arabinogalactan, Mannanoligosaccharides, Champex Champignon extract. Other ingredients: Vegetable Stearic Acid, Silica, Vegetable Magnesium Stearate, Vita-Coat brand (vegetable resin, alpha-lipoic acid).

Fiber Perfect - Jarrow Formulas
Six capsules contain: Fibers 2 g: Psyllium (plantago ovata), Beet (beta-vulgaris), Inulin - FOS (cichorium intybus) • Beneficial Bacteria Metabolites 200 mg: Metabolin brand Metabolites of Propionibacterium Shermani, Green Algae • Chlorella Yaeyama (chlorella vulgaris) 20 mg • Proprietary Blend 1420 mg: Fennel seed (foeniculum vulgare), Rhubarb root 4:1 extract (rheum palmatum), Ginger root (zingiber officinale, freeze dried), Slippery Elm bark (unmus rubra), Dandelion (taraxacum officinale), Peppermint leaves (mentha piperita). Other Ingredients: Celluose, Silicon Dioxide, Magnesium Stearate, Gelatin.

Fiber Plan - Shaklee
2 teaspoons (5 g) contain: Dietary fiber 4 g • Vitamin C 48 mg. Other Ingredients: Psyllium Husk, Pectin, Guar Gum, Locust Bean Gum, Maltodextrin, Ascorbic Acid.

Fiber Plan Daily Crunch - Shaklee
15 g contain: Dietary fiber 5 g • Soluble fiber 2 g • Insoluble fiber 2 g • Protein 1 g • Calcium 60 mg • Iron 0.8 mg • Sodium 25 mg. Other Ingredients: Rice Flour, Soy Fiber, Oat Bran, Psyllium Husk, Acacia Gum, Brown Rice Syrup, Pectin, Fructose, Guar Gum, Calcium Carbonate, Trisodium Phosphate.

Fiber Plan Daily Mix - Shaklee
2 tablespoons (15 g) contain: Dietary fiber 5 g • Soluble fiber 2 g • Insoluble fiber 2 g • Sugars 1 g • Protein 1 g • Calcium 60 mg • Iron 0.8 mg • Sodium 25 mg. Other Ingredients: Rice Flour, Soy Fiber, Oat Bran, Psyllium Husk, Acacia Gum, Brown Rice Syrup, Pectin, Fructose, Guar Gum, Calcium Carbonate, Trisodium Phosphate.

Fiber Plus Capsules - Ortho Molecular Products
Each capsule contains: Proprietary Blend 750 mg: Psyllium seed husks, Psyllium seeds, Rice Bran, Apple Pectin, Fig fruit, Prune fruit, Lactobacillus Acidophilus. Other Ingredients: Natural Vegetable Capsules, Ascorbyl Palmitate, Microcrystalline Cellulose, Silicon Dioxide.

Fiber Plus powder - Ortho Molecular Products
Each 1 tbsp serving contains: Proprietary Blend 11 g: Psyllium seed husks, Psyllium seeds, Rice Bran, Apple Pectin, Fig fruit, Prune, Lactobacillus Acidophilus.

Fiber Soy-Pro - The Vitamin Shoppe
SUPRO Soy Protein Isolate and BeneFiber Soluble Fiber. Orange citrus natural flavor.

Fiber4Life - 4 Life
Each packet contains: Vitamin A (75% from beta carotene, 25% from palmitate) 1000 IU • Vitamin C (as ascorbic acid) 102 mg • Vitamin D 24 IU • Vitamin E (as D-alpha tocopheryl acetate) 6 IU • Thiamin (as thiamine mononitrate) 300 mcg • Riboflavin 340 mcg • Niacin (as niacinamide) 4 mg • Vitamin B6 (as pyridoxine hydrochloride) 400 mcg • Vitamin B12 (as cyanocobalamin) 1.2 mcg • Biotin 60 mcg • Zinc (from zinc amino acid chelate) 3 mg • Selenium (as selenomethionine) 14 mcg • Chromium (from chromium polynicotinate amino acid chelate) 100 mcg • Sodium (from salt) 40 mg • Transfer Factor E-XF from Bovine Colostrum 100 mg • Alpha Lipoic Acid 10 mg • Lagerstroemia Speciosa (banaba leaf extract, 1% corosolic acid) 4 mg. Other Ingredients: Fiber Blend (maltodextrin fiber, soy fiber, cellulose gum, arabinogalactan), Maltodextrin, Citric Acid, Salt, Inulin, Beta Carotene, Soy Extract, Stevia Extract, Potato Maltodextrin.

Fiberall brand - Heritage Consumer Products
Psyllium.
See Editor's Note No. 44.

FiberChoice - CNS, Inc.
Each chewable tablet contains: Fructan 2 g • Magnesium Stearate 25 mg. Other Ingredients: Citric Acid and other natural flavors.

FiberCon - Whitehall-Robins Healthcare
Each caplet contains: Calcium Polycarbophil 625 mg. Other Ingredients: Calcium Carbonate, Caramel, Crospovidone, Hydrocypropyl Methylcellulose, Magnesium Stearate, Microcrystalline Cellulose, Mineral Oil, Povidone, Silica Gel, Sodium Lauryl Sulfate.

Fibergy Drink (almond creme flavor) - USANA Health Sciences
Two scoops contain: Fiber Blend: Soy Fiber, Gum Arabic, Oat Bran, Wheat Bran, Cellulose Gum, Pea Fiber, Xanthan Gum, Corn Bran, Locust Bean Gum, Carrageenan, Citrus Pectin, Oligofructose, Inulin, Apple Fiber • Crystalline • Fructose • Corn Syrup Solids • Rich Syrup Solids • Soy Protein Isolate • High Oleic Sunflower Oil • Natural and Artificial Flavors • Potassium Chloride • Dipotassium Phosphate • Salt • Beta Carotene (color) • Sodium Caseinate (a milk derivative) • Tricalcium Phosphate • Magnesium Oxide • Ascorbic Acid (Vitamin C) • Mono and Diglycerides • Soy Lecithin • Ferric Orthophosphate • Folic Acid • Thiamin Mononitrate (Vitamin B1).

Fibergy Drink (peach mango flavor) - USANA Health Sciences
Two scoops contain: Fiber Blend: Gum Arabic, Soy Fiber, Oat Bran, Wheat Bran, Inulin, Pea Fiber, Oat Fiber, Sugar Beet Fiber, Cellulose Gum, Xanthan Gum, Oligofructose, Citrus Pectin, Stabilized Rice Bran, Apple Fiber • Crystalline Fructose • Natural and Artificial Flavors • High Oleic Sunflower Oil • Corn Syrup Solids • Salt • Beet Juice Powder (color) • Sodium Caseinate (a milk derivative) • Beta Carotene (color) • Mono and Diglycerides • Dipotassium Phosphate • Soy Lecithin.

Fiberific - Nature's Plus
Each 1.4 oz. bar contains: Calories 120 • Calories from Fat 18 • Total Fat 2 g • Saturated Fat 0 g • Cholesterol 0 mg • Total Carbohydrate 23 g • Complex Carbohydrate 14 g • Sugars 9 g • Dietary Fiber 8 g • Soluble Fiber 3.6 g • Insoluble Fiber 4.4 g • Protein 3 g • Sodium 43 mg • Potassium 196 mg. Ingredients: Rolled Oats, Wheat Germ, Brown Rice, Apples, Prunes & Oat Bran. Naturally flavored with Fruit Juice & Honey. No tropical oils.

FiberPlus - PhytoPharmica
Two capsules contain: FiberPlus Proprietary Blend 1000 mg: Psyllium hydrophilic muciloid, Grapefruit pectin, Oat (Avena sativa) fiber, Beet fiber, Carrot fiber, Fructooligosaccharides (FOS; from Jerusalem artichoke), Prune fiber, Ginger (Zingiber officinale) root and rhizome extract, Fenugreek (Trigonella foenum-graecum) seed extract 4:1, Goldenseal (Hydrastis canadensis) root and rhizome extract (standardized to contain 5% total alkaloids including berberine, hydrastine, and canadine), Chamomile (Matricaria recutita) root extract, Marshmallow (Althaea officinalis) root extract 4.25:1, Aloe Vera (Aloe barbadensis) leaf extract, and Cascara sagrada (Rhamnus purshiana) bark, trunk, and branch extract.

FiberSMART Capsules - Renew Life Formulas, Inc.
Four capsules contain: Flax seed (linum usitatissimum) • Borage seed oil (borago officinalis) • FOS (fructooligosaccharides) • Guar gum • Fennel seed (foeniculum vulgare) • L-Glutamine • Marshmallow root (althaea officinalis) • Probiotic Proprietary Blend: Lactobacillus Acidophilus, Bifidobacterium Bifidum, Bifidobacterium Infantis • Slippery Elm bark (ulmus rubra) • Triphala Blend: Indian Gooseberry fruit, Belleric Myrobalan fruit, Tropical Almond fruit. Other Ingredients: Gelatin, Water.

FiberSMART Powder - Renew Life Formulas, Inc.
Each scoop contains: Flax seed (linum usitatissimum) • Borage seed oil (borago officinalis) • FOS (fructooligosaccharides) • Guar gum • Fennel seed (foeniculum vulgare) • L-Glutamine • Marshmallow root (althaea officinalis) • Probiotic Proprietary Blend: Lactobacillus Acidophilus, Bifidobacterium Bifidum, Bifidobacterium Infantis • Slippery Elm bark (ulmus rubra) • Triphala blend: Indian Gooseberry fruit, Belleric Myrobalan fruit, Tropical Almond fruit • Stevia Rebaudiana leaf.

Fibersol - TwinLab
Each rounded teaspoonful contains: Fiber Blend Concentrate [from Psyllium Seed Husks, Guar Gum, Apple Pectin] 4 g • Vitamin C 100 mg.

FiberThin - FiberThin, LLC
Glucomannan (from konjac root).

Fiber-Time - Atrium Biotechnologies
Twelve ounces contain: Bran Fiber • Cascara Sagrada bark • Citrus Fiber • Karaya Gum • Apple Pectin • Prune powder • Psyllium Plantago Ovata Blond • Rhubarb root • Rice Fiber • Sweet Whey.

FiberWise - Melaleuca
Ingredients: Psyllium Husk • Rice Bran • Fructooligosaccharides • Maltodextrin • Apple fiber • Oat fiber • Lactobacillus Sporogenes (acidophilus) • Coenzyme Q10 • Green Tea extract • Grape Seed extract • Aloe Vera extract • Garlic • Ginger root • Licorice root • Burdock • Peppermint • Slippery Elm • Fructose • Soy Lecithin • Natural Flavor • Calcium Carbonate • Malic Acid • Calcium Silica • Beta Carotene • Acesulfame Potassium • Ascorbic Acid • D-Alpha Tocopheryl Acetate • Beet juice powder • Vitamin A Palmitate.

Fiberzyme - Young Living Essential Oils
Each capsule contains: Proprietary Blend: Cellulase, Bee Pollen, Tarragon (artemisia dracunculus) oil, Ginger (zingiber officinale) oil, Peppermint (mentha piperita) oil, Juniper (juniperus osteosperma and/or j. scopulorum) oil, Fennel (foeniculum vulgare) oil, Lemongrass (cymbopogon flexuosus) oil, Anise (pimpinella anisum) oil, Patchouli (pogostemon cablin) oil.

FiboTane - Advocare International
Three capsules contain: Vitamin E (as d-alpha tocopheryl succinate) 15 IU • Chromium (as polynicotinate - ChromeMate) 25 mcg • Chitosan 600 mg • Guar Gum 750 mg • Taurine 300 mg • Beta-Sitosterol 100 mg • Odorless Garlic (bulb - allium sativum) 100 mg • Yellow Dock extract (root - rumex crispus) 100 mg • Niacinamide Ascorbate 50 mg • Buckthorn extract (bark - frangula alnus) 30 mg •Ascorbyl Palmitate 15 mg. Other Ingredients: Silicon Dioxide, Magnesium Stearate, Gelatin.

Fibre and Chlorophyll Toxin Fighter - Hillestad
Two tablets contain: Oat Bran (outer seed coat) 300 mg • Beet root fiber 300 mg • Psyllium seed husk 200 mg • Prune fruit 200 mg • Aloe Vera leaf (from freeze-dried concentrate) 150 mg • Flax seed 100 mg • Cascara Sagrada bark 100 mg • Guar Gum seed 100 mg • Rice husk fiber 50 gm • Deodorized Garlic bulb 50 mg • Bentonite

(colloidal mineral) 100 mg • Black Walnut leaf 30 mg • Chlorophyllin leaf 40 mg • Papain (papaya fruit) 200 mg • Bromelain (pineapple fruit) 50 mg. Other Ingredients: Oyster Shell, Gum Acacia, Cellulose, Magnesium Stearate.

Fibre System Plus - 4 Life
Each packet contains: Psyllium (plantago afra, seed) 600 mg • Black Walnut (juglans regia, hulls) 400 mg • Cranberry (fruit) 250 mg • Cascara Sagrada (bark) 100 mg • Ginger (root) 100 mg • Apple (fruit) 100 mg • Gentian (root) 85 mg • Alder Buckthorn (bark) 75 mg • Slippery Elm (bark) 60 mg • Licorice (root) 50 mg • Sage (leaves) 50 mg • Parsley (leaf) 50 mg • Papain (from Papaya fruit) 50 mg • Bromelain (from Pineapple fruit) 50 mg • Prune (fruit) 50 mg • Red Wheat Fiber (seed) 50 mg • Marshmallow (root) 40 mg • Hops (flower) 30 mg • Frangula extract (bark) 25 mg • Irish Moss (Chondruscrispus, aerial parts) 25 mg • Bee Pollen 25 mg • English Chamomile (flower) 25 mg • Pineapple (fruit) 20 mg • Papaya (fruit) 20 mg • Hawaiian Spirulina Pacifica 10 mg • Goldenseal (root) 10 mg. Other Ingredients: Gelatin Capsule, Rice Bran, Xanthan Gum, Locust Bean Gum, Magnesium Stearate.

Fibre-Max powder - Hillestad
Each 2 tsp serving contains: Dietary Fiber from Psyllium husk 1.68 g • Calcium (as calcium citrate) 100 mg • Magnesium (oxide) 50 mg • Vitamin C (ascorbic acid) 100 mg. Other Ingredients: Orange Juice Powder, Non-Dairy Creamer, Natural Vanilla Flavor, Xanthan Gum.

FibreNet - Pharmanex
Four capsules contain: Chitosan (from shellfish) PolmerPlex 1000 mg. Other Ingredients: Calcium Carbonate, Magnesium Stearate.

FibreNet Plus - Pharmanex
Each scoop contains: Vitamin A (85% Beta-Carotene) 6877 IU • Vitamin C 12 mg • Vitamin D 80 IU • Vitamin E 4 IU • Thiamin 0.30 mg • Riboflavin 0.34 mg • Niacin 4 mg • Vitamin B6 0.40 mg • Folate 80 mcg • Vitamin B12 1.2 mg • Biotin 60 mcg • Pantothenic Acid 2 mg • Calcium 187 mg • Iron 3.8 mg • Phosphorus 100 mg • Iodine 30 mcg • Magnesium 60 mg • Zinc 3 mg • Copper 0.40 mg • Sodium 60 mg • Potassium 190 mg • PolmerPlex 1000 mg.
Ingredients: Crystalline Fructose, Oat Bran, Stabilized Rice Bran, Gum Arabic, Natural and Artificial Flavors, PolmerPlex, High Oleic Sunflower Oil, Corn Syrup Solids, Tricalcium Phosphate, Citric Acid, Beta-Carotene, Dipotassium Phosphate Cellulose Gum, Sugar Beet Fiber, Potassium Citrate, Sodium Caseinate, Magnesium Oxide, Soy Fiber, Salt, Pea Fiber, Xanthan Gum, Ground Psyllium Husks, Ascorbic Acid, dl-Alpha Tocopheryl Acetate, Dicalcium Phosphate, Soy Lecithin, Vitamin A Palmitate, Niacinamide, Zinc Oxide, Electric Iron, Copper Gluconate, d-Calcium Pantothenate, Cholecalciferol, Pyridoxine Hydrochloride, Riboflavin, Thiamine Mononitrate, Cyanocobalamin, Folic Acid, Biotin, Potassium Iodide.

Fibresonic - Matol Botanical International Ltd
Each scoop contains: Fructose • Finely Ground Soya Cotyledon • Finely Ground Sugar Beet pulp • Vegetable oil powder preparation: Non-Hydrogenated Sunflower oil, Corn syrup solids, Sodium Caseinate, Mono- and Diglycerides, Potassium Phosphate Dibasic, Tribasic Calcium Phosphate, Lecithin, Tocopherols • Dehydrated Low Fat Yogurt (fermented skim milk, bacterial culture, silicon dioxide) • Sorbitol • Wheat Bran • Corn Bran • Oat Bran • Calcium Caseinate • Vanilla flavor with other flavors • Almond flavor with other flavors • Carob Bean Gum • Guar Gum • Gum Arabic • Cellulose Gel and Gum • Lecithin • Xanthan Gum • Pectin • Pea hull fiber • Ascorbic Acid • Ascorbyl Palmitate • Carotene • Lactobacillus Acidophilus.

Fibro AMJ Day-Time Formula - 4 Life
Three capsules contain: Vitamin B6 (as pyridoxine hydrochloride) 10 mg • Magnesium (as oxide) 200 mg • Malic Acid 400 mg • Glucosamine Hydrochloride 800 mg • Bovine Cartilage (natural concentrations of mucopolysaccharides and chondroitin sulfates) 200 mg • Proprietary Blend 437 mg: Methyl Sulfonyl Methane (MSM), Boswellia Serrata (20-25% boswellic acids, 70% totally organic acids), N-Acetyl Cysteine, Bromelain (400 GDU), L-Cysteine, Grape extract (vitis vinifera seed, skin and stems with natural concentrations of polyphenols, antho-cyanidins, catechins, proanthocyanidols and resveratrol), Devil's Claw root (harpagophytum procumbens with 1.5%-2.5% harpagosides), Alpha Lipoic Acid, Boron (as citrate). Other Ingredients: Peppermint Leaf, Peppermint Oil, Vegetable Oil, Silica.

Fibro AMJ Night-Time Formula - 4 Life
Each capsule contains: Vitamin B6 (as pyridoxine hydrochloride) 15 mg • Melatonin 2 mg • Pregnenolone 10 mg • 5-Hydroxytryptophan (griffonia simplicifolia seed) 15 mg • Proprietary Blend 595 mg: Creatine Monohydrate, N-Acetyl Cysteine, Cysteine, Pau D'arco inner bark 4:1 extract (tabebuia impetiginosa), Valerian root (valerian officinalis root with 0.8% valerinic acids), Kava kava root (piper methysticum 30% extract), Grape seed, skin, and stem extract (vitis vinifera seed), Alpha Lipoic Acid. Other Ingredients: Peppermint Leaf, Vegetable Oil.

Fibro Complete Multi with Malic Acid - Pro Health
Each tablet contains: Vitamin A (natural fish liver oil) 7500 IU • Beta-Carotene 10,000 IU • Vitamin B1 (thiamine HCl) 50 mg • Vitamin B2 (riboflavin) 50 mg • Vitamin B3 (niacinamide) 50 mg • Vitamin B5 (pantothenic acid) 50 mg • Vitamin B6 (pyridoxine HCl) 50 mg • Vitamin B12 (cyanocobalamin) 250 mcg • Biotin 100 mcg • Folic Acid 400 mcg • Vitamin C (ascorbic acid) 250 mg • Vitamin D (natural fish liver oil) 400 IU • Vitamin E (100% d-alpha) 150 IU • Calcium (amino acid chelate, oystershell) 100 mg • Magnesium Oxide (amino acid chelate) 60 mg • Zinc (amino acid chelate) 15 mg • Copper (amino acid chelate) 1 mg • Iodine (kelp) 150 mcg • Iron (amino acid chelate) 10 mg • Choline (bitartrate) 100 mg • Inositol 75 mg • PABA 30 mg • Rutin 25 mg • Citrus Bioflavonoids 100 mg • Betaine (HCl) 25 mg • Glutamic Acid 25 mg • Potassium (amino acid chelate) 10 mg • Manganese (amino acid chelate) 5 mg • Selenium (amino acid chelate) 200 mcg • Chromium (yeast-free gtf) 250 mcg • Boron (amino acid chelate) 500 mcg • Molybdenum (amino acid chelate) 50 mcg • Nucleic Acid 50 mg • Malic Acid 100 mg • Magnesium Hydroxide 25 mg • IP-6 100 mg • Nova Soy brand Soy 50 mg. Other Ingredients: Alfalfa, Parsley, Lecithin, Rose Hips, Di-Calcium Phosphate, Cellulose, Stearic Acid, Silica.
This product was formerly known as CFS/FM Multi.

Fibro Energy Formula - Pro Health
Three capsules contain: Vitamin B12 (as cyanocobalamin) 500 mcg • Pantothenic Acid (as D-calcium pantothenate) 25 mg • Magnesium (as potassium magnesium aspartate, dihydrate) 30 mg • Potassium (as potassium magnesium aspartate, dihydrate) 98 mg • 7-Keto brand DHEA (3-Acetyl-7-oxo-dehydroepiandrosterone) 10 mg • Acetyl-L-Carnitine HCl 500 mg • Borage oil (borago officinalis dried herb) 130.5 mg • Gamma Linolenic Acid (GLA) 15 mg • Alpha Lipoic Acid 200 mg • Coenzyme Q10 (as ubidicarenone) 100 mg • D-Ribose 50 mg • L-Taurine 500 mg • Malic Acid from Apple 200 mg • Panax Ginseng root powder 200 mg. Other Ingredients: Gelatin, Calcium Silicate, Magnesium Stearate, Water.
This product was formerly known as CFS/FM Energy Formula.

Fibro Freedom - Pro Health
Six capsules contain: White Willow bark extract (standardized to 15% salicin) 30 mg • 5 HTP 100 mg • Malic Acid 1200 mg • Magnesium Hydroxide 300 mg • Glucosamine Sulfate 1500 mg • Chondroitin 200 mg • MSM 1000 mg • Boswellin 150 mg • Curcumin (95% curcuminoids) 50 mg. Other Ingredients: Magnesium Stearate, Gelatin, Water.
This product was formerly known as FM relief. See Editor's Note No. 15.

Fibro Plus - Aspen Group, Inc.
Two capsules contain: Elemental Magnesium 200 mg • Malic Acid 300 mg • Glyciante 50 mg.

FibroLeve **-** PharmAssure
Four tablets contain: Vitamin B6 (as Pyridoxine Hydrochloride) 15 mg • Magnesium (as Magnesium Oxide) 400 mg • Manganese (as Manganese Sulfate) 10 mg • Malic Acid 1200 mg • Boswellin serrata Resin Extract (65% Boswellic Acid=75 mg) 115 mg. Other Ingredients: Cellulose.

FibroMalic **-** Pure Encapsulations
Each vegetable capsule contains: Malic Acid 200 mg • Magnesium (aspartate) 40 mg • L-Carnitine (free-form, from 344 mg of L-carnitine fumarate) 200 mg.

Fibromyalgin **-** Olympia Nutrition
Glucosamine, Collagen, Mag. Malate.

Fibro-My-DMG **-** DaVinci Laboratories
Each tablet contains: Magnesium (as magnesium malate) 50 mg • Dimethylglycine HCl 300 mg • Malic Acid 200 mg • Gamma-Aminobutyric Acid (GABA) 150 mg • Nicotinamide Adenine Dinucleotide (NADH) 5 mg. Other Ingredients: Microcrystalline Celulose, Stearic Acid, Vegetable Stearate, Croscarmellose Sodium, Silicon Dioxide, Hydroxypropyl Methylcellulose.

Fibroplex **-** Metagenics
Two tablets contain: Thiamine (as thiamin mononitrate) 50 mg • Vitamin B6 (as pyridoxine hydrochloride) 50 mg • Magnesium (as magnesium bis-glycinate) 150 mg • Manganese (as manganese glycinate) 5 mg • Malic Acid 600 mg.

Fibro-Response **-** Source Naturals
Three tablets contain: Vitamin A (as beta carotene) 5000 IU • Vitamin C (as ascorbic acid & magnesium ascorbate) 50 mg • Vitamin D (D3, as cholecalciferol) 200 mg • Thiamin (vitamin B1) 30 mg • Riboflavin (vitamin B2) 30 mg • Niacin 37.5 mg • Niacinamide 12. 5mg • Vitamin B6 (as pyridoxine HCl) 40 mg • Folate (as folic acid) 200 mcg • Pantothenic Acid (as calcium D-pantothenate) 50 mg • Magnesium (as magnesium malate, oxide & ascorbate) 300 mg • Zinc (as zinc citrate & monomethionine, OptiZinc brand) 15 mg • Selenium (as L-selenomethionine & sodium selenite) 100 mcg • Copper (as copper sebacate) 1 mg • Manganese (as manganese citrate) 12 mg • Chromium (as chromium polynicotinate, ChromeMate brand) 100 mcg • Molybdenum (as molybdenum chelate) 90 mcg • Malic Acid (as malic acid and magnesium malate) 1.2 g • MSM (methylsulfonylmethane) 1.12 g • Hops extract (yilding 60 gm Humulex brand alpha-acids) 200 mg • GABA (gamma-aminobutyric acid) 150 mg • Milk Thistle seed extract (yielding 70 mg silymarin) 84 mg • N-Acetyl Cysteine 75 mg • Ginkgo Biloba leaf 50:1 extract 60 mg • Dandelion root extract 50 mg • Dandelion root 50 mg • Alpha-Lipoic Acid 50 mg • Bupleurum extract 30 mg • Panax Ginseng root extract 25 mg • Kudzu root 15 mg • Astragalus extract 15 mg • Ginger root 15 mg • Skullcap aerial parts 15 mg • Cassia bark 15 mg • Coenzyme Q10 (ubiquinone) 15 mg • Licorice root extract 10 mg • Bioperine brand Black Pepper extract 3 mg. Other Ingredients: Stearic ACid, Acacia, Modified Cellulose Gum, Colloidal Silicon Dioxide, Magnesium Stearate.

Fibro-X **-** Olympian Labs
Two capsules contain: Malic Acid 600 mg • Shark Cartilage 600 mg • White Willow Bark 50 mg • Valerian root 20 mg • Grape Seed extract 40 mg • Magnesium Glycinate 100 mg • Manganese Glycinate 5 mg.

Fields of Nature Coenzyme Q-10 **-** Inverness Medical Innovations, Inc.
Each capsule contains: Coenzyme Q-10 30 mg. Other Ingredients: Microcrystalline Cellulose, Gelatin, Magnesium Stearate.

Fields of Nature ProtoChol Chewables **-** Inverness Medical Innovations, Inc.
Each tablet contains: Phytosterol Concentrate 400 mg (as Beta-Sitosterol 172 mg, Campesterol 100 mg, Stigmasterol 44 mg). Other Ingredients: Dextrose, Magnesium Stearate, Adipic Acid, Aspartame, Natural and artificial flavors, Artificial colors (FD&C Red No. 40 Lake).

Finally...The Solution for Women **-** Blue Chip Marketing, Inc
Deionzied Water • Aloe Barbadensis gel • Caprylic/Capric Triglyceride • Octyl Palmitate • Cetearyl Alcohol • Polysorbate 60 • Glycerin • Glyceryl Stearate • PEG-100 Stearate • Hydroxyethylcellulose • Xanthan Gum • Dimethicone • Benzyl Nicotinate • Penoxyethanol • Methylparaben • Butylparaben • Ethylparaben • Propylparaben • Chlorphensin • Ylang Ylang oil (cananga odorata) • Lavender oil (lavandula angustifolia).

Finest Acidophilus 10 mg **-** Walgreens
Each capsule contains: Lactobacillus Acidophilus 10 mg. Other Ingredients: Rice Flour, Gelatin, Magnesium Stearate.

Finest B-Complex & C **-** Walgreens
Each caplet contains: Vitamin C 300 mg • Thiamin (vitamin B1) 15 mg • Riboflavin (vitamin B2) 10.2 mg • Niacin 50 mg • Vitamin B6 5 mg • Pantothenic Acid 10 mg. Other Ingredients: Dicalcium Phosphate, Microcrystalline Cellulose, Hydroxypropyl Methylcellulose, Stearic Acid, Croscarmellose Sodium, Crospovidone, Calcium Silicate, Magnesium Stearate, Titanium Dioxide, Polyethylene Glycol.

Finest Chromium Picolinate 400 mcg **-** Walgreens
Each tablet contains: Chromium (from chromium picolinate) 400 mcg. Other Ingredients: Microcrystalline Cellulose, Silicon Dioxide, Magnesium Stearate.

Finest E Blend Vitamin 1000 I.U. **-** Walgreens
Each softgel contains: Vitamin E (dL-alpha tocopheryl acetate, D-alpha tocopheryl acetate) 1000 IU. Other Ingredients: Gleatin, USP Water, Glycerin, Soybean Oil.

Finest E Blend Vitamin 200 I.U. **-** Walgreens
Each softgel contains: Vitamin E (dL-alpha tocopheryl acetate, D-alpha tocopheryl acetate) 200 IU. Other Ingredients: Gelatin, USP Water, Glycerin, Soybean Oil.

Finest E Blend Vitamin 400 I.U. **-** Walgreens
Each softgel contains: Vitamin E (dL-alpha tocopheryl acetate, D-alpha tocopheryl acetate) 400 IU. Other Ingredients: Gelatin, USP Water, Glycerin, Soybean Oil.

Finest Fish Oil Liquid Omega 3 **-** J. R. Carlson Laboratories, Inc.
Each 1 tsp serving contains: Vitamin E (as D-alpha tocopherol) 10 IU • Other Omega-3 Fatty Acids 300 mg • Omega-3 Fatty Acids (from fish oil) 1600 mg • Antioxidant Blend 14 mg • DHA (docosahexaenoic acid) 500 mg • EPA (eicosapentaenoic acid) 800 mg.

Finest Garlic & Parsley **-** Walgreens
Each softgel contains: Garlic bulb oil 0.2 mg • Parsley seed oil 1.0 mg. Other Ingredients: Soybean Oil, Gelatin, Glycerin, Purified Water.

Finest Gelatin caplets **-** Walgreens
Two caplets contain: Gelatin 1300 mg. Other Ingredients: Dicalcium Phosphate, Magnesium Stearate, Hydroxypropyl Methylcellulose, Hydroxypropyl Cellulose, Polyethylene Glycol, Artificial Flavor.

Finest Glucosamine MSM Double Strength **-** Walgreens
Each tablet contains: Glucosamine HCl 500 mg • MSM (methyl sulfonyl methane) 500 mg. Other Ingredients: Dicalcium Phosphate, Microcrystalline Cellulose, Glyceryl Monostearate, Silicon Dioxide, Croscarmellose Sodium, Magnesium Stearate.

Finest L-Carnitine 250 mg **-** Walgreens
Each capsule contains: L-Carnitine-L-Tartrate 250 mg. Other Ingredients: Rice Flour, Gelatin, Silicon Dioxide, Magnesium Stearate.

Finest MSM 500 mg **-** Walgreens
Each capsule contains: MSM (methyl sulfonyl methane) 500 mg. Other Ingredients: Gelatin, Rice, Flour, Magnesium Stearate.

Finest Natural B-100 - Walgreens
Each caplet contains: Thiamin (vitamin B1) 100 mg • Riboflavin (vitamin B2) 100 mg • Niacin 100 mg • Vitamin B6 100 mg • Folate 400 mcg • Vitamin B12 100 mcg • Biotin 100 mcg • Pantothenic Acid 100 mg. Other Ingredients: Calcium Carbonate, Microcrystalline Cellulose, Dicalcium Phosphate, Stearic Acid, Acacia, Modified Cellulose gum, Silicon Dioxide, Crospovidone, Magnesium Stearate, Hydroxypropoyl Methylelcellulose, Polyethylene Glycol.

Finest Natural B-50 - Walgreens
Each caplet contains: Thiamin (vitamin B1) 50 mg • Riboflavin (vitamin B2) 50 mg • Niacin 50 mg • Vitamin B6 50 mg • Folate 400 mcg • Vitamin B12 50 mcg • Biotin 50 mcg • Pantothenic Acid 50 mg. Other Ingredients: Dicalcium Phosphate, Microcrystalline Cellulose, Crospovidone, Stearic Acid, Silicon Dioxide, Magnesium Stearate, Acacia.

Finest Natural Balanced B Complex & C - Walgreens
Each caplet contains: Vitamin C 500 mg • Thiamin (vitamin B1) 50 mg • Riboflavin (vitamin B2) 50 mg • Niacin 50 mg • Vitamin B6 50 mg • Folate 400 mcg • Vitamin B12 50 mcg • Biotin 50 mcg • Pantothenic Acid 50 mg. Other Ingredients: Microcrystalline Cellulose, Hydroxypropyl Methylcellulose, Maltodextrin, Stearic Acid, Magnesium Stearate, Cellulose, Rice Bran, Rose Hips, Mineral Oil, Polyethylene Glycol, Carnauba Wax, Crospovidone.

Finest Natural Beta Carotene 25,000 IU - Walgreens
Each softgel contains: Beta Carotene 25,000 IU. Other Ingredients: Soybean Oil, Gelatin, Corn Oil, Glycerin, Yellow Beeswax, Purified Water, Silica, Lecithin.

Finest Natural Brewer's Yeast - Walgreens
Four tablets contain: Thiamin (vitamin B1) 0.24 mg • Riboflavin (vitamin B2) 0.08 mg • Niacin 0.58 mg • Sodium 5 mg. Other Ingredients: Silicon Dioxide.

Finest Natural C Vitamin 500 mg - Walgreens
Each tablet contains: Vitamin C 500 mg • Sodium 39 mg. Other Ingredients: Sugar, Sorbitol, Stearic Acid, Natural Flavor, Magnesium Stearate, Silicon Dioxide.

Finest Natural C Vitamin 500 mg with Acerola Chewable - Walgreens
Each tablet contains: Vitamin C (from asorbic acid, acerola, lemon bioflavonoid, rose hips) 500 mg • Sodium 29 mg. Other Ingredients: Sugar, Sorbitol, Stearic Acid, Natural Flavor, Magnesium Stearate, Silicon Dioxide.

Finest Natural C Vitamin with Rose Hips 500 mg - Walgreens
Each tablet contains: Vitamin C (from ascorbic acid, rose hips) 500 mg. Other Ingredients: Microcrystalline Cellulose, Sodium Starch Glycolate, Stearic Acid, Silicon Dioxide, Magnesium Stearate.

Finest Natural Calcium 250 + D - Walgreens
Two tablets contain: Vitamin D (as cholecalciferol) • Calcium (as calcium carbonate) 500 mg. Other Ingredients: Microcrystalline Cellulose, Stearic Acid, Croscarmellose Sodium, Sodium Lauryl Sulfate.

Finest Natural Calcium 500 - Walgreens
Each tablet contains: Calcium (as calcium carbonate) 500 mg. Other Ingredients: Croscarmellose Sodium, Hydroxypropyl Methylcellulose, Sodium Lauryl Sulfate, Titanium Dioxide, Magnesium Stearate, Polyethylene Glycol, Carnauba Wax.

Finest Natural Calcium 500 + D - Walgreens
Each tablet contains: Vitamin D (as cholecalciferol) • Calcium (as calcium carbonate) 500 mg. Other Ingredients: Croscarmellose Sodium, Sodium Lauryl Sulfate, Hydroxypropyl Methylcellulose, Titanium Dioxide, Magnesium Stearate, Polyethylene Glycol, Carnauba Wax.

Finest Natural Calcium 600 - Walgreens
Each tablet contains: Calcium (as calcium carbonate) 600 mg. Other Ingredients: Croscarmellose Sodium, Hydroxypropyl Methylcellulose, Sodium Lauryl Sulfate, Titanium Dioxide, Magnesium Stearate, Polyethylene Glycol, Carnauba Wax.

Finest Natural Calcium 600 + D - Walgreens
Each tablet contains: Vitamin D (as cholecalciferol) • Calcium (as calcium carbonate) 600 mg. Other Ingredients: Croscarmellose Sodium, Hydroxypropyl Methylcellulose, Sodium Lauryl Sulfate, Titanium Dioxide, Magnesium Stearate, Polyethylene Glycol, Carnauba Wax, Annatto Color, Carmine Color.

Finest Natural Calcium Citrate + D - Walgreens
Two caplets contain: Vitamin D (as cholecalciferol) • Calcium (as calcium citrate) 630 mg. Other Ingredients: Stearic Acid, Croscarmellose Sodium, Magnesium Stearate, Hydroxypropyl Methylcellulose, Polyethylene Glycol.

Finest Natural Calcium Magnesium - Walgreens
Each tablet contains: Calcium (as calcium carbonate) 333 mg • Magnesium (as magnesium oxide) 167 mg. Other Ingredients: Microcrystalline Cellulose, Hydroxypropyl Methylcellulose, Croscarmellose Sodium, Titanium Dioxide, Stearic Acid, Magnesium Stearate, Sodium Lauryl Sulfate, Polyethylene Glycol, Carnauba Wax.

Finest Natural Calcium Magnesium & Zinc - Walgreens
Each tablet contains: Calcium (as calcium carbonate) 333 mg • Magnesium (as magnesium oxide) 133 mg • Zinc (as zinc gluconate) 5 mg. Other Ingredients: Microcrystalline Cellulose, Crospovidone, Hydroxypropyl Methylcellulose, Titanium Dioxide, Magnesium Stearate, Sodium Lauryl Sulfate, Polyethylene Glycol, Carnauba Wax.

Finest Natural Chromium Picolinate - Walgreens
Each tablet contains: Chromium (from chromium picolinate) 200 mcg. Other Ingredients: Microcrystalline Cellulose, Silicon Dioxide, Magnesium Stearate.

Finest Natural Coral Calcium Plus Minerals & Vitamin D capsules - Walgreens
Three capsules contain: Vitamin A (as palmitate) • Vitamin C (as ascorbic acid) 80 mg • Vitamin D (as cholecalciferol) • Vitamin E (as D-alpha tocopherol) • Calcium (from 1475 mg of coral calcium) 530 mg • Magnesium (from magnesium oxide and coral calcium) 265 mg • Zinc (as zinc oxide) 15 mg • Copper (as copper oxide) 3 mg • Coral Calcium (in a proprietary base) 1475 mg. Other Ingredients: Soybean Oil, Gelatin, USP Water, Glycerin, Yellow Beeswax, Lecithin, Silicon Dioxide, Titanium Dioxide.

Finest Natural Coral Calcium Plus Minerals & Vitamin D softgels - Walgreens
Three softgels contain: Vitamin A (as palmitate) • Vitamin C (as ascorbic acid) 80 mg • Vitamin D (as cholecalciferol) • Vitamin E (as D-alpha tocopherol) • Calcium (from 1475 mg of coral calcium) 530 mg • Magnesium (from magnesium oxide and coral calcium) 265 mg • Zinc (as zinc oxide) 15 mg • Copper (as copper oxide) 3 mg • Coral Calcium (in a proprietary base) 1475 mg. Other Ingredients: Soybean Oil, Gelatin, USP Water, Glycerin, Yellow Beeswax, Lecithin, Silicon Dioxide, Titanium Dioxide.

Finest Natural Cranberry - Walgreens
Each tablet contains: Cranberry extract (vaccinium vitis) 250 mg. Other Ingredients: Dicalcium Phosphate, Microcrystalline Cellulose, Glyceryl Monostearate, Croscarmellose Sodium, Silicon Dioxide, Magnesium Stearate, Aqueous Coating.

Finest Natural E Vitamin 1000 I.U. d-Alpha - Walgreens
Each softgel contains: Vitamin E (D-alpha tocopheryl acetate) 1000 IU. Other Ingredients: Gelatin, USP Water, Soybean Oil, Glycerin.

Finest Natural E Vitamin 200 I. U. d-Alpha - Walgreens
Each softgel contains: Vitamin E (D-alpha tocopheryl acetate) 200 IU. Other Ingredients: Gelatin, USP Water, Soybean Oil, Glycerin.

Some Brand Name Natural Products - What they Contain

www.NaturalDatabase.com contains MANY more listings than appear here.
Editor's Notes are located on pages 2155-2163.

BRAND NAMES

Finest Natural E Vitamin 400 I. U. d-Alpha - Walgreens
Each softgel contains: Vitamin E (D-alpha tocopheryl acetate) 400 IU. Other Ingredients: Gelatin, USP Water, Glycerin.

Finest Natural Echinacea 125 mg - Walgreens
Each tablet contains: Echinacea leaf extract (echinacea purpurea) 125 mg. Other Ingredients: Dicalcium Phosphate, Microcrystalline Cellulose, Glyceryl Monostearate, Croscarmellose Sodium, Silicon Dioxide, Magnesium Stearate, Aqueous Coating.

Finest Natural Echinacea and Goldenseal 200 mg - Walgreens
Each tablet contains: Echinacea leaf extract (echiancea purpurea) 100 mg • Goldenseal root extract (hydrastis canadensis) 100 mg. Other Ingredients: Dicalcium Phosphate, Microcrystalline Cellulose, Glyceryl Monostearate, Croscarmellose Sodium, Silicon Dioxide, Magnesium Stearate, Aqueous Coating.

Finest Natural Ester-C 1000 mg Vitamin C - Walgreens
Each caplet contains: Vitamin C 1000 mg. Other Ingredients: Microcrystalline Cellulose, Stearic Aid, Croscarmellose Sodium, Magnesium Stearate, Silicon Dioxide, Hydroxypropyl Methylcellulose, Carnauba Wax, Polyethylene Glycol.

Finest Natural Ester-C wth Bioflavonoids 500 mg Vitamin C - Walgreens
Each caplet contains: Vitamin C 500 mg • Bioflavonoids 200 mg • Hesperidin 10 mg • Rutin 10 mg. Other Ingredients: Croscarmellose Sodium, Stearic Acid, Ethylcellulose, Silicon Dioxide, Magnesium Stearate, Hydroxypropyl Methylcellulose, Carnauba Wax.

Finest Natural Fish Oil Concentrate 1000 mg - Walgreens
Two softgels contain: Omega-3 Fatty Acids 600 mg • EPA (eicospentaenoic acid) 360 mg • DHA (docoshexaenoic acid) 240 mg. Other Ingredients: Gelatin, Glycerin, Purified Water, D-Alpha Tocopherol.

Finest Natural Fish Oil Concentrate 1760 mg - Walgreens
Two softgels contain: Fish Oil concentrate 1.76 g • Omega-3 Fatty Acids 870 mg • EPA (eicosapentaenoic aid) 520 mg • DHA (docosahexaenoic acid) 350 mg.

Finest Natural Flax Seed Oil 1000 mg - Walgreens
Each softgel contains: Flax seed oil 1 g • Alpha-Linolenic Acid (omega-3) 557 mg • Linoleic Acid (omega-6) 146 mg • Oleic Acid (omega-9) 190 mg. Other Ingredients: Gelatin, Glycerin.

Finest Natural Garlic - Walgreens
Each tablet contains: Calcium (as dicalcium phosphate and calcium carbonate) 50 mg • Garlic bulb powder 400 mg. Other Ingredients: Microcrystalline Celluose, Modified Cellulose Gum, Pharmaceutical Glaze, Stearic Acid, Hydroxypropyl Methylcellulose, Titanium Dioxide, Talc, Anise Oil.

Finest Natural Garlic Oil - Walgreens
Each softgel contains: Garlic bulb 3 mg. Other Ingredients: Soybean Oil, Gleatin, Glycerin.

Finest Natural Ginkgo Biloba 60 mg - Walgreens
Each tablet contains: Ginkgo Biloba leaf extract (standardized to contain 24% ginkgo flavone glycosides, 6% terpene lactones) 60 mg. Other Ingredients: Dicalcium Phosphate, Microcrystalline Cellulose, Glyceryl Monostearate, Croscarmellose Sodium, Silicon Dioxide, Magnesium Stearate, Aqueous Coating.

Finest Natural Glucosamine 500mg Chondroitin 400mg Double Strength - Walgreens
Each capsule contains: Glucosamine HCl 500 mg • Chondroitin Sulfate 400 mg. Other Ingredients: Gelatin, Rice Flour, Magnesium Stearate.

Finest Natural Glucosamine Chondroitin Double Strength - Walgreens
Each capsule contains: Glucosamine HCl 500 mg • Chondroitin Sulfate 400 mg. Other Ingredients: Gelatin, Rice Flour, Magnesium Stearate.

Finest Natural Glucosamine Chondroitin Triple Strength - Walgreens
Each tablet contains: Glucosamine HCl 750 mg • Chondroitin Sulfate 600 mg. Other Ingredietns: Cellulose, Stearic Acid, Croscarmellose Sodium, Silicon Dioxide, Magnesium Stearate.

Finest Natural Glucosamine Chondrotin - Walgreens
Each capsule contains: Glucosamine HCl 500 mg • Chondroitin Sulfate 400 mg. Other Ingredients: Gelatin, Rice Flour, Magnesium Stearate.

Finest Natural Glucosamine Sulfate 500 mg - Walgreens
Each capsule contains: Glucosamine Sulfate 500 mg. Other Ingredients: Gelatin, Rice Flour, Magnesium Stearate.

Finest Natural Glucosamine Sulfate 750 mg - Walgreens
Each tablet contains: Glucosamine Sulfate 750 mg. Other Ingredients: Microcrystalline Cellulose, Stearic Acid, Silicon Dioxide, Magnesium Stearate.

Finest Natural Grapeseed 50 mg - Walgreens
Each tablet contains: Grapeseed & Grape skin extract (vitis vinifera, standardized to contain 90% polyphenols) 50 mg. Other Ingredients: Dicalcium Phosphate, Microcrystalline Celluose, Glyceryl Monostearate, Croscarmellose Sodium, Silicon Dioxide, Magnesium Stearate, Aqueous Coating.

Finest Natural High Potency Zinc 50 mg - Walgreens
Each caplet contains: Zinc (zinc gluconate) 50 mg. Other Ingredients: Microcrystalline Cellulose, Dicalcium Phosphate, Modified Cellulose Gum, Stearic Acid, Hydroxypropyl Methylcellulose, Hydroxypropyl Cellulose, Magnesium Stearate, Polyethylene Glycol.

Finest Natural Magnesium 250 mg - Walgreens
Each tablet contains: Calcium 42 mg • Magnesium 250 mg. Other Ingredients: Microcrystalline Celluose, Modified Cellulose Gum, Stearic Acid, Citric Acid, Magnesium Stearate, Talc, Sodium Lauryl Sulfate.

Finest Natural Menopause Relief - Walgreens
Each tablet contains: Black Cohosh root and rhizome extract 20 mg.

Finest Natural Multi Vitamin & Mineral Supplement - Walgreens
Each caplet contains: Vitamin C 120 mg • Thiamin (vitamin B1) 5 mg • Riboflavin (vitamin B2) 5 mg • Niacin 30 mg • Vitamin B6 5 mg • Folic Acid 400 mg • Vitamin B12 10 mcg • Biotin 10 mcg • Pantothenic Acid 10 mg • Calcium 100 mg • Iron 18 mg • Phosphorus 78 mg • Iodine 150 mcg • Magnesium 100 mg • Zinc 15 mg • Copper 2 mg • Chloride 15 mg • Potassium 15 mg. Other Ingredients: Dicalcium Phosphate, Microcrystalline Cellulose, Gelatin, Stearic Acid, Croscarmellose Sodium, Crospovidone, Hydroxypropyl Methylellulose, Hydroxypropyl Cellulose, Magnesium Stearate, Polyethylene Glycol, Starh, Gluten, Sodium Bisulfite.

Finest Natural Potassium Gluconate - Walgreens
Each tablet contains: Potassium 99 mg. Other Ingredients: Stearic Acid, Magnesium Stearate.

Finest Natural Saw Palmetto - Walgreens
Each softgel contains: Saw Palmetto berry extract (serenoa repens, standardized to contain 85-95% fatty acids, 85-95% sterols) 160 mg. Other Ingredients: Olive Oil, Gelatin, Glycerin.

Finest Natural Selenium 100 mcg - Walgreens
Each tablet contains: Selenium 100 mcg. Other Ingredients: Dicalcium Phosphate, Microcrystalline Cellulose, Stearic Acid, Modified Cellulose Gum, Magnesium Stearate.

Finest Natural Selenium 200 mcg - Walgreens
Each tablet contains: Selenium 200 mcg. Other Ingredients: Dicalcium Phosphate, Microcrystalline Cellulose, Stearic Acid, Croscarmellose Sodium, Magnesium Stearate, Hydroxyproylmethyl Cellulose, Hydroxypropyl Cellulose, Polyethylene Glycol.

Finest Natural Siberian Eleuthero Root - Walgreens
Each tablet contains: Siberian Eleuthero root extract (eleutherococcus senticosus, standardized to contain 0.8% eleutherosides) 200 mg. Other Ingredients: Dicalcium Phosphate, Microcrystalline Cellulose, Glyceryl Monostearate, Croscarmellose Sodium, Silicon Dioxide, Magnesium Stearate, Aqueous Coating.

Finest Natural St. John's Wort 300 mg - Walgreens
Each tablet contains: St. John's Wort extract 300 mg. Other Ingredients: Dicalcium Phosphate USP, Silica Dioxide, Microcrystalline Cellulose, Croscarmellose Sodium NF, Glyceryl Monostearate, Magnesium Stearate.

Finest Natural Timed Release Vitamin C with Rose Hips 1000 mg - Walgreens
Each caplet contains: Vitamin C (from ascorbic acid, rose hips) 1000 mg. Other Ingredients: Hydroxypropyl Methylcellulose, Talc, Stearic Acid, Silicon Dioxide, Magnesium Stearate, Colloidal Silicon Dioxide, Carbauba Wax.

Finest Natural Valerian 250 mg - Walgreens
Each tablet contains: Valerian root extract (valeriana officinalis, standardized to ontain 0.8% valerenic acid) 250 mg. Other Ingredients: Dicalcium Phosphate, Microcrystalline Cellulose, Glyceryl Monostearate, Croscarmellose Sodium, Silicon Dioxide, Magnesium Stearate, Aqueous Coating.

Finest Natural Vitamin A & D - Walgreens
Each softgel contains: Soybean Oil • Skip Jack oil • Fish oil. Other Ingredinets: Gelatin, Glycerin, Water.

Finest Natural Vitamin A & D Cod Liver Oil - Walgreens
Each softgel contains: Cod Liver oil. Other Ingredients: Soybean Oil, Gelatin, Glycerin.

Finest Natural Vitamin C with Rose Hips 1000 mg - Walgreens
Each tablet contains: Vitamin C (from ascorbic acid, rose hips) 1000 mg. Other Ingredients: Microcrystalline Cellulose, Croscarmellose Sodium, Stearic Acid, Powdered Cellulose, Magnesium Stearate, Hydroxypropyl Methylcellulose, Colloidal Silicon Dioxide, Polyethylene Glycol, Carnauba Wax.

Finest Natural Vitamin E Natural 400 IU - Walgreens
Each softgel contains: Vitamin E (as D-alpha tocopheorl) 400 IU • D-Gamma Tocopherol 75 g • Other Tocopherols (D-beta, D-delta) 37 g. Other Ingredients: Soybean Oil, Gelatin, USP Water, Glycerin.

Finest Natural Vitamin Folic Aid 400 mcg - Walgreens
Each tablet contains: Folate 400 mcg. Other Ingredients: Dicalcium Phosphate, Calcium Carbonate, Stearic Acid, Croscarmellose Sodium, Sodium Bicarboante, Magnesium Stearate.

Finest Time Relase Vitamin B-12 - Walgreens
Each tablet contains: Vitamin B12 (cobalamin) 1000 mcg. Other Ingredients: Calcium Sulfate Dihydrate, Whey, Modified Cellulose Gum, Stearic Acid, Ethylcellulose, Calcium Stearate, Silicon Dioxide, Methylcellulose, Purified Water.

Finest Vitamin B-12 - Walgreens
Each tablet contains: Vitamin B12 (cyanocobalamin) 500 mcg. Other Ingredients: Dicalcium Phosphate, Microcrystalline Cellulose, Stearic Acid, Croscarmellose Sodium, Crospovidone, Magnesium Stearate, Silicon Dioxide.

Finest Vitamin B-6 100 mg - Walgreens
Each tablet contains: Vitamin B6 (pyridoxine hydrochloride) 100 mg. Other Ingredients: Dicalcium Phosphate, Microcrystalline Cellulose, Magnesium Stearate.

Fingerprinted Alfalfa - GNC
Each capsule contains: Alfalfa herb powder (Medicago sativa) 500 mg. Other Ingredients: Gelatin.

Fingerprinted Astragalus - GNC
Each capsule contains: Astragalus root powder (as astragalus membranceus) 250 mg. Other Ingredients: Cellulose, Gelatin, Calcium Carbonate.

Fingerprinted Bilberry - GNC
Each capsule contains: Bilberry fruit powder (vaccinium myrtillus L.) 500 mg. Other Ingredients: Gelatin, Cellulose.

Fingerprinted Black Cohosh - GNC
Each capsule contains: Black Cohosh root powder (cimicifuga racemosa) 200 mg. Other Ingredients: Cellulose, Gelatin.

Fingerprinted Black Walnut Hulls - GNC
Each capsule contains: Black Walnut hulls powder (juglans nigra) 300 mg. Other Ingredients: Gelatin, Cellulose, Calcium Carbonate.

Fingerprinted Burdock Root - GNC
Each capsule contains: Burdock root powder (arctium lappa) 500 mg. Other Ingredients: Gelatin.

Fingerprinted Butcher's Broom 100 mg - GNC
Each capsule contains: Butcher's Broom root powder (ruscus aculaetus) 100 mg. Other Ingredients: Cellulose, Calcium Carbonate, Gelatin.

Fingerprinted Butcher's Broom 500 mg - GNC
Each capsule contains: Butcher's Broom root powder (ruscus aculaetus) 500 mg. Other Ingredients: Gelatin, Cellulose.

Fingerprinted Cayenne - GNC
Each capsule contains: Cayenne Pepper powder (capsicum frutescens) 500 mg. Other Ingredients: Gelatin, Cellulose.

Fingerprinted Chickweed - GNC
Each capsule contains: Chickweed powder (stellaria media) 500 mg. Other Ingredients: Gelatin.

Fingerprinted Chlorophyll - GNC
Each capsule contains: Soybean Oil 453 mg • Chlorophyll 60 mg. Other Ingredients: Gelatin, Glycerin, Caramel Color, Titanium Dioxide.

Fingerprinted Dong Quai - GNC
Each capsule contains: Dong Quai 500 mg.

Finocarbo Herbal Tea - Aboca USA, Inc
Each bag contains: Fennel fruit (foeniculum vulgare) 6 mg • Star Anise fruit (illicium verum) 6 mg • Licorice root (glycyrrhiza glabra) 3 mg • Chamomile flowering top (matricaria recutita) 0.2 mg • Peppermint leaf (mentha piperita) 0.1 mg • Caraway fruit (carum carvi) 0.1 mg • Cumin fruit (cuminum cyminum) 0.06 mg • Lemon Balm leaf (melissa officinalis) 0.04 mg.

FinoCarbo Plus - Aboca USA, Inc
Two capsules contain: Vegetable Charcoal 174 mg • Fennel fruit Whole Phytocomplex Concentrate (WPC) (foeniculum vulgare, standardized to 2% essential oil) 116 mg • Cumin fruit powder (cuminum cyminum, standardized to 2% essential oil) 87 mg • Chamomile flower freeze-dried extract (matricaria recutita, flavonoids apigenin-like minimum 1%) 87 mg • Star Anise fruit powder (illcium verum, essential oil minimum 7%) 40.6 mg • Lemon Balm leaf freeze-dried extract (melissa officianlis, standardized to 14% rosmarinic acid) 29 mg • Caraway fruit powder (carum carvi, essential oil minimum 2.2%) 29 mg. Other Ingredients: Gelatin (capsule), Essential Oils Of Fennel, Peppermint, Marjoram.

Fired Up! - FreeLife International
Each packet contains: Vitamin C (as ascorbic and isoascorbic acids) 200 mg • Thiamin (as thiamin hydrochloride) 3 mg • Riboflavin 3.4 mg • Niacin (as niacinamide and niacin) 40 mg • Vitamin B6 (as

BRAND NAMES

pyridoxine HCl) 10 mg • Folate (as folic acid) 100 mcg • Vitamin B12 (as cyanocobalamin) 50 mcg • Biotin 100 mcg • Pantothenic Acid (as D-calcium pantothenate) 20 mg • Phosphorus (as dipotassium phosphate) 24 mg • Chromium (as chromium dinicotinate glycinate) 120 mcg • Potassium (as dipotassium phosphate and potassium citrate) 99 mg • Lipitol brand Complex 600 mg: Green Tea leaf extract, Cinnamon twig extract, Galangal root extract • L-Phenylalanine 500 mg • Taurine 200 mg • Glycine 100 mg • Panax Ginseng root standardized extract 100 mg • DMAE (dimethylaminoethanol) Bitartrate 75 mg. Other ingredients: Natural Flavors, Maltodextrin, Citric Acid, Sucralose, Silica, Beta Carotene (for color).

Firm Foundation Calcium Blend - Physicians Laboratories
Four capsules contain: Calcium 500 mg • Boron Citrate 3 mg.

Firm Foundation Multivitamin & Multimineral - Physicians Laboratories
Six capsules contain: Vitamin A (as beta carotene/a acetate) 5000 IU • Vitamin C (as calcium ascorbate) 60 mg • Vitamin D (as D cholecalciferol) 400 IU • Vitamin E (as E succinate) 30 IU • Vitamin K (as K phytonadione) 80 mcg • Thiamin (as thiamin HCl) 1.5 mg • Riboflavin 1.7 mg • Niacin (as niacinamide, inositol hexaniacinate) 20 mg • Vitamin B12 (as cyanocobalamin) 2 mg • Biotin 400 mcg • Pantothenic Acid (as d-calcium pantothenate) 6 mcg • Iodine (as kelp) 150 mcg • Magnesium (as magnesium aspartate, malate, citrate) 400 mg • Zinc (as zinc monomethionine) 15 mg • Selenium (as selenomethionine) 70 mcg • Copper (as copper chelate, citrate) 2 mg • Manganese (as manganese citrate) 2 mg • Chromium (as chromium polynicotinate) 120 mcg • Molybdenum (as molybdenum chelate) 75 mcg • Calcium 24 mg • Silicon (as sodium meta silicate) 2 mg • Vanadium (as vanadyl sulfate) 10 mcg • Proprietary Enzyme Blend 25 mg: Amyloglecoside, Amylase, Protease, Acid Protease, Cellulase, Lipase, Lactase.

Firm Foundation Vitamin E - Physicians Laboratories
Each capsule contains: Vitamin E (as d-alpha tocopheryl acetate) 400 IU • Ginger rhizome, Supercritical CO2 extract (zingiber officinale) 4 mg.

Firm Lotion - Mannatech
Water • Parrafin • Caprylic/Capric Triglycerides • C 12-15 Alkyl Benzoate • Cetyl Alcohol • Propylene Glycol • Dimethicone • Germaben II (propylene glycol, diazolidinyl urea, methylparaben, propylparaben) • Amino Methylpropanol • Ambrotose Complex (patent pending; naturally occurring plant saccharides including freeze-dried aloe vera gel complex - manapol powder) • Lactic Acid • Niacinamide • Emu Oil • Stearic Acid • Cholesterol • Lavender Oil • Carbomer • Herbal Complex: Barley extract, Clover extract, Ivy extract, Butcherbroom extract, Camellia Oleifera extract, Lady's Thistle extract • Wild Yam extract.

First Call - Natural Bridges Products
Each capsule contains: Proprietary Blend 420 mg: Artichoke extract, Sarsaparilla extract.

Fish Body Oil - Health Center for Better Living
Each softgel contains: EPA 180 mg • DHA 120 mg • Vitamin E 5 IU.

Fish Body Oils 1000 - GNC
Each capsule contains: EPA (Eicosapentaenoic Acid) 180 mg •DHA (Docosahexaenoid Acid) 120 mg. Other Ingredients: Gelatin, Glycerin, Vitamin E.

Fish Body Oils 1000 Deodorized - GNC
Each capsule contains: EPA (Eicosapentaenoic Acid) 180 mg • DHA (Docosahexaenoic Acid) 120 mg. Other Ingredients: Gelatin, Glycerin.

Fish Body Oils with GLA - GNC
Each capsule contains: Vitamin E (as d-alpha Tocopherol) 3 IU • EPA (Eicosapentaenoic Acid) 180 mg • DHA (Docosahexaenoic Acid) 120 mg • GLA (gamma Linolenic Acid) 23 mg. Other Ingredients: Fish body oil, Gelatin, Glycerin, Borage Oil (Borago officinalis), Enteric Coating: Hydroxypropyl Methylcellulose Phthalate, Titanium Dioxide, Flax seed oil, triacetin.

Fish Oil - Benepure, Inc
Each softgel capsule contains: Vitamin E 5 IU • Marine Lipid Concentrate (yielding 300 mg eicosapentaenoic acid [EPA], and 200 mg docosahexaenoic acid [DHA]) 1000 mg. Other Ingredients: Gelatin, Glycerin.

Fish Oil - Optimum Nutrition
Each softgel contains: Fish Oil 1000 mg • EPA (eicosapentaenoic acid) 180 mg • DHA (docosahexaenoic acid) 120 mg. Other Ingredients: Gelatin, Glycerin.

Fish Oil 180 EPA/120 DHA - Vital Nutrients
Each softgel contains: Pure Fish Oil 1000 mg: EPA 180 mg, DHA 120 mg.

Fish Oil Multi - J. R. Carlson Laboratories, Inc.
Two softgels contain: Lutein (FloraGlo brand) 500 mcg • Vitamin A (as beta carotene) 10,000 IU • Vitamin C (as calcium ascorbate) 500 mg • Vitamin D (D3, from fish liver oil) 600 IU • Vitamin E (as D-alpha tocopherol) 400 IU • Thiamin (vitamin B1, as thiamin hydrochloride) 25 mg • Riboflavin (vitamin B2) 25 mg • Niacin (vitamin B3, as niacinamide) 25 mg • Vitamin B6 (as pyridoxine hydrochloride) 25 mg • Folate (folic acid) 800 mcg • Vitamin B12 (cyanocobalamin) 100 mcg • Biotin 300 mcg • Pantothenic Acid (as di-calcium pantothenate) 25 mg • Calcium (as calcium ascorbate) 50 mg • Iodine (from kelp) 150 mcg • Magnesium (as magnesium oxide) 100 mg • Zinc (as zinc gluconate) 15 mg • Selenium (as L-selenomethionine) 200 mcg • Copper (as copper gluconate) 2 mg • Manganese (as manganese gluconate) 3 mg • Chromium 200 mcg • DHA (docosahexaenoic acid) 90 mg • EPA (eicosapentaenoic acid) 130 mg • Phosphatidyl Choline 50 mg • Phosphatidyl Ethanolamine 10 mg • Phosphatidyl Inositol 3 mg • Fish oil concentrate 770 mg • Lecithin 60 mg • Lemon Bioflavonoids complex 25 mg.

Fish Oil Q - J. R. Carlson Laboratories, Inc.
Each softgel contains: Vitamin E (as D-alpha tocopherol) 10 IU • Omega-3 Fatty Acids (from fish oil) 250 mg • DHA (docosahexaenoic acid) 100 mg • EPA (eicosapentaenoic acid) 150 mg • Co-Q10 (coenzyme Q10) 50 mg • L-Carnitine (as L-carnitine tartrate) 50 mg.

Fisol - Nature's Way
Each softgel contains: Fish Oil 500 mg • Vitamin E (d-alpha tocopheryl) 1 IU. Other Ingredients: Aqueaous Coating Solution, Gelatin, Glycerin, Water.

FIT - Agel
Each packet contains: Super Citrimax brand Garcinia Cambogia extract [60% (-)hydroxycitric acid extract of garcinia cambogia fruit) 1300 mg • Apple Cider Vinegar 00 mg. Other Ingredients: Water, Proprietary Sweetening Blend (inulin, xylitol, neotame, acesulfame-K, lactobacillus acidophilus), Fructose, Natural Flavoring, Guar Gum, Grapefruit Seed Extract, Xanthan Gum, Sodium Benzoate.

FIT Advanced Calcium - Apex Fitness Group
Two tablets contain: Elemental Calcium 1000 mg • Vitamin D 200 IU • Elemental Magnesium 500 mg.

FIT Bar (assorted flavors) - Apex Fitness Group
Corn Syrup • High Fructose Corn Syrup • Calcium Caseinate • Sugar • Fractionated Palm kernal oil • Whey Protein Isolate • Soy Protein Isolate • Nonfat Milk • Lactose • Natural and Artificial flavor • Cellulose gel • Salt • Dextrose • Coconut oil and/or Palm oil • Soy Lecithin • Partially Hydrogenated Soybean oil • Calcium Phosphate • Sodium Ascorbate • Ferric Orthophosphate • Alpha Tocopherol Acetate • Niacinamide • Zinc Oxide • Calcium Pantothenate • Coffee • Vitamin A Palmitate • Pyridoxine Hydrochloride • Riboflavin • Thiamin Mononitrate • Folic Acid • Biotin • Potassium Iodide • Vitamin B12. Chocolate Almond Toffee flavor also contains: Almonds • Cocoa (processed with alkali) • High Oleic Sunflower oil •

Tocopherols • Butter (cream, salt) • Guar Gum • Coffee. Chocolate Chip Cookie Dough flavor also contains: Cocoa (processed with alkali), High Oleic Sunflower oil • Tocopherols • Canola oil • Guar gum. Chocolate Mint flavor also contains: High Maltose Corn syrup • Cocoa (processed with alkali), Canola oil • Color Blend (yellow 5 lake, blue 1 lake). Chocolate Peanut Butter Cup flavor also contains: Partially defatted Peanut Flour • Ground Peanuts • Cocoa (processed with alkali) • Oat Fiber • Sunflower Oil • Guar Gum. Cookies 'N Cream flavor also contains: High Maltose Corn syrup • Cocoa (processed with alkali) • Canola Oil • Nonfat Yogurt Powder (cultured whey, nonfat milk) • Titanium Dioxide. Oatmeal Raisin flavor also contains: Raisins • Rolled Oats • Brown Sugar • Nonfat Yogurt Powder (cultured whey, nonfat milk) • Spice • High Oleic Safflower Oil • Honey • Titanium Dioxide • Guar Gum.
This product was formerly called "Nutrition Bar."

***FIT Chromemate* - Apex Fitness Group**
Each tablet contains: Trivalent Chromium (from niacin-bound chromium polynicotinate) 200 mcg. Other Ingredients: Calcium Phosphate, Microcrystalline Cellulose, Croscarmellose, Stearic Acid, Magnesium Stearate.

***FIT Drink Mix (assorted flavors)* - Apex Fitness Group**
Nonfat Milk • Calcium Caseinate • Fructose • Maltodextrin • Whey • Medium Chain Triglycerides • Malted Milk powder (wheat flour and barley malt extract, milk, salt, sodium bicarbonate) • Sodium Citrate • Natural and Artificial Flavor • Salt • Potassium Citrate • Egg White • Soy Lecithin • Magnesium Oxide • Choline Bitartrate • Potassium Chloride • Cellulose Gum • Rice Maltodextrin • Aspartame • Inottiol • Ascorbic Acid • Ferrous Fumarate • Alpha - Tocopherol Acetate • Niacinamide • Zinc Oxide • Manganese Sulfate • Calcium Pantothenate • Copper Sulfate • Vitamin A Palmitate • Pyridoxine Hydrochloride • Riboflavin • Thiamin Mononitrate • Folic Acid • Sodium Molybdate • Chromium Chloride • Biotin • Potassium Iodide • Sodium Selenite • Phytonadione • Vitamin D (D3) • Vitamin B12. Chocolate flavor also contains: Cocoa (processed with alkali). Strawberry flavor also contains: Red Beet Juice, Malic Acid, Beta Carotene.
This product was formerly called "High Performance."

***FIT Ginkgo* - Apex Fitness Group**
Two capsules contain: Phosphatidyl Serine 100 mg • Ginkgo Biloba 60 mg (standardized to 24% ginkgosides & 7% terpenes) 60 mg • Proprietary Blend 365 mg: Green Tea, Guarana, Yerba Mate extract (providing 100 mg caffeine) • Proprietary Cocoa extract (providing PEA (phenylethylamine) and tyramine plus 7.2 mg theobromine) 180 mg. Other Ingredients: Talc, Magnesium Stearate.
This product was formerly called "Instant Einstein."

***FIT Joint Support* - Apex Fitness Group**
Each tablet contains: Glucosamine Sulfate 500 mg • Chondroitin Sulfate A 400 mg. Other Ingredients: Calcium Carbonate, Microcrystalline Cellulose, Magnesium Stearate, Silica, Vegetable Stearate.
See Editor's Note No. 15.

***FIT Multivitamin Children's* - Apex Fitness Group**
Each tablet contains: Beta Carotene (pro vitamin A) 2000 IU • Vitamin A (palmitate) 500 IU • Vitamin C (ascorbic acid) 30 mg • Calcium (calcium phosphate) 20 mg • Iron (fumarate) 9 mg • Vitamin D (D3, cholecalciferol) 200 IU • Vitamin E (natural D-alpha tocopheryl succinate) 15 IU • Vitamin B1 (thiamine HCl) 0.75 mg • Vitamin B2 (riboflavin) 0.85 mg • Niacinamide 10 mg • Vitamin B6 (pyridoxine HCl) 1 mg • Folic Acid 200 mcg • Vitamin B12 (cyanocobalamin) 3 mcg • Phosphorus 15 mg • Magnesium (oxide) 2.5 mg • Zinc (oxide) 1.1 mg. Other Ingredients: Fructose, Natural Cherry & Natural Vanilla Flavor, Vegetable Stearate, Magnesium Stearate, Natural Flavor and Color.
This product was formerly called "Children's Chewables."

***FIT Multivitamin Profiles 1 & 2 (High Carb/Vegan)* - Apex Fitness Group**
Each tablet contains: Vitamin A (beta carotene) 7000 IU • Vitamin C (ascorbic acid) 300 mg • Calcium (elemental) 100 mg • Iron (ferronyl) 5 mg • Vitamin D (ergocalciferol) 400 IU • Vitamin E (D-alpha tocopheryl succinate) 133.33 IU • Vitamin B1 (thiamine HCl) 6.67 mg • Vitamin B2 (riboflavin) 6.67 mg • Niacinamide 20 mg • Vitamin B6 (pyridoxine HCl, pyridoxal 5 phosphate) 6 mg • Folic Acid 266.67 mcg • Vitamin B12 (cyanocobalamin) 4 mcg • Biotin 40 mcg • Pantothenic Acid (calcium pantothenate) 4 mg • Iodine (kelp) 50 mcg • Magnesium (elemental) 66.67 mg • Zinc (elemental) 10 mg • Selenium (L-selenomethionine) 66.67 mcg • Copper (elemental) 1 mg • Manganese 2 mg • Chromium (polynicotinate) 50 mcg • Potassium (elemental) 50 mg. Other Ingredients: Calcium Phosphate, Microcrystalline Cellulose, Vegetable Stearate, Croscarmellose, Magnesium Stearate.

***FIT Multivitamin Profiles 3 & 4 (Balanced Diet)* - Apex Fitness Group**
Each tablet contains: Vitamin A (beta carotene) 7000 IU • Vitamin C (ascorbic acid) 300 mg • Calcium (elemental) 100 mg • Iron (ferronyl) 5 mg • Vitamin D (ergocalciferol) 400 IU • Vitamin E (D-alpha tocopheryl succinate) 133.33 IU • Vitamin B1 (thiamine mononitrate) 4 mg • Vitamin B2 (riboflavin) 4 mg • Niacinamide 20 mg • Vitamin B6 (pyridoxine HCl, pyridoxal 5 phosphate) 6 mg • Folic Acid 266.67 mcg • Vitamin B12 (cyanocobalamin) 12 mcg • Biotin 150 mcg • Pantothenic Acid (calcium pantothenate) 10 mg • Iodine (kelp) 50 mcg • Magnesium (elemental) 100 mg • Zinc (elemental) 7.5 mg • Selenium (L-selenomethionine) 66.67 mcg • Copper (elemental) 1 mg • Manganese 2 mg • Chromium (polynicotinate) 50 mcg • Potassium (elemental) 50 mg. Other Ingredients: Calcium Phosphate, Vegetable Stearate, Croscarmellose, Magnesium Stearate.

***FIT Premenstrual Formula* - Apex Fitness Group**
Each tablet contains: Ascorbic Acid 250 mg • Calcium (phosphate, ascorbate, citrate) 100 mg • D Alpha Tocopherol 200 IU • Riboflavin 5' Phosphate 20 mg • Niacin 20 mg • Pyridoxal-5-Phosphate 50 mg • Calcium Pantothenate (B5) 50 mg • Magnesium (citrate) 200 mg • Zinc 5 mg • Borage oil (40 mg GLA) 180 mg • Alfalfa concentrate 100 mg • Dioscorea Villosa 200 mg • Uva Ursi 400 mg • Uncaria Gambir 100 mg • Kava Kava extract 100 mg. Other Ingredients: Calcium Phosphate, Microcrystalline Cellulose, Vegetable Stearate, Magnesium Stearate, Croscarmellose.

***FIT Prenatal Extra Formula* - Apex Fitness Group**
Each tablet contains: Vitamin A (beta carotene) 5000 IU • Vitamin C (buffered calcium ascorbate) 100 mg • Calcium (from gluconate, aspartate, carbonate, histidinate, ascorbate, citrate, fumarate, succinate, malate and ketoglutarate) 150 mg • Iron (from bisglycinate, chelate, histidinate, citrate, fumarate, succinate, aspartate, gluconate, ascorbate, malate and ketoglutarate) 30 mg • Vitamin D (ergocalciferol) 200 IU • Vitamin E (D-alpha tocopheryl succinate)100 IU • Vitamin B1 (thiamine hydrochloride) 12.5 mg • Vitamin B2 (riboflavin) 12.5 mg • Niacinamide 12.5 mg • Vitamin B6 (pyridoxine HCl) 12.5 mg • Folic Acid 400 mcg • Vitamin B12 (cyanocobalamin) 25 mcg • Biotin 100 mcg • Pantothenic Acid (calcium pantothenate) 12.5 mg • Iodine (potassium iodine) 75 mcg • Magnesium (from oxide, histidinate, aspartate, gluconate, ascorbate, citrate, fumarate, succinate, malate, and ketoglutarate) 50 mg • Zinc (from histidinate, aspartate, gluconate, ascorbate, picolinate, monomethionine, citrate, succinate, malate, fumarate, and ketoglutarate) 7.5 mg • Copper (copper gluconate) 0.05 mg • Manganese (from chelate, gluconate, citrate, histidinate, aspartate, ascorbate) 0.5 mg • Potassium (from gluconate, citrate, histidinate, aspartate, ascorbate, fumarate, succinate, malate, and ketoglutarate) 5 mg • Inositol 12.5 mg • Choline (from bitartrate) 12.5 mg • PABA (para amino benzoic acid) 12.5 mg. Other Ingredients: Vegetable Stearate, Calcium Phosphate, Microcrystalline Cellulose, Xanthan Gum, Magnesium Stearate.

Some Brand Name Natural Products - What they Contain

www.NaturalDatabase.com contains MANY more listings than appear here.
Editor's Notes are located on pages 2155-2163.

FIT Soy Bars (assorted flavors) **-** Apex Fitness Group
Non-GMO Soy Protein Isolate • High Fructose Corn syrup • Maltitol Syrup • Corn Syrup • Natural and Artificial flavor • Dicalcium Phosphate • Salt • Ascorbic Acid • DL-Alpha Tocopherol Acetate • Niacinamide • Zinc Oxide • Electrolytic Iron • Vitamin A Palmitate • Calcium Pantothenate • Pyridoxine Hydrochloride • Riboflavin • Thaimin Mononitrate • Vitamin B12 • Folic Acid • Bitoin • Potassium Iodide. Chocolate Peanut Butter Cup flavor also contains: Confectionary Coating (sugar, fractionated palm kernal oil, cocoa powder, whey powder, nonfat milk powder, soy lecithin, vanilla) • Non-GMO Soynuts • Non-GMO Soy Crisp (soy protein isolate, rice flour, malt, salt) • Peanut Flour • Peanut Butter. Cookies 'N Cream flavor also contains: Cookie pieces (wheat flour, sugar, cocoa powder, soy protein isolate, fractionated palm kernal oil, corn flour, corn syrup, dried milk powder, artificial flavors, salt, sodium bicarbonate, soy lecithin) • Cocoa powder • Soybutter (roasted soybeans, naturally pressed soybean oil, soy concentrate, soy lecithin, salt) • Non-GMO Soy crisp (soy protein isolate, rice flour, malt, salt). Oatmeal Raisin flavor also contains: Soy blend (non-GMO soy protein isolate, non-GMO soy crisp (soy protein isolate, rice flour, malt, salt)), Yogurt coating (sugar, fractionated palm kernal oil, whey powder, nonfat milk powder, yogurt powder, soy lecithin, vanilla) • High Maltose Corn Syrup • Raisin paste • Rolled Oats • Date Paste • Brown Sugar • Cinnamon.

FIT Soy Drink Mix (chocolate and vanilla flavors) **-** Apex Fitness Group
Soy Protein Isolate • Fructose • Maltodextrin • Natural and Artificial flavor (includes milk) • Soy Lecithin • Calcium Phosphate • Medium Chain Triglycerides • Guar gum • Oat fiber • Cellulose • Salt • Xanthan gum • Magnesium Oxide • Potassium Phosphate • Aspartame • Alpha Tocopherol Acetate • Ascorbic Acid • Ferrous Fumarate • Niacinamide • Zinc Oxide • Manganese Sulfate • Calcium Pantothenate • Vitamin A Palmitate • Copper Sulfate • Pyridoxine Hydrochloride • Riboflavin • Thiamin Hydrochloride • Vitamin B12 • Vitamin D (D3) • Folic Acid • Biotin • Potassium Iodide. Chocolate flavor also contains: Cocoa (processed with alkali) • Milk • Salt. Vanilla flavor also includes: Potassium Citrate.

FIT Super Anti-Oxidant **-** Apex Fitness Group
Each tablet contains: Alpha Carotene 1.5 mg • Lutein 6 mg • Lycopene 6 mg • Zeaxanthin 4 mg • CoQ10 30 mg • Alpha Lipoic Acid 25 mg. Other Ingredients: Calcium Phosphate, Magnesium Stearate, Vegetable Stearate, Croscarmellose, Silica.

FIT Vitamin C **-** Apex Fitness Group
Each tablet contains: Vitamin C (ascorbic acid) 1000 mg. Other Ingredients: Calcium Phosphate, Vegetable Stearate, Croscarmellose, Magnesium Stearate.

FIX Crisp Bars (assorted flavors) **-** Apex Fitness Group
Corn Syrup • Soy Protein Isolate • High Fructose Corn Syrup • Sugar • Fractionated Palm kernal oil • Rolled Oats • Fructose • Rice Flour • Barley Malt extract • Glycerine • Calcium Caseinate • Nonfat Milk • Lactose • Whey Protein Isolate • Natural flavor • High Fructose Corn Syrup • Calcium Phosphate • Salt • Soybean oil • Dextrose • Soy Lecithin • Honey • Sodium Ascorbate • Ferric Orthophosphate • Alpha Tocopherol Acetate • Niacinamide • Zinc Oxide • Calcium Pantothenate • Vitamin A Palmitate • Pyridoxine Hydrochloride • Riboflavin • Thiamin Mononitrate • Folic Acid • Biotin • Potassium Iodide • Vitamin B12. Chocolate Peanut Butter flavor also contains: Peanuts • Paritally defatted Peanut Flour • Ground Peanuts • Cocoa (processed with alkali) • Caramel. Citrus flavor also contains: Fructooligosaccharides • Polydextrose • Orange puree from concentrate • Lemon juice from concentrate • Nonfat Yogurt powder (cultured whey, nonfat milk) • Titanium Dioxide • Annatto • Sodium Benzoate • Sulfur Dioxide. Oatmeal Raisin flavor also contains: Raisins • Polydextrose • Fructooligosaccharides • Nonfat Yogurt powder (cultured whey, nonfat milk) • Spice • Caramel • Titanium Dioxide.

Fizzees **-** Advocare International
Each wafer contains: Vitamin C (as ascorbic acid) 240 mg • Wild Schisandra extract (fruit - schisandra chinensis) 30 mg • Echinacea extract (root - echinacea purpurea) 30 mg • Licorice extract (root - glycyrrhiza glabra) 20 mg • Spikenard extract (root and rhizome - Aralia mandshurica) 10 mg. Other Ingredients: Dextrose, Potassium Bicarbonate, Citric Acid, Sucralose, Natural Flavors.

Flash Fighters **-** Puritan's Pride
Three tablets contain: Soy concentrate (yielding 65 mg total Isoflavones) 2,100 mg • Black Cohosh extract (Cimicifuga racemosa) root (2.5% triterpene glycosides) 160 mg • Dong Quai (Angelica sinensis) root 150 mg • Licorice (Glycyrrhiza glabra) root 150 mg • Vitex extract (Vitex agnus-castus) fruit 100 mg.

Flash-Ease Time Release **-** Nature's Sunshine
Each tablet contains: Proprietary Blend 280 mg: Black Cohosh root and rhizome (cimicifuga racemosa, standardized to contain a minimum of 2.5% total triterpene glycosides, calculated as 27-deoxyactein), Dong Quai root (angelica sinensis). Other Ingredients: Maltodextrin, Cellulose, Stearic Acid, Di-Calcium Phosphate, Magnesium Stearate.

Flavay **-** VMAH
Two capsules contain: Masquelier's Oligomeric Proanthocyanidins seed/bark standardzed complex • Macrozyme Active Enzyme Blend 20 mg: Amylase, Cellulase, Lactase, Lipase, Protease, Maltase, Invertase.

Flavay Plus **-** VMAH
Two capsules contain: Vitamin A (100% as beta-carotene) 5000 IU • Vitamin C (ester-c calcium ascorbate) 60 mg • Vitamin E (d-alpha tocopherol succinate) 100 IU • Vitamin B1 (thiamin) 3 mg • Vitamin B2 (riboflavin) 6 mg • Vitamin B6 (pyridoxine) 10 mg • Vitamin B12 (cyanocobalamin) 20 mcg • Zinc Orotate 10 mg • Selenium (organically bound) 20 mcg • Phosphatidyl Serine 100 mg • GABA (gamma amino butyric acid) 60 mg • Ginkgo Biloba leaf standardized extract (24% ginkgo flavone glycosides, 6% terpene lactones) 50 mg • Masquelier's Oligomeric Proanthocyanidins seed/bark extract 50 mg.

Flav-O-Grams **-** Alacer
Each tablet contains: Vitamin C (as calcium-mineral ascorbate) 100 mg • Proprietary Bioflavonoid mix 900 mg • Quercetin 100 mg • Grape seed extract.

Flavoplex C **-** InterPlexus
Two capsules contain: Vitamin C (as calcium ascorbate) 420 mg • Calcium (as ascorbate) 48 mg • Hesperidin 300 mg • Hesperidin Methyl Chalcone 200 mg • Grape seed extract 100 mg • Winter Cherry extract 180 mg • Naringin 100 mg. Other Ingredients: Cellulose.

Flax 1000 mg **-** Jamieson
Each capsule contains: Alpha Linolenic Acid (ALA) 500 mg.

Flax Borage Combo **-** Health From The Sun
Three capsules contain: Alpha-Linolenic Acid (ALA)(Omega-3) 825 mg • Gamma-Linolenic Acid (Omega-6) 72 mg • Linoleic Acid (Omega-6) 320 mg • Oleic Acid (Omega-9) 260 mg. Other Ingredients: Certified Organic Flax seed oil, Borage seed oil, Gelatin, Glycerine, Water, Carob powder.

Flax Essence **-** Jarrow Formulas
Each capsule contains: Lignan from 200 mg of LinumLife Extra brand Flaxseed extract (linum usitatissimum, standardized at 20% SDG) 40 mg. Other Ingredients: Magnesium Stearate.

Flax Lignan Gold **-** Health From The Sun
Each 1 tsp serving contains: 100% Certified Organic Flax seed oil & Particulate with Rosemary extract • Mixed Tocopherols (Vitamin E) • Ascorbyl Palmitate (Vitamin C) • Citric Acid to protect freshness.

Flax Liquid Gold **-** Health From The Sun
Each 1 tsp serving contains: 100% Certified Organic Flax seed oil with Rosemary extract • Mixed Tocopherols (Vitamin E) • Ascorbyl Palmitate (Vitamin C) • Citric Acid to protect freshness.

Flax Oil **-** Vital Nutrients
Each softgel contains: Flax oil (certified organic and cold pressed) 1000 mg.

Flax Oil **-** Swanson Health Products
Each softgel contains: Calories 10 • Calories from Fat 9 • Total Fat 1 g • Organic Flax Oil 1 g.

Flax Oil **-** Metabolic Response Modifiers
Each softgel contains: Flax oil 1,000 mg • Linolenic acid (Omega-3) 550 mg • Linoleic acid (Omega-6) 170 mg • Oleic acid (Omega-9) 170 mg • Mixed short chain fatty acids 110 mg.

Flax Oil 1300 mg **-** Nature's Plus
Each softgel contains: Flax seed oil (linum usitatissimum, standardized 58% alpha linolenic acid) 1300 mg. Other Ingredients: Gelatin, Glycerin, Purified Water.

Flax Seed Oil **-** Pro Health
Each softgel contains: Vitmain A (100% as beta-carotene) 430 IU • Organic Flax Seed Oil (unrefined, from Washington flax seed) 1000 mg • Omega-3 Fatty Acids (as alpha-linolenic acid) 560 mg • Omega-6 Fatty Acids (as linoleic acid) 170 mg • Omega-9 Fatty Acids (as oleic acid) 172 mg. Other Ingredients: Gelatin, Glycerin, Carob Powder, Water.

Flax Seed Oil **-** Mass Quantities, Inc.
Each tablespoon contains: Omega-3 Alpha Lineolic Acid 6.2 g • Omega-6 Lineolic Acid 1.8 g • Omega-9 Oleic Acid 2 g.

Flax Seed Oil 1000 mg **-** Jamieson
Each capsule contains: Alpha Linolenic Acid (ALA) (from Flax seed oil) 500 mg.

Flax Seed Oil 1000 mg **-** The Vitamin Shoppe
Each softgel contains: 1000 mg of 100% pure, organically grown cold-pressed, unrefined virgin flax oil providing the following approximate essential fatty acids: Alpha-Linolenic Acid 550 mg • Linoleic Acid 150 mg • Oleic Acid 190 mg • natural Vitamin E 1 IU.

Flax Seed Oil Caps **-** Ortho Molecular Products
Each soft gel contains: Organic Flax seed oil 1000 mg. Other Ingredients: Natural Gelatin Capsules, Glycerin, Purified Water, Carob Extract.

Flax Seed Oil with Borage Oil **-** Pro Health
Each softgel contains: Flax Seed oil (from wheat) 840 mg • Borage Oil 160 mg • Gamma Linoleic Acid (GLA) 35 mg • Omega-3 Fatty Acids (as linolenic acid) 455 mg • Omega-6 Fatty Acids (as linoleic acid) 190 mg • Omega-9 Fatty Acids (as oleic acid) 175 mg. Other Ingredients: Gelatin, Water, Glycerin, Natural Carob Coating.

Flax/Borage Oil **-** Pure Encapsulations
Each softgel capsule contains: Flax seed oil 500 mg • Borage oil (providing omega-3 285 mg, omega-6 117 mg, omega-9 106 mg, gamma linolenic acid [GLA] 23 mg) 100 mg • Vitamin E (D-alpha-tocopherol) 10 IU. Other Ingredients: Carob.

Flax/Borage Oil **-** Vital Nutrients
Each softgel contains: Flax oil 500 mg • Borage oil 100 mg.

Flax-O-Mega **-** Flora Inc.
Cold pressed Flax Seed oil 1000 mg.

Flaxseed & Cod Liver Oil **-** Puritan's Pride
Each softgel contains: Cold-Pressed Linseed oil 500 mg • Vitamin A (from Cod Liver Oil) 1250 IU • Vitamin D (from Cod Liver Oil) 135 IU.

Flaxseed Oil **-** Golden Glow Natural Health Products
Each capsule contains: Flaxseed oil (linseed oil) 1 g: Oleic Acid 175 mg, Linoleic Acid 175 mg, Linolenic Acid 575 mg.

Flaxseed Oil **-** Optimum Nutrition
Each softgel contains: Flaxseed Oil 1000 mg. Other Ingredients: Gelatin, Glycerin, St. John's Bread Extract.

Flaxseed Oil **-** Jarrow Formulas
Each softgel contains: Flaxseed oil 1000 mg: Alpha-Linolenic Acid (omega-3) 540 mg, Linoleic Acid (omega-6) 150 mg, Oleic Acid (omega-9) 210 mg, Other Lipids 100 mg. Other Ingredients: Gelatin, Glycerin, Water, Carob.

Flaxseed Oil 1000mg **-** Nature's Own
Each tablet contains: Flaxseed oil (linum usitatissimum) 1000 mg: Alpha-Linolenic Acid 450 mg • Linoleic Acid 100 mg • Oleic Acid 100 mg.

Flaxseed Oil 1200 MG **-** PhysioLogics
Each softgel contains: Flaxseed Oil 1200 mg (typically contains alpha-linolenic acid 702 mg) • Linoleic Acid 180 mg • Oleic Acid 210 mg • Other Fatty Acids, Phytonutrients 108 mg. Other Ingredients: Gelatin, Glycerin.

Flex Able Advanced Bone & Joint **-** Amerifit Nutrition
Six caplets contain: Vitamin C (ascorbic acid) 100 mg • Calcium (as dicalcium phosphate) 650 mg • Phosphorus (as dicalcium phosphate) 500 mg • Zinc (as zinc nitrate) 15 mg • Copper (as copper gluconate) 2 mg • Glucosamine Hydrochloride 1500 mg • Chondroitin Sulfate 1200 mg • Citrus Bioflavonoids 500 mg. Other Ingredients: Microcrystalline Cellulose, Croscarmellose Sodium, Vegetable Stearic Acid, Silica, Vegetable Magnesium Stearate, Natural Vegetable Coating.

Flex Able Advanced Formula with Curcumin **-** Amerifit Nutrition
Two caplets contain: Glucosamine HCl 850 mg • Curcumin extract (curcuma longa, turmeric rhizome providing 95% curcuminoids) 300 mg • MSM (methylsulfonylmethane) 250 mg • Ginger root standardized extract (zingiber officinalis, 5% gingerols) 100 mg • Bioperine brand Black Pepper extract (standardized piper nigrum) 2.5 mg. Other Ingredients: Microcrystalline Cellulose, Croscarmellose Sodium, Stearic Acid, Silica, Magneseium Stearate, Pharmaceutical Glaze.
See Editor's Note No. 21.

Flex Able Maximum Strength **-** Amerifit Nutrition
Each capsule contains: Glucosamine Hydrochloride 500 mg • Chondroitin Sulfate 400 mg. Other Ingredients: Gelatin (capsule) Silica, Magnesium Stearate.

Flex Able Natural Chewables **-** Amerifit Nutrition
Each chewable wafer contains: Vitamin C 30 mg • Glucosamine HCl 750 mg • Chondroitin Complex 600 mg: Hydrolyzed Gelatin 500 mg, Chondroitin Sulfate 100 mg. Other Ingredients: Natural Cane Sugar, Dried Vegetable Oil Complex, Vegetable Cellulose, Citric Acid, Vegetable Stearic Acid, Natural Fruit Flavors, Silica, Turmeric (color), Vegetable Magnesium Stearate, Methylsulfonylmethane (MSM).

Flex Able Sugar-Free Chewables **-** Amerifit Nutrition
Each chewable wafer contains: Vitamin C 30 mg • Glucosamine HCl 750 mg • Chondroitin Complex 600 mg: Hydrolyzed Gelatin 500 mg, Chondroitin Sulfate 100 mg. Other Ingredients: Sorbitol, Citric Acid, Vegetable Stearic Acid, Cellulose, Natural Flavors, Turmeric (color), Vegetable Stearate, Silica, Methylsulfonylmethane, Acesulfame, Aspartame (contains phenylalanine).

Flex Able Sugar-Free Orange Drink Mix **-** Amerifit Nutrition
Each packet contains: Protein 1 g • Vitamin C 60 mg • Glucosamine HCl 1500 mg • Chondroitin Sulfate 200 mg • Hydrolyzed Gelatin 1000 mg. Other Ingredients: Citric Acid, Natural Flavor, Aspartame (contains phenylalanine), Beta Carotene Color, Silica.

Some Brand Name Natural Products - What they Contain

www.NaturalDatabase.com contains MANY more listings than appear here.
Editor's Notes are located on pages 2155-2163.

Flex JSH - VitaCube Systems (V3S)
Each tablet contains: D-Glucosamine HCl 500 mg • Chondroitin Sulfate 250 mg • Methylsulfonylmethane (MSM) 250 mg • VitaCube Activating System Proprietary Blend 10 mg: Orange fruit Bioflavonoid Complex, Grapefruit Bioflavonoid Complex, Alfalfa leaf, Ginkgo Biloba leaf, Spirulina algae, Cayenne, Apple Pectin, Odorless Garlic, 7-Isopropoxy Isoflavone, L-Glutathione, Lemon fruit Bioflavonoid Complex, Lycopene 1%, Dimethylglycine, Potassium Glycerophosphate • Boswellia Serrata gum extract 5 mg • Capsicum fruit 5 mg • Turmeric root extract 5 mg. Other Ingredients: Cellulose, Stearic Acid, Croscarmellose Sodium, Silicon Dioxide, Magnesium Stearate, Light Yellw Cellulose Film Coat containing Titanium Dioxide and Riboflavin.

Flex4Life Capsules - 4 Life
Three capsules contain: CetylFlex (proprietary blend of fatty acid esters) 600 mg • Glucosamine (as hydrochloride) 825 mg • Chondroitin (as sulfate) 225 mg. Other Ingredients: Gelatin.

Flex4Life Cream - 4 Life
Purified Water • Saturated Fatty Acid Cetyl Ester • Polyethylene Glycol Monostearate • Glycerin • Glycerol Esters of Fatty Acids • Benzyl Alcohol • L-Menthol • Lecithin • Carboxyvinyl Polymer • Peppermint extract • Natural Vitamin E • Potassium Hydroxide.

FLEXAGEN (FLEXGEN) - New Vitality
Three softgels contain: Celadrin brand CMO Proprietary Blend 1050 mg. Other Ingredients: Soy Lecithin, Fish Oil.

FlexAgility - PhytoPharmica
Each softgel contains: EV.EXT 77 Extract Proprietary Blend 255 mg: Ginger rhizome extract (zingiber officinale), Greater Galangal rhizome extract (alpinia galanga). Other Ingredients: Gelatin, Medium Chain Triglycerides, Glycerin, Beeswax, Silicon Dioxide.

Flexaherb - Wild Rose
Each vegetable capsule contains: Corydalis root 80 mg • White Peony root 80 mg • Licorice root 80 mg • Black Cohosh 80 mg • Cramp bark 40 mg • Cayenne fruit (40,000 HU) 40 mg • Ginger root 40 mg • Lobelia herb 40 mg • Red Clover 40 mg.

Flexa-Herb - Dial Herbs
Kava Kava • Cramp bark • Cayenne • Ginger • Lobelia • Lady Slipper • Red Clover.

Flex-A-Min - Arthritis Research Corp.
Three tablets contain: Glucosamine Sulfate 1500 mg • Chondroitin Sulfate 1200 mg • MSM 500 mg. Other Ingredients: Cellulose, Vegetable Magnesium Stearate, Silica, Titanium Dioxide Color.
See Editor's Note No. 15.

FlexAnew - Natrol, Inc.
Two tablets contain: Calcium (as Calcium Carbonate) 330 mg • Glucosamine Sulfate 750 mg • Chondroitin Sulfate 300 mg • Nexrutine (Phellodendron Amurense bark extract) 250 mg.
See Editor's Note No. 15.

Flexanol - NorthStar Nutritionals
Each capsule contains: Glucosamine HCL 300 mg • Methylsulfonylmethane (MSM) 100 mg • Boswellia Serrata 100 mg • Vitamin C (ascorbyl palmitate) 2 mg • Vitamin E (d-alpha tocopheryl acetate) 2 IU • Vitamin D (cholecalciferol) 20 IU • Eicosapentaenoic Acid (EPA) 24 mg • Docosahexaenoic Acid (DHA) 16 mg • Borage Oil 6 mg • Ginger root 24 mg • Sea Cucumber 20 mg.

Flexaplex - Progressive Labs
Three capsules contain: Vitamin A 3000 IU • Vitamin B6 150 mg • Vitamin B12 300 mcg • Magnesium 300 mg • Copper 3 mg • Potassium 25 mg • Adrenal (Bovine) 30 mg • Valerian root 150 mg • Slippery Elm 30 mg • Gentian root 30 mg • Cape Aloes 30 mg • Skullcap 30 mg • Rue powder 30 mg.
See Editor's Note No. 14.

Flexcin - Flexcin International, Inc.
Three capsules contain: CM8 Cetyl Myristoleate 750 mg • Type II Collagen 120 mg • Glucosamine Sulfate Potassium 550 mg • MSM complex (methylsulfonylmethane) 150 mg • Enzyme Blend 52 mg. Other Ingredients: Manganese, Zinc, Copper, Vitamin C, Calcium, Boron, Bromelain.

FlexCreme - Pharmanex
Menthol 1.25% • Benzyl Alcohol • Butylparaben • Carbomer • Cetyl Myristate • Cetyl Oleate • Cetyl Laurate • Ethylparaben • Glycerin • Glyceryl Stearate • Isobutylparaben • Lecithin • Mentha Piperita (peppermint oil) • Methylparaben • Olea Europaea (olive fruit oil) • PEG-100 Phenoxyethanol • Potassium Hydroxide • Propylparaben • Tocopheryl Acetate • Aqua (water).

Flexicose - DTC Health, Inc.
Each 1/2 tbsp serving contains: Vitamin A (as retinyl palmitate) 1250 IU • Vitamin C (as ascorbic acid) 15 mg • Vitamin E (as D-alpha tocopheryl acetate) 7.5 IU • Manganese (as manganese sulfate) 0.7 mg • Glucosamine HCl & Glucosamine Sulfate 1500 mg • Chondroitin Sulfate 120 mg • Flexibility Complex 1600 mg: Aloe Vera gel, MSM, Omega 3 Fatty Acids (7.5% EPA and DHA), Niacinamide, Yucca root, Bromelain, Boswellia Serrata resin extract.
See Editor's Note No. 15.

Flexile Plus - Aspen Group, Inc.
Three capsules contain: Glucosamine HCl 99% 1500 mg • Chondroitin Sulfate (purified chondroitin sulfate 95%, mixed glycosominoglycans 5%) 1200 mg • Manganese Ascorbate 240 mg • Bromelain 100 mg • Boswellia Serrata extract 100 mg.
See Editor's Note No. 15.

Flexi-Licious Glucosamine Chews - Bronson Laboratories
Each chew contains: Glucosamine 500 mg.

Flexosil - Pure Encapsulations
Each vegetable capsule contains: Devil's Claw root extract (harpagophytum procumbens, standardized to contain a minimum of 5% harpagosides) 500 mg • Vitamin C (ascorbyl palmitate) 5 mg.

FlexTend - Nature's Way
Three caplets contain: Vitamin C (Ascorbic Acid) 180 mg • Vitamin E Acetate 60 IU • Iron 0.78 mg • Sodium 160 mg • Glucosamine Sulfate (sodium salt) 1.5 g. Other Ingredients: Microcrystalline Cellulose, Maltodextrin, Croscarmellose Sodium, Stearic Acid, Magnesium Stearate, Silicon Dioxide, Hydroxypropyl Methylcellulose, Titanium Dioxide, Polyethylene Glycol, Caramel, Polysorbate 80.

Flex-Zyme - Jarrow Formulas
Each tablet contains: Flex-Zyme Complex 300 mg: Protease, Peptizyme SP from Sp. Serratia, Papain, Bromelain, Amylase, Lipase, Rutin, Amla. Other Ingredients: Dicalcium Phosphate, Cellulose, Stearic Acid, Modified Cellulose Gum, Magnesium Stearate.

Flintstones Plus Iron Children's Multivitamin - Bayer
Each chewable tablet contains: Vitamin A 2500 IU • Vitamin C 60 mg • Vitamin D 400 IU • Vitamin E 15 IU • Thiamin 1.05 mg • Riboflavin 1.2 mg • Niacin 13.5 mg • Vitamin B-6 1.05 mg • Folic Acid 300 mcg • Vitamin B-12 4.5 mcg • Iron 15 mg.

Flite Tabs - Aidan Products, LLC
Each capsule contains: Pinokinase Proprietary Blend 250 mg: Pycnogenol, Nattokinase.

Flor*Essence - Flora Inc.
Burdock root • Sheep Sorrel • Slippery Elm • Turkish Rhubarb • Watercress • Kelp • Blessed Thistle • Red Clover.

Flora - DaVinci Laboratories
Two capsules contain: Lactobacillus Acidophilus (yielding 3 billion colony forming units) 540 mg. Other Ingredients: Maltodextrin, Cellulose, Gelatin, Vegetable Stearate.

Flora Vision **-** Flora Inc.
Bilberry extract 250mg • Blueberry.

Floradix Iron and Herbs **-** Dial Herbs
Vitamin B1 • Vitamin B2 • Vitamin B6 • Folic Acid • Vitamin B12 • Vitamin C • Iron • Aqueous Extract from Carrot • Nettle Worth • Spinach • Quitch roots • Angelica root • Fennel • Ocean Kelp • African Allow blossom • Orange peel • Juice concentrates: Pear, Red Grape, Blackcurrant, Orange, Blackberry, Cherry, Beetroot • Yeast (saccharomyces cerevisiae) Extract • Honey • Rose Hip extract • Wheat Germ extract • Natural Flavor.

Flora-Elite **-** InterPlexus
Each caplet contains: Proprietary Blend 2 billion organisms: Lactobacillus Acidophilus, Bifidobacterium Bifidum, Lactobacillus Salivarius. Other Ingredients: Rice Maltodextrin, Micro Crystalline and Cross Linked Cellulose, Stearic Acid/Magnesium Stearate, Turmeric.

Florafiber **-** Herbalife International of America, Inc.
Each tablet contains: Dietary Fiber 0.9g: Cellulose, Apple Pectin (pyrus malus), Blonde Psyllium seed husk, Croscarmellose Sodium, Glucomanna • Calcium (as dicalcium phosphate and calcium silicate) 29 mg • Lactobacillus Acidophilus 6 mg. Other Ingredients: Microcrystalline Cellulose, Stearic Acid, Hydroxypropyl Methylcellulose, Magnesium Stearate, Silicon Dioxide, Hydrogenated Vegetable Oil, Polyethylene Glycol.

FloraGLO brand **-** Kemin Foods
Lutein.

FloraMORE **-** Renew Life Formulas, Inc.
Two capsules contain: Lactobacillus Acidophilus • Lactobacillus Salivarius • Bifidobacterium Bifidum • Bifidobacterium Infantis • Bifidobacterium Longum • FOS (fructooligosaccharides) • L-Glutamine • N-Acetyl D-Glucosamine. Other Ingredients: Rice flour, Gelatin, Water.

FloraSMART **-** Renew Life Formulas, Inc.
Each tablet contains: Lactobacillus Acidophilus • Bifidobacterium Bifidum • Lactobacillus Rhamnosus • Lactobacillus Salivarius • Bifidobacterium Longum • Lactobacillus Casei • Lactococcus Lactis. Other Ingredients: Cellulose, Sodium Carbonate, Pectin, Stearic Acid, Tumeric.

Florastor **-** Xymogen
Each capsule contains: Saccharomyces boulardii 50 mg.

Florastor 250 mg **-** Biocodex, Inc.
Each capsule contains: Saccharomyces Boulardii lyo 5 billion cells. Other Ingredients: Magnesium Stearate, Lactose, Hydroxy-Propyl-Methyl-Cellulose, Titanium Dioxide.

Florastor 50 mg **-** Biocodex, Inc.
Each capsule contains: Saccharomyces Boulardii lyo 1 billion cells. Other Ingredients: Magnesium Stearate, Lactose, Hydroxy-Propyl-Methyl-Cellulose, Titanium Dioxide.

Florastor Extra Strength **-** Xymogen
Each capsule contains: Saccharomyces boulardii 250 mg.

Flower Mix **-** Professional Complementary Health Formulas
Adrenal 3X, 4X • ACTH 6X, 30X • Histamine 12X • Liver 6X, 12X • Aster, Camellia, Carnation, Chrysantehmum, Daffodil, Daisy, Daphne, Gardenia, Gentian, Fladiola, Honeysuckle, Iris, Lilac, Lily, Larkspur, Lupine, Marigold, Oleander, Pansy, Petunia, Peony, Poppy, Rose, Snapdragon, Tulip 6X, 12X, 60X, 100X • Purified Water • 20% USP Alcohol.
See Editor's Note No. 1.

Flu **-** Hyland's
Eupatorium Perfoliatum 3X HPUS • Bryonia 3X HPUS • Gelsemium Sempervirens 3X HPUS • Euphrasia Officinalis 3X HPUS • Kali Iodatum 3X HPUS • Anas Barbariae Hepatis et Cordis extractum 200C HPUS • Lactose USP.
See Editor's Note No. 1.

Flu & Cold Formula **-** HERBALmax
Jinyin flowers • Lianqiao fruits • Sang leaves • Niupangzi fruits.

Flu Guard Nasal Spray **-** Jamieson
Each 1 ml dose contains: 42 mg of active ingredients: Echinacea Angustifolia • Baptista Tinctoria • Thuja Occidentalis • Astragalus Membranaceus • Plantago Lanceolata • Scutellaria Baicalensis.

Flu Resist **-** NatraBio
Active ingredients: Influenzinum 12X • Adrenalinum 6X • Aconitum Napellus 6X • Baptisia Tinctoria 6X • Eupatorium Perfoliatum 6X • Euphrasia Officinarum 6X • Gelsemium Sempervirens 6X • Sticta Pulmonaria 6X • Rhus Toxicodendron 12X. Inactive ingredients: Purified Water, Sodium Chloride, Sodium Phosphate, Benzalkonium Chloride, Benzyl Alcohol, Potassium Chloride, Potassium Phosphate.
See Editor's Note No. 1.

Flu Solve **-** American Biologics
Each drop contains: Abenitum 4X • Bryonia 4X • Eupatorium Pert 3X • Gelsamium 6X • Causticum 6X • Camphora 3X • Eucalyptus 3X • Baptista 4X • Fen. Phos. 8X • Sabadilla 6X. Other Ingredients: 20% Alcohol, Distilled Water.
See Editor's Note No. 1.

Flu, Cold & Cough Formula **-** HERBALmax
Pipa leaves • Baibu root • Jiegeng root • Huangqin radix • Lianqiao fruit.

FLUIDjoint **-** Patent Health, LLC
Two chewable tablets contain: Proprietary Blend 2000 mg: Milk Protein Concentrate, Fructose, Canola Oil, Stearic Acid, Natural French Vanilla Flavor, Caramel Flavor, Magnesium Stearate, Sucrolose, Vitamin B1, Vitamin B2.

Flush Free Niacin **-** Puritan's Pride
Each capsule contains: Niacin 400 mg • Inositol 100 mg.

Flush Free Niacin Inositol Hexanicotinate 500 mg **-** Nature's Bounty
Each capsule contains: Niacin (as inositol hexanicotinate) 400 mg • Inositol (as inositol hexanicotinate) 100 mg. Other Ingredients: Gelatin, Vegetable Magnesium Stearate, Silica.

Flush-Free HexaNiacin **-** Enzymatic Therapy
Each capsule contains: Niacin (Inositol hexaniacinate) contains 500 mg elemental Niacin 650 mg.

Flush-Free Niacin **-** PhytoPharmica
Each capsule contains: Niacin (flush-free Inositol hexaniacinate) 590 mg.

Flush-Free Niacin 500 mg **-** Nature's Life
Each tablet contains: Niacin (Inositol, Hexaniacinate) 500 mg.

FM Herbal Complex **-** Pro Health
Each capsule contains: Proprietary Blend 700 mg: Angelica Sinensis, Citrus Sinensis, Typha Angustifolia, Ligusticum Sinense, Saussura Costus, Gentiana Macrophylla, Carthamus Tinctorius, Bupleurum Chinense, Rheum Palmatum, Alisma Plantago Aquatica, Rehmannia Glutinosa, Achyranthes Bidentata, Paeonia Obovata, Glycyrrhiza Glabra, Commiphora Myrrha, Cyperus Rotundus, Isatis Indigotica, Paeonia Lactiflora, Eleutherococcus, Sessiliflorus, Loranthus Parasiticus, Platycoden Grandiflorum, Notopterygium Forbesii, Belamcanda Chinensis, Sargassum Pallidum, Phellodendron Chinense, Andrographis Paniculata, Sanguisorba Officinalis, Mentha Canadensis.

Focus Child **-** Source Naturals
Two tablets contain: Magnesium (from Magnesium Aspartate and Oxide) 100 mg • Zinc (as Zinc Picolinate) 2 mg • L-Aspartate (from Magnesium Aspartate) 310 mg • DMAE (as DMAE Bitartrate) 100 mg • Standardized Soybean Lecithin (LECI-PS) 50 mg • Yielding 40% Phosphatidylserine 20 mg • Phosphatidylcholine 6 mg • Phosphatidylethanolamine 3.5 mg • Phosphatidylinositol 1 mg • DHA (Docosahexaenoic Acid (Neuromins)) 15 mg • Grape Seed extract 15 mg.

Focus DHA - Source Naturals
Each softgel contains: Docosahexaenoic Acid (DHA) (from Alga Oil [Neuromins]) 100 mg.

Focus Factor - Vital Basics, Inc.
Four tablets contain: Vitamin A (from natural beta-carotene and mixed carotenoids) 4,000 IU • Vitamin C (as ascorbic acid, sodium ascorbate, calcium ascorbate, potassium ascorbate, zinc ascorbate, and ascorbyl palmitate) 250 mg • Vitamin D (as cholecalciferol) 100 IU • Vitamin E (as natural d-alpha- tocopheryl succinate) 30 IU • Thiamin (as thiamin mononitrate) 3mg • Riboflavin 1.7 mg • Niacin (from inositol hexanicotinate and 50% as niacinamide) 25 mg • Vitamin B6 (as pyridoxal-alpha-ketoglutarate, pyridoxal 5-phosphate) 15 mg • Folate (as folic acid) 400 mcg • Vitamin B12 (as cyanocobalamin) 20 mcg • Biotin 300 mcg • Pantothenic acid (as D-calcium pantothenate) 12 mg • Calcium (as calcium citrate, calcium succinate and calcium ascorbate) 50 mg • Iron (as Ferronly carbonyl Iron) 5 mg • Iodine (as potassium iodide and kelp (Ascophyllum nodosum)) 15 mcg • Magnesium (as magnesium citrate, magnesium malate and magnesium taurinate) 100 mg • Zinc (as zinc citrate and zinc ascorbate) 10 mg • Selenium (as selenomethionine) 20 mcg • Copper (as copper citrate and copper Chelazome) 0.4 mg • Manganese (as manganese citrate) 2 mg • Chromium (as chromium polynicotinate) 100 mcg • Molybdenum (as molybdenum amino acid chelate) 10 mcg • Potassium (as potassium citrate, potassium aspartate, and potassium ascorbate) 50 mg • Synergistic and proprietary formulation: L-Glutamine, DMAE (as DMAE bitartrate), L-pyroglutamic acid, phosphatidylserine, DHA concentrate (15% DHA from fish body oil), choline (as choline bitartrate), inositol, pyridoxal-alpha-ketoglutarate, N-acetyltyrosine, Bacopin (Bacopa monnieri extract) (leaf), bilberry fruit standardized extract (25% anthocyansides), GABA, pine bark and Activin (grape seed extract), vinpocetine, Trace-Lyte Electrolyte concentrate, Huperzine (extract of Huperzia serrata) (whole plant), boron (as boron chelate), vanadium (as vanadyl sulfate) 471 mg. Other Ingredients: Dicalcium Phosphate, Microcrystalline Cellulose, Croscarmellose Sodium, Stearic Acid, Silica, Magnesium Stearate and Pharmaceutical Glaze.

Focus Factor Children's Chewable - Vital Basics, Inc.
Four wafers contain: Vitamin A (from natural beta-carotene and mixed carotenoids) 4,000 UI • Vitamin C (as ascorbic acid, sodium ascorbate and zinc ascorbate) 250 mg • Vitamin D (as cholecalciferol) 100 UI • Vitamin E (as natural d-alpha-tocopheryl succinate) 30 UI • Thiamin (as thiamin mononitrate) 3 mg • Riboflavin 1.7 mg • Niacin (from inositol hexanicotinate and 50% as niacinamide) 25 mg • Vitamin B6 (as pyridoxal alpha ketoglutarate) 5 mg • Folate (as folic acid) 40 mcg • Vitamin B12 (as cyanocobalamin) 20 mcg • Biotin 300 mcg • Pantothenic Acid (as D-calcium pantothenate) 12 mg • Calcium (as calcium citrate, calcium ascorbate, calcium malate and calcium succinate) 100 mg • Iron (as ferrocus glycinate) 10 mg • Iodine (as potassium iodide and kelp) 15 mcg • Magnesium (as magnesium citrate, magnesium malate and magnesium taurinate) 100 mg • Zinc (as zinc aspartate and zinc ascorbate) 10 mg • Selenium (as selenomathionine) 20 mcg • Copper (as copper citrate and copper Chelazome) 400 mcg • Manganese (as manganese citrate) 2 mg • Chromium (as chromium polynicotinate) 100 mcg • Potassium (as potassium citrate, potassium ascorbate and potassium aspartate) 50 mg • Synergistic and proprietary formulation, Phosphatidyl serine / soya lecithin complex, DMAE (as DMAE birartrate), Neuromins (Martex Docosahexaenoic acid concentrate), L-glutamine, L-pyroglutamic acid, pyridoxial alpha ketoglutarate, trace mineral complex, N-acetyl-tyrosine, GABA, Inositol, Bilberry (from 100:1 concentrate), Proanthocyanidin blend from Pine Bark and Activin (grape seed extract), Bacopin (Bacopa monnieri extract), Coenzyme Q-10, Huperzine (extract of huperzia serrata), Boron (as boron citrate), Vanadium (as vanadyl sulfate) 640 mg. Other Ingredients: Simple and Complex Carbohydrates from corn, Organic Sucanat with honey, Mixed Fruit, and Cherry Crystals, Cellulose, Magnesium Stearate and Silica.

FolaPro - Metagenics
Each tablet contains: Folate (Metafolin as L-5-methyl tetrahydrofolate) 800 mcg.

Folate - Pure Encapsulations
Each vegetable capsule contains: Folic Acid 800 mg.

Folgard - Upsher-Smith Laboratories
Each tablet contains: Folic Acid 800 mcg • Vitamin B-6 10 mg • Vitamin B-12 115 mcg.

Folic Acid - Benepure, Inc
Each capsule contains: Folic Acid (folnic acid from calcium folinate) 800 mcg. Other Ingredients: Microcrystalline Cellulose, Vegetable Stearate.

Folic Acid - Jarrow Formulas
Each capsule contains: Folic Acid 800 mcg. Other Ingredients: Cellulose, Magnesium Stearate, Gelatin.

Folic Acid - Nature's Bounty
Each tablet contains: Folic Acid 400 mcg. Other Ingredients: Dicalcium Phosphate, Vegetable Stearic Acid, Croscarmellose, Silica, Vegetable Magnesium Stearate.

Folic Acid - Source Naturals
Each tablet contains: Folate (as folic acid) 800 mcg.

Folic Acid - Arrowroot
Each tablet contains: Folic Acid 800 mcg.

Folic Acid - GNC
Each tablet contains: Folic Acid 400 mcg. Other Ingredients: Dextrose, Whole Brown Rice Powder (Oryza Sativa).

Folic Acid - Leiner Health Products
Each tablet contains: Folate (Folic Acid) 400 mcg. Other Ingredients: Dicalcium Phosphate, Cellulose, Stearic Acid, Croscarmellose Sodium, Magnesium Stearate.

Folic Acid - Pro Health
Each tablet contains: Folic Acid (from biologically fermented yeast) 800 mcg • Vitamin B12 (cyanocobalamin) 25 mcg. Other Ingredients: Cellulose, Stearic Acid, Magnesium Stearate.

Folic Acid - Walgreens
Each tablet contains: Folate (folic acid) 400 mcg. Other Ingredients: Dicalcium Phosphate, Calcium Carbonate, Stearic Acid, Croscarmellose Sodium, Sodium Bicarbonate, Magnesium Stearate.

Folic Acid - Golden Glow Natural Health Products
Each tablet contains: Folic Acid 500 mcg.

Folic Acid 0.4 mg - Jamieson
Each tablet contains: Folic Acid 0.4 mg (400 mcg).

Folic Acid 1 mg - Trophic
Each tablet contains: Folic Acid 1 mg.

Folic Acid 1 mg - Jamieson
Each tablet contains: Folic Acid USP 1 mg.

Folic Acid 400 mcg - Nature Made
Each tablet contains: Folate (from folic acid) 400 mcg. Other Ingredients: Dibasic Calcium Phosphate, Croscarmellose Sodium, Magnesium Stearate.
See Editor's Note No. 45.

Folic Acid 400 mcg - Sunmark
Each tablet contains: Folic Acid 400 mcg. Other Ingredients: Dicalcium Phosphate, Calcium Carbonate, Modified Cellulose Gum, Stearic Acid, Acacia, Sodium Bicarbonate, Magnesium Stearate.
See Editor's Note No. 45.

Folic Acid 400 mcg - Schiff
Each tablet contains: Folate (as folic acid) 400 mcg • Calcium (as dibasic calcium phosphate) 25 mg. Other Ingredients: Dextrose, Corn Syrup, Silicon Dioxide, Magnesium Stearate.

Folic Acid 400 mcg - GNC
Each tablet contains: Folic Acid (50%) 400 mcg. Other Ingredients: Dextrose, Whole Brown Rice Powder (oryza sativa).

Folic Acid 400 mcg - J. R. Carlson Laboratories, Inc.
Each tablet contains: Folate (folic acid) 400 mcg.

Folic Acid 500mcg - Nature's Own
Each tablet contains: Folic Acid 500 mcg.

Folic Acid 5mg - Ortho Molecular Products
Each capsule contains: Folic ACid 5 mg • Vitamin B12 (as methylcobalamin) 200 mcg. Other Ingredients: Natural Vegetable Capsules, Ascorbyl Palmitate, Microcrystalline Cellulose, Silicon Dioxide.

Folic Acid 800 - GNC
Each tablet contains: Folic Acid 800 mcg. Other Ingredients: Whole Brown Rice powder (Oryza Sativa).

Folic Acid 800 mcg - Nature's Valley
Each tablet contains: Folic Acid 800 mcg. Other Ingredients: Dicalcium Phosphate, Cellulose, Croscarmellose Sodium, Stearic Acid, Starch, Magnesium Stearate, Silicon Dioxide.
See Editor's Note No. 45.

Folic Acid 800 mcg - J. R. Carlson Laboratories, Inc.
Each tablet contains: Folate (folic acid) 800 mcg.

Folic Acid 800 mcg - Nature's Plus
Each tablet contains: Folic Acid 800 mcg. Other Ingredients: Di-calcium Phosphate, Microcrystalline Cellulose, Rice Bran, Stearic Acid, Magnesium Stearate, Riboflavin, Pharmaceutical Glaze, Silica.

Folic Acid B12 - Standard Process, Inc.
Each tablet contains: Proprietary Blend 374 mg: Carrot root, Calcium Lactate, Porcine Stomach Parenchyma, Defatted Wheat germ, Bovine Spleen, Ovine Spleen, Bovine Adrenal Cytosol extract, Oat flour, Ascorbic Acid • Folate 400 mcg • Vitamin B12 6 mcg. Other Ingredients: Honey, Cellulose.
See Editor's Note No. 14.

Folic Acid Capsules - Optimum Nutrition
Each capsule contains: Folic Acid 400 mcg. Other Ingredients: Microcrystalline Cellulose, Gelatin, Magnesium Stearate.

Folic Acid Dophilus Plus B-12 - Dial Herbs
Two wafers contain: Folic Acid 800 mcg • Vitamin B12 400 mcg • Lactobacillus acidophilus • Lactobacillus plantarum • Lactobacillus bulgaricus • Lactobacillus casei 200 mcg.

Folic Acid Hearts - Nature's Plus
Each tablet contains: Vitamin B6 (as pyridoxine HCl) 5 mg • Folic Acid 400 mcg • Vitamin B12 (as cyanocobalamin) 15 mcg. Other Ingredients: Di-calcium Phosphate, Microcrystalline Cellulose, Stearic Acid, Silica, Magnesium Stearate, Riboflavin, Pharmaceutical Glaze.

Folic Acid Liquid - Pure Encapsulations
Five drops contain: Folic Acid 800 mcg. Other Ingredients: Distilled Water (70%), Glycerol (30%).

Folic Acid Plus B12 - Life Extension
Each tablet contains: Pure Folic Acid 800 mcg • Vitamin B12 300 mcg.

Folic Acid with Vitamin C - Westcoast Naturals
Each capsule contains: Folic Acid 1000 mcg • Vitamin C (ascorbic acid) 30 mg.

FolliGro System 1 Fenugreek Extract - FolliGro Ltd.
Each capsule contains: Fenugreek extract 260 mg • Calcium Pantothenate 10 mg • Nicotinamide 10 mg • Vitamin B6 2 mg • Vitamin B2 1.5 mg • Folate (as folic acid) 95 mcg.

FolliGro System 2 Biospray - FolliGro Ltd.
Each spray contains: Niacinamide 6 mg • Zinc Gluconate 1 mg • D-Alpha-Tocopherol 6 IU. Other Ingredients: Purified Water, Glycerine, Lecithin.

Foltx - Pan American Laboratories, Inc.
Each tablet contains: Folic Acid USP (Folacin) 2.5 mg • Cyanocobalamin USP (B-12) 1 mg • Pyridoxine HCl (B-6) 25 mg.

Food Enzymes - Nature's Sunshine
Two capsules contain: Betaine HCl 324 mg • Bile Salt 80 mg • Bromelain 100 mg • Lipase 30 IU • Alpha Amylase (mycozyme) 180 mg • Pancreatin (8X USP) 45 mg • Papain 90 mg • Pepsin (1:10,000) 120 mg. Other Ingredients: Cellulose, Magnesium Stearate, Silicon Dioxide, Gelatin, Water.

Foot Revival Soak - Abra Therapeutics
Sodium Borate • Sodium Sulfate • Sodium Chloride • Sodium Sesquicarbonate • Olive oil • Peppermint oil • Sage oil • Tea Tree oil • Rosemary oil • Eucalyptus oil • Clove oil • Peru Balsam oil • Arnica flower extract • White Willow bark extract • Lemon Balm extract • Chromium Oxide • Trace Mineral Salts.

For Men Only - Doctor's Best, Inc.
Each tablet contains: L-Glycine 135 mg • L-Alanine 135 mg • L-Glutamic Acid 135 mg • Raw Prostate concentrate 100 mg • Saw Palmetto 100 mg • Golden Rod 50 mg • Pumpkin seed concentrate 10 mg • Vitamin E 10 IU • Zinc 5 mg • Flax Seed Oil 3 mg.
See Editor's Note No. 14.

Formula 1 - Enzymes, Inc.
Two capsules contain: Protease 80,000 HUT • Amylase 9000 DU • Lipase 168 LU • Cellulase 160 CU. Other Ingredients: Plant Fiber, Gelatin, Water.

Formula 100 - Puritan's Pride
Each tablet contains: Vitamin A (as retinyl palmitate and 20% as beta carotene) 10,000 IU • Vitamin C (as ascorbic acid and rose hips) 250 mg • Vitamin D (as cholecalciferol) 400 IU • Vitamin E (as d-alpha tocopheryl acid succinate) 150 IU • Thiamin (Vitamin B1; as thiamine mononitrate) 100 mg • Riboflavin (Vitamin B2) 100 mg • Niacin (as niacinamide) 100 mg • Vitamin B6 (as pyridoxine hydrochloride) 100 mg • Folic Acid 300 mcg • Vitamin B12 (as cyanocobalamin) 100 mcg • Biotin 100 mcg • Pantothenic Acid (as d-calcium pantothenate) 100 mg • Calcium (as calcium carbonate) 100 mg • Iron (as ferrous fumarate) 18 mg • Iodine (as kelp) 150 mcg • Magnesium (as magnesium oxide) 50 mg • Zinc (as zinc oxide) 15 mg • Selenium (as sodium selenate) 25 mcg • Copper (as cupric oxide) 0.5 mg • Manganese (as manganese sulfate) 6.1 mg • Chromium (as GTF chromium yeast) 200 mcg • Potassium (as potassium citrate) 10 mg • PABA (para-aminobenzoic acid) 100 mg • Choline Bitartrate 100 mg • Inositol 100 mg • Rutin 25 mg • Lemon Bioflavonoids 50 mg • Hesperidin 12.5 mg • Betaine Hydrochloride 30 mg • Octacosanol 50 mcg • Proprietary Blend 5 mg: Alfalfa Leaf, Watercress, Parsley Leaf, Rice Bran, Lecithin.

Formula 11 - Enzymes, Inc.
Two capsules contain: Vitamin C (Ascorbic acid) 100 mg • Citrus Bioflavonoids 200 mg • Acerola Cherries (Malpighia punicifolia) 50 mg • Rose Hips (Rosa canina) 50 mg • Amylase 500 DU. Other Ingredients: Plant Fiber, Gelatin, Water.

Formula 113 - Enzymes, Inc.
Two capsules contain: Vitamin C (Ascorbic acid) 50 mg • Amylase 12,000 DU • Citrus Bioflavonoids 110 mg • Wheat Germ 100 mg • Protease 40,000 HUT • Acerola Cherries (Malpighia puncifolia) 25 mg • Rose Hips (Rosa canina) 25 mg • Sucrase (Invertase) 0.2 IAU • Malt Diastase 270 DP • Lipase 38 LU • Cellulase 320 CU • Lactase 480 ALU. Other Ingredients: Plant Fiber, Gelatin, Water.

Formula 12 - Enzymes, Inc.
Three capsules contain: Burdock root (Arctium lappa) 450 mg • Citrus Bioflavonoids 450 mg • Cellulase 1800 CU • Amylase 3600 DU • Protease 7500 HUT • Lipase 15 LU. Other Ingredients: Gelatin, Plant Fiber, Water.

BRAND NAMES

Formula 13 - Enzymes, Inc.
Two capsules contain: Wheat Germ 200 mg • Lecithin 100 mg • Sea Kelp (Macrocystis pyrifera) 20 mg • Amylase 1400 DU • Lipase 38 LU • Protease 4000 HUT • Cellulase 20 CU. Other Ingredients: Plant Fiber, Gelatin, Water.

Formula 14 - Enzymes, Inc.
Two capsules contain: Kelp (Laminaria digitata) 200 mg • Irish Moss 100 mg • Protease 50,000 HUT • Amylase 3000 DU • Lipase 48 LU • Cellulase 400 CU • Potassium Iodide 0.6 mg. Other Ingredients: Plant Fiber, Gelatin, Water.

Formula 15 - Enzymes, Inc.
Two capsules contain: Spirulina Pratensis 150 mg • Alfalfa juice concentrate (Medicago sativa) 150 mg • Parsley leaf (Petroselinum crispum) 100 mg • Protease 21,400 HUT • Amylase 2100 DU • Lipase 16 LU • Cellulase 28 CU. Other Ingredients: Plant Fiber, Gelatin, Water.

Formula 16 - Enzymes, Inc.
Two capsules contain: Calcium (as Calcium Lactate) 60 mg • Protease 12,200 HUT • Amylase 2000 DU • Lipase 24 LU. Other Ingredients: Plant Fiber, Gelatin, Water.

Formula 17 - Enzymes, Inc.
Two capsules contain: Pau D'arco bark (Tabebuia spp.) 200 mg • Yellow Dock root (Rumex crispus) 200 mg • Echinacea root (Echinacea purpurea) 180 mg • Mullein leaf (Verbascum thapsus) 20 mg • Protease 10,000 HUT • Amylase 1600 DU • Lipase 36 LU • Cellulase 60 CU. Other Ingredients: Gelatin, Plant Fiber, Water.

Formula 18 - Enzymes, Inc.
Two capsules contain: Lipase 386 LU • Amylase 9000 DU • Protease 30,500 HUT • Glucoamylase 27 AG • Cellulase 120 CU. Other Ingredients: Plant Fiber, Gelatin, Water.

Formula 19 - Enzymes, Inc.
Two capsules contain: Calcium (as Calcium Gluconate) 41 mg • Magnesium (as Magnesium Gluconate) 9 mg • Protease 4060 HUT • Amylase 666 DU • Lipase 16 LU. Other Ingredients: Plant Fiber, Gelatin, Water, Silica.

Formula 2 - Enzymes, Inc.
Two capsules contain: Amylase 12,000 DU • Protease 49,180 HUT • Glucoamylase 27 AG • Lactobacillus Acidophilus 27 mg • Lipase 96 LU • Cellulase 120 CU. Other Ingredients: Plant Fiber, Gelatin, Water.

Formula 20 - Enzymes, Inc.
Two capsules contain: Amylase 6800 DU • Protease 19,600 HUT • Lipase 72 LU • Cellulase 80 CU. Other Ingredients: Plant Fiber, Gelatin, Water.

Formula 21 - Enzymes, Inc.
Two capsules contain: Protease 40,000 HUT • Amylase 4000 DU • Malt Diastase 540 DP • Sucrase (Invertase) 0.4 IAU • Lipase 72 LU • Cellulase 400 CU • Lactase 900 ALU. Other Ingredients: Plant Fiber, Gelatin, Water, Silica.

Formula 3 - Enzymes, Inc.
Three capsules contain: Amylase 27,000 DU. Other Ingredients: Plant Fiber, Gelatin, Water.

Formula 301 - Enzymes, Inc.
Two capsules contain: Rose Hips (Rosa canina) 180 mg • Alfalfa juice concentrate (Medicago sativa) 130 mg • Echinacea root (Echinacea purpurea) 90 mg • Lipase 136 LU • Protease 16,394 HUT • Mullein leaf (Verbascum thapsus) 10 mg • Amylase 1000 DU • Cellulase 80 CU. Other Ingredients: Plant Fiber, Gelatin, Water.

Formula 4 - Enzymes, Inc.
Three capsules contain: Protease 240,000 HUT. Other Ingredients: Plant Fiber, Gelatin, Water.

Formula 401 - Enzymes, Inc.
Two capsules contain: Horsetail aerial part (Equisetum arvense) 80 mg • Lactobacillus Acidophilus 57 mg • Lipase 138 LU • Protease 20,000 HUT • Cellulase 80 CU. Other Ingredients: Plant Fiber, Gelatin, Water.

Formula 416 - Enzymes, Inc.
Four capsules contain: Calcium (as Calcium Lactate) 60 mg • Protease 332,000 HUT • Amylase 2000 DU • Lipase 24 LU. Other Ingredients: Plant Fiber, Gelatin, Water.

Formula 419 - Enzymes, Inc.
Four capsules contain: Calcium (as Calcium Gluconate) 20 mg • Magnesium (as Magnesium Gluconate) 4 mg • Protease 332,000 HUT • Amylase 400 DU • Lipase 8 LU. Other Ingredients: Plant Fiber, Gelatin, Water.

Formula 4SX For Men - Abundance Marketing
Vitamin E • Zinc • Tribulus Terrestris • Green Tea leaf extract • Panax Ginseng • Muira Puama • Oat straw • Nettle leaf • Full spectrum Chinese herbal concentrates: Cnidium seed, Cistanche stem, Chinese Dodder seed, Chinese Senega root, Japanese Teasel root, Tangerine peel, Schisandra berry. Other Ingredients: Hydrolyzed Vegetable Protein, Dicalcium Phosphate, Microcrystalline Cellulose, Croscarmellose Sodium, Stearic Acid, Silica, Magnesium Stearate, Pharmaceutical Glaze.

Formula 4SX For Women - Abundance Marketing
Hydrolyzed Vegetable Protein • Ginkgo Biloba leaf extract • Chaste Tree berry extract • Mixed Vegetable Phytosterols • Panax Ginseng • Damiana leaf 4:1 extract • Muira Puama stem 4:1 extract • Jujube date.

Formula 5 - Enzymes, Inc.
Three capsules contain: Lipase 360 LU. Other Ingredients: Plant Fiber, Gelatin, Water.

Formula 501 - Enzymes, Inc.
Two capsules contain: Yucca aerial part (Yucca spp.) 175 mg • Alfalfa juice concentrate (Medicago sativa) 175 mg • Safflower petals (Carthamus tinctorius) 150 mg • Oat straw (Avena sativa) 50 mg • Protease 10,000 HUT • Amylase 1500 DU • Cellulase 200 CU • Lipase 12 LU. Other Ingredients: Gelatin, Plant Fiber, Water.

Formula 560 - Immunity Today, LLC.
Each capsule contains: Vitamin C 30 mg • Coenzyme Q10 5 mg • Proprietary Blend of Transfer Factor derived from Bovine Colostrum 165 mg.

Formula 6 - Enzymes, Inc.
Two capsules contain: Marshmallow root (Althaea Officinalis) 450 mg • Rose Hips (Rosa Canina) 150 mg • Amylase 10,000 DU • Protease 37,000 HUT • Cellulase 400 CU • Lipase 24 LU. Other Ingredients: Gelatin, Water, Plant Fiber.

Formula 600 Plus for Men - Nature's Life
Two capsules contain: Saw Palmetto berry (Serenoa repens B.) 600 mg • Active Aminos (l-Glutamic Acid, Glycine & L-Alanine) 170 mg • Zinc (Picolinate) 15 mg • Pumpkin seed (Curcurbita pepo) 50 mg • Pygeum africanum H. bark extract [(150:1) equivalent to 300 mg whole herb] 2 mg • Burdock root (Arctium lappa L.) 5 mg • Cayenne fruit (Capsicum annuum L. var. annuum) 5 mg • Goldenseal root (Hydrastis canadensis L.) 5 mg • Gravel root (Eupatorium purpureum L.) 5 mg • Juniper berry (Juniperus oxycedrus L.) 5 mg • Marshmallow root (Althaea officinalis L.) 5 mg • Parsley leaf (Petroselinum crispum(Mill) Nym.ex. A.W. Hill) 5 mg • White Pond Lily root (Nymphaea odorata) 5 mg • Vitamin B6 (Pyridoxine HCl) 5 mg • Copper (Gluconate) 1 mg • Nature's Life Active Aminos is an exclusive free-form blend of l-Glutamic Acid, l-Alanine & Glycine.

Formula 601 - Enzymes, Inc.
Two capsules contain: Comfrey leaf (Symphytum officinale) 400 mg • Papaya leaf (Carica papaya) 200 mg • Amylase 10,000 DU • Cellulase 400 CU • Lipase 24 LU. Other Ingredients: Gelatin, Water, Plant Fiber.

Formula 7 - Enzymes, Inc.
Two capsules contain: Safflower petals (Carthamus Tinctorius) 300 mg • Amylase 7200 DU • Lipase 138 LU • Protease 11,400 HUT • Cellulase 40 CU. Other Ingredients: Plant Fiber, Gelatin, Water.

Formula 701s - Enzymes, Inc.
Two capsules contain: Collinsonia root part (Collinsonia canadensis) 200 mg • Hawthorn berry (Crataegus oxycanthus) 200 mg • Protease 24,242 HUT • Amylase 3000 DU • Lipase 48 LU • Cellulase 40 CU. Other Ingredients: Gelatin, Plant Fiber, Water.

Formula 75 - Futurebiotics LLC
Vitamin C (Rose hips) 250 mg • Vitamin A (palmitate 10,000 IU, beta carotene 7500 IU) 17,500 IU • Vitamin E (natural) 150 IU • Vitamin D (cholecalciferol) 400 IU • Riboflavin 75 mg • Thiamin 75 mg • Vitamin B6 (pyridoxine HCl) 75 mg • Niacinamide 75 mg • Vitamin B12 (cyanocobalamin) 75 mcg • Folic Acid 400 mcg • Pantothenic Acid 75 mg • Biotin 75 mcg • Iron (chelate) 1.3 mg • Calcium (chelate) 20 mg • Magnesium (chelate) 10 mg • Iodine (kelp) 150 mcg • Selenium (chelate) 25 mcg • Zinc (chelate) 10 mg • Manganese (chelate) 1 mg • Copper (chelate) 1 mg • Molybdenum (chelate) 25 mcg • Chromium (picolinate) 25 mcg • Boron (chelate complex) 0.5 mg • Potassium (chelate complex) 1.8 mg • Inositol 75 mg • Choline (bitartrate) 31 mg • Rutin 25 mg • Para Amino Benzoic Acid (PABA) 75 mg • Hesperidin complex 5 mg • Citrus bioflavonoid complex 25 mg • Betaine HCl 25 mg. In a Green Foods base of: Alfalfa, Barley & Chlorella.

Formula 8 - Enzymes, Inc.
Two capsules contain: Lactobacillus Acidophilus 53 mg • Lactase 1500 ALU • Amylase 1000 DU. Other Ingredients: Plant Fiber, Gelatin, Water.

Formula 801 - Enzymes, Inc.
Each teaspoon contains: Cellulase 75,000 CU • Lactobacillus Acidophilus 900 mg • Bifidobacterium Longum 500 mg. Other Ingredients: Plant Fiber, Silica.

Formula 9 - Enzymes, Inc.
Two capsules contain: Alfalfa juice concentrate (Medicago Sativa) 280 mg • Parsley leaf (Petroselinum Crispum) 134 mg • Horsetail aerial part (Equisetum Arvense) 120 mg • Rose Hips (Rosa Canina) 100 mg • Protease 30,500 HUT • Amylase 3400 DU • Lipase 29 LU. Other Ingredients: Plant Fiber, Gelatin, Water.

Formula HGH - HealthMinded
Four capsules contain: Formula HGH 2715 mg: Amino Peptide complex, Colostrum, Tribulus Terrestris, Citrus complex, Chrysin, Phosphatidyl Serine, Phosphatidyl Choline. Other Ingredients: Stearic Acid, Magnesium Stearate.

Formula IV - GNLD International, LLC.
Two capsules contain: Vitamin A (from fish liver oil) 4000 IU • Vitamin C (as ascorbic acid and from acerola cherry fruit (malpighia punicifolia)) 90 mg • Vitamin D (from fish liver oil) 400 IU • Vitamin E (as D-alpha tocopherol) 10 IU • Thiamine (as thiamine mononitrate and from yeast) 10 mg • Riboflavin (as riboflavin and from yeast) 10 mg • Niacin (as niacinamide and from yeast) 50 mg • Vitamin B6 (as pyridoxine hydrochloride and from yeast) 10 mg • Folic Acid 400 mcg • Vitamin B12 (as cyanocobalamin) 10 mcg • Pantothenic Acid (as calcium pantothenate and from yeast) 12 mg • Iron (as iron peptonate and from parsley leaves (petroselinum crispum)) 25 mg • Iodine (from kelp and as potassium iodide) 100 mcg • Magnesium (as magnesium oxide) 35 mg • Copper (as copper gluconate and from kelp) 2 mg • Manganese (as manganese gluconate) 10 mg • Potassium (as potassium gluconate) 10 mg • Linoleic Acid (from safflower oil) 176 mg • Inositol (as inoitol and from soy lecithin) 65 mg • Lecithin (from soy) 30 mg • Para-Aminobenzoic Acid 30 mg • Betaine Hydrochloride 10 mg • Mixed Tocopherols (non-alpha) 1 mg • TRE-EN-EN Grain Concentrate Blend 450 mg: Rice bran oil, Soy bean oil, Wheat germ oil • Phyto Enzyme Blend 45 mg: Lipase, Protease, Diastate, Amylase. Other Ingredients: Gelatin, Glycerin, Wax, Water, Hydrolyzed Collagen Protein, Titanium Dioixde, Natural Color.

Formula IV Plus - GNLD International, LLC.
Each packette contains: Vitamin A (from retinyl palmitate) 4000 IU • Vitamin C (as ascorbic acid and from acerola cherry fruit (malpighia punicifolia)) 90 mg • Vitamin D (from fish liver oil) 400 IU • Vitamin E (as D-alpha tocopherol) 10 IU • Thiamine (as thiamine mononitrate and from yeast) 10 mg • Riboflavin (as riboflavin and from yeast) 10 mg • Niacin (as niacinamide and from yeast) 50 mg • Vitamin B6 (as pyridoxine hydrochloride and from yeast) 10 mg • Folic Acid 400 mcg • Vitamin B12 (as cyanocobalamin) 10 mcg • Pantothenic Acid (as calcium pantothenate and from yeast) 12 mg • Iodine (from kelp and as potassium iodide) 100 mcg • Magnesium (as magnesium oxide) 35 mg • Zinc (as zinc oxide) 15 mg • Selenium (as sodium selenite) 40 mcg • Copper (as copper gluconate and from kelp) 2 mg • Manganese (as manganese gluconate) 10 mg • Chromium (chelated) 20 mcg • Molybdenum (as molybdenum trioxide) 30 mcg • Potassium (as potassium gluconate) 10 mg • Inositol 65 mg • Lecithin (from soy) 30 mg • Betaine Hydrochloride 10 mg • Mixed Tocopherols (non-alpha) 2 mg • Tre-En-En Grain Concentrate Blend 675 mg: Rice Bran oil, Soy bean oil, Wheat Germ oil • Phyto Enzyme Blend 45 mg: Lipase, Protease, Diastase, Amylase. Other Ingredients: Microcrystalline Celluose, Gelatin, Glycerin, Yellow Beeswax, Sodium Croscarmellose, Hydroxypropyl Methylcellulose, Water, Rice Bran, Wheat Bran, Silicon Dioxide, Magnesium Stearate, Titanium Dioixde, Natural Color, Triacetin.

Formula NT-OX - Jamieson
Each caplet contains: Vitamin A (as Retiyl Palmitate (5000 IU) and 67% (10,000 IU) as Beta Carotene) 15,000 IU • Vitamin C (as Ascorbic Acid) 500 mg • Vitamin E (as D-Alpha Tocopheryl Succinate) 100 IU • Selenium (from Yeast) 50 mcg • In a base of Borage Oil, Sunflower Oil, Rosehips, Rutin, Hesperidin, Citrus Bioflavonoids, Acerola, Kelp, Parsley, Watercress, Alfalfa, Bromelain, Papain, Amylase, Lipase, Cellulase.

Formula SF722 - Thorne Research Inc.
Each gelcap contains: 10-Undecenoic Acid derived from Castor Bean oil 50 mg. Other Ingredients: Extra Virgin Olive Oil, Gelatin, Glycerin, Water.

Formu-Leane - SupraLife
Each capsule contains: ChromeMate Chromium Polynicotinate 75 mcg • Proprietary Blend 485 mg: Ma Huang rhizome/roots, Advantra-Z Citrus Aurantium extract (6%), Guarana seed, Ginkgo Biloba leaf, Gymnema Sylvestre leaf, Gotu Kola leaf extract, Ci Wu Jia root (eleutherococcus senticosus), Green Tea leaf extract, Bladderwrack herb (fucus versiculosus), RiboCell D-Ribose. Other Ingredients: Gelatin, Magnesium Stearate.
See Editor's Note No. 30 and No. 40.

Formu-Leane Z - SupraLife
Each capsule contains: ChromeMate Chromium Polynicotinate 75 mcg • Proprietary Blend 697 mg: Advantra-Z Citrus Aurantium extract (6%), Guarana seed, Ginkgo Biloba leaf, Gymnema Sylvestre leaf, Gotu Kola leaf extract, Ci Wu Jia root (eleutherococcus senticosus), Green Tea leaf extract, Bladderwrack herb (fucus versiculosus), RiboCell D-Ribose, Porio Cocos extract, Creatine, Cayenne, Juniper berry extract, Dandelion root extract, Butcher's Broom extract (ruscus aculeatus), Uva Ursi leaf extract, Bioperine brand Black Pepper extract. Other Ingredients: Gelatin, Magnesium Stearate.
See Editor's Note No. 40.

ForSight - Resource Wellness
Three caplets contain: Vitamin A (89% as Beta Carotene) 15,000 IU • Vitamin C (Ascorbis Acid) 300 mg • Vitamin E Acetate 400 IU • Calcium 650 mg • Iron 0.74 mg • Sodium 10 mg • Lutein/Zeaxanthin 6 mg • Alpha Carotene 2 mg • Grape Seed extract 50 mg. Other Ingredients: Dicalcium Phosphate, Microcrystalline Cellulose, Croscramellose Sodium, Calcium Silicate, Magnesium Stearate, Stearic Acid, Hydroxypropyl Methylcellulose, Propylene Glycol, Polyethylene Glycol, Titanium Dioxide, FD&C Yellow No. 6 Lake, FD&C Red No. 40 Lake, FD&C Blue No. 2 Lake.

Some Brand Name Natural Products - What they Contain

www.NaturalDatabase.com contains MANY more listings than appear here.

Editor's Notes are located on pages 2155-2163.

BRAND NAMES

Forskolin Extract - PhytoPharmica
Each capsule contains: Coleus Forskohlii extract (standardized to contain 18% forskolin [9 mg per capsule]) 50 mg.

ForsLean brand - Sabinsa Corporation
Coleus Forskohlii.

Forslean Extreme - America's Finest
Each capsule contains: Forslean brand 10% extract, providing 25 mg Forskohlin 250 mg.

Forten-Zyme 550 - Atrium Biotechnologies
Each tablet contains: Maxistrength Pancreatin 550 mg (which has been prepared by the lyophilization method to insure the preservation & concentration of natural occuring factors such as Amylase, Lipase & Protease enzyme activity. Proteolytic activity is ensured as specific Chymotrypsin & Trypsin content.). This formula is compounded in a buffered base of Amino Acids for maximum stability.
See Editor's Note No. 14.

Fortified Cod Liver Oil - Nature's Own
Each tablet contains: Fortified Cod Liver oil 160 mg: Vitamin A (retinyl palmitate) 88 IU • Vitamin A (retinyl palmitate) 3912 IU • Vitamin D (D3, as cholecalciferol 10 mcg) 400IU.

Fortified Mineral Neutralizer - The Master's Miracle
Electrically Engineered Stabilized Oxygenated Water • Potassium • Calcium • Magnesium • Lauryl Glucoside.

Fortified Pycnogenol - Puritan's Pride
Three tablets contain: Vitamin A (100% as Beta-Carotene) 25,000 IU • Calcium 340 mg • Selenium (from Selenium Yeast Chelate) 100 mcg • Pine bark extract (Pinus maritmus) 25 mg • Coenzyme Q-10 10 mg • Grape Seed extract (Vitis vinifera) 100 mcg • Whole Food Phytonutrient Blend: Broccoli (entire plant), Carrot (root), Spinach (leaf), Tomato (fruit) 120 mg.

For-Til B12 - Standard Process, Inc.
Each capsule contains: Proprietary Blend 278 mg: Tillandsia Usneoides, Calcium Lactate, Defatted Wheat germ, Oat flour, Calcium Phosphate, Bovine Spleen, Ovine Spleen, Ascorbic Acid, Magnesium Citrate • Vitamin B12 3 mcg. Other Ingredients: Gelatin, Water, Colors, Cellulose.
See Editor's Note No. 14.

Forza-T - InStone Nutrition
Three capsules contain: Vitamin B6 3.5 mg • Magnesium 150 mg • Zinc 10 mg • 6-OXO 300 mg • Tribulus Terrestris (protodioscin 20%) 190 mg. Other Ingredients: Gelatin, Microcrystalline Cellulose, Magnesium Stearate.

FOS (fructooligosaccharides) capsules - Pure Encapsulations
Each vegetable capsule contains: Fructooligosaccharides 750 mg • Vitamin C (as ascorbyl palmitate) 15 mg.

FOS (fructooligosaccharides) powder - Pure Encapsulations
EAch 1 tsp serving contains: Fructooligosaccharides 3000 mg.

FOS + Fiber Fructooligosaccharides - Nikken Inc.
Two tablets contain: Dietary Fiber (as cellulose, legume fiber, apple pectin) 1.5 g • FOS (fructooligosaccharides) 500 mg. Other Ingredients: Acacia Gum, Silicon Dioxide, Croscarmellose Sodium, Magnesium Stearate, Cellulose Coating (hydroxypropyl cellulose, ethyl cellulose, hydroxypropyl methylcellulose, guar gum, propylene glycol, vegetable oil), Brazil Wax.

FOS Daily - Health Smart Vitamins
Each caplet contains: Fructooligosaccharides (FOS) 500 mg • Lactobacillus acidophilus 180 mg • Lactobacillus bulgaricus 30 mg • Streptococcus thermophilus 30 mg.

Fosfree - Mission Pharmacal
Two tablets contain: Vitamin A 3,000 IU • Vitamin C 100 mg • Vitamin D (as Vitamin D3) 300 IU • Thiamine 9 mg • Riboflavin 4 mg • Niacin 21 mg • Vitamin B6 5 mg • Vitamin B12 4 mcg • Pantothenic Acid 2 mg • Calcium 351 mg • Iron 29 mg. Other Ingredients: Sugar, Polyethylene Glycol, Color, Croscarmellose Sodium, Povidone, Food Glaze, Cyanocobalamin, Magnesium Stearate, Yellow 5 Lake, Carnauba Wax, White Beeswax, Sodium Benzoate.

Four-In-One - Goldshield Elite
Each capsule contains: Vitamin C (as Calcium Ascorbate) 120 mg • Aloe 200:1 concentrate leaf gel 200 mg • Wild Yam root (Mexican Yam) 50 mg • Cat's Claw root bark (Uncaria tomentosa) 300 mg • DHEA (Dehydroepiandrosterone) 5 mg. Other Ingredients: Gelatin, Magnesium Stearate, Calcium Stearate, and Silica.

Free Amino - Atrium Biotechnologies
Full Spectrum - Composed of 22 Free Form Pure Amino Acids.

Free Aminos - Allergy Research Group
Each capsule contains: L-Alanine 41 mg • L-Arginine 62 mg • L-Cysteine 14 mg • L-Cystine 62 mg • L-Glutamine 28 mg • Glycine 28 mg • L-Histidine 49 mg • L-Isoleucine 69 mg • L-Leucine 69 mg • L-Lysine 98 mg • L-Methionine 14 mg • L-Phenylalanine 7.5 mg • L-Serine 14 mg • Taurine 4 mg • L-Threonine 56 mg • L-Tyrosine 28 mg • L-Valine 28 mg. Other Ingredients: Cellulose, Magnesium Stearate, Silicon Dioxide.

Free-B - Atrium Biotechnologies
Each tablet contains: Vitamin B1 (Thiamine HCL) 100 mg • Vitamin B2 (Riboflavin) 50 mg • Vitamin B6 (Pyridoxine HCL) 50 mg • Vitamin B12 (Cyanocobalamin) 100 mcg • Niacinamide 150 mg • Pantothenic Acid 100 mg • Biotin 150 mcg • Calcium (Dicalcium Phosphate) 20 mg • Copper (Gluconate) 1 mg • Phosphorus (Dicalcium Phosphate) 20 mg • Zinc (Aspartate) 30 mg.

Freedom Patch (eaZy Patch) - Unknown
Fucus Vesiculosus • Guarana extract • Garcinia Cambogia • Menthol.

Freeze-Dried Garlic - Jarrow Formulas
Each capsule contains: Freeze-Dried Garlic 400 mg • Chlorophyllin 100 mg. Other Ingredients: Magnesium Stearate, Gelatin, Modified Cellulose, Triethyl Citrate, Polyethylene Glycol.

Freeze-Dried Ginger - Jarrow Formulas
Each capsule contains: Freeze-Dried Ginger (zingiber officinale) 500 mg. Other Ingredients: Rice Powder, Silicon Dioxide, Magnesium Stearate, Gelatin.

French Paradox (French Parad'ox) - Arkopharma
Each capsule contains: Red Wine Marc extract (standardized to 25% anthocyanosides (62.5 mg) and 0.02% resveratrol (50 mcg)) 250 mg. Other Ingredients: Cellulose Derivative, Magnesium Stearate, Silica.

Fresh Green Black Walnut Wormwood Complex - NOW Foods
Two droppersful (16 ml) contain: Proprietary blend: Green Black Walnut hulls (Juglans species) 1.6 ml • Wormwood herb (Artemisia absinthium) • Clove buds (Carophyllus species) extracts. Other Ingredients: Grain Alcohol, Distilled Water.

Fresh Harvest - FreeLife International
Two caplets contain: Vitamin A (as mixed carotenes from dunaliella salina algae) 5000 IU • Vitamin C (as ascorbic acid) 150 mg • Vitamin E (as dL-alpha tocopheryl succinate) 6 IU • Vitamin B1 (as thiamin mononitrate) 1 mg • Vitamin B2 (as riboflavin) 0.5 mg • Niacin 3 mg • Vitamin B6 (as pyridoxine HCl) 0.5 mg • Calcium (from fruit and vegetable concentrates) 300 mg • Magnesium (as magnesium oxide) 25 mg • (Rapid-Release: Gold Half) 10X Fruit Concentrate 900 mg: Apple, Apricot, Banana, Black Currant, Blueberry, Cantaloupe, Cranberry, Grapefruit, Guava, Kiwi, Lemon, Lime, Mango, Orange, Papaya, Peach, Pineapple, Red Raspberry, Red Wine Grape, Strawberry, Tomato • Proprietary Plant Enzyme Complex 46,082 units: Protease, Lipase, Acid Protease, Amylase, Glucoamylase, Cellulase, Hemicellulase, Maltase, Sucrase • (Time-Released: Green Half) 10X Vegetable Concentrate 700 mg: Alfalfa, Barley grass, Beet, Broccoli, Brussels sprouts, Cabbage, Carrot,

Cayenne, Fennel, Garlic, Green Bell Pepper, Kale, Oat grass, Onion, Parsley, Spinach, Squash, Turnip, Watercress • Global Algae Blend 300 mg: Klamath Spirulina, Hawaiian Spirulina, Chlorella (broken cell wall), Kombu seaweed, Nori seaweed, Phenalgin brand Cystoseira Canariensis phlorotannin extract, Main coast Ascophyllum kelp, Irish moss, Giant Pacific kelp, Dunaliella Salina, Nova Scotia Dulse • Soluble and Insoluble Fiber 250 mg: Plant Cellulose, Apple Pectin, Citrus Pectin. Other Ingredients: Vegetable Stearic Acid, Silica, Vegetable Magnesium Stearate, Calcium Hydrogen Phosphate, Vita-Coat (vegetable resin, alpha-lipoic acid).

Fresh Nettle Leaf - Gaia Herbs
Nettle leaf (2% caffeic acids and derivatives). Standardized Full Spectrum 100 mg of extract per capsule. Guaranteed Potency 50 mg of extract per capsule.

Friendly Fiber - NSI - Nutraceutical Sciences Institute
Each six capsules contain: Apple Pectin 2.1 g • Oat Bran 2.1 g.

Friendly Flora - Nutri-Quest Rx
Each capsule contains: Jerusalem Artichoke (rich source of Fructooligosaccarides) 200 mg • Cellulase 1200 CU • Lactobacillus Acidophilus 400 million • Acerola extract 25 mg • Rose Hips 25 mg • Bifidobacterium Bifidum 200 million • Bifidobacterium Longum 200 million • Protease 7500 HUT • Lipase 52 LU • Lactobacillus Casei 100 million • Lactobacillus Plantarum 100 million • Lactobacillus Rueteri 100 million • Lactobacillus Salicarius 100 million • Amylase 275 DU • EDS Mineral Mix: Kelp, Calcium Ascorbate, Magnesium Citrate, Zinc Gluconate, Manganese Gluconate. In a base of pure plant fiber.

From The Earth - The Vitamin Shoppe
Three tablets contain: Vitamin A 15000 IU • Vitamin D 400 IU • Vitamin E 200 IU • Vitamin C 1000 mg • Vitamin B1 25 mg • Vitamin B2 25 mg • Vitamin B6 25 mg • Vitamin B12 500 mcg • Vitamin B3 25 mg • Inositol 25 mg • Choline 50 mg • PABA 25 mg • Pantothenic Acid 25 mg • Biotin 50 mcg • Folic Acid 400 mcg • Citrus Bioflavonoids Complex 125 mg • Rutin 25 mg • Quercetin 25 mg • Hesperidin 25 mg • Calcium 200 mg • Magnesium 100 mg • Potassium 99 mg • Zinc 15 mg • Manganese 5 mg • Molybdenum 50 mcg • Iodine 150 mcg • Copper 500 mcg • Selenium 50 mcg • Chromium 200 mcg • Boron 1 mg • Silica 5 mg • RNA 35 mg • DNA 10 mg • Carotenoids 4 mg • Chlorophyll 4 mg • Borage, Flax Seed, and Sunflower Oils 200 mg • L-Glutathione 5 mg • Spirulina 1000 mg • Wheat Grass 100 mg • Barley Grass 100 mg • Chlorella 100 mg • Bee Pollen 100 mg • Korean Ginseng root 50 mg • Garlic 10 mg • Bee Propolis extract 10 mg • Royal Jelly 5 mg • Bromelain 50 mg • Betaine HCl 50 mg • Papain 50 mg • Amylase 5 mg • Lipase 5 mg • Cellulase 5 mg • Lactobacillus Acidophilus, B. bifidum, L-bulgaricus (dairy free) 50 mg • Oat Bran 50 mg • Apple Pectin 50 mg • A unique blend of: Echinacea, Milk Thistle, Goldenseal, Ginger root, Ginkgo Biloba, Capsicum 50 mg.

From The Sea - Puritan's Pride
Three capsules contain: Glucosamine Sulfate (Aminomonosaccharide) 1000 mg • Sea Cucumber (Beche De-Mer) 1000 mg • Shark Cartilage 500 mg.

Fruit Max - Swanson Health Products
Two tablets contain: Apple fruit powder 80 mg • Apricot fruit powder 80 mg • Cherry fruit powder 80 mg • Lemon peel powder 80 mg • Orange peel powder 80 mg • Papaya powder 80 mg • Peach fruit powder 80 mg • Strawberry fruit powder 80 mg • Freeze-Dried Grape juice 50 mg • Freeze-Dried Orange juice 50 mg • Freeze-Dried Pineapple juice 50 mg • Prune juice powder 40 mg • Cranberry juice concentrate 20 mg.

Fruit Punch Phosphagen HP - EAS, Inc.
Each 43 gram serving contains: Phosphagen 5.25 g • Taurine 1000 mg. Ingredients: Dextrose • Phosphagen (HPCE pure Creatine Monohydrate), Taurine • Natural & Artificial Flavor • Citric Acid • Beet Powder for color • Magnesium Phosphate • Disodium Phosphate •Potassium Phosphate.

Fruit4Life - Swanson Health Products
Two tablets contain: Apple fruit powder 80 mg • Apricot fruit powder 80 mg • Cherry fruit powder 80 mg • Lemon peel powder 80 mg • Orange peel powder 80 mg • Papaya powder 80 mg • Peach fruit powder 80 mg • Strawberry fruit powder 80 mg • Freeze-Dried Grape juice 50 mg • Freeze-Dried Orange juice 50 mg • Freeze-Dried Pineapple juice 50 mg • Prune juice powder 40 mg • Cranberry juice concentrate 20 mg.

Fruit-Easy - Progressive Labs
Two tablets contain: A blend of the following 1400 mg: Apples • Cranberry powder • Orange juice powder • Pineapple juice powder • Siberian Ginseng • Ginkgo Biloba • Peaches • Dates • Bromelain • Papain • Lipase • Amylase • Protease • Cellulase • Powdered Cellulose • Apple pectin • Citris pectin • Prune powder • Glucomannan • Lactobacillus Acidophilus • Calcium Gluconate • Green Tea.

Fruitplex - HealthWatchers System
Apple • Lemon • Strawberry • Blueberry • Plum • Cantaloupe • Pear • Cherry • Grapefruit • Raspberry • Grape • Orange • Peach • Watermelon • Pineapple • Papaya

Fruits of Life Potent Cellular Protection - Garden of Life, Inc.
Each tablespoon (10 g) contains: Antioxidant Fruit Organic Concentrate Blend 3000 mg: Blueberry, Raspberry, Strawberry, Blackberry, Prune, Raisin • Mineral Matrix Proprietary Blend 7000 mg: biologically active Alkalinizing Minerals, Enzymes, Probiotics from Goat's Milk.

Fuel for Thought Neuro Nutrition - Nature's Plus
Two tablets contain: L-Glutamine free form amino acid 250 mg • Soy Lecithin 250 mg • RNA (ribonucleic acid) 200 mg • L-Tyrosine free form amino acid 200 mg • L-Phenylalanine free form amino acid 100 mg • Phosphatidylcholine 100 mg • Raw Pituitary concentrate 25 mg • Vitamin B6 (pyridoxine HCl) 10 mg.
See Editor's Note No. 31.

Full Spectrum Cinnamon Extract - Planetary Formulas
Two tablets contain: Calcium 50 mg • Cinnamomum Aromaticum bark extract 10:1 (yielding 8% flavonoids) 300 mg • Cinnamomum Aromaticum bark 100 mg. Other Ingredients: Dibasic Calcium Phosphate, Stearic Acid, Modified Cellulose Gum, Colloidal Silicon Dioxide.

Full Spectrum Jiaogulan - Planetary Formulas
Each tablet contains: Calcium 127 mg • Jiaogulan extract (gynostemma pentaphyllum, standardized to 10% gypenosides) 375 mg. Other Ingredients: Dibasic Calcium Phosphate, Stearic Acid, Colloidal Silicon Dioxide, Modified Cellulose Gum, Magnesium Stearate.

Full Spectrum Life Minerals - Pro Health
Two tablets contain: Vitamin D (as cholecalciferol) 200 IU • Calcium (from carbonate, amino acid chelate, citrate) 1000 mg • Iron (as amino acid chelate) 20 mg • Iodine (from kelp) 150 mcg • Magnesium (from magnesium oxide, amino acid chelate, citrate) 500 mg • Chromium (yeast-free) 100 mcg • Molybdenum (as amino acid chelate) 50 mcg • Potassium (as amino acid chelate) 99 mg • Zinc (as amino acid chelate) 22.5 mg • Selenium (as selenomethionine) 50 mcg • Copper (as amino acid chelate) 1 mg • Manganese (as amino acid chelate) 5 mg • L-Glutamic Acid (HCl) 50 mg • Boron (as amino acid chelate) 3 mg • Vanadium (as amino acid chelate) 50 mcg. Other Ingredients: Cellulose, Silica, Magnesium Stearate.

Full Spectrum Mineral Caps - NOW Foods
Four capsules contain: Vitamin D (as Cholecalciferol) 4000 IU • Calcium (from Hydroxapatite) 500 mg • Phosphorus (from Hydroxapatite) 193 mg • Iodine (from Kelp) 225 mcg • Magnesium (as Magnesium Oxide and Citrate) 500 mg • Zinc (as Amino Acid Chelate) 15 mg • Selenium (as l-Selenomethionine) 100 mcg • Copper (as Amino Acid Chelate) 2 mg • Manganese (as Amino Acid

BRAND NAMES

Chelate) 5 mg • Chromium (as Chromium Chelavite) 200 mcg • Molybdenum (as Amino Acid Chelate) 100 mcg • Potassium (as Amino Acid Chelate) 99 mg • Boron (as Amino Acid Chelate) 3 mg • Vanadium (as Amino Acid Chelate) 50 mcg. Other Ingredients: Gelatin (capsule), Rice Flour, Magnesium Stearate.

Full Spectrum Minerals - NOW Foods
Each tablet contains: Calcium (Carbonate, Amino Acid Chelate, Citrate) 1000 mg • Magnesium (Oxide, Amino Acid Chelate, Citrate) 500 mg • Zinc (Amino Acid Chelate) 22.5 mg • Iron (Amino Acid Chelate) 20 mg • Copper (Amino Acid Chelate) 1 mg • Potassium (Proteinate) 99 mg • Manganese (Amino Acid Chelate) 5 mg • Selenium (L-Selenium Methionine) 50 mcg • Chromium (yeast-free, Proteinate) 100 mcg • Molybdenum (Amino Acid Chelate) 59 mcg • Vanadium (Amino Acid Chelate) 50 mcg • Iodine (Kelp) 150 mcg • L-Glutamic Acid (HCL) 50mg • Vitamin D (Cholecalciferol) 200 IU • Boron 3 mg.

Full Spectrum Pycnogenol - Life Extension
Each capsule contains: Pycnogenol 5 mg • Pine bark extract (4:1, source of high potency proanthocyanidins & leucocyanidins) 30 mg • Grape Seed extract 100 mg • Quercetin 5 mg.

Fungal Defense Candida & Yeast Cleanse -
Garden of Life, Inc.
Each caplet contains: Wild Oregano concentrate (6% volatile oils) 342 mg • Fungal Defense N•Zime Blend 233 mg: Protease 20,000 HUT, Cellulase 20,000 CU • Poten-Zyme D. Salina extract 120 mg • Olive leaf extract (20% oleuropin) 100 mg • Poten-Zyme Garlic juice extract (20:1) 95 mg • Ionic Fulvic Acid mineral blend 80 mg • HSO Probiotic Blend 800 Million CFU: L. Acidophilus, L. Bulgaricus, L. Lactis, L. Plantarum, L. Caseii, S. Boulardii, B. Bifidum, B. Subtilis, B. Lichenformis • Poten-Zyme Yucca juice extract (20:1) 30 mg. Other Ingredients: Cellulose, Stearates (vegetable source).

FuraMag - InterPlexus
Each capsule contains: Magnesium (as fumarate) 140 mg. Other Ingredients: Cellulose.

Furosterol Extreme - America's Finest
Each capsule contains: Tribulus extract 45% 280 mg • Fenusterol extract 50% 280 mg • Diosgenin extract 95% 280 mg. Other Ingredients: Dicalcium Phosphate, Cellulose, Magnesium Stearate, Magnesium Trisilicate.

FUZE Healthy Infuzions Diet White Tea -
FUZE Beverage, LLC
Filtered Water • Natural Pomegranate Passionfruit flavor with other Natural Flavors • White Tea solids • Malic Acid • White Tea extract • Ascorbic Acid • Acesulfame Potassium • Citric Acid • Sucralose • Niacin (vitamin B3) • Calcium Pantothenate • Vitamin E Acetate • Pyridoxine Hydrochloride (vitamin B6) • Folic Acid • Cyanocobalamin.

FUZE Healthy Infuzions Energize (blackberry grape) -
FUZE Beverage, LLC
Filtered Water • Crystalline Fructose • Apple juice concentrate • Pear puree • Natural Flavor • Citric Acid • Blackberry juice concentrate • Pectin • Ascorbic Acid (vitamin C) • Guarana extract 100 mg • Siberian Ginseng extract 100 mg • Red Cabbage extract • Niacin (vitamin B3) • Cyanocobalamin (vitamin B12).

FUZE Healthy Infuzions Energize (exotic punch) -
FUZE Beverage, LLC
Filtered Water • Crystalline Fructose • Orange juice concentrate • Aronia concentrate • Pineapple juice concentrate • Citric Acid • Pectin • Natural Flavor • Ascorbic Acid (vitamin C) • Siberian Ginseng 100 mg • Guarana extract 100 mg • Natural Color • Niacin (vitamin B3) • Papaya puree • Cyanocobalamin (vitamin B12).

FUZE Healthy Infuzions Energize (mojo mango) -
FUZE Beverage, LLC
Filtered Water • Crystalline Fructose • Orange juice concentrate • Mango puree • Passion Fruit juice concentrate • Citric Acid • Pectin • Natural Flavor • Ascorbic Acid (vitamin C) • Siberian Ginseng extract • Guarana extract • Natural Color • Niacin (vitamin B3) • Cyanocobalamin (vitamin B12).

FUZE Healthy Infuzions Focus (orange mango) -
FUZE Beverage, LLC
Filtered Water • Crystalline Fructose • Orange juice concentrate • Mango puree • Passion Fruit juice • Citric Acid • Pectin • Natural Flavor • Ascorbic Acid (vitamin C) • Niacin (vitamin B3) • Calcium Pantothenate (vitamin B5) • Vitamin E Acetate • Pyridoxine Hydrochloride (vitamin B6) • Vitamin A Palmitate • Cyanocobalamin (vitamin B12).

FUZE Healthy Infuzions Green Tea - FUZE Beverage, LLC
Filtered Water • Crystalline Fructose • Honey • Green Tea extract • Citric Acid • Ascorbic Acid • Green Tea solids • Vitamin E Acetate • Niacin (vitamin B3) • Calcium Pantothenate • Siberian Ginseng root extract • Pyridoxine Hydrochloride (vitamin B6) • Folic Acid • Cyanocobalamin (vitamin B12).

FUZE Healthy Infuzions Lemon AID -
FUZE Beverage, LLC
Filtered Water • Crystalline Fructose • Lemon juice concentrate • Pectin • Gum Acacia • Ascorbic Acid (vitamin C) • Citric Acid • Malic Acid • Ester Gum • Vitamin E Acetate • Zinc Picolinate • Sucralose • Vitamin A Palmitate.

FUZE Healthy Infuzions Refresh (banana colada) -
FUZE Beverage, LLC
Filtered Water • Crystalline Fructose • Skim Milk • Banana puree • Apple juice concentrate • Natural Flavor • Sugar • Tricalcium Phosphate • Cream • Lactic Acid • Pectin • Citric Acid • Ascorbic Acid • Niacin • Calcium Pantothenate • Vitamin E Acetate • Sucralose • Pyridoxine Hydrochloride • Vitamin A Palmitate • Cyanocobalamin.

FUZE Healthy Infuzions Refresh (mixed berry) -
FUZE Beverage, LLC
Filtered Water • Crystalline Fructose • Skim Milk • Apple juice concentrate • Sucrose • Tricalcium Phosphate • Cream • Pectin • Citric Acid • Propylene Glycol • Narural Flavor • Black Currant extract • Cherry extract • Blueberry extract • Elderberry concentrate • Ascorbic Acid • Lactic Acid • Niacin • Calcium Pantothenate • Vitamin E Acetate • Sucralose • Pyridoxine Hydrochloride • Vitamin A Palimate • Cyanocobalamin.

FUZE Healthy Infuzions Refresh (peach mango) -
FUZE Beverage, LLC
Filtered Water • Crystalline Fructose • Skim Milk • Apple juice concentrate • Natural Flavor • Sucrose • Cream • Lactic Acid • Pectin • Citric Acid • Ascorbic Acid • Niacin • Calcium Pantothenate • Vitamin E Acetate • Sucralose • Pyridoxine Hydrochloride • Vitamin A Palmitate • Cyanocobalamin.

FUZE Healthy Infuzions Refresh (strawberry guava) -
FUZE Beverage, LLC
Filtered Water • Crystalline Fructose • Skim Milk • Apple juice concentrate • Sugar • Tricalcium Phosphate • Cream • Lactic Acid • Pectin • Citric Acid • Natural Strawberry Flavor with other Natural Flavors • Ascorbic Acid (vitamin C) • Black Carrot Juice concentrate • Niacin (vitamin B3) • Calcium Pantothenate (vitamin B5) • Sucralose • Vitamin E Acetate • Pyridoxine Hydrochloride (vitamin B6) • Vitamin A Palmitate • Cyanocobalamin (vitamin B12).

Some Brand Name Natural Products - What they Contain

www.NaturalDatabase.com contains MANY more listings than appear here.
Editor's Notes are located on pages 2155-2163.

FUZE Healthy Infuzions Slenderize (cranberry-raspberry) - FUZE Beverage, LLC
Filtered Water • Plum juice concentrate • Raspberry juice concentrate • Cranberry juice concentrate • Malic Acid • Natural Flavor • Garcinia Cambogia rind extract • Ascorbic Acid • Grape juice concentrate • Acesulfame Potassium • Sucralose • L-Carnitine • Chromium Polynicotinate.

FUZE Healthy Infuzions Slenderize (strawberry melon) - FUZE Beverage, LLC
Filtered Water • Apple juice concentrate • Malic Acid • Garcinia rind extract • Natural Strawberry • Watermelon flavor • Natural Flavors • Ascorbic Acid (vitamin C) • Acesulfame Potassium • Black Carrrot juice concentrate (color) • L-Carnitine • Sucralose • Chromium Polynicotinate.

FUZE Healthy Infuzions Slenderize (tropical punch) - FUZE Beverage, LLC
Filtered Water • Pineapple juice concentrate • Malic Acid • Mango juice concentrate • Natural Flavor • Garcinia Cambogia rind extract • Purple Carrot juice concentrate • Ascorbic Acid • Acesulfame Potassium • Dragonfruit extract • Sucralose • L-Carnitine • Chromium Polynicotinate.

FUZE Healthy Infuzions White Tea - FUZE Beverage, LLC
Filtered Water • Crystalline Fructose • Honey • Natural Orange Ginger Flavor with other Natural Flavors • White Tea solids • Malic Acid • Ascorbic Acid (vitamin C) • White Tea extract • Niacin (vitamin B3) • Calcium Pantothenate • Vitamin E Acetate • Pyridoxine Hydrochloride (vitamin B6) • Folic Acid • Cyanocobalamin (vitamin B12).

FX-Chrysin - GEN - Genetic Evolutionary Nutrition
Each capsule contains: Chrysin 250 mg • LPC (lysophosphatidyl choline) 200 mg.

FYI For Your Inflammation - Garden of Life, Inc.
Three caplets contain: Chicken Collagen Type II 805 mg • Wild Oregano concentrate (6% volatile oils) 465 mg • Poten-Zyme Cat's Claw extract 375 mg • Systemic Enzyme Blend 350 mg: Bromelain 80,000 HUT, Papain 2,100,00 FCCPU, Protease blend 250,000 FCCPU, Amylase 4000 DU, Lipase 1750 FCCLU, Cellulase 500 CU • Rhododendron Caucasicum extract (40% polyphenols) 150 mg • Poten-Zyme Ginger extract 115 mg • Poten-Zyme Turmeric extract 115 mg • Poten-Zyme Green Barley juice extract 115 mg • Phytosterol blend 60 mg • Laminaria extract (5% algae phenolics) 50 mg • Ulva extract (5% algae phenolics) 50 mg • Bayberry bark extract (77% myricetin) 50 mg. Other Ingredients: Cellulose, Stearates (vegetable source).

G.H.3. Romanian Youth Formula - TheraCeuticals
Each capsule contains: Vitamin A (as beta-carotene) 1200 IU • Thiamin (as thiamin mononitrate) 10 mg • Vitamin B3 (as niacinamide) 80 mg • Vitamin B6 (as pyridoxine hydrochloride) 20 mg • Zinc (as PhytoZinc and zinc gluconate) 2.6 mg • Copper (as copper gluconate) 0.8 mg • Procaine (dimethylaminoethanol bitartrate 200 mg, para-aminobenzoic acid 75 mg) • Ginkgo leaf extract (24% flavone glycosides, 6% terpenes) 50 mg. Other Ingredients: Gelatin, Silicon Dioxide, Magnesium Stearate.

G.I. Fortify - Pure Encapsulations
Each scoop contains: Vitamin C (as ascorbyl palmitate) 30 mg • Psyllium husk powder (plantago indica, providing insoluble fiber 360 mg, soluble fiber 3 g) 4 g • Flax seed powder (providing insoluble fiber 531 mg, soluble fiber 264 mg, lignans 11. 5mg) 2.25 g • L-Glutamine (free-form) 1 g • Deglycyrrhizinated Licorice root extract 600 mg • Marshmallow root 8:1 extract (althaea officinalis) 400 mg • Unripe Plantain banana fruit (musa paradisiaca) 300 mg • Slippery Elm root extract (ulmus fulva) 200 mg • Triphala Proprietary Blend 90 mg: Terminalia Chebula, Terminalis Belerica, Emblica Officinalis.

G.I. Gel: Gastro-Intestinal Tonic - The Herbalist
Slippery Elm bark • Marshmallow root.

G.I. Support - NOW Foods
Three capsules contain: Vitamin A (as Retinol Palmitate) 5000 IU • Vitamin B3 (as Niacinamide) 40 mg • Vitamin B5 (as Calcium Pantothenate) 50 mg • Biotin 1000 mcg • Folic Acid (Folate) 400 mcg • Zinc (as Zn Monomethionine) 15 mg • Selenium (as Selenomethionine) 140 mcg • L-Glutamine 500 mg • Apple Pectin 300 mg • N-Acetyl Glucosamine (NAG) 250 mg • Methylsulfonylmethane (MSM) 250 mg • Deglycyrrhizinated Licorice (DGL) 100 mg • Licorice extract 4:1 root 100 mg • Cat's Claw extract 15:1 bark 100 mg • Ginger powder root 100 mg • Aloe Vera concentrate 200:1 leaf (equivalent to 5000 mg fresh Aloe Vera) 25 mg • Pepsin Enzymes NF 1:10000) 50 mg • Pepsin (2000 USP papaya) 50 mg.

G.I.2 Enhance - Pure Encapsulations
Each vegetable capsule contains: Dried Fish Protein Hydrolyzate 425 mg • L-Glutamine (free-form) 425 mg. Other Ingredients: Rosemary Extract.

G/C 1000 - Progressive Labs
Each capsule contains: Vitamin C (from manganese ascorbate) 60 mg • Manganese (from manganese ascorbate) 15 mg • Glucosamine Hydrochloride 750 mg • Chondroitin Sulfate 250 mg.
See Editor's Note No. 15.

GABA - Enzymatic Therapy/PhytoPharmica
Each capsule contains: Gamma-Aminobutyric Acid (GABA) 250 mg. Other Ingredients: Gelatin, Cellulose, Magnesium Stearate, Silicon Dioxide, Titanium Dioxide Color.

GABA - Pro Health
Each tablet contains: GABA (gamma amino butyric acid) 750 mg. Other Ingredients: Dibasic Calcium Phosphate, Stearic Acid, Sorbitol, Modified Cellulose Gum, Colloidal Silicon Dioxide, Fiber, Magnesium Stearate.

GABA - Source Naturals
Each tablet contains: GABA (gamma amino butyric acid) 750 mg.

GABA (Gamma Aminobutyric Acid) 500 mg - Solgar
Each capsule contains: Calcium (as dicalcium phosphate) 45 mg • GABA (as gamma aminobutyric acid) 500 mg. Other Ingredients: Dicalcium Phosphate, Vegetable Cellulose, Microcrystalline Cellulose, Vegetable Magnesium Stearate, Silica, Water, Vegetable Glycerin.

GABA 375 - Pain & Stress Center
Each capsule contains: GABA (as gamma amino butyric acid) 375 mg • Glycine 100 mg. Other Ingredients: Gelatin Capsule.

GABA 750 MG - Pain & Stress Center
Each capsule contains: GABA (as gamma amino butyric acid) 750 mg • Glycine 25 mg. Other Ingredients: Gelatin Capsule.

GABA Calm - Source Naturals
Each tablet contains: GABA (Gamma Amino Butyric Acid) 100 mg • Glycine 50 mg • Magnesium Taurinate (Yielding 3 mg of Elemental Magnesium) 40 mg • N-Acetyl-L-Tyrosine 25 mg.

GABAnol - Ortho Molecular Products
Two capsules contain: Vitamin B6 (as pyridoxine HCl USP) 50 mg • Magnesium (as ascorbate) 15 mg • GABA 250 mg • Glycine USP 225 mg • Cramp bark 200 mg • Dong Quai root extract (standardized to cotnain 1% ligustilides) 150 mg. Other Ingredients: Natural Vegetable Capsules, Ascorbyl Palmitate, Magnesium Stearate, Microcrystalline Cellulose, Silicon Dioxide.

Gabatein brand - Cyvex Nutrition, Inc.
Green Tea extract.

GABA-Val - Progressive Labs
Each capsule contains: Gamma Amino Butyric Acid (GABA) 50 mg • Valerian root extract (Valeriana officinalis) 300 mg • Thiamine HCl (Vitamin B1) 25 mg • Niacinamide 25 mg • Magnesium (amino acid chelate) 25 mg • Inositol 175 mg • Lupulin (hops pollen) 50 mg •

Passion flower (Passiflora incarnata) 25 mg • Glutamic Acid 25 mg • Brain tissue 25 mg.
See Editor's Note No. 31.

Gainers Fuel (Anabolic Weight Gain Formula) - TwinLab
Each serving contains: Calories 531. Each serving also contains Branched Chain Amino Acids (including Peptide Bonded & Free Amino Acids) 21 g, Essential Vitamins, Minerals, Trace Elements, Key Metabolic Optimizers & Lipotropic Factors.

Gainers Fuel 1000 (Super Anabolic Weight Gain Formula) - TwinLab
Each serving contains: Predigested Proteins & Amino Acids (Complex Carbohydrates, Anabolic Branched Chain Amino Acids) • Vitamins & Minerals •Pharmaceutical Grade Pancreatic digests of Whey Protein (Lactalbumin) & Egg White Protein (Albumin) • Chromium 400 mcg • Boron • L-Carnitine • Beta-Carotene • Kreb's Cycle Mineral Complexes (including Citrates, Aspartates, Succinates & Alpha-Ketoglutarates).

Gainers Fuel 2500 - TwinLab
Whey & Egg White Proteins • Branched Chain Amino Acids: L-Leucine, L-Isoleucine, and L-Valine • Essential Vitamins & Minerals • Chromium Picolinate • L-Carnitine.

Galagen brand - Proventra
Colostrum.

GalantaMind - Life Enhancement Products, Inc.
Each capsule contains: Vitamin B5 (from calcium pantothenate) 100 mg • Galantamine Hydrobromide extract (from lycoris radiata) 8 mg • Choline (from choline dihydrogen citrate) 200 mg.

GalantaMind Plus - Life Enhancement Products, Inc.
Two capsules contain: Vitamin C (as calcium ascorbate) 600 mg • Vitamin E (as D-alpha-tocopheryl acetate) 133 mg • Vitamin B6 (as pyridoxine hydrochloride) 5 mg • Folic Acid 166 mcg • Vitamin B12 (cyanocobalamin) 166 mcg • Pantothenic Acid (vitamin B5 as calcium pantothenate) 100 mg • Turmeric root (powder) 233 mg • Green Tea leaf extract 233 mg • Galantamine Hydrochloride (extracted from galanthus nivalis) 8 mg • Lithium (as lithium carbonate) 2.3 mg.

Gall & Liver Tablets - Life Brand
Agrimony herb 100.1 mg • Goose Grass 100.1 mg • Horehound herb 72.8 mg • Senna leaf 18.2 mg • Woodruff herb 81.25 mg • Wormwood herb 18.2 mg • Yarrow 81.9 mg. Excipients: Corn Starch, Sodium Bicarbonate, Silicon Dioxide, Magnesium Stearate, Methyl Paraben, Propyl Paraben.

Gallbladder - Enzymes, Inc.
Each capsule contains: Proprietary Herbal Blend 400 mg: Globe Artichoke leaf extract, Dandelion root extract, Turmeric root extract, Lecithin, Dandelion leaf extract • Lipase 100 mg. Other Ingredients: Plant Cellulose, Water.

Gallexier Herbal Bitters - Flora Inc.
Artichoke • Dandelion • "other bitter herbs".

Gamma E-Gems - J. R. Carlson Laboratories, Inc.
Each softgel contains: Vitamin E (as D-alpha tocopherol) 90 IU • D-Gamma Tocopherol 500 mg • D-Delta Tocopherol 150 mg • D-Beta Tocopherol 11 mg.

Gamma Oryzanol - Source Naturals
Each tablet contains: Gamma Oryzanol 30 mg.

GammaFrac - Source Naturals
Each tablet contains: Famma Oryzanol 25 mg • FRAC (Ferulic Acid Complex) 50 mg.

Gammalen In Oil Of Primrose - Life Extension
Each 560 mg capsule contains: Linoleic Acid 350 mg • Gamma Linoleic Acid 40 mg • Gamma Linolenic Acid 40 mg • Vitamin E 13.6 IU.

Gandha - 750 - Jarrow Formulas
Each capsule contains: Withania Somnifera (2.5% withanolides) 750 mg.

Garcinia 1000 - Source Naturals
Two tablets contain: Citrin Garcinia cambogia extract [yielding 1,000 mg of (-) Hydroxycitric Acid as Calcium Hydroxycitrate] 2,000 mg • Chromium (150 mcg from ChromeMate GTF Yeast-Free Polynicotinate and 150 mcg from Yeast-Free Chromium Picolinate) 300 mcg.

Garcinia Cambogia - ProThera
Each capsule contains: Garcinia Cambogia fruit dried extract (min. 50% (-) hydroxycitric acid, CitriMax brand) 500 mg. Other Ingredients: Cellulose, Water, Silicon Dioxide, Magnesium Stearate.

Garcinia Cambogia Plus - Atrium Biotechnologies
Each capsule contains: Garcinia cambogia (standardized to contain 50% Hydroxycitric Acid) 340 mg • Atractylodes 80 mg • Citrus aurantii 80 mg • Chromium Picolinate 500 mcg • Chromium Arginate 160 mcg.

Garcinia Plus - Source Naturals
Two tablets contain: Garcinia cambogia Extract (Citrin, yielding 1,000 mg of (-) hydroxycitric acid as calcium hydroxycitrate) 2,000 mg • L-Phenylalanine 200 mg • Chromium (100 mcg from ChromeMate GTF yeast-free polynicotinate and 100 mcg from yeast-free chromium picolinate) 200 mcg.

Garlic - Benepure, Inc
Each tablet contains: Calcium 60 mg • Phosphorus 45 mg • Magnesium 10 mg • Garlic root extract (allium sativum, yielding allicin 4 mg) 400 mg. Other Ingredients: Dicalcium Phosphate, Microcrystalline Cellulose, Croscarmellose Sodium, Stearic Acid, Sodium Lauryl Sulfate, Silicon Dioxide, Magnesium Stearate.

Garlic - Pharmanex
Each caplet contains: Garlic clove powder (Allium sativum) 650 mg. Other Ingredients: Excipients, Binders, Caplet Coating.

Garlic - Olympian Labs
Each capsule contains: Garlic 500 mg.

Garlic - Standard Process, Inc.
Each capsule contains: Garlic bulb 550 mg • Parsley leaf 30 mg. Other Ingredients: Gelatin, Water, Colors, Calcium Stearate.

Garlic - Plus - Aspen Group, Inc.
Each tablet contains: High Potency Garlic (standardized to contain 2500 mcg of allicin) 300 mg • Enzyme Complex 60 mg • Rice Protein-Calcium complex 40 mg.

Garlic & Golden Seal - Nutrivention
Two fl oz contains: Garlic oil • Goldenseal root • Safflower oil • cold-pressed Olive oil • Tocopherol (natural Vitamin E).

Garlic & Parsley - Jamieson
Each tablet contains: Garlic Oil (equivalent to 350 mg fresh garlic) 0.59 mg • Parsley Leaf Powder 50 mg.

Garlic (Allicin-Rich) - Life Brand
Garlic extract powder 500 mg (equivalent to 1500 mg of fresh Garlic cloves). Contains Allicin potential yield of 1.5 mg/g, Thiosulphonates 1.6 mg/g, Allicin 10 mg/g, Gamma Glutamylcysteines 20 mg/g. Other Ingrendients: Cellulose, Calcium Phosphate, Stearic Acid, Magnesium Stearate, Aqueous base film coat.

Garlic + C, Horseradish, Fenugreek & Marshmallow - Nature's Own
Each tablet contains: Arizona odourless Garlic powder (allium sativum), equivalent to fresh bulb 300 mg • Vitamin C (ascorbic acid) 500 mg • Fenugreek extract (trigonella foenum-graecum), equivalent to dry seed 50 mg • Horseradish extract (amoracia rusticana), equivalent to dry root 500 mg • Marshmallow extract (althaea officinalis), equivalent to dry root 50 mg.

Garlic 100:1 extract **-** Pure Encapsulations
Each vegetable capsule contains: Garlic 100:1 extract (odorless, contains a minimum of 5.3 mg scordinin) 250 mg.

Garlic 1000mg **-** Nature's Own
Each tablet contains: Garlic powder (allium sativium) equivalent to fresh bulb 1000 mg.

Garlic 600 **-** J. R. Carlson Laboratories, Inc.
Each tablet contains: Garlic bulb (allium sativum, odorless) 600 mg.

Garlic 6000 **-** Vital Nutrients
Each caplet contains: Allium Sativum (garlic extract) 650 mg: Allicin yield 6000 mcg • Thiosulfinates 6000 mcg • Allicin 13,200 mcg.

Garlic and Apple Vinegar capsules **-** Susan Ambrosino's Herb Club, Inc.
Each capsule contains: Deodorized Garlic 331 mg • Apple Vinegar 331 mg.

Garlic Bulb **-** Aboca USA, Inc
Each capsule contains: Garlic bulb WPC (whole phytocomplex concentrate, allium sativum, standardized to 0.45% allicin, yielding 1.44 mg per capsule) 320 mg. Other Ingredients: Gelatin.

Garlic Complex **-** Shaklee
Two tablets contain: Garlic powder (Allium sativum) clove 1 g • Spearmint oil (Mentha spicata) leaf 3 mg • Rosemary extract (Rosmarinus officinalis) herb 50 mg. Other Ingredients: Maltodextrin, Microcrystallline Cellulose, Carbohydrate gum, Hydroxylated Soy Lecithin, Ascorbyl Palmitate, Mixed Tocopherols Concentrate, Rosemary Extract.

Garlic EC **-** USANA Health Sciences
Each tablet contains: Garlic powder (standardized to 6,000 g allicin yield) 650 mg. Inactive Ingredients: Microcrystalline Cellulose, Dibasic Calcium Phosphate, Hydroxypropyl Methylcellulose Phthalate, Colloidal Silicon Dioxide, Magnesium Silicate, Glycerol Triacetate, Croscarmellose Sodium, Vegetable-derived Stearic Acid, Vegetable-derived Magnesium Stearate.

Garlic Echinacea Goldenseal+ **-** Futurebiotics LLC
Two tablets contain: Echinacea angustifolia leaf powder extract (standardized for 4% (5 mg) echinacosides) 125 mg • Echinacea purpurea leaf powder 80 mg • Echinacea angustifolia leaf powder 20 mg • Goldenseal root powder 225 mg • Garlic bulb powder extract (odorless) 200 mg • Chinese Cinnamon root powder 30 mg • Black Pepper bud powder 20 mg • Clove flower powder 50 mg • Astragalus root powder 50 mg • Ginger root powder 50 mg • Peppermint leaf powder 10 mg • Parsley leaf powder 100 mg • Chamomile flower powder 100 mg • Bayberry bark powder 100 mg • Cayenne fruit powder 25 mg • Barberry bark powder 50 mg • Myrrh resin powder 50 mg. Other Ingredients: Dicalcium phosphate, Cellulose, Stearic acid, Magnesium stearate, Silica.

Garlic Extract 300 mg **-** Vital Nutrients
Each capsule contains: Allium Sativum (garlic extract) 300 mg: Allicin yield 12,000 mcg/g.

Garlic Ginger **-** Jarrow Formulas
Each capsule contains: Odor Modified Garlic 500 mg • Freeze-Dried Ginger 6:1 extract 200 mg. Other Ingredients: Magnesium Stearate, Gelatin.

Garlic HP **-** PhysioLogics
Each tablet contains: Garlic bulb (10000 mcg Allicin/gram) 400 mg.

Garlic HP 650 MG **-** PhysioLogics
Each tablet contains: Garlic bulb powder (allium sativum) 650 mg (standardized to contain a minimum: allicin yield 6500 mcg, total thiosulfinates yield 6500 mcg, alliin yield 14,500 mcg, gamma-glutamylcysteines 5200 mcg). Other Ingredients: Cellulose (plant origin), Calcium Carbonate, Food Glaze, Vegetable Stearic Acid, Croscarmellose, Silica, Vegetable Magnesium Stearate, Cellulose coating.

Garlic Oil **-** Nature's Own
Each tablet contains: Garlic oil (allium sativum) 1000 mcg, equivalent to fresh bulb 3000 mg.

Garlic Oil **-** Golden Glow Natural Health Products
Each capsule contains: Garlic oil 1 mg (equivalent to allium sativum bulb 3 g).

Garlic Oil **-** GNC
Each capsule contains: Garlic Oil (Allium sativa) 0.65 mg. Other Ingredients: Soybean Oil, Gelatin, Glycerin, Corn Oil, Dill Oil, Wheat Germ Oil.

Garlic with High Allicin Complex **-** Nikken Inc.
Each caplet contains: Whole Garlic powdered extract 600 mg Providing: Gamma Glutamylcysteines 12,000 mcg, Alliin 6000 mcg, Sulfur 4800 mcg, Thiosulfinates 1200 mcg, Allicin Yield 1200 mcg. Other Ingredients: Dicalcium Phosphate, Microcrystalline Cellulose, Croscarmellose Sodium, Silicon Dioxide, Stearic Acid, Magnesium Stearate, Enteric Coating (cellulose acetate phthalate, diethyl phthalate).

Garlic/Parsley Formula **-** Nature's Way
Two capsules contain: Proprietary Formula: Garlic bulb • Parsley herb. Other Ingredients: Gelatin.

Garlic-Go! **-** Wakunaga of America
Each caplet contains: Aged Garlic extract powder (bulb) 1000 mg. Other Ingredients: Cellulose, Silica, Magnesium Stearate (vegetable source).

Garlic-Gold **-** Olympian Labs
Each caplet contains: Garlic extract (alium satium) 600 mg • Allicin 7200 mcg.

Garlicin **-** Nature's Way
Each tablet contains: Garlicin alliinaise-rich garlic powder 300 mg. Other Ingredients: Aqueous Coating Solution, Cellulose, Modified Cellulose Gum, Silica, Stearic Acid, Xylitol.

Garlicin HC **-** Nature's Way
Each tablet contains: Calcium 26 mg • Cayenne pepper fruit 15 mg • Garlic bulb 259 mg • Hawthorn dried extract (19% oligomeric procyanidins) 25 mg • Rutin 12 mg • Vitamin E (d-alpha tocopheryl) 15 IU. Other Ingredients: Aqueous Coating Solution, Cellulose, Maltodextrin, Modified Cellulose Gum, Silica, Stearic Acid.

Garlife **-** Life Extension
Each tablet contains: Pure Garlic extract (odor suppressed, standardized to 10,000 ppm allicin) 900 mg.

Garlinase 4000 **-** Enzymatic Therapy
Each tablet contains: Garlic extract, equal to 4000 mg of fresh garlic, standardized to contain a minimum of 3.4% (11000 mcg) of Allicin per tablet by a unique patented process to assure maximum Allicin production in your body 320 mg.

Garliplex 2000 **-** Golden Glow Natural Health Products
Each tablet contains: Allium Sativum extract (equivalent to approx. 2 g garlic bulb) 2000 mg: Allicin 3.71 mg.

GarliPure Daily Formula **-** Natrol, Inc.
Each vegetarian capsule contains: Garlic (Allium sativum) powdered extract bulb 600 mg containing: Gamma Glutamylcysteines 12000 mcg • Allicin 6000 mcg • Sulfur 4800 mcg • Thiosulfinates 1200 mcg • Allicin Yield 1200 mcg. Other Ingredients: 100% Vegetarian capsule Shell made of Kosher Vegetable Cellulose & Water, Magnesium Stearate.

GarliPure Formula 500 **-** Natrol, Inc.
Two tablets contain: Garlic (Allium sativum) powdered extract bulb 1000 mg containing: Gamma Glutamylcysteines 20000 mcg • Allicin 10000 mcg • Sulfur 8000 mcg • Thiosulfinates 1600 mcg • Allicin Yield 1500 mcg. Other Ingredients: Dicalcium Phosphate, Microcrystalline Cellulose, Stearic Acid, Magnesium Stearate, aqueous base film coat.

Some Brand Name Natural Products - What they Contain

www.NaturalDatabase.com contains MANY more listings than appear here.
Editor's Notes are located on pages 2155-2163.

GarliPure Maximum Allicin Formula - Natrol, Inc.
Each caplet contains: Garlic (Allium sativum) powdered extract bulb 600 mg: Gamma Glutamylcysteines 12000 mcg • Allicin 4800 mcg • Sulfur 3900 mcg • Thiosulfinates 3800 mcg • Allicin Yield 3600 mcg. Other Ingredients: Microcrystalline Cellulose, Stearic Acid, Dicalcium Phosphate, Magnesium Stearate Silicon Dioxide, Aqueous base film coat.

GarliPure Once Daily Potency - Natrol, Inc.
Each tablet contains: Garlic (Allium sativum) 600 mg Powdered extract bulb containing: Allicin 13800 mcg • Thiosulfinates 6060 mcg • Allicin Yield 6000 mcg • Gamma Glutamylcysteines 4800 mcg • Sulfur 3900 mcg. Other Ingredients: Dicalcium Phosphate, Microcrystalline Cellulose, Croscarmellose Sodium, Silicon Dioxide, Stearic Acid, Magnesium Stearate.

GarliPure Organic Formula - Natrol, Inc.
Two capsules contain: Garlic (Alium sativum), organically grown powdered extract bulb 1000 mg containing: Gamma Glutamylcysteines 15000 mcg • Allicin 10000 mcg • Sulfur 7000 mcg • Thiosulfinates 1600 mcg • Allicin Yield 1500 mcg. Other Ingredients: 100% Vegetarian capsule Shell made of Kosher Vegetable Cellulose & Water, Silicon Dioxide, Magnesium Stearate.

GarliPure Selenium Plus Formula - Natrol, Inc.
Each capsule contains: Selenium 67 mcg • Garlic (Allium sativum) powdered extract bulb 400 mg: Gamma Glutamylcysteines 8000 mcg • Allicin 4400 mcg • Sulfur 3200 mcg • Thiosulfinates 2040 mcg • Allicin Yield 2000 mcg. Other Ingredients: Gelatin.
See Editor's Note No. 21.

Garlique - Chattem, Inc.
Each tablet contains: Calcium 26 mg • Iron 3 mg • Garlic bulb powder (not less than 5000 mcg of allicin yield) 400 mg. Other Ingredients: Dicalcium Phosphate, Microcrystalline Cellulose, Croscarmellose Sodium, Stearic Acid, Magnesium Stearate, Sodium Lauryl Sulfate, Colloidal Silicon Dioxide, Hydroxypropyl Methylcellulose Phthalate, Talc, Titanium Dioxide, Triacetin, Pharmaceutical glaze (214-112).

Garlite - Nature's Plus
Each capsule contains: Garlic clove (allium sativum) 500 mg. Other Ingredients: Silica, Vegetable Cellulose, Vegetable Glycerin, Purified Water.

Garlitrin 4000 - PhytoPharmica
Each tablet contains: Garlic extract (Allium sativum) bulb extract (standardized to contain a minimum of 3.4% [11,000 mcg] of alliin per tablet) 320 mg.

GarliX - Xymogen
Each capsule contains: Garlic extract: Allicin 6500 mcg, Alliin 14,300 mcg.

Gas - Hyland's
Two tablets contain: Nux Moshata 3X • Asafetida 3X • Ignatia Amara 3X • Lycopodium Clavatum 6X. Base: Lactose USP.

Gas Ease - Enzymes, Inc.
Each capsule contains: n-zimes Proprietary Enzyme Blend 239 mg: alpha-Galactosidase, Amylase, Glucoamylase, Malt Diastase, CereCalase Plus, Cellulase, Xylanase, Pectinase, Lipase, Protease (alkaline, neutral and acid proteases plus peptidase) • Proprietary Herbal Blend 260 mg: Peppermint leaf extract (4:1) plus whole leaf, Fennel seed extract (4:1) plus whole seed, Caraway seed. Other Ingredients: Plant Cellulose, Rice Bran, Water, Lecithin.

GasSTOP - Renew Life Formulas, Inc.
Two capsules contain: Amylase 20,000 DU • Alpha Galactosidase 1000 GAL • Cellulase 3000 CU • Phytase 40 U • Lipase 1200 LU • Protease 10,000 HUT • Invertase 500 SU. Other Ingredients: Vegetable Fiber, Water, Cellulose.

GastrAcid - Xymogen
Each capsule contains: Glutamic Acid 350 mg • Betaine HCl 300 mg • Pepsin (porcine) 100 mg • Gentian root (gentiana lutea) 20 mg.

Gastrex - Standard Process, Inc.
Two capsules contain: Proprietary Blend 590 mg: Okra, Bentonite (montmorillonite), Tillandsia Usenoides, Bovine Liver, Anise seed, Porcine Stomach, Choline Bitartrate, Alginic Acid, Calcium Lactate, Porcine Duodenum, Allantoin, Defatted Wheat germ, Exsiccated Disodium Phosphate, Oat straw extract, Porcine Brain • Vitamin C 3.4 mg • Niacin 6.4 mg • Vitamin B6 0.1 mg • Sodium 5 mg • Potassium 5 mg. Other Ingredients: Gelatin, Water, Calcium Stearate, Colors.
See Editor's Note No. 14.

Gastricin - Gero Vita International
Each capsule contains: Proprietary Blend 510 mg: Codonopsis Pilosula root 4:1 extract, Atractylodes Macrocephala rhizome 8:1 extract, Citrus Sacrodactylus fruit 8:1 extract, Cyperus Rotundus rhizome 8:1 extract, Pinellia Ternata tuber 8:1 extract, Amomum Villosum fruit 8:1 extract, Gardenia Jasminoides fruit 8:1 extract • PhytoSel 30 mg. Other Ingredients: Gelatin, Tricalcium Phosphate, Silicon Dioxide, Magnesium Stearate, Rice Flour, ACF 223.

Gastritix Formula - Nature's Way
Two capsules contain: Chamomile flower 62.5 mg • Fennel seed 237.5 mg • Ginger 237.5 mg • Marshmallow root 50 mg • Slippery Elm bark 125 mg • Wild Yam root 237.5 mg. Other Ingredients: Gelatin, Magnesium Stearate, Maltodextrin.

Gastro - Enzymedica
Each capsule contains: Amylase Thera-Blend 2500 DU • Lipase Thera-Blend 121 FCCFIP • Marshmallow root 95 mg • Gotu Kola 48 mg • Papaya leaf 95 mg • Prickly Ash bark 55 mg • Cellulase Thera-Blend 400 CU.

Gastro Calm - Enzymes, Inc.
Each capsule contains: Proprietary Herbal Blend 355 mg: Marshmallow root extract, Deglycyrrhizinized Licorice root extract, Ginger root extract, Quercetin • Proprietary Enzyme Blend 146 mg: Amylase, Peptidase, Lipase, CereCalase, Invertase, Cellulase, Glucoamylase, Catalase, Malt Diastase, alpha-Galactosidase, Lactase, Pectinase. Other Ingredients: Plant Cellulose, Water.

Gastro-Ad - PhysioLogics
Two tablets contain: Gastro-Ad powder (lactobacillus delbrueckii fermented soy protein) 1000 mg. Other Ingredients: Fructose, Sorbitol, Cellulose (plant origin), Natural Pineapple Flavor, Vegetable Magnesium Stearate, Vegetable Stearic Acid, Silica.

GastroCare - TriLight Herbs
Artichoke leaf extract.

Gastro-Fiber - Standard Process, Inc.
Three capsules contain: Proprietary Blend 1260 mg: Psyllium husk powder, Collinsonia root powder, Apple Pectin, Fennel seed, Fenugreek seed powder. Other Ingredients: Cellulose, Water.

Gastro-Relief - PhytoPharmica
Each chewable tablet contains: Calcium Carbonate 250 mg • Deglycyrrhizinated Licorice (DGL) root extract (Glycyrrhiza glabra) 380 mg • Glycine (Amino Acid) 50 mg.

GastroSoothe - Enzymatic Therapy
Each tablet contains: Calcium Carbonate 250 mg • Deglycyrrhizinated Licorice (DGL) root extract (Glycyrrhiza glabra) 380 mg • Glycine (Amino Acid) 50 mg.

GastroSoothe Chocolate-Mint - Enzymatic Therapy
Each tablet contains: Calcium Carbonate 250 mg • Deglycyrrhizinated Licorice (DGL) root extract (Glycyrrhiza glabra) 380 mg • Glycine (Amino Acid) 50 mg. Flavored with Dutch Cocoa powder, Creme Flavor, & Peppermint.

Some Brand Name Natural Products - What they Contain

www.NaturalDatabase.com contains MANY more listings than appear here.

Editor's Notes are located on pages 2155-2163.

GBE 24/6 brand **-** Soft Gel Technologies, Inc.
Ginkgo Biloba leaf extract.
See Editor's Note No. 44.

GBLVR - Nutri-Quest Rx
Proprietary blend 500 mg: Bayberry • Red Beet root • Yellow Dock • Dandelion root • Fennel seeds • Peppermint • Ginger root • Wild Yam • Blessed Thistle • Garlic 500 mg. In a base of 6X tissue salts: Calc Fluor.

Ge-132 (100 mg) - Jarrow Formulas
Each capsules contains: Germanium 100 mg. Other Ingredients: Cellulose, Magnesium Stearate, Gelatin.

Ge-132 (150 mg) - Jarrow Formulas
Each capsules contains: Germanium 150 mg. Other Ingredients: Cellulose, Magnesium Stearate, Gelatin.

Ge-132 (30 mg) - Jarrow Formulas
Each capsules contains: Germanium 30 mg. Other Ingredients: Cellulose, Magnesium Stearate, Gelatin.

Ge-132 powder - Jarrow Formulas
Each 1/32 tsp serving contains: Bis Beta Carboxyethyl Germanium Sesquioxide 100 mg.

Gelly-Bees Royal Jelly - Nikken Inc.
Two tablets contain: Royal Jelly powder 200 mg • Fructooligosaccharides 200 mg. Other Ingredients: Dextrin, Corn Starch, Crystalline Cellulose, Magnesium Stearate.

GelStat Migraine - GelStat Corporation
Each OraDose dispenser (2 mL) contains: Ginger 2X • Feverfew 3X. Other Ingredients: Ascorbic Acid, Glycerin, Potassium Sorbate, Purified Water, Sorbitol, Xanthan Gum.
See Editor's Note No. 1.

GEN Andro*Gen - GEN - Genetic Evolutionary Nutrition
Each capsule contains: Androstenedione 100 mg.
See Editor's Note No. 47.

GEN CM Relief - GEN - Genetic Evolutionary Nutrition
Each capsule contains: CMO (Cetyl-Myristoleate) 500 mg.

GEN Multi*GenX - GEN - Genetic Evolutionary Nutrition
Each six capsules contain: Antioxidants: Vitamin C (Ascorbic Acid) 1000 mg • Vitamin E (natural d-Alpha Tocopherol) 40 IU • Propanthocyanidins (Grape seed extract) 25 mg • Citrus bioflavonoids 100 mg • Lipoic Acid 50 mg. Vitamins: Vitamin A (Retinol Palmitate) 5000 IU • Vitamin A (Beta Carotene) 20000 IU • Vitamin D (as Vitamin D3, Cholecalciferol) 400 IU • Vitamin B1 (Thiamine HCL) 50 mg • Vitamin B2 (Riboflavin) 50 mg • Vitamin B3 (Niacinamide) 50 mg • Vitamin B5 (Calcium d-Pantothenate) 50 mg • Vitamin B6 (Pyroxine HCL) 50 mg • Vitamin B12 (Cyanocobalamin) 40 mcg • Folic Acid 400 mcg • Biotin 300 mcg. Minerals: Calcium (from Citrate) 400 mg • Magnesium (from Citrate) 200 mg • Iron (from Fe glycinate) 9 mg • Potassium (from Chloride) 150 mg • Zinc (from Monomethionate-OptiZinc) 15 mg • Manganese (from Citrate) 10 mg • Iodine (from Kelp) 100 mcg • Copper (from Co Gluconate) 270 mcg • Chromium (from Cr Nicotinate/Glycinate) 200 mcg • Molybdenum (from Sodium Molybdate) 150 mcg • Selenium (from Amino Acid Chelate) 200 mcg. Lean Muscle Enhancement: RNA (Sodium Ribonucleic Acid) 150 mg • Inositol 40 mg • L-Carnitine 35 mg • Taurine (HCL) 75 mg • L-Glutamine 25 mg • MSM (Methyl Sulfonylmethane) 100 mg • Coenzyme Q10 (Ubiquinone) 30 mg.

GEN Pyruvate Burn - GEN - Genetic Evolutionary Nutrition
Each capsule contains: MED-PRO licensed Pyruvate, from a Pyruvic Acid Complex with Dihydroxyacetone 500 mg. Pyruvic Acid is stabilized with Calcium, Sodium, Potassium or Magnesium to form Pyruvate.

GEN Thermogen - GEN - Genetic Evolutionary Nutrition
Two capsules contain: Ma Huang extract standardized at 6%: 334 (334 x .06 = 20 mg) •Caffeine 200 mg •Naringin 40 mg •White Willow bark extract 75 mg •Potassium (Phosphate) 50 mg •Cayenne 35 mg.
See Editor's Note No. 30.

General Arthritis Remedy (formerly HP 18) - Metagenics
Each drop contains: Hecla Lava 12X • Rhus Toxicodendron 6X • Stellaria Media 6X • Actaea Spicata 6X • Bryonia 12X.
See Editor's Note No. 1.

General Cough Remedy (formerly HP 11) - Metagenics
Each drop contains: Bryonia 6X • Causticum 3X • Hepar Sulphuris Calcareum 30X • Antimonium Tartaricum 12X.
See Editor's Note No. 1.

General Prostate Health Support - Weil Lifestyle, LLC
Each Saw Palmetto Complex tablet contains: Selenium 25 mcg • Saw Palmetto 160 mg • Green Tea 50 mg • Pumpkin seed oil 48 mg • Ginger 40 mg • Urtica Dioica 50 mg • Rosemary leaf supercritical extract 5 mg.

GeniKinoko - Quality of Life Labs
Six capsules contain: Proprietary Blend 2010 mg: GCP (fermented soybean isoflavone extract, polysaccharides from basidiomycetes mushrooms), Cyclodextrin • Genistein 540 mg. Other Ingredients: Gelatin.

GeniSoy Soy Protein Shake (chocolate flavor) - MLO/GeniSoy Products, Inc.
IP Isolated Soy Protein • Fructose • Dutch Processed Cocoa • Guar Gum • Natural Flavor • Canola oil • Cellulose gum • Tricalcium Phosphate • Potassium Chloride • Magnesium Oxide • Ascorbic Acid • Ferrous Fumarate • Vitamin E • Niacinamide • Zinc Oxide • Copper Gluconate • Calcium Pantothenate • Vitamin A Palmitate • Pyridoxine Hydrochloride • Riboflavin • Thiamine Hydrochloride • Folic Acid • Biotin • Selenomethionine • Potassium Iodide • Cyanocobalamin.

GeniSoy Soy Protein Shake (natural flavor) - MLO/GeniSoy Products, Inc.
IP Isolated Soy Protein • Guar gum • Rice flour • Canola oil • Cellulose Gum • Natural Flavors • Tricalcium Phosphate • Potassium Chloride • Magnesium Oxide • Ascorbic Acid • Ferrous Fumarate • Vitamin E • Niacinamide • Zinc Oxide • Copper Gluconate • Calcium Pantothenate • Vitamin A Palmitate • Pyridoxine Hydrochloride • Riboflavin • Thiamine Hydrochloride • Folic Acid • Biotin • Selenomethionine • Potassium Iodide • Cyanocobalamin.

GeniSoy Soy Protein Shake (strawberry banana flavor) - MLO/GeniSoy Products, Inc.
IP Isolated Soy Protein • Fructose • Guar Gum • Natural Flavor • Canola oil • Cellulose gum • Citric Acid • Beet powder • Tricalcium Phosphate • Potassium Chloride • Magnesium Oxide • Ascorbic Acid • Ferrous Fumarate • Vitamin E • Niacinamide • Zinc Oxide • Copper Gluconate • Calcium Pantothenate • Vitamin A Palmitate • Pyridoxine Hydrochloride • Riboflavin • Thiamine Hydrochloride • Folic Acid • Biotin • Selenomethionine • Potassium Iodide • Cyanocobalamin.

GeniSoy Soy Protein Shake (vanilla flavor) - MLO/GeniSoy Products, Inc.
IP Isolated Soy Protein • Fructose • Maltodextrin • Guar Gum • Natural Flavors • Canola oil • Cellulose gum • Tricalcium Phosphate • Potassium Chloride • Magnesium Oxide • Ascorbic Acid • Ferrous Fumarate • Vitamin E • Niacinamide • Zinc Oxide • Copper Gluconate • Calcium Pantothenate • Vitamin A Palmitate • Pyridoxine Hydrochloride • Riboflavin • Thiamine Hydrochloride • Folic Acid • Biotin • Selenomethionine • Potassium Iodide • Cyanocobalamin.

Genistein - Source Naturals
Four tablets contain: Soybean powder 4000 mg • Genistein 11.6 mg • Daidzein 42.4 mg • Glycitein 32 mg • Total Isoflavones 86 mg.

Genix **-** Gero Vita International
Each capsule contains: Zinc (zinc gluconate) 5mg • Tribulus fruit extract (45% steriod sopanins, tribulus terrestris) 400 mg • Barrenwort herb extract (epimedium grandiflorum) 100 mg • Policios Fruticosum root extract 100 mg • English Walnut semen extract (juglans regia) 67 mg • Nutmeg fruit extract (1% essential oils, myristica fragrans) 33 mg. Other Ingredients: Silica, Magnesium Stearate.

Gentle Cleansing Pads **-** FreeLife International
Water • Citrus Aurantium var. Dulcis flower waters (orange) • Epilobium Angustifolium extract (willowherb) • Cucumis Sativus fruit extract (cucumber) • Ulmus Fulva bark extract (slippery elm) • Algae extract (ahnfeltia concinna) • Decyl Glucoside • Glycerin • Hydroxyethylcellulose (plant cellulose) • Lonicera Japonica extract (Japanese honeysuckle) • Potassium Sorbate • Chlorphenesin.

Gentle Fibers **-** Jarrow Formulas
Flax seed meal 31% • Rice Bran 30% • Orange pulp and peel 30% • Grapefruit pulp and peel 6% • Lemon peel 3%.

Gentle Iron 25 mg **-** Solgar
Each capsule contains: Iron (as iron bisglycinate) 25 mg. Other Ingredients: Microcrystalline Cellulose, Vegetable Cellulose, Vegetable Magnesium Stearate, Water, Vegetable Glycerin.

Genuine Nzimes Dr. Howell's Original Formula 1 **-** Enzymes, Inc.
Two capsules contain: n-zimes Proprietary Enzyme Blend 400 mg: Protease, Amylase, Lipase, Cellulase. Other Ingredients: Plant Fiber, Gelatin, Water.

Genuine Nzimes Dr. Howell's Original Formula 10 **-** Enzymes, Inc.
Two capsules contain: n-zimes Proprietary Enzyme Blend 400 mg: Protease, Amylase, Lipase, Cellulase. Other Ingredients: Plant Fiber, Gelatin, Water.

Genuine Nzimes Dr. Howell's Original Formula 10 powder **-** Enzymes, Inc.
Each 1/4 tsp serving contains: n-zimes Proprietary Enzyme Blend 530 mg: Protease, Amylase, Lipase, Cellulase.

GeOxy-132 150 mg **-** American Biologics
Each capsule contains: Organic Germanium 150 mg. Other Ingredients: Rice Powder, Magnesium Stearate.

GeOxy-132 25 mg **-** American Biologics
Each capsule contains: Organic Germanium 25 mg. Other Ingredients: Rice Powder, Magnesium Stearate.

Geriforte Syrup **-** The Himalaya Drug Company
Each 1 tsp (5 mL) serving contains: Chyavanprash concentrate 100 mg: Aegle Marmelos, Clerodendrum Phlomidis, Oroxylum Indicum, Gmelina Arborea, Stereospermum Chelonoides, Sida Cordifolia, Desmodium Gangeticum, Uraria Picta, Phaseolus Trilobus, Teramnus Labialis, Piper Longum, Tribulus Terrestris, Solanum Indicum, Solanum Xanthocarpum, Pistacia Integerrima, Phyllanthus Amarus, Vitis Vinifera, Leptadenia Reticulata, Inula Racemosa, Aquilaria Malaccensis, Terminalia Chebula, Tinospora Cordifolia, Dioscorea Bulbifera, Microstylis Muscifera, Microstylis Wallichi, Hedychium Spicatum, Cyperus Rotundus, Boerhaavia Diffusa, Polygonatum Cirrihfolium, Elettaria Cardamomum, Santalum Album, Nymphaea Stellata, Pueraria Tuberosa, Adhatoda Vasica, Lilium Polyphyllum, Pentatropsis Capensis, Emblica Officinalis • Shilajeet (mineral pitch, purified) 20 mg • Kumkuma (crocus sativus) 5 mg • Himsra (capparis spinosa) 20 mg • Kasani (cichorium intybus) 20 mg • Daruharidara (berberis aristata) 15 mg • Vasaka (adhatoda vasica syn. a.zeylanica) 15 mg • Kakamachi (solanum nigrum) 10 mg • Arjuna (terminalia arjuna) 10 mg • Ashvagandha (withania somnifera) 10 mg • Guduchi (tinospora cordifolia) 10 mg • Draksha (vitis vinifera) 10 mg • Punarnava (boerhaavia diffusa) 10 mg • Kharjura (phoenix dactylifera) 10 mg • Birangasipha (achillea millefolium) 5 mg • Jhavuka (tamarix gallica) 5 mg • Kasamarda (cassia occidentalis) 5 mg • Shatavari (asparagus racemosus) 5 mg • Yashti-Madhu (glycyrrhiza glabra) 5 mg • Mandukaparni (centella asiatica) 5 mg • Haritaki (terminalia chebula) 5 mg • Vidana (embelia ribes) 5 mg • Mundi (sphaeranthus indicus) 5 mg • Gokshura (tribulus terrestris) 5 mg • Kapikachchhu (mucuna pruriens) 2.5 mg • Jatiphalam (myristica fragrans) 2.5 mg • Pippali (piper longum) 2.5 mg • Jaatipatree (myristica fragrans, mace) 2.5 mg • Lavanga (syzygium aromaticum) 2.5 mg • Ela (elettaria cardamomum) 2.5 mg • Yawani (carum copticum syn. trachyspermum ammi) 2.5 mg • Haridra (curcuma longa) 2.5 mg • Musali (asparagus adscendens) 2.5 mg • Udakiryaka (caesalpinia digyna) 2.5 mg • Bhringaraja (eclipta alba syn. e.prostrata) 2.5 mg • Jyothishmati (celastrus paniculatus) 2.5 mg • Vriddadaru (argyreia nervosa) 2.5 mg.
See Editor's Note No. 39.

Geriforte Tablets **-** The Himalaya Drug Company
Each tablet contains: Chyavanprash concentrate 100 mg: Aegle Marmelos, Clerodendrum Phlomidis, Oroxylum Indicum, Gmelina Arborea, Stereospermum Chelonoides, Sida Cordifolia, Desmodium Gangeticum, Uraria Picta, Phaseolus Trilobus, Teramnus Labialis, Piper Longum, Tribulus Terrestris, Solanum Indicum, Solanum Xanthocarpum, Pistacia Integerrima, Phyllanthus Amarus, Vitis Vinifera, Leptadenia Reticulata, Inula Racemosa, Aquilaria Malaccensis, Terminalia Chebula, Tinospora Cordifolia, Dioscorea Bulbifera, Microstylis Muscifera, Microstylis Wallichi, Hedychium Spicatum, Cyperus Rotundus, Boerhaavia Diffusa, Polygonatum Cirrihfolium, Elettaria Cardamomum, Santalum Album, Nymphaea Stellata, Pueraria Tuberosa, Adhatoda Vasica, Lilium Polyphyllum, Pentatropsis Capensis, Emblica Officinalis • Himsra (capparis spinosa) 13.8 mg • Kasani (cichorium intybus) 13.8 mg • Daruharidra (berberis aristata) 10 mg • Vasaka (adhatoda vasica) 10 mg • Kakamachi (solanum nigrum) 6.4 mg • Arjuna (terminalia arjuna) 6.4 mg • Biranjasipha (achillea millefolium) 3.2 mg • Kasamarda (cassia occidentalis) 3.2 mg • Jhavuka (tamarix gallica) 3.2 mg • Ashvagandha (withania somnifera) 30 mg • Shatavari (asparagus racemosus) 20 mg • Yashti-Madhu (glycyrrhiza glabra) 20 mg • Mandukaparni (centella asiatica) 20 mg • Shilajeet (mineral pitch, purified) 20 mg • Haritaki (terminalia chebula) 15 mg • Makardhwaj (sulphide of mercury) 10 mg • Musali (asparagus adscendens) 10 mg • Udakiryaka (caesalpinia digyna) 10 mg • Kapikachchhu (mucuna pruriens) 10 mg • Jatiphalam (myristica fragrans) 10 mg • Pippali (piper longum) 10 mg • Jaatipatree (myristica fragrans, mace) 10 mg • Bhringaraja (eclipta alba syn. e.prostrata) 10 mg • Vriddadaru (argyreia speciosa) 10 mg • Abhrak Bhasma (powdered talc, biotite calx) 10 mg • Jasad Bhasma (zinc calx) 10 mg • Kumkuma (crocus sativus) 7 mg • Mandur Bhasma (ferric oxide calx) 5 mg • Lavanga (sysygium aromaticum) 5 mg • Ela (elettaria cardamomum) 5 mg • Yawani (carum copticum syn. trachyspermum ammi) 5 mg • Haridra (curcuma longa) 5 mg • Jyothishmati (celastrus paniculatus) 5 mg • Loh Bhasma (iron calx) 5 mg.
See Editor's Note No. 39.

Geritol Complete **-** SmithKline Beecham
Each tablet contains: Vitamin A 6000 IU • Vitamin C 60 mg • Vitamin D 400 IU • Vitamin E 30 IU • Vitamin K 25 mcg • Thiamin (B1) 1.5 mg • Riboflavin (B2) 1.7 mg • Niacin (B3) 20 mg • Vitamin B6 2 mg • Folate, Folic Acid, Folacin 0.45 mcg • Vitamin B12 6 mcg • Biotin 0.045 mcg • Pantothenic Acid 10 mg • Calcium 162 mg • Iron 18 mg • Phosphorus 125 mg • Iodine 174 mcg • Magnesium 100 mg • Zinc 15 mg • Selenium 15 mcg • Copper 2 mg • Manganese 2.5 mg • Chromium 15 mcg • Molybdenum 15 mg • Chloride 35 mg • Potassium 40 mg • Nickel 5 mcg • Tin 10 mcg • Silicon 80 mg • Vanadium 10 mcg. Other Ingredients: Microcrystalline Cellulose, Gelatin, Hydrolyzed Protein, Beta Carotene, Stearic Acid, Crospovidone, Hydroxypopyl Methylcellulose, Hydroxypropyl Cellulose, Glycerides of Stearic and Palmitic Acid, Polyethylene Glycol, Magnesium Stearate, Silica, Titanium Dioxide, FD&C Blue #2, FD&C Red #40, FD&C Yellow #6.

Geritol Extend - SmithKline Beecham
Each tablet contains: Vitamin A (40% beta carotene) 3333 IU • Vitamin D 200 IU • Vitamin E 13 IU • Vitamin C 55 mg • Folic Acid 0.2 mg • Thiamin (B1) 1.2 mg • Riboflavin (B2) 1.3 mg • Niacin 15 mg • Vitamin B6 2 mg • Vitamin B12 2.5 mcg • Vitamin K 80 mcg • Iron 9.5 mg • Zinc 14 mg • Iodine 130 mg • Magnesium 32 mg • Calcium 126 mg • Phosphorus 98 mg • Potassium 0.054 mg • Selenium 35 mcg.

Geritol Tonic - SmithKline Beecham
Thiamin (B1) 2.5 mg • Riboflavin (B2) 2.5 mg • Niacin 50 mg • Pantothenic Acid 2 mg • Vitamin B6 0.5 mg • Methionine 25 mg • Choline Bitartrate 50 mg • Sugars 7 g • Iron 18 mg.

Gero-Vita G.H.3. - Gero Vita International
Two tablets contain: Vitamin A (as beta-carotene) 4000 IU • Vitamin C (as ascorbyl palmitate) 42 mg • Vitamin E (as dl-alpha-tocopheryl acetate) 200 IU • Thiamin (as thiamin mononitrate) 100 mg • Riboflavin 100 mg • Vitamin B3 (as niacin) 20 mg • Vitamin B6 (as pyridoxine hydrochloride) 50 mg • Folic Acid 800 mcg • Vitamin B12 (as cyanocobalamin) 20 mcg • Calcium (as calcium carbonate) 76 mg • Magnesium (as magnesium oxide) 100 mg • Zinc (as zinc picolinate) 1.2 mg • Selenium (as selenium amino acid chelate) 100 mcg • Chromium (as chromium polynicotinate) 20 mcg • St. John's Wort extract (entire plant, 0.3% hypericin) 400 mg • Procaine (dimethylaminoethanol bitartrate 200 mg, para-aminobenzoic acid 100 mg) • Ginkgo Biloba leaf powder 50 mg • L-Glutathione 4 mg. Other Ingredients: Microcrystalline Cellulose, Vegetable Stearic Acid, Croscarmellose Sodium, Silicon Dioxide, Gum Acacia, Vegetable Magnesium Stearate.
See Editor's Note No. 20.

Gerovital (GH3) - Nutraceutics Corp.
Two caplets contain: Vitamin B6 5 mg • Folic Acid 400 mcg • Vitamin B12 20 mcg • Pantothenic Acid 50 mg • Procaine (p-aminobenzoic acid 400 mg, 2-dimethylaminoethanol bitartrate 200 mg) • Gingko Biloba extract 500 mg • Proprietary Blend 300 mg: Proteusterone, Schizandra berry, Panax Ginseng root, Gotu Kola leaves.

Gest-Tonic - The Herbalist
Angelica root • Gentian root • Oregon Grape root • Bayberry root bark • Fennel seed • Prickly Ash bark • Ginger root.

GH Fuel - TwinLab
Six capsules contain: L-Ornithine Alpha-Ketoglutarate 3000 mg • Ma Huang extract (standardized for 6% Ephedrine) 334 mg •Kola extract (standardized for 12% Caffeine) 1000 mg • L-Carnitine 100 mg • Chromium (from Chromic Fuel patented Chromium Picolinate) 400 mcg.
See Editor's Note No. 30.

GH Fuel Cocktail - TwinLab
Two tablespoonfuls contain: L-Arginine 6 g • L-Ornithine 1 g • Taurine 250 mg • L-Carnitine 200 mg • Beta-Carotene 10000 IU • Vitamin D 100 IU • Vitamin C 1000 mg • Natural Vitamin E 400 IU • Vitamin B1 1.5 mg • Vitamin B2 1.9 mg • Vitamin B6 2 mg • Niacinamide 20 mg • Vitamin B12 12 mcg • Pantothenic Acid 500 mg • Folic Acid 400 mcg • Biotin 300 mcg • Choline 700 mg • Inositol 250 mg • Calcium (from KrebMins Calcium) 250 mg • Magnesium (from KrebMins Magnesium) 100 mg • Potassium (from KrebMins Potassium) 325 mg • Zinc (from Zinc Picolinate & KrebMins Zinc) 15 mg • Manganese (from KrebMins Manganese) 2 mg • Copper (from KrebMins Copper) 1 mg • Iodine (from Kelp) 10 mcg • Molybdenum (from KrebMins Molybdenum) 50 mcg • Chromium (from Chromium Picolinate) 100 mcg • Selenium (from KrebMins Selenium) 50 mcg • Boron (from Tri-Boron citrate, Aspartate & Glycinate) 1.5 mg. Natural orange flavor 100%.

GH Release - Nature's Plus
Two capsules contain: L-Ornithine free form amino acid 500 mg • L-Arginine free form amino acid 150 mg • Raw Pituitary concentrate 100 mg • Vitamin B6 (pyridoxine HCl) 50 mg.
See Editor's Note No. 31.

GH3 (GH-3, GH 3) - Gero Vita International
Each tablet contains: Hypericum Perforatum extract (0.3% hypericin) 400 mg • Procaine (2-dimethyl aminoethanol bitartrate (DMAE) 100 mg, Para-aminobenzoic acid (PABA) 50 mg) • Calcium Carbonate 100 mg • Thiamine Mononitrate 50 mg • Riboflavin 50 mg • Ascorbyl Palmitate 50 mg • Ginkgo Biloba 50 mg • Pyridoxine HCl 25 mg • Niacin 10 mg • Zinc Picolinate 3 mg • L-Glutathione 2 mg • Chromium Polynicotinate 0.1 mg • Folic Acid 400 mcg • Selenium (amino acid chelated) 50 mcg • Cobalamin 10 mcg • Beta-Carotene 2000 IU • Vitamin E 100 IU.

GH3 Natural Enhancer - Vitamin & Mineral Therapies International (VMTI)
Two tablets contain: Vitamin A (as beta carotene) 5000 IU • Vitamin E (as d-alpha tocopheryl) 200 IU • Thiamin (vitamin B1, as thiamin mononitrate) 50 mg • Riboflavin (as vitamin B2) 50 mg • Folic Acid 800 mcg • Calcium (as carbonate) 200 mg • Zinc (as amino acid chelate) 10 mg • Selenium (as amino acid chelate) 10 mg • Chromium (as polynicotinate) 60 mcg • St. John's Wort leaf 4:1 extract (hypercium perforatum) 400 mg • Glutathione 6 mg. Other Ingredients: Cellulose, Magnesium Stearate, Vegetable Stearins.

GH3 Natural Formula - Vitamin & Mineral Therapies International (VMTI)
Two tablets contain: Vitamin A 5000 IU • Ester C Calcium Ascorbate (vitamin C) 100 mg • Magnesium 100 mg • Folic Acid 800 mcg • Vitamin B12 (cyanocobalamin) 200 mcg • Vitamin B6 (pyridoxine) 30 mg • Vitamin E 90 IU • Glutamic Acid Base 200 mg • L-Tyrosine 200 mg • Procaine (DMAE (dimethylaminoethanol bitartrate) 200 mg, PABA (para amino benzoic acid) 100 mg) • Glucosamine HCl 130 mg • Choline Bitartrate 100 mg • L-Taurine 100 mg • Ginkgo Biloba powder 50 mg. Other Ingredients: Cellulose, Vegetable Stearins, Magnesium Stearate.

GH3 Original Formula - Millenium Health
Each tablet contains: Procaine Hydrochloride 100 mg • Benzoic Acid 6 mg • Potassium Metabisulphite 5 mg • Di-Sodium Phosphate 0.5 mg. Other Ingredients: Natural Orange Coloring.

GH3XL - HealthWatchers System
L-Glutamic Acid • L-Tyrosine • L-Taurine • Glucosamine HCL • Choline Bitartrate • Magnesium • Vitamin B6 • Vitamin Bee pollen • Kelp • Dulse • Irish Moss • Ginseng • Nettles • Alfalfa • Fo-Ti • Pau d'Arco • Fennel Seed • Schizandra • Barley Grass • Acacia Gum • Saussurea • Cat's Claw • Ginger • Licorice.

GHR (HGHR) Gold - Linda Wade Herbal Products
Four capsules contain: Anterior Pituitary (bovine source) 80 mg • Hypothalamus 20 mg • Amino Acids blend (essential amino acids) 1200 mg • Phytosterol Complex 40 mg: Beta Sitosterol, Campesterol, Stigmasterol • Soy Phospholipid Complex 80 mg: Phosphatidyl Serine 40%, Phosphatidyl Choline, Phosphatidyl Ethanolamine, Phosphatidylinositol • Panax Ginseng 80 mg • Vitamin B1 (thiamin) 20 mg • Vitamin B2 (riboflavin) 12 mg • Vitamin B6 (pyridoxine) 40 mg • Vitamin B12 (cobalamin) 100 mg.
See Editor's Note No. 31.

GHR-15 - BIE Health
Two scoops contain: Anterior Pituitary (bovine source) 56 mg • Hypothalamus 8 mg • Saccharides (mono, poly, & oligo) 2500 mg • L-Glutamine 100 mg • L-Arginine 100 mg • L-Pyroglutamate 100 mg • L-Glycine 300 mg • L-Lysine 200 mg • L-Tyrosine 200 mg • GABA 100 mg.
See Editor's Note No. 31 and No. 63.

GI Repair Nutrients - Vital Nutrients
Two capsules contain: L-Glutamine 600 mg • N-Acetyl Glucosamine 400 mg • Larch Arabinogalactan 150 mg • Quercetin 100 mg • Gamma Oryzanol 80 mg • Deglycyrrhized Licorice (DGL) 80 mg • Lactobacillus Sporogenes 50 mg • Ginkgo Biloba 50:1 extract 40 mg.

Ginger - Nature's Way
Two capsules contain: Ginger 1.1 g. Other Ingredients: Gelatin.

Some Brand Name Natural Products - What they Contain

www.NaturalDatabase.com contains MANY more listings than appear here.

Editor's Notes are located on pages 2155-2163.

Ginger - Leiner Health Products
Each softgel contains: Ginger extract (Zingiber officinale) root 125 mg. Other Ingredients: Canola Oil, Gelatin, Glycerin, Yellow Beeswax, Lecithin, Caramel, Turmeric, Titanium Dioxide, Red 40, Annatto, Blue 1.

Ginger - Pharmanex
Each capsule contains: Ginger (Zingiber officinalis, root extract, 20:1) 125 mg. Other Ingredients: Soybean Oil, Gelatin, Purified Water, Glycerin, Beeswax, Carob.

Ginger & Curcumin Joint-Ease - Nature's Life
Four capsules contain: Ginger root (Zingiber officinale) 1300 mg • Curcumin [from Turmeric root (Curcuma longa) providing 90-95% Curcuminoids] 1300 mg.

Ginger Aid - Traditional Medicinals
Ginger rhizome • Blackberry leaf • Stevia leaf • natural Lemon flavor.

Ginger extract - Pure Encapsulations
Each vegetable capsule contains: Ginger extract (zingiber officinale, standardized to contain 5% gingerols) 500 mg.

Ginger Root - Aboca USA, Inc
Each capsule contains: Ginger root WPC (whole phytocomplex concentrate, zingiber officinale, standardized to 0.8% total gingerols, yielding 2.4 mg per capsule) 300 mg. Other Ingredients: Gelatin.

Ginger Root (Zingiber officinale) - Solgar
Each capsule contains: Ginger root 4:1 extract 5 mg • Raw Ginger root powder 500 mg. Other Ingredients: Vegetable Cellulose, Vegetable Magnesium Stearate, Water, Vegetable Glycerin.

Ginger Root Extract - NOW Foods
Each Vcap contains: Ginger root extract (zingiber officinale, standardized to min. 5% gingerols) 250 mg • Ginger root powder (zingiber officinale) 225 mg. Other Ingredients: Cellulose (capsule), Starch, Magnesium Oxide, Magnesium Carbonate, Stearic Acid (vegetable source), Silica, Magnesium Stearate (vegetable source).

Gingerall - Enzymatic Therapy
Each capsule contains: Ginger root extract (Zingiber officinale) standardized to contain 20% pungent compounds calculated as 6-Gingerol & 6-Shogaol 100 mg.

GingerMax - PhytoPharmica
Each capsule contains: Ginger (Zingiber officinale) root extract (standardized to contain 20% pungent compounds calculated as 6-Gingerol and 6-Shogaol) 100 mg.

Gingko Plus - MK Supplements
Each capsule contains: Ginkgo Biloba extract 60 mg • Vinpocetine 5 mg • MSM (methyl sulfonyl methane) 60 mg.

Ginkai - Lichtwer Pharma
Each tablet contains: LI 1370 Ginkgo Biloba leaf extract, standardized to 25% ginkgo flavonoids & 6% terpenoids 50 mg.

Ginkgo + III - Matol Botanical International Ltd
Two tablets contain: Bilberry standardized extract 100 mg • Garlic standardized extract 60 mg • Ginseng standardized extract 50 mg • Ginkgo Biloba standardized extract 40 mg.

Ginkgo 120 - Ortho Molecular Products
Each capsule contains: Ginkgo Biloba leaf extract (standardized to contain 24% ginkgo flavonglycosides and 6% triterpene lactones) 120 mg. Other Ingredients: Natural Vegetable Capsules, Ascorbyl Palmitate, Magnesium Stearate, Microcrystalline Cellulose, Silicon Dioxide.

Ginkgo 250 - Pure Encapsulations
Each vegetable capsule contains: Ginkgo Biloba 8:1 extract (unstandardized 8:1 extract) 250 mg.

Ginkgo 32/9 160 mg - Pure Encapsulations
Each vegetable capsule contains: Ginkgo Biloba 67:1 extract (standardized to contain 32% ginkgoheterosides and 9% terpene lactones, typically providing ginkgolida A 2.5%, ginkgolide B 0.8%, ginkgolide C 1.5%, bilobalides 4.2%) 160 mg.

Ginkgo 32/9 80 mg - Pure Encapsulations
Each vegetable capsule contains: Ginkgo Biloba 67:1 extract (standardized to contain 32% ginkgoheterosides and 9% terpene lactones, typically providing ginkgolida A 2.5%, ginkgolide B 0.8%, ginkgolide C 1.5%, bilobalides 4.2%) 80 mg.

Ginkgo 5 - Pharmline
Active Ingredients: Ginkgo Biloba extract 24/6, standardized to not less than 24% total Ginkgo flavone glycosides & not less than 6% total terpene lactones.

Ginkgo 50 160 mg - Pure Encapsulations
Each vegetable capsule contains: Ginkgo Biloba 50:1 extract (standardized to contain 24% ginkgoheterosides and 6% terpene lactones, typically providing ginkgolida A 1.2%, ginkgolide B 0.8%, ginkgolide C 1.0%, bilobalides 2.5%) 160 mg.

Ginkgo 50 80 mg - Pure Encapsulations
Each vegetable capsule contains: Ginkgo Biloba 50:1 extract (standardized to contain 24% ginkgoheterosides and 6% terpene lactones, typically providing ginkgolida A 1.2%, ginkgolide B 0.8%, ginkgolide C 1.0%, bilobalides 2.5%) 80 mg.

Ginkgo 50:1 & Grape Seed OPC Extract - Jarrow Formulas
Each capsule contains: Ginkgo Biloba leaf 50:1 standardized extract 60 mg • Ginkgoflavonglycosides 24% min • Terpene Lactones 6% min: Ginkgolide A 1.2%, Ginkgolide B 0.8% • Grape seed 100:1 (95% polyphenols) 50 mg. Other Ingredients: Cellulose, Magnesium Stearate, Gelatin.

Ginkgo 50:1 Extract - Vital Nutrients
Each capsule contains: Ginkgo Biloba 50:1 extract (standardized to 24% ginkgo heterosides and 6% terpene lactones) 80 mg.

Ginkgo 7500 - Golden Glow Natural Health Products
Each capsule contains: Ginkgo Biloba leaf 7500 mg • Panax Ginseng root 150 mg • Crataegus Laevigata flowering herb top 150 mg • Centella Asiatica herb 100 mg • Lecithin 100 mg • Glutamine 25 mg • Tyrosine 25 mg.

Ginkgo Alert Formula - PhysioLogics
Each capsule contains: Niacin 5 mg • Vitamin B6 (as pyridoxine hydrochloride) 5 mg • Vitamin B12 (as cyanocobalamin) 250 mcg • Calcium (as dicalcium phosphate) 7 mg • L-Tyrosine 100 mg • DMAE (dimethylaminoethanol) 56 mg • L-Glutamine 150 mg • L-Pyroglutamic Acid 100 mg • Choline (as choline bitartrate) 50 mg • Ginkgo Biloba leaf extract (standardized to contain 24% alkaloids, 9.6 mg) 40 mg • Korean Ginseng root extract (panax ginseng, standardized to contain 14% ginsenosides, 3.5 mg). Other Ingredients: Gelatin, Silica, Vegetable Magnesium Stearate.

Ginkgo B - Metabolic Response Modifiers
Each capsule contains: Ginkgo biloba extract (100:1) 60 mg.

Ginkgo Biloba - CVS Pharmacy
Each softgel contains: Ginkgo Biloba extract (standardized to 24% lavone glyosides; 6% terpene lactones) 60 mg. Other Ingredients: Soybean Oil, Gelatin, Purified Water, Glycerin, Yellow Beeswax, Lecithin, Annatto, Titanium Dioxide, FD&C Yellow #5, FD&C Blue #1, FD&C Red #40.

Ginkgo Biloba - Olympian Labs
Each capsule contains: Ginkgo Biloba extract 120 mg.

Ginkgo Biloba - Rexall - Sundown
Two capsules contain: Ginkgo Biloba leaf extract 40 mg • Ginkgo Biloba leaf 400 mg.

Ginkgo Biloba - Life Extension
Each capsule contains: Ginkgo Biloba extract 120 mg.

Ginkgo Biloba - Puritan's Pride
Each tablet contains: Ginkgo Biloba Extract (standardized for a minumum of 24% Ginkgo Flavone Glycosides and 6% terpenes) 60 mg. Other Ingredients: Dicalcium Phosphate, Cellulose (Plant Origin), Vegetable Stearic Acid, Cellulose Coating, Croscarmellose, Silica, Vegetable Magnesium Stearate.

Ginkgo Biloba - Natrol, Inc.
Each capsule contains: Ginkgo Biloba leaf 50:1 extract (24% ginkgo flavonglycosides) (6% terpene lactone) 120 mg.

Ginkgo Biloba - Celestial Seasonings
Two capsules contain: Proprietary Blend 1700 mg: Ginkgo Biloba (leaves), Ginkgo Biloba (standardized extract, standardized to 24% ginkgoflanonone glycosides, 6% ginkgolides). Other Ingredients: Dicalcium Phosphate, Gelatin, Rice Flour, Stearic Acid, Magnesium Stearate, Silicon Dioxide.

Ginkgo Biloba - Jamieson
Each tablet contains: Ginkgo extract (50:1) Ginkgo biloba leaf (24% flavoglycosides) 40 mg.

Ginkgo Biloba - Nature's Bounty
Each tablet contains: Ginkgo Biloba extract (Standardized for a minimum of 24% Ginkgo Flavone Glycosides and 6% terpenes) 30 mg.

Ginkgo Biloba - NOW Foods
Each Vcaps contains: Ginkgo Biloba extract (50:1 standardized extract containing 24% ginkgoflavonglycosides) 120 mg • Gotu Kola (Centella asiatica) (leaf) 200 mg • Siberian Ginseng (Eleutherococcus senticosus) (root) 150 mg.

Ginkgo Biloba - Benepure, Inc
Each capsule contains: Ginkgo Biloba leaf extract (yielding gingko flavone glycosides 14.4 mg) 60 mg. Other Ingredients: Gelatin, Vegetable Stearate, Rice Flour.

Ginkgo Biloba - DreamPharm
Each capsule contains: Ginkgo Biloba leaf 300 mg • Sclerotium Poriae Cocos 100 mg • Dioscorea Oppositae rhizoma 100 mg.

Ginkgo Biloba - Nature's Bounty
Each tablet contains: Ginkgo Biloba extract 30 mg. Other Ingredients: Dicalcium Phosphate, Cellulose, Vegetable Stearic Acid, Cellulose Coating, Silica, Vegetable Magnesium Stearate.

Ginkgo Biloba (50:1 extract) - Atrium Biotechnologies
Each capsule contains: Ginkgo Biloba, 50:1 extract (24% Ginkgocides) 60 mg.

Ginkgo Biloba 100 mg - Nature's Plus
Each capsule contains: Ginkgo Biloba leaf (standardized 24% ginkgo flavone-glycosides, 6% terpene lactones) 100 mg. Other Ingredients: Microcrystalline Cellulose, Silica, Gelatin, Purified Water.

Ginkgo Biloba 120 mg - Pro Health
Each capsule contains: Ginkgo Biloba leaf 50:1 Concentrate 120 mg. Other Ingredients: Cellulose, Magnesium Stearate, Silicon Dioxide.

Ginkgo Biloba 2000 - Golden Glow Natural Health Products
Each tablet contains: Ginkgo Biloba leaf 2000 mg: Ginkgo Flavonglycosides 10.68 mg, Ginkgolides and Bilobalide 2.68 mg.

Ginkgo Biloba 24% - Enzymatic Therapy
Each capsule contains: Ginkgo Biloba leaf extract (ginkgo biloba folia, standardized to contain 24% ginkgoflavonglycosides, 6% terpene lactones, and 2% bilobalide) 40 mg.

Ginkgo Biloba 24% - Swanson Health Products
Each capsule contains: Ginkgo Biloba leaf extract (24% flavone glycosides, 6% terpene lactones) 60 mg.

Ginkgo Biloba 24% Standardized Extract - NOW Foods
Each capsule contains: Ginkgo Biloba leaf powder 300 mg • Ginkgo Biloba extract (50:1 standardized extract containing 24% ginkgoflavonglycosides) 60 mg. Other Ingredients: Stearic Acid.

Ginkgo Biloba 250 - Enzymatic Therapy
Each capsule contains: Ginkgo (ginkgo biloba, leaf powder and extract standardized to contain 6 mg ginkgoflavonglycosides) 250 mg.

Ginkgo Biloba 40 mg - Leiner Health Products
Each tablet contains: Ginkgo Biloba extract (Ginkgo biloba) leaf 40 mg. Other Ingredients: Calcium Carbonate, Maltodextrin, Cellulose, Hydroxypropyl Methylcellulose, Polyethylene Glycol 3350, Crospovidone, Silicon Dioxide, Hydroxypropyl Cellulose, Titanium Dioxide, Magnesium Stearate, Yellow 5 Lake, Polysorbate 80, Yellow 6 Lake, Blue 2 Lake, Sodium Citrate.

Ginkgo Biloba 40 mg 50:1 - Jarrow Formulas
Three tablets contain: Ginkgo Biloba 50:1 standardized extract 120 mg • Ginkgoflavonglycosides 24% min • Terpene Lactones 6% min: Ginkgolide A 1.3%, Ginkgolide B 1%, Ginkgolide C 1.2%, Bilobalide 2.7%. Other Ingredients: Calcium Phosphate, Cellulose, Modified Cellulose Gum, Stearic Acid, Magnesium Stearate (vegetable source).

Ginkgo Biloba 50:1 (120 mg) - Jarrow Formulas
Each capsule contains: Ginkgo Biloba 50:1 standardized extract 120 mg • Ginkgoflavonglycosides 24% min • Terpene Lactones 6% min: Ginkgolide A 1.3%, Ginkgolide B 1%, Ginkgolide C 1.2%, Bilobalide 2.7%. Other Ingredients: Rice Powder, Magnesium Stearate, Silicon Dioxide, Gelatin.

Ginkgo Biloba 50:1 (60 mg) - Jarrow Formulas
Two capsules contain: Ginkgo Biloba 50:1 standardized extract 60 mg • Ginkgoflavonglycosides 24% min • Terpene Lactones 6% min: Ginkgolide A 1.3%, Ginkgolide B 1%, Ginkgolide C 1.2%, Bilobalide 2.7%. Other Ingredients: Rice Powder, Magnesium Stearate, Silicon Dioxide, Gelatin.

Ginkgo Biloba 50:1 liquid - Jarrow Formulas
Each 1 mL serving contains: Ginkgo Biloba standardized liquid extract 60 mg: Ginkgoflavonglycosides 24.0% min, Terpene Lactones 6.0% min: Ginkgolide A 1.3%, Ginkgolide B 1.0%, Ginkgolide C 1.2%, Bilobalide 2.7%. Other Ingredients: Water, Alcohol (32% by volume).

Ginkgo Biloba 60 mg - Pro Health
Each capsule contains: Ginkgo Biloba leaf extract (standardized for 24% ginkgoflavonglycosides and 6% total terpene lactones) 60 mg. Other Ingredients: Rice Flour, Gelatin, Water.

Ginkgo Biloba 60 mg - Leiner Health Products
Each caplet contains: Ginkgo Biloba leaf extract (ginkgo biloba) 60 mg. Other Ingredients: Calcium Carbonate, Cellulose, Maltodextrin, Hydroxypropyl Methylcellulose, Silicon Dioxide, Polyethylene Glycol 3350, Croscarmellose Sodium, Hydroxypropyl Cellulose, Yellow 5 Lake, Blue 1 Lake, Pharmaceutical Glaze, Crospovidone, Magnesium Stearate, Polysorbate 80, Titanium Dioxide.

Ginkgo Biloba 60 mg - Puritan's Pride
Each tablet contains: Ginkgo Biloba extract (standardized for a minimum of 24% ginkgo flavone glycosides and 6% terpenes) 60 mg. Other Ingredients: Dicalcium Phosphate, Cellulose (plant origin), Vegetable Stearic Acid, Cellulose Coating, Croscarmellose, Silica, Vegetable Magnesium Stearate.

Ginkgo Biloba Complex - Vitamin World
Each capsules contains: Ginkgo Biloba leaf extract (standardized to contain 24% flavone glycosides, 9.6 mg) 40 mg • Ginkgo Biloba leaf 400 mg • Herbal Complex 320 mg: Eleuthero root (eleutherococcus senticosus), Citrus Bioflavonoids, Bilberry fruit 4:1 extract (vaccinium myrtillus). Other Ingredients: Gelatin, Rice Powder, Silica, Vegetable Magnesium Stearate.

BRAND NAMES

Ginkgo Biloba Double Strength **- NOW Foods**
Each Vcap contain: Ginkgo Biloba extract leaf (50:1 standardized extract containing 24% ginkgoflaconglycosides) 120 mg • Gotu Kola (Centella Asiatica) leaf 200 mg • Siberian Ginseng (Eleutherococcus Senticoscus) root 150 mg. Other Ingredients: Stearic Acid.

Ginkgo Biloba Extended Release 120 mg **- Nature's Plus**
Each extended-release tablet contains: Ginkgo Biloba leaf (standardized 24% ginkgo flavone-glycosides, 6% terpene lactones) 120 mg. Other Ingredients: Di-calcium Phosphate, Stearic Acid, Microcrystalline Cellulose, Hydroxypropyl Methylcellulose, Magnesium Stearate, Silica, Pharmaceutical Glaze.

Ginkgo Biloba Extra Strength, 60mg **- Nature Made**
Each capsule contains: Ginkgo Biloba leaf extract 60 mg: Flavone Glycosides 14.4 mg, Terpene Lactones 3.6 mg.

Ginkgo Biloba Extract **- Nature's Bounty**
Each tablet contains: Ginkgo Biloba extract (standardized for a minimum of 24% ginkgoflavoneglycosides, 6% terpenes) 30 mg. Other Ingredients: Dicalcium Phosphate, Cellulose (plant origin), Vegetable Stearic Acid, Cellulose Coating, Silica, Vegetable Magnesium Stearate.

Ginkgo Biloba Extract **- NSI - Nutraceutical Sciences Institute**
Each capsule contains: Ginkgo Biloba extract (standardized to 24% ginkgoflavoneglycosides and 6% terpene lactones) 120 mg.

Ginkgo Biloba Extract **- Quest**
Each caplet contains: Ginkgo Biloba leaf extract (Ginkgo biloba) (provided by 60 mg P.E. 1:50 standardized to contain 24% Ginkgosides) 3000 mg • Citrus Bioflavonoids 200 mg providing Hesperidin 50 mg. Other Ingredients: Calcium Phosphate, Microcrystalline Cellulose, Croscarmellose Sodium, Vegetable Stearin, Magnesium Stearate (vegetable source).

Ginkgo Biloba Extract **- NOW Foods**
Each dropperful (0.8 ml) contains: Ginkgo Biloba extract 0.8 ml. Other Ingredients: Gotu Kola (centella asiatica), Siberian Ginseng (eleutherococcus senticosus), in a base of Distilled Water, Vegetable Glycerine, and Grain Alcohol.

Ginkgo Biloba Extract 60 mg **- The Vitamin Shoppe**
Each capsule contains: Ginkgo Biloba leaf extract (ginkgoselect, standardized to 24% ginkgoflavoglycosides 14 mg, 6% terpene lactones 3.5 mg.) 60 mg.

Ginkgo Biloba Leaf Extract 50:1 **- GNC**
Each tablet contains: Ginkgo Biloba leaf extract 50:1 50 mg. Other Ingredients: Dicalcium Phosphate, Cellulose, Stearic Acid, Magnesium Stearate, Food Glaze.

Ginkgo Biloba Plus **- J. R. Carlson Laboratories, Inc.**
Each softgel contains: Ginkgo Biloba leaves (24% ginkgoflavone glycosides) 40 mg • L-Glutamine 200 mg.

Ginkgo Biloba Plus **- Wakunaga of America**
Each capsule contains: Aged Garlic bulb extract powder 200 mg • Siberian Ginseng root extract 5:1 80 mg • Ginkgo Biloba leaf 50:1 extract (standardized to 24% ginkgoflavonglycosides & 6% terpene lactones) 40 mg. Other Ingredients: Cellulose, Magnesium Stearate (vegetable source).

Ginkgo Biloba Time-Release **- Nature's Sunshine**
Each time-release tablet contains: Ginkgo leaf, dried extract (24% ginkgo flavone glycosides 29 mg, 6% terpene lactones 7 mg) 120 mg. Other Ingredients: Maltodextrin, Cellulose, Stearic Acid, Magnesium Stearate, Silicon Dioxide.

Ginkgo Biloba Tincture **- Jamieson**
Each 1 ml (15 drops) contains: Ginkgo Biloba Leaf 500 mg.

Ginkgo Biloba Xtra **- Sundown**
Each tablet contains: Ginkgo Biloba leaf extract (standardized to 24% flavonol glycosides, 14.4 mg, standardized to 6% terpene lacones, 3.6 mg) 60 mg • Xtra Premium Blend 90 mg: Ashwagandha root, Gotu Kola (aerial parts), Siberian Ginseng root (eleuthero). Other Ingredients: Maltodextrin, Cellulose, Croscarmellose Sodium, Silica, Magnesium Stearate, Dextrin, Titanium Dioxide, Hydroxypropyl Methylcellulose, PEG, Acacia Gum, Guar Gum, Hydroxypropyl Cellulose, Dextrose Monohydrate, Soya Lecithin, Riboflavin (colorant), Yellow 6 Lake, Blue 2 Lake.

Ginkgo Biloba/Gotu Kola **- Futurebiotics LLC**
Each capsule contains: Ginkgo Biloba leaf powder extract (standardized for 24% (29 mg) ginkgo heterosides) 120 mg • Gotu Kola leaf powder extract (standardized for 16% (32 mg) triterpenes) 200 mg. Other Ingredients: Gelatin, Water.

Ginkgo Booster **- Puritan's Pride**
Two tablets contain: Ginkgo Biloba extract (24%) 60 mg • L-Glutamine 100 mg • Lecithin 100 mg • L-Tyrosine 50 mg • Choline (Bitartrate) 100 mg • DMAE (2-Di Methylaminothanol) 40 mg • Vitamin B1 (Thiamine HCl) 20 mg • Vitamin B2 (Riboflavin) 20 mg • Vitamin B12 (Sobalamin/Dibencozide) 50 mcg • Niacin 10 mg • Niacinamide 40 mg • Pantothenic Acid (Calcium d-Pantothenate) 50 mg • Folic Acid 200 mcg • Biotin 50 mcg • Inositol 20 mg • Vitamin C (Ascorbic Acid) 50 mg • Iodine 50 mcg • Betaine HCl 20 mg. In a base of Fo-Ti and Siberian Ginseng.

Ginkgo Concentrate (120 mg) **- Life Enhancement Products, Inc.**
Each capsule contains: Ginkgo Biloba leaf extract 120 mg: Ginkgo Flavone Glycosides 28,800 mcg, Terpene Lactones 7200 mcg, Ginkgolide A 1440 mcg, Ginkgolide B 960 mcg, Ginkgolide C 1200 mcg, Bilobalide 3000 mcg.

Ginkgo Concentrate (60 mg) **- Life Enhancement Products, Inc.**
Each capsule contains: Ginkgo Biloba leaf extract 60 mg: Ginkgo Flavone Glycosides 14,400 mcg, Terpene Lactones 3600 mcg, Ginkgolide A 720 mcg, Ginkgolide B 480 mcg, Ginkgolide C 600 mcg, Bilobalide 1500 mcg.

Ginkgo DHA Mind **- The Vitamin Shoppe**
Each capsule contains: Ginkgo Biloba leaf 24% ginkgoflavoglycosides 6% terpene 60 mg • DHA 50 mg.

Ginkgo Energizer **- The Vitamin Shoppe**
Each capsule contains: Ginkgo Biloba leaf standardized to 24% ginkgoflavoglycosides 6% ginkgolides-bilobalides 60 mg • CoQ10 30 mg.

Ginkgo Gotu Kola Supreme **- Gaia Herbs**
Thirty drops contain: Proprietary Blend 130 mg: Gotu Kola leaf and root (centella asiatica), Eleuthero root (eleutherococcus senticosus), Ginkgo leaf (ginkgo biloba), Fresh Wild Oats milky seed (avena sativa), Chinese Fo-Ti root (he shou wu, polygonum multiflorum), Peppermint leaf (mentha piperita), Rosemary leaf (rosmarinus officinalis), 30-40% Pure Grain Alcohol USP, Spring Water.

Ginkgo Leaf **- Aboca USA, Inc**
Two capsules contain: Ginkgo leaf WPC (whole phytocomplex concentrate, ginkgo biloba, standardized to 0.72% terpene lactones, yielding 2 mg per capsule and to 2.16% ginkgo flavone glycosides, yielding 6 mg per capsule) 554 mg. Other Ingredients: Gelatin.

Ginkgo Leaf **- Gaia Herbs**
Two capsules contain: Ginkgo leaf (ginkgo biloba) 128 mg. Other Ingredients: Vegetable Glycerin, Vegetable Cellulose (capsule).

Ginkgo Leaf (Ginkgo biloba) **- Solgar**
Two capsules contain: Iron 2 mg • Ginkgo Biloba leaf 50:1 extract (standardized to minimum 24% ginkgoflavoglycosides) 20 mg • Raw Ginkgo Biloba leaf powder 600 mg. Other Ingredients: Vegetable Cellulose, Vegetable Magnesium Stearate, Water, Vegetable Glycerin.

Ginkgo Max 120 - Jamieson
Each caplet contains: Ginkgo Biloba Leaf Extract (40 mg of 1:50 extract, equivalent to 2000 mg of whole herb. Standardized to 24% Flavoglycosides with minimum 10 % Quercitin. Other active marker compounds established are, but not standardized to, proanthocyanidins, kaempferol, ginkgolides, bilobalides) 2000 mg.

Ginkgo Neuro-Mind - The Vitamin Shoppe
Each tablet contains: Vitamin B12 (as cyanocobalamin) 0.25 mcg • Vitamin B6 (as pyridoxine HCl) 10 mg • Ginkgo Biloba (Ginkgo biloba) leaf standardized to 24% ginkgoflavoglycosides 6% terpene lactones 50 mg • Phosphatidylserine (LECI-PS) 50 mg • DHA (Docosahexaenoic acid) (Neuromins) 50 mg.

Ginkgo Phytosome - PhytoPharmica
Each softgel capsule contains: Ginkgo (ginkgo biloba leaf phytosome; one part ginkgo extract, standardized to contain 24% ginkgoflavonglycosides and 6% terpene lactones including 2% bilobalide, bound to two parts phosphatidylcholine) 80 mg. Other Ingredients: Soybean Oil, Gelatin, Glycerin, Beeswax, Lecithin.

Ginkgo Sharp - Celestial Seasonings
Two capsules contain: Vitamin B3 (as niacinamide) 40 mg • Proprietary Blend 930 mg: Ginkgo Biloba (leaf), Ginkgo Biloba (standardized to 24% ginkgoflavonone glycosides and 6% ginkgolides.), DHA (50 mg as docohexaenoic acid). Other Ingredients: Dicalcium Phosphate, Gelatin, Rice Flour, Stearic Acid, Magnesium Stearate, Silicon Dioxide.

Ginkgo Synergy - Standard Process, Inc.
Each capsule contains: Proprietary Blend 280 mg: Gotu Kola leaf (centella asiatica), Buckwheat leaf juice, Buckwheat seed, Soybean Lecithin powder • Ginkgo Biloba leaf extract (24% flavoglycosides) 60 mg • Ginkgo Biloba whole leaf 40 mg • Grape seed extract (Masquelier's Original OPC brand) 20 mg. Other Ingredients: Cellulose, Water.

Ginkgo/Co Q10 - Pro Health
Each vegetarian capsule contains: Ginkgo Biloba leaf extract (24% flavone glycosides, 6% terpene lactones) 60 mg • Coenzyme Q10 50 mg. Other Ingredients: Hydroxypropyl Methylcellulose, Rice Flour, Microcrystalline Cellulose, Magnesium Stearate, Water.

Ginkgo/Gotu Kola - Gaia Herbs
Ginkgo and Gotu Kola standardized for 12% flavonoid glycosides & 2.5% triterpenoids. Standardized Full Spectrum 100 mg of extract per capsule. Guaranteed Potency 50 mg of extract per capsule.

Ginkgo-24 - Source Naturals
Each tablet contains: Ginkgo Biloba leaf extract (50:1) (Yielding 24% Ginkgo Flavone Glycosides and 6% Terpene Lactones from 2,000 mg of Ginkgo biloba leaf) 40 mg.

Ginkgo-Combo - Nature's Plus
Each vegetarian capsule contains: Vitamin E (as D-alpha tocopheryl succinate) 50 IU • Ginkgo Biloba leaf 8:1 extract (ginkgoaceae) 120 mg • Capsicum fruit (capsicum frutescens) 80 mg • Gotu Kola root (centella asiatica root) 80 mg. Other Ingredients: Microcrystalline Cellulose, Silica, Vegetable Cellulose, Purified Water.

Ginkgo-Go! - Wakunaga of America
Each caplet contains: Ginkgo Biloba standardized extract 50:1 (leaf) standardized with 24% Ginkgo flavonglycosides & 6% Terpene lactones 120 mg. Inactive Ingredients: Cellulose, Vegetable Starch, Magnesium Stearate (vegetable source), Silica.

Ginkgold - Nature's Way
Each tablet contains: Egb 761 Ginkgo Biloba leaf extract; standardized to 24% Ginkgo flavone glycosides & 6% terpene lactones 60 mg.

Ginkgolidin - PhytoPharmica
Each capsule contains: Ginkgo Biloba leaves extract (Ginkgo biloba folia; standardized to contain 24% ginkgoflavonglycosides, 6% terpene lactones & 2% bilobalide) 40 mg.

GinkgoPlus for Memory - Aboca USA, Inc
Two capsules contain: Ginkgo leaf freeze-dried extract (ginkgo biloba, standardized to 1% terpene lactones, 3% ginkgo flavone glycosides) 160 mg • Bacopa aerial part Whole Phytocomplex Concentrate (WPC)(bacopa monnieri) 160 mg • Siberian Ginseng root (eleutherococcus senticosus, standardized to 0.7% eleutherosides B+E, WPC) 155 mg • Zinc Yeast (saccharomices cerevisiae with zinc, 10%, organically bound) 25 mg. Other Ingredients: Gelatin (capsule).

Ginkgo-PS - USANA Health Sciences
Each tablet contains: Ginkgo Biloba (Standardized Leaf Extract) 25 mg • Lecithin Enriched with Phosphatidylserine 125 mg. Other Ingredients: Dextrose, Hydroxypropyl Methylcellulose, Titamium Dioxide, Ascorbyl Palmitate, Carnauba Wax, Collodial Silicon Dioxide, Croscarmellose Sodium.

Ginkgo-RoseOx - Metagenics
Each tablet contains: RoseOx brand Rosemary leaf extract (rosmarinus officinalis, standardized to 6% carnosic acid) 125 mg • Ginkgo leaf extract (ginkgo biloba, standardized to 24% ginkgoflavonglycosides and 6% terpene lactones) 60 mg.

GinkgoSense - The AIM Companies
Each capsule contains: Ginkgo Biloba extract (standardized to contain 24% ginkgoflavonglycosides and 6% terpene lactones) 120 mg • Bilberry fruit extract (standardized to contain 25% anthocyanosides) 40 mg • Marigold extract: Lutein 400 mcg, Zeaxanthin 18 mcg • DHA (as fish oil) 2.5 g.

Ginko Biloba - HealthWatchers System
Two capsules contain: Standard Ginkgo Biloba 120 mg • Ginko Biloba Powder equivalent to 6000 mg.

Ginkoba - Boehringer Ingelheim
Each tablet contains: Standardized Ginkgo Biloba leaf extract (50:1) 40 mg. Other Ingredients: Hydroxypropyl Methylcellulose, Lactose, Talc, Polyethylene Glycol, Magnesium Stearate, Titanium Dioxide, Synthetic Iron Oxides.

Ginkoba M/E - Boehringer Ingelheim
Each capsule contains: Panax Ginseng Extract (standardized G115) 100 mg • Ginkgo Biloba Extract (standarized GK501) 60 mg. Other Ingredients: Mannitol, Gelatin, Sicon dioxide, Magnesium Stearate.

Ginsana - Pharmaton Natural Health Products
Each capsule contains: Standardized G115 Ginseng root extract (Panax Ginseng, C.A. Meyer) 100 mg. Other Ingredients: Sunflower oil, gelatin, glycerin, lecithin, beeswax, chlorophyll.

Ginsana Chewy Squares - Pharmaton Natural Health Products
Each chewy square contains: Vitamin C • Standardized G115 Ginseng root extract (Panax Ginseng, C.A. Meyer) 50 mg. Other Ingredients: Sucrose, Glucose, Palm kernel oil, Gelatin, Citric Acid, Ascorbic Acid, Lecithin, Natural Flavoring & Coloring.

Ginsana Gold Formula - Pharmaton Natural Health Products
Each tablet contains: Vitamin A (10% as beta carotene) 2500 IU • Vitamin C 60 mg • Vitamin D 400 IU • Vitamin E 30 IU • Vitamin K 80 mcg • Thiamine (vitamin B1) 1.5 mg • Riboflavin (vitamin B2) 1.7 mg • Niacin (vitamin B3) 20 mg • Vitamin B6 2 mg • Folic Acid 400 mcg • Vitamin B12 6 mcg • Calcium (carbonate) 200 mg • Iron 18 mg • Phosphorous 160 mg • Magnesium Oxide 20 mg • Zinc (oxide) 15 mg • Copper 2 mg • Manganese 2 mg • Panax Ginseng root extract 80 mg.

GinsanaSport - Pharmaton Natural Health Products
Each capsule contains: Standardized G-115 Panax Ginseng Extract (Panax Ginseng, C.A. Meyer) (root) 200 mg. Other Ingredients: Sunflower oil, gelatin, glycerin, beeswax, lecithin, turmeric, titanium dioxide, FD&C Green No. 3.

BRAND NAMES

Ginseng - Leiner Health Products
Each softgel contains: Ginseng extract (Panax ginseng) root 100 mg. Other Ingredients: Gelatin, Soybean Oil, Vegetable Oil, Lecithin, Palm Oil, Glycerin, Sorbitol, Yellow Beeswax, Hydrogenated Coconut Oil, Titanium Dioxide, Yellow 5, Blue 1, Red 40, Green 3, Chlorophyll.

Ginseng - Source Naturals
Each tablet contains: Panax Ginseng root 648 mg.

Ginseng - Celestial Seasonings
Two capsules contain: Proprietary Blend 180 mg: Panax Ginseng (root), Panax Ginseng (standardized to 7% ginsenosides). Other ingredients: Dicalcium phosphate, gelatin, rice flour, stearic acid, magnesium stearate and silicon dioxide.

Ginseng - Benepure, Inc
Each capsule contains: Korean White Panax Ginseng root (yielding ginsenosides 30 mg) 150 mg. Other Ingredients: Rice Powder, Vegetable Stearate.

Ginseng Energy - Celestial Seasonings
Two capsules contain: Vitamin E (as d-alpha tocopherol acetate) 10 IU • Vitamin B12 (as cyanocobalamin) 30 mcg • Proprietary Blend 1590 mg: Siberian Ginseng (root), Siberian Ginseng (standardized extract), Panax Ginseng (root), Panax Ginseng (standardized extract) • Coenzyme Q10 (as ubiquinone) 10 mg. Other Ingredients: Dicalcium Phosphate, Gelatin, Rice Flour, Stearic Acid, Magnesium Stearate, Silicon Dioxide. One serving size is equivalent to: Panax Ginseng 200 mg standardized to 7% ginsenosides, Siberian Ginseng 250 mg standardized to 0.8% eleutherosides.

Ginseng Extract - The Vitamin Shoppe
Each softgel contains: 100 mg Panax Ginseng extract standardized for 8% ginsenosides.

Ginseng Phytosome - PhytoPharmica
Each capsule contains: Panax Ginseng root phytosome (bound to phosphatidylcholine under patent) 50 mg.

Ginseng Schizandra Supreme - Gaia Herbs
Thirty drops contain: Proprietary Blend 100 mg: Eleuthero root (eleutherococcus senticosus), Chinese Schizandra berry (schizandra chinensis), Damiana leaf (turnera diffusa), Cola nut (cola nitida), Fresh Wild Oats milky seed (avena sativa), Licorice root (glycyrrhiza glabra), Fresh Skullcap herb (scutellaria lateriflora), Prickly Ash bark (xanthoxylum clava-herculis), 30-40% Pure Grain Alcohol USP, Spring Water.

Ginseng Supreme - Gaia Herbs
Thirty drops contain: Proprietary Blend 80 mg: Fresh Woods Grown American Ginseng (panax quinquefolium), Eleuthero root (eleutherococcus senticosus), Spring Water, 30-35% Pure Grain Alcohol USP.

Ginseng, Korean White, 560mg - Nature Made
Two capsules contain: Korean White Ginseng root 1.12 g: Ginsenosides 22.4 mg.

Ginseng/Aloe Capsules - Aloe Farms
Siberian Ginseng powder 150 mg, Aloe Vera powder 100 mg.

Ginseng/Collagen Firming Creme - Derma E
Ginseng • Collagen (contains 22 amino acids).

Ginseng-Go! - Wakunaga of America
Each capsule contains: Korean Ginseng extract powder (root) 300 mg. Other Ingredients: Cellulose, Magnesium Stearate (vegetable source).

Ginseven - Leiner Health Products
Each caplet contains: American Ginseng extract (Panax quinquefolius) root 75 mg • Ashwagandha extract (Withania somnifera) root 50 mg • Notoginseng extract (Panax notoginseng) root 50 mg • Panax Ginseng extract (Panax ginseng) root 100 mg • Schisandra extract (Schisandra chinensis) fruit 75 mg • Siberian Ginseng extract (Eleutherococcus senticosus) root 75 mg • Suma extract (Pfaffia paniculata) root 100 mg. Other Ingredients: Cellulose, Dicalcium Phosphate, Stearic Acid, Magnesium Stearate, Silicon Dioxide, Sodium Starch Glycolate, Polyethylene Glycol 3350.

GinSting - Futurebiotics LLC
Two tablets contain: Korean Ginseng 1000 mg • Bee Pollen 500 mg.

GinSwee Tea - HerbaSway
Ginger • Panax Ginseng • Blackberry • HerbaSwee (Cucurbitaceae fruit).

GKG - EAS, Inc.
Each capsule contains: Alpha-Ketoglutaric Acid 250 mg • L-Glutamine 275 mg • Taurine 150 mg • Calcium 63 mg • Potassium 25 mg • Magnesium 25 mg • RNA 9.5 mg • Manganese 400 mcg.

GLA - J. R. Carlson Laboratories, Inc.
Two softgels contain: Blackcurrant seed oil (ribes nigrum) 1000 mg • ALA (alpha-linolenic acid) 120 mg • GLA (gamma linolenic acid) 150 mg.

GLA Complex - Shaklee
Each capsule contains: Vitamin E (as D-alpha tocopherol concentrate) 15 IU • Gamma-Linolenic acid (from borage seed oil (Borago officinalis)) 90 mg • Linoleic acid (from sunflower seed oil (Helianthus annus) and borage seed oil (Borago officinalis)) 216 mg. Other Ingredients: Ascorbyl Palmitate, Mixed Tocopherols Concentrate, Rosemary Extract, Gelatin, Glycerin, Water.

GLA Forte - Nature's Plus
Two softgels contain: GLA (Gamma Linolenic Acid) from Borage seed oil & Black Currant Seed oil, 100 mg • Vitamin E (d-Alpha Tocopherol) 200 IU • Vitamin C corn free 100 mg • Vitamin B6 (Pyridoxine HCL) 50 mg • Niacinamide 25 mg • Zinc (Gluconate) 5 mg. In a base containing safflower oil, octacosanol, lecithin & rapeseed.

GLA Forte - Metagenics
Each capsule contains: Borage oil 1000 mg • Gamma-Linolenic Acid 240 mg • Vitamin E (as D-alpha tocopherol acetate) 10 IU.

GLA Mega-260 - Progressive Labs
Each softgel contains: Borage oil 1300 mg which supplies no less than Gamma Linolenic Acid (GLA) 260 mg and Vitamin E 1.5 IU. Fatty Acid Composition: Gamma Linolenic Acid 260 mg • Linoleic Acid 494 mg • Oleic Acid 221 mg.

Glaceau Vitamin Water (balance cran-grapefruit flavor) - Energy Brands, Inc.
Vapor Distilled Water • Crystalline Fructose • Citric Acid • Natural Flavor • Calcium Chloride • Magnesium Chloride • Potassium Bicarbonate • Gum Arabic • Ascorbic Acid (vitamin C) • Natural Color • Cranberry • Black Currant concentrate • Raspberry juice concentrate • Zinc Picolinate • Vitamin E Acetate • Yerba Mate extract • Niacin (vitamin B3) • Pantothenic Acid (vitamin B5) • Ester Gum • Ginkgo Biloba extract • Vitamin A Palmitate • Pyridoxine Hydrochloride (vitamin B6) • Caramel Color • Selenium • Cyanocobalamin (vitamin B12).

Glaceau Vitamin Water (defense flavor) - Energy Brands, Inc.
Vapor Distilled/Deionized Water • Crystalline Fructose • Citric Acid • Vegetable Juice • Natural Flavor • Ascorbic Acid (vitamin C) • Natural Flavor • Vitamin E Acetate • Magnesium Lactate • Calcium Lactate • Zinc Picolinate • Monopotassium Phosphate • Niacin (vitamin B3) • Pantothenic Acid (vitamin B5) • Pyridoxine Hydrochloride (vitamin B6) • Cyanocobalamin (vitamin B12).

Glaceau Vitamin Water (endurance peach mango flavor) - Energy Brands, Inc.
Vapor Distilled Water • Crystalline Fructose • Natural Flavor • Citric Acid • Ribose • Ascorbic Acid (vitamin C) • Magnesium Lactate • Calcium Lactate • Vitamin E Acetate • Monopotassium Phosphate •

Niacin (vitamin B3) • Pantothenic Acid (vitamin B5) • Pyridoxine Hydrochloride (vitamin B6) • Canthaxanthin • Cyanocobalamin (vitamin B12).

Glaceau Vitamin Water (energy tropical citrus flavor) - Energy Brands, Inc.
Vapor Distilled Water • Crystalline Fructose • Citric Acid • Caffeine • Ascorbic Acid (vitamin C) • Gum Arabic • Natural Flavor • Calcium, Magnesium, and Potassium Electrolytes • Gum Ester • Zinc Picolinate • Vitamin E Acetate • Vitamin A Palmitate • Niacin (vitamin B3) • Pantothenic Acid (vitamin B5) • Beta Carotene • Siberian Ginseng extract 25 mg • Guarana extract 25 mg • Cyanocobalamin (vitamin B12) • Caramel Color • Pyridoxine Hydrochloride (vitamin B6).

Glaceau Vitamin Water (essential orange-orange flavor) - Energy Brands, Inc.
Vapor Distilled Water • Crystalline Fructose • Citric Acid • Natural Flavor • Calcium Lactate • Potassium • Gum Arabic • Ascorbic Acid (vitamin C) • Magnesium Electrolyte • Gum Ester • Vitamin A Palmitate • Vitamin E Acetate • Niacin (vitamin B3) • Pantothenic Acid (vitamin B5) • Iron • Cyanocobalamin (vitamin B12) • Beta Carotene • Pyridoxine Hydrochloride (vitamin B6) • Selenium.

Glaceau Vitamin Water (focus kiwi-strawberry flavor) - Energy Brands, Inc.
Vapor Distilled Water • Crystalline Fructose • Citric Acid • Ascorbic Acid (vitamin C) • Gum Arabic • Calcium, Magnesium, and Potassium Electrolytes • Vitamin E Acetate • Gum Ester • Vitamin A Palmitate • Niacin (vitamin B3) • Pantothenic Acid (vitamin B5) • Gotu Kola 25 mg • Siberian Ginseng extract 25 mg • Ginkgo Biloba extract 25 mg • Cyanocobalamin (vitamin B12) • Pyridoxine Hydrochloride (vitamin B6).

Glaceau Vitamin Water (formula 50 flavor) - Energy Brands, Inc.
Vapor Distilled Water • Crystalline Fructose • Natural Flavor • Citric Acid • Ascorbic Acid (vitamin C) • Vitamin E Acetate • Fruit and Vegetable Juice • Magnesium Lactate • Niacin (vitamin B3) • Monopotassium Phosphate • Pantothenic Acid (vitamin B5) • Pyridoxine Hydrochloride (vitamin B6) • Cyanocobalamin (vitamin B12) • Folic Acid.

Glaceau Vitamin Water (multi-v lemonade flavor) - Energy Brands, Inc.
Vapor Distilled Water • Crystalline Fructose • Natural Flavor • Citric Acid • Ascorbic Acid (vitamin C) • Calcium 20 mg • Magnesium and Potassium Electrolytes • Vitamin A Palmitate • Vitamin E Acetate.

Glaceau Vitamin Water (power-c dragonfruit flavor) - Energy Brands, Inc.
Distilled/Deionized Water • Crystalline Fructose • Citric Acid • Natural Flavor • Ascorbic Acid (vitamin c) • Natural Flavor extract • Calcium, Magnesium and Potassium Eelectrolytes • Vitamin E Acetate • Zinc Picolinate • Taurine 3 mg • Vitamin A Palmitate • Niacin (vitamin B3) • Pantothenic Acid (vitamin B5) • Siberian Ginseng extract 25 mg • Chromium Polynicotinate • Cyanocobalamin (vitamin B12) • Pyridoxine Hydrochloride (vitamin B6) • Dragonfruit juice concentrate.

Glaceau Vitamin Water (rescue green tea flavor) - Energy Brands, Inc.
Vapor Distilled Water • Crystalline Fructose • Citric Acid • Green Tea • Natural Flavor • Ascorbic Acid (vitamin C) • Calcium, Magnesium, and Potassium Electrolytes • Rosemary extract 20 mg • Chamomile extract 20 mg • Hibiscus extract 20 mg • Lavender extract 20 mg • Rose Hip extract 20 mg • Niacin (vitamin B3) • Cyanocobalamin (vitamin B12) • Pyridoxine Hydrochloride (vitamin B6).

Glaceau Vitamin Water (revive fruit punch flavor) - Energy Brands, Inc.
Vapor Distilled Water • Crystalline Fructose • Natural Flavor • Citric Acid • Grape Juice • Calcium Chloride • Magnesium Chloride • Potassium Bicarbonate • Grape skin extract • Ascorbic Acid (vitamin C) • Gum Arabic • Gotu Kola extract 25 mg • Vitamin E Acetate • American Ginseng extract 25 mg • Niacin (vitamin B3) • Pantothenic Acid (vitamin B5) • Ester Gum • Vitamin A Palmitate • Pyridoxine Hydrochloride (vitamin B6) • Cyanocobalamin.

Glaceau Vitamin Water (stress b lemon-lime flavor) - Energy Brands, Inc.
Vapor Distilled Water • Crystalline Fructose • Citric Acid • Natural Flavor • Ascorbic Acid (vitamin C) • Gum Arabic • Calcium, Magnesium, and Potassium Electrolytes • Gum Ester • St. John's Wort extract 25 mg • Kava Kava extract 25 mg • Niacin (vitamin B3) • Pantothenic Acid (vitamin B5) • Riboflavin (vitamin B2) • Cyanocobalamin (vitamin B12) • Pyridoxine Hydrochloride (vitamin B6).

Glaceau Vitamin Water (vital-t flavor) - Energy Brands, Inc.
Vapor Distilled/Deionized Water • Crystalline Fructose • Natural Flavor • Citric Acid • Ascorbic Acid (vitamin C) • Rooibos Tea extract • Vitamin E Acetate • Magnesium Lactate • Calcium Lactate • Monopotassium Phosphate • Niacin (vitamin B3) • Pantothenic Acid (vitamin B5) • Pyridoxine Hydrochloride (vitamin B6) • Cyanocobalamin (vitamin B12).

Glan-Fem Plus - Atrium Biotechnologies
Each tablet contains: Ovary 80 mg • Adrenal 20 mg • Thyroid (thyroxin free) 20 mg • Pituitary 10 mg • Vitamin B1 15 mg • Vitamin B2 17 mg • Vitamin B6 16 mg • Vitamin C 120 mg • Niacinamide 60 mg • Folic Acid 200 mcg • Vitamin E (D-alpha tocopherol) 60 IU • Manganese (protein chelated) 5 mg • Selenium 20 mcg.
See Editor's Note No. 31.

Glan-Male Plus - Atrium Biotechnologies
Each tablet contains: Orchic 80 mg • Adrenal 20 mg • Pituitary 10 mg • Vitamin B1 15 mg • Vitamin B2 17 mg • Vitamin B6 16 mg • Vitamin C 120 mg • Niacinamide 60 mg • Folic Acid 200 mcg • Vitamin E (D-alpha tocopherol) 60 IU • Manganese (protein chelated) 5 mg • Selenium 20 mcg.
See Editor's Note No. 14.

Gla-Plus - Atrium Biotechnologies
Each capsule contains: Gamma Linolenic Acid (from Black Currant) 40 mg • Vitamin E (d-Alpha Tocopheryl Acetate) 10 IU.

GliSODin - NOW Foods
Each vegetarian capsule contains: GliSODin brand vegetarian complex 100 mg: SOD (enzyme activity = 100 IU), Gliadin • Wheat grass (triticum aestivum) 250 mg.

GliSODin - Bluebonnet
Each capsule contains: GliSODin complex 100 mg: SOD (superoxide dismutase 100 IU), Glisodin. Other Ingredients: Wheat Maltodextrin, Magnesium Stearate.

GliSODin brand - Isocell
SOD (superoxide dismutase, from cucumis melo extract) • Gliadin (triticum vulgare extract). Other Ingredients: Mannitol, Silica, Magnesium Stearate, Hydroxypropylmethycellulose, Titanium Dioxide.
See Editor's Note No. 44.

Glowing Skin 700 Mega - Susan Ambrosino's Herb Club, Inc.
Each capsule contains: Proprietary Blend 700 mg: DMAE, Alpha Lipoic Acid, Ascorbyl Palmitate.

Glucaherb - Wild Rose
Each tablet contains: Juniper berry 133.3 mg • Uva Ursi leaf 66.6 mg • Licorice root 66 mg • Mullein leaf 66 mg • Cayenne fruit (80,000 HU) 66 mg.

Gluca-Herb - Dial Herbs
Cedar berries • Uva Ursi • Licorice • Mullein • Cayenne.

GlucoBalance - Biotics Research Corporation
Six capsules contain: Vitamin A (as retinyl acetate) 5000 IU • Vitamin C (as calcium ascorbate and ascorbic acid) 500 mg • Vitamin D (as cholecalciferol) 100 IU • Vitamin E (as D-alpha tocopheryl acetate) 400 IU • Thiamin (B1, as thiamin mononitrate) 50 mg • Vitamin B2 (as riboflavin) 25 mg • Niacin (as niacinamide and niacin) 150 mg • Vitamin B6 (as pyridoxine hydrochloride) 30 mg • Folic Acid 800 mcg • Vitamin B12 (as cobalamin) 50 mcg • Biotin 3000 mcg • Pantothenic Acid (as calcium pantothenate) 100 mg • Calcium (as ascorbate, citrate and carbonate) 200 mg • Magnesium (as aspartate, citrate and oxide) 400 mg • Zinc (as zinc picolinate and zinc citrate) 30 mg • Selenium (as selenomethionine) 150 mcg • Copper (as copper gluconate) 2 mg • Manganese (as manganese aspartate) 20 mg • Chromium (as chromium aspartate) 1000 mcg • Potassium (as potassium aspartate) 99 mg • Vanadium (as vanadium aspartate) 20 mcg.

Glucobetic - Flourish The Wellness Company
Each capsule contains: Zinc (gluconate) 15 mg • Chromium GTF (polynicotinate) 240 mcg • Vanadyl Sulfate 10 mg • Gymnema Sylvestre extract 200 mg • Bitter Melon extract (momordica charantia) 200 mg • Fenugreek extract (trigonella foenum-graecum) 100 mg • Bilberry extract (vaccinium myritllus) 40 mg • Cinnamon extract (cinnamomum verum) 30 mg • Jambolan (syzgium cumini) 75 mg • Pterocarpus Marsupium 200 mg • Gulvel (tinospora cordifolia) 50 mg.

GlucoChrom - The AIM Companies
Two capsules contain: Vanadium Citrate 0.394 mg (75 mcg vanadium) • Bitter Melon fruit powder 450 mg • Gymnema Sylvestre leaf extract 500 mg • LeafBrand brand Barley 168 mg (400 mcg chromium).

Gluco-Essentials - Viable Herbal Solutions
Two capsules contain: Proprietary Blend 1200 mg: Bilberry (vaccinium myrtillus), Bitter Melon (momordica charantia), Cinnamon (cinnamomum zeylanicum), Citrus Bioflavonoids, Fenugreek seed (trigonellum foenum-graecum), American Ginseng (panax quinquefolium), Korean Ginseng (panax ginseng), Glucomannan (amorphophallus konjac), Goldenseal root (hydrastis canadensis), Gymnema (gymnema sylvestre), Holy Basil (ocimum basilicum), Jerusalem Artichoke (cynara scolymus), Mistletoe (viscum album), Olive leaf (olea europaea), Psyllium (plantago ovata), Quercetin, Suma root (pfaffia paniculata), Uva Ursi (arctosatphylos uva-ursi).

Gluco-Factors - Metagenics
Each tablet contains: Raw Liver concentrate (bovine) 150 mg • Raw Pancreas concentrate (porcine) 100 mg • Thiamin (as thiamin mononitrate) 100 mg • Zinc (as zinc glycinate) 10 mg • Magnesium (as magnesium bis-glycinate) 25 mg • Niacin 25 mg • Manganese (as manganese gluconate) 2 mg • Chromium (as chromium dinicotinate glycinate) 45 mcg.

GlucoFlex PM - Windmill Health Products
Two caplets contain: Calcium (as calcium carbonate) 250 mg • Magnesium (as magnesium oxide) 100 mg • Glucosamine HCl 500 mg • Herbal Pain Relief Blend 350 mg: Feverfew leaf extract (0.2% parthenolide), White Willow bark, Turmeric Rhizome, Ginger root extract (5% gingerols) • Valerian root extract (0.8% valerenic acid) 200 mg • Hops (strobile) 100 mg. Other Ingredients: Microcrystalline Cellulose, Croscarmellose Sodium, Stearic Acid, Magnesium Stearate, Pharmaceutical Glaze.

Glucogen Ace - ANS - Applied Nutrition Sciences
Glucose • Vitamin A • Vitamin C • Vitamin E.

Glucogen Sport - ANS - Applied Nutrition Sciences
"Vitamins & Minerals enriched Glucose Drink for Sports people."

GlucoLean - Nutripeak
Two tablets contain: Selenium (as selenium amino acid chelate) 50 mcg • Chromium (as chromium polynicotinate) 200 mcg • Guggul extract 1000 mg • Gymnema Sylvestre leaf 150 mg • Coleus Forskohlii extract 130 mg • Alpha-Lipoic Acid 100 mg • D-Pinitol 25 mg • Bitter Melon extract fruit, seed 18.8 mg. Other Ingredients: Cellulose, Stearic Acid, Magnesium Stearate, Silica.

Glucomannan 500 Mg - Natrol, Inc.
Two capsules contain: Hemicellulose 913 mg • Cellulose 61 mg • Pectin Substance 25 mg • Lignin 1 mg. From Amorphophallus Konjac root.

Glucomannan+ - Swanson Health Products
Three capsules contain: Chromium (50% from Chromax® chromium picolinate, 50% from chromium polynicotinate) 150 mcg • Psyllium husk fiber 600 mg • Konjac Glucomannan 450 mg • Apple Pectin • 300 mg • Chitosan (93% deacetylated) 300 mg • Guar Gum 300 mg • Oat Bran fiber 300 mg • Gymnema sylvestre extract (25% gymnemic acids) 75 mg • L-Carnitine (as tartrate) 30 mg.

Glucomine - Body Wise International, Inc.
Three capsules contain: Glucosamine Sulfate 1500 mg • Chondroitin Sulfate 150 mg • Boswellia Gum Std. Extract (Boswellia serrata) 25 mg • White Willow Bark (Salix alba) 25 mg • Devils Claw-Inner Bark (Harpagophytum procumbens) 25 mg • Tea Tree Oil (Melaleuca alternifolia) 25 mg • Una de Gato (Uncaria tomentosa) 25 mg.
See Editor's Note No. 15.

GlucoPrep - HealthMinded
Each tablet contains: Calcium (as citrate) 37 mg • Glucosamine HCl 750 mg • Chondroitin Sulfate 600 mg. Other Ingredients: Dicalcium Phosphate, Stearic Acid, Croscarmellose Sodium, Magnesium Stearate, Micro Crystalline Celluose, Silicon Dioxide.
See Editor's Note No. 15.

Gluco-Pro 900 - Thompson Nutritional Products
Each tablet contains: Glucosamine HCl 500 mg • Chondroitin Sulfate 400 mg.
See Editor's Note No. 15.

Glucoril - PhytoPharmica
Two capsules contain: Vitamin C (ascorbic acid) 100 mg • Vitamin E (mixed tocopherols) 50 IU • Vitamin B6 (pyridoxine HCl) 10 mg • Vitamin B12 (cyanocobalamin) 250 mcg • Biotin 1,000 mcg • Magnesium (Krebs chelate) 100 mg • Zinc (picolinate) 5 mg • Selenium (L-selenomethionine) 40 mcg • Manganese (Krebs chelate) 10 mg • Chromium (picolinate) 50 mcg • Blueberry (Vaccinium myrtillus fructus) extract 5:1 300 mg • Gymnema Sylvestre leaf extract 6:1 (standardized to contain 24% gymnemic acid) 150 mg • Bitter Melon (Momordica charantia) whole fruit extract 100 mg • Fenugreek (Trigonella foenum-graecum) seed extract 4:1 100 mg.

Glucosalage SO4 - Olympian Labs
Each capsule contains: Shark Cartilage 200 mg • Cat's Claw (uncaria tomentosa) 200 mg • Glucosamine Sulfate 2 KCl 200 mg.

Glucosalage SO4 (Extra Strength) - Olympian Labs
Two capsules contain: Shark Cartilage 400 mg • Cat's Claw 400 mg • Glucosamine Sulfate 400 mg • Proprietary Blend: Protease, Amylase, Lipase 100 mg. In a base of White Willow Bark, Valerian Root, Devil's Claw, and Black Willow.

GlucosaMend - Source Naturals
Three tablets contain: Vitamin A (as palmitate) 6000 IU • Vitamin C (as magnesium & manganese ascorbates) 900 gm • Vitamin E (as natural D-alpha tocopheryl) 180 IU • Niacinamide 240 mg • Vitamin B6 (as pyridoxal-5'-phosphate, coenzymated) 10 mg • Manganese (as manganese ascorbate) 9 mg • Magnesium (as mangesium ascorbate) 67 mg • Zinc (as zinc monomethionine, OptiZinc brand) 18 mg • Selenium (as L-selenomethionine) 120 mcg • Copper (as copper sebacate) 1 mg • NAG (N-ascetyl glucosamine) 720 mg • Boswellia

Serratta gum resin extract (yielding 293 mg of boswellic acids) 450 mg • L-Proline 300 mg • L-Lysine (HCl) 300 mg • Quercetin 300 mg • Glucosamine Sulfate (as glucosamine sulfate potassium chloride) 180 mg • Grape seed extract (Proanthodyn brand, with a procyanidolic vlaue of 95) 60 mg. Other Ingredients: Stearic Acid, Modified Cellulose Gum, Colloidal Silicon Dioxide, Magnesium Stearate.

Glucosamine - Nature Made
Each tablet contains: Glucosamine 500 mg.

Glucosamine - Matol Botanical International Ltd
Each 1 tbsp serving contains: Glucosamine Sulfate 500 mg • Methyl Sulfonyl Methane (MSM) 500 mg • Devil's Claw root 1:10 extract 150 mg. Other Ingredients: Purified Water, Glycerin, Fructose, Fish Collagen Hydrolysate, Citric Acid, Natural Flavor, Sodium Citrate, Sodium Benzoate, Potassium Sorbate.

Glucosamine & Boswellin Blend - America's Finest
Each tablet contains: Proprietary Blend 625 mg: Glucosamine Sulphate, Boswellin brand Boswellia Serrata gum extract (65% boswellic acids, curcuminoids), Chondroitin Sulphate, Bromelain enzyme, Digezyme brand Enzyme complex, Bioperine brand Black Pepper fruit extract. Other Ingredients: Cellulose, Stearic Acid, Magnesium Citrate, Magnesium Stearate, Natural Color Glaze.

Glucosamine & Chondroitin - Pro Health
Four capsules contain: Glucosamine HCl 1500 mg • Chondroitin Sulfate 1200 mg • ConcenTrace brand Trace Minerals 800 mg. Other Ingredients: Gelatin, Magnesium Stearate, Silicon Dioxide, Alfalfa.

Glucosamine & Chondroitin - Vital Nutrients
Each capsule contains: Glucosamine Sulfate (from 469 mg of glucosamine sulfate 2KLC) 375 mg • Chondroitin Sulfate 300 mg.

Glucosamine & Chondroitin 500/400 - NOW Foods
Each capsule contains: Sodium 40 mg • Potassium (as Potassium Chloride) 60 mg • Glucosamine Sulfate (from 500 mg Glusocamine Potassium Sulfate complex) 375 mg • Chondroitin Sulfate (min. 90%) (Bovine Source) 400 mg • MSM 100 mg.
See Editor's Note No. 15.

Glucosamine & Chondroitin Combo - Swanson Health Products
Each capsule contains: Glucosamine Sulfate (2KCl) 500 mg • Chondroitin Sulfate 250 mg.
See Editor's Note No. 15.

Glucosamine & MSM - Arrowroot
Each tablet contains: Glucosamine Sulfate 500 mg • MSM 500 mg • Potassium 88 mg.

Glucosamine & MSM Complex - Puritan's Pride
Three tablets contain: Glucosamine Sulfate 1500 mg • MSM 1000 mg • Ginger (Standardized 4% Volatile Oil) 100 mg • Vitamin C (Ascorbic Acid) 60 mg • Manganese 5 mg • White Willow 100 mg.

Glucosamine & UC II Complex - PhysioLogics
Two capsules contain: Glucosamine 2KCl 1500 mg • Undenatured Type II Collagen (from UC II undenatured type II collagen complex 40 mg) 10 mg. Other Ingredients: Rice Powder, Gelatin, Potassium Chloride, Silica, Vegetable Magnesium Stearate.

Glucosamine + Chondroitin - Jarrow Formulas
Four capsules contain: Vitamin C (ascorbic acid) 60 mg • Manganese (as manganese gluconate) 1 mg • Glucosamine Sulfate 2KCl 2000 mg: Glucosamine Sulfate 1500 mg, Potassium Chloride 500 mg • Chondroitin Sulfate (from 1333 mg chondroitin sulfate sodium) 1200 mg. Other Ingredients: Rice Powder, Magnesium Stearate, Gelatin.

Glucosamine 500 mg / Chondroitin 400 mg Capsules - GNC
Three capsules contain: D-Glucosamine HCl 1500 mg • Chondroitin Sulfate Sodium 1200 mg. Other Ingredients: Soybean Oil, Gelatin, Glycerin, Caramel Color, Titanium Dioxide.
See Editor's Note No. 15.

Glucosamine 500 mg / Chondroitin 400 mg Tablets - GNC
Each tablet contains: D-Glucosamine Hydrochloride 500 mg • Chondroitin Sulfate, Sodium 400 mg. Other Ingredients: Red Beet root juice powder.
See Editor's Note No. 15.

Glucosamine 750 mg / Chondroitin 600 mg Tablets - GNC
Each tablet contains: D-Glucosamine HCl 750 mg • Chondroitin Sulfate 600 mg. Other Ingredients: Red Beet root juice powder.
See Editor's Note No. 15.

Glucosamine and MSM - NOW Foods
Two capsules contain: Glucosamine HCl (vegetarian source) 1000 mg • MSM 1000 mg. Other Ingredients: Cellulose (capsule), Magnesium Stearate (vegetable source), Stearic Acid (vegetable source), Silica.

Glucosamine Chondroitin - Arrowroot
Each tablet contains: Glucosamine Sulfate 500 mg • Chondroitin Sulfate 400 mg.Other Ingredients: Potasium 90 mg.
This product was formerly known as Nutra-disc. See Editor's Note No. 15.

Glucosamine Chondroitin & MSM - Pro Health
Two tablets contain: Chondroitin Sulfate (bovine) 600 mg • Glucosamine Sulfate (as D-glucosamine sulfate 2KCl) 750 mg • Methylsulfonylmethane (OptiMSM brand) 1000 mg. Other Ingredients: Magnesium Stearate, Croscarmellose Sodium, Silicon Dioxide, Pharmaceutical Glaze.
See Editor's Note No. 15.

Glucosamine Chondroitin & MSM - Natrol, Inc.
Three tablets contain: Glucosamine Sulfate 1500 mg • Chondroitin Sulfate 1200 mg • MSM (methylsulfonylmethane) 250 mg • Organic Sulfur 83 mg. Other Ingredients: Cellulose, Stearic Acid, Silica, Cellulose Gum, Magnesium Stearate, Methylcellulose, Glycerine.
See Editor's Note No. 15.

Glucosamine Chondroitin & MSM - Puritan's Pride
Three tablets contain: Glucosamine Sulfate (2KCl) 1500 mg • Chondroitin Sulfate 1200 mg • Methylsulfonylmethane (MSM) 500 mg. Other Ingredients: Cellulose (plant origin), Cellulose Coating, Vegetable Magnesium Stearate, Silica, Titanium Dioxide Color.
See Editor's Note No. 15.

Glucosamine Chondroitin Complex with MSM - Source Naturals
Three tablets contain: Vitamin C (as ascorbic acid) 250 mg • Molybdenum (as molybdenum chelate) 320 mcg • Glucosamine Sulfate 1,500 mg • Chondroitin Sulfate 1,200 mg • MSM (methylsulfonylmethane) 800 mg.
See Editor's Note No. 15.

Glucosamine Chondroitin HP - PhysioLogics
Three tablets contain: Glucosamine Hydrochloride 1500 mg • Chondroitin Sulfate 1200 mg. Other Ingredients: Povidone, Beet Root Juice, Vegetable Magnesium Stearate, Silica, Cellulose (plant origin).
See Editor's Note No. 15.

Glucosamine Chondroitin MSM and Astaxanthin TABS - TwinLab
Each tablet contains: MSM 500 mg • Glucosamine 750 mg • Chondroitin 600 mg • Bio-Astin Astaxanthin 8 mg.
See Editor's Note No. 15.

Glucosamine Chondroitin Sulfate - HealthWatchers System
Glucosamine Sulfate • Chondroitin Sulfate • Vitamin C.
See Editor's Note No. 15.

Glucosamine Chondroitin with Manganese - Pure Encapsulations
Each vegetable capsule contains: Glucosamine HCl (shellfish, 99%) 500 mg • Chondroitin Sulfate (bovine, 95%) 400 mg • Manganese (from manganese ascorbate) 5 mg • Ascorbate (from manganese ascorbate) 33 mg • Vitamin C (as ascorbyl palmitate) 5 mg.

BRAND NAMES

Some Brand Name Natural Products - What they Contain

www.NaturalDatabase.com contains MANY more listings than appear here.
Editor's Notes are located on pages 2155-2163.

BRAND NAMES

Glucosamine Chondroitin with MSM - Pure Encapsulations
Each vegetable capsule contains: Glucosamine HCl (shellfish, 99%) 300 mg • Chondroitin Sulfate (bovine, 95%) 300 mg • MSM (methylsulfonylmethane, 99%) 300 mg • Vitamin C (as ascorbyl palmitate) 5 mg.

Glucosamine Complex - Natrol, Inc.
Each capsule contains: Glucosamine Sulfate 100 mg • Glucosamine HCl 300 mg • Glucosamine N-Acetyl 100 mg. Other Ingredients: Rice powder, Silicon Dioxide, Magnesium Stearate, Gelatin.

Glucosamine Complex - Pure Encapsulations
Each vegetable capsule contains: Glucosamine Sulfate (shellfish, from 333 mg of glucosamine sulfate 2KCl, sodium free) 250 mg • Glucosamine HCl (shellfish, from 278 mg of glucosamine HCl) 250 mg • N-Acetyl-D-Glucosamine (from 312 mg of N-acetyl-D-glucosamine) 250 mg • Vitamin C (as ascorbyl palmitate) 15 mg • Manganese (ascorbate) 5 mg.

Glucosamine Complex 1000 mg - Schiff
Two tablets contain: Proprietary Blend 2000 mg: Glucosamine Hydrochloride, Glucosamine Sulfate, N-Acetyl D-Glucosamine. Other Ingredients: Cellulose, Copolyvidone, Magnesium Stearate, Silicon Dioxide, Potassium Chloride.

Glucosamine Complex Syn-flex Liquid Formula - Activex America, Inc.
Each 1/4 oz serving contains: Proprietary Blend 1250 mg: Glucosamine HCl, Glucosamine Sulfate • Shark Cartilage (20% chondroitin sulfate) 25 mg • Boswellin 8 mg • Yucca powder 3 mg • Manganese (ascorbate) 5 mg • Bromelain 1 mg • Vitamin C 5 mg • Omega 3 Fatty Acid 5 mg • Omega 6 Fatty Acid 5 mg • Vitamin A 80 IU • Vitamin E 2 IU.
See Editor's Note No. 15.

Glucosamine Complex With Chondroitin - Puritan's Pride
Two capsules contain: Vitamin C (as ascorbic acid) 200 mg • Manganese (as manganese sulfate) 2 mg • Sodium (as chondroitin sulfate) 30 mg • Glucosamine Sulfate (KCl) 500 mg • Chondroitin Sulfate 400 mg. Other Ingredients: Gelatin, Cellulose (plant origin), Vegetable Magnesium Stearate, Silica.
See Editor's Note No. 15.

Glucosamine Formula - Symmetry
Each packet contains: Glucosamine • Chondroitin Sulfate • Hydrolyzed gelatin • Boswellia • Curcumin • Bilberry • Grape Seed extract • Grape Skin extract • Tumeric extract.
See Editor's Note No. 15.

Glucosamine Fuel - TwinLab
Two tablets contain: Glucosamine Sulfate (Pure Pharmaceutical Grade) 1500 mg • Chondroitin Sulfate (Pure Pharmaceutical Grade) 1200 mg • Glycerol Fuel (contains 99.7% Pure Pharmaceutical Grade Glycerol).

Glucosamine HCl - Pure Encapsulations
Each vegetable capsule contains: Glucosamine (shellfish-free, from 904 mg glucosamine HCl) 750 mg.

Glucosamine HCl Chondroitin - Pure Encapsulations
Each vegetable capsule contains: Glucosamine HCl (shellfish-free, 98%) 500 mg • Chondroitin Sulfate (bovine, 95%) 400 mg • Vitamin C (as ascorbyl palmitate) 10 mg.

Glucosamine HCl Mega 1000 - Jarrow Formulas
Each tablet contains: Glucosamine HCl 1000 mg. Other Ingredients: Cellulose, Dicalcium Phosphate, Modified Cellulose Gum, Stearic Acid, Magnesium Stearate.

Glucosamine HCl, Chondroitin & MSM - Swanson Health Products
Three tablets contain: Glucosamine HCl 750 mg • Chondroitin Sulfate 600 mg • OptiMSM (methylsulfonylmethane) 450 mg.
See Editor's Note No. 15.

Glucosamine MSM - Pure Encapsulations
Two vegetable capsules contain: Glucosamine Sulfate (shellfish, from 666 mg of glucosamine sulfate 2KCl [sodium free]) 500 mg • MSM (methylsulfonylmethane) 500 mg • Ginger extract (zingiber officinale, standardized to contain 5% gingerols) 250 mg • Turmeric extract (curcuma longa, standardized to contain 97% cucuminoids) 250 mg • Vitamin C (as ascorbyl palmitate) 16 mg.

Glucosamine MSM Complex Joint Support Formula - Puritan's Pride
Three tablets contain: Vitamin C (as ascorbic acid) 60 mg • Manganese (as manganese sulfate) 5 mg • Glucosamine Sulfate (2KCl) 1500 mg • MSM (mehtylsulfonylmethane, 340 mg organic sulfur) 1000 mg • Ginger root extract (zingiber officinale, standardized to contain 4% volatile oils) 100 mg • White Willow bark (salix alba) 100 mg. Other Ingredients: Cellulose (plant origin), Vegetable Stearic Acid, Croscarmellose, Silica, Cellulose Coating, Vegetable Magnesium Stearate.

Glucosamine PLUS Calcium with D3 & K1 - Nature's Own
Each tablet contains: Calcium (from calcium carbonate 625 mg) 250 mg • Glucosamine Sulfate / Potassium Chloride Complex 375 mg • Vitamin D (D3, as cholecalciferol 2.5 mcg) 100 IU • Vitamin K (K1, as phytomenadione) 20 mcg.

Glucosamine Plus CSA - Optimum Nutrition
Two capsules contain: Glucosamine Sulfate 1000 mg • Chondroitin Sulfate 800 mg. Other Ingredients: Gelatin, Microcrystalline Cellulose, Magnesium Stearate.

Glucosamine Sulfate - Swanson Health Products
Each capsule contains: Glucosamine Sulfate (2KCl) 500 mg.

Glucosamine Sulfate - Olympian Labs
Each capsule contains: Glucosamine Sulfate (yielding Glucosamine Sulfate 500 mg and Potassium Chloride 170 mg) 670 mg.

Glucosamine Sulfate - Ortho Molecular Products
Each capsule contains: Glucosamine Sulfate 750 mg. Other Ingredients: Natural Vegetable Capsules, Ascorbyl Palmitate, Microcrystalline CEllulose, Silicon Dioxide.

Glucosamine Sulfate - Optimum Nutrition
Each capsule contains: Glucosamine (as glucosamine sulfate potassium) 750 mg. Other Ingredients: Gelatin, Microcrystalline Cellulose, Magnesium Stearate.

Glucosamine Sulfate - Arrowroot
Each tablet contains: Glucosamine Sulfate 500 mg (from natural seafood extract).

Glucosamine Sulfate - Metagenics
Two tablets contain: D-Glucosamine Sulfate 1000 mg • Vitamin C (as ascorbic acid) 60 mg.

Glucosamine Sulfate - PhytoPharmica
Each capsule contains: Glucosamine Sulfate 500 mg.

Glucosamine Sulfate & Shark Cartilage - Swanson Health Products
Each tablet contains: Glucosamine Sulfate (2KCl) 500 mg • Shark Cartilage 250 mg.

Glucosamine Sulfate 1,000 mg - Pure Encapsulations
Each vegetable capsule contains: Glucosamine Sulfate (shellfish, from 1333 mg of glucosamine sulfate 2KCl [sodium free]) 1000 mg • Vitamin C (as ascorbyl palmitate) 16 mg.

Glucosamine Sulfate 1,000 mg - GNC
Each tablet contains: Glucosamine Sulfate (as D-Glucosamine Sulfate.2.NaCl) 1000 mg. Other Ingredients: Cellulose, Dicalcium Phosphate, Stearic Acid, Food Glaze, Silica, Magnesium Stearate.

Glucosamine Sulfate 1000 - GNC
Each tablet contains: Glucosamine Sulfate (as D-Glucosamine Sulfate.2NaCl) 1000 mg. Other Ingredients: Cellulose, Dicalcium Phosphate, Food Glaze.

Glucosamine Sulfate 1000 - Jarrow Formulas
Each tablet contains: Glucosamine Sulfate 2KCl 1340 mg: Glucosamine Sulfate 1000 mg, Potassium Chloride 340 mg (net potassium 178 mg, 5%). Other Ingredients: Cellulose, Modified Cellulose Gum, Stearic Acid, Magnesium Stearate.

Glucosamine Sulfate 1000 MG - PhysioLogics
Each capsule contains: Glucosamine Sulfate 2KCl 1000 mg. Other Ingredients: Gelatin, Vegetable Magnesium Stearate, Silica.

Glucosamine Sulfate 500 - Jarrow Formulas
Each capsule contains: Glucosamine Sulfate 2KCl 670 mg: Glucosamine Sulfate 500 mg, Potassium Chloride 170 mg. Other Ingredients: Magnesium Stearate, Gelatin, Titanium Dioxide.

Glucosamine Sulfate 500 mg - Vitamin World
Each capsule contains: Glucosamine Sulfate (2 KCl) 500 mg. Other Ingredients: Cellulose, Gelatin, Hydroxypropyl Methycellulose, Vegetable Magnesium Stearate.

Glucosamine Sulfate 500 MG - Puritan's Pride
Each capsule contains: Glucosamine Sulfate (2KCl) 500 mg. Other Ingredients: Calcium Phosphate, Gelatin, Vegetable Magnesium Stearate, Silica.

Glucosamine Sulfate 500 mg - Vital Nutrients
Each capsule contains: Glucosamine Sulfate (from 666 mg of glucosamine sulfate 2KCL) 500 mg.

Glucosamine Sulfate 500 MG - PhysioLogics
Each capsule contains: Glucosamine Sulfate 2KCl 500 mg. Other Ingredients: Calcium Phosphate, Gelatin, Vegetable Magnesium Stearate.

Glucosamine Sulfate 500mg & Chondroitin 400mg - Nature's Own
Each tablet contains: Glucosamine Sulfate / Potassium Chloride Complex 500 mg • Chondroitin Sulfate (shark) 400 mg • Copper (from gluconate) 7 mcg • Manganese (from sulfate monohydrate) 3.25 mg • Ascorbic Acid 50 mg.

Glucosamine Sulfate 550 - GNC
Each capsule contains: Glucosamine Sulfate (as D-Glucosamine Sulfate.2NaCl) 550 mg. Other Ingredients: Cellulose, Gelatin.

Glucosamine Sulfate 550 mg - GNC
Each capsule contains: Glucosamine Sulfate (as D-Glucosamine Sulfate.2NaCl) 550 mg. Other Ingredients: Cellulose, Gelatin, Magnesium Stearate.

Glucosamine Sulfate 650 mg - Pure Encapsulations
Each vegetable capsule contains: Glucosamine Sulfate (shellfish, from 866 mg of glucosamine sulfate 2KCl [sodium free]) 650 mg • Vitamin C (as ascorbyl palmitate) 8 mg.

Glucosamine Sulfate 750 - Metagenics
Two tablets contain: D-Glucosamine Sulfate 1500 mg • Vitamin C (as ascorbic acid) 60 mg.

Glucosamine Sulfate 750 mg - Vital Nutrients
Each capsule contains: Glucosamine Sulfate (from 940 mg of glucosamine sulfate 2KCL) 750 mg.

Glucosamine Sulfate 750 mg - Pro Health
Two capsules contian: Potassium (as potassium chloride) 187 mg • Glucosamine Sulfate (as glucose potassium sulfate) 1500 mg. Other Ingredients: Gelatin, Magnesium Stearate, Microcrystalline Cellulose, Silicon Dioxide, Rice Flour.

Glucosamine Sulfate Capsules - J. R. Carlson Laboratories, Inc.
Each capsule contains: Chloride 124 mg • Sodium 80 mg • Glucosamine Sulfate 750 mg.

Glucosamine Sulfate Capsules - PhytoPharmica
Three capsules contain: Stabilized Glucosamine Sulfate 1500 mg • Chloride (from glucosamine sulfate) 234 mg.

Glucosamine Sulfate Chewable - J. R. Carlson Laboratories, Inc.
Each tablet contains: Glucosamine Sulfate (providing sulfur 35 g) 500 mg.

Glucosamine Sulfate Chondroitin Sulfate - Progressive Natural Products
Each 1 tbsp serving contains: Glucosamine Sulfate 500 mg • Vitamin C 500 mg • Chondroitin Sulfate 150 mg • Shark Cartilage 50 mg • CMO 25 mg • Cherry extract 25 mg • Sea Cucumber 25 mg • Manganese Aspartate 5 mg • Zinc Citrate 5 mg • Boron Citrate 1 mg. See Editor's Note No. 15.

Glucosamine Sulfate Complex - PhytoPharmica
Three capsules contain: Vitamin C (ascorbic acid) 1,000 mg • Chloride (from glucosamine sulfate) 156 mg • Sodium 100 mg •Stabilized Glucosamine Sulfate 1,000 mg •L-Tyrosine 500 mg. See Editor's Note No. 21.

Glucosamine Sulfate Packets - PhytoPharmica
Each packet contains: Chloride (from glucosamine sulfate) 234 mg • Glucosamine Sulfate (stabilized) 1500 mg.

Glucosamine Sulfate Packets (orange flavor) - PhytoPharmica
Each packet contains: Carbohydrate <1 gm • Chloride (from glucosamine sulfate) 234 mg • Sodium (from glucosamine sulfate) 150 mg •Stabilized Glucosamine Sulfate (equivalent to three, 500 mg capsules) 1,500 mg.

Glucosamine Sulfate, 750 mg Complex, Superior Joint Support - NOW Foods
Two capsules contain: Potassium (as potassium chloride) 245 mg • Glucosamine Sulfate (from glucosamine potassium sulfate complex 2040 mg) 1500 mg. Other Ingredients: Gelatin (capsule), Magnesium Stearate.

Glucosamine Sulfate-750 - PhytoPharmica
Two tablets contain: Chloride (from glucosamine sulfate) 234 mg • Glucosamine Sulfate (stabilized) 1500 mg • Sodium 150 mg. Other Ingredients: Cellulose, Modified Cellulose, Magnesium Stearate, Lecithin, Carnauba Wax.

Glucosamine Synergy - Standard Process, Inc.
Each capsule contains: Proprietary Blend 31 mg: Calcium Lactate, Nutritional Yeast, Carbamide, Bovine Bone meal, Veal bone PMG extract, Bovine Liver, Defatted Wheat germ, Magnesium Citrate, Oat flour, Calcium Stearate, Inositol, Carrot root powder, Pea vine juice, Tillandsia Usneoide powder, Ribonucleic Acid, Beet root powder, Bovine Spleen, Ovine Spleen, Bovine Adrenal Cytosol extract, Bovine Kidney, Mushroom powder, Bovine Liver fat extract, Flaxseed oil extract, Mixed Tocopherols, Para-Aminobenzoate, Ascorbic Acid, Rice Bran, Soybean Lecithin, Vitamin A Palmitate, Cellulose, Cyanocobalamin, Cholecalciferol • Manganese 1 mg • Sodium 40 mg • Glucosamine Sulfate (from crab shells) 500 mg • Boswellia Serrata extract 60 mg. Other Ingredients: Gelatin, Water, Colors.
See Editor's Note No. 14.

Glucosamine With MSM - Nature's Way
Two tablets contain: Methylsulfonylmethane (MSM) 750 mg • Glucosamine Sulfate Potassium Chloride (providing glucosamine sulfate 750 mg) 1050 mg. Other Ingredients: Maltodextrin, Cellulose, Stearic Acid, Modified Cellulose, Silica, Glycerin.

BRAND NAMES

Glucosamine, Chondroitin & MSM - Swanson Health Products
Each tablet contains: Glucosamine Sulfate (2KCl) 500 mg • Chondroitin Sulfate 400 mg • OptiMSM (methylsulfonylmethane) 200 mg.

Glucosamine/Chondroitin With Support Nutrients - Benepure, Inc
Each capsule contains: Vitamin C 45 mg • Manganese 5 mg • Glucosamine Sulfate 500 mg • Chondroitin Sulfate 400 mg. Other Ingredients: Manganese Ascorbate, Calcium Ascorbate, Gelatin, Silicon Dioxide, Vegetable Stearate.

Glucosamine/Chondroitin/MSM - Doctor's Best, Inc.
Two capsules contain: Sodium (from chondroitin sulfate) 28 mg • Chondroitin Sulfate 600 mg • MSM (Lignisul MSM) 500 mg • Chloride (from glucosamine sulfate KCl) 84 mg • Glucosamine Sulfate KCl 750 mg • Potassium (from glucosamine sulfate KCl) 91 mg. Other Ingredients: Cellulose, Magnesium Stearate, Gelatin Capsule.
See Editor's Note No. 15.

Glucosamine/MSM Complex - Vitamin World
Three tablets contain: Vitamin C (as ascorbic acid) 60 mg • Manganese (as manganese sulfate) 5 mg • Glucosamine Sulfate (2KCl) 1500 mg • MSM (methylsulfonylmethane, 340 mg organic sulfur) 1000 mg • Ginger extract (zingiber officinale root, standardized for 4% volatile oils) 100 mg • White Willow (salix alba bark) 100 mg. Other Ingredients: Cellulose, Food Glaze, Vegetable Stearic Acid, Croscarmellose, Silica, Vegetable Magnesium Stearate.

Glucosamine-Bromelain Mega - Susan Ambrosino's Herb Club, Inc.
Each capsule contains: Glucosamine Sulfate 750 mg • Bromelain 125 mg.

Glucosamine-Sea Cucumber Mega - Susan Ambrosino's Herb Club, Inc.
Each capsule contains: Glucosamine Sulfate 500 mg • Sea Cucumber 150 mg • Shark Cartilage 150 mg • Bromelain 100 mg.

Glucosa-Plex - Progressive Labs
Each capsule contains: Vitamin C 50 mg • Vitamin E (succinate) 25 IU • Pantothenic Acid 50 mg • Glucosamine Sulfate 100 mg • N-Acetyl Glucosamine 50 mg • L-Glutathione 2 mg • N-Acetyl Cysteine 5 mg • L-Cysteine 50 mg • L-Glutamic Acid 50 mg • L-Glycine 50 mg • L-Taurine 25 mg • Soluble Trachea (16% pure chondroitin sulfate-A) 25 mg • Milk Thistle (silybum marianum) 100 mg • Silymarin 5 mg • Green Lipped Mussel 25 mg (natural source of mucopolysaccharides and superoxide dismutase).
See Editor's Note No. 15.

Glucosatrin - Market America, Inc.
Three tablets contain: Vitamin C (ascorbic acid) 100 mg • Zinc (as zinc sulfate) 10 mg • Copper (as copper gluconate) 30 mcg • Manganese (as manganese sulfate) 5 mg • Glucosamine HCl 1500 mg • Scutellaria Baicalensis root (Chinese skullcap) 150 mg • Oleanolic Acid 150 mg • Boswellia Gum resin extract 200 mg • Hops strobile extract 350 mg. Other Ingredients: Microcrystalline Cellulose, Stearic Acid, Croscarmellose Sodium, Magnesium Stearate, Silica, Pharmaceutical Glaze.

Glucos-Bal - Nutri-Quest Rx
Each tablet contains: Vanadyl Sulfate 3 mg • Chromium (Picolinate) 200 mcg • Vitamin B1 10 mg • Vitamin B2 5 mg • Vitamin B6 5 mg • Vitamin B12 10 mcg • Folic Acid 200 mcg • Biotin 500 mcg • Pantothenic Acid (D-Calcium Pantothenate) 20 mg • Niacinamide 20 mg • Niacin 6 mg • Magnesium Aspartate 100 mg • Calcium Ascorbate 100 mg • Manganese Aspartate 4 mg • Zinc (Picolinate) 1 mg • Selenium (Chelate) 30 mcg.

Gluco-Science - Source Naturals
Two tablets contain: Vitamin C (as ascorbic acid) 333 mg • Vitamin E (as D-alpha tocopheryl) 118 IU • Magnesium (as magnesium citrate, oxide & malate) 50 mg • Zinc (as zinc citrate) 3 mg • Thiamin (vitamin B1) 8 mg • Riboflavin (vitamin B2) 8 mg • Niacinamide 66 mg • Vitamin B6 (as pyridoxine HCl) 33 mg • Folate (as folic acid) 200 mcg • Vitamin B12 (as methylcobalamin) 500 mcg • Biotin 2 mg • Vitamin B5 (as pantothenic acid and pantethine) 16 mg • Selenium (as L-selenomethionine and sodium selenite) 33 mcg • Manganese (as manganese cirate) 1 mg • Chromium (as chromium picolinate and ChromeMate brand) 133 mcg • Gymnema Sylvestre extract (25% gymnemic acids) 214 mg • Alpha Lipoic Acid 200 mg • N-Acetyl Cysteine 166 mg • Bitter Melon fruit extract 150 mg • Taurine 100 mg • Garlic clove 83 mg • Hawthorn berry 66 mg • American Ginseng extract 66 mg • Maitake fruiting bodies 66 mg • Pterocarpus Marsupium extract (5% pterostilbene) 66 mg • Eleutherococcus Senticosus root extract 66 mg • L-Glutamine 66 mg • Bilberry fruit extract (37% anthocyanosides) 40 gm • Blueberry leaf extract (20% chlorogenic acid) 33 mg • Fenugreek extract 33 mg • Grape seed extract (Proanthodyn brand) 33 mg • Quercetin 33 mg • Inositol 16 mg • Myricetin 16 mg • Coenzyme Q10 3.3 mg • Vanadium (as bis-glycinateo oxo vanadium) 33 mcg. Other Ingredients: Stearic Acid, Hydroxypropyl Cellulose, Modified Cellulose Gum, Colloidal Silicon Dioxide, Magnesium Stearate.

Glucose M1 - Progressive Health Nutraceuticals
Magnesium 100 mg • Chromium 200 mcg • Zinc 10 mg • Folic Acid 400 mcg • Selenium 500 mcg • Biotin 500 mcg • Vanadium 500 mcg • Alpha Lipoic Acid 600 mg • Bitter Melon extract 500 mg • Taurine 250 mg • Fenugreek 150 mg • Gymnema Sylvestris extract 100 mg.

Glucose M2 - Progressive Health Nutraceuticals
Magnesium 250 mg • Chromium 100 mg • Zinc 10 mg • Calcium 500 mg • Vanadium 500 mg • Alpha Lipoic Acid 300 mg • Bitter Melon extract 500 mg • Gymnema Sylvestris 100 mg.

Glucose Metabolism Factors - Michael's Naturopathic Programs
Nine tablets contain: Vitamin C (as calcium ascorbate) 300 mg • Thiamin 300 mg • Niacin (as niacinamide and 20% as nicotinic acid) 300 mg • Pantothenic Acid (as calcium pantothenate) 210 mg • Calcium (as calcium amino acid chelate) 150 mg • Iodine (from kelp) 675 mcg • Magnesium (as magnesium amino acid chelate) 300 mg • Zinc (as zinc monomethionine) 90 mg • Manganese (as manganese amino acid chelate) 60 mg • Chromium (as chromium polynicotinate) 450 mcg • Proprietary Blend 3900 mg: Essential Fatty Acids (from flax seed; 7% gamma linolenic acid, 64% linoleic acid), Nopales Opuntia cactus, Cedar berry (thuja occidentalis), Glutamine (as L-glutamine), Golden Seal root (hydrastis candensis), Gymnema Sylvestre leaf, Milk Thistle seed extract (silybum marianum, 80% silymarin, 240 mg), Blueberry leaf (vaccinium myrtillus), Bitter Melon seed (momordica charantia), Ginger root (zingiber officinale), Vanadium (vanadyl sulfate). Other Ingredients: Dicalcium Phosphate, Terra Alba (calcium sulfate), Maltodextrin, Magnesium Stearate, Stearic Acid.

Glucose Optimizer - Jarrow Formulas
Four tablets contain: Vitamin C (ascorbic acid) 300 mg • Niacinamide 300 mg • Vitamin B1 (thiamine mononitrate) 5 mg • Vitamin B5 (pantothenic acid) 25 mg • Vitamin B6 (pyrioxine HCl) 5 mg • Vitamin B12 (methylcobalamin) 100 mcg • Biotin 1000 mcg • Vitamin E (as tocopheryl succinate) 100 IU • Folic Acid (folate) 400 mcg • Magnesium (as oxide) 200 mg • Selenium (as methylselenocysteine) 50 mcg • Chromium (from 100 mg of saccharomyces cerevisiae nutritional yeast) 200 mcg • Alpha Lipoic Acid 200 mg • GlucoTrim Crepe Myrtle extract 48 mg • Gymnema Sylvestre (75% gymnemic acids) 300 mg • Bilberry (vaccinium myrtillus, 25% anthocyanosides) 40 mg • Green Tea 5:1 extract (camellia sinensis, 45% polyphenols) 200 mg • Bitter Melon (momordica charantia) 200 mg • Fenugreek fiber extract (trigonella

graecum) 150 mg • Eucalyptus leaf extract (eucalyptus globulus) 100 mg • Taurine 300 mg. Other Ingredients: Cellulose, Dicalcium Phosphate, Modified Cellulose Gum, Stearic Acid, Magnesium Stearate.

Glucose Regulation Complex - Shaklee
Two capsules contain: Magnesium (as Magnesium oxide) 200 mg • Zinc (as Zinc gluconate) 5 mg • Chromium (as Chromium polynicotinate) 400 mcg • Taurine 500 mg • Vanadium (as Vanadium amino acid chelate) 100 mcg • Alpha Lipoic Acid 10 mg • Banaba leaf extract (Lagerstroemia speciosa, standardized to contain 1% colosolic acid). Other Ingredients: Maltodextrin, Gelatin, Water.

Glucose Support Formula - Pure Encapsulations
Each vegetable capsule contains: Maitake 4:1 extract (grifola frondosa) 200 mg • Alpha Lipoic Acid (thioctic acid) 100 mg • Panax Ginseng extract (standardized to contain 27-30% ginsenosides) 100 mg • Eleuterhococcus Senticosus extract (standardized to contain 0.8% eleutheroside E & B) 100 mg • Gymnema Sylvestre extract (standardized to contain 75% gymnemic acids) 75 mg • Chromium (polynicotinate, providing nicotinic acid 1480 mcg, chromium 200 mcg).

Glucose Tabs - PhytoPharmica
Each tablet contains: Dextrose • Cellulose • Natural Raspberry Flavor • Citric Acid • Magnesium Stearate.

Glucosol - Olympian Labs
Each softgel contains: Glucosol brand Corosolic acid 1% standardized extract (lagerstroemia speciosa L., yeilding 240 mcg of corosolic acid) 24 mg.

Glucosol - Life Extension Foundation
Each softgel capsule contains: Corosolic Acid extract (from lagestroemia speciosa L.) 24 mg. Other Ingredients: Rice Bran oil, Gelatin, Glycerin, Silica, Carob extract, Water, Titanium Dioxide.

Glucosol - NOW Foods
Each softgel contains: Glucosol brand Corosolic Acid (lagerstroemia speciosa L. standardized to 1% corosolic acid) 24 mg. Other Ingredients: Gelatin, Glycerol, Carob extract, Water, Titanium Dioxide.

Glucosol - NSI - Nutraceutical Sciences Institute
Each capsule contains: Lagerstroemia Speciosa L. extract (glucosol) 24 mg. Other Ingredients: Cellulose, Magnesium Stearate.

Glucosol brand - Soft Gel Technologies, Inc.
Corosolic Acid.

Glucotize - Medical Research Instituite (MRI)
Each tablet contains: A-Lipoic Acid (thioctic acid) 300 mg. Other Ingredients: Calcium Phosphate, Cellulose Esthers & composites, Magnesium Stearate.

GlucoTrim Rx-Blood Sugar - Nature's Plus
Each softgel contains: GlucoTrim brand Lagerstroemia Speciosa L. (standardized 1% (480 mcg) corosolic acid) 48 mg. Other Ingredients: Rice Bran Oil, Gelatin, Glycerin, Silica, Water, Carob Extract.

Glucovite - TheraNutria
Six tablets contain: Vitamin A (67% as Beta-Carotene, 33% as Vitamin A Palmitate) 7500 IU • Vitamin C (Calcium Ascorbate) 1000 mg • Vitamin D (as Vitamin D3) 400 IU • Vitamin E (natural d-alpha, d-beta, d-gamma, d-delta-tocopherols) 100 IU • Vitamin K (as Vitamin K1) (Phylloquinone) 40 mcg • Thiamine (Mononitrate) 4.5 mg • Riboflavin 3.4 mg • Niacin (50% Niacin, 50% Niacinamide) 40 mg • Vitamin B6 (Pyridoxine HCl) 10 mg • Folic Acid 600 mcg • Vitamin B12 (Cyanocobalamin) 60 mcg • Biotin 200 mcg • Pantothenic Acid (D-Calcium Pantothenate) 20 mg • Calcium (Ascorbate, Propionate, Carbonate) 300 mg • Magnesium (Amino Acid Chelate) 200 mg • Iron (Amino Acid Chelate) 3.6 mg • Iodine (Potassium Iodide) 150 mcg • Zinc (Amino Acid Chelate) 15 mg • Copper (Amino Acid Chelate) 2 mg • Manganese (Amino Acid Chelate) 2 mg • Selenium (50% L-Selenomethionine, 50% Sodium Selenite) 140 mcg • Chromium (Glycine-Niacin Chelate) 600 mcg • Molybdenum (Amino Acid Chelate) 75 mcg • Boron (Citrate) 3 mg • Silicon (Sodium Metasilicate) 3 mg • Vanadium (Vanadyl Sulfate) 100 mcg • Citrus Bioflavonoids 10 mg • Quercetin 10 mcg • Glucosol Banaba leaf extract (L. speciosa L., min. 1% corosolic acid) 2 mg • Alpha-Lipoic acid (Thioctic acid). Other Ingredients: Modified Cellulose Gum, Cellulose, Vegetable Stearine, Silicon Dioxide, Magnesium Stearate, Hydroxymethyl Propylcellulose, Titanium Dioxide, Chlorophyll.

Glutagen - ANS - Applied Nutrition Sciences
Pure Glutamine.

Glutagenics - Metagenics
Each 1 tsp (4.33 g) serving contains: L-Glutamine 3500 mg • Deglycyrrhizinized Licorice root 10:1 extract (glycyrrhiza glabra) 500 mg • Aloe leaf extract (aloe barbadensis) 50 mg.

GlutAloeMine - Xymogen
Each 1 tsp serving contains: L-Glutamine 3 g • Arabinogalactan 2 g • Aloe leaf extract (standardized to 50% polysaccharides) 100 mg.

Glutamine - Golden Glow Natural Health Products
Each tablet contains: Glutamine 500 mg.

Glutamine - Life Enhancement Products, Inc.
Each capsule contains: L-Glutamine 750 mg. Other Ingredients: Silicon Dioxide, Gelatin, Magnesium Stearate.

Glutamine 1000 mg - Vital Nutrients
Each capsule contains: L-Glutamine 1000 mg.

Glutamine 500 mg - Pain & Stress Center
Each capsule contains: Glutamine 500 mg. Other Ingredients: Gelatin Capsule.

Glutamine Caps - Optimum Nutrition
Each capsule contains: L-Glutamine 1000 mg. Other Ingredients: Gelatin, Magnesium Stearate.

Glutamine Capsules - Universal Nutrition
Each capsule contains: L-Glutamine 750 mg • Manganese Sulfate 400 mcg • Potassium Phosphate 30 mg.

Glutamine Flora - Nutri-Quest Rx
Each tablet contains: Combined stabilized microencapsulated freeze-dried Lactobacillus Acidophilus, Bulgaricus & Bifidus 4.5 million IU • L-Glutamine 500 mg • Chlorophyll 20 mg • natural Vitamin E Succinate 5 IU.

Glutamine Fuel Capsules - TwinLab
Two capsules contain: L-Glutamine 1500 mg.

Glutamine Fuel Powder - TwinLab
Each teaspoonful contains: L-Glutamine 4500 mg (4.5 g).

Glutamine Powder - Vital Nutrients
Each 1 tsp serving contains: L-Glutamine 3500 mg.

Glutamine Powder - ProLab
Each 1 tsp (4.5 g) serving contains: L-Glutamine 4500 mg.

Glutamine Powder - Optimum Nutrition
Each 1 tsp (4.5 g) serving contains: L-Glutamine 4.5 g.

Glutathione (Reduced) 100 mg - Vital Nutrients
Each capsule contains: Glutathione (reduced) 100 mg.

Glutathione Booster - J. R. Carlson Laboratories, Inc.
Two capsules contain: Vitamin C (as ascorbic acid) 200 mg • Vitamin E (as D-alpha tocopheryl succinate) 100 IU • Riboflavin (vitamin B2) 5 mg • Selenium (as L-selenomethionine) 200 mcg • Milk Thistle seeds extract (silybum marianum) 140 mg • Asparagus concentrate (asparagus officinalis) 25 mg • Alpha Lipoic 50 mg • Garlic bulb (allium sativum, odorless) 100 mg • Glutathione 10 mg • L-Cysteine (N-acetyl) 200 mg • L-Glutamine 50 mg • L-Glycine 50 mg.

Glutathione Plus - Atrium Biotechnologies
Each capsule contains: L-Glutathione 50 mg • L-Glutamine 200 mg.

Glycemic Balance - Jarrow Formulas
Two scoops (48 g) contain: Vitamin A (as palmitate) 2500 IU • Vitamin C (as sodium ascorbate) 30 mg • Vitamin D (as ergocalciferol) 160 IU • Vitamin E (as D-alpha tocopheryl acetate) 15 IU • Thiamine (as thiamine mononitrate) 1 mg • Riboflavin 1 mg • Niacin (as niacinamide) 11 mg • Vitamin B6 (as pyridoxine hydrochloride) 1 mg • Folate (as folic acid) 208 mcg • Vitamin B12 (as cyanocobalamin) 3 mcg • Biotin 155 mcg • Pantothenic Acid (as D-calcium pantothenate) 5 mg • Calcium (as tricalcium phosphate) 334 mg • Iron (naturally occuring) 3 mg • Phosphorous 186 mg • Iodine (as potassium iodine) 30 mcg • Magnesium (as magnesium oxide) 215 mg • Zinc (as zinc gluconate) 8 mg • Selenium (as selenomethionine) 34 mcg • Copper (as copper gluconate) 1 mg • Manganese (as manganese gluconate) 1 mg • Chromium (as chromium polynicotinate) 120 mcg • Molybdenum (as sodium molybdate) 40 mcg • Sodium (from sodium ascorbate) 190 mg • Potassium (as potassium chloride) 600 mg • Inositol 110 mg • Choline (as choline bitartrate) 38 mg • Alpha Lipoic Acid 40 mg • Rice Protein • Non-GMO Soy Protein Isolate • Rice-X brand solubles (high antioxidant rice bran solubles) • Glutamine Peptides • EnergySmart brand Grape and Brown Rice concentrate • Coconut • Flaxseed Meal • Inulin - FOS (natural extract of chicory) • Lecithin • Carrageenan gum • Natural Flavor • Lo Han Kuo exract (momordica grosvenori).

Glycentials Antioxidant - Mannatech
Two tablets contain: Vitamin A (as dunaliella salina isolate [alpha-, beta-carotene, cryptoxanthin, zeaxanthin, lutein] in PNC) 2500 IU • Vitamin C (as ascorbic acid in PNC) 250 mg • Vitamin D (as cholecalciferol in PNC) 200 IU • Vitamin E (as d-alpha tocopheryl succinate, mixed d-alpha-, d-beta-, d-delta-, d-gamma-tocopherols, tocotrienols PNC) 200 IU • Thiamin (as thiamin mononitrate in PNC) 750 mcg • Riboflavin (as riboflavin in PNC) 850 mcg • Niacin (as niacinamide in PNC) 10 mg • Vitamin B6 (as pyridoxine hydrochloride, pyridoxal 5-phosphate in PNC) 4 mg • Folate (as folic acid in PNC) 400 mcg • Vitamin B12 (as cyanocobalamin in PNC) 12 mcg • Biotin (as biotin in PNC) 150 mcg • Pantothenic Acid (as d-calcium pantothenate in PNC) 5 mg • Calcium (as calcium carbonate, calcium citrate-malate-glycinate in ambroglycin) 500 mg • Iodine (as potassium iodide in ambroglycin) 75 mcg • Magnesium (as magnesium oxide, magnesium glycinate in ambroglycin) 250 mg • Zinc (as zinc glycinate in ambroglycin) 7.5 mg • Selenium (as selenomethionine in ambroglycin) 100 mcg • Copper (as copper glycinate in ambroglycin) 1 mg • Manganese (as manganese glycinate in ambroglycin) 1 mg • Chromium (as chromium dinicotinate-glycinate in ambroglycin) 100 mcg • Molybdenum (as molybdenum glycinate in ambroglycin) 37.5 mcg • Boron (as boron glycinate in ambroglycin) 1 mg • Silica (as silica glycinate in ambroglycin) 1 mg • Vanadium (as vanadium glycinate in ambroglycin) 25 mcg • Proprietary Blend Ambroglycin 240 mg: Glycinated Multiminerals Combined with Watercress (leaves), Spinach (leaves), Green Peas (fruit), Ginger (root), Ambrotose Complex (patent pending), Arabinogalactan (larix decidua gum) Manapol Aloe Vera gel extract (inner leaf gel), Gum Ghatti, Gum Tragacanth • Phytonutrient Complex 2 (PNC) 25 mg: Acerola Cherry (fruit), Orange (peel), Rice Bran, Rose Hips, Soy Protein containing Isoflavones • Inositol 12.5 mg • Choline (as choline bitartrate) 11 mg • Alpha-Lipoic Acid 25 mg • Quercetin 5 mg • Coenzyme Q10 4.5 mg. Other Ingredients: Microcrystalline Cellulose, Silicon Dioxide, Croscarmellose Sodium, Stearic Acid, Magnesium Stearate, Dibasic Calcium Phosphate, Pharmaceutical Glaze.

Glycerin and Rosewater - Walgreens
Water • Glycerin • Methylparaben • Fragrance.

Glycine - J. R. Carlson Laboratories, Inc.
Each 1 tsp serving contains: Glycine 2300 mg.

Glycine - Pure Encapsulations
Each vegetable capsule contains: Glycine (free-form) 500 mg • Vitamin C (as ascorbyl palmitate) 20 mg.

Glycine 500 mg - Solgar
Each capsule contains: Glycine (as aminoacetic acid) 500 mg. Other Ingredients: Vegetable Cellulose, Microcrystalline Cellulose, Vegetable Magnesium Stearate, Vegetable Stearic Acid, Water, Vegetable Glycerin.

Glycine 500 mg - Pain & Stress Center
Each capsule contains: Glycine 500 mg. Other Ingredients: Gelatin Capsule.

Glycine Powder - Pain & Stress Center
Each 1/8 tsp serving contains: Glycine 500 mg.

GLYCO-8 - Pharmagel
Glycolic Acid • Alpha Hydroxy Acids • Antioxidants.

Glyco-B - Atrium Biotechnologies
Each tablet contains: Vitamin B1 35 mg • Vitamin B2 35 mg • Vitamin B6 35 mg • Vitamin B12 35 mcg • Vitamin C 180 mg • Pantothenic Acid 80 mg • Niacinamide 180 mg • Folic Acid 135 mcg • Choline Bitartrate 25 mg • Inositol 10 mg • Biotin 10 mcg • L-Lysine HCL 10 mg • Brewer's Yeast 50 mg • Pancrelipase 20 mg • Selenium 2 mcg • Adrenal 4 mg • Brain 4 mg • Liver 7 mg • Pancreas 2 mg.
See Editor's Note No. 31.

Glycobar: Chocolate Chip - Pharmanex
Each bar contains: Honey • Peanut Butter: Peanuts, Salt • Semi Sweet Chocolate Chips: Sugar, Chocolate Liquor, Cocoa Butter, Soy Lecithin, Vanilla • Brown Sugar • Date Puree • Prune Puree • Rolled Oats • Sugar Beet Fiber • Brown Crisp Rice: Rice Flour, Rice Bran, Rosemary Extract • Modified Guar Gum • Oat Bran • Peanuts • Barley Flakes • Rye Flakes • Soybean Oil • Soy Lecithin • Whey Powder.

Glycobar: Peanut Butter and Jelly - Pharmanex
Each bar contains: Honey • Peanut Butter: Peanuts, Salt • Brown Sugar • Date Puree • Prune Puree • Rolled Oats • Strawberry and Blueberry Fruit Chips: Sugar, Strawberries, Blueberries, Glucose, Pectin, Citric Acid, Sodium Citrate, Natural Flavor • Brown Crisp Rice: Rice Flour, Rice Bran, Rosemary Extract • Modified Guar Gum • Oat Bran • Peanuts • Yogurt Chips: Sugar, Hydrogenated Palm Kernel Oil, Milk Solids, Color (Titanium Dioxide), Soy Lecithin, Vanilla • Barley Flakes • Rye Flakes • Soybean Oil • Soy Lecithin • Whey Powder.

GlycoBears with Ambrotose Complex (GlycoBears, Glyco Bears, Glyco-Bears) - Mannatech
Two tablets contain: Vitamin A (as retinyl palmitate, beta carotene and dunaliella salina extract [alpha carotene cryptoxanthin zeaxanthin leutin] in PNC) 2500 IU • Vitamin C (as ascorbic acid, sodium ascorbate and acerola cherry in PNC) 30 mg • Vitamin D3 (as cholecalciferol in PNC) 200 IU • Vitamin E (as d-alpha-tocopherol succinate and mixed d-alpha-, d-beta-, d-delta-, and d-gamma-tocopherols in PNC) 15 IU • Thiamin (as thiamin mononitrate in PNC) 0.75 mg • Riboflavin 0.85 mg • Niacin (as niacinamide in PNC) 10 mg • Vitamin B6 (as pyridoxine hydrochloride in PNC) 1 mg • Folate (as folic acid in PNC) 200 mcg • Vitamin B12 (as cyanocobalamin in PNC) 3 mcg • Biotin 150 mcg • Pantothenic Acid (as d-calcium pantothenate in PNC) 5 mg • Calcium (as calcium carbonate and calcium citrate in PNC) 12.5 mg • Iodine (as potassium iodide and kelp in PNC [ascophyllum nodosum - whole plant]) 37.5 mcg • Magnesium (as magnesium glycinate in PNC) 2 mg • Zinc (as zinc citrate in PNC) 3.75 mg • Selenium (as selenomethionine in PNC) 17.5 mcg • Copper (as cupric oxide and copper glycinate) 0.5 mg • Manganese (as manganese citrate in PNC) 0.5 mg • Chromium (as chromium niacinate diglycinate) 30 mcg • Molybdenum (as sodium molybdate in PNC) 20 mcg • Potassium (as potassium citrate in PNC) 2 mg • Choline (as choline bitartrate in

PNC) 0.4 mg • Inositol 1 mg • PABA (p-aminobenzoic acid in PNC) 200 mcg • Vanadium (as vanadium glycinate) 10 mcg • Bioflavonoids 10 mcg • Proprietary Blend Ambrotose Complex (patent pending) 12.5 mg: Arabinogalactan (larix decidua gum), Manapol Aloe Vera gel extract (inner leaf gel), Gum Ghatti, Gum Tragacanth • Phytonutrient Complex (PNC) 25 mg: Pineapple, Broccoli, Carrot, Apple, Orange, Tomato, Cauliflower, Brussels Sprout, Beet, Blueberry, Celery, Grape, Grapefruit, Kale, Plum, Raspberry, Spinach, Strawberry, Watermelon, Radish, Lemon, Lime, Cantaloupe, Cherry, Leek or Yellow Pepper, Onion, Papaya, Peach, Pear, Ginger, Green Peas. Other Ingredients: Sorbitol, Stearic Acid, Fructo-Oligosaccharides, Natural Flavors (berry burst only), Dibasic Calcium Phosphate, Turmeric (tropical zing only), Natural Flavors (tropical zing only), Citric Acid, Magnesium Stearate, Malic Acid (berry burst only), Silicon Dioxide, Rice Syrup Solids, Carmine (berry burst only).

Glycogenics **-** Metagenics
Each tablet contains: Vitamin C (as ascorbic acid) 125 mg • Thiamin (as thiamin mononitrate) 14 mg • Riboflavin 16 mg • Niacin (as niacin and niacinamide) 200 mg • Vitamin B6 (as pyridoxine hydrochloride) 22 mg • Folate (as folic acid, L-5-methyl tetrahydrofolate, 5-formyl tetrhydrofolate) 400 mcg • Vitamin B12 (as cyanocobalamin) 250 mcg • Biotin 250 mg • Pantothenic Acid (as D-calcium pantothenate) 75 mg • Choline (as choline bitartrate) 100 mg • Inositol 94 mg • Para-Aminobenzoic Acid (PABA) 15 mg.

GlycoLEAN Accelerator **-** Mannatech
Country Mallow (contains ephedrine) • Proprietary Blend of antioxidants, digestive enzymes, and nutrients.
See Editor's Note No. 17 and No. 39.

GlycoLEAN Accelerator 2 **-** Mannatech
Two capsules contain: Chromium (as chromium dinicotinate glycinate, chromium polynicotinate) 30 mcg • Proprietary Herbal/ Botanical Blend 582 mg: Bitter Orange extract (fruit), Green Tea extract (leaves), American Ginseng (root), Guarana extract (seed), Gotu Kola (leaves), Eleutherococcus Senticosus extract (root), Cinnamon (bark), Curcumin (root), Milk Thistle extract (seed), Bladderwrack (whole plant), Dandelion root, Cayenne (fruit) • Ambrotose Complex (patent pending): Arabinogalactan (larix decidua gum), Manapol Aloe Vera gel extract (inner leaf gel), Gum Ghatti, Gum Tragacanth • Piperine 2.5 mg. Other Ingredients: Gelatin, Microcrystalline Cellulose, Silicon Dioxide, Magnesium Stearate, Stearic Acid.
See Editor's Note No. 40.

GlycoLEAN Catalyst **-** Mannatech
Two tablets contain: Vitamin A (as dunaliella salina isolate [alpha-, beta-carotene, cryptoxanthin, zeaxanthin lutein] in PNC) 2500 IU • Vitamin C (as ascorbic acid in PNC) 180 mg • Vitamin D (as cholecalciferol in PNC) 200 IU • Vitamin E (as d-alpha tocopheryl succinate, mixed d-alpha-, d-beta-, d-delta-, d-gama-tocopherols, and tocotrienols in PNC) 30 IU • Thiamin (as thiamin mononitrate in PNC) 3 mg • Riboflavin (as riboflavin in PNC) 3.4 mg • Niacin (as niacinamide in PNC) 10 mg • Vitamin B6 (as pyridoxine hydrochloride, pyridoxine-5 phosphate in PNC) 4 mg • Folate (as folic acid in PNC) 200 mcg • Vitamin B12 (as cyanocobalamin in PNC) 12 mcg • Biotin (as biotin in PNC) 150 mcg • Pantothenic Acid (as d-calcium pantothenate in PNC) 20 mg • Calcium (as calcium carbonate, calcium citrate-malate-glycinate in ambroglycin) 500 mg • Iodine (as potassium iodide in ambroglycin) 75 mcg • Magnesium (as magnesium oxide, magnesium glycinate, in ambroglycin) 245 mg • Zinc (as zinc glycinate in ambroglycin) 7.5 mg • Selenium (as selenomethionine in ambroglycin) 100 mcg • Copper (as copper glycinate in ambroglycin) 1 mg • Manganese (as manganese glycinate in ambroglycin) 1 mg • Chromium (as chromium dinicotinate glycinate in ambroglycin) 200 mcg • Molybdenum (as molybdenum glycinate in ambroglycin) 37.5 mcg • Blue Green Algae (as spirulina pratensis) 100 mg • Proprietary Blend Ambroglycin 248 mg: Glycinated Multiminerals Combined with Watercress (leaves), Spinach (leaves), Green Peas (fruit), Ginger (root), Ambrotose Complex (patent pending), Arabinogalactan (larix decidua gum), Manapol Aloe Vera gel extract (inner leaf gel), Gum Ghatti, Gum Tragacanth • Choline (as choline bitartrate) 25 mg • Inositol 12.5 mg • Phytonutrient Complex 2 (PNC) 18 mg: Acerola Cherry (fruit), Orange (peel), Rice Bran, Rose Hips, Soy Protein Containing Isoflavones • Alpha-Lipoic Acid 7.5 mg • Coenzyme Q10 6 mg • Boron (as boron glycinate in ambroglycin) 1 mg • Vanadium (as vanadyl glycinate in ambroglycin) 100 mcg. Other Ingredients: Microcrystalline Cellulose, Croscarmellose Sodium, Stearic Acid, Silicon Dioxide, Magnesium Stearate, Dibasic Calcium Phosphate, Pharmaceutical Glaze.

GlycoLEAN Fiber Full **-** Mannatech
Each capsule contains: Magnesium (as magnesium aspartate, magnesium citrate, magnesium oxide) 50 mg • Proprietary Blend 450 mg: Glucomannan, Arabinogalactan (larix decidua), Aloe Vera gel extract (inner leaf gel) • Flax (seed) 50 mg • Spirulina Platensis 50 mg • Gotu Kola (leaves) 25 mg • Lactobacillus Sporogenes 25 mg • Lipase 5 mg. Other Ingredients: Gelatin, Magnesium Stearate, Silicon Dioxide, Cellulose.

GlycoLEAN GlycoSlim Drink Mix (chocolate flavor) **-** Mannatech
Soy Protein Isolate • Fructose • Inulin • Safflower Oil (non-hydrogenated) • Corn Syrup solids (non-hydrogenated) • Cocoa • Fructo-Oligosaccharides • Natural Flavors • Dicalcium Phosphate • Gum Blend: Cellulose Gum, Xanthan Gum, Carrageenan • Ascorbic Acid • Ferrous Fumarate • Magnesium Oxide • Silicon Dioxide • Beta Carotene • Biotin • Sodium Caseinate • Monoglycerides • Diglycerides • Dipotassium Phosphate • Sodium Chloride • D-Alpha-Tocopheryl Acetate • Lecithin • Zinc Citrate • Sodium Molybdate • Niacinamide • D-Calcium Pantothenate • Rice Protein concentrate • Pea Protein concentrate • Manganese Sulfate • Folic Acid • Copper Citrate • Chromium Dinicotinate-Glycinate • Selenomethionine • Pyridoxine Hydrochloride • Cholecalciferol • Thiamin Hydrochloride • Riboflavin • Cyanocobalamin • Potassium Iodide.

GlycoLEAN GlycoSlim Drink Mix (French vanilla flavor) **-** Mannatech
Soy Protein Isolate • Non-Dairy Creamer (safflower oil, corn syrup solids, sodium caseinate, dipotassium phosphate, monoglycerides, diglycerides, lecithin, tocopherols, natural flavors, silicon dioxide) • Fructose • Inulin • Natural Flavors •Fructo-Oligosaccharides • Dicalcium Phosphate • Gum Blend: Cellulose Gum, Xanthan Gum, Carrageenan • Magnesium Oxide • Beta Carotene • Silicon Dioxide • Rice Protein concentrate • Ascorbic Acid • Ferrous Fumarate • Zinc Citrate • D-Alpha-Tocopheryl Acetate • Sodium Molybdate • Biotin • Niacinamide • Selenomethionine • D-Calcium Pantothenate • Pea Protein concentrate • Manganese Sulfate • Copper Citrate • Folic Acid • Chromium Dinicotinate-Glycinate • Cholecalciferol • Pyridoxine Hydrochloride • Thiamin Hydrochloride • Riboflavin • Cyanocobalamin • Potassium Iodide.

GlycoLEAN Manager **-** Mannatech
Bitter Orange (contains synephrine) • Proprietary Blend of antioxidants, digestive enzymes, and nutrients.
See Editor's Note No. 17 and No. 40.

GlycoLoad **-** Optimum Nutrition
Each heaping scoop (59 g) contains: Proprietary GlycoLoad Carbohydrate Blend: Dextrose, Maltodextrin, Fructose • Non-GMO Soy Protein Isolate • Citric Acid • Calcium Citrate • Natural Flavor • Potassium Chloride • Natural Beet Color • Salt • Magnesium Oxide • Ascorbic Acid • D-Alpha Tocopheryl Succinate (natural vitamin E) • Dicalcium Phosphate • Biotin • Zinc Oxide • Niacinamide • Vitamin A Palmitate • D-Calcium Pantothenate • Folic Acid • Pyridoxine Hydrochloride • Riboflavin • Selenomethionine • Thiamin Mononitrate • Cyanocobalamin.

Glycoplex **-** Progressive Labs
Three capsules contain: Vitamin C 500 mg • Thiamin (Vitamin B1) 100 mg • Riboflavin (Vitamin B2) 100 mg • Niacinamide 500 mg • Vitamin B6 100 mg • Folate (folic acid) 300 mcg • Vitamin B12

50 mcg • Biotin 15 mcg • Pantothenic Acid (calcium pantothenate) 250 mcg • Chromium (chromium picolinate) 200 mcg • Inositol 50 mg • Pancrelipase 50 mg • Choline Bitartrate 50 mg • Pyloric substance 45 mg • Para Amino Benzoic Acid (PABA) 60 mg • L-Lysine Monohydrochloride 30 mg. Other Ingredients: Raw Adrenal, Raw Pancreas, Raw Brain and Raw Liver concentrates. See Editor's Note No. 31.

Glycyrrhizinate Forte - Jarrow Formulas
Each capsule contains: Monoammonium Glycyrrhizinate 75 mg • Glycyrrhetinic Acid 98% 75 mg • Glycine 75 mg • L-Methionine 75 mg. Other Ingredients: Celluose, Stearic Acid, Silicon Dioxide, Gelatin.

Goatein IG - Garden of Life, Inc.
Five caplets contain: Poten-Zyme Pure Goat's Milk Protein 4550 mg • Pure Goat's Milk Colostrum 450 mg. Other Ingredients: Cellulose, Stearates (vegetable source).

Goatein Pure Goat's Milk Protein - Garden of Life, Inc.
Each heaping tablespoon (15 g) contains: Goat's Milk Protein concentrate, Pre-digested Goat's Milk Protein concentrate containing a proprietary probiotic blend, Natural Vanilla.

Goat's Rue - Motherlove Herbal Co.
Each 2 oz bottle contains: Goat's Rue. Base: Certified Kosher Alcohol, Glycerin.

Go-Go Caps - Susan Ambrosino's Herb Club, Inc.
Each capsule contains: Proprietary Blend 650 mg: Cordyceps, Bee Pollen, Wild Yam, Tienchi, Licorice root, Hawthorne berry, Royal Jelly 3.5% extract.

Gold Label Noni Juice - Global Health Trax
Two tablespoons (1 fl oz) contain: Vitamin C 10 mg. Other Ingredients: Purified Water, Noni Fruit Juice Concentrate, Raspberry Juice Concentrate, Natural Flavors, Citric Acid, Kelp.

Gold Quest - Nulab, Inc.
Three capsules contain: Vitamin A (as acetate) 5000 IU • Beta Carotene 1 mg • Vitamin D (as vitamin D3) 600 IU • Vitamin E (as dl-alpha tocopheryl acetate) 45 IU • Vitamin C (as ascorbic acid) 90 mg • Thiamine (vitamin B1) 3 mg • Riboflavin (as vitamin B2) 3 mg • Niacinamide (as vitamin B3) 30 mg • Vitamin B6 (as pyridoxine HCL) 4 mg • Folate (as folic acid) 400 mcg • Vitamin B12 (as cyanocobalamin) 6 mg • Biotin 300 mcg • Pantothenic Acid (as calcium pantethonate) 10 mg • Calcium (as dicalcium phosphate) 30 mg • Magnesium (from magnesium oxide) 15 mg • Zinc (zinc aminoate) 15 mg • Copper (copper gluconate) 2 mg • Manganese (manganese aminoate) 7 mg • Iodine (potassium iodine) 150 mcg • Selenium (selenium aspartate) 100 mcg • Protein Blend 300 mg: Rice Protein, Egg-White Protein • Proprietary Herb Blend 432 mg: Maral root extract (leuzea carthamoides), Oat Straw extract (avena sativa), Black Currant powder (ribes nigrum). Other Ingredients: Gelatin, Water.

Gold Specifics Cardio Support - Solgar
Each three tablets contain: Calcium 175 mg • Magnesium (glycinate, oxide) 200 mg • Taurine 800 mg • Trimethylglycine (TMG, from beets) 800 mg • Soy Isoflavone Concentrate (seed) 500 mg • L-Carnitine 300 mg • Standardized Hawthorne extract (leaf/flower, vitexin 2 mg, 1.8%) 125 mg • Cayenne Powder (fruit) 100 mg • Coenzyme Q-10 (as ubiquinone) 60 mg • Grape Seed extract (phenolics 48 mg, 95%) 50 mg. Inactive Ingredients: Microcrystalline Cellulose, Vegetable Stearic Acid, Vegetable Cellulose, Methacrylic Acid, Silica, Vegetable Magnesium Stearate, Titanium Dioxide, Grapeskin, Natural Vitamin E (mixed tocopherols), Natural Beta Carotene, Other Carotenoids, Rosemary extract (aerial), Vitamin C (l-ascorbic acid), Vegetable Glycerin, Glyceryl Triacetate.

Gold Specifics Prostate Support - Solgar
Each two vegicaps contain: Calcium 25 mg • Zinc (as zinc glycinate) 10 mg • Selenium (as l-selenomethionine) 25 mcg • Sodium 15 mg • Modified Citrus Pectin 200 mg • Standardized Pygeum Africanum extract (bark, phytoesterols 3-5 mg, 2-3%) 150 mg • Standardized Saw Palmetto extract (berry, free fatty acids 68-75 mg, 45-50%) 150 mg • Standardized Stinging Nettles extract (leaf, silic acid 2 mg, 1%) 150 mg • Pumpkin powder (seed) 100 mg • Soy Isoflavone Concentrate (seed) 100 mg • Lycopene (from tomato) 7 mg. Inactive Ingredients: Microcrystalline Cellulose, Vegetable Cellulose, Vegetable Magnesium Stearate, Titanium Dioxide, Natural Vitamin E (mixed tocopherols), Natural Beta Carotene, Other Carotenoids, Rosemary extract (aerial), Vitamin C (l-ascorbic acid), Vegetable Glycerin, Riboflavin, Caramel, Water.

Goldcare Capsules - Vitabiotics
Each capsule contains: Vitamin A 900 mcg • Vitamin D 10 mcg • Vitamin E 20 mg • Vitamin C 80 mg • Vitamin B1 (thiamin) 12 mg • Vitamin B2 (riboflavin) 5 mg • Vitamin B3 (niacin) 20 mg • Vitamin B6 (pyridoxine HCl) 20 mg • Folic Acid 500 mcg • Vitamin B12 (cyanocobalamin) 20 mcg • Pantothenic Acid 10 mg • Iron 6 mg • Magnesium 75 mg • Zinc 15 mg • Iodine 130 mcg • Manganese 2 mg • Copper 1.2 mg • Boron 1 mg • Chromium 100 mcg • Selenium 150 mcg • Citrus Bioflavonoids 16 mg • Natural Mixed Carotenoids 3 mg • Ginkgo Biloba extract 10 mg.

Golden Aloe - J. R. Carlson Laboratories, Inc.
Each softgel contains: Aloe Vera 200:1 concentrate 100 mg.

Golden Ener-Z - DreamPharm
Two capsules contain: Proprietary Blend: Cornu Cervi Parvum, Cardamom, Atractylodes, Codonopsis Pilosula, Angelica root, Licorice, Peony White root, Dolichos nut, Poria Cocos, Oryza Sativae germinatus, Barley sprouts, Ligustrum seed, Euryale seed, Deer Antler, Ginseng root, Dioscorea root, Crataegus fruit, Massa Medicata fermentata, Rehmannia cooked, Cnidium root, Cornus fruit, Polygonatum root, Psoralea Sorylifolia fruit, Astragalus root.

Golden Flax Meal - Nature's Life
Two tablespoons (17 g) contain: Low fat Omegaflo Flax seed meal (certified organic by Farm Verified Organic). Naturally occuring fatty acids: Alpha Linolenic Acid (Omega-3) 1710 mg • Linoleic Acid (Omega-6) 480 mg • Oleic Acid (Omega-9) 50 mg • Lignin Fiber 1003 mg • Lignan 13.6 mg.

Golden Flax Oil - Nature's Life
Each 1 tbsp serving contains: Lipid profile, based on a typical analysis of : Omega-3 as Alpha-Linolenic Acid EFA 8.6 g •Omega-6 as Alpha- Linoleic Acid EFA 2.7 g • Omega-9 as Oleic (Monounsaturated Fatty Acid) 2.4 g.

Golden Flax Oil 1000 mg - Nature's Life
Each capsule contains: 100% pure Flax oil (Certified Organically Grown) (Omegaflo Process fresh, unrefined, unfiltered, unbleached, virgin seed oil; Organically grown & processed according to California Organic Foods Act of 1990; Farm Verified Organic). Lipid profile based on a typical analysis: Omega-3 EFA as Alpha-Lenolenic Acid 570 mg • Omega-6 EFA as Linoleic Acid 180 mg • Omega-9 as Oleic Acid 160 mg • Vitamin A (from naturally occuring Beta Carotene) 286 IU • Vitamin E (from naturally occuring Tocopherols) 1 IU.

Golden Flower Blood Cleanser - Grandma's Herbs
Each capsule contains: Proprietary Blend 0.480 g: Burdock root, Pau d'Arco bark, Cleavers herb, Slippery Elm bark, Licorice root, Buckthorn bark, Cascara, Black Walnut hulls, Canaigre herb, Calendula flower, Aloe herb.

Golden Oolong Tea - Tea's Tea - Ito En (North America)
Each 16.9 fl oz bottle contains: Purified Water, Oolong Tea, Vitamin C (ascorbic acid).

Golden Primrose - J. R. Carlson Laboratories, Inc.
Each softgel contains: Evening Primrose oil (oenothera biennis) 1300 mg • GLA (gamma linolenic acid) 110 mg • Linoleic Acid (omega-6, cis) 850 mg • Oleic Acid (omega-9, cis) 80 mg.

BRAND NAMES

Some Brand Name Natural Products - What they Contain

www.NaturalDatabase.com contains MANY more listings than appear here.
Editor's Notes are located on pages 2155-2163.

Golden Seal 500mg - Nature's Own
Each tablet contains: Golden Seal extract (hydrastis canadensis) equivalent to dry root 500 mg.

Golden Spleen 500 - Enzymatic Therapy
Each capsule contains: Spleen Polypeptides 375 mg: A mixture of highly purified bovine-derived spleen polypeptides naturally present in the spleen, including Tuftsin, Splenopentin, Splenin, & Leukokinin • Goldenseal root extract 125 mg: (Hydrastis canadensis) standardized to contain 5% total Alkaloids including: Berberine, Hydrastine, & Canadine.
See Editor's Note No. 14.

Golden Years Tablets - Nature's Plus
Six tablets contain: Vitamin A (as beta carotene) 10,000 IU • Vitamin C (as ascorbic acid) 250 mg • Vitamin D (as ergocalciferol) 400 IU • Vitamin E (as D-alpha tocopheryl succinate) 100 IU • Thiamin (vitamin B1, as thiamine HCl) 25 mg • Riboflavin (vitamin B2) 25 mg • Niacin (as niacinamide) 50 mg • Vitamin B6 (as pyridoxine HCl) 25 mg • Folate (as folic acid) 400 mcg • Vitamin B12 (as cyanocobalamin) 100 mcg • Biotin 100 mcg • Pantothenic Acid (as calcium pantothenate) 50 mg • Calcium (as amino acid chelate/ complex) 300 mg • Iron (as amino acid chelate/complex) 18 mg • Phosphorus (as amino acid complex) 75 mg • Iodine (from kelp) 150 mcg • Magnesium (as amino acid chelate/complex) 150 mg • Zinc (as amino acid chelate/complex) 20 mg • Selenium (as amino acid complex) 50 mcg • Copper (as amino acid chelate) 0.5 mg • Manganese (as amino acid chelate/complex) 10 mg • Chromium (as amino acid chelate) 50 mcg • Potassium (as amino acid complex) 15 mg • Betaine HCl (from beet molasses) 175 mg • Phosphatidylcholine 100 mg • Unsaturated Fatty Acids from Safflower oil (vitamin F) 100 mg • Inositol 75 mg • RNA (ribonucleic acid) 75 mg • L-Glutamine (free form amino acid) 50 mg • Choline (as bitartrate) 32 mg • Citrus Bioflavonoids (from citrus sinensis, citrus limon) 25 mg • PABA (para-aminobenzoic acid) 20 mg • Rutin (from saphora japonica leaf) 10 mg • L-Glutathione 10 mg • Hesperidin (from citrus sinensis, citrus limon fruit) 10 mg • DNA (deoxyribonucleic acid) 7.5 mg. Other Ingredients: Microcrystalline Cellulose, Stearic Acid, Rice Bran, Magnesium Stearate, Rose Hips, Silica, Lecithin, Alfalfa, Papaya, Bromelain (from pineapple fruit), Watercress (rorippa nasturtium-aquaticum), Parsley, Green Cabbage leaf (brassica oleracea), Pharmaceutical Glaze.

Goldenseal - Pharmanex
Each capsule contains: Goldenseal root extract (Hydrastis canadensis) (4:1) 250 mg. Other Ingredients: Rice Flour, Gelatin, Magnesium Stearate, Silicon Dioxide.

Goldenseal - Leiner Health Products
Each caplet contains: Golden Seal extract (Hydrastis canadensis) root 100 mg. Other Ingredients: Calcium Carbonate, Cellulose, Maltodextrin, Hydroxypropyl Methylcellulose, Silicon Dioxide, Polyethylene Glycol 3350, Croscarmellose Sodium, Hydroxypropyl Cellulose, Pharmaceutical Glaze, Crospovidone, Magnesium Stearate, Yellow 5 Lake, Red 40 Lake, Blue 2 Lake, Titanium Dioxide, Polysorbate 80.

Goldenseal - Olympian Labs
Each capsule contains: Goldenseal root 500 mg.

Goldenseal & Echinacea - Olympian Labs
Each capsule contains: Goldenseal 225 mg • Echinacea 225 mg.

Goldenseal and Myrrh - Dial Herbs
Goldenseal • Myrrh.

Goldenseal Plus - Vital Nutrients
Each capsule contains: Hydrastis Canadensis root extract (goldenseal, standardized to 5% berberine/hydrastine) 100 mg • Goldthread 10:1 extract (coptis chinensis) 200 mg.

Goldenseal Root - NOW Foods
Two capsules contain: Goldenseal root powder (hydrastis canadensis) 1000 mg.

Goldenseal Root 500 - Jarrow Formulas
Each capsule contains: Goldenseal root (hydrastis canadensis) 500 mg. Other Ingredients: Magnesium Stearate, Gelatin.

Goldenseal Salve - Dial Herbs
Goldenseal • Myrrh • Shavegrass • Echinacea • Comfrey • Slippery Elm • Lobelia. In a base of Bees Wax , Glycerine & Cold Pressed Olive oil.

Goldenseal-Myrrh Virtue - Blessed Herbs
Goldenseal root • Myrrh Gum • Propolis • Grain alcohol & Distilled Water.

GolfoFlex - Pharmessen
Each capsule contains: Rosemary oil (rosmarinus officinalis) 6.5 mg • Clove oil (eugenia caryophyllata, bud) 2.5 mg. Other Ingredients: Methylcellulose, Avicel, Olive Oil, Aerosil (food grade certified), Capsule (100% vegetarian, certified Kosher & Pareve, & Halal).

GO-lite/am (Appetite Manager) - Enviro-Tech Nutritionals
Griffonia simplicifolia (Containing 5-hydroxytryptophan) • St. John's Wort.

GO-lite/fm (Fat Metabolizer) - Enviro-Tech Nutritionals
Chitosan • Vitamin C • Iodine • Chromium • Thermal Herbal Blend: Sida Cordifolia, Bitter Orange Peel • Yerba Mate leaf • Chitosan.
See Editor's Note No. 39 and No. 40.

Good Dream - DreamPharm
Each capsule contains: Proprietary Blend: Semen Zizyphi Spinosae, Albizziae Julibrissin, Caulis Polygoni Multiflori, Rhizoma Coptidis, Fructus Mori Albae, Fructus Schisandrae Chinensis, Radix Salviae Miltiorrhizzae, Radix Glycyrrhizae, Melatonin.
See Editor's Note No. 16.

Good Morning (Zetox) - Global Health Products
Two capsules contain: Zeolite 765 mg • Vitamin A 200 mcg • Vitamin C 15 mg • Vitamin D 1.25 mcg • Vitamin E 2.5 mg • Niacin 4.5 mg • Folic Acid 50 mcg • Pantothenic Acid 1.5 mg • Vitamin B6 0.5 mg • Riboflavin 0.4 mg • Thiamin 0.35 mg • Biotin 0.037 mg • Vitamin B12 0.25 mcg.

Good-Nite - Goldshield Elite
Each caplet contains: Melatonin 3 mg • Kava Kava root standardized extract (30% kavalactones) 250 mg • Herbal Extract Blend 275 mg: Valerian root standardized extract (0.8% valerenic acids), Catnip aerial parts, Chamomile flower, Hops stobile, Passion flower aerial parts, Skullcap root. Other Ingredients: Dicalcium Phosphate, Vegetable cellulose, Fractionated vegetable oil, Silica, Soy polysaccharides, and Vegetable resin glaze.
See Editor's Note No. 16.

Gotu Kola - Nature's Way
Two capsules contain: Gotu Kola (stem, leaf) 870 mg.

Gotu Kola - NOW Foods
Two capsules contain: Sodium 10 mg • Total Carbohydrate 540 mg • Gotu Kola leaf (Centella Asiatica) 900 mg. Other Ingredients: Stearic Acid.

Gotu Kola - FoodScience of Vermont
Each capsule contains: Gotu Kola (centella asiatica, yielding triterpenes 45 mg) 450 mg.

Gotu Kola - DaVinci Laboratories
Each capsule contains: Gotu Kola (centella asiatica, yielding triterpenes 45 mg) 450 mg.

Gotu Kola - Olympian Labs
Each capsule contains: Gotu Kola 450 mg.

Gotu Kola 500mg - Nature's Own
Each tablet contains: Gotu Kola extract (centella asiatica) equivalent to whole dry plant 500 mg.

Gram-Two Vitamin C - The Vitamin Shoppe
Two tablets contain: Vitamin C 2000 mg: as Ascorbic Acid and as mineral ascorbates of Calcium, Magnesium, Zinc, and Manganese • Bioflavonoids 250 mg: Hesperidin, Rose Hips, Acerola Cherry, Pectin, Orange, Grapefruit, Lemon, Rutin.

Grape Pip 100 mg - Pure Encapsulations
Each vegetable capsule contains: Grape seed extract (vitis vinifera, standardized to contain 92% polyphenols) 100 mg • Vitamin C (as ascorbyl palmitate) 3 mg.

Grape Pip 200 mg - Pure Encapsulations
Each vegetable capsule contains: Grape seed extract (vitis vinifera, standardized to contain 92% polyphenols) 200 mg • Vitamin C (as ascorbyl palmitate) 4 mg.

Grape Pip 50 mg - Pure Encapsulations
Each vegetable capsule contains: Grape seed extract (vitis vinifera, standardized to contain 92% polyphenols) 50 mg • Vitamin C (as ascorbyl palmitate) 3 mg.

Grape Pip 500 mg - Pure Encapsulations
Each vegetable capsule contains: Grape seed extract (vitis vinifera, standardized to contain 92% polyphenols) 500 mg • Vitamin C (as ascorbyl palmitate) 8 mg.

Grape Seed - Pharmanex
Each capsule contains: Grape seed extract (Vitis vinifera) (100:1) 75 mg. Other Ingredients: Rice Flour, Gelatin, Magnesium Stearate, Silicon Dioxide.

Grape Seed (PCO) Extract - PhytoPharmica
Each capsule contains: Grape Seed extract (standardized to contain 95% procyanidolic oligomers (PCOS)) 50 mg. Other Ingredients: Cellulose, Gelatin, Magnesium Stearate, Silicon Dioxide, Titanium Dioxide Color.
See Editor's Note No. 21.

Grape Seed (PCO) Phytosome - PhytoPharmica
Each capsule contains: Grape seed phytosome (vitis vinifera, standardized to contain 95% procyanidolic oligomers [PCOs]) bound to Phosphatidylcholine 50 mg.

Grape Seed 12g - Golden Glow Natural Health Products
Each tablet contains: Grape seed extract (vitis vinifera) 12 g.

Grape Seed 50 mg - Nature's Plus
Each capsule contains: Grape seed (vitis vinifera, standardized to 95% proanthocyanidins) 50 mg. Other Ingredients: Silica, Vegetable Cellulose, Purified Water.

Grape Seed Antioxidant - NOW Foods
Each capsule contains: Grape seed extract (95%) 60 mg • Citrus Bioflavonoids (40%) 300 mg.

Grape Seed Extract - Pro Health
Each capsule contains: Grape seed extract (vitis vinifera seed standardized for 95% proanthocyanidins) 105.3 mg. Other Ingredients: Rice Flower Powder, Silica Dioxide, Magnesium Stearate.

Grape Seed Extract - J. R. Carlson Laboratories, Inc.
Each tablet contains: Bioflavonoids 50 mg • Grape seed extract 130 mg.

Grape Seed Extract - Leiner Health Products
Each tablet contains: Grape seed extract (Vitis vinifera) seed 100 mg. Other Ingredients: Calcium Carbonate, Maltodextrin, Cellulose, Silicon Dioxide, Polyethylene Glycol 3350, Croscarmellose Sodium, Crospovidone, Magnesium Stearate, Hydroxypropyl Methylcellulose, Hydroxypropyl Cellulose, Polysorbate 80.

Grape Seed Extract - Metabolic Response Modifiers
Each capsule contains: Grape Seed extract (85-95% OPC's - offering a minimum 100 mg of OPC's with 20 mg of other vital flavonoids) 120 mg.

Grape Seed Extract - Olympian Labs
Each capsule contains: Grape Seed extract (120:1, consists of 85% Oligomeric Procyanidins) 100 mg.

Grape Seed Extract 100 mg - Vital Nutrients
Each capsule contains: Grape seed 60:1 extract 100 mg.

Grape Seed Extract Extra Strength with MAT - Olympian Labs
Each capsule contains: Grape Seed extract (120:1, consists of 85% Oligomeric Procyanidins) 200 mg. Other Ingredients: MAT (proprietary blend of nutritional ingredients).

Grape Seed Extract Formula - Quest
Each caplet contains: Grape Seed powder (Vitis vinffera) (Provided by 25 mg P.E. 1:100 standardized to contain not less than 95% leucoanthocyanins) 2500 mg • Citrus Bioflavonoids 200 mg providing Hesperidin 50 mg • Rutin powder 25 mg. Other Ingredients: Calcium Phosophate, Microcrystalline Cellulose, Vegetable Stearin, Croscarmellose Sodium, Magnesium Stearate (vegetable source).

Grape Seed Extract Plus - Atrium Biotechnologies
Each capsule contains: Grape seed extract (Leucocyanidins) 50 mg • Bioflavonoids 200 mg.

Grape Seed Liquid Suspension - Nature's Plus
Each dropperful (1 mL) contains: Grape seed (vitis vinifera, standardized 95% (23.75 mg) proanthocyanidins) 25 mg. Other Ingredients: Vegetable Glycerin, Purified Water, Potassium Sorbate, Stevia.

Grape Seed PCO Phytosome 100 mg - Enzymatic Therapy/ PhytoPharmica
Each capsule contains: Grape Seed phytosome (vitis vinifera, standardized to contain 95% procyanidolic oligomers (PCOs) from grape-seed extract bound to phosphatidylcholine) 100 mg. Other Ingredients: Gelatin, Magnesium Stearate, Silicon Dioxide, Titanium Dioxide Color.

Grape Seed Seed - Aboca USA, Inc
Each capsule contains: Grape Seed WPC (whole phytocomplex concentrate, vitis vinifera, standardized to 37.5% proanthocyanidins, yielding 108.75 mg per capsule) 290 mg. Other Ingredients: Gelatin.

Grapefruit Concentrate With Fiber & Herbs - Natrol, Inc.
Two capsules contain: Grapefruit concentrate 10:1 300 mg • Psyllium Husk fiber 100 mg • Rice Bran fiber 100 mg • Oat Bran fiber 100 mg • Licorice root 100 mg • Uva Ursi 100 mg • Apple Cider vinegar 50 mg • Deep Ocean Kelp 50 mg • Lecithin 50 mg • Spirulina 50 mg • Vitamin B6 (Pyridoxine HCL) 25 mg • L-Phenylalanine 25 mg • Cascara Sagrada 20 mg. This is a 10 time concentration of the equivalent of 3000 mg of Whole Grapefruit. Other Ingredients: Silicon Dioxide, Magnesium Stearate, Gelatin, Microcrystalline Cellulose.

Grapefruit Extract - NutriBiotic
Grapefruit extract.

Grapefruit Pectin - J. R. Carlson Laboratories, Inc.
Three tablets contain: Grapefruit Pectin 3 g.

Grapefruit Seed extract - Pure Encapsulations
Each vegetable capsule contains: Grapefruit seed extract (standardized to contain 49% polyphenols) 250 mg • Vitamin C (as ascorbyl palmitate) 10 mg.

Grapeseed Extract - Swanson Health Products
Each capsule contains: Grapeseed extract (95% proanthocyanidins) 50 mg.

Grapeseed Extract - PhysioLogics
Each capsule contains: Grapeseed extract 100 mg • Citrus Bioflavonoid (citrus sinensis) 300 mg. Other Ingredients: Gelatin, Vegetable Magnesium Stearate, Silica.

Some Brand Name Natural Products - What they Contain

www.NaturalDatabase.com contains MANY more listings than appear here.
Editor's Notes are located on pages 2155-2163.

Grapeseed Extract 100 mg **-** Puritan's Pride
Each capsule contains: Grapeseed extract 100 mg • Citrus Bioflavonoids 300 mg.

Grapeseed Extract 50 mg **-** Puritan's Pride
Each capsule contains: Grapeseed extract 50 mg • Citrus Bioflavonoids 500 mg.

Green 15 **-** Grandma's Herbs
Each capsule contains: Proprietary Blend 0.448 g: Wheat Grass herb, Alfalfa root, Red Raspberry leaf/pulp, Parsley herb, Barley Green herb, Spirulina herb, Horsetail Grass herb, Yucca root, Oat Straw herb, Nettle herb, Chia seed, Bee Pollen, Canaigre root, Ginseng root, Cayenne Pepper, Bladderpod herb, Aloe Vera herb. Other Ingredients: Gelatin.

Green Barley powder **-** Golden Glow Natural Health Products
Each 1 tsp serving contains: Barley powder (55%) • Rice powder • Kelp powder • Wheat leaf powder • Chlorella powder.

Green Black Walnut Wormwood Complex **-** NOW Foods
Two droppersful (16 mL) contains: 1.6 mL proprietary blend of Green Black Walnut hulls (Juglans species) • Wormwood herb (Artemisia absinthium) • Clove buds (Carophyllus species) extracts. Other Ingredients: Grain Alcohol, Distilled Water.

Green Chlorella **-** Wild Rose
Each tablet contains: Chlorella (chlorella pyrenoidosa) 200 mg.

Green Defense **-** Nature's Plus
Each scoop (8.5 g) contains: Yaeyama Chlorella (chlorella vulgaris) 500 mg • Spirulina (spirulina microalgae) 500 mg • Wheat grass juice (triticum vulgare) 400 mg • Barley grass juice (hordeum distichon) 400 mg • Green Kamut juice (triticum durum) 420 mg • Quinoa (chendopidium quinoa) 300 mg • Spinach (spinacia oleracea) 100 mg • Broccoli (brassica oleracea) 100 mg • Parsley (petroselinum sativum) 300 mg • Kale (brassica species) 80 mg • Green Tea extract (camellia sinensis, 45% polyphenols, 30# catechins) 30 mg • Milk Thistle (silybum marianum, 80% silymarin) 50 mg • Grape seed 100:1 extract (vitis vinifera, 95% polyphenols) 20 mg • Ginkgo Biloba 50:1 extract (24/6 ginkgoflavoneglycose/terpene lactones, <5 ppm ginkgolic acid) 30 mg • Bilberry 100:1 extract (vaccinium myrtillus) 20 mg • Licorice root extract (glycyrrhiza glabra, 10% glycyrrhizin) 50 mg • Inulin - FOS (chicory extract, cichorium intybus) 200 mg • Bioflavonoids (35%) 25 mg • Lecithin 500 mg • Rice Essence brand Rice Bran solubles 500 mg • Beet (beta vulgaris) 200 mg • Tomato (lyopersicon esculentum) 300 mg • Apple fiber (malus domestica) 800 mg • Ginger 50:1 (zingiber officinale, freeze-dried) 30 mg • Metabolin brand Propionibacterium Shermani metabolites and cell walls 100 mg. Other Ingredients: Rice Syrup Solids, Lo Han Kuo (momordica grosvenori), Guar Gum, Natural Flavor.

Green Hornet Liquid **-** Cytotec Solutions, Inc.
Unknown.
See Editor's Note No. 49.

Green Magma **-** Green Foods Corp.
Each 5.3 oz box contains: Proprietary Blend 150 g: Young Barley Grass powdered juice, Maltodextrin, Brown Rice.

Green Mate **-** Jarrow Formulas
Each capsule contains: Green Mate 5:1 extract (ilex paraguariensis, minimum 20% caffeoylguinic acid) 500 mg. Other ingredients: Cellulose, Magnesium Stearate, Silicon Dioxide, Gelatin.

Green Max Powder **-** Swanson Health Products
Each tablespoon (8.5 grams) contains: Vitamin A (as beta-carotene 40 mg) 66,666 IU • Soy Lecithin 2,142 g • Spirulina powder 1,356 g • Apple Fiber 1.35 g • Wheat Grass powder 445 mg • Alfalfa leaf powder 435 mg • Barley bran powder 435 mg • Brown Rice powder 350 mg • Chlorella (broken cell wall) 350 mg • Soy sprout powder 350 mg • Beet powder 335 mg • Lactobacillus probiotic culture 200 mg • Bee Pollen powder 150 mg • Royal Jelly powder 150 mg • Acerola cherry powder 115 mg • Barley grass powder 97 mg • Licorice root powder 60 mg • Dulse Thallus powder 20 mg • Ginkgo Biloba leaf powder 20 mg • Grape Seed extract (90% proanthocyanidins) 20 mg • Green Tea extract (50% polyphenols) 20 mg • Milk Thistle seed extract (80% silymarin) 20 mg • Astragalus root powder 10 mg • Bilberry powder 10 mg • Echinacea root powder 10 mg • Siberian Ginseng root powder 10 mg.

Green Multi **-** Nature's Life
Three tablets contain: Beta Carotene (equivalent to 25000 IU Vitamin A) 15 mg • Vitamin C 1000 mg • Vitamin E (d-Alpha Tocopheryl Succinate) 300 IU • Vitamin B1 (Thiamine Mononitrate) 25 mg • Vitamin B2 (Riboflavin, Riboflavin 5'-Phosphate) 25 mg • Vitamin B3 (Niacin) 25 mg • Pantothenic Acid (Calcium Pantothenate, Pantetheine-5' -Phosphate) 25 mg • Vitamin B6 (Pyridoxine HCl, Pyridoxal-5'-Phosphate) 25 mg • Folic Acid (Folacin) 400 mcg • Vitamin B12 100 mcg • Biotin (d-Biotin) 60 mcg • Choline (Bitartrate) 14 mg • Inositol (Niacinate) 20 mg • PABA (Para Aminobenzoic Acid) 25 mg • Boron (Citrate, Nature's Life Greens) 100 mg • Calcium (Carbonate, Citrate/Malate) 250 mg • Chromium (Picolinate, Polynicotinate) 100 mcg • Copper (Citrate, Gluconate) 1 mg • Iodine (Potassium Iodine, Nature's Life Greens) 75 mcg • Iron (Glycinate, Nature's Life Greens) 10 mg • Magnesium (Oxide, Nature's Life Greens) 125 mg • Manganese (Gluconate, Citrate) 6 mg • Molybdenum (Molybdate, Nature's Life Greens) 50mcg • Potassium (Gluconate, Iodide, Nature's Life Greens) 90 mg • Selenium (Selenite, Cysteine) 100 mcg • Vanadium (Vanadyl Sulfate) 25 mcg • Zinc (Picoliante, Monomethionine) 15 mg • Lemon Bioflavonoids Complex (50% active) 100 mg • Quercetin (Saphora japonica) 25 mg • Rutin (Sapora japonica) 25 mg • Hesperidin (Citrus fruit peel) 25 mg • Bromelain from Pineapple (2000 GDU/g) 25 mg • Papain from Papaya (2000 USP units/g) 25 mg • Betaine HCl, beets 25 mg • Amylase (30000 SKB IU/g) 6 mg • Lipase 10000 Usp IU/g) 6 mg • Cellulase (10000 USP IU/g) 6 mg • Nature's Life Greens powder 1000 mg.

Green Phytofoods **-** NOW Foods
Each nine gram serving contains: Lecithin fine powder 2000 mg • Spirulina (Hawaiian) 1000 mg • Alfalfa juice concentrate 700 mg • Wheat grass powder organic 500 mg • Barley grass powder organic 500 mg • Carrot powder 500 mg • Barley Malt powder 400 mg • Broccoli powder 350 mg • Brown Rice Bran 350 mg • Apple fiber 350 mg • Apple Pectin 300 mg • Oat Bran 300 mg • Chlorella powder 300 mg • Red Beet powder 300 mg • Panax ginseng root powder (min 5% Ginsenosides) 250 mg • Siberian Ginseng root powder (Eleutherococcus senticosus) 100 mg • Peppermint powder 150 mg • Green Tea extract (Camellia sinensis) (40% Catechins) 100 mg • Royal Jelly powder (min 5% 10-HDA) 100 mg • Fructo Oligo Saccharides (NutraFlora FOS) 100 mg • Trace Mineral concentrate 100 mg • Milk Thistle extract (80% Silymarin) 80 mg • Kelp powder 50 mg • Ginkgo Biloba extract (24% Ginkgo Flavonglycosides) 20 mg • Grape seed extract (95% Polyphenols) 20 mg • Bilberry extract (25% Anthocyanidins) 20 mg • Plant Based Enzymes 100 mg: Protease 12500 HUT, Lipase 200 LU, Lactase 200 LAC, Bromelain 5000 FCC, Amylase 2500 DU, Cellulase 500 CMC, Papain 6000 PU • Coenzyme Q10 10 mg • Alpha Lipoic Acid 10 mg • Stevia extract 10 mg.

Green Source **-** Puritan's Pride
Three tablets contain: Vitamin A (100% as Beta Carotene) 15,000 IU • Vitamin C 1000 mg • Vitamin D 400 IU • Vitamin E 250 IU • Thiamin (Vitamin B-1) 25 mg • Riboflavin (Vitamin B-2) 25 mg • Niacin 25 mg • Vitamin B-6 25 mg • Folic Acid 400 mcg • Vitamin B-12 25 mcg • Biotin 50 mcg • Pantothenic Acid 25 mg • Calcium 250 mg • Iron 15 mg • Iodine 150 mcg • Magnesium 125 mg • Zinc 15 mg • Selenium 25 mcg • Copper 500 mcg • Manganese 4 mg • Chromium 100 mcg • Molybdenum 50 mcg • Potassium 50 mg • Boron 1 mg • Choline Bitartrate 50 mg • Inositol 25 mg • PABA (Para-Aminobenzoic Acid) 25 mg • Citrus Bioflavonoids Complex (Orange) 100 mg • Quercetin 25 mg • Rutin 25 mg • Hesperidin (Orange) 10 mg • Bromelain (Pineapple-2000 GDU/gm) 20 mg •

Betaine Hydrochloride 20 mg • Papain (Papaya) 20 mg • Amylase 5 mg • Lipase 5 mg • Protease 1 mg • Cellulase 2.5 mg • Proprietary Lactobacillus blend 25 mg: L. Acidophilus, L. Bifidus, L. Bulgaricus (Milk-Free: minimum 1 billion viable micro-organisms per gram) • Oat Bran 25 mg • Pectin (Apple) 25 mg • RNA 35 mg • DNA 10 mg • Carotenoids 10 mg • Chlorophyll 4 mg • Vegetable Oil as Borage and Sunflower (dry, cold-pressed - providing Essential Fatty Acids, GLA) 100 mg • L-Glutathione 5 mg • Spirulina 1000 mg • Wheat grass juice (dry) 100 mg • Sprouted Barley juice (dry) 100 mg • Flaxseed Oil (dry) 100 mg • Chlorella (broken cell wall) 100 mg • Bee Pollen 100 mg • Siberian Ginseng (Eleutherococcus senticosus) root 50 mg • Dehydrated Garlic (allium sativum) bulb 10 mg • Proprietary herbal blend 60 mg: Echinacea (Echinacea purpurea) aerial, Milk Thistle (Silybum marianum) seed, Goldenseal (Hydrastis canadensis) root, Ginger root (Zingiber officinale), Ginkgo Biloba (Ginkgo biloba) leaf, Cayenne Pepper (Capsicum annuum) fruit. Other Ingredients: Cellulose (plant origin), Acacia Gum, Croscarmellose, Vegetable Stearic Acid, Vegetable Magnesium Stearate, Cellulose Coating.

Green Source Iron Free - Vitamin World
Three tablets contain: Vitamin A (100% as Beta Carotene) 15,000 IU • Vitamin C 1000 mg • Vitamin D 400 IU • Vitamin E 250 IU • Thiamin (Vitamin B-1) 25 mg • Riboflavin (Vitamin B-2) 25 mg • Niacin 25 mg • Vitamin B-6 25 mg • Folic Acid 400 mcg • Vitamin B-12 25 mcg • Biotin 50 mcg • Pantothenic Acid 25 mg • Calcium 250 mg • Iodine 150 mcg • Magnesium 125 mg • Zinc 15 mg • Selenium 25 mcg • Copper 0.5 mg • Manganese 4 mg • Chromium 100 mcg • Molybdenum 50 mcg • Potassium 50 mg • Boron 1 mg • Choline Bitartrate 50 mg • Inositol 25 mg • PABA (Para-Aminobenzoic Acid) 25 mg • Citrus Bioflavonoids Complex (Orange) 100 mg • Quercetin 25 mg • Rutin 25 mg • Hesperidin (Orange) 10 mg • Bromelain (Pineapple-2000 GDU/gm) 20 mg • Betaine Hydrochloride 20 mg • Papain (Papaya) 20 mg • Amylase 5 mg • Lipase 5 mg • Protease 1 mg • Cellulase 2.5 mg • Proprietary Lactobacillus blend 25 mg: L. Acidophilus, L. Bifidus, L. Bulgaricus (Milk-Free: minimum 1 billion viable micro-organisms per gram) • Oat Bran 25 mg • Pectin (Apple) 25 mg • RNA 35 mg • DNA 10 mg • Carotenoids 10 mg • Chlorophyll 4 mg • Vegetable Oil as Borage and Sunflower (dry, cold-pressed - providing Essential Fatty Acids, GLA) 100 mg • L-Glutathione 5 mg • Spirulina 1000 mg • Wheat grass juice (dry) 100 mg • Sprouted Barley juice (dry) 100 mg • Flaxseed Oil (dry) 100 mg • Chlorella (broken cell wall) 100 mg • Bee Pollen 100 mg • Siberian Ginseng (Eleutherococcus senticosus) root 50 mg • Dehydrated Garlic (allium sativum) bulb 10 mg • Proprietary herbal blend 60 mg: Echinacea (Echinacea purpurea) aerial, Milk Thistle (Silybum marianum) seed, Goldenseal (Hydrastis canadensis) root, Ginger root (Zingiber officinale), Ginkgo Biloba (Ginkgo biloba) leaf, Cayenne Pepper (Capsicum annuum) fruit. Other Ingredients: Cellulose (plant origin), Acacia Gum, Croscarmellose, Vegetable Stearic Acid, Vegetable Magnesium Stearate, Cellulose Coating.

Green Stuff - Gary Null & Associates (GNA)
Green Mix: Green Kamut juice, Wheat Grass juice, Barley Green juice, Alfalfa leaf, Oat grass juice, Broccoli, Parsley, Kale • Flaxseed • Raw Brown Rice • Fruit Juice Mix: Pineapple, Lemon, Lime • Carrot juice • Earthrise Farms Spirulina • Yucca root • Black Licorice root extract.

Green Tea - 70 - DaVinci Laboratories
Each capsule contains: Green Tea extract (camellia sinensis, yielding total polyphenols 450 mg, epigallo-catechin-3-gallate 350 mg) 500 mg. Other Ingredients: Rice Flour, Vegetable Cellulose.

Green Tea 500 mg - Jarrow Formulas
Each capsule contains: Green Tea 5:1 extract. Other Ingredients: Cellulose, Silicon Dioxide, Magnesium Stearate, Gelatin.

Green Tea Antioxidant - Enzymatic Therapy
Each capsule contains: Green Tea leaf extract (camellia sinensis, standardized to contain 47-52% polyphenols [catechin, epicatechin, epicatechin gallate, epigallocatechin gallate], 5-10% caffeine) 250 mg. Other Ingredients: Cellulose, Gelatin, Magnesium Stearate, Silicon Dioxide, Titanium Dioxide Color.

Green Tea Barley Essence - Green Foods Corp.
Each 5.3 oz jar contains: Proprietary Blend 150 g: Young Barley Grass powdered juice, Maltodextrin, Green Tea, Brown Rice, Natural Flavors.

Green Tea Bath - Abra Therapeutics
Sodium Borate • Sodium Sulfate • Sodium Chloride • Sodium Sesquicarbonate • Olive Oil • Herbal Extract Blend: Organic Whole Leaf Green Tea, Calendula, Chamomile flowers • Essential Oils Blend: Lemongrass oil, Grapefruit oil, Sweet Orange oil, Sweet Marjoram oil.

Green Tea Body Lotion - Abra Therapeutics
Organic Green Tea tips in spring water • Aloe Vera juice • Apricot • Coconut • Jojoba oil • Vegetable Emulsifying wax • Vegetable Glycerin • Shea Butter • Extract of Organic Green Tea leaf • Calendula flowers • Chamomile flowers • Rosehips Bioflavonoids • Natural Vitamin E • Essential Oils Blend: Lemongrass oil, Grapefruit oil, Sweet Orange oil, Sweet Marjoram oil, Sweet Fennel oil, Sage oil.

Green Tea Complex - Leiner Health Products
Each tablet contains: Vitamin C (Ascorbic Acid) 120 mg • Green Tea extract (Camellia sinensis) leaf 100 mg. Other Ingredients: Calcium Carbonate, Cellulose, Hesperidin Complex, Rutin, Maltodextrin, Quercetin, Silicon Dioxide, Polyethylene Glycol 3350, Croscarmellose Sodium, Starch, Crospovidone, Magnesium Stearate, Hydroxypropyl Methylcellulose, Hydroxypropyl Cellulose, Polysorbate 80.

Green Tea Diet - Schiff
Each tablet contains: Green Tea extract EGCG (epigallocatechin gallate) 270 mg • Caffeine 150 mg.

Green Tea Diet, Timed Release - Schiff
Each tablet contains: Green Tea leaf extract (camellia sinensis) 225 mg • EGCG (epigallocalechin gallate) 90 mg • Caffeine (as caffeine anhydrous) 50 mg. Other Ingredients: Cellulose, Dextrose, Dextrin, Titanium Dioxide, Hydroxypropyl Methylcellulose, Polyethylene Glycol, Soy Lecithin, Caramel Color, Dextrose, Riboflavin, Croscarmellose Sodium, Magnesium Stearate.

Green Tea Essence - Life Enhancement Products, Inc.
Each tablet contains: Green Tea leaf extract 500 mg. Other Ingredients: Gelatin, Silicon Dioxide.

Green Tea Extract - Benepure, Inc
Each capsule contains: Green Tea extract (camellia sinensis, yielding epigallo-catechin-3-gallate [EGCG] 70 mg) 500 mg. Other Ingredients: Rice Flour, Vegetable Cellulose.

Green Tea extract - Pure Encapsulations
Each vegetable capsule contains: Green Tea extract (standardized to contain a minimum of 90% total tea catechins, providing epigallocatechin gallate [EGCG] 70%, caffeine <0.42%) 100 mg • Vitamin C (as ascorbyl palmitate) 3 mg.

Green Tea Extract - Pro Health
Each capsule contains: Green Tea extract 500 mg. Other Ingredients: Gelatin, Magnesium Trisillicate, Magnesium Stearate.

Green Tea Extract - PhytoPharmica
Each capsule contains: Green Tea leaf extract(camellia sinensis, standardized to contain 47%-52% polyphenols [catechin, epicatechin, epicatechin gallate, and epigallocatechin gallate] and 5%-10% Caffeine) 250 mg.

Green Tea Extract - Nature's Way
Each capsule contains: Green Tea dried extract 170 mg • Red Clover blossoms 315 mg. Other Ingredients: Gelatin.

Green Tea Extract - HealthWatchers System
Green Tea Extract • Green Tea Powder. Each capsule is the equivalent of 700 mg of Green Tea Powder.

Some Brand Name Natural Products - What they Contain

www.NaturalDatabase.com contains MANY more listings than appear here.
Editor's Notes are located on pages 2155-2163.

Green Tea Extract - Olympian Labs
Each capsule contains: Green Tea extract 500 mg.

Green Tea Extract - NSI - Nutraceutical Sciences Institute
Each capsule contains: Green Tea extract (standardized 98% polyphenols, 80% Catechins, and 45% EGCG) 500 mg.

Green Tea Extract 275 mg - Vital Nutrients
Each capsule contains: Camellia Sinensis (green tea extract, 80% catechins) 275 mg: 30-50% EGCG (epigallocatechin gallate), 30-50% epicatechin, epicatechin gallate epigallocatechin.

Green Tea Formula GT80 - Jamieson
Each capsule contains: Green Tea Phytosome (Camellia sinensis) 80 mg • Synergistic Antioxidant Nutrients Derived from Vitamin C, Grape Seed Extract, Bioflavonoids 30 mg.

Green Tea Leaf - Aboca USA, Inc
Two capsules contain: Green Tea leaf WPC (whole phytocomplex concentrate, camellia sinensis, standardized to 7% epigallocatechin gallate, yielding 19.6 mg per capsule) 560 mg. Other Ingredients: Gelatin.

Green Tea Phytosome - Enzymatic Therapy/PhytoPharmica
Each capsule contains: Green Tea leaf phytosome (camellia sinensis) bound to Phosphatidylcholine 100 mg. Other Ingredients: Cellulose, Gelatin, Modified Cellulose Gum, Titanium Dioxide Color, Magnesium Stearate.

Green Tea Remedy - Puritan's Pride
Each caplet contains: Green Tea extract 200 mg • Reishi mushroom 25 mg • Maitake mushroom 25 mg • Shiitake mushroom 25 mg • Astragalus 100 mg • Ligustrum 50 mg • Cat's Claw 100 mg • Vitamin C 60 mg • Selenium 50 mcg • Zinc 6 mg • Spirulina 50 mcg • Super-Oxide Dismutase 10 mg • N-acetyl Cysteine 25 mg.

Green Tea Salt Glow - Abra Therapeutics
Purified Water • Aloe Vera • Coconut oil • Olive oil • Kukui oil • Jojoba oil • Stearic Acid • Glycerin • Glyceryl Stearate • Cetyl Alcohol • St. John's Wort extract • Wild Yam extract • French Lavender essential oil • Boswellia Olibanum essential oil • Sodium PCA • Allantoin • Lecithin • Methylparaben • Propylparaben.

Green Tea Salt Scrub - Abra Therapeutics
20% Volcanic Ash • Natural Mineral Blend: Sodium Borate, Sodium Sulfate, Sodium Chloride • Organic Oils Blend: Almond, Olive, Sunflower, Jojoba, Lemongrass, Grapefruit, Sweet Orange, Sweet Marjoram • Organic whole leaf Green Tea.

Green-Lipped Mussel - Quest
Each capsule contains: Freeze-dried Green Lipped Mussel (Perna canaliculus) 625 mg.

Grime Bar - All Terrain Company
Sodium Palmate • Sodium palm kernelate • Water • Glycerin • Pumice • Peppermint oil • Sodium Chloride • Hemp seed oil • Rosemary leaf oil • Tetrasodium EDTA • Chlorophyll / Copper Complex.

Gripe Water Alcohol Free - R.W. Packaging, Ltd.
Each 5 mL contains: Sodium Bicarbonate 50 mg.

Gripe Water Liquid - R.W. Packaging, Ltd.
Each 5 mL contains: Sodium Bicarbonate 50 mg.

Gripp-Heel - Heel/BHI, Inc.
Aconitum Napellus 4X • Bryonia Alba 4X • Eupatorium Perfoliatum 3X • Phosphorus 5X • Lachesis Mutus 12X.
See Editor's Note No. 1.

Gro Pro - Universal Nutrition
Ten capsules contain: Creatine Monohydrate 5000 mg • L-Glutamine 2000 mg • Acetyl L-Carnitine 500 mg • L-Leucine (BCAA) 250 mg • L-Isoleucine (BCAA) 250 mg • L-Valine (BCAA) 250 mg • N-Acetyl-Cysteine (NAC) 200 mg • Tribulus Terrestris L. 250 mg • DHEA 50 mg • Zinc 15 mg.

Growth Fuel - TwinLab
Nine capsules contain: B-Hydroxy B-Methylbutyrate Monohydrate (HMB) 3000 mg • L-Glutamine 2000 mg • Creatine Monohydrate 5000 mg • N-Acetyl-Cysteine (NAC) 200 mg • Acetyl-L-Carnitine 50 mg • Zinc (from Zinc Picolinate) 30 mg • DHEA (Dehydroepiandrosterone) 50 mg.

Growth Hormone Support - Pure Encapsulations
Each vegetable capsule contains: Arginine HCl 500 mg • Ornithin Alpha-Ketoglutarate 250 mg.

GS 750 - Xymogen
Each capsule contains: Glucosamine Sulfate 750 mg.

GS- Similase - Tyler
Two capsules contain: Plant Enzymes 525 mg: Protease (I, II, III, IV), Amylase, Cellulase (I, II), Lipase (I, II), Phytase, Lactase (I, II), Sucrase (invertase), Maltase (malt diastase). Other Ingredients: Microcrystalline Cellulose, Gelatin, Water.

GS-500 - Enzymatic Therapy
Three capsules contain: Chloride (from glucosamine sulfate) 234 mg • Sodium (from glucosamine sulfate) 150 mg • Glucosamine Sulfate (stabilized) 1500 mg. Other Ingredients: Gelatin, Magnesium Stearate, Silicon Dioxide, Titanium Dioxide Color.

GS-500 and Chondroitin - Enzymatic Therapy
Three tablets contain: Chloride 234 mg • Sodium 250 mg • Glucosamine Sulfate 1500 mg • Chondroitin Sulfate 1200 mg.
See Editor's Note No. 15.

GSC (Glandular Stress Complex) - Progressive Labs
Each capsule contains: Vitamin B12 24 mcg • Raw Bovine Adrenal 15 mg • Raw Bovine Liver 15 mg • Raw Bovine Thymus 60 mg • Raw Bovine Spleen 15 mg • Raw Bovine Stomach 15 mg.
See Editor's Note No. 14.

GS-Complex - Enzymatic Therapy
Three capsules contain: Vitamin C (ascorbic acid) 1000 mg • Chloride (from glucosamine sulfate) 156 mg • Sodium 100 mg • Glucosamine Sulfate (stabilized) 1000 mg • L-Tyrosine 500 mg. Other Ingredients: Gelatin, Silicon Dioxide, Magnesium Stearate, Titanium Dioxide Color.

GTF Chromium 200 mcg - Jamieson
Each tablet contains: GTF Chromium (Derived from Brewer's Yeast) 200 mcg.

Guar Gum - Atrium Biotechnologies
Each tablet contains: Pure Guar Gum 1000 mg.

Guarana Chai - Traditional Medicinals
Assam Black leaf Tea • Cardamom seed • Ginger rhizome • Roasted Chicory root • Nutmeg seed • Organic Black Peppercorn • Guarana seed dry extract • Stevia leaf • Vanilla Bean dry extract • Clove stem • Rose petal • Cinnamon bark oil.

Guarana Energizer - Source Naturals
Each tablet contains: Guarana 900 mg.

Guarana-Gotu Kola Virtue - Blessed Herbs
Ma Huang • Siberian Ginseng root • Guarana seed • Gotu Kola • Licorice root • Grain alcohol & Distilled Water.
See Editor's Note No. 30.

Guaraviton - On Time International Corporation
Filtered Water • Sucarose • Acai Extract • Panax Ginseng root • Caramel Extract • Color C • Citric Acid • Sodiumbenzoate • Ascorbic Acid.

Guggal Extra Strength - R-U Ved U.S.A.
Guggal standardized extract (25 mg of Z & E guggalsterones) • Amla • Harar • Bahera • Magnesium • Vitamin B6.

Guggul E&Z Extract 99% - Vital Nutrients
Two capsules contain: Guggul extract (commiphora mukul, 99% E&Z guggulsterones) 75 mg.

BRAND NAMES

Some Brand Name Natural Products - What they Contain

www.NaturalDatabase.com contains MANY more listings than appear here.
Editor's Notes are located on pages 2155-2163.

BRAND NAMES

Guggul extract - Pure Encapsulations
Each vegetable capsule contains: Guggul gum resin extract (commiphora mukul, standardized to contain 2.5% Z and E guggulsterones) 500 mg.

Guggulbolic - Syntrax Innovations
Each capsule contains: Guggulsterones 30 mg.

Guggulbolic Extreme - Syntrax Innovations
Each capsule contains: Guggul EZ100 30 mg • Guggul Resin extract (standardized for 30 mg total guggulsteroids) 30 mg. Other Ingredients: Microcrystalline Cellulose, Gelatin, Titanium Dioxide, Yellow #5, Red #40.

Gugulipid Plus Lactospore - America's Finest
Each tablet contains: Gugulipid brand extract with 2.5% Z&E Guggulsterones 1000 mg • Lactospore brand Lactobacillus Sporogenes (min. guaranteed) 100 million. Other Ingredients: Cellulose, Stearic Acid, Magnesium Silicate, Magnesium Stearate, Pharmaceutical Glaze.

GugulPlex - PhytoPharmica
Each tablet contains: Niacin 250 mg • Vitamin C 100 mg • Chromium 50 mcg • Guggul extract 250 mg • Ginger root extract 200 mg.

GugulPlus - Enzymatic Therapy
Each tablet contains: Niacin (Inositol hexaniacinate) 250 mg • Vitamin C (Potassium Ascorbate) 100 mg • Chromium (Chromium Polynicotinate) (ChromeMate brand of patented Niacin-bound GTF Chromium) 50 mcg • Other Ingredients: Guggul extract (Commiphora Mukul) standardized to contain Guggulsterones 25 mg/gram) 250 mg • Ginger root extract 6.5:1 (Zingiber officinale) 200 mg.

Gui Pi Tang Plus - Secara
Organic Licorice root (gan cao) 294 mg • Organic Ginger rhizome (gan jian) 195 mg • Atractylodes rhizome 5:1 extract (bai zhu) 195 mg • Asian Ginseng root 4:1 extract (ren shen) 195 mg • Hoelen sclerotium 5:1 extract (fu ling) 195 mg • Reishi mushroom fruit body (10% polysaccharides (19 mg)) 195 mg • Astragalus root 5:1 extract (huang qi) 156 mg • California Poppy 4:1 extract 156 mg • Dong Quai root 5:1 extract (dang qui) 156 mg • Jujube seeds 5:1 extract (suan zao ren) 117 mg • Jujube fruit 5:1 extract (da zao) 99 mg • Longan fruit 5:1 extract (long yan rou) 99 mg • Polygala root 5:1 extract (yuan zhi) 99 mg • Rhodiola herb 5:1 extract 99 mg.

Gum Weed Salve - Dial Herbs
Gum Weed • Licorice • Myrrh • Goldenseal • Arnica • Strawberry • Lobelia • Cayenne. In a base of Bees Wax, Glycerine & Cold Pressed Olive oil.

Gum-Ease - The Herbalist
Echinacea root • Myrrh Gum • Blood root • Bayberry root bark • Peppermint oil (essential) • Cinnamon oil (essential) • Clove oil (essential).

Gurmar - 4 Life
Each capsule contains: Gymnema leaf (gymnema sylvestris) 365 mg • Gymnema extract (24% gymnemic acid) 35 mg. Other Ingredients: Gelatin, Magnesium Stearate.

Gymnema Leaf - Aboca USA, Inc
Each capsule contains: Gymnema leaf WPC (whole phytocomplex concentrate, gymnema sylvestre, standardized to 4.5% total gymnemasaponins, yielding 11.25 mg per capsule) 250 mg. Other Ingredients: Gelatin.

Gymnema Sylvestre - Puritan's Pride
Each tablet contains: Gymnema Sylvestre 400 mg • Citrus Fiber 200 mg.

Gymnema Sylvestre 250 mg - Vital Nutrients
Each capsule contains: Gymnema Sylvestre extract (standardized to 25% gymnemic acids) 250 mg.

Gymnema Sylvestre 400 mg - NOW Foods
Each capsule contains: Gymnema Sylvestre leaves extract (GS4 brand, 25% glycemic acid) 400 mg. Other Ingredients: Rice Flour, Magnesium Stearate, Silica.

Gymnema Sylvestre 75 - Pure Encapsulations
Each vegetable capsule contains: Gymnema Sylvestre extract (standardized to contain 75% gymnemic acids) 250 mg • Vitamin C (as ascorbyl palmitate) 10 mg.

Gymnema-75 - Jarrow Formulas
Each capsule contains: Gymnema Sylvestris (gymnemic acids 75%) 500 mg.

Gynecrine - Progressive Labs
Each capsule contains: Vitamin A 1000 IU • Vitamin C 100 mg • Vitamin E (DL-alpha tocopherol) 50 IU • Thiamin (vitamin B1) 10 mg • Riboflavin (vitamin B2) 10 mg • Vitamin B6 (pyridoxine) 18 mg • Iodine (as potassium iodide) 150 mcg • Magnesium (as magnesium oxide) 100 mg • Manganese (as manganese gluconate) 10 mg • Ovary concentrate (bovine) 20 mg • Mammary concentrate 10 mg • Pancreas concentrate 10 mg • Adrenal concentrate 10 mg • Pituitary concentrate 10 mg • Lecithin 10 mg • Flax seed oil 10 mg. See Editor's Note No. 31.

Gypsy Cold Care - Traditional Medicinals
Each 1 cup serving contains: Menthol 5 mg (as it naturally occurs in the peppermint leaf, mentha x piperita). Other Ingredients: Rose Hip, Cinnamon Bark, Yarrow Flower, Ginger Rhizome, Elder Flower, Safflower Petal, Clover Stem, Hyssop Herb, Licorice Root Dry Extract.

Hair & Skin Formula - Nature's Way
Four capsules contain: Biotin (Biotin Triurate) 1.6 mg • Calcium 50 mg • Cayenne pepper fruit 160 mg • Fizyme Enzyme Formula 100 mg • Fo-Ti root 160 mg • Glucosamine HCL 400 mg • Horsetail grass 160 mg • Kelp (whole Thallus) 160 mg • MSM (Methyl Sulfonyl Methane) 600 mg • Nettle herb 160 mg • Oatstraw stem, leaf 160 mg • Rosemary herb 160 mg. Other Ingredients: Gelatin, Magnesium Stearate, Millet.

Hair & Skin Nutrition - Enzymatic Therapy
Each capsule contains: Vitamin A (Fish Liver oil) 1666 IU • Vitamin D (Fish Liver oil) 333 IU • Vitamin E (D-Alpha Tocopherol) 33 IU • Vitamin C (Ascorbic Acid) 100 mg • Niacin/Niacinamide 33 mg • Zinc (Chelate) 15 mg • Vitamin B6 (Pyridoxine HCL) 10 mg • Pantothenic Acid (D-Calcium Pantothenate) 8.3 mg • Riboflavin (Vitamin B2) 1.7 mg • Biotin 333 mcg • Folic Acid 33 mcg • Other ingredients: Unsaturated Free Fatty Acids (Linoleic, Arachidonic & Linolenic from Unrefined Germ oil & Safflower seed oil) 300 mg • Lecithin (Soy) 200 mg • Choline Bitartrate 50 mg • Intrinsic Glandular Lipids 50 mg • Inositol 33 mg. In a base of L-Cysteine as a natural amino acid synergistic component.
See Editor's Note No. 14.

Hair Clean 1-2-3 Lice Remover - Quantum, Inc.
Coconut Oil • Anise Oil • Ylang Ylang Oil • Isopropyl Alcohol.

Hair Formula - Pharmanex
Each capsule contains: Vitamin E (as D-Alpha Tocopheryl Acetate) 3 IU • Riboflavin (as Riboflavin-5-Phosphate) 0.75 mg • Vitamin B6 (as Pyridoxine Hydrochloride) 3 IU • Biotin (as Biotin) 200 mcg • Pantothenic Acid (as Calcium Pantothenate) 25 mg • DL-Methionine 200 mg • L-Cysteine 105 mg • Lactalbumin Hydrolysate 25 mg • Millet Extract 20 mg. Other Ingredients: Gelatin, Maltodextrin, Starch, Vanillin, Stearic Acid (Vegetable Derived), Silicon Dioxide.

Hair Genesis - HairGenesis
Each softgel contains: Beta Sitosterol 50 mg • Saw Palmetto Berry extract (85/95% liposterolic standardized) 200 mg • Lecithin 50 mg • Inositol 100 mg • Phosphatidyl Choline 25 mg • Niacin 15 mg • Biotin 100 mcg. Other Ingredients: Alcohol SDA-40, Propylene Glycol, Deionized Water, Polysorbate-80, Isoceteth-20, Hydrolyzed Mucopolysaccharides, Beta-Sitosterol, Biotin, Citric Acid.

Hair Million - DreamPharm
Each capsule contains: Proprietary Blend: Radix Angelicae Sinensis, Radix Bupleuri Chinensis, Sclerotium Poriae Cocos, Atractylodes Rhizoma, Paeoniae Radix, Glycyrrhizae Radix, Fructus Ligustri Lucidi, Fructus Lycii Chinensis, Radix Polygoni Multiflori, Radix Paeoniae Rubra, Herba Artemisiae Capillaris, Cortex Cinnamomi Cassiae, Eucommiae Ulmoides Bark, Rhizoma Gastrodiae Elatae, Radix Morindae Officinalis, Rhizoma Ligustici, Codonopsitis Sinensis, Fructus Liquidambaris, Uncaria Sinensis, Fructus Chaenomelis, Vaccaria Pyramidata, Hedyotis Diffusa, Laminaria Japonica, Tulipa Edulis, Eisenia Bicyclis.

Hair No More - Ultra Herbal, LLC
Aloe Vera • Glycerin • Chamomile extract • Water • Calcium Hydroxide • Calcium Thioglycolate Trihydrate • Isopropyl Palmitate • Cetyl Alcohol • Pro-Vitamin Antioxidant Complex: Vitamin E, Vitamin A, Pro-Vitamin E, Vitamin K, Green Tea extract, Herbal Extracts • Forestal • Willow bark • Butcher's Broom extract • Hydrocotyle • Hydrolyzed Milk Protein • Calendula Officinalis • Hydrolyzed Yeast Protein • Horse Chestnut extract • Licorice extract • Phenoxethanol • Fragrance.

Hair Nutrients - Biotech Corp.
Three tablets contain: Shen Min [a proprietary blend of 12:1 standardized He Shou Wu (Fo Ti) root extract and He Shou Wu root powder] 1755 mg • Bioperine brand Black Pepper extract 3 mg.

Hair Support for Men - Futurebiotics LLC
Two capsules contain: Vitamin A (5000 IU as fish liver oil, 5000 IU as beta carotene) 10000 IU • Vitamin C (ascorbic acid) 250 mg • Vitamin D (ergocalciferol) 200 IU • Vitamin E (d-alpha tocopherol succinate) 30 IU • Vitamin B1 (thiamine HCl) 10 mg • Vitamin B2 (riboflavin) 10 mg • Vitamin B6 (pyridoxine HCl) 10 mg • Vitamin B12 (cyanocobalamin) 16 mcg • Folic Acid 400 mcg • Biotin (d-biotin) 500 mcg • Pantothenic Acid (calcium pantothenate) 100 mg • Zinc (amino acid chelate) 25 mg • Selenium (amino acid chelate) 100 mcg • Para Aminobenzoic Acid (PABA) 30 mg • Boron (amino acid chelate) 3 mg • MSM (methyl-sulfonyl-methane) 500 mg • Horsetail leaf powder extract (4:1) 50 mg • Saw Palmetto berry extract (4:1) powder 50 mg • Hair Support Herbal Base 200 mg: Citrus Bioflavonoids, Saw Palmetto berry powder, Schizandra berry extract powder, Horsetail leaf powder. Other Ingredients: Gelatin, Water.

Hair, Skin & Nails - Health Factor
Each capsule contains: Choline Bitartrate 100 mg • DL Methionine 100 mg • Borage Seed 150 mg • Flax Seed 150 mg • Gelatin 150 mg • Lecithin 100 mg.

Hair, Skin & Nails Advanced MSM Formula - Solgar
Each two tablets contain: Vitamin C (as l-ascorbic acid) 120 mg • Calcium 90 mg • Zinc (as zinc citrate) 15 mg • Copper (as copper glycinate) 2 mg • MSM (as methylsulfonylmethane) 1000 mg • Silicon (as silica, as L-corallioides [red algae powder]) 50 mg • L-Proline 50 mg • L-Lysine (as l-lysine HCl) 50 mg. Inactive Ingredients: Microcrystalline Cellulose, Vegetable Cellulose, Silica, Vegetable Stearic Acid, Vegetable Magnesium Stearate, Vegetable Glycerin.

Hair, Skin & Nails for Men - Futurebiotics LLC
Three tablets contain: Beta Carotene 10,000 IU • Vitamin C 120 mg • Vitamin B2 (Riboflavin) 10 mg • Vitamin B1 (Thiamin) 10 mg • Calcium 600 mg • Iron (Amino Acid Chelate) 6 mg • Vitamin D (Fish Liver Oil) 200 IU • Vitamin E (Natural Mixed Tocopherols) 30 IU • Vitamin B6 (Pyridoxine) 10 mg • Folic Acid 400 mcg • Vitamin B12 16 mcg • Phosphorus 300 mg • Iodine (Kelp) 225 mcg • Magnesium (Oxide) 200 mg • Zinc (Gluconate) 25 mg • Biotin 400 mcg • Pantothenic Acid (Calcium Salt) 30 mg • Choline (Bitartrate) 150 mg • Inositol 60 mg • Para Amino Benzoic Acid (PABA) 50 mg • Selenium (Amino Acid Chelate) 25 mcg • Manganese (Amino Acid Chelate) 10 mg • Niacinamide 50 mg • In a special potentiating base containing: Gelatin, Cysteine, Methionine, Ribonucleic Acid (RNA), Bioflavonoids, Betaine HCl, Oat Straw, Horsetail Extract, Saw Palmetto Berry, Smilax Extract, Siberian Ginseng Extract, Standardized Panax Ginseng Extract & Rutin.

Hair, Skin & Nails for Women - Futurebiotics LLC
Three tablets contain: Vitamin A (Beta Carotene) 10,000 IU • Vitamin C 120 mg • Thiamin (B1) 10 mg • Riboflavin 10 mg • Niacinamide 50 mg • Calcium 600 mg • Iron (Amino Acid Chelate) 6 mg • Vitamin D (Fish Liver Oil) 200 IU • Vitamin E (Natural Mixed Tocopherols) 30 IU • Vitamin B6 (Pyridoxine) 10 mg • Folic Acid 400 mcg • Vitamin B12 16 mcg • Phosphorus 300 mg • Iodine (Kelp) 225 mcg • Magnesium (Oxide) 200 mg • Zinc (Gluconate) 15 mg • Biotin 400 mcg • Pantothenic Acid (Calcium Salt) 30 mg • Choline (Bitartrate) 150 mg • Inositol 60 mg • Para Amino Benzoic Acid (PABA) 50 mg • Selenium (Amino Acid Chelate) 25 mcg • Manganese (Amino Acid Chelate) 10 mg • Ribonucleic Acid (RNA) 60 mg • Bioflavonoids 50 mg • Rutin 25 mg • Betaine HCl 50 mg • In a base containing L-Cysteine, L-Methionine, Gelatin, Papain, Oat Straw, Echinacea, Horsetail, Asparagus.

Hair, Skin & Nails Formula w/2500 mcg Biotin - GNC
Two tablets contain: Vitamin A (as retinyl acetate) 5000 IU • Vitamin C (as ascorbic acid) 120 mg • Vitamin D (as cholecalciferol) 200 IU • Vitamin E (as d-alpha tocopheryl succinate) 60 IU • Thiamin B1 (as thiamin mononitrate) 1.5 mg • Riboflavin B2 (vitamin B2) 1.7 mg • Niacin B3 (as niacinamide) 20 mg • Folate (folic acid, folacin) 200 mcg • Biotin 2500 mcg • Calcium (as calcium citrate malate) 200 mg • Phosphorus (as dicalcium phosphate) 100 mg • Zinc (as zinc oxide) 15 mg • Boron (as boron citrate) 1 mcg • MSM (methylsulfonyl-methane) 100 mg • Hydrolyzed Gelatin 100 mg • L-Cysteine 100 mg • L-Methionine 50 mg • Horsetail Rush Herb Extract (equisetum arvense) 2 mg • Lutein 500 mcg. Other Ingredients: Cellulose, Titanium Dioxide (natural mineral whitener), Vegetable Acetoglycerides, Chlorophyllin.

Hair, Skin, & Nails - Health Smart Vitamins
Each capsule contains: Vitamin A (as beta carotene) 5,000 IU • MSM (methylsulfonylmethane) 233 mg • Tea green leaf (50% polyphenols, 60 mg) 120 mg • Horsetail stem (7% silica, 3.15 mg) 45 mg • Gotu Kola whole plant (10% triterpenes, 4 mg) 40 mg • Blueberry fruit (5% anthocyanins, 1.5 mg) 30 mg • Dandelion root 10 mg.

HairPrep capsules - HealthMinded
Four capsules contain: Folic Acid 800 mcg • Biotin 1400 mcg • Pantothenic Acid (as D-calcium pantothenate) 300 mg • Iodine (as potassium iodide/Atlantic kelp) 150 mcg • Zinc (as monomethionine) 15 mg • HairPrep Proprietary Blend 1705 mg: Fo-ti root, Fo-ti root dried extract, Saw Palmetto berry dried extract, Silica (as silicon dioxide), Kelp (whole thallus), Soybean dried extract (standardized to 40% isoflavones), Kudzu root, Black Pepper fruit. Other Ingredients: Gelatin, Stearic Acid, Magnesium Stearate.

HairPro - HealthMinded
Folate (as folic acid) • Pantothenic Acid (as dicalcium pantothenate) • Biotin • Iodine (from kelp) • Zinc (as zinc methionine) • He Shou Wu root (polygonum multiflorum) • Isoflavones (from soy/glycine max) • Kudzu (pueraria lobata) • Saw Palmetto berries • Silica • Black Pepper extract (piper nigrum, standardized).

Halibut-Liver Oil - Golden Glow Natural Health Products
Each softgel contains: Halibut Liver oil 145 mg • Cholecalciferol (vitamin D3) 10 mcg • Retinyl Palmitate (vitamin A) 4000 IU.

Hangover Over - Golden Glow Natural Health Products
Each tablet contains: Tangerine peel 50 mg • Cardamon fruit 100 mg • Tangerine fruit 100 mg • Plantago root and rhizome 100 mg • Ginger root 82 mg • Polyporus Umbellatus fruit 82 mg • Atractylodes Lancea root and rhizome 80 mg • Kudzu 940 mg • Panax Ginseng 82 mg • Cayenne 26 mg. Other Ingredietns: Gluten.

Hangover Relief - Hangover Solutions Inc.
Each tablet contains: Sodium (carbonates) 333 mg • Magnesium (oxide) 20 mg • Vitamin C (ascorbic acid) 200 mg • Vitamin B-1 4.5 mg • Vitamin B-2 5.1 mg • Niacinamide 60 mg • Pantothenic

BRAND NAMES

Acid (d-calcium pantothenate) 30 mg • Vitamin B-6 (pyridoxine) 6 mg • Vitamin B-12 18 mcg • Biotin 200 mcg • Folic Acid 400 mcg • Choline (bitartrate) 100 mg • Inositol 1 mg • PABA 1 mg • Acerola Cherry extract 50 mg • Ginger extract 50 mg • White Willow Bark 100 mg • L-Glutamine 600 mg • Yerba Mate 50 mg. Other Ingredients: Citric Acid, Sorbitol, Natural Orange Flavor, Acosulfame Potassium, Canola Oil, Docusate Sodium.

Hapizen Daytime Formula - Newtell, Inc.
Each capsule contains: Proprietary Blend 200 mg: Valerian root, Hops, Catnip, Passionflower, Chamomile.

Hapizen Nighttime Formula - Newtell, Inc.
Each capsule contains: Proprietary Blend 250 mg: Passionflower, Hops, Catnip, L-Valine, L-Tyrosine, White Willow bark, Inositol.

Happy Bunny Spaz Juice - XL Distro
Carbonated Pure Water • High Fructose Corn Syrup and/or Sugar • Citric Acid • Taurine 1000 mg • Natural and Artificial Flavors • Sodium Benzoate • Potassium Sorbate • Caffeine 50 mg • Inositol 50 mg • Guarana • Ginseng • Niacin • D-Calcium Pantothenate • Pyridoxine Hydrochloride (vitamin B6) • Blue 1 • Cyanocobalamin (vitamin B12).

Happy Camper - Natural Balance
Two capsules contain: Proprietary blend 840 mg: Passion Flower • Kava Kava • Siberian Ginseng • Gotu Kola • Schisandra • Wood Betony • Lavender.

Happy Colon Mega - Susan Ambrosino's Herb Club, Inc.
Each capsule contains: Goldenseal 5% extract • Milk Thistle 80% extract • Cascara Sagrada • Flax seed • Marshmallow root • Cat's Claw inner bark • Fenugreek • Ginger.

HAS Original Formula - Nature's Way
Two capsules contain: Proprietary Formula: Brigham Tea herb • Burdock root • Cayenne pepper fruit • Cleavers herb • Elecampane • Goldenseal root • Marshmallow root • Parsley herb • Rosemary herb. Other Ingredients: Gelatin.

Hawaiian Noni Juice - Youngevity
Purified Water • Morinda citrifolia • Lecithin • Potassium Sorbate • Artificial Flavoring • Vilcabamba Mineral Essence: Potassium, Calcium, Magnesium, Zinc, Chromium, Selenium, Iron, Copper, Molybdenum, Vanadium, Iodine, Cobalt, Manganese.

Hawthorn - Leiner Health Products
Each caplet contains: Hawthorn extract (Crataegus spp.) leaves and flowers 250 mg. Other Ingredients: Calcium Carbonate, Glucose, Cellulose, Maltodextrin, Silicon Dioxide, Hydroxypropyl Methylcellulose, Polyethylene Glycol 3350, Croscarmellose Sodium, Pharmaceutical Glaze, Crospovidone, Magnesium Stearate, Hydroxypropyl Cellulose, Red 40 Lake, Polysorbate 80, Titanium Dioxide, Povidone.

Hawthorn - Pharmanex
Each capsule contains: Hawthorn flowers & leaves (5.5:1) extract (Crategus oxyacantha) 125 mg. Other Ingredients: Rice Flour, Gelatin.

Hawthorn - PhysioLogics
Each capsule contains: Hawthorn leaf, flower extract (crataegus oxyacantha, standardized to contain 2% vitexin, 3 mg) 150 mg. Other Ingredients: Maltodextrin, Gelatin, Vegetable Magnesium Stearate, Silica.

Hawthorn - Jarrow Formulas
Each capsule contains: Hawthorn 5:1 concentrate (minimum 1.8% vitexin 4'-rhamnoside) 500 mg. Other Ingredients: Rice Powder, Silicon Dioxide, Magnesium Stearate, Gelatin.

Hawthorn extract - Pure Encapsulations
Each vegetable capsule contains: Hawthorn extract (crataegus oxycantha, standardized to contain 2% vitexins) 500 mg.

Hawthorn Flowering Top - Aboca USA, Inc
Two capsules contain: Hawthorn flowering top WPC (whole phytocomplex concentrate, crataegus monogyna, standardized to 3.1% total flavonoids, yielding 7.7 mg per capsule) 496 mg. Other Ingredients: Gelatin.

Hawthorn Phytosome - Enzymatic Therapy/PhytoPharmica
Two capsules contain: Hawthorn leaf/flower phytosome (crataegus oxyacantha) bound to Phosphatidylcholine 200 mg. Other Ingredients: Cellulose, Gelatin, Magnesium Stearate, Silicon Dioxide, Titanium Dioxide Color.

Hawthorn Supreme - Gaia Herbs
Forty drops contain: Proprietary Blend 300 mg: Hawthorn berry solid extract, Hawthorn flower buds, Hawthorn leaf (crataegus spp.), 50% Vegetable Glycerin, 20-25% Pure Grain Alcohol USP, Spring Water.

Hawthorn Supreme - Gaia Herbs
Two capsules contain: Hawthorn leaf and flower (crataegus spp.) 100 mg • Hawthorn berry (crataegus spp.) 240 mg. Other Ingredients: Vegetable Glycerin, Vegetable Cellulose (capsule).

Hawthorne - Factor VR25 - Jamieson
Each caplet contains: Hawthorne Flower 1250 mg.

Hawthorne Berry Extract - Ortho Molecular Products
Each capsule contains: Hawthorne leaf and flower extract (standardized to contain 1.8% vitexn-2"-O-rhamnoside) 250 mg • Hawthorne berry extract 200 mg. Other Ingredients: Natural Vegetable Capsules, Ascorbyl Palmitate, Magnesium Stearate, Microcrystalline Cellulose, Silicon Dioxide.

Hawthorne Extract - Vital Nutrients
Each capsule contains: Crataegus Oxyacantha leaf and flower extract (hawthorne, standardized to 1.8 - 2% vitexin) 450 mg.

Hay Relief - Rainbow Light
Each caplet contains: Nettle tops 260 mg • Goldenseal rhizome and root powder 40 mg • Licorice root 40 mg • Lemon • Thyme herb 30 mg • Dong Quai root 20 mg • Eyebright herb 8 mg. Other Ingredients: Cellulose, Gum Arabic, Vegetable Stearin, and Silica.

HCA Citrimax - Bronson Laboratories
Each capsule contains: Calcium (as calcium carbonate) 36 mg • CitriMax brand Garcinia Cambogia fruit extract (providing 250 mg of (-) hydroxycitric acid (HCA)) 500 mg.

HCL and Pepsin - J. R. Carlson Laboratories, Inc.
Each tablet contains: Pepsin 250 mg • Betaine (as betaine hydrochloride) 500 mg.

H-Complex - Progressive Labs
Each capsule contains: Vitamin E 15 IU • Stone root (Collinsonia canadensis) 400 mg • Comfrey root (Symphytum officinale) 50 mg • Bayberry bark (Myrica cerifera) 50 mg • Goldenseal root (Hydrastis canadensis) 40 mg • Green Beet leaf powder 25 mg • Betony (Betonica officinalis) 10 mg.

HDT Andros-D 100 - Human Development Technologies (HDT)
Each capsule contains: Androstenedione 100 mg • Zinc 15 mg • Bioperine brand Black Pepper extract 2.5 mg.
See Editor's Note No. 47.

HDT GLX-37.5 - Human Development Technologies (HDT)
Each capsule contains: Vanadyl Sulfate (yielding 7.5 mg elemental Vanadium) 37.5 mg • Taurine 600 mg • Magnesium 200 mg • Selenium 33 mcg • Ginger 20 mg • Cinnamon 20 mg • Chromium Picolinate 200 mcg.

Head Relief - NOW Foods
Two capsules contain: Feverfew leaf (tanacetum parthenium) (min. 0.9% Parthenolide) 400 mg • Kava root extract (piper methysticum) (30% kavalactones) 100 mg • Ginger root extract (zingiber officinale)

5% standardized 50 mg • Proprietary Blend 50 mg: Purple Willow bark (salix purpurea), Meadow Sweet (filipendula ulmaria), Wintergreen (gaultheria procumbens).

Headacha - HerbaSway
Ginkgo Biloba • Dong Quai • Ginger • Kudzu • Bupleurum • Coptis • Blackberry • HerbaSwee (Cucurbitaceae fruit).

Headache - Hyland's
Two tablets contain: Iris Versicolor 3X • Gelsemium Sempervirens 3X • Ipecac 3X • Belladonna 6X. Base: Lactose USP.
See Editor's Note No. 1.

Headache Relief - New Chapter, Inc.
Each capsule contains: Feverfew stem, leaf & flower, supercritical extract (1% parthenolide- 1.25 mg) 125 mg • Green Tea leaf extract (50% polyphenols- 50 mg) (7% caffeine) 100 mg • Wintergreen leaf extract, salicylic acid derivatives 75 mg • Ginger (rhizome) certified organic (minimum 20% pungent compounds- 10 mg, 4% zingiberene- 2 mg) 50 mg • Meadowsweet herb, extract, salicylic acid derivatives 38 mg • Purple Willow bark (Salix purpurea) extract salicylic acid derivatives 38 mg • California Poppy whole plant, extract 5:1(leaf & essential oil), supercritical extract (23% total phenolic antioxidants - 2.3 mg) 20 mg • Rosemary leaf & essential oil, supercritical extract (23% total phenolic antioxidants - 2.3 mg) 10 mg • Ginger rhizome, certified organic (post - supercritical ethanolic extract) (3% pungent compounds - 0.3 mg) 10 mg • Lavender flower, supercritical extract (25% linalool - 2.5 mg) 10 mg • Hops strobiles, supercritical extract (35% humulones - 1.7 mg) (12% lupulones - 0.6 mg) 5 mg • Valerian root (Valeriana officinalis & Valerians mexicanus) supercritical extract (60% valepotrates - 3 mg) 5 mg. Other Ingredients: Olive Oil certified organic, Yellow Beeswax, Gelatin, Vegetable Glycerine, Purified Water, Carob.

Headache Remedy - PhytoPharmica
Twenty drops contain: Ruta graveolens 8x • Argentum nitricum 6x • Digitalis purpurea 6x • Cimicifuga racemosa 4x • Gelsemium sempervirens 4x • Sanguinaria canadensis 4x • Chelidonium majus 3x • Cyclamen europaeum 3x • Iris versicolor 3x • Melilotus 3x. In a base of 40% USP alcohol by volume.
See Editor's Note No. 1 and No. 21.

Headache Remedy - Lehning Laboratories
Ruta graveolens 8X • Argentum nitricum 6X • Digitalis purpurea 6X • Cimicifuga racemosa 4X • Gelsemium sempervirens 4X • Sanguinaria canadensis 4X • Chelidonium majus 3X • Cyclamen europaeum 3X • Iris versicolor 3X • Melilotus 3X. In a base of 40% USP alcohol by volume.
See Editor's Note No. 1.

Headmed - Baywood International
Each capsule contains: Riboflavin (Vitamin B2) 850 mg • Proprietary Blend 275 mg: Petasites Hybridus extract (40:1), Ginkgo Biloba leaf.

Heal-All Salve - Blessed Herbs
Goldenseal root • Heal-All • Comfrey root • German Chamomile flower • Plantain leaf • Echinacea Angustifolia root • Yarrow flower • Gotu Kola • St. John's Wort flower • Calendula flower • Organic Cold-Pressed Olive oil & Essential oil of Lavender.

Health Fitness - Vidafit
Each serving contains: Folate 300 mcg • Niacin 16 mg • Pantothenic Acid 5 mg • Riboflavin 1.3 mg • Thiamine 1.2 mg • Vitamin A 3300 mg • Vitamin B12 2.4 mcg • Vitamin B6 1.3 mg • Vitamin C 75 mg • Vitamin D 200 IU • Vitamin E 10 IU • Calcium 500 mg • Chromium 50 mcg • Copper 1 mg • Iodine 150 mcg • Magnesium 420 mg • Phosphorus 500 mg • Potassium 100 mg • Selenium 50 mcg • Zinc 15 mg • Whey Protein 2 grams.

Health Pak - Optimum Nutrition
Each pak (4 capsules) contains: Vitamin A (as Betatene natural mixed carotenoids) 25,000 IU • Vitamin C (as ascorbic acid) 1000 mg • Vitamin D (as cholecalciferol) 400 IU • Vitamin E (as D-alpha tocopherol succinate) 400 IU • Thiamin (as thiamin hydrochloride) 50 mg • Riboflavin 50 mg • Niacin (as niacinamide) 50 mg • Vitamin B6 (as pyridoxine hydrochloride) 50 mg • Folic Acid 400 mcg • Vitamin B12 (as cyanocobalamin) 50 mcg • Biotin 300 mcg • Pantothenic Acid (as D-calcium pantothenate) 50 mg • Calcium (as calcium carbonate, citrate) 500 mg • Iron (as ferrous fumarate) 5 mg • Iodine (as kelp) 5 mg • Magnesium (as magnesium oxide, aspartate) 250 mg • Zinc (as zinc picolinate) 15 mg • Selenium (as selenomethionine) 200 mcg • Copper (as copper AA chelate) 1 mg • Manganese (as manganese gluconate) 5 mg • Chromium (as chromium GTF) 100 mcg • Molybdenum (as molybdenum AA chelate) 250 mcg • Potassium (as potassium citrate, aspartate) 50 mg • Choline (as choline bitartrate) 50 mg • Inositol 50 mg • PABA (as para-aminobenzoic acid) 50 mg • Alpha-Carotene 467 mcg • Zeaxanthin 97 mcg • Cryptoxanthin 119 mcg • Lutein 76 mcg. Other Ingredients: Gelatin, Magnesium Stearate, Silica.

HealthPak 100 AM Packet - USANA Health Sciences
Each packet contains: Vitamin A (as Beta Carotene) 10000 IU • Vitamin C (as Calcium, Potassium, Magnesium, and Zinc Ascorbates) 1166 mg • Vitamin D (Vitamin D3 as Cholecalciferol) 350 IU • Vitamin E (as D-Alpha Tocopheryl Succinate) 300 IU • Vitamin K (as Phylloquinone) 40 mcg • Thiamine (as Thiamine HCl) 18 mg • Riboflavin 18 mg • Niacin (as Niacin and Niacinamide) 26.6 mg • Vitamin B6 (as Pyridoxine HCl) 18 mg • Folate (as Folic Acid) 666 mcg • Vitamin B12 (as Cyanocobalamin) 40 mcg • Biotin 200 mcg • Pantothenic Acid (as D-Calcium Pantothenate) 60 mg • Calcium (as Calcium Citrate) 225 mg • Iodine (as Potassium Iodide) 75 mcg • Magnesium (as Magnesium Citrate, Amino Acid Chelate) 190 mg • Zinc (as Zinc Citrate) 6.7 mg • Selenium (as L-Selenomethionine and Amino Acid Complex) 67 mcg • Copper (as Amino Acid Chelate) 1 mg • Manganese (as Manganese Gluconate) 1.7 mg • Chromium (as Chromium Picolinate and Polynicotinate) 100 mcg • Molybdenum (as Molybdenum Citrate) 16.7 mcg • Bioflavonoid Complex: Rutin, Quercetin, Hesperidin (Citrus SPP. L.) Fruit, Green Tea Extract - Decaffeinated (Camellia Sinensis Hunt)(Leaves), Bilberry Extract (Vaccinium Myrtillus L.) Fruit 129 mg • Inositol 100 mg • Choline Bitartrate 66.6 mg • N-Acetyl-L-Cysteine 43.4 mg • Bromelain 33.4 mg • Alpha Lipoic Acid 10 mg • Coenzyme Q10 8 mg • Turmeric Extract (Curcuma Longal)Root 10 mg • Glutathione 6.6 mg • Broccoli Concentrate (Brassica Oleracea V. Botrytis L.) Flower 10 mg • Lutein (Tagetes Erecta L., Flower) 400 mcg • Lycopene 700 mcg • Boron (as Boron Citrate) 1.33 mg • Silicon (as Amino Acid Complex) 3.25 • Vanadium (as Vanadyl Sulfate) 10 mcg • Ultra Trace Minerals 1 mg • Grape Seed Extract 90 mg • Olive Extract (Olea Europaea L., Fruit) 20 mg. Other Ingredients: Microcrystalline Cellulose, Pregelatinized Starch, Croscarmellose Sodium, Ascorbyl Palmitate, Dextrin, Collodial Silicon Dioxide, Dextrose.

HealthPak 100 PM Packet - USANA Health Sciences
Each packet contains: Vitamin A (as Beta Carotene) 5000 IU • Vitamin C (as Calcium, Potassium, Magnesium, and Zinc Ascorbates) 433 mg • Vitamin D (Vitamin D3 as Cholecalciferol) 350 IU • Vitamin E (as D-Alpha Tocopheryl Succinate) 300 IU • Vitamin K (as Phylloquinone) 20 mcg • Thiamine (as Thiamine HCL) 9 mg • Riboflavin 9 mg • Niacin (as Niacin and Niacinamide) 13.3 mg • Vitamin B6 (as Pyridoxine HCl) 9 mg • Folate (as Folic Acid) 333 mcg • Vitamin B12 (as Cyanocobalamin) 20 mcg • Biotin 100 mcg • Pantothenic Acid (as D-Calcium Pantothenate) 30 mg • Calcium (as Calcium Citrate) 315 mg • Iodine (as Potassium Iodide) 150 mcg • Magnesium (as Magnesium Citrate, Amino Acid Chelate) 290 mg • Zinc (as Zinc Citrate)13.4 mg • Selenium (as L-Selenomethionine and Amino Acid Complex) 134 mcg • Copper (as Amino Acid Chelate) 2 mg • Manganese (as Manganese Gluconate) 3.4 mg • Chromium (as Chromium Picolinate and Polynicotinate) 200 mcg • Molybdenum (as Molybdenum Citrate) 33.4 mcg • Bioflavonoid Complex: Rutin, Quercetin, Hesperidin (Citrus SPP. L.) Fruit, Green Tea Extract - Decaffeinated (Camellia Sinensis Hunt)(Leaves), Bilberry Extract (Vaccinium Myrtillus L.) Fruit 90 mg • Inositol 50 mg • Choline Bitartrate 33.3 mg • N-Acetyl

L-Cysteine 21.7 mg • Bromelain 16.7 mg • Alpha Lipoic Acid 5 mg • Coenzyme Q10 4 mg • Turmeric Extract (Curcuma Longal)Root 130 mg • Glutathione 3.3 mg • Broccoli Concentrate (Brassica Oleracea V. Botrytis L.) Flower 5 mg • Lutein (Tagetes Erecta L., Flower) 200 mcg • Lycopene 350 mcg • Resveratrol (Polygonum Cuspidatum Sieb. & Zucc., Root and Rhizome) 1000 mcg • Rosemary Extract (Rosmarinus Officinalis L., Leaves) 50 mg • Boron (as Boron Citrate) 2.33 mg • Silicon (as Amino Acid Complex) 4.25 • Vanadium (as Vanadyl Sulfate) 20 mcg • Ultra Trace Minerals 2 mg • Olive Extract (Olea Europaea L., fruit) 10 mg. Other Ingredients: Microcrystalline Cellulose, Pregelatinized Starch, Croscarmellose Sodium, Ascorbyl Palmitate, Dextrin, Collodial Silicon Dioxide, Dextrose.

HealthSmiles - Health Smart Vitamins
Two tablets contain: Vitamin A (as beta-carotene) 5,000 IU • Vitamin C (as ascorbic acid) 60 mg • Vitamin D (as ergocalciferol) 400 IU • Vitamin E (d-alpha tocopheryl acetate) 30 IU • Thiamin (as thiamin HCl) 1.5 mg • Riboflavin 1.7 mg • Niacin (as niacinamide) 20 mg • Vitamin B6 (as pyridoxine HCl) 2 mg • Folate (as folic acid) 10 mcg • Vitamin B12 (cyanocobalamin) 6 mcg • Biotin 50 mcg • Pantothenic acid (as calcium pantothenate) 10 mg • Calcium (as calcium amino acid chelate) 20 mg • Iron (as iron amino acid chelate) 5 mg • Iodine (from kelp) 100 mcg • Magnesium (as magnesium amino acid chelate) 10 mg • Zinc (as zinc amino acid chelate) 3 mg • Copper (as copper amino acid chelate) 50 mcg • Manganese (as maganese amino acid chelate) 50 mcg • Potassium (as potassium amino acid chelate) 1 mg • Apple fruit 50 mg • Papaya fruit 50 mg • Pineapple fruit 50 mg • Lemon Bioflavonoids 20 mg • Spirulina 20 mg • Sunflower oil seed 20 mg • Rice bran 10 mg • Beet Greens leaf 5 mg • Broccoli aerial parts 5 mg • Brown rice 5 mg • Carrot root 5 mg • Dog Rose (rose hips) 5 mg • Mango fruit 5 mg • Spinach leaf 5 mg • West Indian Cherry (fruit, Malpighia pruncifolia) 5 mg • Para-aminobenzoic acid (PABA) 400 mcg • Choline (as choline bitartrate) 10 mcg • Inositol 10 mcg.

Healthy Aging Formula - Waiora
Two caplets contain: Calcium 22 mg • Proprietary Y.E. Blend/ Complex 1100 mg: Bioactive Hyperimmune Milk Protein Concentrate, 3Beta-Acetoxy-Androst-5-ene-7,17-dione. Other Ingredients: Dicalcium Phosphate, Xylitol, Sodium Starch Glycolate, Magnesium Stearate, Silicon Dioxide.

Healthy Aging with High Potency NT Factor - Nutritional Therapeutics, Inc.
Two tablets contain: NT Factor complex 1300 mg: Phosphoglycolipids with Phosphatidylcholine and Glycolipids, Bifidobacterium, Lactobacillus, L. Acidophilus, Rice Bran extract, Arginine, Beet root fiber, Black Strap Molasses, Glycine, Magnesium Sulfate, Para-Aminobenzoic Acid, Leek, Pantethine, Taurine, Garlic, Calcium Borogluconate, Potassium Citrate, Calcium Sulfate, Spirulina, Bromelain, Natural Vitamin E, Calcium Ascorbate, Alpha-Lipoic Acid, Oligosaccharides, Vitamin B6, Niacinamide, Riboflavin, Inositol, Niacin, Calcium Pantothenate, Thiamin, Vitamin B12, Folic Acid, Chromium Picolinate • Mitochondrial Fuel Blend 200 mg: Potassium Pyruvate, Alpha-Ketoglutaric Acid, L-Carnitine-L-Tartrate, Creatine Phosphate. Other Ingredients: Microcrystalline Cellulose, Croscarmellose Sodium, Methyl Cellulose, Magnesium Stearate, Silica.

Healthy Antioxidants - Health Smart Vitamins
Three tablets contain: Vitamin A (as beta-carotene) 20,000 IU • Vitamin C (ascorbic acid) 60 mg • Vitamin E (as d-alpha tocopheryl acetate) 30 IU • Calcium (as dicalcium phosphate) 3.5 mg • Selenium (as selenomethionine) 60 mcg • Garlic bulb (>=10,000 mcg allicin/g, >=4 mg) 400 mg • Tomato fruit (1% lycopene, 3 mg) 300 mg • Oregano leaf 150 mg • Rosemary leaf (>=6% carnosic acid, >=9 mg) 150 mg.

Healthy Breathing Support - Weil Lifestyle, LLC
Each Vitamin C tablet contains: Vitamin C 1000 mg. Each Lung Support Formula softgel contains: Turmeric 190 mg • Green Tea 150 mg • Clove 7.5 mg • Ginger 7.5 mg • Parsley 7.5 mg • Peppermint 7.5 mg • Rosemary 7.5 mg.

Healthy Cells Breast - Enzymatic Therapy/PhytoPharmica
Each tablet contains: Folic Acid 200 mcg • Vitamin B12 (cyanocobalamin) 500 mcg • Calcium D-Glucarate 200 mg • Iodine (as potassium iodide) 213 mcg • Broccoli floret and stalk concentrate (brassica oleracea, standardized to contain a minimum of 125 mcg sulforaphane) 125 mg • Green Tea (camellia sinensis) leaf extract (decaffeinated; standardized to contain a minimum of 70% polyphenols) 50 mg • Maitake mushroom powder (grifola frondosa) 50 mg • Maitake mushroom extract (grifola frondosa, standardized to contain a minimum of 28% D-fraction compound) 5 mg.

Healthy Cells Prostate - Enzymatic Therapy/PhytoPharmica
Each tablet contains: Calcium D-Glucarate 200 mg • Selenium (L-selenomethionine) 200 mcg • Broccoli floret and stalk concentrate (brassica oleracea, standardized to contain a minimum of 125 mcg of sulforaphane) 125 mg • Green Tea leaf extract (camillia sinensis, decaffeinated) 50 mg • Maitake mushroom powder (grifola frondosa) 50 mg • Maitake mushroom extract (grifola frondosa, standardized to contain a minimum of 28% D-fraction compound) 5 mg • Lycopene 2.5 mg.

Healthy Cholesterol - NSI - Nutraceutical Sciences Institute
Each four capsules contain: Gamma Oryzanol 300 mg • Gugulipids (standardized for 2.5% guggul sterones) 1000 mg • Beta Sitosterol 150 mg • Green Tea extract (standardized 98% polyphenols, 80% catechins, 45% EGCG) 300 mg • Artichoke extract (standardized for 5% cynarine) 600 mg • Grape seed extract (Activinf) 200 mg • Chromium (as chromium polynicotinate, Chromemates) 400 mcg • Pantethine 450 mg • Policosanol 20 mg.

Healthy Digestion - Health Smart Vitamins
Each capsule contains: Digestive Enzyme Blend: Ox Bile, Protease, Amylase, Lipase, Cellulase, Bromelain, Papain 138 mg • Plant Fiber Base: Sugar Beet Fiber, Rice Bran, Beech cellulose, Spruce cellulose 77 mg.
See Editor's Note No. 14.

Healthy Eyes - Health Smart Vitamins
Each capsule contains: Vitamin A (as beta-carotene) 6,000 IU • Vitamin E (as dl-alpha-tocopheryl acetate) 50 IU • Zinc (as zinc citrate) 25 mg • Selenium (as selenomethionine) 40 mcg • Copper (as copper citrate) 2 mg • Bilberry fruit (36% anthocyanosides, 21.6 mg) 60 mg.

Healthy Eyes - DaVinci Laboratories
Each capsule contains: Vitamin A (100% as beta-carotene) 5000 IU • Vitamin C (ascorbate; ascorbic acid) 250 mg • Vitamin E (D-alpha tocopheryl succinate) 30 IU • Riboflavin 5 mg • Vitamin B12 (methylcobalamin) 10 mcg • Zinc 5 mg • Selenium (L-selenomethionine) 25 mcg • Lutein 6.7 mg • Lycopene 5 mg • Zeaxanthin 700 mcg • L-Glutathione 10 mg • Taurine 50 mg • Alpha Lipoic Acid 25 mg • Quercetin 30 mg • Eyebright whole herb extract (euphrasia officinalis) 60 mg • Bilberry fruit (vaccinium myrtillus L.) 40 mg. Other Ingredients: Rice Flour, Vegetable Stearate, Vegetable Cellulose.

Healthy Eyes Super 100 - Susan Ambrosino's Herb Club, Inc.
Each capsule contains: Proprietary Blend 600 mg: Ginkgo 24/6 extract, Bilberry 4:1 concentrate, Ginkgo leaf, Eyebright, African Bird pepper.

Healthy Hair, Skin, & Nails (60) - Rainbow Light
Each capsule contains: Beta-Carotene 5000 IU • Vitamin E natural 100 IU • Tomato Paste concentrate (Lycopene)300 mg • Vitamin C (Zinc & Copper Ascorbates) 180 mg • Rice Bran 150 mg • Inositol 150 mg • Horsetail herb 4:1 extract 150 mg • Nettles tops 4:1 extract 120 mg • Ginger rhizome 4:1 extract 120 mg • L-Cysteine 100 mg

• Spirulina 100 mg • PABA (Para Aminobenzioc Acid) 75 mg • Red Pepper fruit 60 mg • Pantothenic Acid (Vitamn B5) 60 mg • Rosemary leaf 4:1 extract 50 mg • Maidenhair Fern 40 mg • Marine Mineral Complex 25 mg • Niacin (Vitamin B3) 20 mg • Zinc (Ascorbate)15 mg • Rosemary oil 3 mg • Pyridoxine (Vitamin B6) 2 mg • Biotin 1800 mcg • Copper (Ascorbate) 1500 mcg • Folic Acid 400 mcg • Cyanocobalamin (Vitamin B12) 6 mcg.

Healthy Hearing - Health Smart Vitamins
Each capsule contains: Vitamin B12 (as cyanocobalamin) 100 mcg • Magnesium (as magnesium aspartate) 50 mg • Black Cohosh root 50 mg • Ginkgo leaf (24% ginkgo flavonglycosides, 7.2 mg; 6% terpene lactones, 1.8 mg) 30 mg • Vinpocetine 5 mg.

Healthy Heart with Folic Acid and B6 - Heritage Health Products
Each tablet contains: Vitamin B6 5 mg • Pyridoxal 5 Phosphate 0.5 mg • Folic Acid 600 mcg • Folinic Acid 1 mcg.

Healthy Immunity - Health Smart Vitamins
Each capsule contains: Astragalus root (70% polysaccharides, 70 mg) 100 mg • Elderberry (European elder berry - 10% anthocyanins, 10 mg) 100 mg • Tea green leaf (90% polyphenols, 90 mg) 100 mg • Shiitake (Mycelia extract, LEM, fruiting body) 60 mg • Reishi mycelica 30 mg • Grifola frondosa (maitake mushroom, fruiting body) 25 mg.

Healthy Joints - Health Smart Vitamins
Each capsule contains: Vitamin C (ascorbic acid) 60 mg • Manganese (as manganese glycinate) 2 mg • Glucosamine Sulfate 200 mg • Chondroitin Sulfate 100 mg • Glucosamine Hydrochloride 100 mg • Sea Cucumber 100 mg.
See Editor's Note No. 15.

Healthy Joints - Pro Health
Two capsules contain: Vitamin B3 (niacinamide) 67 mg • Vitamin B5 (pantothenic acid) 67 mg • Vitamin B6 (as pyridoxine HCl) 33 mg • Vitamin C (ascorbic acid) 67 mg • Magnesium (amino acid chelate) 133 mg • Zinc (picolinate) 10 mg • Manganese (amino acid chelate) 5 mg • Copper (amino acid chelate) 2 mg • Glucosamine HCl 667 • Boswellin brand standardized herbal extract of Boswellia Serrata 200 mg • Sea Cucumber 100 mg • Bromelain (2000 GDU activity from pineapple) 100 mg • PABA (para-aminobenzoic acid) 67 mg • Alfalfa juice concentrate 67 mg. Other Ingredients: Gelatin, Stearic Acid, Magnesium Stearate.

Healthy Legs Horse Chestnut Seed Extract - Leiner Health Products
Each caplet contains: Citrus Bioflavonoids complex 15 mg • Ginger powder (Zingiber officinale) root 100 mg • Gotu Kola (Centella asiatica) leaf 33 mg • Grape Seed extract (Vitis vinifera) seed 2 mg • Horse Chestnut extract (Aesculus hippocastanum) seed 300 mg. Other Ingredients: Dicalcium Phosphate, Hydroxypropyl Methylcellulose, Stearic Acid, Dextrin, Titanium Dioxide, Magnesium Stearate, Polyethylene Glycol 8000, Lecithin.

Healthy Liver - NSI - Nutraceutical Sciences Institute
Each six capsules contain: Vitamin C (as magnesium ascorbate) 750 mg • Vitamin E (as d-alpha tocopherols succinate and mixed tocopherols) 250 IU • Thiamine (vitamin B1) 500 mg • Riboflavin (vitamin B2) 10 mg • Niacinamide (vitamin B3) 100 mg • Pyridoxine HCl (vitamin B6) 50 mg • Folic Acid 800 mcg • Vitamin B12 (methylcobalamin) 2 mg • Biotin 3 mg • Pantothenic Acid (vitamin B5) 50 mg • Magnesium (as ascorbate, Ester C) 51 mg • Zinc (as Opti-Zinc) 15 mg • Selenium (selenomethionine) 400 mcg • Chromium (Chrimate, as chromium polynicotinate) 200 mg • Molybdenum (as chelate, AAC) 150 mcg • Potassium (as citrate) 99 mg • Co-enzyme Q10 30 mg • Alpha Lipoic Acid 600 mg • Milk Thistle extract (80% silymarin) 900 mg • N-Acetyl-Cysteine 300 mg • Phosphatidylcholine (LeciPC35P) 400 mg.

Healthy Meal - Vidafit
Each serving contains: Folate 300 mcg • Niacin 16 mg • Pantothenic Acid 5 mg • Riboflavin 1.3 mg • Thiamine 1.2 mg • Vitamin A 2600 IU • Vitamin B12 2.4 mcg • Vitamin B6 1.3 mg • Vitamin C 75 mg • Vitamin D 200 IU • Vitamin E 10 IU • Calcium 500 mg • Chromium 50 mcg • Copper 1 mg • Iodine 150 mcg • Magnesium 420 mg • Phosphorus 500 mg • Potassium 100 mg • Selenium 50 mcg • Zinc 15 mg • Capsicum 5 mg • Glucomannan 500 mg • Soy Protein 6 grams • Whey Protein 12 grams.

Healthy Mood Body Benefits Pak - Leiner Health Products
Each packet contains: Kava Kava extract (Piper methysticum) root 200 mg • Lecithin 45 mg • Licorice extract (Glycyrrhiza glabra) root 60 mg • Siberian Ginseng extract (Eleutherococcus senticosus) root 150 mg • Siberian Ginseng powder (Eleutherococcus senticosus) root 45 mg • St. John's Wort extract (Hypericum perforatum) aerial parts 900 mg. Other Ingredients: Cellulose, Dicalcium Phosphate, Calcium Carbonate, Croscarmellose Sodium, Silicon Dioxide, Stearic Acid, Maltodextrin, Magnesium.

Healthy Prostate - Health Smart Vitamins
Each softgel contains: Saw Palmetto berry (85-95% fatty acids and sterols, 136-152 mg)160 mg • Pygeum africanum bark (>13% total sterols, >6.5 mg) 50 mg • Pumpkin seed oil 40 mg.

Healthy Snack - Vidafit
Each serving contains: Folate 300 mcg • Niacin 16 mg • Pantothenic Acid 5 mg • Riboflavin 1.3 mg • Thiamine 1.2 mg • Vitamin A 2600 IU • Vitamin B12 2.4 mcg • Vitamin B6 1.3 mg • Vitamin C 75 mg • Vitamin D 200 IU • Vitamin E 10 IU • Calcium 500 mg • Chromium 50 mcg • Copper 1 mg • Iodine 150 mcg • Magnesium 420 mg • Phosphorus 500 mg • Potassium 100 mg • Selenium 50 mcg • Zinc 15 mg • Capsicum 5 mg • Glucomannan 300 mg • Soy Protein 3 grams • Whey Protein 6 grams.

Healthy Soy Chocolate - Nature's Life
Each scoop (35 g) contains: Supro Soy Protein Isolate (with less than 2% Lecithin) • Rice Syrup Solids • Fructose • Cocoa powder (with less than 2% Lecithin) • Fructooligosaccharides • Magnesium Citrate • Calcium Carbonate • Glycine • Apple Pectin • Ascorbic Acid • d-Alpha Tocopherol Acetate • Zinc Citrate • Niacinamide • Copper Gluconate • d-Calcium Pantothenate • Manganese Gluconate • Vitamin A Palmitate • l-Selenomethionine • Cholecalciferol • Chromium Niacinate • Pyridoxine HCl • Thiamine Mononitrate • Riboflavin • Folic Acid • Biotin • Potassium Iodide • Sodium Selenite • Sodium Molybdate • Cyanocobalamin.

Healthy Soy Formula - Health Smart Vitamins
Each capsule contains: Soy bean (10% isoflavones, 30 mg) 300 mg • Red Clover aerial parts (8% isoflavones, 16 mg) 200 mg.

Healthy Soy Vanilla - Nature's Life
Each scoop (33 g) contains: Supro Soy Protein Isolate (with less than 2% lecithin) • Maltodextrin • Rice Syrup Solids • Fructose • Fructooligosaccharides • Magnesium Citrate • Calcium Carbonate • Glycine • Apple Pectin • natural Flavors • Ascorbic Acid • d-Alpha Tocopherol Acetate • Zinc Citrate • Niacinamide • Copper Gluconate • d-Calcium Pantothenate • Manganese Gluconate • Vitamin A Palmitate • l-Selenomethionine • Cholecalciferol • Chromium Niacinate • Pyridoxine HCl • Thiamine Mononitrate • Riboflavin • Folic Acid • Biotin • Potassium Iodide • Sodium Selenite • Sodium Molybdate • Cyanocobalamin.

Healthy Vein Support - Health Smart Vitamins
Each capsule contains: Vitamin C (ascorbic acid) 50 mg • Horse Chestnut aerial parts (15% escin, 33.75 mg) 225 mg • Butcher's Broom root (10% ruscogennis, 16.7 mg) 167 mg • Rutin 90 mg • Hesperidin (35% bioflavonoids, 26.25 mg) 75 mg.

Healthy Weight - Health Smart Vitamins
Two capsules contain: Calcium (as calcium salt of hydroxy citric acid) 79 mg • Chromium (as chromium picolinate) 100 mcg • Garcinia cambogia fruit (50% (-) hydroxy citric acid [HCA], 250 mg) 500 mg • L-carnitine (as L-carnitine tartrate) 166 mg.

BRAND NAMES

Healthy Whey - Nature's Life
Three tablespoons (or each rounded scoop, 23 g) contain: Whey Protein concentrate • Natural Flavor composed of Di, Tri, Oligo & Polypeptides (providing 58% B-lactoglobulin, 22% A-Lactalbumin, 10% Immunoglobulin, 10% Minor Proteins & Lactoferrin).

Healthy Woman Soy Menopause - Personal Products
Each tablet contains: Soy Standardized extract 320 mg • Includes Isoflavones 55 mg.

Healthy-Thin - BodyHealth
McB-E60 100 mg • Herbal extract blend 275 mg: Hoodia Gordonii extract, Simmondsia Chinensis extract, Phaseolus Vulgaris extract, Salacia Reticulata, Banaba PE (1% corsolic acid) • Herbal blend 160 mg: Buchu extract, Corn Silk extract, Dandelion root extract, Parsley extract • Vitamin B6 (pyridoxine) 20 mg.

HearAll - NaturalCare
Two capsules contain: Thiamine (B1, as thiamine mononitrate) 1.5 mg • Riboflavin (B2) 1.7 mg • Niacin (B3, as inositol hexanicinate, non-flush) 20 mg • Vitamin B6 (as pyridoxine HCl) 2 mg • Folic Acid 800 mcg • Vitamin B12 (as methylcobalamin) 500 mcg • Magnesium (as amino acid chelate) 93 mg • Zinc (as amino acid chelate) 10 mg • Proprietary Blend 415 mg: Acetyl L-Carnitine, N-Acetylcysteine, Butcher's Broom root (at 10% ruscogenin), Ginkgo Biloba leaf (at 24% flavoglycosides/6% terpenes), Vinpocetine, CoQ10, Alpha Lipoic Acid. Other Ingredients: Gelatin, Purified Water, Glycerin, Titanium Dioxide.

Heart Actives - VitaStore
Six tablets contain: Coenzyme Q-10 5 mg • Chitosan 500 mg • Hawthorne 200 mg • Chromium 100 mcg • Green Tea Extract 200 mg • Fiber Complex (Oat Bran & Psyllium) 1000 mg • Lecithin 500 mg • Vitamin B3 (Niacin) 50 mg • Calcium 500 mg • L-Carnitine 250 mg • Ginger 200 mg • EFA Complex (Essential Fatty Acids) 500 mg • Selenium 150 mcg • Vitamin B1 (Thiamine) 1.5 mg.

Heart Bran - Gero Vita International
Three capsules contain: OatVantage 50% Oat Beta-Glucan 1.5 g • Blue-Max Vaccinium Angustifolium extract 90 mg • Bil-Max Vaccinium Myrtillus 90 mg • Grape-Max Vitis labrusco 90 mg • Apple-Max Mallus Pumila 90 mg. Other Ingredients: Gelatin, Rice Flour, Magnesium Stearate, Silicon Dioxide, Titanium Dioxide.

Heart Energy - J. R. Carlson Laboratories, Inc.
Each 1-2 gels contain: Vitamin E (as D-alpha tocopherol) 60 mg • Vitamin B12 (cyanocobalamin) 200 mcg • Mixed Tocopherols 60 mg • Omega-3 Fish oil concentrate 1000 mg • DHA (docosahexaenoic acid) 125 mg • EPA (eicosapentaenoic acid) 200 mg • Alpha Lipoic 50 mg • Co-Q10 (coenzyme Q10) 100 mg • L-Carnitine 400 mg.

Heart Essentials - Health Smart Vitamins
Two caplets contain: Vitamin A (as 83% beta-carotene, 17% palmitate) 15,000 IU • Vitamin C (as ascorbic acid) 250 mg • Vitamin D (as cholecalciferol) 400 IU • Vitamin E (as d-alpha tocopheryl) 400 IU • Thiamin (as thiamin mononitrate) 25 mg • Riboflavin 25 mg • Niacin (as 50% nicotinic acid, 50% niacinamide) 50 mg • Vitamin B6 (as pyridoxine HCl) 25 mg • Folate (folic acid) 400 mcg • Vitamin B12 (as cyanocobalamin) 100 mcg • Biotin 300 mcg • Pantothenic Acid (as calcium pantothenate) 25 mg • Calcium (as 71% calcium carbonate, 24% dicalcium phosphate, 5% mixed calcium complexes) 269 mg • Phosphorus (as dicalcium phosphate) 10 mg • Iodine (as potassium iodide) 150 mcg • Magnesium (as 90% magnesium oxide, 5% magnesium citrate, 5% magnesium glycinate) 100 mg • Zinc (as zinc ascorbate) 15 mg • Selenium (as selenomethionine) 100 mcg • Copper (as copper citrate) 2 mg • Manganese (as manganese gluconate) 2 mg • Chromium (as chromium polynicotinate) 200 mcg • Molybdenum (as molybdenum amino acid chelate) 50 mcg • Potassium (as potassium citrate) 99 mg • Chondroitin Sulfate 50 mg • Betaine HCl 25 mg • Bioflavonoids 25 mg • Choline (as bitartrate) 25 mg • Garlic bulb (250 mcg allicin) 25 mg • Hawthorn leaf, flower (1.8% vitexin - 2" - rhamnoside) 0.45 mg • Inositol 25 mg • L-Carnitine 25 mg • Lecithin (from soybean) 25 mg • Bromelain (from pineapple, 6,000 PU/g, 120 PU) 20 mg • Coenzyme Q10 10 mg • Lipase (from fermentation of Aspergillus niger) 10 mg • Alpha Lipoic acid 10 mg • Papain (from latex of fruit) 10 mg • Para-aminobenzoic acid (PABA) 10 mg • Rutin 5 mg • Boron (as boron asparate) 2 mg • Silicon (as silicon dioxide) 2 mg • Vanadium (as vanadium amino acid chelate) 10 mcg.
See Editor's Note No. 15.

Heart Essentials - Swanson Health Products
Each tablet contains: Vitamin C (as ascorbic acid) 100 mg • Vitamin E (as d-alpha tocopheryl succinate) 33.3 IU • Niacin 9 mg • Vitamin B-6 (as pyridoxine HCl) 17 mg • Folic Acid 135 mcg • Vitamin B-12 (as cyanocobalamin) 33.3 mcg • Calcium (from amino acid chelate) 33.3 mg • Magnesium (from amino acid chelate) 33.3 mg • Selenium (as selenomethionine) 50 mcg • Chromium (ChromeMate) 33 mcg • Potassium (from amino acid chelate) 33 mg • Taurine 100 mg • Trimethylglycine 84 mg • Odor-Controlled Garlic bulb (PureGar 10,000 ppm allicin potential) 34 mg • Hawthorn berry extract (1.8% vitexin-2' rhamnosides) 17 mg • L-Carnitine 17 mg • Lecithin 17 mg • Coenzyme Q10 10 mg • Ginger root extract (5% gingerols) 8.4 mg.

Heart Formula - Nature's Way
Two capsules contain: Betaine Anhydrous 200 mg • Coenzyme Q10 (Ubiquinone) 15 mg • Folic Acid (Folate) 300 mc • Hawthorne dried extract (1.8%-2.2% Vitexin) 350 mg • Niacin (Vitamin B3) 20 mg • Potassium (Aspartate, Chloride) 20 mg • Pyridoxine HCL 50 mg • Reishi dried extract (10% Polysaccharides) 25 mg • Siberian Ginseng root 250 mg • Vitamin B12 (Cyanocobalamin) 400 mcg • Vitamin E (d-Alpha Tocopheryl) 50 IU. Other Ingredients: Gelatin, Magnesium Stearate, Millet.

Heart Formula - HERBALmax
Danshen radix • Danggui radix • Sanleng rhizoma • Ezhu rhizoma • Chuanxiong rhizoma • Shanzha fruits • Renshen.

Heart Health Essential Omega III - Market America, Inc.
Two capsules contain: 100% Natural Vitamin E (D-alpha tocopherol) 15 IU • Fish Body Oil (50% purity) 3000 mg: EPA (eicosapentaenoic omega-3 fatty acid) 900 mg, DHA (docosahexaenoic omega-3 fatty acid) 600 mg. Other Ingredients: Gelatin, Glycerin, Natural Lemon Flavor.

Heart Health LipiTrim Ultra - Market America, Inc.
Two capsules contain: Tocotrienol Complex (from 167 mg NuTriene 30% tocotrienol oil) 50 mg • Policosanol (from 11.2 mg Marcosanol 90% policosanol complex) 10 mg. Other Ingredients: Soybean Oil, Gelatin, Glycerin, Soy Lecithin, Beeswax, Chlorophyll, Titanium Dioxide.

Heart Health Support - Weil Lifestyle, LLC
Each Magnesium Glycinate tablet contains: Magnesium Glycinate 200 mg.
Each CoQ10 softgel contains: Coenzyme Q10 60 mg.
Each L-Arginine capsule contains: L-Arginine 500 mg.

Heart Health TriActive - Market America, Inc.
Two tablets contain: Thiamin (vitamin B1 as thiamin mononitrate) 2.6 mg • Riboflavin (vitamin B2) 3 mg • Niacin (vitamin B3 as niacinamide) 25 mg • Pantothenic Acid (vitamin B5 as calcium D-pantothenate) 12.5 mg • Vitamin B6 (as pyridoxine hydrochloride) 15 mg • Vitamin B12 (as cyanocobalamin) 500 mcg • Biotin 150 mcg • Folate (as Metafolin) 300 mcg • Zinc (as zinc oxide) 7.5 mg • Garlic (allium sativum, minimum 1% allicin) 450 mg • Beta-Sitosterol (from 637.5 mg 40% beta-sitosterol plant sterols, as Cholestatin) 250 mg • Hawthorn berry 75 mg • Cassia Nomame (minimum 6% flavonoids) 50 mg • Guggulsterones (from 95% guggulsterones granules) 5 mg. Other Ingredients: Calcium Carbonate, Croscarmellose Sodium, Calcium Silicate, Microcrystalline Cellulose, Magnesium Stearate, Crospovidone, Dextrose, Hydroxypropylmethyl Cellulose, Colloidal Silicon Dioxide, Carnauba Wax, Vegetable Acetoglycerides, Polyethylene Glycol, Polysorbate 80.

Heart Power - Gero Vita International
Each capsule contains: Vitamin E (D alpha tocopheryl succinate) 25 IU • Acetyl-L-carnitine 500 mg • Coenzyme Q10 100 mg • Alpha Lipoic Acid 50 mg. Other Ingredients: Gelatin, Silicon Dioxide, Magnesium Stearate.

Heart ReNew - NOW Foods
Each 2 tbsp serving contains: Thiamine (vitamin B1 from thiamine HCl) 3 mg • Riboflavin (vitamin B2) 3 mg • Niacin (vitamin B3 from inositol nicotinate, flush-free) 100 mg • Vitamin B6 (from pyridoxine HCl) 3 mg • Folate (as folic acid) 400 mcg • Vitamin B12 (as cyanocobalamin) 20 mcg • Pantothenic Acid (vitamin B5 from calcium d-pantothenate) 10 mg • Calcium 20 mg • Sodium 35 mg • Potassium 210 mg • Soy based Phospholipids 10 g (typically provides phosphtidylcholine 2.2 g, phosphatidylethanolamine 2 g, phosphatidylinositol 1.4 g, other phospholipids 1.5 g) • Choline 300 mg • Inositol (from phospholipids/inositol nicotinate) 240 mg • Soy Protein isolate (non-GE) 4 g • L-Carnitine (from L-carnitine tartrate) 500 mg • Trimethylglycine (TMG) 40 mg • Stevia Rebaudiana leaf extract (standardized to min. 80% rebaudioside A) 42 mg. Other Ingredients: Fructose, Natural Orange and Vanilla Flavors.

Heart Science - Source Naturals
Six tablets contain: Vitamin A (Beta Carotene) 45000 IU • Vitamin B1 (Thiamin) 50 mg • Inositol Hexanicotinate 500 mg • Vitamin B6 (Pyridoxine HCl) 25 mg • Coenzymated B6 (Pyridoxal-5'-Phosphate)(Yielding 16.9 mg of Vitamin B6) 25 mg • Vitamin B12 (Cyanocobalamin) 500 mcg • Folic Acid 800 mcg • Vitamin C (Magnesium Ascorbate) 1500 mg • Vitamin E (D-Alpha Tocopheryl) (Natural) 400 IU • Chromium (ChromeMate Polynicotinate 150 mcg and Chromium Picolinate 150 mcg) 300 mcg • Copper (Sebacate) 750 mcg • Magnesium (Ascorbate, Taurinate and Oxide) 300 mg • Potassium (Citrate) 99 mg • Selenium (L-Selenomethionine) 200 mcg • Silica (from 400 mg of Horsetail Extract) 28 mg • Coenzyme Q10 (Ubiquinone) 60 mg • L-Carnitine L-Tartrate 500 mg • Hawthorn berry extract 400 mg • Proanthodyn (grape seed extract)(with a Proanthocyanidolic Value of 95) 100 mg • L-Proline 500 mg • L-Lysine (HCl) 500 mg • N-A-G (N-Acetyl Glucosamine) 500 mg • Bromelain (2000 GDU per g) 1200 mg • Taurine (Magnesium Taurinate) 500 mg • Inositol (Hexanicotinate) 50 mg.

Heart Sense - NorthStar Nutritionals
Four tablets contain: Niacin (as flush-free inositol hexanicotinate) 100 mg • Vitamin B6 (as pyridoxine HCl) 8 mg • Active Garlic extract (deodorized, equivalent to approximately 1500 mg of garlic power) 900 mg • Chromium (as ChromeMate brand chromium polynicotinate) 100 mcg • Bioactive Base Blend 40 mg: Soya Lecithin, Cholestatin brand purified Soy Phytosterols, Uva Ursi leaf, Papaya leaf, Papain, Bromelain, Betaine Hydrochloride, L-Glutamic Acid, Selenium Chelate, Alfalfa leaf, Apple Pectin, Citrus pulp, Capsicum pepper, Yucca bark, Wild Cherry bark, Chlorophyll, Hawthorn berry. Other Ingredietns: Dicalcium Phosphate, Sodium Starch Glycolate, Magnesium Stearate, Stearic Acid, Pharmaceutical Glaze.

Heart Source Bars, Honey Nut Crunch - Advocare International
Rice Syrup • Crisp Rice (rice flour, malt extract, rice bran) • Toasted Rolled Oats • Peanuts • Ground Peanuts • Sesame Seeds • Glycerin • Figs • Natural Flavor • Artificial Flavor • Beta Glucan extract (from yeast) • Phytosterol • High Fructose Corn Syrup • Flax (seed) Oil • Guar Gum • Soybean Oil • Salt • Honey • Sucralose • Mixed Tocopherols (vitamin E) • L-Carnitine • Beta-Carotene • Soy Lecithin • Lipoic Acid • Folic Acid • Chromium Polynicotinate • TBHQ (added to protect flavor).

Heart Support - Olympia Nutrition
CoQ10 • Alpha Lipoic Acid • Garlic • Hawthorn • Cayenne • Magnesium.
See Editor's Note No. 14.

Heart Support - NOW Foods
Three tablets contain: Vitamin B1 (Thiamine HCL) 50 mg • Vitamin B6 (Pyridoxine HCL) 50 mg • Vitamin B12 (Cyanocobalamin) 1000 mcg • Folic Acid 800 mcg • Magnesium (Oxide/Aspartate) 200 mg • Potassium (Chloride/Aspartate) 200 mg • Iodine (Kelp extract) 300 mcg • Selenium (Selenomethionine) 140 mcg • Coenzyme Q10, pure 30 mg • L-Carnitine 400 mg • Pure-Gar Garlic 1000 mg • Hawthorne berry extract (standardized to contain 1.25% Vitexin-4' Rhamnoside) 150 mg • Alpha Lipoic Acid 20 mg • Ginger root 250 mg • Cayenne pepper (40000 Heat units) 150 mg.

Heart Support - Nutri-Quest Rx
Each tablet contains: Heart 100 mg • Spleen 40 mg • Co-Enzyme Q-10 2 mg • Vitamin C (Sago Palm) 100 mg • Vitamin E (Succinate) 100 IU • L-Carnitine HCL 20 mg.

Heartbeat Elite Scientifically Complete - J. R. Carlson Laboratories, Inc.
Six tablets contain: Vitamin A (as beta carotene from algae) 6000 IU • Vitamin C (as calcium ascorbate) 2000 mg • Vitamin D (D3, cholecalciferol) 600 IU • Vitamin E (as D-alpha tocopheryl succinate) 600 IU • Thiamin (vitamin B1, as thiamin mononitrate) 60 mg • Riboflavin (vitamin B2) 12 mg • Niacin (vitamin B3, as niacin and niacinamide) 100 mg • Vitamin B6 (as pyridoxine hydrochloride) 60 mg • Folate (folic acid) 1000 mcg • Vitamin B12 (cyanocobalamin) 300 mcg • Biotin 300 mcg • Pantothenic Acid (as di-calcium pantothenate) 60 mg • Calcium (as di-calcium pantothenate, ascorbate) 300 mg • Iodine (from kelp) 150 mcg • Magnesium (as magnesium glycinate chelate) 300 mg • Zinc (as zinc glycinate chelate) 18 mg • Selenium (as L-selenomethionine) 180 mcg • Copper (as copper glycinate chelate) 2 mg • Manganese (as manganese glycinate chelate) 6 mg • Chromium (as chromium glycinate chelate) 300 mcg • Molybdenum (as molybdenum glycinate chelate) 120 mcg • Potassium (as potassium chloride) 99 mg • Lutein 1 mg • Lycopene 3 mg • Alpha Lipoic 30 mg • Boron (as boron citrate) 3 mg • Co-Q10 (coenzyme Q10) 30 mg • Grape seed extract 10 mg • L-Arginine 120 mg • L-Carnitine 300 mg.

Heartburn Free - Enzymatic Therapy
Each softgel contains: Orange (citrus sinesis, peel extract standardized to contain 98.5% d-limonene) 1000 mg.

Heartburn STOP - Renew Life Formulas, Inc.
Each tablet contains: Ellagic Acid (from pomegranate and raspberry fruit) • Raspberry fruit • Green Tea • Turmeric root • Fava bean • Mastic gum • Lecithin powder • Apple Pectin • Gastric Mucin • Vitamin C • Vitamin E (D-alpha tocopherol succinate) • Vitamin A (beta carotene) • Zinc (amino acid chelate) • Calcium (carbonate) • Magnesium (carbonate) • Sodium Bicarbonate.

HeartCare - Nature's Way
Each tablet contains: Hawthorn dried extract (19% oligomeric procyanidins) 80 mg.

HeartOption - BioImmune, Inc.
Each 20 gram scoop contains: Vitamin A (as beta-carotene) 1000 IU • Vitamin C 600 mg • Vitamin D (D3) 80 IU • Vitamin E (mixed tocopherols) 200 IU • Thiamin (vitamin B1) 20 mg • Riboflavin (vitamin B2) 20 mg • Vitamin B3 (inositol hexaniacinate) 60 mg • Vitamin B3 (niacinamide) 100 mg • Folic Acid 800 mcg • Vitamin B6 50 mg • Vitamin B12 (hydroxycobalamin) 300 mcg • Biotin 150 mcg • Pantothenic Acid (calcium) 90 mg • Calcium (gluconate) 50 mg • Magnesium (glycinate) 200 mg • Zinc (arginate) 15 mg • Selenium (methionate) 70 mcg • Manganese (citrate) 1 mg • Chromium (picolinate) 100 mcg • Molybdenum (glycinate) 50 mcg • Potassium (gluconate) 50 mg • Boron 0.5 mg • Vanadium (pentoxide) 70 mcg • Germanium Sesquioxide 25 mg • Alpha-Carotene 10 mg • Pregnenolone 5 mg • DHEA 3 mg • CoEnzyme Q10 50 mg • Cordyceps Sinensis 200 mg • Inositol 30 mg • Choline 40 mg • Para Amino Benzoic Acid 15 mg • Lecithin 600 mg • L-Alanine 76 mg • L-Arginine 400 mg • L-Aspartic Acid 204 mg • L-Carnitine 200 mg • L-Cystine 200 mg • L-Glutamic Acid 3.4 mg • L-Glycine 74 mg •

BRAND NAMES

L-Histidine 46 mg • L-Isoleucine 86 mg • L-Leucine 144 mg • L-Lysine 910 mg • L-Methionine 154 mg • L-Ornithine HCl 150 mg • L-Phenylalanine 92 mg • L-Proline 390 mg • L-Serine 92 mg • L-Taurine 600 mg • L-Threonine 66 mg • L-Tyrosine 66 mg • L-Tryptophan 11 mg • L-Valine 88 mg • N-Acetyl-Cysteine 50 mg • Glutathione 50 mg • Pancreatin 8X 2.5 mg • Papain 10 mg • Bromelain 25 mg • Grape Skin Extract 150 mg • Hawthorne Berry Extract 175 mg • Garlic (1% alicin) 80 mg • Tocotrienols 15 mg • Trimethyl Glycine 600 mg • Methylsulfonylmethane 50 mg • Alpha Lipoic Acid 50 mg. In a base of Oat Bran, Rice Bran, ISO Malt, Freeze-dried Pineapple, Pineapple Flavoring, Stevia, Silicon Dioxide.

Heart's Ease - The Herbalist
Hawthorn berry, leaf & flower • Dandelion root, leaf & flower • Skullcap herb • Yarrow flower • Horsetail herb • Lemon Balm herb • Prickly Ash bark • Cayenne pepper.

HeartVin - Life Enhancement Products, Inc.
Each capsule contains: Vitamin C (from ascorbyl palmitate) 64 mg • Resveratrol 20% (polygonum cuspidatum root) 10 mg • Green Tea (90% polyphenols, 6% caffeine) 400 mg • Quercetin 40 mg. Other Ingredients: Gelatin Capsule, Rice Flour, Silicon Dioxide.

Heat - The Sports Nutrition Source, Inc.
Each capsule contains: Ma Huang concentrate 24 mg • Caffeine USP 80 mg • Guarana seed concentrate 75 mg • White Willow bark concentrate 75 mg • Cayenne fruit 60 mg • Ginger root 40 mg.
See Editor's Note No. 30.

Heavenly Skin & Hair Care - Gary Null & Associates (GNA)
Whole leaf Aloe Vera concentrate, Jojoba oil, Licorice and Grape seed extracts, Tri-Silica complex, MSM, Antioxidant Botanical extracts, Liposomal Vitamins, Oat Bran glucan, Tissue Respiratory Factor, and more.

Heavy Metal CLEANSE - Renew Life Formulas, Inc.
Mineral Support Formula: Two capsules contain: Vitamin C (ascorbic acid) 500 mg • Vitamin B1 (thiamine hydrochloride) 25 mg • Vitamin B2 (riboflavin) 25 mg • Vitamin B3 (no flush-inositol hexanicotinate) 25 mg • Vitamin B6 (pyridoxine HCl) 25 mg • Folic Acid 400 mcg • Vitamin B12 (cyanocobalamin) 100 mcg • Biotin 300 mcg • Vitamin B5 (calcium pantothenate) 25 mcg • Calcium (calcium carbonate) 50 mg • Magnesium (magnesium aspartate) 100 mg • Zinc (zinc gluconate) 15 mg • Selenium (selenium amino acid chelate/ selenomethionine) 200 mcg • Copper (copper citrate) 2 mg • Manganese (manganese citrate) 8 mg • Chromium (chromium glycinate) 100 mcg • Molybdenum (molybdenum citrate) 50 mcg • Boron (boron citrate) 100 mcg • Vanadium (vanadium citrate) 50 mcg • Other Ingredients: Gelatin, Water.
Organ Cleanse Formula: Two capsules contain: Chlorella (cracked shell) 300 mg • Cilantro 100 mg • Sodium Alginate (laminaria) 100 mg • Spirulina 100 mg • Bladderwrack (fucus vesiculosus) 50 mg • Garlic (1500 ppm allicin) 50 mg • Kelp (ascophyllumnodosum) 50 mg • L-Leucine 50 mg • NAC (N-acetyl-cysteine) 50 mg • Alpha Lipoic Acid 20 mg. Other Ingredients: Hypromellose, Water.

Heavyweight Gainer 900 - Champion Nutrition
Each serving contains: Metacarb-III (branching complex carbohydrates extracted from Corn Hybrids including Maltodextrins) • Peptol-III: pre-digested highly efficient protein blend consisting of Whey Protein Concentrate, Fat-Free, Cholesterol-Free, Red-Muscle Protein Complex, Debitterized Enzyme Digest of Lactalbumin, & Egg White Protein • extra grade Whey • Fructose • low-fat Cocoa powder • MCT's • Metavite-III [Champion Nutrition's advanced Vitamin/ Mineral formula consisting of di-Calcium Pantothenate, Potassium, Citrate, Magnesium Gluconate, Potassium Chloride, Choline Bitartrate, Inositol, Ascorbic Acid, D-Calcium Pantothenate, Niacin, Zinc Gluconate, d-Alpha Tocopherol Succinate, Molybdenum Aspartate, Selenium Aspartate, Manganese Gluconate, Chromemate-GTF (Chromium Polynicotinate), Copper Gluconate, Pyridoxal-5-Phosphate, Thiamine HCL, D-Biotin, Potassium Iodide, Ergocalciferol, Folic Acid, Cyanocobalamin] • Cellulose Gum • Xanthan • Natural & Artificial Flavors • Lecithin • Sunnette Brand of Acesulfame-K • Carrageenan • Aspartame. Contains Phenylalanine.

HeightMax Concentrate - Sunny Health Nutrition Technology & Products, Inc.
Each serving contains: Vitamin A (50% palmitate; 50% beta-carotene) 15,000 IU • Vitamin C (as ascorbic acid) 300 mg • Vitamin D (as cholecalciferol) 400 IU • Vitamin E (as D-alpha tocopheryl succinate) 150 IU • Thiamin (as thiamin mononitrate) 75 mg • Riboflavin 75 mg • Niacin 35 mg • Vitamin B6 (as pyridoxine HCl) 75 mg • Folic Acid 400 mcg • Vitamin B12 (as cobalamin) 75 mcg • Biotin 75 mcg • Pantothenic Acid 75 mcg • Korean Ginseng extract 50 mg • American Ginseng extract 50 mg • Siberian Ginseng extract 50 mg • Ginkgo Biloba extract 50 mg • Gotu Kola extract 30 mg.

HeightMax Plus - Sunny Health Nutrition Technology & Products, Inc.
Each tablet contains: Calcium (as calcium carbonate and gluconate-chelate) 1000 mg • Iron 12 mg • Iodine 150 mg • Magnesium 500 mg • Zinc 10 mg • Selenium (as L-selenomethionine) 50 mg • Copper (as chelate and copper oxide) 1 mg • Manganese (as glycinate amino-acid chelate) 1 mg • Chromium (as niacin amino-acid chelate) 30 mcg • Molybdenum (glycine amino-acid chelate) 25 mcg • Potassium (as potassium amino acid complex) 1.8 mg • Inositol 100 mg • Choline (as choline bitartrate) 50 mg • Betaine HCl 25 mg • Biotin 25 mg • Citrus Bioflavonoids 25 mg • Hesperidin 10 mg • Boron (as amino acid chelate) 3 mg • Carotenoids 100 mcg • 5-HTP (hydroxytryptophan) 50 mg • Lysine 50 mg • Branched Chain Amino Acids (BCAA, 1:1:1 parts of leucine, isoleucine, and valine) 150 mg • Taurine 250 mg • L-Arginine 250 mg • L-Ornithine 125 mg • GABA (gamma amino butyric acid) 100 mg • Gamma-Oryzanol 125 mg.

Hemagenics - Metagenics
Each tablets contain: Iron (as iron glycinate) 29 mg • Vitamin B6 (as pyridoxine hydrochloride) 5 mg • Thiamin (as thiamin mononitrate) 5 mg • Folate (as folic acid, L-5-methyl tetrahydrofolate, 5-formyl tetrahydrofolate) 600 mcg • Vitamin B12 (as cyanocobalamin) 350 mcg • Succinic Acid 100 mg • Glycine 100 mg • Copper (as copper glycinate) 1 mg.

Hemaplex - Progressive Labs
Each capsule contains: Iron (from 200 mg iron peptonate) 32 mg • Vitamin C (ascorbic acid) 200 mg • Thiamin HCl (Vitamin B1) 2 mg • Riboflavin (Vitamin B2) 2 mg • Niacin 13 mg • Niacinamide 15 mg • Vitamin B6 (pyridoxine HCl) 2 mg • Folate (folic acid) 400 mcg • Vitamin B12 (cyanocobalamin) 50 mcg • Base 50 mg: Raw Duodenum, Raw Liver, Raw Stomach, Red Bone Marrow, Beef Peptone, Citrus Pectin, Betaine HCl, Bile Salts, Rose Hips, Alfalfa, Wheat Germ.
See Editor's Note No. 14.

Hem-Care - PhytoPharmica
Two capsules contain: Butcher's Broom root and rhizome extract (ruscus aculeatus, standardized to contain 9-11% saponins calculated as ruscogenins) 100 mg • Calcium (as calcium lactate) 20 mg • Choline Bitartrate 150 mg • Glycosaminoglycans (GAGs) 25 mg • Sophora Japonica flower bud (standardized to contain 95% rutin) 100 mg • Phosphorus (as tricalcium phosphate) 25 mg • Stone Root root and rhizome (collinsonia canadensis) 500 mg • Vitamin C (ascorbic acid) 100 mg • Vitamin E (as D-alpha tocopheryl acid succinate) 30 IU.
See Editor's Note No. 14.

HemHalt - TriLight Herbs
Blue Cohosh • Bayberry • Yarrow • Capsicum.

Hem-Mend: Hemorrhoid Support - The Herbalist
Stone root fresh dried (Collinsonia canadensis) • Celandine fresh-flowering herb (Chaelidonium majus) • Witch Hazel fresh-dried leaf (Hamamelis virginiana) • Horse Chestnut fresh nut (Aesculus hippocastanum).

Hemo-Plus - Atrium Biotechnologies
Each tablet contains: Vitamin C 300 mg • Vitamin B1 10 mg • Vitamin B2 10 mg • Vitamin B6 10 mg • Vitamin B12 250 mcg • Folic Acid 800 mcg • Niacinamide 20 mg • Iron Peptonate 113 mg • Manganese (Proteinate Chelated) 5 mg • Liver 75 mg.
See Editor's Note No. 14.

Hemorrhoid Remedy - PhytoPharmica
Twenty drops contain: Aloe socotrina 4x • Sulphur 4x • Collinsonia canadensis 3x •Narum nitricum 3x • Nux vomica 3x • Paeonia officinalis 3x •Teucrium scorodonia 3x • Verbascum thapsus 2x • Aesculus hippocastanum 1x • Boldo 1x • Hamamelis virginiana 1x. In a base of 45% USP alcohol by volume.
See Editor's Note No. 1.

Hemorrhoids - Hyland's
Two tablets contain: Aesculus Hippocastanum 3X • Ratanhia 3X • Nux Vomica 3X (0.0012% alkaloids) • Calcarea Fluorica 6X. Base: Lactose USP.
See Editor's Note No. 1.

Hemorrhol - Xymogen
Active Ingredients: Witch Hazel (hammamelis virginiana) 10% • Glycerin 10% • Cod Liver oil 3%. Other Ingredients: Deionized Water, Aloe Vera Gel, Shea Butter, Sunflower Seed Oil, Caprylic/ Capric Triglycerides, Cetyl Alcohol, Polyacrylamide and C13-C14 Isoparaffin and Laureth-7, Stearic Acid, Cetearyl Alcohol and Ceteareth-20, Hydroxypropylmethylcellulose, Disodium EDTA, Carbomer, TEA, Croton lechleri Extract, Uncaria spp, Green Tea Extract, Allantoin, Methyl Paraben, Propyl Paraben, Diazolidinyl.

HemoStream - DreamPharm
Two capsules contain: Proprietary Blend: Chitosan, Barley Grass, Rehmannia radix, Angelica Sinensis radix, Cinnamomi Ramulus, Ligustici Wallchii rhizoma, Carthami Flos, Mass Medicata Fermentata, Scirpi rhizoma, Salivae Miltiorrhizae rhizoma, Zedoaria, Malt, Licorice, Crataegus fructus, Mastic, Agrimony, Burdock.

Hem-Tone - Enzymatic Therapy
Two capsules contain: Vitamin E (D-Alpha Tocopherol Succinate) 30 IU • Calcium Lactate 130 mg • Vitamin C (Ascorbic Acid) 100 mg • Phosphorus (Tricalcium Phosphate) 25 mg • Other Ingredients: Colinsonia root (Stone root) 500 mg • Choline Bitartrate 150 mg • Butchers Broom extract (Ruscus aculeatus) standardized to contain 10% Saponins (calculated as Ruscogenin) 100 mg • Rutin (Buckwheat) 100 mg • Glycosaminoglycans 25 mg: A mixture of highly purified bovine-derived Glycosaminoglycans naturally present in the aorta including Dermatan Sulfate, Heparan Sulfate, Hyaluronic Acid, Chondroitin Sulfate, & related Hexosaminoglycans.
See Editor's Note No. 15.

Hep - Mushroom Blend - Wild Rose
Each vegetable cap contains: Maitake 4:1 extract 95 mg • Shiitake 8:1 extract 70 mg • Coriolus mushroom 8:1 extract 45 mg • Dandelion root 70 mg • Black Radish root 35 mg • Burdock root 35 mg.

Hep Support - Gaia Herbs
Two capsules contain: Astragalus root (astragalus membranaceus) 200 mg • Chinese Skullcap root (scutellaria baicalensis) 100 mg • Chinese Bupleurum root (bupleurum falcatum) 60 mg • Reishi mushroom (ganoderma lucidum) 30 mg • Maitake mushroom (grifola frondosa) 20 mg • Licorice root (glycyrrhiza glabra) 20 mg. Other Ingredients: Vegetable Glycerin, Vegetable Cellulose (capsule).

Hepastat - BotanicLab
Bupleurum Chinense DC (bupleurum; chai-hu) • Scutellaria Baicalensis Georgi (scute; huang-chin) • Paeonia Lactiflora Pall (white peony root; chih-shao) • Isatis Indigotica Fort (isatidis; ta-ching-yeh) • Astragalus Membranaceus (astragalus; huang-chi) • Silybum Marianum Gaertn (milk thistle; shui-fei-fi) • Apis Mellifera (honey bee) L. (royal jelly; fon-hwang-chiang) • Glycyrrhiza Glabra L. (licorice; gan-cao).

Hepatacin - Metagenics
Two tablets contain: Proprietary Blend 550 mg: Picrorhiza root 8:1 extract (picrorhiza kurroa, containing kutkins), Andrographis leaf 16:1 extract (andrographis paniculata), Amla fruit 3:1 extract (emblica officinalis, containing tannins), Arjuna bark 5:1 extract (terminalia arjuna, containing tannin), Cinnamon bark (cinnamomum cassia).

Hepatic Factors - Michael's Naturopathic Programs
Three tablets contain: Vitamin A (as beta carotene) 1500 IU • Vitamin E (as D-alpha tocopheryl succinate) 150 IU • Vitamin K (as phylloquinone) 45 mcg • Thiamin (as thiamin hydrochloride) 30 mg • Niacin (as nicotinic acid) 30 mg • Vitamin B12 (as cyanocobalamin) 300 mcg • Pantothenic Acid (as D-calcium pantothenate) 30 mg • Proprietary Blend 2153 mg: Lecithin (from soy), Choline (as choline bitartrate), Inositol, Dandelion root 4:1 extract (taraxacum officinale), Methionine (as L-methionine hydrochloride), Threonine (as L-threonine), Butternut root bark (juglans cinerea), Milk Thistle seed 20:1 extract (silybum marianum, 80% silymarin, 60 mg), Yellow Dock root (rumex crispus), Burdock root 4:1 extract (arcitum lappa). Other Ingredients: Microcrystalline Cellulose, Calcium Carbonate, Stearic Acid, Magnesium Stearate.

Hepatic Support - Zone Labs
Six capsules contain: Vitamin C (ascorbic acid) 100 mg • Organic Spirulina 700 mg • Barley juice powder 100 mg • Alfalfa juice powder 100 mg • Chlorella powder 50 mg • Milk Thistle extract (silymarin) 50 mg • Lecithin 50 mg • Hesperidin complex 50 mg • Rutin 50 mg • Indole 3 Carbinol 100 mg • Alpha Lipoic Acid 100 mg • L-Methionine 50 mg • L-Cysteine 50 mg • L-Carnitine (as fumarate) 25 mg • Choline (as choline bitartrate) 55 mg • Glutathione 50 mg • NAC (N-acetyl cysteine) 100 mg. Other Ingredients: Gelatin, Microcrystalline Celluose, FOS, Magnesium Stearate, Silica, Purified Water, Broccoli Extract, Brussels Sprout Extract, Cabbage Extract, Maitake Mushrooms, Sodium Lauryl Sulfate.

Hepato-C - Pacific BioLogic
Salvia root • Heydyotis • Scutellaria (barbat skullcap) • Peony root (red) • Codonopsis root (natural) • Lycium fruit • Dryopteris rhizome • Rhodiole Sachelanensi root • Polygonum root (thin) • Magnolia bark • Knotweed rhizome (bushy) • Astragalus root (Grade 1) • Capillaris shoots & leaves • Bitter Orange (ripened fruit) • Polyporus Sclerotium.
See Editor's Note No. 40.

Hepato-Detox - Pacific BioLogic
Salvia root • Codonopsis root (natural) • Lycium fruit • Polygonatum rhizome • Astragalus root (Grade 1) • Reishi Mushroom • Privet fruit (ligustrum) • Ginseng root (red ji lin) • Cherry (cornelian asiatic).

Hepatox - PhytoPharmica
Three tablets contain: Barberry bark of root 6:1 extract (berberis vulgaris) 150 mg • Beet root (beta vulgaris) 300 mg • Betaine HCl 75 mg • Biotin 200 mcg • Boldo leaf 2:1 extract (peumus boldus) 150 mg • Celandine aerial part (chelidonium majus) 135 mg • Choline Bitartrate 850 mg • Evening Primrose seed oil (oenothera biennis, standardized to contain 4.5% gamma-linoleic acid (GLA) 30 mg • Fringe Tree bark (chionanthus virginicus) 135 mg • Inositol 50 mg • Liver (desiccated) 40 mg • L-Methionine 250 mg • Niacin (as nicain and nicainamide) 40 mg • Ox Bile extract 90 mg • Vitamin A (as retinyl acetate) 4500 IU • Vitamin B12 (as cyanocobalamin) 3 mcg • Vitamin C (ascorbic acid and from rose hips) 25 mg.
See Editor's Note No. 14.

Hepatrophin PMG - Standard Process, Inc.
Each tablet contains: Bovine Liver PMG extract 320 mg. Other Ingredients: Honey, Calcium Stearate.
See Editor's Note No. 14.

Hepol - ProJoba
Each tablet contains: Botanical Glutathione Yeast extract YH 85 mg • Aloe Vera extract 45 mg • Polbax extract 40 mg. Other Ingredients: Lacrose Alfa, Microcrystalline Cellulose, Magnesium Stearate, Colloidal Silicon Dioxide, Talc, Natural Resin.

Her Pleasure Sexual Enhancing Gel - Eve's Accents
L-Arginine • Menthol • Epimedium • Guarana seed extract • Damiana • Wild Yam (Mexican) • Purified Water.

Her Stuff - Blue Stuff, Inc.
Each 4 oz bottle contains: Whole leaf Aloe Vera • Purified Water • Yam extract • Polyglycerylmethacylate • Propylene Glycol • Carbomer-940 • Safflower oil • Emu oil • Isopropyl Palmitate • Natural Progesterone extract • Laureth-4 • Gluceryl Stearate • PEG-100 Stearate • Siberian Ginseng root extract • Black Cohosh root extract • Burdock root extract • Licorice root extract • Hops extract • Alfalfa extract • Tansy extract • Dang Gui extract • Sweet Almond oil • Jojoba oil • Avocado oil • Triethanolamine • Rosemary oil • Fragrance • Chamomile extract • Tetrasodium EDTA • Sodium Hydroxymethylglycinate • Tocopherol.

Herba Fuel - TwinLab
Three capsules contain: Ma Huang extract (standardized for 6% Ephedrine) 334 mg • Chinese Green Tea extract (standardized for 7% Caffeine & 20% Polyphenols) 1500 mg. In a natural base of Siberian Ginseng (Eleutherococcus senticosus).
See Editor's Note No. 30.

HerbaCoral Coral Calcium & 72 Coral Minerals - HerbaLab
Three capsules contain: Vitamin C (as ascorbic acid) 15 mg • Vitamin D (as cholecalciferol) 1200 IU • Calcium (from coral) 690 mg • Magnesium (amino acid chelate & coral) 168 mg • Coral Powder 672 mg • Malic Acid 30 mg • Betaine Hydrochloride 15 mg.

Herbal Aloe Drink - Herbalife International of America, Inc.
Water • Aloe Vera concentrate • Citric Acid • Chamomile extract • Potassium Sorbate • Sodium Benzoate • Sodium Citrate • Lemon Juice concentrate.

Herbal Armor Lotion - All Terrain Company
Active Ingredients: Citronella Oil 12% • Peppermint Oil 2.5% • Cedar Oil 2% • Lemongrass Oil 1% • 0.05% Geranium Oil. Other Ingredients (82.45%): Water, Beeswax, Soybean Oil, Steareth-100, Aloe Vera Gel, Glycerin, Sorbitol, Sorbitan, Tristearate, Xanthan Gum, Silica, Methylparaben, Propylparaben.

Herbal Armor SPF 15 - All Terrain Company
Active Ingredients: Zinc Oxide • Octyl Methoxycinnamate. Other Ingredients: Water, Beeswax, Soybean Oil, Glycerin, Aloe Vera Gel, Bentonite, Steareth-100, Sorbitan Tristearate, Xanthan Gum, Methylparaben, Propylparaben.

Herbal Armor Spray - All Terrain Company
Active Ingredients: Citronella Oil 12% • Peppermint Oil 2.5% • Cedar Oil 2% • Lemongrass Oil 1% • Geranium Oil 0.05%. Other Ingredients (82.45%): Water, Beeswax, Soybean Oil, Steareth-100, Sorbitan Tristearate.

Herbal Biotic - Vital Nutrients
Two capsules contain: Coptis Chinensis 10:1 extract 100 mg • Forsythia Suspensa 20:1 extract 50 mg • Lonicera Japonica 7:1 extract 150 mg • Allium Sativum extract (garlic) 200 mg • Myrrh powder 200 mg • Echinacea extract (4% phenolics) 250 mg • Citrus Bioflavonoid Complex 200 mg • Zinc (citrate) 10 mg • Vitamin A (acetate) 10,000 IU • Vitamin C 500 mg.

Herbal Breath - DreamPharm
Two capsules contain: Rhizoma Polygonati Odoranti 100 mg • Herba Menthae Haplocalysis 100 mg • Herba Agastaches Seu Pogostemi 100 mg • Spearmint leaf 100 gm • Semen Pruni Armeniacae 50 mg • Fructus Amomi Kravanh 50 mg.

Herbal CA - Nature's Sunshine
Each capsule contains: Proprietary Blend 385 mg: Alfalfa aerial parts (medicago sativa), Horsetail stem and strobilus (equisetum arvense), Oat straw stem (avena sativa), Great Plantain leaf (plantago major), Marshmallow root (althaea officinalis), Wheat grass aerial parts (triticum aestivum), Hops flower (humulus lupulus). Other Ingredients: Gelatin, Water.

Herbal Cold - Puritan's Pride
Each tablet contains: Vitamin C (calcium ascorbate) 500 mg • Calcium (calcium ascorbate) 50 mg • Poplar Bud extract 25 mg • Senega extract 10 mg • Oil of Thyme 5 mg • Oil of Eucalyptus 5 mg • Hore Hound powdered 10 mg • Coltsfoot powdered 10 mg • Licorice root powdered 15 mg • Capsicum powdered 10 mg • Cubeb powdered 10 mg • Slippery Elm bark powdered 10 mg • Fennel powdered 10 mg • Jamaican Ginger powdered 10 mg • Honey 10 mg • Lemon Juice 1 mg • Rutin 10 mg • Bee Pollen 10 mg • Bee Propolis 50 mg.

Herbal Cold Relief - Jamieson
Each capsule contains: Ephedra stem extract (Ephedra sinensis, equivalent to 10.2 mg of ephedrine) 62.5 mg • Grindelia aerial parts 1:4 extract (Grindelia Camporum) 0.5 mg • Eucalyptus oil (Eucalypyus Globulus) 0.05 mg • Echinacea Root (Echinacea purpurea) 100 mg.
See Editor's Note No. 30.

Herbal Cold Season Defense - Quantum, Inc.
Three capsules contain: Vitamin C 250 mg • Echinacea angustifolia standardized to 4% phenolic compounds 100 mg • Elderberry (10:1) extract 100 mg • Goldenseal root (3:1) extract 25 mg. Other Ingredients: Vegetable Sterine, Magnesium Stearate, Micro Crystalline Cellulose.
See Editor's Note No. 21.

Herbal Colon Cleanser & Tonic - Grandma's Herbs
Each capsule contains: Proprietary Blend .450 g: Cascara Sagrada, Senna pods, Psyllium seeds/hulls, Licorice root, Aloes, Turkey Rhubarb, Buckthorn, Prunes, Dandelion, Barberry, Slippery Elm, Marshmallow, Alfalfa, Calmus root, Plantain, Black Walnut, Butternut, Gentian root, Red Clover, Flax Seed, Sage Brush, Chicory, Fennel, Ginger, Chamomile, Calendula, Wahoo, Blue Vervain, Blue Flag, Red Raspberry leaf, Yucca.

Herbal Complex for Eyes - Hillestad
Each tablet contains: Eye Bright herb 400 mg • Bilberry fruit extract (from concentrate) 200 mg • Taurine (amino acid) 100 mg • Carrot taproot 30 mg. Other Ingredients: Oyster Shell, Cellulose, Ethyl Cellulose, Silica, Magnesium Stearate.

Herbal Complex for Immune System - Hillestad
Each tablet contains: Elderberry flower 300 mg • Echinacea whole plant extract (from concentrate) 300 mg • Goldenseal root 12.5 mg • Zinc (gluconate) 15 mg. Other Ingredients: Oyster Shell, Cellulose, Ethyl Cellulose, Magnesium Stearate.

Herbal Complex for Men - Hillestad
Each tablet contains: Vitamin C (ascorbic acid) 250 mg • Muira Puama root extract (from concentrate) 100 mg • Yohimbe bark exract (from concentrate) 50 mg • Ginkgo Biloba leaf extract 40 mg • Saw Palmetto fruit extract (from concentrate) 25 mg. Other Ingredients: Oyster Shell, Calcium Phosphate, Ethyl Cellulose, Cellulose, Magnesium Stearate, Silica.

Herbal Complex for Stress - Hillestad
Each tablet contains: Valerian root 400 mg • Hops flower 150 mg • Kava-Kava root 150 mg • Passionflower 150 mg • Licorice root 100 mg. Other Ingredients: Oyster Shell, Cellulose, Ethyl Cellulose, Magnesium Stearate.

Herbal Decongestant Expectorant Capsules - Life Brand
Ma Huang (Ephedra) 50 mg as a standardized extract 1:10 (equivalent to 500 mg Ma Huang) with 4 mg of total Ephedrines • Wild Horehound leaf 150 mg • Thyme herb extract (1:4) 100 mg (equivalent to 400 mg of Thyme) • Coltsfoot leaf 50 mg • Mullein leaf 50 mg • Cayenne 1.125 mg • Marshmallow root 9 mg • Slippery Elm bark 9 mg. Other Ingredients: Gelatin, Water.
See Editor's Note No. 30.

Herbal Diuretic - Progressive Labs
Each capsule contains: Proprietary blend 120 mg: Buchu leaves (Barsoma crenata) • Couch Grass root (Triticum repens) • Proprietary blend 330 mg: Hydrangea root (Hydrangea arborescens), Corn Silk

(Stigmata maidis), Juniper berry (Juniperus communis), Burdock root (Arctium lappa), Uva Ursi leaf (Arctostaphylos Uva-Ursi), Ginger root (Zingiber officinale) Parsley (Petroselium sativum), Marshmallow root (Althaea officinalis).

Herbal Diuretic - Jamieson
Each capsule contains: Uva Ursi 200 mg • Buchu Leaves 100 mg.

Herbal Diuretic Formula - Quest
Each caplet contains: Uva Ursi leaf (Arctostaphylos uva-ursi) (Provided by 50 mg P.E. 1:4) 200 mg • Juniper berry extract (Junuperus communis) (Provided by 80 mg P.E. 1:4) 320 mg • Parsley root (Petroselinum crispum) (Provided by 40 mg P.E. 1:4) 160 mg. Other Ingredients: Buchu leaves, Cayenne, Corn Silk, Kelp, Parsley leaf, Pumpkin seed, Saw Palmetto berries, Calcium Phosphate, Vegetable Stearin, Croscarmellose Sodium, Magnesium Stearate (vegetable source).

Herbal Diuretic Tablets - Life Brand
Buchu leaf extract (1:4) 25 mg (equivalent to 100 mg Buchu leaf) • Uva Ursi leaf extract (1:3) 33.3 mg (equivalent to 100 mg Uva Ursi leaf) • Juniper berry extract (1:2) 50 mg (equivalent to 100 mg of Juniper berries) • Celery seed 75 mg • Parsley root 75 mg. Excipients: Microcrystalline Cellulose, Tricalcium Phosphate, Corn Starch, Magnesium Stearate.

Herbal Douche - Dial Herbs
Mineral Water • Aloe Vera • White Oak bark • Slippery Elm • Uva Ursi • Cayenne.

Herbal Ecstacy - Global World Media
Each pill contains: Ephedra • Ma Huang • Guarana • Gingko biloba • Cola Nut • Gotu-Kola • Fo-Ti-Tient (Fo-Ti) • Green Tea • Rou Gui (Chinese Nutmeg).
See Editor's Note No. 5 and No. 30.

Herbal Enhancer - Pentabosol
Two tablets contain: Cinnamon bark 150 mg • Green Tea leaf extract (36% catechin and polyphenols) 100 mg • Cloves 50 mg • Brewer's Yeast 100 mg • Flax Seed 100 mg • Cumin seed 25 mg • Garlic extract (odor controlled) 25 mg • Gymnema Sylvestre leaf 150 mg • Fenugreek seed 150 mg • Coriander 50 mg • Bilberry leaf 10 mg. Other Ingredients: Dicalcium Phosphate, Microcrystalline Cellulose, Croscarmellose Sodium, Stearic Acid, Magnesium Stearate, Silica, Pharmaceutical Glaze.

Herbal Exfoliating Scrub - FreeLife International
Purified Water • Walnut shell powder (juglans regia) • Vegetable Glycerin • Algae extract • Orange water (citrus aurantium dulcis) • Luffa Cylindrica • Xanthan gum • Jojoba beads • Sodium Stearoyl Lactylate • Sodium Lactate • Sodium PCA • Sorbitol • Proline • Allantoin • Camellia Oleifera seed extract • Luffa Cylindrica extract • Mate extract (ilex paraguariensis) • Bergamot oil (citrus aurantium bergamia) • Basil oil (ocimum basilicum) • Eucalyptus oil (eucalyptus globulus) • Shea Butter (butyrospermum parkii) • Chlorphenesin • Benzoic Acid • Chlorophyllin - Copper Complex.

Herbal Expector-Aid - Quantum, Inc.
Each softgel contains: Vitamin C (ascorbic acid) 200 mg • Elderberry extract berry standardized to 5% flavonoids 200 mg • Fenugreek powder seed (4:1) extract 100 mg • Horehound powder flower, leaf, stem (4:1) extract 100 mg • Anise seed (4:1) extract 100 mg • Marshmallow root (4:1) extract 60 mg • Anise seed oil 40 mg • Echinacea extract flower, leaf (4:1 PE) 40 mg • Menthol Crystals 20 mg • Eucalyptus Oil 10 mg. Other Ingredients: Gelatin Shell: Gelatin, Glycerin, St. John's Bread, Titanium Dioxide; Liquid Fill: Sunflower Seed Oil, Beeswax, Lecithin.
See Editor's Note No. 21.

Herbal Fem - Nutri-Quest Rx
Golden Seal root, Dong Quai, Blessed Thistle, Red Raspberry leaves, Squaw Vine, Scullcap, Cayenne, Blue Cohosh, Licorice root, Wild Yam root, Passion Flower 408 mg. In a base of 6X tissue salts: Calc Fluor, Calc Phos, Calc Sulph, Kali Mur, Kali Phos, Kali Sulph, Mag Phos, Nat Mur, Nat Phos, Nat Sulph, Silica.

Herbal Formula I - Hillestad
Each tablet contains: Magnesium Oxide 25 mg • Celery seed 125 mg • Garlic (deodorized) 200 mg • Hawthorn berries 25 mg • Chamomile (various parts) 25 mg • Cayenne herb 25 mg• Valerian root 25 mg • Black Cohosh root 50 mg • Ginseng root 25 mg • Gotu Kola herb 25 mg • CoEnzyme Q10 5 mg. Other Ingredients: Oyster Shell, Lecithin, Glycerol Monostearate, Stearic Acid, Magnesium Stearate, Silicon Dioxide.

Herbal Formula II - Hillestad
Each tablet contains: Glucosamine (glucosamine sulfate) 125 mg • Chondroitin Sulfate (cartilage) 75 mg • Yucca leaf extract 50 mg • Chaparral leaf 25 mg • Cayenne fruit 25 mg • Garlic (deodorized) 15 mg • Red Clover flower 25 mg • Feverfew leaf extract 25 mg • Willow bark 25 mg • Sarsaparilla root 25 mg • Citric Acid (fruit) 50 mg. Other Ingredients: Magnesium Oxide, Ethyl Cellulose, Cellulose, Stearic Acid, Magnesium Stearate.
See Editor's Note No. 15.

Herbal Formula III - Hillestad
Each tablet contains: Sodium Caprylate 120 mg • Pau d'Arco bark 50 mg • Horseradish root 12.5 mg • Clover extract oil 800 mcg • Goldenseal root 50 mg • Buchu leaves 50 mg • Caprylic acid 75 mg. Other Ingredients: Dicalcium Phosphate, Silicon Dioxide, Magnesium Stearate.

Herbal Formula IX - Hillestad
Each tablet contains: Buchu leaf extract (from concentrate) 500 mg • Uva Ursi leaf 25 mg • Goldenseal root 25 mg • Bilberry fruit 25 mg • American Ginseng root 25 mg • Dahlia powder 75 mg • Guar Gum 25 mg • Chromium GTF 50 mcg.

Herbal Formula V - Hillestad
Three tablets contain: Vitamin C (ascorbic acid) 100 mg • Vitamin E (D-alpha tocopherol) 200 IU • Vitamin B6 (pyridoxine hydrochloride) 150 mg • Pantothenic Acid (calcium pantothenate) 500 mg • Calcium (oyster shell) 219 mg • Magnesium (magnesium oxide) 250 mg • Zinc (zinc chelate) 10 mg • Manganese (manganese chelate) 10 mg • Potassium (potassium gluconate) 105 mg • Choline (choline bitartrate) 20 mg • Gamma Oryzanol (rice bran extract) 150 mg • Lecithin 50 mg • Dong Quai root 250 mg • Black Cohosh root 150 mg • Licorice root 125 mg • Dandelion root 100 mg • Ginseng root 50 mg • Gotu-Kola leaves 75 mg. Other Ingredients: Oyster Shell, Magnesium Stearate.

Herbal Formula VI - Hillestad
Two tablets contain: Vitamin C (ascorbic acid) 400 mg • Vitamin E (D-alpha tocopherol) 160 IU • Niacin 8.3 mg • Folic Acid 67 mcg • Calcium (oyster shell) 48.7 mg • Magnesium (magnesium oxide) 100 mg • Selenium (molasses culture) 16.7 mcg • Potassium (potassium aspartate) 33 mg • L-Carnitine 100 mg • CoEnzyme Q10 20 mg • Citrus Bioflavonoids 100 mg • Lecithin 33 mg • Bromelain 33 mg • Lipase 12 mg • Amylase 12 mg • Papain 12 mg • Hawthorne berries 34 mg • Garlic (odorless) 34 mg • Bilberry berries 33.7 mg • Cayenne fruit 33.7 mg • Butcher's Broom root 34 mg. Other Ingredients: Oyster Shell, Cellulose, Magnesium Stearate.

Herbal Formula VII - Hillestad
Four tablets contain: Biotin 400 mcg • Pantothenic Acid (calcium pantothenate) 32 mg • Calcium (bone meal, oyster shell) 732 mg • Phosphorous (bone meal) 300 mg • Iodine (kelp) 250 mcg • Magnesium (magnesium oxide) 333 mg • Zinc (zinc chelate) 15 mg • Selenium 25 mcg • Inositol 60 mg • PABA 50 mg • RNA 60 mg • Bioflavonoids 50 mg • Rutin 26 mg • Betaine Hydrochloride 50 mg • L-Cysteine 150 mg • Methionine 100 mg • Papain 50 mg • Alfalfa leaves 45 mg • Echinacea root 75 mg • Horsetail (whole herb) 150 mg • Asparagus shoots 50 mg • Rose Hips 50 mg. Other Ingredients: Oyster Shell, Gelatin, Magnesium Stearate, Silicon Dioxide.

Herbal Formula VIII - Hillestad
Four tablets contain: Vitamin A (beta carotene) 7500 IU • Vitamin C (ascorbic acid) 1000 mg • Vitamin B12 75 mcg • Pantothenic Acid (D-calcium pantothenate) 10 mg • Magnesium (oxide) 300 mg •

Potassium (aspartate) 45 mg • Bioflavonoids 300 mg • Ginkgo Biloba leaf 45 mg • Goldenseal root 45 mg • Nettle leaf 45 mg • Echinacea root 225 mg • Licorice root 45 mg • Bee Pollen 225 mg. Other Ingredients: Oyster Shell, Cellulose, Magnesium Sterate, Silicon Dioxide.

Herbal Gargle **-** Dial Herbs
Sage • Myrrh • Goldenseal • Bayberry • Cayenne • Ginger • pure Apple cider vinegar aged in wood.

Herbal GI **-** PhysioLogics
Each capsule contains: Glucosamine (HCl) 150 mg • Gamma Oryzanol 200 mg • Chamomile (1.2% Apigenin, 1.8 mg; 0.5% Essential oil, 0.75 mg) 150 mg • Aloe Vera 100 mg • Wild Yam (6% total Saponins, 4.5 mg) 75 mg.

Herbal Gold Cigarettes **-** Alternative Cigarettes Inc
Each cigarette contains: Marshmallow • Yerba Santa • Damiana • Passion Flower • Jasmine • Ginseng. Regular, menthol, vanilla, and cherry are available.
See Editor's Note No. 6.

Herbal Grobust **-** HomeCure, Inc.
Sabal • Damiana • Dong Quai • Blessed Thistle • Kava Kava • Dandelion root • Oat Bran • Wild Yam • Mother's Wort.

Herbal Immune Complex **-** Solgar
Standardized Astragalus root (glucosides 0.5 mg [0.5%], polysaccharides 70 mg [70%]) 100 mg • Standardized Cat's Claw extract inner bark (mitraphylline 3 mg [3%], polyphenols 15 mg [15%]) 100 mg • Standardized Echinacea purpurea extract root, leaf (echinacosides 4 mg [4%], polysaccharides 15 mg [15%]) 100 mg • Standardized Deglycyrrhized Licorice extract root (glycyrrhizin<1 mg [1%]) 100 mg • Standardized Elderberry extract berry (polyphenols 30 mg [30%]) 100 mg • Standardized Olive Leaf extract leaf (oleuropein 6 mg [6%]) 100 mg • Raw Elderberry powder flower 20 mg • Raw Echinacea powder root, leaf 20 mg • Raw Licorice powder root 20 mg • Raw Olive Leaf powder 20 mg • Raw Astragalus powder root 20 mg. Other Ingredients: Vegetable Cellulose, Vegetable Stearic Acid, Vegetable Magnesium Stearate, Vegetable Glycerin, PhytO2X Blend containing: Natural Vitamin E (mixed tocopherols), Natural Beta Carotene and other Carotenoids, Rosemary extract aerial, Vitamin C (L-ascorbic-acid), Water.

Herbal Insomnia Tablets **-** Life Brand
Valerian root extract (1:4) 50 mg (equivalent to 200 mg Valerian root) • Passion Flower herb 80 mg • Chamomile flower extract (1:4) 15 mg (equivalent to 60 mg Chamomile flowers) • Mistletoe herb 50 mg • Hops flower 50 mg • Wild Lettuce leaf 40 mg. Excipients: Tricalcium Phosphate, Corn Starch, Silicon dioxide, Magnesium Stearate.

Herbal Klenz **-** Progressive Labs
Each capsule contains: Vitamin A 3500 IU • Echinacea (Echinacea angustifolia) 200 mg • Golden Seal (Hydrastis canadensis) 125 mg • Irish Moss (Chondrus crispus) 40 mg • Ginger root (Zingiber officinale) 35 mg • Burdock root (Arctium lappa) 35 mg • Peony root (Paeonia officinalis) 35 mg • Peony root skin (Paeonia officinalis) 35 mg • Licorice root (Glycyrrhiza glabra) 25 mg • Red Clover flower (Trifolium pratense) 20 mg.

Herbal Laxative **-** Holista
Each capsule contains: Cascara Sagrada extract 200 mg • Senna leaves 250 mg.

Herbal Laxative (Stomach-Ease) Tablets **-** Life Brand
Senna leaves 240 mg • Cascara Sagrada bark 150 mg • Licorice root 30 mg • Juniper berries 8 mg • Rhubarb root 8 mg • Gentian root 8 mg • Buchu leaves 4 mg. Excipients: Corn Starch, Sodium Bicarbonate, Silicon Dioxide, Magnesium Stearate, oil of Peppermint.

Herbal Laxative Formula **-** Quest
Each caplet contains: Cascara Sagrada bark (Rhamnus purshiana) (Provided by 50 mg P.E. 7:1) 350 mg • Rhubarb root (Rheum officinale L.) (Provided by 30 mg P.E. 1:4) 120 mg. Other Ingredients: Cayenne, Ginger root, Licorice root, Marshmallow root, Calcium Phosphate, Croscarmellose Sodium, Microcrystalline Cellulose, Magnesium Stearate (vegetable source), Vegetable Stearin.

Herbal Lite **-** BioTreasures Inc.
Each caplet contains: Calcium Pyruvate 1050 mg • L-Phenylalanine 116 mg • Manganese Chelate 6 mcg • Chromium Polynicotinate 500 mcg • Proprietary Herbal Blend 1830 mg: Citrus Aurantium, Garcinia Cambogia, St. John's Wort, Green Tea, Gotu Kola, Siberian Ginseng, Stevia.
See Editor's Note No. 40.

Herbal Liver Complex **-** Solgar
Each vegicap contains: Standardized Milk Thistle extract aerial, seed (silymarin 80 mg [80%]) 100 mg • Standardized Dandelion extract whole plant (vitexin 3 mg [3%]) 100 mg • Standardized Turmeric extract root (curcuminoids 71 mg [95%]) 75 mg • Standardized Schisandra extract fruit (schisandrins 0.5 mg [1%]) 50 mg • Standardized Picrorizha kurroavv extract Picroliv (kutkin 3 mg [3.5%]) 75 mg • Standardized Phyllanthus amarus extract leaf (sesquiterpenes>2 mg [4%]) 50 mg • Phosphatidylcholine 100 mg • Raw Milk Thistle powder aerial 75 mg • Raw Dandelion powder root 75 mg. Other Ingredients: Microcrystalline Cellulose; Vegetable Cellulose; Vegetable Stearic Acid; Vegetable Magnesium Stearate; Vegetable Glycerin; PhytO2X Blend containing Natural Vitamin E (mixed tocopherols), Natural Beta Carotene and other Carotenoids, Rosemary extract aerial, Vitamin C (L-ascorbic acid), Water.

Herbal Male Complex **-** Solgar
Each vegicap contains: Standardized Saw Palmetto extract berry (FFA 34 mg-38 mg [45%-50%]) 75 mg • Standardized Nettles extract leaf (silic acid 0.75 mg [1%]) 75 mg • Standardized Astragalus extract root (glucosides 0.38 mg [0.5%], polysaccharides 53 mg [70%]) 75 mg • Standardized Korean Panax Ginseng extract root (eleutherosides 0.6 mg [0.8%]) 75 mg • Soy Isoflavone extract seed 75 mg • Raw Astragalus powder root 50 mg • Raw Korean Ginseng powder root 25 mg • Raw Siberian Ginseng powder root 25 mg • Raw Nettles powder leaf 25 mg. Other Ingredients: Microcrystalline Cellulose; Vegetable Cellulose; Vegetable Stearic Acid; Vegetable Magnesium Stearate; Vegetable Glycerin; PhtO2X blend containing Natural Vitamin E (mixed tocopherols), Natural Beta Carotene and Other Carotenoids, Rosemary extract aerial, Vitamin C (L-ascorbic acid), Water.

Herbal Migraine Formula **-** Quest
Each caplet contains: Feverfew powder (Tanacetum parthenium) (contains no less than 0.2% parthenolides) 125 mg. Other Ingredients: Calcium Phosphate, Croscarmellose Sodium, Microcrystalline Cellulose, Vegetable Stearin, Magnesium Stearate (vegetable source).

Herbal Nerve Tablets **-** Life Brand
Valerian root extract (1:4) 50 mg (equivalent to 200 mg Valerian root) • Skullcap herb 100 mg • Hops flowers 50 mg. Excipients: Tricalcium Phosphate, Corn Starch, Magnesium Stearate, Silicon Dioxide.

Herbal Niagra **-** Young Again Nutrients
Three capsules contain: Bulgarian Tribulus Terrestris 750 mg • Ginseng Panax 500 mg • Yohimbe Bark 300 mg • Saw Palmetto (25%) 100 mg • Vitamin B3 (Niacinamide) 50 mg.

Herbal Nightcap **-** Trader Joe's
Passion flower 150 mg • Chamomile 4 mg • Hops 60 mg.

Herbal Oxy Forte **-** American Biologics
Each capsule contains: Pycnogenol 10 mg • Grape pip extract 50 mg • Quercetin 100 mg • Milk Thistle 10 mg • Ginkgo Biloba 20 mg • Green Tea extract 75 mg. Other Ingredients: Dicalcium Phosphate, Cellulose, Sodium Starch Glyconate, Silicon Dioxide.

Herbal Pain and Fever Relief **-** Holista
Each capsule contains: White Willow bark powder 300 mg • Meadowsweet extract 250 mg.

Some Brand Name Natural Products - What they Contain

www.NaturalDatabase.com contains MANY more listings than appear here.
Editor's Notes are located on pages 2155-2163.

Herbal Pain Relief Formula - Quest
Each caplet contains: White Willow bark (Salix alba) (Provided by 250 mg P.E. 1:12 standardized to contain 11% Salicin) 3000 mg. Other Ingredients: Blue Vervain, Kelp, Red Raspberry leaf, Skullcap and Wood Betony. Calcium Phosphate, Magnesium Stearate (vegetable source), Microcrystalline Cellulose, Vegetable Stearin.

Herbal Phen Fen Stage 2 - HPF L.L.C.
Two tablets contain: St. John's Wort 400 mg • Ma Huang 250 mg • Green Tea leaf extract 450 mg. Other Ingredients: Dicalcium Phosphate, Microcrystalline Cellulose, Croscarmellose Sodium, Stearic Acid, Silica, Magnesium Stearate, Pharmaceutical glaze. See Editor's Note No. 30.

Herbal Re:Store - Source Naturals
Three tablets contain: Vitamin C (as ascorbic acid) 156 mg • L-Glutamine 300 mg • Oregon Grape root 225 mg • Blessed Thistle leaves & flowers 180 mg • Plantain leaf 180 mg • Red Clover flower 180 mg • Cloves fruit 180 mg • Artemesia leaf & stem 150 mg • Black Walnut hull extract 150 mg • Bupleurum root 150 mg • Burdock root 150 mg • Ginger root 150 mg • Grapefruit seed extract 150 mg • Licorice root 150 mg • Quercetin 150 mg • Slippery Elm bark 150 mg • Yellow Dock root 150 mg • Dandelion root 150 mg • Cat's Claw bark 100 mg • Dandelion root extract 100 mg • Milk Thistle seed extract (yielding 75 mg silymarin) 90 mg • Bioflavonoid complex 75 mg • Garlic root 75 mg • Sarsaparilla root 75 mg • Turmeric root 75 mg. Other Ingredients: Stearic Acid, Colloidal Silicon Dioxide, Modified Cellulose Gum, Magnesium Stearate.

Herbal Regulator - VitaStore
Two tablets contain: Potassium (as gluconate) 25 mg • Hydrangea root 100 mg • Graminis Rhizoma root 50 mg • Cornsilk 50 mg • Parsley whole herb 25 mg • Uva Ursi leaves 75 mg.

Herbal Relaxant Formula - Quest
Each caplet contains: Valerian root (Valeriana officinalis) (Provided by 100 mg P.E. 1:5 standardized to contain 0.8% Valerenic Acid) 500 mg • Chamomile flower (Chamomilla recutita L.) (Provided by 50 mg P.E. 1:4 standardized to contain 1% Apigenin) 200 mg. Other Ingredients: Ginger root, Hops, Marshmallow root, Skullcap, Calcium Phosphate, Croscarmellose Sodium, Magnesium Stearate (vegetable source), Microcrystalline Cellulose, Vegetable Stearin.

Herbal Rescue - Viable Herbal Solutions
Each capsule contains: Proprietary blend 600 mg: Capsicum (capsicum annuum), Dandelion root (taraxacum officinale), Gentian (gentiana lutea), Ginkgo Biloba, Milk Thistle (silybum marianum), Prickly Pear Cactus (opuntia ficus indica), Skullcap (scutellaria laterifolia), White Willow bark (salix alba), Vitamin B1 (thiamine), Vitamin B2 (riboflavin), Vitamin B3 (niacin), Vitamin B5 (pantothenic acid), Vitamin B6 (pyridoxine), Vitamin B12 (cyanocobalamin), Biotin, Folic Acid.

Herbal Seltzer - Dial Herbs
Sodium • White Willow bark • Fever Few • Ginger • Mint • Stevia • Potassium Bicarbonate • Sodium Bicarbonate • Citric Acid. Flavored & sweetened with natural orange flavorings, natural fruit flavors & dextrose.

Herbal Serenity Show of Hands - BeautiControl Inc.
Sodium Chloride • Persea Gratissima oil (avocado) • Sea salt (Dead Sea salt) • Canola oil • Macadamia Ternifolia seeds oil • Carthamus Tinctorius seed oil (hybrid safflower) • Mentha Piperita oil (peppermint) • Mentha Viridis leaf oil (spearmint) • Citrus Aurantium var. Dulcis oil (orange) • Melaleuca Alternifolia leaf oil (tea tree) • Keratin Amino Acids • Tocopheryl Acetate • Benzophenone-3 • Fragrance • Red 17.

Herbal Slim - Nature's Way
Four capsules contain: Proprietary formula: Black Walnut hulls • Burdock root • Chickweed leaf & stem • Echinacea Purpurea stem, leaf, flower • Fennel seed • Hawthorne berry • Kelp (whole Thallus) • Licorice root • Papaya leaves • Parsley herb • Safflower flower. Other Ingredients: Gelatin.

Herbal Throat Lozenges Sugar Free - Natureworks
Two lozenges contain: Menthol 6 mg • Peppermint Oil 2 mg. Other Ingredients: Bee Propolis, Chlorophyll, Capsicum, Wild Cherry Bark, Horehound, Rose Hips, Cocillana Bark, Euphorbia, Echinacea, Slippery Elm, Mullein, Lemon Balm, Black Cherry Flavor, Magnesium Stearate, Calcium Stearate, Silica.

Herbal Tranquility - Optimum Nutrition
Valerian root • Passionflower extract.

Herbal Tranquility Complex - Solgar
Each vegicap contains: Standardized Kava Kava extract root (kavalactones 30 mg [30%]) 100 mg • Standardized Valerian extract root (valernic acid 0.8 mg [0.8%]) 100 mg • Standardized Passionflower extract aerial (isovitexin 2mg-3mg [3%-4%]) 75 mg • Standardized Schisandra extract fruit (schisandrins 0.75 mg [1%]) 75 mg • Standardized St. John's Wort extract aerial (hypericin 0.23 mg [0.3%]) 75 mg • Standardized American Ginseng extract root (ginsenosides 5 mg [10%]) 50 mg • Raw Kava Kava powder root 50 mg • Raw St. John's Wort powder aerial 50 mg • Raw Valerian powder root 50 mg. Other Ingredients: Microcrystalline Cellulose; Vegetable Cellulose; Vegetable Stearic Acid; Vegetable Magnesium Stearate; Vegetable Glycerin; PhytO2X Blend containing Natural Vitamin E (mixed tocopherols), Natural Beta Carotene and other Carotenoids, Rosemary extract aerial, Vitamin C (L-ascorbic acid), Water.

Herbal Treasures - BioTreasures Inc.
Each caplet contains: Kelp 40 mg • Reishi Mushroom 40 mg • Papain (from Papaya) 40 mg • Alfalfa 200 mg • Vitamin A (Beta Carotene) 5000 IU • Vitamin C (Ester-C Calcium Ascorbate) 75 mg • Vitamin E (D-Alpha Tocopheryl Acetate) 30 IU • Vitamin B1 (Thiamine) 1.5 mg • Vitamin B2 (Riboflavin) 1.7 mg • Vitamin B3 (Niacin) 20 mg • Vitamin B5 (Pantothenic Acid) 10 mg • Vitamin B6 (Pyridoxine) 2 mg • Vitamin B12 (Cyanocobalamin) 6 mcg • Folic Acid 400 mcg • Calcium (Calcium Chelate) 400 mg • Magnesium (Ascorbate) 150 mg • Zinc (Zinc Chelate) 74 mg • Chromium (Chromium Polynicotate) 1000 mcg • Proprietary Herbal Blend 610 mg: Grape Seed extract, Garlic extract, Ginkgo biloba extract, Green Tea extract, Siberian Ginseng, Silymarin (Milk Thistle extract), Astragalus extract, Hawthorne berries extract, Horsetail extract, Ashwaganda extract, Stevia extract.

Herbal Up Formula - Nature's Way
Two capsules contain: Bee Pollen • Cayenne pepper fruit • Gotu Kola stem, leaf • Proprietary Blend (840 mg) • Siberian Ginseng root. Other Ingredients: Gelatin.

Herbal UR-Kidney - Nutri-Quest Rx
Proprietary blend 430 mg: Juniper Berries • Parsley • Uva Ursi, Marshmallow • Ginger • Golden Seal root • Corn Silk • Cleavers root. In a base of 6X tissue salts: Mag Phos, Nat Sulph, Calc Phos, Calc Sulph.

Herbal V - Ultra-V
Two tablets contain: Yohimbe extract 2% 250 mg • Avena Sativa extract 10:1 150 mg • Androstenedione 90 mg • Saw Palmetto extract 4:1 100 mg • Guarana extract 22% 300 mg • Taurine 200 mg • Siberian Ginseng extract 35:1 30 mg • Tribulus Terrestris extract 40% 50 mg. Other Ingredients: Dicalcium Phosphate, Microcrystalline Cellulose, Magnesium Sterate, Stearic Acid. See Editor's Note No. 47.

Herbal V: Women's Formula - VitaZip, Inc.
Avena Sativa 10:1 Extract • Kava Kava 30% • Muira Puama 4:1 Extract • St. John's Wort 3% • Ginkgo Biloba 24%/6%.

Herbal Virility - Herbal Groups
Yohimbe bark • Maca tuber • Catuaba bark • Muira Puama bark • Tribulus herb • L-Arginine HCl • Cola seed • Oatstraw grassy stalks • Stinging Nettle leaves • Pumpkin seed • Cayenne fruit (25,000 HU) • Ginger root • American Ginseng root • Eleuthero root • Asian Ginseng root • Sarsaparilla root • Orchic substance (bovine) • Boron Citrate. See Editor's Note No. 17.

Herbal Vivid Maximum Gain - Unknown
Three tablets contain: Niacin 75 mg • Zinc (as zinc oxide) 40 mg • Yohimbe bark 700 mg • Maca tuber 500 mg • Catuaba bark 125 mg • Muira Puama bark 125 mg • Tribulus aerial 100 mg • L-Arginine HCl 100 mg • Cola seed 75 mg • Oatstraw grassy stalks 75 mg • Stinging Nettle leaf 75 mg • Pumpkin seed 75 mg • Cayenne fruit (25,000 HU) 60 mg • Ginger root 60 mg • American Ginseng root 50 mg • Eleuthero root 50 mg • Asian Ginseng root 50 mg • Sarsaparilla root 50 mg • Orchic substance (bovine) 30 gm • Boron citrate 10 mg. Other Ingredients: Cellulose, Modified Cellulose, Gum Arabic (acacia), Silicon Dioxide, Vegetable Magnesium Stearate, Vegetable Stearic Acid, FD&C Blue #2/Indigo Carmine Lake.
See Editor's Note No. 14.

Herbal Water Control - Jamieson
Two capsules contain: Calcium (as Calcium Sulfate) 54 mg • Uva Ursi leaf (Arctostaghylos uva-ursi (L) Spreng) 400 mg • Buchu leaf (Barosma Betulina Bartl. Et Wendl.) 200 mg.

Herbal Women's Formula - Quest
Each caplet contains: White Willow bark powder (Salix alba) (Provided by 85 mg P.E. 1:12 standardized to contain 11% Salicin) 1000 mg • Valerian root (Valeriana officinalis) (Provided by 40 mg P.E. 1:5 standardized to contain 0.8% Valerenic Acid) 200 mg • Chamomile flower (Chamomilla recutita L.) (Provided by 20 mg P.E. 1:4 standardized to contain 1% Apigenin) 80 mg • Uva Ursi leaf (Arctostaphylos uva-ursi) (Provided by 50 P.E. 1:4 standardized to contain 10% Arbutin) 200 mg • Juniper berry (Juniperus communis) (Provided by 80 mg P.E. 1:4) 320 mg • Parsley root (Petroselinum crispum) (Provided by 40 mg P.E. 1:4) 160 mg. Other Ingredients: Calcium Phosphate, Croscarmellose Sodium, Magnesium Stearate (vegetable source), Microcrystalline Cellulose, Silicon Dioxide.

Herbal World Ginseng Complex - Vitamin World
Each capsule contains: American Ginseng root (Panax quinquefolius) 200 mg • Korean Ginseng root (Panax ginseng) 200 mg • Red Chinese Ginseng root (Panax ginseng) 200 mg • Siberian Ginseng root (eleutherococcus senticosus) 200 mg • Royal Jelly (57.14 mg of a 3.5:1 extract) 200 mg. Other Ingredients: Gelatin, Vegetable Magnesium Stearate, Silica.

Herbalax - Health Factor
Each capsule contains: Cascara Sagrada (Rhamnus purshiana) 260 mg • Peppermint (Menta piperita) 90 mg.

Herbal-Biotic - The Herbalist
Oregon Grape Root • Golden Seal root • Yerba Mansa root.

Herbal-F - Progressive Labs
Each capsule contains: Vitamin B6 (as pyridoxine HCl) 20 mg • Magnesium (as magnesium oxide/soy protein complex) 15 mg • Damiana leaf (Turnera aphrodisiaca) 60 mg • Passion flower (Passiflora incarnata) 40 mg • Black Cohosh root (Cimicifuga racemosa) 20 mg • Blue Cohosh root (Caulophyllum thalictroides) 20 mg • Ginger root (Zingiber officinale) 60 mg • Cramp bark (Viburnum opulus) 75 mg • Wild Yam root (Dioscorea villosa) 40 mg • False Unicorn root (Chamaelirium luteum) 40 mg • Squaw vine (Mitchella repens) 40 mg • Blackhaw bark (Viburnum punifolium) 40 mg • Prickly Ash bark (Zanthoxylum americanum) 40 mg • White Birch bark (Betula alba) 40 mg • Ovarian substance 10 mg.
See Editor's Note No. 14.

Herbalifeline - Herbalife International of America, Inc.
Each softgel contains: Vitamin E (as D-alpha tocopherol) 8 IU • Fish oil (marine lipid complex) 500 mg. Other Ingredients: Gelatin, Glycerin, Soybean Oil, White Thyme Oil, Clove Oil, Peppermint Oil, Ethyl Vanillin.

Herbalist's Choice - The Herbalist
Gotu Kola herb • Guarana seed • Kola Nut • American Ginseng root • Licorice root • Damiana leaf • Echinacea root • Osha root • Cinnamon bark • Ginger root • Cayenne pepper.

HerbalKidz KidZinc Lozenges - Nature's Plus
Each lozenge contains: Zinc (as aspartate, monomethionine and proprionate) 8 mg • Botaniplex 100 mg: Echinacea root & rhizome extract (echinacea angustifolia), Olive leaf extract (olea europa), Slippery Elm bark (ulmus rubra), Ginger root extract (zingiber officinale). Other Ingredients: Fructose, Natural Flavors, Citric Acid, Stearic Acid, Guar Gum, Magnesium Stearate, Silica, Natural Color.

Herbal-M - Progressive Labs
Each capsule contains: Vitamin E 30 IU • Zinc (as zinc oxide) 15 mg • Damiana leaf (Turnera aphrodesiaca) 60 mg • Siberian Ginseng/ Korean Ginseng blend (Eleutherococcus senticosus & Panax ginseng) • Cayenne (Capsicum annuum) 50 mg • Dong Quai (Angelica sinensis) 25 mg • Yohimbe (Pausinystalia johimbe) 10 mg • Muira Puama (Pytchopetalum olacoides) 10 mg • Goldenrod (Solidago virguarea) 10 mg • Orchic Substance 10 mg.
See Editor's Note No. 14.

Herbaretic - Suddenly Slender
Each tablet contains: Alfalfa 50 mg • Buchu 50 mg • Uva Ursi 50 mg • Couch Grass 50 mg • Parsley 50 mg • Juniper berries 50 mg • Asparagus 50 mg • Watermelon seed powder 50 mg • Cubebs 50 mg • Shave Grass 50 mg • Corn Silk 50 mg • Golden Rod 50 mg • Cranberries 50 mg.

Herbasaurs Bedwetting - Nature's Sunshine
Ammonium Carbonicum (ammonium carbonate) 6X • Cina (wormseed) 6X • Equisetum Hyemale (scouring rush) 6X • Benzoicum Acidum (benzoic acid) 8X • Causticum (Hahnemann's causticum) 8X • Verbascum Thapsus (mullein) 8x. Other ingredients: Purified Water, Glycerin.
See Editor's Note No. 1.

HerbaSlim - HerbaSway
St. John's Wort • Bitter Orange • Green Tea • Cassia tora • Panax Ginseng • Kudzu • Knotweed • Lycium • Cayenne pepper • Blackberry • HerbaSwee (Cucurbitaceae fruit).
See Editor's Note No. 40.

Herbetom Pulm - Bioserum Laboratory
Each 10 mL contains: Proprietary Blend: Aloe Vera juice, Propolis, Elder extract, Beta Carotene, Pine bud extract, Thyme, Plantain, Golden Sun, Echinacea, Eucalyptus.

Herb-Lax - Shaklee
Each four tablets contain: Dietary fiber 1 g • Calcium 20 mg • Iron 0.36 mg • Herb-Lax Proprietary Blend 1.7 g: (standardized to contribute 16 mg total sennosides) Senna powder (Cassia augustifolia) leaf, Buckthorn powder (Rhamnus frangula) bark, Licorice powder (Glycyrrhiza glabra) root, Alfalfa powder (Medicago sativa) leaf, Fennel powder (Foeniculum vulgare) seed, Anise powder (Pimpinella anisum) seed, Rhubarb powder (Rheum palmatum) root, Blue malva powder from Malva Sylvestris flower, Culver's root powder (Veronicastrum virginicum) root. Other Ingredients: Microcrystalline Cellulose, Karaya Gum, Corn Syrup Solids, Malt Extract, Barley Extract.

Herbolax - The Himalaya Drug Company
Each capsule/tablet contains: Trivruth (ipomoea turpethum syn. operculina turpethum) 70 mg • Haritaki (terminalia chebula) 50 mg • Kasani (cichorium intybus) 50 mg • Kasamarda (cassia occidentalis) 50 mg • Kakamachi (solanum nigrum) 40 mg • Yashti-Madhu (glycyrrhiza glabra) 40 mg • Sunthi (zingiber officinale) 45 mg • Vidanga (embelia ribes) 10 mg.

Herbs & Prunes Formula - Nature's Life
Each tablet contains: Senna leaf (Senna alexandrina) 400 mg • Rhubarb root (Rheum officinale) 10 mg • Chinese Asparagus root (Tian dong, Asparagus cochinchinensis) 5 mg • Beet leaf (Beta vulgaris rubra) 5 mg • Buckthorn bark (Rhamnus frangula) 5 mg • Cabbage leaf (Brassica oleracea capitata) 5 mg • Cascara Sagrada (Rhamnus purshiana) 5 mg • Celery leaf (Apium graveolens) 5 mg • Cranberry (Vaccinium macrocarpon) 5 mg • Culvers root (Leptandra

virginica) 5 mg • Dried Prune (Prunus aractus) 5 mg • Parsley leaf (Petroselinum crispum) 5 mg • Spinach leaf (Spinacia oleracea) 5 mg.

Herbs For Kids Echinacea/GoldenRoot Orange - Botanical Laboratories
Each 1 mL serving contains: Echinacea Purpurea root extract • Oregon Grape root extract. Other Ingredients: Kosher Coconut and/or Palm Kernal Glycerine, Purified Water, Natural Orange extract, Citric Acid.

Herbs For Kids Feverfew Blend - Botanical Laboratories
Each 1 mL serving contains: Meadowsweet herb extract • Feverfew herb • Yarrow flowers • Echinacea Purpurea root • Skullcap herb • Lemon Balm herb • Wild Oat tops. Other Ingredients: Kosher Coconut and/or Palm Kernal Glycerine, Purified Water, Citric Acid.

Herbs For Kids St. John's Wort Blend - Botanical Laboratories
Each 1 mL serving contains: St. John's Wort flowering tops extract • Lemon Balm herb • Chamomile flowers • Wild Oat tops • Skullcap herb • Peppermint leaf • Lavender flowers. Other Ingredients: Kosher Coconut and/or Palm Kernal Glycerine, Purified Water, Citric Acid.

Herbs For Kids Sweet Echinacea - Botanical Laboratories
Each 1 mL serving contains: Echinacea Purpurea root. Other Ingredients: Kosher Coconut and/or Palm Kernal Glycerine, Purified Water, Citric Acid.

Herbs For Kids Valerian Extract - Botanical Laboratories
Each 1 mL serving contains: Valerian root extract. Other Ingredients: Kosher Coconut and/or Palm Kernal Glycerine, Purified Water, Citric Acid.

Herbulk - Metagenics
Each level scoop (20 g) contains: Rice Flour • Psyllium seed powder • Psyllium husk powder • Prune fiber concentrate • Guar Gum • Cellulose Gum • Ascorbic Acid.

Herpanacine - Diamond-Herpanacine Associates
Six capsules contain: L-Lysine 1500 mg • A-Beta-Carotene 25,000 IU • L-Tyrosine 500 mg • E-D-Alpha 200 IU • Selenium 100 mcg • Dandelion leaf • Sarsaparilla • Astragalus • Ligustrum • Echinacea.

Herpe-Caps - Life Extension
Each capsule contains: L-Lysine 500 mg • L-Glysine 20 mg.

Herp-Eeze - Olympian Labs
Each capsule contains: Larreastat 50 mg • Ascorbic Acid 250 mg.

HerpeStat Cold Sore Lip Shield - Origin BioMedicinals
Shea Butter • Bees Wax • Polyphenon 70 Green Tea catechin extract • Avena Sativa Oil • Zinc Oxide • Peppermint Oil • Geranium Oil • Prunella Vulgaris extract • Tea Tree Oil • Bergamot Oil • Vitamin C • Vitamin E.

HerpeStat Medicated Cream - Origin BioMedicinals
Active Ingredient: Prunella vulgaris 1% extract.

Herpilyn - Enzymatic Therapy
Active ingredient: Allantoin 1%. Other Ingredients: Melissa extract (Lemon Balm) 70:1, White Soft Paraffin, Benzyl Alcohol.

Hesperidine Plus - Pure Encapsulations
Each vegetable capsule contains: Hesperidin Methyl Chalcone 250 mg • Bromelain (2400 gdu/gram) 125 mg • Vitamin C (as ascorbyl palmitate) 9 mg.

HGH Activator - Gero Vita International
Six sprays contain: Excell Activator (micro molecular polypeptide complex) 3000 mg. Other Ingredients: Purified Water, Phospholipids, Glycerin, Wheat Germ Oil, Sodium Citrate, Citric Acid, Potassium Sorbate, Maltodextrin, Methylparaben, Propylparaben, Glycine, Orange-Mint Natural Flavor.

HGH at Night - Global Health Trax
Two tablespoons (1 fl oz) contain: Potassium (from potassium sorbate) 35 mg • Collagen Hydrosylate 2 g • Fructo Oligo Saccharides (FOS) 200 mg • Conjugated Linoleic Acid (CLA) 100 mg • Trace Element Complex 500 mg • Amino Acid Complex 1250 mg: Glutamic Acid, Glutathione, Arginine, L-Carnitine, Ornithine, Methionine, L-Glutamine. Other Ingredients: Purified Water, Citric Acid, Sodium Benzoate, Berry Flavoring, Glycerin.

HGH Booster - Life Extension
Three sprays contain: L-Arginine 200 mg • L-Ornithine 100 mg • DHEA 1000 mcg • Glutamine 5 mcg • L-Lysine 5 mcg • Polymer Matrix 2 mcg.

HGH Energizer - Ultra Herbal, LLC
Two caplets contain: Vitamin B6 (pyridoxine as pyridoxine hydrochloride) 20 mg • Tribulus fruit (tribulus terrestris) 250 mg • L-Arginine Hydrochloride 150 mg • L-Leucine 150 mg • L-Glutamine 140 mg • L-Lysine Hydrochloride 90 mg • Gamma-Amino Butyric Acid 75 mg • L-Isoleucine 60 mg • L-Valine 55 mg • Colostrum (standardized to contain 30% immunoglobins) 25 mg • L-Ornithine Hydrochloride 25 mg • L-Glycine 10 mg. Other Ingredients: Calcium Carbonate, Dibasic Calcium Phosphate, Tribasic Calcium Phosphate, Microcrystalline Cellulose, Fructose, Dextrose, Scurose, Maltodextrin, Croscarmellose Sodium, Stearic Acid, Magnesium Stearate, Silicon Dioxide, Sodium Starch Glycolate, Modified Cellulose, Citric Acid, Xylitol, Sucralose, Natural and Artificial Flavors, Acacia Gum, Shellac, Sodium Lauryl Sulfate, Sorbitol, Gelatin, Hydroxypropyl Methylcellulose, Hydroxypropyl Cellulose, Hydroxypropyl Ethylcellulose, Pharmaceutical Glaze, Food Glaze, Starch, Talc, Titanium Dioxide, Vegetable Oil, FD&C Red 40, FD&C Red Red Lake, FD&C Blue 40, FD&C Blue Lake, FD&C Yellow 40, FD&C Yellow Lake, Water.

HGH Release - NewLibido
Each two capsules contain: Arginine (L-arginine HCl) 200 mg • Ornithine (L-ornithine HCl) 150 mg • Lysine (L-lysine HCl) 50 mg • Glutamine (L-glutamine HCl) 150 mg • Colostrum (bovine) 100 mg • Anterior Pituitary extract 50 mg • Orinthine Alphaketoglutarate 50 mg • Glycine (L-glycine HCl) 50 mg. Other Ingredients: Gelatin, Dicalcium Phosphate, Magnesium Stearate, Stearic Acid.
See Editor's Note No. 14.

hGH SecreatGAIN - I Force
Three capsules contain: B6 (pyridoxal 5' phosphate) 10 mg • Zinc Monomethionine 20 mg • 2-Amino-5-Guanidinopentanoic Acid-5 Oxo L-Proline 1000 mg • 2,6-Diaminohexanoic Acid 100 mg • 2-Amino-4-(methylthio) Butanoic Acid 500 mg • Alpha Glyceryl-Phosphorylcholine 200 mg • Coleus Forskohlii (95% forskolin) 50 mg. Other Ingredients: Gelatin, Microcrystalline Cellulose, Magnesium Stearate, Silica.

HGH15 - HealthMinded
Four capsules contain: HGH15 Complex 1500 mg: Anterior Pituitary, Hypothalamus, Amino Acid blend, Phytosterol complex, Beta Sitosterol, Campesterol, Stigmasterol, Soy Phosphatides complex, Phosphatidyl Serine, Phosphatidyl Choline, Phosphatidyl Ethanolamine, Phosphatidyl Inositol, Panax Ginseng. Other Ingredients: Stearic Acid, Magnesium Stearate.
See Editor's Note No. 31.

Hi Energy Multi for Men - Futurebiotics LLC
Three tablets contain: Beta Carotene 25,000 IU • Vitamin C • (Ascorbic Acid, Palmitate) 250 mg • Vitamin D 200 IU • Vitamin E 60 IU • Vitamin B1 (Thiamin) 25 mg • Vitamin B2 (Riboflavin) 25 mg • Niacinamide 50 mg • Pantothenic Acid 25 mg • Vitamin B6 25 mg • Vitamin B12 100 mcg • Biotin 300 mcg • Folic Acid 400 mcg • Phosphatidyl Choline 100 mg • Inositol 75 mg • Ribonucleic Acid (RNA) 75 mg • Para Amino Benzoic Acid (PABA) 75 mg • Zinc (Monomethionine) 30 mg • Calcium (Phosphate, Citrate, Amino Acid Chelate) 200 mg • Magnesium (Citrate, Amino Acid Chelate) 200 mg • Iron (Gluconate) 6 mg • Potassium (Citrate) 99 mg • Chromium

(Polynicotinate) 200 mcg • Copper (Gluconate) 2 mg • Iodine (Kelp) 200 mcg • Manganese (Proteinate) 5 mg • Molybdenum (Amino Acid Chelate) 25 mcg • Selenium (Selenomethionine) 200 mcg. In a base of herbal extracts, powders & nutritional concentrates equivalent to 2,000 mg: Active Ginsenosides (from Standardized Ginseng Extract), Saw Palmetto, Avena Sativa, Ginseng, Hawthorn, Garlic (Odorless Extract), Bee Pollen, Foti, Adrenal Concentrate, Octacosanol (Wheat Free), Alfalfa Juice Concentrate, Spirulina.
See Editor's Note No. 14.

Hi Potency B-Stress Tab - Arrowroot
Two tablets contain: Vitamin B1 50 mg • Choline 100 mg • Vitamin B2 50 mg • Inositol 100 mg • Vitamin B6 100 mg • Vitamin C 750 mg • Vitamin B12 125 mcg • Calcium 100 mg • Niacinamide 200 mg • Magnesium 100 mg • Biotin 150 mcg • Chromium 50 mcg • Folic Acid 400 mcg • Valerian 10 mg • Pantothenic Acid 200 mg • Skullcap 10 mg • PABA 50 mg • Passiflora 10 mg.

Hi-B 100 Complex Vegetarian Formula - Nature's Life
Each tablet contains: Vitamin B1 (Thiamine Hydrochloride) 100 mg • Vitamin B2 (Riboflavin) 100 mg • Vitamin B6 (Pyridoxine Hydrochloride) 100 mg • Vitamin B12 (Cobalamin concentrate) 100 mcg • Folic Acid 400 mcg • Biotin 100 mcg • Niacinamide 100 mg •Pantothenic Acid (d-Calcium Pantothenate) 100 mg • Choline (Bitartrate) 100 mg • PABA (Para Aminobenzoic Acid) 100 mg •Inositol 100 mg. In a natural base of Alfalfa, Parsley, Rice Bran & Watercress.

Hi-B-100 Complex - Nature's Life
Each capsule contains: Vitamin B1 (Thiamine HCl) 100 mg • Vitamin B2 (Riboflavin) 100 mg • Vitamin B6 (Pyridoxine HCl) 100 mg • Vitamin B12 (Cobalamin concentrate) 100 mcg • Niacinamide 100 mg • Pantothenic Acid (d-Calcium Pantothenate) 100 mg • Choline (Bitartrate) 100 mg • Inositol 100 mg • Biotin 100 mcg • Folic Acid 400 mcg • PABA (Para-Aminobenzioc Acid) 100 mg. In a natural base of Rice Bran.

Hi-Fiber - J. R. Carlson Laboratories, Inc.
Each rounded tsp contains: Calcium 11 mg • Iron 1 mg • Psyllium (as psyllium seed husk) 6 g.

High Absorption Calcium - Doctor's Best, Inc.
Each tablet contains: Vitamin D (as cholecalciferol) 100 IU • Calcium (as calcium bis-glycinate) 250 mg • Zinc (as zinc bis-glycinate) 3.75 mg • Copper (as copper bis-glycinate) 0.5 mg • Manganese (as manganese bis-glycinate) 0.5 mg • Boron (as boron glycinate) 125 mcg • Bioperine brand Black Pepper extract 2 mg. Inactive Ingredients: Stearic Acid, Cellulose, Croscarmellose Sodium, Magnesium Stearate, Silicon Dioxide.

High Five - Pharmanex
Each tablet contains: Boswellia Serrata Extract (stem) 125 mg • Fungal Protease (Aspergillus Oryzae) 100 mg • Bromelain (from Pineapple extract) 50 mg • Quercetin 25 mg • Papain (from Papaya extract) 10 mg. Other Ingredients: Dicalcium Phosphate, Microcrystalline Cellulose, Cellulose Powder, Silica, Magnesium Stearate.

High Gamma Tocopherol - PhysioLogics
Each softgel contains: Vitamin E (as d-alpha tocopherol) 200 IU • D-Gamma-Tocopherol 200 mg • Other Tocopherols (d-delta, d-beta tocopherol) 78 mg • Tocotrienols 2 mg. Other Ingredients: Gelatin, Glycerin, Non-GMO Soybean Oil.

High Lignan Flax Seed Oil - Pure Encapsulations
Each softgel capsule contains: Organic high lignan Flax seed oil (typically contains alpha-linolenic acid 456-684 mg, linoleic acid 128-192 mg, oleic acid 144-240 mg, palmitic acid, stearic acid 72-108 mg, lignans 4 mg) 1000 mg. Other Ingredients: Gelatin, Glycerin, Caramel Color.

High Nutrition - Natrol, Inc.
Each capsule contains: Vitamin C (as Ascorbic Acid) 60 mg • Niacin (as Niacinamide) (Vitamin B3) 2 mg • Vitamin B6 (as Pyridoxine HCl) 2 mg • Thiamine (Vitamin B1) 1.5 mg • In a specially formulated base containing: Winter Berry root 4:1 • Country Malva leaf 5:1, Siberian Ginseng root, Ginger root, Licorice root. Other Ingredients: Silicon Dioxide, Magnesium Stearate, Gelatin.

High Performance Creatine - Puritan's Pride
Each serving contains: Creatine Monohydrate 5.25 g • Taurine 1000 mg.

High Potency Apple Cider Vinegar - NOW Foods
Two capsules contain: Apple Cider Vinegar powder 900 mg. Other Ingredients: Gelatin (capsule), Magnesium Stearate, Silica.

High Potency B Compound - Trophic
Each caplet contains: Vitamin B1 (as thiamine mononitrate) 55 mg • Vitamin B2 55 mg • Niacinamide 55 mg • Vitamin B6 (as pyridoxine HCl) 55 mg • Vitamin B12 55 mcg • Biotin 55 mcg • Folic Acid 1 mg • D-Pantothenic Acid (as calcium pantothenate) 55 mg • PABA 55 mg • Vitamin C 55 mg • Choline 55 mg • Inositol 55 mg.

High Potency B-Complex with Vitamin C - Puritan's Pride
Each caplet contains: Vitamin C (as ascorbic acid) 300 mg • Thiamin (Vitamin B1; as thiamine mononitrate) 15 mg • Riboflavin (Vitamin B2) 10.2 mg • Niacin (as niacinamide) 50 mg • Vitamin B6 (as pyridoxine hydrochloride) 5 mg • Pantothenic Acid (as d-calcium pantothenate) 10 mg. Other Ingredients: Dicalcium Phosphate, Cellulose (Plant Origin), Cellulose Coating, Croscarmellose, Vegetable Magnesium Stearate, Silica, FD&C Yellow No.5 Aluminum Lake, Titanium Dioxide Color, Vegetable Stearic Acid, Guar Gum.

High Potency Calcium 500 - Walgreens
Each tablet contains: Calcium (as calcium carbonate from oyster shell) 500 mg. Other Ingredients: Croscarmellose Sodium, Hydroxypropyl Methylcellulose, Sodium Lauryl Sulfate, Titanium Dioxide, Magnesium Stearate, Polyethylene Glycol, Carnauba Wax, FD&C Blue No. 1 Lake, FD&C Yellow No. 5 Lake Tartrazine.

High Potency Calcium 500+D - Walgreens
Each tablet contains: Vitamin D (as cholecalciferol) • Calcium (as calcium carboante from oyster shell) 500 mg. Other Ingredients: Croscarmellose Sodium, Hydroxypropyl Methylcellulose, Sodium Lauryl Sulfate, Titanium Dioxide, Magnesium Stearate, Polyethylene Glycol, Carnauba Wax, FD&C Blue No. 1 Lake, FD&C Yellow No. 5 Lake, Tartrazine.

High Potency Calcium 600 - Walgreens
Each tablet contains: Calcium (as calcium carbonate) 600 mg. Other Ingredients: Croscarmellose Sodium, Hydroxypropyl Methylcellulose, Sodium Lauryl Sulfate, Titanium Dioxide, Magnesium Stearate, Polyethylene Glycol, Carnauba Wax.

High Potency Calcium 600+D - Walgreens
Each tablet contains: Vitamin D (as cholecalciferol) • Calcium (as calcium carboante) 600 mg. Other Ingredients: Croscarmellose Sodium, Hydroxypropyl Methylcellulose, Sodium Lauryl Sulfate, Titanium Dioxide, Magnesium Stearate, Polyethylene Glycol, Carnauba Wax, FD&C Yellow No. 6 Lake.

High Potency Calcium+Minerals - Walgreens
Each tablet contains: Vitamin D (as cholecalciferol) • Calcium (as calcium carbonate) 600 mg • Magnesium (as magnesium oxide) 40 mg • Zinc (as zinc oxide) 7.5 mg • Copper (as cupric oxide) 1 mg • Manganese (as manganese sulfate) 1.8 mg • Boron (as sodium borate) 250 mcg. Other Ingredients: Microcrystalline Cellulose, Crospovidone, Hydroxypropyl Methylcellulose, Titanium Dioxide, Sodium Lauryl Sulfate, Magnesium Stearate, Triacetin, Polysorbate 80, FD&C Red No.40 Lake, FD&C Yellow No. Lake, FD&C BLue No. 1 Lake.

High Potency Cal-Mag Plus - Quest
Each tablet contains: Calcium (Citrate) 250 mg • Magnesium (Oxide) 250 mg • Vitamin C (Ascorbic Acid) 150 mg • Vitamin D (as Vitamin D3) 100 IU • Zinc (Citrate) 10 mg. Other Ingredients: Croscarmellose Sodium, Magnesium Stearate (vegetable source), Microcrystalline Cellulose, Silicon Dioxide, Vegetable Stearin.

High Potency Garlic - Nature's Sunshine
Each tablet contains: Calcium (as dicalcium phosphate) 58 mg • Phosphorus (as dicalcium phosphate) 46 mg • Garlic bulb (allium sativum) 400 mg. Other Ingredients: Cellulose, Broccoli Flowers (brassica oleracea), Stearic Acid, Turmeric Root (curcuma longa), Red Beet Root (beta vulgaris), Rosemary Leaf (rosmarinus officinalis), Carrot Root (daucus carota), Tomato Fruit (solanum lycopersicum), Chinese Cabbage Leaf (brassica rapa), Cabbage Leaf (brassica oleracea), Orange and Grapefruit Bioflavonoids, Hesperidin.

High potency Glucosamine Sulfate 1000mg - Nature's Own
Each tablet contains: Glucosamine Sulfate / Potassium Chloride Complex 1000 mg

High Potency Grapine - Nature's Sunshine
Each tablet contains: Calcium (di-calcium phosphate) 60 mg • Phosphorous (di-calcium phosphate) 50 mg • Grapine proanthocyanidins from Grape seed & Pine bark 60 mg. Inactive Ingredients: Cellulose (plant fiber), Stearic Acid, Silicon Dioxide (powdered silica), Magnesium Stearate (vegetable).

High Potency Iron from Ferrous Sulfate - Leiner Health Products
Each tablet contains: Iron (Ferrous Sulfate) 27 mg. Other Ingredients: Calcium Carbonate, Starch, Maltodextrin, Cellulose, Croscarmellose Sodium, Tricalcium Phosphate, Hydroxypropyl Methylcellulose, Polyethylene Glycol 3350, Silicon Dioxide, Talc, Magnesium Stearate, Hydroxypropyl Cellulose, Red 40 Lake, Polysorbate 80, Titanium Dioxide, Povidone.

High Potency Magnesium 500 mg - Puritan's Pride
Each tablet contains: Magnesium (as magnesium oxide) 500 mg. Other Ingredients: Cellulose (plant origin), Starch, Povidone, Magnesium Silicate, Cellulose Coating, Titanium Dioxide Color, Vegetable Magnesium Stearate, Propylene Glycol.

High Potency Soft Multiple - Swanson Health Products
Each softgel contains: Vitamin A (as beta-carotene) 5000 IU •Vitamin C USP (as ascorbic acid) 150 mg • Vitamin D (as cholecalciferol) 200 IU •Vitamin E (as d-alpha tocopherol) 100 IU •Thiamin USP (as thiamin mononitrate; vitamin B-1) 25 mg • Riboflavin USP (vitamin B-2) 25 mg • Niacin (as niacin 5 mg; as niacinamide 25 mg) 30 mg • Vitamin B-6 (as pyridoxine HCl) 25 mg • Folic Acid 200 mcg • Vitamin B-12 (as cyanocobalamin) 25 mcg • Biotin 25 mcg • Pantothenic Acid (as d-calcium pantothenate) 25 mg • Calcium (from calcium carbonate) 100 mg • Iron (as ferrous fumarate) 7.5 mg • Iodine (as potassium iodide) 75 mcg • Magnesium (from magnesium oxide) 50 mg • Zinc (from zinc oxide) 7.5 mg • Selenium (from selenomethionine) 12.5 mcg • Copper (from copper gluconate) 0.5 mg • Manganese (from manganese sulfate) 5 mg • Chromium (from Chromax chromium picolinate) 12.5 mcg • Molybdenum (sodium molybdate) 12.5 mcg. Lecithin 40 mg • Choline (as choline bitartrate) 25 mg • Inositol 25 mg • PABA (para-aminobenzoic acid) 25 mg, Boron (from calcium borogluconate) 0.5 mg • Silica (from silicon dioxide) 0.25 mg • Vanadium (from vanadyl sulfate) 5 mcg.

High Strength Aloe Vera - Puritan's Pride
Each tablet contains: Aloe Vera(200:1 Extract, Aloe Barbadensis Miller) 100 mg. Other Ingredients: Dicalcium Phosphate, Cellulose (Plant Origin), Vegetable Stearic Acid, Croscarmellose, Cellulose Coating, Silica, Vegetable Magnesium Stearate.

High Strength Cod Liver Oil - Nature's Bounty
Each softgel contains: Vitamin A (as Cod Liver Oil and Retinyl Palmitate) 2664 IU • Vitamin D (as Cod Liver Oil and Cholecalciferol) 200 IU • Cod Liver Oil 1000 mg • Eicosapentaenoic Acid 110 mg • Docosahexaenoic Acid 100 mg. Other Ingredients: Gelatin, Glycerin.

High Stress B & C - Source Naturals
Each four tablets contain: Vitamin C (ascorbic acid) 666 mg • Vitamin D (vitamin D3 from cholesalceferol) 68 IU • Thiamin (vitamin B1) 66 mg • Riboflavin (vitamin B2) 40 mg • Niacin (as niacinamide 133 mg and niacin 33 mg) 166 mg • Vitamin B6 (pyridoxide HCl) 53 mg • Folate (as folate acid) 560 mcg • Vitamin B12 (as cyanocobalamin) 133 mcg • Biotin 133 mcg • Pantothenic Acid (as calcium d-pantothenate) 333 mg • Calcium 133 mg • Magnesium (as magnesium oxide & taurinate) 323 mg • Potassium (as potassium citrate) 33 mg • Valerian Root 400 mg • Catnip Leaf 333 mg • Zizyphus Seed 266 • Hops Flower 233 mg • Skullcap Leaf and Stem 233 mg • Chamomile Flower 200 mg • Passion Flower 200 mg • GABA (gamma amino butyric acid) 200 mg • Spirulina 200 mg • Wood Betony Leaf, Stem, and Flower 166 mg • Inositol 133 mg • Ginger Root 100 mg • Phosphatidyl Choline (as lecithin) 89 mg • Licorice Root 66 mg • L-Tyrosine 66 mg • Choline (as bitartrate) 66 mg • PABA (para amino benzoic acid) 53 mg.

High Thyroid - Enzymes, Inc.
Each capsule contains: Proprietary Herbal Blend 270 mg: Bugleweed herb extract, Lemon Balm herb extract, Flaxseed, Passionflower herb extract • Proprietary Blend 57 mg: Protease, CereCalase. Other Ingredients: Cellulose, Water.

Higher Mind - Source Naturals
Four tablets contain: Phosphatidyl Serine (Leci-PS) 150 mg • Vitamin B1 (Thiamin) 100 mg • Vitamin B2 (Riboflavin) 25 mg • Vitamin B3 (Inositol Hexanicotinate 100 mg and Niacin 50 mg) 150 mg • Vitamin B5 (Pantothenic Acid) 50 mg • Vitamin B6 (PAK and Pyridoxine HCl) 100 mg • Vitamin B12 50 mcg • Folic Acid 800 mcg • Biotin 50 mcg • Vitamin C (Calcium and Zinc Ascorbates) 200 mg • Calcium (Ascorbate, Carbonate, Malate, Succinate) 100 mg • Magnesium (Malate, Succinate, Taurinate, Oxide) 200 mg • Zinc (Ascorbate) 10 mg • Manganese (Citrate) 5 mg • L-Pyroglutamic Acid 750 mg • L-Glutamine 500 mg • Acetyl L-Carnitine 300 mg • DMAE (Bitartrate) 100 mg • Taurine (Magnesium Taurinate) 200 mg • DLPA (DL-Phenylalanine) 200 mg • Phosphatidyl Choline 157.5 mg • Phosphatidyl Ethanolamine 105 mg • N-Acetyl L-Tyrosine 100 mg • GABA (Gamma Amino Butyric Acid) 100 mg • PAK (Pyridoxine Alpha-Ketoglutarate) 100 mg • Ginkgo Biloba extract 24% (50:1) 50 mg • Phosphatidyl Inositol 45 mg • Alpha-Lipoic Acid (Thioctic Acid) 20 mg • Coenzyme Q10 (Ubiquinone) 10 mg • Inositol 10 mg.

Hi-Lignan Flax Oil - Jarrow Formulas
Each 1 tbsp serving contains: Average analysis: Alpha-Linolenic Acid (omega-3) 7980 mg • Linoleic Acid (omega-6) 2240 mg • Oleic Acid (omega-9) 2520 mg • Lignans 8764 mcg • Mixed Carotenoids 1000 mcg.

Himalayan Diet Breakthrough - AVS Marketing
Nepalese Mineral Pitch • Tribulus Terrestris • Boerhaavia • Cardamon • Commiphora Mukul • Emblica Officinalis • Terminalia Chebula • Terminalia Bellirica.

Himalayan Goji Juice - FreeLife International
Reconstituted Goji juice (from whole lycium barbarum fruit) • Grape juice concentrate • Pear juice concentrate • Apple juice concentrate • Pear puree • Natural flavor • Sodium Benzoate • Potassium Sorbate.

Himalayan Green Tea - R-U Ved U.S.A.
100% Himalayan Green Tea.

Himcocid - The Himalaya Drug Company
Each 1 tsp (5 mL) serving contains: Varatika (syn. cowrie bhasma, cowrie shell calx/ash) 70 mg • Dugdhapashana (soft stone/magnesium silicate) 70 mg • Mouktika Sukti (syn. mouktika bhasma, pearl oyster shell calx) 15 mg • Yashtimadhu (glycyrrhiza glabra) 5 mg.

Some Brand Name Natural Products - What they Contain

www.NaturalDatabase.com contains MANY more listings than appear here.
Editor's Notes are located on pages 2155-2163.

BRAND NAMES

Himcolin Gel - The Himalaya Drug Company
Each 1 gm serving contains: Jyotishmati oil (celastrus paniculatus) 200 mg • Lathakasthuri oil (hibiscus abelmoschus) 150 mg • Vathada oil (prunus amygdalus) 100 mg • Nirgundi oil (vitex negundo) 100 mg • Karpasa oil (gossypium herbaceum) 50 mg • Mukulaka oil (pistacia vera) 50 mg • Jatiphalam oil (myristica fragrans) 30 mg • Jaatipatree oil (myristica fragrans, mace) 30 mg • Lavanga oil (syzygium aromaticum) 30 mg • Taja oil (cinnamomum cassia) 3 mg.

Himcospaz - The Himalaya Drug Company
Each capsule contains: Sati (curcuma zedoaria) 25.5 mg • Sunthi (zingiber officinale) 24 mg • Ajamoda (apium graveolens) 96 mg.

Himplasia - The Himalaya Drug Company
Each tablet contains: Gokshura (tribulus terrestris) 140 mg • Putikaranja (caesalpinia bonducella) 120 mg • Puga (areca catechu) 100 mg • Shatavari (asparagus racemosus) 80 mg • Varuna (crataeva nurvala) 80 mg • Akika Pishti (processed agate) 80 mg.

Hi-Potent-C (powdered) - Nutri-Quest Rx
Each level teaspoonful contains: Vitamin C 1500 mg •Mannitol 1355 mg •Rose Hips 250 mg •Lemon Bioflavonoids 130 mg •Hesperidin Complex 50 mg •Rutin 35 mg •Acerola concentrate 35 mg •natural Flavor.

Hista-Block - Nature's Sunshine
Two capsules contain: Proprietary Blend 540 mg: Stinging Nettle leaf (urtica dioica), Quercetin (dihydrate), Citrus Aurantium (fructus aurantia immaturi), Bromelain fruit (ananas comosus). Other Ingredients: Di-Calcium Phosphate, Cellulose, Maltodextrin, Magnesium Stearate, Silicon Dioxide, Gelatin, Water.
See Editor's Note No. 40.

Historal - Progressive Health Nutraceuticals
Methylsulfonyl Methane 1000 mg • Vitamin C 500 mg • Echinacea Purpurea 100 mg • Vitamin E 30 IU • Quercetin 50 mg • Grape seed extract 25 mg • Stinging Nettle 25 mg • Coleus Forskolin 15 mg.

Hives - Hyland's
Two tablets contain: Apis Mellifica Ca 3X • Urtica Urens 3X • Natrum Muriaticum 6X • Arsenicum Album 6X. Base: Lactose.
See Editor's Note No. 1.

HMB - EAS, Inc.
Each 4 capsule serving contains: HMB 1000 mg • Potassium Phosphate 200 mg.

HMB Caps - Optimum Nutrition
Each capsule contains: Hydroxymethyl Butyrate (HMB, as calcium beta-hydroxy beta-methylbutyrate monohydrate) 1000 mg. Other Ingredients: Gelatin, Microcrystalline Cellulose, Magnesium Stearate.

HMF Forte - Genestra - Seroyal
Each capsule contains: L. Acidophilus 4 billion CFU • L. Bifidus 1 billion CFU • FOS (Fructo-oligo-saccharides) 100 mg.

HMF Forte - InterPlexus
Each capsule contains: Proprietary Blend 6 billion organisms: Lactobacillus Acidophilus, Bifidobacterium Bifidus, Bifidobacterium Brevis. Other Ingredients: Chickory Fructooligosaccharides (FOS), Cellulose.

HMF Powder - Genestra - Seroyal
Each quarter teaspoon (1 g) contains: L. Acidophilus 3 billion CFU • L. Bifidus 3 billion CFU • FOS (fructo-oligo-saccharides) 450 mg.

HMF Replete - Genestra - Seroyal
Each packet contains: L. Acidophilus 10 billion CFU • L. Bifidus 10 billion CFU • L. Bulgaricus 10 billion CFU • FOS (fructo-oligo-saccharides) 9 g.

HMS 90 - Immunotec Research, Ltd.
Undenatured Whey Protein.

Holista Echinacea - Holista
Each capsule contains: Echinacea angustifolia/purpurea (root) (16:1 extract) 500 mg.

Holista Echinacea Tincture - Holista
Each mL contains: Echinacea angustifolia dried root 1:1 standardized extract in alcohol 45% 200 mg.

Holista Evening Primrose Oil 1000 mg - Holista
Each capsule contains: Evening Primrose Oil 1000 mg, containing 10% gamma-linolenic acid and 70% linoleic acid.

Holista Evening Primrose Oil 500 mg - Holista
Each capsule contains: Evening Primrose Oil (not less than 50 mg of gamma-linolenic acid and 350 mg of lenoleic acid) standardized to 10% GLA 500 mg.

Holista Feverfew - Holista
Each capsule contains: Feverfew (Tanacetum parthenium) standardized to a minimum of 0.2% parthenolide 125 mg.

Holista Lactase enzyme - Holista
Each capsule contains: Food Chemical Codex Lactase 3000 units.

Holista Milk Thistle - Holista
Each capsule contains: Milk Thistle (Silybum marianum) standardized to silymarin 80% 150 mg.

Holista Milk Thistle Tincture - Holista
Each mL contains: Milk Thistle seed from 1:1 fluid extract in 65% alcohol 0.2 mg.

Holista Saw Palmetto - Holista
Each caplet contains: Saw Palmetto (Serenoa repens) extract from berries 10:1 160 mg.

Holista Saw Palmetto Tincture - Holista
Each mL contains: Saw Palmetto dried berries of Seronoa repens 1:1 in 45% alcohol 0.2 mg.

Holista Tea Tree Oil 20% Lotion - Holista
Tea Tree oil (Melaleuca alternifolia) 0.2 mL. Other Ingredients: Water, Alcohol.

Holista Valerian - Holista
Each capsule contains: Valerian Root Extract standardized to 0.8% Valerenic Acid 500 mg.

Holista Valerian Tincture - Holista
Each mL contains: Valerian Root from the rhizome and roots of Valeriana officianalis 1:1 in 60% alcohol 0.2 mg.

Holista Zinc Lozenges - Holista
Each lozenge contains: Zinc (citrate) 5 mg • Echinacea 50 mg • Vitamin C 50 mg.

Homeopathic Bug Bite Relief - Hyland's
Active Ingredients: Apis Mellifica 3X HPUS • Calendula Officinalis 3X HPUS • Echinacea Angustifolia 3X HPUS • Ledum Palustre 3X HPUS • Urtica Dioica 3X HPUS. Inactive Ingredients: Petrolatum USP, Beeswax USP, Citronella Oil, Methylparaben USP, Propylparaben USP.
See Editor's Note No. 1.

Homeopathic Nasal Swab - Western Research Laboratories
Aloe • Glycerin • Arnica • Histamine • Luffa Officinalis • Euphorbium Officinaurm • Hepar Sulphuricum • Bryonia • Mercurius Iodatus Flavus • Mucosa Nasalis • Sabadilla • Lemna Minor • Lachesis.
See Editor's Note No. 1.

Homocysteine Control - Nature's Way
Each capsule contains: Betaine Anhydrous 500 mg • Folic Acid (folate) 800 mcg • Pyridoxine HCl 20 mg • Vitamin B-12 (cyanocobalamin) 400 mcg. Other Ingredients: Cellulose, Gelatin, Magnesium stearate, Millet.

Homocysteine De-Crease - Nutri-Quest Rx
Each tablet contains: Trimethylglycine 300 mg • Pyridoxal 5 Phosphate 5 mg (enteric coated) • Vitamin B12 200 mcg • Dimethyl Glycine 25 mg • Niacinamide 20 mg • Cysteine 15 mg • Molybdenum Chelate 30 mcg • Selenium Chelate 15 mcg • Vitamin B6 15 mg (enteric coated) • Folic Acid 275 mg • Vitamin E Succinate 10 IU • Red Beet root 25 mg • Choline Bitartrate 10 mg • Magnesium Chelate 100 mg • Zinc Chelate 10 mg.

Homocysteine Factors - Pure Encapsulations
Each vegetable capsule contains: Pyridoxal 5' Phosphate (activated B6) 75 mg • Folic Acid 800 mcg • Methylcobalamin (B12) 400 mcg • Trimethylglycine (anhydrous betaine) 1000 mg • Vitamin C (as ascorbyl palmitate) 10 mg.

Homocysteine Formula - Nature's Life
Each capsule contains: Vitamin B6 (Pyridoxine HCl) 10 mg • Folic Acid 800 mcg • Vitamin B12 400 mcg • Choline (Bitartrate) 50 mg • Betaine HCl 50 mg.

Homocysteine Guard Elite - J. R. Carlson Laboratories, Inc.
Three tablets contain: Vitamin B6 (as pyridoxine hydrochloride) 25 mg • Folate (folic acid) 1000 mcg • Vitamin B12 (cyanocobalamin) 1000 mcg • NAC (N-acetyl cysteine) 1800 mg.

Homocysteine PF - Jarrow Formulas
Each tablet contains: Vitamin B6 (pyridoxine HCl) 15 mg • Vitamin B12 (methylcobalamin) 150 mcg • Folic Acid 400 mcg • Trimethylglycine (TMG, anhydrous betaine) 500 mg. Other Ingredients: Cellulose, Dicalcium Phosphate, Stearic Acid (vegetable source), Modified Cellulose Gum, Magnesium Stearate, Silicon Dioxide.

Homocysteine Regulators - NOW Foods
Each Vcap contains: Vitamin B6 (as Coenzyme Pyridoxyl-5-Phosphate) 20 mg • Vitamin B12 (as Cyanocobalamin) 250 mcg • Folic Acid 800 mcg • Trimethylglycine (Betaine) 400 mg.

HomocystexPlus with TMG & TroxeRutin - Natrol, Inc.
Each capsule contains: Riboflavin (Vitamin B2) 25 mg • Vitamin B6 (as pyridoxine HCl) 25 mg • Folic Acid 800 mcg • Vitamin B12 (as cobalamin) 500 mcg • Betaine TMG (as betaine trimethylglycine) 500 mg • TroxeRutin 100 mg • Choline (as choline bitartrate) 25 mg. Other Ingredients: Silicon Dioxide, Magnesium Stearate, Gelatin.

Honey Apple Double Ginseng - Traditional Medicinals
Asian Ginseng root (Panax ginseng) • American Ginseng root (Panax quinquefolius) • Siberian Ginseng root (Eleutherococcus senticosus) • Chamomile flower • Licorice root • Orange peel • dried Apples • Prince Ginseng rootlets (Pseudostellada heterophylla) • Natural Honey & Apple flavors.

Honey C Chews Chewable C 100 mg - Nature's Life
Each wafer contains: Vitamin C (buffered) 100 mg • Rose Hips powder (Rosa canina) 50 mg • Acerola berry powder (Malpighia glabra) 25 mg.

Honey C Chews Chewable C 300 mg - Nature's Life
Each wafer contains: Vitamin C (buffered) 300 mg • Rose Hips powder (Rosa canina) 50 mg • Acerola berry powder (Malpighia glabra) 25 mg.

Honey-B-Anise "Old Tyme" Sore Throat Syrup - Thayers Natural Pharmaceuticals
Vegetable Glycerin • Honey • Purified Water • Propylene Glycol • Anise Oil • Bee Propolis.

Hoodia Diet Tabs - Nature's Rx
Each tablet contains: Hoodia Gordonii (20:1) 50 mg • Calcium Pyruvate 300 mg • Calcium (from calcium pyruvate) 48 mg • Citrus Pectin 40 mg • Prune 30 mg • Grapefruit seed extract 30 mg • Chromium 100 mcg.

Hoodia Gordonii Cactus - Planet Hoodia
Each capsule contains: Hoodia Gordonii 400 mg.

Hoodia Weight-Loss - VitaSalveo
Three tablets contain: Chromium Polynicotinate 10% 100 mcg • Calcium Pyruvate 48 mg • Hoodia Gordonii powder 50 mg • Citrus Pectin 40 mg • Grapefruit seed extract (4:1) 30 mg • Prune powder 30 mg. Other Ingredients: Rice Bran Powder, Magnesium Stearate (NF/FCC vegetable grade, kosher).

HoodiaLean - Phytobase, Inc.
Two vegetable capsules contain: Hoodia Gordonii 20:1 extract 850 mg • Proprietary Blend 250 mg: Standardized Cocoa Almond blend, Suma root, Gymnema Sylvestre extract, Naringin, Cayenne pepper extract.

HooDiat Mints - Life Enhancement Products, Inc.
Fructose • Hoodia Gordonii whole plant concentrate • Peppermint • Menthol • Citric Acid • Stearic Acid • Silicon Dioxide • Magnesium Stearate.

Hoodoba Diet Pills - Hoodoba
Two capsules contain: Vitamin B6 (as pyridoxal-5-phosphate) 3 mg • Manganese (as manganese sulfate) 2 mg • Chromium (chelated) 150 mcg • Hoodoba Proprietary Blend 1529 mg: Garcinia Cambogia fruit extract (50% hydroxycitric acid), Hoodia Gordonii Cactus, Citrus Aurantium extract (immature peel), Green Tea leaf extract (20% polyphenols), Nut Grass extract, Banaba leaf extract (1% corosolic acid), Red Panax Ginseng root, Vanadium (vanadyl sulfate), Bioperine brand Black Pepper extract. Other Ingredients: Gelatin, Microcrystalline Cellulose, Magnesium Stearate, Silica.

Hops, Valerian & Scullcap - Dial Herbs
Hops • Valerian • Scullcap.

Hormogen - Atrium Biotechnologies
Each capsule contains: Lecithin 200 mg • Safflower oil 200 mg • Wheat Germ oil (Cold Pressed) 66.667 mg • Rice Bran oil 66.667 mg • Soybean oil 66.667 mg.

Hormone Harmony - iVillage Inc.
Two softgels contain: Schizandra berry extract (wu-wei-zi, 2% schizandrins, 3.2 mg) 160 mg • Ginger rhizome supercritical extract (certified organic, 30% pungent compounds, 8.1 mg; 8% zingiberene, 2.1 mg; 23 mg post-supercritical ethanolic (PSE) extract, 2% pungent compounds, 0.46 mg) 50 mg • Black Cohosh berry root & rhizome extract (8% triterpene glycosides, 3.2 mg) 40 mg • Chastetree berry extract (vitus agnus-castus, 0.6% aucubin, 0.2 mg; 0.5% agnuside, 0.2 mg) 40 mg • Rosemary leaf supercritical extract (23% total phenolic antioxidants, 2.3 mg) 10 mg. Other Ingredients: Evening Primrose Seed Oil Supercritical Extract, Olive Oil - Extra Virgin, Maltodextrin, Yellow Beeswax, Gelatin, Vegetable Glycerine, Purified Water, Carob.

Hormone Nutrients - Wellness for Women
Each capsule contains: Vitamin B-6 (as pyridoxine HCl) 50 mg • Magnesium (from amino acid chelate) 75 mg • Motherwort (5:1 concentrate) 100 mg • Vitex Chasteberry extract (0.5% agnusides) 100 mg • Dong Quai extract (1% ligustilides) 75 mg • SoyLife brand Soy protein extract (1% soy isoflavones) 75 mg • Black Cohosh extract (2.5% triterpene-glycosides) 50 mg.

Horny Goat Weed - ProLab
Two capsules contain: Horny Goat weed (epimedium sagittatum, epimedium brevicornum, standardized to 10% icariin) 500 mg • Maca Pure (lepidium meyenii, standardized to 0.6% macamides & macaenes) 250 mg • Macuna Pruriens (standardized to 15% L-dopa) 33.3 mg • Polypodium Vulgare (standardized to 8% 20-hydroxyecdysone) 25 mg.

Horse Chestnut - Jamieson
Each caplet contains: Horse Chestnut Seed 1100 mg.

Horse Chestnut Extract - Enzymatic Therapy/PhytoPharmica
Each capsule contains: Horse Chestnut seed extract (aesculus hippocastanum, standardized to contain 20% triterpene glycosides calculated as escin) 250 mg. Other Ingredients: Gelatin, Cellulose, Magnesium Stearate, Silicon Dioxide, Titanium Dioxide Color.

Horse Chestnut Herbal Balm - Nature's Life
Deionized Water • Horse Chestnut seed extract [(Aesculus hippocastanum L.) standardized to 2% aescin] • Phospholipids from Safflower & Sunflower seed oil • Caprylic/Capric Triglyceride • Apricot Kernel oil • Soy Lecithin • Glycerine (Vegetable) • Tocopherol (natural Vitamin E) • Arnica extract • Panthenol • Saccharide Isomerate • Xanthan Gum • Carrageenan (Irish Moss) • Dimethicone • Lauroyl Lysine • Natural Fragrant Essential Oils Blend • Sodium Hydroxymethylglycinate.

Horsechestnut Extract 300 mg - Vital Nutrients
Each capsule contains: Aesculus Hippocastanum seed extract (horsechesnut, standardized to 20% escin) 300 mg.

Horsetail Aerial Part - Aboca USA, Inc
Two capsules contain: Horsetail aerial part WPC (whole phytocomplex concentrate, equisetum maximum, standardized to contain 0.95% total flavonoids calculated as isoquercitrin, yielding 2.5 mg per capsule) 524 mg. Other Ingredients: Gelatin.

Horsetail Extract Formula - Quest
Each caplet contains: Horsetail powder (Equisetum arvense) (provided by 125 mg 1:4 Aqueous Extract) 500 mg • Rosehips powder (Rose canina) 50 mg • Burdock root powder (Arctium lappa) 30 mg • Marshmallow root powder (Althaea officinalis) 30 mg • Parsley leaf powder (Plantago major) 30 mg • Slippery Elm bark powder (Ulmus fulva) 30 mg. Other Ingredients: Calcium Phosphate, Microcrystalline Cellulose, Croscarmellose Sodium, Magnesium Stearate (vegetable source), Vegetable Stearin.

Horsetail Plus Fo-Ti - The Herbalist
Horsetail fresh-dried herb (Equisetum arvense) • Fo-Ti fresh-dried root (Polygonum multiflorum) • Nettles fresh-dried leaf (Urtica dioica) • Red Clover fresh-dried blossom (Trifolium pratense) • Burdock fresh-dried root (Arctium lappa).

Hot Back Support Pak - Ortho Molecular Products
Each packet contains: Vitamin C (as ascorbic acid USP, acerola fruit extract) 430 mg • Vitamin B6 (as pyridoxine HCl USP) 50 mg • Magnesium (as ascorbate) 15 mg • Bromelain 2400 GDU/g) 890 mg • Turmeric root extract (standardized to contain 95% curcumin) 660 mg • Panreatin 6X 400 mg • Quercetin Dihydrate 310 mg • GABA 250 mg • Papain 230 mg • Glycine USP 225 mg • Cramp bark 200 mg • Rutin 160 mg • Acerola fruit extract (standardized to contain 17% vitamin C) 100 mg • Thymus 70 mg • Trypsin 70 mg • Dong Quai root extract (standardized to contain 1% ligustilides) 150 mg • Hesperidin complex 50 mg • Hibiscus flowers 50 mg • Amylase 30 mg • Lipase 30 mg • Lysozyme 20 mg • Cellulase 4 mg • Alpha Chymotrypsin 2 mg.

Hot Flash - Source Naturals
Three tablets contain: Soy concentrate, yielding 65 mg Isoflavones 2100 mg • Black Cohosh 160 mg • Dong Quai extract 150 mg • Licorice root extract 150 mg • Vitex extract 100 mg.

Hot Flashex - Natrol, Inc.
Each tablet contains: Vitamin E (as d-alpha tocopherol) 50 IU • Calcium (as tri-calcium phosphate) 70 mg • Licorice 100 mg • Black Cohosh root 60 mg, Triterpenes (2.5%) 15 mg • Chamomile extract 50 mg • Kava Kava root 30 mg, Kavalactones (30%) 9 mg. Other Ingredients: Mono & Di-Glycerides, Croscarmellose Sodium, Silicon Dioxide, Stearic Acid, Magnesium Stearate.

Hot Mommies Essential 3 - Goldshield Elite
Four tablets contain: Chromium (as chromium dinicotinate glycinate) 400 mcg • Citrus Aurantium extract (bitter orange) 1300 mg • Green Tea leaf extract 600 mg • Kudzu root extract 100 mg • Rhubarb root extract 160 mg • Carthamus Tinctorius seed 70 mg • Siberian Ginseng (eleuthero) 38 mg • Gypenosides from Gynostema pentaphyllum plant extract 21 mg • Proprietary Blend 1413 mg: Polygonum Multiflorium root extract, Lycium berry extract, Lotus seed, Dong Quai root extract, Ligusticum Wallichi root, White Atractylodes rhizome, Astragalus root extract, White Peony root extract, Sicklepod Senna seed (cassia tora), Crataegus Oxyacantha berry and leaf extract, Gymnema Sylvestre leaf extract, Licorice root extract. Other Ingredients: Dicalcium Phosphate, Microcrystalline Cellulose, Croscarmellose Sodium, Stearic Acid, Anise Oil, Magnesium Stearate, Silica, Calcium Silicate, Pharmaceutical Glaze. See Editor's Note No. 40.

Hot Plants For Her - Enzymatic Therapy
Two capsules contain: MacaPure brand Maca root extract (lepidium meyenii standardized to contain 0.6% macaenes and macamides) 400 mg • Ashwagandha root extract (withania somnifera standardized to contain 4% withanolides) 250 mg • Rhodiola root extract (rhodiola rosea standardized to contain 3% rosavins and 1% salidroside) 150 mg • Eleuthero root extract (eleutherococcus senticosus standardized to contain a minimum of 0.8% eleutherosides E and B) 150 mg • Catuaba bark 4:1 extract (erythroxylum catuaba) 100 mg. Other Ingredients: Gelatin, Cellulose, Magnesium Stearate, Titanium Dioxide Color, Silicon Dioxide.

Hot Plants For Him - Enzymatic Therapy
Two capsules contain: MacaPure brand Maca root extract (lepidium meyenii standardized to contain 0.6% macaenes and macamides) 400 mg • Yohimbe bark extract (pausinystalia yohimbe standardized to contain 4% yohimbines) 200 mg • Rhodiola root extract (rhodiola rosea standardized to contain 3% rosavins and 1% salidroside) 150 mg • Horny Goat Weed aerial part extract (epimedium sagittatum standardized to contain 10% flavonoids calculated as icariin) 100 mg • Panax Ginseng root extract (standardized to contain a minimum of 7% ginsenosides) 100 mg • LJ100 Tongkat Ali brand Tongkat Ali root 100:1 extract (eurycoma longifolia) 50 mg. Other Ingredients: Gelatin, Cellulose, Magnesium Stearate, Titanium Dioxide Color, Silicon Dioxide.

Hot-Rox - BioTest Laboratories, LLC
Two capsules contain: Thiamin (vitamin B1) 20 mg • Niacin (vitamin B3) 20 mg • Pantothenic Acid 20 mg • Pyridoxal-5-Phosphate 50 mg • Vitamin B12 (methylcobalamin) 995 mcg • HOT-ROX Thermogenic Formula 950 mg: N-Acetyl-L-Tyrosine, MDX complex: Androst-5-ene-7-one-317-diethl-carbonate, Sclaremax propreitary Salvia Sclarea extract, Guggulsterone Z, Guggulsterone E; Caffeine, 5-Hydroxy - L-Tryptophan.

Hoxsey Formula - The Herbalist
Red Clover fresh-dried blossoms (trifolium pratense) • Chaparral fresh-dried leaf (larrea tridentata) • Licorice fresh-dried root (glycyrrhiza glabra) • Oregon Grape fresh-dried root (berberis nervosa)• Burdock fresh-dried root (arctium lappa) • Sarsaparilla fresh-dried root (smilax ornata) • Echinacea fresh root (echinacea angustifolia) • Prickly Ash fresh-dried bark (xanthoxylum americanum).

Hoxsey Red Clover Supreme - Gaia Herbs
Forty drops contain: Proprietary Blend 50 mg: Red Clover blossoms (trifolium pratense), Buckthorn bark (rhamnus fragula), Barberry root bark (berberis vulgaris), Burdock root (arctium lappa), Stillingia root (stillingia silvatica), Poke root (phytolacca americana), Fresh Nettle leaf (urtica dioica), Cascara Sagrada bark (rhamnus purshiana), Licorice root (glycyrrhiza glabra), Prickly Ash bark (xanthoxylum clava-herculis), Sweet Orange essential oil, Spring Water, 35-45% Pure Grain Alcohol USP.

HPF Hangover Prevention Formula - Perfect Equation
Each capsule contains: Tex-OE brand Opuntia Indica Cactus fruit standardized extract 800 IU • Vitamin B1 (as thiamin mononitrate) 3 mg • Riboflavin 3.4 mg • Niacin (as inositol hexaniacinate) 40 mg •

Vitamin B6 (as pyridoxine hydrochloride) 4 mg • Pantothenic Acid (as D-calcium pantothenate) 20 mg. Other Ingredients: Mannitol, Gelatin, Tricalcium Phosphate, Silica, Magnesium Stearate.

HPX Hydrating Gel - Nu Skin Enterprises
Water • Kukui nut oil • Propylene Glycol • Human Placental Protein • Tocopheryl Acetate • Phospholipids • Tocopherol • Carbomer • Triethanolamine • Methylparaben • Disodium EDTA • Phenoxyethanol • BHT.

HTP Calm - Natural Balance
Two capsules contain: Vitamin B6 (as pyridoxine hydrochloride) 20 mg • Proprietary Blend 500 mg: Passion Flower (aerial portion extract), Gotu Kola (aerial portion extract), Kava Kava (root, rhizome extract) • St. John's Wort flower extract (standardized to 0.3% hypericin) 300 mg • 5-HTP (5-hydroxytryptophan from griffonia simplicifolia seed extract) 50 mg. Other Ingredients: Gelatin, Magnesium Stearate.

HTP10 Complex - Pain & Stress Center
Each capsule contains: Vitamin C (ascorbyl palmitate) 2 mg • Vitamin B6 (pyridoxal 5' phosphate) 0.6 mg • Magnesium (magnesium oxide) 25 mg • Alpha-Ketoglutaric Acid 15 mg • 5-Hydroxytryptophan (5-HTP) 10 mg • Proprietary Blend 109 mg: Glycine, Gamma Amino Butyric Acid (GABA), Glutamine, Lysine, Taurine. Other Ingredients: Gelatin Capsule.

Hua Fo - Shenlong Natural International, Inc.
Each tablet contains: Panax Ginseng 18 mg • Ligustrum lucidum fruit (Privet fruit) 72 mg • Curculigoo orchiodes (Golden-Eye Grass rhizome) 54 mg. Other Ingredients: Epimemdium grandiflorum (Licentious Goat Wort) 84 mg, Polygonium multiflorum (Black Haired Mr. He) 72 mg.
See Editor's Note No. 3.

Hua Fo VIGOR-MAX - Shenlong Natural International, Inc.
Each tablet contains: Epimedium Macranthum 84 mg • Polygonum Multiflorum 72 mg • Ligustrum Lucidum 72 mg • Curculigo Orchioides 54 mg • Panax Ginseng 18 mg.
See Editor's Note No. 23.

Huang Lian Jie Du Tang Plus - Secara
Chinese Skullcap root 5:1 extract (huang qin) 525 mg • Gardenia fruit 5:1 extract (zhi zi) 535 mg • Phellodendron bark 5:1 extract (huang bai) 535 mg • Coptis rhizome 5:1 extract (huang lian) 269 mg • Organic Goldenseal rhizome 252 mg • Organic Oregano leaf 113 mg • Organic Oregano oil 11 mg.

Human Growth Complex - Ultra Lab
Each tablet contains: Somatotrophine (GH) 12X • Insulin-Like Growth Factor-1 (IGF-1) 12X • Alfalfa 3X • Arnica Montana 15X • Arsenicum Album 15X • Baptisia 15X • Bryonia 15X • China Officinalis 15X • Gelsemium Sempervirens 15X • Lacticum Acidum 15X • Lycopodium Clavatum 15X • Phosphorus 15X • Rhus Toxicodendron 15X • Ruta Graveolens 10X.
See Editor's Note No. 1.

Human Growth Hormone (HGH) - Youngevity
Each capsule contains: L-Lysine HCL • L-Arginine • L-Ornithine • L-Glutamine • L-Tyrosine • Vilcabamba Mineral Essence: Potassium, Calcium, Magnesium, Zinc, Chromium, Selenium, Iron, Copper, Molybdenum, Vanadium, Iodine, Cobalt, Manganese.

HumanoVar - GEN - Genetic Evolutionary Nutrition
Each capsule contains: Vitamin E 30 IU • Selenium (from amino acid chelate) 50 mcg • Proteic Embryo Extract (from fertilized chicken eggs) 100 mg. Inactive Ingredients: Gelatine, Magnesium Stearate, Silicon Dioxide.

Huperzine A - Life Enhancement Products, Inc.
Each capsule contains: Huperzine A 50 mcg.

Huperzine A - Pro Health
Each tablet contains: Huperzine A 50 mcg. Other Ingredients: Calcium Phosphate, Cellulose, Stearic Acid, Croscarmellose Sodium, Magnesium Stearate, Silicon Dioxide.

Huperzine A Complex - Puritan's Pride
Each tablet contains: Folic Acid 200 mcg • Vitamin B12 (as cyanocobalamin) 6 mcg • DMAE (from DMAE bitartrate) (dimethylaminoethanol) 50 mg • Panax ginseng (root standardized extract: provides 5 mg ginsenosides) 125 mg • Huperzine A (from standardized Huperiza serrata) leaf extract 50 mcg • L-Tyrosine 75 mg • Bioperine brand Black Pepper extract (from standardized piperine) 2.5 mg.

Huperzine A Complex - PhysioLogics
Each tablet contains: Folic Acid 200 mg • Vitamin B12 (as cyanocobalamin) 6 mcg • DMAE (dimethylaminoethanol, from dmae bitartrate) 50 mg • Ginseng root (panax ginseng, standardized extract providing 5 mg ginsenosides) 100 mg • Huperzine A (from standardized extract of huperzia serrate leaf) 50 mcg • L-Tyrosine 75 mg • Piper Nigrum fruit (from standardized piperine) 2.5 mg. Other Ingredients: Silica, Vegetable Magnesium Stearate, Vegetable Stearic Acid, Dicalcium Phosphate, Cellulose (plant origin), Croscarmellose.

Huperzine A Ginkgo/Ginseng - Nutrapharm, Inc.
Each capsule contains: Huperzine A 50 mcg • Ginkgo biloba extract 60 mg • Panax ginseng extract 150 mg. Other Ingredients: Malto dextrin, magnesium stearate, microcrystalline cellulose, & silica. Free of sugar, yeast, milk, artificial colors, flavors & dyes.

Huperzine A w/Ginkgo - Nutrapharm, Inc.
Each capsule contains: Huperzine A 50 mcg • Ginkgo biloba extract 60 mg. Other Ingredients: Malto dextrin, magnesium stearate, microcrystalline cellulose, & silica. Free of sugar, yeast, corn, milk, artificial colors, flavors & dyes.

Huperzine A w/Ginseng - Nutrapharm, Inc.
Each capsule contains: Huperzine A 50 mcg • Panax ginseng extract (standardized to 8% ginsenosides) 150 mg. Other Ingredients: Malto dextrin, magnesium stearate, microcrystalline cellulose, & silica. Free of sugar, yeast, corn, milk products, artificial colors, flavors & dyes.

Huperzine A w/Vitamin E - Nutrapharm, Inc.
Each capsule contains: Huperzine A 50 mcg • Vitamin E (D-alpha tocopheryl acetate) 100 IU. Other Ingredients: Malto dextrin, magnesium stearate, & silica. Free of sugar, yeast, corn, milk, artificial colors, flavors & dyes.

Huperzine Rx-Brain - Nature's Plus
Each tablet contains: Huperzine-A (from huperzia serrata) 50 mcg. Other Ingredients: Di-calcium Phosphate, Microcrystalline Cellulose, Stearic Acid, Magnesium Stearate, Silica, Pharmaceutical Glaze.

HVP - Nature's Sunshine
Each capsule contains: Proprietary Blend 390 mg: Valerian root, Skullcap herb, Hops flowers.

HY 2 - Pacific BioLogic
St. John's Wort.

Hyaluronic Acid - Pure Encapsulations
Each vegetable capsule contains: Hyaluronic Acid powder (providing a minimum of 9% hyaluronic acid) 70 mg.

Hyaluronic Acid - Source Naturals
Two tablets contain: Protein 1 g • Calcium 167 mg • BioCell brand Collagen II 1 g: Type II Collagen 600 mg, Chondroitin Sulfate 200 mg, Hyaluronic Acid 100 mg. Other Ingredients: Dibasic Calcium Phosphate, Stearic Acid, Hydroxypropyl Cellulose, Modified Cellulose Gum, Natural Peppermint Flavor, Colloidal Silicon Dioxide.

Hyaluronic Acid - Vitamin World
Each capsule contains: Hyaluronic Acid (sodium hyaluronate) 20 mg. Other Ingredients: Rice Powder, Gelatin, Silica.

BRAND NAMES

Hyben Vital **-** Hyben Vital International
Wild Dog Rose Hips (hips and kernals, dried and powdered). Available in Denmark.

HY-C **-** Nature's Sunshine
Three capsules contain: Proprietary Blend 1395 mg: Glehnia root (glenia littoralis), Eucommia bark (eucommia ulmoides), Rehmannia root tuber (rehmannia glutinosa), Ophiopogon root tuber (ophiopogon japonicus), Pueraria root (pueraria lobata), Trichosanthes root (trichosanthes kirilowii), Achyranthes root (achyranthes bidentata), Alisma rhizome (alisma plantago aquatica), Anemarrhena rhizome (anemarrhena asphodeloides), Asparagus root tuber (asparagus cochinchinesis), Poria Cocos (hoelen sclerotium), Moutan root bark (paeonia suffruticosa), Cornus fruit (cornus officinalis, seedless), Licorice root (glycyrrhiza uralensis), Phellodendron stem bark (phellodendron amurense), Schizandra fruit (schisandra chinensis). Other Ingredients: Gelatin, Water.

Hydra Cleanse **-** Pharmagel
Aloe Vera • a complex of marine-based extracts of Seaweed, Algae, and Spirulina • Oat extract • Beta Glucan • Panthenol.

Hydra Fuel **-** TwinLab
Glucose Polymers & Glucose (approximately 5%) • Fructose (about 2%). Replenishes important Electrolytes & Minerals: Sodium, Potassium, Magnesium, Chloride, Chromium, Phosphorus.

Hydra Joint BASIC **-** Renutra Natural Health Products
Purified Water • Glucosamine Sulfate • MSM • Vitamin C (as ascorbic acid) • Citric Acid • Carrageenan • Natural Flavors • Potassium Sorbate • Sodium Benzoate • Stevia leaf extract.

Hydra Joint TOTAL **-** Renutra Natural Health Products
Purified Water • Glucosamine Sulfate • Chondroitin Sulfate • Citric Acid • MSM • Vitamin C (as ascorbic acid) • Natural Flavors • Stevia leaf extract • Carrageenan • Potassium Sorbate • Sodium Benzoate.

Hydramax Ginkgo Biloba PhytoSerum **-** Abra Therapeutics
Aloe Vera juice • ABRA4 PhytoSerum Complex: Ginkgo Biloba extract, White Willow bark extract, Ivy extract, Horsetail extract, Mallow extract, Comfrey extract, Chamomile extract • Vegetable Glycerin • Jojoba nut oil • Avocado oil • Kukui nut oil • Macadamia nut oil • Glyceryl Stearate • Time Release Ginkgo Biloba Phytoliposomes (standardized ginkgo flavonglycosides from ginkgo) • Stearic Acid • Sorbitol • Allantoin • Panthenol (pro-vitamin B5) • Borage Seed oil • Alpha-Tocopherol (vitamin E) • Beta Carotene (pro-vitamin A) • Ascorbyl Palmitate (vitamin C) • Ylang Ylang oil • Geranium oil • Methylparaben • Propylparaben.

Hydrated Bentonite **-** Nature's Sunshine
Purified Water • Bentonite USP.

Hydrating Cleanser **-** Abra Therapeutics
Deionized Water • Extract of Orange Blossom • Rose Bud • Bulgarian Chamomile • Horsetail • French Lavender • Vegetable Glycerine • Kukui nut • Macadamia nut • Glyceryl Stearate • Aloe Vera gel • Stearic Acid • Jojoba nut oil • Sorbital • Avocado seed oil • Cucumber extract • Allantoin • Panthenol • Borage seed oil • Vitamin E • Vitamin A • Vitamin C • Essential Oils of Geranium and Ylang-Ylang • Methylparaben • Propylparaben.

Hydravax **-** Metabolic Nutrition, Inc.
Three capsules contain: Dandelion root (20%) 2010 mg • Uva Ursi (20% arbutin) 1050 mg • Green Tea leaf (50%/35%) 900 mg • Cranberry powder 300 mg • Magnesium Citrate 180 mg • Couch Grass 150 mg • Corn Silk 150 mg • Buchu leaf (4:1) 90 mg • Juniper berry (4:1) 90 mg • Hydrangea root (4:1) 90 mg.

Hydrochloric Acid **-** American Biologics
Each tablet contains: Betaine HCl 150 mg • Pepsin 12 N.F. 10 mg • Ammonium Chloride 35 mg • Glutamic Acid HCl 50 mg • Vitamin B6 2 mg • Pancreatin (4X, N.F.) 10 mg. Other Ingredients: Calcium Carbonate, Magnesium Stearate, Dicalcium Phosphate.

Hydroderm **-** Life Extension
Collagen (marine) • Distilled Water/Igepal • Cephene • Methyl Paraben • Ethyl Paraben • Propyl Paraben • Butyl Paraben • Isobutyl Paraben • Synasol • Serum Protein • Purified Water • PRE complex • Sodium Methylparaben • Imidazolidinyl Urea • Trisodium EDTA • Potassium Sorbate • Citric Acid • Ascorbic Acid.

HydroEye SoftGels **-** ScienceBased Health
Two capsules contain: Vitamin A (from retinyl palmitate) 1040 IU • Vitamin C (from calcium ascorbate, ester-c) 90 mg • Vitamin B6 (from pyridoxal 5 phosphate) 6.3 mg • Magnesium (from magnesium sulfate) 20 mg • Black Currant seed oil (15.6% gamma linolenic acid, [GLA]) 750 mg • Mucin Complex (60% mucin) 250 mg • Cod Liver oil 1.6 mg. Other Ingredients: Gelatin, Water, Vegetable Shortening, Glycerine, Lecithin, Beeswax, Titanium Dioxide, Caramel Color.

HydroTest **-** NutraBolics
Six milliliters contain: Liquid German Tribulus Terrestris (80% proctodioscin) 40 mg • Designer Pro-Testosterone Complex 500 mg: Eurycoma Longifolia (50:1), Avena Sativa (10:1), Rhodiola Rosea (3% rosavins, 39% salidorosides), Fenugreek 4-Hydroxy Isoleucine (30%).

Hydroxy Ripped **-** Puritan's Pride
Four capsules contain: Chromium 300 mcg • Hydroripped 2000 (Garcinia cambogia) fruit rind (containing 1,000 of HCA) 1,667 mg • Guarana extract (Paullina cupana) seed (standardized for 22% caffeine) 1,000 mg • Ma Huang extract (Ephedra sinica) aerial (standardized for 21 mg of ephedra alkaloids) 360 mg • Salicin complex (from White Willow Bark) Salix alba (containing 15% salicin) 150 mg • L-Carnitine 150 mg.
See Editor's Note No. 21 and No. 30.

Hydroxycitrate Plus **-** Metagenics
Each tablet contains: L-Carnitine 100 mg • Niacin (as niacinamide) 50 mg • Pantothenic Acid (as D-calcium pantothenate) 25 mg • Riboflavin 10 mg • Manganese (as manganese arginine) 750 mcg • Chromium (as chromium nicotinate glycinate) 75 mcg • Garcinia fruit extract (garcinia cambogia) 500 mg.

Hydroxycut **-** MuscleTech
Four capsules contain: Hydroxagen (supplying 100 mg of Hydroxycitric Acid) 2000 mg • Ma Huang extract 334 mg • Guarana extract 910 mg • Willow bark extract 100 mg • L-Carnitine 100 mg • Chromium Picolinate 300 mcg.
See Editor's Note No. 21 and No. 30.

Hydroxycut (ephedra free) **-** MuscleTech
Three capsules contain: Calcium (as hydroxycitrate) 152 mg • ChromaTech brand Chromium (as polynicotinate) 133 mcg • Potassium (as chloride/hydroxycitrate) 225 mg • Hydroxagen Plus Proprietary Blend 1.7 g: Super CitriMax brand Garcinia Cambogia fruit & rind extract (standardized for (-) hydroxycitric acid), Gymnema Sylvestre leaf extract (standardzed for gymnemic acid), Glucomannan (amorphallus konjac), Alpha Lipoic Acid, Willow Bark extract (purple & white, standardized for salicin), L-Carnitine (as tartarate) • HydroxyTea 393 mg: Green Tea Leaf extract (standardized for 95% polyphenols: 70% catechins: 45% epigallocatechin gallate - 90 mg EGCG), Caffeine (as caffeine anhydrous), Guarana seed extract (standardized for 200 mg of caffeine). Other Ingredients: Gelatin, Magnesium Stearate, Silica, Cellulose.
See Editor's Note No. 68.

Hydroxycut Caffeine-Free **-** MuscleTech
Three capsules contain: Calcium (as calcium hydroxycitrate) 152 mg • Chromium (as polynicotinate) 133 mcg • Potassium (as hydroxycitrate) 225 mg • Hydroxagen Plus Blend 1.71 g: Garcinia Cambogia fruit/rind extract (standardized for hydroxycitric acid), Gymnema Sylvestre leaf extract (standardized for gymnemic acid), Glucomannan (amorphophallus konjac), Alpha Lipoic Acid, Willow bark extract (purple & white, standardized for salicin), L-Carnitine (as tartrate) • Hydroxy Tea I Caffeine-free Green Tea leaf extract

(standardized for 95% polyphenols, 70% catechins, 45% epigallocatechin gallate, 90 mg) 200 mg. Other Ingredients: Gelatin, Magnesium Stearate, Silica, Cellulose.

Hyperbalance - Gero Vita International
Each capsule contains: Uncaria rhynchophylla (Chinese cat's claw) extract 100 mg • Heal-All (Prunella vulgaris) extract (herb) 100 mg • Apocynum venetum (plant) extract 100 mg • Eucommia (bark) extract 100 mg • Sickle Pod Senna (seed) extract 100 mg • Gastrodia (rhizome) extract 50 mg • Wild Chrysanthemum (flower) extract 50 mg • Rauwolfia yunnanenis (root) extract 15 mg. Other Ingredients: Dicalcium Phosphate, Silicon Dioxide, Vegetable Magnesium Stearate, Gelatin.

HyperiCalm - Enzymatic Therapy
Each capsule contains: St. John's Wort (Hypericum perforatum) extract standardized to 0.3% hypericins (900 mcg) & 4% hyperforin (12 mg), verified by HPLC 300 mg.

Hypericum 0.3 300 mg - Pure Encapsulations
Each vegetable capsule contains: Hypericum extract (St. John's wort, standardized to contain 0.3% hypericin, 3% hyperforin) 300 mg • Vitamin C (as ascorbyl palmitate) 3 mg.

Hypericum 0.3 600 mg - Pure Encapsulations
Each vegetable capsule contains: Hypericum extract (St. John's wort, standardized to contain 0.3% hypericin, 3% hyperforin) 600 mg • Vitamin C (as ascorbyl palmitate) 6 mg.

Hypericum Extract 0.3% 300 mg - Vital Nutrients
Each capsule contains: Hypericum Perforatum extract (St. John's wort, standardized to 0.3% hypericin and 3-5% hyperforin) 300 mg.

HyperiMed - PhytoPharmica
Each capsule contains: St. John's Wort extract (hypericum perforatum, standardized to 0.3% hypericins (900 mcg) & 4% hyperforin (12 mg)), 300 mg.

Hypertrol Rx-Blood Pressure - Nature's Plus
Two tablets contain: Magnesium (as amino acid chelate/complex) 400 mg • Chromium (as polynicotinate) 200 mcg • Hypertrol Proprietary Botanical Extract Complex 1120 mg: Kudzu root (radix puerariae), Horse Chestnut seed (aesculus hippocastanum), English Hawthorne berry (crataegus laevigata), Grape seed (vitis vinifera), Coleus Forskohlii root, Bilberry fruit (vaccinium myrtillus) • Garlic clove (odor-modified allium sativum, standardized 1% (3 mg) allicin potential) 300 mg • Bioflavonoids (from citrus limon exocarp) 100 mg • Polygonum Cuspidatum root extract 8 mg. Other Ingredients: Di-Calcium Phosphate, Microcrystalline Cellulose, Stearic Acid, Silica, Magnesium Stearate, Pharmaceutical Glaze.

Hypo-Ade - Enzymatic Therapy
Two tablets contain: Vitamin A (53% as beta carotene and as retinyl acetate) 5000 IU • Vitamin C (ascorbic acid) 200 mg • Thiamin (as thiamin HCl, vitamin B1) 25 mg • Riboflavin (vitamin B2) 25 mg • Niacin (as niacinamide and niacin) 115 mg • Vitamin B6 (as pyridoxine HCl) 25 mg • Vitamin B12 (as cyanocobalamin) 25 mcg • Pantothenic Acid (as calcium D-pantothenate) 100 mg • Zinc (as zinc gluconate) 10 mg • Manganese (as manganese gluconate) 2.3 mg • Chromium (as chromium polynicotinate) 267 mcg • Sodium 5 mg • Potassium (as potassium aspartate) 50 mg • Inositol 200 mg • Pancreas extract (freeze-dried) 150 mg • Choline Bitartrate 100 mg • L-Methionine 100 mg • Beet root (beta vulgaris) 100 mg • Adrenal extract 65 mg • Betaine HCl 50 mg • Wild Yam root (dioscorea villosa) 50 mg • Barberry bark of root 6:1 extract (berberis vulgaris) 30 mg. Other Ingredients: Cellulose, Modified Cellulose Gum, Magnesium Stearate, Modified Cellulose, Dandelion Leaf, Goldenseal Root, Liver, Lecithin, Carnauba Wax, Lung, Pancreas, Heart, Kidney, Spleen.
See Editor's Note No. 14.

Hypo-Ade Capsules - Enzymatic Therapy
Two capsules contain: Vitamin A (53% as beta carotene, retinyl acetate) 5000 IU • Vitamin C (ascorbic acid) 200 mg • Thiamin (as thiamin HCl, vitamin B1) 25 mg • Riboflavin (vitamin b2) 25 mg • Niacin (as niacinamide, niacin) 115 mg • Vitamin B6 (as pyridoxine HCl) 25 mg • Vitamin B12 (as cyanocobalamin) 25 mcg • Pantothenic Acid (as calcium d-pantothenate) 100 mg • Zinc (as zinc gluconate) 10 mg • Manganese (as manganese gluconate) 2.3 mg • Chromium (as chromium picolinate) 267 mcg • Potassium (as potassium aspartate) 50 mg • Inositol 200 mg • Pancreas extract (freeze-dried) 150 mg • Choline Bitartrate 100 mg • L-Methionine 100 mg • Beet root (beta vulgaris) 100 mg • Adrenal extract (freeze-dried) 65 mg • Betaine HCl 50 mg • Wild Yam root (dioscorea villosa) 50 mg • Pituitary extract 40 mg • Barberry root bark 6:1 extract (berberis vulgaris) 30 mg. Other Ingredients: Gelatin, Magnesium Stearate, Silicon Dioxide, Titanium Dioxide Color, Dandelion Leaf, Goldenseal Root, Liver, Lung, Pancreas, Heart, Kidney, Spleen.
See Editor's Note No. 31.

HypoAllergenic Taurine - Kirkman Laboratories
Each capsule contains: Taurine 325 mg. Inactive Ingredients: Plant Cellulose.

Hyporil - PhytoPharmica
Two tablets contain: Adrenal extract 65 mg • Barberry bark of root 6:1 extract (berberis vulgaris) 30 mg • Beet root (beta vulgaris) 100 mg • Betaine HCl 50 mg • Choline Bitartrate 100 mg • Chromium (as chromium polynicotinate) 267 mg • Inositol 200 mg • L-Methionine 100 mg • Manganese (as manganese gluconate) 2.3 mg • Niacin (as niacinamide and niacin) 115 mg • Pancreas extract (freeze-dried) 150 mg • Pantothenic Acid (as calcium D-pantothenate) 100 mg • Potassium (as potassium aspartate) 50 mg • Riboflavin (vitamin B2)25 mg • Thiamin (as thiamin HCl, vitamin B1) 25 mg • Vitamin A (53% as beta carotene and as retinyl acetate) 5000 IU • Vitamin B12 (as cyanocobalamin) 25 mcg • Vitamin B6 (as pyridoxine HCl) 25 mg • Vitamin C (ascorbic acid) 200 mg • Wild Yam (dioscorea villosa) 50 mg • Zinc (as zinc gluconate) 10 mg.
See Editor's Note No. 14.

Hypothalamus PMG - Standard Process, Inc.
Each tablet contains: Proprietary Blend 205 mg: Bovine Hypothalamus PMG extract, Magnesium Citrate • Calcium 20 mg • Sodium 10 mg. Other Ingredients: Cellulose.
See Editor's Note No. 31.

Hypothalamus, Organic Glandular - Allergy Research Group
Each capsule contains: Hypothalamus tissue (bovine) 500 mg. Other Ingredients: Cellulose, Stearic Acid.
See Editor's Note No. 31.

Hypothalmex - Standard Process, Inc.
Each tablet contains: Proprietary Blend 200 mg: Bovine Hypothalamus Cytosol extract, Magnesium Citrate • Calcium 20 mg. Other Ingredients: Cellulose.
See Editor's Note No. 31.

Hypothyroid Remedy (formerly HP 26) - Metagenics
Each tablet contains: Thyroidinum 6X.
See Editor's Note No. 1.

Hythiol-C - SSP Co., Ltd.
Six tablets contain: L-Cysteine 240 mg • Vitamin C 300 mg • Calcium Pantothenate (vitamin B5) 34 mg

I.B.S. Intestinal Bowel SUPPORT - Renew Life Formulas, Inc.
Intestinal Lining Support: Two capsules contain: L-Glutamine • N-Acetyl Glucosamine • Gamma Oryzanol • Proprietary Herbal Blend: Cranesbill root (geranium maculatum), Ginger root (zingiber officinale), Marigold flower (calendula officinalis), Marshmallow root (althaea officinalis). Other Ingredients: Hypromellose, Water.
Bowel Support: Slippery Elm bark (ulmas rubra) • German Chamomile flower (matricaria recutita) • Fenugreek seed (trigonella foenum-graecum) • Fennel seed (foeniculum vulgare) • Skullcap herb (scutellaria lateriflora) • Cranberry fruit (vaccinium macrocarpon) • Peppermint leaf (mentha piperita) • Proprietary Chinese Herbal

Extract Blend: Atractylodes root (bai zhu), Yin Chen Hao (capillary artemisia herb), Codonopsis root (dang shen), Jobs Tears seed (yi yi ren), Schisandra fruit (wu wei zi), Huo Xiang (agastache whole plant), Chinese Licorice root (zi gan cao), Chinese Thoroughwax (chai hu), Ginger root (pao jiang), Korean Ash branch, bark (qin pi), Magnolia bark (hou po), Phellodendron bark (huang bai), Poria Cocos root (fu ling), Psyllium seed (che qian zi), Chinese Goldthread (huang lian), Chinese White Peony root (bai shao), Costus root (mu xiang), Siler root (fang feng), Tangerine peel (chen pi), Angelica root (bai zhi) • MSM (methylsulfonylmethane). Other Ingredients: Hypromellose, Water.

I3C Rx - Xymogen
Each capsule contains: Indole-3-Carbinol 150 mg • SulFoPlex Proprietary blend 375 mg: Cabbage powder, Rosemary leaf extract (11% carnosic acid), Broccoli extract, Brussel sprout extract, Green Tea leaf extract (40% catechins), Ascorbyl Palmitate.

Iberogast - Enzymatic Therapy/PhytoPharmica
A 100 mL bottle contains: German Chamomile flower (matricaria recutita) 20 mL • Clown's Mustard plant (iberis amara) 15 mL • Angelica root and rhizome (angelica archangelica) 10 mL • Caraway fruit (carum carvi) 10 mL • Milk Thistle fruit (silybum marianum) 10 mL • Lemon Balm leaf (melissa officinalis) 10 mL • Celandine aerial part (chelidonium majus) 10 mL • Licorice root (glycyrrhiza glabra) 10 mL • Peppermint leaf (mentha x piperita) 5 mL.
See Editor's Note No. 69.

ICaps AREDS Formula - Alcon Laboratories
Two tablets contain: Vitamin C 226 mg • Vitamin E 200 IU • Zinc 34.8 mg • Copper 0.8 mg • Vitamin A 14,320 IU. Other Ingredients: Microcrystalline Cellulose, Dicalcium Phosphate, Gelatin, Hydroxypropyl Methylcellulose, Silicon Dioxide, Magnesium Stearate, Stearic Acid, Polyethylene Glycol, Sucrose, Dextrin, Titanium Dioxide, Corn Starch, FD&C Red #40 Lake, Dextrose Monohydrate, Lecithin, Ascorbyl Palmitate, FD&C Yellow #6 Lake, dl-Alpha Tocopherol, Sodium Ascorbate, Sorbic Acid, Sodium Benzoate, Polysorbate 80.

ICaps Lutein & Zeaxanthin Formula - Alcon Laboratories
Two tablets contain: Vitamin A (as beta carotene) 6600 IU • Vitamin C (as ascorbic acid) 400 mg • Vitamin E 150 IU • Riboflavin (B2) 10 mg • Zinc (as zinc acetate) 60 mg • Selenium 40 mcg • Copper 4 mg • Manganese 10 mg • Lutein & Zeaxanthin 4 mg. Other Ingredients: Hydroxypropyl Methylcellulose, Gelatin, Microcrystalline Cellulose, Dicalcium Phosphate, Silicon Dioxide, Magnesium Stearate, Corn Starch, Titanium Dioxide, Polyethylene Glycol, Ascorbyl Palmitate, Sodium Ascorbate, Sorbic Acid, Polysorbate 80, Sodium Benzoate, Carnauba Wax.

Iced Lemon Fibergy Bar - USANA Health Sciences
Each bar contains: Rolled Oats, Dextrose, Oat Fiber, Fractionated Palm Kernel Oil, Oat Flour, Citric Acid, Lemon Oil, Gum Arabic, Soy Lecithin, Crystalline Fructose, Inulin (Natural Extract of Chicory), High Fructose Corn Syrup, Dehydrated Cane Juice, Oat Bran, Barley Flour, Date Puree, Brown Crisp Rice (Rice Flour, Rice Bran, Rosemary Extract), Vegetable Glycerin, Oat Flour, Rolled Barley, Flax Seed Meal, Soy Lecithin, Natural Flavors, Baking Soda, Corn Starch, Gelatin.

Ideas - Starlight International
Each four tablets contain: St. John's Wort, 0.3% (hypericum perforatum, flowering parts) 400 mg • Gingko biloba extract, 4:1 (leaf) 100 mg • Basil / Tulsi extract, 4:1 (ocimum sanctum, leaf) 150 mg • Lemon Balm (melissa officinalis, leaf) 150 mg • Siberian Ginseng extract, 4:1 (eleutherococcus senticosus, root) 200 mg • Gotu Kola extract, 4:1 (cantella asiatica, plant) 150 mg • Bacopa Monneria (water hyssop extract, 4:1, plant) 150 mg • Spirulina 5 mg • Rosemary (rosmarinus officinalis, leaf) 5 mg • English Lavender (lavandula officinalis, flower) 5 mg. Inactive Ingredients: Dicalcium Phosphate, Microcrystalline Cellulose, Stearic Acid, Croscarmellose Sodium, Magnesium Stearate, Silicon Dioxide, Dextrin, Dextrose, Lecithin, Carboxymethylcellulose Sodium, Sodium Citrate.

IF-C - Nature's Sunshine
Four capsules contain: Proprietary Blend 1860 mg: Lonicera flower (lonicera japonica), Forsythia fruit (forsythia suspensa), Chrysanthemum flower (chrysanthemum morifolium), Gardenia fruit (gardenia jasminoides), Cnidium rhizome (ligusticum wallichii), Peony root without bark (paeonia officinalis and lactiflora), Platycodon root (platycodon grandiflorum), Schizonepeta flower (schizonepeta tenuifolia), Scute root (scutellaria baicalensis), Arctium seed (arctium lappa), Bupleurum root (bupleurum chinense), Dong Quai root (angelica sinensis), Phellodendron stem bark (phellodendron amurense), Siler root (siler divaricatum), Vitex fruit (vitex rotundifolia), Carthamus Tinctorius flower, Coptis rhizome (coptis chinensis), Licorice root (glycyrrhiza uralensis). Other Ingredients: Gelatin, Water.

IGF Fuel - TwinLab
Two capsules contain: DHEA (dehydroepiandrosterone) 50 mg • Zinc (from zinc picolinate) 50 mg • L-Glutamine 2000 mg.

IGF-1 Advantage Plus - Alternecare Health Products
Two sprays contain: Deer Velvet extract (cervidae parvum cornu) 11 mg • Stevia leaf extract 1.6 mg.

IgG 2000 DF capsules - Xymogen
Four capsules contain: IgG 2000 DF (serum-derived immunoglobulin concentrate) 2500 mg • Immunoglobulin G (IgG) 1000 mg • Other Immunoglobulins (IgA, IgM, IgE, IgD) 300 mg.

IgG 2000 DF powder - Xymogen
Each 1 tbsp serving contains: IgG 2000 DF (serum-derived immunoglobulin concentrate) 5000 mg • Immunoglobulin G (IgG) 2000 mg • Other Immunoglobulins (IgA, IgM, IgE, IgD) 600 mg.

IgG Boost - Pharmanex
Two capsules contain: Colostrum MFT (minimum 50% IgG content) 250 mg.

IgG Pure - Xymogen
Two scoops (20 g) contain: Calcium 60 mg • Phosphorus 60 mg • Magnesium 10 mg • Sodium 40 mg • Potassium 120 mg • Immunoglobulins 1.5 g.

Illumination - Amazon Herb
Ua de Gato • Jatoba • Pau d'Arco • Tayuya • Fucus • Suma • Star Anise • Pedra Hume Ca • Carqueja • Horsetail • Artichoke • Boldo • Bitter Orange • Alfalfa • Quebra Pedra • Jurubeba • Passion Flower • Mulungu • Espinhiera Santa • Cajueiro • Muira Puama • Catuaba • Yerba Mate • Cornsilk • Lemon Balm • Peppermint • Lemon Grass • Pata de Vaca • Sarsaparilla • Chamomile • Stevia • Chuchuhuasi • Sangre de Drago.
See Editor's Note No. 40.

Image Recovery Cream - Life Extension
Aloe, D.I. Water, Fruit Citric Acid, Glycolic Acid, Emulsifying Wax, Collagen, Protein, Squalene, Soybean oil, Calendula oil, Jojoba oil, Lemon extract, Keratin, Germaben 2.

IMM Formula - Pure Encapsulations
Each vegetable capsule contains: Astragalus Membranaceus 8:1 extract 200 mg • Echinacea Angustifolia extract (standardized to contain 4% echinacosides) 100 mg • Thymus extract (bovine) 200 mg • Ligustrum Lucidum 5:1 extract 200 mg.

Imm-Gest - Aidan Products, LLC
Each capsule contains: Zinc (zinc aspartate, 1.5 mg elemental zinc) 10 mg • Biodiastase 2000 Blend 45 mg: Cellulase, Amylase, Protease • Newlase Blend 30 mg: Protease, Lipase • Lactobacillus Sporagenes 5 mg • Transglucosidase 10 mg • Lipase AP-12 10 mg • Ginger root (zingiber officinale) 100 mg • L-Glutamine 240 mg • Lactobacillus Fermentum extract • Papaya fruit powder 40 mg. Other Ingredients: Vegetable Capsule.

Imm-Kine - Aidan Products, LLC
Each capsule contains: Lactobacillus Fermentum extract 250 mg • Beta 1,3 Glucans (from saccharomyces cerevisiae) 50 mg.

Some Brand Name Natural Products - What they Contain

www.NaturalDatabase.com contains MANY more listings than appear here.
Editor's Notes are located on pages 2155-2163.

Immortale for Men - Roex
Each tablet contains: Tribulus Terrestris 250 mg • Panax ginseng 50 mg • Damiana 50 mg • Avena sativa 100 mg • Sarsaparilla 50 mg.

Immortale for Women - Roex
Each tablet contains: Tribulus Terrestris 250 mg • Panax ginseng 50 mg • Damiana 50 mg • Avena sativa 100 mg • Dong Quai 50 mg.

ImmPower - American Biosciences
Two capsules contain: A.H.C.C. (active hexose correlated compound) Proprietary Blend 1 g: Mushroom Mycelia extract, Candelilla wax, Cyclodextrin, Microcrystalline Cellulose. Other Ingredients: VCap Plant-Derived Cellulose, Water, Silica, Glycerin.

IMMU-C - Nutri-Quest Rx
Each tablet contains: Vitamin C (Sago Palm) 500 mg • Rutin 15 mg • Lemon Bioflavonoids 15 mg • Hesperidin Complex 15 mg • Tissue concentrates (not extracts) of Bovine Source from Lymph, Thymus, Spleen • 5X Propolis 2 mg.
See Editor's Note No. 14.

Immugel - Young Living Essential Oils
Deionized Water • Methylcellulose • Hydrolized Vegetable Protein • German Chamomile Extract • Cinnamon Oil • Clove • Rosemary • Lemon • Thyme • Oregano.

Immuguard - Optimum Nutrition
Echinacea Angustifolia extract • Goldenseal root.

ImmuHerbs - Pure Encapsulations
Three vegetable capsules contain: Arabinogalactan extract (larix spp.) 500 mg • Elderberry (standardized to contain 28% anthocyanins) 500 mg • Olive leaf extract (olea europaea l, standardized to contain 17-23% oleuropein) 500 mg • Maitake mushroom 4:1 extract (grifola frondosa) 250 mg • Garlic 100:1 extract (odorless, providing scordinin 5.3 mg) 250 mg • Vitamin C (as ascorbyl palmitate) 30 mg.

ImmunACE - Nature's Plus
Two tablets contain: Vitamin A (as beta carotene) 20,000 IU • Vitamin C (as ascorbic acid) 1000 mg • Vitamin E (as D-alpha tocopheryl succinate) 400 IU • Folic Acid 200 mcg • Iron (as amino acid chelate) 18 mg • Zinc (as amino acid chelate) 30 mg • Selenium (as amino acid complex) 200 mcg • L-Cysteine (free form amino acid) 200 mg. Other Ingredients: Microcrystalline Cellulose, Di-Calcium Phosphate, Silica, Stearic Acid, Magnesium Stearate, Riboflavin, Chlorophyll, Echinacea Angustifolia Root and Rhizome, Pau d'Arco, Thyme Leaf, Juniper (juniperus communis fruit), Korean Ginseng Root, Irish Moss (chondrus crispus), Rosemary Leaf, Pharmaceutical Glaze.

Immunace (Immunance) - Vitabiotics
Two capsules contain: Vitamin A 800 mcg • Vitamin D 10 mcg • Vitamin E 110 mg • Vitamin C 300 mg • Vitamin B1 (thiamin) 14 mg • Vitamin B2 (riboflavin) 8 mg • Vitamin B6 20 mg • Folic Acid 500 mcg • Vitamin B12 14 mcg • Pantothenic Acid 20 mg • Vitamin K 95 mcg • Betacarotene 6 mg • Iron 6 mg • Magnesium 100 mg • Zinc 15 mg • Iodine 200 mcg • Copper 2 mg • Manganese 4 mg • Selenium 200 mcg • Chromium 100 mcg • Cystine 40 mg • Methionine 40 mg • Bioflavonoids 30 mg.
See Editor's Note No. 32.

ImmunActin Throat Spray - Nature's Plus
Purified Water • Exclusive Liposomal Herbal Complex:Olivir (Olea europa leaf extract) (supplying purified Calcium Elenolate), Kava Kava extract (Piper methysticum root) (standardized 4% Kavalactones), Echinacea extract (Echinacea angustifolia root & rhizome) (standardized 4% Echinacosides), Elderberry extract (Sambucus canadensis fruit) (standardized 30% Flavonoids), Ginger (Zingiber officinale root) (standardized 4% Volatile oils) • Wild Clover Honey • Oil of Peppermint.

ImmunActin Throat Syrup - Nature's Plus
Vegetable Glycerine • Exclusive Liposomal Herbal Complex: Elderberry extract (Sambucus canadensis fruit) (standardized 30% Falvonoids), Echinacea extract (Echinacea angustifolia root & rhizome) (standardized 4% Echinacosides), Slippery Elm (Ulmus rubra bark) (naturally rich in Phytosterols, Sesquitepenes & Mucilage), Goldenseal extract (Hydrastis canadensis root) (standardized 10% Alkaloids, 5% Hydrastine), White Willow extract (Salix alba bark) (standardized 7-9% Salicin), Astragalus extract (Astragalus membranaceus root) (standardized 0.4% 4'-Hydroxy-3'-Methoxyisoflavone 7-Sug), Schisandra extract (Schisandra chinensis fruit) (standardized 9% schisandrins), Zinc Gluconate • Wild Clover • Honey • Methol • Natural Cherry flavor.

ImmunActinB - Nature's Plus
Two capsules contain: Vitamin C corn free 300 mg • Vitamin E natural 100 IU • Echinacea [(Echinacea angustifolia root & rhizome) standardized 4% Echinacosides] 50 mg • Astragalus [(Astragalus membranaceus root) standardized 0.4% 4'-Hydroxy-3'-Methoxyisoflavone 7-Sug] 50 mg • Chinese Green Tea [(Camellia sinensis leaf) decaffeinated, standardized 20% Polyphelols] 50 mg • Tumeric [(Curcuma longa rhizome) standardized 95% Curcumin] 50 mg • Garlic odor-modified [(Allium sativum clove) standardized 0.35% Allicin, 0.65% Allicin, 0.40% Thiosulfinates, 0.085% Allyl Mercaptan] 50 mg • Schisandra [(Schisandra chinensis fruit) standardized 9% Schisandrins] 25 mg • Pau D'Arco [(Tabebuia impetiginosa bark) standardized 3% Naphthoquinones] 25 mg • Goldenseal [(Hydrastis canadensis root & rhizome) standardized 10% Alkaloids, 5% Hydrastine] 25 mg • Shiitake Mushroom [(Lentinus edodes mycelia) standardized 3.2% KS-2 Polysaccharides (peptidomannan)] 15 mg • Zinc (Monomethionine) 15 mg • Beta Carotene (supplying 10000 IU of Vitamin A activity) 6 mg • Grape seed [(Vitis vinifera) standardized 95% Proanthocyanidins] 5 mg • Bioperine brand Black Pepper extract (piper nigrum fruit, standardized to 95% 1-Piperoylpiperidine) 5 mg.

Immun'Age - PhytoPharmica
Each packet contains: Fermented Papaya 3 g.

ImmunAssure - Schiff
Two tablets contain: Vitamin C (as ascorbic acid) 60 mg • Immunoglobulin G 500 mg • Proprietary Blend 72.5 mg: Andrographis Paniculata leaf extract, Echinacea Purpurea extract. Other Ingredients: Cellulose, Croscarmellose Sodium, Hydroxypropyl Methylcellulose, Maltodextrin, Polyethylene Glycol, Magnesium Stearate, Silicon Dioxide.

Immune - Orenda International
Two capsules contain: Calcium d-Glucarate 300 mg • Lactobacillus fementum extract (muramyl peptides) 200 mg • Oat Straw extract (beta 1,3 glucan) 50 mg. Other Ingredients: Cellulose, Rice Bran, Magnesium Sillicate, Silicon Dioxide.

Immune 7-Keto - GNC
Each tabet contains: 7-Keto-DHEA 25 mg. Other Ingredients: Dicalcium Phosphate, Cellulose.

Immune Actives - VitaStore
Each tablet contains: Echinacea 500 mg • Goldenseal 250 mg • Beta Carotene (Vitamin A) 2500 IU • Zinc Gluconate 30 mg • Vitamin C 120 mg • Licorice 150 mg • Astragalus 145 mg • Grape Seed extract 50 mg • Green Tea 200 mg • Garlic 300 mg • L-Lysine 500 mg.

Immune Booster - Vidafit
Each serving contains: Biotin 30 mcg • Folate 400 mcg • Niacin 20 mg • Pantothenic Acid 10 mg • Riboflavin 1.7 mg • Thiamine 1.5 mg • Vitamin A 2600 IU • Vitamin B12 6 mcg • Vitamin B6 2 mg • Vitamin C 120 mg • Vitamin D 200 IU • Vitamin E 30 IU • Boron 1 mg • Calcium 500 mg • Chromium 120 mcg • Copper 2 mg • Iodine 150 mcg • Magnesium 400 mg • Phosphorus 500 mg • Potassium 100 mg • Selenium 70 mcg • Zinc 30 mg • Acidophilus 50 mg • Astragalus 300 mg • Echinacea Extract 75 mg • Garlic 10 mg • Siberian Ginseng 100 mg • Soy Protein 2 g.

Immune Booster Body Benefits Pak - Leiner Health Products
Each packet contains: Zinc Gluconate 50 mg • Vitamin C 740 mg • Echinacea extract (Echinacea augustifolia, Echinacea purpurea) root 200 mg • Garlic (Allium sativum) clove 200 mg • Propolis 100 mg.

BRAND NAMES

Other Ingredients: Ascorbic Acid, Dicalcium Phosphate, Starch, Hydroxypropyl Methylcellulose, Maltodextrin, Croscarmellose Sodium, Silicon Dioxide, Cellulose, Stearic Acid, Rose Hips, Sodium Starch Glycolate, Magnesium.

Immune Builder - JHS Natural Products
Each capsule contains: Coriolus Versicolor extract 75 mg • Reishi fruit body extract 75 mg • Maitake fruit body extract 75 mg • Shiitake (lentinula edodes) extract 75 mg • Cordyceps Sinensis Cs-4 Mycelial extract 75 mg.

Immune Building Complex - Shaklee
Two caplets contain: Mach-4 Proprietary Blend of Macrophage Activating Chinese Herbs 500 mg: Pumpkin seed extract (Cucurbita moschata), Safflower extract (Carthamus tinctorius) flower, Asian plantain extract (plantago asiatica) seed, Japanese Honeysuckle extract (Lonicera japonica) flower. Microcrystalline Cellulose, Dicalcium Phosphate, Silicon Dioxide, Croscarmellose Sodium, Hydroxypropyl Methylcellulose, Titanium Dioxide, Soy Lecithin, Caramel Color, Carnauba Wax.

Immune Formula - Pharmanex
Each capsule contains: Vitamin C (as calcium ascorbate) 200 mg • Echinacea root 6:1 extract (echinacea purpurea) 225 mg • Goldenseal root 4:1 extract (hydrastis canadensis) 125 mg • Arabinogalactan 100 mg • Beta-Sitosterol 30 mg. Other Ingredients: Gelatin, Microcrystalline Cellulose, Magnesium Stearate, Silicon Dioxide.

Immune Formula - Nature's Life
Three tablets contain: Antioxidant Vitamins: Beta Carotene [(Dunaliella salina) equivalent to 25000 IU Vitamin A] 15 mg • Other naturally occurring carotenoids in D. salina: Alpha Carotene (equivalent to 393 IU Vitamin A) 473 mcg • Cryptoxanthin (equivalent to 96 IU Vitamin A) 116 mcg • Zeaxanthin 95 mcg • Lutein 74 mcg • Vitamin C (Calcium Ascorbate) 1000 mg • Vitamin E (d-Alpha Tocopheryl Succinate) 200 IU. Other Nutrients: Vitamin A (Retinyl Palmitate) 8000 IU • Vitamin B6 (Pyridoxine HCl) 50 mg • Vitamin B12 (Cobalamin) 100 mcg • Folic Acid 400 mcg • Selenium (I-Selenomethionine) 100 mcg • Zinc (Citrate) 25 mg • Copper (Citrate) 2 mg • Medical Herbs: Echinacea purpurea root (Trout Lake Farm Certified Organically Grown) 500 mg • Korean Ginseng root extract [(Panax ginseng) standardized to 10% ginsenosides] 100 mg • Natural Base: Lemon Bioflavonoid Complex (50% active flavonols) 100 mg.

Immune Formula - 4 Life
Each capsule contains: Licorice (root) 54 mg • Echinacea Purpurea (aerial parts) 54 mg • Schizandra (fruit) 54 mg • Siberian Ginseng (root) 54 mg • Astragalus (root) 54 mg • Gotu Kola (aerial parts) 54 mg • Immune Proprietary Extract Blend 45 mg: Astragalus extract (root), Echinacea Purpurea extract (aerial parts), Schizandra extract (fruit), Korean Ginseng extract (root), Siberian Ginseng extract (root), Licorice extract (root), Gotu Kola extract (aerial parts) • Korean Ginseng (root) 31 mg.

Immune Health Formula - Metabolife International, Inc.
Each caplet contains: Forsythia Suspensa (forsythia) • Isatis Tinctoria (isatis) • Astragalus Membranaceus (astragalus) • Lonicera Dasystyla (honeysuckle) • Belamcanda Chinensis (blackberry lily) • Paeonia Veitchii (Chinese peony).

Immune Multi Nutrients - Vital Nutrients
Six capsules contain: Betatene brand Beta Carotene with Mixed Carotenoids 100,000 IU • Vitamin D (from lanolin) 200 IU • D-Alpha-Tocopheryl Succinate (natural vitamin E) 500 IU • Thiamine (vitamin B1) 150 mg • Riboflavin 5' Phosphate (activated vitamin B2) 150 mg • Niacinamide 100 mg • Inositol Hexaniacinate (niacin) 30 mg • Pyridoxal-5-Phosphate (activated vitamin B6) 50 mg • Folic Acid (pure powder) 1 mg • Methylcobalamin (pure vitamin B12) 1 mg • Biotin (pure powder) 9 mg • Pantothenic Acid (vitamin B5) 150 mg • Magnesium (citrate) 200 mg • Zinc (picolinate) 35 mg • Copper (glycinate) 1 mg • Selenium (selenomethionine) 500 mcg • Molybdenum (citrate) 200 mcg • N-Acetyl Cysteine 1000 mg • Coenzyme Q10 100 mg • Lipoic Acid (thioctic acid) 100 mg • Phytonadione (vitamin K1) 1 mg • Pancreatic Enzymes (full strength uncut) 100 mg • Phosphatidyl Choline 30% 150 mg.

Immune Protectors - TwinLab
Four hard gelatin capsules contain: Dry Vitamin A (from vitamin A acetate) 5000 IU • Dry Beta-Carotene (pro-vitamin A) 20,000 IU • Zinc (from zinc gluconate) 50 mg • Copper (from copper gluconate) 2 mg • Dry Vitamin E (D-alpha tocopheryl succinate) 400 IU • Selenium (from selenomethionine & selenite) 200 mcg • CoQ10 (coenzyme Q10) 5 mg • Vitamin B6 100 mg • Vitamin C 2000 mg • Citrus Bioflavonoids 100 mg • Quercetin (non-citrus bio-active bioflavonoid) 25 mg • L-Glutathione (reduced) 50 mg • Vitamin B12 250 mcg • Folic Acid 800 mcg • Pantothenic Acid 50 mg • Biotin 100 mcg • Vitamin B2 10 mg • Manganese (from manganese gluconate) 10 mg • Vitamin B3 (niacinamide) 10 mg. Base: Pau d'Arco, Onion, Garlic, Black Walnut, Echinacea, Golden Seal root.

Immune Rx - Alternecare Health Products
Two tablets contain: Bee Propolis 50 mg • Shiitake Mushroom 50 mg • Reishi Mushroom 50 mg • Garlic 25 mg • Suma 25 mg •Red Clover 25 mg • Pau d'Arco 25 mg • Milk Thistle 25 mg • Shark Cartilage 15 mg • Golden Seal 25 mg • Siberian Ginseng 25 mg • Echinacea 25 mg • Astragalus 25 mg • N-Acetyl Cysteine 15 mg • Zinc 15 mg • L-Glutathione 15 mg • CO Q10 5 mg.

Immune Stimulator - Nature's Sunshine
Each capsule contains: Beta Glucans (saccharomyces cerevisiae) 200 mg • Arabinogalactan (larix sp.) 100 mg • Proprietary Blend 110 mg: Colostrum, Cordyceps (cordyceps sinensis), Reishi mushroom (ganoderma lucidum), Maitake mushroom (grifola frondosa). Other Ingredients: Cellulose, Gelatin, Water.

Immune Support - Vital Nutrients
Each capsule contains: Astragalus 15:1 extract 200 mg • Echinacea extract 4% Phenolics 100 mg • White Atractylodes 15:1 extract 100 mg • Siler 12:1 extract 100 mg • Isatis root 14:1 extract 50 mg • Ginger root 5:1 extract 50 mg • Glycyrrhiza Glabra root extract (licorice) 50 mg.

Immune Support - Eidon Inc.
Each 1 tbsp serving contains: Zinc 3 mg • Selenium 0.11 mg • Sulfur 3 mg • Silica 31.5 mg. Other Ingredients: Purified Water.

Immune System - Nutrivention
Each tablet contains: Vitamin A 5000 IU • Pantothenic Acid 25 mg • Vitamin B6 25 mg • Vitamin C 20 mg • Vitamin B1 18 mg • Vitamin B2 18 mg • Vitamin E 15 IU • Inositol 15 mg • Choline 8 mg • Magnesium 5 mg • Zinc 5 mg • Folic Acid 400 mcg • Selenium 50 mcg • Echinacea 100 mg • Astragalus 100 mg • L-Cysteine 100 mg • Suma 100 mg • Codonopsis 75 mg • Rei-Shi Mushroom 75 mg • White Astractylodes 50 mg • Schizandra berries 50 mg • Privet berries 50 mg • Watercress 50 mg • Shiitake Mushroom 50 mg • Juniper berries 50 mg.

Immune System Booster Formula - Cambridge Nutraceuticals
Each serving contains: Glutamine 10 g • Vitamin A (as mixed carotenoids) 6500 IU • Vitamin C 200 mg • Vitamin E 125 IU • Selenium 70 mcg • N-Acetyl-Cysteine 600 mg.

Immune26 Wellness Bar (almond delight) - Legacy for Life
Rice syrup • Organic Egg White Protein • Organic Almond Butter • Egg powder with immune components • Organic crispy brown rice • Sliced Almonds • Raisins • Pure Vanilla • Sesame seeds • Spirulina • Almond extract • Kosher Sea Salt.

Immune26 Wellness Bar (peppermint brownie) - Legacy for Life
Rice syrup • Organic Egg White Protein • Organic Almond Butter • Egg powder with immune components • Chocolate Liquor • Organic crispy brown rice • Sliced Almonds • Raisins • Natural Flavoring • Pure Vanilla • Sesame seeds • Spirulina • Almond extract • Kosher Sea Salt.

Some Brand Name Natural Products - What they Contain

www.NaturalDatabase.com contains MANY more listings than appear here.
Editor's Notes are located on pages 2155-2163.

Immune-Action **-** Nature's Plus
Each capsule contains: Astragalus root 200 mg • Ligustrum berries 100 mg • Schisandra berries 100 mg • Shiitake Mushrooms 100 mg • Echinacea root 100 mg • Young Barley leaves 50 mg • Pau D'Arco bark 50 mg.

Immunectar **-** Nature's Plus
Each 2 tbsp serving contains: Vitamin A 40,000 IU • Vitamin C 1000 mg • Calcium 250 mg • Vitamin E 400 IU • Egg yolk Lecithin 2000 mg • Phosphatidyl Choline 250 mg • Colostrum 150 mg • Suma brand Pfaffia Paniculata (Martius) Kuntze root 150 mg • Chlorella 150 mg • Astragalus root (astragalus membranaceus) 75 mg • Ligustrum berry (ligustrum lucidum) 75 mg • Echinacea root powder (echinacea angustifolia) 75 mg • Schisandra berry (schisandra chinensis) 75 mg • Shiitake mushroom (lentinus edodes) 75 mg • Coenzyme Q10 15 mg. Other Ingredients: Nonfat Milk Protein, Fructose, Natural Vanilla Flavor, Natural Graham Flavor, Cinnamon, Natural Dried Honey.

Immun-Eeze **-** Allergy Limited
Each capsule and lozenge together contain: Vitamin C (as ascorbic acid) 250 mg • Thiamin (as thiamine mononitrate) 25 mg • Riboflavin 25 mg • Niacin (as niacinamide) 20 mg • Vitamin B6 (as pyridoxine HCl) 25 mg • Vitamin B12 (as cyanocobalamin) 3 mg • Manganese (as manganese citrate) 6 mg. Other Ingredients: Maltodextrin, Sucrose, Gelatin, Vegetable-derived Magnesium Stearate, Croscarmellose Sodium, Silicon Dioxide.

Immunene **-** PhysioLogics
Each capsule contains: Astragalus root (astragalus membranaceus, standardized to contain 0.5% flavonglycosides, 0.5 mg) 100 mg • Cat's Claw bark (uncaria tomentosa, standardized to contain 4% triterpenes, 2 mg) 50 mg • Reishi Mushroom extract aerial parts (ganoderma lucidum, standardized to contain 4% triterpenes, 2 mg) 50 mg • Shiitake Mushroom aerial parts (lentinula edodes) 50 mg • Maitake Mushroom aerial parts (grifola frondosa) 10 mg • Shiitake Mushroom extract (lentinula edodes, standardized to contain 1.5% PPPT 1/0.3% EP3). Other Ingredients: Rice Powder, Gelatin, Vegetable Magnesium Stearate, Silica.

ImmunePrep **-** HealthMinded
Two capsules contain: 1-3,1-6-Beta-Glucan (beta-1,3/1, 6-glucan, highly purified Norwegian beta glucan-NBG) 750 mg. Other Ingredients: Gelatin, Stearic Acid, Magnesium Stearate.

ImmuneTune **-** Young Living Essential Oils
Each capsule contains: Tumeric Extract • Magnesium Citrate • Yucca Root • Potassium Citrate • Echinacea Root • Calcium Citrate • Wild Yam • Pantothenic Acid • Grape Seed Extract • Selenium • Chromium • Alpha Lipoic Acid • Ginger Extract • Orange Oil • Pine Oil • Ravensara Oil • Lemon Oil • Fir Oil • Cistus Oil • Gelatin.

Immunitril **-** Optimal Therapeutics
Each capsule contains: Vitamin C (as calcium ascorbate) 250 mg • Calcium 30 mg • Vitamin E (as dL-alpha tocopheryl) 30 IU • Zinc (as oxide) 20 mg • Selenium 200 mcg • Arabinogalactan 1300 mg • Echinacea Purpurea leaf 350 mg • Elderberry fruit powder 180 mg • Astragalus 150 mg • Golden Seal 125 mg • Maitake mushroom 4:1 extract 50 mg. Other Ingredients: Gelatin, Cellulose, Magnesium Stearate.

Immuno Chews **-** Global Health Trax
Three tablets contain: Vitamin A 294 IU • Vitamin C 3 mg • Calcium 66 mg • Iron 1 mg • Bovine Colostrum 1350 mg. Other Ingredients: Fructose, Pineapple Flavoring, Magnesium.

Immuno Complex **-** Quality of Life Labs
Two capsules contain: Astragalus 850 mg • Echinacea 450 mg • Vitamin C 120 mg • A.H.C.C. Mushroom Mycelia extract Proprietary Blend 50 mg. Other Ingredients: Gelatin, Silicon Dioxide, Magnesium Stearate.

Immuno Support Complex **-** Nutrition Dynamics, Inc.
Each capsule contains: Vitamin C 200 mg • Pantothenic Acid 10 mg • Vitamin A 10,000 IU • Vitamin B12 10 mcg • Calcium Chelate 60 mg • Zinc Chelate • RNA 60 mg • Thymus 50 mg · Lemon Bioflavonoids 40 mg • Lymph 25 mg • Spleen 25 mg • Bromelain 20 mg. Other Ingredients: Bee Pollen, Dehydrated Pineapple.
See Editor's Note No. 14.

ImmunoBlend **-** Rexall - Sundown
Each capsule contains: Turmeric Rhizome extract (standardized to 95% curcuminoids, 95 mg) 100 mg • Echinacea Purpurea extract (standardized to 4% phenolic compounds, 4 mg) 100 mg • Immuno Proprietary Blend: Garlic bulb, Astragalus root, Reishi Mushroom, Cat's Claw Bark 175 mg. Other Ingredients: Gelatin.

Immunoboost **-** Shawnee Moon
Peony root • Gotu Kola • Chrysanthemum • Astragalus • Licorice • Kelp • Suma • Pau d'arco • Red Clover.

Immunocal **-** Immunotec Research, Ltd.
100% Milk Whey Protein.

Immunocil **-** Laub Biochem Co.
Each tablet contains: Humic / Fulvic extract 250 mg. Other Ingredients: Microcrystalline, Cellulose, Colloidal Silicone Dioxide, Gelatin, Magnesium Stearate.

ImmunoFin **-** LaneLabs
G-E Lipids 50 mg • Shark Liver Oil 250 mg.

Immunogarl-1 **-** Olympian Labs
Three capsules contain: Garlic extract 600 mg • Ginkgo Biloba leaf extract 120 mg •Proprietary Blend 600 mg: Amylase, Protease, Lipase • Ascorbic Acid 240 mg •L-Glutamine 450 mg •Maitake Mushroom 30 mg.

ImmunoGuard **-** Advocare International
Four capsules contain: Vitamin C (as ascorbic acid) 240 mg • Maitake extract (d-fraction - grifola frondosa) 100 mg • Reishi extract (fruit - ganoderma lucidum) 150 mg • Shiitake extract (mycelium - lentinus edodes) 200 mg • Broccoli extract (stem/flower/leaf - brassica oleracea) 300 mg • Green Tea extract (leaf - camellia sinensis) 150 mg • Curcumin extract (root - curcuma longa) 100 mg • Astragalus extract (root - astragalus membranaceus) 50 mg • Mixed Citrus Flavonoids 200 mg. Other Ingredients: Silicon Dioxide, Magnesium Stearate, Gelatin.

ImmunoKinoko **-** Quality of Life Labs
Two capsules contain: Proprietary Blend 1000 mg: Mushroom Mycelia extract, Candelilla Wax, Cyclodextrin, Microcrystalline Cellulose. Other Ingredients: Silica, Gelatin, Glycerin.

ImmunoMax Allergy **-** NorthStar Nutritionals
Two capsules contain: Methylsulfonylmethane (MSM) 250 mg • Acerola berry extract 50 mg • Apple skin extract 50 mg • Rhododendron Caucasicum 50 mg • Magnesium 100 mg • Pantothenic Acid 50 mg.

ImmunoShield **-** PhytoPharmica
Each tablet contains: Vitamin A (as acetate) 10,000 IU • Vitamin C (ascorbic acid) 200 mg • Vitamin D (as cholecalciferol) 35 IU • Vitamin B12 (as cyanocobalamin) 50 mcg • Pantothenic Acid (as calcium D-pantothenate) 25 mg • Calcium (as calcium lactate) 41 mg • Magnesium (as magnesium citrate) 6.7 mg • Zinc (as zinc gluconate) 10.5 mg • European Elder berry 4:1 extract (sambucus nigra) 100 mg • Alfalfa (medicago sativa) aerial part extract 10:1 50 mg • Astragalus root(astragalus membranaceus, extract standardized to conatin a minimum of 0.5% 4'-hydroxy-3'-methoxyisoflavone-7-glucoside) 50 mg • Mixed Citrus Bioflavonoids 50% (from citrus fruits) 30 mg • Proprietary Trace Mineral Blend 24 mg: Selenium (as selenium yeast), Silicon (as magnesium trisilicate), Boron (as sodium borate), Nickel (as nickel chelate), Tin (as tin chelate), Molybdenum (as sodium molybdate), Vanadium (as vanadyl sulfate). Other Ingredients: Cellulose, Modified Cellulose, Magnesium Stearate, Carnauba Wax, Lecithin.

Immuno-SP - Benepure, Inc
Each tablet contains: Dimethylglycine HCl 300 mg • Maitake PD-Fraction extract (grifola frondosa, yielding D-fraction 5 mg) 17 mg • Larix Occidentalis extract (larch tree, yielding arabinogalactan polysaccharides 222.5 mg) 227 mg • Beta 1,3 Glucans (from baker's yeast cell walls) 100 mg. Other Ingredients: Microcrystalline Cellulose, Stearic Acid, Vegetable Stearate, Croscarmellose Sodium, Silicon Dioxide, Hydroxypropyl Methylcellulose.

ImmunoSTART - Mannatech
Each tablet contains: Colostrum (bovine) 150 mg • Beta-1,3 / 1,6 Glucans 2 20 mg • Lactoferrin 10 mg • Citrus Pectin 5 mg. Other Ingredients: Glucose, Stearic Acid, Natural Flavors, Citric Acid, Magnesium Stearate, Silicon Dioxide.

Immunosure Extra Strength Day-Time Drink Mix - Schiff
Each packet contains: Immunoglobulins (derived from cow's blood) 1000 mg • Vitamin C 60 mg • Echinacea 132 mg • Andrographis 1 mg.
This product was formerly known as ImmunoLin.

Immunosure Extra Strength Night-Time Drink Mix - Schiff
Each packet contains: Immunoglobulins (derived from cow's blood) 1000 mg • Vitamin C 60 mg • Echinacea 132 mg • Andrographis 1 mg • Melatonin 1 mg.
This product was formerly known as ImmunoLin. See Editor's Note No. 26.

Immunosure Tablets - Schiff
Each two tablets contains: Immunoglobulins (derived from cow's blood) 500 mg • Vitamin C 60 mg • Echinacea 132 mg • Andrographis 1 mg.
This product was formerly known as ImmunoLin.

ImmunPlex - Pro Health
Each scoop (approx. 10.2 g) contains: Provon Undenatured Whey Protein Isolate (typical protein composition: beta-lactoglobulin 51%, gamma-lactalbumin 23%, glycomacropeptides 18%, bovine serum albumin and immunoglobulins 5%, lactoferrin, lactoperoxidase and others 2%) • Natural Vanilla flavor.

Immuplex - Standard Process, Inc.
Two capsules contain: Proprietary Blend 565 mg: Bovine Liver (PMG) extract, Veal Bone extract, Nutritional Yeast, Bovine Spleen (PMG) extract, Bovine Thymus (PMG) extract, Bovine Thymus (Cytosol) extract, Bovine Liver, Bovine Spleen, Ovine Spleen, Calcium Lactate. Other Ingredients: Gelatin, Zinc Liver Chelate, Ascorbic Acid, Iron Liver Chelate, Water, Chromium Yeast, Copper Liver Chleate, Selenium Yeast, Mixed Tocopherols, Natural Colors, Pyridoxine Hydrochloride, Calcium Stearate, Vitamin A Palmitate, Folic Acid, Cyanocobalamin.
See Editor's Note No. 14.

IMMU-Power - Nutri-Quest Rx
Each tablet contains: Tissue concentrate (not an extract) from Thymus 60 mg • Vitamin A (palmitate) 300 IU • Vitamin B6 15 mg • Niacin 10 mg • Pantothenic Acid 55.5 mg • Vitamin B12 200 mcg • Folic Acid 150 mcg • Vitamin C (sago palm) 150 mg • Natural Vitamin E (succinate) 70 IU • Suma 7 mg • ISB Complex 107 mg: Magnesium, Selenium, SOD Type G, Zinc, Echinacea purpurea, Goldenseal, L-Cysteine HCl, L-Ornithine, Ferric Phosphate, Garlic • L- Aspartic Acid • Natural Flavor.
See Editor's Note No. 14.

Immutol - Immunocorp
Each capsule contains: Beta Glucan 375 mg.

I-MNS - Dial Herbs
Black Cohosh • Blue Cohosh • Red Raspberry • Catnip • Wild Yam • Wild Carrot • Motherwort • Pennyroyal • St. John's Wort.

Imperial Garlic 6500 - Puritan's Pride
Each tablet contains: Garlic bulb powder (allium sativum) 650 mg standardized to contain a minimum: Allicin yeild 6500 mcg, total thiosulfinates yield 6500 mcg, Alliin yield 14,500 mcg, Gamma-Glutamylcysteines 5200 mcg. Other Ingredients: Dicalcium Phosphate, Cellulose (plant origin), Food Glaze, Calcium Carbonate, Croscarmellose, Vegetable Stearic Acid, Hydroxypropyl Methylcellulose, Titanium Dioxide Color, Magnesium Silicate, Anise Oil (pimpinella anisum, seed).

Imperial Green Tea - Jamieson
Each tea bag contains: Chinese Green Tea leaf (Camellia sinensis) • Ginger root (Singiber officinale) • Leechee fruit (Litchi chinensis).

Imucell WGP - Biothera
Each capsule contains: Beta Glucan (naturally derived from Saccromyces cerevisae) 250 mg. Other Ingredients: Microcrystalline Cellulose, Gelatin, Water.

ImuDrops - FreeLife International
Each 1 mL serving contains: Herbal Formula 500 mg: Elderberry, Echinacea Purpurea root, Fresh Osha root, Goldenseal root, Propolis, Lomatium root, Ginger root, American Feverfew root, Yin Chiao Formula: Isatis root, Pubescent Holly root, Chrysanthemum flower, Forsythia fruit, Honeysuckle flower, Lophatherum herb, Kudzu root, Schizonepeta herb. Other Ingredients: Deionized Water, Vegetable Glycerin, Grain Alcohol (20% by volume), Honey, Natural Flavors.

Imumax - FreeLife International
Each tablet contains: Patented EV.EXT 10 standardized American Feverfew (Parthenium integrifolium) root 75 mg • standardized Echinacea (Echinacea purpurea) root 25 mg. Other Ingredients: Calcium Hydrogen Phosphate, Microcrystalline Cellulose, Silica Dioxide, Hydrous Magnesium Silicate, Magnesium Stearate, Zein, Alginates.

Imun-Comp - Aspen Group, Inc.
Two tablets contain: Vitamin C (ascorbic acid) 250 mg • Vitamin B1 (thiamin HCl) 30 mg • Vitamin E (D-alpha tocopherol) 200 IU • Beta Carotene 5000 IU • Copper (gluconate) 300 mcg • Selenium Chelate 25 mcg • Zinc (gluconate) 15 mg • Bone Marrow 65 mg • Lymph 65 mg • Papain 50 mg • Pituitary Whole 15 mg • Spleen 130 mg • Thymus 550 mg • Bromelain 50 mg • Echinacea extract 300 mg • L-Lysine HCl 250 mg • Trypsin 1:75 25 mg • Blue Flag 130 mg • Fennel 70 mg • Goldenseal herb 70 mg.
See Editor's Note No. 31.

Indigestion - Hyland's
Two tablets contain: Cinchona Officinalis 3X HPUS • Hydrastis Canasensis 3X HPUS • Phosphoricum Acidum 3X HPUS • Kali Bichrominum 3X HPUS. Base: Lactose USP.
See Editor's Note No. 1.

Indigestion Remedy - PhytoPharmica
Twenty drops contain: Podophyllum peltatum 4x • Carduus marianus 3x • Dolichos pruriens 3x • Leptandra virginica 3x • Lycopodium clavatum 3x • Nux vomica 3x • Boldo 1x • Chelidonium majus 1x. In a base of 50% USP alcohol by volume.
See Editor's Note No. 1.

Indium XL - East Park Research, Inc.
Indium Sulfate Anhydrous (.9999% pure) • Distilled Water.

Indium-Energy - East Park Research, Inc.
Each tablet contains: Indium Sulfate (.9999% pure) 24 mg • Trace Minerals: Zinc Oxide, Copper Oxide, Selenium, Chromium, Manganese, Potassium Iodide, Dicalcium Phosphate. Other Ingredients: Microcrystalline Cellulose, Stearic Acid, Silicon Dioxide, Magnesium Stearate.

Indole Pro - MMS Pro
Each three capsules contain: Vitamin A 100 IU • Vitamin E (as d-alpha tocopheryl succinate) 13 IU • Potassium 10 mg • Proprietary Blend (BioResponse-DIM containing 25% diindolylmethane) 150 mg: Starch, Diindolylmethane, Natural Vitamin E, Phosphatidylcholine, Silica • Proprietary Blend (Protectamins) 150 mg: Spinach powder, Cabbage powder, concentrated Broccoli powder. Inactive Ingredients: Cellulose, Gelatin, Chlorophyll.

Indole-3-Carbinol 200 mg - Pure Encapsulations
Each vegetable capsule contains: Indole-3-Carbinol 200 mg.

Indole-3-Carbinol 400 mg - Pure Encapsulations
Each vegetable capsule contains: Indole-3-Carbinol 400 mg.

Indolplex - PhytoPharmica
Each tablet contains: Diindolylmethane (DIM) 30 mg.
See Editor's Note No. 21.

Indolplex - Tyler Encapsulations
Four capsules contain: Vitamin E 22 IU • Indolplex Proprietary Blend 240 mg: Food Grade Starch, Diindolylmethane, Tocophersolan, Phosphatidylcholine, Silica. Other Ingredients: Microcrystalline Cellulose, Ascorbyl Palmitate, Gelatin, Water.

Indolplex with DIM - Enzymatic Therapy/PhytoPharmica
Each tablet contains: Proprietary Blend 120 mg: Modified Food Starch, 25% Diindolylmethane (DIM), D-Alpha-Tocopheryl Succinate, Silicon Dioxide, Phosphatidylcholine. Other Ingredients: Calcium Carbonate, Modified Cellulose Gum, Modified Cellulose, Titanium Dioxide Color, Lecithin, Carnauba Wax.

InflamActin - Nature's Plus
Two capsules contain: Boswellin (Boswellia serrata gum resin) (standardized 65% Boswellic Acids) 250 mg • Bromelain (standardized 90 GDU) 150 mg • DLPA (dl-Phenylalanine) (Free Form Amino Acid) 100 mg • Turmeric (Curcuma longa rhizome) standardized 95% Curcumin 75 mg • Vitamin C (corn free) 60 mg • St. John's Wort (Hypericum perforatum flower) (standardized 0.3-0.5% Hypericin) 50 mg • Chamomile (Matricaria recutita flower) (standardized 1% Apigenin, 0.5% Essential oil) 50 mg • Feverfew (Tanacetum parthenium leaf) (standardized 0.7% Parthenolide) 50 mg • Goldenseal (Hydrastis canadensis root & rhizome) (standardized 10% Alkaloids, 5% Hydrastine) 25 mg • Ginger (Zingiber officinale root) standardized 4% Volatile oils 25 mg.

InflamActin Cream - Nature's Plus
Active ingredient: Methyl Salicylate 18%. Other Ingredients: Exclusive Liposomal Herbal Complex: Boswellin (Boswellia serrata gum resin extract) (standardized 65% Boswellic Acids), Tumeric rhizome extract (Curcuma longa) (standardized 95% Curcumin), Gorgonian extract (Pseudopterogoria elisbethae leaf) (standardized 4% Pseudopterosin), Natural Vitamin E. In a vanishing Liposomal Cream Base.

Inflama-Rest - Source Naturals
Three tablets contain: Magnesium (as magnesium chelate) 300 mg • Zinc (as zinc monomethionine, OptiZinc brand) 10 mg • Selenium (as L-selenomethionine, SelenoPure brand, and sodium selenite) 100 mcg • Manganese (as manganese succinate) 5 mg • Turmeric extract (95% curcumin) 525 mg • Ginger root 500 mg • Ginger root 4:1 extract (5% gingerols) 375 mg • Ashwagandha 5:1 extract 300 mg • Quercetin 200 mg • Milk Thistle seed extract (80% silymarin) 160 mg • Chinese Skullcap root extract (30% flavones) 150 mg • S.O.D. (superoxide dismutase, GliSODin brand) 120 mg • Oregon Grape root 120 mg • Bromelain (2000 GDU per gram) 100 mg • Chinese Skullcap root extract (80% baicalin) 80 mg • Green Tea extract (95% polyphenols) 80 mg • Feverfew 4:1 extract 80 mg • Stinging Nettles 16:1 extrat 60 mg • White Willow bark extract (15% salicin) 60 mg • Boswellia extract (20% boswellic acids) 60 mg • Rosemary extract (20% diterpenes) 50 mg • Tocotrienols extract 15 mg • Resveratrol (polygonum cuspidatum extract) 10 mg • Bioperine brand Black Pepper extract 10 mg. Other Ingredients: Modified Cellulose Gum, Stearic Acid, Acacia Gum, Collodial Silicon Dioxide.

Inflamase - Progressive Labs
Each capsule contains: Enteric release phase: Pancreatin 100 mg • Lipase 10 mg • Amylase 10 mg • Trypsin 200 mg • Alpha Chymotrypsin 2 mg. Gastric release phase: Bromelain 100 mg • Catalase 25 mcg • Superoxide Dismutase 25 mcg.
See Editor's Note No. 14.

Inflamma-bLOX - Ortho Molecular Products
Six capsules contain: Skullcap root extract (scutellaria baicalensis, standardized to contain 30% isoflavones) 1400 mg • Bee Propolis extract 2X 950 mg • Turmeric root extract (standardized to contain 95% curcumin) 850 mg • Graminex C60 brand Pollen extract 700 mg. Other Ingredients: Natural Vegetable Capsules, Ascorbyl Palmitate, Magnesium Stearate, Microcrystalline Cellulose, Silicon Dioxide.

Inflammation Formula - HERBALmax
Huangqin radixs • Longdancao • Chuanxilian • Lianqiao fruits • Jinyin flowers.

Inflammex - American Biologics
Each drop contains: Apis Met. 4X • Belladonna 4X • Mercur. Corr 5X • Baryta Mur 6X • Lachesis 12X • Calc. Iod 4X • Hepar Mur 6X • Kali Bichrom 4X • Marum Verum 6X • Phytolacca 4X • Magnesium (as citrate) 100 mg. Other Ingredients: 20% Alcohol, Distilled Water.
See Editor's Note No. 1.

Inflamzyme - PhytoPharmica
Each tablet contains: Vitamin C (ascorbic acid) 100 mg • Magnesium (carbonate) 25 mg •Bromelain (1800 MCU/g) 125 mg • Quercetin 125 mg • Mixed Citrus Bioflavonoids complex (50% concentrate) 100 mg • L-Cysteine (HCl) 75 mg.

Infla-Profen - Gaia Herbs
Two capsules contain: Devil's Claw root (harpagophytum procumbens) 300 mg • Feverfew tops (chrysantehmum parthenium; 0.5% (2.25 mg) parthenolide) 300 mg • Turmeric rhizome (curcuma longa) 100 mg • Yucca root (yucca spp.) 46 mg • Burdock root and seed (arctium lappa) 32 mg • Celery seed (apium graveolens) 16 mg • Jamaican Dogwood bark (piscidia erythrina) 12 mg • Nettle leaf (urtica dioica) 8 mg • Ginger rhizome, supercritical CO2 extract (zingiber off.) 8 mg. Other Ingredients: Vegetable Glycerin, Lecithin, Vegetable Cellulose (capsule).

Inflavonoid - Metagenics
Each tablet contains: Lemon Bioflavonoid complex (standardized to 50% full spectrum bioflavonoids) 250 mg • Vitamin C (as ascorbic acid) 100 mg • Turmeric rhizome (curcuma longa) 450 mg • Ginger rhizome (zingiber officinale) 150 mg.

Inflavonoid Intensive Care - Metagenics
Two tablets contain: Lemon Bioflavonoid complex (standardized to 50% (100 mg) full spectrum bioflavonoids) 200 mg • Quercetin 100 mg • Vitamin C (as ascorbic acid) 200 mg • Boswellia gum extract (boswellia serrata, standardized to 70% (280 mg) boswellic acids) 400 mg • Turmeric rhizome extract (curcuma longa, standardized to 95% (285 mg) curcuminoids) 300 mg • Ginger rhizome extract (zingiber officinale, standardized to 5% (10 mg) gingerols) 200 mg • Cayenne Pepper fruit (capsicum annuum) 50 mg.

Influenzinum 30C - Washington Homeopathics
Flu Vaccine, 2005 strain 30C.
See Editor's Note No. 1.

Influenzinum 30X - Washington Homeopathics
Flu Vaccine, 2005 strain 30X.
See Editor's Note No. 1.

Inholtra - Omni Nutraceuticals
Two Quicksorb gels contain: Vitamin C (as ascorbyl palmitate) 1 mg • Vitamin E (as D-alpha tocopherol) 7 IU • Manganese (as manganese aspartate) 0.60 mg • Omega-3 fatty acid (eicosapentainoic acid 400 mg and docosahexaenoic acid 300 mg) 465 mg • D-Glucosamine Sulfate 335 mg • N-Acetyl D-Glucosamine 335 mg • Omega-6 fatty acid (as gamma-linolenic acid) 135 mg. Other Ingredients: Vegetable Oil, Fish Oil, Gelatin, Glycerin, Carob, Water.

BRAND NAMES

Inholtra Natural Pain Relief Formula - Omni Nutraceuticals
Three quicksorb gels contain: Glucosamine Sulfate 500 mg • N-Acetyl D-Glucosamine 500 mg • Chondroitin Sulfate (as Chondroitin Sulfates A & B) 200 mg • EPA 400 mg • DHA 300 mg • GLA 300 mg • Vitamin E 10 IU • Ascorbyl Palmitate 5 mg • Manganese 1 mg.
See Editor's Note No. 15.

Inner Sun - 4 Life
Each capsule contains: Thiamin (as thiamine mononitrate) 0.95 mg • Riboflavin (vitamin B2) 1.1 mg • Niacin (as niacinamide) 12.6 mg • Vitamin B6 (as pyridoxine hydrochloride) 1.3 mg • Folic Acid 29 mcg • Vitamin B12 (as cyanocobalamin) 4.3 mcg • Biotin 21.6 mcg • Pantothenic Acid (as calcium pantothenate) 7.2 mg • St. John's Wort aerial parts (0.3% hypericin) 300 mg • English chamomile flower 20 mg • English Hawthorn berry 20 mg • Choline (as choline bitartrate) 18.8 mg • Hops flower 10 mg • Rosemary leaf 10 mg • Inositol 9.45 mg • Para-Aminobenzoic Acid (PABA) 0.95 mg. Other Ingredients: Gelatin, Rice Bran, Magnesium Stearate.

Innerclean Herbal Laxative Inner Tabs - At Last Naturals, Inc.
Two tablets contain: Senna 640 mg. Other Ingredients: Buckthorn, Psyllium Husk, Anise Seed, Fennel Seed, Psyllium Seed.

Innerclean Herbal Laxative Powder - At Last Naturals, Inc.
Each 1/2 tsp serving contains: Senna 610 mg. Other Ingredients: Buckthorn, Psyllium Husk, Anise Seed, Fennel Seed, Psyllium Seed.

InnerPower (assorted flavors) - Life Enhancement Products, Inc.
Each 1 tbsp serving contains: Vitamin A (as beta-carotene) 802 mcg • Vitamin C (ascorbic acid) 500 mg • Vitamin E (as dL-alpha-tocopheryl acetate) 120 IU • Pantothenic Acid (vitamin B5 as calcium pantothenate) 500 mg • Calcium (as calcium pantothenate and calcium borate) 47 mg • Zinc (as zinc gluconate) 3 mg • Copper (as copper gluconate) 400 mcg • Chromium (as chromium aspartate) 25 mcg • L-Arginine 6 g • Choline (as choline dihydrogen citrate) 667 mg • Taurine 200 mg • Glycine 150 mg • Boron (as calcium borate) 2 mg. Other Ingredients: Malic Acid, Natural Flavors, Citric Acid, Silicon Dioxide, Fumaric Acid, Acesulfame K. Citrus and Tropical flavors also contain: Stevia. Cherry flavor also contains: Xylitol.

InoCell brand - Unknown
Inositol • Cal-Mag IP6.
See Editor's Note No. 44.

Inositol - Puritan's Pride
Each tablet contains: Inositol 650 mg.

Inositol - Nature's Bounty
Each tablet contains: Inositol 650 mg. Other Ingredients: Cellulose, Vegetable Stearic Acid, Food Glaze, Talc, Magnesium Silicate, Vegetable Magnesium Stearate.

Inositol - Source Naturals
Each 1/4 teaspoon contains: Inositol powder 600 mg.

Inositol - Standard Process, Inc.
Each tablet contains: Inositol 405 mg. Other Ingredients: Honey, Calcium Stearate.

Inositol - J. R. Carlson Laboratories, Inc.
Each tablet contains: Inositol 500 mg.

Inositol 650 mg - Solgar
Each tablet contains: Calcium (as dicalcium phosphate) 65 mg • Inositol 650 mg. Other Ingredients: Dicalcium Phosphate, Microcrystalline Cellulose, Vegetable Cellulose, Vegetable Stearic Acid, Titanium Dioxide, Silica, Vegetable Glycerin, Carnauba Wax.

Inositol 650 mg - Vitamin World
Each tablet contains: Inositol 650 mg. Other Ingredients: Cellulose (plant orign), Vegetable Stearic Acid, Food Glaze, Magnesium Silicate, Vegetable Magnesium Stearate.

Inositol capsules - Jarrow Formulas
Each capsule contains: Inositol 750 mg. Other Ingredients: Cellulose, Magnesium Stearate, Gelatin.

Inositol crystalline powder - Jarrow Formulas
Each 1/4 tsp serving contains: Inositol 600 mg.

Inositol Hexaniacinate - Ortho Molecular Products
Each capsule contains: Inositol Hexaniacinate 650 mg. Other Ingredients: Natural Vegetable Capsules, Ascorbyl Palmitate, Microcrystalline Cellulose, Silicon Dioxide.

Inositol HexaNicotinate - Life Enhancement Products, Inc.
Each capsule contains: Niacin (from inositol hexanicotinate) 195 mg. Other Ingredients: Gelatin Capsule, Silicon Dioxide.

Inositol Hexaphosphate - Olympian Labs
Two capsules contain: Inositol Hexaphosphate 1000 mg • Kelp 100 mg • Wheat Grass 60 mg.

Inositol Powder - Vital Nutrients
Each 1 slightly rounded tsp serving contains: 100% Pure Inositol powder 4000 mg.

Inositol Powder - Puritan's Pride
Each 1/4 teaspoon contains: Inositol powder 600 mg.

Inositol Powder - Optimum Nutrition
Each 1/4 level tsp (600 mg) serving contains: Inositol 600 mg.

Inositol Powder - GNC
Each 1/4 teaspoon contains: Inositol 600 mg.

Inositol Powder - Vitamin World
Each 1/4 tsp (1g) serving contains: Inositol 1000 mg.

Inositol Powder - Standard Process, Inc.
Each 1/4 tsp serving contains: Inositol 700 mg.

InosoPhate 6 (IP6-Inositol Complex) - EcoNugenics
Each capsule contains: Inositol 280 mg • Inositol Hexaphosphate 230 mg. Other Ingredients: Gelatin, Magnesium Stearate, Silica.

Inspired By Nature Chelated Potassium 99 mg - Puritan's Pride
Each caplet contains: Potassium (as potassium gluconate) 99 mg. Other Ingredients: Crospovidone, Vegetable Stearic Acid, Silica, Vegetable Magnesium Stearate, Cellulose Coating.

Inspired By Nature Chelated Zinc Lozenges 23 mg - Puritan's Pride
Each lozenge contains: Zinc (as zinc citrate and zinc gluconate) 23 mg. Other Ingredients: Fructose, Sorbitol, Honey Powder, Vegetable Stearic Acid, Citric Acid, Silica, Vegetable Magnesium Stearate, Natural Lemon Flavor, Orange Flavor.

Inspired By Nature DHEA 25 mg - Puritan's Pride
Each tablet contains: DHEA (dehydroepiandrosterone) 25 mg. Other Ingredients: Cellulose (plant origin), Dicalcium Phosphate, Croscarmellose, Vegetable Stearic Acid, Vegetable Magnesium Stearate, Silica.

Inspired By Nature DHEA 5 mg - Puritan's Pride
Each tablet contains: DHEA (dehydroepiandrosterone) 5 mg. Other Ingredients: Dicalcium Phosphate, Cellulose (plant origin), Silica, Vegetable Magnesium Stearate.

Inspired By Nature Magnesium 250 mg - Puritan's Pride
Each tablet contains: Magnesium (as magnesium oxide) 250 mg. Other Ingredients: Cellulose (plant origin), Vegetable Stearic Acid, Vegetable Magnesium Stearate, Silica.

Some Brand Name Natural Products - What they Contain

www.NaturalDatabase.com contains MANY more listings than appear here.
Editor's Notes are located on pages 2155-2163.

Inspired By Nature Milk Free Probiotic Acidophilus **-** Puritan's Pride
Each capsule contains: Lactobacillus blend 40 mg: Lactobacillus Acidophilus, Lactobacillus Rhamnosus, Lactobacillus Bifidus. Other Ingredients: Dicalcium Phosphate, Cellulose (plant origin), Hydroxypropyl Methylcellulose, Vegetable Stearic Acid, Silica, Vegetable Magnesium Stearate.

Inspired By Nature Probiotic Acidophilus with Pectin **-** Puritan's Pride
Two capsules contain: Proprietary Blend of Cultures 180 mg: Lactobacillus Acidophilus, L. Brevis, L. Salivarius, L. Helveticus, L. Bulgaricus, Bifidobacterium Bifidum • Citrus Pectin 200 mg. Other Ingredients: Dicalcium Phosphate, Gelatin, Cellulose (plant origin), Silica, Vegetable Magnesium Stearate.

Inspired By Nature Salmon Oil 500 mg **-** Puritan's Pride
Two softgels contain: Salmon Oil 1000 mg • Eicosapentaenoic Acid (EPA) 80 mg • Docosahexaenoic Acid (DHA) 120 mg. Other Ingredients: Gelatin, Glycerin.

Inspired By Nature Sam-e 200 mg **-** Puritan's Pride
Two tablets contain: S-Adenosylmethionine 400 mg. Other Ingredients: Cellulose (plant origin), Croscarmellose, Polymethacrylate, Silica, Vegetable Magnesium Stearate, Triethyl Citrate, Vegetable Stearic Acid, Citric Acid, Ascorbic Acid, Riboflavin.

Inspired By Nature Vitamin C-1000 mg Tablets with Rose Hips **-** Puritan's Pride
Each tablet contains: Vitamin C with Rose Hips 1000 mg.

Inspired By Nature Vitamin C-500 mg Softgels with Rose Hips **-** Puritan's Pride
Each softgel contains: Vitamin C with Rose Hips 500 mg. Other Ingredients: Soybean Oil, Gelatin, Lecithin, Beeswax, St. John's Bread extract, Caramel Color.

Instant Brewer's Yeast **-** GNC
Two tablespoons contain: Thiamin 0.75 mg • Riboflavin 1.2 mg •Niacin 8 mg •Vitamin B6 1.8 mg • Folate, Folic Acid, Folacin 20 mcg • Vitamin B12 0.12 mcg •Biotin 12 mcg •Pantothenic acid 0.6 mg • Iron 1.8 mg • Phosphorus 20 mg • Magnesium 28 mg •Zinc 2.25 mg • Copper 0.9 mg. Ingredients: Brewer's Yeast, Psyllium husk powder, Guar Gum, Citrus Pectin powder.

Instant Soy'n Whey **-** Next Nutrition
Water-Extracted Soy Protein concentrate • Non-Denatured Whey Protein concentrate • Fructose • Natural Vanilla flavoring • Lecithin • Modified Food starch • Malic acid • Cellulose gum • Kudzu extract • Momordica extract • Stevia • Vitamin E.

Insulean Rice **-** Xymogen
Two scoops (55 g) contain: Vitamin A (mixed carotenoids) 2500 IU • Vitamin D (D3, as cholecalciferol) 200 IU • Vitamin E (D-alpha tocopherol succinate) 15 IU • Vitamin C (ascorbic acid) 30 mg • Vitamin B1 (thiamine) 750 mcg • Vitamin B2 (riboflavin) 850 mcg • Vitamin B3 (niacinamide) 10 mg • Vitamin B6 (pyridoxine HCl) 1 mg • Folate (folic acid & 5-formyl tetrahydrofolate) 200 mcg • Vitamin B12 (cyanocobalamin) 3 mcg • Biotin 150 mcg • Pantothenic Acid (calcium) 55 mg • Calcium (citrate) 500 mg • Magnesium (citrate, glycinate) 200 mg • Phosphorus 500 mg • Potassium 175 mg • Chromium (aspartate) 60 mcg • Zinc (aspartate and bisglycinate chelate) 15 mg • Selenium (selenomethionine) 35 mcg • Manganese (aspartate) 1 mg • Iodine (potassium) 75 mcg • Molybdenum (aspartate) 37.5 mcg • L-Glutamine 1000 mg • L-Taurine 1000 mg • Aminogen brand Proteolytic Enzyme 300 mg • OptORAC brand Antioxidant blend 350 mg.

Insulean Soy **-** Xymogen
Two scoops (55 g) contain: Vitamin A (mixed carotenoids) 2500 IU • Vitamin D (D3, as cholecalciferol) 200 IU • Vitamin E (D-alpha tocopherol succinate) 15 IU • Vitamin C (ascorbic acid) 30 mg • Vitamin B1 (thiamine) 750 mcg • Vitamin B2 (riboflavin) 850 mcg • Vitamin B3 (niacinamide) 10 mg • Vitamin B6 (pyridoxine HCl) 1 mg • Folate (folic acid & 5-formyl tetrahydrofolate) 200 mcg • Vitamin B12 (cyanocobalamin) 3 mcg • Biotin 150 mcg • Pantothenic Acid (calcium) 55 mg • Calcium (citrate) 500 mg • Magnesium (citrate, glycinate) 200 mg • Phosphorus 500 mg • Potassium 175 mg • Chromium (aspartate) 60 mcg • Zinc (aspartate and bisglycinate chelate) 15 mg • Selenium (selenomethionine) 35 mcg • Manganese (aspartate) 1 mg • Iodine (potassium) 75 mcg • Molybdenum (aspartate) 37.5 mcg • L-Glutamine 1000 mg • L-Taurine 1000 mg • Aminogen brand Proteolytic Enzyme 300 mg • OptORAC brand Antioxidant blend 350 mg • Isoflavones 24 mg.

Insulean Whey **-** Xymogen
Two scoops (55 g) contain: Vitamin A (mixed carotenoids) 2500 IU • Vitamin D (D3, as cholecalciferol) 200 IU • Vitamin E (D-alpha tocopherol succinate) 15 IU • Vitamin C (ascorbic acid) 30 mg • Vitamin B1 (thiamine) 750 mcg • Vitamin B2 (riboflavin) 850 mcg • Vitamin B3 (niacinamide) 10 mg • Vitamin B6 (pyridoxine HCl) 1 mg • Folate (folic acid & 5-formyl tetrahydrofolate) 200 mcg • Vitamin B12 (cyanocobalamin) 3 mcg • Biotin 150 mcg • Pantothenic Acid (calcium) 55 mg • Calcium (citrate) 500 mg • Magnesium (citrate, glycinate) 200 mg • Phosphorus 500 mg • Potassium (whey formula) 300 mg • Chromium (aspartate) 60 mcg • Zinc (aspartate and bisglycinate chelate) 15 mg • Selenium (selenomethionine) 35 mcg • Manganese (aspartate) 1 mg • Iodine (potassium) 75 mcg • Molybdenum (aspartate) 37.5 mcg • L-Glutamine 1000 mg • L-Taurine 1000 mg • Aminogen brand Proteolytic Enzyme 300 mg • OptORAC brand Antioxidant blend 350 mg.

InsuLeanR **-** NutraBolics
Two capsules contain: D-Pinitol 20 mg • R- ALA 200 mg • Gymnema Sylvestre 200 mg • Banaba leaf extract (1% corosolic acid (glucosol)) 40 mg.

InsuLife **-** Life Enhancement Products, Inc.
Three capsules contain: Vitamin C (as 75% ascorbic acid and 25% ascorbyl palmitate) 200 mg • Vitamin E (as 50% D-A-tocopheryl succinate and 50% mixed tocopherols: A, B and Y) 100 IU • Vitamin K (as phylloquinone) 90 mcg • Vitamin B6 (pyridoxine) 10 mg • Chromium (as chromium aspartate) 1 mg • Alpha-Lipoic Acid 600 mg • EGCG (epigallocatechin gallate, from green tea) 240 mg • N-Acetylcysteine 75 mg • Goat's Rue leaf extract (galega officinalis, 20% guanylhydraine) 20 mg • MHCP (methylhydroxychalcone polymer, from cinnamon) 12 mg • Vanadium (as vanadyl sulfate) 1 mg.

Intact Colostrum **-** GNC
Each packet (20.4 grams) contains: Bovine Colostrum powder (standardized for minumum 15% IgG content). Other Ingredients: Artificial Vanilla Flavoring, Acesulfame Potassium.

IntakeLean **-** InStone Nutrition
Each scoop (30 g) contains: EssentialPro 18 g: Calcium Caseinate, Whey Protein concentrate, Milk Protein concentrate, Hydrolyzed Wheat Gluten (as a source of glutamine peptides), Whey Protein Isolate, Hydrolyzed Whey Protein Concentrate • Ultra W3 Fatty Acid Blend 2.5 g: High-Oleic Sunflower Creamer, Conjugated Linoleic Acid, Flax Seed powder, Vegetable DHA powder • Dutch processed Cocoa • FiberZyme 3 g: Fibersol-2 Fiber, Digestive Enzyme blend • Natural and Artificial Flavors • Inulin • Vitamin and Mineral blend • Cellulose Gum • Tri-Calcium Phosphate • Xanthan Gum • Guar Gum • Acesulfame Potassium • Sucralose.

IntakePerformance **-** InStone Nutrition
Each packet contains: EssentialPro 45 g: Calcium Caseinate, Whey Protein concentrate, Milk Protein concentrate, Hydrolyzed Wheat Gluten (as a source of glutamine peptides), Whey Protein Isolate, Hydrolyzed Whey Protein Concentrate • Ultra W3 Fatty Acid Blend 6 g: High-Oleic Sunflower Creamer, Conjugated Linoleic Acid, Flax Seed powder, Vegetable DHA powder • Dutch processed Cocoa •

FiberZyme: Fibersol-2 Fiber, Digestive Enzyme blend • Natural and Artificial Flavors • Inulin • Vitamin and Mineral blend • Cellulose Gum • Tri-Calcium Phosphate • Xanthan Gum • Guar Gum • Acesulfame Potassium • Sucralose.

IntegritE Max Capsules - E'OLA
Four capsules contain: Glucosamine Sulfate 1500 mg • MSM (Methylsulfonylmethane) 750 mg • Proprietary Blend 480 mg: Boswellia (bark), Sea Cucumber, L-Cysteine, Horsetail (shoots), Bromelain. Other Ingredients: Rice Flour, Gelatin, Magnesium Stearate.

Intelectol - Memory Secret
Each tablet contains: Vinpocetine (from periwinkle seed extract) 5 mg. Other Ingredients: Lactose, Hydroxypropylcellulose, Magnesium Stearate, Talc.

IntelleQ - Advocare International
Two capsules contain: Niacin 20 mg • Vitamin C (as potassium ascorbate) 60 mg • Choline (as bitartrate) 100 mg • Taurine 200 mg • Boron (as amino acid complex) 700 mcg • Ribonucleic Acid 1 mg • Phospholipid Complex (standardized phosphatidylserine) 150 mg • Ginkgo Biloba extract (leaf - ginkgo biloba) 100 mg • Gotu Kola extract (leaf/stem/flower - centella asiatica) 150 mg • Grape extract (seed/skin - vitis vinifera Activin) 5 mg • Bacopa extract (leaf/stem - Bacopa monniera) 400 mg. Other Ingredients: Silicon Dioxide, Magnesium Stearate, Gelatin.

Intensive Eye Complex - Nu Skin Enterprises
Water • Aloe Barbadensis gel • Propylene Glycol Stearate SE • Squalane • Butylene Glycol • Caprylic/Capric Triglyceride • Octyl Stearate • Glycerin • Cetearyl Alcohol • Biosaccharide Gum-1 • Stearic Acid • Ceteareth-20 • Barrier Repair Complex: Linoleic Acid, Soy Stearols, Soy Phospholipids, Tocopherol, Ascorbyl Palmitate • Carrot extract (daucus carota sativis) • Shea Butter (butyrospermem perkii) • Kukui nut oil (aleurites moluccana) • Stearyl Glycyrrhetinate • Ginkgo Biloba extract • Allantoin • Phospholiids • Octyl Palmitate • Dioctyl Adipate • Aminomethyl Propanol • Methylparaben • Phenoxyethanol • Chlorphenesin • Phenylethyl Alcohol • Propylparaben • Disodium EDTA • Chlorhexidine Gluconate.

Interex - Benson Pendant
Each capsule contains: Epimedium Grandiflorum extract 187.50 mg • Muira Puama 4:1 extract (ptychopetalum) 75 mg • Maca 75 mg • L-Arginine Hydrochloride USP 75 mg • Cnidium Monnier extract 37.50 mg • Xanthroparmelia Scabrosa extract 37.50 mg • Tribulus Terrestris extract 37.50 mg • Mucuna Pruriens extract (15% levo-dopa) 37.5 mg • Coleus Forskolin 10% (ForsLean) 37.5 mg. Other Ingredients: Microcrystalline Cellulose, Silica, Dicalcium Phosphate, Talcum, Magnesium Stearate, Gelatin.

Internal Sweep powder (World's Best Internal Klenz) - Nature's Medicine Corporation
Alfalfa powder • Aloe Vera • Althaea root powder • Buchu leaf • Burdock root powder • Capsicum fruit powder • Chickweed leaf • Cinnamon bark powder • Citrus Pectin • Clove seed powder • Corn Silk • Dandelion root powder • Echinacea root powder • Fenugreek seed powder • Fennel seed powder • Flax seed powder • Fructooligosaccharides • Garlic powder (odorless) • Ginger root powder • Goldenseal root • Grapefruit Pectin • Guar gum • Irish Moss • Licorice root • Peppermint leaf • Rhubarb root bark powder • Stevia Rebaudiana • Papaya fruit powder • Pumpkin seed powder • Psyllium husks • Red Clover • Rhubarb root • Slippery Elm • Uva Ursi leaf. Other Ingredients: Acidophilus, Natural Banana Flavor, Natural Lemon Flavor, Fructose.

Intesol - Metagenics
Each softgel contains: Chamomile flower extract (matricaria recutita, standardized to 2.5%-5.5% apigenin glycosides) 250 mg • Peppermint oil (mentha x piperita, supplying a minimum of 50% total menthol) 200 mg • English Lavender flower oil (lavandula angustifolia) 20 mg.

IntestaLife - Holista
Each capsule contains: 4 billion active cells specially cultured strains of Lactobacillus Rhamnosus • Lactobacillus acidophilus • Bifido longum.

Intestamend - Health From The Sun
Three capsules contain: Protein 1 g • Calcium 24 mg • Glutamine 200 mg • Lysine 132 mg • Leucine 103 mg • Methionine 49 mg • Threonine 59 mg • Valine 69 mg • Trypophane 11 mg • Isoleucine 60 mg • Phenylalanine 48 mg. Ingredients: Deep-Ocean White Fish, Gelatin, Glycerine, Water, natural Rosemary flavor.

IntestiCalm - TriLight Herbs
Meadowsweet • German Chamomile • Slippery Elm • Ginger • Blackberry • Red Raspberry • Cinnamon.

Intestinal Bowel Soother - Renew Life Formulas, Inc.
Two capsules contain: Slippery Elm bark (ulmas rubra) 200 mg • German Chamomile flower (matricaria recutita) 200 mg • Fenugreek seed (trigonella foenum-graefcum) 100 mg • Fennel seed (Foeniculum vulgare) 100 mg • Skullcap herb (scutellaria lateriflora) 100 mg • Cranberry fruit (vaccinium macrocarpon 25:1) 50 mg • Peppermint leaf (mentha piperita) 50 mg • Proprietary Chinese Herbal Blend 12:1 Extract 600 mg: Atractylodes root (bai zhu), Yin Chen Hao (capillary artemisia herb), Codonopsis root (dang shen), Job's Tears seed (yi yi ren), Schisandra fruit (wu wei zi), Huo Xiang (agastache whole plant), Chinese Licorice root (zhi gan cao), Chinese Thoroughwax (chai hu), Ginger root (pao jiang), Korean Ash branch and bark (gin pi), Magnolia bark (hou po), Phellodendron bark (huang bai), Poria Cocos root (fu ling), Psyllium seed (che qian zi), Chinese Goldthread (huang lian), Chinese White Peony root (bai shao), Costus root (mu xiang), Siler root (fang feng), Tangerine peel (chen pi), Angelica root (bai zhi) • MSM (methylsulfonylmethane) 200 mg. Other Ingredients: Hypromellose, Water.

Intestinal Fortitude - Nutri-Quest Rx
Each tablet contains: L-Glutamine 150 mg • Buffered Vitamin C (Sago) 25 mg • N-Acetyl Glucosamine 75 mg • Vitamin E Succinate 10 IU • Lipoic Acid 2 mg • Ginkgo Biloba extract 2 mg • Deglycerrized Licorice 50 mg • Slippery Elm 100 mg • Lactobacillus Acidophilus 1 million IU • Cats Claw 15 mg • Ginkgo Biloba herb 50 mg • Jerusalem Artichoke 25 mg • Zinc Chelate 5 mg • Lactobacillus Bifidus 1 million IU.

Intestinal Freedom - American Biologics
Each capsule contains: Black Walnut hulls 225 mg • Black Walnut extract 45 mg • Ficin (fig enzyme) 45 mg • Jerusalem Oak seed 45 mg • Bromelain (pineapple enzyme) 45 mg • Papain (papaya enzyme) 45 mg • Cascara Sagrada bark 45 mg • Sage 45 mg • Male Fern 45 mg. Other Ingredients: Garlic (odorless), Green Ginger, Culver's Root, Violet Leaves, Pomegranate Bark, Pumpkin Seed, Tansy Seed, White Oak Bark.

Intestinal Rescue - The Herbalist
Psyllium seed & husk • Guar gum • Ginger root • Medical Grade Pectin • Bentonite clay • Rhubarb root • Cinnamon bark.

IntestiNEW - Renew Life Formulas, Inc.
Each scoop contains: L-Glutamine • N-Acetyl-Glucosamine • Gamma Oryzanol • Proprietary Herbal Blend: Cranesbill root (geranium maculatum), Ginger root (zingiber officinale), Marigold flower (calendula officinalis), Marshmallow root (althaea officinalis).

Intestive - Proper Nutrition - PNI
Four capsules contain: Vitamin B12 0.23 mcg • Sodium 5 mg • Potassium 30 mg • White Fish 1.8 g • Omega-3 19 mg • Colostrum (casein- & lactose-free, bovine) 160 mg • Boswellia 40 mg. Other Ingredients: Gelatin.

Intimate Health with VASX - EnerGreens, Inc.
Each capsule contains: VASX brand Proprietary Blend 475 mg: Cassia tree, Dodder seed, Epimedium, Wolfberry, Saling, Cistanche, Magnolia vine fruit, Red Raspberry, Narrow Leaved Polygia,

Rehmannia root, Eucommia bark, Hindo Lotus seed, Bidernate Achyranthes, Oleaster bark, Milk Vetch seed, Cherokee Rose, Aborvitae seed • American Ginseng 15 mg • Ginkgo Biloba 10 mg. Other Ingredients: Calcium Carbonate, Microcrystalline Cellulose, Stearic Acid, Silicon Dioxide, Magnesium Stearate, Pharmaceutical Coating.

Intimate Response - Source Naturals
Each tablet contains: Vitamin B6 (as pyridoxine HCl) 5 mg • Folate (as folic acid) 50 mcg • Wild Oats 150 mg • L-Arginine 100 mg • Dong Quai root extract 75 mg • Yohimbe bark standardized extract (yielding 2.5 mg yohimbines) 63 mg • Ginkgo Biloba leaf (24%, 50:1 extract) 60 mg • Panax Ginseng root extract 38 mg • Nettle root extract 25 mg • Epimedium Bicorum leaf extract 15 mg • Boron (as boron chelate) 1.5 mg • Pregnenolone 1.25 mg.

Intlecs Huperzine A - Intlecs
Each tablet contains: Huperzine A (Chinese club moss, Huperzia serrata) 50 mcg.

Intrasound Cleanse Formula - TriStar Online
Each scoop contains: Maltodextrin • Calcium Citrate • Natural Flavors • Magnesium Citrate • Gum • Citric Acid • Beta Carotene Gum • Stevia • Rebaudiana Extract • Soy Lecithin • Beet Powder • Lactobacillus Acidophilus • Lactobacillus Bifidus • Fructooligosaccharides • Papaya Powder • Prune Powder • Ascorbic Acid • Barley Sprout Powder • Wheat Sprout Powder • Oat Sprout Powder • Fenugreek. Fiber blend: Oat Fiber, Cellulose Gel/Cellulose, Purified Cellulose, Partially Hydrolyzed Soy Fiber, Psyllium Husk, Rice Bran, Citrus Pectin.

Intrasound Energy Drink - TriStar Online
Whole leaf aloe • Purified water • Natural Flavor • Fructose • Kaolin Clay • Trace Minerals • Citric Acid • Stevia • Xanthan Gum • Fiber • Ginseng Extract • Sage Extract • Dandelion Extract • Potassium Gluconate • Sodium Benzoate • Potassium Sorbate.

Intrasound Enzyme Formulas - TriStar Online
Each capsule contains: Amylase • Lipase • Protease • Cellulase • Intervase or Sucrase • Lactase • Malt Diastase • Calcium Citrate • Kaolin Clay • Beef Gelatin Capsule.

Intrasound Gel - TriStar Online
Generic Conductive Gel • Kaolin Clay.

Intrasound Herbal Accelerator - TriStar Online
Each capsule contains: Lipase • Cellulase • Amylase • Protease • Chromium Picolinate • Chromium Polynicotinate • Garcinia Cambogia Extract • Sida Cordifolia Herb • Yerba Mate • Kola Nut • Bladderwrack Algae • Cayenne Pepper • Siberian Ginseng Root. See Editor's Note No. 39.

Intrasound Mouth Rinse - TriStar Online
Whole leaf aloe • Purified Water • Natural Flavor • Kaolin Clay • Chlorophyll • Stevia • Sodium Benzoate.

Intrasound Powder - TriStar Online
Kaolin Clay.

Intrasound Tooth Gel - TriStar Online
Whole Leaf Aloe • Purified Water • Glycerin • Carrageenan (seaweed) • Hydrated Silica • Sodium Lauroyl Sarcosinate • Chlorophyll • Kaolin Clay • Natural Flavor • Stevia • Potassium Sorbate.

Intrinsi B12/Folate - Metagenics
Each tablet contains: Vitamin B12 (as cyanocobalamin) 500 mcg • Folate (as folic acid, L-5-methyl tetrahydrofolate, 5-formyl tetrahydrofolate) 800 mcg • Intrinsic Factor (porcine) 20 mg.

Intrinsic Plus - Progressive Labs
Each capsule contains: Vitamin B12 (cyanocobalamin) 500 mcg • Folate (folic acid) 800 mcg • Pancreatic enzyme concentrate 50 mg • Porcine Stomach 250 mg • Pyloric Substance 60 mg. See Editor's Note No. 14.

Invigorate II - Cytotec Solutions, Inc.
Some ingredients include: Proprietary Blend: Kryukova, Water, Natural Fruit Flavor, Citric Acid, Acesulfame Potassium, FD&C Red. The complete ingredients for this product are unknown. See Editor's Note No. 49.

Invigorex - Austin Research Institute
Two capsules contain: Vitamin B6 (as pyridoxine HCl) 12.5 mg • Niacin (as niacinamide) 10 mg • Natural Vitamin E 15 IU • Zinc (as oxide) 7.5 mg • L-Arginine HCl 750 mg • Tribulus Terrestris extract (20%) 200 mg • Muira Puama extract (4:1) 150 mg • Jujube dates (ziziphus jujuba) 100 mg • Avena Sativa extract 100 mg • Peruvian Maca root 50 mg • Stinging Nettle extract (5:1) 25 mg • Horny Goat Weed powder 100 mg • Siberian Ginseng powder 100 mg • Saw Palmetto powder 50 mg. Other Ingredients: Gelatin, Microcrystalline Cellulose, Magnesium Stearate, Water.

Iodine (potassium iodide) - Pure Encapsulations
Each vegetable capsule contains: Iodine (potassium iodide) 225 mcg.

Iodine and Tyrosine - Pure Encapsulations
Each vegetable capsule contains: Iodine (potassium iodide) 225 mcg • L-Tyrosine (free-form) 500 mg.

Iodine Mineral Supplement - Eidon Inc.
Each 1 tsp serving contains: Iodine (providing approx. 15 ppm iodine) 75 mcg. Other Ingredients: Purified Water.

Iodomere - Standard Process, Inc.
Each tablet contains: Proprietary Blend 338 mg: Conch (stombus gigas), Carrot root, Bovine Liver, Echinacea root • Iodine 200 mcg • Potassium 5 mg. Other Ingredients: Honey, Calcium Stearate. See Editor's Note No. 14.

Ios-Rich Soy (vegetarian) - Jarrow Formulas
Soy Protein Isolate (non-GMO) • Natural Vanilla flavor.

IP6 - Pure Encapsulations
Each vegetable capsule contains: IP6 (inositol hexaphosphate, purified brown rice extract) 500 mg.

IP-6 - PhysioLogics
Two capsules contain: Inositol Hexaphosphate 1020 mg. Other Ingredients: Cellulose (plant origin), Gelatin, Silica, Vegetable Magnesium Stearate.

IP6 capsules - Jarrow Formulas
Each capsule contains: Calcium-Magnesium Inositol Hexaphosphate 615 mg: IP6 500 mg, Calcium 85 mg, Magnesium 30 mg. Other Ingredients: Rice powder, Magnesium Stearate, Gelatin.

IP6 Optimizer - Jarrow Formulas
Each capsule contains: IP6•Ca•Mg 367 mg: IP6 300 mg, Calcium 51 mg, Magnesium 16 mg • Gamma Oryzanol 50 mg • Ferulic Acid 50 mg. Other Ingredients: Rice Powder, Magnesium Stearate, Gelatin.

IP6 powder - Jarrow Formulas
Each scoop contains: Calcium-Magnesium Inositol Hexaphosophate 1230 mg: IP6 (extracted from rice bran) 1000 mg, Calcium 170 mg, Magnesium 60 mg.

Iplex - Standard Process, Inc.
Two capsules contain: Proprietary Blend 967 mg: Arrowroot flour, Inositol, Calcium Lactate, Porcine Eye PMG extract, Phosphoric Acid, Dried Buckwheat leaf juice, Buckwheat seed, Veal Bone PMG extract, Carrot root, Bovine Liver, Magnesium Citrate, Porcine Stomach, Choline Bitartrate, Nutritional Yeast, Bovine Adrenal, Defatted Wheat germ, Alfalfa flour, Bovine Kidney, Dried Alfalfa juice, Allantoin, Mushroom, Manganese Glycerophosphate, Bovine Adrenal Cytosol extract, Porcine Brain, Bovine Bone, DL-Methionine, Oat flour, Soybean Lecithin, Veal Bone meal, Mixed Tocopherols, Carrot oil, Peanut bran • Vitamin A 520 IU • Vitamin C 6.2 mg • Riboflavin 0.4 mg • Niacin 4.8 mg • Vitamin B6 0.2 mg. Other Ingredients: Gelatin, Water, Colors, Calcium Stearate. See Editor's Note No. 14.

IpriBone - GNC
Two tablets contain: Vitamin D (as Cholecalciferol) 400 IU • Calcium (as Calcimate Calcium Citrate Malate) 200 mg • 7-Isopropoxy Isoflavone (Ostivone) 600 mg.

Ipriflavone 200 - Jarrow Formulas
Each capsule contains: Ipriflavone (7-isopropoxyflavone) 200 mg. Other Ingredients: Cellulose, Magnesium Stearate, Silicon Dioxide, Gelatin.

Ipriflavone 300 mg - Vital Nutrients
Each capsule contains: Ipriflavone 300 mg.

Ipriflavone with Vitamin D3 - Pure Encapsulations
Each vegetable capsule contains: Ipriflavone 300 mg • Vitamin D (D3) 200 IU.

Iromin-G - Mission Pharmacal
Each tablet contains: Vitamin A 4000 IU • Vitamin C 100 mg • Vitamin D (as Vitamin D3; Cholecalciferol) 400 IU • Vitamin B1 4.8 mg • Vitamin B2 (Cyanocobalamin) 2 mg • Vitamin B3 10 mg • Vitamin B6 20 mg • Folate 0.8 mg • Vitamin B12 2 mcg • Vitamin B5 1 mg • Calcium 57 mg • Iron 29.5 mg. Other Ingredients: Sugar, Microcrystalline Cellulose, Color, Croscarmellose Sodium, Magnesium Stearate, Povidone, Red 40 Lake, Food Glaze, Carnauba Wax, Sodium Benzoate, White Beeswax, Yellow 6 Lake.

Iron - Source Naturals
Each tablet contains: Iron (from 250 mg of Iron Amino Acid Chelate) 25 mg.

Iron 18 mg Timed Release - GNC
Each tablet contains: Iron (as ferrochel) 18 mg. Other Ingredients: Dicalcium Phosphate, Cellulose.

Iron 35 mg Timed Release - Jamieson
Each caplet contains: Elemental Iron 35 mg.

Iron 40 mg - Nature's Plus
Two tablets contain: Iron (as amino acid chelate) 40 mg. Other Ingredients: Di-calcium Phosphate, Microcrystalline Cellulose, Stearic Acid, Magnesium Stearate, Pharmaceutical Glaze, Silica.

Iron 50 mg Slow Release tablets - Sunmark
Each time-release tablet contains: Iron 50 mg (as 160 mg of ferrous sulfate). Other Ingredients: Maltodextrin, Calcium Carbonate, Hypromellose, Stearic Acid, Magnesium Stearate, Silicon Dioxide, Pregelatinized Corn Starch, Titanium Dioxide, Triethyl Citrate, Mineral Oil, Polysorbate 80, Carnauba Wax.
See Editor's Note No. 45.

Iron 50 mg Timed Release - Jamieson
Each caplet contains: Elemental Iron 50 mg.

Iron 65 mg - Nature Made
Each tablet contains: Iron 65 mg.
See Editor's Note No. 45.

Iron All Organic Iron Plus Liver, B-Complex, Vitamin C - Puritan's Pride
Two tablets contain: Vitamin C (as ascorbic acid and rose hips) 67 mg • Thiamin (vitamin B1 as thiamin hydrochloride) 1.5 mg • Riboflavin (vitamin B2) 3 mg • Niacin (as niacinamide) 0.5 mg • Vitamin B6 (as pyridoxine hydrochloride) 17 mcg • Folic Acid 11 mcg • Vitamin B12 (as cyanocobalamin) 8 mcg • Biotin (as D-biotin) 0.5 mcg • Pantothenic Acid (as D-calcium pantothenate) 45 mcg • Iron (as ferrous gluconate) 38 mg • Desiccated Liver 67 mg • L-Lysine (as L-lysine hydrochloride) 20 mg • Inositol 2 mg • Choline (as choline bitartrate) 1.5 mg • PABA (para-aminobenzoic acid) 10 mcg. Other Ingredients: Dicalcium Phosphate, Cellulose (plant origin), Croscarmellose, Vegetable Stearic Acid, Cellulose Coating, Vegetable Magnesium Stearate, Silica.
See Editor's Note No. 14.

Iron Caps - TwinLab
Each capsule contains: Iron (from Chelated Ferrous Fumarate) 18 mg.

Iron Complex - PhytoPharmica
Two capsules contain: Vitamin C (ascorbic acid) 120 mg • Folic Acid 400 mcg • Vitamin B12 (cyanocobalamin) 200 mcg • Iron (ferrous succinate) 50 mg • Liquid Liver fractions (predigested soluble concentrate) 500 mg • Chlorophyll (fat-soluble) 10 mg.
See Editor's Note No. 14.

Iron Complex - Nature's Life
Each capsule contains: Iron (Peptonate) 25 mg • Vitamin C 20 mg • Niacinamide 10 mg • Vitamin B1 (Thiamine HCl) 1 mg • Vitamin B2 (Riboflavin) 1 mg • Vitamin B6 (Pyridoxine HCl) 1 mg • Folic Acid 30 mcg • Vitamin B12 (Cobalamin concentrate) 15 mcg • Copper (Gluconate) 100 mcg • Manganese (Gluconate) 1 mg • Betaine HCl 15 mg. In a natural base of Rose Hips concentrate.

Iron Free Multi - Arrowroot
Four tablets contain: Beta Carotene 10,000 IU • Vitamin C (from ester C) 100 mg • Vitamin E 60 IU • Vitamin D (D3) 200 IU • Vitamin B1 10 mg • Vitamin B2 12 mg • Niacin 5 mg • Niacinamide 20 mg • Vitamin B6 12 mg • Vitamin B12 25 mcg • Folic Acid 400 mg • Biotin 30 mg • Pantothenic Acid 30 mg • Choline 10 mg • Inositol 10 mg • PABA 10 mg • Calcium 30 mg • Phosphorus 20 mg • Manganese 10 mg • Zinc 10 mg • Copper 1 mg • Magnesium 10 mg • Iodine 75 mcg • Selenium 50 mcg • Chromium 50 mcg.

Iron Plex - PhysioLogics
Each capsule contains: Vitamin C (as ascorbic acid) 60 mg • Folic Acid 400 mcg • Vitamin B12 (as cyanocobalamin) 8 mcg • Iron (as ferrous bis-glycinate) 28 mg. Other Ingredients: Maltodextrin, Gelatin, Vegetable Magnesium Stearate, Silica.

Iron Plus - Golden Glow Natural Health Products
Each tablet contains: Ferrous Fumarate 16 mg: Iron 5 mg • Folic Acid 95 mcg • Cyanocobalamin (vitamin B12) 50 mcg • Pyridoxine Hydrochloride (vitamin B6) 5 mg • Calcium Ascorbate Dihydrate 121 mg: Ascorbic Acid (vitamin C) 100 mg.

Iron Plus - Nutri-Quest Rx
Each tablet contains: Iron (Ferrous Fumurate) 50 mg • Vitamin C 100 mg • L-Glycine 100 mg • Niacinamide 15 mg • Betaine HCL 15 mg • Vitamin E (Succinate) 15 IU • D-Calcium Pantothenate (Pantothenic Acid) 13 mg • Vitamin B2 4 mg • Vitamin B1 3 mg • Vitamin B6 2 mg • Folic Acid 200 mcg • Vitamin B12 25 mcg • Choline Bitartrate 12.5 mg.

Iron Plus C Complex - Shaklee
Each tablet contains: Vitamin C (as Ascorbic acid) 60 mg • Calcium (as Dicalcium and Tricalcium phosphate) 130 mg • Iron (as Ferrous fumarate) 18 mg • Phosphorus (as Dicalcium and Tricalcium phosphate) 100 mg. Other Ingredients: Maltodextrin, Modified Cellulose Gum, Beet Powder, Acacia Gum, Spinach Powder, Barley Flour, Locust Bean Gum, Agar-Agar.

Iron Tablets 325 mg - Sunmark
Each tablet contains: Iron (as ferrous sulfate) 325 mg. Other Ingredients: Dicalcium Phosphate, Microcrystalline Cellulose, Hydroxypropyl Methylcellulose, Modified Cellulose Gum, Stearic Acid, Crospovidone, Alginic Acid, Magnesium Stearate, Artificial Colors (including FD&C blue no. 1, FD&C yellow no. 6, titanium dioxide), Silicon Dioxide, Polyethylene Glycol.
See Editor's Note No. 45.

Iron Woman - Traditional Medicinals
Yellow Dock root • Burdock root • Dandelion root • Licorice root • Nettle leaf • Prune fruit • Astragalus root • Stevia leaf.

Iron-C - Pure Encapsulations
Each vegetable capsule contains: Iron (glycinate) 7.5 mg • Iron (aspartate) 7.5 mg • Pure Ascorbic Acid 175 mg • Vitamin C (as ascorbyl palmitate) 3 mg.

Ironchel 18 mg - GNC
Each capsule contains: Iron (as ferrochel) 18 mg. Other Ingredients: Cellulose, Dicalcium Phosphate, Gelatin.

Iron-Free MultiLogics - PhysioLogics
Each caplet contains: Vitamin A (as 83% beta carotene, vitamin a palmitate) 15,000 IU • Vitamin C (as acorbic acid) 250 mg • Vitamin D (as cholecalciferol) 400 IU • Vitamin E (as d-alpha tocopheryl acetate) 150 IU • Thiamine (vitamin B1, as thiamin mononitrate) 75 mg • Riboflavin (vitamin B2) 75 mg • Niacin (as niacinamide) 75 mg • Vitamin B6 (as pyridoxine hydrochloride) 75 mg • Folic Acid 400 mcg • Vitamin B12 (as cyanocobalamin) 75 mcg • Biotin 300 mcg • Pantothenic Acid (as d-calcium pantothenate) 75 mg • Calcium (as dicalcium phosphate, lithothamnium) 92 mg • Iodine (as potassium iodide) 150 mg • Magnesium Chelate 10 mg • Zinc Chelate 10 mg • Selenium (as selenomethionate) 25 mcg • Copper (as copper amino acid chelate) 1 mg • Manganese (as manganese amino acid chelate) 1 mg • Chromium (as chromium amino acid chelate) 25 mcg • Molybdenum (as molybdenum amino acid chelate) 27 mcg • Boron (as boron amino acid chelate) 500 mcg • Inositol 75 mg • PABA (para-aminobenzoic acid) 75 mg • Choline (as choline bitartrate) 31 mg • Betaine Hydrochloride 25 mg • Citrus Bioflavonoids (citrus spp., fruit) 25 mg • Rutin (dimorphandra mollis, fruit) 25 mg • Hesperidin Complex (citrus aurantium, citrus spp., fruit) 5 mg. Other Ingredients: Cellulose (plant origin), Gelatin, Croscarmellose, Vegetable Stearic Acid, Silica, Vegetable Magnesium Stearate, Cellulose Coating.
See Editor's Note No. 40.

IronSorb - Jarrow Formulas
Each capsule contains: Iron (from 360 mg iron protein succinylate) 18 mg. Other Ingredients: Celluose, Silicon Dioxide, Magnesium Stearate.

I-Sight - Xymogen
Two capsules contain: Zinc (as amino acid chelate) 35 mg • L-Taurine 400 mg • Alpha Lipoic Acid 150 mg • Lycopene extract (providing 0.18 mg lycopene) 6 mg • Lutein extract (providing 0.9 mg lutein) 30 mg • Bilberry extract (standardized to contain 25% anthocyanidins) 180 mg • N-Acetyl Cysteine 200 mg • Quercetin 100 mg • Turmeric root extract (standardized to contain 95% curcuminoids) 100 mg.

Iso D3 - Metagenics
Each tablet contains: Vitamin D (as cholecalciferol) 2000 IU • Soybean concentrate 64 mg • Total Isoflavones (containing all forms of genistin, daidzin, and glycitin) 25 mg.

IsoBolic - NutraBolics
Two scoops (55 g) contain: Isobolic Advanced Protein Matrix: Cross-Flow Micro-Filtrated Whey Protein Isolate, Micellar Casein, Egg Isolate (egg albumin), Whey Protein Concentrate • CLA • Bromazyme • Flaxseed powder • Sucralose • Natural/Artificial Flavors.

Isochrome - Market America, Inc.
Each capful (3.33 g) contains: Boron (chelate) 2 mg • L-Carnitine 20 mg • Chromium (picolinate) 100 mcg • Chromium (argininate) 115 mcg • Coenzyme Q10 60 mg • Lipase 5 mg • Vitamin B2 (riboflavin) 3 mg • Vitamin B6 (pyridoxine HCl) 2 mg • Potassium (bicarbonate) 95 mg. Other Ingredients: Fructose, Glucose, Citric Acid, Maltodextrin, Silica, Calcium Sulfate, Natural Lemon-Lime Flavor.

IsoFlav - Ortho Molecular Products
Each capsule contains: Novasoy brand Soybean extract (standardized to cotnain 40% isoflavones) 250 mg • LinumLife brand Flax hull concentrate (standardized to contain 3.5% lignans) 220 mg • Alfalfa leaf 8:1 extract 125 mg • Red Clover blossom extract (standardized to contain 8% isoflavonoids) 100 mg. Other Ingredients: Natural Vegetable Capsules, Magnesium Stearate, Microcrystalline Cellulose.

Isolase Enzymes - Physicians Laboratories
Each capsule contains: Xylanase, Beta-Glucanase (from trichderma longibrachiatum) 224 IsoU.

IsoProtein Plus (French vanilla flavor) - Pure Encapsulations
One and one-half scoops contain: Calcium (naturall occurring) 778 mg • Vitamin D (D3) 200 IU • Soy Isoflavone concentrate 1700 mg • Flax seed powder 6.7 g • Soy Lecithin 5 g • Citrus peel pectin 2 g • L-Glutamine (free-form) 1 g • Red Beet fruit 1 g • Beta Glucan (1,3 beta-d-glucan) 500 mg • Green Tea leaf extract (standardized to contain 60% polyphenols) 500 mg • Reduced Glutathione (free-form) 50 mg • Stevia 57 mg. Other Ingredients: Calcium Enriched Soy Protein Isolate, Lo Han Fruit Extract (momordica grosvenori).

IsoProtein Plus (original flavor) - Pure Encapsulations
One and one-half scoops contain: Calcium (naturall occurring) 778 mg • Vitamin D (D3) 200 IU • Soy Isoflavone concentrate 1700 mg • Flax seed powder 6.7 g • Soy Lecithin 5 g • Citrus peel pectin 2 g • L-Glutamine (free-form) 1 g • Red Beet fruit 1 g • Beta Glucan (1,3 beta-d-glucan) 500 mg • Green Tea leaf extract (standardized to contain 60% polyphenols) 500 mg • Reduced Glutathione (free-form) 50 mg • Stevia 17 mg. Other Ingredients: Calcium Enriched Soy Protein Isolate.

IsoProtein Plus (strawberry banana flavor) - Pure Encapsulations
One and one-half scoops contain: Calcium (naturall occurring) 778 mg • Vitamin D (D3) 200 IU • Soy Isoflavone concentrate 1700 mg • Flax seed powder 6.7 g • Soy Lecithin 5 g • Citrus peel pectin 2 g • L-Glutamine (free-form) 1 g • Red Beet fruit 1 g • Beta Glucan (1,3 beta-d-glucan) 500 mg • Green Tea leaf extract (standardized to contain 60% polyphenols) 500 mg • Reduced Glutathione (free-form) 50 mg • Stevia 57 mg. Other Ingredients: Calcium Enriched Soy Protein Isolate, Lo Han Fruit Extract (momordica grosvenori).

IsoPure - Nature's Best
Each serving contains: Creamy Vanilla Ingredients: Ion Exchanged Whey Protein Isolate, Maltodextrin, Vitamin, Mineral & Amino Acid Blend, Natural & Artificial Flavor, Xanthan Gum, Aspartame, Acesulfame K. Dutch Chocolate Ingredients: Ion Exchange Whey Protein Isolate, Maltodextrin, Vitamin, Mineral & Amino Acid Blend, Cocoa, Xanthan Gum, Natural & Artificial Flavor, Aspartame, Acesulfame K. Orange Creamsicle Ingredients: Ion Exchange Whey Protein Isolate, Maltodextrin, Vitamin, Mineral & Amino Acid Blend, Natural & Artificial Flavor, Xanthan Gum, Aspartame, Acesulfame K, Artificial Color (Yellow #6). Strawberries & Cream Ingredients: Ion Exchange Whey Protein Isolate, Maltodextrin, Vitamin, Mineral & Amino Acid Blend, Natural & Artificial Flavor, Freeze-Dried Strawberry Crystals, Xanthan Gum, Aspartame, Acesulfame K, Artificial Color (Red #3). Chocolate Peanut Butter Swirl Ingredients: Ion Exchange Whey Protein Isolate, Maltodextrin, Vitamin, Mineral & Amino Acid Blend, Cocoa, Natural & Artificial Flavor, Xanthan Gum, Aspartame, Acesulfame K.

Iso-Rich Soy Greens - Jarrow Formulas
Non-GMO Soy Protein Isolate • Yaeyama Chlorella • Bromelain • Spirulina • Papain • Non-GMO Lecithin • Lo Han Kuo extract (momordica grosvenorii) • Natural Vanilla flavor.

Iso-Soy (chocolate caramel flavor) - Solgar
Isoflavone Soy Protein Isolate • Crystalline Fructose • Soy Concentrate • Natural Flavors • Dutch Cocoa • Maltodextrin • Vegetable gum.

Iso-Soy (vanilla bean flavor) - Solgar
Isoflavone Soy Protein Isolate • Isoflavone Soy Concentrate • Maltodextrin • Crystalline Fructose • Natural Vanilla Bean flavor • Vegetable Fiber.

Isotonix B-12 Special Formula - Market America, Inc.
Each capful contains: Vitamin B2 (riboflavin-5-phosphate) 3 mg • Vitamin B12 (cyanocobalamin) 120 mcg • Folic Acid 400 mcg • Magnesium (carbonate) 40 mg • Potassium (bicarbonate) 94 mg. Other Ingredients: Fructose, Glucose, Citric Acid, Maltodextrin, Silica, Pectin, Calcium Sulfate, Natural Lemon-Lime Flavor.

Isotonix Calcium Plus Formula - Market America, Inc.
Each capful contains: Calcium (gluconate) 166.6 mg • Calcium (chloride) 166.6 mg • Calcium (lactate) 166.6 mg • Magnesium (bicarbonate) 40 mg • Vitamin D (D3) 400 IU • Potassium (bicarbonate) 99 mg • Boron (chelate) 1 mg. Other Ingredients: Malic Acid, Citric Acid, Calcium Sulfate, Beta-Carotene (vitamin A precursor), Silica, Natural Lemon Lime Flavor.

Isotonix Coenzyme Q10 - Market America, Inc.
Each capful (3.33 g) contains: Coenzyme Q10 100 mg • Vitamin E (acetate) 200 IU • Lipase 5 mg • Vitamin B2 (riboflavin) 3 mg • Potassium (bicarbonate) 108 mg. Other Ingredients: Fructose, Glucose, Citric Acid, Silica, Calcium Sulfate, Maltodextrin, Natural Lemon-Lime Flavor.

Isotonix Digestive Enzyme Formula with Probiotics - Market America, Inc.
Each capful (3.33 g) contains: DigeZyme 100 mg: Amylase 2400 U, Protease 600 U, Cellulase 20 U, Lactase 400 U, Lipase 100 U • Maltase 125 MWU • Sucrase 400 SU • Magnesium (carbonate) 24 mg • Potassium (bicarbonate) 88 mg • Lactobacillus Sporogenes (Lactospore) 150,000,000 CFU. Other Ingredients: Fructose, Glucose, Citric Acid, Maltodextrin, Silica, Apple Pectin, Calcium Sulfate, Natural Lemon-Lime Flavor.

Isotonix Formula MultiTech - Market America, Inc.
Each capful (3.3 g) contains: Beta-Carotene 10,000 IU • Vitamin B1 2.6 mg • Vitamin B2 3 mg • Niacin 40 mg • Pantothenic Acid 20 mg • Vitamin B6 4 mg • Vitamin B12 75 mcg • Folic Acid 400 mcg • Biotin 300 mcg • Vitamin C 150 mg • Vitamin D (D3) 400 IU • Vitamin E (d-alpha-tocopheryl succinate) 60 IU • Vitamin K 100 mcg • Calcium 50 mg • Chromium 120 mcg • Copper 1000 mcg • Iodine 150 mcg • Magnesium 25 mg • Potassium 108 mg • Selenium 55 mcg • Silicon 2 mg • Zinc 7.5 mg. Other Ingredients: Fructose, Citric Acid, Orange Fruit Powder, Mandarin Fruit Powder, Malic Acid, Glucose, Natural Orange Flavor, Tricalcium Phosphate, Sucralose.

Isotonix Formula MultiTech with Iron - Market America, Inc.
Each capful (3.3 g) contains: Beta-Carotene 10,000 IU • Vitamin B1 2.6 mg • Vitamin B2 3 mg • Niacin 40 mg • Pantothenic Acid 20 mg • Vitamin B6 4 mg • Vitamin B12 75 mcg • Folic Acid 400 mcg • Biotin 300 mcg • Vitamin C 150 mg • Vitamin D (D3) 400 IU • Vitamin E (d-alpha-tocopheryl succinate) 60 IU • Vitamin K 100 mcg • Calcium 50 mg • Chromium 120 mcg • Copper 1000 mcg • Iodine 150 mcg • Iron 15 mg • Magnesium 25 mg • Potassium 108 mg • Selenium 55 mcg • Silicon 2 mg • Zinc 7.5 mg. Other Ingredients: Fructose, Citric Acid, Orange Fruit Powder, Mandarin Fruit Powder, Malic Acid, Glucose, Natural Orange Flavor, Tricalcium Phosphate, Sucralose.

Isotonix Maximum ORAC Formula - Market America, Inc.
Each capful (3.33 g) contains: Potassium (bicarbonate) 125 mg • Vitamin C (ascorbic acid) 100 mg • Cranberry 200 mg • Blueberry 100 mg • Grape 93 mg • Raspberry 90 mg • Elderberry 40 mg • Black Currant 40 mg • Pomegranate 40 mg • Plum 20 mg • Choke Cherry 20 mg • Natural Tocopherol (d-gamma 70%, d-delta 21%, d-alpha 7%, d-beta 2%) 30 mg • Tocotrienols (mixed isomers) 20 mg • Bioperine brand Black Pepper extract 56 mcg. Other Ingredients: Fructose, Citric Acid, Maltodextrin, Glucose, Silica.

Isotonix Might-a-Mins - Market America, Inc.
Each capful contains: Beta-Carotene (vitamin A precursor) 2500 IU • Vitamin B1 (thiamin HCl) 0.75 mg • Vitamin B2 (riboflavin) 0.85 mg • Vitamin B3 (niacin/niacinamide 1:4) 10 mg • Vitamin B5 (calcium d-pantothenate) 5 mg • Vitamin B6 (pyridoxine HCl) 1 mg • Vitamin B12 (cyanocobalamin) 3 mcg • Biotin 33 mcg • Vitamin C (ascorbic acid) 30 mg • Vitamin D (D3) 200 IU • Vitamin E (as d-alpha-tocopheryl succinate) 15 IU • Calcium (lactate, carbonate, sulfate, phosphate, citrate) 30 mg • Chromium (amino acid chelate) 10 mcg • Copper (gluconate) 182.2 mcg • Iodine (potassium iodide) 75 mcg • Magnesium (carbonate) 5 mg • Manganese (sulfate) 1 mg • Selenium (amino acid chelate) 20.6 mcg • Silicon (dioxide) 20 mg • Potassium (bicarbonate, citrate) 120 mg • Zinc (gluconate) 5.7 mg • Proprietary Phytonutrient Blend 1.04 g: Apple, Broccoli, Carrot, Cranberry, Grape, Kiwi, Lemon, Lime, Orange, Peach, Pineapple, Raspberry, Spinach, Strawberry, Tomato • Lactobacillus Sporogenes (Lactospore) 50,000,000 CFU. Other Ingredients: Fructose, Citric Acid, Malic Acid, Glucose, Natural Mandarin Orange Flavor, Sucralose.

Isotonix OPC-3 - Market America, Inc.
Each capful (3.33 g) contains: Grape seed extract 25 mg • Red Wine extract 30 mg • Pine bark extract (Pycnogenol) 25 mg • Bilberry extract 25 mg • Citrus Bioflavonoids extract 93 mg • Potassium (bicarbonate) 93 mg. Other Ingredients: Fructose, Glucose, Citric Acid, Maltodextrin, Silica, Calcium Sulfate, Pectin.

Isotonix Vision Formula with Lutein - Market America, Inc.
Each capful (3.33 g) contains: Beta Carotene 5000 IU • Vitamin C (ascorbic acid) 75 mg • Vitamin E (d, l-alpha-tocopheryl acetate) 33 IU • Potassium (bicarbonate) 150 mg • Zinc (lactate) 7 mg • Chromium (arginate) 100 mcg • Copper (gluconate) 100 mcg • Bilberry 50 mg • Taurine 42 mg • Quercetin 25 mg • Eyebright 10 mg • Lutein 7 mg • Lycopene 2 mg • Zeaxanthin 1.4 mg. Other Ingredients: Fructose, Natural Orange Powder, Citric Acid, Natural Orange Flavor, Malic Acid, Calcium Phosphate, Glucose, Silica, Sucralose.

Isotonix Vitamin C Formula - Market America, Inc.
Each capful (3.33 g) contains: Vitamin C (ascorbic acid) 500 mg • Beta-Carotene (vitamin A precursor) 800 IU • Potassium (bicarbonate) 101 mg. Other Ingredients: Fructose, Glucose, Maltodextrin, Malic Acid, Natural Orange Flavor, Silica, Citric Acid.

ISSF - AIE Pharmaceuticals
Glycyrrhiza Glabra • Milk Thistle • Cynara Scolymus • Bupleurum • Berberis Vulgaris • Magnolia vine • Astragali radix • Gentiana Lutea • Salvia Miltiorrhiza • Lycium Barbarum • Peony • Taraxacum Officinale • Wild Yam • Rumex Crispus • Arctium Lappa • Magnesium Stearate • Brown Rice powder • Gelatin • Water.

Itch Nix - Quantum
Purified Water • Aloe Vera gel • Propylene Glycol • Echinacea extract • Glycerine • Calendula extract (marigold) • Witch Hazel extract • Comfrey extract • Nettles extract • Clove bud oil • Menthol • Camphor • Thiamin (vitamin B1) • Riboflavin (vitamin B2) • Pyridoxine (vitamin B6) • Cyanocobalamin (vitamin B12) • Ferric Ammonium Citrate (iron) • Allantoin • Cellulose Gum.

IVC-Max - Aidan Products, LLC
Each capsule contains: Vitamin C 50 mg • Vitamin K (phytoquinone, from vitamin K1 1% on mannitol) 1.25 mg • Niacinamide 50 mg • Biotin 100 mcg • Selenium (from selenium amino acid chelate, 1% Se) 100 mcg • Alpha Lipoic Acid 150 mg • Quercetin 125 mg • Grape Seed Extract 25 mg.

Ivy Calm - PhytoPharmica
Each 2 tsp serving contains: English Ivy leaf extract (hedera helix, standardized to contain hedaracoside C 9 mg) 33 mg. Other Ingredients: Purified Water, Glycerol, Fructose, Natural Flavors, Sucrose Laurate, Potassium Sorbate, Citric Acid.

Ivy Extract - Enzymatic Therapy/PhytoPharmica
Two tablets contain: English Ivy leaf extract (hedera helix 4:1) 50 mg. Other Ingredients: Lactose, Cellulose, Stearic Acid, Magnesium Stearate, Silica.

Jambrulin - Unjha Ayurvedic Pharmacy
Each tablet contains: Jamungiri extract 20% • Tribung Bhasma 20% • Refined Shilajet (mineral pitch) 20% • Mamejave extract 10% • Bili Patra 10% • Gudmar 10% • Nim Patra 10%.

Jarro-Dophilus + Colostrum - Jarrow Formulas
Each capsule contains: Lactobacillus Rhamnosus R049 20% 672 million • Lactobacillus Casei R215 20 % 672 million • Lactobacillus Plantarum R202 20% 672 million • Lactobacillus Acidophilus R052

10% 336 million • Bifidobacterium Longum R023 20% 672 million • Bifidobacterium Breve R070 10% 336 million • Colostrum 500 mg. Other Ingredients: Ascorbic Acid, Magnesium Stearate.

Jarro-Dophilus + FOS capsules - Jarrow Formulas
Each capsule contains: FOS (fructooligosaccharides) 210 mg • Lactobacillus Rhamnosus R-011 20% 670 million • Lactobacillus Casei R0256/R0215 20% 670 million • Lactobacillus Plantarum R0202/R1012 10% 360 million • Lactobacillus Acidophilus R-052 20% 670 million • Bifidobacterium Longum BB536 670 million • Bifidobacterium Breve R-070 10% 360 million • Vitamin C 1 mg. Other Ingredients: Maltodextrin, Magnesium Stearate, Gelatin.

Jarro-Dophilus + FOS powder - Jarrow Formulas
Each 1/4 tsp serving contains: FOS (fructooligosaccharides) 400 mg • Lactobacillus Rhamnosus R011 20% 2.4 billion • Lactobacillus Casei R256 20% 2.4 billion • Lactobacillus Plantarum R202 10% 1.2 billion • Lactobacillus Acidophilus R052 20% 2.4 billion • Bifidobacterium Longum BB536 (morinaga strain) 20% 2.4 billion • Bifidobacterium Breve R070 10% 1.2 billion • Vitamin C 1 mg. Other Ingredients: Maltodextrin.

Jarro-Dophilus + Lactoferrin - Jarrow Formulas
Each capsule Contains: Lactobacillus Rhamnosus R049 20% 672 million • Lactobacillis Casei R215 20 % 672 million • Lactobacillus Plantarum R202 20% 672 million • Lactobacillus Acidophilus R052 10% 336 million • Bifidobacterium Longum R023 20% 672 million • Bifidobacterium Breve R070 10% 336 million • Lactoferrin 200 mg. Other Ingredients: Ascorbic Acid, Magnesium Stearate.

Jarro-Dophilus EPA - Jarrow Formulas
Each capsule contains: Probiotic Bacteria 4.4 billion organisms: Lactobacillus Rhamnosus R0011 15.4% 680 million, Lactobacillus Casei R0256 15.4% 680 million, Lactobacillus Plantarum R0202 7.7% 340 million, Lactobacillus Acidophilus R0052 15.4% 680 million, Bifidobacterium Longum BB536 (morinaga strain) 15.4% 680 million, Bifidobacterium Breve R0070 7.7% 340 million, Pediococcus Acidilactici R1001 15.3% 670 million, Lactococcus Diacetylactis R0100 7.6% 330 million. Other Ingredients: Potato Starch, Magnesium Stearate, Ascorbic Acid, Cellulose, Hydroxypropyl Methylcellulose, Magnesium Silicate, Methacrylate Copolymer.

Jarro-Dophilus Original - Jarrow Formulas
Each capsule contains: Probiotic Bacteria 3.36 billion organisms: Lactobacillus Rhamnosus R-011 40% 1.344 billion, Lactobacillus Rhamonosus R-049 25% 840 million, Lactobacillus Acidophilus R-052 10% 336 million, Lactobacillus Plantarum R-202 10% 336 million, Bifidobacterium Longum BB356 (Morinaga strain) 10% 336 million, Bifidobacterium Breve 070 5% 168 million • Vitamin C 1 mg. Other Ingredients: Maltodextrin, Microcrystalline Cellulose, Magnesium Stearate, Gelatin.

Jarro-Gar 800 - Jarrow Formulas
Each capsule contains: Garlic 800 mg: Allicin 1.2 mg, Allin 8 mg, Diallyldisulphides 64 mg, Selenium 6 mcg, Amino Acids 29 mg, Sulfur compounds 0.8 mg. Other Ingredients: Rice Powder, Magnesium Stearate, Gelatin.

Jarrow Pak Plus - Jarrow Formulas
Each packet contains: Yang Minerals (two larger white oval tablets): Calcium (from bovine hydroxyapatite) 600 mg • Phosphorus (from bovine hydroxyapatite) 219 mg • Magnesium (from oxide) 180 mg • Potassium (from potassium oxide) 99 mg • Zinc (from monomethionate) 7.5 mg • Manganese (from citrate) 0.5 mg • Selenium (50/50 L-selenomethionine and sodium selenate) 200 mcg • GTF Chromium (from nicotinate/citrate) 150 mcg • Molybdenum (from sodium molybdate) 100 mcg • Iodine (from potassium iodide) 225 mcg • Vitamin D (D3, cholecalciferol) 400 IU • Vitamin A (as palmitate) 5000 IU.
Yin Mineral Tablets (two green speckled tablets): Vitamin C (ascorbic acid) 250 mg • Calcium (from bovine hydroxyapatite) 400 mg • Phosphorus (from bovine hydroxyapatite) 146 mg • Magnesium (from oxide) 300 mg • Zinc (as zinc monomethionine) 7.5 mg • Manganese (as citrate) 1.5 mg • GTF Chromium (from nicotinate/citrate) 100 mcg.
Fat Soluble Vitamins: Beta Carotene (reddish softgel) 10,000 IU • Vitamin E (natural D-alpha tocopherol succinate, dry E; white capsule) 400 IU.
B-Right Complex (bright yellow oval tablet): Vitamin B1 (thiamin HCl) 25 mg • Vitamin B2 (riboflavin) 25 mg • Vitamin B3 (niacin) 25 mg • Vitamin B3 (niacinamide) 100 mg • Vitamin B5 (D-calcium pantothenate) 100 mg • Pantethine (vitamin B5 derivative) 25 mg • Vitamin B6 (pyridoxine HCl) 25 mg • Vitamin B6 (pyridoxal 5-phosphate) 10 mg • Vitamin B12 (as methylcobalamin) 100 mcg • Folic Acid 400 mcg • Biotin 300 mcg • PABA (para-aminobenzoic acid) 30 mg • Choline Bitartrate 50 mg • Inositol 50 mg.
C+ Herbs (two brown speckled tablets): Vitamin C (ascorbic acid) 500 mg • Silymarin 30:1 concentrate (standardized to 80% silybin) 75 mg • Astragalus root 6:1 extract 150 mg • Schisandra 5:1 extract 75 mg • Picrorrhiza Kurroa (PicroLiv brand, 3.5-4% kutkin) 50 mg • Skullcap root 4:1 extract (scutellaria) 300 mg. Other Ingredients: Capsule: Cellulose, Silicon Dioxide, Magnesium Stearate, Gelatin, Titanium Dioxide.
Tablet: Modified Cellulose Gum, Cellulose, Calcium Phosphate, Stearic Acid, Silicon Dioxide, Magnesium Stearate, Calcium Stearate, Sodium Copper Chlorophyllin.
Softgel: Soybean Oil, Glycerin, Lecithin, Gelatin, Vitamin E Mixed Tocopheryl, Water, Annatto, Titanium Dioxide.

Jarro-Zymes Plus - Jarrow Formulas
Each capsule contains: Porcine Pancreatic Enzymes 400 mg: Lipase (porcine) 10,000 USP units, Protease (porcine) 50,000 USP units, Amylase (porcine) 50,000 USP units • Alpha Galactosidase (aspergillus niger fermentation) 25 mg/625 AGS units. Other Ingredients: Rice Powder, Magnesium Stearate, Silicon Dioxide, Gelatin.

Jarsin 300 - Lichtwer Pharma
Each tablet contains: Dry St. John's Wort extract 300 mg. Other Ingredients: Lactose Monohydrate, Silicon Dioxide, Cellulose powder, Magnesium Stearate, Vanillin, Dimeticon Emulsion, Hypromellose, Macrogol 4000, Saccharin Sodium, Talcum, Titanium Dioxide, Iron Oxide Hydrate.

Jarsin 750 - Lichtwer Pharma
Each tablet contains: -arzneilich wirksamer Bestandteil: Trockenextrakt aus Johanniskraut (3-6:1) 750 mg • Auszugsmittel: Menthol 80% (V/V). Inactive Ingredients: Hochdisperses Siliciumdioxid, Mikrokristalline Cellulose, Vanillin, Hypromellose, Stearinsaure, Eisenoxid Gelb (E 172), Titandioxid (E 171), Lactose-Monohydrat, Hoherkettige, Partialglyceride, Sojapolysaccharid.

Javaan 50 - Javaan Corporation
Each tablet contains: Beta Carotene 26,666 IU • Vitamin A 1333 IU • Vitamin D 160 IU • Vitamin E 44 IU • Vitamin C 80 mg • Folate (folic acid) 400 mcg • Vitamin B1 (thiamin mononitrate) 2.2 mg • Vitamin B2 (riboflavin) 1.5 mg • Niacin 16 mg • Vitamin B6 3 mg • Vitamin B12 4 mcg • Calcium 200 mg • Iodine 200 mcg • Iron 16 mg • Magnesium 100 mg • Zinc 14 mg • Copper 1.4 mg • Selenium 20 mcg.

Jen Fe Patch - Nexagen USA
ForsLean brand Coleus Forskohlii extract (forskolin) • ChromeMate brand Chromium Poly-Nicotinate • Guarana (paullina cupana) • Cosmoperine brand extract of Black Pepper and Long Pepper.

JenFe Patch - Nexagen USA
ForsLean brand Coleus Forskohlii extract (forskolin) • ChromeMate brand Chromium Poly-Nicotinate • Guarana (paullina cupana) • Cosmoperine brand extract of Black Pepper and Long Pepper.

Jen-Fe Patch - Nexagen USA
ForsLean brand Coleus Forskohlii extract (forskolin) • ChromeMate brand Chromium Poly-Nicotinate • Guarana (paullina cupana) • Cosmoperine brand extract of Black Pepper and Long Pepper.

Some Brand Name Natural Products - What they Contain

www.NaturalDatabase.com contains MANY more listings than appear here.
Editor's Notes are located on pages 2155-2163.

BRAND NAMES

Jiaogulan - Solaray
Two capsules contain: Jiaogulan root/rhizome extract (gynostemma pentaphyllum, guaranteed 98% gypenosides) 804 mg • Jiaogulan aerial parts (gynostemma pentaphyllum) 200 mg.

Jiaogulan Gynostemma - Paradise Herbs
Each vcap contains: Gynostemma Pentaphyllum whole plant extract 12:1 (equivalent to whole plant 3000 mg) 250 mg • 30% Gypenosides 75 mg. Other Ingredients: Capsules (vegetable cellulose).

Jin Gui Shen Qi Wang Plus - Secara
Rhemannia root tuber 5:1 extract (sheng di huang) 470 mg • Organic Cinnamon bark (rou gui) 416 mg • Asiatic Dogwood fruit 5:1 extract (shan zhu yu) 235 mg • Chinese Yam rhizome 5:1 extract (shan yao) 235 mg • Saw Palmetto fruit (10% fatty acids (23 mg)) 225 mg • Asian Water Plantain rhizome 5:1 extract (ze xie) 176 mg • Poria Sclerotium 5:1 extract (fu ling) 176 mg • Tree Peony root bark 5:1 extract (mu dan pi) 176 mg • Cordyceps mycelia 5:1 extract 135 mg • Cinnamon oleo resin 6 mg.

JIN-ZHI Thermo Drops - E'OLA
Fifteen drops contain: Zhi Shi (Citrus Aurantium) 250 mg • Proprietary Blend 18 mg: Caffeine, Guarana Herb, Ginseng Root, Licorice Root. Other Ingredients: Water, Glycerin, Citric Acid, Sodium Benzoate.
See Editor's Note No. 40.

Joint & Muscle Pain Cream - Shaklee
Active Ingredients: Menthol (5%). Inactive Ingredients: Aloe Barbadensis leaf gel (aloe vera), Butylene Glycol, Carbomer, Cetyl Alcohol, Cyclomethicone, Dimethicone, Glyceryl Stearate, Imidazolidinyl Urea, Methylparaben, PEG-12 Glyceryl Distearate, PEG-100 Stearate, Phenoxyethanol, Propylparaben, Prunus Amygdalus dulcis oil (sweet almond), Purified Water, Triethanolamine, Xanthan Gum.

Joint Actives - VitaStore
Six tablets contain: Glucosamine HCl 1500 mg • Shark Cartilage 500 mg • Salix Alba 200 mg • Boswellia 250 mg • Green Lipped Mussel 250 mg • Quercetin 300 mg • Manganese 5 mg • L-Methionine 100 mg • Zinc Gluconate 25 mg • Turmeric 250 mg • Bromelain 200 mg • Vitamin C 300 mg • Vitamin E 90 IU.

Joint Aid - Optimum Nutrition
Six capsules contain: Vitamin C (as ascorbic acid) 1000 mg • Vitamin D (as cholecalciferol) 400 IU • Vitamin E (as DL-alpha tocopherol acetate) 200 IU • Calcium (as calcium carbonate, citrate) 500 mg • Magnesium (as magnesium oxide, aspartate) 250 mg • Zinc (as zinc picolinate) 20 mg • Glucosamine (as glucosamine sulfate potassium) 1500 mg • Chondroitin (as chondroitin sulfate) 150 mg • Turmeric rhizome extract (curcuma longa, standardized to 95% curcuminoids) 1500 mg • Quercetin (as quercetin dihydrate) 100 mg • Borage oil 50 mg • Marine Lipids 50 mg. Other Ingredients: Gelatin, Magnesium Stearate, Silica.

Joint Armor - All Terrain Company
Three capsules contain: Vitamin E 30 IU • Zinc (from zinc sulfate) 15 mg • Glucosamine Sulfate 1200 mg • Chondroitin Sulfate 300 mg • Eicosapentaenoic Acid (EPA Omega-3) 260 mg • Docosahexaenoic Acid (DHA Omega-3) 170 mg • Gamma Linolenic Acid (GLA Omega-3)120 mg • Linoleic Acid (LA Omega-6) 210 mg • Omega-9 Oleic Acid 270 mg • Other Ingredients: Fish Oil, Glucosamine Sulfate, Borage Oil, Chondrotin Sulfate, Zinc Sulfate, Vitamin E (D-Alpha Tocopheryl), Gelatin, Glycerin, Purified Water, Unbleached Lecithin, Beeswax, Acrosil, Caramel.

Joint Builder - Jarrow Formulas
Two tablets contain: Glucosamine Sulfate (from 2000 mg 2GS 2KCl) 1500 mg • MSM (methylsulfonylmethane) 500 mg • Manganese (as gluconate) 1 mg • Vitamin C (calcium ascorbate) 100 mg • Vitamin D (D3, cholecalciferol) 100 IU. Other Ingredients: Calcium Phosphate, Cellulose, Stearic Acid, Magnesium Stearate, Modified Cellulose Gum, Silicon Dioxide.

Joint Complex - Puritan's Pride
Three capsules contain: Glucosamine Sulfate 500 mg • Vitamin C 250 mg • Bromelain (2400 GDU per gram) 250 mg • Boswellin (Boswellia Serrata) 250 mg • Curcumin (Curcuma Longa) 50 mg • Zinc (Amino Acid Chelate) 10 mg • Chondroitin Sulfate A 10 mg • White Willow Bark 100 mg • Shark Cartilage 500 mg • Vervain 100 mg.
See Editor's Note No. 15.

Joint Cream - The Vitamin Shoppe
Glucosamine • Boswellin • Capsaicin.

Joint Ease - Vital Nutrients
Two capsules contain: Harpagophytum Procumbens extract (devil's claw) 200 mg • Boswellia Serrata extract (25% boswellic acids by HPLC) 200 mg • Bromelain 2400 GDU/g (pure uncut bromelain) 200 mg • Curcuma Longa extract (90% curcuminoids by HPLC) 200 mg • Feverfew (0.7% parthenolide by HPLC) 200 mg • Glycyrrhiza Glabra root extract (licorice) 100 mg • Urtica Dioica leaf 5:1 extract (nettle) 100 mg.

Joint Essentials - Swanson Health Products
Three capsules contain: Vitamin C (as ascorbic acid) 250 mg • Zinc (from amino acid chelate) 15 mg • Manganese 5 mg • Glucosamine Sulfate (2KCl) 500 mg • Boswellian Boswellia Serrata Resin (65% boswellic acid) 250 mg • Bromelain (2400 GDU) 250 mg • Chondroitin Sulfate 200 mg • OptiMSM (methylsulfonylmethane) 100 mg • White Willow Bark 100 mg • Curcumin 50 mg • Devil's Claw powder 25 mg • Quercetin 25 mg • Sea Cucumber 25 mg • Yucca root extract 25 mg.
See Editor's Note No. 15.

Joint Fitness - Celestial Seasonings
Two capsules contain: Vitamin C (as ascorbic acid) 225 mg • Pantothenic Acid (as calcium pantothenate) 15 mg • Glucosamine Sulfate/HCl 150 mg • Flax Seed 225 mg • Turmeric (standardized to 95% curcuminoids) extract 185 mg. Other Ingredients: Dicalcium Phosphate, Gelatin, Rice Flour, Stearic Acid, Magnesium Stearate, Silicon Dioxide.

Joint Formula - PharmAssure
Two tablets contain: Sodium 140 mg • Vitamin C (as Ascorbic Acid) 60mg • Selenium (as Selenium Chelate) 100 mcg • D-Glucosamine Sulfate 750 mg • .2NaCl Chondroitin Sulfate, Sodium 600 mg • Boswellin serrate Resin Extract (65% Boswellic Acid=200 mg) 308 mg • Bromelain 200 GDU. Other Ingredients: Cellulose, Croscarmellose Sodium, Dicalcium Phosphate
See Editor's Note No. 15.

Joint Free Plus - Schiff
Each slightly rounded scoop (12.6 g) contains: Hydrolyzed Collagen 10 g • Glucosamine Hydrochloride 1500 mg • Chondroitin Sulfate 500 mg • Methylsulfonylmethane (MSM) 500 mg. Other Ingredients: Silicon Dioxide.

Joint Fuel - TwinLab
Six capsules contain: Glucosamine Sulfate 1500 mg • Chondroitin Sulfate A (CSA) 100 mg • Zinc (from Chelated Zinc Picolinate) 30 mg • Manganese (from Chelated Manganese Gluconate) 5 mg • Vitamin C 1000 mg • Natural Vitamin E (Succinate) 800 IU • Selenium (from Selenomethionine) 200 mcg • Turmeric extract (Curcuma longa) (standardized for 95% Curcumin) 1300 mg • Quercetin (Bioflavonoid) 100 mg • Bromelain 200 mg.
See Editor's Note No. 15.

Joint Fuel Liquid Concentrate - TwinLab
Each tablespoon contains: Glucosamine HCl 500 mg • Chondroitin Sulfate 400 mg • Betaine 166 mg • Hydrolyzed Collagen 33 mg • Chicken Type II Collagen 33 mg • Vitamin B6 3.3 mg • Folic Acid 400 mcg • Vitamin B12 166 mcg.
See Editor's Note No. 15.

Joint Health - One-A-Day - Bayer
Each tablet contains: Vitamin C 30 mg • Vitamin E 30 IU • Manganese 1.5 mg • Lecithin 10 mg • Glucosamine Sulfate powder (includes Dipotassium Cl 125 mg) 500 mg • Devil's Claw Standardized extract (Harpagophytum procumbens) root 134 mg.
See Editor's Note No. 21.

Joint Health Complex - Shaklee
Three capsules contain: Zinc (as Zinc gluconate) 1.5 mg • Copper (as Copper gluconate) 0.2 mg • Manganese (as Manganese gluconate) 0.2 mg • Glucosamine hydrochloride 1.4 g • Osteokinetics Enhanced Proprietary Blend 450 mg: Devil's Claw extract (Harpagophytum procumbens) root, Alfalfa concentrate (Medicago sativa) leaf • Boron (as Boron protein hydrolysate) 0.5 mg. Other Ingredients: Maltodextrin, Gelatin, Water.

Joint Juice (Lemon Iced Tea) - Joint Juice, Inc.
Each 8 fl oz serving contains: Vitamin C 60 mg • Glucosamine HCl 1500 mg.

Joint Juice (Orange-Tangerine) - Joint Juice, Inc.
Each 8 fl oz serving contains: Vitamin C 60 mg • Glucosamine HCl 1500 mg.

Joint Juice (Tropical) - Joint Juice, Inc.
Each 8 fl oz serving contains: Vitamin C 60 mg • Glucosamine HCl 1500 mg.

Joint Maintenance - Puritan's Pride
Three softgels contain: Manganese (from manganese aspartate) 1 mg • Glucosamine Sulfate (2KCl) 1500 mg • Chondroitin Sulfate 1200 mg • Citrus Bioflavonoids (citrus sinensis, fruit) 45 mg. Other Ingredients: Soybean Oil, Gelatin, Glycerin, Lecithin, Caramel Color, Beeswax (yellow).
See Editor's Note No. 15.

Joint Movement Glucosamine & Chondrotin with MSM and Collagen - Symtec
Two tablespoons (30 mL) contain: Sodium 75 mg • Vitamin C (as ascorbic acid) 60 mg • Vitamin D (as vitamin D3-cholecalciferol) 400 IU • Glucosamine HCl 2000 mg • Chondroitin Sulfate (as chondroitin sulfate disodium) 1200 mg • MSM 500 mg • Collagen 50 mg.
See Editor's Note No. 15.

Joint Performance - Metabolic Response Modifiers
Four capsules contain: Glucosamine Sulfate 1000 mg • MSM (Methyl-Sulfonyl-Methane) 500 mg • Noto-Gin (Panax Ginseng 45% saponins) 100 mg • Chondroitin complex 280 mg • Collagen complex 200 mg • Sea Cucumber 100 mg • CMO (25%) 100 mg • Boswellia 200 mg • Bromelain (2400 GDU) 100 mg • White Willow bark (0.1% salicylates) 80 mg • Tumeric (95% curcuminoids) 75 mg • Manganese (citrate) 8 mg.
See Editor's Note No. 15.

Joint Power Rx - Physician Formulas
Four capsules contain: Glucosamine Sulfate (from shellfish) 1500 mg • Chondroitin Sulfate 700 mg • MSM 400 mg • CMO complex 100 mg • Boswellia Serrata extract 100 mg • Curcumin 50 mg • Cat's Claw extract 50 mg • Devil's Claw extract 50 mg • Grape seed extract 20 mg • Sea Cucumber 20 mg. Other Ingredients: Gelatin (capsule).

Joint Principles - Life Enhancement Products, Inc.
Each capsule contains: Glucosamine Sulfate 375 mg • Chondroitin 4,6-Sulfate 150 mg.
See Editor's Note No. 15.

Joint Rejuvenator - BioTreasures Inc.
Each caplet contains: Glucosamine Sulfate 1500 mg • Chondroitin Sulfate 750 mg • Turmeric 750 mg • Devil's Claw 400 mg • Bromelain 100 mg.
See Editor's Note No. 15.

Joint Rescue - TwinLab
Three softgels contain: Vitamin E (from d-Alpha Tocopherols) 400 IU • Glucosamine HCl & Glucosamine Sulfate 750 mg • Chondroitin Sulfate 50 mg • Turmeric powder extract (standardized for 95% Curcumin) 650 mg • Boswellin (Boswellia serrata extract) (standardized for 65% Boswellic Acids) 13 mg • Ginger root extract 50 mg • EPA 750 mg • DHA 750 mg • Borage Oil 100 mg.
See Editor's Note No. 15.

Joint Rescue Formula with Glucosamine+ - Health Tech Industries (Dr. Bussan's)
Each capsule contains: Glucosamine sulfate 500 mg • Herbal Extract Complex 125 mg: Wild Yam, Licorice root, Aloe Vera, Pfaffia root, Red Poppy flower, Tumeric, White Peony root, Yucca, Corydalis rhizome, Super Dioxide Dismutase (SOD), Catalase Oxidants • Methionine 75 mg • Malic Acid 50 mg • Polyascorbic Acid (vitamin c) 25 mg • Niacinamide 10 mg • Pantothenic Acid (vitamin B5) 5 mg • Manganese Gluconate Chelate 5 mg.

Joint Rx - Xymogen
Four capsules contain: Green Lipped Mussel (perna canaliculus) 1000 mg • MSM (methylsulfonylmethane) 1000 mg • Glucosamine HCl 600 mg • Chondroitin Sulfate 600 mg • Vitamin C 75 mg • Hyaluronic Acid 30 mg • Manganese (as manganese bis-glycinate chelate) 10 mg.

Joint Soother - Vitamin World
Three tablets contain: Glucosamine Sulfate (2KCl) 1500 mg • Chondroitin Sulfate 1200 mg • MSM (methylsulfonylmethane) 500 mg. Other Ingredients: Cellulose, Titanium Dioxide Color, Cellulose Coating, Vegetable Stearic Acid, Vegetable Magnesium Stearate, Silica.

Joint Support - NOW Foods
Three capsules contain: Vitamin B3 (Niacinamide) 100mg • Vitamin B5 (Pantothenic Acid) 100 mg • Vitamin B6 (Pyridoxine HCl) 50 mg • Vitamin C (Ascorbic Acid) 100 mg • Magnesium (Oxide) 200 mg • Zinc (Picolinate) 15 mg • Manganese (Amino Acid Chelate) 7 mg • Copper (Amino Acid Chelate) 3 mg • Glucosamine HCl 1000 mg • Boswellin standardized herbal extract of Boswellia serrata 300 mg • Sea Cucumber 300 mg • Bromelain (2000 GDU activity from pineapple) 150 mg • PABA (Para-Aminobenzoic Acid) 10 mg • Devil's Claw (Harpagophytum procumbens) 100 mg.

Joint Support - Futurebiotics LLC
Four tablets contain: Devil's Claw 400 mg • Yucca 300 mg • Horsetail 200 mg • Ginger 200 mg • Alfalfa juice concentrate 200 mg • Chinese Cinnamon 250 mg • Magnesium: (oxide, chloride, ascorbate) 400 mg • Beta Carotene 250 mg • Vitamin C (ascorbic acid, Rose hips) 120 mg • Niacin 8 mg • Niacinamide 250 mg • Vitamin D (Fish oils) 200 IU • Vitamin E (natural) 25 IU • Vitamin B6 (pyridoxine HCl) 8 mg • Vitamin B12 (cyanocobalamin) 12 mcg • Zinc (sulfate) 15 mg • Copper (gluconate) 750 mcg • Biotin 80 mcg • Pantothenic Acid 35 mg • Selenium (methionate) 120 mcg • Glutamic Acid HCl 100 mg • Lecithin 100 mg • Betaine HCl 75 mg • Para Amino Benzoic Acid (PABA) 25 mg • Potassium (sulfate) 20 mg.

Joint Support - Olympia Nutrition
Glucosamine • Boswellin • Sea Cucumber • Bromelain • Yucca • Alfalfa.

Joint Support - Eidon Inc.
Each 1 tbsp serving contains: Silica 62.5 mg • Sulfur 10 mg. Other Ingredients: Purified Water.

Joint Support - Arrowroot
Each tablet contains: Vitamin C (as ascorbic acid) 100 mg • Niacin (as niacinamide) 25 mg • Pantothenic Acid (as D-calcium pantothenate) 25 mg • Manganese (as amino acid chelate) 25 mg • Glucosamine Sulfate (from 1333 mg of glucosamine sulfate potassium chloride) 1000 mg • Chondroitin Sulfate Complex 100 mg • Boswellia Serrata extract (standardized to 40% boswellic acids) 100 mg • MSM (methylsulfonylmethane) 100 mg • Turmeric root

BRAND NAMES

extract (standardized to 95% curcumin) 50 mg • Bromelain (standardized to 1800 GDU) 25 mg • Grape seed extract 10 mg • Quercetin 10 mg • Ginger root powder 50 mg • L-Proline 50 mg. Other Ingredients: Magnesium Stearate, Cellulose, Vegetable Stearin, Dicalcium Phosphate, Silica.
See Editor's Note No. 15.

Joint Support **-** Herbalife International of America, Inc.
Each tablet contains: Glucosamine Sulfate, Potassium Salt 500 mg • Methylsulfonylmethane (MSM) 250 mg • Dried Boswellia gum extract (boswellia serrata) 75 mg • Enzyme HL2-491 40 mg: Peptizyme SP brand Endopeptidase, Bromelain fruit • Dried Turmeric root extract 20 mg • Bioperine brand dried Black Pepper fruit extract 1 mg. Other Ingredients: Microcrystalline Cellulose, Maltodextrin, Stearic Acid, Croscarmellose Sodium, Silicon Dioxide, Soy Lecithin, Hydroxypropyl Methylcellulose, Dextrose, Carboxymethylcellulose, Magnesium Stearate, Polyethylene Glycol, Sodium Citrate.

Joint Support **-** Weil Lifestyle, LLC
Each Glucosamine capsule contains: Glucosamine Sulfate 500 mg. Each Joint Support Formula softgel contains: Holy Basil 50 mg • Ginger SBSC 50 mg • Green Tea 50 mg • Rosemary 50 mg • Turmeric 50 mg • Hu Zhang 40 mg • Barberry 20 mg • Chinese Goldthread 20 mg • Oregano 20 mg • Scutellaria Baicalensis 10 mg.

Joint Support Formula **-** Health Smart Vitamins
Each capsule contains: Methylsulfonylmethane (MSM) 333 mg • Glucosamine Sulfate 200 mg • Chondroitin Sulfate 67 mg.
See Editor's Note No. 15.

Joint Synergy **-** Olympia Nutrition
Glucosamine Sulfate • Sea Cucumber • MSM • Hydrolyzed Cartilage.

Joint Synergy + **-** Metabolic Response Modifiers
Four capsules contain: Glucosamine Sulfate (KCl) 1000 mg • MSM (methyl-sulfonyl-methane) 500 mg • Panax Pseudoginseng (noto-panax ginseng, 50-60% Saponins supplying 45% Ginsenosides) 100 mg • Chondroitin complex 280 mg • Collagen complex 200 mg • Sea Cucumber (25% mucopolysaccharides) 100 mg • CMO (25%) 100 mg • Boswellia serrata 200 mg • Bromelain (2400 GDU) 100 mg • White Willow bark (0.1% salicylates) 80 mg • Tumeric (95% curcuminoids) 75 mg • Manganese (citrate) 8 mg.
See Editor's Note No. 15.

Joint2Life **-** Mosaic Nutraceuticals Corp
Each chew contains: Glucosamine 500 mg • Celadrin brand Cetylated Fatty Acids oil 200 mg. Other Ingredients: Corn Syrup, Sugar, Natural and Artificial Flavors, Mono & Diglycerides, Soya Lecithin, Salt, FD&C Red 1, FD&C Blue 1, Fulvic Acid.

Jointace Capsules **-** Vitabiotics
Two capsules contain: Glucosamine Sulfate 400 mg • Omega-3 Fish Oil 400 mg • Cod Liver Oil 400 mg • Vitamin D 10 mcg • Vitamin E 80 mg • Vitamin C 60 mg • Folic Acid 500 mcg • Vitamin B12 20 mcg • Zinc 15 mg • Manganese 3 mg • Copper 2 mg • Selenium 160 mcg • Boron 1.5 mg • Lecithin 30 mg.

Jointace Fizz **-** Vitabiotics
Each tablet contains: Glucosamine Sulfate 675 mg • Chondroitin Sulfate 100 mg • Vitamin C 60 mg • Magnesium 25 mg • Ginger extract 40 mg.
See Editor's Note No. 15.

Jointace Tablets **-** Vitabiotics
Two tablets contain: Glucosamine Sulfate 1000 mg • Chondroitin Sulfate 400 mg • Vitamin D 10 mcg • Vitamin E 40 mg • Vitamin C 60 mg • Folic Acid 400 mcg • Vitamin B12 20 mcg • Zinc 10 mg • Manganese 4 mg • Copper 1 mg • Selenium 120 mcg • Ginger root extract 80 mg.
See Editor's Note No. 15.

JointFlex **-** SmartScience Laboratories, Inc.
Active Ingredient: Camphor (3.1%). Inactive Ingredients: Acetylated lanolin, acrylates/C10-30, alkyl acrylate, crosspolymer, aloe vera, C12-15 alkyl benzoate, chondroitin sulfate, purified water, diazolidnyl urea, dimethicone, dimethiconol stearate, disodium EDTA, dl panthenol, glucosamine sulfate, glycerin, glycerol stearate, glycosaminoglycans, hydroxylated lanolin, hydroxypropylene methylcellulose, lodopropynyl, butylcarbomate, methyl gluceth-20, methyl glucose, sesquistearate, peppermint oil, polysorbate 20, potassium carbomer, tocopheryl acetate.
See Editor's Note No. 15.

JointPower **-** Trimedica
Six capsules contain: Glucosamine Sulfate 1500 mg • Vitamin C 1000 mg • natural Vitamin E (Succinate) 800 IU • Manganese (Chelated Manganese Gluconate) 5 mg • Zinc (Chelated Zinc Picolinate) 15 mg • Copper (Chelated Copper Gluconate) 1.5 mg • Tumeric (Curcuma longa) extract (standardized for 95% Curcumin) 1300 mg • Boswellia serrata extract (standardized for 60-65 Boswellic Acids) 100 mg • Bromelain 100 mg • Selenium (from Selenomethionine) 200 mcg.

Joint-Ritis **-** Naturopathic Labs Intl., Inc.
Active Ingredient: Natural Menthol 16%. Inactive Ingredients: Lanolin, Eucalyptus Oil, Copaiba Oil, Lavender Oil, Glucosamine Sulfate, Chondroitin Sulfate.
See Editor's Note No. 15.

Joints Formula **-** Nature's Way
Three capsules contain: Alfalfa concentrate 125 mg • Boswellia dried extract 300 mg • Copper (Amino Acid Chelate) 1 mg • Glucosamine HCL 750 mg • Grape seed dried extract 48 mg • Manganese Amino Acid Chelate 5 mg • Nettle root 250 mg • Wild Yam root 75 mg • Zinc Amino Acid Chelate 7.5 mg. Other ingredients: Gelatin, Magnesium Stearate, Millet.

Jojoba & E Skin Oil **-** Derma E
90% Jojoba • 10% Vitamin E oil.

Juice Plus+ Garden Blend **-** NSA International
Two capsules contain: Proprietary Blend 1500 mg: Vegetable juice powder and pulp from Carrots, Parsley, Beets, Kale, Broccoli, Cabbage, Spinach, and Tomato; Lipase, Amylase, Protease, Cellulase, Beet Fiber, Barley Bran, Oat Bran, Cabbage Fiber, Glucomannan, Plant Cellulose, dried Plant Fiber, Lactobacillus Acidophilus, Anthocyanins, Allicin, Lycopene, Polyphenol Catechins, Dunaliella Salina, Indole Carbinols.
See Editor's Note No. 35.

Juice Plus+ Orchard Blend **-** NSA International
Two capsules contain: Proprietary Blend 1500 mg: Fruit juice powder and pulp from Apple, Orange, Pineapple, Cranberry, Peach, Acerola Cherry, Papaya, Bromelain, Papain, Lipase, Amylase, Protease, Cellulase, Apple Pectin, Citrus Pectin, Date Fiber, Prune Powder, Glucomannan, Citrus Bioflavonoids, Dried Plant Fiber, Lactobacillus Acidophilus, Anthocyanins, Polyphenol Catechins, Dunaliella Salina, Indole Carbinoles.
See Editor's Note No. 36.

JuiceRX **-** Harcourt & Johnston
100% pure whole leaf Aloe Vera juice, Honey, Eleuthero Ginseng, Wild Cherry, Cultivated Seaweed (alaria valida, costaria costata, fucus gardneri, gigartina, laminaria, nereocysts, phodymprhenia pertusa, ulva latuca, ulva linza), Citric Acid, Spirulina, Potassium Benzoate, Potassium Sorbate.

Juicy Fruit-C **-** Metagenics
Each tablet contains: Vitamin C (as ascorbic acid) 500 mg • Citrus Bioflavonoid Complex 7 mg.

Jungamals **-** Pharmanex
Each capsule contains: Vitamin A (as vitamin A palmitate, 50% as beta-carotene) 2500 IU • Vitamin C (sodium ascorbate) 150 mg • Vitamin D (D3, as cholecalciferol) 200 IU • Vitamin E (D-alpha tocopheryl acetate) 30 IU • Vitamin K (phytonadione) 20 mcg • Thiamin (thiamin mononitrate) 0.75 mg • Riboflavin (riboflavin) 0.85 mg • Niacin (niacinamide) 10 mg • Vitamin B6 (as pyridoxine

hydrochloride) 1 mg • Folate (as folic acid) 200 mcg • Vitamin B12 (as cyanocobalamin) 3 mcg • Biotin (as biotin) 150 mcg • Pantothenic Acid (as D-calcium pantothenate) 5 mg • Calcium (calcium carbonate, calcium citrate) 150 mg • Iron (iron chelate) 4.5 mg • Iodine (as potassium iodide) 37.5 mcg • Magnesium (magnesium aspartate, magnesium oxide) 100 mg • Zinc (zinc chelate) 3.75 mg • Selenium (L-selenomethionine, sodium selenite) 35 mcg • Copper (as copper chelate, copper oxide) 0.5 mg • Manganese (as manganese chelate) 0.5 mg • Chromium (as chromium chelate) 60 mcg • Molybdenum (as molybdenum chelate) 37.5 mcg • Silicon (as sodium metasilicate) 1 mg. Other Ingredients: Fructose, Sorbitol, Sucrose, Natural Flavors, Citric Acid, Stearic Acid, Tumeric (for color), Carrageenan Gum, Microcrystalline Cellulose, Malic Acid, Carmine (for color).

Juniper Berry Supreme **- Gaia Herbs**
Thirty drops contain: Proprietary Blend 70 mg: Juniper berry extract (juniperis communis), Spring Horsetail herb (equisetum arvense), Corn Silk (zea mays), Goldenrod leaf and tops (solidago odora/ canadensis), Cleavers herb (galium aparine), Marshmallow root (althaea officinalis) • 45-55% Pure Grain Alcohol, USP • Spring Water.

Just An Ounce Calcium/Magnesium Lead Free **- Trimedica**
Each fluid ounce contains: Calcium 1200 mg • Magnesium 600 mg • Iron 5 mg • Zinc 5 mg • Manganese 5 mg • Copper 1 mg • Chromium 0.2 mg • Selenium 0.2 mg • Molybdenum 0.2 mg • Vanadium 0.1 mg • Potassium 90 mg • Iodine 0.15 mg • Boron 0.05 mg • Vitamin D 400 IU. Other Ingredients: Purified Water, Glycerine, Calcium, Carbonate, Magnesium Hydroxide, Mineral Extracts, Additional Trace Mineral Blend: Silver, Antimony, Barium, Beryllium, Bismuth, Bromine, Carbon, Cerium, Cesium, Chlorine, Cobalt, Dysprosium, Erbium, Europium, Fluorine, Gadolinium, Gallium, Gold, Hafnium, Holmium, Niobium, Nitrogen, Osmium, Oxygen, Palladium, Phosphorus, Platinum, Praseodymium, Rhenium, Ruthenium, Samarium, Scandium, Silicon, Sodium, Strontium, Sulfur, Tantalum, Tellurium, Terbium, Thallium, Thorium, Thulium, Tin, Titanium, Tungsten, Ytterbium, Zirconium.

Just Natural Timed Release Vitamin C with Rose Hips 1000 mg **- Walgreens**
Each caplet contains: Vitamin C (from ascorbic acid, rose hips) 1000 mg. Other Ingredients: Hydroxypropyl Methylcellulose, Talc, Stearic Acid, Silicon Dioxide, Magnesium Stearate, Colloidal Silicon Dioxide, Carnauba Wax.

Just Once B-Complete **- Rainbow Light**
Each tablet contains: Thiamin (vitamin B1) 50 mg • Riboflavin (vitamin B2) 50 mg • Niacinamide (vitamin B3) 50 mg • Pyridoxine HCl (vitamin B6) 50 mg • Folic Acid 400 mcg • Cyanocobalamin (vitamin B12) 50 mcg • Biotin 300 mcg • Pantothenic Acid (vitamin B5) 50 mg • Choline 42 mg • Inositol 50 mg • PABA (para-aminobenzoic acid) 50 mg • Rice Bran 50 mg • Rice Bran 4:1 extract (equivalent to 100 mg of rice bran powder) 25 mg • Spirulina 30 mg • Siberian Ginseng root 100 mg • Vegetables, Herbs & Greens 4:1 extracts (equivalent to 60 mg of whole food powder) 15 mg: Astragalus root, Beet, Broccoli, Carrot, Celery, Green Beans, Horsetail herb, Jujube fruit, Stinging Nettle tops, Parsley, Seaweed, Spinach. Inactive Ingredients: Vegetable Gum, Modified Cellulose, Cellulose, Silica, Stearic Acid (vegetable), Magnesium Stearate, Vegetable Food Glaze.

Just Once Daily Herbs **- Rainbow Light**
Each tablet contains: 2:1 Herbal extracts (equivalent to 900 mg of herbal powder) 450 mg: Reishi herb, Siberian Ginseng root, Milk Thistle seed, Ginger root, Schisandra fruit, Vegetarian Cordyceps herb, Gentian root • Siberian Ginseng root 400 mg • Spirulina 100 mg. Inactive Ingredients: Vegetable Gum, Microcrystalline Cellulose, Silica, Stearic Acid (vegetable), Magnesium Stearate, Vegetable Food Glaze.

Just Once Food-Based C-1000 **- Rainbow Light**
Each tablet contains: Vitamin C (ascorbic acid) 1000 mg • Citrus Bioflavonoids 50 mg • Whole Food Blend 40 mg: Orange, Guava, Broccoli • Elderberry fruit (2:1 extract, equivalent to 30 mg of herbal powder) 15 mg • Spirulina 10 mg. Inactive Ingredients: Cellulose, Stearic Acid (vegetable), Modified Cellulose, Silica, Magnesium Stearate, Vegetable Food Glaze.

Just Once Food-Based Calcium **- Rainbow Light**
Each tablet contains: Calcium (carbonate, amino acid chelate, citrate-malate) 500 mg • Magnesium (oxide, aspartate) 250 mg • Vitamin D 100 IU • Stinging Nettles tops 20 mg • Horsetail whole herb 20 mg • Spirulina 20 mg • Glutamic Acid HCl 20 mg. Inactive Ingredients: Cellulose, Stearic Acid (vegetable), Modified Cellulose Gum, Silica, Magnesium Stearate, Vegetable Food Glaze.

Just Once Food-Based Magnesium **- Rainbow Light**
Each tablet contains: Magnesium (oxide) 400 mg • Chlorella 20 mg • Spirulina 20 mg • 2:1 Herbal extracts (equivalent to 50 mg of herbal powder) 25 mg: Fennel seed, Peppermint leaf. Inactive Ingredients: Microcrystalline Cellulose, Stearic Acid (vegetable), Modified Cellulose Gum, Silica, Magnesium Stearate, Vegetable Food Glaze.

Just Once Iron-Free Multivitamin **- Rainbow Light**
Each tablet contains: Vitamin A (beta-carotene) 10,000 IU • Vitamin C (ascorbic acid, magnesium ascorbate) 200 mg • Vitamin D 100 IU • Vitamin E (dl-alpha tocopheryl succinate) 60 IU • Vitamin K (phytonadione) 30 mcg • Thiamin (vitamin B1) 6 mg • Riboflavin (vitamin B2) 6 mg • Niacinamide (vitamin B3) 30 mg • Pyridoxine (vitamin B6) 6 mg • Folic Acid 400 mcg • Cyanocobalamin (vitamin B12) 25 mcg • Biotin 300 mcg • Pantothenic Acid (vitamin B5) 30 mg • Calcium (amino acid chelate) 30 mg • Iodine (from kelp) 100 mcg • Magnesium (glycinate, ascorbate) 30 mg • Zinc (citrate, monomethionine) 5 mg • Selenium (selenomethionine) 25 mcg • Copper (glycinate) 500 mcg • Manganese (glycinate) 2.5 mg • Chromium (dinicotinate) 50 mcg • Molybdenum (aspartate) 12 mcg • Potassium (chloride, citrate) 20 mg • Boron (citrate, asparate, glycinate) 50 mcg • Vanadium (vanadyl sulfate) 8 mcg • Bioflavonoids (from lemon) 60 mg • Choline 15 mg • Inositol 15 mg • Rutin 15 mg • Hesperidin 10 mg • PABA (para-aminobenzoic acid) 5 mg • Protease 332 HUT • Amylase 113 DU • Lipase 1.2 LU • Cellulase 1.3 CU • Apple Pectin 20 mg • Green Papaya 12 mg • Spirulina 100 mg • Siberian Ginseng root 75 mg • Tomato Paste powder 40 mg • Ginkgo leaf 30 mg • Wheat Sprouts Complex 20 mg • Vegetable & Herbs Concentrates 20 mg: Horsetail herb, Jujube fruit, Carrots, Broccoli, Spinach, Parsley, Stinging Nettles tops, Celery, Astragalus root, Beets, Green Beans, Seaweed. Inactive Ingredients: Stearic Acid (vegetable), Modified Cellulose, Microcrystalline Cellulose, Silica, Magnesium Stearate, Vegetable Food Glaze.

Just Once Kid's One MultiStars **- Rainbow Light**
Each tablet contains: Vitamin A (as palmitate, beta-carotene) 400 IU • Vitamin C (ascorbic acid) 10 mg • Vitamin D (cholecalciferol) 400 IU • Vitamin E (d-alpha tocopheryl succinate) 10 IU • Vitamin K (phylloquinone) 20 mcg • Thiamin (vitamin B1) 2 mg • Riboflavin (vitamin B2) 2 mg • Niacinamide (vitamin B3) 13 mg • Pyridoxine (vitamin B6) 2 mg • Folic Acid 200 mcg • Cyanocobalamin (vitamin B12) 1 mcg • Biotin 25 mcg • Pantothenic Acid (vitamin B5) 4 mg • Calcium (carbonate) 100 mg • Iron (carbonyl) 5 mg • Iodine (kelp) 25 mcg • Magnesium (oxide) 50 mg • Zinc (oxide) 2.5 mg • Selenium (amino acid chelate) 20 mcg • Copper (amino acid chelate) 250 mcg • Mangenese (citrate) 1.5 mg • Chromium (glycinate, dinicotinate) 30 mcg • Molybdenum (amino acid chelate) 30 mcg • Potassium (citrate) 15 mg • Citrus Bioflavonoids 25 mg • PABA (para-aminobenzoic acid) 1 mg • Spirulina 10 mg • 2:1 Herbal extracts (equivalent to 100 mg of herbal powder) Proprietary Blend 50 mg: Stinging Nettles tops, Ginger rhizome, Peppermint herb, German Chamomile flowers • Organic Vegetables Extracts (equivalent to 50 mg of vegetable powder) Proprietary Blend 12.5 mg: Kamut leaf juice, Barley Grass juice, Oat Grass juice, Alfalfa leaf juice, Dandelion greens, Carrots, Collards, Cauliflower, Stinging Nettles, Parsley, Onions. Inactive Ingredients: Fructose, Dextrates, Natural Orange, Pineapple & Cherry Flavors, Vegetable Stearine, Silica, Magnesium Stearate, Citric Acid.

Just Once Men's One Multivitamin - Rainbow Light
Each tablet contains: Vitamin A (palmitate, beta-carotene) 10,000 IU • Vitamin C (ascorbic acid) 120 mg • Vitamin D (vitamin D3, cholecalciferol) 50 IU • Vitamin E (dl-alpha tocopheryl succinate) 100 IU • Vitamin K (phytonadione) 100 mcg • Thiamin (vitamin B1) 25 mg • Riboflavin (vitamin B2) 25 mg • Niacinamide (vitamin B3) 25 mg • Pyridoxine HCl (vitamin B6) 25 mg • Folic Acid 400 mcg • Cyanocobalamin (vitamin B12) 25 mcg • Biotin 150 mcg • Pantothenic Acid (vitamin B5) 25 mg • Calcium (citrate-malate) 50 mg • Magnesium (oxide) 25 mg • Zinc (citrate) 20 mg • Selenium (selenomethionine, amino acid chelate) 200 mcg • Copper (amino acid chelate) 2 mg • Chromium (amino acid chelate) 200 mcg • Molybdenum (amino acid chelate) 75 mcg • Choline (bitartrate) 25 mg • PABA (para-aminobenzoic acid) 25 mg • Inositol 25 mg • Citrus Bioflavonoids 25 mg • Saw Palmetto berry (2:1 extract equivalent to 100 mg of herbal powder) 50 mg • Tomato Paste Concentrate (providing lycopene) 50 mg • Spirulina 50 mg • Protease 664 HUT • Amylase 226 DU • Lipase 2.4 LU • Cellulase 2.7 CU. Inactive Ingredients: Vegetable Cellulose, Microcrystalline Cellulose, Stearic Acid (vegetable), Magnesium Stearate, Silica, Vegetable Food Glaze.

Just Once Multivitamin - Rainbow Light
Each tablet contains: Vitamin A (beta-carotene) 10,000 IU • Vitamin C (ascorbic acid, magnesium ascorbate) 240 mg • Vitamin D 100 IU • Vitamin E (d-alpha tocopheryl) 60 IU • Vitamin K 30 mcg • Thiamin (vitamin B1) 6 mg • Riboflavin (vitamin B2) 6 mg • Niacinamide (vitamin B3) 30 mg • Pyridoxine (vitamin B6) 6 mg • Folic Acid 400 mcg • Cyanocobalamin (vitamin B12) 25 mcg • Biotin 300 mcg • Pantothenic Acid (vitamin B5) 30 mg • Calcium (amino acid chelate) 30 mg • Iron (glycinate) 2 mg • Iodine (from kelp) 100 mcg • Magnesium (glycinate, ascorbate) 30 mg • Zinc (citrate, monomethionine) 5 mg • Selenium (selenomethionine) 25 mcg • Copper (glycinate) 500 mcg • Manganese (glycinate) 2 mg • Chromium (dinicotinate) 50 mcg • Molybdenum (aspartate) 10 mcg • Potassium (chloride, citrate) 20 mg • Boron (glycinate) 50 mcg • Vanadium (vanadyl sulfate) 8 mcg • Bioflavonoids (from lemon) 60 mg • Rutin 15 mg • Choline 15 mg • Inositol 15 mg • Hesperidin 10 mg • PABA (para-aminobenzoic acid) 5 mg • Protease 1189 HUT • Amylase 93 DU • Lipase 1 LU • Cellulase 1 CU • Apple Pectin 20 mg • Green Papaya 10 mg • Spirulina 100 mg • Siberian Ginseng root 70 mg • Ginkgo leaf 30 mg • Wheat sprouts 20 mg • Stinging Nettles tops (4:1 extract) 10 mg • Carotene Complex 10 mg: Carrot root, Parsley leaf • Spinach leaf 10 mg. Inactive Ingredients: Microcrystalline Cellulose, Silica, Stearic Acid (vegetable), Modified Starch, Magnesium Stearate, Vegetable Food Glaze.

Just Once Prenatal One Multivitamin - Rainbow Light
Each tablet contains: Vitamin A (as palmitate 3500 IU, beta-carotene 2500 IU) 6000 IU • Vitamin C (ascorbic acid) 100 mg • Vitamin D (vitamin D3, cholecalciferol) 400 IU • Vitamin E (dl-alpha tocopheryl succinate) 100 IU • Thiamin (vitamin B1) 10 mg • Riboflavin (vitamin B2) 10 mg • Niacinamide (vitamin B3) 20 mg • Pyridoxine (vitamin B6) 15 mg • Folic Acid 800 mcg • Cyanocobalamin (vitamin B12) 25 mcg • Biotin 300 mcg • Pantothenic Acid (vitamin B5) 15 mg • Calcium (carbonate, citrate-malate) 200 mg • Iron (amino acid chelate) 30 mg • Iodine (kelp) 150 mcg • Magnesium (oxide) 100 mg • Zinc (citrate) 15 mg • Copper (amino acid chelate) 2 mg • Vitamin K (phytonadione) 65 mcg • Selenium (selenomethionine) 100 mcg • Manganese (citrate) 2 mg • Chromium (amino acid chelate) 120 mcg • Molybdenum (amino acid chelate) 75 mcg • Potassium (citrate) 10 mg • Citrus Bioflavonoids 25 mg • Choline (bitartrate) 10 mg • Inositol 10 mg • PABA (para-aminobenzoic acid) 10 mg • Boron (glycinate) 1 mg • Protease 660 HUT • Amylase 226 DU • Lipase 2.4 LU • Cellulase 2.8 CU • Spirulina 20 mg • Ginger root (fresh juice, 10:1 extract equivalent to 200 mg of herbal powder) 20 mg • Red Raspberry leaf (2:1 extract equivalent to 100 mg of herbal powder) 50 mg. Inactive Ingredients: Microcrystalline Cellulose, Stearic Acid (vegetable), Modified Cellulose, Magnesium Stearate, Silica, Vegetable Food Glaze.

Just Once Total Antioxidant Protection - Rainbow Light
Each tablet contains: Vitamin A (as beta-carotene from D. salina) 5000 IU • Vitamin C (ascorbic acid) 500 mg • Vitamin E (dl-alpha tocopheryl succinate) 100 IU • Zinc (citrate) 10 mg • Selenium (selenomethionine, amino acid chelate) 100 mcg • Copper (amino acid chelate) 1 mg • Dunaliella Salina 51 mg • 4:1 Herbal Extracts Proprietary Blend (equivalent to 280 mg of herb powder) 70 mg: Bilberry herb, Marigold flowers, Turmeric herb • Tomato Paste powder (providing lycopene) 50 mg • Vegetables, Herbs & Greens 4:1 extracts Proprietary Blend (equivalent to 300 mg of powder) 75 mg: Astragalus root, Beet, Broccoli, Carrot, Celery, Green Beans, Horsetail herb, Jujube herb, Stinging Nettle tops, Parsley, Seaweed, Spinach • Rosemary leaf oil 0.5 mg • Spirulina 40 mg. Other Ingredients: Cellulose, Stearic Acid (vegetable), Silica, Magnesium Stearate, Vegetable Food Glaze.

Just Once Veggies & Greens - Rainbow Light
Each tablet contains: Vitamin A beta-carotene from spirulina) 2338 IU • Vitamin C (from vegetables) 5 mg • Vitamin B12 (from spirulina) 1.1 mcg • Iron (from spirulina and vegetables) 0.7 mg • Spirulina 500 mg • Chlorella 50 mg • Barley Grass 50 mg • Wheat Grass 50 mg • Vegetables, Herbs & Greens 4:1 extracts (equivalent to 600 mg of powder) 150 mg: Astragalus root, Beet, Broccoli, Carrot, Celery, Green Beans, Horsetail herb, Jujube fruit, Stinging Nettles tops, Parsley, Seaweed, Spinach • Broccoli powder 125 mg • Cabbage powder 125 mg • Tomato Paste Concentrate (providing lycopene) 125 mg • Rosemary leaf oil 0.5 mg • Ginger root 50 mg. Inactive Ingredients: Stearic Acid (vegetable), Silica, Modified Cellulose, Cellulose, Magnesium Stearate, Vegetable Food Glaze.

Just Once Women's One Multivitamin - Rainbow Light
Each tablet contains: Vitamin A (palmitate, beta-carotene) 10,000 IU • Vitamin C (ascorbic acid) 120 mg • Vitamin D (vitamin D3, cholecalciferol) 100 IU • Vitamin E (d-alpha tocopheryl succinate) 100 IU • Vitamin K (phytonadione) 100 mcg • Thiamin (vitamin B1) 25 mg • Riboflavin (vitamin B2) 25 mg • Niacinamide (vitamin B3) 25 mg • Pyridoxine HCl (vitamin B6) 25 mg • Folic Acid 400 mcg • Cyanocobalamin (vitamin B12) 25 mcg • Biotin 150 mcg • Pantothenic Acid (vitamin B5) 25 mg • Calcium (carbonate, citrate-malate) 200 mg • Iron (amino acid chelate) 6 mg • Magnesium (oxide) 100 mg • Zinc (citrate) 10 mg • Selenium (selenomethionine, amino acid chelate) 200 mcg • Copper (amino acid chelate) 1 mg • Manganese (citrate) 2 mg • Chromium (amino acid chelate) 200 mcg • Molybdenum (amino acid chelate) 75 mcg • Choline (bitartrate) 25 mg • PABA (para-aminobenzoic acid) 25 mg • Inositol 25 mg • Boron (glycinate) 1 mg • Citrus Bioflavonoids 25 mg • Non-GMO Soy Isoflavones (2.5%) 25 mg • Red Clover blossoms (2:1 extract, equivalent to 50 mg of herbal powder) 25 mg • Dong Quai root (4:1 extract, equivalent to 200 mg of herbal powder) 50 mg • Spirulina 50 mg • Protease 664 HUT • Amylase 226 DU • Lipase 2.4 LU • Cellulase 2.7 CU. Inactive Ingredients: Vegetable Cellulose, Microcrystalline Cellulose, Stearic Acid (vegetable), Silica, Magnesium Stearate, Vegetable Food Glaze.

Just Vitamins - Nature's Plus
Each sustained-release tablet contains: Vitamin A (as beta carotene) 25,000 IU • Vitamin C (as ascorbic acid) 250 mg • Vitamin D (as ergocalciferol) 1000 IU • Vitamin E (as D-alpha tocopheryl succinate) 200 IU • Thiamin (vitamin B1 as thiamine HCl) 125 mg • Riboflavin (vitamin B2) 125 mg • Niacin (as niacinamide) 80 mg • Vitamin B6 (as pyridoxine HCl) 125 mg • Folate (as folic acid) 400 mcg • Vitamin B12 (as cyanocobalamin) 250 mcg • Biotin 125 mcg • Pantothenic Acid (as calcium pantothenate) 125 mg • Inositol 100 mg • PABA (para-aminobenzoic acid) 80 mg • Choline (as bitartrate) 42 mg. Other Ingredients: Microcrystalline Cellulose, Stearic Acid, Di-calcium Phosphate, Hydroxypropyl Methylcellulose, Magnesium Stearate, Rose Hips, Rice Bran, Carob, Papaya, Watercress, Parsley, Pacific Kelp, Alfalfa, Green Cabbage, Acerola Cherry, Pharmaceutical Glaze, Silica.

Just-Whey - SportPharma
Each serving contains: Non-denatured specially filtered Whey Protein concentrate • Ion-exchanged Whey Protein • Natural & Artificial Vanilla Flavors • Acesulfame K.

Juven - MTI BioTech
Each 23 gram packet contains: Arginine (free-base) 7 g • Glutamine 7 g • HMB (calcium-beta-hydroxy-beta-methylbutyrate) 1.5 g. Inactive Ingredients: Citric Acid, Natural & Artificial Flavors, Sugar, Dipotassium Phosphate, Aspartame, Acesulfame Potassium, FD&C Yellow #6 or FD&C Blue Lake #2 and FD&C Red #40.

Juvenon Energy Formula - Juvenon, Inc.
Each tablet contains: Calcium (from calcium carbonate) 78 mg • Alpha Lipoic Acid 200 mg • Acetyl-L-Carnitine HCl 500 mg. Inactive Ingredients: Calcium Carbonate, Stearic Acid, SIlicon Dioxide, Croscarmellose Sodium, Acacia, Magnesium Stearate, White Cellulose Film-coat containing Titanium Dioxide.

K & MG Aspartate - Atrium Biotechnologies
Each tablet contains: Potassium Aspartate (which yields potassium 78 mg & l-aspartic acid 209 mg) 261 mg • Magnesium Aspartate (which yields magnesium 28 mg & l-aspartic acid 242 mg) 278 mg.

K & U - MMS Pro
Each capsule contains: Juniper berries • Parsley herb • Ginger root • Uva Ursi leaves • Marshmallow root • Cramp bark • Golden Seal root.

KAL Beyond Calcium - Nutraceutical Corp.
Each five tablets contain: Vitamin D (as Vitamin D3) (as natural Cholecalciferol) 400 IU • Calcium (as Calcium Citrate) 1000 mg • Magnesium (as Magnesium Citrate) 400 mg • Boron (as Boron Amino Acid Chelate) 6 mg • Horsetail 20 mg • Guaranteed Potency Soy Isoflavones (from NovaSoy supplying 25 mg (40%) Isoflavones and 12.5 mg (20%) Genistin) 62.5 • Ipriflavone (as 7-Isopropoxy - Isoflavone from Ostivone) 200 mg • ActiSorb Base 10 mg: Bioperine brand Black Pepper extract (piper longum), Cayenne (capsicum frutecens), Turmeric (curcuma longa), Rosemary (rosmarinus officinalis), Ginger (zingiber officinale). Other Ingredients: Cellulose, Stearic Acid, Silica, and Magnesium Stearate.

KAL Magnesium Glycinate 400 Vegetarian Formulation - Nutraceutical Corp.
Each tablet contains: Magnesium (as magnesium glycinate) 200 mg. Other Ingredients: Cellulose, Stearic Acid, Magnesium Stearate.

Kalm-Assure - Nature's Plus
Each tablet contains: Rapid Release Layer: Pantothenic Acid (Vitamin B5) 50 mg • GABA (Gamma Aminobutyric Acid) 25 mg • Magnesium (Citrate) 25 mg • Pyridoxal-5-Phosphate (P5P) 5 mg. Sustained Release Layer: Kava (Piper methysticum root) standardized 30% kavalactones 100 mg • Passion Flower (Passiflora incarnata) standardized 4% Isovitexin 75 mg • Hops fruit (Humulus lupulus) standardized 5.2% bitter acids 10 mg • Siberian Ginseng (Eleutherococcus senticosus) standardized 0.8% Eleutherosides 25 mg • Chamomile (Matricaria recutita flower) standardized 1% Apigenin 25 mg.

Kamatone - R-U Ved U.S.A.
Ashwagandha standardized extract • Mucuna Pruriens standardized extract • Tribulus standardized extract • Saffron standardized extract • Amla standardized extract • Shilajeet standardized extract (purified mineral pitch) • Pipli standardized extract • Licorice standardized extract • Bacopa Monnieri (standardized to 50% bacopasides) • Bala standardized extract • Talmakhana standardized extract • Akarkara standardized extract • Muira Puama standardized extract • Colchicum standardized extract • Yohimbe standardized extract.
See Editor's Note No. 39.

Kan Jang (Kanjang) - Swedish Herbal Institute
Each tablet contains: Standardized Andrographis paniculata root extract (4% Andrographolides) 300 mg. Other Ingredients: Mycrocrystalline, Sodium Starch Glyconate, Magnesium Stearate, Zien.

Kaprex - Metagenics
Each tablet contains: Proprietary Blend 440 mg: Luduxin from reduced iso-alpha acids from humulus lupulus extract and magnesium salt, Oleanolic Acid from olive leaf extract (olea europaea), Rosemary leaf extract (rosmarinus officinalis).

Kava 30% - Nature's Way
Each capsule contains: Kava dried extract (30% kavalactones) 350 mg • Passion Flower stem, leaf, fruit & flower 500 mg.

Kava Extract - NSI - Nutraceutical Sciences Institute
Each softgel contains: Kava (Kaviar, kavalactones 84%) 75 mg.

Kava Extract 250 mg - Vital Nutrients
Each capsule contains: Piper Methysticum root extract (kava kava, standardized to 30% kavalactones) 250 mg.

Kava Kava - Olympian Labs
Each capsule contains: Kava extract 500 mg.

Kava Kava - Gaia Herbs
Three capsules contain: Kava Kava rhizome (piper methysticum) 409 mg. Other Ingredients: Lecithin, Vegetable Glycerin, Vegetable Cellulose (capsule).

Kava Kava - Puritan's Pride
Each capsule contains: Kava Kava root (in a millet grain base) 300 mg.

Kava Kava - Leiner Health Products
Each caplet contains: Kava Kava extract (Piper methysticum) root 200 mg. Other Ingredients: Calcium Carbonate, Cellulose, Maltodextrin, Hydroxypropyl Methylcellulose, Silicon Dioxide, Polyethylene Glycol 3350, Croscarmellose Sodium, Hydroxypropyl Cellulose, Crospovidone, Magnesium Stearate, Yellow 6 Lake, Red 40 Lake, Blue 2 Lake, Pharmaceutical Glaze, Polysorbate 80, Titanium Dioxide.

Kava Kava - Pharmanex
Each softgel contains: Kava Kava root (11:1) extract (Piper methysticum) 175 mg. Other Ingredients: Soybean Oil, Gelatin, Glycerin, Maltodextrin, Beeswax, Lecithin, Carob.

Kava Kava - Gaia Herbs
Kava Kava standardized for 5% kavalactones. Standardized Full Spectrum 136 mg of extract per capsule. Guaranteed Potency 68 mg of extract per capsule.

Kava Kava - Quest
Each capsule contains: Kava Kava (provided by 150 mg P.E. 1:12 standardized to 30% Kavalactones) 1800 mg. Other Ingredients: Microcrystalline Cellulose, Magnesium Stearate (vegetable source).

Kava Kava 3000 mg - Jamieson
Each capsule contains: Kava Kava root (Piper methysticum, 250 mg powdered extract 1:12) 3000 mg. Other Ingredients: Gelatin, Calcium Sulfate, Maltodextrin, Cellulose, Magnesium Stearate, Silica.

Kava Kava Plus - The Herbalist
Kava Kava root • Siberian Ginseng root • St. John's Wort flowering tops • Oat seed • Skullcap herb.

Kava Kava Root Extract - Source Naturals
Each softgel contains: Kava Kava root extract (Piper methysticum) (standardized to 40% Kavalactones, yielding 70 mg of Kavalactones) 175 mg. In a base of Soybean Oil, Lecithin and Beeswax.

Kava Kava XTRA - Sundown
Each capsule contains: Kava Kava root extract (standardized to 30% kavalactones, 75 mg) 250 mg • XTRA Premium Blend 100 mg: Hops (strobiles), German Chamomile flower heads, Passionflower flowers/fruit. Other Ingredients: Gelatin, Natural Vegetable Fiber.

Kava Kava-Valerian Virtue - Blessed Herbs
Kava Kava root • Scullcap • Valerian root • St. John's Wort flower • Lobelia • Arnica flower & herb • Grain alcohol & Distilled Water.

Kava Oasis - New Chapter, Inc.
Each softgel contains: Kava root, supercritical extract, (60% kavapyrones- 75 mg) 125 mg • Valerian root, (Valeriana officinalis & Valeriana mexicanus) supercritical extract, (60% valepotriates- 3 mg) 5 mg • Lavender flower, supercritical extract (25% Linalool- 1.2 mg) 5 mg • Passion Flower herb, extract, (3% vitexin- 0.15 mg) 5 mg • Chastetree berry, extract (0.6% aucubin- 0.03 mg) (0.5% agnuside- 0.025 mg) 5 mg • Gotu Kola leaf, extract, (10% asiaticoside- 0.5 mg) (3.% triterpenes- 1.5 mg) 5 mg • Ginger supercritical broad spectrum complex (rhizome), certified organic, (minimum 20% pungent compounds- 1 mg, 4% zingiberene- 0.2 mg) 5 mg • Chamomile flower, supercritical extract (minimum 25% alpha-bisabolol- 1.2 mg) 5 mg. Other Ingredients: Olive Oil (certified organic), Yellow Beeswax.

Kava-30 - PhytoPharmica
Each capsule contains: Kava (Piper methysticum) root and rhizome extract (standardized to contain 30% kavalactones [75 mg of kavalactones]) 250 mg.
See Editor's Note No. 21.

Kava-55 - PhytoPharmica
Each capsule contains: Kava (Piper methysticum) root (rhizome) extract (standardized to contain 55% kavalactones [82.5 mg kavalactones]) 150 mg.
See Editor's Note No. 21.

Kava-77 - Source Naturals
Each softgel contains: Kava Kava root extract (Piper methysticum) (standardized to 55% Kavalactones yielding 75 mg of Kavalactones) 140 mg. In a base of Rice Bran Oil, Lecithin, Silicon Dioxide and Beeswax.

Kavacin - PhytoPharmica
Each capsule contains: Kava root extract (Piper methysticum) 200 mg standardized to contain 30% kavalactones (60 mg per capsule) • Oat Straw extract 10:1 (Avena sativa) 100 mg • Pyridoxine-Alpha-Ketoglutarate (PAK) 50 mg • Pantothenic Acid 50 mg • Nicotinamide 50 mg • Thiamine HCL (Vitamin B1) 25 mg.
See Editor's Note No. 21.

KaValerian Caplet - Leiner Health Products
Each caplet contains: Magnesium Citrate 10 mg • Chamomile extract (Matricaria recutita) flower 50 mg • Kava Kava extract (Piper methysticum) root 75 mg • Lecithin 15 mg • Valerian extract (Valeriana officinalis) root 200 mg. Other Ingredients: Dicalcium Phosphate, Cellulose, Stearic Acid, Magnesium Stearate, Dextrin, Silicon Dioxide, Dextrose, Sodium Carboxymethylcellulose, Sodium Citrate.

Kavatime - Bodyonics, Ltd.
Each tablet contains: Kava Kava Root (Piper Methysticum) 350 mg • Kava Kava Powdered Extract 150 mg • Herbolics Support Complex 50 mg: Barley Malt Flour, Brewers Yeast (saccharomyces cerevisiae), Hops (humulus lupulus), Ginger root extract (zingiber officinale). Other Ingredients: Calcium Phosphate, Magnesium Stearate, Gelatin.

KavaTone - Enzymatic Therapy
Each capsule contains: Kava root extract (Piper methysticum) (standardized to contain 30% Kavalactones 60 mg per capsule) 200 mg • Oat Straw extract 10:1 (Avena sativa) 100 mg • Pyridoxine-Alpha-Ketoglutarate (PAK) 50 mg • Pantothenic Acid 50 mg, Nicotinamide 50 mg • Thiamin HCl (Vitamin B1) 25 mg.

Kavatrol - Natrol, Inc.
Each capsule contains: Kava root extract (30% Kavalactones) 200 mg • In an exclusive base of complementary herbs: Passion flower, Chamomile flower, Hops flower, Schizandra fruit. Other Ingredients: Magnesium Stearate, Silicon Dioxide, Gelatin.

K-B Herb - Wild Rose
Each tablet contains: Uva Ursi leaf 3:1 extract 345 mg • Juniper berry 12 mg • Buchu leaf 57 mg • Parsley leaf 57 mg • Marshmallow root 57 mg • Ginger root 57 mg.

KB-C - Nature's Sunshine
Three capsules contain: Proprietary Blend 1500 mg: Eucommia bark (eucommia ulmoides), Cis-Tan-Che stem (cistanche salsa), Achyranthes root (achyranthes bidentata), Dipsacus root (dipsacus asper), Drynaria rhizome (drynaria fortunei), Poria Cocos (hoelen sclerotium), Morinda root (morinda officinalis), Rehmannia root tuber (rehmannia glutinosa), Astragalus root (astragalus membranaceus), Cornus fruit (cornus officinalis), Dong Quai root (angelica sinensis), Dioscorea rhizome (dioscorea batatas), Epimedium leaf (epimedium macranthum), Ligustrum fruit (ligustrum licidium), Liquidamber fruit (liquidamber taiwaniana), Lycium fruit (lycium chinense), Panax Ginseng root, Atractylodes rhizome (atractylodes macrocephala). Other Ingredients: Gelatin, Water.

Kelp - Jamieson
Each tablet contains: Pacific Kelp 650 mg (Iodine from Kelp not less than 650 mcg).

Kelp - J. R. Carlson Laboratories, Inc.
Each tablet contains: Iodine (from kelp) 150 mcg • Alfalfa leaves powder (medicago sativa) 10 mg.

Kelp 1000mg - Golden Glow Natural Health Products
Each tablet contains: Fucus Vesiculosus herb (kelp) 1000 mg • Iodine 100 mcg.

KetoCal - SHS North America
Each 100 mL of powder contains: Vitamin A 253 IU • Vitamin D (as vitamin D3) 41.6 IU • Vitamin E 2.2 IU • Vitamin K 8 mcg • Thiamin 0.13 mg • Riboflavin 0.13 mg • Vitamin B6 0.13 mg • Vitamin B12 0.26 mcg • Niacin 1.5 mg • Folic Acid 38 mcg • Pantothenic Acid 0.52 mg • Biotin 2.5 mcg • Vitamin C 12 mg • Choline 96 mg • Inositol 27 mg • Calcium 160 mg • Phosphorous 130 mg • Magnesium 22 mg • Iron 2.2 mg • Zinc 1.2 mg • Manganese 0.32 mg • Copper 120 mcg • Iodine 16.4 mcg • Molybdenum 5.2 mcg • Chromium 3.8 mcg • Selenium 6.8 mcg • Sodium 60 mg • Potassium 216 mg • Chloride 100 mg. Ingredients: Hydrogenated Soybean Oil, Dry Whole Milk, Refined Soybean Oil, Soy Lecithin, Corn Syrup Solids, Tripotassium Citrate, Tricalcium Citrate, Potassium Chloride, Tricalcium Phosphate, Choline Bitartrate, Magnesium Hydrogen Phosphate, Calcium Phosphate, Magnesium Acetate, Trisodium Citrate, M-Inositol, L-Isoleucine, L-Tryptophan, Ethyl Vanillin (artificial flavor), L-Ascorbic Acid, Ferrous Sulfate, Aspartame (artificial sweetener), L-Carnitine, Taurine, Zinc Sulfate, DL-Alpha Tocopheryl, Nicotinamide, Manganese Sulfate, Calcium-D-Pantothenate, Copper Sulfate, Beta Carotene (artificial color), Thiamin Hydrochloride, Pyridoxine Hydrochloride, Riboflavin, Vitamin A Acetate, Folic Acid, Chromium Sulfate, Potassium Iodide, Sodium Molybdate, Sodium Hydrogen Selenite, Phylloquinone, D-Biotin, Vitamin D3, Cyanocobalamin.

KETOjuice Tablets - Nature's Plus
Two bi-layered tablets contain: Vitamin A (as beta carotene) 15,000 IU • Vitamin C (as ascorbic acid) 270 mg • Vitamin E (as D-alpha tocopheryl succinate) 4.3 IU • Thiamin (vitamin B1, as thiamine mononitrate) 0.4 mg • Riboflavin (vitamin B2) 0.4 mg • Niacin (as nicotinic acid) 4.5 mg • Vitamin B6 (as pyridoxine HCl) 0.8 mg • Folate (as folic acid) 189.2 mcg • Vitamin B12 (as cyanocobalamin) 6 mcg • Biotin 13.4 mcg • Pantothenic Acid (as calcium pantothenate) 2 mg • Zinc (as zinc citrate) 1.4 mg • Copper (as copper citrate) 0.7 mg • Manganese (as manganese citrate) 1.6 mg • KETOfruit Proprietary Blend 1000 mg: Whole Fruit 10X Concentrates of Apple, Apricot, Banana, Black Currant, Camu-Camu, Cranberry, Orange, Peach, Red Raspberry, Strawberry, Tomato; Standardized Extracts of Papaya, Pineapple, Red Wine Grape • KETOveg Proprietary Blend 1000 mg: Whole 10X Concentrates of Alfalfa sprout, Barley grass juice, Cabbage leaf, Cayenne (capsicum frutescens fruit), Onion bulb, Parsley leaf, Shiitake Mushroom (lentinus edodes mycelia); Celery seed 4X Concentrate; Standardized Extracts of Broccoli floret, Carrot root, Garlic clove, Reishi Mushroom (ganoderma lucidum), Spinach leaf, Spirulina (spirulina platensis) • KETOfiber Proprietary Blend

140 mg: Vegetable Cellulose, Apple Pectin, Modified Citrus Pectin • KETObolic AA Proprietary Blend 100 mg: Isoleucine, Leucine, Lysine, Tyrosine • KETOzyme Proprietary Blend (supplies 11,121 total enzyme units) 50 mg: Bromelain (from pineapple fruit), Papain (from papaya fruit), Amylase (aspergillus oryzae), Lipase (A. oryzae), Cellulase (A. niger), Protease (A. oryzae) KETOflora Proprietary Blend 20 mg: Lactospore brand culture of B. coagulans, Dahlulin PB brand lactic flora growth accelerant and energy enhancer from Dahlia Inulin and Chicory root (cichorium intybus). Other Ingredients: Di-calcium Phosphate, Stearic Acid, Magnesium Stearate, Silica, Pharmaceutical Glaze, Fructooligosaccharides (FOS), Polyphenols, Lutein, Beta-cryptoxanthin, Lycopene, Alpha Carotene, Sulforaphane, Allicin, Gamma-Glutamylcysteines, Triterpenes, Polysaccharides, KS-2 peptidomannan, Chlorophyll.

KETOslim Chocolate Peanut Bar - Nature's Plus
Protein Blend: Soy Protein Nuggets (soy protein isolate, rice starch, brown rice flour) • Whey Protein Isolate • Calcium Caseinate • Vita-Sweet brand Proprietary Blend: Maltitol, FOS (fructooligosaccharides) • Sugar Free Chocolate Coating: Maltitol, Palm Kernel Oil, Nonfat Dry Milk, Dutch Cocoa, Soy Lecithin, Salt, Natural Flavor • Ground Peanuts (peanut butter, peanut oil, peanut flour, dry roasted peanuts) • High Fructose Complex: Fruit Concentrate, Corn and/or Malt • Guar Gum, Natural Flavor • Tri-Calcium Phosphate • Magnesium Oxide • Ascorbic Acid • Niacinamide • Ferrous Fumarate • Vitamin E Acetate • Zinc Oxide • Copper Gluconate • Vitamin A Palmitate • Calcium Pantothenate • Pyridoxine Hydrochloride • Riboflavin • Thiamine Mononitrate • Folic Acid • Biotin • Selenium Amino Acid Chelate • Potassium Iodide • Cyanocobalamin • Super CitriMax brand Garcinia Cambogia extract • Carnitine • Taurine • Apple Cider Vinegar • Phenalgin • Spirulina • Chlorella • Red Kelp • Brown Kelp • Ulva • Red Seaweed • Dulse • Alfalfa Sprout • Barley grass juice • Parsley • Broccoli floret • Olive leaf • Spinach • Beet greens • Irish Moss • Green Oats • Kale leaf • Chicory • Artichoke flower • Collards • Parsnips • Green Zucchini • Dandelion greens • Turnip greens • Peas • Mustard greens • Green Tea • Cabbage leaf • Cayenne • Onion bulb • Shiitake mushroom • Celery seed • Carrot root • Garlic clove • Reishi mushroom • Apple • Apricot • Banana • Black Currant • Camu-Camu • Cranberry • Orange • Peach • Red Raspberry • Strawberry • Tomato • Papaya • Pineapple • Red Wine Grape • Bromelain • Papain • Protease • Lactobacillus Acidophilus • Bifidobacterium Longum • B. Bifidum • Lecithin • Hawthorne • Gugulipid brand Guggulu extract.

KETOslim Shake (assorted flavors) - Nature's Plus
Two scoops (33 g) contain: Vitamin A 3333 IU • Vitamin C 167 mg • Calcium 100 mg • Iron 1.5 mg • Vitamin D 67 IU • Vitamin E 67 IU • Vitamin K 1.7 mcg • Thiamin 8.3 mg • Riboflavin 8.3 mg • Niacin 8.3 mg • Vitamin B6 8.3 mg • Folic Acid 266 mcg • Vitamin B12 333 mcg • Biotin 100 mcg • Pantothenic Acid 20 mg • Phosphorus 67 mg • Iodine 50 mcg • Magnesium 50 mg • Zinc 8.3 mg • Selenium 21 mcg • Copper 0.67 mg • Manganese 1.7 mg • Chromium 100 mcg • Molybdenum 10 mcg • Critical Metabolism blend 50 mg: Super Citrimax brand Garcinia Cambogia, Carnitine, Taurine, Apple Cider Vinegar • Critical Green Whole Food Blend 33 mg: Phenalgin, Spirulina, Chlorella, Red Kelp, Brown Kelp, Ulva, Red Seaweed, Dulse, Alfalfa Sprout, Barley grass juice, Parsley, Broccoli floret, Olive leaf, Spinach, Beet greens, Irish Moss, Green Oats, Kale leaf, Chicory, Artichoke flower, Collards, Parsnip, Green Zucchini, Dandelion greens, Turnip greens, Peas, Mustard greens, Green Tea, Cabbage leaf, Cayenne, Onion bulb, Shiitake Mushroom, Celery seed, Carrot root, Garlic clove, Reishi Mushroom, Apple, Apricot, Banana, Black Currant, Camu-Camu, Cranberry, Orange, Peach, Red Raspberry, Strawberry, Tomato, Papaya, Pineapple, Red Wine Grape • Citrus Bioflavonoids (from citrus limon exocarp) 33 mg • Critical Enzyme blend 17 mg: Bromelain, Papain, Protease • Inositol 17 mg • PABA (para-aminobenzoic acid) 17 mg • Choline (as bitartrate) 7 mg • Critical Flora blend 17 million cells: Lactobacillus Acidophilus, Bifidobacterium Longum and B. Bifidum • Base: Lecithin, Hawthorne, Gugulipid. Other Ingredients: Non-GMO Isolated Soy Protein, Fructooligosaccharides (FOS), Microcrystalline Cellulose, Psyllium seed husk, Bee Pollen. Banana flavor also contains: Banana Flavor. Cappuccino flavor also contains: Cappuccino flavor. Vanilla flavor also contains: Natural Vanilla Flavor. Chocolate flavor also contains: Cocoa. Strawberry flavor also contains: Strawberry Flavor, Beet Juice.

KETOsnax High Protein Gourmet Chips Nacho Cheese - Nature's Plus
Non-GMO Soy Protein Concentrate • Tapioca • High Oleic Safflower or Mid Oleic Sunflower oil • Salt • Non-GMO Defatted Soy flour • Cheddar Cheese powder (cheddar cheese, di-sodium phosphate) • Onion powder • Garlic powder • Whey powder • Tomato powder • Spices • Natural Cheese Flavor • Cane juice powder • Cultured Whey (maltodextrin) • Lactic Acid powder (lactic acid, calcium lactate) • Yeast extract • Paprika extract • Citric Acid • Dehydrated Jalapeno powder.

KETOsnax High Protein Gourmet Chips Savory Ranch - Nature's Plus
Non-GMO Soy Protein Concentrate • Tapioca • High Oleic Safflower or Mid Oleic Sunflower oil • Salt • Non-GMO Defatted Soy flour • Buttermilk powder • Onion powder • Garlic powder • Nonfat Dry Milk • Whey powder • Cane juice powder • Spices • Natural Butter flavor (flavor in soybean oil) • Jalapeno powder • Lactic Acid powder (lactic acid, calcium lactate) • Citric Acid • Yeast extract.

KETOsnax High Protein Gourmet Chips Zesty Barbecue - Nature's Plus
Non-GMO Soy Protein Concentrate • Tapioca • High Oleic Safflower or Mid Oleic Sunflower oil • Salt • Non-GMO Defatted Soy flour • Cane Juice powder • Tomato powder • Dehydrated Molasses (refinery syrup, cane mill molasses and cane caramel) • Natural Flavor (gum arabic, natural vinegar flavor) • Onion powder • Garlic powder • Spices • Natural Smoke Flavor (flavor, maltodextrin) • Paprika • Concentrated Bell Peppers • Yeast extract • Partially Hydrogenated Cottonseed oil and/or Soy Bean oil • Citric Acid • Caramel Color.

KETOtropic Tablets - Nature's Plus
Two tablets contain: Vitamin B6 (as pyridoxine HCl) 50 mg • Copper (as gluconate) 2 mg • Chromium (as polynicotinate) 100 mcg • Rice Bran 100 mg • L-Methionine (free form amino acid) 100 mg • Phytosterol Complex 100 mg • L-Carnitine (L-carnitine-L-tartrate, supplying 51% beta sitosterol, 18% campesterol and 20% stigmasterol) 100 mg • Chinese Green Tea leaf (camellia sinensis, decaffeinated, standardized to 50% polyphenols) 100 mg • Super CitriMax brand Garcinia Cambogia fruit (standardized to 60% [-]hydroxycitrate (HCA) 100 mg • Critical Metabolism Blend 100 mg: Garcinia Cambogia, Carnitine, Taurine, Apple Cider Vinegar • Eleuthero root (eleutherococcus senticosus) 75 mg • Rhodiola root (rhodiola rosea, standardized to 2.3% rosavins, 2.8% salidroside, 70% polyphenols, 5.4% beta-vicianosides, 1.4% rosin, 1.2% rosarin) 75 mg • Gotu Kola root (centella asiatica) 75 mg • Fo-ti root (polygonum multiflorum) 75 mg • Choline (as bitartrate) 50 mg • Inositol 50 mg • Metabromine brand Cacao fruit extract (theobroma cacao, theobromine 2.4 mg, caffeine 0.6 mg) 40 mg • Proteolytic Enzyme Blend 25 mg: Bromelain, Papain, Protease. Other Ingredients: Di-calcium Phosphate, Stearic acid, Magnesium Stearate, Silica, Pharmaceutical Glaze.

KETOzyme Capsules - Nature's Plus
Each capsule contains: Copper (as gluconate) 2 mg • Rice Bran 150 mg • Aminogen (aspergillus niger and aspergillus oryzae complex) 100 mg • Fructooligosaccharides from Dahlia Inulin and Chicory root 100 mg • Lipase (from brown rice fermentation) 50 mg • Protease (from brown rice fermentation) 50 mg • Oxidase (from brown rice fermentation) 50 mg • Bromelain (from pineapple fruit) 50 mg • Lactospore brand microencapsulated pure culture of B. Coagulans (provides 300 million viable cells) 50 mg • Papain (from papaya fruit) 25 mg. Other Ingredients: Silica, Microcrystalline Cellulose, Gelatin, Purified Water.

Key To Sun - Nikken Inc.
Two tablets contain: Chitin Chitosan Powder 300 mg. Other Ingredients: Dextrin, Crystalline Cellulose, Magnesium Stearate.

Key-E 200 IU - J. R. Carlson Laboratories, Inc.
Each tablet contains: Vitamin E (as D-alpha tocopheryl succinate) 200 IU.

Key-E 400 IU - J. R. Carlson Laboratories, Inc.
Each tablet contains: Vitamin E (as D-alpha tocopheryl succinate) 400 IU.

Key-E Cream - J. R. Carlson Laboratories, Inc.
Each gram contains: Vitamin E (as D-alpha tocopheryl acetate) 30 IU.

Key-E Ointment - J. R. Carlson Laboratories, Inc.
Each gram contains: Vitamin E (as D-alpha tocopheryl acetate) 30 IU.

Key-E Powder - J. R. Carlson Laboratories, Inc.
Each 1/4 level tsp serving contains: Vitamin E (as D-alpha tocopheryl succinate) 700 IU.

Key-E-Kaps 200 IU - J. R. Carlson Laboratories, Inc.
Each tablet contains: Vitamin E (as d-alpha tocopheryl succinate) 200 IU.

Key-E-Kaps 400 IU - J. R. Carlson Laboratories, Inc.
Each capsule contains: Vitamin E (as D-alpha tocopheryl succinate) 400 IU.

K-Factors - Alacer
Four tablets contain: Vitamin C (as ascorbates) 780 mg • Vitamin B6 (pyridoxine HCl) 10 mg • Calcium (ascorbate) 50 mg • Magnesium (ascorbate) 20 mg • Manganese (ascorbate) 2 mg • Potassium (citrate and aspartate) 396 mg • Chromium (ascorbate) 25 mcg.

KIC Fuel - TwinLab
Each capsule contains: KIC 500 mg.

Kid Vits - NOW Foods
Two tablets contain: Beta-Carotene 4000 IU • Vitamin A (as Palmitate) 1000 IU • Vitamin B1 (Thiamine HCL) 3 mg • Vitamin B2 (Riboflavin) 3.4 mg • Vitamin B3 (Niacinamide) 20 mg • Vitamin B5 (Pantothenic Acid) 15 mg • Vitamin B6 (Pyridoxine HCL) 4 mg • Vitamin B12 (Cyanocobalamin) 10 mcg • Biotin 100 mcg • Folic Acid 400 mcg • Vitamin C (Ascorbic Acid, Calcium Ascorbate) 120 mg • Vitamin D (Cholecalciferol) 200 IU • Vitamin E (d-Alpha Tocopheryl Succinate) 30 IU • Calcium (Carbonate, Ascorbate) 30 mg • Magnesium (Oxide, Amino Acid Chelate) 20 mg • Zinc (Amino Acid Chelate) 5 mg • Iron (Ferrochel Iron Bisglycinate) 5 mg • Copper (Amino Acid Chelate) 0.2 mg • Iodine (Kelp) 75 mcg • Manganese (Amino Acid Chelate) 1 mg • Selenium (Amino Acid Chelate) 10 mcg • Chromium (Chelavite) 60 mcg • Molybdenum (Amino Acid Chelate) 15 mcg • Acerola 25 mg • Bioflavonoids (40 % Hesperidin) 25 mg • Choline 10 mg • Inositol 10 mg • PABA 4 mg.

Kid-Alert - The Herbalist
Ginkgo fresh leaf (Ginkgo biloba) • Gotu Kola fresh herb (Hydrocotyle asiatica) • Lemon Balm fresh leaf (Melissa officinalis) • St. John's Wort fresh flower tops (Hypericum perf.) • Siberian Ginseng fresh-dried root (Eleuthero sent.). In a base of kosher glycerine, distilled water, and Grapefruit seed extract.

Kidalin Adult Formula - Herbs, Etc.
Catnip leaf • Damiana • Kola Nut • Lavender flowers • Chamomile flowers • Periwinkle herb • Lemon Balm • Licorice root • Oat seed • Grain Alcohol.

Kidalin Child Formula - Herbs, Etc.
Catnip leaf • Damiana • Kola Nut • Lavender flowers • Chamomile flowers • Periwinkle herb • Lemon Balm • Licorice root • Oat seed • Grain Alcohol • Vegetable Glycerin • Orange peel oil • Natural Flavorings.

KidCalm St. John's Wort Complex - Enzymatic Therapy
Two capsules contain: Magnesium (Krebs Cycle Chelate) 50 mg • Vitamin B6 (Pyridoxal-5-Phosphate) 15 mg • Zinc (Krebs Cycle chelate) 15 mg. Other Ingredients: St. John's Wort extract (Hypericum perforatum) standardized to contain 0.3% Hypericin, verified by HPLC 100 mg • Valerian root extract (Valerian officinalis) standardized to contain a minimum of 0.8% Valerenic acids 100 mg • GABA (Gamma-Aminobutyric Acid) 100 mg • L-Tyrosine 100 mg • Kava root extract (Piper methysticum) standardized to contain 30% Kavalactones 50 mg • Melissa extract (Melissa officinalis) standardized to contain a minimum of 5% Rosmarinic Acid 50 mg • Grape seed (PCO) extract standardized to contain 95% Procyanidolic Oligomers (PCOs) 20 mg.

Kid-Ease - The Herbalist
Lemon Balm fresh leaf (Melissa officinalis) Valerian fresh root (Valeriana officinalis) • St. John's Wort fresh flower tops (Hypericum perf.). In a base of kosher glycerine and Grapefruit seed extract.

Kidney Activator - Nature's Sunshine
Four capsules contain: Proprietary Blend 1880 mg: Poria Cocos (hoelen), Sileris root (ledebouriella seseloides), Chaenomeles fruit (chaenomeles lagenaria), Morus root bark (morus alba), Astragalus root (astragalus membranaceus), Psyllium seed (plantago asiatica), Alisma rhizome (alisma plantago aquatica), Peony root without bark (paeonia lactiflora), Atractylodes rhizome (atractylodes lancea), Magnolia bark (magnolia liliflora and officinalis), Polyporus plant (polyporus umbellata), Cinnamon twig (cinnamomum cassia), Citrus Aurantium peel, Ginger rhizome (zingiber officinale), Typhonium rhizome (typhonium flagelliforme), Licorice root (glycyrrhiza glabra). Other Ingredients: Gelatin, Water.
See Editor's Note No. 40.

Kidney Bladder Formula - Nature's Way
Two capsules contain: Proprietary formula: Cramp bark • Ginger • Goldenseal root • Juniper berries • Marshmallow root • Parsley herb • Uva Ursi leaves. Other Ingredients: Gelatin.

Kidney Blend - The Herbalist
Dandelion root • Burdock seed • Uva Ursi leaf • Corn Silk • Echinacea root • St. John's Wort flower • Yarrow flower • Cayenne pepper.

Kidney Factors - Michael's Naturopathic Programs
Three tablets contain: Vitamin D (as calciferol) 300 IU • Niacin (as niacinamide) 60 mg • Vitamin B6 (as pyridoxine) 6 mg • Vitamin B12 (as cobalamin) 30 mcg • Calcium (as calcium amino acid chelate) 75 mg • Magnesium (as magnesium amino acid chelate) 150 mg • Proprietary Blend 2640 mg: Celery seed (apium graveolens), Gravel root (eupatorium purpureum), Hydrangea root (hydrangea arborescens), Juniper berry (juniperus communis), Glutamine (as L-glutamine), Glycine (as L-glycine), Parsley leaf (petroselinum sativum), Buchu leaf (barosma betulina), Uva ursi leaf (arctostaphylos uva ursi), Bromelain (from pineapple). Other Ingredients: Dicalcium Phosphate, Maltodextrin, Magnesium Stearate, Stearic Acid.

Kidney Plus - The Herbalist
Uva Ursi leaf • Juniper berry • Buchu leaf • Echinacea root • Pipsissewa leaf • St. John's Wort flower • Yarrow flower • Cayenne pepper.

Kidney Tea: Soothing Diuretic Tea - The Herbalist
Marshmallow root • Juniper berry • Plantain leaf • Dandelion root • Parsley root • Mullein leaf • Horsetail herb • Nettles leaf • Rosehips.

Kidney/Urinary Tract - Enzymes, Inc.
Each capsule contains: Vitamin A (100% as Beta Carotene from Dunalelia) 4500 IU • Proprietary Herbal Blend 342 mg: Uva Ursi leaves extract, Cornsilk extract, Wild Hydrangea root extract, Goldenrod leaves extract • Protease 75 mg. Other Ingredients: Cellulose, Water.

Kidneycare - PhysioLogics
Two capsules contain: Potassium 50 mg • Dandelion root 300 mg • Astragalus root (70% Polysaccharides, 175 mg) 250 mg • Corn silk 150 mg • Yarrow 150 mg.

Kidney-Liver Complex - Enzymatic Therapy
Two capsules contain: Kidney-Liver Complex (Predigested Soluble concentrate) 500 mg • Artichoke extract (Cynara solymus) standardized to contain 15% Caffeylquinic Acids 100 mg • Multi-Glandular Complex 100 mg: Raw Liver, Raw Lung, Raw Pancreas, Raw Heart, Raw Kidney, Raw Spleen, Raw Brain.
See Editor's Note No. 21 and No. 31.

Kids Be Well - The Herbalist
Astragalus fresh root (Astragalus membranaceous) • Echinacea fresh root (Echinacea angustifolia) • Lemon Balm fresh leaf (Melissa officinalis) • St. John's Wort fresh flower tops (Hypericum perf.) • Ginkgo fresh leaf (Ginkgo biloba). In a base of kosher glycerine and grapefruit seed extract.

Kid's Choice Multi - Golden Glow Natural Health Products
Each tablet contains: Retinyl Palmitate 1.375 mg: Vitamin A 2500 IU • Cholecalciferol (vitamin D3) 10 mcg • Thiamine Nitrate (vitamin B1) 1 mg • Riboflavin (vitamin B2) 1.2 mg • Nicotinamide (vitamin B3) 13.5 mg • Pyridoxine Hydrochloride (vit B6) 1.05 mg • Ascorbic Acid (vitamin C) 60 mg • D-Alpha-Tocopheryl Acid Succinate 1.24 mg:: Natural Vitamin E 1.5 IU • Choline Bitartrate 1 mg • Inositol 1 mg • Cyanocobalamin (vitamin B12) 4.5 mcg • Folic Acid 30 mcg • Biotin 50 mcg • Calcium Pantothenate (vitamin B5) 8.25 mg • Iron (as fumarate) 1 mg • Potassium (as citrate) 2 mg • Zinc (as amino acid chelate) 100 mcg • Copper (as sulfate-anhydrous) 3 mcg • Fucus Vesiculosus extract (kelp) 50 mg: Iodine 4 mcg • Rosa Canina extract (rosehips) 6 mg • Lecithin 5 mg • Calcium (as hydrogen phosphate and dolomite) 12.2 mg • Magnesium (as dolomite) 900 mcg. Other Ingredients: Gluten (from maltodextrin, derived from wheat).

Kid's Choice: Versatile Herbal for Children - The Herbalist
Echinacea root • Lemon Balm leaf • Goldenseal root.

Kid's Herbal Armor - All Terrain Company
Active Ingredients: Citronella oil • Peppermint oil • Cedar leaf oil • Lemongrass oil • Geranium oil. Other Ingredients: Water, Beeswax, Soybean Oil, Aloe Vera Gel, Vegetable Glycerin, Sorbitol, Potassium Sorbate, Citric Acid, Vitamin C, Vitamin E.

Kid's Herbal Armor SPF 15 - All Terrain Company
Active Ingredients: Citronella oil • Peppermint oil • Cedar leaf oil • Lemongrass oil • Geranium oil • Titanium Dioxide. Other Ingredients: Water, Beeswax, Aloe Vera Gel, Bentonite, Vegetable Glycerin, Sorbitol, Lecithin, Potassium Sorbate, Citric Acid, Vitamin C, Vitamin E.

Kids Multi - Jarrow Formulas
Four tablets contain: Vitamin A (as palmitate/beta-carotene; 50/50) 2500 IU • Vitamin C (as ascorbic acid) 100 mg • Vitamin D (as cholecalciferol) 200 IU • Vitamin E (D-alpha tocopheryl succinate) 40 IU • Vitamin B1 (as thiamin mononitrate) 3 mg • Vitamin B2 (as riboflavin) 3 mg • Vitamin B3 (as niacin) 10 mg • Vitamin B6 (as pyridoxine hydrochloride) 2 mg • Folic Acid 200 mcg • Vitamin B12 (as cyanocobalamin) 6 mcg • Biotin 300 mcg • Pantothenic Acid (as calcium pantothenic) 10 mg • Calcium (from milk minerals) 140 mg • Phosphorus (from milk minerals) 60 mg • Iron (from iron protein succinylate) 6 mg • Iodine (potassium iodide) 100 mcg • Magnesium (as citrate) 60 mg • Zinc (as amino acid chelate) 8 mg • Selenium (as L-selenomethionine/sodium selenate 80/20) 50 mcg • Copper (as oxide) 1 mg • Manganese (as citrate) 1 mg • Chromium (as yeast chromium) 60 mcg • Potassium (as potassium chloride) 5 mg • Lutein (from lutein ester) 3 mg • Inositol 20 mg. Other Ingredients: Xylitol, Microcrystalline Cellulose, Sorbitol, Natural Orange and Tangerine Flavor, Beta-Carotene, Citric Acid, Silicon Dioxide, Orange Powder, Orange Juice Powder, Glycerin, MogroPure brand Lo Han Fruit Juice Concentrate (momordica grosvenori).

KidSoothe - PhytoPharmica
Two capsules contain: Vitamin B6 (pyridoxal-5-phosphate) 15 mg • Magnesium (Krebs cycle chelate) 50 mg • Zinc (Krebs cycle chelate) 15 mg • St. John's Wort (Hypericum perforatum) flower head extract (standardized to contain a minimum of 0.3% hypericin and 4% hyperforin) 100 mg• Valerian (Valeriana officinalis) root extract (standardized to contain a minimum of 0.8% valerinic acids) 100 mg • GABA (Gamma-aminobutyric acid) 100 mg • L-Tyrosine 100 mg • Kava (Piper methysticum) root extract (standardized to contain 30% kavalactones) 50 mg • Melissa (Melissa officinalis) leaf extract (standardized to contain a minimum of 5% rosmarinic acid) 50 mg • Grape Seed (PCO) extract (standardized to contain 95% procyanidolic oligomers [PCOs]) 20 mg.
See Editor's Note No. 21.

Killer MRP - Impact Nutrition
ProSpectrum Proprietary Protein Blend: Whey Protein Isolate, Soy Protein Isolate, Egg Albumin, Calcium Caseinate • Soy Lecithin • Maltodextrin • Natural and Artificial Flavors • Fibersol-2 brand Maltodextrin • Vitamin and Mineral Blend: Dicalcium Phosphate, Potassium Chloride, Magnesium Oxide, Ascorbic Acid, DL-Alpha Tocopheryl Acetate, Ferric Orthophosphate, Niacinamide, Zinc Oxide, Copper Gluconate, Vitamin A Palmitate, D-Calcium Pantothenate, Pyridoxine Hydrochloride, Riboflavin, Thiamin Hydrochloride, Vitamin D (D2), Folic Acid, Biotin, Potassium Iodide, Cyanocobalamin • Flaxseed oil powder • Sunflower seed oil powder • L-Glutamine • Sucralose • Branched Chain Amino Acids • Aminogen brand Enzymes.

Kinder Love Children's Multivitamin - Dial Herbs
Vitamin A • Vitamin C • Vitamin B from Yeast extract • Vitamin E • Thiamin • Niacin • Vitamin B6 • Calcium • Phosphorus • Magnesium • Aqueous extract from: Carrots, Anise, Licorice root, Milfoil herb, Horsetail herb, Chamomile flowers, Peppermint Leaves, Watercress, Wheat Germ, Coriander seeds, Nettles, Spinach, Orange peel • Orange juice • Pear juice concentrate • Malt extract • Yeast extract • Maple Syrup • Honey • Rose Hip extract • Wheat Germ extract • Natural Flavor.

Kindermins micellized liquid - Herbalife International of America, Inc.
Each dropper (1 mL) contains: Vitamin A (as retinyl palmitate) 2500 IU • Vitamin C (as ascorbic acid) 40 mg • Vitamin D (as cholecalciferol) 400 IU • Vitamin E (as D-alpha tocopherol) 15 IU • Thiamin (as thiamine hydrochloride) 1 mg • Riboflavin (as riboflavin-5-phosphate) 1.2 mg • Niacin (as niacinamide) 10 mg • Vitamin B6 (as pyridoxine hydrochloride) 1 mg • Vitamin B12 (as biotin) 150 mcg • Pantothenic Acid (as D-panthenol) 5 mg. Other Ingredients: Purified Water, Fructose, Glyceirn, Natural Grape Flavor, Polysorbate 80, Potassium Sorbate, Sucralose, Sodium Benzoate, Alfalfa Extract, Rosehips Extract, Acerola Extract, Chamomile Extract.

Kindervital - Flora Inc.
Vitamin A • Vitamin B Complex • Vitamin C • Vitamin D • Vitamin E.

Kinder-Vites - Atrium Biotechnologies
Two chewable tablets contain: Vitamin A (Palmitate) 2500 IU • Vitamin D (as Vitamin D3) 200 IU • Vitamin E 10 IU • Vitamin K 10 mcg • Vitamin B1 3.2 mg • Vitamin B2 3 mg • Vitamin B6 3.2 mg • Vitamin B12 10 mcg • Vitamin C 100 mg • Niacinamide 13.5 mg • Folic Acid 200 mcg • Pantothenic Acid 5 mg • Biotin 60 mcg. Minerals: Calcium 12 mg • Magnesium 3.2 mg • Manganese 2.5 mg • Copper 100 mcg • Zinc 8 mg • Iron 12 mg • Iodine 100 mcg • Selenium 10 mcg • Chromium 10 mcg • Molybdenum 5 mcg • Vanadium 5 mcg • Citrus Bioflavonoids, Rutin, & Hesperidin 60 mg • Choline 10 mg • Inositol 2 mg • PABA 10 mg. Formulated in a base of pleasant tasting, natural source flavoring & excipients.

Some Brand Name Natural Products - What they Contain

www.NaturalDatabase.com contains MANY more listings than appear here.
Editor's Notes are located on pages 2155-2163.

BRAND NAMES

Kinerase Cream **-** Valeant Pharmaceuticals International
N(6)furfuryladenine (0.1%) • Purified Water • Propylene Glycol • Stearic Acid • Isopropyl Palmitate • Glyceryl Stearate • Laureth 23 Cetyl Alcohol • Safflower oil • Stearyl Alcohol • Soy Sterol • Panthenol • Aloe Vera gel • Hydrolyzed Elastin • Dimethicone • Methylparaben • Propylparaben • Imidazolidinyl Urea • Carbomer • Triethanolamine • Sodium Hydroxide • Ascorbic Acid.

Kinerase Intensive Eye Cream **-** Valeant Pharmaceuticals International
Purified Water • Glyceryl Stearate • Laureth-23 • Isopropyl Palmitate • Propylene Glycol • Stearic Acid • Cetyl Alcohol • Carthamus Tinctorius seed oil (safflower) • Soya Sterol • Stearyl Alcohol • Dimethicone • Imidazolidinyl Urea • Citric Acid • Sodium Hydroxide • Methylparaben • Soluble Collagen • Carbomer • N(6)furfuryladenine • Panthenol • Propylparaben • Triethanolamine • Ascorbic Acid • Hydrolyzed Elastin • Aloe Barbadensis leaf juice.

Kinerase Lotion **-** Valeant Pharmaceuticals International
Purified Water • Glycerin • Stearyl Alcohol • Glyceryl Stearate • PEG-100 Stearate • Safflower Oil • Octyl Hydroxystearate • Cetyl Alcohol • Aloe Barbadensis gel • Dimethicone • Diazolidinyl Urea • Carbomer • Methylparaben • Soy Sterol • Triethanolamine • Panthenol • Propylparaben • Tocopheryl Acetate • Sodium Hydroxide • Ascorbic Acid • Retinyl Palmitate • Cholecalciferol • Corn Oil • N(6)furfuryladenine.

Kinoko **-** Quality of Life Labs
Four capsules contain: AHCC Proprietary Blend 1000 mg: Mushroom Mycelia extract, Candelilla Wax, Cyclodextrin, Microcrystalline Cellulose. Other Ingredients: Silica, Gelatin, Glycerin.

Kinotakara **-** K-Link International
Each packet contains: Tourmaline • Chitosan • Wood Vinegar • Pearl powder • Silica • Dextrin • Glycol.

Kira **-** Lichtwer Pharma US
Each tablet contains: St. John's Wort (Hypericum perforatum, extract LI 160, standardized to contain 0.3% hypericin) 300 mg. Other Ingredients: Sucrose, Lactose, Talc, Powdered Cellulose, Hydroxypropyl Methylcellulose, Polyethylene Glycol, Castor Oil, Magnesium Stearate, Polyvinylpyrrolidone (pvp), Silicon Dioxide, Gelatin, Titanium Dioxide, Carnauba Wax.

Kirkland Signature B-50 Formula **-** Kirkland
Each tablet contains: Vitamin C (from ascorbic acid) 500 mg • Vitamin E (from dL-alpha tocopheryl acetate) 30 IU • Thiamin (vitamin B1, from thiamin mononitrate) 50 mg • Riboflavin (vitamin B2) 50 mg • Niacin (from niacinamide) 50 mg • Vitamin B6 50 mg • Folate (folic acid) 400 mcg • Vitamin B12 (from cyanocobalamin) 50 mcg • Biotin 300 mcg • Pantothenic Acid (from D-calcium pantothenate) 50 mg • Iron (as ferrous fumarate) 18 mg • Zinc (as zinc oxide) 15 mg • Selenium (as sodium selenate) 25 mcg • Copper (as cupric sulfate) 2 mg. Other Ingredients: Calcium Carbonate, Dibasic Calcium Phosphate, Corn Starch, Cellulose Gel, Gelatin, Maltodextrin, Hydroxypropyl Methylcellulose, Crospovidone, Croscarmellose Sodium, Magnesium Stearate, Silicon Dioxide, Polyethylene Glycol.
See Editor's Note No. 45.

Kirkland Signature Calcium with Vitamin D **-** Kirkland
Each tablet contains: Vitamin D (as cholecalciferol) 200 IU • Calcium (as calcium carbonate) 500 mg. Other Ingredients; Maltodextrin, Hydroxypropyl Methylcellulose, Talc, Pregelatinized Starch, Croscarmellose Sodium, Acacia, Hydroxypropyl Cellulose, Silicon Dioxide, Titanium Dioxide, Magnesium Stearate, Polysorbate 80, Yellow 5 Lake, Blue 1 Lake, Polyethylene Glycol 3350, Povidone, Sodium Citrate.
See Editor's Note No. 45.

Kirkland Signature Calcium, Vitamin D, Magnesium & Zinc **-** Kirkland
Each tablet contains: Vitamin D 134 IU • Calcium (from calcium carbonate) 334 mg • Magnesium (from magnesium oxide) 134 mg • Zinc (from zinc oxide) 5 mg • Copper (from cupric oxide) 0.66 mg • Manganese (from manganese sulfate) 1.2 mg • Boron (from sodium borate) 168 mcg. Other Ingredients: Maltodextrin, Croscarmellose Sodium, Hydroxypropyl Methylcellulose, Titanium Dioxide, Magnesium Stearate, Polyethylene Glycol, Silicon Dioxide, Triethyl Citrate, Polysorbate 80.
See Editor's Note No. 45.

Kirkland Signature Chewable Children's **-** Kirkland
Each tablet contains: Vitamin A (from vitamin A acetate, beta carotene) 5000 IU • Vitamin C (from sodium ascorbate, ascorbic acid) 250 mg • Vitamin D (from ergocalciferol) 400 IU • Vitamin E (from D-alpha tocopheryl acetate) 30 IU • Thiamin (vitamin B1,from thiamine mononitrate) 1.7 mg • Riboflavin (vitamin B2) 1.7 mg • Niacin 20 mg • Vitamin B6 2 mg • Folic Acid 400 mcg • Vitamin B12 (from cyanocobalamin) 6 mcg • Biotin (USP method 2) 40 mcg • Pantothenic Acid (from D-calcium pantothenate) 10 mg • Calcium (from tricalcium phosphate, calcium silicate) 200 mg • Phosphorus (from dicalcium phosphate) 100 mg • Iodine 150 mcg • Magnesium (from magnesium oxide) 20 mg • Zinc (from zinc oxide) 15 mg • Copper (from cupric oxide) 2 mg. Other Ingredients: Sorbitol, Dicalcium Phosphate, Mannitol, Natural & Artificial Flavors (cherry, grape, orange), Mono- & Diglycerides, Magnesium Stearate, Stearic Acid, Corn Starch, Paritally Hydrogenated Soybean Oil, Sucralose (SPLENDA brand), Gelatin, Red 40 Lake, Orange Juice Powder, Yellow 6 Lake, Lactose, Blue 2 Lake.
See Editor's Note No. 45.

Kirkland Signature Chewable Vitamin C 500 mg **-** Kirkland
Each tablet contains: Vitamin C (from sodium ascorbate, ascorbic acid) 500 mg. Other Ingredients: Sorbitol, Natural Orange Juice Powder, Natural and Artificial Flavors, Magnesium Stearate, Sucrose, Sucralose, Yellow No. 6 Lake.
See Editor's Note No. 45.

Kirkland Signature Daily Multi Vitamins & Minerals **-** Kirkland
Each tablet contains: Vitamin A (as vitamin A acetate) 5000 IU • Vitamin C (as ascorbic acid) 120 mg • Vitamin D 400 IU • Vitamin E (as dL-alpha tocopheryl acetate) 60 IU • Vitamin K (as phylloquinone) 25 mcg • Thiamin (vitamin B1, as thiamin mononitrate) 1.5 mg • Riboflavin (vitamin B2) 1.7 mg • Niacin (as niacinamide) 20 mg • Vitamin B6 (as pyridoxine hydrochloride) 2 mg • Folate (folic acid) 400 mcg • Vitamin B12 (as cyanocobalamin) 6 mcg • Biotin 30 mcg • Pantothenic Acid (as D-calcium pantothenate) 10 mg • Calcium 162 mg • Iron (as ferrous fumarate) 18 mg • Phosphorus 109 mg • Iodine (as potassium iodide) 150 mcg • Magnesium (as magnesium oxide) 100 mg • Zinc (as zinc oxide) 22.5 mg • Selenium (as selenium dioxide) 45 mcg • Copper (as copper oxide) 3 mg • Manganese (as manganese sulfate) 2.5 mg • Chromium (as chromium sulfate, chromium chloride) 120 mcg • Molybdenum (as sodium molybdate) 75 mcg • Chloride 72 mg • Potassium (as potassium chloride) 80 mg • Silicon (as sodium metasilicate) 2 mg • Boron (as sodium borate) 150 mcg • Tin (as stannous chloride) 11 mcg • Vanadium (as sodium metavanadate) 10 mcg • Nickel (as nickelous sulfate) 5 mcg • Lutein 275 mcg. Other Ingredients: Dibasic Calcium Phosphate, Cellulose Gel, Gelatin, Croscarmellose Sodium, Crospovidone, Magnesium Stearate, Hydroxypropyl Methylcellulose, Silicon Dioxide, Corn Starch, Corn Oil, Polyethylene Glycol, Modified Food Starch.
See Editor's Note No. 45.

Kirkland Signature Daily Multi-Vitamin **-** Pharmavite Corp.
Each tablet contains: Vitamin A (25% as beta carotene) 10000 IU • Vitamin C 120 mg • Vitamin D 400 IU • Vitamin E 60 IU • Vitamin K 25 mcg • Thiamin 1.5 mg • Riboflavin 1.7 mg • Niacin 20 mg • Vitamin B-6 2 mg • Folic Acid 400 mcg • Vitamin B-12 6 mcg

• Biotin 30 mcg • Pantothenic Acid 10 mg • Calcium 162 mg • Iron 9 mg • Phosphorus 109 mg • Iodine 150 mcg • Magnesium 100 mg • Zinc 22.5 mg • Selenium 45 mcg • Copper 3 mg • Manganese 2.5 mg • Chromium 100 mcg • Molybdenum 25 mcg • Chloride 36.3 mg • Potassium 40 mg • Nickel 5 mcg • Tin 10 mcg • Silicon 2 mg • Vanadium 10 mcg • Boron 150 mcg.

Kirkland Signature Daily Multivitamin & Mineral with Lycopene - Kirkland
Each tablet contains: Vitamin A (25% as beta carotene) 5000 IU • Vitamin C 120 mg • Vitamin D 400 IU • Vitamin E 60 IU • Vitamin K 25 mcg • Thiamin (vitamin B1) 1.5 mg • Riboflavin (vitamin B2) 1.7 mg • Niacin 20 mg • Vitamin B6 2 mg • Folate 400 mcg • Vitamin B12 6 mcg • Biotin 30 mcg • Pantothenic Acid 10 mg • Calcium 162 mg • Iron 18 mg • Phosphorus 109 mg • Iodine 150 mcg • Magnesium 100 mg • Zinc 22.5 mg • Selenium 45 mcg • Copper 3 mg • Manganese 2.5 mg • Chromium 120 mcg • Molybdenum 75 mcg • Chloride 72 mg • Potassium 80 mg • Boron 150 mcg • Nickel 5 mcg • Tin 11 mcg • Silicon 2 mg • Vanadium 10 mcg • Lycopene 300 mcg. Other Ingredients: Cellulose, Gelatin, Croscarmellose Sodium, Crospovidone, Magnesium Stearate, Stearic Acid, Starch, Dextrin, Mannitol, Acacia, Vegetable Oil and Oleoresins, Dextrose, Resin, Sodium Carboxymethylcellulose, Sucrose.
See Editor's Note No. 45.

Kirkland Signature Fish Oil Concentrate 1000 mg - Kirkland
Two softgels contain: Natural Fish Oil concentrate 2000 mg: EPA (eicosapentaenoic acid) 360 mg • DHA (docosahexaenoic acid) 240 mg. Other Ingredients: Gelatin, Glycerin, D-Alpha Tocopherol, Water.
See Editor's Note No. 45.

Kirkland Signature Glucosamine & Chondroitin - Kirkland
Three tablets contain: Glucosamine HCl 500 mg • Chondroitin Sulfate 400 mg. Other Ingredients: Cellulose, Hydroxypropyl Methylcellulose, Croscarmellose Sodium, Red Beet Juice Powder, Silicon Dioxide, Magnesium Stearate.
See Editor's Note No. 45.

Kirkland Signature High Energy Packets - Kirkland
Each packet contains: Vitamin A (29% as beta carotene) 3500 IU • Vitamin C 1060 mg • Vitamin D 400 IU • Vitamin E 460 IU • Vitamin K 10 mcg • Thiamin (vitamin B1) 51.5 mg • Riboflavin (vitamin B2) 51.7 mg • Niacin 70 mg • Vitamin B6 53 mg • Folate (folic acid) 800 mcg • Vitamin B12 80 mcg • Biotin 80 mcg • Pantothenic Acid 60 mg • Calcium 1200 mg • Phosphorus 48 mg • Iodine 150 mcg • Magnesium 100 mg • Zinc 15 mg • Selenium 20 mcg • Copper 2 mg • Manganese 3.5 mg • Chromium 350 mcg • Molybdenum 160 mcg • Chloride 72 mg • Sodium 10 mg • Potassium 80 mg • Boron 300 mcg • Nickel 5 mcg • Silicon 2 mg • Vanadium 10 mcg • Lutein 275 mcg • Lycopene 300 mcg • Panax Ginseng root extract 100 mg. Other Ingredients: Cellulose, Gelatin, Maltodextrin, Croscarmellose Sodium, Glycerin, Soybean Oil, Lecithin, Corn Starch, Palm Oil, Hypromellose, Magnesium Stearate, Acacia, Crospovidone, Silicon Dioxide, Coconut Oil, Yellow Beeswax, Stearic Acid, Sodium Starch Glycolate, Sorbitol, Polyethylene Glycol, Mineral Oil, Rose Hips, Titanium Dioxide, Povidone, Talc, Resin, Hydroxypropyl Cellulose, Sucrose, Talc, Sorbitol, Yellow Beeswax, Hydrogenated Hydroxypropyl Cellulose, Kelp Powder, Polyethylene Glycol, Dextrin, Polysorbate 80, Brewer's Yeast, Rice Bran, Glucose, Sodium Lauryl Sulfate, Alfalfa Powder, Para-Aminobenzoic Acid, Parsley Powder, Watercress, Sodium Molybdate, Yellow 5, Blue 1, Carnauba Wax, Red 40, Green 3, Chlorophyll.
See Editor's Note No. 45.

Kirkland Signature High Potency Calcium Vitamin D, Magnesium & Zinc - Kirkland
Each tablet contains: Vitamin D (as cholecalciferol) 134 IU • Calcium (as calcium carbonate) 334 mg • Magnesium (as magnesium oxide) 134 mg • Zinc (as zinc oxide) 5 mg • Copper (as cupric oxide) 0.66 mg • Manganese (as manganese sulfate) 1.2 mg • Boron (as sodium borate) 168 mcg. Other Ingredients: Maltodextrin, Starch, Hydroxypropyl Methylcellulose, Propylene Glycol, Acacia, Talc, Titanium Dioxide, Croscarmellose Sodium, Hydroxypropyl Cellulose, Silicon Dioxide, Polysorbate 80, Magnesium Stearate, Polyethylene Glycol 3350, Povidone.
See Editor's Note No. 45.

Kirkland Signature Mature Adults Daily Multi - Kirkland
Each tablet contains: Vitamin A (50% as beta carotene, 50% as vitamin A acetate) 5000 IU • Vitamin C (as ascorbic acid) 60 mg • Vitamin D 400 IU • Vitamin E (as dL-alpha tocopheryl acetate) 60 IU • Vitamin K (as phylloquinone) 10 mcg • Thiamin (vitamin B1, as thiamin mononitrate) 1.5 mg • Riboflavin (vitamin B2) 1.7 mg • Niacin (as niacinamide) 20 mg • Vitamin B6 (as pyridoxine hydrochloride) 3 mg • Folate (folic acid) 400 mcg • Vitamin B12 (as cyanocobalamin) 30 mcg • Biotin 30 mcg • Pantothenic Acid (as D-calcium pantothenate) 10 mg • Calcium (as calcium carbonate) 200 mg • Phosphorus 48 mg • Iodine (as potassium iodide) 150 mcg • Magnesium (as magnesium oxide) 100 mg • Zinc (as zinc oxide) 15 mg • Selenium (as sodium selenate) 20 mcg • Copper (as copper oxide) 2 mg • Manganese (as manganese sulfate) 3.5 mg • Chromium (as chromium chloride) 150 mcg • Molybdenum (as sodium molybdate) 160 mcg • Chloride 72 mg • Potassium (as potassium chloride) 80 mg • Boron (as sodium borate) 300 mcg • Nickel (as nickelous sulfate) 5 mcg • Silicon (as sodium metasilicate) 2 mg • Vanadium (as sodium metavanadate) 10 mcg • Lutein 275 mcg. Other Ingredients: Dibasic Calcium Phosphate, Cellulose Gel, Gelatin, Croscarmellose Sodium, Magnesium Stearate, Hydroxypropyl Methylcellulose, Silicon Dioxide, Corn Starch, Modified Food Starch, Corn Oil, Polyethylene Glycol.
See Editor's Note No. 45.

Kirkland Signature Natural Fish Oil Concentrate - Kirkland
Each softgel contains: Natural Fish Oil Concentrate 1000 mg: EPA (eicosapentaenoic acid) 180 mg, DHA (docosahexaenoic acid) 120 mg. Other Ingredients: Gelatin, Glycerin, D-Alpha Tocopherol.
See Editor's Note No. 45.

Kirkland Signature Premium Performance - Kirkland
Each tablet contains: Vitamin A (66% as beta carotene) 5000 IU • Vitamin C 120 mg • Vitamin D 400 IU • Vitamin E 75 IU • Vitamin K 80 mcg • Thiamin (vitamin B1) 5.25 mg • Riboflavin (vitamin B2) 6 mg • Niacin 50 mg • Vitamin B6 10 mg • Folic Acid 400 mcg • Vitamin B12 25 mcg • Biotin 60 mcg • Pantothenic Acid 10 mg • Calcium 165 mg • Iron 9 mg • Phosphorus 130 mg • Iodine 150 mcg • Magnesium 50 mg • Zinc 15 mg • Selenium 200 mcg • Copper 3.5 mg • Manganese 7.5 mg • Chromium 200 mcg • Molybdenum 75 mcg • Chloride 90 mg • Potassium 100 mg • Boron 60 mcg • Nickel 6.5 mcg • Silicon 4 mg • Tin 10 mcg • Vanadium 10 mcg • Lutein 250 mcg • Lycopene 300 mcg • Panax Ginseng root extract 55 mg • Ginkgo Biloba leaf extract (standardized to 24% (14.4 mg) ginkgo flavone glycosides) 60 mg. Other Ingredients: Cellulose, Gelatin, Croscarmellose Sodium, Magnesium Stearate, Corn Starch, Glucose, Hupromellose, Povidone, Polyethylene Glycol, Acacia, Sucrose.
See Editor's Note No. 45.

Kirkland Signature Vitamin C 1000 mg - Kirkland
Each tablet contains: Vitamin C (from ascorbic acid, rose hips, hesperidin complex, acerola, lemon bioflavonoids complex, rutin) 1000 mg • Citrus Bioflavonoids Complex 100 mg. Other Ingredients: Microcrystalline Cellulose, Corn Starch, Sodium Starch Glycollate, Magnesium Stearate, Hydroxypropyl Methylcellulose, Stearic Acid, Silicon Dioxide, Carnauba Wax, Polyethylene Glycol.
See Editor's Note No. 45.

Kirkland Signature Vitamin C 1000 mg with Rose Hips - Kirkland
Each tablet contains: Vitamin C 1000 mg • Rose Hips • Citrus Bioflavonoid complex 100 mg. Other Ingredients: Microcrystalline Cellulose, Corn Starch, Sodium Starch Glycollate, Magnesium Stearate, Hydroxypropyl Methylcellulose, Stearic Acid, Silicon Dioxide, Carnauba Wax, Polyethylene Glycol, Acerola, Lemon Bioflavonoids Complex.
See Editor's Note No. 45.

BRAND NAMES

Kirkland Signature Vitamin E 1000 I.U. **- Kirkland**
Each softgel contains: Vitamin E (from dL-alpha tocopheryl acetate) 1000 IU. Other Ingredients: Gelatin, Glycerin, Vegetable Oil.
See Editor's Note No. 45.

Kirkland Signature Vitamin E 400 I.U. **- Kirkland**
Each softgel contains: Vitamin E (as dL-alpha tocopheryl acetate) 400 IU. Other Ingredients: Gelatin, Glycerin, Water.
See Editor's Note No. 45.

KLB6 Grapefruit Diet **- Puritan's Pride**
Four tablets contain: Grapefruit extract 800 mg • Glucomannan 800 mg • Vitamin B6 20 mg • Lecithin 200 mg • Kelp 75 mg • Cider Vinegar 100 mg • Uva Ursi 25 mg • L-Phenylalanine 25 mg.

KlenzTea (World's Best Internal Klenz) **- Nature's Medicine Corporation**
Buckthorn bark • Chamomile flower • Cinnamon bark • Fennel seeds • Ginger root • Milk Thistle • Natural Lemon flavor • Cat's Claw bark • Peppermint leaf • Rose Hip fruit • Senna leaf • Passion fruit • Uva Ursi leaf.

K-Mag Aspartate **- Source Naturals**
Each tablet contains: Potassium (from 565.7 mg of Potassium Aspartate HCl) 99 mg • Magnesium (from 1,027.4 mg of Magnesium Aspartate HCl) 75 mg.

K-Mag C **- Source Naturals**
Each tablet contains: Potassium (Citrate and Ascorbate) 99 mg • Magnesium (Malate and Ascorbate) 75 mg • Vitamin C (Magnesium and Potassium Ascorbates) 500 mg.

K-Mag KG **- Source Naturals**
Each tablet contains: Potassium (from 285 mg Potassium alpha-Ketoglutarate) 99 mg • Magnesium (from 715 mg Magnesium alpha-Ketoglutarate) 100 mg.

Knock Out **- Schiff**
Each tablet contains: Melatonin 3 mg • Valerian extract (valerian officinalis, root) 100 mg • Valerenic Acid 0.8 mg • GABA (gamma aminobutyric acid) 100 mg • L-Theanine 50 mg • Vitamin B6 0.5 mg • Calcium 200 mg • Magnesium 10 mg • Glycine 40 mg.
See Editor's Note No. 26.

Koflet **- The Himalaya Drug Company**
Each lozenge contains: Khadira (acacia catechu) 35 mg • Lavanga (syzygium aromaticum) 20 mg • Haritaki (terminalia chebula) 25 mg • Ela (elattaria cardamomum) 2.5 mg • Tvak (cinnamomum zeylanicum) 2.5 mg • Trikatu 9 mg: Piper Nigrum, Piper Longum, Zingiber Officinale.

Koflet Syrup **- The Himalaya Drug Company**
Each 1 tsp (5 mL) serving contains: Madhu (mel despumatum syn. mel depuratum, purified) 1.25 mg • Guggulu (balsamodendron mukul syn. commiphora wightii, purified) 35 mg • Draksha (vitis vinifera) 35 mg • Vishnupriya (ocimum sanctum, syn. o.tenuiflorum) 25 mg • Jufa (hyssopus officinalis) 25 mg • Guduchi (tinospora cordifolia) 20 mg • Vasaka (adhatoda vasica syn. a.zeylanica) 15 mg • Jaatipatree (myristica fragrans, mace) 15 mg • Yashti-Madhu (glycyrrhiza glabra) 10 mg • Gojihva (onosma bracteatum) 10 mg • Neelapuspha (viola odorata) 10 mg • Triphala 9 mg: Emblica Officinalis, Terminalia Chebula, Terminalia Bellirica • Trikatu 9 mg: Piper Nigrum, Piper Longum, Zingiber Officinalis • Vidanga (embelia ribes) 8 mg • Kantakari (solanum xanthocarpum syn. s.surattense) 8 mg • Taja (cinnamomum cassia) 8 mg • Navasagara (ammonii chloridum) 3 mg.

Kolorex capsules **- Forest Herbs Research**
Horopito (pseudowintera colorata) 175 mg • Anise seed (pimpinella nisum) 175 mg • Gelatine capsules 90 mg.

Kolorex Cream **- Forest Herbs Research**
Horopito (pseudowintera colorata) • Water (aqua) • Cetyl Alcohol • Apricot kernal oil (p. armeniaca) • Tea Tree oil (m. alternifolia) • Ceto Steryl Alcohol • Emulgin B2 (ceteareth-20) • Vitamin E • Aloe Vera extract 200% • Lemon Tea Tree oil • Potassium Sorbate • Lactic Acid.

Kolorex Extra Strength capsules **- Forest Herbs Research**
Horopito (pseudowintera colorata) 350 mg • Anise seed (pimpinella anisum) 450 mg • Vegecap capsule 90 mg.

Kolorex Honey Skin Care Cream **- Forest Herbs Research**
Horopito (pseudowintera colorata) • Water (aqua) • Cetyl Alcohol • Apricot kernal oil (p. armeniaca) • Tea Tree oil (m. alternifolia) • Ceto Steryl Alcohol • Emulgin B2 (ceteareth-20) • Vitamin E • Aloe Vera extract 200% • Lemon Tea Tree oil • Potassium Sorbate • Lactic Acid • Manuka Honey.

Kolorex liquid filled capsules **- Forest Herbs Research**
Horopito (pseudowintera colorata) 175 mg • Anise seed (pimpinella nisum) 175 mg • Virgin Olive oil • Non-GM Lecithin • Plant Derived Cellulose.

Kolorex Mouth & Throat Care **- Forest Herbs Research**
Each 1.7 g sachet contains: Horopito leaf (pseudowintera colorata) • Anise seed (pimpinella anisum) • Lemon grass (cymbopogon citratus).

Kong **- KMS**
Two tablets contain: Damiana leaf powder 400 mg • Ashwaganda root powder 200 mg • Catuaba bark powder 220 mg • Tribulus fruit extract (20% steroid saponina) 200 mg • Muira Puama root powder 200 mg • Horny Goat Weed powder 300 mg • Suma root powder 150 mg • Passion Flower powder 100 mg • Dutch Cocoa powder 100 mg • Yohimbe bark powder 70 mg. Other Ingredients: Microcrystalline Cellulose (plant fiber), Dicalcium Phosphate, Croscarmellose Sodium, Stearic Acid, Magnesium Stearate, Silica, Pharmaceutical Glaze, Talc.

Kong Black Voodoo **- KMS**
Two capsules contain: Catuaba bark 4:1 extract 300 mg • Muira Puama root/stem 4:1 extract 150 mg • Damiana leaf 4:1 extract 150 mg • Maca root extract (lepidium meyenii, standardized 0.6% macamides and macaenes) 100 mg • L-Arginine base 100 mg • Proprietary Virility Blend 300 mg: Saw Palmetto fruit 4:1 extract, Horny Goat weed leaf 5:1 extract (epimedium grandiflorum), Cucostta seed 4:1 extract.

Konsyl Bulk Forming Fiber Laxative tablets **- Konsyl Pharmaceuticals**
Each tablet contains: Calcium Polycarbophil 625 mg. Other Ingredients: Calcium Carbonate, Hydroxypropyl Methylcellulose, Microcrystalline Cellulose, Powdered Cellulose, Polyplasdone, Croscarmellose Sodium, Colloidal Silicon Dioxide, Caramel Color, Magnesium Stearate.

Konsyl Natural Fiber Laxative **- Konsyl Pharmaceuticals**
Each 1 tsp serving contains: Psyllium Hydrophilic Mucilloid 6 g.

Korean Ginseng **- GNC**
Each capsule contains: Korean Ginseng root powder 648 mg. Other Ingredients: Gelatin.

Korean Ginseng 100 mg **- Nature's Bounty**
Each capsule contains: Korean Ginseng root (Panax ginseng, standardized to contain 7% ginsenosides, 7 mg) 100 mg. Other Ingredients: Maltodextrin, Cellulose (plant origin), Gelatin, Vegetable Magnesium Stearate, Silica.

Korean Ginseng 500 **- Golden Glow Natural Health Products**
Each capsule contains: Panax Ginseng root powder 500 mg.

Korean Ginseng 500mg **- Nature's Own**
Each tablet contains: Korean Ginseng root powder (panax ginseng) 500 mg.

Korean Ginseng capsules **- Eu Yan Sang**
Each capsule contains: Radix Panax Ginseng 420 mg.

Korean Ginseng Extended Release 1000 mg - Nature's Plus
Each extended-release tablet contains: Korean Ginseng root (panax ginseng root, standardized 15% ginsenosides) 1000 mg. Other Ingredients: Di-calcium Phosphate, Stearic Acid, Hydroxypropyl Methylcellulose, Microcrystalline Cellulose, Magnesium Stearate, Silica, Pharmaceutical Glaze.

Korean Ginseng Rush - GNC
Each capsule contains: Korean Ginseng root 500 mg • Guarana seed extract (Paullinia cupana) 95 mg. Other Ingredients: Gelatin.

Korean Ginseng Standardized - Sundown
Each capsule contains: Korean (Asian) Ginseng root extract (standardized to 7% ginsenosides, 7 mg) 100 mg. Other Ingredients: Gelatin, Natural Vegetable Fiber.

Korean Red Ginseng - Jamieson
Each caplet contains: Calcium 65 mg • Korean Red Ginseng root (Panax Ginseng) 4% ginsenosides saponins 250 mg.

Korean Red Panax Mega - Susan Ambrosino's Herb Club, Inc.
Each capsule contains: Red Panax Ginseng 384 mg • White Panax Ginseng 20% 96 mg • Siberian Ginseng 0.8% 96 mg.

Korean White Ginseng - Nature's Way
Two capsules contain: Korean Ginseng root 1.02 g. Other Ingredients: Gelatin, Magnesium stearate.

Kosher Omega-3 Liquid (lemon) - Nordic Naturals
Each 1/2 tsp (2.5 mL) serving contains: Vitamin E (mixed tocopherols) 35 IU • Omega-3 Fatty Acids 875 mg (EPA 450 mg, DHA 300 mg, other Omega-3 125 mg).

Krebs Calcium-Magnesium Chelate - Enzymatic Therapy/ PhytoPharmica
Each tablet contains: Calcium (chelated with citrate, fumarate, malate, succinate, alpha ketoglutarate [CFMSA chelate]) 200 mg • Magnesium (as CFMSA chelate) 120 mg. Other Ingredients: Stearic Acid, Cellulose, Magnesium Stearate, Silicon Dioxide.
See Editor's Note No. 21.

Krebs Cycle Chelates (Vegetarian) - Enzymatic Therapy
Four tablets contain: Calcium (chelated with citrate, fumarate, malate, succinate, alpha ketoglutarate [CFMSA chelate]) 600 mg • Iron (as CFMSA chelate) 5 mg • Iodine (from marine organic minerals) 100 mcg • Magnesium (as CFMSA chelate) 400 mg • Zinc (as CFMSA chelate) 15 mg • Selenium (as CFMSA chelate) 15 mg • Copper (as CFMSA chelate) 1 mg • Manganese (as CFMSA chelate) 2 mg • Chromium (as CFMSA chelate) 100 mcg • Molybdenum (as CFMSA chelate) 25 mcg • Potassium (as CFMSA chelate) 99 mg • Boron (as CFMSA chelate) 4 mg • Vanadium (as CFMSA chelate) 50 mcg. Other Ingredients: Cellulose, Modified Cellulose Gum, Stearic Acid, Silicon Dioxide, Magnesium Stearate, Modified Cellulose, Maltodextrin.

Krebs Ionized Calcium - PhytoPharmica
Two tablets contain: Calcium 250 mg.
See Editor's Note No. 21.

Krebs Ionized Chelates - PhytoPharmica
Four tablets contain: Calcium (chelated (Krebs) with citrate, fumarate, malate, succinate, alpha-ketoglutarate; CFMSA chelate) 600 mg • Iron (CFMSA chelate) 5 mg • Iodine (from marine organic minerals) 100 mcg • Magnesium (CFMSA chelate) 400 mg • Zinc (CFMSA chelate) 15 mg • Selenium (CFMSA chelate) 75 mcg • Copper 1 mg (CFMSA chelate) • Manganese (CFMSA chelate) 2 mg • Chromium (CFMSA chelate) 100 mcg • Molybdenum (CFMSA chelate) 25 mcg • Potassium (CFMSA chelate) 99 mg • Boron (CFMSA chelate) 4 mg • Vanadium (CFMSA chelate) 50 mcg.

Krebs Ionized Zinc - PhytoPharmica
Each tablet contains: Zinc 15 mg.
See Editor's Note No. 21.

Krebs Magnesium-Potassium Chelates - PhytoPharmica
Each tablet contains: Magnesium (as chelated (Krebs) with citrate, fumarate, malate, succinate, and alpha ketoglutarate) 250 mg • Potassium (as chelated (Krebs) with citrate, fumarate, malate, succinate, and alpha ketoglutarate) 100 mg.

Krill-plex - Pure Encapsulations
Two softgel capsules contain: Krill oil providing Vitamin A (naturally occurring all-trans retinol) 100 IU, Vitamin E (naturally occurring) 0.5 IU, Omega-3 Fatty Acids 300 mg, EPA 150 mg, DHA 90 mg, Omega-6 Fatty Acids 20 mg, Omega-9 Fatty Acids 85 mg, Phospholipids 400 mg, Astaxanthin 1.5 mg) 1000 mg. Other Ingredients: Gelatin, Glycerin, Water.

Kudja - HerbaSway
Kudzu • Ginkgo Biloba • Blackberry • Green Tea • HerbaSwee (Cucurbitaceae fruit).

Kuff-Soothe - R-U Ved U.S.A.
Cardamom • Piper Longum • Bamboo Manna • Cinnamon. Base: Honey, Sugar.

Kwai ACE - Lichtwer Pharma
Each tablet contains: Dried Garlic (guaranteed 0.6% allicin yield, 1800 mcg) 300 mg • Vitamin A 450 mcg • Vitamin C 80 mg • Vitamin E 20 mg.

Kwai Every Day - Lichtwer Pharma
Each tablet contains: Garlic clove powder 450 mg (allium sativum L). Other Ingredients: Maltitol, Hydroxypropyl Methylcellulose, Calcium Carbonate, Cellulose, Silica, Acacia, Magnesium Stearate, Carnauba Wax.

Kwai Heart Fit - Lichtwer Pharma
Each tablet contains: Garlic powder sucrose 300 mg • Vitamin C (Ascorbic Acid Sorbitol) 80 mg • Vitamin E (Tocopherol Acetate) 20 IU • Vitamin A (Acetate) 2640 IU. Other Ingredients: Talc, Corn Starch, Hydroxypropylmethylcellulose, Polivinylpyrrolidone, Silicon Dioxide, Stearic Acid, Castor oil, Magnesium Stearate, Powdered Cellulose, Glucose Syrup, Titanium Dioxide, Carnauba Wax, Bees Wax, Riboflavin, Beta-Carotene.

Kwai Odor-Free Garlic - Lichtwer Pharma
Each tablet contains: Dried Garlic clove powder (yielding 900 mcg of allicin) 150 mg. Other Ingredients: Hydroxypropylmethylcellulose, Silicon Dioxide, Maltitol, Magnesium Stearate, Magnesium Silicate, Carnauba Wax, Powdered Cellulose, Castor Oil, Gum Arabic.

Kwai One-A-Day - Lichtwer Pharma
Each tablet contains: Dried Garlic (guaranteed 0.6% allicin yield, 1800 mcg) 300 mg.

Kwai Original - Lichtwer Pharma
Each tablet contains: Dried Garlic (guaranteed 0.6% allicin yield, 600 mcg) 100 mg.

Kwik Size XXXL - Labrada Bodybuilding Nutrition
Each serving contains: Kwik Carb: Maltodextrin and Polydextrose • Kwik Pro: Whey Protein Concentrate, Calcium Caseinate, Soy Protein Concentrate • Cocoa powder (dutch processed) • Natural & Artificial flavors • Vitamin & Mineral Blend • Xanthan gum • Dipotassium Phosphate • Aspartame • Peptigen Proprietary Blend: Alpha Amylase, Malt Diatase, Protease, and Lactase • Medium Chain Triglycerides.

Kyno-H - Harcourt & Johnston
Each capsule contains: Adenosine Monophosphate (AMP) 370 mg • 3-0-Methal-Chiroinositol 50 mg • Potassium Phosphate 275 mg • Magnesium Gluconate 30 mg • Cnidium Monnier 3.5 mg • Selenium 0.007 mg • Vitamin B5 (pantothenic acid) 14 mg • Vitamin B12 0.00625 mg.

Kyo-Chlorella - Wakunaga of America
Each six tablets contain: 100% pure broken cell wall Chlorella powder 3 g.

Some Brand Name Natural Products - What they Contain

www.NaturalDatabase.com contains MANY more listings than appear here.
Editor's Notes are located on pages 2155-2163.

BRAND NAMES

Kyo-Chrome Aged Garlic Extract Cholesterol Formula - Wakunaga of America
Two capsules contain: Aged Garlic extract powder 400 mg • Niacin 20 mg • Chromium (as Chromium Picolinate) 200 mcg. Other Ingredients: Microcrystalline Cellulose, Magnesium Stearate (vegetable source).

Kyo-Dophilus L. Acidophilus; B. Bifidum; B. Longum - Wakunaga of America
Each capsule contains: L. Acidophilus [Lactobacillus Acidophilus], B. Bifidum [Bifidobacterium Bifidum], and B. Longum [Bifidobacterium Longum] 1.5 billion cells. Other Ingredients: Vegetable Starch Complex.

Kyo-Green - Wakunaga of America
Each teaspoon contains: Kyo-Green Proprietary Blend 2.5 g • Barley Grass Powder • Cooked Brown Rice • Wheat Grass Powder • Bulgarian Chlorella • Pacific Kelp.

Kyolic - Wakunaga of America
Each caplet contains: Aged Garlic extract powder 600 mg. Other Ingredients: Microcrystalline Cellulose • Magnesium Stearate • Silicon Dioxide.

Kyolic Aged Garlic Extract Enriched with Vitamin B1 and B12 - Wakunaga of America
Each capsule contains: Vitamin B1 (thiamine hydrochloride) 8 mg • Vitamin B12 (cyanocobalamin) 1 mcg. Other Ingredients: Aged Garlic Extract, Liver Extract, Water, Residual Alcohol from extraction.
See Editor's Note No. 14.

Kyolic Aged Garlic Extract Garlic Plus - Wakunaga of America
Two capsules (or tablets) contain: Aged Garlic extract powder 540 mg • Brewer's Yeast 54 mg • Kelp 18 mg. Other Ingredients: Whey, Brewer's Yeast, Alginic Acid (seaweed), Kelp, Collodial Silica, Magnesium Stearate (vegetable source).

Kyolic Aged Garlic Extract Kyolic HI-PO - Wakunaga of America
Two capsules (or tablets) contain: Aged Garlic extract powder (bulb) 600 mg. Other Ingredients: Whey, Alginic Acid (seaweed), Silica, Cellulose, Magnesium Stearate (vegetable source).

Kyolic Aged Garlic Extract Plus Enzyme - Wakunaga of America
Two tablets contain: Aged Garlic powder 700 mg • KYOLIC Enzyme Complex (Amylase, Protease, Cellulose, and Lipase from Aspergillus oryzae and A. niger) 60 mg • Rice Protein-Calcium Complex 40 mg. Other Ingredients: Alginic Acid (seaweed), Colloidal Silica, and Magnesium Stearate (vegetable source).

Kyolic Aged Garlic Extract Plus Lecithin - Wakunaga of America
Two capsules contain: Aged Garlic extract powder (bulb) 600 mg • Lecithin 380 mg. Other Ingredients: Silica, Magnesium Stearate (vegetable source).

Kyolic Aged Garlic Extract Vitamin A, C, E, Selenium - Wakunaga of America
Two capsules contain: Vitamin A (from 12 mg of beta-carotene) 20000 IU • Vitamin C (calcium ascorbate) 240 mg • Vitamin E (d-alpha-tocopheryl succinate) 120 IU • Selenium (L-selenomethionine) 50 mcg • Aged Garlic extract powder (bulb) 400 mg • Green Tea powder (leaf) 89 mg. Other Ingredients: Silica, Magnesium Stearate (vegetable source).

Kyolic Aged Garlic Extract Vitamin C, Astragalus - Wakunaga of America
Two capsules contain: Vitamin C (Ester C) 210 mg • Calcium (citrate polyascorbate) 46 mg • Aged Garlic extract powder (bulb) 440 mg • Astragalus extract powder (root) 200 mg. Other Ingredients: Calcium Citrate, Magnesium Stearate (vegetable source).

Kyolic Aged Garlic Extract Vitamin E, Cayenne, Hawthorn Berry - Wakunaga of America
Two capsules contain: Vitamin E (d-alpha-tocopheryl succinate) 200 IU • Aged Garlic extract powder (bulb) 600 mg • Hawthorn berry (fruit) 100 mg • Cayenne Pepper (fruit) 20 mg. Other Ingredients: Cellulose, Magnesium Stearate (vegetable source), Silica.

Kyolic brand - Wakunaga of America
Garlic.
See Editor's Note No. 44.

Kyolic Cardio Logic - Wakunaga of America
Each capsule contains: Vitamin E (as d-alpha-tocopheryl acid succinate) 50 IU • Vitamin B6 5 mg • Folate (as folic acid) 200 mcg • Vitamin B12 100 mcg • Aged Garlic bulb extract powder 200 mg • L-Carnitine 30 mg • Coenzyme Q10 30 mg • Alpha-Lipoic Acid 30 mg. Other Ingredients: Cellulose, Colloidal Silica, Magnesium Stearate (vegetable source).

Kyolic Echinacea Aged Garlic Extract - Wakunaga of America
Two capsules contain: Aged Garlic powder (bulb) 600 mg • Echinacea extract powder (root) 100 mg. Other Ingredients: Cellulose (pine), Magnesium Stearate (vegetable source).

Kyolic Estro Logic - Wakunaga of America
Each capsule contains: Black Cohosh root extract (standardized to 2.5% triterpene glycosides) 100 mg • Soybean Isoflavones (seed) (standardized to 40% isoflavones) 50 mg • Wild Yam root extract (standardized to 6% total saponins) 33.3 mg • Sage leaf extract 25 mg • Chaste Tree berry extract 12.5 mg • Vervain leaf extract 12.5 mg • Astragalus root extract 12.5 mg • Motherwort leaf extract 12.5 mg. Other Ingredients: Cellulose, Silica, Magnesium Stearate (vegetable source).

Kyolic Formula 100 - Wakunaga of America
Two capsules contain: Aged Garlic extract powder (bulb) 600 mg. Other Ingredients: Cellulose, Magnesium Stearate (vegetable source).

Kyolic Liquid Aged Garlic Extract - Wakunaga of America
Each 1/4 tsp serving contains: Aged Garlic extract (bulb) 1 mL. Other Ingredients: Water, Residual Alcohol from Extraction.

Kyolic Neuro Logic - Wakunaga of America
Two capsules contain: Folate (as folic acid) 200 mcg • Vitamin B12 100 mcg • Aged Garlic bulb powder 400 mg • Lecithin 200 mg • Ginkgo Biloba leaf extract 60 mg • Phosphatidylserine (30%) 50 mg • Acetyl-L-Carnitine 25 mg. Other Ingredients: Cellulose, Colloidal Silica, Magnesium Stearate (vegetable source).

Kyolic One Per Day - Life Extension
Each caplet contains: Aged Garlic bulb powder 1000 mg. Other Ingredients: Cellulose, Silica, Magnesium Stearate (vegetable source).

Kyolic Prosta Logic - Wakunaga of America
Each capsule contains: Zinc (as Zinc Picolinate) 7.5 mg • Saw Palmetto berry extract 160 mg • Aged Garlic bulb extract powder 100 mg • Pumpkin seed oil extract 50 mg • Pygeum Africanum bark extract 50 mg • Lycopene (as tomato oleoresin) 2.5 mg. Other Ingredients: Wheat Germ Oil, Beeswax, Soft Gelatin Capsule.

Kyolic Reserve Aged Garlic Extract - Wakunaga of America
Each capsule contains: Aged Garlic extract powder (bulb) 600 mg. Other Ingredients: Vegetable Protein, Magnesium Stearate (vegetable source), Silica.

Kyolic-EPA Aged Garlic Extract - Wakunaga of America
Two capsules contain: EPA (eicosapentaenoic acid) 560 mg • DHA (docosahexaenoic acid) 240 mg • Aged Garlic powder 240 mg • Vitamin E (mixed tocopherol) 10 mg. Other Ingredients: Glycerin, Soft Gelatin Capsule.

L & V Formula - Dial Herbs
Wild Lettuce • Valerian • Wood Betony.

L. Acidophilus - Nature's Sunshine
Two capsules contain: Lactobacillus Acidophilus (milk free, providing 200,000,000 L. acidophilus) 840 mg. Other Ingredients: Gelatin, Water.

L. Reuteri - Nature's Sunshine
Each chewable tablet contains: L. Reuteri (lactobacillus reuteri) 100 million. Other Ingredients: Mannitol, Xylitol, Lactulose, Mono- & Diglycerides, Malic Acid, Natural Lemon Flavor, Zein (corn protein), Riboflavin Phosphate.

L.B.T. Caps: Lower Bowel Tonic - The Herbalist
Cascara Sagrada fresh-dried bark (rhamnus purshiana) • Barberry root bark (berberis vulgaris) • Fennel fresh-dried seed (foeniculum vulgare) • Bayberry fresh-dried root bark (myrica cerifera) • Ginger fresh root (zingiber officinale) • Turkey Rhubarb fresh-dried root (rheum palmatum) • Lobelia fresh-dried herb (lobelia inflata) • Cayenne fresh-dried pepper (capsicum annum).

Labor Prep - TriLight Herbs
Blue Cohosh • Squaw Vine • False Unicorn • Black Haw.

Lacidofil Defense DF - Xymogen
Each capsule contains: Lactobacillus Acidophilus Rosell-52 3 billion live organisms • Lactobacillus Rhamnosus Rosell-11 1 billion live organisms • Bifidobacterium Longum Rosell-175 1 billion live organisms • Zinc 2 mg • Selenium 12.5 mcg. Other Ingredients: Gelatin, Potato Starch, Magnesium Stearate, Ascorbic Acid.

Lacidofil DF - Xymogen
Each capsule contains: Lactobacillus Acidophilus Rosell-52 and Lactobacillus Rhamnosus Rosell-11 2 billion live organisms.

Lactaid Ultra (tablets & caplets) - McNeil Nutritionals LLC
Each caplet contains: Sodium 5 mg • Lactase enzyme 9000 FCC lactase units.

Lactase Enzyme - Nature's Way
Three capsules contain: Lactase enzyme 690 mg. Other Ingredients: Gelatin, Magnesium stearate, Maltodextrin.

Lact-Enz - Standard Process, Inc.
Two capsules contain: Proprietary Blend 1000 mg: Maltodextrin, Amylase, Protease, Cellulase, Lipase, Lactobacillus Acidophilus, Bifidobacterium Longum. Other Ingredients: Gelatin, Water, Colors, Calcium Stearate.

Lactic Acid Yeast - Standard Process, Inc.
Each wafer contains: Proprietary Blend 899 mg: Corn, Whey, Malt Syrup, Saccharomyces Cerevisiae (yeast). Other Ingredients: Glycerin, Honey, Arabic gum, Cellulose, Calcium Stearate.

Lactium - Ingredia
Milk Protein Hydrolysate.

Lacto - Enzymedica
Each capsule contains: Lactase 9500 ALU • Amylase Thera-Blend 7500 DU • Protease Thera-Blend 25,000 HUT • Glucoamylase 25 AG • Lipase Thera-Blend 600 FCCFIP • Maltase 350 DP • Cellulase Thera-Blend 300 CU • Alpha-Galactosidase 50 GALU • Invertase 25 INVU.

Lactobacillus Acidophilus - Pure Encapsulations
Each vegetable capsule contains: Lactobacillus Acidophilus (providing 1.5 billion CFU of the patented LA-1 strain) 150 mg.

Lactobacillus Acidophilus Milk-Base - Nature's Life
Each capsule contains: Lactobacillus species (Combined L. Acidophilus, L. Bulgaricus & L. Caucasious) 250 mg.

Lactobacillus Acidophilus Milk-Free - Nature's Life
Each capsule contains: Lactobacillus acidophilus 500 mg.

Lactobacillus Sporogenes - Pure Encapsulations
Each vegetable capsule contains: Lactobacillus Sporogenes (providing 1.5 billion CFU) 150 mg • Vitamin C (as ascorbyl palmitate) 8 mg.

LactoCalcium brand - Cyvex Nutrition, Inc.
Essential Milk Minerals containing <25% Calcium.
See Editor's Note No. 44.

Lactoferon Chewable Colostrum - Nature's Plus
Two chewable tablets contain: Colostrum 500 mg. Other Ingredients: Fructose, Stearic Acid, Malted Milk, Milk Protein Concentrate, Vanilla Flavor, Magnesium Stearate, Silica.

Lactoferrin - Jarrow Formulas
Each capsule contains: Lactoferrin 250 mg. Other Ingredients: Rice Powder, Magnesium Stearate, Silicon Dioxide, Gelatin, Titanium Dioxide.

Lactoferrin Plus - Pro Health
Each capsule contains: Lactoferrin 100 mg • Colostrum 250 mg • Lysozyme 5 mg. Other Ingredients: Gelatin, Magnesium Stearate.

Lactoferrin with Colostrum - The Vitamin Shoppe
Each capsule contains: Lactoferrin (from whey) 100 mg • Colostrum (from bovine) providing 20% immunoglobulins 250 mg • Lysozyme (from whey) 5 mg.

Lactoviden - Metagenics
Each capsule contains: Proprietary Blend 15 billion live oragnisms: Lactobacillus Acidophilus NCFM Strain, Lactobacillus Salivarius Ls-33, Lactobacillus Paracasei Lpc-37, Lactobacillus Plantarum Lp-115, Streptococcus Thermophilus St-21.

LactoZYME - Renew Life Formulas, Inc.
Each capsule contains: Lactase 9000 FCCALU • Lipase 600 LU • Papain 90,000 PU. Other Ingredients: Vegetable Fiber, Water, Cellulose.

Lady V - Ultra-V
Three capsules contain: Vitamin D (as Cholecalciferol) 21 IU • Niacin (as Niacinamide) 20 mg • Vitamin B6 (as Pyridoxine HCl) 2.4 mg • Folic Acid (as Folacin) 6.4 mg • Vitamin B12 (as Cyancolalamine) 6 mg • Avena Sativa extract 10:1 150 mg • Kava Kava 10 mg • Guarana 300 mg • White Willow bark 10 mg • Muira Puama 4:1 20 mg • St. John's Wort 250 mg • Siberian Ginseng 35:1 30 mg • Ginkgo Biloba 40 mg • Cordyceps 100 mg • Damiana 20 mg • L-Taurine 200 mg.

Lakota Joint Care Formula - Teton Tasunke Pejuta, Inc.
Elk Velvet Antler • Collagen Type II • Hyaluronic Acid • Neutrophils • Pantocrine • Alkaline Phosphatase • Bone Morphogenetic Protein • Glucosamine Sulfate • Herparan Sulfate • Dermatan Sulfate • Keratan Sulfate • Chondroitin Sulfate • Glucosamine Hydrochloride • Sulfur • Uronic Acid • Boswellia Serrata • White Willow bark • Yucca root • Sarsaparilla • Feverfew • Devil's Claw • L-Proline • Bromelain • Omega 3 Fatty Acids & Omega 6 Fatty Acids • All Essential Amino Acids • Calcium • Iron • Phosphorus • Zinc.
See Editor's Note No. 15 and No. 17.

L-Alanine - J. R. Carlson Laboratories, Inc.
Each 1 tsp serving contains: L-Alanine 1500 mg.

Lambert's Green Lipped Mussel Extract - Lambert
Each capsule contains: Green Lipped Mussel extract 350 mg. Other Ingredients: Gelatin.

Land, Lake & Sea - Great Life Labs
Two tablets contain: Vitamin A (as beta-carotene and as mixed carotenoids from D. salina algae) 5000 IU • Vitamin C (as ascorbic acid) 100 mg • Vitamin D (as cholecalciferol) 400 IU • Vitamin E (as DL-alpha-tocopheryl acetate) 50 IU • Thiamin (as thiamin mononitrate) 10 mg • Riboflavin (riboflavin) 10 mg • Niacin (niacin) 25 mg • Vitamin B6 (as pyridoxine hydrochloride) 5 mg • Folate (as folic acid) 400 mcg • Vitamin B12 (as cyanocobalamin) 25 mcg • Biotin (as biotin) 300 mcg • Pantothenic Acid (as calcium pantothenate) 10 mg • Calcium (as dibasic calcium phosphate) 225 mg • Iodine (from sea kelp (ascophyllum nodosum)) 150 mcg • Magnesium (as magnesium oxide) 25 mg • Zinc (as zinc citrate) 7.5 mg • Selenium (as selenomethionine) 70 mcg • Copper (as copper

BRAND NAMES

gluconate) 1 mg • Manganese (as manganese gluconate) 2 mg • Chromium (as niacin bound dinicotinate glycinate) 120 mcg • Molybdenum (as molybdenum chelate) 75 mcg • Pine bark (pinus strobus) and Grape seed (vitis vinifera) 50/50 blend 50 mg • Fruit and Vegetable Phytonutrient Concentrate Blend 500 mg: Alfalfa sprouts, Asparagus, Broccoli, Brussels sprouts, Cabbage, Cauliflower, Garlic, Kale, Mustard Greens, Soybean, Spinach, Papaya, Pineapple, Cantaloupe, Carrot, Cherry, Grapefruit, Lemon, Orange, Peach, Pear, Red Grape, Red Pepper, Strawberry, Tomato, Yellow Squash, Wheat Grass • Shiitake mushroom 10 mg • California Blue Green Algae (spirulina pratensis) 50 mg • Bulgarian Green Algae (chlorella pyrinoides) 50 mg • Dunaliella Red Algae (dunaliella salina) 20 mg • Phenalgin extract of Cystoseira Canariensis (1% phlorotannin) 50 mg • Maine Coast Sea Kelp (ascophyllum nodosum) 37.25 mg • Irish Moss extract (chondrus crispus) 5 mg. Other Ingredients: Cellulose, Croscarmellose Sodium, Vegetable Stearic Acid, Vegetable Magnesium Stearate, Silica, Pharmaceutical Glaze.

L-Arginine - Allergy Research Group
Each capsule contains: L-Arginine 500 mg. Other Ingredients: Cellulose, Silicon Dioxide, Stearic Acid.

l-Arginine - Pure Encapsulations
Each vegetable capsule contains: L-Arginine HCl 750 mg.

L-Arginine - Nature's Plus
Each capsule contains: L-Arginine (free form amino acid) 500 mg. Other Ingredients: Silica, Microcrystalline Cellulose, Glycerin, Purified Water.

L-Arginine - Ortho Molecular Products
Each capsule contains: L-Arginine USP 750 mg. Other Ingredients: Natural Vegetable Capsules, Ascorbyl Palmitate, Microcrystalline Cellulose, Silicon Dioxide.

L-Arginine - PhysioLogics
Each capsule contains: L-Arginine 500 mg. Other Ingredients: Gelatin, Vegetable Magnesium Stearate, Silica.

L-Arginine 500 - GNC
Each capsule contains: L-Arginine 500 mg. Other Ingredients: Gelatin.

L-Arginine 500 mg - Nature's Bounty
Each capsule contains: L-Arginine 500 mg. Other Ingredients: Gelatin, Vegetable Magnesium Stearate, Silica.

L-Arginine 500 mg - Solgar
Each capsule contains: L-Arginine 500 mg. Other Ingredients: Microcrystalline Cellulose, Vegetable Magnesium Stearate, Water, Vegetable Glycerin.

L-Arginine capsules - J. R. Carlson Laboratories, Inc.
Each capsule contains: L-Arginine 675 mg.

L-Arginine powder - J. R. Carlson Laboratories, Inc.
Each 1 tsp serving contains: L-Arginine 3000 mg.

L-Arginine/L-Ornithine 500/250 - Solgar
Each capsule contains: L-Arginine 500 mg • L-Ornithine (as L-ornithine HCl) 250 mg. Other Ingredients: Vegetable Cellulose, Vegetable Magnesium Stearate, Silica, Water, Vegetable Glycerin.

Larix 1000 - Jarrow Formulas
Each tablet contains: Arabinogalactan Polysaccharide (larix occidentalis) 1000 mg. Other Ingredients: Cellulose, Stearic Acid, Modified Cellulose Gum, Magnesium Stearate (vegetable source), Silicon Dioxide.

L-Asparagine - J. R. Carlson Laboratories, Inc.
Each 1 tsp serving contains: L-Asparagine (monohydrate) 1500 mg.

L-Aspartic Acid - J. R. Carlson Laboratories, Inc.
Each 1 tsp serving contains: L-Aspartic Acid 1500 mg.

Lauricidin (monolaurin) - Med-Chem Labs
Each pellet contains: Highly purified Monolaurin lipid.

Lava - Universal Nutrition
Each 83 g serving contains: Creatine Monohydrate 5.5 g • Chromium 75 mcg • Glutamine 2.5 g • Taurine 1.2 g • Sodium 180 mg • Potassium 360 mg. Ingredients: Ultra & Micro-Filtrated Whey Protein Concentrate (Containing Whey Peptide-Rich Lactoglobulins, Lactalbumin, Immunoglobulins & Lactoferrin) • GlycoCarb Complex (Dextrose & Glucose Polymers) • Maltodextrin • 100% Pure Creatine Monohydrate • Glutamine • Taurine • Magnesium Oxide • Disodium Phosphate • Potassium Phosphate • Fruit Flavor • Lecithin • Ascorbic Acid • Vitamin E Succinate • Niacin • Citric Acid • Aspartame • Carmine (for color) • Chromium (GTF).

Lavigra - Lavigra
Eurycoma Longifola • Cistanche Deserticola • Epimedium Sagitatum • Panax Ginseng • Cuscutae Chinensis semen • Polygonum Multiflorum • Lycium Chinense • Schisandra Chinensis • Rehmannia Glutinosa • Cnidium Monnier • Yohimbe • Long Jack • Zingiber Officinale • Bioperine-R brand Black Pepper extract.

Laxaco - Jamieson
Each capsule contains: Calcium (as Calcium Sulfate) 25 mg • Senna leaf (Cassia senna L.) 240 mg • Cascara Sagrada bark (Rhamnus purshiana DC) 150 mg.

Laxaco - Jamieson
Each capsule contains: Cascara Sagrada 150 mg • Senna Leaves 240 mg.

LaxaColon - DreamPharm
Each capsule contains: Proprietary Blend: Senna leaf, Aloe, Prune powder.

LaxActin - Nature's Plus
Each capsule contains: Cascara Sagrada (Rhamnus purshiana bark) (standardized 25-30% Hydroxyanthracene derivatives - HAD) 100 mg • Passion Flower [(Passiflora incarnata flower) standardized 3.5-4% Flavonoids] 100 mg • Senna [(Cassia senna leaf) standardized 5% Sennosides] 50 mg.

Laxaherb - Dial Herbs
Cascara Sagrada • Buckthorn • Ginger • Bayberry • Goldenseal • Raspberry • Fennel • Lobelia • Rhubarb.

Laxaherb - Wild Rose
Each tablet contains: Cascara Sagrada bark 200 mg • Buckthorn bark 50 mg • Barberry root bark 35 mg • Turkey Rhubarb root 75 mg • Red Raspberry leaf 35 mg • Ginger root 75 mg • Fennel seed 35 mg • Cayenne fruit (40,000 HU) 10 mg.

LBS II - Nature's Sunshine
Four capsules contain: Proprietary Blend 1700 mg: Cascara Sagrada bark (rhamnus purshiana), Buckthorn bark (rhamnus frangula), Licorice root (glycyrrhiza glabra), Capsicum fruit (capsicum annuum), Ginger root (zingiber officinale), Oregon Grape root (berberis aquifolium), Turkey Rhubarb root (rheum officinale), Couch Grass herb (agropyron repens), Red Clover tops (trifolium pratense). Other Ingredients: Kosher Gelatin, Water.

LBT 3 - Wild Rose
Each tablet contains: Ginger root 52.2 mg • Lobelia herb 34 mg • Cascara Sagrada bark 104.2 mg • Barberry root bark 34.8 mg • Fennel seed 34.8 mg • Goldenseal root 34.8 mg • Red Raspberry leaf 34.8 mg • Turkey Rhubarb root 34.8 mg • Cayenne fruit (80,000 HU) 17.4 mg.

L-Carnitine - Olympian Labs
Two capsules contain: L-Carnitine Fumarate 1000 mg.

L-Carnitine - BioGenesis Nutraceuticals
Each veggie capsule contains: L-Carnitine Tartrate (67%, yields 500 mg of elemental L-carnitine) 750 mg.

Some Brand Name Natural Products - What they Contain

www.NaturalDatabase.com contains MANY more listings than appear here.
Editor's Notes are located on pages 2155-2163.

L-Carnitine - GNC
Each capsule contains: L-Carnitine (as L-Carnitine Fumarate) 250 mg. Other Ingredients: Gelatin, Magnesium Stearate.

L-Carnitine - Nature's Plus
Each capsule contains: L-Carnitine (as L-carnitine-L-tartrate) 300 mg. Other Ingredients: Silica, Gelatin, Purified Water.

L-Carnitine - Swanson Health Products
Two capsules contain: L-Carnitine (from tartrate and free-form) 500 mg.

L-Carnitine - New Hope Health Products
Each capsule contains: L-Carnitine 500 mg • Vitamin B5 15 mg • Vitamin B6 5 mg.

L-Carnitine - Source Naturals
Each capsule contains: L-Carnitine 250 mg.

L-Carnitine - Metabolic Response Modifiers
Each capsule contains: L-Carnitine 500 mg • Vitamin B5 15 mg • Vitamin B6 5 mg.

L-Carnitine - Ortho Molecular Products
Each capsule contains: L-Carnitine (as L-tartrate) 500 mg. Other Ingredients: Natural Vegetable Capsules, Ascorbyl Palmitate, Magnesium Stearate, Microcrystalline Cellulose, Silicon Dioxide.

L-Carnitine - Pure Encapsulations
Each vegetable capsule contains: L-Carnitine (free-form, from 500 mg of L-carnitine-L-tartrate) 340 mg • Vitamin C (as ascorbyl palmitate) 12 mg.

L-Carnitine - DaVinci Laboratories
Each caplet contains: Calcium 280 mg • L-Carnitine Hydrochloride 250 mg. Other Ingredients: Calcium Carbonate, Cellulose, Silica, Vegetable Stearate, Stearic Acid.

L-Carnitine (250 mg) - Allergy Research Group
Each tablet contains: L-Carnitine 250 mg. Other Ingredients: Cellulose, Dicalcium Phosphate, Silicon Dioxide, Magnesium Stearate, Stearic Acid.

L-Carnitine (500 mg) - Allergy Research Group
Each tablet contains: L-Carnitine 500 mg. Other Ingredients: Cellulose, Dicalcium Phosphate, Silicon Dioxide, Magnesium Stearate, Stearic Acid.

L-Carnitine 250 - GNC
Each capsule contains: L-Carnitine (as L-carnitine fumarate) 250 mg. Other Ingredients: Gelatin.

L-Carnitine 250 - Jarrow Formulas
Each capsule contains: L-Carnitine (from 375 mg L-carnitine tartrate) 250 mg. Other Ingredients: Cellulose, Magnesium Stearate, Silicon Dioxide, Gelatin.

L-Carnitine 250 MG - PhysioLogics
Each capsule contains: L-Carnitine (as l-carnitine fumarate) 250 mg. Other Ingredients: Gelatin, Rice Powder, Silica, Vegetable Magnesium Stearate.

L-Carnitine 250 mg - Pro Health
Two capsules contain: L-Carnitine (from L-carnitine tartrate) 500 mg. Other Ingredients: Magnesium Stearate, Calcium Carbonate, Gelatin.

L-Carnitine 250 mg - Solgar
Each capsule contains: Vitamin B6 (as pyridoxine HCl) 2.5 mg • L-Carnitine 250 mg. Microcrystalline Cellulose, Vegetable Cellulose, Vegetable Stearic Acid, Vegetable Magnesium Stearate, Silica, Water, Vegetable Glycerin.

L-Carnitine 500 - Jarrow Formulas
Each capsule contains: L-Carnitine (from 750 mg L-carnitine tartrate) 500 mg. Other Ingredients: Cellulose, Magnesium Stearate, Silicon Dioxide, Gelatin.

L-Carnitine 500 - Optimum Nutrition
Each tablet contains: Calcium (as dicalcium phosphate) 96 mg • Phosphorus (as dicalcium phosphate) 74 mg • L-Carnitine (as L-carnitine tartrate) 500 mg. Other Ingredients: Pharmaceutical Glaze, Stearic Acid, Silica, Magnesium Stearate, Croscarmellose Sodium (disintegrant).

L-Carnitine 500 - GNC
Each capsule contains: L-carnitine (as L-carnitine L-tartrate) 500 mg. Other Ingredients: Gelatin.

L-Carnitine 500 MG - PhysioLogics
Each tablet contains: L-Carnitine 500 mg. Other Ingredients: Cellulose (plant origin), Dicalcium Phosphate, Vegetable Stearic Acid, Silica, Croscarmellose, Cellulose Coating, Vegetable Magnesium Stearate, Titanium Dioxide Color, Food Glaze, Magnesium Silicate, Vanillin.

L-Carnitine 500 mg - Pro Health
Each vegetarian capsule contains: L-Carnitine (free-form) 500 mg. Other Ingredients: FloGard, Maltodextrin, Magnesium Stearate, Dicalcium Phosphate, Cellulose, Acidisol.

L-Carnitine capsules - J. R. Carlson Laboratories, Inc.
Each capsule contains: L-Carnitine (as L-carnitine tartrate) 300 mg.

l-Carnitine fumarate - Pure Encapsulations
Each vegetable capsule contains: L-Carnitine (free-form from 586 mg L-carnitine fumarate) 340 mg • Vitamin C (as ascorbyl palmitate) 12 mg.

L-Carnitine powder - J. R. Carlson Laboratories, Inc.
Each 1 tsp serving contains: L-Carnitine 2000 mg.

L-Carnitine with Chromium - Metagenics
Each tablet contains: L-Carnitine 250 mg • Chromium (as chromium aspartate) 50 mcg.

L-Carnosine - Ortho Molecular Products
Each capsule contains: L-Carnosine 500 mg. Other Ingredients: Natural Vegetable Capsules, Ascorbyl Palmitate, Magnesium Stearate, Microcrystalline Cellulose, Silicon Dioxide.

L-Carnosine - Pure Encapsulations
Each vegetable capsule contains: L-Carnosine (beta-alanyl-L- histidine) 500 mg.

L-Carnosine 500 - Jarrow Formulas
Each capsule contains: L-Carnosine (alanylhistidine) 500 mg. Other Ingredients: Rice Powder, Magnesium Stearate, Silicon Dioxide, Gelatin.

L-Citrulline - Allergy Research Group
Each 1-1/4 tsp (3 g) serving contains: L-Citrulline 3 g.

L-Cysteine 500 - GNC
Each tablet contains: L-Cysteine 500 mg. Other Ingredients: Cellulose, Dicalcium Phosphate.

L-Cysteine 500 mg - Solgar
Each capsule contains: L-Cysteine (as L-cysteine HCl) 500 mg. Other Ingredients: Vegetable Cellulose, Vegetable Magnesium Stearate, Silica, Microcrystalline Cellulose, Water.

LDL-RX - Athletic Technologies Inc.
Two capsules contain: Red Yeast Rice 1000 mg • Niacin 50 mg • Guggulipids 50 mg • Beta-Sisterol 50 mg • Capiscum 50 mg • Garlic 50 mg • Lecithin 200 mg.

Lean "4" - The Vitamin Shoppe
Each six tablets contain: Lecithin 1200 mg • Vitamin B6 (pyridoxine HCl) 50 mg • Iodine (kelp) 210 mcg • Cider Vinegar Powder 240 mg • Grapefruit Powder 300 mg.

BRAND NAMES

Some Brand Name Natural Products - What they Contain

www.NaturalDatabase.com contains MANY more listings than appear here.
Editor's Notes are located on pages 2155-2163.

Lean & Clean **-** The Sports Nutrition Source, Inc.
Each capsule contains: Proprietary Blend 470 mg: Papaya fruit, Echinacea root, Black Walnut leaves, Fennel seeds, Parsley plant, Norwegian Kelp plant, Safflower flowers, Burdock root, Chickweed herb, Hawthorn berries, Cayenne fruit.

Lean Body **-** Labrada Bodybuilding Nutrition
LeanPro: Cross flow ultrafiltered Whey Protein concentrate, ion exchange Whey Protein isolate, cross flow microfiltered Whey Protein isolate, hydrolyzed Whey Protein isolate peptides, Milk Protein isolate, Caseinate, L-Glutamine, Taurine, Magnesium Alpha Keto Glutarate • Maltodextrin • Vitamin and Mineral Blend: Dicalcium Phosphate, Magnesium Oxide, Ascorbic Acid, Vitamin E Acetate, Niacinamide, Electrolytic Iron, Zinc Oxide, Sodium Chloride, D-Calcium Pantothenate, Pyridoxine HCl, Copper Gluconate, Manganese Citrate, Vitamin A Acetate, Thiamine Mononitrate, Riboflavin, Folic Acid, Manganese Sulfate, Potassium Iodide, Chromium Picolinate, Cholecalciferol, Sodium Molybdate, Cyanocobalamin, Sodium Selenite • Natural & Artificial Flavors • Polydextrose • Medium Chain Triglycerides • Xanthan Gum • Cellulose Gum • Aspartame.

Lean Connection **-** The Coral Connection
Three capsules contain: Calcium (as hydroxycitrate) 165 mg • Chromium (as polynicotate) 133 mcg • Potassium (as hydroxycitrate) 240 mg • Garcinia Cambogia fruit extract 1500 mg • (-) Hydroxycitric Acid 900 mg • Gymnema Sylvestre leaf extract 133 mg • Gymnemic Acids 33 mg • Phaseolamin 2250 330 mg • Green Tea (50% polyphenols) 180 mg • Oat Bran 105 mg • Psyllium husk 105 mg. Other Ingredients: Hydroxypropyl Cellulose, Glycerine, Magnesium Stearate, Silicon Dioxide.

Lean Dreams **-** The Sports Nutrition Source, Inc.
Each tablet contains: Vitamin B-6 (Pyridoxine) 15 mg • Niacin (niacinamide) 50 mg • L-Ornithine 500 mg • L-Glycine 667 mg • Valerian root extract 150 mg • Hops powder 20 mg.

LEAN Drink Mix (chocolate and vanilla flavors) **-** Apex Fitness Group
Fructose • Whey Protein Concentrate • Calcium Caseinate • Soy Protein Isolate • Whey • Nonfat Milk • Oat Fiber • Natural and Artificial Flavor • Cellulose • Maltodextrin • Guar Gum • Partially Hydrogenated Soybean oil and Cottonseed oil • Soy Lecithin • Carrageenan • Potassium Phosphate • Egg White • Rice Maltodextrin • Magnesium Oxide • Salt • Asparatame • Calcium Phosphate • Ascorbic Acid • Ferrous Fumarate • Alpha Tocopherol Acetate • Niacinamide • Zinc Oxide • Manganese Sulfate • Calcium Pantothenate • Copper Sulfate • Vitamin A Palmitate • Pyridoxine Hydrochloride • Riboflavin • Thiamin Hydrochloride • Folic Acid • Biotin • Potassium Iodide • Vitamin D (D3) • Vitamin B12. Chocolate flavor also contains: Cocoa (processed with alkali).
This product was formerly called "High Performance Lite."

LEAN Fat Burn 1 **-** Apex Fitness Group
Three tablets contain: Niacinamide 10 mg • Pyridoxine 5' Phosphate 10 mg • Choline Bitartrate 1000 mg • Inositol 1000 mg • Taurine 300 mg • Methionine 300 mg • Betaine HCl 150 mg • L-Carnitine 150 mg • Herbal Base 100 mg: Papain, Sarsaparilla, Shave Grass, Hawthorne berries, Capsicum, Gotu Kola, Hyssop, Valerian root, Myrrh gum. Other Ingredients: Calcium Phosphate, Microcrystalline Cellulose, Magnesium Stearate, Vegetable Stearate, Croscarmellose, Vanilla Flavor, Silica.
This product was formerly called "Lipotropic & Transport."

LEAN Fat Burn 2 **-** Apex Fitness Group
Two tablets contain: Pyruvate-1000 brand Pyruvate (from calcium, potassium and sodium salts of pyruvic acid) 1000 mg. Other Ingredients: Calcium Carbonate, Xanthan Gum, Inulin, Stearic Acid, Magnesium Stearate, Silica.
This product was formerly called "Pyruvate 1000."

LEAN Fat Burn 2 **-** Apex Fitness Group
Each tablet contains: Pyruvate 1000 brand: Calcium, Potassium and Sodium Salts of Pyruvic Acid 100 mg. Other Ingredients: Calcium Carbonate, Xanthan Gum, Inulin, Vegetable Stearate, Magnesium Stearate, Silica.

LEAN Fat Burn 3 **-** Apex Fitness Group
Two capsules contain: Guarana and Green Tea extracts (standardized for caffeine 390 mg, theophylline 20 mg, theobromine 1 mg) • Bitter Orange (standardized for synephrine 5 mg) • L-Tyrosine 300 mg • L-Theanine 30 mg • Synergistic Thermo Complex: Maca, Jeevani, Pyruvate, Peptide GPX, D-Ribose 100 mg. Other Ingredients: Calcium Phosphate, Talc, Magnesium Stearate, Gelatin.
This product was formerly called "T-2 Lean."
See Editor's Note No. 40.

Lean Formula with Advantra Z **-** USANA Health Sciences
Two tablets contain: Sour Orange Extract (Citrus Aurantium L. fruit) 650 mg • Green Tea Extract (Camellia Sinensis Kuntze leaf) 50 mg • Guarana Extract (Paullinia Cupana Bonpl. & Kunth. fruit) 50 mg • Cayenne (Capsicum Annum L. fruit) 30 mg. Other Ingredients: Microcrystalline Cellulose, Croscarmellose Sodium, Ascorbyl Palmitate, Collodial Silicon Dioxide, Dextrin, Dextrose.
See Editor's Note No. 40.

Lean Gainer **-** Champion Nutrition
Each serving contains: Peptol-C: Whey Protein Concentrate, Creatine Monohydrate, Amino Acids, L-Leucine, L-Glutamine • Metabarb-V (blend of Simple & Complex Carbohydrates containing Glucose Polymers & Whey) • Low Fat Cocoa powder •Natural & Artificial Flavors • Metavite IV (Vitamin-Mineral Complex) • FIBR3: Cellulose, Oat Fiber, Psyllium husks • Aspartame • Succinate ETF: Potassium Succinate, L-Glutamic Acid, Inosine, Magnesium Succinate, Calcium Succinate • Bromelain •Papain • Defatted Peanut Flour •Sunette (Brand of Acesulfame-K) • Vanadyl Polynicotinate. Contains Phenylalanine.

Lean Image Carb Blocker **-** Pro Star International
Two tablets contain: Wheat Amylase Inhibitor 10 mg • Pro Carb Blend 300 mg: Gymnema Sylvestre leaf and extract, Fenugreek seed, Lycium berry, Vanadium (from vanadyl sulfate) • Banaba leaf extract (1% corosolic acid) 16 mg. Other Ingredients: Dicalcium Phosphate, Microcrystalline Cellulose, Croscarmellose Sodium, Stearic Acid, Magnesium Stearate, Silica, Pharmaceutical Glaze.
See Editor's Note No. 37.

Lean Machine **-** The Sports Nutrition Source, Inc.
Two scoops contain: Sodium 85 mg • Potassium 85 mg • Protein 37 g • Creatine Monohydrate 3000 mg • L-Glutamine 2000 mg • Methylsulfonylmethane 1000 mg • Glucosamine Sulfate 500 mg • Chondroitin Sulfate 350 mg • White Willow Bark extract 75 mg • Ascorbic Acid 100 mg • Bromelain 100 mg.
See Editor's Note No. 15.

LEAN Resist 1 **-** Apex Fitness Group
Three tablets contain: Vitamin B6 (pyridoxine HCl) 30 mg • Manganese (gluconate) 15 mg • Chromium (polynicotinate) 200 mcg • Citrimax brand Garcinia Cambogia extract (containing 50% (-) hydroxycitric acid) 1500 mg • L-Carnitine Tartrate 350 mg • Vanadyl Sulfate (provides 1.89 mg of elemental vanadium) 10 mg • GLA (gamma linolenic acid) 100 mg • Thermogenic Complex Herbs 60 mg: Gymnema Sylvestre, Bitter Melon, Cloves, Tumeric. Other Ingredients: Calcium Phosphate, Microcrystalline Cellulose, Vegetable Stearate, Croscarmellose, Magnesium Stearate, Silica.
This product was formerly called "Thermo-Transport Formula."

LEAN Resist 2 **-** Apex Fitness Group
Each tablet contains: Cholecystokinin (CCK) 100 mg. Other Ingredients: Calcium Phosphate, Microcrystalline Cellulose, Vegetable Stearate, Magnesium Stearate, Croscarmellose, Silica.
This product was formerly called "CCK."

***LEAN Resist 3* - Apex Fitness Group**
Two tablets contain: Griffonia Simplicifolia providing 10% 5-HTP (5-hydroxy-L-tryptophan, 100 mg) 1000 mg • Herbolics Support Complex 100 mg: Jatoba, Maca, Para Todo, Guarana. Other Ingredients: Calcium Phosphate, Microcrystalline Cellulose, Vegetable Stearate, Croscarmellose, Magnesium Stearate.
This product was formerly called "5 HTP."

***Lean System 7* - PPI, Inc.**
Three capsules contain: Yerba Mate leaves (ilex paraguanensis) 500 mg • Guarana seed extract (paullinia cupana, standardized to 22% alkaloids as caffeine, 154 mg) 700 mg • Citrus Aurantium fruit extract (standardized for 6% synephrine, 18 mg) 300 mg • ForsLean Coleus Forskohlii root extract (standardized for 20% forskolin, 30 mg) 150 mg • 7-Keto (3-acetyl-7-oxo-dehydroepiandrosterone) 50 mg • Dandelion leaf and root powder (taraxacum officinale) 250 mg • Bioperine brand Black Pepper extract (piper nigrum fruit, standardized to 98% piperine, 4.9 mg) 5 mg.
See Editor's Note No. 40.

***Lean Tabs* - Fizogen Precision Technologies Inc.**
Three tablets contain: Dexafenadrine (hybrid thermogenic fusion) 785 mg: Caffeine Anhydrous, Green Tea extract, Yerba Mate root extract, Green Coffee bean extract, Cordia Salicifolia extract, Cocoa extract, Taurine, Citrus Naringin, Vinpocetine • Hydropropol (water removal complex) 462 mg: Horse Tail extract, Dandelion root extract, Uva Ursi extract • Carboxen (cabo-metabolic driving agent) 250 mg: Garcinia Cambogia extract (HCA), L-Carnitine • C-AMP SCB (cyclic AMP triggering agent) 140 mg: Clary Sage extract, Bergenin • Myotonal (muscle tone enhancer) 130 mg: Mucuna Pruriens extract, Cyanotis Vaga extract, Rhodiola Rosea extract • Neurotrol (appetite controlling blend) 130 mg: Hoodia Gordonii cactus extract, Caralluma cactus extract, Simthin Jojoba seed extract, Griffonia Simplicifolia seed extract • Tetravlain (thyroid T3/T4 secretagogue) 130 mg: L-Tyrosine, Olive leaf extract, Guggulsterones E&Z • Degestol (hyper digestive fusion) 75 mg: Terminalia Chebula fruit extract, Terminalia Belerica fruit extract, Emblica Officinalis fruit extract • Egc-Heat (thermobolic accelerator) 67 mg: Evodium extract, Ginger root extract, Cayenne extract.

***Lean Tea Complex* - Optimum Nutrition**
Each capsule contains: Green Tea leaf extract (camellia sinensis, standardized to 20% caffeine & 35% EGCG, epigallo-catechin-gallate) 700 mg • Black Tea powdered leaf 10 mg • Oolong Tea powdered leaf 10 mg • Bioperine brand Black Pepper extract (piper nigrum fruit, standardized to 95% piperine) 5 mg. Other Ingredients: Gelatin, Magnesium Stearate.

***Lean Xtreme* - Designer Supplements**
Each capsule contains: 7-OH (7-hydroxy-dehydroepiandrosterone) 50 mg. Other Ingredients: Maltodextrin, Gelatin, Silicon Dioxide, Magnesium Stearate.

***LeanFire* - InStone Nutrition**
Three capsules contain: Vitamin C 120 mg • L-Tyrosine 650 mg • Green Tea 300 mg • Caffeine Anhydrous 300 mg • Evo-Lean Blend 255 mg: Rhodiola Rosea root, Evodia Rutaecarpa, E & Z Guggulsterones • 7-Keto 50 mg. Other Ingredients: Gelatin, Silicon Dioxide, Magnesium Stearate.

***Learner's Edge Pure Kids* - Integrative Therapeutics**
Three capsules contain: Selenium (from l-selenomethionine) 25 mcg • Milk Thistle seed extract (silybum marianum, 80% silymarin) 150 mg • NAC (as n-acetyl-l-cysteine) 25 mg • D-Glucarate Calcium D-glucarate 100 mg • Trimethylglycine (as betaine) 150 mg • Alpha-Ketoglutaric Acid 250 mg • Taurine 100 mg • L-Glutathione, reduced 25 mg • L-Methionine 100 mg • Choline (from choline bitartrate) 100 mg • MSM (methylsulfonylmethane) 100 mg. Other Ingredients: Microcrystalline Cellulose, Ascorbyl Palmitate, Capsule (gelatin, water).

***Learner's Edge System ChildEssence* - Integrative Therapeutics**
Four capsules contain: Vitamin A (67% from retinyl acetate & 33% as natural beta-carotene with mixed carotenoids) 7500 IU • Vitamin C (as ascorbic acid) 200 mg • Vitamin D (as cholecalciferol) 200 IU • Vitamin E (from natural mixed tocopherols) 100 IU • Thiamin (from thiamine pyrophosphate) 10 mg • Riboflavin (as riboflavin-5'-phosphate) 10 mg • Niacin (as niacinamide) 40 mg • Vitamin B6 (from pyridoxal-5'-phosphate) 25 mg • Folate (as folic acid) 200 mcg • Vitamin B12 (as methylcobalamin) 200 mcg • Biotin 100 mcg • Pantothenic Acid (from calcium pantothenate) 20 mg • Calcium (50% from calcium glycinate, 50% from calcium citrate/malate complex) 200 mg • Iron (from ferrous succinate) 10 mg • Iodine (from potassium iodide) 150 mcg • Magnesium (50% from magnesium glycinate and 50% from calcium citrate/malate complex) 200 mg • Zinc (from zinc sulfate) 7.5 mg • Selenium (from l-selenomethionine) 30 mcg • Chromium (from chromium nicotinate) 50 mcg • Molybdenum (from molybdenum citrate) 25 mcg • Citrus Bioflavonoids 25 mg. Other Ingredients: Microcrystalline Cellulose, Ascorbyl Palmitate, Capsule (gelatin & water).

***Learner's Edge System DigestRight* - Integrative Therapeutics**
Two capsules contain: Proprietary Enzyme Blend 315 mg: Protease (provides dipeptidylpeptidase IV, exopeptidase, endopeptidase, peptide peptidohydrolase activity) 14,500 USP/20,200 PC/34, 300 HUT/2000 CFAU, Amylase 6700 USP/6000 DU/6000, Lipase 630 LU/300 LU, Lactase 2400 LacU, Cellulase 124 CU, Phytase 0.64 PU, Sucrase (invertase) 300 INVU, Maltase (malt diastase) 10,800 DP. Other Ingredients: Microcrystalline Cellulose, Ascorbyl Palmitate, Capsule (gelatin, water).

***Learner's Edge System ImmunoKids* - Integrative Therapeutics**
Three capsules contain: Vitamin C (as ascorbic acid) 500 mg • Calcium (from calcium magnesium phytate) 65 mg • Zinc (from zinc sulfate) 10 mg • IP-6 (inositol hexaphosphate, from calcium magnesium phytate) 400 mg • Inositol 110 mg • Leucoselect Phytosome 83 mg: Grape seed Polyphenols (including procanidolic oligomers (vitis vinifera)) 26 mg, Phosphatidylcholine (from soy bean) 55 mg • Pine bark extract (pinus maritima, 95% polyhenols, including procyanidolic oligomers) 25 mg • Savantero Cat's Claw bark extract (uncaria tomentosa, 1.3% pentacyclic oxindole alkaloids, free of tetracyclic oxindole alkaloids) 10 mg • Aloe Vera inner leaf gel powder 20 mg • Citrus Bioflavonoids 50 mg • Monolaurin (as glyceryl monolaurate) 10 mg. Other Ingredients: Microcrystalline Cellulose, Ascorbyl Palmitate, Capsule (gelatin & water).

***Learner's Edge System Learner's Edge* - Integrative Therapeutics**
Three capsules contain: Vitamin E (from d-alpha tocopheryl succinate) 10 IU • DMAE (as dimethylaminoethanol bitartrate) 200 mg • L-Theanine 25 mg • Acetyl-L-Carnitine (from acetyl l-carnitine HCl) 300 mg • L-Carnosine 400 mg • Vitaline Coenzyme Q10 Blend (coenzyme Q10 as ubiquinone 30 mg) 175 mg • Ginkgo Biloba leaf extract (24% flavone glycosides, 6% terpene lactones) 50 mg • American Ginseng root extract (panax quinquefolium, 5% ginsenosides) 200 mg. Other Ingredients: Microcrystalline Cellulose, Ascorbyl Palmitate, Micosolle (vegetable fatty acids, silicon dioxide, magnesium sulfate), Capsule (gelatin, water).

***Leci-Choline brand* - Degussa Food Ingredients/BL BioActives**
PhosphatidylCholine.

***Leci-Key* - J. R. Carlson Laboratories, Inc.**
Two level teaspoons contain: Vitamin E (naturally occurring) 1 IU • Calcium 111 mg • Iron 0 mg • Phosphorus 480 mg • Potassium 180 mg • Linoleic Acid 4 g • Phosphatidyl Choline 525 mg • Phopshatidyl Inositol 300 mg • Linolenic Acid 0.5 g • Essential Polyunsaturated Fatty Acids 5 g.

Some Brand Name Natural Products - What they Contain

www.NaturalDatabase.com contains MANY more listings than appear here.
Editor's Notes are located on pages 2155-2163.

Leci-Plus **-** Atrium Biotechnologies
Each capsule contains: Raw Unbleached Lecithin 650 mg • Choline Bitartrate 50 mg • Inositol 50 mg • Biotin 60 mcg • Niacinamide 30 mg • Vitamin B6 2 mg • Magnesium Glycero Phosphate 100 mg • Magnesium 12 mg • Phosphorus 16 mg.

Leci-PS brand **-** Degussa Food Ingredients/BL BioActives
PhosphatidylSerine.

Lecithin **-** Health Center for Better Living
"Rich source of choline, a B-complex nutrient," HCBL Lecithin derived from soybeans

Lecithin **-** NOW Foods
Four softgels contain: Phosphatidyl Choline 560 mg • Phosphatidyl Ethanolamine 128 mg • Phosphatidyl Inositol 16 mg. Other Ingredients: Soybean Lecithin, Gelatin, Glycerine, Water.

Lecithin **-** Jamieson
Each capsule contains: Lecithin derived from Pure Soy 1200 mg.

Leci-Thin **-** Nature's Plus
Each wafer contains: Lecithin 1500 mg derived from natural Soybean, rich in Choline, Inositol & Phosphorus • Wheat Bran 500 mg • Vegetable Cellulose 200 mg • Protein, vegetable soy & peanut 150 mg. Made from the finest quality Lecithin, containing 95% Soy Phosphatides. In an all natural base of carob, coconut & vanilla bean.

Lecithin & Milk powder **-** Nature's Life
Two heaping tablespoons contain: Linoleic Acid (omega-6) 3681 mg • Linolenic Acid (omega-3) 438 mg • Oleic Acid (omega-9) 575 mg • Palmitic Acid 1269 mg • Stearic Acid 288 mg • Phosphatidyl Choline 2.8g • Phosphatidyl Ethanolamine 2.5 g • Phosphatidyl Inositol 1.8 g • Choline 378 mg • Inositol 275 mg • Calcium 132 mg • Iron 1 mg • Magnesium 11 mg • Phosphorus 471 mg • Potassium 276 mg • Sodium 57 mg • Alanine 103 mg • Arginine 137 mg • Aspartic Acid 213 mg • Cysteine 11 mg • Glutamic Acid 779 mg • Glycine 68 mg • Histidine (essential amino acid) 99 mg • Isoleucine (essential amino acid) 216 mg • Leucine (essential amino acid) 334 mg • Lysine (essential amino acid) 270 mg • Methionine (essential amino acid) 110 mg • Phenylalanine (essential amino acid) 190 mg • Proline 407 mg • Serine 209 mg • Threonine (essential amino acid) 148 mg • Tryptophan (essential amino acid) 49 mg • Tyrosine 209 mg • Valine (essential amino acid) 243 mg.

Lecithin 1200 mg **-** J. R. Carlson Laboratories, Inc.
Each softgel contains: Choline (as phosphatidyl choline) 26 mg • Inositol (as phosphatidyl inositol) 19 mg • Lecithin 1200 mg.

Lecithin 1200 mg **-** Arrowroot
Each capsule contains: Lecithin 1200 mg.

Lecithin Choline **-** PhysioLogics
Each softgel contains: Phosphatidyl Choline (from soy lecithin concentrate 1200 mg) 420 mg. Other Ingredients: Gelatin, Glycerin.

Lecithin Plus **-** GNC
Two capsules contain: Niacin 20 mg • Chromium (as chromium picolinate) 200 mcg • Garlic powder (allium sativum) 500 mg •Phosphatidyl Choline (as liquid soy lecithin) 141 mg. Other Ingredients: Gelatin, Soybean oil, Glycerin, Caramel Color, Titanium Dioxide.

Leg Cramps Ointment **-** Hyland's
Active Ingredients: Aconitum Nap. 3X • Arnica Montana 3X • Ledum Pal. 3X • Magnesia Phosphorica 10X • Rhus Toxicodendron 6X • Viscum. Album 3X. Inactive Ingredients: Olive Oil N.F., Stearyl Alcohol, Natural Wintergreen Oil, Kokam Butter, Glyceryl Monostearate, Soy Lecithin, Methylparaben, Propylparaben, Butylparaben.
See Editor's Note No. 1.

Leg Cramps with Quinine **-** Hyland's
Two tablets contain: Cinchona Officinalis 3X (quinine) • Viscum Album 3X • Gnaphalium Polycephalum 3X • Rhus Toxicodendron 6X • Aconitum Napellus 6X • Ledum Palustre 6X • Magnesia Phosphorica 6X. Base: Lactose NF.
See Editor's Note No. 1.

Leg Vein Essentials **-** Swanson Health Products
Two time-release capsules contain: Vitamin C (as calcium ascorbate) 120 mg • Horse Chestnut extract (22% escin) 400 mg • Butcher's Broom extract (10% saponins calculated as ruscogenin) 150 mg • Gotu Kola extract (10% asiaticosides) 100 mg • Hesperidin (40% bioflavonoids) 100 mg • Bilberry extract (25% anthocyanidins) 20 mg • Grapeseed extract (90%-95% proanthocyanidins) 20 mg • Hawthorn berry extract (2% vitexin-2' rhamnosides) 20 mg.

Leg Veins Formula **-** Nature's Way
Two capsules contain: Butcher's Broom root 200 mg • Cayenne pepper fruit 50 mg • Dandelion leaf 250 mg • Grape seed dried extract 37.5 mg • Horse chestnut dried extract 200 mg • Prickly Ash bark 100 mg • Vitamin C (Ascorbic Acid) 30 mg. Other Ingredients: Gelatin, Magnesium Stearate, Millet.

Leg-Aid **-** Futurebiotics LLC
Two capsules contain: Niacin (as flush free niacin) 20 mg • MSM (methyl-sulfonyl-methane) 400 mg • Citrus Bioflavonoids 220 mg • Glucosamine sulfate 400 mg • Grape Seed powder extract (standardized for 95% (24 mg) proanthocyanidins) 25 mg • Horse Chestnut (standardized at 18-22% (50-62 mg) aescin) 280 mg • Butcher's Broom root powder 200 mg • Prickly Ash bark powder 125 mg • Ginkgo Biloba leaf powder 30 mg. Other Ingredients: Magnesium stearate, Gelatin, Water.

Lemon/Lime C 500 mg **-** Nature's Plus
Each chewable tablet contains: Vitamin C (as ascorbic acid) 500 mg. Other Ingredients: Fructose, Natural Flavors, Magnesium Stearate, Silica, Natural Colors, Lemon Bioflavonoids (from citrus limon fruit), Rutin, Hesperidin, Acerola Cherry (malpighia glabra fruit), Rose Hips (rosa canina fruit), Papaya Fruit, Green Pepper Extract (from capsicum annuum fruit), Black Currant Fruit Concentrate, Dolomite, Stearic Acid.

Lemon-Lime Multi-Vitamin For Adults **-** LiFizz Effervescent Vitamins
Each tablet contains: Magnesium 80 mg • Calcium 200 mg • Zinc 5 mg • Iron 6 mg • Vitamin A 5000 IU • Vitamin E 15 IU • Vitamin C 60 mg • Vitamin B2 (Riboflavin) 1.7 mg • Vitamin B6 (Pyridoxine) 2 mg • Vitamin B12 (Cyanocobalamin) 6 mcg • Vitamin B1 (Thiamin) 1.5 mg • Niacin (Vitamin PP or B3) 20 mg • Pantothenic Acid 10 mg • Free Folic Acid 400 mcg • Biotin 300 mcg • Vitamin D 400 IU.

Leptoprin **-** A.G. Waterhouse
Two capsules contain: Calcium (amino acid chelate) 264 mg • Vitamin B6 25 mg • Leptoprin Proprietary Blend 989 mg: Acetylsalicyclic Acid 324 mg, Caffeine (34 mg from standardized kola nut 280 mg) 200 mg • Green Tea leaf extract (standardized for polyphenols/catechins content), L-Tyrosine, Kelp (0.15% iodine 100 mg), Ephedrine Alkaloids (exclusive 10% extract from whole plant ma huang 200 mg) 20 mg, Cayenne fruit. Other Ingredients: Rice Flour.

Leptoprin-SD **-** A.G. Waterhouse
Two capsules contain: Niacin 20 mg • Calcium (as calcium amino acid chelate) 39 mg • Copper (from copper amino acid chelate) 0.5 mg • Leptoprin-SD Proprietary Blend 1188 mg: Yerba Mate leaf standardized extract (SE), Guarana seed SE, Caffeine, Damiana leaf SE, L-Tyrosine, Acetylsalicylic Acid 81 mg, Green Tea leaf SE, Kola Nut SE, Eucommia bark, Schizonepeta Spica SE, Piper Nigrum fruit, Hoelen, Polygonum root, Turmeric rhizome.

Leptoprin-SF **-** A.G. Waterhouse
Two capsules contain: Calcium (amino acid chelate) 132 mg • Leptoprin-SF Proprietary Blend 1493.5 mg: Calcium Phosphate, Commiphora Mukul extract, Garcinia Cambogia (HCA 125 mg),

BRAND NAMES

L-Tyrosine, Acetylsalicylic Acid 162.5 mg, Dipotassium Phosphate, Sodium Phosphtae, Disodium Phosphate, Phosphatidyl Choline, Scutellaria root, Bupleurum root, Epimedium herb. Other Ingredients: Rice Flour.

LessTerol - Omega Alpha Pharmaceuticals
Each capsule contains: Policosanol 10 mg • Red Rice Yeast 100 mg • Guggulipid 10 mg • Niacin (inositol hexanicotinate) 250 mg • Folic Acid 500 mcg.

Level 90 Blood Sugar Stabilizer - Market America, Inc.
Two tablets contain: Niacin 7 mg • Niacinamide 10 mg • Magnesium (oxide) 17 mg • Chromium (amino acid chelate) 100 mcg • Cyanocobalamin (vitamin B12) 50 mcg • Glucomannan (amorphophallus tuber extract) 175 mg • L-Glutamic Acid 100 mg • L-Carnitine 50 mg • Coenzyme Q10 10 mg • Vanadium (amino acid chelate) 15 mcg. Other Ingredients: Microcrystalline Cellulose, Stearic Acid, Magnesium Stearate, Silicon Dioxide, Croscarmellose Sodium, Dicalcium Phosphate.

L-Glutamic Acid - J. R. Carlson Laboratories, Inc.
Each 1 tsp serving contains: L-Glutamic Acid 4000 mg.

L-Glutamic Acid 500 mg - Solgar
Each tablet contains: L-Glutamic Acid 500 mg. Other Ingredients: Microcrystalline Cellulose, Vegetable Stearic Acid, Vegetable Cellulose, Silica, Vegetable Magnesium Stearate.

L-Glutamine - Ortho Molecular Products
Each capsule contains: L-Glutamine USP 700 mg Other Ingredients: Natural Vegetable Capsules, Ascorbyl Palmitate, Magnesium Stearate, Microcrystalline Cellulose, Silicon Dioxide.

L-Glutamine - PhysioLogics
Each tablet contains: L-Glutamine 500 mg. Other Ingredients: Cellulose (plant origin), Dicalcium Phosphate, Hydroxypropyl Cellulose, Vegetable Stearic Acid, Povidone, Silica, Croscarmellose, Vegetable Magnesium Stearate, Cellulose Coating.

L-Glutamine - J. R. Carlson Laboratories, Inc.
Each capsule contains: L-Glutamine 750 mg.

L-Glutamine - Jarrow Formulas
Each scoop (2 g) contains: L-Glutamine 2 g.

L-Glutamine - J. R. Carlson Laboratories, Inc.
Each 1 tsp serving contains: L-Glutamine 3000 mg.

L-Glutamine 1000 - GNC
Each tablet contains: L-glutamine 1000 mg. Other Ingredients: Dicalcium Phosphate, Cellulose.

L-Glutamine 1000 - Jarrow Formulas
Each tablet contains: L-Glutamine 1000 mg. Other Ingredients: Cellulose, Modified Cellulose Gum, Stearic Acid, Magnesium Stearate, Silicon Dioxide.

l-Glutamine 1000 mg - Pure Encapsulations
Each vegetable capsule contains: L-Glutamine (free-form) 1000 mg • Vitamin C (as ascorbyl palmitate) 10 mg.

L-Glutamine 500 - GNC
Each capsule contains: L-Glutamine 500 mg. Other Ingredients: Dicalcium Phosphate, Gelatin.

L-Glutamine 500 mg - Arrowroot
Each capsule contains: L-Glutamine 500 mg.

l-Glutamine 500 mg - Pure Encapsulations
Each vegetable capsule contains: L-Glutamine (free-form) 500 mg • Vitamin C (as ascorbyl palmitate) 5 mg.

L-Glutamine 500 mg - Solgar
Each capsule contains: L-Glutamine 500 mg. Other Ingredients: Vegetable Cellulose, Microcrystalline Cellulose, Vegetable Magnesium Stearate, Vegetable Stearic Acid, Water, Vegetable Glycerin.

L-Glutamine 500 mg - Pro Health
Each capsule contains: L-Glutamine (free form) 500 mg. Other Ingredients: Rice Flour, Gelatin, Magnesium Stearate.

L-Glutamine 500mg - Nature's Own
Each tablet contains: Glutamine 500 mg.

L-Glutamine 750 - Jarrow Formulas
Each capsule contains: L-Glutamine 750 mg. Other Ingredients: Rice Powder, Magnesium Stearate, Silicon Dioxide, Gelatin.

L-Glutamine Plus - Atrium Biotechnologies
Each tablet contains: L-Glutamine (an essential amino acid) 300 mg • L-Tryosine (an essential amino acid) 100 mg • Raw Bovine Adrenal concentrate 50 mg • Calcium Ascorbate (Vitamin C) 100 mg. See Editor's Note No. 14.

L-Glutamine powder - Ortho Molecular Products
Each scoop contains: L-Glutamine USP 3 g.

l-Glutamine powder - Pure Encapsulations
Each 1 level tsp serving contains: L-Glutamine (free-form) 3 g.

L-Glutamine Powder - PhysioLogics
Each level teaspoon (3.3 g) contains: L-Glutamine 3.3 g.

L-Glutathione - Ortho Molecular Products
Each capsule contains: Reduced L-Glutathione 75 mg. Other Ingredients: Natural Vegetable Capsules, Ascorbyl Palmitate, Magnesium Stearate, Microcrystalline Cellulose, Silicon Dioxide.

L-Glutathione (Reduced) - Alpine Pharmaceuticals
Each capsule contains: L-Glutathione 200 mg.

L-Glutathione 250 mg - Solgar
Each capsule contains: L-Glutathione 250 mg. Other Ingredients: Microcrystalline Cellulose, Vegetable Cellulose, Vegetable Magnesium Stearate, Silica, Water, Vegetable Glycerin.

L-Glutathione 50 mg - Solgar
Each capsule contains: L-Glutathione 50 mg. Other Ingredients: Microcrystalline Cellulose, Vegetable Cellulose, Vegetable Magnesium Stearate, Water, Vegetable Glycerin.

LHB (Lipase Herbal Blend) - Global Health Trax
Each capsule contains: Chromium (as chromium picolinate, chromium polynicotinate) 50 mcg • Garcinia (whole plant) 125 mg • Bladderwrack (algae) 38 mg • California Nettles (whole plant) 38 mg • Plantain leaf 38 mg • Northern Prickly Ash bark 38 mg • Nature's Turn Enzyme Blend 73 mg: Protease 4.5 (30,000 HUT), Lipase (200 FCCLU), Amylase (3000 DU), Cellulase • Fenugreek seed 20 mg. Other Ingredients: Soy Lecithin Oil Blend, Gelatin, Water.

Libilov for Men - Nutrica, Inc.
Each tablet contains: Tribulus Terrestris leaf extract 250 mg • Ginkgo Biloba leaf extract 20 mg. Other Ingredients: Corn Starch, Hydroxypropyl Methylcellulose (HPMC), Colloidal Silicon Dioxide, Microcrystalline Cellulose, Dibasic Calcium Phosphate Dihydrate, Croscarmellose Sodium, Methyl Paraben, Propyl Paraben, Magnesium Stearate, Titanium Dioxide, Talc, Polyethylene Glycol.

Libilov with L-Arginine - Nutrica, Inc.
Each tablet contains: Tribulus Terrestris leaf extract 250 mg • Gingko Biloba leaf extract 20 mg • L-Arginine 250 mg. Other Ingredients: Corn Starch, Hydroxypropyl Methylcellulose (HPMC), Colloidal Silicon Dioxide, Microcrystalline Cellulose, Dibasic Calcium Phosphate Dihydrate, Croscarmellose Sodium, Methyl Paraben, Propyl Paraben, Magnesium Stearate, Titanium Dioxide, Talc, Polyethylene Glycol.

Libracol - Magistral Biotech
Each capsule contains: Enzymatic Polychitosamine Hydrolisat 30 kDa from Chitosan (HEP-30, a specific deacetylated low molecular weight compound) 800 mg. Other Ingredients: Gelatin.

Lice Treatment & Prevention: Herbal Hair Oil - The Herbalist
Pure essential oils of Rosemary • Lavender • Bay • Sage • Formulated with botanical extracts of Nettles leaf • Burdock root • Red Clover blossom • Chaparral leaf. In a base of cold-pressed oils of Sweet Almond and Jojoba.

Licorice - Nature's Way
Three capsules contain: Licorice root 1.35 g. Other Ingredients: Gelatin.

Licorice Garlic - Atrium Biotechnologies
Each capsule contains: Licorice root 250 mg • Garlic 260 mg.

Licorice Plus - Metagenics
Three tablets contain: Licorice root extract (glycyrrhiza glabrra, standardized to 13.5% glycyrrhizic acid) 900 mg • Ashwagandha root extract (withania somnifera) 150 mg • Proprietary Herbal Blend 4:1 extract 750 mg: Rehmannia root (rehmannia glutinosa), Chinese Yam root (dioscorea oppositifolia).

Licorice Root 400 mg - Vital Nutrients
Each capsule contains: Licorice root extract (glycyrrhiza glabra, glycyrrhizin minimum 16% by HPLC) 400 mg.

Licorice Root Extract - Ortho Molecular Products
Each capsule contains: Licorice root extract (standardized to contain 12% glycyrrhizin) 450 mg. Other Ingredients: Natural Vegetable Capsules, Magnesium Stearate, Microcrystalline Cellulose.

Licorice Root Liquid - Ortho Molecular Products
Each drop contains: Licorice root extract (glycyrrhiza glabra, extracted in spring water and USP pure grain alcohol, standardized to contain 7.5% glycyrrhizin, minimum fresh herb strength ration 2:1) 10 mg. Other Ingredients: Glycerin, Water.

Life Essentials Dietary Supplement - Pharmanex
Each capsule contains: Vitamin A (as vitamin A palmitate) 2500 IU • Beta Carotene (from dunaliella salina) 1000 IU •Vitamin C (as ascorbic acid, acerola cherry extract) 70 mg •Vitamin D (D3 as cholecalciferol) 200 IU •Vitamin E (as D-alpha tocopheryl succinate, beta, gamma, delta tocopherols) 30 IU •Thiamin (as thiamine mononitrate) 0.75 mg •Riboflavin 0.85 mg •Niacin (as niacinamide) 10 mg •Vitamin B-6 (as pyridoxine hydrochloride, pyridoxal-5-phosphate) 1 mg • Folic Acid 200 mcg •Vitamin B-12 (as cyanocobalamin) 3 mcg •Biotin 75 mcg • Pantothenic Acid (as D-calcium pantothenate) 5 mg •Calcium (as calcium carbonate, calcium chelate) 100 mg •Iron (as iron chelate) 1.5 mg •Iodine (as potassium iodide) 37.5 mcg •Magnesium (as magnesium chelate, magnesium citrate, magnesium oxide) 50 mg •Zinc (as zinc chelate) 7.5 mg •Selenium (as L-selenomethionine) 17.5 mcg • Copper (as copper chelate) 1 mg •Manganese (as manganese chelate) 1.75 mg •Chromium (as chromium chelate) 60 mcg •Molybdenum (as molybdenum chelate) 37.5 mcg •Potassium (as potassium chloride) 40 mg •Boron (as boron citrate) 0.5 mg •Horsetail extract 75 mg.

Life Extension 7-Keto DHEA - Life Extension
Each capsule contains: 7-Keto DHEA (3-acetyl-7-oxo-dehydroepiandrosterone) 25 mg. Other Ingredients: Rice Flour, Gelatin.

Life Extension Mix Caps - Life Extension
Fourteen capsules contain: Vitamin A (50% as natural D. salina beta-carotene/mixed carotenoids, 50% as acetate) 10,000 IU • Alpha-Carotene 89 mcg • Zeaxanthin 18 mcg • Cryptoxanthin 24 mcg • Lutein 12 mcg • Vitamin C (as ascorbic acid, calcium ascorbate, ascorbyl palmitate, magnesium ascorbate, niacinamide ascorbate, acerola juice powder) 2605 mg • Vitamin D (D3, as cholecalciferol) 400 IU • Vitamin E (as natural d-alpha tocopheryl succinate) 400 IU • Thiamine (vitamin B1, as thiamine hydrochloride) 125 mg • Riboflavin (vitamin B2, with riboflavin 5-phosphate coenzyme 2 mg) 50 mg • Niacin (vitamin B3, as 53% niacinamide, 40% niacin, 7% niacinamide ascorbate) 187 mg • Vitamin B6 (as pyridoxine HCl with pyridoxal 5' phosphate coenzyme 2.5 mg) 100 mg • Folic Acid 800 mcg • Vitamin B12 (as 42% cyanocobalamin, 42% hydroxylcobalamin, 14% ion exchange resin) 600 mcg • Biotin 3000 mcg • Pantothenic Acid (as d-calcium pantothenate with pantethine 5 mg) 600 mg • Calcium (as calcium ascorbate, calcium pantothenate, calcium d-glucarate) 227 mg • Iodine (as potassium iodine) 75 mg • Magnesium (oxide 260.96 elemental, citrate 15.66 elemental, aspartate 19.62 mg elemental, glycinate 11.74 mg elemental, taurinate 7.83 mg elemental, arginate 5.87 mg elemental, ascorbate 3.40 mg elemental) 325 mg • Zinc (as methionate, zinc succinate) 35 mg • Selenium (as 50% se-methylselenocysteine, 25% selenomax, l-selenomethionine in a base of dicalcium phosphate, 25% sodium selenate) 200 mcg • Copper (as copper amino acid chelate) 1 mg • Manganese (as manganese gluconate) 3 mg • Chromium (as chromium polynicotinate) 200 mcg • Molybdenum (as sodium molybdate) 125 mcg • Potassium (as potassium chloride, aspartate) 37.4 mg • Lysine (as l-lysine HCl) 500 mg • N-Acetyl-Cysteine (NAC) 600 mg • Taurine 500 mg • Choline (as choline bitartrate) 117.5 mg • Inositol 250 mg • Phosphatidylcholine (from soy) 150 mg • Bromelain (from pineapple, 2400 GDU per gram) 15 mg • Para-Aminobenzoic Acid (PABA) 200 mg • Trimethylglycine (TMG, as betaine anhydrous, from sugar beets) 100 mg • Bilberry berry extract (baccinium myrtillus, standardized for 25% anthocyanidins 7.5 mg) 30 mg • Citrus Bioflavonoid complex (hesperidin, citrus aurantium 470 mg, naringin 140 mg, naringenin 7-b-rutinoside/others 10 mg) 1300 mg • Ascorbyl Palmitate (fat soluble vitamin C) 250 mg • Ginger root extract (zingiber officinale, 5% gingerols 10 mg) 200 mg • Grapeseed extract (vitis vinifera, inner core of fruit, 95% proanthocyanidins 23.75 mg) 25 mg • Grape extract (vitis vinifera L.) 25 mg providing the following typical profile of active ingredients: proanthycyanidins [95%, includes dimeric procyanidins 1.25 mg] 23.75 mg, anthocyanidins [5%] 1.25 mg, trans-resveratrol >500 ppm, cis-resveratrol <100 ppm) 25 mg • Milk Thistle seeds extract (silybum marianus, standardized for 85% silymarin 85 mg) 100 mg • Dilaurylthiodipropionate 25 mg • Thiodiproprionic Acid 25 mg • Acerola juice powder extract 1:4 (malpighia punicifolia l.) 300 mg • Alpha-Carotene 1000 IU • Broccoli concentrate complex (proprietary blend: broccoli concentrate, calcium d-glucarate, providing sulphoraphane 1.5 mg) 500 mg • Calcium D-Glucarate 200 mg • Boron (as boron citrate/asparate/glycinate) 3 mg • Labiatae plants extract (from rosemary, thyme, sage) 300 mg • Typical Profile (to equal 4.5-8.5% total flavones, 13.5-25.5 mg): Apigenin-7-Glucoside (3.5-5%) 10.5-15 mg, Apigenin (0.0-1%) 0-3 mg, Luteolin (0.5-1%) 1.5-3 mg, Other Flavones (0.5-1.5%) 1.4-4.5 mg • Lutein (purified concentrate from marigold flowers, tagetes erecta, providing zeaxanthin 99 mcg) 15 mg • Lycopene (from tomato skin extract) 3 mg • Raspberry leaf extract (rubus idaeus, standardized for 38.45% ellagic acid 50 mg) 130 mg. Other Ingredients: Magnesium Stearate. See Editor's Note No. 40.

Life Extension Mix Powder w/Stevia - Life Extension
Fourteen capsules contain: Vitamin A (50% as natural D. salina beta-carotene/mixed carotenoids, 50% as acetate) 10,000 IU • Alpha-Carotene 89 mcg • Zeaxanthin 18 mcg • Cryptoxanthin 24 mcg • Lutein 12 mcg • Vitamin C (as ascorbic acid, calcium ascorbate, ascorbyl palmitate, magnesium ascorbate, niacinamide ascorbate, acerola juice powder) 2605 mg • Vitamin D (D3, as cholecalciferol) 400 IU • Vitamin E (as natural d-alpha tocopheryl succinate) 400 IU • Thiamine (vitamin B1, as thiamine hydrochloride) 125 mg • Riboflavin (vitamin B2, with riboflavin 5-phosphate coenzyme 2 mg) 50 mg • Niacin (vitamin B3, as 53% niacinamide, 40% niacin, 7% niacinamide ascorbate) 187 mg • Vitamin B6 (as pyridoxine HCl with pyridoxal 5' phosphate coenzyme 2.5 mg) 100 mg • Folic Acid 800 mcg • Vitamin B12 (as 42% cyanocobalamin, 42% hydroxylcobalamin, 14% ion exchange resin) 600 mcg • Biotin 3000 mcg • Pantothenic Acid (as d-calcium pantothenate with pantethine 5 mg) 600 mg • Calcium (as calcium ascorbate, calcium pantothenate, calcium d-glucarate) 227 mg • Iodine (as potassium iodine) 75 mg • Magnesium (oxide 260.96 elemental, citrate 15.66 elemental, aspartate 19.62 mg elemental, glycinate 11.74 mg

elemental, taurinate 7.83 mg elemental, arginate 5.87 mg elemental, ascorbate 3.40 mg elemental) 325 mg • Zinc (as methionate, zinc succinate) 35 mg • Selenium (as 50% se-methylselenocysteine, 25% selenomax, l-selenomethionine in a base of dicalcium phosphate, 25% sodium selenate) 200 mcg • Copper (as copper amino acid chelate) 1 mg • Manganese (as manganese gluconate) 3 mg • Chromium (as chromium polynicotinate) 200 mcg • Molybdenum (as sodium molybdate) 125 mcg • Potassium (as potassium chloride, aspartate) 37.4 mg • Lysine (as l-lysine HCl) 500 mg • N-Acetyl-Cysteine (NAC) 600 mg • Taurine 500 mg • Choline (as choline bitartrate) 117.5 mg • Inositol 250 mg • Phosphatidylcholine (from soy) 150 mg • Bromelain (from pineapple, 2400 GDU per gram) 15 mg • Para-Aminobenzoic Acid (PABA) 200 mg • Trimethylglycine (TMG, as betaine anhydrous, from sugar beets) 100 mg • Bilberry berry extract (baccinium myrtillus, standardized for 25% anthocyanidins 7.5 mg) 30 mg • Citrus Bioflavonoid complex (hesperidin, citrus aurantium 470 mg, naringin 140 mg, naringenin 7-b-rutinoside/others 10 mg) 1300 mg • Ascorbyl Palmitate (fat soluble vitamin C) 250 mg • Ginger root extract (zingiber officinale, 5% gingerols 10 mg) 200 mg • Grapeseed extract (vitis vinifera, inner core of fruit, 95% proanthocyanidins 23.75 mg) 25 mg • Grape extract (vitis vinifera L.) 25 mg providing the following typical profile of active ingredients: proanthycyanidins [95%, includes dimeric procyanidins 1.25 mg] 23.75 mg, anthocyanidins [5%] 1.25 mg, trans-resveratrol >500 ppm, cis-resveratrol <100 ppm) 25 mg • Milk Thistle seeds extract (silybum marianus, standardized for 85% silymarin 85 mg) 100 mg • Dilaurylthiodipropionate 25 mg • Thiodiproprionic Acid 25 mg • Acerola juice powder extract 1:4 (malpighia punicifolia l.) 300 mg • Alpha-Carotene 1000 IU • Broccoli concentrate complex (proprietary blend: broccoli concentrate, calcium d-glucarate, providing sulphoraphane 1.5 mg) 500 mg • Calcium D-Glucarate 200 mg • Boron (as boron citrate/asparate/glycinate) 3 mg • Labiatae plants extract (from rosemary, thyme, sage) 300 mg • Typical Profile (to equal 4.5-8.5% total flavones, 13.5-25.5 mg): Apigenin-7-Glucoside (3.5-5%) 10.5-15 mg, Apigenin (0.0-1%) 0-3 mg, Luteolin (0.5-1%) 1.5-3 mg, Other Flavones (0.5-1.5%) 1.4-4.5 mg • Lutein (purified concentrate from marigold flowers, tagetes erecta, providing zeaxanthin 99 mcg) 15 mg • Lycopene (from tomato skin extract) 3 mg • Raspberry leaf extract (rubus idaeus, standardized for 38.45% ellagic acid 50 mg) 130 mg. Other Ingredients: Stevia, Natural Orange Color, Lecithin Powder. See Editor's Note No. 40.

Life Extension Mix Tabs - Life Extension
Nine tablets contain: Vitamin A (50% as natural D. salina beta-carotene/mixed carotenoids, 50% as acetate) 10,000 IU • Alpha-Carotene 89 mcg • Zeaxanthin 18 mcg • Cryptoxanthin 24 mcg • Lutein 12 mcg • Vitamin C (as ascorbic acid, calcium ascorbate, ascorbyl palmitate, magnesium ascorbate, niacinamide ascorbate, acerola juice powder) 2605 mg • Vitamin D (D3, as cholecalciferol) 400 IU • Vitamin E (as natural d-alpha tocopheryl succinate) 400 IU • Thiamine (vitamin B1, as thiamine hydrochloride) 125 mg • Riboflavin (vitamin B2, with riboflavin 5-phosphate coenzyme 2 mg) 50 mg • Niacin (vitamin B3, as 53% niacinamide, 40% niacin, 7% niacinamide ascorbate) 187 mg • Vitamin B6 (as pyridoxine HCl with pyridoxal 5' phosphate coenzyme 2.5 mg) 100 mg • Folic Acid 800 mcg • Vitamin B12 (as 42% cyanocobalamin, 42% hydroxylcobalamin, 14% ion exchange resin) 600 mcg • Biotin 3000 mcg • Pantothenic Acid (as d-calcium pantothenate with pantethine 5 mg) 600 mg • Calcium (as calcium ascorbate, calcium panothenate, calcium d-glucarate) 227 mg • Iodine (as potassium iodine) 75 mg • Magnesium (oxide 260.96 elemental, citrate 15.66 elemental, aspartate 19.62 mg elemental, glycinate 11.74 mg elemental, taurinate 7.83 mg elemental, arginate 5.87 mg elemental, ascorbate 3.40 mg elemental) 325 mg • Zinc (as methionate, zinc succinate) 35 mg • Selenium (as 50% se-methylselenocysteine, 25% selenomax, l-selenomethionine in a base of dicalcium phosphate, 25% sodium selenate) 200 mcg • Copper (as copper amino acid chelate) 1 mg • Manganese (as manganese gluconate) 3 mg • Chromium (as chromium polynicotinate) 200 mcg • Molybdenum (as sodium molybdate) 125 mcg • Potassium (as potassium chloride, aspartate) 37.4 mg • Lysine (as l-lysine HCl) 500 mg • N-Acetyl-Cysteine (NAC) 600 mg • Taurine 500 mg • Choline (as choline bitartrate) 117.5 mg • Inositol 250 mg • Phosphatidylcholine (from soy) 150 mg • Bromelain (from pineapple, 2400 GDU per gram) 15 mg • Para-Aminobenzoic Acid (PABA) 200 mg • Trimethylglycine (TMG, as betaine anhydrous, from sugar beets) 100 mg • Bilberry berry extract (baccinium myrtillus, standardized for 25% anthocyanidins 7.5 mg) 30 mg • Citrus Bioflavonoid complex (hesperidin, citrus aurantium 470 mg, naringin 140 mg, naringenin 7-b-rutinoside/others 10 mg) 1300 mg • Ascorbyl Palmitate (fat soluble vitamin C) 250 mg • Ginger root extract (zingiber officinale, 5% gingerols 10 mg) 200 mg • Grapeseed extract (vitis vinifera, inner core of fruit, 95% proanthocyanidins 23.75 mg) 25 mg • Grape extract (vitis vinifera L.) 25 mg providing the following typical profile of active ingredients: Proanthocyanidins (95%, includes dimeric procyanidins 1.25 mg) 23.75 mg, Anthocyanidins (5%) 1.25 mg, Trans-Resveratrol >500 ppm, Cis-Resveratrol <100 ppm • Milk Thistle seeds extract (silybum marianus, standardized for 85% silymarin 85 mg) 100 mg • Dilaurylthiodipropionate 25 mg • Thiodiproprionic Acid 25 mg • Acerola juice powder extract 1:4 (malpighia punicifolia l.) 300 mg • Alpha-Carotene 1000 IU • Broccoli concentrate complex (proprietary blend: broccoli concentrate, calcium d-glucarate, providing sulphoraphane 1.5 mg) 500 mg • Calcium D-Glucarate 200 mg • Boron (as boron citrate/asparate/glycinate) 3 mg • Labiatae plants extract (from rosemary, thyme, sage) 300 mg • Typical Profile (to equal 4.5-8.5% total flavones, 13.5-25.5 mg): Apigenin-7-Glucoside (3.5-5%) 10.5-15 mg, Apigenin (0.0-1%) 0-3 mg, Luteolin (0.5-1%) 1.5-3 mg, Other Flavones (0.5-1.5%) 1.4-4.5 mg • Lutein (purified concentrate from marigold flowers, tagetes erecta, providing zeaxanthin 99 mcg) 15 mg • Lycopene (from tomato skin extract) 3 mg • Raspberry leaf extract (rubus idaeus, standardized for 38.45% ellagic acid 50 mg) 130 mg. Other Ingredients: Microcrystalline Cellulose, Stearic Acid, Magnesium Stearate, Croscarmellose Sodium, Silica, Pharmaceutical Glaze.

Life Extension One-Per-Day Tablets - Life Extension
Each tablet contains: Vitamin A (as beta-carotene 20, as palmitate 80%) 5000 IU • Vitamin C (as niacinamide and calcium ascorbates, ascorbic acid) 500 mg • Vitamin D (as cholecalciferol) 200 IU • Vitamin E (as D-alpha-tocopheryl succinate) 200 IU • Thiamine (vitamin B1, as thiamine HCl) 75 mg • Riboflavin (vitamin B2) 50 mg • Niacin (vitamin B3, as niacinamide ascorbate) 50 mg • Vitamin B6 (as pyridoxine HCl) 75 mg • Folate (as folic acid) 800 mcg • Vitamin B12 (as cyanocobalamin) 300 mcg • Pantothenic Acid (as D-calcium pantothenate) 100 mg • Calcium (from D-calcium pantothenate, calcium ascorbate) 20 mg • Iodine (from Atlantic kelp) 150 mcg • Magnesium (as magnesium oxide) 100 mg • Zinc (as OptiZinc R zinc DL-methionine complex) 30 mg • Selenium (as L-selenomethionine) 100 mcg • Manganese (as manganese gluconate) 2 mg • Chromium (as chromium polynicotinate) 200 mcg • Molybdenum (as molybdenum amino acid chelate) 100 mcg • Potassium (as potassium citrate) 25 mg • Alpha-Carotene 50 mcg • Boron (as boron amino acid chelate) 3 mg • Choline (bitartrate) 22.9 mg • Inositol 50 mg • Xantopina R plus Lutein extract (from marigold cempasuchil flowers (tagetes erectus L.) standardized for 40% lutein (5 mg), 4% zeaxanthin (0.5 mg)) 12.5 mg • Lycopene (as Lyc-O-Mato tomato extract) 2 mg • PABA (para-aminobenzoic acid) 2 mg • Biotin 300 mcg. Other Ingredients: Dicalcium Phosphate, Microcrystalline Cellulose, Maltodextrin, Stearic Acid, Magnesium Stearate, Croscarmellose Sodium, Silicon Dioxide, Purified Water, Methylcellulose, Propylene Glycol.

Life Extension Two-Per-Day Tablets - Life Extension
Two tablets contain: Vitamin A (as beta-carotene 20, as palmitate 80%) 5000 IU • Vitamin C (as niacinamide and calcium ascorbates, ascorbic acid) 500 mg • Vitamin D (as cholecalciferol) 400 IU • Vitamin E (as D-alpha-tocopheryl succinate) 200 IU • Thiamine (vitamin B1, as thiamine HCl) 75 mg • Riboflavin (vitamin B2) 50 mg • Niacin (vitamin B3, as niacinamide ascorbate) 50 mg • Vitamin B6 (as pyridoxine HCl) 75 mg • Folate (as folic acid)

800 mcg • Vitamin B12 (as cyanocobalamin) 300 mcg • Biotin 300 mcg • Pantothenic Acid (as D-calcium pantothenate, calcium ascorbate) 20 mg • Iodine (from Atlantic kelp) 150 mcg • Magnesium (as magnesium oxide) 100 mg • Zinc (as OptiZinc zinc DL-methionine complex) 30 mg • Selenium (as L-selenomethionine) 100 mcg • Manganese (as manganese gluconate) 2 mg • Chromium (as chromium polynicotinate) 200 mcg • Molybdenum (as molybdenum amino acid chelate) 100 mcg • Potassium (as potassium citrate) 25 mg • Alpha-Carotene 50 mcg • Boron (as boron amino acid chelate) 3 mg • Choline (bitartrate) 22.9 mg • Inositol 50 mg • Xantopina plus Lutein extract (from marigold cempasuchil flowers (tagetes erectus L.), standardized for 40% lutein (5 mg), 4% zeaxanthin (0.5mg)) 12.5 mg • Lycopene (as Lyc-O-Mato tomato extract) 2 mg • PABA (para-aminobenzoic acid) 30 mg. Other Ingredients: Dicalcium Phosphate, Microcrystalline Cellulose, Maltodextrin, Stearic Acid, Magnesium Stearate, Croscarmellose Sodium, Silicon Dioxde, Purified Water, Methylcellulose, Propylene Glycol.

Life Force Multiple - Source Naturals
Two tablets contain: Vitamin A (beta carotene) 7500 IU • Vitamin A (palmitate) 5000 IU • Total Vitamin A activity 12500 IU • Vitamin B-1 (thiamin) 50 mg • Vitamin B-2 (riboflavin) 50 mg • Niacinamide 35 mg • Niacin 15 mg • Vitamin B-5 (pantothenic acid) 50 mg • Vitamin B-6 (pyridoxine HCl) 50 mg • Vitamin B-12 (cyanocobalamin) 100 mcg • Biotin 150 mcg • Folic Acid 400 mcg • Vitamin C (ascorbic acid crystals, ascorbyl palmitate) 500 mg • Vitamin D-3 (cholecalciferol) 200 IU • Vitamin E D-alpha Tocopheryl (natural) 200 IU • Boron (amino acid chelate) 2 mg • Calcium (chelate, citrate, malate) 100 mg • Chromium (ChromeMate yeast-free polynicotinate) 100 mcg • Copper (sebacate) 1 mg • Iodine (from kelp) 100 mcg • Iron (fumarate) 6 mg • Magnesium (chelate, citrate, oxide) 100 mg • Manganese (citrate) 3 mg • Molybdenum (amino acid chelate) 100 mcg • Potassium (citrate) 50 mg • Selenium (L-Selenomethionine and sodium selenite) 100 mcg • Zinc (citrate and OptiZinc monomethionine) 15 mg. Other Ingredients: Coenzyme Q10 (ubiquinone) 20mg, Alpha-Lipoic Acid (thioctic acid) 25 mg, N-Acetyl Cysteine 100 mg, DMAE (bitartrate) 30 mg, Silymarin (milk thistle seed extract) 60 mg, Ginkgo Biloba 24% (50:1 extract) 20 mg, Choline (bitartrate) 50 mg, Inositol 50mg , Hawthorn berry 75 mg, Turmeric root 75 mg, Bilberry fruit extract standardized to 25% anthocyanidins 10 mg, Proanthodyn (grape seed extract) 25 mg, L-Tyrosine 50 mg, Methylsulfonylmethane 25 mg, Bioperine brand Black Pepper extract 3 mg.

Life Force Multiple No Iron - Source Naturals
Two tablets contain: Vitamin A (beta carotene) 7500 IU • Vitamin A (palmitate) 5000 IU • Total Vitamin A activity 12500 IU • Vitamin B-1 (thiamin) 50 mg • Vitamin B-2 (riboflavin) 50 mg • Niacinamide 35 mg • Niacin 15 mg • Vitamin B-5 (pantothenic acid) 50 mg • Vitamin B-6 (pyridoxine HCl) 50 mg • Vitamin B-12 (cyanocobalamin) 100 mcg • Biotin 150 mcg • Folic acid 400 mcg • Vitamin C (ascorbic acid crystals, ascorbyl palmitate) 500 mg • Vitamin D-3 (cholecalciferol) 200 IU • Vitamin E D-alpha Tocopheryl (natural) 200 IU • Boron (amino acid chelate) 2 mg • Calcium (chelate, citrate, malate) 100 mg • Chromium (ChromeMate yeast-free polynicotinate) 100 mcg • Copper (sebacate) 1 mg • Iodine (from kelp) 100 mcg • Magnesium (chelate, citrate, oxide) 100 mg • Manganese (citrate) 3 mg • Molybdenum (amino acid chelate) 100 mcg • Potassium (citrate) 50 mg • Selenium (L-Selenomethionine and sodium selenite) 100 mcg • Zinc (citrate and OptiZinc monomethionine) 15 mg. Other Ingredients: Coenzyme Q10 (ubiquinone) 20mg, Alpha-Lipoic Acid (thioctic acid) 25 mg, N-Acetyl Cysteine 100 mg, DMAE (bitartrate) 30 mg, Silymarin (milk thistle seed extract) 60 mg, Ginkgo Biloba 24% (50:1 extract) 20 mg, Choline (bitartrate) 50 mg, Inositol 50mg , Hawthorn berry 75 mg, Turmeric root 75 mg, Bilberry fruit extract standardized to 25% anthocyanidins 10 mg, Proanthodyn (grape seed extract) 25 mg, L-Tyrosine 50 mg, Methylsulfonylmethane 25 mg, Bioperine brand Black Pepper extract 3 mg.

Life Minerals - Source Naturals
Four tablets contain: Calcium (Citrate, Fumarate, Malate, Succinate and alpha-Ketoglutarate) 480 mg • Magnesium (Citrate, Fumarate, Malate, Succinate and alpha-Ketoglutarate) 480 mg • Potassium (Citrate, Malate, Fumarate, Succinate, and alpha-Ketoglutarate) 99 mg • Zinc (OptiZinc Zinc Monomethionine 20 mg and Ascorbate 10 mg) 30mg • Chromium (ChromeMate GTF Chromium Polynicotinate) 300 mcg • Selenium (Selenomethionine and Sodium Selenite) 200 mcg • Iron (Fumarate, Citrate and Succinate) 15 mg • Boron(Amino Acid Chelate) 3 mg • Silica (Horsetail Silica extract) 4.5 mg • Iodine (from Kelp) 150 mcg • Copper (Sebacate) 2 mg • Molybdenum (Chelate) 300 mcg • Vitamin B-6 (Pyridoxine HCl) 10 mg • Vitamin C (Zinc and Manganese Ascorbates) 78 mg • Vitamin D-3 (Cholecalciferol) 200 IU.

Life Minerals-No Iron - Source Naturals
Four tablets contain: Calcium (Citrate, Fumarate, Malate, Succinate and alpha-Ketoglutarate) 480 mg • Magnesium (Citrate, Fumarate, Malate, Succinate and alpha-Ketoglutarate) 480 mg • Potassium (Citrate, Malate, Fumarate, Succinate, and alpha-Ketoglutarate) 99 mg • Zinc (OptiZinc Zinc Monomethionine 20 mg and Ascorbate 10 mg) 30 mg • Chromium (ChromeMate GTF Chromium Polynicotinate) 300 mcg • Selenium (Selenomethionine and Sodium Selenite) 200 mcg • Boron (Amino Acid Chelate) 3 mg • Silica (Horsetail Silica extract) 4.5 mg • Iodine (from Kelp) 150 mcg • Copper (Sebacate) 2 mg • Molybdenum (Chelate) 300 mcg • Vitamin B-6 (Pyridoxine HCl) 10 mg • Vitamin C (Zinc and Manganese Ascorbates) 78 mg • Vitamin D-3 (Cholecalciferol) 200 IU.

Life Spark - Source Naturals
Four tablets contain: Vitamin B1 (Thiamin) 30 mg • Vitamin B2 (Riboflavin) 30 mg • Vitamin B3 (Niacin 25 mg and Niacinamide 125 mg) 150 mg • Vitamin B5 (Pantothenic Acid) 100 mg • Vitamin B6 (Pyridoxine HCl) 25 mg • Vitamin B12 (Cyanocobalamin) 100 mcg • Vitamin E (D-Alpha Tocopheryl) (Natural) 150 IU • Magnesium (Oxide, Citrate) 250 mg • Potassium (Citrate) 99 mg • Glycine 500 mg • Tyrosine 250 mg • Coenzyme Q10 (Ubiquinone) 50 mg • Alpha-Lipoic Acid 25 mg • Herbal Blend 1170 mg: Siberian Ginseng, Panax Ginseng, Polygonum Multiflori (Fo Ti), Cyperus, Panax Ginseng extract, Tien Chi, and Siberian Ginseng extract.

LifeGuard Advanced Antioxidant - Starlight International
Each two tablets contain: Vitamin A (as beta carotene) 5000 IU • Vitamin C (as asorbic acid) 300 mg • Vitamin E (as d-alpha tocopheryl succintate) 30 IU • Zinc (as zinc picolinate) 50 mg • Selenium (as sodium selenite) 60 mcg • Bilberry extract 4:1 (vaccinium myrtillus, fruit) 400 mg • Green Tea extract 4:1 (carmellia sinensis, leaf) 150 mg • Turmeric (curcuma longa, rhizome) 150 mg • Pine Bark extract (pinus strobus, bark) 40 mg • Ginkgo Biloba extract (leaf) 24% Ginkgo flavone glycosides, 6% terpene lactones 20 mg • Garlic (allim salivum, root) deodorized 10 mg • Echinacea purpurea (plant) 10 mg • Goldenseal (hydrastis caradensis, plant) 2 mg. Inactive Ingredients: Croscarmellose Sodium, Dicalcium Phosphate, Hydroxpropylcellulose, Stearic Acid, Magnesium Stearate, Microcrystalline Cellulose, Calcium Carbonate, Calcium Sulfate, Silicon Dioxide, Dextrin, Dextrose, Lecithin, Sodium Citrate.

LifeGuard Cholesterol Control - Starlight International
Two tablets contain: Red Rice Yeast (Monascus purpureus, Plant) 800 mg • Fo-Ti (Polygonum multiforum, Plant) 50 mg • Soy 80 mg • Beta Sitosterol 100 mg • English Hawthorn (Crataegus laevigata, Fruit) 30 mg. Other Ingredients: Calcium Carbonate, Microcrystalline Cellulose, Stearic Acid, Croscarmellose Sodium, Magnesium Stearate, Silicon Dioxide, Hydroxypropylcellulose, Dextrin, Dextrose, Lecithin, Sodium Citrate.

LifeGuard Joint Formula - Starlight International
Three tablets contain: Manganese (as manganese ascorbate) 6 mg • Glucosamine HCl 750 mg • Chondroitin Sulfate, 95% 250 mg • MSM (methyl-sulfonyl-methane) 100 mg • Sulfate (sodium-sulfate) 30 mg • Turmeric, 90% curcumin (curcuma longa, root) 25 mg • Boswellia Serrata extract, 65% (boswellic acid, trunk) 25 mg. Other Ingredients: Dicalcium Phosphate, Microcrystalline Cellulose, Stearic Acid, Croscarmellose Sodium, Silicon Dioxide, Magnesium Stearate, Dextrin, Dextrose, Lecithin, Sodium Carboxymethylcellulose, Sodium Citrate.
See Editor's Note No. 15.

LifeGuard Junior **-** Starlight International
Each two tablets contain: Vitamin A (as beta carotene) 1000 IU • Vitamin C (as sodium ascorbate) 100 mg • Vitamin E (as d-alpha tocopheryl acetate) 20 IU • Bilberry extract 4:1 (vaccinium myrtillus, fruit) 100 mg • Vegetable complex (tomato, carrot, cabbage, broccoli, and green pepper powder) 100 mg • Acerola (malpighia glabra, fruit) 75 mg • Rosehips powder (rosa canina, fruit) 25 mg • Grape Seed extract, 95% flavanols (vitis vinifera seed) 2 mg.

LifePak anti-aging formula **-** Pharmanex
Each packet contains: Vitamin A (as vitamin A palmitate, 83% as beta carotene from palm fruit and blakeslea trispora extracts) 7500 IU • Vitamin C (as calcium ascorbate) 250 mg • Vitamin D (as cholecalciferol) 200 IU • Vitamin E (as D-alpha tocopheryl acetate, beta, gamma, delta tocotrienols, tocotrienols) 150 IU • Vitamin K (as phytonadione) 20 mcg • Thiamin (as thiamine mononitrate) 3.75 mg • Riboflavin (as riboflavin) 4.25 mg • Niacin (as niacin, niacinamide) 20 mg • Vitamin B6 (as pyridoxine hydrochloride) 5 mg • Folate (as folic acid) 300 mcg • Vitamin B12 (as cyanocobalamin) 15 mcg • Biotin (as biotin) 150 mcg • Pantothenic Acid (as D-calcium pantothenate) 15 mg • Calcium (as calcium carbonate, calcium ascorbate, calcium propionate) 250 mg • Iodine (as potassium iodide) 50 mcg • Magnesium (as magnesium chelate, magnesium oxide) 125 mg • Zinc (as zinc chelate) 7.5 mg • Selenium (as L-selenomethionine, sodium selenite) 70 mcg • Copper (as copper chelate) 0.5 mg • Manganese (as manganese chelate) 1 mg • Chromium (as chromium chelate) 100 mcg • Molybdenum (as molybdenum chelate) 37.5 mcg • Polyphenol and Flavonoid Blend 97.5 mg • Catechins (from camellia sinensis leaf 20:1 extract) 45 mg • Quercetin 25 mg • Grape seed extract (with min. 95% polyphenols) 12.5 mg • Citrus Bioflavonoids (from citrus fruits) 12.5 mg • Isoflavones (from soy extract) 2.5 mg • Alpha-Lipoic Acid 15 mg • Inositol (as inositol) 5 mg • Carotenoid Blend (other than beta-carotene) 4.5 mg • Lycopene (from lycopene) 2. 5mg • Alpha Carotene (from palm fruit extract) 1 mg • Lutein (from marigold flower extract) 1 mg • Boron (as boron citrate) 1.5 mg • Silicon (as sodium metasilicate) 1.5 mg • Vanadium (as vanadyl sulfate) 10 mcg.

LifePak Prenatal **-** Pharmanex
Each vitamin/phytonutrient capsule contains: Vitamin A (vitamin A palmitate, 50% as beta carotene from dunaliella salina) 5000 IU • Vitamin C (calcium ascorbate) 150 mg • Vitamin D (D3, cholecalciferol) 200 IU • Vitamin E (D-alpha tocopheryl succinate) 75 IU • Vitamin K (K1, phytonadione) 20 mcg • Thiamin (thiamine mononitrate) 1.7 mg • Riboflavin (riboflavin) 2 mg • Niacin (niacin, niacinamide) 20 mg • Vitamin B6 (pyridoxine hydrochloride) 2.5 mg • Folate (folic acid) 400 mcg • Vitamin B12 (cyanocobalamin) 8 mcg • Biotin (biotin) 150 mcg • Pantothenic Acid (D-calcium pantothenate) 10 mg • Inositol 250 mcg • Lutein (from marigold flower extract) 1 mg • Lycopene (from tomato extract) 0.5 mg.
Two mineral capsules contain: Calcium (calcium carbonate, calcium citrate, calcium chelate) 325 mg • Iron (iron chelate) 15 mg • Iodine (potassium iodide) 37.5 mcg • Magnesium (magnesium aspartate, magnesium oxide, magnesium chelate) 175 mg • Zinc (zinc chelate) 10 mg • Selenium (1-selenomethionine) 35 mcg • Copper (copper chelate) 1 mg • Manganese (manganese chelate) 1.5 mg • Chromium (chromium chelate) 90 mcg • Molybdenum (molybdenum chelate) 37.5 mcg • Inositol 250 mcg • Lycopene (from tomato extract) 0.5 mg • Lutein (from marigold flower extract) 1 mg • Boron (as boron citrate) 1.5 mg • Silicon (sodium metasilicate) 1.5 mg • Vanadium (vanadyl sulfate) 10 mcg. Other Ingredients: Maltodextrin, Sodium Carboxymethylcellulose, Magnesium Stearate.

LifePak Prime **-** Pharmanex
Each packet contains: Vitamin A (as vitamin A palmitate, 83% as beta carotene from palm fruit and blakeslea trispora extracts) 7500 IU • Vitamin C (as calcium ascorbate) 250 mg • Vitamin D (as cholecalciferol) 300 IU • Vitamin E (as D-alpha tocopheryl acetate, beta, gamma, delta tocopherols, tocotrienols) 150 IU • Vitamin K (as phytonadione) 20 mcg • Thiamin 3.75 mg • Riboflavin (as riboflavin) 4.25 mg • Niacin (as niacin, niacinamide) 20 mg • Vitamin B6 (as pyridoxine hydrochloride) 5 mg • Folate (as folic acid) 300 mcg • Vitamin B12 (as cyanocobalamin) 30 mcg • Biotin (as biotin) 150 mcg • Pantothenic Acid (as D-calcium pantothenate) 15 mg • Calcium (as calcium carbonate, calcium ascorbate, tricalcium phosphate, calcium propionate) 500 mg • Phosphorus (as tricalcium phosphate) 100 mg • Iodine (as potassium iodide) 50 mcg • Magnesium (as magnesium chelate, magnesium oxide) 250 mg • Zinc (as zinc chelate) 10 mg • Selenium (as L-selenomethionine, sodium selenite) 70 mcg • Copper (as copper chelate) 0.5 mg • Manganese (as manganese chelate) 1 mg • Chromium (as chromium chelate) 100 mcg • Molybdenum (as molybdenum chelate) 37.5 mcg • Polyphenol and Flavonoid blend 100 mg • Catechins from Camellia Sinensis leaf extract (20:1) 45 mg • Grape seed extract (min. 92% polyphenols) 25 mg • Quercetin 25 mg • Citrus Bioflavonoids (from citrus fruits) 12.5 mg • Isoflavones (from soy extract) 2.5 mg • Glucosamine Hydrochloride 100 mg • Alpha-Lipoic Acid 25 mg • N-Acetyl-L-Cysteine 25 mg • Milk Thistle fruit extract (silybum marianum 80% silymar) 25 mg • Ginkgo Biloba 27/7 leaf extract (ginkgo biloba) 20 mg • Coenzyme Q-10 (ubiquinone) 10 mg • Inositol (as inositol) 5 mg • Silicon (as sodium metasilicate) 5 mg • Reduced L-Glutathione 5 mg • Lycopene (as lycopene) 2.5 mg • Alpha-Carotene (from palm fruit extract) 1 mg • Lutein (from marigold flower extract) 1 mg • Boron (as boron citrate) 1.5 mg • Vanadium (as vanadyl sulfate) 10 mcg. Other Ingredients: Gelatin, Microcrystalline Cellulose, Magnesium Stearate, Silicon Dioxide.

LifePak Teen **-** Pharmanex
Two capsules contain: Vitamin A (as vitamin A palmitate, 50% as beta carotene from blakeslea trispora) 5000 IU • Vitamin C (as calcium ascorbate) 100 mcg • Calcium (as calcium carbonate, calcium ascorbate) 250 mg • Iron (as iron chelate) 4.5 mg • Vitamin D (as cholecalciferol) 200 IU • Vitamin E (as mixed natural tocopherols) 50 IU • Vitamin K1 (as phytonadione) 20 mcg • Thiamin (as thiamine mononitrate) 1.5 mg • Riboflavin (as riboflavin) 1.7 mg • Niacin (as niacin, niacinamide) 20 mg • Vitamin B6 (as pyridoxine hydrochloride) 5 mg • Folate (as folic acid) 200 mcg • Vitamin B12 (as cyanocobalamin) 15 mcg • Biotin (as biotin) 150 mcg • Pantothenic Acid (as D-calcium pantothenate) 15 mg • Iodine (as potassium iodide) 37.5 mcg • Magnesium (as magnesium oxide, magnesium chelate) 100 mg • Zinc (as zinc chelate) 7.5 mg • Selenium (as L-selenomethionine, sodium selenite) 35 mcg • Copper (as copper chelate) 1 mg • Manganese (as manganese chelate) 2 mg • Chromium (as chromium chelate) 60 mcg • Molybdenum (as molybdenum chelate) 60 mcg • Boron (as boron citrate) 1.5 mg • Silicon (as sodium metasilicate) 1.5 mg • Vanadium (as vanadyl sulfate) 10 mcg. Other Ingredients: Microcrystalline Cellulose, Sodium Carboxymethyl Cellulose, Magnesium Stearate, Silicon Dioxide.

LifePak Trim (LifePak and TrimPak) **-** Pharmanex
Each LifePak packet contains: Vitamin A (as vitamin A palmitate, 6250 as beta carotene from palm fruit and blakeslea trispora extracts) 1250 IU • Vitamin C (as calcium ascorbate) 250 mg • Vitamin D (as cholecalciferol) 200 IU • Vitamin E (as D-alpha tocopheryl acetate, beta, gamma, delta tocopherols, tocotrienols) 150 IU • Vitamin K (as phytonadione) 20 mcg • Thiamin (as thiamine mononitrate) 2.75 mg • Riboflavin (as riboflavin) 4.25 mg • Niacin (as niacin, niacinamide) 20 mg • Vitamin B6 (as pyridoxine hydrochloride) 5 mg • Folate (as folic acid) 300 mcg • Vitamin B12 (as cyanocobalamin) 15 mcg • Biotin (as biotin) 150 mcg • Pantothenic Acid (as D-calcium pantothenate) 15 mg • Calcium (as calcium carbonate, calcium ascorbate, calcium propionate) 250 mg • Iodine (as potassium iodide) 50 mcg • Magnesium (as magnesium chelate, magnesium oxide) 125 mg • Zinc (as zinc chelate) 7.5 mg • Selenium (as L-selenomethionine, sodium selenite) 70 mcg • Copper (as copper chelate) 0.5 mg • Manganese (as manganese chelate) 1 mg • Chromium (as chromium chelate) 100 mcg • Molybdenum (as molybdenum chelate) 37.5 mcg.
Each TrimPak packet contains: Chromium (as chromium chelate, chromium picolinate) 100 mcg • Garcinia Cambogia with Hydroxy Citric Acid 375 mg • Chitosan (from shellfish) PolmerPlex 1000 mg.

Other Ingredients: Calcium Carbonate, Sodium Carboxymethylcellulose, Cellulose Powder, Magnesium Stearate, Maltodextrin.

LifePak Women Anti-Aging formula - Pharmanex
Each packet (1 vitamin capsule, 2 phytonutrient capsules, 3 mineral capsules) contains: Vitamin A (83% as beta carotene from palm fruit and blakeslea trispora extracts, vitamin A palmitate) 7500 IU • Vitamin C (as calcium ascorbate) 250 mg • Vitamin D (as cholecalciferol) 200 IU • Vitamin E (as D-alpha tocopheryl acetate, beta, gamma, delta tocopherols, tocotrienols) 150 IU • Vitamin K (as phytonadione) 20 mcg • Thiamin (as thiamine mononitrate) 3.75 mg • Riboflavin (as riboflavin) 4.25 mg • Niacin (as niacin, niacinamide) 20 mg • Vitamin B6 (as pyridoxine hydrochloride) 10 mg • Folate (as folic acid) 300 mcg • Vitamin B12 (as cyanocobalamin) 15 mcg • Biotin (as biotin) 150 mc g • Pantothenic Acid (as D-calcium pantothenate) 15 mg • Calcium (as calcium carbonate, tricalcium phosphate, calcium propionate, calcium ascorbate) 500 mg • Phosphorus (as tricalcium phosphate) 100 gm • Iron (as iron chelate) 5 mg • Iodine (as potassium iodide) 50 mcg • Magnesium (as magnesium chelate, magnesium oxide) 250 mg • Zinc (as zinc chelate) 7.5 mg • Selenium (as L-selenomethionine, sodium selenite) 70 mcg • Copper (as copper chelate) 0.5 mg • Manganese (as manganese chelate) 1 mg • Chromium (as chromium chelate) 100 mcg • Molybdenum (as molybdenum chelate) 37.5 mcg • Inositol (as inositol) 125 mg • Cranberry powder 200 mg • Polyphenol and Flavonoid Blend 95 mg: Catechins as Camellia Sinensis leaf 20:1 extract, 45 mg, Quercetin 25 mg, Grape seed (min. 95% polyphenols) 12.5 mg, Citrus Bioflavonoids (from citrus fruits) 12.5 mg, Isoflavones (from soy extract) 12.5 mg • Evening Primrose Oil powder with Gamma Linolenic Acid 75 mg • Borage Seed oil powder with Gamma Linolenic Acid 75 mg • Alpha-Lipoic Acid 15 mg • Carotenoid Blend (other than beta-carotene) 4.5 mg • Lycopene (as lycopene) 2.5 mg • Alpha-Carotene (from plam fruit extract) 1 mg • Lutein (from marigold flower extract) 1 mg • Boron (as boron citrate) 1.5 mg • Silicon (as sodium metasilicate) 1.5 mg • Vanadium (as vanadyl sulfate) 10 mcg. Other Ingredients: Gelatin, Microcrystalline Celluose, Magnesium Stearate, Silicon Dioxide.

Life's Greens - Puritan's Pride
Each scoop (8.8 g) contains: Green Organic Gluten-Free Grasses: Wheat Grass powder 350 mg • Barley grass powder 350 mg • Alfalfa grass powder 350 mg • Oat grass powder 350 mg. Blue-Green And Sea Algae: Spirulina 1,000 mg • Chlorella (cracked-cell) 350 mg • Dunaliella salina 40 mg • Nova Scotia Dulse 30 mg. Adapogenic And Support Herbs: Licorice root 100 mg • Siberian Ginseng (Eleuthrococcus senticosus) 60 mg • Suma (Pfaffia paniculata) 60 mg • Astragalus membraneceus 60 mg • Echinacea purpurea 60 mg • Powdered Ginger root 5 mg. Nutrient-Rich Superfoods: Lecithin 99% oil-free 2,000 mg • Wheat sprout powder 350 mg • Acerola berry juice powder 200 mg • Beet juice powder 200 mg • Spinach octacosanol 150 mg • Royal Jelly (5% 10-HDA) 150 mg • Bee Pollen 150 mg • Vitamin E (d'alpha tocopheryl succinate) 100 IU. Dairy-Free Probiotic Cultures (Total count, Non-dairy culture: 5.0 billion): actoacillus group (L. rhamnosus A, L. rhamnosus B, L. acidophilus, L. casei, L. delbrueckii subsp. bulgaricus) 3.5 billion • Bifidobacterium group (B. longum, B. breve) 1.0 billion • Streptococcus salivarius subsp. thermophilus 500 million. Natural Fibers: Flaxseed meal 500 mg • Apple Pectin and fiber 500 mg • Fructooligosaccharides (FOS) 500 mg. Standardized Bioflavonoid Extracts: Milk Thistle extract (silybum marianum: standardized for 80% silymarin) 60 mg • Ginkgo Biloba extract (standardized for 6% terpene: lactones & 24 % ginkgo flavoglycosides) 20 mg • Green Tea catechins (standadized for 60% catechins) 20 mg • Grape pip extract (92% proanthocyanidins) 20 mg • Bilberry extract (standardized to 25% anthocyanidins) 20 mg.

LifeSPRINGS CALMAX Dietary Supplement - Golden Glow Natural Health Products
Each 7 g serving contains: Calcium Gluconate 4.55 g: Calcium 406 mg • Magnesium Carbonate 791 mg: Magnesium 202 mg • Ascorbic Acid 756 mg • Citric Acid 903 mg.

LifeStyle DailyFoods - MegaFood
Six tablets contain: Vitamin A (from 21 mg FoodState) 5000 IU • Vitamin C (from 1050 mg FoodState) 250 mg • Vitamin D (D3, from 4 mg FoodState) 200 IU • Vitamin E (from 840 mg FoodState) 200 IU • Vitamin K (K1, from 6 mg FoodState) 60 mcg • Thiamine (B1, from 92 mg FoodState) 22 mg • Riboflavin (B2, from 189 mg FoodState) 18 mg • Niacinamide (from 210 mg FoodState) 50 mg • Vitamin B6 (from 116 mg FoodState) 22 mg • Folic Acid (from 62 mg FoodState) 600 mcg • Vitamin B12 (from 19 mg FoodState) 90 mcg • Biotin (from 63 mg FoodState) 300 mcg • Pantothenic Acid (from 193 mg FoodState) 46 mg • Calcium (from 2000 mg FoodState) 100 mg • Iron (from 180 mg FoodState) 9 mg • Iodine (From 10 mg FoodState) 150 mcg • Magnesium (from 2000 mg FoodState) 100 mg • Zinc (from 300 mg FoodState) 15 mg • Selenium (from 100 mg FoodState) 100 mcg • Copper (from 20 mg FoodState) 200 mcg • Manganese (from 60 mg FoodState) 200 mcg • Chromium (GTF, from 50 mg FoodState) 100 mcg • Molybdenum (from 12 mg FoodState) 25 mcg • Beta Carotene 5000 IU • Bioflavonoids (from FoodState vitamin C) 105 mg • Choline 30 mg • Potassium 25 mg • Inositol 20 mg • PABA 5 mg • Boron 1 mg • Vanadium 20 mcg • Hydrilla Verticillata 50:1 250 mg • Barley grass concentrate 200 mg • Alfalfa 100 mg • Carrot 25 mg • Green Papaya 5:1 25 mg • Beet root 5:1 25 mg • Cranberry 25:1 5 mg • Tomato 4:1 5 mg • Broccoli 5 mg • Cabbage 5 mg • Orange peel 5 mg • Acerola 4:1 5 mg • Eleuthero root 5:1 25 mg • Ginger rhizome 5:1 25 mg • Astragalus root 4:1 25 mg • Schizandra fruit 4:1 25 mg • Turmeric root 10:1 20 mg • Ginkgo leaf 8:1 10 mg • Licorice root 4:1 10 mg • Nettle leaf 4:1 10 mg • Fo-Ti root 5:1 10 mg • Reishi mushroom mycelia 7:1 10 mg • Shiitake mushroom 4:1 10 mg • Hawthorn berry 4:1 10 mg • Milk Thistle seed 4:1 10 mg • Wild Green Oats seed 4:1 10 mg • Spring Horsetail leaf 5:1 10 mg • Kudzu root 10:1 10 mg • Dandelion leaf 4:1 5 mg • Dandelion root 4:1 5 mg. Other Ingredients: Vegetable Lubricant, Food Glaze.

Lifezyme Digestive Enzyme Complex - Life Extension
Each tablet contains: Acidophilus 75 mg • Bromelain 115 mg • Pepsin 30 mg • Papaya 105 mg • Malt Diastase 30 mg • Cellulase 10 mg • Lactase 2 mg • Amylase 15 mg • Protease 10 mg • Lipase 100 mg.

Lift Visage - Jevene (Jeven)
Aloe Vera • Aluminum Silicate • BHT • Ceteareth 20 • Cetearyl Alcohol • Cetyl Alcohol • Diazolidinyl Urea • Dimethicone • EDTA • Fragrance • Glycerin • Glyceryl Stearate • Glycolic Acid • Jojoba oil • Lactic Acid • Methylparaben • Mineral oil • Octyl Methoxycinnamate • PEG-40 Stearate • Potassium Hydroxide • Propylene Glycol • Propylparaben • Salicylic Acid • Sodium Borate • Tocopheryl Acetate • Water • Xanthan Gum.

Lifting Cream - FreeLife International
Neroli Hydrolate (orange blossom water) • Botanical extracts in Purified Water: Willowherb, Green Tea • Pure Grain Alcohol • Lavender oil • Corn Starch (aluminum-free) • Vegetable Glycerin • Oat Beta Glucan • DL Panthenol • Caprylic/Capric Tri Glycerides • Glyceryl Monostearate • Jojoba oil • Gatuline Lifting Complex: Lupin extract, Wild Thyme • Olive Squalane • Pure Clover Honey • Sodium Lauryl Lactylate • Alpha-Lipoic Acid • Bisabolol • Cetyl Alcohol • Liposome Complex: Lecithin, Lauryl Alcohol, Palmitic Acid, Deanol Bitartrate (DMAE), Tocopheryl Acetate (vitamin E), Methylsulfonylmethane (MSM), Grape Seed oil • Gum Arabic • Guar Gum • Xanthan Gum • Phenoxyethanol (phenolic compound/ phenoxetol) • Benzyl Alcohol • Lonicera Japonica (Japanese honeysuckle).

Light & Fit Energy Shake (Chocolate) - Earthrise Nutritionals, LLC.
Isolated Soy Protein • Rice Maltodextrin • Dutch processed Cocoa • Acacia Gum • Sucanat unrefined Sugar Cane juice • Natural Flavors • Tribasic Calcium Phosphate • Magnesium Oxide • Earthrise Spirulina • Soy Fiber • Dipotassium Phosphate • Xanthan Gum • Potassium Citrate • Soy Lecithin • Lemon Bioflavonoids • Microcrystalline Cellulose • Celluose Gum • Choline Bitartrate • Bee Pollen • Vitamin C (ascorbic acid) • Inositol • Stevia • Vitamin E (D-alpha tocopherol succinate) • Apple Pectin • Rice Bran • Oat Fiber • Genestra powdered whole Beer concentrate • Papain • Bromelain • Vitamin B3 (niacinamide) • Hesperidin complex • Rutin • Magna Sweet Licorice extract • PABA (para amino benzoic acid) • Zinc Oxide • Manganese Sulfate • Vitamin A Palmitate • D-Calcium Pantothenate • Ferrous Fumarate • Copper Sulfate • Vitamin B6 (pyridoxine HCl) • Vitamin B2 (riboflavin) • Vitamin B1 (thiamin HCl) • Grapefruit extract • Vitamin D (D3) • Folic Acid • Biotin • Chromium Chloride • Potassium Iodide • Sodium Molybdate • Sodium Selenite • Vitamin K • Vitamin B12 (cyanocobalamin).

Light & Fit Energy Shake (Vanilla) - Earthrise Nutritionals, LLC.
Isolated Soy Protein • Rice Maltodextrin • Acacia Gum • Sucanat Sugar Cane juice • Natural Flavors • Tribasic Calcium Phosphate • Magnesium Oxide • Earthrise Spirulina • Soy Fiber • Potassium Phosphate • Xanthan Gum • Potassium Citrate • Soy Lecithin • Lemon Bioflavonoids • Microcrystalline Cellulose • Celluose Gum • Choline Bitartrate • Bee Pollen • Vitamin C (ascorbic acid) • Inositol • Stevia • Vitamin E (D-alpha tocopherol succinate) • Apple Pectin • Rice Bran • Oat Fiber • Genestra powdered whole Beer concentrate • Papain • Bromelain • Vitamin B3 (niacinamide) • Hesperidin complex • Rutin • Magna Sweet Licorice extract • PABA (para amino benzoic acid) • Zinc Oxide • Manganese Sulfate • Vitamin A Palmitate • D-Calcium Pantothenate • Ferrous Fumarate • Copper Sulfate • Vitamin B6 (pyridoxine HCl) • Vitamin B2 (riboflavin) • Vitamin B1 (thiamin HCl) • Grapefruit extract • Vitamin D (D3) • Folic Acid • Biotin • Chromium Chloride • Potassium Iodide • Sodium Molybdate • Sodium Selenite • Vitamin K • Vitamin B12 (cyanocobalamin).

Light Appetite Formula - Earthrise Nutritionals, LLC.
Three caplets contain: Vitamin A 100 IU • Vitamin C 30 mcg • Thiamin 1.5 mg • Riboflavin 1.7 mg • Niacin 20 mg • Vitamin B6 30 mg • Vitamin B12 15 mcg • Calcium 20 mcg • Iron 1 mg • Iodine 225 mcg • Chromium 50 mcg • Sodium 24 mg • Potassium 26 mg • Proprietary Blend: Earthrise Spirulina, Natural Alfalfa Powder, Soy Lecithin, Apple Cider Vinegar, Sea Kelp, Bladderwrack, Plantain, L-Phenylalanine, Bromelain, Ascorbic Acid, Pyridoxine HCl, Gymnema Sylvester, Thiamin Mononitrate, Chromium Picolinate, Cyanocobalamin. Other Ingredients: D-Calcium Phosphate, Glyceryl Monostearate, Magnesium Stearate, Silica.

Lightly Lemon - J. R. Carlson Laboratories, Inc.
Each softgel contains: Vitamin A (from cod liver oil) 150 IU • Vitamin D (from cod liver oil) 80 IU • Vitamin E (as D-alpha tocopherol) 2 IU • Omega-3 Fatty Acids (from cod liver oil) 230 mg.

Limbrel (flavocoxid) - Primus Pharmaceuticals, Inc
Each capsule contains: Flavocoxid; Scutellaria Baicalensis extract (baicalin), Acacia Catechu extract (catechin) 250 mg.
See Editor's Note No. 73.

Linden Hawthorn Supreme - Gaia Herbs
Thirty drops contain: Proprietary Blend 200 mg: Dried Linden flowers (tilia spp.), Dried Hawthorn berry, Hawthorn leaf and flower, Mistletoe herb (viscum flavescnes), Valerian root (valeriana officinalis), Spring Water, 40-50% Pure Grain Alcohol USP.

Line Assist Creme - Aspen Group, Inc.
Each gram contains: Tocopheryl Acetate 1% • Panthenol 1% • Ascorbyl Palmitate 0.3% • Water • Diisopropyl Adipate • Cetearyl Alcohol • Potassium Cetyl Phosphate • Retinyl Palmitate • Palmitate • Tocopherol • Dimethicone • Carbomer • Ammonium Hydroxide • Quaternium-15 • Disodium EDTA.

Lingzhi Cracked Spores Powder Capsules - Eu Yan Sang
Pure Lingzhi 'Cracked' Spores Powder.

Liniment Virtue - Blessed Herbs
St. John's Wort flower • Comfrey root • Angelica root • Valerian root • Lobelia herb • Ginger root • Calendula flower • Arnica flower & herb • Cayenne pepper • Essential oils of Myrrh, Hyssop, Rosemary, Lavender & German Chamomile • Grain alcohol & Distilled Water.

Linum B6 - Standard Process, Inc.
Each perle contains: Vitamin B6 2 mg • Flaxseed oil 630 mg. Other Ingredients: Gelatin, Glycerin, Beeswax, Water, Carob.

LinumLife - Pure Encapsulations
Each vegetable capsule contains: Flaxseed hull (standardized to contain 3.5-6% lignans) 800 mg • Omega-3 Fatty Acids 48-64 mg • Omega-6 Fatty Acids 8-24 mg.

Lioness Women's Sexual Libido Enhancer - Universal Products
Three capsules contain: Tribulus 667 mg • Muira Puama 427 mg • Catuaba bark 352 mg • Androstenedione 127 mg • L-Arginine 127 mg • Ginseng (Korean) 60 mg • Avena Sativa 60 mg • Natural Vitamin E 37 IU. Other Ingredients: Magnesium Stearate, Gelatin.
See Editor's Note No. 47.

Lipidyn - Progressive Health Nutraceuticals
Vitamin C 250 mg • Vitamin E 200 IU • Vitamin B5 100 mg • Chromium 50 mcg • Beta Sitosterol 100 mg • Inositol 100 mg • Policosanol 25 mg • Gum Guggul extract 25 mg • Garlic 200 mg • Psyllium 500 mg.

Lipitrol - Ortho Molecular Products
Three capsules contain: Chromium (as ChromeMate brand) 200 mcg • Inositol Hexaniacinate 1350 mg • Gugul resin (standardized to contain 2.5% gugulsterones) 500 mg • Guar gum 225 mg • Artichoke leaf extract (standardized to contain 5% cynarin) 150 mg. Other Ingredients: Natural Vegetable Capsules, Ascorbyl Palmitate, Magnesium Stearate, Microcrystalline Cellulose, Silicon Dioxide.

Lipo 6 - Nutrex, Inc.
Two liqui-caps contain: Synephrine HCl 20 mg • synthetic 99% Guggulsterones Z&E 1:1 20 mg • Yohimbe HCl 3 mg • Caffeine Anhydrous USP 200 mg • Bioperine brand Black Pepper extract 5 mg. Other Ingredients: Sesame Oil, Oleic Acid, Gelatin.
See Editor's Note No. 21.

Lipo 6 Ephedra Free - Nutrex, Inc.
Two capsules contain: Citrus Aurantium 335 mg (total amines 7.5%, individual amines: synephrine 6%, N-methyl tyramine 0.9-1.6%, tyramine 0.2-0.4%, hordenine 0.2-0.4%, octopamine 0.2-0.4%) • Caffeine anhydrous USP 200 mg• Yohimbe HCl 250 mg • Coleus Forskohlii (standardized to 20% forskolin) 100 mg • Carnitrex L-Carnitine 100 mg • Bioperine brand Black Pepper extract 5 mg. Other Ingredients: Gelatin, L-Tartrate, Maltodextrin, Magnesium Stearate.
See Editor's Note No. 40.

Lipo Rx Metabolism Booster - Athletic Technologies Inc.
Each capsule contains: Vitamin B6 25 mg • Iodine 150 mcg • Chromium 100 mcg • Guarana 300 mg • Theobromine 100 mg • Yerba Mate extract 50 mg • Green Tea extract 50 mg • Garcinia Cambogia 250 mg • Chitosan 250 mg • Gymnema Sylvestre 50 mg • Banaba 25 mg • Calcium Pyruvate 50 mg • Apple Cider Vinegar 25 mg • Grapefruit powder 25 mg • Coleus Forskohlii 25 mg • White Willow bark 25 mg • Uva Ursi 25 mg • Juniper berry 25 mg • Buchu leaf 25 mg • Cayenne Pepper 10 mg.

Lipo Trim - NOW Foods
Three tablets contain: Choline 1000 mg • Inositol 1000 mg • L-Methionine 500 mg • Taurine 250 mg • L-Carnitine 100 mg • Pyridoxine (B6) 10 mg • Chromium Picolinate 200 mcg.

BRAND NAMES

Lipo-AMP **-** E'OLA
Each 0.7 mL spray contains: Vitamin B12 10 mcg • Proprietary Blend 188 mg: Ephedra (branch) Extract, Guarana (seed) Extract, Caffeine, Stevia (leaf) Extract, White Willow Bark Extract, Atractylodes (herb) Extract, Licorice (root) Extract, Dimethyl Amino Ethanol Bitartrate, Dibencozide. Other Ingredients: Purified Water, Fructose, Hydrochloric Acid, Natural and Artificial Peppermint Flavor, Lecithin, Potassium Sorbate, Sodium Benzoate.
See Editor's Note No. 30.

Lipo-Complex **-** Progressive Labs
Each capsule contains: Pancreatic enzyme concentrate 400 mg (equivalent in enzymatic activity to 4X USP) • Pepsin 1:3000 (from Pepsin 1:10,000) 100 mg • Green Beet leaf powder 100 mg • Raw Liver concentrate 10 mg • Ox bile 10 mg.
See Editor's Note No. 14.

Lipodrene **-** High Tech Pharmaceuticals
Each tablet contains: Proprietary Blend 660 mg: Sida Cordifolia leaves extract (supplying 25 mg ephedrine group alkaloides), Citrus Aurantium fruit 10%, Caffeine 100 mg, 5-Hydroxytryptophan (5HTP), Melatonin (5-methoxytryptamine), Green Tea leaves extract, Cassia Nomame whole plant, Hoodia cactus 12:1 extract, Yohimbe bark 8% extract, Naringen fruit.
See Editor's Note No. 16, No. 21, No. 30 and No. 39.

Lipodrene-SR **-** High Tech Pharmaceuticals
Each tablet contains: Proprietary Blend 272.5 mg: Citrus Aurantium fruit (12.5 mg synephrine), Hoodia cactus extract, Cassia Nomame extract, 6,6 Dihydroxy Bergaottin fruit, Yohimbe bark extract (1 mg yohimbe alkaloids), Naringen fruit, Commiphora Mukul root/resin, Coleus Forskolin root, Pilocarpus, Jaborandi leaves extract, L050 Hydroxy Tryptophan, 5-Hydroxy Tryptamine HCl • Caffeine (anhydrous) 75 mg • Thermo-RX Complex 250 mg: Green Tea leaves RM7343 extract, Acacia leaves 70% extract, Theobroma, Cocoa seed extract, Phenylethylamine HCl.
See Editor's Note No. 40.

Lipoflavonoid **-** Numark Laboratories
Three caplets contain: Vitamin C 300 mg • Thiamine 1 mg • Riboflavin 1 mg • Niacin 10 mg • Vitamin B6 1 mg • Vitamin B12 5 mcg • Pantothenic Acid 5 mg • Choline 334 mg • Bioflavonoids 300 mg • Inositol 334 mg.

Lipo-Gen **-** Metagenics
Two tablets contain: Choline (as choline bitartrate) 300 mg • Inositol 150 mg • Taurine 100 mg • L-Methionine 100 mg • Vitamin C (as ascorbic acid) 100 mg • Betaine Hydrochloride 100 mg • Magnesium (as magnesium oxide) 50 mg • Vitamin B6 (as pyridoxine hydrochloride) 10 mg • Folate (as folic acid) 100 mcg • Vitamin B12 (as cyanocobalamin) 10 mcg • Proprietary Blend: Artichoke leaf extract (cynara scolymus, containing cynarin and chlorogenic acid) • Chen Pi 5:1 extract (citrus reticulata, containing bioflavonoids including hesperidin, nobiletin, citral) • Fumitory 4-6:1 extract (fumaria officinalis, containing alkaloids as protopine).

Lipoic Acid **-** Life Enhancement Products, Inc.
Each capsule contains: Alpha Lipoic Acid 100 mg. Other Ingredients: Rice Flour, Gelatin.

Lipoic Acid 100 **-** Ortho Molecular Products
Each capsule contains: Biotin 100 mcg • Lipoic Acid 100 mg. Other Ingredients: Natural Vegetable Capsules, Magnesium Stearate, Microcrystalline Cellulose.

Lipoic Acid 150 mg **-** Vital Nutrients
Each capsule contains: Lipoic Acid (thioctic acid) 150 mg.

Lipoic Acid 300 **-** Ortho Molecular Products
Each capsule contains: Biotin 300 mcg • Lipoic Acid 300 mg. Other Ingredients: Natural Vegetable Capsules, Magnesium Stearate, Microcrystalline Cellulose.

Lipoic Acid 300 mg **-** Vital Nutrients
Each capsule contains: Lipoic Acid (thioctic acid) 300 mg.

Lipoic Acid 50 mg **-** Vital Nutrients
Each capsule contains: Lipoic Acid (thioctic acid) 50 mg.

Lipoicare **-** PhysioLogics
Each capsule contains: Taurine 200 mg • Alpha-Lipoic Acid 25 mg • Calendula flower, Marigold (5% Lutein 3 mg; > 0.22% Zeaxanthin, 0.13 mg) 60 mg.

LipoKinetix **-** Syntrax Innovations
Each capsule contains: Phenylpropanolamine (PPA) 25 mg • Caffeine 100 mg • Yohimbine 3 mg • Diiodothyronine 100 mg • Sodium Usniate 100 mg.
See Editor's Note No. 11.

Liposamal Progesterone Liquid **-** MK Supplements
Progesterone USP 15 mg.

Liposin **-** Metabolic Nutrition, Inc.
Each capsule contains: Chitosan, pH modified 3000 mg • Psyllium husk 600 mg • Ascorbic acid 600 mg • L-Carnitine 450 mg • Glucomannan 150 mg.
See Editor's Note No. 37.

Lipotain **-** Metagenics
Two tablets contain: Niacin (as inositol hexanicotinate) 1000 mg • Guggul resin extract (commiphora mukul, containing guggulsterones) 750 mg.

Lipo-THIN **-** E'OLA
Each 0.7 mL spray contains: Chromium (as Chromium Chloride) 200 mcg • Proprietary Blend 132 mg: L-Carnitine, Green Tea (leaf) Extract, Dibencozide. Other Ingredients: Purified Water, Glycerin, Fructose, Polyglyceryl-10 Oleate, Hydroxylated Soy Lecithin, Potassium Sorbate, Natural and Artificial Flavors.

Lipotrene **-** Mosaic Nutraceuticals Corp
Each chew contains: Policosanol 10 mg. Other Ingredients: Hydrogenated Starch Hydrolysate, Cream, Palm Kernal Oil, Artificial Flavors, Citric Acid, Mono & Diglycerides, Soya Lecithin, Sucralose, FD&C Red 40, Fulvic Acid.

LipoTrol **-** Advocare International
Two caplets contain: Pyridoxine (as HCl) 2 mg • Zinc (as monomethionine - OptiZinc) 1 mg • Chromium (as polynicotinate - ChromeMate) 50 mcg • Garcinia extract (fruit - Garcinia cambogia) 1000 mg • Tulsi extract (leaf - ocimum sanctum) 25 mg • Taurine 25 mg • Beta-Sitosterol 12.5 mg • L-Carnitine 12.5 mg • Gymnema extract (leaf - gymnema sylvestre) 5 mg • Vanadium (as bis-maltolato-oxovanadium) 100 mcg. Other Ingredients: Dicalcium Phosphate, Silicon Dioxide, Cellulose, Stearic Acid, Magnesium Stearate.

Lipotrope **-** Progressive Labs
Each capsule contains: Vitamin C 50 mg • Vitamin B6 5 mg • Folate (folic acid) 200 mcg • Vitamin B12 200 mcg • Pantothenic Acid 60 mg • Magnesium Aspartate 25 mg • Milk Thistle (Silybum marianum) 100 mg • Choline Bitartrate 150 mg • Inositol 75 mg • Betaine HCl 60 mg • DL-Methionine 50 mg • Black Radish (Raphanus nigra) 50 mg • Green Beet leaf powder 50 mg • Celandine (Chelidonium majus) 15 mg • Chionanthus (Chionanthus virginica) 15 mg • PABA 25 mg.

Lipotropic **-** Ortho Molecular Products
Five capsules contain: Choline Bitartrate 1800 mg • L-Methionine USP 900 mg • Inositol 575 mg.

Lipotropic Action **-** Puritan's Pride
Each capsule contains: Iodine (as potassium iodide) 25 mcg • Magnesium (as magnesium amino acid chelate) 8.3 mg • Selenium (as selenomethionine) 0.33 mcg • Manganese (as manganese amino acid chelate) 1.6 mg • Molybdenum (as molybdenum amino acid chelate) 8.33 mg • Potassium (as potassium amino acid chelate) 16.5 mg • Boron (as boron chelate) 0.33 mcg • Vanadium (as vanadium amino acid chelate) 0.33 mcg • Choline Bitartrate 35.46 mg • Inositol 25 mg • Ginger (zingiber officinale) root 25 mg • L-Methionine 16.67 mg • L-Carnitine (as L-carnitine fumarate) 16.67 mg • Beta Sitosterol 16.67 mg • Dandelion root (taraxacum

officinale) 12.5 mg • Barberry (berberis vulgaris) root 12.5 mg • Turmeric (curcuma longa) root 12.5 mg • Milk Thistle (silybum marianum) seed 12.5 mg • Cinnamon (cinnamonum verum) bark 12.5 mg • Siberian Ginseng (eleutherococcus senticosus) root 8.33 mg • Gotu Kola (centella asiatica) aerial 8.33 mg • Fo-Ti (polygonum multiflorum) root 8.33 mg • Cayenne pepper (capsicum annuum) fruit 4.16 mg • DigeZyme enzyme complex: Anylase (1:2,000), Neutral Protease, Cellulase, Galactohydrolase Lactase, Lipase 50 mg.

Lipotropic Complex - Nature's Life
Three tablets contain: L-Methionine (free-form amino acid) 1000 mg • Choline (from 2040 mg choline bitartrate) 1000 mg • Inositol 1000 mg • Betaine HCl (sugar beets) 250 mg • Milk Thistle (silybum marianum) 50 mg • Vitamin B6 (pyridoxine hydrochloride) 10 mg • L-Taurine (free-form amino acid) 10 mg • L-Carnitine (free-form amino acid) 10 mg • Lecithin (soy, 61% phosphatides) 10 mg • Beet root powder (beta vulgaris rubra) 5 mg • Dandelion root powder (taraxacum officinale) 5 mg • Culvers root powder (leptandra virginica) 5 mg • Apple Cider Vinegar 5 mg • Barberry root bark (berberis vulgaris) 5 mg • Chromium (Nutrition 21 brand, picolinate) 25 mcg.

Lipotropic Complex - Tyler Encapsulations
Two capsules contain: Vitamin B6 (as pyridoxine hydrochloride USP) 25 mg • Folic Acid USP 100 mcg • Vitamin B12 (as cyanocobalamin USP) 25 mcg • Magnesium (as magnesium aspartate, oxide USP) 34 mg • L-Methionine USP 333 mg • Choline (as choline bitartrate) 192 mg • Black Radish root (raphanus sativus-niger) 133 mg • Beet leaf (beta vulgaris) 133 mg • Inositol 125 mg • Fringe Tree root bark (chionanthus virginicus) 100 mg • Dandelion root (taraxacum officinale) 100 mg • Milk Thistle seed (silybum marianum) 100 mg • Celandine aerial parts extract (chelidonium majus, 2.3% alkaloids) 37 mg • Ox Bile extract 25 mg • Milk Thistle seed extract (silybum marianum, 80% silymarin) 12.7 mg. Other Ingredients: Ascorbyl Palmitate, Gelatin, Water.
See Editor's Note No. 14.

Lipotropic Fuel - TwinLab
Five capsules contain: Choline 500 mg • Inositol 250 mg • L-Methionine 100 mg • Vitamin B12 100 mcg • Betaine 100 mg • L-Carnitine 100 mg • Milk Thistle extract (standardized for 80% Silymarin) 500 mg • Natural Vitamin E (Succinate) 400 IU • Vitamin C 1000 mg • Vitamin B1 25 mg • N-Acetyl Cysteine (NAC) 250 mg • L-Glutathione 100 mg • Vitamin B2 25 mg • Selenium (from Selenomethionine) 150 mcg • Zinc (from Mono-Methionine) 15 mg.

Lipotropic Plus - Vitamin Express
Three tablets contain: Niacin (as nicotinic acid) 100 mg • Vitamin B12 (as cobalamin) 50 mcg • Betaine HCl 50 mg • Choline (as choline bitartrate) 450 mg • Clove 90 mg • DL-Methionine 1000 mg • Hawthorn Berry 30 mg • Inositol 1000 mg • Liver (from desiccated whole liver) 6 mg • Yucca 30 mg. Other Ingredients: Calcium Phosphate, Calcium Stearate, Cellulose, Lecithin, Silica, Stearic Acid.
See Editor's Note No. 14.

LipotropiX - Xymogen
Four capsules contain: Greater Celandine 4:1 extract 100 mg • Dandelion 4:1 extract 150 mg • Guggul extract (10%) 75 mg • Choline (citrate) 400 mg • Taurine 200 mg • Inositol Hexanicotinate 1000 mg • Methionine 400 mg.

Lipovarin - Sterling-Grant Laboratories
Three tablets contain: Metabromine fruit extract (theobroma cacao, 6% theobromine 20 mg) 330 mg • 6% Theobromine 20 mg • Advantra Z Citrus Aurantium (10% total amines 35 mg) 350 mg • Green Tea leaf extract (camellia sinensis, 30% tea polyphenols 30 mg, 20% tea catechins 20 mg) 100 mg • Serotain (18.5% 5-hydroxytryptophan 45 mg) 250 mg • Caffeine 200 mg • Glucuronolactone 300 mg • Taurine 200 mg • L-Carnitine L-Tartrate 15 mg • 7-Keto (7-keto-dehydroepiandrosterone acetate) 50 mg • Coral Calcium 200 mg.
See Editor's Note No. 40.

Lipovitan B3 Energy Drink - Taisho Pharmaceutical CA. Inc.
Carbonated Water • Sugar • Citric Acid • Taurine • Artificial Flavor • Sodium Citrate • Anhydrous Caffeine • Royal Jelly extract • Niacinamide • Riboflavin - 5 - Phosphorous (sodium) • Pyridoxine Hydrochloride • Thiamine Mononitrate.

Lipoxinol - Sci-Core Research
Four capsules contain: Selenium 100 mcg • Chromium (as chromium dinicotinate glycinate) 100 mcg • Calcium Sulfate 152 mg • Proprietary Fiberzide Blend 1800 mg: Glucomannan, Zanthan gum • Proprietary Thermazene Blend 789 mg: Green Tea leaf extract (50% catechins and 35% polyphenols), Caffeine, Forslean brand Forskolin, Vinpocetine, Bioperine brand Black Pepper extract • Proprietary Thyrotril Blend 85 mg: Pure Synthetic E+Z Guggulsterones, Sclareolide 96%, Atlantic Kelp. Other Ingredients: Gelatin, Cellulose, Magnesium Stearate.

Lipozyme - Young Living Essential Oils
Each capsule contains: Proprietary Blend: Lipase, Bee Pollen, Pancreatin, Tarragon Oil, Ginger Oil, Peppermint Oil, Juniper Oil, Fennel Oil, Lemongrass Oil, Anise Oil, Patchouli Oil.

Liqiang 4 - Liqiang Research Institute
Unknown.
See Editor's Note No. 65.

Liqua B Complex 50 - GNC
Each capsule contains: Vitamin E (as d-alpha tocopherol) 2 IU • Thiamin (as thiamin mononitrate) 50 mg • Riboflavin 50 mg • Niacin (as niacinamide) 50 mg • Vitamin B6 (as pyridoxine hydrochloride) 50 mg • Folate (folic acid, folacin) 400 mcg • Vitamin B12 (as cyanocobalamin) 50 mcg • Biotin 50 mcg • Pantothenic Acid (as calcium d-pantothenate) 50 mg • Choline Bitartrate 50 mg • Inositol 50 mcg • Para-aminobenzoic Acid (PABA) 50 mg. Other Ingredients: Soybean Oil, Gelatin, Glycerin, Lecithin, Caramel Color, Titanium Dioxide, Korean Ginseng (panax ginseng).

Liqua Thin - E'OLA
Each 10 drops contain: Chromium 200 mcg • Proprietary Blend 155 mg: L-Carnitine, Green Tea (leaf) extract, Atractylodes (herb) extract, Choline Bitartrate, Dibencozide. Inactive Ingredients: Water, Hydrochloric Acid, Citric Acid, Glycerine, Sodium Benzoic Acid.

Liqui Lea - Shaklee
Each 1 tsp serving (5 mL) contains: Vitamin A (as vitamin A palmitate) 5000 IU • Vitamin D (as cholecalciferol) 400 IU • Vitamin E (as D-A-tocopheryl acetate) 15 IU • Thiamin (as thiamin hydrochloride) 2.1 mg • Riboflavin (as riboflavin sodium phosphate) 1.8 mg • Niacin (as niacinamide) 20 mg • Vitamin B6 (as pyridoxine hydrochloride) 2 mg • Vitamin B12 (as cyanocobalamin) 9 mcg • Biotin (as D-biotin) 300 mcg • Pantothenic Acid (as D-panthenol) 5 mg • Iron (as ferric ammonium citrate) 18 mg. Other Ingredients: Sorbitol, Natural Flavor, Glycerin, Purified Water, Sesame Oil, Soy Lecithin, Gum Ghatti, Citric.

Liquid Aminos - Puritan's Pride
Each softgel contains: L-Alanine 30 mg • L-Arginine 54 mg • L-Aspartic Acid 83 mg • L-Cysteine 10 mg • L-Glutamic Acid 145 mg • L-Glycine 33 mg • L-Histidine 20 mg • L-Isoleucine 35 mg • L-Leucine 60 mg • L-Lysine 59 mg • L-Methionine 9 mg • L-Phenylalanine 41 mg • L-Proline 38 mg • L-Serine 39 mg • L-Threonine 32 mg • L-Tryptophan 7 mg • L-Tyrosine 22 mg • L-Valine 33 mg.

Liquid Anti-Oxidant - Natrol, Inc.
Two teaspoons (10 ml) contain: Anti-Oxidant Vitamins & Trace Minerals: Vitamin A (beta carotene) 10000 IU • Vitamin C (Calcium ascorbate) 500 mg • Vitamin E (acetate) 200 IU • Selenium (monomethionine) 90 mcg • Advanced Flavonoids: GP Complex+ 80 mg • Rutin, Quercetin, & Hesperidin 10 mg • Tropical fruit extracts from: Acerola, Cashew fruit, Passion fruit, Orange, Lime & Mango in a specially formulated base of: Purified Water, Brown Rice Syrup, Honey & Citric Acid.

Liquid B Complex with Iron - Nature's Plus
Each 1 tbsp (15 mL) serving contains: Thiamin (vitamin B1 as thiamine HCl) 20 mg • Riboflavin (vitamin B2) 15 mg • Niacin (as niacinamide) 50 mg • Vitamin B6 (as pyridoxine HCl) 25 mg • Vitamin B12 (as cyanocobalamin) 100 mcg • Biotin 25 mcg • Pantothenic Acid (as panthenol) 50 mg • Iron (as gluconate) 50 mg • Choline (as bitartrate) 21 mg • Inositol 50 mg. Other Ingredients: Water, Honey, Ginseng, Blackstrap Molasses, Beet Root, Fo-Ti (polygonum multiflorum), Gotu Kola Root (centella asiatica).

Liquid B-Complex - GNC
Each dropperful (1 ml) contains: Riboflavin (as riboflavin-5-phosphate) 1.7 mg • Vitamin B6 (as pyrifoxine hydrochloride) 2 mg • Vitamin B12 (as cyanocobalamin) 1000 mcg • Pantothenic acid (as dexpanthenol) 30 mg. Other Ingredients: Purified Water, Glycerin, Fructose, Sorbitol, Natural Orange, Lemon, and Lime Flavors, Citric Acid, Stevia, Sodium Benzoate.

Liquid Cal-600 - J. R. Carlson Laboratories, Inc.
Each softgel contains: Calcium (as DL-calcium phosphate) 600 mg.

Liquid Calcium - J. R. Carlson Laboratories, Inc.
Three softgels contain: Vitamin D (D3, cholecalciferol) 1000 IU • Calcium (as di-calcium phosphate) 1000 mg • Phosphorus (as Dicalcium phosphate) 774 mg.

Liquid Calcium - Nature's Bounty
Three softgels contain: Vitamin A (as Retinyl Palmitate) 825 IU • Vitamin D (as Cholecalciferol) 180 IU • Calcium (as Calcium Carbonate) 600 mg. Other Ingredients: Soybean Oil, Gelatin, Glycerin, Lecithin, Titanium Dioxide Color.

Liquid Calcium - Nature's Plus
Each 2 tbsp (30 mL) serving contains: Vitamin D (as cholecalciferol) 100 IU • Calcium (as carbonate, gluconate) 1000 mg • Magnesium (as carbonate, gluconate) 200 mg. Other Ingredients: Vanilla, Malt, Nonfat Milk, Honey, Blackstrap Molasses.

Liquid Calcium Magnesium Citrate - Puritan's Pride
Each teaspoon (15 ml) contains: Calcium (Citrate, Lactate, Gluconate) 600 mg • Magnesium (Citrate) 300 mg • Vitamin D (Cholecalciferol) 400 IU.

Liquid Calcium/Magnesium Dietary Supplement - N.V. Perricone M.D. Cosmeceuticals
Each softgel contains: Vitamin D (as cholecalciferol 0.83 mcg) 33 IU • Vitamin K (as phytonadione) 3.3 mcg • Calcium (as calcium carbonate, calcium aspartate, calcium citrate, calcium gluconate, calcium hydroxyapatite, and calcium malate) 333 mg • Magnesium (as magnesium oxide, magnesium aspartate, and magnesium citrate) 133 mg • Boron (as boron gluconate) 0.33 mg • Horsetail extract (aerial parts) 8.33 mg. Other Ingredients: Soybean Oil, Gelatin, Glycerin, Soy Lecithin, Evening Primrose Oil, Titanium Dioxide, Silica.

Liquid Cal-Mag - J. R. Carlson Laboratories, Inc.
Two softgels contain: Vitamin D (D3, cholecalciferol) 1000 IU • Calcium (as calcium carbonate) 400 mg • Magnesium (as magnesium oxide) 200 mg.

Liquid Carnitine 1000 - Jarrow Formulas
Each 1 tbsp (15 mL) serving contains: Pantothenic Acid (vitamin B5 as D-calcium pantothenate) 10 mg • L-Carnitine (USP grade, elemental free base) 1000 mg. Other Ingredients: Purified Water, Vegetable Glycerine, Natural Vanilla Flavor, Grapefruit Seed Extract, Potassium Sorbate.

Liquid Children's Multiple - Natrol, Inc.
Two teaspoons contain: Essential Vitamins: Vitamin A (beta carotene) 2,500 IU • Vitamin C (calcium ascorbate & ascorbic acid) 100 mg • Vitamin D (as Vitamin D3) (calciferol) 400 IU • Vitamin E (Acetate) 30 IU • Thiamine (Vitamin B1) 1 mg • Riboflavin (Vitamin B2) 1 mg • Niacin (Niacinamide) 12 mg • Vitamin B6 (pyridoxine HCl) 1.4 mg • Vitamin B12 (cyanocobalamin) 2.5 mcg • Pantothenic Acid (calcium d-pantothenate) 6 mg • Folic Acid 100 mcg • Biotin 20 mcg • Flavonoid: Hesperidin, Acerola, Cashew fruit, Passion fruit, Orange & Lime 10 mg • Tropical fruit extracts from: Lemon, Orange, Lime, Mango • Other extracts from: natural Vanilla Bean extract • Herbal extracts: Anise Seed, Licorice root, Millefolium plant, Horsetail Grass plant, Chamomile leaf & flowers, Peppermint leaf, Nettles plant, Spinach leaf & Sodium Benzoate (0.1% added to help protect flavor). In a base of Purified Water, Brown Rice Syrup, Glycerine & Citric Acid.

Liquid Children's Multi-Vitamin - Natrol, Inc.
Two teaspoons (10 ml) contain: Essential Vitamins: Vitamin A (beta carotene) 2500 IU • Vitamin C (calcium ascorbate & ascorbic acid) 100 mg • Vitamin D (as Vitamin D3) (calciferol) 400 IU • Vitamin E (Acetate) 30 IU • Vitamin B1 (Thiamine) 1 mg • Vitamin B2 (Riboflavin) 1 mg • Niacin (Niacinamide) Vitamin B3 12 mg • Vitamin B6 (pyridoxine HCl) 1.4 mg • Vitamin B12 (cyanocobalamin) 2.5 mcg • Pantothenic Acid (calcium D-pantothenate) 6 mg • Folic Acid 100 mcg • Biotin 20 mcg • Flavonoid: Hesperidin 10 mg • Tropical fruit extracts from: Lemon, Orange, Lime, Mango • Other extracts from: natural Vanilla Bean extract • Herbal extracts: Anise Seed, Licorice root, Millefolium plant, Plantain root, Horsetail Grass plant, Chamomile leaf & flowers, Peppermint leaf, Nettles plant, Spinach leaf & Sodium Benzoate (0.1% added to help protect flavor). In a base of: Purified Water, Brown Rice Syrup, Glycerine & Citric Acid.

Liquid Chlorophyll - Nature's Sunshine
Each 1 tsp serving contains: Chlorophyllin (sodium copper chlorophyllin, derived from alfalfa) 15 mg. Other Ingredients: Purified Water, Methylparaben, Spearmint Oil (mentha spicata and cardiaca), Propylparaben.

Liquid Chlorophyll Concentrate - American Biologics
Each drop contains: Sodium Copper Chlorophyllin 2.5 mg • Natrum Phosphoricum 6.5 mg. Other Ingredients: Glycerin.

Liquid Colloidal Mineral Energy - World Nutrition
Each fluid ounce contains: Magnesium 100 mg • Calcium 25 mg • Potassium 15 mg • Manganese 5 mg • Silica 1100 mcg • Selenium 50 mcg • Chromium 50 mcg • Vitamin B12 1000 mcg • Biotin 200 mcg • 72 Polycolloidal Mineral Blend (including aluminum) Approximately 1.7 ppm: Antimony, Arsenic, Barium, Beryllium, Bismuth, Boron, Bromine, Cadmium, Cerium, Cesium, Chloride, Cobalt, Copper, Dysprosium, Erbium, Europium, Fluoride, Gadolinium, Gallium, Germanium, Gold, Hafnium, Holmium, Indium, Iodine, Iridium, Iron, Lanthanum, Lead, Lithium, Lutetium, Mercury, Molybdenum, Neodymium, Osmium, Palladium, Phosphorus, Platinum, Praseodymium, Rhenium, Rhodium, Rubidium, Ruthenium, Samarium, Scandium, Silver, Sodium, Strontium, Sulfur, Tantalum, Tellurium, Terbium, Thalium, Thorium, Thulium, Tin, Titanium, Tungsten, Vanadium, Ytterbium, Yttrium, Zirconium. Other Ingredients: Purified Water, Sorbitol, Magnesium Citrate/Gluconate/Sulfate, Polycolloid Minerals (calcium sulfate, diatomaceous earth), Citric Acid, Calcium Citrate/Levulinate, Natural Flavor, Zinc Gluconate/Citrate, Sodium Benzoate (as a preservative), Caramel Color, Manganese Citrate/Sulfate, Potassium Gluconate/Citrate/Chloride, Sodium Metasilicate, Cyanocobalamin, Chromium Picolinate/Chloride, Biotin, Selenium Complex (selenomethionine, sodium selenite).

Liquid Coral Calcium - Utrition Inc.
Each fluid ounce contains: Vitamin D (cholecalciferol) 400 IU • Coral Calcium 1000 mg • Magnesium (citrate) 200 mg • Manganese (gluconate) 1 mg • Boron (sodium bicarbonate) 2 mg • Lysine 10 mg. Other Ingredients: Purified Water, Glycerin USP (vegetable), Crystalline Fructose, Citric Acid, Natural Flavors, Colloidal Silver, Xanthan Gum, Potassium Benzoate, Potassium Sorbate, Stevia Extract.

Liquid Ester-C - Natrol, Inc.
Two teaspoons (10 ml) contain: Vitamin C (from Ester-C calcium ascorbate) 250 mg • Calcium (from Ester-C calcium ascorbate) 25 mg • Pure Bioflavonoids containing: Rutin, Quercetin, & Hesperidin 10 mg • Tropical fruit extracts from: Acerola, Cashew fruit, Passion

fruit, Orange, Lime & Mango. In a specially formulated base of: Purified Water, Brown Rice Syrup, Honey, natural Vanilla Bean extract, Citric Acid & Sodium Benzoate (0.1% added to help protect flavor).

Liquid Iron Ferrochel - Natrol, Inc.
Four teaspoons (20 mL) contain: Iron & Vitamins: Iron (Ferrochel chelate) 14.5 mg • Vitamin C (Calcium Ascorbate) 100 mg • Vitamin B1 (Thiamine) 1 mg • Vitamin B6 (Pyridoxine HCl) 2 mg • Vitamin B12 (Cyanocobalamin) 3 mcg • Niacinamide 13 mg • Herbal extracts: Nettles, Kelp, Spinach, Yarrow, Angelica, Horsetail Grass, Siberian Ginseng, Yellow Dock, Burdock root, Pau D'Arco, Rose Hips & Alfalfa • Tropical fruit extracts from: Acerola, Pineapple, Cashew fruit, Passion fruit, Lime & Mango. In a specially formulated base of: Purified Water, Brown Rice Syrup, Honey & natural fruit flavors.

Liquid Joint Repair (pineapple/orange flavor) - Utrition Inc.
Two tablespoons contain: Sodium 30 mg • Vitamin C 60 mg • Glucosamine Sulfate 2000 mg • Chondroitin Sulfate 1200 mg • Opti-Methyl Sulfonyl Methane 500 mg. Other Ingredients: Purified Water, Fructose, Citric Acid, Collagen, Red Beet Color, Natural Flavors, Potassium Citrate, Potassium Benzoate, Potassium Sorbate.
See Editor's Note No. 15.

Liquid Kalm With Kava Kava root extract - Natrol, Inc.
Two teaspoons (10 ml) contain: Guaranteed Potency Herbal extracts: Kava Kava root extract standardized to contain 30% Kavalactones 25 mg • Passion flower Herb extract standardized to Contain 3.5% Isovitexin 20 mg • Chamomile flower extract standardized to Contain 0.5% Apigenin 25 mg • Hops Cone extract standardized to Contain 0.35% Flavonoids 25 mg • Vitamin: Vitamin B6 2 mg • Herbal extract blend: Lemon Balm leaf, Oat Straw, Marjoram leaf, Cowslip herb, Rosemary leaf, Scullcap herb. Other ingredients: Honey & Brown Rice Syrup, natural Lemon & Ginger flavor, Cashew fruit & Passion fruit powder, Citric Acid, Sodium Benzoate (0.1% added to protect flavor).

Liquid L-Carnitine 1000 - Optimum Nutrition
Each 2 tbsp (30 mL) serving contains: L-Carnitine 1000 mg • Pantothenic Acid (from D-calcium pantothenic acid) 20 mg.

Liquid Liver Extract - Enzymatic Therapy
Two softgels contain: Vitamin B12 (as cyanocobalamin) 200 mcg • Iron 2 mg • Liquid Liver Fractions (predigested soluble concentrate) 1100 mg. Other Ingredients: Soybean Oil, Gelatin, Glycerin, Lecithin, Caramel Color, Beeswax, Titanium Dioxide Color.
See Editor's Note No. 14.

Liquid Magnesium - J. R. Carlson Laboratories, Inc.
Each softgel contains: Magnesium (as magnesium oxide) 400 mg.

Liquid Multi Colloidal Minerals - GNC
Two tablespoons contain: Deionized/Distilled Water, Colloidal Mineral Clay, Methylparaben, Antimony, Barium, Beryllium, Bismuth, Boron, Calcium, Cerium, Cesium, Chromium, Cobalt, Copper, Dysprosium, Erbium, Europium, Gadolinium, Gallium, Gold, Hafnium, Holmium, Indium, Iridium, Iron, Lanthanum, Lithium, Lutetium, Magnesium, Manganese, Molybdenum, Neodymium, Nickel, Niobium, Palladium, Platinum, Phosphorus, Potassium, Praseodymium, Rhenium, Rhodium, Rubidium, Ruthenium, Samarium, Scandium, Selenium, Silica, Silver, Sulfur, Tantalum, Tellurium, Terbium, Thallium, Thorium, Thulium, Titanium, Tungsten, Uranium, Vanadium, Ytterbium, Yttrium, Zinc, Zirconium.

Liquid Multiple Minerals - J. R. Carlson Laboratories, Inc.
Three softgels contain: Calcium (from calcium carbonate and glycinate chelate) 500 mg • Iron (as iron glycinate chelate) 18 mg • Iodine (from kelp) 100 mcg • Magnesium (as magnesium oxide & magnesium glycinate) 250 mg • Zinc (as zinc glycinate chelate) 15 mg • Selenium (from kelp) 77 mcg • Copper (as copper glycinate chelate) 2 mg • Manganese (as manganese glycinate chelate) 7 mg • Chromium (from kelp) 75 mcg • Molybdenum (from kelp) 5 mcg • Potassium (from potassium sulfate) 99 mg • Boron (as boron glycinate chelate) 1 mg.

Liquid Multi-Vitamin - Natrol, Inc.
Two teaspoons (10 ml) contain: Vitamins & Minerals: Vitamin A (beta carotene) 10000 IU • Vitamin C (Calcium Ascorbate) 200 mg • Vitamin D (cholecalciferol) 400 IU • Vitamin E (Acetate) 100 IU • Vitamin B1 (Thiamine) 7.5 mg • Vitamin B2 (Riboflavin) 8.5 mg • Niacin (Niacinamide) Vitamin B3 20 mg • Vitamin B6 (Pyridoxine HCl) 17 mg • Vitamin B12 (cyanocobalamin) 50 mcg • Pantothenic Acid (calcium d-pantothenate) 50 mg • Inositol 25 mg • Folic Acid 400 mcg • Biotin 300 mcg. Advanced Flavonoids: GP Flavonoids Complex+ 50 mg • Rutin, Quercetin, & Hesperidin 10 mg • Herbal extracts: Nettles, Kelp, Parsley, Ginger, Oats, Alfalfa, Hops, Peppermint, Rose Hips, Spinach & Echinacea, Natural Vanilla Bean flavor, natural Ginger flavor • Tropical fruit extracts from: Acerola, Pineapple, Cashew fruit, Passion fruit, Mango, Orange, Lime & Lemon. In a Specially Formulated Base of: Purified Water, Brown Rice Syrup, Honey, Glycerine, Citric Acid, Sodium Benzoate to help protect flavor, Milk Thistle & Citrus fruits.

Liquid Multi-Vitamin - Puritan's Pride
Each tablespoonful (15 ml) contains: Vitamin A (as Retinyl Palmitate) 5,000 IU • Vitamin C (as Ascorbic Acid) 250 mg • Vitamin D (as Cholecalciferol) 400 IU • Vitamin E (as d-Alpha Tocopheryl plus Mixed Tocopherols) 125 IU • Thiamin (Vitamin B1; as Thiamine Mononitrate) 25 mg • Riboflavin (Vitamin B2; as Riboflavin-5'-Phosphate Sodium) 25 mg • Niacin (as Niacinamide) 150 mg • Vitamin B-6 (as Pyridoxine Hydrochloride) 50 mg • Folic Acid 400 mcg • Vitamin B-12 (as Cyanocobalamin) 50 mcg • Biotin (as D-Biotin) 50 mcg • Pantothenic Acid (as Dexpanthenol) 150 mg • PABA (Para-Aminobenzoic Acid) 25 mg • Choline Bitartrate 200 mg • Inositol 100 mg.

Liquid NewBust (Liquid New Bust) - Tiger-One.com
Water • Saw Palmetto • Extra Virgin Olive Oil • Dong Quai • Damiana • Glycerin • Foenugreek seed • Blessed Thistle • Violet • Wild Yam • Fennel Seed • Althea root • Cumin seed • Hops.
See Editor's Note No. 17.

Liquid Pantothenic Acid - J. R. Carlson Laboratories, Inc.
Each 1 tsp serving contains: Pantothenic Acid (as di-calcium pantothenate) 200 mg.

Liquid Propolis Extract With Herbs - TwinLab
Ten drops contain: Propolis 500 mg • Proprietary Herbal Blend 500 mg: Golden Seal root, Echinacea root, Myrrh, Black Walnut leaves, Marshmallow root, Licorice root, Garlic, Capsicum.

Liquid Serotonin 1X - Pain & Stress Center
Serotonin 1X. Other Ingredients: Distilled Water.
See Editor's Note No. 1.

Liquid Speed - Cytotec Solutions, Inc.
Unknown.
See Editor's Note No. 49.

Liquid Stevia - Physicians Laboratories
Each 1/8 teaspoon contains: Stevia Rebaudiana Bertoni leaves 15 mg.

Liquid Vitamin B-12 - GNC
Each dropperful (1ml) contains: Vitamin B12 (as cyanocobalamin) 1000 mcg. Other Ingredients: Purified Water, Propylene Glycol, Sorbitol, Natural Cherry Flavor, Methylparaben, Stevia, Propylparaben.

Liqui-Lieve - Gaia Herbs
Three capsules contain: Dandelion leaf and root (taraxacum officinalis) 200 mg • Parsley seed, leaf and root (petroselinum crispum) 108 mg • Juniper berry (juniperus communis) 134 mg • Fenugreek seed (trigonella foenum-graecum) 96 mg • Cascara Sagrada (rhamnus purshiana) 72 mg • Fennel seed (foeniculum vulgare) 16 mg • Bladderwrack fronds (fucus vesiculosus) 16 mg • Coriander leaf (coriandrum sativum) 14 mg. Other Ingredients: Vegetable Glycerin, Vegetable Cellulose (capsule).

Some Brand Name Natural Products - What they Contain

www.NaturalDatabase.com contains MANY more listings than appear here.

Editor's Notes are located on pages 2155-2163.

Listol - Progressive Health Nutraceuticals
Magnesium 300 mg • DMAE Bitartrate 350 mg • N-Acetyl L-Cysteine HCl 400 mg • Olive leaf extract 15 mg • Pyridoxal-5-Phosphate 15 mg • Folic Acid 400 mcg • Huperzine A extract 100 mcg • Lecithin 25 mg.

Lithinase - Progressive Labs
Each capsule contains: Lithium Amino Acid Chelate 25 mg • Elemental Lithium 50 mcg • Pea powder 25 mg • Buckwheat 25 mg • Millet flour 25 mg • Lentil powder 25 mg (carefully dried to preserve their natural nutrient content).

Lithium - American Biologics
Each capsule contains: Lithium (in a specially grown biologically active vegetable culture containing naturally associated and organically bound lithium) 50 mcg. Other Ingredients: Magnesium Stearate.

Lithium Orotate - Life Link
Each tablet contains: Lithium Orotate (elemental lithium 5.8 mg) 135 mg.

Lithium Orotate - Ortho Molecular Products
Each capsule contains: Lithium (as lithium orotate) 10 mg. Other Ingredients: Natural Vegetable Capsules, Ascorbyl Palmitate, Magnesium Stearate, Microcrystalline Cellulose, Silicon Dioxide.

Little One Children's Multiple - Metabolic Products
Each tablet contains: Vitamin A (Palmitate) 2500 IU • Vitamin A (Natural Mixed Carotenoids) 2500 IU • Vitamin C (Hypoallergenic from Beet sugar and Ascorbyl Palmitate) 100 mg • Vitamin E (D-Alpha, Natural) 60 IU • Vitamin B1 (Thiamin Mononitrate) 5 mg • Vitamin B2 (Riboflavin) 5 mg • Vitamin B3 (Niacinamide) 25 mg • Vitamin B5 (D-Calcium Pantothenate) 25 mg • Vitamin B6 (Pyridoxine) 5 mg • Vitamin B12 (Cyanocobalamin) 10 mcg • Folic Acid 400 mcg • Biotin 300 mcg • Vitamin D (Cholecalciferol) 400 IU • Iron (Carbonyl) 9 mg • Iodine (K-Iodine) 100 mcg • Copper (Gluconate) 2 mg • Manganese (Gluconate) 1 mg • Zinc (Citrate) 15 mg • Molybdenum (Sodium Molybdate) 25 mcg • Chromium (GTF-Polynicotinate) 100 mcg • Selenium (L-Selenomethionine, Sodium Selenite) 100 mcg.

Liu Wei Di Huang Wan Plus - Secara
Rehmannia tuber 5:1 extract (shu di huang) 561 mg • Asiatic Dogwood ruit 5:1 extract (shan zhu yu) 270 mg • Asian Water Plantain rhizome 5:1 extract (ze xie) 225 mg • Chinese Yam rhizome 5:1 extract (shan yao) 225 mg • Hoelen sclerotium 5:1 extract (fu ling) 225 mg • Siberian Ginseng root/rhizome (0.8% eleutherosides) 225 mg • Tree Peony root bark 5:1 extract (mu dan pi) 225 mg • Ginkgo leaf extract (24% flavone glycosides) 180 mg • Organic American Ginseng root (xi yang shen) 114 mg.

Liv.52 DS - The Himalaya Drug Company
Each tablet contains: Himsra (capparis spinosa) 130 mg • Kasani (cichorium intybus) 130 mg • Mandur Bhasma (ferric oxide calx) 66 mg • Kakamachi (solanum nigrum) 64 mg • Arjuna (terminalia arjuna) 64 mg • Kasamarda (cassia occidentalis) 32 mg • Biranjasipha (achillea millefolium) 32 mg • Jhavuka (tamarix gallica) 32 mg.

Liv.52 Syrup - The Himalaya Drug Company
Each 1 tsp (5 mL) serving contains: Himsra (capparis spinosa) 17 mg • Kasani (cichorium intybus) 17 mg • Kakamachi (solanum nigrum) 8 mg • Arjuna (terminalia arjuna) 8 mg • Kasamarda (cassia occidentalis) 4 mg • Biranjasipha (achillea millefolium) 4 mg • Jhavuka (tamarix gallica) 4 mg.

Liv.52 tablets - The Himalaya Drug Company
Each tablet contains: Himsra (capparis spinosa) 65 mg • Kasani (cichorium intybus) 65 mg • Mandur Bhasma (ferric oxide calx) 33 mg • Kakamachi (solanum nigrum) 32 mg • Arjuna (terminalua arjuna) 32 mg • Kasamarda (cassia occidentalis) 16 mg • Biranjasipha (achillea millefolium) 16 mg • Jhavuka (tamarix gallica) 16 mg.

Livaplex - Standard Process, Inc.
Each capsule contains: Proprietary Blend 598 mg: Bovine Liver extract, Spanish Black Radish (root), Bovine Liver, Calcium Lactate, Beet (root), Carrot (root), Tillandsia Usneoides, Dried Beet (leaf) juice, Betaine Hydrochloride, Magnesium Citrate, Choline Bitartrate, Soy (bean), Oat Flour, Bovine Kidney, Bovine Prostate, Bovine Adrenal extract, Defatted Wheat (germ), Bovine Liver Fat extract, Bovine Orchic extract, Ascorbic Acid, Flaxseed Oil extract, Mixed Tocopherols • Gelatin • Zinc Liver Chelate 5.5 mg • Iron Liver Chelate 2.7 mg • Water • Potassium Bicarbonate • Calcium Stearate • Niacinamide 2.8 mg • Copper Liver Chelate 109 mcg • Colors • Pyridoxine Hydrochloride 0.8 mg • Vitamin A Palmitate 1260 IU • Prolamine Iodine (zein) 9.6 mcg.
See Editor's Note No. 14.

Liv-A-Tox - Enzymatic Therapy
Three tablets contain: Vitamin A (from fish liver oil) 4500 IU • Vitamin C (ascorbic acid and from rose hips) 25 mg • Niacin 40 mg • Vitamin B12 (as cyanocobalamin) 3 mcg • Biotin 200 mcg • Sodium 5 mg • Choline Bitartrate 850 mg • Red Beet root 300 mg • L-Methionine 250 mg • Barberry bark of root (berberis vulgaris) 150 mg • Boldo leaf extract (peumus boldus, 2:1) 150 mg • Celandine whole plant (chelidonium majus) 135 mg • Fringe Tree bark (chionanthus virginicus) 135 mg • Ox Bile extract 90 mg • Betaine HCl 75 mg • Inositol 50 mg. Other Ingredients: Cellulose, Calcium Carbonate, Stearic Acid, Modified Cellulose Gum, Silicon Dioxide, Magnesium Stearate, Chlorophyll Color, Anise Oil.
See Editor's Note No. 14.

Live Calm Sleep Deep - Cocoon Nutrition
Each capsule contains: L-Tetrahydropalmatine 30 mg • Magnesium Chloride 12.6 mg. Other Ingredients: Microcrystalline Cellulose.

Liver - Nutrivention
Each tablet contains: Inositol 100 mg • Choline Bitartrate 100 mg • Vitamin E 50 IU • Vitamin B1 10 mg • Niacin 10 mg • Pantothenic Acid 10 mg • Vitamin A (Beta Carotene) 500 IU • Vitamin B12 100 mcg • Vitamin K 15 mcg • Lecithin 300 mg • Milk Thistle (Cardus marianus) 200 mg • Dandelion root 200 mg • Burdock root 50 mg • L-Methionine 50 mg • L-Theronine 30 mg • Yellow Dock 25 mg • Butternut root bark 25 mg.

Liver - Enzymes, Inc.
Each capsule contains: Vitamin C (100% from Acerola Cherries) 8.5 mg • Proprietary Herbal Blend 421 mg: Milk Thistle seed extract, Chinese Thoroughwax root extract, Beet root extract, Rehmannia root extract, Rice Bran, Dandelion root extract, Safflower petals powder • Proprietary Enzyme Blend 65 mg: pHysioProtease, CereCalase. Other Ingredients: Plant Cellulose, Water.

Liver & Gallbladder Remedy (formerly HP 23) - Metagenics
Each drop contains: Chelidonium Majus 3X • Cinchona Officinalis 6X • Lycopodium Clavatum 30X • Colocynthis 12X • Chionanthus Virginica 3X.
See Editor's Note No. 1.

Liver Agents - Sojourn Health
Three capsules contain: Vitamin B6 (pyridoxine HCl) 80 mg • Selenium 50 mg • Proprietary Base 2450 mg: Artichoke powder (cynara floridanum), Sarsaparilla root extract, DL-Methionine, Milk Thistle extract, Beet greens (freeze-dried), Choline (bitartrate), N-Acetyl Cysteine, Astragalus root powder (astragalus membranaceus). Other Ingredients: Rice Powder, Magnesium Stearate, Gelatin.

Liver Balance - Nature's Sunshine
Four capsules contain: Proprietary Blend 1940 mg: Bupleurum root (bupleurum chinese), Peony root (paeonia officinalis), Typhonium rhizome (typhonium flagelliforme), Cinnamon twig (cinnamomum cassia), Dong Quai root (angelica polymorpha), FuShen sclerotium with root (poria cocos), Scute root (scutellaria baicalensis), Citrus Aurantium fruit, Atractylodes rhizome (atractylodes lancea), Panax Ginseng root, Ginger rhizome (zingiber officinale), Licorice root (glycyrrhiza uralensis). Other Ingredients: Gelatin, Water.
See Editor's Note No. 40.

Liver Chelate - Atrium Biotechnologies
Each tablet contains: Ferrous Fumarate as Chelated Proteinates 55 mg • Copper 1 mg • Folic Acid 40 mcg • Vitamin B12 20 mcg • Raw Liver concentrate (not an extract) of Bovine source 190 mg. See Editor's Note No. 14.

Liver Detox - Renew Life Formulas, Inc.
Part I (Morning Formula): Two capsules contain: Selenium (L-selenomethionine) • Milk Thistle seed • Phosphatidyl Choline (soy lecithin) • Dandelion root 4:1 extract • L-Methionine • L-Taurine • NAC (N-acetyl-cysteine) • Alpha Lipoic Acid • Artichoke leaf 4:1 extract (2% cynarin) • Green Tea leaf (50% polyphenols) • Tumeric root (95% curcumin). Other Ingredients: Hypromellose, Water.
Part II (Evening Formula): Two capsules contain: Belleric Myrobalan fruit (terminalia bellerica) • Boerhavia Diffusa root and herb • Eclipta Alba root and herb (4.5% waldelactones) • Tinospora Cordifolia stem • Andrographis Paniculata leaf p.e. tt (10% andrographolides) • Picrorhiza Kurroa root. Other Ingredients: Hypromellose, Water.

Liver DTX Complex - Shaklee
Three caplets contain: Milk Thistle extract (Silybum marianum) seed 300 mg • DTX Enhanced Proprietary Blend 900 mg: Schizandra extract (Schizandra chinensis) fruit, Dandelion extract (Taraxacum officinale) root and leaf, Reishi Mushroom extract (Ganoderma lucidum) cap and stalk, Turmeric extract (Curcuma longa) rhizome, Artichoke extract (Cynara scolymus) leaf. Other Ingredients: Maltodextrin, Cellulose, Acacia Gum, CrosCarmellose Sodium, Silicon Dioxide.

Liver Essentials - Swanson Health Products
Two capsules contain: Milk Thistle seed extract (85% silymarin) 350 mg • Dandelion root 170 mg • Burdock root 120 mg • Parsley root 120 mg • Picroliv Picrorhiza Kurroa 100 mg • Black Radish root 70 mg • N-Acetyl Cysteine 50 mg • Trimethylglycine (as betaine anhydrous) 50 mg • Alpha Lipoic Acid 20 mg.

Liver Extract - PhytoPharmica
Two softgels contain: Iron 2 mg • Liquid Liver Fractions (predigested soluble concentrate) 1100 mg • Sodium 5 mg • Vitamin B12 (as cyanocobalamin) 200 mcg. Other Ingredients: Soybean Oil, Gelatin, Glycerin, Lecithin, Beeswax, Caramel Color, Titanium Dioxide Color. This product was formerly known as Aqueous Liver Extract. See Editor's Note No. 14.

Liver Extract with Eleuthero - PhytoPharmica
Two softgels contain: Eleuthero root 20:1 extract (eleutherococcus senticosus, standardized to contain a minimum of 0.5% eleutheroside E) 50 mg • Iron 2 mg • Liquid Liver Fractions (predigested soluble concentrate) 1100 mg • Sodium 5 mg • Vitamin B12 (as cyanocobalamin) 200 mcg. Other Ingredients: Soybean Oil, Gelatin, Glycerin, Lecithin, Beeswax, Caramel Color, Titanium Dioxide color. This product was formerly known as Aqueous Liver Extract with Siberian Ginseng. See Editor's Note No. 14.

Liver Formula - HERBALmax
Gentian root • Isatis root • Curcuma root • Wormwood herb • Gambir plant • Selfheal fruit-spike • Cassia seed.

Liver Glandular - American Biologics
Each tablet contains: Raw Liver concentrate (bovine origin) 450 mg. Other Ingredients: Dicalcium Phosphate, Magnesium Stearate. See Editor's Note No. 14.

Liver Guard - Source Naturals
Two tablets contain: Vitamin B1 (Thiamin) 7.5 mg • Vitamin B2 (Riboflavin) 7.5 mg • Niacinamide and Niacin 50 mg • Vitamin B5 (Pantothenic Acid) 15 mg • Vitamin B6 (Pyridoxine HCl) 10 mg • Vitamin B12 (Cyanocobalamin) 25 mcg • Folic Acid 200 mcg • Vitamin C (Ascorbic Acid and Zinc Ascorbate) 527 mg • Fat-Soluble Vitamin C (from 238 mg of Ascorbyl Palmitate) 100 mg • Vitamin E (D-Alpha Tocopheryl) (Natural) 75 IU • Magnesium (Oxide, Malate) 60 mg • Potassium (Citrate) 49.5 mg • Selenium (as L-Selenomethionine) 50 mcg • Zinc (OptiZinc Zinc Monomethionine 10 mg and Zinc Ascorbate 5 mg) 15 mg • Silymarin (from Milk Thistle seed extract) 200 mg • N-Acetyl Cysteine 200 mg • Dandelion root extract 125 mg • • Turmeric extract (95% Curcumin) 76 mg • Choline (Bitartrate) 50 mg • Inositol 50 mg • Alpha-Lipoic Acid (Thioctic acid) 25 mg • Coenzyme Q10 (Ubiquinone) 12.5 mg.

Liver Health - Gaia Herbs
Two capsules contain: Milk Thistle seed (silybum marianum) 100 mg • Turmeric rhizome (curcuma longa) 100 mg • Schizandra berry (schizandra chinensis) 100 mg • MSM (methylsulfonylmethane) 100 mg • Chinese Skullcap root (scutellaria baicalensis) 56 mg • Licorice root (glycyrrhiza glabra) 20 mg. Other Ingredients: Vegetable Glycerin, Lecithin, Vegetable Cellulose (capsule).

Liver Health - Enzymes, Inc.
Two capsules contain: n-zimes Proprietary Enzyme Blend 64 mg: pHysioProtease (177,600 pHysio-U), CereCalse Plus • Proprietary Herbal Blend 380 mg: Milk Thistle seed extract (standardized to contain 80% silymarin), Beet root extract (equivalent to 400 mg raw herb), Schizandra fruit extract (equivalent to 320 mg raw herb), Rice Bran, Dandelion root extract (equivalent to 80 mg raw herb), Turmeric root extract (standardized to contain 95% curcumin). Other Ingredients: Plant Cellulose, Water.

Liver Maintenance Formula - PhysioLogics
Each capsule contains: Dandelion root (taraxacum officinale) 50 mg • Milk Thistle seed (silybum marinum, standardized to contain 80% silymarin, 80 mg) 100 mg • Alpha Lipoic Acid 75 mg • Trimethyl Glycine 175 mg • N-Acetyl Cysteine 100 mg. Other Ingredients: Gelatin, Rice Powder, Silica, Magnesium Stearate.

Liver Performance - Metabolic Response Modifiers
Each capsule contains: N-Acetyl-Cysteine (NAC) 400 mg • Alpha Lipoic Acid 100 mg • Choline Bitartrate 100 mg • Silymarin (32 mg of milk thistle extract standardized to 80% silymarin) 100 mg • Picrorhiza Kurroa 25 mg • Andographis Paniculata 25 mg • Vitamin E 40 IU • Vitamin B12 (methylcobalamin) 20 mcg.

Liver Protect - Xymogen
Each capsule contains: Alpha-Lipoic Acid 200 mg • Silymarin (from milk thistle seed extract, standardized to 80% silymarin) 210 mg • Selenium (from selenomethionine) 100 mcg • N-Acetyl-L-Cysteine 200 mg.

Liver Support - Vital Nutrients
Two capsules contain: Dandelion root 4:1 extract 200 mg • Artichoke leaf 6:1 extract 200 mg • Curcumin 20:1 extract 200 mg • Milk Thistle seed extract (silybin, silicristin, silidianin, silymarin minimum 80% by HPLC) 200 mg • Schisandra 20:1 extract 100 mg • Bupleurum 10:1 extract 100 mg • Rehmannia 6:1 extract 100 mg • Choline Bitartrate 160 mg • L-Methionine 100 mg.

Liver Support II - Vital Nutrients
Two capsules contain: Picrorhiza Kurroa 5:1 extract 360 mg • Milk Thistle extract 250 mg • Silybin A & B extract 50 mg • Artichoke leaf 5:1 extract 300 mg • Curcumin extract 300 mg • Dandelion root 4:1 extract 100 mg.

Liver-Enhancer - HerbaSway
Reishi • Poria • Cordyceps • Maitake • Shiitake • Hericium • Schisandra • Lycium • Milk Thistle • Blackberry • HerbaSwee (Cucurbitaceae fruit).

LiverRight - Pro Health
Two capsules contain: L-Methionine 350 mg • Betaine (trimethylglycine) 200 mg • Green Tea leaf 50% extract (camellia sinensis standardized to provide 100 mg of polyphenols) 200 mg • Turmeric 95% extract (curcuma domestica standardized to provide 190 mg curcuminoids) 200 mg • Artichoke leaf 5% extract (cynara scolymus standardized to provide 5 mg of sesquiterpene lactones) 100 mg • Milk Thistle seed 80% extract (silybum marianum standardized to provide 80 mg silymarin) 100 mg • Schisandra powder (schisandra chinensis) 250 mg • Defatted Liver Concentrate (hormone free) 250 mg. Other Ingredients: Gelatin, Dicalcium Phosphate, Magnesium Stearate, Magnesium Trisillicate. See Editor's Note No. 14.

BRAND NAMES

LiveRx **-** Metabolic Response Modifiers
Each capsule contains: N-Acetyl-Cysteine (NAC) 400 mg • Alpha Lipoic Acid 100 mg • Choline 100 mg • Silymarin 100 mg • Picrorhiza kurroa 25 mg • Andrographis Paniculata 25 mg • Vitamin E 40 IU • Vitamin B12 (methylcobalamin) 20 mcg.

Living B Complex **-** Garden of Life, Inc.
Three caplets contain: Thiamine (vitamin B1) 9 mg • Riboflavin (vitamin B2) 10 mg • Niacin (vitamin B3) 60 mg • Vitamin B6 12 mg • Folic Acid 800 mcg • Vitamin B12 500 mcg • Biotin 300 mcg • Pantothenic Acid 60 mg • Inositol 50 mg • PABA (para-aminobenzoic acid) 10 mg • Choline 30 mg • Poten-Zyme Superfood Blend (25-1) 1650 mg: Brown Rice Bran, Spirulina, Alfalfa grass juice • Poten-Zyme 11 "No Stress" Blend 900 mg: Rhodiola Rosea, Ganoderma Lucidum, Grifola Frondosa, Lentinula Edodes, Agaricus Blazei, Trametes Versicolor, Cordyceps Sinensis, Hericium Erinaceus, Poria Cocos, Tremella Fuciformia, Polyporus Umbellatus, Blakesleo Trispora. Other Ingredients: Cellulose, Stearates (vegetable source).

Living Calcium Homeostatic Calcium **-** Garden of Life, Inc.
Three caplets contain: Calcium 600 mg • Vitamin C 60 mg • Vitamin D 400 IU • Iodine 150 mcg • Magnesium 150 mg • Zinc 6 mg • Copper 1 mg • Manganese 2 mg • Silica 90 mg • Boron 2 mg • Organic Trace Mineral Blend 1050 mg • Poten-Zyme Organic Green Food Blend (25-1) 930 mg: Alfalfa grass juice, Barley grass juice, Wheat grass juice, Oat grass juice, Rye grass juice • Poten-Zyme Ocean Vegetable Blend 300 mg: Ecloria Radiata, Ascophyllum Nodosum, Laminaria Japonica, Macrocystis Pyrifera, Alaria Esculenta. Other Ingredients: Cellulose, Stearates (vegetable source).

Living Energy **-** Futurebiotics LLC
Four tablets contain: Chlorella 500 mg • Bee Pollen 1000 mg • Ginseng 4:1 extract equivalent to 250 mg • Royal Jelly (freeze dried) 25 mg • Schizandra 4:1 extract equivalent to 250 mg • Astragalus 4:1 extract equivalent to 250 mg • Spirulina 500 mg • Alfalfa juice concentrate 1200 mg.

Living Multi Iron Free Formula with Homeostatic Nutrients **-** Garden of Life, Inc.
Nine caplets contain: Vitamin A (beta carotene) 15,000 IU • Vitamin C 225 mg • Vitamin D 400 IU • Vitamin E 225 IU • Vitamin K 60 mcg • Thiamine (vitamin B1) 9 mg • Riboflavin (vitamin B2) 10 mg • Niacin (vitamin B3) 60 mg • Vitamin B6 12 mg • Vitamin B12 500 mcg • Biotin 300 mcg • Pantothenic Acid 60 mg • Calcium 250 mg • Iodine 150 mcg • Magnesium 150 mg • Zinc 15 mg • Selenium 200 mcg • Copper 200 mcg • Manganese 3 mg • Chromium 200 mcg • Potassium 99 mg • Molybdenum 100 mcg • Boron 1 mg • Vanadium 100 mcg • Inositol 50 mg • PABA (para-aminobenzoic acid) 10 mg • Choline 30 mg • Bioflavonoids 100 mg • Lycopene 5 mg • Lutein 5 mg • Alpha Lipoic Acid 150 mg • Poten-Zyme 20 Antioxidant Veggie Juice Blend (25-1) 3150 mg: Alfalfa grass, Barley grass, Wheat grass, Rye grass, Oat grass, Broccoli, Cauliflower, Kale, Collard Greens, Brussels Sprouts, Carrot, Beet, Spinach, Parsley, Cucumber, Asparagus, Celery, Cabbage, Onion, Garlic • Organic Trace Mineral Blend 2900 mg • Poten-Zyme 9 Ocean Vegetable Blend 2000 mg: Spirulina Platensis, Chlorella Vulgaris, Lithothamnion Calcereum, Dunaliella Salina, Ecloria Radiata, Ascophyllum Nodosum, Laminaria Japonica, Macrocystis Pyrifera, Alaria Esculenta • Poten-Zyme 23 Antioxidant Fruit Blend (60-1) 1800 mg: Acerola Cherry, Blueberry (fruit, leaf), Pomegranate, Apple (fruit, skin), Black Currant, Apricot, Nectarine, Prune, White Cherry, Elderberry, Grape (fruit, seed, skin, leaf), Peach, Mango, Strawberry, Raspberry, Blackberry, Orange, Grapefruit, Lemon, Lime, Cranberry, Pineapple, Papaya • Poten-Zyme 11 Tonic Mushroom Blend 800 mg: Ganoderma Lucidum, Grifola Frondosa, Lentinula Edodes, Agaricus Blazei, Trametes Versicolor, Cordyceps Sinensis, Hericium Erinaceus, Poria Cocos, Tremella Fuciformia, Polyporus Umbellatus, Blakesleo Trispora • Poten-Zyme 6 Botanical Blend (40-1) 250 mg: Rhododendron Caucasicum, Yucca, Rosemary, Ginger, Turmeric, Wild Oregano. Other Ingredients: Cellulose, Stearates (vegetable source).

Living Multi Optimal Formula **-** Garden of Life, Inc.
Nine caplets contain: Vitamin A (beta carotene) 15,000 IU • Vitamin C 225 mg • Vitamin D 400 IU • Vitamin E 225 IU • Vitamin K 60 mcg • Thiamine (vitamin B1) 9 mg • Riboflavin (vitamin B2) 10 mg • Niacin (vitamin B3) 60 mg • Vitamin B12 500 mcg • Biotin 300 mcg • Pantothenic Acid 60 mg • Calcium 250 mg • Iron 9 mg • Iodine 150 mcg • Magnesium 150 mg • Zinc 15 mg • Selenium 200 mcg • Copper 200 mcg • Manganese 3 mg • Chromium 200 mcg • Potassium 99 mg • Molybdenum 100 mcg • Boron 1 mg • Vanadium 100 mcg • Inositol 50 mg • PABA (para-aminobenzoic acid) 10 mg • Choline 30 mg • Bioflavonoids 100 mg • Lycopene 5 mg • Lutein 5 mg • Alpha Lipoic Acid 150 mg • Poten-Zyme 20 Antioxidant Veggie Juice Blend (25-1) 3150 mg: Alfalfa grass, Barley grass, Wheat grass, Rye grass, Oat grass, Broccoli, Cauliflower, Kale, Collard Greens, Brussels Sprouts, Carrot, Beet, Spinach, Parsley, Cucumber, Asparagus, Celery, Cabbage, Onion, Garlic • Organic Trace Mineral Blend 2900 mg • Poten-Zyme 9 Ocean Vegetable Blend 2000 mg: Spirulina Platensis, Chlorella Vulgaris, Lithothamnion Calcereum, Dunaliella Salina, Ecloria Radiata, Ascophyllum Nodosum, Laminaria Japonica, Macrocystis Pyrifera, Alaria Esculenta • Poten-Zyme 23 Antioxidant Fruit Blend (60-1) 1800 mg: Acerola Cherry, Blueberry (fruit, leaf), Pomegranate, Apple (fruit, skin), Black Currant, Apricot, Nectarine, Prune, White Cherry, Elderberry, Grape (fruit, seed, skin, leaf), Peach, Mango, Strawberry, Raspberry, Blackberry, Orange, Grapefruit, Lemon, Lime, Cranberry, Pineapple, Papaya • Poten-Zyme 11 Tonic Mushroom Blend 800 mg: Ganoderma Lucidum, Grifola Frondosa, Lentinula Edodes, Agaricus Blazei, Trametes Versicolor, Cordyceps Sinensis, Hericium Erinaceus, Poria Cocos, Tremella Fuciformia, Polyporus Umbellatus, Blakesleo Trispora • Poten-Zyme 6 Botanical Blend (40-1) 250 mg: Rhododendron Caucasicum, Yucca, Rosemary, Ginger, Turmeric, Wild Oregano. Other Ingredients: Cellulose, Stearates (vegetable source).

Living Multi Optimal Men's Formula with Homeostatic Nutrients **-** Garden of Life, Inc.
Six caplets contain: Vitamin A (beta carotene) 10,000 IU • Vitamin C 50 mg • Vitamin D 400 IU • Vitamin E 225 IU • Vitamin K 60 mcg • Thiamine (vitamin B1) 9 mg • Riboflavin (vitamin B2) 10 mg • Niacin (vitamin B3) 60 mg • Vitamin B6 12 mg • Folic Acid 800 mcg • Vitamin B12 500 mcg • Biotin 300 mcg • Pantothenic Acid 60 mg • Calcium 250 mg • Iron 9 mg • Iodine 150 mcg • Magnesium 150 mg • Zinc 20 mg • Selenium 200 mcg • Copper 200 mcg • Manganese 3 mg • Chromium 200 mcg • Potassium 99 mg • Molybdenum 100 mcg • Boron 1 mg • Vanadium 100 mcg • Inositol 50 mg • PABA (para-aminobenzoic acid) 10 mg • Choline 30 mg • Bioflavonoids 100 mg • Lycopene 5 mg • Lutein 5 mg • Alpha Lipoic Acid 150 mg • Poten-Zyme 20 Antioxidant Veggie Juice Blend (25-1) 750 mg: Alfalfa grass, Barley grass, Wheat grass, Rye grass, Oat grass, Broccoli, Cauliflower, Kale, Collard Greens, Brussels Sprouts, Carrot, Beet, Spinach, Parsley, Cucumber, Asparagus, Celery, Cabbage, Onion, Garlic • Organic Trace Mineral Blend 800 mg • Poten-Zyme 9 Ocean Vegetable Blend 2050 mg: Spirulina Platensis, Chlorella Vulgaris, Lithothamnion Calcereum, Dunaliella Salina, Ecloria Radiata, Ascophyllum Nodosum, Laminaria Japonica, Macrocystis Pyrifera, Alaria Esculenta • Poten-Zyme 23 Antioxidant Fruit Blend (60-1) 1650 mg: Acerola Cherry, Blueberry (fruit, leaf), Pomegranate, Apple (fruit, skin), Black Currant, Apricot, Nectarine, Prune, White Cherry, Elderberry, Grape (fruit, seed, skin, leaf), Peach, Mango, Strawberry, Raspberry, Blackberry, Orange, Grapefruit, Lemon, Lime, Cranberry, Pineapple, Papaya • Poten-Zyme 11 Tonic Mushroom Blend 750 mg: Ganoderma Lucidum, Grifola Frondosa, Lentinula Edodes, Agaricus Blazei, Trametes Versicolor, Cordyceps Sinensis, Hericium Erinaceus, Poria Cocos, Tremella Fuciformia, Polyporus Umbellatus, Blakesleo Trispora • Poten-Zyme 5 Botanical Blend (40-1) 100 mg: Yucca, Rosemary, Ginger, Turmeric, Wild Oregano • Poten-Zyme 5 Men's Herbal Blend (40-1) 1075 mg: Maca, Rhodiola Rosea, Rhododendron Caucasicum, Bee Pollen, Aralia Racemosa. Other Ingredients: Cellulose, Stearates (vegetable source).

Living Multi Optimal Women's Formula with Homeostatic Nutrients - Garden of Life, Inc.
Six caplets contain: Vitamin A (beta carotene) 10,000 IU • Vitamin C 150 mg • Vitamin D 400 IU • Vitamin E 225 IU • Vitamin K 60 mcg • Thiamine (vitamin B1) 9 mg • Riboflavin (vitamin B2) 10 mg • Niacin (vitamin B3) 60 mg • Vitamin B6 12 mg • Folic Acid 800 mcg • Vitamin B12 500 mcg • Biotin 300 mcg • Pantothenic Acid 60 mg • Calcium 250 mg • Iron 18 mg • Iodine 75 mcg • Magnesium 150 mg • Zinc 15 mg • Selenium 200 mcg • Copper 200 mcg • Manganese 3 mg • Chromium 200 mcg • Potassium 99 mg • Molybdenum 100 mcg • Boron 1 mg • Vanadium 100 mcg • Inositol 50 mg • PABA (para-aminobenzoic acid) 10 mg • Choline 30 mg • Bioflavonoids 100 mg • Lycopene 5 mg • Lutein 5 mg • Alpha Lipoic Acid 150 mg • Poten-Zyme 20 Antioxidant Veggie Juice Blend (25-1) 900 mg: Alfalfa grass, Barley grass, Wheat grass, Rye grass, Oat grass, Broccoli, Cauliflower, Kale, Collard Greens, Brussels Sprouts, Carrot, Beet, Spinach, Parsley, Cucumber, Asparagus, Celery, Cabbage, Onion, Garlic • Organic Trace Mineral Blend 800 mg • Poten-Zyme 9 Ocean Vegetable Blend 1975 mg: Spirulina Platensis, Chlorella Vulgaris, Lithothamnion Calcereum, Dunaliella Salina, Ecloria Radiata, Ascophyllum Nodosum, Laminaria Japonica, Macrocystis Pyrifera, Alaria Esculenta • Poten-Zyme 23 Antioxidant Fruit Blend (60-1) 1650 mg: Acerola Cherry, Blueberry (fruit, leaf), Pomegranate, Apple (fruit, skin), Black Currant, Apricot, Nectarine, Prune, White Cherry, Elderberry, Grape (fruit, seed, skin, leaf), Peach, Mango, Strawberry, Raspberry, Blackberry, Orange, Grapefruit, Lemon, Lime, Cranberry, Pineapple, Papaya • Poten-Zyme 11 Tonic Mushroom Blend 750 mg: Ganoderma Lucidum, Grifola Frondosa, Lentinula Edodes, Agaricus Blazei, Trametes Versicolor, Cordyceps Sinensis, Hericium Erinaceus, Poria Cocos, Tremella Fuciformia, Polyporus Umbellatus, Blakesleo Trispora • Poten-Zyme 5 Botanical Blend (40-1) 100 mg: Yucca, Rosemary, Ginger, Turmeric, Wild Oregano • Poten-Zyme 5 Women's Herbal Blend (40-1) 1075 mg: Maca, Rhodiola Rosea, Rhododendron Caucasicum, Aralia Racemosa, Schizandra. Other Ingredients: Cellulose, Stearates (vegetable source).

Living Vitamin C - Garden of Life, Inc.
Three caplets contain: Vitamin C 500 mg • Bioflavonoids 150 mg • Poten-Zyme Whole Food Vitamin C Blend 2100 mg: Acerola Cherry, Camu Camu (myrciaria dubla), Indian Gooseberry (emblic officinalis) • Poten-Zyme Organic Whole Citrus Blend 750 mg: Orange, Grapefruit, Lemon, Lime (fruit, pulp, peel, seeds) • Poten-Zyme Organic Green Blend (25-1) 450 mg: Alfalfa grass juice, Wheat Grass juice, Oat grass juice, Barley grass juice, Rye grass juice • Organic Trace Mineral Blend 450 mg • Poten-Zyme Organic Fermented Fruit Blend 150 mg: Raspberry, Strawberry, Blueberry, Blackberry, Prune, Grape (fruit, skin, seeds). Other Ingredients: Cellulose, Stearates (vegetable source).

Livr D-Tox - Nutri-Quest Rx
Each tablet contains: Glucuronic Acid 10 mg • Liver 5 mg • Vitamin A 1000 IU • Vitamin C 25 mg • Vitamin B1 5 mg • Vitamin E 10 IU • Black Currant seed oil 5 mg • Cellulase 50 mg • Amylase 50 mg • Lipase 50 mg • Protease 50 mg • Lipoic Acid 2 mg • Phosphatidyl Choline 5.75 mg • Choline Bitartrate 15 mg • DL-Methionine 5 mg • Calcium Chelate 50 mg • Magnesium 50 mg • Zinc Chelate 5 mg • Selenium Chelate 25 mcg • Manganese 1 mg • Milk Thistle 100 mg • Silymarin 5 mg • Garlic 50 mg • Beet root 25 mg • Beet leaf 25 mg. See Editor's Note No. 14.

Liv-R-Actin Milk Thistle Blend in Vegetarian Capsules - Nature's Plus
Two Vegicaps contain: Herbal Blend, 600 mg: Dandelion, Barberry, Goldenseal, Wild Oregon Grape & Celery seed 600 mg • Milk Thistle extract, providing 70%, 98 mg of the active flavonoid Silymarin 140 mg.

Livral - AIE Pharmaceuticals
Each capsule contains: Proprietary Blend 750 mg: Milk Thistle extract, Phyllanthus amarus, Dandelion root (taraxacum officinale), Grape seed extract (vitis vinifera), Artichoke, Choline, Inositol.

Livral Complex - AIE Pharmaceuticals
Each capsule contains: Proprietary Blend 750 mg: Milk Thistle extract, Phyllanthus Amarus, Dandelion root (taraxacum officinale), Cat's Claw bark, Licorice root, Tribulus terrestris, Culver's root, Oregon Grape root, Yellow Dock, Burdock root, Echinacea root, Grape seed extract (vitis vinifera), Artichoke, Catechin.

Livtone - R-U Ved U.S.A.
Phyllanthus Niruri standardized extract • Andrographis Paniculata standardized extract • Apple juice concentrate standardized extract • Belleric Myrobalan standardized extract • Berberis Aristata standardized extract • Boerhavia Diffusa standardized extract • Eclipta Alba standardized extract • Picrorhiza Kurroa standardized extract • Solanum Nigrum standardized extract • Tephrosia Purpurea standardized extract • Terminalia Chebula standardized extract • Tinospora Cordifolia standardized extract • Raphanus Sativum standardized extract • Silybum Marianum.

l-Lysine - Pure Encapsulations
Each vegetable capsule contains: L-Lysine (free-form) 500 mg • Vitamin C (as ascorbyl palmitate) 10 mg.

L-Lysine - J. R. Carlson Laboratories, Inc.
Each capsule contains: L-Lysine (as L-lysine monohydrochloride) 500 mg.

L-Lysine - J. R. Carlson Laboratories, Inc.
Each 1 tsp serving contains: L-Lysine 1200 mg.

L-Lysine - Ortho Molecular Products
Each capsule contains: L-Lysine HCl USP 500 mg Other Ingredients: Natural Vegetable Capsules, Ascorbyl Palmitate, Magnesium Stearate, Microcrystalline Cellulose, Silicon Dioxide.

L-Lysine - PhysioLogics
Each tablet contains: L-Lysine (as l-lysine hydrochloride) 500 mg. Other Ingredients: Cellulose (plant origin), Food Glaze, Croscarmellose, Vegetable Magnesium Stearate, Silica, Magnesium Silicate.

L-Lysine 1000 - GNC
Each tablet contains: L-lysine (as L-Lysine Monohydrochloride) 1000 mg. Other Ingredients: Povidone.

L-Lysine 1000 mg - Solgar
Each tablet contains: Sodium 5 mg • L-Lysine (as L-lysine HCl) 1000 mg. Other Ingredients: Microcrystalline Cellulose, Vegetable Cellulose, Vegetable Stearic Acid, Silica, Vegetable Glycerin, Carnauba Wax.

L-Lysine 500 - Jarrow Formulas
Each capsule contains: L-Lysine (from 625 mg L-lysine HCl) 500 mg. Other Ingredients: Magnesium Stearate, Rice Powder, Gelatin.

L-Lysine 500 - GNC
Each tablet contains: L-lysine (as L-Lysine Monohydrochloride) 500 mg. Other Ingredients: Cellulose.

L-Lysine 500 mg - Rexall - Sundown
Each caplet contains: L-Lysine HCl 500 mg. Other Ingredients: Microcrystalline Cellulose, Hydrogenated Cottonseed Oil, Croscarmellose Sodium.

L-Lysine 500 mg - Sunmark
Each tablet contains: L-Lysine (hydrochloride) 500 mg. Other Ingredients: Microcrystalline Cellulose, Dicalcium Phosphate, Stearic Acid, Calcium Silicate, Magnesium Stearate.
See Editor's Note No. 45.

L-Lysine 500 mg - Pro Health
Each tablet contains: L-Lysine (from L-lysine hydrochloride) 500 mg. Other Ingredients: Cellulose, Silica, Magnesium Stearate.

L-Lysine 500 mg - Solgar
Each capsule contains: L-Lysine (as L-lysine HCl) 500 mg. Other Ingredients: Vegetable Cellulose, Microcrystalline Cellulose, Vegetable Magnesium Stearate, Water, Vegetable Glycerin.

BRAND NAMES

L-Lysine 500 mg Capsules - Arrowroot
Each capsule contains: L-Lysine 500 mg.

L-Lysine 500 mg Tablets - Arrowroot
Each tablet contains: L-Lysine 500 mg.

L-Lysine Plus - Atrium Biotechnologies
Each tablet contains: L-Lysine HCl (an essential amino acid) 500 mg • Ascorbic Acid (Vitamin C) 100 mg.

L-Methionine - J. R. Carlson Laboratories, Inc.
Each capsule contains: L-Methionine 500 mg.

L-Methionine - J. R. Carlson Laboratories, Inc.
Each 1 tsp serving contains: L-Methionine 3000 mg.

l-Methionine - Pure Encapsulations
Each vegetable capsule contains: L-Methionine (free-form) 375 mg.

Lo Han Sweet - Jarrow Formulas
Two scoops contain: Xylitol • MogroPure brand Momordica Grosvenorii (lo han fruit juice concentrate). Other Ingredients: Inulin-FOS (fructooligosaccharide), Silicon Dioxide.

Lobelia and Cayenne - Dial Herbs
Lobelia • Cayenne.

Lobelia Herb, 425 mg - Nature's Way
Each capsule contains: Lobelia (stem, leaf, flower) 425 mg. Other Ingredients: Gelatin, Magnesium Stearate.

Lomatium Osha Supreme - Gaia Herbs
Two capsules contain: Garlic bulb (allium sativum) 40 mg • Osha root (ligusticum porterii) 34 mg • Lomatium root (lomatium dissectum) 30 mg • Grindelia floral bud (grindelia robusta) 22 mg • Irish Moss (chondrus crispus) 20 mg • Hyssop flowers (hyssopus off.) 10 mg • Barberry root (berberis vulgaris) 8 mg • Oregon Grape root (berberis aquifolium) 8 mg • Goldenseal rhizome (hydrastis canadensis) 8 mg • Mullein leaf (verbascum olympicum) 8 mg • Lobelia herb and seed (lobelia inflata) 6 mg • St. John's Wort flower bud (hypericum perforatum) 6 mg • Echinacea Purpurea root 4 mg • Echinacea Pupurea flowering top 4 mg • Echinaacea Angustifolia root 3 mg • Echinacea purpurea seed 0.7 mg. Other Ingredients: Vegetable Glycerin, Vegetable Cellulose (capsule).

Lomatium-Goldenseal Virtue - Blessed Herbs
Lomatium root • Astragalus root • Osha root • Echinacea Angustifolia root • Goldenseal root • Siberian Ginseng root • Licorice root • Reishi mycelium • Shitake mycelium • Grain alcohol & Distilled Water.

Long Dan Xie Gan Tang Plus - Secara
Milk Thistle extract (80% silymarin) 384 mg • Dong Quai root 5:1 extract (dang gui) 345 mg • Organic Psyllium seed 345 mg • Rehmannia tuber 5:1 extract (shu di huang) 345 mg • Organic Licorice root (gan cao) 234 mg • Baikal Skullcap root 5:1 extract (huang qin) 192 mg • Asian Water Plantain rhizome 5:1 extract (ze xie) 171 mg • Bupleurum root 5:1 extract (chai hu) 78 mg • Gardenia fruit 5:1 extract (zhi zi) 78 mg • Scabrous Gentian root & rhizome 5:1 extract (long dan) 78 mg.

Longdan Xie Gan Wan - KwangChow First Chinese Medicine Factory
Unknown.
See Editor's Note No. 46.

Longdan Xie Ganwan - Unknown
Unknown.
See Editor's Note No. 46.

Longdan Ziegan Wan - China Beijing Tong-Ren Tang
Unknown.
See Editor's Note No. 46.

Longest Living Acidophilus - Futurebiotics LLC
Each capsule contains: Acidophilus fortified with Rhamnosus, encapsulated in a base of Rice powder & Beet fiber. 1 billion Live Organisms per capsule.

Longevinex - Resveratrol Partners, LLC
Each capsule contains: Proprietary Longevinex Blend 100 mg: providing not less than 15 mg Resveratrol from Giant Knotweed leaf extract (polygonum cuspidatum), Red Grape skin extract (vitis vinifera) • Quercetin 75 mg • Phytic Acid 25 mg • Lecithin 100 mg. Other Ingredients: Gelatin.

Longe-Vit-E - Holista
Each capsule contains: Vitamin C (Ester-C) 250 mg • Beta Carotene 10000 IU • Vitamin E (d-alpha tocopherol) 200 IU • Selenium 50 mcg • Vitamin B6 25 mg • Magnesium 50 mg • Manganese 1.5 mg • Copper 1.0 mg.

Longevity - Young Living Essential Oils
Clove Oil • Orange Oil • Thyme Oil • Frankincense Oil.

Longevity 2AEP + HGHR - Urban Nutrition Inc
Three capsules contain: Calcium 2-AEP (2-amino ethanol phosphate; 50 mg elemental calcium) 510 mg • Magnesium 2-AEP (32 mg elemental calcium) 510 mg • Potassium 2-AEP (43 mg elemental calcium) 255 mg • HGHR (human growth hormone releaser): Anterior Pituitary gland 75 mg, L-Arginine 45 mg • L-Glutamine 45 mg • L-Lysine 45 mg • L-Tyrosine 15 mg. Other Ingredients: Duratex, Pure Food Glaze, Avicel, Magnesium Stearate, Cab-O-Sil.
See Editor's Note No. 14.

Longevity Crystal - Sante International
Each tablet contains: Herbal Extract-Based Blend 500 mg: Gynostemma Pentaphyllum, Crataegus Pinnatifida (hawthorn leaves/berries), Camellia Sinensis (green tea).

Longevity Multi - Jarrow Formulas
Six capsules contain: Vitamin A (as retinyl palmitate) 2000 IU • Beta Carotene (pro-vitamin A) 3 mg • Vitamin C (ascorbic acid) 500 mg • Vitamin D (D3, cholecalciferol from fish liver oil) 600 IU • Vitamin E (D-alpha tocopherol succinate) 200 IU • Vitamin B1 (as thiamin mononitrate) 50 mg • Vitamin B2 (riboflavin) 50 mg • Vitamin B3 (niacinamide) 100 mg • Vitamin B6 (pyridoxine HCl) 20 mg • Folic Acid 400 mcg • Methyl Vitamin B12 (cobalamin concentrate) 100 mcg • Vitamin K (phylloquinone) 100 mcg • Biotin 300 mcg • Choline (as choline bitartrate) 25 mg • Pantothenic Acid (D-calcium pantothenate) 250 mg • Calcium (elemental, from 1850 mg calcium phosphate from milk) 500 mg • Iodine (from potassium iodide) 150 mcg • Magnesium (as magnesium oxide) 400 mg • Zinc (from zinc monomethionate) 15 mg • Selenium (as L-selenomethionine/sodium selenate 50/50) 200 mcg • Copper (as copper gluconate) 2 mg • Manganese (as manganese citrate) 1 mg • Chromium GTF (bound to saccharomyces cerevisiae) 200 mcg • Molybdenum (as trivalent sodium molybdate) 75 mcg • Potassium (as potassium chloride) 99 mg • Gamma Tocopherol 100 mg • Lutein (tagetes erecta) 5 mg • Lycopene (from GMO-free tomatoes) 5 mg • Silymarin (silybum marianum 30:1, 80% extract) 75 mg • Grape seed OPCs 50 mg • Rosemary extract (rosmarinus officinalis) 50 mg • Inositol 150 mg • Para-Aminobenzoic Acid (PABA) 250 mg. Other Ingredients: Calcium Phosphate, Modified Cellulose Gum, Stearic Acid, Silicon Dioxide, Magnesium Stearate, Modified Cellulose.

Longevity Signal A.M. Formula - Oasis Wellness Network
Each capsule contains: N-Acetyl-Cysteine 100 mg • Acetyl-L-Carnitine 60 mg • Alpha Lipoic Acid 50 mg • Chlorella powder (whole plant) 50 mg • Fo-Ti root extract 50 mg • Wolfberry fruit extract 50 mg • MaxCell Proprietary Blend 25 mg: Zisyphus Jujube, Piper Nigrum, Aloe Vera, Glycyrrhiza Glabra • 7-Keto DHEA 15 mg • DHEA 7.5 mg. Other Ingredients: Cellulose, Dicalcium Phosphate, Magnesium Stearate, Silica.

Longevity Signal P.M. Formula - Oasis Wellness Network
Each capsule contains: Wolfberry fruit extract 200 mg • Chlorella powder (whole plant) 150 mg • Fo-Ti root extract 100 mg • N-Acetyl-Cysteine 50 mg • Alpha Lipoic Acid 50 mg • MaxCell Proprietary Blend 25 mg: Zisyphus Jujube, Piper Nigrum, Aloe Vera, Glycyrrhiza Glabra • DIM (diindolylmethane) 25 mg • Active Aloe (200:1) 20 mg • 7-Keto DHEA 12.5 mg • DHEA 5 mg • R5P (riboflavin-5-phosphate) 3 mg • P5P (pyridoxal-5-phosphate) 3 mg •

Methylcobalamin 800 mcg. Other Ingredients: Cellulose, Dicalcium Phosphate, Magnesium Stearate, Silica.

LongoVital **-** Paramedical A/S
Three tablets contain: Proprietary Blend 462 mg: Paprika, Rosemary, Peppermint, Hawthorn, Pumpkin seeds, Yarrow flowers • Vitamin A 800 mcg • Thiamin (B1) 1.4 mg • Riboflavin (B2) 1.6 mg • Vitamin B6 2 mg • Niacin 18 mg • Pantothenic Acid 6 mg • Vitamin C 60 mg • Vitamin D 5 mcg • Vitamin E 10 mg.

Longs Natural Magnesium 250 mg **-** Longs
Each tablet contains: Magnesium (as magnesium oxide) 250 mg. Other Ingredients: Cellulose, Talc, Sodium Starch Gycolate, Starch, Silicon Dioxide, Croscarmellose Sodium, Polyethylene Glycol, Kelp, Magnesium Stearate.

Long-Term Adrenal **-** Enzymes, Inc.
Each capsule contains: Vitamin C (100% from Acerola Cherries) 10 mg • Proprietary Herbal Blend 385 mg: Codonopsis root extract, Chinese Thoroughwax root extract, Rice Bran, Astragalus root extract • Proprietary Enzyme Blend 80 mg: pHysioProtease, CereCalase. Other Ingredients: Plant Cellulose, Water.

Looking Young **-** FreeLife International
Two caplets contain: Vitamin A (100% from beta-carotene, alpha-carotene, cryptoxanthin, zeaxanthin, lutein) 2500 IU • Vitamin C (from glycosyl flavonebound isoascorbic acids 130 mg) 100 mg • Vitamin E (as natural d-alpha-tocopheryl succinate) 30 IU • Biotin 100 mcg • Pantothenic Acid (as D-calcium pantothenate) 10 mg • Calcium (from calcium hydrogen phosphate) 150 mg • Zinc (as patented OptiZinc zinc monomethionine) 5 mg • Manganese (as patented Chelazome glycine amino acid chelate) 2.5 mg • Glucosamine / Aloe Mucopolysaccharides Complex 1000 mg: Glucosamine Hydrochloride, Vegetable Beta-Polysaccharides, Aloe Vera 40x concentrate • Microencapsulated Lactobacillus Sporogenes 100 million cells • Catalase 1000 units • Proprietary Blend 130 mg: Ascorbic Acid, Sodium Isoascorbate, Citrus Glycosyl Flavones (cirantin, isosakuranetin-7-beta-uritinoside, narirutin, eriocitrin, noblietin, tangeretin, heptamethoxyflavone) • Sea Vegetable Marine Protein/Fiber concentrate (from Irish moss and algae extract) 100 mg • Red Grape skin standardized extract 100 mg • MSM (methylsulfonylmethane) 100 mg • Purified Soy Phosphatides 100 mg • Proprietary Blend 100 mg: RNA (ribonucleic acid), DNA (deoxyribonucleic acid) complex. Proprietary Blend 2500 Units: Soy Polysaccharides, Plant Enzymes. Proprietary Blend 50 mg: Artichoke leaf standardized extract (2% cynarin), Chamomile flower, Citrus Pectin, Gentian root, Milk Thistle seed, Wild Yam root • Silica (colloidal, from N. Atlantic Sea kelp) 30 mg. Other Ingredients: Calcium Hydrogen Phosphate, Cellulose, Vegetable Stearic Acid, Calcium Carbonate, Vegetable Magnesium Stearate, Calcium Silicate, Vita-Coat (vegetable resin, alpha-lipoic acid).

L-Ornithine 500 mg **-** Solgar
Each capsule contains: L-Ornithine (as L-ornithine HCl) 500 mg. Other Ingredients: Vegetable Cellulose, Microcrystalline Cellulose, Vegetable Magnesium Stearate, Silica, Vegetable Stearic Acid, Water, Vegetable Glycerin.

L-Ornithine Caps **-** Nature's Plus
Each capsule contains: L-Ornithine (free form amino acid) 500 mg. Other Ingredients: Microcrystalline Cellulose, Silica, Gelatin, Purified Water.

Love Bites **-** Nature's Plus
Each chewable tablet contains: Vitamin A (as beta carotene) 5000 IU • Vitamin C (as ascorbic acid) 75 mg • Vitamin D (as ergocalciferol) 400 IU • Vitamin E (as D-alpha-tocopheryl acetate) 30 IU • Thiamin (vitamin B1, as thiamine HCl) 5 mg • Riboflavin (vitamin B2) 5 mg • Niacin (as niacinamide) 10 mg • Vitamin B6 (as pyridoxine HCl) 5 mg • Folate (as folic acid) 10 mcg • Vitamin B12 (cyanocobalamin) 10 mcg • Biotin 50 mcg • Pantothenic Acid (as calcium pantothenate) 10 mg • Calcium (as gluconate) 20 mg • Iron (as gluconate) 10 mg • Iodine (from kelp) 100 mcg • Magnesium (as gluconate) 10 mg • Zinc (as gluconate) 3 mg • Manganese (as gluconate) 2 mg • Potassium (as gluconate) 4 mg • Choline (as bitartrate) 2 mg • Inositol 2 mg • PABA (para-aminobenzoic acid) 0.6 mg. Other Ingredients: Fructose, Acacia Gum, Di-Calcium Phosphate, Microcrystalline Cellulose, Stearic Acid, Silica, Freeze-Dried Pineapple Fruit, Tangerine Fruit, Rose Hips (rosa canina).

Love Dust for Men **-** Susan Ambrosino's Herb Club, Inc.
Each capsule contains: Proprietary Blend 500 mg: Ginkgo 24/7 extract, Panax Ginseng 20% extract, Damiana 4:1 concentrate, Muira Puama 4:1 concentrate, Ginger, Wild Yam, Suma, L-Arginine.

Love Me Dew for Women **-** Susan Ambrosino's Herb Club, Inc.
Each capsule contains: Proprietary Blend 500 mg: Panax Ginseng 20% extract, Damiana 4:1 concentrate, Ginger, Wild Yam, Suma, L-Arginine.

Love-Berries **-** Nature's Plus
Each pill contains: Cranberry concentrate 45X 200 mg • Vitamin C corn free 60 mg. Sweetened with VitaSweet.

Loving You **-** Life Enhancement Products, Inc.
Medium Chain Triglycerides • Butylated Hydroxytoluene.

Low Carb CLEANSE I **-** Renew Life Formulas, Inc.
Vegetable Formula: Two capsules contain: Chlorella • Spirulina • Alfalfa juice powder • Barley grass and juice powder • Beet leaf, root and juice powder • Broccoli powder • Brussel Sprouts powder • Cabbage powder • Carrot powder • Garlic powder • Kale powder • Spinach powder. Other Ingredients: Hypromellose, Water.

Low Carb CLEANSE II **-** Renew Life Formulas, Inc.
Two capsules contain: Magnesium (as magnesium hydroxide) • Cape Aloe gel (aloes ferox) • Rhubarb root (rheum officinalis) • Slippery Elm bark (ulmas fulva) • Marshmallow root (althaea officinalis) • Fennel seed (foeniculum vulgare) • Ginger root (zingiber officinale) • Triphala blend: Indian Gooseberry fruit (phyllanthus emblica), Belleric Myrobalan fruit (terminalia bellerica), and Tropical Almond fruit (terminalia chebula). Other Ingredients: Hypromellose, Water.

Low Thyroid **-** Enzymes, Inc.
Each capsule contains: Proprietary Herbal Blend 390 mg: Bladderwrack kelp extract, Rice Bran, Coleus root extract, Ginger root extract, Black Currant seed extract • Proprietary Herbal Blend 115 mg: pHysioProtease, CereCalase. Other Ingredients: Plant Cellulose, Water.

LowCarb ENZYME **-** Renew Life Formulas, Inc.
Two capsules contain: Betaine HCl 650 mg • Plant Enzyme Blend 525 mg • Protease 200,000 HUT • Lipase 10,000LU.

Lowcarb OIL **-** Renew Life Formulas, Inc.
Three capsules contain: Vitamin E (as D-alpha tocopherol) 30 IU • Alpha Linolenic Acid (ALA) 495 mg • Eicosapentaenoic Acid (EPA) 162 mg • Docosahexaenoic Acid (DHA) 108 mg • Gamma Linolenic Acid (GLA) 180 mg • Linoleic Acid 468 mg • Oleic Acid 408 mg • Lipase 15 mg.

LPC **-** OSMO Therapy
Each capsule contains: Lysophosphatidyl Choline 300 mg.

LPC Serum **-** The Vitamin Factory
Each 1 oz serving contains: Pycnogenol • Vitamin C.

L-Phenylalanine 500 mg **-** Arrowroot
Each capsule contains: L-Phenylalanine 500 mg.

L-Phenylalanine 500 mg **-** Solgar
Each capsule contains: L-Phenylalanine 500 mg. Other Ingredients: Cellulose, Dicalcium Phosphate, Magnesium Stearate, Water.

L-Proline **-** J. R. Carlson Laboratories, Inc.
Each capsule contains: L-Proline 500 mg.

l-Proline **-** Pure Encapsulations
Each vegetable capsule contains: L-Proline (free- form) 750 mg • Vitamin C (as ascorbyl palmitate) 15 mg.

Some Brand Name Natural Products - What they Contain

www.NaturalDatabase.com contains MANY more listings than appear here.
Editor's Notes are located on pages 2155-2163.

L-Proline **-** J. R. Carlson Laboratories, Inc.
Each 1 tsp serving contains: L-Proline 3000 mg.

L-Proline 500 mg **-** Solgar
Each capsule contains: L-Proline 500 mg. Other Ingredients: Vegetable Cellulose, Vegetable Magnesium Stearate, Water, Vegetable Glycerin.

L-Proline/L-Lysine 500/500 mg **-** Solgar
Each tablet contains: L-Proline 500 mg • L-Lysine (as L-lysine HCl) 500 mg. Other Ingredients: Microcrystalline Cellulose, Vegetable Cellulose, Titanium Dioxide, Silica, Vegetable Magnesium Stearate, Vegetable Glycerin, Carnauba Wax.

L-Pyroglutamic Acid **-** Source Naturals
Each tablet contains: L-Pyroglutamic acid 1,000 mg.

L-Serine **-** J. R. Carlson Laboratories, Inc.
Each 1 tsp serving contains: L-Serine 2000 mg.

L-T **-** Pain & Stress Center
Each capsule contains: L-Theanine (Suntheanine brand) 100 mg • L-Glycine 180 mg • L-Glutamine 180 mg. Other Ingredients: Gelatin Capsule.

L-Taurine 500 mg **-** Pro Health
Each capsule contains: L-Taurine (free-form) 500 mg. Other Ingredients: Rice Flour, Gelatin.

L-Theanine **-** FoodScience of Vermont
Each capsule contains: L-Theanine (Suntheanine brand) 200 mg. Other Ingredients: Rice Flour, Vegetable Stearate, Gelatin, Water.

L-Theanine **-** PhysioLogics
Each capsule contains: L-Theanine 100 mg. Other Ingredients: Cellulose (plant origin), Dicalcium Phosphate, Gelatin, Vegetable Magnesium Stearate, Magnesium Silicate, Silica.

l-Theanine **-** Pure Encapsulations
Each vegetable capsule contains: L-Theanine 200 mg.

L-Theanine **-** PhytoPharmica
Each capsule contains: L-Theanine 100 mg. Other Ingredients: Cellulose, Gelatin, Magnesium Stearate, Titanium Dioxide Color.

L-Theanine Calm-Plex **-** Pro Health
Each capsule contains: L-Theanine 100 mg • GABA 275 mg • 5-HTP 10 mg. Other Ingredients: Stearic Acid, Silicon Dioxide, Cellulose, Gelatin.

L-Threonine **-** J. R. Carlson Laboratories, Inc.
Each 1 tsp serving contains: L-Threonine 2000 mg.

L-Threonine 500 mg **-** Solgar
Each capsule contains: L-Threonine 500 mg. Other Ingredients: Vegetable Cellulose, Vegetable Stearic Acid, Vegetable Magnesium Stearate, Water, Vegetable Glycerin.

l-Tyrosine **-** Pure Encapsulations
Each vegetable capsule contains: L-Tyrosine (free form) 800 mg.

L-Tyrosine **-** J. R. Carlson Laboratories, Inc.
Each capsule contains: L-Tyrosine 500 mg.

L-Tyrosine **-** J. R. Carlson Laboratories, Inc.
Each 1 tsp serving contains: L-Tyrosine 1700 mg.

L-Tyrosine **-** DaVinci Laboratories
Each capsule contains: L-Tyrosine 500 mg. Other Ingredients: Silicon Dioxide, Vegetable Stearate, Cellulose, Vegetable Cellulose.

L-Tyrosine **-** Ortho Molecular Products
Each capsule contains: L-Tyrosine USP 500 mg Other Ingredients: Natural Vegetable Capsules, Ascorbyl Palmitate, Magnesium Stearate, Microcrystalline Cellulose, Silicon Dioxide.

L-Tyrosine 500 **-** GNC
Each tablet contains: L-Tyrosine 500 mg. Other Ingredients: Cellulose, Acacia.

L-Tyrosine 500 **-** Jarrow Formulas
Each capsule contains: L-Tyrosine 500 mg. Other Ingredients: Rice Powder, Magnesium Stearate, Silicon Dioxide, Gelatin.

L-Tyrosine 500 mg **-** Solgar
Each capsule contains: L-Tyrosine 500 mg. Other Ingredients: Vegetable Cellulose, Microcrystalline Cellulose, Vegetable Magnesium Stearate, Vegetable Stearic Acid, Water, Vegetable Glycerin.

L-Tyrosine 500 mg **-** Nature's Plus
Each capsule contains: Vitamin B6 (pyridoxine HCl) 50 mg • L-Tyrosine (free form amino acid) 500 mg. Other Ingredients: Silica, Gelatin, Purified Water.

Lubriflex3 **-** Schiff
Two tablets contain: Glucosamine Hydrochloride 1500 mg • Hyaluronic Acid 3.3 mg • Proprietary Herbal Extract 250 mg: Chinese Skullcap root (scutellaria baicalensis), Black Catechu bark (acacia catechu). Other Ingredients: Cellulose, Hydroxypropyl Methylcellulose, Polydextrose, Triacetin, Titanium Dioxide, Polyethylene Glycol, Riboflavin, Stearic Acid, Copolyvidone, Magnesium Stearate, Silicon Dioxide.

Lukol **-** The Himalaya Drug Company
Each tablet contains: Dhataki (woodfordia fruticosa) 40 mg • Kokilaksha (hygrohila auriculata syn. asteracantha longifolia) 40 mg • Shatavari (asparagus racemosus) 40 mg • Sarpagandha (rauwolfia serpentina) 20 mg • Punarnava (boerhaavia diffusa) 10 mg • Vasaka (adhatoda zeylanica) 20 mg • Puga (areca catechu) 20 mg • Jatiphalam (myristica fragrans) 16 mg • Ela (elattaria cardamomum) 11 mg • Nagkesara (mesua ferrea) 11 mg • Jeeraka (cuminum cyminum) 10 mg • Chandana (santalum album) 10 mg • Bilva (aegle marmelos) 5 mg • Sunthi (zingiber officinale) 5 mg • Triphala 5 mg: Emblica Officinalis, Terminalia Chebula, Terminalia Bellirica • Maricha (piper nigrum) 5 mg • Hyamarka (wrightia tinctoria) 5 mg • Guggulu (commiphora wightii) 5 mg • Palasa (butea frondosa syn. b.monosperma) 4 mg • Shilajeet (mineral pitch, purified) 9 mg • Praval Bhasma (coral calx) 7 mg • Loh Bhasma (iron calx) 5 mg • Trivang 5 mg: Lead (naga), Tin (vanga), Zinc (yasada).

Lukol DS **-** The Himalaya Drug Company
Each tablet contains: Dhataki (woodfordia fruticosa) 80 mg • Kokilaksha (hygrophila auriculata syn. asteracantha longifolia) 80 mg • Shatavari (asparagus racemosus) 80 mg • Sarpagandha (rauwolfia serpentina) 40 mg • Punarnava (boerhaavia diffusa) 20 mg • Vasaka (adhatoda zeylanica) 20 mg • Puga (areca catechu) 40 mg • Jatiphalam (myristica fragrans) 32 mg • Ela (elattaria cardamomum) 22 mg • Nagkesara (mesua ferrea) 22 mg • Jeeraka (cuminum cyminum) 20 mg • Chandana (santalum album) 20 mg • Bilva (aegle marmelos) 10 mg • Sunthi (zingiber officinale) 10 mg • Triphala 10 mg: Emblica Officinalis, Terminalia Chebula, Terminalia Bellirica • Maricha (piper nigrum) 10 mg • Hyamaraka (wrightia tinctoria) 10 mg • Guggulu (commiphora wightii) 10 mg • Palasa (butea frondosa syn. b.monosperma) 8 mg • Shilajeet (mineral pitch, purified) 18 mg • Praval Bhasma (coral calx) 14 mg • Loh Bhasma (iron calx) 10 mg • Trivang 10 mg: Lead (naga), Tin (vanga), Zinc (yasada).

Lullaby Nighttime Formula **-** Starlight International
Each two tablets contain: Niacin (Niacinamide) 50 mg • Vitamin B6 (pyridoxine HCl) 20 mg • Calcium (as calcium lactate) 10 mg • Magnesium (as magnesium oxide) 114 mg • Kava Kava extract, 4:1 (piper methysticum, root) 200 mg • Valerian extract, 4:1 (valeriana officinalis, root) 150 mg • Lemon Balm (melissa officinalis, leaf) 150 mg • Passion Flower (passiflora incarnata, plant) 150 mg • Melatonin 5 mg. Inactive Ingredients: Dicalcium Phosphate, Microcrystalline Cellulose, Stearic Acid, Gum Acacia, Croscarmellose Sodium, Silicon Dioxide, Magnesium Stearate, Pharmaceutical Glaze, Ethylcellulose, Dextrin, Dextrose, Lecithin, Sodium Citrate.

Luna Chai Tea - Clif Bar Inc
Ingredients: Soy Protein Isolate • Rice Flour • Malt Extract • Rolled Oats • Roasted Soybean • Soy Flour • Milled Flaxseed • Brown Rice Syrup • Evaporated Cane Juice • Fractionated Palm Kernel Oil • Soy Flour • Soy Lecithin • Soy Milk • Green Tea Extract • Ground Ginger • Green Tea Leaves • Cloves • Anise • Cinnamon • Cardamom • Sea Salt • Natural Flavors.

Luna Cherry Covered Chocolate - Clif Bar Inc
Ingredients: Soy Protein Isolate • Rice Flour • Cocoa • Rolled Oats • Roasted Soybean • Milled Flaxseed • Brown Rice Syrup • Evaporated Cane Juice • Fractionated Palm Kernel Oil • Soy Flour • Soy Lecithin • Oat Flour • Beet Juice (for coloring) • Dried Plums • Cherries • Sea Salt • Natural Flavors.

Luna Chocolate Pecan Pie - Clif Bar Inc
Ingredients: Soy Protein Isolate • Rice Flour • Malt Extract • Rolled Oats • Roasted Soybean • Soy Flour • Milled Flaxseed • Brown Rice Syrup • Pecans • Sea Salt • Cinnamon • Evaporated Cane Juice • Fractionated Palm Kernel Oil • Decaffeinated Green Tea Extract • Cocoa • Soy Lecithin • Natural Flavors.

Luna Chocolate Peppermint Stick - Clif Bar Inc
Ingredients: Soy Protein Isolate • Rice Flour • Cocoa • Rolled Oats • Roasted Soybean • Milled Flaxseed • Brown Rice Syrup • Evaporated Cane Juice • Fractionated Palm Kernel Oil • Soy Flour • Soy Lecithin • Peppermint Oil • Oat Flour • Sea Salt • Natural Flavors • Red Cabbage extract (for coloring) • Sunflower Oil • Unsweetened Chocolate • Salt • Baking Soda.

Luna Key Lime Pie - Clif Bar Inc
Ingredients: Soy Protein Isolate • Rice Flour • Malt Extract • Rolled Oats • Soy Protein Isolate • Soybean • Soy Flour • Milled Flaxseed • Brown Rice Syrup • Evaporated Cane Juice • Fractionated Palm Kernel Oil • Oat Fiber • Oat Flour • Gum Arabic • Citric Acid • Soy Lecithin • Sea Salt • Green Tea Extract • Soy Milk • Natural Flavors • Freeze-dried Lime • Spinach Extract.

Luna LemonZest - Clif Bar Inc
Ingredients: Soy Protein Isolate • Rice Flour • Malt Extract • Rolled Oats • Roasted Soybean • Soy Flour • Milled Flaxseed • Brown Rice Syrup • Evaporated Cane Juice • Fractionated Palm Kernel Oil • Oat Fiber • Oat Flour • Gum Arabic • Citric Acid • Lemon Oil • Soy Lecithin • Soy Milk • Decaffeinated Green Tea Extract • Sea Salt • Natural Flavors.

Luna Nuts Over Chocolate - Clif Bar Inc
Ingredients: Soy Protein Isolate • Rice Flour • Malt Extract • Rolled Oats • Roasted Soybean • Soy Flour • Milled Flaxseed • Brown Rice Syrup • Evaporated Cane Juice • Fractionated Palm Kernel Oil • Peanut Flour • Peanut Butter • Cocoa • Soy Lecithin • Soy Milk • Decaffeinated Green Tea Extract • Sea Salt • Natural Flavors.

Luna Orange Bliss - Clif Bar Inc
Ingredients: Soy Protein Isolate • Rice Flour • Malt Extract • Rolled Oats • Soy Protein Isolate • Soybean • Soy Flour • Milled Flaxseed • Brown Rice Syrup • Evaporated Cane Juice • Fractionated Palm Kernel Oil • Oat Fiber • Oat Flour • Citric Acid • Gum Arabic • Soy Lecithin • Paprika Extract • Salt • Sea Salt • Green Tea Extract • Soy Milk • Natural Flavors • Annatto.

Luna Peanut Butter 'N Jelly - Clif Bar Inc
Ingredients: Soy Protein Isolate • Rice Flour • Malt Extract • Cocoa • Rolled Oats • Roasted Soybean • Milled Flaxseed • Brown Rice Syrup • Evaporated Cane Juice • Fractionated Palm Kernel Oil • Soy Flour • Soy Lecithin • Sunflower Oil • Oat Flour • Beet Juice (for coloring) • Strawberry Puree • Cranberries • Apple Juice • Blueberry Juice • Blueberry Extract • Peanut Butter • Peanut Flour • Glucose • Pectin • Citric Acid • Sea Salt • Natural Flavors.

Luna Sesame Raisin Crunch - Clif Bar Inc
Ingredients: Soy Protein Isolate • Rice Flour • Malt Extract • Rolled Oats • Roasted Soybean • Soy Flour • Milled Flaxseed • Brown Rice Syrup • Raisins • Toasted Sesame Seeds • Dry Roasted Sunflower Seeds • Decaffeinated Green Tea Extract • Sea Salt • Natural Flavors.

Luna S'mores - Clif Bar Inc
Ingredients: Soy Protein Isolate • Rice Flour • Malt Extract • Rolled Oats • Roasted Soybean • Soy Flour • Milled Flaxseed • Brown Rice Syrup • Evaporated Cane Juice • Fractionated Palm Kernel Oil • Soy Flour • Soy Lecithin • Oat Fiber • Oat Flour • Gum Arabic • Decaffeinated Green Tea Extract • Sea Salt • Natural Marshmallow & Graham Cracker Flavors • Citric Acid • Cocoa.

Luna Sweet Dreams - Clif Bar Inc
Ingredients: Soy Protein Isolate • Rice Flour • Cocoa • Rolled Oats • Roasted Soybean • Milled Flaxseed • Brown Rice Syrup • Evaporated Cane Juice • Fractionated Palm Kernel Oil • Soy Flour • Soy Lecithin • Peanuts • Defatted Peanut Flour • Sea Salt • Natural Flavors.

Luna Toasted Nuts 'N Cranberry - Clif Bar Inc
Ingredients: Soy Protein Isolate • Rice Flour • Malt Extract • Rolled Oats • Roasted Soybean • Soy Flour • Milled Flaxseed • Brown Rice Syrup • Cashews • Almonds • Pumpkin Seeds • Cranberries • Apple Juice • Decaffeinated Green Tea Extract • Natural Flavors.

Luna Tropical Crisp - Clif Bar Inc
Ingredients: Soy Protein Isolate • Rice Flour • Malt Extract • Rolled Oats • Roasted Soybean • Soy Flour • Milled Flaxseed • Brown Rice Syrup • Evaporated Cane Juice • Fractionated Palm Kernel Oil • Soy Flour • Soy Lecithin • Soy Milk • Toasted Coconut • Coconut Milk Powder • Dried Pineapple • Decaffeinated Green Tea Extract • Freeze-Dried Pineapple • Natural Flavors.

Lung Support - Nature's Sunshine
Three capsules contain: Proprietary Blend 1560 mg: Astragalus root (astragalus membranaceus), Aster root (aster tataricus), Qinjiao root (gentiana macrophylla), Platycodon root (platycodon grandiflorum), Anemarrhena rhizome (anemarrhena asphodeloides), Bupleurum root (bupleurum chinense), Dong Quai root (angelica polymorpha), Lycium bark (lycium chinense), Ophiopogon root tuber (ophiopogon japonicus), Panax Ginseng root, Atractylodes rhizome (atractylodes lancea), Blue Citrus peel (citrus reticulata), Citrus Aurantium peel, Typhonium rhizome (typhonium flagelliforme), Schizandra fruit (schisandra chinensis), Licorice root (glycyrrhiza uralensis). Other Ingredients: Gelatin, Water.
See Editor's Note No. 40.

Lung Support Formula - Gero Vita International
Astragalus membranaceus • Cordyceps sinensis • Ophiopogon japonicus.

Lung Tan Xie Gan pills - Kwangchow Pharmaceutical Industry Co.
Unknown.
See Editor's Note No. 46.

Lung Tonic - TriLight Herbs
Mullein • Wild Cherry bark • Chestnut • Astragalus root • Peppermint • Plantain • Chickweed • Pleurisy root • Elecampane • Horehound. Base: Glycerine, Distilled Purified Water.

Lung-Mend - The Herbalist
Elecampane root • Grindelia herb • Pleurisy root • Butterbur root • Marshmallow root • Usnea lichen • Yerba Santa leaf • Lobelia leaf • Yerba Mansa root.

Lungs - Enzymes, Inc.
Two capsules contain: Vitamin C (100% from Acerola Cherries) 17 mg • Proprietary Herbal Blend 490 mg: Mullein herb extract, Thyme herb extract, Sundew herb extract, Ginkgo Biloba leaf extract, Green Tea extract • Proprietary Enzyme Blend 440 mg: Amylase, pHysioProtease. Other Ingredients: Plant Cellulose, Water.

Luprinol - Klein-Becker
Two capsules contain: Ephedrine alkaloids from Ma Huang extract 20 mg • Caffeine (34 mg from standardized kola nut 280 mg) 200 mg • Acetylsalicylic acid 324 mg • DHEA 8.4 mg • Schizonepeta (spica) 250 mg. Other Ingredients: Rice Flour.
See Editor's Note No. 30.

BRAND NAMES

Lustre **-** Source Naturals
Six tablets contain: Vitamin A (Beta Carotene) 15000 IU • Vitamin A (Palmitate) 5000 IU • Vitamin B1 (Thiamin) 10 mg • Vitamin B2 (Riboflavin) 10 mg • Niacinamide 30 mg • Vitamin B5 (Calcium D-Pantothenate) 50 mg • Vitamin B6 (Pyridoxine HCl) 20 mg • Vitamin B12 (Cyanocobalamin) 30 mcg • Biotin 2000 mcg • Folic Acid 800 mcg • Vitamin C (Magnesium, Zinc and Manganese Ascorbates) 1000 mg • Vitamin E (D-Alpha Tocopheryl)(Natural) 200 IU • Copper (Sebacate) 1.5 mg • Magnesium (Ascorbate) 59 mg • Silica (Horsetail Silica Extract) 36 mg • Manganese (Ascorbate) 6 mg • Selenium (as L-Selenomethionine and Sodium Selenite) 200 mcg • L-Proline 600 mg • Inositol 500 mg • L-Cysteine (HCl) 400 mg • Choline (Bitartrate) 100 mg • L-Methionine 100 mg • N-Acetyl Cysteine 100 mg • PABA (Para Amino Benzoic Acid) 100 mg.

Lutein **-** Pure Encapsulations
Each softgel capsule contains: Lutein (from 100 mg marigold flower extract) 20 mg • Vitamin E (mixed tocopherols) 1 IU.

Lutein **-** Jarrow Formulas
Each softgel contains: Lutein (from 40 mg esters, tagetes erecta, marigold petal extract) 20 mg • Zeaxanthin (as esters, tagetes erecta, marigold petal extract) 1 mg. Other Ingredients: Soybean Oil, Beeswax, Gelatin, Glycerin, Water.

Lutein **-** NSI - Nutraceutical Sciences Institute
Each softgel contains: Lutein 20 mg.

Lutein **-** PhysioLogics
Each softgel contains: Lutein 20 mg. Other Ingredients: Corn Oil, Gelatin, Glycerin, Yellow Beeswax, Lecithin.

Lutein **-** Sundown
Each softgel contains: Lutein 6 mg • Healthy Eye Blend 2.3 mg: Bilberry fruit extract 4:1, Spinach leaf, Zeaxanthin. Other Ingredients: Rice Bran Oil, Gelatin, Glycerin, Corn Oil, Water.

Lutein & Bilberry Complex **-** PhysioLogics
Each capsule contains: Lutein (containing naturally occurring zeaxanthin) 6 mg • Bilberry fruit extract (vacciunum myrtillus, standardized to contain 25% anthocyanosides) 20 mg. Other Ingredients: Dicalcium Phosphate, Cellulose (plant origin), Gelatin, Vegetable Stearic Acid, Silica, Vegetable Magnesium Stearate.

Lutein & Zeaxanthin Complex **-** Vitamin World
Each softgel contains: Vitamin A (as beta carotene) 14,320 IU • Vitamin C (as ascorbic acid) 226 mg • Vitamin E (as DL-alpha tocopherol acetate) 200 IU • Zinc (as zinc oxide) 34.8 mg • Copper (as copper oxide) 0.8 mg • Lutein 4 mg • Zeaxanthin 172 mcg. Other Ingredients: Soybean Oil, Gelatin, Glycerin, Partially Hydrogenated Corn Oil, Corn Oil, Soy Lecithin, Titanium Dioxide Color, Yellow 6 Lake, Red 40 Lake, Blue 1 Lake.

Lutein 15 mg with Kale **-** J. R. Carlson Laboratories, Inc.
Each capsule contains: Lutein (FloraGlo brand, from marigolds) 15 mg • Zeaxanthin (FloraGlo brand, from marigold flowers) 900 mcg.

Lutein 20 **-** Pain & Stress Center
Each softgel contains: Lutein (from 40 mg esters, tagetes erecta) 20 mg • Zeaxanthin (as esters, tagetes erecta) 1 mg. Other Ingredients: Soybean Oil, Beeswax.

Lutein 20 mg **-** Allergy Research Group
Each softgel contains: Vitamin E (as mixed tocopherols) 1 IU • Lutein 20 mg • Zeaxanthin 900 mcg. Other Ingredients: Safflower Oil, Yellow Beeswax, Corn Oil.

Lutein 20 mg Natural Carotenoid **-** Nature's Bounty
Each softgel contains: Lutein 20 mg. Other Ingredients: Corn Oil, Gelatin, Glycerin, Yellow Beeswax, Lecithin.

Lutein 20 mg Natural Carotenoid **-** Puritan's Pride
Each softgel contains: Lutein 20 mg. Other Ingredients: Corn Oil, Gelatin, Glycerin, Yellow Beeswax, Lecithin.

Lutein 6 mg **-** J. R. Carlson Laboratories, Inc.
Each softgel contains: Vitamin E (as D-alpha tocopherol) 1 IU • Lutein (FloraGlo brand, from marigolds) 6 mg • Zeaxanthin (FloraGlo brand, from marigold flowers) 264 mg.

Lutein 6 mg Natural Carotenoid **-** Puritan's Pride
Each softgel contains: Lutein 6 mg. Other Ingredients: Corn Oil, Gelatin, Glycerin, Beeswax.

Lutein 6 mg Natural Carotenoid **-** Nature's Bounty
Each softgel contains: Lutein 6 mg. Other Ingredients: Corn Oil, Gelatin, Glycerin, Yellow Beeswax.

Lutein Carotenoid Complex **-** Solgar
Each capsule contains: Vitamin A (100% natural beta carotene) 2500 IU • Lutein (from marigold flower) 15 mg • Carotenoid Mix 29 mcg: Alpha Carotene, Lutein, Zeaxanthin, Cryptoxanthin. Other Ingredients: Vegetable Cellulose, Microcrystalline Cellulose, Vegetable Glycerin, Vegetable Magnesium Stearate, Annatto, Titanium Dioxide, Caramel, Carnauba Wax, Water.

Lutein i care **-** Nature's Life
Each capsule contains: Lutein (FloraGLO) [from Marigold petals (Tagetes erecta)] 5 mg • Beta Carotene [(Dunaliella salina) equivalent to 5000 IU Vitamin A] 3 mg • Other naturally occurring carotenoids in D. salina: Zeaxanthin (T. erecta, D. salina) 370 mcg • Alpha Carotene 106 mcg • Cryptoxanthin 20 mcg • Zinc (Gluconate) 5 mg • Copper (Gluconate) 2.5 mg.

Lutein Lycopene Carotene Complex **-** Solgar
Each capsule contains: Vitamin A (100% beta carotene from carrot oil and D. salina) 10,000 IU • Lutein (from marigold flower) 5 mg • Lycopene (from tomato) 5 mg • Alpha Carotene (from carrot and D. salina) 1.72 mg • Zeaxanthin (from marigold flower) 263 mcg • Phytoene (from lycopene) 134 mcg • Phytofluene (from lycopene) 45 mcg. Other Ingredients: Vegetable Cellulose, Microcrystalline Cellulose, Vegetable Magnesium Stearate, Titanium Dioxide, Vegetable Glycerin, Caramel, Grapeskin, Carnauba Wax, Water.

Lutein Plus **-** Puritan's Pride
Each capsule contains: Lutein (with 240-600 mcg Zeaxanthin) 6 mg • In a 330 mg base of: Spinach, Blueberry Powder and Bilberry extract.

Lutein Rx-Eye **-** Nature's Plus
Each capsule contains: Vitamin A (as beta carotene) 20,000 IU • Vitamin C (as ascorbic acid, ascorbyl palmitate) 500 mg • Vitamin E (as d-alpha tocopheryl succinate) 200 mg • Vitamin B2 (as riboflavin) 25 mg • Zinc (as monomethionine) 20 mg • Selenium (as amino acid complex) 50 mcg • Chromium (as polynicotinate) 120 mcg • Citrus Bioflavonoid Complex 125 mg • MSM (methylsulfonylmethane) 100 mg • Lutein (active carotenoid from marigold flower extract) 20 mg • Bilberry (vaccinium myrtillus fruit, standardized 25% [5 mg] anthocyanosides) 20 mg • L-Glutathione (free form amino acid) 5 mg • Zeaxanthin (from marigold flower extract) 876 mcg.

Lutein Z **-** Jamieson
Each capsule contains: Lutein and Zeaxanthin Complex (derived from Marigold flowers) 50 mg • CyanoSome 3 Botanical Complex 4600 mg: European Grape Seed 2500 mg, Ginkgo Biloba Leaf 2000 mg, Bilberry Fruit 100 mg, Green Tea Extract 2.5 mg.

Lutein-20 **-** DreamPharm
Each capsule contains: Lutein (5% powder containing zeaxanthin, extracted from marigold flower) 20 mg • Vitamin C 60 mg • Buckwheat powder 500 mg.

Lutein-6 **-** DreamPharm
Two capsules contain: Lutein (5% powder containing zeaxanthin, extracted from marigold flower) • Vitamin C 60 mg. Other Ingredients: Buckwheat Powder.

LVR Formula **-** Pure Encapsulations
Each vegetable capsule contains: Milk Thistle extract (silybum marianum, standardized to contain 80% silymarin) 100 mg • Artichoke (cynara scolymus, standardized to contain 3% caffeylquinic acids) extract 150 mg • Turmeric extract (curcuma

longa, standardized to contain 97% curcuminoids) 150 mg • Greater Celandine 4:1 extract (chelidonium majus) 100 mg • Barberry 6:1 extract (berberis vulgaris) 75 mg • Vitamin C (as ascorbyl palmitate) 12 mg.

Lycobeads brand - H. Reisman Corporation
Lycopene.
See Editor's Note No. 44.

Lyc-o-matic 15 mg - Natrol, Inc.
Each tablet contains: Calcium (as calcium carbonate) 46 mg • Lycopene (from natural tomato powder, tomato extract) 15 mg • Tomato powder 535 mg. Other Ingredients: Cellulose, Stearic Acid, Cellulose Gum, Silica, Magnesium Stearate.

LYC-O-MATO 15 mg Soft Gel Capsules (Olive oil) - Healthy Origins
Each softgel contains: Lyc-O-Mato 250 mg • Vitamin A (as natural beta-carotene) 333 IU • Vitamin E (as d-alpha tocopherol) 5.5 IU • Lycopene 15 mg • Phytoene 1 mg • Phytofluene 1 mg • Phytosterols 1 mg. Other Ingredients: Olive Oil, Gelatin, Glycerin, Purified Water, Annatto.

LYC-O-MATO 15 mg Soft Gel Capsules (Soybean oil) - Healthy Origins
Each softgel contains: Lyc-O-Mato 250 mg • Vitamin A (as natural beta-carotene) 333 IU • Vitamin E (as d-alpha tocopherol) 5.5 IU • Lycopene 15 mg • Phytoene 1 mg • Phytofluene 1 mg • Phytosterols 1 mg. Other Ingredients: Soybean Oil, Gelatin, Glycerin, Purified Water, Annatto.

LYC-O-MATO 5 mg Soft Gel Capsules (Soybean oil) - Healthy Origins
Each softgel contains: Lycopene 5 mg. Other Ingredients: Soybean Oil, Gelatin, Glycerin, Purified Water, Annatto.

Lyc-O-Mato brand - LycoRed Natural Products Industries, Ltd.
Tomato extract.
See Editor's Note No. 44.

LYC-O-MATO Clinical Trio (Olive oil) - Healthy Origins
Each softgel contains: Lyc-O-Mato 250 mg • Vitamin A (as natural beta-carotene) 333 IU • Vitamin E (as d-alpha tocopherol) 200 IU • Selenium 100 mcg • Lycopene 15 mg • Phytoene 1 mg • Phytofluene 1 mg • Phytosterols 1 mg. Other Ingredients: Gelatin, Glycerin, Olive Oil, Purified Water, Annatto.

LYC-O-MATO PLUS Seleno Excell Soft Gel Capsules - Healthy Origins
Each softgel contains: Lyc-O-Mato 250 mg • Vitamin A (as natural beta-carotene) 333 IU • Seleno Excell Selenium 100 mcg • Vitamin E (as d-alpha tocopherol) 5.5 IU • Lycopene 15 mg • Phytoene 1 mg • Phytofluene 1 mg • Phytosterols 1 mg. Other Ingredients: Soybean Oil, Gelatin, Glycerin, Purified Water, Annatto.

Lycopene - Nature's Way
Each softgel capsule contains: Tomato seed oil standardized to (Lycopene) 5000 mcg • Canola oil • Beeswax • Lecithin • natural Vitamin E (d-Alpha Tocopheryl).

Lycopene - NSI - Nutraceutical Sciences Institute
Each softgel contains: Lycopene 15 mg • Rice Bran oil 231 mg.

Lycopene - Olympian Labs
Two capsules contain: Tomato Lycopene 300 mg • Vegetable Enzymes (amylase, lipase, protease) 100 mg.

Lycopene - Nature's Life
Each capsule contains: Lycopene 6 mg • Carrot Carotenoids 2 mg providing: Beta Carotene (Vitamin A equivalent 2500 IU) 1500 mcg, Alpha Carotene (Vitamin A equivalent 417 IU) 500 mcg, Phytoene 39 mcg, Phytofluene 13 mcg.

Lycopene - Quest
Each capsule contains: Lyc-o-Mato brand Lycopene 5000 mcg. Other Ingredients: Rice Bran Oil, Sunflower Oil, Vegetable Stearin, Beeswax, Lecithin.

Lycopene - EcoNugenics
Each softgel contains: Lycopene 15 mg • Tomato Lipids 205 mg. Other Ingredients: Rice Bran Oil, Gelatin, Glycerin, Water, Triglycerides, Beeswax, Silica.

Lycopene - PhysioLogics
Each softgel contains: Lycopene 10 mg. Other Ingredients: Soybean Oil, Gelatin, Beeswax / Soybean Oil Mixture, Glycerin.

Lycopene 10 mg - Pure Encapsulations
Each softgel capsule contains: Lycopene 10 mg.

Lycopene 10 mg - Puritan's Pride
Each softgel contains: Lycopene 10 mg.

Lycopene 10 mg (from tomatoes) - J. R. Carlson Laboratories, Inc.
Each softgel contains: Lycopene 10 mg.

Lycopene 15mg - J. R. Carlson Laboratories, Inc.
Each softgel contains: Lycopene 15 mg.

Lycopene 20 mg - Pure Encapsulations
Each softgel capsule contains: Lycopene 20 mg.

Lycopene 5 mg - Pure Encapsulations
Each softgel capsule contains: Lycopene 5 mg.

Lycopene 5 mg - Puritan's Pride
Each softgel contains: Lycopene 5 mg.

Lycopene Carotenoid Complex - Solgar
Each capsule contains: Vitamin A (beta carotene) 2500 IU • Lycopene 15 mg • Carotenoid Mix 29 mcg: Alpha Carotene, Lutein, Zeaxanthin, Crytoxanthin. Other Ingredients: Microcrystalline Cellulose, Titanium Dioxide, Vegetable Magnesium Stearate, Vegetable Glycerin, Caramel, Grape Skin, Carnauba Wax, Water.

Lycopene Plus - Life Enhancement Products, Inc.
Each capsule contains: Lycopene (from tomato extract) 10 mg.

Lycopene Softgels - Optimum Nutrition
Each softgel contains: Lycopene 5 mg. Other Ingredients: Gelatin, Soybean Oil, Glycerine, Vegetable Oil, Yellow Beeswax.

Lycopene-Rich Tomato Concentrate - Jamieson
Each caplet contains: Organic Ripe Tomato Concentrate 100 mg • Lycopene Nutritional Factor 10 mg.

Lycoplex - Pain & Stress Center
Two softgels contain: Folic Acid 400 mcg • Zinc Aspartate, 20% 75 mg • Saw Palmetto extract 320 mg • Pumpkin seed oil 80 mg • Lycopene 7% 150 mg • Vegetable oil 671 mg • Beeswax 70 mg • Silica 30 mg. Other Ingredients: Gelatin Capsule, Glycerin, Water, Carob Extract, Titanium Dioxide.

Lyco-Sorb - Jarrow Formulas
Each softgel contains: Lycopene 10 mg • Phytoene 1 mg • Phytofluene 1 mg • Gamma Tocopherol 4 mg. Other Ingredients: Lecithin, Medium Chain Triglycerides (MCTs), Soybean Oil, Beeswax, Gelatin, Glycerin, Water, Carob.

Lycosoy - TwinLab
Two softgels contain: Vitamin D 400 IU • Vitamin E 200 IU • Selenium 200 mcg • Omega-3 Fish Oil conc. 460 mcg • Soy Bean extract 150 mg • Lycopene 5 mg • Green Tea leaf extract 2 mg.

Lymph - Enzymes, Inc.
Each capsule contains: Proprietary Herbal Blend 390 mg: Burdock root extract, Wild Indigo root extract, Cleavers herb extract, Yellow Dock root extract, Figwort herb powder • Proprietary Enzyme Blend 110 mg: pHysioProtease, Amylase, Lipase, CereCalase. Other Ingredients: Plant Cellulose, Water.

Lymphatone - The Herbalist
Echinacea root • Red root • Cleavers herb • Yellow Dock root • Burdock root • Wild Indigo root • Poke root.

Lympho-Clear - Enzymatic Therapy
Each capsule contains: Red Clover extract 4:1 (Trifolium pratense) 200 mg • Burdock root extract 4:1 (Arctium lappa) 200 mg • Oregon Grape root extract 6:1 (Berberis aquifolium) 100 mg • Licorice root extract (Glycyrrhiza glabra) standardized to contain 5% Glycyrrhizic Acid 50 mg • Goldenseal root extract (Hydrastis canadensis) standardized to contain 5% total Alkaloids including: Berberine, Hydrastine & Canadine 50 mg.

Lymphotend - American Biologics
Each drop contains: Xanthoxylum 0X • Sarsaparilla 6X • Phytolacca 0X • Sillinia 0X • Trifolium Prat. 0X • Lappa Arct. 0X • Amygdalus 0X • Cascara Sag. 0X • Berberis 0X • Glycyrrhiza 0X • Larre Diyaicata 0X. Other Ingredients: 20% Alcohol, Distilled Water.
See Editor's Note No. 1.

Lymph-Spleen Soluble Fractions - PhytoPharmica
Each capsule contains: Lymph-Spleen Complex (predigested soluble concentrate) 250 mg • Multi-Glandular Complex 100 mg: Raw Liver, Raw Lung, Raw Pancreas, Raw Heart, Raw Kidney, Raw Spleen & Raw Brain. All organs and glands derived from bovine sources except raw pancreas (porcine).
See Editor's Note No. 21 and No. 31.

Lypo - Enzymedica
Each capsule contains: Lactase 300 ALU • Lipase Thera-Blend 2000 FCCFIP • Amylase Thera-Blend 5500 DU • Protease Thera-Blend 20,000 HUT.

Lyprinol - Tyler Encapsulations
Two softgel capsules contain: Marine Lipid extract from Perna Canaliculus 100 mg. Other Ingredients: Olive Oil, D-Alpha Tocopherol, Gelatin, Sorbitol, Glycerin.

Lysine - Pain & Stress Center
Each capsule contains: Vitamin C (as ascorbyl palmitate) 6 mg • L-Lysine (L-lysine HCl 625 mg) 500 mg. Other Ingredients: Gelatin.

Lysine 500 mg - Vital Nutrients
Each capsule contains: L-Lysine 500 mg.

Lysozyme Plus - Atrium Biotechnologies
Each tablet contains: Pancreatin 200 mg • Papain 100 mg • Bromelain 75 mg • Rutin 60 mg • Trypsin 35 mg • Thymus 35 mg • Amylase 15 mg • Lipase 15 mg • Lysozyme 10 mg • Cellulase 2 mg • Zinc Gluconate 4 mg • a-Chymotrypsin 1 mg.
See Editor's Note No. 14.

M.C.H.C. Capsules - Progressive Labs
Each capsule contains: Calcium 250 mg, from 500 mg M.C.H.C. 125 mg, from 500 mg Calcium Citrate 125 mg • Iron (from M.C.H.C.) 0.3 mg • Vitamin K 20 mcg • Phosphorus (from M.C.H.C) 65 mg • Magnesium (from M.C.H.C.) 4 mg • Zinc (from M.C.H.C.) 0.075 mg • Copper (from M.C.H.C.) 0.01 mg • Manganese (from M.C.H.C.) 0.045 mg • Potassium (from M.C.H.C.) 0.035 mg • Protein (from M.C.H.C. as collagen glycosaminoglycans) 125 mg • Boron (as boron aspartate) 0.75 mg • Fluorapatite (from M.C.H.C.) 31 mcg • Silicon (from M.C.H.C.) 19 mcg • Strontium (from M.C.H.C.) 10 mcg.

M.C.H.C. Tablets - Progressive Labs
Each tablet contains: Calcium (elemental) 250 mg, from 500 mg M.C.H.C. 125 mg, from 500 mg. Calcium Citrate 125 mg • Iron (from M.C.H.C.) 0.3 mg • Vitamin K 20 mcg • Phosphorum (from M.C.H.C.) 65 mg • Magnesium (from M.C.H.C.) 4 mg • Zinc (from M.C.H.C.) 0.075 mg • Copper (from M.C.H.C.) 0.01 mg • Manganese (from M.C.H.C.) 0.045 mg • Potassium (from M.C.H.C.) 0.035 mg • Protein (from M.C.H.C. as collagen glycosaminoglycans) 125 mg • Boron (as aspartate) 750 mcg • Fluorapatite (from M.C.H.C.) 31 mcg • Silicon (from M.C.H.C.) 19 mcg • Strontium (from M.C.H.C.) 10 mcg.

M.V. Teen - Futurebiotics LLC
100% or more of the USRDA for 16 vitamins and minerals, 100 mcg of chromium and selenium.

M/R/S Mushroom Formula - Pure Encapsulations
Each vegetable capsule contains: Shiitake mushroom extract (lentinus edodes, standardized to contain 6% polysaccharides) 250 mg • Reishi mushroom extract (ganoderma lucidum, standardized to contain 10% polysaccharides and 4% triterpenes) 250 mg • Maitake mushroom 4:1 extract (grifola frondosa) 250 mg • Vitamin C (as ascorbyl palmitate) 8 mg.

M1T - Higher Power
Each capsule contains: Methyl-1-Testosterone 5 mg. Other Ingredients: Maltodextrin, Magnesium Stearate, Gelatin.

MA II Juice Enhancer - Alacer
Two measurefuls (1.5 g) contain: Vitamin C (as ascorbates) 2000 mg • Potassium (citrate, aspartate, ascorbate) 80 mg • Calcium (ascorbate) 70 mg • Magnesium (ascorbate, citrate) 70 mg • Zinc (ascorbate) 10 mg • Manganese (ascorbate) 2 mg • Molybdenum (ascorbate) 100 mcg • Chromium (ascorbate, niacinate) 100 mcg • Quercetin 25 mg • Natural Lime flavor. Other Ingredients: Acacia Gum, Magnesium Stearate, Vegetable Stearic Acid, Cellulose, Psyllium Husks, Parsley Seed, Silicon Dioxide, Chlorophyll, Titanium Dioxide, Polyethylene Glycol.

MA III Juice Enhancer - Alacer
Two measurefuls (1.5 g) contain: Vitamin C (as ascorbates) 2000 mg • Potassium (citrate, aspartate, ascorbate) 80 mg • Calcium (ascorbate) 70 mg • Magnesium (ascorbate, citrate) 70 mg • Zinc (ascorbate) 10 mg • Manganese (ascorbate) 2 mg • Molybdenum (ascorbate) 100 mcg • Chromium (ascorbate, niacinate) 100 mcg • Quercetin 25 mg • Mixed Bioflavonoids 25 mg • Vitamin B1 (thiamine HCl) 1.5 mg • Vitamin B2 (riboflavin) 1.7 mg • Vitamin B3 (as niacinates of potassium, calcium, magnesium, zinc, manganese, molybdenum, chromium) 20 mg • Vitamin B6 (pyridoxine HCl) 10 mg • Vitamin B12 (cyanocobalamin) 6 mcg • Vitamin E (tocopheryl acetate) 15 IU • Pantothenic Acid 10 mg • MSM (methylsulfonyl methane) 20 mg • D-Biotin 300 mcg • Folic Acid 400 mcg • Beta Carotene Complex (from D. salina) 5000 IU • Selenium (L-selenomethionine) 100 mcg • Iodine (potassium iodide) 25 mcg • Ginkgo Biloba extract • Grape seed extract. Other Ingredients: Acacia Gum, Magnesium Stearate, Vegetable Stearic Acid, Cellulose, Psyllium Husks, Parsley Seed, Silicon Dioxide, Chlorophyll, Titanium Dioxide, Polyethylene Glycol.

Maalox Max Maximum Strength plus Antigas - Novartis
Each tablet contains: Calcium Carbonate 1000 mg • Simethicone 60 mg. Other Ingredients: Acesulfame K, Colloidal Silicon Dioxide, Croscarmellose Sodium, D&C Red #30 Lake, D&C Yellow #10 Aluminum Lake, Dextrose, FD&C Red #40 Aluminum Lake, FD&C Yellow #6 Aluminum Lake, Flavors, Magnesium Stearate, Maltodextrin, Mannitol, Pregelatinized Starch.

Maca - Source Naturals
Three tablets contain: Maca root extract (MacaPure) (Lepidium meyenii) Standardized to 0.6% macamides and macaenes yielding 4.5 mg macamides and macaenes 750 mg.

Maca - NutraMedix
Two capsules contain: Maca root (lepidium meyenii) 1 g. Other Ingredients: Gelatin Capsule, Magnesium Stearate.

MACA Capsules - Golden Glow Natural Health Products
Each tablet contains: 100% pure Maca (lipidium peruvianum) 500 mg.

Maca Standardized - NutraMedix
Two capsules contain: Maca root (lepidium meyenii, 0.5% total glucosinolates) 5 mg. Other Ingredients: Gelatin Capsule, Magnesium Stearate.

Some Brand Name Natural Products - What they Contain

www.NaturalDatabase.com contains MANY more listings than appear here.

Editor's Notes are located on pages 2155-2163.

Macerat Drainer Elixir - PhytoPharma
Aqueous extracts blend: Anis seeds, Bardane root, Birch leaves, Black Currant leaves, Black Radish, Cherry stems, Commen, Dandelion roots and leaves, Fennel seeds, Fumitory, Green Tea, Heather, Mint, Nettle, Parsley, Sage, Watercress.

Macerat Purgative Elixir - PhytoPharma
Aqueous extracts blend: Artichoke, Black Radish, Camu Cane, Cardamon, Celery, Chrysantellum Indicum, Muscade.

MacroForce Plus C - ImmuDyne, Inc.
Each capsule contains: Vitamin C (as Calcium Ascorbate) 394 mg • Calcium (as Calcium Carbonate) 44 mg • Beta-1,3-D-glucan (from cell walls of yeast, Saccharomyces cerevisiae) 7.5 mg.

Macro-Min - Atrium Biotechnologies
Each tablet contains: Calcium Aspartate 600 mg • Magnesium Gluconate 300 mg • Potassium Aspartate 88.3 mg • Manganese Aspartate 50 mg • Vitamin D (as Vitamin D3) 250 IU.

Macro-Mineral Complex - Advocare International
Two caplets contain: Calcium (as citrate and hydroxyapatite) 220 mg • Magnesium (amino acid chelate and ascorbate) 200 mg • Vitamin D (ergocalciferol) 40 IU • Vitamin C (magnesium ascorbate) 60 mg • Pyridoxine (as HCl) 3 mg • Manganese (amino acid chelate) 1 mg • Zinc (monomethionine, OptiZinc brand) 2 mg • Copper (amino acid chelate) 200 mcg • Silicon (amino acid chelate) 300 mcg • Boron (as amino acid chelate) 200 mcg • Potassium Bicarbonate 500 mg • Shave Grass herb extract (equisetum arvense) 50 mg • Green Tea leaf extract (camellia sinensis) 50 mg • Ginger root extract (zingiber officinale) 25 mg. Other Ingredients: Dicalcium Phosphate, Silicon Dioxide, Cellulose, Stearic Acid, Magnesium Stearate.

Macu Care - PhysioLogics
Each capsule contains: Taurine 200 mg • Calendula flower (calendula officinalis, 5% lutein, 3 mg, 0.22% zeaxanthin, 132 mcg) 60 mg • Alpha Lipoic Acid 25 mg • Mixed Xanthophylis (from calendula flower) 2 mg. Other Ingredients: Rice Powder, Gelatin, Vegetable Magnesium Stearate, Silica.

Macula Support Drops - Natural Ophthalmics
Active Ingredients: Calcarea Fluorica HPUS 10x • Calcarea Phosphorica HPUS 10x • Kali Phosphoricum HPUS 6x • Natrum Muriaticum HPUS 6x • Carboneum Sulphuratum HPUS 6x. Inactive Ingredients: Sterile Water, Sodium Chloride, Sodium Citrate, Citrate, Polysorbate 80.

Macular Support Formula - Pure Encapsulations
Two vegetable capsules contain: N-Acetyl-L-Cysteine (free-form) 250 mg • Reduced Glutathione (free-form) 50 mg • Bilberry extract (vaccinium myrtillus, standardized to contain 25% anthocyanosides) 80 mg • Grape seed extract (vitis vinifera, standardized to 92% oligomeric proanthocyanidins) 50 mg • FloraGLO brand Lutein (from 120 mg of marigold flower extract) 6 mg • Betatene brand Mixed Carotenoids 25,000 IU: Beta Carotene 14280 mcg, Alpha Carotene 450 mcg • Zeaxanthin 90 mcg, Cryptoxanthin 110 mcg, Lutein 70 mcg • Vitamin C (as ascorbic acid) 800 mg • Vitamin C (as ascorbyl palmitate) 100 mg.

MaculaRx Plus - ScienceBased Health
Two capsules contain: Vitamin A (50% from retinyl palmitate and 50% from beta carotene) 2500 IU • Vitamin C (from ascorbic acid) 250 mg • Vitamin E (as d-alpha tocopheryl succinate) 200 IU • Zinc (from zinc ascorbate) 40 mg • Selenium (from selenium amino acid chelate) 35 mcg • Copper (from copper gluconate) 1 mg • Other Carotenoids (Xanthophylls) 7.875 mg • Lutein 7.5 mg • Zeaxanthin 375 mcg. Other Ingredients: Gelatin, Water, Rice Flour.

MacuVision - Health Smart Vitamins
Two capsules contain: Taurine 400 mg • Calendula (5% Lutein, 6 mg; >0.22% Zeaxanthin, 264 mcg) 120 mg • Alpha-Lipoic Acid 50 mg.

Mag Chlor 85 - Pain & Stress Center
Twenty-five drops contain: Magnesium (as magnesium chloride) 85 mg • Chloride 245 mg. Other Ingredients: Demineralized Water.

Mag Citrate - Metagenics
Two tablets contain: Magnesium (as magnesium citrate) 200 mg • Calcium (as calcium citrate) 40 mg.

Mag Glycinate - Metagenics
Two tablets contain: Magnesium (as magnesium bis-glycinate) 200 mg.

Mag Link - Pain & Stress Center
Two tablets contain: Calcium (Calcium Carbonate) 225 mg • Magnesium (Magnesium Chloride Hexahydrate) 130 mg • Chloride 375 mg.

Mag-Ascorbs - Alacer
Two tablets contain: Vitamin C (as calcium and magnesium ascorbate) 940 mg • Magnesium (magnesium ascorbate) 60 mg • Vitamin B6 (pyridoxine HCl) 4 mg • Mixed Bioflavonoids 100 mg.

Magic Cigarettes - Alternative Cigarettes Inc
Each cigarette contains: Marshmallow • Yerba Santa • Damiana • Passion Flower • Jasmine • Ginseng. Regular and menthol are available.
See Editor's Note No. 6.

Magma Plus - Green Foods Corp.
Each 5.3 oz jar contains: Proprietary Blend 150 g: Young Barley Grass powdered juice, Carrot, Wheat Grass, Alfalfa, Lettuce, Cabbage, Daikon Radish, Bean Sprouts, Celery, Tomato, Spinach, Kale, Maltodextrin, Lecithin, Honey, Bee Pollen, Royal Jelly, Apple, Banana, Pineapple, Papaya, Mango, Raspberry, Chicory root extract, Wheat Germ extract, L. Bifidus, L. Acidophilus, L. Planatarum, Spirulina, Chlorella, Licorice root extract, Coix extract, Vitamin E, Acerola extract, Brown Rice, Red Beet extract, Milk Thistle extract, Echinacea Purpurea extract, Siberian Ginseng extract, American Ginseng extract, Astragalus extract, Aloe Vera, Green Tea extract, Ginger root extract, Stevia extract, Reishi Mushroom extract, Cayenne Pepper, Garlic, Cat's Claw extract, Yucca root extract, Ginkgo Biloba extract, Garcinia Cambogia extract, Glucomannan, Bilberry extract, Grape Seed extract, Lipase, Amylase, Protease.

MagmaSLIM - Green Foods Corp.
Four capsules contain: Super Citrimax brand Garcinia Cambogia (hydroxycitric acid) 535 mg • Clarinol brand CLA (conjugated linoleic acid) 535 mg • Green Magma: Barley Grass juice, Maltodextrin 235 mg • Green Tea extract (camellia sinensis) 214 mg.

Magna Pac Daily Basics - Swanson Health Products
Each packet (three softgels, five tablets) contains: Vitamin A (as beta-carotene) 25000 IU • Vitamin C USP (as ascorbic acid) 1 g • Vitamin D (from fish liver oil) 400 IU •Vitamin E (as d-alpha tocopheryl acetate) 400 IU • Thiamin (as thiamin HCl; vitamin B-1) 50 mg • Riboflavin (vitamin B-2) 50 mg • Niacin (as niacinamide) 50 mg • Vitamin B-6 (as pyridoxine HCl) 50 mg • Folic Acid USP 40 mcg • Vitamin B-12 (as Cyanocobalamin) 50 mcg • Biotin USP 50 mcg • Pantothenic Acid (as d-calcium pantothenate) 50 mg • Calcium (500 mg from oyster shell, 500 mg from carbonate, aspartate, citrate) 1 g • Iron (from Albion amino acid chelate) 18 mg • Iodine (from kelp) 150 mcg • Magnesium (from magnesium oxide) 250 mg • Zinc 50 mg • Selenium (from selenomethionine) 50 mcg • Copper 2 mg • Manganese 10 mg • Chromium 50 mcg •Potassium (from potassium proteinate) 99 mg • Lecithin 1.2 g • 72 Trace Mineral compound 72 mg • Betaine HCl 50 mg • Choline (as choline bitartrate) 50 mg • Inositol FCC 50 mg • PABA (para-aminobenzoic acid) 50 mg • Rose Hips (from concentrate) 50 mg.

Magna Pac for Cardio - Swanson Health Products
Each packet (four capsules, three softgels) contains: Vitamin E (D-alpha tocopherol from mixed tocopherols) 400 IU • Thiamin (as thiamin HCl; vitamin B-1) 100 mg • Riboflavin (vitamin B-2) 100 mg • Niacinamide USP 100 mg • Vitamin B-6 USP (as pyridoxine HCl) 100 mg • Folic Acid 400 mcg • Vitamin B-12 USP (as cyanocobalamin) 100 mcg • Biotin USP 100 mcg • Pantothenic Acid (as d-calcium pantothenate) 100 mg • Flaxseed Oil 1 g • Trimethylglycine (as betaine anhydrous) 1 g • Standardized Hawthorn berry extract (1.8% vitexin-2' rhamnosides) 250 mg • Hawthorn berry

powder 250 mg • Choline (as choline bitartrate) 100 mg • Inositol 100 mg • PABA (para-aminobenzoic acid) 100 mg • Coenzyme Q10 30 mg • Garlic (500:1 concentrate equal to 500 mg of fresh garlic) 1 mg.

Magna Pac for Joints - Swanson Health Products
Each packet (seven capsules, one softgel) contains: Manganese (Albion amino acid chelate) 40 mg • Glucosamine Sulfate (2KCl) 1.5 g • Borage Oil (24% GLA) 1 g • Chondroitin Sulfate 1 g • OptiMSM (methylsulfonylmethane) 1 g • Boswellia Serrata powder 300 mg • Boswellia Serrata (65% boswellic acid) 200 mg • Optimum Abzorption Complex Proprietary Blend: Ginger (root), Piper longum, Piper nigrum 45 mg.
See Editor's Note No. 15.

Magna Pac for Menopause - Swanson Health Products
Each packet (six capsules, two softgels) contains: Vitamin C (ascorbic acid) 1 g • Vitamin E (as d-alpha tocopherol from mixed tocopherols) 400 IU • Borage Oil (24% GLA) 1 g • Black Cohosh powder 860 mg • SoyLife Soy extract (3% soy isoflavones) 750 mg • Dong Quai herb powder 300 mg • Licorice root extract (15% glycyrrhizic acid) 300 mg • Dong Quai extract (1% ligustilides) 200 mg • Licorice root powder 170 mg • Rose Hips (from concentrate) 60 mg • Black Cohosh (5% triterpene glycosides calculated as 27-deoxyactein) 40 mg.

Magna Pac for Prostate - Swanson Health Products
Each packet (five capsules, one tablet) contains: Vitamin E (D-alpha tocopherol from mixed tocopherols) 400 IU • Zinc (from zinc gluconate) 50 mg • Selenium (L-selenomethionine) 50 mcg • Pumpkin Seed oil 1 g • Saw Palmetto (25% fatty acids) 1 g • Pygeum powder 400 mg • Beta Sitosterol (Cholestatin) 120 mg • Pygeum extract (6.5% phytosterols) 100 mg • Lycopene (Lyc-O-Mato) 5 mg.

Magna Rx+ - NEP Products
Each tablet contains: Pygeum Africanum bark 250 mg • Maca root (lepidium meyenii) 125 mg • Horny Goat Weed (epimedium sagittatum) 75 mg • Oat Straw 75 mg • Catuaba 50 mg • Oriental Ginseng root 50 mg • L-Arginine 50 mg • Stinging Nettle leaf 37.5 mg • Cayenne fruit 25 mg • Muira Puama whole herb 25 mg • Orchic substance 25 mg • Oyster extract 25 mg • Tribulus Terrestris L (aerial parts) 25 mg • Smilax Officinalis root 12.5 mg • Astragalus root 10 mg • Licorice root 10 mg • Pumpkin seed 10 mg • Boron (as boron citrate) 1 mg.

MagnaCal - Holista
Each capsule contains: Calcium from citrate (equivalent to 625 mg) 125 mg • Magnesium from oxide (equivalent to 206 mg) 125 mg • Vitamin D (as Vitamin D3) 100 IU.

MagneBind 200 - Nephro-Tech, Inc.
Each tablet contains: Magnesium Carbonate (57 mg elemental) 200 mg • Calcium Carbonate (160 mg elemental) 400 mg.

MagneBind 300 - Nephro-Tech, Inc.
Each tablet contains: Magnesium Carbonate (85 mg elemental) 300 mg • Calcium Carbonate (100 mg elemental) 250 mg.

MagneBind 400 Rx - Nephro-Tech, Inc.
Each tablet contains: Magnesium Carbonate (114 mg elemental) 400 mg • Calcium Carbonate (80 mg elemental) 200 mg • Folic Acid 1 mg.

Magnesium - J. R. Carlson Laboratories, Inc.
Each capsule contains: Magnesium (as magnesium oxide) 350 mg.

Magnesium - Source Naturals
Each tablet contains: Magnesium (from 500 mg of magnesium amino acid chelate) 100 mg.

Magnesium - DaVinci Laboratories
Each capsule contains: Magnesium (as magnesium citrate) 140 mg. Other Ingredients: Rice Flour, Vegetable Stearate, Vegetable Cellulose.

Magnesium - Eidon Inc.
Each 1 tbsp serving contains: Magnesium (providing approx. 553 ppm magnesium) 8 mg. Other Ingredients: Purified Water.

Magnesium - PhysioLogics
Each caplet contains: Magnesium (as magnesium oxide) 250 mg. Other Ingredients: Dicalcium Phosphate, Cellulose (plant origin), Starch, Magnesium Silicate, Cellulose Coating, Vegetable Magnesium Stearate.

Magnesium (aspartate) - Pure Encapsulations
Each vegetable capsule contains: Magnesium (aspartate) 75 mg • Vitamin C (as ascorbyl palmitate) 9 mg.

Magnesium (citrate) - Pure Encapsulations
Each vegetable capsule contains: Magnesium (citrate) 150 mg • Vitamin C (as ascorbyl palmitate) 11 mg.

Magnesium (citrate) 150 mg - Vital Nutrients
Each capsule contains: Magnesium (citrate) 150 mg.

Magnesium (citrate/malate) - Pure Encapsulations
Each vegetable capsule contains: Magnesium (citrate/malate) 120 mg • Vitamin C (as ascorbyl palmitate) 10 mg.

Magnesium (glycinate) - Pure Encapsulations
Each vegetable capsule contains: Magnesium (glycinate) 120 mg • Vitamin C (as ascorbyl palmitate) 10 mg.

Magnesium (glycinate) 120 mg - Vital Nutrients
Each capsule contains: Magnesium (glycinate) 120 mg.

Magnesium 100 mg - Jamieson
Each tablet contains: Magnesium 100 mg.

Magnesium 100mg - Sundown
Four caplets contain: Magnesium (as magnesium oxide, magnesium gluconate) 400 mg. Other Ingredients: Microcrystalline Cellulose, Crospovidone, Silica, Lactose, Hydroxypropyl Methyl-Cellulose, Titanium Dioxide (color), Magnesium Stearate, Triacetin, Stearic Acid.

Magnesium 200 mg - Nature's Plus
Each tablet contains: Magnesium (as amino acid chelate) 200 mg. Other Ingredients: Di-calcium Phosphate, Stearic Acid, Microcrystalline Cellulose, Magnesium Stearate, Pharmaceutical Glaze, Silica.

Magnesium 250 - GNC
Each tablet contains: Magnesium (as magnesium oxide and magnesium gluconate) 250 mg. Other Ingredients: Dicalcium Phosphate, Cellulose.

Magnesium 250 mg - Nature Made
Each tablet contains: Magnesium (from magnesium oxide) 250 mg. Other Ingredients: Cellulose Gel, Croscarmellose Sodium, Magnesium Stearate.
See Editor's Note No. 45.

Magnesium 250 mg - Sunmark
Each tablet contains: Magnesium (oxide) 250 mg. Other Ingredients: Calcium Carbonate, Microcrystalline Cellulose, Modified Cellulose Gum, Stearic Acid, Citric Acid, Magnesium Stearate, Talc, Sodium Lauryl Sulfate.
See Editor's Note No. 45.

Magnesium 50 mg - Jamieson
Each tablet contains: Magnesium 50 mg.

Magnesium 500 - GNC
Each capsule contains: Magnesium (as magnesium oxide) 500 mg. Other Ingredients: Gelatin.

Magnesium 500 mg - Puritan's Pride
Each tablet contains: Magnesium (as magnesium oxide) 500 mg. Other Ingredients: Cellulose (plant origin), Starch, Magnesium Silicate, Cellulose Coating, Titanium Dioxide Color, Vegetable Magnesium Stearate.

Some Brand Name Natural Products - What they Contain

www.NaturalDatabase.com contains MANY more listings than appear here.
Editor's Notes are located on pages 2155-2163.

Magnesium Aspartate - Life Enhancement Products, Inc.
Each capsule contains: Magnesium (as magnesium aspartate) 100 mg.

Magnesium Aspartate 667 mg - American Biologics
Each tablet contains: Magnesium Aspartate 667 mg. Other Ingredients: Dicalcium Phosphate, Cellulose, Magnesium Stearate.

Magnesium Caps - TwinLab
Each hard gelatin capsule contains: Elemental Magnesium (from magnesium oxide and magnesium aspartate) 400 mg.

Magnesium Chelate - Golden Glow Natural Health Products
Each tablet contains: Magnesium Amino-Acid Chelate 500 mg: Magnesium 100 mg.

Magnesium Chelate - PhysioLogics
Each caplet contains: Calcium (as dicalcium phosphate, calcium stearate) 15 mg • Magnesium (as magnesium glycinate, magnesium oxide) 200 mg. Other Ingredients: Cellulose (plant origin), Crocarmellose, Silica, Vegetable Stearic Acid, Cellulose Coating.

Magnesium Citrate - Solgar
Two tablets contain: Magnesium (as mangesium citrate) 400 mg. Other Ingredients: Microcrystalline Cellulose, Vegetable Cellulose, Dicalcium Phosphate, Silica, Vegetable Magnesium Stearate, Vegetable Glycerin, Carnauba Wax.

Magnesium Complex - Klaire Laboratories
Each capsule contains: Magnesium Glycinate (Amino Acid Chelate) 100 mg.

Magnesium hGH Release - For Youthful Health
Each packet contains: Maximum hGH Release Amino Acid Blend 7300 mg: L-Glutamine, Lysine Monohydrochloride, L-Arginine, Gamma Aminobutyric Acid (GABA), Glutamine peptides, L-Tyrosine. Maximum hGH Release Glycoamino Acid-Glucose Complex 4950 mg • Maximum hGH Release Secretagogue Proprietary Blend 3100 mg: Alpha Lipoic Acid (ALA), Glycine, Acetyl L-Carnitine Hydrochloride, Alpha-Glycerylphosphorylcholine.

Magnesium Lactate - Standard Process, Inc.
Three capsules contain: Magnesium 210 mg • Soy bean 310 mg. Other Ingredients: Gelatin, Calcium Stearate, Water, Colors.

Magnesium Malate - Source Naturals
Each tablet contains: Magnesium Malate 1000mg • Malic Acid 825 mg • Magnesium 152 mg.

Magnesium Multi-Min - Nutri-Quest Rx
Each tablet contains: As an Aspartic Acid Chelate (amino acid Chelate): Phosphorus 10 mg • Calcium 100 mg • Magnesium 500 mg • Iron 5 mg • Potassium 200 mg • Zinc 30 mg • Copper 250 mcg • Manganese 30 mg • Chromium 500 mcg • Molybdenum 10 mcg • Selenium 25 mcg • Vanadium 60 mcg • Silicon 0.33 mcg • Lithium 0.05 mcg.

Magnesium Optimizer - Jarrow Formulas
Each tablet contains: Magnesium (as citrate) 100 mg • Potassium (as chloride) 49.5 mg • Taurine 350 mg. Other Ingredients: Cellulose, Dicalcium Phosphate, Stearic Acid, Modified Cellulose Gum, Magnesium Stearate.

Magnesium Plus - Pro Health
Each tablet contains: Magnesium (as magnesium amino acid chelate) 200 mg. Other Ingredients: Cellulose, Vegetable Stearine, Silica, Magnesium Stearate.

Magnesium Potassium Aspartate - Pro Health
Each tablet contains: Magnesium (as magnesium aspartate complex) 100 mg • Potassium (as potassium aspartate complex) 99 mg. Other Ingredients: Cellulose, Stearic Acid, Modified Cellulose Gum, Methylcellulose, Magnesium Stearate, Silica.

Magnesium With Vitamin B6 - Solgar
Three tablets contain: Vitamin B6 (as pyridoxine HCl) 25 mg • Calcium (as dicalcium phosphate) 230 mg • Magnesium (as magnesium oxide) 400 mg • Sodium 5 mg. Other Ingredients: Dicalcium Phosphate, Microcrystalline Cellulose, Vegetable Cellulose, Vegetable Stearic Acid, Vegetable Magnesium Stearate.

Magnesium-Potassium Aspartate - The Vitamin Shoppe
Magnesium 100 mg • Potassium 100 mg.

Maharishi Amrit Kalash Ambrosia - Maharishi Ayurveda Products
Meda Milkweed • Black Musale • Heart-Leaved Moonseed • East Indian Globe Thistle • Butterfly Pea • Licorice • Vanda Orchid • Elephant Creeper • Indian Wild Pepper.

Maharishi Amrit Kalash Nectar - Maharishi Ayurveda Products
Whole Cane Sugar • Indian Gooseberry • Indian Gallnut • Ghee • Honey • Cardamom • Cinnamon • Dried Catkins • Indian Pennywort • Cyperus • Nutgrass • White Sandalwood • Aloeweed • Butterfly Pea • Shoe Flower • Licorice • Turmeric. Processed in the aqueous extract of: Castor root • Country Mallow • Thatch Grass • Eragrostis cynosuroides • Sugar Cane • Indian Asparagus • Spreading Hogweed • Giant Potato • Winter Cherry • Indian Kudju • Trumpet flower • Premna Integrifolia • Desmodium gangeticum • Uraria picta • Yellow-berried Night Shade • Small Caltrops • Phaseolus trilobus • Teramnus labialis • Bengal Quince • Cashmere bark.
See Editor's Note No. 39.

Maharishi Amrit Kalash Sugar-Free Nectar - Maharishi Ayurveda Products
Indian Gooseberry • Indian Gallnut • Cardamom • Cinnamon • Dried Catkins • Indian Pennywort • Cyperus • Nutgrass • White Sandalwood • Aloeweed • Butterfly Pea • Shoe Flower • Licorice • Turmeric. Processed in the aqueous extract of: Castor root • Country Mallow • Thatch Grass • Eragrostis Cynosuroides • Sugar Cane • Indian Asparagus • Spreading Hogweed • Giant Potato • Winter Cherry • Indian Kudju • Trumpet flower • Premna Integrifolia • Desmodium gangeticum • Uraria picta • Yellow-berried Night Shade • Small Caltrops • Phaseolus trilobus • Teramnus labialis • Bengal Quince • Cashmere bark.
See Editor's Note No. 39.

Maitake D-Fraction - Pure Encapsulations
Each vegetable capsule contains: Maitake D-fraction extract (grifola frondosa, standardized to contain 30% D-Fraction) 20 mg • Whole Maitake fruit (grifola frondosa) 250 mg • Vitamin C (as ascorbyl palmitate) 25 mg • Vitamin C (pure ascorbic acid) 25 mg.

Maitake Mushroom - Pure Encapsulations
Each vegetable capsule contains: Maitake mushroom 4:1 extract (grifola frondosa) 500 mg.

Maitake Supreme - Gaia Herbs
Two capsules contain: Patented Maitake extract (griffola frondosa) 60 mg. Other Ingredients: Vegetable Glycerin, Vegetable Cellulose.

MaitakeGold 404 Capsules - Natural Factors
Each capsule contains: MaitakeGold 404 powdered extract 15 mg • Multi Mycelia Blend 85 mg: Shiitake, Agaricus Blazei, Schizophyllum Commune, Cordyceps Sinensi, Tremella Fuciformis, Ganoderma Lucidum, Coriolus Versicolor, Pria Cocos, Hericum Einaceus, Grifola Frondosa. Other Ingredients: Rice Powder, Gelatin Capsule (gelatin, purified water), Magnesium Stearate.

MaitakeGold 404 Drops - Natural Factors
Seven tenths milliliters contain: Vitamin C (as ascorbic acid) 21 mg • MaitakeGold 404 powdered extract 23 mg. Other Ingredients: Vegetable Glycerin, Water.

MALE - Life Enhancement Products, Inc.
Five capsules contain: Magnesium (as magnesium aspartate) 50 mg • Zinc (as zinc citrate) 30 mg • Selenium (as sodium selenite) 25 mcg • Copper (as copper gluconate) 2 mg • Potassium (as potassium

aspartate) 50 mg • L-Arginine 2800 mg • Muira Puama root extract 1000 mg • Tribulus Terrestris leaf extract 750 mg • Urtica Dioica leaf extract 500 mg • Avena Sativa extract (top) 300 mg • Ashwagandha root extract 300 mg • Choline (as choline citrate) 250 mg • Panax Ginseng radix extract 250 mg • Ginkgo Biloba leaf extract 50 mg.

Male Activator **-** The Sports Nutrition Source, Inc.
Two capsules contain: Niacin 20 mg • Wild Oats extract 200 mg • Yohimbe 250 mg • Damiana leaf 150 mg • Siberian Ginseng root 100 mg • Bee Pollen 100 mg • Cordyceps 50 mg • Cayenne 50 mg.

Male Advantage **-** Body Wise International, Inc.
Three capsules contain: Zinc (Krebs Cycle Chelate) 15 mg • Saw Palmetto berry fruit extract 4:1 (Equivalent to 1000 mg Saw Palmetto) 250 mg • Kava Kava root 250 mg • Alpha-Ketoglutaric Acid 200 mg • Flaxseed 100 mg • Pumpkin seed 75 mg • Korean Ginseng root 75 mg • Siberian Ginseng root 75 mg • Turmeric root extract (95% Curcumin) 50 mg • Damiana leaf 50 mg • L-Alanine 50 mg • L-Glutamic Acid 50 mg • Glycine 50 mg • Pygeum Africana Bark wet extract 150:1 50 mg • Gotu Kola whole plant 50 mg • Bromelain 50 mg. Other Ingredients: Gelatin, Magnesium Stearate, Cellulose, Dicalcium Phosphate, Silicon Dioxide.

Male Drive **-** Dial Herbs
Vitamin E • Yohimbe • Green Oats • Zinc • Siberian Ginseng • L-Histidine. In a base of Velvet Antler, Rehmanniae, Cormus Wolfberries, Astragalus seed, Epimedii, Vaccriae, Cyperi.

Male Factor 1000 **-** Herbalife International of America, Inc.
Each capsule contains: Vitamin C (as ascorbic acid) 50 mg • Calcium (as calcium carbonate and dicalcium phosphate) 96 mg • Sodium 10 mg • Swissoats A111 Blend 500 mg: Dried Oat seed extract, Dried Nettle root extract, Sea Buckthorn fruit, Glycine, Glucose, Citric Acid, Silicon Dioxide, Dried Oriental Ginseng root extract, Dried Eleuthero root extract. Other Ingredients: Gelatin, Acacia, Magnesium Stearate, Titanium Dioxide.

Male Formula **-** Oasis Wellness Network
Each tablet contains: Calcium 25 mg • Vitamin E (as d-alpha tocopherol acetate) 50 IU • Selenium (yeast) 25 mcg • L-Glutamine 200 mg • MaxCell Proprietary Blend 125 mg: Zisyphus Jujube, Piper Nigrum, Aloe Vera, Glycyrrhiza Glabra • Glucosamine Sulfate 100 mg • Epimedium Grandiflorum leaf extract 100 mg • Tribulus Terrestris fruit extract 75 mg • American Ginseng root extract 50 mg • Lycopene 2.5 mg. Other Ingredients: Cellulose, Stearic Acid, Calcium Sulfate, Magnesium Stearate, Silica.

Male Formula **-** 4 Life
Each capsule contains: Damiana leaf 85 mg • Sarsaparilla root 80 mg • Siberian Ginseng root 57 mg • Saw Palmetto fruit 55 mg • Pumpkin seed 55 mg • Male Proprietary Extract Blend 45 mg: Pumpkin seed extract, Muira Puama bark extract, Saw Palmetto frui), Sarsaparilla root extract, Damiana leaf extract • Pygeum bark (pygeum africanum, 25% phytosterols) 23 mg. Other Ingredients: Gelatin Capsule, Magnesium Stearate.

Male Fuel **-** TwinLab
Six capsules contain: Yohimbe bark extract (standardized for Yohimbine) 800 mg • L-Arginine HCl 2800 mg • Ginkgo Biloba extract (standardized for 24% flavonoid glycosides) 60 mg • Natural Vitamin E 400 IU • Zinc (from Zinc Picolinate) 30 mg • L-Tyrosine 100 mg • Vitamin B6 50 mg • Choline Bitartrate 200 mg • Vitamin B5 (Pantothenic Acid) 100 mg • Saw Palmetto (Serenoa repens) extract 120 mg • Phytosterol Complex (providing Beta-Sitosterol 60 mg) 120 mg.

Male Libido **-** Gaia Herbs
Three capsules contain: Maca tuber (lepidium meyenii) 120 mg • Horny Goat Weed (epimedium grandiflorum) 54 mg • Saw Palmetto, supercritical CO2 extract (serenoa repens) 54 mg • Tribulus bark (tribulus terrestris) 45 mg • Yohimbe bark (coryanthe yohimbe) 30 mg • Sarsaparilla root (smilax off. v. omata) 15 mg • Muira Puama root (ptychopetalum olacoides) 15 mg • Fo Ti root (polygonum multiflorum) 15 mg • Wild Oats milky seed (avena sativa) 15 mg. Other Ingredients: Vegetable Glycerin, Vegetable Cellulose.

Male Multi Vitamins **-** Health Center for Better Living
Each tablet contains: Vitamin A (as retinyl palmitate and 50% from beta-carotene) 5,000 IU • Vitamin C (as ascorbic acid) 150 mg • Vitamin D (as cholecalciferol) 100 IU • Vitamin E (as dl-alpha-tocopheryl acetate) 50 IU • Vitamin K (as phytonadione) 10 mcg • Thiamin (as thiamin HCl) 10 mg • Riboflavin 10 mg • Niacin (as niacinarnide) 30 mg • Vitamin B6 (as pyridoxine HCl) 5 mg • Folate (as folic acid) 100 mcg • Vitamin B12 (as cyanocobalamin) 10 mcg • Biotin 100 mcg• Pantothenic Acid (as D-calcium patothenate) 5 mg • Calcium (as calcium carbonate and dicalcium phosphate) 150 mg • Iodine (from Kelp) 50 mcg • Magnesium (as magnesium oxide) 25 mg • Zinc (as zinc citrate) 5 mg • Selenium (as selenomethionine) 100 mcg • Copper (as copper oxide) 1 mg • Manganese (as manganese sulfate) 1 mg • Chromium (as chromium dinicotinate glycinate) 100 mcg • Molybdenum (as sodium molybdate) 20 mcg • Boron (as boron chelate) 300 mcg • Grape seed extract (40% proanthocyanidins) 10 mg • Citrus bioflavonoids complex 15 mg • Rutin 10 mg • Silica (from horsetail herb) 5 mg • Montmorillonite (source of 72 trace minerals) 25 mg • Octacosanol (from rice bran) 2 mg • Saw palmetto berry 50 mg.

Male Performax **-** PhysioLogics
Each capsule contains: Muira Puama root (ptychopetalum olacoides, from 4:1 extract) 500 mg • Korean Ginseng root (panax ginseng, standardized to contain 14% ginsenosides, 3.5 mg) 25 mg • Ginkgo Biloba leaf extract (standardized to contain 24% ginkgo flavonglycosides, 3.2 mg, 6% terpenes, 0.8 mg) 13.3 mg. Other Ingredients: Rice Powder, Gelatin, Vegetable Magnesium Stearate, Silica.

Male Potential **-** Health Smart Vitamins
Each capsule contains: Muira Puama bark 500 mg • Panax Ginseng root (14% ginsenosides, 3.5 mg) 25 mg • Ginkgo leaf (24 % ginkgo glavonglycosides 3.2 mg; 6% terpene lactones, 0.8 mg) 13 mg.

Male Power **-** Futurebiotics LLC
Panax Ginseng (active standardized ginsenosides) 5 mg • Siberian Ginseng 50:1 extract 750 mg • Avena Sativa (wild oats) 200 mg • Smilax (sarsaparilla) 200 mg • Saw Palmetto extract 200 mg • Mexican Yam extract 200 mg • Polygonum Multiflorum extract 250 mg • Astragalus extract 250 mg • Schizandra extract 250 mg • Alfalfa 500 mg • Licorice root extract 500 mg • Muira Puama 150 mg • Deer Antler 50 mg • Kelp 150 mg • Spirulina 100 mg • Black Cohosh 100 mg • Mullein 100 mg • Ginger 35 mg • Bee Pollen 500 mg • Royal Jelly 30 mg • Vitamin B12 500 mcg • Zinc (citrate) 25 mg • Glandulars: Pancreas 100 mg, Orchic 90 mg, Thymus 90 mg, Adrenal 80 mg, Heart 75 mg, Lymph 35 mg, Prostate 35 mg, Spleen 20 mg, Pituitary 15 mg.
See Editor's Note No. 31.

Male Power Plus (Sophora Flavescens) **-** Spectrum Partners Inc.
Each capsule contains: Proprietary Blend 550 mg: Eurycoma Longifolia Jack 20:1 extract, Epimedium 50% standardized, Maca 4:1 extract, Cnidium Monnier extract 50%, Sophora Flavescens extract, Ginkgo Biloba extract, Butea Superba proprietary extract, Tribulus Terrestris 40% standardized, Macuna Pruriens 20% standardized.
See Editor's Note No. 70.

Male Response **-** Source Naturals
Three tablets contain: Vitamin E (as Natural D-Alpha Tocopheryl) 100 IU • Vitamin B6 (Pyridoxine HCl) 25 mg • Pantothenic Acid (Vitamin B5) 50 mg • Zinc (as OptiZinc Monomethionine) 15 mg • Selenium (as L-Selenomethionine and Selenium Chelate) 150 mcg • Copper (as Copper Sebacate) 1 mg • Tribulus leaf, stem and flower (Yielding 200 mg of Furostanol Saponins) 500 mg • Maca root extract (Lepidium Meyenii) 300 mg • Yohimbe bark standardized extract 4% (Yielding 9 mg of Yohimbine) 225 mg • Muira Puama stem extract 200 mg • Oat Straw leaf extract (Avena sativa) 200 mg • Siberian Ginseng root 200 mg • Damiana leaf and stem 200 mg • Saw Palmetto berry 200 mg • Mexican Sarsaparilla root 200 mg • Ashwagandha root 150 mg • Panax Ginseng root standardized extract

8% (Yielding 8 mg of Ginsenosides) 100 mg • Ginkgo Biloba leaf extract (50:1) (Yielding 14 mg of Ginkgo Flaconglycosides) 60 mg • Stinging Nettle root extract (16:1) 60 mg • Ginger root 60 mg.

MalePrep **-** HealthMinded
Each capsule contains: Vitamin A (as retinol palmitate) 1250 IU • Vitamin E (as dL-alpha tocopheryl acetate) 8 IU • Cernitine Flower pollen complex 400 mg. Other Ingredients: Gelatin, Stearic Acid, Magnesium Stearate.

MaleRatio **-** Life Enhancement Products, Inc.
Four capsules contain: Vitamin C (ascorbic acid and ascorbigen) 110 mg • Vitamin B12 (cyanocobalamin) 400 mcg • Iodine (potassium iodine) 100 mcg • Selenium (sodium selenite) 250 mcg • Chrysin 750 mg • Indole-3-Carbinol 200 mg • Diindolylmethane 120 mg • DHEA 25 mg • Lycopene 30 mg. Other Ingredients: Magnesium Stearate, Gelatin.

Malic Acid + **-** PhysioLogics
Each capsule contains: Magnesium (as magnesium oxide, magnesium aspartate) 100 mg • Potassium (as potassium aspartate) 10 mg • Malic Acid 250 mg • Coenzyme Q10 15 mg. Other Ingredients: Rice Powder, Gelatin, Vegetable Magnesium Stearate, Silica.

Malic Acid 250 mg **-** Pro Health
Two tablets contain: Malic Acid 500 mg. Other Ingredients: Microcrystalline Cellulose, Dibasic Calcium Phosphate, Stearic Acid, Colloidal Silicon Dioxide, Magnesium Stearate.

Malic Acid Plus **-** Pain & Stress Center
Two capsules contain: Malic Acid 800 mg • Boswellia Serrata 300 mg • Magnesium 100 mg • Chromium Picolinate 50 mcg • Vitamin C 10 mg • Vitamin B6 5 mg. Other Ingredients: Gelatin Capsule.

Malic Acid+ **-** PhysioLogics
Each capsule contains: Magnesium (Oxide, Aspartate) 100 mg • Potassium (Aspartate) 10 mg • Malic Acid 250 mg • Coenzyme Q10 15 mg.

Maltsupex **-** Wallace Laboratories
Each level scoop contains: Malt Soup Extract derived from natural barley malt 8 g.

Mammary PMG **-** Standard Process, Inc.
Each tablet contains: Proprietary Blend 185 mg: Bovine Mammary PMG extract, Magnesium Citrate • Calcium 20 mg • Sodium 10 mg. Other Ingredients: Cellulose.
See Editor's Note No. 14.

Manganese **-** Source Naturals
Each tablet contains: Manganese (from 150 mg of manganese amino acid chelate) 15 mg.

Manganese **-** GNC
Each tablet contains: Manganese (as manganese gluconate) 10 mg. Other Ingredients: Dicalcium Phosphate, Cellulose.

Manganese (aspartate/citrate) **-** Pure Encapsulations
Each vegetable capsule contains: Manganese (aspartate) 5 mg • Manganese (citrate) 5 mg.

Manganese 50 mg **-** Nature's Plus
Each tablet contains: Manganese (as amino acid chelate) 50 mg. Other Ingredients: Di-Calcium Phosphate, Microcrystalline Cellulose, Stearic Acid, Magnesium Stearate, Pharmaceutical Glaze, Silica.

Manganese B12 **-** Standard Process, Inc.
Each tablet contains: Proprietary Blend 133 mg: Carrot root, Bovine Bone • Vitamin C 9.2 mg • Vitamin B12 5 mcg • Iron 1 mg • Zinc 1.9 mg • Copper 0.2 mg • Manganese 34 mg. Other Ingredients: Honey, Cellulose.

Manganese Extra **-** Olympian Labs
Each capsule contains: Manganese Chelate 30 mg • Huckleberry 100 mg • Blueberry 100 mg • Lady Slipper 50 mg • Black Walnut 50 mg.

Mangaplex **-** Progressive Labs
Each tablet contains: Vitamin C (ascorbic acid) 80 mg • Vitamin D (as Vitamin D3) (cholecalciferol) 50 IU • Vitamin E (d-alpha tocopheryl succinate) 10 IU • Thiamin HCl (Vitamin B1) 5 mg • Vitamin B6 (pyridoxine HCl) 10 mg • Vitamin B12 (cyanocobalamin) 10 mcg • Calcium (calcium lactate 175 mg) 26 mg • Manganese (manganese sulfate 200 mg) 73 mg • Choline Bitartrate 30 mg • Bioflavonoids 20 mg • Horsetail 100 mg • Rose Hips 5 mg • Green Pea concentrate 200 mg • Raw Liver concentrate 10 mg.
See Editor's Note No. 14.

Mangosteen Plus **-** Perfect Health
Reconstituted Garcinia Mangostana puree (from tropical mangosteen whole fruit) • Sweet Pear juice and puree concentrates • Dark Red Grape juice concentrate • Plump Blueberry juice concentrate • Bright Red Sour Cherry juice concentrate • Pacific Pineapple juice concentrate • Crimson Cranberry juice concentrate • Exotic Thai Lychee fruit juice concentrate • Shimmering Starfruit juice concentrate • Garcinia Mangostana peel extract • Ascorbic Acid (vitamin C).

MannaBar Protein Formula **-** Mannatech
Each bar contains: Solnuts Soybeans, Soya, toasted Soya pieces • roasted Cashew Butter with Safflower oil • Rice Syrup (partially polished brown rice, koji, water) • Isolated Soy Protein • Dried Apricots • Dried Cranberries (sweetened with apple juice) • Date paste • Natural Vegetable Glycerin • Raspberry flavor • Energy Smart (fruit juice, natural grain dextrins) • Honey Granola: quick Oats, Canola Oil, Honey, Lecithin • Supro Plus Nuggets (isolated soy protein, rice flour, malt, salt) • Pear juice concentrate • Nonfat dry milk solids • Rolled Oats • Flax seed • Whey Protein concentrate • Wheat Bran • Calcium Caseinate • Ambrotose complex (naturally occurring plant saccharides including freeze-dried aloe vera gel extract - Manapol powder) • Phytosterols from Wild Yam root • Phyt•Aloe flash-dried complex: Broccoli, Brussels Sprouts, Cabbage, Carrot, Cauliflower, Garlic, Kale, Onion, Tomato, Turnip, Papaya, Pineapple • Citric Acid • Natural Flavoring.

MannaBAR, Vanilla Yogurt-Coated Apple Crunch **-** Mannatech
Each bar contains: Coating: dehydrated Cane juice, fractionated Palm Kernel Oil, nonfat Milk powder, Yogurt powder, Lactic Acid, Soy Lecithin, natural Vanilla • Dry Roasted Soybeans • Toasted Cashew Butter with Safflower oil • Dried Apple Pieces • Rice Syrup (partially polished brown rice, koji, water) • Isolated Soy Protein • Date Paste • Natural Vegetable Glycerin • Honey Granola: quick Oats, Canola Oil, Honey, Lecithin • Energy Smart (fruit juice, natural grain dextrins) • Apple Flavor • Supro Plus Nuggets (isolated soy protein, rice flour, malt, salt) • Rolled Oats • Apple Juice Concentrate • Nonfat Dry Milk Solids • Flax Seed • Whey Protein Concentrate • Wheat Bran • Calcium Caseinate • Natural Flavoring • Cinnamon • Ambrotose Complex (naturally occurring plant saccharides including freeze-dried aloe vera inner leaf gel extract - Manapol powder) • Phytosterols from Wild Yam Root • Phyt•Aloe dehydrated Complex: Broccoli, Brussels Sprouts, Cabbage, Carrot, Cauliflower, Garlic, Kale, Onion, Tomato, Turnip, Papaya, Pineapple.

Manna-C **-** Mannatech
Two capsules contain: Vitamin C (from Acerola fruit) 53 mg • Proprietary Blend Ambrotose Complex (patent pending) 84 mg: Arabinogalactan (larix decidua gum), Manapol Aloe Vera gel extract (inner leaf gel), Gum Ghatti, Gum Tragacanth • Herbal Blend 398 mg: Boneset (aerial part), Lemon Verbena (leaves), Sage (leaves), Catnip (aerial part), Peppermint (leaves), Yarrow (flowers), Horehound (aerial part). Other Ingredients: Gelatin, Sodium Starch Glycolate, Stearic Acid.

MannaCLEANSE **-** Mannatech
Two caplets contain: Proprietary Fiber Blend 750 mg: Oat fiber, Black Currant fiber, Psyllium (seed husk), Carrageenan, Glucomannan • Essential Oils/Botanical Blend 145 mg: Fenugreek (seed), Fennel (seed), Ginger (root), Rosemary (leaves), Neroli Orange (blossom), Peppermint (leaves) • Fatty Acid Blend 120 mg:

Flax (seed), Sodium Caprylate, Rice (bran), Lecithin, Borage (seed) • Flora Growth Promotants 80 mg: Inulin-Oligosaccharide Complex, Beta-Glucans • Probiotic Flora Blend 24 mg: Lactobacillus Sporogenes, L. Acidophilus, L. Plantarum, L. Casei, Bifidobacterium Bifidum • Enzyme Blend 20 mg: Amylase, Protease, Lactase, Lipase, Cellulase • Ambrotose Complex (patent pending) 2 mg: Arabinogalactan (larix decidua gum), Manapol Aloe Vera gel extract (inner leaf gel), Gum Ghatti, Gum Tragacanth. Other Ingredients: Dibasic Calcium Phosphate, Microcrystalline Cellulose, Croscarmellose Sodium, Stearic Acid, Silicon Dioxide, Magnesium Stearate, Natural Flavor. Film Coat Ingredients: Hydroxypropyl Methycellulose, Hydroxypropyl Cellulose, Polyethylene Glycol.

Mannatonin **-** Mannatech
Each tablet contains: Melatonin 1 mg • Proprietary Blend Ambrotose Complex (patent pending) 10 mg: Naturally Occurring Plant Saccharides (including freeze-dried aloe vera inner leaf gel extract - manapol powder) • Valerian root 100 mg • Lecithin 50 mg. Other Ingredients: Dibasic Calcium Phosphate, Microcrystalline Cellulose, Tribasic Calcium Phosphate, Molasses, Wheat Germ, Croscarmellose Sodium, Magnesium Stearate, Silicon Dioxide, Calcium Silicate, Coating (shellac, talc, gelatin, sucrose, calcium sulfate, kaolin, titanium dioxide, carnauba wax).

Mannose Powder **-** Vital Nutrients
Each 1/2 tsp serving contains: D-Mannose powder 1000 mg.

Man-Rx **-** Athletic Technologies Inc.
Two tablets contain: Androstenedione 100 mg • Yohimbe 250 mg • Avena Sativa 150 mg • Saw Palmetto 100 mg • Guarana extract 300 mg • Taurine 200 mg • Siberian Ginseng 30 mg • Tribulus Terrestris 50 mg • Panax Ginseng 30 mg • Rhodiola Rosea 10 mg • Wild Yam extract 250 mg • Maca 100 mg • Arginine 100 mg • Niacin 10 mg.
See Editor's Note No. 47.

Marapuama **-** Holistic International, Inc.
Each capsule contains: Ptychopetalum Olacoides (marapuama) 5:1 500 mg.

Marine Beta Carotene **-** Jarrow Formulas
Each softgel contains: Beta Carotene (from dunaliella salina, equivalent to 25,000 IU of pro-vitamin A) 15 mg • Vitamin E 5 IU. Other Ingredients: Soybean Oil, Gelatin, Glycerin, Purified Water.

Marine Beta Carotene **-** Jarrow Formulas
Each softgel contains: Beta Carotene (from Dunaliella salina) (Equivalent to 25000 IU of pro Vitamin A) activity 15 mg • Vitamin E 5 IU. Other Ingredients: Soybean Oil, Lecithin.

Marine Beta Carotene 25,000 IU **-** Nature's Life
Each capsule contains: Beta Carotene (Dunaliella salina, vitamin A equivalent 25,000 IU) (Other natural Carotenoids occuring in D. Salina) 15 mg • Alpha Carotene 500 mcg • Cryptoxanthin 130 mcg • Zeaxanthin 100 mcg • Lutein 86 mcg. Vitamin E (d-Alpha Tocopherol) 1.5 IU.

Marine Carotene **-** The Vitamin Shoppe
Each softgel contains: Natural Beta-Carotene 15 mg (equivalent to 25,000 IU Vitamin A activity) providing other naturally occurring Carotenoids: Alpha-carotene, Lutein, Cryptoxanthin, and Zeaxanthin.

Marine Omega **-** Pharmanex
Two softgels contain: Vitamin E (as natural mixed tocopherols) 10 IU • Marine Lipid concentrate 2000 mg • Omega 3 Fatty Acids 100 mg: EPA 300 mg, DHA 200 mg, Other Omega 3 Fatty Acids • NKO Krill oil 100 mg. Other Ingredients: Gelatin, Glycerin, Purified Water, Natural Lemon Oil, Vanillin.

Marshmallow **-** Nature's Way
Two capsules contain: Marshmallow root 910 mg. Other Ingredients: Gelatin.

Martrim **-** VitaStore
Cayenne • Ginseng (Siberian) • Guarana (Paullinia Cupana) • Gymnema Sylvestre • Kelp • Phenylalanine • Pullulan • Sidacordifilia Extract • Zingiber • Vitamin A • Vitamin B1 • Vitamin B6 • Vitamin B12 • Vitamin C • Vitamin D • Vitamin E (d-alpha tocopherol) • Folic Acid • Iodine (Kelp) • Niacin • d-Biotin • Pantothenic Acid • Potassium Gluconate.

Masculex **-** Enzymatic Therapy
Two capsules contain: Vitamin E (D-Alpha Tocopherol) 100 IU. Other Ingredients: Muira Puama Powdered extract 6:1 (Ptychopetalum olacoides) 250 mg • Liquid Liver Fractions (predigested soluble concentrate) 250 mg • Wheat Germ oil concentrate 100 mg • Beta-Sitosterol 100 mg • Mexican Damiana leaves extract (Tunera diffusa) 100 mg • Saw Palmetto Berry extract (Serenoa repens) standardized to contain 85%-95% fatty acids & biologically active sterols 40 mg • Cola Nut extract (Cola nitida) (contains 4.8 mg Caffeine) 40 mg • Panax ginseng extract standardized to contain 7% Saponins (calculated as Ginsenoside Rg1) 40 mg • Ginkgo Biloba leaves extract (Ginkgo biloba folia) standardized to contain 24% ginkgoflavonglycosides 20 mg.
See Editor's Note No. 14.

Masculex for Men **-** Enzymatic Therapy
Each two softgel capsules contain: Vitamin E (as d-alpha tocopherol) 100 IU • Liquid Liver Fractions (predigested soluble concentrate) 250 mg • Muira Puama (ptychopetalum olacoides, root extract 6:1) 250 mg • Wheat Germ Oil 100 mg • Beta-Sitosterol 100 mg • Damiana (turnera diffusa, leaf extract 5:1) 100 mg • Saw Palmetto (serenoa repens, berrry extract standardized to contain 88-95% fatty acids, 0.2-0.4% total sterols, 0.1-0.3% beta-sitosterol) 40 mg • Cola (cola nitida, nut extract containing 4.8 mg caffeine) 40 mg • Korean Ginseng (panax ginseng, root extract standardized to contain a minimum of 7% ginsenosides) 40 mg • Ginkgo (ginkgo biloba, leaf extract standardized to contain 24% ginkgoflavonglycosides, 6% terpene lactones, and 2% bilobalide) 20 mg.

MascuPlex **-** PhytoPharmica
Two softgel capsules contain: Cola nut extract (cola nitida, standardized to contain 4.8 mg caffeine) 40 mg • Damiana leaf 5:1 extract (turnera diffusa) 100 mg • Ginkgo leaf extract (ginkgo biloba, standardized to contain 24% ginkgoflavonglycosides, 6% terpene lactones, and 2% bilobalide) 20 mg • Liquid Liver Fractions (predigested soluble concentrate) 250 mg • Muira Puama root 6:1 extract (ptychopetalum olacoides) 250 mg • Panax Ginseng root extract (standardized to contain a minimum of 7% ginsenosides) 40 mg • Proprietary Phytosterol Blend 100 mg: Beta Sitosterol, Campesterol, Stigmasterol • Saw Palmetto berry extract (standardized to contain 85-95% fatty acids, 0.2-0.4% total sterols, and 0.1-0.3% beta sitosterol) 40 mg • Vitamin E (as D-alpha tocopherol) 100 IU • Wheat Germ oil 100 mg.
See Editor's Note No. 14.

Mass Fuel **-** TwinLab
High Biological-Quality Milk & Egg Proteins • Branched Chain Amino Acids (L-Leucine, L-Isoleucine & L-Valine) • L-Glutamine • Alpha-Ketoglutarates • Keto-Isocaproate (KIC) • L-Ornithine Alpha-Ketoglutarate • L-Carnitine • Creatine Monohydrate • High Potencies Of Vitamins & Minerals • Potassium 2000 mg • Chromium 300 mcg (from patented Chromic Fuel Chromium Picolinate).

Masters **-** Pharmanex
Two capsules contain: Vitamin A (100% as Beta-Carotene)(Beta-Carotene, Dunaliella Salina) 3750 IU • Vitamin C (as Ascorbic Acid) 150 mg • Vitamin D (as Vitamin D3)(as Cholecalciferol) 200 IU • Vitamin E (as d-Alpha Tocopheryl Succinate) 150 IU • Riboflavin (as Riboflavin) 0.85 mg • Vitamin B6 (as Pyridoxine Hydrochloride) 1 mg • Folate (as Folic Acid) 200 mcg • Vitamin B12 (as Cyanocobalamin) 3 mcg • Calcium (Calcium Carbonate, Calcium Chelate, Calcium Citrate) 250 mg • Magnesium (Magnesium Oxide, Magnesium Chelate) 100 mg • Zinc (Zinc Chelate) 7.5 mg • Chromium (Chromium Chelate, Chromium Picolinate) 100 mcg • Korean Panax Ginseng with Ginsenosides 25 mcg • Siberian Ginseng

extract with Eleutherosides 25 mg • Ginkgo Biloba Powder with Ginkgoflavonglycosides 20 mg • Echinacea Purpurea Powder with Echinacosides 20 mg • Cranberry Concentrate with Quinnic Acid 12.5 mg • Bilberry Powder with Anthocyanosides 10 mg.

Mastic Gum 500 - Jarrow Formulas
Two capsules contain: Mastic gum (pistacia lentiscus) 1000 mg. Other Ingredients: Cellulose, Magnesium Stearate, Titanium Dioxide, Silicon Dioxide, Gelatin.

Mastic Gum Extract - Source Naturals
Two capsules contain: Calcium (from coral) 68 mg • Mastic Gum extract (pistacia lentiscus, yielding 25% alpha and masticonic acids) 1 g. Other Ingredients: Gelatin, Dibasic Calcium Phsophate, Maltodextrin, Colloidal Silicon Dioxide, Magnesium Stearate.

Mastitix - TriLight Herbs
Echinacea herb • German Chamomile • Red root • Baptesia root • Boneset • Yarrow • Elderflower • Usnea.

Matol - Matol Botanical International Ltd
Each 1 mL serving contains: Potassium (citrate) 25.8 mg • Potassium (glycerophosphate) 0.16 mg • Iron (glycerophosphate) 0.09 mg • Iodine (potassium iodide) 0.0015 mg • Magnesium Glycerophosphate 0.84 mg. Base: Camomile herb, Sarsaparilla root, Celery seed, Angelica root, Dandelion root, Horehound herb, Licorice root, Polygala Senega root, Passion flower herb, Thyme herb, Gentian root, Saw Palmetto berry, Alfalfa herb.

Matol Kaps - Matol Botanical International Ltd
Each capsule contains: Potassium (citrate) 172 mg • Potassium (glycerophosphate) 1.067 mg • Iron (glycerophosphate) 0.60 mg • Magnesium (glycerophosphate) 5.6 mg. Base: Camomile herb, Sarsaparilla root, Celery seed, Angelica root, Dandelion root, Horehound herb, Licorice root, Polygala Senega root, Passion flower herb, Thyme herb, Gentian root, Saw Palmetto berry, Alfalfa herb.

Matol Kosher - Matol Botanical International Ltd
Each 1 mL serving contains: Potassium (citrate) 25.8 mg • Potassium (glycerophosphate) 0.16 mg • Iron (glycerophosphate) 0.09 mg • Iodine (potassium iodide) 0.0015 mg • Magnesium glycerophosphate 0.84 mg. Base: Camomile herb, Sarsaparilla root, Celery seed, Angelica root, Dandelion root, Horehound herb, Licorice root, Polygala Senega root, Passion flower herb, Thyme herb, Gentian root, Saw Palmetto berry, Alfalfa herb.

Matrixx - Allergy Research Group
Two capsules contain: Vitamin C (as ascorbic acid) 33 mg • Vitamin E (as D-alpha-tocopheryl acid succinate) 55 IU • Calcium (calcium citrate) 27 mg • Magnesium (as magnesium citrate) 40 mg • Zinc (as zinc citrate) 4 mg • Selenium (as sodium selenite/selenomethionine) 33 mcg • Copper (as copper sebacate) 0.27 mg • Manganese (as manganese citrate) 4.7 mg • Molybdenum (as sodium molybdate) 330 mcg • Boron (as boron citrate) 1.2 mg • N-Acetyl-D-Glucosamine 67 mg • Chondroitin Sulfate 130 mg • Glucosamine Sulfate 500 mg • L-Lysine 67 mg • L-Proline 107 mg • Hawthorne dried extract (crataegus oxyacantha) 295 mg • Horsetail dried extract (equisetum arvense) 6.7 mg • Bromelain 10 mg. Other Ingredients: Cellulose, Magnesium Stearate, Ethyl Vanillin.

MAX Creatine - Apex Fitness Group
Each tablet contains: Creatine Monohydrate 200 mg • Glutamine peptide 400 mg. Other Ingredients: Calcium Phosphate, Croscarmellose, Vegetable Stearate, Magnesium Stearate.
This product was formerly called "Creatine & Glutamine Peptide Complex."

Max DHA - Jarrow Formulas
Each softgel contains: Fish Oil (source of omega-3) 600 mg: DHA (docosahexaenoic acid) 250 mg, EPA (eicosapentaenoic acid) 36 mg, Other Omega-3 72 mg • Gamma Tocopherol 5 mg • Ascorbyl Palmitate 2 mg. Other Ingredients: Gelatin, Glycerine, Water, Carob.

MAX DHEA - Apex Fitness Group
Each tablet contains: Dehydroepiandrosterone (DHEA) 25 mg. Other Ingredients: Calcium Phosphate, Stearic Acid, Magnesium Stearate, Croscarmellose.
This product was formerly called "Ergogen DHEA."

MAX Drink Mix (chocolate and vanilla flavors) - Apex Fitness Group
Whey Protein Concentrate • Maltodextrin • Milk Protein Isolate • Calcium Caseinate • Natural and Artificial flavor (includes milk) • Salt • Potassium Phosphate • Soy Lecithin • Potassium Chloride • Cellulose gum • Aspartame • Taurine • L-Glutamine • Calcium Alpha-Ketoglutarate • Xanthan Gum • Magnesium Oxide • Potassium Citrate • Medium Chain Triglycerides • Sodium Caseinate • Egg White • Beta Carotene • Ascorbic Acid • Ferrous Fumarate • Alpha Tocopherol Acetate • Niacinamide • Zinc Oxide • Manganese Sulfate • Calcium Pantothenate • Copper Sulfate • Vitamin A Palmitate • Pyridoxine Hydrochloride • Riboflavin • Thiamin Mononitrate • Folic Acid • Sodium Molybdate • Chromium Chloride • Biotin • Potassium Iodide • Sodium Selenite • Phytonadione • Vitamin D (D3) • Vitamin B12. Chocolate flavor also contains: Cocoa (processed with alkali).
This product was formerly called "Ergogen High Performance X-Treme."

Max GLA - PhysioLogics
Each softgel contains: Linolenic Acid 375 mg • Gamma-Linolenic Acid (GLA) 229 mg •Oleic Acid 190 mg • Palmitic Acid 114 mg • Stearic Acid 41 mg •Palmitoleic Acid 3 mg.

Max GLA - Pro Health
Each softgel contains: Borage Oil 1 g • Gamma Linolenic Acid (GLA) 240 mg • Linoleic Acid 400 mg • Oleic Acid 200 mg • Palmitic Acid 100 mg • Stearic Acid 60 mg. Other Ingredients: Gelatin, Glycerin, Water.

Max HGH - Unknown
Two tablets contain: L-Glutamine 125 mg • Glycine 233 mg • L-Arginine HCl 125 mg • L-Ornithine HCl 50 mg • Pepsin 1:3000 100 mg • Peptide 100 mg. Other Ingredients: Di-Calcium Phosphate, Microcrystalline Cellulose, Croscarmellose Sodium, Stearic Acid, Silica, Magnesium Stearate, Pharmaceutical Glaze.

MAX Protein - Apex Fitness Group
Two tablets contain: L-Phenylalanine 84 mg • L-Tryptophan 30.1 mg. Other Ingredients: Calcium Phosphate, Vegetable Stearate, Croscarmellose, Gelatin, Magnesium Stearate, Silica.

MAX Recovery (formerly BCAA) - Apex Fitness Group
Each tablet contains: L-Leucine 450 mg • L-Isoleucine 50 mg • L-Valine 100 mg. Other Ingredients: Calcium Phosphate, Microcrystalline Cellulose, Vegetable Stearate, Croscarmellose, Magnesium Stearate, Povidone.
This product was formerly called "BCAA", or "Branched Chain Amino Acids."

MAX Volumizer - Apex Fitness Group
Ten tablets contain: Taurine 2 g • L-Glutamine 2 g • Creatine 6 g • Glycine 1000 mg • L-Alanine 500 mg • Betaine HCl 500 mg • Inositol 1000 mg. Other Ingredients: Calcium Phosphate, Sorbitol, Vegetable Stearate, Magnesium Stearate, Croscarmellose.
This product was formerly called "Ergogen Muscle Cell Volumizer."

MAX Whey Drink Mix (chocolate and vanilla flavors) - Apex Fitness Group
Whey Protein Concentrate • Maltodextrin • Whey Protein Isolate • Natural and Artificial flavor (includes milk) • Hydrolyzed Whey Protein • Cellulose gum • Glutamine peptide from Hydrolyzed Wheat Protein • Xanthan gum • Aspartame • Acesulfame K • Magnesium Oxide • Ascorbic Acid • Ferrous Fumarate • Alpha Tocopherol Acetate • Niacinamide • Zinc Oxide • Manganese Sulfate • Calcium Pantothenate • Copper Sulfate • Vitamin A Palmitate • Pyridoxine Hydrochloride • Riboflavin • Thiamin Mononitrate • Folic Acid • Sodium Molybdate • Chromium Chloride • Bitoin • Potassium Iodide • Sodium Selenite • Phytonadione • Vitamin D (D3) • Vitamin B12.

Chocolate flavor also contains: Cocoa (processed with alkali). Vanilla flavor also contains: Annatto (added for color).
This product was formerly called "Apex High Performance Better Whey."

MAX Workout - Apex Fitness Group
Six tablets contain: Potassium Magnesium Aspartate/Citrate 4500 mg • Green Tea / Guarana / Cocoa extract (providing caffeine 300 mg, theobromine 1.5 mg, theophylline 30 mg) 742 mg • American Ginseng (standardized to contain 8% ginsenosides) 300 mg. Other Ingredients: Calcium Phosphate, Microcrystalline Cellulose, Vegetable Stearate, Croscarmellose, Lecithin, Magnesium Stearate.

Maxadrine with Ephedra - D & E Pharmaceuticals
Two capsules contain: Pantothenic Acid 40 mg • Citrus Aurantium (standardized to 4% synephrine) 125 mg • Ma Huang plant (standardized to 12.5 mg ephedrine) 208 mg • Guarana seed extract (standardized to 200 mg caffeine) 910 mg • White Willow bark extract (standardized to 15 mg salicin) 105 mg • Acetyl L-Carnitine 100 mg • L-Tyrosine 80 mg • Ginger root 50 mg. Other Ingredients: Calcium Phosphate, Talc, Gelatin, Magnesium Stearate.
See Editor's Note No. 30 and No. 40.

Max-A-Mins - Arrowroot
Two tablets contain: Vitamin D (D3 as cholecalciferol) 200 IU • Calcium (calcium carbonate) 1,000 mg • Magnesium (magnesium oxide, amino acid chelate) 500 mg • Iron (iron peptonate) 18 mg • Zinc (zinc oxide, amino acid chelate) 50 mg • Selenium (selenium oxide) 100 mcg • Copper (copper gluconate, amino acid chelate) 2 mg • Manganese (carbonate, amino acid chelate) 10 mg • Chromium (chromium chloride) 100 mcg • Potassium (potassium chloride) 99 mg • Betaine HCl 100 mg • Glutamic Acid HCl 100 mg. Base: Boron, Lithium, Molybdenum, Silicon, Sulfur, Vanadium.

Maxativa - Futurebiotics LLC
Two tablets contain: Oat extract (4:1) 300 mg • Nettles extract (4:1) 150 mg • Glycine 100 mg • Vitamin C 100 mg • Smilax-Ginseng-Damiana Complex 400 mg • Bee Pollen (Lyophilized) 350 mg • Zinc (Oxide, Gluconate) 15 mg • Royal Jelly (Lyophilized) 45 mg • Niacinamide 15 mg.

MaxEPA - Puritan's Pride
Each softgel contains: Eicosapentaenoic Acid (EPA) 180 mg • Docosahexaenoic Acid (DHA) 120 mg. Contains not less than 30% Omega-3 polyunsaturates.

MaxEPA 1000 - Golden Glow Natural Health Products
Each capsule containss: MaxEPA brand Natural Fish oil 1 g: Omega-3 Marine Triglycerides 300 mg: Eicosapentaenoic Acid 171 mg, Docosahexaenoic Acid 114 mg.

MaxEPA 1000 mg - Nature's Life
Each capsule contains: MaxEPA 1000 mg providing the following naturally occuring essential nutrients: EPA (Eicosapentaneoic Acid) 180 mg • DHA (Docosahexaenoic Acid) 180 mg • Vitamin E (D-Alpha Tocopherol) 30 IU. In a natural base of certified organic Safflower oil.

Maxi B-Caps with Taurine - Country Life Vitamins
Each capsule contains: Thiamin (vitamin B1, as thiamine HCl, thiamine cocarboxylase) 25 mg • Riboflavin (vitamin B2, as riboflavin, riboflavin 5' phosphate) 25 mg • Niacin (as 52% niacinamide & 48% niacin) 50 mg • Vitamin B6 (as pyridoxine HCl, pyridoxide alpha-ketoglutarate, pyridoxal 5' phosphate) 63.75 mg • Folic Acid 800 mcg • Vitamin B12 (as dibencozide) 500 mcg • D-Biotin 300 mg • Pantothenic Acid (as d-calcium pantothenate, pantethine) 200 mg • Inositol 100 mg • Taurine (free form) 100 mg • Choline (from 100 mg of choline bitartrate) 46 mg • PAK (pyridoxine alpha-ketoglutarate) 25 mg • PABA (para-aminobenzoic acid) 25 mg. Inactive Ingredients: Cellulose, Magnesium Stearate, Silica.

Maxi L-Carnitine 500 mg - Solgar
Each tablet contains: Calcium (as dicalcium phosphate) 40 mg • L-Carnitine 500 mg. Other Ingredients: Microcrystalline Cellulose, Dicalcium Phosphate, Vegetable Cellulose, Vegetable Stearic Acid, Silica, Titanium Dioxide, Vegetable Magnesium Stearate, Vegetable Glycerin, Carnauba Wax.

Maxi-Boz - Jarrow Formulas
Each capsule contains: Boswellia Serrata (boswellic acids 65%) 500 mg. Other Ingredients: Microcrystalline Cellulose.

Maxi-Complete - Atrium Biotechnologies
Each tablet contains: Vitamin A Palmitate 10000 IU • Vitamin D (as Vitamin D2 Fish oil) 400 IU • Vitamin B1 Thiamine HCL 10 mg • Vitamin B2 Riboflavin 10 mg • Vitamin B6 Pyridoxine HCL 10 mg • Vitamin B12 Cyanocobalamin 15 mcg • Vitamin C Ascorbic Acid 150 mg • Vitamin E Acetate 60 IU • Biotin 6 mcg • Niacin-Niacinamide 50 mg • Pantothenic Acid 25 mg • Folic Acid 400 mcg • Calcium Amino Acid Chelate 30 mg • Iodine 100 mcg • Iron Amino Acid Chelate 50 mg • Magnesium Amino Acid Chelate 20 mg • Manganese Amino Acid Chelate 6 mg • Phosphorus 20 mg • Zinc Amino Acid Chelate 5 mg • Choline Bitartrate 100 mg • Inositol 100 mg • PABA 30 mg • Rutin 25 mg. In a base of Alfalfa, Bone Meal, Bromelain, Kelp, Papaya, Rose Hips.

MaxiFlex Glucosamine Formula - Medical Ophthalmics
Two capsules contain: Glucosamine Sulfate 1500 mg • Vitamin C (ascorbic acid) 90 mg.

MaxiFlex Joint & Cartilage Formula - Medical Ophthalmics
Three capsules contain: Glucosamine Sulfate 1500 mg • Chondroitin Sulfate 1200 mg • Vitamin C (ascorbic acid) 90 mg.

MaxiFlex Multinutrient Formula - Medical Ophthalmics
Four capsules contain: Glucosamine Sulfate 1500 mg • Chondroitin Sulfate 1200 mg • Vitamin A (beta-carotene) 2500 IU • Vitamin B3 (niacin) 20 mg • Vitamin B5 (pantothenic acid) 10 mg • Vitamin B6 (pyridoxine) 2 mg • Vitamin C (ascorbic acid) 90 mg • Vitamin D 200 IU • Vitamin E (D-alpha tocopherol) 30 IU • Alpha-Lipoic Acid 10 mg • Boron 2 mg • Calcium 100 mg • Magnesium 50 mg • MSM 300 mg • Selenium 75 mcg • Silicon 3 mg • White Willow bark 30 mg.
See Editor's Note No. 15.

Maximal Sterol Complex - Aspen Group, Inc.
Six tablets contain: Fucosterol 6963 mcg • Beta Sitosterol 5148 mcg • Campestrol 3069 mcg • Stigmatero 1749 mcg • Other Naturally Occuring Sterols 9174 mcg (26103 mcg of sterols) • Liver 2600 mg • Orchic 1000 mg • Thymus 200 mg • Heart 200 mg • Lung 200 mg • Kidney 200 mg • Adrenal 150 mg • Prostate 120 mg • Pituitary 150 mg • Hypothalamus 60 mg • Pancreas 120 mg • Bee pollen 1000 mg • Korean Ginseng 100 mg • Royal Jelly 30 mg • Calcium 200 mg • Magnesium 100 mg • Potassium 99 mg • Octacosanol 1650 mcg • RNA 60 mg • DNA 30 mg • Linoleic Acid 1040 mg • Oleic Acid 698 mg • Palmitic Acid 263 mg • Linolenic Acid 109 mg • Stearic Acid 56 mg • Lignoceric Acid 14 mg • Arachidonic Acid 13 mg • Elcoanoic Acid 11 mg • Behenic C Acid 6 mg • Myristic Acid 5 mg • Capsicum 100 mg • Alfalfa 100 mg • Dandelion root 100 mg • Garlic 100 mg • Yellow Dock 100 mg • Gota Kola 100 mg • Licorice root 100 mg • Arginine 1200 mg • Lysine 600 mg • Ornithine 600 mg • Leucine 40 mg • Valine 38 mg • Lysine 34 mg • Isoleucine 30 mg • Phenylalanine 30 mg • Theronine 24 mg • Methionine 20 mg • Tryptophan 8 mg • Trace Minerals.
See Editor's Note No. 31.

Maximum Anti-Oxidant Formula - Nature's Bounty
Two tablets contain: Vitamin A (as Beta Carotene) 15000 IU • Vitamin C (as Calcium Ascorbate and Ascorbyl Palmitate) 500 mg • Vitamin E (as d-Alpha Tocopheryl Succinate) 400 IU • Zinc (as Zinc Picolinate) 7.5 mg • Selenium (as L-Selenomethionine) 50 mcg • Copper (as Copper Lysinate) 1 mg • Manganese (as Manganese Arginate) 2.5 mg • Coenzyme Q-10 1000 mcg • Pycnogenol 3000 mcg • Quercetin 15 mg • Citrus Bioflavonoid Complex 50 mg • L-Glutathione 1000 mcg • N-Acetyl Cysteine 5000 mcg • L-Cysteine Hydrochloride 50 mg • Green Tea extract aerial 500 mcg • Echinacea root 25 mg • Bilberry leaf 25 mg • Schizandra berry 25 mg • Barley Juice powder 2 mg • Broccoli powder 2.5 mg • Spirulina 2 mg • Chlorella 2.5 mg • Citrus Fiber 50 mg. Other Ingredients:

BRAND NAMES

Cellulose, Dicalcium Phosphate, Vegetable Stearic Acid, Food Glaze, Magnesium Silicate, Vegetable Magnesium Stearate, Silica, Croscarmellose.

Maximum Anti-Oxidant Formula vegetarian - Puritan's Pride
Two tablets contain: Vitamin A (as beta carotene) 15,000 IU • Vitamin C (as calcium ascorbate & ascorbyl palmitate) 500 mg • Vitamin E (as d-alpha tocopheryl succinate) 400 IU • Selenium (as l-selenomethionine) 50 mcg • Coenzyme Q10 1000 mcg • Pycnogenol 3000 mg • Quercetin 15 mg • Citrus Bioflavonoids Complex 50 mg • L-Glutathione 1000 mcg • N-Acetyl-Cysteine 5000 mcg • L-Cysteine HCl 50 mg • Copper (as copper lysinate) 1 mg • Manganese (as manganese arginate) 2.5 mg • Zinc (as zinc picolinate) 7.5 mg • Green Tea extract 500 mcg • Echinacea 25 mg • Bilberry 25 mg • Schizandra 25 mg. In a natural base of Broccoli powder 2.5 mg, Spirulina 2 mg, Chlorella 2.5 mg, Barley juice powder 2 mg, and Citrus fiber 50 mg.

Maximum Fat Burners - Optimum Nutrition
CitriMax brand Garcinia Cambogia extract 500 mg • L-Carnitine • Choline • Inositol • Methionine.

Maximum Strength Glucosamine Chondroitin - Puritan's Pride
Three tablets contain: Glucosamine Hydrochloride 1500 mg • Chondroitin Sulfate 1200 mg.
See Editor's Note No. 15.

Maximum Wellness Formula - Pro Health
Each scoop (10.2 g) contains: Vitamin A (beta carotene) 7500 IU • Vitamin C (ascorbic acid) 500 mg • Vitamin D (cholecalciferol) 400 IU • Vitamin E (D-alpha tocopheryl succinate) 200 IU • Thiamin (vitamin B1) 100 mg • Riboflavin (vitamin B2) 100 mg • Niacin (vitamin B3 as inositol hexaniacinate) 35 mg • Vitamin B6 (pyridoxine HCl) 80 mg • Folic Acid 800 mcg • Vitamin B12 (cyanocobalamin) 1000 mcg • Biotin 300 mcg • Pantothenic Acid (D-calcium pantothenate) 25 mg • Calcium (calcium carbonate, amino acid chelate) 600 mg • Iodine (from kelp) 150 mcg • Magnesium (magnesium glycinate, aspartate) 300 mg • Zinc (zinc picolinate) 25 mg • Selenium (selenium amino acid chelate) 300 mcg • Copper (copper gluconate) 1 mg • Manganese (manganese glycinate) 4 mg • Chromium (as ChromeMate brand chromium polynicotinate) 200 mcg • Molybdenum (molybdenum amino acid chelate) 300 mcg • Potassium (potassium aspartate) 110 mg • Alpha Lipoic Acid 100 mg • Boron (boron amino acid chelate) 1.5 mg • ColostruMune brand Colostrum (from bovine) 1000 mg • Fructo-Oligosaccharides (cichorium intybus root) 250 mg • Korean Ginseng powder (panax ginseng root) 200 mg • Inositol 1000 mg • Malic Acid from Apple 900 mg • OptiMSM brand Methylsulfonylmethane 500 mg • Whey Protein Hydrosylate 5.4 g • Alanine 273 mg • Arginine 143 mg • Aspartic Acid 520 mg • Cysteine 122 mg • Glutamic Acid 83 mg • Glycine 98 mg • Histidine 88 mg • Isoleucine 253 mg • Leucine 617 mg • Lysine 483 mg • Methionine 117 mg • Phenylalanine 179 mg • Proline 246 mg • Serine 209 mg • Threonine 241 mg • Tryptophan 95 mg • Tyrosine 206 mg • Valine 262 mg.

Maxine Gentle Iron-Free - Country Life Vitamins
Each two capsules contain: Vitamin A (as beta-carotene, natural mixed carotenoids, retinyl palmitate) 5000 IU • Vitamin C (as calcium ascorbate, potassium ascorbate, ascorbyl palmitate, magnesium ascorbate) 300 mg • Vitamin D (as ergocalciferol) 200 IU • Vitamin E (as d-alpha tocopheryl acid succinate) 200 IU • Vitamin K (as phytonadione) 50 mcg • Thiamin (vitamin B1 as thiamine HCl) 25 mg • Riboflavin (vitamin B2) 25 mg • Niacin 30 mg • Vitamin B6 200 mg • Folic Acid 800 mcg • Vitamin B12 (as cyanocobalamin) 500 mcg • d-Biotin 300 mcg • Pantothenic Acid (as d-calcium pantothenate) 200 mg • Calcium (as calcium hydroxyapatite, tricalcium phosphate, ascorbate, citrate) 200 mg • Phosphorous (as calcium hydroxyapatite) 84 mg • Iodine (from kelp) 225 mcg • Magnesium (as rice chelate, oxide, ascorbate) 300 mg • Zinc (as zinc monomethionine) 15 mg • Selenium (as l-selenomethionine) 100 mcg • Copper (as citrate) 1 mg • Manganese (as citrate) 5 mg • Chromium (as chromium picolinate) 100 mcg • Molybdenum (as molybdenum citrate) 50 mcg • Potassium (as potassium citrate, ascorbate) 99 mg • Inositol 100 mg • L-Tyrosine (free form) 100 mg • Chaste Berry extract (4:1) 50 mg • Choline (from 100 mg choline bitartrate) 45 mg • PABA (para-aminobenzoic acid) 30 mg • Ashwagandha extract (8:1, root) 25 mg • Grape Skin extract 25 mg • Grape Seed extract 25 mg • Enzyme Blend 25 mg: Papain 10525 PU, Lipase 300 LU, Protease 12 SAPU, Lactase 7 LACU, Alpha-Galactosidase 3 AGSU, Phytase 3 PHU, Bromelain 1 STU, Alpha-Amylase 1 SKBU • Marigold extract 20 mg • Black Pepper extract (bioprene) 2 mg • Boron (as boron citrate) 1 mg • Vanadium (from 2.8 mg of BGOV) 500 mcg. Inactive Ingredients: Cellulose, Silica, Gum Acacia, Magnesium Stearate.

Maxi-Sorb Carni Q-Gel + E - Country Life Vitamins
Each softgel contains: Vitamin C (as ascorbyl palmitate) 12 mg • Vitamin E (as dl-alpha tocopherol) 75 IU • L-Carnitine (from 440 mg of l-carnitine fumerate) 250 mg • Coenzyme Q10 30 mg. Inactive Ingredients: Medium Chain Triglycerides, Polysorbate 80, Triacetin, Lecithin, Gelatin, Glycerin, Sorbitol, Purified Water, Annatto Seed Extract Color, Carob Pod Extract, Beeswax, Titanium Dioxide Color.

Maxi-Sorb CoQ10 with 150 IU of Vitamin E - Country Life Vitamins
Each softgel contains: Vitamin E (as dl-tocopheryl acetate) 150 IU • Coenzyme Q-10 60 mg. Inactive Ingredients: Polysorbate 80, Gelatin, Medium Chain Triglycerides, Glycerin, Lecithin, Sorbitol, Triacetin, Purified Water, Titanium Dioxide, Color, Annatto Seed Extract Color.

Maxogenol - Nutraceutics Corp.
Two caplets contain: Proprietary Blend 300 mg: Grape seed extract, Grape skin extract, Green Tea extract, Coastal White Pine extract, Bilberry, Alpha Tocotrienol, Gamma Tocotrienol, Carotinoids, Co Enzyme Q6-10.

MaxoPlex - Pharmessen
Each capsule contains: Cinnamon leaf oil 3.5 mg • Mountain Savory oil (satureja montana) 3.5 mg • Clove oil 3.5 mg • Headed Savory oil (thymus capitatus) 1.75 mg. Other Ingredients: Methylcellulose, Avicel, Olive Oil, Aerosil, Capsule (Kosher & Pareve, and Halal).

MaxStar - Johnston-Keay Laboratories, Inc
Each tablet contains: Vitamin B6 (from pyridoxine hydrochloride) 5 mg • Magnesium Aspartate 50 mg • Green Tea leaf (camellia sinensis, 50% polyphenols, 4-9% caffeine) 325 mg • Fructose 1-6 Diphosphate 125 mg • Panax Ginseng root (8% ginsenoside) 60 mg • Ginkgo Biloba leaf (24%/6%) 40 mg • Yerba Mate leaf (iled paraguariensis) 40 mg • Guarana seeds (paullinia cupana) 40 mg • Thermogenic Herbal Concentrate 40 mg: Peppermint leaf, Verbena herb, Cinnamon bark, Ginger root, Orange peel, Cayenne pepper, Chicory root. Other Ingredients: Calcium Carbonate, Microcrystalline Cellulose, Croscarmellose Sodium, Stearic Acid, Magnesium Stearate, Pharmaceutical Glaze.

MaxxLength3 - MK Supplements
Two tablets contain: Zinc (as zinc oxide) 20 mg • Yohimbe bark 225 mg • Maca 120 mg • Epimedium Sagittatum 120 mg • Oat straw 45 mg • Catuaba • Ginseng root • L-Arginine • Nettle leaf • Cayenne (fruit) • Muira Puama whole herb • Orchic Substance • Oyster meat powder • Tribulus Terrestris • Sarsaparilla • Astragalus root • Pumpkin seed • Boron (as boron citrate).
See Editor's Note No. 14.

MBX (Meta-Burn Xtreme) - Metabolic Response Modifiers
Each capsule contains: Caffeine (USP) 90 mg • 1R, 2S-norephedrine (HCl) 25 mg • Coleus Forskohlii (20% forskolin) 25 mg • Naringin 5 mg • Yohimbine (HCl) 2.75 mg.

MCHC Calcium - Progressive Labs
Each capsule contains: Vitamin D (D3, as cholecalciferol) 100 IU • Vitamin K (phytonadione) 20 mcg • Calcium (elemental from microcrystalline calcium hydroxyapatite - MCHC - 500 mg, calcium citrate 500 mg) 250 mg • Phosphorus (from MCHC) 65 mg • Magnesium (from MCHC) 4 mg • Zinc (from MCHC) 0.075 mg • Copper (from MCHC) 0.01 mg • Manganese (from MCHC) 0.045 mg • Potassium (from MCHC) 0.035 mg • Protein (from MCHC as

collagen glycosaminoglycans) 125 mg • Boron (as aspartate) 750 mg • Fluorapatite (from MCHC) 31 mg • Silicon (from MCHC) 19 mg • Strontium (from MCHC) 10 mcg. Other Ingredients: Magnesium Stearate, Gelatin.

MCH-Cal **- Natrol, Inc.**
Two capsules contain: Vitamin D (as Cholecalciferol) 200 IU • Calcium (as calcium hydroxyapatite) 125 mg • Magnesium (as Magnesium oxide) 300 mg. Other Ingredients: Magnesium Stearate, Silicon Dioxide, Gelatin.

MCT Fuel (Emulsified Medium-Chain Triglycerides) **- TwinLab**
Emulsified Medium Chain Triglycerides (MCTs) • Emulsified Vitamin E. Contains: 100% natural Orange flavor & small amounts of Lecithin & Apple Pectin.

MD6 **- BioTest Laboratories, LLC**
Two capsules contain: L-Tyrosine 200 mg • Alpha Lipoic Acid 200 mg • Caffeine 100 mg • 5hydroxy L-Tryptophan 25 mg • Yohimbe HCl 5 mg • Ephedra Sinica extra 335 mg. Other Ingredients: Gelatin, Magnesium Stearate, Cellulose.
See Editor's Note No. 21 and No. 30.

Meal Shakes (Bavarian cocoa flavor) **- Shaklee**
Nonfat Dry Milk, Fructose, Acacia Gum, Calcium Sodium Caseinate, Lowfat Cocoa Processed with Alkali, Maltodextrin, Natural Flavors, Magnesium Oxide, Soy Lecithin, Xanthan Gum, Ascorbic Acid, Selenium Yeast, Chromium Yeast, Ferrous Fumarate, D-alpha Tocopheryl Acetate, Molybdenum Yeast, Niacinamide, Vitamin A Palmitate, Zinc Oxide, Copper Gluconate, Calcium Pantothenate, Manganese Sulfate, Vitamin B12, Pyridoxine Hydrochloride, Vitamin D, Thiamin Mononitrate, Folic Acid, Biotin, Riboflavin, Potassium Iodide.

Meal Shakes (French vanilla flavor) **- Shaklee**
Nonfat Dry Milk, Fructose, Maltodextrin, Acacia Gum, Calcium Sodium Caseinate, Natural Flavors, Magnesium Oxide, Soy Lecithin, Xanthan Gum, Ascorbic Acid, Selenium Yeast, Chromium Yeast, Ferrous Fumarate, D-alpha Tocopheryl Acetate, Molybdenum Yeast, Niacinamide, Vitamin A Palmitate, Zinc Oxide, Copper Gluconate, Calcium Pantothenate, Manganese Sulfate, Vitamin B12, Pyridoxine Hydrochloride, Vitamin D, Thiamin Mononitrate, Folic Acid, Biotin, Riboflavin, Potassium Iodide.

Meda C-Block **- MedaBiotics**
Two capsules contain: Chromium (as chromium dinicotinate glycinate) 100 mcg • Phaseolamin White Kidney bean extract 700 mg • Green Tea leaf extract (50% catechins and 35% polyphenols) 200 mg. Other Ingredients: Gelatin, Dicalcium Phosphate, Magnesium Stearate, Silica.

Meda F-Block **- MedaBiotics**
Two capsules contain: Vitamin C (as ascorbic acid) 100 mg • Chitosan (marine fiber concentrate) 1000 mg • Calcium 150 mg • Vegetable Cellulose 100 mg. Other Ingredients: Gelatin, Dicalcium Phosphate, Magnesium Stearate, Silica.

MedCaps DPO **- Xymogen**
Four capsules contain: Calcium D-Glucarate 100 mg • Vitamin B6 (as pyridoxal 5'-phosphate) 50 mg • Folate (as folic acid) 800 mcg • Vitamin B12 (as methylcobalamin) 200 mcg • Artichoke leaf extract 600 mg • Watercress powder 500 mg • Silymarin (from milk thistle seed extract) 210 mg • Alpha Lipoic Acid 200 mg • N-Acetyl Cysteine 200 mg • Sodium Sulfate 200 mg • Catechins from Green Tea leaf extract 150 mg • Ellagic Acid from Pomegranate fruit extract 150 mg • MSM (methylsulfonylmethane) 100 mg. Other Ingredients: Cellulose, Stearic Acid, Silicon Dioxide.

MedCaps GI **- Xymogen**
Four capsules contain: Pantothenic Acid (as calcium D-pantothenate) 100 mg • Zinc (as bis-glycinate chelate) 15 mg • Inulin 800 mg • L-Glutamine 500 mg • Aloe leaf extract 50 mg.

MedCaps IS **- Xymogen**
Two capsules contain: Thiamine (as thiamine hydrochloride) 100 mg • Niacin (as niacinamide) 100 mg • Biotin 10 mg • Chromium (as chromium polynicotinate) 1000 mcg • Fenugreek seed 15:1 extract 300 mg • Bitter Gourd extract 2.5% 150 mg • Gymnema Sylvestre extract 25% 100 mg • Vanadium (as vanadyl sulfate) 5 mg.

MedCaps Menopause **- Xymogen**
Four capsules contain: Panax Ginseng root powder 400 mg • Hesperidin 200 mg • Para Amino Benzoic Acid (PABA) 200 mg • Licorice root extract (12% glycyrrhizin) 150 mg • Wild Yam root 10:1 extract 100 mg • Black Cohosh root extract (2.5% triterpenes) 100 mg • Dong Quai root extract 100 mg • Isoflavones (as kudzu root extract) 100 mg • Resveratrol 2000 mcg • Boron (as boron citrate) 100 mcg.

MedCaps PMS **- Xymogen**
Four capsules contain: Vitamin B6 (as pyridoxal-5'-phosphate) 50 mg • Folate (as folic acid and calcium folinate) 800 mcg • Vitamin B12 (as methylcobalamin) 100 mcg • Magnesium (as magnesium chelate) 200 mg • Chelazome brand Zinc 15 mg • Calcium D-Glucarate 100 mg • Chasteberry extract (vitex) 100 mg • Ashwaganda root powder 100 mg • Indole 3 Carbinol 100 mg • RoseOx brand Rosemary leaf extract 25 mg • Resveratrol 2 mg.

MedCaps T3 **- Xymogen**
Four capsules contain: Vitamin A (as retinyl palmitate) 3000 IU • Vitamin D (as cholecalciferol) 400 IU • Vitamin E (as D-alpha tocopherol succinate) 100 IU • Iodine (as atlantic kelp) 150 mcg • Zinc (as zinc citrate) 10 mg • Selenium (as L-selenomethionine) 400 mcg • Guggulsterones (from guggul extract) 100 mg • Rosemary leaf extract 100 mg • Ashwaganda root powder 100 mg.

Mederma **- Merz Pharmaceuticals**
Purified Water • PEG-4 • Onion (Allium cepa) extract • Xanthan Gum • Allantoin • Fragrance • Methylparaben • Sorbic Acid.

Medicated Cold Sore Balm w/Bee Propolis **- Thayers Natural Pharmaceuticals**
Camphor • Peppermint Oil (menthol source). A gentle base of Castor Oil, Beeswax, Wheat Germ Oil, Carnuba Palm Wax, Lanolin, Propolis, Vitamin E.

MediHerb Albizia 1:2 **- Standard Process, Inc.**
Each 5 mL serving contains: Albizia 1:2 extract 5 mL. Other Ingredients: Purified Water, 25% alcohol.

MediHerb Albizia Complex **- Standard Process, Inc.**
Each tablet contains: Baikal Skullcap root 3:1 extract (from scutellaria baicalensis) 800 mg • Albizia bark 4:1 extract (from albizia lebbek) 800 mg • Feverfew leaf powder (tanacetum parthenium) 50 mg • Calcium 40 mg. Other Ingredients: Calcium Acid Phosphate, Cellulose, Sodium Starch Glycollate, Silica, Hypromellose, Magnesium Stearate.

MediHerb Aloe Vera 4.5:1 **- Standard Process, Inc.**
Each 25 mL serving contains: Aloe Vera leaf (from aloe barbadensis, 4.5:1, containing acemannan 281 mg) 25 mL • Stevia leaf 1:2 extract (from stevia rebaudiana leaf 250 mg) 500 mcL. Other Ingredients: Natural Citrus Flavors, Purified Water.

MediHerb Andrographis Complex **- Standard Process, Inc.**
Each tablet contains: Echinacea root 4:1 extract (from echinacea angustifolia 500 mg) 125 mg • Holy Basil leaf 4:1 extract (from ocimum tenuiflorum 500 mg) 125 mg • Andrographis herb 10:1 extract (from andrographis paniculata 1 g, containing andrographolide 10 mg) 100 mg • Holy Basil leaf essential oil (ocimum tenuiflorum) 10 mg • Calcium 40 mg. Other Ingredients: Calcium Acid Phosphate, Cellulose, Hypromellose, Silica, Sodium Starch Glycollate, Magnesium Stearate.

MediHerb Ashwaganda 1:2 **- Standard Process, Inc.**
Each 5 mL serving contains: Ashwaganda root 1:2 extract (from withania somnifera root 2.5 g) 5 mL. Other Ingredients: Purified Water, 45% Alcohol.

Some Brand Name Natural Products - What they Contain

www.NaturalDatabase.com contains MANY more listings than appear here.
Editor's Notes are located on pages 2155-2163.

MediHerb Astragalus 1:2 **-** Standard Process, Inc.
Each 5 mL serving contains: Astragalus root 1:2 extract (from astragalus membranaceus 2.5 g,) 5 mL. Other Ingredients: Purified Water, 25% Alcohol.

MediHerb Astragalus Complex **-** Standard Process, Inc.
Each tablet contains: Astragalus root 4:1 extract (from astragalus membranaceus 850 mg) 212.5 mg • Echinacea root 6:1 extract (from echinacea purpurea 650 mg) 108.3 mg • Eleuthero root 10:1 extract (from eleutherococcus senticosus 750 mg, containing eleutheroside E 570 mcg) 75 mg • Calcium 40 mg. Other Ingredients: Cellulose, Calcium Acid Phosphate, Silica, Sodium Starch Glycollate, Hypromellose, Magnesium Stearate.

MediHerb Bacopa 1:2 **-** Standard Process, Inc.
Each 5 mL serving contains: Bacopa herb 1:2 extract (from bacopa monnieri 2.5 g) 5 mL. Other Ingredients: Purified Water, 25% Alcohol.

MediHerb Bacopa Complex **-** Standard Process, Inc.
Each tablet contains: Schisandra fruit 4:1 extract (from schisandra chinensis 650 mg) 162.5 mg • Eleuthero root 10:1 extract (from eleutherococcus senticosus 500 mg, containing eleutheroside E 380 mcg) 50 mg • Bacopa herb 50:1 extract (from bacopa monnieri herb 1.5 g, containing bacosides 15 mg) 30 mg • Rosemary oil 10 mg • Calcium 40 mg. Other Ingredients: Calcium Acid Phosphate, Cellulose, Hypromellose, Magnesium Stearate, Silica, Sodium Starch Glycollate.

MediHerb Baical Skullcap 1:2 **-** Standard Process, Inc.
Each 5 mL serving contains: Baikal Skullcap root 1:2 extract (from scutallaria baicalensis root 2.5 g) 5 mL. Other Ingredients: Purified Water, 60% alcohol.

MediHerb Bilberry 1:1 **-** Standard Process, Inc.
Each 5 mL serving contains: Bilberry fruit fresh 1:1 extract (from vaccinium myrtillus fruit fresh 5 g) 5 mL. Other Ingredients: Purified Water, 25% Alcohol.

MediHerb Bilberry 6000 mg **-** Standard Process, Inc.
Each tablet contains: Bilberry fruit fresh 100:1 extract (from vaccinium myrtillus fruit fresh 6 g, containing anthocyanosides 15 mg) 60 mg • Calcium 20 mg. Other Ingredients: Calcium Acid Phosphate, Cellulose, Magnesium Stearate, Sodium Starch Glycollate, Silica.

MediHerb Black Cohosh 1:2 **-** Standard Process, Inc.
Each 2.5 mL serving contains: Black Cohosh root 1:2 extract (from cimicifuga racemosa 1.25 g) 2.5 mL. Other Ingredients: Purified Water, 60% Alcohol.

MediHerb Black Haw 1:2 **-** Standard Process, Inc.
Each 5 mL serving contains: Black Haw bark 1:2 extract (from viburnum prunifolium 2.5 g) 5 mL. Other Ingredients: Purified Water, 30% Alcohol.

MediHerb Black Walnut Hulls 1:10 **-** Standard Process, Inc.
Each 5 mL serving contains: Black Walnut hulls 1:10 extract (from juglans nigra 500 mg) 5 mL. Other Ingredients: Purified Water, 60% Alcohol.

MediHerb Bladderwrack 1:1 **-** Standard Process, Inc.
Each 5 mL serving contains: Bladderwrack herb 1:1 extract (from fucus vesiculosus 5 g) 5 mL. Other Ingredients: Purified Water, 25% Alcohol.

MediHerb Blue Cohosh 1:2 **-** Standard Process, Inc.
Each 2.5 mL serving contains: Blue Cohosh root 1:2 extract (from caulophyllum thalictroides 1.25 g) 2.5 mL. Other Ingredients: Purified Water, 70% alcohol.

MediHerb Boswellia Complex **-** Standard Process, Inc.
Each tablet contains: Boswellia gum resin 4:1 extract (from boswellia serrata 1.2 g, containing boswellic acids 180 mg) 300 mg • Celery seed fruit 6:1 extract (from apium graveolens 1 g) 166.7 mg • Ginger rhizome 5:1 extract (from zingiber officinales 300 mg) 60 mg • Turmeric rhizome 25:1 extract (from curcuma longa 2 g, containing curcuminoids 70.4 mg) 80 mg • Calcium 40 mg. Other Ingredients: Calcium Acid Phosphate, Cellulose, Hypromellose, Magnesium Stearate, Silica, Sodium Starch Glycollate.

MediHerb Broncafect **-** Standard Process, Inc.
Two tablets contain: Licorice root 3.5:1 extract (from glycyrrhiza glabra 1.5 g) 428.6 mg • Pleurisy root 4:1 extract (from asclepias tuberosa 750 mg) 187.5 mg • Echinacea Purpurea root 6:1 extract (from echinacea purpurea 750 mg) 125 mg • White Horehound herb 4:1 extract (from marrubium vulgare 360 mg) 90 mg • Ginger rhizome 5:1 extract (from zingiber officinale 360 mg) 72 mg • Thyme oil 20 mg • Calcium 80 mg. Other Ingredients: Calcium Acid Phosphate, Hypromellose, Silica, Sodium Starch Glycollate, Magnesium Stearate, Cellulose.

MediHerb Broncafect Phytosynergist **-** Standard Process, Inc.
Each 5 mL serving contains: Echinacea root 1:2 extract (from echinacea angustifolia 500 mg) 1 mL • Licorice root 1:1 extract (from glycyrrhiza glabra 1 g) 1 mL • Pleurisy root 1:2 extract (from asclepias tuberosa 500 mg) 1 mL • Thyme leaf 1:2 extract (from thymus vulgaris 500 mg) 1 mL • Ginger rhizome 1:2 extract (from zingiber officinale 250 mg) 500 mcL • White Horehound herb 1:2 extract (from marrubium vulgare 250 mg) 500 mcL. Other Ingredients: Purified Water, 43% Alcohol.

MediHerb Buchu 1:2 **-** Standard Process, Inc.
Each 5 mL serving contains: Buchu leaf 1:2 extract (from barosma betulina 2.5 g) 5 mL. Other Ingredients: Purified Water, 60% Alcohol.

MediHerb Bugleweed 1:2 **-** Standard Process, Inc.
Each 5 mL serving contains: Bugleweed herb extract (from lycopus virginicus 2.5 g) 5 mL. Other Ingredients: Purified Water, Alcohol.

MediHerb Bupleurum 1:2 **-** Standard Process, Inc.
Each 5 mL serving contains: Bupleurum root 1:2 extract (from bupleurum falcatum 2.5 g) 5 mL. Other Ingredients: Purified Water, 45% Alcohol.

MediHerb Burdock 1:2 **-** Standard Process, Inc.
Each 5 mL serving contains: Burdock root 1:2 extract (from arctium lappa 2.5 g) 5 mL. Other Ingredients: Purified Water, 25% Alcohol.

MediHerb Burdock Complex **-** Standard Process, Inc.
Each tablet contains: Burdock root powder (arctium lappa) 242 mg • Sheep Sorrel herb powder (rumex acetosella) 130 mg • Slippery Elm stem bark powder (ulmus rubra) 32 mg • Rhubarb root powder (rheum palmatum) 8 mg • Calcium 40 mg. Other Ingredients: Calcium Acid Phosphate, Cellulose, Hypromellose, Magnesium Stearate, Silica, Sodium Starch Glycollate.

MediHerb Calendula 1:2 **-** Standard Process, Inc.
Each 5 mL serving contains: Calendula flower 1:2 extract (from calendula officinalis 2.5 g) 5 mL. Other Ingredients: Purified Water, 90% Alcohol.

MediHerb Californian Poppy 1:2 **-** Standard Process, Inc.
Each 5 mL serving contains: California Poppy herb 1:2 extract (from eschscholtzia californica 2.5 g) 5 mL. Other Ingredients: Purified Water, 45% Alcohol.

MediHerb Capsella Complex Phytosynergist **-** Standard Process, Inc.
Each 5 mL serving contains: Dong Quai root 1:2 extract (from angelica sinensis 750 mg) 1.5 mL • False Unicorn root 1:2 extract (from chamaelirium luteum 625 mg) 1.25 mL • Shepherd's Purse herb 1:2 extract (from capsella bursa-pastoris 625 mg) 1.25 mL • White Peony root 1:2 extract (from paeonia lactiflora root 500 mg) 1 mL. Other Ingredients: Purified Water, 40% Alcohol.

MediHerb Cat's Claw 1:2 **-** Standard Process, Inc.
Each 5 mL serving contains: Cat's Claw inner bark 1:2 extract (from uncaria tomentosa 2.5 g) 5 mL. Other Ingredients: Purified Water, 60% Alcohol.

Some Brand Name Natural Products - What they Contain

www.NaturalDatabase.com contains MANY more listings than appear here.
Editor's Notes are located on pages 2155-2163.

BRAND NAMES

MediHerb Cat's Claw Complex - Standard Process, Inc.
Each tablet contains: Cat's Claw inner stem bark 5:1 extract (from uncaria tomentosa 1.5 g) 300 mg • Pau d'Arco inner stem bark 5:1 extract (from tabebuia avellanedae 500 mg) 100 mg • Echinacea root 6:1 extract (from echinaca purpurea 500 mg) 83.3 mg • Calcium 40 mg. Other Ingredients: Calcium Acid Phosphate, Cellulose, Hypromellose, Magnesium Stearate, Silica, Sodium Starch Glycollate.

MediHerb Celery Seed 1:2 - Standard Process, Inc.
Each 5 mL serving contains: Celery seed fruit 1:2 extract (from apium graveolens 2.5 g) 5 mL. Other Ingredients: Purified Water, 60% Alcohol.

MediHerb Chamomile High Grade 1:2 - Standard Process, Inc.
Each 5 mL serving contains: Chamomile flower 1:2 extract (from matricaria recutita 2.5 g, containing bisabolol 2 mg) 5 mL. Other Ingredients: Purified Water, 60% Alcohol.

MediHerb Chaste Tree - Standard Process, Inc.
Each tablet contains: Chaste Tree fruit 6:1 extract (from vitex agnus-castus 500 mg) 83.3 mg • Calcium 60 mg. Other Ingredients: Calcium Acid Phosphate, Cellulose, Hypromellose, Magnesium Stearate, Silica, Sodium Starch Glycollate.

MediHerb Chaste Tree 1:2 - Standard Process, Inc.
Each 1 mL serving contains: Chaste Tree fruit 1:2 extract (from vitex agnus-castus 500 mg) 1 mL. Other Ingredients: Purified Water, 60% Alcohol.

MediHerb Cinnamon Quills 1:2 - Standard Process, Inc.
Each 5 mL serving contains: Cinnamon quills stem bark 1:2 extract (from cinnamomum zeylanicum 2.5 g) 5 mL. Other Ingredients: Purified Water, 70% Alcohol.

MediHerb Cleavers 1:2 - Standard Process, Inc.
Each 5 mL serving contains: Cleavers herb 1:2 extract (from galium aparine 2.5 g) 5 mL. Other Ingredients: Purified Water, 25% Alcohol.

MediHerb Colax - Standard Process, Inc.
Each tablet contains: Cascara stem bark 4:1 extract (from rhamnus purshiana 560 mg) 140 mg • Dandelion root 4:1 extract (from taraxacum officinale 375 mg) 93.75 mg • Yellow Dock root 4:1 extract (from rumex crispus 375 mg) 93.75 mg • Dill seed 4:1 extract (from anethum graveolens 375 mg) 93.75 mg • Chamomile flower 4:1 extract (from matricaria recutita 280 mg) 70 mg • Calcium 40 mg. Other Ingredients: Calcium Acid Phosphate, Cellulose, Hypromellose, Magnesium Stearate, Silica, Sodium Starch Glycollate.

MediHerb Coleus 1:1 - Standard Process, Inc.
Each 5 mL serving contains: Coleus Forskohlii root 1:1 extract (from coleus forskholii 5 g, containing forskolin 12.5 mg) 5 mL. Other Ingredients: Purified Water, 50% Alcohol.

MediHerb Corn Silk 1:1 - Standard Process, Inc.
Each 5 mL serving contains: Corn Silk styles and stigma 1:1 extract (from zea mays 5 g) 5 mL. Other Ingredients: Purified Water, 25% Alcohol.

MediHerb Cramp Bark 1:2 - Standard Process, Inc.
Each 5 mL serving contains: Cramp bark 1:2 extract (from viburnum opulus 2.5 g) 5 mL. Other Ingredients: Purified Water, 30% Alcohol.

MediHerb Cramplex - Standard Process, Inc.
Two tablets contain: Corydalis tuber 5:1 extract (from corydalis ambigua 1.2 g) 240 mg • Raspberry leaf 4:1 extract (from rubus ideaus 800 mg) 200 mg • Wild Yam root and rhizome 4:1 extract (from dioscorea villosa 800 mg) 200 mg • Cramp Bark stem bark 5:1 extract (from viburnum opulus 800 mg) 160 mg • Ginger rhizome 6:1 extract (from zingiber officinalis 800 mg) 133.3 mg • Calcium 124 mg. Other Ingredients: Calcium Acid Phosphate, Cellulose, Silica, Sodium Starch Glycollate, Magnesium Stearate, Hypromellose.

MediHerb Cranberry Complex - Standard Process, Inc.
Each tablet contains: Buchu leaf 4:1 extract (from barosma betulina 600 mg) 150 mg • Crataeva stem bark 8:1 extract (from crataeva nurvula 1 g) 125 mg • Uva Ursi leaf 4:1 extract (from arctostaphylos uva-ursi 500 mg) 125 mg • Cranberry fruit juice concentrate 25:1 (from vaccinium macrocarpon fruit fresh 2.5 g) 100 mg. Other Ingredients: Calcium Acid Phosphate, Cellulose, Hypromellose, Magnesium Stearate, Silica, Sodium Starch Glycollate.

MediHerb Cranesbill Root 1:2 - Standard Process, Inc.
Each 5 mL serving contains: Cranesbill root 1:2 extract (from geranium maculatum 2.5 g) 5 mL. Other Ingredients: Purified Water, 45% Alcohol.

MediHerb Damiana 1:2 - Standard Process, Inc.
Each 5 mL serving contains: Damiana leaf 1:2 extract (from turnera diffusa 2.5 g) 5 mL. Other Ingredients: Purified Water, 60% Alcohol.

MediHerb Dandelion Leaves 1:1 - Standard Process, Inc.
Each 5 mL serving contains: Dandelion leaf 1:1 extract (from taraxacum officinale 5 g) 5 mL. Other Ingredients: Purified Water, 25% Alcohol.

MediHerb Dandelion Root 1:2 - Standard Process, Inc.
Each 5 mL serving contains: Dandelion root 1:2 extract (from taraxacum officinale 2.5 g) 5 mL. Other Ingredients: Purified Water, 25% Alcohol.

MediHerb DermaCo - Standard Process, Inc.
Each tablet contains: Oregon Grape root and rhizome 4:1 extract (from berberis aquifolium (mahonia aquifolium) 360 mg) 90 mg • Sarsaparilla root and rhizome 4:1 extract (from smilax ornata 360 mg) 90 mg • Cleavers herb 5:1 extract (from galium aparine 360 mg) 72 mg • Burdock root 4:1 extract (from arctium lappa 270 mg) 67.5 mg • Yellow Dock root 4:1 extract (from rumex crispus 270 mg) 40 mg • Calcium 40 mg. Other Ingredients: Calcium Acid Phosphate, Cellulose, Hypromellose, Magnesium Stearate, Silica, Sodium Starch Glycollate.

MediHerb DiaCo Phytosynergist - Standard Process, Inc.
Each 5 mL serving contains: Echinacea root 1:2 extract (from echinacea angustifolia 500 mg) 1 mL • Elder flower 1:2 extract (from sambucus nigra 500 mg) 1 mL • Lime flower 1:2 extract (from tilia species 500 mg) 1 mL • Yarrow herb 1:2 extract (from achillea millefolium 500 mg) 1 mL • Ginger rhizome 1:2 extract (from zingiber officinale 250 mg) 500 mcL • Licorice root 1:1 extract (from glycyrrhiza glabra 500 mg) 500 mcL. Other Ingredients: Purified Water, 43% Alcohol.

Mediherb DiGest - Standard Process, Inc.
Each tablet contains: Dandelion root 4:1 extract (from taraxacum officinale 500 mg) 125 mg • Tangerine fruit peel 5:1 extract (from citrus reticulata 500 mg) 100 mg • Milk Thistle fruit 70:1 extract (from silybum marianum 2.1 g, containing flavanolignans calculated as silybin 24 mg) 30 mg • Ginger rhizome 5:1 extract (from zingiber officinale 100 mg) 20 mg • Gentian root 5:1 extract (from gentiana lutea 100 mg) 20 mg • Tangerine fruit peel oil (citrus reticulata) 12.5 mg • Chamomile flower essential oil (matricaria recutita) 5 mg • Calcium 52 mg. Other Ingredients: Cellulose, Calcium Acid Phosphate, Silica, Sodium Starch Glycollate, Hypromellose, Magnesium Stearate.

MediHerb DiGest Phytosynergist - Standard Process, Inc.
Each 5 mL serving contains: Chamomile flower 1:2 extract (from matricaria recutita 750 mg) 1.5 mL • Dandelion root 1:2 extract (from taraxacum officinale 500 mg) 1.5 mL • Echinacea root 1:2 extract (from echinacea angustifolia 500 mg) 1 mL • Milk Thistle seed 1:1 extract (from silybum marianum 1 g) 1 mL • Gentian root 1:2 extract (from gentiana lutea 100 mg) 200 mcL. Other Ingredients: Purified Water, 43% Alcohol.

MediHerb Dong Quai - Standard Process, Inc.
Each tablet contains: Dong Quai root 4:1 extract (from angelica sinensis 1 g) 250 mg • Calcium 20 mg. Other Ingredients: Calcium Acid Phosphate, Cellulose, Silica, Sodium Starch Glycollate, Hypromellose, Magnesium Stearate.

Some Brand Name Natural Products - What they Contain

www.NaturalDatabase.com contains MANY more listings than appear here.
Editor's Notes are located on pages 2155-2163.

MediHerb Dong Quai 1:2 - Standard Process, Inc.
Each 5 mL serving contains: Dong Quai root 1:2 extract (from angelica sinensis 2.5 g) 5 mL. Other Ingredients: Purified Water, 45% Alcohol.

MediHerb Echinacea Premium - Standard Process, Inc.
Each tablet contains: Echinacea root 4:1 extract (from echinacea angustifolia 600 mg, containing aklylamides 2 mg) 150 mg • Echinacea root 6:1 extract (from echinacea purpurea 675 mg, containing alkylamides 2.1 mg) 112.5 mg • Calcium 60 mg. Other Ingredients: Calcium Acid Phosphate, Cellulose, Silica, Sodium Starch Glycollate, Hypromellose, Magnesium Stearate.

MediHerb Echinacea Purpurea 1:2 - Standard Process, Inc.
Each 5 mL serving contains: Echinacea Purpurea root 1:2 extract (from echinacea purpurea 2.5 g) 5 mL. Other Ingredients: Purified Water, 60% Alcohol.

MediHerb Echinacea Purpurea 1:3 Glycetract - Standard Process, Inc.
Each 5 mL serving contains: Echinacea Purpurea root 1:3 extract (from echinacea purpurea 1.67 g) 5 mL. Other Ingredients: Purified Water, Glycerol, Potassium Sorbate.

MediHerb Echincea Premium Blend 1:2 - Standard Process, Inc.
Each 5 mL serving contains: Echinacea root 1:2 extract (from echinacea purpurea 1.5 g) 3 mL • Echinacea root 1:2 extract (from echinacea angustifolia 1 g, total alkylamides from both extracts 7.5 mg) 2 mL. Other Ingredients: Purified Water, 60% Alcohol.

MediHerb Eleuthero - Standard Process, Inc.
Each tablet contains: Eleuthero root 10:1 extract (from eleutherococcus senticosus 1.25 g, containing eleutheroside E 950 mcg) 125 mg • Calcium 20 mg. Other Ingredients: Calcium Acid Phosphate, Cellulose, Magnesium Stearate, Sodium Starch Glycollate.

MediHerb Eleuthero 1:2 - Standard Process, Inc.
Each 5 mL serving contains: Eleuthero 1:2 extract (from eleutherococcus senticosus 2.5 g, containing eleutheroside E 2.5 mg) 5 mL. Other Ingredients: Purified Water, 25% Alcohol.

MediHerb Euphrasia Complex - Standard Process, Inc.
Each tablet contains: Eyebright herb 4:1 extract (from euphrasia officinalis 650 mg) 162.5 mg • Golden Rod herb 4:1 extract (from solidago virgaurea 650 mg) 162.5 mg • Echinacea purpurea root 6:1 extract (from echinacea purpurea 370 mg) 61.67 mg • Golden Seal root and rhizome 3:1 extract (from hydrastis canadensis 125 mg) 41.67 mg • Cayenne fruit 4:1 extract (from capsicum annuum 10 mg) 2.5 mg • Calcium 60 mg. Other Ingredients: Calcium Acid Phosphate, Cellulose, Hypromellose, Magnesium Stearate, Silica, Sodium Starch Glycollate.

MediHerb Evening Primrose Oil - Standard Process, Inc.
Each capsule contains: Evening Primrose Oil (from oenothera biennis seed, containing gamma-linolenic acid 100 mg) 1 g. Other Ingredients: Gelatin.

MediHerb Eyebright 1:2 - Standard Process, Inc.
Each 5 mL serving contains: Eyebright herb 1:2 extract (from euphrasia officinalis 2.5 g) 5 mL. Other Ingredients: Purified Water, 45% Alcohol.

MediHerb Fe-Max Iron Tonic - Standard Process, Inc.
Each 5 mL serving contains: Iron (from ferrous gluconate) 5 mg • Vitamin C (ascorbic acid) 25 mg • Vitamin B6 (pyridoxine hydrochloride) 2.5 mg • Vitamin B2 (riboflavin) 2.5 mg • Vitamin B1 (thiamine hydrochloride) 2.5 mg • Folic Acid 150 mcg • Vitamin B12 (cyanocobalamin) 1.5 mcg • Codonopsis root 1:2 extract (from codonopsis pilosula 500 mg) 1 mL • Nettle leaf 1:2 extract (from urtica dioica 500 mg) 1 mL • Ashwaganda root 2:1 extract (from withania somnifera 500 mg) 1 mL • Vervain herb 2:1 extract (from verbena officinalis 250 mg) 500 mcL • Licorice root 2:1 extract (from glycrrhiza glabra 500 mg) 143 mg • Ginger rhizome 1:2 extract (from zingiber officinale 50 mg) 100 mcL • Stevia leaf 1:2 extract (from stevia rebaudiana 50 mg) 100 mcL. Other Ingredients: Glycerol, Purified Water, Fruit & Vegetable Juices: Beet Root, Grape, Pear, Apple, Carrot, Lemon.

MediHerb Feverfew - Standard Process, Inc.
Each tablet contains: Feverfew leaf powder (tanacetum parthenium, containing parthenolide 900 mcg) 150 mg • Calcium 60 mg. Other Ingredients: Calcium Acid Phosphate, Cellulose, Sodium Starch Glycollate, Silica, Magnesium Stearate.

MediHerb Ganoderma & Shiitake - Standard Process, Inc.
Each tablet contains: Shiitake mushroom 4:1 extract (from lentinula edodes 800 mg) 200 mg • Reishi mushroom 66:1 extract (from ganoderma lucidum 6.6 g) 100 mg • Calcium 60 mg. Other Ingredients: Calcium Acid Phosphate, Cellulose, Sodium Starch Glycollate, Silica, Hypromellose, Magnesium Stearate.

MediHerb Garlic 1:1 - Standard Process, Inc.
Each 5 mL serving contains: Garlic bulb fresh 1:1 extract (from allium sativum 5 g) 5 mL. Other Ingredients: Purified Water, 45% Alcohol.

MediHerb Garlic 5000mg - Standard Process, Inc.
Each tablet contains: Garlic bulb 6.5:1 extract (from allium sativum 1.04 g, containing alliin 4.3 mg) 160 mg • Allium Sativum bulb powder (containing alliin 1.4 mg) 100 mg • Calcium 20 mg. Other Ingredients: Calcium Acid Phosphate, Cellulose, Hypromellose, Magnesium Stearate, Enteric Coating, Sodium Starch Glycollate.

MediHerb Gentian 1:2 - Standard Process, Inc.
Each 1 mL serving contains: Gentian root 1:2 extract (from gentiana lutea 500 mg) 1 mL. Other Ingredients: Purified Water, 45% Alcohol.

MediHerb Ginger 1:2 - Standard Process, Inc.
Each 2.5 mL serving contains: Ginger rhizome 1:2 extract (from zingiber officinale 1.25 g) 2.5 mL. Other Ingredients: Purified Water, 90% Alcohol.

MediHerb Ginkgo 2:1 - Standard Process, Inc.
Each 1 mL serving contains: Ginkgo leaf 2:1 extract (from ginkgo biloba 2 g, containing ginkgo flavone glycosides 9.6 mg) 1 mL. Other Ingredients: Purified Water, 50% Alcohol.

MediHerb Ginkgo 2000mg - Standard Process, Inc.
Each tablet contains: Ginkgo Biloba leaf 50:1 extract (from ginkgo biloba 2 g, containing ginkgo flavone glycosides 10.68 mg, containing ginkgolides and bilobalide 2.68 mg) 40 mg • Calcium 40 mg. Other Ingredients: Calcium Acid Phosphate, Cellulose, Magnesium Stearate, Sodium Starch Glycollate.

MediHerb Globe Artichoke 1:2 - Standard Process, Inc.
Each 5 mL serving contains: Globe Artichoke leaf 1:2 extract (from cynara scolymus 2.5 g) 5 mL. Other Ingredients: Purified Water, 60% Alcohol.

MediHerb Golden Seal 1:3 - Standard Process, Inc.
Each 5 mL serving contains: Golden Seal root and rhizome 1:3 extract (from hydrastis canadensis 1.67 g, containing hydrastine 40 mg and berberine 40 mg) 5 mL. Other Ingredients: Purified Water, 45% Alcohol.

MediHerb Golden Seal 500mg - Standard Process, Inc.
Each tablet contains: Golden Seal root and rhizome 3:1 extract (from hydrastis canadensis 500 mg) 166.7 mg • Calcium 40 mg. Other Ingredients: Calcium Acid Phosphate, Cellulose, Hypromellose, Magnesium Stearate, Silica, Sodium Starch Glycollate.

MediHerb Gotu Kola 1:2 - Standard Process, Inc.
Each 5 mL serving contains: Gotu Kola herb 1:2 extract (from centella asiatica 2.5 g) 5 mL. Other Ingredients: Purified Water, 45% Alcohol.

MediHerb Grindelia 1:2 - Standard Process, Inc.
Each 5 mL serving contains: Grindelia herb 1:2 extract (from grindelia camporum 2.5 g) 5 mL. Other Ingredients: Purified Water, 60% Alcohol.

MediHerb Gymnema 1:1 **- Standard Process, Inc.**
Each 5 mL serving contains: Gymnema leaf 1:1 extract (from gymnema sylvestre 5 g) 5 mL. Other Ingredients: Purified Water, 25% Alcohol.

MediHerb Gymnema 4g **- Standard Process, Inc.**
Each tablet contains: Gymnema Sylvestre leaf 10:1 extract (from gymnema sylvestre 4 g, containing gymnemic acids 100 mg) 400 mg • Calcium 60 mg. Other Ingredients: Calcium Acid Phosphate, Cellulose, Hypromellose, Magnesium Stearate, Enteric Coating, Sodium Starch Glycollate.

MediHerb Hawthorn **- Standard Process, Inc.**
Each tablet contains: Hawthorn herb flowering top 3:1 extract (from crataegus monogyna 1 g, containing vitexin-2-rhamnoside 6.68 mg and catechin polymers 15 mg) 334 mg • Calcium 60 mg. Other Ingredients: Calcium Acid Phosphate, Cellulose, Hypromellose, Magnesium Stearate, Sodium Starch Glycollate.

MediHerb Hawthorn Berries 1:2 **- Standard Process, Inc.**
Each 5 mL serving contains: Hawthorn fruit 1:2 extract (from crataegus monogyna 2.5 g, containing oligomeric procyanidins 26 mg) 5 mL. Other Ingredients: Purified Water, 45% Alcohol.

MediHerb Herbal Throat Spray Phytosynergist **- Standard Process, Inc.**
Four sprays contain: Echinacea root 1:2 extract (from echinacea angustifolia 10 mg) 20 mcL • Calendula flower 1:2 extract (from calendula officinalis 10 mg) 20 mcL • Marshmallow root 1:5 extract (from althaea officinalis 40 mg) 200 mcL • Sage herb 1:2 extract (from salvia officinalis 30 mg) 60 mcL • Myrrh resin 1:5 extract (from commiphora mol-mol stem oleo-gum-resin 1 mg) 5 mcL • Clove oil (syzgium aromaticum) 1.25 mcL. Other Ingredients: Glycerol, Menthol, Propyl Hydroxybenzoate, Methyl Hydroxybenzoate, Purified Water, 16.25% Ethanol.

MediHerb HiPep Phytosynergist **- Standard Process, Inc.**
Each 5 mL serving contains: Licorice root 1:1 extract (from glycyrrhiza glabra 1.5 g) 1.5 mL • Meadowsweet herb 1:2 extract (from filipendula ulmaria 625 mg) 1.25 mL • Chickweed fresh herb succus (from stellaria media 1 g) 1 mL • Echinacea root 1:2 extract (from echinacea angustifolia 375 mg) 750 mcL • Golden Seal root and rhizome 1:3 extract (from hydrastis canadensis 167 mg) 500 mcL. Other Ingredients: Purified Water, 34% Alcohol.

MediHerb Horsechestnut 1:2 **- Standard Process, Inc.**
Each 5 mL serving contains: Horse Chestnut seed 1:2 extract (from aesculus hippocastanum 2.5 g) 5 mL. Other Ingredients: Purified Water, 35% Alcohol.

MediHerb HorseChestnut Complex **- Standard Process, Inc.**
Each tablet contains: Butcher's Broom root and rhizome 4:1 extract (from ruscus aculeatus 800 mg, containing ruscogenin 20 mg) 200 mg • Horse Chestnut seed 6:1 extract (from aesculus hippocastanum 1.2 g, containing escin 40 mg) 200 mg • Ginkgo Biloba leaf 50:1 extract (from ginkgo biloba 1.5 g, containing ginkgo flavone glycosides 7.3 mg and ginkgolides and bilobalide 1.8 mg) 30 mg • Calcium 20 mg. Other Ingredients: Calcium Acid Phosphate, Cellulose, Hypromellose, Magnesium Stearate, Silica, Sodium Starch Glycollate, Enteric Coating.

MediHerb Horsetail 1:2 **- Standard Process, Inc.**
Each 5 mL serving contains: Horsetail herb 1:2 extract (from equisetum arvense 2.5 g) 5 mL. Other Ingredients: Purified Water, 25% Alcohol.

MediHerb Hydrangea 1:2 **- Standard Process, Inc.**
Each 5 mL serving contains: Hydrangea root 1:2 extract (from hydrangea arborescens 2.5 g) 5 mL. Other Ingredients: Purified Water, 45% Alcohol.

MediHerb Jamaican Dogwood 1:2 **- Standard Process, Inc.**
Each 5 mL serving contains: Jamaican Dogwood root bark 1:2 extract (from piscidia erythrina 2.5 g) 5 mL. Other Ingredients: Purified Water, 60% Alcohol.

MediHerb Korean Ginseng 1:2 **- Standard Process, Inc.**
Each 2.5 mL serving contains: Korean Ginseng main root 1:2 extract (from Panax ginseng 1.25 g, containing ginsenosides as Rg1 and Rb1 27.5 mg) 2.5 mL. Other Ingredients: Purified Water, 60% Alcohol.

MediHerb Licorice 1:1 **- Standard Process, Inc.**
Each 2.5 mL serving contains: Licorice root 1:1 extract (from glycyrrhiza glabra 2.5 g) 2.5 mL. Other Ingredients: Purified Water, 20% Alcohol.

MediHerb Licorice High Grade 1:1 **- Standard Process, Inc.**
Each 2.5 mL serving contains: Licorice root 1:1 extract (from glycyrrhiza glabra 2.5 g, containing glycyrrhizin 75 mg) 2.5 mL. Other Ingredients: Purified Water, 20% Alcohol.

MediHerb LivCo **- Standard Process, Inc.**
Each tablet contains: Schisandra fruit (4:1 extract from schisandra chinensis fruit 1 g) 250 mg • Rosemary leaf (5:1 extract from rosmarinus officinalis leaf 500 mg) 100 mg •Milk Thistle seed (70:1 extract from silybum marianum seed 2 g, containing flavanoligans calc. as silybin 24 mg) 28.6 mg • Calcium 20 mg. Inactive Ingredients: Calcium Acid Phosphate, Cellulose, Sodium Starch Glycollate, Hypromellose, Magnesium Stearate.

MediHerb Livton Complex **- Standard Process, Inc.**
Each tablet contains: Globe Artichoke leaf 4:1 extract (from cynara scolymus 800 mg) 200 mg • Dandelion root 4:1 extract (from taraxacum officinale 400 mg) 100 mg • Milk Thistle fruit 70:1 extract (from silybum marianum 7 g, containing flavanolignans calculated as silybin 84 mg) 100 mg • Greater Celandine herb 5:1 extract (from chelidonium majus 200 mg) 50 mg • Fringe Tree root bark 5:1 extract (from chionanthus virginicus 160 mg) 32 mg • Calcium 40 mg. Other Ingredients: Calcium Acid Phosphate, Cellulose, Hypromellose, Magnesium Stearate, Silica, Sodium Starch Glycollate.

MediHerb Marshmallow root 1:5 Glycetract **- Standard Process, Inc.**
Each 5 mL serving contains: Marshmallow root 1:5 extract (from althaea officinalis root 1 g) 5 mL. Other Ingredients: Purified Water, Glycerol, Citrus Seed Extract.

MediHerb Milk Thistle 1:1 **- Standard Process, Inc.**
Each 5 mL serving contains: Milk Thistle seed 1:1 extract (from silybum marianum 5 g, containing flavanolignans calculated as silybin 125 mg) 5 mL. Other Ingredients: Purified Water, 70% Alcohol.

MediHerb Milk Thistle 1:1 Glycetract **- Standard Process, Inc.**
Each 5 mL serving contains: Milk Thistle seed 1:1 extract (from silybum marianum 5 g, containing flavanolignans calculated as silybin 50 mg) 5 mL. Other Ingredients: Purified Water, Glycerol, Citrus Seed Extract.

MediHerb Mistletoe 1:2 **- Standard Process, Inc.**
Each 5 mL serving contains: Mistletoe herb 1:2 extract (from viscum album 2.5 g) 5 mL. Other Ingredients: Purified Water, 45% Alcohol.

MediHerb Motherwort 1:2 **- Standard Process, Inc.**
Each 5 mL serving contains: Motherwort herb 1:2 extract (from leonurus cardiaca 2.5 g) 5 mL. Other Ingredients: Purified Water, 25% Alcohol.

MediHerb Nettle Leaf 1:2 **- Standard Process, Inc.**
Each 5 mL serving contains: Nettle leaf 1:2 extract (from urtica dioica 2.5 g) 5 mL. Other Ingredients: Purified Water, 25% Alcohol.

MediHerb Nettle Root 1:2 **- Standard Process, Inc.**
Each 5 mL serving contains: Nettle root 1:2 extract (from urtica dioica 2.5 g) 5 mL. Other Ingredients: Purified Water, 25% Alcohol.

MediHerb Nevaton **- Standard Process, Inc.**
Each tablet contains: Schisandra fruit 4:1 extract (from schisandra chinensis 675 mg) 168.8 mg • Damiana leaf 4:1 extract (from turnera diffusa 625 mg) 156.3 mg • Skullcap herb 4:1 extract (from scutellaria lateriflora 500 mg) 125 mg • St. John's Wort herb

flowering top 6:1 extract (from hypericum perforatum 750 mg, containing hypericins 413 mcg) 125 mg • Calcium 40 mg. Other Ingredients: Calcium Acid Phosphate, Cellulose, Hypromellose, Magnesium Stearate, Silica, Sodium Starch Glycollate.

MediHerb Oats Seed 1:1 - Standard Process, Inc.
Each 5 mL serving contains: Oats seed 1:1 extract (from avena sativa 5 g) 5 mL. Other Ingredients: Purified Water, 25% Alcohol.

MediHerb Oregon Grape 1:2 - Standard Process, Inc.
Each 5 mL serving contains: Oregon Grape root and rhizome 1:2 extract (from berberis aquifolium (mahonia aquifolium) 2.5 g) 5 mL. Other Ingredients: Purified Water, 25% Alcohol.

MediHerb Pasque Flower 1:2 - Standard Process, Inc.
Each 2.5 mL serving contains: Pasque Flower herb 1:2 extract (from anemone pulsatilla 1.25 g) 2.5 mL. Other Ingredients: Purified Water, 25% Alcohol.

MediHerb Pau d'Arco 1:2 - Standard Process, Inc.
Each 5 mL serving contains: Pau d'Arco bark 1:2 extract (from tabebuia avellanedae 2.5 g) 5 mL. Other Ingredients: Purified Water, 45% Alcohol.

MediHerb Poke Root 1:5 - Standard Process, Inc.
Each 1 mL serving contains: Poke Root root 1:5 extract (from phytolacca decandra 200 mg) 1 mL. Other Ingredients: Purified Water, 45% Alcohol.

MediHerb Prickly Ash 1:2 - Standard Process, Inc.
Each 2.5 mL serving contains: Prickly Ash bark 1:2 extract (from zanthoxylum clava-herculis 1.25 g) 2.5 mL. Other Ingredients: Purified Water, 45% Alcohol.

MediHerb PulmaCo - Standard Process, Inc.
Each tablet contains: Chinese Skullcap root 3:1 extract (from scutellaria baicalensis 500 mg) 166.7 mg • Malabar Nut Tree leaf 5:1 extract (from adhatoda vasica 750 mg) 150 mg • Grindelia herb 4:1 extract (from grindelia camporum 300 mg) 75 mg • Turmeric rhizome 25:1 extract (from curcuma longa 1 g, containing curcuminoids 38 mg) 40 mg • Ginkgo leaf 50:1 extract (from ginkgo biloba 1 g, containing ginkgo flavonglycosides 4.8 mg) 20 mg • Sweet Fennel seed essential oil (foeniculum vulgare) 5 mg • Calcium 40 mg. Other Ingredients: Cellulose, Calcium Acid Phosphate, Silica, Sodium Starch Glycollate, Hypromellose, Magnesium Stearate.

MediHerb Red Clover 1:2 - Standard Process, Inc.
Each 5 mL serving contains: Red Clover flower 1:2 extract (from trifolium pratense 2.5 g) 5 mL. Other Ingredients: Purified Water, 25% Alcohol.

MediHerb Rehmannia 1:2 - Standard Process, Inc.
Each 5 mL serving contains: Rehmannia root 1:2 extract (from rehmannia glutinosa 2.5 g) 5 mL. Other Ingredients: Purified Water, 25% Alcohol.

MediHerb Rehmannia Complex - Standard Process, Inc.
Each tablet contains: Rehmannia root 2.5:1 extract (from rehmannia glutinosa 350 mg) 140 mg • Bupleurum root 4.5:1 extract (from bupleurum falcatum 700 mg) 155.5 mg • Hemidesmus root 5:1 extract (from hemidesmus indicus 500 mg) 100 mg • Feverfew leaf and stem 3:1 extract (from tanacetum parthenium 165 mg) 55 mg • Calcium 59 mg. Other Ingredients: Cellulose, Calcium Hydrogen Phosphate, Silica, Sodium Starch Glycollate • Magnesium Stearate.

MediHerb ResCo - Standard Process, Inc.
Each tablet contains: Licorice root 3.5:1 extract (from glycyrrhiza glabra 500 mg) 142.9 mg • Mullein leaf 4:1 extract (from verbascum thapsus 470 mg) 117.5 mg • Euphorbia herb 4:1 extract (from euphorbia hirta 280 mg) 70 mg • Grindelia herb 4:1 extract (from gindelia camporum 280 mg) 70 mg • Ginger rhizome 5:1 extract (from zingiber officinale 180 mg) 36 mg • Fennel oil (fruit essential oil, foeniculum vulgare) 12 mg • Thyme oil (leaf essential oil, from thymus vulgaris) 12 mg • Calcium 40 mg. Other Ingredients: Calcium Acid Phosphate, Cellulose, Hypromellose, Magnesium Stearate, Silica, Sodium Starch Glycollate.

MediHerb ResCo Phytosynergist - Standard Process, Inc.
Each 5 mL serving contains: Mullein leaf 1:2 extract (from verbascum thapsus 625 mg) 1.25 mL • Licorice root 1:1 extract (from glycyrrhiza glabra 1 g) 1 mL • Elecampane root 1:2 (from inula helenium 375 mg) 750 mcL • Euphorbia herb 1:2 extract (from euphorbia hirta 375 mg) 750 mcL • Grindelia herb 1:2 extract (from grindelia camporum 375 mg) 750 mcL • Ginger rhizome 1:2 extract (from zingiber officinale 250 mg) 500 mcL • Fennel oil (foeniculum vulgare) 15 mcL. Other Ingredients: Purified Water, 46% Alcohol.

MediHerb Rhodiola & Ginseng Complex - Standard Process, Inc.
Each tablet contains: Rhodiola root 20:1 extract (from rhodiola rosea root 3 g containing rosavins 4.5 mg and salidroside 1.5 mg) 150 mg • Korean Ginseng root 5:1 extract (from panax ginseng root 500 mg containing ginsenosides as Rg1 and Rb1 8.4 mg) 100 mg. Other Ingredients: Cellulose, Calcium Acid Phosphate, Sodium Starch Glycollate, Hypromellose, Magnesium Stearate.

MediHerb Sage 1:2 - Standard Process, Inc.
Each 5 mL serving contains: Sage herb 1:2 extract (from salvia officinalis 2.5 g) 5 mL. Other Ingredients: Purified Water, 60% Alcohol.

MediHerb Saligesic - Standard Process, Inc.
Each tablet contains: White Willow stem bark 20:1 extract (from salix spp 8 g, containing salicin 60 mg) 400 mg • Calcium 30 mg.

MediHerb Sarsaparilla 1:2 - Standard Process, Inc.
Each 5 mL serving contains: Sarsaparilla root and rhizome 1:2 extract (from smilax ornata 2.5 g) 5 mL. Other Ingredients: Purified Water, 45% Alcohol.

MediHerb Saw Palmetto 1:2 - Standard Process, Inc.
Each 5 mL serving contains: Saw Palmetto fruit 1:2 extract (from serenoa serrulata 2.5 g) 5 mL. Other Ingredients: Purified Water, 45% Alcohol.

MediHerb Schisandra 1:2 - Standard Process, Inc.
Each 5 mL serving contains: Schisandra fruit 1:2 extract (from schisandra chinensis 2.5 g) 5 mL. Other Ingredients: Purified Water, 45% Alcohol.

MediHerb Serenoa Complex - Standard Process, Inc.
Each capsule contains: Saw Palmetto fruit 10:1 extract (from serenoa serrulata 1.6 g, containing serenoa serrulata fatty acids 144 mg) 160 mg. Other Ingredients: Pumpkin Seed Oil, Soya Oil, Gelatin, Glycerol.

MediHerb Silymarin - Standard Process, Inc.
Each tablet contains: Milk Thistle fruit 70:1 extract (from silybum marianum 14 g, containing flavonolignans calculated as silybin 168 mg) 200 mg • Calcium 20 mg. Other Ingredients: Calcium Acid Phosphate, Cellulose, Sodium Starch Glycollate, Silica, Magnesium Stearate.

MediHerb Skullcap 1:2 - Standard Process, Inc.
Each 5 mL serving contains: Skullcap 1:2 extract (from scutellaria lateriflora 2.5 g) 5 mL. Other Ingredients: Purified Water, 45% Alcohol.

MediHerb St. John's Wort 1.8g - Standard Process, Inc.
Each tablet contains: St. John's Wort herb flowering top 6:1 extract (from hypericum perforatum 1.8 g, containing hypericins 990 mcg and hyperforin 9 mg) 300 mg • Calcium 60 mg. Other Ingredients: Calcium Acid Phospahte, Cellulose, Hypromellose, Magnesium Stearate, Silica, Sodium Starch Glycollate.

MediHerb St. John's Wort 1:2 - Standard Process, Inc.
Each 5 mL serving contains: St. John's Wort herb flowering top 1:2 extract (from hypericum perforatum 2.5 g, containing hypericins 1 mg) 5 mL. Other Ingredients: Purified Water, 45% Alcohol.

MediHerb St. John's Wort High Grade 1:2 **- Standard Process, Inc.**
Each 5 mL serving contains: St. John's Wort flowering herb 1:2 extract (from hypericum perforatum 2.5 g, containing hypericins 2 mg) 5 mL. Other Ingredients: Purified Water, 60% Alcohol.

MediHerb Thyroid Complex **- Standard Process, Inc.**
Each tablet contains: Bladderwrack whole plant 3.5:1 extract (from fucus vesiculosus 1.05 g, containing iodine 600 mcg) 300 mg • Withania (ashwaganda) root 5:1 extract (from withania somnifera 600 mg) 120 mg • Bacopa herb 50:1 extract (from bacopa monnieri 2.5 g, containing bacosides 25 mg) 50 mg • Calcium 52 mg. Other Ingredients: Calcium Acid Phosphate, Cellulose, Sodium Starch Glycollate, Hypromellose, Silica, Magnesium Stearate.

MediHerb Tienchi Ginseng 1:2 **- Standard Process, Inc.**
Each 5 mL serving contains: Tienchi Ginseng root 1:2 extract (from Panax notoginseng 2.5 g) 5 mL. Other Ingredients: Purified Water, 45% Alcohol.

MediHerb Tribulus **- Standard Process, Inc.**
Each tablet contains: Tribulus herb 4.5:1 extract (from tribulus terrestris 2.79 g, containing furostanol saponins 100 mg) 620 mg • Calcium 24 mg. Other Ingredients: Calcium Acid Phosphate, Cellulose, Hypromellose, Magnesium Stearate, Sodium Starch Glycollate.

MediHerb Turmeric 1:1 **- Standard Process, Inc.**
Each 5 mL serving contains: Turmeric rhizome 1:1 extract (from curcuma longa 5 g) 5 mL. Other Ingredients: Purified Water, 45% Alcohol.

MediHerb UriCo Phytosynergist **- Standard Process, Inc.**
Each 5 mL serving contains: Couch Grass rhizome 1:1 extract (from agropyron repens 1.5 g) 1.5 mL • Echinacea root 1:2 extract (from echinacea angustifolia 625 mg) 1.25 mL • Licorice root 1:1 extract (from glycyrrhiza glabra 1.25 mg) 1.25 mL • Buchu leaf 1:2 extract (from barosma betulina 500 mg) 1 mL. Other Ingredients: Purified Water, 36% Alcohol.

MediHerb Uva Ursi 1:2 **- Standard Process, Inc.**
Each 5 mL serving contains: Uva Ursi leaf 1:2 extract (from arctostaphylos uva-ursi 2.5 g) 5 mL. Other Ingredients: Purified Water, 45% Alcohol.

MediHerb Valerian 1:2 **- Standard Process, Inc.**
Each 5 mL serving contains: Valerian root 1:2 extract (from valeriana officinalis 2.5 g) 5 mL. Other Ingredients: Purified Water, 45% Alcohol.

MediHerb Valerian Complex **- Standard Process, Inc.**
Each tablet contains: Spiny Jujube seed 5:1 extract (from zizyphus spinosa 900 mg) 180 mg • Valerian root and rhizome 5:1 extract (from valeriana officinalis 700 mg) 140 mg • Passion Flower herb 5:1 extract (from passiflora incarnata 500 mg) 100 mg • Calcium 40 mg. Other Ingredients: Calcium Acid Phosphate, Hypromellose, Magnesium Stearate, Silica, Sodium Starch Glycollate.

MediHerb Vervain 1:2 **- Standard Process, Inc.**
Each 5 mL serving contains: Vervain herb 1:2 extract (verbena officinalis) 5 mL. Other Ingredients: Purified water, 25% Alcohol.

MediHerb Vitanox **- Standard Process, Inc.**
Each tablet contains: Rosemary leaf 5:1 extract (from rosmarinus officinalis 1 g) 200 mg • Green Tea 6:1 extract (From camelia sinensis 1g, containing catechins 83.35 mg) 166.7 mg • Turmeric rhizome 25:1 extract (from curcuma longa 2 g, containing curcuminoids 70.4 mg) 80 mg • Grape seed 120:1 extract (from vitis vinifera 6 g, containing procyanidins 42.5 mg) 50 mg • Calcium 40 mg. Other Ingredients: Calcium Acid Phosphate, Cellulose, Hypromellose, Magnesium Stearate, Silica, Sodium Starch Glycollate.

MediHerb White Peony 1:2 **- Standard Process, Inc.**
Each 5 mL serving contains: White Peony root 1:2 extract (from paeonia lactiflora 2.5 g) 5 mL. Other Ingredients: Purified Water, 45% Alcohol.

MediHerb Wild Yam 1:2 **- Standard Process, Inc.**
Each 5 mL serving contains: Wild Yam root and rhizome 1:2 extract (from discorea villosa 2.5 g, containing steroidal saponins as dioscin 75 mg) 5 mL. Other Ingredients: Purified Water, 60% Alcohol.

MediHerb Wild Yam Complex **- Standard Process, Inc.**
Each tablet contains: False Unicorn root 4:1 extract (from chamaelirium luteum 360 mg) 90 mg • Wild Yam root and rhizome 4:1 extract (from discorea villosa 360 mg) 90 mg • Sage herb 5:1 extract (from salvia officinalis 290 mg) 58 mg • Korean Ginseng root 5:1 extract (from Panax ginseng 75 mg, containing ginsenosides as Rg1 and Rb1 1.4 mg) 15 mg • St. John's Wort herb flowering top 6:1 extract (from hypericum perforatum 360 mg, containing hypericins 198 mcg) 60 mg • Calcium 60 mg. Other Ingredients: Calcium Acid Phosphate, Cellulose, Hypromellose, Magnesium Stearate, Silica, Sodium Starch Glycollate.

MediHerb Withania Complex **- Standard Process, Inc.**
Each tablet contains: Licorice root 3.5:1 extract (from glycyrrhiza glabra 750 mg) 214 mg • Withania (ashwaganda) root 5:1 extract (from withania somnifera 950 mg) 190 mg • Skullcap herb 4:1 extract (from scutellaria lateriflora 470 mg) 117.5 mg • Korean Ginseng root 5:1 extract (from Panax ginseng 100 mg, containing ginsenosides as Rg1 and Rb1 1.86 mg) 20 mg • Calcium 40 mg. Other Ingredients: Calcium Acid Phosphate, Cellulose, Silica, Sodium Starch Glycollate, Hypromellose, Magnesium Stearate.

MediHerb Withania Complex Phytosynergist **- Standard Process, Inc.**
Each 5 mL serving contains: Korean Ginseng root 5:1 extract (from panax ginseng root 125 mg, containing ginsenosides as Rg1 and Rb1 2.32 mg) 25 mg • Ashwaganda root 1:2 extract (from withania somnifera root 1.25 g) 2.5 mL • Skullcap herb 1:2 extract (from scutellaria lateriflora herb 625 mg) 1.25 mL • Licorice root 1:1 extract (from glycyrrhiza glabra root 1 g) 1 mL. Other Ingredients: Purified Water, 41% Alcohol.

MediHerb Wormwood 1:5 **- Standard Process, Inc.**
Each 1 mL serving contains: Wormwood herb 1:5 extract (from artemisia absinthium 200 mg) 1 mL. Other Ingredients: Purified Water, 45% Alcohol.

MediHerb Wormwood Complex **- Standard Process, Inc.**
Each tablet contains: Stemona root 3:1 extract (from stemona sessilifolia 1000 mg) 333 mg • Black Walnut green hulls 4:1 extract (from juglans nigra 100 mg) 25 mg • Wormwood herb 4:1 extract (from artemisia absinthium 100 mg) 25 mg • Clove oil 20 mg • Calcium 18 mg. Other Ingredients: Cellulose, Silica, Calcium Acid Phosphate, Sodium Starch Glycollate, Hypromellose, Magnesium Stearate.

MediHerb Yellow Dock 1:2 **- Standard Process, Inc.**
Each 5 mL serving contains: Yellow Dock root 1:2 extract (from rumex crispus 2.5 g) 5 mL. Other Ingredients: Purified Water, 25% Alcohol.

MediTropin **- Nutraceutics Corp.**
Three effervescent tablets contain: Proprietary Blend Glycoamino Acid Complex 6230 mg: Symbiotropin, Anterior Pituitary Peptides (porcine), Protein Growth Factors, GHRH Decapeptides (porcine) • Polyose Complex (mono, poly and oligo saccharides) 3075 mg. Other Ingredients: Citric Acid, Potassium Bicarbonate, Glucose, L-Glutamine, L-Arginine, L-Pyroglutamate, Sodium Bicarbonate, L-Lysine Monohydrochloride, L-Leucine, Glycine, Polyethylene Glycol, Sodium Carbonate, Mixed Berry Flavor, L-Tyrosine, Gamma Aminobutyric Acid, Inositol Hexanicotinate, Sodium Benzoate Powder.

Meditropin Anti-Aging Therapy with Symbiotropin Plus + - Nutraceutics Corp.
Three effervescent tablets contain: Glycoamino Acid Proprietary Complex 6230 mg: Symbiotropin, Anterior Pituitary Peptides (porcine), Protein Growth Factors, GHRH Decapeptides (porcine) • Polyose complex 3075 mg: Monosaccharides, Polysaccharides, Oligosaccharides. Other Ingredients: Citric Acid, Potassium Bicarbonate, Glucose, L-Glutamine, L-Arginine, L-Pyrogluatamate, Sodium Bicarbonate, L-Lysine Monohydrochloride, L-Leucine, Glycine, Polyethylene Glycol, Sodium Carbonate, Mixed Berry Flavor, L-Tyrosine, Gamma Aminobutyric Acid, Inositol Hexanicotinate, Sodium Benzoate Powder.

Medphen - Olympian Labs
Six capsules contain: Proprietary Blend 3000 mg: Green Tea extract, Garcinia Cambogia, Ginger, Mustard Seed, Cayenne, Astragalus, White Willow Bark, Uva Ursi, Siberian Ginseng, Gotu Kola.

Medroid - Sports One
19-Nor-4-Androstenediol • 19-Norandrostenedione • Androstenedione • 4-Androstenediol • 5-Androstenediol • Tribulus Terrestris • Acetyl-L-Carnitine • Thermogenic Formula using a proprietary half-life enzymatic conversion excelerator. Capsule 1: Tribulus Terrestris 250 mg, 5-Androstene-3B,17B-Diol 50 mg.
Capsule 2: Androstenedione 100 mg, Acetyl L-Carnitine 100 mg, 4-Androstene-3, 17-Diol 100 mg. Capsule 3 (Proprietary half-life excelerator): Ma Huang herb 10:1 extract, Green Tea leaf 10:1 extract, White Willow bark, Secret Half Life Enzymatic Conversion Excelerator. Capsule 4: 5-Androstene-3B,17B-Diol 50 mg, 19-Nor-4-Androstene-3B, 17B-Diol 50 mg, 19-Norandrostenedione 100 mg.
See Editor's Note No. 30, No. 47 and No. 54.

MEG-3 brand - Ocean Nutrition Canada
Omega-3 fatty acids from purified Fish Oil: EPA (eicosapentaenoic acid) • DHA (docosahexaenoic acid).
See Editor's Note No. 44 and No. 45.

Mega B-100 sustained release tablets - Nature's Plus
Each tablet contains: Thiamin (vitamin B1, as thiamine hydrochloride) 100 mg • Riboflavin (vitamin B2) 100 mg • Niacin (as niacinamide) 100 mg • Vitamin B6 (as pyridoxine HCl) 100 mg • Folate (as folic acid) 100 mcg • Vitamin B12 (as cyanocobalamin) 100 mcg • Biotin 100 mcg • Pantothenic Acid (as calcium pantothenate) 100 mg • Inositol 100 mg • Choline (as bitartrate) 42 mg • PABA (as para-aminobenzoic acid) 30 mg. Other Ingredients: Di-calcium Phosphate, Stearic Acid, Hydroxypropyl Methylcellulose, Rice Bran, Magnesium Stearate, Alfalfa, Watercress, Parsley, Silica, Pharmaceutical Glaze.

Mega B-125 - The Vitamin Shoppe
Each sustained-release tablet contains: Vitamin B1 (thiamin) 125 mg • Vitamin B2 (riboflavin) 125 mg • Vitamin B6 (pyridoxine HCl) 125 mg • Vitamin B12 (cobalamin concentrate) 125 mcg • Niacinamide 125 mg • Folic Acid 400 mcg • Pantothenic Acid (D-calcium pantothenate) 125 mg • D-Biotin 125 mcg • Choline Bitartrate 125 mg • Inositol 125 mg • PABA 125 mg. In a base of Alfalfa, Watercress, Parsley, and Rice Concentrate.

Mega B-150 sustained release tablets - Nature's Plus
Each tablet contains: Thiamin (vitamin B1, as thiamine hydrochloride) 150 mg • Riboflavin (vitamin B2) 150 mg • Niacin (as niacinamide) 150 mg • Vitamin B6 (as pyridoxine HCl) 150 mg • Folate (as folic acid) 250 mcg • Vitamin B12 (as cyanocobalamin) 150 mcg • Biotin 150 mcg • Pantothenic Acid (as calcium pantothenate) 150 mg • Inositol 150 mg • PABA (para-aminobenzoic acid) 150 mg • Choline (as bitartrate) 63 mg. Other Ingredients: Microcrystalline Cellulose, Stearic Acid, Di-calcium Phosphate, Rice Bran, Hydroxypropyl Methylcellulose, Magnesium Stearate, Silica, Watercress, Alfalfa, Parsley, Pharmaceutical Glaze.

Mega Cal Calcium - Jamieson
Each tablet contains: Elemental Calcium 650 mg.

Mega Cal Calcium and Magnesium - Jamieson
Each caplet contains: Elemental Calcium (from microbound formula of carbonate and Krebs cycle sources of Citrate, Fumarate, Malate, Succinate, and Glutamate) 333 mg • Elemental Magnesium (from Oxide and Krebs cycle sources of Citrate, Fumarate, Malate, Succinate, and Glutamate) 167 mg.

Mega Cal Calcium and Magnesium with Zinc - Jamieson
Each tablet contains: Elemental Calcium 333 mg • Elemental Magnesium 167 mg • Elemental Zinc Gluconate 20 mg.

Mega Cal Calcium Chewy Swiss (chocolate flavor) - Jamieson
Each square contains: Elemental Calcium 650 mg • Vitamin D (as Vitamin D3) Cholecalciferol 200 IU.

Mega Cal Calcium Citrate with Vitamin D - Jamieson
Each caplet contains: Elemental Calcium (from Calcium Citrate) 250 mg • Vitamin D (as Vitamin D3 Cholecalciferol) 50 IU.

Mega Cal Calcium with Vitamin D - Jamieson
Each caplet contains: Elemental Calcium 650 mg • Vitamin D 200 IU.

Mega Cal Calcium/Magnesium with Vitamin D - Jamieson
Each caplet contains: Elemental Calcium 333 mg • Elemental Magnesium 167 mg • Vitamin D 133 IU.

Mega Cal Chewable Calcium 350 mg - Jamieson
Each tablet contains: Elemental Calcium 350 mg.

Mega C-B-R - Source Naturals
Each tablet contains: Vitamin C (as ascorbic acid) 1000 mg • Calcium (from citrus bioflavonoid complex) 125 mg • Citrus Bioflavonoid Complex 500 mg • Rutin 52 mg • Hesperidin Complex 50 mg • Acerola 10 mg.

Mega C-Complex 1000 - The Vitamin Shoppe
Each tablet contains: Vitamin C (fortified with rose hips) 1000 mg • Citrus Bioflavonoids 500 mg • Hesperidin Complex 50 mg • Rutin 50 mg • Acerola 10 mg.

Mega Chromic Fuel (Chromium Picolinate) 500 mcg - TwinLab
Each capsule contains: Trivalent Chromium (from Pure Crystalline Chromium Picolinate) 500 mcg.

Mega Chromium Picolinate - Source Naturals
Each tablet contains: Trivalent Chromium (from Chromax brand of yeast-free Chromium Picolinate) 300 mcg.

Mega CLA 1200 - Nature's Plus
Each softgel contains: Conjugated Linoleic Acid (CLA) 1200 mg • st. 1:1 c9-t11:t10-c12 888 mg. Other Ingredients: Gleatin, Glycerin, Purified Water, Natural Coloring.

Mega CoQ10 - TwinLab
Each capsule contains: Coenzyme Q10 30 mg.

Mega CoQ10 300 mg - Life Extension
Each softgel contains: Coenzyme Q10 (Japanese pharmaceutical grade) 300 mg • Rice Bran oil 475 mg • Rosemary extract 3 mg. Other Ingredients: Gelatin, Glycerin, Water, Beeswax, Lecithin.

Mega Creatine Fuel - TwinLab
Each capsule contains: University-Tested Pure Creatine Monohydrate 1200 mg.

Mega Diet Caps - Puritan's Pride
Three capsules contain: Ma Huang extract (standardized for 6% ephedra) 334 mg • Guarana extract (standardized for 22% caffeine) 910 mg • CitriMax brand Garcinia Cambogia (hydroxycitrate) 500 mg • Chromium (picolinate) 200 mcg • L-Carnitine 100 mg • Potassium Phosphate 50 mg • Magnesium Phosphate 50 mg • Green Tea 10 mg • Citrus Bioflavonoids 10 mg • Ginger root 10 mg • Cayenne 10 mg.
See Editor's Note No. 21 and No. 30.

Mega Fat Burners - Optimum Nutrition
Two tablets contain: Calcium (as dicalcium phosphate) 241 mg • Phosphorus (as dicalcium phosphate) 186 mg • Chromium (as chromium picolinate) 400 mcg • Garcinia rind extract (garcinia cambogia, standardized to 50% hydroxycitric acid) 500 mg • L-Carnitine (as L-carnitine tartrate) 100 mg • Choline (as choline bitartrate) 400 mg • Inositol 200 mg. Other Ingredients: Pharmaceutical Glaze, Stearic Acid, Croscarmellose Sodium, Magnesium Stearate, Silica.

Mega G - CCA Industries, Inc.
Each caplet contains: Grapefruit extract 75 mg • Glucomannan (konjac root) 600 mg • Gymnema Sylvestre (25% standardized) 50 mg. Other Ingredients: Microcrystalline Cellulose, Calcium Carbonate, Stearic Acid, Magnesium Stearate, Croscarmellose.

Mega Garlic Plus - Herbalife International of America, Inc.
Each tablet contains: Vitamin C (as ascorbic acid) 70 mg • Calcium (from dicalcium phosphate) 35 mg • Phosphorus (from dicalcium phosphate) 34 mg • Garlic clove powder 612 mg. Other Ingredients: Microcrystalline Cellulose, Methacrylic Acid Copolymer, Croscarmellose Sodium, Hypromellose, Stearic Acid, Talc, Titanium Dioxide, Triethyl Citrate, Magnesium Stearate, Cellulose, Vegetable Acetoglycerides, Silicon Dioxide, Polyethylene Glycol, Polysorbate 80, Methyl Paraben, Propyl Paraben, FD&C Blue #1, FD&C Yellow #5.

Mega Ginseng Blend - Herbalife International of America, Inc.
Each tablet contains: Dried Panax Ginseng root extract 25 mg • Dried Eleuthero root extract 25 mg • Dried Gynostemma Pentaphyllum root extract 12.5 mg • Dried Ashwagandha root extract 12.5 mg • Dried Panax Notoginseng root extract (5% ginsenosides) 12.5 mg • Bio-Absorption Complex-5 11.5 mg: Soy Lecithin, Ascorbyl Palmitate, Plant Cellulose Enzyme, Cinnamon bark powder, Dried Black Pepper fruit extract. Other Ingredients: Dicalcium Phosphate, Microcrystalline Cellulose, Silicon Dioxide, Hypromellose, Croscarmellose Sodium, Magnesium Stearate, Hydroxypropyl Cellulose, Polysorbate, Polyethylene Glycol.

Mega Glucosamine 750 - Swanson Health Products
Each capsule contains: Glucosamine Sulfate (2KCl) 750 mg.

Mega Manna 500 mg - Nature's Life
Each capsule contains: Glucomannan (Amorphophallus konjac) 500 mg.

Mega Max - Aspen Group, Inc.
Each tablet contains: Vitamin C 250 mg • Vitamin E 150 IU • Vitamin A 25,000 USP Units • Vitamin D 1000 USP Units • Vitamin B1 75 mg • Vitamin B2 75 mg • Vitamin B6 75 mg • Vitamin B12 75 mg • Niacinamide 75 mg • Choline 75 mg • Inositol 75 mg • Para Aminobenzoic Acid 75 mg • Pantothenic Acid 75 mg • Biotin 75 mg • Folic Acid 400 mcg • Rutin 25 mg • Citrus Bioflavonoids Complex 25 mg • Hesperidin Complex 5 mg • Betaine HCl 25 mg • Glutamic Acid 25 mg • Iodine 15 mg • Calcium 50 mg • Potassium 10 mg • Iron 10 mg • Magnesium 7.2 mg • Manganese 6.1 mg • Zinc 15 mg • Selenium 10 mcg • Amino Acids: Arginine, Aspartic Acid, Alanine, Cystine, Glutamic Acid, Glycine, Histidine, Isoleucine, Lucine, Lysine, Methionine, Ornithine, Phenylalanine, Proline, Serine, Threonine, Tyrosine, Tryptophan, Valine. Natural Base of: Alfalfa, Parsley, Golden Seal root, Buckthorn root, Rosemary, Watercress, Mandrake root, Spinach, Lovage, Kelp, Kale, Ginseng, Rhubarb root.

Mega Mind - Source Naturals
Four tablets contain: Vitamin B1 (Thiamin) 500 mg • Vitamin B2 (Riboflavin) 50 mg • Vitamin B3 (150 mg Niacinamide and 50 mg Niacin) 200 mg • Vitamin B5 (Pantothenic Acid) 50 mg • Vitamin B6 (Pyridoxine HCl) 50 mg • Vitamin B12 (Cyanocobalamin) 50 mcg • Folic Acid 800 mcg • Biotin 500 mcg • Vitamin C (Calcium and Zinc Ascorbates) 197 mg • Calcium (Ascorbate, Carbonate, Malate, Succinate) 100 mg • Magnesium (Malate, Succinate, Taurinate, Oxide) 200 mg • Zinc (Ascorbate) 10 mg • Manganese (Citrate) 5 mg • L-Pyroglutamic Acid 1000 mg • L-Glutamine 500 mg • DMAE (Bitartrate) 160 mg • Acetyl L-Carnitine 400 mg • N-Acetyl L-Tyrosine 300 mg • Taurine (Magnesium Taurinate) 198 mg • Ginkgo Biloba 24% with a Proanthocyanidolic value of 95 (50:1 Extract) 120 mg • Proanthodyn (from Grape Seed extract) 100 mg • GABA (Gamma Amino Butyric Acid) 100 mg • Coenzyme Q10 (Ubiquinone) 15 mg • Alpha-Lipoic Acid (Thioctic Acid) 15 mg.

Mega Mineral Plus - Global Health Trax
One tablespoon (16 fl oz) contains: Vitamin D (as cholecalciferol) 200 IU • Calcium (as calcium citrate, tricalcium phosphate) 600 mg • Magnesium (as magnesium citrate) 200 mg • Zinc (as zinc gluconate) 5 mg • Selenium (as selenium amino acid chelate) 25 mcg • Manganese (as manganese gluconate) 2.5 mg • Chromium (as chromium polynicotinate) 125 mcg • Molybdenum (as sodium molybdate) 62.5 mcg • Potassium (as potassium citrate) 50 mg • Boron (as boron amino acid chelate) 1 mg • Chondroitin Sulfate 37.5 mg • Glucosamine Sulfate 75 mg • Silica (from nyacol silica) 200 mg • Glucono Delta Lactone (GDL) 1000 mg • Trace Mineral Blend (from sea mineral salts) 1750 mg. Other Ingredients: Purified Water, Glycerin, Natural Orange Flavor, Natural Vanilla Flavor, Vegetable Gum, Sucralose, Potassium Sorbate, Sodium Benzoate. See Editor's Note No. 15.

Mega Minerals - Nature's Life
Four capsules contain: Boron (Citrate) 1 mg • Calcium (Carbonate, Citrate/Malate) 1000 mg • Chromium (Picolinate {US Patent #33988}, Polynicotinate) 200 mcg • Copper (Glyconate, Citrate) 1 mg • Iodine (Kelp) 25 mcg • Iron (Fumerate, Peptonate) 15 mg • Magnesium (Oxide, Citrate) 500 mg • Manganese (Citrate) 10 mg • Molybdenum (Sodium Molybdate) 20 mcg • Potassium (Citrate) 99 mg • Selenium (l-Selenomethionine) 100 mcg • Silicon Dioxide 20 mg • Vanadium 20 mcg • Zinc (Picolinate, Citrate) 15 mg • Vitamin D 200 IU • Betaine HCl 100 mg • Glutamic Acid 100 mg.

Mega Multiple III - Pro Health
Nine tablets contain: Beta Carotene 24,000 IU • Vitamin A (acetate) 10,000 IU • Alpha Carotene 1000 IU • Vitamin B1 (thiamine) 100 mg • Vitamin B2 (riboflavin) 100 mg • Niacin 25 mg • Niacinamide 75 mg • Vitamin B6 (pyridoxine) 200 mg • Vitamin B12 (cyanocobalamin) 200 mcg • Biotin 300 mcg • Folic Acid 1 mg • Pantothenic Acid 200 mg • Vitamin C (ascorbic acid) 500 mg • Vitamin C (calcium ascorbate) 500 mg • Vitamin D (as cholecalciferol) 400 IU • Vitamin E (as dL-alpha tocopheryl acetate) 600 IU • Vitamin K 100 mcg • Calcium (as calcium citrate) 25 mg • Iodine (kelp) 50 mcg • Molybdenum (sodium molybdate) 500 mcg • Selenium (dioxide) 100 mcg • Selenium (selenomethionine) 100 mcg • Magnesium Oxide 700 mg • Calcium Chelate 500 mg • Choline Bitartrate 500 mg • L-Taurine 500 mg • Acerola juice 300 mg • Citrus Bioflavonoids 260 mg • Hesperidin Complex 260 mg • Inositol 250 mg • Lycopene 250 mg • Betaine HCl (trimethylglycine) 250 mg • Calcium Citrate 175 mg • Phosphatidyl Choline (lecithin) 150 mg • Alfalfa leaf 121.68 mg • Ascorbyl Palmitate 100 mg • Broccoli Powder 100 mg • Magnesium Aspartate 100 mg • Magnesium Chelate 100 mg • Magnesium Succinate 100 mg • Malic Acid 100 mg • N-Acetyl Cysteine 100 mg • Trace Minerals 100 mg • Barley grass 83.34 mg • Chlorella 83.34 mg • Oat grass 83.34 mg • Spirulina 83.34 mg • Spinach 83.34 mg • Wheat germ 83.34 mg • Wheat grass 83.34 mg • Bromelain 50 mg • OptiZinc brand Zinc 50 mg • PABA 50 mg • Potassium Aspartate 50 mg • Zinc Succinate 50 mg • Potassium Chloride 49 mg • Blue Green Algae 45 mg • Betaine Hydrochloride 25 mg • Bilberry extract 25 mg • Calcium Hydroxyapatite 25 mg • L-Glutathione 25 mg • Grape seed extract 25 mg • Papain (papaya enzymes) 25 mg • Rutin 25 mg • Milk Thistle extract 20 mg • Amylase 10 mg • Fructooligosaccharides 10 mg • Green Tea (decaffeinated) 10 mg • Lipase 10 mg • Manganese Gluconate 10 mg • Pepsin 10 mg • Protease 10 mg • Lutein extract 6.6 mg • Dilauryl Thiodipropionate 5 mg • Superoxide Dismutase (SOD) 5 mg • Boron (Citrate) 1 mg • Copper Chelate 1 mg • Chromium Picolinate 100 mcg • Chromium Polynicotinate 100 mcg. Other Ingredients: Microcrystalline Cellulose, Calcium Phosphate Dibasic, Stearic Acid, Silicon Dioxide, Croscarmellose Sodium, Calcium Stearate, Hydroxypropyl Cellulose, Magnesium Stearate, Talc, Magnesium Carbonate, Sodium Lauryl Sulfate, Ethylcellulose.

Some Brand Name Natural Products - What they Contain

www.NaturalDatabase.com contains MANY more listings than appear here.
Editor's Notes are located on pages 2155-2163.

Mega N-R-G Thirty **-** Progressive Labs
Four tablets contain: Vitamin A (50% as beta carotene) 15000 IU • Vitamin C 600 mg • Vitamin D (as Vitamin D3) 100 IU • Vitamin E 200 IU • Thiamin (Vitamin B1) 25 mg • Riboflavin (Vitamin B2) 15 mg • Niacin (Vitamin B3) 50 mg • Niacinamide (Vitamin B3) 100 mg • Vitamin B6 25 mg • Folate (folic acid) 400 mcg • Vitamin B12 100 mcg • Biotin 300 mcg • Pantothenic Acid (as calcium pantothenate) 250 mg • Calcium (as aspartate) 120 mg • Iodine (from kelp) 150 mcg • Magnesium (as aspartate) 120 mg • Zinc Gluconate 15 mg • Selenium (as aspartate) 200 mcg • Manganese (as aspartate) 2 mg • Chromium (as aspartate) 200 mcg • Potassium (as aspartate) 9.9 mg • Choline 100 mg • Inositol 100 mg • Bioflavonoids 300 mg • PABA 100 mg • L-Methionine 75 mg • L-Lysine 75 mg.

Mega Once-A-Day **-** Progressive Labs
Each tablet supplies: Vitamin A (as palmitate and beta carotene) 25000 IU • Vitamin C 250 mg • Vitamin D 500 IU • Vitamin E 150 IU • Thiamin (Vitamin B1) 75 mg • Riboflavin (Vitamin B2) 75 mg • Niacinamide 75 mg • Vitamin B6 (pyridoxine) 75 mg • Folate (folic acid) 400 mcg • Vitamin B12 (cyanocobalamin) 75 mcg • Biotin 75 mcg • Pantothenic Acid 75 mg • Calcium (amino acid chelate) 50 mg • Iron (amino acid chelate) 10 mg • Iodine (from kelp) 225 mcg • Magnesium (amino acid chelate) 7 mg • Zinc (amino acid chelate) 15 mg • Selenium (amino acid chelate) 15 mcg • Copper (amino acid chelate) 25 mcg • Manganese (amino acid chelate) 6 mg • Silicon (amino acid chelate) 15 mg • Chromium (amino acid chelate) 10 mg • Molybdenum (amino acid chelate) 5 mcg • Potassium 10 mg • Boron (as boron gluconate) 750 mcg • Choline Bitartrate 75 mg • Inositol 75 mg • Para Amino Benzoic Acid (PABA) 75 mg • Betaine HCl 25 mg • Glutamic Acid HCl 25 mg • Rutin 25 mg • Lemon bioflavonoid complex 25 mg • Hesperidin complex 25 mg. Natural base of: Oat fiber, Alfalfa, Lecithin, Parsley, Bee Pollen, Royal Jelly, and Albumin.

Mega Pak Multiple **-** Nature's Life
Each packet of nine capsules contains: Vitamin A (Fish Liver oil) 7500 IU • Beta Carotene (equivalent to 7500 IU Vitamin A) 4.5 mg • Vitamin B1 (Thiamine HCl) 100 mg • Vitamin B2 (Riboflavin) 100 mg • Vitamin B6 (Pyridoxine HCl) 100 mg • Vitamin B12 (Cobalamin) 100 mcg • Folic Acid 400 mcg • Niacinamide 100 mg • Pantothenic Acid (d-Calcium Pantothenate) 100 mg • Choline (Bitartrate) 100 mg • Inositol 100 mg • Biotin (d-Biotin) 100 mcg • PABA (Para Aminobenzoic Acid) 100 mg • Vitamin C 1000 mg • Lemon Bioflavonoids Complex (TESTLAB) 25 mg • Rose Hips (Rosa canina)15 mg • Acerola (Malpighia glabra) 5 mg • Hesperidin Conplex (Citrus) 5 mg • Rutin (Saphora japonica) 5 mg • Vitamin E (d-Alpha Tocopherol, Beta, Delta & Gamma Tocopherols) 400 IU • Boron (Citrate) 1 mg • Calcium (Carbonate, Citrate/Malate) 1000 mg • Chromium (Picolinate, Polynicotinate) 200 mcg • Copper (Gluconate, Citrate) 1 mg • Iodine (Kelp) 25 mcg • Iron (Fumerate, Peptonate) 15 mg • Magnesium (Oxide, Citrate) 500 mg • Manganese (Citrate) 10 mg • Molybdenum (Sodium Molybdate) 20 mcg • Potassium (Citrate) 99 mg • Selenium (l-Selenomethionine) 100 mcg • Silicon Dioxide 20 mg • Vanadium (Vanadyl Sulfate) 20 mcg • Zinc (Picolinate • Citrate) 15 mg • Vitamin D (as Vitamin D3) (Cholecalciferol) 200 IU • Betaine HCl 100 mg • Glutamic Acid HCl 100 mg • Bromelain (Proteolytic Enzyme from Pineapple, activity: 225 MCU) 250 mg • Papain (Proteolytic Enzyme from Papaya, acivity 17.5 MCU) 250 mg. In a natural base of Lecithin, Rice Bran & Soy oil.

Mega PC-35 **-** Jarrow Formulas
Two softgels contain: Choline (from 35% PC lecithin) 114 mg • Lecithin 2400 mg: Phosphatidylcholine 840 mg, Phosphatidylethanolamine 120 mg. Other Ingredients: Gelatin, Glycerin, Water.

Mega Plus **-** Swanson Health Products
Each tablet contains: Vitamin A (from fish liver oil) 10,000 IU • Vitamin C USP (as ascorbic acid) 250 mg • Vitamin D (from fish liver oil) 400 IU • Vitamin E (as d-alpha tocopheryl succinate) 100 IU • Thiamin USP (as thiamin HCl; vitamin B-1) 75 mg • Riboflavin USP (vitamin B-2) 75 mg • Niacinamide 100 mg • Vitamin B-6 (as pyridoxine HCl) 75 mg • Folic Acid USP 400 mcg • Vitamin B-12 (as cyanocobalamin) 250 mcg • Biotin 150 mcg • Pantothenic Acid (as d-calcium pantothenate) 100 mg • Calcium (from bone meal) 150 mg • Iron (as ferrous fumarate) 18 mg • Phosphorus (from bone meal) 72 mg • Iodine (from kelp) 225 mcg • Magnesium (from magnesium oxide) 75 mg • Zinc (from zinc gluconate) 10 mg • Selenium (from amino acid chelate) 50 mcg • Copper (from copper gluconate) 2 mg • Manganese (from manganese carbonate sulfate) 7 mg • Chromium (from amino acid chelate) 20 mcg • Choline (as choline bitartrate) 100 mg.

Mega Potency Fat Burner **-** Optimum Nutrition
L-Carnitine • CitriMax brand Chromium Picolinate • Chromium Polynicotinate.

Mega Primrose **-** Source Naturals
Each softgel contains: Evening Primrose Oil 1300 mg.

Mega Probiotic **-** DaVinci Laboratories
Each capsule contains: Probiotic Bacteria Complex 5 billion cells: Lactobacillus Casei HA-108 (20%) 1 billion, Lactobacillus Rhamnosus HA-111 (20%) 1 billion, Lactobacillus Acidophilus HA-122 (15%) 750 million, Lactobacillus Lactis HA-136 (15%) 750 million, Bifidobacterium Breve HA-129 (10%) 500 million, Bifidobacterium Longum HA-135 (10%) 500 million, Bifidobacterium Bifidum HA-132 (5%) 250 million, Streptococcus Thermophilus HA-110 (5%) 250 million • Fructooligosaccharides (FOS) 440 mg. Other Ingredients: Magnesium Stearate, Ascorbic Acid, Vegetable Cellulose.

Mega Senior Plus **-** AIE Pharmaceuticals
Vitamin A (as retinyl acetate and 50% as beta-carotene) • Vitamin C (as ascorbic acid) • Vitamin D (as cholecalciferol) • Vitamin E (as DL-alpha tocopheryl acetate) • Vitamin K (as phytonadione) • Thiamin (as thiamin mononitrate) • Riboflavin • Niacin (as niacinamide) • Vitamin B6 (as pyridoxine hydrochloride) • Folic Acid • Vitamin B12 (as cyanocobalamin) • Biotin • Pantothenic Acid (as calcium pantothenate) • Calcium (from calcium carbonate and dibasic calcium phosphate) • Iron (from ferrous fumarate) • Phosphorus (from dibasic calcium phosphate) • Iodine (from potassium iodide) • Magnesium (from magnesium oxide) • Zinc (from zinc oxide) • Selenium (from selenium selenate) • Copper (from cupric oxide) • Manganese (from manganese sulfate) • Chromium (from chromium chloride) • Molybdenum (from sodium molybdate) • Potassium (from potassium chloride) • Nickel (from nickelous sulfate) • Boron (from sodium borate and potassium borate) • Silicon (from sodium metasilicate and silicon dioxide) • Vanadium (from sodium metavanadate). Other Ingredients: Stearic Acid, Croscarmellose Sodium, Cellulose, Titanium Dioxide, Polysorbate 80, Natural Color, Hydroxypropyl Methylcellulose, Polyethylene Glycol, Magnesium Stearate.

Mega Soy Extract **-** Life Extension
Two capsules contain: Soybean powdered extract 270 mg (standardized to supply genistein/isoform genistin 51.6 mg, Daidzein/ isoform daidzin 50 mg, Glycitein/isoform glycitin 9.4 mg). Other Ingredients: Gelatin, Water.

Mega Vim 75 **-** Jamieson
Each caplet contains: Vitamin A (from Acetate) 8500 IU • Beta-Carotene (Provitamin A) 1500 IU • Vitamin D 400 IU • Vitamin C (Ascorbic Acid) 250 mg • Vitamin E (from Succinate) 150 IU • Vitamin B1 (Thiamin Mononitrate) 75 mg • Vitamin B2 (Riboflavin) 75 mg • Vitamin B6 (Pyridoxine HCl) 75 mg • Vitamin B12 (Cyanocobalamin) 75 mcg • Niacinamide 75 mg • Vitamin B5 (Pantothenic Acid from Calcium D-Pantothenate) 75 mg • Biotin (D-Biotin) 75 mcg • Folic Acid 0.4 mg • Chelated Calcium, Calcium (Carbonate) 130 mg • Chelated Iron 4 mg • Chelated Copper 1 mg • Iodine (from Kelp) 0.15 mg • Chelated Magnesium, Magnesium (Oxide) 50 mg • Chelated Manganese 0.61 mg • Chelated Zinc 1.5 mg • Chelated Potassium 2 mg • Chelated Chromium 10 mcg • Chelated Selenium 10 mcg • Choline Bitartrate 75 mg • Inositol 75 mg.

Mega Vim Level 4 Potency Multivitamin - Jamieson
Each caplet contains: Vitamin A (from Acetate) 5000 IU • Beta Carotene 1500 IU • Vitamin D 400 IU • Vitamin C 250 mg • Vitamin E 150 IU • Vitamin B1 75 mg • Vitamin B2 75 mg • Vitamin B3 (No Flush Niacinamide) 75 mg • Vitamin B5 75 mg • Vitamin B6 75 mg • Vitamin B12 75 mg • Folic Acid 400 mcg • Biotin 75 mcg • Calcium 150 mg • Iron 4 mg • Copper 1 mg • Iodine 0.1 mg • Magnesium 75 mg • Zinc 10 mg • Vanadium 1 mcg • Molybdenum 1mcg • Lutein 300 mcg • Lycopene 300 mcg • Ginseng 10 mg • Soy Phosphotidyl Complex 5 mg • Digestive Enzyme Absorption Factors derived from: Peppermint, Bromelaine, Papain, Amylase, Lipase, Cellulose 4000 mg.

Mega Vita Gel - Puritan's Pride
Two softgels contain: Vitamin A (as fish liver oil and 40% beta carotene) 10,000 IU • Vitamin C (as ascorbic acid and rose hips) 300 mg • Vitamin D (as fish liver oil) 400 IU • Vitamin E (as mixed tocopherols) 300 IU • Thiamin (Vitamin B1; as thiamine mononitrate) 50 mg • Riboflavin (Vitamin B2) 50 mg • Niacin (as niacinamide) 50 mg • Vitamin B6 (as pyridoxine hydrochloride) 50 mg • Folic Acid 400 mcg • Vitamin B12 (as cyanocobalamin) 50 mcg • Biotin (as d-biotin) 50 mcg • Pantothenic Acid (as d-calcium pantothenate) 50 mg • Calcium (as calcium carbonate and dicalcium phosphate) 200 mg • Iron (as ferrous fumarate) 15 mg • Phosphorus (as dicalcium phosphate) 50 mg • Iodine (as kelp) 150 mcg • Magnesium (as magnesium oxide) 50 mg • Zinc (as zinc citrate) 15 mg • Selenium (as selenium yeast) 25 mcg • Copper (as copper gluconate) 2 mg • Manganese (as manganese carbonate) 10 mg • Chromium (as chromium picolinate) 3.1 mcg • Potassium (as potassium citrate) 30 mg • Boron (as boron amino acid chelate) 1 mg • Rutin 10 mg • Citrus Bioflavonoids 30 mg • PABA 50 mg • Royal Jelly 5 mg • Choline Bitartrate 50 mg • Inositol 50 mcg • Garlic oil 135 mg • Lecithin 80 mg • Octacosanol 10 mcg • RNA 2 mg • DNA 2 mg • Coenzyme Q10 100 mcg.

Mega Vita Liquid - Puritan's Pride
Each 15ml tablespoonful contains: Vitamin A (as retinyl palmitate) 5,000 IU • Vitamin C (as ascorbic acid) 250 mg • Vitamin D (as cholecaliferol) 400 IU • Vitamin E (as d-alpha tocopherol plus mixed tocopherols) 125 IU • Thiamin (Vitamin B1) (as thiamine mononitrate) 25 mg • Riboflavin (Vitamin B2) (as Riboflavin 5'-Phosphate Sodium) 25 mg • Niacin (as niacinamide) 150 mg • Vitamin B6 (as pyridoxine hydrochloride) 50 mg • Folic Acid 400 mcg • Vitamin B12 (as cyanocobalamin) 50 mcg • Biotin (as D-biotin) 50 mcg • Pantothenic Acid (as dexpanthenol) 150 mg • PABA (para-aminobenzoic acid) 25 mg • Choline Bitartrate 200 mg • Inositol 100 mg.

Mega Vita Min for Teens - Puritan's Pride
Three tablets contain: Vitamin A (100% as beta carotene) 5, 000 IU • Vitamin C (as ascorbic acid) 350 mg • Vitamin D (as cholecalciferol) 400 IU • Vitamin E (as d-alpha tocopheryl succinate) 30 IU • Vitamin K (as phytonadione) 10 mcg • Thiamin (Vitamin B1; as thiamine mononitrate) 4.5 mg • Riboflavin (Vitamin B2) 5.1 mg • Niacin (as niacinamide) 20 mg • Vitamin B6 (as pyridoxine hydrochloride) 6 mg • Folic Acid 400 mcg • Vitamin B12 (as cyanocobalamin) 1 mcg • Biotin (as d-biotin) 45 mcg • Pantothenic Acid (as d-calcium pantothenate) 10 mg • Calcium (as dicalcium phosphate and calcium citrate) 100 mg • Iron (as ferrous fumarate) 18 mg • Phosphorus (as dicalicum phosphate) 20 mg • Iodine (as potassium iodide) 150 mcg • Magnesium (as Magnesium oxide) 50 mg • Zinc (as zinc oxide) 15 mg • Selenium (as selenium yeast) 5 mcg • Copper (as copper sulfate) 2 mg • Manganese (as manganese sulfate) 2 mg • Chromium (as GTF chromium yeast) 20 mcg • Molybdenum (as molybdenum yeast) 20 mcg • Choline (as choline bitartrate) 50 mcg • Inositol 50 mcg. Other Ingredients: Cellulose (Plant Origin), Vegetable Stearic Acid, Cellulose Coating, Croscarmellose, Silica, Guar Gum, Mannitol.

Mega Vita Min for Women - Puritan's Pride
Two tablets contain: Vitamin A (as retinyl palmitate and beta carotene) 10,000 IU • Vitamin C (as ascorbic acid and rose hips) 250 mg • Vitamin D (as cholecalciferol) 400 IU • Vitamin E (as D-alpha tocopheryl acetate) 125 IU • Thiamin (Vitamin B1) 80 mg • Riboflavin (Vitamin B2) 80 mg • Niacin 80 mg • Vitamin B6 80 mg • Folic Acid 400 mcg • Vitamin B12 80 mcg • Biotin 300 mcg • Pantothenic Acid 80 mg • Calcium (as calcium carbonate and calcium phosphate) 500 mg • Iron 15 mg • Phosphorus 225 mg • Iodine 150 mcg • Magnesium 200 mg • Zinc 15 mg • Selenium 100 mcg • Copper 2 mg • Manganese 2 mg • Chromium 100 mcg • Molybdenum 25 mcg • Chloride 10 mg • Potassium 10 mg • Boron 2 mg • Silica 2 mg • Cranberry 25 mg • Deordorized Garlic (Allium sativum) bulb 25 mg • Dong Quai (Angelica sinensis) root 25 mg • Black Cohosh (Cimicifuga racemosa) root 25 mg • Red Clover (Trifolium pratense) blossom 25 mg • Wild Yam (Discorea villosa) root 25 mg • Vitex extract (Vitex agnus castus) fruit 25 mg • Chamomile (Matricaria chamomilla) flower 25 mg • Soy isoflavones 25 mg • Ipriflavone 25 mg • Bee Pollen 25 mg • Royal Jelly 5 mg • Barley Grass 5 mg • Choline 10 mg • Inositol 10 mg • Para Aminobenzoic acid 10 mg • Rutin 25 mg • Citrus Bioflavonoids Complex 25 mg • Hesperine Complex 5 mg • Betaine Hydrochloride 25 mg • Coenzyme Q10 500 mcg • Pycnogenol (Pinus maritima) bark 500 mcg.

Mega Vitamin B6 250 mg - Trophic
Each caplet contains: Vitamin B6 (pyridoxine HCl) 250 mg.

Mega Zinc Plus - Golden Glow Natural Health Products
Each tablet contains: Zinc Amino Acid Chelate 50 mg: Zinc 10 mg • Magnesium Amino Acid Chelate 100 mg: Magnesium 20 mg • Manganese Amino Acid Chelate 50 mg: Manganese 5 mg • Pyridoxine Hydrochloride (vitamin B6) 15 mg • Beta Carotene 3 mg • D-Alpha-Tocopheryl Acid Succinate 41.3 mg: Natural Vitamin E 50 IU • Folic Acid 100 mcg.

Mega-16 Permathene Maximum Strength - CCA Industries, Inc.
Each tablet contains: Phenylpropanolamine HCl 75 mg. Other Ingredients: Croscarmellose, D&C Yellow #10, Dicalcium Phosphate, FD&C Blue #1, FD&C Yellow #6, Lactose, Magnesium Stearate, Methylcellulose , Microcrystalline Cellulose, Stearic Acid, Titanium Dioxide.

Mega-Cal Calcium 650 mg - Jamieson
Each caplet contains: Vitamin D (as Cholecalciferol) 200 IU • Calcium (as Calcium Carbonate, Calcium Citrate, Calcium Fumarate, Calcium Malate, Calcium Succinate, Calcium Glutamate) 650 mg.

Mega-Chel - Nature's Sunshine
Six tablets contain: Vitamin A (beta-carotene, palmitate) 20,000 IU • Vitamin C (ascorbic acid) 2000 mg • Vitamin D 325 IU • Vitamin E (D-alpha tocopherol) 200 IU • Vitamin B1 (thiamine) 100 mg • Vitamin B2 (riboflavin) 25 mg • Niacin 50 mg • Vitamin B6 (pyridoxine HCl) 75 mg • Folic Acid 200 mcg • Vitamin B12 (cyanocobalamin) 125 mcg • Biotin 50 mcg • Pantothenic Acid (D-calcium pantothenate) 250 mg • Calcium (amino acid chelate, Di-calcium phosphate, D-calcium pantothenate) 200 mg • Iron (ferrous fumarate) 5 mg • Phosphorus (di-calcium phosphate) 145 mg • Iodine (potassium iodide) 63 mcg • Magnesium (amino acid chelate, magnesium oxide) 200 mg • Zinc (gluconate, oxide) 15 mg • Selenium (amino acid chelate) 125 mcg • Copper (copper gluconate) 125 mcg • Manganese (amino acid chelate) 2.5 mg • Chromium (amino acid chelate) 100 mcg • Potassium (gluconate) 200 mg • P-Aminobenzoic Acid (PABA) 125 mg • Inositol 20 mg • Coenzyme Q10 5 mg • Cysteine HCl 375 mg • Methionine 88 mg. Other Ingredients: Stearic Acid, Cellulose, Magnesium Stearate, Magnesium Silicate, Citrus Bioflavonoids, Rutin, Silicon Dioxide, Adrenal Substance, Spleen Substance, Thymus Substance, Ginkgo Leaf (ginkgo biloba), Hawthorn Berry (crataegus oxyacanthoides).

Mega-Energy - Puritan's Pride
Two tablets contain: Total Carbohydrate 1 g • Calcium 67 mg • Sodium 10 mg • Guarana extract 8:1 seed 225 mg • Kola Nut extract 8:1 seed 200 mg • Royal Jelly 65 mg • Korean Ginseng extract 15:1 root 64 mg • Gotu Kola extract 6:1 aerial parts 23 mg • Alfalfa Parsley blend (Alfalfa aerial parts, Parsley leaf) 16 mg • Barley Grass aerial parts 16 mg • Bee Pollen 16 mg • Disodium Inosinate 16 mg •

Suma root 16 mg • Wheat Grass aerial parts 16 mg • Beta-Sitosterol 8.8 mg • Stigmasterol 4 mg • Campesterol 3.2 mg • Octacosanol 1 mg.

Mega-Kid Multiple - Source Naturals
Two tablets contain: Vitamin A (beta-carotene) 6000 IU • Vitamin B-1 (thiamin) 3 mg • Vitamin B-2 (riboflavin) 3 mg • Niacinamide 10 mg • Vitamin B-5 (calcium D-Pantothenate) 8 mg • Vitamin B-6 (pyridoxine HCl) 3 mg • Vitamin B-12 (cyanocobalamin) 10 mcg • Biotin 100 mcg • Folic acid 200 mcg • Vitamin C (calcium and manganese ascorbates) 200 mg • Vitamin D-3 (cholecalciferol) 400 IU • Vitamin E (natural D-alpha) 30 IU • Vitamin K (phytonadione) 20 mcg • Calcium (ascorbate) 21.28 mg • Chromium (ChromeMate yeast-free polynicotinate) 10 mcg.

MegaMam - TriLight Herbs
Milk Thistle • Chaste Tree berries • Fennel • Borage • Red Raspberry • Lemon Balm.

MegaMind - Source Naturals
DMAE • Acetyl L-Carnitine • GABA • Pyroglutamic • Ginkgo • Lipoic • CoQ10.

Mega-Mins - Nature's Plus
Two tablets contain: Calcium (as amino acid chelate/complex) 1000 mg • Phosphorus (as amino acid complex) 200 mg • Iodine (from kelp) 225 mcg • Magnesium (as amino acid chelate/complex) 500 mg • Zinc (as amino acid complex) 50 mg • Selenium (as amino acid complex) 4 mcg • Manganese (as amino acid chelate/complex) 10 mg • Chromium (as amino acid chelate) 4 mcg • Potassium (as amino acid complex) 99 mg. Other Ingredients: Stearic Acid, Isolated Soy Protein, Microcrystalline Cellulose, Magnesium Stearate, Carob.

MegaMuscle - Life Extension
Six tablets contain: L-Arginine 5000 mg • L-Ornithine 2500 mg • Vitamin C 200 mg • Hypothalamus Gland 10x 50 mg • Pituitary Gland 10x 50 mg • Vitamin B6 20 mg.
See Editor's Note No. 31.

MegaNutrition - DreamPharm
Each tablet contains: Vitamin A 560 IU • Beta-Carotene 470 IU • Vitamin D 38 IU • Vitamin E Succinate 40 IU • Ascorbic Acid (vitamin C) 18 mg • Thiamin 5 mg • Riboflavin 4 mg • Pyridoxine 6 mg • Niacin 4 mg • Niacinamide 4 mg • Di-Calcium Phosphate 10.3 mg • Vitamin B12 6.5 mg • Folic Acid 12.5 mg • Biotin 4.8 mg • Choline 10 mg • Inositol 1.3 mg • Para-Aminobenzoic Acid 11.3 mg • Calcium 250 mg • Magnesium 60 mg • Iron 2.5 mg • Iodine 1.5 mcg • Copper 40 mcg • Zinc 3.5 mg • Chromium 4 mcg • Selenium 1.3 mcg • Potassium 15 mg • Manganese 1.5 mg • Pancreatin 25.2 mg • Pancrillipase 6.3 mg • Bromelain 3.8 mg • Ox Bile extract 12.5 mg • Glutamic Acid 10 mg • Cellulose 127 mg • Hydrogenated Vegetable oil 54 mg • Silica 21 mg • Magnesium Stearate 5 mg.
See Editor's Note No. 14.

Mega-Polyzyme - InterPlexus
Each capsule contains: Protease 50,000 HUT • Amylase 10,000 SKB • Lipase 5000 LU • Bromelain 100 GDU • Papain 2,000,000 PU • Cellulase 600 CU. Other Ingredients: Gelatin.

Megasorb B-Complex "50" - Solgar
Each tablet contains: Thiamin (as thiamin mononitrate) 50 mg • Riboflavin 50 mg • Niacin (as niacin, niacinamide) 50 mg • Vitamin B6 (as pyridoxine HCl) 50 mg • Folic Acid 400 mcg • Vitamin B12 (as cobalamin) 50 mcg • • Biotin (as D-biotin) 50 mcg • Pantothenic Acid (from D-calcium pantothenate) 50 mg • Magnesium (as magnesium citrate) 20 mg • Choline (as choline bitartrate) 21 mg • Lecithin 50 mg • Inositol 50 mg • Cocarboxylase 5 mg • Pantethine 5 mg • Pyridoxal-5-Phosphate 5 mg • Riboflavin-5-Phosphate 5 mg. Other Ingredients: Microcrystalline Cellulose, Silica, Vegetable Magnesium Stearate, Cellulose, Vegetable Glycerin, Carnauba Wax.

Megasorb Vitamin B12 500 mcg - Solgar
Each nugget contains: Vitamin B12 (as cobalamin) 5000 mcg • Dibencozide 100 mcg. Other Ingredients: Mannitol, Vegetable Magnesium Stearate, Silica, Natural Cherry Flavor.

Mega-Stress Complex - Nature's Plus
Each tablet contains: Vitamin C (as ascorbic acid) 500 mg • Thiamin (vitamin B1, as thiamine HCl) 60 mg • Riboflavin (vitamin B2) 60 mg • Niacin (as niacinamide) 125 mg • Vitamin B6 (as pyridoxine HCl) 100 mg • Folate (as folic acid) 400 mcg • Vitamin B12 (as cyanocobalamin) 250 mcg • Biotin 75 mcg • Pantothenic Acid (as calcium pantothenate) 200 mg • Calcium (as amino acid chelate/complex) 100 mg • Magnesium (as amino acid chelate/complex) 50 mg • Zinc (as amino acid chelate/complex) 25 mg • Inositol 100 mg • Valerian root (valeriana officinalis) 50 mg • Choline (as bitartrate) 32 mg • PABA (para-aminobenzoic acid) 30 mg • Chamomile flower (matricaria recutita) 25 mg. Other Ingredients: Stearic Acid, Microcrystalline Cellulose, Rose Hips (rosa canina), Isolated Soy Protein, Hydroxypropyl Methylcellulose, Silica, Magnesium Stearate, Rice Bran, Pharmaceutical Glaze.

MegaTropin - Urban Biologics
Each packet contains: Vitamin C 100 mg • Niacin 50 mg • Vitamin B6 8 mg • Glycoamine Acid-Glucose Complex 2197 mg • Novel Polyose Complex 2030 mg • Megatropin Amino Acid Complex 7450 mg: Glycine, L-Glutamine, L-Arginine, L-Lysine, GABA, Pyroglutamic Acid, L-Ornithine, L-Tyrosine • Mucuna Pruriens 200 mg • Colostrum 100 mg • Alpha GPC 100 mg • Milk Thistle 4:1 extract 70 mg • 5-HTP 50 mg. Other Ingredients: Natural Flavors, Sodium Bicarbonate, Potassium Bicarbonate, Beta Carotene Color.

Megavital Forte - Futurebiotics LLC
One tablet contains: Vitamin C 60 mg • Vitamin B1 (thiamin HCl) 10 mg • Vitamin B2 (riboflavin) 10 mg • Niacinamide 25 mg • Vitamin E 15 IU • Vitamin B6 (pyridoxine Hcl) 10 mg • Folic Acid 400 mcg • Vitamin B12 (cyanocobalamin) 50 mcg • Magnesium (oxide, gluconate) 25 mg • Zinc (gluconate) 15 mg • Biotin 201 mcg • Pantothenic Acid 20 mg • Choline Bitartrate 100 mg • Inositol 40 mg • Iodine (potassium iodide) 180 mcg • Sodium Phosphate 500 mcg • Phosphatidylcholine (55% strength) 50 mg • Papain 15 mg • Lecithin 25 mg • Selenium (yeast) 100 mcg • Chromium (polynicotinate) 25 mcg • Betaine HCl 25 mg. In a biological base containing a special blend of: Selenium Rich Yeast, Soy protein, Power Green complex (Barley grass, Chlorella, Alfalfa juice concentrate) & Para Amino Benzoic Acid (PABA).

Mega-Vita-Min - Puritan's Pride
Each tablet contains: Vitamin A (as Retinyl Palmitate) 8,000 IU • Vitamin C (as Ascorbic Acid) 250 mg • Vitamin D (as Cholecalciferol) 400 IU • Vitamin E (as d-Alpha Tocopheryl Acetate) 125 IU • Thiamin (Vitamin B-1; as Thiamine Mononitrate) 80 mg • Riboflavin (Vitamin B-2) 80 mg • Niacin (as Niacinamide) 80 mg • Vitamin B-6 (as Pyridoxine Hydrochloride) 80 mg • Folic Acid 400 mcg • Vitamin B-12 (as Cyanoccobalamin) 80 mcg • Biotin 80 mcg • Pantothenic Acid (as-d-Calcium Panothenate) 80 mg • Calcium (as Calcium Carbonate) 8 mg • Iron (as Ferrous Gluconate) 2 mg • Iodine (as Kelp) 150 mcg • Magnesium (as Magnesium Oxide) 6 mg • Zinc (as Zinc Gluconate) 1.4 mg • Selenium (as Sodium Selenate) 25 mcg • Copper (as Copper Gluconate) 0.07 mg • Manganese (as Manganese Gluconate) 0.12 mg • Chromium (as Chromium Picolinate) 25 mcg • Molybdenum (as Sodium Molybdate) 25 mcg • Potassium (as Potassium Gluconate) 1.6 mg • Boron (as Sodium Borate) 0.5 mg • Choline Bitartrate 80 mg • Inositol 80 mg • PABA 80 mg • Rutin 30 mg • Citrus Bioflavonoid Complex 25 mg • Hesperidin Complex 5 mg • Betaine Hydrochloride 25 mg • Coenzyme Q-10 500 mcg • Deodorized Garlic 1 mg • Korean Ginseng 1 mg • Pycnogenol 500 mcg.

Mega-Vita-Min Multiple - Nature's Life
Each tablet contains: Beta Carotene (Vitamin A equivalent to 5000 IU) 3 mg • Vitamin B1 (Thiamine HCl) 10 mg • Vitamin B2 (Riboflavin) 10 mg • Vitamin B6 (Pyridoxine HCl) 10 mg • Vitamin B12 (Cobalamin concentrate) 100 mcg • Niacin 10 mg • Pantothenic Acid (D-Calcium Pantothenate) 20 mg • Folic Acid 400 mcg • Choline (Bitartrate) 90 mg • Inositol 90 mg • Biotin (D-Biotin) 50 mcg • PABA (Para Aminobenzoic Acid) 20 mg • Lemon Bioflavonoids Complex (Testlab) 15mg • Vitamin C 100 mg • Vitamin E (d-Alpha Tocopherol mixed with Tocopherols) 10 IU •

BRAND NAMES

Boron (Full-Ranged Amino Acid Chelated) 25 mg • Calcium (Full-Ranged Amino Acid Chelated) 50 mg • Chromium (Nutrition 21 Picolinate) 50 mcg • Copper (Full-Ranged Amino Acid Chelated) 200 mcg • Iodine (Icelandic Kelp) 225 mcg • Magnesium (Full-Ranged Amino Acid Chelated) 50 mg • Manganese (Full-Ranged Amino Acid Chelated) 2 mg • Molybdenum (Proteinate) 25 mcg • Phosphorus (Full-Ranged Amino Acid Chelated & Complexed) 19 mg • Potassium (Proteinate) 15 mg • Selenium (Nutrition 21 Selenomethionine) 25 mcg • Silicon (Dioxide) 25 mcg • Vanadium (Full-Ranged Amino Acid Chelated) 25 mcg • Zinc (Nutrition 21 Picolinate) 2 mg • Betaine HCl 30 mg • Nucleic Acids (RNA & DNA from Yeast) 30 mg • CoQ10 (Co-Enzyme Ubiquione) 500 mcg, Essential Fatty Acids (Soy, Spirulina) 25 mg • Super Green Pro 96 (Soy Protein Super Food) 330 Mg. In a natural base containing: Rose Hips concentrate, Acerola, Rutin, Hesperidin, Lecithin, Milk-Free Lactobacillus Acidophilus, Alfalfa leaf, Watercress, Parsley, "72 Trace Minerals, Rice Bran, Spirulina, Barley Green, Psyllium, Apple Pectin, Oat Bran, Bromelain, Papain, Chlorella & Chlorophyll.

MegaVitamins - Matol Botanical International Ltd
Each caplet contains: Vitamin A (retinyl palmitate, 10% as beta carotene) 1250 IU • Vitamin C (ascorbic acid) 45 mg • Vitamin D (cholecalciferol) 100 IU • Vitamin E (DL-alpha-tocopheryl acetate) 22.5 IU • Thiamin (mononitrate) 0.375 mg • Riboflavin 0.425 mg • Niacin 6.25 mg • Vitamin B6 (pyridoxine HCl) 0.5 mg • Folate (folic acid) 100 mcg • Vitamin B12 (cyanocobalamin) 1.5 mcg • Biotin 75 mcg • Pantothenic Acid (D-calcium pantothenate) 2.5 mg • Calcium (carbonate) 50 mg • Iron (ferrous fumarate) 4.5 mg • Iodine (from kelp) 40 mcg • Magnesium (glycinate) 50 mg • Zinc (glycinate) 3.75 mg • Selenium 17.5 mcg • Copper (glycinate) 0.5 mg • Manganese (glycinate) 0.5 mg • Chromium 30 mcg • Molybdenum (glycinate) 18.75 mcg • Quercetin 12.5 mg • Choline Bitartrate 12.5 mg • Inositol 12.5 mg • Alpha-Lipoic Acid 12.5 mg • Olive leaf 4:1 extract (olea europaea) 12.5 mg • Milk Thistle seed extract (silybum marianum L., 80% as silymarin) 12.5 mg. Other Ingredients: Sprout Blend: Barley Sprouts, Millet Sprouts, Oat Sprouts, Wheat Sprouts, White Soy Sprouts and Broccoli Sprouts, Fruit and Vegetable Blend: Pineapple, Broccoli, Carrot, Apple, Orange, Tomato, Brussles Sprouts, Cauliflower, Beet, Blueberry, Celery, Grape, Grapefruit, Kale, Lemon, Lime, Plum, Raspberry, Strawberry, Watermelon, Radish, Cantaloupe, Cherry, Leek, Onion, Papaya, Peach, and Pear, Dicalcium Phosphate, Microcrystalline Cellulose, Croscarmellose Sodium, Stearic Acid, Magnesium Stearate, Slicia.

Mega-Vite 85 Multiple - Source Naturals
Each tablet contains: Vitamin A (palmitate 10000 IU, beta carotene 2000 IU) 12000 IU • Vitamin C (calcium, zinc and manganese ascorbates) 250 mg • Vitamin B-1 (thiamin) 85 mg • Vitamin B-2 (riboflavin) 85 mg • Niacinamide 85 mg • Vitamin B-6 (pyridoxine HCl) 85 mg • Folic acid 420 mcg • Vitamin B-12 (cyanocobalamin) 85 mcg • Biotin 85 mcg • Vitamin B-5 (calcium D-Pantothenate) 85 mg • Vitamin D-3 (cholecalciferol) 400 IU • Vitamin E (D-alpha tocopheryl) 100 IU • Calcium (ascorbate, citrate) 30 mg • Iron (fumarate) 12 mg • Iodine (from kelp) 150 mcg • Magnesium (citrate, oxide) 20 mg • Zinc (ascorbate) 15 mg • Copper (sebacate) 1 mg • Potassium (citrate) 10 mg • Manganese (ascorbate) 6 mg • Chromium (amino acid chelate) 100 mcg • Selenium (amino acid chelate) 50 mcg • Molybdenum (amino acid chelate) 100 mcg • Boron (amino acid chelate) 1 mg. Other Ingredients: PABA (para amino benzoic acid) 85 mg, Choline Bitartrate 85 mg, Inositol 85 mg, Bioflavonoid complex 25 mg, Rutin 20 mg, Hesperidin complex 5 mg.

Mega-Vites 75 - The Vitamin Shoppe
Each tablet contains: Vitamin D 400 IU • Vitamin A Activity 10000 IU • Vitamin C 250 mg • Vitamin E 150 IU • Vitamin B1 75 mg • Vitamin B2 75 mg • Vitamin B6 75 mg • Vitamin B12 75 mcg • Niacinamide 75 mg • PABA 75 mg • Pantothenic Acid 75 mg • Choline Bitartrate 75 mg • Inositol 75 mg • D-Biotin 75 mcg • Folic Acid 400 mcg • Rutin 25 mg • Citrus Bioflavonoid Complex 5 mg • Hesperidin 5 mg • Betaine Hydrochloride 25 mg • L-Glutamic Acid 25 mg • Iodine 150 mcg • Calcium 50 mg • Potassium 10 mg • Iron 10 mg • Magnesium 10 mg • Manganese 6.1 mg • Zinc 15 mg • Chromium 10 mcg • Selenium 10 mcg.

Mega-Zyme - Enzymatic Therapy
Two tablets contain: Pancreatic Enzymes 10X full strength, undiluted & uncut 325 mg: Units of Activity: Protease 96580, Amylase 98780, Lipase 24496 • Trypsin 75 mg • Papain 50 mg • Bromelain (1200 MCU) 50 mg • Amylase 10 mg • Lipase 10 mg • Lysozyme 10 mg • Chymotrypsin 2 mg.
See Editor's Note No. 14.

Mela-Cal - Melaleuca
Two tablets contain: Vitamin C 30 mg • Vitamin D 400 IU • Calcium 650 mg • Phosphorous 493 mg • Magnesium 158 mg.

Melancor (melancor-nh) - Melancor Consumer Healthcare
Each capsule contains: Calcium 75 mg • Vitamin B2 12 mg • Vitamin B6 12 mg • Vitamin B12 50 mcg • Folic Acid 200 mcg • Biotin 250 mcg • Pantothenic Acid 100 mg • Iodine 75 mcg • Zinc 20 mg • Proprietary Blend 1200 mg: Bromelain, PABA, Choline, Inositol, L-Cysteine, Collagen.

Mela-T - Alacer
Each lozenge contains: Melatonin 0.5 mg • Glycine 600 mg • Sorbitol 100 mg • Vitamin C (as calcium-magnesium ascorbate) 80 mg • Vitamin B6 (pyridoxine HCl) 10 mg • Zinc Ascorbate 100 mcg • Magnesium Citrate 35 mg • Proprietary Niacin Complex 2 mg • Banana flavor 2 mg.
See Editor's Note No. 26.

Melatonin - New Hope Health Products
Each capsule contains: Melatonin (5-methoxy-tryptamine) 3 mg.
See Editor's Note No. 16.

Melatonin - Benepure, Inc
Each capsule contains: Melatonin 3 mg. Other Ingredients: Rice Flour, Gelatin.
See Editor's Note No. 26.

Melatonin - Life Extension
Each capsule contains: Melatonin (pure pharmaceutical grade) 3 mg.
See Editor's Note No. 26.

Melatonin - Olympian Labs
Each capsule contains: Melatonin 3 mg.
See Editor's Note No. 16.

Melatonin - GNC
Each tablet contains: Vitamin B6 (as Pyridoxine Hydrochloride) 2 mg • Melatonin 3 mg. Other Ingredients: Dicalcium Phosphate, Cellulose.
See Editor's Note No. 26.

Melatonin - Optimum Nutrition
Each tablet contains: Melatonin 3 mg.
See Editor's Note No. 16.

Melatonin - BioDynamax
Each capsule contains: Melatonin 3 mg.
See Editor's Note No. 16.

Melatonin - Xymogen
Each sublingual tablet contains: Melatonin 3 mg.
See Editor's Note No. 26.

Melatonin - American Biologics
Each tablet contains: Melatonin 3 mg • Vitamin B6 6 mg • Niacin (vitamin B3) 5 mg. Other Ingredients: Natural Orange Base, Fructose, Sorbitol, Magnesium Stearate, Cellulose.
See Editor's Note No. 26.

Melatonin - AIE Pharmaceuticals
Each tablet contains: Melatonin 3 mg • Vitamin B6 10 mg.

Melatonin - Metabolic Response Modifiers
Each capsule contains: Melatonin (5-methoxy-tryptamine) 3 mg.
See Editor's Note No. 16.

Melatonin (100 mcg) - Life Enhancement Products, Inc.
Each capsule contains: Vitamin B6 (as pyridoxal-5-phosphate) 50 mcg • Melatonin 100 mcg.

Some Brand Name Natural Products - What they Contain

www.NaturalDatabase.com contains MANY more listings than appear here.
Editor's Notes are located on pages 2155-2163.

Melatonin (3 mg) - Life Enhancement Products, Inc.
Each capsule contains: Vitamin B6 (as pyridoxal-5-phosphate) 450 mcg • Melatonin 3 mg.

Melatonin (300 mcg) - Life Enhancement Products, Inc.
Each capsule contains: Vitamin B6 (as pyridoxal-5-phosphate) 50 mcg • Melatonin 300 mcg.

Melatonin 0.5 mg - Pure Encapsulations
Each vegetable capsule contains: Melatonin 0.5 mg.

Melatonin 1 mg - PhysioLogics
Each tablet contains: Melatonin (as n-acetyl-5-methoxytryptamine) 1 mg. Other Ingredients: Dicalcium Phosphate, Cellulose (plant origin), Vegetable Stearic Acid, Croscarmellose, Magnesium Stearate.

Melatonin 1 mg - Nature's Bounty
Each tablet contains: Melatonin (as N-acetyl-5-methoxytryptamine) 1 mg. Other Ingredients: Dicalcium Phosphate, Cellulose (plant origin), Vegetable Stearic Acid, Croscarmellose, Magnesium Stearate.
See Editor's Note No. 26.

Melatonin 1 Sublingual - GNC
Each tablet contains: Melatonin 1 mg. Other Ingredients: Sorbitol, Mannitol, Natural Flavor.
See Editor's Note No. 26.

Melatonin 10 mg - Vital Nutrients
Each capsule contains: Melatonin 10 mg.
See Editor's Note No. 26.

Melatonin 1mg Tablets - Ortho Molecular Products
Each tablet contains: Melatonin 1 mg. Other Ingredients: Sorbitol, Xylitol, Stearic Acid, Silicon Dioxide, Magnesium Stearate.

Melatonin 2.5 mg Sublingual - Pro Health
Each sublingual tablet contains: Melatonin 2.5 mg • Coenzymated Vitamin B6 (as pyridoxal-5-phosphate) 500 mcg. Other Ingredients: Sorbitol, Natural Lemon Flavor, Stearic Acid, Magnesium Stearate.
See Editor's Note No. 26.

Melatonin 20 mg - Vital Nutrients
Each capsule contains: Melatonin 20 mg.
See Editor's Note No. 26.

Melatonin 20 mg - Pure Encapsulations
Each vegetable capsule contains: Melatonin 20 mg.

Melatonin 3 - GNC
Each tablet contains: Vitamin B6 (as pyridoxine hydrochloride) 2 mg • Melatonin 3 mg. Other Ingredients: Dicalcium Phosphate, Cellulose.
See Editor's Note No. 26.

Melatonin 3 mg - TwinLab
Each tablet contains: Melatonin 3 mg.
See Editor's Note No. 26.

Melatonin 3 mg - Schiff
Each tablet contains: Vitamin B6 (as pyridoxine hydrochloride) 10 mg • Calcium (as calcium carbonate) 86 mg • Melatonin 3 mg. Other Ingredients: Cellulose, Croscarmellose Sodium, Magnesium Stearate.
See Editor's Note No. 26.

Melatonin 3 mg - PhysioLogics
Each tablet contains: Melatonin (as n-acetyl-5-methoxytryptamine) 3 mg. Other Ingredients: Dicalcium Phosphate, Cellulose (plant origin), Vegetable Magnesium Stearate, Vegetable Stearic Acid, Silica, Croscarmellose.

Melatonin 3 mg - Pro Health
Each tablet contains: Melatonin 3 mg. Other Ingredients: Dicalcium Phosphate, Sodium Starch Glycolate, Stearic Acid, Magnesium Stearate.
See Editor's Note No. 26.

Melatonin 3 mg - Nature's Bounty
Each tablet contains: Melatonin (as N-acetyl-5-methoxytryptamine) 3 mg. Other Ingredients: Dicalcium Phosphate, Cellulose (plant origin), Vegetable Magnesium Stearate, Vegetable Stearic Acid, Silica, Croscarmellose.
See Editor's Note No. 26.

Melatonin 3 mg - Puritan's Pride
Each tablet contains: Melatonin (as N-acetyl-5-methoxytryptamine) 3 mg. Other Ingredients: Dicalcium Phosphate, Cellulose (plant origin), Vegetable Magnesium Stearate, Vegetable Stearic Acid, Silica, Croscarmellose.

Melatonin 3 mg - Vital Nutrients
Each capsule contains: Melatonin 3 mg.
See Editor's Note No. 26.

Melatonin 3 mg - Pure Encapsulations
Each vegetable capsule contains: Melatonin 3 mg.

Melatonin 3 mg - Vivitas
Each capsule contains: Melatonin (synthetic N-acetyl-5-methoxytryptamine) 3 mg. Other Ingredients: Tricalcium Phosphate, Gelatin, Magnesium Stearate, Silicon Dioxide.
See Editor's Note No. 26.

Melatonin 3 mg - Vitamin World
Each tablet contains: Melatonin (as N-acetyl-5-methoxytryptamine) 3 mg. Other Ingredients: Dicalcium Phosphate, Cellulose (plant origin), Vegetable Magnesium Stearate, Vegetable Stearic Acid, Silica, Croscarmellose.

Melatonin 3 Timed Release - GNC
Each tablet contains: Melatonin 3 mg. Other Ingredients: Dicalcium Phosphate, Cellulose.
See Editor's Note No. 26.

Melatonin 3mg Capsules - Ortho Molecular Products
Each capsule contains: Melatonin 3 mg. Other Ingredients: Natural Gelatin Capsules, White Rice Flour.

Melatonin 500 mcg - Nature's Way
Each lozenge contains: Melatonin 500 mcg. Other Ingredients: Magnesium Stearate, Sorbitol.
See Editor's Note No. 16.

Melatonin Caps - TwinLab
Each capsule contains: Melatonin 3 mg. Other Ingredients: Potato Starch, Cellulose, Gelatin, Purified Water, Magnesium Stearate, MCT.
See Editor's Note No. 26.

Melatonin Controlled Release 2 mg - TwinLab
Each tablet contains: Melatonin 2 mg.
See Editor's Note No. 26.

Melatonin Forte - PhytoPharmica
Two capsules contain: Kava (Piper methysticum) root extract (standardized to contain 30% kavalactones) 210 mg • Valerian (Valeriana officinalis) root extract (standardized to contain a minimum of 0.8% valerenic acids) 150 mg • Melatonin 500 mcg.
See Editor's Note No. 21.

Melatonin PM Complex - Anabolic Laboratories
Each tablet contains: Melatonin 1 mg • Vitamin B6 (pyridoxine HCl) 5 mg • Vitamin B2 (riboflavin) 3 mg • Vitamin B3 (niacinamide) 10 mg • Vitamin B12 (ion-exchange resin) 12.5 mcg • Calcium (lactate) 40 mg • Magnesium (oxide) 30 mg • Chinese Herbal Complex 195 mg: Valerian Root extract, Ziziphus Spinosa seed, Salviae Miltiorrhiza root, Succinum (Amber), Biotae Orientalis seed, Coptis Chinensis rhizome, Chamomile flower, Hops Strobile, Passion Flower, Skullcap herb. Other Ingredients: Cellulose, Stearic Acid, Magnesium Stearate, Vanillin, Vegetable Oil, Silica.
See Editor's Note No. 16.

Melatonin Spray **-** Nature's Plus
Each spray contains: Melatonin (N-Acetyl-5-Methoxytryptamine) 1.5 mg • GABA (Gamma Aminobutyric Acid) 2500 mcg • Pyridoxal-5-Phosphate (P5P) 2500 mcg. In a proprietary liposomal complex of Essential Metabolic Factors, Purified Water, Vegetable Glycerine, Purified Lecithin, Citrus seed extract (Citrus sinensis), Vitamin E & natural Peppermint flavor.
See Editor's Note No. 16.

Melatonin Sustain **-** Jarrow Formulas
Each tablet contains: Vitamin B6 (pyridoxine HCl) 2 mg • Magnesium (from oxide) 100 mg • Melatonin 1 mg. Other Ingredients: Calcium Phosphate, Cellulose, Modified Cellulose, Modified Cellulose Gum, Stearic Acid, Magnesium Stearate, Silicon Dioxide, Vanilla.

Melatonin Tablets, Accurate Release, 1 mg **-** Nature's Bounty
Each tablet contains: Melatonin (n-Acetyl-5 Methoxytryptamine) 1 mg. Other Ingredients: Dicalcium Phosphate, Microcrystalline, Cellulose, Vegetable Magnesium Stearate, Croscarmellose Sodium.
See Editor's Note No. 26.

Melatonin Tablets, Accurate Release, 200 mcg **-** Nature's Bounty
Each tablet contains: Pure Melatonin 200 mcg.
See Editor's Note No. 26.

Melatonin Time Release 1 mg **-** Natrol, Inc.
Each tablet contains: Calcium (as Dicalcium Phosphate) 40 mg • Melatonin 1 mg. Other Ingredients: Time Release Agent (Hydrogenated Vegetable Oil), stearic acid, silica, magnesium stearate.
See Editor's Note No. 26.

Melatonin Time Release 3 mg **-** Natrol, Inc.
Each tablet contains: Calcium (as Calcium Carbonate) 63 mg • Melatonin 3 mg. Other Ingredients: Cellulose, Silica, Stearic Acid, Cellulose Gum, Magnesium Stearate.
See Editor's Note No. 26.

Melatonin Ultra **-** FreeLife International
One-half teaspoon contains: Proprietary Blend 400 mg: Fructose, Dextrates, Sorbitol, Natural Orange/Lemon Flavor, Polynesian Kava root extract, German Chamomile leaf extract, European Hops extract (strobile), English Lemon Balm leaf powder, Japanese Peppermint leaf Powder, North American Scullcap (aerial parts), European Valerian root extract • Melatonin (n-acteyl-5-methoxytryptamine) 1 mg. Other Ingredients: Silicon Dioxide, Magnesium Stearate, RapidSorb (exclusive flavoring and transport system).

Melatonin, Time Released 5 mg **-** Pro Health
Two capsules contain: Vitamin C (as niacinimide ascorbate) 223 mg • Niacin (as niacinamide ascorbate) 73 mg • Vitamin B12 (as cyanocobalamin) 100 mcg • Calcium (as calcium citrate) 48 mg • Magnesium (as magnesium oxide) 120 mg • Chromium (as ChromeMate brand chromium polynicotinate) 50 mcg • Inositol 100 mg • Melatonin (50% immediate release, 50% time-released) 5 mg • Pyridoxal Phosphate 10 mg. Other Ingredients: Gelatin, Rice Flour, Magnesium Stearate.

Melbrosia **-** Pronatura
Each capsule contains: Flower Pollen (including bee bread - perga) • Gelatin capsule shell • Royal Jelly (lyophilised) • Acerola extract.

Melissa Supreme **-** Gaia Herbs
Fifteen drops contain: Proprietary Blend 60 mg: Lemon Balm (melissa off.), German Chamomile flowers (matricaria recutita), Passionflower vine (passiflora incarnata), Fresh Skullcap herb (scutellaria lateriflora), Fresh Wild Oats milky seed (avena sativa), Gotu Kola concentrated glycerite (centella asiatica), Mineral Salts extracted from Kelp, 45-55% Pure Grain Alcohol USP, Spring Water.

Mellow Tonin **-** Jarrow Formulas
Each capsule contains: Vitamin B6 2 mg • Melatonin 3 mg. Other Ingredients: Rice Powder, Magnesium Stearate.

MeltRX 24 Ultra **-** Unknown
Two capsules contain: Vitamin B6 (as pyridoxal-5-phosphate) 5 mg • Vitamin B12 (as methylcobalamin) 25 mcg • Manganese (as manganese sulfate) 3 mg • Chromium (as chromium dinicotinate glycinate) 150 mcg • Meltpro Proprietary Blend 1499 mg: Glucomannan (from konjac root), Cocoa extract (standardized for theobromine), Green Tea leaf extract (standardized for EGCG and polyphenols), Hoodia Gordonii cactus stem 20:1 extract, Nut Grass extract (cyperus rotundus, standardized for octopamine), 5-HTP (from griffonia simplicifolia seed), Coleus Forskolin tubers extract, Alpha-Lipoic Acid (standardized for thioctic acid), Banaba leaf extract (lagerstromia speciosa, standardized for corosolic acid), Naringin (from grapefruit rind), Vanadium (as vanadyl sulfate), Bioperine brand Black Pepper extract. Other Ingredients: Dicalcium Phosphate, Microcrystalline Cellulose, Croscarmellose Sodium, Stearic Acid, Magnesium Stearate, Silica, Pharmaceutical Glaze.

Mel-Vita **-** Melaleuca
Three tablets contain: Vitamin A 10,000 IU • Vitamin C 135 mg • Vitamin D 250 IU • Vitamin E 30 IU • Vitamin K 25 mcg • Thiamin 15 mg • Riboflavin 17 mg • Niacin 75 mg • Vitamin B6 21 mg • Folate 400 mcg • Vitamin B12 15 mcg • Biotin 30 mcg • Pantothenic Acid 18 mg • Calcium 250 mg • Iron 18 mg • Phosphorous 192 mg • Iodine 150 mcg • Magnesium 240 mg • Zinc 15 mg • Selenium 200 mcg • Copper 3 mg • Manganese 5 mg • Chromium 15 mcg • Molybdenum 200 mcg • Potassium 45 mg.

MemBrain Essentials **-** Life Enhancement Products, Inc.
Each dropper contains: Vitamin C (from ascorbyl palmitate) 5 mg • Vitamin E (from DL-alpha tocopherol) 10 IU • Phosphatidylserine 100 mg • Phosphatidylcholine 25 mg. Other Ingredients: Medium-Chain Triglycerides, Ethanol, Butylated Hydroxytoluene.

Membrin **-** Ortho Molecular Products
Each capsule contains: Ginkgo Biloba leaf extract (standardized to contain 24% ginkgoflavoneglycosides and 6% terpene lactones) 120 mg • Vinpocetine 30 mg • Huperzin alkaloids (from huperzia seratta leaf extract 100 mcg. Other Ingredients: Natural Vegetable Capsules, Ascorbyl Palmitate, Microcrystalline Cellulose, Silicon Dioxide.

MemorAble **-** Resource Wellness
Two softgels contain: Vitamin B6 (Pyridoxine HCl) 2 mg • Vitamin B12 (Cyanocobalamin) 6 mcg • Ginkgo Biloba extract (leaves) 120 mg • Lecithin 1200 mg. Other Ingredients: Gelatin, Soybean Oil, Glycerin, Beeswax, Titanium Dioxide, FD&C Yellow No. 6, FD&C Red No. 40, FD&C Blue No. 1.

MemorActin **-** Nature's Plus
Two capsules contain: Phosphatidylcholine 250 mg • Inositol 125 mg • Ginkgo Biloba leaf (standardized 24% Ginkgo Flavone-Glycosides, 6% Terpene Lactones) 100 mg • Vitamin C corn free 100 mg • Pantothenic Acid (Calcium Pantothenate) 50 mg • Phosphatidylserine 25 mg • Bilberry (Vaccinium myrtillus fruit) standardized 25% Anthocyanosides 10 mg • Beta Carotene pro-Vitamin A (supplying 10000 IU of Vitamin A activity) 6 mg • Coenzyme Q10 (Ubiquinone) 2.5 mg.

MemorAll **-** Xymogen
Two capsules contain: Vitamin B6 (as P5P) 10 mg • Vitamin B12 (as methylcobalamin) 200 mcg • Folate (as folic acid and calcium folinate) 400 mcg • N-Acetyl Cysteine 200 mg • Acetyl-L-Carnitine 500 mg • Phosphatidylserine 100 mg • Ginkgo Biloba 24:6 extract 120 mg • Bacopa Monniera standardized extract 100 mg • Vinpocetine 10 mg • Huperzine A 200 mcg • Resveratrol 2 mg.

Memorall **-** PharmAssure
Each softgel contains: Vitamin E 50 IU • Huperzine A 50 mcg. Other Ingredients: Soybean Oil, Gelatin, Glycerin, Caramel Color, Titanium Dioxide.

Memorall (Preventive Nutrition) **-** GNC
Two softgels contain: Vitamin A (as beta-carotene) 2333 IU • Vitamin C (as ascorbic acid) 60 mg • Vitamin E (as D-alpha tocopheryl acetate) 30 IU • Folate, Folic Acid, Folacin 400 mcg • Vitamin B12

(as cyanocobalamin) 12 mcg • EPA (eicosapentaenoic acid, as fish body oil) 200 mg • DHA (docosahexaenoic acid, as fish body oil) 150 mg • Ginkgo Biloba leaves extract 120 mg • Phosphatidyl Serine (as soy lecithin) 25 mg • Coenzyme Q-10 10 mg • Citrus Bioflavonoids 10 mg • Huperzine A 100 mcg. Other Ingredients: Soybean Oil, Gelatin, Glycerin, Caramel Color, Titanium Dioxide.

Memoren **-** R-U Ved U.S.A.
Bacopa Monnieri (standardized to 50% bacopasides) • Ashwagandha • Centella Asiatica • Convolvulus Pleuricalis • Ginkgo Biloba.

Memory 2000 **-** Natural Balance
Two tablets contain: Niacin 40 mg • Ginkgo leaf standardized extract 120 mg • Phosphatidylserine 100 mg • DMAE 100 mg • Acetyl-L-Carnitine 20 mg • Vinpocetine 5 mg.

Memory Balm **-** Life Enhancement Products, Inc.
Four capsules contain: Pantothenic Acid (vitamin B5 as calcium pantothenate) 400 mg • Lemon Balm leaf (melissa officinalis) 1600 mg • Choline (as choline dihydrogen citrate) 800 mg.

Memory Formula **-** Youngevity
Ginkgo biloba leaf • Gotu Kola herb • Cayenne pepper • Siberian Ginseng • Magnesium • Lecithin • L-Glutamine • L-Tyrosine • Vitamin B6 • Vitamin B3 • Vilcabamba Mineral Essence: Potassium, Calcium, Magnesium, Zinc, Chromium, Selenium, Iron, Copper, Molybdenum, Vanadium, Iodine, Cobalt, Manganese.

Memory Mate **-** FreeLife International
Each caplet contains: Thiamin (as thiamin hydrochloride) 3 mg • Folate (as folic acid) 200 mcg • Vitamin B12 (cyanocobalamin) 12 mcg • Pantothenic Acid (as D-calcium pantothenate) 25 mcg • Zinc (as zinc citrate) 5 mg • Brahmi leaf and stem standardized extract (bacopa monniera, 20% bacosides A & B) 100 mg • Herbal Brain Factors Proprietary Blend 150 mg: Fo-ti root, Ginger root, Gotu Kola leaf, Schizandra berry, Eleuthero root • Soy Activation Complex 50 mg: Phosphatidylcholine, Phosphatidylinositol, Phosphatidylethanolamine, Phosphatidylcephalin, Phosphatidylserine • DMAE (dimethylaminoethanol bitartrate) 75 mg • Ginkgo Biloba leaf standardized extract (27% ginkgo flavonglycosides, 7% sesquiterpene lactones) 60 mg • L-Glutamine 50 mg • Vinpocetine 5 mg • Huperzine A (from huperzia serrata whole plant) 100 mcg • UltraSoy Delivery System Soy Polysaccharides and Plant Enzymes 2500 units. Other Ingredients: Calcium Hydrogen Phosphate, Cellulose, Cellulose Gum, Vegetable Stearic Acid, Silica, Calcium Silicate, Vegetable Magnesium Stearate, Vita-Coat.

Memory Power **-** The Vitamin Shoppe
Two tablets contain: Ginkgo Biloba extract standardized to contain 24% ginkgoflavonglycosides • L-Phenylalanine • L-Glutamine • RNA • Choline • Gotu Kola • Lecithin • Ginkgo Biloba leaf powder.

Memory Support Complex **-** Leiner Health Products
Each caplet contains: Vitamin B12 (Cyanocobalamin) 6 mcg • Ginkgo Biloba extract (Ginkgo biloba) leaf 60 mg • Gotu Kola extract (Centella asiatica) leaf 10 mg • Phosphatidylserine 25 mg • Phosphatidylserine complex 83 mg. Other Ingredients: Calcium Carbonate, Maltodextrin, Cellulose, Silicon Dioxide, Polyethylene Glycol 3350, Croscarmellose Sodium, Tricalcium Phosphate, Crospovidone, Magnesium Stearate, Hydroxypropyl Methycellulose, Resin, Hydroxypropyl Cellulose, Polysorbate 80.

Memory Upgrade **-** Life Enhancement Products, Inc.
Each 1 tbsp serving contains: Vitamin C (as niacinamide ascorbate) 78 mg • Vitamin E (as D,L-alpha-tocopheryl acetate) 30 IU • Thiamine (vitamin B1 as thiamine hydrochloride) 3 mg • Riboflavin (vitamin B2) 3 mg • Niacin (vitamin B3 as niacinamide ascorbate) 75 mg • Vitamin B6 (as pyridoxine hydrochloride) 5 mg • Vitamin B12 (cyanocobalamin) 100 mcg • Biotin 300 mcg • Pantothenic Acid (vitamin B5 as calcium pantothenate) 500 mg • Calcium (as calcium pantothenate) 46 mg • Zinc (as zinc gluconate) 3 mg • Copper (as copper gluconate) 420 mcg • Chromium (as chromium aspartate) 25 mcg • Glycine 150 mg • Choline 1 g • Taurine 200 mg.

Memory Upgrade II **-** Life Enhancement Products, Inc.
Each rounded teaspoon contains: Vitamin C (as niacinamide ascorbate) 78 mg • Vitamin E (as D,L-alpha tocopheryl acetate) 30 IU • Thiamine (vitamin B1) 3 mg • Riboflavin (vitamin B2) 3 mg • Niacin (vitamin B3 as niacin and niacinamide ascorbate) 75 mg • Vitamin B6 (as pyridoxine hydrochloride) 5 mg • Vitamin B12 (as cyanocobalamin) 100 mcg • Biotin 300 mcg • Pantothenic Acid (vitamin B5 as calcium pantothenate) 500 mg • Calcium (as pantothenate) 46 mg • Zinc (as gluconate) 3 mg • Copper (as gluconate) 420 mcg • Chromium (as aspartate) 25 mcg • Glycine 150 mg • Choline 1 g • Taurine 1 g.

Memorya **-** HerbaSway
Ginkgo Biloba • Dong Quai • Kudzu • Rehmannia • Panax Ginseng • Schisandra • Knotweed • Blackberry • HerbaSwee (Cucurbitaceae fruit).

Men Plus Ester C **-** Nutrivention
Two tablets contain: Vitamin C 300 mg • Vitamin E 200 IU • Choline Bitartrate 150 mg • Inositol 150 mg • Niacinamide 150 mg • Pantothenic Acid 150 mg • Essential Fatty Acids 100mg • Vitamin A 1500 IU • Vitamin B6 75 mg • Vitamin B2 75 mg • Vitamin B1 75 mg • Vitamin D 1000 IU • Biotin 500 mcg • Vitamin B12 500 mcg • Folic Acid 400 mcg • Iodine (Kelp) 150 mcg • Saw Palmetto berry 200 mg • Sarsaparilla 200 mg • Bioflavonoids 150 mg.

Men-Applause **-** The Herbalist
Dong Quai root • Black Cohosh root • Chaste Tree berry • Siberian Ginseng root • Oat seed • Wild Yam root.

Menastil **-** Claire Ellen Products
Active Ingredient: Calendula Oil 1X. Inactive Ingredients: Menthyl Acetate, Beta-Pinene, Alpha-Pinene, Coriander Oil, Rosemary Oil, Pennyroyal Oil, White Camphor, Cornmint Oil, Almond Oil, Orange Oil, Mineral Oil.
See Editor's Note No. 1.

MenoCare **-** The Himalaya Drug Company
Each tablet contains: Proprietary Blend 900 mg: Cinnamon (cinnamonum cassia), Haritaki (terminalia chebula), Ashwagandha (withania somnifera), Licorice (glycyrrhiza glabra), Arjuna (terminalia arjuna), Shatavari (asparagus racemosus), Asoka Tree (saraca indica), Gotu Kola (centella asiatica).

MenoEase **-** Wellness for Women
Each capsule contains: Black Cohosh (5% triterpene glycosides calculated as 27-deoxyactein) 20 mg • Black Cohosh powder 430 mg.

Menofem **-** Vitamin Plus Company
HGH Somatotropin • Liver • Pituitary L.A. • Estrone • Black Cohosh extract (cimicifuga racemosa) • Red Clover extract (trifolium pratense) • L-Arginine • L-Glutamine • Glycine • L-Histidine • L-Isoleucine • L-Leucine • L-Lysine • L-Methionine • L-Ornithine • L-Phenylalanine • L-Threonine • L-Tryptophan • L-Valine.
See Editor's Note No. 56.

Menoflash **-** Olympian Labs
Two capsules contain: Black Cohosh extract 100 mg. In a base of Dong Quai, Siberian Ginseng, and Passion Flower.

Menopace Tablets **-** Vitabiotics
Each tablet contains: Vitamin A (2500 IU) 750 mcg • Vitamin D (200 IU) 5 mcg • Vitamin E (natural source) 30 mg • Vitamin C 45 mg • Vitamin B1 (thiamin) 10 mg • Vitamin B2 (riboflavin) 5 mg • Vitamin B3 (niacin) 20 mg • Vitamin B6 (pyridoxine HCl) 40 mg • Folic Acid 500 mcg • Vitamin B12 (cyanocobalamin) 9 mcg • Biotin 30 mcg • Pantothenic Acid 30 mg • PABA (para-aminobenzoic acid) 25 mg • Iron 6 mg • Magnesium 100 mg • Zinc 15 mg • Iodine 225 mcg • Manganese 2 mg • Copper 1 mg • Chromium 50 mcg • Selenium 100 mcg • Soy Isoflavone extract 20 mg: Diadzein 1.1 mg, Glycetine 0.77 mg, Genistein 0.33 mg, Boron 2 mg.

Menopausal Formula **-** Nature's Herbs
Each capsule contains: Dong Quai 75 mg • Siberian Ginseng 100 mg.

Menopause **-** Nutrivention
Each tablet contains: Pantothenic Acid 50 mg • Vitamin B6 50 mg • Vitamin C 50 mg • Vitamin E 100 IU • PABA 50 mg • Calcium 50 mg • Iodine (Kelp) 150mcg • Borage GLA concentrate 150 mg • Mexican Wild Yam root 150 mg • Chaste Tree berry 150 mg • Dong Quai root 150 mg • Licorice root 100 mg • Unicorn root 100 mg • Black Cohosh root 50 mg • Passion flower 50 mg.

Menopause Balance Complex **-** Shaklee
Two capsules contain: Black Cohosh extract (Cimifuga racemosa) root (Standardized to contain 2.5% total triterpene glycosides as 27-deoxyactein) 80 mg • Soy Isoflavones 30 mg • Flaxseed extract (Linum usitatissimum) seed 333 mg • Flaxseed Oil 600 mg • Phytofem Proprietary Blend 100 mg: Dong Quai extract (Angelica sinensis) root, Red Clover extract (Trifolium pratense) herb, Licorice extract (Glycyrrhiza glabra) root. Other Ingredients: Soybean Oil, Beeswax, Soy Lecithin, Ascorbyl Palmitate, Mixed Tocopherols Concentrate, Rosemary Extract, Gelatin, Glycerin, Water, Annatto.

Menopause Bath **-** Abra Therapeutics
Sodium Borate • Sodium Sulfate • Sodium Chloride • Sodium Sesquicarbonate • Olive oil • Chamomile oil • Clary Sage oil • Jasmine oil • Fennel oil • Mace oil • Marjoram oil • Peru Balsam oil • Poppy extract • English Ivy leaf extract • Willow bark extract • Chromium Oxide • Trace Mineral Salts.

Menopause Formula **-** Nature's Life
Four capsules contain: Black Cohosh root extract (Cimicifuga racemosa) (standardized to provide 2.5% or 4 mg Triterpene Glycosides as 27-Deoxyactein) 160 mg • Vitamin C (Calcium Ascorbate) 1200 mg • Vitamin E (d-Alpha Tocopheryl Succinate) 200 IU • Hesperidin (plant source flavonols) 1200 mg • Women's Phyto-Estrogen Blend 100 mg: Soy bean, Wild Yam, Rice Flour, Flax seed & Amaranth.

Menopause Formula **-** Natrol, Inc.
Three capsules contain: Calcium (as calcium carbonate) 250 mg • Magnesium (as magnesium oxide) 125 mg • Soy Isoflavones 100 mg (genistein (10%) 10 mg) • Kava Kava 100 mg (kavalactones (30%) 30 mg) • Red Raspberry 100 mg • Mexican Wild Yam 50 mg • Licorice root 50 mg • Red Clover 50 mg • Horse Chestnut 50 mg • Dong Quai 50 mg • Black Cohosh root 40 mg • Damiana 30 mg • Vitex (agnus-castus) 25 mg • Gingko Biloba 24:6 25 mg • Gotu Kola 25 mg • Gamma Oryzanol 20 mg. Other Ingredients: Rice powder, Silicon Dioxide, Magnesium Stearate, Gelatin.

Menopause Formula **-** Pharmanex
Each capsule contains: Isoflavones from Soy extract 25 mg • Kava Lactones (from Kava Kava root extract) 25.5 mg • Black Cohosh root powder 50 mg. Other Ingredients: Calcium Carbonate, Maltodextrin, Magnesium Stearate, Silicon Dioxide.

Menopause Formula **-** Pharmanex
Each capsule contains: Isoflavones (from soy extract) 25 mg • L-Theanine extract 70:1 (from camellia sinensis) 50 mg • Black Cohosh root powder 50 mg. Other Ingredients: Gelatin, Microcrystalline Cellulose, Stearic Acid, Silicon Dioxide.

Menopause Formula **-** HERBALmax
Horny Goat weed leaves • Scrophularia root • Hares Ear root • Mandarin Orange • Chinese Angelica root.

Menopause Formula **-** Schiff
Three tablets contain: Vitamin K (as phytonadione) 40 mcg • Vitamin B6 (as pyridoxine hydrochloride) 15 mg • Folate (folic acid, folacin) 400 mcg • Vitamin B12 (as cyanocobalamin) 12 mcg • Calcium (as calcium carbonate) 500 mg • Magnesium (as magnesium oxide) 200 mg • Sage leaf (salvia officinalis) 100 mg • Black Cohosh root standardized extract (cimifuga racemosa, 2.5% triterpenoidglycosides) 80 mg • Soy Isoflavones 50 mg • Boron 2 mg • Giant Knotweed root (polygonum cuspidatum, reservatrol 1 mg) 5 mg. Other Ingredients: Microcrystalline Cellulose, Stearic Acid, Croscarmellose Sodium, Hydroxypropyl Methylcellulose, Maltodextrin, Magnesium Stearate, Methylcellulose, Mannitol, Acacia, Polyethylene Glycol, Hydroxypropyl Cellulose.

Menopause Multiple **-** Source Naturals
Six tablets contain: SoyLife genistein-rich Soy concentrate (Yielding 62 mg of Isoflavones: Daidzein 34 mg, Glycitein 20 mg, Genistein 8 mg) • CimiPure Black Cohosh standardized extract 2.5% (Yielding 4 mg Triterpene Glycosides) (Containing 27-Deoxyactein) 160 mg • Vitex extract (Vitex Agnus-Castus) 150 mg • Dong Quai extract (Angelica sinensis) 100 mg • Licorice root extract (Glycyrrhiza glabra) 15 mg • Taurine (Magnesium taurinate) 455 mg • N-Acetyl Cysteine 100 mg • Silymarin (Milk Thistle seed extract) 60 mg • Alpha-Lipoic Acid (Thioctic Acid) 30 mg • Ginkgo Biloba 24% (50:1 Extract) 20 mg • Coenzyme Q10 (Ubiquinone) 15 mg • Vitamin A (Beta Carotene) 13000 IU • Vitamin A (Palmitate) 7000 IU • Vitamin B1 (Thiamin) 50 mg • Vitamin B2 (Riboflavin) 50 mg • Niacinamide 50 mg • Vitamin B5 (Calcium D-Pantothenate) 70 mg • Vitamin B6 (Pyridoxine HCl) 50 mg • Vitamin B12 (Cyanocobalamin) 50 mcg • Biotin 200 mcg • Folic Acid 600 mcg • Vitamin C (Ascorbic Acid, Calcium and Magnesium Ascorbates) 1000 mg • Vitamin D (as Vitamin D3) (Cholecalciferol) 400 IU • Vitamin E (D-Alpha Tocopheryl) (Natural) 400 IU • Boron (Chelate) 3 mg • Calcium (Carbonate, Citrate and Ascorbate) 300 mg • ChromeMate brand Chromium Polynicotinate 100 mcg • Chromium Picolinate 100 mcg 200 mcg • Magnesium (Oxide, Taurinate, Malate, and Ascorbate) 400 mg • Manganese (Citrate) 2 mg • Selenium (L-Selenomethionine) 200 mcg • OptiZinc brand Zinc Monomethionine 12 mg.

Menopause Nutritional System 1 **-** Schiff
Four caplets contain: Vitamin A (as 50% Acetate & 50% Beta Carotene) 5000 IU • Vitamin C (as Ascorbic Acid) 500 mg • Vitamin D (as Cholecalciferol) 200 IU • Vitamin E (as d-Alpha Tocopheryl Succinate) 400 IU • Thiamin (as Thiamin Hydrochloride) 25 mg • Riboflavin 25 mg • Niacin (Niacinamide) 25 mg • Vitamin B6 (as Pyridoxine Hydrochloride) 15 mg • Folate (as Folic Acid) • Vitamin B12 (as Cyanocobolamin) 25 mcg • Biotin 100 mcg • Pantothenic Acid (as d-Calcium Pantothenate) 25 mg • Calcium (as Citrate) 500 mg • Iron (as Ferrous Fumerate) 7.5 mg • Iodine (from Kelp) 75 mcg • Magnesium (as Oxide) 250 mg • Zinc (as Gluconate) 7.5 mg • Selenium (as L-Selenomethionine) 12.5 mg • Copper (as Gluconate) 1 mg • Manganese (as Gluconate) 5 mg • Chromium (as Polynicotinate) 50 mcg. Potassium (as Gluconate) 50 mg • Choline (as Bitartrate) 25 mg • Inositol 25 mg • PABA (Para AminoBenzioc Acid) 25 mg • Boron (as Amino Acid Chelate) 1.5 mg • Bromelain 50 mg • Papain 32.5 mg • Citrus Bioflavonoids 400 mg #8226; Rutin 100 mg. Other Ingredients: Cellulose, Maltodextrin, Stearic Acid, Sillica, Magnesium Sterate, Plyethylene Glycol.

Menopause Nutritional System 2 **-** Schiff
Four caplets contain: Fennel fruit (foeniculum vulgare) 100 mg • Black Cohosh root (cimicifuga racemosa) 100 mg • Anise seed (pimpinella anisum) 100 mg •Blessed Thistle herb (cnicus benedictus) 100 mg.

Menopause Support **-** Vital Nutrients
Each capsule contains: Black Cohosh extract (cimicifuga racemosa, standardized to 27-deoxyactein by HPLC) 40 mg • Dong Quai root 7:1 extract (angelica sinensis) 150 mg • Rehmannia 6:1 extract 100 mg • Wild Yam root 10:1 extract (dioscorea villosa) 100 mg • Sage leaf 4:1 extract (salvia officinalis) 100 mg • Chaste Tree berry extract (vitex agnus castus, 0.5% agnuside) 50 mg • Ginkgo Biloba 50:1 extract 40 mg • Licorice root extract (16% glycyrrhizin) 25 mg.

Menopause Support Formula **-** Body Language Vitamin Co.
Each capsule contains: Black Cohosh extract (Cimicifuga racemosa root, standardized to contain 2.5% triterpine glycosides) 200 mg • Dong Quai (Angelica sinensis root) 150 mg • Red Clover extract (Trifolium pratense flower) 75 mg • Novasoy Phytoestrogen extract (yields 32.5 mg soy isoflavones, genistein and dadzein) 70 mg • Wild Yam 50 mg • Chasteree berry (Vitex agnus-cactus fruit) 50 mg • Hops 50 mg • Fenugreek 50 mg • Damiana (Turnera diffusa leaves) 25 mg. Other Ingredients: Vegetable Cellulose Capsule, Rice Powder, Magnesium Stearate.

Some Brand Name Natural Products - What they Contain

www.NaturalDatabase.com contains MANY more listings than appear here.
Editor's Notes are located on pages 2155-2163.

Menophase - Futurebiotics LLC
Complex of 4:1 extracts & powders (equivalent to 1700 mg of raw herbs) 450 mg containing: Foti, Peony Root, Withania Somnifera, Dong Quai, Chinese Sage & Carlina Ancalis • Pantothenic Acid (Vitamin B5) 75 mg • Ribonucleic Acid (RNA) 40 mg • Pyridoxine (Vitamin B6) 15 mg • Zinc (from gluconate) 7.5 mg.

MenoPrep - HealthMinded
Three capsules contain: MenoPrep Proprietary Blend 760 mg: Soy Isoflavones (non-GE, min. 20% isoflavones), Wild Yam root extract (dioscorea villosa, 6% diosgenin), Licorice root 4:1 extract (glycyrrhiza glabra), Dong Quai root powder (angelica sinensis), Red Raspberry leaves powder (rubus ideaus L.), Black Cohosh root extract (cimicifuga racemosa, 2.5% triterpene glycosides), Chasteberry fruit 10:1 extract (vitex agnus-castus), Ginger root & rhizome powder (zingiber officinale), Red Clover flower (trifolium pratens, 8% isoflavones), Ginkgo leaf standardized extract (ginkgo biloba, 24% ginkgoflavoneglycosides, 6% terpene lactones). Other Ingredients: Gelatin, Stearic Acid, Magnesium Stearate.

MenoPro - HealthMinded
Two capsules contain: Vitamin E 30 IU • Vitamin B6 10 mg • Folic Acid (100%) 400 mcg • Vitamin B12 25 mg • Calcium 500 mg • Magnesium 50 mg • Chromium 200 mcg • MenoPro Propreitary Blend 344.5 mg: Shen Min (he shou wu standardized extract 10%), Wild Yam root, Isoflavones (genestein0rich phytonutrients from soy), Dong Quai extract, Black Cohosh root, Chasteberry standardized extract, Boron Amino Acid Chelate. Other Ingredients: Stearic Acid, Magnesium Stearate.

Menopryn - Rx Vitamins
Black Cohosh (standardized) 50 mg • Isoflavone complex.

Menosan - The Himalaya Drug Company
Each tablet contains: Ashoka (saraca indica) 130 mg • Shatavari (asparagus racemosus) 110 mg • Kukkutandatvak Bhasma (hen's egg shell calx) 125 mg • Zahar Mohra Bhasma (calx serpentine, magnesium silicate) 125 mg • Haritaki (terminalia chebula) 110 mg • Bala (sida cordifolia) 105 mg • Yashtimadhu (glycyrrhiza glabra) 100 mg • Mandukaparni (centella asiatica) 50 mg • Vasaka (adhatoda vasica) 30 mg • Amalaki (emblica officinalis) 130 mg • Durva (cynodon dactylon) 30 mg • Nagkesara (mesua ferrea) 60 mg • Lajjalu (mimosa pudica) 30 mg • Lodhra (symplocos racemosa) 65 mg • Chandana (santalum album) 65 mg • Anantamul (hemidesmus indicus) 65 mg • Praval Pishti (processed coral) 130 mg • Sourashtri Bhasma (alum) 30 mg • Trinakantamani Pishti 30 mg. See Editor's Note No. 39.

Menovamp - Aboca USA, Inc
Each capsule contains: Chaste tree fruit powder (vitex agnus-castus, standardized to 0.1% agnuside) 121.2 mg • Hawthorne flower and leaf WPC (whole phytocomplex concentrate, crataegus oxycantha, standardized to 1% total flavonoids) 113.1 mg • Black Cohosh rhizome freeze-dried extract (cimicifuga racemosa, standardized to 1.5% acteine + 27% deoxiacteine) 68.7 mg • Motherwort WPC (leonurus cardiaca, aerial part) 40.4 mg • Passiflo 2-LMF brand Passionflower leaf (passiflora incarnata, multifraction freeze-dried extract, standardized to 8% total flavonoids) 40.4 mg • Sage leaf WPC (salvia officinalis, standardized to 1.6% rosmarinic acid) 20.2 mg. Other Ingredients: Gelatin.

Menovin - Biotech Corp.
Two tablets contain: Natural Vitamin E (dl-alpha tocopherol succinate) 30 IU • Vitamin B6 (pyridoxine HCl) 10 mg • Vitamin B12 (cyanocobalamin) 25 mg • Folate (as folic acid) 400 mg • Calcium (as calcium carbonate, dicalcium phosphate) 500 mg • Magnesium (as magnesium oxide, stearate) 50 mg • Chromium (as patented dinicotinate glycinate) 200 mcg • Shen Min (he shou wu, 12:1 standardized extract to 10% chrysophanics, 1.8% anthraquiones) 100 mg • Isoflavones (genestein-rich phytonutrients from soy (glycine max) and kudzu (peuraria)) 50 mg • Black Cohosh root (cimicifuga racemosa, 4:1 standardized extract) 40 mg • Chasteberry (vitex agnus castus, standardized to 5% vitexin) 75 mg • Dong Quai root (angelica sinensis, 4:1 extract) 50 mg • Kava Kava root (piper methysticum, 30% kavalactones) 100 mg • Wild yam root (discorea villosa) 65 mg • Boron (as boron chelates) 2 mg. Other Ingredients: Microcrystalline Cellulose, Croscarmellose Sodium, Stearic Acid, Silica, Magnesium Stearate, Pharmaceutical Glaze.

Men's ArginMax - GNC
Six tablets contain: Vitamin A (as retinyl palmitate) 5000 IU • Vitamin C (as ascorbic acid) 60 mg • Vitamin E (as d-alpha tocopherol succinate) 30 IU • Thiamin (as thiamin mononitrate) 1.5 mg • Riboflavin (B2) 1.7 mg • Niacin (as niacinamide) 20 mg • Vitamin B-6 (pyridoxine hydrochloride) 2 mg • Folic Acid 400 mcg • Vitamin B-12 (cyanocobalamin) 6 mcg • Biotin 300 mcg • Pantothenic Acid (as calcium d-pantothenate) 10 mg • Zinc (gluconate) 15 mg • Selenium 70 mcg • L-Arginine 3000 mg •Korean Ginseng extract aerial parts and roots 100 mg • American Ginseng root 100 mg • Ginkgo Biloba extract leaf 50 mg. Other Ingredients: Microcrystallin Cellulose, Magnesium Stearate, Hydroxypropyl Methylcellulose, Silica, Titanium Dioxide, PEG, Polysorbate 80.

Men's Formula - Nature's Sunshine
Three capsules contain: Zinc (gluconate) 15 mg • Proprietary Blend 1512 mg: Saw Palmetto fruit extract (serenoa repens), Gotu Kola aerial parts (hydrocotyle asiatica), Pygeum bark extract (prunus africana), Stinging Nettle root extract (urtica dioica), Standarized Lycopene concentrate. Other Ingredients: Gelatin, Water.

Men's Formula - Rexall - Sundown
Two capsules contain: Vitamin A (100% as beta-carotene, 20% of which is from Dunaliella salina algae) 5000 IU • Vitamin D (as cholecalciferol) 40 IU • Vitamin E (as dl-alpha-tocopheryl acetate and d-alpha-tocopheryl succinate) 60 IU • Niacin (as niacinamide) 10 mg • Vitamin B-6 (as pyridoxine HCl and pyridoxal 5-phosphate) 2 mg • Folic Acid 200 mcg • Vitamin B-12 (as cyanocobalamin) 12 mcg • Biotin 50 mcg • Pantothenic Acid (as calcium d-pantothenate) 20 mg • Calcium (as calcium carbonate, calcium malate, calcium citrate, and hydroxyapatite) 100 mg • Magnesium (as magnesium oxide, magnesium citrate and magnesium chelate) 150 mg • Zinc (as zinc chelate, zinc gluconate and zinc citrate) 7.5 mg • Selenium (as L-selenomethionine and sodium selenate) 50 mcg • Copper (as copper chelate, copper citrate, and copper aspartate) 1 mg • Manganese (as manganese chelate and manganese aspartate) 1 mg • Chromium (as chromium chelate, chromium glutathionate and chromium nicotinate) 100 mcg • Molybdenum (as molybdenum aspartate and molybdenum chelate) 25 mcg • Potassium (as potassium chloride, potassium aspartate and potassium citrate) 50 mg • Saw Palmetto fruit 200 mg • Dry Fish Oil (omega-3 fatty acids) 50 mg • L-Arginine 50 mg • Bromelain 25 mg • L-Carnitine 25 mg • L-Glutamine 25 mg • Papain 25 mg • Taurine 25 mg • Coenzyme Q-10 2.5 mg • Glutathione 2.5 mg • Vanadium (as vanadium aspartate and vanadium chelate) 10 mcg • Men's Formula Blend: Nettle aerial parts, Oats, Pumpkin Seed (curcubita pepo), Tomato, Alfalfa Juice Concentrate aerial parts, Spirulina pacifica blue-green algae, Grape Seed extract, Lycopene, Alpha-Lipoic Acid, Lutein 205 mg. Other Ingredients: Gelatin, Maltodextrin, Magnesium Stearate.

Men's Formula 800+ Prostate Support - Nature's Life
Two capsules contain: Saw Palmetto berry extract (Serenoa repens B. standardized to 85% Liposterolic Acids equivalent to 1600 mg whole herb) 160 mg • Stinging Nettle plant (Urtica dioica L.) 150 mg • Pygeum africanum H. bark extract (concentrated 130:1; equivalent to 6500 mg whole herb) 50 mg • Beta Sitosterol (Soy oil) 10 mg • Zinc (Gluconate, Citrate, Picolinate) 15 mg • Copper (Gluconate, Citrate) 1 mg • Flax seed oil (Linum usitatissimum L.) 235 mg • (Omegaflo Process Certified Organically Grown) Providing naturally occuring Omega 3 Essential Fatty Acid: Alpha Linolenic Acid 133 mg.

Men's Formula Plus - Swanson Health Products
Two softgels contain: Zinc (from zinc gluconate) 15 mg • Saw Palmetto extract (85% free fatty acids) 320 mg • Pumpkin Seed oil 80 mg • Lycopene (tomato) 10 mg.

Men's Longevity Essentials Plus **-** EcoNugenics
Six capsules contain: Vitamin A (as beta-carotene, palmitate) 15,000 IU • Vitamin C (as ascorbic acid, calcium ascorbate, magnesium ascorbate) 1000 mg • Vitamin D (as cholecalciferol) 400 IU • Vitamin E (as alpha tocopherol succinate) 400 IU • Vitamin K 80 mcg • Vitamin B1 (as thiamine hydrochloride) 5 mg • Vitamin B2 (as riboflavin-5-phosphate) 10 mg • Vitamin B3 (as niacin, niacinamide) 50 mg • Vitamin B6 (as pyridoxine hydrochloride, pyridoxal-5-phosphate) 22 mg • Folic Acid 800 mcg • Vitamin B12 (as cyanocobalamin) 50 mcg • Biotin 300 mcg • Vitamin B5 (as calcium pantothenate) 30 mg • Calcium (as citrate, aspartate) 100 mg • Iodine (as potassium iodide) 150 mcg • Magnesium (as oxide, citrate, aspartate) 200 mg • OptiZinc Zinc 15 mg • Selenium (as selenomethionine) 100 mcg • Copper (as sebacate) 2 mg • Manganese (as sulfate) 3 mg • ChromeMate Chromium 120 mcg • Molybdenum (as sodium molybdate) 75 mcg • Potassium (as citrate, aspartate) 30 mg • Men's Longevity Supernutrient Blend 221 mg: Inositol, Taurine, PABA (para-aminobenzoic acid), Phosphatidylcholine, Choline, Acetyl-l-Carnitine, Ginkgo leaf extract, DMAE (2-dimethylaminoethanol bitartrate), Bilberry berry extract, Boron • Men's Longevity Liver Health Blend 170 mg Glycine, Broccoli extract • Garlic bulb concentrate, Milk Thistle seed extract, Turmeric extract, Oregon Grape root • Men's Longevity Antioxidant Blend 145 mg: Alpha-Lipoic Acid, Hesperidin complex, Citrus Bioflavonoid complex, Quercetin, Grape Seed extract, L-Glutathione, Lutein • Men's Longevity Prostate Health Blend 625 mg: Saw Palmetto berry extract, Oat spiklet extract, Korean Ginseng root, Pygeum bark extract, Stinging Nettle herb, Damiana leaf, Pumpkin seed, Lycopene.

Men's Longevity ProstaCare PC **-** EcoNugenics
Six capsules contain: Vitamin C (as ascorbic acid, calcium ascorbate, magnesium ascorbate) 250 mg • Vitamin D (D3, as cholecalciferol) 600 IU • Vitamin E (as D-alpha tocopherol succinate) 400 IU • Zinc (as orotate, methionine) 40 mg • Selenium (as selenomethionine, sodium selenate) 200 mcg • Turmeric rhizome extract (curcuma longa, 95% curcumin) 500 mg • Saw Palmetto berry (serenoa repens, 45%-50% fatty acids, sterols) 360 mg • Stinging Nettle root extract (urtica dioica) 300 mg • Royal Jelly concentrate 250 mg • PectaSol Modified Citrus Pectin 250 mg • Broccoli extract (brassica oleoracea, 22:1) 200 mg • Garlic bulb concentrate (allium sativum) 150 mg • Alpha-Lipoic Acid 150 mg • Calcium D-Glucarate 150 mg • Quercetin 100 mg • Pumpkin seed extract (curcurbita pepo) 100 mg • Pygeum bark extract (13% sterols) 100 mg • Mushrooms 250 mg: Reishi, Coriolus, Polyporus • L-Glutathione 100 mg • Indole-3-Carbinol 75 mg • Citrus Bioflavonoid complex 50 mg • Green Tea leaf extract (camellia sinensis) 50 mg • Lycopene 30 mg • Lutein 20 mg • Men's Longevity Prostate Protection Blend 330 mg: Heal-All spiklets, Codonopsis root, Smilax Glabra rhizome, Oldelandia Diffusa herb, Job's Tears seed, Eleuthero root • Men's Longevity Prostate Blend 160 mg: Licorice root extract, Laminaria Japonica herb, Sargassum Fusiforme herb • Men's Longevity Liver Care Blend 115 mg: Taraxaci Mongolici herb/root, Baikal Skullcap root, Mum flower, Chinese Thoroughwax root. Other Ingredients: Gelatin, Dicalcium Phosphate, Silica, Magnesium Stearate.

Men's Mood-Enhancer **-** HerbaSway
St. John's Wort • Ginkgo biloba • He Sho Wu • Horny Goat Weed • Schisandra • Knotweed • Astragalus • Lycium • Skullcap • Blackberry • Bupleurum • HerbaSwee (Cucurbitaceae fruit).

Men's Nutra-Pack **-** Nature's Plus
Each pack contains: Vitamin A (as beta carotene) 25,000 IU • Vitamin C (as ascorbic acid) 1100 mg • Vitamin D (as ergocalciferol) 1000 IU • Vitamin E (as D-alpha tocopheryl succinate) 300 IU • Thiamin (vitamin B1, as thiamine HCl) 100 mg • Riboflavin (vitamin B2) 100 mg • Niacin (as niacinamide) 100 mg • Vitamin B6 (pyridoxine HCl) 100 mg • Folate (as folic acid) 400 mcg • Vitamin B12 (as cyanocobalamin) 100 mcg • Biotin 100 mcg • Pantothenic Acid (as calcium pantothenate) 100 mg • Calcium (as amino acid chelate/complex) 540 mg • Iron (as amino acid chelate/complex) 38.5 mg • Phosphorus (as amino acid complex) 100 mg • Iodine (from kelp) 262.5 mcg • Magnesium (as amino acid chelate/complex) 270 mg • Zinc (as amino acid chelate/complex) 75 mg • Selenium (as amino acid complex) 35 mcg • Manganese (as amino acid chelate/complex) 11.1 mg • Chromium (as amino acid chelate) 65 mcg • Potassium (as amino acid complex) 64.5 mg • Citrus Bioflavonoids (from citrus spp. exocarp) 525 mg • Pancreatin 4X (equivalent to USP 650 mg) 162.5 mg • Rutin (from saphora japonica leaf) 125 mg • Hesperidin (from citrus limon exocarp) 105 mg • Glutamic Acid HCl 100 mg • Inositol 100 mg • PABA (para-aminobenzoic acid) 100 mg • Acidophilus (lactobacillus, bulgaricus, bifidus) 75 mg • Ox Bile extract 60 mg • Acerola 50 mg • Bromelain (1:10, from pineapple fruit) 50 mg • Choline (as bitartrate) 42 mg • Pepsin 1:15,000 (equivalent to pepsin NF 150 mg) 32.5 mg • Papain (from papaya) 32.5 mg • Malt Diastase 32.5 mg • Betaine HCl (from beet molasses) 25 mg • Cellulase 10 mg • Hemicellulase 2.5 mg • Lactase 2.5 mg. Other Ingredients: Di-calcium Phosphate, Microcrystalline Cellulose, Stearic Acid, Rose Hips (rosa canina fruit), Magnesium Stearate, Silica, Isolated Soy Protein, Hydroxypropyl Methylcellulose, Rice Bran, Parsley, Peppermint Leaf, Fennel Seed, Ginger Root, Rosemary Leaf, Watercress, Alfalfa, Green Cabbage, Wheat Germ Flour, Pacific Kelp, Papaya, Date, Apple Pectin, Black Currant Seed, Garlic, Broccoli, Chinese Cabbage Leaf (brassica campestris), Fig, Brown Rice, Barley Grass, Bee Pollen, Oat Bran, Spinach, Chlorella, Spirulina, Carrot, Sunflower Oil, Lecithin, Pharmaceutical Glaze, Gelatin, Glycerin, Purified Water.

Men's One A Day Multi **-** Golden Glow Natural Health Products
Each capsule contains: Thiamine Nitrate (vitamin B1) 15 mg • Riboflavin (vitamin B2) 15 mg • Pyridoxine Hydrochloride (vitamin B6) 15 mg • Nicotinamide (vitamin B3) 15 mg • Ascorbic Acid (vitamin C) 100 mg • Calcium (as hydrogen phosphate) 40 mg • Magnesium (as sulfate trihydrate) 20 mg • Manganese (as sulfate monohydrate) 1 mg • Beta Carotene 1.5 mg • Cholecalciferol (vitamin D3 100 IU) 2.5 mcg • Cyanocobalamin (vitamin B12) 25 mcg • Calcium Pantothenate (vitamin B5) 15 mg • Biotin 25 mcg • Folic Acid 100 mcg • DL-Alpha-Tocopheryl Acetate 25 mg: Vitamin E 25 IU • Potassium (as sulfate) 2 mg • Zinc (as sulfate monohydrate) 10 mg • Siberian Ginseng root extract (eleutherococcus senticosus) 100 mg • Saw Palmetto extract serenoa serrulata 100 mg: Fatty Acids 7.08 mg.

Men's Potency Support **-** NAI - Natural Alternatives International
Four capsules contain: Maca root (lepidium meyenii) 900 mg • Tribulus Terrestris whole plant 500 mg • Cordyceps mycelia (cordyceps sinensis) 200 mg • Asian Ginseng root (Panax ginseng) 250 mg • Epimedium (epimedium sagittatum) 50 mg • Muira Puama bark (ptychopetalus olacoides) 200 mg.

Men's Prime Multi **-** Swanson Health Products
Each tablet contains: Vitamin A (as beta-carotene) 3000 IU • Vitamin C (as ascorbic acid) 100 mg • Vitamin D (as cholecalciferol) 50 IU • Vitamin E (as d-alpha tocopheryl succinate) 60 IU • Thiamin (as thiamin HCl; vitamin B-1) 5 mg • Riboflavin (vitamin B-2) 5 mg • Vitamin B-6 (as pyridoxine HCl) 5 mg • Folic Acid 200 mcg • Vitamin B-12 (as cyanocobalamin) 5 mcg • Biotin 5 mcg • Pantothenic Acid (as d-calcium pantothenate) 5 mg • Iron (from Albion amino acid chelate) 5 mg • Iodine (from kelp) 50 mcg • Magnesium (from magnesium oxide) 50 mg • Zinc (from Albion amino acid chelate) 15 mg • Selenium (from Albion amino acid chelate) 100 mcg • Chromium (from Albion amino acid chelate) 25 mcg • Green Tea powder 50 mg • Pygeum powder 50 mg • Saw Palmetto Extract (5% fatty acids) 50 mg • Rutin 25 mg • Muira Puama 20 mg • Tribulus Terrestris (20% saponins) 20 mg • Yohimbe powder (4:1) 20 mg • Korean Ginseng powder (5% ginsenosides) 15 mg • Nettle Concentrate (4:1) 15 mg • Pumpkin Seed powder 15 mg • Inositol 10 mg, Bilberry powder (25% anthocyanidins) 5 mg • Choline (as choline bitartrate) 5 mg • Ginkgo Biloba leaf extract (24% flavone glycosides, 6% terpene lactones) 5 mg • PABA (para-aminobenzoic acid) 5 mg • Coenzyme Q10 2 mg • Lycopene Complex 100 mcg.

Men's Support - Rainbow Light
Each tablet provides: Sarsaparilla root 50 mg • Wild Oat green tops 100 mg • Damiana oxide 100 mg • Kava Kava rhizome 75 mg • Saw Palmetto fruit 50 mg • Pumpkin seed 25 mg • Ginseng 25 mg • Selenium 25 mg • Wood Betony 50 mg • Blue Vervain 50 mg • Ginger rhizome 100 mg • Vitamin A 1000 IU • Vitamin E 25 IU • Zinc 5 mg.

Men's Virility Power - NOW Foods
Two capsules contain: Epimedium extract 375 mg • Muira Puama 100 mg • Maca 100 mg • Tribulus extract 75 mg • Panax Ginseng 50 mg • Damiana 50 mg • Ginkgo Biloba 30 mg • Cayenne 25 mg. Other Ingredients: Cellulose, Stearic Acid, Silica, Magnesium Stearate.

MenstraCalm - Jarrow Formulas
Four tablets contain: Vitamin C (calcium ascorbate) 100 mg • Vitamin D (D3) 100 IU • Natural Vitamin E (D-alpha-tocopheryl succinate) 100 IU • Vitamin B6 (pyridoxine) 25 mg • Folic Acid 200 mcg • Calcium (as calcium citrate) 132 mg • Magnesium (as magnesium oxide) 60 mg • Potassium (as potassium chloride) 99 mg • Dong Quai root 5:1 extract (angelica sinensis) 500 mg • Xiang Fu tuber 5:1 extract (cyperus rotundus) 500 mg • Shu Di Huang 5:1 (rehmannia glutinosa) 400 mg • Lindera 5:1 (lindera stychnifolin) 200 mg • Chaste Tree fruit 5:1 extract (vitex agnus-castus) 300 mg • Dandelion root (taraxacum officinale) 200 mg. Other Ingredients: Magnesium Stearate, Gelatin.

Menstru-Care - Natrol, Inc.
Two tablets contain: Vitamin B12 (as cobalamin) 75 mcg • Folic Acid 100 mcg • Calcium (as calcium carbonate) 299 mg • Iron (as iron glycinate) 30 mg • Chasteberry 75 mg • CrampBark 4:1 (Viburnum opulus) 75 mg • Dong Quai 75 mg, Ferulic Acid (1%) 750 mcg • Uva Ursi 50 mg • Kava Kava 50 mg, Kavalactones (30%) 15 mg • Squaw Vine 50 mg • Black Cohosh 20 mg, Triterpenes (2.5%) 0.5 mg. Other Ingredients: Mono & Di-Glycerides, Stearic Acid, Croscarmellose Sodium, Silicon Dioxide, Magnesium Stearate.

Menta-FX - CV Technologies Inc.
St. John's Wort 200 mg • HT-1001 (extract of American Ginseng) 100 mg • Ginkgo Biloba 25 mg.

Mental Acuity Formula - PhytoPharmica
Two capsules contain: Alpha Lipoic Acid 600 mg • Bacopa aerial part extract (bacopa monnieri, standardized to contain 20% bacosides) 300 mg • Folic Acid 800 mcg • Ginkgo leaf extract (ginkgo biloba, standardized to contain 24% ginkgoflavonglycosides, 6% terpene lactones, and 2% bilobalide) • Vitamin B12 (as cyanocobalamin) 500 mcg • Vitamin B6 (as pyridoxine HCl) 15 mg. Other Ingredients: Gelatin, Modified Cellulose Gum, Magnesium Stearate, Silicon Dioxide, Titanium Dioxide Color.

Mental Advantage + Ginkgo - PhytoPharmica
Each chewable tablet contains: Plumbum metallicum 8x • Ambra grisea 5x • Kali phosphoricum 5x • Ginkgo 1x • Magnesia muriatica 1x • Magnesia phosphorica 1x.
See Editor's Note No. 1.

Mental Alertness - Gaia Herbs
Two capsules contain: Eleuthero root (eleutherococcus senticosus) 80 mg • Ginkgo leaf (ginkgo biloba) 40 mg • Gotu Kola herb (centella asiatica) 40 mg • Fo Ti (polygonum multiflorum) 26 mg • Wild Oats milky seed (avena sativa) 22 mg • Peppermint herb (mentha piperita) 20 mg • Vinpocetine (from coacanga seed) 10 mg • Rosemary leaf, supercritical CO2 extract (rosmarinus off.) 8 mg. Other Ingredients: Vegetable Glycerin, Vegetable Cellulose (capsule).

Mental Clarity - Sundown
Two capsules contain: Ginkgo Biloba leaf extract (standardized to 24% flavonol glycosides, 6% terpene lactones) 40 mg • Ginkgo Biloba leaf 400 mg • Herbal Complex Blend 280 mg: Siberian Ginseng root, Bilberry fruit 4:1 extract. Other Ingredients: Gelatin.

Mental Edge - Source Naturals
Four tablets contain: Phosphatidyl Choline 350 mg • Choline (Bitartrate) 100 mg • DMAE (Bitartrate) 160 mg • Ginkgo Biloba leaf extract (50:1) 20 mg • Vitamin B1 (Thiamin) 50 mg • Vitamin B2 (Riboflavin) 20 mg • Vitamin B3 (80 mg Niacinamide and 40 mg Niacin) 120 mg • Vitamin B5 (Calcium D-Pantothenate) 120 mg • Vitamin B6 (Pyridoxine HCl) 25 mg • Vitamin B12 (Cyanocobalamin) 50 mcg • Folic Acid 400 mcg • Biotin 50 mcg • Inositol 30 mg • Vitamin C (Ascorbic Acid, Zinc and Magnesium Ascorbates) 150 mg • Calcium (Citrate) 60 mg • Magnesium (Oxide, Citrate) 120 mg • Potassium (Citrate) 99 mg • Zinc (Ascorbate) 10 mg • Manganese (Ascorbate) 5 mg • L-Pyroglutamic Acid 500 mg • L-Glutamine 500 mg • L-Tyrosine 275 mg • L-Phenylalanine 125 mg • Taurine 100 mg • Herbal Formula 595 mg: Siberian Ginseng 225 mg, Gotu Kola 150 mg, Schizandra 80 mg, Ginger root 80 mg, Cayenne 60 mg.

Mentalin - Metagenics
Two tablets contain: Proprietary Blend 500 mg: Bacopa leaf 4:1 extract (bacopa monnieri, containing bacosides A & B), Gotu Kola leaf 8:1 extract (centella asiatica, containing asiaticosides), Amla fruit 3:1 extract (emblica officinalis, containing tannins), Ashwagandha root 5:1 extract (withania somnifera, containing withanolides).

Mentat - The Himalaya Drug Company
Each tablet contains: Brahmi (bacopa monnieri) 136 mg • Manduk Parani (centella asiatica) 70 mg • Ashvagandha (withania somnifera) 52 mg • Vishnukrantha (evolvulus alsinoides) 52 mg • Jatamansi (nardostachys jatamansi) 52 mg • Tagara (valeriana wallichii syn. v.jatamansi) 50 mg • Vidanga (embelia ribes) 50 mg • Vatadha (prunus amygdalus) 50 mg • Vacha (acorus calamus) 42 mg • Haritaki (terminalia chebula) 36 mg • Amalaki (emblica officinalis) 36 mg • Guduchi (tinospora cordifolia) 36 mg • Jyotishmati (celastrus paniculatus) 32 mg • Shyonaka (oroxylum indicum) 32 mg • Brahmi (bacopa monnieri) 80 mg • Kapikachchhu (mucuna pruriens) 18 mg • Ela (elattaria cardamomum) 18 mg • Arjuna (terminalia arjuna) 18 mg • Shatapuspha (foeniculum vulgare) 18 mg • Vidari (ipomoea digitata) 18 mg • Salabmisri (orchis mascula) 18 mg • Sunthi (zingiber officinale) 14 mg • Vibhitaki (terminalia belirica syn. t.bellirica) 14 mg • Jatiphalam (myristica fragrans) 14 mg • Lavanga (syzygium aromaticum) 10 mg • Mukta Pishti (processed pearl) 3 mg.

Mentat Syrup - The Himalaya Drug Company
Each 1 tsp (5 mL) serving contains: Brahmi (bacopa monnieri) 144 mg • Manduk Parani (centella asiatica) 70 mg • Ashvagandha (withania somnifera) 52 mg • Vishnukrantha (evolvulus alsinoides) 52 mg • Jatamansi (nardostachys jatamansi) 52 mg • Tagara (valeriana wallichii syn. v.jatamansi) 50 mg • Vidanga (embelia ribes) 50 mg • Vatadha (prunus amygdalus) 50 mg • Vacha (acorus calamus) 42 mg • Haritaki (terminalia chebula) 36 mg • Amalaki (emblica officinalis) 36 mg • Guduchi (tinospora cordifolia) 36 mg • Jyotishmati (celastrus paniculatus) 32 mg • Shyonaka (oroxylum indicum) 32 mg • Kapikachchhu (mucuna pruriens) 1.8 mg • Ela (elattaria cardamomum) 1.8 mg • Arjuna (terminalia arjuna) 1.8 mg • Shatapuspha (foeniculum vulgare) 1.8 mg • Vidari (ipomoea digitata) 1.8 mg • Salabmisri (orchis mascula) 1.8 mg • Sunthi (zingiber officinale) 1.4 mg • Vibhitaki (terminalia belirica syn. t.bellirica) 1.4 mg • Jatiphalam (myristica fragrans) 1.4 mg • Lavanga (syzygium aromaticum) 1 mg.

Mentharil - PhytoPharmica
Each enteric-coated softgel capsule contains: Peppermint oil extract (mentha piperita, from leaf) 0.2 mL • Rosemary leaf and stem oil extract (rosmarinus officinalis) 0.02 mL • Thyme oil extract (thymus vulgaris, from whole plant) 0.02 mL.

Mephyton (phytonadione) Vitamin K1 - Merck & Co., Inc.
Each tablet contains: Phytonadione 5 mg. Other Ingredients: Acacia, Calcium Phosphate, Collodial Silicon Dioxide, Lactose, Magnesium Stearate, Starch, Talc.

MeraCap Coral Calcium - Merazon Health Products, Inc.
Each capcule contains: Coral powder 600 mg • Calcium Citrate 5 mg • Vitamin D 400 IU. Other Ingedients: Malic Acid, Betaine HCl.

Meso Vision **-** PhysioLogics
Each softgel contains: Proprietary Blend 20 mg: Lutein, Meso - Zeaxanthin, Zeaxanthin. Other Ingredients: Soybean Oil, Gelatin, Glycerin, Beeswax (yellow).

Mesosilver **-** Purest Colloids, Inc.
Each 5 mL contains: Colloidal Silver • Deionized Water.

MESO-Tech **-** MuscleTech
Each packet contains: MesoPro: Whey Protein Concentrate, Ion-Exchanged Whey Protein • Maltodextrin • Glutamine Blend • Natural & Artificial Flavors • Cellulose gum • Vitamin & Mineral Blend • Phenylalanine • Taurine • Guar gum • Xanthan gum • Acesulfame Potassium • Aspartame • Carrageenan • Essential Fatty Acid Blend: Borage oil, Lecithin, Flax seed oil • Phenylalanine.

Meta Boost **-** EnerGreens, Inc.
Each capsule contains: New Zealand Adrenal Glandular 200 mg • Proprietary Blend 300 mg: Citrus Aurantium standardized extract, Siberian Ginseng, Schisandra berries, Korean Ginseng, Cayenne pepper, Bladderwrack. Other Ingredients: Gelatin.
See Editor's Note No. 14 and No. 40.

Meta EPO **-** Metagenics
Each softgel contains: Evening Primrose oil: Gamma-Linolenic Acid 50 mg • Linoleic Acid 366 mg.

Meta I 3 C **-** Metagenics
Each capsule contains: Indole-3-Carbinol 150 mg • Rosemary leaf extract (rosemarinus officinale, standardized to 11% carnosic acid derivatives) 50 mg.

Meta Lipoate **-** Metagenics
Two tablets contain: Alpha-Lipoic Acid 200 mg.

Meta Lipoate 300 **-** Metagenics
Each tablet contains: Alpha-Lipoic Acid 300 mg.

MetaBerry **-** Oasis Wellness Network
Each ounce (30 mL) contains: Fruit Concentrates Blend 0.5 oz: Cranberry, Cherry, Blueberry, Grape • Active Aloe (200:1) 102 mg • Ginkgo Biloba leaf extract (24%) 20 mg • Alpha Lipoic Acid 20 mg • MaxCell Proprietary Blend 5 mg: Zisyphus Jujube, Piper Nigrum, Aloe Vera, Glycyrrhiza Glabra. Other Ingredients: Sodium Benzoate, Potassium Sorbate.

Metabo Taffy Ephedra Free Starch Neutralizer **-** The Natural One
Each soft chew contains: Phase-2 extract from White Kidney Bean (Phaseolus vulgaris) 500 mg. Other Ingredients: Glucose Syrup, Sucrose, Sweetened Condensed Milk (whole milk, sugar), Palm Kernel Oil, Whey, Chocolate, Mono and Diglycerides, Soya Lecithin, Natural Flavors.

Metabol X **-** BioGenesis Nutraceuticals
Two level scoops (42.8 g) contain: Vitamin A (Betatene brand mixed carotenoids, beta carotene, vitamin A palmitate) 3000 IU • Vitamin C (ascorbic acid) 500 mg • Vitamin D (cholecalciferol) 200 IU • Vitamin E (D-alpha toocpherol acetate) 100 IU • Vitamin B1 (thiamin mononitrate) 50 mg • Vitamin B2 (riboflavin) 0.9 mg • Niacin (niacinamide) 10 mg • Vitamin B6 (90% pyridoxal 5' phosphate, 10% pyridoxine hydrochloride) 21 mg • Folate (folic acid) 200 mcg • Vitamin B12 (cyanocobalamin) 200 mcg • Biotin 6000 mcg • Pantothenic Acid (D-calcium pantothenate) 5 mg • Calcium (calcium glycinate) 350 mg • Iron (ferrous fumarate) 4 mg • Phosphorus (potassium phosphate) 470 mg • Iodine (potassium iodide) 75 mcg • Magnesium (magnesium glycinate) 330 mg • Zinc (zinc citrate) 15 mg • Selenium (selenomethionine) 100 mcg • Copper (copper gluconate) 1 mg • Manganese (manganese gluconate) 2.5 mg • Chromium (chromium nicotinate) 300 mcg • Molybdenum (sodium molybdate) 37.5 mcg • Sodium (sodium sulfate) 30 mg • Potassium (potassium phosphate) 660 mg • Vanadium (vanadyl sulfate) 500 mcg • L-Leucine 225 mg • L-Isoleucine 100 mg • L-Valine 175 mg • Glycine 1000 mg • L-Carnitine (L-carnitine tartrate) 100 mg • Coenzyme Q-10 10 mg • L-Glutamine 500 mg • L-Tyrosine 500 mg • Choline (choline dihydrogen citrate) 50 mg • Inositol 30 mg • Alpha Lipoic Acid 100 mg • Gamma Oryzanol 100 mg • Malic Acid 600 mg • NADH 5 mg • Grape seed extract (95% proanthocyanidins) 10 mg • Fenugreek seed 4:1 extract 100 mg • American Ginseng root extract (5% ginsenosides) 60 mg • Ginkgo Biloba leaf extract (24% ginkgo flavone glycosides) 20 mg • 5 Hydroxytryptophan (5-HTP) 25 mg • Lecithin powder (23% phosphatidylcholine, 20% phosphatidylethanolamine, 14% phosphatidylinositol) 2530 mg. Other Ingredients: Rice Protein, Fibersol-2 brand Soluble Fiber Glucose Polymer Complex, Beflora Plus brand Natural Flavors, Potassium Phosphate, Gum Blend (xanthan, cellulose, carrageenan), Xylitol, Silica, Sodium Chloride.

Metabolean **-** Premier Marketing
Each caplet contains: Ginger • Magnesium • Vitamin E • Zinc • Mahuang • Astragalus • Guarana • Bee Pollen • Chromium Picolinate • Siberian Ginseng • Sarsaparilla • Goldenseal • Nettles • Gotu Kola • Lecithin • Damiana • Royal Jelly • Bladderwrack • Blue Green Algae • Licorice.
See Editor's Note No. 30.

Metabolic Action **-** Puritan's Pride
Each capsule contains: Vitamin B6 (as Pyridoxine Hydrochloride) 10 mg • Vitamin B12 (as Cyanocoballamin) 6.67 mcg • Chromium (as Chromium Picolinate) 66 mcg • PABA (Para-Aminobenzoic Acid) 16.67 mg • Licorice (Glycyrrhiza glabra) root 116.67 mg • Siberian Ginseng (Eleutherococcus senticosus) root 66.67 mg • Bee Pollen 66.67 mg • L-Glutamine 33.33 mg • L-Tyrosine 33.33 mg • DMAE (as Dimethylaminoethanol Bitartrate) 33.33 mg • L-Taurine 33.33 mg • Korean Ginseng (Panax ginseng) root 33.33 mg • Suma (Pfaffia paniculata) root 33.33 mg • Schizandra (Schisandra chinensis) fruit 33.33 mg • Chlorella plant 33.33 mg • Gymnema (Gymnema Sylvestre) leaf 33.33 mg • American Ginseng (Panax quinquefolius) root 16.67 mg.

Metabolic Booster **-** Pentabosol
Each tablet contains: Vitamin C (as ascorbic acid) 100 mg • Niacin (from 100 mg of inositol hexanicotinate) 80 mg • Vitamin B6 (as pyridoxine HCL) 50 mg • L-Carnitine (as l-carnitine L-tartrate) 20 mg • Glycine 300 mg • Sodium Pyruvate 125 mg. Other Ingredients: Dicalcium Phosphate, Microcrystalline Cellulose, Croscarmellose Sodium, Stearic Acid, Magnesium Stearate, Silica, Pharmaceutical Glaze.

Metabolic Digestive Support **-** Zone Labs
Two capsules contain: Green Tea extract 250 mg • Bromelain (600 GDU) 600 mg • Quercetin 50 mg • M.E. Complex 3000 mcg: Papain, Lipase, Pancreatin, Ajowan extract, Fennel extract, Lactase, Multi Enzyme complex. Other Ingredients: Gelatin, Microcrystalline Cellulose, Magnesium Stearate, Silica.

Metabolic Fat Loss **-** Olympian Labs
Two capsules contain: Chromium Picolinate 100 mcg • L-Carnitine Fumarate 150 mg • Garcinia Cambogia 500 mg • Uva Ursi 150 mg • Vitamin B6 25 mg • White Willow Bark 20 mg. In a natural base of Guarana.

Metabolic Rx **-** Alternecare Health Products
Three tablets contain: Choline Bitartrate 500 mg • Inositol 500 mg • Acetyl L-Carnitine 500 mg • L-Methionine 500 mg • Taurine 500 mg • Phosphatidyl Choline 200 mg • Betaine HCl 200 mg • Dandelion root 4:1 extract 200 mg • Milk Thistle seed (70% Silymarin) 100 mg • Bayberry bark 100 mg • Artichoke leaf extract (cynara scolymus) 50 mg • Potassium 50 mg • Yellow Dock 50 mg • Vitamin B6 (as pyridoxine alpha-ketoglutarate and pyridoxyl phosphate) 10 mg • Chromium (as chromium polynicotinate and chromium picolinate) 200 mcg.

Metabolic Thyrolean **-** ProLab
Each capsule contains: Phosphatidyl Choline 12.5 mg • Calcium Phosphate 125 mg • Dipotassium Phosphate 75 mg • Sodium Phosphate 37.5 mg • Disodium Phosphate 37.5 mg • Gum Guggul extract (Guggelsterone) 125 mg • Garcinia cambogia 125 mg • L-Tyrosine 125 mg.

Some Brand Name Natural Products - What they Contain

www.NaturalDatabase.com contains MANY more listings than appear here.
Editor's Notes are located on pages 2155-2163.

Metabolife 356 - Metabolife International, Inc.
Each tablet contains: Vitamin E 6 IU • Magnesium (as magnesium chelate) 75 mg • Zinc (as zinc chelate) 5 mg • Chromium (as chromium picolinate) 75 mcg • Proprietary Blend: Guarana Concentrate seed (40 mg naturally-occurring caffeine), Ma Huang concentrate aerial part (12 mg naturally-occurring ephedrines), Bee Pollen, Ginseng root, Ginger root, Lecithin, Bovine Complex, Damiana leaf, Sarsaparilla root, Golden Seal aerial part, Nettles leaf, Gotu Kola aerial part, Spirulina Algae, Royal Jelly 728 mg. Other Ingredients: Methocel, Silica, Croscarmellose Sodium, Magnesium Stearate.
See Editor's Note No. 14, No. 21 and No. 67.

Metabolife Complete - Metabolife International, Inc.
Pre-Breakfast & Pre-Lunch Formula: Two caplets contain: Thiamin (as thiamin mononitrate) 1.5 mg • Riboflavin 1.7 mg • Niacin (as niacinamide) 20 mg • Vitamin B6 (as pyridoxine hdyrochloride) 5 mg • Pantothenic Acid (as D-calcium pantothenate) 10 mg • Calcium (as hydroxycitrate and di-calcium phosphate) 115 mg • Chromium (as chromium polynicotinate) 113 mcg • Sodium 60 mg • Potassium 150 mg • Proprietary Blend 1770 mg: Super CitriMax brand Garcinia fruit extract (standardized for hydroxycitric acid), Guarana seed extract (standardized for caffeine). Other Ingredients: Maltodextrin, Modified Cellulose, Caffeine, Dicalcium Phosphate, Stearic Acid, Silica, Dextrin, Dextrose, Lecithin, Sodium Carboxymethylcellulose, Sodium Citrate.
Pre-Dinner Formula: Two caplets contain: Thiamin (as thiamin mononitrate) 1.5 mg • Riboflavin 1.7 mg • Niacin (as niacinamide) 20 mg • Vitamin B6 (as pyridoxine hydrochloride) 5 mg • Pantothenic Acid (as D-calcium pantothenate) 10 mg • Calcium (as hydroxycitrate) 75 mg • Chromium (as chromium polynicotinate) 133 mcg • Sodium 60 mg • Potassium 150 mg • Proprietary Blend 1556 mg: Super CitriMax brand Garcinia fruit extract (Standardized for hydroxycitric acid). Other Ingredients: Modified Cellulose, Maltodextrin, Stearic Acid, Silica, Dexrin, Titanium Dioxide, Polyehtylene Glycol, Lecithin, Dextrose, Sodium Carboxymethylcellulose, FD&C Yellow #5, FD&C Red #40, Sodium Citrate, FD&C Blue #2.

Metabolife Ephedra Free - Metabolife International, Inc.
Two tablets contain: Sodium 60 mg • Potassium 30 mg • Calcium 50 mg • Chromium (as chromium picolinate) 150 mcg • Proprietary Blend 1132 mg: Green Tea extract leaf (standardixed for EGCG and total catechins), Super Citrimax Garcinia Cambogia extract fruit (standardized for hydroxycitric acid), Guarana seed extract (standardized for caffeine), Yerba Mate extract leaf (standardized for caffeine). Other Ingredients: Modified Cellulose, Maltodextrin, Caffeine, Dicalcium Phosphate, Stearic Acid, Sodium Bicarbonate, Silica, Dextrin, Citric Acid, Dextrose, Lecithin, Sodium Carboxymethylcellulose, Sodium Citrate.

Metabolife Ultra - Metabolife International, Inc.
Two caplets contain: Thiamin (vitamin B1, as thiamin mononitrate) 1.5 mg • Riboflavin (vitamin B2) 1.7 mg • Niacin (vitamin B3, as niacinamide) 20 mg • Vitamin B6 (as pyridoxine hydrochloride) 5 mg • Pantothenic Acid (as d-calcium pantothenate) 10 mg • Calcium (as hydroxycitrate, dicalcium phosphate) 60 mg • Magnesium (as magnesium oxide) 100 mg • Potassium 80 mg • Garcinia fruit extract (standardized for hydroxycitric acid) 850 mg • Proprietary Blend 292 mg: Guarana seed extract (standardized for caffeine 54 mg), Bitter Orange fruit extract (citrus aurantium amara, standardized for synephrine 6.6 mg). Other Ingredients: Modified Cellulose, Maltodextrin, Caffeine, Dicalcium Phosphate, Stearic Acid, Dextrin, Dextrose, Lecithin, Sodium Carboxymethylcellulose, Magnesium Stearate, Sodium Citrate.
See Editor's Note No. 40.

Metabolife Ultra Caffeine Free - Metabolife International, Inc.
Two caplets contain: Thiamin (vitamin B1, as thiamin mononitrate) 1.5 mg • Riboflavin (vitamin B2) 1.7 mg • Niacin (vitamin B3, as niacinamide) 20 mg • Vitamin B6 (pyridoxine hydrochloride) 5 mg • Pantothenic Acid (as d-calcium pantothenate) 10 mg • Calcium (as hydroxycitrate) 75 mg • Chromium (as chromium picolinate) 133 mcg • Potassium 150 mg. Other Ingredients: Modified Cellulose, Maltodextrin, Stearic Acid, Silica, Dextrin, Titanium Dioxide, Polyethylene Glycol, Lecithin, Dextrose, Sodium Carboxymethylcellulose, FD&C Yellow 5, FD&C Red 40, Sodium Citrate, FD&C Blue 2.

Metabolift - TwinLab
Two capsules contain: Ma Huang extract 334 mg • Guarana extract (standardized for 22% Caffeine) 910 mg • Chromium (from Chromic Fuel patented Chromium Picolinate) 200 mg. In a concentrated herbal base of White Willow bark extract & Cayenne.
See Editor's Note No. 30.

Metabolift MaHuang Free Formula - TwinLab
Two tablets contain: Guarana seed extract (standardized for 22% caffeine) 800 mg • Citrus Aurantium extract (standardized for 6% synephrine alkaloids) 325 mg • Proprietary Blend 360 mg: St. John's Wort (9 mg, standardized for hypericin), L-Phenylalanine, Green Tea leaf extract (standardized for epigallocatechin gallate), Quercetin Dihydrate, Citrus Bioflavonoid Complex (containing naringin), Ginger root, Cayenne fruit.
See Editor's Note No. 40.

Metabolite - 4 Life
Each capsule contains: Bladderwrack leaf 140 mg • Red Wheat Fiber seed 70 mg • Hawaiian Spirulina Pacifica 40 mg • Sage leaf 35 mg • Frangula bark extract 20 mg • Papaya 18 mg • Pineapple 18 mg • Papain from Papaya fruit 17 mg • Bromelain from Pineapple fruit 17 mg • Artichoke leaf 15 mg. Other Ingredients: Gelatin, Xanthan Gum, Locust Bean Gum, Rice Bran.

Metab-O-Lite - Richardson Labs
One tablet contains: Vitamin E 6 IU • Magnesium (as Magnesium chelate) 75 mg • Zinc (as Zinc chelate) 5 mg • Chromium (as Chromium Picolinate) 75 mcg • Proprietary Blend 728 mg: Ephedra (Ma Huang) concentrate (aerial part, 12 mg naturally-occurring ephedrines) • Bee Pollen • Siberian Ginseng root • Ginger root • Lecithin • Bovine Cartilage • Damiana leaf • Sarsaparilla root • Goldenseal aerial part • Nettles leaf • Gotu Kola aerial part • Spirulina Algae • Royal Jelly. Other Ingredients: Cellulose, Croscarmellose Sodium, Hydroxypropyl Cellulose, Silica, Hydroxypropyl Methylcellulose, DL-Alpha-Tocopheryl Acetate, Magnesium Stearate, Maltodextrin, PEG.
See Editor's Note No. 30.

Metab-O-LITE Ephedra Free - Rexall - Sundown
Two caplets contain: Vitamin C 50 mg • Proprietary Blend 1 g: Black Tea Extract (leaf), Caffeine (from guarana extract seed and caffeine), Rutin, Ginger Extract (root), Dill Extract 20:1 (aerial part). Other Ingredients: Dextrose, Microcrystalline Cellulose, Crospovidone, Maltose, Dextrin, Hydroxypropyl Methylcellulose, Titanium Dioxide (color), Magnesium Stearate, PEG, Riboflavin (color), Soy Lecithin, Blue 2 Lake, Yellow 6 Lake, Red 40 Lake.

Metabolol II - Champion Nutrition
Each serving contains: Metacarb Plus (complex carbohydrates from corn hybrids) • Peptol PER4 + protein formulation: Enzyme Modified Egg Albumin, Whey Protein Concentrate, Potassium Caseinate, Peptides from Enzyme Modified Lactalbumin, & Pharmaceutical Grade Amino Acids: L-Leucine, L-Isoleucine, L-Valine, L-Cystine, L-Phenylalanine, L-Methionine, L-Threonine, L-Lysine, L-Glutamic Acid • Polylactate • Medium Chain Triglycerides • Metavite bioactive vitamin mineral formula: Calcium Carbonate, Pyridoxine Alpha-Ketoglutarate (PAK), Choline Bitartrate, Inositol, Di-Calcium Phosphate, Calcium Lactate, Calcium Citrate, Magnesium Oxide, Magnesium Citrate, Zinc Picolinate, Ester-C, (Esterified Calcium Polyascorbate), Potassium Phosphate, D-Alpha Tocopherol Succinate Esterified Zinc Polyascorbate, Molybdenum Aspartate, Iron Succinate, Manganese Citrate, Niacin, Calcium Pantothenate, Copper Glycinate, Chromium-Polynicotinate • Pyridoxal-5-Phosphate • Retinyl Palmitote, Riboflavin-5-Phosphate • Thiamine HCL • D-Biotin • Potassium Iodide • Ergocalciferol • Folic Acid • Cyanocobalamin • Intrinsic Factor Complex • Succinate ETF

Complex: Potassium Succinate, Magnesium Succinate, Calcium Succinate, L-Glutamic Acid, Inosine, & Pyridoxine Alpha-Ketoglutarate (PAK) Inosine, Lecithin, Natural Flavors, L-Carnitine, Lipoic Acid, Selenium Aspartate.

Metaboloss **- NFI Dietary Supplements**
Ginger • Magnesium • Vitamin E • Zinc • Ma Huang • Astragalus • Bee Pollen • Chromium Picolinate • Siberian Ginseng • Sarsaparilla • Goldenseal • Nettles • Gotu Kola • Lecithin • Damiana • Royal Jelly • Bladderwrack • Blue Green Algae • Licorice.
See Editor's Note No. 30.

MetabolStim **- BioGenesis Nutraceuticals**
Each veggie capsule contains: Thiamine Mononitrate (B1) 2 mg • Riboflavin (B2) 2 mg • Niacinamide (B3) 20 mg • Pyridoxine (P5P, HCl, B6) 5 mg • Iodine (fucus vesiculosus, bladderwrack) 67 mcg • Zinc (citrate/malate, aspartate) 5 mg • Manganese (aspartate) 1 mg • Selenium (selenomethionine) 40 mcg • Vanadium (aspartate) 300 mcg • L-Aspartic Acid 175 mg • L-Glutamic Acid 100 mg • N-Acetyl L-Cysteine 50 mg • N-Acetyl L-Tyrosine 100 mg.

MetaboMax **- Nature's Sunshine**
Each tablet contains: Chinese Ephedra (12 mg total ephedra alkaloids) • Bee Pollen • Siberian Ginseng • Ginger • Lecithin • Cordyceps • Kelp • Damiana • Sarsaparilla • Golden Seal • Nettle • Gotu Kola • Spirulina • Royal Jelly.
See Editor's Note No. 30.

MetaboMax EF **- Nature's Sunshine**
Two tablets contain: Vitamin E (D-alpha tocopherol) 12 IU • Chromium (amino acid chelate) 150 mcg • Proprietary Blend 1274 mg: Garcinia fruit (garcinia cambogia 50% HCA), Bitter Orange fruit (fructus aurantia, synephrine 6% extract), Lotus leaf extract (folium nelumbinis), Green Tea extract (camellia sinensis, decaffeinated, 60% EGCG), Bee Pollen, Eleuthero root (eleutherococcus senticosus), Cordyceps powder, L-Carnitine, Kelp leaf and stem (ascophyllum nodosum and laminaria digitata), Spirulina (algae). Other Ingredients: Cellulose, Di-Calcium Phosphate, Stearic Acid, Magnesium Stearate, Silicon Dioxide.
See Editor's Note No. 40.

MetaBoost **- Advocare International**
Two caplets contain: Vitamin C (as potassium/magnesium/sodium ascorbates) 600 mg • Iodine (as potassium iodide) 50 mcg • Guarana extract (seed - paullinia cupana) 150 mg • Oolong Tea extract (leaf - camellia sinensis) 200 mg • Eleuthero extract (root - eleutherococcus senticosus) 50 mg. Other Ingredients: Dicalcium Phosphate, Silicon Dioxide, Cellulose, Stearic Acid, Magnesium Stearate, Vanillin.

Meta-Booster **- Nu-Creations**
Each capsule contains: Vitamin E 6 IU • Magnesium 75 mg • Zinc 5 mg • Chromium Picolinate 75 mcg • Meta-Booster Proprietary Blend 803 mg: Guarana, Ma Huang concentrate, Bee Pollen, Siberian Ginseng, Ginger, Lecithin, Bovine Complex, Damiana, Sarsaparilla, Goldenseal, Canadensis, Nettle, Gotu Kola, Spirulina, Royal Jelly. Other Ingredients: Dicalcium Phosphate, Pharmaceutical Glaze, Magnesium Stearate.
See Editor's Note No. 14. and No. 30.

Metabosurge **- Puritan's Pride**
Each tablet contains: Vitamin C (as Ascorbic Acid) 20 mg • Vitamin E (as dl-Alpha Tocopheryl Acetate) 6 IU • Magnesium (as Magnesium Oxide) 75 mg • Zinc (as Zinc Oxide) 5 mg • Chromium (as Chromium Picoline) 75 mcg • Proprietary Blend: Ma Huang (Ephedra sinica) aerial (standardized for 12 mg ephedra alkaloids), Guarana extract, Citrus Aurantium, Bee Pollen, Korean Ginseng, Ginger, Lecithin, White Willow, Damiana, Sarsaparilla, Golden Seal, Nettles, Gotu Kola, Spirulina, Green Tea extract, Bladderwrack extract 750 mg.
See Editor's Note No. 21, No. 30 and No. 40.

Metabosurge Ephedra Free Formula **- Puritan's Pride**
Two tablets contain: Calcium (from hydroxycitrate and dicalcium phosphate) 50 mg • Chromium (as chromium picolinate) 150 mcg • Proprietary Blend 1132 mg: Green Tea leaf extract (camellia sinensis, standardized to contain polyphenols, EGCG, catechins), Super CitriMax Garcinia Cambogia fruit extract (standardized to contain hydroxycitric acid), Guarana bark extract (paullinia cupana, standardized to contain caffeine), Yerba Mate leaf (ilex paraguariensis, standardized to contain caffeine). Other Ingredients: Cellulose, Silica, Vegetable Stearic Acid, Acacia Gum, Vegetable Magnesium Stearate, Cellulose Coating.

Metabotrim **- Pharmanex**
Each capsule contains: Vitamin C (Calcium Ascorbate) 75 mg • Niacin (Niacinamide) 10 mg • Vitamin B6 (Pyridoxine Hydrochloride, Pycodoxal-5-Phosphate) 3 mg • Vitamin B12 (Cyanocobalamin, Dibencozide) 6 mcg • Magnesium (Magnesium Asparate, Magnesium Citrate, Magnesium Chelate) 20 mg • Chromium (Chromium Chelate, Chromium Picolinate) 100 mcg • Potassium (Potassium Asparate, Potassium Citrate) 20 mg • Carnitine (L-Carnitine L-Tartrate) 100 mg. Other Ingredients: Cellulose, Magnesium Stearate, Vanillin, Silicon Dioxide.

MetaboTrim **- VitaStore**
Each tablet contains: Vitamin E 6 IU • Magnesium (as Magnesium Chelate) 75 mg • Zinc (as Zinc Chelate) 5 mg • Chromium (as Chromium Picolinate) 75 mcg. Blended Formula 728 mg: Guarana Concentrate (seed) (40 mg Naturally-occurring caffeine), Ma Huang Concentrate (herb: aerial part) (12 mg naturally-occurring ephedrine), Bee Pollen, Ginseng (root), Lecithin (vitamin), Bovine Complex, Damiana (leaf), Sarsaparilla (root), Goldenseal (aerial part), Nettles (leaf), Gotu Kola (aerial part), Spirulina Algae, Royal Jelly. Other Ingredients: Methocel, Silica, Croscarmellose Sodium, Magnesium Stearate.
See Editor's Note No. 14 and No. 30.

MetaBurn **- Oasis Wellness Network**
Each capsule contains: Calcium (from carbonate, citrate) 75 mg • Green Tea leaves extract (70% polyphenols, 25% EGCG, 5% L-theanine) 300 mg • Bitter Orange fruit extract (6% synephrine) 150 mg • BioResponse DIM Complex 50 mg: Starch, Diindolylmethane, D-Alpha-Tocopheryl Succinate, Phosphatidylcholine, Silica • MaxCell Proprietary Blend 12.5 mg: Jujube fruit extract, Black Pepper fruit extract, Aloe Vera dried gel, Chinese Licorice root. Other Ingredients: Magnesium Stearate, Silica, Gelatin.
See Editor's Note No. 40.

Meta-Burn **- Metabolic Response Modifiers**
Two capsules contain: Garcinia cambogia (50%) HCA 500 mg • Ma Huang (8% ephedra) 225 mg • Green Tea (50% caffeine) 100 mg • Caffeine (anhydrous) 100 mg • White Willow bark (2%salicylates) 60 mg • Naringin 20 mg • L-Tyrosine 50 mg • Choline bitartrate 100 mg • Chromium (chelate 10%) 200 mcg • Vanadium (sulfate) 3 mg • Alpha Lipoic Acid 50 mg • Vitamin B5 (pantothenic acid) 50 mg • Potassium (phosphate) 74 mg • Iodine (as potassium iodide) 750 mcg • Cayenne Pepper 10 mg.
See Editor's Note No. 30.

Meta-Burn EF **- Metabolic Response Modifiers**
Four capsules contain: Garcinia cambogia (50%) HCA 2000 mg • Citrus aurantium (6% synephrine) 350 mg • Green Tea (40% caffeine) 225 mg • Phosphate (potassium phosphate) 124 mg • White Willow bark (1% salicylates) 60 mg • Coleus Forskohlii (10% Forskolin) 50 mg • Naringin 20 mg • Alpha Lipoic Acid 25 mg • Cayenne Pepper 20 mg • Potassium (potassium phosphate) 101 mg • Iodine (Iodine USP) 750 mcg • Chromium (as chelate) 300 mcg.
See Editor's Note No. 40.

Meta-CLA **- E'OLA**
Each capsule contains: Tonalin 500 mg • Aloe-Min E'OLA Mineral Blend 25 mg: Active Aloe, Calcium Gluconate Monohydrate.

MetaCort Spray **- DermaBolics Laboratories**
Five sprays contain: Androstenetrione 100 mg • 7-OXO-DHEA 100 mg. Other Ingredients: Isopropyl Alcohol, Propylene Glycol, Octyl Salicylate, Triglyceride Complex, Water, D-Limonene.

Meta-Dream - Meta-Sure Health
Two caplets contain: Potassium (as potassium phosphate) 160 mg • Calcium (as calcium phosphate) 30 mg • Cellulex Blend: Borage extract seed, Bladderwrack extract, Sweet Clover extract, Grape Seed extract, Lecithin (soy), Ginkgo Biloba extract 250 mg • L-Carnitine 25 mg • L-Tyrosine 70 mg • Collagen Complex 120 mg • Valerian powder root 15 mg • Skullcap powder root 10 mg • Passion Flower powder leaf 10 mg •5-HTP seed 750 mcg • Melatonin 250 mcg. See Editor's Note No. 16.

MetaFiber - Metagenics
Rice Bran • Beet Fiber • Oat Fiber • Apple Fiber • Cellulose • Olive Oil • D-Alpha Tocopheryl Acetate.

Metafolin - Source Naturals
Each tablet contains: Folate as Metafolin (L-methylfolate) 800 mcg. Other Ingredients: Microcrystalline Cellulose, Stearic Acid, Colloidal Silicon Dioxide.

MetaFuel (chocolate flavor) - Oasis Wellness Network
Two scoops (45 g) contain: Vitamin A (as vitamin A palmitate) 2250 IU • Vitamin C (as ascorbic acid) 30 mg • Vitamin D (as cholecalciferol) 180 IU • Vitamin E (as alpha-tocopheryl acetate) 15 IU • Vitamin K (phytonadione) 5 mcg • Thiamin (as thiamin mononitrate) 1 mg • Riboflavin (USP) 1 mg • Niacin (as niacinamide) 9 mg • Vitamin B6 (as pyridoxine hydrochloride) 1 mg • Folic Acid (USP) 180 mcg • Vitamin B12 (as cyanocobalamin) 3 mcg • Biotin (USP) 120 mcg • Pantothenic Acid (as d-calcium pantothenate) 4.5 mg • Calcium 250 mg • Iron 1 mg • Phosphorus 150 mg • Iodine (as potassium iodide) 30 mcg • Magnesium (as magnesium oxide) 80 mg • Zinc (as zinc oxide) 3 mg • Selenium 32 mcg • Copper (as copper sulfate) 0.4 mg • Manganese (as manganese sulfate) 1 mg • Chromium (as chromium polynicotinate) 42 mcg • Molybdenum (as molybdenum glycinate) 19 mcg • Sodium 280 mg • Potassium 640 mg • MaxCell Proprietary Blend 25 mg: Jujube extract, Aloe Vera gel, Black Pepper extract, Chinese Licorice. Other Ingredients: Protein Blend: Whey Protein, Soy Protein Isolate • Dutch Cocoa • Fiber Blend: Cellulose, Gum Acacia, Xanthan Gum, Flax Seed Powder, Cellulose Gum, Oat Fiber • Inulin • High Oleic Safflower Oil • Natural/Artificial Flavors • Lecithin • Enzyme Blend: Protease, Lipase, Cellulase, Amylase, Bromelain, Papain • Sucralose • Stevia Extract.

MetaFuel (vanilla flavor) - Oasis Wellness Network
Two scoops (45 g) contain: Vitamin A (as vitamin A palmitate) 2250 IU • Vitamin C (as ascorbic acid) 30 mg • Vitamin D (as cholecalciferol) 180 IU • Vitamin E (as alpha-tocopheryl acetate) 15 IU • Vitamin K (phytonadione) 5 mcg • Thiamin (as thiamin mononitrate) 1 mg • Riboflavin (USP) 1 mg • Niacin (as niacinamide) 9 mg • Vitamin B6 (as pyridoxine hydrochloride) 1 mg • Folic Acid (USP) 180 mcg • Vitamin B12 (as cyanocobalamin) 3 mcg • Biotin (USP) 120 mcg • Pantothenic Acid (as d-calcium pantothenate) 4.5 mg • Calcium 3000 mg • Iron 1 mg • Phosphorus 150 mg • Iodine (as potassium iodide) 30 mcg • Magnesium (as magnesium oxide) 40 mg • Zinc (as zinc oxide) 3 mg • Selenium 32 mcg • Copper (as copper sulfate) 0.4 mg • Manganese (as manganese sulfate) 1 mg • Chromium (as chromium polynicotinate) 42 mcg • Chloride (as potassium chloride) 25 mg • Molybdenum (as molybdenum glycinate) 19 mcg • Sodium 280 mg • Potassium 640 mg • MaxCell Proprietary Blend 25 mg: Jujube extract, Aloe Vera gel, Black Pepper extract, Chinese Licorice. Other Ingredients: Protein Blend: Whey Protein, Soy Protein Isolate • Fiber Blend: Cellulose, Gum Acacia, Xanthan Gum, Flax Seed Powder, Cellulose Gum, Oat Fiber • Inulin • High Oleic Safflower Oil • Natural/Artificial Flavors • Lecithin • Enzyme Blend: Protease, Lipase, Cellulase, Amylase, Bromelain, Papain • Sucralose • Stevia Extract.

Metagest - Metagenics
Two tablets contain: Betaine Hydrochloride 1300 mg • Pepsin (porcine) 90 mg • Gentian root (gentiana lutea) 40 mg.

MetaGlycemX - Metagenics
Two tablets contain: Vitamin C (as ascorbic acid) 300 mg • Vitamin E (as d-alpha-tocopheryl succinate) 200 IU • Thiamin (as thiamin mononitrate) 15 mg • Riboflavin 9 mg • Niacin (as niacinamide) 90 mg • Pantothenic Acid (as d-calcium pantothenate) 30 mg • Vitamin B6 (as pyridoxine hydrochloride) 9 mg • Vitamin B12 (as cyanocobalamin) 150 mcg • Biotin 2 mg • Folate (as folic acid) 400 mcg • Zinc (as zinc glycinate) 9 mg • Copper (as copper lysinate hydrochloride) 0.75 mg • Manganese (as manganese citrate) 1.2 mg • Chromium (as chromium polynicotinate) 600 mcg • Selenium (as selenomethionine) 90 mcg • Vanadium (as vanadyl sulfate) 0.5 mg • Alpha-Lipoic Acid 100 mg • L-Carnosine 50 mg • Taurine 300 mg • Chinese Cinnamon bark (cinnamomum cassia) 500 mg • Catechins 100 mg • Epigallocatechin Gallate (EGCG, from decaffeinated green tea leaf, camellia sinensis) 66.5 mg.

MetaGreens - Oasis Wellness Network
Each tablespoon (6 g) contains: Alfalfa juice (organic, 33:1) 1200 mg • Spirulina (organic) 1200 mg • Inulin 1000 mg • Rice Solubles 500 mg • Kamut (whole leaf, organic, 5:1) 416 mg • Barley (whole leaf, organic, 5:1) 416 mg • Oat (whole leaf, organic, 5:1) 416 mg • Pineapple 250 mg • Cruciferous Vegetable Blend 200 mg • L-Glutamine 100 mg • Nopal Cactus 100 mg • Eleuthero extract 100 mg • Kyo-Dophilus 40 mg • Kelp (wildcrafted) 30 mg • Dulse (wildcrafted) 30 mg • Stevia 20 mg • Aloe Vera gel (organic, 200:1) 10 mg • MaxCell Proprietary Blend 10 mg: Zisyphus Jujube, Piper Nigrum, Aloe Vera gel, Glycyrrhiza Glabra.

Meta-HGH - E'OLA
One scoop contains: Niacin 16 mg • Proprietary Blend 4.18 g: Glutamine, Glycine, Gum Guggul, Forskolin, E'OLA Mineral Blend.

Metal Cleanse - BioGenesis Nutraceuticals
Each 1 tsp serving (5 mL) contains: Sodiumedetate 3X • Calcare Flourica 3X, 6X • Calcarea Phosphorica 3X, 6X • Calcarea Sulfica 3X, 6X • Ferrum Phosphoricum 3X, 6X • Kalium Muriaticum 3X, 6X • Kalium Phosphoricum 3X, 6X • Kalium Sulfuricum 3X, 6X • Magnesia Phosphorica 3X, 6X • Natrum Muriaticum 3X, 6X • Naturm Phosphoricum 3X, 6X • Silicea 3X, 6X • Mercurius 9C • Polubum Metallicum 9C • Natrum Sulfurica 3X, 6X • Arsenicum Album 9C • Alumina 9C • CAdium Metallicum 9C • Stannum Metallicum 9C • Berberis Aquifollum 6C • Taraxicum Officinalls 6C • Lycopodium Clavatum 6C • Phytolacca Decanda 6C • 80% Reversed Osmosis Water • 20% Alcohol.
See Editor's Note No. 1.

Metal Magnet - PhytoPharmica
Each capsule contains: Proprietary Humifulvate Complex 75 mg: Humic Acid, Fulvic Acid, Phenolic Acid. Other Ingredients: Cellulose, Gelatin, Magnesium Stearate.

Metal-Free - BodyHealth
Proprietary Blend 330 mcg: Microactivated Algae, Lactobacillus extract, Bifidus extract, Peptidylgluconase, Glycine, Ionic sea minerals, Hydrated Colloidal Silica, Glutathione, Vitamin C, Hyaluronic Acid, Fulvic Acid, Ferulic Acid, Lipoic Acid, Chlorella, Acetylcysteine.

Metalogic - PhysioLogics
Each capsule contains: Vitamin C (ascorbic acid) 250 mg • Zinc 15 mg • Copper (glycinate) 500 mcg • N-Acetyl Cysteine 200 mg • L-Methionine 30 mg • Alpha-Lipoic Acid 25 mg • L-Glutathione 5 mg • Selenium (selenomethionine) 75 mcg.

Metamucil capsules - Proctor & Gamble
Six capsules contain: Psyllium husk 0.52 g. Other Ingredients: Gelatin, Polysorbate 80, Caramel Color.

Metamucil Fiber Wafers - Proctor & Gamble
Each wafer contains: Psyllium husk 3.4 g. Other Ingredients: Ascorbic Acid, Brown Sugar, Cinnamon, Corn Oil, Flavors, Fructose, Lecithin, Modified Food Starch, Molasses, Oat Hull Fiber, Sodium Bicarbonate, Sucrose, Water, Wheat Flour.

Metamucil powder - Proctor & Gamble
Each rounded teaspoon contains: Pure Psyllium Husk Fiber 3.4 g. Other Ingredients: Sucrose.

Metamucil Sugar Free **-** Proctor & Gamble
Each packet contains: Pure Psyllium husk fiber 3.4 g. Other Ingredients: Aspartame, Citric Acid, Maltodextrin, Yellow #6.

MetaPlex **-** Allergy Research Group
Three tablets contain: Vitamin B6 (as pyridoxal-5-phosphate and pyridoxine hydrochloride) 22.5 mg • Calcium (as pyruvate and dicalcium phosphate) 68 mg • Chromium (as nicotinate) 6 mcg • Chitosan 600 mg • L-Carnitine 150 mg • Arthred Hydrolyzed Collagen 450 mg • Garcinia Cambogia fruit extract (75% hydroxycitric acid) 300 mg • Pyruvate (as calcium pyruvate) 320 mg. Other Ingredients: Dicalcium Phosphate, Modified Cellulose, Stearic Acid, Magnesium Stearate, Silicon Dioxide, Ethyl Vanillin.

MetaPower **-** Oasis Wellness Network
Each softgel contains: Vitamin E 6 IU • Marine Lipid oil 1 g • EPA 300 mg • DHA 200 mg • Coenzyme Q10 3.5 mg • Maxcell Powder Proprietary Blend 8.33 mg: Jujube fruit extract, Black Pepper fruit extract, Aloe Vera gel (dried), Chinese Licorice. Other Ingredients: Gelatin, Glycerin, Beeswax, Water, Lecithin, Titanium Dioxide, Chlorophyllin, Beta-Carotene.

Meta-Sitosterol **-** Metagenics
Three tablets contain: Beta-Sitosterol 1000 mg • Campesterol 500 mg • Stigmasterol 275 mg • Other Plant Sterols 225 mg • Folate (as folic acid, L-5-methyl tetrahydrofolate, 5-formyl tetrahydrofolate) 800 mcg.

Meta-Sure Metagizer **-** Meta-Sure Health
Each caplet contains: Vitamin E (as d-alpha Tocopheryl) 7 IU • Niacin 5 mg • Vitamin B6 5 mg • Folic Acid 50 mcg • Vitamin B12 10 mcg • Magnesium (as Magnesium Chelate, Magnesium Salicylate) 11 mg • Zinc (as Zinc Chelate) 3 mg • Chromium (as Chromium Aspartate, Chromium Picolinate) 75 mcg • SurePlex Blend: Guarana concentrate seed (contains 46 mg naturally occuring caffeine), Ma Huang concentrate aerial part (contains 12 mg naturally occuring ephedrines), Taurine, Potassium Citrate, Siberian Ginseng root, Spirulina algae, Ginger root, Green Tea concentrate leaf (contains 2 mg naturally occuring caffeine), Lecithin, Farcinia Cambogia concentrate fruit, Bladderwrack leaf, Inositol, Nettle leaf, Royal leaf, Sarsaparilla root, Cayenne fruit, White Willow bark, Naringen fruit, Hawthorne fruit, L-Methionine, Ginkgo Biloba leaf, Gotu Kola (aerial part) 700 mg. Other Ingredients: Croscarmellose Sodium, Magnesium Stearate, Methocel, Microcrystalline Cellulose, Silica.
See Editor's Note No. 30.

Meta-Thin **-** New Hope Health Products
Two capsules contain: Garcinia cambogia (50%) HCA 750 mg • Ma Huang (8% ephedra) 225 mg • Green Tea (50% caffeine) 125 mg • Caffeine (anhydrous) 100 mg •White Willow bark (2% salicylates) 60 mg • Naringin 20 mg • L-Tyrosine 50 mg • Choline bitartrate 100 mg • Chromium (chelate 10%) 200 mcg • Vanadium (sulfate) 3 mg • Alpha-lipoic acid 50 mg • Vitamin B-5 (Pantothenic acid) 50 mg • Potassium (Phosphate) 74 mg • Iodine (as Potassium iodide) 750 mcg • Cayenne Pepper 10 mg.
See Editor's Note No. 30.

MetaTox Oral **-** PhysioLogics
Each capsule contains: Vitamin C (Ascorbic Acid) 250 mg • N-Acetylcysteine 200 mg • L-Methionine (Zn/Se Monomethionine) 52.5 mg • Alpha-Lipoic Acid (USP) 5 mg • L-Glutathione (USP) 5 mg • Zinc (as Zinc Monomethionine) 15 mg • Copper (Glycinate) 0.5 mg • Selenium (Methionine) 75 mcg.

Metazyme **-** Metagenics
Each tablet contains: Protease 3600 PU • Amylase 4400 AU • Lipase 990 LU • Cellulase 200 CU.

Methionine **-** Pain & Stress Center
Each capsule contains: Vitamin C (ascorbyl palmitate) 5 mg • L-Methionine 500 mg. Other Ingredients: Gelatin Capsule.

Methionine Detox Complex **-** Pro Health
Each capsule contains: Riboflavin 1.7 mg • Vitamin B6 (as pyridoxine HCl) 0.8 mg • Folic Acid 400 mcg • Calcium (as calcium carbonate) 50 mg • DL-Methionine 500 mg • Betaine 100 mg • L-Taurine 50 mg. Other Ingredients: Gelatin, Silica, Magnesium Stearate, Rice Flour.

Methoxy Complex Caps **-** Optimum Nutrition
Each capsule contains: 5-Methyl-7-Methoxy-Isoflavone 200 mg • 7-Isopropoxyisoflavone (ipriflavone) 150 mg • Grapefruit extract (standardized to 20% naringin) 50 mg. Other Ingredients: Gelatin, Microcrystalline Cellulose, Magnesium Stearate, Silica.

Methoxy-7 **-** BioTest Laboratories, LLC
Two teaspoons contain: 5-Methyl-7-Methoxy-Isoflavone 400 mg • Cholesterol 520 mg. Other Ingredients: Purified Water, Fatty-Acid Ethyl Esters, Polysorbate 60, Lecithin, Natural and Artificial Flavors, Potassium Sorbate, Methyl Paraben, Disodium EDTA, Butylated Hydroxyanisole, Sucralose, Vegetable Gum.

MethOxyvone **-** Metabolic Response Modifiers
Each capsule contains: 5-methyl-7-methoxyisoflavone 150 mg • 7-isopropoxyisoflavone 40 mg • Lysophosphatidylcholine 40 mg.

Methyl 1-Test **-** Legal Gear
Each tablet contains: 17-Methyl-1-Androstene-17b-ol-3one 10 mg. Other Ingredients: Microcrystalline Cellulose, Magnesium Stearate, Gelatin.

Methyl 1-Testosterone Xtreme **-** IDS
Each capsule contains: 17-Alpha-Methyl 1-Testosterone 10 mg • Bergamottin (6,7,-dihydroxybergamottin (DHB)) 100 mg • Proprietary Blend 255 mg: Bupleurum, Hoelen, Cayenne • Vitamin B6 2 mg • Vitamin B12 6 mcg • Niacin 20 mg. Other Ingredients: Gelatin, Magnesium Stearate, Silica.

Methyl B-12 1000 **-** Jarrow Formulas
Each lozenge contains: Methylcobalamin (methyl B12) 1000 mcg. Other Ingredients: Sorbitol, Mannitol, Fructose, Lemon Flavor, Citric Acid, Stearic Acid, Magnesium Stearate.

Methyl B-12 5000 **-** Jarrow Formulas
Each lozenge contains: Methylcobalamin (methyl B12) 5000 mcg. Other Ingredients: Sorbitol, Mannitol, Fructose, Microcrystalline Cellulose, Magnesium Stearate, Cherry Flavor.

Methyl Protect **-** Xymogen
Each capsule contains: Vitamin B12 (as methylcobalamin) 1000 mcg • Vitamin B6 (as pyridoxal 5'-phosphate) 10 mg • Folate (as folic acid and 5 formyl tetrahydrofolate) 1000 mcg • Trimethylglycine (as anhydrous betaine) 250 mg.

Methylcobalamin **-** Pure Encapsulations
Each vegetable capsule contains: Methylcobalamin (vitamin B12) 1000 mcg.

methylCOBALAMIN 1 mg **-** Source Naturals
Each tablet contains: Vitamin B12 (as methylcobalamin) 1 mg.

methylCOBALAMIN 5 mg **-** Source Naturals
Each tablet contains: Vitamin B12 (as methylcobalamin) 5 mg.

MET-Rx Arthro-HCP **-** Rexall - Sundown
Fourteen grams contain: Arthred (Hydrolyzed Collagen Protein) 10 g • Maltodextrin • Glucosamine Hydrochloride & Glucosamine Sulfate 1.5 g.
See Editor's Note No. 21.

MET-Rx Hy-Gear **-** Rexall - Sundown
Each 40 g serving contains: Creatine Monohydrate 5 g • Carbohydrate 34 g. Ingredients: Citrus Mist flavor: CeraSport (Rice Syrup Solids, Sodium Chloride, Potassium Chloride & Trisodium Citrate) • Fructose • Creatine Monohydrate • Glucose • Natural & Artificial Flavors • Citric Acid • Malic Acid • Beta Carotene & Beet juice powder for color. Strazzyberry Flavor: CeraSport (Rice Syrup Solids, Sodium Chloride, Potassium Chloride & Trisodium Citrate) • Fructose • Creatine Monohydrate • Glucose • Natural & Artificial Flavors • Beet juice powder for color.

Some Brand Name Natural Products - What they Contain

www.NaturalDatabase.com contains MANY more listings than appear here.
Editor's Notes are located on pages 2155-2163.

MET-Rx Keto Pro - Rexall - Sundown
Milk Protein Isolates, Caseinate, Whey Protein Concentrate, Glutamine, Calcium-B-Hydroxy B-Methylbutyrate Monohydrate, Lactoferrin • Medium Chain Triglycerides • Natural & Artifical Flavor • Cellulose • Maltodextrin • Dipotassium Phosphate • Potassium Chloride & Citrate • Carrageenan • Salt • Sodium Citrate.

MET-Rx Mass Action - Rexall - Sundown
Each serving contains: Micronized Creatine 5 g • HMB 1.5 g • Trimethylglycine (TMG) 500 mg • Improved Nutrient Uptake. Ingredients: Glucose • Creatine Monohydrate • HMB • Trimethylglycine • Natural & Artificial Flavors • Beta Carotene & Beet juice powder for colors • Xanthan Gum • Aspartame.

MET-Rx Meal Replacement for the Best Shape of Your Life - Rexall - Sundown
Each powdered packet contains: Extreme Chocolate: METAMYOSYN: Milk Protein Isolates, Caseinate, Glutamine, Whey Protein Concentrate, Egg White • Maltodextrin • Dutch Cocoa (alkali processed) • Vitamins & Minerals: Dicalcium Phosphate, Potassium Chloride, Dipotassium Phosphate, Potassium Citrate, Salt, Sodium Citrate, Magnesium Oxide, Choline Bitartrate, Ascorbic Acid, D-Alpha-Tocopheryl Acetate, Ferrous Fumarate, Niacinamide, Vitamin A Palmitate, Zinc Oxide, Calcium Pantothenate, Vitamin K, Manganese Sulfate, Vitamin D (as Vitamin D3), Copper Sulfate, Pyridoxine Hydrochloride, Riboflavin, Thiamine Hydrochloride, Chromium Picolinate, Cobalamin Concentrate (Vitamin B12), Folic Acid, Biotin, Sodium Molybdate, Sodium Selenite, Potassium Iodide • Natural & Artificial Flavors • Partially Hydrogenated Coconut oil • Corn Syrup Solids • Cellulose Gum • Xanthan Gum • Aspartame • Carrageenan • Beta Carotene • Acesulfame Potassium • Lecithin • Mono & Diglycerides. Original: METAMYOSYN: Milk Protein Isolates, Caseinate, Glutamine, Whey Protein Concentrate, Egg White, Maltodextrin • Vitamins & Minerals: Dicalcium Phosphate, Potassium Chloride, Dipotassium Phosphate, Potassium Citrate, Salt, Sodium Citrate, Magnesium Oxide, Choline Bitartrate, Ascorbic Acid, d-Alpha-Tocopheryl Acetate, Ferrous Fumarate, Niacinamide, Vitamin A Palmitate, Zinc Oxide, Calcium Pantothenate, Vitamin K, Manganese Sulfate, Vitamin D (as Vitamin D3), Copper Sulfate, Pyridoxine Hydrochloride, Riboflavin, Thiamine Hydrochloride, Chromium Picolinate, Cobalamin Concentrate (Vitamin B12), Folic Acid, Biotin, Sodium Molybdate, Sodium Selenite, Potassium Iodide • Natural & Atrificial Flavors • Corn Syrup Solids • Cellulose Gum • Xanthan Gum • Aspartame • Carrageenan • Beta Carotene • Acesulfame Potassium • Lecithin • Mono & Diglycerides. White Chocolate Mocha: METAMYOSYN: Milk Protein Isolates, Caseinate, Glutamine, Whey Protein Concentrate, Egg White, Maltodextrin • Vitamins & Minerals: Dicalcium Phosphate, Potassium Chloride, Dipotassium Phosphate, Potassium Citrate, Salt, Sodium Citrate, Magnesium Oxide, Choline Bitartrate, Ascorbic Acid, d-Alpha-Tocopheryl Acetate, Ferrous Fumarate, Niacinamide, Vitamin A Palmitate, Zinc Oxide, Calcium Pantothenate, Vitamin K, Manganese Sulfate, Vitamin D (as Vitamin D3), Copper Sulfate, Pyridoxine Hydrochloride, Riboflavin, Thiamine Hydrochloride, Chromium Picolinate, Cobalamin Concentrate (Vitamin B12), Folic Acid, Biotin, Sodium Molybdate, Sodium Selenite, Potassium Iodide • Natural & Artificial Flavors • Soluble Coffee • Dutch Cocoa (alkali processed) • Partially Hydrogenated Coconut oil • Corn Syrup Solids • Cellulose Gum • Xanthan Gum • Aspartame • Carrageenan • Beta Carotene • Acesulfame Potassium • Lecithin • Mono & Diglycerides.

MET-Rx Thermicore - Rexall - Sundown
Three capsules contain: Ma Huang extract 250 mg • Caffeine 200 mg • Bitter Orange extract 400 mg. Other Ingredients: Cellulose, Polyvinylpyrrolidone & Gelatin.
See Editor's Note No. 30 and No. 40.

Mexican Yam Extract - Enzymatic Therapy
Two capsules contain: Wild Yam root extract (dioscorea villosa, standardized to contain 10% diosgenin) 480 mg • Adrenal extract (freeze-dried) 200 mg • Beta Sitosterol 42 mg. Other Ingredients: Gelatin, Cellulose, Magnesium Stearate, Titanium Dioxide Color.
See Editor's Note No. 14.

Mg/K Aspartate - Metagenics
Each tablet contains: Magnesium 50 mg • Potassium 80 mg.

MGN3 (MGN-3, MGN 3) - LaneLabs
Two capsules contain: MGN-3 proprietary blend 500 mg: Rice Bran, Hyphomycetes Mycelia extract, Beet Root Fiber, Calcium Phosphate, Silica, Magnesium Stearate, Gelatin, Water, Glycerin.
See Editor's Note No. 9 and No. 21.

MiBrain - Jarrow Formulas
Four softgels contain: Vitamin B2 (riboflavin) 200 mg • Magnesium (as citrate/oxide 50/50) 300 mg • Chromium (from saccharomyces cerevisiae) 200 mcg • Omega 3 Fatty Acids (from sardine oil, providing 125 mg DHA and 50 mg EPA) 210 mg • Feverfew (tanacetum parthenium) 100 mg • Butterbur 30:1 extract (petasites hybridus) 50 mg • Ginger rhizome (zingiber officinale, 5% gingerols and shogaols) 250 mg • Devil's Claw (harpagophytum procumbens, 5% iridoid glycosides) 250 mg • White Willow bark (salicis cortex, 15% salicin) 200 mg • Green Tea (camellia sinensis, 60% polyphenols) 150 mg. Other Ingredients: Soybean Oil, Gelatin, Glycerin, Purified Water, Carob Extract Concentrate, Lecithin, Beeswax, Carob Powder, Gelatin, Glycerin, Water.

MicroDefense - Pure Encapsulations
Each vegetable capsule contains: Black Walnut hull 10:1 extract (juglans nigra L.) 75 mg • Olive leaf extract (olea europaea L., standardized to contain 17-23% oleuropein) 100 mg • Artemisia whole plant extract (artemisia annua L., standardized to contain 5% artemisinin) 200 mg • Clove (syzygium aromaticum) 75 mg • Grapefruit seed extract (standardized to contain 49% polyphenols) 85 mg • Vitamin C (as ascorbyl palmitate) 5 mg.

Microhydrin - Royal BodyCare
Each capsule contains: Silica hydride powder 250 mg • Flanaga Microclusters (Silica, Potassium Carbonate, Magnesium Sulfate) • Rice flour • Rice Bran oil.

Micronized Creatine - AST Sports Science
Each 1 tsp serving contains: Creatine Monohydrate 5 g.

Micronutrient Supplement - Alotek Supplement Company
Two capsules contain: Vitamin C 120 mg • Proprietary Blend 1000 mg: Spirulina, Olive leaf extract, Red Marine Algae, Bovine Colostrum. Other Ingredients: Microcrystalline Cellulose, Gelatin.

Mid-Life - Aspen Group, Inc.
Each tablet contains: Cimicifuga Racemosa root and rhizome (the compounds Triterpine Glycosides, standardized at 1 mg) 40 mg.

Midlife Care - Health Factor
Each capsule contains: Oat Straw extract (10:1) (Avena sativa) 250 mg • Dong Quai extract (4:1) (Angelica sinensis) 100 mg • Black Cohosh extract (4:1) (Cimicifuga racemosa) 80 mg • Licorice extract (4:1) (Glycyrrhiza glabra) 70 mg • Chasteberry (Vitex agnus-castus) 50 mg • Pomegranate (Punica granatum) 39.5 mg.

Mid-Life Creme - Aspen Group, Inc.
Aloe Vera gel in Distilled Water with Catalyst Altered Normalizer • D-Alpha-Tocopherol & mixed Tocopherols • Cetyl Alcohol • Almond oil • Ociyl Palmitate • Panthenol • Peg 8 Stearate • Hydrogenated Vegetable oil • Glycerine • extract of Wild Yam • Micronized Progesterone • Polysorbate 60 • Propylene Glycol • Hyaluronic Acid • oil of Lemon • Keratin • Carbomer 940 • Grapefruit seed extract.

Midlife Ease - Jarrow Formulas
Three capsules contain: Linum Usitatissimum (LinumLife Extra brand flax extract) 40 mg • Vitex 10:1 extract (vitex agnus castus) 100 mg • Dong Quai 7:1 extract (angelica sinensis) 200 mg • Black Cohosh extract (cimicifuga racemosa, 2.5% triterpene) 80 mg • Eleuthero 50:1 (ci wu jia, eleutherococus senticosus) 100 mg • Valerian root 5:1 extract (valeriana officinalis) 200 mg • Licorice root 4:1 extract (glycyrrhiza uralensis) 200 mg • Bupleurum Chinense 4:1 extract (chai hu) 200 mg • Wu Wei Zi 10:1 extract (schizandra chinensis) 200 mg. Other Ingredients: Magnesium Stearate (vegetable source), Hydroxypropylmethylcellulose (HPMC).

Mid-Life Plus - Aspen Group, Inc.
Each caplet contains: Vitamin E (as natural d-alpha tocopherol succinate) 30 IU • Vitamin C 60 mg • Thiamin (as thiamin mononitrate) 2 mg • Riboflavin 2 mg • Niacin (niacinamide) 20 mg • Vitamin B6 (as pyridoxine HCl) 10 mg • Vitamin B12 (as cyanocobalamin) 6 mcg • Folate (as folic acid) 400 mcg • Calcium (from calcium carbonate) 150 mg • Selenium (from L-Selenomethionine) 70 mcg • Boron (chelate) 1.5 mg • Purified Isoflavones from soybean & pueraria root 50 mg • Kava Kava root standardized extract (30% kavalactones) 100 mg • Black Cohosh root 40 mg.

Midnight Stallion - NVE Pharmaceuticals
Each capsule contains: Proprietary Blend 250 mg: Ephedra extract (leaves, stems, 25 mg ephedrine group alkaloids), Kola Nut (seeds, <1 mg caffeine group alkaloids), Green Tea (leaves, <1 mg caffeine group alkaloids), Mate (leaves, <1 mg caffeine group alkaloids), Gotu Kola (leaves), Rhodiola (root) • Caffeine (anhydrous) 300 mg • Other Ingredients: Gelatin, Stearic Acid, Magnesium Stearate, Di Basic Calcium Phosphate, Titanium Dioxide, FD&C Blue #1, FD&C Red #40.
See Editor's Note No. 30.

Mighty Lean - Nature's Plus
Three capsules contain: Vitamin B12 [as cyanocobalamin] 500 mcg • Chromium (as chromium polynicotinate, chloride) 120 mcg • Proprietary Mighty Lean Herbal Blend 620 mg: Guarana seed, Spirulina, Cacao fruit (theobroma cacao), Green Tea leaf (camellia sinensis) • Rhodiola Rosea root (with standardized rosavin, salidroside, polyphenols, beta-vicianosides, rosin and rosarin) 300 mg • Korean Ginseng root (panax ginseng, standardized to 15% ginsenosides) 250 mg • CitriMax brand Garcinia Cambogia fruit extract, standardized to 50% [-]hydroxycitrate 100 mg • ForsLean brand Coleus Forskohlii extract (with standardized forskolin) 100 mg • Conjugated Linoleic Acid (CLA, standardized 1:1 c9-t11:t10-c12) 100 mg • Eleuthero root (eleutherococcus senticosus, standardized to 0.8% eleutherosides) 50 mg • Bioperine brand Black Pepper (piper nigrum fruit, standardized to 95% 1-piperoylpiperdine) 1 mg. Other Ingredients: Energy Blend (creatine monohydrate, alpha lipoic acid, glutamine, S-adenosylmethionine), Gelatin, Silica, Purified Water.

Mighty One 3000 - Optimum Nutrition
Four scoops (224 g) contain: Proprietary Protein Blend: Whey Protein Concentrate, Soy Protein Isolate • Complex Carbohydrates • Crystalline Fructose • Cocoa • Artificial Flavor • Mighty One Vitamin Mineral Blend: Ascorbic Acid, DL-Alpha Tocopherol Acetate, Ferrous Fumarate, Niacinamide, Vitamin A Palmitate, Potassium Iodide, D-Calcium Pantothenate, Zinc Oxide, Vitamin D (D3), Copper Sulfate, Pyridoxine Hydrochloride, Riboflavin, Thiamin Mononitrate, Folic Acid, Biotin, Cyanocobalamin (vitamin B12).

MigraActin - Nature's Plus
Two capsules contain: Feverfew (Tanacetum parthenium leaf) standardized 1.2% Parthenolide 700 mg • Pantothenic Acid 50 mg • Ginkgo Biloba leaf (standardized 24% Ginkgo Flavone-Glycosides, 6% Terpene Lactones) 10 mg • Bioperine brand Black Pepper extract (piper nigrum fruit, standardized 95% 1-piperoylpiperidine) 5 mg • Trimethylglycine (TMG) 5 mg.

Migraban Feverfew - Jamieson
Each tablet contains: Dried Feverfew leaf (Tanacetum parthenium L.) (Equivalent to 250 mcg of Parthenolide with a complete active sesquiterpene lactone complex) 125 mg.

Migracare - Enzymatic Therapy
Each capsule contains: Feverfew extract (Tanacetum parthenium) standardized to contain 0.6% Parthenolide 100 mg.

MigraClear - MK Supplements
Each capsule contains: Vitamin B2 (riboflavin) 400 mg • Ginger (zingiber officinale, standardized to contain 5% gingerols) 100 mg • Feverfew (gerardia pedicularia) 100 mg.

MigraDaily - NatureWell Inc.
Each tablet contains: Magnesium (as magnesium oxide) 180 mg • Vitamin B-2 (riboflavin) 200 mg •Vitamin B-1 (thiamin) 15 mg • Feverfew extract (leaf, standardized to 0.8% Parthenolide) 25 mg • White Willow extract (bark, standardized to 15% Salacin) 15 mg. Other Ingredients: Cellulose, Silicon Dioxide, Vegetable Stearine, Titanium Dioxide, Magnesium Stearate.

Migra-Ease - Optimum Nutrition
Feverfew • White Willow.

MigraHealth - Health Assure
Each caplet contains: Riboflavin (vitamin B2) 200 mg • Magnesium (oxide/citrate) 150 mg • Feverfew leaf (Puracol) 50 mg. Other Ingredients: Vegetable Gum, Cellulose, Vegetable Stearine, Silicon Dioxide, Dextrose, Sodium Starch Glycolate, Titanium Dioxide, Caramel, Carmine, Magnesium Stearate.

Migraherb - Wild Rose
Each capsule contains: Feverfew leaf 78 mg • Ginger root 100 mg • White Willow bark 50 mg • Cayenne fruit 50 mg.

Migraine Relief - Hyland's
Each tablet contains: Glonoinum 12X • Belladonna 6X • Gelsemium 6X • Nux Vomica 6X • Iris Versicolor 6X • Sanguinaria Canadensis 6X. Other Ingredients: Lactose N.F.
See Editor's Note No. 1.

Migra-Lieve - Natural Science Corp. of America
Two caplets contain: Feverfew Extract (Tanacetum parthenium, standardized to 0.7% Parthenolide) 100 mg • Magnesium (Citrate/ Oxide 1:1) 300 mg •Riboflavin (Vitamin B2) 400 mg.

Migraplex - PharmAssure
Two tablets contain: Riboflavin (B2) 50mg • Magnesium (as Magnesium stearate) 200 mg • Ginger Root Extract (Zingiber officinale) 150 mg • Feverfew Leaves Extract (Tanacetum parthenium; 0.5% Parthenolide=0.75mg) 150 mg. Other Ingredients: Dicalcium Phosphate, Cellulose.

Migra-Profen - Gaia Herbs
Two capsules contain: Feverfew leaf (tanacetum parthenium; 0.5% (1.8 mg) parthenolide) 360 mg • Chinese Skullcap root (scutellaria baicalensis) 110 mg • Kava Kava (piper methysticum; 55% (38.5 mg) kavalactones) 70 mg • Valerian root (valeriana officinalis) 30 mg • Jamaican Dogwood bark (piscidia eruthrina) 20 mg • Rosemary leaf, supercritical extract (rosmarinus off.) 8 mg • Ginger rhizome, supercritical CO2 extract (zingiber off.) 8 mg. Other Ingredients: Vegetable Glycerin, Vegetable Cellulose (capsule).

MigraSpray - NatureWell Inc.
Each spray contains: Proprietary Homeopathic Blend: Feverfew leaf and flower (tanacetum parenthenium) 3X • Goldenseal rhizome and root (hydrastis) 3X • Dandelion root (taraxicum denleonis) 3X • Polyporus Officinalis (polyporus umbellatus, sclerotium) 3X. Inactive Ingredients: Distilled Water, Glycerin, Ascorbic Acid, Potassium Sorbate, Disodium EDTA.
See Editor's Note No. 1.

Migraway - PhysioLogics
Each capsule contains: Riboflavin (Vitamin B2) 100 mg • Vitamin B6 (as Pyridoxine Hydrochloride) 20 mg • Ginger root (5% Gingerols, 7.5 mg) 150 mg • Feverfew leaf (1.2% Parthenolides, 0.6 mg) 50 mg • White Willow bark (7.5% Salicin, 3.75 mg) 50 mg • Ginkgo leaf (24% Ginkgoflavonglycosides, 9.6 mg; 6% Terpene Lactones, 2.4 mg) 40 mg.

Migra-X - Olympian Labs
Two capsules contain: Feverfew extract 600 mg. In a 300 mg natural base of Ginkgo Biloba extract, Gotu Kola, and White Willow Bark.

Migrelief - PR Osteo
Two caplets contain: Puracol Feverfew (whole herb and extract) 100 mg • Riboflavin 400 mg • Magnesium 360 mg.

BRAND NAMES

Some Brand Name Natural Products - What they Contain

www.NaturalDatabase.com contains MANY more listings than appear here.
Editor's Notes are located on pages 2155-2163.

MigRelief - Quantum
Two caplets contain: Riboflavin 400 mg • Magnesium 300 mg • Puracol brand Feverfew whole leaf 100 mg.

Milagro For Men - Goldshield Elite
Four caplets contain: Zinc (from Zinc Citrate) 30 mg • L-Arginine Hydrochloride 2800 mg • African Yohimbe bark standardized extract (2% yohimbine) (Pausinystalia johimbe) 800 mg • DHEA (Dehydroepiandrosterone) 50 mg • Global Male Herbal Blend 300 mg: Damiana leaf (Turnera aphrodisiaca), Muira Puama bark (Ptychopetalum olacoides), Jamaica Ginger root (Zingiber officinale), Mucuna pruriens seed, Withania somnifera root, Tinospora cordifolia leaf, Licorice root (Glycyrrhiza uralensis), Tribulus terrestris root, Nutmeg fruit (Myristica fragans), Korean Ginseng (Panax ginseng), Siberian Ginseng (Acanthopanax senticosus), Chinese Red Panax Ginseng (Panax ginseng), Manchurian Tienchi Ginseng (Panax notoginseng), Oat Straw (Avena sativa), Stinging Nettle (Urtica dioica). Other Ingredients: Calcium Phosphate, Vegetable Cellulose, Fractionated Vegetable Oil, Silica, and Vita-Lok brand resin glaze.

Milagro For Women - Goldshield Elite
Four caplets contain: Vitamin E (as natural D-alpha tocopherol succinate) 400 IU • Soy Phytoestrogens Concentrate (providing 80 mg isoflavones as daidzin and daidzein, genistin and genistein, glycitin and glycetein) 2670 mg • DHEA (dehydroepiandrosterone) 50 mg • Global Female Herbal Blend 500 mg: Wild Yam (discorea villosa), Red Clover blossom (trifolium pratense), Damiana leaf (turnera aphrodisiaca), Squaw Vine (mitchella repens), Jamaica Ginger root (zingiber officinale), Tribulus Terrestris root, Licorice root (glycyrrhiza uralensis), Fennel seed (foeniculum vulgare), Magnolia bark (magnolia officinalis), Korean Ginseng root (panax ginseng), Siberian Ginseng root (acanthopanax ginseng), Chinese Red Panax Ginseng root (panax ginseng), Manchurian Tienchi Ginseng (panax notoginseng), Black Cohosh root (cimicifuaga racemosa), Oat Straw (avena sativa), Stinging Nettle (urtica dioica). Inactive Ingredients: Dicalcium Phosphate, Vegetable Cellulose, Fractionated Vegetable Oil, Silica, Vita-Lok.

Mild Child - The Herbalist
Catnip leaf • Fennel seed • Chamomile flower • Lemon Balm leaf.

Mild-C capsules - J. R. Carlson Laboratories, Inc.
Each capsule contains: Vitamin C (as calcium ascorbate) 500 mg • Calcium (as calcium ascorbate) 56 mg.

Mild-C Chewable - J. R. Carlson Laboratories, Inc.
Each tablet contains: Vitamin C (as calcium ascorbate) 250 mg • Calcium (as calcium ascorbate) 25 mg.

Mild-C Crystals - J. R. Carlson Laboratories, Inc.
Each 1 tsp serving contains: Vitamin C (as calcium ascorbate) 3600 mg • Calcium (as calcium ascorbate) 400 mg.

Mild-C Timed-Release - J. R. Carlson Laboratories, Inc.
Each tablet contains: Vitamin C (as calcium ascorbate) 1000 mg • Calcium (as calcium ascorbate) 111 mg.

Milk Thistle - PhysioLogics
Each capsule contains: Milk Thistle seed extract (silybum marianum, standardized to contain a minimum of 80% silymarin) 250 mg. Other Ingredients: Maltodextrin, Gelatin, Magnesium Silicate, Vegetable Magnesium Stearate, Silica.

Milk Thistle - BioDynamax
Each tablet contains: Milk Thistle 175 mg.

Milk Thistle - Pharmanex
Each capsule contains: Milk Thistle extract 175 mg. Other Ingredients: Rice Flour, Magnesium Stearate, Silicon Dioxide.

Milk Thistle - Jamieson
Each caplet contains: Milk Thistle 4500 mg.

Milk Thistle - Sundown
Each capsule contains: Milk Thistle seed extract (standardized to 80% silymarin 140 mg) 175 mg. Other Ingredients: Gelatin.

Milk Thistle - Leiner Health Products
Each softgel contains: Milk Thistle extract (Silybum marianum) fruit 150 mg. Other Ingredients: Soybean Oil, Gelatin, Glycerin, Yellow Beeswax, Lecithin, Polysorbate 80, Caramel, Titanium Dioxide, Red 40, Blue 1.

Milk Thistle - GNC
Each capsule contains: Milk Thistle seed extract (Silybum marianum) 200 mg. Other Ingredients: Gelatin, Celulose, Dicalcium Phosphate, Magnesium Stearate.

Milk Thistle (Silymarin) - DaVinci Laboratories
Each capsule contains: Milk Thistle seed extract (silybum marianum, yielding silymarin 240 mg) 300 mg. Other Ingredients: Rice Flour, Vegetable Stearate, Vegetable Cellulose.

Milk Thistle 7000 - Golden Glow Natural Health Products
Each tablet contains: Milk Thistle fruit extract (silybum marianum) 7000 mg: Flavanolignins (as silybin) 84 mg.

Milk Thistle Combination - Swanson Health Products
Each capsule contains: Milk Thistle seed extract (standardized to 80% silymarin) 175 mg • Dandelion root 85 mg • Black Radish root 60 mg • Burdock root 60 mg • Ginger root 60 mg • Parsley root 35 mg.

Milk Thistle Complex - Pro Health
Each capsule contains: Silymarin from Milk Thistle seed extract 112 mg • Choline Bitartrate 50 mg • Inositol 50 mg • Ascorbic Acid (as vitamin C) 100 mg • Vitamin E (as natural D-alpha tocopherol succinate) 25 IU. Other Ingredients: Silica, Cellulose, Magnesium Stearate.

Milk Thistle Extract 250 mg - Vital Nutrients
Each capsule contains: Silybum Marianum seed extract (silybin, silicristin, silidianin, silymarin minimum 80% by HPLC) 250 mg.

Milk Thistle Extract- NSI - NSI - Nutraceutical Sciences Institute
Each capsule contains: Milk Thistle (standardized to 80% silymarin) 300 mg.

Milk Thistle Formula - Quest
Each caplet contains: Milk Thistle seed powder (Silybum marianum) (provided by 60 mg of P.E. 1:8) 480 mg • Butternut bark of root powder (Juglans cineraria) 155 mg • Dandelion root powder (Taraxacum oficinale) 155 mg • Licorice root powder (Glycyrrhiza glabra) 40 mg • Wild Yam root powder (Dioscorea villosa) 10 mg. Other Ingredients: Calcium Phosphate, Microcrystalline Cellulose, Vegetable Stearin, Croscarmellose Sodium, Magnesium Stearate (vegetable source).

Milk Thistle Fruit - Aboca USA, Inc
Two capsules contain: Milk Thistle fruit WPC (whole phytocomplex concentrate, silybum marianum, standardized to contain 11.12% silymarin calculated as silybin, yielding 30 mg per capsule) 540 mg. Other Ingredients: Gelatin.

Milk Thistle Healthy Liver - DreamPharm
Each capsule contains: Milk Thistle seed extract (80% silymarin) 200 mg • Artemisia Vulgaris 100 mg • Corydalis Turtschaninovii rhizome 100 mg • Cyperus Rotundus rhizome 100 mg.

Milk Thistle Mega - Susan Ambrosino's Herb Club, Inc.
Each capsule contains: Milk Thistle full spectrum extract 330 mg • Milk Thistle 80% Silymarin guaranteed potency extract 330 mg.

Milk Thistle Plus - Wild Rose
Each capsule contains: Milk Thistle seed 175 mg • Dandelion root 85 mg • Ginger root 60 mg • Burdock root 60 mg • Parsley root 35 mg • Black Radish root 60 mg.

Milk Thistle Seed - Gaia Herbs
Two capsules contain: Milk Thistle (silybum marianum) 300 mg. Other Ingredients: Lecithin, Vegetable Glycerin, Vegetable Cellulose.

Some Brand Name Natural Products - What they Contain

www.NaturalDatabase.com contains MANY more listings than appear here.
Editor's Notes are located on pages 2155-2163.

BRAND NAMES

Milk Thistle Seed - Gaia Herbs
Milk Thistle seed (standardized for 80% silymarins). Standardized Full Spectrum 150 mg of extract per capsule.

Milk Thistle X - Enzymatic Therapy
Two capsules contain: Milk Thistle fruit extract (silybum marianum, standardized to contain 80% silymarin 240 mg, calculated as silybin) 300 mg • Dandelion root extract (taraxacum officinale, 4:1) 20 mg • Artichoke leaf extract (cynara scolymus, standardized to contain 13-18% caffeylquinic acids calculated as chlorogenic acid) 20 mg • Licorice root extract (glycyrrhiza glabra, standardized to contain 5% glycyrrhizic acid) 20 mg. Other Ingredients: Cellulose, Gelatin, Magnesium Stearate, Titanium Dioxide Color, Silicon Dioxide.

Milk Thistle XTRA - Sundown
Two capsules contain: Milk Thistle seed extract (standardized to 80% silymarin 192 mg) 240 mg • XTRA Premium Blend 560 mg: Dandelion root, Fennel seed, Licorice root. Other Ingredients: Gelatin.

Milk Thistle Yellow Dock - Gaia Herbs
Forty drops contain: Proprietary Blend 50 mg: Milk Thistle seed (silybum marianum), Yellow Dock root (rumex crispus), Burdock root (arctium lappa), Echinacea Supreme: Echinacea Angustifolia root, Echinacea Purpurea root, flower head and seed, Sarsaparilla root (smilax ornata), Oregon Grape root (berberis aquifolium), 45-55% Pure Grain Alcohol USP, Spring Water.

Milk-Based Soy-Free Lactobacillus Acidophilus - Nature's Life
Two tablespoons (1 fl.oz or 29.6 ml) contain: Purified Water • Non-fat Milk powder • viable Lactobacillus Acidophilus Culture.

Milk-Free Chewable Calcium - Nature's Plus
Four chewable tablets contain: Vitamin D (as ergocalciferol) 200 IU • Calcium (as gluconate, aspartate, carbonate) 1000 mg. Other Ingredients: Fructose, Acacia Gum, Microcrystalline Cellulose, Stearic Acid, Silica, Natural Spearmint Flavor.

Milk-Zyme - Atrium Biotechnologies
Each capsule contains: Lactase 30 mg • Rennin 10 mg.

MIN - Agel
Each packet contains: Vitamin A (as retinyl palmitate) 5000 IU • Vitamin C (as ascorbic acid) 60 mg • Vitamin D (as cholecalciferol) 400 IU • Vitamin E (as mixed tocopherols) 30 IU • Thiamin (as thiamin hydrochloride) 1.5 mg • Riboflavin (as riboflavin) 1.7 mg • Vitamin B3 (as niacinamide) 20 mg • Vitamin B6 (as pyridoxine hydrochloride) 2 mg • Folate (as folic acid) 400 mcg • Vitamin B12 (as cyanocobalamin) 6 mcg • Biotin (as biotin) 300 mcg • Pantothenic Acid (as calcium pantothenate) 10 mg • Calcium (as calcium chelate, calcium phosphate) 150 mg • Phosphorus (as calcium phosphate) 150 mg • Iodine (as potassium iodide) 75 mcg • Magnesium (as magnesium chelate) 40 mg • Zinc (as zinc chelate) 1.5 mg • Selenium (as selenium chelate) 14 mcg • Copper (as copper chelate) 0.5 mg • Manganese (as manganese chelate) 1 mg • Chromium (as chromium chelate) 60 mcg • Molybdenum (as molybdenum chelate) 37.5 mcg • Vanadium (as vanadium chelate) 5 mcg • Inositol (as inositol) 100 mg • Apple Cider Vinegar 400 mg. Other Ingredients: Water, Proprietary Sweetening Blend (inulin, xylitol, neotame, acesulfame-K, lactobacillus acidophilus), Fructose, Natural Flavoring, Guar Gum, Grapefruit Seed Extract, Xanthan Gum, Sodium Benzoate.

Min-Chex - Standard Process, Inc.
Each capsule contains: Bovine Orchic Cytosol extract 95 mg • Niacinamide 25 mg • Vitamin B6 5 mg. Other Ingredients: Calcium lactate, Kelp powder, Vacuum Dried Bovine and Ovine Spleen, Magnesium citrate, Manganese lactate, Bone Liver powder, Vacuum Dried Porcine Stomach, Processed Soy Bean powder, Potassium Para-Aminobenzoate, Pyridoxine Hydrochloride, Defatted Wheat Germ, Vacuum Dried Bovine Brain, and Ascorbic acid.
See Editor's Note No. 31.

Mind & Memory - Health Factor
Each capsule contains: Ginkgo Biloba 4:1 extract (standardized to 24% gingkoflavonglycosides) 160 mg • Gotu Kola 4:1 extract (hydrocotyle asaitica) 150 mg • Rosemary 150 mg.

MindPrep - HealthMinded
Four capsules contain: Vitamin A (as acetate) 4000 IU • Vitamin C (ascorbic acid) 250 mg • Vitamin D (as cholecalciferol) 100 IU • Vitamin E (as D-alpha tocopheryl succinate) 30 IU • Thiamin (as thiamin mononitrate) 4 mg • Riboflavin (vitamin B2) 2 mg • Niacin (as nicotinic acid) 26 mg • Vitamin B6 (as pyridoxine HCl) 6 mg • Folic Acid 400 mcg • Vitamin B12 (as cyanocobalamin) 20 mcg • Biotin (as triturate) 300 mcg • Pantothenic Acid (as D-calcium pantothenate) 12 mg • Calcium (as citrate) 50 mg • Iron (as fumarate) 6 mg • Magnesium (as oxide) 100 mg • Zinc (as citrate) 10 mg • Selenium (as amino acid chelate) 20 mcg • Copper (as gluconate) 400 mcg • Manganese (as citrate) 2 mg • Chromium (as polynicotinate) 100 mcg • Molybdenum (as amino acid chelate) 10 mcg • Potassium (as citrate) 50 mg • MindPrep Proprietary Blend 704 mg: DMAE (bitartrate), L-Glutamine, Ginkgo Biloba leaf dried extract, Bacopa aerial parts dried extract, L-Pyroglutamic Acid, Phosphatidylserine (from soy lecithin), Fish Oil (30% EPA/DHA), Choline (bitartrate), Inositol, Pyridoxine Alpha Ketoglutarate, Asian Ginseng root dried extract, N-Acetyl-L-Tyrosine, Bilberry fruit dried extract, GABA, Grape skin dried extract, Grape seed dried extract, Vinpocetine (from periwinkle herb dried extract), Trace Mineral Complex, Huperzine-A (from toothed clubmoss whole plant dried extract), Boron (as citrate), Vanadium (as sodium meta-vanadate), Kelp whole thallus. Other Ingredients: Gelatin, Stearic Acid, Magnesium Stearate.

MindPro - HealthMinded
Four capsules contain: Vitamin A 4000 IU • Vitamin C 250 mg • Vitamin D 100 IU • Vitamin E 30 IU • Thiamin 3 mg • Riboflavin 2 mg • Niacin 25 mg • Vitamin B6 5 mg • Folic Acid 400 mcg • Vitamin B12 20 mcg • Biotin 300 mcg • Pantothenic Acid 12 mg • Calcium 50 mg • Iron 5 mg • Iodine (kelp) 15 mcg • Magnesium 100 mg • Zinc 10 mg • Selenium 20 mcg • Copper 0.4 mg • Manganese 2 mg • Chromium 100 mcg • Molybdenum 10 mcg • Potassium 50 mg • MindPro Proprietary Blend 2000 mg: DMAE Bitartrate, L-Glutamine, Ginkgo Biloba extract, Bacopa Monniera standardized extract, L-Pyroglutamic Acid, Phosphatidylserine, DHA (fish oil concentrate 15%), Choline Bitartrate, Inositol, Pyridoxine Alpha Ketoglutarate, Panax Ginseng standardized extract, N-Acetyl-L-Tyrosine, Trace Mineral Complex or Kelp, Huperzine A, Boron Citrate, Vanadium (as vanadyl sulfate). Other Ingredients: Stearic Acid, Magnesium-Stearate.

Mineral 650 - Pure Encapsulations
Six vegetable capsules contain: Calcium (citrate) 300 mg • Magnesium (citrate) 250 mg • Manganese (aspartate) 10 mg • Zinc (picolinate) 25 mg • Potassium (aspartate) 99 mg • Copper (glycinate) 2 mg • Iron (glycinate) 10 mg • Selenium (selenomethionine) 200 mcg • Chromium (polynicotinate) 200 mcg • Vanadium (aspartate) 100 mcg • Molybdenum (aspartate) 100 mcg • Iodine (potassium iodide) 100 mcg • Boron (glycinate) 2 mg • Vitamin C (as ascorbyl palmitate) 84 mg.

Mineral 650 without iron & copper - Pure Encapsulations
Six vegetable capsules contain: Calcium (citrate) 300 mg • Magnesium (citrate) 250 mg • Manganese (aspartate) 10 mg • Zinc (picolinate) 25 mg • Potassium (aspartate) 99 mg • Selenium (selenomethionine) 200 mcg • Chromium (polynicotinate) 200 mcg • Vanadium (aspartate) 100 mcg • Molybdenum (aspartate) 100 mcg • Iodine (potassium iodide) 100 mcg • Boron (glycinate) 2 mg • Vitamin C (as ascorbyl palmitate) 84 mg.

Mineral Balance - Jarrow Formulas
Six capsules contain: Vitamin A (as palmitate) 5000 IU • Vitamin D (D3, as cholecalciferol) 400 IU • Calcium (as hydroxyapatite) 1000 mg • Iodine (from potassium iodide) 225 mcg • Magnesium (as magnesium oxide) 600 mg • Zinc (as monomethionate) 15 mg • Selenium (as selenomethionine) 100 mcg • Copper (as gluconate)

2 mg • Manganese (as citrate) 1 mg • Chromium (from saccharomyces cerevisiae) 200 mcg • Molbybdenum (trivalent sodium molybdate) 200 mcg • Potassium (as chloride) 99 mg. Other Ingredients: Rice Powder, Magnesium Stearate, Silicon Dioxide, Gelatin.

Mineral Health - Metagenics
Each 1 tsp serving contains: Calcium (as calcium glycinate) 100 mg • Magnesium (as magnesium bis-glycinate) 100 mg • Malic Acid 87 mg • Citric Acid 87 mg • Glycine 72 mg. Other Ingredients: Fructose, Natural Apple Flavor, Methylcellulose.

Mineral Milk Powder - Global Health Trax
Each gram contains: Calcium (from coral) 375 mg • Magnesium (from coral) 7 mg.

Minerogen - ANS - Applied Nutrition Sciences
Each capsule contains: Calcium 200 mg • Magnesium 75 mg • Copper 250 mcg • Chromium 25 mcg • Manganese 100 mcg • Molybdenum 50 mcg • Selenium 25 mcg • Potassium 100 mg • Vanadium 25 mcg • Boron 1 mg • Zinc 7.5 mg.

Minimal and Essential - Vital Nutrients
Each capsule contains: Vitamin A (acetate) 2500 IU • Betatene brand natural Beta Carotene 5000 IU • Vitamin D (D3, as cholecalciferol) 200 IU • Vitamin E (D-alpha tocopheryl succinate) 200 IU • Vitamin C (100% ascorbic acid) 400 mg • Vitamin B1 (thiamine HCl) 25 mg • Vitamin B2 (riboflavin) 25 mg • Vitamin B5 (calcium pantothenate) 25 mg • Vitamin B6 (pyridoxine HCl) 25 mg • Vitamin B12 (hydroxocobalamin) 200 mcg • Inositol Hexaniacinate (no-flush niacin) 25 mg • Folic Acid 400 mcg • Biotin 200 mcg • Zinc (citrate) 10 mg • Manganese (aspartate) 5 mg • Copper (glycinate) 1 mg • Chromium (polynicotinate) 100 mcg • Selenium (selenomethionine) 100 mcg.

Mini-Multi - J. R. Carlson Laboratories, Inc.
Each tablet contains: Vitamin A (as beta carotene) 5000 IU • Vitamin C (as calcium ascorbate) 120 mg • Vitamin D (D3, cholecalciferol) 400 IU • Vitamin E (as D-alpha tocopheryl succinate) 60 IU • Thiamin (vitamin B1, as thiamin mononitrate) 1 mg • Riboflavin (vitamin B2) 1 mg • Niacin (vitamin B3, as niacinamide) 20 mg • Vitamin B6 (as pyridoxine hydrochloride) 2 mg • Folate (folic acid) 400 mcg • Vitamin B12 (cyanocobalamin) 6 mcg • Biotin 30 mcg • Pantothenic Acid (as di-calcium pantothenate) 10 mg • Calcium (as calcium carbonate and calcium ascorbate) 20 mg • Iodine (from kelp & potassium iodide) 75 mcg • Magnesium (as magnesium oxide) 40 mg • Zinc (as zinc citrate) 15 mg • Selenium (from kelp) 25 mcg • Copper (as copper gluconate) 2 mg • Manganese (as manganese gluconate) 2 mg • Chromium (from kelp) 25 mcg.

Minor Pain Comfort - Source Naturals
Two tablets contain: Calcium 50 mg • Vitamin C (as ascorbic acid) 100 mg • Hops extract (yielding 300 mg Humulex brand alpha-acids) 1 g. Other Ingredients: Sorbitol, Microcrystalline Cellulose, Modified Cellulose Gum, Colloidal Silicon Dioxide, Stearic Acid.

Mintacin - Enzymatic Therapy
Each capsule contains: Simethicone 25 mg. Other Ingredients: Peppermint oil extract (Mentha piperita) 0.2 mL.

Min-Tran - Standard Process, Inc.
Four tablets contain: Calcium 120 mg • Iodine 200 mcg • Magnesium 19 mg • Sodium 16 mg. Other Ingredients: Alfalfa, Water.

Minute Maid Premium Heart Wise - The Coca-Cola Company
Water • Concentrated Orange Juice • Plant Sterols • Vitamin E (alpha-tocopheryl acetate) • Vitamin B6 (pyridoxine hydrochloride) • Vitamin B12 • Beta Carotene.

Mioplex Pure Extract - Boland Naturals, Inc.
Each tablet contains: Proprietary Blend: Bee Pollen, Flower Pollen.

Mirac - Berean Development
Two capsules contain: Vitamin C (as ascorbic acid) 500 mg • Calcium (from calcium carbonate) 78 mg • Sodium 2 mg • Bioflavonoid Complex 500 mg • Bromelain 500 mg. Other Ingredients: Cellulose, Stearic Acid, Croscarmellose Sodium, Silicon Dioxide, Magnesium Stearate.

Miracle II Neutralizer - Tedco, Inc.
Some ingredients include: Energized Stabilized Oxygenated Water • Ash of Dedecyl solution • Calcium • Potassium • Magnesium.

Mission Prenatal - Mission Pharmacal
Each tablet contains: Vitamin A 4000 IU • Vitamin C 100 mg • Vitamin D (as Vitamin D3) 400 IU • Vitamin B1 4.7 mg • Vitamin B2 2 mg • Vitamin B3 10 mg • Vitamin B6 2.8 mg • Folate 0.4 mg • Vitamin B12 2 mcg • Vitamin B5 1 mg • Calcium 50 mg • Iron 29.5 mg. Other Ingredients: Sugar, Microcrystalline Cellulose, Color, Povidone, Croscarmellose Sodium, Magnesium Stearate, FD & C Red 40 Lake, Food Glaze, Carnauba Wax, Cholecalciferol, White Beeswax, Sodium Benzoate, Cyanocobalamin.

Mission Prenatal FA - Mission Pharmacal
Each tablet contains: Vitamin A 4000 IU • Vitamin C 100 mg • Vitamin D (as Vitamin D3) 400 IU • Vitamin B1 4.7 mg • Vitamin B2 2 mg • Vitamin B3 10 mg • Vitamin B6 10 mg • Folate 0.8 mg • Vitamin B12 2 mcg • Vitamin B5 1 mg • Calcium 50 mg • Iron 29.5 mg • Zinc 15 mg. Other Ingredients: Sugar, Microsrystalline Cellulose, Color, Magnesium Stearate, Croscarmellose Sodium, Povidone, Food Glaze, Blue 1 Lake, Carnauba Wax, Sodium Benzoate, White Beeswax, Cholecalciferol, Cyanocobalamin.

Mission Prenatal HP - Mission Pharmacal
Each tablet contains: Vitamin A 4000 IU • Vitamin C 100 mg • Vitamin D (Vitamin D3; Cholecalciferol) 400 IU • Vitamin B1 4 mg • Vitamin B2 2 mg • Vitamin B3 10 mg • Vitamin B6 20 mg • Folate 0.8 mg • Vitamin B12 (Cyanocobalamin) 2 mcg • Vitamin B5 1 mg • Calcium 50 mg • Iron 29.5 mg. Other Ingredients: Sugar, Microcrystalline Cellulose, Color, Magnesium Stearate, Croscarmellose Sodium, Povidone, FD & C Yellow 5 Lake, Food Glaze, FD & C Blue 1 Lake, Sodium Benzoate, Carnauba Wax, FD & C Yellow 6 Lake, White Beeswax.

MI-T-Cell - Progressive Labs
Each capsule contains: Vitamin C (ascorbyl palmitate) 50 mg • Vitamin E Succinate 30 mg • Thiamin HCl (Vitamin B1) 5 mg • Riboflavin (Vitamin B2) 5 mg • Magnesium (as magnesium malate) 50 mg • L-Glutathione 50 mg • N-Acetyl-Carnitine 30 mg • N-Acetyl Cysteine 50 mg • CoEnzyme Q10 10 mg • Lipoic Acid 50 mg • L-Isoleucine 225 mcg • Red Grape skin (Vitis vinifera) 50 mg.

Mitochondria Ignite with NT Factor - Pro Health
Two tablets contain: Calcium (as phosphate, sulfate, pyruvate) 160 mg • Phosphorus (as calcium phosphate) 50 mg • Magnesium (as sulfate) 50 mg • Carnitine Fumarate 140 mg • Creatine Monohydrate 100 mg • Pantethine 50 mg • NT Factor proprietary blend 1350 mg: Phosphoglycolipids - includes polyunsaturated Phosphatidylcholine, Glycolipids and other Polyunsaturated Phosphatidyl nutrients. Other Ingredients: Microcrystalline Cellulose, Croscarmellose Sodium, Methyl Cellulose, Magnesium Stearate, Silica.

Mitochondrial Resuscitate - Metagenics
Each tablet contains: Vitamin C (as ascorbyl palmitate) 50 mg • Vitamin E (as D-alpha tocopheryl succinate) 36 IU • Thiamin (as thiamin mononitrate) 5 mg • Riboflavin 5 mg • Magnesium (as magnesium malate) 50 mg • Creatine (as creatine monohydrate) 100 mg • N-Acetylcysteine 50 mg • L-Glutathione 50 mg • Alpha-Lipoic Acid 50 mg • Acetyl-L-Carnitine Hydrochloride 30 mg • Coenzyme Q10 5 mg • Red Grape Skin extract (vitis vinifera) 5 mg.

Mixed Greens - Health Smart Vitamins
Each capsule contains: Broccoli aerial parts (2% glucosinolates, 2 mg) 100 mg • Tea green, leaf (50% polyphenols) 100 mg • Tomato fruit (1% lycopene) 50 mg • Calendula flower (5% lutein) 38 mg • Garlic bulb (10,000 mcg allicin/g) 25 mg • Ginger root (5% gingerols) 25 mg • Milk Thistle seed (80% silymarin) 25 mg • Red Grape (Vitis vinifera skin, 30% anthocyanidins) 25 mg • Soy Isoflavones bean (5% isoflavones) 25 mg • Turmeric root (95% curcumin) 25 mg.

Mixed Vegetable Phytonutrients - Leiner Health Products
Two tablets contain: Lutein 3000 mcg • Lycopene 1000 mcg • Sulforaphane 33 mcg • Zeaxanthin 150 mcg. Other Ingredients: Calcium Carbonate, Broccoli, Carrot, Spinach, Tomato, Cellulose, Maltodextrin, Gelatin, Lutein/Lycopene Suspension, Sucrose, Starch, Hydroxypropyl Methylcellulose, Titanium Dioxide, Hydroxypropyl Cellulose, Crospovidone, Silicon Dioxide, Pharmaceutical Glaze, Polyethylene Glycol 3350, Ascorbyl Palmitate, Tocopherols, Magnesium Stearate, Polysorbate 80, Yellow 6 Lake, Blue 2 Lake.

Mixed Vegetables - Nature's Plus
Three tablets contain: Broccoli floret (Brassica oleracea) naturally rich in sulorophane & indole-3-carbinol equivalent to 10000 mg fresh broccoli 1000 mg • Spinach leaf (Spinacia oleracea) naturally rich in monoterpenes equivalent to 1000 mg fresh Spinach 100 mg • Carrot root (Daucus carota) naturally rich in carotenoids, coumarins & Polyacetylenes equivalent to 1000 mg fresh Carrot 100 mg • Cabbage leaf (Brassica chinensis) naturally rich in Sterols, Phenolic Acids & Indoles equivalent to 1000 mg. fresh Cabbage 100 mg.

MNS Gold - Advocare International
Two white packets contain: Vitamin A (as palmitate) 2500 IU • Vitamin A (as beta-carotene) 12,500 IU • Vitamin C (as ascorbic acid/ mineral ascorbates) 600 mg • Vitamin D (as cholecalciferol) 400 IU • Vitamin E (as D-alpha tocopheryl succinate) 150 IU • Thiamine 9 mg • Riboflavin 10.2 mg • Niacin (as niacinamide/niacin) 120 mg • Vitamin B6 (as pyridoxine HCl) 12 mg • Folic Acid 800 mcg • Vitamin B12 (as cyanocobalamin) 36 mcg • Biotin 300 mcg • Pantothenic Acid 40 mg • Calcium (as amino acid chelate) 150 mg • Phosphorus (as amino acid chelate) 100 mg • Iodine (from kelp) 150 mcg • Magnesium (as amino acid chelate/phosphate) 200 mg • Zinc (as zinc monomethionine) 15 mg • Selenium (L-selenomethionine) 80 mcg • Copper (as amino acid chelate) 2 mg • Manganese (as amino acid chelate) 4 mg • Chromium (as chromium polynicotinate) 100 mcg • Molybdenum (as amino acid chelate) 50 mcg • Potassium (as amino acid chelate/phosphate) 100 mg • Inositol 6 mg • Choline (as bitartrate) 60 mg • Boron (as amino acid chelate) 300 mcg • Vanadium (as bis-gylcinate-oxovanadium) 50 mcg • Silicon (as amino acid chelate) 500 mcg • Coenzyme Q-10 150 mcg • Octacosanol 2 mg • Ribonucleic Acid (RNA) 2 mg • Odorless Garlic bulb powder (allium sativum) 50 mg • L-Glutathione 5 mg • Gamma-Oryzanol 5 mg • Citrus Flavonoids 100 mg • Grape Seed extract (vitis vinifera) 5 mg • Milk Thistle fruit extract (silybum marianum) 5 mg • Ginkgo leaf extract (ginkgo biloba) 10 mg • Eicosapentaenoic Acid (from marine lipids) 180 mg • Docosahexaenoic Acid (from marine lipids) 120 mg • D-Limonene powder 300 mg • Grapefruit juice powder 200 mg • 5-Hydroxytryptophan (griffonia simplicifolia seed) 25 mg.
Two gold packets contain: Vitamin A (as beta-carotene) 2000 IU • Vitamin C (as ascorbic acid/mineral ascorbates) 600 mg • Niacin (as niacinamide/niacin) 40 mg • Vitamin B6 (as pyridoxine HCl) 4 mg • Iodine (from kelp) 50 mcg • Magnesium (as amino acid chelate/ phosphate) 50 mg • Zinc (as zinc monomethionine) 2 mg • Chromium (as chromium polynicotinate) 100 mcg • Potassium (as amino acid chelate/phosphate) 100 mg • Vanadium (as bis-gylcinate-oxovanadium) 200 mcg • Garcinia fruit extract (garcinia cambogia) 2000 mg • Tulsi leaf extract (ocimum sanctum) 50 mg • Taurine 50 mg • Beta-Sitosterol 25 mg • L-Carnitine 25 mg • Gymnema leaf extract (gymnema sylvestre) 10 mg • Oolong Tea leaf extract (camellia sinensis) 200 mg • Guarana seed extract (paullinia cupana) 550 mg • Eleuthero root extract (eleutherococcus senticosus) 50 mg • Green Tea leaf extract (camellia sinensis) 20 mg • Green Orange pericarp extract (citrus aurantium) 1000 mg. Other Ingredients: Dicalcium Phosphate, Silicon Dioxide, Cellulose, Stearic Acid, Magnesium Stearate, Peppermint Extract, Vanillin, Beet Root Powder (for color), Gelatin, Glycerin, Water.
See Editor's Note No. 40.

MNS Platinum - Advocare International
Two white packets contain: Vitamin A (as palmitate) 2500 IU • Vitamin A (as beta-carotene) 12,500 IU • Vitamin C (as ascorbic acid/ mineral ascorbates) 600 mg • Vitamin D (as cholecalciferol) 400 IU • Vitamin E (as D-alpha tocopheryl succinate) 150 IU • Thiamine 9 mg • Riboflavin 10.2 mg • Niacin (as niacinamide/niacin) 120 mg • Vitamin B6 (as pyridoxine HCl) 12 mg • Folic Acid 800 mcg • Vitamin B12 (as cyanocobalamin) 36 mcg • Biotin 300 mcg • Pantothenic Acid 40 mg • Calcium (as amino acid chelate) 150 mg • Phosphorus (as amino acid chelate) 100 mg • Iodine (from kelp) 150 mcg • Magnesium (as amino acid chelate) 200 mg • Zinc (as zinc monomethionine) 15 mg • Selenium (L-selenomethionine) 80 mcg • Copper (as amino acid chelate) 2 mg • Manganese (as amino acid chelate) 4 mg • Chromium (as chromium polynicotinate) 100 mcg • Molybdenum (as amino acid chelate) 50 mcg • Potassium (as amino acid chelate) 100 mg • Inositol 6 mg • Choline (as bitartrate) 60 mg • Boron (as amino acid chelate) 300 mcg • Vanadium (as bis-gylcinate-oxovanadium) 50 mcg • Silicon (as amino acid chelate) 500 mcg • Coenzyme Q-10 150 mcg • Octacosanol 2 mg • Ribonucleic Acid (RNA) 2 mg • Odorless Garlic powder (allium sativum bulb) 50 mg • L-Glutathione 5 mg • Gamma-Oryzanol 5 mg • Citrus Flavonoids 100 mg • Grape Seed extract (vitis vinifera) 5 mg • Milk Thistle fruit extract (silybum marianum) 5 mg • Ginkgo leaf extract (ginkgo biloba) 10 mg • Eicosapentaenoic Acid (from marine lipids) 180 mg • Docosahexaenoic Acid (from marine lipids) 120 mg.
Two platinum packets contain: Vitamin C (as ascorbic acid/mineral ascorbates) 600 mg • Niacin (as niacinamide/niacin) 10 mg • Vitamin B6 (as pyridoxine HCl) 4 mg • Iodine (from kelp) 50 mcg • Zinc (as zinc monomethionine) 2 mg • Chromium (as chromium polynicotinate) 100 mcg • Vanadium (as bis-gylcinate-oxovanadium) 200 mcg • Garcinia fruit extract (garcinia cambogia) 2000 mg • Tulsi leaf extract (ocimum sanctum) 50 mg • Taurine 50 mg • Beta-Sitosterol 25 mg • L-Carnitine (as tartrate) 25 mg • Gymnema leaf extract (gymnema sylvestre) 10 mg • Oolong Tea leaf extract (camellia sinensis) 800 mg • Kola Nut extract (cola acuminata) 500 mg • Guarana seed extract (paullinia cupana) 150 mg • Coleus Forskohlii root extract 30 mg • Resveratrol (from polygonum cuspidatum) 25 mg • Eleuthero root extract (eleutherococcus senticosus) 50 mg • White Willow bark extract (salix alba) 60 mg • L-Tyrosine 800 mg • L-Glutamine 1600 mg. Other Ingredients: Dicalcium Phosphate, Silicon Dioxide, Cellulose, Stearic Acid, Magnesium Stearate, Peppermint Extract, Vanillin, Beet Root Powder (for color), Gelatin, Glycerin, Water.

MNS Yellow - Advocare International
Two white packets contain: Vitamin A (as palmitate) 2500 IU • Vitamin A (as beta-carotene) 12,500 IU • Vitamin C (as ascorbic acid/ mineral ascorbates) 600 mg • Vitamin D (as cholecalciferol) 400 IU • Vitamin E (as D-alpha tocopheryl succinate) 150 IU • Thiamine 9 mg • Riboflavin 10.2 mg • Niacin (as niacinamide/niacin) 120 mg • Vitamin B6 (as pyridoxine HCl) 12 mg • Folic Acid 800 mcg • Vitamin B12 (as cyanocobalamin) 36 mcg • Biotin 300 mcg • Pantothenic Acid 40 mg • Calcium (as amino acid chelate) 150 mg • Phosphorus (as amino acid chelate) 100 mg • Iodine (from kelp) 150 mcg • Magnesium (as amino acid chelate/phosphate) 200 mg • Zinc (as zinc monomethionine) 15 mg • Selenium (selenomethionine) 80 mcg • Copper (as amino acid chelate) 2 mg • Manganese (as amino acid chelate) 4 mg • Chromium (as chromium polynicotinate) 100 mcg • Molybdenum (as amino acid chelate) 50 mcg • Potassium (as amino acid chelate/phosphate) 100 mg • Inositol 6 mg • Choline (as bitartrate) 60 mg • Boron (as amino acid chelate) 300 mcg • Vanadium (as bis-gylcinate-oxovanadium) 50 mcg • Silicon (as amino acid chelate) 500 mcg • Coenzyme Q-10 150 mcg • Octacosanol 2 mg • Ribonucleic Acid (RNA) 2 mg • Odorless Garlic bulb powder (allium sativum) 50 mg • L-Glutathione 5 mg • Gamma-Oryzanol 5 mg • Citrus Flavonoids 100 mg • Grape Seed extract (vitis vinifera) 5 mg • Milk Thistle fruit extract (silybum marianum) 5 mg • Ginkgo leaf extract (ginkgo biloba) 10 mg • Eicosapentaenoic Acid (from marine lipids) 180 mg • Docosahexaenoic Acid (from marine lipids) 120 mg.
Two yellow packets contain: Vitamin A (as beta-carotene) 2000 IU • Vitamin C (as ascorbic acid/mineral ascorbates) 600 mg • Niacin (as niacinamide/niacin) 40 mg • Vitamin B6 (as pyridoxine HCl) 4 mg • Iodine (from kelp) 50 mcg • Magnesium (as amino acid chelate/ phosphate) 100 mg • Zinc (as zinc monomethionine) 2 mg • Chromium (as chromium polynicotinate) 100 mcg • Potassium (as amino acid chelate/phosphate) 200 mg • Vanadium (as bis-gylcinate-

oxovanadium) 200 mcg • Garcinia fruit extract (garcinia cambogia) 2000 mg • Tulsi leaf extract (ocimum sanctum) 50 mg • Taurine 50 mg • Beta-Sitosterol 25 mg • L-Carnitine 25 mg • Gymnema leaf extract (gymnema sylvestre) 10 mg • Oolong Tea leaf extract (camellia sinensis) 200 mg • Guarana seed extract (paullinia cupana) 550 mg • Eleuthero root extract (eleutherococcus senticosus) 50 mg • Green Tea leaf extract (camellia sinensis) 20 mg • Cayenne fruit extract (capsicum annuum) 32 mg • Proprietary Blend ThermoGen-HC 224 mg: Gotu Kola (whole plant), Cassia bark, Peppermint leaf, Peppermint stem, Lemon Verbena leaf, Lemon Verbena flower, Chamomile leaf, Chamomile flower, Ginger root, Chinese Licorice root, Sweet Orange peel, Chicory root. Other Ingredients: Dicalcium Phosphate, Silicon Dioxide, Cellulose, Stearic Acid, Peppermint Extract, Vanillin, Gelatin, Glycerin, Water.

Modrenal GF - PhysioLogics
Three caplets contain: Vitamin B1 (Thiamine HCl) 40 mg • Vitamin B2 (Riboflavin) 30 mg • Vitamin B5 (Calcium Pantothenate) 150 mg • Vitamin B6 (pyridoxine HCl) 25 mg • Vitamin B12 (cyanocobalamin) 30 mcg • Vitamin C (Ascorbic Acid) 200 mg • Vitamin E (D-Alpha Tocopherol) 100 IU • Vitamin B3 (Niacinamide) 50 mg • Iron (Ferrous Succinate) 10 mg • Magnesium (Citrate) 200 mg • Calcium (Citrate) 250 mg • Folic Acid 100 mcg • Biotin 20 mcg • Siberian Ginseng (Eleutherococcus senticosus; GPH: 0.3% eleutherosides b & e) 75 mg • Lemon Bioflavonoids 50 mg • Passion Flower 50 mg • Chamomile 50 mg • Skullcap 50 mg • Choline 40 mg • PABA 10 mg • Inositol 10 mg • Chromium GTF (Nicotinate) 250 mcg.

ModuCare Grape Chewabe Tablets - Purity Life International
Each tablet contains: Sterols (from pinus martima, pinus pinaster) 20 mg • Sterolins (from pinus martima, pinus pinaster) 0.2 mg. Other Ingredients: Zylitol (natural birch sweetener), Natural Grape Flavor, Citric Acid, Malic Acid, Inulin, Silicon Dioxide, Magnesium Stearate.

Moducare Sterinol - Essential Phytosterolins, Inc.
Each capsule contains: Plant Sterols 20 mg • Plant Sterolins 200 mcg. Other Ingredients: White Rice Flour, Magnesium Silicate, Gel Cap.

ModuCare Vegetarian Capsules - Purity Life International
Each capsule contains: Sterols (from pinus martima, pinus pinaster) 20 mg • Sterolins (from pinus martima, pinus pinaster) 0.2 mg. Other Ingredients: Rice Flour, Magnesium Silicate, Vegetable Cellulose, Water, Vegetable Glycerin, Silicon.

ModuChol - Purity Life International
Each capsule contains: Phytosterols Esters (from vegetable oil) 650 mg.

ModuProst - Purity Life International
Each capsule contains: Harzol (providing sterols 10 mg, sterolins 0.1 mg) 112 mg • Saw Palmetto extract 150 mg • Nettles extract (1:10) 100 mg • Green Tea 50 mg • Lycopene 0.25 mg.

Moisture Restore Day Protective Lotion (combination to oily) - Nu Skin Enterprises
Water • Octyldodecyl Neopentanoate • Glycerin • Cyclomethicone • Clyceryl Stearate • PEG-100 Stearate • Cetyl Alcohol • Algae extract • Tocopheryl Acetate • Calendula Officinalis flower extract • Anthemis Nobilis flower extract • Tilia Cordata flower extract • Centaurea Cyanus flower extract • Hypericum Perforatum extract • Allantoin • Hydrogenated Lecithin • Dimethicone • Butylene Glycol • Polyacrylamide • Laureth-7 • Disodium EDTA • Myristyl Myristate • C13-14 Isoparrifin • Phenoxyethanol • Chlorphenesin • Propylparaben • Methylparaben • Benzoic Acid • Fragrance.

Moisture Restore Day Protective Lotion (normal to dry) - Nu Skin Enterprises
Water • Octyldodecyl Neopentanoate • Glycerin • Cyclomethicone • Cetyl Alcohol • Glyceryl Stearate • PEG-75 Stearate • Algae extract • Butyrosperum Parkii extract (shea butter) • Oenothera Biennis oil (evening primrose oil) • Tocopheryl Acetate • Calendula Officinalis flower extract • Anthemis Nobilis flower extract • Tilia Cordata flower extract • Centaurea Cyanus flower extract • Chamomilla Recutita flower extract (matricaria) • Hypericum Perforatum extract • Limnanthes Alba seed oil • Allantoin • Hydrogenated Lecithin • Dimethicone • Butylene Glycol • Polyacrylamide • Laureth-7 • Ceteth-20 • Steareth-20 • Tetrasodium EDTA • Myristyl Myristate • C13-14 Isoparrifin • Phenoxyethanol • Chlorphenesin • Propylparaben • Methylparaben • Benzoic Acid • Fragrance.

Moisture Restore Intense Moisturizer - Nu Skin Enterprises
Aqua • Aloe Barbadensis • C12-15 Alkyl Benzoate • Glyceryl Stearate • Milk Lipids (lactis lipida) • Cetearyl Alcohol • Butyrospermum Parkii • Butylene Glycol • Caprylic/Capric Triglycerides • Urea • Sodium Behenoyl Lactylate • Glycerin • Pistacia Vera • Helianthus Annuus • Methyl Gluceth-10 • Sodium PCA • Glycine • Alanine • Proline • Serine • Threonine • Lysine • Arginine • Glutamic Acid • Sorbitol • Betaine • Dimethicone • Tocopheryl Acetate • Tocopherol • Parfum • Chlorphenesin • Methylparaben • Disodium EDTA • Propylparaben.

Moisture Revival Lotion - Abra Therapeutics
Purified Water • Aloe Vera • Coconut oil • Olive oil • Kukui oil • Jojoba oil • Stearic Acid • Glycerin • Glyceral Stearate • Cetyl Alcohol • St. John's Wort extract • Wild Yam extract • Lavender oil • Boswellia oil • Sodium PCA • TEA • Allantoin • Lecithin • Methylparaben • Propylparaben.

Moisture Therapy Bath - Abra Therapeutics
Sodium Borate • Sodium Sulfate • Sodium Chloride • Sodium Sesquicarbonate • Olive Oil • Essential Oils Blend: Rose, Palmarosa, Olibanum, Chamomile, Peru Balsam, Ylang Ylang • Herbal Extracts Blend: Calendula flower, Kukui nut oil, Aloe Vera gel • Chromium Oxide • Trace Mineral Salts.

Moistur-Eyes - J. R. Carlson Laboratories, Inc.
Three softgels contain: Vitamin A (as beta carotene) 5000 IU • Vitamin C (as ascorbic acid) 240 mg • Vitamin D (D3, cholecalciferol) 200 IU • Vitamin E (as D-alpha tocopherol) 60 IU • Vitamin B6 (as pyridoxine hydrochloride) 20 mg • Biotin 300 mcg • Zinc (as zinc gluconate) 7 mg • Salmon oil 1000 mg • GLA (gamma linolenic acid) 220 mg • DHA (docosahexaenoic acid) 120 mg • EPA (eicosapentaenoic acid) 180 mg • Borage oil 1000 mg.

Moisturizing Cleansing Creme - Aspen Group, Inc.
Each gram contains: Tocopheryl Acetate 1% • Panthenol 1% • Water • Mineral Oil • Steareth-2 • PPG-15 • Stearyl Ether • Tocopheryl Acetate • Octyl Palmitate • Isoceteth-20 • Cetearyl Octanoate • Carbomer • Dimethicone • Ammonium Hydroxide • Propylene Glycol • Diazolidinyl Urea • Methylparaben • Propylparaben.

MoloCure - Molo-Cure Research, Inc.
Each capsule contains: Proprietary blend 500 mg: Stabilized Aloe Mucilaginous Polysaccharide molecules • L-Glutamine powder.

Moly-B - J. R. Carlson Laboratories, Inc.
Each tablet contains: Molybdenum (as molybdenum glycinate chelate) 500 mcg.

Molymin - Progressive Labs
Each capsule contains: Molybdenum (amino acid chelate) 50 mcg • Pea powder 150 mg • Lentil powder 75 mg • Buckwheat 75 mg • Millet flour 75 mg.

MonaVie - Monarch
Reconstituted Puree from Proprietary Blend: Acai fruit, White Grape, Nashi Pear, Acerola, Pear, Aronia, Purple Grape, Cranberry, Passion fruit, Banana, Apricot, Prune, Kiwi, Blueberry, Bilberry, Camu Camu, Wolfberry, Pomegranate, Lychee fruit. Other Ingredients: Citric Acid, Natural Flavor, Sodium Benzoate.

MonaVie Active - Monarch
Reconstituted Puree from Proprietary Blend: Acai fruit, White Grape, Nashi Pear, Acerola, Pear, Aronia, Purple Grape, Cranberry, Passion fruit, Banana, Apricot, Prune, Kiwi, Blueberry, Bilberry, Camu Camu, Wolfberry, Pomegranate, Lychee fruit • Glucosamine • Celadrin brand CMO. Other Ingredients: Citric Acid, Natural Flavor, Sodium Benzoate.

Some Brand Name Natural Products - What they Contain

www.NaturalDatabase.com contains MANY more listings than appear here.
Editor's Notes are located on pages 2155-2163.

BRAND NAMES

Monobrex - Selmedica Healthcare
Each capsule contains: Proprietary Blend 500 mg: Astragalus root, Cleavers, Dandelion root, Echinacea Angustifolia, Echinacea Purpurea, Eucalyptus leaf, Feverfew, Garlic, Gentain, Ginkgo Biloba, Goldenseal root, Hops, Maitake Mushroom, Milk Thistle, Oats, Oregon Grape root, Pau D'Arco, Peppermint leaf, Poke root, White Willow bark, Yellow Dock, Citrus Bioflavonoids, Vitamin B12.

Monolaurin (Coconut Extract) - Olympia Nutrition
Coconut extract 300 mg.

Monolaurin (Lauric Acid) 300 mg - Ecological Formulas
Each capsule contains: Lauric Acid from Coconut oil 300 mg. Base: Inosine 7.5 mg, Calcium (phosphate) 106 mg. Other Ingredients: Dicalcium Phosphate, Cellulose Powder, Silicon Dioxide.

Monthly Comfort - Source Naturals
Six tablets contain: Vitamin A (Palmitate) 6000 IU • Vitamin C (Ascorbic Acid and Zinc Ascorbate) 600 mg • Vitamin E (D-Alpha Tocopheryl) (Natural) 150 IU • Vitamin B1 (Thiamin) 20 mg • Vitamin B2 (Riboflavin) 20 mg • Niacinamide 100 mg • Vitamin B5 (Calcium D-Pantothenate) 30 mg • Vitamin B6 (Pyridoxine HCl) 150 mg • Vitamin B12 (Cyanocobalamin) 30 mcg • Folic Acid 800 mcg • Calcium (Carbonate, Citrate) 200 mg • Chromium (ChromeMate GTF Yeast-Free Polynicotinate) 300 mcg • Magnesium (Oxide, Citrate) 450 mg • Zinc (Ascorbate) 20 mg • Taurine 500 mg • N-Acetyl Cysteine 300 mg • DLPA (DL-Phenylalanine) 250 mg • Choline (Bitartrate) 100 mg • Inositol 100 mg • Herbal Formula 1350 mg • Chasteberry 400 mgl • Dong Quai root 200 mg • Black Cohosh root 175 mg • Blue Cohosh root 175 mg • Silymarin (Milk Thistle seed extract) 100 mg • Cyperus rhizome 100 mg • Dong Quai root extract 100 mg • Dandelion root extract 100 mg.

Montmorency CherryFlex - Flavonoid Sciences
Each softgel contains: Cherry Flex brand Tart Cherries: Anthocyanins 100 mg, Flavones 20 mg. Other Ingredients: Olive Oil, Gelatin, Glycerin, Purified Water, Beeswax.

Mood & Fatigue Formula - HERBALmax
Mandarin Orange • Chinese Angelica root • White Peony root • Wild Tumeric root • Ginseng • Tuber Ophiopogonis Japonici.

Mood Actives - VitaStore
Four tablets contain: St. John's Wort (0.3% Hypericin) 450 mg • Kava Kava 325 mg • Ginseng 200 mg • Valerian 200 mg • Licorice Root 150 mg • L-Methionine 100 mg • L-Phenylalanine 200 mg • L-Tyrosine 500 mg • L-Taurine 500 mg • Folic Acid 0.4 mg • Vitamin C 300 mg • Vitamin B6 (Pyridoxine) 4 mg • Vitamin B12 12 mcg • Zinc 50 mg.

Mood Aid Formula - Nature's Way
Each capsule contains: Korean Ginseng dried extract 33.3 mg • L-5 Hydroxytryptophan (Griffonia bean extract) 3.33 mg • Niacin (Vitamin B3) 3.33 mg • Riboflavin (Vitamin B2) 284 mcg • Scullcap herb 100 mg • St. John's Wort dried extract (0.3% Dianthrones measures as Hypercin) 300 mg • Thiamine (Vitamin B1) 350 mcg • Vitamin B12 (Cyanocobalamin) 1 mcg • Vitamin B6 (Pyridoxine HCl) 330 mcg. Other Ingredients: Gelatin, Magnesium Stearate, Millet.

Mood Balance - Source Naturals
Each three tablets contain: Vitamin C (as zinc ascorbate) 54 mg • Thiamin (vitamin B1) 22 mg • Riboflavin (vitamin B2) 25 mg • Niacinamide 50 mg • Vitamin B6 (as pyridoxine HCl) 50 mg • Folate (as folic acid) 400 mcg • Vitamin B12 (as cyanocobalamin) 30 mcg • Biotin 300 mcg • Pantothenic Acid (as calcium d-pantothenate) 25 mg • Magnesium (as magnesium oxide & taurinate) 194 mg • Zinc (zinc ascorbate) 10 mg • Manganese (as manganese citrate) 3 mg • St. John's Wort (0.3%, yielding 2.7 mg hypericin) 900 mg • L-Tyrosine 200 mg • Lemon Balm leaf 100 mg • Valerian root extract 100 mg • L-Phenylalanine 100 mg • Taurine (as magnesium taurinate) 87 mg • Kava root extract (30%, yielding 26 mg kavalactones) 85 mg • DMAE (as bitartrate) 60 mg • N-Acetyl L-Tyrosine 50 mg.

Mood Food - Xymogen
Each capsule contains: Vitamin B6 (as pyridoxine 5-phosphate) 4 mg • GABA 250 mg • Magnesium (glycinate and taurate) 50 mg • Folate (as folic acid and calcium folinate) 800 mcg • Vitamin B12 (as methylcobalamin) 1000 mcg • 5-HTP 50 mg.

Mood Mender - Celestial Seasonings
Two capsules contain: Vitamin B6 (as pyridoxine HCL) 6 mg • Folic Acid 200 mcg • Vitamin B12 (as cyanocobalamin) 12 mcg • Selenium (as methionine chelate) 140 mcg • Chromium (as polynicotinate) 120 mcg • Proprietary Blend 1930 mg: St. John's Wort (leaf,stem,flower), St. John's Wort (standardized extract), Siberian Ginseng (root), Siberian Ginseng (standardized extract). Other Ingredients: May contain Dicalcium Phosphate, Gelatin, Rice Flour, Stearic Acid, Magnesium Stearate, Silicon Dioxide.

Mood Optimizer - Alacer
Each tablet contains: St. John's Wort extract (0.3% hypericum) 300 mg • Kava Kava extract (30%) 100 mg • Vitamin C (as calcium magnesium ascorbate) 60 mg • Vitamin B6 (pyridoxine HCl) 10 mg • Melatonin 25 mcg • Magnesium Citrate 20 mg • Vitamin B3 (magnesium niacinate) 100 mg • Zinc Ascorbate 100 mcg • Ginkgo Biloba 24:6 extract 10 mg • Flower Pollen extract 10 mg • Ginseng root powder 10 mg • L-Tyrosine 60 mg • L-Phenylalanine 30 mg • DL-Phenylalanine 30 mg • Folic Acid 50 mcg • Valerian root 0.8 extract 5 mg • 5-hydroxytryptophan 10 mg.
See Editor's Note No. 26.

Mood Support with St. John's Wort - Natrol, Inc.
One capsule contains: Guaranteed Potency St. John's Wort supplying 0.3% Hypericin 300 mg • Ginseng supplying 8% Ginsenosides 100 mg • L-Tyrosine 50 mg • Lemon Balm 25 mg • DMAE (Di Methyl Amino Ethanol Bitartrate) 25 mg • Vitamin E (d-Alpha Tocopheryl Acetate) 30 IU • Folic Acid 400 mcg • Vitamin B12 (Cyanocobalamin) 50 mcg • Selenium (l-Selenomethionine) 25 mcg. Other Ingredients: Silica, Magnesium Stearate, Gelatin.

Mood Sync - Pain & Stress Center
Each capsule contains: Vitamin C 6 mg • Vitamin B6 (pyridoxine HCl) 5 mg • L-Tyrosine 200 mg • Gamma Amino Butyric Acid (GABA) 125 mg • L-Taurine 110 mg • L-Glutamine 75 mg • 5-Hydroxytryptophan (5-HTP) 25 mg. Other Ingredients: Gelatin.

MoodPlex - PharmAssure
Three capsules contain: St. John's Wort with Flowers Extract (Hypericum perforatum; 0.3% Hypericin) 900 mg • Griffonia Simplicifolia Seed Extract (20% 5-Hydroxy-Tryptopan) 100 mg • D,L-Phenylalanine 100 mg. Other Ingredients: Cellulose, Gelatin, Calcium Carbonate.

MoodPrep - HealthMinded
Three capsules contain: Vitamin C (ascorbic acid) 15 mg • Thiamine (as thiamin HCl) 60 mg • Riboflavin (vitamin B2) 45 mg • Niacin (as nicotinic acid) 30 mg • Vitamin B6 (as pyridoxine HCl) 60 mg • Folic Acid 390 mcg • Vitamin B12 (as cyanocobalamin) 150 mcg • Calcium (as citrate) 15 mg • MoodPrep Proprietary blend 1111 mg: St. John's Wort herb dried extract, Ginkgo Biloba leaf dried extract, DHA, 5-HTP (from griffonia bean), Inositol, Cayenne Pepper fruit, SAMe. Other Ingredients: Gelatin, Stearic Acid, Magnesium Stearate.

MoodPro - HealthMinded
Three capsules contain: Vitamin B1 (thiamine) 60 mg • Vitamin B2 (riboflavin) 45 mg • Vitamin B3 (niacin) 30 mg • Vitamin B6 (pyridoxine) 60 mg • Vitamin B9 (folic acid) 390 mcg • Vitamin B12 150 mcg • 5-HTP 30 mg • DHA 60 mg • Ginkgo Biloba 90 mg • St. John's Wort (3%) 900 mg • MoodPro Proprietary Blend 105 mg: Inositol, Calcium Citrate, Ascorbic Acid, Lemon Balm, Basil, Cayenne, Clove Oil. Other Ingredients: Stearic Acid, Magnesium Stearate.

Mor-Andro 200 - OSMO Therapy
Each capsule contains: 4-Androstene-3Beta,17Beta-Diol (androdiol) 100 mg • 4-Androstene-3,17-Dione (androstenedione) 100 mg • Zinc Gluconate 5 mg • Niacin (nicotinic acid) 20 mg.
See Editor's Note No. 47.

More - Puritan's Pride
Six tablets contain: Vitamins: Vitamin A 10,000 IU • Vitamin C (w/ Rose Hips) 500 mg • Vitamin D 400 IU •Vitamin E 100 IU • Thiamine (B-1) 10 mg • Riboflavin (B-2) 15 mg • Niacinamide (B-3) 100 mg • Vitamin B-6 10 mg • Vitamin B-12 25 mcg • Biotin 150 mcg • Choline Bitartrate 250 mg • Folic Acid 400 mcg • Inositol 25 mg • PABA 30 mg • Pantothenic Acid 100 mg. Minerals: Calcium 750 mg • Copper 2 mg • Iodine 0.15 mg • Iron 30 mg • Magnesium 40 mg • Manganese 5 mg • Phosphorus 350 mg • Potassium 50 mg • Sodium 0.3 mg • Zinc 30 mg • Trace amounts of chlorine, flourine, sulphur, silicon, molybdenum, boron, etc. Amino Acids (from yeast and liver): Arginine 6.6 mg • Cysteine 2.8 mg • Glutamic Acid 8 mg • Histidine 3.2 mg • Isoleucine 11 mg • Leucine 12.4 mg • Lysine 13 mg • Methionine 4.2 mg • Phenylalanine 7.4 mg • Threonine 2.25 mg • Tyrosine 9.2 mg • Valine 8.8 mg. Additional Ingredients: Algin 150 mg • Bee Pollen 10 mg • Desiccated Liver 100 mg • Hesperidin 25 mg • Lemon Bioflavonoid complex 50 mg • Red Bone Marrow 60 mg • Rutin 40 mg • Yeast 100 mg. Formulated in a natural food base of vegetable concentrate of watercress, tomato, onion, celery, celery seed, garlic.
See Editor's Note No. 14.

More Milk - Motherlove Herbal Co.
Each 2 oz bottle contains: Blessed Thistle • Nettles • Fennel seed. In a base of certified kosher alcohol and glycerin.

More Milk Plus - Motherlove Herbal Co.
Each 2 oz bottle contains: Fenugreek • Blessed Thistle • Nettles • Fennel seed. In a base of certified kosher alcohol and glycerin.

More Milk Two - Motherlove Herbal Co.
Each 2 oz bottle contains: Raspberry leaf • Nettles • Alfalfa. Base: Certified Kosher Alcohol, Glycerin.

More Than A Diet - American Health
Three duotabs contain: Chromium (as chromium picolinate and chromium polynicotinate) 100 mcg • Lipoactive Factors Proprietary Blend 344 mg: L-Carnitine Tartrate, Pyruvate, Inositol, Choline Bitartrate, L-Methionine, Lecithin, Phosphatidyl Choline (PC), Phosphatidyl Serine (PS), Taurine, Betaine Hydrochloride, Vanadium (as vanadyl sulfate) • Amino Factors Proprietary Blend 350 mg: Creatine Monohydrate, L-Lysine, L-Leucine, Glycine, Glutathione, L-Phenylalanine, L-Tyrosine • Herbal Thermo Factors Proprietary Blend 232 mg: Capsicum fruit, Ginger root, Licorice root, Mustard seed, Green Tea leaf, American Ginseng root, Cinnamon bark, Korean Ginseng root, Siberian Ginseng root, Piper Longum fruit, Guggulipid, Suma root, Schizandra fruit, Astragalus root, Hawthorn berry, Kola nut seed, Guarana seed • Fiber Factors Proprietary Blend 500 mg: Oat Bran Fiber, Citrus Pectin Fiber, Pulp Cellulose, Vegetable Cellulose, Beet Fiber • Herbal Fluid Factors Proprietary Blend 190 mg: Uva Ursi leaf, Buchu leaf, Couch Grass rhizome, Corn Silk stigma, Hydrangea root, Juniper berry • Essential Fatty Acids Factors Proprietary Blend 90 mg: Gotu Kola (aerial), Milk Thistle seed (silymarin), Chickweed (aerial), Borage seed oil, Black Currant fruit, Primrose seed oil, Flax seed oil, Conjugated Linoleic Acid, Dandelion root • Appetite Factors Proprietary Blend 550 mg: Citrimax HCA (from garcinia cambogia), Chitosan (shellfish fiber), OP's (wheat oligio peptides), Gymnema Sylvestre leaf, Apple Cider Vinegar, Phaseolus Vulgaris pods • Green Super Food Factors Proprietary Blend 500 mg: Spirulina, Chlorella, Barley Grass juice, Wheat Grass, Kelp, Alfalfa leaf • Enzyme Factors Proprietary Blend 220 mg: Coenzyme Q-10, Bromelain, Lipase, Protease, Cellulase, Aspergillus Niger, Aspergillus Oryzae, Fructooligosaccharides (FOS), Pancreatin • Fruit Extract Factors Proprietary Blend 67.5 mg: Apple, Apricot, Banana, Cranberry, Orange, Lemon, Lime, Papaya, Pineapple, Strawberry, Watermelon, Grapeseed (OPC), Grapefruit • Vegetable Extract Factors Proprietary Blend 50 mg: Cabbage, Celery, Broccoli, Brussel Sprouts, Yams, Carrots, Kale, Collard Greens, Spinach, Cauliflower. Other Ingredients: Dicalcium Phosphate, Cellulose (plant origin), Vegetable Magnesium Stearate, Xanthan Gum, Cellulose Coating, Silica.

Morning Soothe - TriLight Herbs
Ginger • Lemon Balm • German Chamomile • Red Raspberry leaf • Peach leaf.

MotherNature Saw Palmetto Berry Extract - Mother Nature
Each softgel contains: Saw Palmetto extract (serenoa repens) 160 mg. Other Ingredients: Olive Oil, Gelatin, Glycerin, Water.

Mother's Milk - Traditional Medicinals
Fennel seed • Anise seed • Coriander seed • Spearmint leaf • Lemongrass leaf • Lemon Verbena leaf • Althea root • Blessed Thistle leaf • Fenugreek seed.

Motion Mate - Nature's Way
Two capsules contain: Ginger • Hyssop herb • Meadowsweet herb • Peppermint leaves • Red Raspberry leaves. Other Ingredients: Gelatin, Magnesium Stearate, Millet.

Motion Sickness - Hyland's
Two tablets contain: Nux Vomica 6X • Tabacum 6X • Petroleum 12X • Cocculus Indicus 30X. Base: Lactose USP.
See Editor's Note No. 1.

Motion Sickness Remedy - PhytoPharmica
Twenty drops contain: Cocculus indicus 8x • Plumbum aceticum 8x • Argentum nitricum 6x • Glonoinum 6x • Zincum valerianicum 6x • Belladonna 4x • Nux vomica 4x • Pulsatilla 4x • Vinca minor 3x • Artemesia Vulgaris 1x. In a base of 45% USP alcohol by volume.
See Editor's Note No. 1.

Mouth-Mend - The Herbalist
Echinacea root • Golden Seal root • Myrrh Gum • Propolis • Spilanthes herb • Yerba Mansa root.

Movana - Boehringer Ingelheim
Each tablet contains: St. John's Wort flower & leaf extract WS-5572 (stabilized minimum hyperforin content 3%, Standardized Hypericin content 0.3%) 300 mg. Other Ingredients: Microcrystalline Cellulose • Corn Starch • Croscarmellose Sodium • Hydroxypropyl Methylcellulose, PEG-4000 • Magnesium Stearate • Silicon Dioxide • Ascorbic Acid • Synthetic Iron Oxide • Titanium Dioxide • Talc • Vanillin.

Move Ease Multi - Pro Health
Two tablets contain: Vitamin A (from natural fish liver oil) 10,000 IU • Beta-Carotene 10,000 IU • Vitamin B1 (thiamine HCl) 30 mg • Vitamin B2 (riboflavin) 30 mg • Vitamin B3 (niacinamide) 30 mg • Vitamin B5 (pantothenic acid) 30 mg • Vitamin B6 (pyridoxine HCl) 30 mg • Vitamin B12 (cyanocobalamin) 250 mcg • Biotin 100 mcg • Folic Acid 400 mcg • Vitamin C (ascorbic acid) 250 mg • Vitamin D (from natural fish liver oil) 400 IU • Vitamin E (100% D-alpha) 150 IU • Calcium (amino acid chelate, oyster shell) 100 mg • Magnesium (oxide, amino acid chelate) 60 mg • Zinc (amino acid chelate) 15 mg • Copper (amino acid chelate) 1 mg • Iodine (kelp) 150 mcg • Choline Bitartrate 100 mg • Inositol 75 mg • PABA 30 mg • Rutin 25 mg • Citrus Bioflavonoids 100 mg • Betaine HCl 25 mg • Glutamic Acid 25 mg • Potassium (amino acid chelate) 10 mg • Manganese (amino acid chelate) 5 mg • Selenium (amino acid chelate) 200 mcg • Chromium (yeast-free GTF) 250 mcg • Boron (amino acid chelate) 500 mcg • Molybdenum (amino acid chelate) 50 mcg • Nucleic Acid 50 mg • Glucosamine HCl 750 mg • MSM 250 mg. Base: Alfalfa, Parsley, Lecithin, Rose Hips, Dicalcium Phosphate, Cellulose, Stearic Acid, Silica.

Move E-Z - TriLight Herbs
Dandelion • Yellow Dock • Ginger • Dark Plum.

Move Free Plus Calcium with Hyaluronic Acid - Schiff
Each tablet contains: Vitamin D (as cholecalciferol) 133 IU • Calcium (as calcium carbonate) 167 mg • Proprietary Blend 500 mg: Glucosamine Hydrochloride, N-Acetyl D-Glucosamine, Glucosamine Sulfate (potassium salt) • Chondroitin Sulfate 400 mg • Hyaluronic Acid. Other Ingredients: Titanium Dioxide Color, Dextrose, Hydrosypropyl Cellulose, Triacetin, Polyethylene Glycol, Maltodextrin, Croscarmellose Sodium, Magnesium Stearate.
This product was formerly called Pain Free.
See Editor's Note No. 15.

BRAND NAMES

Some Brand Name Natural Products - What they Contain

www.NaturalDatabase.com contains MANY more listings than appear here.
Editor's Notes are located on pages 2155-2163.

BRAND NAMES

Move Free Plus MSM with Hyaluronic Acid - Schiff
Four tablets contain: Proprietary Blend 1.5 g: Glucosamine Hydrochloride, N-Acetyl D-Glucosamine, Glucosamine Sulfate • Chondroitin 1.2 g • MSM 1.5 g • Hyaluronic Acid. Other Ingredients: Cellulose, Titanium Dioxide, Polydextrose, Hydroxypropyl Methylcellulose, Triacetin, Polyethylene Glycol, Copolyvidone, Silicon Dioxide, Magnesium Stearate, Potassium Chloride.

Move Free Plus SAMe with Hyaluronic Acid - Schiff
Three tablets contain: Proprietary Blend 1.5 g: N-Acetyl D-Glucosamine, Glucosamine Sulfate, Glucosamine Hydrochloride • S-Adenosyl-L-Methionine (SAMe) 400 mg • Hyaluronic Acid. Other Ingredients: Cellulose, Hydroxypropyl Methylcellulose Phthalate, Titanium Dioxide, Mannitol, Stearic Acid, Triacetin, Sodium Starch Glycolate, Modified Cellulose Gum, Citric Acid, Silicon Dioxide, Potassium Chloride.

Move Free Triple Strength with Hyaluronic Acid - Schiff
Two gelcaps contain: Proprietary Blend 1.5 g: Glucosamine Hydrochloride, N-Acetyl D-Glucosamine, Glucosamine Sulfate • Chondroitin 1.2 g • Hyaluronic Acid. Other Ingredients: Gelatin, Water, Glycerin, Titanium Dioxide, Caramel Color, Cellulose, Polydextrose, Hydroxypropyl Methylcellulose, Titanium Dioxide, Polydextrose, Triacetin, Polyethylene Glycol, Copolyvidone, Silicon Dioxide, Magnesium Stearate, Potassium Chloride.
See Editor's Note No. 15.

Move Free with Hyaluronic Acid - Schiff
Each caplet contains: Glucosamine Complex 500 mg: Glucosamine Hydrochloride, N-Acetyl D-Glucosamine, Glucosamine Sulfate • Chondroitin Sulfate 400 mg • Hyaluronic Acid. Other Ingredients: Cellulose, Titanium Dioxide, Dextrose, Hydroxypropyl Methylcellulose, Polyethelyne Glycol, Sodium Carboxymethyl Cellulose, Mineral Oil, Sodium Citrate, Polysorbate 80, Dextrin, Copolyvidone, Silicon Dioxide, Magnesium Stearate.
See Editor's Note No. 14.

Mo-Zyme - Biotics Research Corporation
Each tablet contains: Molybdenum (from vegetable culture) 50 mcg.

MP Max - E'OLA
Two capsules contain: Saw Palmetto (berry) 8:1 604 mg • Proprietary Blend 350 mg: Pumpkin (seed), Pygeum (bark), Tomato (fruit), Nettle (root). Other Ingredients: Gelatin, Millet Flour, Magnesium Stearate, Silicon Dioxide.

MPC Maximum Prostate Care - Market America, Inc.
Two tablets contain: Zinc Citrate 30 mg • Selenium (as selenomethionine) 100 mcg • Saw Palmetto berry (serenoa repens small) 400 mg • Pygeum Africanum bark extract (standardized to contain 14% beta sitosterol and 0.5% docosanol) 100 mg • Prostate Health Proprietary Blend 425 mg: Chrysanthemum flower (dendranthema morifolium tzvel.), San-Qi Ginseng root (Panax notoginseng burk.), Dyer's Woad leaf (isatis indigotica fort.), Baikal Skullcap root (scutellaira baicalensis georgi), Reishi stem (ganoderma lucidum karst), Rhabdosia leaf (rhabdosia rubescens hara), Licorice root (glycyrrhiza uralensis fisch). Other Ingredients: Microcrystalline Cellulose, Stearic Acid, Magnesium Stearate, Silicon Dioxide, Croscarmellose Sodium, Dicalcium Phosphate.

MPF - Progressive Labs
Six capsules contain: Vitamin A 25000 IU • Vitamin E 180 IU • Folic Acid 780 mcg • Zinc Picolinate 60 mg • L-Glutamine 1500 mg • N-Acetyl Glucosamine 1050 mg • Gamma Oryzanol 360 mg • Cat's Claw (Uncaria tomentosa) 450 mg.

MPRX - AST Sports Science
Two capsules contain: Vitamin B6 22 mg • Magnesium (as magnesium salicylate) 100 mg • Pro-Therm Green Tea leaf extract (standardized for epigallocatechin gallate EGCG, l-phenylalanine, L-tyrosine, caffeine as caffeine anhydrous and theobromine HCl) 1400 mg.

MRP-44 - Human Development Technologies (HDT)
Each serving contains: L-Glutamine 2 g • Taurine 1 g • MRP1000 blend: Micro Ultra Filtered Whey Protein concentrate • Egg Albumen • Micro Ultra Filtered Whey Protein Isolate, Ion Exchanged Whey Protein Isolate • Maltodextrin • natural & artificial flavorings • L-Glutamine • Di-Calcium Phosphate • Taurine • Inulin • Cellulose Gum • Xanthan Gum • Magnesium Oxide • Lecithin • Fructose • Stevia • Acesulfame Potassium • Ascorbic Acid • Vitamin A Acetate • Vitamin E Acetate • Niacinamide • Iron Electrolytic • Zinc Oxide • D-Calcium Pantothenate • Ergocalciferol • Pyridoxine HCL • Copper Gluconate • Riboflavin • Thiamine Mononitrate • Folic Acid • Biotin • Potassium Ionide • Cyanocobalamin.

MSM - Trimedica
Each capsule contains: Methylsulfonylmethane 99.9% • Water 0.1%.

MSM - NOW Foods
Two capsules contain: Lignisul MSM (methylsulphonylmethane) 2 g. Other Ingredients: Magnesium Stearate, Stearic Acid.

MSM - Nature's Bounty
Each capsule contains: Methylsulfonylmethane (255 mg organic sulfur) 750 mg. Other Ingredients: Dicalcium Phosphate, Gelatin, Vegetable Magnesium Stearate, Silica.

MSM - Natural Balance
Each tablet contains: MSM (methylsulfonylmethane) 1000 mg. Other Ingredients: Cellulose, Silicon Dioxide, Stearic Acid, Magnesium Stearate.

MSM - Olympian Labs
Each capsule contains: MSM (methylsulfonylmethane) 500 mg.

MSM - Quest
Each caplet contains: Lignisul brand MSM 1000 mg. Other Ingredients: Croscarmellose Sodium, Silicon Dioxide, and Magnesium Stearate.

MSM - Swanson Health Products
Two capsules contain: OptiMSM Methylsulfonylmethane 1 g.

MSM - Metabolic Response Modifiers
Each capsule contains: MSM (methyl-sulfonyl-methane) 750 mg.

MSM - PhytoPharmica
Each tablet contains: MSM (methylsulfonylmethane) 1000 mg.

MSM - Nature's Sunshine
Two tablets contain: Methylsulfonylmethane (MSM) 1500 mg. Other Ingredients: Cellulose, Maltodextrin, Stearic Acid, Magnesium Stearate.

MSM - Enzymatic Therapy
Each tablet contains: MSM (methylsulfonylmethane) 1000 mg. Other Ingredients: Cellulose, Modified Cellulose, Titanium Dioxide Color, Magnesium Stearate, Lecithin, Carnauba Wax.

MSM & Glucosamine Cream - PhysioLogics
Purified Water • Stearic Acid • MSM (methylsulfonylmethane) • Cetyl Alcohol • Glyceryl Stearate • Polysorbate 80 • Ceteary1 Alcohol • Aloe Vera gel (aloe barbadensis, leaf) • Tocopheryl Acetate • Fragrance • Glucosamine Sulfate • Ceteareth-20 • Triethanolamine • Diazolidinyl Urea • Sweet Almond oil (prunus amygdalus dulcus) • Carbomer • Methylparaben • Propylparaben • Sodium Benzoate • Jojoba oil (simmondsia chinensis) • Cayenne extract (capsicum frutescens) • Arnica extract (arnica montana) • Matricaria Recutita extract (chamomilla recutita) • Ginger extract (zingiber officinale) • Comfrey extract (symphytum officinale).

MSM (Methylsulfonylmethane) - Pro Health
Two capsules contain: OptiMSM brand MSM (methylsulfonylmethane) 2000 mg. Other Ingredients: Magnesium Stearate, Gelatin.

MSM (OptoMSM) - NSI - Nutraceutical Sciences Institute
Each capsule contains: MSM (methyl sulfonyl methane, OptiMSM) 1000 mg.

MSM 1000 - Jarrow Formulas
Each capsule contains: Methylsulfonylmethane (providing 341 mg of organic sulfur) 1000 mg. Other Ingredients: Dicalcium Phosphate, Cellulose, Magnesium Stearate, Modified Cellulose Gum, Modified Cellulose, Stearic Acid, Silicon Dioxide.

MSM 1000 - GNC
Each capsule contains: MSM (Methylsulfonyl-Methane) 1000 mg. Other Ingredients: Gelatin.

MSM 1000 - Aspen Group, Inc.
Each capsule contains: 100% pure MSM (methyl sulfonyl methane) 1000 mg.

MSM 1000 - Jamieson
Each caplet contains: MSM (Methylsulfonylmethane) 1000 mg.

MSM 1000 MG - PhysioLogics
Each capsule contains: MSM (methylsulfonylmethane, organic sulfur 340 mg) 1000 mg. Other Ingredients: Gelatin, Calcium Stearate.

MSM 1000 mg - Vital Nutrients
Each capsule contains: Methylsulfonylmethane (MSM) 1000 mg.

MSM 1500 - GNC
Each tablet contains: MSM (methylsulfonyl-methane) 1500 mg. Other Ingredients: Cellulose, Titanium Dioxide, Caramel Color, Imitation Vanilla.

MSM 1500 mg - Vitamin World
Each tablet contains: Methylsulfonylmethane 1500 mg. Other Ingredients: Dicalcium Phosphate, Silica, Vegetable Magnesium Stearate, Cellulose Coating.

MSM 500 / Glucosamine 500 - GNC
Each capsule contains: MSM (Methylsulfonyl-Methane) 500 mg • Glucosamine Sulfate (as D-Glucosamine Sulfate .2KCl) 500 mg. Other Ingredients: Gelatin.

MSM 500 mg - Rexall - Sundown
Two tablets contain: Calcium 36 mg • MSM (methylsulfonylmethane) 1 g. Other Ingredients: Dicalcium Phosphate, Stearic Acid, Silica.

MSM 500 mg - PhysioLogics
Each capsule contains: Methylsulfonylmethane (organic sulfur 170 mg) 500 mg. Other Ingredients: Gelatin, Magnesium Stearate, Silica.

MSM 750 - Pain & Stress Center
Each capsule contains: MSM (methyl sulfonyl methane) 750 mg. Other Ingredients: Magnesium Stearate, Gelatin Capsule.

MSM Caps - Optimum Nutrition
Each capsule contains: Methylsulfonylmethane (as glucosamine sulfate potassium) 1 g. Other Ingredients: Gelatin, Magnesium Stearate.

MSM capsules - Pure Encapsulations
Each vegetable capsule contains: MSM (methylsulfonylmethane) 850 mg.

MSM Cream - At Last Naturals, Inc.
Aloe Vera gel • MSM (Dimethyl Sulfone) • Soybean oil • Stearic Acid • Cetyl Alcohol • Triethanolamine • Glycerin • Calendula Officinalis extract • Tocopherol (vitamin E) • Retinyl Palmitate (vitamin A) • Lecithin • Methylparaben • Propylparaben.

MSM Cream - Vitamin World
Water • MSM (methylsulfonylmethane) • Stearic Acid • Propylene Glycol • Cetyl Alcohol • Glyceryl Stearate • Cetyl Esters • Polysorbate 80 • Quaternium-15 • Triethanolamine • Magnesium Aluminum Silicate • Sunflower oil • Jojoba oil • Sweet Almond oil • Methylparaben • Carbomer • Propylparaben • Disodium EDTA • Panthenol • Hydrolyzed Collagen • Korean Ginseng (panax ginseng) • Tocopheryl Acetate • Cholecalciferol • Rosemary oil • Essential Oil Blend: Lavender oil (lavendula angustifolia), Petitgrain oil (citrus aurantium), Thyme oil (thymus vulgaris), Rosemary oil (rosmarinus officinalis), Chamomile oil (matricaria chamomilla), Sweet Birch oil (betula lenta) • Aloe Vera Gel (aloe barbadensis) • Ginkgo Biloba (ginkgo biloba) • Lecithin • Retinyl Palmitate.

MSM Extra Strength - Olympian Labs
Each tablet contains: MSM (methylsulfonylmethane) 1300 mg.

MSM Formula with White Willow - Health Smart Vitamins
Two capsules contain: Vitamin C (as ascorbyl palmitate) 30 mg • MSM (methylsulfonylmethane) 500 mg • Chondroitin Sulfate 300 mg • White Willow bark (3% salicins, 1.5 mg) 50 mg.
See Editor's Note No. 15.

MSM Herbal Moisturizing Soap Bar - At Last Naturals, Inc.
Aloe Vera gel • MSM • Chamomile extract • Calendula extract • Vitamin A • Vitamin C • Vitamin E.

MSM Liquid - Trimedica
Each teaspoon contains: MSM 390 mg. Other Ingredients: Purified Water.

MSM Plex - PharmAssure
Each capsule contains: MSM (methyl-sulfonyl-methane) 500 mg • Glucosamine Sulfate 500 mg.

MSM Plus - Progressive Labs
Each capsule contains: Vitamin C (as magnesium ascorbate) 100 mg • Magnesium (as magnesium ascorbate) 7 mg • Methyl Sulfonyl Methane (MSM) 800 mg.

MSM Plus Glucosamine - Optimum Nutrition
Each tablet contains: Methylsulfonylmethane (MSM) 1 g • Glucosamine (as glucosamine sulfate potassium) 500 mg. Other Ingredients: Pharmaceutical Glaze, Stearic Acid, Magnesium Stearate, Croscarmellose Sodium (disintegrant).

MSM Powder - Vitamin World
One-half teaspoon contains: MSM (methylsulfonylmethane, 1023 mg organic sulfur) 3000 mg. Other Ingredients: Silica.

MSM Powder - Natural Balance
Each teaspoon contains: Vitamin C (as ascorbic acid) 240 mg • MSM (methylsulfonylmethane) 4000 mg. Other Ingredients: Silicon Dioxide.

MSM powder - Pure Encapsulations
Each scoop contains: MSM (methylsulfonylmethane) 3 g.

MSM Rejuvenator - Progressive Labs
Ingredients: Stabilized Aloe Vera gel • Methylsulfonyl Methane • Glycerine • Caprylic/Capric Triglycerides • Jojoba oil • Polyquanterium-32 (colloidal polymers) • Evening Primrose oil • Cetyl Alcohol • Steryl Alcohol • Tetrahexyldecyl Ascorbate (lipid soluble Vitamin C) • Tocopheryl Acetate (Vitamin E) • Ginseng extract • Chamomile extract. Extracts of: Grape seed, Willow bark, Calendula, White Lily, Japanese Green Tea, Gum Mint, Cucumber, Soapbark, Balm of Gilead, Bee Propolis: Betaglucans. Essential oils of: Lemongrass, Rosemary, Sage, Cedarwood, Tetrasodium EDTA, Methylparaben, Propylparben, Diazolidiny Lurea.

MSM Sulfur - J. R. Carlson Laboratories, Inc.
Each capsule contains: MSM (methylsulfonylmethane) 1000 mg • Sulfur 334 mg.

MSM Sulfur - J. R. Carlson Laboratories, Inc.
Each capsule contains: MSM (methylsulfonylmethane) 900 mg • Sulfur 334 mg.

MSM Sulfur capsules - Jarrow Formulas
Each capsule contains: Methyl-Sulfonyl-Methane (MSM, providing 340 mg of organic sulfur) 1000 mg. Other Ingredients: Magnesium Stearate, Gelatin.

MSM Sulfur powder - Jarrow Formulas
Each scoop contains: Methyl-Sulfonyl-Methane (MSM, providing 340 mg of organic sulfur) 1000 mg.

Some Brand Name Natural Products - What they Contain

www.NaturalDatabase.com contains MANY more listings than appear here.
Editor's Notes are located on pages 2155-2163.

BRAND NAMES

MSM Ultra Caplets **-** FreeLife International
Each caplet contains: Vitamin C (from glycerol flovone-bound ascorbic and isoascorbic acids) 60 mg • Methylsulfonylmethane (MSM) 1000 mg • Proprietary Blend 100 mg: Ascorbic Acid, Isoascorbic Acid, Citrus Glycosyl Flavones (cirantin, isosakuranetin-7-beta-rutinoside, narirutin, eriocitrin, nobiletin, tangeretin, hepatamethoxyflavone). Other Ingredients: Cellulose, Cellulose Gum, Vegetable Stearic Acid, Silica, Vegetable Magnesium Stearate, Vita-Coat (vegetable resin, alpha-lipoic acid).

MSM Ultra Powder **-** FreeLife International
One-half teaspoon (2.24 g) contains: Vitamin C (from glycosyl flavone-bound ascorbic and isoascorbic acids 200 mg) 120 mg • MSM (methylsulfonylmethane) 2000 mg • Propreitary Blend 200 mg: Ascorbic Acid, Sodium Isoascorbate, Citrus Glycosyl Flavones • Stevia leaf extract (stevia rebaudiana) 40 mg.

MSM Ultra Power Punch **-** FreeLife International
Two rounded teaspoons (16.5 g) contain: Vitamin C from Citri-C brand Complex 60 mg • Eleuthero root 400 mg • Dahlulin brand Complex Carbohydrate (from Dahlia variabilis) 250 mg • Patented MSM (purified methylsulfonylmethane) 1000 mg • Proprietary Citri-C Complex Blend 100 mg: Ascorbic Acid, Iso-Ascorbic Acid, Citrus Glycosyl Flavones (cirantin, isosakuranetin-7-betarutinoside, narirutin, eriocitrin, nobiletin, tangeretin, heptamethoxyflavone). Other Ingredients: Raspberry Juice Concentrate, Maltodextrin, Citric Acid, Stevia Extract, Natural Flavors, Beet Juice Color.

MSM Ultra Therapeutic Lotion **-** FreeLife International
Aloe Vera • Willow Bark • Grapefruit seed • Green Tea • Rosemary • Purified Water • Methylsulfonylmethane in Soybean Lecithin (MicroSoy brand) • Glycerin • Stearic DiEster • Palmityl Alcohol • Palmityl Esters • Glyceryl Monoester (stearate) • Silica Fluid • Safflower oil • Coconut oil • Soybean oil • Methyl Glucose Sesquistearate • Retinyl Palmitate • Lipoic Acid • Alpha Bisabalol • Ascorbic Acid (vitamin C from sugar beet) • Bioflavonoid Complex • Mixed Tocopherols (alpha, beta, gamma, delta) • Coconut Esters Gel • Collagen Amino Acids • Hydrolized Silk Protein • L-Glutathione • Thyme oil • Musk oil • Jasmine oil • Natural Fragrance.

MSM with Glucosamine Cream **-** Vitamin World
Purified Water • Stearic Acid • MSM (methylsulfonylmethane) • Cetyl Alcohol • Glyceryl Stearate • Propylene Glycol • Polysorbate 80 • Cetearyl Alcohol • Aloe Vera Gel (aloe barbadensis leaf) • Tocopheryl Acetate • Fragrance • Glucosamine Sulfate • Ceteareth-20 • Diazolidinyl Urea • Triethanolamine • Sweet Almond oil (prunus amygdalus dulcis) • Carbomer • Methylparaben • Propylparaben • Sodium Benzoate • Jojoba oil (simmondsia chinensis) • Capsicum Frutescens extract • Arnica Montana extract • Chamomilla Recutita extract (matricaria) • Ginger extract (zingiber officinale) • Comfrey extract (symphytum officinale).

MSM with Glucosamine Sulfate **-** PhytoPharmica
Each capsule contains: Chloride (from glucosamine sulfate) 78 mg • Sodium (from glucosamine sulfate) 50 mg • Stabilized Glucosamine Sulfate 500 mg • MSM (methylsulfonylmethane) 250 mg.

MSM with GS-500 (OptiMSM) **-** Enzymatic Therapy
Each capsule contains: Chloride (from glucosamine sulfate) 78 mg • Sodium (from glucosamine sulfate) 50 mg • Glucosamine Sulfate (stabilized) 500 mg • MSM (methylsulfonylmethane) 250 mg. Other Ingredients: Gelatin, Magnesium Stearate, Silicon Dioxide, Titanium Dioxide Color.

MSM, Methylsulfonylmethane **-** Allergy Research Group
Each capsule contains: Methylsulfonylmethane 500 mg • Molybdenum 10 mcg. Other Ingredients: Cellulose, Silicon Dioxide, Stearic Acid.

MSM900 **-** Ortho Molecular Products
Each capsule contains: Methylsulfonylmethane 900 mg. Other Ingredients: Natural Vegetable Capsules, Ascorbyl Palmitate, Magnesium Stearate, Microcrystalline Cellulose, Silicon Dioxide.

Mucho Mate **-** Traditional Medicinals
Green & Roasted Yerba Mate leaf • Ginger rhizome • Lemon peel • natural Lemon flavor • Stevia leaf.

Mucoplex **-** Progressive Labs
Each capsule contains: Comfrey root (Symphytum officinale) 225 mg • Pepsin (1:3000) 65 mg • Bromelain 50 mg • Raw Duodenum 10 mg. See Editor's Note No. 14.

Muco-Plex **-** Enzymatic Therapy
Two tablets contain: Niacin 30 mg • Vitamin B6 (pyridoxine HCl) 10 mg • Iodine (potassium iodide) 75 mcg • Marshmallow 8:1 extract (althea officinalis, mucilage content 30-40%) 450 mg • Raw Duodenum Tissue 450 mg • Pancreatic Enzymes 3X 100 mg • L-Methionine 100 mg • Gastric Mucin powder 100 mg • Pepsin 1:10000 65 mg • Pituitary extract 15 mg. Base: Crude Licorice extract (glycyrrhiza glabra), Allantoin-Methionine (comfrey) Complex, Acidophilus, Aloe Vera.
See Editor's Note No. 31.

Mucosagen **-** Ortho Molecular Products
Two capsules contain: Biotin 250 mcg • L-Glutamine USP 500 mg • Quercetin 335 mg • N-Acetyl Cysteine USP 85 mg • Bromelain (2400 GDU/g) 85 mg • Gamma Oryzanol 85 mg • Tumeric root extract (standardized to contain 95% curcumin) 85 mg • N-Acetyl-D-Glucosamine 70 mg • Milk Thistle seed extract (standardized to contain 80% silymarin) 45 mg. Other Ingredients: Natural Vegetable Capsules, Ascorbyl Palmitate, Magnesium Stearate, Microcrystalline Cellulose, Silicon Dioxide.

MucoStop **-** Enzymedica
Each capsule contains: Amylase Thera-Blend 14,850 DU • Protease Thera-Blend 45,000 HUT • Glucoamylase 50 AG • Betaglucanase 60 BGU • Lipase Thera-Blend 500 FCCFIP • Alpha-Galactosidase 100 GalU • Cellulase Thera-Blend 400 CU • Xylanase 550 XU • Seaprose 15 mg • Pectinase with Phytase 350 endo-Pgu • Hemicellulase 30 HCU • Invertase 5 INVU.

Mullein Lobelia **-** Atrium Biotechnologies
Each capsule contains: Mullein leaves 375 mg • Lobelia 125 mg.

Multi 1-to-3 **-** Jarrow Formulas
Three tablets contain: Vitamin A (palmitate) 3000 IU • Beta Carotene (15,000 % RDI IU) 5000 IU • Vitamin C (from calcium ascorbate) 500 mg • Vitamin D (D3, cholecalciferol) 400 IU • Natural Vitamin E (D-alpha tocopheryl succinate) 200 IU • Vitamin B1 (thiamin) 50 mg • Vitamin B2 (riboflavin) 50 mg • Vitamin B3 (niacin) 50 mg • Vitamin B3 (niacinamide) 50 mg • Vitamin B6 (pyridoxine HCl) 50 mg • Folic Acid 400 mcg • Vitamin B12 (cobalamin concentrate) 50 mcg • Biotin 300 mcg • Pantothenic Acid (D-calcium pantothenate) 100 mg • Calcium (450 mg from bovine hydroxyapatite, 50 mg from calcium ascorbate) 450 mg • Iodine (from kelp) 225 mcg • Magnesium (as oxide) 300 mg • Zinc (from monomethionate) 15 mg • Selenium (as L-selenomethionine/sodium selenate 50/50) 100 mcg • Copper (from gluconate) 2 mg • Manganese (from citrate) 2 mg • Chromium (from nicotinate-citrate complexed to niacin) 200 mcg • Molybdenum (from sodium molybdate) 200 mcg • Potassium (from potassium chloride) 99 mg • Lutein 3 mg • Bilberry (1.8% anthocyanosides) 80 mg • Ginger 50 mg • MSM 25 mg • Rosemary extract 110 mg • Choline (from choline bitartrate) 48 mg • Inositol 100 mg. Other Ingredients: Cellulose, Silicon Dioxide, Stearic Acid, Magnesium Stearate (vegetable source), Modified Cellulose Gum.

Multi Caps **-** Progressive Labs
Three capsules contain: Vitamin A 10000 IU • Vitamin C 120 mg • Vitamin D (as Vitamin D3) 400 IU • Vitamin E 15 IU • Thiamin (Vitamin B1) 10 mg • Riboflavin (Vitamin B2) 10 mg • Niacinamide 100 mg • Vitamin B6 10 mg • Folate (folic acid) 400 mcg • Vitamin B12 50 mcg • Biotin 25 mcg • Pantothenic Acid 40 mg • Calcium 200 mg • Iron 15 mg • Magnesium 100 mg • Zinc 15 mg • Selenium 25 mcg • Manganese 20 mg • Iodine 150 mcg • Chromium 20 mcg • Potassium 99 mg • Choline 75 mg • Inositol 75 mg • PABA 30 mg • Citrus bioflavonoids 100 mg • Rutin 25 mg • Hesperidin 25 mg •

Glutamic Acid 30 mg • L-Lysine 50 mg • DL-Methionine 50 mg • Pancreatin 60 mg • Bile Salts 5 mg • RNA (Brain) 50 mg • Unsaturated Fatty Acids 50 mg. Other Ingredients: Rose Hips, Ginseng, Goldenseal, Fo Ti Teng, Gotu Kola, Sarsaparilla, Watercress, Kelp, Green Cabbage, Rice polishings, Raw Stomach substance (not an extract), Alfalfa, Parsley, Papaya.
See Editor's Note No. 31.

Multi Carotene - Puritan's Pride
Each softgel contains: Beta Carotene (Pro-Vitamin A Activity) 25,000 IU • Alpha-Carotene 1 mg • Lycopene 5 mg • Lutein 6 mg • Zeaxanthin 0.3 mg.

Multi Chelate - Progressive Labs
Six capsules contain: Calcium 500 mg • Iron 15 mg • Magnesium 250 mg • Zinc 10 mg • Iodine 150 mcg • Selenium 25 mcg • Copper 1 mg • Manganese 10 mg • Chromium 50 mcg • Molybdenum 150 mcg • Potassium 99 mg • Vanadium 150 mcg • Silicone 2 mg • Raw Glandular concentrate 200 mg. The raw glandular materal in this product is prepared by a special process which does not exceed physiological temperature (37 Celcius). Guaranteed free of chemical pesticides and synthetic hormones.
See Editor's Note No. 14.

Multi Easy Powder - Jarrow Formulas
Each scoop (or 2 tsp, or 10 g) contains: Vitamin A (as retinol palmitate) 1500 IU • Beta-Carotene) from natural dunaliella salina) 5000 IU • Vitamin C (as calcium ascorbate) 500 mg • Vitamin D (ergocalciferol) 400 IU • Vitamin E (natural D-alpha tocopheryl succinate) 400 IU • Vitamin K (phylloquinone) 50 mcg • Vitamin B1 (as thiamine mononitrate) 25 mg • Vitamin B2 (riboflavin) 25 mg • Vitamin B3 (niacin) 10 mg • Niacinamide 50 mg • Vitamin B6 (as pyridoxine hydrochloride) 25 mg • Folic Acid 400 mcg • Vitamin B12 (cyanocobalamin) 100 mcg • Biotin 300 mcg • Vitamin B5 (calcium pantothenate) 100 mg • Calcium (as calcium citrate) 540 mg • Iodine (as potassium iodide) 150 mcg • Magnesium (as magnesium citrate) 250 mg • Zinc (as monomethionate) 15 mg • Selenium (as selenomethionine/sodium selenate) 100 mcg • Copper (as copper gluconate) 1 mg • Manganese (as manganese gluconate) 1 mg • Chromium (as chromium picolinate) 120 mcg • Molybdenum (as sodium molybdate) 75 mcg • Potassium (as potassium chloride) 99 mg • Boron (as citrate) 1 mg • Choline 55 mg • Inositol 100 mg • Rice Essence brand Rice Bran Concentrate 3 g • Lecithin 500 mg. Other Ingredients: Natural Vanilla Flavor, Lo Han Extract (momordica grosvenorii).

Multi Fiber Complex - Naturade
Each capsule contains: Psyllium seed husk 400 mg • Guar Gum 50 mg • Slippery Elm bark 50 mg • Licorice root 50 mg • Apple Pectin 50 mg • Grapefruit Pectin 50 mg • Glucomannan 50 mg. Other Ingredients: Magnesium Stearate, Silicon Dioxide, Gelatin.

Multi for Seniors - Health Center for Better Living
Each tablet contains: Vitamin A (as retinyl acetate and beta-carotene) 6,000 IU • Vitamin C (as ascorbic acid) 60 mg • Vitamin D (as cholecalciferol) 400 IU • Vitamin E (as dl-alpha-tocopheryl acetate) 45 IU • Vitamin K (as phytonadione) 10 mcg • Vitamin B1 (as thiamin mononitrate) 1.5 mg • Vitamin B2 (as riboflavin) 1.7 mg • Niacin (as niacinarnide) 20 mg • Vitamin B6 (as pyridoxine HCl) 3 mg • Folate (as folic acid) 200 mcg • Vitamin B12 (as cyanocobalamin) 25 mcg • Biotin 30 mcg • Pantothenic Acid (as D-calcium patothenate) 10 mg • Calcium (as calcium carbonate and dicalcium phosphate) 200 mg • Iron (as ferrous fumarate) 9 mcg • Phosphorus (as dicalcium phosphate) 48 mcg • Iodine (as potassium iodide) 150 mcg • Magnesium (as magnesium oxide) 100 mg • Zinc (as zinc oxide) 15 mg • Selenium (as sodium selenate) 25 mcg • Copper (as cupric oxide) 2 mg • Manganese (as manganese sulfate (2.5 mg) • Chromium (as chromium amino acid chelate) 100 mcg • Molybdenum (as sodium molybdate) 25 mcg • Potassium (as postassium chloride)80 mg • Nickel (as nickelous sulfate) 5 mcg • Silicon (as sodium metasilicate) 10 mcg • Vanadium (as sodium metavanadate) 10 mcg.

Multi Ginseng 1000 mg, Concentrated - GNC
Each capsule contains: Multi-Ginseng Root (from 50 mg of multi-ginseng extract 20:1) 1000 mg. Other Ingredients: Soybean Oil, Gelatin, Glycerin, Caramel Color, Titanium Dioxide (natural mineral whitener).

Multi Glandular - American Biologics
Each tablet contains: Spleen 257 mg • Brain 68 mg • Liver 45 mg • Heart 32 mg • Kidney 32 mg • Pancreas 9 mg • Duodenum 9 mg • Thymus 8 mg • Adrenal 8 mg • Pituitary 2 mg (all of bovine origin). Other Ingredients: Dicalcium Phosphate, Magnesium Stearate.
See Editor's Note No. 31.

Multi Health Plus - Sojourn Health
Eight capsules contain: Beta Carotene (pro-vitamin A) 20,000 IU • Vitamin D (activated ergosterol) 100 IU • Vitamin E (mixed tocopherols & D-alpha from natural vegetable sources) 400 IU • Vitamin B1 (thiamine HCl) 100 mg • Vitamin B2 (riboflavin) 75 mg • Niacinamide 150 mg • Vitamin B5 (pantothenic acid) 150 mg • Vitamin B6 (pyridoxine HCl) 75 mg • Vitamin B12 150 mcg • Folic Acid 800 mcg • Biotin 200 mcg • Vitamin C (sago palm) 1000 mg • Calcium (amino acid chelate) 900 mg • Magnesium (oxide, amino acid chelate) 450 mg • Zinc (amino acid chelate) 45 mg • Copper (amino acid chelate) 3 mg • Iodine (kelp) 225 mcg • Selenium (amino acid chelate) 70 mcg • Chromium (amino acid chelate) 150 mcg • Manganese (amino acid chelate) 20 mg • Vitamin B10 (PABA) 75 mg • Choline (bitartrate) 50 mg • Inositol 50 mg • Betaine (HCl) 150 mg • Bioflavonoids 200 mg • Rutin 20 mg • Hesperidin 15 mg • Potassium (amino acid chelate) 99 mg. Other Ingredients: Rice Powder, Magnesium Stearate, Gelatin.

Multi Mega Minerals - GNC
Two tablets contain: Vitamin D (as cholecalciferol) 400 IU • Calcium (as calcium carbonate) 1000 mg • Iron (as hydrolyzed protein chelate) 18 mg • Iodine (as kelp) 150 mcg • Magnesium (as magnesium oxide) 500 mg • Zinc (as hydrolyzed protein chelate) 22.5 mg • Copper (as hydrolyzed protein chelate) 3 mg • Manganese (as hydrolyzed protein chelate) 10 mcg • Chromium (as hydrolyzed protein chelate) 100 mcg • Chloride (as potassium chloride) 90 mg • Potassium (as potassium chloride) 95 mg • Betaine Hydrochloride 100 mg. Other Ingredients: Cellulose.

Multi Mineral Citrate Complete - Puritan's Pride
Four capsules contain: Calcium (Citrate, Carbonate, Aspartate) 1000 mg • Magnesium (Citrate, Oxide, Aspartate) 500 mg • Potassium 99 mg • Zinc 50 mg • Iron (Fumarate) 10 mg • Manganese 10 mg • Copper (Gluconate) 2 mg • Selenium (Chelate) 100 mcg • Chromium (Chelate) 200 mcg • Molybdenum (Chelate) 100 mcg • Silica (Chelate) 10 mcg • Boron 3 mg.

Multi Oral-Chelate - Sojourn Health
Three capsules contain: EDTA 75 mg • Proprietary Base 1337.5 mg: Bentonite Clay, Garlic powder, Cysteine HCl, Homeopathic Hawthorne berry (crataegus) 6X, Grape seed, L-Carnitine, L-Methionine, L-Phenylalanine, L-Lysine, Malic Acid, Methyl Sulfonyl Methane (MSM), Ginkgo Biloba, Artichoke powder (cynara floridanum), Bromelain, Milk Thistle extract (silybum marianum), Alpha-Lipoic Acid (thioctic), Chondroitin Sulfate, Lipase, CoQ10, Green Tea (camellia sinensis), Catalase, Boron. Other Ingredients: Rice Powder, Magnesium Stearate, Gelatin.

Multi Pro 32X - AST Sports Science
Each caplet contains: Vitamin A (as beta carotene/vitamin A acetate) 10,000 IU • Vitamin C (as ascorbic acid) 200 mg • Vitamin D (as vitamin D3) 400 IU • Vitamin E (as dL-alpha tocopheryls) 60 IU • Vitamin K 25 mcg • Thiamin 30 mg • Riboflavin 30 mg • Niacin (as niacinamide) 30 mg • Vitamin B6 30 mg • Folic Acid 400 mcg • Vitamin B12 30 mcg • Biotin 60 mcg • Pantothenic Acid 30 mg • Calcium (as di-calcium phosphate) 75 mg • Iron (as ferrous fumarate) 18 mg • Phosphorus (as di-calcium phosphate) 45 mg • Iodine (as potassium iodine) 150 mcg • Magnesium (as magnesium oxide) 100 mg • Zinc (as zinc chelate) 30 mg • Selenium (as selenium chelate) 25 mcg • Copper (as copper chelate) 2 mg • Manganese (as manganese sulfate) 5 mg • Chromium (as chromium chelate) 25 mcg

• Molybdenum (as molybdenum chelate) 25 mcg • Chloride (as potassium chloride) 36 mg • Potassium (as potassium chloride) 40 mg • Silicon 30 mg • Tin (as tin chelate) 10 mcg • Vanadium (as vanadium chelate) 10 mcg • Boron (as boron chelate) 150 mcg • Nickel (as nickel chelate) 25 mcg. Other Ingredients: Croscarmellose Sodium, Magnesium Stearate, Microcrystalline Cellulose.

Multi Ultra Mega - GNC
Each tablet contains: Vitamin A (50% as beta-carotene, 50% as acetate) 10,000 IU • Vitamin C (as ascorbic acid) 200 mg • Vitamin D (as cholecalciferol) 400 IU • Vitamin E (as d-alpha tocopheryl succinate) 100 IU • Thiamin (as thiamin mononitrate) 75 mg • Riboflavin 75 mg • Niacin (as niacinamide) 75 mg • Vitamin B6 (as pyridoxine hydrochloride) 75 mg • Folate, Folic Acid, Folacin, 400 mcg •Vitamin B12 (as cyanocobalamin) 75 mcg • Biotin 75 mcg • Pantothenic Acid (as calcium d-pantothenate) 75 mg • Calcium (as calcium carbonate) 100 mg • Iron (as ferrous fumarate) 18 mg • Iodine (as kelp) 150 mcg • Magnesium (as magnesium oxide) 7 mg • Zinc (as zinc oxide) 15 mg • Selenium (as hydrolyzed protein chelate) 10 mcg • Copper (as copper sulfate) 250 mcg • Manganese (as manganese sulfate) 6 mg • Chromium (as hydrolyzed protein chelate) 10 mcg • Molybdenum (as hydrolyzed protein chelate) 10 mcg • Potassium (as potassium chloride) 10 mg •Boron (as boron citrate) 100 mcg • Silica (as silicon dioxide) 10 mcg • Choline (as choline bitartrate) 35 mg • Inositol 75 mcg • Para-Aminobenzoic Acid (PABA) 75 mg • Trimethylglycine (TMG) 10 mg • Rutin powder 25 mg • Citrus Bioflavonoid Complex (as 6.25 mg citrus bioflavoniod complex 4x) 25 mg • Hesperidin Complex 5 mg • N-Acetyl-L-Cysteine (NAC) 500 mcg • Alpha-Lipoic Acid 1 mg • Green Tea leaves (camellia sinensis). Other Ingredients: Cellulose, Food Glaze, Rose Hips powder (rosina canina), Soy Protein, Papain, Alfalfa powder (medicagn sativa), Watercress powder (nasturtium officinale), Parsley herb powder (petroselinum crispum), Lecithin powder, Whole Brown Rice powder (oryza sativa).

Multi Ultra Mega Gold Timed Release - GNC
Two tablets contain: Vitamin A (75% as Betatene beta-Carotene; 25% as Acetate) 20,000 IU • Vitamin C (as Ascorbic Acid) 500 mg • Vitamin D (as Cholecalciferol) 400 IU • Vitamin E (as d-alpha Tocopheryl Succinate) 300 IU • Thiamin (as Thiamin Mononitrate) 100 mg • Riboflavin 100 mg • Niacin (as Niacinamide) 100 mg • Vitamin B6 (as Pyridoxine Hydrochloride) 100 mg • Folate, Folic Acid, Folacin 400 mcg • Vitamin B12 (as Cyanocobalamin) 150 mcg • Biotin 100 mcg • Pantothenic Acid (as Calcium d-Pantothenate) 100 mg • Calcium (as Calcium Carbonate) 50 mg • Iron (as Ferrous Fumarate) 10 mg • Iodine (as Kelp) 100 mcg • Magnesium (as Magnesium Oxide) 50 mg • Zinc (as Zinc Oxide) 15 mg • Selenium (as Selenium Yeast) 150 mcg • Copper (as Cupric Oxide) 2 mg • Manganese (as Manganese Gluconate) 10 mg • Chromium (as GTF Chromium Yeast) 150 mcg • Molybdenum (as Molybdenum Yeast) 150 mcg • Potassium (as Potassium Chloride) 10 mg • Boron (as Boron Gluconate) 1 mg • Chlorine Bitartrate 50 mg • Inositol 25 mg • Para-Aminobenzoic Acid 50 mg • Trimethylglycine (TMG) 25 mg • Citrus Bioflavonoid Complex 25 mg • Rutin powder 10 mg • Hesperidin Complex 5 mg • Quercetin Dihydrate 10 mg • Natural Carotenoid Complex 15 mg • N-Acetyl-L-cysteine (NAC) 10.5 mg • Amylase 10 mg • Lipase 5 mg • Protease 2 mg • Cellulase 5 mg • Lycopene 200 mcg • Alpha-lipoic Acid 4.5 mg • Green Tea leaves (Camellia sinensis) 15 mg. Other Ingredients: Cellulose, Vegetable Acetoglycerides, Titanium Dioxide, Chlorophyll.

Multi Ultra Mega Gold Without Iron - GNC
Two tablets contain: Vitamin A (75% as Betatene Beta-Carotene; 25% as Acetate) 20,000 IU • Vitamin C (as Ascorbic Acid) 500 mg • Vitamin D (as Cholecalciferol) 400 IU • Vitamin E (as d-alpha Tocopheryl Succinate) 300 IU • Thiamin (as Thiamin Mononitrate) 100 mg • Riboflavin 100 mg • Niacin (as Niacinamide) 100 mg • Vitamin B6 (as Pyridoxine Hydrochloride) 100 mg • Folate, Folic Acid, Folacin 400 mcg • Vitamin B12 (as Cyanocobalamin) 150 mcg • Biotin 100 mcg • Pantothenic Acid (as Calcium d-Pantothenate) 100 mg • Calcium (as Calcium Carbonate) 50 mg • Iodine (as Kelp) 100 mcg • Magnesium (as Magnesium Oxide) 50 mg • Zinc (as Zinc Oxide) 15 mg • Selenium (as Selenium Yeast) 150 mcg • Copper (as Cupric Oxide) 2 mg • Manganese (as Manganese Gluconate) 10 mg • Chromium (as GTF Chromium Yeast) 100 mcg • Molybdenum (as Molybdenum Yeast) 150 mcg • Potassium (as Potassium Chloride) 10 mg • Boron (as Boron Gluconate) 1 mg • Chlorine Bitartrate 50 mg • Inositol 25 mg • Para-Aminobenzoic Acid (PABA) 50 mg • Trimethylglycine (TMG) 25 mg • Citrus Bioflavonoid Complex 25 mg • Rutin powder 10 mg • Hesperidin Complex 5 mg • Quercetin Dihydrate 10 mg • Natural Carotenoid Complex 15 mg • N-Acetyl-L-Cysteine (NAC) 10.5 mg • Amylase 10 mg • Lipase 5 mg • Protease 2 mg • Cellulase 5 mg • Lycopene 200 mcg • Alpha-lipoic Acid 4.5 mg • Green Tea leaves (Camellia sinensis) 15 mg. Other Ingredients: Cellulose, Vegetable Actoglycerides, Titanium Dioxide, Chlorophyll.

Multi Ultra Mega Green - GNC
Three tablets contain: Vitamin A (75% as beta-Carotene, 25% as Retinyl Acetate) 20,000 IU • Vitamin C (as Ascorbic Acid) 500 mg • Vitamin D (as Cholecalciferol) 400 IU • Vitamin E (as d-alpha Tocopheryl Succinate) 300 IU • Thiamin (as Thiamin Mononitrate) 25 mg • Riboflavin 25 mg • Niacin (as Niacinamide) 25 mg • Vitamin B6 (as Pyridoxine Hydrochloride) 25 mg • Folate, Folic Acid, Folacin 400 mcg • Vitamin B12 (as Cyanocobalamin) 250 mcg • Biotin 50 mcg • Pantothenic Acid (as Calcium d-Pantothenate) 25 mg • Calcium (as Calcium Carbonate and Hydrolyzed Protein Chelate) 50 mg • Iron (as Hydrolyzed Protein Chelate and Ferrous Fumarate) 10 mg • Iodine (as kelp) 100 mcg • Magnesium (as Magnesium Oxide and Hydrolyzed Protein Chelate) 50 mg • Zinc (as Hydrolyzed Protein Chelate) 15 mg • Selenium (as L-Selenomethionine) 50 mcg • Copper (as Cupric Oxide and Hydrolyzed Protein Chelate) 2 mg • Manganese (as Hydrolyzed Protein Chelate) 10 mg • Chromium (as Hydrolyzed Protein Chelate and Chromium Picolinate) 100 mcg • Molybdenum (as Hydrolyzed Protein Chelate) 150 mcg • Spirulina powder 400 mg • Green Tea leaf powder (camellia sinesis) 250 mg • Citrus Bioflavonoid Complex 100 mg • Safflower oil 100 mg • Flaxseed oil 100 mg • Borage oil 100 mg • Wheat Grass powder (Triticum aestivum) 100 mg • Barley Grass powder (Hordeum vulgare) 100 mg • Bee Pollen 100 mg • Trimethylglycine 100 mg • Choline Bitartrate 50 mg • Para Aminobenzoic Acid (PABA) 50 mg • Chlorella powder 50 mg • Siberian Ginseng root powder (Eleutheroccus senticosus) 50 mg • RNA (Yeast Free) 35 mg • Inositol powder 25 mg • Rutin powder 25 mg • Quercetin Dihydrate 25 mg • Oat Bran powder (Avena sativa) 25 mg • Apple Pectin 25 mg • Betaine Hydrochloride 20 mg • Papain 20 mg • Bromelain 20 mg •N-Acetyl L-Cysteine 15 mg • DNA (Yeast Free) 10 mg • Odorless Garlic powder (allium sativum) 10 mg • Echinacea root powder (Echinacea angustifolia) 10 mg • Milk Thistle extract (Silybum marianum) 10 mg • Goldenseal root powder (hydrastis canadensis) 10 mg • Ginkgo Biloba extract 50:1 (24% ginkgo flavone glycosides) 10 mg • Cayenne Pepper powder (Capsicum frutescens) 10 mg • Alpha Lipoic Acid 10 mg • Hesperidin Complex 5 mg • L-Glutathione 5 mg • Alpha Amylase 5 mg • Lipase 5 mg • Carotenoids (as natural carotenoid powder) 4 mg • Cellulase 2.5 mg • Boron (as protein chelate and boron gluconate powder) 1 mg • Silicon 1 mg • Lycopene 500 mcg. Other Ingredients: Maltodextrin, Cellulose, Povidone, Vegetable Acetoglycerides, Titanium Dioxide, Chlorophyll, Rose Hips powder.

Multi Vitamin - Oasis Wellness Network
Each tablet contains: Vitamin A (50% palmitate, 50% beta carotene) 2500 IU • Vitamin C (as ascorbic acid, calcium ascorbate) 125 mg • Vitamin D (as cholecalciferol) 200 IU • Vitamin E (as d-alpha-tocopherol acetate) 30 IU • Vitamin B1 (as thiamin mononitrate) 5 mg • Vitamin B2 (as riboflavin) 5 mg • Vitamin B3 (as niacinamide) 8 mg • Vitamin B6 (as pyridoxine HCl) 10 mg • Folate (as folic acid) 200 mcg • Vitamin B12 (as cyanocobalamin) 25 mcg • Biotin 100 mcg • Pantothenic Acid (as calcium pantothenate) 8 mg • Calcium (as calcium and citrate) 75 mg • Iron (as glycinate) 5 mg • Iodine (as potassium iodide) 75 mcg • Magnesium (as magnesium citrate) 50 mg • Zinc (as monomethionine) 8 mg • Selenium (as sodium selenite) 13 mcg • Copper (as amino acid chelate) 1 mg • Manganese (amino acid chelate) 3 mg • Chromium (as yeast) 25 mcg • Molybdenum (as amino acid chelate) 25 mcg • Potassium (as

citrate) 38 mg • Choline (as bitartrate) 25 mg • Betaine (as HCl) 13 mg • Inositol 10 mg • Bioflavonoid Complex 18 mg • MaxCell Proprietary Blend 60 mg: Zisyphus Jujube, Piper Nigrum, Aloe Vera gel, Glycyrrhiza Glabra. Other Ingredients: Stearic Acid, Cellulose, Magnesium Stearate, Silicon Dioxide.

Multi Vitamin Energy Plus for Women - Futurebiotics LLC
Two tablets contain: Beta Carotene 8500 IU • Vitamin C (Acerola, Ascorbic Acid) 225 mg • Thiamin 12.5 mg • Riboflavin 12.5 mg • Niacinamide 50 mg • Calcium (Phosphate, Carbonate) 625 mg • Iron (Amino Acid Chelate) 8 mg • Vitamin D 400 IU • Vitamin E (Natural Mixed Tocopherols) 30 IU • Vitamin B6 15 mg • Folic Acid 400 mcg • Vitamin B12 30 mcg • Biotin 300 mcg • Pantothenic Acid 25 mg • Para Amino Benzoic Acid (PABA) 85 mg • Choline 150 mg • Inositol 30 mg • Iodine (Kelp) 150 mcg • Magnesium (Oxide, Ascorbate) 150 mg • Zinc (Amino Acid Chelate) 15 mg • Ribonucleic Acid (RNA) 50 mg • Chromium (Polynicotinate) 60 mcg • Potassium (Amino Acid Chelate) 90 mg • Selenium (Selenomethionine) • In a base of Peony Root, Dong Quai, Aloe Vera, Methionine, Chamomile, Rosemary, American Ginseng, Chlorella, Bee Pollen, Sea Vegetable, Dandelion root, Betaine HCl, Chinese Licorice & Raw Alfalfa Juice Concentrate.

Multi Vitamin/Mineral Formula - Body Language Vitamin Co.
Three tablets contain: Beta Carotene 5000 IU • Magnesium 175 mg • Vitamin B1 25 mg • Calcium 200 mg • Vitamin B2 25 mg • Selenium 25 mcg • Vitamin B5 25 mg • Manganese 1mg • Vitamin B6 25 mg • Zinc 5 mg • Niacinamide 25 mg • Iodine 150 mcg • Vitamin B12 12 mcg • Copper 2 mg • Folic Acid 400 mcg • Molybdenum 10 mcg • Vitamin D (as vitamin D3) 400 IU • Vanadium 10 mcg • Vitamin K 25 mcg • Boron 150 mcg • Vitamin E 100 IU • Taurine 250 mg • Vitamin C 100 mg • Choline 105 mg • Biotin 600 mcg • Chromium 25 mcg • Pine Bark extract 10 mg • Potassium Chloride 37.5 mg • Green Tea extract 25 mg • Phosphoglycolipids 100 mg • Inositol 40 mg • Betaine 25 mg • Burdock 50 mg • Horsetail 50 mg • Sage 50 mg.

MultiBite Plus Iron - GNC
Each tablet contains: Vitamin A (14% as Beta Carotene, 86% as Retinyl Acetate) 2500 IU • Vitamin C (as sodium ascorbate) 60 mg • Vitamin D (as cholecaliferol) 400 IU • Vitamin E (as d-alpha tocopheryl acetate) 15 IU • Thiamin (as thiamin mononitrate) 1.05 mg • Riboflavin 1.2 mg • Niacin (as niacinamide) 13.5 mg • Vitamin B-6 (as pyridoxine hydrochloride) 1.05 mg • Folic Acid 300 mcg • Vitamin B-12 (as cyanocobalamin) 4.5 mcg • Iron (as carbonyl iron) 15 mg. Other Ingredients: Fructose, Sorbitol, Natural Flavors, Carmine Color.

Multi-Carotene - PhysioLogics
Each softgel contains: Beta-Carotene (pro-vitamin A activity) 25,000 IU • Vitamin E (as mixed tocopherols) 3 IU • Alpha-Carotene 1 mg • Lycopene 5 mg • Lutein 6 mg • Zeaxanthin 0.3 mg • Proprietary Blend 5 mg: Carrot, Tomato, Spinach concentrates, Medium Chain Triglycerides (MCT's). Other Ingredients: Gelatin, Glycerin, Beeswax and Soybean Oil Mixture, Lecithin, St. John's Bread Extract, Caramel Color.

Multi-Carotene Antioxidant - Nature's Way
Each softgel contains: Alpha Carotene 9900 mcg • Beta Carotene 18,600 mcg • Gamma Carotene 1200 mcg • Lycopene 30 mcg.

Multi-Chelated Boron 3 mg - Solgar
Each vegetable capsule contains: Sodium 5 mg • Boron (as boron citrate, glycinate, aspartate chelate) 3 mg. Other Ingredients: Microcrystalline Cellulose, Vegetable Cellulose, Vegetable Stearic Acid, Water.

Multi-Enzyme Formula - Puritan's Pride
Each tablet contains: Betaine 200 mg • Pepsin 50 mg • Bromelain 50 mg • Amylase 100 mg • Lipase 25 mg • Cellulase 10 mg • Papain 50 mg • Protease 100 mg • Ox Bile 30 mg • Pancrease Substance 200 mg.
See Editor's Note No. 14.

Multi-Gel - J. R. Carlson Laboratories, Inc.
Six softgels contain: Vitamin A (as beta carotene) 6000 IU • Vitamin C (as calcium ascorbate) 1200 IU • Vitamin D (D3, cholecalciferol) 1200 IU • Vitamin E (as D-alpha tocopherol) 400 IU • Vitamin K 40 mcg • Thiamin (vitamin B1, as thiamin mononitrate) 50 mg • Riboflavin (vitamin B2) 50 mg • Niacin (vitamin B3, as niacinamide) 50 mg • Vitamin B6 (as pyridoxine hydrochloride) 50 mg • Folate (folic acid) 600 mcg • Vitamin B12 (cyanocobalamin) 100 mcg • Biotin 300 mcg • Pantothenic Acid (as di-calcium pantothenate) 50 mg • Calcium (carbonate & ascorbate) 1000 mg • Iron (as iron glycinate chelate) 18 mg • Iodine (from potassium iodide) 18 mg • Magnesium (as magnesium oxide) 400 mg • Zinc (as zinc citrate) 15 mg • Selenium (as L-selenomethionine) 105 mcg • Copper (as copper gluconate) 2 mg • Manganese (as citrate) 2 mg • Lutein 600 mg • Papaya concentrate 60 mg • Phosphatidyl Choline 107 mg • Phosphatidyl Inositol 7 mg • Chromium (as amino acid chelate) 180 mcg • Rutin 60 mg • Alpha Lipoic 12 mg • Bioflavonoids 60 mg • CoQ10 (coenzyme Q10) 12 mg • Lecithin 60 mg.

Multigenics - Metagenics
Six tablets contain: Vitamin A (25% as retinyl acetate and 75% as beta-carotene) 20,000 IU • Vitamin E (as D-alpha tocopheryl succinate) 100 IU • Vitamin D (as cholecalciferol) 20 IU • Vitamin C (as ascorbic acid) 1200 mg • Niacin (as niacinamide, niacin) 420 mg • Betaine Hydrochloride 325 mg • Choline (as choline bitartrate) 200 mg • Inositol 188 mg • Pantothenic Acid (as D-calcium pantothenate) 200 mg • Citrus Bioflavonoid Complex 100 mg • Para-Aminobenzoic Acid (PABA) 50 mg • Vitamin B6 (as pyridoxine hydrochloride) 40 mg • Riboflavin 34 mg • Thiamin (as thiamin mononitrate) 30 mg • Folate (as folic acid) 800 mcg • Biotin 300 mcg • Vitamin B12 (as cyanocobalamin) 200 mcg • Calcium (as calcium citrate) 500 mg • Magnesium (as magnesium bis-glycinate, citrate) 250 mg • Potassium (as potassium aspartate) 99 mg • Iron (as iron glycinate) 10 mg • Zinc (as zinc aspartate) 20 mg • Manganese (as manganese aspartate) 1 mg • Copper (as copper lysinate) 2 mg • Chromium (as chromium dinicotinate glycinate) 200 mcg • Selenium (as selenium aspartate) 200 mcg • Iodine (as potassium iodide) 150 mcg • Molybdenum (as molybdenum aspartate) 100 mcg • Vanadium (as vanadyl sulfate) 39 mcg • Quercetin (as quercetin dihydrate) 25 mg • Alpha-Carotene 162 mcg • Cryptoxanthin 43 mcg • Zeaxanthin 23 mcg • Lutein 23 mcg.

Multigenics Chewable - Metagenics
Each tablet contains: Vitamin A (50% as retinyl acetate and 50% as beta-carotene) 2500 IU • Vitamin C (as magnesium ascorbate and ascorbic acid) 100 mg • Vitamin D (as cholecalciferol) 100 IU • Vitamin E (as D-alpha tocopheryl succinate) 20 IU • Thiamin (as thiamin mononitrate) 1.4 mg • Riboflavin 1.6 mg • Niacin (as niacinamide) 20 mg • Vitamin B6 (as pyridoxine hydrochloride) 1.4 mg • Folate (as folic acid) 300 mcg • Vitamin B12 (as cyanocobalamin) 6 mcg • Biotin 38 mcg • Pantothenic Acid (as D-calcium pantothenate) 10 mg • Calcium (as calcium citrate malate) 15 mg • Iron (as iron glycinate) 2 mg • Iodine (as potassium iodide) 70 mcg • Magnesium (as magnesium citrate, ascorbate) 15 mg • Zinc (as zinc gluconate) 2 mg • Copper (as copper lysinate) 100 mcg • Manganese (as manganese aspartate) 200 mcg • Quercetin (as quecetin dihydrate) 2 mg • Alpha-Carotene 13 mcg • Cryptoxanthin 4 mcg • Zeaxanthin 2 mcg • Lutein 2 mcg. Other Ingredients: Fructose, Xylitol, Sorbitol, Stearic Acid, Natural Flavors, Silica, Licorice Extract, Guar Gum, Malic Acid, Citric Acid.

Multigenics Intensive Care Formula - Metagenics
Eight tablets contain: Vitamin A (25% as retinyl acetate and 75% as beta-carotene) 20,000 IU • Vitamin D (as cholecalciferol) 400 IU • Vitamin E (as D-alpha tocopheryl succinate) 100 IU • Vitamin C (as ascorbic acid) 1200 mg • Thiamin (as thiamin mononitrate) 30 mg • Riboflavin 34 mg • Niacin (as niacin and niacinamide) 420 mg • Pantothenic Acid (as D-calcium pantothenate) 200 mg • Vitamin B6 (as pyridoxine hydrochloride) 40 mg • Folate (as folic acid, L-5-methyl tetrahydrofolate, 5-formyl tetrahydrofolate) 800 mcg • Vitamin B12 (as cyanocobalamin) 200 mcg • Biotin 200 mcg • Betaine Hydrochloride 175 mg • Choline (as choline bitartrate) 125 mg • Inositol 120 mg • Para-Aminobenzoic Acid (PABA) 50 mg •

Citrus Bioflavonoid Complex 100 mg • Calcium (as calcium citrate, MCHC, and calcium glycinate) 500 mg • Magnesium (as magnesium bis-glycinate, citriate) 250 mg • Potassium (as potassium aspartate) 99 mg • Iron (as iron glycinate) 10 mg • Phosphorus (as MCHC) 115 mg • Iodine (as potassium iodide) 150 mcg • Chromium (as chromium dinicotinate glycinate) 200 mcg • Selenium (as selenium aspartate) 200 mcg • Molybdenum (as molybdenum aspartate) 100 mcg • Vanadium (as vanadyl sulfate) 39 mcg • L-Glutamine 100 mg • Quercetin (as quercetin dihydrate) 25 mg • Alpha-Carotene 194 mcg • Cryptoxanthin 55 mcg • Zeaxanthin 27 mcg • Lutein 27 mcg • SOD Precursor Blend: Copper (as copper lysinate) 2 mg, Zinc (as zinc glycinate, histidinate) 20 mg, Manganese (as manganese glycinate) 1 mg.

Multigenics Intensive Care Formula without Iron - Metagenics
Eight tablets contain: Vitamin A (25% as retinyl acetate and 75% as beta-carotene) 20,000 IU • Vitamin D (as cholecalciferol) 400 IU • Vitamin E (as D-alpha tocopheryl succinate) 100 IU • Vitamin C (as ascorbic acid) 1200 mg • Thiamin (as thiamin mononitrate) 30 mg • Riboflavin 34 mg • Niacin (as niacin and niacinamide) 420 mg • Pantothenic Acid (as D-calcium pantothenate) 200 mg • Vitamin B6 (as pyridoxine hydrochloride) 40 mg • Folate (as folic acid, L-5-methyl tetrahydrofolate, 5-formyl tetrahydrofolate) 800 mcg • Vitamin B12 (as cyanocobalamin) 200 mcg • Biotin 200 mcg • Betaine Hydrochloride 175 mg • Choline (as choline bitartrate) 125 mg • Inositol 120 mg • Para-Aminobenzoic Acid (PABA) 50 mg • Citrus Bioflavonoid Complex 100 mg • Calcium (as calcium citrate, MCHC, and calcium glycinate) 500 mg • Magnesium (as magnesium bis-glycinate, citrate) 250 mg • Potassium (as potassium aspartate) 99 mg • Phosphorus (as MCHC) 115 mg • Iodine (as potassium iodide) 150 mcg • Chromium (as chromium dinicotinate glycinate) 200 mcg • Selenium (as selenium aspartate) 200 mcg • Molybdenum (as molybdenum aspartate) 100 mcg • Vanadium (as vanadyl sulfate) 39 mcg • L-Glutamine 100 mg • Quercetin (as quercetin dihydrate) 25 mg • Alpha-Carotene 194 mcg • Cryptoxanthin 55 mcg • Zeaxanthin 27 mcg • Lutein 27 mcg • SOD Precursor Blend: Copper (as copper lysinate) 2 mg, Zinc (as zinc glycinate, histidinate) 20 mg, Manganese (as manganese glycinate) 1 mg.

Multigenics Powder - Metagenics
Each rounded scoop (12 g) contains: Vitamin A (66% as beta-carotene and 33% [5000 IU] as retinyl acetate) 15,000 IU • Vitamin D (as cholecalciferol) 10 IU • Vitamin E (as D-alpha tocopheryl succinate) 100 IU • Vitamin C (as calcium ascorbate) 600 mg • Niacin (as niacinamide and niacin) 210 mg • Thiamin (as thiamin mononitrate) 15 mg • Riboflavin 17 mg • Vitamin B6 (as pyridoxine hydrochloride) 30 mg • Pantothenic Acid (as D-calcium pantothenate) 80 mg • Para-Aminobenzoic Acid (PABA) 25 mg • Folate (as folic acid) 400 mcg • Biotin 180 mcg • Vitamin B12 (as cyanocobalamin) 66 mcg • Betaine Hydrochloride 166 mg • Calcium (as calcium citrate, malate, ascorbate) 300 mg • Phosphorus (as rice fiber) 150 mg • Magnesium (as magnesium bis-glycinate) 60 mg • Potassium (as potassium aspartate) 130 mg • Sodium 10 mg • Iodine (as potassium iodide) 75 mcg • Zinc (as zinc aspartate) 10 mg • Iron (as iron glycinate) 2 mg • Copper (as amino acid chelate) 1 mg • Manganese (as manganese aspartate) 500 mcg • Selenium (as selenium aspartate) 102 mcg • Chromium (as chromium dinicotinate glycinate) 99 mcg • Vanadium (as vanadyl sulfate) 50 mcg • Molybdenum (as molybdenum aspartate) 50 mcg • Choline (as choline bitartrate) 102 mg • Inositol 97 mg • Lemon Bioflavonoid Complex 50 mg • Sulforaphane (as broccoli powder) 20 mcg • Lutein (as spinach powder) 8 mcg • Quercetin 17 mg • Lycopene (as tomato powder) 5 mcg • Stevia leaves (stevia rebaudiana) 60 mg. Other Ingredients: Rice Fiber Concentrate, Rice Syrup Solids, Guar Gum, Citric Acid, Natural Flavor, Rice Protein.

Multigenics Without Iron - Metagenics
Six tablets contain: Vitamin A (25% [5000 IU] as retinyl acetate and 75% as beta-carotene) 20,000 IU • Vitamin E (as D-alpha tocopheryl succinate) 100 IU • Vitamin D (as cholecalciferol) 20 IU • Vitamin C (as ascorbic acid) 1200 mg • Niacin (as niacinamide, niacin) 420 mg • Betaine Hydrochloride 325 mg • Choline (as choline bitartrate) 200 mg • Inositol 188 mg • Pantothenic Acid (as D-calcium pantothenate) 200 mg • Citrus Bioflavonoid Complex 100 mg • Para-Aminobenzoic Acid (PABA) 50 mg • Vitamin B6 (as pyridoxine hydrochloride) 40 mg • Riboflavin 34 mg • Thiamin (as thiamin mononitrate) 30 mg • Folate (as folic acid) 800 mg • Biotin 300 mcg • Vitamin B12 (as cyanocobalamin) 200 mcg • Calcium (as calcium citrate) 500 mg • Magnesium (as magnesium bis-glycinate, citrate) 250 mg • Potassium (as potassium aspartate) 99 mg • Zinc (as zinc aspartate) 20 mg • Manganese (as manganese aspartate) 1 mg • Copper (as copper lysinate) 2 mg • Chromium (as chromium dinicotinate glycinate) 200 mcg • Selenium (as selenium aspartate) 200 mcg • Iodine (as potassium iodide) 150 mcg • Molybdenum (as molybdenum aspartate) 100 mcg • Vanadium (as vandyl sulfate) 39 mcg • Quercetin (as quercetin dihydrate) 25 mg • Alpha-Carotene 162 mcg • Cryptoxanthin 43 mcg • Zeaxanthin 23 mcg • Lutein 23 mcg.

Multiglan Chelate - Atrium Biotechnologies
Six tablets contain: Calcium 500 mg • Magnesium 250 mg • Potassium 99 mg • Manganese 10 mg • Iron 18 mg • Silicon 2 mg • Zinc 15 mg • Iodine (Kelp) 150 mcg • Chromium 200 mcg • Selenium 25 mcg • Molybdenum 150 mcg • Vanadium 150 mcg • Chelated Proteinates, together in a base of of Raw Tissue concentrates (not extracts): Spleen 144 mg, Brain 30 mg, Liver 20 mg, Heart 14 mg, Thymus 4 mg, Adrenal 4 mg, Pancreas 4 mg, Duodenum 4 mg, Pituitary 2 mg) 240 mg.
See Editor's Note No. 31.

Multiglan Plus - Atrium Biotechnologies
Each tablet contains: Spleen 256.5 mg • Brain 67.5 mg • Liver 45 mg • Heart 31.5 mg • Kidney 31.5 mg • Thymus 8 mg • Adrenal 8 mg • Pituitary 2 mg • Pancreas 9 mg • Duodenum 9 mg.
See Editor's Note No. 31.

MultiLogics - PhysioLogics
Each caplet contains: Vitamin A (83% as beta carotene, 17% as retinyl palmitate) 15,000 IU • Vitamin C (as ascorbic acid) 250 mg • Vitamin D (as cholecalciferol) 400 IU • Vitamin E (as d-alpha tocopherol acetate) 150 IU • Thiamin (vitamin B1, as thiamin mononitrate) 75 mg • Riboflavin (vitamin B2) 75 mg • Niacin (as niacinamide) 75 mg • Vitamin B6 (as pyridoxine hydrochloride) 75 mg • Folic Acid 400 mcg • Vitamin B12 (as cyanocobalamin) 75 mcg • Biotin 300 mcg • Pantothenic Acid (as d-calcium pantothenate) 75 mg • Calcium (as lithothamnium coralloids, dicalcium phosphate) 57 mg • Iron (as iron amino acid chelate) 1 mg • Iodine (as potassium iodide) 150 mcg • Magnesium (as magnesium amino acid chelate, magnesium oxide) 11mg • Zinc (as zinc amino acid chelate) 10 mg • Selenium (as selenomethionate) 25 mcg • Copper (as copper amino acid chelate) 1 mg • Manganese (as manganese amino acid chelate) 1 mg • Chromium (as chromium amino acid chelate) 25 mcg • Molybdenum (as molybdenum amino acid chelate, molybdenum yeast) 27 mcg • Boron (as boron amino acid chelate) 500 mcg • Inositol 75 mg • PABA (para-aminobenzoic acid) 75 mg • Choline (as choline bitartrate) 31 mg • Betaine Hydrochloride 25 mg • Citrus Bioflavonoids (citrus spp., fruit) 25 mg • Rutin (dimorphandra mollis, fruit) 25 mg • Hesperidin complex (citrus aurandum, citrus spp., fruit) 5 mg. Other Ingredients: Cellulose (plant origin), Croscarmellose, Vegetable Stearic Acid, Silica, Cellulose Coating.

MultiLogics for Children - PhysioLogics
Two tablets contain: Vitamin A (as 67% Beta-Carotene, 33% Fish Liver oil) 7500 IU • Vitamin C (as Ascorbic Acid) 180 mg • Vitamin D (as Vitamin D3)(from Fish Liver oil) 200 IU • Vitamin E (as D-Alpha Tocopherol Succinate) 90 IU • Vitamin K (as Phytonadione) 30 mcg • Thiamine (as Thiamine Mononitrate) 3 mg • Riboflavin (Vitamin B2) 3.4 mg • Niacin (as Niacinamide) 20 mg • Vitamin B6 (as Pyridoxine HCl) 4 mg • Folic Acid 400 mcg • Vitamin B12 12 mcg • Biotin 300 mcg • Pantothenic Acid (as d-Calcium Panthothenate) 20 mg • Calcium (as Calcium Citrate-Aspartate Complex) 100 mg • Iron (as Iron Carbonyl) 4.5 mg • Iodine (as Potassium Iodide, Kelp) 75 mcg • Magnesium (as Magnesium Citrate-Aspartate Complex) 100 mg • Zinc (as Amino Acid Zinc

Chelate) 5 mg • Selenium (as Amino Acid Selenium Complex) 50 mcg • Copper (as Copper Gluconate) 400 mcg • Manganese (as Amino Acid Manganese Chelate) 1 mg • Chromium (as Chromium Polynicotinate) 50 mcg • Molybdenum (as Amino Acid Molybdenum Chelate) 50 mcg • Black Currant seed 5 mg • Choline (Bitartate) 5 mg • Boron (Aspartate-Citrate) 1 mg.

MultiLogics for Men - PhysioLogics
Three tablets contain: Vitamin E (d-alpha tocopherol acetate) 250 IU • Calcium (aquamins, carbonate) 530 mg • Magnesium (amino acid chelate/oxide) 140 mg • Zinc (amino acid chelate) 15 mg • Iron (ferrous bisglycinate) 5 mg • Copper (amino acid chelate) 1 mg • Chromium (amino acid chelate) 175 mcg • Selenium (amino acid complex) 175 mcg • Tomato extract (1% lycopene, 1.6 mg) 160 mg • Saw Palmetto berry (20-25% fatty acids & lipid sterols 15-18.75 mg) 75 mg • Bioflavonoids (citrus spp.) 50 mg • Rutin 50 mg • Hesperidin 50 mg • Green Tea leaf (45% Polyphenols, 22.5 mg) 50 mg • Betaine HCl 50 mg • Ginkgo Biloba leaf (24% ginkgo flavonglycosides, 9.6 mg; 6% terpene lactones, 24 mg) 40 mg • Nettles (1-2% silica, 300-600 mcg) 30 mg • Beta Sitosterol 30 mg • Black Cohosh root (cimicifuga racemosa) 25 mg • Grapeseed extract (vitis vinifera, standardized to contain 50% proanthocyanidins)25 mg • Tomato concentrate (lycopersicon esculentum, equivalent to tomato 108 mg) 10.8 mg • Black Pepper (piper nigrum) 5 mg • Lutein 3 mg • Tomato extract (blakelea trispora, standardized to cotain 3% lycopenes) 1.6 mg. Other Ingredients: Cellulose (plant origin), Croscarmellose, Vegetable Stearic Acid, Polyvinylpyrrolidone, Silica, Vegetable Magnesium Stearate, Cellulose Coating.

MultiLogics for Women - PhysioLogics
Three caplets contain: Vitamin E (as d-alpha tocopheryl acetate) 250 IU • Calcium (as lithothamnium coralliodes, calcium carbonate) 530 mg • Iron (as ferrous bisglycinate) 5 mg • Magnesium (as magnesium amino acid chelate, magnesium oxide) 130 mg • Zinc (as zinc amino acid chelate) 15 mg • Selenium (as selenium amino acid chelate) 174 mcg • Copper (as copper amino acid chelate) 1 mg • Chromium (as chromium amino acid chelate) 174 mcg • Boron (as boron amino acid chelate) 500 mcg • Betaine Hydrochloride 50 mg • Citrus Bioflavonoids (fruit) 50 mg • Green Tea extract (Camellia sinensis, leaf, standardized to contain 50% polyphenols 25 mg) 50 mg • Hesperidin Complex (citrus aurantium and citrus spp., fruit) 50 mg • Rutin (dimorphandra mollis, fruit) 50 mg • Ginkgo Biloba extract (leaf, standardized to contain 24% alkaloids 9.6 mg) 40 mg • Black Cohosh (cimicifuga racemosa, root) 25 mg • Chasteberry extract (vitex agnus castus fruit, standardized to contain 0.5% agmisode 1.26 mg) 25 mg • Dong Quai (angelica sinensis root, 1% ligustilides) 25 mg • Grape seed extract (vitis vinifera leaf, standardized to contain 50% proantocyanids 12.5 mg) 25 g • Choline (as choline bitartrate) 20 mg • Kudzu extract (pueraria thomsonii root, standardized to contain 1% daidzein 0.12 mg) 13 mg • Tomato concentrate (lycopersicon esculentum fruit, equivalent to 108 mg of tomato) 11 mg • Black Pepper (piper nigrum fruit) 5 mg • Lutein 3 mg • Lycopene (from tomato, blakeslea trispora, standardized to contain 3% lycopenes 0.02 mg) 2 mg. Other Ingredients: Cellulose, Croscarmellose, Vegetable Stearic Acid, Polyvinylpyrrolidone, Silica, Vegetable Magnesium Stearate, Cellulose Coating, Potassium Amino Acid Chelate.

Multi-Mega Minerals - Puritan's Pride
Two tablets contain: Calcium 1,000 mg • Magnesium 500 mg • Iron 30 mg • Manganese 10 mg • Potassium 95 mg • Chromium 100 mcg • Vitamin D 400 IU • Iodine 150 mcg • Copper 3 mg • Zinc 22.5 mg. Other Components: Betaine Hydrochloride 100 mg • Glutamic Acid Hydrochloride 100 mg • Chloride 90 mg.

Multi-Min Chelate - Metagenics
Each tablet contains: Calcium (as calcium citrate, tricalcium phosphate, MCHC) 83 mg • Magnesium (as magnesium citrate, magnesium bis-glycinate) 67 mg • Potassium (as potassium chloride, iodide) 33 mg • Phosphorus (as tricalcim phosphate, MCHC) 7 mg • Iron (as iron glycinate) 7 mg • Zinc (as zinc glycinate) 7 mg • Copper (as copper lysinate) 1 mg • Magnanese (as manganese glycinate) 1 mg • Iodine (as potassium iodide) 50 mcg • Selenium (as selenium aspartate) 33 mcg • Chromium (as chromium dinicotinate glycinate) 30 mcg • Vanadium (as vanadium maltol complex) 17 mcg • Molybdenum (as molybdenum aspartate) 17 mcg • Vitamin C (as ascorbic acid) 125 mg • Vitamin D (as cholecalciferol) 33 IU • Betaine Hydrochloride 108 mg • Horsetail aerial part (equisetum arvense, natural source of silica) 8.25 mg.

Multimineral - Benepure, Inc
Each tablet contains: Calcium 333 mg • Iron 6.7 mg • Iodine (from kelp) 50 mcg • Magnesium 167 mg • Zinc 10 mg • Selenium 17 mcg • Copper 0.7 mg • Chromium 33 mcg • Potassium 33 mg. Other Ingredients: Microcrystalline Cellulose, Croscarmellose Sodium, Silica, Stearic Acid, Vegetable Stearate.

Multi-Mineral Citrate Complete - The Vitamin Shoppe
Eight capsules contain: Calcium 1000 mg • Magnesium 500 mg • Potassium 99 mg • Zinc 50 mg • Boron 3 mg • Copper 2 mg • Selenium 100 mcg • Chromium 200 mcg • Molybdenum 100 mcg • Iron 10 mg • Manganese 10 mg.

Multi-Minerals - The Vitamin Shoppe
Three tablets contain: Calcium 1000 mg • Zinc 22.5 • Copper 1 mg • Selenium 50 mcg • Chromium 100 mcg • Vanadium 50 mcg • Glutamic Acid 50 mg • Magnesium 500 mg • Iron 20 mg • Potassium 99 mg • Manganese 5 mg • Boron 3 mg • Molybdenum 50 mcg • Iodine 150 mcg • Vitamin D 200 IU.

Multi-Minerals Citrate Formula - Vital Nutrients
Four capsules contain: Calcium (citrate/malate) 300 mg • Magnesium (citrate) 270 mg • Potassium (citrate) 90 mg • Zinc (citrate) 21 mg • Manganese (citrate) 4 mg • Boron (citrate) 3 mg • Chromium (polynicotinate) 200 mcg • Selenium (selenomethionine) 150 mcg • Vanadium (citrate) 10 mcg • Iodine (potassium iodide) 120 mcg • Molybdenum (citrate) 90 mcg.

Multi-Minerals Complex - Schiff
Three tablets contain: Vitamin D (as cholecalciferol) 400 IU • Calcium (as calcium carbonate) 1.2 g • Iron (as ferrous fumarate) 18 mg • Iodine (from kelp) 150 mcg • Magnesium (as magnesium oxide) 600 mg • Zinc (as zinc citrate) 30 mg • Selenium (as L-selenomethionine) 100 mcg • Copper (as copper gluconate) 2 mg • Manganese (as manganese gluconate) 10 mg • Chromium (as amino acid chelate) 100 mcg • Molybdenum (as amino acid chelate) 100 mcg • Potassium (as potassium citrate) 99 mg • Proprietary Mineral Transport Blend 64 mg: Citrates, Fumerates, Succinates, Gluconates, Aspartates, Ascorbates, Amino Acid Chelates, Ketoglutarates, Picolinates • Boron (as boron aspartate) 3 mg. Other Ingredients: Cellulose, Croscarmellose Sodium, Stearic Acid, Methylcellulose Polyethylene Glycol, Magnesium Stearate.

Multi-mune - Purity Life International
Three capsules contain: Vitamin A (as palmitate) 1605 IU • Vitamin C (as calcium ascorbate, magnesium ascorbate) 1 g • Vitamin E (as D-alpha tocopherol succinate) 1000 IU • Vitamin B6 (as pyridoxal-5-phosphate) 45 mg • Magnesium (as glycinate, ascorbate) 100 mg • Zinc (as citrate) 15 mg • Selenium (as selenomethionine) 100 mcg • Coenzyme Q10 (ubiquinone) 30 mg • Reduced L-Gluthione 45 mg • Alpha Lipoic Acid (thioctic acid) 30 mg. Other Ingredients: Gelatin.

Multi-Nutrients - Vital Nutrients
Six capsules contain: VItamin A (acetate) 5000 IU • Betatene brand natural Beta Carotene (with mixed carotenoids) 20,000 IU • Vitamin D (D3, from lanolin) 400 IU • Natural Vitamin E (D-alpha tocopheryl succinate) 400 IU • Ascorbic Acid 1000 mg • Thiamine HCl (vitamin B1) 100 mg • Riboflavin (pure powder) 50 mg • Riboflavin 5-Phosphate (activated vitamin B2) 10 mg • Niacinamide 100 mg • Inositol Hexaniacinate (no-flush niacin) 50 mg • Pyridoxine HCl (vitamin B6) 50 mg • Pyridoxal-5-Phosphate (activated vitamin B6) 15 mg • Vitamin B5 (calcium pantothenate) 400 mg • Hydroxocobalamin (pure vitamin B12) 500 mcg • Folic Acid 800 mcg • Biotin 400 mcg • Calcium (50% citrate/malate, 50% carbonate) 400 mg • Calcium (pantothenate) 33 mg • Magnesium (50% citrate, 50% oxide) 300 mg • Potassium (chloride) 99 mg • Zinc (citrate) 25 mg • Manganese (aspartate) 5 mg • Copper (glycinate)

2 mg • Boron (citrate) 500 mcg • Chromium (polynicotinate) 200 mcg • Selenium (selenomethionine) 200 mcg • Vanadium (vanadyl sulfate) 200 mcg • Molybdenum (aspartate) 100 mcg.

Multi-Nutrients (veg caps) - Vital Nutrients
Six veggie capsules contain: VItamin A (acetate) 5000 IU • Betatene brand natural Beta Carotene (with mixed carotenoids) 20,000 IU • Vitamin D (D3, from lanolin) 400 IU • Natural Vitamin E (D-alpha tocopheryl succinate) 400 IU • Ascorbic Acid 1000 mg • Thiamine HCl (vitamin B1) 100 mg • Riboflavin (pure powder) 50 mg • Riboflavin 5-Phosphate (activated vitamin B2) 10 mg • Niacinamide 100 mg • Inositol Hexaniacinate (no-flush niacin) 50 mg • Pyridoxine HCl (vitamin B6) 50 mg • Pyridoxal-5-Phosphate (activated vitamin B6) 15 mg • Vitamin B5 (calcium pantothenate) 400 mg • Hydroxocobalamin (pure vitamin B12) 500 mcg • Folic Acid 800 mcg • Biotin 400 mcg • Calcium (50% citrate/malate, 50% carbonate) 400 mg • Calcium (pantothenate) 33 mg • Magnesium (50% citrate, 50% oxide) 300 mg • Potassium (chloride) 99 mg • Zinc (citrate) 25 mg • Manganese (aspartate) 5 mg • Copper (glycinate) 2 mg • Boron (citrate) 500 mcg • Chromium (polynicotinate) 200 mcg • Selenium (selenomethionine) 200 mcg • Vanadium (vanadyl sulfate) 200 mcg • Molybdenum (aspartate) 100 mcg.

Multi-Nutrients II Citrate Formula (Copper, no Iron) - Vital Nutrients
Six capsules contain: Betatene brand natural Beta Carotene (with mixed carotenoids) 20,000 IU • Ascorbic Acid 850 mg • Vitamin D (D3, from lanolin) 400 IU • Natural Vitamin E (D-alpha tocopheryl succinate) 400 IU • Thiamine HCl (vitamin B1) 50 mg • Riboflavin (pure powder) 15 mg • Riboflavin 5-Phosphate (activated vitamin B2) 10 mg • Niacinamide 150 mg • Inositol Hexaniacinate (no-flush niacin) 10 mg • Pyridoxine HCl (vitamin B6) 15 mg • Pyridoxal-5-Phosphate (activated vitamin B6) 10 mg • Folic Acid 800 mcg • Hydroxocobalamin (pure vitamin B12) 500 mcg • Biotin 400 mcg • Vitamin B5 (calcium pantothenate) 450 mg • Iodine (potassium iodide) 225 mcg • Calcium (96% citrate/malate, 4% pantothenate) 400 mg • Magnesium (citrate) 285 mg • Zinc (citrate) 15 mg • Copper (glycinate) 2 mg • Selenium (selenomethionine) 200 mcg • Manganese (citrate) 6 mg • Chromium (polynicotinate) 200 mcg • Molybdenum (citrate) 100 mcg • Potassium (citrate) 90 mg • Boron (citrate) 3 mg • Vanadium (citrate) 100 mcg.

Multi-Nutrients III Citrate Formula (without Copper & Iron) - Vital Nutrients
Six capsules contain: Betatene brand natural Beta Carotene (with mixed carotenoids) 20,000 IU • Ascorbic Acid 850 mg • Vitamin D (D3, from lanolin) 400 IU • Natural Vitamin E (D-alpha tocopheryl succinate) 400 IU • Thiamine HCl (vitamin B1) 50 mg • Riboflavin (pure powder) 15 mg • Riboflavin 5-Phosphate (activated vitamin B2) 10 mg • Niacinamide 150 mg • Inositol Hexaniacinate (no-flush niacin) 10 mg • Pyridoxine HCl (vitamin B6) 15 mg • Pyridoxal-5-Phosphate 10 mg • Folic Acid 800 mcg • Hydroxocobalamin (pure vitamin B12) 500 mcg • Biotin 400 mcg • Vitamin B5 (calcium pantothenate) 450 mg • Iodine (potassium iodide) 225 mcg • Calcium (96% citrate/malate, 4% pantothenate) 400 mg • Magnesium (citrate) 285 mg • Zinc (citrate) 15 mg • Selenium (selenomethionine) 200 mcg • Manganese (citrate) 6 mg • Chromium (polynicontinate) 200 mcg • Molybdenum (citrate) 100 mcg • Potassium (citrate) 90 mg • Boron (citrate) 3 mg • Vanadium (citrate) 100 mcg.

Multi-Nutrients IV (Citrate Formula) - Vital Nutrients
Six capsules contain: Betatene brand natural Beta Carotene (with mixed carotenoids) 20,000 IU • Ascorbic Acid 850 mg • Vitamin D (D3, from lanolin) 400 IU • Natural Vitamin E (D-alpha tocopheryl succinate) 400 IU • Thiamine HCl (vitamin B1) 50 mg • Riboflavin (pure powder) 15 mg • Riboflavin 5-Phosphate (activated vitamin B2) 10 mg • Niacinamide 150 mg • Inositol Hexaniacinate (no flush niacin) 10 mg • Pyridoxine HCl (vitamin B6) 15 mg • Pyridoxal-5-Phosphate (activated vitamin B6) 10 mg • Folic Acid 800 mcg • Hydroxocobalamin (pure vitamin B12) 500 mcg • Biotin 400 mcg • Vitamin B5 (calcium pantothenate) 450 mg • Iodine (potassium iodide) 225 mcg • Calcium (96% citrate/malate, 4% pantothenate) 400 mg • Magnesium (citrate) 285 mg • Zinc (citrate) 15 mg • Copper (glycinate) 2 mg • Iron (aspartate) 10 mg • Selenium (selenomethionine) 200 mcg • Manganese (citrate) 6 mg • Chromium (polynicotinate) 200 mcg • Molybdenum (citrate) 100 mcg • Potassium (citrate) 90 mg • Boron (citrate) 3 mg • Vanadium (citrate) 100 mcg.

Multi-Nutrients V (No Boron or Copper) - Vital Nutrients
Four capsules contain: Vitamin A (acetate) 2500 IU • Betatene brand natural Beta Carotene (with mixed carotenoids) 15,000 IU • Vitamin D (D3, from lanolin) 400 IU • Natural Vitamin E (D-alpha tocopheryl succinate) 300 IU • Ascorbic Acid 250 mg • Thiamine HCl (vitamin B1) 25 mg • Riboflavin (pure powder) 50 mg • Niacinamide 100 mg • Vitamin B5 (calcium pantothenate) 100 mg • Pyridoxine HCl (vitamin B6) 25 mg • Pyridoxal-5-Phosphate (activated vitamin B6) 5 mg • Hydroxocobalamin (pure vitamin B12) 1000 mcg • Folic Acid 800 mcg • Biotin 300 mcg • Quercetin 100 mg • Calcium (citrate/malate) 250 mg • Magnesium (citrate) 200 mg • Zinc (citrate) 30 mg • Manganese (citrate) 5 mg • Molybdenum (aspartate) 100 mcg • Iodine (potassium iodide) 150 mcg • Chromium (polynicotinate) 200 mcg • Selenium (selenomethionine) 400 mcg • Vanadium (vanadyl sulfate) 10 mcg.

Multi-Nutrients with Iron and Iodine - Vital Nutrients
Six capsules contain: Vitamin A (acetate) 5000 IU • Iron (aspartate) 18 mg • Iodine (from kelp) 150 mcg • Betatene brand natural Beta Carotene (with mixed carotenoids) 20,000 IU • Vitamin D (D3, from lanolin) 400 IU • Natural Vitamin E (D-alpha tocopheryl succinate) 400 IU • Ascorbic Acid 1000 mg • Thiamine HCl (vitamin B1) 100 mg • Riboflavin (pure powder) 50 mg • Riboflavin 5-Phosphate (activated vitamin B2) 10 mg • Niacinamide 100 mg • Inositol Hexaniacinate (no-flush niacin) 50 mg • Pyridoxal-5-Phosphate (activated vitamin B6) 15 mg • Pyridoxine HCl (vitamin B6) 50 mg • Vitamin B5 (calcium pantothenate) 400 mg • Hydroxocobalamin (pure vitamin B12) 500 mcg • Folic Acid 800 mcg • Biotin 400 mcg • Calcium (50% citrate/malate, 50% carbonate) 400 mg • Calcium (pantothenate) 33 mg • Magnesium (50% citrate, 50% oxide) 300 mg • Potassium (chloride) 99 mg • Zinc (citrate) 25 mg • Manganese (aspartate) 5 mg • Copper (glycinate) 2 mg • Boron (citrate) 500 mcg • Chromium (polynicotinate) 200 mcg • Selenium (selenomethionine) 200 mcg • Vanadium (vanadyl sulfate) 200 mcg • Molybdenum (aspartate) 100 mcg.

MULTI-One - Westcoast Naturals
Each tablet contains: Vitamin A (palmitate) 10,000 IU • Vitamin B1 (thiamine HCl) 52 mg • Vitamin B2 (riboflavin) 52 mg • Vitamin B6 (pyridoxine HCl) 52 mg • Vitamin B12 (cyanocobalamin) 52 mcg • Vitamin C (ascorbic acid) 150 mg • Vitamin D (D3 as cholecalciferol) 400 IU • Vitamin E (D-alpha tocopheryl acetate) 50 IU • Folic Acid 0.2 mg • D-Pantothenic Acid (calcium D-pantothenate) 52 mg • Niacinamide 52 mg • Biotin (D-biotin) 52 mcg • Calcium (carbonate HVP chelate) 125 mg • Iron (HVP chelate) 4 mg • Magnesium (oxide HVP chelate) 50 mg • Zinc (gluconate) 10 mg • Manganese (HVP chelate) 1 mg • Copper (gluconate) 1 mg • Iodine (potassium iodide from kelp) 0.1 mg • Chromium (HVP chelate) 25 mg • Selenium (HVP chelate) 25 mg • Choline (bitartrate) 53 mg • Inositol 52 mg • DL-Methionine 52 mg. Base: Kelp, Flavonoids, Rutin, Spirulina, Hesperidin Complex, Alfalfa.

Multiple Mineral - Eidon Inc.
Each 1 tbsp serving contains: Boron 13.5 mcg • Calcium 2250 mcg • Chromium 0.9 mcg • Copper 9 mcg • Iodine 0.675 mcg • Iron 22.5 mcg • Magnesium 2250 mcg • Manganese 45 mcg • Potassium 445.5 mcg • Selenium 0.9 mcg • Silica 75000 mcg • Sulfur 6000 mcg • Zinc 135 mcg. Other Ingredients: Purified Water.

Multiple Mineral (Amino Acid) Chelate - Trophic
Each tablet contains: Calcium (amino acid chelate) 83.33 mg • Magnesium (amino acid chelate) 41.67 mg • Phosphorus (as proteinate) 33.33 mg • Potassium (as proteinate) 16.50 mg • Iron (amino acid chelate) 1.67 mg • Manganese (amino acid chelate) 1.67 mg • Zinc (amino acid chelate) 1.67 mg • Iodine (kelp) 25 mcg.

Multiple One - Pro Health
Each tablet contains: Vitamin A as Beta-Carotene 10,000 IU • Vitamin A (as retinyl palmitate) 10,000 IU • Vitamin C (ascorbic acid) 250 mg • Vitamin D (from natural fish liver oil) 400 IU • Vitamin E (as natural D-alpha tocopheryl succinate) 150 IU • Thiamine (as thiamine HCl) 75 mg • Riboflavin (vitamin B2) 75 mg • Niacin (as niacinamide) 75 mg • Vitamin B6 (pyridoxine HCl) 75 mg • Folate (folic acid) 400 mcg • Vitamin B12 (cyanocobalamin) 100 mcg • Biotin 100 mcg • Pantothenic Acid (from calcium pantothenate) 75 mg • Calcium (amino acid chelate, oyster shell) 100 mg • Iron (from amino acid chelate) 10 mg • Iodine (from kelp) 150 mcg • Magnesium (oxide, amino acid chelate) 60 mg • Zinc (amino acid chelate) 15 mg • Selenium (amino acid chelate) 25 mcg • Copper (amino acid chelate) 1 mg • Manganese (amino acid chelate) 5 mg • Chromium (yeast-free GTF) 50 mcg • Molybdenum (amino acid chelate) 50 mcg • Potassium (chloride) 10 mg • Boron (amino acid chelate) 500 mcg • Choline (bitatrate) 100 mg • Inositol 75 mg • PABA 30 mg • Rutin 25 mg • Betaine HCl 25 mg • Glutamic Acid 25 mg • Nucleic Acid 50 mg • Citrus Bioflavonoids (37% hesperidin) 100 mg. Base: Alfalfa, Parsley, Lecithin, Rose Hips, Dicalcium Phosphate, Cellulose, Stearic Acid, Silica.

Multiple Vitamin Essentials - Sunmark
Each tablet contains: Vitamin A 5000 IU • Vitamin B6 2 mg • Vitamin B12 6 mcg • Vitamin C 60 mg • Vitamin D 400 IU • Vitamin E 30 IU • Thiamin (vitamin B1) 1.5 mg • Riboflavin (vitamin B2) 1.7 mg • Niacin 20 mg • Folic Acid 400 mcg • Pantothenic Acid 10 mg. Other Ingredients: Gelatin, Starch, Microcrystalline Cellulose, Crospovidone, Dextrin, Stearic Acid, Hypromellose, FD&C Red No. 40 Lake, Polyethylene Glycol, Dextrose, Magnesium Stearate, Titanium Dioxide, Lecithin, Gluten, Beta Carotene, FD&C Yellow No. 6 Lake, FD&C Blue No. 2 Lake, Sodium Bisulfite.
See Editor's Note No. 45.

Multiple Vitamin Women's Formula - Sunmark
Each tablet contains: Vitamin A 2500 IU • Vitamin B6 2 mg • Vitamin B12 6 mcg • Vitamin C 60 mg • Vitamin D 400 IU • Vitamin E 30 IU • Thiamin (vitamin B1) 1.5 mg • Riboflavin (vitamin B2) 1.7 mg • Niacin 10 mg • Folic Acid 400 mcg • Magnesium 50 mg • Zinc 15 mg • Pantothenic Acid 5 mg • Calcium 450 mg • Iron 18 mg. Other Ingredients: Acacia, Gelatin, Modified Cellulose Gum, Stearic Acid, Titanium Dioxide, Dextrin, Hypromellose, Magnesium Stearate, Polyethylene Glycol, Dextrose, Sodium Lauryl Sulfate, Lecithin, Beta Carotene, FD&C Yellow No. 5 Lake, FD&C Yellow No. 6 Lake, FD&C Blue No. 2 Lake, Gluten.
See Editor's Note No. 45.

Multiple Vitamins & Minerals - Trophic
Each tablet contains: Vitamin A 10,000 IU • Vitamin D (as D3) 400 IU • Vitamin C 100 mg • Vitamin E 10 IU • Vitamin B1 10 mg • Vitamin B2 10 mg • Vitamin B6 10 mg • PABA 10 mg • D-Pantothenic Acid 10 mg • Citrus Bioflavonoids 10 mg • Rutin 10 mg • Glutamic Acid 10 mg • Papain 10 mg • Rose Hips 10 mg • Bromelain 10 mg • Niacin 25 mg • Choline Bitartrate 25 mg • Inositol 25 mg • Vitamin B12 10 mcg • Biotin 10 mcg • Folic Acid 10 mcg.

Multiple Vitamins & Minerals - GNC
Each tablet contains: Vitamin A (as beta-carotene) 5000 IU • Vitamin C (as Ascorbic Acid) 60 mg • Vitamin D (as Cholecalciferol) 400 IU • Vitamin E (as dl-alpha Tocopheryl Acetate) 30 IU • Thiamin (as Thiamin Mononitrate) 1.5 mg • Riboflavin 1.7 mg • Niacin (as Niacinamide) 20 mg •Vitamin B6 (as Pyridoxine Hydrochloride) 2 mg • Folate, Folic Acid, Folacin 400 mcg • Vitamin B12 (as Cyanocobalamin) 6 mcg • Biotin 30 mcg • Pantothenic Acid (as Calcium d-Pantothenate) 10 mg • Calcium (as Dicalcium Phosphate) 162 mg • Iron (as Carbonyl Iron) 18 mg •Phosphorus (as Cicalcium Phosphate) 100 mg • Iodine (as Potassium Iodine) 150 mcg • Magnesium (as Magnesium Oxide) 100 mg • Zinc (as Zinc Sulfate) 15 mg • Selenium (as Sodium Selenate) 20 mg • Copper (as Copper Oxide) 2 mg • Manganese (as Manganese Sulfate) 7.5 mg • Chromium (as Chromium Chloride) 15 mcg • Molybdenum (as Sodium Molybdate) 15 mcg • Nickel (as Nickerl Sulfate) 5 mcg • Tin (as Stannous Chloride) 10 mcg • Silicon (as Sodium MetaSilicate) 2 mg • Vanadium (as Sodium MetaVanadate) 10 mcg • Boron (as Sodium Borate Decahydrate) 150 mcg. Other Ingredients: Cellulose, Vegetable Acetoglycerides, Stearic Acid, Titanium Dioxide.

Multiplex Formula - 4 Life
Each capsule contains: Vitamin A (as beta carotene) 5000 IU • Vitamin C (as ascorbic acid) 150 mg • Vitamin E (as D-alpha tocopheryl succinate) 30 IU • Thiamin (as thiamine mononitrate) 15 mg • Riboflavin (Vitamin B2) 17 mg • Niacin (as niacinamide) 33 mg • Vitamin B6 (as pyridoxine HCl) 8 mg • Folic Acid 600 mcg • Vitamin B12 (as cyanocobalamin) 15 mcg • Biotin 300 mcg • Pantothenic Acid (as calcium pantothenate) 22 mg • Zinc (as zinc fluconate) 10 mg • Selenium (as selenomethionine) 60 mcg • Chromium (as chromium picolinate) 75 mcg • Potassium (as potassium citrate) 33 mg • Hawaiian Spirulina Pacifica 90 mg • Citrus Bioflavanoids (from citrus fruit) 40 mg • Choline (as choline bitartrate) 27 mg • Para-Aminobenzoic (PABA) 25 mg • Inositol 24 mg • Lysine (as L-lysine monohydrochloride) 20 mg • Histidine (as L-histidine HCl monohydrate) 18 mg • Isoleucine (as L-isoleucine) 15 mg • Phenylanine (as DL-phenylalanine) 15 mg • Catnip leaf 15 mg • Rose Hips (Rosa canina) fruit 15 mg • English Hawthorn (berry) 10 mg • Licorice (root) 10 mg.

MULTI-Plus - Westcoast Naturals
Each caplet contains: Beta Carotene (as pro-vitamin A) 10,000 IU • Vitamin B1 4.5 mg • Vitamin B2 2.5 mg • Vitamin B6 2.5 mg • Vitamin B12 5 mcg • Vitamin C 100 mg • Vitamin D (as D3) 400 IU • Vitamin E 10 IU • Folic Acid 0.05 mg • D-Pantothenic Acid 5 mg • Niacinamide 20 mg • Biotin 10 mcg • Calcium 125 mg • Iron 4 mg • Magnesium 50 mg • Zinc 1 mg • Manganese 1 mg • Copper 1 mg • Iodine 0.10 mg • Potassium 10 mg • Choline Bitartrate 15 mg • Inositol 15 mg • DL-Methionine 20 mg • Glutamic Acid HCl 15 mg • Betaine HCl 10 mg • Bromelain 5 mg • Pepsin 5 mg • Lemon Bioflavonoids 25 mg • Para Aminobenzoic Acid (PABA) 15 mg • Rutin 10 mg • Echinacea 5 mg • Quercetin 5 mg • Apple Pectin 5 mg.

Multi-Quest - Nutri-Quest Rx
Three tablets contain: Vitamin A (Palmitate) 2000 IU • Vitamin D (as Vitamin D3) 400 IU • Vitamin E (Succinate) 200 IU • Vitamin C (Sago Palm) 1000 mg • Lemon Bioflavonoids 100 mg • Rutin 25 mg • Hesperidin Complex 50 mg • Vitamin B6 25 mg • Vitamin B1 13 mg • Vitamin B2 10 mg • Niacin 45 mg • Vitamin B12 30 mcg • Pantothenic Acid (Calcium Pantothenate) 50 mg • Folic Acid 200 mcg • Choline Bitartrate 100 mg • Inositol 100 mg • Biotin 400 mcg • PABA 50 mg • L-Glycine 9.66 mg • Calcium Gluconate 15.36 mg • Vitamin F 5 mg • Chlorophyll 16 mg • Calcium Aspartate 500 mg • Magnesium Aspartate 250 mg • Phosphorus Chelate 200 mg • Potassium Proteinate 30 mg • Copper Chelate 1 mg • Zinc Aspartate 5 mg • Manganese Aspartate 15 mg • Molybdenum Chelate 50 mcg • Chromium Chelate 25 mcg • Selenium Chelate 30 mcg • Iodine (kelp) 50 mcg • Sodium Proteinate 30 mcg • Rubidium Chelate 15 mcg • Lithium Chelate 8 mcg • L-Phenylalanine 13 mg • L-Histidine 6 mg • L-Tyrosine 9 mg • L-Lysine 13 mg • L-Valine 15 mg • DL-Methionine 9 mg • L-Isoleucine 13 mg • L-Leucine 18 mg • L-Threonine 9 mg • L-Glutamic Acid 2 mg • Goldenseal root 45 mg • Siberian Ginseng 45 mg • Garlic 40 mg • Tillandsia 30 mg • Rice Bran 176 mg • Almond Meal 150 mg.

Multiron Capsules - Vitabiotics
Each capsule contains: Vitamin A 750 mcg • Vitamin B1 (thiamin) 10 mg • Vitamin B2 (riboflavin) 2 mg • Vitamin B3 (niacin) 18 mg • Folic Acid 500 mcg • Vitamin B12 (cyanocobalamin) 10 mcg • Vitamin D 5 mcg • Vitamin B6 (pyridoxine HCl) 5 mg • Pantothenic Acid 4 mg • Vitamin E 5 mg • Vitamin C 30 mg • Iron 18 mg • Iodine 140 mcg • Magnesium 50 mg • Zinc 15 mg • Copper 1 mg • Manganese 2 mg • Selenium 100 mcg • Chromium 50 mg • Ginseng 40 mg • Citrus Bioflavonoids 30 mg.

Some Brand Name Natural Products - What they Contain

www.NaturalDatabase.com contains MANY more listings than appear here.
Editor's Notes are located on pages 2155-2163.

BRAND NAMES

Multi-Scorb - Progressive Labs
Each tablet contains: Vitamin C (as mineral ascorbates) 1000 mg • Calcium (ascorbate) 50 mg • Magnesium (ascorbate) 30 mg • Zinc (ascorbate) 3 mg • Manganese (ascorbate) 3 mg • Potassium (ascorbate) 60 mg • Citrus BioFlavonoid 5X complex 125 mg (as undiluted hesperidin, naringin and rutin).

Multivit Syrup - Hadas Natural Products
Vitamin A 2000 IU • Vitamin D (D3) 400 IU • Vitamin B1 1.25 mg • Vitamin B2 1.5 mg • Vitamin B6 1.25 mg • Vitamin B12 1 mcg • Rose Hip extract 100 mg • Folic Acid 75 mcg • Calcium Pantothenate 10 mg • Nicotinamide 12 mg.

MultiVitamin - HealthMinded
Three tablets contain: Vitamin A (beta carotene & palmitate) 21,000 IU • Vitamin C (ascorbic acid) 900 mg • Vitamin D (water dispensable) 1200 IU • Vitamin E (D-alpha tocopheryl succinate) 400 IU • Vitamin K 80 mcg • Vitamin B1 (thiamine mononitrate) 12 mg • Vitamin B2 (riboflavin) 12 mg • Niacinamide 60 mg • Vitamin B6 (pyridoxine HCl, pyridoxal 5 phos.) 18 mg • Folic Acid 800 mcg • Vitamin B12 (cyanocobalamin) 36 mcg • Biotin 450 mcg • Pantothenic Acid (calcium pantothenate) 30 mg • Calcium (elemental) 300 mg • Iron (elemental) 15 mg • Iodine (kelp) 150 mcg • Magnesium (elemental) 400 mg • Zinc (elemental) 22.5 mg • Selenium (L-selenomethionine) 200 mcg • Copper (elemental) 3 mg • Manganese (elemental) 6 mg • Chromium (plynicotinate) 150 mcg • Molybdenum 75 mcg • Potassium (elemental) 105 mg. Other Ingredients: Di Calcium Phosphate, Stearic Acid, Croscarmellose Sodium, Magnesium Stearate, Micro Crystalline Cellulose, Silicon Dioxide.

Multizyme - Standard Process, Inc.
Each capsule contains: Proprietary Blend 337 mg: Fig fruit, Defatted Almonds, Pancreatin 3X, Fatty Acids, Bromelain, Lipase, Cellulase, Papain, Amylase. Other Ingredients: Gelatin, Lactose, Water, Colors, Calcium Stearate.

Munit-E - Holista
Each capsule contains: Beta Carotene 10000 IU • Vitamin A 5000 IU • Vitamin C 500 mg • Vitamin B6 25 mg • Zinc 20 mg • Echinacea (angustifolia/purpurea) 300 mg • Bioflavonoids 100 mg • Garlic 50 mg • Ginger 50 mg.

Muscle - Gary Null & Associates (GNA)
Composed of plant sources. Fortified with Methionine, Leucine, Valine, Isoleucine, and Lysine.

Muscle Builder - Aspen Group, Inc.
Four tablets contain: Gamma Oryzanol 50 mg • Inosine 200 mg • Testicular Glan 600 mg • L-Ornithine 700 mg • Beta-Sitosterol 200 mg • Adrenal 400 mg • Thymus 400 mg.
See Editor's Note No. 14.

Muscle Dynamo - Source Naturals
Four tablets contain: Vitamin B1 (Thiamin) 30 mg • Vitamin B2 (Riboflavin) 30 mg • Niacinamide (125 mg) and Niacin (25 mg) 150 mg • Vitamin B5 (Calcium D-Pantothenate) 100 mg • Vitamin B6 (Pyridoxine HCl) 25 mg • Vitamin B12 (Cyanocobalamin) 100 mcg • Folic Acid 400 mcg • Vitamin E D-Alpha Tocopheryl (Natural) 100 IU • Magnesium (Citrate and Succinate) 181 mg • Potassium (Succinate) 99 mg • Calciium (Succinate) 89 mg • Succinate Complex (Magnesium/Calcium/Potassium Succinates) 1,300 mg • Inosine 500 mg • PAK (Pyridoxine alpha-Ketoglutarate) 100 mg • Coenzyme Q10 (Ubiquinone) 30 mg • Alpha-Lipoic Acid (Thioctic Acid) 25 mg • l-Isoleucine 120 mg • L-Leucine 360 mg • L-Valine 120 mg • Glycine 500 mg • L-Tyrosine 150 mg • Korean Ginseng root 250 mg • Siberian Ginseng root extract 100 mg.

Muscle Dynamo II - Source Naturals
One oz contains: Vitamin A 1,250 IU • Vitamin C (Ascorbic Acid) 30 mg • Thiamin (Vitamin B1) 380 mcg • Riboflavin (Vitamin B2) 430 mcg • Niacin 20 mg • Calcium 150 mg • Iron 1 mg • Vitamin D 100 IU • Vitamin E 15 IU • Vitamin B6 500 mcg • Folic Acid 100 mcg • Vitamin B12 3 mcg • Phosphorus 150 mcg • Iodine 25 mcg • Magnesium 50 mg • Zinc 7.5 mg • Copper 250 mcg • Biotin 75 mcg • Pantothenic Acid 2.5 mg • Potassium 300 mg • Manganese 2 mg • Chromium 150 mcg • Molybdenum 50 mcg • Selenium 30 mcg.

Muscle Mass - Source Naturals
Two tablets contain: Vitamin C (Ascorbic Acid) 50 mg • Vitamin B5 (Calcium D-Pantothenate) 20 mg • Vitamin B6 (Pyridoxine HCl) 20 mg • Iodine (from kelp) 56 mcg. Other Ingredients: Arginine Pyroglutamate 718 mg, L-Lysine HCl 718 mg, L-Ornithine (Ornithine HCl) 200 mg, Branched Chain Amino Acids (BCAAs) 174 mg (L-Leucine 100 mg, L-Isoleucine 30 mg and L-Valine 44 mg), Lipotropic Factors 360 mg (Choline Bitartrate 200 mg, Inositol 100 mg, L-Methionine 30 mg and Betaine HCl 30 mg), Glycine 50 mg, Trans-Ferulic Acid 50 mg, L-Carnitine (L-Carnitine L-Tartrate) 10 mg, Special Herbal Blend 590 mg: Saw Palmetto, Sarsaparilla, Wild Yam Root, Astragalus, Kelp, Ginseng, Pueraria, Licorice Root.

Muscle Milk - CytoSport
Two scoops (or one packet) contain: EVOPRO: Micellar Alpha and Beta Caseins and Casseinates, Whey concentrates, Whey isolates, Whey peptides, Purified Bovine Colostrum extract (secretory IgA and IGF-1), Glutamine peptides, L-Taurine, Lactoferrin • LEANLIPIDES: Canola oil, BETAPOL Enzyme Engineered Polyunsaturated Long-Chain Vegetable Oils, MCT, L-Carnitine • Maltodextrin • CYTOVITE I Vitamin and Mineral premix: Vitamin A Acetate, Cholecalciferol, D-Alpha-Tocopherol Acetate, Ascorbic Acid, Folate, Thiamine Monohydrate, Riboflavin, Niacinamide, Pyridoxine HCl, Cyanocobalamin, Biotin, Pantothenic Acid, Di-Calcium Phosphate, Potassium Iodide, Potassium Chloride, Ferrous Fumarate, Magnesium Oxide, Copper Gluconate, Zinc Oxide • Gum Arabic • ENDOCREATINE Creatine Precursor: Glycocyamine, Betaine Anhydrous, SAMe (S-adenosylmethionine) • Natural and Artificial Flavors • Lecithin • Sucralose.

Muscle Nitrous - VPX Sports
Each 10 cc serving contains: A-AKG Arginine Alpha-Ketoglutarate 3000 mg • Magnesium Peroxide (MgO2) 50 mg. Other Ingredients: Highly Purified Water, Lecithin, Propylene Glycol, Polyethylene Glycol, Glycerine, Lipoject Technologies Proprietary Polylipid, Delivery Matrix, Vegetable Gum, Sucralose, Potassium Sorbate, Natural and Artificial Flavors, EDTA, Phosphoric Acid.

Muscle Optimeal - Jarrow Formulas
Muscle Optimeal Tri-Protein Blend: Whey Protein concentrate and isolate, Rice Protein concentrate, Partially Hydrolyzed Rice Protein and Milk Protein • MultiCarb/MultiFiber Complex Carbohydrate Blend: Fibersol-2 brand complex Maltodextrin Fiber, Xylitol, Rice Starch, Stabilized Rice Bran, Rice Bran Solubles • Fructose • Cellulose Gel • Cellulose Gum • Multi-Vitamin/Mineral Blend: Potassium Chloride, Dicalcium Phosphate, Magnesium Oxide, Ascorbic Acid, Ferric Orthophosphate, D-Alpha Tocopheryl Acetate, Niacinamide, Zinc Oxide, Copper Gluconate, Vitamin A Palmitate, D-Calcium Pantothenate, Manganese Sulfate, Pyridoxine Hydrochloride, Riboflavin, Thiamin Mononitrate, Chromium Picolinate, Vitamin D (D3), Folic Acid, Biotin, Potassium Iodide, Sodium Molybdate, Vitamin K, Sodium Selenate, Cyanocobalamin • Lo Han natural sweetener • Carrageenan • Lecithin.

Muscle Spasm Remedy (formerly HP 17) - Metagenics
Each tablet contains: Hypericum Perforatum 6X • Cocculus Indicus 6X • Kali Phosphoricum 6X • Magnesia Phosphorica 3X • Mezereum 3X • Rhus Toxicodendron 30X • Arsencium Album 6X • Hammamelis Virginana 3X • Conium Maculatum 6X • Colocynthis 12X.
See Editor's Note No. 1.

Muscle Therapy Bath - Abra Therapeutics
Sodium Borate • Sodium Sulfate • Sodium Chloride • Sodium Sesquicarbonate • Olive oil • Eucalyptus oil • Rosemary oil • Bergamot oil • Juniper oil • Lemongrass oil • Fir oil • Peru Balsam oil • Pepperwood leaf extract • Bearberry leaf extract • Sage leaf extract • Chromium Oxide • Trace Mineral Salts.

Some Brand Name Natural Products - What they Contain

www.NaturalDatabase.com contains MANY more listings than appear here.
Editor's Notes are located on pages 2155-2163.

***MusclEase* - PhysioLogics**
Two capsules contain: Magnesium (as magnesium aspartate) 100 mg • Calcium (as calcium citrate) 45 mg • Valerian root (valeriana officinalis, standardized to contain 0.8% valernic acid, 0.8 mg) 100 mg • Kava Kava root (piper methysticum, standardized to contain 30% kavalactones, 30 mg) 100 mg • Passion Flower plant (passiflora incarmata, standardized to contain 3.5% flavonoids, 3.5 mg) 100 mg. Other Ingredients: Gelatin, Rice Powder, Vegetable Magnesium Stearate, Silica.

***MuscleSoothe* - Vita Pharmica - formerly Neopharmica**
Two tablets contain: Proprietary Blend 2000 mg: San-Qi Ginseng root, Dong-Quai root, Sichuan Teasel rhizome, Safflower Flower, Astilbe Chinensis plant.

***MuscleTech* - MuscleTech**
Six capsules contain: Acetyl-L-Carnitine 1000 mg • Glutamine 2000 mg • L-Leucine 1000 mg • L-Valine 250 mg • L-Isoleucine 250 mg • OKG 100 mg • Zinc 60 mg • Taurine 1000 mg.

***MusculoSkeletal Formula* - 4 Life**
Each capsule contains: Gotu Kola 54 mg • Alfalfa leaf 54 mg • Devil's Claw root 54 mg • Turmeric root 54 mg • Ginger root 54 mg • Saw Palmetto berry 54 mg • MusculoSkeletal Proprietary Extract Blend 45 mg: Devil's Claw root extract, Saw Palmetto berry extract, Wild Yam root extract, Gotu Kola leaf extract, Alfalfa leaf extract, Horsetail extract, Ginger root extract • Wild Yam root 31 mg. Other Ingredients: Gelatin, Magnesium Stearate.

***Mushroom Immune Defense* - Source Naturals**
Two tablets contain: Vitamin C (ascorbic acid) 100 mg • Shiitake mycelia biomass 200 mg • Reishi mycelia biomass 200 mg • Maitake mycelia biomass 200 mg • Turkey Tail mycelia biomass 150 mg • Proprietary blend 1.3 g: Agaricus Blazei mycelica biomass, Hericium Erinaceous mycelica biomass, Flammulina Velutipes mycelica biomass, Tremella mycelica biomass, Schizophyllum Commiune mycelica biomass, Artist's Conk mycelica biomass, Poria mycelica biomass, Zhu Ling mycelica biomass, Pleurotus Ostreatus mycelica biomass, Cordycops Sinensis mycelica biomass, Cordyceps Militaris mycelica biomass, Armilleria Mellea mycelica biomass, Shiitake mushroom extract, Reishi mushroom extract, Maitake mushroom extract, Turkey Tail mushroom extract, Cordyceps Sinensis CS-4 standardized extract (0.1% adenosine), Agaricus Blazei mushroom extract, Maitake (beta-glucan) fraction. Other Ingredients: Stearic Acid, Colloidal Silicon Dioxide, Modified Cellulose Gum.

***Mushroom Optimizer capsules* - Jarrow Formulas**
Three capsules contain: Folic Acid and Methyl Folate 90 mcg • Cordyceps Sinensis 300 mg • Tremella Fuciformis (white wood ear) 225 mg • Coriolus Versicolor (turkey tail, yun zhi) 200 mg • Ganoderma Lucidum (fing-zhi, reishi) 200 mg • Grifola Frondosa (maitake) 200 mg • Lentinula Edodes 200 mg • Agaricus Blazei 175 mg. Other Ingredients: Rice Powder, Magnesium Stearate, Gelatin.

***Mushroom Optimizer powder* - Jarrow Formulas**
Each scoop (1.5 g) contains: Folic Acid and Methyl Folate 90 mcg • Cordyceps Sinensis (cordyceps) 300 mg • Tremella Fuciformis (white wood ear) 225 mg • Coriolus Versicolor (turkey tail, yun zhi) 200 mg • Ganoderma Lucidum (fing-zhi, reishi) 200 mg • Grifola Frondosa (maitake) 200 mg • Lentinula Edodes (shitake) 200 mg • Agaricus Blazei 175 mg.

***Mustard Salve* - Dial Herbs**
Mustard • Wintergreen • Comfrey • Arnica • Camphor • Cayenne. In a base of Beeswax , Glycerine & Cold Pressed Olive oil.

***MVP* - Mannatech**
Each caplet contains: Ephedrine (from country mallow) 10 mg • Caffeine (from kola nut) 40 mg • Wild Yam root (standardized for phytoserols) • Kola Nut seed • Country Mallow (sida cortifolia aerial) • Atlantic Kelp whole plant •Cayenne Pepper fruit • Ambrotose Complex: naturally occuring plant polysaccharides including freeze-dried Aloe Vera inner leaf gel extract - Manapol powder. Other Ingredients: Cellulose, Calcium Carbonate, Silicon Dioxide, Hydroxypropyl Methylcellulose, Croscarmellose Sodium, Stearic Acid, Magnesium Stearate.
See Editor's Note No. 17 and No. 39.

***My Defense* - Natrol, Inc.**
Three capsules contain: Vitamin C (as calcium ascorbate) 60 mg • Arabinogalactan 1.5 g • Maitake extract (4:1) 50 mg • Cranberry juice powder 250 mg • Astragalus root powder 100 mg • Papain 100 mg. Other Ingredients: Silica, Magnesium Stearate, Gelatin.

***My Favorite Multiple — The Pill Companion* - Natrol, Inc.**
Two tablets contain: Vitamin A (as d-salina beta-carotene) 5000 IU • Vitamin C (as ascorbic acid) 300 mg • Vitamin D (as cholecalciferol) 200 IU • Vitamin E (as d-alpha tocopherol succinate) 30 IU • Vitamin K (as phytonadione) 40 mcg • Thiamin (vitamin B1) 5 mg • Riboflavin (vitamin B2) 5 mg • Niacin (vitamin B3) 20 mg • Vitamin B6 (as pyridoxine HCl) 15 mg • Folic Acid 600 mcg • Vitamin B12 (as cyanocobalamin) 24 mcg • Biotin 150 mcg • Pantothenic Acid (as calcium d-pantothenate) 5 mg • Calcium (as calcium citrate) 100 mg • Iron (as iron amino acid chealate) 4.5 mg • Magnesium (as magnesium oxide) 300 mg • Zinc (as zinc amino acid chelate) 30 mg • Selenium (as selenium amino acid chelate) 35 mcg • Copper (as copper amino acid chelate) 0.5 mg • Manganese (as manganese amino acid chelate) 0.5 mg • Chromium (as chromium picolinate) 60 mcg • Molybdenum (as molybdenum amino acid chelate) 38 mcg • Boron (as boron amino acid chelate) 1 mg • Soy extract 10 mg • Soy Isoflavones 4 mg. Other Ingredients: Cellulose, Stearic Acid, Silica, Cellulose Gum, Magnesium Stearate, Methylcellulose, Glycerine.

***My Favorite Multiple Original capsules* - Natrol, Inc.**
Six capsules contain: Vitamin A (as beta carotene & Vitamin A palmitate) 10000 IU • Vitamin C (as calcium ascorbate) 250 mg • Vitamin D (as cholecalciferol) 400 IU • Vitamin E (as d-alpha tocopheryl succinate) 400 IU • Thiamine (as thiamin HCl) (Vitamin B1) 50 mg • Riboflavin (Vitamin B2) 50 mg • Niacin (as niacin & niacinamide) 50 mg • Vitamin B6 (as pyridoxine HCl) 50 mg • Folic Acid 400 mcg • Vitamin B12 (as cyanocobalamin) 50 mcg • Biotin 300 mcg • Pantothenic Acid (as d-calcium pantothenate) 50 mg • Calcium (as calcium carbonate & calcium citrate) 1 g • Iron (as iron glycinate) 18 mg • Iodine (from kelp) 150 mcg • Magnesium (as magnesium citrate & magnesium oxide) 400 mg • Zinc 25 mg • Selenium 200 mcg • Copper 2 mg • Manganese (as manganese gluconate) 2 mg • Chromium 200 mcg • Molybdenum 50 mcg • Potassium (as potassium chloride) 99 mg • Betaine (as betaine TMG trimethylglycine) 300 mg • MultiEnzyme Blend: Amylase, Papain, Protease, Bromelain, Lipase 110 mg • GP Flavonoid Complex + 100 mg extracted from: Rose Hips fruit, Tumeric root, Acerola berries, Bilberry berries, Hawthorne berries, Grape skin, Milk Thistle seed, & Citrus fruit • PABA (as para amino benzoic acid) 50 mg • Choline (as choline bitartrate) 50 mg • Inositol 50 mg • Hesperidin 25 mg • Rutin 25 mg • Siberian Ginseng 4:1 extract root 1 mg • Boron 200 mcg. Other Ingredients: Silicon Dioxide, Magnesium Stearate, Gelatin.

***My Favorite Multiple Original tablets* - Natrol, Inc.**
Four tablets contain: Vitamin A (as d-Salina beta carotene & Vitamin A palmitate) 10000 IU • Vitamin C (as calcium ascorbate) 250 mg • Vitamin D (as cholecalciferol) 400 IU • Vitamin E (as d-alpha tocopheryl succinate) 400 IU • Thiamine (as Thiamine HCl) (Vitamin B1) 50 mg • Riboflavin (Vitamin B2) 50 mg • Niacin (as Niacin & Niacinamide) 50 mg • Vitamin B6 (as pyridoxine HCl) 50 mg • Folic Acid 400 mcg • Vitamin B12 (as cyanocobalamin) 50 mcg • Biotin 300 mcg • Pantothenic Acid (as d-calcium pantothenate) 50 mg • Calcium (as calcium carbonate & calcium citrate) 1 g • Iron (as iron glycinate) 18 mg • Iodine (from kelp) 150 mcg • Magnesium (as magnesium citrate & magnesium oxide) 400 mg • Zinc 25 mg • Selenium 200 mcg • Copper 2 mg • Manganese (as manganese gluconate) 2 mg • Chromium 200 mcg • Molybdenum 50 mcg • Potassium (as potassium chloride) 99 mg • Betaine (as betaine TMG trimethylglycine) 300 mg • Multi Enzyme Blend: amylase, papain, protease, bromelain, lipase 110 mg • GP Flavonoid Complex 100 mg extracted from: Rose Hips fruit, Tumeric root, Acerola berries, Bilberry berries, Hawthorne berries, Grape skin, Milk Thistle Seed, &

citrus fruit • PABA (as para amino benzoic acid) 50 mg • Choline (as choline bitartrate) 50 mg • Inositol 50 mg • Hesperidin 25 mg • Rutin 25 mg • Siberian Ginseng 4:1 extract root 15 mg • Boron 200 mcg. Other Ingredients: Microcrystalline Cellulose, Mono & Di-Glycerides, Silicon Dioxide, Magnesium Stearate, Stearic Acid, Croscarmellose Sodium.

My Favorite Multiple Prime - Natrol, Inc.
Six capsules contain: Vitamin A (from retinal acetate, 60% beta carotene [from natural carotenoid blend, d-salina]) 7500 IU • Vitamin C (from calcium ascorbate) 180 mg • Vitamin D (as cholecalciferol) 600 IU • Vitamin E (as d-alpha tocopherol succinate) 120 IU • Thiamin (as thiamin HCl, vitamin B1) 3 mg • Riboflavin (vitamin B2) 3.4 mg • Niacin (niacinamide) 40 mg • Vitamin B6 (as pyridoxine HCl) 4 mg • Folic Acid 600 mcg • Vitamin B12 (as cyanocobalamin) 100 mcg • Biotin 600 mcg • Pantothenic Acid (as D-calcium pantothenate) 20 mg • Calcium (as calcium: citrate, carbonate, ascorbate) 700 mg • Iron (as iron amino acid chelate) 18 mg • Iodine (from kelp) 150 mcg • Magnesium (as magnesium oxide) 400 mg • Zinc (as zinc amino acid chelate) 30 mg • Selenium (as selenium amino acid chelate) 140 mcg • Copper (as copper amino acid chelate) 4 mg • Manganese (as manganese gluconate) 4 mg • Chromium (as chromium amino acid chelate) 120 mg • Molybdenum (as molybdenum amino acid chelate) 75 mcg • Boron (as boron amino acid chelate) 200 mcg • 50+ Supporting Nutrient Blend 580 mg: Coenzyme Q10 30 mg, Glucosamine HCl 500 mg, Acetyl L-Carnitine 25 mg, Green Tea (50% polyphenols) 10 mg, Bilberry extract (25% anthocyanins) 15 mg • Natrol's Ultra Green Blend 100 mg: Alfalfa juice (leaf), Barley grass, Spirulina (algae), Parsley (leaf), Spinach (leaf), Peppermint (leaf), Spearmint (leaf) • Enzyme Blend 100 mg: Amylase, Papain, Protease, Bromelain, Lipase • Carotenoid Blend 75 mg: Tomato, Marigold, Palm Oil • Beta Carotene 1830 mcg • Lutein 630 mcg • Lycopene 360 mcg • Alpha Carotene 120 mcg • Cryptoxanthin 24 mcg • Zeaxanthin 24 mcg • Inositol 5 mg • Choline Bitartrate 5 mg. Other Ingredients: Silica, Magnesium Stearate, Gelatin.

My Favorite Multiple Take One - Natrol, Inc.
One tablet contains: Vitamin A (as beta carotene) 10000 IU • Vitamin C (as calcium ascorbate) 100 mg • Vitamin D (as cholecalciferol) 400 IU • Vitamin E (as d-alpha tocopheryl succinate) 100 IU • Thiamine (as thiamin HCl) (Vitamin B1) 15 mg • Riboflavin (Vitamin B2) 17 mg • Niacin 20 mg • Vitamin B6 (as pyridoxine HCl) 17 mg • Folic Acid 400 mcg • Vitamin B12 (as cyanocobalamin) 50 mcg • Biotin 300 mcg • Pantothenic Acid (as D-calcium pantothenate) 50 mg • Calcium 25 mg • Iron 18 mg • Iodine 150 mcg • Magnesium 10 mg • Zinc 15 mg • Selenium 200 mcg • Copper 2 mg • Manganese 5 mg • Chromium 200 mcg • Molybdenum 50 mcg • Potassium 5 mg • Silica 10 mg • Vanadium 10 mcg • Boron 3 mg • GP Flavonoid Complex + 100 mg, extracted from: Rose Hips fruit, Tumeric root, Acerola berries, Bilberry berries, Hawthorne berries, Grape skin, Milk Thistle Seed & Citrus fruit • UltraGreen Blend concentrate extract 100 mg from: Alfalfa juice leaf, barley grass, spirulina algae, parsley leaf, spinach leaf, peppermint leaf, & spearmint leaf • Lecithin 50 mg • Choline (as choline bitartrate) 50 mg • PABA (as para amino benzoic acid) 25 mg • Inositol 25 mg. Other Ingredients: Mono & Di-Glycerides, Silicon Dioxide, Stearic Acid, Croscarmellose Sodium, Magnesium Stearate.

My Favorite Multiple Take One Without Iron tablets - Natrol, Inc.
Each tablet contains: Vitamin A (as beta carotene) 10000 IU • Vitamin C (as calcium ascorbate) 100 mg • Vitamin D (as cholecalciferol) 400 IU• Vitamin E (as d-alpha tocopheryl succinate) 100 IU •Thiamine (as thiamin HCl) (Vitamin B1) 15 mg •Riboflavin (Vitamin B2) 17 mg • Niacin 20 mg • Vitamin B6 (as pyridoxine HCl) 17 mg • Folic Acid 400 mcg • Vitamin B12 (as cyanocobalamin) 50 mcg • Biotin 300 mcg • Pantothenic Acid (as D-calcium pantothenate) 50 mg • Calcium 25 mg • Iodine 150 mcg • Magnesium 10 mg • Zinc 15 mg • Selenium 200 mcg • Copper 2 mg • Manganese 5 mg • Chromium 200 mcg • Molybdenum 50 mcg • Potassium 5 mg • Silica 10 mg • Vanadium 10 mcg • Boron 3 mg • GP Flavonoids 100 mg, extracted from: Rose Hips fruit, Tumeric root, Acerola berries, Bilberry berries, Hawthorne berries, Grape skin, Milk Thistle seed, & Citrus fruit • UltraGreen Blend 100 mg concentrate extract from: Alfalfa juice leaf, Barley grass, Spirulina algae, Parsley leaf, Spinach leaf, Peppermint leaf, & Spearmint leaf • Lecithin 50 mg • Choline (as choline bitartrate) 50 mg • PABA (as para amino benzoic acid) 25 mg • Inositol 25 mg. Other Ingredients: Mono & Di-Glycerides, Silicon Dioxide, Stearic Acid, Croscarmellose Sodium, Magnesium Stearate.

My Favorite Multiple With Coral Calcium & Zeaxanthin - Natrol, Inc.
Two capslues contain: Vitamin A (as retinal acetate, 10% beta carotene) 5000 IU • Vitamin C (as calcium ascorbate) 60 mg • Vitamin D (as cholecalciferol) 400 IU • Vitamin E (as d-alpha tocopheryl succinate) 30 IU • Vitamin K (as phytonadione) 40 mcg • Riboflavin (vitamin B2) 1.7 mg • Niacin (as niacinamide) 20 mg • Vitamin B6 (as pyridoxine HCl) 2 mg • Folic Acid 400 mcg • Vitamin B12 (as cyanocobalamin) 6 mcg • Biotin 300 mcg • Pantothenic Acid 10 mg • Calcium (from coral and calcium ascorbate) 250 mg • Zinc (as zinc oxide) 15 mg • Selenium (as selenium amino acid chelate) 70 mcg • Copper (as copper sulfate) 2 mg • Manganese (as manganese gluconate) 2 mg • Chromium (as chromium picolinate) 120 mcg • Molybdenum (as amino acid chelate) 75 mcg • Boron (as boron amino acid chelate) 200 mcg • Zeaxanthin 2 mg. Other Ingredients: Gelatin, Silica, Magnesium Stearate.

My Favorite Multiple Without Iron capsules - Natrol, Inc.
Six capsules contain: Vitamin A (as beta carotene & Vitamin A palmitate) 10000 IU • Vitamin C (as calcium ascorbate) 250 mg • Vitamin D (as cholecalciferol) 400 IU • Vitamin E (as d-alpha tocopheryl succinate) 400 IU • Thiamine (as thiamin HCl) (Vitamin B1) 50 mg • Riboflavin (Vitamin B2) 50 mg • Niacin (as niacin & niacinamide) 50 mg • Vitamin B6 (as pyridoxine HCl) 50 mg • Folic Acid 400 mcg • Vitamin B12 (as cyanocobalamin) 50 mcg • Biotin 300 mcg • Pantothenic Acid (as d-calcium pantothenate) 50 mg • Calcium (as calcium carbonate & calcium citrate) 1 g • Iodine (from kelp) 150 mcg • Magnesium (as magnesium citrate & magnesium, oxide) 400 mg • Zinc 25 mg • Selenium 200 mcg • Copper 2 mg • Manganese (as manganese gluconate) 2 mg • Chromium 200 mcg • Molybdenum 50 mcg • Potassium(as potassium chloride) 99 mg • Betaine (as betaine TMG trimethylglycine) 300 mg • MultiEnzyme Blend 110 mg: amylase, papain, protease, bromelain & lipase • GP Flavonoid Complex + 100 mg extracted from: Rose Hips fruit, Tumeric root, Acerola berries, Bilberry berries, Hawthorne berries, Grape skin, Milk Thistle Seed & Citrus fruit • PABA (as para amino benzoic acid) 50 mg • Choline (as choline bitartrate) 50 mg • Inositol 50 mg • Hesperidin 25 mg • Rutin 25 mg • Siberian Ginseng 4:1 extract root 15 mg • Boron 200 mcg. Other Ingredients: Silicon Dioxide, Magnesium Stearate, Gelatin.

My Favorite Multiple Without Iron tablets - Natrol, Inc.
Four tablets contain: Vitamin A (as d-Salina beta carotene & Vitamin A palmitate) 10000 IU • Vitamin C (as calcium ascorbate) 250 mg • Vitamin D (as cholecalciferol) 400 IU • Vitamin E (as d-alpha tocopheryl succinate) 400 IU • Thiamine 50 mg • Riboflavin (Vitamin B2) 50 mg • Niacin (as Niacin & Niacinamide) 50 mg • Vitamin B6 (as pyridoxine HCl) 50 mg • Folic Acid 400 mcg • Vitamin B12 (as cyanocobalamin) 50 mcg • Biotin 300 mcg • Pantothenic Acid (as D-calcium pantothenate) 50 mg • Calcium (as calcium carbonate & calcium citrate) 1 g • Iodine (from kelp) 150 mcg • Magnesium (citrate & oxide) 400 mg • Zinc 25 mg • Selenium 200 mcg • Copper 2 mg • Manganese (as manganese gluconate) 2 mg • Chromium 200 mcg • Molybdenum 50 mcg • Potassium (chloride) 99 mg • Betaine (TMG trimethylglycine) 300 mg • MultiEnzyme Blend 110 mg consisting of: Amylase, Papain, Protease, Bromelain & Lipase • GP Flavonoid Complex 100 mg extracted from: Rose Hips fruit, Tumeric root, Acerola berries, Bilberry berries, Hawthorne berries, Grape skin, Milk Thistle seed & Citrus fruit • PABA (as para amino benzoic acid) 50 mg • Choline (as choline bitartrate) 50 mg • Inositol 50 mg • Hesperidin 25 mg • Rutin 25 mg • Siberian Ginseng 4:1 extract root 15 mg • Boron 200 mcg. Other Ingredients: Microcrystalline Cellulose, Mono & Di-Glycerides, Silicon Dioxide, Magnesium Stearate, Stearic Acid, Croscarmellose Sodium.

Mycelia Immunity Formula **-** PhysioLogics
Each capsule contains: Mycelia Complex Blend 500 mg: Shiitake Mushroom Mycelia extract, Rice Bran. Other Ingredients: Gelatin, Silica, Vegetable Magnesium Stearate.

Mycelized Children's Multi-Vitamin **-** Metagenics
Each 1 mL serving (one full dropper) contains: Vitamin A (as retinyl palmitate) 1250 IU • Vitamin D (as cholecalciferol) 200 IU • Vitamin E (as D-alpha tocopherol acetate) 10 IU • Thiamin (as thiamin mononitrate) 1.4 mg • Riboflavin (as riboflavin-5-phosphate) 1.6 mg • Niacin (as niacinamide) 18 mg • Vitamin B6 (as pyridoxine hydrochloride) 1.4 mg • Biotin 300 mcg • Vitamin B12 (as cyanocobalamin) 6 mcg • Pantothenic Acid 10 mg • Vitamin C (as ascorbic acid) 80 mg. Other Ingredients: Deionized Water, Ethoxylated Castor Bean Oil, Glycerin, Citric Acid, Potassium Sorbate, Sodium Benzoate.

Mycelized Vitamin A **-** Metagenics
Each drop contains: Vitamin A (as retinyl palmitate) 5000 IU. Other Ingredients: Deionized Water, Castor Bean Oil, Glycerin, Citric Acid, Potassium Sorbate, Sodium Benzoate.

Mycelized Vitamin E **-** Metagenics
Each one mL serving (20 drops) contains: Vitamin E (as D-alpha tocopherol acetate) 150 IU. Other Ingredients: Deionized Water, Ethoxylated Castor Bean Oil, Glycerin, Citric Acid, Potassium Sorbate, Sodium Benzoate.

MycoCeutics MycoPhyto Complex Capsules **-** EcoNugenics
Six capsules contain: MycoCeutics MycoPhyto Proprietary Blend 3840 mg: Reishi (ganoderma lucidum), Coriolus (coriolus versicolor), Umbellatus (polyporus umbellatus), Agaricus (agaricus blazei), Cordyceps (cordyceps sinensis), Maitake (grifola frondosa) • Beta-1,3-Glucan (from purified yeast) 100 mg.

MycoCeutics MycoPhyto Complex Powder **-** EcoNugenics
Each heaping scoop (4 g) contains: MycoCeutics MycoPhyto Proprietary Blend 3840 mg: Reishi (ganoderma lucidum), Coriolus (coriolus versicolor), Umbellatus (polyporus umbellatus), Agaricus (agaricus blazei), Cordyceps (cordyceps sinensis), Maitake (grifola frondosa) • Beta-1,3-Glucan (from purified yeast) 100 mg • Beta-Glucan 337 mg.

MycoCeutics Ten Mushroom Formula **-** EcoNugenics
Four Capsules contain: MycoCeutics 10 Mushroom Proprietary Blend 2400 mg: Reishi (ganoderma lucidum), Poria Cocos, Cordyceps (cordyceps sinensis), Tremella Fuciformia, Umbellatus (polyporus umbellatus), Coriolus (coriolus versicolor), Maitake (grifola frondosa), Shitake (lentinula edodes), Wood Ear (auricularia auricula), Hericium Erinaceus • Beta-1,3-Glucan (from purified yeast) 30 mg • Beta-Glucan 275 mg. Other Ingredients: Gelatin, Magnesium Stearate, Silica.

Mycoferon **-** Metagenics
Fifteen drops (0.5 mL) contain: Proprietary Mycelial Mushroom Biomass Blend 500 mg: Reishi extract (ganoderma lucidum), Tochukaso extract (cordyceps sinensis), Hakumokuji extract (tremella fuciformis), Shiitake extract (lentinus edodes), Maitake extract (grifola frondosa), Kawaratake extract (coriolus versicolor), Choreimaitake extract (polyporus umbellatus). Other Ingredients: Ethanol, Organic Brown Rice, 25%-30% Alcohol by volume.

Myco-Feron Supreme Blend **-** Wild Rose
Each vegetable cap contains: Reishi 15:1 extract 40 mg • Reishi mushroom powder 40 mg • Cordyceps 40 mg • Maitake 4:1 extract 40 mg • Maitake mushroom powder 40 mg • Shiitake mushroom powder 40 mg • Chaga mushroom 8:1 extract 40 mg • Poria mushroom 40 mg • Polyporus (zhu ling) 40 mg • Agaricus mushroom 40 mg.

Myelin-MS **-** Olympia Nutrition
Spingomyelin- pharmaceutical grade.

MygraFew Standardized Feverfew Extract **-** Nature's Way
Each tablet contains: Dried Feverfew Extract (leaf, standardized Feverfew Extract delivering 600 mcg parthenolide, 5% parthenolide) 12 mg.

MygrAid Formula **-** Nature's Way
Each capsule contains: Feverfew leaves 100 mg • Feverfew dried extract 33.3 mg • Lavender flower 50 mg • Linden leaf & flower 70 mg • Magnesium Amino Acid Chelate 33.3 mg. Other Ingredients: Gelatin, Magnesium Stearate, Millet.

Mylanta Calci Tabs Extra Strength **-** Johnson & Johnson
Two tablets contain: Calcium 600 mg. Other Ingredients: Dextrose, Maltodextrin, Microcrystalline Cellulose, Magnesium Stearate, Starch, Cellulose, Citric and Fumaric Acids, Natural and Artificial Flavors, Mineral Oil, Sucrose, FD&C Yellow #6, FD&C Yellow #5, FD&C Blue #1, FD&C Red #27, Ethylmaltol, Crospovidone, Hydroxypropyl Methylcellulose, Stearic Acid.

Mylanta Calci Tabs Ultra Strength **-** Johnson & Johnson
Two tablets contain: Calcium Carbonate 1000 mg. Other Ingredients: Dextrose, Maltodextrin, Microcrystalline Cellulose, Magnesium Stearate, Starch, Cellulose, Citric and Fumaric Acids, Natural and Artificial Flavors, Mineral Oil, Sucrose, FD&C Yellow #6, FD&C Yellow #5, FD&C Blue #1, FD&C Red #27, Ethylmaltol, Crospovidone, Hydroxypropyl Methylcellulose, Stearic Acid.

Myo Malate **-** Ortho Molecular Products
Each capsule contains: Vitamin B6 (as pyridoxine HCl USP) 25 mg • Magnesium (as malate) 60 mg • Malic Acid (as malic acid, magnesium malate) 600 mg. Other Ingredients: Natural Vegetable Capsules, Ascorbyl Palmitate, Magnesium Stearate, Microcrystalline Cellulose, Silicon Dioxide.

Myo-Blast **-** Cytodyne LLC
Each two capsules contain: Cystoseira Canariensis (as MyoZap CSP3) 600 mg • Rhodiola Rosea extract (standardized for 5% rosavin) 200 mg • Rhaponticum Carthomoides extract (standardized for 25% 20-hydroxyecdysone) 62.5 mg • Anabolic Amino Acid Complex 485 mg: Taurine, Carnosine, L-Leucine.

MyoCalm **-** Metagenics
Two tablets contain: Magnesium (as magnesium citrate) 100 mg • Calcium (as calcium lactate) 50 mg • Passionflower (passiflora incarnata) 180 mg • Passionflower 5.35:1 extract (passiflora incarnata) 20 mg • Valerian root (valeriana officinalis) 90 mg • Valerian root 6.15:1 extract (valeriana officinalis) 10 mg.

MyoCalm P.M. **-** Metagenics
Three tablets contain: Magnesium (as magnesium citrate) 150 mg • Calcium (as calcium lactate) 75 mg • Passion Flower (passiflora incarnata) 270 mg • Passion Flower 5.35:1 extract (passiflora incarnata) 30 mg • Valerian root (valeriana officinalis) 135 mg • Valerian root 6.15:1 extract (valeriana officinalis) 15 mg • Hops flower, strobile (humulus lupulus) 270 mg • Hops cone 7.5:1 extract (humulus lupulus) 30 mg • Lemon Balm leaf 5:1 extract (melissa officinalis) 150 mg.

Myo-Comp **-** PhytoPharmica
Two tablets contain: Vitamin C (ascorbic acid) 120 mg • Vitamin D (cholecalciferol) 266 IU • Vitamin E (D-alpha tocopheryl succinate) 20 IU • Thiamin (thiamin HCl, vitamin B1) 10 mg • Riboflavin (vitamin B2) 10 mg • Niacin 10 mg • Vitamin B6 (pyridoxine HCl) 12 mg • Vitamin B12 (cyanocobalamin) 20 mcg • Calcium (bone meal) 360 mg • Magnesium (chelate) 60 mg • Manganese (chelate) 3 mg • Potassium Chloride 50 mg • Choline Bitartrate 100 mg • Muscle extract 100 mg • Inositol 100 mg • Betaine HCl 60 mg • Ammonium Chloride 60 mg • RNA powder 6 mg.

Myoplex Lite Nutrition Shake (chocolate caramel flavor) **-** EAS, Inc.
Each packet (53 g) contains: Prolean II (whey protein from concentrate/isolate, calcium caseinate, soy protein isolate, l-glutamine, taurine) • Corn Syrup solids • Natural and Artificial Flavors • Vitamin & Mineral Blend: Tricalcium Phosphate, Calcium

BRAND NAMES

Citrate, Potassium Chloride, Disodium Phosphate, Magnesium Oxide, Dipotassium Phosphate, Choline Bitartrate, Beta Carotene, Ascorbic Acid, Dl-Alpha Tocopheryl Acetate, Niacinamide, Ferrous Fumarate, Manganese Gluconate, Biotin, Zinc Oxide, Boron Proteinate, Thiamine Hydrochloride, D-Calcium Pantothenate, Vitamin A Palmitate, Copper Sulfate, Chromium Citrate, Pyridoxine Hydrochloride, Riboflavin, Selenium Amino Acid Chelate, Molybdenum Amino Acid Chelate, Folic Acid, Cyanocobalamin, Potassium Iodide • Oat fiber • Cocoa (processed with alkali) • Maltodextrin • Cellulose Gum • Salt • High Oleic Sunflower Oil • Sucralose (Splenda brand) • Mono- and Diglycerides • Soy Lecithin.

Myoplex Lite Nutrition Shake (chocolate mint flavor) **-** EAS, Inc.
Each packet (53 g) contains: Prolean II (whey protein from concentrate/isolate, calcium caseinate, soy protein isolate, L-glutamine, taurine) • Corn Syrup solids • Vitamin & Mineral Blend: Tricalcium Phosphate, Calcium Citrate, Potassium Chloride, Disodium Phosphate, Magnesium Oxide, Dipotassium Phosphate, Choline Bitartrate, Beta Carotene, Ascorbic Acid, Dl-Alpha Tocopheryl Acetate, Niacinamide, Ferrous Fumarate, Manganese Gluconate, Biotin, Zinc Oxide, Boron Proteinate, Thiamine Hydrochloride, D-Calcium Pantothenate, Vitamin A Palmitate, Copper Sulfate, Chromium Citrate, Pyridoxine Hydrochloride, Riboflavin, Selenium Amino Acid Chelate, Molybdenum Amino Acid Chelate, Folic Acid, Cyanocobalamin, Potassium Iodide • Oat fiber • Chocolate chips (sugar, partially hydrogenated vegetable oil (palm kernal, cottonseed oil), cocoa (processed with alkali), corn syrup solids, soy lecithin, artifical flavor, salt) • Cellulose Gum • Salt • High Oleic Sunflower Oil • Natural Flavors • Sucralose (Splenda brand) • Mono and Diglycerides • Soy Lecithin.

Myoplex Lite Nutrition Shake (chocolate peanut butter flavor) **-** EAS, Inc.
Each packet (53 g) contains: Prolean II (whey protein from concentrate/isolate, calcium caseinate, soy protein isolate, l-glutamine, taurine) • Corn Syrup solids • Vitamin & Mineral Blend: Tricalcium Phosphate, Calcium Citrate, Potassium Chloride, Disodium Phosphate, Magnesium Oxide, Dipotassium Phosphate, Choline Bitartrate, Beta Carotene, Ascorbic Acid, Dl-Alpha Tocopheryl Acetate, Niacinamide, Ferrous Fumarate, Manganese Gluconate, Biotin, Zinc Oxide, Boron Proteinate, Thiamine Hydrochloride, D-Calcium Pantothenate, Vitamin A Palmitate, Copper Sulfate, Chromium Citrate, Pyridoxine Hydrochloride, Riboflavin, Selenium Amino Acid Chelate, Molybdenum Amino Acid Chelate, Folic Acid, Cyanocobalamin, Potassium Iodide • Oat fiber • Natural and Artificial Flavors • Cocoa (processed with alkali) • Maltodextrin • Cellulose Gum • Salt • High Oleic Sunflower Oil • Natural Flavors • Sucralose (Splenda brand) • Mono- and Diglycerides • Soy Lecithin.

Myoplex Lite Nutrition Shake (dark chocolate flavor) **-** EAS, Inc.
Each packet (53 g) contains: Prolean II (whey protein from concentrate/isolate, calcium caseinate, soy protein isolate, L-glutamine, taurine) • Corn Syrup solids • Cocoa (processed with alkali) • Vitamin & Mineral Blend: Tricalcium Phosphate, Calcium Citrate, Potassium Chloride, Disodium Phosphate, Magnesium Oxide, Dipotassium Phosphate, Choline Bitartrate, Beta Carotene, Ascorbic Acid, Dl-Alpha Tocopheryl Acetate, Niacinamide, Ferrous Fumarate, Manganese Gluconate, Biotin, Zinc Oxide, Boron Proteinate, Thiamine Hydrochloride, D-Calcium Pantothenate, Vitamin A Palmitate, Copper Sulfate, Chromium Citrate, Pyridoxine Hydrochloride, Riboflavin, Selenium Amino Acid Chelate, Molybdenum Amino Acid Chelate, Folic Acid, Cyanocobalamin, Potassium Iodide • Oat fiber • Natural and Artificial Flavors • Maltodextrin • Cellulose Gum • Salt • High Oleic Sunflower oil • Sucralose (Splenda brand) • Mono- and Diglycerides • Soy Lecithin.

Myoplex Low Carb-Chocolate Cream **-** Nutripeak
Each packet contains: Protein 50 g • Vitamin A Palmitate (35% as Beta Carotene) 7500 IU • Vitamin D (Cholecalciferol) 400 mg • Niacin (Niacinamide) 10 mg • Biotin 150 mcg • Magnesium Oxide 240 mg • Manganese Sulfate 2 mg • Vitamin C (Ascorbic Acid) 90 mg • Vitamin E (dl-Alpha Tocopheryl Acetate) 45 IU • Vitamin B6 (Pyridoxine Hydrochloride) 1 mg • Pantothenic Acid (D-Calcium Pantothenate) 5 mg • Zinc Oxide 7.5 mg • Chromium Citrate 96 mcg • Calcium (Tricalcium Phosphate and Dipotassium Phosphate) 0.5 mg • Thiamin Hydrochloride 0.75 mcg • Folic Acid 200 mcg • Phosphorus 0.35 g • Selenium Amino Acid Chelate 32 mcg • Molybdenum Amino Acid Chelate 52.5 mcg • Iron (ferrous fumarate) 9 mg • Riboflavin 0.83 mg • Vitamin B12 (cyanocobalamin) 3 mcg • Iodine (Potassium Iodide) 74 mg • Copper Sulfate 1 mg. Other Ingredients: Protein Blend: Calcium Caseinate, Whey Protein Concentrate, Milk Protein Isolate, Whey Protein Isolate, Sodium Caseinate; Dutch Processed Cocoa; Partially Hydrogenated Canola Oil; Corn Syrup Solids; Natural and Artificial Flavors; Fibersol (Maltodextrin); Salt; Soy Lecithin; Aspartame; Xanthan Gum; Cellulose Gum; Medium Chain Triglycerides; Carrageenan; Mono & Diglycerides.

Myoplex Original **-** EAS, Inc.
Each packet (76 g) contains: MyoPro: Whey Protein concentrate (from specially filtered and ion-exchanged whey protein), Calcium Caseinate, Milk-Protein isolate, Taurine, L-Glutamine, Sodium Caseinate, Egg Albumin, Alpha-Ketoglutaric Acid (AKG) • Calcium Caseinate • Corn Syrup Solids • Maltodextrin • Cocoa • Oat Fiber • Vitamin and Mineral Blend: Dipotassium Phosphate, Potassium Chloride, Magnesium Oxide, Choline Bitartrate, Disodium Phosphate, Beta Carotene, DL-Alpha Tocopheryl Acetate, Potassium Citrate, Ascorbic Acid, Ferrous Fumarate, Manganese Gluconate, Biotin, Tricalcium Phosphate, Niacinamide, Zinc Oxide, D-Calcium Pantothenate, Vitamin A Palmitate, Copper Sulfate, Chromium Citrate, Cyanocobalamin, Selenium Amino Acid Chelate, Molybdenum Amino Acid Chelate, Folic Acid, Pyridoxine Hydrochloride, Riboflavin, Thiamine Hydrochloride, Potassium Iodide • Sunflower oil • Natural and Artificial Flavors • Salt • Sucralose • Mono and Diglcyerides • Medium Chain Triglycerides • Soy Lecithin.

Myoplex Plus (vanilla flavor) **-** EAS, Inc.
Each 76 gram serving contains: Potassium 550 mg • Fiber < 1 g • Myopro [A unique blend of Whey Protein Isolate from specially filtered & ion-exchanged Whey Protein, Calcium Caseinate, Milk Protein Isolate, Taurine, L-Glutamine, Sodium Caseinate, Egg Albumin, & Calcium Alpha-Ketoglutarate (AKG)] • Maltodextrin • Corn Syrup Solids • Vitamin & Mineral Blend [Potassium Chloride, Disodium Phosphate, Calcium Phosphate, Magnesium Oxide, Potassium Citrate, Potassium Phosphate, Choline Bitartrate, Beta-Carotene, Ascorbic Acid, Dl-Alpha Tocopheryl Acetate, Ferrous Fumarate, Molybdenum Amino Acid Chelate, Boron Proteinate, Manganese Gluconate, Selenium Amino Acid Chelate, Niacinamide, Zinc Oxide, Calcium Pantothenate, Chromium Citrate, Copper Sulfate, Vitamin A Palmitate, Pyridoxine Hydrochloride, Riboflavin, Thiamine Hydrochloride, Vitamin D (as Vitamin D3), Folic Acid, Biotin, Potassium Iodide, & Cyanocobalamin] • Natural & Artificial Flavor • Partially Hydrogenated Canola oil • Aspartame • Citrimax brand Garcinia Cambogia extract • Salt • Medium-Chain Triglycerides • Xanthan Gum • Soy Lecithin • Cellulose Gum • Mono & Diglycerides • Borage oil. Contains Phenylalanine.

Myoplex Plus Deluxe **-** EAS, Inc.
Each 83 g Vanilla serving contains: Choline 100 mg • Molybdenum 50 mcg • Boron 1 mcg • Manganese 400 mcg • Selenium 33 mcg • Chromium 100 mcg • Vanadyl Sulfate 10 mg • Conjugated Linoleic Acid 1000 mg • Sodium RNA 9.5 mg • MyoPro Proprietary Protein Blend: Whey Protein Isolate (from ion-exchanged whey, milk protein isolate, calcium caseinate, sodium caseinate, & egg albumin) • Maltodextrin GKG Proprietary Blend: L-Glutamine, Calcium Alpha-Ketoglutarate (AKG), Taurine, Potassium Chloride, Potassium Phosphate, Magnesium Phosphate, Magnesium Oxide, Sodium RNA, Manganese Glycinate • CLA (conjugated linoleic acid from sunflower oil) • Natural & Artificial Flavors • Partially Hydrogenated Canola oil • Xanthan Gum • V2G Proprietary Blend: Taurine, Vanadyl Sulfate, Sodium Selenate • Vitamin & Mineral Blend: Choline Bitartrate, Beta-Carotene, Ascorbic Acid, Dl-Alpha Tocopheryl Acetate, Ferrous

Fumarate, Molybdenum Amino Acid Chelate, Boron Proteinate, Niacinamide, Zinc Oxide, Calcium Pantothenate, Chromium Citrate, Copper Sulfate,Vitamin A Palmitate, Pyridoxine Hydrochloride, Riboflavin, Thiamine Hydrochloride, Vitamin D (D3), Folic Acid, Biotin, Potassium Iodide, Cyanocobalamin • Corn Syrup Solids • Salt • Soy Lecithin • Asparatame • Cellulose Gum • Carrageenan • Citrimax brand Garcinia Cambogia extract • Medium-Chain Triglycerides • Mono & Diglycerides • Borage oil • Phenylalanine.

Myoplex Plus Deluxe Bar - EAS, Inc.
Gral & Artificial Flavors • Nonfat Milk • Milk • Cocoa • Unsweetened Chocolate • GKG [A proprietary blend containing L-Glutamine, Calcium Alpha-Ketoglutarate (AKG), Taurine, Potassium Chloride, Potassium Phosphate, Magnesium Oxide, Magnesium Phosphate, Sodium RNA, & Manganese Glycinate] • V2G: A proprietary blend containing Taurine, Vanadyl Sulfate, Sodium Selenate • Vitamin & Mineral Blend [Dicalcium Phosphate, Sodium Ascorbate, Ferric Orthophosphate, Dl-Alpha Tocopherol Acetate, Niacinamide, Zinc Oxide, Copper Gluconate, Calcium Pantothenate, Chromium Citrate, Vitamin A Palmitate, Pyridoxine Hydrochloride, Riboflavin, Thiamine Mononitrate, Folic Acid, Chromium Chloride, Sodium Molybdate, Biotin, Potassium Iodide, Phylloquinone, Cholecalciferol, & Cyanocobalamin] • CLA (Calcium Conjugated Linoleic Acid from Sunflower oil) • Lecithin.

Myo-Plus - Standard Process, Inc.
Two tablets contain: Proprietary Blend 626 mg: Bovine Heart PMG extract, Bovine Liver, Choline Bitartrate, Calcium Lactate, Porcine Stomach, Bovine Orchic extract, Tillandsia Usneoides powder, Defatted Wheat germ, Nutritional Yeast, Allantoin, Inositol, Bovine Spleen, Ovine Spleen, Bovine Adrenal Cytosol extract, Porcine Brain, Oat flour • Vitamin C 14.5 mg • Vitamin E 2 IU • Riboflavin 1.6 mg • Niacin 14 mg • Vitamin B6 0.5 mg • Selenium 2.8 mcg • Potassium 5 mg. Other Ingredients: Honey, Arabic Gum, Glycerin.
See Editor's Note No. 14.

MyoSport - Pharmalogic
Each pouch contains: Phosphorous 179 mg • Magnesium 60 mg • Potassium 80 mg • Creatine Monohydrate 10 g. Other Ingredients: Dextrose, SynChros TD (time released creatine monohydrate), Agave Nectar, Pure Creatine Monohydrate, Disaccharide, Cocoa, Saturated Polyglycolysed Glycerides, Lecithin, Sodium Citrate, Magnesium Citrate, Natural Flavors, Artificial Flavors, Disodium Phosphate, Potassium Phosphate, Gum Acacia, Xantham Gum, Guar Gum, Gum Arabic, Silicon Dioxide.

Myostat - BioTest Laboratories, LLC
Each capsule contains: CSP-3 (Sulfo-Polysaccharide Extract from Cultured Cystoseria Canariensis) 500 mg. Other Ingredients: Gelatin, Cellulose, Magnesium Stearate.

Myo-Tone - Enzymatic Therapy
Each tablet contains: Vitamin D (Fish Liver oil) 133 IU • Vitamin E succinate/Wheat Germ) 10 IU • Calcium (Bone Meal) 180 mg • Manganese (Chelate) 63 mg • Vitamin C (Ascorbic Acid/Rose Hips) 60 mg • Potassium Chloride 50 mg • Magnesium (Chelate) 30 mg • Vitamin B6 (Pyridoxine HCl) 6 mg • Thiamine HCL (Vitamin B1) 5 mg • Niacin 5 mg • Riboflavin (Vitamin B2) 5 mg • Vitamin B12 (Cyanocobalamin) 10 mcg • Other Ingredients: Choline Bitartrate 50 mg • Muscle extract 50 mg • Inositol 50 mg • Betaine HCl 30 mg • Ammonium Chloride 30 mg, RNA Powder 3 mg.
See Editor's Note No. 14.

Myotrophin PMG - Standard Process, Inc.
Each tablet contains: Proprietary Blend 185 mg: Bovine Muscle PMG extract, Magnesium Citrate • Calcium 20 mg. Other Ingredients: Cellulose.
See Editor's Note No. 14.

MyoVive - Nutricia
One pack (4 fl oz) contains: Vitamin A 1113 IU • Vitamin C 125 mg • Vitamin D 100 IU • Vitamin E 400 IU • Thiamin (Vitamin B1) 13 mg • Riboflavin (Vitamin B2) 1.5 mg • Niacin (Vitamin B3) 10 mg • Vitamin B6 3 mg • Folic Acid 300 mcg • Vitamin B12 1.5 mcg • Biotin 50 mcg • Pantothenic Acid (Vitamin B5) 2 mg • Calcium 126 mg • Iron 0.4 mg • Phosphorus 74 mg • Iodine 40 mcg • Magnesium 9 mg • Zinc 6 mg • Selenium 20 mcg • Copper 0.6 mg • Manganese 1.2 mg • Chromium 13 mcg • Molybdenum 20 mcg • Chloride 81 mg • Sodium 50 mg • Potassium 300 mg • Cysteine 115 mg • Choline 40 mg • Coenzyme Q10 68 mg • L-Carnitine 1.4 g • Creatine 875 mg • Taurine 1.4 g • Fluoride 0.4 mg.

Myrrh Salve - Dial Herbs
Myrrh • White Poplar • Balsam Fir • Black Walnut • Cayenne. In a base of Beeswax, Glycerine & Cold Pressed Olive oil.

Myrrh-Goldenseal Plus Formula - Nature's Way
Two capsules contain: Proprietary formula: Cayenne pepper fruit • Goldenseal root • Myrrh Gum (Oleo-Gum Resin from stems). Other Ingredients: Gelatin.

Myrrh-Prickly Ash Bark Virtue - Blessed Herbs
Echinacea Angustifolia root • Goldenseal root • Myrrh Gum • Propolis • Prickly Ash bark • Grain alcohol & Distilled Water.

N A C (N-Acetyl Cysteine) - J. R. Carlson Laboratories, Inc.
Each 1 tsp serving contains: N-Acetyl Cysteine 1700 mg.

N A C (N-Acetyl Cysteine) - J. R. Carlson Laboratories, Inc.
Each capsule contains: L-Cysteine (N-acetyl) 500 mg.

NAC - Pain & Stress Center
Each capsule contains: Vitamin C (ascorbyl palmitate) 5 mg • N-Acetyl Cysteine 600 mg. Other Ingredients: Gelatin Capsule.

NAC - Xymogen
Each capsule contains: N-Acetyl Cysteine 600 mg.

N-A-C - Jarrow Formulas
Each capsule contains: N-Acetyl-L-Cysteine 500 mg. Other Ingredients: Cellulose, Magnesium Stearate, Silicon Dioxide, Gelatin.

NAC (N-Acetyl-L-Cysteine) 600 mg - Solgar
Each capsule contains: NAC (as N-acetyl-L-cysteine) 600 mg. Other Ingredients: Vegetable Cellulose, Vegetable Magnesium Stearate, Silica, Water, Vegetable Glycerin.

NAC (N-Acetyl-L-Cysteine) 600 mg - Vital Nutrients
Each capsule contains: N-Acetyl-L-Cysteine 600 mg.

NAC 600 - GNC
Each capsule contains: N-Acetyl-L-Cysteine 600 mg. Other Ingredients: Gelatin, Cellulose, Dicalcium Phosphate.

NAC 600 & Glutathione 100 - GNC
Each capsule contains: N-Acetyl-L-Cysteine 600 mg • L-Glutathione 100 mg. Other Ingredients: Gelatin.

NAC 600 mg - Pure Encapsulations
Each vegetable capsule contains: N-Acetyl-L-Cysteine (free-form) 600 mg • Vitamin C (as ascorbyl palmitate) 5 mg.

NAC 900 mg - Pure Encapsulations
Each vegetable capsule contains: N-Acetyl-L-Cysteine (free-form) 900 mg • Vitamin C (as ascorbyl palmitate) 10 mg.

NAC Fuel - TwinLab
Each capsule contains: Highest Quality Pharmaceutical Grade NAC (N-Acetyl-Cysteine) 600 mg.

N-A-C Sustain - Jarrow Formulas
Each tablet contains: N-Acetyl-L-Cysteine 600 mg. Other Ingredients: Polyacrylate, Calcium Phosphate, Cellulose, Stearic Acid, Magnesium Stearate, Silicon Dioxide.

N-Acetyl Cysteine - DaVinci Laboratories
Each capsule contains: N-Acetyl Cysteine 500 mg. Other Ingredients: Rice Flour, Gelatin (vegetable source), Vegetable Stearate.

N-Acetyl Cysteine - PhysioLogics
Each capsule contains: N-Acetyl Cysteine 600 mg. Other Ingredients: Maltodextrin, Gelatin, Silica, Vegetable Magnesium Stearate.

Some Brand Name Natural Products - What they Contain

www.NaturalDatabase.com contains MANY more listings than appear here.

Editor's Notes are located on pages 2155-2163.

BRAND NAMES

N-Acetyl Cysteine **- Ortho Molecular Products**
Each capsule contains: N-Acetyl Cysteine USP 500 mg.Other Ingredients: Natural Vegetable Capsules, Ascorbyl Palmitate, Magnesium Stearate, Microcrystalline Cellulose, Silicon Dioxide.

N-Acetyl Cysteine **- Pro Health**
Each capsule contains: Calcium 24 mg • N-Acetyl Cysteine 600 mg. Other Ingredients: Stearic Acid, Microcrystalline Cellulose, Colloidal Silicon Dioxide, Modified Cellulose Gum, Magnesium Stearate.

N-Acetyl Glucosamine **- Allergy Research Group**
Each capsule contains: N-Acetyl-D-Glucosamine 500 mg. Other Ingredients: Cellulose, Stearic Acid.

N-Acetyl Tyrosine **- Jarrow Formulas**
Each capsule contains: Vitamin B6 (as pyridoxine hydrochloride) 5 mg • N-Acetyl Tyrosine 350 mg. Other Ingredients: Rice Powder, Magnesium Stearate, Silicon Dioxide, Gelatin.

N-A-G 750 **- Jarrow Formulas**
Each capsule contains: N-Acetyl-Glucosamine 750 mg. Other Ingredients: Magnesium Stearate, Gelatin.

Nails Special Formulation **- Vitamin World**
Each capsule contains: Vitamin B-6 (as pyridoxine hydrochloride) 6 mg • Magnesium (as magnesium aspartate) 17 mg • Potassium (as potassium aspartate) 45 mg • Amino Acid (from casein) 1500 mg. Other Ingredients: Cellulose (plant origin), Dicalcium Phosphate, Croscamellose, Vegetable Stearic Acid, Polyvinylpyrrolidone, Silica, Cellulose Coating.

NaPCA Moisture Mist **- Nu Skin Enterprises**
Water (aqua) • Aloe Vera gel • Glycerin • Propylene Glycol • Sodium PCA • Lactic Acid • Citric Acid • Hyaluronic Acid • Sodium Lactate • Niacinamide • Glycine • Inositol • Urea • Fructose • Octyl Methoxycinnamate • Polysorbate 20 • Methylparaben • Diazolidinyl Urea • 2-Bromo-2-Nitropropane-1,3-Diol • Sodium Benzoate.

NaPCA Moisturizer **- Nu Skin Enterprises**
Water • Aloe Vera gel • Stearic Acid • Propylene Glycol • Glyceryl Stearate SE • Sodium PCA • Tocopheryl Linoleate • Tocopheryl Acetate • Hyaluronic Acid • Algae extract • Sorbitol • Allantoin • Retinyl Palmitate • Cholecalciferol • Royal Jelly • RNA • Octyl Methoxycinnamate • Octyl Stearate • Octyl Palmitate • Dioctyl Adipate • Cetearyl Alcohol • Ceteareth-20 • Carbomer • Triethanolamine • Fragrance • Diazolidinyl Urea • Methylparaben • Propylparaben • Disodium EDTA • Iron Oxides.

Nasal Spray **- NutriBiotic**
Contains 0.1% Grapefruit extract, combined with Sodium Ascorbate (buffered Vitamin C).

NatCell Adrenal **- Allergy Research Group**
Each bottle (7 mL) contains: NatCell Adrenal (bovine aqueous extract) 7 mL.

NatCell Liver **- Allergy Research Group**
Each bottle (7 mL) contains: NatCell Liver (bovine liver aqueous extract) 7 mL.
See Editor's Note No. 14.

NatCell Liver **- Atrium Biotechnologies**
Each 7 mL vial contains: Water • Liver and Mescenchyme extracts of Bovine Embryos.
See Editor's Note No. 14.

NatCell Mesenchyme **- Allergy Research Group**
Each bottle (7 mL) contains: NatCell Mesenchyme (bovine mesenchyme aqueous extract) 7 mL.

Naticor **- Generation+**
Three vegetable capsules contain: Nattokinase 108 mg • Serrapeptase 45 mg • Protease 72 mg • Lipoic Acid 105 mg. Other Ingredients: Rutoside, Calcium Citrate, Magnesium Citrate, Zinc Methionate.

Natrapel Plus Insect Repellent **- Tender Corporation**
Active Ingredients: Citronella oil 5% • Geraniol 2% • 2-Phenethyl Propionate 2% • Sodium Lauryl Sulfate 1.74% • Potassium Sorbate 0.20%. Inactive Ingredients: Purified Water, Sorbitol, Wintergreen Oil, Mineral Oil, Sodium Bicarbonate, Xanthan Gum.

Natria Irish Moss Lotion **- Nature's Sunshine**
Water • Butylene Glycol • Cetearyl Alcohol • Glycerin • Sodium Stearoyl Lactylate • Glyceryl Stearate • Chondrus Crispus extract (Irish moss) • Cetraria Islandica extract (Iceland moss) • Carthamus Tinctorius seed oil (safflower) • Glycine Soja seed extract • Glycine Soja lipids • Squalane • Biosaccharide Gum-1 • Retinyl Palmitate (vitamin A) • Panthenyl Triacetate (vitamin B) • Tetrahexyldecyl Ascorbate (vitamin C) • Tocopheryl Acetate (vitamin E) • Aloe Barbadensis • Camellia Oleifera leaf extract (green tea) • Chamomilla Recutita flower extract (matricaria) • Ginkgo Biloba leaf extract • Panax Ginseng root extract • Ulva Lactuca extract (sea lettuce) • Vitis Vinifera seed extract (grape) • Zea Mays oil (corn) • Morinda Citrifolia extract (noni) • Fragrance • Sodium PCA • Ergothioneine • Sodium Hyaluronate • Dipotassium Glycyrrhizate • Hydrogenated Vegetable Oil • Caprylic/Capric Triglyceride • Xanthan Gum • Tetrasodium EDTA • Carbomer • Diemthicone • Phenoxyethanol • Methylparaben • Butylparaben • Ethylparaben • Propylparaben.

Natto-K **- Enzymedica**
Each capsule contains: Nattokinase NSK-SD 800 FU • Amylase Thera-Blend 3600 DU • Protease Thera-Blend 16,000 HUT • Bromelain 96 GDU • Mineral Blend 40 mg • Glucoamylase 40 AGU • Cellulase Thera-Blend 1000 CU • Lipase Thera-Blend 600 FCCFIP.

Nattokinase **- Source Naturals**
Two softgels contain: Nattokinase (providing 1440 fibrinolytic units (FU) of activity) 72 mg. Other Ingredients: Soybean Oil, Gelatin, Glycerin, Beeswax, Glycerin Fatty Acid Ester, Soybean Lecithin.

Nattokinase **- Ortho Molecular Products**
Each softgel contains: Vitamin E 10 IU • Nattokinase (at least 20,000 fibrynoliyic units per gram at time of manufacture) 50 mg. Other Ingredients: Rice Bran Oil, Gelatin, Glycerin, Purified Water, Lecithin, Yellow Beeswax, Turmeric Powder, Titanium Dioxide.

Nattokinase **- Springboard**
Two capsules contain: Nattokinase 1440 FU (72 mg). Other Ingredients: Soybean Oil, Soybean Lecithin.

Nattokinase **- Advanced Orthomolecular Research (AOR)**
Each softgel contains: Nattokinase 38 mg. Other Ingredients: Soy, Lecithin, Soybean Oil, Bees Wax, Glycerin Fatty Acid Ester, Gelatin, Glycerin.

NattoKinase **- Xymogen**
Each capsule contains: NSK-SD brand Nattokinase (active enzyme at 20,000 FU/g) 40 mg. Other Ingredients: Cellulose, Magnesium Stearate.

Nattokinase 100 MG **- Solaray**
Each capsule contains: Nattokinase 100 mg. Other Ingredients: Rice Flour, Gelatin Capsule, Cellulose, Glyceryl Triacetate, Magnesium Stearate, Silica.

Nattokinase 100 mg (2,000 FU) **- NSI - Nutraceutical Sciences Institute**
Each capsule contains: Nattokinase (providing 2000 fibrinolytic units (FU) of activity (NSK-SD)) 100 mg. Other Ingredients: Kosher Gelatin, Cellulose, Magnesium Stearate.

Nattokinase 1500 **- Naturally Vitamins**
Two tablets contain: Nattokinase (providing 1500 FU, 20,000 FU/gm) 75 mg • Rutin Bioflavonoid Complex (vitamin P) 100 mg. Other Ingredients: Plant Fiber, Modified Cellulose Gum, Colloidal Silica, Vegetable Magnesium Stearate, Vegetable Stearic Acid, pH-Resistant Enteric Coating.

Nattokinase Formula **- Aidan Products, LLC**
Each capsule contains: Nattokinase (NSK-SD) 36.7 mg. Other Ingredients: Soybean Oil, Lecithin, Gelatin, Glycerin, Beeswax.

Some Brand Name Natural Products - What they Contain

www.NaturalDatabase.com contains MANY more listings than appear here.
Editor's Notes are located on pages 2155-2163.

Nattokinase Plus **-** Vesta Pharmaceuticals
Two capsules contain: Vitamin E 400 IU • Nattokinase 200 mg (3600 FU). Other Ingredients: Microcrystalline Cellulose, Magnesium Stearate, Silicon Dioxide.

NattoQ10 **-** World Nutrition
Each capsule contains: NattoVega Propriety Blend 20 mg • Reishi mushroom 250 mg • Hydro soluble Coenzyme Q10 complex 60 mg. Other Ingredients: Vegetable Cellulose, Water, Rice Bran.

Natura Mix Adult (Caps) **-** Aboca USA, Inc
Each capsule contains: Asian Ginseng root Whole Phytocomplex Concentrate (WPC) (panax ginseng, standardized to 4% total ginsenosides) 94.5 mg • Royal Jelly (10 hydroxydecenoic acid minimum 2%) 94.5 mg • Siberian Ginseng root WPC (eleutherococcus senticosus, standardized to 0.7% eleutherosides B+E) 40.5 mg • Bee Pollen powder 40.5 mg. Other Ingredients: Gelatin (capsule).

Natura Mix Adult (Vials) **-** Aboca USA, Inc
Each vial contains: Bilberry fruit juice concentrate (vaccinium myrtillus, total anthocyanidins minimum 0.2%) 8.3 g • Acacia Honey 6 g • Royal Jelly (10 hydroxydecenoic acid minimum 1%) 0.5 g • Asian Ginseng root freeze-dried extract (panax ginseng, standardized to 15% total ginsenosides) 0.12 g • Bee Pollen freeze-dried extract 0.03 g • Siberian Ginseng root freeze-dried extract (eleutherococcus senticosus, standardized to 1.5% eleutherosides B+E) 0.023 g • Brewer's Yeast freeze-dried extract 0.027 g.

Natura Mix Child **-** Aboca USA, Inc
Each vial contains: Acacia Honey 9.9 g • Bilberry fruit juice complex (vaccinium myrtillus, total anthocyanosides minimum 0.2%) 4 g • Royal Jelly (10 hydroxydecenoic acid minimum 1%) 0.5 g • Blackberry fruit juice concentrate (rubus fruticosus) 0.45 g • Acerola fruit freeze-dried extract (malpighia glabra) 0.04 g • Bee Pollen freeze-dried extract 0.04 g • Brewer's Yeast freeze-dried extract 0.02 g. Other Ingredients: Natural Strawberry Flavoring.

Natura Mix Senior **-** Aboca USA, Inc
Each vial contains: Acacia Honey 7.7 g • Bilberry fruit juice concentrate (vaccinium myrtillus, total anthocyanidins minimum 0.2%) 6.5 g • Royal Jelly (10 hydroxydecenoic acid minimum 1%) 0.5 g • Ginkgo leaf freeze-dried extract (ginkgo biloba, standardized to 1% terpene lactones, 3% ginkgo flavone glycosides) 0.15 g • Bee Pollen freeze-dried extract 0.06 g • Schisandra fruit (schisandra chinensis, standardized to 1% schizandrins) 0.045 g • Acerola fruit freeze-dried extract (malpighia glabra) 0.035 g. Other Ingredients: Natural Lemon Flavoring.

Naturafed **-** Pacific BioLogic
Angelica root (dahurica) • Peppermint (field mint) • Bupleurum root (natural) • Cnidium root • Ligusticum root (Chinese) • Astragalus root (Grade 1) • Scute root • Platycodon root • Honeysuckle flower • Schizonepta stem • Gentian root (Chinese) • Ephedra Herba (aerial) • Jasmine fruit (cape) • Magnolia flower • Houtuynia.
See Editor's Note No. 30.

Natural Advanced Carotenoid Complex **-** Solgar
Each softgel contains: Vitamin A (100% as natural beta carotene) 25,000 IU • Zinc (as zinc oxide) 1.2 mg • Alpha Carotene 10 mg • Lutein (from marigold flower) 2 mg • Carotenoids 750 mcg • Gamma-Carotene 400 mcg • Annatto seed extract 3 mg • Zeaxanthin (from marigold flower) 55 mcg • Lecithin (from soy) 6 mg. Other Ingredients: Corn Oil, Gelatin, Glycerin, Yellow Beeswax, D-Alpha Tocopherol, Water.

Natural B100 Complex **-** Sunmark
Each tablet contains: Thiamin 100 mg • Riboflavin 100 mg • Niacin 100 mg • Vitamin B6 100 mg • Folate 400 mcg • Vitamin B12 100 mcg • Biotin 100 mcg • Pantothenic Acid 100 mg. Other Ingredients: Dicalcium Phosphate, Microcrystalline Cellulose, Modified Cellulose Gum, Stearic Acid, Silicon Dioxide, Magnesium Stearate, Crospovidone, Hydroxypropyl Methylcellulose, Hydroxypropyl Cellulose, Polyethylene Glycol.
See Editor's Note No. 45.

Natural B-12 with Liver **-** Leiner Health Products
Each tablet contains: Vitamin B12 (Cyanocobalamin) 1000 mcg. Other Ingredients: Dicalcium Phosphate, Stearic Acid, Liver, Croscarmellose Sodium, Yeast, Silicon Dioxide, Magnesium Stearate.

Natural B50 Complex **-** Sunmark
Each tablet contains: Thiamin 50 mg • Riboflavin 50 mg • Niacin 50 mg • Vitamin B6 (pyridoxine HCl) 50 mg • Folate 400 mcg • Vitamin B12 50 mcg • Biotin 50 mcg • Pantothenic Acid 50 mg. Other Ingredients: Dicalcium Phosphate, Microcrystalline Cellulose, Calcium Pantothenate, Modified Cellulose Gum, Stearic Acid, Silicon Dioxide, Magnesium Stearate.
See Editor's Note No. 45.

Natural B6 100 mg **-** Sunmark
Each tablet contains: Vitamin B6 (pyridoxine hydrochloride) 100 mg. Other Ingredients: Dicalcium Phosphate, Microcrystalline Cellulose, Magnesium Stearate.
See Editor's Note No. 45.

Natural Balance B-100 Complex **-** Leiner Health Products
Each tablet contains: Thiamin Mononitrate (Vitamin B1) 100 mg • Riboflavin (Vitamin B2) 100 mg • Vitamin B6 (Pyridoxine Hydrochloride) 100 mg • Niacin 100 mg • Biotin 100 mcg • Vitamin B12 100 mcg • Pantothenic Acid 100 mg • Folate 400 mcg. Other Ingredients: Calcium Carbonate, Cellulose, Maltodextrin, Croscarmellose Sodium, Silicon Dioxide, Polyethylene Glycol 3350, Dicalcium Phosphate, Crospovidone, Tricalcium Phosphate.

Natural Balance B-50 Complex **-** Leiner Health Products
Each tablet contains: Vitamin B12 50 mcg • Pantothenic Acid (D-calcium pantothenate) 50 mg • Thiamin Mononitrate (vitamin B1) 50 mg • riboflavin (Vitamin B2) 50 mg • Vitamin B6 (pyridoxine hydrochloride) 50 mg • Niacin (niacinamide) 50 mg • Folate 100 mcg • Biotin 50 mcg. Other Ingredients: Calcium Carbonate, Cellulose, Maltodextrin, Croscarmellose Sodium, Sodium Starch Glycolate, Silicon Dioxide, Polyethylene Glycol 3350, Tricalcium Phosphate.

Natural Balanced B Complex + C **-** Leiner Health Products
One tablet contains: Vitamin B12 50 mcg • Vitamin C (Ascorbic Acid) 500 mg • Pantothenic Acid (d-Calcium Pantothenate) 50 mg • Thiamin Mononitrate (Vitamin B1) 50 mg • Riboflavin (Vitamin B2) 50 mg • Vitamin B6 (Pyridoxine Hydrochloride) 50 mg • Niacin 50 mg • Biotin 50 mcg • Folate 400 mcg. Other Ingredients: Calcium Carbonate, Yeast, Cellulose, Croscarmellose Sodium, Sodium Starch Glycolate, Silicon Dioxide, Rose Hips, Polyethylene Glycol 3350, Cyanocobalamin.

Natural Bee Pollen **-** Lichtwer Pharma US
Each tablet contains: Bee Pollen 500 mg. Other Ingredients: Sorbitol, Calcium Carbonate, Sodium Starch Glycolate, Silicon Dioxide, Maltodextrin, Crospovidone, Hydroxypropyl Methylcellulose, Stearic Acid, Hydroxypropyl Cellulose, Magnesium Stearate, Polysorbate 80, Polyethylene Glycol 3350.

Natural Beta Carotene **-** Leiner Health Products
Each softgel contains: Vitamin A 25000 IU. Other Ingredients: Soybean Oil, Gelatin, Glycerin, Partially Hydrogenated Cottonseed and Soybean oils, Yellow Beeswax, Beta Carotene, Carrot Oil.

Natural Beta Carotene **-** Vital Nutrients
Each capsule contains: Beta Carotene (natural beta carotene, mixed carotenes, naturally derived from d. salina) 25,000 IU.

Natural Beta-Carotene 25,000 IU **-** Arrowroot
Each gelcap contains: Beta-Carotene 25,000 IU (from D. salina).

Natural Breath Pearls **-** Golden Glow Natural Health Products
Each liquid-filled gelcap contains: Peppermint oil 20 mg • Parsley seed oil 16 mg.

Natural Brewer's Yeast **-** Leiner Health Products
Two tablets contain: Vitamin B1 0.12 mg • Vitamin B2 0.04 mg • Niacin 0.30 mg • Vitamin B6 0.02 mg. Other Ingredients: Brewer's Yeast, Cellulose, Guar Gum, Silicon Dioxide.

Natural Bronchial Syrup - Tom's of Maine
Each teaspoon (5 ml) contains: Thyme extract (Thymus vulgaris L) 190 mg • Pine extract (Pinus strobus L) 125 mg • Marshmallow aqueous extract (Althaea officinalis L) 103 mg • Licorice extract (Glycyrrhiza glabra L) 75 mg. Other Ingredients: Honey, Natural Black Cherry extract, Natural Almond extract, Xanthan Gum, or Natural Benzoic Acid.

Natural Calcium & Magnesium - Leiner Health Products
Each tablet contains: Magnesium Oxide 167 mg • Calcium 334 mg. Other Ingredients: Oyster Shell, Maltodextrin, Cellulose, Talc, may contain less than 2% of Mineral Oil, Soy Fiber, Croscarmellose Sodium, Sodium Starch Glycolate, Crospovidone, Magnesium Stearate, Stearic Acid.

Natural Calcium Magnesium & Zinc - Leiner Health Products
Each tablet contains: Calcium Carbonate 333 mg • Magnesium Oxide 133 mg • Zinc Sulfate 5 mg. Other Ingredients: Maltodextrin, Starch, Cellulose, Croscarmellose Sodium, Tricalcium Phosphate, Talc, Sodium Starch Glyolate, Hydroxypropyl Methylcellulose, Silicon Dioxide, Magnesium Stearate, Hydroxypropyl Cellulose, Egg.

Natural Chewable Acidophilus - Puritan's Pride
Each tablet contains: Lactobacillus Acidophilus 10 mg. Other Ingredients: Sucrose, Dextrose, Sweet Whey, Maltodextrin, Cellulose (Plant Origin), Carrageenan, Dried Banana Powder, Vegetable Magnesium Stearate, Silica, Vanilla Flavor, Malt Flavor.

Natural Cholesterol Formula - Xtend-Life Nutraceuticals Inc.
Two soft gels contain: Policosanol (from sugar cane) 25 mg • Policosanol (rice bran) 25 mg • Phytosterols (beta sitosterol) 330 mg • Guggulipid extract 150 mg • Theaflavin extract (from green tea) 200 mg • Proprietary Natural Oil Blend 1320 mg: Oryzanol Rice Bran oil, D-Limonene oil, Pumpkin seed oil, Vitamin E oil, Lecithin oil.

Natural Coenzyme Q10 - Nature's Bounty
Each softgel contains: Coenzyme Q-10 30 mg. Other Ingredients: Rice Bran Oil, Gelatin, Glycerin, Beeswax, Soybean Oil Mixture, Lecithin.

Natural Curves - Biotech Corp.
Two tablets contain: Proprietary Blend 493 mg: Saw Palmetto berry (sabal serrulata), Damiana leaves (turnera aphrodisiaca), Dong Quai root (angelica sinensis), Dandelion root (taraxacum officinale), Blessed Thistle leaves (cnicus benedictus), Kava Kava root (piper methysticum), Wild Yam root (dioscorea villosa), Motherwort leaves (leonurus carduaca), Fenugreek seed (trigonella foenum-graecum), Black Cohosh (cimicifuga racemosa), Fennel seed (foeniculum vulgare), Chasteberry root (vitex agnus castus), Panax Ginseng, Soy Isoflavones (glycine max), Bioperine brand Black Pepper (piper nigrum). Other Ingredients: Oat Bran Filler, Anise Oil.

Natural Curves Instant Bust Firming Gel - Biotech Corp.
Deionized Water • Propylene Glycol • Niacin • Hydroxypropyl Methylcellulose • Polysorbate 20 • Sodium Hydroxide • DMDM Hydantoin • Iodopropynyl Butylcarbamate • Algae extract • Calendula Officinalis flower extract • Benzophenone-4 • Tocopherol • Blue 1 • Red 33.

Natural D-Hist - Ortho Molecular Products
Each capsule contains: Vitamin C (as ascorbic acid) 150 mg • Quercetin 200 mg • Stinging Nettles leaf powder 200 mg • Bromelain (2400 GDU/g) 50 mg • N-Acetyl Cysteine USP 25 mg. Other Ingredients: Natural Vegetable Capsules, Magnesium Stearate, Microcrystalline Cellulose.

Natural Dolomite with Bone Meal - Puritan's Pride
Six tablets contain: Calcium (from Dolomite and Bone Meal) 1,287 mg • Magnesium (from Dolomite) 303 mg • Phosphorus 294 mg.

Natural E - GNC
Each capsule contains: Vitamin E 400 IU. Other Ingredients: Calcium Sulfate, Gelatin.

Natural E 1000 d-alpha Form - GNC
Each capsule contains: VItamin E (as d-alpha tocopheryl acetate) 1000 IU. Other Ingredients: Gelatin, Soybean Oil, Glycerin.

Natural E 1000 Natural Mixed Tocopherols - GNC
Each capsule contains: Vitamin E (as d-alpha tocopherols) 1000 IU. Other Ingredients: Soybean Oil, Gelatin, Glycerin.

Natural E 200 - GNC
Each capsule contains: Vitamin E (as d-alpha tocopherol) 200 IU. Other Ingredients: Gelatin, Soybean Oil, Glycerin.

Natural E 400 IU - GNC
Each capsule contains: Vitamin E 400 IU. Other Ingredients: Calcium Sulfate, Gelatin.

Natural E 400 IU - Sunmark
Each softgel contains: Vitamin E 400 IU. Other Ingredients: Gelatin, Glycerin, Soybean Oil, Purified Water.
See Editor's Note No. 45.

Natural E 400 Natural Mixed Tocopherols - GNC
Each capsule contains: Vitamin E (as d-alpha tocopherol) 400 IU. Other Ingredients: Soybean Oil, Gelatin, Glycerin.

Natural E 400 Softgel Capsules - GNC
Each capsule contains: Vitamin E (as d-alpha tocopheryl acetate) 400 IU. Other Ingredients: Gelatin, Soybean oil, Glycerin.

Natural E 400 with Selenium - GNC
Each capsule contains: Vitamin E (as d-alpha tocopheryl acetate) 400 IU • Selenium (as yeast) 100 mcg. Other Ingredients: Soybean oil, Gelatin, Glycerin, Carob extract, Titanium Dioxide.

Natural E Mixed Tocopherols - Ortho Molecular Products
Each soft gel contains: Vitamin E (as D-alpha tocopherol) 400 IU • Total non alpha Tocopherols forms 200 mg: Gamma Tocopherol 146 mg, Delta Tocopherols 33 mg. Other Ingredients: Mixed Tocopherol Blen, Gelatin, Glycerin, Purified Water.

Natural E-400 - Jarrow Formulas
Each softgel contains: Vitamin E (as D-alpha tocopheryl acetate) 400 IU. Other Ingredients: Soybean Oil, Gelatin, Glycerin, Water.

Natural Emulsified Vitamin E 500IU - Golden Glow Natural Health Products
Each capsule contains: D-Alpha-Tocopherol 335 mg: Natural Vitamin E 500 IU.

Natural Facelift Capsule - Healthy Revelations Inc.
Meadowfoam seed oil (limnanthes alba) • Cyclomethicone • Tocopheryl Acetate • Isopropyl Alcohol • Isostearoyl Hydrolyzed Collagen • Retinyl Palmitate • Placental Lipids • Alcohol • Calendula Officinalis extract • Olive Oil Unsaponifiables • Soybean Oil Unsaponifiables • Wheat Germ Oil Unsaponifiables • Pollen extract • Isodecyl Citrate • Tripropylene Glycol Citrate • Juniperus Communis extract • Rosemary extract (rosmarinus officinalis) • Eucalyptus extract (eucalyptus globules) • Fenugreek extract (trigonella foenum graecum) • Peppermint extract (mentha piperita) • Propylparaben • Salicylic Acid • Clary extract (salvia sclarea) • Bitter Orange extract (citrus aurantium) • Coenzyme Q10 • N-Stearoyl-DL-Sphinganine • Allantoin • Dibutyl Lauroyl Glutamide • FD&C Green #3.

Natural Facelift Facial Mask - Healthy Revelations Inc.
Water • Carbomer • Panthenol • Urea • Aloe extract (aloe barbadensis) • Glycerin • Glyceryl Stearate • Glucose • Caprylic/Capric Triglyceride • Hydrolyzed Elastin • Hydrolyzed Collagen • Soluble Collagen • Lactoyl Methylsilanol Elastinate • Hops extract • Placental Enzymes • Dimethylsilanol Hyaluronate • Methylsilanol Hydroxproline Asparate • Licorice extract • Hydrocotyl extract • Butcherbroom extract • Green Tea extract • Coenzyme Q10 • Tocopheryl Acetate • Meadowfoam seed oil • Placental Lipids • Retinyl Palmitate • Ivy extract • Bearberry extract • Glycosaminoglycans • Arnica extract • Juniper extract • Myrrh extract • Sorbitol • Stearic Acid • Polysorbate 60 • PEG 7 Glyceryl Cocoate • Stearyl Alcohol • Coneflower extract • Methylparaben • Horsetail

extract • Propylparaben • Niacinamide • PCA Ethyl Cocoyl Arginate • PVM/MA Decadiene Crosspolymer • Cabbage Rose extract • Dibutyl Lauroyl Glumatide • Tocopherol • Ascorbyl Palmitate • Lecithin • Glyceryl Oleate • Citric Acid • Adenosine Phosphate • Adenosine Triphosphate • Propylene Glycol • Fragrance • FD&C Red #40.

Natural Fast Release Lysine **-** Leiner Health Products
Each tablet contains: L-Lysine Monohydrochloride 500 mg. Other Ingredients: Dicalcium Phosphate, Cellulose, Croscarmellose Sodium, Stearic Acid, Silicon Dioxide, Magnesium Stearate.

Natural Fish Oil Concentrate **-** Leiner Health Products
Two softgels contain: Natural Fish Oil concentrate 2000 mg • EPA (eicosapentaenoic acid) 360 mg • DHA (docosahexaenoic acid) 240 mg. Other Ingredients: Gelatin, Glycerin, D-Alpha Tocopherol.

Natural Form GH-3 **-** Life Extension
Each tablet contains: DMAE 100 mg • Tyrosine 100 mg • Chondroitin Sulfate 65 mg • PABA (para-aminobenzoic acid) 50 mg • Glutamine 50 mg • Phosphatidyl Choline 50 mg • Taurine 50 mg • Magnesium 50 mg • Ascorbyl Palmitate 50 mg • Ginkgo Biloba 25 mg • Vitamin E 30 mg • Vitamin B6 15 mg • Vitamin B12 1 mg.
See Editor's Note No. 15.

Natural Gain Plus **-** Ultra Herbal, LLC
Two tablets contain: Niacin 50 mg • Zinc (as zinc oxide) 26 mg • Maca tuber 333 mg • Catuaba bark 83 mg • Muira Puama bark 83 mg • L-Arginine HCl 67 mg • Heart-Leaf Sida (entire plant) 80 mg • Barrenwort (aerial parts) 73 mg • Tribulus herb 67 mg • Cola seed 50 mg • Oat straw 50 mg • Stinging Nettle leaf 50 mg • Pumpkin seed 50 mg • Ginger root 40 mg • Cayenne (25,000 HU) 40 mg • American Ginseng root 33 mg • Eleuthero root 33 mg • Asian Ginseng root 33 mg • Sarsaparilla root 33 mg • Orchic Substance (bovine) 20 mg • Boron Citrate 7 mg. Other Ingredients: Cellulose, Gum Arabic (acacia), Vegetable Stearic Acid, Modified Cellulose, Silicon Dioxide, Vegetable Magnesium Stearate, FD&C Blue #2, FD&C Indigo Carmine Lake.
See Editor's Note 14 and No. 39.

Natural Garlic Oil **-** Leiner Health Products
Each softgel contains: Garlic oil 3 mg. Other Ingredients: Vegetable Oil, Gelatin, Glycerin.

Natural Herbal Cleanse **-** Abundance Marketing
Each scoop contains: Herbal Cleanse Blend 650 mg: Cassia seed, Juniper berry powder, Rhubarb root, Buchu leaf, Cascara Sagrada bark, Corn Silk powder, Date powder, Fig fruit, Ginger root, Slippery Elm powder bark, Tamarind fruit extract • Fiber Blend 7500 mg: Fibresol-2 brand Glucose Polymer Complex, Apple Pectin, Guar Gum, Oat Bran, Oat Fiber, Psyllium Fiber, Rice Fiber • Stevia leaf extract 66 mg. Other Ingredients: Beflora Plus with 50% Fructooligosaccharides, 47.5% Soy extract and 2.5% Potato starch, Natural Flavors, Citric Acid, Malic Acid, Beet Juice Powder, Silica.

Natural Herbal Energizer Caps **-** Leiner Health Products
Each caplet contains: Ginseng concentrate (American Ginseng, Korean Ginseng, Chinese Panax Ginseng) 200 mg • Herbal Blend 740 mg. Other Ingredients: Yerba Mate Extract, Croscarmellose Sodium, Gotu Kola, Guarana Extract, Dicalcium Phosphate, Stearic Acid, Magnesium Stearate, Silicon Dioxide, Cellulose, Hydroxypropyl Methylcellulose, Polyethylene Glycol 3350, Hydroxypropyl Cellulose, Damiana, Fo-Ti, Green Tea Extract, Jamaican Ginger.

Natural High Potency Iron **-** Leiner Health Products
Each softgel contains: Iron (Ferrous Fumarate) 27 mg. Other Ingredients: Vegetable Oil, Gelatin, Vegetable Shortening (Partially hydrogenated Soybean and Palm Oils), Glycerin, Blackstrap Molasses, Yellow Beeswax, Hydrogenated Soybean Oil, Lecithin, Polysorbate 80, Caramel Color, Titanium Dioxide.

Natural High Potency Multivitamin/Mineral **-** Leiner Health Products
Each tablet contains: Thiamin (Vitamin B1) 10 mg • Riboflavin (Vitamin B2) 10 mg • Phosphorus 40 mg • Biotin 10 mcg • Magnesium Oxide 100 mg • Vitamin B12 12 mcg • Vitamin C (Ascorbic Acid)100 mg • Calcium Carbonate 62 mg • Iron (Ferrous Fumarate) 27 mg • Vitamin A 7500 IU • Vitamin B6 3 mg • Selenium 10 mcg • Copper 2 mg • Folate 400 mcg • Iodine 150 mcg • Niacin (Niacinamide) 20 mg • Pantothenic Acid 10 mg • Vitamin D 400 IU • Vitamin E (dl-Alpha Tocopheryl Acetate) 30 IU • Zinc Sulfate 15 mg. Other Ingredients: Dicalcium Phosphate, Cellulose, Gelatin, Starch, Maltodextrin, Croscarmellose Sodium, Sodium Starch Glycolate, Kelp, Silicon Dioxide.

Natural Imperial Ginseng **-** Leiner Health Products
Each tablet contains: Ginseng (Siberian) root 250 mg. Other Ingredients: Dicalcium Phosphate,Vegetable Oil, Croscarmellose Sodium, Silicon Dioxide, Magnesium Stearate, Hydroxopropyl Methylcellulose, Hydroxypropyl Cellulose, Polysorbate 80, Polyethylene Glycol 3350.

Natural Iron-Free Multivitamin/Mineral Formula **-** Leiner Health Products
Each tablet contains: Molybdenum (Sodium Molybdate) 25 mcg • Vitamin K (Phytonadione) 25 mcg • Selenium (Sodium Selenate) 20 mcg • Magnesium Oxide 100 mg • Chromium Chloride 25 mcg • Calcium Carbonate 162 mg • Manganese Sulfate 2.5 mg • Phosphorus 109 mg • Copper (Cupric Oxide) 2 mg • Folate (Folic Acid) 400 mcg • Iodine 150 mcg • Niacin (Niacinamide) 20 mg • Pantothenic Acid (d-Calcium Pantothenate) 10 mg • Riboflavin (Vitamin B2) 1.7 mg • Thiamin Mononitrate (Vitamin B1) 1.5 mg • Vitamin A Acetate 5000 IU • Vitamin B12 (Cyanocobalamin - USP Method 2) 6 mcg • Vitamin B6 (Pyridoxine Hydrochloride) 2 mg • Vitamin C (Ascorbic Acid) 60 mg • Vitamin D (Ergocalciferol) 400 IU • Vitamin E (dl-Alpha Tocopheryl Acetate) 30 IU • Zinc Oxide 15 mg • Biotin (USP Method 2) 30 mcg • Chloride 36.3 mg • Potassium Chloride 40 mg • Nickel (Nickelous Sulfate) 5 mcg • Silicon 2 mg • Tin (Stannous Chloride) 10 mcg • Vanadium (Sodium Metavanadate) 10 mcg. Other Ingredients: Dicalcium Phosphate, Gelatin, Cellulose, Croscarmellose Sodium, Sodium Starch Glycolate, Hydroxypropyl Methylcellulose, Starch, Sodium Metasilicates & Oxides, Pharmaceutical Glaze, Polyethylene Glycol 3350, Magnesium Stearate, Maltodextrin, Hydroxypropyl Cellulose, Mannitol, Sodium & Potassium Borates, Polysorbate 80, Beta Carotene, Resin.

Natural KLB6 **-** Puritan's Pride
Two softgels contain: Vitamin B6 (Pyridoxine HCl) 7 mg • Lecithin 200 mg • Kelp 50 mg • Cider Vinegar 80 mg.

Natural L-Formula Lysine **-** Leiner Health Products
Each tablet contains: L-Lysine Monohydrochloride 500 mg. Other Ingredients: Cellulose, Polyethylene Glycol 3350, Croscarmellose Sodium, Silicon Dioxide, Magnesium Stearate.

Natural Light **-** Cell Tech
Each capsule contains: Chromium 50 mcg • Proprietary Algae Blend 80 mg: Blue-Green Algae (aphanizomenon flos-aquae), Bladderwrack Algae, Kelp 1:10 extract • Proprietary Enzyme Blend 40 mg: Lipase, Amylase, CereCalase, Protease, Pectinase • Cell Tech Herbal Weight Loss Blend 577 mg: Garcinia rind extract, Kola nut extract (10% caffeine), Gotu Kola (aerial part), Siberian Ginseng root, Fo-ti root, Gymnema sylvestre leaf extract (25% gymnemic acid), St. John's Wort (aerial part), Bitter Orange standardized extract, Guarana 4:1 extract (seed), Hawthorn extract (leaf and flower), Maca root, Green Tea extract 80/60, Cascara Sagrada bark, Ginkgo Biloba leaf 50:1 extract, Ginger (rhizome), White Willow bark, Cayenne Pepper fruit, Chromium Polynicotinate • Lecithin 15 mg. Other Ingredients: Vegetable Cellulose, Rice Bran, Water.
See Editor's Note No. 40.

Natural Lutein 6 MG **-** CVS Pharmacy
Each softgel contains: Lutein 6 mg. Other Ingredients: Corn Oil, Gelatin, Glycerin, Yellow Beeswax.

Natural Magnesium **-** Leiner Health Products
Each tablet contains: Magnesium Oxide 250 mg. Other Ingredients: Cellulose, Talc, Sodium Starch Glycolate, Starch, Silicon Dioxide, Croscarmellose Sodium, Polyethylene Glycol, Magnesium Stearate.

Some Brand Name Natural Products - What they Contain

www.NaturalDatabase.com contains MANY more listings than appear here.
Editor's Notes are located on pages 2155-2163.

BRAND NAMES

Natural Man - NDS Nutrition
Two capsules contain: Vitamin A (beta carotene with mixed carotenoids) 10,000 IU • Vitamin D (cholecalciferol) 400 IU • Vitamin E (D-alpha tocopheryl) 100 IU • Vitamin K 80 mcg • Vitamin C (calcium ascorbate) 600 mg • Vitamin B1 (thiamine) 50 mg • Vitamin B2 (riboflavin) 49 mg • Vitamin B3 (niacinamide) 50 mg • Vitamin B5 (calcium pantothenate) 50 mg • Vitamin B6 (pyridoxine) 50 mg • Vitamin B12 200 mcg • Biotin 400 mcg • Folic Acid 400 mcg • Calcium (milk calcium complex) 180 mg • Magnesium (citrate) 90 mg • Zinc (aspartate) 30 mg • Copper (gluconate) 2 mg • Iodine (potassium iodine) 150 mcg • Vanadium (asparate) 10 mcg • Boron (aspartate) 250 mcg • Manganese (citrate) 2 mg • Selenium (methionine) 100 mcg • Molybdenum (aspartate) 75 mcg • Chromium (nicotinate) 100 mcg. Other Ingredients: Brown Rice, Magnesium Stearate, Gelatine, Water.

Natural Mixed Carotenoids - Golden Glow Natural Health Products
Each softgel contains: Natural Mixed Carotenoids 30 mg.

Natural Multi-Amino Acid - GNC
Three capsules contain: L-Alanine 88.7 mg • L-Arginine 80.7 • L-Aspartic Acid 108 mg • L-Cystine 4.6 mg • L-Glutamic Acid 272.7 mg • Glycerine 142.2 mg • L-Histidine 25.6 mg • L-Isoleucine 33.3 mg • L-Leucine 99 mg • L-Lysine 88.3 mg • L-Methionine 29.2 mg • L-Phenylalanine 60 mg • L-Proline 169.8 mg • L-Serine 71.7 mg • L-Threonine 40.1 mg • L-Tryptophan 10.3 mg • L-Tyrosine 49.7 mg • L-Valine 48.4 mg • Hydroxylysine 5.6 mg • Hydroxyproline 78.9 mg • Protein (as calcium caseinate & gelatin) 2 g • Vitamin E (as d-alpha tocopherol) 1.5 IU • Liquid Soy Lecithin 22.5 mg. Other Ingredients: Soybean Oil, Glycerin, Titanium Dioxide.

Natural Multi-Minerals - Solgar
Two tablets contain: Vitamin D (as cholecalciferol) 200 IU • Calcium (from bone meal and dolomite) 374 mg • Iron (as ferrous gluconate) 10 mg • Phosphorus 118 mg • Iodine (from kelp) 50 mcg • Magnesium (from bone meal and dolomite) 76 mg • Copper (gluconate) 0.5 mg • Manganese (gluconate) 0.1 mg • Sodium 10 mg • Herbal Blend 10 mg: Acerola berry, Rose Hips fruit, Alfalfa whole plant, Parsley aerial, Watercress whole plant, Kelp whole plant. Other Ingredients: Microcrystalline Cellulose, Vegetable Cellulose, Silica, Potassium Gluconate, Glycerin, Zinc Gluconate, Carnauba Wax.

Natural Orange Flavour C-1000mg - Golden Glow Natural Health Products
Each tablet contains: Ascorbic Acid (vitamin C, from sodium ascorbate 563 mg and ascorbic acid 500 mg) 1000 mg. Other Ingredients: Saccharin Sodium, Gluten (from maltodextrin, derived from wheat).

Natural Orange Flavour C-500mg - Golden Glow Natural Health Products
Each tablet contains: Ascorbic Acid (vitamin C, from sodium ascorbate 281.23 mg and ascorbic acid 250 mg) 500 mg. Other Ingredients: Saccharin Sodium, Gluten (from maltodextrin, derived from wheat).

Natural Oyster Shell Calcium - Leiner Health Products
Each tablet contains: Calcium 500 mg. Other Ingredients: Oyster Shell, Maltodextrin, Acacia Gum, Croscarmellose Sodium, Tricalcium Phosphate, Magnesium Stearate.

Natural Oyster Shell Calcium with D - Leiner Health Products
Each tablet contains: Vitamin D 200 IU • Calcium 500 mg. Other Ingredients: Oyster Shell, Maltodextrin, Acacia, may contain less than 2% of Cellulose, Mineral Oil, Croscarmellose Sodium, Tricalcium Phosphate, Soy Fiber, Magnesium Stearate, Ergocalciferol, Crospovidone, Stearic Acid.

Natural Potassium Gluconate - Leiner Health Products
Each tablet contains: Potassium Gluconate 90 mg. Other Ingredients: Cellulose, Croscarmellose Sodium, Sodium Starch Glycolate, Starch, Polyethylene Glycol 3350, Silicon Dioxide, Magnesium Stearate.

Natural Progesterone Cream - DaVinci Laboratories
Soy • Saw Palmetto • Dong Quai • Cramp Bark • Sarsaparilla • Rosemary extract • Vitamin A • Vitamin E (tocopherol) • Avocado oil • Carrot oil • Lemon Grass oil.

Natural Prostate Formula - Life Extension
Each softgel contains: Saw Palmetto berries CO2 extract (serenoa repens) 160 mg • Free Fatty Acids/Sterols (85-95% from saw palmetto extract) 136 mg • Stinging Nettle root extract (urtica dioica) 120 mg • Pygeum bark extract (pygeum africanum) 50 mg • Sterols (from pygeum extract) 6.5 mg • Lycopene (from tomato extract) 5 mg • Boron (from boron citrate, glycinate/aspartate) 1.5 mg • Rosemary extract (rosmarinus officinalis) 400 mcg. Other Ingredients: Gelatin, Pumpkin Seed Oil, Glycerin, Water, Carob.

Natural Quit - JBS Natural Products
Denicotizing Formula: Alfalfa leaf • Barberry bark • Buckthorn bark • Burdock root • Cascara Sagrada • Chaparral • Dandelion root • Goldenseal root • Hyssop • Kelp • Oregon Grape root • Pau D'Arco • Prickly Ash • Yellow Dock root • Yucca root. Anti-Addiction Formula: Anise seed • Barberry bark • Bee Pollen • Blue Cohosh root • Catnip herb • Cayenne 40M • Chamomile • Echinacea angustifolia herb • Eleutherococcus • Fennel seed • Gentian root • Gotu Kola • Hops flower • Lemongrass • Licorice root • Lobelia herb • Myrrh gum • Passionflower • Peppermint leaf • Safflower • Sarsaparilla •Skullcap herb • Slippery Elm bark • Valerian root • Wood Betony. Aromatherapy Formula: Camphor • Eucalyptus • Denatured Alcohol 40 • Peppermint • Rosemary • Ylang Ylang.

Natural Radiance Cream - Life Extension
Vitamin A, Vitamin E, Vitamin C, Green Tea extract, Deionized Water, Grape Seed oil, Cetyl Palmitate, Isocetyl Stearate, Glycerin, Cetyl Alcohol, Polyacrylamide, C13-14 Isoparafin, Laureth-7, Phenyl Trimethicone, Dimethicone, Laurether-16.

Natural Relief Cold & Flu Chewable with Zinc - Boericke & Tafel
Each tablet contains: Aconitum Napellus 4X 25 mg • Bryonia Alba 4X 25 mg • Eucalyptus Globulus 2X 10 mg • Eupatorium Perfoliatum 2X 25 mg • Gelsemium Sempervirens 4X 25 mg • Ipecacuanha 3X 25 mg • Phosphorus 6X 25 mg.
See Editor's Note No. 1.

Natural Rest - Hillestad
Each tablet contains: Niacin (niacinamide) 50 mg • Vitamin B6 (pyridoxine hydrochloride) 10 mg • Calcium (oyster shell and calcium lactate) 100 mg • Magnesium (oxide) 80 mg • Glycine (amino acid) 100 mg • GABA (gamma-amino butyric acid) 50 mg • Taurine (L-taurine amino acid) 100 gm • Inositol 150 mg • Chamomile flower 50 mg • Hops fruit 50 mg • Passion Flower flower 50 mg • Valerian root 50 mg • Skullcap herb 50 mg. Other Ingredients: Gum Arabic, Cellulose, Ethyl Cellulose, Magnesium Stearate, Silica.

Natural SAM-e 200 - Jarrow Formulas
Each tablet contains: S-Adenosyl Methionine (from 400 mg of SAM-e tosylate disulfate) 200 mg. Other Ingredients: Microcrystalline Cellulose, Enteric Coating (methacrylate copolymers), Glycerol Behenate, Magnesium Silicate, Triethyl Citrate, Glycerol Palmitostearate, Medium Chain Triglycerides, Magnesium Stearate, Silicon Dioxide, Mannitol, Sodium Starch Glycolate, Titanium Dioxide, Yellow Iron Oxide.

Natural SAM-e Joint - Jarrow Formulas
Each tablet contains: S-Adenosyl Methionine (from 400 mg of SAM-e tosylate disulfate) 200 mg • Glucosamine HCl 525 mg. Other Ingredients: Microcrystalline Cellulose, Enteric Coating (methacrylate copolymers), Glycerol Behenate, Silicon Dioxide, Magnesium Silicate, Triethyl Citrate, Glyceryl Palmitostearate, Medium Chain Triglycerides, Magnesium Stearate, Titanium Dioxide, Sorbitan Oleate, Yellow Iron Oxide, Red Iron Oxide.

Some Brand Name Natural Products - What they Contain

www.NaturalDatabase.com contains MANY more listings than appear here.
Editor's Notes are located on pages 2155-2163.

Natural Sensation - Strategic Science & Technology
Water • Choline Chloride • L-Arginine • Sodium Chloride • Mineral Oil • Zinc Chloride • Glyceryl Stearate SE • Squalene • Cetyl Alcohol • Magnesium Chloride • Propylene Glycol Stearate SE • Wheat Germ Oil • Glyceryl Stearate • Isopropyl Myristate • Stearyl Stearate • Polysorbate-60 • Propylene Glycol • Oleic Acid • Tocopherol Acetate • Collagen • Sorbitan Stearate • Vitamin A • Vitamin D • Triethanolamine • Methylparaben • Aloe Vera extract • Imidazolidinyl Urea • Propylparaben • BHA.

Natural Source Calcium & Magnesium - Leiner Health Products
Each tablet contains: Magnesium Oxide 167 mg • Calcium Carbonate 333 mg. Other Ingredients: Maltodextrin, Cellulose, Talc, Croscarmellose Sodium, Mineral Oil, Hydroxypropyl Methylcellulose, Soy Polysaccharide, Citric Acid, Starch Silicon Dioxide, Polyethylene Glycol, Magnesium Stearate, Crospovidone, Gum Arabic Stearic Acid.

Natural Source Calcium + Vitamin D - Leiner Health Products
Each tablet contains: Calcium Carbonate 500 mg • Vitamin D (Cholecalciferol) 125 IU. Other Ingredients: Maltodextrin, Talc, Pregelatinized Starch, Croscarmellose Sodium, Acacia, Hydroxypropyl Methylcellulose, Silicon Dioxide, Magnesium Stearate, Hydroxypropyl Cellulose, Polysorbate 80, Polyethylene Glycol 3350.

Natural Source Calcium + Vitamin D - Leiner Health Products
Each tablet contains: Vitamin D (Cholecalciferol) 125 IU • Calcium Carbonate 250 mg. Other Ingredients: Maltodextrin, Talc, Pregelatinized Starch, Croscarmellose Sodium, Acacia, Silicon Dioxide, Magnesium Stearate.

Natural Source Calcium Pharmaceutical Grade - Leiner Health Products
Each tablet contains: Calcium Carbonate 500 mg. Other Ingredients: Maltodextrin, Acacia, Starch, Croscarmellose Sodium, Cellulose, Hydroxypropyl Methylcellulose, Talc, Silicon Dioxide, Mineral Oil, Soy Polysaccharide, Magnesium Stearate, Polyethylene Glycol 3350, Hydroxypropyl Cellulose, Polysorbate 80, Crospovidone, Stearic Acid.

Natural Source Calcium, Magnesium, & Zinc - Leiner Health Products
Each tablet contains: Calcium Carbonate 333 mg • Magnesium Oxide 133 mg • Zinc Sulfate 5 mg. Other Ingredients: Maltodextrin, Cellulose, Croscarmellose Sodium, Talc, Hydroxypropyl Methylcellulose, Acacia, Soy Polysaccharide, Mineral Oil, Silicon Dioxide, Starch, Magnesium Stearate, Stearic Acid, Citric Acid, Sodium Starch Glycolate, Polyethylene Glycol, Hydroxypropyl Cellulose, Polysorbate 80, Crospovidone.

Natural Source DHEA - Life Extension
Each tablet contains: Discorea Villosa (wild yam) 250 mg • GABA (gamma-aminobutyric acid) 75 mg • Alpha Ketoglutaric Acid 75 mg • Glycine 75 mg • Saw Palmetto 75 mg.

Natural Soya Lecithin - Leiner Health Products
Each softgel contains: Soya Lecithin 1200 mg. Other Ingredients: Gelatin, Glycerin.

Natural Sport Creatine Chewable with FOS - Nutraceutical Corp.
Each two wafers contain: Creatine Monohydrate 3 g • Proprietary FOS Fiber Blend (BeFlora) (265 mg Fructo-oligosaccharides) 530 mg. Inactive Ingredients: Guar Gum, Cellulose, Natural Tangerine flavor, Citric Acid, Stearic Acid, Maltose, Natural Orange flavor, Silica, Magnesium Stearate.

Natural Sports Extreme Cordyceps - Nutraceutical Corp.
Each capsule contains: Cordyceps CS-4 mycelial biomass (Cordyceps sinensis, 36 mg Cordycepic acid) 525 mg • Cordyceps mycelial biomass (cordyceps sinensis, minimum 10 mg cordydepic acid, minimum 1 mg cordycepin) 100 mg • Reishi mushroom (ganoderma lucidum) 75 mg • Maitake mushroom (grifolia fondosa) 75 mg. Other Ingredients: Gelatin, Magnesium Stearate, Silica, Brown Rice.

Natural Sterol Complex - Universal Nutrition
Two tablets contain: Mexican Wild Yam root 1000 mg • Smilax officinalis extract 1000 mg • Muira puama 1000 mg • Gotu Kola 515 mg • Boron 3 mg • Gamma Oryzanol 500 mg • Fucosterol 7959 mcg • Beta Sitosterol 5663 mcg • Campesterol 3376 mcg • Stigmasterol 1924 mcg • "other Sterols" 1009 mcg • Bee Pollen 1000 mg • Guarana 500 mg • Korean Ginseng 100 mg • Cytochrome C 100 mg • Dimethylglycine 100 mg • Inosine 100 mg • Royal Jelly 30 mg • Kola Nut 25 mg • Calcium 200 mg • Magnesium 100 mg • Potassium 99 mg • Linoleic Acid 1040 mg • Oleic Acid 698 mg • Palmitic Acid 263 mg • Linoleic Acid 109 mg • Stearic Acid 56 mg • Lignoceric Acid 14 mg • Arachidonic Acid 13 mg • Behenic Acid 6 mg • Myristic Acid 5 mg • Octacosanol 1650 mcg • RNA 60 mg • DNA 30 mg • Capsicum 100 mg • Alfalfa 100 mg • Dandelion root 100 mg • Garlic 100 mg • Yellow Dock 100 mg • Licorice root 100 mg • Hops 100 mg • Milk Thistle 10 mg.

Natural Time Release B-12 - Leiner Health Products
Each tablet contains: Vitamin B12 (Cyanocobalamin) 1000 mcg. Other Ingredients: Dicalcium Phosphate, Hydrogenated Vegetable Oil, Cellulose, Magnesium Stearate, Silicon Dioxide.

Natural Time Release B-6 - Leiner Health Products
Each tablet contains: Vitamin B6 (Pyridoxine Hydrochloride) 200 mg. Other Ingredients: Dicalcium Phosphate, Hydrogenated Vegetable Oil, Silicon Dioxide, Stearic Acid, Magnesium Stearate, Yeast, Rose Hips, Watercress.

Natural Time Release Balanced B-100 - Leiner Health Products
Each tablet contains: Thiamin Mononitrate (Vitamin B1) 100 mg • Riboflavin (Vitamin B2) 100 mg • Vitamin B6 (Pyridoxine Hydrochloride) 100 mg • Niacin (Niacinamide) 100 mg • Biotin 100 mcg • Vitamin B12 100 mcg • Pantothenic Acid 100 mg • Folate 400 mcg. Other Ingredients: Dicalcium Phosphate, Hydrogenated Vegetable Oil, Stearic Acid, Silicon Dioxide, Magnesium Stearate, Resin, Gum Acacia, Wheat Bran, Cellulose, Para Aminobenzoic Acid.

Natural Time Release Balanced B-50 - Leiner Health Products
Each tablet contains: Vitamin B12 50 mcg • Pantothenic Acid (d-Calcium Pantothenate) 50 mg • Thiamin Mononitrate (Vitamin B1) 50 mg • Riboflavin (Vitamin B2) 50 mg • Vitamin B6 (Pyridoxine Hydrochloride) 50 mg • Niacin (Niacinamide) 50 mg • Biotin 50 mcg • Folate 400 mcg. Other Ingredients: Dicalcium Phosphate, Hydrogenated Vegetable Oil, Stearic Acid, Cellulose, Magnesium Stearate, Silicon Dioxide, Resin, Gum Acacia, Hydroxypropyl Cellulose.

Natural Time Release Complete Multivitamin/Mineral - Leiner Health Products
Each tablet contains: Selenium 5 mcg • Calcium 62.5 mg • Magnesium 25 mg • Molybdenum 5 mcg • Vitamin B12 35 mcg • Copper 1 mg • Vitamin C (Ascorbic Acid) 250 mg • Chromium 5 mcg • Pantothenic Acid (d-Calcium Pantothenate) 30 mg • Manganese 5 mg • Thiamin Mononitrate (Vitamin B1) 35 mg • Riboflavin (Vitamin B2) 35 mg • Potassium Chloride 99 mg • Vitamin B6 (Pyridoxine Hydrochloride) 35 mg • Niacin 35 mg • Iodine 225 mcg • Vitamin A 7500 IU • Folate 400 mcg • Iron (Ferrous Sulfate) 18 mg • Vitamin D 400 IU • Vitamin E 30 IU • Zinc 15 mg • Biotin 5 mcg. Other Ingredients: Dicalcium Phosphate, Hydrogenated Vegetable Oil, Cellulose, Stearic Acid, Gelatin, Silicon Dioxide.

Natural Time Release Maximum Choice - Leiner Health Products
Two tablets contain: Chloride 18 mg • Potassium 20 mg • Vitamin B12 50 mcg • Vitamin C (Ascorbic Acid) 400 mg • Vitamin E (D-Alpha Tocopheryl Acid Succinate) 200 IU • Pantothenic Acid (D-Calcium Pantothenate) 50 mg • Iron 8.2 mg • Chromium 50 mcg •

Selenium 25 mcg • Thiamin Mononitrate (Vitamin B1) 50 mg • Riboflavin (Vitamin B2) 50 mg • Calcium 260 mg • Vitamin B6 (Pyridoxine Hydrochloride) 50 mg • Niacin (Niacinamide) 50 mg • Magnesium Oxide 100 mg • Vitamin A 10000 IU • Molybdenum 15 mcg • Phosphorus 200 mg • Zinc Sulfate 25 mg • Biotin 50 mcg • Copper 3 mg • Iodine 225 mcg • Manganese 3 mg • Folate 400 mcg • Vitamin D 400 IU. Other Ingredients: Dicalcium Phosphate, Hydrogenated Vegetable Oil, Beta Carotene, Stearic Acid.

Natural Time Release Vitamin C with Rose Hips - Leiner Health Products
Each tablet contains: Vitamin C 500 mg. Other Ingredients: Dicalcium Phosphate, Hydrogenated Vegetable Oil, Stearic Acid, Rose Hips, Silicon Dioxide, Magnesium Stearate, Starch, Ethylcellulose.

Natural Ultra E 1000 - GNC
Each capsule contains: Vitamin A 1000 IU •Vitamin E 1000 IU. Other Ingredients: Soybean oil, Gelatin, Glycerin, Caramel Color, Titanium Dioxide.

Natural Ultra E 400 - GNC
Each capsule contains: Vitamin A (as beta-carotene) 400 IU • Vitamin E (as d-alpha tocopherol) 400 IU. Other Ingredients: Gelatin, Soybean Oil, Glycerin, Caramel Color, Titanium Dioxide.

Natural Vitamin A - Benepure, Inc
Each capsule contains: Vitamin A (as fish liver oil) 25,000 IU.

Natural Vitamin A - Leiner Health Products
Each softgel contains: Vitamin A 8000 IU. Other Ingredients: Vegetable Oil, Gelatin, Glycerin, Fish Liver Oil.

Natural Vitamin A & D (Cod Liver Oil) USP - Leiner Health Products
Each softgel contains: Vitamin D 135 IU • Vitamin A 1250 IU. Other Ingredients: Cod Liver Oil, Gelatin, Glycerin, and may contain Water.

Natural Vitamin B-Complex with Vitamin C - Sunmark
Two tablets contain: Vitamin C 300 mg • Thiamin 10 mg • Riboflavin 10 mg • Niacin 100 mg • Vitamin B6 10 mg • Folate 400 mcg • Vitamin B12 75 mcg • Biotin 30 mcg • Pantothenic Acid 50 mg. Other Ingredients: Dicalcium Phosphate, Microcrystalline Cellulose, Modified Cellulose Gum, Stearic Acid, Hydroxypropyl Methylcellulose, Magnesium Stearate, Crospovidone, Polyethylene Glycol, Brewer's Yeast, Choline, Inositol, PABA, Rice Bran.
See Editor's Note No. 45.

Natural Vitamin C - Benepure, Inc
Each tablet contains: Vitamin C 500 mg • Mixed Citrus Bioflavonoids 96 mg • Pectin 84 mg. Other Ingredients: Cellulose, Magnesium Stearate, Stearic Acid.

Natural Vitamin C 1000 Mg With Rose Hips - Nature's Valley
Each tablet contains: Vitamin C from Rose Hips 1000 mg. Other Ingredients: Hydrogenated Vegetable Oil, Stearic Acid, Silicon Dioxide, Starch, Magnesium Stearate, Ethylcellulose, Hydroxypropyl Methylcellulose, Dicalcium Phosphate, Hydroxypropyl Cellulose, Polysorbate 80, Polyethylene Glycol 3350.
See Editor's Note No. 45.

Natural Vitamin C with Rose Hips - Leiner Health Products
Each tablet contains: Vitamin C 250 mg. Other Ingredients: Ascorbic Acid, Calcium Carbonate, Cellulose, Rose Hips, Silicon Dioxide, Talc, Polyethylene Glycol 3350, Tricalcium Phosphate, Crospovidone, Magnesium Stearate.

Natural Vitamin E - Optimum Nutrition
Each softgel contains: Vitamin E (as D-alpha tocopherol acetate) 400 IU. Other Ingredients: Gelatin, Soy Oil.

Natural Vitamin E - NSI - Nutraceutical Sciences Institute
Each softgel contains: Vitamin E 400 IU.

Natural Vitamin E - Puritan's Pride
Each softgel contains: Vitamin E (as d-alpha tocopheryl acetate) 400 IU. Other Ingredients: Gelatin, Glycerin, Soybean Oil.

Natural Vitamin E - Nutritional Therapeutics, Inc.
Each tablet contains: Vitamin E 200 IU • Pantethine (Coenzyme A Precursor) 25 mg • Selenium 12.5 mg • NT Factor tablet base 47.5 mg.

Natural Vitamin E - Leiner Health Products
Each softgel contains: Vitamin E (dl-Alpha Tocopheryl Acetate and D-Alpha Tocopherol) 200 IU. Other Ingedients: Gelatin, Glycerin, Vegetable Oil.

Natural Vitamin E - Swanson Health Products
Eash softgel contains: Natural Vitamin E (as d-alpha tocopheryl acetate) 400 IU.

Natural Vitamin E & Lecithin - Golden Glow Natural Health Products
Each capsule contains: D-Alpha-Tocopherol 337 mg: Natural Vitamin E 500 IU • Lecithin 500 mg.

Natural Vitamin E 1000 IU - Arrowroot
Each softgel contains: Vitamin E 1000 IU (D-alpha tocopheryl acetate from soy).

Natural Vitamin E 1000IU - Golden Glow Natural Health Products
Each capsule contains: D-Alpha-Tocopherol 671 mg: Natural Vitamin E 1000 IU.

Natural Vitamin E 200 IU - Arrowroot
Each softgel contains: Vitamin E 200 IU (D-alpha tocopheryl acetate from soy).

Natural Vitamin E 250IU - Golden Glow Natural Health Products
Each capsule contains: D-Alpha-Tocopherol 167.6 mg: Natural Vitamin E 250 IU.

Natural Vitamin E 400 IU - Leiner Health Products
Each softgel contains: Vitamin E (dl-Alpha Tocopheryl Acetate and D-Alpha Tocopherol) 400 IU. Other Ingredients: Gelatin, Glycerin, Vegetable Oil.

Natural Vitamin E 400 IU - Nature's Valley
Each softgel contains: Vitamin E as DL-Alpha Tocopheryl Acetate 400 IU. Other Ingredients: Gelatin, Soybean Oil, Glycerin.
See Editor's Note No. 45.

Natural Vitamin E 400 IU - Pro Health
Each softgel contains: Vitamin E 400 IU. Other Ingredients: Vegetable Oil Concentrate, Gelatin, Glycerin, Water.

Natural Vitamin E 400 IU - Arrowroot
Each softgel contains: Vitamin E 400 IU (D-alpha tocopheryl acetate from soy).

Natural Vitamin E 400 IU with Mixed Tocopherols - Vital Nutrients
Each softgel contains: Vitamin E 400 IU: D-Alpha Tocopherol 268.5 mg, D-Beta, D-Gamma and D-Delta Tocopherols 60 mg.

Natural Vitamin E 400IU - Vital Nutrients
Each softgel contains: Vitamin E (D-alpha tocopherol) 400 IU.

Natural Vitamin E 500IU - Golden Glow Natural Health Products
Each capsule contains: D-Alpha-Tocopherol 335 mg: Natural Vitamin E 500 IU.

Natural Vitamin E d-Alpha - Leiner Health Products
Each softgel contains: Vitamin E (d-Alpha Tocopheryl Acetate) 400 IU. Other Ingredients: Vegetable Oil, Gelatin, Glycerin, Water.

Some Brand Name Natural Products - What they Contain

www.NaturalDatabase.com contains MANY more listings than appear here.
Editor's Notes are located on pages 2155-2163.

Natural Vitamin E Mixed Tocopherols - GNC
Each capsule contains: Vitamin E (as d-alpha Tocopherol) 200 IU. Other Ingredients: Soybean Oil, Gelatin, Glycerin.

Natural Vitamin E With Mixed Tocopherols - Benepure, Inc
Each capsule contains: Vitamin E (as D-alpha tocopherol) 400 IU • Mixed Tocopherols (yielding D-beta 4 mg, D-gamma 42 mg, D-delta 21 mg) 67 mg. Other Ingredients: Soybean Oil, Gelatin, Glycerin.

Natural Whole Herb Aloe Vera Gel - Vitamin World
Each softgel contains: Aloe Vera gel 200:1 extract 25 mg. Other Ingredients: Soybean Oil, Gelatin, Glycerin, Cottonseed Oil, White Beeswax.

Natural Whole Herb Avena Sativa Complex 500 mg - Vitamin World
Two capsules contain: Proprietary Blend 1000 mg: Eleuthero root (eleutherococcus senticosus), Oat extract (avena sativa), Nettle leaf extract (urtica dioica). Other Ingredients: Gelatin, Silica, Vegetable Magnesium Stearate.

Natural Whole Herb Saw Palmetto 1000 mg - Vitamin World
Each softgel contains: Saw Palmetto berry (serenoa repens, from 250 mg of 4:1 extract) 1000 mg. Other Ingredients: Soybean Oil, Gelatin, Glycerin, Yellow Beeswax, Soy Lecithin, Caramel Color.

Natural Woman - NDS Nutrition
Three capsules contain: Vitamin A (beta carotene with mixed carotenoids) 10,000 IU • Vitamin D (cholecalciferol) 400 IU • Vitamin E (D-alpha tocopheryl) 100 IU • Vitamin K 80 mcg • Vitamin C (calcium ascorbate) 500 mg • Vitamin B1 (thiamine) 50 mg • Vitamin B2 (riboflavin) 49 mg • Vitamin B3 (niacinamide) 50 mg • Vitamin B5 (calcium pantothenate) 50 mg • Vitamin B6 (pyridoxine) 50 mg • Vitamin B12 200 mcg • Biotin 400 mcg • Folic Acid 400 mcg • Calcium (milk calcium complex) 400 mg • Magnesium (citrate) 200 mg • Iron (fumerate) 10 mg • Zinc (aspartate) 20 mg • Copper (gluconate) 2 mg • Iodine (potassium iodine) 150 mcg • Vanadium (aspartate) 10 mcg • Boron (aspartate) 250 mcg • Manganese (citrate) 2 mg • Selenium (methionine) 100 mcg • Molybdenum (aspartate) 75 mcg • Chromium (nicotinate) 100 mcg. Other Ingredients: Brown Rice, Magnesium Stearate, Gelatine, Water.

Natural Wonder Woman - DreamPharm
Two capsules contain: Dong Quai root (angelica sinensis) 300 mg • Black Cohosh root (cimicifuga racemosa) 150 mg • Blue Cohosh root (caulophyllum thalictroides) 100 mg.

Natural Zinc Gluconate - Leiner Health Products
Each tablet contains: Zinc Gluconate 50 mg. Other Ingredients: Starch, Croscarmellose Sodium, Sodium Starch Glycolate, Magnesium Stearate.

Natural ZZZ's - Ortho Molecular Products
Two capsules contain: Valerian root extract (standardized to cotnain 0.8% valerenic acids) 450 mg • Jujube seed extract (standardized to contain 2% triterpene saponins) 300 mg • Passionflower aerial portion extract (standardized to contain 3.5% flavonoids) 200 mg • L-Theanine 100 mg. Other Ingredients: Natural Vegetable Capsules, Magnesium Stearate, Microcrystalline Cellulose.

Naturally Blended Vitamin E - GNC
Each capsule contains: Vitamin E (as dl-alpha Tocopheryl Acetate and D-alpha Tocopherol) 400 IU. Other Ingredients: Gelatin, Glycerin.

Naturally Clear Cleansing Scrub - Nature's Life
Ingredients: Distilled Water • Niacinamide • Disodium Oleth-3 Sulfosuccinate (from coconut oil) • Walnut Shell powder • Cetyl Alcohol (from vegetable oils) • Sucrose Cocoate • Apricot Kernel Oil • Citric Acid • Sodium PCA • Aloe Vera gel • Beta Carotene.

Naturally Clear Dietary Supplement - Nature's Life
Each two capsules contain: Vitamin A (as palmitate) 5000 IU • Vitamin C (as ascorbic acid and ascorbyl palmitate) 200 mg • Vitamin D (vitamin D3, as cholecalciferol) 133 IU • Vitamin E (as D-alpha tocopheryl succinate) 100 IU • Thiamine (vitamin B1, as thiamine HCl) 5 mg • Riboflavin (vitamin B2) 5 mg • Vitamin B3 (as niacinamide) 10 mg • Vitamin B6 (as pyridoxine HCl) 10 mg • Folic Acid 133 mcg • Vitamin B12 (as cyanacobalamin) 50 mcg • Biotin (as d-biotin) 100 mcg • Pantothenic Acid (as d-calcium pantothenate) 10 mg • Zinc (from zinc picolinate) 15 mg • Selenium (as selenomethionine/sodium selenite) 100 mcg • Copper (from copper gluconate) 1 mg • Chromium (from chromium nicotinate) 100 mcg • Proprietary Blend 840 mg: L-Lysine HCl, L-Arginine, L-Cysteine HCl, L-Glutamine. Inactive Ingredients: Gelatin Capsule.

Naturally Clear Nourishing Spray - Nature's Life
Ingredients: Distilled Water • Niacinamide • Aloe Vera • Sodium PCA.

Naturally Herbal Phen - Optimum Nutrition
St. John's Wort • Bitter Orange.
See Editor's Note No. 40.

Naturally Inspired Absorbable Calcium with Vitamin D - Vitamin World
Two softgels contain: Vitamin D (as cholecalciferol) 100 IU • Calcium (as calcium carbonate) 1000 mg. Other Ingredients: Soybean Oil, Gelatin, Glycerin, Lecithin, Titanium Dioxide Color.

Naturally Inspired Adult Chewable Pineapple Flavored - Vitamin World
Each tablet contains: Vitamin A (as beta carotene) 5000 IU • Vitamin C (as ascorbic acid and rose hips) 150 mg • Vitamin D (as cholecalciferol) 400 IU • Vitamin E (as D-alpha tocopheryl acetate) 100 IU • Thiamin (vitamin B1, as thiamine hydrochloride) 15 mg • Riboflavin (vitamin B2) 15 mg • Niacin (as niacinamide) 25 mg • Vitamin B6 (as pyridoxine hydrochloride) 15 mg • Folic Acid 100 mcg • Vitamin B12 (as cyanocobalamin) 15 mcg • Biotin (as D-biotin) 20 mcg • Pantothenic Acid (as D-calcium pantothenate) 20 mg • Calcium (as calcium carbonate) 10 mg • Iron (as ferrous fumarate) 5 mg • Iodine (as potassium iodide) 100 mcg • Magnesium (as magnesium gluconate) 145 mcg • Zinc (as zinc gluconate) 325 mcg • Copper (as copper gluconate) 50 mcg • Manganese (as manganese gluconate) 17 mcg • Soy Lecithin 25 mg • Choline Bitartrate 5 mg • Hesperidin Complex (citrus limon exocarp) 5 mg • Betaine Hydrochloride 5 mg • Rutin (saphora japonica leaf) 2.5 mg • Bioflavonoids (citrus limon exocarp) 2.5 mg • PABA (para-aminobenzoic acid) 2.5 mg • Inositol 2.5 mg. Other Ingredients: Fructose, Cellulose, Natural and Artficial Pineapple Flavor, Silica, Vegetable Magnesium Stearate, Sucralose, Rice Bran.

Naturally Inspired Alfalfa 500 mg (7 1/2 grain) - Vitamin World
Three tablets contain: Alfalfa leaf (medicago sativa) 1500 mg. Other Ingredients: Dicalcium Phosphate, Vegetable Stearic Acid, Vegetable Magnesium Stearate, Croscarmellose.

Naturally Inspired Amino Complex 600 mg - Vitamin World
Each tablet contains: L-Arginine (as L-arginine hydrochloride) 50 mg • L-Cysteine (as L-cysteine hydrochloride) 50 mg • L-Histidine 50 mg • L-Isoleucine 50 mg • L-Leucine 50 mg • L-Lysine (as L-lysine hydrochloride) 50 mg • L-Methionine 50 mg • L-Ornithine (as L-ornithine hydrochloride) 50 mg • L-Phenylalanine 50 mg • L-Threonine 50 mg • L-Tyrosine 50 mg • L-Valine 50 mg. Other Ingredients: Povidone, Vegetable Stearic Acid, Cellulose, Croscarmellose, Food Glaze, Vegetable Magnesium Stearate, Silica.

Naturally Inspired Astaxanthin 4 mg - Vitamin World
Each softgel contains: Astaxanthin 4 mg. Other Ingredients: Soybean Oil, Gelatin, Glycerin.

Naturally Inspired B-100 Complex capsules - Vitamin World
Each tablet contains: Thiamin (vitamin B1) 100 mg • Riboflavin (vitamin B2) 100 mg • Niacin (as niacinamide) 100 mg • Vitamin B6 (as pyridoxine hydrochloride) 100 mg • Folic Acid 400 mcg • Vitamin B12 (as cyanocobalamin) 100 mcg • Biotin (as D-biotin) 100 mcg • Pantothenic Acid (as D-calcium pantothenate) 100 mg • Choline Bitartrate 100 mg • PABA (para-aminobenzoic acid) 100 mg •

Inositol 100 mg • Proprietary Blend 7.5 mg: Alfalfa, Watercress, Parsley, Lecithin, Rice Bran. Other Ingredients: Gelatin, Vegetable Magnesium Stearate, Silica.

Naturally Inspired B-100 Ultra B-Complex tablets - Vitamin World
Each tablet contains: Thiamin (vitamin B1) (as thiamine mononitrate) 100 mg • Riboflavin (vitamin B2) 100 mg • Niacin (as niacinamide) 100 mg • Vitamin B6 (as pyridoxine hydrochloride) 100 mg • Folic Acid 100 mcg • Vitamin B12 (as cyanocobalamin) 100 mcg • Biotin (as D-biotin) 100 mcg • Pantothenic Acid (as D-calcium pantothenate) 100 mg • Inositol 100 mg • PABA (para-aminobenzoic acid) 100 mg • Choline Bitartrate 100 mg • Proprietary Blend 5 mg: Parsley leaf powder, Rice Bran powder, Watercress leaf powder, Alfalfa leaf powder, Lecithin granules. Other Ingredients: Cellulose, Vegetable Stearic Acid, Croscarmellose, Cellulose Coating, Dicalcium Phosphate, Silica, Guar Gum.

Naturally Inspired B-150 Mega B-Complex - Vitamin World
Each tablet contains: Thiamin (vitamin B-1, as thiamin mononitrate) 150 mg • Riboflavin (vitamin B-2) 150 mg • Niacin (as niacinamide) 150 mg • Vitamin B-6 (as pyridoxine hydrochloride) 100 mg • Folic Acid 400 mcg • Vitamin B-12 (as cyanocobalamin) 150 mcg • Biotin (as D-biotin) 150 mcg • Pantothenic Acid (as D-calcium pantothenate) 150 mg • Choline Bitartrate 150 mg • PABA (para-aminobenzoic acid) 150 mg • Inositol 150 mg • Proprietary Blend 7.5 mg: Alfalfa (medicago sativa), Watercress (nasturtium officinale), Parsley leaf (petroselinum crispum), Soy Lecithin, Rice Bran. Other Ingredients: Cellulose, Hydroxypropyl Cellulose, Mannitol, Vegetable Magnesium Stearate, Cellulose Coating.

Naturally Inspired B-50 B-Complex Vitamin - Vitamin World
Each tablet contains: Thiamin (vitamin B-1, as thiamin mononitrate) 50 mg Riboflavin (vitamin B-2) 50 mg • Niacin (as niacinamide) 50 mg • Vitamin B-6 50 mg (as pyridoxine hydrochloride) • Folic Acid 400 mcg • Vitamin B-12 (as cyanocobalamin) 50 mcg • Biotin (as D-biotin) 50 mcg • Pantothenic Acid (as D-calcium pantothenate) 50 mg • PABA (para-aminobenzoic acid) 50 mg • Inositol 50 mg • Choline Bitartrate 50 mg • Proprietary Blend 2.5 mg: Alfalfa, Watercress, Parsley, Lecithin, Rice Bran. Other Ingredients: Cellulose (Plant Origin), Dicalcium Phosphate, Vegetable Stearic Acid, Croscarmellose, Cellulose Coating, Silica, Mannitol, Vegetable Magnesium Stearate.

Naturally Inspired B-Complex and B-12 USP - Vitamin World
Each tablet contains: Thiamin (vitamin B-1, (as thiamin hydrochloride and brewers yeast) 7 mg • Riboflavin (vitamin B-2 (as riboflavin and brewers yeast) 14 mg • Niacin (as niacin and brewers yeast) 4.5 mg • Vitamin B-12 (as cyanocobalamin and brewers yeast) 25 mcg • Protease (as papain powder) 10 mg. Other Ingredients: Dicalcium Phosphate, Cellulose, Vegetable Stearic Acid, Croscaremellose, Silica, Mannitol, Vegetable Magnesium Stearate.

Naturally Inspired Bee Pollen 500 mg - Vitamin World
Each tablet contains: Bee Pollen 500 mg. Other Ingredients: Cellulose, Vegetable Stearic Acid, Acacia Gum, Silica, Croscarmellose, Vegetable Magnesium Stearate.

Naturally Inspired Bee Pollen Complex 1000 Plus - Vitamin World
Each tablet contains: Bee Pollen 1000 mg • Bee Propolis 10 mg • Royal Jelly (2.9 mg of a 3.5:1 extract) 10 mg. Other Ingredients: Cellulose, Stearic Acid, Hydroxypropyl Cellulose, Croscarmellose, Silica, Acacia, Cellulose, Vegetable Magnesium Stearate.

Naturally Inspired Bee Pollen Granules - Vitamin World
Each 1 level tsp (3 g) serving contains: Bee Pollen Granules 3 g.

Naturally Inspired Bee Propolis 500 mg - Vitamin World
Each capsule contains: Bee Propolis (from 125 mg of concentrate) 500 mg. Other Ingredients: Dicalcium Phosphate, Cellulose, Gelatin, Silica, Vegetable Magnesium Stearate.

Naturally Inspired Beta Sitosterol - Vitamin World
Two softgels contain: Sterol Esters (from soybeans) 1000 mg • Beta Sitosterol 250 mg • Campesterol 120 mg • Stigmasterol 80 mg. Other Ingredients: Soybean Oil, Citrus Pectin, Gelatin, Glycerin, Titanium Dioxide Color.

Naturally Inspired Beta-Carotene 15 mg - Vitamin World
Each softgel contains: Vitamin A, 100% as Beta-Carotene 25,000 IU. Other Ingredients: Soybean Oil, Gelatin, Glycerin, Yellow Beeswax, Soy Lecithin.

Naturally Inspired Beta-Carotene 6 mg - Vitamin World
Each softgel contains: Vitamin A, 100% as Beta-Carotene 10,000 IU. Other Ingredients: Soybean Oil, Gelatin, Glycerin, Yellow Beeswax, Soy Lecithin.

Naturally Inspired Betaine Hydrochloride 400 mg - Vitamin World
Each tablet contains: Betaine Hydrochloride 400 mg. Other Ingredients: Cellulose, Dicalcium Phosphate, Vegetable Stearic Acid, Croscarmellose, Silica, Vegetable Magnesium Stearate, Cellulose Coating.

Naturally Inspired Black Currant Oil - Vitamin World
Each softgel contains: Black Currant seed oil (providing gamma linolenic acid (GLA) 80 mg) 535 mg. Other Ingredients: Gelatin, Glycerin.

Naturally Inspired Borage Oil 1000 mg - Vitamin World
Each softgel contains: Borage oil (borago officinalis seed oil) 1000 mg: Gamma Linolenic Acid (GLA) 240 mg, Linoleic Acid (LA) 360 mg. Other Ingredients: Gelatin, Glycerin.

Naturally Inspired C & E - Vitamin World
Each softgel contains: Vitamin C (ascorbic acid and rose hips) 500 mg • Vitamin E (D-alpha tocopherol plus D-beta, D-gamma and D-delta tocopherols) 400 IU. Other Ingredients: Gelatin, Glycerin, Soybean Oil, Soy Lecithin, Caramel Color, Yellow Beeswax.

Naturally Inspired Certified Pure Apple Pectin 500 mg with Vitamin C - Vitamin World
Three tablets contain: Vitamin C (as ascorbic acid) 30 mg • Apple Pectin 1500 mg. Other Ingredients: Croscarmellose, Cellulose, Lactose, Corn Starch, Cellulose Coating, Silica, Vegetable Magnesium Stearate.

Naturally Inspired C-Ester Ascorbyl Palmitate 500 mg - Vitamin World
Each capsule contains: Vitamin C (from 500 mg of ascorbyl palmitate) 212 mg. Other Ingredients: Gelatin, Povidone, Silica, Vegetable Magnesium Stearate.

Naturally Inspired Chelated Potassium 99 mg - Vitamin World
Each caplet contains: Potassium (as potassium gluconate) 99 mg. Other Ingredients: Crospovidone, Vegetable Stearic Acid, Silica, Vegetable Magnesium Stearate, Cellulose Coating.

Naturally Inspired Chelated Zinc Lozenges 23 mg - Vitamin World
Each lozenge contains: Zinc (as zinc citrate and zinc gluconate) 23 mg. Other Ingredients: Fructose, Sorbitol, Honey Powder, Vegetable Stearic Acid, Citric Acid, Natural and Artificial Flavors, Silica, Vegetable Magnesium Stearate.

Naturally Inspired Chewable ProBiotic Acidophilus - Vitamin World
Each wafer contains: Lactobacillus blend 100 mg: Lactobacillus Acidophilus, Lactobacillus Bifidus. Other Ingredients: Sucrose, Dextrose, Fructose, Cellulose, Natural Flavor, Vegetable Stearic Acid, Blueberry Fruit Powder, Vegetable Magnesium Stearate, Beet Juice, Silica.

Naturally Inspired Chewable Vitamin C-500 mg **-** Vitamin World
Each tablet contains: Vitamin C (as sodium ascorbate, ascorbic acid, and rose hips) 500 mg. Other Ingredients: Sugar, Sorbitol, Vegetable Stearic Acid, Natural Orange Flavor, Silica, Vegetable Magnesium Stearate.

Naturally Inspired Children's Chewable Animal Chews **-** Vitamin World
Each tablet contains: Vitamin A (as retinyl palmitate, beta carotene) 2500 IU • Vitamin C (as calcium ascorbate) 60 mg • Vitamin D (as cholecalciferol) 200 IU • Vitamin E (as D-alpha tocopheryl acid succinate) 15 IU • Vitamin K (as phytonadione) 1 mcg • Thiamin (vitamin B1, as thiamin mononitrate) 0.75 mg • Riboflavin (vitamin B2) 0.85 mg • Niacin (as niacinamide) 10 mg • Vitamin B6 (as pyridoxine hydrochloride) 1 mg • Folic Acid 200 mcg • Vitamin B12 (as cyanocobalamin) 3 mcg • Biotin (as D-biotin) 150 mcg • Pantothenic Acid (as D-calcium pantothenate) 5 mg • Calcium (as carbonate, citrate, and ascorbate) 125 mg • Iron (as ferrous fumarate) 2 mg • Iodine (as potassium iodide, kelp) 37.5 mcg • Magnesium (as oxide and ascorbate) 50 mg • Zinc (as zinc amino acid chelate) 3.75 mg • Copper (as copper gluconate) 0.5 mg • Manganese (as manganese gluconate) 0.5 mg • Chromium (as chromium polynicotinate) 7.5 mcg • Molybdenum (as sodium molybdate) 5 mcg • Boron (as calcium borogluconate) 5 mcg • Vanadium (as vanadyl sulfate) 2.5 mcg • Nickel (as nickelous sulfate) 1 mcg • Tin (as stannous chloride) 1 mcg • Choline Phosphatides (as lecithin) 2.5 mg • Inositol Phosphatides (as lecithin) 2.5 mg • Rutin 2.5 mg • Green Barley juice powder 1.5 mg • Chlorella powder 1.5 mg • Spirulina powder 2.5 mg • Alfalfa juice powder 2.5 mg • Rice Bran powder 5 mg • Carrot juice powder 2.5 mg • Natural Licorice root 2 mg. Other Ingredients: Sucrose, Dextrose, Dried Raspberry Juice, Cellulose, Fructose, Glycerides of Stearic and Palmitic Acids, Vegetable Magnesium Stearate, Dried Honey Powder, Citric Acid, Carrageenan, Guar Gum, Cranberry Juice Concentrate, Raspberry Flavor, Silica, Mannitol.

Naturally Inspired Children's Chewable Animal Chews with Calcium **-** Vitamin World
Each tablet contains: Vitamin A (as retinyl palmitate and 50% as beta carotene) 2500 IU • Vitamin C (as calcium ascorbate and rose hips) 60 mg • Vitamin D (as cholecalciferol) 200 IU • Vitamin E (as D-alpha tocopheryl acid succinate) 15 IU • Thiamin (vitamin B1, as thiamin mononitrate) 0.75 mg • Riboflavin (vitamin B2) 0.85 mg • Niacin (as niacinamide) 10 mg • Vitamin B6 (as pyridoxine hydrochloride) 1 mg • Folic Acid 200 mcg • Vitamin B12 (as cyanocobalamin) 3 mcg • Biotin (as D-biotin) 50 mcg • Pantothenic Acid (as D-calcium pantothenate) 5 mg • Calcium (as carbonate, citrate, ascorbate) 125 mg • Proprietary Blend 415 mg: Raspberry juice concentrate, Dried Grape juice, Dried Pear juice, Dried Black Currant juice, Powdered Apricots, Powdered Peaches, Powdered Dates, Acerola juice extract. Other Ingredients: Sugar, Fructose, Cellulose, Natural Flavors, Mono- and Diglycerides, Acacia Gum, Adipic Acid, Beet Juice Concentrate Powder, Vegetable Magnesium Stearate, Mannitol, Silica.

Naturally Inspired Coral Calcium 500 mg **-** Vitamin World
Two capsules contain: Calcium (from 1000 mg of coral calcium) 370 mg. Other Ingredients: Gelatin, Rice Powder, Silica, Vegetable Magnesium Stearate.

Naturally Inspired Easy Iron **-** Vitamin World
Each capsule contains: Vitamin C (as ascorbic acid) 60 mg • Folic Acid 400 mcg • Vitamin B12 (as cyanocobalamin) 8 mcg • Iron (as ferrous bis-glycinate) 28 mg. Other Ingredients: Maltodextrin, Gelatin, Vegetable Magnesium Stearate, Silica.

Naturally Inspired EPA Natural Fish Oil 1000 mg **-** Vitamin World
Each softgel contains: Vitamin E (as D-alpha tocopherol plus D-beta, D-gamma and D-delta) 1.1 IU • Fish Oil 1000 mg • EPA (eicosapentaenoic acid) 180 mg • DHA (docosahexaenoic acid) 120 mg. Other Ingredients: Gelatin, Glycerin.

Naturally Inspired Ester-C 1000 mg with Bioflavonoids **-** Vitamin World
Each tablet contains: Vitamin C (as Ester-C calcium ascorbate) 1000 mg • Calcium (as Ester-C calcium ascorbate) 110 mg • Citrus Bioflavonoid fruit (citrus spp.) 100 mg • Rutin fruit (dimorphandra mollis) 20 mg • Hesperidin fruit complex (citrus spp.) 20 mg. Other Ingredients: Cellulose (plant origin), Vegetable Stearic Acid, Croscarmellose, Silica, Vegetable Magnesium Stearate, Cellulose.

Naturally Inspired Ester-C 500 mg with Bioflavonoids **-** Vitamin World
Each capsule contains: Vitamin C (from Ester-C calcium ascorbate) 500 mg • Calcium (as Ester-C calcium ascorbate) 55 mg • Citrus Bioflavonoid fruit (citrus sinensis) 100 mg • Rutin fruit (dimorphandra mollis) 5 mg • Hesperidin fruit complex (citrus spp.) 5 mg. Other Ingredients: Gelatin, Cellulose (plant origin), Silica, Vegetable Magnesium Stearate.

Naturally Inspired Evening Primrose Oil 1000 mg **-** Vitamin World
Each softgel contains: Evening Primrose Oil 1000 mg: Cis-Linoleic Acid (LA) 700 mg, Gamma-Linolenic Acid (GLA) 90 mg. Other Ingredients: Gelatin, Glycerin.

Naturally Inspired Evening Primrose Oil 1300 mg **-** Vitamin World
Each softgel contains: Evening Primrose Oil 1300 mg: Cis-Linoleic Acid (LA) 949 mg, Gamma-Linolenic Acid (GLA) 117 mg. Other Ingredients: Gelatin, Glycerin.

Naturally Inspired Evening Primrose Oil 500 mg **-** Vitamin World
Each softgel contains: Evening Primrose Oil 500 mg: Cis-Linoleic Acid 365 mg, Gamma-Linolenic Acid (GLA) 45 mg. Other Ingredients: Gelatin, Glycerin.

Naturally Inspired Herba Vision Lutein and Bilberry Complex **-** Vitamin World
Each capsule contains: Lutein (containing naturally occurring zeaxanthin) 6 mg • Bilberry fruit extract (vaccinium myrtillus, standardized to contain 25% anthocyanosides) 20 mg. Other Ingredients: Dicalcium Phosphate, Cellulose (plant origin), Gelatin, Vegetable Stearic Acid, Silica, Vegetable Magnesium Stearate.

Naturally Inspired High Potency Calcium 600 + Vitamin D **-** Vitamin World
Two tablets contain: Vitamin D (as cholecalciferol) 400 IU • Calcium (as calcium carbonate) 1200 mg • Soy Isoflavones 50 mg. Other Ingredients: Acacia Gum, Maltodextrin, Croscarmellose, Cellulose Coating, Vegetable Magnesium Stearate.

Naturally Inspired High Potency Magnesium 500 mg **-** Vitamin World
Each tablet contains: Magnesium (oxide) 500 mg. Other Ingredients: Cellulose, Starch, Povidone, Magnesium Silicate, Cellulose Coating, Titanium Dioxide Color, Magnesium Stearate, Propylene Glycol.

Naturally Inspired L-Arginine 1000 mg **-** Vitamin World
Each tablet contains: L-Arginine (hydrochloride) 1000 mg. Other Ingredients: Cellulose, Povidone, Stearic Acid, Silica, Cellulose, Magnesium Stearate.

Naturally Inspired Lutein 20 mg **-** Vitamin World
Each softgel contains: Lutein 20 mg. Other Ingredients: Corn Oil, Gelatin, Glycerin, Yellow Beeswax, Lecithin.

Naturally Inspired Macu Vision **-** Vitamin World
Each capsule contains: Taurine 200 mg • Lutein 3 mg • Alpha Lipoic Acid 25 mg. Other Ingredients: Rice Powder, Gelatin, Vegetable Magnesium Stearate, Silica.

Naturally Inspired Magnesium 250 mg **-** Vitamin World
Each caplet contains: Magnesium (oxide) 250 mg. Other Ingredients: Cellulose, Starch, Cellulose Coating, Titanium Dioxide Color, Magnesium Silicate, Vegetable Magnesium Stearate.

Some Brand Name Natural Products - What they Contain

www.NaturalDatabase.com contains MANY more listings than appear here.
Editor's Notes are located on pages 2155-2163.

BRAND NAMES

Naturally Inspired Magnesium Citrate - Vitamin World
Each tablet contains: Magnesium (as magnesium citrate) 100 mg. Other Ingredients: Cellulose (plant origin), Vegetable Stearic Acid, Croscarmellose, Silica, Vegetable Magnesium-Stearate, Cellulose Coating.

Naturally Inspired Mega B-50 High Potency Formula - Vitamin World
Each capsule contains: Thiamin (vitamin B-1, as thiamin mononitrate) 50 mg • Riboflavin (vitamin B-2) 50 mg • Niacin (as niacinamide) 50 mg • Vitamin B-6 (as pyridoxine hydrochloride) 50 mg • Folic Acid 400 mcg • Vitamin B-12 (as cyanocobalamin) 50 mcg • Biotin (as D-biotin) 50 mcg • Pantothenic Acid (as D-calcium pantothenate) 50 mg • Choline Bitartrate 50 mg • Inositol 50 mg • PABA (para-aminobenzoic acid) 50 mg • Proprietary Blend 5 mg: Alfalfa leaf, Watercress, Parsley leaf, Soy Lecithin, Rice Bran. Other Ingredients: Gelatin, Magnesium Stearate, Mannitol, Silica.

Naturally Inspired Mega Vita-Min - Vitamin World
Each tablet contains: Vitamin A (retinyl palmitate) 8000 IU • Vitamin C (ascorbic acid and rose hips) 250 mg • Vitamin D (cholecalciferol) 400 IU • Vitamin E (D-alpha tocopheryl acetate) 125 IU • Thiamin (vitamin B1) 80 mg • Riboflavin (vitamin B2) 80 mg • Niacin (niacinamide) 80 mg • Vitamin B6 (pyridoxine HCl) 80 mg • Folic Acid 400 mcg • Vitamin B12 (cyanocobalamin) 80 mcg • Biotin (as D-biotin) 80 mcg • Pantothenic Acid (D-calcium pantothenate) 80 mg • Calcium (carbonate) 8 mg • Iron (ferrous gluconate) 2 mg • Iodine (kelp) 150 mcg • Magnesium (oxide) 6 mg • Zinc (gluconate) 1.4 mg • Selenium (sodium selenite) 25 mcg • Copper (gluconate) 0.07 mg • Manganese (gluconate) 0.12 mg • Chromium (picolinate) 25 mcg • Molybdenum (sodium molybdate) 25 mcg • Potassium (gluconate) 1.6 mg • Boron (sodium borate) 0.5 mg • Choline Bitartrate 80 mg • Inositol 80 mg • PABA (para-aminobenzoic acid) 80 mg • Rutin fruit (dimorphandra mollis) 30 mg • Citrus Bioflavonoids fruit (citrus sinensis) 25 mg • Hesperidin 5 mg • Betaine Hydrochloride 25 mg • Coenzyme Q-10 500 mg • Deodorized Garlic bulb (allium sativum) 1 mg • Korean Ginseng root (Panax ginseng) 1 mg • Pycnogenol 500 mcg • Proprietary Blend 4 mg: Alfalfa leaf, Watercress, Parsley leaf, Rice Bran, Lecithin. Other Ingredients: Cellulose (plant origin), Vegetable Stearic Acid, Croscarmellose, Silica, Mannitol, Vegetable Magnesium Stearate, Cellulose Coating, Starch.

Naturally Inspired Milk Free ProBiotic Acidophilus - Vitamin World
Each capsule contains: Lactobacillus Blend 40 mg: Lactobacillus Acidophilus, Lactobacillus Rhamnosus, Lactobacillus Bifidus. Other Ingredients: Dicalcium Phosphate, Cellulose (plant origin), Hydroxypropyl Methylcellulose, Vegetable Stearic Acid, Silica, Vegetable Magnesium Stearate.

Naturally Inspired MSM 750 mg - Vitamin World
Each capsule contains: MSM (methylsulfonylmethane, organic sulfur 255 mg) 750 mg • Other Ingredients: Dicalcium Phosphate, Gelatin, Vegetable Magnesium Stearate, Silica.

Naturally Inspired Natural Vitamins A & D from Fish Liver Oils - Vitamin World
Each softgel contains: Vitamin A 5000 IU • Vitamin D 400 IU. Other Ingredients: Gelatin, Glycerin.

Naturally Inspired Sublingual B-12 Microlozenges 500 mcg - Vitamin World
Each microlozenge contains: Vitamin B-12 500 mcg (as cyanocobalamin). Other Ingredients: Mannitol, Sucrose, Cellulose, Croscarmellose, Silica, Hydrogenated Cottonseed Oil, Natural Cherry Flavor, Vegetable Magnesium Stearate.

Naturally Inspired Sublingual Vitamin B-12 2500 mcg - Vitamin World
Each tablet contains: Vitamin B-12 (as cyanocobalamin) 2500 mcg. Other Ingredients: Mannitol, Vegetable Stearic Acid, Hydroxypropyl Methylcellulose, Natural Cherry Flavor, Croscarmellose, Vegetable Magnesium Stearate, Silica.

Naturally Inspired Sublingual Vitamin B-12 5000 mcg - Vitamin World
Each tablet contains: Vitamin B-12 (as cyanocobalamin) 5000 mcg • Coenzyme B-12 (as dibencozide) 100 mcg. Other Ingredients: Sucrose, Cellulose, Croscarmellose, Hydrogenated Vegetable Oil, Natural Cherry Flavor, Hydroxypropyl Cellulose, Natural Flavor, Silica, Vegetable Magnesium Stearate.

Naturally Inspired Super Alfalfa 250 mg - Vitamin World
Each tablet contains: Alfalfa Juice Concentrate (medicago sativa) 250 mg. Other Ingredients: Acacia, Cellulose, Oil of Spearmint, Oil of Peppermint.

Naturally Inspired Time Release B-50 Vitamin B-Complex - Vitamin World
Each tablet contains: Thiamin (vitamin B-1, as thiamin mononitrate) 50 mg • Riboflavin (vitamin B-2) 50 mg • Niacin (as niacinamide) 50 mg • Vitamin B-6 (as pyridoxine hydrochloride) 50 mg • Folic Acid 400 mcg • Vitamin B-12 (as cyanocobalamin) 50 mcg • Biotin (as D-biotin) 50 mcg • Pantothenic Acid (as D-calcium pantothenate) 50 mg • Proprietary Blend 50 mg: Inositol, Choline Bitartrate, PABA (para-aminobenzoic acid), Alfalfa, Watercress, Parsley, Lecithin, Rice Bran. Other Ingredients: Dicalcium Phosphate, Cellulose, Cellulose Coating, Vegetable Stearic Acid, Silica, Vegetable Magnesium Stearate, Mannitol.

Naturally Inspired Time Release B-Complex plus C - Vitamin World
Each tablet contains: Vitamin C (as ascorbic acid and rose hips) 300 mg • Thiamin (vitamin B-1, as thiamin mononitrate) 18 mg • Riboflavin (vitamin B-2) 10 mg • Niacin (as niacinamide) 50 mg • Vitamin B-6 (as pyridoxine hydrochloride) 5 mg • Folic Acid 400 mcg • Vitamin B-12 (as cyanocobalamin) 10 mcg • Biotin 50 mcg • Pantothenic Acid (as D-calcium pantothenate) 10 mg. Other Ingredients: Cellulose, Dicalcium Phosphate, Hydroxy Methylcellulose, Vegetable Stearic Acid, Silica, Cellulose Coating, Vegetable Magnesium Stearate, Mannitol.

Naturally Inspired Time Release Mega Vita-Min - Vitamin World
Each tablet contains: Vitamin A (as retinyl palmitate) 8000 IU • Vitamin C (as ascorbic acid and rose hips) 250 mg • Vitamin D (as cholecalciferol) 400 IU • Vitamin E (as D-alpha tocopheryl acetate) 125 IU • Thiamin (vitamin B1, as thiamine mononitrate) 80 mg • Riboflavin (vitamin B2) 80 mg • Niacin (as niacinamide) 80 mg • Vitamin B6 (as pyridoxine hydrochloride) 80 mg • Folic Acid 400 mcg • Vitamin B12 (as cyanocobalamin) 80 mcg • Biotin (as D-biotin) 80 mcg • Pantothenic Acid (as D-calcium pantothenate) 80 mg • Calcium (as calcium carbonate) 8 mg • Iron (as ferrous gluconate) 2 mg • Iodine (as kelp) 150 mcg • Magnesium (as magnesium oxide) 6 mg • Zinc (as zinc gluconate) 1.4 mg • Selenium (as sodium selenite) 25 mcg • Copper (as copper gluconate) 0.07 mg • Manganese (as manganese gluconate) 0.12 mg • Chromium (as chromium picolinate) 25 mcg • Molybdenum (as sodium molybdate) 25 mcg • Potassium (as potassium gluconate) 1.6 mg • Boron (as sodium borate) 0.5 mg • Choline Bitartrate 80 mg • Inositol 80 mg • PABA (para-aminobenzoic acid) 80 mg • Rutin fruit (dimorphandra mollis) 30 mg • Citrus Bioflavonoids fruit (citrus sinensis) 25 mg • Hesperidin fruit (citrus spp.) 5 mg • Betaine Hydrochloride 25 mg • Coenzyme Q-10 500 mg • Deodorized Garlic bulb (allium sativum) 1 mg • Korean Ginseng root (Panax ginseng) 1 mg • Pycnogenol 500 mcg • Proprietary Blend 4 mg: Alfalfa leaf, Watercress, Parsley leaf, Rice Bran, Lecithin. Other Ingredients: Methylcellulose, Vegetable Stearic Acid, Silica, Mannitol, Vegetable Magnesium Stearate, Cellulose Coating, Starch.

Naturally Inspired Time Release Vitamin B-12 1000 mcg Ener-B - Vitamin World
Each tablet contains: Ener-B brand Vitamin B-12 (as cyanocobalamin) 1000 mcg. Other Ingredients: Dicalcium Phosphate, Cellulose, Hydroxypropyl Methylcellulose, Vegetable Stearic Acid, Silica, Vegetable Magnesium Stearate.

Naturally Inspired Time-Release B-100 Ultra B-Complex - Vitamin World
Each time-release tablet contains: Thiamin (vitamin B1 as thiamin mononitrate) 100 mg • Riboflavin (vitamin B2) 100 mg • Niacin (as niacinamide) 100 mg • Vitamin B6 (as pyridoxine hydrochloride) 100 mg • Folic Acid 400 mcg • Vitamin B12 (as cyanocobalamin) 100 mcg • Biotin (as D-biotin) 100 mcg • Pantothenic Acid (as D-calcium pantothenate) 100 mg • PABA (para-aminobenzoic acid) 100 mg • Inositol 100 mg • Choline Bitartrate 100 mg • Proprietary Blend 1 mg: Alfalfa, Watercress, Parsley, Soy Lecithin, Rice Bran. Other Ingredients: Hydroxy Methylcellulose, Cellulose, Calcium Silicate, Mannitol, Cellulose Coating, Magnesium Stearate, Silica.

Naturally Inspired Tine-Release Vitamin B-12 1500 mcg - Vitamin World
Each tablet contains: Vitamin B12 (as cyanocobalamin) 1500 mcg. Other Ingredients: Dicalcium Phosphate, Hydroxypropyl Methylcellulose, Vegetable Stearic Acid, Cellulose Coating, Vegetable Magnesium Stearate, Silica, Mannitol.

Naturally Inspired Vitamin B-1 100 mg - Vitamin World
Each tablet contains: Vitamin B1 (as thiamin hydrochloride) 100 mg. Other Ingredients: Dicalcium Phosphate, Cellulose, Vegetable Stearic Acid, Silica, Vegetable Magnesium Stearate, Cellulose Coating, Glycerin, Sodium Citrate.

Naturally Inspired Vitamin B-1 250 mg - Vitamin World
Each tablet contains: Vitamin B1 (as thiamin hydrochloride) 250 mg. Other Ingredients: Cellulose, Vegetable Stearic Acid, Cellulose Coating, Croscarmellose, Silica, Vegetable Magnesium Stearate.

Naturally Inspired Vitamin B-12 100 mcg - Vitamin World
Each tablet contains: Vitamin B-12 (as cyanocobalamin) 100 mcg. Other Ingredients: Dicalcium Phosphate, Cellulose, Mannitol, Vegetable Stearic Acid, Silica, Vegetable Magnesium Stearate.

Naturally Inspired Vitamin B-12 250 mcg - Vitamin World
Each tablet contains: Vitamin B-12 (as cyanocobalamin) 250 mcg. Other Ingredients: Dicalcium Phosphate, Cellulose (Plant Origin), Mannitol, Vegetable Stearic Acid, Silica, Magnesium Stearate.

Naturally Inspired Vitamin B-12 500 mcg capsules - Vitamin World
Each capsule contains: Vitamin B-12 (as cyanocobalamin) 500 mcg. Other Ingredients: Rice Powder, Gelatin, Vegetable Magnesium Stearate, Silica.

Naturally Inspired Vitamin B-12 500 mcg tablets - Vitamin World
Each tablet contains: Vitamin B-12 (as cyanocobalamin) 500 mcg. Other Ingredients: Dicalcium Phosphate, Cellulose, Croscarmellose, Vegetable Stearic Acid, Silica, Vegetable Magnesium Stearate.

Naturally Inspired Vitamin B-2 (Riboflavin) 100 mg - Vitamin World
Each tablet contains: Riboflavin (vitamin B2) 100 mg. Other Ingredients: Dicalcium Phosphate, Cellulose, Croscarmellose, Vegetable Stearic Acid, Vegetable Magnesium Stearate, Cellulose Coating, Guar Gum, Silica.

Naturally Inspired Vitamin B-6 100 mg - Vitamin World
Each tablet contains: Vitamin B-6 (as pyridoxine hydrochloride) 100 mg • Calcium 27 mg • Phosphorus 20 mg. Other Ingredients: Dicalcium Phosphate, Cellulose, Croscarmellose, Vegetable Stearic Acid, Silica, Vegetable Magnesium Stearate.

Naturally Inspired Vitamin B-6 50 mg - Vitamin World
Each tablet contains: Vitamin B-6 (as pyridoxine hydrochloride) 50 mg • Calcium 45 mg. Other Ingredients: Dicalcium Phosphate, Cellulose, Croscarmellose, Vegetable Stearic Acid, Silica, Vegetable Magnesium Stearate.

Naturally Inspired Vitamin C & Zinc Lozenges - Vitamin World
Each lozenge contains: Vitamin C (as ascorbic acid and rose hips) 300 mg • Zinc (as zinc citrate) 7 mg • Natural Food Base 30 mg: Rutin, Hesperidin, Acerola, Citrus Bioflavonoid, Black Currant. Other Ingredients: Sucrose, Dextrose, Maltodextrin, Cottonseed Oil, Starch, Natural Flavor, Vegetable Magnesium Stearate.

Naturally Inspired Vitamin C-1000 mg with Rose Hips - Vitamin World
Each tablet contains: Vitamin C (as ascorbic acid and rose hips) 1000 mg. Other Ingredients: Cellulose (plant origin), Croscarmellose, Vegetable Stearic Acid, Silica, Cellulose Coating, Vegetable Magnesium Stearate.

Naturally Inspired Vitamin C-500 mg with Rose Hips - Vitamin World
Each tablet contains: Vitamin C (as ascorbic acid and rose hips) 500 mg. Other Ingredients: Cellulose (plant origin), Cellulose Coating, Croscarmellose, Vegetable Stearic Acid, Vegetable Magnesium Stearate, Silica.

Naturally Inspired Vitamins A & D - Vitamin World
Each softgel contains: Vitamin A 10,000 IU • Vitamin D 400 IU. Other Ingredients: Gelatin, Glycerin, Soybean Oil.

Naturally Inspired Yeast Free Chromium Picolinate - Vitamin World
Each tablet contains: Chromium (as Chromium Picolinate) 200 mcg. Other Ingredients: Dicalcium Phosphate, Cellulose (Plant Origin), Vegetable Stearic Acid, Silica, Vegetable Magnesium Stearate.

Naturally Inspired Zinc Picolinate 25 mg - Vitamin World
Each caplet contains: Zinc (as zinc picolinate) 25 mg. Other Ingredients: Dicalcium Phosphate, Cellulose (plant origin), Vegetable Stearic Acid, Vegetable Magnesium Stearate.

Naturally Kids' Calcees Chewable Calcium + D - Naturally Vitamins
Each tablet contains: Calcium 300 mg • Vitamin D (cholecalciferol) 50 IU. Other Ingredients: Fruit concentrate, Vanilla powder.

Naturally Lean Matrix - ProLab
Three capsules contain: Proprietary Blend 2 g: 3-Hydroxy-L-Tyrosine from Mucuna Pruriens, Guggul gum resin (E-guggulsterones, Z-guggulsterones), Caffeine, Green Tea leaf extract (epigallocatechin gallate, polyphenols), Coleus Forskohlii root, Naringin, Evodia Rutaecarpa fruit, Chaste Tree berries (Vitex agnus-castus fruit), Bitter Orange extract (citrus aurantium, synephrine, N-methyl-tyramine, hordenine, octopamine, tyramine). Other Igredients: Gelatin, Silica, Magnesium Stearate.
See Editor's Note No. 40.

Naturally Phen - Optimum Nutrition
DL-Phenylalanine L-5-Hydroxytryptophan Tyrosine.

Naturally Ripped - Optimum Nutrition
Ma Huang • Guarana • L-Carnitine • Chromium Picolinate.
See Editor's Note No. 21 and No. 30.

NaturalMax OstiBone - NaturalMax - Nutraceutical
Each capsule contains: Calcium (as Calcium Carbonate) 120 mg • Ostivone (as Isoproproxy Isoflavone) 200 mg. Inactive ingredients: Gelatin, Cellulose, Magnesium Stearate.

Natural-Source d-Alpha Vitamin E brand - ADM
Vitamin E.
See Editor's Note No. 44.

NaturalSoy - Vital Nutrients
Each 3 tbsp serving contains: Vitamin A 153 IU • Vitamin E 1.27 IU • Vitamin C 25 mg • Vitamin B1 (thiamine) 0.37 mg • Vitamin B2 (riboflavin) 0.15 mg • Vitamin B3 (niacin) 1.4 mg • Folic Acid 140 mcg • Calcium 167 mg • Copper 0.1 mg • Iron 3 mg • Phosphorus 164 mg • Selenium 1.4 mcg • Zinc 0.84 mg.

Some Brand Name Natural Products - What they Contain

www.NaturalDatabase.com contains MANY more listings than appear here.
Editor's Notes are located on pages 2155-2163.

BRAND NAMES

NaturalTrim **-** Starlight International
Each capsule contains: Chromium (as chromium picolinate) 6 mcg • Magnesium Gluconate 7 mg • Calcium Gluconate 5 mg • Ma Huang (ephedra sinica, plant) 275 mg • Total Ephedrine Alkaloids 22 mg • Bladderwrack (fucus vesiculosus, plant) 35 mg • Uva Ursi extract, 4:1 (arctostaphylosuva ursi, leaf) 25 mg • Couch Grass (agropyron repens, rhizome) 8.75 mg • Dandelion (taraxacum officinale, root) 8.75 mg • Hydrangea (hydrangea arborescans, root) 8.75 mg • Nettle (urtica dioica, leaf) 8.75 mg • Buchu (carosma betulina, leaf) 8.75 mg • Parsley extract, 4:1 (petroselinum crispum, leaf) 8 mg • Corn Silk (zea mays, flower pistil) 7 mg • Fumitory (fumaria officinalis, plant) 6 mg • Goldenrod (solidago odora, leaf) 6 mg • English Hawthorn (crataegus laevigata, berry) 5 mg • Licorice (glycyrrhiza glabra, root) 5 mg • Marshmallow (althea officinalis, root) 5 mg • Apple Pectin 5 mg. Other Ingredients: Silicon Dioxide, Magnesium Stearate, Dicalcium Phosphate, Gelatin.
See Editor's Note No. 21 and No. 30.

NaturalTrim Ephedra Free **-** Starlight International
Each capsule contains: Proprietary Blend 520 mg: Guarana seed extract (paullinia cupana, containing 72 mg caffeine), Rhododendron Caucasicum leaf extract, Arctic root (rhodiola rosea), Corn Silk (zea mays, flower pistil), Buchu leaf (agathosma betulina). Other Ingredients: Silicon Dioxide, Magnesium Stearate, Gelatin.

Naturatussin 1 **-** Pacific BioLogic
Platycodon root (balloon flower) • Licorice root • Cynanchum root • Red Date (Chinese jujube) • Sophora root • Burdock fruit (great) • Fritillaria bulb (tendrilled) • Peppermint (field mint) • Ephedra Herba (aerial) • Apricot kernal (northern) • Aster root (purple).
See Editor's Note No. 30.

Naturatussin 2 **-** Pacific BioLogic
Houttuynia Herba • Platycodon root (balloon flower) • Hogfennel root (peucedanum) • Aster root (purple) • Honeysuckle flower • Cynanchum root • Trichosanthes fruit peel • Peach kernal • Momordica Fruit (arhat) • Fritillaria bulb (tendrilled) • Burdock fruit.

Natura-UR **-** Pacific BioLogic
Angelica root (dahurica) • Citrus peel (tangerine) • Andrographis • Isatis leaf • Licorice root • Scute root • Platycodon root • Honey Suckle flower • Chrysanthemum flower • Forsynthia fruit • Burdock fruit • Notopterygium root & rhizome.

Naturcoksinum **-** Homeolab
Each vial contains: Anas Barbariae Hepatis et Cordis extractum (autolysed liver & heart of duck) 200C.
See Editor's Note No. 1.

Nature Cleanse BotaniCleanse **-** Nature's Plus
Each tablet contains: Botanical Proprietary Blend 500 mg: Butternut bark (Juglans cinera), Yellow Dock root (Rumex crispus), Blessed Thistle flower (Cnicus benedictus), Red Clover leaf (Trifolium pratense), Clove bud (Eugenia caryophyllata), Milk Thistle seed (Silybum marianum), Uva Ursi leaf (Arctostaphylos uva-ursi), Cranberry fruit (Vaccinium macrocarpon), Ginger root (Zingiber officinale), Cascara Sagrada bark (Rhamnus purshiana) Hibiscus flower (Hibiscus abelmoschus), Juniper berry (Juniperus oxycedrus), Senna leaf (Cassia senna), Slippery Elm bark (Ulmus rubra), Fennel seed (Foeniculum vulgare), Cayenne fruit (Capsicum frutescens), Dandelion root (Taraxacum officinale), Parsley leaf (Petroselinum crispum), Alfalfa leaf (Medicago sativa), Fenugreek seed (Trigonella foenum-graecum), Aloe Vera, Apple Cider Vinegar • Green Food Proprietary Blend 100 mg: Chlorophyll, Chlorella, broken cell Blue-Green Micro-Algae, Spirulina Algae (Spirulina platensis), Irish Moss (Chondrus crispus), Barley Grass juice (Hordeum vulgare), Pacific Kelp (Laminaria) • Vitamin C (corn free) 100 mg.

Nature Cleanse Fiber Diet **-** Nature's Plus
Nine capsules contain: Oat Bran (87% Fiber) 1912.5 mg • Psyllium husks (80% Fiber) 1912.5 mg • Apple pectin (84% Fiber) 180 mg • Vitamin C 157.5 mg • Butcher's Broom (15% Fiber) 135 mg • Bentonite U.S.P. grade 90 mg • Cellulose (100% Fiber) 90 mg • Lactobacillus acidophilus 90 million viable cells 22.5 mg.

Nature Cleanse PuriFiber Powder **-** Nature's Plus
Each teaspoon (3.75g) contains: Fiber Complex 3500 mg containing a proprietary blend of fiber rich concentrates: Psyllium husks (Plantago ovata), Apple pectin (Malus sylvestris), Butcher's Broom rhizome (Ruscus aceleatus), Bentonite, modified citrus pectin, Cellulose, Rice fiber (Oryza sativa), Slippery Elm bark (Ulmus rubra), Oat bran (Avena sativa), Beet juice & fiber (Beta vulgaris), Prune fiber (Prunus) • Chitosan, vegetarian 50 mg • FOS (Fructooligosaccharides) Lactic flora growth accelerant 50 mg • Lipase fat-digesting enzyme 50 mg • Peptide FM bioactive oligopeptide 25 mg • Lactospor micro-encapsulated pure culture of B. Coagulans, provides 1 million viable cells 1.7 mg.

Nature Derm Skin Care System **-** PhytoPharmica
Two capsules contain: Bromelain (1200 MCU/g) 200 mg • Burdock root 4:1 extract (arctium lappa) 10 mg • Calcium (lactate) 11 mg • Magnesium (oxide) 72 mg • Niacin 10 mg • Pantothenic Acid (as clacium D-pantothenate) 10 mg • Potassium (as potassium chloride) 105 mg • Ribonucleic Acid (RNA) 20 mg • Sulfur (sublimed) 25 mg • Thymus 25 mg • Vitamin A (as retinyl acetate) 10,000 IU • Vitamin B12 (cyanocobalamin) 3 mcg • Vitamin B6 (pyridoxine HCl) 8 mg • Vitamin C (ascorbic acid) 200 mg • Zinc (chelate) 30 mg.
See Editor's Note No. 14.

Nature Derm Skin Care System Acne Cream **-** PhytoPharmica
Each application contains: Sulfur 3%. Other Ingredients: Purified Water, Zinc, Sage Extract, Silymarin Phytosome, Hawthorne Extract, Chamomile Extract, 18-Beta-Glycyrrhetinic Acid, Essential Oil of Rosemary, Urea, and Vitamin E (Tocopherol), Natural and Hypoallergenic Fragrance.

Nature Force **-** Rexall - Sundown
Two tablets contain: Vitamin A (100% beta-carotene) 10000 IU • Vitamin C 300 mg • Vitamin E (dl-alpha-tocopheryl acid succinate) 90 IU • Calcium 255 mg • Selenium (from selenium amino acid chelate) 50 mcg • Sodium 5 mg • Nature Force Proprietary Blend: Mixed Berry Skin extract, Alfalfa aerial parts, Tomato, European Wine Grape concentrate (vitis vinifera), Plant Enzymes (glucose oxidase, peroxidase, catalase), Cruciferous Vegetable concentrate (cabbage head, cauliflower flower head, broccoli flower head), Green Tea leaf extract, Garlic, Rose Hips, and Seeds extract (rosa canina), Freeze-Dried Carrot root juice 188 mg. Other Ingredients: Dicalcium Phosphate, Croscarmellose Sodium, Silica, Magnesium Stearate.

Nature Made Adult Multi-Vitamin Chewable **-** Pharmavite Corp.
Each tablet contains: Vitamin A (as beta-carotene) 5000 IU • Vitamin C 250 mg • Vitamin D 400 IU • Vitamin E 30 IU • Thiamin 1.5 mg • Riboflavin 1.7 mg • Niacin 20 mg • Vitamin B6 2 mg • Folic Acid 400 mcg • Vitamin B12 6 mcg • Biotin 40 mcg • Pantothenic Acid 10 mg • Calcium 200 mg • Phosphorous 100 mg • Iodine 150 mcg • Magnesium 20 mg • Zinc 15 mg • Copper 2 mg • Sodium 15 mg. Inactive Ingredients: Sorbitol, Fructose, Xylitol, Stearic Acid, Mono & Diglycerides of Fatty Acids, Carrageenan, Gelatin, Aspartame, Yellow 6 Lake, Corn Starch, Citric Acid, Natural & Artificial Flavors, Modified Food Starch, Aluminum Oxide, Red 40 Lake.

Nature Made Balanced B-150 Complex **-** Pharmavite Corp.
Each tablet contains: Thiamin mononitrate (Vitamin B1) 150 mg • Riboflavin (Vitamin B2) 150 mg • Niacin (Niacinamide, Vitamin B3) 150 mg • Vitamin B6 (Pyridoxine Hydrochloride) 150 mg • Folate (Folic Acid, Folacin, as Folate) 400 mcg • Vitamin B12 (Cyanocobalamin) 150 mcg • Biotin 150 mcg • Pantothenic Acid 150 mg. Other Ingredients: Dibasic Calcium Phosphate, Hydroxypropyl Methylcellulose, Magnesium Stearate, Polyethylene Glycol, Carnauba Wax.

Nature Made Cal Burst **-** Pharmavite Corp.
Each soft chew contains: Calcium Carbonate (providing elemental calcium 500 mg) 1250 mg •Vitamin D 200 IU. Other Ingredients: Corn Syrup, Calcium Carbonate, Sugar, Hydrogenated Coconut Oil, Cocoa (flavor), Nonfat Dried Milk, Glycerin, Corn Starch, Salt, Lecithin, Natural and Artificial Flavors.

Some Brand Name Natural Products - What they Contain

www.NaturalDatabase.com contains MANY more listings than appear here.
Editor's Notes are located on pages 2155-2163.

Nature Made Calcium and Magnesium with Zinc - Pharmavite Corp.
Each tablet contains: Calcium Carbonate 333 mg • Magnesium Oxide 133 mg • Zinc Sulfate 5 mg. Other Ingredients: Maltodextrin, Croscarmellose Sodium, Silicon Dioxide, Magnesium Stearate, Hydroxypropyl Methylcellulose, Cellulose, Polyethylene Glycol.

Nature Made Magnesium 250 mg - Pharmavite Corp.
Each tablet contains: Magnesium (as magnesium oxide) 250 mg. Inactive Ingredients: Cellulose, Croscarmellose Sodium, Magnesium Stearate.

Nature Made Rekindle - Pharmavite Corp.
Each two tablets contain: Calcium 250 mg • L-Arginine 1250 mg • Asian Ginseng (Korean) root extract 50 mg • Damiana leaf 25 mg • Ginkgo leaf extract 25 mg. Other Ingredients: L-Arginine Hydrochloride, Calcium Carbonate, Cellulose Gel, Hydroxypropyl Methylcellulose, Stearic Acid, Silicon Dioxide, Magnesium Stearate, Titanium Dioxide, Red 40 Lake, Polyethylene Glycol, Triethyl Citrate, Polysorbate 80, Blue 2 Lake.

Nature Made SAM-e - Pharmavite Corp.
Two tablets contain: S-adenosylmethionine 400 mg • 4-butanedisulfonate • Cellulose • Sodium Starch Glycolate • Methacrylic Acid Copolymer • Talc • Polyethylene Glycol • Silica • Magnesium Stearate • Polysorbate 80 • Sodium Hydroxide • Iron Oxide • Simethicone.

Nature Made Soy Isoflavones 50 mg - Pharmavite Corp.
Each tablet contains: Soy Isoflavones 50 mg. Other Ingredients: Dibasic Calcium Phosphate, Cellulose, Soy Extract, Croscarmellose Sodium, Magnesium Stearate, Silicon Dioxide.

Nature Made Vinpocetine - Pharmavite Corp.
Each tablet contains: Vinpocetine 5 mg.

Nature Made Vitamin C - 1000 - Pharmavite Corp.
Each tablet contains: Vitamin C 1000 mg. Other Ingredients: Ascorbic Acid, Corn Starch, Cellulose, Magnesium Stearate, Stearic Acid, Silica Gel.

Nature Made Vitamin E - Pharmavite Corp.
Each softgel contains: Vitamin E 400 IU. Other Ingredients: DL-Alpha Tocopheryl Acetate, Gelatin, Glycerin, Water.

Nature's Collagen - DaVinci Laboratories
Each tablet contains: Hydrolyzed Collagen Type II 500 mg • Methylsulfonylmethane 400 mg • Glucosamine HCl 300 mg. Other Ingredients: Rice Flour, Vegetable Stearate.

Nature's Cure Two-Part Acne Treatment System for Males - Nature's Cure
This is a 2 component product that includes tablets and a cream. Each tablet contains: Calendula officinalis (marigold) 6x • Hydrastis canadensis (golden seal) 6x • Juglans regia (walnut) 6x • Antimonium crudum (antimonius sulfide) 12x • Echinacea angustifolia (cone flower) 12x • Ledum palustre (wild rosemary) 12x • Orchitimun (glandular) 12x • Sarsaparilla (wild licorice) 12x • Hepar Sulfuris Calcareum (calcium sulfide) 24x • Carbo Vegetabilis (vegetable carbon) 30x. Other Ingredients: Lactose. The cream contains: Benzoyl Peroxide (5%). Other Ingredients: Purified Water, Carbomer 940, Allantoin, Aloe Vera concentrate, Diazolidinyl Urea, Disodium Edetate, Dioctyl Sodium Sulfosuccinate, Sodium Hydroxide.
See Editor's Note No. 1.

Nature's Cure Two-Part Acne Treatment System, Cream, for Females - Nature's Cure
Active Ingredients: Benzoyl Peroxide (5%). Inactive Ingredients: Purified Water, Carbomer 940, Alantoin, Aloe Vera concentrate, Diazolidinyl Urea, Disodium Edetate, Dioctyl Sodium Sulfosuccinate, Sodium Hydroxide.

Nature's Cure Two-Part Acne Treatment System, Tablets, for Females - Nature's Cure
Each tablet contains: Juglans regia (walnut) 6x • Antimonium Crudum (antimonius sulfide) 12x • Candida albicans (yeast) 12x, 30x, 60x, 200x • Echinacea angustifolia (cone flower) 12x • Kali Bromatum (potassium bromide) 12x • Ledum palustre (wild rosemary) 12x • Oophorunum (glandular) 12x • Hepar Sulfuris Calcareum (calcium sulfide) 24x • Carbo Vegetabilis (vegetable carbon) • Cimicifuga racemosa (black cohosh) 30x • Cistus canadensis (frost weed) 30 x • Graphites (graphite) 30x. Other Ingredients: Lactose.
See Editor's Note No. 1.

Nature's Fingerprint - GNC
Each capsule contains: Wild Yam root 150 mg • Evening Primrose 90 mg • Chaste Tree berry 50 mg.

Nature's Life Greens capsules - Nature's Life
Each 500 mg capsule contains: Green Peas (Pisum sativum) • Celery (Apium graveolens) Cabbage (Brassica oleracea capitata) • Cauliflower (Brassica oleracea botrutis) • Broccoli (Brassica oleracea italica) • Spinach (Spinacia oleracea) • Green Bell Peppers (Capsicum frutescens) • Green Onions (Allium cepa) • Hawaiian grown Spirulina plantesis • Parsley (Petroselinum crispum) • Green Chili Peppers (Capsicum annum) • Green Garlic sprouts (Allium sativum) • Jalepeno Peppers (Capsicum annum) • Green Tea leaves (Camellia sinensis) • Alfalfa (Medicago sativa) • Barley Grass (Hordeum vulgare) • Dunaliella salina • Chlorella • Pacific Alaria (Alaria marginata) • Kelp (Laminaria species) • Pacific Nori (Porphyra tenera) Dulse (Phodymenia palmata) • Kombu (Laminaria setchellii) • Sea Lettuce (Ulva lactuca) • Sea Palm (Pastelsi palmaeformis).

Nature's Life Greens powder - Nature's Life
Five grams of powder contain: Green Peas (Pisum sativum) • Celery (Apium graveolens) Cabbage (Brassica oleracea capitata) • Cauliflower (Brassica oleracea botrutis) • Broccoli (Brassica oleracea italica) • Spinach (Spinacia oleracea) • Green Bell Peppers (Capsicum frutescens) • Green Onions (Allium cepa) • Hawaiian grown Spirulina plantesis • Parsley (Petroselinum crispum) • Green Chili Peppers (Capsicum annum) • Green Garlic sprouts (Allium sativum) • Jalepeno Peppers (Capsicum annum) • Green Tea leaves (Camellia sinensis) • Alfalfa (Medicago sativa) • Barley Grass (Hordeum vulgare) • Dunaliella salina • Chlorella • Pacific Alaria (Alaria marginata) • Kelp (Laminaria species) • Pacific Nori (Porphyra tenera) Dulse (Phodymenia palmata) • Kombu (Laminaria setchellii) • Sea Lettuce (Ulva lactuca) • Sea Palm (Pastelsi palmaeformis).

Nature's Lining - LaneLabs
Each chewable tablet contains: Zinc (from PepZin GI zinc-carnosine) 8 mg • L-Carnosine (from PepZin GI zinc-carnosine) 29.5 mg. Other Ingredients: Fructose, Guar Gum, Microcrystalline Cellulose, Magnesium Stearate, Corn Starch, Peppermint Oil.

Nature's Noni - Nature's Sunshine
Reconstituted Morinda fruit (morinda citrifolia) • Grape juice Concentrate • Pear juice concentrate • Grape skin extract • Malic Acid • Tartaric Acid • Citric Acid • Ascorbic Acid.

Nature's Resource Ginkgo Biloba - Pharmavite Corp.
Each capsule contains: Ginkgo Biloba leaf extract (standardized to 24% ginkgo flavone glycosides) 60 mg. Other Ingredients: Rice Flour, Gelatin, Water.

Nature's White Cross - D & E Pharmaceuticals
Each tablet contains: pure Ephedra extract 400 mg.
See Editor's Note No. 30.

Nature's Youth HGH - Nature's Youth, LLC
Each 13 g packet contains: Proprietary Amino Acid Blend: Glycine, L-Glutamine, L-Tyrosine, GABA, L-Arginine HCl, L-Lysine HCl, Pyroglutamic Acid • Glycoamino Acid Complex • Glucose Polymers • Anterior Pituitary Peptides • Broad Bean (l-dopa).
See Editor's Note No. 31.

Nature-Slim Tea - Triple Leaves Brand
Malva Verticellata.

Naturex Multi II - Swanson Health Products
Each capsule contains: Vitamin A (as palmitate) 5000 IU • Vitamin C USP (as ascorbic acid) 150 mg • Vitamin D (as cholecalciferol) 200 IU • Vitamin E (as D-alpha tocopheryl succinate) 75 IU • Thiamin HCl (vitamin B1) 50 mg • Riboflavin (vitamin B2) 50 mg • Niacinamide 50 mg • Vitamin B-6 (as pyridoxine HCl) 50 mg • Folic Acid 200 mcg • Vitamin B-12 (as cyanocobalamin) 20 mcg • Biotin 25 mcg • Pantothenic Acid (as d-calcium pantothenate) 50 mg • Iron (from ferrous gluconate) 0.5 mg • Iodine (from potassium iodide) 75 mcg • Zinc (from zinc gluconate) 1.5 mg • Selenium (as selenomethionine) 5 mcg • Copper (from copper gluconate) 0.5 mg • Manganese (from manganese gluconate) 0.5 mg • Chromium (from amino acid chelate) 50 mcg • Choline (as choline bitartrate) 25 mg • Inositol 25 mg • PABA (para-aminobenzoic acid) 25 mg • Betaine HCl 12.5 mg • Lemon Bioflavonoid Complex 12.5 mg • L-Glutamic Acid 12.5 mg • Rutin 12.5 mg • Hesperidin Complex 2.5 mg.

Natur-Leaf - Lifeline, Inc.
Each capsule contains: Blend of sprout phytochemicals 300 mg: Wild African Potato root • Lupins sprouts • Fenugreek sprouts • Barley sprouts • Wheat sprouts • Soybean sprouts • African Sunflower sprouts. Blend of enzymes 50 mg: Enzyme Mineral blend • Protease • Amylase • Lipase • Cellulase • Sucrase • Maltase • Lactase • Bromelain • Ionic Mineral blend.

Naturvite - Solgar
Each tablet contains: Vitamin B12 (cobalamin) 250 mcg • Vitamin A (palmitate) 10,000 IU • Vitamin D (cholecalciferol) 400 IU • Vitamin B1 (thiamine mononitrate) 25 mg • Vitamin B2 (riboflavin) 25 mg • Vitamin B6 (pyridoxine HCl) 25 mg • Vitamin C (ascorbic acid) 150 mg • Niacinamide 100 mg • Calcium Pantothenate 50 mg • Vitamin E (D-alpha tocopheryl succinate) 25 IU • Biotin 20 mcg • Folic Acid 100 mcg • Iron (gluconate) 6 mg • Iodine (kelp) 100 mcg • Zinc (gluconate) 180 mcg • Calcium (bone meal) 13.5 mg • Magnesium (gluconate) 388 mcg • Copper (gluconate) 35 mcg • Potassium 1.6 mg • Manganese (gluconate) 670 mcg • Choline (bitartrate) 62 mg • Inositol 150 mg • Rutin 25 mg • PABA (para aminobenzoic acid) 25 mg • Citrus Bioflavonoid complex 25 mg • Betaine HCl 25 mg • Hesperidin 5 mg • Desiccated Liver 50 mg • L-Lysine HCl 10 mg. Other Ingredients: Vegetable Cellulose, Silica, Vegetable Stearic Acid, Alfalfa, Acerola, Kelp, Parsley, Rose Hips, Watercress.
See Editor's Note No. 14.

Naudicelle - Key Pharmaceuticals
Each softgel contains: Evening Primrose oil with 10% GLA (gammalinolinic acid).

Nazanol - Metagenics
Two tablets contain: Proprietary Blend 2500 mg: Chinese Skullcap root (scutellaria baicalensis), Schizonepeta whole plant (schizonepeta tenuifolia), Fragrant Angelica root (angelica dahurica), Chinese Cinnamon twig (cinnamon aromaticum), Xanthium fruit (xanthium sibiricum), Astragalus root (astragalus membranaceus), Bai-Zhu Atractylodes rhizome (atractylodes macrocephala), Siler root (ledebouriella divaricata).

NeoCell - PhysioLogics
Two tablets contain: Raw Anterior Pituitary Concentrate 25 mg • GABA (gamma-aminobutyric acid) 125 mg • Phytosterol Complex (soy, rice) 100 mg • Soy Phosphatide Complex (24% phosphatidylcholine, 20% phosphatidylethanolamine, 14% phosphatidylinositol, 13% photoglycolipids) 200 mg • DMG Complex 50 mg: Trimethylglycine Hydrochloride, N,N-Dimethylglycine • Amino Acid Complex 700 mg: L-Glycine, L-Lysine Hydrochloride, L-Tyrosine, L-Arginine Hydrochloride, L-Ornithine Hydrochloride, L-Glutamine. Other Ingredients: Lecithin, Cellulose (plant origin), Silica, Vegetable Stearic Acid, Hydroxy Methylcellulose, Croscarmellose, Vegetable Magnesium Stearate, Cellulose Coating.
See Editor's Note No. 31.

NeoProstate B-300 - BCN - Beachwood Canyon, Naturally, Ltd.
Each caplet contains: Beta-sitosterol 300 mg • Zinc Citrate 15 mg. Ingredients: Mixed Sterols including Beta-sitosterol (at least 50%), Stig-masterol, Campesterol, Lupeol, Cycloartenon, Famesol, Phytol and Zinc.

NephPlex Rx - Nephro-Tech, Inc.
Each tablet contains: Ascorbic Acid 60 mg #8226; Thiamine 1.5 mg • Riboflavin 1.7 mg • Pyridoxine 10 mg • Cyanocobalamin 6 mcg • Pantothenic Acid 10 mg • Biotin 300 mcg • Niacinamide 20 mg • Zinc 12.5 mg • Folic Acid 1 mg.

Nephron FA - Nephro-Tech, Inc.
Two tablets contain: Ferrous Fumarate 200 mg • Ascorbic Acid 40 mg • Thiamine 1.5 mg • Riboflavin 1.7 mg • Pyridoxine 10 mg • Niacinamide 20 mg • Cyanocobalamin 6 mcg • Pantothenic Acid 10 mg • Biotin 300 mcg • Docusate Sodium 75 mg • Folic Acid 1 mg.

Nervaherb - Wild Rose
Each vegetable capsule contains: Valerian root 4:1 extract 100 mg • Oat seed 100 mg • Hops 2:1 extract 100 mg • Skullcap herb 100 mg • Black Cohosh 75 mg • Passion flower 50 mg.

Nerve Guard - Flora Inc.
St. John's Wort.

Nervous Tension Remedy (formerly HP 22) - Metagenics
Each tablet contains: Magnesia Phosphorica 3X • Colocynthis 12X • Kali Phosphoricum 30X • Hyoscyamus Niger 12X • Ignatia Amara 6X • Passiflora Incarnata 3X • Avena Sativa tincture.
See Editor's Note No. 1.

Ness Digest Chewables - Enzymes, Inc.
Each tablet contains: n-zimes Proprietary Enzyme Blend 204 mg: Protease, Lipase, Amylase, Glucoamylase, Malt Diastase, Lactase, Invertase, alpha-Galactosidase, CereCalase, Cellulase, Pectinase. Other Ingredients: Dextrose (Corn Sugar), Fructose (Fruit Sugar), Natural Raspberry Flavor, Silica (mineral), Plant Cellulose, Citric Acid, Veg. Magnesium Sterate, Proprietary Plant-derived Sweetener.

Ness Formula 10 - Enzymes, Inc.
Two capsules contain: Brewers Yeast 200 mg • Sucrase (Invertase) 3.6 IAU • Gotu Kola aerial part (Cantella Asiatica) 100 mg • Amylase 6000 DU • Protease 30,000 HUT • Rose Hips (Rosa Canina) 50 mg • Lipase 24 LU • Cellulase 200 CU. Other Ingredients: Gelatin, Plant Fiber, Water.

Nettle - Nature's Way
Two capsules contain: Nettle herb 870 mg. Other Ingredients: Gelatin.

Nettle & Pygeum with Pumpkin - Enzymatic Therapy
Each capsule contains: Nettle root extract 16:1 (Urticae dioica radix) 300 mg • Pumpkin seed oil (Cucurbita pepo) 175 mg • Pygeum africanum extract standardized to contain 13% total sterols 25 mg.

Nettle and Perilla Flavonoid Complex (Allercept 450) - Jamieson
Each caplet contains: Nettle leaf 1:6 extract (urtica dioica) • Perilla Fruit 1:37 extract (perilla frutescens) 450 mg.

Nettle Leaf - Gaia Herbs
Two capsules contain: Nettle leaf (urtica dioica) 100 mg. Other Ingredients: Vegetable Glycerin, Vegetable Cellulose (capsule).

Nettle-Pygeum Complex - PhytoPharmica
Each capsule contains: Pumpkin seed oil (cucurbita pepo) 175 mg • Pygeum Africanum bark extract (prunus africana, standardized to contain 13% total sterols) 25 mg • Stinging Nettle root 16:1 extract (urtica dioica) 300 mg.

Nettle-Reishi Virtue - Blessed Herbs
Nettle • Reishi mycelium • Chinese Ephedra • Yerba Santa leaf • Propolis • Ginkgo leaf • Licorice root • Grain alcohol & Distilled Water.
See Editor's Note No. 30.

Neuragen **-** Origin BioMedicinals
Geranium Oil extract • Lavender Oil extract • Bergamot Oil extract • Eucalyptus Oil extract • Tea Tree Oil extract.

Neural Support Formula **-** The Vitamin Factory
Each tablet contains: Vitamin E (D-alpha tocopheryl-succinate) 100 IU • Neuromins (13% DHA powder) 100 mg • Phosphatidylserine Complex 20% 50 mg • Ginkgo Biloba leaf extract (24/6) 40 mg • Bacopin extract (Bacopa monniera, min. 20% Bacosides) 25 mg • Pycnogenol (Maritime Pine bark extract) 15 mg.

NeuRecover-DA (Depressant Abuse) **-** Natural Distributors International, Inc.
Six capsules contain: Vitamin A 2000 IU • Vitamin C 600 mg • Vitamin B1 14.5 mg • Vitamin B2 5 mg • Niacin (niacinamide ascorbate) 200 mg • Calcium (chelate) 150 mg • Iron 9 mg • Vitamin E 30 IU • Vitamin B6 18 mg • Folic Acid 0.4 mg • Vitamin B12 0.03 mg • Magnesium 150 mg • Zinc 15 mg • Biotin 0.3 mg • Pantothenic Acid 90 mg • Chromium (picolinate) 0.06 mg • DL-Phenylalanine 2760 mg • L-Glutamine 150 mg.

NeuRecover-SA (Stimulant Abuse) **-** Natural Distributors International, Inc.
Six capsules contain: Vitamin C 600 mg • Vitamin B1 10 mg • Vitamin B2 15 mg • Niacin (Niacinamide) 100 mg • Calcium (chelate) 150 mg • Iron 9 mg • Vitamin B6 (pyridoxal-5-phosphate) 20 mg • Folic Acid 0.4 mg • Vitamin B12 0.03 mg • Magnesium (oxide) 150 mg • Zinc (chelate) 30 mg • Pantothenic Acid 90 mg • Chromium (picolinate) 0.06 mg • DL-Phenylalanine 1500 mg • L-Tyrosine 900 mg • L-Glutamine 300 mg.

Neuro B-12, Methylcobalamin 1 mg **-** Pro Health
Each sublingual tablet contains: Methylcobalamin 1 mg. Other Ingredients: Sorbitol, Mannitol, Microcrystalline Cellulose, Natural and Artificial Strawberry Flavor, Croscarmellose Sodium, Magnesium Stearate, Silicon Dioxide, Pharmaceutical Glaze.

Neuro B-12, Methylcobalamin 5 mg **-** Pro Health
Each sublingual tablet contains: Methylcobalamin 5 mg. Other Ingredients: Sorbitol, Mannitol, Microcrystalline Cellulose, Natural and Artificial Strawberry Flavor, Croscarmellose Sodium, Magnesium Stearate, Silicon Dioxide, Pharmaceutical Glaze.

Neuro Care-Rx **-** Alternecare Health Products
Each capsule contains: Cayenne 125 mg • Ginger 125 mg • St. John's Wort 125 mg • Ginko Biloba 40 mg • Malic Acid 100 mg • Vitamin B3 100 mg • Vitamin C 60 mg • Manganese 10 mg • Copper 1 mg • Vitamin B6 50 mg.

Neuro Defense **-** Jarrow Formulas
Four capsules contain: Niacinamide 500 mg • Apigenin 100 mg • Silymarin (80% silybin) 150 mg • Grape seed (vitis vinifera) 100 mg • Green Tea (camellia sinensis, 40% polyphenols) 300 mg • Phosphatidycholine 130 mg. Other Ingredients: Rice Powder, Magnesium Stearate.

Neuro Optimizer **-** Jarrow Formulas
Four capsules contain: CDP Choline (cytidine 5'-diphoscholine) 300 mg • Phosphatidyl Serine (PS) 100 mg • Acetyl L-Carnitine 500 mg • L-Glutamine 500 mg • Alpha Lipoic Acid 50 mg • Taurine 500 mg • Phosphatidylcholine 135 mg. Other Ingredients: Silicon Dioxide, Magnesium Stearate, Gelatin.

Neuro-Boost Spray **-** Nature's Plus
Each spray contains: Phosphatidylserine-rich purified Lecithin concentrate supplying Activated Phosphatides 50 mg: Phosphatidylserine (PS) 10 mg, Phosphatidylcholine (PC) 10 mg, Cephalin (Phosphatidylethanolamine) 6 mg, Phosphoinositides 3 mg • DMAE (2-Dimethylaminoethanol Bitartrate) 12.5 mg • N-Acetyl-Tyrosine pharmaceutical grade free form amino acid 5 mg • Pantothenic Acid 5 mg • Korean Ginseng root (Panax ginseng CA Meyer) standardized 15% ginsenosides 5 mg • Chinese Green Tea leaf (camellia sinensis) standardized 50% polyphenols 5 mg • Chinese Green Tea leaf standardized 24% ginkgo flavone glycosides, 6% terpene lactones 1000 mcg. In a proprietary Liposomal Complex of Essential Metabolic Factors, Purified Water, Vegetable Glycerine, Purified Lecithin, Citrus seed extract (Citrus sinensis), Vitamin E & (natural Root Beer) Sarsaparilla flavor.

Neuro-DHA **-** Metabolic Response Modifiers
Each sofgel contains: Fish Oil concentrate 500 mg • Min. 50% DHA 250 mg • Max. 20% EPA 100 mg • 20% Mixed fatty acids 100 mg • 10% stearidonic acid 50 mg • Vitamin C (Ascorbyl palmitate) 2 mg • Vitamin E (mixed-tocopherols) 4 mg.

Neurodyne **-** Life Extension
Each tablet contains: Acetyl Choline (synaptic factor, herbal proteinomeric neuro-transmitter release agent) 10 mg • Guarana (potentiating factor) 775 mg.

NeuroGenic **-** Nature's Plus
Two tablets contain: Vitamin C (as ascorbic acid) 150 mg • Pantothenic Acid (as calcium pantothenate) 100 mg • Phosphatidylcholine 250 mg • L-Glutamine (free form amino acid) 200 mg • Ginkgo Biloba leaf (standardized 24% ginkgo flavone-glycosides and 6% terpene lactones) 60 mg • L-Phenylalanine 100 mg • Ashwagandha root (withania somnifera, standardized 1.5% withanolids) 50 mg • Chinese Green Tea leaf (camellia sinensis, standardized 20% polyphenols) 20 mg • Bilberry fruit (vaccinium myrtillus, standardized 25% anthocyanosides) 15 mg • Pyridoxine Alpha-Ketoglutarate (PAK) 10 mg • Coenzyme Q10 (ubiquinone) 5 mg. Other Ingredients: Di-calcium Phosphate, Microcrystalline Cellulose, Magnesium Stearate, Stearic Acid, Silica.

Neurological Formula **-** Xtend-Life Nutraceuticals Inc.
Six tablets contain: 5-HTP (5-hydroxytryptophan) 50 mg • Alpha Lipoic Acid 200 mg • Betaine HCl 100 mg • Choline Bitartrate 100 mg • DMAE (dimethylaminoethanol) 275 mg • Huperzine A 300 mcg • Phosphatidyl Choline (as lecithin) 160 mg • Phosphatidyl Serine (phosphatidyl-L-serine) 100 mg • Quercetin 50 mg • Resveratrol 30 mg • SAMe (S-adenosylmethionine) 100 mg • Vinpocetine 15 mg • Acetyl L-Carnitine 150 mg • D-Phenylalanine 80 mg • L-Carnosine 150 mg • L-Carnitine Tartrate 150 mg • L-Glutamine 50 mg • L-Histidine 50 mg • L-Taurine 50 mg • L-Threonine 20 mg • L-Tyrosine 100 mg • L-Valine 50 mg • Amylase 50 mg • Bromelain 50 mg • Biotin 2 mg • Folic Acid 600 mcg • Inositol Hexaphosphate 75 mg • Piperine 10 mg • Selenium 500 mcg • Vitamin B6 20 mg • Vitamin D (D3, as cholecalciferol) 400 IU • Bacopin 50 mg • Bilberry 50 mg • Blueberry 50 mg • Chamomile 50 mg • Dandelion root 100 mg • Ginkgo Biloba 100 mg • Gotu Kola 50 mg • Green Tea 100 mg • Hawthorn berry 50 mg • Hops 60 mg • Passion Flower 50 mg • Pomegranate 80 mg • Grape seed 100 mg • Rhodiola Rosea 100 mg • Rosemary 50 mg • Schizandra 50 mg • Siberian Ginseng 50 mg • Silymarin (milk thistle) 100 mg • Yucca root 50 mg.

Neuro-Max **-** New Hope Health Products
Two capsules contain: Phospholipid Complex (containing 100 mg Phosphatidylserine) 500 mg • Ashwagandha Extract 80 mg • Bacopa Monniera Extract 80 mg • Ginkgo Biloba Extract 60 mg • Cytidine diphosphate choline 12 mg • Vinpocetine 5 mg • Niacin 10 mg.

Neuro-Max **-** Olympia Nutrition
Phosphatidylserine 50 mg • Ashwaganda 50 mg • Ginkgo 20 mg • Pregnenolone 25 mg.

Neuro-Max **-** Metabolic Response Modifiers
Two capsules contain: Phospholipid Complex 500 mg • Ashwaganda extract 100 mg • Ginkgo Biloba extract 40 mg • Pregnenolone 50 mg.

Neuro-Max for Children **-** Dr. Venessa's Formulas
Each three wafers contain: Lecithin 500 mg • Ginkgo Biloba extract (standardized 24%) 100 mg • Grape Seed extract (standardized 95%) 10 mg • Gotu Kola 100 mg • L-Glutamic Acid 100 mg • L-Glutamine 50 mg • Dimethylglycine 50 mg • Phosphatidylserine 25 mg • L-Tyrosine 50 mg • Folic Acid 100 mcg • Biotin 100 mcg • GABA 50 mg • Choline 20 mg • Inositol 20 mg • Vitamin B1 20 mg • Vitamin B2 20 mg • Vitamin B5 20 mg • Vitamin B6 200 mg • Vitamin B12 50 mg. Inactive Ingredients: Fructose, Natural Flavors, Stearic Acid, Magnesium Stearate.

Neuro-Max II - Metabolic Response Modifiers
Each capsule contains: Phospholipid complex (containing 100 mg Phosphatidlyserine) 500 mg • Ashwagandha extract 80 mg • Ginkgo Biloba extract (28/11) 60 mg • Cytidine diphosphate choline 12 mg • Vinpocetine 5 mg • Niacin 10 mg.

Neuromins - 200 - Martek Biosciences Corp.
Each capsule contains: DHA (docosahexaenoic acid) 200 mg. Inactive Ingredients: High Oleic Sunflower Oil, Ascorbyl Palmitate (vitamin C), Mixed Natural Tocopherol (vitamin E), Natural Mixed Carotenoids, Gelatin, Turmeric, Carmine, Water, Glycerine.

Neuromins 100 mg - Pure Encapsulations
Each softgel capsule contains: DHA (docosahexaenoic acid) 100 mg • High oleic Sunflower oil 400 mg • Vitamin E (as mixed tocopherols) 0.18 mg • Vitamin C (as ascorbyl palmitate) 0.125 mg.

Neuromins 200 mg - Pure Encapsulations
Each softgel capsule contains: DHA (docosahexaenoic acid) 200 mg • High oleic Sunflower oil 300 mg • Vitamin E (as mixed tocopherols) 0.18 mg • Vitamin C (as ascorbyl palmitate) 0.125 mg.

Neuromins DHA - Martek Biosciences Corp.
Each capsule contains: DHA (docosahexaenoic acid from algae oil) 100 mg. Inactive Ingredients: High Oleic Sunflower Oil, Ascorbyl Palmitate (vitamin C), Mixed Natural Tocopherol (vitamin E), Natural Mixed Carotenoids, Gelatin, Water, Glycerine.

Neuromins DHA - Source Naturals
Each softgel contains: Docosahexaenoic Acid (DHA) (Derived rom algal oil (oceanic phytophankton), in a base of high-oleic sunflower oil, vitamin C (ascorbyl palmitate) and vitamin E (mixed tocopherols) as antioxidants) 100 mg.

Neuromins DHA - Nature's Way
Each softgel contains: Neruomins DHA 100 mg. Other Ingredients: Gelatin, Glycerin, Sunflower Oil, Vitamin C, Vitamin E D-alpha tocopheryl, Water.

Neuromins DHA brand - Martek Biosciences Corp.
Docosahexaenoic Acid.
See Editor's Note No. 44.

Neuromins DHA Chewables - Martek Biosciences Corp.
Each capsule contains: DHA (docosahexaenoic acid from algal oil) 100 mg. Inactive Ingredients: High Oleic Sunflower Oil, Sugar, Yellow Beeswax, Natural Flavor, Ascorbyl Palmitate (Vitamin C), Mixed Natural Tocoperol (Vitamin E), Mixed Carotenoids, Gelatin, Glycerine, Caramel Color, Titanium Dioxinde.

Neuromins for Kids - Martek Biosciences Corp.
Eah capsule contains: DHA (docosahexaenoic acid) 100 mg. Inactive Ingredients: High Oleic Sunflower Oil, Ascorbyl Palmitate, (vitamin C), Mixed Natural Tocopherol (vitamin E), Natural Mixed Carotenoids, Gelatin, Water, Glycerine.

Neuromins PL - Martek Biosciences Corp.
Each capsule contains: DHA (docosahexaenoic acid) 200 mg. Inactive Ingredients: High Oleic Sunflower Oil, Ascorbyl Palmitate (vitamin C), Mixed Natural Tocopherol, Natural Mixed Carotenoids, Gelatin, Turmeric, Carmine, Water, Glycerine.

Neuropeptide Eye Contour Cream - N.V. Perricone M.D. Cosmeceuticals
CLB-253 Neuropeptide • CLS-72 Neuropeptide • Hyaluronic Acid • CLF-835 Neuropeptide • Glyceryl Stearate • PEG-100 Stearate • CLM-287 Neuropeptide • CLA-744 Neuropeptide • Magnesium Asparate • Zinc Gluconate • Copper Gluconate • Simmondsia Chinensis seed oil (jojoba) • CLE-935 Neuropeptide • Lecithin • DMAE (dimethyl MEA) • L-Tyrosine • Thioctic Acid (alpha lipoic acid) • Phenoxyethanol • Methylparaben • Ethylparaben • Butylparaben • Propylparaben • Isopropylparaben • Cetyl Alcohol • Dimethicone • Isopropyl Palmitate • C12-15 Alkyl Benzoate • Glycerin • Citric Acid • Triethanolamine • Carbomer • Betaglucan • BHT • Tetrasodium EDTA.

Neurophine - Progressive Health Nutraceuticals
Vitamin B6 20 mg • Vitamin C 100 mg • Potassium 99 mg • Magnesium 200 mg • Zinc 15 mg • Chromium 100 mcg • Copper 500 mcg • Manganese 1 mg • Boswellia Serrata 50 mg • Turmeric 25 mg • Cayenne pepper 5 mg • Methylsulfonyl Methane 500 mg • Chondroitin Sulfate 300 mg • Hyaluronic Acid 150 mg • BioCell brand Type II Collagen 1500 mg.
See Editor's Note No. 15.

Neuroplex - Standard Process, Inc.
Two capsules contain: Proprietary Blend 696 mg: Tillandsia Usneoides, Bovine Orchic Cytosol extract, Bovine Spleen, Porcine Brain PMG extract, Defatted Wheat germ, Bovine Hypothalamus, Bovine Anterior Pituitary, Calcium Lactate, Bovine Liver, Potassium Para-Aminobenzoate, Bovine Pituitary PMG extract, Porcine Brain, Ascorbic Acid • Thiamine 0.9 mg • Riboflavin 0.9 mg • Niacin 40 mg • Vitamin B6 8.9 mg • Iron 8.9 mg • Zinc 17.7 mg • Copper 0.3 mg • Sodium 15 mg. Other Ingredients: Gelatin, Water, Colors.
See Editor's Note No. 31.

NeuroShield - Life Enhancement Products, Inc.
Each capsule contains: Ginkgo Biloba 120 mg • Resveratrol 10 mg.

Neurosol - Metagenics
Each softgel contains: Gamma-Linoleic Acid (GLA, from borage seed oil) 160 mg • Vitamin A (as beta-carotene) 2000 IU • Vitamin C (as Ultra Potent-C brand) 133 mg • Niacin (as niacinamide ascorbate) 10 mg • Vitamin B6 (as pyridoxine hydrochloride) 25 mg • Folate (as 5-formyl tetrahydrofolate) 267 mcg • Vitamin B12 (as methylcobalamin) 167 mcg • Intrinsic Factor (porcine) 6.7 mg.

Neuro-SP - Benepure, Inc
Each tablet contains: Magnesium (as magnesium aspartate) 10 mg • Manganese (as amino acid chelate) 1000 mcg • Dimethylglycine HCl 250 mg • Glutamine 200 mg • Acetyl-L-Carnitine 175 mg • Phosphatidylserine 100 mg • Phosphatidylcholine 50 mg. Other Ingredients: Microcrystalline Cellulose, Stearic Acid, Vegetable Stearate, Croscarmellose Sodium, Silicon Dioxide, Hydroxypropyl Methylcellulose.

NeuroSyn - PharmAssure
Two softgel capsules contain: Vitamin E (as Natural d-alpha tocopheryl Acetate) 30 IU • High Choline Soy Lecithin (35% Phosphatidylcholine) 500 mg • DHA (Docosahexaenioc Acid;as Marine Microalgae Oil) 100 mg • Ginkgo Biloba Leaves Extract (24% Ginkgo Flavonglycosides, 6% Terpene Lactones) 120 mg • Vinpocetine 5 mg. Other Ingredients: Gelatin, Soybean Oil, Glycerin, Caramel Color, Titanium Dioxide.

Neurotrophin PMG - Standard Process, Inc.
Each tablet contains: Proprietary Blend 205 mg: Porcine Brain PMG extract, Magnesium Citrate • Calcium 10 mg • Sodium 10 mg. Other Ingredients: Cellulose.

Neurovar - Optimal Therapeutics
Each capsule contains: Vitamin C 100 mg • Cognizin brand Citicoline 250 mg • Neurovar Proprietary Complex 210 mg: Phosphatidylserine, Bacopa Monniera (20% bacosides), Alpha GPC (L-alpha-glycerylphosphorylcholine), Ginkgo Biloba, Acetyl-L-Carnitine, Vinpocetine. Other Ingredients: Gelatin, Cellulose, Magnesium Stearate.

Neurozan - Vitabiotics
Each capsule contains: Vitamin D (as D3 200 IU) 5 mcg • Vitamin E (natural source) 60 mg • Vitamin C 30 mg • Vitamin B1 (thiamin) 20 mg • Vitamin B2 (riboflavin) 3.2 mg • Vitamin B3 (niacin) 18 mg • Vitamin B6 (pyridoxine HCl) 25 mg • Folacin (as folic acid) 500 mcg • Vitamin B12 (cyanocobalamin) 50 mcg • Pantothenic Acid 12 mg • Iron 7 mg • Zinc 15 mg • Manganese 4 mg • Copper 1.5 mg • Selenium 200 mcg • Chromium 50 mcg • L-Arginine 40 mg • Glutamine 10 mg • Glutathione 5 mg • Omega-3 DHA (docosahexaenoic acid, 50%) 100 mg • Co-enzyme Q10 6 mg • Phosphatidylserine 10 mg • Phosphatidylcholine 10 mg • Natural Mixed Carotenoids 2 mg • Lecithin 17 mg.

Neurozyme - New Chapter, Inc.
Each softgel contains: DHA (Docosahexaenoic acid), supercritical extract (from Arctic fish oil- 100 mg) (DPA min. 10%- 10 mg, EPA min. 5%- 5 mg) 50 mg • Rosemary leaf, supercritical extract (23% total phenolic antioxidants- 7 mg) 30 mg • Ginger (rhizome), certified organic, supercritical extract (minimum 20% pungent compounds, 5% zingiberence- 1.5 mg) 30 mg • Sage leaf, supercritical extract (38%- 42% total phenolic antioxidants- 6 mg) 15 mg • Chamomile flower, supercritical extract (25% alpha-bisabolol -3.8 mg) 15 mg • Clove bud, supercritical extract (65% euaenol -6.5 mg) 10 mg • Potency Assured Extracts, Ginkgo leaf (12% flavone glycosides) 120 mg • Gotu Kola leaf (10% asiaticoside -12 mg, 30% triterpenes- 36 mg) 120 mg • Club Moss, Chinese Huperzia serrata (0.5% Huperzine A -0.3 mg) 60 mg • Ashwaganda root (extract 4:1) 60 mg • Cat's Claw root (extract 4:1) (3% alkaloids- 1.5 mg) 50 mg • Lemon Balm, Melissa officinalis leaf (5% rosemarininc acid- 1.5 mg) 30 mg • Bacopin, Bacopa monniera (Brahil leaf extract), (Bacosides A and B 20.65%- 6.2 mg), (0.6% alkaloids- 0.2 mg) 30 mg • Paeonia, Eurpoean (extract 5:1) 20 mg • Holy Basil, Ocimum sanctum (leaf) (2.5% ursalic acid- 0.5 mg) 20 mg • Turmeric (rhizome) (7-9% curcumin- 1.6 mg) 20 mg • Red Wine, (30% total polyphenols- 6 mg) 20 mg • Chamomile flower (extract 5:1) 15 mg • Vitamin E 2 IU. Other Ingredients: Olive Oil - certified organic, Yellow Beeswax.

Neutra-Gas - PhytoPharmica
Each capsule contains: Simethicone 25 mg • Peppermint oil extract (Mentha piperita) 0.2 ml. Chlorophyll is used as a natural coloring agent.
See Editor's Note No. 21.

Neutralis - BotanicLab
Scutellaria Baicalensis Georgi (scute; huang-chin) • Bupleurum Chinense DC (bupleurum; chai-hu) • Dendranthema Morifolium Tzvel (chrysanthemum; chu-hua) • Pinctada Martensii Dunker (pearl; chen-chu) • Isatis Indigotica Fort (isatidis; ta-ching-yeh) • Glycyrrhiza Glabra L. (licorice; gan-cao).

New Choice - The Herbalist
Gingko leaf • Gotu Kola herb • Guarana seed • American Ginseng root • Siberian Ginseng root • Jamaican Sarsaparilla root • Kola Nut • Licorice root • Cinnamon bark • Ginger root • Cayenne pepper.

New Life Colostrum - Symbiotics, Inc.
100% Bovine Colostrum

New Life Colostrum Capsules - Symbiotics, Inc.
Two capsules contain: 100% Bovine Colostrum from New Zealand cows 960 mg • Vitamin A 336 IU • Vitamin C 2.8 mg • Iron 1.4 mg • Calcium 10 mg.

New Life Colostrum High-IG - Symbiotics, Inc.
Two capsules contain: 100% Bovine Colostrum 960 mg • Vitamin A 504 IU • Vitamin C 4.2 mg • Iron 2.1 mg • Calcium 15 mg • Immunoglobulin 288 mg.

New Life Colostrum Powder - Symbiotics, Inc.
One teaspoon contains: 100% Bovine Colostrum from New Zealand cows 1440 mg • Vitamin A 504 IU • Vitamin C 4.2 mg • Iron 2.1 mg • Calcium 15 mg • Immunoglobulin 246 mg.

New Life Hair - Sundown
Each tablet contains: Vitamin E 5 IU • Niacin (as niacinamide) 15 mg • Folic Acid 400 mcg • Vitamin B12 (as cyanocobalamin) 6 mcg • Pantothenic Acid (as calcium d-pantothenate) 92 mg • Calcium 100 mg • Iron (as ferrous fumarate) 1 mg • Iodine (as potassium iodide) 150 mcg • Zinc (as zinc gluconate) 15 mg • Manganese (as manganese gluconate) 10 mg • Choline (as choline bitartrate) 120 mg • Silica 26 mg. Other Ingredients: Dicalcium Phosphate, Microcrystalline Cellulose, Croscarmellose Sodium, Hydroxypropyl Methylcellulose, Hydrogenated Vegetable Oil, Magnesium Stearate, Pharmaceutical Glaze, Titanium Dioxide, Dl-Alpha-Tocopheryl Acetate, Riboflavin (colorant), PEG, Polysorbate 80, Yellow 6 Lake.

New Man Tea - The Herbalist
Damiana leaf • Fo-ti root • Sassafras bark • Licorice root • Cinnamon bark • Saw Palmetto berry • Sarsaparilla bark • Parsley root • Marshmallow root • Orange peel.

New Woman Tonic - The Herbalist
Chaste Tree berry • Black Cohosh root • Black Haw bark • Motherwort herb • Cramp bark • Skullcap herb • Ginger root.

NewBust (New Bust) - Tiger-One.com
Saw Palmetto • Dong Quai • Damiana • Fenugreek seed • Blessed Thistle • Violet • Wild Yam • Fennel seed • Althea root • Cumin seed • Hops.
See Editor's Note No. 17.

NewBust Lotion (New Bust Lotion) - Tiger-One.com
Water • Saw Palmetto • Extra Virgin Olive Oil • Dong Quai • Damiana • Glycerin • Foenugreek seed • Blessed Thistle • Violet • Wild Yam • Fennel seed • Althea root • Cumin seed • Hops.
See Editor's Note No. 17.

NewCurves Breast Beautifying Formula capsules - Rozge Cosmeceutical
Sabal fruits • Sabal Serrulata • Dong Quai • Fennel seed powder • Rodiola Rosea • Black Cohosh • Methylsulfonylmethane • Natural Vegetable Glycerin Capsules.

NewCurves Breast Beautifying Formula creme - Rozge Cosmeceutical
Aloe Vera gel • Glycerine • Isopropyl Myristate • Safflower oil • Glyceryl Stearate • Propylene Glycol • Stearic Acid • Stearyl Alcohol • Honey • Squalane • Dimethicone • Hydroxyethyl Cellulose • DL-Alpha Tocopherol (vitamin E) • Calendula extract • Damiana extract • Saw Palmetto berry extract • Dong Quai extract • Black Cohosh extract • Potassium Sorbate • Methylparaben • Propylparaben.

Nexcite - Nordic Drinks
Each 100 mL serving contains: Carbonated Water 93 g • Sugar 8.5 g • Citric Acid 0.2 g • Damiana (extract) 59 mg • Schizandra (extract) 58 mg • Mate (extract) 57 mg • (Guarana extract) 56 mg • Caffeine 30 mg • Flavoring 23 mg • Ginseng (extract) 18 mg • Sodium benzoate (E211) 15 mg • Colour (E133) 65 pg.

Nexrutine - Solanova
Each capsule contains: Nexrutine (a patent pending plant extract from Phellodendron amurense) 250 mg. Other Ingredients: Snow White Filler, Microcrystalline Cellulose, Magnesium Stearate, Silicon Dioxide, Gelatin, Glycerin, Purified Water.

NF Formulas Liquid Calcium Magnesium - Integrative Therapeutics
Each tablespoon (15 mL) contains: Vitamin D (as ergocalciferol) 100 IU • Calcium (as calcium carbonate) 500 mg • Magnesium (as magnesium oxide) 500 mg • Boron (as boron oxide) 250 mcg. Other Ingredients: Deionized Water, Glycerin, Cellulose Gum, Methyl Paraben, Propyl Paraben, Ethyl Vanillin.

NF Formulas pectra Probiotic with Cofactors - Integrative Therapeutics
Three capsules contain: Spectra Probiotic Proprietary Blend 600 mg: Lactobacillus Acidophilus, Bifidobacterium Bifidum, Bifidobacterium Infantis, Bifidobacterium Longum, Lactobacillus Blugaricus, Lactobacillus Casei, Lactobacillus Salivarius, Streptococcus Thermophilus • FOS (fructooligosaccharides) 270 mg • NAG (N-acetyl-glucosamine) 105 mg. Other Ingredients: Rice Flour, Gelatin, Water.

NF Formulas Prenatal Forte - Integrative Therapeutics
Two tablets contain: Vitamin A (as retinyl acetate, beta-carotene) 3334 IU • Vitamin C (as calcium ascorbate) 166 mg • Vitamin D (as ergocalciferol) 134 IU • Vitamin E (as dl-alpha tocopheryl acetate) 134 IU • Vitamin K (as phytonadione) 10 mcg • Thiamin (as thiamine hydrochloride) 8 mg • Riboflavin 8 mg • Niacin (as niacinamide) 8 mg • Vitamin B6 (as pyridoxine HCl) 16 mg • Folic Acid 267 mcg • Vitamin B12 (as cyanocobalamin) 50 mcg • Biotin 100 mcg •

Pantothenic Acid (as calcium pantothenate) 16 mg • Calcium (as calcium carbonate, citrate, and ascorbate) 400 mg • Iron (as iron citrate) 16 mg • Iodine (kelp source, Ascophyllum nodosum) 50 mcg • Magnesium (as magnesium oxide and citrate) 200 mg • Zinc (as zinc citrate) 8 mg • Selenium (as selenium chelate) 34 mcg • Copper (as copper citrate) 1 mg • Manganese (as manganese citrate) 3.4 mg • Chromium (as chromium chelate) 24 mcg • Potassium (as potassium citrate) 34 mg • Citrus Bioflavonoids Complex 66 mg • L-Glutamic Acid HCl 34 mg • Soy Lecithin 34 mg • Alfalfa leaf (Medicago sativa) 26 mg • Raspberry leaf (Rubus idaeus) 26 mg • Yellow Dock root (Rumex crispus) 26 mg • Cranberry fruit extract (Vaccimium macrocarpon, 25:1) 16 mg • Dandelion root (Taraxacum officinale) 16 mg • Papaya leaf (Carica papaya) 16 mg • Stinging Nettle leaf (Urtica diocia) 16 mg • Choline (as choline bitartrate) 8 mg • Inositol 8 mg • Lactobacillus Acidophilus 8 mg • PhytoZyme Enzyme Blend 6 mg: Amylase, Cellulase, Glucoamylase, Invertase, Lipase, Pectinase with Phytase, Protease, Lactase • Hesperidin Complex 4 mg • Rutin 4 mg • Boron (as boron citrate) 84 mcg. Other Ingredients: Microcrystalline Cellulose, Croscarmellose Sodium, Stearic Acid, Silicon Dioxide, Hydroxypropyl Methocellulose, Magnesium Silicate.

NFA-500 **- Human Development Technologies (HDT)**
Each capsule contains: L-Tyrosine 500 mg • Acetylcholine 25 mg • DMAE 25 mg • St. John's Wort 60 mg. Additional Ingredients: DLPA • Ginkgo Biloba • Vitamin B12 • Vitamin B6 • Vitamin B1 • Vitamin C • Copper Sulfate • Folic Acid • Phosphorus • Zinc • Bioperine brand Black Pepper extract.

N-FLAM Plus **- Nutri-Quest Rx**
Each enteric coated tablet contains: Pancreatin 170 mg • Papain 100 mg • Bromelain 80 mg • Trypsin 40 mg (Chymotrypsin 8 mg) • Lipase 15 mg • Amylase 17 mg • Rutin 85 mg • Calf Thymus 45 mg • Zinc Gluconate 4 mg • Partoid concentrate 1 mg.
See Editor's Note No. 14.

NG-Rx **- Maxam Nutraceutics**
Distilled Water • Microactivated peptite fractions of Phosphatidylcholine, Phosphatidylserine, N-Acetyl-L-Carnitine, DMAE, Acetyl Serine, L-Tyrosine, Amino Acids, Ginkgo extract, and Mucuna extract in a Colloidal Matrix.

Niacin **- Leiner Health Products**
Each tablet contains: Niacin (Nicotinic acid) 100 mg. Other Ingredients: Lactose, Starch, Stearic Acid, Silicon Dioxide, Magnesium Stearate.

Niacin **- PhytoPharmica**
Each capsule contains: Niacin (as inositol hexaniacinate) 590 mg. Other Ingredients: Gelatin, Magnesium Stearate, Titanium Dioxide Color, Silicon Dioxide.

Niacin **- Nature's Bounty**
Each tablet contains: Niacin 100 mg. Other Ingredients: Cellulose, Dicalcium Phosphate, Vegetable Stearic Acid, Povidone, Vegetable Magnesium Stearate, Silica.

Niacin **- Source Naturals**
Each tablet contains: Niacin 100 mg.

Niacin 100 mg **- Arrowroot**
Each tablet contains: Niacin 100 mg.

Niacin 100 mg **- Westcoast Naturals**
Each capsule contains: Niacin (as vitamin B3) 100 mg.

Niacin 100 mg **- J. R. Carlson Laboratories, Inc.**
Each tablet contains: Niacin (vitamin B3) 100 mg.

Niacin 100 mg Tablets **- Nature's Plus**
Each tablet contains: Niacin (as nicotinic acid) 100 mg. Other Ingredients: Microcrystalline Cellulose, Di-calcium Phosphate, Stearic Acid, Rice Bran, Magnesium Stearate, Pharmaceutical Glaze, Silica.

Niacin 100mg **- Ortho Molecular Products**
Each capsule contains: Niacin 100 mg.

Niacin 250 **- GNC**
Each tablet contains: Niacin 250 mg. Other Ingredients: Dicalcium Phosphate, Cellulose, Whole Brown Rice powder (Oryza sativa).

Niacin 250 mg **- Sunmark**
Each time-release tablet contains: Niacin (as nicotinic acid) 250 mg. Other Ingredients: Carnauba Wax, Dicalcium Phosphate, Glyceryl Behenate, Talc, Magnesium Stearate.
See Editor's Note No. 45.

Niacin 50 mg **- J. R. Carlson Laboratories, Inc.**
Each tablet contains: Niacin (vitamin B3) 50 mg.

Niacin 500 **- GNC**
Each tablet contains: Niacin 500 mg. Other Ingredients: Dicalcium Phosphate, Cellulose, Food Glaze, Whole Brown Rice powder (Oryza Sativa).

Niacin 500 mg **- Arrowroot**
Each tablet contains: Niacin 500 mg.

Niacin 500 mg **- J. R. Carlson Laboratories, Inc.**
Each tablet contains: Niacin (vitamin B3) 500 mg.

Niacin 500 mg **- Jamieson**
Each caplet contains: Niacin 500 mg.

Niacin 500 mg **- Westcoast Naturals**
Each capsule contains: Niacin (as vitamin B3) 500 mg.

Niacin 500 mg PR **- Arrowroot**
Each prolonged-release tablet contains: Niacin 500 mg.

Niacin 500 mg Timed **- Rexall - Sundown**
Each caplet contains: Niacin 500 mg • Calcium 106 mg. Other Ingredients: Dicalcium Phosphate, Hydroxypropyl Methylcellulose, Hydrogenated Cottonseed Oil, Stearic Acid, Magnesium Stearate.

Niacin Easy 200 **- Life Enhancement Products, Inc.**
Each capsule contains: Vitamin C (from ascorbyl palmitate) 2 mg • Niacin (from niacin) 200 mg • Magnesium (from magnesium hydroxide) 26.7 mg.

Niacin Flush Free **- Nature's Bounty**
Each capsule contains: Niacin (as Inositol Hexanicotinate) 400 mg • Inositol (as Inositol Hexanicotinate) 100 mg. Other Ingredients: Gelatin, Dicalcium Phosphate, Vegetable Magnesium Stearate, Silica.

Niacin Non-Flush **- Westcoast Naturals**
Each capsule contains: Niacin (inositol nicotinate) 500 mg • Inositol (inositol hexaniacinate) 120 mg.

Niacin Time Release **- Puritan's Pride**
Each capsule contains: Niacin 250 mg.

Niacin with Cholestatin **- Futurebiotics LLC**
Each tablet contains: Niacin 400 mg • Cholestatin 400 mg.

Niacin+ **- PhysioLogics**
Each capsule contains: Niacin (as inositol hexanicotinate) 400 mg • Vitamin C (as magnesium ascorbate) 100 mg • Chromium (as chromium amino acid chelate) 6 mcg. Other Ingredients: Gelatin, Rice Powder, Vegetable Magnesium Stearate, Silica.

Niacinamide **- Nature's Bounty**
Each tablet contains: Niacin (as Niacinamide) 500 mg. Other Ingredients: Cellulose, Dicalcium Phosphate, Vegetable Stearic Acid, Silica, Vegetable Magnesium Stearate.

Niacinamide 1000 mg Sustained Release tablets **- Nature's Plus**
Each timed-release tablet contains: Niacin (as niacinamide) 1000 mg. Other Ingredients: Stearic Acid, Di-calcium Phosphate, Rice Bran, Hydroxypropyl Methylcellulose, Magnesium Stearate.

Niacin-Amide 500 mg **- J. R. Carlson Laboratories, Inc.**
Each tablet contains: Niacin (vitamin B3, as niacinamide) 500 mg.

Niacinamide 500 mg Tablets **-** Nature's Plus
Each tablet contains: Niacin (as niacinamide) 500 mg. Other Ingredients: Microcrystalline Cellulose, Di-calcium Phosphate, Stearic Acid, Rice Bran, Magnesium Stearate, Pharmaceutical Glaze, Silica.

Niacinamide B6 **-** Standard Process, Inc.
Each capsule contains: Proprietary Blend 433 mg: Bovine Liver, Porcine Stomach, Calcium Lactate, Soy bean, Bovine Spleen, Ovine Spleen, Defatted Wheat germ, Potassium Para-Aminobenzoate, Porcine Brain, Ascorbic Acid • Niacin 50 mg • Vitamin B6 9 mg. Other Ingredients: Gelatin, Water, Colors.
See Editor's Note No. 14.

Niacinamide flush free 250 mg **-** Jarrow Formulas
Each capsule contains: Niacinamide 250 mg. Other Ingredients: Rice Powder, Magnesium Stearate, Gelatin.

Niacin-Time **-** J. R. Carlson Laboratories, Inc.
Each tablet contains: Niacin (vitamin B3) 500 mg.

Niacitol 500 mg **-** Pure Encapsulations
Each vegetable capsule contains: Inositol Nicotinate 625 mg: Niacin (vitamin B3) 500 mg • Inositol 125 mg • Vitamin C (as ascorbyl palmitate) 15 mg.

Niacitol 725 mg **-** Pure Encapsulations
Each vegetable capsule contains: Inositol Nicotinate 906 mg: Niacin (vitamin B3) 725 mg • Inositol 181 mg • Vitamin C (as ascorbyl palmitate) 30 mg.

Niacor **-** Upsher-Smith Laboratories
Each tablet contains: Niacin (as nicotinic acid) 500 mg. Other Ingredients: Colloidal Silicon Dioxide, Corn Starch, Lactose, Microcrystalline Cellulose, Povidone (K-25), Purified Stearic Acid.

Niagra ACTRA-Rx **-** Shenyang Chang Gang Yibao Alcohol Co., Ltd.
Proprietary Blend 450 mg: Proline, Histidine, Glutamic Acid, Arginine, Aspartic Acid, Tyrosine, Phenylalanine, Lysine, Leucine, Glycosine, Threonine, Iso-Leucine, Alanine, Serine, Methionine, Tryptophan, Cystis Acid • Lycium fruit • Epimedium herb • Cistanche root • Vitamin B1 • Vitamin B2 • Minerals.
See Editor's Note No. 58.

Nicodrops **-** Nicodrops Company
Each 4 g lozenge contains: Peppermint Flavor • Ginseng • Ginseng flavor • Sugar • Corn Syrup • Valerian fluid extract • St. John's wort fluid extract.

Nicodrops - Canada **-** Nicodrops Company
Each lozenge contains: Medicinal Ingredients: Lobelia aerial parts (Lobelia inflata) 65 mg. Non-medicinal Ingredients: Peppermint flavor, sugar, corn syrup, Ginseng flavor, Gingeng root (Panax japonicum, Valerian root (Valerian officinalis), St. John's Wort flower tops (Hypericum proforatum).

Nico-End **-** PhytoPharmica
Each tablet contains: Nux vomica 8x • Lobelia 6x • Staphysagria 6x • Tabacum 6x.
See Editor's Note No. 1 and No. 21.

Nicorette fresh mint (2 mg) **-** GlaxoSmithKline (GSK)
Each piece contains: Nicotine 2 mg. Other Ingredients: Chewing Gum Base, Xylitol, Sodium Carbonate, Peppermint Oil, Menthol, Polacrilin, Magnesium Oxide, Sodium Bicarbonate, Talc, Butylated Hydroxy Toluene (E321).

Nicorette fresh mint (4 mg) **-** GlaxoSmithKline (GSK)
Each piece contains: Nicotine 4 mg. Other Ingredients: Chewing Gum Base, Xylitol, Sodium Carbonate, Peppermint Oil, Menthol, Polacrilin, Magnesium Oxide, Sodium Bicarbonate, Talc, Butylated Hydroxy Toluene (E321).

Nicotine Relief **-** Gaia Herbs
Two capsules contain: Licorice root (glycyrrhiza uralensis and glycyrriza glabra) 315 mg • Lobelia herb and seed (lobelia inflata) 48 mg • Wild Oats milky seed (avena sativa) 38 mg • St. John's Wort flower buds (hypericum perforatum) 36 mg • Calamus root (acorus calamus) 30 mg • Passionflower flowering vine (passiflora incarnata) 26 mg. Other Ingredients: Vegetable Glycerin, Vegetable Cellulose.

Night Loss **-** Abundance Marketing
Chromium • Cleansing Herbal Infusion: Aloe Vera juice, Licorice root extract (13% glycyrrhizin), Fenugreek seed, Garcinia Cambogia fruit extract, Buchu leaf, Rhubarb root, Sarsaparilla root, Gentian root • P.M. Herbal Blend: Aloe Vera leaf juice, Chamomile (flowering tops), Passion Flower, Skullcap (aerial parts), Hops strobile • Bioflavonoid Blend: Cherry juice crystals, Citrus Bioflavonoids, Rutin, Hesperidin, Acerola berry. Other Ingredients: Purified Water, Fructose, Potassium Sorbate, Vegetable Glycerin, Citric Acid, Potassium Benzoate, Natural Cherry Flavor, Carmel Color.

Night Nervine **-** Grandma's Herbs
Each capsule contains: Proprietary Blend 0.426 g: Hops flower, Valerian root, Blue Vervain herb, Scullcap herb, St. John's Wort herb, Black Cohosh root, Lady's Slipper root, Lily of the Valley herb, Bladdderpod herb, Mistletoe herb, Spearmint root. Other Ingredients: Gelatin.

Night Supply Nourishing Cream **-** Nu Skin Enterprises
Water • Caprylic/Capric Triglycerides • Cyclomethicone • Cetyl Alcohol • Glycerin • Macadamia Ternifolia seed oil • Glyceryl Stearate • Squalane • PEG-75 Stearate • Phosphatidylcholine • Oenothera Biennis oil (evening primrose) • Butyrospermum Parkii extract (shea butter) • Anthemis Nobilis flower extract • Calendula Officinalis flower extract • Tilia Cordata flower extract • Centaurea Cyanus flower extract • Chamomilla Recutita flower extract (matricaria) • Hypericum Perforatum extract • Limnanthes Alba seed oil (meadowfoam) • Hydrogenated Lecithin • Tocopheryl Acetate • Dimethicone • Butylene Glycol • Polyacrylamide • Ceteth-20 • Steareth-20 • C12-14 Isoparaffin • Laureth-7 • Myristyl Myristate • Neopentyl Glycol Diheptanoate • Fragrance (parfum) • Tetrasodium EDTA • Phenoxyethanol • Methylparaben • Isopropylparaben • Butylparaben • Chlorphenesin.

Night Supply Nourishing Lotion **-** Nu Skin Enterprises
Water • Cyclomethicone • Ethoxydiglycol • Glycerin • Panthenol • Caprylic/Capric Triglyceride • Hydrogenated Polyisobutene • Glyceryl Stearate • PEG-100 Stearate • Phosphatidylcholine • Sodium PCA • Tocopheryl Acetate • Carbomer • Didecene • Glycol Stearate • Cetyl Alcohol • Triethanolamine • Fragrance (parfum) • Phenoxyethanol • Methylparaben • Ethylparaben • Propylparaben • Butylparaben.

Night Time Formulation **-** Olympian Labs
Each capsule contains: Valerian root 200 mg • Passion Flower 200 mg • Skullcap 50 mg • L-Tyrosine 25 mg • Parsley 50 mg • Peppermint 75 mg • Calcium Citrate 80 mg • Pantothenic Acid 20 mg.

NightRest **-** Source Naturals
Two tablets contain: Melatonin 4 mg • Magnesium (Magnesium Glycinate and Magnesium Taurinate) 200 mg • Glycine (Magnesium Glycinate and Glycine) 502 mg • Taurine (Magnesium Taurinate) 435 mg • Passionflower 120 mg • GABA (Gamma Amino Butyric Acid) 100 mg • Skullcap 70 mg • Chamomile extract (4:1) 60 mg.
See Editor's Note No. 16.

NightTime Complex with Melotonin **-** Pharmanex
Each capsule contains: Valerian root extract 75 mg • Passion Flower extract 37.5 mg • Kava Lactones (from Kava Kava root extract) 7.5 mg • Hops Strobile powder (fruit) 25 mg • Chamomile flower powder 25 mg • Melissa officinalis powder (leaf & flower) 25 mg • Mixed Tocopherols 0.5 mg • Melatonin 0.5 mg. Other Ingredients: Maltodextrin, Magnesium, Silicon Dioxide.
See Editor's Note No. 26.

NightTime Formula **-** Pharmanex
Each capsule contains: Valerian root extract 75 mg • Passion flower extract 37.5 mg • L-Theanine (from camellia sinensis) 25 mg • Hops Strobils fruit powder 25 mg • Chamomile flower powder 25 mg • Lemon Balm powder (melissa officinalis) 25 mg • Melatonin 0.5 mg. Other Ingredients: Gelatin, Microcrystalline Cellulose, Magnesium Stearate, Silicon Dioxide.
See Editor's Note No. 26.

Nighty Night **-** Traditional Medicinals
Passionflower • Spearmint leaf • Chamomile herb • Lemon Verbena leaf • Licorice root • Lilia Star flower • Lemon peel • Lemongrass leaf • Catnip leaf • Hop Strobile.

Nimbicidin **-** Jarrow Formulas
Each capsule contains: Neem 10:1 (azadirachraindica) 500 mg.

Niteworks **-** Herbalife International of America, Inc.
Two scoops (approx. 9.7 g) contain: Vitamin C (ascorbic acid) 500 mg • Vitamin E (D-alpha tocopheryl acetate) 400 IU • Folic Acid (folate & calcium folinate) 400 mcg • Proprietary Blend 5.2 g: L-Arginine, L-Citrulline • Lemon Balm extract 50 mg • Alpha Lipoic Acid 10 mg. Other Ingredients: Natural Flavor, Sucralose.

Nitric Boost **-** Optimum Nutrition
Three caplets contain: Arginine Alpha-Ketoglutarate (A-AKG) 3 g. Other Ingredients: Dicalcium Phosphate, Microcrystalline Cellulose, Stearic Acid, Solutab, Magnesium Stearate, Silica.

Nitrix **-** BSN Inc.
Three tablets contain: L-Arginine Alpha-Ketoglutarate (AAKG) 3000 mg • CRTS2 (controlled release technology & support system) 1897 mg: Methocel (micro-polymer hydrophilic ether matrix), Phosphoplexx (calcium phosphate, di-potassium phosphate, sodium phosphate), 2CM (dicreatine malate), L-Citruline, NAD (nicotinamide adenine dinucleotide), Folic Acid (folate). Other Ingredients: Magnesium Stearate.

Nitro Fuel (Ion Exchange Whey Protein Powder) **-** TwinLab
Each serving contains: Pure Protein 25 g.

Nitro Fuel (The Ultimate Anti-Catabolic Amino Acid Drink) **-** TwinLab
Protein (Amino Acids) & Carbohydrates • Whey Protein Concentrate [a source of Branched Chain Amino Acids (L-Leucine, L-Isoleucine, L-Valine)] • Chromium Picolinate • Alpha-Ketoglutarates.

NitrOGenX **-** PharmaGenX
Each 4 cc serving contains: L-Arginine Alpha-Ketoglutarate 1500 mg. Other Ingredients: Water, Natural Vegetable Glycerin, Emulsifiers, Phospholipids, Medium Chain Triglycerides, Sucralose, Potassium Sorbate Benzoate, Natural and Artificial Flavors.

Nitro-Tech **-** MuscleTech
Whey Peptides • Whey Protein Concentrate • Guar gum • D-Myo-Inositol • Glucomannan • Taurine • Alpha Lipoic Acid • D-Pinitol • Glycosidal Saponins • Folic Acid • Natural & Artificial Flavors • L-Glutamine Peptides • Calcium Alpha Ketoglutarate • Dipotassium Phosphate • Lecithin • Magnesium Oxide • N-Acetyl-Cysteine • DL-Tocopherol Acetate • Acesulfame Potassium • Aspartame • Pyridoxine Hydrochloride.

Nitroxy3 **-** Iovate Health Sciences U.S.A. Inc.
Five capsules contain: Vasodilase 3 g: L-Arginine Hydrochloride, L-Arginine Alpha Ketoglutarate • Stimugrow 1.7 g: Creatine Monohydrate, L-Leucine, L-Valine. Other Ingredients: Potassium Chloride, Celluose, Dextrose, Stearic Acid, Silica, Mangesium Stearate, Ethyl Cellulose, Titanium dioxide, Dicalcium Phosphate.

NKO (Neptune Krill Oil) **-** Jamol Laboratories
Two softgels contain: Vitamin A 100 IU • Vitamin E 0.5 IU • Choline 73 mg • Phospholipid - Omega 3 Complex 400 mg: Omega 3 Fatty Acids 300 mg, EPA (eicosapentaenoic acid) 150 mg, DHA (docosahexaenoic acid) 90 mg • Omega 6 Fatty Acids 20 mg • Astaxanthin 1.5 mg. Other Ingredients: Gelatin, Glycerin, Water.

NK-Stim **-** Ortho Molecular Products
Two capsules contain: Zinc (as Chelazome brand amino acid chelate) 10 mg • Arabinogalactan Heartwood (from Western larch tree) 640 mg • Olive leaf extract (standardized to contain 20% oleuropein) 400 mg • Aloe Vera leaf exudate 200:1 concentrate) 160 mg. Other Ingredients: Natural Vegetable Capsules, Magnesium Stearate, Microcrystalline Cellulose.

NO Jet-Lag **-** Miers Laboratories
Active Ingredients: Arnica Montana (leopard's bane) 30C • Bellis Perennis (daisy) 30C • Chamomilla (wild chamomile) 30C • Ipecacuanha (ipecac) 30C • Lycopodium (clubmoss) 30C. Inactive Ingredients: Sorbitol, Magnesium Stearate, Sterilized Talc.
See Editor's Note No. 1.

No. 1 GARLIC PLUS ESTER-C & FOS **-** Dial Herbs
Two capsules contain: Pure-Gar deodorized Garlic concentrate 300 mg • FOS Micro Flora Growth concentrate 300 mg • Vitamin C from Ester-C 200 mg.

No. 56 K KIDNEY **-** Systemic Formulas
Rose Hips • RNA/DNA Kidney Factors • Gelatin • Magnesium Sulfate • Vitamin C • Ch de Bugre • Fish Liver Oil (Source of Vitamins A and D) • Sete Sangrias • Calcium Carbonate • RNA/DNA Adrenal Factors • Hesperidin • Serine • RNA/DNA Thalamus Factors • Tyrosine • Spearmint Oil • Rose Petal Essence • Aloe Vera.
See Editor's Note No. 31.

NO2 **-** Medical Research Instituite (MRI)
Three capsules contain: Arginine Alpha-Ketoglutarate (A-AKG) 3000 mg.

Noni **-** Source Naturals
Each capsule contains: Hawaiian Noni (Morinda citrifolia) 375 mg.

Noni (morinda citrifolia) Juice Concentrate **-** NutraMedix
Five drops contain: Proprietary Blend 0.25 mL: Noni (morinda citrifolia), Noni extract, Mineral water, Ethanol.

Noni Juice **-** Golden Glow Natural Health Products
100% pure Noni fruit juice (morinda citrifolia).

Non-Stipation Syrup **-** Hadas Natural Products
Sorbitol Syrup • Plums • Figs • Psyllium • Fennel • Caraway • Ginger • Coriander.

Nopal Strepta (Prickly Pear Cactus) **-** Cactu-Life
Each capsule contains: 100% Opuntia Streptacantha 450 mg.

Nopalacrin **-** 4R Health Products
Each capsule contains: Nopal 500 mg.

NoPhedra **-** Absolute Nutrition
Two capsules contain: Green Tea leaf extract (standardized for 90 mg epigallocatechin gallate and 28.8 mg caffeine) 360 mg • Advantra-Z brand Citrus Aurantium fruit, root (8 mg synephrine) 200 mg • Guarana seed (standardized at 44 mg caffeine) 200 mg • L-Tyrosine (as L-tyrosine hydrochloride) 150 mg • Flavanex-Er brand Bioflavanoid Matrix 150 mg: Quercetin, Naringin, Fisetin • Forslean brand Forskolin (standardized at 20% coleus forskohlii) 50 mg • 5-HTP 25 mg. Other Ingredients: Dicalcium Phosphate Dihydrate, Magnesium Stearate.
See Editor's Note No. 40.

Norabol **-** Mass Quantities, Inc.
Each capsule contains: 19-Nor-4-androstenedione 100 mg • Silymarin 20 mg • Niacin 10 mg • Zinc 5 mg.

NorCycloDiol-4 (Sports One Cycloplex Pro-Hormone) **-** Sports One
Each lozenge contains: Nor- 4-Androstenediol Cycloplex (cyclodextrin complex) 10 mg.
See Editor's Note No. 54.

Some Brand Name Natural Products - What they Contain

www.NaturalDatabase.com contains MANY more listings than appear here.
Editor's Notes are located on pages 2155-2163.

NorCycloDione (Sports One Cycloplex Pro-Hormone) **-** Sports One
Each lozenge contains: 19-Nor-4-Androstenedione Cycloplex (cyclodextrin complex) 25 mg.

Nordisk of Denmark Propolis **-** Health From The Sun
Each capsule contains: 50% Propolis • 50% Bee Pollen in a natural mineral base of Calcium Phosphate.

Norexin **-** Biotech Corp.
Two tablets contain: Natural Vitamin E (as d-alpha tocopheryl succinate) 30 IU • Niacin (as niacinamide) 20 mg • Selenium (as selenomethionine) 35 mcg • Chromium (as chromium dinicotinate glycinate) 200 mcg • Ma Huang herb extract (15 mg ephedrine alkaloids) 150 mg • Green Tea leaf extract (VerdOx, yielding 150 mg natural caffeine, 90 mg polyphenols including EGCG) 600 mg • French Grape Seed extract (AdipoVin) 40 mg • Neurothermic Modulator Proprietary Blend 523 mg: Magnesium Citrate, Glycine, L-Theanine.
See Editor's Note No. 21 and No. 30.

Norexin Ephedra Free **-** Biotech Corp.
Two tablets contain: Natural Vitamin E (as natural d-alpha tocopheryl succinate) 30 IU • Niacin (as niacinamide) 20 mg • Magnesium (as magnesium citrate) 50 mg • Selenium (as selenomethionine) 35 mcg • Chromium (as chromium dinicotinate glycinate) 200 mcg • Citrus Aurantium rind (yielding 8 mg of synephrine) 200 mg • VerdOx standardized Green Tea leaf extract (camellia sinensis, yielding 150 mg of natural caffeine and 90 mg of polyphenols, including EGCG) 600 mg • AdipoVin exclusive French Grape seed (vitis vinifera) 40 mg • Neurothermic Modulator Proprietary Blend 523 mg: Magnesium Citrate, Glycine, L-Theanine. Other Ingredients: Dicalcium Phosphate, Microcrystalline Cellulose, Croscarmellose Sodium, Stearic Acid, Magnesium Stearate, Silica, Peppermint Oil (in coating), Calcium Silicate, Pharmaceutical Glaze.
See Editor's Note No. 40.

Norexin Slim Sculpt **-** Biotech Corp.
Each 15 mL serving contains: Chromium from Picolinate 15 mcg • Garcinia Cambogia extract (50% HCA) 50 mg • Conjugated Linoleic Acid 45 mg. Other Ingredients: Purified Water, Hydrolyzed Collagen, Glycerin, Citric Acid, Natural Flavor, Aloe Vera Concentrate, Acesulfame Potassium, Xanthan Gum, Sodium Citrate, Potassium Sorbate, Sodium Benzoate, Ethyl Maltol, Chromium Picolinate, Calcium Pyruvate.

North Atlantic Kelp **-** Solgar
Each tablet contains: Calcium (as dicalcium phosphate) 45 mg • Iodine (from 142 mg of dehydrated North Atlantic kelp) 225 mcg • Sodium 5 mg. Other Ingredients: Dicalcium Phosphate, Microcrystalline Cellulose, Silica, Vegetable Cellulose, Vegetable Stearic Acid, Vegetable Magnesium Stearate.

Norwegian Cod Liver Oil **-** Puritan's Pride
Each softgel contains: Natural Vitamin A 1,250 IU • Natural Vitamin D (from Cod Liver Oil) 135 IU.

Norwegian Cod Liver Oil **-** Nature's Bounty
Each softgel contains: Vitamin A (from Cod Liver Oil) 1250 IU • Vitamin D (from Cod Liver Oil) 135 IU. Other Ingredients: Cod Liver Oil, Soybean Oil, Gelatin, Glycerin.

Norwegian Cod Liver Oil **-** Solgar
Each softgel contains: Vitamin A 1250 IU • Vitamin D 135 IU • EPA (as eicosapentaenoic acid 12%) 49 mg • DHA (as docosahexaenoic acid 8%) 32 mg. Other Ingredients: Gelatin, Glycerin, Water.

Norwegian Salmon Oil **-** J. R. Carlson Laboratories, Inc.
Two softgels contain: Vitamin E (as D-alpha tocopherol) 20 IU • Omega-3 Fatty Acids (from salmon oil) 750 mg • DHA (docosahexaenoic acid) 250 mg • EPA (eicosapentaenoic acid) 360 mg.

NOS High Performance Energy Drink **-** High Performance Beverage Co.
Carbonated Water • High Fructose Corn Syrup • Citric Acid • Taurine • Sodium Citrate • Natural Passion Fruit Flavor with other Natural Flavors • D-Ribose • L-Carnitine • Caffeine • Sodium Hexametaphosphate • Pectin • Ascorbic Acid (vitamin C) • Inositol • Gum Arabic • Monopotassium Phosphate • Sodium Benzoate • Potassium Sorbate • Ester Gum • Panax Ginseng root extract • Calcium Disodium Salt of EDTA • Sucralose • Pyridoxine Hydrochloride (vitamin B6) • Beta-Carotene • Cyanocobalamin (vitamin B12).

Nose & Throat **-** Enzymes, Inc.
Two capsules contain: Vitamin C (100% from Acerola Cherries) 70 mg • Zinc (100% as Zinc Citrate) 10 mg • Proprietary Herbal Blend 360 mg: Elder Flower tops extract, Garlic bulb extract, Wild Indigo root extract, Quercetin, Grape seed extract • Proprietary Enzyme Blend 320 mg: Amylase, pHysioProtease, Peptidase. Other Ingredients: Plant Cellulose, Water.

Nourishing Body Bar **-** FreeLife International
Sodium Palmate • Sodium Cocoate/Sodium Palm Kernelate • Purified Water • Vegetable Glycerin • Lavender oil • Grapefruit oil • Ylang Ylang oil • Coconut oil • Methylsulfonylmethane (MSM) • Sodium Gluconate • Coconut fatty acid • BioEnhanced Grapefruit seed extract (BGSE) • Olive oil • Grape seed oil.

Nourishing Body Cleanser **-** FreeLife International
Purified Water • Sodium Lauroyl Sarcosinate • Decyl Glucoside • Vegetable Glycerine • Guar Gum • Pure Honey • Aloe Vera gel • Methylsulfonylmethane (MSM) • Hibiscus flower (sabdariffa extract) • Anthemis Nobilis oil (chamomile) • Citrus Aurantium var. Dulcis oil (orange) • Lavandula Angustifolia oil (lavender) • Citrus Limonum oil (lemon) • Azadirachta Indica extract (neem) • Panthenol (vitamin B5) • Allantoin • Citric Acid • Sodium Hydroxymethylglycinate.

Novasoy brand **-** ADM
Soybean extract powdered compound.
See Editor's Note No. 44.

Now Sports Amino 1000 **-** NOW Foods
Four capsules contain: Vitamin B6 13 mg • Proprietary Blend 4 g: Amino Acids from Soy Protein Isolate, Predigested Casei, Predigested Lactalbumin, Carnitine, Ornithine and Gelatin. Other Ingredients: Gelatin (capsule), Magnesium Stearate.

Now Sports Amino 1500 **-** NOW Foods
Three chewable tablets contain: Vitamin B6 (as pyridoxine HCl) 3.2 mg • Proprietary Blend 4.5 g: Amino Acids, Proteins sourced from Whey Protein • Stevia Rebaudiana leaf extract. Other Ingredients: Magnesium Stearate, Cellulose, Stearic Acid, Cellulose, Fructose, Natural Flavor.

Now Sports L-glutamine 1000 mg **-** NOW Foods
Each capsule contains: L-Glutamine (free-form) 1 g. Other Ingredients: Gelatin (capsule), Stearic Acid, Magnesium Stearate, Silica.

Now Sports L-Glutamine Free Form Vegetarian **-** NOW Foods
Each 1/4 level tsp serving contains: L-Glutamine 750 mg.

Now Sports L-Glutamine Powder **-** NOW Foods
Each 1/4 level tsp serving contains: L-Glutamine 750 mg.

Now Sports ZMA **-** NOW Foods
Three capsules contain: Vitamin B6 15 mg • Magnesium 450 mg • Zinc 30 mg • ZMA (zinc magnesium aspartate) 2.4 g (2400 mg). Other Ingredients: Gelatin (capsule), Magnesium Stearate.

NOX3 **-** Universal Nutrition
Three tablets contain: NO Complex 3000 mg: Arginine Alpha-Ketoglutarate, Arginine Ketoisocaproate • NO Booster 100 mg: Ornithine Alpha-Ketoglutarate. Other Ingredients: Beta-Cyclodextrin, Calcium Phosphate, Xanthan, Cellulose, Inulin, Magnesium Stearate.

NO-Xplode - BSN Inc.
Each scoop (20.5 g) contains: Vitamin B6 (pyridoxine HCl) 25 mg • Vitamin B12 (cyanocobalamine) 120 mcg • Folic Acid 400 mcg • Magnesium 360 mg • Phosphorus 500 mg • Calcium 75 mg • NO-Xplode Proprietary Blend 20,500 mg: L-Arginine AKG, Citral-M Citruline Malate, L-Citruline AKG, L-Histidine AKG, RC-NOS Rutacarpine 95%, Gynostemma Pentaphyllum (95% gypenosides), NAD (nicotinamide adenine dinuleotide), 2CM Dicreatine Malate, Betapure Trimethylglycine, Glycovol Glycocyamine, GuaniPro Guanidino Proplonic Acid, Cinnulin PF Aqueous Cinnamon extract, Keto-Isocaproate Potassium, L-Tyrosine, Taurine, Endurlac Glucuronolactone, L-Tyrosine AKG, Methylxanthines (caffeine), MCT (medium chain triglycerides), Vinpocetine 99%, Vincamine 99%, Vinburnine 99%, Calcium Phosphate, Magnesium Oxide, Potassium Phosphate, Sodium Phosphate, Potassium Glycerophosphate, Magnesium Glycerophosphate, Glycerola Stearate. Other Ingredients: Maltodextrine, Citric Acid, Sodium Bicarbonate, Lemon Juice Powder, Malic Acid, Potassium Citrate, Natural and Artificial Flavors, Aspartame, Acesulfame Potassium, FD&C Red 40, FD&C Blue 1.

NoxyLane4 - LaneLabs
Four veggie capsules (or two double strength capsules) contain: MGN3 Proprietary Blend (arabinoxylane compound) 1000 mg: Rice Bran, Hyphomycetes Mycelia enzyme from Shiitake mushroom • HAI (heated algal ingredient) Amino Acid extract (from sea algae) <1 mg. Other Ingredients: Microcrystalline Cellulose, Hypromellose, Magnesium Stearate, Silica.
See Editor's Note No. 21.

NOZ - NutraBolics
Nineteen grams contain: Tricreatine Malate 3 g • Arginine Alpha-KetoGlutarate 1 g • R- ALA 100 mg • N-Acetyl-L-Glutamine 1 g • Glycocyamine 1.5 g. Other Ingredients: Designer Complex Carbohydrates, Glucose Polymers (derived from vegetable sources), Sucralose, Natural/Artificial Flavor.

NRG Formula (NR Glow) - TriLight Herbs
Echinacea Angustifolia herb • Oregon Grape root • Pau d'Arco • Red root • Red Clover • Peppermint leaf • Buchu leaf • Licorice root • Thyme leaf • Ginger root • Capsicum.

N-R-G Protein Powder - Naturade
Each 1 oz serving contains: Isolated Soy Protein • Calcium Caseinate • Sweet Dairy whey • Carrageenan • Soy Lecithin • Enzymatically Predigested Lactalbumin • Egg albumin • Papain & Natural Vanilla flavor.

NSC-100 Immunition Extra Strength - NSC
Each capsule contains: Beta Glucan (MG Beta-1,3/1,6-Glucan) 10 mg.

NSC-24 Allergy Immunition - NSC
Two capsules contain: Beta Glucan (MG Beta-1,3/1,6-Glucan) 3 mg • Vitamin C 300 mg • Quercetin 300 mg • Hydrastus Canadensis 160 mg • Astragalus 60 mg • OPC (grape seed extract) 30 mg • Vitamin A (palmitate) 9000 IU • Beta Carotene 18 mg • Lemon Bioflavonoids 10 mg • Rutin 10 mg • Hesperidin 10 mg • Rose Hips 10 mg • Acerola Cherry 10 mg • Zinc (picolinate) 4 mg.

NSC-24 Caprylic Acid Immunition - NSC
Four gelatin capsules contain: Beta Glucan (Beta-1,3/1,6-Glucan) 4 mg • Caprylic Acid 360 mg.

NSC-24 Circulatory Immunition - NSC
Six capsules contain: Beta Glucan (Beta-1,3/1,6-Glucan) 6 mg • Vitamin C 1568.16 mg • Bromelain 140 mg • Coenzyme Q10 50 mg • Potassium Ascorbate 245.52 mg • Potassium Aspartate 308.88 mg • Magnesium Aspartate 205.92 mg • Magnesium Ascorbate 245.52 mg • L-Lysine 605.88 mg • L-Proline 605.88 mg.

NSC-24 Immunition Original Formula - NSC
Each capsule contains: Beta Glucan (MG Beta-1,3/1,6-Glucan) 3 mg.

NSK-SD - Pure Encapsulations
Each vegetable capsule contains: Nattokinase 50 mg (1000 FU).

NSK-SD brand - Japan Bio Science Laboratory Co., Ltd.
Proprietary Nattokinase extract.
See Editor's Note No. 44.

N-Snor - Abundance Marketing
Purified Water • Vegetable Glycerin • Safflower Oil • Lecithin • Almond Oil • Polysorbate 80 • Peppermint Oil • Potassium Sorbate • Citric Acid • Sodium Benzoate • Methylparaben • Propylparaben • Sodium EDTA • Natural Orange Flavor.

N-TENSE - Raintree Nutrition, Inc.
Each capsule contains: Proprietary Blend 650 mg: Graviola, Mullaca, Vassourinha, Espinheira Santa, Mutamba, Bitter Melon, Suma, Cat's Claw.

Nu Colour Eye Makeup Remover - Nu Skin Enterprises
Water • Cyclomethiocone • Cetearyl Octanoate • C13-14 Isoparaffin • PPG-2 Myristyl Ether Propionate • Jojoba oil (buxus chinensis) • Rice bran oil (oryza sativa) • Polyacrylamide • Polysorbate 20 • Laureth-7 • Tocopherol • Tocopheryl Acetate • Bisabolol • Phenoxyethanol • Methylparaben • Butylparaben • Ropylparaben • Ethylparaben.

Nu Knees - The Sports Nutrition Source, Inc.
Three capsules contain: Glucosamine Sulfate 1000 mg • Chondroitin Sulfate 750 mg • MSM 750 mg • White Willow Bark 150 mg • Bromelain 100 mg • Vitamin C 90 mg.
See Editor's Note No. 15.

Nu Skin 180 Face Wash (180 Face Wash) - Nu Skin Enterprises
Glycerin • Ascorbic Acid • Sesame oil (sesamum indicum) • C12-15 Alkyl Benzoate • Sodium Cocoyl Isethionate • Hydrogenated Soybean oil • Sodium C14-16 Olefin Sulfonate • Grape seed extract (vitis vinifera) • Ginkgo Biloba • Ginseng extract (Panax ginseng) • Stearyl Glycyrrhetinate • Carbomer • Titanium Dioixde • Fragrance (parfum).

NuBiotic - PhytoPharmica
Each tablet contains: Vitamin A (fish liver oil) 10,000 IU •Vitamin C (ascorbic acid) 200 mg • Vitamin D (fish liver oil) 35 IU • Vitamin B12 (cyanocobalamin) 2.5 mcg • Pantothenic Acid (calcium D-pantothenate) 25 mg •Calcium (lactate) 41 mg •Magnesium (citrate) 6.7 mg • Zinc (gluconate) 10.5 mg • RNA powder 60 mg • Alfalfa (Medicago sativa) leaf and stem juice powder 50 mg • Lemon Bioflavonoids 30 mg •Spleen extract 30 mg • Thymus extract 25 mg • Trace Mineral Concentrate (kelp) 25 mg •Unsaturated free fatty acids (oil of evening primrose) 15 mg • Lung extract 10 mg.
See Editor's Note No. 21 and No. 53.

Nucleic Acid with RNA and DNA - Quest
Each tablet contains: RNA (Ribonucleic Acid) 200 mg • DNA (Deoxyribonucleic Acid) 60 mg • Brewer's Yeast 190 mg. Other Ingredients: Dibasic Calcium Phosphate, Microcrystalline Cellulose, Vegetable Stearin, Magnesium Stearate, Silicon Dioxide.

NuFem - Enzymatic Therapy
Each tablet contains: Black Cohosh (standardized to contain 2.5% triterpene glycosides calculated as 27-deocyacetin) 20 mg. Other Ingredients: Microcrystalline Cellulose, Lactose, Stearic Acid, Silicon Dioxide, Potato Starch, Magnesium Stearate.
Available in Canada.

NuFem Plus Soy - Enzymatic Therapy
Each tablet contains: Black Cohosh (standardized to contain 2.5% triterpene glycosides calculated as 27-deocyacetin) 20 mg • Soy bean extract (standardized to contain 15% isoflavones calculated as genistein and daidzein, non-GMO) 100 mg. Other Ingredients: Microcrystalline Cellulose, Calcium Carbonate, Stearic Acid, Croscarmellose Sodium, Silicon Dioxide, Magnesium Stearate, Water-Soluble Coating (hydroxypropyl methylcellulose, hydroxypropyl cellulose, polyethylene glycol).
Available in Canada.

Some Brand Name Natural Products - What they Contain

www.NaturalDatabase.com contains MANY more listings than appear here.
Editor's Notes are located on pages 2155-2163.

NuFem Plus St. John's Wort - Enzymatic Therapy
Each tablet contains: Black Cohosh (standardized to contain 2.5% triterpene glycosides calculated as 27-deocyacetin) 20 mg • St. John's Wort extract (standardized to contain a minimum of 0.3% hypericin and 4% hyperforin) 100 mg. Other Ingredients: Microcrystalline Cellulose, Stearic Acid, Silicon Dioxide, Croscarmellose Sodium, Magnesium Stearate, Water-Soluble Coating (hydroxypropyl methylcellulose, titanium dioxide, polyethylene glycol, maltodextrin, sodium citrate, polysorbate 80, chlorophyll).
Available in Canada.

Nugest 900 - Nutraceutics Corp.
Purified Water • Ethoxydiglycol • Progesterone USP • C-12-15 • Alkyl Benzoate • Caprylic/Capric Triglyceride • Demasterone (bioactive multi wild yam species complex) • Trans-V-DS (lipo copolymer complex) • Dimethicone • Tocopheryl Acetate • Essence • Methylparaben • Propylparaben • Polysorbate 40 • Imidazolidinyl Urea • Disodium EDTA.

Nugest Serum - Nutraceutics Corp.
Purified Water • Demasterone (bioactive multi wild yam species complex) • Ethoxydiglycol • Protein Oligopeptide Biofactors • Caprylic/Capric Triglyceride • Trans-V-DS (lipo copolymer complex) • Glyceryl Stearate • PEG-100 Stearate • Caprylic/Capric/Stearic Triglyceride • Progesterone USP • Methyl-Paraben • Phenoxyethanol • Diazolidinly Urea • Disodium EDTA • Polysorbate 20 • Sodium Alginate • Essence.

Nugestrone - Nutraceutics Corp.
Aloe Vera • Glycerin • Canola Oil • Stearic Acid • Safflower Oil • Glyceryl Stearate Se • Wild Mexican Yam Extract • Octyl Palmitate • Deionized Water • Cetyl Alcohol • Glyceryl Stearate • PEG-100 Stearate • Progesterone USP • Polysorbate 60 • Sorbitan Sesquioleate • Methyl Glyceth-20 • Imidazolidinyl Urea • DMDM Hydantoin • Methylparaben • Propylparaben • Citric Acid.

NuHair Hair Regrowth Tablets for Men - Biotech Corp.
Two tablets contain: Folate (as folic acid) 800 mcg • Pantothenic Acid (as dicalcium pantothenate) 200 mg • Biotin 1400 mcg • Iodine (from kelp) 150 mg • Zinc (as zinc monomethionine) 15 mg • He Shou Wu (12:1 standardized extract) 450 mg • He Shou Wu root powder (polygonum multiflorum) 870 mg • Shen Min Herb Blend 433 mg: Saw Palmetto berries (sabal serrulata), Beta Sitosterol, Isoflavones (from pueraria lobata root and soybeans) • Silica (from colloidals) 40 mg • Bioperine brand Black Pepper extract (piper nigrum standardized extract) 5 mg. Other Ingredients: Microcrystalline Cellulose, Croscarmellose Sodium, Stearic Acid, Magnesium Stearate, Pharmaceutical Glaze.

NuHair Hair Regrowth Tablets for Women - Biotech Corp.
Two tablets contain: Vitamin A (as retinyl palmitate) 5000 IU • Niacin (as nicotinic acid) 20 mg • Vitamin B6 (pyridoxine HCl) 10 mg • Biotin 1400 mcg • Pantothenic Acid 200 mg • He Shou Wu root standardized extract (12:1) 450 mg • Soy Isoflavones (glycine max, from 50 mg 40% standardized soybean extract) 20 mg • Black Cohosh root standardized extract 40 mg • Horse Chestnut standardized extract 50 mg • Hydrolyzed Collagen 250 mg • Silica 100 mg • Gingko Biloba leaf 100 mg • Uva Ursi root standardized extract 50 mg • Burdock root extract (4:1) 25 mg • Cayenne pepper (80,000 scoville heat units) 25 mg • Bioperine brand Black Pepper extract (piper nigrum standardized extract) 5 mg. Other Ingredients: Microcrystalline Cellulose, Croscarmellose Sodium, Stearic Acid, Magnesium Stearate, Dicalcium Phosphate, Pharmaceutical Glaze.

NuHair Thinning Hair Serum - Biotech Corp.
Alcohol SD40 • Purified Water • Propylene Glycol • Jojoba oil • Herbal Blend Hair Complex: Henna, Horsetail, Rosemary, Tormentil, Burdock, Honey, Goldenseal • Lecithin • PEG-40 Stearate • Steareth-20 • Tilisina Complex • Cholesterol • Trichopeptide • Retinyl Palmitate • Tocopheryl Acetate • He Shou Wu extract • Saw Palmetto extract • Nettle extract • Propyl Gallate • Biotin • Polysorbate 20 • Chamomile extract • Carbomer • Disodium EDTA • Aminomethyl Propanol • Phenoxyethanol • Methylparaben • Butylparaben • Ethylparaben • Propylparaben.

NuLung - The Council On Natural Health
Two tablets contain: Vitamin A (as beta-carotene, with natural mixed carotenoids) 5000 IU • Vitamin C (as ascorbic acid) 100 mg • Vitamin B12 (as cyanocobalamin) 1.25 mcg • Pantothenic Acid (as D-calcium pantothenate) 3.5 mg • Zinc (as zinc gluconate) 0.6 mg • Calcium Lactate 30 mg • Ribonucleic Acid 30 mg • Lemon Bioflavonoid Complex 15 mg • Thymus substance (porcine) 12.5 mg • Chinese Ging Fei Tang Herbal Bland 500 mg: Skullcap root, Gardenia fruit, Dong Quai root, Licorice root, Ophiopogon tuber, Asparagus root, Schisandra berry, Tritillary bulb, Monus root bark, Platycodon root, Hoelen Scierotium, Bamboo stalk (barrbusa brenflora), Jujube date, Citrus peel (citrus leiocarpus) • Jade Windscreen Herbal Blend 50 mg: Atractylodes rhizome, Astragalus root, Ledebourilla root, Ginger root. Bio-active Base Blend 35 mg: Alfalfa leaf, Barley Malt extracts, Wheat Germ, Rose Hips, Lymphatic Substance (bovine), Chlorophyll (from alfalfa leaf). Other Ingredients: Dicalcium Phosphate, Microcrystalline Cellulose, Croscarmellose Sodium, Stearic Acid, Silica, Magnesium Stearate, Pharmaceutical Glaze.
See Editor's Note No. 14.

Numovil - Berkeley Premium Nutraceuticals
Two tablets contain: Thiamin (as thiamin mononitrate) 10 mg • Ginkgo Biloba leaf standardized extract 120 mg • Alpha-Lipoic Acid 50 mg • Vinpocetine 10 mg • Huperzine-A 100 mcg • Purified Phospholipids 100 mg: Phosphatidylcholine 39 mg, Phosphatidylethanolamine 33 mg, Phosphatidylinositol 23 mg, Phosphatidylserine 5 mg • Green Tea leaf extract (providing 100 mg naturally-occurring caffeine) 500 mg. Other Ingredients: Dicalcium Phosphate, Microcrystalline Celluose, Croscarmellose Sodium, Stearic Acid, Magnesium Stearate, Silica, Film Coat Ingredients (hypromellose, hydroxypropyl cellulose, polyethylene glycol with colors to be determined).

Nuproxi - Berkeley Premium Nutraceuticals
Each tablet contains: Vitamin A (as retinyl palmitate and 50% as beta-carotene) 5000 IU • Vitamin C (as Ester-C brand calcium ascorbate) 250 mg • Vitamin D (as cholecalciferol) 400 IU • Vitamin E (as natural D-alpha-tocopheryl succinate) 100 IU • Folate (as folic acid) 400 mcg • Biotin 300 mcg • Zinc (as zinc citrate) 15 mg • Selenium (as sodium selenate) 70 mcg • Copper (as copper gluconate) 2 mg • Nuproxi Proprietary Blend 402 mg: Glucosamine HCl, Collagen, Grape Seed standardized extract, Alpha-Lipoic Acid, Lycopene. Other Ingredients: Dicalcium Phosphate, Microcrystalline Cellulose, Croscarmellose Sodium, Stearic Acid, Magnesium Stearate, Silica, Film Coat Ingredients (hypromellose, hydroxypropyl cellulose, polyethylene glycol, propylene glycol, titanium dioxide, riboflavin).

Nutraceutics ABC & Tea - Nutraceutics Corp.
Each tablet contains: Potassium (bicarbonate) 120 mg • Vitamin A (palmitate) 250 IU • Vitamin C (ascorbic acid) 1000 mg • Calcium (carbonate) 70 mg • Thiamine Mononitrate 15 mg • Riboflavin (as 5-phosphate) 16 mg • Niacinamide 50 mg • Pyridoxine HCl 8 mg • Vitamin B12 (cyanocobalamin) 10 mcg • Biotin 150 mcg • Pantothenic Acid (calcium pantothenate) 25 mg • Green Tea extract 70 mg. Other Ingredients: Sorbitol, Citric Acid, Sodium Bicarbonate, Polyethylene Glycol, Natural and Artificial Flavors, Sodium Benzoate, Sodium Carbonate, Sucralose.

Nutra-Flax - Pure Encapsulations
Each vegetable capsule contains: Flax seed powder 750 mg: Omega-3 Fatty Acids 52 mg • Omega-6 Fatty Acids 14 mg • Omega-9 Fatty Acids 20 mg • Lignans 3.8 mg.

NutraFlora Powder - Source Naturals
Three tablets contain: NutraFlora Fructooligosaccharides (FOS) 3000 mg.

NutraFloraFOS - Natrol, Inc.
One capsule contains: FOS (Fructooligosaccharides) 500 mg. Other Ingredients: Magnesium Stearate, Gelatin.

Some Brand Name Natural Products - What they Contain

www.NaturalDatabase.com contains MANY more listings than appear here.
Editor's Notes are located on pages 2155-2163.

Nutragel **-** Nutraceutics Corp.
Active Ingredients: Purified Water • Dermasterone (bioactive multi wild yam species) • Protein Oligopeptide Biofactors • Caprylic/Capric Triglyceride • Trans-V-DS (lipo copolymer complex). Inactive Ingredients: Methylparaben, Phenoxyethanol, Diazolidinyl Urea, Disodium EDTA, Polysorbate 20, Sodium Alginate.

NutraGreens **-** Earthrise Nutritionals, LLC.
Twenty tablets contain: Vitamin A 5000 IU • Vitamin C 90 mg • Vitamin D 80 IU • Vitamin E (d-alpha-tocopherol acetate) 30 IU • Thiamin (Vitamin B-1) 1.5 mg • Riboflavin (Vitamin B-12) 1.7 mg • Niacin (Vitamin B-3) 20 mg • Vitamin B6 2 mg • Folic Acid 400 mcg • Vitamin B12 7.2 mcg • Biotin 300 mcg • Pantothenic Acid 10 mg • Calcium (Citrate) 24 mg • Iron (Gluconate) 2.7 mg • Iodine (Kelp) 30 mcg • Magnesium (Citrate) 18 mg • Zinc (Methionine) 10 mg • Selenium (Aminoate) 18 mcg • Copper (Gluconate) 1 mg • Manganese (Gluconate) 2 mg • Chromium (Aminoate) 50 mcg • Potassium (Spirulina & Asparatate) 25 mg • Proprietary Blend: Earthrise Spirulina, Lecithin, Natural Apple Concentrate, Prune Powder, Boron (Aminoate), Licorice extract (DGL), Sarsaparilla root, Siberian Ginseng extract (35:1, root), Ginkgo Biloba extract (24% Flavone Glycosides, 6% Terpene Lactones), Milk Thistle extract (80% Silymarin), Royal Jelly, Kelp, Dulse, Astragalus root, Stevia leaf, Ginger root extract (5%), Green Tea extract (50% Polyphenols), Broccoli Powder, Carrot Powder, Beet Powder, Celery Powder, Grape Seed extract (95% OPC), Octacosanol, Pine Bark extract (50% OPC), Cayenne Pepper fruit, Coenzyme Q-10 4242 mg • Proprietary Digestive Complex: Gum Arabic, Lactobacillus acidophilus DDS, Bifidobacterium longum, Aloe Vera, Amylase, Cellulase 253 mg.

NutraJoint Plus Glucosamine **-** KNOX
Each scoop contains: Sodium 30 mg • Protein 9 g • Vitamin C (as ascorbic acid) 60 mg • Vitamin D (as cholecalciferol) 80 IU • Vitamin E (as dl-alpha tocopheryl acetate) 6 IU • Vitamin K (as phytonadione) 16 mcg • Calcium 300 mg • Zinc (as zinc gluconate) 3 mg • Copper (as copper gluconate) 0.4 mg • Manganese (as manganese sulfate) 0.4 mg • Gelatine 10 g • Glucosamine Hydrochloride 1500 mg.

NutraMetrix B Complex Plus **-** Market America, Inc.
Each capful (3.33 g) contains: Vitamin B2 (riboflavin-5-phosphate) 3 mg • Vitamin B12 (cyanocobalamin) 120 mcg • Folic Acid 400 mcg • Potassium (bicarbonate) 94 mg • Magnesium (carbonate) 40 mg. Other Ingredients: Fructose, Glucose, Citric Acid, Maltodextrin, Silica, Pectin, Calcium Sulfate, Natural Lemon-Lime Flavor.

NutraMetrix Blood Sugar Maintenance **-** Market America, Inc.
Each tablet contains: Biotin 1.3 mg • Magnesium (oxide) 67 mg • Zinc (gluconate) 2.5 mg • Chromium (nicotinate) 67 mcg • Glucomannan 400 mg • Alpha-Lipoic Acid 200 mg • Gymnema Sylvestre 133 mg • American Ginseng 33 mg • Vanadium (amino acid chelate) 15 mcg. Other Ingredients: Dicalcium Phosphate, Microcrystalline Cellulose, Stearic Acid, Magnesium Stearate, Croscarmellose Sodium, Silicon Dioxide.

NutraMetrix Calcium Complete **-** Market America, Inc.
Two capfuls (6.67 g) contain: Calcium (carbonate, lactate, phosphate, sulfate, citrate) 750 mg • Magnesium (oxide, carbonate) 200 mg • Manganese (sulfate) 1 mg • Vitamin B2 (riboflavin-5-phosphate) 2 mg • Vitamin C (ascorbic acid) 58 mg • Vitamin D (D3, cholecalciferol) 400 IU • Boron (sodium borate) 1 mg • Potassium (bicarbonate, citrate) 225 mg. Other Ingredients: Fructose, Glucose, Orange Powder, Citric Acid, Apple Pectin, Malic Acid, Natural/ Orange Flavor.

NutraMetrix Coenzyme Q10 100 **-** Market America, Inc.
Each capful (3.33 g) contains: Coenzyme Q10 100 mg • Vitamin E (acetate) 200 IU • Lipase 5 mg • Vitamin B2 (riboflavin) 3 mg • Potassium (bicarbonate) 108 mg. Other Ingredients: Fructose, Glucose, Citric Acid, Silica, Calcium Sulfate, Maltodextrin, Natural Lemon-Lime Flavor.

NutraMetrix Digestive Enzymes with Probiotics **-** Market America, Inc.
Each capful (3.33 g) contains: DigeZyme 100 mg: Amylase 2400 U, Protease 600 U, Cellulase 20 U, Lactase 400 U, Lipase 100 IU • Maltase 125 MWU • Sucrase 400 SU • Magnesium 24 mg • Potassium 88 mg • Lactobacillus Sporogenes 150,000,000 CFU. Other Ingredients: Fructose, Glucose, Citric Acid, Maltodextrin, Silica, Apple Pectin, Calcium Sulfate, Natural Lemon-Lime Flavor.

NutraMetrix Female Support Formula **-** Market America, Inc.
Two tablets contain: Thiamin HCl (vitamin B1) 20 mg • Riboflavin (vitamin B2) 20 mg • Niacin (vitamin B3) 20 mg • D-Calcium Pantothenate (vitamin B5) 11.8 mg • Pyridoxine HCl (vitamin B6) 10 mg • Folic Acid 400 mcg • Cyanocobalamin (vitamin B12) 200 mcg • D-Alpha-Tocopherol (vitamin E) 50 IU • Soy extract (soy isoflavones, 3%) 200 mg • Dong Quai root 1% extract 200 mg • Evening Primrose oil 200 mg • Wild Yam 180 mg • Black Cohosh root 2.5% extract 160 mg • Chaste berry extract (vitex agnus-castus) 150 mg • Horsetail 150 mg • Red Clover 140 mg • Passiflora 120 mg • Valerian root 120 mg • Sage 100 mg • St. John's Wort 70 mg. Other Ingredients: Dicalcium Phosphate, Microcrystalline Cellulose, Stearic Acid, Magnesium Stearate, Croscarmellose Sodium, Silicon Dioxide.

NutraMetrix Glucosatrin **-** Market America, Inc.
Three tablets contain: Vitamin C (ascorbic acid) 100 mg • Zinc (as zinc sulfate) 10 mg • Copper (as copper gluconate) 30 mcg • Manganese (as manganese sulfate) 5 mg • Glucosamine HCl 1500 mg • Scutellaria Baicalensis root (Chinese skullcap) 150 mg • Oleanolic Acid 150 mg • Boswellia Gum resin extract 200 mg • Hops strobile extract 350 mg. Other Ingredients: Microcrystalline Cellulose, Stearic Acid, Croscarmellose Sodium, Magnesium Stearate, Silica.

NutraMetrix Herbal Antioxidant **-** Market America, Inc.
Two capsules contain: Vitamin A (as beta-carotene) 5000 IU • Vitamin C (as ascorbic acid) 200 mg • Vitamin E (as D-alpha tocopheryl succinate) 30 IU • Selenium (as SelenoExcell brand yeast) 200 mcg • Green Tea extract 300 mg • Ginkgo Biloba leaf extract (24% ginkgo flavoglycosides/6% terpene lactones) 50 mg • Milk Thistle 50 mg • L-Glutathione 1 mg • Bilberry powder 50 mg. Other Ingredients: Rice Powder, Silica, Magnesium Stearate, Gelatin.

NutraMetrix Isochrome **-** Market America, Inc.
Each capful (3.33 g) contains: Vitamin B2 (riboflavin) 3 mg • Vitamin B6 (pyridoxine HCl) 2 mg • Chromium (picolinate) 100 mcg • Chromium (argininate) 115 mcg • Potassium (bicarbonate) 95 mg • Coenzyme Q10 60 mg • L-Carnitine 20 mg • Lipase 5 mg • Boron (chelate) 2 mg. Other Ingredients: Fructose, Glucose, Citric Acid, Maltodextrin, Silica, Calcium Sulfate, Natural Lemon-Lime Flavor.

NutraMetrix Maximum ORAC Formula **-** Market America, Inc.
Each capful (3.33 g) contains: Potassium (bicarbonate) 125 mg • Vitamin C (ascorbic acid) 100 mg • Cranberry 200 mg • Blueberry 100 mg • Grape 93 mg • Raspberry 90 mg • Elderberry 40 mg • Black Currant 40 mg • Pomegranate 40 mg • Plum 20 mg • Choke Cherry 20 mg • Natural Tocopherol (d-gamma 70%, d-delta 21%, d-alpha 7%, d-beta 2%) 30 mg • Tocotrienols (mixed isomers) 20 mg • Bioperine brand Black Pepper extract 56 mcg. Other Ingredients: Fructose, Citric Acid, Maltodextrin, Glucose, Silica.

NutraMetrix Multivitamins & Multiminerals With Iron **-** Market America, Inc.
Each capful (3.3 g) contains: Beta-Carotene 10,000 IU • Vitamin B1 2.6 mg • VItamin B2 3 mg • Niacin 40 mg • Pantothenic Acid 20 mg • Vitamin B6 4 mg • Vitamin B12 75 mcg • Folic Acid 400 mcg • Biotin 300 mcg • Vitamin C 150 mg • Vitamin D (D3) 400 IU • Vitamin E 66 IU • Vitamin K 100 mcg • Calcium 50 mg • Chromium 120 mcg • Copper 1000 mcg • Iodine 150 mcg • Iron 1.5 mg • Magnesium 25 mg • Potassium 108 mg • Silicon 2 mg • Selenium 55 mcg • Zinc 7.5 mg. Other Ingredients: Fructose, Citric Acid, Orange Fruit Powder, Mandarin Fruit Powder, Malic Acid, Glucose, Orange Flavor, Tricalcium Phosphate, Sucralose.

Some Brand Name Natural Products - What they Contain

www.NaturalDatabase.com contains MANY more listings than appear here.
Editor's Notes are located on pages 2155-2163.

NutraMetrix Multivitamins & Multiminerals Without Iron - Market America, Inc.
Each capful (3.3 g) contains: Beta-Carotene 10,000 IU • Vitamin B1 2.6 mg • Vitamin B2 3 mg • Niacin 40 mg • Pantothenic Acid 20 mg • Vitamin B6 4 mg • Vitamin B12 75 mcg • Folic Acid 400 mcg • Biotin 300 mcg • Vitamin C 150 mg • Vitamin D (D3) 400 IU • Vitamin E (d-alpha-tocopheryl succinate) 66 IU • Vitamin K 100 mcg • Calcium 50 mg • Chromium 120 mcg • Copper 1000 mcg • Iodine 150 mcg • Magnesium 25 mg • Potassium 108 mg • Selenium 55 mcg • Silicon 2 mg • Zinc 7.5 mg. Other Ingredients: Fructose, Citric Acid, Orange Fruit Powder, Mandarin Fruit Powder, Malic Acid, Glucose, Natural Orange Flavor, Tricalcium Phosphate, Sucralose.

NutraMetrix OPC-3 - Market America, Inc.
Each capful (3.33 g) contains: Grape seed extract 25 mg • Red Wine extract 25 mg • Pine bark extract 25 mg • Bilberry extract 25 mg • Citrus Bioflavonoids extract 25 mg • Potassium (bicarbonate) 93 mg. Other Ingredients: Fructose, Glucose, Citric Acid, Maltodextrin, Silica, Calcium Sulfate, Pectin.

NutraMetrix Prostate Health Formula - Market America, Inc.
Two tablets contain: Zinc Citrate 30 mg • Selenium (as selenomethionine) 100 mcg • Saw Palmetto berry (serenoa repens) 400 mg • Pygeum Africanum bark extract (standardized to contain 14% beta-sitosterol and 0.5% docosanol) 100 mg • Prostate Health Proprietary Blend 425 mg: Chrysanthemum flower (dendranthema morifolium tzvel.), San-Qi Ginseng root (Panax notoginseng burk.), Dyer's Woad leaf (isatis indigotica fort.), Baikal Skullcap root (scutellaria baicalensis georgi), Reishi stem (ganoderma lucidum karst), Rhabdosia leaf (rhabdosia rubescens hara), Licorice root (glycyrrhiza uralensis fisch). Other Ingredients: Microcrystalline Cellulose, Stearic Acid, Magnesium Stearate, Silicon Dioxide, Croscarmellose Sodium, Dicalcium Phosphate.

NutraMetrix Vision Support Formula - Market America, Inc.
Each capful (3.33 g) contains: Beta Carotene 5000 IU • Vitamin C (ascorbic acid) 75 mg • Vitamin E (d, l-alpha-tocopheryl acetate) 33 IU • Potassium (bicarbonate) 150 mg • Zinc (lactate) 7 mg • Chromium (arginate) 100 mcg • Copper (gluconate) 100 mcg • Bilberry 50 mg • Taurine 42 mg • Quercetin 25 mg • Eyebright 10 mg • Lutein 7 mg • Lycopene 2 mg • Zeaxanthin 1.4 mg. Other Ingredients: Fructose, Natural Orange Powder, Citric Acid, Natural Orange Flavor, Malic Acid, Calcium Phosphate, Glucose, Silica, Sucralose.

NutraMetrix Vitamin C - Market America, Inc.
Each capful (3.33 g) contains: Vitamin C (ascorbic acid) 500 mg • Beta-Carotene (vitamin A precursor) 800 IU • Potassium (bicarbonate) 101 mg. Other Ingredients: Fructose, Glucose, Maltodextrin, Malic Acid, Natural Orange Flavor, Silica, Citric Acid.

Nutramin Body System - Informulab
One Capsule contains: Vitamin A (Beta Carotene) 1562 IU • Vitamin C 125 mg • Vitamin E 25 IU • Vitamin B-1 (Thiamine Mononitrate) 2.5 mg • Vitamin B2 (Riboflavin) 2.5 mg • Vitamin B6 (Pyridoxine HCl) 2.5 mg • Vitamin B12 (Cyanocobalamin) 2.5 mcg • Vitamin B3 (Niacinimide) 5 mg • Vitamin B5 (Pantothenic Acid) 10 mg • Vitamin B8 (Folic Acid) 50 mcg • Biotin (Water soluble Vit. B) 12.5 mcg • Vitamin D 50 IU • Calcium (Amino acid chelate) 62.5 mg • Phosphorus (Di-calcium phosphate) 6.25 mg • Magnesium (Amino acid chelate) 37.5 mg • Iron (Amino acid chelate) 2.25 mg • Zinc (Amino acid chelate) 1.875 mg • Manganese (Amino acid chelate) 0.625 mg • Copper (Amino acid chelate) 0.25 mg • Chromium Chelavite 18.75 mcg • Selenium (Amino acid chelate) 0.625 mcg • Potassium (Amino acid chelate) 3.125 mg • Iodine (as Potassium iodine) 18.75 mcg • Horsetail Herb 3.125 mg • White Willow Bark 3.125 mg • Bee Pollen 3.125 mg • Hops Flower 3.125 mg • Licorice Root 3.125 mg • Skullcap 3.125 mg • Valerian 3.125 mg • Garlic (Bulb-odorless) 3.125 mg • Citrus Bioflavonoids 3.125 mg • Rosehips 3.125 mg • Rutin 3.125 mg • Ginseng Root (Siberian) 3.125 mg • Alfalfa Herb 3.125 mg • Ginkgo Leaf 3.125 mg • Hawthorne Berry 3.125 mg • Beet Root 3.125 mg • Cayenne Fruit 3.125 mg • L-Lysine 3.125 mg • L-Proline 3.125 mg • L-Glutamine 3.125 mg • Live Food Enzyme Blend (vegetable source Protease, Lipase and Amylase) 6.25 mg • Pycnogenol 0.25 mg.

Nutramine - Calwood Nutritionals
Each scoop contains: L-Histidine 280 mg • L-Isoleucine 360 mg • L-Leucine 560 mg • L-Lysine 410 mg • L-Methionine 560 mg • L-Phenylalanine 560 mg • L-Threonine 250 mg • L-Tryptophan 130 mg • L-Valine 410 mg.

Nutramine T - Calwood Nutritionals
Two scoops contain: L-Histidine 220 mg • L-Isoleucine 290 mg • L-Leucine 440 mg • L-Lysine 310 mg • L-Methionine 440 mg • L-Phenylalanine 340 mg • L-Threonine 320 mg • L-Tryptophan 120 mg • L-Valine 360 mg • L-Tyrosine 660 mg.

NutraSleep - Source Naturals
Four tablets contain: Niacinamide 10 mg • Vitamin B6 (Pyridoxine HCl) 2 mg • Calcium (citrate and carbonate) 250 mg • Magnesium (citrate, oxide and taurinate) 450 mg • Taurine (Magnesium taurinate) 1000 mg • Inositol 700 mg • GABA (Gamma Amino Butyric Acid) 600 mg • Skullcap 250 mg • Passionflower 200 mg • Valerian root 200 mg • Chamomile extract 100 mg.

NutraSpray Quercetin - Source Naturals
Each spray contains: Quercetin 50 mg.

NutraStart Meal Replacement Drink (Vanilla, Chocolate) - 4 Life
Two scoops contain: Vitamin A (as palmitate) 2500 IU • Vitamin C (as ascorbic acid) 144 mg • Vitamin D (as cholecalciferol) 200 IU • Vitamin E (as D-alpha tocopheryl acetate) 15 IU • Thiamin (as thiamin mononitrate) 800 mcg • Riboflavin 900 mcg • Niacin (as niacinamide) 10 mg • Vitamin B6 (as pyridoxine hydrochloride) 1 mg • Folate (as folic acid) 200 mcg • Vitamin B12 (as cyanocobalamin) 3 mcg • Biotin 150 mcg • Pantothenic Acid (as D-calcium pantothenate) 5 mg • Calcium (Vanilla flavor 74 mg, Chocolate flavor 75 mg) • Iron (from iron amino acid chelate and soy protein isolate) 3 mg • Iodine (from potassium iodide) 75 mg • Zinc (from zinc amino acid chelate) 3 mg • Copper (as copper amino acid chelate and soy protein isolate) 1 mg • Transfer Factor E-XF from Bovine Colostrum and Egg yolk. Other Ingredients: Crystalline Fructose, Soy Protein Isolate, Maltodextrin, Whey Protein Concentrate, Soy Fiber, Maltodextrin Fiber, Sunflower Oil, Corn Syrup Solids, Natural Flavors, Cellulose Gum, Sodium Caseinate, Mono- and Diglycerides, Dipotassium Phoshpate, Dicalcium Phosphate.

Nutra-Support Bone - J. R. Carlson Laboratories, Inc.
Three softgels contain: Vitamin D (D3, cholecalciferol) 2000 IU • Calcium (from calcium carbonate and glycinate c) 1000 mg • Magnesium (as magnesium oxide and magnesium gly) 400 mg • Manganese (as manganese glycinate chelate) 2 mg • Boron (as boron glycinate chelate) 3 mg.

Nutra-Support Energy - J. R. Carlson Laboratories, Inc.
Two capsules contain: Thiamin (vitamin B1, as thiamin mononitrate) 15 mg • Riboflavin (vitamin B2) 17 mg • Niacin (vitamin B3, as niacinamide) 20 mg • Vitamin B6 (as pyridoxine hydrochloride) 20 mg • Folate (folic acid) 400 mcg • Vitamin B12 (cyanocobalamin) 60 mcg • Pantothenic Acid (as di-calcium pantothenate) 100 mg • Magnesium (as magnesium oxide) 100 mg • American Ginseng (10% ginsenosides) 600 mg • Co-Q10 (coenzyme Q10) 30 mg • L-Carnitine 30 mg.

Nutra-Support Immune - J. R. Carlson Laboratories, Inc.
Two capsules contain: Vitamin C (as ascorbic acid) 200 mg • Vitamin E (as D-alpha tocopheryl succinate) 100 IU • Riboflavin (vitamin B2) 5 mg • Selenium (as L-selenomethionine) 200 mcg • Milk Thistle seeds extract (silybum marianum) 140 mg • Asparagus concentrate (asparagus officinalis) 25 mg • NAC (N-acetyl cysteine) 200 mg • Alpha Lipoic 50 mg • Garlic bulb (allium sativum, odorless) 100 mg • Glutathione 10 mg • L-Glutamine 50 mg • L-Glycine 50 mg.

Some Brand Name Natural Products - What they Contain

www.NaturalDatabase.com contains MANY more listings than appear here.
Editor's Notes are located on pages 2155-2163.

Nutra-Support Joint Cartilage Builder - J. R. Carlson Laboratories, Inc.
Three tablets contain: Vitamin C (as calcium ascorbate) 60 mg • MSM (methylsulfonylmethane) 240 mg • Potassium (supplied by glucosamine) 190 mg • Cartilage (US source, bovine) 1000 mg • Glucosamine Sulfate (KCl) 1500 mg.

Nutra-Support Memory - J. R. Carlson Laboratories, Inc.
Two softgels contain: Phosphatidyl Serine (from soybeans) 100 mg • Ginkgo Biloba leaves (24% ginkgoflavone glycosides) 100 mg • Acetyl-L-Carnitine 100 mg • DHA (docosahexaenoic acid) 200 mg • L-Glutamine 200 mg.

Nutra-Support Prostate - J. R. Carlson Laboratories, Inc.
Two softgels contain: Selenium (as L-selenomethionine) 200 mcg • Zinc (as zinc amino acid chelate) 30 mg • Gamma Tocopherol 50 mg • Glycine 100 mg • Beta Sitosterol 60 mg • Stinging Nettle root (standardized to 30PPM scopoletin) 100 mg • Pygeum Africanum (standardized to 25% sterols) 50 mg • Lycopene 10 mg • Saw Palmetto berry extract (serenoa repens, 90% fatty acids) 320 mg • Boron (as boron glcyinate chelate) 3 mg • L-Alanine 100 mg • L-Glutamine 100 mg.

Nutri Fiber - Progressive Labs
One tablespoon contains: Calcium 10.2 mg • Iron 0.35% • Thiamin (Vitamin B1) 0.36 mg • Riboflavin (Vitamin B2) 0.18 mg • Niacin 1.89 mg • Vitamin B6 1.66 mg • Pantothenic Acid 044 mg • Phosphorus 11.5 mg • Magnesium 31.8 mg • Zinc 2.42 mg • Copper 0.26 mg • Manganese 0.13 mg • Sodium 0.6% • Potassium 34.2 mg • Linolenic Acid (omega 3) 1.36 g.

Nutri Plex - The Sports Nutrition Source, Inc.
One and a half scoops contain: Sodium 200 mg • Potassium 680 mg • Protein 25 g • Vitamin A 2500 IU • Vitamin C 30 mg • Calcium 800 mg • Iron 9 mg • Vitamin D 200 IU • Vitamin E 15 IU • Pantothenic Acid 5 mg • Vitamin B-1 75 mg • Vitamin B-2 85 mg • Vitamin B-3 10 mg • Vitamin B-6 1 mg • Vitamin B-12 3 mcg • Biotin 125 mcg • Zinc 7.5 mcg • Copper 1 mg • Magnesium 200 mg • Manganese 2 mg • Iodine 75 mcg • Phosphorus 160 mg • Selenium 32 mcg • Molybdenum 60 mcg • Chromium 78 mcg.

Nutri/Digest - Hillestad
Each tablet contains: Amylase (fungal) 60 mg • Lipase 75 mg • Papain / Papaya leaf 60 mg • Pineapple 25 mg • Angelica (from extract concentrate) 100 mg • Parsley leaf (from extract concentrate) 100 mg • Annatto seed 25 mg • Aloe Vera leaf (from concentrate) 1000 mg. Other Ingredients: Sorbitol, Fructose, Celluose, Ethyl Cellulose, Magnesium Stearate, Stearic Acid.

Nutri/Vein - Hillestad
Each tablet contains: Vitamin C (ascorbic acid) 125 mg • Calcium (oyster shell and calcium citrate) 150 mg • Butchers Broom root 150 mg • Gotu-Kola leaf (from extract concentrate) 50 mg • Horse Chestnut seed 50 mg • Hawthorn berries 50 mg • Grape seed extract 30 mg • Witch Hazel leaf & bark 25 mg • Rutin flower 100 mg • Citrus Bioflavonoid fruit 50 mg. Other Ingredients: Cellulose, Ethyl Cellulose, Magnesium Stearate, Glyceryl Stearate, Silicon Dioxide.

Nutri-1000 - The Vitamin Shoppe
Each tablet contains: Vitamin D 400 IU • Vitamin A 25000 IU • Vitamin C 100 mg • Vitamin E 100 IU • Vitamin B1 100 mg • Vitamin B2 100 mg • Vitamin B6 100 mg • Vitamin B12 100 mcg • Niacinamide 100 mg • PABA 100 mg • Pantothenic Acid 100 mg • Choline 100 mg • Inositol 100 mg • Biotin 100 mcg • Folic Acid 400 mcg • Rutin 25 mg • Citrus Bioflavonoid Complex 25 mg • Hesperidin Complex 5 mg • Betaine Hydrochloride 25 mg • Glutamic Acid 25 mg • Iodine 150 mcg • Calcium 50 mg • Potassium 15 mg • Iron 25 mg • Magnesium 20 mg Manganese 6.1 mg • Zinc 20 mg • Chromium 15 mcg • Selenium 10 mcg. In a whole-food base of rice concentrate, parsley, kelp, alfalfa, green cabbage, acerola, sarsaparilla, watercress, and golden seal.

Nutri-All Multiple Powder - Nature's Life
Each scoop (about 15 g) contains: Vitamin A (Beta Carotene) 20,000 IU • Vitamin E (d-Alpha Tocopheryl Acetate) 390 IU • Vitamin B1 (Thiamine Mononitrate) 30 mg • Vitamin B2 (Riboflavin) 30 mg • Vitamin B3 (Niacinamide) 110 mg • Vitamin B6 (Pyridoxine HCl) 30 mg • Vitamin B12 (Cobalamin concentrate) 30 mcg • Folic Acid 400 mcg • Biotin 30 mcg • Pantothenic Acid (D-Calcium Pantothenate) 110 mg • Inositol 110 mg • Choline (Citrate) 110 mg • Vitamin C 510 mg • Lemon Bioflavonoids (TESTLAB 50% Flavonoids) 100 mg • Rutin 30 mg • Boron (Proteinate) 25 mcg • Calcium (Carbonate, Ascorbate, Citrate/Malate) 800 mg • Chromium (Polinicotinate, Aspartate) 60 mcg • Copper (Citrate) 1 mg • Iodine (Kelp) 22.5 mg • Iron (Fumerate) 8 mg • Magnesium (Oxide, Citrate) 400 mg • Manganese (Citrate) 4 mg • Molybdenum (Molybdate) 60 mcg • Potassium 99 mg • Selenium (selenomethionine) 60 mcg • Silicone (Dioxide) 10 mg • Zinc (Picolinate) 20 mg. In a natural base of Protein powder, Oat Fiber, Rice Syrup solids, Psyllium husks & natural Orange flavor. Contains 10 mg of naturally occurring Sodium.

Nutri-All Multiple Softgel - Nature's Life
Six softgel capsules contain: Beta Carotene (Vitamin A equivalent 10000 IU) 6 mg • Vitamin A (Fish Liver oil) 10000 IU • Vitamin D (as Vitamin D3) (Cholecalciferol) 400 IU • Vitamin B1 (Thiamine Mononitrate) 80 mg • Vitamin B2 (Riboflavin) 80 mg • Vitamin B3 (Niacinamide) 80 mg • Vitamin B6 (Pyridoxine HCl) 80 mg • Folic Acid 400 mcg • Vitamin B12 (Trituration of concentrate) 100 mcg • Biotin 50 mcg • Pantothenic Acid (d-Calcium Pantothenate) 80 mg • Choline Bitartrate 50 mg • Inositol 50 mg • Vitamin E (d-Alpha Tocopherol) 400 IU • Vitamin C (Ascorbic Acid & Rose Hips) 500 mg • Lemon Bioflavonoids (50% TESTLAB) 50 mg • Rutin Complex (Dimorphandra mollis) 25 mg • Hesperidin Complex (Citrus) 25 mg • Calcium (Carbonate) 1000 mg • Chromium (Picolinate, Nutrition 21) 200 mcg • Copper (Gluconate) 1 mg • Iodine (Potassium Iodide) 225 mcg • Magnesium (Oxide) 600 mg • Manganese (Citrate) 10 mg • Molybdenum (Molybdate) 20 mcg • Potassium (Citrate) 50 mg • Selenium (l-Selenomethionine) 50 mcg • Vanadium (Vanadyl Sulfate) 20 mcg • Zinc (Citrate) 15 mg • Betaine HCl 25 mg • CoEnzyme Q10 5 mg • Chlorophyll (oil-soluble) 100 mg. In a natural base of Safflower oil, Lecithin & Soy.

NutriBiotic Capsules Plus - NutriBiotic
Grapefruit extract • Echinacea extract • Artemisa annua extract.

NutriBiotic Tablets - NutriBiotic
Grapefruit extract 100 mg.

Nutri-Cal Hearts - Nature's Plus
Two chewable tablets contain: Vitamin D (as ergocalciferol) 100 IU • Calcium (as lactate, aspartate, gluconate, carbonate) 500 mg • Magnesium (as gluconate, aspartate, hydroxide) 250 mg. Other Ingredients: Fructose, Acacia Gum, Stearic Acid, Silica, Malted Milk, Nonfat Milk, Vanilla, Whey.

Nutri-Calm - Nature's Sunshine
Each tablet contains: Vitamin C (ascorbic acid) 400 mg • Vitamin B1 (thiamine) 20 mg • Vitamin B2 (riboflavin) 20 mg • Niacin (niacinamide) 40 mg • Vitamin B6 (pyridoxine) 20 mg • Folic Acid 125 mcg • Vitamin B12 (cyanocobalamin) 34 mcg • Biotin 100 mcg • Pantothenic Acid (D-calcium pantothenate) 80 mg. Other Ingredients: Schisandra Fruit (schisandra chinensis), Choline (bitartrate), Wheat Germ Flour, Inositol, Bee Pollen, Para Aminobenzoic Acid (PABA), Lemon Bioflavonoid, Valerian Root Concentrate (valeriana officinalis), Passion Flower Concentrate (passiflora incarnata), Hops Flower Concentrate (humulus lupulus), Di-Calcium Phosphate, Cellulose, Stearic Acid, Silicon Dioxide, Magnesium Stearate.

NutriClean Aloe - Market America, Inc.
Two tablets contain: Aloe Ferox leaf 860 mg • Aloe Barbadensis leaf 200 mg. Other Ingredients: Dicalcium Phosphate, Microcrystalline Cellulose, Croscarmellose Sodium, Stearic Acid, Magnesium Stearate, Silica, Pharmaceutical Glaze.

NutriClean Fiber Powder **-** Market America, Inc.
Each scoop (15.7 g) contains: Vitamin A (as beta-carotene) 2000 IU • L-Glutamine 1000 mg • NutriClean Fiber Blend 13.3 g: Soy Fiber, Soluble Fiber complex, Alfalfa leaf, Beet root fiber, Flax seed fiber, Guar Gum, Inulin, Oat Bran, Psyllium seed husk • Probiotic Blend 1.5 billion CFU: Lactobacillus Acidophilus, Lactobacilllus Plantarum, Lactobacillus Sporogenes (Lactospore brand encapsulated L. sporogenes), Bifidobacterium Bifidum, Lactobacillus Casei. Other Ingredients: Citric Acid, Natural Flavors, Acesulfame Potassium, Silica, Sucralose.

NutriClean HepatoCleanse **-** Market America, Inc.
Two capsules contain: Proprietary Blend 1260 mg: Milk Thistle seed extract (standardized to 80% silymarin), N-Acetyl-L-Cysteine, Dandelion root, Garlic bulb, Hawthorn berry extract, Schizandra Chinensis fruit and seed extract, Yellow Dock root, Burdock root, Licorice root, Barberry bark, Rosemary leaf, Ginger root, Bayberry root bark, Green Tea leaf extract, Hyssop (aerial parts), Red Clover flower, Curcumin root extract. Other Ingredients: Calcium Sulfate, Gelatin, Magnesium Stearate, Silica.

NutriClean Release **-** Market America, Inc.
Two tablets contain: Proprietary Blend 1160 mg: Rhubarb root, Buckthorn bark, Cascara Sagrada bark extract (20% hydroxyanthrocene derivatives, calculated as cascaroside A), Gentian root, Anise seed, Fennel seed, Black Walnut bark, Oregon Grape root, Scutellaria root extract, Goldenseal aerial parts, Peppermint leaf. Other Ingredients: Dicalcium Phosphate, Microcrystalline Cellulose, Croscarmellose Sodium, Stearic Acid, Silica, Magnesium Stearate, Pharmaceutical Glaze.

Nutri-Cleanse **-** Nu-Creations
Each tablet contains: Aloe Vera resin 430 mg • Aloe Vera leaf 200 mg. Other Ingredients: Anise, Fennel, Psyllium, Rhubarb, Kelp, Flax, Dicalcium Phosphate, Pharmaceutical Glaze, Magnesium Stearate.

NutriCology 5HTP, 5-L-Hydroxytryptophan **-** Allergy Research Group
Each capsule contains: 5HTP (5-L-hydroxytryptophan) 50 mg. Other Ingredients: Cellulose, Stearic Acid, Silicon Dioxide.

NutriCology Acetyl-L-Carnitine (250 mg) **-** Allergy Research Group
Each capsule contains: Acetyl-L-Carnitine 250 mg. Other Ingredients: Cellulose, Silicon Dioxide, Stearic Acid.

NutriCology Acetyl-L-Carnitine (500 mg) **-** Allergy Research Group
Each capsule contains: Acetyl-L-Carnitine 500 mg. Other Ingredients: Cellulose, Silicon Dioxide, Stearic Acid.

NutriCology Adrenal Cortex, Organic Glandular **-** Allergy Research Group
Each capsule contains: Adrenal Cortex tissue (bovine). Other Ingredients: Cellulose, Magnesium Stearate.
See Editor's Note No. 14.

NutriCology Adrenal, Organic Glandular **-** Allergy Research Group
Each capsule contains: Adrenal tissue (bovine) 300 mg. Other Ingredients: Cellulose, Silicon Dioxide, Stearic Acid.
See Editor's Note No. 14.

NutriCology Aller-Aid Formula II **-** Allergy Research Group
Each capsule contains: Iodine (from kelp) 30 mcg • Selenium (from kelp) 200 mcg • Macrocystis Pyrifera (kelp) 200 mg. Other Ingredients: Silicon Dioxide, Magnesium Stearate.

NutriCology AngioBlock **-** Allergy Research Group
Four capsules contain: Convolvulus Arvensis leaves extract 1000 mg. Other Ingredients: Maltodextrin.

NutriCology AntiOx, Cysteine Free **-** Allergy Research Group
Each capsule contains: Vitamin A (40% as retinyl palmitate and 60% as beta-carotene) 12,500 IU • Vitamin C (as ascorbyl palmitate) 4 mg • Vitamin E (as DL-alpha-tocopheryl acetate) 100 IU • Thiamin (as thiamin hydrochloride) 10 mg • Riboflavin (80% as riboflavin and 20% as riboflavin-5-phosphate) 12.5 mg • Niacin (50% as niacinamide) 10 mg • Vitamin B6 (80% as pyridoxine hydrochloride and 20% as pyridoxal-5-phosphate) 12.5 mg • Folic Acid 100 mcg • Vitamin B12 (as cyanocobalamin) 100 mcg • Pantothenic Acid (as calcium pantothenate) 25 mg • Zinc (as zinc citrate) 7.5 mg • Selenium (87% as sodium selenite and 13% as selenomethionine) 75 mcg • Copper (as copper sebacate) 0.5 mg • Manganese (as manganese citrate) 5 mg • Glutathione (reduced) 50 mg • L-Methionine 75 mg • Taurine 75 mg • Trimethylglycine 50 mg • Coenzyme Q10 10 mg • Proanthocyanidins, as Grape seed extract 1.25 mg. Other Ingredients: Magnesium Stearate, Silicon Dioxide.

NutriCology Arthred Collagen Formula **-** Allergy Research Group
Two level scoops (10.5 g) contain: Hydrolyzed Collagen 10.5 g.
See Editor's Note No. 14.

NutriCology BestCafe **-** Allergy Research Group
Each 2 mL (60 drops) serving contains: Proprietary Blend 2 mL: Ginkgo Biloba, Catechins, Resveratrol, Ginsenoside. Other Ingredients: Natural Coffee Flavor, Glycerin, Purified Water.

NutriCology Bone Calcium Complex **-** Allergy Research Group
Three capsules contain: Vitamin C (as ascorbic acid) 67 mg • Vitamin D (as cholecalciferol) 130 IU • Vitamin K (as phytonadione) 67 mcg • Vitamin B6 (as pyridoxine hydrochloride and pyridoxal-5'-phosphate) 4.3 mg • Folic Acid 130 mcg • Calcium (as calcium hydroxyapatite) 270 mg • Magnesium (as magnesium citrate) 170 mg • Zinc (as zinc citrate) 3.3 mg • Copper 0.17 mg • Manganese (as manganese citrate) 2 mg • Chromium (as chromium nitrate) 50 mcg • Boron (as glycerol borate) 1 mg • Chondroitin Sulfate 130 mg • Horsetail dried stem extract (equisetum arvense) 8.3 mg • Dong Quai dried root extract (angelica sinensis) 83 mg • Licorice dried root extract (glycyrrhiza glabra) 83 mg • Alfalfa dried leaf extract (medicago sativa) 83 mg. Other Ingredients: Cellulose, Silicon Dioxide.
See Editor's Note No. 15.

NutriCology Brain Aid **-** Allergy Research Group
Each tablet contains: Vitamin A (as beta-carotene) 1000 IU • Vitamin C (as ascorbic acid) 5 mg • Vitamin E (as D-alpha-tocopheryl acid succinate) 5 IU • Thiamin (67% as thiamin hydrochloride and 33% as TTFD) 7.5 mg • Riboflavin (67% as riboflavin hydrochloride and 33% as riboflavin-5-phosphate) 7.5 mg • Niacin (86% as niacinamide) 17.5 mg • Vitamin B6 (75% as pyridoxine hydrochloride and 25% as pyridoxal-5-phosphate) 10 mg • Folic Acid 50 mcg • Vitamin B12 (as dibencoside) 25 mcg • Biotin 50 mcg • Pantothenic Acid (as calcium pantothenate) 20 mg • Zinc (as zinc citrate) 5 mg • Selenium (90% as sodium selenite and 10% as selenomethionine) 25 mcg • Copper (as copper sebacate) 0.5 mg • Chromium (as chromium nicotinate) 25 mcg • Molybdenum (as sodium molybdate) 25 mcg • Boron (as boron citrate) 250 mcg • Ginkgo Biloba extract 15 mg • Siberian Ginseng extract 15 mg • Korean Ginseng extract 20 mg • Gotu Kola extract 50 mg • L-Glutamine 125 mg • L-Tyrosine 100 mg • Acetyl-L-Carnitine 25 mg • Choline Bitartrate 40 mg • Inositol 25 mg • DMAE (dimethylaminoethanol) 125 mg • Phosphatidylcholine 125 mg • Phosphatidylserine 10 mg • Quercetin 25 mg • Cayenne pepper 25 mg. Other Ingredients: Dicalcium Phosphate, Cellulose, Magnesium Stearate, Silicon Dioxide, Stearic Acid.

NutriCology BrainWave Plus **-** Allergy Research Group
Each capsule contains: Acetyl-L-Carnitine 100 mg • L-Glutamine 80 mg • Choline Bitartrate 40 mg • Phosphatidylserine 30 mg • Ginkgo Biloba extract (standardized to 24% ginkgo flavonglycosides and 6% terpene lactones) 24 mg • Siberian Ginseng 15:1 extract 20 mg • Panax Ginseng extract (standardized to 7% ginsenosides) 20 mg • Ashwaganda extract 20 mg • Gotu Kola (powdered) 10 mg • Royal

BRAND NAMES

Jelly 20 mg • Bacopa Monniera extract (standardized to 30% bacosides) 20 mg • Vinpocetine 2 mg • CDP - Choline 50 mg • Huperzine A 20 mcg • Thymus 20 mg • DMAE (dimethylaminoethanol) 20 mg. Other Ingredients: Cellulose, Magnesium Stearate, Silicon Dioxide.

NutriCology Buffered Vitamin C capsules - Allergy Research Group
Two capsules contain: Vitamin C (as ascorbic acid) 1000 mg • Calcium (as calcium carbonate) 190 mg • Magnesium (as magnesium carbonate) 104 mg • Potassium (as potassium carbonate) 16 mg. Other Ingredients: Cellulose, Stearic Acid.

NutriCology Buffered Vitamin C powder - Allergy Research Group
Each 1 tsp (4.7 g) serving contains: Vitamin C (as ascorbic acid) 2135 mg • Calcium (as calcium carbonate) 405 mg • Magnesium (as magnesium carbonate) 215 mg • Potassium (as potassium carbonate) 90 mg. Other Ingredients: Cellulose.

NutriCology ButyrEn - Allergy Research Group
Each tablet contains: Calcium (as calcium/magnesium butyrate) 100 mg • Magnesium (as calcium/magnesium butyrate) 100 mg • Butyrate 815 mg. Other Ingredients: Dicalcium Phosphate, Celluose, Magnesium Stearate, Silicon Dioxide.

NutriCology Calcium Citrate - Allergy Research Group
Each capsule contains: Calcium (as calcium citrate) 150 mg. Other Ingredients: Stearic Acid.

NutriCology Calcium Magnesium Citrate - Allergy Research Group
Each capsule contains: Calcium (as calcium citrate) 100 mg • Magnesium (as magnesium citrate) 100 mg. Other Ingredients: Stearic Acid, Cellulose.

NutriCology Calcium Pyruvate - Allergy Research Group
Each capsule contains: Calcium (as calcium pyruvate) 110 mg • Pyruvate 530 mg. Other Ingredients: Stearic Acid.

NutriCology Children's Multi-Vi-Min - Allergy Research Group
Each capsule contains: Vitamin A (as retinyl palmitate) 800 IU • Vitamin E (as DL-alpha-tocopheryl-acetate) 16 IU • Thiamin (as thiamin hydrochloride) 4 mg • Riboflavin (as riboflavin-5-phosphate) 2 mg • Niacin (as niacinamide) 2 mg • Vitamin B6 (as pyridoxine hydrochloride and pyridoxal-5-phosphate) 6.2 mg • Folic Acid 12 mcg • Vitamin B12 32 mcg • Biotin 16 mcg • Pantothenic Acid (as calcium pantothenate) 20 mg • Iron (as ferric ammonium citrate) 0.7 mg • Magnesium (as magnesium citrate) 10 mg • Zinc (as zinc citrate) 1.1 mg • Selenium (as sodium selenite) 8 mcg • Copper (as copper citrate) 60 mcg • Manganese (as manganese citrate) 0.6 mcg • Chromium (as amino acid complex) 16 mcg • Molybdenum (as sodium molybdate) 8 mcg • Potassium (as potassium chloride) 4 mg • Vanadium (as vanadium pentoxide) 8 mcg • PABA (para-aminobenzoic acid) 8 mg • Glutamic Acid 8 mg. Other Ingredients: Cellulose, Magnesium Stearate, Silicon Dioxide.

NutriCology Chitosan - Allergy Research Group
Two capsules contain: Chitosan 1 g. Other Ingredients: Stearic Acid.

NutriCology Chromium Complex with ChromeMate - Allergy Research Group
Each capsule contains: Niacin 50 mg • Vitamin B6 (as pyridoxine hydrochloride) 20 mg • Chromium (as chromium nicotinate) 250 mcg • L-Glutathione (reduced) 2.5 mg • Guar Gum (cyamopsis tetragonolobus, galactomannan) 450 mg. Other Ingredients: Cellulose, Magnesium Stearate, Silicon Dioxide.

NutriCology Coagulase Oxygenation Formula, Fibrenase II - Allergy Research Group
Each tablet contains: Proprietary Blend 500 mg: Panax Notoginseng root, Crataegus Oxyacantha fruit, Centella Asiatica leaves, Salvia Miltiorrhiza root. Other Ingredients: Cellulose, Stearic Acid.

NutriCology Complete Heart - Allergy Research Group
Each scoop (20 g) contains: Vitamin A (as beta-carotene) 2000 IU • Vitamin C (as ascorbic acid) 500 mg • Vitamin D (D3) 100 IU • Vitamin E (as D-alpha-tocopherol) 320 IU • Vitamin K 80 mcg • Thiamin (vitamin B1) 30 mg • Riboflavin (vitamin B2) 30 mg • Niacin 160 mg • Vitamin B6 16 mg • Folic Acid 320 mg • Vitamin B12 80 mcg • Biotin 240 mcg • Pantothenic Acid 100 mg • Calcium (as calcium citrate/gluconate) 280 mg • Magnesium (as magnesium glycinate/gluconate) 160 mg • Zinc (as zinc arginate) 12 mg • Selenium (as sodium selenite/selenomethionine) 80 mcg • Copper (as copper glycinate) 0.8 mg • Manganese (as manganese glycinate) 1 mg • Chromium (as chromium polynicotinate) 160 mcg • Molybdenum (as sodium molybdate) 40 mcg • Potassium (as potassium gluconate) 40 mg • Boron (as boron citrate) 0.4 mg • Vanadium (as vanadium pentoxide) 80 mcg • Alpha-Carotene 8 mg • Pregnenolone 6 mg • Dehydroepiandrosterone (DHEA) 6 mg • Coenzyme Q10 60 mg • Inositol 50 mg • Choline 50 mg • Para-Aminobenzoic Acid (PABA) 20 mg • Lecithin (26% phosphatidylcholine) 500 mg • L-Alanine 30 mg • L-Arginine 480 mg • L-Aspartic Acid 85 mg • L-Carnitine 200 mg • L-Cystine 10 mg • L-Glutamine 600 mg • Glycine 30 mg • L-Histidine 20 mg • L-Isoleucine 35 mg • L-Leucine 60 mg • L-Lysine 45 mg • L-Methionine 160 mg • L-Ornithine 200 mg • L-Phenylalanine 38 mg • L-Proline 38 mg • L-Serine 38 mg • Taurine 500 mg • L-Threonine 28 mg • L-Tyrosine 220 mg • L-Valine 40 mg • N-Acetyl-L-Cysteine 200 mg • Glutathione 100 mg • Pancreatin 10 mg • Papain 16 mg • Bromelain 20 mg • Grape skin extract 200 mg • Hawthorn berry extract 200 mg • Garlic (1% allicin) 100 mg • Lutein 2 mg • Lycopene 0.4 mg • Tocotrienols 20 mg • Trimethylglycine 200 mg • Methylsulfonylmethane 80 mg • Eicosapentaenoic Acid (EPA) 145 mg • Docosahexaenoic Acid (DHA) 95 mg • Gamma-Linolenic Acid 90 mg • Linolenic Acid 220 mg • Oleic Acid 85 mg • Palmitic Acid 65 mg • Stearic Acid 25 mg • Flax Seed oil 400 mg • Lipoic Acid 30 mg. Other Ingredients: Oat Bran, Honey Powder, Rice Bran, Psyllium Bran, Apple Fiber, Lemon Flavor, Stevia.

NutriCology Complete Heart II without Hormones - Allergy Research Group
Each scoop (20 g) contains: Vitamin A (as beta-carotene) 2000 IU • Vitamin C (as ascorbic acid) 500 mg • Vitamin D (D3) 100 IU • Vitamin E (as D-alpha-tocopherol) 320 IU • Vitamin K 80 mcg • Thiamin (vitamin B1) 30 mg • Riboflavin (vitamin B2) 30 mg • Niacin 160 mg • Vitamin B6 16 mg • Folic Acid 320 mg • Vitamin B12 80 mcg • Biotin 240 mcg • Pantothenic Acid 100 mg • Calcium (as calcium citrate/gluconate) 280 mg • Magnesium (as magnesium glycinate/gluconate) 160 mg • Zinc (as zinc arginate) 12 mg • Selenium (as sodium selenite/selenomethionine) 80 mcg • Copper (as copper glycinate) 0.8 mg • Manganese (as manganese glycinate) 1 mg • Chromium (as chromium polynicotinate) 160 mcg • Molybdenum (as sodium molybdate) 40 mcg • Potassium (as potassium gluconate) 40 mg • Boron (as boron citrate) 0.4 mg • Vanadium (as vanadium pentoxide) 80 mcg • Alpha-Carotene 8 mg • Coenzyme Q10 60 mg • Inositol 50 mg • Choline 50 mg • Para-Aminobenzoic Acid (PABA) 20 mg • Lecithin (26% phosphatidylcholine) 500 mg • L-Alanine 30 mg • L-Arginine 480 mg • L-Aspartic Acid 85 mg • L-Carnitine 200 mg • L-Cystine 10 mg • L-Glutamine 600 mg • Glycine 30 mg • L-Histidine 20 mg • L-Isoleucine 35 mg • L-Leucine 60 mg • L-Lysine 45 mg • L-Methionine 160 mg • L-Ornithine 200 mg • L-Phenylalanine 38 mg • L-Proline 38 mg • L-Serine 38 mg • Taurine 500 mg • L-Threonine 28 mg • L-Tyrosine 220 mg • L-Valine 40 mg • N-Acetyl-L-Cysteine 200 mg • Glutathione 100 mg • Pancreatin 10 mg • Papain 16 mg • Bromelain 20 mg • Grape skin extract 200 mg • Hawthorn berry extract 200 mg • Garlic (1% allicin) 100 mg • Lutein 2 mg • Lycopene 0.4 mg • Tocotrienols 20 mg • Trimethylglycine 200 mg • Methylsulfonylmethane 80 mg • Eicosapentaenoic Acid (EPA) 145 mg • Docosahexaenoic Acid (DHA) 95 mg • Gamma-Linolenic Acid 90 mg • Linolenic Acid 220 mg • Oleic Acid 85 mg • Palmitic Acid 65 mg • Stearic Acid 25 mg • Flax Seed oil 400 mg • Lipoic Acid 30 mg. Other Ingredients: Oat Bran, Honey Powder, Rice Bran, Psyllium Bran, Apple Fiber, Lemon Flavor, Stevia.

NutriCology Complete Immune - Allergy Research Group
Each serving scoop (20 g) provides: Co-Enzyme Q10 75 mg • Grape seed extract (95%) 250 mg • Alpha Carotene 5 mg • Beta Carotene (from mixed carotenoids) 7500 IU • Lycopene 1.5 mg • Vitamin E (mixed tocopherols) 200 IU • Vitamin C 1175 mg • Folic Acid 400 mcg • Vitamin A 2500 IU • Vitamin B1 23 mg • Vitamin B2 23 mg • Vitamin B3 (niacinamide) 150 mg • Vitamin B3 (niacin) 10 mg • Vitamin B5 150 mg • Vitamin B6 25 mg • Vitamin B12 200 mcg • Biotin 200 mcg • Inositol hexaphosphate 175 mg • Choline 63 mg • Germanium Sesquioxide 50 mg • N-Acetyl Cysteine 375 mg • Glutathione 175 mg • L-Carnitine 100 mg • Calcium (carbonate, glycinate) 50 mg • Magnesium (carbonate, glycinate) 75 mg • Vitamin D (as Vitamin D3) 200 IU • Zinc (arginate) 15 mg • Copper (glycinate) 1 mg • Potassium (ascorbate) 50 mg • Chromium (picolinate) 100 mcg • Molybdenum 125 mcg • Manganese 1.25 mg • Selenium 100 mcg • EPA 500 mg • Iron (aspartate) 1.5 mg • Iodine 75 mcg • MSM 100 mg • Borage oil 150 mg • Genistein from soy isolate 5 mg • Tocotrienol 25 mg • Biofavonoid complex 50 mg • Trimethyl Glycine 250 mg • Sulforaphane (broccoli) 50 mg • Beta Glucan (1-3) 25 mg • Green Tea extract 50 mg • Mushroom extract 1500 mg • Bromelain 163 mg • Turmeric 100 mg • Panax Ginseng 50 mg • Astragalus 50 mg • Taurine 250 mg • Lactoferrin 50 mg • In a base of Wheat bran, Whey protein, Oat bran, Rice bran, Psyllium bran, Apple fiber, Lemon flavor, Stevia, Lemon oil & Lime oil. This product was formerly known as Total Immune.

NutriCology Complete Nerve - Allergy Research Group
Each scoop (20 g) contains: Vitamin A (as beta-carotene) 1680 IU • Vitamin C (as ascorbic acid) 440 mg • Vitamin D (D3) 130 IU • Vitamin E (as mixed tocopherols) 360 IU • Vitamin K 45 mcg • Thiamin (vitamin B1) 22 mg • Riboflavin (vitamin B2) 22 mg • Niacin (as inositol hexanicotinate) 180 mg • Vitamin B6 22 mg • Folic Acid 350 mcg • Vitamin B12 22 mcg • Biotin 130 mcg • Pantothenic Acid 110 mg • Calcium (as calcium citrate/gluconate) 310 mg • Magnesium (as magnesium glycinate/gluconate) 130 mg • Zinc (as zinc arginate) 13 mg • Selenium (as sodium selenite/ selenomethionine) 90 mcg • Copper (as copper glycinate) 0.9 mg • Chromium (as chromium picolinate) 180 mcg • Potassium (as potassium gluconate) 45 mg • Alpha-Carotene 7 mg • Dehydroepiandrosterone (DHEA) 7 mg • Coenzyme Q10 67 mg • Inositol 22 mg • Choline 22 mg • Para-Aminobenzoic Acid 22 mg • Lecithin (26% phosphotidylcholine) 1440 mg • L-Alanine 35 mg • L-Arginine 110 mg • L-Aspartic Acid 95 mg • L-Carnitine 110 mg • L-Cystine 11 mg • L-Glutamine 67 mg • Glycine 67 mg • L-Histidine 22 mg • L-Isoleucine 45 mg • L-Lysine 50 mg • L-Methionine 180 mg • L-Ornithine Hydrochloride 220 mg • L-Phenylalanine 45 mg • L-Proline 45 mg • L-Serine 42 mg • Taurine 670 mg • L-Threonine 45 mg • L-Tyrosine 440 mg • N-Acetyl-L-Cysteine 440 mg • Glutathione (reduced) 110 mg • Pancreatin 13 mg • Papain 22 mg • Bromelain 22 mg • Grape skin extract 220 mg • Garlic (1% allicin) 45 mg • Lutein 1.8 mg • Lycopene 1.3 mg • Eicosapentaenoic Acid (EPA) 160 mg • Docosahexaenoic Acid (DHA) 110 mg • Palmitic Acid 130 mg • Stearic Acid 40 mg • Flax Seed Oil 440 mg • Lipoic Acid 45 mg • Methylsulfonylmethane 45 mg. Other Ingredients: Oat Bran, Rice Bran, Psyllium Bran, Stevia, Apple Fiber, Flavoring.

NutriCology Connection - Allergy Research Group
Two capsules contain: Vitamin C (as ascorbic acid) 33 mg • Vitamin E (as D-alpha-tocopheryl acid succinate) 55 IU • Calcium (as calcium citrate) 27 mg • Magnesium (as magnesium citrate) 40 mg • Zinc (as zinc citrate) 4 mg • Selenium (as sodium selenite/selenomethionine) 33 mcg • Copper (as copper sebacate) 0.27 mg • Manganese (as manganese citrate) 4.7 mg • Molybdenum (as sodium molybdate) 330 mcg • Boron (as boron citrate) 1.2 mg • N-Acetyl-D-Glucosamine 67 mg • Chondroitin Sulfate 130 mg • Glucosamine Sulfate 500 mg • L-Lysine 67 mg • L-Proline 107 mg • Hawthorne dried extract (crataegus oxyacantha) 295 mg • Horsetail dried extract (equisetum arvense) 6.7 mg • Bromelain 10 mg. Other Ingredients: Cellulose, Magnesium Stearate, Ethyl Vanillin.
See Editor's Note No. 15.

NutriCology Copper Sebacate - Allergy Research Group
Each capsule contains: Copper (as copper sebacate) 4 mg. Other Ingredients: Cellulose, Dicalcium Phosphate, Magnesium Stearate, Silicon Dioxide.

NutriCology DietEz Meal Replacement Powder - Allergy Research Group
Two scoops (40 g) contain: Vitamin A (56% as beta-carotene, 22% as vitamin A palmitate, 22% as carotenoid (mix)) 9000 IU • Vitamin C (as magnesium ascorbate) 300 mg • Calcium (as calcium citrate and phosphate) 300 mg • Iron (as ferric ammonium citrate) 3 mg • Vitamin D (D3, as cholecalciferol) 130 IU • Vitamin E (as mixed tocopherols) 100 IU • Thiamin (as thiamin hydrochloride) 15 mg • Riboflavin (as riboflavin-5-phosphate) 10 mg • Niacin (as niacinamide) 15 mg • Vitamin B6 (as pyridoxine hydrochloride) 15 mg • Folic Acid 100 mcg • Vitamin B12 (as methylcobalamin) 50 mcg • Biotin 150 mcg • Pantothenic Acid 200 mg • Phosphorus (as calcium phosphate and potassium phosphate) 142 mg • Iodine (as potassium iodide) 25 mcg • Magnesium (as magnesium citrate) 200 mg • Zinc (as zinc picolinate) 10 mg • Selenium (as selenomethionine) 50 mcg • Copper (as copper gluconate) 1 mg • Manganese (as manganese gluconate) 1.3 mg • Chromium (as chromium polynicotinate) 75 mcg • Molybdenum (as sodium molybdate) 50 mcg • Potassium (as potassium iodide and potassium phosphate) 120 mg • Boron (as sodium borate) 250 mcg • Vanadium (as sodium vanadate) 1000 mcg • N-Acetyl-L-Cysteine 50 mg • L-Glutathione (reduced) 50 mg • Glycine 1800 mg • Taurine 200 mg • L-Glutamine 1000 mg • Alpha-Lipoic Acid 20 mg • MSM (methylsulfonylmethane) 100 mg • Quercetin 100 mg • Green Tea extract (standardized to 40% catechins) 15 mg • Grape seed & skin extract (standardized to 95% polyphenols) 25 mg • Lactobacillus Sporogenes 300 million. Other Ingredients: Rice Protein Concentrate, Rice Syrup Solids, Cellulose, Natural Cherry Flavor.

NutriCology DietPlex - Allergy Research Group
Three tablets contain: Vitamin B6 (as pyridoxal-5-phosphate and pyridoxine hydrochloride) 22.5 mg • Calcium (as calcium pyruvate and dicalcium phosphate) 68 mg • Chromium (as chromium nicotinate) 6 mcg • Chitosan 600 mg • L-Carnitine 150 mg • Arthred (hydrolyzed collagen) 450 mg • Garcinia Cambogia fruit extract (75% hydroxycitric acid) 300 mg • Pyruvate (as calcium pyruvate) 320 mg. Other Ingredients: Dicalcium Phosphate, Modified Cellulose, Stearic Acid, Magnesium Stearate, Silicon Dioxide, Ethyl Vanillin.

NutriCology Enzocaine - Allergy Research Group
Two capsules contain: Zinc (as zinc methionate) 10 mg • Selenium (50% as sodium selenite and 50% as selenomethionine) 40 mcg • Copper (as coper sebacate) 1 mg • Molybdenum (as sodium molybdate) 300 mcg • MSM (methylsulfonylmethane) 500 mg • Boswellia Serrata gum extract (standardized to 70% boswellic acid) 200 mg • Turmeric (95% curcumin) 400 mg • Bromelain (3600 MCU/g) 400 mg • Ginger (5% gingerols) 40 mg • White Willow bark extract (salix alba, standardized to 15% salicin) 50 mg. Other Ingredients: Cellulose, Stearic Acid.

NutriCology EPO Evening Primrose Oil - Allergy Research Group
Each softgel contains: Evening Primrose Oil 500 mg providing Gamma-Linolenic Acid (omega-6) 45 mg and Linoleic Acid (omega-6) 375 mg.

NutriCology Ester-C Magnesium - Allergy Research Group
Each capsule contains: Vitamin C (as magnesium ascorbate) 500 mg • Magnesium (as magnesium ascorbate) 35 mg. Other Ingredients: Cellulose.

NutriCology Esterol with Ester-C - Allergy Research Group
Each capsule contains: Vitamin C (as calcium ascorbate) 675 mg • Calcium (as calcium ascorbate) 75 mg • Rutin 50 mg • quercetin 25 mg • Proanthocyanidins 2.5 mg. Other Ingredients: Magnesium Stearate, Silicon Dioxide.

NutriCology Flax Seed Oil liquid - Allergy Research Group
Each 1 tbsp (approx. 14 g) serving contains: Flax seed oil 14 g providing Alpha-Linolenic Acid (omega-3) 8.1 g, Linoleic Acid (omega-6) 2.3 g, Oleic Acid (omega-9) 2.2 g. Other Ingredients: Rosemary, Mixed Tocopherol, Ascorbyl Palmitate, Citric Acid.

NutriCology Flax Seed Oil softgels - Allergy Research Group
Each softgel contains: Flax Seed Oil 1000 mg providing Alpha-Linolenic Acid (omega-3) 570 mg, Linoleic Acid (omega-6) 155 mg, Oleic Acid (omega-9) 185 mg.

NutriCology Flax Seed powder - Allergy Research Group
Each 1 tbsp (approx. 9 g) serving contains: Flax seed powder 9 g providing Lignans 43 mg, Omega-3 Fatty Acids 670 mg, Omega-6 Fatty Acids 190 mg, Omega-9 Fatty Acids 210 mg.

NutriCology Free Aminos - Allergy Research Group
Each capsule contains: L-Alanine 41 mg • L-Arginine 62 mg • L-Cysteine 14 mg • L-Cystine 62 mg • L-Glutamine 28 mg • Glycine 28 mg • L-Histidine 49 mg • L-Isoleucine 69 mg • L-Leucine 69 mg • L-Lysine 98 mg • L-Methionine 14 mg • L-Phenylalanine 7.5 mg • L-Serine 14 mg • Taurine 4 mg • L-Threonine 56 mg • L-Tyrosine 28 mg • L-Valine 28 mg. Other Ingredients: Cellulose, Magnesium Stearate, Silicon Dioxide.

NutriCology Ginkgo Complex - Allergy Research Group
Each capsule contains: Vitamin B6 (as pyridoxal-5-phosphate) 5 mg • Folic Acid 400 mcg • Vitamin B12 (as cyanocobalamin) 400 mcg • L-Glutamine 200 mg • L-Phenylalanine 100 mg • L-Tyrosine 100 mg • Ribonucleic Acid (RNA) 18 mg • Ginkgo Biloba extract 70 mg. Other Ingredients: Magnesium Stearate, Silicon Dioxide.

NutriCology GLA Borage Oil - Allergy Research Group
Each softgel contains: Borage Oil 1.3 g • Gamma-Linolenic Acid (omega-6) 300 mg • Linoleic Acid (Omega-6) 480 mg.

NutriCology Glucosamine Sulfate - Allergy Research Group
Each capsule contains: Glucosamine Sulfate (sodium) 250 mg • Glucosamine Sulfate (potassium) 250 mg. Other Ingredients: Cellulose, Stearic Acid.

NutriCology IndoleGard - Allergy Research Group
Four capsules contain: BioResponse DIM (a patented diindolylmethane complex), Starch, DIM (25% min.), Vitamin E Succinate, Phosphatidylcholine, Silica 300 mg. Other Ingredients: Cellulose, Carbowax, Silicon Dioxide.

NutriCology L-Arginine - Allergy Research Group
Each capsule contains: L-Arginine 500 mg. Other Ingredients: Cellulose, Silicon Dioxide, Stearic Acid.

NutriCology L-Carnitine (250 mg) - Allergy Research Group
Each tablet contains: L-Carnitine 250 mg. Other Ingredients: Cellulose, Dicalcium Phosphate, Silicon Dioxide, Magnesium Stearate, Stearic Acid.

NutriCology L-Citruline - Allergy Research Group
Each 1-1/4 tsp (3 g) serving contains: L-Citruline 3 g.

NutriCology L-Glutamine (500 mg) - Allergy Research Group
Each capsule contains: L-Glutamine 500 mg. Other Ingredients: Cellulose, Stearic Acid.

NutriCology Liquid Molybdenum - Allergy Research Group
Each drop contains: Molybdenum (as ammonium molybdate) 25 mcg. Other Ingredients: Distilled Water.

NutriCology Liver, Organic Glandular - Allergy Research Group
Each capsule contains: Liver tissue (bovine) 500 mg. Other Ingredients: Silicon Dioxide, Magnesium Stearate.
See Editor's Note No. 14.

NutriCology L-Lysine - Allergy Research Group
Each capsule contains: L-Lysine 500 mg. Other Ingredients: Cellulose, Silicon Dioxide, Stearic Acid.

NutriCology L-Methionine - Allergy Research Group
Each capsule contains: L-Methionine 500 mg. Other Ingredients: Cellulose, Stearic Acid.

NutriCology L-Tyrosine - Allergy Research Group
Each capsule contains: L-Tyrosine 500 mg. Other Ingredients: Cellulose, Silicon Dioxide, Stearic Acid.

NutriCology Lutein 20 mg - Allergy Research Group
Each softgel contains: Vitamin E (as mixed tocopherols) 1 IU • Lutein 20 mg • Zeaxanthin 900 mcg. Other Ingredients: Safflower Oil, Yellow Beeswax, Corn Oil.

NutriCology Mathake Herb Tea - Allergy Research Group
Each bag contains: Mathake herb (teminalia catappa).

NutriCology Melatonin - Allergy Research Group
Each capsule contains: Melatonin 1.3 mg. Other Ingredients: Cellulose, Stearic Acid.
See Editor's Note No. 26.

NutriCology Modified Citrus Pectin capsules - Allergy Research Group
Three capsules contain: Modified Citrus Pectin 1.5 g.

NutriCology Modified Citrus Pectin powder - Allergy Research Group
Each 1 tsp (5 g) serving contains: Modified Citrus Pectin 5 g.

NutriCology MSM, Methylsulfonylmethane - Allergy Research Group
Each capsule contains: Methylsulfonylmethane 500 mg • Molybdenum 10 mcg. Other Ingredients: Cellulose, Silicon Dioxide, Stearic Acid.

NutriCology NAC, N-Acetyl-Cysteine - Allergy Research Group
Each tablet contains: N-Acetyl-L-Cysteine 500 mg. Other Ingredients: Dicalcium Phosphate, Cellulose, Magnesium Stearate, Silicon Dioxide, Stearic Acid.

NutriCology Nattokinase Fibrenase I - Allergy Research Group
Two capsules contain: Nattokinase 276 mg. Other Ingredients: Soybean Oil, Soybean Lecithin, Glycerin Fatty Acid Ester, Beeswax.

NutriCology Nattokinase with Vitamin E - Allergy Research Group
Two capsules contain: Vitamin E (D-alpha-tocopherol) 20 IU • Nattokinase (1600 FU) 80 mg. Other Ingredients: Rice Bran Oil, Lecithin, Yellow Beeswax.

NutriCology NattoZyme Nattokinase 50 mg - Allergy Research Group
Two vegetarian capsules contain: Nattokinase (2000 FU) 100 mg. Other Ingredients: Cellulose, Magnesium Stearate.

NutriCology No-Flush Niacin - Allergy Research Group
Each capsule contains: Niacin (as inositol hexanicotinate) 430 mg. Other Ingredients: Cellulose, Silicon Dioxide, Stearic Acid.

NutriCology NutriBalance Children's Formula - Allergy Research Group
Two scoops (5 g) contain: Vitamin A (71% as beta-carotene) 3500 IU • Vitamin E (as d-alpha-tocopheryl acid succinate) 100 IU • Thiamin (as thiamin hydrochloride) 4.5 mg • Riboflavin (as riboflavin-5-phosphate) 4.5 mg • Niacin 15 mg • Vitamin B6 (as pyridoxine hydrochloride and pyridoxal-5-phosphate) 9.3 mg • Folic Acid 40 mcg • Vitamin B12 20 mcg • Biotin 20 mcg • Pantothenic Acid 25 mg • Calcium (as calcium carbonate) 100 mg • Magnesium (as magnesium carbonate) 250 mg • Chromium (as chromium nitrate) 25 mcg • Para-Aminobenzoic Acid 10 mg • Inositol 10 mg • Choline 25 mg • L-Glutamine 1.5 g • Flax meal 500 mg • Stevia leaves, dried extract 10 mg • Soy protein powder 1.5 g • Cellulose 250 mg • Total Count Probiotic Cultures 1 billion: Lactobacillus group (L.

rhamnosus A, L. rhamnosus B, L. acidophilus, L. casei, L. bulgaricus) 700 million • Bifidobacterium goup (B. longum, B. breve) 200 million • Streptococcus Thermophilus 100 million.

NutriCology OcuDyne - Allergy Research Group
Two capsules contain: Vitamin A (23% as retinyl palmitate and 77% as beta-carotene) 8125 IU • Vitamin C (as ascorbic acid) 125 mg • Vitamin E (as DL-alpha-tocopheryl acetate) 100 IU • Thiamin (as thiamin hydrochloride) 5 mg • Riboflavin 6.25 mg • Niacin (83% as niacinamide) 15 mg • Vitamin B6 (as pyridoxine hydrochloride) 7.5 mg • Folic Acid 200 mcg • Vitamin B12 12.5 mcg • Pantothenic Acid 25 mg • Calcium (as calcium citrate) 25 mg • Magnesium (as magnesium citrate) 62.5 mg • Zinc (as zinc picolinate) 12.5 mg • Selenium (as sodium selenite and selenomethionine) 50 mcg • Copper (as copper sebacate) 0.75 mg • N-Acetyl-L-Cysteine 62.5 mg • Glycine 12.5 mg • L-Methionine 50 mg • Taurine 125 mg • Glutamic Acid 12.5 mg • Quercetin 75 mg • Ginkgo Biloba dried leaves extract 15 mg • Bilberry dried fresh berries extract (vaccinium myrtillus) 10 mg. Other Ingredients: Cellulose, Stearic Acid.

NutriCology OcuDyne II with Lutein and Added Minerals - Allergy Research Group
Two capsules contain: Vitamin A (23% as retinyl palmitate and 77% as beta-carotene) 8125 IU • Vitamin C (as ascorbic acid) 125 mg • Vitamin E (as DL-alpha-tocopheryl acetate) 50 IU • Thiamin (as thiamin hydrochloride) 5 mg • Riboflavin 6.25 mg • Niacin (86% as niacinamide) 15 mg • Vitamin B6 (as pyridoxine hydrochloride) 7.5 mg • Folic Acid 200 mcg • Vitamin B12 12.5 mcg • Pantothenic Acid 25 mg • Calcium (as calcium citrate) 25 mg • Iodine (as potassium iodide) 5 mcg • Magnesium (as magnesium citrate) 62.5 mg • Zinc (as zinc citrate) 12.5 mg • Selenium (as sodium selenite and selenomethionine) 50 mcg • Copper (as copper sebacate) 0.75 mg • Manganese (as manganese citrate) 2.5 mg • Chromium (as chromium nicotinate) 50 mcg • Molybdenum (as sodium molybdate) 30 mcg • Potassium (as potassium chloride) 25 mg • Boron (as boron citrate) 150 mcg • N-Acetyl-L-Cysteine 62.5 mg • Glycine 12.5 mg • L-Methionine 50 mg • Taurine 125 mg • Glutamic Acid 12.5 mg • Lutein 2.5 mg • Zeaxanthin 125 mcg • Quercetin 75 mg • Ginkgo Biloba dried leaves extract 15 mg • Bilberry dried fresh berries extract (vaccinium myrtillus) 10 mg. Other Ingredients: Cellulose, Magnesium Stearate.

NutriCology Original AntiOx - Allergy Research Group
Each capsule contains: Vitamin A (as beta-carotene) 7500 IU • Vitamin C (as ascorbic acid) 45 mg • Vitamin E (as DL-alpha-tocopheryl-acetate) 150 IU • Thiamin (as thiamin hydrochloride) 19 mg • Riboflavin (as riboflavin-5-phosphate) 19 mg • Niacin (as niacinamide) 16.5 mg • Vitamin B6 (as pyridoxal-5-phosphate) 4.5 mg • Pantothenic Acid (as calcium pantothenate) 16.5 mg • Zinc (as zinc sulfate) 11 mg • Selenium (as sodium selenite) 56 mcg • L-Cysteine 75 mg • Glutathione (reduced) 37.5 mg • Trimethylglycine 30 mg. Other Ingredients: Cellulose, Magnesium Stearate, Silicon Dioxide.

NutriCology Pancreas, Organic Glandular (LAMB) - Allergy Research Group
Each capsule contains: Pancreas gland, lamb 425 mg. Other Ingredients: Cellulose, Stearic Acid.
See Editor's Note No. 14.

NutriCology Pancreas, Organic Glandular (PORK) - Allergy Research Group
Each capsule contains: Pancreas gland, pork 425 mg. Other Ingredients: Cellulose, Stearic Acid.
See Editor's Note No. 14.

NutriCology Pantothenic Acid - Allergy Research Group
Each capsule contains: Pantothenic Acid (as calcium pantothenate) 500 mg • Calcium (as calcium pantothenate) 42 mg. Other Ingredients: Silicon Dioxide.

NutriCology PhosSerine Complex - Allergy Research Group
Three softgels contain: Vitamin C (as ascorbic acid) 10 mg • Phosphatidylserine and Lysophosphatidylserine 100 mg • Other Phospholipids and Glycerides 380 mg • Soy Oil 200 mg.

NutriCology PMS Nutritional Support - Allergy Research Group
Each capsule contains: BioResponse DIM (a patented diindolylmethane complex), Starch, DIM (25% min.), Vitamin E Succinate, Phosphatidylcholine, Silica 75 mg • Green Tea extract (decaffeinated, standardized to 60% catechins) 600 mg • Vitex Agnus-Castus berry extract 20 mg. Other Ingredients: Stearic Acid.

NutriCology Pregnenolone (100 mg) - Allergy Research Group
Each tablet contains: Pregnenolone 100 mg. Other Ingredients: Cellulose, Magnesium Stearate, Silica Gel, Fatty Acids, Silicon Dioxide.

NutriCology Pregnenolone (50 mg) - Allergy Research Group
Each tablet contains: Pregnenolone 50 mg. Other Ingredients: Cellulose, Magnesium Stearate, Silica Gel, Fatty Acids, Silicon Dioxide.

NutriCology Prostate Nutritional Support - Allergy Research Group
Two softgels contain: Zinc (as zinc citrate) 10 mg • Pumpkin seed oil 893 mg • Saw Palmetto berry extract (standardized to 85-95% fatty acids) 320 mg • BioResponse DIM 320 mg: Diindolylmethane complex, starch, DIM (25% min.), Vitamin E Succinate, Phosphatidylcholine, Silica • Nettle root extract 16:1 300 mg • Beta-Sitosterol 120 mg • Lycopene 15 mg. Other Ingredients: Yellow Beeswax.

NutriCology Pure Vitamin C capsules - Allergy Research Group
Each capsule contains: Vitamin C (as ascorbic acid) 1000 mg. Other Ingredients: Stearic Acid.

NutriCology Pure Vitamin C powder - Allergy Research Group
Each 1/4 tsp (1 g) serving contains: Vitamin C (as ascorbic acid) 1000 mg.

NutriCology Pyridoxine P5P Vitamin B6 - Allergy Research Group
Each capsule contains: Vitamin B6 (91% as pyridoxine hydrochloride and 9% as pyridoxal-5-phosphate) 275 mg. Other Ingredients: Cellulose, Stearic Acid, Silicon Dioxide.

NutriCology Quercetin 300 - Allergy Research Group
Each capsule contains: Vitamin C (as calcium ascorbate) 75 mg • Vitamin E (as Dl-alpha-tocopheryl acetate) 70 IU • Quercetin 300 mg. Other Ingredients: Cellulose, Stearic Acid.

NutriCology Quercetin with Bioflavonoids - Allergy Research Group
Each capsule contains: Lemon Bioflavonoid complex 400 mg • Quercetin 50 mg • Hesperidin 50 mg • Rutin 50 mg. Other Ingredients: Cellulose, Stearic Acid.

NutriCology Saw Palmetto Complex with Lycopene - Allergy Research Group
Two softgels contain: Zinc (as zinc citrate) 10 mg • Pumpkin seed oil 1.5 g • Saw Palmetto berry extract (serenoa repens standardized to 85-95% fatty acids) 320 mg • Beta-Sitosterol 120 mg • Lycopene 15 mg. Other Ingredients: Silicon Dioxide.

NutriCology Selenium Solution - Allergy Research Group
Each 1/2 tsp (2.5 mL) serving contains: Selenium (as sodium selenite) 100 mcg. Other Ingredients: Distilled Water.

NutriCology SkinGlow **-** Allergy Research Group
Three softgels contain: Hyaluronic Acid powder (9% min. hyaluronic acid) 210 mg. Other Ingredients: Rice Bran Oil, Yellow Beeswax, Titanium Dioxide.

NutriCology Stabilium 200 **-** Allergy Research Group
Two capsules contain: Garum Armoricum 210 mg • Virgin Sunflower Oil 170 mg • Lecithin 20 mg.

NutriCology Superior Kava Kava **-** Allergy Research Group
Each softgel contains: Kava Kava root (piper methysticum forst, minimum 80% kavalactone extract standardized to 75 mg kavalactones). Other Ingredients: Soybean Oil, Beeswax, Glycerin Fatty Acid Ester, Polysorbate 80.
See Editor's Note No. 21.

NutriCology Taurine (#70620) **-** Allergy Research Group
Each capsule contains: Taurine 500 mg. Other Ingredients: Celluose, Silicon Dioxide, Stearic Acid.

NutriCology Taurine (#73920) **-** Allergy Research Group
Each capsule contains: Taurine 1000 mg. Other Ingredients: Cellulose, Silicon Dioxide, Stearic Acid.

NutriCology The New AntiOx, Cysteine Free **-** Allergy Research Group
Each capsule contains: Vitamin A (40% as retinyl palmitate and 60% as beta-carotene) 12,500 IU • Vitamin C (as ascorbyl palmitate) 4 mg • Vitamin E (as DL-alpha-tocopheryl acetate) 100 IU • Thiamin (as thiamin hydrochloride) 10 mg • Riboflavin (80% as riboflavin and 20% as riboflavin-5-phosphate) 12.5 mg • Niacin (50% as niacinamide) 10 mg • Vitamin B6 (80% as pyridoxine hydrochloride and 20% as pyridoxal-5-phosphate) 12.5 mg • Folic Acid 100 mcg • Vitamin B12 (as cyanocobalamin) 100 mcg • Pantothenic Acid (as calcium pantothenate) 12.5 mg • Zinc (as zinc citrate) 7.5 mg • Selenium (87% as sodium selenite and 13% as selenomethionine) 75 mcg • Copper (as copper sebacate) 0.5 mg • Manganese (as manganese citrate) 5 mg • Glutathione (reduced) 50 mg • L-Methionine 50 mg • Taurine 50 mg • Trimethylglycine 50 mg • Proanthocyanidins, as Grape seed extract 12.5 mg • Coenzyme Q10 15 mg • Lipoic Acid 12. 5mg • Ginkgo Biloba extract 20 mg. Other Ingredients: Magnesium Stearate.

NutriCology Well Mind **-** Allergy Research Group
Each capsule contains: Zinc (as zinc valerate) 60 mcg • St. John's Wort dried leaves and flowers extract (hypericum perforatum) 125 mg • Kava Kava dried root extract (piper methysticum) 60 mg • Valerian dried root extract 30 mg • Passionflower dried leaves extract (passiflora incarnata) 30 mg • Schizandra dried berries extract (schizandra chinensis) 30 mg • Gotu Kola powdered herb (centella asiatica) 15 mg • Cypripedium dried root extract (cypripedium pubescens) 2.5 mg. Other Ingredients: Cellulose, Magnesium Stearate, Silicon Dioxide.

NutriCology WomanPrime **-** Allergy Research Group
Each capsule contains: Vitamin A (as vitamin A palmitate) 1250 IU • Vitamin C (as ascorbic acid) 25 mg • Vitamin E (as D-alpha-tocopheryl acid succinate) 125 IU • Vitamin B6 (as pyridoxine hydrochloride) 6.25 mg • Folic Acid 200 mcg • Vitamin B12 5 mcg • Pantothenic Acid (as calcium pantothenate) 70 mg • Magnesium (as magnesium aspartate) 8.25 mg • Selenium (as selenomethionine) 12.5 mcg • Boron (as boron citrate) 250 mcg • Hesperidin 125 mg • PABA (para-aminobenzoic acid) 75 mg • Adrenal 31 mg • Korean Ginseng extract 25 mg • Black Cohosh extract 25 mg. Other Ingredients: Cellulose, Magnesium Stearate, Silicon Dioxide.

NutriCology ZenMind **-** Allergy Research Group
Two capsules contain: GABA (gamma-aminobutyric acid) 550 mg • L-Theanine 200 mg. Other Ingredients: Silicon Dioxide, Carbowax.

Nutrient 280 **-** Pure Encapsulations
Six vegetable capsules contain: Ascorbic Acid 300 mg • Vitamin C (as ascorbyl palmitate) 36 mg • Mixed Carotenoids 4500 IU: Beta Carotene 2570 mcg, Alpha Carotene 81 mcg, Zeaxanthin 16 mcg, Cryptoxanthin 20 mcg, Lutein 13 mcg • Vitamin D (as D3) 120 IU • Vitamin E (D-alpha tocopheryl succinate) 120 IU • Thiamine HCl (vitamin B1) 30 mg • Riboflavin (vitamin B2) 15 mg • Riboflavin 5' Phosphate (vitamin B2) 7.5 mg • Pyridoxine HCl (vitamin B6) 7.5 mg • Pyridoxal 5' Phosphate (vitamin B6) 7.5 mg • Niacinamide 30 mg • Inositol Hexaniacinate (no-flush niacin) 27 mg • Folic Acid 240 mcg • Biotin 240 mcg • Pantothenic Acid (calcium pantothenate 120 mg • Methylcobalamin (vitamin B12) 300 mcg • Calcium (citrate) 90 mg • Magnesium (citrate) 60 mg • Potassium (aspartate) 30 mg • Zinc (picolinate) 7.5 mg • Manganese (aspartate) 3 mg • Iron (glycinate) 3 mg • Boron (glycinate) 600 mcg • Copper (glycinate) 600 mcg • Iodine (potassium iodide) 60 mcg • Chromium (polynicotinate) 60 mcg • Selenium (selenomethionine) 60 mcg • Vanadium (aspartate) 60 mcg • Molybdenum (aspartate) 30 mcg.

Nutrient 950 **-** Pure Encapsulations
Six vegetable capsules contain: Ascorbic Acid 1000 mg • Vitamin C (as ascorbyl palmitate) 120 mg • Mixed Carotenoids 15000 IU: Beta Carotene 8568 mcg, Alpha Carotene 270 mcg, Zeaxanthin 54 mcg, Cryptoxanthin 66 mcg, Lutein 42 mcg • Vitamin D (as D3) 400 IU • Vitamin E (D-alpha tocopheryl succinate) 400 IU • Thiamine HCl (vitamin B1) 100 mg • Riboflavin (vitamin B2) 50 mg • Riboflavin 5' Phosphate (activated B2) 25 mg • Pyridoxine HCl (vitamin B6) 25 mg • Pyridoxal 5' Phosphate (activated B6) 25 mg • Niacinamide 100 mg • Inositol Hexaniacinate (no-flush niacin) 90 mg • Folic Acid 800 mcg • Biotin 800 mcg • Pantothenic Acid (calcium pantothenate) 400 mg • Methylcobalamin (vitamin B12) 1000 mcg • Calcium (citrate) 300 mg • Magnesium (citrate) 200 mg • Potassium (aspartate) 99 mg • Zinc (picolinate) 25 mg • Manganese (aspartate) 10 mg • Iron (glycinate) 10 mg • Boron (glycinate) 2 mg • Copper (glycinate) 2 mg • Iodine (potassium iodide) 200 mcg • Chromium (polynicotinate) 200 mcg • Selenium (selenomethionine) 200 mcg • Vanadium (aspartate) 200 mcg • Molybdenum (aspartate) 100 mcg.

Nutrient 950 with NAC **-** Pure Encapsulations
Six vegetable capsules contain: Ascorbic Acid 1000 mg • Vitamin C (as ascorbyl palmitate) 120 mg • Mixed Carotenoids 15000 IU: Beta Carotene 8568 mcg, Alpha Carotene 270 mcg, Zeaxanthin 54 mcg, Cryptoxanthin 66 mcg, Lutein 42 mcg • Vitamin D (as D3) 400 IU • Vitamin E (D-alpha tocopheryl succinate) 400 IU • Thiamine HCl (vitamin B1) 100 mg • Riboflavin (vitamin B2) 50 mg • Riboflavin 5' Phosphate (activated B2) 25 mg • Pyridoxine HCl (vitamin B6) 25 mg • Pyridoxal 5' Phosphate (activated B6) 25 mg • Niacinamide 100 mg • Inositol Hexaniacinate (no-flush niacin) 90 mg • Folic Acid 800 mcg • Biotin 800 mcg • Pantothenic Acid (calcium pantothenate) 400 mg • Methylcobalamin (vitamin B12) 1000 mcg • Calcium (citrate) 300 mg • Magnesium (citrate) 200 mg • Potassium (aspartate) 99 mg • Zinc (picolinate) 25 mg • Manganese (aspartate) 10 mg • Iron (glycinate) 10 mg • Boron (glycinate) 2 mg • Copper (glycinate) 2 mg • Iodine (potassium iodide) 200 mcg • Chromium (polynicotinate) 200 mcg • Selenium (selenomethionine) 200 mcg • Vanadium (aspartate) 200 mcg • Molybdenum (aspartate) 100 mcg • N-Acetyl-L-Cysteine 1000 mcg.

Nutrient 950 without copper & iron **-** Pure Encapsulations
Six vegetable capsules contain: Ascorbic Acid 1000 mg • Vitamin C (as ascorbyl palmitate) 120 mg • Mixed Carotenoids 15000 IU: Beta Carotene 8568 mcg, Alpha Carotene 270 mcg, Zeaxanthin 54 mcg, Cryptoxanthin 66 mcg, Lutein 42 mcg • Vitamin D (as D3) 400 IU • Vitamin E (D-alpha tocopheryl succinate) 400 IU • Thiamine HCl (vitamin B1) 100 mg • Riboflavin (vitamin B2) 50 mg • Riboflavin 5' Phosphate (activated B2) 25 mg • Pyridoxine HCl (vitamin B6) 25 mg • Pyridoxal 5' Phosphate (activated B6) 25 mg • Niacinamide 100 mg • Inositol Hexaniacinate (no-flush niacin) 90 mg • Folic Acid 800 mcg • Biotin 800 mcg • Pantothenic Acid (calcium pantothenate) 400 mg • Methylcobalamin (vitamin B12) 1000 mcg • Calcium (citrate) 300 mg • Magnesium (citrate) 200 mg • Potassium (aspartate) 99 mg • Zinc (picolinate) 25 mg • Manganese (aspartate) 10 mg • Boron (glycinate) 2 mg • Iodine (potassium iodide) 200 mcg • Chromium (polynicotinate) 200 mcg • Selenium (selenomethionine) 200 mcg • Vanadium (aspartate) 200 mcg • Molybdenum (aspartate) 100 mcg.

Nutrient 950 without copper, iron & iodine - Pure Encapsulations
Six vegetable capsules contain: Ascorbic Acid 1000 mg • Vitamin C (as ascorbyl palmitate) 120 mg • Mixed Carotenoids 15000 IU: Beta Carotene8568 mcg, Alpha Carotene 270 mcg, Zeaxanthin 54 mcg, Cryptoxanthin 66 mcg, Lutein 42 mcg • Vitamin D (as D3) 400 IU • Vitamin E (D-alpha tocopheryl succinate) 400 IU • Thiamine HCl (vitamin B1) 100 mg • Riboflavin (vitamin B2) 50 mg • Riboflavin 5' Phosphate (activated B2) 25 mg • Pyridoxine HCl (vitamin B6) 25 mg • Pyridoxal 5' Phosphate (activated B6) 25 mg • Niacinamide 100 mg • Inositol Hexaniacinate (no-flush niacin) 90 mg • Folic Acid 800 mcg • Biotin 800 mcg • Pantothenic Acid (calcium pantothenate) 400 mg • Methylcobalamin (vitamin B12) 1000 mcg • Calcium (citrate) 300 mg • Magnesium (citrate) 200 mg • Potassium (aspartate) 99 mg • Zinc (picolinate) 25 mg • Manganese (aspartate) 10 mg • Boron (glycinate) 2 mg • Chromium (polynicotinate) 200 mcg • Selenium (selenomethionine) 200 mcg • Vanadium (aspartate) 200 mcg • Molybdenum (aspartate) 100 mcg.

Nutrient 950 without iron - Pure Encapsulations
Six vegetable capsules contain: Ascorbic Acid 1000 mg • Vitamin C (as ascorbyl palmitate) 120 mg • Mixed Carotenoids 15000 IU: Beta Carotene 8568 mcg, Alpha Carotene 270 mcg, Zeaxanthin 54 mcg, Cryptoxanthin 66 mcg, Lutein 42 mcg • Vitamin D (as D3) 400 IU • Vitamin E (D-alpha tocopheryl succinate) 400 IU • Thiamine HCl (vitamin B1) 100 mg • Riboflavin (vitamin B2) 50 mg • Riboflavin 5' Phosphate (activated B2) 25 mg • Pyridoxine HCl (vitamin B6) 25 mg • Pyridoxal 5' Phosphate (activated B6) 25 mg • Niacinamide 100 mg • Inositol Hexaniacinate (no-flush niacin) 90 mg • Folic Acid 800 mcg • Biotin 800 mcg • Pantothenic Acid (calcium pantothenate) 400 mg • Methylcobalamin (vitamin B12) 1000 mcg • Calcium (citrate) 300 mg • Magnesium (citrate) 200 mg • Potassium (aspartate) 99 mg • Zinc (picolinate) 25 mg • Manganese (aspartate) 10 mg • Boron (glycinate) 2 mg • Copper (glycinate) 2 mg • Iodine (potassium iodide) 200 mcg • Chromium (polynicotinate) 200 mcg • Selenium (selenomethionine) 200 mcg • Vanadium (aspartate) 200 mcg • Molybdenum (aspartate) 100 mcg.

Nutri-Essence Digest Chewables - Enzymes, Inc.
Each tablet contains: n-zimes Proprietary Enzyme Blend 204 mg: Protease (alkaline, neutral and acid proteases plus peptidase), Lipase, Amylase, Glucoamylase, Malt Diastase, Lactase, Invertase, alpha-Galactosidase, CereCalase, Cellulase, Pectinase. Other Ingredients: Dextrose (Corn Sugar), Fructose (Fruit Sugar), Natural Raspberry Flavor, Silica (Mineral) Plant Cellulose, Citric Acid, Veg. Magnesium Sterate, Proprietary Plant-derived Sweetener.

Nutri-Essence Digestion - Enzymes, Inc.
Each capsule contains: n-zimes Proprietary Blend 364 mg: Protease (alkaline, neutral and acid proteases plus peptidase), Lipase, Amylase, Glucoamylase, Malt Diastase, Lactase, Invertase, alpha-Galactosidase, CereCalase Plus, Cellulase, Xylanase, Pectinase • Proprietary Herbal Blend 155 mg: Ginger root extract (5% gingerols) plus whole root, Gentian root, Caraway seed, Peppermint leaf extract (4:1) plus whole leaf. Other Ingredients: Plant Cellulose, Water, Lecithin, Rice Bran.

Nutri-Fast Trim - Nu-Creations
Three tablets contain: Chromium 400 mcg. Other Ingredients: Guar Gum, Gum Karaya, American Desert Herb, Guarana, Korean Ginseng, Bee Pollen, White Willow, Bladderwrack, Gotu Kola, Licorice, Reishi Mushroom, Chickweed, Mate, Gymnema Sylvestis, Fennel, Astragalus, Ginger, Rehmannia, Dicalcium Phosphate, Pharmaceutical Glaze, Magnesium Stearate.

NutriFi - Pharmanex
Each teaspoon contains: Oat Fiber • Maltodextrin • Dextrose (Glucose) • Cellulose • Citrus Pectin • Psyllium Fiber • Gum Arabic.

Nutri-Genic Softgels - Nature's Plus
Two softgels contain: Vitamin A (as beta carotene) 10,000 IU • Vitamin C (as calcium ascorbate) 500 mg • Vitamin D (as cholecalciferol) 400 IU • Vitamin E (as D-alpha tocopheryl succinate) 200 IU • Thiamin (vitamin B1, as thiamine HCl) 50 mg • Riboflavin (vitamin B2) 40 mg • Niacin (as niacinamide) 75 mg • Vitamin B6 (as pyridoxine HCl) 50 mg • Folate (as folic acid) 400 mcg • Vitamin B12 (as cyanocobalamin) 75 mcg • Biotin 50 mcg • Pantothenic Acid (as calcium pantothenate) 75 mg • Calcium (as ascorbate) 50 mg • Iron (as gluconate) 10 mg • Magnesium (as gluconate, sulfate) 25 mg • Zinc (as gluconate) 15 mg • Manganese (as gluconate) 6 mg • Potassium (as citrate) 10 mg • Inositol 75 mg • Choline (as bitartrate) 32 mg • Citrus Bioflavonoids (from citrus limon exocarp) 25 mg • Betaine HCl (from beet molasses) 25 mg • Rutin (from saphora japonica leaf) 20 mg • PABA (para-aminobenzoic acid) 15 mg • Papain (from carica papaya fruit) 10 mg • Hesperidin (from saphora japonica leaf) 5 mg. Other Ingredients: Safflower Oil, Gelatin, Glycerin, Rice Bran, Purified Water.

Nutri-Genic Tablets - Nature's Plus
Two tablets contain: Vitamin A (as beta carotene) 10,000 IU • Vitamin C (as calcium ascorbate) 500 mg • Vitamin D (as ergocalciferol) 400 IU • Vitamin E (as D-alpha tocopheryl succinate) 200 IU • Thiamin (vitamin B1, as thiamine HCl) 50 mg • Riboflavin (vitamin B2) 40 mg • Niacin (as niacinamide) 75 mg • Vitamin B6 (as pyridoxine HCl) 50 mg • Folate (as folic acid) 400 mcg • Vitamin B12 (as cyanocobalamin) 75 mcg • Biotin 50 mcg • Pantothenic Acid (as calcium pantothenate) 75 mg • Calcium (as ascorbate) 50 mg • Iron (as gluconate) 10 mg • Magnesium (as gluconate) 25 mg • Zinc (as gluconate) 15 mg • Manganese (as gluconate) 6 mg • Potassium (as citrate) 10 mg • Inositol 75 mg • Choline (as bitartrate) 32 mg • Citrus Bioflavonoids (from citrus limon exocarp) 25 mg • Betaine HCl (from beet molasses) 25 mg • Rutin (from saphora japonica leaf) 20 mg • PABA (para-aminobenzoic acid) 15 mg • Papain (from papaya) 10 mg • Hesperidin (from saphora japonica leaf) 5 mg. Other Ingredients: Microcrystalline Cellulose, Stearic Acid, Magnesium Stearate, Rice Bran, Silica, Pharmaceutical Glaze.

Nutrilite A+Zinc - Quixtar, Inc.
Each tablet contains: Vitamin A 10000 IU • Zinc Oxide 15 mg • Zinc Gluconate 15 mg.

Nutrilite Antioxidant Complex with Pycnogenol - Quixtar, Inc.
Each capsule contains: Pycnogenol 60 mg • Grape Seed extract 30 mg • Green Tea extract (Decaffeinated) 300 mg • Alpha-Lipoic Acid 45 mg • Glutathione 60 mg • Turmeric extract 75 mg.

Nutrilite Bilberry with Lutein - Quixtar, Inc.
Each softgel contains: Bilberry extract • Lutein • Zeaxanthin • DHA.

Nutrilite Bio C Plus - Quixtar, Inc.
Each tablet contains: Vitamin C (from ascorbic acid and acerola concentrate) 250 mg • Calcium (from calcium carbonate and tricalcium phosphate) 50 mg • Acerola concentrates 200 mg: Acerola Cherry fruit extract (malpighia emarginata L.), Maltodextrin, Silicon Dioxide 200 mg • Citrus Multiflavonoid Complex 35 mg: Grapefruit, Mandarin, Lemon (fruit and peel). Other Ingredients: Calcium Carbonate, Microcrystalline Cellulose, Corn Starch, Sodium Carboxymethylcellulose, Tricalcium Phosphate, Hydroxypropyl Methylcellulose, Magnesium Stearate, Maltodextrin, Glycerin.

Nutrilite Black Cohosh and Soy - Quixtar, Inc.
Each tablet contains: Black Cohosh extract 120 mg • Soy Protein 300 mg • Isoflavones 49.8 mg • Acerola Cherry Concentrate 30 mg • Calcium 60 mg.

Nutrilite Calcium Magnesium Plus - Quixtar, Inc.
Each tablet contains: Calcium 651 mg • Magnesium 324 mg • Zinc 10 mg • Copper 2 mg • Manganese 2.5 mg • NUTRILITE Alfalfa Concentrate with Phytofactors Plant Compounds.

Nutrilite ChromPic Extra - Quixtar, Inc.
Each capsule contains: Chromium 300 mcg (providing Chromium picolinate 2400 mcg) • Vanadium 220 mcg • Gymnema sylvestre 100 mcg.

Nutrilite CoEnzyme Q10 Complex - Quixtar, Inc.
Each capsule contains: CoEnzyme Q10 30 mg • L-Carnitine 100 mg • Taurine 125 mg • Bioflavonoids 25 mg.

Nutrilite Concentrated Fruits and Vegetables - Quixtar, Inc.
Each tablet contains: Lycopene 1.5 mg • Lutein 3 mg • Quercetin 75 mg • Ellagic Acid 20 mg • Hesperidin 3 mg • EGCG 45 mg • Nutrilite Phytonutrient Concentrate 55 mg: Phytonutrients from Blueberries, Elderberries, Rosemary, Acerola Cherries, Broccoli, Carrots, Spinach.

Nutrilite Daily Free - Quixtar, Inc.
Each tablet contains: Vitamin A (20% as beta carotene) 5000 IU • Vitamin C 90 mg • Vitamin D 400 IU • Vitamin E 30 IU • Thiamin 2.3 mg • Riboflavin 2.6 mg • Niacin 20 mg • Vitamin B6 2 mg • Folic Acid 400 mcg • Vitamin B12 9 mcg • Biotin 300 mcg • Pantothenic Acid 10 mg • Calcium 200 mg • Phosphorus 20 mg • Iodine 150 mcg • Magnesium 100 mg • Zinc 15 mg • Selenium 70 mcg • Copper 2 mg • Manganese 2 mg •Chromium 120 mcg • Molybdenum 75 mcg • Nutrilite Watercress concentreate 100 mg.

Nutrilite Daily Multivitamin and Multimineral - Quixtar, Inc.
Each tablet contains: Vitamin A (20% as beta carotene) 5000 IU • Vitamin C 90 mg • Vitamin D 400 IU •Vitamin E 30 IU • Vitamin K 80 mcg • Thiamin 2.3 mg • Riboflavin 2.6 mg • Niacin 20 mg • Vitamin B-6 2 mg • Folic Acid 400 mcg • Vitamin B-12 9 mcg • Biotin 300 mcg • Pantothenic Acid 10 mg • Calcium 200 mg • Iron 6 mg • Phosphorus 45 mg • Iodine 150 mcg • Magnesium 100 mg • Zinc 15 mg • Selenium 70 mcg • Copper 2 mg • Manganese 2 mg • Chromium 120 mcg • Molybdenum 75 mcg • Nutrilite 518 mg.

Nutrilite Digestive Enzyme Complex - Quixtar, Inc.
Each capsule contains: Lipase 31 mg • Lactase 40 mg • Amylase 20 mg • Alpha-Galactosidase 10 mg • Ginger root extract 150 mg • NUTRILITE Parsley Concentrate with Phytofactors Compounds.

Nutrilite Double X - Quixtar, Inc.
Each tablet contains: Vitamin A (75% as beta carotene) 5000 IU • Vitamin C (from ascorbic acid, acerola powder) 250 mg • Vitamin D 200 IU • Vitamin E (d-alpha tocopheryl succinate) 150 IU • Vitamin K (from phytonadione) 40 mcg • Thiamin 12.5 mg • Riboflavin 12.5 mg • Niacin 35 mg •Vitamin B-6 25 mg • Folic Acid 400 mcg • Vitamin B-12 50 mcg •Biotin (from d-biotin) 150 mcg • Pantothenic Acid 25 mg • Calcium (from calcium carbonate) 450 mg • Phosphorous (from calcium phosphate) 10 mg •Iodine 75 mcg • Magnesium (from magnesium oxide) 225 mg • Zinc (from zinc gluconate) 10 mg • Selenium (from sodium selenite) 50 mcg • Copper (from copper gluconate) 1 mg • Manganese (from manganese gluconate) 2.5 mg • Chromium (from chromium chloride) 60 mcg • Molybdenum (from sodium molybdate) 37.5 mcg • Potassium (from potassium chloride) 40 mg • Alpha Lipoic Acid 5 mg • MSM (methylsulfonyl methane) 30 mg • Lycopene 0.5 mg • Lutein 0.5 mg • Quercetin 50 mg •Spirulina 25 mg • Boron (from boron aspartate) 500 mcg • Vanadium (from vanadyl sulfate) 10 mcg. Other Ingredients: Alfalfa extract, Parsley Dehydrate, Acerola concentrate, Citrus Bioflavonoid concentrate, Methylsulfonyl Methane, Brassica concentrate, Horseradish root, Mixed Tocopheryls, Calcium Pantothenate, Pyridoxine Hydrochloride, Niacinamide, Spirulina, Thiamine Mononitrate.

Nutrilite Echinacea with Astragalus - Quixtar, Inc.
Each tablet contains: Echinacea extract 200.1 mg • Astragalus extract 50.1 mg • Chlorella powder 50.1 mg.

Nutrilite Garlic & Licorice - Quixtar, Inc.
Each tablet contains: Garlic 1000 mg • Licorice extract 21 mg.

Nutrilite Garlic Heart Care Formula - Quixtar, Inc.
Two tablets contain: Garlic bulb powder (allium sativum) 600 mg: Alliin (minimum) 13,500 mcg, Allicin yield (minimum 45% of alliin) 6000 mcg • Peppermint leaves extract 30 mg. Other Ingredients: Microcrystalline Cellulose, Stearic Acid, Lac Resin, Natural Peppermint Flavor, Sodium Starch Glycolate, Sodium Carboxymethylcellulose, Silicon Dioxide, Methylcellulose.

Nutrilite Ginkgo Biloba and DHA - Quixtar, Inc.
Each softgel contains: Standardized Ginkgo Biloba extract 160 mg • DHA 180 mg • Gotu Kola 68 mg.

Nutrilite Glucosamine HCl with Boswellia - Quixtar, Inc.
Two tablets contain: Glucosamine HCl 750 mg • Boswellia 60 mg • Bromelain 80 mg. Other Ingredients: Nutrilite Acerola Concentrate, Lemon Bioflavonoid Concentrate (with phytonutrients).

Nutrilite IntestiFlora - Quixtar, Inc.
Each stick pack (1.4 g) contains: Bifidobacterium Longum 500,000,000 CFU • Lactobacillus Acidophilus 500,000,000 CFU • Fructooligosaccharides (FOS) 1 g. Other Ingredients: Coconut and Palm Oil, Gelatin, Glycerin, Lecithin, Citrus Pectin.

Nutrilite Iron-Folic Plus - Quixtar, Inc.
Each tablet contains: Folate 133 mcg • Iron 15 mg • Calcium 40 mg.

Nutrilite Iron-Folic Plus - Quixtar, Inc.
Each tablet contains: Folic Acid 133 mcg • Calcium (from calcium carbonate) 40 mg • Iron (from spinach concentrate and ferrous fumarate) 15 mg • Spinach concentrate (spinach dehydrate, spinacla oleracea L. leaf and stem, ferrous gluconate) 142 mg. Other Ingredients: Dextrose, Maltodextrin, Microcrystalline Cellulose, Corn Starch, Sodium Carboxymethylcellulose, Hydroxypropyl Methylcellulose, Silicon Dioxide, Magnesium Stearate, Glycerin.

Nutrilite Kids Chewables Multivitamin Multimineral - Quixtar, Inc.
Each tablet contains: Vitamin A (from vitamin A palmitate and 25% from beta carotene) 2500 IU • Vitamin C (from ascorbic acid and tropical fruit concentrate) 40 mg • Vitamin D (cholecalciferol) 200 IU • Vitamin E (from D-alpha tocopheryl acid succinate) 20 IU • Vitamin K (phytonadione) 40 mcg • Thiamin (mononitrate) 0.75 mg • Riboflavin 0.85 mg • Niacin (niacinamide) 10 mg • Vitamin B6 (pyridoxine hydrochloride) 1 mg • Folate (folic acid) 200 mcg • Vitamin B12 (cyanocobalamin) 3 mcg • Biotin 150 mcg • Pantothenic Acid (calcium pantothenate) 5 mg • Calcium (calcium carbonate) 75 mg • Iron (ferrous fumarate) 3 mg • Iodine (potassium iodide) 75 mcg • Magnesium (oxide) 38 mg• Zinc (oxide) 7.5 mg • Selenium (selenite) 35 mcg • Copper (cupric oxide) 1 mg • Manganese (citrate) 1 mg • Chromium (chloride) 60 mcg • Molybdenum (from sodium molybdate) 38 mcg • Tropical Fruit Concentrate 50 mg: Acerola Cherry fruit extract (malpighia emarginata L.), Passion fruit (passiflora edulis), Pineapple fruit (bromelia ananas), Guava fruit (psidium guajava), Cashew fruit (anacardium occidentale), Maltodextrin, Dextrin. Other Ingredients: Xylitol, Sorbitol, Partially Hydrogenated Soy Oil, Microcrystalline Cellulose, Natural Flavor, Mono and Diglycerides, Dicalcium Phosphate, Silicon Dioxide, Maltodextrin, Magnesium Stearate, Citric Acid, Sodium Carboxymethylcellulose, Carminic Acid.

Nutrilite LeadingEdge Heart Pack - Quixtar, Inc.
Each packet contains: CoEnzyme Q10 • Garlic • Licorice • Omega 3 Complex • Natural B Complex.

Nutrilite Lecithin-E - Quixtar, Inc.
Each tablet contains: Lecithin (from Soybean Oil) 290 mg • Vitamin E 30 IU.

Nutrilite Milk Thistle and Dandelion - Quixtar, Inc.
Each tablet contains: Milk Thistle extract (Silybin Extract 228 mg) 468 mg • Dandelion root extract 375 mg • Turmeric extract 225 mg • Lemon Bioflavonoids • Acerola Cherry Concentrate.

Nutrilite Natural B Complex - Quixtar, Inc.
Each tablet contains: Thiamin 1.2 mg • Riboflavin 1.2 mg • Niacin 6.67 mg • Vitamin B6 1.2 mg • Folic Acid 133.33 mcg • Vitamin B12 2 mcg • Pantothenic Acid 5 mg • Inositol 3.6 mg • Para-Aminobenzoic Acid 3 mg. Other Ingredients: Dicalcium Phosphate, Yeast, Microcrystalline Cellulose, Lactose, Hydroxypropyl Methylcellulose, Calcium Stearate, Silicon Dioxide, Glycerin.

Nutrilite OceanEssentials - Quixtar, Inc.
Each softgel contains: EPA (eicosapentaenoic acid) 150 mg • DHA (docosahexaenoic acid) 150 mg.

Some Brand Name Natural Products - What they Contain

www.NaturalDatabase.com contains MANY more listings than appear here.
Editor's Notes are located on pages 2155-2163.

Nutrilite Omega 3 Complex **-** Quixtar, Inc.
Each softgel contains: Vitamin E (from mixed tocopherols) 30 IU • Omega-3 Fatty Acids (from salmon and flaxseed oils) 300 mg • Alpha Linolenic Acid (from flaxseed oil) 185 mg • EPA (eicosapentaenoic acid, from salmon oil) 65 mg • DHA (docosahexaenoic acid, from salmon oil) 45 mg. Other Ingredients: Gelatin, Glycerin, Yellow Bees Wax, Soy Lecithin, Soybean Oil, Caramel Color, Lemon Oil.

Nutrilite Parselenium-E **-** Quixtar, Inc.
Each tablet contains: Vitamin E (from vitamin E succinate) 400 IU • Calcium (from tricalcium phosphate) 110 mg • Phosphorous (from tricalcium phosphate) 50 mg • Selenium (from selenium yeast) 10 mcg • Parsley leaf, stem concentrate (nasturium spp.) 77 mg. Other Ingredients: Microcrystalline Cellulose, Hydroxypropyl Methylcellulose, Silicon Dioxide, Magnesium Stearate, Modified Cellulose Gum, Glycerin.

Nutrilite Passionflower with Chamomile **-** Quixtar, Inc.
Each tablet contains: Passionflower 129.9 mg • Chamomile 81.3 mg • Hops 18.75 mg.

Nutrilite PriMroSe Plus **-** Quixtar, Inc.
Each softgel contains: Vitamin A (100% as betacarotene) 100 IU • Evening Primrose Oil (oenothera biennis, seed) 125 mg • Borage Oil (borago officinalis, seed) 125 mg • Ginger extract (zingiber officinale, root) 32 mg • Chasteberry extract (vitus agnus-castus, fruit) 15 mg • Dong Quai extract (angelica sinensis, root) 15 mg • Lemon Bioflavonoid concentrate (citrus limon L., fruit) 25 mg. Other Ingredients: Gelatin, Glycerin, Yellow Beeswax, Soybean Oil, Maltodextrin, Lecithin, Canola Oil, Corn Oil, Natural Caramel Color.

Nutrilite Saw Palmetto with Nettle Root **-** Quixtar, Inc.
Each softgel contains: Saw Palmetto 318 mg • Pumpkin seed oil 480 mg • Nettle root 240 mg.

Nutrilite Siberian Ginseng with Ginkgo Biloba **-** Quixtar, Inc.
Each capsule contains: Siberian Ginseng extract 200 mg • Ginkgo Biloba extract 133.6 mg • NUTRILITE Acerola Cherry and Citrus Bioflavonoid Concentrates.

Nutrilite St. John's Wort with Lemon Balm **-** Quixtar, Inc.
Each capsule contains: St. John's Wort (0.3% Hypericin) 900 mg • Lemon Balm 78 mg • Lemon Bioflavonoid Concentrate 72 mg • Vitamin C (from Acerola Cherry Concentrate) 10 mg.

Nutrilite Trim Advantage Weight Management Support Pack **-** Quixtar, Inc.
Each strip containing four capsules contains: Calcium (from oyster shells) 80 mg • Chromium (from chromium picolinate) 100 mcg • Garcinia Cambogia fruit 633 mg •Conjugated Linoleic Acid (from sunflower oil) 600 mg • Kola Nut extract seed 100 mg • L-Carnitine (from l-carnitine fumarate) 100 mg • Lemon Bioflavonoid extract (citrus lemon peel) 106 mg •Parsley dehydrate stem and leaves 66 mg • Gymnema Sylvestre leaves 33 mg • Vanadium (from vanadium glycinate) 6.7 mcg. Inactive Ingredients: Gelatin, Cellulose, Magnesium Stearate, Beeswax, Lecithin, Caramel Coloring.

Nutrilite Triple Guard Echinacea **-** Quixtar, Inc.
Three tablets contain: Triple Guard Echinacea Blend 506 mg: Purpurea root and arial parts, Angustifolia root • Citrus Multiflavonoid Complex 100 mg: Grapefruit, Royal Mandarin, Lemon (fruit and peel). Other Ingredients: Corn Starch, Microcrystalline Cellulose, Maltodextrin, Stearic Acid, Sodium Carboxymethyl Cellulose, Silicon Dioxide, Methylcellulose, Glycerin.

Nutrilite Valerian and Hops **-** Quixtar, Inc.
Three tablets contain: Standardized Valerian root extract (0.8% valerenic acid) 450 mg • Valerian whole root extract 150 mg • Lemon Balm leaf extract 150 mg • Hops cone extract 100 mg • Citrus Bioflavonoid concentrate 100 mg: Grapefruit, Mandarin, Lemon. Other Ingredients: Microcrystalline Cellulose, Maltodextrin, Corn Starch, Stearic Acid, Sodium Carboxymethylcellulose, Hydroxypropyl Methylcellulose, Silicon Dioxide, Glycerin, Natural Flavor.

Nutrilite Women's GLA Blend with Evening Primrose Oil **-** Quixtar, Inc.
Each softgel contains: Evening Primrose • Borage Oil • Black Currant seed oil • Chasteberry • Dong Quai • Ginger Extract.

Nutrimeal (Dutch chocolate flavor) **-** USANA Health Sciences
Two scoops contain: Soy Protein • Dutch Cocoa • High Oleic Sunflower Oil • Gum Arabic • Vitamin and Mineral Blend: Dicalcium Phosphate, Magnesium Phosphate, Dipotassium Phosphate, Niacinamide (Niacin), Ascorbic Acid (vitamin C), Ferric Orthophosphate, Zinc Oxide, D-Alpha Tocopheryl Acetate (natural vitamin E), Vitamin A Palmitate, Riboflavin (vitamin B2), Pyridoxine Hydrochloride (Vitamin B6), Thiamin Mononitrate (Vitamin B1), Cholecalciferol (Vitamin D3), Folic Acid, Cyanocobalamin (Vitamin B12), Potassium Iodide • Inulin • Corn Syrup Solids • Rice Syrup Solids • Natural and Artificial Flavors • Cellulose • Oat Fiber • Sodium Caseinate (a milk derivative) • Salt • Cellulose Gum • Mono and Diglycerides • Xanthan Gum • Soy Lecithin • Oligofructose.

Nutrimeal (French vanilla flavor) **-** USANA Health Sciences
Two scoops contain: Soy Protein Isolate • Fructose • High Oleic Sunflower Oil • Gum Arabic • Inulin • Corn Syrup Solids • Vitamin and Mineral Blend: Dicalcium Phosphate, Magnesium Phosphate, Dipotassium Phosphate, Niacinamide (niacin), Ascorbic Acid (vitamin C), Ferric Orthophosphate, Zinc Oxide, D-Alpha Tocopheryl Acetate (natural vitamin E), Vitamin A Palmitate, Riboflavin (vitamin B2), Pyridoxine Hydrochloride (vitamin B6), Thiamin Mononitrate (vitamin B1), Cholecalciferol (vitamin D3), Folic Acid, Cyanocobalamin (vitamin B12), Potassium Iodide • Rice Syrup Solids, Natural Flavors • Cellulose • Oat Fiber • Sodium Caseinate • Cellulose Gum • Salt • Mono and Diglycerides • Xanthan Gum • Soy Lecithin • Oligofructose.

Nutrimeal (wild strawberry flavor) **-** USANA Health Sciences
Two scoops contain: Soy Protein Isolate • Fructose • Gum Arabic • Inulin • High Oleic Sunflower oil • Corn Syrup Solids • Vitamin and Mineral Blend: Dicalcium Phosphate, Magnesium Phosphate, Dipotassium Phosphate, Niacinamide, Ascorbic Acid (vitamin C), Ferric Orthophosphate, Zinc Oxide, D-Alpha Tocopheryl Acetate (natural vitamin E), Vitamin A Palmitate, Riboflavin (vitamin B2), Pyridoxine Hydrochloride (vitamin B6), Thiamin Mononitrate (Vitamin B1), Cholecalciferol (vitamin D3), Folic Acid, Cyanocobalamin (vitamin B12), Potassium Iodide • Natural and Artificial Flavors • Cellulose • Sodium Caseinate • Oat Fiber • Beet Juice Powder • Xanthan Gum • Mono and Diglycerides • Salt • Soy Lecithin • Oligofructose.

Nutrimere **-** Standard Process, Inc.
Two capsules contain: Proprietary Blend 397 mg: Conch (strombus gigas), Carrot root. Other Ingredients: Gelatin, Water, Colors.

Nutrimmune Chews **-** Pharmanex
Each chew contains: Colostrum Microfiltrate 500 mg • Calcium 250 mg. Other Ingredients: Vitamin D.

Nutri-Plex **-** Nu-Creations
Three tablets contain: Vitamin A 5000 IU • Vitamin C 180 mg • Vitamin D 400 IU • Vitamin E 50 IU • Vitamin K 80 mcg • Vitamin B1 1.5 mg • Vitamin B2 1.7 mg • Niacin 20 mg • Vitamin B6 2 mg • Folic Acid 400 mg • Vitamin B12 6 mcg • Biotin 300 mcg • Pantothenic Acid 10 mg • Calcium 100 mg • Phosphorus 100 mg • Iodine 100 mcg • Magnesium 150 mcg • Zinc 50 mg • Selenium 15 mg • Copper 70 mcg • Manganese 2 mg • Chromium 2 mg • Molybdenum 400 mcg • Vanadium 75 mcg • Boron 1 mcg • Potassium 79 mg • Choline 10 mg • Inositol 10 mg • Garcinia cambogia 300 mg • Korean Ginseng 100 mg • Siberian Ginseng 200 mg. Other Ingredients: Anise, Fennel, Psyllium, Rhubarb, Kelp, Flax, Dicalcium Phosphate, Magnesium Stearate.

Nutri-Shield **-** Nu-Creations
Two capsules contain: Vitamin A 25,000 mg • Vitamin C 1000 mg • Vitamin E 400 mg • Vitamin B6 25 mg • Zinc 25 mg • Selenium 100 mg • Copper 2 mg • Chromium 25 mg • Bioflavonoid Complex

BRAND NAMES

150 mg • Rutin 40 mg • Quercetin 10 mg • Superoxide 100 mg • Astragalus 50 mg • Ginkgo biloba 15 mg • Rosemary 50 mg • Alpha Lipoic Acid 20 mg • Silymarin 50 mg • Lutein 6 mg • Spirulina 100 mg • Grape Seed extract 25 mg • Pine Bark extract 25 mg • Coenzyme Q-10 20 mg • L-Glutathione 10 mg • L-Glycerine 100 mg • Siberian Ginseng 50 mg • Reishi Mushroom 50 mg • Curcumin 50 mg. Other Ingredients: Dicalcium Phosphate, Pharmaceutical Glaze, Magnesium Stearate.

NutrisorbA **- InterPlexus**
Each drop (0.05 mL) contains: Vitamin A (as retinol palmitate) 10,000 IU. Other Ingredients: Water.

NutrisorbB12 **- InterPlexus**
Each drop (0.05 mL) contains: Vitamin B12 (as hydroxycobalamine) 50 mcg. Other Ingredients: Water.

Nutrition Bar (double chocolate flavor) **- USANA Health Sciences**
One bar contains: Protein Blend: Roasted Soybeans, Soy Protein Isolate, Whey Protein Concentrate • High Fructose Corn Syrup • Coating: Sugar, Palm Kernel Oil, Cocoa Powder, Whey Protein, Nonfat Milk Powder, Lecithin, Natural Flavors • Maltitol Syrup • Fructose • Cocoa • Natural Flavors • Lecithin • Palm Kernel Oil.

Nutrition Bar (peanut butter crunch flavor) **- USANA Health Sciences**
One bar contains: Protein Blend: Roasted Soybeans, Soy Protein Isolate, Textured Soy Flour, Whey Protein Concentrate • High Fructose Corn Syrup • Coating: Sugar, Palm Kernel Oil, Cocoa Powder, Whey Powder, Nonfat Milk Powder, Lecithin, Natural Flavors • Maltitol Syrup • Fructose • Peanut Flour • Peanut Butter.

Nutrition Warehouse Boron Complex Plus **- Puritan's Pride**
Four capsules contain: Boron 3 mg • MCHA (microcrystalline hydroxyapatite) 2000 mg • Calcium (from MCHA) 520 mg • Phosphorous (from MCHA) 260 mg • Magnesium carbonate elemental 160 mg • Magnesium aspartate elemental 40 mg • Vitamin D (as Vitamin D3) 260 IU • Vitamin K 120 mcg • Manganese 10 mg • Silica 100 mg. Other Ingredients: Magnesium, Potassium, Zinc, Selenium, Manganese, Iron, Collagen, Glycosaminoglycans, substituent Amino Acids.
See Editor's Note No. 21.

Nutrition Warehouse Multi Minerals with Boron **- Puritan's Pride**
Three tablets contain: Calcium (Carbonate, Citrate) 1000 mg • Magnesium (Oxide, Citrate) 500 mg • Zinc 22.5 mg • Iron 20 mg • Copper 1 mg • Potassium 99 mg • Manganese 5 mg • Selenium 50 mcg • Chromium (yeast-free) 100 mcg • Molybdenum 50 mcg • Vanadium 50 mcg • Iodine (Kelp) 150 mcg • L-Glutamic Acid (HCL) 50 mg • Vitamin D (Cholecalciferol) 200 IU • Boron Citrate 3 mg.
See Editor's Note No. 21.

Nutri-Vit **- Progressive Labs**
One tablespoon (15 ml) contains: Vitamin A 3750 IU • Vitamin C 60 mg • Vitamin D 600 IU • Vitamin E 15 IU • Thiamin (B1) 1.05 mg • Riboflavin (B2) 1.2 mg • Niacin 13.5 mg • Vitamin B6 1.05 mg • Folate (folic acid) 300 mcg • Vitamin B12 4.5 mcg • Biotin 225 mcg • Pantothenic Acid 7.5 mg • Iron 15 mg • Zinc 12 mg.

Nutrizyme **- Tyler Encapsulations**
Three capsules contain: Vitamin A (as natural beta-carotene with mixed carotenoids, palmitate) 10,000 IU • Vitamin C (from Poly-C ascorbates) 150 mg • Vitamin D (as cholecalciferol) 50 IU • Vitamin E (as D-alpha tocopheryl succinate) 25 mg • Vitamin K (as phytonadione) 25 mcg • Thiamine (as thiamine hydrochloride) 25 mg • Riboflavin (as riboflavin 12.6 mg, riboflavin-5'-phosphate 5.1 mg) 17.7 mg • Niacin (as Niacinol brand) 25 mg • Vitamin B6 (as pyridoxine HCl 37.5 mg, pyridoxal-5'-phosphate 5.1 mg) 42.6 mg • Folic Acid 200 mcg • Vitamin B12 (as cyanocobalamin) 100 mcg • Biotin 150 mcg • Pantothenic Acid (as calcium pantothenate) 25 mg • Calcium (as calcium citrate, malate, ascorbate) 200 mg • Magnesium (as magnesium citrate, ascorbate) 200 mg • Zinc (as zinc picolinate, ascorbate) 10 mg • Selenium (as selenium aspartate) 50 mcg • Copper (as copper aspartate) 0.5 mg • Manganese (as manganese aspartate) 5 mg • Chromium (from GlucoChrome brand) 75 mcg • Molybdenum (as molybdenum aspartate) 25 mcg • Potassium (as potassium citrate, ascorbate) 25 mg • Plant Enzymes 62 mg: Protease (I, II, IV), Amylase, Cellulase (I), Lipase (II), Lactase (II), Sucrase (invertase), Maltase (malt diastase) • Bioflavonoids 37.5 mg • Choline (as choline bitartrate) 25 mg • Inositol 25 mg • Gamma-Oryzanol (from rice bran oil) 20 mg • Rutin 12.5 mg • Pro-Flora 5 mg • L-Glutathione (reduced) 750 mcg • Boron (as boron aspartate, citrate) 0.5 mg • Vanadium (as vanadium aspartate) 25 mcg. Other Ingredients: Microcrystalline Cellulose, Gelatin, Water.

NxTrim **- Nova Pharmaceutical, Inc.**
Two tablets contain: Vitamin C (ascorbic acid) 200 mg • Niacin 10 mg • Vitamin B6 (as pyridoxine hydrochloride) 4 mg • Vitamin B12 (as cyanocobalamin) 166 mcg • Calcium (as dibasic calcium phosphate) 55 mg • Chromium (as chromium polynicotinate) 100 mcg • Phenylalanine (as L-phenylalanine hydrochloride) 300 mg • Glutamine (as L-glutamine hydrochloride) 50 mg • Tyrosine (as L-tyrosine hydrochloride) 100 mg • St. John's Wort extract 50 mg • L-Carnitine 20 mg • Korean Ginseng powdered root 70 mg • Uva Ursi powdered leaves 50 mg. Other Ingredients: Whey, Stearic Acid, Magnesium Stearate, Pharmaceutical Glaze.

Nytex **- Tharos Laboratories, Inc.**
Two capsules contain: Vitamin E 20 IU • Vitamin B3 30 mg • Vitamin B6 30 mg • Vitamin B12 250 mcg • Magnesium 100 mg • Valerian root extract 400 mg • Procidin-GB Proprietary Blend 50 mg: Grape extract, Blueberry extract • Suntheanine brand L-Theanine 50 mg • Melatonin 3 mg.

Nytol **- GlaxoSmithKline (GSK)**
Each capsule contains: Diphenhydramine Hydrochloride 25 mg. Other Ingredients: Corn Starch, Lactose, Microcrystalline Cellulose, Silica, Stearic Acid.

O.U.T. (Ovarian Uterine Tonic) **- The Herbalist**
Chaparral leaf • Pipsissewa leaf • False Unicorn root • Prickly Ash bark • Cramp bark • Licorice root • Saw Palmetto berry • Red Clover.

OA Plus **- BotanicLab**
Paeonia Lactiflora Pall (white peony root; chih-shao) • Panax Ginseng C.A. Meyer (ginseng; jen-sheng) • Glycyrrhiza Glabra L. (licorice; gan-cao) • Food Mycophyta (food mycophyta; shiyong-zhen-jun) • Apis Mellifera (honey bee) L. (royal jelly; fon-hwang-chiang) • Apis Cerana (honey; feng-mi) • Ostrea Gigas Thunberg (oyster shell; mu-li).

Oasis A.M. **- Oasis Wellness Network**
Each tablespoon contains: Potassium 42 mg • Protein 1 g • Calcium 28 mg • Iron 1 mg • Siberian Ginseng root extract 58 mg • Gotu Kola extract (whole plant) 48 mg. Other Ingredients: Roasted Carob, Barley, Chicory Root, Almond, Fig, Dates, Natural Coffee Flavor.

Oats-Scullcap Virtue **- Blessed Herbs**
Oats in milk stage • Scullcap • St. John's Wort flower • Lemon Balm • Lavender flower • Rosemary & Blackberry brandy.

Occuplex **- Puritan's Pride**
Eight capsules contain: Vitamin A 32,800 IU • Vitamin C (ascorbic acid) 500 mg • Vitamin E (as DL-alpha tocopheryl acetate) 400 IU • Thiamin 20 mg • Riboflavin 25 mg • Niacin (niacinamide and niacin) 60 mg • Vitamin B6 30 mg • Folic Acid 800 mcg • Vitamin B12 50 mcg • Pantothenic Acid 100 mg • Calcium 100 mg • Magnesium 250 mg • Zinc 30 mg • Selenium 200 mcg • Copper 3 mg •Lutein 10 mg • N-Acetyl-Cysteine 250 mg • Bilberry leaf 40 mg • Ginkgo Biloba 24% extract 60 mg • Quercetin 300 mg • L-Taurine 500 mg • L-Methionine 200 mg • Glutamic acid 50 mg • L-Glycine 50 mg.

Octa-Carotene **- Nature's Plus**
Each softgel contains: Vitamin A (as beta-carotene, carrot oil extract) 10,000 IU • Lutein (marigold flower extract) 6 mg • Lycopene 5 mg • Alpha Carotene (carrot oil extract) 1.7 mg • Zeaxanthin (marigold flower extract) 263 mcg • Phytoene (colorless carrot oil extract) 134

mcg • Astaxanthin (Antarctic crustacea extract) 102 mcg • Phytofluene (colorless carrot oil extract) 45 mcg •

OcuActin **- Nature's Plus**
Two capsules contain: Vitamin C corn free 100 mg • Citrus Bioflavonoid Complex 100 mg • Vitamin E natural 50 IU • Zinc (Monomethionine) 30 mg • Bilberry [(Vaccinium myrtillus fruit) standardized 25% Anthocyanosides] 25 mg • Goldenseal [(Hydrastis canadensis root & rhizome) standardized 10% Alkaloids, 5% Hydrastine] 25 mg • Echinacea [(Echinacea angustifolia root & rhizome) standardized 4% Echinacosides] 25 mg • Chinese Green Tea [(Camellia sinensis leaf) decaffeinated, standardized 50% Polyphenols] 25 mg • Grape Seed [(Vitis vinifera) standardized 95% Proanthocyanidins] 10 mg Glutathione (pharmaceutical grade Free Form Amino Acid) 10 mg • Beta Carotene (supplying 15000 IU of Vitamin A activity) 9 mg • Lutein (active Carotenoid from Marigold flower extract) 6 mg • Coenzyme Q10 (Ubiquinone) 5 mg • Copper (Glycinate) 2 mg • Zeaxanthin (active Carotenoid from Marigold flower extract) 263 mcg • Vitamin A (Retinol) 5000 IU • Selenium (Selenomethionine) 50 mcg.

Ocu-Care **- Nature's Plus**
Two tablets contain: Strengthening Nutrients: Bilberry standardized 25% Anthocyanosides 30 mg • Citrus Bioflavonoid Complex supplying: (Active Flavonones with Hesperidin & Eriocitrin 24%, Active Flavonols & Flavones, Pectin, Cellulose & Narigen 20%) 250 mg • Rutin (Saphora japonica) 100 mg. Protectant Nutrients: Pantothenic Acid 100 mg • L-Lysine free form amino acid 50 mg. Antioxidant Nutrients: Beta Carotene pro-Vitamin A, supplying 20000 IU Vitamin A activity • Vitamin A Fish Liver oil 5000 IU • Vitamin E natural 200 IU • NAC (N-Acetyl-Cysteine) 50 mg • Zinc (Monomethionine) 20 mg.

OcuDyne **- Allergy Research Group**
Two capsules contain: Vitamin A (23% as retinyl palmitate and 77% as beta-carotene) 8125 IU • Vitamin C (as ascorbic acid) 125 mg • Vitamin E (as DL-alpha-tocopheryl acetate) 100 IU • Thiamin (as thiamin hydrochloride) 5 mg • Riboflavin 6.25 mg • Niacin (83% as niacinamide) 15 mg • Vitamin B6 (as pyridoxine hydrochloride) 7.5 mg • Folic Acid 200 mcg • Vitamin B12 12.5 mcg • Pantothenic Acid 25 mg • Calcium (as calcium citrate) 25 mg • Magnesium (as magnesium citrate) 62.5 mg • Zinc (as zinc picolinate) 12.5 mg • Selenium (as sodium selenite and selenomethionine) 50 mcg • Copper (as copper sebacate) 0.75 mg • N-Acetyl-L-Cysteine 62.5 mg • Glycine 12.5 mg • L-Methionine 50 mg • Taurine 125 mg • Glutamic Acid 12.5 mg • Quercetin 75 mg • Ginkgo biloba leaves, dried extract 15 mg • Bilberry fresh berries dried extract (vaccinium myrtillus) 10 mg. Other Ingredients: Cellulose, Stearic Acid.

OcuDyne II with Lutein and Added Minerals **- Allergy Research Group**
Two capsules contain: Vitamin A (23% as retinyl palmitate and 77% as beta-carotene) 8125 IU • Vitamin C (as ascorbic acid) 125 mg • Vitamin E (as D-alpha-tocopheryl acid succinate) 50 IU • Thiamin (as thiamin hydrochloride) 5 mg • Riboflavin 6.25 mg • Niacin (86% as niacinamide) 15 mg • Vitamin B6 (as pyridoxine hydrochloride) 7.5 mg • Folic Acid 200 mcg • Vitamin B12 12.5 mcg • Pantothenic Acid 25 mg • Calcium (as calcium citrate) 25 mg • Iodine (as potassium iodide) 5 mcg • Magnesium (as magnesium citrate) 62.5 mg • Zinc (as zinc citrate) 12.5 mg • Selenium (as sodium selenite and selenomethionine) 50 mcg • Copper (as copper sebacate) 0.75 mg • Manganese (as manganese citrate) 2.5 mg • Chromium (as chromium nicotinate) 50 mcg • Molybdenum (as sodium molybdate) 30 mcg • Potassium (as potassium chloride) 25 mg • Boron (as boron citrate) 150 mcg • N-Acetyl-L-Cysteine 62.5 mg • Glycine 12.5 mg • L-Methionine 50 mg • Taurine 125 mg • Glutamic Acid 12.5 mg • Lutein 2.5 mg • Zeaxanthin 125 mcg • Quercetin 75 mg • Horsetail extract (equisetum arvense) 2.5 mg • Ginkgo Biloba leaves extract 15 mg • Bilberry fresh berries extract (vaccinium myrtillus) 10 mg. Other Ingredients: Cellulose, Magnesium Stearate.

Ocular Defense **- PhysioLogics**
Two capsules contain: Vitamin A (as 80% beta-carotene, retinyl palmitate) 12,500 IU •Vitamin E (as d-alpha tocopherol succinate) 100 IU •Riboflavin (vitamin B2) 10 mg •Vitamin B6 (as pyridoxine HCl) 10 mg •Zinc (as zinc copper amino acid chelate) 15 mg • Selenium (as selenium amino acid chelate) 50 mcg •Copper (as copper amino acid chelate) 8 mg • Chromium (as chromium amino acid chelate) 100 mcg •Taurine 200 mg •N-Acetyl Cysteine 100 mg • Bilberry fruit extract (vaccinum myrtillus, standardized to contain 25% anthocyanosides) 60 mg •Quercetin root (dimorphandra gardina) 60 mg •L-Glutathione 25 mg. Other Ingredients: Rice Powder, Gelatin, Vegetable Magnesium Stearate, Silica.

Ocular Defense Formula **- Herbalife International of America, Inc.**
Each tablet contains: Vitamin A (as mixed carotene) 500 IU • Vitamin C (as ascorbic acid) 150 mg • Calcium (as calcium carbonate) 68 mg • Zinc (as zinc amino acid chelate) 2.5 mg • Selenium (as selenium amino acid chelate) 25 mcg • Copper (as cupric oxide) 0.5 mg • Manganese (as manganese amino acid chelate) 1 mg • Citrus Bioflavonoids 75 mg • Dried Bilberry fruit extract 50 mg • Dried Turmeric rhizome extract 10 mg • Lutein (5% from tagetes erecta flower) 4 mg • N-Acetyl Cysteine 2 mg. Other Ingredients: Microcrystaline Cellulose, Magensium Taurate • Croscarmellose Sodium, Maltodextrin, Quercetin, Curcuma Longa, Cellulose, Stearic Acid, Silicon Dioxide, Magnesium Stearate, Hydroxypropyl Celluose, Alpha-Lipoic Acid, Sodium Carboxymethylcellulose, Dextrin, Dextrose, Soy Lecithin, Sodium Citrate.

Ocular Defense Plus **- PhysioLogics**
Four capsules contain: Vitamin A (as beta-carotene) 40,000 IU • Vitamin C (as ascorbic acid) 1500 mg • Vitamin E (as d-alpha tocopherol succinate) 400 IU • Riboflavin (vitamin B2) 50 mg • Zinc (as zinc picolinate) 25 mg • Selenium (as selenomethionine) 100 mcg • Chromium (as gtf chromium yeast) 200 mcg • Quercetin fruit (from dimorphandra mollis) 100 mg • Bilberry leaf extract (vaccinium myrtillus, standardized to conatin 25% anthocyanosides) 10 mg • Rutin fruit (dimorphandra mollis) 100 mg • Citrus Bioflavonoid fruit complex (citrus sinensis) 250 mg • Taurine 200 mg • N-Acetyl Cysteine 200 mg • L-Glutathione 10 mg • Lutein 20 mg. Other Ingredients: Gelatin, Silica, Vegetable Magnesium Stearate.

OculoNutrients **- Pure Encapsulations**
Six vegetable capsules contain: Ascorbic Acid 1000 mg • Vitamin C (as ascorbyl palmitate) 120 mg • Mixed Carotenoids 15000 IU: Beta Carotene 8568 mcg, Alpha Carotene 270 mcg, Zeaxanthin 54 mcg, Cryptoxanthin 66 mcg, Lutein 42 mcg • Zeaxanthin 2 mg • Lutein (from 200 mg marigold flower extract) 10 mg • Vitamin D (as D3) 400 IU • Vitamin E (D-alpha tocopherol succinate) 400 IU • Thiamine HCl (vitamin B1) 100 mg • Riboflavin (vitamin B2) 50 mg • Riboflavin 5' Phosphate (activated B2) 25 mg • Pyridoxine HCl (vitamin B6) 25 mg • Pyridoxal 5' Phosphate (activated B6) 25 mg • Niacinamide 100 mg • Inositol Hexaniacinate (no-flush niacin) 90 mg • Folic Acid 800 mcg • Biotin 800 mcg • Pantothenic Acid (calcium pantothenate) (vitamin B5) 400 mg • Methylcobalamin (vitamin B12) 1000 mcg • Calcium (citrate) 300 mg • Magnesium (citrate) 200 mg • Potassium (aspartate) 99 mg • Zinc (picolinate) 25 mg • Manganese (aspartate) 10 mg • Boron (glycinate) 2 mg • Copper (glycinate) 2 mg • Iodine (potassium iodide) 200 mcg • Chromium (polynicotinate) 200 mcg • Selenium (selenomethionine) 200 mcg • Vanadium (aspartate) 200 mcg • Molybdenum (aspartate) 100 mcg.

Oculotrophin PMG **- Standard Process, Inc.**
Each tablet contains: Proprietary Blend 191 mg: Bovine Eye PMG extract, Magnesium Citrate • Calcium 20 mg • Sodium 15 mg. Other Ingredients: Cellulose.

Ocu-Plus **- Aspen Group, Inc.**
Two tablets contain: Beta-Carotene 25,000 IU • Vitamin E (D-alpha tocopherol) 400 IU • Vitamin C 1000 mg • Citrus bioflavonoid complex 250 mg • Quercetin 100 mg • Bilberry extract (25% anthocyanosides) 80 mg • Rutin 100 mg • Zinc (gluconate) 50 mg • Copper (gluconate) 2 mg • Selenium (selenomethionine) 50 mcg •

N-Acetyl L-Cysteine (glutathione precursor) 200 mg • L-Glutathione 10 mg • Eyebright 50 mg • Alpha-Lipoic Acid 50 mg • Chromium Picolinate 200 mcg • Lutein (containing zeaxanthin) 6 mg • Ginkgo Biloba 25 mg.

OcuPower **-** NSI - Nutraceutical Sciences Institute
Three capsules contain: Vitamin A (retinyl palmitate) 2500 IU • Betatene Natural Mixed Carotenoids 15,000 IU: Beta Carotene, Alpha-Carotene, Lutein, Zeaxanthin, Cryptoxanthin • Lutein (from 200 mg standardized FloraGlo with zeaxanthin) 10 mg • Lycopene (from 12 mg Lyc-O-Mato) 600 mcg • Vitamin B1 (thiamin) 50 mg • Vitamin B2 (riboflavin) 10 mg • Vitamin B3 (niacinamide) 70 mg • Vitamin B5 (d-calcium pantothenate) 50 mg • Vitamin B6 (pyridoxine HCl) 50 mg • Vitamin B12 (methylcobalamin) 500 mcg • Folic Acid (folacin) 800 mcg • Biotin 300 mcg • Vitamin C (Ester-C) 1500 mg • Vitamin D (D3, cholecalciferol) 400 IU • Vitamin E (natural d-alpha, beta, delta, gamma forms) 500 IU • Calcium (from over 1200 mg of citrate, malate, ascorbate) 256 mg • Magnesium (from taurinate, citate) 300 mg • Zinc (L-OptiZinc) 25 mg • Selenium (l-selenomethionine) 200 mcg • Boron (chelate) 2 mg • Copper (chelate) 1 mg • Manganese (chelate) 2 mg • Chromium (glucose tolerance factor ChromeMate) 200 mcg • Iodine (kelp) 75 mcg • Molybdenum (chelate) 75 mcg • Bioperine brand Black Pepper extract 5 mg • Enzymes 50 mg: Amylae, Cellulase, Protease, Lipase, Lactase • Citrus Bioflavonoids 250 mg • Quercetin Bioflavonoids 100 mg • Rutin Bioflavonoids 100 mg • Bilberry extract (standardized 25% anthocyanosides) 160 mg • Alpha Lipoic Acid 150 mg • Taurine (magnesium taurate) 900 mg • N-Acetyl-Cysteine 200 mg • L-Glutathione 10 mg • L-Glycine 100 mg.

OcuSense **-** Natrol, Inc.
Two capsules contain: Vitamin A (from beta-carotene) 5000 IU • Vitamin C (as calcium ascorbate) 60 mg • Vitamin E (as d-alpha tocopheryl succinate) 30 IU • Zinc (as zinc methionate) 15 mg • Selenium (as l-selenomethioine) 70 mcg • Copper (as copper amino acid chelate) 2 mg • Lutein (from marigold flowers) 13 mg • Zeaxanthin (from marigold flowers) 3 mg • Bilberry fruit extract 2 mg • Anthocyanosides 500 mcg • Carrot powder 10 mg • Carotenoid Blend 10 mg: Tomato, Marigold flowers, Palm seed • Beta-Carotene 295 mcg • Alpha-Carotene 19 mcg • Cryptoxanthin 4 mcg. Other Ingredients: Gelatin, Silica, Magnesium Stearate.

Ocutabs - Walgreens
Two tablets contain: Vitamin A (beta-carotene) • Vitamin C (ascorbic acid) 226 mg • Vitamin E (dL-alpha tocopheryl acetate) • Zinc (zinc oxide) 34.8 mg • Copper (cupric oxide) 0.8 mg. Other Ingredients: Lactose, Microcrystalline Cellulose, Gelatin, Silica, Croscarmellose Sodium, Pharmaceutical Glaze, Stearic Acid, Hydroxypropylmethylcellulose, Sucrose, Polyvinylpyrrolidone, Titanium Dioxide, Crospovidone, Magnesium Silicate, Starch, Triacitin, Magnesium Stearate, FD&C Yellow No. 6 Lake, Mineral Oil, Ascorbyl Palmitate, Sodium Ascorbate, FD&C Red No. 40.

Ocutabs with Lutein - Walgreens
Each tablet contains: Vitamin A (100% as beta carotene) • Vitamin C (ascorbic acid) 200 mg • Vitamin E (dL-alpha tocopheryl acetate) • Zinc (zinc oxide) 40 mg • Copper (cupric oxide) 2 mg • Lutein 2 mg. Other Ingredients: Dicalcium Phosphate, Microcrystalline Cellulose, Calcium Carbonate, Gelatin, Croscarmellose Sodium, Sucrose, Corn Starch, Silica, Hydroxypropylmethylcellulose, Stearic Acid, Polyvinylpyrrolidone, Titanium Dioxide, Crospovidone, Magnesium Silicate, Acacia, Maltodextrin, Triacitin, Magnesium Stearate, Mineral Oil, Mixed Tocopherols, Sodium Ascorbate, Ascorbyl Palmitate, FD&C Yellow No. 6 Lake, Tricalcium Phosphate.

Ocuvite - Bausch & Lomb
Each tablet contains: Vitamin A (100% as beta carotene) 5000 IU • Vitamin C (ascorbic acid) 60 mg • Vitamin E (dl-alpha tocopherol acetate) 30 IU • Zinc (from zinc oxide) 40 mg • Selenium (from sodium selenate) 40 mcg • Copper (from cupric oxide) 2 mg. Other Ingredients: Dibasic Calcium Phosphate, Microcrystalline Cellulose, Calcium Carbonate, Crospovidone, Hydroxypropyl Methylcellulose, Titanium Dioxide, Silica Gel, Magnesium Stearate, Stearic Acid, FD&C Yellow No. 6, Triethyl Citrate, Sodium Lauryl Sulfate.

Ocuvite Extra - Bausch & Lomb
Each tablet contains: Vitamin A (beta carotene) 1000 IU • Vitamin C (ascorbic acid) 300 mg • Vitamin E (dl-alpha tocopherol acetate) 100 IU • Riboflavin (B2) 3 mg • Niacin (B3, niacinamide) 40 mg • Zinc (from zinc oxide) 40 mg • Selenium (from sodium selenate) 55 mcg • Copper (from cupric oxide) 2 mg • Manganese 5 mg • L-Glutathione 5 mg • Lutein 2 mg. Other Ingredients: Dibasic Calcium Phosphate, Microcrystalline Cellulose, Calcium Carbonate, Crospovidone, Hydroxypropyl Methylcellulose, Titanium Dioxide, Silicon Dioxide, Magnesium Stearate, Stearic Acid, FD&C Yellow No. 6, Triethyl Citrate, Polysorbate 80, Sodium Lauryl Sulfate.

Ocuvite Lutein - Bausch & Lomb
Each capsule contains: Vitamin C (ascorbic acid) 60 mg • Vitamin E (dl-alpha tocopherol acetate) 30 IU • Zinc (from zinc oxide) 15 mg • Copper (from cupric oxide) 2 mg • Lutein 6 mg. Other Ingredients: Lactose Monohydrate, Crospovidone, Magnesium Stearate, Silicon Dioxide.

Ocuvite PreserVision - Bausch & Lomb
Two tablets contain: Vitamin A (beta-carotene) 14,320 IU • Vitamin C (ascorbic acid) 226 mg • Vitamin E (dl-alpha tocopheryl acetate) 200 IU • Zinc (zinc oxide) 34.8 mg • Copper (cupric acid) 0.8 mg. Other Ingredients: Lactose Monohydrate, Microcrystalline Cellulose, Crospovidone, Stearic Acid, Magnesium Stearate, Silicon Dioxide, Polysorbate 80, Triethyl Citrate, FD&C Red #40.

ODex - Pure Encapsulations
Each vegetable capsule contains: Champignon extract (agaricus bisporis) 53 mg • Malic Acid 23 mg • Dextrin 175 mg.

Odor-Free Imperial Garlic 6500 - Vitamin World
Each tablet contains: Garlic bulb powder (allium sativum) 650 mg standardized to contain a minimum: Allicin yield 6500 mcg, total Thiosulfinates yield 6500 mcg, Alliin yield 14,500 mcg, Gamma-Glutamylcysteines 5200 mcg. Other Ingredients: Dicalcium Phosphate, Cellulose (plant origin), Food Glaze, Calcium Carbonate, Croscarmellose, Vegetable Stearic Acid, Hydroxypropyl Methylcellulose, Ttianium Dioxide Color, Magnesium Silicate, Anise Oil (pimpinella anisum, seed).

Odorless Garlic - Jamieson
Each capsule contains: Garlic Bulb Powder - equivalent to 500 mg of fresh garlic.

Odorless Garlic - Schiff
Each softgel contains: Freeze Dried 5x Garlic bulb powder (allium sativum) 100 mg • Garlic bulb oil (allium sativum) 1 mg • Hawthorne berry (crataegus spp.) 20 mg • Parsley leaf (petroselinum crispum) 10 mg. Other Ingredients: Gelatin, Glycerin, Water, Soybean Oil, Hardened Vegetable Oil Coating (cellulose acetate phithalate, food glaze, beeswax, methyl cellulose, ethyl cellulose, acetylated monoglycerides), Lecithin, Titanium Dioxide.

Odorless Garlic 1000 mg - Nature's Bounty
Each softgel contains: Odorless Garlic (allium sativum, from 10 mg garlic oil concentrate, equivalent to 1000 mg of fresh garlic bulb) 1000 mg. Other Ingredients: Soybean Oil, Gelatin, Glycerin, Silica.

Odourless Cod Liver Oil - Golden Glow Natural Health Products
Each softgel contains: Cod Liver oil 275 mg: Vitamin A 632 IU, Vitamin D (D3, as cholecalciferol 1.58 mcg) 63.2 IU.

Odourless Fish Oil - Golden Glow Natural Health Products
Each capsule contains: Natural Fish oil (salmon) 1000 mg: Omega-3 Marine Triglycerides 300 mg, Eicosapentaenoic Acid 180 mg; Docosahexaenoic Acid 120 mg.

Odourless Garlic 3000 - Golden Glow Natural Health Products
Each capsule contains: Garlic oil (equivalent to allium sativum bulb 3000 mg) 1 mg. Other Ingredients: Soya Oil, Peppermint Oil, Polysorbate 80, Sorbitan Mono-Oleate, Gelatin, Glycerol, Water.

Some Brand Name Natural Products - What they Contain

www.NaturalDatabase.com contains MANY more listings than appear here.
Editor's Notes are located on pages 2155-2163.

OFF! Botanicals Insect Repellent Lotion - S. C. Johnson & Son, Inc.
Active Ingredients: P-Menthane-3,8-Diol (cis/trans isomer ratio: min. 60% [+/-] cis and max 40% [+/-] trans) 10%.

Ogoplex Pure Extract - Boland Naturals, Inc.
Each tablet contains: Proprietary Blend: Bee Pollen, Flower Pollen, Vitamin A, Vitamin E.

OHM - Agel
Each packet contains: Vitamin C (as ascorbic acid) 60 mg • Thiamin (as thiamin hydrochloride) 0.75 mg • Riboflavin (as riboflavin) 1.7 mg • Vitamin B3 (as niacinamide) 20 mg • Vitamin B6 (as pyridoxine hydrochloride) 2 mg • Vitamin B12 (as cyanocobalamin) 18 mcg • Pantothenic Acid (as calcium pantothenate) 10 mg • Chromium (as chromium chelate) 60 mcg • Vanadium (as vanadium chelate) 10 mcg • Inositol (as inositol) 50 mg • Proprietary Blend: Taurine, D-Ribose, Schizandra fruit, Apple Cider Vinegar, Korean Ginseng root, Rhodiola root. Other Ingredients: Water, Proprietary Sweetening Blend (inulin, xylitol, neotame, acesulfame-K, lactobacillus acidophilus), Fructose, Natural Flavoring, Guar Gum, Grapefruit Seed Extract, Xanthan Gum, Sodium Benzoate.

Oil of Oregano - Gaia Herbs
Two capsules contain: Oregano leaf, supercritical CO2 extract (origanum vulgare) 400 mg. Other Ingredients: Lecithin, Vegetable Cellulose (capsule).

OilSMART - Renew Life Formulas, Inc.
Three capsules contain: Flaxseed oil 300 mg • Borage seed oil 300 mg • Fish oil 300 mg • Lipase 15 mg. Other Ingredients: Gelatin, Glycerin, Purified Water, Silicon Dioxide, Natural Caramel Color, Lecithin.

OKG Fuel Capsules OKG (L-Ornithine Alphaketoglutarate) - TwinLab
Each capsule contians: OKG 650 mg.

OKG Fuel Powder - TwinLab
Each teaspoonful contains: OKG 3.5 grams (3500 mg).

Okra Pepsin E3 - Standard Process, Inc.
Each capsule contains: Proprietary Blend 227 mg: Okra, Tillandsia Usneoides extract, Bovine Orchic extract, Pepsin 1:10,000 extract, Carbamide, Alginic Acid, Allantoin. Other Ingredients: Gelatin, Lactose, Water, Calcium stearate, Colors.

Ola Loa - Aarisse Health Care
Each packet contains: Vitamin C (ascorbic acid) 1000 mg • Vitamin B1 (thiamine) 2 mg • Vitamin B2 (riboflavin) 1 mg • Vitamin B3 (niacinamide) 10 mg • Vitamin B6 (pyridoxine) 10 mg • Folic Acid 600 mcg • Vitamin B12 (hydroxycobalamin) 100 mcg • Pantothenic Acid 10 mg • Biotin 100 mcg • Vitamin D (vitamin D3, cholecalciferol) 200 IU • Vitamin E (D-alpha tocopherol acetate) 30 IU • Vitamin K (vitamin K1, phylloquinone) 20 mcg • Coenzyme Q10 25 mg • Vitamin A 1000 IU • Lipoic Acid 1 mg • Choline Bitartrate 10 mg • Potassium (bicarbonate) 200 mg • Sodium (bicarbonate) 27 mg • Calcium (carbonate/ascorbate) 29 mg • Magnesium (ascorbate) 25 mg • Zinc (picolinate) 5 mg • Manganese (picolinate) 1.5 mg • Copper (aspartate) 500 mcg • Molybdenum (trioxide) 75 mcg • Selenium (selenite) 50 mcg • Chromium (picolinate) 100 mcg • Potassium Iodide 50 mcg • Boron (citrate) 1 mg • N-Acetyl-Cysteine (NAC) 50 mg • Arginine 100 mg • Lysine 100 mg • Glycine 1000 mg • TMG (Betaine) 1000 mg • Glutamine 100 mg • Bromelain 10 mg • Pineapple Bioflavonoids 100 mg. Other Ingredients: Fructose, Citric Acid, Aspartic Acid, Tartaric Acid, Malic Acid, Natural Fruit Flavors, Stevia.

Ola Loa Orange Energy - Ola Loa, LLC
Each packet contains: Vitamin C 1000 mg • Vitamin B1 2 mg • Vitamin B2 1 mg • Vitamin B3 10 mg • Vitamin B6 10 mg • Folic Acid 600 mcg • Vitamin B12 100 mcg • Pantothenic Acid 10 mg • Biotin 100 mcg • Vitamin D (D3) 200 IU • Vitamin E 30 IU • Vitamin K (K1) 20 mcg • Coenzyme Q10 25 mg • Vitamin A 1000 IU • Lipoic Acid 1 mg • Choline Bitartrate 10 mg • Beta Carotene 3333 IU • Potassium (bicarbonate) 200 mg • Sodium (bicarbonate) 27 mg • Calcium (carbonate, ascorbate) 29 mg • Magnesium (ascorbate) 25 mg • Zinc (picolinate) 5 mg • Manganese (picolinate) 1.5 mg • Copper (aspartate) 500 mcg • Molybdenum (trioxide) 75 mcg • Selenium (selenite) 50 mcg • Chromium (picolinate) 100 mcg • Iodide (potassium iodide) 50 mcg • Boron (citrate) 1 mg • N-Acetyl Cysteine (NAC) 50 mg • Arginine 100 mg • Lysine 100 mg • Glycine 1000 mg • TMG - Betaine 1000 mg • Glutamine 100 mg • Bromelain 10 mg • Pineapple Bioflavonoids 100 mg. Other Ingredients: Fructose, Citric Acid, Aspartic Acid, Tartaric Acid, Malic Acid, Natural Fruit Flavors, Stevia.

Ola Loa Orange Repair - Ola Loa, LLC
Each packet contains: Vitamin A (palmitate) 3000 IU • Vitamin A (as beta carotene) 833 IU • Vitamin C 500 mg • Vitamin D (D3, cholecalciferol) 400 IU • Vitamin K 200 mcg • Calcium (carbonate) 25 mg • Magnesium (oxide) 250 mg • Zinc (citrate) 5 mg • Potassium (bicarbonate) 99 mg • Selenium (l-methionine) 50 mcg • Copper (gluconate) 500 mcg • Manganese (gluconate) 3 mg • Molybdenum (amino acid chelate) 200 mcg • Sodium (sodium bicarbonate) 140 mg • Vanadium (vanadyl sulfate) 1 mg • Boron (boron citrate) 500 mcg • Citrus Bioflavonoids 30 mg • Bromelain (from pineapple) 30 mg • Gotu Kola extract 50 mg • Stevia extract 30 mg • Ginger root extract (10:1) 50 mg • L-Glycine 500 mg • Taurine 250 mg • L-Lysine 100 mg • L-Arginine 100 mg • L-Carnitine 100 mg • Glucosamine Sulfate 500 mg • Betaine TMG 500 mg • Inositol Hexanicotinate 100 mg • Calcium Pyruvate 30 mg. Other Ingredients: Fructose, Citric Acid, Natural Orange Flavor.

Olay Essential Bone Health Formula - Avon
Each tablet contains: Vitamin D 200 IU • Calcium (535 mg from calcium carbonate, 65 mg from dibasic calcium phosphate) 600 mg • Phosphorus 50 mg • Magnesium 40 mg. Other Ingredients: Acacia Gum, Hydroxypropyl Methylcellulose, Croscarmellose Sodium, Titanium Dioxide (artificial color), Polyethylene Glycol, Triethyl Citrate, Polysorbate 80, Sodium Citrate, Corn Starch.

Olay Ester-C Alpha Lipoic Collagen Support - Avon
Each tablet contains: Vitamin C Ester-C (calcium ascorbate) 500 mg • Alpha Lipoic Acid 50 mg. Other Ingredients: Cellulose Gel, Croscarmellose Sodium, Magnesium Stearate, Hydroxypropyl Methylcellulose, Titanium Dioxide (artificial color), Yellow 6 Lake, Polyethylene Glycol, Polysorbate 80.

Olay Super B-Stress Defense - Avon
Each tablet contains: Vitamin C 500 mg • Vitamin E 30 IU • Thiamin (vitamin B1) 10 mg • Riboflavin (vitamin B2) 10 mg • Niacin (vitamin B3) 100 mg • Vitamin B6 5 mg • Folate, Folic Acid, Folacin 400 mcg • Vitamin B12 12 mcg • Biotin 100 mcg • Pantothenic Acid 20 mg. Other Ingredients: Gelatin, Corn Starch, Cellulose Gel, Hydroxypropyl Methylcellulose, Polyethylene Glycol.

Olay Vitamin A Retinol/Beta Carotene - Avon
Each softgel contains: Vitamin A (63% as beta carotene) 8000 IU • Vitamin D 200 IU. Other Ingredients: Soybean Oil, Gelatin, Glycerin, Yellow Beeswax, Corn Oil, Cottonseed Oil, Water.

Olay Vitamins Beauty Nutrients - Avon
Each packet contains: Vitamin A 5000 IU • Vitamin C 120 mg • Vitamin D 400 IU • Vitamin E 460 IU • Thiamin (vitamin B1) 3 mg • Riboflavin (vitamin B2) 3.4 mg • Niacin (vitamin B3) 20 mg • Vitamin B6 4 mg • Folate, Folic Acid, Folacin 400 mcg • Vitamin B12 25 mcg • Biotin 30 mcg • Pantothenic Acid 10 mg • Calcium 250 mg • Phosphorus 48 mg • Iodine 150 mcg • Magnesium 120 mg • Zinc 22 mg • Selenium 50 mcg • Copper 5 mg • Manganese 2 mg • Chromium 120 mcg • Molybdenum 25 mcg • Chloride 72 mg • Potassium 80 mg • Nickel 5 mcg • Silicon 2 mg • Vanadium 10 mcg • Boron 150 mcg • Alpha Lipoic Acid 50 mg • CoEnzyme Q-10 32 mg • Green Tea Leaf extract (polyphenols 25 mg) 50 mg. Other Ingredients: Soybean Oil, Glycerin, Cellulose Gel, Water, Lactose, Hydroxypropyl Methylcellulose, Acacia, Crospovidone, Kelp, Silicon Dioxide, Polyethylene Glycol, Artificial Colors, Corn Starch, Triethyl Citrate, Blue 2 Lake, Red 40 Lake, Yellow 6 Lake,, Sodium Borate, Yellow 5 Lake, Lutein, Blue 1 Lake.

OLAY Vitamins Ultra CoQ10 150 mg - Pharmavite Corp.
Each softgel contains: Vitamin E 100 IU • Coenzyme Q10 150 mg. Other Ingredients: Soybean Oil, Gelatin, Glycerin, Sorbitol, Water, Polysorbate 80, Red 40, Titanium Dioxide, Blue 1.

Olde World Icelandic Cod Liver Oil (lemon mint flavor) - Garden of Life, Inc.
Each teaspoon (5 mL) contains: Vitamin A 4500 IU • Vitamin D 480 IU • Vitamin E 5 IU • Total Omega-3 Fatty Acids 962 mg: DHA 453 mg, EPA 320 mg, Other Omega-3 189 mg. Other Ingredients: Natural Lemon Essence, Natural Mint Essence.

Oliceutic-20 - Nature's Plus
Each capsule contains: Oliceutic-20 brand Olea Europaea leaf (standardized 20-25% (50-62.5 mg) oleuropein) 250 mg. Other Ingredients: Maltodextrin, Silica, Gelatin, Purified Water.

Olimmune - PhysioLogics
Three capsules contain: Licorice DGL (1% Glycyrrhizin, 7.6 mg) 760 mg • Astragalus (70% Polysaccharides, 140 mg) 200 mg • Ligusticum 200 mg • N-Acetyl-Cysteine (NAC) 135 mg • Olive leaf extract (17% Oleuropein, 17 mg) 100 mg.

Olive Balm (Royal Image Cosmetics) - InterPlexus
Aloe Barbadensis gel • Olive extract • Olive Squalane • Shea Butter • Rose Hip oil • Olive oil • Coconut oil • Spikenard • Extracts blend: Arnica, Comfrey, Ginkgo, Ginseng, Bioflavonoids • Glycerin • Olibanum • Hyaluronic Acid • Natural Essences • Azulene • Allantoin • Menthol • Turmeric extract • Tocopherol (vitamin E) • Retinyl Palmitate (vitamin A) • Cholecalciferol (vitamin D3) • Citric Acid.

Olive Leaf - Gaia Herbs
Two capsules contain: Olive leaf (olea europaea) 500 mg. Other Ingredients: Vegetable Glycerin, Lecithin, Vegetable Cellulose (capsule).

Olive Leaf - Jamieson
Each caplet contains: European Concentrate Olive Leaf 1250 mg.

Olive Leaf Extract - Olympian Labs
Each capsule contains: Olive Leaf extract 500 mg.

Olive Leaf extract - Pure Encapsulations
Each vegetable capsule contains: Olive leaf extract (olea europaea, standardized to contain 17-23% oleuropein) 500 mg.

Olive Leaf Extract - Ortho Molecular Products
Each capsule contains: Olive leaf extract (standardized to contain 20% oleuropein) 500 mg. Other Ingredients: Natural Vegetable Capsules, Magnesium Stearate, Microcrystalline Cellulose.

Olive Leaf Extract - Swanson Health Products
Each capsule contains: Olive leaf extract (15% oleuropein) 500 mg.

Olive Leaf Extract (15% Oleuropein) - Pro Health
Each Vcap contains: Olive leaf extract (oleo europea L. standardized for 15% oleuropein) 500 mg. Other Ingredients: Vegetable Cellulose, Magnesium Stearate, Silicon Dioxide, Glycerin.

Olive Leaf Extract with Hawthorn - PhytoPharmica
Two capsules contain: Olive leaf extract (olea europaea, standardized to contain 17%-23% oleuropein) 500 mg • Hawthorn leaf and flower extract (crataegus oxyacantha, standardized to contain 1.8% vitexin-2'-rhamnoside) 300 mg.

Olive Leaf Liquid Suspension - Nature's Plus
Each 1 ml serving contains: Olive leaf extract (olea europa, standardized 6% oleuropein) 125 mg. Other Ingredients: Purified Water, Vegetable Glycerin, Xanthan Gum, Citric Acid, Potassium Sorbate.

Olive Leaf Plus - Golden Glow Natural Health Products
Each tablet contains: Olive leaf extract (olea europaea) 1650 mg • Pau d'Arco inner stem bark (tabebuia avellanedae) 200 mg • Allium Sativum powder (garlic) 1000 mg.

Olive Leaf Plus - Health Smart Vitamins
Four capsules contain: Echinacea Blend: Echinacea purpurea root, leaf, Echinacea angustifolia root (4% total phenolic compounds, 10 mg) 1000 mg • Olive leaf, (Olea europaea: 17% oleuropein, 136 mg) 800 mg • Una de Gato inner bark, (Uncaria tomentosa; 2% oxindole alkaloids 1.3 mg) 80 mg.

Olivenol Capsules - CreAgri
Each capsule contains: Proprietary Organic Olive oil extract (containing polyphenols, including 5 mg Hidrox hydroxytyrosol) 300 mg. Other Ingredients: Maltodextrin, Cellulose (plant fiber), 100% Vegetarian Capsule.

Olivenol Tablets - CreAgri
Each tablet contains: Proprietary Olive oil Water Blend (containing polyphenols, including 5 mg Hidrox hydroxytyrosol) 300 mg. Other Ingredients: Calcium Carbonate, Maltodextrin, Microcrystalline Cellulose, Stearic Acid, Silicon Dioxide, Croscarmellose Sodium, Magnesium Stearate, Dextrin, Dextrose, Lecithin, Sodium Carboxymethylcellulose, Sodium Citrate.

Olympian Energy - Olympian Labs
Two capsules contain: Eleutherococcus Senticosus 200 mg • Gotu Kola (centellia asiatica) 200 mg • Guarana (paullinia cupana) 200 mg • Kola nut (cola acuminata) 200 mg • Korean Ginseng (panax ginseng) 200 mg • Cayenne (capsicum annum) 20 mg • Vitamin B6 (pyridoxine HCl) 10 mg.

Oly-Zymes - Olympian Labs
Each capsule contains: Proprietary Blend: Amylase, Protease, Lipase 200 mg.

Omega 3 Basic Master Nutrient Formula - Designing Health, Inc.
Each tablespoon contains: Vitamin A (90% as beta carotene) 55 IU • Thiamine (Vitamin B1) 0.1 mg • Calcium 22 mg • Iron 0.7 mg • Omega-3 1000 mg • Omega-6 450 mg • Omega-9 400 mg • Hesperidin 80 mg • Spirulina 8 mg • Kelp (macrocystis pyrifuri) 6 mg. Other Ingredients: Flax Seed, Blackstrap Molasses, Rice Bran, Nutritional Yeast, Sunflower Seed, Alfalfa, Carrot, Apple, Sesame Seed, Licorice Root, Broccoli, Cherry, Parsely, Sprouted Green Barley, Nettle, Vanilla Bean, Ginger Root, Sage, Rosemary, Garlic, and Yucca Schidigera Extract.

Omega 3 Fatty Acids - Trader Joe's
EPA (eicosapentaenoic acid) 300 mg • DHA (docosahexaenoic acid) 200 mg.

Omega 3 Fish Oils - Olympian Labs
Each softgel contains: Marine Lipid concentrate 1000 mg • EPA (eicosapentaenoic acid) 180 mg • DHA (docasahexaenoic acid) 120 mg • Vitamin E (d-alpha tocopherol) 1 mg.

Omega 3/DHA Esters - Xtend-Life Nutraceuticals Inc.
Each soft gel contains: Fish Oil esters 1000 mg: Omega 3 Fatty Acids 440 mg, DHA (docosahexaenoic acid) 250 mg, EPA (eicosapentaenoic acid) 110 mg, Vitamin E 1.5 IU.

Omega 3-6-9 - Pro Health
Two softgels contain: Flax Seed oil (cold pressed) 1400 mg • Evening Primrose oil (cold pressed) 300 mg • Canola oil (cold pressed) 260 mg • Black Currant oil 20 mg • Pumpkin Seed oil 20 mg. Other Ingredients: Gelatin, Glycerin, Water, Carob, Natural Vitamin E.

Omega 3-6-9 - The Vitamin Shoppe
Two softgels contain the Omega 3-6-9 essential fatty acids from 100% pure cold-pressed vegetable seed oils of: Borage 500 mg • Flaxseed 150 mg • Safflower 50 mg • Canola 200 mg • Olive 100 mg. Plus 150 mg of Omega-3 components (EPA-DHA) naturally present in Salmon Oil, providing the following: A/Gamma Linolenic Acid (Omega-3) 220 mg • Linoleic Acid (Omega-6) 290 mg • Oleic Acid (Omega-9) 306 mg.

Omega Balance - Jarrow Formulas
Each softgel contains: Fish Oil (60% omega-3) 500 mg: DHA (docosahexaenoic aicd) 235 mg, EPA (eicosapentaenoic acid) 45 mg, Stearidonic Acid 20 mg • GLA (derived from borage oil) 25 mg • CLA (conjugated linoleic acid) 100 mg • Gamma Tocopherol 4 mg. Other Ingredients: Gelatin, Glycerin, Water, Carob.

Omega Combination - Vital Nutrients
Each softgel contains: Natural Vitamin E 15 IU • Evening Primrose oil 415 mg • Gamma Linolenic Acid (GLA) 37 mg • Cis-Linoleic Acid (LA) 308 mg • Fish oil 135 mg.

Omega Complete - Body Wise International, Inc.
Each two capsules contain: EPA (eicosapentaenoic acid) 300 mg • DHA (docosahexaenoic acid) 200 mg • Other Omega-3 Fatty Acids 80 mg • GLA (gamma linolenic acid) 36 mg • Other Omega-6 Fatty Acids 74 mg • Omega-9 Fatty Acids 150 mg • Basil Oil (Ocimum basilicum) 10 mg • Thyme Oil (Thymus vulgaris) 10 mg • Turmeric Oil (Curcuma longa) 10 mg • Proprietary Blend 6 mg: Rosemary extract, Ascorbyl Palmitate, Natural Tocopherols.

Omega III Essential Fatty Acids - Nature's Life
Three capsules contain: Eicosapentaenoic Acid (EPA) (Fish Body oils) 540 mg • Docosahexaenoic Acid (DHA) (Fish Body oils) 360 mg • Garlic extract (1000:1)(Allium sativum) 150 mg • Vitamin C (Ascorbate Palmitate) 10 mg • Vitamin E (d-Alpha Tocopherol) 30 IU. In a natural base of certified organic Safflower oil.

Omega Plex - American Biologics
Each capsule contains: Soluble Sodium Salt of Butyric Acid 700 mg.

Omega Protect - Jamieson
Each capsule contains: Flax Oil 400 mg • Borage Oil 400 mg • Fish Oil 400 mg • Natural Vitamin E 10 IU • Alpha Linolenic Acid 53% 12 mg • Eicosapentaenoic (EPA) 18% 72 mg • Docosahexaenoic (DHA) 12% 48 mg • Linoleic Acid 207 mg • Gamma Linolenic Acid 18% 76 mg • Oleic Acid 173 mg.

Omega Woman - Nordic Naturals
Two softgels contain: Vitamin E (mixed tocopherols) 30 IU • EPA (eicosapentaenoic acid) 36 mg • DHA (docosahexaenoic acid) 24 mg • Evening Primrose Oil 800 mg • GLA (gamma linolenic acid) 82 mg. Other Ingredients: Purified Deep Sea Fish Oil, Soft Gel Capsule, (gelatin, water, glycerin, natural lemon oil), Antioxidant Blend (lecithin, ascorbyl palmitate).

Omega-3 - Natrol, Inc.
Two softgels contain: Omega-3 Fish Oil 2 g • EPA (eicosapentaenoic acid, 18%) 360 mg • DHA (docosahexaenoic acid, 12%) 240 mg. Other Ingredients: Gelatin, Glycerin, Mixed Tocopherols (natural).

Omega-3 Complex - PhysioLogics
Each softgel contains: Fish Oil 1000 mg: EPA (eicosapentaenoic acid) 180 mg, DHA (docosahexaenoic acid) 120 mg. Other Ingredients: Gelatin, Glycerin.

Omega-3 Complex 1200 MG - PhysioLogics
Each softgel contains: Fish Oil 1200 mg: EPA (eicosapentaenoic acid) 216 mg, DHA (docosahexaenoic acid) 144 mg. Other Ingredients: Gelatin, Glycerin.

Omega-3 Complex HP - PhysioLogics
Each softgel contains: Fish Oil 1000 mg: EPA (eicosapentaenoic acid) 300 mg, DHA (docosahexaenoic acid) 200 mg. Other Ingredients: Gelatin, Glycerin.

Omega-3 Dietary Supplement - N.V. Perricone M.D. Cosmeceuticals
Each softgel contains: Vitamin E (as natural D-alpha tocopherol 4 mg) 5 IU • Vitamin B6 (as pyridoxine HCl) 1.6 mg • Folate (as folic acid) 66.6 mcg • Vitamin B12 (cyanocobalamin) 8.3 mcg • Marine Lipid Concentrate 500 mg: Eicosapentaenoic Acid (EPA) 150 mg, Docosahexaenoic Acid (DHA) 100 mg, Other Omega-3 Fatty Acids from Flaxseed oil 25 mg • High-Allicin odor controlled Garlic 150 mg • Turmeric rhizome extract (95% curcuminoids) 42 mg • Ginger root oil 8.3 mg • Dried Ginger root 1.6 mg • Ginger standardized extract 4 mg • Rosemary leaf extract 25 mg • Tocotrienols concentrate (Nutriene brand) 4 mg. Other Ingredients: Gelatin, Glycerin, Medium Chain Triglycerides, Soy Lecithin, Beeswax, Titanium Dioxide.

Omega-3 Glucosamine - Natrol, Inc.
Three softgels contain: Glucosamine HCl 1.5 g • Chondroitin Sulfate 100 mg • Fish Oil concentrate 1 g • EPA (eicosapentaenoic acid) 300 mg • DHA (docosapentaenoic acid) 200 mg • Borage Oil 500 mg • GLA (gamma-linolenic acid) 95 mg. Other Ingredients: Soybean Lecithin, Natural Tocopherol, Beeswax, Gelatin, Glycerin, Purified Water, Caramel, Carob.
See Editor's Note No. 15.

Omega-3 HeartFelt - Life Enhancement Products, Inc.
Each capsule contains: Marine Lipid Concentrate 1000 mg: EPA (eicosapentaenoic acid) 180 mg, DHA (docosahexaenoic acid) 120 mg.

Omega-EFA - Metagenics
Each capsule contains: EPA (eicosapentaenoic acid) 150 mg • DHA (docosahexaenoic acid) 120 mg • GLA (gamma-linolenic acid) 90 mg • Vitamin E (as D-alpha tocopherol) 15 IU.

Omega-H3 Capsules - Vitabiotics
Each capsule contains: Betacarotene 5 mg • Vitamin A 750 mcg • Vitamin D 5 mcg • Vitamin B1 (thiamin) 20 mg • Vitamin B2 (riboflavin) 5 mg • Vitamin B3 (nicotinamide) 25 mg • Calcium Pantothenate 10 mg • Vitamin B6 (pyridoxine HCl) 10 mg • Vitamin B12 (cyanocobalamin) 9 mcg • Biotin 30 mcg • Folic Acid 500 mcg • Vitamin C 60 mg • Vitamin E 20 mg • PABA (para-aminobenzoic acid) 30 mg • Pollen extract 2 mg • Lecithin 40 mg • Wheat Germ Oil 100 mg • Cod Liver Oil 50 mg • Omega-3 Oil 50 mg • Ginseng 4 mg • L-Lysine 40 mg • Methionine 60 mg • Zinc 15 mg • Manganese 2 mg • Inositol 30 mg • Iron 15 mg • Iodine 150 mcg • Copper 2 mg • Magnesium 30 mg • Selenium 100 mcg • Chromium 50 mcg • Molybdenum 50 mcg • Garlic 20 mg • Rutin 10 mg.

OmegaPlex - Advocare International
Three softgels contain: Vitamin E (as D-alpha tocopherol) 15 IU • Eicosapentaenoic Acid 900 mg • Docosahexaenoic Acid 600 mg. Other Ingredients: Gelatin, Water, Glycerin.

OmegaPure 300 - Xymogen
Each softgel contains: Vitamin E (as mixed tocopherols) 10 IU • Natural Marine Lipid Concentrate 1 g • EPA (eicosapentaenoic acid) 180 mg • DHA (docosahexaenoic acid) 120 mg.

OmegaPure 600 - Xymogen
Each softgel contains: Vitamin E (as mixed tocopherols) 10 IU • Natural Marine Lipid Concentrate 1.2 g • EPA (eicosapentaenoic acid) 360 mg • DHA (docosahexaenoic acid) 240 mg.

OmegaPure EFA - Xymogen
Each softgel contains: Vitamin E (as D-alpha tocopherol) 5 IU • Flaxseed oil 400 mg • Borage seed oil 400 mg • Fish oil. Fatty Acid profile: Omega-3 Fatty Acids 420 mg: Alpha Linolenic Acid 220 mg, Eicosapentaenoic Acid (EPA) 120 mg, Docosahexaenoic Acid (DHA) 80 mg • Omega-6 Fatty Acids 276 mg: Linolenic Acid 180 mg, Gamma Linolenic Acid (GLA) 96 mg • Omega-9 Fatty Acids 152 mg. Other Ingredients: Gelatin, Glycerin.

OmegaTru Organic Flaxseed Oil - Swanson Health Products
Each tablespoon (1/2 oz) contains: Alpha Linolenic Acid 7 g • Linoleic Acid 2 g • Oleic Acid 2.8 g.

Omega-Zyme (-Zyme) Digestive Enzyme Blend Caplets - Garden of Life, Inc.
Each caplet contains: Proprietary N-zimes Blend 535 mg: Protease blend 74,750 HUT, Bromelain 230,000 FCCPU, Papain 287,500 FCCPU, Lipase 3450 FCCLU, Amylase 23,000 DU, Glucoamylase 30 AGU, Malt Diastase 193 DP, Invertase 64 SU, Lactase 863 ALU, Alpha-Galactosidase 504 GaLU, Cellulase 690 CU, Pectinase 16 endo-PG, Xylanase 575 XU, CereCalase 115 MU • Poten-Zyme Botanical Blend 300 mg: Ginger, Cat's Claw, Yucca juice, Turmeric, Probiotic cultures, Barley Grass juice. Other Ingredients: Cellulose.

Omega-Zyme (-Zyme) Digestive Enzyme Blend Powder - Garden of Life, Inc.
Each scoop contains: Proprietary N•zimes Blend 500 mg: Protease blend 65,000 HUT, Bromelain 200,000 FCCPU, Papain 250,000 FCCPU, Lipase 3000 FCCLU, Amylase 20,000 DU, Glucoamylase 25.8 AGU, Malt Diastase 168 DP, Invertase 56 SU, Lactase 750 ALU, Alpha-Galactosidase 438 GaLU, Cellulase 1500 CU, Pectinase 14 endo-PG, Xylanase 500 XU, CereCalase 100 MU • Soluble extract of Rice Bran 400 mg.

O'My O Clitoral Stimulating Gel - O'My Products, Inc.
Water • Vegetable Glycerin • Grapefruit seed extract • Hemp seed oil • Benzyl Nicotinate • Sodium Benzoate • Potassium Sorbate • Menthol • L-Arginine • Aminophylline • Citric Acid.

On Target Magnesium Plus - Life Enhancement Products, Inc.
Each capsule contains: Vitamin C 20 mg • Magnesium (as magnesium aspartate) 133 mg.

Oncolyn - Sante International
Each tablet contains: Herbal Extract-Based Blend 750 mg: Gynostemma Pentaphyllum, Crataegus Pinnatifida (hawthorn leaves/berries), Camellia Sinensis (green tea).

Oncotax - American Metabolic Institute
Unknown
See Editor's Note No. 19.

Oncovite - Mission Pharmacal
Each tablet contains: Vitamin A 9,000 IU • Vitamin C 500 mg • Vitamin D (as Vitamin D3) 400 IU • Vitamin E 100 IU • Thiamine 0.34 mg • Riboflavin 0.5 mg • Niacin 5 mg • Vitamin B6 25 mg • Folate 0.4 mg • Vitamin B12 1.6 mcg • Pantothenic Acid 2.3 mg • Zinc 7.5 mg. Other Ingredients: Microcrystalline Cellulose, Color, Acrylic Resin, Croscarmellose Sodium, Magnesium Silicate, Magnesium Stearate, Ethylcellulose, Silicon Dioxide, Polyethylene Glycol, Food Glaze, Ethyl Vanallin, Cholecalciferol, Cyanocobalamin.

One - Puritan's Pride
Each tablet contains: Vitamin A (as Retinyl Palmitate and Beta Carotene) 10,000 IU • Vitamin C (as Ascorbic Acid with Rose Hips) 250 mg • Vitamin D (as Cholecalciferol) 400 IU • Vitamin E (as D-Alpha Tocopheryl Acetate) 30 IU • Thiamin (Vitamin B-1; as Thiamine Hydrochloride) 25 mg • Riboflavin (Vitamin B-2) 25 mg • Niacin (as Niacinamide) 50 mg • Vitamin B-6 (as Pyridoxine Hydrochloride) 50 mg • Folic Acid 400 mcg • Vitamin B-12 (as Cyanocobalamin) 50 mcg • Biotin (as D-Biotin) 50 mcg • Pantothenic Acid (as D-Calcium Pantothenate) 50 mg • Calcium (as Bone Meal) 50 mg • Iron (as Ferrous Fumarate) 10 mg • Phosphorus (as Bone Meal) 23 mg • Iodine (as Potassium Iodide) 150 mcg • Magnesium (as Magnesium Oxide) 100 mg • Zinc (as Zinc Sulfate) 15 mg • Selenium (as Selenium Yeast) 25 mcg • Copper (as Copper Sulfate) 2 mg • Manganese (as Manganese Sulfate) 5 mg • Chromium (as Chromium Chloride) 100 mcg • Molybdenum (as Sodium Molybdate) 15 mcg • Chloride (as Potassium Chloride) 1 mg • Potassium (as Potassium Chloride) 1 mg • PABA (Para-Aminobenzoic Acid) 50 mg • Inositol 15 mg • Choline Bitartrate 15 mg. Base: Bioflavonoids, Rutin, Rose Hip, Yeast, Kelp, Dolomite.

One Daily - Leiner Health Products
Each tablet contains: Folate (Folic Acid) 400 mcg • Niacin (Niacinamide) 20 mg • Pantothenic Acid (d-Calcium Pantothenate) 10 mg • Riboflavin (Vitamin B2) 1.7 mg • Thiamin Mononitrate (Vitamin B1) 1.5 mg • Vitamin A Acetate 5000 IU • Vitamin B12 (Cyanocobalamin - USP Mehtod 2) 6 mcg • Vitamin B6 (Pyridoxine Hydrochloride) 2 mg • Vitamin C (Ascorbic Acid) 60 mg • Vitamin D (Ergocalciferol) 400 IU • Vitamin E (dl-Alpha Tocopheryl Acetate) 30 IU. Other Ingredients: Calcium Carbonate, Gelatin, Maltodextrin, Hydroxypropyl Methylcellulose, Starch, Cellulose, Croscarmellose Sodium, Sodium Starch Glycolate, Silicon Dioxide, Hydroypropyl Cellulose, Red 40 Lake, Polyethylene Glycol 3350, Magnesium Stearate, Polysorbate 80, Resin, Titanium Dioxide, Povidone.

One Daily - The Vitamin Shoppe
Each tablet contains: Vitamin A 10000 IU • Vitamin D (as Vitamin D3) 400 IU • Vitamin C 100 mg • Citrus Bioflavonoids 25 mg • Rutin 5 mg • Hesperidin Complex 5 mg • Vitamin E 150 IU • Vitamin B1 25 mg • Vitamin B2 25 mg • Vitamin B6 25 mg • Vitamin B12 100 mcg • Calcium Pangamate 25 mg • Pantothenic Acid 25 mg • Biotin 50 mcg • Folic Acid 400 mcg • Niacinamide 25 mg • Inositol 25 mg • Choline 25 mg • PABA 25 mg • Calcium 100 mg • Magnesium 50 mg • Potassium 25 mg • Manganese 5 mg • Zinc 15 mg • Iron 18 mg • Selenium 50 mcg • GTF Chromium 50 mcg • Iodine 150 mcg • Copper 2 mg • Molybdenum 100 mcg • Vitamin K 25 mcg • SOD 25 mcg • Octacosanol 100 mcg • L-Carnitine 5 mg • CoQ10 10 mcg • GLA 5 mg • Korean Ginseng 10 mg • Bee Pollen 10 mg • Royal Jelly 5 mg • Betaine HCl 10 mg • Pepsin 10 mg • Bromelain 10 mg • Papain 10 mg • Lecithin 25 mg • L-Glutathione 5 mg • L-Cysteine 5 mg • L-Methionine 5 mg • EPA & DHA 50 mg.

One Daily + Minerals - Leiner Health Products
Each tablet contains: Chromium Yeast 10 mcg • Magnesium Hydroxide100 mg • Selenium Yeast 10 mcg • Calcium 130 mg • Molybdenum Yeast 10 mcg • Manganese Sulfate 2.5 mg • Copper (Cupric Sulfate) 2 mg • Folate (Folic Acid) 400 mcg • Iodine (Potassium Iodide) 150 mcg • Iron (Ferrous Fumarate) 18 mg • Niacin (Niacinamide) 20 mg • Pantothenic Acid (d-Calcium Pantothenate) 10 mg • Riboflavin (Vitamin B2) 1.7 mg • Thiamin Mononitrate (Vitamin B1) 1.5 mg • Vitamin A Acetate 5000 IU • Vitamin B12 (Cyanocobalamin - USP Method 2) 6 mcg • Vitamin B6 (Pyridoxine Hydrochloride) 2 mg • Vitamin C (Ascorbic Acid) 60 mg • Vitamin D (Ergocalciferol) 400 IU • Vitamin E (dl-Alpha Tocopheryl Acetate) 30 IU • Zinc Sulfate 15 mg • Biotin (USP Method 2) 30 mcg • Phosphorus 100 mg • Chloride 34 mg • Potassium Chloride 37.5 mg. Other Ingredients: Dicalcium Phosphate, Gelatin, Pregelatinized Starch, Cellulose, Sodium Starch Glycolate, Hydroxypropyl Methylcellulose, Croscarmellose Sodium, Silicon Dioxide, Tricalcium Phosphate, Red 40 Lake, Polyethylene Glycol 3350, Hydroxypropyl Cellulose, Pharmaceutical Glaze, Magnesium Stearate, Crospovidone, Polysorbate 80, Titanium Dioxide, Beta Carotene, Resin, Povidone.

One Daily 50+ - Leiner Health Products
Each tablet contains: Vitamin B12 (Cyanocobalamin) 30 mcg • Thiamin Mononitrate (Vitamin B1) 4.5 mg • Vitamin B6 (Pyridoxine Hydrochloride) 6 mg • Magnesium Hydroxide 100 mg • Vitamin K (Phytonadione) 20 mcg • Manganese Sulfate 4 mg • Riboflavin (Vitamin B2) 3.4 mg • Vitamin C (Ascorbic Acid) 120 mg • Vitamin E (dl-Alpha Tocopheryl Acetate) 60 IU • Chromium Chloride 180 mcg • Pantothenic Acid (d-Calcium Pantothenate) 15 mg • Selenium (Sodium Molybdate) 105 mcg • Zinc Sulfate 22.5 mg • Molybdenum (Sodium Molybdate) 93.75 mcg • Calcium Carbonate 120 mg • Copper (Cupric Sulfate) 2 mg • Folate (Folic Acid) 400 mcg • Iodine (Potassium Iodide) 150 mcg • Niacin (Niacinamide Ascorbate) 20 mg • Vitamin A Acetate 5000 IU • Vitamin D (Cholecalciferol) 400 IU • Biotin (USP Method 2) 30 mcg • Chloride 34 mg • Potassium Chloride 37.5 mg. Other Ingredients: Starch, Cellulose, Dicalcium Phosphate, Maltodextrin, Hydroxypropyl Methylcellulose, Croscarmellose Sodium, Gelatin, Titanium Dioxide, Calcium Silicate, Crospovidone, Pharmaceutical Glaze, Magnesium Stearate, Hydroxypropyl Cellulose, Resin, Mannitol, Polyethylene Glycol 3350, Polysorbate 80, Yellow 6 Lake, Blue 2 Lake, Beta Carotene.

One Daily Men's Formula - Leiner Health Products
Each tablet contains: Magnesium Hydroxide 100 mg • Manganese Sulfate 3.5 mg • Riboflavin (Vitamin B2) 2.55 mg • Thiamin Mononitrate (Vitamin B1) 2.25 mg • Vitamin B12 (Cyanocobalamin - USP Mehtod 2) 9 mcg • Vitamin B6 (Pyridoxine Hyrochloride) 3 mg • Vitamin C (Ascorbic Acid) 90 mg • Vitamin E (dl-Alpha Tocopheryl Acetate) 45 IU • Chromium Chloride 150 mcg • Selenium (Sodium Selenate) 87.5 mcg • Copper (Cupric Sulfate) 2 mg • Folate (Folic Acid) 400 mcg • Iodine (Potassium Iodide) 150 mcg • Molybdenum (Sodium Molybdate) 75 mcg • Niacin (Niacinamide Ascorbate) 20 mg • Pantothenic Acid (d-Calcium Pantothenate) 10 mg • Vitamin A 5000 IU • Vitamin D (Cholecalciferol) 400 IU • Zinc Sulfate 15 mg • Chloride 34 mg • Potassium Chloride 37.5 mg. Other Ingredients:

Starch, Cellulose, Dicalcium Phosphate, Gelatin, Croscarmellose Sodium, Hydroxypropyl Methylcellulose, Calcium Silicate, Crospovidone, Hydroxypropyl Cellulose, Pharmaceutical Glaze, Polyethylene Glycol 3350, Yellow 6 Lake, Titanium Dioxide, Resin, Beta Carotene, Polysorbate 80.

One Daily Multiple - Nature's Life
Each capsule contains: Beta Carotene (Vitamin A equivalent to 10,000 IU) 6 mg • Vitamin D (as Vitamin D3) (Cholecalciferol) 200 IU • Vitamin E (d-Alpha Tocopheryl Succinate) 100 IU • Vitamin B1 (Thiamine Mononitrate) 25 mg • Vitamin B2 (Riboflavin & Riboflavin 5'-Phosphate) 25 mg • Vitamin B6 Pyridoxine HCl & Pyridoxine 5'-Phosphate) 25 mg • Niacinamide 50 mg • Vitamin B12 (Cyancobalamin) 100 mcg • Folic Acid 400 mcg • Pantothenic Acid (d-Calcium Pantothenate) 50 mg • Biotin (d-Biotin) 300 mcg • Choline (Bitartrate) 25 mg • Inositol 25 mg • PABA (Para Aminobenzoic Acid) 25 mg • Vitamin C 100 mg • Boron (Citrate) 50 mcg • Calcium (Carbonate, Citrate/ Malate) 50 mg • Chromium (Picolinate) 100 mcg • Copper (Gluconate, Citrate) 1 mg • Magnesium (Oxide,Citrate) 10 mg • Manganese (Gluconate) 5 mg • Molybdenum (Sodium Molybdate) 150 mcg • Potassium (Chloride) 5 mg • Selenium (Selenomethionine) 100 mcg • Silicon (Dioxide) 10 mg • Vanadium(Vandyl Sulfate) 25 mcg • Zinc (Picolinate) 15 mg.

One Daily with Calcium, Iron, & Zinc - Leiner Health Products
Each tablet contains: Calcium Carbonate 45 mg • Iron (Ferrous Fumarate) 27 mg • Folate (Folic Acid) 400 mcg • Niacin (Niacinamide) 20 mg • Pantothenic Acid (d-Calcium Pantothenate) 10 mg • Riboflavin (Vitamin B2) 1.7 mg • Thiamin Mononitrate (Vitamin B1) 1.5 mg • Vitamin A Acetate 5000 IU • Vitamin B12 (Cyanocobalamin - USP Method 2) 6 mcg • Vitamin B6 (Pyridoxine Hydrochloride) 2 mg • Vitamin C (Ascorbic Acid) 60 mg • Vitamin D (Cholecalciferol) 400 IU • Vitamin E (dl-Alpha Tocopheryl Acetate) 30 IU • Zinc Oxide 15 mg. Other Ingredients: Maltodextrin, Gelatin, Hydroxypropyl Methylcellulose, Croscarmellose Silicon Dioxide, Propylene Glycol, Titanium Dioxide, Hydroxypropyl Cellulose, Polyethylene Glycol 3350, Pharmaceutical Glaze, Starch, Magnesium Stearate, Yellow 5 Lake, Yellow 6 Lake, Polysorbate 80, Beta Carotene, Povidone, Resin.

One Daily without Iron - The Vitamin Shoppe
Each tablet contains: Vitamin A 10000 IU • Vitamin D (as Vitamin D3) 400 IU • Vitamin C 100 mg • Citrus Bioflavonoids 25 mg • Rutin 5 mg • Hesperidin Complex 5 mg • Vitamin E 150 IU • Vitamin B1 25 mg • Vitamin B2 25 mg • Vitamin B6 25 mg • Vitamin B12 100 mcg • Calcium Pangamate 25 mg • Pantothenic Acid 25 mg • Biotin 50 mcg • Folic Acid 400 mcg • Niacinamide 25 mg • Inositol 25 mg • Choline 25 mg • PABA 25 mg • Calcium 100 mg • Magnesium 50 mg • Potassium 25 mg • Manganese 5 mg • Zinc 15 mg • Selenium 50 mcg • GTF Chromium 50 mcg • Iodine 150 mcg • Copper 2 mg • Molybdenum 100 mcg • Vitamin D 25 mcg • SOD 25 mcg • Octacosanol 100 mcg • L-Carnitine 5 mg • CoQ10 10 mcg • GLA 5 mg • Korean Ginseng 10 mg • Bee Pollen 10 mg • Royal Jelly 5 mg • Betaine HCl 10 mg • Pepsin 10 mg • Bromelain 10 mg • Papain 10 mg • Lecithin 25 mg • L-Glutathione 5 mg • L-Cysteine 5 mg • L-Methionine 5 mg • EPA & DHA 50 mg.

One Step - Progressive Labs
Each level scoop (approx 31 g) contains: Vitamin A 5000 IU • Ester C brand Vitamin C 177 mg • Vitamin D 200 IU • Covitol brand Vitamin E 70 IU • Vitamin K 40 mcg • Thiamin (vitamin B1) 3 mg • Riboflavin (vitamin B2) 3 mg • Niacinamide (vitamin B3) 13 mg • Vitamin B6 (pyridoxine HCl) 30 mg • Folate (folic acid) 446 mcg • Vitamin B12 250 mcg • Biotin 150 mcg • Pantothenic Acid 23 mg • Calcium 326 mg • Iron 3 mg • Phosphorus 266 mg • Iodine 38 mcg • Magnesium 255 mg • Zinc (as ascorbate) 8 mg • Selenium 40 mcg • Copper (as amino acid chelate) 2 mg • Manganese (as ascorbate) 6 mg • Chromium (as nicotinate) 100 mcg • Molybdenum 13 mg • Chloride 175 mg • Ultralec brand Lecithin 1000 mg • Glucosamine HCl 750 mg • Nopal 750 mg • Trimethylglycine 250 mg • MSM (methyl sulfonyl methane) 250 mg • Beta 1,3 Glucans 250 mg • L-Cysteine 175 mg • Inulin (fructo-oligosaccharides) 170 mg • Gamma Oryzanol 150 mg • L-Glutamine 125 mg • L-Ornithine 100 mg • L-Taurine 100 mg • Citri-Max brand Garcinia Cambogia 75 mg • Globulin Protein 75 mg • Citrus Bioflavonoid 5X Complex 50 mg • Aloe Isolate 50 mg • Inositol 25 mg • Creatine Pyruvate 25 mg • Siberian Ginseng root extract (eleutherococcus senticosus) 25 mg • Betatene brand Lycopene 25 mg • Alpha Lipoic Acid 25 mg • Soy Isoflavones (from 63 mg NovaSoy brand) 25 mg • Guggulipid extract (commiphora mukul) 13 mg • Leci-PS brand Phosphatidyl Serine 11 mg • L-Glutathione 10 mg • Quercetin 10 mg • FloraGlo brand Lutein 8 mg • Ginkgo Biloba leaf extract 5 mg • Grape seed extract (vitis vinifera) 5 mg • Grape skin extract (vitis vinifera) 5 mg • Bioperine brand Black Pepper extract 5 mg • Mixed Tocotrienols 2 mg • Coenzyme Q10 1 mg • Pycnogenol brand Oligomeric Proanthocyanidins 1 mg • Boron 250 mcg. Other Ingredients: Arcon VF Brand Soy Protein Concentrate, Rice Bran, Guar Gum, Natural Vanilla, Other Natural Flavors, Stevia.

One-A-Day 50 Plus Formula - Bayer
Each tablet contains: Vitamin A 5000 IU • Vitamin C 120 mg • Vitamin D 400 IU • Vitamin E 60 IU • Vitamin K 20 mcg • Thiamin (B1) 4.5 mg • Riboflavin (B2) 3.4 mg • Niacin 20 mg • Vitamin B6 6 mg • Folic Acid 400 mcg • Vitamin B12 30 mcg • Biotin 30 mcg • Pantothenic Acid 15 mg • Calcium (elemental) 120 mg • Iodine 150 mcg • Magnesium 100 mg • Zinc 22.5 mg • Selenium 105 mcg • Copper 2 mg • Manganese 4 mg • Chromium 180 mcg • Molybdenum 93.75 mcg • Chloride 34 mg • Potassium 37.5 mg.

One-A-Day Active Formula - Bayer
Each tablet contains: Vitamin A 5000 IU • Vitamin C 120 mg • Vitamin D 400 IU • Vitamin E 60 IU • Vitamin K 25 mcg • Thiamin (vitamin B1) 4.5 mg • Riboflavin (vitamin B2) 5.1 mg • Niacin 40 mg • Vitamin B6 6 mg • Folic Acid 400 mcg • Vitamin B12 18 mcg • Biotin 40 mcg • Pantothenic Acid 10 mg • Calcium (elemental) 110 mg • Iron 9 mg • Phosphorus 48 mg • Iodine 150 mcg • Magnesium 40 mg • Zinc 15 mg • Selenium 45 mcg • Copper 2 mg • Manganese 2 mg • Chromium 100 mcg • Molybdenum 25 mcg • Chloride 180 mg • Potassium 200 mg • Nickel 5 mcg • Tin 10 mcg • Silicon 6 mg • Vanadium 10 mcg • Boron 150 mcg • American Ginseng root standardized extract (panax quinquefolius) 55 mg.

One-A-Day Bedtime & Rest - Bayer
Each two tablets contain: Calcium 450 mg • Magnesium 80 mg • Lecithin 20 mg • Kava Kava standardized extract (piper methysticum) root 100 mg • Valerian Standardized extract (valeriana officinalis) root 200 mg • Rosemary Standardized extract (rosmannus officinalis) leaf 10 mg.
See Editor's Note No. 21.

One-A-Day Bone Strength - Bayer
Each tablet contains: Vitamin D 100 IU • Calcium (precipitated) 500 mg • Soy bean standardized extract 28 mg.
See Editor's Note No. 21.

One-A-Day CarbSmart - Bayer
Each tablet contains: Vitamin A (100% as beta carotene) 2500 IU • Vitamin C 90 mg • Vitamin D 400 IU • Vitamin E 45 IU • Vitamin K 25 mcg • Thiamin (vitamin B1) 2.2 mg • Riboflavin (vitamin B2) 2.5 mg • Niacin 25 mg • Vitamin B6 3 mg • Folic Acid 400 mcg • Vitamin B12 9 mcg • Biotin 450 mcg • Pantothenic Acid 15 mg • Calcium 200 mg • Phosphorus 154 mg • Magnesium 100 mg • Zinc 22.5 mg • Selenium 105 mcg • Copper 2 mg • Manganese 2 mg • Chromium 200 mcg • Molybdenum 75 mg • Potassium 99 mg. Other Ingredients: Cellulose, Croscarmellose Sodium, Titanium Dioxide, Magnesium Stearate, Gelatin, Dextrose, Hypromellose, Corn Starch, Silicon Dioxide, Crospovidone, Dextrin, Polyethylene Glycol, Sodium Carboxymethylcellulose, Glucose, FD&C Yellow #5 (tartrazine) Lake, Mineral Oil, Sodium Citrate, Resin, Acacia, Lecithin, Polysorbate 80, FD&C Yellow #6 Lake.

One-A-Day Cholesterol Health - Bayer
Each two tablets contain: Vitamin E 200 IU • Lecithin 100 mg • Garlic (Allium sativum) freeze dried/bulb 30 mg • Soy Standardized extract (Glycine max or spp.) bean 140 mg.
See Editor's Note No. 21.

Some Brand Name Natural Products - What they Contain

www.NaturalDatabase.com contains MANY more listings than appear here.
Editor's Notes are located on pages 2155-2163.

BRAND NAMES

One-A-Day Cold Season - Bayer
Each tablet contains: Vitamin C 500 mg • Zinc 7.5 mg • Echinacea Standardized extract (Echinacea purpurea) whole plant/root 50 mg. See Editor's Note No. 21.

One-A-Day Energy Formula - Bayer
Each tablet contains: Thiamin (B1) 2.25 mg • Niacin 20 mg • Vitamin B6 3 mg • Folic Acid 200 mcg • Pantothenic Acid 10 mg • Chromium (as Picolinate) 100 mcg • Ginseng Standardized extract (Panax ginseng) root 200 mg.

One-A-Day Maximum Formula - Bayer
Each tablet contains: Vitamin A Acetate 5000 IU • Vitamin C (Ascorbic Acid) 60 mg • Vitamin D 400 IU • Vitamin E Acetate 30 IU • Vitamin K (Phytonadione) 25 mcg • Thiamin Mononitrate 1.5 mg • Riboflavin (Vitamin B2) 1.7 mg • Niacin (Vitamin B3) 20 mg • Vitamin B6 (Pyridoxine Hydrochloride) 2 mg • Folate (Folic Acid, Folacin) 400 mcg • Vitamin B12 6 mcg • Biotin 30 mcg • Pantothenic Acid (Calcium Pantothenate) 10 mg • Calcium Carbonate 162 mg • Iron (Ferrous Fumarate) 18 mg • Phosphorus 109 mg • Iodine (Potassium Iodide) 150 mcg • Magnesium Hydroxide 100 mg • Zinc Sulfate15 mg • Selenium (Sodium Selenate) 20 mcg • Copper (Cupric Sulfate) 2 mg • Manganese 3.5 mg • Chromium Chloride 65 mcg • Molybdenum (Sodium Molybdate) 160 mcg • Chloride 72 mg • Potassium Chloride 80 mg • Nickel (Nickelous Sulfate) 5 mcg • Tin (Stannous Chloride)10 mcg • Silicon (Sodium Metasilicate) 2 mg • Vanadium (Sodium Metavanadate) 10 mcg • Boron (Disodium Borate) 150 mcg. Other Ingredients: Cellulose, Modified Cellulose Gum, Gelatin, Citric Acid, Hydroxypropyl Methylcellulose, Magnesium Stearate, Artificial Color, Silicon Dioxide, Disodium Borate, Beta Carotene.

One-A-Day Memory & Concentration - Bayer
Each tablet contains: Vitamin B6 1 mg • Vitamin B12 3 mcg • Choline 60 mg • Ginkgo Standardized extract (Ginkgo biloba) leaf 60 mg.

One-A-Day Menopause Health - Bayer
Each tablet contains: Vitamin E 15 IU • Calcium (precipitated) 250 mg • Lecithin 15 mg • Black Cohosh Standardized extract (Cimicifuga racemosa) root 10 mg • Soy Standardized extract (Glycine max or spp.) bean 42 mg.
See Editor's Note No. 21.

One-A-Day Men's Health Formula - Bayer
Each tablet contains: Vitamin A (vitamin A acetate, 14% as beta carotene) 3500 IU • Vitamin C (ascorbic acid, ascorbyl palmitate) 90 mg • Vitamin D (ergocalciferol) 400 IU • Vitamin E (DL-alpha tocopherol acetate) 45 IU • Vitamin K (phytonadione) 20 mcg • Thiamin (B1, thiamine mononitrate) 1.2 mg • Riboflavin (B2) 1.7 mg • Niacin (B3, niacinamide) 16 mg • Vitamin B6 (pyridoxine hydrochloride) 3 mg • Folate, Folic Acid, Folacin 400 mcg • Vitamin B12 (cyanocobalamin) 18 mcg • Biotin 30 mcg • Pantothenic Acid (D-calcium pantothenate) 5 mg • Calcium (elemental, calcium carbonate) 210 mg • Magnesium (magnesium oxide) 120 mg • Zinc (zinc oxide) 15 mg • Selenium (sodium selenate) 105 mcg • Copper (cupric oxide) 2 mg • Manganese (manganese sulfate) 2 mg • Chromium (chromium chloride) 120 mcg • Potassium (potassium chloride) 100 mg • Lycopene (lycopersicon esculentum fruit) 0.6 mg. Other Ingredients: Cellulose, Gelatin, Croscarmellose Sodium, Acacia, Dicalcium Phosphate, Stearic Acid, Silicon Dioxide, Dextrin, Magnesium Stearate, Starch, Calcium Silicate, Sucrose, Mannitol, Hydroxypropyl Methylcellulose, Resin, Dextrose, Lecithin, Sodium Carboxymethylcellulose, Sodium Ascorbate, Sodium Citrate.

One-A-Day Prostate Health - Bayer
Two softgels contain: Zinc Gluconate 15 mg • Pumpkin Seed Oil Standardized extract 80 mg • Saw Palmetto Standardized extract (Serenoa repens) berry 320 mg. Other Ingredients: Gelatin, Glycerin, Vegetable Oil, Beeswax, Lecithin, Titanium Dioxide, FD&C Red #40 (Tartrazine), FD&C Yellow #6, FD&C Blue #1, FD&C Yellow #5 (Tartrazine).

One-A-Day Tension & Mood - Bayer
Each tablet contains: Vitamin C 60 mg • Thiamin (B1) 1.125 mg • Niacin 10 mg • Folic Acid 100 mcg • Pantothenic Acid 5 mg • Lecithin 15 mg • Kava Kava root/rhizome standardized extract (piper methysticum) 100 mg • St. John's Wort leaf/flower standardized extract (hypericum perforatum) 225 mg.
See Editor's Note No. 21.

One-A-Day Women's Formula - Bayer
Each tablet contains: Vitamin A 2500 IU • Vitamin C 60 mg • Vitamin D 400 IU • Vitamin E 30 IU • Thiamin (Vitamin B1) 1.5 mg • Riboflavin (Vitamin B2) 1.7 mg • Niacin 10 mg • Vitamin B6 2 mg • Folic Acid 400 mcg • Vitamin B12 6 mcg • Pantothenic Acid 5 mg • Calcium (elemental) 450 mg • Iron 18 mg • Magnesium 50 mg • Zinc 15 mg.

One-Gram C - J. R. Carlson Laboratories, Inc.
Each tablet contains: Vitamin C (as ascorbic acid) 1000 mg.

One-Per-Meal Radical Shield - Life Enhancement Products, Inc.
Each capsule contains: Vitamin A (as vitamin A palmitate) 1667 IU • Vitamin A (as beta-carotene) 10 mg • Vitamin C (as calcium ascorbate and niacinamide ascorbate) 300 mg • Vitamin D (as cholecalciferol) 300 IU • Vitamin E (as D,L-alpha-tocopheryl acetate) 67 IU • Vitamin K (as phytonadione) 47 mcg • Thiamine (vitamin B1 as thiamine hydrochloride) 5.2 mg • Riboflavin (vitamin B2) 6.7 mg • Niacin (vitamin B3 as niacinamide ascorbate) 40 mg • Vitamin B6 (as pyridoxine hydrochloride) 15 mg • Folic Acid 267 mcg • Vitamin B12 (cyanocobalamin) 33 mcg • Biotin 167 mcg • Pantothenic Acid (vitamin B5 as calcium pantothenate) 43 mg • Calcium (as calcium ascorbate and calcium pantothenate) 31 mg • Iodine (as potassium iodide) 50 mcg • Zinc (as zinc gluconate) 12 mg • Selenium (as sodium selenite) 57 mcg • Copper (as copper gluconate) 1 mg • Manganese (as manganese gluconate) 833 mcg • Chromium (as chromium aspartate) 67 mcg • Molybdenum (as molybdenum gluconate) 167 mcg • Taurine 50 mg • L-Cysteine Hydrochloride 33 mg • Quercetin 17 mg • Boron (as calcium borate) 1 mg.

OneSource - Health Smart Vitamins
Each caplet contains: Vitamin D (cholecalciferol) 400 IU • Vitamin A (60% retinyl acetate, 40% beta-carotene) 5,000 IU • Vitamin C (ascorbic acid) 60 mg • Vitamin E (DL-alpha-tocopheryl acetate) 30 IU • Vitamin K (phytonadione) 25 mcg • Thiamin (thiamin mononitrate) 1.5 mg • Riboflavin 1.7 mg • Niacin (niacinamide) 20 mg • Vitamin B6 (pyridoxine HCl) 2 mg • Folate (folic acid) 400 mcg • Vitamin B12 (cyanocobalamin) 6 mcg • Biotin 30 mcg • Pantothenic Acid (D-calcium pantothenate) 10 mg • Calcium (dicalcium phosphate) 162 mg • Iron (ferrous fumarate) 18 mg • Phosphorus (dicalcium phosphate) 125 mg • Iodine (potassium iodide) 150 mcg • Magnesium (90% oxide, 10% amino acid chelate) 100 mg • Zinc (amino acid chelate) 15 mg • Selenium (selenomethionine) 20 mcg • Copper (sulfate) 2 mg • Manganese (sulfate) 2.5 mg • Chromium (picolinate) 25 mcg • Molybdenum (sodium molybdenate) 25 mcg • Chloride (potassium chloride) 36 mg • Potassium (chloride) 40 mg • Silica (dioxide) 2 mg • Boron (sodium borate) 150 mcg • Tin (stannous chloride) 10 mcg • Vanadium (amino acid chelate) 10 mcg • Nickel (sulfate) 5 mcg.

OneSource Complete Prenatal - Perrigo
Two caplets contain: Vitamin A (25% as beta carotene) 4800 IU • Vitamin C 120 mg • Vitamin D 400 IU • VItamin E 30 IU • Thiamin 1.84 mg • Riboflavin 2 mg • Niacin 20 mg • Vitamin B6 20 mg • Folic Acid 800 mcg • Vitamin B12 12 mcg • Calcium 300 mg • Iron 28 mg • Iodine 150 mcg • Zinc 25 mg • Copper 2 mg. Other Ingredients: Microcrystalline Cellulose, Acacia, Gelatin, Modified Cellulose Gum, Sucrose Ester, Dextrin, Titanium Dioxide, Hypromellose, Polyethylene Glycol, Lecithin (soy), FD&C Red #40 Lake, DExtrose, FD&C Yellow #6 Lake, Gluten.

OPC - Pain & Stress Center
Each capsule contains: Oligomeric Proanthocyanidin 95% extract (from grape seeds) 30 mg. Other Ingredients: Gelatin Capsule.

Some Brand Name Natural Products - What they Contain

www.NaturalDatabase.com contains MANY more listings than appear here.
Editor's Notes are located on pages 2155-2163.

OPC Synergy - Standard Process, Inc.
Each capsule contains: Proprietary Blend 295 mg: Buckwheat juice powder, Green Tea leaf powder, Carrot powder • Grape seed extract 50 mg • Red Wine extract 25 mg • Green Tea extract 25 mg • Bilberry 25 mg. Other Ingredients: Gelatin, Water, Calcium Stearate, Colors.

OPCs + II - Matol Botanical International Ltd
Two capsules contain: Beta-1,3-D-Glucan 700 mg • Acerola Cherry extract 200 mg • Masquelier's brand Grape seed extract 100 mg.

OPCs +95 (100 mg) - Jarrow Formulas
Each softgel contains: Grape Seed 100:1 extract (95% polyphenols consisting of: catechins, epicatechins 10 mg, dimers 15 mg, oligomers 67 mg, gallic acid 3 mg) 100 mg. Other Ingredients: Rice Powder, Magnesium Stearate, Silicon Dioxide, Gelatin.

OPCs +95 (50 mg) - Jarrow Formulas
Each capsule contains: Grape seed 100:1 extract (from grape seed, 95% polyphenols consisting of approximately: catechins, epicatechins 5 mg, dimers 7.5 mg, oligomers 33.5 mg, gallic acid 1.5 mg) 50 mg. Other Ingredients: Rice Powder, Magnesium Stearate, Silicon Dioxide, Gelatin.

Ophthacare - The Himalaya Drug Company
Yawani (carum copticum syn. trachyspermum ammi) • Vibhitaki (terminalia belerica syn. t.bellirica) • Amalaki (emblica officinalis) • Haridra (curcuma longa) • Vishu Priya (ocimum sanctum syn. o.tenuiflorum) • Satapatri (rosa damascena syn. r.centifolia) • Karpoora (cinnamomum camphora) • Madhu (mel despumatum syn. mel despumatum, purified) • Phenyl Mercuric Nitrate (as preservative).

Ophthaplus - Atrium Biotechnologies
Each tablet contains: Raw Eye concentrate 120 mg • Raw Brain concentrate 20 mg • Eyebright 150 mg • Rutin 125 mg • Hesperidin Complex 20 mg.
See Editor's Note No. 31.

OptaFlex brand - Cargill Health & Food Technologies
Chondroitin.
See Editor's Note No. 4, No. 44 and No. 45.

Optein - Solgar
Each level scoop (35 grams) contains: Vitamin A (3600 IU palmitate 18%, 1400 IU as natural beta carotene from Dunaliella salina) 5000 IU • Vitamin C (as L-ascorbic-acid) 45 mg • Vitamin D (as cholecalciferol) 300 IU • Vitamin E (as D-alpha tocopheryl acetate) 23 IU • Thiamin (as thiamin mononitrate) 1.1 mg • Riboflavin 1.3 mg • Niacin (as niacinamide) 15 mg • Vitamin B6 (as pyridoxine hydrochloride) 1.5 mg • Folic Acid 300 mcg • Vitamin B12 (as cyanocobalamin) 5 mcg • Biotin (as D-biotin) 200 mcg • Pantothenic Acid (as D-calcium pantothenate) 7.5 mg • Calcium (as calcium carbonate, calcium from proteinate) 200 mg • Iron (as reduced iron, iron from proteinate) 9 mg • Iodine (as potassium iodide, brown seaweed extract) 115 mcg • Magnesium (as magnesium oxide, magnesium from proteinate) 100 mg • Zinc (as zinc oxide) 11 mg • Selenium (selenium from proteinate) 14 mcg • Copper (as copper gluconate) 1.5 mg • Manganese (as manganese from proteinate) 0.4 mg • Chromium (as chromium polynicotinate) 24 mcg • Molybdenum (molybdenum from proteinate) 15 mcg • Sodium 120 mg • Potassium (from malted oat cereal solids) 70 mg • Lecithin (from lecithin oil) 500 mg • Dried Red Beet powder 50 mg • Dried Broccoli powder (Brassica aleracea) aerial 50 mg • Dried Carrot powder (Daucus carota) root 40 mg • Spirulina powder 50 mg • Alfalfa Sprouts powder (Medicago sativa) aerial 50 mg • Kamut Grass powder (triticum durham egyptum) aerial 50 mg • Wheat Grass powder (Tritizum vulgare) aerial 50 mg • Barley Grass powder (Hordeum vulgare) aerial 50 mg • Reishi Mushroom extract (Ganoderma lucidum) 20 mg • Maitake Mushroom extract (Gifola frondosa) 20 mg • Shiitake Mushroom powder (Lentinus edodes) 20 mg • Brown Seaweed Extract 30 mg • Isoflavones from Soy concentrate 20 mg • Octacosanol (from wheat germ oil) 250 mcg • Lactoferrins 10 mg • Glutamine Peptides 100 mg • Astragalus extract (Astragalus membranaceus) root 20 mg • Schisandra extract (Schizandra chinensis) fruit 20 mg • American Ginseng extract (Panax quinquefolium) root 20 mg • Siberian Ginseng extract (Acanthopanax seticosus) root 20 mg • Korean Ginseng extract (Panax ginseng) root 20 mg • Rhodiola extract (Rhodiola rosea) root 20 mg • Elderberry extract (Sambucus nigra, canadensis) berry 20 mg • Fruit Polyphenols (from apple, apricot, nectarine, cherry, prune, pomegranate) 20 mg • Beta Glucan (from oat fiber) 25 mg • Dried Colostrum powder 50 mg • Cytidine Monophosphate 5 mg • Adenosine Monophosphate 5 mg • Uridine Monophosphate 5 mg • Guanosine Monophosphate 5 mg • Phosphatidylcholine (from lecithin oil) 100 mg • Phosphatidylinositol (from lecithin oil) 20 mg. Other Ingredients: Malted Oat Cereal Solids, Crystalline Fructose, Soy Protein Isolate, Whey Protein Isolate, Whey Protein Concentrate, Dried Malt, Oat Fiber, Natural Chocolate Flavor, Dutch Cocoa, Soy Concentrate, Apple Fiber, Gum Arabic, Apple Pectin, Dried Cream, Black Currant Fiber, Lemon Fiber, Rice Fiber Concentrate, Fruit Concentrate.

Opti Fuel (The Ultimate Metabolic Optimizer) - TwinLab
Each serving contains: Pharmaceutical Grade Pep-Tide Bonded & Free Amino Acids [derived from the natural Pancreatic digests of Whey Protein (Lactalbumin) & Egg White Protein (Albumin)] 15 g • Branched Chain Amino Acids (L-Leucine, L-Isoleucine & L-Valine) • Carbohydrates & Medium Chain Triglycerides (MCTs) • High Potency Metabolic Activator Vitamins & Minerals • Electro-Lytes • Antioxidants • Stress B Complex • Lipotropic Factors • Methyl Donors • TMG (Trimethylglycine) • Siberian Ginseng • Octacosanol • Gamma-Oryzanol & Synergistic Metabolic Optimizers (such as Inosine) • L-Carnitine • CoQ10 • Lipoic Acid • Pantetheine • Pyridoxine-Alpha-Ketoglutarate • Soluble Potassium Phosphate & Mineral Succinates • Aspartates • Citrates • Fumarates • Malates • Alpha-Ketoglutarates.

Opti Fuel 2 - TwinLab
Each serving contains: Carbohydrates (derived primarily from Glucose Polymers & Glucose with small amounts of 100% Pure Crystalline Fructose) 100 g • Predigested Whey Protein • Extra Branched Chain Amino Acids (L-Leucine, L-Isoleucine, L-Valine) • Vitamin C • Vitamin E • Beta-Carotene • Other Important Antioxidant Nutrients such as: Selenium, Coenzyme Q10 & Alpha Lipoic Acid, High Potency B Complex Vitamins, Calcium, Magnesium, Potassium, Zinc & Chromium Picolinate • Carni Fuel (L-Carnitine Magnesium Citrate).

OptiBerry - Pure Encapsulations
Each vegetable capsule contains: Proprietary Blend 50 mg: Malvidin, Cyanidin, Delphinidin, Petunidin, Wild Blueberry extract (vaccinium angustifolium), Strawberry powder (fragaria chiloensis), Cranberry powder (vaccinium macrocarpon), Wild Bilberry fruit extract (vaccinium myritillus), Elderberry fruit extract (sambucus nigra), Raspberry seed powder (rubus idaeus) • Vitamin C (as ascorbyl palmitate) 5 mg.

OptiBerry Essence - Vitamin Power
Each capsule contains: OptiBerry Proprietary Blend 30 mg: Wild Blueberry fruit extract (vaccinium angustifolium), Strawberry fruit concentrate (gragaria chilonesis), Cranberry fruit concentrate (vaccinium macrocarpon), Bilberry fruit extract (vaccinium myrtillus), Elderberry fruit extract (sambucus nigra), Raspberry seed powder (rubus idseus) • Citrus Bioflavonoids 100 mg.

Opti-Cherry - Hillestad
Each tablet contains: Sour Cherry 250 mg • Vitamin C (ascorbic acid) 150 mg • Kelp plant 25 mg • Burdock root 25 mg • Dandelion root 25 mg • Chamomile flower 25 mg • Fennel seed 25 mg • Yucca root 25 mg • Red Clover flower 25 mg • Gentian root 25 mg. Other Ingrdients: Egg Shell, Cellulose, Calcium Phosphate, Silica, Magnesium Stearate, Ethyl Cellulose, Aloe Vera, Folic Acid.

OptiCleanse GHI - Xymogen
Two scoops (52 g) contain: Vitamin A (as mixed carotenoids) 2500 IU • Vitamin C (as sodium ascorbate) 250 mg • Calcium (as calcium citrate) 300 mg • Vitamin D (as cholecalciferol) 100 IU • Vitamin E (as D-alpha tocopherol acetate) 125 IU • Thiamin (as

thiamin HCl) 15 mg • Riboflavin (as riboflavin 5'-phosphate) 5 mg • Niacin (as niacinamide) 200 mg • Vitamin B6 (as pyridoxal 5'-phosphate) 5 mg • Folic Acid (as folic acid and calcium folinate) 400 mcg • Vitamin B12 (as methylcobalamin) 50 mcg • Biotin 150 mg • Pantothenic Acid (as D-calcium pantothenate) 35 mg • Phosphorus (as dipotassium phosphate and monopotassium phosphate) 200 mg • Iodine (as potassium iodide) 60 mcg • Magnesium (as magnesium citrate and magnesium malate) 250 mg • Zinc (as zinc aspartate) 10 mg • Selenium (as selenomethionine) 100 mcg • Manganese (as manganese gluconate) 2 mg • Chromium (as chromium aspartate) 60 mcg • Molybdenum (as molybdenum amino acid chelate) 30 mcg • L-Glycine 1500 mg • Lysine 500 mg • Betaine (as trimethylglycine) 150 mg • L-Glutamine 1200 mg • Hesperidin 250 mg • Quercetin 250 mg • Rutin 200 mg • Curcumin 200 mg • Taurine 175 mg • N-Acetyl Cysteine 150 mg • Ginger root powder 150 mg • Methylsulfonylmethane 120 mg • Alpha Lipoic Acid 100 mg • Watercress herb powder 100 mg • Ellagic Acid (as pomegranate extract) 100 mg • Choline (as choline bitartrate) 100 mg • Green Tea extract (60% catechins) 55 mg • Preventium brand Potassium D-Glucarate 250 mg • Aminogen brand 300 mg • L-Threonine 35 mg. Other Ingredients: Rice Protein Concentrate, Rice Syrup Solids, Lignamax brand, Olive Oil, Natural Flavors, Xanthan Gum.

OptiCleanse Plus - Xymogen
Two scoops contain: Vitamin A 5000 IU • Vitamin D 65 IU • Vitamin B1 5.5 mg • Niacin 11 mcg • Folate 110 mg • Biotin 160 mg • Iron 4.5 mg • Phosphorus 260 mg • Magnesium 135 mg • Selenium 55 mcg • Manganese 1.65 mg • Molybdenum 165 mg • Vitamin C 220 mg • Vitamin E 110 IU • Vitamin B2 2.2 mg • Vitamin B6 6 mg • Vitamin B12 22 mcg • Pantothenic Acid 5.5 mcg • Calcium 174 mg • Iodine 55 mcg • Zinc 11.5 mg • Copper 1.2 mg • Chromium 55 mcg • Chloride 48 mg • N-Acetyl-L-Cysteine 55.5 mg • L-Glutathione 28 mg • L-Threonine 28 mg • Linoleic Acid 150 mg • L-Glycine 1500 mg • L-Cysteine 55.5 mg • L-Lysine 333 mg • Alpha Linolenic Acid 538 mg • Oleic Acid 125 mg • Preventium brand Potassium Hydrogen Glucarate 250 mg.

OptiFiber SCFA - Xymogen
Each scoop (15 g) contains: Vitamin A (100% as beta carotene) 1250 IU • Vitamin C (as ascorbic acid) 30 mg • Vitamin E (as D-alpha tocopherol succinate) 15 IU • Stevia leaf 22.5 mg.

Optiflora Prebiotic Complex - Shaklee
Each teaspoon (4 g) contains: Dietary fiber 3 g • Optiflora Proprietary Prebiotic Blend 3 g: Inulin, Fructooligosaccharides (FOS) • Mixed tocopherols 32 mg. Other Ingredients: Fructose, Maltodextrin, Natural Flavors.

Optiflora Probiotic Complex - Shaklee
Each capsule contains: Bifidobacterium longum 250 million • Lactobacillus acidophilus 250 million. Other Ingredients: Palm Oil, Gelatin, Glycerin, Soy Lecithin, Pectin.

Opti-Lean - Optimum Nutrition
Citrimax Garcinia Cambogia extract 500 mg.

OptiMag 125 - Xymogen
Each capsule contains: Magnesium (as magnesium glycinate/lysinate and dimagnesium malate) 125 mg.

Optimal Life Factors - FreeLife International
Each scoop (12 g) contains: PF3 (PreBiotic Factors 3X) 7 g: Inulin Heteroglycans from Chicory root (cichoria intybus), Indian Cluster Bean (cyamopsis tetragonolobus), Larch bark (Larix siberica), Colloidal Silica • L-Glutamine 5 g.

Optimal Performance - Rexall - Sundown
Each tablet contains: Zinc (as zinc gluconate) 7.5 mg • Spirulina (spirulina pacifica) 125 mg • Bee Pollen 100 mg • Royal Jelly 100 mg • Siberian Ginseng root 75 mg • Octacosanol 0.5 mg. Other Ingredients: Corn Syrup solids, Croscarmellose Sodium, Alfalfa leaf, Hydrogenated Vegetable Oil, Silica, Magnesium Stearate.

Opti-Men - Optimum Nutrition
Two tablets contain: Vitamin A (as CaroCare natural mixed carotenoids) 7500 IU • Vitamin C (as ascorbic acid) 300 mg • Vitamin D (as cholecalciferol) 200 IU • Vitamin E (as D-alpha tocopheryl succinate) 200 IU • Vitamin K (as phytonadione) 75 mcg • Thiamin (as thiamin hydrochloride) 30 mg • Riboflavin 30 mg • Niacin (as niacinamide) 30 mg • Vitamin B6 (as pyridoxine hydrochloride) 30 mg • Folic Acid 400 mcg • Vitamin B12 (as cyanocobalamin) 100 mcg • Biotin 250 mcg • Pantothenic Acid (as D-calcium pantothenate) 30 mg • Calcium (as calcium carbonate, citrate) 200 mg • Iodine (as kelp) 150 mcg • Magnesium (as magnesium oxide, aspartate) 100 mg • Zinc (as zinc citrate) 30 mg • Selenium (as selenomethionine) 70 mcg • Copper (as copper gluconate) 2 mg • Manganese (as manganese gluconate) 5 mg • Chromium (as chromium GTF) 120 mcg • Molybdenum (as molybdenum AA chelate) 80 mcg • Raw Oyster concentrate 50 mg • Saw Palmetto powdered berries 100 mg • Pygeum Africanum powdered bark 70 mg • Damiana powdered leaf 100 mg• Nettles powdered leaf 30 mg • Lycopene (as LYC-O-MATO natural tomato lycopene) 250 mcg • Alpha-Carotene 140 mcg • Cryptoxanthin 34 mcg • Zeaxanthin 28 mcg • Lutein 250 mcg • Alpha Lipoic Acid 25 mg • Citrus Bioflavonoids fruit 70 mg • Grape Seed extract (vitis vinifera, standardized to 95% polyphenols) 25 mg • Deodorized Garlic powdered bulb 50 mg • Ginkgo Biloba powdered leaf 70 mg • Korean Ginseng powdered root 100 mg • PABA (para-aminobenzoic acid) 10 mg • Choline (as choline bitartrate) 10 mg • Inositol 10 mg. Other Ingredients: Stearic Acid, Hydroxy Propyl Methyl Cellulose, Calcium Phosphate, Croscarmellose Sodium (disintegrant), Gelatin, Magnesium Stearate, Gum Acacia, Silica.

OptimEyes - Body Wise International, Inc.
Three tablets contain: Beta Carotene (Dunaliella salina algae) 9 mg (Equivalent to Vitamin A 15000 IU) • Vitamin C (as Ascorbic Acid) 1000 mg • Vitamin E (as D-Alpha Tocopheryl Succinate and Mixed Tocopherols-Alpha, Beta, Gamma and Delta) 100 IU • Zinc (Krebs Cycle Chelate) 20 mg • Selenium (as L-Selenomethionine) 250 mcg • Copper (Krebs Cycle Chelate) 2 mg • Taurine 500 mg • N-Acetyl-L-Cysteine 200 mg • Bilberry fruit extract 100:1 (25% Anthocyanidins) 80 mg • Ginkgo Biloba leaf extract 50:1 (24% Flavonglycosides) 60 mg • Alpha Lipoic Acid 25 mg • Lutein 6 mg.

Optimized Lecithin 500 - GNC
Each capsule contains: Vitamin E (as D-alpha tocopherol) 5 IU • Lecithin (as liquid soy lecithin) 500 mg. Other Ingredients: Gelatin, Glycerin, Rosemary oil (Rosmarinus offcinalis).

OptiMSM brand - Cardinal Nutrition
Methysulfonylmethane.
See Editor's Note No. 44.

Optimum Foods - MegaFood
Six tablets contain: Vitamin A (2000 IU from 10 mg FoodState, 5000 IU beta carotene from B. trispora) 7000 IU • Vitamin C (from 1050 mg FoodState) 250 mg • Vitamin D (D3, from 4 mg FoodState) 200 IU • Vitamin E (from 420 mg FoodState) 10 mg • Vitamin K (K1, from 5 mg FoodState) 45 mcg • Thiamine (B1, from 84 mg FoodState) 20 mg • Riboflavin (B2, from 105 mg FoodState) 10 mg • Niacinamide (B3, from 147 mg FoodState) 35 mg • Vitamin B6 (from 52 mg FoodState) 10 mg • Folic Acid (from 63 mg FoodState) 600 mcg • Vitamin B12 (from 13 mg FoodState) 65 mcg • Biotin (from 63 mg FoodState) 300 mcg • Pantothenic Acid (from 104 mg FoodState) 25 mg • Calcium (from 2000 mg FoodState) 100 mg • Iron (from 160 mg FoodState) 8 mg • Iodine (from 7 mg FoodState) 100 mcg • Magnesium (from 2000 mg FoodState) 100 mg • Zinc (from 300 mg FoodState) 15 mg • Selenium (from 100 mg FoodState) 100 mcg • Copper (from 12 mg FoodState) 125 mcg • Manganese (from 60 mg FoodState) 3 mg • Chromium (GTF, from 50 mg FoodState) 100 mcg • Molybdenum (from 12 mg FoodState) 25 mcg • Wild Blueberry 50:1 75 mg • Pomegranate 40:1 50 mg • Raspberry 15:1 50 mg • Strawberry 15:1 45 mg • Elderberry 15:1 45 mg • Prune 8:1/Plum 45 mg • Papaya 3:1 30 mg • Cranberry 15:1 20 mg • Broccoli 20:1 75 mg • Spinach 12:1 50 mg • Tomato 15:1 50 mg • Garlic 10:1 50 mg • Onion 17:1 50 mg • Okra 10:1 50 mg • Cabbage

sprout 10:1 45 mg • Carrot 15:1 45 mg • Kale 15:1 45 mg • Beet root 5:1 35 mg • Parsley 12:1 25 mg • Bioperine brand extract from Piper Nigrum 2 mg • Green Papaya 4:1 25 mg • Shiitake mushroom 4:1 (lentinus edodes) 50 mg • Cordyceps mycelia 4:1 (cordycpes sinensis) 50 mg • Reishi mushroom mycelia 7:1 (ganoderma lucidum) 40 mg • Lutein (from marigold) 5 mg • Lycopene (from tomato) 3 mg • Capsanthin (from marigold & capsicum spp.) 1 mg • Zeaxanthin (from marigold & capsicum spp.) 1 mg • Gamma Carotene (from B. trispora) 90 mcg • Citroxanthin (from B. trispora) 45 mcg • Beta Zeacarotene (from B. trispora) 18 mcg • Laminaria seaweed (kelp) 75 mg • Watercress 50 mg • Whole Concord Grape with Grape seed 45 mg • Apricot 35 mg • Mango 35 mg • Pineapple 35 mg • Celery 30 mg • Lemon peel 20 mg • Bioflavonoids (from 395 FoodState vitamin C) 250 mg • Choline (from 126 mg FoodState) 30 mg • Potassium (from 400 mg FoodState) 20 mg • Inositol (form 42 mg FoodState) 10 mg • Boron (from 100 mg FoodState) 3 mg • Vanadium (from 25 mg FoodState) 25 mcg. Other Ingredients: Vegetable Lubricant, Guar Gum, Silica, Food Glaze.

Optimum Nutrition - Optimum Nutrition
Hawthorn Berry • Garlic Extract.

Optimum Omega - Pharmanex
Each capsule contains: Vitamin E (as D-alpha tocopheryl acetate) 5 IU • Marine Lipid Concentrate 1000 mg: Omega 3 Fatty Acids: EPA 180 mg, DHA 120 mg, Other Omega 3 Fatty Acids 50 mg • Garlic oil 1 mg. Other Ingredients: Gelatin, Glycerin, Water.

Optimune - Rx Vitamins
Pharmaceutical Grade Arabinogalactan 250 mg • Phosphoric Nucleotides 4000 mcg.

Opti-Pro Meal - Optimum Nutrition
Two heaping scoops (73 g) contain: Proprietary Nitroplex Protein Blend: Whey Protein Concentrate, Calcium Caseinate, Egg Albumen, Whey Protein Isolate • Proprietary Polysaccharide Matrix: Maltodextirn, Cellulose Gum, Xanthan Gum, Corn Syrup Solids, Amylopectin (waxy corn starch), High Amylose Corn Starch • Cocoa • Vitaplus Blend: Calcium Citrate, DiPotassium Phosphate, Magnesium Oxide, DiCalcium Phosphate, Choline Bitartrate, Potassium Chloride, Ascorbic Acid, DL-Alpha Tocopheryl Acetate, Ferrous Fumarate, Niacinamide, Vitamin A Palmitate, Zinc Oxide, Potassium Iodide, D-Calcium Pantothenate, Phytonadione, Copper Sulfate Pentahydrate, Manganese Sulfate, Cholecalciferol, Pyridoxine Hydrochloride, Molybdenum Glycinate, Riboflavin, Thiamin Mononitrate, Selenium Glycinate, Chromium Picolinate, Folic Acid, Biotin, Cyanocobalamin • Natural and Artificial Flavor • Medium Chain Triglycerides • Canola oil • Aspartame • Soy Lecithin • Acesulfame Potassium.

Opti-Pro Meal Bars - Optimum Nutrition
Each bar (75 g) contains: Corn Syrup • Protein Blend: Soy Protein Isolate, Whey Protein Isolate, Calcium Caseinate • Milk Chocolate (sugar, palm kernal oil, non-fat dry milk solids, cocoa powder, salt) • Cocoa • Maltodextrin • Raisins • Fructose • Glycerol • Lecithin • Inulin • Artificial Flavor • Vitamin/Mineral Blend: Magnesium Oxide, Ascorbic Acid, Chromium GTF Polynicotinate, Niacinamide, Biotin, D-Alpha Tocopheryl Succinate, Vitamin A Palmitate, Copper Gluconate, Zinc Oxide, D-Calcium Pantothenate, Cholecalciferol, Folic Acid, Pyridoxine Hydrochloride, Riboflavin, Thiamin Mononitrate, Cyanocobalamin • Carbogen • Aminogen.

OptiSight - Advocare International
Two capsules contain: Zinc (as monomethionine OptiZinc) 3 mg • Vitamin C (as potassium ascorbate) 60 mg • Lutein (as esters from tagetes sp.) 20 mg • Zeaxanthin (as free-form and esters from tagetes sp.) 2 mg • Astaxanthin (from Haematococcus sp.) 10 mg • Bilberry extract (fruit - vaccinium myrtillus) 150 mg • Alpha-Lipoic Acid 50 mg • N-Acetyl Cysteine 75 mg • Taurine 200 mg • Mixed Tocotrienols (from seed - glycine max) 30 mg •Curcumin extract (root - curcuma longa) 50 mg • L-Glutathione 5 mg • Beta-Carotene (from D. salina mixed carotenoids) 1.5 mg. Other Ingredients: Silicon Dioxide, Magnesium Stearate, Gelatin.

Opti-Soy - Optimum Nutrition
Each scoop (32 g) contains: Non-GMO Soy Protein Isolate • Vitamin/Mineral Blend: Calcium Citrate, Magnesium Oxide, Ascorbic Acid, D-Alpha Tocopheryl Succinate (natural vitamin E), Niacinamide, Maltodextrin, D-Calcium Pantothenate, Molybdenum Amino Acid Chelate, Zinc Oxide, Selenomethionine, Vitamin A Palmitate, Riboflavin, Thiamin Mononitrate, Manganese Sulfate, Pyridoxine Hydrochloride (vitamin B6), Folic Acid, Chromium Picolinate, Potassium Iodide, Cyanocobalamin • Cocoa • Natural and Artificial Flavor • Salt • Sucralose.

OptiVision - PhysioLogics
Two capsules contain: Vitamin A (Beta-Carotene) 10000 IU • Vitamin A (Palmitate) 2500 IU • Taurine 200 mg • Bilberry (GPH: 36% anthocyanosides) 100 mg • Vitamin E (D-Alpha Tocopherol) 100 IU • N-Acetylcysteine 100 mg • Quercetin (GPH: 98% Bioflavonoids) 50 mg • Glutathione 25 mg • Vitamin B2 (Riboflavin) 10 mg • Vitamin B6 (Pyridoxine HCl) 10 mg • Zinc (Glycinate) 15 mg • Copper (Glycinate) 2 mg • Chromium (Niacin/Glycine Chelate) 100 mcg • Selenium (Selenomethionine) 50 mcg.

OptiVision Forte - Similasan
Four caplets contain: Vitamin A (45% (1,650 IU) as Beta Carotene) 3,650 IU • Vitamin C 150 mg • Vitamin D (cholecalciferol) 200 IU • Vitamin E (d-alpha tocopheryl acetate) 75 IU • Thiamin (Vitamin B-1) 25 mg • Riboflavin (Vitamin B-2) 38 mg • Niacin 20 mg • Vitamin B6 (from 25 mg pyridoxyl-5 phosphate) 17 mg • Folic Acid 400 mcg • Vitamin B12 (dibencozide) 84 mcg • Biotin 100 mcg • Pantothenic Acid (from d-calcium panthothenate) 25 mg • Calcium (rice protein chelate) 75 mg • Magnesium (rice protein chelate) 75 mg • Zinc (rice protein chelate) 19 mg • Selenium (rice protein chelate) 50 mcg • Manganese (rice protein chelate) 10 mg • Chromium (rice protein chelate) 25 mcg • Bioflavinoids (citrus) 75 mg • Alpha-Lipoic Acid 30 mg • Lutein (from Calendula officinalis flowers) 5,065 mcg • Coenzyme Q-10 (emulsified) 2.5 mg • Alpha-Carotene 415 mcg • Zeaxanthine 333 mcg • Lycopene 300 mcg • Cryptoxanthine 100 mcg • Proprietary Blend 1130 mg: Eye Bright Herb, Taurine, L-Cysteine, L-Arginine, Cayenne, Garlic Bulb, Ginger Root, Ginkgo Biloba leaf, L-Glutamine, Glycine, Bilberry 5:1 extract, Inositol, L-Histidine, Raw Eye Concentrate, L-Glutathione, Lecithin, and SuperOxide Dismutase (SOD). Other Ingredients: Special Plant Cellulose, Vegtable Stearates, Acacia, Gum Tragacanth, Natural Silica, and Magnesium Stearate. See Editor's Note No. 14.

Opti-Vitamins - Sunmark
Each tablet contains: Vitamin A (as beta carotene) 1000 IU • Vitamin C (as ascorbic acid) 200 mg • Vitamin E (as dL-alpha tocopheryl acetate) 60 IU • Zinc (as zinc oxide) 40 mg • Selenium (from sodium selenate) 55 mcg • Copper (as cupric oxide) 2 mg • Lutein 2 mg. Other Ingredients: Microcrystalline Cellulose, Gelatin, Modified Cellulose Gum, Crospovidone, Dextrin, Titanium Dioxide, Hypromellose, Magnesium Stearate, Stearic Acid, Polyethylene Glycol, Dextrose, Lecithin, FD&C Yellow No. 6 Lake, Gluten. See Editor's Note No. 45.

Opti-Vites - Optimum Nutrition
Each capsule contains: Vitamin A (as beta-carotene, vitamin A palmitate) 5000 IU • Vitamin C (as ascorbic acid) 90 mg • Vitamin D (as cholecalciferol) 400 IU • Vitamin K (as phytonadione) 50 mcg • Thiamin (as thiamin hydrochloride) 2.25 mg • Riboflavin 2.55 mg • Niacin (as niacinamide) 20 mg • Vitamin B6 (as pyridoxine hydrochloride) 3 mg • Biotin 150 mcg • Pantothenic Acid (as D-calcium pantothenate) 10 mg • Calcium (as dicalcium phosphate) 60 mg • Iron (as ferrous fumarate) 3.6 mg • Phosphorus (as dicalcium phosphate) 45 mg • Iodine (as kelp) 150 mcg • Magnesium (as magnesium oxide) 100 mg • Zinc (as zinc citrate) 15 mg • Selenium (as selenomethionine) 87.5 mcg • Copper (as copper AA chelate) 2 mg • Manganese (gluconate) 1 mg • Chromium (picolinate) 150 mcg • Molybdenum (as molybdenum AA chelate) 75 mcg • Chloride (as potassium chloride) 63 mg • Potassium (as potassium chloride) 70 mg. Other Ingredients: Gelatin, Magnesium Stearate, Silica.

BRAND NAMES

Some Brand Name Natural Products - What they Contain

www.NaturalDatabase.com contains MANY more listings than appear here.
Editor's Notes are located on pages 2155-2163.

BRAND NAMES

Opti-Vue **-** The Vitamin Shoppe
Two capsules contain: Vitamin A 10000 IU • Vitamin C 200 mg • Vitamin E 50 IU • Potassium 100 mg • Niacin 30 mg • Zinc 5 mg • Riboflavin 3 mg • Selenium 50 mcg • Lutein 6 mg • Zeaxanthin 240-600 mcg • Eyebright Extract 200 mg • Raw Eye Tissue 160 mg • Raw Muscle Tissue 100 mg • Inositol 100 mg • Alfalfa concentrate 50 mg • Citrus Bioflavonoids 50 mg • Quercetin 200 mg • Rutin 25 mg • Bilberry extract 40 mg • Glutathione 5 mg • N-Acetyl Cysteine 50 mg. Base: Rice Carrot Parsley, Spinach Concentrate.
See Editor's Note No. 14.

Opti-Women **-** Optimum Nutrition
Two capsules contain: Vitamin A (as CaroCare natural mixed carotenoids, vitamin A palmitate) 5000 IU • Vitamin C (as ascorbic acid) 250 mg • Vitamin D (as cholecalciferol) 600 IU • Vitamin E (as D-alpha tocopheryl succinate) 100 IU • Vitamin K (as phytonadione) 80 mcg • Thiamin (as thiamin hydrochloride) 20 mg • Riboflavin 20 mg • Niacin (as niacinamide) 20 mg • Vitamin B6 (as pyridoxine hydrochloride) 20 mg • Folic Acid 600 mcg • Vitamin B12 (as cyanocobalamin) 100 mcg • Biotin 250 mcg • Pantothenic Acid (as D-calcium pantothenate) 150 mg • Calcium (as calcium carbonate, citrate) 150 mg • Iron (as iron AA chelate) 18 mg • Iodine (as kelp) 200 mcg • Magnesium (as magnesium aspartate) 75 mg • Zinc (as zinc citrate) 15 mg • Selenium (as selenomethionine) 70 mcg • Copper (as copper gluconate) 2 mg • Manganese (as manganese gluconate) 5 mg • Chromium (as chromium GTF) 120 mcg • Molybdenum (as molybdenum AA chelate) 70 mcg • Ostivone Isopropoxy Isoflavone 10 mg • Soy Isoflavones (as NovaSoy) 2 mg • Lycopene (as LYC-O-MATO natural tomato lycopene) 250 mcg • Alpha-Carotene 93.5 mcg • Zeaxanthin 18.7 mcg • Cryptoxanthin 22.8 mcg • Lutein 250 mcg • Chasteberry 4:1 berry extract (vitus agnus-castus) 50 mg • Grape Seed extract (vitis vinifera, standardized to 95% polyphenols) 10 mg • Dong Quai 4:1 root extract (angelica sinensis) 80 mg • Horse Chestnut root extract (aesculus hippocastanum, standardized to 20% aescin) 25 mg • Butchers Broom powdered root 15 mg • Garcinia rind extract (garcinia cambogia, standardized to 52% HCA) 50 mg • Uva Ursi powdered leaf 50 mg • Alpha Lipoic Acid 20 mg • Deodorized Garlic powdered bulb 10 mg • Citrus Bioflavonoids fruit 10 mg. Other Ingredients: Calcium Phosphate, Gelatin, Magnesium Stearate, Silica.

OptiZinc **-** Source Naturals
Each tablet contains: Zinc (from 150 mg of OptiZinc zinc monomethionine) 30 mg • Copper (sebacate) 300 mcg.

Optizinc **-** Natrol, Inc.
One capsule contains: Zinc (Monomethionine) 30 mg. Other Ingredients: Microcrystalline Cellulose, Magnesium Stearate, Gelatin.

OptiZinc brand **-** Cardinal Nutrition
Zinc.
See Editor's Note No. 44.

Opti-Zyme **-** Goldshield Elite
One caplet contains: Calcium (from 500 mg Calcium Carbonate) 180 mg • Amylase 4250 DU • Protease 10255 HUT • Cellulase 630 CU • Lactase 350 Lac U • Lipase 65 LU • Invertase 0.6 IAU • Glucoamylase 15 AG • Multi-algae blend: Spirulina algae, Bladderwrack kelp, Klamath Lake algae, Canary Island algae, Chlorella algae, Maine coast kelp, and Sargassi seaweed • Supporting herbal blend: Turmeric rhizome, Fennel seed, Ginger root, and Soy sprouts. Other Ingredients: Vegetable cellulose, Fractionated vegetable oil, Soy polysaccharides, Silica, and Vegetable resin glaze.

Opti-Zyme Pro **-** Goldshield Elite
One capsule contains: Amylase 3400 SKB • Lipase 2250 LU • Cellulase 5400 C-ase • Protease 10200 HUT • Amyloglucosidase 22 AG • Acid stable protease 340 APU • Invertase 102 Sumner U • Lactase 351 LAU • Lactobacillus acidophilus 100 million CFU • Bifidobacterium bifidum 50 million CFU • Dulse algae 50 mg • Trace mineral complex (Montmorillonite) 100 mg • Spirulina blue-green algae 50 mg • Bromelain 50 mg. Other Ingredients: Gelatin, Calcium Sulfate, Magnesium Stearate, and Silica.

OptOmega **-** USANA Health Sciences
Two teaspoons contain: Certified Organic Cold Pressed Flaxseed, Sunflower Seed, Pumpkin Seed Oil, Mixed Tocopherols, D-Alpha-Tocopherol, Tumeric Extract.

Oraflow Plus **-** Nutrition for Life International
Ten tablets contains: Vitamin A 40,000 IU • Vitamin D 400 IU • Vitamin E 650 IU • Vitamin C 4,500 mg • Folic Acid 400 mcg • Vitamin B1 200 mg • Vitamin B2 (Riboflavin) 30 mg • Niacin 100 mg • Vitamin B6 160 mg • Vitamin B12 200 mcg • Biotin 100 mcg • Pantothenic Acid 3.76 mg • Calcium 300 mg • Iodine 125 mcg • Magnesium 300 mg • Zinc 30 mg • Copper 250 mcg • Potassium 275 mg • Manganese 5 mg • Choline 725 mg • Inositol 40 mg • Chromium 150 mcg • Sodium 15 mg • Selenium 250 mcg • L-Arginine 1 g • L-Methionine 200 mg • N-Acetyl-L-Cysteine 750 mg • Marine Lipids 50 mg • Bioflavonoids 100 mg • PABA 300 mg • Adrenal 50 mg • Spleen 50 mg • Thymus 50 mg • Hawthorne berry 26 mg • Butchers Broom 16 mg.
See Editor's Note No. 14.

Oral Nutrient Chelates **-** Enzymatic Therapy
Six tablets contain: Vitamin C (ascorbic acid) 1.5 g • Niacin (as niacinamide, niacin) 630 mg • Vitamin B6 (as pyridoxine HCl) 150 mg • Calcium (from calcium chloride 291 mg) 105 mg • Iodine (from kelp) 600 mcg • Magnesium (from magnesium orotate 1.8 g, magnesium ascorbate 300 mg) 146 mg • Zinc (from zinc ascorbate 45 mg) 9 mg • Selenium (from selenium ascorbate 30 mg) 300 mcg • Copper (from copper gluconate 750 mcg) 113 mcg • Manganese (from manganese ascorbate) 6 mg • Sodium 5 mg • Potassium (from potassium orotate 150 mg, potassium aspartate 105 mg, potassium phosphate 30 mg, potassium chloride 30 mg) 80 mg • Beta-Sitosterol 450 mg • Taurine 300 mg • Mucopolysaccharide (soluble) 300 mg • Betaine HCl 300 mg • Ammonium Chloride 291 mg • L-Methionine 195 mg • Bromelain (1800 M.C.U./g) 150 mg. Other Ingredients: Cellulose, Fennel (foeniculum vulgare), Stearic Acid, Modified Cellulose Gum, Magnesium Stearate, Silicon Dioxide, Titanium Dioxide Color, Peppermint (mentha x piperita).

Oralmat Drops **-** Schumacher Pharmaceuticals of Melbourne
Each 10 mL contains: Rye (secale cereale) Extract.

Orange Burst **-** Advocare International
Two tablets contain: Vitamin A (as palmitate) 1000 IU • Vitamin C (as ascorbic acid and sodium ascorbate) 450 mg • Vitamin E (as D-alpha tocopheryl succinate) 17.5 IU • Folic Acid 100 mcg • Sodium 5 mg • Mixed Carotenoids (from D. salina) 600 mcg • Grape extract (seed/skin - vitis vinifera, Activin brand) 20 mg. Other Ingredients: Fructose, Xylitol, Stearic Acid, Natural Orange Flavor, Magnesium Stearate, Silicon Dioxide, Guar Gum, Turmeric Extract.

Orange Butterfly **-** Cytotec Solutions, Inc.
Unknown.
See Editor's Note No. 49.

Orange Juice Cee **-** Arrowroot
Three wafers contain: Vitamin C 500 mg • Bioflavonoids 25 mg.

Orange Juice Jr. **-** Nature's Plus
Each chewable tablet contains: Vitamin C (as ascorbic acid) 100 mg. Other Ingredients: Fructose, Natural Orange Flavor, Magnesium Stearate, Silica, Beet Juice, Stearic Acid, Lemon Bioflavonoids (from citrus limon fruit), Rutin, Hesperidin, Acerola Cherry Fruit (malpighia glabra), Rose Hips Fruit (rosa canina), Papaya Fruit, Green Pepper Extract (from capsicum annuum), Black Currant Fruit Concentrate, Dolomite.

Ora-Pops **-** Alacer
Each lozenge contains: Vitamin C (as ascorbates) 250 mg • Vitamin B1 (as thiamine HCl) 0.13 mg • Vitamin B2 (as riboflavin) 0.69 mg • Vitamin B3 (as niacin complexes) 1.25 mg • Vitamin B6 (as pyridoxine HCl) 2.5 mg • Folic Acid 125 mcg • Vitamin B12 (as cyanocobalamin) 6.25 mcg • Pantothenic Acid (as calcium pantothenate) 0.63 mg • Calcium 12.5 mg • Magnesium 10 mg • Zinc (as zinc ascorbate) 0.5 mg • Manganese 0.5 mg • Chromium (as chromium ascorbate) 5 mcg • Sodium 15 mg • Potassium 100 mg.

Other Ingredients: Ascorbic Acid, Carbonates of Potassium, Sodium, Magnesium and Calcium, Citric, Malis, Aspartic, and Tartaric Acids, Phosphates of Potassium, Sodium, and Calcium, PEG, Povidone, Magnesium Stearate, Magnesium Hydroxide, Quercetin, Manganese Gluconate, Natural Flavors.

Oraxinol **- Xymogen**
Two capsules contain: Oraxinol Proprietary blend 1000 mg (standardized to provide 6000 trolox equivalents per gram): RosemarinX brand Rosemary extract • Berr-X brand Anthocyanin extract.

Orchex **- Standard Process, Inc.**
Each capsule contains: Proprietary Blend 470 mg: Bovine Liver, Bovine Orchic Cytosol extract, Calcium Lactate, Manganese Lactate, Porcine Stomach, Bovine Spleen, Ovine Spleen, Soy bean, Defatted Wheat germ, Magnesium Citrate, Porcine Brain, Ascorbic Acid • Niacin 25 mg • Vitamin B6 5 mg. Other Ingredients: Gelatin, Water. See Editor's Note No. 14.

Orchic PMG **- Standard Process, Inc.**
Each tablet contains: Proprietary Blend 220 mg: Bovine Orchic PMG extract, Magnesium Citrate • Calcium 20 mg • Sodium 25 mg. Other Ingredients: Cellulose.

Oregano Oil Complex **- Pro Health**
Each softgel contains: Oregano oil (origanum vulgare, minimum 5.5% carvacrol) 181 mg • Ginger oil (zingiber officinale) 17.6 mg • Fennel oil (foeniculum vulgare) 19.3 mg. Other Ingredients: Gelatin, Soybean Oil, Glycerin, Enteric Coating, Water, Carob.

Oregano Plus **- EnerGreens, Inc.**
Each capsule contains: Proprietary Blend 625 mg: Oregano, Siberian Ginseng, American Ginseng, Schisandra berries, Bladderwrack, Ginkgo Biloba standardized extract. Other Ingredients: Gelatin.

Orexis (pervalidus obduro) **- Urban Nutrition Inc**
Tribulus Terrestris • Epimedium • Yohimbe extract • Muira Puama • Panax Ginseng • Catuaba bark extract • Damiana (turnera aphrodisiaca).

Organic Alfalfa **- Jamieson**
Each caplet contains: Alfalfa 650 mg.

Organic Flax 1000 **- Health From The Sun**
Two capsules contain: Alpha-Linolenic Acid (ALA) (Omega-3) 1.1 g • Linoleic Acid (Omega-6) 280 mg • Oleic Acid (Omega-9) 290 mg. Ingredients: Certified Organic Flax seed oil, Gelatin, Glycerine, Water, Carob powder.

Organic Flax Oil 1000 mg **- Nature's Bounty**
Each softgel contains: Flax seed oil 1000 mg: Alpha-Linoleic Acid 585 mg, Linoleic Acid 150 mg, Oleic Acid 175 mg, Other Fatty Acids and Phytonutrients 90 mg. Other Ingredients: Gelatin, Glycerin, Caramel Color.

Organic Flax Oil Cold Pressed **- Nature's Bounty**
Each 1 tsp (5 mL) serving contains: Flax seed oil 4650 mg: Alpha-Linolenic Acid 2558 mg, Linoleic Acid 691 mg, Oleic Acid 983 mg, Palmitic Acid 235 mg, Stearic Acid 151 mg.

Organic Flax Seed Oil **- Benepure, Inc**
Each capsule contains: Flax seed oil (yielding alpha-linolenic acid 585 mg, linoleic acid 150 mg, oleic acid 175 mg, palmitic acid 55 mg, stearic acid 35 mg) 1000 mg. Other Ingredients: Gelatin, Glycerin, Carob Extract, Croscarmellose.

Organic Flax Seed Oil 1000 mg **- Arrowroot**
Each softgel contains: Flax Seed oil 1000 mg.

Organic Flaxseed Oil **- PhysioLogics**
Each softgel contains: Organic Flaxseed oil 1000 mg (typically contains alpha-linolenic acid 585 mg) • Linoleic Acid 150 mg • Oleic Acid 175 mg • Other Fatty Acids, Phytonutrients 90 mg. Other Ingredients: Gelatin, Glycerin, Caramel Color.

Organic Flaxseed Oil **- Vitamin World**
Each 1 tsp (5 mL) serving contains: Organic Flaxseed oil 4650 mg: Alpha-Linolenic Acid 2720 mg, Linoleic Acid 698 mg, Oleic Acid 814 mg, Other Fatty Acids and Phytonutrients 418 mg.

Organic Flaxseed Oil 1000 mg **- Vitamin World**
Each softgel contains: Flaxseed oil 1000 mg: Alpha-Linolenic Acid 585 mg, Linoleic Acid 150 mg, Oleic Acid 175 mg, Other Fatty Acids and Phytonutrients 90 mg. Other Ingredients: Gelatin, Glycerin, Caramel Color.

Organic High Lignan Flaxseed Oil **- Vitamin World**
Each 1 tsp (5 mL) serving contains: Organic high lignan Flaxseed oil 4650 mg: Alpha-Linolenic Acid 2650.5 mg, Linoleic Acid 744 mg, Oleic Acid 837 mg, Palmitic Acid, Stearic Acid 418.5 mg.

Organic Mineral Formula **- Golden Glow Natural Health Products**
Each tablet contains: Calcium Amino Acid 250 mg: Calcium 50 mg • Magnesium Amino Acid Chelate 100 mg: Magnesium 20 mg • Zinc Amino Acid Chelate 50 mg: Zinc 5 mg • Manganese Amino Acid Chelate 25 mg: Manganese 2.5 mg • Chromium Picolinate 16 mcg: Chromium 2 mcg • Potassium Aspartate 66.68 mg: Potassium 15 mg • Iron Amino Acid Chelate 10 mg: Elemental Iron 1 mg • Potassium Iodide 26 mcg: Iodine 20 mcg, Potassium 6 mcg • Copper Sulphate (anhydrous) 2 mg: Copper 795 mcg.

Organic Wild Yam Deodorant **- Avalon Natural Products**
Certified Organic Lavender Floral Water (lavandula officinalis) • Certified Organic Extracts Blend: Wild Yam root (discorea villasa), Echinacea (echinacea purpurea), Golden Seal (hydrastis canadensis), Sage (sage officinales) • Organic Myrrh (comminphora myrrha) • Certified Organic Aloe Barbadensis • Vegetable Cellulose • Grapefruit seed extract (citrus grandis) • Castor oil (ricinus communis) • Tocopherol (vitamin E) • Methyl/Propylparaben • Pure Essential Oils.

Organically Bound Minerals **- Standard Process, Inc.**
Each tablet contains: Iodine 250 mcg • Potassium 15 mg • Dried Alfalfa juice 295 mg • Kelp 95 mg. Other Ingredients: Calcium Stearate.

Oricid **- Ortho Molecular Products**
Each scoop contains: Potassium (from proprietary blend) 270 mg • Proprietary Blend 1.17 g: Potassium Sorbate, Aloe Vera leaf exudate 200:1 concentrate.

Original Apple Cider Vinegar Diet **- Vitamin World**
Three tablets contain: Vitamin B6 (as pyridoxine hydrochloride) 25 mg • Chromium (as chromium proteinate) 200 mcg • Apple Cider Vinegar 900 mg • Apple Pectin 150 mg • Gymnema Sylvestre leaf 600 mg. Other Ingredients: Dicalcium Phosphate, Cellulose, Vegetable Stearic Acid, Croscarmellose, Silica, Vegetable Magnesium Stearate, Cellulose Coating.

Ornidex **- Biocodex, Inc.**
Each two capsules contain: L-Ornithine 300 mg. Inactive Ingredients: Dibasic Calcium Phosphate, Colloidal Silica, Magnesium Stearate, Hydroxy-proptyl-methyl-cellulose, Titanium Dioxide (E 171).

Orotates and Chelated Minerals **- Nature's Own**
Each tablet contains: Calcium (from amino acid chelate) 50 mg • Magnesium (from amino acid chelate) 20 mg • Zinc (from amino acid chelate) 5 mg • Manganese (from amino acid chelate) 2.5 mg • Iron (from amino acid chelate) 1 mg • Chromium (from chromium picolinate) 2 mcg • Potassium (from potassium aspartate) 15 mg • Iodine (from potassium iodine) 20 mcg • Copper (from cupric sulfate anhydrous) 795 mcg.

Ortho Adrene Forte **- Ortho Molecular Products**
Two capsules contain: Vitamin A (as betatene brand natural mixed carotenoids) 500 IU • Vitamin C (as sodium ascorbate USP) 125 mg • Vitamin E (as D-alpha tocopherol acid succiante) 20 IU • Niacin USP 20 mg • Vitamin B6 (as pyridoxine HCl and pyridoxal 5 phosphate) 30 mg • Vitamin B12 (as methylcobalamin) 50 mcg • Pantothenic Acid (as D-calcium pantothenate) 90 mg • Calcium (as Citrimal

BRAND NAMES

brand) 50 mg • Magnesium (as citrate) 15 mg • Manganese (as citrate) 5 mg • Herbal Base Blend 450 mg: Wild Yam root 4:1 extract, German Chamomile flower, Dandelion root 4:1 extract, Eleuthero root extract (siberian ginseng, standardized to contain 0.8% eleutherocides), Licorice root extract (standardized to contain 12% glycyrrhizin) • Adrenal concentrate (bovine) 220 mg • Whole Pituitary (bovine) 15 mg. Other Ingredients: Natural Vegetable Capsules, Magnesium Stearate, Microcrystalline Cellulose.
See Editor's Note No. 31.

Ortho B Complex - Ortho Molecular Products
Each capsule contains: Thiamine (B1 from thiamine HCl USP) 50 mg • Vitamin B2 (as riboflavin USP and riboflavin 5 phosphate) 50 mg • Niacin (as niacinamide USP) 50 mg • Vitamin B6 (as pyridoxine HCl USP and pyridoxal 5 phosphate) 50 mg • Folic Acid 800 mcg • Vitamin B12 (as methylcobalamin) 200 mcg • Biotin 75 mcg • Pantothenic Acid (as D-calcium pantothenate) 50 mg • Choline Bitartrate 50 mg • Inositol 50 mg. Other Ingredients: Natural Vegetable Capsules, Ascorbyl Palmitate, Magnesium Stearate, Microcrystalline Cellulose, Silicon Dioxide.

Ortho Biotic - Ortho Molecular Products
Each capsule contains: Proprietary Blend 7 billion CFU: Bifidobacterium Longum, Bifidobacterium Bifidum, Lactobacillus Acidophilus, Lactobacillus Casei • Fructooligosaccharides 163 mg. Other Ingredients: Natural Vegetable Capsules, Ascorbyl Palmitate, Magnesium Stearate, Microcrystalline Cellulose, Silicon Dioxide.

Ortho Derma - Ortho Molecular Products
Three capsules contain: Vitamin A (as Betatene brand natural mixed carotenoids, palmitate) 15,000 IU • Vitamin D (D3, as cholecalciferol) 400 IU • Vitamin E (as D-alpha tocopherol succinate) 300 IU • Thiamine (vitamin B1 from thiamine HCl USP) 10 mg • Riboflavin (vitamin B2 USP) 10 mg • Niacin USP 20 mg • Vitamin B6 (as pyridoxine HCl USP) 20 mg • Pantothenic Acid (as D-calcium pantothenate) 25 mg • Zinc (as Chelazome brand amino acid chelate) 15 mg • Chromium (as ChromeMate brand) 100 mcg • Burdock root 4:1 extract 400 mg • L-Proline USP 250 mg • Stinging Nettles leaf 250 mg • Dandelion root 4:1 extract 150 mg • Gotu Kola aerial portion 4:1 extract 50 mg • Milk Thistle seed extract (standardized to contain 80% silymarin) 50 mg • ActiVin brand Grape seed extract 25 mg • Silicon 10 mg. Other Ingredients: Natural Vegetable Capsules, Magnesium Stearate, Microcrystalline Cellulose.

Ortho Digestzyme - Ortho Molecular Products
Each tablet contains: Glutamic Acid 110 mg • Betaine HCl 100 mg • Pancreatin 6X 100 mg • Pepsin 100 mg • Ox Bile extract 60 mg • Pancrelipase 50 mg • Papain 50 mg • Bromelain 40 mg • Amylase 30 mg. Other Ingredients: Dicalcium Phosphate, Magnesium Stearate, Sorbitol.

Ortho DTX - Ortho Molecular Products
Two capsules contain: Guar Gum 200 mg • Radish root 200 mg • Beet leaf 100 mg • Citrus Pectin 100 mg • Elder flower 100 mg • L-Cysteine HCl Monohydrate USP 100 mg • L-Methionine USP 100 mg • Activated Carbon 50 mg • Choline Bitartrate 50 mg • Inositol 50 mg • Milk Thistle seed extract (standardized to contain 80% silymarin) 50 mg • Pancreatin 6X USP 50 mg • Betaine HCl USP 25 mg • L-Glutathione 25 mg. Other Ingredients: Natural Vegetable Capsules, Magnesium Stearate, Microcrystalline Cellulose.

Ortho Kidney Forte - Ortho Molecular Products
Each capsule contains: Cranberry juice concentrate 250 mg • Dandelion root 4:1 extract 100 mg • Sweet Goldenrod aerial portion 100 mg • Red Clover blossom 80 mg • Celery seed 4:1 extract 65 mg • Kidney (bovine) 40 mg. Other Ingredients: Magnesium Stearate, Microcrystalline Cellulose.

Ortho Liver Forte - Ortho Molecular Products
Three capsules contain: Vitamin A (as palmitate) 6000 IU • Vitamin C (as ascorbic acid USP) 30 mg • Niacin USP 45 mg • Vitamin B12 (as methylcobalamin) 45 mcg • Bitoin 180 mcg • Choline Bitartrate 600 mg • L-Methionine USP 300 mg • Beet leaf 225 mg • Inositol 210 mg • Milk Thistle seed extract (standardized to 80% silymarin) 210 mg • N-Acetyl Cysteine 150 mg • Barberry root bark 150 mg • Ox Bile extract NF 90 mg • Radish root 75 mg • Artichoke leaf extract (standardized to 5% cynarin) 60 mg • Liver (bovine) 60 mg. Other Ingredients: Gelatin, Magnesium Stearate, Microcrystalline Cellulose.

Ortho Spleen Forte - Ortho Molecular Products
Each capsule contains: Bovine Spleen 350 mg • Bovine Thymus 25 mg • Bovine Lymph 25 mg • Goldenseal root extract (standardized to contain 5% alkaloids) 25 mg • Red Clover blossom 75 mg • Hesperidin complex 50 mg • Rutin 50 mg. Other Ingredients: Natural Gelatin Capsules, Magnesium Stearate, Microcrystalline Cellulose.

Ortho Thymus Forte - Ortho Molecular Products
Two capsules contain: Vitamin A (as palmitate) 1000 IU • Zinc (as Chelazome brand amino acid chelate) 8 mg • Thymus (bovine) 750 mg • Eleuthero root extract (siberian ginseng, standardized to contain 0.8% eleutherosides) 80 mg • Echinacea Angustifolia root extract (standardized to contain 4% echinacosides) 60 mg • Lymph (bovine) 50 mg • Spleen (bovine) 50 mg • St. John's Wort flower extract (standardized to contain 0.3% hypericin and 3% hyperforin) 50 mg • Adrenal concentrate (bovine) 25 mg. Other Ingredients: Natural Gelatin Capsules, Magnesium Stearate, Microcrystalline Cellulose.

Ortho Worcid Forte - Ortho Molecular Products
Each capsule contains: Proprietary Blend 610 mg: Black Walnut hull powder, Artemesia Annua herb powder, Slippery Elm bark powder, Garlic bulb powder, Senna leaves powder. Other Ingredients: Natural Vegetable Capsules, Magnesium Stearate, Microcrystalline Cellulose.

Orthoflex - Pacific BioLogic
Siberian Ginseng • Angelica root (Chinese) • Angelica root (pubescent) • Eucommia bark • Siler root • Cinnamon Twig • Astragalus root • Homalomena rhizome • Notopterygium root & rhizome • Gentiana root • Pseudoginseng root • Teasal root • Ginger.

Orthomega Fish Oil - Ortho Molecular Products
Each soft gel contains: EPA 420 mg • DHA 300 mg. Other Ingredients: Purified Marine Triglyceride Concentrate, Vitamin E Mixed Tocopherols, Gelatin, Glycerin, Purified Water.

OS-Cal - SmithKline Beecham
Each tablet contains: Calcium Carbonate 500 mg. Other Ingredients: Dextrose Monohydrate, Maltodextrin, Microcrystalline Cellulose, Magnesium Stearate, Artificial Flavors, Sodium Chloride.

Oscillococcinum (Oscillo) - Boiron
Active Ingredients: Anas Barbariae Hepatis et Cordis extractum (duck liver extract) HPUS 200 CK. Inactive Ingredients: Sucrose 0.85 g, Lactose 0.15 g.
See Editor's Note No. 1.

OSF Plus - Matol Botanical International Ltd
Each capsule contains: Ai/E10 brand Colostrum and Whey Protein extract 100 mg • Astragalus root 200 mg • Base: Rice Powder.

Osha-Lomatium Virtue - Blessed Herbs
Osha root • Lomatium root • Pau d'Arco bark • Propolis • Shitake mycelium • Echinacea Angustifolia root • Goldenseal root • Licorice root • Grain alcohol & Distilled Water.

Osporo - BotanicLab
Acanthopanax Senticosus (siberian ginseng; wu-chia-pi) • Psoralea Corylifolia L. (scurfy pea; bu-gu-zhi) • Epimedium Brevicornum Maxim (epimedium; yin-yang-huo) • Ostrea Gigas Thunberg (oyster shell; mu-li) • Paeonia Lactiflora Pall (white peony root; chih-shao) • Glycyrrhiza Glabra L. (licorice; gan-cao) • Apis Mellifera (honey bee) L. (royal jelly; fon-hwang-chiang).

Oss Aide - InterPlexus
Three capsules contain: Vitamin A (as palmitate) 2500 IU • Vitamin D (as cholecalciferol) 200 IU • Vitamin K (as phytonadione) 1.6 mg • Folic Acid 800 mcg • Calcium (as malate) 400 mg • Magnesium (as malate) 100 mg • Zinc (as malate) 5 mg • Copper (as citrate) 0.5 mg • Boron (as aspartate) 2 mg. Other Ingredients: Cellulose.

Ossopan MD - Xymogen
Four capsules contain: Calcium (as MCHC and di-calcium malate) 800 mg • Magnesium (as di-magnesium malate and magnesium glycinate) 400 mg • Vitamin D (as cholecalciferol) 200 IU.

Ostarplex - Standard Process, Inc.
Each capsule contains: Proprietary Blend 407 mg: Alfalfa flour, Nutritional Yeast, Veal Bone PMG extract, Betaine Hydrochloride, Arrowroot flour, Ammonium Chloride, Soy bean, Choline Bitartrate, Bovine Liver, Phosphoric Acid, Porcine Stomach, Calcium Lactate, Manganese Glycerophosphate, Bovine Adrenal, Magnesium Citrate, Bovine Spleen, Ovine Spleen, Licorice root, Defatted Wheat germ, Inositol, Allantoin, Porcine Brain, Ascorbic Acid • Riboflavin 0.1 mg • Niacin 1.3 mg • Vitamin B6 0.2 mg. Other Ingredients: Gelatin, Water, Colors.
See Editor's Note No. 14.

Osteo - Aspen Group, Inc.
Each tablet contains: Calcium Orotate 376 mg • Magnesium Orotate 200 mg • Calcium Aspartate 24 mg • Vitamin D 400 mg.

Osteo Bi-Flex - Rexall - Sundown
Three caplets contain: Vitamin C 60 mg • Vitamin D 400 IU • Calcium 500 mg • Glucosamine HCl 1500 mg • Chondroitin Sulfate 1200 mg. Other Ingredients: Red Beet Juice powder, Crospovidone, Magnesium Stearate, Croscarmellose Sodium, Silica.
See Editor's Note No. 15.

Osteo Bi-Flex: Double Strength Caplets - Rexall - Sundown
Three caplets contain: Vitamin C (as ascorbic acid) 60 mg • Manganese (as manganese sulfate) 2 mg • Sodium 105 mg • Glucosamine HCl 1500 mg • Chondroitin Sulfate 1200 mg • Boron (as sodium tetraborate) 3 mg. Other Ingredients: Microcrystalline Cellulose, Sodium Carboxymethylcellulose, Crospovidone, Red 40 Lake, Yellow 5 Lake, Maltodextrin, Magnesium Stearate, Dextrose, Yellow 6 Lake, Soy Lecithin, Sodium Citrate, Blue 1 Lake.
See Editor's Note No. 15.

Osteo Bi-Flex: Double Strength Softgels - Rexall - Sundown
Three softgels contain: Sodium 100 mg • Glucosamine HCl 1500 mg • Chondroitin Sulfate 1200 mg. Other Ingredients: Soybean Oil, Gelatin, Soy Lecithin, Yellow Beeswax, Silica, Sodium Tripoly-Phosphate, Red 40, Titanium Dioxide, Blue 1.
See Editor's Note No. 15.

Osteo Bi-Flex: Fast-Acting Caplets - Rexall - Sundown
Two caplets contain: Sodium 45 mg • Willow Bark extract (salix spp.) 800 mg • Glucosamine HCl 750 mg • Chondroitin Sulfate 600 mg • Boron 1.5 mg. Other Ingredients: Microcrystalline Cellulose, Hydroxypropyl Methylcellulose, Crospovidone, Boron Amino Acid Chelate (hydrolyzed rice protein, boric acid, glycine, aspartic acid, hydrolyzed soy protein), Pharmaceutical Glaze, Silica, Magnesium Stearate, Titanium Dioxide (color), Yellow 5 Lake, Red 40 Lake, Blue 1 Lake, Yellow 6 Lake, Soy Lecithin.
See Editor's Note No. 15.

Osteo Bi-Flex: Performance Caplets - Rexall - Sundown
Two caplets contain: Vitamin C (as ascorbic acid) 500 mg • Niacin (as niacinamide) 10 mg • Vitamin B12 (as cyanocobalamin) 10 mcg • Sodium 5 mg • Glucosamine HCl 750 mg • L-Arginine 750 mg • Boron 1.5 mg. Other Ingredients: L-Arginine Monohydrochloride, Microcrystalline Cellulose, Corn Starch, Calcium Silicate, Crospovidone, Boron Amino Acid Chelate (hydrolyzed rice protein, boric acid, glycine, aspartic acid, hydrolyzed soy protein), Hydroxypropyl Methylcellulose, Magnesium Stearate, PEG, Dextrin, Titanium Dioxide (color), Dextrose, Soy Lecithin, Blue 2 Lake, Red 40 Lake, Blue 1 Lake, Yellow 6 Lake.

Osteo Bi-Flex: Plus Calcium Caplets - Rexall - Sundown
Three caplets contain: Vitamin C (as ascorbic acid) 60 mg • Vitamin D (as cholecalciferol) 400 IU • Calcium (as calcium carbonate) 500 mg • Sodium 110 mg • Glucosamine HCl 1500 mg • Chondroitin Sulfate 1200 mg. Other Ingredients: Microcrystalline Cellulose, Sodium Carboxymethylcellulose, Crospovidone, Titanium Dioxide, Maltodextrin, Magnesium Stearate, Yellow 5 Lake, Dextrose, Soy Lecithin, Sodium Citrate, Red 40 Lake, Blue 1 Lake, Yellow 6 Lake.
See Editor's Note No. 15.

Osteo Bi-Flex: Plus MSM Caplets - Rexall - Sundown
Four caplets contain: Sodium 115 mg • Glucosamine HCl 1500 mg • Chondroitin Sulfate 1200 mg • Methylsulfonylmethane (MSM) 1000 mg. Other Ingredients: Microcrystalline Cellulose, Sodium Carboxymethylcellulose, Yellow 5 Lake, Crospovidone, Magnesium Stearate, Yellow 6 Lake, Maltodextrin, Dextrose, Soy Lecithin, Sodium Citrate, Red 40 Lake, Blue 1 Lake.
See Editor's Note No. 15.

Osteo Bi-Flex: Triple Strength Caplets - Rexall - Sundown
Two caplets contain: Vitamin C (as ascorbic acid) 60 mg • Manganese (as manganese sulfate) 2 mg • Sodium 105 mg • Glucosamine HCl 1500 mg • Chondroitin Sulfate 1200 mg • Boron (as sodium tetraborate) 3 mg. Other Ingredients: Microcrystalline Cellulose, Sodium Carboxymethylcellulose, Crospovidone, Red 40 Lake, Yellow 5 Lake, Maltodextrin, Magnesium Stearate, Dextrose, Yellow 6 Lake, Soy Lecithin, Sodium Citrate, Blue 1 Lake.
See Editor's Note No. 15.

Osteo Formula - Quest
Each tablet contains: Calcium (HVP Chelate) 125 mg • Magnesium (HVP Chelate) 125 mg • Vitamin C 50 mg • Vitamin D (as Vitamin D3) 50 IU • Silicon (HVP Chelate) 125 mcg • N-Acetyl Glucosamine (NAG) 125 mg • Betaine HCl 25 mg. Other Ingredients: Croscarmellose Sodium, Magnesium Stearate (vegetable source), Microcrystalline Cellulose, Vegetable Stearin.

Osteo Plex - Olympian Labs
Four capsules contain: Calcium Citrate 800 mg • Magnesium (oxide) 400 mg • Boron (proteinate) 400 mcg • Zinc (amino acid chelate) 10 mg.

Osteo Protector - The Vitamin Shoppe
Each tablet contains: Vitamin D (as cholecalciferol) 100 IU • Calcium (as carbonate, hydroxyapatite) 500 mg • Magnesium (as oxide, citrate) 250 mg • Ipriflavone (7-Isopropoxy Isoflavone (Ostivone)) 200 mg.

Osteo-Aid - Futurebiotics LLC
Six capsules contain: Vitamin D 400 IU • Calcium (as calcium citrate) 1000 mg • Magnesium (as magnesium amino acid chelate) 400 mg • Boron (as amino acid chelate) 1.5 mg • Ostivone Ipriflavone (7-isopropoxy isoflavone) 100 mg • Soy Isoflavone extract powder (standardized for 10% (5 mg) phytoestrogen isoflavones) 50 mg. Other Ingredients: Gelatin, Water.

OsteoBalance - Pure Encapsulations
Seven vegetable capsules contain: Calcium (microcrystalline hydroxyapatite) 600 mg • Calcium (citrate/malate) 600 mg • Horsetail 5:1 extract (equisetum arvense) 300 mg • Magnesium (aspartate) 115 mg • Manganese (aspartate) 10 mg • Zinc (picolinate) 30 mg • Copper (glycinate) 2.5 mg • Boron (glycinate) 2 mg • Vitamin C (as ascorbyl palmitate) 102 mg • Vitamin D (as D3) 400 IU.

Osteocare - Puritan's Pride
Two capsules contain: Vitamin D (as cholecalciferol) 133 IU • Calcium (as calcium citrate) 400 mg • Ipriflavone (as 7-isopropoxy isoflavone) 200 mg.

Osteocare Fizz - Vitabiotics
Each tablet contains: Calcium 400 mg • Magnesium 50 mg • Zinc 5 mg • Copper 0.5 mg • Manganese 0.75 mg • Selenium 25 mcg • Vitamin C 60 mg • Vitamin D 2.5 mcg.

Osteocare Liquid - Vitabiotics
Two teaspoons contain: Calcium 300 mg • Magnesium 150 mg • Zinc 6 mg • Vitamin D 3.8 mcg.

Osteocare Tablets - Vitabiotics
Two tablets contain: Calcium 800 mg • Magnesium 300 mg • Zinc 10 mg • Vitamin D 5 mcg • Manganese 1.5 mg • Selenium 50 mcg • Boron 0.6 mg • Copper 1 mg.

BRAND NAMES

Some Brand Name Natural Products - What they Contain

www.NaturalDatabase.com contains MANY more listings than appear here.
Editor's Notes are located on pages 2155-2163.

Osteo-Citrate - Metagenics
Each tablet contains: Calcium (as calcium citrate) 200 mg • Magnesium (as magnesium oxide) 150 mg.

Osteo-Genics - Metagenics
Two tablets contain: Microcrystalline Hydroxyapatite Concentrate (MCHC) 400 mg • Calcium (as MCHC, calcium citrate malate) 300 mg • Phosphorus (as MCHC) 47 mg • Magnesium (as magnesium oxide) 200 mg • Betaine Hydrochloride 200 mg • Raw Kidney concentrate (bovine) 100 mg • Vitamin D (as cholecalciferol) 100 IU • Vitamin C (as ascorbic acid) 40 mg • Horsetail aerial parts (equisetum arvense, natural source of silica) 100 mg.

OsteoGuard - Advocare International
Four caplets contain: Calcium (as amino acid chelate) 400 mg • Magnesium (as amino acid chelate) 200 mg • Vitamin D (as ergocalciferol) 200 IU • Zinc (as amino acid chelate) 7.5 mg • Copper (as amino acid chelate) 1 mg • Manganese (as amino acid chelate) 800 mcg • Vitamin K (as phytonadione) 80 mcg • Green Tea extract (leaf - camellia sinensis) 50 mg • Ginger extract (root - zingiber officinale) 100 mg • Boron (as amino acid chelate) 1 mg • Silicon (as amino acid chelate) 800 mcg • Ipriflavone (Ostivone) 600 mg. Other Ingredients: Dicalcium Phosphate, Silicon Dioxide, Cellulose, Stearic Acid, Magnesium Stearate.

Osteo-Joint - Leiner Health Products
Each caplet contains: Deoiled Lecithin (Glycine max) bean 25 mg • Devil's Claw extract 40 mg • Glucosamine Sulfate powder 500 mg • Methylsulfonylmethane 25 mg • Rice Starch (Oryza sativa) 25 mg. Other Ingredients: Calcium Carbonate, Cellulose, Methylcellulose, Maltodextrin, Deoiled Lecithin, Rice Starch, Silicon Dioxide, Croscarmellose Sodium, Stearic Acid, Dextrin, Crospovidone, Magnesium Stearate.

Osteologic - PhysioLogics
Four tablets contain: Vitamin D (as Cholecalciferol) 400 IU • Vitamin K (as Phytonadione) 80 mcg • Vitamin B6 (as Pyridoxine HCl) 2 mg • Folate (Folic Acid) 400 mcg • Pantothenic Acid (as D-Calcium Pantothenate) 10 mg • Calcium (as Calcium Carbonate) 1000 mg • Iodine (from Kelp) 471 mcg • Magnesium (as 58% Magnesium Oxide, 25% Magnesium Glycinate, 17% Magnesium Carbonate) 400 mg • Zinc (as Zinc Citrate) 15 mg • Selenium (from natural salts) 3 mcg • Copper (as Copper Aspartate) 2 mg • Manganese (as mixed Manganese salts) 378 mcg • Chromium (from natural salts) 38 mcg • Molybdenum (from natural salts) 115 mcg • Silicon (as Silicon Dioxide) 20 mg • Boron (as 98% Boron Aspartate, 2% natural salts) 3 mg.

OsteoLogic 2000 - PhysioLogics
Three caplets contain: Vitamin D (as cholecalciferol) 400 IU • Vitamin K (as phytonadione) 80 mcg • Calcium (as hydroxyapatite phosphate, dicalcium phosphate) 1020 mg • Phosphorus (as hydroxyapatite phosphate, dicalcium phosphate) 524 mg. Other Ingredients: Cellulose (plant origin), Croscarmellose, Silica, Vegetable Stearic Acid, Cellulose Coating, Vegetable Magnesium Stearate.

OsteoLogic Pro - PhysioLogics
Two tablets contain: Vitamin D (as cholecalciferol) 150 IU • Vitamin K (as phytonadione) 28 mcg • Calcium (as calcium citrate, calcium hydroxyapatite, dicalcium phosphate) 400 mg • Phosphorus (as calcium hydroxyapatite, dicalcium phosphate) 112 mg • Magnesium (as magnesium citrate, magnesium oxide) 134 mg • Zinc (as zinc glycinate) 5 mg • Manganese (as manganese amino acid chelate) 0.7 mg • Boron (as boron amino acid chelate) 360 mcg • Silica (as silicon dioxide) 35 mg. Other Ingredients: Cellulose (plant origin), Croscarmellose, Vegetable Stearic Acid, Cellulose Coating, Vegetable Magnesium Stearate.

OsteoMax - Nutraceutics Corp.
Each tablet contains: Calcium 500 mg • Magnesium 200 mg • Vitamin D3 200 IU • Lysine 100 mg. Other ingredients: Citric Acid, Calcium Carbonate, Sodium Bicarbonate, Magnesium Oxide, Orange Flavor, Sodium Carbonate, Polysorbate 80.

Osteo-Max - Metabolic Response Modifiers
Each capsule contains: Ipriflavone 200 mg • MCHC (yielding 167 mg elemental calcium) 667 mg.

Osteo-Nutrients - Vital Nutrients
Six capsules contain: Calcium (50% citrate/malate, 50% carbonate) 1200 mg • Magnesium (50% citrate, 50% oxide) 400 mg • Horsetail 200 mg • Lysine 200 mg • Vitamin D (D3, as cholecalciferol) 200 IU.

Osteo-Nutrients II - Vital Nutrients
Four capsules contain: Calcium (carbonate/citrate, malate) 1000 mg • Magnesium (oxide/citrate) 500 mg • Horsetail extract 100 mg • Lysine 100 mg • Boron (citrate) 3 mg • Vitamin D (D3, as cholecalciferol) 200 IU.

OsteoPeak Men - Osteogenic Care Technologies (OST)
Two capsules contain: Vitamin D (as cholecalciferol) 200 IU • Calcium (as calcium citrate) 90 mg • Organic Kosher Certified OsteoPeak Proprietary Blend 250 mg: Rehmannia Glutinosa Libosch, Eleutherococcus Senticosus Max. Other Ingredients: Gelatin Capsule, Organic Maltodextrin.

OsteoPeak Menopause - Osteogenic Care Technologies (OST)
Three capsules contain: Vitamin D (as cholecalciferol) 300 IU • Calcium (as calcium citrate) 180 mg • Organic, Kosher Certified OsteoPeak Proprietary Blend 500 mg: Rehmannia Glutinosa Libosch, Eleutherococcus Senticosus Max. Other Ingredients: Gelatin Capsule, Organic Maltodextrin.

OsteoPeak Natural - Osteogenic Care Technologies (OST)
Three capsules contain: Organic, Kosher Certified OsteoPeak Proprietary Blend 750 mg: Rehmannia Glutinosa Libosch, Eleutherococcus Senticosus Max. Other Ingredients: Gelatin Capsule, Organic Maltodextrin.

OsteoPeak Osteorus - Osteogenic Care Technologies (OST)
Two gummy dinosaurs contain: Vitamin D (cholecalciferol) 400 IU • Calcium (as tricalcium phosphate) 20 mg • Organic, Kosher Certified OsteoPeak Proprietary Blend 50 mg: Rehmannia Glutinosa Libosch, Eleutherococcus Senticosus Max. Other Ingredients: Organic Sugar, Organic Corn Syrup, Pectin, Fuamric Acid, Citric Acid, Natural Flavors/Colors (turmeric, annatto, black carrot juice concentrate, grape skin extract), Fractionated Coconut Oil, Carnauba Wax.

OsteoPeak Premenopause - Osteogenic Care Technologies (OST)
Each capsule contains: Vitamin D (as cholecalciferol) 100 IU • Calcium (as calcium citrate) 55 mg • Organic, Kosher Certified OsteoPeak Proprietary Blend 150 mg: Rehmannia Glutinosa Libosch, Eleutherococcus Senticosus Max. Other Ingredients: Gelatin Capsule, Organic Maltodextrin.

Osteo-Plus - Nutri-Quest Rx
Each tablet contains: Boron (special organic complex) 1 mg • Magnesium Chelate 400 mg • Calcium Chelate 100 mg • Calcium Aspartate 100 mg • Calcium Giuconate 50 mg • Calcium (Hydroxyapatite) 156 mg • Calcium (Veal Bone) 39 mg • Red Bone Marrow 10 mg • Calcium Citrate 50 mg • Vitamin C 25 mg • Vitamin D 50 IU • L-Glutamic Acid HCL 15 mg • Betaine HCL 10 mg • Salmiac 10 mg • Parathyroid 2 mg. In a base containing Horsetail Rush (Shave grass), Source of Natural Silicon 15 mg, Calcium Fluoride (Cell Salt) Safflower herb 25 mg.
See Editor's Note No. 14.

Osteoporosis Formula - Nature's Life
Each four capsules contain: Calcium (Citrate/Malate, Carbonate) 1000 mg • Magnesium (Oxide, Citrate) 500 mg • Vitamin C (Ascorbic Acid) 40 mg • Betaine HCl 40 mg • Zinc (Picolinate) 15 mg • Manganese (Gluconate) 5 mg • Boron (Citrate) 2 mg • Vitamin K (as Vitamin K1) mg • Copper (Gluconate) 1 mg • Silicon (Dioxide) 1 mg • Vitamin D (as Vitamin D3) (Cholecalciferol) 400 IU. In a natural base of Springtime Horsetail herb (Equisetum arvense).

OsteoPrev - Ortho Molecular Products
Four capsules contain: Vitamin D (D3, as cholecalciferol) 1000 IU • Vitamin K (as phytonadione) 1 mg • Folic Acid 800 mcg • Calcium (as hydroxyapatite, Citrimal brand) 200 mg • Phosphorus (as chelate) 15 mg • Magnesium (as buffered amino acid chelate, citrate) 150 mg • Selenium (as amino acid complex) 200 mcg • Copper (as lysinate) 1 mg • Manganese (as Chelazome brand) 10 mg • Molybdenum (as amino acid chelate) 150 mcg • Ipriflavone 600 mg • Strontium Citrate 200 mg • Montmorillonite 150 mg • Boron (as proteinate) 5 mg. Other Ingredients: Natural Vegetable Capsules, Turmeric Root Extract, Ascorbyl Palmitate, Magnesium Stearate, Microcrystalline Cellulose, Silicon Dioxide.

OsteoPrime - Enzymatic Therapy
Four tablets contain: Vitamin D 200 IU • Calcium (Aspartate, Citrate, Succinate, Fumarate, Carbonate, Lactate, Malate) 600 mg • Magnesium (Aspartate, Oxide) 250 mg • Vitamin C (Ascorbic Acid) 100 mg • Vitamin B6 (Pyridoxine) 25 mg • Niacinamide 20 mg • Zinc (Picolinate) 15 mg • Manganese (Aspartate) 15 mg • Thiamine HCl (Vitamin B1) 10 mg • Riboflavin (Vitamin B2) 10 mg • Pantothenic Acid (D-Calcium Pantothenate) 10 mg • Copper (Gluconate) 1.5 mg • Folic Acid 400 mcg • Vitamin K (Phytonadione) 150 mcg • Chromium (Aspartate) 100 mcg • Selenium sodium Selenite) 100 mcg • Molybdenum (Sodium Molybdate) 50 mcg • Vitamin B12 (Cyanocobalamin) 10 mcg. Other Ingredients: Betaine HCl 20 mg • Silicon Sodium Metasilicate 1 mg • Boron (Chelated) 750 mcg • Strontium (Nonradioactice) 500 mcg.

OsteoPrime Fort - PhytoPharmica
Four tablets contain: Betaine HCl 20 mg • Boron (as boron Krebs cycle chelates) 2 mg • Calcium (from tricalcium phosphate, clacium carbonate, calcium Krebs cycle chelates, and calcium citrate) 600 mg • Chromium (as chromium aspartate) 200 mcg • Copper (as copper gluconate) 2 mg • Folic Acid 800 mcg • Magnesium (as magnesium oxide and magnesium aspartate) 250 mg • Manganese (as mananese aspartate) 7 mg • Molybdenum (as sodium molybdate) 50 mcg • Niacin (as niacinamide) 50 mg • Pantothenic Acid (as calcium D-pantothenate) 20 mg • Phosphorus (from tricalcium phosphate) 130 mg • Riboflavin (vitamin B2) 20 mg • Selenium (as sodium selenite) 100 mcg • Silicon (as magnesium trisilicate) 1 mg • Strontium (as strontium chloride) 1 mg • Thiamin (as thiamin HCl, vitamin B1) 20 mg • Vitamin B12 (as cyanocobalamin) 20 mcg • Vitamin B6 (as pyridoxine HCl) 25 mg • Vitamin C (ascorbic acid) 100 mg • Vitamin D (as cholecalciferol) 300 IU • Vitamin K (as phytonadione) 300 mcg • Zinc (as zinc picolinate) 20 mg.

OsteoPure - Marathon Nutrifoods
Each two capsules contain: Red Yeast Rice (monascus purpureus went) 200 mg. Inactive Ingredients: Whey, Gelatin, Magnesium Stearate.

OsteoPure + - Marathon Nutrifoods
Each two capsules contain: Red Yeast Rice (monascus purpureus went) 200 mg • Pueraria root (pueraria lobata) 300 mg. Inactive Ingredients: Whey, Dicalcium Phosphate, Gelatin, Magnesium Stearate.

OsteoSoy - FreeLife International
Four caplets contain: Vitamin D (as cholecalciferol) 125 IU • Vitamin K (as phylloquinone) 30 mcg • Vitamin B6 (as pyridoxine HCl) 5 mg • Folate (as folic acid) 400 mcg • Vitamin B12 (as cyanocobalamin) 25 mcg • Calcium (as hydroxyapatite, calcium hydrogen phosphate, citramal calcium-citrate-malate-glycinate) 1100 mg • Phosphorus (as hydroxyapatite, calcium hydrogen phosphate) 350 mg • Magnesium (as magnesium oxide, chelazome magnesium glycinate, magnesium citrate) 400 mg • Zinc (as chelazome zinc citrate, zinc glycinate) 15 mg • Copper (as chelazome copper glycinate) 1 mg • Manganese (as chelazome manganese glycinate) 2 mg • Chaste berry (from standardized extract 5:1, 5% vitexicarpin, 1% vitricin 50 mg) 250 mg • Dong Quai (from standardized extract 5:1, 10,000 ppm ligustilide 50 mg) 250 mg • Licorice root (from 50 mg standardized extract 4:1, 13% glycyrrihizin 50 mg) 200 mg • Silica (colloidal) 70 mg • Isoflavones (genistein, daidzein, puerarin from kudzu root, soybean) 40 mg • Boron (as boron chelate) 2 mg • Soyatab (caplet disintegration accelerant from soy polysaccharides) 180 mg. Other Ingredients: Cellulose, Cellulose Gum, Vegetable Stearic Acid, Vegetable Magnesium Stearate, Vita-Coat (vegetable resin, alpha-lipoic acid).

Osteosupport - Health Factor
Four tablets contain: Calcium (Citrate/Hydroxylapatite) 850 mg • Vitamin D (as Vitamin D3) (Cholecalciferol) 100 IU • Iodine (Kelp) 100 mcg • Magnesium (Citrate) 650 mg • Boron (Citrate) 2 mg • Silicon (Citrate) 500 mcg • Vanadium (Pentoxide) 75 mcg • Betaine HCl 65 mg • Glutamic Acid 65 mg.

Osteo-Support - The Vitamin Shoppe
Two tablets contain: Calcium 500 mg • Magnesium 250 mg • Vitamin D 100 IU.

Ostivone - Enzymatic Therapy
Each capsule contains: Ostivone Ipriflavone 200 mg.

Ostivone - Anabolic Laboratories
Each tablet contains: Ipriflavone (ostivone 7-isopropoxy isoflavone) 200 mg.

Ostivone - Natrol, Inc.
Each capsule contains: 7-Isopropoxy-Isoflavone 100 mg. Other Ingredients: Rice Powder, Magnesium Stearate, Gelatin.

Ostivone - Source Naturals
One tablet contains: Ipriflavone (Ostivone) 300 mg.

Ostivone - PhytoPharmica
Each capsule contains: Ipriflavone (Ostivone brand) 200 mg.

O-Tropin - Orenda International
Active Ingredients: Lipotropin Complex Proprietary Blend 200 mg: Alpha GPC (alpha glycerlphosphoryl choline), GABA (gamma amino butyric acid), Mucuna Pruiens (l-dopa bean extract), Moomiyo extract (Russian mumie) • HGH Stimulator Proprietary Blend 300 mg: Ornithine Alpha Ketoglutarate, L-Glutamine, L-Arginine, L-Lysine, L-Valine, L-Isoleucine, L-Tyrosine, Glycine. Other Ingredients: Purified Water, Lecithin Phospholipids, Sodium Citrate, Citric Acid, Potassium Sorbate, Maltodextrin, Sodium Benzoate, Methylparaben, Natural Flavors, Artificial Flavors.

Ouch Ointment - Earth Science
Each 100 mL tube contains: Water • Tea Tree oil • Glyceryl Stearate • Capric Caprylic Triglycerides • Echinacea extract • Witch Hazel extract • Steareth-20 • Glycerine • Calendula extract • Saccharomyces Lysate • St. John's Wort • Dimethicone • Plantain extract • Potassium Sorbate • Sodium Carbomer 940 • Peppermint oil • Mont-Morillonite Clay • Grape extract.

Our Daily Fish - Functional Products
Six softgels contain: Vitamin E 0.33 IU • Vitamin B1 0.09 mg • Vitamin B2 0.15 mg • Vitamin B3 3.5 mg • Vitamin B6 0.3 mg • Folic Acid 12 mcg • Pantothenic Acid 0.15 mg • Calcium 260 mg • Iron 1 mg • Phosphorus 200 mg • Iodine 60 mcg • Magnesium 25 mg • Zinc 0.3 mg • Selenium 30 mcg • Copper 0.1 mg • Potassium 250 mg • Arginine 200 mg • Histidine 250 mg • Isoleucine 200 mg • Leucine 30 mg • Lysine 200 mg • Methionine 200 mg • Phenylalanine 200 mg • Threonine 100 mg • Tyrosine 200 mg • Valine 200 mg • Omega 6 Linoleic Acid 300 mg • Omega 3 ALA 85 mg • Omega 3 EPA 230 mg • Omega 3 DHA 450 mg. Ingredients: Fish Oil, Di-Calcium Phosphate, Glycerin (Kosher), Water, Potassium Sulfate, Salmon Oil, Docosahexaenoic Acid, L-Leucine, Linoleic Acid, L-Histidine, L-Arginine, L-Isoleucine, L-Lysine, L-Methionine, L-Phenylalanine, L-Tyrosine, L-Valine, Eicosapentaenoic Acid, Flax Seed Oil, Soybean Lecithin, Safflower Oil, Bees Wax, L-Threonine, Alpha-Linolenic Acid, Magnesium Oxide, Selenium Yeast, Niacinamide, Ferrous Sulfate, Zinc Oxide, Pyridoxine HCl, D-Alpha Tocopherol, Curpric Sulfate, Calcium Phantothenate, Riboflavin, Thiamine HCl, Potassium Iodide, Retinol Palmitate, Folic Acid.

Some Brand Name Natural Products - What they Contain

www.NaturalDatabase.com contains MANY more listings than appear here.
Editor's Notes are located on pages 2155-2163.

BRAND NAMES

Our Daily Fruit - Functional Products
Three softgels contain: Vitamin A 511 IU • Vitamin C 112 mg • Vitamin E 0.36 IU • Vitamin K 10 mcg • Vitamin B1 0.05 mg • Vitamin B2 0.06 mg • Vitamin B3 0.5 mg • Vitamin B6 0.1 mg • Folic Acid 10 mcg • Pantothenic Acid 0.21 mg • Calcium 30 mg • Iron 0.5 mg • Phosphorus 23 mg • Magnesium 20 mg • Zinc 0.17 mg • Copper 0.2 mg • Manganese 0.5 mg • Potassium 250 mg • Omega 6 Linoleic Acid 150 mg • Omega 3 ALA 30 mg. Ingredients: Potassium Sulfate • Gelatin • Vegetable Oil • Safflower Oil • Linoleic Acid • Alpha-Linolenic Acid • Gamma-Linolenic Acid • Glycerin (Kosher) • Ascorbic Acid • Di-Calcium Phosphate • Evening Primrose Oil • Water • Flax Seed Oil • Soybean Lecithin • Bees Wax • Magnesium Oxide • Annatto Seed • Bilberry Extract • Natural Beta Carotene • Ferrous Sulfate • Manganese Sulfate • Phytonadione • Niacinamide • Cupric Sulfate • d-Alpha Tocopheryl • Calcium Pantothenate • Zinc Oxide • Pyridoxine HCl • Riboflavin • Thiamine HCl • Folic Acid.

Our Daily Veggies - Functional Products
Three softgels contain: Vitamin A 1916 IU • Vitamin C 39 mg • Vitamin E 0.6 mg • Vitamin K 50 mcg • Vitamin B1 0.12 mg • Vitamin B2 0.1 mg • Vitamin B3 1 mg • Vitamin B6 0.23 • Folic Acid 40 mcg • Pantothenic Acid 0.37 mg • Calcium 88 mg • Iron 2 mg • Phosphorus 70 mg • Magnesium 35 mg • Zinc 0.7 mg • Selenium 10 mcg • Copper 0.1 mg • Manganese 0.5 mg • Potassium 400 mg • Omega 6 Linoleic Acid 670 mg • Omega 3 ALA 100 mg • Omega 3 GLA 20 mg • Soy Isoflavone 0.2 mg • Lutein 0.39 mg • Lycopene 0.18 mg. Ingredients: Safflower Oil, Potassium, Sulfate, Gelatin, Glycerin (Kosher), Di-Calcium Phosphate, Evening Primrose Oil, Flax Seed Oil, Vegetable Oil, Gamma-Linolenic Acid, Alpha-Linolenic Acid, Linoleic Acid, Water, Magnesium Oxide, Soybean Lecithin, Bees Wax, Ascorbic Acid, Tomato Concentrate, Ferrous Sulfate, Natural Beta Carotene, Phytonadione, Selenium Yeast, Lutein, Manganese Sulfate, Lycopene, Niacinamide, Zinc Oxide, D-Alpha Tocopherol, Soy Isoflavone, Calcium Pantothenate, Pyridoxine HCl, Cupric Sulfate, Thiamine HCl, Riboflavin, Folic Acid.

Ovary-Uterus Complex - Enzymatic Therapy
Each capsule contains: Ovary-Uterus complex (predigested soluble concentrate) 250 mg • Multi-Glandular Complex 100 mg: Raw Liver, Raw Lung, Raw Pancreas, Raw Heart, Raw Kidney, Raw Spleen, & Raw Brain.
See Editor's Note No. 21 and No. 31.

Ovatrophin PMG - Standard Process, Inc.
Each tablet contains: Proprietary Blend: 190 mg: Bovine Ovary PMG extract, Magnesium Citrate • Calcium 20 mg • Sodium 20 mg. Other Ingredients: Cellulose.
See Editor's Note No. 14.

Overdrive - Pharmanex
Each capsule contains: Vitamin A (100% as Beta-Carotene from Dunaliella Salina, Beta-Carotene) 2500 IU • Vitamin C (as Ascorbic Acid) 300 mg • Vitamin E (d-Alpha Tocopheryl Succinate) 75 IU • Thiamin (as Thiamine Mononitrate) 0.75 mg • Riboflavin (as Riboflavin) 0.85 mg • Vitamin B6 (as Pyridoxine Hydrochloride) 1 mg • Folate (as Folic Acid) 100 mcg • Vitamin B12 (as Cyanocobalamin) 3 mcg • Pantothenic Acid (as d-Calcium Pantothenate) 5 mg • Magnesium (as Magnesium Asparate, Magnesium Oxide) 60 mg • Selenium (as L-Selenomethionine) 35 mcg • Chromium (as Chromium Chelate, Chromium Picolinate) 100 mcg • Bromelain (from Pineapple extract) 50 mg • Papain (from Papaya extract) 50 mg • Citrus Bioflavonoid Complex 50 mg • Hydromins (from Sea Salt extract) 50 mg • N-Acetyl-L-Cysteine 20 mg • Quercetin 12.5 mg • Grape Seed Extract with Leucoanthocyanin 2.5 mg.

Ovex - Standard Process, Inc.
Each tablet contains: Proprietary Blend 185 mg: Bovine Ovary Cytosol extract, Magnesium Citrate, Mixed Tocopherols • Vitamin C 2 mg. Other Ingredients: Calcium Lactate, Cellulose, Calcium Stearate, Gelatin.
See Editor's Note No. 14.

Ovex P - Standard Process, Inc.
Each tablet contains: Proprietary Blend 185 mg: Porcine Ovary Cytosol extract, Magnesium Citrate, Mixed Tocopherols • Vitamin C 2 mg. Other Ingredients: Cellulose, Gelatin.

Ox - SAN Nutrition
Three caplets contain: Citruline-Malate 3000 mg • Regall Biosorb 5 mg. Other Ingredients: Cellulose, Stearic Acid, Magnesium Stearate.

Oxi Nutrients - Vital Nutrients
Six capsules contain: Natural Beta Carotene (with mixed carotenoids) 80,000 IU • Natural Vitamin E (D-alpha tocopheryl succinate) 400 IU • Vitamin C (ascorbic acid) 4000 mg • Selenium (selenomethionine) 200 mcg • Green Tea extract (80% catechins) 100 mg • Quercetin 150 mg • Grape seed extract (proanthocyanidins 95%) 40 mg.

Oxitrol - Ortho Molecular Products
Two capsules contain: Vitamin A (as Betatene brand natural mixed carotenoids) 7500 IU • Vitamin C (as ascorbic acid USP) 500 mg • Vitamin E (as D-alpha tocopherol succinate) 300 IU • Selenium (as amino acid complex) 100 mcg • N-Acetyl Cysteine USP 200 mg • Green Tea extract (standardized to contain 50% polyphenols) 100 mg • Lipoic Acid 100 mg • Quercetin 100 mg • ActiVin brand Grape seed extract 75 mg. Other Ingredients: Natural Vegetable Capsules, Ascorbyl Palmitate, Magnesium Stearate, Microcrystalline Cellulose, Silicon Dioxide.

Oxy 17 - Progressive Health Nutraceuticals
Magnesium 20 mg • L-Glutamine 500 mg • Cordyceps 500 mg • Noni extract 500 mg • Coleus Forskolin 15 mg • Grape seed extract 10 mg • Vitamin B6 20 mg • Vitamin B12 500 mcg • Vitamin C 60 mg.

Oxy Shield - Futurebiotics LLC
Three tablets contain: Vitamin E (natural d-alpha tocopherol) 400 IU • Beta Carotene 25,000 IU • Vitamin C 1000 mg • N-Acetyl Cysteine 125 mg • Cysteine 125 mg • Zinc (citrate, gluconate) 25 mg • Copper 1 mg • Selenium (selenomethionine) 150 mcg • Garlic (Pure-Gar) 400 mg • Green Tea 400 mg • Rosemary extract 50 mg • Licorice extract 700 mg • Astragalus extract 350 mg • Tricosanthes extract 150 mg • Siberian Ginseng extract 750 mg • Pau D'Arco 50 mg • Cayenne 30 mg • Methionine 50 mg • Red Clover flowers 100 mg • Barley grass powder 100 mg • Chamomile 100 mg • Ribonucleic Acid (RNA) 50 mg • Kelp 100 mg • Iodine (kelp) 150 mcg • Molybdenum 20 mcg.

Oxy-5000 Forte - American Biologics
Each tablet contains: Catalase 10,000 units • Superoxide Dismutase (SOD) 5000 units • Glutathione, reduced 10 mg • N-Acetyl Cysteine (NAC) 10 gm • L-Cysteine (as the hydrochloride) 10 mg • Vitamin B2 (riboflavin) 5 mg • Vitamin E (natural) 5 IU • Thioproline 1000 mcg • Folic Acid 60 mcg • Selenium (from 25 mcg sodium selenite) 11 mcg. Other Ingredients: Dicalcium Phosphate, Cellulose, Magnesium Stearate.

Oxydrene - Klein-Becker
Two capsules contain: Crenulin-RCC Proprietary Blend 500 mg: Sedum Crenulata root, Hoppophae fruit, Fructus Lychii Chinensis fruit. Other Ingredients: Rice Flour.

Oxy-G2 - Body Wise International, Inc.
Two capsules contain: Beta Carotene (Vitamin A 6250 IU) 3.75 mg • Vitamin C 75 mg • Vitamin E (as d-alpha Tocopheryl Succinate) 30 IU • Pantothenic Acid (from Calcium Pantothenate) 50 mg • Selenium (as L-Selenomethionine) 100 mcg • Molybdenum (Krebs Cycle Chelate) 100 mcg • Organic Germanium 100 mg • Ginkgo Biloba Leaf 100 mg • Milk Thistle Seed Std. Extract (80% Silymarin) 50 mg • Echinacea Purpurea Root 50 mg • Cytochrome C Oxidase 50 mg • Krebs Cycle Chelated Replenished Factors 50 mg • L-Glutathione 50 mg • Ascorbyl Palmitate 50 mg • L-Cysteine 25 mg • L-Tyrosine 25 mg • Pau D'Arco (Taheebo Tea Bark) 25 mg • Chlorophyll 20 mg.

Some Brand Name Natural Products - What they Contain

www.NaturalDatabase.com contains MANY more listings than appear here.
Editor's Notes are located on pages 2155-2163.

Oxygen Elements Plus - Global Health Trax
Seven drops contain: Global Health Trax Proprietary Blend 326 mg: Ionic Trace Elements, Citric Acid, Gluconic Acid, Rice Vinegar, Hydrogen Sulfate, Purified Water, Amino Acid Blend, Enzyme Blend.

Oxygen Plus - Market America, Inc.
Two capsules contain: Vitamin A (as beta carotene) 5000 IU • Vitamin C (as ascorbic acid) 200 mg • Vitamin E (as d-alpha tocopherol succinate) 30 IU • Selenium (as SelenoPrecise yeast bound selenium) 200 mcg • Green Tea extract 300 mg • Ginko Biloba leaf extract (24% ginko flavoglycosides/6% terpene lactones) 50 mg • Milk Thistle 50 mg • L-Glutathione 1 mg • Bilberry powder 50 mg. Other Ingredients: Rice Powder, Silica, Magnesium Stearate, Gelatin.

Oxygenics - Metagenics
Each tablet contains: Vitamin A (35% as retinyl acetate and 65% as beta-carotene) 7500 IU • Vitamin C (as Ultra-Potent-C brand) 70 mg • Niacin (as niacinamide ascorbate) 5.6 mg • Vitamin E (as D-alpha tocopheryl succinate) 100 IU • Thiamin (as thiamin mononitrate) 1.5 mg • Selenium (as selenomethionine) 25 mcg • D-Mannitol 25 mg • Glutathione 5 mg • N-Acetylcysteine 50 mg • Sorbic Acid 25 mg • Alpha-Lipoic Acid 200 mcg • Alpha-Carotene 58 mcg • Cryptoxanthin 16 mcg • Zeaxanthin 8 mcg • Lutein 8 mcg • SOD Precursor Blend: Zinc (as zinc glycinate, histidine) 5 mg, Copper (as copper lysinate) 500 mcg, Manganese (as manganese glycinate) 1 mg • Milk Thistle seed extract (silybum marianum, standardized to 70% silymarin) 29 mg • Quercetin 8 mg • Turmeric rhizome extract (curcuma longa, standardized to 95% curcuminoids) 6 mg • Grape seed extract (vitis vinifera) 5 mg.

Oxy-Moxy - En Garde Health Products
Twenty drops contain: Proprietary Blend 0.7 g: Deionized Water • Norwegian Seaweed extract from Seawrack & Bladderwrack • Citric Acid • Menthol • Mint leaf extract (Menta viridis).

Oxy-Nectar Ten-Stage Antioxidant Beverage - Nature's Plus
Each scoop (33 g) contains: Vitamin A 10,000 IU • Vitamin C 600 mg • Vitamin E 200 IU • Zinc 15 mg • Selenium 50 mcg • Citrus Bioflavonoids (active flavonols, flavonones, flavones, naringen) 50 mg • Quercetin (saphora japonica) 25 mg • Rutin (saphora japonica) 25 mg • Hesperidin 5 mg • Eriocitrin 5 mg • Pycnogenol (pinus maritima, standardized to 85-95% proanthocyanidins) 5 mg • Astragalus root (astragalus membranaceus) 150 mg • Ligustrum berry (ligustrum lucidum) 150 mg • Shiitake mushroom (lentinus edodes) 100 mg • Echinacea root (echinacea purpurea) 100 mg • Schisandra fruit (schisandra chinensis) 100 mg • Ginkgo Biloba 50:1 (standardized to 24% ginkgo flavone-glycosides) 10 mg • Broccoli 10:1 (brassica oleracea) 150 mg • Spinach 10:1 (spinacia oleracea) 50 mg • Chinese Cabbage 10:1 (brassica chinensis) 50 mg • Carrot 10:1 (daucus carota) 50 mg • Tomato 50 mg • Garlic (odorless) 25 mg • Mixed Wild Berry extract (European red wine grape, blackberry, red raspberry and black raspberry) 250 mg • Bilberry (standardized to 25% anthocyanosides) 10 mg • NAC (N-acetyl-cysteine) 15 mg • L-Methionine 10 mg • L-Glutathione 10 mg • Spirulina (blue-green micro-algae) 50 mg • Dried Green Barley juice 50 mg • Chlorella 25 mg • Oxidase 10 mg • Catalase 5 mg • Peroxidase 5 mg • Chlorophyll (spirulina, chlorella, barley grass) 685 mcg • Carotenoids (spirulina, chlorella, barley grass) 4 mcg. Other Ingredients: Fructose, Non-GMO Isolated Soy Protein, Maltodextrin, Natural Vanilla Flavor, Rose Hips, Eriocitrin, Guava, West Indian Cherry, Mango.

Oxy-Pro - Progressive Labs
Each capsule contains: Vitamin A (as beta carotene) 12500 IU • Vitamin C 150 mg • Vitamin E (d-alpha tocopheryl succinate) 100 IU • Riboflavin (B2) 12.5 mg • Niacinamide 12.5 mg • Vitamin B6 10 mg • Zinc (glycinate) 7.5 mg • Selenium (as selenomethionine) 100 mcg • Copper (lysinate) 0.5 mg • Manganese (as manganese glycinate) 4 mg • Molybdenum (as sodium molybdate) 5 mcg • Quercetin 50 mg • N-Acetyl Cysteine 50 mg • Glutathione 2.5 mg.

OxyTech - Dulwich Health
Magnesium Peroxide 500 mg • Vitamin C 75 mg • Bioflavonoids 25 mg.

Oyster Calcium - Nature's Bounty
Two tablets contain: Vitamin A (as Retinyl Acetate) 1600 IU • Vitamin D (as Cholecalciferol) 400 IU • Calcium (as Oyster Shell) 750 mg. Other Ingredients: Maltodextrin, Acacia, Cellulose, Croscarmellose, Cellulose Coating, Vegetable Magnesium Stearate.

Oyster Calcium - Puritan's Pride
Each tablet contains: Vitamin A (as Retinyl Acetate) 1600 IU • Vitamin D (as Cholecalciferol) 400 IU • Calcium (as Oyster Shell) 750 mg.

Oyster Shell Calcium - Nature's Bounty
Each tablet contains: Calcium (as Oyster Shell Powder) 500 mg. Other Ingredients: Maltodextrin, Acacia Gum, Cellulose, Croscarmellose, Cellulose Coating, Vegetable Magnesium Stearate.

Oystercal 500 - Puritan's Pride
Each tablet contains: Calcium (as Calcium Carbonate from Oyster Shell) 500 mg.

Oystercal 500 + D - Puritan's Pride
Each tablet contains: Vitamin D (as Ergocalciferol) 125 IU • Calcium (as Oyster Shell) 500 mg.

P5'P - Pain & Stress Center
Each capsule contains: Vitamin C (ascorbic acid & ascorbyl palmitate) 250 mg • Vitamin B6 (as 50 mg pyridoxal 5'phosphate) 30 mg. Other Ingredients: Gelatin Capsule.

P-5-P 50 mg - Solgar
Each tablet contains: Calcium (as dicalcium phosphate) 65 mg • Pyridoxal-5-Phosphate 50 mg. Other Ingredients: Dicalcium Phosphate, Vegetable Cellulose, Methacrylic Acid, Vegetable Magnesium Stearate, Vegetable Glycerin, Riboflavin, Titanium Dioxide, Glyceryl Tricetate, Carnauba Wax.

P5P 50 activated B6 - Pure Encapsulations
Each vegetable capsule contains: Pyridoxal 5' Phosphate (activated B6) 50 mg • Vitamin C (as ascorbyl palmitate) 3 mg.

PABA - Source Naturals
Each tablet contains: PABA (para-Aminobenzoic Acid) 100 mg.

PABA 1000 mg Sustained Release tablets - Nature's Plus
Each tablet contains: PABA (para-aminobenzoic acid) 1000 mg. Other Ingredients: Stearic Acid, Di-calcium Phosphate, Rice Bran, Hydroxypropyl Methylcellulose, Magnesium Stearate, Silica, Pharmaceutical Glaze.

PABA 500 - GNC
Each tablet contains: Para-Aminobenzoic Acid (PABA) 500 mg. Other Ingredients: Cellulose, Whole Brown Rice powder (Oryza Sativa).

PABA 500 mg PR - Arrowroot
Each prolonged-release tablet contains: Para Aminobenzoic Acid (PABA) 500 mg.

Pacific Kelp - Quest
Each tablet contains: Pacific Kelp 650 mg. Other Ingredients: Calcium Carbonate, Silicon Dioxide, Magnesium Stearate (vegetable source).

Padma 28 - Padma A.G.
Each tablet contains: Saussuria 40 mg • Iceland Moss 40 mg • Margosa 35 mg • Myrobalan 30 mg • Red Sandalwood 30 mg • Cardamom 30 mg • Allspice 25 mg • Bengal Quince 20 mg • Potentilla Golden Seal 15 mg • Licorice 15 mg • Ribwort 15 mg • Columbine 15 mg • Knot grass 15 mg • Cloves 12 mg • Gingerlily 10 mg • Heartleaved Sida 10 mg • Valerian 10 mg • Wild Lettuce 6 mg • Marigold 5 mg • Camphor 4 mg • Aconite 1 mg • Calcium sulfate 20 mg • Sorbitol 73 mg • Cilicum dioxide 12 mg. See Editor's Note No. 39.

Some Brand Name Natural Products - What they Contain

www.NaturalDatabase.com contains MANY more listings than appear here.
Editor's Notes are located on pages 2155-2163.

BRAND NAMES

Padma Basic - EcoNugenics
Two tablets contain: Padma Basic Proprietary Blend 804 mg: Iceland Moss (cetraria islandica L. Ach.), Costus root, Margose fruit (azadirachtaindica A. juss), Cardamom fruit, Red Sandalwood heart wood, Tropical Almond fruit, Allspice fruit, Bengal Quince fruit (aegle marmelos (L.) correa), Calcium Sulfate, Columbine aerial part (aquilegia vulgaris L.), English Plantain aerial part (polygonum aviculare L.), Licorice root, Knotgrass aerial part, Golden Cinquefoil aerial part (potentilla aurea L.), Clove flower, Gingerlily rhizome (hedychium spicatum buch.-Ham.), Heartleaved Sida Cordifolia aerial part (sida cordifolia L.), Valerian root, Lettuce leaf (lactuca sativa L.), Calendula flower, Natural Camphor. Other Ingredients: Sorbitol, Silicon Dioxide.
See Editor's Note No. 39.

Pain & Inflammation Remedy (formerly HP 1) - Metagenics
Each tablet contains: Apis Mellifica 12X • Belladonna 6X • Mercurius Corrosivus 12X • Ferrum Phosphoricum 3X • Rhus Toxicodendron 12X • Croton Tiglium 3X.
See Editor's Note No. 1.

Pain Away - Dr. Mike's Vitamins
Menthol • Deionized Water • Sesame oil • Canola oil • Borage Seed oil • Ricinoleic Acid (from castor oil) • Emu oil • TEA • MSM • Herbal Extract Blend: Witch Hazel, Feverfew, Marigold, Capsicum, St. John's Wort, Arnica, Rue, Chamomile • Aloe Vera Gel • Carbomer 940 • Methyl Paraben • Propyl Paraben • Fragrance.

Pain Control - Pain & Stress Center
Each capsule contains: Vitamin B6 (pyridoxine HCl) 2 mg • DL-Phenylalanine 250 mg • GABA (gamma amino butyric acid) 100 mg • Boswellia Serrata 200 mg • Ashwagandha herb powder 100 mg. Other Ingredients: Gelatin Capsule.

Pain Relief Complex - Shaklee
Three caplets contain: Boswellia resin extract (boswellia serrata, standardized to 40% totoal boswellic acids) 1000 mg • Safflower flower extract (carthamus tinctorius) 150 mg. Other Ingredients: Microcrystalline Cellulose, Sorbitol, Calcium Stearate, Croscarmellose Sodium.

Pain Stop - Flora Inc.
Willow bark.

PainDefense Joint & Muscle Formula - PharmTech
Each capsule contains: Manganese (as manganese citrate) 4 mg • Glucosamine Sulfate (KCl) 500 mg • MSM (methyl-sulfonyl-methane) 250 mg • Panax Notoginseng (50-60 saponins supplying 45% ginsenosides) 50 mg • Chondroitin Complex 140 mg • Collagen Complex 100 mg • Sea Cucumber (25% mucopolysaccharides) 50 mg • Cetyl Myristoleate (CMO) 50 mg • Boswellia Serrate (25% boswellic acid) 50 mg • Bromelain (2400 GDU) 50 mg • White Willow bark (1% salicylates) 40 mg • Turmeric (95% curcuminoids) 34.5 mg.
See Editor's Note No. 15.

PainFactor - HealthMinded
Water, Glycerin, Glyceryl Stearate, Cetearyl Alcohol, Sodium Stearoyl Lactylate, Caprylic/Capric Triglyceride, Menthol, Dimethicone, PainFactor, Capsicum Frutescens Resin, Phenoxyethanol, Methylparaben, Butylparaben, Ethylparaben, Propylparaben, Propylene Glycol, Diazolidnyl Urea, Peppermint leaf oil, Carbomer, Xanthan gum, Tetrasodium EDTA, Tocopheryl Acetate, Sodium PCA, Camellia Sinensis extract, Panax Ginseng root extract, Chamomilla Recutita (matricaria) flower extract, Ginkgo Biloba extract, Aloe Barbadensis leaf juice, Panthenyl Triacetate, Tetrahexyldecyl Ascorbate, Squalane, Retinyl Palmitate, Retinyl.

Paingon - R-U Ved U.S.A.
Boswellia Serrata standardized extract • Ashwagandha standardized extract • Curcuma Longa standardized extract • Ginger standardized extract • Glucosamine Sulphate standardized extract • Chondroitin Sulphate standardized extract • Colchicum standardized extract.
See Editor's Note No. 15.

Paingon Cream - R-U Ved U.S.A.
Capsaicin - derived plant extract (0.025%) • Boswellia Serrata • Menthol • Deionized Water • Carbomer • Titanium Dioxide • Herbal oils, extract • TEA • Methylparaben • Propyl Paraben.

Pain-Less - The Herbalist
White Willow bark • Feverfew herb • Jamaican Dogwood root bark • Black Cohosh root • Passionflower herb • Butterbur root • St. John's Wort flower.

Pain-Less Rub - The Herbalist
Oils of Sweet Almond, Aloe Vera, St. John's Wort flower, Calendula flower & Arnica flower • Essential oils of French Lavender, Peppermint, Lemon Grass, Wintergreen, Nutmeg, Bergamot & Camphor • Comfrey root extract, Echinacea root extract, White Willow bark extract, Cayenne pepper extract.

Palmcia - Magistral Biotech
Each 10 mL serving contains: Saw Palmetto berries extract 400 mg. Other Ingredients: Spring Water, Glycerine, Natural Flavours.

Palmetto Plus - USANA Health Sciences
Each capsule contains: Saw Palmetto Extract (Serenoa Repens) fruit standardized to contain a minimum of 85% fatty acids 320 mg • Lycopene (Solanium Lycopersicum) fruit 5 mg • Soy Isoflavones (Glycine Max) seed 25 mg. Other Ingredients: Gelatin, Glycerin, Purified Water, Natural Carob Color, Beeswax, Lecithin, Titanium Dioxide.

Palmettoplex - Standard Process, Inc.
Three capsules contain: Proprietary Blend 278 mg: Bovine Prostate PMG extract, Glutamic Acid, Tomato fruit powder, Alanine, Glycine • Zinc 7.5 mg • Sodium 40 mg • Saw Palmetto berry extract (serenoa repens) 160 mg • Saw Palmetto berry powder 320 mg • Stinging Nettle root extract (uritca dioica) 220 mg • Pygeum extract 24 mg. Other Ingredients: Maltodextrin, Gelatin, Water, Silica, Honey, Colors, Calcium Stearate, Corn Starch.
See Editor's Note No. 14.

Palmitol - Flora Inc.
Saw Palmetto berries • Zinc 50 mg • Vitamin B6 120 mg.

Palmvitee - LaneLabs
Two capsules contain: Vitamin E 350 IU (as gamma tocotrienol, alpha tocotrienol, delta tocotrienol, & d-alpha tocopherol). Other Ingredients: Gelatin, water, & glycerin.

Panax Ginseng - Ortho Molecular Products
Each capsule contains: Panax Ginseng root extract (standardized to contain 10% ginsenosides) 300 mg. Other Ingredients: Natural Vegetable Capsules, Magnesium Stearate, Microcrystalline Cellulose.

Panax Ginseng - Pharmanex
Each capsule contains: Ginseng Panax root (5:1) extract (Panax Ginseng C.A. Meyer) 100 mg. Other Ingredients: Rice Flour, Gelatin.

Panax Ginseng 27/30 - Pure Encapsulations
Each vegetable capsule contains: Panax Ginseng extract (standardized to contain 27-30% total ginsenosides) 250 mg.

Panax Ginseng Extract - Enzymatic Therapy
Each capsule contains: Korean Ginseng root extract (panax ginseng, standardized to 7% ginsenosides) 100 mg. Other Ingredients: Cellulose, Gelatin, Magnesium Stearate, Titanium Dioxide Color.

Panax Ginseng Phytosome - Enzymatic Therapy
Each capsule contains: Korean Ginseng root Phytosome (panax ginseng, bound to phosphatidylcholine) 50 mg. Other Ingredients: Gelatin, Magnesium Stearate, Silicon Dioxide, Titanium Dioxide Color.

Panaxin - PhytoPharmica
Each capsule contains: Korean Ginseng (Panax ginseng) root extract (standardized to contain 7% ginsenosides) 100 mg.

Pancreas Chelate Plus - Atrium Biotechnologies
Each tablet contains: Zinc (Protein Chelated) 15 mg • Chromium (Protein Chelated) 200 mcg • Pancreas Substance (from total maxi strength Pancreatin 75 mg, Raw Pancreas concentrate 75 mg) 150 mg. To insure the naturally occuring factors as well as the concentrated forms of Lipase & Amylase Enzymes.
See Editor's Note No. 14.

Pancreas Glandular - American Biologics
Each tablet contains: Raw Pancreas concentrate 330 mg. Other Ingredients: Dicalcium Phosphate, Magnesium Stearate.
See Editor's Note No. 14.

Pancreas Plus - Nutri-Quest Rx
Each tablet contains: Pancreatin 270 mg • Pancreas 130 mg [Tissue concentrate (not extract) of Bovine Source]. Natural occuring factors as well as concentrated forms of Protease, Lipase, & Amylase enzymes.
See Editor's Note No. 14.

Pancreatic Enzyme Formula - Pure Encapsulations
Each vegetable capsule contains: Pure Pancreatin (porcine) 500 mg: Lipase 17,500 USP units, Protease 110,000 USP units, Amylase 120,000 USP units.

Pancreatic Enzymes 500mg (full strength) - Vital Nutrients
Each capsule contains: Pancreatin 500 mg: Protease 111,500; Amylase 122,500; Lipase 17,750.

Pancreatic VegEnzymes - Pure Encapsulations
Each vegetable capsule contains: Proprietary Blend of Plant Enzymes 200 mg (providing 200 PAU): Amylase, Lipase, Protease • Vitamin C (as ascorbyl palmitate) 2 mg.

Pancreatic VegEnzymes L - Pure Encapsulations
Each vegetable capsule contains: Proprietary Blend of Plant Enzymes 200 mg (providing 200 PALU): Amylase, Lipase, Protease • Vitamin C (as ascorbyl palmitate) 2 mg.

Pancreatin - Life Enhancement Products, Inc.
Each capsule contains: Pancreatin 4X USP (porcine panreas glandular concentrate) 500 mg: Protease 50,000 USP units, Amylase 50,000 USP units, Lipase 4000 USP units. Other Ingredients: Silicon Dioxide, Gelatin Capsule.

Pancreatin & Ox Bile Extract - Vital Nutrients
Each vegetarian capsule contains: Pancreatin 250 mg: Protease 55,700 USP units; Amylase 61,250 USP units; Lipase 8875 USP units; Ox Bile extract (45%-50% cholic acid) 100 mg.

Pancreatrophin PMG - Standard Process, Inc.
Each tablet contains: Proprietary Blend 425 mg: Bovine Pancreas PMG extract, Dried Alfalfa juice, Nutritional Yeast, Porcine Duodenum, Defatted Wheat germ, Dried Buckwheat leaf juice, Buckwheat seed. Other Ingredients: Arabic Gum, Calcium Stearate.
See Editor's Note No. 14.

Panoderm Forte - American Biologics
Short Chain Fatty Acid Precursors.

Panoderm I - American Biologics
Squalene • Short Chain Fatty Acid Precursors.

Panoderm II - American Biologics
Squalene • Short Chain Fatty Acid Precursors.

Pantethine - Puritan's Pride
Each tablet contains: Pantethine 165 mg.

Pantethine - PhytoPharmica
Each tablet contains: Pantethine 300 mg.

Pantethine - Pure Encapsulations
Each vegetable capsule contains: Pantethine 250 mg.

Pantethine - Jarrow Formulas
Each softgel contains: Pantethine 300 mg. Other Ingredients: Gelatin, Glycerin, Water, Natural Annatto, Caramel.

Pantethine Coenzyme A - Pro Health
Each softgel contains: Pantethine 300 mg. Other Ingredients: Gelatin, Glycerin, Water, Natural Annatto, Carob.

Pantethine Complex - The Vitamin Shoppe
Each tablet contains 300 mg of Pantethine Complex supplying: Pantethine (coenzyme A precursor) 150 mg • Pantothenic Acid (D-calcium pantothenate) 150 mg.

Pantethine Liquid Capsules - Ortho Molecular Products
Two capsules contain: Pantethine 900 mg. Other Ingredients: Natural Vegetable Capsules, Vegetable Glycerine.

Pantethine/Policosanol - Pure Encapsulations
Each vegetable capsule contains: Pantethine 250 mg • Policosanol 10 mg: 1-octacosanol 6-8 mg, 1-triacontanol 0-2 mg, 1-hexacosanol 0.2-3 mg, 1-tetracosanol 0-1 mg, 1-nonacosanol 0-1 mg, 1-dotriacontanol 0.01-1 mg, 1-tetratriacontanol 0.01-1 mg, 1-heptacosanol 0-0.06 mg • Vitamin C (ascorbyl palmitate) 10 mg.

Pantethine-Time - J. R. Carlson Laboratories, Inc.
Each tablet contains: Pantethine (from pantesin) 300 mg.

Pantothenic Acid - Nature's Bounty
Each tablet contains: Pantothenic Acid (as d-Calcium Pantothenate) 200 mg. Other Ingredients: Cellulose, Vegetable Stearic Acid, Starch, Croscarmellose, Silica, Vegetable Magnesium Stearate.

Pantothenic Acid - Source Naturals
Each tablet contains: Pantothenic Acid (vitamin B5, as calcium D-pantothenate) 100 mg.

Pantothenic Acid 100 mg - Puritan's Pride
Each tablet contains: Calcium Pantothenate 109 mg.

Pantothenic Acid 1000 mg Sustained Release tablets - Nature's Plus
Each tablet contains: Pantothenic Acid (as calcium pantothenate) 1000 mg. Other Ingredients: Microcrystalline Cellulose, Stearic Acid, Hydroxypropyl Methylcellulose, Silica, Rice Bran, Magnesium Stearate, Pharmaceutical Glaze.

Pantothenic Acid 200 mg - Puritan's Pride
Each tablet contains: Calcium Pantothenate 218 mg.

Pantothenic Acid 250 - GNC
Each tablet contains: Pantothenic Acid (as calcium d-pantothenate) 250 mg. Other Ingredients: Dicalcium Phosphate, Gelatin, Cellulose, Whole Brown Rice powder (Oryza sativa).

Pantothenic Acid 250 mg - Arrowroot
Each tablet contains: Pantothenic Acid 250 mg.

Pantothenic Acid 500 - GNC
Each capsule contains: Pantothenic Acid 500 mg. Other Ingredients: Gelatin, Cellulose, Whole Brown Rice powder (Oryza sativa).

Pantothenic Acid 500 mg - Vital Nutrients
Each capsule contains: Pantothenic Acid 500 mg (calcium pantothenate) • Calcium 45 mg.

Pantothenic Acid 500 mg capsules - Nature's Plus
Each capsule contains: Pantothenic Acid (as calcium pantothenate) 500 mg. Other Ingredients: Microcrystalline Cellulose, Rice Bran, Silica, Vegetable Cellulose, Purified Water.

Pantothenic Acid 500 mg PR - Arrowroot
Each prolonged-release tablet contains: Pantothenic Acid 500 mg.

Pantothenic Acid 500 mg tablets - Nature's Plus
Each tablet contains: Pantothenic Acid (as calcium pantothenate) 500 mg. Other Ingredients: Di-calcium Phosphate, Stearic Acid, Magnesium Stearate, Rice Bran, Pharmaceutical Glaze, Silica.

Pantothenic Acid B5 - Jarrow Formulas
Each capsule contains: Pantothenic Acid (from D-calcium pantothenate) 500 mg. Other Ingredients: Cellulose, Magnesium Stearate, Gelatin.

Some Brand Name Natural Products - What they Contain

www.NaturalDatabase.com contains MANY more listings than appear here.

Editor's Notes are located on pages 2155-2163.

BRAND NAMES

Pantothenic Acid Time **-** J. R. Carlson Laboratories, Inc.
Each tablet contains: Pantothenic Acid (as di-calcium pantothenate) 500 mg.

PanXyme pH **-** Xymogen
Each capsule contains: Calcium (as calcium carbonate) 60 mg • Proprietary Enzyme Blend 85 mg: Biodiastase brand, Newlase, Lipase. Other Ingredients: Cellulose, Magnesium Stearate.

Papaya **-** Leiner Health Products
Each tablet contains: Total Carbohydrate 1 g • Papain 10 mg • Papaya fruit powder 250 mg • Pineapple juice solid powder 150 mg. Other Ingredients: Compressible Sugar, Stearic Acid, Mannitol, Cellulose, Magnesium Stearate, Silicon Dioxide, Artificial Pineapple Flavor.

Para Thyrolate **-** Progressive Labs
Each capsule contains: Calcium 100 mg • Iodine 225 mcg • Phosphorus 40 mg • Parathyroid concentrate 500 mcg • Thyroid concentrate (thyroxin-free) 25 mg. Other Ingredients: Dicalcium Phosphate, Cellulose, Protein Conjugate, Pacific Sea Kelp, Calcium Carbonate, Papain, Guar Gum, Stearic Acid, Gelatin.
See Editor's Note No. 14.

Para-Cid **-** Atrium Biotechnologies
Each tablet contains: Betaine HCL 250 mg • Pepsin 20 mg. In a slow release matrix.

Paracid Forte **-** Ortho Molecular Products
Each capsule contains: Sweet Wormwood aerial portion 175 mg • Olive leaf extract (standardized to contain 20% oleuropein) 110 mg • Oregano leaf 10:1 extract 85 mg • Grapefruit seed extract (Citricidal brand) 75 mg • Goldenseal root extract (standardized to contain 4.8% hydrastine) 60 mg • Berberine sulfate 50 mg. Other Ingredients: Natural Vegetable Capsules, Magnesium Stearate, Microcrystalline Cellulose, Silicon Dioxide.

Paraclear **-** PhysioLogics
Two capsules contain: Sweet Annie leaf, stem 400 mg • Garlic bulb (10,000 mcg alliin/g, 2 mg) 200 mg • Pau D'Arco bark 200 mg • Goldthread root (10% alkaloids, 15 mg) 150 mg • Black Walnut husk 100 mg • Ficin (from fig) 10 mg. Other Ingredients: Gelatin.

Para-Clens **-** Nutri-Quest Rx
Each tablet contains: Artemisia Annua 50 mg • Garlic powder 50 mg • Black Walnut 50 mg • Pumpkin seed 50 mg • Oregano oil 1 mg • Tea Tree 2 mg • Grapefruit seed extract 50 mg • Bromelain 50 mg • Papain 50 mg.

ParaFree **-** Young Living Essential Oils
Sesame Seed Oil • Cumin Oil • Olive Oil • Thyme Oil • Clove • Anise • Nutmeg • Fennel • Vetiver • Idaho Tansy • Melaleuca Alternifolia • Bay Laurel.

ParaGONE **-** Renew Life Formulas, Inc.
Part I: Two capsules contain: Undecylenic Acid (from coconut and Castor bean) • Black Walnut hull and seed • Quassia • Wormwood leaf and stem • Bismuth Citrate • Caprylic Acid (as magnesium caprylate) • Cape Aloe gel • Garlic bulb • Pau d'Arco bark 5:1 extract • Clove seed • Grapefruit seed and rind • Pumpkin seed • Piper Longum seed • Rosemary leaf and stem 4:1 extract • Thyme leaf and stem 4:1 extract. Other Ingredients: Hypromellose, Water.
Part II: 15 Drops contain: Black Walnut hull and seed • Marshmallow root • Orange peel • Wormwood leaf and stem • Clove seed. Other Ingredients: Filtered Water, Ethyl Alcohol 35%-45% USP.

ParaNix (World's Best Internal Klenz) **-** Nature's Medicine Corporation
Black Walnut hulls • Clove buds • Chlorophyll • Diatomaceous Earth • Elecampane plant (inula helenium) • False Unicorn root • Fenugreek seeds • Garlic bulb • Gentian root • Grapefruit seed extract • Hyssop • Myrrh gum • Peppermint leaf • Prickly Ash bark • Pumpkin seeds • Turmeric root • Wormwood • Yellow Dock.

Paraplex **-** Standard Process, Inc.
Each tablet contains: Proprietary Blend 199 mg: Magnesium Citrate, Bovine Pancreas PMG extract, Dried Alfalfa juice, Nutritional Yeast, Porcine Duodenum, Bovine Adrenal PMG extract, Bovine Pituitary PMG extract, Bovine Thyroid PMG extract (processed to remove thyroxine), Defatted Wheat germ, Dried Buckwheat leaf juice • Calcium 20 mg. Other Ingredients: Cellulose.
See Editor's Note No. 31.

Paraprost **-** Nikken Kagakusha
Each capsule contains: L-Glutamic Acid 265 mg • L-Alanine 100 mg • Aminoacetic Acid 45 mg.
Available in Japan.

Para-relief **-** Enzymatic Therapy
Two capsules contain: Citricidal extract (citrus paradisi, macfad., grapefruit seed) 100 mg • Goldenseal root (hydrastis canadensis, 5% hydrastine extract) 100 mg • Sweet Annie (artemisia annua, aerial parts) 100 mg • Quassia bark (picrasma excelsa extract 4:1) 100 mg • Black Walnut green outer hull (juglans nigra extract 4:1) 100 mg • Garlic bulb (allium sativum, 0.8% allicin extract) 100 mg • Clove buds (syzygium aromaticum) 100 mg • Pure Plant Enzymes Blend 41 mg: Protease I, II, III (USP XXIII, pH7.5) 3265 USP, FCC IV (pH7.0) 5235 PC, FCC IV (pH4.7) 5440 HUT, Amylase (USP XXI, pH6.8) 3300 USP, FCC IV (pH4.8) 1430 DU, Cellulase II (FCC IV pH4.5) 101 CU, Lipase II (FCC III pH6.5) 43 LU.

Parasillan **-** Olympian Labs
Each capsule contains: Proprietary Blend 700 mg: Plaintain, Barberry Bark, Chaparral, Citrus Bioflavonoids, Lobelia, Black Walnut, Wormwood, Psyllium Hull, Cayenne Pepper.

Parasites & Worms **-** Grandma's Herbs
Each capsule contains: Proprietary Blend 0.496 g: Tansy herb, Wormwood leaf, Black Walnut hulls, Garlic herb, Pomegranate rind/bark, Hyssop herb, Pumpkin seed, Blue Vervain herb, Senna leaf, Chaparral herb, Bayberry bark.

ParaStat **-** Premier Research Labs
Each Vcap contains: Proprietary Blend 515 mg: Holarrhena Antidysenterica bark and seed, Protease, Lipase, Amylase, Cellulase, Invertase, Lactase, Maltase. Other Ingredients: Vegetable Capsule.

Para-Tech **-** Wild Rose
Each capsule contains: Sweet Annie 300 mg • Grapefruit seed 7:1 extract 150 mg • Black Walnut hull 75 mg.

Parathyroid **-** Atrium Biotechnologies
Each tablet contains: Parathyroid (Bovine) 10 mg • Thyroid (Thyroxin free) 30 mg • Stomach (Bovine) 32 mg • Dulse 300 mg • Calcium 50 mg • Phosphorus 22 mg • Vitamin D (as Vitamin D3) 100 IU • Vitamin B12 20 mcg • Folic Acid 440 mcg • Beet 50 mg • Carrot 50 mg. Calcium, Phosphorus, Beet & Carrot powders, Iodine.
See Editor's Note No. 14.

ParaZYME **-** Renew Life Formulas, Inc.
Each capsule contains: Betaine Hydrochloride • Borage seed (borago officinalis) • Flax seed (linum usitatissimum) • L-Glutamine • Soy Lecithin • Butyric Acid (as calcium butyrate) • FOS (fructooligosaccharides) • Para Plant Enzyme Blend: Amylase 417 DU, Protease 2083 HUT, Lipase 17 LU, Lactase 58 LacU, Cellulase 167 CU, Invertase 0.08 IAU, Maltase 1.87 DP, Pectinase with Phytase 6.25 endo PGU, Pepsin • Probiotic Blend: Lactobacillus Acidophilus, Bifidobacterium Bifidum, Bifidobacterium Infantis • Quercetin 2400 gdu/gm • Bromelain 3600 mcu/gm • Gamma Oryzanol • N-Acetyl D-Glucosamine • Papain. Other Ingredients: Gelatin, Water.

Parex Intensive Care **-** Metagenics
Two tablets contain: Pumpkin seed (curcubita pepo) 300 mg • Sweet Wormwood (artemisia annua) 240 gm • Plantain leaf (plantago major) 200 gm • Gentian root (gentiana lutea) 150 mg • Barberry root (berberis vulgaris) 300 mg • Oregon Grape root extract (mahonia aquifolium) 100 mg • Goldenseal root (hydrastis canadensis) 50 mg • Bromelain 26 mg • Peptidase (Peptizyme SP) 10 mg.

Some Brand Name Natural Products - What they Contain

www.NaturalDatabase.com contains MANY more listings than appear here.
Editor's Notes are located on pages 2155-2163.

Parotid PMG **-** Standard Process, Inc.
Each tablet contains: Proprietary Blend 244 mg: Bovine Parotid PMG extract, Magnesium Citrate. Other Ingredients: Calcium Lactate, Cellulose, Calcium Stearate.
See Editor's Note No. 14.

Party Pill II **-** Life Enhancement Products, Inc.
Three capsules contain: Vitamin C (calcium ascorbate and niacinamide ascorbate) 831 mg • Vitamin D (cholecalciferol) 133 IU • Vitamin E (D,L-alpha-tocopheryl acetate) 133 IU • Thiamine (vitamin B1) 21 mg • Riboflavin (vitamin B2) 40 mg • Niacin (vitamin B3 as niacinamide ascorbate) 83 mg • Vitamin B6 (as pyridoxine hydrochloride) 22 mg • Folic Acid 400 mcg • Vitamin B12 (cyanocobalamin) 33 mcg • Biotin 67 mcg • Pantothenic Acid (vitamin B5 as calcium pantothenate) 77 mg • Calcium (as calcium citrate and calcium pantothenate) 77 mg • Zinc (gluconate) 27 mg • Selenium (as sodium selenate) 67 mcg • Copper (as copper gluconate) 1 mg • Chromium (aspartate) 200 mcg • Taurine 367 mg • L-Cysteine Hydrochloride 367 mg • Quercetin 67 mg • Hesperidin 67 mg.

Passion Rx **-** Physician Formulas
Ashwagandha • Catuaba • Cnidium Monnieri • Coleus Forskohlii • Damiana • Horny Goat Weed • Maca • Mucuna Pruriens • Muira Puama • Passion Flower • Pfaffia Paniculata • Rehmannia • Rhodiola • Shilajit (mineral pitch) • Tongkat Ali • Tribulus Terrestris.

Passionflower Leaf **-** Aboca USA, Inc
Two capsules contain: Passionflower leaf Phytocomplex Concentrate, passiflora incarnata, standardized to 5% total flavonoids, yielding 15.25 mg per capsule) 610 mg. Other Ingredients: Gelatin.

Patented CLAPure CLA **-** Ultimate Nutrition
Each softgel contains: CLAPure CLA (proprietary blend providing 75-80% conjugated linoleic acid) 1000 mg. Other Ingredients: Gelatin, Glycerin, Natural Caramel Color.

PatentLEAN **-** Patent Health, LLC
Each capsule contains: 3-acetyl-7-oxo-dehydroepiandrosterone 100 mg.

Pau d'Arco **-** Golden Glow Natural Health Products
Each tablet contains: Pau d'Arco extract 500 mg.

Pau D'Arco **-** Source Naturals
Each tablet contains: Pau d'Arco extract (Tabebuia altissima) 500 mg • Pau d'Arco (Inner Bark) 25 mg • Vitamin C (Ascorbic Acid) 10 mg • Pro-Vitamin A (Beta Carotene) 500 IU.

Pau d'Arco-Black Walnut Virtue **-** Blessed Herbs
Pau d'Arco bark • Usnea lichen • Calendula flower • Echinacea Angustifolia root • Black Walnut hull • Goldenseal root • Myrrh Gum • Grain alcohol & Distilled Water.

Paw Paw Cell-Reg **-** Nature's Sunshine
Each capsule contains: Standardized Pawpaw twig extract (asimina triloba) 12.5 mg. Other Ingredients: Cellulose, Magnesium Stearate, Silicon Dioxide, Gelatin, Water.

PB8 **-** Nutrition Now
Two capsules contain: Proprietary Blend 1200 mg: FOS • Lactobacillus acidophilus • Lactobacillus plantarum • Lactobacillus rhamnosus • Lactobacillus casei • Lactobacillus bulgaricus • Streptococcus thermophilus • Bifidobacterium bifidum • Bifidobacterium longum.

PBGS+ **-** 4 Life
Proprietary OPC Extract • Grape seed • Maritime Pine bark • Grape skin • Citrus Bioflavonoids • Digestive Enzyme Blend.

PC Calm **-** High Life Formulas
Three capsules contain: Proprietary Blend 2365 mg: Sterolins (400 mg), Cernitin 63, Scutellaria Baicalensis, Serenoa Repens (standardized 45%), Quercetin, Rabdosia Rubescens, Ganoderma Lucidum, Taraxacum Mongolicum, Isatis Indigotica, Patrinia Villosa, Panax Notoginseng, Oldenlandia Diffusa, Dendranthema Morifolium, Trifolium Pratense (4:1), Glycyrrhiza Uralensis.

PC Hope **-** Rephe Products
Two capsules contain: Magnesium (as oxide) 200 mg • Sterolins 400 mg • Quercetin 100 mg • Proprietary Blend 500 mg: Reishi (as ganoderma lucidum), Baikal Skullcap (as scutellaira baicalensis), Rabdosia (as rabdosia rubescens Hara), Dyer's Woad (as isatis indigotica Fortune), Mum (as dendranthema morifolium Tzelev), Saw Palmetto (as serenoa repens), San-Qi Ginsing (as panax notoginseng), Licorice (as glycyrrhiza glabra L). Other Ingredients: Gelatin, Starch, Water.

PC SPES **-** BotanicLab
Each capsule contains: Proprietary Blend 320 mg: Da Qing Ye (Isatis indigotica), Licorice (glycyrrhiza glabra, glycyrrhiza uralensis), San Qi (panax pseudoginseng), Reishi Mushroom (ganoderma lucidum), Baikal Skullcap (scutellaria baicalensis), Chrysanthemum (dendranthema morifolium), Rabdosia Rubescens, Saw Palmetto (serenoa repens).
See Editor's Note No. 7.

PC-55 **-** LaneLabs
Each 1 tsp serving contains: Phosphatidyl Choline 1.43 g • Choline 210 mg. Other Ingredients: Phosphatidyl Ethanolamine, Inositol Phosphatides, Related Phospholipids.

PCA-Rx **-** Maxam Nutraceutics
Unknown.
See Editor's Note No. 17 and No. 41.

Peaceful Nights **-** Pro Health
Four tablets contain: Niacinamide 10 mg • Vitamin B6 (as pyridoxine HCl) 2 mg • Calcium (as calcium citrate & carbonate) 260 mg • Iron 560 mcg • Magnesium (as magnesium citrate, oxide and taurinate) 436 mg • Inositol 700 mg • GABA (gamma amino butyric acid) 600 mg • Taurine (as magnesium taurinate) 433 mg • Skullcap leaf and stem 250 mg • Passion Flower 200 mg • Valerian root 200 mg • Chamomile flower extract 100 mg. Other Ingredients: Stearic Acid, Modified Cellulose Gum, Magnesium Stearate.

Peach Drinkable Yogurt **-** Stonyfield Farm
Each 10 fl oz bottle contains: Active Live Cultures: S. Thermophilus • L. Bulgaricus • L. Acidophilus • Bifidus • L. Casei • L. Reuteri. Ingredients: Cultured Pasturized Low Fat Milk • Organic Sugar • Organic Nonfat Dry Milk • Inulin • Pectin • Beet Juice Concentrate • Organic Peach Puree • Natural Flavors.

Peach Stuff **-** Blue Stuff, Inc.
Each jar contains: Whole leaf Aloe Vera concentrate • Purified Water • Glyceryl Stearate • PEG 100 Stearate • Propylene Glycol • Glycerth-26 • Cetyl Alcohol • Stearic Acid • Hydrolyzed Elastin • Hydrolyzed Mucipolysaccharides • Revitalin • Polysorbate-20 • Carbomer-940 • Triethanolamine • Methylparaben • Fragrance • Imidazolidinyl Urean • Propylparaben • Retinol • Tocopherol • FD&C Red No. 33 • FD&C Yellow No. 6.

Peak Performance **-** FreeLife International
Three capsules contain: Vitamin C (ascorbic acid) 500 mg • L-Glutamine 1000 mg • Rhodiola rosea root standardized extract (5% rosavin, 2% salidroside) 100 mg • Alpha-Lipoic Acid 100 mg. Other ingredients: Gelatin, Cellulose, Vegetable Magnesium Stearate, Silica.

Peanut Butter StandardBar **-** Standard Process, Inc.
Protein blend: Whey protein concentrate, Egg white, Rice Protein • Maltitol syrup • Peanut Butter • Glycerin • Brown Rice syrup • Whey crisps (whey protein and rice flour) • Natural Flavors • Peanuts • Grape seed oil • Peanut flour • Soybean Lecithin oil • Wheat germ oil.

PectaSol brand **-** EcoNugenics
Modified Citrus Pectin.
See Editor's Note No. 44.

PectaSol Modified Citrus Pectin capsules **-** Pure Encapsulations
Each vegetable capsule contains: Modified Citrus Pectin 800 mg • Vitamin C (as ascorbyl palmitate) 16 mg.

Some Brand Name Natural Products - What they Contain

www.NaturalDatabase.com contains MANY more listings than appear here.
Editor's Notes are located on pages 2155-2163.

BRAND NAMES

PectaSol Modified Citrus Pectin Capsules - EcoNugenics
Six capsules contain: PectaSol Modified Citrus Pectin 4.8 g • Dietary Fiber 3.4 g • Sodium 90 mg • Potassium 600 mg.

PectaSol Modified Citrus Pectin powder - Pure Encapsulations
Each scoop contains: Modified Citrus Pectin 5 g.

PectaSol Modified Citrus Pectin Powder - EcoNugenics
Each scoop (five grams) contains: PectaSol Modified Citrus Pectin 5 g • Dietary Fiber 3.5 g • Sodium 90 mg • Potassium 600 mg.

Pedi-Active A.D.D. Chewables - Nature's Plus
Two tablets contain: LECI-PS (Phosphatidylserine-rich purified Lecithin concentrate) 100 mg • DMAE (2-dimethylaminoethanol bitartrate) 100 mg.

Pedi-Active Spray - Nature's Plus
Each spray contains: DMAE (2-Dimethylaminoethanol Bitartrate) 50 mg • LECI-PS Phosphatidylserine-rich purified Lecithin concentrate supplying Activated Phosphatides: [Phosphatidylserine 10 mg, Phosphatidylcholine 10 mg, Cephalin (Phosphatidylethanolamine) 6 mg, Phosphoinositides 3 mg] 50 mg. In a proprietary liposomal complex of Essential Metabolic Factors, Purified Water, Vegetable Glycerine, Purified Lecithin, Citrus seed extract (Citrus sinensis), Vitamin E & natural Wild Berry flavor.

Pedi-ADD - Aspen Group, Inc.
Each chewable tablet contains: Phosphatidylserine - Purified Lecithin concentrate supplying Activated Phosphatides 50 mg: Phosphatidylserine 10 mg • Phosphatidylcholine 10 mg • Cephalin (phosphatidylethanolamine) 6 mg • Phosphoinositides 5 mg • DMAE (2-dimethylaminoethanol bitartrate) 50 mg.

PediaLean - Klein-Becker
Each capsule contains: Pediatropin Proteinophallus Rivieri / Araceae tuber extract 500 mg.

PediaNutrients capsules - Pure Encapsulations
Four vegetable capsules contain: Vitamin A (acetate) 2500 IU • Ascorbic Acid 60 mg • Vitamin C (as ascorbyl palmitate) 20 mg • Calcium (citrate) 130 mg • Iron (glycinate) 16 mg • Vitamin D (as D3) 400 IU • Vitamin E (D-alpha tocopherol succinate) 16 IU • Thiamin HCl (vitamin B1) 1.4 mg • Riboflavin (vitamin B2) 1.2 mg • Niacinamide 16 mg • Pyridoxine HCl (vitamin B6) 1.4 mg • Folic Acid 100 mcg • Methylcobalamin (vitamin B12) 1.4 mcg • Biotin 66 mcg • Pantothenic Acid (calcium pantothenate) 6 mg • Iodine (potassium iodide) 90 mcg • Magnesium (citrate) 40 mg • Zinc (citrate) 10 mg • Selenium (selenomethionine) 30 mcg • Copper (glycinate) 2 mg • Manganese (aspartate) 2 mg • Chromium (polynicotinate) 120 mcg • Molybdenum (aspartate) 60 mcg.

PediaNutrients powder - Pure Encapsulations
Two scoops contain: Vitamin A (acetate) 2500 IU • Ascorbic Acid 60 mg • Calcium (citrate) 130 mg • Vitamin D (as D3) 400 IU • Vitamin E (D-alpha tocopherol succinate) 16 IU • Thiamin HCl (vitamin B1) 1.4 mg • Riboflavin (vitamin B2) 1.2 mg • Niacinamide 16 mg • Pyridoxine HCl (vitamin B6) 1.4 mg • Folic Acid 100 mcg • Methylcobalamin (vitamin B12) 1.4 mcg • Biotin 66 mcg • Pantothenic Acid (calcium pantothenate) 6 mg • Iodine (potassium iodide) 90 mcg • Magnesium (citrate) 40 mg • Zinc (citrate) 10 mg • Selenium (selenomethionine) 30 mcg • Copper (glycinate) 2 mg • Manganese (aspartate) 2 mg • Chromium (polynicotinate) 120 mcg • Molybdenum (aspartate) 60 mcg. Other Ingredients: Xylitol, Natural Flavors, Hypo-allergenic Plant Fiber.

Pediatric Nutritional Drink (strawberry and vanilla flavors) - Bright Beginnings
Water • Sugar (sucrose) • Maltodextrin (corn) • Sodium Caseinate • Calcium Caseinate • High-Oleic Safflower Oil • Soy Oil • Fractionated Coconut Oil (medium-chain triglycerides) • Whey Protein Concentrate • Natural and Artificial Flavors • Calcium Phosphate Tribasic • Monopotassium Phosphate • Potassium Citrate • Magnesium Chloride • Potassium Chloride • Soy Lecithin • Mono- and Diglycerides • Carrageenan • Choline Chloride • Ascorbic acid • Sodium Ascorbate • M-Inositol • Vitamin E Acetate • Taurine • Zinc Sulfate • Niacinamide • Calcium Pantothenate • Ferrous Sulfate • L-Carnitine • Vitamin A Palmitate • Vitamin D (D3) • Pyridoxine Hydrochloride • Thiamine • Phylloquinone • Riboflavin • Manganese Sulfate • Copper Sulfate • Cyanocobalamin • Folic Acid • Biotin • Chromium Chloride • Potassium Iodide • Sodium Molybdate • Sodium Selenite. Strawberry Flavor contains FD&C Red #3.

Pediatri-Vite - Genestra - Seroyal
Each teaspoon (5 mL) contains: Vitamin A (palmitate) 1700 IU • Vitamin D (D3, cholecalciferol) 170 IU • Vitamin E (mixed tocopherols) 10 IU • Vitamin C (ascorbic acid) 50 mg • Thiamin Hydrochloride (vitamin B1) 800 mcg • Riboflavin (vitamin B2) 800 mcg • Niacin (vitamin B3) 4 mg • Pantothenic Acid (d-calcium pantothenate) 2 mg • Pyridoxine Hydrochloride (vitamin B6) 1 mg • Cyanocobalamin (vitamin B12) 10 mcg • Folic Acid 70 mcg • Biotin 70 mcg • Calcium (chloride) 25 mg • Potassium (aspartic acid chelate) 10 mg • Magnesium (aspartic acid chelate) 5 mg • Iron (aspartic acid chelate) 4 mg • Zinc (aspartic acid chelate) 4 mg • Manganese (aspartic acid chelate) 800 mcg • Copper (aspartic acid chelate) 500 mcg • Iodine (potassium iodide) 25 mcg • Molybdenum (aspartic acid chelate) 85 mcg • Vanadium (aspartic acid chelate) 85 mcg • Chromium (chloride) 35 mcg • Selenium (selenomethionine) 35 mcg • Choline (bitartrate) 10 mg • Inositol 800 mcg. Other Ingredients: Natural Cherry Flavor, Fructose.

Pedia-Vit - Progressive Labs
Two teaspoons (10 ml) contain: Vitamin A 2500 IU • Vitamin C 40 mg • Vitamin D 400 IU • Vitamin E 10 IU • Thiamin (B1) 0.7 mg • Riboflavin (B2) 0.8 mg • Niacin (B3) 9 mg • Vitamin B6 0.7 mg • Folate (folic acid) 200 mcg • Vitamin B12 3 mcg • Biotin 150 mcg • Pantothenic Acid 5 mg • Iron 10 mg • Zinc 8 mg.

Pedi-Vites Multiple - Aspen Group, Inc.
Each tablet contains: Vitamin A Palmitate 180 IU • Vitamin D (as Vitamin D3) 150 IU • Vitamin E 10 IU • Vitamin B1 2 mg • Vitamin B2 2 mg • Vitamin B6 2 mg • Vitamin B12 6 mcg • Vitamin C 60 mg • Niacinamide 5 mg • Folic Acid 100 mcg • Pantothenic Acid 3 mg • Biotin 30 mcg • Calcium (carbonate) 10 mg • Magnesium (gluconate) 2 mg • Manganese (gluconate) 1 mg • Selenium (selenium aspartate) 5 mcg • Chromium (chromium ACP) 5 mcg • Molybdenum (sodium molybdate) 2 mcg • Vanadium (vanadium sulfate) 2 mcg • Chlorophyll 1 mg • Boron (boron citrate) 50 mcg.

Penetran Plus - Transdermal Technologies
Active Ingredients: strong Ammonia solution 2.5%. Inactive Ingredients: Allantoin, Ascorbyl Palmitate, Benzethonium Chloride, Cetyl Palmitate, Cold Pressed Lemon Oil, Decanoic Acid Triglyceride, De-Ionized Water, Dexpanthenol, Glycerol Monolaurete, Imidazolinium, Methyl Sulphate, Merguard 1200, Methylsulfonylmethane, Olive Oil, Sorbitan Monopalmitate, Tocopherol Acetate.

Penetrin - White-Broadman, Inc.
Each capsule contains: Zinc 10 mg • L-Arginine 1125 mg • Cnidium Monnier extract 30 mg • Xanthoparmelia extract 30 mg • Gamma Amino Butyric Acid 30 mg • Naringh extract 25 mg • Quebracho extract 60 mg.

Pentabosol Powder - Pentabosol
Each 5.3 g scoop contains: Riboflavin 1 mg • Biotin 600 mcg • Chromium Polynicotinate 400 mcg • Proprietary Blend 4510 mg: L-Aspartic Acid, Garcinia Cambogia extract (fruit, 50% (-) hydroxycitric acid), L-Carnitine Tartrate. Other Ingredients: Guar Gum, Maltodextrin, Sucralose, Citric Acid.

Pepogest - Nature's Way
Each softgel contains: Peppermint oil 0.2 ml • Soybean oil 0.1 ml.

PepperCare - SiCap Industries, LLC
Cayenne extract • Shea butter • Kukui oil (aleurites moluccana) • Grapeseed oil extract • Yuca root (yucca schidigera) • Vitamin E (T-50) • Rosemary oleoresin • Green Tea extract • Nettle oil extract • Black Pepper oil extract (piper nigrum) • Jojoba oil (simmondsia chinensis) • Grapefruit seed extract • Ylang Ylang oil • Calendula oil.

Peppermint Essential Oil **-** Golden Glow Natural Health Products
Mentha Piperita herb essential oil.

Peppermint Plus **-** Enzymatic Therapy
Each enteric-coated capsule contains: Peppermint oil extract (Mentha piperita) 0.2 ml • Rosemary oil extract (Rosemarinus officinalis) 0.02 ml • Thyme oil extract (Thymus vulgaris) 0.02 ml.

PeppermintZ Intestinal Aid **-** Nature's Life
Each gel contains: Senna leaf (senna alexandria) 400 mg • Peppermint leaf oil (mentha piperita) 180 mg • Caraway seed oil (carum carvi) 50 mg • Proprietary Blend 100 mg: Lemon Balm extract (melissa officinalis), Chamomile flower extract (matricaria chamomilla), Fennel seed extract, Ginger root extract (zingiber officinale). Inactive Ingredients: Safflower Oil, Beeswax, Lecithin.

PeptiTonic **-** DreamPharm
Each tablets contains: Proprietary Blend: Atractylodes Lanceae Rhizoma, Magnoliae Cortex, Citri Sinensis Exocarpium, Atractylodes Macrocephala Rhizoma, Sclerotium Poriae Cocos, Alismatis Rhizoma, Polyporus Umbellatus, Cinnamomi Cortex, Zingiberis Rhizoma, Zizyphus Jujuba Fructus, Papaya Leaf, Acidophilus, Montmorillanite.

PepZin-GI **-** GNC
Each capsule contains: PepZin GI brand Zinc-Carnosine 37.5 mg. Other Ingredients: Calcium Carbonate, Gelatin, Cellulose, Magnesium Stearate.

Perfect Antioxidant **-** Sundown
Each caplet contains: Vitamin A (100% as beta-carotene) 7500 IU • Vitamin C (from ascorbic acid, rose hips with seeds) 250 mg • Vitamin E (as dl-alpha-tocopheryl acetate, d-alpha-tocopheryl acid succinate) 200 IU • Calcium (as calcium carbonate) 48 mg • Zinc (as zinc citrate) 7.5 mg • Selenium (as selenium amino acid chelate) 15 mcg • Copper (as cupric sulfate) 1 mg • Manganese (as manganese sulfate) 1.5 mg. Other Ingredients: Microcrystalline Cellulose, Croscarmellose Sodium, Crospovidone, Silica, Hydroxypropyl Methylcellulose, Magnesium Stearate, PEG.

Perfect Cal **-** Futurebiotics LLC
Four tablets contain: Calcium (from Hydroxyappatite crystal) 400 mg • Calcium Complex (Citrate, Carbonate) 600 mg • Magnesium (Citrate, Oxide, Hydroxyappatite) 600 mg • Vitamin D 200 IU • Boron 1.5 mg • Horsetail (from extract) 750 mg.

Perfect Food Original Super Green Formula **-** Garden of Life, Inc.
Two heaping tablespoons (10 g) contain: Perfect Green Blend 5200 mg: 33:1 pure juice concentrates of certified organic Kamut grass, Barley grass, Oat grass, Alfalfa grass, Dandelion grass, Spirulina, Chlorella, Dunalellia, Sea Kelp, Sea Dulse, Sea Vegetables • Perfect Whole Food Matrix 2500 mg: RiceX Solubles, Certified Organic Pre-digested concentrates of Amaranth, Millet, Buckwheat (containing 22 amino acids, 90 antioxidants, EFAs) • Perfect Seed Blend 1500 mg: Certified Organic raw, naturally stabilized Flax seeds, Chia seeds, Sesame seeds, Sunflower seeds • Perfect Digestion, Detox and Immunity Blend 500 mg: Lactobacillus Acidophilus, L. Bulgaricus, L. Leichmanni, L. Lactis, L. Delbreukii, L. Casei, L. Caucasicus, L. Fermenti, L. Plantarum, L. Brevis, L. Helveticus, Bifidobacterium Bifidum, Bacilus Subtilis, B. Ichenformis, Live Enzymes (protease, amylasae, lipase, cellulase), PhytoSterolins • Perfect Vegetable Blend 300 mg: Certified Organic Carrot, Tomato, Beet, Broccoli, Cauliflower, Kale, Cabbage, Brussles Sprouts, Parsley, Spinach, Asparagus, Celery, Cucumber, Green Bell Pepper, Garlic, Onion, Ginger. Other Ingredients: Cellulose, Vegetable Coating.

Perfect Food Super Green Formula Caplets **-** Garden of Life, Inc.
Five caplets contain: Perfect Green Blend 2600 mg: 100% pre-digested blend of Barley grass juice, Wheat grass juice, Oat grass juice, Alfalfa grass juice • Perfect Protein-Mineral Blend 1000 mg: Spirulina, Chlorella, Dunaleila, Kelp, Dulse • Perfect Whole Food Matrix 1000 mg: Flax seeds, Pumpkin seeds, Sesame seeds, Sunflower seeds, Chia seeds, Garbanzo beans, Red Lentils, Miso, Kidney beands, Adzuki beans, Millet, Brown Rice, Maize, Buckwheat (gluten, phytate free) • Perfect Veggie Blend 200 mg: Carrot juice, Beet juice, Tomato juice, Sweet Potato, Broccoli, Kale, Cabbage, Cauliflower, Brussels Sprouts, Parsley, Spinach, Asparagus, Celery, Cucumber, Green Bell Pepper, Garlic, Ginger, Onion • Acerola Cherry 200 mg. Other Ingredients: Cellulose.

Perfect Food Super Green Formula Powder **-** Garden of Life, Inc.
Two heaping tablespoons (10 g) contain: Perfect Green Blend 6000 mg: Barley grass juice, Wheat grass juice, Oat grass juice, Alfalfa grass juice • Perfect Protein-Mineral Blend 2563 mg: 50% pre-digested blend of Spirulina, Chlorella, Dunaliella, Kelp, Dulse • Perfect Whole Food Matrix 975 mg: 50% pre-digested blend of Brown Rice, Flax seeds, Pumpkin seeds, Sesame seeds, Sunflower seeds, Chia seeds, Garbanzo beans, Red Lentils, Miso, Kidney beans, Adzuki beans, Millet, Buckwheat (gluten free) • Perfect Veggie Blend 250 mg: 50% pre-digested blend of Carrot juice, Beet juice, Tomato juice, Sweet Potato, Broccoli, Kale, Cabbage, Cauliflower, Brussels Sprouts, Parsley, Spinach, Asparagus, Celery, Cucumber, Green Bell Pepper, Garlic, Ginger, Onion • Acerola Cherry 200 mg.

Perfect Meal Shake, Chocolate **-** Advocare International
Each packet contains: L-Lysine 1000 mg • L-Glutamine 500 mg • Choline 5 mg • Inositol 5 mg • Whole Carrot powder 100 mg • Oat Grass powder 100 mg. Other Ingredients: PM-Ultra Protein Complex (modified casein, soy protein powder, whey protein concentrate, di-peptides, tri-peptides), Fructose, Maltodextrin, Cocoa Powder, Purified Cellulose, Canola Oil, Hydrolyzed Guar Gum, Corn Syrup Solids, L-Lysine Monohydrochloride, Potassium Chloride, L-Glutamine, Calcium Carbonate, Magnesium Oxide, Soy Lecithin, Dicalcium Phosphate, Natural Flavors, Artificial Flavors, Carrot Powder, Oat Grass Powder, Lactobacillus Acidophilus, Acesulfame, Medium Chain Triglycerides, Papain, Bromelain, Rice Syrup Solids, Choline Citrate, Ascorbic Acid, Vitamin E Acetate, Inositol, Ferrous Fumarate, Niacinamide, Zinc Oxide, Calcium Pantothenate, Vitamin A Palmitate, Copper Sulfate, Manganese Sulfate, Vitamin D, Pyridoxine Hydrochloride, Riboflavin, Thiamine Mononitrate, Chromium Polynicotinate, Folic Acid, Biotin, Sodium Selenite, Sodium Molybdate, Potasssium Iodide, Vitamin K, Cyanocobalamin.

Perfect Protein **-** Metagenics
Each scoop (23 g) contains: Calcium 95 mg • Sodium 88 mg • Potassium 48 mg • Phophorus 38 mg • Magnesium 14 mg • Alanine 0.92 g • Arginine 0.33 g • Aspartic Acid 2.02 g • Cysteine 0.42 g • Glutamic Acid 3.12 g • Glycine 0.33 g • Histidine 0.3 g • Isoleucine (BCAA) 1.08 g • Leucine (BCAA) 1.86 g • Lysine 1.58 g • Methionine 0.4 g • Phenylalanine 0.53 g • Proline 0.98 g • Serine 0.81 g • Threonine 1.23 g • Tryptophan 0.33 g • Tyrosine 0.54 g • Valine (BCAA) 1.03 g • Whey Protein Isolate (containing beta-lactoglobulin-51%, alpha-lactalbulmin-26%, other constituents of whey protein isolate-23%) • Whey Protein Hydrolysate • Fructose • Apple Pectin • Guar Gum • Natural Vanilla Flavor • Soy Lecithin.

Perfectil Tablets **-** Vitabiotics
Each tablet contains: Vitamin D 5 mcg • Vitamin E (natural source) 40 mg • Vitamin C 60 mg • Vitamin B1 (thiamin) 8 mg • Vitamin B2 (riboflavin) 4 mg • Vitamin B3 (niacin) 18 mg • Vitamin B6 (pyridoxine HCl) 20 mg • Folic Acid 500 mcg • Vitamin B12 (cyanocobalamin) 9 mcg • Biotin 0.045 mg • Pantothenic Acid 40 mg • Iron 12 mg • Magnesium 75 mg • Zinc 15 mg • Iodine 200 mcg • Manganese 2 mg • Copper 2 mg • Silicon 15 mg • Chromium 50 mcg • Selenium 100 mcg • Cystine 10 mg • Natural Mixed Carotenoids 4 mg • Echinacea extract 195 mg • Burdock extract 80 mg.

Perfecting Serum **-** FreeLife International
Neroli Hydrolate (orange blossom water) • Aloe Barbadensis gel • Botanical Extracts in Purified water: Bearberry, Licorice, Green Tea • Vegetable Glycerin • Plant Cellulose • DL Panthenol • Magnesium Ascorbyl Phosphate (vitamin C) • Olive Squalane • Pure Clover

Honey • Deanol Bitartrate (DMAE) • Alpha-Lipoic Acid • Oat Beta Glucan • Gatuline Lifting Complex: Lupin extract, Wild Thyme • Tocopheryl Acetate (vitamin E) • Grape Seed oil • Phenoxyethanol (phenolic compound/phenoxetol) • Benzyl Alcohol • Benzoic Acid • Lonicera Japonica (Japanese honeysuckle).

Performance Enhancer Creatine Fuel - TwinLab
Each capsule contains: Creatine Monohydrate 700 mg.

Performance Gold - Advocare International
Two caplets contain: Moomiyo 100 mg • Golden Root extract (rhodiola rosea) 25 mg • Siberian Ginseng root extract (eleutherococcus senticosus) 50 mg • Inosine 500 mg • Hydrolyzed Whey Peptides 1000 mg. Other Ingredients: Dicalcium Phosphate, Silicon Dioxide, Cellulose, Stearic Acid, Magnesium Stearate.

Perfor-Max - Goldshield Elite
One caplet contains: Grape seed extract (vitis vinifera) 25 mg • Pine bark extract (Pinus pinaster) 25 mg • Turmeric rhisome extract 25 mg • Botanical Blend 50 mg: Green Tea leaf extract (36% catechin & polyphenols), Hawthorn berry extract (5% flavonoid glycosides), and Rosemary leaf extract. Other Ingredients: Dicalcium Phosphate, Vegetable cellulose, Vegetable oil, Soy polysaccharides, Silica.

PerforMAXX - Optimum Nutrition
Two capsules contain: Vitamin A (as vitamin A acetate, beta carotene) 10,000 IU • Vitamin C (as ascorbic acid) 300 mg • Vitamin D (as cholecalciferol) 300 IU • Vitamin E (as D-alpha tocopheryl succinate) 200 IU • Thiamin (as thiamin mononitrate) 75 mg • Riboflavin 75 mg • Niacin (as niacinamide) 75 mg • Vitamin B6 (as pyridoxine hydrochloride) 7.5 mg • Folic Acid 400 mcg • Vitamin B12 (as cyanocobalamin) 75 mcg • Biotin 75 mcg • Pantothenic Acid (as D-calcium pantothenate) 75 mg • Calcium (as calcium phosphate) 20 mg • Iron (as ferrous fumarate) 9 mg • Iodine (as potassium iodide) 150 mcg • Magnesium (as magnesium oxide, magnesium citrate) 10 mg • Zinc (as zinc oxide, zinc gluconate) 10 mg • Selenium (as selenomethionine) 35 mcg • Copper (as copper gluconate) 1 mg • Manganese (as manganese sulfate) 1 mg • Chromium (as chromium GTF) 60 mcg • Molybdenum (as sodium molybdate) 25 mcg • Potassium (as potassium chloride) 1.8 mg • Proprietary PerforMAXX Blend 334 mg: Inositol, PABA (para-aminobenzoic acid), N-Acetyl Cysteine, Choline (as choline bitartrate), Ginkgo Biloba leaf extract (ginkgo biloba L., standardized to 24% flavone glycosides, 6% terpene lactones), Korean Ginseng root powder, Rutin, Citrus Bioflavonoid powder, Hesperidin complex, Astaxanthin, Boron (as boron citrate), Lycopene, Lutein, Tocotrienols, Alpha Carotene, Cryptoxanthin, Zeaxanthin. Other Ingredients: Gelatin, Microcrystalline Cellulose, Magnesium Stearate, Stearic Acid, Silica.

Perfusia-SR - Thorne Research Inc.
Each sustained-release capsule contains: L-Arginine 350 mg.

Peridin-C - Beutlich Pharmaceuticals
Each tablet contains: Ascorbic Acid (Vitamin C) 200 mg • Hesperidin Complex (Bioflavonoid) 150 mg • Hesperidin Methyl Chalcone (Bioflavonoid) 50 mg.

Perika St. John's Wort - Nature's Way
Each tablet contains: Perika (WS 5572) dried St. John's Wort extract 300 mg.

Perimine - Metagenics
Each tablet contains: Perilla seed extract 100 mg.

PermaSlim - Momentum
Two capsules contain: Vitamin B12 100 mcg • Vitamin B6 16 mg • Proprietary Blend 600 mg: Citrus Aurantium, Green Tea extract. Other Ingredients: Cellulose, Magnesium Stearate, Silicon Dioxide. See Editor's Note No. 40.

Permathene-16 Maximum Strength Caffeine Free - CCA Industries, Inc.
Each tablet contains: Phenylpropanolamine HCl 75 mg. Other Ingredients: Croscarmellose, D&C Yellow #10, Dicalcium Phosphate, FD&C Blue #1, FD&C Yellow #6, Lactose, Magnesium Stearate, Methylcellulose, Microcrystalline Cellulose, Stearic Acid, Titanium Dioxide.

Permea Plus - Arden Healthcare
Each tablet contains: Vitamin D 2.5 mcg • Vitamin E 40 mg • Vitamin C 30 mg • Vitamin B1 8 mg • Vitamin B2 4 mg • Vitamin B3 18 mg • Vitamin B6 9 mg • Vitamin B12 9 mcg • Folic Acid 500 mcg • Biotin 45 mg • Pantothenic Acid 40 mg • Iron 12 mg • Calcium 168 mg • Magnesium 50 mg • Zinc 15 mg • Iodine 200 mcg • Manganese 2 mg • Copper 2 mg • Silicon 10 mg • Chromium GTF 50 mcg • Selenium 100 mcg • Cystine 10 mg • Betacarotene 3 mg • Lutein 30 mcg • PABA 20 mg • Citrus Bioflavonoids 15 mg.

Permeability Factors - Tyler Encapsulations
Two softgel capsules contain: Vitamin E (as d-alpha tocopheryl acetate) 11 IU • L-Glutamine 500 mg • NAG (n-acetyl glucosamine) 250 mg • Gamma Linolenic Acid (as borage seed oil) 133 mg • Phosphatidylcholine 56 mg. Other Ingredients: Safflower Oil, Lecithin, Beeswax, Gelatin, Glycerin, Titanium Dioxide, Carob.

Persic-GLA - Atrium Biotechnologies
Each capsule contains: Borage oil 100 mg • Cold Processed Persic oil yielding the following Lipid Acids: Vitamin F Factors 370 mg, Oleic 192 mg, Linoleic 109 mg, Gamma Linolenic 30 mg, Palmitic 18 mg, Palmitoleic 5 mg, Stearic 4 mg, Linolenic 701 mcg, Heptodecanoic 409 mcg, Arachadic 330 mcg, Arachidonic 111 mcg • Potassium 113 mcg • Magnesium 7 mcg • Phosphorus 4 mg • Calcium 4 mcg.

Personal Radical Shield capsules - Life Enhancement Products, Inc.
Three capsules contain: Vitamin A (as vitamin A palmitate) 1250 IU • Vitamin A (as beta-carotene) 1.9 mg • Vitamin C (as ascorbic acid and ascorbyl palmitate) 813 mg • Vitamin D (as cholecalciferol) 250 IU • Vitamin E (as D,L-alpha-tocopheryl acetate) 200 mg • Vitamin K (as phytonadione) 35 mcg • Thiamine (vitamin B1 as thiamine hydrochloride) • Riboflavin (vitamin B2) 25 mg • Niacin (vitamin B3) 125 mg • Vitamin B6 (as pyridoxine hydrochloride) 16.7 mg • Folic Acid 200 mcg • Vitamin B12 (cyanocobalamin) 50 mcg • Biotin 750 mcg • Pantothenic Acid (vitamin B5 as calcium panothenate) 150 mg • Calcium (as calcium citrate and calcium pantothenate) 105 mg • Iodine (as potassium iodide) 37.5 mcg • Zinc (as zinc gluconate) 12.5 mg • Selenium (as sodium selenite) 50 mcg • Copper (as copper gluconate) 750 mcg • Manganese (as manganese gluconate) 1 mg • Chromium (as chromium aspartate) 50 mcg • Molybdenum (as molybdenum glycinate) 62.5 mcg • Taurine 312.5 mg • L-Cysteine Hydrochloride 125 mg • Quercetin 32.5 mg • Hesperidin 30 mg • Boron (as calcium borate) 750 mcg.

Personal Radical Shield powder - Life Enhancement Products, Inc.
Each 1 tsp serving contains: Vitamin A (as vitamin A palmitate) 1250 IU • Vitamin A (as beta-carotene) 1.9 mg • Vitamin C (as ascorbic acid and ascorbyl palmitate) 813 mg • Vitamin D (as cholecalciferol) 250 IU • Vitamin E (as D,L-alpha-tocopheryl acetate) 200 mg • Vitamin K (as phytonadione) 35 mcg • Thiamine (vitamin B1 as thiamine hydrochloride) • Riboflavin (vitamin B2) 25 mg • Niacin (vitamin B3) 125 mg • Vitamin B6 (as pyridoxine hydrochloride) 16.7 mg • Folic Acid 200 mcg • Vitamin B12 (cyanocobalamin) 50 mcg • Biotin 750 mcg • Pantothenic Acid (vitamin B5 as calcium panothenate) 150 mg • Calcium (as calcium citrate and calcium pantothenate) 105 mg • Iodine (as potassium iodide) 37.5 mcg • Zinc (as zinc gluconate) 12.5 mg • Selenium (as sodium selenite) 50 mcg • Copper (as copper gluconate) 750 mcg • Manganese (as manganese gluconate) 1 mg • Chromium (as chromium aspartate) 50 mcg • Molybdenum (as molybdenum glycinate) 62.5 mcg • Taurine 312.5 mg • L-Cysteine Hydrochloride 125 mg • Quercetin 32.5 mg • Hesperidin 30 mg • Boron (as calcium borate) 750 mcg.

Petadolex - Pure Encapsulations
Each softgel capsule contains: Butterbur 28-44:1 root extract (petasites hybridus, standardized to contain 7.5 mg of petasin and isopetasin) 50 mg.

Some Brand Name Natural Products - What they Contain

www.NaturalDatabase.com contains MANY more listings than appear here.
Editor's Notes are located on pages 2155-2163.

Petadolex - PhytoPharmica
Each softgel contains: Purple Butterbur root extract (petasites hybridus - Petadolex brand, standardized to contain 7.5 mg petasins and to be free of pyrrolizidine alkaloids (PAs)). Other Ingredients: Medium Chain Triglycerides, Gelatin, Glycerin, Water, Riboflavin.

Petadolex - Weber & Weber
Each capsule contains: Petasites Hybridus extract (butterbur root, 30:1) 50 mg • Petasin and Isopetasin 7.5 mg. Other Ingredients: Natural Coloring, Carmine, Glycerole, Gelatin, Titanoxide.

Petaforce - Bioforce Canada Inc
Each capsule contains: Butterbur root 30:1 dry extract (petasites hybridus) 25 mg. Other Ingredients: Triglycerides, Gelatin, Glycerol, Sorbitol (from natural plant source), Black and Red Iron Oxides.

Pevonia Anti-Aging Marine Collagen Cream - Pevonia Skin Care
Active Ingredients: Collagen • Hyaluronic Acid • Begetal Squalene Oil • Jonquil Essential Oil • Arnica • Micronized Titanium Dioxide.

pH Balance Mattefying Toner (combination to oily skin) - Nu Skin Enterprises
Water (aqua) • Hamamelis Virginiana distillate (witch hazel) • Butylene Glycol • Fragaria Vesca fruit (strawberry) • Foeniculum Vulgare fruit extract (fennel) • Copper PCA • Silica • Boron Nitride • Hypericum Perforatum extract • Anthemis Nobilis flower extract • Calendula Officinalis flower extract • Centaurea Cyanus flower extract • Chamomilla Recutita flower extract (matricaria) • Tilia Cordata flower extract • Glycerin • PEG-40 Hydrogenated Castor oil • Fragrance (parfum) • Tetrasodium EDTA • Benzoic Acid • Phenoxyethanol • Chlorphenesin • Methylparaben • Ethylparaben.

pH Balance Toner (normal to dry skin) - Nu Skin Enterprises
Water (aqua) • Aloe Barbadensis • Hamamelis Virginiana distillate (witch hazel) • Glycerin • Butylene Glycol • Fragaria Vesca fruit (strawberry) • Camphor • Fucus Vesiculosus extract • Gellidiela Acerosa extract (algae) • Hypnea Musciformis extract • Sargassum Filipendula extract (algae) • Hyaluronic Acid • Sodium PCA • Royal Jelly • Sorbitol • Citric Acid • Triethanolamine • Disodium EDTA • Phenoxyethanol • Methylparaben • Caramel.

PharmaPure PharmaFlex 500 - Pure Tek Corp.
Each three tablets contain: Glucosamine 1500 mg • Chondroitin 600 mg • Phellodendron bark extract (Nexrutine) 500 mg.
See Editor's Note No. 15.

PharmaPure PharmaFlex 750 - Pure Tek Corp.
Each two tablets contain: Glucosamine 1500 mg • Phellodendron bark extract (Nexrutine) 750 mg.

Pharmaton Antistax - Boehringer Ingelheim
Each capsule contains: Red Vine leaf extract 180 mg. Other Ingredients: Gelatin, Dried Glucose Syrup, Silicon Dioxide, Talc, Maize Starch, Magnesium Stearate, Colours (E 172, E 171).

Pharmaton Flexium Joint Comfort - Boehringer Ingelheim
Two tablets contain: SAM-e (as S-adenosylmethionine 1,4-butanedisulfonate) 400 mg. Other Ingredients: Microcrystalline Cellulose, Sodium Startch Glycolate, Methacrylic Acid Copolymer, Talc, Polyethylene Glycol 6000, Colloidal Silica, Magnesium Stearate, Polysorbate 80, Sodium Hydroxide, Iron Oxide, Simethicone.

Pharmaton Flexium Joint Comfort & Cartilage Renewal - Boehringer Ingelheim
Each tablet contain: SAM-e (as S-adenosylmethionine 1,4-butanedisulfonate) 200 mg • Glucosamine HCl 500 mg. Other Ingredients: Microcrystalline Cellulose, Sodium Starch Glycolate, Povidone, Methacrylic Acid Copolymer, Talc, Polyethylene Glycol 6000, Magnesium Stearate, Colloidal Silica, Polysorbate 80, Sodium Hydroxide, Iron Oxide, Simethicone.

Phase 2 - Swanson Health Products
Two capsules contain: Phaseolamin 2250 Phaseolus vulgaris L. from White Kidney Bean (dried bean fraction) 1 g. Other Ingredients: Gelatin, Magnesium Stearate.

Phase 2 Starch Neutralizer - Pure Encapsulations
Each vegetable capsule contains: Phaseolus Vulgaris (dried bean fraction) 500 mg • Vitamin C (as ascorbyl palmitate) 10 mg.

Phase'oLean Forte - Life Plus
Each tablet contains: Kidney Bean (Phaseolus vulgaris L.) protein concentrate 500 mg.

PH-Basic - Enzymedica
Each capsule contains: Amylase Thera-Blend 2500 DU • Cellulase Thera-Blend 600 CU • Protease Thera-Blend 1000 HUT • Lipase Thera-Blend 190 FCCFIP • Pectinase with Phytase 200 endo-Pgu • Mineral Blend: Potassium Bicarbonate, Sodium Bicarbonate, Magnesium Citrate.

PhenCal 106 - Great American Nutrition
Six tablets contain: Vitamin B6 (as pyridoxal-5-phosphate) 30 mg • Chromium (as picolinate) 200 mcg • DL-Phenylalanine 2700 mg • L-Tyrosine 300 mg • L-Glutamine 150 mg • L-5-Hydroxytryptophan 15 mg • L-Carnitine 60 mg.

Phen-First - Life Extension
Each tablet contains: Ma Huang extract 150 mg • Guarana extract 350 mg • L-Carnitine Fumerate 50 mg • Chromium Picolinate 200 mcg • St. John's Wort 150 mg • Uva Ursi 12.5 mg • Korean Ginseng 12.5 mg • Phenylalanine 12.5 mg • Ginkgo Biloba 12.5 mg • Vitamin B6 5 mg • Vitamin B12 5 mg • Calcium Pyruvate 50 mg • Green Tea extract 12.5 mg.
See Editor's Note No. 30.

Phen-Free - EAS, Inc.
Four capsules contain: Caffeine 99 mg • Citrus aurantium 300 mg (Bitter Orange peel standardized to 6% Synephrine) • Yohimbe 100 mg • Cordyceps 500 mg (standardized to 7% Cordyceptic Acid) • L-Tyrosine 500 mg • St. John's Wort 200 Mg (standardized to 0.3% Hypericin) • Cayenne Pepper powder 30 mg.
See Editor's Note No. 40.

Phenolox - Metabolic Nutrition, Inc.
Six capsules contain: Green Tea leaf (50%/35%) 1800 mg • Advantra Z Citrus Aurantium (6%) 900 mg • Di Potassium Phosphate 600 mg • L-Carnitine 510 mg • L-Phenylalanine 300 mg • Cayenne pepper extract 300 mg • Coleus Forskohlii (20%) 270 mg • Yohimbe (3%) 180 mg • Chromium Picolinate 750 mcg.
See Editor's Note No. 40.

Phen-Rx - Athletic Technologies Inc.
Each capsule contains: Magnesium 75 mg • Vitamin E 3 IU • Zinc 1 mg • Chromium Picolinate 10 mcg • Guarana extract (33%) 300 mg • Theobromine 100 mg • Cocoa powder 200 mg • Konjac root 20 mg • Ginger root powder 5 mg • Spirulina 5 mg • Damiana powder 5 mg • Garcinia Cambogia (50% HCA) 5 mg • Gotu Kola 5 mg • Lecithin powder 5 mg.

PhenSafe - Applied Nutrition
Three capsules contain: St. John's Wort (.3% hypericin) 300 mg • L-Glutamic Acid HCl 100 mg • B6 Pyridoxine HCl 20 mg • Niacinamide (B3) 10 mg • Zinc 8 mg • Folic Acid 200 mcg • ChromeMate 125 mcg • B12 100 mcg • Selenium 75 mcg • Proprietary Blend 640 mg: Advantra Z brand Citrus Aurantium, Licorice root powder, Ginger root powder, Cayenne powder, Mustard seed powder, Green Tea extract, Fennel seed powder, Bioperine brand Black Pepper extract.
See Editor's Note No. 40.

Phenylalanine - Pain & Stress Center
Each capsule contains: Vitamin C (as ascorbyl palmitate) 5 mg • Vitamin B6 (as pyridoxine HCl) 10 mg • L-Phenylalanine 500 mg. Other Ingredients: Gelatin Capsule.

Some Brand Name Natural Products - What they Contain

www.NaturalDatabase.com contains MANY more listings than appear here.
Editor's Notes are located on pages 2155-2163.

BRAND NAMES

Phenyltropic X - Mass Quantities, Inc.
Each capsule contains: Proprietary blend 650 mg: Sida Cordifolia • Synephrine • Guarana • White Willow Bark • Commiphora Mukul. See Editor's Note No. 39 and No. 40.

Phoenaz - Dazzle, Inc.
Three tablets contain: Vitamin E 60 mg • Vitamin B6 • Calcium carbonate granularV Proprietary Blend 3012 mg: Rye Flour, Malt powder diastatic, Barley Grass, Wheat Grass powder, Blessed Thistle, Wild Yam extract, Corn powder, Damiana leaf powder, Saw Palmetto extract, Soy Isoflavones, European Hops.

Phoenaz - Phoenaz, Inc.
Six tablets contain: Calcium (as Calcium Carbonate) 36 mg • Proprietary Blend 520 mg: L-Arginine, Mucuna Pruriens (15% L-Dopa), Ashwaganda, Basil, Alpha GPC, Tribulis Terrestrial extract 40%, Cordyceps Sinesis extract, Optizine. Other Ingredients: Magnesium Stearate, Silicone Dioxide, Gelatin.

Phos Fuel - TwinLab
Four capsules contain: Sodium Phosphate (Dibasic) 4000 mg • Potassium Bicarbonate 816 mg • L-Carnosine 50 mg • Lipoic Acid 100 mcg • Vitamin B1 1.5 mg • Vitamin B2 1.9 mg • Vitamin B3 (Niacinamide) 20 mg • Vitamin B6 2 mg • Pantothenic Acid 10 mg • Biotin 300 mcg.

Phosfood Liquid - Standard Process, Inc.
Ten drops contain: Phosphorus 40 mg. Other Ingredients: Water, Ortho-Phosphoric Acid, Inositol, Riboflavin.

PhosLo Gelcaps - Nabi Biopharmaceuticals
Each gelcap contains: Calcium Acetate 667 mg • Polyethylene Glycol (PEG 8000) 10 mg. Other Ingredients: FD&C Blue #1, D&C Red #28, Titanium Dioxide, Gelatin.

PhosLo Tablets - Nabi Biopharmaceuticals
Each tablet contains: Calcium Acetate 667 mg • Polyethylene Glycol (PEG 8000) 10 mg.

Phosoplex - Optimal Therapeutics
Four capsules contain: Copper (as copper gluconate) 3 mg • Boron (as boron aspartate citrate) 3 mg • BioCell Collagen II brand Collagen Type II 1000 mg • Hydrolyzed Collagen Type II 600 mg • Chondroitin Sulfate 200 mg • Hyaluronic Acid 100 mg • Hyaluronic Acid (from Biocell collagen type II) 200 mg • Chondroitin Sulfate (from Biocell collagen type II) 200 mg • D-Glucosamine Sulfate KCl 750 mg • MSM (methylsulfonylmethane) 375 mg • Bromelain 250 mg • Horsetail extract 250 mg • Nextrutine brand Phellodendron Amurense extract 250 mg. Other Ingredients: Gelatin, Cellulose, Magnesium Stearate.

PhosphaGems - EAS, Inc.
Each 42 gram serving contains: Phosphagen (HPCE pure Creatine Monohydrate) 5.2 g • TriCarb Complex (Sucrose, High-Dextrose Corn Syrup & Dextrose) • Phosphagen (HPCE pure Creatine Monohydrate) • Modified Starch • Natural & Artificial Flavor • Disodium Phosphate • Malic Acid • Colored with Cochineal extracts.

Phosphagen - EAS, Inc.
Each 5 gram serving contains: Phosphagen 5 g.

Phosphatide I-C-E - Progressive Labs
Each softgel contains: Phosphatidylcholine 420 mg • Phosphatidylethanolamine 210 mg • Phosphatidylinositol 120 mg • Total Phosphatides 750 mg.

Phosphatidyl Choline - Pro Health
Each softgel contains: Phosphatidyl Choline 420 mg. Other Ingredients: Gelatin, Glycerin, Water.

Phosphatidyl Choline - J. R. Carlson Laboratories, Inc.
Each softgel contains: Phosphatidyl Choline 1280 mg • Phosphatidyl Choline 460 mg • Phosphatidyl Ethanolamine 102 mg • Phosphatidyl Inositol 32 mg.

Phosphatidyl Choline - Source Naturals
Each softgel contains: Soy lecithin 1,200 mg • Phosphatidyl Choline 420 mg.

Phosphatidyl Choline Complex - Nature's Life
Each capsule contains: Phosphatidyl Choline Complex 120 mg: Phosphatides: Phosphatidyl Choline (contains 65 mg Choline) 420 mg • Phosphatidyl Ethanolamine 108 mg • Phosphatidyl Inositol (contains 6 mg Inositol) 24 mg • Phosphatidic Acid 36 mg • Linoleic Acid (Omega-6) 313 mg • Linolenic Acid (Omega-3) 24 mg • Oleic Acid (Omega-9) 73 mg • Palmitic Acid 78 mg • Stearic Acid 24 mg.

Phosphatidyl Serine - Pro Health
Each softgel contains: Phosphatidyl Serine 100 mg • Soybean Oil 30 mg. Other Ingredients: Gelatin, Glycerin, Water.

Phosphatidyl Serine - J. R. Carlson Laboratories, Inc.
Each softgel contains: Phosphatidyl Serine (from soybeans) 100 mg.

Phosphatidyl Serine - Life Enhancement Products, Inc.
Each capsule contains: Phosphatidylserine 100 mg • Phosphatidylcholine 45 mg • Phosphatidylethanolamine 25 mg • Phosphatidylinositol 5 mg.

Phosphatidyl Serine - Progressive Labs
Each softgel contains: Phospholipids: Phosphatidylserine (soy phospholipid) 100 mg • Phosphatidylcholine (soy phospholipid) 45 mg • Phosphatidylethanolamine (soy phospholipid) 10 mg • Phosphatidylinositol (soy phospholipid) 10 mg. Fatty Acids: Linoleic Acid 113 mg • Linolenic Acid 11 mg • Oleic Acid 12 mg • Stearic Acid 1 mg • Palmitic Acid 24 mg • Capric Acid 49 mg • Caprylic Acid 130 mg. Minerals: Phosphorus 8 mg • Potassium 3 mg.

Phosphatidyl Serine 50 - GNC
Each capsule contains: Phosphatidyl Serine 50 mg. Other Ingredients: Soybean oil, Gelatin, Glycerin.

Phosphatidylcholine - Pure Encapsulations
Each softgel capsule contains: Phosphatidylcholine (from 1200 mg of soy lecithin concentrate) 420 mg. Other Ingredients: Gelatin, Glycerin.

Phosphatidylserine - Ortho Molecular Products
Each softgel contains: Phosphatidylserine 100 mg • Phosphatidylcholine 35 mg • Phosphatidylethanolamine 10 mg • Phosphatidylinositol 5 mg. Other Ingredients: Soybean Oil, Natural Gelatin Capsules, Glycerine, Purified Water.

Phosphatidylserine - PhysioLogics
Two capsules contain: Phosphatidylserine Complex 500 mg. Phospholipids: Phosphatidylserine 100 mg • Phosphatidylcholine 100 mg • Phosphatidylethanolamine 60 mg • Phosphatidylinositol 30 mg. Fatty Acids: Linoleic Acid 135 mg • Linolenic Acid 30 mg • Oleic Acid 25 mg • Stearic Acid 15 mg • Palmitic Acid 45 mg. Minerals: Phosphorus 15 mg • Potassium 5 mg.

Phosphatidylserine Complex - The Vitamin Shoppe
Each softgel contains: 500 mg Phospholipids providing 100 mg of Phosphatidylserine and 400 mg other Phospholipids.

Phosphatidylserine Complex - NSI - Nutraceutical Sciences Institute
Each softgel contains: Phosphatidylserine 100 mg • Phosphatidylcholine 45 mg • Phosphatidylehtnaolamine 10 mg • Phosphatidylinositol 5 mg.

Phosphatidylserine Complex - Solgar
Each tablet contains: Calcium (as dl-calcium phosphate) 40 mg • Phosphatidylserine Complex 500 mg • Phosphatidylserine 100 mg • Phosphatidylcholine 100 mg • Phosphatidylethanolamine 60 mg • Phosphatidylinositol 30 mg.Other Ingredients: Soy Lecithin powder (phosphatidylserine complex), Microcrystalline Cellulose, Dicalcium Phosphate, Vegetable Cellulose, Vegetable Stearic Acid, Vegetable Magnesium Stearate, Silica, Vegetable Glycerin.

Phosphatidylserine Complex - PhysioLogics
Each softgel contains: Vitamin C (as ascorbic acid) 5 mg • Phospholipid Complex 500 mg: Soy Lecithin standardized to contain 20% phosphatidylserine 100 mg, Phosphatidic Acid, Phosphatidylinositol, Soy Phospholipids/Glycerides, Phosphatidylcholine, Phosphatidylethanolamine. Other Ingredients: Gelatin, Glycerin, Caramel Color, Sorbitol, Titanium Dioxide Color.

Phosphatidyl-Serine Complex - Olympian Labs
Each softgel contains: Phospholipids 500 mg: Phosphatidylserine (soy phospholipid), Phosphatidylcholine (soy phospholipid), Phosphatidylethanolamine (soy phospholipid), Phosphatidylinositol (soy phospholipid) • Fatty Acids 748 mg: Caprylic Acid, Linoleic Acid, Capric Acid, Oleic Acid, Palmitic Acid, Linolenic Acid, Stearic Acid. Other Ingredients: Gelatin, Glycerin, Borage Oil, Water.

Phosphatidylserine Complex With Ginkgo - PhysioLogics
Each softgel contains: Vitamin C (as ascorbic acid) 5 mg • Phospholipid Complex from Soy Lecithin 500 mg: standardized to contain 20% Phosphatidylserine 100 mg, Phosphatidic Acid, Phosphatidylinositol, Soy Phospholipids/Glycerides, Phosphatidylcholine, Phosphatidylethanolamine • Ginkgo Biloba extract (standardized to contain 24% ginkgoflavoneglycosides, 7.2 mg) 30 mg. Other Ingredients: Gelatin, Glycerin, Lecithin, Yellow Beeswax, Caramel Color, Sorbitol, Titanium Dioxide Color.

Phosphatidylserine/DMAE Complex - Nature's Plus
Two capsules contain: Activated Soy Phosphatides (from soy) 550 mg • Phosphatidylcholine 200 mg • Cephalin (phosphatidylethanolamine) 150 mg • Phosphoinositides 100 mg • Glycosphingolipids 100 mg • Phosphatidylserine (from soy) 100 mg • DMAE (as 2-dimethylaminoethanol bitartrate) 100 mg. Other Ingredients: Silica, Magnesium Stearate, Gelatin, Titanium Dioxide, Purified Water.

Phospholoba Q10 - Olympian Labs
Two capsules contain: Phophatidylserine Complex 500 mg • Ginkgo Biloba 30 mg • Coenzyme Q10 15 mg • Fatty Acids & Minerals 270 mg.

Physician's Super Antioxidant - N.V. Perricone M.D. Cosmeceuticals
Two caplets contain: Vitamin A (as natural beta-carotene and with natural mixed carotenoids 600 mcg) 2000 IU • Vitamin C (as buffered ascorbic acid) 250 mg • Vitamin D (as cholecalciferol 2.5 mcg) 200 IU • Vitamin E (as D-alpha-tocopherol acid succinate 41.3 mg) 100 IU • Thiamin (as thiamin HCl) 10 mg • Riboflavin (as riboflavin) 10 mg • Niacin (as niacinamide) 10 mg • Vitamin B6 (as pyridoxine HCl and pyridoxal-5'-phosphate) 10 mg • Folate (as folic acid) 400 mcg • Vitamin B12 (as cyanocobalamin) 10 mcg • Biotin 75 mcg • Pantothenic Acid (as D-calcium pantothenate) 12.5 mg • Calcium (as calcium carbonate) 166 mg • Iodine (as kelp) 37.5 mcg • Magnesium (as magnesium oxide) 100 mg • Zinc (as zinc gluconate) 7.5 mg • Selenium (as L-selenomethionine) 50 mcg • Copper (as copper gluconate) 0.075 mg • Manganese (as manganese gluconate) 0.5 mg • Chromium (as chromium polynicotinate) 50 mcg • Molybdenum (as sodium molybdate) 37.5 mcg • Potassium (as potassium citrate) 25 mg • Boron (as calcium borogluconate) 250 mcg • Vanadium (as vanadyl sulfate) 250 mcg • Trace Mineral complex (mineralized sea weed) 15 mg • Silica (vegetable source) 45 mcg • Choline (as choline bitartrate) 25 mcg • Inositol 25 mg • Betaine HCl 7.5 mg • L-Carnitine (as L-carnitine tartrate) 6.25 mg • Papain (papaya enzyme) 12.5 mg • Bromelain (80 GDU/g, pineapple enzyme) 12.5 mg • Aloe Vera gel (200x) 0.62 mg • N-Acetyl-L-Cysteine 50 mg • L-Arginine HCl 50 mg • L-Glutathione 3.75 mg • L-Lysine (as L-lysine HCl) 5 mg • Taurine 7.5 mg • DL-Methionine 7.5 mg • Citrus Bioflavonoid complex 5 mg • Rutin 5 mg • Hesperidin complex 5 mg • Green Tea leaf extract (polyphenol catechins) 5 mg • Licorice root extract 2.5 mg • Grape seed extract (proanthocyanidins) 5 mg • Bilberry fruit extract (anthocyanidins) 5 mg • Chlorophyllins (chlorophyll) 10 mg • Ginkgo Biloba leaf extract (flavoglycosides) 5 mg • Lutein (marigold flower extract) 2.5 mg • Alpha Lipoic Acid 25 mg • Co-Enzyme Q-10 6.25 mg • Quercetin dihydride 5 mg • Probiotic Blend 1,000,000 CFU: Lactobacillus Sporogenes, L. Acidophilus, L. Bulgaricus, Bifidobacterium Bifidus • Vegetable Actives Blend 100 mg: Broccoli, Carrot, Tomato, Brussels sprout, Cauliflower, Beet, Celery, Kale, Radish, Leek, Onion • Fruit Actives Blend 100 mg: Pineapple, Apple, Orange, Blueberry, Grape, Grapefuit, Lemon, Lime, Plum, Raspberry, Strawberry, Watermelon, Cantaloupe, Cherry, Papaya, Peach, Pear • Nut and Grain Actives Blend 100 mg: Almond oil powder, Evening Primrose seed oil (4.8% GLA), Flax seed, Olive leaf extract, Plant Sterol Concentrate: Beta-Sitosterol (45%), Campesterol (25%), and Stigmasterol (18%), Soy Isoflavones (1% total isoflavones as genistein, genistin, daidzin, daidzein), Soy Lecithin, Soy Polysaccharides, Tocopherols (D-alpha-, beta-, gamma-, delta-) • Herbal Actives Blend 100 mg: Alfalfa aerial parts, Capsicum fruit, Chamomile flower, Fennel seed, Fenugreek seed, Ginger root, Gotu Kola leaf, Green Pepper fruit, Hawthorne berry, Hyssop aerial parts, Myrrh gum, Peppermint leaf, Sarsaparilla root. Other Ingredients: Microcrystalline Cellulose, Croscarmellose Sodium, Stearic Acid, Magnesium Stearate, Pharmaceutical Glaze.

PhysioKids MultiLogics Chewable - PhysioLogics
Two tablets contain: Vitamin A (as beta carotene) 5000 IU • Vitamin C (ascorbic acid) 60 mg • Vitamin D (as ergocalciferol) 400 IU • Vitamin E (as d-alpha tocopherol acetate) 30 IU • Thiamin (as thiamine HCl) 1.5 mg • Riboflavin 1.7 mg • Niacin (as niacinamide) 20 mg • Vitamin B6 (as pyridoxine HCl) 2 mg • Folate (folic acid) 10 mcg • Vitamin B12 (as cyanocobalamin) 6 mcg • Biotin 50 mcg • Pantothenic Acid (as calcium pantothenate) 10 mg • Calcium (as calcium amino acid chelate) 20 mg • Iron (as iron amino acid chelate) 5 mg • Iodine (from kelp) 100 mcg • Magnesium (as magnesium amino acid chelate) 10 mg • Zinc (as zinc amino acid chelate) 3 mg • Copper (as copper amino acid chelate) 0.05 mg • Manganese (as manganese amino acid chelate) 0.05 mg • Potassium (as potassium amino acid chelate) 1 mg • Apple (fruit) 50 mg • Papaya (fruit) 50 mg • Pineapple (fruit) 50 mg • Lemon Bioflavonoids 20 mg • Spirulina 20 mg • Sunflower Oil (seed) 20 mg • Rice Bran 10 mg • Beet Greens (leaf) 5 mg • Broccoli (aerial parts) 5 mg • Brown Rice 5 mg • Carrot (root) 5 mg • Dog Rose (rose hips) 5 mg • Mango (fruit) 5 mg • Spinach (leaf) 5 mg • West Indian Cherry (malpighia prunicifolia, fruit) 5 mg • Para-aminobenzoic Acid (PABA) 400 mcg • Choline (as choline bitartrate) 10 mcg • Inositol 10 mcg. Other Ingredients: Fructose, Maple Crystals, Honey, Molasses, Natural Cherry Flavor, Silica, Beet Juice, Magnesium Stearate, Fruit Juices.

PhysioSoy Powder (chocolate flavor) - PhysioLogics
Each scoop (31 g) contains: Potassium 180 mg • Dietary Fiber <2g • Protein 25 g • L-Alanine 1035 mg • L-Arginine 1847 mg • L-Aspartic Acid 2826 mg • L-Cysteine 307 mg • L-Glutamic Acid 4646 mg • L-Glycine 1035 mg • L-Histidine 643 mg • L-Isoleucine 1203 mg • L-Leucine 1987 mg • L-Lysine 1539 mg • L-Methionine 307 mg • L-Phenylalanine 1259 mg • L-Proline 1231 mg • L-Serine 1259 mg • L-Threonine 923 mg • L-Tryptophan 335 mg • L-Tyrosine 923 mg • L-Valine 1231 mg • Isoflavone Blend 50 mg: Genistein 30 mg, Daidzein 17 mg, Glycitein 3 mg. Other Ingredients: Isolated Soy Protein, Cocoa Powder, Natural/Artificial Flavors, Soy Lecithin, Acesulfame Potassium, Salt.

PhysioSoy Powder (natural flavor) - PhysioLogics
Each scoop (31 g) contains: Potassium 30 mg • Protein 24 g • L-Alanine 1036 mg • L-Arginine 1848 mg • L-Aspartic Acid 2828 mg • L-Cysteine 308 mg • L-Glutamic Acid 4648 mg • L-Glycine 1036 mg • L-Histidine 644 mg • L-Isoleucine 1204 mg • L-Leucine 1988 mg • L-Lysine 1540 mg • L-Methionine 308 mg • L-Phenylalanine 1260 mg • L-Proline 1232 mg • L-Serine 1260 mg • L-Threonine 924 mg • L-Tryptophan 336 mg • L-Tyrosine 924 mg • L-Valine 1232 mg • Isoflavone Blend 50 mg: Genistein 30 mg, Daidzein 17 mg, Glycitein 3 mg. Other Ingredients: Isolated Soy Protein (with <2% lecithin).

PhysioSoy Powder (vanilla flavor) - PhysioLogics
Each scoop (29 g) contains: Potassium 70 mg • Protein 25 g • L-Alanine 1050 mg • L-Arginine 1874 mg • L-Aspartic Acid 2827 mg • L-Cysteine 312 mg • L-Glutamic Acid 4713 mg • L-Glycine 1050 mg • L-Histidine 653 mg • L-Isoleucine 1221 mg • L-Leucine 2016 mg •

L-Lysine 1561 mg • L-Methionine 312 mg • L-Phenylalanine 1277 mg • L-Proline 1249 mg • L-Serine 1277 mg • L-Threonine 937 mg • L-Tryptophan 340 mg • L-Tyrosine 937 mg • L-Valine 1249 mg • Isoflavone Blend 50 mg: Genistein 30 mg, Daidzein 17 mg, Glycitein 3 mg. Other Ingredients: Isolated Soy Protein, Natural/Artificial Flavors, Soy Lecithin, Acesulfame Potassium.

PhysioWhey Powder - PhysioLogics
Two rounded scoops (28 g) contain: Calcium 70 mg • Phosphorus 70 mg • Magnesium 10 mg • Sodium 55 mg • Potassium 150 mg • L-Glutamine 100 mg • L-Isoleucine 100 mg • L-Leucine 100 mg • L-Valine 100 mg • Stevia leaf extract (stevia rebaudiana) 80 mg. Other Ingredients: Whey Protein Concentrate, Natural Flavors, Fructose, Xanthan Gum.

Phyt•Aloe, Capsules (PhytAloe, Phyt Aloe, Phyt-Aloe) - Mannatech
Each capsule contains: Proprietary Blend Phyt Aloe Complex 490 mg: Broccoli, Brussels Sprout, Cabbage, Carrot, Cauliflower, Garlic, Kale, Onion, Tomato, Turnip, Papaya, Pineapple • Ambrotose Complex (patent pending) 50 mg: Arabinogalactan (larix decidua gum), Manapol Aloe Vera gel extract (inner leaf gel), Gum Ghatti, Gum Tragacanth. Other Ingredients: Gelatin, Magnesium Stearate.

PhytAloe, Powder (PhytAloe, Phyt Aloe, Phyt-Aloe) - Mannatech
Each one-half teaspoon contains: Proprietary Blend Phyt•Aloe Complex 907 mg: Broccoli, Brussels Sprout, Cabbage, Carrot, Cauliflower, Garlic, Kale, Onion, Tomato, Turnip, Papaya, Pineapple • Ambrotose Complex 93 mg: Arabinogalactan (larix decidua gum), Manapol Aloe Vera gel extract, Gum Ghatti, Gum Tragacanth.

Phyto Complete capsules - Metagenics
Twenty tablets contain: Vitamin A (100% as beta-carotene) 3500 IU • Soy Lecithin 700 mg • Tofu powder 400 mg • Rice Starch 150 mg • Vitamin C (as ascorbic acid) 60 mg • Citrus Bioflavonoid complex 50 mg • Sodium (as sea salt) 25 mg • Cellulase enzyme 25 mg • Vitamin E (as D-alpha tocopheryl succinate) 12 IU • Amylase enzyme 8 mg • Zinc (as zinc glycinate) 4 mg • Pycnogenol 900 mcg • Carrot powder (daucus carota) 1150 mg • Tomato powder (solanum lycopersicum) 100 mg • Broccoli powder (brasicca oleracea var. italica) 600 mg • Pollen plant extract 130 mg • Schisandra fruit extract (schisandra chinensis) 130 mg • White Cabbage leaf powder (brassica oleracea var. capitata) 100 mg • Apple Pectin powder (malus domestica) 100 mg • Green Tea leaf extract (camellia sinensis) 50 mg • Barley Grass powder (hordeum bulgare) 50 mg • Wheat Grass powder (triticum aestivum) 50 mg • Chlorella leaf powder (chlorella spp.) 20 mg • Spirulina algae powder (spirulina platensis) 20 mg • Milk Thistle seed extract (silybum marianum) 10 mg • Siberian Ginseng root extract (eleutherococcus senticosus) 10 mg • Astragalus root extract 8 mg • Aloe leaf extract (aloe barbadensis) 5 mg • Beet root powder (beta vulgaris rubra) 5 mg • Ginger rhizome extract (zingiber officinale) 5 mg • Rose Hips powder (rosa canina) 5 mg • Sunflower seed oil powder (helianthus annus) 5 mg • Bilberry fruit extract (vaccinium myrtillus) 4 mg • Gingko Biloba leaf extract (ginkgo biloba) 2.5 mg • Grape seed extract (vitis vinifera) 1.5 mg • Ginger root powder (zingiber officinale) 1 mg • Turmeric rhizome powder 1 mg • Curcumin (from turmeric rhizome extract, curcuma longa) 5 mg • Horseradish root powder (amoracia lapathifolia) 200 mcg • Cayenne powder (capsicum annuum) 200 mcg.

Phyto Complete powder - Metagenics
Each scoop (5 g) contains: Vitamin A (100% as beta-carotene) 3500 IU • Soy Lecithin 700 mg • Tofu powder 400 mg • Rice Starch 150 mg • Vitamin C (ascorbic acid) 60 mg • Citrus Bioflavonoid complex 50 mg • Sodium (as sea salt) 25 mg • Cellulase enzyme 25 mg • Vitamin E (as D-alpha tocopheryl succinate) 12 IU • Amylase enzyme 8 mg • Zinc (as zinc glycinate) 4 mg • Pycnogenol 900 mcg • Carrot powder (daucus carota) 1150 mg • Tomato powder (solanum lycopersicum) 100 mg • Broccoli powder (brasicca oleracea var. italica) 600 mg • Pollen plant extract (cracked) 130 mg • Schisandra fruit extract (schisandra chinensis) 130 mg • White Cabbage leaf powder (brassica oleracea var. capitata) 100 mg • Apple Pectin powder (malus domestica) 100 mg • Green Tea leaf extract (camellia sinensis) 50 mg • Barley Grass powder (hordeum bulgare) 50 mg • Wheat Grass powder (triticum aestivum) 50 mg • Chlorella leaf powder (chlorella spp.) 20 mg • Spirulina algae powder (spirulina platensis) 20 mg • Milk Thistle seed extract (silybum marianum) 10 mg • Siberian Ginseng root extract (eleutherococcus senticosus) 10 mg • Astragalus root extract (astragalus membranaceus) 8 mg • Aloe leaf extract (aloe barbadensis) 5 mg • Beet root powder (beta vulgaris rubra) 5 mg • Ginger rhizome extract (zingiber officinale) 5 mg • Rose Hips powder (rosa canina) 5 mg • Sunflower seed oil powder (helianthus annus) 5 mg • Bilberry fruit extract (vaccinium myrtillus) 4 mg • Gingko Biloba leaf extract (ginkgo biloba) 2.5 mg • Grape seed extract (vitis vinifera) 1.5 mg • Ginger root powder (zingiber officinale) 1 mg • Turmeric rhizome powder (curcuma longa) 1 mg • Curcumin (from turmeric rhizome extract, curcuma longa) 5 mg • Horseradish root powder (amoracia lapathifolia) 200 mcg • Cayenne fruit powder (capsicum annuum) 200 mcg.

Phyto Estrogen Power - Nature's Herbs
Four capsules contain: Soy Germ Isoflavone concentrate 1400 mg • Kudzu root extract 100 mg • Certified Potency Korean Ginseng extract 100 mg • Certified Potency Dong Quai extract 100 mg • Mexican Wild Yam extract 100 mg • Boron 3 mg • Natural Vitamin E 800 IU. In a base of Chasteberry powder and Arrowroot.

Phyto Flavonoids - Olympia Nutrition
Contains the extracts of Silymarin, Curcumin, Green Tea, Quercetin, Rosemary, Bilberry, Hawthorn, Ginger, Ginkgo Biloba, Bromelain, Cranberry.

Phyto Quench Supreme - Gaia Herbs
Thirty drops contain: Proprietary Blend 80 mg: Dried Green Tea leaf (camellia sinensis), Fresh Turmeric root (curcuma longa), Fresh Ginkgo leaf (ginkgo biloba), Dried Licorice root (glycyrrhiza glabra), Dried Siberian Ginseng root (eleutherococcus senticosus), Dried Rosemary leaf (rosmarinus officinalis), Dried Thyme leaf (thymus vulgaris), Dried Schizandra berry (schisandra chinensis), Fresh Ginger rhizome (zingiber officinale), Spring Water, 50-60% Pure Grain Alcohol USP.

Phyto Surge - PhytoPharmica
One tablespoon contains: Arsenicum album 6x • Nux vomica 3x • Podophyllum peltatum 3x • Cinchona officinalis 2x • Rhamnus frangula 2x • Artemisia vulgaris 1x • Avena sativa 1x • Cinnamomum 1x • Gentiana lutea 1x • Sterculia acuminata 1x. In a base of 20% USP alcohol by volume.
See Editor's Note No. 1 and No. 21.

Phyto•Bears (Phyto-Bears, Phyto Bears, PhytoBears) - Mannatech
Each Phyto-Bear contains: Phyt•Aloe Complex 40 mg: Broccoli, Brussels Sprout, Cabbage, Carrot, Cauliflower, Garlic, Kale, Onion, Tomato, Turnip, Papaya, Pineapple • Ambrotose Complex 4 mg: naturally occurring plant polysaccharides including freeze-dried Aloe Vera inner leaf gel extract - Manapol powder. Other Ingredients: Corn syrup, Sucrose water, Gelatin, Citric acid, Grape juice concentrate, Natural flavors, Natural colors, Olive oil, Beeswax.
See Editor's Note No. 17.

Phyto•Bears w/Ambrotose Complex (Phyto-Bears, PhytoBears, Phyto Bears) - Mannatech
Each bear contains: Proprietary Blend Phyt Aloe Complex 40 mg: Broccoli, Brussels Sprout, Cabbage, Carrot, Cauliflower, Garlic, Kale, Onion, Tomato, Turnip, Papaya, Pineapple • Ambrotose Complex (patent pending) 4 mg: Naturally Occurring Plant Polysaccharides (including freeze-dried aloe vera inner leaf gel extract - manapol powder). Other Ingredients: Corn Syrup, Sucrose, Water, Gelatin, Citric Acid, Grape Juice Concentrate, Natural Flavors, Natural Colors, Olive Oil, Beeswax.

Phyto-ADR - Pure Encapsulations
Each vegetable capsule contains: Calcium Pantothenate (vitamin B5) 150 mg • Panax Ginseng root extract (standardized to contain 2730% total ginsenosides) 150 mg • Eleutherococcus Senticosus root extract

(standardized to contain 0.8% eleutheroside E & B) 100 mg • Ashwagandha extract (withania somnifera, standardized to contain 5% withanolides) 150 mg • Rhodiola Rosea root extract (standardized to contain 3% total rosavins and min. 1% salidrosides) 50 mg • Astragalus Membranaceus 8:1 root extract 150 mg • Vitamin C (as ascorbyl palmitate) 15 mg.

PhytoBalance - Pure Encapsulations
Each vegetable capsule contains: Alfalfa 10:1 extract (medicago sativa) 100 mg • Rehmanniae 6:1 extract 100 mg • Dong Quai 6:1 extract (angelica sinesis) 100 mg • Licorice root extract (glycyrrhiza, standardized to contain 12% glycyrrhizic acid) 100 mg • Motherwort 4:1 extract (leonurus cardiaca) 50 mg • Chaste tree 5:1 extract (vitex) 50 mg • Wild Yam 10:1 extract (dioscorea) 50 mg • Black Cohosh extract (cimicifuga racemosa, standardized to contain 2.5% triterpene glycosides) 50 mg.

Phyto-Biotic - Enzymatic Therapy
Each capsule contains: Barberry Bark of root extract 6:1 (berberis vulgaris) 200 mg • Oregon Grape root extract 6:1 (berberis aquifolium) 200 mg • Goldenseal root extract (hydrastis canadensis, standardized to contain 5% total alkaloids including berberine, hydrastine & canadine) 50 mg.

Phyto-Clear - Phytohealing Inc.
Aloe Vera gel, Huang Lian herb extract, Huang Qin herb extract, Glucose, Cellulose, Thickening Agents.

PhytoDefense - GNLD International, LLC.
Each packette contains: Vitamin A (as beta-carotene) 7500 IU • Vitamin C (as ascorbic acid) 100 mg • Vitamin E (as D-alpha-tocopherol) 18 IU • Lycopene 1200 mcg • Lutein / Zeaxanthin 410 mcg • Carotenoid Complex Blend 900 mg: Wild Carrot root oleoresin (daucus carota), Red Bell Pepper fruit oleoresin (capsicum frutescens), Tomato fruit oleoresin (lycopersicon esculentum), Spinach leaves oleoresin (spinacia oleracea), Apricot fruit concentrate (prunus armeniacea), Strawberry fruit concentrate (fragaria vesca), Peach fruit concentrate (prunus persica) • Flavonoid Complex Blend 654 mg: Cranberry fruit extract (vaccinium macrocarpus), Kale leaves concentrate (brassica oleracea acephala), Green Tea leaves extract (camellia sinensis), Beet root concentrate (beta vulgaris), Elderberry fruit extract (sambucus nigra), Red Grape Skin extract (vitis vinifera), Black Grape Skin extract (vitis vinifera), Orange fruit extract (citrus aurantium), Lemon fruit (citrus limon), Grapefruit fruit extract (citrus paradisi) • Cruciferous Complex Blend 525 mg: Soymilk powder, Broccoli leaves extract (brassica oleracea botrytis), Radish root extract (raphanus sativus), Kale leaves extract (brassica oleracea acephala), Orange fruit extract (citrus aurantium), Black Mustard fruit extract (brassica nigra), Licorice root extract (glycyrrhiza glabra), Brown Mustard fruit concentrate (brassica nigra), Watercress leaves and stem concentrate (rorippa nasturtium officinale). Other Ingredients: Microcrystalline Celluose, Gelatin, Olive Oil, Glycerin, Yellow Beeswax, Calcium Carbonate, Purified Water, Lecithin, Sodium Croscarmellose, Stearic Acid, Starch, Silicon Dioxide, Hydroxypropyl Methylcellulose, Soybean Oil, Triacetin, Natural Colors, Simethicone.

Phytodolor - PhytoPharmica
Active Ingredients: Common ash (Fraxinus excelsior) bark (4.5:1) 0.20 ml • Aspen (populus tremula) leaves & bark (4.5:1) 0.60 ml • Goldenrod (solidago virgaurea) aerial (4.8:1) 0.20 ml. Other Ingredients: Water, Alcohol (45.6%).
See Editor's Note No. 21.

Phytodolor - Enzymatic Therapy
Each drop contains: Common Ash 0.20 ml • Aspen leaf and bark 0.60 ml • Goldenrod 0.20 ml. Other Ingredients: Water, Alcohol 45.6%.

Phytoestrin - USANA Health Sciences
Each tablet contains: Soy Isoflavones (Glycine Max) seed 14.0 mg • Black Cohosh extract (Cimicifuga Racemosa) root 50.0 mg • Chasteberry powder (Vitex Agnus-Castus) fruit 50.0 mg • Licorice root extract (Glycyrrhiza Glabrera) 30.0 mg • Dong Quai extract (Angelica Sinensis) root 15.0 mg. Other Ingredients: Dextrose, Ascorbyl Palmitate, Croscarmellose Sodium, Dextrin (Modified Food Starch), Colloidal Silicon Dioxide.

Phyto-Estrogen - Gaia Herbs
Three capsules contain: Alfalfa leaf (medicago sativa) 300 mg • Vitex berry (vitex agnus-castus) 90 gm • Black Cohosh rhizome (cimicifuga racemosa) 27 mg • Red Clover blossoms (trifolium pratense) 21 mg • Wild Oats milky seed (avena sative) 21 mg • Blue Vervain herb (verbena hastata) 18 mg • Dandelion leaf and root 12 mg • St. John's Wort flower bud (hypericum perforatum) 12 mg • Sage leaf 12 mg. Other Ingredients: Glycerin, Lecithin, Vegetable Cellulose.

Phyto-Estrogen Cream - Nature's Herbs
Each one oz serving contains: Active Ingredients: Liposomal Soy Isoflavone extract 60 mg • Pomegranate seed juice extract 150 mg • Red Clover tops extract 80 mg • Black Cohosh root extract 80 mg • Dong Quai root extract 25 mg. Inactive Ingredients: Purified Water, Lecithin Phospholipid, Aloe Vera Gel, Caprylic/Capric Triglyceride, Glyceryl Stearate, Glycerin, Cetearyl Alcohol, Ceteareth-20, Cetyl Alcohol, Stearic Acid, Tocopheryl Acetate (natural vitamin E), Cocoa Butter, Grapefruit seed extract, Methylparaben, Propylparaben, Dowicil, Sorbic Acid, Xanthan Gum, Rosemary Oil, Fragrance.

Phyto-Flavonoids - Futurebiotics LLC
Two capsules contain: Procyanidol • Whole Grape extract* 50 mg • Green Tea powder concentrate 150 mg • Citrus bioflavonoids 500 mg • Rutin 75 mg • Quercetin 150 mg • Soy isoflavone extract 500 mg • Berry blend (Raspberry, Blackberry, Blueberry) 200 mg • Cruciferous Vegetable powder blend 200 mg.

Phyto-Fruit - Olympia Nutrition
Guava • Papaya • Mango • Raspberry • Blueberry • Grapefruit • Grape • Ginseng.

PhytoFruit Concentrates - NOW Foods
Two V Caps contain: Grape seed extract (95% Polyphenols) 20 mg • Concentrated fruit extract powders: Acerola Cherry 50 mg, Cranberry 50 mg, Guava 50 mg, Papaya 50 mg, Raspberry 50 mg, Blueberry 50 mg, Grapefruit 50 mg, Mango 50 mg, Pineapple 50 mg, Strawberry 50 mg • Panax ginseng (5% Ginsenosides) 50 mg • Bromelain (2000 GDU from pineapple) 50 mg • Protease (100 SAP Units) 50 mg • Amylase (3000 DU Units) 50 mg • Lipase (100 LU Units) 50 mg • Cellulase (500 CMC Units) 50 mg.

PhytoGreens - Genestra - Seroyal
Each tablespoon contains: Wheat Grass juice 400 mg • Barley Grass juice 400 mg • Alfalfa Grass juice 400 mg • Green Papaya juice 400 mg • Red Beet juice 200 mg • Acerola berry juice 25 mg • Spirulina 1000 mcg • Chlorella 600 mg • Broccoli 600 mg • Cauliflower 600 mg • Lecithin 2000 mg • Phosphatidylcholine 480 mg • Wheat sprout 400 mg • Octacosanol 250 mg • Spinach 250 mg • Dunaliella Salina 50 mg • Dandelion 50 mg • Celandine (chelidonium majus) 50 mg • Ginkgo 50:1 extract (standardized to 24% ginkgoflavoglycosides, 6% terpene lactones) 40 mg • Bilberry (vaccinium myrtillus, standardized 25% anthocyanins) extract 40 mg • Grape seed extract (standardized 85% proanthocyanidins) 40 mg • FOS (fructo-oligo-saccharides) 1000 mg • Apple Pectin 25 mg • Bromelain (pineapple) 25 mg • Parsley (petroselinum sativum) 25 mg • Celery (apium graveolens) 25 mg • Watercress (nasturtium officinale) 25 mg • Papain (papaya) 25 mg • Bee Pollen 200 mg.

Phytokids Formula - Body Language Vitamin Co.
Two chewable tablets contain: Beta Carotene 2500 IU • Magnesium 25 mg • Vitamin B1 1.5 mg • Calcium 50 mg • Vitamin B2 1.7 mg • Selenium 50 mcg • Vitamin B5 10 mg • Manganese 1 mg • Vitamin B6 2 mg • Zinc 5 mg • Niacinamide 10 mg • Iodine 50 mcg • Vitamin B12 6 mcg • Copper 500 mcg • Folic Acid 200 mcg • Molybdenum 2 mcg • Vitamin D (vitamin D3) 400 IU • Vanadium 2 mcg • Vitamin K 80 mcg • Boron 25 mcg • Vitamin E 60 IU • Silica 5 mg • Vitamin C 100 mg • Choline 50 mg • Biotin 200 mcg • Grape Seed extract 1 mg • Pine Bark extract 1 mg • Green Tea extract 20 mg • Flavonoids 50 mg • Lycopene 50 mg • Quercetin 10 mg • Allicin 10 mg • Soy Lecithin 25 mg • Phosphatidylcholine 25 mg.

Phytolax - 4 Life
Each capsule contains: Alder Buckthorn (bark) 100 mg • Cascara Sagrada (bark) 95 mg • Ginger (root) 90 mg • Parsley (leaf) 35 mg • Black Walnut (hull) 30 mg • Frangula extract (bark) 20 mg. Other Ingredients: Xanthum Gum, Gelatin Capsule, Magnesium Stearate.

PhytoMax - PhytoPharmica
Two capsules contain: St. John's Wort (hypericum perforatum) flower head extract (standardized to contain 0.3% hypericin and 4% hyperforin) 500 mg • Valerian (valeriana officinalis) root extract (standardized to contain a minimum of 0.8% valerenic acids) 30 mg • Passion Flower (passiflora incarnata) dried aerial part 4:1 extract 30 mg.
See Editor's Note No. 21.

Phytonutrient Based B-Complex - Arrowroot
Each tablet contains: Vitamin B1 (thiamine, brown rice bran) 15 mg • Folic Acid (folic acid, brown rice bran) 400 mcg • Vitamin B2 (riboflavin, brown rice bran) 20 mg • Pantothenic Acid (D-calcium pantothenate, brown rice bran) 50 mg • Vitamin B6 (pyridoxine HCl, brown rice bran) 20 mg • PABA (PABA, brown rice bran) 10 mg • Vitamin B12 (cobalamin concentrate, greens) 150 mcg • Choline (bitartrate, brown rice bran) 10 mg • Niacinamide (niacinamide, brown rice bran) 12.5 mg • Inositol (inositol, brown rice bran) 10 mg • Niacin (niacin, brown rice bran) 12.5 mg • Biotin (biotin, brown rice bran) 300 mcg.

Phytonutritional - Natural Connections, Inc.
Each 9500 mg contains: Wheat Grass juice powder 400 mg • Barley Grass juice powder 400 mg • Alfalfa Grass juice powder 400 mg • Green Papaya 400 mg • Blue Green Algae & Spirulina 800 mg • Chlorella (cracked-cell) 800 mg • Broccoli freeze-dried powder 800 mg • Cauliflower freeze-dried powder 800 mg • Lecithin (with phosphatidylcholine) 2000 mg • Wheat Sprout powder (gluten-free) 400 mg • Acerola berry juice powder 300 mg • Beet juice powder 200 mg • Spinach & Octacosanol powder 500 mg • Dunaliella Salina 50 mg • Green Tea extract (60% catechins) 50 mg • Milk Thistle (silybum marianum, 80% silymarin) 50 mg • Ginkgo Biloba (24% ginkgoflavonglycosides, 6% terpenes) 50 mg • Bilberry (25% anthocyanidins) 40 mg • Proanthocyanidins as grape seed extract OPC 85+ and pine bark extract OPC 85 40 mg • Probiotic Cultures (dairy free) 10 billion CFU: L-Acidophilus (DDS-1), L-Rhamnosus, L-Bifidus, S, Lactis, Bifidobacterium longum, B. Bifidim, S. Thermophilus • Fructooligosaccharides (FOS) 1000 mg. Inactive Ingredients: Apple Pectin, Bromelain (lower stem, pineapple plants, parsley, celery and watercress).

Phyto-Proz Supreme - Gaia Herbs
Forty drops contain: Proprietary Blend 240 mg: Kava Kava root professional strength (piper methysticum), St. John's Wort flower buds professional strength (hypericum perforatum), Passion Flower vine (passiflora incarnata), Gotu Kola leaf and root (centella asiatica), Schizandra berry (schizandra chinensis), Eleuthero root (eleutherococcus senticosus), Fresh Wild Oats milky seed (avena sativa), Stinging Nettle seed (urtica dioica), Calamus root (aconus calamus), Prickly Ash bark (xanthoxylum clava-herculis), 60% Pure Grain Alcohol USP, Spring Water.

Phyto-Proz Supreme capsules - Gaia Herbs
Three capsules contain: St. John's Wort flower bud (hypericum perforatum) 105 mg • Kava Kava rhizome (piper methysticum) 103 mg • Schizandra berry (schizandra chinensis) 90 mg • Siberian Ginseng root (eleutherococcus senticosus) 45 mg • Passionflower vine (passiflora incarnata) 27 mg • Wild Oats milky seed (avena sativa) 21 mg • Gotu Kola herb (centella asiatica) 18 mg • Prickly Ash bark (xanthoxylum clava-herculis) 9 mg • Nettle seed (uritca dioica) 6 mg • Calamus root (acorus calamus) 3 mg. Other Ingredients: Vegetable Glycerin, Vegetable Cellulose (capsule).

Phytoslim Active - Aboca USA, Inc
Each capsule contains: Bitter Orange freeze-dried extract (citrus aurantium, standardized to 5% synephrine) 242 mg • Green Tea leaf powder (camellia sinensis, standardized to 3% caffeine, to 6% EGCG) 157 mg • Chromium Yeast (saccharomices cerevisiae with chromium, 0.2%) 25 mg. Other Ingredients: Gelatin.
See Editor's Note No. 40.

Phytoslim Purifier - Aboca USA, Inc
Each tea bag (two grams) contains: Java Tea leaf (orthosiphon stamineus) 0.4 g • Licorice root (glycyrrhiza glabra) 0.4 g • Fennel fruit (foeniculum vulgare) 0.34 g • European Goldenrod flowering top (solidago virgaurea) 0.2 g • Certified Organic Peppermint leaf (mentha piperita) 0.2 g • Certified Organic Dandelion root (taxacum officinale) 0.16 g • Turmeric root (curcuma longa) 0.1 g • Horsetail top (equisetum arvense) 0.1 g • Certified Organic Stinging Nettle leaf (urtica dioica) 0.1 g.

Phytoslim Reduce - Aboca USA, Inc
Each packet contains: Dietary Fiber 2110 mg • Glucomannan micronized tuber (amorphophallus konjac, standardized to 76% fiber) 1500 mg • Tangerine fruit dehydrated juice (citrus reticulata blanco) 1000 mg • Mannite (micronized) 900 mg • Chicory root (cichorium intybus, inulin extracted from the root standardized to 89% fiber) 750 mg • Orange fruit dehydrated juice (citrus sinensis) 500 mg • Psyllium (plantago ovata, micronized, standardized to 98% fiber) 250 mg • Flax seed freeze-dried mucilage (linum usitatissimum) 30 mg • Linden flower freeze-dried mucilage (tilla platyphilos) 30 mg • Marshmallow root freeze-dried mucilage (althaea officinalis) 30 mg. Other Ingredients: Natural Lemon Flavoring.

Phytosterol Complex - Progressive Labs
Each capsule contains: Niacin (vitamin B3) 20 mg • Beta-Sitosterol 106 mg • Campesterol 52 mg • Stigmasterol 42 mg.

Phytotality - PhysioLogics
Each capsule contains: Broccoli extract (2% Glucosinolates, 2 mg) 100 mg • TeaGreen leaf (50 % polyphenols, 50 mg) 100 mg • Tomato extract (1% lycopene, 500 mcg) 50 mg • Calendula flower Marigold (5% Lutein, 150 mcg) 3 mg • Soy Isoflavones extract (5 % Isoflavones, 1.25 mg) 25 mg • Red Grape skin extract (30% Anthocyanidins, 7.5 mg) 25 mg • Garlic bulb (10000 mcg Allicin/g, 250 mcg) 25 mg • Turmeric (95% Curcumin, 1.9 mg) 2 mg • Ginger root (5% Gingerols, 100 mcg) 2 mg • Milk Thistle seed (80% Silymarin, 20 mg) 25 mg • Onion 2 mg • Carrot 2 mg • Beet root 2 mg • Celery 2 mg • Leek 2 mg •Garlic 2 mg •Cauliflower 2 mg • Asparagus 2 mg • Broccoli 2 mg • Cabbage 2 mg.

Phytotality Daily - PhysioLogics
Three tablets contain: Vitamin A (100% as beta carotene) 15,000 IU • Vitamin C 1000 mg • Vitamin D 400 IU • Vitamin E 250 IU • Thiamin (vitamin B1) 25 mg • Riboflavin (vitamin B2) 25 mg • Niacin 25 mg • Vitamin B6 25 mg • Folic Acid 400 mcg • Vitamin B12 25 mcg • Biotin 50 mcg • Pantothenic Acid 25 mg • Calcium 250 mg • Iron 15 mg • Iodine 150 mcg • Magnesium 125 mg • Zinc 15 mg • Selenium 25 mcg • Copper 500 mcg • Manganese 4 mg • Chromium 100 mcg • Molybdenum 50 mcg • Potassium 50 mg • Boron 1 mg • Choline Bitartrate 50 mg • Inositol 25 mg • PABA (para-aminobenzoic acid) 25 mg • Citrus Bioflavonoid complex (citrus sinensis) 100 mg • Quercetin (from dimorphandra mollis) 25 mg • Rutin fruit (dimorphandra mollis) 25 mg • Hesperidin Complex 10 mg: Citrus Aurandium, Citrus Spp. • Bromelain (pineapple 2000 GDU/gm) 20 mg • Betaine Hydrochloride 20 mg • Papain (papaya) 20 mg • Amylase 5 mg • Lipase 5 mg • Protease 1 mg • Cellulase 2.5 mg • Proprietary Lactobacillus Blend 25 mg: Lactobacillus Acidophilus, Lactobacillus Bifidus, Lactobacillus Bulgaricus (milk-free: minimum 1 billion viable micro-organisms per gram, at time of manufacture) • Oat Bran husk (avena sativa) 25 mg • Pectin (apple) 25 mg • RNA 35 mg • DNA 10 mg • Carotenoids 10 mg • Chlorophyll 4 mg • Vegetable Oil (borage/sunflower, dry, cold-pressed providing essential fatty acids, GLA) 100 mg • L-Glutathione 5 mg • Spirulina 1000 mg • Wheat Grass juice (dry) 100 mg • Sprouted Barley juice (dry) 100 mg • Flaxseed oil (dry) 100 mg • Chinese Chlorella (broken cell wall) 100 mg • Bee Pollen 100 mg • Eleuthero root (eleutherococcus senticosus) 50 mg • Dehydrated Garlic bulb (allium sativum) 10 mg • Proprietary Herbal Blend 60 mg: Echinacea fruit (echinacea purpurea), Milk Thistle seed (silybum marianum), Goldenseal root (hydrastis canadensis), Ginger root (zingiber officinale), Ginkgo Biloba leaf (ginkgo biloba),

Cayenne Pepper fruit (capsicum annuum). Other Ingredients: Silica, Cellulose (plant origin), Acacia Gum, Croscarmellose, Vegetable Stearic Acid, Ferrous Fumarate, Vegetable Magnesium Stearate, Kelp, Sodium Copper Chlorophyllin, Ester-C Cupric Gluconate, Cellulase, Riboflavin 5' Phosphate, Pantethine, Chromium Picolinate, Pyridoxyl 5' Phosphate, Molybdenum Chelates, Coenzyme B12, Calcium Amino Acid Chelates, Calcium Ascorbate, Calcium Aspartate, Calcium Bisglycinate, Calcium Citrate, Calcium Gluconate, Calcium Histidinate, Calcium Ketoglutarate, Calcium Malate, Calcium Spirulina Chelates, Calcium Succinate, Cupric Amino Acid Chelates, Cupric Ascorbate, Cupric Aspartate, Cupric Bisglycinate, Cupric Histidinate, Cupric Ketoglutarate, Cupric Malate, Cupric Spirulina Chelates, Cupric Succinate, Ferrous Amino Acid Chelates, Ferrous Ascorbate, Ferrous Aspartate, Ferrous Bisglycinate, Ferrous Citrate, Ferrous Gluconate, Ferrous Histidinate, Ferrous Ketoglutarate, Ferrous Malate, Iron Spirulina Chelates, Ferrous Succinate, Magnesium Amino Acid Chelates, Magnesium Ascorbate, Magnesium Aspartate, Magnesium Bisglycinate, Magnesium Citrate, Magnesium Gluconate, Magnesium Histidinate, Magnesium Ketoglutarate, Magnesium Malate, Magnesium Spirulina Chelates, Magnesium Succinate, Manganese Amino Acid Chelates, Manganese Ascorbate, Manganese Aspartate, Manganese Bisglycinate, Manganese Histidinate, Manganese Ketoglutarate, Manganese Malate, Manganese Spirulina Chelates, Manganese Succinate, Potassium Amino Acid Chelates, Potassium Ascorbate, Potassium Aspartate, Potassium Bisglycinate, Potassium Gluconate, Potassium Histidinate, Potassium Ketoglutarate, Potassium Malate, Potassium Spirulina Chelates, Potassium Succinate, Zinc Amino Acid Chelates, Zinc Ascorbate, Zinc Aspartate, Zinc Bisglycinate, Zinc Citrate, Zinc Gluconate, Zinc Histidinate, Zinc Ketoglutarate, Zinc Malate, Zinc Spirulina Chelates, Zinc Succinate, Ergocalciferol.

Phytotality Powder - PhysioLogics
Each scoop (9 g) contains: Sodium 35 mg • Potassium 75 mg • Protein 1 g • Vitamin E (as d-alpha tocopheryl acid succinate) 100 IU • Green Organic Gluten-Free Grass Complex: Wheat Grass powder 350 mg, Barley Grass powder 350 mg, Alfalfa Grass powder 350 mg, Oat Grass powder 350 mg • Blue-Green Algae / Sea Algae Complex: Spirulina (arthospire plantensis, microalgae) 1000 mg, Chlorella (chlorella pyrenoidosa, microalgae) 350 mg, Dunaliella Salina 40 mg, Nova Scotia Dulse (palmaria palmata, seaweed) 30 mg • Adaptogenic/Support Herb Complex: Licorice root (glycyrrhiza glabra) 100 mg, Eleuthero root (eltutherococcus senticosus) 60 mg, Suma root (pfaffia paniculata) 60 mg, Astragalus root (astragalus membranaceus) 60 mg, Echinacea leaf (echinacea purpurea) 60 mg, Ginger root (zingiber officinale 5 mg • Nutrient-Rich Superfood Complex: Lecithin (99% oil-free) 2000 mg, Wheat sprout powder 350 mg, Acerola berry juice powder 200 mg, Beet juice powder 200 mg, Spinach Octacosanol 150 mg, Royal Jelly (5% 10-DHA) 150 mg, Bee Pollen 150 mg • Dairy-Free Probiotic Culture Complex 3.5 Billion (total count, non-dairy culture at time of manufacture 5 billion): Lactobacillus Rhamnosus A, Lactobacillus Rhamnosus B, Lactobacillus Acidophilus, Lactobacillus Casei, Lactobacillus Delbrueckii Subsp., Lactobacillus Bulgaricus, Bifidobacterium Longum / Bifidobacterium Breve 1 billion, Streptococcus Salivarius Subsp., Thermophilus 500 million • Natural Fiber Complex: Flaxseed meal 500 mg, Apple Pectin, Apple Fiber 500 mg, Fructooligosaccharides (FOS) 500 mg • Standardized Bioflavonoid Extract Blend: Milk Thistle seed (silybum marianum, standardized for 80% silymarin) 60 mg, Ginkgo Biloba leaf (ginkgo biloba, standardized for 24% ginkgo flavone glycosides) 20 mg, Green Tea Catechins leaf (camellia sinensis, standardized for 60% catechins) 20 mg, Grapeseed (92% proanthocyanidins) 20 mg, Bilberry fruit (myrtilli frucus, standardized to 25% anthocyanidins) 20 mg.

PhytoxyActin - Nature's Plus
Two capsules contain: Vitamin C corn free 250 mg • Broccoli (standardized 0.035% lutein, 0.004% B-cryptoxanthin, 0.0025% lycopene, 0.0025% alpha carotene, 0.0025% beta carotene, 0.004% sulforaphane) 100 mg • Carrot root (standardized 0.003% lutein, 0.0010% lycopene, 0.0063% alpha carotene, 0.0075% beta carotene) 100 mg • Vitamin E 100 IU • Spinach (standardized 0.0043% lutein, 0.0024% lycopene, 0.0043% beta carotene, 0.0038% B-cryptoxanthin) 75 mg • Tomato (standardized 0.0075% lutein, 0.0155% lycopene, 0.0015% beta carotene) 75 mg • Echinacea (standardized 4% echinacosides) 75 mg • Astragalus (standardized 0.4% 4'-hydroxy-3'-methoxyisoflavone 7-sug) 50 mg • Green Tea (standardized 50% polyphenols) 50 mg • Red Wine concentrate (alcohol free, standardized 20% polyphenols) 50 mg • Turmeric (standardized 95% curcumin) 50 mg • Garlic (standardized 0.35% allicin, 0.65% allicin, 0.40% thiosulfinates, 0.085% allyl mercaptan) 50 mg • Shiitake mushroom (standardized 3.2% KS-2 polysaccharides) 25 mg • Grape seed extract (standardized 95% proanthocyanidins) 25 mg • Beta Carotene pro-Vitamin A (naturally supplying 25000 IU of Vitamin A activity) 15 mg.

Pick-Me-Up Formula - Bee-Alive Inc.
Royal Jelly (non-freeze dried) • Damiana leaf extract • Saw Palmetto fruit extract • Cayenne fruit extract • Asian Ginseng root • Vegetable Glycerin • Clover Honey • Deionized Water • Natural Almond Flavor.

Pilex Ointment - The Himalaya Drug Company
Lajjalu (mimosa pudica) • Bhringaraja (eclipta prostrata syn. e.alba) • Nirgundi (vitex negundo) • Zergul (calendula officinalis) • Karpoora (cinnamomum camphora) • Tankana (sodium biborate) • Yashad Bhasma (zinc calx).

Pilex Tablets - The Himalaya Drug Company
Each tablet contains: Guggulu (commiphora wightii syn. balsamodendron mukul) 0.26 mg • Shilajeet (mineral pitch, purified) 32 mg • Nimba seed (melia azadirachta syn. azadiractha indica) 14 mg • Daruharidra (berberis aristata) 64 mg • Amalaki (emblica officinalis) 32 mg • Haritaki (terminalia chebula) 32 mg • Vibhitaki (terminalia bellirica syn. t.belerica) 32 mg • Aragvadha (cassia fistula) 32 mg • Kanchanara (bauhinia variegata) 32 mg • Nagkesara (mesua ferrea) 6 mg.

PimpJuice - Fillmore Street Brewery LLC.
Water • High Fructose Corn Syrup and/or Sucrose • Apple Juice Concentrate • Citric Acid • Natural Flavor • D-Ribose • Malic Acid • Ascorbic Acid • Inositol • Maltodextrin • Guarana seed extract (paullinia cupana) • Niacin • Calcium Pantothenate • Taurine • Pyridoxine Hydrochloride • Yellow #5 • Riboflavin • Blue #1 • Cyanocobalamin.

Pinadol - Berkeley Premium Nutraceuticals
Each tablet contains: Vitamin C (as ascorbic acid) 250 mg • Thiamin (as thiamin HCl) 25 mg • Riboflavin 25 mg • Niacin (as niacinamide) 25 mg • Vitamin B6 (as pyridoxine HCl) 25 mg • Folate (as folic acid) 400 mcg • Vitamin B12 (as cyanocobalamin) 25 mcg • Pantothenic Acid (as D-calcium pantothenate) 25 mg • Magnesium (as magnesium oxide) 200 mg • Magnolia bark standardized extract 30 mg • L-Tyrosine 100 mg • Eleuthero root standardized extract 200 mg. Other Ingredients: Dicalcium Phosphate, Microcrystalline Cellulose, Croscarmellose Sodium, Stearic Acid, Magnesium Stearate, Silica.

Pineal Concentrate - Progressive Labs
Each capsule contains: Veal bone concentrate 100 mg • Flaxseed oil 20 mg • Pineal concentrate 7 mg • Pituitary concentrate 3 mg. See Editor's Note No. 31.

Pineal Plus - Atrium Biotechnologies
Each tablet contains: Raw Pineal Tissue concentrate (Bovine) 8 mg • Raw Whole Pituitary concentrate (Bovine) 20 mg • Raw Calf Bone concentrate (Bovine) 150 mg • Cold Pressed Flaxseed oil 10 mg. See Editor's Note No. 14.

Pinna-Cal - Goldshield Elite
Six caplets contain: Vitamin D (as Cholecalciferol) 125 IU • Vitamin K (as Phytonadione) 80 mcg • Calcium (as purified Calcite, Hydroxyapatite, Calcium Citrate, and Calcium Lactate) 1000 mg • Magnesium (as Magnesium Citrate and Oxide) 400 mg • Boron (as Boron Citrate) 2 mg • Ipriflavone 600 mg. Other Ingredients: Vegetable cellulose, Fractionated vegetable oil, Silica, Soy polysaccharides, and Vita-Lok vegetable resin glaze.

BRAND NAMES

Pinnacle 5-HTP Tryptobol - Bodyonics, Ltd.
Two capsules contain: Griffonia Simplicifolia (providing 10% (100 mg) 5-HTP (5-Hydroxy-L-Tryptophan)) 1000 mg • Herbolics Support Complex (from Jatoba, Maca, Para Todo, Yerba Mate) 100 mg. Other Ingredients: Calcium Phosphate, Microcrystalline Cellulose, Magnesium Stearate, Gelatin.

Pinnacle Andro-150 Poppers - Bodyonics, Ltd.
Two tabs contain: Balanced Andro Complex 150 mg: 4-AD 128 mg, 4-AD-EC 15 mg, NOR-4-AD 5 mg, A1-E 2 mg. Other Ingredients: Fructose, Sorbitol, Natural Flavor, Stearic Acid, Magnesium Stearate, Cellulose, Croscarmellose, Sucralose.
See Editor's Note No. 47.

Pinnacle Androstat 100 - Bodyonics, Ltd.
Each tablet contains Androstenedione 100 mg. Other Ingredients: Calcium Phosphate, Lecithin, Xanthan Gum, Stearic Acid, Magnesium Stearate.
See Editor's Note No. 47.

Pinnacle Androstat Pro Six - Bodyonics, Ltd.
Each tablet contains: 4-androstenediol (4-androstene-3, 17-diol) 125 mg • 4-androstene-3,17-dione (4-androstenedione) 5 mg • 5-androstene-3, 17-dione (5-androstenedione) 5 mg • 5-androstene-3beta,17beta-diol (5-androstenediol) 5 mg • 19-nor-5-androstene-3, 17-diol (19-nor 5-androstendiol) 5 mg. Other Ingredients: Calcium Phosphate, Lecithin, Xanthan Gum, Stearic Acid, Magnesium Stearate.
See Editor's Note No. 47 and No. 54.

Pinnacle Androstat100 Poppers (cool mint flavor) - Bodyonics, Ltd.
Two tablets contain: 4-androstene-3, 17-diol (4-androstenediol) 83.33 mg • 4-androstenedione-3,17-dione (4-androstenedione) 3.33 mg • 5-androstene-3, 17-dione (5-androstenedione) 3.33 mg • 5-androstene-3beta,17beta-diol (5-androstenediol) 3.33 mg • 19-nor-5-androstene-3, 17-diol (19-nor 5-androstendiol) 3.33 mg. Other Ingredients: Fructose, Sorbitol, Natural Flavor, Stearic Acid, Magnesium Stearate, Cellulose, Croscarmellose, Sucralose.
See Editor's Note No. 47 and No. 54.

Pinnacle Androstat100 Poppers (licorice flavor) - Bodyonics, Ltd.
Two tablets contain: 4-androstene-3, 17-diol (4-androstenediol) 83.33 mg • 4-androstene-3,17-dione (4-androstenedione) 3.33 mg • 5-androstene-3, 17-dione (5-androstenedione) 3.33 mg • 5-androstene-3beta,17beta-diol (5-androstenediol) 3.33 mg • 19-nor-5-androstene-3, 17-diol (19-nor 5-androstendiol) 3.33 mg. Other Ingredients: Fructose, Sorbitol, Natural Flavor, Stearic Acid, Magnesium Stearate, Cellulose, Croscarmellose, Sucralose.
See Editor's Note No. 47 and No. 54.

Pinnacle Androstat100 Poppers (wild berry flavor) - Bodyonics, Ltd.
Two tablets contain: Balanced Andro Complex: 4-androstene-3, 17-diol (4-androstenediol) 83.33 mg • 4-androstene-3,17-dione (4-androstenedione) 3.33 mg • 5-androstene-3, 17-dione (5-androstenedione) 3.33 mg • 5-androstene-3beta,17beta-diol (5-androstenediol) 3.33 mg • 19-nor-5-androstene-3, 17-diol (19-nor 5-androstendiol) 3.33 mg. Other Ingredients: Fructose, Sorbitol, Natural Flavor, Stearic Acid, Magnesium Stearate, Cellulose, Croscarmellose, Sucralose.
See Editor's Note No. 47 and No. 54.

Pinnacle Androstat6 - Bodyonics, Ltd.
Two tablets contain: Balanced Andro Complex: 4-androstene-3, 17-diol (4-androstenediol) 125 mg • 4-androstene-3,17-dione (4-androstenedione) 5 mg • 5-androstene-3, 17-dione (5-androstenedione) 5 mg • 5-androstene-3beta,17beta-diol (5-androstenediol) 5 mg • 19-nor-5-androstene-3, 17-diol (19-nor 5-androstendiol) 5 mg. Other Ingredients: Fructose, Sorbitol, Natural Licorice Flavor, Stearic Acid, Magnesium, Stearate and 100% Natural Beta Cyclodextrins.
See Editor's Note No. 47 and No. 54.

Pinnacle Beta Activated Protein with HMB - Bodyonics, Ltd.
Twelve tablets contain: Calcium B-Hydroxy B-Methylbutyrate Monohydrate (HMB) 3 g • Beta Peptide (a proprietary blend of very distinct cosein, whey and aligopeptides) 12 g • Alanine 392 mg • Arginine 419 mg • Aspartic Acid 713 mg • Cystine 74 mg • Glutamic Acid 2806 mg • Glycine 232 mg • Isoleucine (BCAA) 635 mg • Leucine (BCAA) 1044 mg • Lysine 906 mg • Methionine 307 mg • Phenylalanine 556 mg • Proline 1178 mg • Serine 617 mg • Threonine 494 mg • Tryptophan 142 mg • Tyrosine 461 mg • Valine (BCAA) 732 mg. Other Ingredients: Calcium Phosphate, Stearic Acid, Magnesium Stearate, Croscarmellose, Silica.

Pinnacle BHP-5 - Bodyonics, Ltd.
Each tablet contains: Hydrolyzed BHP5 (Pregnenolone) 15 mg. Other Ingredients: Calcium Phosphate, Stearic Acid, Magnesium Stearate, Croscarmellose.

Pinnacle Chrysinex 250 - Bodyonics, Ltd.
Each tablet contains: Chrysin Complex [Derived from a custonized blend of 98% pure 5,7-Dihydroxyflavone and natural powered extract poplar bud (Populus candicans)] 250 mg • Cruciferous Vegetable Concentrate (Standardized to contain 10% Indole 3-Carbinol) 25 mg. Other Ingredients: Calcium Phosphate, Stearic Acid, Magnesium Stearate, Lecithin, Xanthan Gum.

Pinnacle Cordyceps 500 - Bodyonics, Ltd.
Each tablet contains: Dong Chong Zia Cao (Cordyceps sinensis-winter bug, summer herb) • Sha Shen (Adenophora tetraphylla) • WuWei Zi (Schisandra chinensis) • Gan Jiang (Zingiber officinale) • Dahlulin (Dahlia inulin juice concentrate). Other Ingredients: Dicalcium Phosphate, Croscarmellose, Magnesium Stearate, Stearic Acid.

Pinnacle Crea Glutide 2400 - Bodyonics, Ltd.
Each tablet contains: Crea-Glutide 2400 mg • Creatine Monohydrate 2 g • Glutamine Peptide 400 mg. Other Ingredients: Calcium Phosphate, Stearic Acid, Magnesium Stearate, Croscarmellose.

Pinnacle Crea-Glutide - Bodyonics, Ltd.
Two tablespoons contains: Dextrose • BioReacted Crea-Glutide Complex • Complex Carbohydrate • Dahlulin (Dry Dahlia Inulin Juice Complex) • Citric Acid • Natural Cranberry Flavor • Xanthan Gum • Stevia Extract • Beet Extract.

Pinnacle CreaRibose ATP Kichers - Bodyonics, Ltd.
Six tablets contain: Creatine Monohydrate 5 grams • D-Ribose 3 g. Other Ingredients: Magnesium Stearate, Cellulose, Calcium Phosphate, Stearic Acid.

Pinnacle Fractionized CCK 100 - Bodyonics, Ltd.
Each tablet contains: Cholecystokinin (CCK) (Derived from a purified blend of edible bovine tissue fractions, providing 1000 picomotes of standardized Cholecystokinin (CCK) a bioactive substance) 100 mg. Other Ingredients: Calcium Phosphate, Microcrystalline Cellulose, Stearic Acid, Magnesium Stearate, Croscarmellose Silica.
See Editor's Note No. 14.

Pinnacle Gro Tropin - Bodyonics, Ltd.
Three capsules contain: Alpha GPC (alpha-glycerylphosphorylcholine) 500 mg • AminoGlutein Peptide Glutamine Peptide (30%) 500 mg • Colostrum (colostral isoform extract) 500 mg • Tribulus Terrestris (40% furostanol saponins) 500 mg • Phoshphatidylserine 500 mcg • Chrysin (98% pure 5,7 dehydroxyflavone) 750 mcg. Other Ingredients: Magnesium Stearate, Gelatin.

Pinnacle Horny Goat Weed - Bodyonics, Ltd.
Two capsules contain: Horny Goat Weed (Epimedium grandiflorum) standardized 10% Icariin 500 mg • Maca Pure (Lepidium meyenii) standardized to 0.6% macamides and macaenes 250 mg • Mucuna pruriens standardized 15% L-Dopa (L-dihydroxyphenylalanine) 33.3 mg • Polypodium vulgare standardized 8% 20-hydroxyecdysone 25 mg. Other Ingredients: Calcium Phosphate, Magnesium Stearate, Gelatin.

Pinnacle NoX2 - Bodyonics, Ltd.
Three tablets contain: Proprietary Blend 3000 mg: Arginine Alpha-Ketoglutarate (A-AKG), Arginine-Ketoisocaproate (A-KIC). Other Ingredients: Beta Cyclodextrin, Cephalins, Xanthan, Inulin, Sorbitol, Calcium Phosphate, Magnesium Stearate, Stearic Acid.

Pinnacle NoX2 Overnight Extender - Bodyonics, Ltd.
Four tablets contain: Citruline-HP (pure l-citruline citrate-malate) 2000 mg • Arginine Alpha-Ketoglutarate (A-AKG) 1500 mg • Arginine-Ketoisocaproate (A-KIC) • Proprietary NoX2 Enhancers 267 mg: Ketoisocaproate Potassium (klC-K), American Ginseng (Panax quinquefolius), Saw Palmetto (serenoa repens). Other Ingredients: Gama Cyclodextrin, Cephalins, Xanthan, Inulin, Sorbitol, Calcium Phosphate, Magnesium Stearate, Stearic Acid.

Pinnacle P-ALC 500 - Bodyonics, Ltd.
Each tablet contains: Phosphorolytic Acetyl L-Carnitine (PALC) (Including Inulin and Succunates) 500 mg. Other Ingredients: Calcium Phosphate, Stearic Acid, Magnesium Stearate, Silica, Croscarmellose.

Pinnacle PS Complex 500 - Bodyonics, Ltd.
Each tablet contains: Cephalized PS (Phosphatidyl Serine Complex) (BioActivated Phospholipid fractions standardized to 55% cephalins phosphatidyl serine, choline, inositol and ethanolamine) 500 mg. Other Ingredients: Microcrystalline Cellulose, Calcium Phosphate, Stearic Acid, Magnesium Stearate, Croscarmellose, Silica.

Pinnacle PYRUVATE 1000 - Bodyonics, Ltd.
Each tablet contains: Sodium 60 mg • Potassium 40 mg • Calcium 100 mg • Stabilized Trimin Pyruvate Complex 1000 mg (From Calcium, Potassium, and Sodium salts of Pyruvic Acid, plus Dihydroxyacetone. Inulinized in a bioactive complex of Phosphorolytic Dahlia Inulin providing a long chain carbohydrate molecule). Other Ingredients: Calcium Phosphate, Stearic Acid, Magnesium Stearate, Silica, Croscarmellose.

Pinnacle PYRUVATE 500 - Bodyonics, Ltd.
Each tablet contains: Sodium 30 mg • Potassium 20 mg • Calcium 50 mg • Stabilized Trimin Pyruvate Complex 500 mg (From Calcium, Potassium, and Sodium salts of Pyruvic Acid, plus Dihydroxyacetone. Inulinized in a bioactive complex of Phosphorolytic Dahlia Inulin providing a long chain carbohydrate molecule). Other Ingredients: Calcium Phosphate, Stearic Acid, Magnesium Stearate, Silica, Croscarmellose.

Pinnacle SAMe - Bodyonics, Ltd.
Each tablet contains SAM-e 200 mg • Vitamin B12 50 mcg • Folic Acid 100 mcg.

Pinnacle Super Crea Glutide A-DS - Bodyonics, Ltd.
Each scoop contains: Creatine Monohydrate 6 g • Glutamine Peptide 2 g • Taurine 2 g • Dahlulin (Dry Dahlia Inulin Juice Complex) 500 mg • Complex Carbohydrate • Natural Flavor • Xanthan Gum • Stevia Extract • Beta Carotene.

Pinnacle Thermophen - Bodyonics, Ltd.
Two tablets contain: St. John's Wort (0.3% hypericin) 150 mg • Citrus Aurantium (Bitter Orange peel) (1.5- 3% synephrine) 200 mg • Kava Kava (40% Kavalactones) 100 mg • Yerba Mate (20% Methylxanthines) 200 mg. Other Ingredients: Calcium Phosphate, Microcrystalline Cellulose, Stearic Acid, Magnesium Stearate, Croscarmellose.
See Editor's Note No. 40.

Pinnacle Tribestrol 250 - Bodyonics, Ltd.
Two captabs contain: Tribulus Terrestris (providing 40% (100 mg) Furostanol Saponins) 250 mg • Herbolics Support Complex (from Catuaga, Muira Puama, Chachuhuasu, Iporuru) 100 mg. Other Ingredients: Calcium Phosphate, Stearic Acid, Magnesium Stearate, Croscarmellose.

Pinnacle Ultra Strength Volumax (chocolate flavor) - Bodyonics, Ltd.
Two scoops contain: Whey Protein Concentrate (Ion Exchange) • Complex Carbohydrate (Maltodextrin) • Creatine Monohydrate • Dutch Cocoa powder • Soy Fiber • Oat Fiber • Natural & Artificial Vanilla Flavor • Glutamine Peptide • Dahluin (Dry Dahlia Inulin Juice Complex) • Whey Protein Hydrolysate • Taurine • Potassium Phosphate • Calcium Phosphate • Magnesium Oxide • Potassium Chloride • Xanthan Gum • Aspartame • Psyllium • Monosodium Phosphate • Ascorbic Acid • Beta Carotene • dl-Alpha Tocopheryl Acetate • Ferrous Fumarate • Niacinamide • Zinc Oxide • Vitamin A Palmitate • D-Calcium Pantothenate • Manganese Sulfate • RNA Powder • Soy Lecithin • Vitamin K (as Vitamin K1) • Copper Sulfate • Pyridoxine Hydrochloride • Riboflavin • Thiamine Hydrochloride • Cyanocobalamin • Vitamin D (D3) • Folic Acid • Chromium Chloride • Biotin • Selenomethionine • Chromium Picolinate • Sodium Molybdate • Potassium Iodide • Sodium Selenate.

Pinnacle Ultra Strength Volumax (vanilla flavor) - Bodyonics, Ltd.
Two scoops contain: Whey Protein Concentrate (Ion Exchange) • Complex Carbohydrate (Maltodextrin) • Creatine Monohydrate • Soy Fiber • Oat Fiber • Natural & Artificial Vanilla Flavor • Glutamine Peptide • Dahluin (Dry Dahlia Inulin Juice Complex) • Whey Protein Hydrolysate • Taurine • Potassium Phosphate • Calcium Phosphate • Magnesium Oxide • Potassium Chloride • Xanthan Gum • Aspartame • Psyllium • Monosodium Phosphate • Ascorbic Acid • Beta Carotene • dl-Alpha Tocopheryl Acetate • Ferrous Fumarate • Niacinamide • Zinc Oxide • Vitamin A Palmitate • D-Calcium Pantothenate • Manganese Sulfate • RNA powder • Soy Lecithin • Vitamin K (as Vitamin K1) • Copper Sulfate • Pyridoxine Hydrochloride • Riboflavin • Thiamine Hydrochloride • Cyanocobalamin • Vitamin D (as Vitamin D3) • Folic Acid • Chromium Chloride • Biotin • Selenomethionine • Chromium Picolinate • Sodium Molybdate • Potassium Iodide • Sodium Selenate.

Pinnacle Whey Ahead (chocolate flavor) - Bodyonics, Ltd.
One scoop contains: Whey Ahead Complex (a blend of Whey Protein Concentrates and Whey Protein Isolates, and Partially Pre-digested Ion Exchanged Whey Protein Hydrolysates) • Creatine Monohydrate • Glutamin Peptide • Dutch Cocoa Powder • Natural and Artifical Vanilla Flavor • Tourine • Dahlulin (Dry Dahlia Inulin Juice Complex) • Xanthan Gum • Beta Carotene • Aspartame.

Pinnacle Whey Ahead (vanilla flavored) - Bodyonics, Ltd.
Each scoop contains: Whey Ahead brand Complex: Whey Protein Concentrates, Whey Protein Isolates, Whey Protein Hydrolysates • Creatine Monohydrate • Glutamine Peptide • Natural and Artifical Vanilla Flavor • Tourine • Dahlulin (Dry Dahlia Inulin Juice Complex) • Xanthan Gum • Beta Carotene • Aspartame.

PinnoThin brand - Loders Croklaan
Pinolenic Acid from Korean Pine (pinus koraiensis).
See Editor's Note No. 44.

Pituitary Glandular - American Biologics
Each tablet contains: Raw Pituitary concentrate (bovine origin) 40 mg. Other Ingredients: Dicalcium Phosphate, Magnesium Stearate.
See Editor's Note No. 31.

Pituitrophin PMG - Standard Process, Inc.
Each tablet contains: Proprietary Blend 118 mg: Magnesium Citrate, Bovine Pituitary extract (45 mg). Other Ingredients: Calcium Lactate, Calcium Stearate, Cellulose.
See Editor's Note No. 31.

Pizazz - Nature's Plus
Each tablespoon contains: L-Phenylalanine free form amino acid 250 mg • Pantothenic Acid 75 mg • Inositol 50 mg • Niacinamide 40 mg • Vitamin B1 (Thiamine) 30 mg • Vitamin B2 (Riboflavin) 30 mg • Vitamin B6 (Pyridoxine HCL) 30 mg • Choline (Bitartrate) 21 mg • Vitamin B12 (from Cobalamin) 100 mcg • Biotin 30 mcg. In a natural high-energy base of Bee Pollen, Ginseng, Gotu Kola, & Fo-Ti. Sweetened with Honey & Blackstrap Molasses.

Placenta Out - TriLight Herbs
Dong Quai (angelica) • Blue Cohosh • Shepherd's Purse.

Plant Enzimase - Nutri-Quest Rx
Each 360 mg capsule contains: Amylase 4500 DU • Protease 15,000 HUT • Lipase 65 IU • Invertase 0.25 IAU • Malt Diastase 150 DPI • Lactase 200 LacU • Cellulase 60 CU. Base: Beet root fiber.

Plantain Buchu Supreme - Gaia Herbs
Thirty drops contain: Proprietary Blend 40 mg: Plantain leaf and corm (plantago lanceolata), Dried Buchu leaves (barosma betulina), Corn Silk (zea mays), Horsetail grass (equisetum arvense), St. John's Wort flower buds (hypericum perforatum), Arnica flowers (arnica latifolia), Thuja leaf (thuja occidentalis) • Spring Water • Pure Grain Alcohol USP.

Plantain Salve - Dial Herbs
Plantain • Chickweed • Mint • Comfrey • Oat Straw. In a base of Bees Wax, Glycerine & Cold Pressed Olive oil.

PLUS Herbal-Amino Acid - Mannatech
Each caplet contains: Iron 1 mg • Wild Yam (root; standardized for 25 mg phytosterols) 200 mg • L-Glutamic Acid 200 mg • Glycine 200 mg • L-Lysine 200 mg • L-Arginine 100 mg • Beta Sitosterol 25 mg • Proprietary Blend 2.5 mg: Arabinogalactan (larix decidua gum), Manapol Aloe Vera gel extract (inner leaf gel), Gum Ghatti, Gum Tragacanth. Other Ingredients: Microcrystalline Cellulose, Stearic Acid, Croscarmellose Sodium, Silicon Dioxide, Magnesium Stearate, Titanium Dioxide Coating.

PM Evening Activator - Slimlife
Two caplets contain: Niacin (as niacinamide) 20 mg • Vitamin B6 (as pyridoxine HCl) 2 mg • Potassium (as gluconate) 100 mg • L-Carnitine HCl 100 mg • Valerian root powder 50 mg. Other Ingredients: Dicalcium Phosphate, Cellulose, Stearic Acid, Magnesium Stearate, Silicone Dioxide, Croscarmellose Sodium, Pharmaceutical Glaze, Talc USP.

PM Herbal Cleansing Program Cleansing Formula - Herbalife International of America, Inc.
Each tablet contains: Calcium (as calcium carbonate) 208 mg • Exclusive Blend 507 mg: Bromelain, Patented Enzyme Complex (from DigeZyme), Aloe leaf, Rutin, Garlic bulb, 4-D Glucohydrolase, Triacylglycerol Aclhydrolase, Dried Fenugreek seed extract, Red Clover flower, Slippery Elm bark, Tang Kuei root, Hippophae Rhamnoides berry, Goldenseal root, Barberry root, Castor seed oil (ricinus communis), Lemon Bioflavonoids (citrus limon), Peppermint leaf, Catalase, Black Walnut leaf, L-Taurine, Dried Milk Thistle seed extract, N-Acetyl Cysteine. Other Ingredients: Stearic Acid, Cross-Linked Sodium Carboxymethylcellulose, Microcrystalline Cellulose, Silicon Dioxide, Hydroxypropyol Cellulose, Magnesium Stearate, Food Grade Shellac.

PM Menopause Formula - PhytoPharmica
PM Formula: Each purple tablet contains: Valerian root extract (valeriana officinalis, standardized to contain a minimum of 0.8% valerenic acids) 200 mg • Hops flower 6.6:1 extract (humulus lupulus) 100 mg • L-Theanine 50 mg • Black Cohosh root and rhizome extract (standardized to contain 2.5% triterpene glycosides calculated as 27-deoxyactein) 20 mg. Other Ingredients: Cellulose, Modified Cellulose, Modified Cellulose Gum, Magnesium Stearate, Carrot and Paprika Extract Color, Lecithin, Carnauba Wax.

PMS - Hyland's
Two tablets contain: Viburnum Opulus 2X • Caulophyllum Thalictroides 3X • Cocculus Indicus 3X • Gelsemium Sempervirens 3X. Base: Lactose USP.
See Editor's Note No. 1.

PMS Day 1-14 - Gaia Herbs
Two capsules contain: Chinese Dong Quai root (angelica sinensis) 164 mg • Black Cohosh root (cimicifuga racemosa) 30 mg • Saw Palmetto berry (serenoa repens) 20 mg • Licorice root (glycyrrhiza glabra) 20 mg • Partridgeberry (mitchella repens) 16 mg • Dandelion root and leaf (taraxacum off.) 14 mg • Ginger rhizome, supercritical CO2 extract (zingiber off.) 8 mg. Other Ingredients: Vegetable Glycerin, Lecithin, Vegetable Cellulose (capsule).

PMS Day 14-28 - Gaia Herbs
Three capsules contain: Chaste Tree berry (vitex agnus-castus) 90 mg • Dong Quai root (angelica sinensis) 54 mg • Kava Kava rhizome (piper methysticum) 42 mg • Licorice root (glycyrrhiza glabra) 30 mg • Black Cohosh rhizome (cimicifuga racemosa) 30 mg • Wild Yam root (dioscorea villosa) 24 mg • St. John's Wort flower bud (hypericum perforatum) 24 mg • Motherwort (leonurus cardiaca) 24 mg • Ginger rhizome, supercritical CO2 extract (zingiber off.) 12 mg. Other Ingredients: Vegetable Glycerin, Vegetable Cellulose.

PMS Escape - Back Bay Scientific
Each packet (50 g) contains: Vitamin C 60 mg • Vitamin B6 0.5 mg • Calcium 50 mg • Magnesium 20 mg. Ingredients: Simple Carbohydrates (dextrose), Complex Carbohydrates (maltodextrin, starch), Citric Acid, Ascorbic Acid, Pyridoxine Hydrochloride, Calcium Lactate, Magnesium Lactate, Natural & Artificial Flavor, FD&C Red #40.

PMS Formula - The Vitamin Shoppe
Each capsule contains: Vitamin B12 25 mcg • Vitamin B6 10 mg • St. John's Wort 150 mg • Siberian Ginseng 100 mg • Korean Ginseng root 50 mg • Chamomile 100 mg.

PMS Formula - Schiff
Three tablets contain: Vitamin E (as D-alpha tocopheryl acetate) 200 IU • Vitamin B1 (as thiamin mononitrate) 35 mg • Vitamin B6 (as pyridoxine hydrochloride) 50 mg • Folate (as folic acid) 400 mcg • Vitamin B12 12 mcg • Calcium (as calcium carbonate) 500 mg • Magnesium (as magnesium oxide) 200 mg • Zinc (as zinc gluconate) 2 mg • Chaste Tree berry extract (vitex agnus-castus) 20 mg • Dandelion 200 mg • Cramp Bark extract 80 mg • Ginger 70 mg. Other Ingredients: Cellusoe, Hydroxypropyl Methylcellulose, Cellulose Gum, Silicon Dioxide, Magnesium Stearate, Acacia, Maltodextrix, Methylcellulose, Gelatin, Polyethylene Glycol, Hydroxypropyl Cellulose.

PMS Formula - Nature's Way
Three capsules contain: Black Cohosh root 150 mg • Cramp bark 250 mg • Dandelion leaf 150 mg • L-5 Hydroxytryptophan (Griffonia bean extract) 5 mg • Lobelia herb 150 mg • Magnesium Amino Acid Chelate 50 mg • Niacin (Vitamin B3) 10 mg • Pyridoxine HCL 76 mg • Riboflavin (Vitamin B2) 852 mcg • Thiamine (Vitamin B1) 750 mcg • Vitamin B12 (Cyanocobalamin) 3 mcg. Other Ingredients: Gelatin, Millet.

PMS Formula - Puritan's Pride
Three tablets contain: Vitamin B-6 354 mg • Folic Acid 400 mcg • Calcium 125 mg • Magnesium 250 mg • Potassium 99 mg • Evening Primrose oil 500 mg • Proprietary Herbal Complex Blend 150 mg: derived from Dong Quai, Black Cohosh, Fo-Ti, Dandelion, Watercress, Parsley, Yellow Dock.

PMS Formula with Indolplex - PhytoPharmica
Two tablets contain: Vitamin D (as cholecalciferol) 250 IU • Calcium (as calcium citrate and calcium carbonate) 200 mg • Iodine (as potassium iodide) 80 mcg • Magnesium (as magnesium aspartate) 100 mg • Chaste Tree (Vitex-agnus castus) berry extract (standardized to contain a minimum of 0.5% agnuside) 20 mg • Diindolylmethane (DIM, as Indolplex brand blend) 14 mg.

PMS Forte - Futurebiotics LLC
Two tablets contain: Thiamin HCl (B1) 12 mg • Riboflavin (B2) 12 mg • Pyridoxine HCl (B6) 65 mg • Niacinamide 50 mg • Vitamin C (ascorbic acid) 60 mg • Dong Quai (extract equal to) 300 mg • Choline Bitartrate 75 mg • Para Amino Benzoic Acid (PABA) 85 mg • Methionine 60 mg • Inositol 50 mg • Iron (ferrous fumarate) 8 mg • Potassium (citrate, gluconate) 60 mg • Magnesium (oxide, amino acid chelate) 350 mg • Vitamin B12 40 mcg • Iodine (potassium, iodide) 150 mcg • Zinc (gluconate) 15 mg • Pantothenic Acid 60 mg • Folic Acid 400 mcg • Calcium (carbonate, phosphate) 300 mg • Vitamin E 30 IU • Ribonucleic Acid (RNA) 40 mg • Biotin 300 mcg. Base: Vitex Agnus Castus, Uva Ursi, Royal Jelly, Raw Alfalfa Juice

Concentrate, Cramp Bark, Betaine HCl, Chamomile, Squawvine, American Ginseng Extract, Chinese Licorice, Melissa, Marjoram, Polygonum Multiflorum.

PMS Multivitamin - Arrowroot
Six tablets contain: Beta Carotene 6250 IU • Bioflavonoids 250 mg • Vitamin A 6250 IU • Rutin 25 mg • Vitamin E 300 IU • Rose Hips 100 mg • Vitamin D (D3) 100 IU • Calcium 200 mg • Vitamin B1 25 mg • Magnesium 400 mg • Vitamin B2 25 mg • Iodine 150 mcg • Vitamin B3 25 mg • Iron 18 mg • Vitamin B6 300 mg • Copper 0.5 mg • Vitamin B12 70 mcg • Zinc 50 mg • Folic Acid 400 mcg • Manganese 10 mg • Biotin 70 mcg • Potassium 99 mg • Pantothenic Acid 100 mg • Selenium 100 mcg • Choline 300 mg • Chromium 100 mcg • Inositol 25 mg • Betaine HCl 100 mg • PABA 25 mg • Fatty Acids 50 mg • Vitamin C 1500 mg.

PMS Relief Formula - Body Language Vitamin Co.
Each capsule contains: Black Cohosh (Cimicifuga racemosa root, standardized to contain 2.5% triterpine glycosides) 200 mg • Dong Quai (Angelica sinensis root) 200 mg • Wild Yam 100 mg • Chastetree berry (Vitex agnus-castus fruit) 100 mg • Damiana (Turnera diffusa leaves) 50 mg • Red Raspberry 100 mg • Feverfew 150 mcg • Juniper berry 50 mg. Other Ingredients: Vegetable Cellulose Capsule, Rice Powder, Magnesium Stearate.

PMS Support - Vital Nutrients
Each capsule contains: Chaste Tree berry extract (vitex agnus castus, 0.5% agnuside) 200 mg • Dong Quai root 7:1 extract (angelica sinensis) 125 mg • Wild Yam root 10:1 extract (dioscorea villosa) 125 mg • Ashwagandha root 5:1 extract 50 mg • Passionflower (passiflora) 50 mg • Licorice root extract (16% glycyrrhizin) 25 mg.

PMS Symptom Free - Enzymatic Therapy
Two tablets contain: Vitamin D (as cholecalciferol) 250 IU • Calcium (as calcium carbonate, calcium citrate) 200 mg • Iodine (as potassium iodide) 80 mcg • Magnesium (as magnesium aspartate) 100 mg • Chaste Tree berry extract (vitex-agnus castus, standardized to contain 0.5% agnuside) 20 mg • Diindolylmethane (DIM) 14 mg. Other Ingredients: Cellulose, Modified Cellulose, Starch (corn), D-Alpha-Tocopheryl Succinate, Titanium Dioxide Color, Phosphatidylcholine, Lecithin, Silicon Dioxide, Carnauba Wax.

PMS Tea - Traditional Medicinals
One tea bag contains: Dandelion root: 500 mg. Other Herbal Ingredients: Roasted Carob pod, Roasted Barley, Roasted Chicory root, Parsley leaf, Oat Straw herb, Nettle leaf, Chickweed herb, Uva Ursi leaf, Cramp bark, Cornsilk style and stigma.

PMS Therapy Bath - Abra Therapeutics
Sodium Borate • Sodium Sulfate • Sodium Chloride • Sodium Sesquicarbonate • Olive oil • Geranium oil • Marjoram oil • Clary Sage oil • Chamomile oil • Nutmeg oil • Fennel oil • Peru Balsam oil • Melissa leaf extract • Vitex berry extract • Wild Yam root extract • Chromium Oxide • Trace Mineral Salts.

PMSOS - Nature's Herbs
Four capsules contain: Vitamin B6 500 mg • natural Vitamin E (D-Alpha Tocopherol Succinate) 400 IU • Uva Ursi extract (concentrated standardized for 10% Arbutin equivalent to 1200 of dried herb) 400 mg • Valerian root extract (standardized for .72-.88% valernic acid = to 1600 mg of dried herb) 400mg • White Willow bark extract (standardized for 15% salicin - White Willow extract 5:1= to 1600 mg of dried herb) 200 mg • Chasteberry extract (Vitex agnus castus - standardized for 11k ppm Glycosides equivalent to 600 mg of dried herb) 100 mg • Ginger root 305 mg • Dong Quai root 200 mg.

Pneumo-Carotene - Metagenics
Each tablet contains: Vitamin A (12% [2000 IU] as retinyl acetate and 88% [15,000 IU] as beta-carotene) 17,000 IU • Vitamin C (as ascorbic acid) 200 mg • Raw Lung concentrate (bovine) 200 mg • Vitamin E (as D-alpha tocopheryl succinate) 20 IU • Folic Acid 200 mcg • Selenium (as selenium aspartate) 10 mcg • Quercetin (as quercetin dihydrate) 25 mg.

Pneumotrate - Progressive Labs
Each capsule contains: Vitamin A 2500 IU • Beta Carotene 2500 IU • Vitamin C 90 mg • Bovine lung concentrate 200 mg.
See Editor's Note No. 14.

Pneumotrophin PMG - Standard Process, Inc.
Each tablet contains: Proprietary Blend 182 mg: Bovine Lung PMG extract, Magnesium Citrate • Calcium 20 mg • Sodium 15 mg. Other Ingredients: Cellulose.
See Editor's Note No. 14.

Poena - BotanicLab
Panax Pseudoginseng Wall (pseudo-ginseng; san-chi) • Achryanthes Bidentata Bl. (achyranthes; niu-hsi) • Corydalis Bulbosa (corydalis; yen-hu-suo) • Cynanchum Paniculatum Kitag (cynanchum; pai-chien) • Isatis Indigotica Fort (isatidis; ta-ching-yeh) • Paeonia Lactiflora Pall (white peony root; chih-shao) • Glycyrrhiza Glabra L. (licorice; gan-cao).

PoisePlus - Atrium Biotechnologies
Six tablets contain: Vitamin A 15000 IU • Vitamin E 140 IU • Vitamin C 1050 mg • Bioflavonoids 300 mg • Chlorophyll (oil) 60 mg • Along with the following Amino Acid chelated minerals: Calcium 500 mg • Magnesium 250 mg • Potassium 99 mg • Manganese 10 mg • Iron 15 mg • Zinc 10 mg • Copper 2 mg • Iodine 150 mcg • Chromium 200 mcg • Selenium 25 mcg • Molybdenum 150 mcg • Vanadium 150 mcg • Silicon 2 mcg. Base: Raw Bovine Tissue concentrates (not extracts): Spleen 150 mg, Brain 30 mg, Liver 25 mg, Heart 15 mg, Kidney 15 mg, Thymus 10 mg, Adrenal 10 mg, Pituitary 10 mg, Pancreas 10 mg, Duodenus 10 mg) 285 mg.
See Editor's Note No. 31.

Poison Ivy/Oak - Hyland's
Two tablets contain: Rhus Toxicodendron 6X • Croton Tiglium 6X • Xerophyllum 6X. Base: Lactose USP.
See Editor's Note No. 1.

Pokemon Children's Multiple Vitamin - Rexall - Sundown
Each chewable tablet contains: Vitamin A 5000 IU • Vitamin C (as sodium ascorbate and ascorbic acid) 60 mg • Vitamin D (as cholecalciferol) 400 IU • Vitamin E (as dl-alpha tocopheryl acetate) 30 IU • Thiamin (as thiamin mononitrate) 1.5 mg • Riboflavin 1.7 mg • Niacin (as niacinamide) 20 mg • Vitamin B-6 (as pyridoxine HCl) 2 mg • Folic Acid 400 mcg • Vitamin B-12 (as cyanocobalamin) 6 mcg • Biotin 40 mcg • Pantothenic Acid (as calcium D-pantothenate) 10 mg • Calcium 150 mg • Iron (as ferrous sulfate) 18 mg • Phosphorous 80 mg • Iodine (as potassium iodide) 150 mcg • Magnesium (as magnesium oxide) 20 mg • Zinc (as zinc oxide) 15 mg • Copper (as cupric oxide) 2 mg.

PoliChol - Life Enhancement Products, Inc.
Each capsule contains: Pantothenic Acid (vitamin B5 as calcium pantothenate) 100 mg • Vitamin C (as ascorbyl palmitate) 20 mg • Choline (as choline dihydrogen citrate) 100 mg • Policosanol 5 mg.

Policosanol - Life Extension Foundation
Each tablet contains: Policosanol (enhanced octasanol extract) 10 mg. Other Ingredients: Cellulose, mannitol, hydroxypropylmethylcellulose, citric acid, sodium starch glycolate, polyethylene glycol, croscarmellose sodium, stearic acid, silica, riboflavin.

Policosanol - Ortho Molecular Products
Each capsule contains: Policosanol (from sugar cane) 20 mg. Other Ingredients: Natural Vegetable Capsules, Ascorbyl Palmitate, Magnesium Stearate, Microcrystalline Cellulose, Silicon Dioxide.

Policosanol - Doctor's Trust Vitamins
Each tablet contains: Calcium (dicalcium phosphate) 82 mg • Policosanol 10 mg. Other Ingredients: Dicalcium Phosphate, Stearic Acid, Magnesium Trisilicate, Magnesium Stearate, Pharmaceutical Glaze.

Policosanol 10 mg - Pure Encapsulations
Each vegetable capsule contains: Policosanol (from sugar cane wax) 10 mg: 1-octacosanol 6-8 mg, 1-triacontanol 0-2 mg, 1-hexacosanol 0.2-3 mg, 1-tetracosanol 0-1 mg, 1-nonacosanol 0-1 mg, 1-dotriacontanol 0.01-1 mg, 1-tetratriacontanol 0.01-1 mg, 1-heptacosanol 0-0.06 mg.

Policosanol 20 mg - Pure Encapsulations
Each vegetable capsule contains: Policosanol (from sugar cane wax) 20 mg: 1-octacosanol 12-15 mg, 1-triacontanol 0-4 mg, 1-hexacosanol 0.4-6 mg, 1-tetracosanol 0-2 mg, 1-nonacosanol 0-2 mg, 1-dotriacontanol 0.02-2 mg, 1-tetratriacontanol 0.02-2 mg, 1-heptacosanol 0-0.1 mg.

Policosanol Cholesterol Complex - Source Naturals
Three tablets contain: Vitamin C (ascorbic acid) 600 mg • Vitamin E (natural D-alpha-tocopheryl) 200 IU • Niacin (inositol hexanicotinate) 500 mg • Iodine (from kelp) 150 mcg • Chromium (chromium picolinate and ChromeMate) 100 mcg • Phytosterols Complex (40% yielding 300 mg beta-sitosterol) 750 mg • Inositol (hexanicotinate) 640 mg • Garlic powder extract (standardized to 8000 ppm allicin) 600 mg • Turmeric extract (95% curcumin) 526 mg • Artichoke extract (standardized to 2.5% cynarins) 250 mg • Methylmethioninesulfonium Chloride (vitamin U) 200 mg • Green Tea extract 95% 100 mg • Soy Bean concentrate (40 mg isoflavones) 100 mg • Guggul Gum resin extract (standardized to 2.5% Gugulipid: guggulsterones Z & E) 100 mg • Ginkgo Biloba leaf 24% (50:1 extract) 60 mg • Dandelion root 4:1 extract 50 mg • Hawthorn berry 4:1 extract 50 mg • Myricetin 30 mg • Policosanol 20 mg. Other Ingredients: Stearic Acid, Modified Cellulose Gum, Hydroxy Propyl Cellulose, Colloidal Silicon Dioxide, Magnesium Stearate.

Polishing Peel - Nu Skin Enterprises
Water (aqua) • Bentonite • Zea Mays starch (corn) • Glycerin • Sorbitol • PEG-40 Hydrogenated Castor oil • Lactobacillus / Cucurbita Pepo fruit ferment extract • Polygonum Cuspidatum root extract • Hamamelis Virginiana water (witch hazel) • Caprylyl Glycol • Polysorbate 80 • Polyvinyl Alcohol • Hexylene Glycol • Ammonium Laureth Sulfate • C20-40 Pareth-10,1,2-Hexanediol • Disodium EDTA • Fragrance (parfum) • Ammonium Silver Zinc Aluminum Silicate • Titanium Dioxide.

Poly C - Golden Glow Natural Health Products
Each 1.25 mL serving (1.03 g) contains: Total Ascorbic Acid (vitamin C) 404.79 mg (from calcium ascorbate 412 mg, potassium ascorbate 41.2 mg, magnesium ascorbate 41.2 mg • Citrus Bioflavonoid extract 2.06 mg • Hesperidin 5.15 mg • Rosehips powder (rosa canina) 2.06 mg. Other Ingredients: Gluten (from maltodextrin, derived from wheat).

Poly C - USANA Health Sciences
Each tablet contains: Vitamin C (as Calcium, Potassium, Magnesium, and Zinc Ascorbates) 600 mg • Citrus Bioflavonoids (Citrus SPP. L.) fruit 65 mg • Rutin 7 mg • Quercetin 3 mg. Other Ingredients: Fumed Silica, Purified Water.

Poly C Mixed Ascorbates - Golden Glow Natural Health Products
Each tablet contains: Ascorbic Acid (vitamin C, from calcium ascorbate dihydrate 330 mg, magnesium ascorbate 350 mg and potassium ascorbate 320 mg) 760.93 mg • Citrus Bioflavonoid extract 100 mg.

Polyerga Plus - Polyerga
Each tablet contains: Peptides from Porcine Spleen 230 mg. Other Ingredients: Sucrose, Talc, Microcrystalline Cellulose, Calcium Carbonate, Clay, Polyvinyl Pyrrolidone, Powdered Cellulose, Acacia, Shellac, Corn Syrup, Titanium Dioxide, Magnesium Stearate, Cornstarch, Silicon Dioxide, Ferric Oxide, Polyethylene Glycol (MW 6000), Montan Glycol Wax, Castor Oil, Polyoxylated Castor Oil, Sodium Lauryl Sulfate.

Poly-MVA - AMARC Enterprises
Two teaspoons contain: Proprietary Blend: Palladium, Molybdenum, Ruthenium, Rhodium, Lipoic Acid, Vitamin B1 (HCl), Vitamin B2, Vitamin B12, Vitamin A, Acetyl Cysteine, Formyl Methionine. See Editor's Note No. 24.

Polyphenon 100 Green Tea Catechin Capsules - Origin BioMedicinals
Polyphenon 70 Green Tea extract (100 mg catechins) • Vitamin E (D-alpha-tocopherol) • Soybean Oil • Wheat Germ Oil • Beeswax • Gelatin • Emulsifier.

Polyphenon Green Tea Acne Cream - Origin BioMedicinals
Jojoba Oil • Bees Wax • Lecithin • Ascorbyl Palmitate (vitamin C) • Sorbic Acid • 3% Polyphenon 70 Green Tea extract • 0.5% Salicylic Acid • 0.2% Tea Tree Oil.

Polyphenon Green Tea Skin Cream - Origin BioMedicinals
Jojoba oil • Aloe Vera • Beeswax • Lecithin • Polyphenon 70 Green Tea extract • Ascorbyl Palmitate • Lavender oil • Tea Tree oil.

Polysorbate 80 - The Vitamin Shoppe
Contains 100% pharmaceutical-grade Polysorbate 80.

Poly-Vi-Sol Chewable Vitamins - Mead Johnson Nutritionals
Each chewable tablet contains: Vitamin A Acetate 2500 IU • Vitamin C (Ascorbic Acid) 60 mg • Vitamin D (Vitamin D3) 400 IU • Vitamin E Acetate 15 IU • Thiamin Mononitrate 1.05 mg • Riboflavin 1.2 mg • Niacin (Niacinamide) 13.5 mg • Vitamin B-6 Hydrochloride 1.05 mg • Folate (Folic Acid) 0.3 mg • Vitamin B-12 4.5 mcg • Iron (Ferrous Fumarate)12 mg • Zinc Oxide 8 mg • Copper (Cupric Oxide) 0.8 mg. Other Ingredients: Dextrates, Sugar, Sodium Ascorbate, Magnesium Stearate, Stearic Acid, Silicon Dioxide, Artificial Flavor and Color (Red 40 Lake), Salt.

PolyVytaMyns - InterPlexus
Two capsules contain: Vitamin A (47% (10,000 IU) as palmitate, 53% (11,400 IU) as beta carotene) 21,400 IU • Vitamin D (as cholecalciferol) 800 IU • Vitamin E (as D-alpha tocopheryl acetate) 80 IU • Vitamin K (as phytonadione) 960 mcg • Thiamin (vitamin B1) 14 mg • Riboflavin (vitamin B2) 14 mg • Niacin (as niacinamide) 66 mg • Vitamin B6 (as pyridoxine) 72 mg • Folic Acid 1600 mcg • Vitamin B12 (as hydroxycobalamine) 140 mcg • Biotin 4000 mcg • Pantothenic Acid (vitamin B5) 270 mg • Iodine (as potassium iodide) 200 mcg • Zinc (as malate) 20 mg • Selenium (AAC) 70 mcg • Copper (as citrate) 2 mg • Manganese (as citrate) 2 mg • Chromium (as polynicotinate) 100 mcg • Molybdenum (as chelate) 400 mcg • Boron (as aspartate) 2 mg • L-Cysteine HCl 152 mg. Other Ingredients: Boswellia, Rosemary Extract, Hesperidin, Hesperidin Methyl Chalcone, Naringin, Cellulose, Natural Oils.

Polyzyme - Young Living Essential Oils
Each capsule contains: Proprietary Blend: Protease, Phylase, Peptidase, Papain, Bromelain, Lipase, Anise Oil, Peppermint Oil, Rosemary Oil.

POM Wonderful Pomegranate Blueberry - POM Wonderful LLC
100% Pomegranate, Blueberry, Pineapple, Blackberry juices (from concentrates and natural flavors).

POM Wonderful Pomegranate Cherry - POM Wonderful LLC
100% Pomegranate, Cherry, Pineapple juices (from concentrates and natural flavors).

POM Wonderful Pomegranate Juice - POM Wonderful LLC
100% Pomegranate juice (from concentrates and natural flavors).

POM Wonderful Pomegranate Mango - POM Wonderful LLC
100% Pomegranate, Mango juices (from concentrates and natural flavors).

Some Brand Name Natural Products - What they Contain

www.NaturalDatabase.com contains MANY more listings than appear here.
Editor's Notes are located on pages 2155-2163.

POM Wonderful Pomegranate Tangerine - POM Wonderful LLC
100% Pomegranate, Orange, Tangerine juices (from concentrates and natural flavors).

PomActive brand - Cyvex Nutrition, Inc.
Pomegranate extract (70% ellagic acid).
See Editor's Note No. 44.

Pomegranate 250 mg - Vitamin World
Each capsule contains: Pomegranate seed (punica granatum) 200 mg • Pomegranate fruit extract (punica granatum, 40% ellagic acid) 50 mg. Other Ingredients: Rice Powder, Gelatin, Vegetable Magnesium Stearate, Silica.

Pomegranate Juice Concentrate - Jarrow Formulas
Each 1 tbsp (15 mL) serving contains: Pomegranate juice concentrate 15 mL: Total Polyphenols 165 mg, Ellagic Acid 21 mg, Gallic Acid 7 mg.

PomEllagic 70 brand - Cyvex Nutrition, Inc.
Pomegranate extract.

PomEllagic Plus - Pure Encapsulations
Each vegetable capsule contains: Pomegranate fruit extract (punica granatum L., standardized to contain 70% ellagic acid) 250 mg • Red Raspberry fruit extract (rubus idaeus, standardized to contain 40% ellagic acid) 100 mg • Vitamin C (as ascorbyl palmitate) 5 mg.

Ponaris Nasal Emollient - Jamol Laboratories
Active Ingredients: Pine Oil, Eucalyptus Oil, Peppermint Oil, Cajeput Oil, Cottonseed Oil as iodized organic oils. Total Iodine 0.5%-0.7%.

Portion Control Formula - Abundance Marketing
Galactomannan/Glucomannane Blend • Caffeine from Guarana seed extract • Green Tea extract • Galangal root extract • Cinnamon twig extract. Other Ingredients: Gelatin, Calcium Sulfate, Magnesium Stearate, Silica.

POS 1 Amino and Herbal Dietary Supplement - Advocare International
Each caplet contains: Niacin 7 mg • Magnesium (as amino acid chelate) 50 mg • Zinc (as monomethionine) 2 mg • Copper (as amino acid chelate) 167 mcg • Moomiyo 33 mg • L-Arginine 400 mg • L-Ornithine 200 mg • Oat Grass leaf/stem extract (avena sativa) 67 mg • Nettle leaf extract (urtica dioica) 17 mg • Eleuthero root extract (eleutherococcus senticosus) 8 mg • Ashwagandha root extract (withania somnifera) 17 mg • Saw Palmetto berry extract (serenoa repens) 33 mg • Wild Yam root extract (dioscorea villosa) 17 mg • Vanadium (as bis-maltolato-oxovanadium) 67 mcg.

POS 2 Drink Mix - Advocare International
Each pouch contains: Choline 50 mcg • Inositol 50 mg • Vanadium 200 mcg • Boron 250 mcg • Gamma Oryzanol 150 mcg • L-Carnitine 25 mg • Inosine 100 mg • Silicon 1 mg • Creatine 2000 mg • DL-Methionine 250 mg • L-Leucine 200 mg • L-Valine 100 mg • L-Isoleucine 100 mg • Maltodextrin • Fructose • Soy Protein powder • Modified Casein • Cocoa powder • MyoForce: Creatine Monohydrate, Creatine Phosphate, Eleuthero root • Soy Lecithin • Canola oil • Dicalcium Phosphate • Carob powder • Salt • Medium Chain Triglycerides • Magnesium Oxide • Calcium Carbonate • DL-Methionine • Natural Flavors • Artificial Flavors • L-Leucine • Potassium Chloride • Xanthan Gum • Silicon Dioxide • Guar Gum • Ascorbic Acid • L-Valine • L-Isoleucine • Inosine • Rice Syrup Solids • Fructooligosaccharides • Citrus Pectin • Inositol • Zinc Gluconate • Calcium Pantothenate • L-Carnitine • Niacinamide • Vitamin E Succinate • Beta Carotene • Manganese Sulfate • Ferrous Fumarate • Selenomethionine • Calcium Borate • Copper Gluconate • Pyridoxine Hydrochloride • Riboflavin • Thiamine Hydrochloride • Vanadyl Sulfate • Chromium Polynicotinate (ChromeMate brand) • Cholecalciferol • Papain • Bromelain • Gamma Oryzanol • Folic Acid • Choline Dihydrogen Citrate • Biotin • Sodium Molybdate • Dibencozide • Cyanocobalamin • Potassium Iodide.

POS 3 - Advocare International
Each pouch contains: Pure Crystalline Fructose • Maltodextrin • Malic Acid • Dextrose • Magnesium Citrate • Sodium Citrate • Potassium Citrate • Calcium Phosphate • L-Glutamine • Ascorbic Acid • Salt • L-Arginine • Potassium Chloride • Natural Flavors • Beta-Carotene • Beet juice concentrate (for color) • Sucralose • Vegetable Gum • Pyridoxine Alpha-Ketoglutarate • Niacinamide • Calcium Pantothenate • Riboflavin • Thiamine Hydrochloride • Chromium Polynicotinate (ChromeMate brand) • L-Glutathione • Coenzyme Q-10.

POS 4 Arginine Power - Advocare International
Each rounded tablespoon contains: Vitamin A (as beta carotene) 1250 IU • Folate 100 mcg • Pantothenic Acid (as calcium salt) 50 mg • Vitamin B12 (as cyanocobalamin) 60 mcg • Chromium (as polynicotinate) 60 mcg • L-Arginine 5 g • -Glycine 1 g • DL-Methionine 150 mg • Choline (as bitartrate) 100 mg.

POS 5 - Advocare International
Three caplets contain: B-Hydroxymethylbutyrate 2000 mg • Suma root extract (pfaffia paniculata) 200 mg • Green Tea leaf extract (camellia sinensis) 120 mg • Moomiyo 50 mg • Ashwagandha root extract (withania somnifera) 100 mg. Other Ingredients: Dicalcium Phosphate, Silicon Dioxide, Cellulose, Stearic Acid, Magnesium Stearate.

POS Muscle Fuel - Advocare International
Each pouch (0.8 oz/22.5 g) contains: Vitamin A (as beta-carotene) 1250 IU • Vitamin C (as ascorbic acid) 180 mg • Folic Acid 100 mg • Vitamin B12 (as cyanocobalamin) 30 mcg • Pantothenic Acid (as calcium pantothenate) 20 mg • Calcium (as calcium citrate) 200 mg • Magnesium (as magnesium citrate) 40 mg • Zinc (as zinc gluconate) 3 mg • Chromium (as chromium citrate) 60 mcg • Sodium (as bicarbonate) 140 mg • Potassium (as bicarbonate) 150 mg • Creatine (as citrate and monohydrate) 3 g • L-Arginine Alpha-Ketoglutarate 2 g • D-Ribose 1.5 g • Green Tea leaf extract (camellia sinensis) 500 mg • Calcium Pyruvate 500 mg • Glycine 500 mg • L-Carnitine 400 mg • L-Citrulline 200 mg • Betaine (as HCl) 100 mg • Caffeine 70 mg • Vanadium (as amino acid chelate) 4 mg • Boron (as amino acid chelate) 100 mcg. Other Ingredients: Maltodextrin, Bicarbonates of Potassium, Sodium and Calcium, Citric Acid, Malic Acid, Tartaric Acid, Aspartic Acid, Calcium Silicate, Natural and Artificial Flavors, Beet Root Juice Powder, Sucralose.

Positive Thoughts - Source Naturals
Three tablets contain: St. John's Wort (Hypericum Perforatum) 900 mg (Yielding 0.3% Hypericin 2.7 mg) • Valerian root extract (Valeriana officinalis) 100 mg (Yielding 0.8% Valerenic Acids 800 mcg) • Kava Root Extract (Piper methysticum) 85 mg (Yielding 30% Kavalactones 25 mg) • Lemon Balm (Melissa officinalis) 100 mg • GABA (Gamma Amino Butyric Acid) 300 mg • Taurine (Magnesium Taurinate) 200 mg • Magnesium (oxide, taurinate) 200 mg • L-Tyrosine 200 mg • N-Acetyl L-Tyrosine 50 mg • L-Phenylalanine 100 mg • DMAE (Dimethylaminoethanol bitartrate) 60 mg • Vitamin C (Zinc ascorbate) 50 mg • Vitamin B1 (Thiamin) 25 mg • Vitamin B2 (Riboflavin) 25 mg • Niacinamide 50 mg • Vitamin B5 (Pantothenic Acid) 25 mg • Vitamin B6 (Pyridoxine HCl) 50 mg • Vitamin B12 (Cyanocobalamin) 25 mg • Biotin 300 mcg • Folic Acid 400 mcg • Manganese 3 mg • Zinc (ascorbate) 10 mg.

Post Laser Surgery - Natural Ophthalmics
Active Ingredients: Arnica 12x • Eyebright (euphrasia) 8x • Staphysagria 6x • Aconite 12x • Hypericum 6x. Inactive Ingredients: Sterile Water, Sodium Chloride, Citrates, Polysorbate 80.

Post-Menopausal Formula - Oasis Wellness Network
Each tablet contains: Vitamin D (cholecalciferol) 67 IU • Vitamin E (D-alpha tocopheryl acetate) 20 IU • MaxCell Proprietary Blend 33 mg: Zisyphus Jujube, Aloe Vera gel, Glycyrrhiza Glabra, Piper Nigrum • Soy Isoflavone extract 8 mg • Black Cohosh root extract 5 mg • Vitamin C (ascorbyl palmitate) 3 mg • Calcium (citrate/malate/phosphate) 24 mg • Flax seed powder 133 mg • Wild Yam root extract 100 mg • Dong Quai root extract 67 mg. Other Ingredients: Stearic Acid, Cellulose, Calcium Sulfate, Magnesium Stearate, Silica.

BRAND NAMES

Some Brand Name Natural Products - What they Contain

www.NaturalDatabase.com contains MANY more listings than appear here.
Editor's Notes are located on pages 2155-2163.

BRAND NAMES

Posture-D - S.C.P.I.
Two tablets contain: Calcium (as tribasic calcium phosphate) 1200 mg • Vitamin D (as cholecalciferol) 250 IU. Other Ingredients: Dextrose, Carboxymethylcellulose Sodium, Magnesium Stearate, Adipic Acid, Natural & Artificial Flavors, FD&C Red #40 Aluminum Lake, FD&C Blue #2 Aluminum Lake, FD&C Yellow #6 Aluminum Lake.

Posture-D - Inverness Medical Innovations, Inc.
Each tablet contains: Vitamin D (as cholecalciferol) 125 IU • Calcium (as tribasic) 600 mg. Other Ingredients: Maltodextrin, Croscarmellose Sodium, Cellulose, Hydroxypropyl Methylcellulose, Citric Acid, Starch, Silicon Dioxide, Magnesium Stearate, Titanium Dioxide, Mineral Oil, Polysorbate 80, Sodium Lauryl Sulfate.

Potassium - Solgar
Each tablet contains: Calcium (as dicalcium phosphate) 70 mg • Potassium (as potassium gluconate) 99 mg. Other Ingredients: Dicalcium Phosphate, Silica, Vegetable Cellulose, Vegetable Magnesium Stearate.

Potassium - Solgar
Each tablet contains: Calcium (as dicalcium phosphate) 70 mg • Potassium (as potassium gluconate) 99 mg. Other Ingredients: Dicalcium Phosphate, Silica, Vegetable Cellulose, Vegetable Magnesium Stearate.

Potassium - Eidon Inc.
Each 1 tbsp serving contains: Potassium 35 mg. Other Ingredients: Purified Water.

Potassium - GNC
Each tablet contains: Potassium (as Potassium Gluconate) 99 mg. Other Ingredients: Dextrose, Stearic Acid, Silica, Magnesium Stearate.

Potassium - Source Naturals
Each tablet contains: Potassium (from 495 mg of potassium amino acid chelate) 99 mg.

Potassium - J. R. Carlson Laboratories, Inc.
Each tablet contains: Potassium 99 mg.

Potassium & Magnesium Aspartate 250 - GNC
Each capsule contains: Magnesium (as Monomagnesium Di-L-Aspartate) 250 mg • Potassium (as Monopotassium Aspartate) 250 mg. Other Ingredients: Gelatin, Cellulose.

Potassium (aspartate) - Pure Encapsulations
Each vegetable capsule contains: Potassium (citrate) 99 mg • Vitamin C (as ascorbyl palmitate) 11 mg.

Potassium (citrate) - Pure Encapsulations
Each vegetable capsule contains: Potassium (citrate) 200 mg • Vitamin C (as ascorbyl palmitate) 11 mg.

Potassium 100 mg Timed Release - Jamieson
Each caplet contains: Potassium 100 mg.

Potassium 50 mg - Jamieson
Each tablet contains: Potassium (as Potassium Gluconate) 50 mg.

Potassium 99 mg - Sunmark
Each caplet contains: Potassium (gluconate) 99 mg. Other Ingredients: Stearic Acid, Magnesium Stearate, Hydroxypropyl Methylcellulose, Hydroxypropyl Cellulose, Polyethylene Glycol. See Editor's Note No. 45.

Potassium Amino Acid Complex - Solgar
Each tablet contains: Potassium (as potassium glycinate amino acid complex) 99 mg. Other Ingredients: Microcrystalline Cellulose, Vegetable Cellulose, Vegetable Stearic Acid.

Potassium and Magnesium Aspartate - Golden Glow Natural Health Products
Each tablet contains: Potassium Aspartate 250 mg: Potassium 54.24 mg • Magnesium Aspartate 250 mg: Magnesium 18.72 mg.

Potassium Caps - TwinLab
Each capsule contains: Potassium (from potassium citrate and potassium aspartate) 99 mg. Other Ingredients: Gelatin, Potato Starch, Purified Water, Magnesium Stearate, MCT, Silica.

Potassium Fuel - TwinLab
Two capsules contain: Potassium Alpha-Ketoglutarate (supplying Elemental Potassium 99 mg) 325 mg • Magnesium Alpha-Ketoglutarate (Elemental Magnesium 100 mg) 700 mg.

Potassium Gluconate - GNC
Each tablet contains: Potassium (as potassium gluconate) 99 mg. Other Ingredients: Dextrose.

Potassium Gluconate 550 mg - Nature Made
Each tablet contains: Potassium 90 mg • Potassium (from 550 mg potassium gluconate) 90 mg. Other Ingredients: Cellulose Gel, Stearic Acid, Magnesium Stearate, Silicon Dioxide, Croscarmellose Sodium. See Editor's Note No. 45.

Potassium Gluconate with Folic Acid - Quest
Each tablet contains: Potassium Gluconate 650 mg • Folic Acid 400 mcg. Other Ingredients: Croscarmellose Sodium, Calcium phosphate, Magnesium Stearate (vegetable source), Microcrystalline Cellulose, Vegetable Stearin.

Potassium Magnesium (aspartate) - Pure Encapsulations
Each vegetable capsule contains: Potassium (citrate) 99 mg • Magnesium (citrate) 70 mg • Vitamin C (as ascorbyl palmitate) 8 mg.

Potassium Magnesium (citrate) - Pure Encapsulations
Each vegetable capsule contains: Potassium (citrate) 140 mg • Magnesium (citrate) 70 mg • Vitamin C (as ascorbyl palmitate) 11 mg.

Potassium Magnesium Aspartate - Solgar
Each capsule contains: Magnesium (as magnesium aspartate) 20 mg • Potassium (as potassium aspartate) 50 mg. Other Ingredients: Vegetable Cellulose, Vegetable Stearic Acid, Vegetable Magnesium Stearate, Water, Vegetable Glycerin.

Potassium Plus - PhytoPharmica
Each tablet contains: Colloidal Alkaline Ash Mineral Concentrate 80 mg: Dulse whole plant (palmaria palmata), Orange fruit (citrus sinesis), Banana fruit (musa paradisiaca), Sugarcane stalk concentrate (saccharum officinarum) • Mojave Yucca stem and root (yucca schidgera) 25 mg • Pantothenic Acid (as calcium D-pantothenate) 5 mg • Potassium (as potassium chloride and potassium citrate) 100 mg • Proprietary Trace Mineral Blend 125 mg: Selenium (as selenium yeast, SelenoExcell brand), Silicon (as magnesium trisilicate), Boron (as sodium borate), Nickel (as nickel chelate), Tin (as tin chelate), Molybdenum (as sodium molybdate), Vanadium (as vanadyl sulfate) • Vitamin B6 (as pyridoxine HCl) 1 mg.

Potassium Plus - Olympian Labs
Each capsule contains: Potassium Gluconate 99 mg • Dandelion 100 mg • Barley Grass 100 mg • Red Clover 50 mg • Basil 50 mg • Mulberry leaf 100 mg • Blessed Thistle 50 mg.

Potassium Plus - Enzymatic Therapy
Each tablet contains: Potassium (Chloride/Citrate) 99 mg • Magnesium Citrate 10 mg • Magnesium Sulfate 5 mg • Pantothenic Acid (D-calcium pantothenate) 5 mg • Vitamin B6 (pyroxidine HCl) 1 mg. Other Ingredients: Colloidal Alkaline Ash Mineral concentrate: Alfalfa juice concentrate, Sea Plant extract, Bio-Min TR8 (Enzymatic Tract Mineral concentrate), Orange juice concentrate, Banana concentrate, Sugar Cane juice concentrate 855 mg, Yucca 25 mg.

Potassium Plus - GNC
Two tablets contain: Vitamin A (beta-carotene) 5000 IU • Vitamin C (ascorbic acid) 60 mg • Riboflavin (B2) 1.7 mg • Pantothenic Acid (calcium D-pantothenate) 5 mg • Calcium (calcium carbonate and dicalcium phosphate) 250 mg • Phosphorus (dicalcium phosphate) 50 mg • Magnesium (oxide) 100 mg • Zinc (citrate) 5 mg • Potassium (gluconate) 99 mg. Other Ingredients: Cellulose, Titanium Dioxide, Vegetable Acetoglycerides, Rose Hips powder (Rosina canina).

Potency Formula - HERBALmax
Lurong • Indian Mulberry root • Eucommia bark • Chinese Angelica root • Peach seed • Ginseng • Ligustri Lucidi fruit.

Potency Plus - Gero Vita International
Each capsule contains: Morinda Officinalis root extract (5% anthroquinones) 70 mg • Curculigo Orchioides rhizome 8:1 extract 70 mg • Epimedium Grandiflorum leaf extract (5% flavonoids) 70 mg • Rubus Chingii berries extract (12% organic acids) 70 mg • Rehmannia Glutinosa root extract (1% catalpol) 30 mg • Dioscorea Opposita root extract (6% diosgenines) 30 mg • Salvia Miltiorrhiza root 8:1 extract 30 mg • Panax Ginseng root extract (20% ginsenosides) 30 mg • Cinnamomum Cassia bark extract (5% cinnamaldehyde) 30 mg • Ligusticum Chuanxiang rhizome extract (5% ligustrazin) 30 mg. Other Ingredients: Dicalcium Phosphate, Cellulose, Sodium Croscarmellose, Stearic Acid, Silica, Magnesium Stearate, Gelatin, ACF 223.

Potent V with Herbs - Vitamin World
Two tablets contain: Niacin 45 mg • Guarana seed extract (paullinia cupana, standardized to 22% caffeine) 300 mg • Yohimbe bark extract (standardized to 2% yohimbine) 250 mg • Taurine 200 mg • Oats aerial 10:1 extract (avena sativa) 150 mg • Saw Palmetto berry 4:1 extract (serenoa repens) 100 mg • Orchic Substance (raw testicular extract) 50 mg • Ginkgo Biloba leaf extract (standardized to 24% ginkgo flavone glycosides) 40 mg • Korean Ginseng root (panax ginseng) 30 mg. Other Ingredients: Cellulose, Dicalcium Phosphate, Croscarmellose, Vegetable Stearic Acid, Acacia Gum, Silica, Vegetable Magnesium Stearate, Polyvinylpyrrolidone, Cellulose.

Potent-C Energy - Nature's Plus
Each packet contains: Vitamin A (as beta carotene) 500 IU • Vitamin C (as ascorbic acid) 1000 mg • Vitamin D (as ergocalciferol) 50 IU • Vitamin E (as acetate) 5 IU • Thiamin (vitamin B1, as thiamine HCl) 1 mg • Riboflavin (vitamin B2) 1 mg • Niacin 10 mg • Vitamin B6 (as pyridoxine HCl) 2 mg • Folate 50 mcg • Vitamin B12 (as cyanocobalamin) 10 mcg • Biotin 10 mcg • Pantothenic Acid (as calcium pantothenate) 5 mg • Calcium (as carbonate) 100 mg • Magnesium (as carbonate) 20 mg • Zinc (as carbonate) 5 mg • Selenium (as selenomethionine) 10 mcg • Manganese (as aminoate complex) 2 mg • Chromium (as amino acid chelate) 10 mcg • Potassium (as bicarbonate) 99 mg. Other Ingredients: Fructose, Natural Orange Flavor, Maltodextrin, Guar Gum, Annatto Seed Extract (natural color), Lemon Bioflavonoids, Rutin, Hesperidin, Rose Hips, Acerola Cherry, CoQ10, Green Tea, Ginger, Bee Pollen, Rare Earth Trace Elements.

Power Fuel (Exercise & Recovery Drink) - TwinLab
Each serving contains: Carbohydrates (derived from Glucose Polymers & Glucose with small amounts of Fructose) 100 g • Anticatabolic Branched Chain Amino Acids (L-Leucine, L-Isoleucine, L-Valine) • L-Glutamine & Alpha-Ketoglutarates • Antioxidant Nutrients: Vitamin E, Vitamin C, & Beta-Carotene • B Vitamins • Chromium (from patented Chromic Fuel Chromium Picolinate) • Coenzyme Q10 • L-Carnitine • Potassium • Magnesium • Phosphate & Creatine • Carni Fuel (L-Carnitine & Magnesium).

Power Generation - Rexall - Sundown
Three capsules contain: L-Tyrosine 750 mg • DMAE (as 2-dimethylaminoethanol L-bitartrate) 200 mg • Korean Ginseng extract root (standardized to 7% ginsenosides, 10 mg) 143 mg • Caffeine (as caffeine citrate) 50 mg • Ginkgo Biloba extract leaf (standardized to 24% ginkgo flavone glycosides, 9.6 mg; standardized to 6% terpene lactones, 2.4 mg) 40 mg • Cayenne fruit 30 mg. Other Ingredients: Gelatin, Citric Acid, Maltodextrin, Magnesium Stearate.

Power Herbs Migracin - Nature's Herbs
Each softgel contains: Vitamin E (d-alpha tocopheryl succinate) 400 IU • Magnesium (from magnesium oxide) 200 mg • Feverfew extract (aerial part, standardized for 0.7% sesquiterpene lactones) 10.5 mg • White Willow Bark extract (standardized for 15% salicin) 25 mg • Ginger root extract (standardized for 5% gingerols) 25 mg. Other Ingredients: Soybean Oil, Gelatin, Glycerin, Purified Water, Lecithin, Yellow Beeswax, Titanium Dioxide, Chlorophyll.

Power L-Glutamine Pro - PureForm
Each 5 g serving contains: L-Glutamine 5 g.

Power Nutrient - Goldshield Elite
Each 2 tbsp serving (1 oz/30 ml) contains: Vitamin A (as 37% Beta-Carotene, 63% Retinyl palmitate) • Vitamin C (as Ascorbic acid) 60 mg • Vitamin D (as Cholecalciferol) 400 IU • Vitamin E (as DL-tocopherol) 30 IU • Thiamin (as Thiamine mononitrate) 1.5 mg • Riboflavin (as Riboflavin monophosphate) 1.7 mg • Niacin (as Niacinamide) 20 mg • Vitamin B6 (as Pyrodoxine HCL) 2 mg • Folate (as Folic acid) 400 mcg • Vitamin B12 (as Cyanocobalamin) 6 mcg • Biotin 300 mcg • Pantothenic acid (Vitamin B5) (as D-calcium pantothenate) 10 mg • Calcium (as Calcium lactate-gluconate) 40 mg • Iron 6 mg. Other Ingredients: Purified water, Fructose, Citric acid, Colloidal mineral blend, Natural Cranberry flavor, Sodium benzoate, Potassium sorbate and Maltodextrin.

Power Nutrient Plus - Goldshield Elite
Each 1 tbsp serving (15 ml) contains: Vitamin A (as 100% Beta-Carotene) 5000 IU • Vitamin C (Ascorbic acid) 60 mg • Vitamin D (as Cholecalciferol) 400 IU • Thiamin (as Thiamin HCl) 1.5 mg • Riboflavin (as Riboflavin-5-phosphate) 1.7 mg • Niacin (as Niacinamide) 5 mg • Vitamin B6 (as Pyridoxine HCl) 2 mg • Folate (Folic acid) 400 mcg • Vitamin B12 (as Cyanocobalamin) 6 mcg • Biotin 300 mcg • Pantothenic acid (as D-calcium pantothenate) 10 mg • Calcium (as Calcium lactate-gluconate) 40 mg • Korean Ginseng root extract 50 mg. Other Ingredients: Purified water, Fructose, Citric acid, Natural flavors, Aloe vera gel, Poly-colloidal organic minerals, Electrolyte complex (Potassium chloride, Magnesium citrate and Sodium citrate), Cellulose gum, Potassium sorbate, and Sodium benzoate.

Power Skin Conditioner For Men - Jamieson
Aloe Vera Gel • Algae Extract • Royal Jelly • Cucumber • Wheat Amino Acids.

Power Thin - Gold Star Nutrition
Ma Huang • Guarana • Magnesium • Chromium • Ginseng • Bladderwrack • Kola Nut • White Willow Bark • Fo-Ti • Ginger root • Gotu Kola • Licorice root • Hawthorne Berries • Saw Palmetto • Ginkgo Biloba • Boron • Spirulina • Potassium Citrate • Vitamin B12 • Folic Acid.
See Editor's Note No. 30.

Power Tropin - For Youthful Health
Each packet contains: Power Tropin Brand Amino Acid Proprietary Blend 9000 mg: L-Glutamine, Glycine, L-Arginine, Gamma Aminobutyric Acid (GABA), Glutamine peptides, L-Tyrosine. Power Tropin Glycoamino Acid-Glucose Complex 4950 mg • Power Tropin Secretagogue Proprietary Blend 1400 mg: L-Lysine Monohydrochloride, Acetyl L-Carnitine Hydrochloride, Alpha Lipoic Acid (ALA), Alpha-Glycerylphosphorylcholine.

Power V with Herbs - Nature's Bounty
Two tablets contain: Yohimbe bark extract (pausinystalie yohimba, standardized to contain 2% yohimbine) 250 mg • Niacin (B3) 45 mg • Oats aerial extract (avena sativa) 150 mg • Ginkgo Biloba leaf extract (ginkgo biloba, standardized to contain 24% ginkgo flavone glycosides) 40 mg • Saw Palmetto berry extract (serenoa repens) 100 mg • Guarana seed extract (paullinia cupana, standardized to 22% caffeine) 300 mg • Taurine 200 mg • Siberian Ginseng root extract (eleutherococcus senticosus) 30 mg • Orchic substance 50 mg.
See Editor's Note No. 14.

Power Vitamins for Men - Jamieson
Three caplets contain: Vitamin B1 (Thiamine Mononitrate) 20 mg • Vitamin B2 (Riboflavin) 20 mg • Vitamin B6 (Pyrodixine HCl) 20 mg • Niacinamide 150 mg • Vitamin B12 (Cyanocobalamin) 50 mcg • Pantothenic Acid (Calcium D-Panthenate) 30 mg • Folic Acid 0.2 mg • Vitamin A (Acetate) 7500 IU • Beta Carotene (Pro-Vitamin A) 1500 IU • Vitamin D 200 IU • Vitamin E (D-Alpha Tocopheryl Succinate) 30 IU • Vitamin C (Ascorbic Acid) 200 mg • Calcium (Carbonate) 250 mg • Magnesium (Oxide) 100 mg • Potassium 50 mg • Zinc 5 mg • Iodine (Kelp) 15 mg • Selenium 10 mcg • Chromium 10

BRAND NAMES

mcg • Siberian Ginseng root (PE 1:8) 100 mg • Astragalus root (PE 1:4) 50 mg • Codonopsis root 50 mg • Damiana leaves (PE 1:6.5) 50 mg • Licorice root (PE 1:2) 50 mg • Fo-Ti root (PE 1:8) 50 mg • Grape Seed (PE 1:5) 50 mg • Citrus Bioflavonoids 50 mg • European Garlic 80 mg • Spirulina 80 mg • Chlorella 80 mg • Wheat Grass 80 mg • Borage 50 mg • Sunflower Oil 50 mg • Coenzyme Q10 (Ubiquinone) 10 mg • Seed Source Protein (Amaranth, Sunflower, Bean, Quinoa, Diu, Radish) 80 mg • Inositol 20 mg • Dl-Methionine 2.2 mg • Bromelain 48.5 mg • Papain 36.4 mg • Amylase 6.1 mg • Lipase 6.1 mg • Cellulase 3.0 mg.

PowerActin **-** Nature's Plus
Two capsules contain: Korean Ginseng [(Panax ginseng root) standardized 15% Ginsenosides] 250 mg • Siberian Ginseng (Eleutherococcus senticosus root, standardized 0.8% Eleutherosides) 150 mg • Cayenne (capsicum frutescens fruit, standardized 100,000 STU) 150 mg • Ashwagandha (withania somnifera root, standardized 1.5% Withanolids) 50 mg • Schisandra (schisandra chinensis fruit, standardized 9% Schisandrins) 50 mg • Coenzyme Q10 (ubiquinone) 5 mg • Vitamin B12 (from cobalamin) 500 mcg.

PowerCLEANSE **-** Renew Life Formulas, Inc.
Organ Support Formula: Two capsules contain: Vitamin A (as vitamin A acetate) 2500 IU • Vitamin C (as ascorbic acid) 240 mg • Vitamin E (as D-alpha tocopheryl succinate) 25 IU • Riboflavin 20 mg • Niacin (as inositol hexanicotinate) 20 mg • Vitamin B6 (as pyridoxine HCl) 20 mg • Folic Acid 800 mcg • Vitamin B12 100 mcg • Zinc (as zinc citrate) 8 mg • Selenium (as selenomethionine) 50 mcg • Copper (as copper gluconate) 1 mg • Manganese (as manganese aspartate) 8 mg • Proprietary Herbal Blend: Garlic bulb (allium sativum) 1500 ppm allicin, Dandelion root (taraxacum officinale), Artichoke root and leaf (cynara scolymus), Turmeric root (curcuma longa, 95% curcumin), Milk Thistle seed (silybum marianum, 80% silymarin), Choline (as choline bitartrate) L-Methionine, L-Taurine, NAC (N-acetyl-cysteine). Other Ingredients: Gelatin, Water.
Colon Cleansing Formula: Two capsules contain: Magnesium (as magnesium hydroxide) • Cape Aloe gel (aloe ferox) • Rhubarb root (rheum officinalis) • Slippery Elm bark (ulmus rubra) • Marshmallow root (althaea officinalis) • Fennel seed (foeniculum vulgare) • Ginger root (zingiber officinale) • Triphala blend: Indian Gooseberry fruit, Belleric Myrobalan fruit, and Tropical Almond fruit. Other Ingredients: Hypromellose, Water.

PoweRelief **-** Pain & Stress Center
Two capsules contain: DLPA (DL-Phenylalanine) 500 mg • GABA 200 mg • Boswellia 300 mg • Passion Flower 150 mg • Magnesium 10 mg • Vitamin B6 4 mg.

PowerKids **-** Advocare International
Two tablets contain: Vitamin A (as palmitate) 500 IU • Vitamin A (as beta-carotene) 5000 IU • Vitamin C (as ascorbic acid) 60 mg • Vitamin D (as ergocalciferol) 200 IU • Vitamin E (as d-alpha tocopheryl succinate) 15 IU • Thiamine (as mononitrate) 1.5 mg • Riboflavin 1.8 mg • Niacin (as niacinamide) 16 mg • Vitamin B6 (as pyridoxine HCl) 2 mg • Folic Acid 200 mcg • Vitamin B12 (as cyanocobalamin) 6 mcg • Biotin 50 mcg • Pantothenic Acid (as calcium pantothenate) 5 mg • Calcium (as amino acid chelate) 50 mg • Iron (as amino acid chelate) 2.5 mg • Iodine (as amino acid chelate) 60 mcg • Magnesium (as amino acid chelate) 50 mg • Zinc (as amino acid chelate) 5 mg • Selenium (as selenomethionine) 35 mcg • Copper (as amino acid chelate) 500 mcg • Manganese (as amino acid chelate) 500 mcg • Chromium (as polynicotinate-ChromeMate) 60 mcg • Molybdenum (as amino acid chelate) 15 mcg • Boron (as amino acid chelate) 100 mcg • Inositol 2.5 mg • Choline (as choline bitartrate) 15 mg • Coenzyme Q-10 50 mcg. Other Ingredients: Fructose, Xylitol, Soybean Oil, Natural Cherry Flavor, Natural Orange Flavor, Stearic Acid, Silicon Dioxide, Magnesium Stearate, Beet Root Powder (for color), Turmeric (for color), Sucralose, Monoammonium Glycyrrhizinate (from licorice), Carrot Powder, Apple Powder.

Power-Plex Sustained Release Tablets **-** Nature's Plus
Each extended-release tablet contains: Vitamin A (as beta carotene) 10,000 IU • Vitamin C (as ascorbic acid) 300 mg • Vitamin D (as ergocalciferol) 400 IU • Vitamin E (as D-alpha tocopheryl succinate) 100 IU • Thiamin (vitamin B1, as thiamine HCl) 25 mg • Riboflavin (vitamin B2) 25 mg • Niacin (as niacinamide) 100 mg • Vitamin B6 (as pyridoxine HCl) 25 mg • Folate (as folic acid) 100 mcg • Vitamin B12 (as cyanocobalamin) 250 mcg • Biotin 20 mcg • Pantothenic Acid (as calcium pantothenate) 46 mg • Calcium (as amino acid chelate/complex) 26 mg • Iron (as amino acid chelate/complex) 25 mg • Phosphorus (as amino acid complex) 13.5 mg • Magnesium (as amino acid chelate/complex) 6.1 mg • Zinc (as amino acid chelate) 0.18 mg • Copper (as amino acid chelate) 0.28 mg • Manganese (as amino acid chelate/complex) 10 mg • Potassium (as amino acid complex) 0.1 mg • Inositol 50 mg • PABA (para-aminobenzoic acid) 25 mg • Betaine HCl (from beet molasses) 25 mg • Soya Lecithin 25 mg • Rutin (from saphora japonica leaf) 25 mg • Citrus Bioflavonoids (from citrus limon exocarp) 25 mg • Choline (as bitartrate) 21 mg • Hesperidin (from citrus limon exocarp) 5 mg. Other Ingredients: Di-calcium Phosphate, Microcrystalline Cellulose, Hydroxypropyl Methylcellulose, Silica, Rose Hips, Stearic Acid, Watercress, Horsetail root, Rice Bran, Isolated Soy Protein, Magnesium Stearate, Papaya, Parsley, Pacific Kelp, Alfalfa, Green Cabbage, Acerola Cherry, Wheat Germ Flour.

Pozitive Energy **-** BodyHealth
Each 1 mL serving contains: Vitamin B12 (cyanocobalamin) 100 mcg • Vitamin B1 (thiamine mononitrate) 0.375 mg • Vitamin B3 (niacin NF, FCC) 1.7 mg • Vitamin B6 (pyridoxine) 2.5 mg • Betaine (trimethylglycine) 1.5 mg • Biotin 4 mcg • Folic Acid 20 mcg • Choline Bitartrate 2.5 mg • Inositol 1.25 mg • L-Cysteine 5 mg • Grape skin extract 3.75 mg • Ginkgo liquid extract 1.25 mg • Zinc Gluconate 0.25 mg • Pyruvate (CWS) 10 mg • Taurine 2 mg • Malic Acid 1.5 mg • Herbal extract blend 49 mg: Ginseng, Green Tea, Yerba Mate. Other Ingredients: Purified Water, Crystalline Frucotse, Stevia, Natural Flavors, Sodium Benzoate, Potassium Sorbate, Xylitol.

Pre **-** Pacific BioLogic
Patrina • Peony root (white) • Bupleurum root (natural) • Ligusticum root • Jack-in-the-Pulpit rhizome • Angelica root (Chinese) • Hornet Nest • Vaccaria seeds • Argimony • Cyperus rhizome • Motherwort (Chinese) • Tumeric tuber • Bitter Orange ripened fruit.
See Editor's Note No. 40.

PreCare Chewables **-** KV Pharmaceutical Co.
Each tablet contains: Vitamin C (as Ester-C) 50 mg • Calcium (carbonate) 250 mg • Iron (as MicroMask ferrous fumerate) 40 mg • Vitamin D (vitamin D3, as cholecalciferol) 6 mcg • Vitamin E (as dl-alpha-tocopheryl acetate) 3.5 mg • Vitamin B6 (as pyridoxine HCl) 2 mg • Folic Acid, USP 1 mg • Magnesium (as magnesium oxide, USP) 50 mg • Zinc (as zinc oxide, USP) 15 mg • Copper (as cupric oxide) 2 mg. Inactive Ingredients: Citric Acid, FD&C Yellow No. 6 Lake, Flow Agents, Sweetening Agents, Natural and Artificial Flavors.

PreCare Conceive **-** KV Pharmaceutical Co.
Each tablet contains: Vitamin C (as Ester-C) 60 mg • Calcium (carbonate) 200 mg • Iron (as ferrous fumarate and carbonyl iron) 30 mg • Vitamin E (as dl-alpha-tocopheryl acetate) 30 IU • Thiamine (as thiamine mononitrate) 3 mg • Riboflavin, USP 3.4 mg • Niacin (as niacinamide, USP) 20 mg • Pyridoxine (as pyridoxine HCl, USP) 50 mg • Folic Acid, USP 1 mg • Magnesium (as magnesium oxide) 100 mg • Cyanocobalamin 12 mcg • Zinc (as zinc oxide) 15 mg • Copper (as cupric oxide) 2 mg. Inactive Ingredients: Cellulose Polymers, Flow Agents, Pigment Natural Wax, FD&C Yellow #10 Aluminum Lake, FD&C Yellow #6 Aluminum Lake, Lactose.

PreCare Prenatal **-** KV Pharmaceutical Co.
Each caplet contains: Vitamin C (as Ester-C) 50 mg • Calcium (carbonate) 250 mg • Iron (ferrous fumerate and carbonyl iron) 40 mg • Vitamin E (DL-alpha-tocopheryl acetate) 3.5 mg • Vitamin D (D3, as cholecalciferol) 6 mcg • Thiamine (thiamine mononitrate, USP) 3 mg • Riboflavin, USP 3.4 mg • Niacin (niacinamide) 20 mg • Pyridoxine (pyridoxine HCl) 20 mg • Folic Acid, USP 1 mg • Cyanocobalamin 12 mcg • Magnesium (magnesium oxide) 50 mg • Zinc (as zinc sulfate, USP) 15 mg • Copper (as cupric sulfate) 2 mg. Inactive Ingredients: Natural Oils, natural Wax, Cellulose Polymers, Flow Agents, FD&C Yellow No. 6 Aluminum Lake.

Pre-Drinking Formula - Sojourn Health
Four capsules contain: Vitamin C (sago palm) 1000 mg • Vitamin D (activated ergosterol) 100 IU • Vitamin E (mixed tocopherols) 400 IU • Vitamin B1 (thiamin HCl) 75 mg • Vitamin B2 (riboflavin) 75 mg • Vitamin B3 (niacinamide) 75 mg • Vitamin B6 (pyridoxine HCl) 75 mg • Folic Acid 400 mcg • Vitami nB12 75 mcg • Biotin 200 mcg • Vitamin B5 (pantothenic acid) 75 mg • Calcium (AA chelate) 900 mg • Selenium (AA chelate) 100 mcg • Copper (AA chelate) 1 mg • Proprietary Base 875 mg: Methionine DL, Bioflavonoids, Betaine (HCl), PABA (B10), Choline (bitartrate), Inositol.

Pregnacare Cream - Vitabiotics
Calendula extract (calendula officinalis) • Evening Primrose Oil (oenothera biennis) • Aloe extract (aloe barbadensis) • Allantoin • Pantothenic Acid (D-panthenol) • Vitamin E (alpha tocopheryl acetate) • Vitamin C (sodium ascorbyl phosphate) • Sodium Chloride • Magnesium Sulphate • Zinc Oxide • Menthol.

Pregnacare Tablets - Vitabiotics
Each tablet contains: Vitamin D (200 IU) 5 mcg • Vitamin E (natural source) 20 mg • Vitamin C 70 mg • Vitamin B1 (thiamin) 3 mg • Vitamin B2 (riboflavin) 2 mg • Vitamin B3 (niacin) 20 mg • Vitamin B6 (pyridoxine HCl) 10 mg • Folic Acid 400 mcg • Vitamin B12 (cyanocobalamin) 6 mcg • Betacarotene (natural source) 3 mg • Vitamin K 70 mcg • Iron 20 mg • Magnesium 150 mg • Zinc 15 mg • Iodine 140 mcg • Copper 1 mg.

Pregnancy Tea - Traditional Medicinals
Spearmint leaf • Red Raspberry leaf • Lemongrass leaf • Strawberry Leaf • Fennel seed • Nettle leaf • Rose Hip • Alfalfa herb • Lemon Verbena leaf.

Pregnancy-6 Formula (Pregnancy 6) - Nature's Way
Each capsule contains Proprietary Formula 425 mg: Black Cohosh root • Blessed Thistle • False Unicorn root • Penny Royal flowering top • Red Raspberry leaves • Squaw Vine vine, leaf, fruit. Other Ingredients: Gelatin.
See Editor's Note No. 8.

Preg-Natal + DHA - Jarrow Formulas
Each packet contains: Vitamin A (as retinyl palmitate, 50% as betacarotene from dunaliella salina) 5000 IU • Vitamin C (from calcium ascorbate) 120 mg • Vitamin D (D3, cholecalciferol) 400 IU • Vitamin E (D-alpha-tocopheryl succinate) 60 IU • Vitamin K (phylloquinone) 80 mcg • Vitamin B1 (as thiamin mononitrate) 3 mg • Vitamin B2 (riboflavin) 3.4 mg • Vitamin B3 (niacinamide) 40 mg • Vitamin B6 (pyridoxine hydrochloride) 4 mg • Folic Acid 800 mcg • Vitamin B12 (methylcobalamin) 12 mcg • Biotin 300 mcg • Pantothenic Acid (as calcium pantothenate) 20 mg • Calcium (from calcium citrate) 1200 mg • Iron (from ferrous gluconate) 25 mg • Iodine (from potassium iodide) 150 mcg • Magnesium (as magnesium oxide) 500 mg • Zinc (as zinc monomethionate) 15 mg • Selenium (as L-selenomethionine/sodium selenate 50/50) 80 mcg • Copper (as copper gluconate) 2 mg • Manganese (as manganese citrate) 2 mg • Chromium (from chromium nicotinate/citrate) 120 mcg • Potassium (as potassium chloride) 99 mg • DHA 250 mg • Choline (as choline bitartrate) 25 mg • Inositol 50 mg • Lutein 3 mg • Ginger 50 mg. Other Ingredients: Stearic Acid, Microcrystalline Cellulose, Calcium Stearate, Hydroxypropyl Cellulose, Croscarmellose Sodium, Silicon Dioxide.

Pregnenolone - Ortho Molecular Products
Each tablet contains: Pregnenolone 10 mg. Other Ingredients: Sorbitol, Xylitol, Sodium Croscarmellose, Stearic Acid, Potassium Bicarbonate, Magnesium Stearate, Silicon Dioxide, Natural Flavors, Cranberry.

Pregnenolone - Metabolic Response Modifiers
Each capsule contains: Pregnenolone 10 mg.

Pregnenolone - GNC
Each capsule contains: Pregnenolone 50 mg. Other Ingredients: Cellulose, Gelatin, Calcium Carbonate.

Pregnenolone (10 mg) - Life Enhancement Products, Inc.
Each capsule contains: Vitamin C (as ascorbyl palmitate) 10 mg • Pregnenolone 10 mg.

Pregnenolone (100 mg) - Life Enhancement Products, Inc.
Each capsule contains: Vitamin C (as ascorbyl palmitate) 10 mg • Pregnenolone 100 mg.

Pregnenolone (25 mg) - Life Enhancement Products, Inc.
Each capsule contains: Vitamin C (as ascorbyl palmitate) 10 mg • Pregnenolone 25 mg.

Pregnenolone (50 mg) - Life Enhancement Products, Inc.
Each capsule contains: Vitamin C (as ascorbyl palmitate) 10 mg • Pregnenolone 50 mg.

Pregnenolone 10 mg - Pure Encapsulations
Each vegetable capsule contains: Pregnenolone (3-alpha-hydroxy-5-beta-pregnen-20-one) 10 mg.

Pregnenolone 25 MG - Pain & Stress Center
Each capsule contains: Pregnenolone 25 mg. Other Ingredietns: Rice Powder, Gelatin Capsule.

Pregnenolone 30 mg - Pure Encapsulations
Each vegetable capsule contains: Pregnenolone (3-alpha-hydroxy-5-beta-pregnen-20-one) 30 mg.

Pregnenolone 30 mg - PhysioLogics
Each capsule contains: Pregnenolone 30 mg. Other Ingredients: Dicalcium Phosphate, Cellulose (plant origin), Gelatin, Silica, Vegetable Magnesium Stearate.

Pregnenolone 5 mg - Pure Encapsulations
Each vegetable capsule contains: Pregnenolone (3-alpha-hydroxy-5-beta-pregnen-20-one) 5 mg.

Pregnenolone 50 MG - Pain & Stress Center
Each capsule contains: Pregnenolone 50 mg. Other Ingredients: Rice Powder, Gelatin Capsule.

Pregnenolone 50 mg - PhysioLogics
Each capsule contains: Pregnenolone 50 mg. Other Ingredients: Rice Powder, Gelatin, Vegetable Magnesium Stearate, Silica.

Pregnenolone-15 - PhytoPharmica
Each capsule contains: Pregnenolone 15 mg.
See Editor's Note No. 21.

PregnonePlus - Xymogen
Deionized Water • Aloe Vera gel • Caprylic/Capric Triglycerides • Shea Butter • Sunflower seed oil • Stearic Acid • Natural Pregnenolone • Glyceryl Stearate • PEG-100-Stearate • Beeswax • Isopropyl Palmitate • MSM • Evening Primrose oil (oenothera biennis) • Burdock root extract • Chamomile extract • Ginseng extract • Lavender extract • Lecithin • Vegetable Glycerin • Stearyl Alcohol or Cetyl Alcohol • Carbomer • Triethanolamine • Xanthan Gum • Hydroxypropylmethylcellulose • Allantoin • Disodium EDTA • Potassium Sorbate • Grape seed extract.

Prelief - AkPharma Inc.
Two tablets contain: Calcium 130 mg • Phosphorus 100 mg. Other Ingredients: Magnesium Stearate.

Prelieve PMS - Boehringer Ingelheim
One mini-tablet contains: Standardized Vitex Agnus-Castus Extract (2:1) (fruit) 20 mg. Other Ingredients: Lactose, magnesium stearate, polyvidone, talc, PEG-100, polymethacrylic acid derivatives, FD&C blue #2, titanium dioxide, synthetic iron oxide.

Pre-Load Creatine Complex - Optimum Nutrition
Each scoop (47 g) contains: Creatine Monohydrate 6 g • L-Glutamine 1 g • Taurine 1 g • L-Isoleucine 500 mg • L-Valine 500 mg • L-Arginine 250 mg • L-Glycine 250 mg • Carbogen 200 mg. Other Ingredients: Dextrose, Natural Color, Magnesium Phosphate, Sodium Phosphate, Potassium Phosphate, Citric Acid, Natural Flavor.

Some Brand Name Natural Products - What they Contain

www.NaturalDatabase.com contains MANY more listings than appear here.
Editor's Notes are located on pages 2155-2163.

Prelox Blue - Herbalife International of America, Inc.
Two tablets contain: Protein 2 g • Prelox Proprietary Blend 1638 mg: L-Arginine HCl, Aspartic Acid, Pycnogenol (dried pine bark extract). Other Ingredients: Microcrystalline Cellulose, Corn Starch, Croscarmellose Sodium, Hypromellose, Magnesium Stearate, Silicon Dioxide, Titanium Dioxide, Triacetin, Acacia Gum (stems and branches), FD&C Blue #1, FD&C Blue #2.

Premence Capsules - Vitabiotics
Each capsule contains: Vitamin A 700 mcg • Vitamin E 30 mg • Vitamin C 60 mg • Vitamin B1 (thiamin) 12 mg • Vitamin B2 (riboflavin) 1.6 mg • Vitamin B3 (niacin) 36 mg • Vitamin B6 (pyridoxine HCl) 10 mg • Folic Acid 400 mcg • Vitamin B12 (cyanocobalamin) 5 mcg • Iron 15 mg • Magnesium 150 mg • Zinc 15 mg • Iodine 100 mcg • Copper 1 mg.

Premens - Ortho Molecular Products
Two capsules contain: Vitamin B6 USP (as pyridoxine HCl USP) 50 mg • Magnesium (as Chelazome brand amino acid chelate, citrate) 200 mg • Turmeric root extract (standardized to contain 95% curcumin) 75 mg • Chaste berry fruit 10:1 extract 20 mg. Other Ingredients: Natural Vegetable Capsules, Magnesium Stearate, Microcrystalline Cellulose.

PremensisRx - KV Pharmaceutical Co.
Each tablet contains: Vitamin B6 (as pyridoxine HCl) 75 mg • Vitamin B12 (as cyanocobalamin) 12 mcg • Folic Acid, USP 1 mg • Calcium (as calcium carbonate) 200 mg. Inactive Ingredients: Natural Waxes, Cellulose Polymers, FD&C Blue No. 1 Aluminum Lake, FD&C Yellow No. 10 Aluminum Lake.

Premenstra - HerbaSway
Dong Quai • Wild Yam • Knotweed • Ginger • Licorice • Blackberry • HerbaSweet (cucurbitaceae fruit).

Premier Formula for Ocular Nutrition - Optim 3
Four capsules contain: Vitamin A (beta carotene) 20,000 IU • Vitamin C (as Ocucel C brand, Ester-C brand MV 200 mg, ascorbic acid 1000 mg) 1200 mg • Vitamin E (as D-alpha tocopheryl succinate) 440 IU • Riboflavin (vitamin B2) 60 mg • Calcium (as calcium carbonate and Ester-C brand MV) 117 mg • Zinc (as zinc sulfate) 60 mg • Selenium (as selenium chelate) 120 mcg • Copper (as copper gluconate) 8 gm • Chromium (as GTF chromium) 200 mcg • Ocucel brand Lutein Complex with FloraGLO brand Lutein 383 mg: FloraGLO brand Lutein 10 mg, Zeaxanthin 500 mcg, Eyebright whole plant, L-Glutathione, Astaxanthin, Bilberry • Citrus Bioflavonoids 200 mg • L-Taurine 200 mg • Quercetin 100 mg • Rutin 100 mg • N-Acetyl-Cysteine 40 mg. Other Ingredients: Magnesium Stearate, Silicon Dioxide, Microcrystalline Cellulose, Gelatin.

Premier One Royal Jelly 2000 - Nutraceutical Corp.
Each capsule contains: Royal Jelly 3.5x (equivalent to 2000 mg) 572 mg.

Premium Calcium - Mosaic Nutraceuticals Corp
Each chew contains: Vitamin D 100 IU • Vitamin K 40 mcg • Calcium 500 mg. Other Ingredients: Hydrogenated Starch Hydrolysate, Palm Kernal OIl, Mono & Diglycerides, Soya Lecithin, Salt, Sucralose, Artificial Flavors, Fulvic Acid.

Premium Cleansing Herbs - Longevity
Three capsules contain: Riboflavin (vitamin B2) 20 mg • Chelated Minerals Proprietary Blend 318 mg: Potassium, Calcium, Magnesium, Zinc, Chromium, Selenium, Iron, Copper, Molybdenum, Vanadium, Iodine, Cobalt, Manganese • Cascara Sagrada bark (rhamnus purshiana) 300 mg • Yucca root (yucca filimentosa) 300 mg • Fennel Seed fruit (foniclum vulgare) 50 mg • Pau D'arco inner bark (tabebuia avellanedae) 50 mg • Peppermint leaf, top (mentha piperita) 50 mg • Yellowdock root (rumex crispus) 50 mg. Other Ingredients: Gelatin, Rice Flour, Magnesium Stearate, Silicon Dioxide.

Premium Echinacea - Holista
Each capsule contains: Echinacea angustifolia (root) from standardized 6.5:1 extract (4% echinacoside) 500 mg.

Premium Echinacea - Olympian Labs
Each capsule contains: Premium Echinacea 400 mg.

Premium HGH Precursors - Youngevity
Six capsules contain: Vitamin B6 (pyridoxine hydrochloride) 6 mg • Manganese (amino acid chelate) 1.5 mg • Chromium (amino acid chelate) 90 mcg • Arginine (L-arginine hydrochloride) 300 mg • Glutamine (L-glutamine) 300 mg • Glycine (L-glycine) 300 mg • Ornithine (L-ornithine) 300 mg • Tyrosine (L-tyrosine) 300 mg • Vilcabamba Mineral Essence Proprietary Blend 300 mg: Potassium, Calcium, Magnesium, Zinc, Chromium, Selenium, Iron, Copper, Molybdenum, Vanadium, Iodine, Cobalt, Manganese • GABA 150 mg • Kelp (Laminaria spp) 150 mg. Other Ingredients: Gelatin, Rice Flour, Magnesium Stearate, Silicon Dioxide.

Premium Korean Ginseng - Olympian Labs
Each capsule contains: Korean Ginseng 650 mg.

Premium Noni Chews - Mosaic Nutraceuticals Corp
Each chew contains: Noni extract 500 mg. Other Ingredients: Corn Syrup, Sugar, Palm Kernal Oil, Natural and Artificial Flavors, Mono & Diglycerides, Soya Lecithin, Salt, FD&C Red 40, FD&C Blue 1, Fulvic Acid.

Premium Soy Protein Isolate Powder - Puritan's Pride
Each serving approximately contains: Total Isoflavones 60 mg • Genistein 36 mg • Daidzein 21 mg • Glycitein 3 mg.

Premium Super Cell Protector - Longevity
Three capsules contain: Chelated Minerals Blend 270 mg: Potassium, Calcium, Magnesium, Zinc, Chromium, Selenium, Iron, Copper, Molybdenum, Vanadium, Iodine, Cobalt, Manganese • Grape seed extract (142.5 mg proanthocyanidins) 150 mg. Other Ingredients: Gelatin, Rice Flour, Magnesium Stearate, Silicon Dioxide.

Pre-Natal - J. R. Carlson Laboratories, Inc.
Four tablets contain: Vitamin A (as palmitate and beta carotene) 8000 IU • Vitamin C (as calcium ascorbate) 300 mg • Vitamin D (D2, calciferol) 400 IU • Vitamin E (as D-alpha tocopheryl succinate) 150 IU • Thiamin (vitamin B1, as thiamin mononitrate) 6 mg • Riboflavin (vitamin B2) 8 mg • Niacin (vitamin B3, as niacinamide) 80 mg • Vitamin B6 (as pyridoxine hydrochloride) 10 mg • Folate (folic acid) 1000 mcg • Vitamin B12 (cyanocobalamin) 32 mcg • Biotin 300 mcg • Iron (as iron glycinate chelate) 36 mg • Calcium (as calcium carbonate citrate) 1000 mg • Iodine (from kelp) 150 mcg • Magnesium (as magnesium oxide) 450 mg • Zinc (as zinc glycinate chelate) 15 mg • Selenium (as L-selenomethionine) 70 mcg • Copper (as copper glycinate chelate) 2 mg • Manganese (as manganese glycinate chelate) 2 mg • Chromium (as chromium glycinate chelate) 120 mcg • Pantothenic Acid (as D-calcium pantothenate) 40 mg • Bioflavonoids 100 mg • Grape seed extract 10 mg.

Pre-Natal - Aspen Group, Inc.
Each tablet contains: Vitamin A (from vitamin A acetate & beta carotene) 4000 IU • Vitamin D (cholecalciferol) 400 IU • Vitamin E (d2-alpha tocopherol acetate) 11 mg • Vitamin C (ascorbic acid) 100 mg • Folic acid 0.8 mg • Vitamin B1 (thiamine mononitrate) 1.84 mg • Vitamin B2 (riboflavin) 1.7 mg • Niacinamide 18 mg • Vitamin B6 (pyridoxine hydrochloride) 2.6 mg • Vitamin B12 (cyanocobalamin) 4 mcg • Calcium (sulfate) 200 mg • Iron 20 mg • Zinc (oxide) 25 mg.

Pre-Natal - Jamieson
Each caplet contains: Vitamin D 1000 IU • Beta Carotene 1800 IU • Vitamin D 200 IU • Vitamin C 150 mg • Vitamin E 30 mg • Vitamin B1 3 mg • Vitamin B2 3.75 mg • Vitamin B6 10 mg • Vitamin B12 10 mcg • Vitamin B3 22 mg • Vitamin B5 10 mg • Biotin 30 mcg • Folic Acid 1 mg • Chelated Calcium 200 mg • Chelated Magnesium 100 mg • Chelated Zinc 20 mg • Chelated Iron 30 mg • Chelated Copper 1 mg • Chelated Chromium 25 mcg • Chelated Manganese 5 mg • Iodine (from kelp) 15 mg. In a base of Rutin, Hesperidin, Acerola, Rosehips, Bioflavonoids, Peppermint, Chamomile, Bromelain, Papain, Amylase, Lipase, Cellulase.

Pre-Natal Caps - NOW Foods
Four capsules contain: Vitamin A (Beta Carotene) 10000 IU • Vitamin B1 (thiamine HCl) 5 mg • Vitamin B2 (riboflavin) 5 mg • Vitamin B3 (niacinamide) 20 mg • Vitamin B5 (pantothenic Acid) 20 mg • Vitamin B6 (pyridoxine HCl) 5 mg • Vitamin B12 (cyanocobalamin) 20 mcg • Biotin 300 mcg • Folic Acid 800 mcg • Vitamin C (calcium ascorbate) 120 mg • Vitamin D (fish liver oil) 400 IU • Vitamin E (D-alpha tocopheryl succinate) 150 IU • Vitamin K 80 mcg • Calcium (carbonate, ascorbate) 1200 mg • Magnesium (oxide) 500 mg • Zinc (amino acid chelate) 15 mg • Iron (bisglycinate) 36 mg • Copper (amino acid chelate) 1 mg • Iodine (kelp) 150 mcg • Manganese (amino acid chelate) 3.5 mg • Selenium (L-selenomethionine) 50 mcg • Chromium (picolinate) 100 mcg • Molybdenum (amino acid chelate) 80 mcg • Potassium (chloride) 50 mg • Vanadium (amino acid chelate) 25 mcg • Choline 10 mg • Inositol 10 mg • PABA 4 mg.

PreNatal Care - Natrol, Inc.
Three tablets contain: Vitamin A (as Vitamin A palmitate & d-Salina beta carotene) 5000 IU • Vitamin C (calcium ascorbate) 100 mg • Vitamin D (as cholecalciferol) 200 IU • Vitamin E (as d-alpha tocopherol) 100 IU • Vitamin K 25 mcg • Thiamine (Vitamin B1) (as Thiamine HCl) 25 mg • Riboflavin (Vitamin B2) 25 mg • Niacinamide 25 mg • Vitamin B6 (pyridoxine HCl) 25 mg • Folic Acid 800 mcg • Vitamin B12 (as cobalamin) 50 mcg • Biotin 100 mcg • Pantothenic Acid (as calcium pantothenate) 50 mg • Calcium (as calcium carbonate) 250 mg • Iron 25 mg • Iodine (from kelp) 150 mcg • Magnesium (as magnesium oxide) 125 mg • Zinc (as zinc gluconate) 15 mg • Selenium (as l-Selenomethionine) 100 mcg • Copper (copper gluconate) 2 mg • Manganese (as manganese gluconate) 50 mcg • Potassium (as potassium proteinate) 99 mg • DHA (docosahexenoic acid) 100 mg • Choline (as choline bitartrate) 50 mg • Betaine (as betaine HCl) 50 mg • Ginger root extract 50 mg • Inositol 25 mg • PABA (para amino benzoic acid) 25 mg • Red Raspberry extract leaf 15 mg • Rosemary extract leaf 15 mg • Squaw Vine powdered aerial part 15 mg. Other Ingredients: Mono & Di-Glycerides, Microcrystalline Cellulose, Stearic Acid, Silicon Dioxide, Magnesium Stearate.

Prenatal Complex - AIE Pharmaceuticals
Each tablet contains: Vitamin A (as palmitate) • Vitamin C (as ascorbic acid) • Vitamin D (as cholecalciferol) • Riboflavin • Thiamin (as thiamin mononitrate) • Vitamin B6 (as pyridoxine hydrochloride) • Niacin (as niacinamide) • Folic Acid • Calcium (from calcium sulfate) • Vitamin B12 (as cyanocobalamin) • Iodine (from kelp powder) • Zinc (from zinc sulfate) • Copper (from cupric sulfate) • Iron (from ferrous fumarate) • Manganese (from manganese sulfate) • Magnesium (from magnesium oxide) • Potassium (from potassium chloride). Other Ingredients: Stearic Acid, Magnesium Stearate, Guar Gum, Dibasic Calcium Phosphate, Croscarmellose Sodium, Silicon Dioxide, Ethylcellulose.

Prenatal Complex - Nature's Plus
Each tablet contains: Vitamin A (as beta carotene) 8000 IU • Vitamin C (as ascorbic acid) 120 mg • Vitamin D (as ergocalciferol) 400 IU • Vitamin E (as d-alpha tocopheryl acetate) 60 IU • Vitamin B1 (as thiamine HCl) 3 mg • Vitamin B2 (as riboflavin) 3.4 mg • Niacin (as niacinamide) 40 mg • Vitamin B6 (as pyridoxine HCl) 4 mg • Folate (as folic acid) 800 mcg • Vitamin B12 (as cyanocobalamin) 12 mcg • Biotin 600 mcg • Pantothenic Acid (as calcium pantothenate) 20 mg • Calcium (as amino acid chelate/complex) 162 mg • Iron (as amino acid chelate/complex) 18 mg • Phosphorous (as amino acid complex) 125 mg • Iodine (from kelp) 300 mcg • Magnesium (as amino acid chelate/complex) 100 mg • Zinc (as gluconate) 7.5 mg • Copper (as gluconate) 4 mg.

Pre-Natal Complex - Puritan's Pride
Four capsules contain: Vitamin A (as retinyl acetate) 8,000 IU • Vitamin C (as ascorbic acid) 120 mg • Vitamin D (as cholecalciferol) 400 IU • Vitamin E (as d-alpha tocopheryl acid succinate) 30 IU • Thiamin (Vitamin B1; as thiamine mononitrate) 1.7 mg • Riboflavin (Vitamin B2) 2.0 mg • Niacin (as niacinamide) 20 mg • Vitamin B6 (as pyridoxine hydrochloride) 2.5 mg • Folate (as folic acid) 800 mcg • Vitamin B12 (as cyanocobalamin) 8 mcg • Biotin 300 mcg • Pantothenic Acid (as d-calcium pantothenate) 10 mg • Calcium (as calcium carbonate and calcium citrate) 1,300 mg • Iron (as ferrous fumarate) 28 mg • Iodine (as potassium iodide) 150 mcg • Magnesium (as magnesium oxide) 450 mg • Zinc (as zinc citrate) 15 mg • Selenium (as sodium selenate) 70 mcg • Copper (as cupric gluconate) 2 mg • Manganese (as manganese gluconate) 2 mg • Chromium (as chromium picolinate) 120 mcg • Molybdenum (as sodium molybdate) 75 mcg • Potassium (as potassium chloride and potassium citrate) 10 mg • Choline (as choline bitartrate) 20 mg • Inositol 20 mg • PABA (as Para-Aminobenzoic acid) 2 mg • Cranberry fruit 60 mg • Peppermint Oil 20 mg • Ginger root 20 mg.

Prenatal Daily - Health Factor
Three capsules contain: Beta Carotene (pro Vitamin A) 2500 IU • Vitamin A (Acetate) 4000 IU • Vitamin B1 (Thiamine HCl) 10 mg • Vitamin B2 (Riboflavin & R5'P) 10 mg • Vitamin B3 (Niacinamide) 20 mg • Calcium (Ascorbate & Carbonate) 250 mg • Iron (Feronyl) 40 mg • Vitamin D (Ergocalciferol) 400 IU • Vitamin E (d-Alpha Tocopheryl) 100 IU • Vitamin B6 (Pyridoxine HCl & P5'P) 30 mg • Folic Acid 800 mcg • Vitamin B12 (Cobalamin) 100 mcg • Iodine (Potassium Iodide) 150 mcg • Magnesium (Oxide) 125 mg • Zinc (Picolinate) 20 mg • Copper (Citrate) 2 mg • Biotin 300 mcg • Vitamin B5 (Pantothenic Acid) 25 mg • Vitamin B10 (PABA) 25 mg • Vitamin K (Phytonadione) 15 mcg • Choline (Bitartrate) 12.5 mg • Inositol 12.5 mg • Chromium (Nichrome-3) 200 mg • Manganese (Citrate) 7 mg • Selenium (Amino Acid Chelate) 100 mcg • Lemon Bioflavonoids 25 mg • Rutin 5 mg • Hesperidin 5 mg • Lactobacillus Acidophilus (3 billion/gm) 20 mg.

Prenatal Formula - Nature Made
Each tablet contains: Vitamin A 4000 IU • Vitamin C 100 mg • Vitamin D 400 IU • Vitamin E 11 IU • Thiamin 1.5 mg • Riboflavin 1.7 mg • Niacin 18 mg • Vitamin B6 2.6 mg • Folate 800 mcg • Vitamin B12 4 mcg • Calcium 20 mg • Iron 27 mg • Zinc 25 mg. Other Ingredients: Cellulose, Acacia, Croscarmellose Sodium, Silicon Dioxide, Corn Starch, Magnesium Stearate, Hydroxypropyl Methylcellulose, Polyethylene Glycol, Peanut Oil.
See Editor's Note No. 45.

Pre-Natal Formula - PhysioLogics
Four capsules contain: Vitamin A (retinyl acetate) 8000 IU • Vitamin C (ascorbic acid) 120 mg • Vitamin D (cholecalciferol) 400 IU • Vitamin E (D-alpha tocopherol acid succinate) 30 IU • Thiamin (vitamin B1, as thiamine mononitrate) 1.7 mg • Riboflavin (vitamin B2) 2 mg • Niacin (niacinamide) 20 mg • Vitamin B6 (pyridoxine hydrochloride) 2.5 mg • Folic Acid 800 mcg • Vitamin B12 (cyanocobalamin) 8 mcg • Biotin (D-biotin) 300 mcg • Pantothenic Acid (D-calcium pantothenate) 10 mg • Calcium (calcium carbonate and citrate) 1300 mg • Iron (ferrous fumarate) 28 mg • Iodine (potassium iodide) 150 mcg • Magnesium (magnesium oxide) 450 mg • Zinc (zinc citrate) 15 mg • Selenium (sodium selenate) 70 mcg • Copper (cupric gluconate) 2 mg • Manganese (manganese gluconate) 2 mg • Chromium (chromium picolinate) 120 mcg • Molybdenum (sodium molybdate) 75 mcg • Potassium (potassium chloride and citrate) 10 mg • Choline (choline bitartrate) 20 mg • Inositol 20 mg • PABA (para-aminobenzoic acid) 2 mg • Cranberry fruit (vaccinium macrocarpon) 60 mg • Peppermint Oil (mentha piperita) 20 mg • Ginger root (zingiber officinale) 20 mg. Other Ingredients: Gelatin, Acacia Gum, Maltodextrin, Vegetable Magnesium Stearate, Silica.

Prenatal Formulation - Olympian Labs
Four tablets contain: Beta Carotene 5000 IU • Vitamin B-1 (thiamine HCl) 1.5 mg • Vitamin B-2 (riboflavin) 1.6 mg • Vitamin B-3 (inositol hexanicotinate) 17 mg • Vitamin B-5 (calcium pantothenate) 10 mg • Vitamin B-6 (pyridoxine HCl) 2.2 mg • Vitamin B-9 (folic Acid) 600 mcg • Vitamin B-12 (cyanocobalamin) 6 mcg • Vitamin C (ascorbic acid) 70 mg • Vitamin D (cholecalciferol) 400 IU • Vitamin E (d-alpha-tocopherol acetate) 30 IU • d-Biotin 300 mcg • Inositol 10 mg • PABA 2 mg • Choline Bitartrate 10 mg • Chromium 25 mcg • Calcium 1200 mg • Copper 2 mg • Iron 30 mg • Magnesium 320 mg • Manganese 2 mg • Potassium 50 mg • Selenium 65 mcg • Zinc 15 mg • Phosphorus 130 mg • Iodine (kelp) 150 mcg.

Some Brand Name Natural Products - What they Contain

www.NaturalDatabase.com contains MANY more listings than appear here.
Editor's Notes are located on pages 2155-2163.

BRAND NAMES

PreNatal Herbal - Vital Nutrients
Two capsules contain: Red Raspberry leaf 4:1 extract 200 mg • Yellow Dock root 4:1 extract 200 mg • Dandelion root 4:1 extract 200 mg • Ginger root 5:1 extract 200 mg • Nettle leaf 5:1 extract 100 mg • Cranberry 25:1 extract 100 mg • Rutin NF 100 mg.

Prenatal Multi - Arrowroot
Four tablets contain: Vitamin A 5000 IU • Biotin 200 mcg • Beta Carotene 3000 IU • Folic Acid 800 mcg • Vitamin D (D3) 400 IU • Copper 2 mg • Vitamin E 60 IU • Iron 60 mg • Vitamin C 120 mg • Magnesium 400 mg • Vitamin B1 3 mg • Calcium 1000 mg • Vitamin B2 3.4 mg • Iodine 150 mcg • Niacinamide 20 mg • Phosphorus 780 mg • Vitamin B6 10 mg • Zinc 20 mg • Vitamin B12 12 mcg • Chromium 25 mcg • Pantothenic Acid 20 mg.

PreNatal Multi-Nutrients - Vital Nutrients
Six capsules contain: Vitamin A (acetate) 5000 IU • Betatene brand Natural Beta Carotene (with mixed carotenoids) 5000 IU • Ascorbic Acid 500 mg • Vitamin D (D3, from lanolin) 400 IU • D-Alpha-Tocopheryl Succinate (natural vitamin E) 400 IU • Thiamine HCl (vitamin B1) 50 mg • Riboflavin (pure powder) 10 mg • Riboflavin 5-Phosphate (activated vitamin B2) 10 mg • Niacinamide 50 mg • Pyridoxine HCl (vitamin B6) 50 mg • Folic Acid 800 mcg • Hydroxocobalamin (pure vitamin B12) 200 mcg • Biotin 300 mcg • Calcium-Pantothenate 100 mg • Iodine (potassium iodide) 225 mcg • Calcium (98% citrate/malate, 2% pantothenate) 500 mg • Magnesium (citrate) 250 mg • Zinc (citrate) 25 mg • Selenium (selenomethionine) 200 mcg • Manganese (citrate) 10 mg • Chromium (polynicotinate) 200 mcg • Molybdenum (citrate) 50 mcg • Potassium (chloride) 90 mg • Boron (citrate) 1 mg • Vanadium (citrate) 50 mcg • Copper (glycinate) 2 mg • Iron (aspartate) 30 mg • Phytonadione (vitamin K1) 100 mcg.

Prenatal Multiple - Nature's Life
Six capsules contain: Beta Carotene (Vitamin A equivalent to 15,000 IU) 9 mg • Vitamin D (Cholecalciferol) 200 IU • Vitamin B1 (Thiamine HCl) 50 mg • Vitamin B2 (Riboflavin) 50 mg • Vitamin B3 (Niacinamide) 50 mg • Vitamin B6 (Pyridoxine HCl) 75 mg • Vitamin B12 (Cyancobalamin concentrate) 50 mcg • Folic Acid 800 mcg • Pantothenic Acid (d-Calcium Pantothenate) 50 mg • Biotin (D-Biotin) 800 mcg • Inositol 50 mg • Choline (Bitartrate) 50 mg • PABA (Para Aminobenzoic Acid) 25 mg • Vitamin C 300 mg • Lemon Bioflavonoids Complex (TESTLAB 50%, Flavonoids, Flavones, Naringen & Eriocitrin) 50 mg • Rutin (Saphora japonica) 25 mg • Vitamin E (d-Alpha Tocopheryl Succinate) 200 IU • Vitamin K (Phylloquinone) 5 mg • Boron (Citrate) 50 mcg • Calcium (Carbonate, Citrate/ Malate) 1000 mg • Chromium (Picolinate, Nutrition 21, US Patent #33988) 200 mcg • Copper (Gluconate, Citrate) 1.5 mg • Iodine (Potassium Iodide) 25 mcg • Iron (Fumarate, Peptonate) 18 mg • Magnesium (Oxide, Citrate) 500 mg • Manganese (Citrate) 10 mg • Molybdenum (Molybdate) 20 mcg • Potassium (Citrate, Iodide) 99 mg • Selenium (l- Selenomethionine) 100 mcg • Silicon (Dioxide) 20 mcg • Vanadium (Vanadyl Sulfate) 20 mcg • Zinc (Picolinate, Methionine) 15 mg • Red Raspberry leaf (Rubus idaeus) 100 mg • Betaine HCl 50 mg.

PreNatal Nutrients - Pure Encapsulations
Four vegetable capsules contain: Ascorbic Acid 70 mg • Vitamin C (as ascorbyl palmitate) 40 mg • Calcium (citrate) 200 mg • Iron (glycinate) 27 mg • Vitamin D (as D3) 400 IU • Vitamin E (D-alpha tocopherol succinate) 18.2 IU • Thiamin HCl (vitamin B1) 1.6 mg • Riboflavin (vitamin B2) 1.7 mg • Niacinamide 20 mg • Pyridoxine HCl (vitamin B6) 2.2 mg • Folic Acid 1 mg • Methylcobalamin (vitamin B12) 2.6 mcg • Biotin 300 mcg • Pantothenic Acid (calcium pantothenate) 6 mg • Iodine (potassium iodide) 150 mcg • Magnesium (citrate) 80 mg • Zinc (citrate) 15 mg • Selenium (selenomethionine) 70 mcg • Copper (glycinate) 2 mg • Manganese (aspartate) 2 mg • Chromium (polynicotinate) 120 mcg • Molybdenum (aspartate) 75 mcg • Betatene brand Mixed Carotenoids 8000 IU: Beta Carotene 4570 mcg, Alpha Carotene 144 mcg, Zeaxanthin 29 mcg, Cryptoxanthin 35 mcg, Lutein 22 mcg • DHA (docosahexaenoic acid) 100 mg. Other Ingredients: Denatured Corn Starch, Hypo-allergenic Plant Fiber.

Prenatal Plus Optizinc - Nutrivention
Four tablets contain: Calcium (Chelate) 1200 mg • Magnesium (Chelate) 300 mg • Vitamin C 300 mg • Phosphorus (Chelate) 150 mg • Niacinamide 100 mg • Vitamin E 100 IU • Potassium 99 mg • Vitamin A 1500 IU • Pantothenic Acid 60 mg • Choline Bitartrate 60 mg • Inositol 50 mg • Vitamin B1 50 mg • Iron (Amino Acid Chelate) 45 mg • Vitamin B1 25 mg • Vitamin B2 25 mg • Zinc 25 mg • Manganese (Amino Acid Chelate) 10 mg • Vitamin D 400 IU • Copper 1 mg • Folic Acid 800 mcg • Biotin 300 mcg • Iodine (Kelp) 150 mcg • Chromium 100 mcg • Selenium 100 mcg • Vitamin B12 100 mcg • Vitamin K 100 mcg • Pumpkin seeds 200 mg • Yellow Dock 200 mg • Alfalfa 100 mg • Bioflavonoids 100 mg • Beet tops 100 mg • Horsetail grass 100 mg • Hesperidin 50 mg • PABA 30 mg • Rutin 25 mg.

Prenatal Tablets - Nature's Plus
Each tablet contains: Vitamin A (as beta carotene) 8000 IU • Vitamin C (as ascorbic acid) 120 mg • Vitamin D (as ergocalciferol) 400 IU • Vitamin E (as D-alpha tocopheryl succinate) 60 IU • Thiamin (vitamin B1 as thiamine HCl) 3 mg • Riboflavin (vitamin B2) 3.4 mg • Niacin (as niacinamide) 40 mg • Vitamin B6 (as pyridoxine HCl) 4 mg • Folate (as folic acid) 800 mcg • Vitamin B12 (as cyanocobalamin) 12 mcg • Biotin 600 mcg • Pantothenic Acid (as calcium pantothenate) 20 mg • Calcium (as amino acid chelate/complex) 162 mg • Iron (as amino acid chelate/complex) 18 mg • Phosphorus (as amino acid complex) 125 mg • Iodine (from kelp) 300 mcg • Magnesium (as amino acid chelate/complex) 100 mg • Zinc (as gluconate) 7.5 mg • Copper (as gluconate) 4 mg. Other Ingredients: Di-calcium Phosphate, Isolated Soy Protein, Microcrystalline Cellulose, Magnesium Stearate, Stearic Acid, Rice Bran, Rose Hips, Pharmaceutical Glaze, Silica.

Prenatal Tablets - Leiner Health Products
Each tablet contains: Niacin (Niacinamide) 18 mg • Riboflavin (Vitamin B2) 1.7 mg • Vitamin A Acetate 4000 IU • Vitamin B12 (Cyanocobalamin - USP Method 2) 4 mcg • Vitamin E (dl-Alpha Tocopheryl Acetate) 11 IU • Vitamin C (Ascorbic Acid) 100 mg • Zinc Oxide 25 mg • Iron (Ferrous Fumarate) 27 mg • Calcium Sulfate 200 mg • Thiamin Mononitrate (Vitamin B1) 1.84 mg • Vitamin B6 (Pyridoxine Hydrochloride) 2.6 mg • Folate (Folic Acid) 800 mcg • Vitamin D (Ergocalciferol) 400 IU. Other Ingredients: Cellulose, Maltodextrin, Starch, Hydroxypropyl Methylcellulose, Croscarmellose Sodium, Sodium Starch Glycolate, Gelatin, Silicon Dioxide, Tricalcium Phosphate, Polyethylene Glycol 3350, Hydroxypropyl Cellulose, Titanium Dioxide, Magnesium Stearate, Phamaceutical Glaze, Polysorbate 80, Lactose, Yellow 6 Lake, Red 40 Lake, Blue 1 Lake, Beta Carotene, Resin.

Prenatal Vitamins - Nature's Bounty
Each tablet contains: Vitamin A (retinyl acetate and beta carotene) 4000 IU • Vitamin C (as Ascorbic Acid) 100 mg • Vitamin D (as Cholecalciferol) 400 IU • Vitamin E (as dl-Alpha Tocopheryl Acetate) 11 IU • Thiamin (as Thiamine Mononitrate) 1.84 mg • Riboflavin (Vitamin B-2) 1.7 mg • Niacin (as Niacinamide) 18 mg • Vitamin B-6 (Pyridoxine Hydrochloride) 2.6 mg • Folic Acid 800 mcg • Vitamin B-12 (as Cyanocobalamin) 4 mcg • Calcium (as Calcium Sulfate) 200 mg • Iron (as Ferrous Fumarate) 27 mg • Zinc (as Zinc Oxide) 25 mg. Other Ingredients: Cellulose, Vegetable Stearic Acid, Croscarmellose, Cellulose Coating, Vegetable Magnesium Stearate, Titanium Dioxide, FD&C Yellow No. 6 Aluminum Lake, FD&C Red No. 40 Aluminum Lake, FD&C Blue No. 1 Aluminum Lake.

Prenatal Vitamins - Sunmark
Each tablet contains: Vitamin A (30% as beta carotene) 4000 IU • Vitamin B6 2.6 mg • Vitamin B12 4 mcg • Vitamin C 100 mg • Vitamin D 400 IU • Vitamin E 11 IU • Thiamin (vitamin B1) 1.84 mg • Riboflavin (vitamin B2) 1.7 mg • Niacin 18 mg • Folate 800 mcg • Calcium 200 mg • Iron 27 mg • Zinc 25 mg. Other Ingredients: Microcrystalline Cellulose, Acacia, Sucrose Ester, Gelatin, Modified Cellulose Gum, Hypromellose, Hydroxypropyl Cellulose, Titanium Dioxide, Polyethylene Glycol, FD&C Yellow No. 6 Lake, FD&C Red No. 40 Lake, Maltodextrin, FD&C Blue No. 1 Lake, Gluten.
See Editor's Note No. 45.

Pre-Nate Oil - The Herbalist
Herbal oils of Sweet Almond, Safflower, Aloe Vera, Vitamin E, St. John's Wort flower, Calendula flower • Essential oils of French Lavender & Lemon.

Prenox D7 - Progressive Health Nutraceuticals
Vitamin A 5000 IU • Vitamin B1 25 mg • Vitamin B12 200 mcg • Vitamin C 250 mg • Vitamin E 45 IU • Selenium 200 mcg • Zinc 20 mg • Beta Carotene 5000 IU • L-Glutamine 500 mg • Milk Thistle extract 100 mg • Betaine 12.5 mg • Reishi mushroom 50 mg • Shitake mushroom 50 mg • Immune Enhancer AG 50 mg • N-Acetyl Cysteine HCl 50 mg • Beta Sitosterol 25 mg • L-Carnitine HCl 10 mg • Olive leaf extract 10 mg • Coenzyme Q10 1 mg.

Pressure-FX - CV Technologies Inc.
Each capsule contains: Shark Cartilage 180 mg • Cordyceps extract 20 mg.

Pressur-Lo - Futurebiotics LLC
Six tablets contain: Vitamin A (as beta-carotene) 6,000 IU • Vitamin C (as ascorbic acid) 360 mg • Vitamin D (as ergocalciferol) 150 IU • Thiamin 12 mg • Riboflavin 12 mg • Niacin (as niacinamide) 180 mg • Vitamin B6 (as pyridoxine hydrochloride) 12 mg • Vitamin B12 (as cyanocobalamin) 30 mcg • Pantothenic Acid (as calcium pantothenate) 120 mg • Calcium (as calcium carbonate, ascorbate) 480 mg • Magnesium (as magnesium oxide, chloride, citrate) 360 mg • Zinc (as zinc gluconate) 18 mg • Selenium (as selenomethionine) 120 mcg • Manganese (as manganese amino acid chelate) 24 mg • Chromium (as chromium polynicotinate) 180 mcg • Potassium (as potassium chloride, citrate) 330 mg • Garlic bulb powder concentrate 480 mg • Hawthorn berry powder extract (4:1) 282 mg • Horsetail leaf powder 180 mg • Juniper berry powder 180 mg • Valerian root powder 180 mg • Cayenne fruit powder 150 mg • Beta-sitosterol complex 210 mg • Rutin 150 mg • Betaine hydrochloride 150 mg • Taurine 480 mg. Other Ingredients: Cellulose, Stearic Acid, Magnesium Stearate, and Silica.

Prevalin - VitaStore
Bee Pollen • Brindal Berry (Hydroxycitric Acid, HCA) • Chromium Picolinate • Ginger • Ginseng • Carnitine • White Willow Bark • Vitamin A • Vitamin B1 • Vitamin B6 • Vitamin B12 • Vitamin C • Vitamin D • Vitamin E (D-Alpha Tocopherol) • Folic Acid • Iodine (Kelp) • Niacin • d-Biotin • Pantothenic Acid • Potassium Gluconate.

Prevent Pro Fiber Formula - Deseret Laboratories
Each scoop (6.6 g) contains: Guar Gum, Gum Arabic, Pectin, Locust Bean Gum, Natural Cherry flavor, Citrus flavor enhancer, Beet powder, Maltodextrin, Sucralose, Policosanol 5 mg.

Prevent Spray - Xtreme Formulations
Five sprays contain: PREVENT Proprietary Blend 0.875 mL: 3,6,17-Androstenetrione, 4-Hydroxyandrostenedione, Caffeine Anhydrous, Synephrine HCl, Octopamine HCl, Tyramine HCl. Other Ingredients: Isopropyl Alcohol, Benzyl Alcohol, Water, N-Methyl-2-Pyrrolidinone, Triglyceride Complex, L-Menthol, Laurocapram, Carbomer.

Preventa Tea - HerbaSway
Soy • Green Tea • Ginger • Blackberry • HerbaSweet (cucurbitaceae fruit).

Preventium brand - Applied Food Sciences, LLC
Potassium Hydrogen Glucarate: Monopotassium D-Glucarate • Potassium Acid Saccharate • Potassium Bisaccharate • Potassium Hydrogen Saccharate.
See Editor's Note No. 44.

Prevent-X - Cambridge Nutraceuticals
Each serving contains: L-Glutamine 10 g • N-Acetyl-Cysteine 4 g • Vitamin A (as mixed carotenoids) 4000 IU • Vitamin C 2000 mg • Vitamin E 700 IU • Folate 300 mcg • Magnesium 300 mg • Selenium 70 mcg • Zinc 10 mg • Copper 0.5 mg.

Previdia - Nutrica, Inc.
Each tablet contains: Tribulus Terrestris leaf extract 250 mg • Black Cohosh root extract 50 mg • Calcium 200 mg. Other Ingredients: Corn Starch, High Grade Plant Cellulose (HPMC), Colloidal Silicon Dioxide, Magnesium Stearate, Methyl Paraben, Propyl Paraben, Dibasic Calcium Phosphate Dihydrate, Croscarmellose Sodium, Titanium Dioxide, Talc, Polyethylene Glycol, Usalake FD&C Blue 1.

Pre-Vites - Puritan's Pride
Each tablet contains: Vitamin A 2500 IU • Vitamin C 60 mg • Vitamin D 400 IU • Vitamin E 15 IU • Thiamin 1.05 mg • Riboflavin 1.2 mg • Niacin 13.5 mg • Vitamin B6 1.05 mg • Folic Acid 0.3 mg • Vitamin B12 4.5 mcg.

Pre-Vites - Nature's Bounty
Each tablet contains: Vitamin A (as Retinyl Acetate) 2500 IU • Vitamin C (as Ascorbic Acid) 60 mg • Vitamin D (as Cholecalciferol) 400 IU • Vitamin E (as d-Alpha Tocopheryl Acetate) 15 IU • Thiamin Mononitrate (Vitamin B1) 1.05 mg • Riboflavin (Vitamin B2) 1.2 mg • Niacin (as Niacinamide) 13.5 mg • Vitamin B-6 (as Pyridoxine Hydrochloride) 1.05 mg • Folic Acid 0.3 mg • Vitamin B-12 (as Cyanocobalamin) 4.5 mcg. Other Ingredients: Sugar, Vegetable Stearic Acid, Natural Orange Flavor, Vegetable Magnesium Stearate, Silica, Mannitol.

Pre-Vites with Iron - Nature's Bounty
Each tablet contains: Vitamin A (as Retinyl Acetate) 2500 IU • Vitamin C (as Ascorbic Acid) 60 mg • Vitamin D (as Cholecalciferol) 400 IU • Vitamin E (as d-Alpha Tocopheryl Acetate) 15 IU • Thiamin Mononitrate (Vitamin B1) 0.05 mg • Riboflavin (Vitamin B2) 1.2 mg • Niacin (as Niacinamide) 13.5 mg • Vitamin B6 (as Pyridoxine Hydrochloride) 1.05 mg • Folic Acid 0.3 mg • Vitamin B12 (as Cyanocobalamin) 4.5 mcg • Iron (as Ferrous Fumarate) 7.5 mg. Other Ingredients: Sugar, Vegetable Stearic Acid, Natural Orange Flavor, Vegetable Magnesium Stearate, Silica, Mannitol.

Prima-C - PhysioLogics
Each capsule contains: Vitamin C (as Calcium Ascorbate) 500 mg • Calcium (as Calcium Ascorbate) 57 mg • Bioflavonoids (from citrus) 7 mg • Hesperidin 10 mg • Rutin 10 mg.

Primaderm - Prime Pharmaceutical Corp. (Canadian)
Active Ingredient: Mahonia Aquifolium.

Primal Defense HSO Probiotic Formula Caplets - Garden of Life, Inc.
Each caplet contains: Poten-Zyme Superfood Blend 800 mg: Barley grass juice, Oat grass juice, Yucca juice • Ionic Plant Based Minerals 100 mg • HSOs Probiotic Blend 1 billion CFU • Iron (fulvic acid source) 1.8 mg. Other Ingredients: Cellulose, Stearate (vegetable source).

Primal Defense HSO Probiotic Formula Powder - Garden of Life, Inc.
Each scoop contains: HSO Probiotic Blend 1 Billion CFU • Poten-Zyme Superfood Blend 800 mg: Dunaliella Salina, Barley grass juice, Oat Grass juice, Yucca juice • Ionic Plant Based Minerals 100 mg • Iron (fulvic acid source) 1.8 mg. Other Ingredients: Cellulose, Stearates (vegetable source).

Primanol Borage Oil - Jamieson
Each capsul contains: CIS-Linoleic Acid: from Borage Seed Oil 140.4 mg • CIS-Linoleic Acid: from Sunflower Seed Oil 75.6 • Gamma Linolenic Acid: from Borage Seed Oil 90 mg • Vitamin E (d-Alpha Tocopheryl Acetate) 10 IU.

Primavar - Unknown
Each capsule contains: 19-Norandrostenedione 100 mg • 4-Androstenediol 100 mg.
See Editor's Note No. 54.

Primavar II - Unknown
Each capsule contains: Bolandiol (Norandrostenediol) 100 mg • 4-Androstenediol 100 mg.
See Editor's Note No. 54.

Some Brand Name Natural Products - What they Contain

www.NaturalDatabase.com contains MANY more listings than appear here.
Editor's Notes are located on pages 2155-2163.

BRAND NAMES

PrimaVu Herbal Eye Drops - Molecular Health Commerce, Inc.
Matricaria Chamomilla L. tincture (German chamomile) HPUS 3X • Euprhasia Officinalis tincture (eyebright) HPUS 3X.
See Editor's Note No. 1.

PrimaVu Herbal Eye Drops Acuta - Molecular Health Commerce, Inc.
Euphrasia Officinalis tincture (eyebright) HPUS 3X • Foeniculum Vulgare tincture (fennel) HPUS 3X • Melilotus Officinalis tincture (yellow sweet clover) HPUS 3X.
See Editor's Note No. 1.

PrimaVu Herbal Eye Wash - Molecular Health Commerce, Inc.
Euphrasia Officinalis tincture (eyebright) HPUS 4X • Matricaria Chamomilla L. tincture (German chamomile) HPUS 4X.
See Editor's Note No. 1.

Prime Advantage Creatine Serum - Muscle Marketing USA
Each serving contains: Damiana • Yohimbe • Pygeum africanum • Glucosamine • Vitamin B12.

Prime Dreamz - Market America, Inc.
Two tablets contain: Magnesium (as magnesium oxide) 400 mg • Proprietary Herbal Blend 840 mg: Wild Jujube seed extract, Mucuna Pruriens seed extract, Passionflower 4:1 extract (aerial parts), Chamomile flower extract, Hops strobile 4:1 extract (humulus lupulus), Lemon Balm leaf extract, Valerian root extract, Melatonin (3 mg). Other Ingredients: Dicalcium Phosphate, Microcrystalline Cellulose, Croscarmellose Sodium, Stearic Acid, Magnesium Stearate, Silica, Film Coat (hypromellose, hydroxypropyl cellulose, polyethylene glycol, propylene glycol, titanium dioxide, carmine.)

Prime Factor for Men - Market America, Inc.
Three tablets contain: Pantothenic Acid (as D-calcium pantothenate) 100 mg • Iodine (from kelp) 75 mcg • Chromium (as chromium dinicotinate glycinate) 50 mcg • Zinc (as zinc arginate) 10 mg • Proprietary Herbal Blend 1571 mg: Silymarin (from milk thistle seed extract), Coleus Forskohlii tuber extract, Fo Ti root extract, Ashwagandha root extract, Astragalus root extract, Panax Ginseng root, L-Alpha-Glycerylphosphorycholine Hydrate (alpha-GPC), Lycium berry extract, Schizandra berry extract, Gamma-Aminobutyric Acid (GABA), Ornithine Alpha Ketoglutarate, Pregnenolone, Dehydroepiandrosterone (DHEA), Red Date fruit extract, RNA/DNA (from brewer's yeast). Other Ingredients: Dicalcium Phosphate, Guar Gum, Calcium Carbonate, Microcrystalline Cellulose, Stearic Acid, Vegetable Stearin, Citrus Pectin, Magnesium Stearate, Silica, Pharmaceutical Glaze.

Prime Factor for Women - Market America, Inc.
Three tablets contain: Pantothenic Acid (as D-calcium pantothenate) 100 mg • Iodine (from kelp) 33 mcg • Chromium (as chromium dinicotinate glycinate) 50 mcg • Zinc (as zinc glycinate) 5 mg • Proprietary Herbal Blend 1720 mg: L-Alpha-Glycerylphosphorycholine Hydrate (alpha-GPC), Silymarin (from milk thistle seed extract), Gamma-Aminobutyric Acid (GABA), Fo Ti root extract, Coleus Forskohlii tuber extract, Ornithine Alpha Ketoglutarate, Dong Quai root, Ashwagandha root extract, Eleuthero root extract, Astragalus root extract, Wild Yam root extract, Lycium berry extract, Red Date fruit, RNA/DNA (from brewer's yeast), Tribulus Terrestris extract (stem and dried fruit), Pregnenolone, Dehydroepiandrosterone (DHEA). Other Ingredients: Dicalcium Phosphate, Guar Gum, Microcrystalline Cellulose, Calcium Carbonate, Stearic Acid, Vegetable Stearin, Citrus Pectin, Magnesium Stearate, Silica, Pharmaceutical Glaze.

Prime Years - Schiff
Each softgel contains: Vitamin A (100% as beta carotene) 5000 IU • Vitamin C (as ascorbic acid, niacinamide ascorbate) 100 mg • Vitamin D (as cholecalciferol) 400 IU • Vitamin E (as d-alpha tocopherol) 60 IU • Vitamin K (as phylloquinone) 10 mcg • Vitamin B1 (as thiamin mononitrate) 5 mg • Vitamin B2 (as riboflavin) 5 mg • Vitamin B3 (as niacinamide ascorbate) 20 mg • Vitamin B6 (as pyridoxine hydrochloride) 5 mg • Folate (as folic acid) 400 mcg • Vitamin B12 (as cyanocobalamin) 25 mcg • Biotin 30 mcg • Pantothenic Acid (as d-calcium pantothenate) 20 mg • Calcium (from tricalcium phosphate) 100 mg • Iron (as ferrous chelate) 4 mg • Phosphorus (from tricalcium phosphate) 47 mg • Iodine (from kelp) 150 mcg • Magnesium (as magnesium oxide) 100 mg • Zinc (as zinc oxide) 15 mg • Selenium (from yeast) 20 mcg • Copper (as copper gluconate) 2 mg • Manganese (as manganese gluconate) 3.5 mg • Chromium (from yeast) 130 mcg • Molybdenum (as sodium molybdate) 75 mcg • Potassium (as potassium citrate) 10 mg • DL-Methionine 15 mg • Boron (as boron amino acid chelate) 1 mg. Other Ingredients: Soybean Oil, Softgel (gelatin, glycerin, St. John's bread), Lecithin, Rice Bran, Betaine Hydrochloride, Caramel Color.

Primo GH Stak - NutraBolics
Four capsules contain: L-Glutamine 1200 mg • Mucuna Pruriens (15% l-dopa) 100 mg • Colostrum 25% 500 mg • Phosphatidyl Choline 250 mg • Ascorbic Acid 500 mg • Passion Flower extract 400 mg • Schizandra 100 mg.

Primo HGH Stack - NutraBolics
Four capsules contain: L-Arginine 800 mg • L-Lysine 800 mg • L-Ornithine 260 mg • IsoLeucine 264 mg • L-Glycine 80 mg • Leucine 264 mg • Vitamin B6 (pyridoxine HCl) 200 mg • Gamma Aminobutyric Acid 400 mg • Valine 264 mg • Passion Flower extract 400 mg • Schizandra 100 mg.

Primobolin - National Urological Group
Each capsule contains: Proprietary Blend 550 mg: Epimedium 20% extract, L-Arginine, S-(2-Boeonethy)-L-Cysteine, Xanthoparmelia Scabrosa, Cnidium Monnier, Cistanches 12% extract, L-Citruline, Quebracho 8% extract, Gamma Amino Butyric Acid.

Primrose - Aspen Group, Inc.
Each softgel contains: Evening Primrose oil 500 mg • Vitamin E (D-alpha tocopherol) 10 IU • Gamma Linolenic Acid 40 mg • Linoleic Acid 350 mg.

Primrose 500 - Jarrow Formulas
Each softgel contains: Evening Primrose oil (oenothera lamarhciana) 500 mg • GLA (gamma linolenic acid) 45 mg • Gamma Tocopherol (a form of vitamin E) 7 mg. Other Ingredients: Gelatin, Glycerin, Water.

Primrose Oil - Atrium Biotechnologies
Each capsule contains: Oil of Evening Primrose 500 mg • Vitamin E (d-Alpha Tocopheryl Acetate) 10 IU • Gamma Linolenic Acid 40 mg • Lenoleic Acid 350 mg.

Prism Cola Green Tea Soda - Long Life Beverages
Carbonated Water • Organic Cane Sugar • Caramel (color) • Green Tea extract • Phosphoric Acid • Caffeine • Citric Acid.

Prism Lemon-Lime Green Tea Soda - Long Life Beverages
Carbonated Water • Organic Cane Sugar • Natural Lemon Lime Flavors • Green Tea extract • Citric Acid • Sodium Citrate.

Pro Blend 55 - Human Development Technologies (HDT)
Two scoops contain: Protein Blend of Micro Ultra Filtered Whey Protein concentrate, Egg Albumen, Calcium Caseinate, Micro Ultra Filtered Whey Protein Isolate, Ion Exchanged Whey Protein Isolate, Hydrolyzed Whey Protein Isolate • Natural & artificial Chocolate Flavorings • Acesulfame Potassium • Stevia.

Pro Bono - Ortho Molecular Products
Two packets contain: Vitamin D (D2, cholecalciferol) 1000 IU • Vitamin K (phytonadione) 1 mg • Folic ACid 800 mcg • Calcium (hydroxyapatite, Citrimal brand) 1000 mg • Phosphorus (chelate) 15 mg • Magnesium (amino acid chelate, citrate, aspartate) 400 mg • Selenium (amino acid complex) 200 mcg • Copper (lysinate) 1 mg • Manganese (Chelazome brand) 10 mg • Molybdenum (amino acid chelate) 150 mcg • Ipriflavone 600 mg • Strontium Citrate 1000 mg • Montmorillonite 150 mg • Boron (proteinate) 5 mg. The Clear/White packet contains 900 mg Calcium. The Clear/Clear packet contains 900 mg Strontium. Other Ingredients: Cranberry Juice Concentrate, Turmeric Root Extract, Ascorbyl Palmitate, Magnesium Stearate, Microcrystalline Cellulose, Silicon Dioxide.

Pro Citravin - Unknown
Each tablet contains: Pantothenic Acid 50 mg • GTF Chromium 60 mcg • Advantra Z Bitter Orange 500 mg • Guarana 4:1 extract (50 mg caffeine) 300 mg • Apple Cider Vinegar 200 mg • Capsicum 50 mg • Ginger root 5:1 extract 50 mg • Panax Ginseng root 5:1 extract 50 mg. Other Ingredients: Cellulose, Stearic Acid.
See Editor's Note No. 40.

Pro Complex APS - Optimum Nutrition
Two scoops (68 g) contain: Proprietary Amino Acid Blend 2 g: Glutamine Peptides, L-Leucine, L-Isoleucine, L-Valine • Aminogen 250 mg • Lactase (standardized to 100,000 FCC units/g) 1 mg • Protein Blend: Whey Protein Isolate, Whey Protein Concentrate, Egg Albumen, Whey Peptides • Natural and Artificial Flavor • Lecithin • Vitamin/Mineral Blend: Ascorbic Acid, Chromium GTF Polynicotinate, D-Alpha Tocopheryl Succinate (natural vitamin E), DiCalcium Phosphate, Biotin, Vitamin A Palmitate, Niacinamide, D-Calcium Pantothenate, Cholecalciferol, Folic Acid, Pyridoxine Hydrochloride, Riboflavin, Cyanocobalamin • Acesulfame Potassium, Sucralose.

Pro Complex Bars - Optimum Nutrition
Each bar (85 g) contains: Proprietary Blend 50 mg: Glutamine Peptides, L-Leucine, L-Isoleucine, L-Valine, Aminogen • Pro Complex Multi-Protein Blend: Calcium Caseinate, Whey Protein Isolate, Soy Protein Isolate • Glycerine • Maltitol • Coating (maltitol, palm kernal oil, cocoa, whey powder, lecithin, natural flavor) • Filtered Water • Natural Flavor • Lecithin • Peanut Flour • Ground Peanuts • Salt • Vitamin/Mineral Blend: Ascorbic Acid, D-Alpha Tocopheryl Succinate (natural vitamin E), Maltodextrin, Niacinamide, D-Calcium Pantothenate, Pyridoxine Hydrochloride, Chromium Polynicotinate, Riboflavin, Vitamin A Palmitate, Biotin, Folic Acid, Cholecalciferol, Cyanocobalamin • Sucralose • Acesulfame Potassium.

Pro Energy - Pro Health
Three capsules contain: Thiamin (vitamin B1, thiamine HCl) 51 mg • Vitamin B6 (as pyridoxine HCl) 51 mg • Magnesium (as magnesium glycinate) 26.3 mg • Malic Acid from Apple 600 mg • L-Tyrosine 75 mg. Other Ingredients: Rice Flour, Gelatin, Microcrystalline Cellulose, Magnesium Stearate, Water.

Pro Fuel (Milk & Egg Protein Drink) - TwinLab
Each serving contains: Pure Milk & Egg Protein 40 g • Extra Branched Chain Amino Acids (L-Leucine, L-Isoleucine, L-Valine) • L-Glutamine • All Essential Vitamins & Minerals including B Complex Vitamins plus Antioxidant Vitamin C & Vitamin E, Calcium & Magnesium. Patented Chromic Fuel Chromium Picolinate including Potassium, Zinc & Chromium.

Pro Lite - Optimum Nutrition
L-Carnitine • Choline • Inositol.

Pro Performance Chewable Creatine Monohydrate Tablets (Lemon-Lime) - GNC
Each tablet contains: Creatine Monohydrate 2.5 g. Other Ingredients: Sucrose, Dextrose, Natural Flavors, Beta-Carotene, Riboflavin Color.

Pro Performance Chewable Creatine Monohydrate Tablets (Orange) - GNC
Each tablet contains: Creatine Monohydrate 2.5 g. Other Ingredients: Sucrose, Dextrose, Natural Flavors, Beta-Carotene, Riboflavin Color.

Pro Performance Creatine Burst Dietary Supplement (Fruit Punch) - GNC
Two scoops (95 g) contain: Vitamin C 250 mg • Riboflavin (B2) 0.85 mg • Vitamin B6 1 mg • Folate, Folic Acid, Folacin 200 mcg • Vitamin B12 3 mcg • Calcium 20 mg • Phosphorus 100 mg • Magnesium 70 mg • Copper 2 mg • Chromium 300 mcg • Potassium 99 mg • Creatine Monohydrate 10 g • Taurine 2 g • L-Serine 1 g • Guanidinoacetate 200 mg. Other Ingredients: Maltodextrin, Natural/Artificial Flavor, Vitamin/Mineral Blend, Citric Acid, Acesulfame Potassium, Sucralose, FD&C Red #40.

Pro Performance Weight Gainer 1850, Strawberry Banana - GNC
Three cups (400 g) contain: Maltodextrin • Corn Syrup Solids • Protein Blend: Calcium Caseinate, Whey Protein Concentrate, Whey Protein Isolate, Sweet Dairy Whey, Egg Albumen • Fructose, Dextrose, Artificial Banana/Strawberry Flavor • Vitamin/Mineral PreMix: Di-Potassium Phosphate, Magnesium Oxide, Calcium Carbonate, Ascorbic Acid, Ferrous Fumarate, Chromium Polynicotinate, Biotin, D-Alpha Tocopheryl Succinate, Vitamin A Palmitate, Niacinamide, Copper Gluconate, Potassium Iodide, Zinc Oxide, D-Calcium Pantothenate, Selenomethionine, Riboflavin, Folic Acid, Cholecalciferol, Pyridoxine Hydrochloride, Manganese Glycinate, Thiamin Mononitrate, Molybdenum Glycinate, Cyanocobalamin • Guar Gum • Natural Beet Color • Citric Acid • Lecithin • Aminogen • Carbogen.

Pro-50 - Enzymatic Therapy
Each capsule contains: Vitamin A (Fish Liver oil) 1500 IU • Zinc (Chelate) 20 mg • Vitamin B6 (Pyridoxine HCL) 10 mg • Other Ingredients: EFA (unrefined Vegetable Lipids) 630 mg • Amino Acid Complex 150 mg • Prostate extract freeze-dried 150 mg • Saw Palmetto Berry extract 4:1 100 mg.
See Editor's Note No. 14.

Proactazyme Plus - Nature's Sunshine
Two capsules contain: Protease 4.5 (for protein) 19,000 HUT • Protease 6.0 (for protein) 3000 HUT • Protease 3.0 (for protein) 16 SAPU • Amylase (for starch) 4200 DU • Glucoamylase (for starch) 10 AGU • Lipase (for fat) 24 LU • Cellulase/Hemicellulase (for fiber) 120 CU • Invertase (for sugar) 220 SU • Malt Diastase (for starch) 550 DP • Alpha-Galactosidase (for sugar) 100 GALU • Peptidase (for protein) 2000 HUT. Other Ingredients: Beet root (beta vulgaris), Potassium Citrate, Caraway Seed (carum carvi), Dandelion Root (taraxacum officinale), Fennel Seed (foeniculum vulgare), Gentian Root (gentiana lutea), Ginger Rhizome (zingiber officinale), Gelatin, Water.

ProAlgen - Nordic Naturals
Each hardgel contains: Sodium 36 mg • Alginate 400 mg • Milk Thistle 40 mg.

Pro-Antho Forte - Progressive Labs
Each capsule contains: Pycnogenol 10 mg • Grape seed extract (vitis vinifera 5:1 concentrate) 50 mg • Ginkgo leaf extract (Ginkgo biloba, 50:1 concentrate) 20 mg • Green Tea leaf extract (Camellia sinensis, 65% standardized extract) 75 mg • Quercetin 100 mg • Milk Thistle (Silibum marianum, 80% standardized extract) 10 mg.

Proantho-C - Metagenics
Each tablet contains: Vitamin C (Ultra Potent-C brand) 250 mg • Niacin 20 mg • Grape Seed extract (vitis vinifera) 25 mg.

Probacillus Plus - ProJoba
Each tablet contans: Proprietary Blend 4 billion cells: Lactobacillus Acidophilus, Bifidobacterium Bifidum. Inactive Ingredients: Inositol, Monoatril Glutamas, Ascorbate, Yeast extract, Polysaccharides, Skim Milk Powder, Magnesium Stearate, Dextrose.

ProBasics (chocolate flavor) - Pure Encapsulations
One and a half scoops (42.1 g) contain: Calcium (naturally occurring) 168 mg • Phosphorous (naturally occurring) 146 mg • Magnesium (naturally occurring) 55 mg • Potassium (naturally occurring) 213 mg • Stevia 20 mg. Other ingredients: Whey Protein Isolate, Rice Protein Concentrate, Natural Flavors, Lo Han fruit extract (momordica grosvenori), Cocoa, Xylitol.

ProBasics (French vanilla flavor) - Pure Encapsulations
One and a half scoops (39.4 g) contain: Calcium (naturally occurring) 164 mg • Phosphorous (naturally occurring) 122 mg • Magnesium (naturally occurring) 38 mg • Potassium (naturally occurring) 110 mg • Stevia 40 mg. Other ingredients: Whey Protein Isolate, Rice Protein Concentrate, Natural Flavors, Lo Han fruit extract (momordica grosvenori).

***ProBasics (stawberry banana creme flavor)* - Pure Encapsulations**
One and a half scoops (38.2 g) contain: Calcium (naturally occurring) 164 mg • Phosphorous (naturally occurring) 122 mg • Magnesium (naturally occurring) 38 mg • Potassium (naturally occurring) 110 mg • Stevia 40 mg. Other ingredients: Whey Protein Isolate, Rice Protein Concentrate, Natural Flavors, Lo Han fruit extract (momordica grosvenori).

***Probiata* - Wakunaga of America**
Each tablet contains: Lactobacillus acidophilus 1 billion live cells in a vegetable starch complex.

***ProBio PCC* - Pharmanex**
Each capsule contains: Lactobacillus Fermentuam P.C.C. 100 mg.

***ProbioKids* - Metagenics**
Each 1/2 tsp serving contains: Proprietary Blend 7.5 billion organisms: Bifidobacterium Lactis BI-01, Bifidobacterium Lactis BI-07, Streptococcus Thermophilus St-21.

***Probioplex* - Metagenics**
Each rounded teaspoon contains: Immunoglobulins from whey protein 200 mg.

***Probioplex Intensive Care powder* - Metagenics**
Each 1 tbsp serving contains: Immunogloblulins from whey protein 241 mg • Lactoferrin 80 mg • Lactoperoxidase 20 mg.

***Probioplex Intensive Care tablets* - Metagenics**
Four tablets contain: Immunogloblulins from whey protein 150 mg • Lactoferrin 53 mg • Lactoperoxidase 13 mg. Other Ingredients: Fructooligosaccharides.

***Probiotic* - Enzymes, Inc.**
Each capsule contains: Proprietary Blend 345 mg: Lactobacillus plantarum, Lactobacillus casei, Bifidobacterium longum, Lactobacillus acidophilus. Other Ingredients: Plant Cellulose, Water.

***Probiotic A.Y.* - Futurebiotics LLC**
Lactobacillus acidophilus 3 billion cells at formulation Fructooligosaccharides (NutraFlora FOS) 600 mg • Inulin FOS 200 mg • Garlic (Pure-Gar 1500TM deodorized concentrate) 75 mg • Pau D'Arco 25 mg • Licorice (4:1 extract) 25 mg • Caprylic Acid (MCT) 100 mg • Echinacea (4:1 extract) 25 mg.

***Probiotic Eleven* - Nature's Sunshine**
Two capsules contain: Lactobacillus Rhamnosus 1.6 billion • Bifidobacterium Bifidus 1.2 billion • Lactobacillus Acidophilus 1.2 billion • Lactobacillus Brevis 1.2 billion • Lactobacillus Bulcaricus 1.2 billion • Lactobacillus Plantarum 1.2 billion • Streptococcus Thermophilus 1.2 billion • Bifidobacterium Infantis 800 million • Bifidobacterium Longum 800 million • Lactobacillus Casei 800 million • Lactobacillus Salivarius 800 million. Other Ingredients: FOS (short and long chain), Kosher Gelatin, Water.

***Probiotic Pearls* - PhytoPharmica**
Each pearl contains: Proprietary Probiotic Blend 1 billion CFU: Lactobacillus Acidophilus, Bifidobacterium Longum. Other Ingredients: Palm Oil, Gelatin, Glycerin, Lecithin, Pectin.

***ProBiotic Restore* - Advocare International**
Two capsules contain: Vitamin A (as beta-carotene) 2000 IU • OptiZinc Zinc (as zinc monomethionine) 1 mg • Lactobacillus Acidophilus 1 billion • Bifidobacterium Bifidum 1 billion • Fructooligosaccharides 500 mg • Moomiyo 50 mg • Aloe Vera rind powder 100 mg. Other Ingredients: Silicon Dioxide, Magnesium Stearate, Gelatin.

***Probiotica* - McNeil Consumer Healthcare**
Each tablet contains: Lactobacillus reuteri 100 million cells. Other Ingredients: Mannitol, Xylitol, Lactulose, Mono- and Diglycerides, Malic Acid, Lemon Flavor, Zein (corn protein), Riboflavin Phosphate.

***Probiotics 24B* - Matol Botanical International Ltd**
Each capsule contains: Lactobacillus Rhamnosus HA-111 6 billion CFU • Lactobacillus Acidophilus HA-122 4.8 billion CFU • Lactobacillus Casei HA-108 4.8 billion CFU • Bifidobacterium Longum HA-135 2.4 billion CFU • Lactococcus Lactis subsp. Lactis HA-136 2.4 billion CFU • Bifidobacterium Bifidum HA-132 1.2 billion CFU • Bifidobacterium Breve HA-129 1.2 billion CFU • Lactobacillus Planturum HA-119 1.2 billion CFU. Other Ingredients: Fructo-Oligosaccharides, Vegetable Capsule, Magnesium Stearate, Ascorbic Acid.

***Probiotics 24B for Women* - Matol Botanical International Ltd**
Each capsule contains: Lactobacillus Acidophilus HA-122 4.8 billion CFU • Lactobacillus Casei HA-108 4.8 billion CFU • Lactobacillus Rhamnosus HA-111 4.8 billion CFU • Streptococcus Thermophilus HA-110 4.8 billion CFU • Bifidobacterium Bifidum HA-132 1.2 billion CFU • Bifidobacterium Breve HA-129 1.2 billion CFU • Bifidobacterium Longum HA-135 1.2 billion CFU. Other Ingredients: Fructo-Oligosaccharides, Vegetable Capsule, Calcium Gluconate, Magnesium Sulfate, Magnesium Stearate, Ascorbic Acid.

***Pro-Body Balance (Pro-Equilibre)* - Abundance Marketing**
Each 1 tbsp serving contains: Proprietary Blend 4000 mg: Proprietary Herbal Complex: Aloe Vera leaf gel, Alfalfa leaf, American Ginseng root, Bioperine brand Black Pepper standardized extract, Buchu leaf, Cinnamon bark, Citrus Bioflavonoids, Corn Silk, Cranberry, Siberian Ginseng root, Goldenrod leaf, Grape seed, Kelp, Parsley, Grape skin, Ginger root, Holy Basil leaf, Honey, Olive leaf, Orange peel, Pomegranate fruit • Superfood Blend: Lycium, Hawaiian Noni juice, Papaya, Apple, Grape, Raspberry, Strawberry • Natural Sea Vegetation Blend: Trace Minerals, Amino Acids • Fruit and Vegetable Blend: Pineapple, Broccoli, Carrots, Orange, Brussels Sprouts, Cauliflower, Beet, Blueberry, Celery, Fig fruit, Grapefruit, Kale, Plum, Spinach, Radish, Watermelon, Lemon, Lime, Leek, Yellow Pepper, Cantaloupe, Onion, Peach, Tomato • Enzyme Blend: Bromelain, Papain, Amylase, Cellulase, Lactase, Lipase, Neutral Protease • Whole Food Greens Blend: Barley greens, Buckwheat, Kamut, Red Beet, Wheat grass, Chlorella, Phenalgin brand Brown algae, Dulse, Seaweed, Nori, Dunaliella Salina algae, Barley malt, Mung bean, Soybean, Wheat berry, Apple Pectin, Carrot fiber, Bee Pollen, Acerola, Astragalus root, Neutral root, Bilberry fruit, Spirulina. Other Ingredients: Purified Water, Fructose, Natural Flavors, Xanthan Gum, Potassium Sorbate, Sodium Benzoate, Citric Acid, Potassium Citrate, Cellulose Gum.

***ProBone-O Drops* - Life Enhancement Products, Inc.**
Each 1/2 dropper contains: Vitamin B12 1 mg • Folic Acid 1 mg • Pluronic Lecithin Organogel (PLO) 1.14 g.

***Pro-Brom* - Atrium Biotechnologies**
Each tablet contains: Bromelain 100 mg • Papayotin 30 mg.

***Procosa II* - USANA Health Sciences**
Two tablets contain: Manganese (as Manganese gluconate) 2.5 mg • Vitamin C (as Calcium Ascorbate) 150 mg • Glucosamine Sulfate 1000 mg • Silicon (as Amino Acid Complex) 1.5 mg • Turmeric Extract (Curcuma Longal root) 250 mg.

***Procylon (dominor centurion)* - Vision Laboratories**
Two tablets contain: Male Vitality Blend 1150 mg: Korean Ginseng root extract (4% ginsenosides), Yohimbe bark (1% yohimbine alkaloids), Saw Palmetto berry, Damiana leaf, L-Glutamic Acid, L-Lysine HCl, Wild Jujube seed extract, Ginkgo Biloba leaf, L-Arginine HCl, L-Alanine. Other Ingredients: Dicalcium Phosphate, Microcrystalline Cellulose, Toasted Wheat Germ, Croscarmellose Sodium, Stearic Acid, Magnesium Stearate, Silica.

***ProDHA (strawberry or unflavored)* - Nordic Naturals**
Two softgels contain: Vitamin E (mixed tocopherols) 12 IU • Omega-3 Fatty Acids 740 mg (DHA 500 mg, EPA 150 mg, other Omega-3 90 mg).

Some Brand Name Natural Products - What they Contain

www.NaturalDatabase.com contains MANY more listings than appear here.
Editor's Notes are located on pages 2155-2163.

Pro-DMG-B15 - PhytoPharmica
Each capsule contains: Calcium Gluconate 31 mg • Magnesium Aspartate 125 mg • Potassium Aspartate 125 mg • Trimethylglycine (TMG) 100 mg • N,N-Dimethylglycine HCl 100 mg • Glycine 25 mg. See Editor's Note No. 21.

Pro-Dophilus with FOS - Pro Health
Each capsule contains: Probiotic Bacteria 3.36 Billion organisms: L. Rhamnosus type B 672 million, L. Casei R215 672 million, L. Plantarum R202 336 million, L. Acidophilus RO52 72 million, Bifidobacterium Longum 672 million, Bifidobacterium Breve 336 million, Fructo-Oligosaccharides 210 mg • Vitamin C 1 mg. Other Ingredients: Maltodextrin, Gelatin.

ProEFA (lemon) - Nordic Naturals
Two soft gels contain: Vitamin E (mixed tocopherols) 27 IU • Omega-3 Fatty Acids 638 mg (EPA 296 mg, DHA 196 mg, Other Omega-3 146 mg) • Borage oil 360 mg (GLA 72 mg).

ProEFA Liquid (lemon) - Nordic Naturals
Each 1/2 tsp (2.5 mL) serving contains: Vitamin E (mixed tocopherols) 34 IU • Omega-3 Fatty Acids 798 mg (EPA 370 mg, DHA 245 mg, Other Omega-3 183 mg) • Borage oil 450 mg (GLA 90 mg).

ProEndorphin - Pharmalogic
Each sachet contains: Thiamine (as thiamine mononitrate) 15 mg • Riboflavin (as riboflavin phosphate) 16 mg • Niacin 50 mg • Vitamin B6 (as pyridoxine hydrochloride) 41 mg • Vitamin B12 (as cyanocohalamin) 300 mcg • Biotin 150 mcg • Pantothenic Acid (as calcium pantothenate) 48 mg • Novel Polyose Complex 700 mg • Proprietary Blend P.E. Complex 400 mg: Phenylalanine (as dl-phenylalanine), Phenylalanine (as d-phenylalanine) • DMAE (2-dimethylaminoethanol bitartrate) 200 mg • Myo-Inositol 100 mg • GNS2 Ginseng Extract (panax ginseng; standardized to 20% ginsenosides) 200 mg • Proprietary Blend NeuroMediating Complex 225 mg: Cola Nitida (seed), Taurine (as l-taurine). Other Ingredients: Citric Acid, Glucose, Beta Cyclodextrins, Natural Orange, Lemon Flavor, Lime Flavor.

ProEndorphin - Nutraceutics Corp.
Each effervescent sachet contains: Thiamine (as thiamine mononitrate) 15 mg • Riboflavin (as riboflavin phosphate) 16 mg • Niacin 50 mg • Vitamin B6 (as pyridoxine hydrochloride) 41 mg • Vitamin B12 (as cyanocobalamin) 300 mcg • Biotin 150 mcg • Pantothenic Acid (as calcium pantothenate) 48 mg • Novel Polyose Complex 700 mg • P.E. Complex 400 mg: Phenylalanine (as DL phenylalanine), Phenylalanine (as D phenylalanine) • DMAE (2-dimethylaminoethanol bitartrate) 200 mg • Myo-Inositol 100 mg • GNS2 Ginseng extract (panax ginseng, standardized to 20% ginsenosides) 200 mg • NeuroMediating Complex Proprietary Blend 225 mg: Cola Nitida seed, Taurine (as l-taurine). Other Ingredients: Citric Acid, Glucose, Beta Cyclodextrins, Natural Orange, Lemon and Lime Flavor.

Proenzi 99 (formerly Pro-Enz 99+) - Abundance Marketing
Ephedra stem (Ephedrine) 8 mg • Bladderwrack herb 15 mg • Astragalus root 15 mg • Rehmannia root 10 mg • White Willow bark 10 mg • Siberian Ginseng 10 mg • Kola nut 85 mg • Reishi Mushroom 5 mg • Dandelion root 5 mg • Ginger root 5 mg • Black Pepper extract 2.5 mg. In a base of Green Tea 85 mg • Bee Pollen 10 mg • Chromium (Chloride) 100 mcg • Niacin 1 mg. See Editor's Note No. 30.

ProEPA (lemon) - Nordic Naturals
Two softgels contain: Vitamin E (mixed tocopherols) 22 IU • Omega-3 Fatty Acids 1200 mg (EPA 900 mg, DHA 200 mg, other Omega-3 100 mg).

Pro-Essence - Flora Inc.
Burdock root • Juniper Berry • Prickley Ash bark • Slippery Elm bark • Uva Ursi.

ProEstron - Nutraceutics Corp.
Two caplets contain: Proprietary Blend Estrasterone 870 mg: Glycyrrhiza Uralensis (root), Isoflavone Complex, Dong Quai root, Black Cohosh root • Titrated Vitex 500 mg: Vitex Agnus-Castus fruit, Dioscorea root blend. Other Ingredients: Magnesium Stearate, DiCalcium Phosphate, Microcrystalline Cellulose.

Pro-F Complex - PhytoPharmica
Two tablets contain: Vitamin A (fish liver oil) 3000 IU • Vitamin D (fish liver oil) 100 IU • Calcium (lactate) 82 mg • Zinc (chelate) 20 mg • Magnesium (citrate) 13 mg • Pacific Sea Kelp 200 mg • Ovarian extract 90 mg • Whole Pituitary extract 60 mg • Adrenal extract 60 mg • Uterus extract 60 mg • RNA powder 60 mg. See Editor's Note No. 21 and No. 31.

Profemme - ProJoba
Each tablet contains: Flower Pollen extract WSI 72 mg • Flower Pollen extract LS1 4 mg. Other Ingredients: Microcrystalline Cellulose, Lactose, Magnesium Stearate, Silicon Dioxide, Natural Resin, Polyethylene Glycol, Talc.

Professional's Care Always Active Aloe Foot Cream - Warren Laboratories
Aloe Vera distillate • Glyceral MonoStearate • Isopropyl Myristate • Stearyl Stearate • Propylene Glycol • Mink oil • Glyceryl Stearate • Cetearyl Alcohol • Ceteareth-20 • Cetyl Alcohol • Ceteth-10 • Fragrance • Propyl Parabens • Methyl Parabens.

Professional's Care Always Active Aloe Gel - Warren Laboratories
Barbadensis Miller Aloe Vera distillate • Carbamer • Methyl Parabens.

Professional's Care Always Active Aloe Herbal Rub - Warren Laboratories
Aloe Vera distillate • 1-Menthol • Steareth-2 • Steareth-21 • Peppermint oil • Spearmint oil • Sodium Carbomer • Clove oil • Propyl Parabens • Methyl Parabens.

Professional's Care Always Active Aloe Liniment Rub - Warren Laboratories
Aloe Vera distillate • SDA 40-A Ethanol • Sodium Carbamer • 1-Menthol • Methyl Parabens • Peppermint oil • FD&C Blue #1.

Professional's Care Always Active Aloe Lotion Plus - Warren Laboratories
Aloe Vera distillate • Isopropyl Myristate • Isopropyl Palamate • Stearyl Alcohol • Ceteareth-20 • Glyceryl Stearate • PEG-100 Stearate • Cotton seed oil • Propylene Glycol • Cetearyl Alcohol • Propyl Parabens • Fragrance • Methyl Parabens • Sodium Carbamer.

Professional's Care Always Active Aloe Oil of Wintergreen - Warren Laboratories
Aloe Vera distillate • Methyl Salicylate • 1-Menthol • Propylene Glycol • Cetearyl Alcohol • Steareth-21 • Steareth-2 • Sodium Carbamer • Propyl Parabens • Methyl Parabens.

Professional's Care Always Active Aloe Ointment - Warren Laboratories
Aloe Vera distillate • Glyceryl Stearate • PEG-100 Stearate • Cetyl Esters • Cetyl Alcohol • Mineral oil • Glycerin • Methyl Parabens • Propyl Parabens.

Professional's Care Always Active Aloe Spray Mister - Warren Laboratories
100% Barbadensis Miller Aloe Vera distillate.

Profile 1 - Mannatech
Three tablets contain: Vitamin A 2500 IU • Vitamin B1 27 mg • Vitamin B12 18 mcg • Vitamin B2 24 mg • Vitamin B6 26 mg • Beta Carotene 100 IU • Bioflavonoids 95 mg • Biotin 36 mcg • Vitamin C 187 mg • Choline 19 mg • Vitamin D 400 IU • Vitamin E 30 IU • Folic Acid 400 mcg • Inositol 90 mcg • Vitamin K 90 mcg • Niacinamide 30 mg • PABA 5 mg • Pantothenic Acid 5 mg • Boron 150 mcg • Calcium 10 mg • Copper 20 mcg • GTF Chromium

150 mcg • Iodine 3 mcg • Iron 5 mg • Magnesium 50 mg • Manganese 12 mg • Molybdenum 70 mcg • Potassium 75 mg • Selenium 15 mcg • Silicon 500 mcg • Vanadium 10 mcg • Zinc 7 mg • Ambrotose Complex (naturally occurring plant polysaccharides including freeze-dried Aloe Vera inner leaf gel extract - Manapol powder) 25 mg.
See Editor's Note No. 17.

Profile 2 - Mannatech
Three tablets contain: Vitamin A 15000 IU • Vitamin B1 2 mg • Vitamin B12 125 mcg • Vitamin B2 5 mg • Vitamin B6 2 mg • Beta Carotene 5000 IU • Bioflavonoids 56 mg • Biotin 57 mcg • Vitamin C 130 mg • Choline 55 mg • Vitamin D 170 IU • Vitamin E 62 IU • Folic Acid 200 mcg • Inositol 25 mg • Vitamin K 50 mcg • Niacinamide 38 mg • PABA 7 mg • Pantothenic Acid 29 mg • Boron 500 mcg • Calcium 75 mg • Copper 700 mcg • GTF Chromium 50 mcg • Iodine 100 mcg • Iron 2 mg • Magnesium 10 mg • Manganese 2 mg • Molybdenum 70 mcg • Potassium 7 mg • Selenium 15 mcg • Silicon 2.5 mcg • Vanadium 10 mcg • Zinc 15 mg • Ambrotose Complex (naturally occurring plant polysaccharides including freeze-dried aloe Vera inner leaf gel extract - Manapol powder) 25 mg.
See Editor's Note No. 17.

Profile 3 - Mannatech
Three tablets contain: Vitamin A 7500 IU • Vitamin B1 7 mg • Vitamin B12 68 mcg • Vitamin B2 8 mg • Vitamin B6 10 mg • Beta Carotene 2500 IU • Bioflavonoids 75 mg • Biotin 52 mcg • Vitamin C 170 mg • Choline 40 mg • Vitamin D 210 IU • Vitamin E 50 IU • Folic Acid 300 mcg • Inositol 20 mcg • Vitamin K 90 mcg • Niacinamide 32 mg • PABA 6 mg • Pantothenic Acid 23 mg • Boron 300 mcg • Calcium 60 mg • Copper 300 mcg • GTF Chromium 80 mcg • Iodine 30 mcg • Iron 3.5 mg • Magnesium 25 mg • Manganese 8 mg • Molybdenum 70 mcg • Potassium 12 mg • Selenium 15 mcg • Silicon 2 mg • Vanadium 10 mcg • Zinc 10 mg • Ambrotose Complex (naturally occurring plant polysaccharides including freeze-dried Aloe Vera inner leaf gel extract - Manapol powder) 25 mg.
See Editor's Note No. 17.

Proflavanol - USANA Health Sciences
Each tablet contains: Vitamin C (as calcium, potasium, magnesium and zinc ascorbates) 100 mg • Grape Seed extract 30 mg • Ascorbyl Palmitate 12 mg. Inactive Ingredients: Microcrystalline Cellulose, Croscarmellose Sodium, Pregelatinized Starch, Dextrin, Colloidal Silicon Dioxide, Dextrose.

Proflavanol 90 - USANA Health Sciences
Each tablet contains: Vitamin C (as calcium, potasium, magnesium and zinc ascorbates) 300 mg • Grape Seed extract 90 mg • Ascorbyl Palmitate 12 mg. Inactive Ingredients: Microcrystalline Cellulose, Croscarmellose Sodium, Pregelatinized Starch, Dextrin, Colloidal Silicon Dioxide, Dextrose.

Proflora - BioBotanical Research
Distilled Water • Lactobacillus Acidophilus (whey fermentation) • Bifidobacterium complex • Aloe Vera • Yucca Schidigera • Lactobacillus Salivarius • Chlorophyll • Herba Mentha Piperita • Radix Zingiber Officinalis • Taraxacum Officinale • Viola Odorata.

ProForm Bars, Peanut Chocolate - Advocare International
SusCarb (fructose, maltodextrin, glycerin) • Protein Blend (soy protein isolate, whey protein concentrate, L-glutomine, L-lysine) • Milk Chocolate flavored coating (sugar, palm kernel oil, nonfat milk, cocoa [processed with alkali], dextrose, lecithin, natural flavor) • Water • Crisp Rice (rice flour, malt extract, rice bran) • Cocoa (processed with alkali) • Natural Flavors • Guarana extract • Walnuts • Choline Bitartrate • Kola Nut extract • Taurine • Green Tea extract • Potassium Chloride • Ascorbic Acid • Creatine Monohydrate • Calcium Pantothenate • Salt • Niacinamide • D-Alpha Tocopheryl Succinate • Pyridoxine Hydrochloride • L-Carnitine • Ginkgo Biloba extract • Folic Acid • Riboflavin • Thiamine Hydrochloride • Beta-Carotene • Chromium Polynicotinate (ChromeMate) • Biotin • Cyanocobalamin.

Pro-G Yam Cream - Nature's Sunshine
Purified Water • Glycerin • Octyl Salicylate • Lanolin Alcohol • Decyl Oleate • Glyceryl Stearate • PEG-40 Hydrogenated Castor oil • Progesterone • PEG-40 Stearate • Phenoxyethanol • Sorbitan Oleate • Wild Yam extract (dioscorea villosa) • Hydrogenated Lecithin • Dimethicone • Acrylates/C10-30 Alkyl Acrylate Crosspolymer • Horsetail extract (equisetum arvense) • Yucca extract (yucca schidigrea) • Chamomile extract (matricaria recutita) • Methylparaben • Tocopheryl Acetate • Sodium Hydroxide • Butylparaben • Menthol • Ethylparaben • Ginkgo Biloba extract • Aloe Barbadensis gel • Propylparaben.

ProGain - Metagenics
Two scoops (78 g) contain: Vitamin A (50% as retinyl palmitate and 50% as beta-carotene) 2500 IU • Vitamin D (cholecalciferol) 100 IU • Vitamin E (D-alpha tocopheryl succinate) 15 IU • Calcium (glycinate) 230 mg • Vitamin C (ascorbic acid) 15 mg • Folate (folic acid) 200 mcg • Vitamin B12 (cyanocobalamin) 3 mcg • Thiamin (mononitrate) 0.75 mg • Riboflavin 1 mg • Niacin (niacinamide) 5 mg • Vitamin B6 (pyridoxine alpha ketoglutarate) 26 mg • Biotin 150 mcg • Pantothenic Acid (D-calcium pantothenate) 41 mg • Inositol 50 mg • Sodium 190 mg • Potassium (phosphate) 310 mg • Phosphorus 104 mg • Magnesium (bis-glycinate) 145 mg • Manganese (arginate) 1 mg • Copper (glycinate) 380 mcg • Zinc (arginate) 3 mg • Iron (glycinate) 3 mg • Molybdenum (aspartate) 5 mcg • Chromium (dinicotinate glycinate) 100 mcg • Boron (citrate, aspartate, glycinate) 245 mcg • Selenium (as selenomethionine) 13 mcg • Betaine Hydrochloride 50 mg • Alpha-Ketoglutarate 21 mg • Alpha-Lipoic Acid 100 mcg. Other Ingredients: Maltodextrin, Fructose, Whey Protein, Natural Flavors.

Pro-Gain - Nature's Life
Two scoops (28.35 g) contain: SUPRO brand soy protein isolate containing Lecithin • Whey • Fructose • Non-fat Dry Milk • natural Vanilla Flavor • Yeast • Egg Albumin • Eggshell powder • Kelp • natural Papain Enzyme concentrate • Cobalamin concentrate (B12). Pro-Gain also contains 34 mg of naturally occuring Isoflavones, including 21 mg Genistein & 10 mg Daidzen.

Progensa - Life-Flo
Each ounce contains: Natural Progesterone USP Grade 480 mg. Other Ingredients: Grape seed extract, aloe vera, vitamin E, & primrose.

Progensa20 - Xymogen
Deionized Water • Aloe Vera gel • Caprylic/Capric Triglycerides • Shea Butter • Sunflower seed oil • Stearic Acid • Natural Progesterone USP • Glyceryl Stearate • PEG-100-Stearate • Beeswax • Isopropyl Palmitate • MSM • Evening Primrose oil (oenothera biennis) • Burdock root extract • Chamomile extract • Ginseng extract • Lavender extract • Lecithin • Vegetable Glycerin • Stearyl Alcohol or Cetyl Alcohol • Flavonoids (extracts of artichoke and sarsaparilla) • Carbomer • Triethanolamine • Xanthan Gum • Hydroxypropylmethylcellulose • Allantoin • Disodium EDTA • Potassium Sorbate • Grape seed extract.

ProgensaPlus - Xymogen
Deionized Water • Aloe Vera gel • Caprylic/Capric Triglycerides • Shea Butter • Sunflower seed oil • Stearic Acid • Natural Progesterone USP • Glyceryl Stearate • PEG-100-Stearate • Beeswax • Isopropyl Palmitate • MSM • PhytoPro brand natural super Phytoestrogen • Red Clover tops extract • Chasteberry extract • Dong Quai extract • Saw Palmetto extract • Lavender extract • Tocotrienols • Lecithin • Vegetable Glycerin • Stearyl Alcohol or Cetyl Alcohol • Flavonoids (from artichoke and sarsaparilla) • Carbomer • Triethanolamine • Xanthan Gum • Hydroxypropylmethylcellulose • Allantoin • Disodium EDTA • Potassium Sorbate • Grape seed extract.

Pro-Gest - PhytoPharmica
Two tablets contain: Niacinamide 20 mg • Betaine HCl 310 mg • L-Glutamic Acid HCl 310 mg • Bromelain (from pineapple) 10:1 200 mg • Papain 200 mg • Mylase Lipase 200 mg • Mycozyme (fungal amylase) 50 mg • Ox Bile extract 32 mg • Pancreas extract 32 mg.
See Editor's Note No. 14.

Pro-Gest Progesterone Cream - Transitions for Health, Inc.
Ingredients: Distilled Water • Aloe Barbadensis gel • Tocopheryl Acetate • Cetyl Alcohol • Octyl Palmitate • Sweet Almond oil (prunus amygdalus dulcis) • Panthenol • PEG-8 Stearate • Stearic Acid • Glycerin • USP Progesterone • Polysorbate 60 • Propylene Glycol • Lemon oil (citrus medica limonum) • Carbomer • Methylparaben • Propylparaben • Triethanolamine • Phenoxyethanol.

Progesta Plus - Aarisse Health Care
Each 3 oz pump contains: Aloe Vera extract • Shea Butter • Phospholipids/Liposomes • Natural Progesterone USP micronized • Wild Yam extract • Polysaccharides • Evening Primrose Oil • Vitamin E • Allantoin • Potassium Sorbate (fron pears and avocados) • Rosemary Oil • Red Clover Isoflavones.

ProgestaCare - Life-Flo
Aloe Vera gel • Caprylic/Capric Triglyceride • natural Progesterone derived from the Mexican Wild Yam root • Evening Primrose oil (Oenothera biennis) • Vitamin E Acetate • Isostearic Acid • Glyceryl Stearate • Siberian Ginseng • Burdock root • Black Cohosh • MSM • Chamomile • Glycerin • Allantoin • Grape seed extract.

Pro-Gest-Ade - Enzymatic Therapy
Each tablet contains: Niacinamide 10 mg. Other Ingredients: Betaine HCl 155 mg • Glutamic Acid HCl 155 mg • Bromelain (600 MCU) 100 mg • Papain 100 mg • Mylase (lipase) 100 mg • Mycozyme (amylase) 25 mg • Ox Bile extract 16 mg • Pancreas extract 16 mg. See Editor's Note No. 14.

Progestaroma - Global Health Trax
Purified Water • Octyl Palmitate (from palm oil) • Glycerine • Ceteayl Glucoside • Tocopheryl Acetate • Progesterone USP (500 mg/oz) • Cetyl Alcohol (from coconut) • Panthenol • Aloe Vera Gel • Wild Yam extract • Ascorbic Acid • Sodium Hyaluronate • Carbomer • Sodium Hydroxide • Potassium Sorbate • Pure Essential Oils Blend: Sandalwood, Lavender, Orange, Geranium • Grapefruit seed extract.

Progesterone Cream - PhysioLogics
Purified Water • Aloe Vera gel • Petrolatum • Tocopheryl Acetate (vitamin E) • Cetearyl Alcohol and Ceteareth-20 • Glyceryl Stearate • C12-15 Alkyl Benzoate • Stearic Acid • Cetyl Alcohol • Glycerin • Progesterone • Triethanolamine • Polysorbate 80 • Keratin Amino Acids • Diazolidinyl Urea • Carbomer • Coconut oil • Almond oil • Grapefruit seed extract (citrus grandis) • Methylparaben • BHA • Lemon oil (citrus medica limonum) • Propylparaben • Panthenol • Sodium Hyaluronate.

Progesterone Cream - Source Naturals
Each ounce contains: Natural Progesterone USP from Soy 500 mg. Inactive Ingredients: Purified Water, Aloe Vera Gel, Cetearyl Glucoside, Caprylic/Capric Triglyceride, Cetyl Alcohol, Glycerin, Wild Yam extract, Tocopheryl Acetate (Natural Vitamin E), Lecithin Phospholipid, Glyceryl Stearate, Jojoba, Squalane, Stearic Acid, Sage leaf extract, Black Cohosh root extract, Ginseng root extract, Marigold tops extract, Grapefruit seed extract, Methylparaben, Propylparaben, Sorbic Acid, Xanthan Gum, Rosemary Oil.

Progesterone Plus Creme - Nutri-Quest Rx
Water • Stearic Acid • Cetyl Alcohol • Sesame oil • Progesterone USP (Homeopathic) • Triethanolame • Arnica oil • Evening Primrose oil • Zinc • Copper • Magnesium • Glyconucleopeptides • Peg 10 Soya Sterol • Hydroxyethycellulose • Disodium EDTA • Cetyl Ricinoleate • Canola oil • Wild Yam • Dex - Panthenol (Vitamin B5) • Progesterone USP • Honey • Lecithin • NaPCA • Silicon • Iron • Peg 7 Glycerol Cocoate • Carrot oil • Carbomer • Phenyldimethicone • Sodium Hydroxymethylglycinate.

Progesterone Transdermal - Life Enhancement Products, Inc.
Aloe Vera gel • Distilled Water • C10-C18 Triglycerides • Tocopherol • Polyethylene Glycol esters • Octyl Palmitate • Glyceryl Stearate • Isopropyl Alcohol • Cetyl Alcohol • USP Progesterone • Emulsifying wax NF • Avocado oil • Glycerine • Panthenol • Hydrolyzed Protein • Hyaluronic Acid • Lemon oil • Carbomer 940 • Methylparaben • Propylparaben.

Progesterone-DP - Life Enhancement Products, Inc.
Aloe Vera gel • Distilled Water • C10-C18 Triglycerides • Tocopherol • Polyethylene Glycol esters • Octyl Palmitate • Glyceryl Stearate • Isopropyl Alcohol • Cetyl Alcohol • USP Progesterone • Emulsifying wax NF • Avocado oil • Glycerine • Pregnenolone • Dehydroepiandrosterone • Panthenol • Hydrolyzed Protein • Hyaluronic Acid • Lemon oil • Carbomer 940 • Methylparaben • Proplyparaben.

ProGram16: Chocolate - Pharmanex
Each bar contains: High Fructose Corn Syrup • Whey Protein Isolate • Soy Protein Isolate • Sugar • Milk Protein Isolate • Cocoa Butter • Unsweetened Chocolate • Lowfat Cocoa (processed with alkali) • Milk • Creatine Monohydrate 1 g • Glycerin • Maltodextrin • Dicalcium Phosphate • Natural and Artificial Flavors • Taurine 250 mg • Magnesium Carbonate • Potassium Chloride • Potassium Citrate • Egg Whites • Ascorbic Acid • Lecithin • D-Alpha Tocopherol Acetate • Beta-Carotene • Niacinamide • Calcium Pantothenate • Zinc Oxide • Chromium Chelate • Carbonyl Iron • Copper Gluconate • Manganese Sulfate • Pyridoxine Hydrochloride • Riboflavin • Thiamine Mononitrate • Folate (folic acid) • Biotin • Potassium Iodide • Sodium Molybdate • Sodium Selenite • Phytonadine • Cholecalciferol • Cyanocobalamin.

ProGram16: Coconut - Pharmanex
Each bar contains: High Fructose Corn Syrup • Whey Protein Isolate • Soy Protein Isolate • Sugar • Partially Defatted Peanut Flour • Milk Protein Isolate • Cocoa Butter • Unsweetened Chocolate • Milk • Creatine Monohydrate 1 g • Glycerin • Natural and Artificial Flavors • Maltodextrin • Dicalcium Phosphate • Potassium Chloride • Taurine 250 mg • Magnesium Carbonate • Egg Whites • Ascorbic Acid • Lecithin • Salt • d-Alpha Tocopherol Acetate • Beta-Carotene • Niacinamide • Calcium Pantothenate • Zinc Oxide • Chromium Chelate • Carbonyl Iron • Copper Gluconate • Manganese Sulfate • Pyridoxine Hydrochloride • Riboflavin • Thiamine Mononitrate • Folate (Folic Acid) • Biotin • Potassium Iodide • Sodium Molybdate • Sodium Selenite • Phytonadine • Cholecalciferol • Cyanocobalamin.

ProGram16: Peanut Butter - Pharmanex
Each bar contains: High Fructose Corn Syrup • Whey Protein Isolate • Soy Protein Isolate • Sugar • Partially Defatted Peanut Flour • Milk Protein Isolate • Cocoa Butter • Unsweetened Chocolate • Milk • Creatine Monohydrate 1 g • Glycerin • Maltodextrin • Dicalcium Phosphate • Natural and Artificial Flavors • Taurine 250 mg • Magnesium Carbonate • Potassium Chloride • Egg Whites • Ascorbic Acid • Lecithin • Salt • d-Alpha Tocopherol Acetate • Beta-Carotene • Niacinamide • Calcium Pantothenate • Zinc Oxide • Chromium Chelate • Carbonyl Iron • Copper Gluconate • Manganese Sulfate • Pyridoxine Hydrochloride • Riboflavin • Thiamine Mononitrate • Folate (Folic Acid) • Biotin • Potassium Iodide • Sodium Molybdate • Sodium Selenite • Phytonadine • Cholecalciferol • Cyanocobalamin.

Progressive 17 - Progressive Natural Products
Vitamin C 60 mg • Vitamin E 30 IU • Phosphatidylserine 20 mg • Acetyl L-Carnitine HCl 50 mg • Ginkgo Biloba extract 25 mg • Huperzine A extract 500 mcg • Vinpocetine 10 mcg • Bacopa extract 50 mcg.

Progressive 27 - Progressive Health Nutraceuticals
Vitamin C 60 mg • Zinc 10 mg • Omega 3 Fatty Acids 50 mg • L-Glutamine 200 mg • L-Arginine HCl 200 mg • Aloe Vera 50 mg • Gotu Kola 100 mg • BioCell brand Type II Collagen 100 mg • Hyaluronic Acid 10 mg • Chondroitin Sulfate 60 mg.
See Editor's Note No. 15.

Progressive 7 - Progressive Health Nutraceuticals
Vitamin E 100 IU • Calcium 500 mg Selenium 150 mcg • Coenzyme Q10 5 mg • Soy Isoflavones 20 mg • Shitake mushroom 50 mg • Immune Enhancer AG 200 mg • Green Tea extract 250 mg • Lecithin 25 mg.

Pro-Guard - Nutralife Health & Fitness (NZ) Ltd.
Each tablet contains: Saw Palmetto Fruit 500 mg • Hydrangea Root and Rhiz. 100 mg • Golden Rod Herb 50 mg • Couch Grass Root 200

BRAND NAMES

mg • Horsetail Herb 100 mg • Panax Ginseng Root 100 mg • Zinc Gluconate (providing 15 mg zinc) 112.5 mg • Magnesium Amino Acid Chelate (Providing magnesium 15 mg) 75 mg • Calcium Ascorbate 250 mg • Pyridoxine Hydrocholoride (Vitamin B6) 15 mg • Glutamine 100 mg • Glycine 100 mg • Alanine 100 mg.

ProHerbs Blood Sugar Balance **- Mason Vitamins, Inc.**
Two tablets contain: Biotin 600 mcg • Magnesium (as Oxide) 200 mg • Zinc (as Sulfate) 30 mg • Gymnema Sylvestre leaves (standardized to 24% Gymnemic Acid) 300 mg • Bitter Melon powder (Momordica charantia fruit) 200 mg • Ginkgo Biloba leaf (standardized to 24% flavonoids glycosides & 6% terpene lactones) 120 mg • Chromium Picolinate 400 mcg • Alpha Lipoic Acid 150 mg • Quercetin 50 mg • Vanadium (as Vanadyl Pentoxide) 40 mcg. Other Ingredients: Dicalcium Phosphate, Microcrystalline Cellulose, Croscarmellose Sodium, Hydroxypropylmethylcellulose, Magnesium Stearate, Mineral Oil, Polyethylene Glycol, Stearic Acid, Titanium Dioxide, Sodium Lauryl Sulfate, FD&C Yellow #6 Lake, Red #40 Lake, Iron Oxide.

ProHerbs Bone & Joints **- Mason Vitamins, Inc.**
Three tablets contain: Vitamin D (D3) 240 IU • Calcium (as Calcium Carbonate) 1005 mg • Isoflavones as Soy standardized extract 60 mg • Glucosamine Sulfate 510 mg • Chondroitin Sulfate 405 mg • Boron 4.5 mg. Other Ingredients: Croscarmellose Sodium, Hydroxypropylmethylcellulose, Magnesium Stearate, Mineral Oil, Polyethylene Glycol, Stearic Acid, Titanium Dioxide, Sodium Lauryl Sulfate, Iron Oxide.
See Editor's Note No. 15.

ProHerbs Breast Health **- Mason Vitamins, Inc.**
Two tablets contain: Vitamin C (as ascorbic acid) 200 mg • Selenium (as selenomethionine) 200 mcg • Broccoli extract (20:1 extract) 170 mg • Curcumin root extract (Curcuma longa standardized to 2% curcuminoids) 600 mg • Genistein from Soy extract 20 mg • Citrus Bioflavonoids 100 mg • Flaxseed powder 400 mg. Other Ingredients: Dicalcium Phosphate, Microcrystalline Cellulose, Croscarmellose Sodium, Stearic Acid, Magnesium Stearate, Hydroxypropylmethylcellulose, Mineral Oil, Triacetin, Titanium Dioxide, FD&C Yellow #6 Lake.

ProHerbs Energy **- Mason Vitamins, Inc.**
Each tablet contains: Thiamin HCl (B1) 25 mg • Riboflavin (B2) 25 mg • Vitamin B6 (Pyridoxine HCl) 25 mg • Vitamin B12 (Cyanocobalamin) 50 mcg • Folic Acid 400 mcg • Korean Ginseng root (Panax Ginseng standardized to 10% ginsenosides) 100 mg • Kola Nut (3:1 extract) (Cola acuminata) 500 mg • Guarana root (Paullina cupana 3:1 extract) 200 mg • Royal Jelly 50 mg. Other Ingredients: Dicalcium Phosphate, Microcrystalline Cellulose, Croscarmellose Sodium, Hydroxypropylmethylcellulose, Magnesium Stearate, Mineral Oil, Stearic Acid, Titanium Dioxide, Triacetin, FD&C Yellow #6 Lake.

ProHerbs Immune Defense **- Mason Vitamins, Inc.**
Two tablets contain: Vitamin C (Ascorbic Acid) 500 mg • Vitamin E (Dl-Alpha Tocopherol Acetate) 400 IU • Zinc (as Sulfate) 15 mg • Selenium (as Selenomethionine) 200 mcg • ActiVin Grape Seed extract (Vitis vinifera seeds standardized to 95% polyphenols) 100 mg • Echinacea root (Echinacea purpurea) 100 mg • Alpha Lipoic Acid (standardized to 4% phenolic compounds) 50 mg. Other Ingredients: Dicalcium Phosphate, Croscarmellose Sodium, Hydroxypropylmethylcellulose, Magnesium Stearate, Microcrystalline Cellulose, Mineral Oil, Polyethylene Glycol, Silicon Dioxide, Stearic Acid, Titanium Dioxide, Sodium Lauryl Sulfate, FD&C Yellow #6 Lake, Yellow #10 Lake.

ProHerbs Leg Vein & Circulation **- Mason Vitamins, Inc.**
Two tablets contain: Vitamin C 240 mg • Green Tea leaf (camellia sinensis standardized to 50% catechins) 100 mg • Horse Chestnut seed (standardized to 18-20% total saponins) 300 mg • Butcher's Broom root (ruscus aculeatus standardized to 10% saponins) 200 mg • Citrus Bioflavonoid complex 200 mg. Other Ingredients: Dicalcium Phosphate, Croscarmellose Sodium, Mineral Oil, Hydroxypropyl Methylcellulose, Magnesium Stearate, Microcrystalline Cellulose, Polyethylene Glycol, Silicon Dioxide, Stearic Acid, Titanium Dioxide, FD&C Red #27 Lake, FD&C Blue #1 Lake.

ProHerbs Memory **- Mason Vitamins, Inc.**
Each tablet contains: Thiamin HCl (B1) 25 mg • Niacin (as Niacinamide) 10 mg • Vitamin B6 (Pyridoxine HCl) 25 mg • Vitamin B12 (Cyanocobalamin) 25 mcg • Ginkgo Biloba extract (Ginkgo biloba leaves standardized to 24% ginkgo flavonoid glycosides & 6% terpene lactones) 120 mg • Memorzine (Huperzia serrata moss extract) 25 mcg • Korean Ginseng (Panax Ginseng root standardized to 4% ginsenosides) 100 mg. Other Ingredients: Dicalcium Phosphate, Microcrystalline Cellulose, Croscarmellose Sodium, Hydroxypropylmethylcellulose, Magnesium Stearate, Mineral Oil, Polyethylene Glycol, Stearic Acid, Titanium Dioxide, Sodium Lauryl Sulfate, FD&C Yellow #10 Lake, FD&C Blue #1 Lake and FD&C Blue #2 Lake.

ProHerbs Prostate **- Mason Vitamins, Inc.**
Two softgels contain: Vitamin E (Dl-Alpha Tocopheryl Acetate) 30 IU • Zinc (as Sulfate) 15 mg • Selenium (as Selenomethionine) 200 mcg • LycoPure (equivalent to 5 mg Lycopene) 71 mg • Saw Palmetto berries (Serenoa repens standardized to 85%-95% free fatty acids) 320 mg • Stinging Nettle root (Urtica dioca L. 2% minimum plant silica) 200 mg • Pumpkin Seed Oil (Cucurbita pepo seeds) 30 mg. Other Ingredients: Soybean Oil, Beeswax, Gelatin, Glycerin, Water, Chlorophyllin, Sodium, Copper, Titanium Dioxide.

ProHerbs Relax & Ease Tension **- Mason Vitamins, Inc.**
Two tablets contain: Thiamine HCl (B1) 50 mg • Riboflavin (B2) 50 mg • Vitamin B6 (Pyridoxine HCl) 50 mg • Vitamin B12 (Cyanocobalamin) 100 mcg • Kava Kava root (Piper methysticum standardized to 30% kavalactones) 300 mg • Passion Flower (Passiflora incarnata standardized to 4% flavonoids) 100 mg • Chamomile flower (Matricaria chamomilla standardized to greater than 1% apigenin) 100 mg. Other Ingredients: Dicalcium Phosphate, Microcrystalline Cellulose, Croscarmellose Sodium, Hydroxypropylmethylcellulose, Magnesium Stearate, Mineral Oil, Polyethylene Glycol, Stearic Acid, Titanium Dioxide, Sodium Lauryl Sulfate, Yellow #6 Lake, FD&C Blue #1 Lake, FD&C Red #40 Lake, FD&C Blue #2 Lake.

ProHerbs Vision Health **- Mason Vitamins, Inc.**
Two tablets contain: Vitamin A (100% Beta Carotene) 2500 IU • Zinc (sulfate) 15 mg • Selenium (selenomethionine) 200 mcg • Copper (cupric oxide) 2 mg • Bilberry extract (vaccinium myrtillus, standardized to 25% anthocyanidins) 160 mg • Lutein 6 mg • Lycopene 5 mg. Other Ingredients: Dicalcium Phosphate, Microcrystalline Cellulose, Croscarmellose Sodium, Hydroxypropyl Methylcellulose, Magnesium Stearate, Mineral Oil, Polyethylene Glycol, Stearic Acid, Titanium Dioxide, Sodium Lauryl Sulfate, FD&C Red #40 Lake, FD&C Blue #1 Lake, FD&C Blue #2 Lake.

PROhGH Sport for Men **- Nutraceutics Corp.**
Each effervescent sachet contains: Symbiotropin Complex 2720 mg: Aminotrope-7, Anterior Pituitary Peptides (porcine) • Novel Polyose Proprietary Complex 1100 mg • Chaperone Molecule Complex 350 mg: Inositol, Tribulus Terrestris. Other Ingredients: Citric Acid, Sodium Bicarbonate, Glucose, L-Glutamine, L-Arginine, L-Pyroglutamate, L-Lysine, Glycine, Gamma Aminobutyric Acid, Alpha-Glycerylphosphorylcholine, Mixed Berry Flavor.

PROhGH Sport for Women **- Pharmalogic**
Each sachet contains: Proprietary Blend Symbiotropin 2720 mg: Aminotrope-7, Anterior Pituitary Peptides (porcine) • Novel Polyose Complex 1100 mg • Chaperone Molecule Complex 320 mg: Inositol, Soy Isoflavones. Base: Citric Acid, Sodium Bicarbonate, Glucose, L-Glutamine, L-Arginine, L-Pyroglutamate, L-Lysine, Glycine, Alpha-glycerylphosphorylcholine, Gamma Aminobutyric Acid.

ProhGH Symbiotropin **- Nutraceutics Corp.**
Two tablets contain: Glycoamino Acid Complex 4200 mg • Aminotrope-7 Anterior Pituitary Peptides Polyose Complex 2300 mg. Other Ingredients: Citric Acid, Potassium Bicarbonate, Glucose, L-Glutamine, L-Arginine, L-Pyroglutamate, Sodium Bicarbonate,

L-Lysine Monohydrochloride, Gamma Aminobutyric Acid, Glycine, Sodium Carbonate, Polyethlene Glycol, Mixed Berry Flavor, Magnesium Stearate, Sodium Benzoate powder.
See Editor's Note No. 31.

PRO-hGH Symbiotropin Growth Hormone Releasing Complex **-** Nutraceutics Corp.
Two tablets contain: Anterior Pituitary Peptides • Aminotrope-7 (a sequenced glycoamino acid complex) 4200 mg • Novel Polyose complex (pharmaceutical mono, poly & oligo saccharides) 2230 mg. Base: L-Glutamine, L-Arginine, L-Pyroglutamate, GABA, L-Glycine, L-Lysine, L-Tyrosine & Vicia Faba Major.
See Editor's Note No. 31.

Prokapha **-** R-U Ved U.S.A.
Black Pepper • Ginger • Cinnamon • Green Cardamom • Pipli • Garlic • Mineral Salt.

Prokapha Tea **-** R-U Ved U.S.A.
Clove • Cardamom • Ginger • Green Tea • Cinnamon.

Prolab CarbPRO **-** ProLab
Granulated Medium Length Complex Carbohydrates (maltodextrin) extracted from grains.

ProLab GlutaMASS **-** ProLab
Each capsule contains: L-Glutamine 275 mg • Alpha-Ketoglutaric Acid 250 mg • Taurine 150 mg • Calcium (AKG) 63 mg • Magnesium (oxide) 25 mg • Potassium (citrate) 25 mg • RNA 9.5 mg • Manganese 400 mcg.

ProLab Lean Rx **-** ProLab
Each 72 g packet contains: Protein Blend of Milk Protein Isolates • Caseinates • Whey Protein Concentrates & Egg Whites • Maltodextrin • Cocoa • Natural Flavors • Dicalcium Phosphate • Potassium Chloride • Dipotassium Phosphate • Potassium Citrate • Sodium Chloride • Sodium Citrate • Magnesium Oxide • Medium Chain Triglycerides • Choline Bitartrate • Vegetable Gum • Aspartame • Lecithin • Betaine • Beta Carotene • Manganese Sulfate • Canola oil • Glutamine • Inositol • Vitamin E Acetate • Vitamin B12 • Vitamin A Palmitate • Thiamine • Riboflavin • Vitamin D • Niacin • Pyridoxine HCL • Calcium Pantothenate • Potassium Iodide • Ferrous Gluconate • Copper Gluconate • Zinc Oxide • Biotin • Folic Acid • Selenium Chelate • Molybdenium Yeast • Vitamin K • Paba • Chromium Picolinate.

ProLab MSM **-** ProLab
Each capsule contains: MSM (Methyl-Sulfonyl-Methane) 1000 mg.

ProLab N-Large 2 (N-Large II) **-** ProLab
Each serving (153 g) contains: Maltodextrin • Cross-Flow Micro-Filtered Cold Processed Ion Exchanged Whey • Fructose • Natural Flavoring.

ProLab Stoked **-** ProLab
Each rounded scoop contains: Caffeine 200 mg • Ephedra alkaloids 20 mg • Guarana 10 mg • Green Tea extract 10 mg • White Willow 75 mg. In a base of Yohimbe bark, Quercetin & Citrus aurantium.
See Editor's Note No. 21, No. 30 and No. 40.

Prolamine Iodine **-** Standard Process, Inc.
Each tablet contains: Calcium 35 mg • Iodine 3 mg. Other Ingredients: Magnesium Citrate, Cellulose.
See Editor's Note No. 14.

Pro-Life Soy Protein **-** Nature's Life
Two scoops (28.35 g) contain: SUPRO brand soy protein isolate containing Lecithin • natural Vanilla Flavor • natural Papain Enzyme concentrate • Cobalamin concentrate.

Prolo Max **-** Ortho Molecular Products
Four capsules contain: Vitamin C 180 mg • Magnesium 40 mg • POtassium 10:1 20 mg • Fo Ti root powder 5:1 500 mg • Methylsulfonylmethane (MSM) 500 mg • L-Prolien USP 5:1 500 mg • Siberian Ginseng root extract (standaradized to contain 5% eleutheroside E) 300 mg • L-Cysteine USP 250 mg • Horsetail leaf powder 250 mg • RNA 250 mg • Gotu Kola leaf 4:1 extract 250 mg • Glucosamine HCl 100 mg.

Pro-Lysine Ascorbs **-** Alacer
Each tablet contains: Vitamin C (as calcium-magnesium ascorbate) 500 mg • L-Proline (amino acid) 250 mg • L-Lysine (amino acid) 250 mg. Other Ingredients: Cellulose, Vegetable Stearic Acid, Magnesium Stearate, Pharmaceutical Glaze, Titanium Dioxide, Polyethylene Glycol.

Promend **-** The Herbalist
Saw Palmetto berry • Goldenrod flower tops • Echinacea root • Horsetail herb • Plantain herb • Ginger root.

Promensil **-** Novogen
Each tablet contains: Isoflavone Phytoestrogens as Red Clover leaf extract 40 mg. Other Ingredients: Dicalcium phosphate, Microcrystalline cellulose, Hydroxypropyl methylcellulose, Magnesium stearate, Mixed tocopherols, Silica, Soy polysaccharide, Titanium dioxide, Polyethylene glycol, & Organic coloring containing: Red 40, Yellow 6, Yellow 5, Blue 1.

Promilin Fenugreek Extract **-** Source Naturals
Each tablet contains: Promilin brand standardized Fenugreek seed extract (yielding 100 mg 4-hydroxyisoleucine) 500 mg • Fenugreek seed 4:1 extract 100 mg. Other Ingredients: Dibasic Calcium Phosphate, Modified Cellulose Gum, Colloidal Silicon Dioxide, Magnesium Stearate, Stearic Acid.

ProMotion **-** Advocare International
Three capsules contain: Glucosamine (as HCl) 1500 mg • Gotu Kola extract (leaf/stem/flower - centella asiatica) 100 mg • Manganese Sulfate (as monohydrate) 10 mg • MSM (methylsulfonyl methane) 100 mg • White Willow bark extract (salix alba) 30 mg. Other Ingredients: Silicon Dioxide, Magnesium Stearate, Gelatin.

ProOmega **-** Nordic Naturals
Each gelcap contains: EPA 173 mg • DHA 123 mg • Other Omega-3 49 mg.

ProOmega (lemon) **-** Nordic Naturals
Two softgels contain: Vitamin E (mixed tocopherols) 11 IU • Omega-3 Fatty Acids 1400 mg (EPA 700 mg, DHA 500 mg, other Omega-3 200 mg).

ProOmega Liquid (lemon) **-** Nordic Naturals
Each 1/2 tsp (2.5 mL) serving contains: Vitamin E (mixed tocopherols) 14 IU • Omega-3 Fatty Acids 1750 mg (EPA 875 mg, DHA 625 mg, other Omega-3 250 mg).

Pro-Optimizer **-** Metagenics
Three scoops (131 g) contain: Vitamin A 2500 IU • Vitamin C 30 mg • Vitamin D 200 IU • Vitamin E 15 IU • Thiamin 0.75 mg • Riboflavin 0.85 mg • Niacin 10 mg • Vitamin B6 1 mg • Folic Acid 0.2 mg • Vitamin B12 3 mcg • Biotin 0.15 mg • Pantothenic Acid 5 mg • Calcium 60 mg • Iron 10 mg • Phosphorus 80 mg • Iodine 75 mcg • Magnesium 231 mg • Zinc 8 mg • Copper 1 mg • Manganese 2 mg • Sodium 320 mg • Potassium 220 mg • Alanine 1500 mg • Arginine 820 mg • Aspartate 2900 mg • Cysteine 740 mg • Glutamic Acid 4490 mg • Glycine 560 mg • Histidine 500 mg • Isoleucine 1550 mg • Leucine 3420 mg • Lysine 2630 mg • Methionine 600 mg • Phenylalanine 980 mg • Proline 1290 mg • Serine 960 mg • Threonine 1260 mg • Tryptophan 530 mg • Tyrosine 1030 mg • Valine 1560 mg.

Propax with NT Factor **-** Nutritional Therapeutics, Inc.
Each packet contains: Vitamin A (as acetate) 4375 IU • Vitamin A (as natural beta-carotene) 3750 IU • Vitamin C (as calcium ascorbate) 150 mg • Vitamin D (D3, as cholecalciferol) 32 IU • Vitamin E (as D-alpha tocopherol) 145 IU • Vitamin K (phytonadione) 2.5 mcg • Vitamin B1 (as thiamin HCl) 6.25 mg • Vitamin B2 (as riboflavin/ribose-5-phosphate) 30 mg • Vitamin B3 (as niacinamide) 60 mg • Vitamin B6 (as pyridoxine/P-5-P) 40 mg • Folic Acid (as folate) 200 mcg • Vitamin B12 (as cyanocobalamin) 25 mcg • Biotin 25 mcg • Pantothenic Acid (as d-calcium pantothenate) 25 mg • Calcium (as phosphate, ascorbate, citrate, sulfate, borogluconate) 360 mg • Iodine

(as kelp) 18.75 mcg • Magnesium (as carbonate, oxide, glycinate, sulfate) 160 mg • Zinc (as methionate) 12.5 mg • Selenium (as selenomethionine) 75 mcg • Copper (as tyrosinate) 300 mcg • Manganese (as glycinate) 2.5 mg • Chromium (as nicotinate) 50 mcg • Molybdenum (as glycinate) 20 mcg • Potassium (as citrate) 12.8 mg • Bioflavonoids (as citrus, rutin, rosehips, quercetin) 165 mg • Boron (as calcium borogluconate) 500 mcg • Co Enzyme Q 10 4 mg • Creatine Monohydrate, Creatine Phosphate 122.5 mg • Grape Seed extract 5 mg • Inositol (inositol/inositol nicotinate) 25 mg • Lactoferrin 4 mg • Pantethine (as coenzyme A precursor) 70 mg • Vanadium (as vanadyl sulfate) 12.5 mcg • Alpha-Keto Glutarate 125 mg • Glutathione (as reduced) 5 mg • L-Tyrosine 60 mg • N-Acetyl-L-Cysteine 25 mg • Taurine 110 mg • Green Tea extract 50 mg • Horsetail (as silica) 12.5 mg • Phosphoglycolipids 160 mg • EPA (as eicosapentaenoic acid) 180 mg • DHA (as docosahexaenoic acid) 120 mg • NT Factor 1400 mg. Other Ingredients: Gelatin, Microcrystalline Cellulose, Methylcellulose, Croscarmellose Sodium, Magnesium Stearate, Silica, Water, Glycerine.

Prophet 3H (Prophet3H) - Prophet 3H
Unknown.
See Editor's Note No. 17.

Propita - R-U Ved U.S.A.
Mango powder • Dried Coriander leaves • Mint • Pomegranate seeds • Fennel • Basil • Cumin • Mineral Salt.

Propita Tea - R-U Ved U.S.A.
Cardamom • Holy Basil • Sandalwood • Licorice • Cinnamon.

Propolene - Obesity Research Institute
Three capsules contain: Proprietary Blend 1500 mg: Glucomannan, Propol brand Konjac root. Other Ingredients: Microcrystalline Cellulose, Gelatin, Stearic Acid, Magnesium Stearate.

Propo-Mune - Atrium Biotechnologies
Each tablet contains: Propolis 5X 92 mg • Thymus 67 mg • Lymph 30 mg • Spleen 25 mg • Brain 25 mg • Folic Acid 400 mcg.
See Editor's Note No. 31.

ProPortion Bars (chocolate peanut butter flavor) - Rexall - Sundown
Each bar contains: Protein 12 g • Vitamin A 2250 IU • Vitamin C 27 mg • Calcium 100 mg • Iron 9 mg • Vitamin D 180 IU • Vitamin E 13.5 IU • Thiamin 0.675 mg • Riboflavin 0.765 mg • Niacin 9 mg • Vitamin B6 0.9 mg • Folate 200 mcg • Vitamin B12 2.7 mcg • Biotin 135 mcg • Pantothenic Acid 4.5 mg • Phosphorus 150 mg • Iodine 67.5 mcg • Magnesium 80 mg • Zinc 6.75 mg • Copper 1 mg • Chromium 52.5 mcg.

Pro-Rite - J. R. Carlson Laboratories, Inc.
Each tablet contains: L-Lysine (as L-lysine monohydrochloride) 500 mg • L-Proline 500 mg.

ProSexual Plus capsules - Life Enhancement Products, Inc.
Six capsules contain: Vitamin C (ascorbic acid) 500 mg • Thiamine (vitamin B1 as thiamine hydrochloride) 25 mg • Niacin (vitamin B3) 50 mg • Vitamin B6 (pyridoxine HCl) 25 mg • Folic Acid 133 mcg • Vitamin B12 (cyanocobalamin) 100 mcg • Zinc (gluconate) 5 mg • Copper (gluconate) 500 mcg • Chromium 30 mcg • L-Arginine 3 g • Glycine 200 mg • Ginkgo Biloba leaf extract 30 mg • Dibencozide 5 mg • Boron (calcium borate) 2 mg.

ProSexual Plus powder - Life Enhancement Products, Inc.
Each rounded tablespoon (21 g) contains: Vitamin C (ascorbic acid) 500 mg • Thiamine (vitamin B1, as thiamine hydrochloride) 25 mg • Niacin (vitamin B3) 50 mg • Vitamin B6 (pyridoxine HCl) 25 mg • Folic Acid 133 mcg • Vitamin B12 (cyanocobalamin) 100 mcg • Zinc (gluconate) 5 mg • Copper (gluconate) 500 mcg • Chromium 30 mcg • L-Arginine 3 g • Glycine 200 mg • Ginkgo Biloba leaf extract 30 mg • Dibencozide 5 mg • Boron (calcium borate) 2 mg.

ProsFlow - Life Enhancement Products, Inc.
Three capsules contain: Saw Palmetto extract (serenoa repens) 320 mg • Stinging Nettle root (urtica dioica) 240 mg.

Prosina - LifeSpan Health Products
Each tablet contains: Beta-Sitosterol 30 mg • Beta-D-Glucosidase 0.1 mg.

ProSoothe - Pure Encapsulations
Each vegetable capsule contains: Chaste tree 5:1 extract (vitex) 100 mg • Wild Yam 10:1 extract (dioscorea) 100 mg • Dandelion root 4:1 extract 100 mg • Bupleurum root 5:1 extract 100 mg • Pyridoxal 5' Phosphate (activated B6) 50 mg • Ginger extract (zingiber officinale, standardized to contain 5% gingerols) 30 mg.

Prosplex - Olympian Labs
Two capsules contain: Inositol Hexaphosphate 400 mg • Quercetin 200 mg • Saw Palmetto 320 mg • Tomato Lycopene 200 mg • Zinc (gluconate) 10 mg • Pumpkin seed 10 mg • Pygeum Aficanum 20 mg.

ProsShield - Life Enhancement Products, Inc.
Two capsules contain: Vitamin D (as cholecalciferol) 133 IU • Vitamin E (as D,L-alpha-tocopheryl acetate) 16.7 IU • Vitamin E (as gamma-tocopherol, in mixed tocopherols) 40 mg • Vitamin E (as mixed tocopherols and tocotrienols) 1.67 mg • Riboflavin (vitamin B2) 20 mg • Zinc (as zinc gluconate) 10 mg • Selenium (as selenomethionine) 17 mcg • Saw Palmetto berries extract (40% free fatty acids and phytosterols) 320 mg • Green Tea leaf extract (90% polyphenols, 60% catechins) 133 mg • Urtica Dioica root extract (stinging nettle) 240 mg • Pygeum Africanum bark extract (2.5% phytosterols) 33 mg • Lycopene 10 mg • Resveratrol (from polygonum cuspidatum root) 3.33 mg • Boron (calcium borate) 1 mg.

Prosta Glan - Progressive Labs
Each capsule contains: Magnesium (as magnesium gluconate) 10 mg • Zinc (as zinc glycinate) 3.3 mg • Raw Bovine prostate concentrate 80 mg • Saw Palmetto 4:1 extract Lipoic Sterolic (Serenoa repens) 100 mg • Pygeum (Prunus africanum) 25 mg • Glutamic Acid 135 mg • Alanine 135 mg • Glycine 135 mg • Uva Ursi leaf (Arctostaphylos uva-ursi) 10 mg • Unsaturated Fatty Acids 10 mg • Pumpkin seed concentrate (Curcurbita pepo) 10 mg • Pollen 5 mg.
See Editor's Note No. 14.

Prosta Kit - Flora Inc.
Formula 1: Palmitol Saw Palmetto berries • Zinc 50 mg • Vitamin B6 120 mg. Formula 2: Flax-O-Mega flax seed oil 1000 mg. Formula 3: Pro-Essence Burdock root • Juniper Berry • Prickly Ash bark • Slippery Elm bark • Uva Ursi.

Prosta Support - Nutri-Quest Rx
Each tablet contains: Vitamin C 10 mg • Vitamin B6 10 mg • Vitamin E (succinate) 5 IU • Zinc Chelate 10 mg • L-Glycine 120 mg • L-Alanine 120 mg • L-Glutamic Acid 120 mg • Saw Palmetto 106 mg • Pygeum Africanus extract 10 mg • Pygeum Africanus herb 20 mg • Pumpkin seed 200 mg • Stinging Nettle leaf 75 mg • Echinacea 25 mg • Ginkgo Biloba 20 mg • Wild Yam 20 mg • Uva Ursi 10 mg.

Prostabs Plus - Futurebiotics LLC
Three tablets contain: Glutamic Acid 390 mg • Glycine 390 mg • Raw Prostate Concentrate 150 mg • Alanine 390 mg • Vitamin B6 7.5 mg • Vitamin C (ascorbate) 15 mg • Zinc (gluconate) 30 mg • Magnesium (oxide) 105 mg • Saw Palmetto berry 4:1 extract 300 mg.
See Editor's Note No. 14.

Prosta-Comp - Atrium Biotechnologies
Each tablet contains: Saw Palmetto berry extract 100 mg • Pumpkin seed oil extract 50 mg • Pygeum africanum extract 25 mg • Uva Ursi 50 mg • Zinc Gluconate 25 mg • Hydrangea extract 150 mg • Panax ginseng extract 100 mg.

ProstActin - Nature's Plus
Two softgels contain: Pygeum [(Prunus africanum bark) standardized 12-13% Phytosterols] 200 mg • Saw Palmetto [(Serenoa repens fruit) standardized 95% Fatty Acids] 80 mg • Glycine (Free form Amino Acid) 50 mg • Alanine (Free Form Amino Acid) 50 mg • Glutamine (Free Form Amino Acid) 50 mg • Turmeric [(Curcuma longa rhizome) standardized 95% Curcumin] 50 mg • Pumpkin Seed oil [(Curcurbita maxima seed) standardized 7% Alpha-Linolenic Acid] 50 mg • Zinc (Zinc Monomethionine) 30 mg • Vitamin E natural 200 IU.

Some Brand Name Natural Products - What they Contain

www.NaturalDatabase.com contains MANY more listings than appear here.
Editor's Notes are located on pages 2155-2163.

Prost-Actin - Nature's Plus
Each tablet contains: Saw Palmetto berries 250 mg • Raw Prostate concentrate 140 mg • Zinc (Monomethionine) 50 mg • Vitamin A (Beta Carotene) 10000 IU • Vitamin E natural 200 IU.
See Editor's Note No. 14.

Prostactive Plus Saw Palmetto - Nature's Way
Each softgel contains: Saw Palmetto berry 12:1 extract 160 mg • Nettle root 10:1 extract 120 mg.

ProstaFlo - Pure Encapsulations
Each vegetable capsule contains: Secale Cereale extract (flower pollen extract, containing water and fat soluble fractions in a 20:1 ratio) 320 mg.

ProstaGuard - PhysioLogics
Each softgel contains: Alphastal Blend 250 mg: Saw Palmetto extract (serenoa repense, berry, standardized to contain 80% fatty acids, sterols), Astaxanthin (from h. pluvialis). Other Ingredients: Gelatin, Glycerin.

Prosta-Health - Aarisse Health Care
Each 3 oz. pump contains: Natural Progesterone • Saw Palmetto extract • Red Clover • Damiana • Tribulus Terrestris • Dong Quai • Vitamin A • Vitamin E • Vitamin B5 • Ginseng • Shea Butter • Aloe Vera.

Prostamax Plus - Woods Supplements
Each capsule contains: Saw Palmetto extract 150 mg • Cranberry 50 mg • Zinc Gluconate 37.5 mg • Magnesium Oxide 10 mg • Vitamin B6 1.1 mg.

ProstaMed - Enzymatic Therapy
Each capsule contains: Saw Palmetto Berry extract 160 mg standardized to contain 85%-95% fatty acids & sterols: 0.15% - 0.3% fatty alcohols, 0.2%-0.4% total sterols, 0.1%-0.3% beta-sitosterol.

Prosta-Metto - The Vitamin Shoppe
Each softgel contains: Saw Palmetto extract 160 mg • Pumpkin seed oil 40 mg • Pygeum Africanum extract 10 mg • Bearberry extract 10 mg • Zinc 15 mg • Vitamin B6 5 mg.

Prosta-Metto Saw Palmetto Complex - Puritan's Pride
Each softgel contains: Saw Palmetto berry extract (Serenoa repens: Standardized to contain 85-95% fatty acids and biologically active sterol compounds) 80 mg • Pumpkin Seed oil extract (Curburbita pepo) 40 mg • Pygeum Africanum extract 10 mg • Bearberry extract (Uva Ursi) 5 mg.

ProStamina - DreamPharm
Two capsules contain: Ginseng radix 30 mg • Angelica Sinensis radix 50 mg • Zingiberis rhizoma 20 mg • Hoelen 40 mg • Licorice root 40 mg • Dioscorea rhizoma 20 mg • Cuscuta semen 30 mg • Schisandra fructus 50 mg • Corni fructus 20 mg • Morindae radix 50 mg • Yohimbe powder 150 mg.

Prosta-Plex - Dr. Donsbach
Two capsules contain: Saw Palmetto extract 250 mg • Pygeum extract 7.5 mg • Stinging Nettle extract 100 mg • Zinc gluconate 5 mg.

Prostaprime - Puritan's Pride
Each tablet contains: Raw Prostate concentrate 100 mg • Saw Palmetto 100 mg • Pygeum extract 75 mg. Other Ingredients: Golden Rod, Pumpkin Seed Concentrate, Flaxseed Oil, Glycine, Glutamic Acid, and Alanine.
See Editor's Note No. 14.

ProstaPro - PhytoPharmica
Each softgel capsule contains: Saw Palmetto berry extract (standardized to contain 85-95% fatty caids, 0.2-0.4% total sterols, and 0.1-0.3% beta sitosterol) 160 mg.

Prosta-Q - Farr Laboratories, LLC
Each capsule contains: Zinc (from zinc gluconate) 5 mg • Proprietary Blend [Quercetin, Cranberry (berry), Saw Palmetto (berry), Bromelain, Papain] 540 mg.

Prostasol formerly PC Plus - Dr. Donsbach
Two capsules contain: Magnesium (as oxide) 200 mg • Sterolins 400 mg • Quercetin 100 mg • Proprietary Blend 500 mg: Reishi (as ganoderma lucidum), Baikal Skullcap (as scutellaria baicalensis), Rabdosia (as rabdosia rubescens hara), Dyer's Woad (as isatis indigotica fortune), Mum (as dendranthema morifolium tzelev), Saw Palmetto (as serona repens), San-Qi Ginseng (as panax notoginseng), Licorice (as glycyrrhiza glabra L.).

ProstaSoy - FreeLife International
Two caplets contain: Zinc (as patented chelazome zinc glycinate) 15 mg • Selenium (as selenomethionine) 100 mcg • Saw Palmetto standardized extract (85%-95% sterols, fatty acids) 320 mg • Proprietary Blend 250 mg: standardized extracts of Soybean, Kudzu root (providing beta sitosterol 60 mg, isoflavones 40 mg) • Proprietary Blend 125 mg: Tomato Lycopene concentrate (2000 mcg/g), Stinging Nettle root 4:1 extract (urtica dioica), African Wild Cherry bark 4:1 extract (pygeum africanum) • Proprietary Blend 2500 Units: Soy Polysaccharides, Plant Enzymes. Other Ingredients: Calcium Hydrogen Phosphate, Cellulose, Vegetable Stearic Acid, Silica, Vegetable Magnesium Stearate, Vita-Coat (vegetable resin, alpha-lipoic acid).

Prostat - ProJoba
Each tablet contains: Standardized extract of Graminae Pollen 70 mg • Fat soluble Gramanie extract EA 10 4 mg. Other Ingredients: Microcrystalline Cellulose, Lactose, Magnesium Stearate, Colloidal Silicon Dioxide, Natural Resin, Talc, Propylene Glycol.

Prostata - Gero Vita International
Each capsule contains: Urtica Dioica extract 16:1 150 mg • Serenoa Serrulata extract 106 mg • Apis Mellifica 83.33 mg • L-Alanine 66.67 mg • Glycine 66.67 mg • L-Glutamic Acid 66.67 mg • Pygeum Africanum extract 50 mg • Vitamin B6 15 mg • Panax Ginseng extract 8.33 mg • Zinc Arginate 7.5 mg • Hydrangea extract 5 mg • Copper 0.5 mg • Beta Carotene 8333 IU.

Prostate 2.1 - Theralogix
Vitamin E (as mixed tocopherols) 100 IU • Vitamin D 800 IU • Selenium (as selenomethionine) 200 mcg • Lycopene (as Lyc-O-Mato brand) 30 mg • Soy Isoflavones (as Novasoy brand) 50 mg.

Prostate 5LX - New Chapter, Inc.
Two softgels contain: Saw Palmetto berry extract (85-95% total fatty acids) 320 mg • Green Tea leaf extract (45% polyphenols) 100 mg • Pumpkin seed oil 96 mg • Ginger rhizome extract (minimum 20% pungent compounds- 16 mg 5% zingiberene) 80 mg • Urtica root 10:1 hydroalcoholic extract (nettle) 50 mg • Urtica root 5:1 aqueous extract (nettle) 50 mg • Selenium 50 mcg • Rosemary leaf and oil extract (23% total phenolic antioxidants) 10 mg. Other Ingredients: Olive Oil, Yellow Beeswax, Gelatin, Vegetable Glycerin, Purified Water, Carob.

Prostate Care - Pro Health
Two tablets contain: Calcium 125 mg • Saw Palmetto berry extract 224 mg • Pumpkin seed oil extract 180 mg • Pygeum bark extract 125 mg • Proprietary Blend 970 mg: Echinacea root, Gardenia fruit, Alisma rhizome, Salvia root, Gravel Root, Codonopsis root, Cuscuta seed, Ligustrum seed, Plantain seed, Dong Quai root. Other Ingredients: Dibasic Calcium Phosphate, Stearic Acid, Acacia Gum, Colloidal Silicon Dioxide, Modified Cellulose Gum, Magnesium Stearate.

Prostate Essentials - Swanson Health Products
Each capsule contains: Zinc (picolinate) 15 mg • Saw Palmetto extract (20% free fatty acids) 160 mg • Stinging Nettle concentrate 120 mg • Korean Ginseng root 50 mg • Pygeum extract (3% sterols) 50 mg • Pumpkin seed concentrate 40 mg • Glycine 25 mg • L-Alanine 25 mg • L-Glutamic Acid 25 mg • Beta Sitosterol 20 mg.

Prostate Factors - Michael's Naturopathic Programs
Four tablets contain: Vitamin C (as calcium ascorbate) 100 mg • Vitamin E (as D-alpha tocopheryl succinate) 100 IU • Magnesium (as magnesium amino acid chelate) 75 mg • Niacin (as niacinamide) 10 mg • Pantothenic Acid (as calcium pantothenate) 20 mg • Zinc (as

zinc monomethionine) 20 mg • Proprietary Blend 1966 mg: Bee Pollen, Alanine (as L-alanine), Parsley leaf (petroselinium sativum), Glutamine (as L-glutamine), Glycine, Echinacea root (echinacea angustifolia), Gravel root (eupatorium purpureum), Soy Isoflavones: Daidzein Glycosides (5.5%), Glycitein Glycosides (3%), Genistein Glycosides (1.9%), Liposterolic extract (from saw palmetto berry), Pygeum bark (pygeum africanum, 1% phytosterols, 250 mcg), Saw Palmetto fruit (serenoa serrulata, 5% fatty acids, 1.3 mg). Other Ingredients: Terra Alba (calcium sulfate), Maltodextrin, Stearic Acid, Magnesium Stearate, Calcium Amino Acid Chelate.

Prostate FLO **-** Xymogen
Each capsule contains: Zinc (as zinc glycinate) 5 mg • Saw Palmetto berry extract (standardized to contain 85% fatty acids) 160 mg • Pygeum Africanum extract (standardized to contain 13% sterols) 80 mg • Nettle leaf extract (standardized to contain 1% silica) 100 mg • Lycopene extract (providing 0.45 mg of lycopene) 15 mg • Pumpkin seed extract 320 mg.

Prostate Formula **-** Nature's Way
Two capsules contain: Beta Glucan 2.2 mg • Calcium 26 mg • Dandelion leaf 230 mg • Lycopene 2.4 mg • Saw Palmetto dried extract 360 mg • Soy Isoflavone dried extract 25 mg • Zinc (amino acid chelate) 7 mg. Other Ingredients: Gelatin, Magnesium Stearate, Millet, Silica.

Prostate Formula **-** Youngevity
Saw Palmetto 400 mg • Pygeum bark 80 mg • Pumpkin seed 80 mg • Atractylodes herb • Licorice root 40 mg • Bupleurum root 40 mg • Vitamin E 100 IU • Vitamin C 60 mg • Vitamin B6 4 mg • Vilcabamba Mineral Essence: Potassium, Calcium, Magnesium, Zinc, Chromium, Selenium, Iron, Copper, Molybdenum, Vanadium, Iodine, Cobalt, Manganese.

Prostate Formula **-** Life Extension
Each tablet contains: Serenoa Serrulta 100 mg • Pygeum Africanum extract 100 mg • Hydrangea extract 85 mg • Silica 85 mg • L-Alanine 67 mg • Glutamic Acid 68 mg • Glycine 67 mg • Panax Ginseng extract 10 mg • Zinc 10 mg • Vitamin A 10,000 IU • Vitamin E (D-alpha tocopherol) 200 IU.

Prostate Formula **-** Pharmanex
Each capsule contains: Selenium (yeast) 100 mcg • Saw Palmetto berry 10:1 extract (sereona repens) 160 mg • Green Tea (camellia sinensis) 85 mg • Lycopene 3 mg. Other Ingredients: Gelatin, Silicon Dioxide, Microcrystalline Cellulose, Magnesium Stearate.

Prostate Health **-** DaVinci Laboratories
Two capsules contain: Vitamin C (as calcium ascorbate and ascorbic acid) 300 mg • Vitamin E (D-alpha tocopheryl succinate) 100 IU • Vitamin B6 (pyridoxal 5-phosphate) 40 mg • Folic Acid 300 mcg • Zinc (as zinc citrate) 5 mg • Saw Palmetto berry extract (serenoa repens, yielding 288 mg free fatty acids) 640 mg • Green Tea extract (yielding epigallo catechin gallate [EGCG] 30 mg) 100 mg • Pumpkin seed oil powder 100 mg • Alpha Lipoic Acid 70 mg • Beta Sitosterol 50 mg • Stinging Nettle leaf extract (urtica dioica) 40 mg • Pygeum Africanum (yielding 4.8 mg phytosterols) 40 mg • Lycopene 30 mg • Resveratrol (as trans-resveratrol) 5 mg. Other Ingredients: Rice Flour, Vegetable Stearate, Vegetable Cellulose.

Prostate Health **-** Enzymes, Inc.
Three capsules contain: Zinc (from Zinc Citrate) 30 mg • n-zimes Proprietary Enzyme Blend 75 mg: pHysioProtease (213,120 pHysio-U), CereCalase Plus • Proprietary Herbal Blend 495 mg: Saw Palmetto berry extract (standardized to contain 45% fatty acids), Pumpkin seed extract (standardized to contain 25% fatty acids), Pygeum bark extract (equivalent to 1350 mg raw herb), Hydrangea root extract (equivalent to 180 mg raw herb), Rice Bran. Other Ingredients: Plant Cellulose, Water.

Prostate Health **-** EnerGreens, Inc.
Each capsule contains: Beta-Sitosterol 150 mg • IP-6 (inositol hexaphosphate) 50 mg • Zinc (from chelate) 15 mg • Copper (from chelate) 2 mg • Vitamin E (D-alpha tocopherol) 33 IU • Quercetin 50 mg • Proprietary Blend 335 mg: Saw Palmetto berry 4:1 powdered extract, Ashwagandha 4:1 powdered extract, He Shou Wu extract, Lycopene standardized extract (min. 3%). Other Ingredients: Gelatin.

Prostate Health **-** Sundown
Two capsules contain: Zinc (as zinc oxide) 5 mg • Saw Palmetto fruit 450 mg • Herbal Complex Blend 100 mg: Nettle root, Pygeum bark. Other Ingredients: Gelatin.

Prostate Health **-** Celestial Seasonings
Two capsules contain: Vitamin E (as d-alpha tocopherol acetate) 90 IU • Zinc (as gluconate) 15 mg • Proprietary Blend 1230 mg: Saw Palmetto (berries), Saw Palmetto (standardized extract), Stinging Nettle root (standardized extract). Other Ingredients: (May contain one or more of the following) Dicalcium Phosphate, Gelatin, Rice Flour, Stearic Acid, Magnesium Stearate, and Silicon Dioxide.

Prostate Health Formula **-** Schiff
Two capsules contain: Vitamin D (as cholecalciferol) 400 IU • Calcium (as calcium silicate, calcium D-glucarate) 29 mg • Zinc (as zinc citrate) 15 mg • Selenium (from high selenium yeast) 70 mcg • Copper (as copper gluconate) 1 mg • Saw Palmetto berry extract (serenoa repens) 667 mg • Free Fatty Acids (from saw palmetto extract) 300 mg • Calcium D-Glucarate 50 mg • Lycopene 12 mg. Other Ingredients: Gelatin, Maltodextrin, Magnesium Stearate, Silicon Dioxide, Titanium Dioxide.

Prostate Optimizer **-** Jarrow Formulas
Two softgels contain: Vitamin D (D3, cholecalciferol) 200 IU • Saw Palmetto (serenoa repens, Sabalselect brand, 85-95% fatty acids and sterols) 320 mg • Lycopene (Lyc-O-Mato brand GMO-free tomato extract) 10 mg • Fish oil (molecular distilled) 600 mg: DHA (docosahexaenoic acid) 252 mg, EPA (eicosapentaenoic acid) 15 mg • Pumpkin seed oil 320 mg • Milk Thistle seed extract (silybum marianum, 30:1 concentrate yielding 80% or 60 mg silymarin) 75 mg • Stinging Nettles extract (urtica dioica) 100 mg • Pollen extract (Cernitin brand) 250 mg • Flaxseed SDG lignans (linum usitatissimum, from 100 mg LinumLife Extract brand 20% SDG extract) 20 mg • Green Tea extract (40% polyphenols) 100 mg • Ascorbyl Palmitate 10 mg • Gamma Tocopherol 3 mg. Other Ingredients: Yellow Beeswax, Carob, Gelatin, Glycerin.

Prostate PMG **-** Standard Process, Inc.
Each tablet contains: Proprietary Blend 242 mg: Bovine Prostate PMG extract, Magnesium Citrate • Calcium 10 mg • Sodium 50 mg. Other Ingredients: Cellulose.
See Editor's Note No. 14.

Prostate Power Rx **-** Physician Formulas
Two capsules contain: Saw Palmetto fruit extract (serenoa repens, standardized to contain 45% fatty acids) 640 mg • Stinging Nettle root 4:1 extract (urtica dioica) 100 mg • Quercetin 100 gm • Rosemary leaf 4:1 extract (rosmarinus officinalis) 100 mg • Beta Sitosterol 60 mg • Pygeum bark 4:1 extract (pygeum africanum) 50 mg • Daidzein (standardized to contain 40% isoflavones) 10 mg • Genistein (standardized to contain 40% isoflavones) 10 mg • Lyc-O-Mato brand Lycopene (lycopersicon escatatum fruit) 10 mg. Other Ingredients: Rice Flour, Gelatin, Glycerin, Magnesium Stearate, Silicon Dioxide, Maltodextrin, Water.

Prostate Support **-** NOW Foods
Each gelcap contains: Saw Palmetto • Pygeum • Stinging Nettle • Lycopene. Other Ingredients: Pumpkin seed oil, Zinc & Vitamin B6.

Prostate Support Formula **-** PhysioLogics
Two capsules contain: Zinc (as zinc glycinate) 15 mg • Copper (as copper amino chelate) 2 mg • Vitamin B6 (as pyridoxine HCl) 100 mg • Beta Sitosterol 60 mg • Pygeum bark extract (pygeum africanum, standardized to contain 2.5% phytosterols 5 mg) 100 mg • Pumpkin seed Oil extract (cucurbita pepo) 100 mg • Stinging Nettle leaf (urtica dioica, standardized to contain 1-2% silica, 4-8 mg) 400 mg. Other Ingredients: Gelatin, Rice Powder, Vegetable Magnesium Stearate, Silica.

Prostate-Duo - Uronat Nutrition Company, Inc.
Each softgel contains: Saw Palmetto extract (minimun 85% free fatty acids & 5% sterols) 160 mg • Pygeum africanum extract (minimum 13% sterols) 50 mg. Other Ingredients: Gelatin, Glycerin, Pumpkin seed oil, Water, Carob.

Prostatonin - PanGeo Health Brands, Inc.
Each capsule contains: Pygeum Africanum 25 mg • Nettle root 300 mg. Other Ingredients: Grape Oil, Gelatin, Triglycerides, Glycerol, Sorbitol, Soya Lecithin, Synthetic Iron Oxides, Titanium Dioxide.

Prostatrol Forte - Ortho Molecular Products
Each capsule contains: Zinc (as Chelazome brand amino acid chelate) 8 mg • Selenium (as amino acid complex) 50 mcg • Copper (as lysinate) 500 mcg • Saw Palmetto fruit extract (standardized to contain 45%-55% fatty acids) 300 mg • Nettles root extrat (standardized to contain 30ppm scopoletin) 120 mg • Pygeum bark extract (standardized to contain 25% phytosterols) 50 mg. Other Ingredients: Natural Vegetable Capsules, Ascorbyl Palmitate, Magnesium Stearate, Microcrystalline Cellulose, Silicon Dioxide.

ProsTect - Advocare International
Three capsules contain: Zinc (monomethionine OptiZinc) 5 mg • Selenium (selenomethionine) 35 mcg • Vitamin D (as ergocalciferol) 40 IU • Red Clover flower/leaf extract (trifolium pratense) 200 mg • Saw Palmetto berry extract (serenoa repens) 50 mg • Cernitin Flower Pollen Extract 400 mg: Secale Cereale, Zea Mays, Phleum Pratence • Green Tea leaf extract (camellia sinensis) 50 mg • Glycine 200 mg • Tomato fruit extract (lycopene, lycopersicon esculentum) 500 mg. Other Ingredients: Silicon Dioxide, Magnesium Stearate, Gelatin.

Prostenil - Aboca USA, Inc
Two capsules contain: Saw Palmetto fruit powder (serenoa repens, standardized to 14% total liposterolic extract) 456 mg • Bearberry leaf freeze-dried extract(arctostaphylos uva-ursi, standardized to 12% arbutin) 60 mg • Stinging Nettle root freeze-dried extract (urtica dioica, standardized to 0.01 scopoletin) 30.6 mg • Echinacea root freeze-dried extract (echinacea pallida standardized to 2% echinacoside) 30 mg • Zinc Yeast (saccharomices cerevisiae, with zinc, 10% organically bound) 22.6 mg. Other Ingredients: Gelatin (capsule), Essential Oils of Cajuput, Italian Cypress.

Prostex - Metabolic Products
Two capsules contain: Proprietary Amino Acid blend 810 mg: Glutamic Acid, Alanine, Aminoacetic Acid (glycine). Other Ingredients: Gelatin, Polyethylene glycol 8000.

ProstGard - Holista
Each capsule contains: Zinc (from gluconate) 15 mg • Vitamin B6 (pyridoxine HCl) 5 mg • Saw Palmetto (Serenoa repens) extract of berries (10:1) 80 mg • Pumpkin Seed Oil 500 mg.

Prostoid - HealthWatchers System
Vitamin C • Vitamin A • Vitamin E • Vitamin B6 • Serenoa Senulata • Pygeum Africanum Extract • Hydrangea Extract • Bee Pollen • Siberian Ginseng Extract • Glutamic Acid • L-Glycine • L-Alanine • Silica • Solidago Fragrans Extract • Zinc • Damiana • Dong Quai • Gotu Kola • Juniper • Copper.

Prost-X - Standard Process, Inc.
Each capsule contains: Proprietary Blend 270 mg: Tillandsia Usneoides, Calcium Glycerophosphate, Bovine Prostate Cytosol extract. Other Ingredients: Gelatin, Honey, Water, Colors.
See Editor's Note No. 14.

Protagest - PhytoPharmica
Three tablets contain: Ammonium Chloride 96 mg • Betaine HCl 975 mg • L-Glutamic Acid HCl 585 mg • Niacin (as niacinamide) 30 mg • Ox Bile extract 45 mg • Pancreatic Enzymez 4X 10 mg • Papain 6X 15 mg • Pepsin 1:3000 292 mg • Potassium (as potassium chloride) 50 mg • Vitamin B6 (as pyridoxine HCl) 1.5 mg.
See Editor's Note No. 14.

Protandim - Lifeline Therapeutics, Inc.
Each caplet contains: Calcium (as calcium carbonate/di-calcium phosphate) 74 mg • Proprietary Blend 675 mg: Milk Thistle seed extract (silybum marianum), Bacopa aerial part extract (bacopa monnieri), Ashwagandha root (withania somnifera), Green Tea leaf extract (camellia sinensis), Turmeric rhizome extract (curcuma longa). Other Ingredients: Croscarmellose Sodium, Magnesium Stearate, Microcrystalline Cellulose, Modified Cellulose, Silica, Stearic Acid.

Protazyme - Enzymatic Therapy
Each tablet contains: Potassium Chloride 32 mg • Niacinamide 10 mg • Vitamin B6 (Pyridoxine HCL) 500 mcg. Other Ingredients: Betaine HCL 325 mg • Glutamic Acid HCL 195 mg • Pepsin 1:10000 97 mg • Ammonium Chloride 32 mg • Papain 6X 30 mg • Ox Bile extract 15 mg • Pancreatic Enzymes 4X 10 mg.
See Editor's Note No. 14.

Protease - Enzymes, Inc.
Each capsule contains: Protease 417 mg • Calcium Citrate 45 mg. Other Ingredients: Plant Cellulose, Water.

Protease Plus - Enzymes, Inc.
Each capsule contains: Calcium (from Calcium Citrate) 27 mg • pHysioProtease 607 mg. Other Ingredients: Plant Cellulose, Water.

Protector Caps - The Vitamin Shoppe
Three capsules contain: Vitamin A (Beta-carotene) 10000 IU • Vitamin E (d-alpha tocopheryl succinate) 200 IU • Ester C 500 mg • Pycnogenol 10 mg • Selenium (L-Selenomethionine) 50 mcg • CoQ10 10 mg • Green Tea extract (30% Polyphenols) 25 mg • Quercetin 25 mg.

Protector SPF 15 - Jason
Vitamin C Complex • Beta Hydroxy Acid.

Protefood - Standard Process, Inc.
Each capsule contains: Proprietary Blend 435 mg: Defatted Wheat germ, Bovine Adrenal, Choline Bitartrate, Carrot root, Ribonucleic Acid, DL-Methionine, L-Lysine Mono-Hydrochloride, Glutamic Acid, Peanut bran • Vitamin C 3.2 mg • Calcium 50 mg. Other Ingredients: Bovine Bone, Gelatin, Veal Bone meal, Water, Colors.

Protein 95 Soy Protein - Nature's Life
Two 2 scoops (28.35 g) contain: SUPRO brand Soy Protein Isolate containing Lecithin • natural Vanilla Flavor • natural Papain Enzyme concentrate.

Protein Boost - Nutri-Quest Rx
Two tablespoons contain: Alanine 646 mg • Arginine 1190 mg • Aspartic Acid 1853 mg • Cystine 187 mg • Glutamic Acid 3060 mg • Glycine 680 mg • Histidine 408 mg • Isoleucine 765 mg • Leucine 1275 mg • Lysine 986 mg • Methionine 221 mg • Phenylalanine 850 mg • Proline 901 mg • Serine 833 mg • Threonine 612 mg • Tyrosine 629 mg • Valine 782 mg. Ingredients: Isolated Soy Protein, Calcium & Sodium Caseinate, Tri Calcium Phosphate, Lecithin, Soybean oil, Magnesium Oxide, Papain, Ascorbic Acid, Ferrous Fumurate, Kelp, Niacin, Calcium Pantothenate, Vitamin A, Pyridoxine HCL, Thiamine HCL, Riboflavin, Vitamin D, Vanilla Flavor.

Protein Cysteine For Hair - Life Extension
Each tablet contains: Primary Dried Yeast Blend 500 mg: Histidine, Lysine, Leucine, Tryptophan, Phenylalanine, Methionine, Valine, Threonine, Isoleucine • Proprietary Blend 300 mg: Vitamin B1, Vitamin B2, Niacin, Biotin, Vitamin B6, Folic Acid • Casein 125 mg • L-Cysteine 100 mg • Di-Methione 3 mg. Other Ingredients: Carotene; In 72 Natural-Trace-Mineral Base.

Protein Digestion - Enzymes, Inc.
Each capsule contains: Proprietary Enzyme Blend 366 mg: Amylase, Protease, Lipase, Peptidase, Glucoamylase, Cellulase. Other Ingredients: Plant Cellulose, Water.

Some Brand Name Natural Products - What they Contain

www.NaturalDatabase.com contains MANY more listings than appear here.
Editor's Notes are located on pages 2155-2163.

Protein Drink Mix (chocolate flavor) - Herbalife International of America, Inc.
Soy Protein Isolate • Vegetable Oil Preparation: Sunflower oil, Maltodextrin, Sodium Caseinate, Mono- and Diglycerides, Soy Lecithin, Mixed Tocopherols as antioxidants, Silicon Dioxide • Calcium Caseinate, Cocoa powder • Vitamin and Mineral mix: Vitamin A Palmitate, Vitamin D (D3), Vitamin E Acetate, Biotin, Folic Acid, Niacinamide, D-Calcium Pantothenate, Thiamin Mononitrate, Cyanocobalamin, Riboflavin, Pyridoxine HCl, Ascorbic Acid, Phytonadione, Chromium Chloride, Copper Gluconate, Potassium Iodide, Reduced Iron, Magnesium Phosphate, Manganese Sulfate, Sodium Molybdate, Selenomethionine, Zinc Sulfate, Dextrose • Natural and Artifical Flavors. Other Ingredients: Maltodextrin, Salt, Tricalcium Phosphate, Xanthan Gum, Potassium Chloride, Guar Gum, Soy Lecithin, Silicon Dioxide, Sucralose, Acesulfame Potassium.

Protein Drink Mix (vanilla flavor) - Herbalife International of America, Inc.
Soy Protein Isolate • Vegetable Oil Preparation: Sunflower oil, Maltodextrin, Sodium Caseinate, Mono- and Diglycerides, Soy Lecithin, Mixed Tocopherols as antioxidants, Silicon Dioxide • Calcium Caseinate, Maltodextrin • Vitamin and Mineral mix: Vitamin A Palmitate, Vitamin D (D3), Vitamin E Acetate, Biotin, Folic Acid, Niacinamide, D-Calcium Pantothenate, Thiamin Mononitrate, Cyanocobalamin, Riboflavin, Pyridoxine HCl, Ascorbic Acid, Phytonadione, Chromium Chloride, Copper Gluconate, Potassium Iodide, Reduced Iron, Magnesium Phosphate, Manganese Sulfate, Sodium Molybdate, Selenomethionine, Zinc Sulfate, Dextrose • Natural and Artifical Flavors. Other Ingredients: Salt, Tricalcium Phosphate, Xanthan Gum, Potassium Chloride, Guar Gum, Soy Lecithin, Silicon Dioxide, Sucralose, Acesulfame Potassium.

ProteinFusion Bar - Metagenics
Each bar contains: Soy Protein Isolate • Whey Protein Isolate • Calcium Caseinate • Glycerin • Polydextrose • Maltitol • Palm kernel oil • Nonfat Milk Solids • Cocoa powder • Lecithin • Salt • Natural Flavor • Hydrolyzed Gelatin • Maltitol Syrup • Rice Flour • Malt • Chocolate Liquor • Canola oil • Water • Whey Protein Hydrolysate • Natural Flavors • Cellulose gel • Mono- and Diglycerides • Guar Gum • Tricalcium Phosphate • Ascorbic Acid • D-Alpha Tocopherol • Niacinamide • Zinc Oxide • Copper Gluconate • Calcium Pantothenate • Pyridoxine Hydrochloride • Thiamin Mononitrate • Manganese Sulfate • Riboflavin • Vitamin A Palmitate • Chromium Chloride • Folic Acid • Biotin • Potassium Iodide • Sodium Molybdate • Sodium Selenite • Cyanocobalamin.

Protogen-A - Life Extension
Each tablet contains: Pure Protogen A 250 mg (natural liver base).

Protrypsin - Metagenics
Two tablets contain: Chymotrypsin 10,000 USP • Trypsin 14,000 UPS • Raw Pancreas concentrate (porcine) 100 mg.

Protykin/Resveratrol - Natrol, Inc.
Two capsules contain: Polygonum cuspidatum extract root 50 mg • Trans-Resveratrol 10 mg Total Reservatrols 12 mg • Emodin 5 mg. Other Ingredients: Rice powder, Magnesium Stearate, Gelatin.

ProV for Men - For Youthful Health
Four tablets contain: Vitamin B6 25 mg • Niacin 20 mg • Vitamin E 30 IU • Zinc 15 mg • L-Arginine HCl 2000 mg • Tribulus Terrestris extract 400 mg • Muira Puama 4:1 extract 300 mg • Yohimbe bark extract (standardized for 8 mg yohimbine alkaloids) 200 mg • Avena Sativa extract 200 mg • Peruvian Maca root 100 mg • Stinging Nettle 5:1 extract 50 mg. Other Ingredients: Dicalcium Phosphate, Cellulose Stearic Acid, Magnesium Stearate, Silicon Dioxide.

ProV for Women - For Youthful Health
Four tablets contain: Vitamin B6 25 mg • Niacin 20 mg • Vitamin E 30 IU • Zinc 15 mg • L-Arginine HCl 2000 mg • Tribulus Terrestris extract 400 mg • Muira Puama 4:1 extract 300 mg • Horny Goat Weed 10% extract 200 mg • Avena Sativa 13% extract 200 mg • L-Taurine 200 mg • Stinging Nettle 5:1 extract 50 mg • Soy Isoflavones 30 mg • American Ginseng 30% extract 30 mg. Other Ingredients: Dicalcium Phosphate, Cellulose, Stearic Acid, Magnesium Stearate, Silicon Dioxide.

Provasca - Endomatrix Inc.
Each capsule contains: Proprietary Blend 240 mg: Green Seaweed leaf extract powder, L-Arginine (as l-arginine hydrochloride).

Provata - R-U Ved U.S.A.
Cardamom • Ginger • Cloves • Cumin • Coriander seeds • Fennel • Mineral Salt.

Provata Tea - R-U Ved U.S.A.
Fennel • Licorice • Ginger • Cinnamon • Black Cardamom • Ajwain.

Provillus - Ultra Herbal, LLC
Two caplets contain: Vitamin B6 (pyridoxine hydrochloride) 5 mg • Biotin 5 mg • Magnesium (oxide) 150 mg • Zinc (oxide) 15 mg • Saw Palmetto fruit (serenoa repens) 1500 mg • Proprietary Blend 30 mg: Nettle leaf (urtica dioica), Gotu Kola (centella asiatica), Pumpkin seed (cucurbita maxima), Eleuthero root (eleutherococcus senticosus), Uva-Ursi root (arctostaphylos uva-ursi), Muira Puama (ptychopetalum olacoides). Other Ingredients: Gelatin, Rice Flour, Magnesium Stearate, Silicon Dioxide, Maltodextrin, Water.

Provitor - Magistral Biotech
Each 1 mL serving contains: Potassium (citrate) 25.8 mg • Potassium (glycerophosphate) 0.16 mg • Magnesium (glycerophosphate) 0.84 mg • Iron (glycerophosphate) 0.09 mg • Iodine (potassium iodine) 0.0015 mg • Proprietary Standardized Extract Blend 385 mg: Ginkgo Biloba leaf, Asian Ginseng root, Guarana seed, Raisin seed • Proprietary Concentrated Extract Blend 680 mg: Damiana leaf, Spirulina algae. Other Ingredients: Spring Water, Glycerine, Calcium Glycerophosphate, Natural Flavours.

Provol - Upsher-Smith Laboratories
Each capsule contains: Pygeum africanum bark extract 50 mg.

ProXeed - Sigma-Tau Pharmaceuticals, Inc.
Each packet contains: Active Ingredients: L-Carnitine Fumarate 1 g • Fructose • Acetyl L-Carnitine HCL 0.5 g • Citric Acid. Inactive Ingredients: Mannitol, polyethylene glycol, artificial flavorings, povidone, & silicone dioxide.

Proxylon - Syntrax Innovations
Each capsule contains: 7-Isopropoxyisoflavone 250 mg.

Prulato - Berkeley Premium Nutraceuticals
Each tablet contains: Zinc (as zinc citrate) 15 mg • Prulato Proprietary Blend 1005 mg: Swedish Flower Pollen, Ho Shou Wu root (polygonum multiflorum), saw Palmetto berry standardized extract, Tomato Lycopene concentrate. Other Ingredients: Calcium Carbonate, Microcrystalline Cellulose, Croscarmellose Sodium, Stearic Acid, Magnesium Stearate, Silica.

PS (Phosphatidylserine) - Metabolic Response Modifiers
Each softgel contains: Phosphatidylserine 100 mg • Other Phospholipids 380 mg • Soy oil 200 mg • Vitamin C 10 mg.

PS 100 - GNC
Each capsule contains: High Serine Soy Lecithin 0.5 g • Phosphatidyl Serine Complex 500 mg • Phosphatidylserine 100 mg • Phosphatidylcholine 45 mg • Phosphatidyethanolamine 10 mg • Phosphatidylinositol 5 mg. Other Ingredients: Gelatin, Glycerin.

PS 100 (standardized phosphatidylserine) - Pure Encapsulations
Each vegetable capsule contains: Phosphatidylserine 100 mg.

PS Memory Care - Rexall - Sundown
Each softgel contains: Phosphatidylserine complex 500 mg Standardized to: Phosphatidylserine 100 mg • Phosphatidylcholine 45 mg • Phosphatidylethanolamine 10 mg • Phosphatidylinositol 5 mg. Other Ingredients: Soya Lecithin, Gelatin, Glycerine, Soybean Oil, Water.

Some Brand Name Natural Products - What they Contain

www.NaturalDatabase.com contains MANY more listings than appear here.
Editor's Notes are located on pages 2155-2163.

PS-100 capsules - Jarrow Formulas
Each capsule contains: Phosphatidylserine (PS) 100 mg • Phosphatidylcholine (PC) 12 mg • Gamma Tocopherol 3 mg. Other Ingredients: Calcium Phosphate, Cellulose, Silicon Dioxide, Magnesium Stearate, Gelatin.

PS-100 softgels - Jarrow Formulas
Each softgel contains: Phosphatidylserine (PS) 100 mg • Phosphatidylcholine (PC) 60 mg • Gamma Tocopherol 4 mg. Other Ingredients: Soybean Oil, Gelatin, Glycerin, Water.

Psoriacin - Dr. Clayton's Naturals
Each tablet contains: Berberis Aquifolium 3X. Other Ingredients: White Oak bark, Marshmallow root, Mullein leaves, Black Walnut leaves or hulls, Gravel root, Red Clover blossoms, Burdock root, Skullcap.

Psorizide Forte - Loma Lux Laboratories
Each tablet contains: Fumaric Acid 30 mg • Potassium Bromide 22 mg • Nickel Sulfate 2.6 mg. Other Ingredients: Lactose, Magnesium Stearate.

Psycles Female Nutrient Support System - Starlight International
Each two tablets contain: Vitamin B6 (as pyridoxine hydrochloride) 30 mg • Magnesium (magnesium oxide) 100 mg • Chaste Tree 4:1 extract (vitex agnus-castus) 200 mg • Black Cohosh root 4:1 extract (cimicifuga racemosa) 200 mg • Dong Quai root 4:1 extract, (angelica polymorpha) 150 mg • Dandelion leaf 4:1 extract (taraxacum officinale) 125 mg • Motherwort 4:1 extract (leonurus cardiaca) 100 mg • Ginger root (zingiber officinalis) 100 mg • Quercetin 25 mg • Red Raspberry leaf (rubus idaeus) 2 mg • Stinging Nettle leaf (urtica dioica) 2 mg • Spirulina 2 mg. Other Ingredients: Maltodextrin, Dicalcium Phosphate, Microcrystalline Cellulose, Croscarmellose Sodium, Stearic Acid, Magnesium Stearate, Silicon Dioxide, Methylcellulose, Microfine Wax, Carbowax.

Psyllium - Metabolic Response Modifiers
Each tablespoon contains: Psyllium husk (dietary fiber 4 g) 5 g.

Psyllium - J. R. Carlson Laboratories, Inc.
Six capsules contain: Psyllium seed husk 3 mg.

Psyllium (Secrets of the Psyllium & Orange Flavored Psyllium Powder) - Trader Joe's
Psyllium husk fiber • Secrets of the Psyllium 85%: Fiber (per heaping tablespoon) 6 g • Orange flavored Psyllium powder 35%: Fiber (per heaping tablespoon) 3 g.

Psyllium Husk - Pro Health
Three capsules contain: Psyllium husk powder (from plantago asiatica seed) 1.5 g. Other Ingredients: Gelatin, Magnesium Stearate.

PTE Support - PhysioLogics
Two capsules contain: Bromelain (2400 GDU) 500 mg • Serratiopeptidase 10 mg.

Pumpkin Power - Pain & Stress Center
Each capsule contains: Pumpkin seed oil (curcubita pepo, entire seed) 1000 mg. Other Ingredients: Gelatin, Glycerol, Water.

Pumpkin Seed Extract - Enzymatic Therapy/PhytoPharmica
Each capsule contains: Pumpkin seed extract (cucurbita pepo, 18:1) 300 mg. Other Ingredients: Gelatin, Magnesium Stearate, Silicon Dioxide, Titanium Dioxide Color.
See Editor's Note No. 21.

Pumpkin Seed Oil - GNC
Each capsule contains: Pumpkin Seed oil 1 g. Other Ingredients: Gelatin, Glycerin.

Pure & Natural Formula - Bee-Alive Inc.
Each 1/5 teaspoon contains: Royal Jelly (non-freeze dried) 1.1 g.

Pure Agility - PhytoPharmica
Three tablets contain: Chloride (from glucosamine sulfate) 234 mg • Chondroitin Sulfate (from marine source, with average molecular weight less than 16,000 daltons) 1200 mg • Glucosamine Sulfate (stabilized) 1500 mg • Sodium 185 mg.

Pure Ascorbic Acid capsules - Pure Encapsulations
Each vegetable capsule contains: Ascorbic Acid 1000 mg • Vitamin C (as ascorbyl palmitate) 20 mg.

Pure Ascorbic Acid powder - Pure Encapsulations
Each 1 tsp serving contains: Ascorbic Acid 3200 mg.

Pure Bovine Cartilage - EcoNugenics
Four capsules contain: Bovine Cartilage 3 g • Calcium 30 mg. Other Ingredients: Gelatin, Magnesium Stearate, Silica.
See Editor's Note No. 14.

Pure Build - PhytoPharmica
Each tablet contains: Indolplex Complex 120 mg: Modified food starch, 25% Diindolylmethane (DIM), D-Alpha-Tocopheryl Succinate, Silicon Dioxide, Phosphatidylcholine.

Pure C Crystals - Nature's Life
Each 1/4 teaspoon contains: Vitamin C (Ascorbic Acid) 1250 mg.

Pure CitriMax 250 mg - Natrol, Inc.
Each capsule contains: Calcium (from (-)hydroxycitric acid) 75 mg • (-) HydroxyCitric Acid (from garcinia cambogia fruit, CitriMax brand) 250 mg. Other Ingredients: Gelatin, Magnesium Stearate.

Pure Cleansing Gel (combination to oily skin) - Nu Skin Enterprises
Water • Ammonium Lauryl Sulfate • Lauryl Betaine • Sodium Lauroyl Sarcosinate • Glycerin • PEG-120 Methyl Glucose Dioleate • Papain • Citrus Limonum fruit extract (citrus medica limonum, lemon) • Foeniculum Vulgare fruit extract (fennel) • Anthenis Nobilis flower extract • Calendula Officinalis flower extract • Centaurea Cyanis flower extract • Chamomilla Recutita flower extract (matricaria) • Geranium Maculatum extract • Hypericum Perforatum extract • Salvia Officinalis leaf extract • Sambucus Nigra flower extract • Tilia Cordata flower extract • Carbomer • Butylene Glycol • PVP • Sodium Chloride • Fragrance (parfum) • Tetrasodium EDTA • Benzoic Acid • Phenoxyethanol • Chlorphenesin • Methylparaben.

Pure Comfort - FreeLife International
Aloe Vera gel • SD-38 Grain Alcohol with Spearmint oil • Methylsulfonylmethane (MSM) • Glyceryl Stearate • Sweet Almond oil • Caprylic/Capric Triglyceride • Cetyl Alcohol • Camphor • Witch Hazel • Sodium Stearoyl Lactylate • Menthol • Glycerin • Hydrogenated Lecithin • Glucosamine Sulfate • Manuka oil • Tea Tree oil • Tocopherol Acetate (vitamin E) • Willowherb extract • Allantoin • Burdock root extract • BioEnhanced Grapefruit seed extract (BGSE) • Hydroxyethylcellulose • Stearic Acid.

Pure Confidence - FreeLife International
Arctium Lappa (burdock root) • Pure Grain Alcohol • Lavender essential oil • Caprylic/Capric Triglyceride (derived from plants) • Zinc Ricinoleat • Hydrogenated Lecithin • Essential Ylang Ylang oil.

Pure Core - PhytoPharmica
Three capsules contain: Biotin 150 mcg • Calcium (lysinate, aspartate, citrate) 150 mg • Choline (as choline bitartrate) 38 mg • Chromium (glycinate, aspartate, lysinate) 75 mcg • Copper (citrate, aspartate, glycinate, lysinate) 563 mcg • Folic Acid 300 mcg • Inositol 38 mg • Magnesium (aspartate, citrate, glycinate, lysinate) 113 mg • Manganese (aspartate, lysinate, citrate, glycinate) 6 mg • Molybdenum (aspartate, glycinate, lysinate) 38 mcg • Niacin (niacinamide, Niacinol brand) 53 mg • Pantothenic Acid (calcium pantothenate) 150 mg • Potassium (chloride) 38 mg • Riboflavin 26 mg • Selenium (aspartate, glycinate, lysinate complexes) 38 mcg • Thiamin (hydrochloride) 38 mg • Vanadium (aspartate, glycinate, lysinate) 38 mcg • Vitamin A (natural beta carotene with mixed carotenoids) 9375 IU • Vitamin B12 (cyanocobalamin) 150 mcg • Vitamin B6 (as pyridoxine HCl 50 mg, pyridoxal-5'-phosphate

10 mg) 45 mg • Vitamin C (ascorbic acid) 281 mg • Vitamin E (D-alpha tocopheryl succinate) 150 IU • Zinc (as zinc picolinate, lysinate, aspartate, glycinate) 9 mg.

Pure Dimension **-** PhytoPharmica
Three softgels contain: Fish Oil Concentrate 1.5 g: EPA (eicosapentaenoic acid) 210 mg, DHA (docosahexaenoic acid) 125 mg.

Pure Energy **-** Montana Naturals, Inc.
Each 800 mg caplet contains: Bee Pollen (Apis pollenus) • Dibaxic Calcium Phosphate • Gotu Kola (Centella asiatica) • Siberian Ginseng (Eleutherococcus senticosus) • Gotu Kola standardized extract • Royal Jelly • Siberian Ginseng standardized extract.

Pure Ephedrene Alkaloid Extract **-** NVE Pharmaceuticals
Each tablet contains: Ephedra extract (leaves, stems, pure phamaceutical grade, supplying ephedrine alkaloids 24 mg) 240 mg. See Editor's Note No. 30.

Pure Eye Drops **-** Heel/BHI, Inc.
Each 0.45 mL vial contains: Cochlearia Officinalis 5X • Echinacea Angustifolia 5X • Euphraisa Officinalis 5X • Pilocarpus 5X. Other Ingredients: Isotonic Saline Solution.
See Editor's Note No. 1.

Pure Fuel **-** PhytoPharmica
Each softgel contains: Eleuthero root 20:1 extract (eleutherococcus senticosus, standardized to contain a minimum of 0.5% eleutheroside E) • Iron 1 mg • Liquid Liver Fractions (predigested soluble concentrate) 550 mg • Vitamin B12 (as cyanocobalamin) 100 mcg.
See Editor's Note No. 14.

Pure Heat **-** VitaCube Systems (V3S)
Two tablets contain: Zinc 2.5 mg • Pure Heat 1010 mg: Boswellia Serrata gum extract (65%), Methylsulfonylmethane, Bromelain 600, Tumeric root extract, Ginger root extract, Lemon Bioflavonoids, Quercetin Dihydrate, Capsicum (80,000 HU) • VitaCube Activating System 20 mg: Orange Bioflavonoids Complex, Alfalfa leaf, Ginkgo Biloba leaf, Spirulina algae, Cayenne, Apple Pectin, Odorless Garlic, 7-Isopropoxy Isoflavone, L-Glutathione, Lemon Bioflavonoids Complex, Lycopene 1%, Dimethylglycine, Potassium Glycerophosphate, Rutin, Bromelain, Lutein 5%. Other Ingredients: Cellulose, Stearic Acid, Croscarmellose Sodium, Silicon Dioxide, Magnesium Stearate, Orange Cellulose Film-Coat.

Pure Relief **-** Kalchem International
Active Ingredient: Menthol.

Pure Skin Clarifying Supplement **-** Murad, Inc.
Two tablets contain: Vitamin A (as palmitate) 4000 IU • Vitamin C (calcium 60% and zinc ascorbate 40%) 300 mg • Vitamin E (natural) 400 IU • Thiamin (vitamin B1, as thiamine HCl) 25 mg • Riboflavin (vitamin B2) 25 mg • Niacin (vitamin B3) 50 mg • Vitamin B6 (pyridoxine HCl) 50 mg • Folic Acid 400 mcg • Biotin 300 mcg • Pantothenic Acid (vitamin B5) 25 mg • Calcium (ascorbate) 62 mg • Magnesium (oxide) 200 mg • Zinc (ascorbate) 15 mg • Selenium (L-selenomethionine) 200 mcg • Beta Carotene 2500 IU • Glucosamine HCl 65 mg • L-Lysine HCl 250 mg • L-Glycine 250 mg • L-Proline 500 mg • Alpha Lipoic Acid 50 mg • Horsetail leaf extract 400 mg: Silica 28 mg • Grape seed extract (38.4%) 50 mg • Lecithin 75 mg • EFA 150 mg • Burdock root powder 83 mg • Yellowdock powder 97 mg. Other Ingredients: Dicalcium Phosphate, Microcrystalline Cellulose, Stearic Acid, Magnesium Stearate, Croscarmellose Sodium, Aerosil, Pharmaceutical Glaze, Talc.

Pure Soy Protein Powder **-** Puritan's Pride
Each scoop (28 g) contains: L-Alanine 1064 mg • L-Arginine 1876 mg • L-Aspartic Acid 2856 mg • L-Cysteine 308 mg • L-Glutamic Acid 4704 mg • L-Glycine 1036 mg • L-Histidine 644 mg • L-Isoleucine 1204 mg • L-Lysine 1540 mg • L-Methionine 336 mg • L-Phenylalanine 1288 mg • L-Proline 1260 mg • L-Serine 1288 mg • L-Threonine 924 mg • L-Tryptophan 308 mg • L-Tyrosine 924 mg • L-Valine 1232 mg.

Pure Symmetry **-** PhytoPharmica
Each chewable tablet contains: Coenzyme Q10 (ubiquinone 10) 100 mg • Vitamin E (as dL-alpha tocopheryl acetate, D-alpha tocopheryl acetate, and mixed tocopherols) 300 IU.

Pure Vitamin C 500 mg **-** Nature's Bounty
Each tablet contains: Vitamin C (as ascorbic acid) 500 mg. Other Ingredients: Cellulose (plant origin), Croscarmellose, Vegetable Magnesium Stearate, Silica, Vegetable Stearic Acid.

PureChoice Beta-S **-** Baywood International
Each tablet contains: Calcium (as dl-calcium phosphate) 42 mg • Phosphorus (as dl-calcium phosphate) 26 mg • Beta-Sitosterol complex 300 mg • Pectin (citrus) 30 mg. Other Ingredients: Microcrystalline Cellulose, Lecithin, Silica, Polyvinylprolidone, Croscarmellose Sodium, Magnesium Stearate, Vinegar (cider).

PureHands Gel **-** The Himalaya Drug Company
Each 1 mL serving contains: Hrivera (coleus vettiveroides) 35 mg • Dhanyaka (coriandrum sativum) 25 mg • Nimbuka (citrus limon) 25 mg • Ushira (vetiveria zizanioides) 20 mg • Nimba (azadirachta indica) 15 mg. Base: Prasanna (rectified spirit, ethyl alcohol).

PureWeigh PREMEAL Beverage (chocolate mint flavor) **-** Pure Encapsulations
Each scoop (28.6 g) contains: Vitamin C (pure ascorbic acid) 83.5 mg • Vitamin C (buffered ascorbic acid, from calcium ascorbate, magnesium ascorbate, potassium ascorbate) 41.5 mg • Vitamin C (ascorbyl palmitate) 10 mg • Vitamin D (as D3) 100 IU • Vitamin E (D-alpha tocopherol succinate) 33.5 IU • Thiamine HCl (vitamin B1) 8.5 mg • Riboflavin (vitamin B2) 4 mg • Riboflavin 5' Phosphate (activated B2) 2 mg • Niacinamide 8.5 mg • Inositol Hexaniacinate (no-flush niacin) 7.5 mg • Pyridoxine HCl (vitamin B6) 2 mg • Pyridoxal 5' Phosphate (activated B6) 2 mg • Folic Acid 100 mcg • Methylcobalamin (vitamin B12) 83.5 mcg • Biotin 1.3 mg • Pantothenic Acid (calcium pantothenate) 33.5 mg • Calcium (naturally occurring, calcium citrate and milk minerals) 374 mg • Phosphorous 178 mg • Magnesium (naturally occurring and magnesium citrate) 63 mg • Zinc (picolinate) 2 mg • Selenium (selenomethionine) 16.5 mcg • Manganese (aspartate) 0.8 mg • Chromium (polynicotinate) 200 mcg • Molybdenum (aspartate) 8.5 mcg • Potassium (naturally occurring and potassium aspartate) 192 mg • Mixed Carotenoids 1250 IU • Vanadium (aspartate) 16.5 mcg • Serotein brand Protein Complex w/ MFR Factors 15 g: Isoflavones 12 mg, Calcium Enriched Soy Protein Isolate, Whey Protein Isolate, Myo-inositol • SloCarb brand Slow Release Carbohydrate Complex 7.5 g: High Amylose Resistant Starch (maltodextrin), High Viscosity Glucomannan (konjac root), High Lignan Flax seed fiber, 1,3 Beta Glucan • LivClear brand 215 mg: Red Beet extract, Milk Thistle extract (80% silymarin), Taurine, Green Tea leaf extract (standardized to contain a minimum of 65% total tea catechins): Epigallocatechin gallate (EGCg) (min) 23%, Caffeine 7% • Stevia 30 mg. Other Ingredients: Soy Protein Isolate, Whey Protein Isolate, Natural Flavors, Lo Han fruit extract (momordica grosvenori), Cocoa, Xylitol.

PureWeigh PREMEAL Beverage (French vanilla flavor) **-** Pure Encapsulations
Each scoop (25.5 g) contains: Vitamin C (pure ascorbic acid) 83.5 mg • Vitamin C (buffered ascorbic acid, from calcium ascorbate, magnesium ascorbate, potassium ascorbate) 41.5 mg • Vitamin C (ascorbyl palmitate) 10 mg • Vitamin D (as D3) 100 IU • Vitamin E (D-alpha tocopherol succinate) 33.5 IU • Thiamine HCl (vitamin B1) 8.5 mg • Riboflavin (vitamin B2) 4 mg • Riboflavin 5' Phosphate (activated B2) 2 mg • Niacinamide 8.5 mg • Inositol Hexaniacinate (no-flush niacin) 7.5 mg • Pyridoxine HCl (vitamin B6) 2 mg • Pyridoxal 5' Phosphate (activated B6) 2 mg • Folic Acid 100 mcg • Methylcobalamin (vitamin B12) 83.5 mcg • Biotin 1.3 mg • Pantothenic Acid (calcium pantothenate) 33.5 mg • Calcium (naturally occurring, calcium citrate and milk minerals) 369 mg • Phosphorous 150 mg • Magnesium (naturally occurring and magnesium citrate) 44 mg • Zinc (picolinate) 2 mg • Selenium (selenomethionine) 16.5 mcg • Manganese (aspartate) 0.8 mg •

Chromium (polynicotinate) 200 mcg • Molybdenum (aspartate) 8.5 mcg • Potassium (naturally occurring and potassium aspartate) 69 mg • Mixed Carotenoids 1250 IU • Vanadium (aspartate) 16.5 mcg • Serotein brand Protein Complex w/ MFR Factors 15 g: Isoflavones 12 mg, Calcium Enriched Soy Protein Isolate, Whey Protein Isolate, Myo-inositol • SloCarb brand Slow Release Carbohydrate Complex 7.5 g: High Amylose Resistant Starch (maltodextrin), High Viscosity Glucomannan (konjac root), High Lignan Flax seed fiber, 1,3 Beta Glucan • LivClear brand 215 mg: Red Beet extract, Milk Thistle extract (80% silymarin), Taurine, Green Tea leaf extract (standardized to 65% total tea catechins): Epigallocatechin gallate (EGCg) • Stevia 30 mg. Other Ingredients: Soy Protein Isolate, Whey Protein Isolate, Natural Flavors, Lo Han fruit extract (momordica grosvenori).

PureWeigh PREMEAL Beverage (original flavor) - Pure Encapsulations
Each scoop (24.2 g) contains: Vitamin C (ascorbic acid) 83.5 mg • Vitamin C (from calcium ascorbate, magnesium ascorbate, potassium ascorbate) 41.5 mg • Vitamin C (ascorbyl palmitate) 10 mg • Vitamin D (D3) 100 IU • Vitamin E (D-alpha tocopherol succinate) 33.5 IU • Thiamine HCl (vitamin B1) 8.5 mg • Riboflavin (vitamin B2) 4 mg • Riboflavin 5' Phosphate (activated B2) 2 mg • Niacinamide 8.5 mg • Inositol Hexaniacinate (no-flush niacin) 7.5 mg • Pyridoxine HCl (vitamin B6) 2 mg • Pyridoxal 5' Phosphate (activated B6) 2 mg • Folic Acid 100 mcg • Methylcobalamin (vitamin B12) 83.5 mcg • Biotin 1.3 mg • Pantothenic Acid (calcium pantothenate) 33.5 mg • Calcium (naturally occurring, calcium citrate and milk minerals) 369 mg • Phosphorous 150 mg • Magnesium (naturally occurring and magnesium citrate) 44 mg • Zinc (picolinate) 2 mg • Selenium (selenomethionine) 16.5 mcg • Manganese (aspartate) 0.8 mg • Chromium (polynicotinate) 200 mcg • Molybdenum (aspartate) 8.5 mcg • Potassium (naturally occurring and potassium aspartate) 69 mg • Mixed Carotenoids 1250 IU • Vanadium (aspartate) 16.5 mcg • Serotein brand Protein Complex w/ MFR Factors 15 g: Isoflavones 12 mg, Calcium Enriched Soy Protein Isolate, Whey Protein Isolate, Myo-inositol • SloCarb brand Slow Release Carbohydrate Complex 7.5 g: High Amylose Resistant Starch (maltodextrin), High Viscosity Glucomannan (konjac root), High Lignan Flax seed fiber, 1,3 Beta Glucan • LivClear brand 215 mg: Red Beet extract, Milk Thistle extract (80% silymarin), Taurine, Green Tea leaf extract (standardized to 65% total tea catechins): Epigallocatechin gallate (EGCg). Other Ingredients: Soy Protein Isolate, Whey Protein Isolate, Natural Flavors, Lo Han fruit extract (momordica grosvenori).

PureWeigh PREMEAL Beverage (pineapple coconut flavor) - Pure Encapsulations
Each scoop (24.7 g) contains: Vitamin C (pure ascorbic acid) 83.5 mg • Vitamin C (from calcium ascorbate, magnesium ascorbate, potassium ascorbate) 41.5 mg • Vitamin C (ascorbyl palmitate) 10 mg • Vitamin D (as D3) 100 IU • Vitamin E (D-alpha tocopherol succinate) 33.5 IU • Thiamine HCl (vitamin B1) 8.5 mg • Riboflavin (vitamin B2) 4 mg • Riboflavin 5' Phosphate (activated B2) 2 mg • Niacinamide 8.5 mg • Inositol Hexaniacinate (no-flush niacin) 7.5 mg • Pyridoxine HCl (vitamin B6) 2 mg • Pyridoxal 5' Phosphate (activated B6) 2 mg • Folic Acid 100 mcg • Methylcobalamin (vitamin B12) 83.5 mcg • Biotin 1.3 mg • Pantothenic Acid (calcium pantothenate) 33.5 mg • Calcium (naturally occurring, calcium citrate and milk minerals) 369 mg • Phosphorous 150 mg • Magnesium (naturally occurring and magnesium citrate) 44 mg • Zinc (picolinate) 2 mg • Selenium (selenomethionine) 16.5 mcg • Manganese (aspartate) 0.8 mg • Chromium (polynicotinate) 200 mcg • Molybdenum (aspartate) 8.5 mcg • Potassium 69 mg • Mixed Carotenoids 1250 IU • Vanadium (aspartate) 16.5 mcg • Serotein brand Protein Complex w/ MFR Factors 15 g: Isoflavones 12 mg, Calcium Enriched Soy Protein Isolate, Whey Protein Isolate, Myo-inositol • SloCarb brand Slow Release Carbohydrate Complex 7.5 g: Maltodextrin, High Viscosity Glucomannan (konjac root), High Lignan Flax seed fiber, 1,3 Beta Glucan • LivClear brand 215 mg: Red Beet extract, Milk Thistle extract (80% silymarin), Taurine, Green Tea leaf extract (standardized to 65% total tea catechins) • Stevia 30 mg. Other Ingredients: Soy Protein Isolate, Whey Protein Isolate, Natural Flavors, Lo Han fruit extract (momordica grosvenori).

PureWeigh PREMEAL Beverage (strawberry banana flavor) - Pure Encapsulations
Each scoop (24.6 g) contains: Vitamin C (pure ascorbic acid) 83.5 mg • Vitamin C (buffered ascorbic acid, from calcium ascorbate, magnesium ascorbate, potassium ascorbate) 41.5 mg • Vitamin C (ascorbyl palmitate) 10 mg • Vitamin D (as D3) 100 IU • Vitamin E (D-alpha tocopherol succinate) 33.5 IU • Thiamine HCl (vitamin B1) 8.5 mg • Riboflavin (vitamin B2) 4 mg • Riboflavin 5' Phosphate (activated B2) 2 mg • Niacinamide 8.5 mg • Inositol Hexaniacinate (no-flush niacin) 7.5 mg • Pyridoxine HCl (vitamin B6) 2 mg • Pyridoxal 5' Phosphate (activated B6) 2 mg • Folic Acid 100 mcg • Methylcobalamin (vitamin B12) 83.5 mcg • Biotin 1.3 mg • Pantothenic Acid (calcium pantothenate) 33.5 mg • Calcium (naturally occurring, calcium citrate and milk minerals) 369 mg • Phosphorous 150 mg • Magnesium (naturally occurring and magnesium citrate) 44 mg • Zinc (picolinate) 2 mg • Selenium (selenomethionine) 16.5 mcg • Manganese (aspartate) 0.8 mg • Chromium (polynicotinate) 200 mcg • Molybdenum (aspartate) 8.5 mcg • Potassium (naturally occurring and potassium aspartate) 69 mg • Mixed Carotenoids 1250 IU • Vanadium (aspartate) 16.5 mcg • Serotein brand Protein Complex w/ MFR Factors 15 g: Isoflavones 12 mg, Calcium Enriched Soy Protein Isolate, Whey Protein Isolate, Myo-inositol • SloCarb brand Slow Release Carbohydrate Complex 7.5 g: High Amylose Resistant Starch (maltodextrin), High Viscosity Glucomannan (konjac root), High Lignan Flax seed fiber, 1,3 Beta Glucan • LivClear brand 215 mg: Red Beet extract, Milk Thistle extract (80% silymarin), Taurine, Green Tea leaf extract (standardized to 65% total tea catechins) • Stevia 30 mg. Other Ingredients: Soy Protein Isolate, Whey Protein Isolate, Natural Flavors, Lo Han fruit extract (momordica grosvenori).

PureWeigh-FM - Pure Encapsulations
Three vegetable capsules contain: Banaba extract (lagerstroemia speciosa L., standardized to contain 1% corosolic acid) 48 mg • Green Tea extract (standardized to 65% total tea catechins) 525 mg: Epigallocatechin gallate (EGCg) 121 mg, Caffeine 37 mg • Taurine (free-form) 450 mg • DHEA Acetate-7-one 150 mg • Biotin 1.5 mg • Magnesium (citrate) 125 mg • Chromium (polynicotinate) 125 mcg • Vitamin C (as ascorbyl palmitate) 45 mg.

Pur-Gar - NOW Foods
Each tablet contains: Pur-Gar 600 mg.

Purified Chondroitin Sulfates - American Biologics
Each capsule contains: Purified Chondroitin Sulfates (as purified extract of bovine trachea tissue) 500 mg • Papain 15 mg. Other Ingredients: Magnesium Stearate.
See Editor's Note No. 15.

Purify - Enzymedica
Each capsule contains: Protease Thera-Blend 132,000 HUT • Calcium Citrate 32 mg.

Purifying Hand Wash - FreeLife International
Aqueous Extract Blend: Hibiscus flower extract, Canadian Willowherb, Purified water • BioEnhanced Grapefruit seed extract (BGSE) 100X • Hesperidin • Pure Grain Alcohol • Decyl Glucoside • Lauryl Glucoside • Vegetable Glycerin • Celulose Gum • Lonicera Japonica (Japanese honeysuckle) • Potassium Sorbate • Citric Acid • Pure Clover Honey • Methylsulfonylmethane (MSM) • Harmonic Essence #3 • Vitamin E Acetate • Essential Grapefruit oil • Essential Orange oil • Benzyl Alcohol • Phenoxyethanol.

Purim - The Himalaya Drug Company
Each tablet contains: Haridra (curcuma longa) 36 mg • Aragvadha (cassia fistula) 36 mg • Bakuchi (psoralea corylifolia) 36 mg • Kushta (saussurea lappa) 36 mg • Katuka (picrorhiza kurroa) 36 mg • Nimba (azadirachta indica syn. melia axadirachta) 32 mg • Guduchi (tinospora cordifolia) 32 mg • Varuna (crataeva magna syn. c.nurvala) 32 mg • Triphala 31 mg: Emblica Officinalis, Terminalia Chebula, Terminalia Bellirica • Vidanga (embelia ribes) 31 mg • Bhringaraja (eclipta alba syn. e.prostrata) 31 mg • Kalamegha (andrographis paniculata) 31 mg.

Some Brand Name Natural Products - What they Contain

www.NaturalDatabase.com contains MANY more listings than appear here.
Editor's Notes are located on pages 2155-2163.

Puristat Absorb - Abbott Industries
Each tablet contains: Chitosan powder 90% HD 278 mg. Other Ingredients: Dicalcium Phosphate Dihydrate (unmilled), Sweet Dairy Whey SD, Croscarmellose Sodium, Stearic Acid, Magnesium Stearate.

Puristat Boost - Abbott Industries
Two tablets contain: Siberian Ginseng (as Eleuthro L.) root 400 mg. Other Ingredients: Dicalcium Phosphate Dihydrous, Magnesium Stearate, Microcrystalline Cellulose, Silicon Dioxide, Stearic Acid, Sweet Dairy Whey.

Puristat Cleanse - Abbott Industries
Six tablets contain: Cascara Sagrada bark 400 mg • Buckthorn bark 200 mg • Rhubarb root 200 mg • Ginger root 150 mg • Goldenseal herb (aerial parts) 75 mg • Raspberry leaf 75 mg • Fennel seed 75 mg • Cayenne Pepper 25 mg • Mult. Fiber Blend 750 mg: Vegetable Cellulose, Beet fiber, Oat fiber, Pea fiber, Apple Pectin, Citrus Pectin. Other Ingredients: Dicalcium Phosphate, Croscarmellose Sodium, Stearic Acid, Silicon Dioxide, Hydroxypropylmethylcellulose (HPMC).

Puristat Restore - Abbott Industries
Three caplets contain: Lactobacillus Acidophilus & Lactospore 2 billion CFO • Aloe leaf 500 mg • Barberry root 150 mg • Black Radish root 150 mg • Marshmallow root 100 mg • Echinacea herb (aerial parts) 100 mg • Red Clover flower 100 mg • Burdock root 100 mg • Mullein leaf 50 mg • Parsley leaf 50 mg • Wood Betony herb (whole plant) 50 mg • Dandelion root 50 mg • Ginger root 50 mg • Cramp bark 50 mg. Other Ingredients: Magnesium Stearate.

Puritron - Puritan's Pride
Six tablets contain: Vitamin A (as Fish Liver Oil) 10,000 IU • Vitamin C (ascorbic acid) 300 mg • Vitamin D (cholecalciferol) 400 IU • Vitamin E (D-alpha tocopheryl acetate) 100 IU • Thiamin mononitrate (vitamin B1) 25 mg • Riboflavin (vitamin B2) 25 mg • Niacin (niacinamide) 25 mg • Vitamin B6 (pyridoxine hydrochloride) 25 mg • Folic Acid 400 mcg • Vitamin B12 (cyanocobalamin) 25 mcg • Biotin 150 mcg • Pantothenic Acid (D-calcium pantothenate) 25 mg • Calcium (bone meal) 800 mg • Iron (ferrous gluconate) 30 mg • Phosphorus (bone meal) 400 mg • Iodine (kelp) 150 mcg • Magnesium (oxide) 100 mg • Zinc (gluconate) 30 mg • Selenium (yeast) 25 mcg • Copper (gluconate) 1 mg • Manganese (gluconate) 0.07 mg • Potassium (gluconate) 40 mg • Brewer's Yeast 600 mg • Choline Bitartrate 24 mg • Inositol 36 mcg • PABA (para-aminobenzoic acid) 40 mcg • Rutin 30 mg • Citrus Bioflavonoid complex 30 mg • Hesperidin complex 25 mg • Nucleic Acid 40 mg • Desiccated Liver 100 mg • Red Bone Marrow 60 mg • Lecithin 60 mg • Wheat Germ Oil 20 mg • Papain 20 mg • Rose Hips 1 mg. Amino Acids from Brewer's Yeast and Desiccated Liver: Alanine 19.3 mg, Arginine 8.1 mg, Aspartic Acid 20 mg, Cysteine 2.7 mg, Glutamic Acid 32.8 mg, Glycine 12.8 mg, Histidine 8 mg, Isoleucine 13.1 mg, Leucine 21.1 mg, Lysine 21.9 mg, Methionine 5.4 mg, Phenylalanine 12.5 mg, Proline 11.9 mg, Serine 13.6 mg, Threonine 13.2 mg, Tryptophan 3.8 mg, Tyrosine 8.9 mg, Valine 12.6 mg.
See Editor's Note No. 14.

Pycnogenol - Pro Health
Two capsules contain: Pycnogenol 60 mg • Citrus Bioflavonoids (40% hesperidin) 600 mg. Other Ingredients: Magnesium Stearate.

Pycnogenol - Leiner Health Products
Each tablet contains: Pycnogenol 50 mg. Other Ingredients: Calcium Carbonate, Maltodextrin, Cellulose, Tricalcium Phosphate, Talc, Polyethylene Glycol 3350, Silicon Dioxide, Crospovidone, Croscarmellose Sodium, Magnesium Stearate.

Pycnogenol - NOW Foods
Each capsule contains: European Pine bark.

Pycnogenol 100 mg - Pure Encapsulations
Each vegetable capsule contains: Pycnogenol (pine bark extract, standardized to contain 65-75% proanthocyanins) 100 mg • Vitamin C (as ascorbyl palmitate) 4 mg.

Pycnogenol 25 Mg - Natrol, Inc.
One capsule contains: Pine Bark extract 25 mg. Other Ingredients: Microcrystalline Cellulose, Magnesium Stearate, Gelatin.

Pycnogenol 25mg - Sundown
Three tablets contain: Vitamin A (100% as beta-carotene) 25,000 IU • Calcium 340 mg • Selenium (as selenium yeast chelate) 100 mg • Maritime Pine bark extract 25 mg • Coenzyme Q-10 10 mg • Grape Seed extract 100 mcg • Whole Food Phytonutrient Blend 120 mg: Broccoli (entire plant), Carrot root, Spinach (entire plant), Tomato fruit. Other Ingredients: Calcium Carbonate, Microcrystalline Cellulose, Croscarmellose Sodium, Magnesium Stearate.

Pycnogenol 50 mg - Pure Encapsulations
Each vegetable capsule contains: Pycnogenol (pine bark extract, standardized to contain 65-75% proanthocyanins) 50 mg • Vitamin C (as ascorbyl palmitate) 2 mg.

Pycnogenol 50 mg - Schiff
Each capsule contains: Maritime Pine Bark extract (pinus maritima) 50 mg. Other Ingredients: Maltodextrin, Capsule (gelatin, lauryl sulfate, silicon dioxide), Magnesium Stearate, Silicon Dioxide.

Pycnogenol 50 Mg - Natrol, Inc.
One capsule contains: Pine Bark extract 50 mg. Other Ingredients: Microcrystalline Cellulose, Magnesium Stearate, Gelatin.

Pycnogenol Capsules - Nature's Plus
Each capsule contains: Pycnogenol (pinus maritima bark standardized to 85-95% [25.5-28.5] proanthocyanidins) 30 mg. Other Ingredients: Silica, Gelatin, Purified Water.

Pycnogenol Plus - Aspen Group, Inc.
Each capsule contains: Bioflavonoids 200 mg • Grape Seed extract 25 mg • Pycnogenol 25 mg.

Pycnogenol With Citrus Bioflavonoids - QualiCeutix
Each tablet contains: Pycnogenol (French martime pine bark extract) 50 mg • Citrus Bioflavonoid complex 250 mg. Other Ingredients: Microcrystalline Cellulose, Dicalcium Phosphate, Stearic Acid, Croscarmellose Sodium, Hydroxypropyl Methylcellulose, Magnesium Stearate, Silicon Dioxide, Polyethlene Glycol.

Pycnogenol with Vitamins C, E, & A - Derma E
Pycnogenol • Vitamin C • Vitamin E • Vitamin A.

Pycno-Plus Protection - HealthWatchers System
Grape Seed Extract • Pine Bark Powder Plus • Beta Carotene • Vitamin C • Cat's Claw Powder • Bioflavonoids • Rutin • Acerola.

Pygeum - Nature's Way
Each capsule contains: Pygeum bark extract concentrate (standardized to 13% sterols 6.5 mg) 50 mg • Vitamin B6 (Pyridoxine HCl) 12.5 mg • Zinc (Citrate) 15 mg • Copper (Citrate) 1.5 mg • Selenium 50 mcg. In a base of Pumpkin seed oil.

Pygeum/Saw Palmetto - Pro Health
Each softgel contains: Saw Palmetto berry extract (serenoa repens fruit) 80 mg • Pygeum Africanum bark extract 25 mg • Pumpkin seed oil 750 mg. Other Ingredients: Gelatin, Glycerin, Carob, Water.

Pyloricil - Ortho Molecular Products
Three capsules contain: Mastic Gum extract 1000 mg • Bismuth Citrate 250 mg • Berberine Sulfate 100 mg • Ginger root extract (standardized to contain 5% gingerols) 100 mg.

Pyridoxal 5-Phosphate Plus - Klaire Laboratories
Each capsule contains: Pyridoxal 5-Phosphate 50 mg • Magnesium (as Magnesium Glycinate Chelate) 100 mg.

Pyridoxal-5' Phosphate - Vital Nutrients
Each capsule contains: Pyridoxal-5-Phosphate (activated vitamin B6) 50 mg.

Pyridoxine B6 50mg - Jarrow Formulas
Each capsule contains: Pyridoxine (as hydrochloride) 50 mg. Other Ingredients: Cellulose, Magnesium Stearate, Gelatin.

BRAND NAMES

Some Brand Name Natural Products - What they Contain

www.NaturalDatabase.com contains MANY more listings than appear here.
Editor's Notes are located on pages 2155-2163.

Pyruvate **-** Aspen Group, Inc.
Each capsule contains: Calcium Pyruvate 750 mg.

Pyruvate Fuel **-** TwinLab
Each capsule contains: Calcium Pyruvate Monohydrate 750 mg.

Pyruvate Powder **-** Source Naturals
Each capsule contains: Calcium Pyruvate Monohydrate 750 mg.

Pyruvate Power **-** Swanson Health Products
Two capsules contain: Calcium (as calcium pyruvate) 244 mg • Pyruvate (as calcium pyruvate) 1.05 g • Cayenne 100 mg.

Python **-** Swedish Herbal Institute
One tablet contains: Damiana 100 mg • Gotu Kola 30 mg • Green Oat Straw seeds 100 mg • Muira Puama 100 mg • Saw Palmetto 100 mg • Ginkgo Biloba 30 mg • Siberian Ginseng 200 mg • Korean Ginseng root 200 mg • Guarana seeds 50 mg • Schisandra fruit/seed 100 mg • Stinging Nettle leaf 200 mg • Tribulus Terrestris 250 mg.

Q-absorb Co-Q10 (100 mg) **-** Jarrow Formulas
Each softgel contains: Co-Enzyme Q10 (ubiquinone) 100 mg • Gamma Tocopherol 4 mg. Other Ingredients: Lecithin, Medium Chain Glycerides (MCGs), Gelatin, Glycerin, Water, Carob.

Q-absorb Co-Q10 (30 mg) **-** Jarrow Formulas
Each softgel contains: Co-Enzyme Q10 (ubiquinone) 30 mg • Gamma Tocopherol 4 mg. Other Ingredients: Lecithin, Medium Chain Glycerides (MCGs), Gelatin, Glycerin, Water, Carob.

Qec 100 **-** Xymogen
Each softgel contains: Vitamin A (as Betatene brand mixed carotenoids) 2334 IU • Vitamin E (as mixed tocopherols) 100 IU • Coenzyme Q10 (ubiquinone) 100 mg. Other Ingredients: Rice Bran Oil, Gelatin, Glycerin, Beeswax, Water, Natural Annatto extract (color), Titanium Dioxide.

Q-Gel 15 mg **-** Tishcon-GelTec
Each softgel capsule contains: Vitamin E 3 IU • Coenzyme Q-10 15 mg. Other Ingredients: Gelatin, Glycerin, Purified Water, Titanium Dioxide, Annatto Seed Extract, Proprietary Biosolv brand base: Polysorbate 80, Lecithin, Sorbitan Monoleate, Medium Chain Triglycerides.
See Editor's Note No. 45.

Q-Gel 15mg **-** N.V. Perricone M.D. Cosmeceuticals
Each softgel contains: Vitamin E (D-alpha toocpherol, conc.) 3 IU • Coenzyme Q-10 (ubidecarenone, USP verified) 15 mg. Other Ingredients: Gelatin, Glycerin, Sorbitol, Purified Water, Titanium Dioxide, Annatto Seed Extract, Polysorbate 80, Lecithin, Triacetin, Medium Chain Triglycerides.

Q-Gel Brand **-** Tishcon-GelTec
Coenzyme Q10.
See Editor's Note No. 44 and No. 45.

Q-Gel Forte 30 mg **-** Tishcon-GelTec
Each softgel capsule contains: Vitamin E 6 IU • Coenzyme Q-10 30 mg. Other Ingredients: Gelatin, Glycerin, Purified Water, Titanium Dioxide, Annatto Seed Extract, Proprietary Biosolv brand base: Polysorbate 80, Lecithin, Sorbitan Monoleate, Medium Chain Triglycerides.
See Editor's Note No. 45.

Q-Gel forte Coenzyme Q10 **-** Solanova
Each softsules contains: Vitamin E (d-alpha tocopherol conc.) 6 IU • Coenzyme Q-10 (ubidecarenone) 30 mg. Other Ingredients: Gelatin, Glycerin, Purified Water, Titanium Dioxide, Annato seed extract, plus a proprietary Bio Solv base (polysorbate 80, lecithin, sorbitan monoleate, medium chain triglycerides).

Q-Gel Mega 100 mg **-** Tishcon-GelTec
Each softgel capsule contains: Vitamin E 150 IU • Coenzyme Q-10 100 mg. Other Ingredients: Gelatin, Sorbitol, Glycerin, Purified Water, Polysorbate 80, Hydroxylated Lecithin, Medium Chain Triglycerides, Annatto Seed Extract, Soybean Oil.
See Editor's Note No. 45.

Q-Gel Ultra 60 mg **-** Tishcon-GelTec
Each softgel capsule contains: Coenzyme Q-10 60 mg • Vitamin E 150 IU. Other Ingredients: Gelatin, Sorbitol, Glycerin, Purified Water, Titanium Dioxide, Annato seed extract, Proprietary Biosolv brand base: Polysorbate 80, Lecithin, Sorbitan Monoleate, Medium Chain Triglycerides.
See Editor's Note No. 45.

Qiang Shen Huo Xue Wan Plus **-** Secara
White Willow bark 10:1 extract (bai liu) 681 mg • Organic Licorice root (gan cao) 249 mg • Myrrh gum resin (mo yao) 210 mg • Achyranthes root 5:1 extract (niu xi) 186 mg • Safflower head 5:1 extract (hong hua) 186 mg • Dong Quai root 5:1 extract (dang gui) 186 mg • Red Peony root 5:1 extract (chi shao) 186 mg • Bitter Orange young fruit 5:1 extract (zhi shi) 102 mg • Ligusticum Wallichii rhizome 5:1 extract (chuang xiong) 102 mg • Bupleurum root 5:1 extract (chai hu) 81 mg • Rehmannia tuber 5:1 extract (shu di huang) 81 mg.
See Editor's Note No. 40.

Qmelt **-** HVL, Inc
Each tablet contains: Natural Coenzyme Q10 60 mg. Other Ingredients: Mannitol, Sorbitol, Citric Acid, Vegetable Stearate, Natural Orange Flavor, Povidone.

QR-4 **-** Ortho Molecular Products
Each capsule contains: Feverfew aerial portion extract (standardized to contain 1% parthenolides) 200 mg • White Willow bark extract (standardized to contain 2.5% salicin) 100 mg • German Chamomile flower 50 mg • Green Tea leaf 50 mg • Rosemary aerial portion 50 mg • Scullcap aerial portion 50 mg. Other Ingredients: Natural Vegetable Capsules, Magnesium Stearate, Microcrystalline Cellulose.

Q-Sorb Co Q-10 60 mg Plus Vitamin E **-** Vitamin World
Each capsule contains: Vitamin E (as D-alpha tocopherol acetate) 300 IU • Coenzyme Q-10 120 mg. Other Ingredients: Polysorbate 80, Gelatin, Medium Chain Triglycerides, Glyceryl Tributyrate, Glycerin, Sorbitol, Soy Lecithin, Annatto Extract, Titanium Dioxide Color.

Q-Sorb Coenzyme Q-10 **-** Nature's Bounty
Each softgel contains: Coenzyme Q-10 50 mg. Other Ingredients: Rice Bran Oil, Gelatin, Glycerin, Mixture of Beeswax and Soybean Oil, Lecithin, Titanium Dioxide Color.

Q-Sorb Coenzyme Q-10 (120 mg) **-** Vitamin World
Each softgel capsule contains: Coenzyme Q-10 120 mg. Other Ingredients: Rice Bran Oil, Gelatin, Glycerin, Mixture of Beeswax and Soybean Oil, Lecithin, Titanium Dioxide Color.

Q-Sorb Coenzyme Q-10 (30 mg) **-** Vitamin World
Each softgel contains: Q-Sorb Coenzyme Q-10 30 mg. Other Ingredients: Rice Bran Oil, Gelatin, Glycerin, Soy Lecithin, Yellow Beeswax, Titanium Dioxide Color.

Q-Sorb Coenzyme Q-10 (50 mg) **-** Vitamin World
Each softgel contains: Q-Sorb Coenzyme Q-10 50 mg. Other Ingredients: Rice Bran Oil, Gelatin, Glycerin, Soy Lecithin, Yellow Beeswax, Titanium Dioxide Color.

Q-Sorb Coenzyme Q-10 (75 mg) **-** Vitamin World
Each softgel capsule contains: Coenzyme Q-10 75 mg. Other Ingredients: Rice Bran Oil, Gelatin, Glycerin, Mixture of Beeswax and Soybean Oil, Lecithin, Titanium Dioxide Color.

Q-Sorb Coenzyme Q-10 200 mg **-** Puritan's Pride
Each softgel contains: Q-Sorb Coenzyme Q-10 200 mg. Other Ingredients: Rice Bran Oil, Gelatin, Glycerin, Lecithin, Titanium Dioxide Color, Beeswax and Soybean Oil mixture.

Q-Sorb CO-Q-10 120 mg **-** Puritan's Pride
Each softgel contains: Q-Sorb Coenzyme Q-10 120 mg. Other Ingredients: Rice Bran Oil, Gelatin, Glycerin, Soy Lecithin, Yellow Beeswax, Titanium Dioxide Color.

Q-Sorb CO-Q-10 75 mg - Puritan's Pride
Each softgel: Q-Sorb Coenzyme Q-10 75 mg. Other Ingredients: Rice Bran Oil, Gelatin, Glycerin, Soy Lecithin, Beeswax and Soybean Oil Mixture, Titanium Dioxide Color.

Quality E - Life Enhancement Products, Inc.
Each capsule contains: Vitamin E (dL-alpha tocopheryl acetate) 200 IU. Other Ingredients: Gelatin, Maltodextrin, Silicon Dioxide.

Quanterra Emotional Balance - Warner-Lambert
Each tablet contains: LI 160 WS (hyperforin stabilized) St. John's Wort standardized extract 300 mg.

Quanterra Mental Sharpness, Ginkgo Biloba - Warner-Lambert
Each tablet contain: Egb 761 Ginkgo Biloba leaf extract; standardized to 24% Ginkgo flavone glycosides & 6% terpene lactones) 60 mg. Other Ingredients: Lactose, microcrystalline cellulose, maize starch, hydroxypropyl methylcellulose, croscarmellose sodium, polyethylene glycol, magnesium stearate, silicon dioxide, artificial color, talc, ferric oxide, & dimethicone.
See Editor's Note No. 21.

Quanterra Prostate, Saw Palmetto - Warner-Lambert
Each softgel contains: Saw Palmetto Berry dried extract (Seronoa repens, berry, dried extract) 160 mg. Other Ingredients: Gelatin, Glycerol, & Ferric Oxide.

Quanterra Sinus Defense - Warner-Lambert
Each tablet contains: Gentian Root (gentian lutea) 9 mg • Elder Flower (sambucus nigra) 29 mg • European Vervain aerial parts (verbena) 29 mg • Primrose Flower (primula veris) 29 mg • Sorrel aerial parts (rumex acesota) 29 mg. Other Ingredients: Sucrose, Talc, Lactose Monohydrate, Calcium Carbonate, Potato Starch, Maize Starch, Maize Swell-Starch Flour, Colloidal Anhydrous Silica, Stearic Palmitic Acid, Titanium Dioxide, Glucose Syrup, Gelatin, Shellac, Magnesium Oxide, Sorbitol, Eudragit E 12.5, Montan Glycol Wax, Povidone, Castor Oil.
See Editor's Note No. 52.

Quanterra Sleep Valerian - Warner-Lambert
Three tablets contain: Valerian (Valeriana officinalis) root, dried extract 300 mg • Lemon Balm (Melissa officinalis) leaf, dried extract 150 mg. Other Ingredients: Sucrose, Castor Oil, Talc, Methylhydroxypropyl Cellulose, Microcrystalline Cellulose, Crospovidone, Silicon Dioxide, Calcium Carbonate, Polyethylene Glycol, Titanium Dioxide, Eudragit L 30 D, Glucose Syrup, Carmellose Sodium, FD&C Blue No. 2 Aluminum Lake, Magnesium Stearate, Polyvidon, Carnauba Wax, Polysorbate 80.

Quanterra Stomach Comfort, Ginger - Warner-Lambert
Two capsules contain: Ginger (Zingiber Officinale, root) 500 mg. Other Ingredients: Gelatin, colloidal anhydrous silica, & sodium laurel sulfate.

QueaseEase - Pacific BioLogic
Pinellia rhizome • Citrus peel • Fritillaria bulb • Poria Plant Fungus (hoelen) • Licorice root • Ginger rhizome • Chrysanthemum flower • Astragalus seed • Gastrodia rhizome • Bamboo shavings • Perilla leaf • Peppermint.

Quercetin - Metabolic Response Modifiers
Each capsule contains: Quercetin 500 mg.

Quercetin - Pure Encapsulations
Each vegetable capsule contains: Quercetin 250 mg.

Quercetin & Vitamin C - NSI - Nutraceutical Sciences Institute
Each capsule contains: Vitamin C (ascorbic acid) 700 mg • Quercetin 250 mg.

Quercetin (250mg) - Vital Nutrients
Each capsule contains: Quercetin Dihydrate 250 mg.

Quercetin + ***C*** - Puritan's Pride
Two capsules contain: Quercetin 500 mg • Vitamin C 1400 mg.

Quercetin 500 - Jarrow Formulas
Each capsule contains: Quercetin 500 mg. Other Ingredients: Cellulose, Silicon Dioxide, Magnesium Stearate, Gelatin.

Quercetin 500 mg - NOW Foods
Each Vcap contains: Quercetin (from quercetin dihydrate) 500 mg. Other Ingredients: Cellulose (capsule), Cellulose, Magnesium Stearate (vegetable source).

Quercetin Plus - Nature's Plus
Two tablets contain: Vitamin C (as ascorbic acid) 300 mg • Quercetin (from saphora japonica leaf) 250 mg • Bromelain (from pineapple fruit) 100 mg. Other Ingredients: Di-calcium Phosphate, Stearic Acid, Silica, Magnesium Stearate, Pharmaceutical Glaze.

Quercetin/Bromelain Complex - Pro Health
Three tablets contain: Vitamin C (as magnesium ascorbate) 600 mg • Magnesium (from magnesium ascorbate) 39 mg • Quercetin Dihydrate (dimorphandra mollis seed) 1000 mg • Bromelain (from pineapple) 300 mg. Other Ingredients: Dicalcium Phosphate, Microcrystalline Cellulose, Stearic Acid, Magnesium Stearate, Croscarmellose Sodium, Pharmaceutical Glaze.

Quercetin-Bromelain - Doctor's Best, Inc.
Each capsule contains: Quercetin 250 mg • Bromelain 125 mg.

Quercezyme-Plus - Enzymatic Therapy
Each capsule contain: Vitamin C (Ascorbic Acid) 100 mg • Magnesium (Carbonate) 25 mg. Other ingredients: Bromelain (1800 MCU) 125 mg, Quercetin 125 mg, Mixed Bioflavonoids Complex 50% concentrate 100 mg, L-Cysteine (HCL) 75 mg.

Quick Bust - Natural Certified Solutions
Three capsules contain: Fenugreek extract 219 mg • Saw Palmetto 168 mg • Fennel seed 162 mg • L-Tyrosine 135 mg • Mexican Wild Yam 96 mg • Kelp powder 90 mg • Damiana 51 mg • Dong Quai 48 mg • Mother's Wort 48 mg • Black Cohosh extract 45 mg • Avena Sativa 42 mg • Blessed Thistle 39 mg • Humulus Lupulus 30 mg.

Quick Dissolve Maalox - Novartis
Each tablet contains: Calcium Carbonate 600 mg. Other Ingredients: Aspartame, Colloidal Silicon Dioxide, Croscarmellose Sodium, Dextrose, Flavors, Magnesium Stearate, Maltodextrin, Mannitol, Pregelatinized Starch, Red #30 Lake.

Quick Dissolve Maalox - Maximum Strength - Novartis
Each tablet contains: Calcium Carbonate 1000 mg • Sodium 2 mg. Other Ingredients: Aspartame, Corn Starch, Croscarmellose Sodium, Dextrose, Flavors, Magnesium Stearate, Maltodextrin, Mannitol, Pregelatinized Starch, Silica, Sodium Chloride, Red #30 Lake.

Quick Trim - Cybergenics America Co.
Each caplet contains: Complex 1: Guarana seed extract • L-Tyrosine • L-Phenylalanine • Garcinia Cambogia (Citrimax) • Griffonia extract • Kola Nut powder • Chinese Ginseng • Cayenne pepper • Phenalgin • Astragalus root • Cinnamon bark • Green Tea • Pacific Kelp. Complex 2: Lecithin • Ginger • Cascara Sagrada • Buchu leaf extract • Uva Ursi leaf • Juniper berry extract • Choline Bitartrate • Inositol • L-Methionine • Chickweed herb • Red Clover powder • Dandelion root extract • Senna leaf extract • Cynarin complex. Complex 3: Chamomile flower • Valerian root extract • Hawthorne extract • Kava Kava root • Immature Orange peel • Lemon Verbena • Skullcap. Complex 4: Enzyme blend • Magnesium Oxide • Calcium Chelate • Selenium Yeast • Zinccitrata • Zinc Picolinate • Ascorbic Acid • Beta Carotene • Niacin • D Alpha Tocopheryl Acetate • Pyridoxine HCl • Riboflavin • Thiamin HCl • Potassium Iodide • Folic Acid • Cyanocobalamin • Chromium Picolinate • Phytonadione • Cholecalciferol.

Qwell - Remington Health Products, LLC
Each 1 fl oz (30 mL) serving contains: Niacin 20 mg • Policosanol 40 mg • Plant Sterols 900 mg • Inositol 50 mg.

R.U. Vedic Energy - R-U Ved U.S.A.
Bacopa standardized extract (standardized to 50% bacopasides) • Green Tea standardized extract • Bala • Amla • Trikatu: Piper Nigrum, Piper Longum, Zingiber Officinale.
See Editor's Note No. 39.

RA Spes - BotanicLab
Acanthopanax Senticosus Harms (siberian ginseng; wu-chia-pi) • Alisma Plantago-Aquatica L. (alisma; tse-hsieh) • Artemisia Capillaris Thunb (artemisia; ai-yeh) • Bupleurum Chinense DC (bupleurum; chai-hu) • Corydalis Bulbosa (corydalis; yen-hu-suo) • Dioscorea Opposita Thunb (dioscorea; shan-yao) • Glycyrrhiza Glabra L. (licorice; gan-cao) • Schisandra Chinensis Baill (schizandra; wu-wei-zi) • Scutellaria Baicalensis (scute; huang-chin).

Radiant Health Basic Essence EFAs - Maximum Efficiency Products
Each capsule contains: Proprietary Blend 725 mg: Essential oils from seeds of Flax, Sunflower, Sesame, Pumpkin, and Borage; and Mixed Tocopherols 725 mg.

Radiant Health Liquid Basic Essence - Maximum Efficiency Products
Each bottle contains: Proprietary Blend 8 fl oz: Essential oils from seeds of Flax, Sunflower, Sesame, Pumpkin, and Borage, and Mixed Tocopherols.

Radical Fruits Antioxidant Formula - Garden of Life, Inc.
Three caplets contain: Poten-Zyme Grape skin/fruit/seed extract (20:1) 975 mg • Poten-Zyme Raspberry fruit/seed extract (20:1) 585 mg • Poten-Zyme Goat's Milk Whey extract (20:1) 300 mg • Prune extract (60% polyphenols) 198 mg • Poten-Zyme Blueberry extract (20:1) 195 mg • Blueberry leaf extract (20% chlorogenic acid) 102 mg • Pomegranate extract (90% polyphenols, 40% elagic acid) 102 mg • Apple skin extract (80% polyphenols, 5% phloridzine) 99 mg • Grape leaf extract (90% polyphenols, 5% astilbine) 99 mg • Cherry extract (60% polyphenols) 51 mg. Other Ingredients: Cellulose, Stearate (vegetable source).

Radical Raiders - Puritan's Pride
Three capsules contain: Vitamin A (beta carotene) 25,000 IU • Vitamin E (d-alpha tocopheryl) 400 IU • Vitamin C (Ester C) 500 mg • Selenium (l-selenomethionine) 50 mcg • Zinc (picolinate) 50 mg • Calcium (Ester C) 50 mg • Coenzyme Q10 3,000 mcg • Pycnogenol 3,000 mcg • Citrus Bioflavonoids complex 50 mg • Quercetin 30 mg • L-Glutathione 1,000 mcg • N-Acetyl-Cysteine 100 mg • Green Tea extract 3,000 mcg • Bilberry extract 30 mg.

Rapid Balance-G.I. - DaVinci Laboratories
Each capsule contains: Mannon Oligosaccharides (MOS) 450 mg • Proprietary Probiotic Blend 50 mg: Lactobacillus Acidophilus, Lactobacillus Rhamnosus, Bifidobacterium Tongum (300 million CFU).

Raspberry - Natrol, Inc.
Each single serving contains: Vitamin C (Ascorbic Acid) 250 mg • Acerola berry extract 20 mg • Echinacea (Purpurea extract 16:1) 12.5 mg • White Willow bark 100 mg • Slippery Elm bark 75 mg • Stevia powder 20 mg. Other Ingredients: Lemon Juice powder, Fructose, natural Raspberry flavor, Honey powder, Citric Acid, Natural Elderberry flavor, Calcium Carbonate.

Raspberry Drinkable Yogurt - Stonyfield Farm
Each 10 fl oz bottle contains: Active Live Cultures: S. Thermophilus • L. Bulgaricus • L. Acidophilus • Bifidus • L. Casei • L. Reuteri. Ingredients: Cultured Pasturized Low Fat Milk • Organic Sugar • Organic Nonfat Dry Milk • Inulin • Pectin • Beet Juice Concentrate • Carrot Juice Concentrate • Organic Raspberry Puree • Natural Flavors.

Raw Adrenal - Enzymatic Therapy
Each two capsules contain: Vitamin C (ascorbic acid/rose hips) 250 mg • Pantothenic Acid (D-calcium pantothenate) 100 mg • Vitamin B6 (pyridoxine HCl) 50 mg • L-Tyrosine 250 mg • Betaine 250 mg • Pituitary extract freeze-dried 120 mg • Adrenal extract (predigested soluble concentrate) 400 mg • Adrenal Cortex extract 33 mg.
See Editor's Note No. 31.

Raw Adrenal II - Enzymatic Therapy
Two tablets contain: Vitamin C (ascorbic acid/rose hips) 250 mg • Pantothenic Acid (D-calcium pantothenate) 250 mg • Vitamin B6 (pyridoxine HCl) 50 mg • L-Tyrosine 500 mg • Betaine 250 mg • Pituitary extract freeze-dried 120 mg • Adrenal extract (predigested soluble concentrate) 100 mg • Ginger root 6.5:1 extract (zingiber officinale) 100 mg • Adrenal cortex extract 33 mg.
See Editor's Note No. 31.

Raw Liver - J. R. Carlson Laboratories, Inc.
Six capsules contain: Thiamin (vitamin B1) 30 mcg • Riboflavin (vitamin B2) 224 mg • Niacin (vitamin B3) 1 mg • Vitamin B12 (cyanocobalamin) 1 mcg • Iron 1 mg • Whole Liver concentrate 3 g.

Reacted Calcium - Ortho Molecular Products
Two capsules contain: Calcium (as hydroxyapatite, Citrimal brand, buffered Chelazome brand, aspartate) 435 mg. Other Ingredients: Natural Vegetable Capsules, Ascorbyl Palmitate, Magnesium Stearate, Microcrystalline Cellulose, Silicon Dioxide.

Reacted Cal-Mag - Ortho Molecular Products
Two capsules contain: Calcium (as Citrimal brand, amino acid chelate, aspartate, hydroxyapatite) 190 mg • Magnesium (as buffered amino acid chelate, citrate) 170 mg. Other Ingredients: Natural Vegetable Capsules, Ascorbyl Palmitate, Magnesium Stearate, Microcrystalline Cellulose, Silicon Dioxide.

Reacted Chromium - Ortho Molecular Products
Each capsule contains: Chromium (as ChromeMate brand, Chelavite brand) 200 mcg. Other Ingredients: Natural Vegetable Capsules, Ascorbyl Palmitate, Magnesium Stearate, Microcrystalline Cellulose, Silicon Dioxide.

Reacted Iron - Ortho Molecular Products
Each capsule contains: Iron (as Ferrochel brand) 29 mg.

Reacted Magnesium - Ortho Molecular Products
Two capsules contain: Magnesium (as citrate, Chelazome brand) 235 mg. Other Ingredients: Natural Vegetable Capsules, Ascorbyl Palmitate, Magnesium Stearate, Microcrystalline Cellulose, Silicon Dioxide.

Reacted Magnesium & Potassium - Ortho Molecular Products
Each capsule contains: Potassium (as citrate, complex) 99 mg. Other Ingredients: Natural Vegetable Capsules, Ascorbyl Palmitate, Magnesium Stearate, Microcrystalline Cellulose, Silicon Dioxide.

Reacted Multimin - Ortho Molecular Products
Four capsules contain: Calcium (as amino acid chelate) 300 mg • Magnesium (as buffered amino acid chelate) 150 mg • Zinc (as Chelazome brand amino acid chelate) 25 mg • Selenium (as amino acid complex) 190 mcg • Copper (as lysinate) 950 mcg • Manganese (as Chelazome brand) 5 mg • Chromium (as ChromeMate brand 190 mcg • Molybdenum (as amino acid chelate) 45 mcg • Potassium (as complex) 90 mg • Betaine HCl USP 45 mg • Vanadyl Sulfate 3 mg • Boron (as proteinate) 45 mcg. Other Ingredients: Natural Vegetable Capsules, Ascorbyl Palmitate, Magnesium Stearate, Microcrystalline Cellulose, Silicon Dioxide.

Reacted Potassium - Ortho Molecular Products
Each capsule contains: Potassium (as citrate, complex) 99 mg. Other Ingredients: Natural Vegetable Capsules, Ascorbyl Palmitate, Magnesium Stearate, Microcrystalline Cellulose, Silicon Dioxide.

Reacted Selenium - Ortho Molecular Products
Each capsule contains: Selenium (as chelate) 200 mcg. Other Ingredients: Natural Vegetable Capsules, Ascorbyl Palmitate, Magnesium Stearate, Microcrystalline Cellulose, Silicon Dioxide.

Reacted Zinc - Ortho Molecular Products
Each capsule contains: Zinc (as Chelazome brand) 54 mg. Other Ingredients: Natural Vegetable Capsules, Ascorbyl Palmitate, Magnesium Stearate, Microcrystalline Cellulose, Silicon Dioxide.

RealSJW - Paragon Laboratories
Each tablet contains: St. John's Wort (0.03% Hypericin, 4% min. Hyperforin) 300 mg • Grape Seed extract (LeucoSelect) 1 mg. Other Ingredients: Calcium Phosphate, Dipacic Microcrystalline Cellulose, Vegetable Oil, Croscarmellose Sodium, Magnesium Stearate, Silicon Dioxide.

REBOUND - Dynamarketing Group Inc.
Two tablets contain: Fumaric Acid 100 mg • Succinic Acid 250 mg • L-Glutamine 250 mg • L-Cysteine (L-cysteine HCl) 15 mg • Crystal Glucose 250 mg • Young Barley Grass juice powder 75 mg • Vitamin C (calcium ascorbate) 45 mg • Vitamin B1 (thiamine hydrochloride) 2 mg • Vitamin B12 (cyanocobalamin) 1200 mcg • Folic Acid 400 mcg. Other Ingredients: Dextrose, Magnesium Stearate, Stearic Acid, Croscarmellose Sodium, FD&C Blue.

Recall - Life Enhancement Products, Inc.
Three capsules contain: Spanish Sage essential oil (salvia lavandulaefolia) 50 mcL • High-Oleic Sunflower oil 450 mL.

Recall Support - The Vitamin Shoppe
Two tablets contain: Ginkgo Biloba Extract 24% ginkgoflavoglycosides 25 mg • Phosphatidylserine 10 mg • L-Phenylalanine 250 mg • L-Glutamine 250 mg • Choline 250 mg • Gotu Kola 200 mg • RNA/DNA 100 mg • Magnesium (citrate, gluconate) 50 mg • Ginseng Extract (Panax Ginseng) 50 mg • B6 10 mg. In a base of Lecithin and Rice concentrate.

Recancostat 400 - Tyler Encapsulations
Each capsule contains: L-Glutathione (reduced) 400 mg • AnthoRedoxin Proprietary Blend 200 mg: Beet root (Beta vulgaris), Black Currant berry (Ribes nigrum), European Elderberry extract (Sambucus nigra), Bilberry berry extract (Vaccinium mytrillus) • L-Cysteine 80 mg. Other Ingredients: Microcrystalline Cellulose, Ascorbyl Palmitate, Gelatin, Water.

Recovazon - Amazon Herb
Dong Quai • Samambaia • Tangerine peel • Aquilaria • Safflower • Manaca • Peach kernel • Dalergia wood • Bitter Orange • Tayuya • Iporuru • Una de Gato.
See Editor's Note No. 40.

Recovery Formula - Sojourn Health
Four capsules contain: Vitamin E (mixed tocopherols) 400 IU • Vitamin B1 (thiamin HCl) 50 mg • Vitamin B2 (riboflavin) 50 mg • Vitamin B3 (niacinamide) 50 mg • Vitamin B6 (pyridoxine HCl) 50 mg • Folic Acid 200 mcg • Vitamin B12 50 mg • Biotin 100 mcg • Vitamin B5 (pantothenic acid) 50 mg • Proprietary Base 2075 mg: Lecithin, Echinacea, N-Acetyl Cysteine, Methionine (DL), L-Carnitine, Vitamin B10 (PABA), Choline (bitartrate), Inositol.

Recovery Gotu Kola PhytoSerum - Abra Therapeutics
Aloe Vera juice • ABRA8 PhytoSerum Complex: Gotu Kola extract, Astragalus extract, Elder flower extract, Calendula extract, Oat straw extract, Alfalfa extract, Raspberry leaf extract • Vegetable Glycerin • Jojoba nut oil • Kukui nut oil • Macadamia nut oil • Time Release Gotu Kola Phytoliposomes (standardized asiaticosides from gotu kola) • Glyceryl Stearate • Stearic Acid • Sorbitol • Avocado seed oil • Allantoin • Panthenol (pro-vitamin B5) • Borage Seed oil • Alpha-Tocopherol (vitamin E) • Beta Carotene (pro-vitamin A) • Ascorbyl Palmitate (vitamin C) • Lavender oil • Neroli oil • Methylparaben • Propylparaben.

Recovery Rub - All Terrain Company
Almond Oil • Arnica • Caprilic-Capric Triglycerides • Ceteareth-20 • Cetyl Alcohol • Cinnamon oil • Citric Acid • Dimethicone • Glycerin • Kava Kava extract • Methylparaben • Olive Oil • Propylparaben • Sweet Clover leaf extract • Shea Butter • Steareth-2 • Water.

Red Bull Energy Drink - Red Bull N.A., Inc.
Each 250 mL can contains: Carbonated Water • Sucrose • Glucose • Sodium Citrate • Taurine • Glucuronolactone • Caffeine • Inositol • Niacinamide • Calcium Pantothenate • Pyridoxine HCl • Vitamin B12 • Artificial Flavors • Colors.
See Editor's Note No. 14 and No. 42.

Red Clover - Nature's Way
Each capsule contains: Red Clover blossoms 430 mg. Other Ingredients: Gelatin.

Red Clover - Wild Rose
Each vegetable cap contains: Red Clover standardized extract 40% 125 mg • Isoflavones 50 mg • Chaste berry (vitex angus-castus) 150 mg • Dandelion root (taraxacum officinale) 100 mg • Black Cohosh root (cimcifuga racemosa) 50 mg.

Red Clover Combination - Nature's Way
Each capsule contains: Barberry bark • Buckthorn bark • Burdock root • Cascara Sagrada bark • Echinacea Purpurea stem, leaf, flower • Licorice root • Peach bark • Prickly Ash bark • Red Clover blossoms • Rosemary • Sarsaparilla root • Sorrell. Other ingredients: Gelatin.

Red Clover Extract - Source Naturals
Each tablet contains: Red Clover leaf extract (8%) 500 mg • Calcium 164 mg • Isoflavones 40 mg.

Red Clover Extract Eternal Woman - Source Naturals
Each tablet contains: Red Clover leaf extract (8%) 500 mg • Calcium 164 mg • Isoflavones 40 mg.

Red Clover Support Complex - Puritan's Pride
Each tablet contains: Vitamin E 10 IU • Red Clover extract (Trifolium pratense) aerial (dried weight equivalent) standardized for 40 mg of isoflavone phytoestrogens (naturally contains: genistein, biochanin A, daidzein, formononetin) 200 mg • Soy Isoflavones 40 mg • Black Cohosh extract (Cimicifuga racemosa) root (standarized to contain 2.5% Triterpene) 50 mg • Wild Yam (Dioscorea villosa) root 50 mg • Horse Chestnut extract (Aesculus hippocastanum) seed (standardized to contain 2.5% aescin) 25 mg • Rosemary extract (Rosmarinus officinalis) leaf 15 mg • Silica 25 mg.

Red Clover Supreme - Gaia Herbs
Forty drops contain: Proprietary Blend 60 mg: Red Clover blossoms (trifolium pratense), Stinging Nettle leaf, Cleavers (galium aparine), Yellow Dock root (rumex crispus), Burdock root (arctium lappa), Yarrow flowers (achillea millefolium), Plantain leaf/corm (plantago lanceolata), Licorice root (glycyrrhiza glabra), Prickly Ash bark (xanthoxylum clava-herculis), Grain Alcohol, Spring Water.

Red Dragon Cold & Flu Relief - Jamieson
Each capsule contains: Honeysuckle (Lonicera japonica Thunb. PE 1:2) 149.3 mg • Forsythia fruit (Forsythia suspensa Thunb. PE 1:2) 149.3 mg • White Mulberry (Morus Alba L.PE 1:2) 119.4 mg • Chrysanthemum flower (Chrysanthemum morifolium Ramat PE 1:2) 89.6 mg • Adenophora root (Adenophora Tetraphylla Thunb PE 1:2) 89.6 mg • Schizonepata stem (Schizonepata tenifolia Briq PE 1:2) 89.6 mg • Ningpo Figwort root (Scrophularia ninpoensis Hemsl PE 1:2) 74.6 mg • Great Burdock fruit (Arctium Lappa L PE 1:2) 74.6 mg • Hogfennel root (Peucedanum praeruptorum Dunn PE 1:2) 74.6 mg • Field Mint leaf (Mentha haplocalyx Briq PE 1:2) 44.8 mg • Licorice root (glycyrrhiza uralensis Fischer PE 1:2) 44.8 mg..

Red Dragon Imperial Ginseng - Jamieson
Each caplet contains: Panax Ginseng (derived from Shiu Chu, Tien Chi and Red Kirin) • 500 mg Roots of: Prince Adenophorae, Salvia, Scrophulara, Codonopsis and Polygonum Ginsengs, Radix Astragail, Canodermae Lucidum, Fructus Lycii Berry.

Red Dragon Imperial Ginseng and Garlic - Jamieson
Each capsule contains: Panax Ginseng (derived from Shiu Chu, Tien Chi and Red Kirin) • Roots of: Prince Adenophorae, Salvia, Scrophulara, Codonopsis and Polygonum Ginseng, Radix Astragail, Canodermae Lucidum, Fructus Lycii Berry 250 mg • Tibetan Plateau Garlic 250 mg.

Some Brand Name Natural Products - What they Contain

www.NaturalDatabase.com contains MANY more listings than appear here.
Editor's Notes are located on pages 2155-2163.

Red Dragon Imperial Ginseng and Royal Jelly **-** Jamieson
Each caplet contains: Panax Ginseng (derived from Shiu Chu, Tien Chi and Red Kirin) • Roots of: Prince Adenophorae, Salvia, Scrophulara, Codonopsis and Polygonum Ginseng, Radix Astragail, Canodermae Lucidum, Fructus Lycii Berry 500 mg • Fresh Royal Jelly 250 mg.

Red Dragon Imperial Green Tea **-** Jamieson
Each tea bag contains: Chinese Green Tea Leaf • Ginger Root • Natural Leechee Fruit Flavour.

Red Dragon Imperial Royal Jelly **-** Jamieson
Each capsule contains: Pure Royal Jelly concentrate equivalent to fresh Royal Jelly 500 mg.

Red Root-Cleavers Virtue **-** Blessed Herbs
Nettle • Horsetail Grass • Red Root • Cleavers • Sage leaf • Mullein leaf • Goldenseal root • Poke root • Ginger root • Grain alcohol & Distilled Water.

Red Stuff **-** Gary Null & Associates (GNA)
Contains a fruit mix including Cranberries, Cherries, Pears, Watermelons, Pink Grapefruit, Lecithin, Apple Pectin, Papayas, and Peaches.

Red Wine Formula **-** Health Smart Vitamins
Each capsule contains: Tea (green, leaf: 90% polyphenols, 180 mg) 200 mg • Vitis vinifera (grape seed: 95% proanthocyanidins, 95 mg or >260 Porter Value Units) 100 mg • Resveratrol (from Polygonum cuspidatum) 4 mg.

Red Yeast Rice **-** Nature's Sunshine
Two capsules contain: Red Yeast Rice (monoascus purpureus) 1200 mg. Other Ingredients: Cellulose, Magnesium Stearate, Gelatin, Water.

RedGidity **-** Life Enhancement Products, Inc.
Each capsule contains: Korean Red Ginseng (panax ginseng extract) 900 mg.

RedLine **-** VPX Sports
Each 5 mL serving contains: Proprietary Blend 637 mg: Caffeine Citrate, Caffeine Anhydrous, Evoburn brand Evodiamine, N-Acetyl-Tyrosine, Guggulsterones E & Z, Yerba Mate, Green Tea, 5-Hydroxy-L-Tryptophan, cAMP (adenosine cyclic 3',5'-monophosphate), Vinpocetine, Yohimbine HCl. Other Ingredients: Highly Purified Water, Lecithin, Propylene Glycol, Polyethylene Glycol, Glycerine, Lipoject Technologies Proprietary Polylipid, Delivery Matrix, Vegetable Gum, Citric Acid, Carmine Red, Liquid Red, Sucralose, Potassium Sorbate, Natural and Artificial Flavor, Natural Colors, EDTA.

RedLine Caps **-** VPX Sports
Three caps contain: Proprietary Blend 910 mg: Caffeine Citrate, Caffeine Anhydrous, Evoburn brand pure Evodiamine, Octapomine, Guggulsterones E & Z, Yerba Mate, Green Tea, Synephrine, cAMP (adenosine cyclic 3',5'-monophosphate), Vinpocetine, Yohimbine HCl. Other Ingredients: Sucralose, Natural Flavor, Colors. See Editor's Note No. 40.

RedLine RED **-** VPX Sports
Caffeine Citrate • Caffeine Anhydrous • Evoburn brand Pure Evodiamine • N-Acetyl-Tyrosine • Yerbe Mate • Green Tea • 5-Hydroxy-L-Tryptophan • CAMP (adenosine cyclic 3'5'-monophosphate) • Vinpocetine • Yohimbine HCl. Other Ingredients: Highly Purified Water, Citric Acid, Carmine Red, Liquid Red, Sucralose, Potassium Sorbate, Natural and Artificial Flavor, Natural Colors.

Reduced Glutathione **-** Pure Encapsulations
Each vegetable capsule contains: L-Glutathione (free-form, reduced) 100 mg.

Reduced Glutathione 500 **-** Jarrow Formulas
Each capsule contains: Reduced Glutathione 500 mg. Other Ingredients: Cellulose, Magnesium Stearate, Silicon Dioxide, Gelatin.

Reduced L-Glutathione 150 mg **-** Klaire Laboratories
Reduced L-Glutathione 150 mg.

Reduced L-Glutathione 250 mg **-** Pro Health
Each capsule contains: Vitamin C (as ascorbic acid) 175 mg • L-Glutathione (reduced L-glutamyl-L-cysteinylglycine) 250 mg. Other Ingredients: Gelatin, Magnesium Stearate, Water.

Reduced L-Glutathione 250 MG **-** PhysioLogics
Each capsule contains: L-Glutathione (reduced) 250 mg. Other Ingredients: Cellulose (plant origin), Gelatin, Acacia Gum, Vegetable Magnesium Stearate, Silica, Vanilla Flavor.

Reduced L-Glutathione 75 mg **-** Klaire Laboratories
Reduced L-Glutathione 75 mg.

Regal Pro-Meal **-** Nature's Life
Two scoops (28.35 g) contain: Supro brand Soy Protein Isolate containing Lecithin • Whey • Fructose • Non-fat Dry Milk • natural Vanilla Flavor • Yeast • Egg Albumin • Eggshell powder • Kelp • natural Papain Enzyme concentrate & Cobalamin concentrate (B12). Regal Pro-Meal also contains 34 mg of naturally occuring Isoflavones including 21 mg Genistein & 10 mg Daidzein.

Regenasure **-** Cargill Health & Food Technologies
Ingredients: 100% vegetarian Corn-derived Glucosamine. See Editor's Note No. 43.

Regenerating Antioxidant Serum **-** Waiora
Certified Organic Floral Water of Juniper berries, Lemon Balm, Lavender • Steam Distilled Water • Chamomile • Angelica • Marshmallow • Oatstraw • Certified Organic Sunflower oil • Vegetable Glycerine • Glyceral STearate • Cetearyl Alcohol • Cetearth-20 • Shea Butter • Certified Organic Coco Butter • Certified Organic Mango Butter • Certified Organic Avocado Butter • Ester-C brand buffered Vitamin C • Panthenol (vitamin B complex factor) • Ceramide III • Alpha Lipoic Acid • Vitamin A • D-Alpha Tocopherol (natural vitamin E) • DMAE • Essential oil blend of Orange oil, Lavender oil, Rosemary oil • Xanthan Gum • Caprylic Acid • Glycine • Methylparaben • Propylparaben.

Regeneration Extreme Repair **-** BeautiControl Inc.
Purified Water • Glycerin • Cetearyl Alcohol • Sodium Cetearyl Sulfate • C12-C15 Alkyl Benzoate • Urea • Stearic Acid • Lanolin Alcohol • Lactic Acid • Citric Acid • Tartaric ACid • Allantoin • Lecithin • Simethicone • DMDM Hydantoin • Iodopropynyl Butylcarbamate • Methylparaben • Propylparaben.

Regeneration Softgels **-** Nature's Plus
Three softgels contain: Vitamin A (as beta carotene) 25,000 IU • Vitamin C (as ascorbic acid) 200 mg • Vitamin D (as ergocalciferol) 400 IU • Vitamin E (as D-alpha tocopherol acetate) 200 IU • Thiamin (vitamin B1, as thiamine HCl) 50 mg • Riboflavin (vitamin B2) 50 mg • Niacin (as niacinamide) 50 mg • Vitamin B6 (as pyridoxine HCl) 50 mg • Folate (as folic acid) 400 mcg • Vitamin B12 (as cyanocobalamin) 100 mcg • Biotin 300 mcg • Pantothenic Acid (as calcium pantothenate) 100 mg • Calcium (as amino acid chelate/complex) 100 mg • Iron (as amino acid chelate/complex) 4.5 mg • Iodine (from kelp) 150 mcg • Magnesium (as amino acid chelate/complex) 50 mg • Zinc (as amino acid chelate/complex) 15 mg • Selenium (as amino acid complex) 20 mcg • Copper (as glycinate) 1 mg • Manganese (as amino acid chelate/complex) 5 mg • Chromium (as polynicotinate) 50 mcg • Molybdenum (as amino acid complex) 20 mcg • Potassium (as glycero-phosphate) 25 mg • Milk Thistle seed (silybum marianum, standardized to 80% silymarin) 75 mg • Parsley leaf (petroselinum crispum) 75 mg • Juniper berry (juniperus communis) 50 mg • Celery seed 4X (apium graveolens) 50 mg • Cayenne fruit (capsicum frutescens) 50 mg • Echinacea root (echinacea purpurea) 50 mg • Citrus Bioflavonoids (from citrus limon exocarp) 50 mg • Choline (as bitartrate) 50 mg • Inositol 50 mg • Korean Ginseng root (panax ginseng, standardized to 5% ginsenosides) 50 mg • Glucosamine Sulfate (aminomonosaccharide) 30 mg • Chinese Green Tea leaf extract (camellia sinensis, standardized to 40% polyphenols) 25 mg • Borage seed oil (borago officinalis, standardized to 25% gamma linolenic acid) 25 mg •

Ginkgo Biloba leaf (standardized to 24%ginkgo flavone-glycosides, 6% terpene lactones) 10 mg • Bilberry fruit (vaccinium myrtillus, standardized to 25% anthocyanosides) 5 mg • Wild Grape seed extract (mahonia aquifolia, standardized to 95-100% leucoanthocyanins) 5 mg • Oleoresin Turmeric rhizome (curcuma longa, standardized to 90-95% curcumin) 5 mg • Vanadium (as vanadyl sulfate) 1 mg. Other Ingredients: Safflower Oil, Gelatin, Glycerin, Purified Water.

RegeniCare - Oasis Wellness Network
Each packet (7 g) contains: Vitamin C (ascorbic acid) 300 mg • Glucosamine Sulfate 1500 mg • MSM (methylsulfonylmethane) 1500 mg • Chondroitin Sulfate 750 mg • Protectin Proprietary Blend 300 mg: Acacia Catechu, Scutellaria Baicalensis • CMO 50 mg • MaxCell Proprietary Blend 20 mg: Zisyphus Jujube, Aloe Vera gel, Piper Nigrum, Glycyrrhiza Glabra. Other Ingredients: Citric Acid, Maltodextrin, Calcium Silicate, Natural Flavors, Stevia.
See Editor's Note No. 15.

Regular Vita-Vim Level 2 Potency Multivitamin - Jamieson
Each caplet contains: Vitamin A (from Acetate) 5000 IU • Beta Carotene 1500 IU • Vitamin D 400 IU • Vitamin C 150 mg • Vitamin E 15 IU • Vitamin B1 2.5 mg • Vitamin B2 2.5 mg • Vitamin B3 (no flush Niacinamide) 25 mg • Vitamin B5 25 mg • Vitamin B6 25 mg • Vitamin B12 25 mg • Folic Acid 400 mcg • Biotin 15 mcg • Calcium 150 mg • Iron 4 mg • Copper 1 mg • Iodine 0.1 mg • Magnesium 75 mg • Zinc 10 mg • Chromium 10 mcg • Selenium 10 mcg • Lutein 300 mcg • Lycopene 300 mcg • Citrus Bioflavonoids 2000 mcg • Soy Phosphotidyl Complex 5 mg • Digestive Enzyme Absorption Factors derived from: Peppermint, Bromelain, Papain, Amylase, Lipase, Cellulose 4000 mg.

Regyon Day - Hadas Natural Products
Each tablet contains: Passiflora Incarnata standardized extract 250 mg • Humulus Lupulus standardized extract 25 mg • Melissa standardized extract 25 mg • Vitamin B1 15 mg • Vitamin B6 15 mg.

Regyon Night - Hadas Natural Products
Each tablet contains: Passiflora Incarnata standardized extract 250 mg • Scutellaria Lateriflora standardized extract 50 mg • Humulus Lupulus standardized extract 50 mg • Melissa standardized extract 25 mg.

Regyon Syrup - Hadas Natural Products
Each 5 mL serving contains: Orange flavored fructose-glucose syrup • Passiflora standardized extract 250 mg • Humulus Lupulus standardized extract 50 mg • Melissa standardized extract 50 mg.

Rehab Forte - Progressive Labs
Two capsules contain: Vitamin C 500 mg • Niacinamide 200 mg • Vitamin B6 (pyridoxine HCl) 50 mg • Calcium (amino acid chelate) 200 mg • Elemental Calcium 40 mg • Magnesium (amino acid chelate) 100 mg • Elemental Magnesium 20 mg • Zinc (amino acid chelate) 30 mg • Elemental Zinc 7.6 mg • Manganese (amino acid chelate) 50 mg • Elemental Manganese 5 mg • Copper (amino acid chelate) 2 mg • Elemental Copper 0.01 mg • Potassium Sulfate 200 mg • Elemental Potassium 90 mg • Chondroitin Sulfate 50 mg • Lemon bioflavonoids 500 mg • Rutin 50 mg.
See Editor's Note No. 15.

Rehmannia Complex - Standard Process, Inc.
Each tablet contains: Rehmannia root extract (2.5:1, rehmannia glutinosa 350 mg) 140 mg • Bupleurum root extract (4.5:1, bupleurum falcatum 700 mg) 155.5 mg • Hemidesmus root extract (hemidesmus indicus 500 mg) 100 mg • Feverfew leaf/stem extract (3:1, tanacetum parthenium 165 mg) 55 mg • Calcium 59 mg. Other Ingredients: Cellulose, Calcium Hydrogen Phosphate, Silica, Sodium Starch Glycolate, Magnesium Stearate.

Rehydration - Vidafit
Each serving contains: Thiamine 1 mg • Vitamin A 100 IU • Vitamin C 1 mg • Calcium 20 mg • Iron 0.5 mg • Phosphorus 22 mg • Potassium 30 mg • Sodium 75 mg • Complex Carbohydrates 50 g.

Reishi 5 - New Chapter, Inc.
Two capsules contain: Vitamin C 60 mg • Ginger extract (rhizome) 5% pungent compounds 50 mg • Mushroom Mycelia Reishi (mycelia), certified organic 200 mg • Shiitake (mycelia), certified organic mushroom extract 200 mg • Reishi (mushroom) minimum 4% triterpenes, 12.5% polysaccharides 40 mg • Maitake (mushroom) minimum 25% total polysaccharides 40 mg • Shiitake (mycelia) LEM, freeze dried, minimum EP3 1.5% PPT1 6% 40 mg • Cordyceps (mycelia) (dong-chong-zia-cao) 4:1 20 mg • Coriolus (mushroom) 8:1 20 mg. Other Ingredients: Vegetable Cellulose.

Reishi Bupleurum Supreme - Gaia Herbs
Thirty drops contain: Proprietary Blend 60 mg: Reishi mushroom (ganoderma lucidum), Bupleurum root (bupleurum chinense), Astragalus root (astragalus membranaceus), St. John's Wort flower buds (hypericum perforatum), Chinese Skullcap root (scutellaria baicalensis), Lomatum root (lomatium dissectum), Red Root (ceanothus americana), Licorice root (glycyrrhiza uralensis and g. glabra), Fresh Thuja leaf (thuja occidenatlis), Prickly Ash bark (xanthoxylum clava-herculis), Spring Water, 45-55% Pure Grain Alcohol USP.

Reishi Cordyceps - Wild Rose
Each vegetable cap contains: Reishi 15:1 extract 50 mg • Cordyceps extract Cs-4 250 mg • Reishi mushroom powder 200 mg.

Reishi Defense - Traditional Medicinals
Red Reishi Mushroom (Ganoderma lucidum) Myccllium & Fruit Body • Ginger rhizome • Astragalus root • Roasted Barley grain • Licorice root • Stevia leaf.

Reishi Extract - Nature's Way
Two capsules contain: Reishi dried extract 376 mg. Other Ingredients: Gelatin, Millet.

Reishi Extract - Wild Rose
Each capsule contains: Organic Reishi mushroom extract (GP 4% triterpenes) 60 mg • Echinacea Angustifolia root 150 mg • Echinacea Purpurea root 150 mg • Ginger root 150 mg • Barberry root bark 75 mg.

Reishi Extract 500mg - Vital Nutrients
Each capsule contains: Reishi mushroom 50:1 extract (ganoderma lucidum, 4% triterpenes and 10% polysaccharides) 500 mg.

Reishi Mushroom - Pure Encapsulations
Each vegetable capsule contains: Reishi mushroom extract (ganoderma lucidum, standardized to contain 10% polysaccharides and 4% triterpenes) 500 mg.

Reishi Premium - Wild Rose
Each vegetable cap contains: Reishi 15:1 extract • Reishi mushroom powder 300 mg.

ReishiMax GLp - Pharmanex
Each capsule contains: Reishi mushroom 20:1 powdered extract with spores (ganoderma lucidum) 500 mg. Other Ingredients: Gelatin.

Reishitaki - Metagenics
Each capsule contains: Shiitake mushroom (lentinus edodes) 400 mg • Reishi mushroom (ganoderma lucidum) 400 mg.

Rejoyn Veromax - American MedTech
Two capsules contain: L-Arginine 200 mg • Zizyphi fructus 200 mg • Siberian Ginseng 200 mg • Saw Palmetto 200 mg • Ginkgo Biloba 75 mg • L-Alanine 75 mg • Glutamic Acid 75 mg • L-Lysine 75 mg. Other Ingredients: Pvp, Dicalcium Phosphate, Cellulose, Croscarmellose Sodium, Vegetable sterine, Magnesium stearate, Silicon dioxide and Pharmaceutical glaze.

Rejuvalean17 - United Healthcare Labs
Three capsules contain: Anterior Pituitary Peptides (from pork) 80 mg • Hypothalamus 20 mg • L-Glutamine 200 mg • L-Ornithine 200 mg • L-Arginine 200 mg • L-Pyroglutamate 200 mg • L-Glycine 500 mg • L-Lysine 200 mg • L-Tyrosine 200 mg • Phytosterol 40 mg • Soy Phosphatides Complex 80 mg • Panax Ginseng 80 mg.

Some Brand Name Natural Products - What they Contain

www.NaturalDatabase.com contains MANY more listings than appear here.

Editor's Notes are located on pages 2155-2163.

RejuVeinate - PhysioLogics
Two capsules contain: Vitamin C (as ascorbic acid) 120 mg • Horse Chestnut seed extract (aesculus hippocastanum, standardized to contain 10% aescin, 30 mg) 300 mg • Butcher's Broom aerial parts (ruscus aculeatus, standardized to contain 10% ruscogenin, 20 mg) 200 mg • Gotu Kola aerial parts (centella asiatica) 120 mg • Citrus Bioflavonoids (citrus spp., standardized to contain 29% hesperidin, 23.2 mg) 80 mg • Bilberry fruit (vaccinium myrtillis, standardized to contain 25% anthocyanidins, 10 mg) 40 mg. Other Ingredients: Gelatin, Rice Powder, Vegetable Magnesium Stearate, Silica.

Rejuvenate cream - BioGenesis Nutraceuticals
Each 1 g serving contains: Estriol USP 0.3%. Base: Water, MSM, Sunflower oil, Chamomile extract, Vitamin A, Vitamin D, Vitamin E, Glycerol Monostearate, Germaben, Essential oils, Lavender, Cedar.

Rejuvenate Dietary Supplement - N.V. Perricone M.D. Cosmeceuticals
Each softgel contains: Vitamin E (as natural D-alpha tocopherol 6 mg) 7.5 IU • Coenzyme Q-10 5 mg • L-Carnitine Fumarate 75 mg • Alpha-Lipoic Acid 25 mg • Tocotrienol concentrate (Nutriene brand) 5 mg. Other Ingredients: Medium Chain Triglycerides, Gelatin, Glycerin, Beeswax, Soy Lecithin, Polysorbate 80, Caramel Color, Titanium Dioxide.

Rejuvenating Cream - Nu Skin Enterprises
Water • Aloe Vera gel • Propylene Glycol • Stearic Acid • Cetearyl Alcohol • Ceteareth-20 • Dioctyl Adipate • Octyl Stearate • Octyl Palmitate • Stearamidopropyl Dimethylamine • Ceteth-2 • Glycol Stearate • Glycerin • Tocopheryl Linoleate • Octyl Methoxycinnamate • Hyaluronic Acid • Algae extract • Sorbitol • Hydrolyzed Elastin • Allantoin • Sodium PCA • Retinyl Palmitate • Cholecalciferol • Tocopheryl Acetate • Biotin • Panthenol • Royal Jelly • Citric Acid • RNA • Fragrance • Caramel • Triethanolamine • Diazolidinyl Urea • Methylparaben • Propylparaben • Disodium EDTA.

Rejuvenex - Life Extension Foundation
Purified Water • Alkoxylated Diester • Isocetyl Steroyl Stearate • Octyl Salicylate • Glycolic Acid • Cetyl Alcohol • Stearyl Alcohol • Dimethicone • Butyl Methoxydibenzoylmethane • Maleated Soybean oil (ceraphyl NGA) • Potato starch (solanum tuberosum) • Safflower oil (carthamus tinctorius) • Dimethylaminoethanol Bitartrate (DMAE) • Retinyl Palmitate (vitamin A) • Ascorbyl Palmitate (vitamin C) • Sodium Ascorbyl Phosphate (vitamin C) • Tocopheryl Acetate (vitamin E) • Tocopherol (vitamin E) • Alpha-Lipoic Acid • Sodium Hyaluronate • Sodium PCA • RNA • Beta Glucan • Kinetin • Lactic Acid • Allantoin • Panthenol (vitamin B) • Glycerin • Squalane • Zinc Oxide • Ginseng extract (panax ginseng) • Arginine • Aloe Barbadensis gel • Glcyeryl Stearate • PEG-100 Stearate • Phenoxyethanol • Urea • Lavender oil • Propylparaben • Methylparaben • Disodium EDTA • Imidazolidinyl Urea • Passion Flower essential oil blend • Ylang Ylang oil (canaga adorata).

Rejuvine - Metabolic Response Modifiers
Two teaspoons contain: DHEA 25 mg • Pregnenolone 25 mg.

Rejuvinol AM - Dermalogics
Purified Water • Cetearyl Alcohol • Glyceryl Stearate • PEG-100 Stearate, Acetyl Hexapeptide-3 (argireline) • Green Tea leaf extract • Chamomile extract • Hyaluronic Acid • Tocopheryl Acetate • Korean Ginseng root extract • Olive leaf extract •oOctyl Methoxy Cinnamate • Sunflower oil • Dimethicone • Ethylhexyl Benzoate • Stearic Acid • Fragrance • Methyl Paraben • Propyl Paraben.

Rejuvox PM - Dermalogics
Purified Water • Cetearyl Alcohol • Glyceryl Stearate • PEG-100 Stearate • Acetyl Hexapeptide-3 (argireline) • Chamomile flower extract • Glycolic Acid • Malic Acid • Hyaluronic Acid • Willowbark extract • Retinyl Palmitate • Calcium Ascorbate • Tocopheryl Acetate • Sunflower oil • Fragrance • Methyl Paraben • Propyl Paraben.

Relacore - Carter-Reed Company
Each capsule contains: Vitamin C 333 mg • Calcium (as carbonate and pantothenate) 21.5 mg • Thiamin (vitamin B1) 5 mg • Riboflavin (vitamin B2) 7 mg • Vitamin B6 17 mg • Vitamin B12 3.5 mcg • Biotin 150 mcg • Pantothenic Acid (as calcium pantothenate) 7.8 mg • Magnesium 67 mg • Relacore Proprietary Blend 266 mg: Magnolia bark SE, Passion Flower herb SE, Scutellaria root SE, Niacinamide, DHEA (< 15 mg), Panax Ginseng root, Pinellia tuber, Poria fungus, Jujuba fruit, Perilla leaf, Phosphatidylserine.

Relacore - Carter-Reed Company
Two capsules contain: Vitamin C 333 mg • Thiamin (vitamin B1) 5 mg • Riboflavin (vitamin B2) 5 mg • Vitamin B6 17 mg • Vitamin B12 3.5 mcg • Biotin 50 mcg • Pantothenic Acid (as calcium pantothenate) 8 mg • Calcium (as carbonate and pantothenate) 33 mg • Magnesium (as oxide) 67 mg • Relacortin Proprietary Blend 265 mg: Passion Flower herb standardized extract, Magnolia bark standardized extract, Scutellaria root standardized extract, Niacinamide, DHEA 15 mg, Panax Ginseng root, Poria fungus, Jujuba fruit, Perilla Frutescens leaf, Phosphatidylserine. Other Ingredients: Rice Flour, Magnesium Stearate, Silicon Dioxide, Gelatin.

Relastyl - Nutraceutics Corp.
Water • Butylene Glycol • Hydrogenated Polyisobutene • Glycerin • Tricaprylin • C12-15 Alkyl Benzoate • Cetyl Alcohol • Glyceryl Stearate • Butyrospermum Parkii fruit (shea butter) • PEG-40 Stearate • Sorbitan Stearate • Dimethicone • Carbomer • Polysorbate 20 • Palmitoyl Pentapeptide-3 • Squalane • Biosaccharide Gum-1 • Oenothera Biennis oil (evening primrose) • Hamamelis Virginiana extract (witch hazel) • Cucumis Sativus fruit extract (cucumber) • Methylparaben • Propylparaben • Phenoxyethanol • Diazolidinyl Urea • Fragrance.

RELAX - Ortho Molecular Products
Each capsule contains: Magnesium (as citrate) 9 mg • German Chamomile flowers 120 mg • Oat Straw stem 10:1 extract 20 mg • Hops strobile powder 20 mg • Valerian root powder 15 mg • Horsetail grass powder 20 mg • Skullcap plant powder 30 mg.

Relax & Sleep - Futurebiotics LLC
Two tablets contain: Calcium (as calcium carbonate, phosphate, amino acid chelate) 150 mg • Magnesium (as magnesium oxide, amino acid chelate) 150 mg • Relax & Sleep Blend 860 mg: Valerian root powder, Chamomile flower powder, Hawthorn berry powder, Fennel seed powder, Passion flower powder, Skullcap leaf powder, Hops flower powder, Lemon Balm herb powder, Oat Straw leaf/stem powder, Red Clover herb powder, Catnip leaf powder, Spearmint leaf powder, Vanilla bean powder. Other Ingredients: Dicalcium phosphate, Stearic acid, Magnesium stearate, Silica.

Relax & Sleep Formula 2 - Futurebiotics LLC
Two tablets contain: Valerian root - A balanced blend of extract & powder equivalent to dried root 500 mg • Chamomile - A balanced blend of extract & powder equivalent to dried blossoms 250 mg • Magnesium (oxide, amino acid chelate) 150 mg • Calcium (carbonate, phosphate, amino acid chelate) 150 mg. Specially formulated in a base of natural, time-tested herbs (in the form of extracts & powders) including: Hawthorn berry, Fennel, Passion flower, Scullcap, Hops, Lemon Balm, Avena Sativa, Red Clover, Catnip, Spearmint leaves & Vanilla.

Relax Now - Health Factor
Each capsule contains: Kava Kava 100 mg • Valerian 100 mg • Scutellaria 100 mg • Passion flower (2:1 extract) 75 mg • Hops 25 mg • Chamomilla 6X • Lady Slipper 3X.

Relax Now - Herbalife International of America, Inc.
Each tablet contains: Calcium (as calcium carbonate) 85 mg • Dried Jujube seed extract 150 mg • Dried Ashwagandha root extract 100 mg • Dried Passionflower aerial parts extract 75 mg • Bio-Absorption Complex-5 21 mg: Soy Lecithin, Ascorbyl Palmitate, Plant Cellulose Enzyme, Cinnamon bark powder, Dried Black Pepper fruit extract. Other Ingredients: Microcrystalline Cellulose, Sodium Starch Glycolate, Stearic Acid, Hypromellose, Maltodexrin, Acacia, Magnesium Stearate, Silicon Dioxide, Cellulose.

Relax-O-Comp - PhytoPharmica
Two tablets contain: Calcium (as calcium citrate) 90 mg • Chamomile flower 4:1 extract (matricaria recutita) 150 mg • Evening Primrose seed oil (oenothera biennis) 20 mg • Hops flower 5:1 extract (humulus lupulus) 60 mg • Magnesium (as magnesium oxide and magnesium gluconate) 105 mg • Niacin (as niacinamide and niacin) 130 mg • Passionflower leaf (passiflora incarnata) 60 mg • Valerian root (valeriana officinalis) 150 mg • Vitamin B6 (as pyridoxine HCl) 20 mg • Vitamin D (as cholecalciferol) 100 IU • Zinc (as zinc chelate) 5 mg.

Relax-U - The Herbalist
Valerian root • Skullcap herb • Passionflower herb.

Release Afternoon - NDS Nutrition
Each capsule contains: Proprietary Blend 850 mg: Caffeine, L-Tyrosine, Magnesium Salicylate, Theobromine, Guarana, Synephrine, Guggulsterones, Yohimbine 3 mg, Hypericum (using St. John's wort at 0.3%), Vitamin B12.
See Editor's Note No. 40.

Release Evening - NDS Nutrition
Each capsule contains: Proprietary Blend 750 mg: Citrin K, Psyllium husk, Valerian root, Ho Shou Wu, Turkey Rhubarb, Cascara Sagrada, Senna extract, Piper Nigrum.

Release Morning - NDS Nutrition
Each capsule contains: Proprietary Blend 895 mg: Caffeine, Magnesium Salicylate, Theobromine, Guarana, Synephrine, Guggulsterones, Yohimbine 4.5 mg, Hypericum (using St. John's wort at 0.3%), Vitamin B12.
See Editor's Note No. 40.

Releve - MHP
Two tablets contain: Baikal Skullcap root extract 200 mg • N-Acetylcysteine 500 mg • Glucosamine Sulfate 2KCl 500 mg • IsoOxygene brand Humulus Lupulus L. extract 500 mg • Alpha Lipoic Acid 100 mg. Other Ingredients: Guar Gum, Dicalcium Phosphate, Stearic Acid, Calcium Carbonate, Microcrystalline Celluose, Citrus Pectin, Magnesium Stearate, Silica, Film Coat (hydroxypropyl methylcellulose, hydroxyethyl cellulose, polyethylene glycol, propylene glycol, FD&C blue #2 lake, titanium dioxide, sodium citrate).

Relief Formula - Pharmanex
Each capsule contains: MSHA TCM extract 450 mg: Magnolia Biondii flower extract (4:1), Saposhnikovia Divaricata root extract (3:1), Hedysarum Polybotrys root extract (2:1), Atractylodes Macrocephaia root extract (1.5:1).

Relief Plus - Health Factor
Each capsule contains: Goldenseal extract (4:1)(Hydrastis canadensis) 125 mg • Chamomile (Matricaria chamomilla) 100 mg • Valerian (Valeriana officinalis) 85 mg • Feverfew (Tanacetum parthenium) 590 mg • Cayenne Pepper 50 mg.

Relief Rx - Athletic Technologies Inc.
Two tablets contain: Glucosamine Sulfate 500 mg • Chondroitin Sulfate 400 mg • Shark Cartilage 750 mg • Green Lipped Mussel 250 mg • MSM 250 mg • L-Histidine 10 mg • Boron 1 mg.
See Editor's Note No. 15.

Reliv Arthaffect - Reliv International
Each scoop (8.5 g) contains: Arthred (hydrolyzed collagen) • Glucosamine Sulfate • Ginkgo Biloba • Borage Oil Powder • Turmeric • Boswellia Serrata • Ashwagandha • Cat's Claw • Sarsaparilla Root • Licorice Root • Kelp • Burdock Root • Alfalfa • Barley Grass • Echinacea Root • Yucca Extract • Devil's Claw Extract • Bilberry Extract • Celery Seed • Capsicum • Aloe Vera • Bioperine brand Black Pepper extract (piper nigrum) • Soy Lecithin.

Reliv Celleboost - Reliv International
Two capsules contain: (-) Hydroxycitric Acid 375 mg • Oatrim brand hydrolyzed Oat flour 360 mg • Chromium 50 mcg.

Reliv Cellebrate - Reliv International
Each scoop contains: (-) Hydroxycitric Acid 375 mg • L-Carnitine 75 mg • Chromium 50 mcg • Choline 50 mg • Inositol 50 mg • Gamma-Linolenic Acid (as borage oil powder) 50 mg • Ginkgo Biloba leaves 33 mg • Coenzyme Q10 15 mg. Other Ingredients: Maltodextrin, Soy Lecithin, Quaker Oatrim (hydrolyzed oat flour).

Reliv Classic - Reliv International
Each scoop (16 g) contains: Soy Protein Isolate • Soy Flour • Brewer's Yeast • Lecithin • Psyllium Fiber • Dicalcium Phosphate • Ascorbic Acid • Methionine • Potassium Chloride • Magnesium Phosphate • Natural Flavor • Licorice Root • Garlic Rhubarb Root • Rose Hips • Cayenne • Kelp • OptiZinc Brand Zinc Momomethionine • Ferrous Fumarate • Calcium Pantothenate • Niacinamide • Vitamin E Acetate • Vitamin A Palmitate • Vitamin D • Copper • Gluconate • Papain • Bromelain • Thiamin HCL • Riboflavin • Beta Carotene • Pyridoxine HCL • Biotin • Folic Acid • Potassium Iodine • Vitamin B12 • Sodium Selenite • ChromeMate Brand of Niacin Bound Chromium Polynicotinate.

Reliv FibRestore - Reliv International
Each scoop (14 g) contains: Vitamin A (100% as mixed carotenoids) 3500 IU • Vitamin C 300 mg • Vitamin E 200 IU • Iron 0.72 mg • Sodium 20 mg • FibRestore Proprietary Blend 154 mg: Oriental Ginseng (panax ginseng), Garlic (allium sativum), Capsicum fruit (capsicum fructescens), Licorice root (glycyrrhiza glabra L.), Kelp (ascophyllum nodosum), Rhubarb root (rheum officinal ballon), Hibiscus flower (hibiscus sabdariffa), Irish Moss (chondrus crispus), Siberian Ginseng (eleutherococus senticosus), Aloe Vera (aloe barbadensis), Chicory root (cichorium intybus), Dandelion root (taraxacum officinale), Chamomile flower (matricaria recutita), Alfalfa herb (medicago sativa), Pearl Barley (hordeum distichon), Cayenne (capsicum annuum), Ginger root (zingiber officinale), Celery seed (apium graveolens L.), Sarsaparilla root (smilax ornata lemaire), Passion flower (passiflora incarnata), Foenugreek seed (trigonelloa foenum graecum L.), Papain (carrica papaya), Bromelain (from pineapple stem, ananas sativas LINNE). Other Ingredients: Oat Fiber, Corn Bran, Apple Fiber, Soy Fiber, Pea Fiber, Citrus Fiber, Carrageenan Gum, Guar Gum, Xanthan Gum, Gum Arabic, Soy Extract, Fructooligosaccharides (FOS), Alpha Tocopheryl Acetate, Ascorbic Acid, Natural Mixed Carotenoids, Natural and Artifical Flavor, Soy Lecithin, Citric Acid.

Reliv Innergize! - Reliv International
Each scoop (19 g) contains: Fructose • Maltodextrin • Citric Acid • Potassium Citrate • Tricalcium Phosphate • Sodium Chloride • Magnesium Oxide • Ascorbic Acid • Beta Carotene • OptiZinc Brand Zinc • ChromeMate brand Chromium Polynicotinate.

Reliv Now - Reliv International
Each scoop (15 g) contains: Whey • Soy Protein Isolate • Fructose • Dicalcium Phosphate • Magnesium Phosphate • Calcium Caseinate • Calcium Carbonate • Natural Flavor • Ascorbic Acid • Potassium Chloride • Lecithin • PABA (para-aminobenzoic acid) • Kelp • OptiZinc Brand of Zinc Monomethionine • Ferrous Fumarate • Calcium Pantothenate • Beta Carotene • Vitamin A Palmitate • Vitamin D (as Vitamin D3) • Thiamin HCl • Riboflavin • Niacinamide • Vitamin E Acetate • Pyridoxine HCl • Folic Acid • Vitamin B12 • Potassium Iodide • Copper Gluconate • Biotin • Sodium Selenite • ChromeMate Brand of Niacin Bound Chromium Polynicotinate • Sodium Molybdate • Vitamin K • Manganese Sulfate • Rutin •Garlic • Cayenne • Butternut Bark • Rhubarb Root •Blue Vervain • Licorice Root • Irish Moss.

Reliv ProVantage - Reliv International
Each scoop (26 g) contains: Soy Protein Isolate • Fructose • Medium Chain Triglycerides • Creatine Monohydrate • Tonalin brand Conjugated Linoleic Acid (CLA) • Lecithin • L-Arginine • L-Glutamine • L-Leucine • L-Lysine • L-Carnitine • L-Alanine • Glycine • Ornithine Alpha Ketoglutarate • Coenzyme Q10 • Activin (Grape Seed extract) • Phosphatidylserine & Phosphatidylcholine • Bioperine brand Black Pepper extract (piper nigrum) • Natural & Artificial Flavors • Alpha-Lipoic Acid.

Reliv ReversAge - Reliv International
Each 16 g scoop contains: Proprietary Blend: Aminotrope-7, Anterior Pituitary Peptides (porcine), Alpha Glycerylphosphorycholine, Chaperone Molecule Complex, 7-KETO (3-Acetyl-7-Oxo Dehydroepiandrosterine), S-Adenosyl-L-Methionine, Omega 3 Fatty Acids, Tri Methyl Glycine, Lactobacillus Acidophilus, Bifidobacterium Bifidum, Fructooligosaccharides, Acetyl L-Carnitine 1855 mg • Proprietary Blend 297.5 mg: N-Acetyl Cysteine, Alpha Lipoic Acid, Gluthione, Resveratrol, CoEnzyme Q10 • Proprietary Blend 250 mg: Ginkgo Biloba leaf, Quercetin Dihydrate, Spirulina plant powder, Maca tuber powder, Wild Yam root powder, Chlorella powder, Diosmin, Nettle leaf powder. Other Ingredients: Maltodextrin, Fructose, Natural Flavors, Artificial Flavors, Citric Acid, Lecitihin, Xanthan Gum, Potassium Citrate, DiPotassium Phosphate, L-Glutamine, L-Arginine Pyrogluamate, L-Lysine Monochloride, Glycine, Gamma Aminobutyric Acid.

Reliv SoySentials - Reliv International
Each scoop (22 g) contains: Soy Protein Isolate • Fructose • Inulin • Dehydrated Cranberries • Calcium Carbonate • Dicalcium Phosphate • Lactobacillus Acidophilus • Lecithin • Natural & Artifical Flavors • Activin brand Grape seed extract • Protykin brand Resveratrol • Ipriflavone • Black Cohosh root • Dong Quai root • Wild Yam • Panax Ginseng • Green Tea extract • Chasteberry • Horse Chestnut • Nettle root • Hops • Licorice root • Coenzyme Q10 • Folic Acid • Ascorbic Acid • Pyridoxine HCL • Alpha Tocopheryl Acetate • Beet powder • Stevia extract • Acesulfame Potassium • Alpha Lipoic Acid.

Reliv Ultrim+Plus - Reliv International
Each scoop (28 g) contains: Soy Protein Isolate • Whey • Fructose • Milk Protein • Nonfat Dry Milk • Xanthan Gum • Dicalcium Phosphate • Magnesium Phosphate • Calcium Carbonate • Natural & Artificial Flavor • Ascorbic Acid • Potassium Chloride • Lecithin • Aspartame • PABA (para-aminobenzoic acid) • Kelp • OptiZinc Brand of Zinc Monomethionine • Ferrous Fumarate • Calcium Pantothenate • Vitamin A Palmitate • Vitamin D (D3) • Thiamin HCl • Riboflavin • Niacinamide • Vitamin E Acetate • Pyridoxine HCl • Folic Acid • Vitamin B12 • Potassium Iodide • Copper Gluconate • Biotin • Sodium Selenite • ChromeMate Brand of Niacin Bound Chromium Polynicotinate • Sodium Molybdate • Vitamin K • Manganese Sulfate • Rutin • Garlic • Cayenne • Butternut Bark • Rhubarb Root • Blue Vervain • Licorice Root • Irish Moss.

Relora - Pure Encapsulations
Each vegetable capsule contains: Relora brand Proprietary Blend 250 mg: Magnolia Officinalis bark extract, Phellodendron Amurense bark extract • Vitamin C (as ascorbyl palmitate) 5 mg. Other Ingredients: Modified Food and Corn Starch, Silicon Dioxide.

Relora - Solanova
Each capsule contains: Relora Magnolia Officinalis and Phellodendron Amurense extract 250 mg. Other Ingredients: Snow White Filler, Magnesium Stearate, Silicon Dioxide, Gelatin, Glycerin, Purified Water.

Relora - Swanson Health Products
Each capsule contains: Proprietary Blend 250 mg: Magnolia Officinalis, Phellodendron Amurense. Other Ingredients: Gelatin, Microcrystalline Cellulose (plant fiber), Magnesium Stearate.

Relora 300mg - NOW Foods
Each Vcap contains: Relora Proprietary Blend 300 mg: Magnolia Officinalis, Phellodendron Amurense. Other Ingredients: Rice Flour, Cellulose (capsule), Modified Food and Corn Starch, Silica, Magnesium Stearate (vegetable source).

Remedief - Natrol, Inc.
Each capsule contains: Boswellia Serrata extract (65% total organic acids) 75 mg • White Willow bark (25% salicylic acid) 160 mg • Phellodendron bark extract (Nexrutine) 75 mg • Kava Kava root extract (30% kavalactones) 100 mg. Other Ingredients: Silica, Magnesium Stearate, Gelatin.

Remember When - Bee-Alive Inc.
Two half droppers (2mL) contain: Ginkgo Biloba leaf extract (standardized to 24% flavone glycosides 14.4 mg, 6% terpene lactones 3.6 mg) 60 mg • Rhodiola Rosea root extract 100 mg • Gotu Kola fresh leaf extract 0.17 ml • Royal Jelly (non-freeze dried) 25 mg. Other Ingredients: Vegetable Glycerin, Deionized Water, Clover Honey, Natural Spearmint Flavor, Xanthan Gum.

Remember! Mental Sharpness Formula - Enzymatic Therapy
Each two capsules contain: Vitamin B6 (as pyridoxine HCl) 15 mg • Folic Acid 800 mcg • Vitamin B12 (as cyanocobalamin) 500 mcg • Alpha Lipoic Acid 600 mg • Bacopa (bacopa monnieri, aerial part extract standardized to 20% bacosides) 300 mg • Ginkgo (ginkgo biloba, leaf extract standardized to 24% ginkgoflavonglycosides, 6% terpene lactones, and 2% bilobalide) 120 mg.

Remember-FX - CV Technologies Inc.
North American Ginseng (panax quinquefolium) 100 mg.

Remi Capsules - MHP
Two capsules contain: Chromium (as picolinate) 100 mcg • Citrus Aurantium extract (6% synephrine) 250 mg • Caffeine (from green tea extract) 100 mg • Theobroma Cacau extract 280 mg. Water Balance Blend: Couchgrass rhizome, Buchu leaf, Uva Ursi leaf, Juniper berry, Hydrangea root, Cornsilk stylus.
See Editor's Note No. 40.

Remi Gel - MHP
Purified Water • SD Alcohol 40 • Lipocel 805: 5% Palmaria Palmata extract, 95% Dipropylene Glycol, 1% Laminaria Digitata, 99% Hydroethylcellulose, 0.5% Mannitol • Polysorbate 20 • Lemon peel extract (citrus medica limonum) • Orange extract (citrus aurantium dulcis) • Grapefruit extract (citrus grandis) • Palmarose extract (cymbopogon martini) • Diazolidinyl Urea • Methylparaben • Propylparaben • Tetrasodium EDTA • Citric Acid • FD&C Blue No. 1 • FD&C Red No. 40 • FD&C Yellow No. 5.

Remifemin - PhytoPharmica
Each tablet contains: Black Cohosh (Cimicifuga racemosa) root and rhizome extract (standardized to contain triterpene glycosides [calculated as 27-deoxyactein]) 20 mg.
See Editor's Note No. 21.

Remifemin Menopause - GlaxoSmithKline (GSK)
Each tablet contains: Black Cohosh (Cimicifuga racemosa) & rhizome extract (standardized to contain 1 mg of triterpene glycosides calculated as 27-Deoxyacetin) 20 mg. Other Ingredients: Lactose, Cellulose, Potato Starch, Magnesium Stearate, Peppermint Flavor.

Remifemin Plus - Enzymatic Therapy/PhytoPharmica
Each tablet contains: Standardized Cimicifuga racemosa (Black Cohosh) root & rhizome extract (standardized for triterpene glycosides content, calculated as 27-Deoxyactein) 20 mg • St. John's Wort extract standardized to contain hypericin 250 mcg.
See Editor's Note No. 21.

Remotiv - Zeller
Each tablet contains: Hypericum extract Ze 117, standardized to a daily amount of 1 mg hypericin (St. John's Wort) 250 mg.

Renafood - Standard Process, Inc.
Each tablet contains: Proprietary Blend 395 mg: Dried Kidney bean juice, Bovine Kidney PMG extract, Bovine Kidney, Lactose, Defatted Wheat germ, Oat flour, Tillandsia Usneoides, Beet root, Carrot root • Vitamin A 770 IU • Vitamin C 1.7 mg • Sodium 15 mg. Other Ingredients: Honey, Arabic Gum, Gelatin.
See Editor's Note No. 14.

Renagen DTX - Metagenics
Each capsule contains: Vitamin B6 (pyridoxine hydrochloride) 10 mg • Vitamin B12 (cyanocobalamin) 125 mcg • Folate (folic acid, L-5-methyl tetrahydrofhoate, 5-formyl tetrahydrofoate) 400 mcg • N-Acetylcysteine 200 mcg • Cordyceps mycelium extract (paecilomyces hepiali) 200 mg • Chinese Salvia root (salvia miltiorrhiza) 200 mg.

Renalka Syrup **-** The Himalaya Drug Company
Each 1 tsp (5 mL) serving contains: Gokshura (tribulus terrestris) 50 mg • Varuna (crataeva magna syn. c.nurvala) 50 mg • Sariva (hemidesmus indicus) 50 mg • Musta (cyperus rotundus) 50 mg • Ushira (vetiveria zizanoides) 50 mg • Shatavari (asparagus racemosus) 50 mg • Trikatu 16.5 mg: Piper Nigrum, Piper Longum, Zingiber Officinale • Ela (elattaria cardamomum) 16.5 mg • Kshara Parpati (ammonium chloride, potash alum, potassium nitrate) 75 mg.

RenaPlex **-** Nephro-Tech, Inc.
Each tablet contains: Ascorbic Acid 60 mg • Thiamine 1.5 mg • Riboflavin 1.7 mg • Pyridoxine 10 mg • Cyanocobalamin 6 mcg • Pantothenic Acid 10 mg • Biotin 300 mcg • Niacinamide 20 mg • Zinc 12.5 mg • Folic Acid 0.8 mg.

Renatrate **-** Progressive Labs
Each capsule contains: Vitamin A 5000 IU • Vitamin C 90 mg • Bovine kidney concentrate 300 mg. The glandular concentrate in this product is prepared by a special process which does not exceed physiological temperature (37º C). Guaranteed free of chemical pesticides and synthetic hormones.
See Editor's Note No. 14.

Renatrophin PMG **-** Standard Process, Inc.
Each tablet contains: Proprietary Blend: 245 mg: Bovine Kidney PMG extract, Magnesium Citrate. Other Ingredients: Calcium Lactate, Cellulose, Calcium Stearate.
See Editor's Note No. 14.

Renewal HGH Advanced **-** Always Young
Each spray contains: HGH 9X/30X (somatropin) • Albumin 3C • Colostrum 30C • MSM (methyl-sulfonyl-methane) 9X • Ornithine 9X • Protease 9X • RNA (ribonucleic acid) 9X • Silica 9X • Zinc Sulphate 3C. Inactive Ingredients: Purified Water, 10% USP Alcohol, 8% USP Vegetable Glycerin.
See Editor's Note No. 1.

Renewal HGH Original **-** Always Young
Active Ingredient: HGH (somatropin) 3X/30X/100X. Base: Purified Water, 10% USP Alcohol, 8% USP Vegetable Glycerin.

Renewal HGH Workout **-** Always Young
Each spray contains: HGH (somatropin) 9X/12C/30X • IGF-1 (insulin-like growth factor-1) 6X/12X/30X • Growth Factors Elk Velvet Antler 9X/9C • Testosterone 30C/100X/1M • Androstenedione 9C/100X • Creatine Monohydrate 9C/100X • Trans-Ferulic Acid 30C/100X • Amino Acid Complex 10X/30X: L-Arginine Pyroglutimate 30X/30C, L-Carnitine 12X/30X, L-Glutamine 12X/30X, L-Isoleucine 9X, L-Leucine 9X, L-Valine 9X, OKG (ornithine alpha-ketoglutarate) 3C • DHEA (dehydroepiandrosterone) 30X/30C • Hyaluronic Acid 9X/30X/9C • NADH (nicotinamide adenine dinucleotide) 30X/100X/15C • Pituitarium 9X/30X/3C • Pregnenolone 9C/12X • Co-Enzyme A 12C/30X • Protease 9X/100X • Ribose 12C/30C • Trypsin 9X/30C • B Complex 30C/100X • Vitamin E 3C/30X • Boron 30X/30C • Chromium 30X/30C • Germanium 30X • Vanadium 9X/30X/30C • Zinc Sulphate 30X • Trace Minerals 30C/100X. Inactive Ingredients: Purified Water, 10% USP Alcohol, 8% USP Vegetable Glycerin.
See Editor's Note No. 1.

Renewal IGF-1 Growth Factor **-** Always Young
Each spray contains: IGF-1 (insulin-like growth factor-1) 12C. Inactive Ingredients: Purified Water, 10% USP Alcohol 8%, USP Vegetable Glycerin.
See Editor's Note No. 1.

Renew-U **-** The Herbalist
Milk Thistle seed • Echinacea root • Oregon Grape root • Dandelion herb • Burdock root • Yellow Dock root • Cleavers herb • Wild Indigo root • Ginger root • Fennel seed.

RenuDerm **-** Mellen Nutraceutical Corp.
Each four capsules contain: Vitamin C (as Ester-C) 400 mg • Selenium (sodium selenite) 100 mcg • BioCell Collagen II (chicken-derived) 2000 mg • Chondroitin Sulfate 400 mg • Hyaluronic Acid 200 mg • Alpha Lipoic Acid 100 mg • Tocotrienol (palm-derived) 30 mg • Kelp 75 mg • Bladderwrack 50 mg.
See Editor's Note No. 15.

Reosto **-** The Himalaya Drug Company
Each tablet contains: Arjuna (terminalia arjuna) 45 mg • Guggulu (commiphora wightii) 235 mg • Ashvagandha (withania somnifera) 4 5mg • Godanti Bhasma (calcium) 120 mg • Bala (sida cordifolia) 45 mg • Rasna (vanda roxburghii) 50 mg • Kukkutandatvak Bhasma (hen's egg shell calx) 35 mg.
See Editor's Note No. 39.

Repagene Emulsion **-** Atrium Biotechnologies
Each teaspoon contains: Squalene 1.5 g (emulsified form).

Repair **-** Enzymedica
Each capsule contains: Protease Thera-Blend 65,000 HUT • Papain 750,000 PU • Bromelain 600 GDU • Amylase Thera-Blend 4000 DU • Lipase Thera-Blend 300 FCCFIP • Catalase 50 Baker.

Repel Lemon Eucalyptus **-** WPC Brands, Inc.
Active Ingredients: Oil of Lemon Eucalyptus 40% (approximately 65% p-menthane-3,8-diol). Other Ingredients: 60%.

Repel Plant Based Lemon Eucalyptus Insect Repellent **-** WPC Brands, Inc.
Active Ingredients: Oil of Lemon Eucalyptus 40% (approximately 65% p-menthane-3,8-diol).

Replenishing Body Lotion **-** FreeLife International
Aqueous Extract Blend: Oat, Hibiscus flower extract, Aloe Barbadensis gel, Algae, Purified Water • Bioenhanced Grapefruit seed extract (BGSE) 100X • Pure Grain Alcohol • Lavender oil • Caprylic/Capric Tri Glycerides • Vegetable Glycerin • Jojoba oil • Olive Squalane • Cetyl Alcohol • Corn Starch • Liposomal Delivery System: Hydrogenated Lecithin, Lauryl Alcohol, Palmatic Acid • Pure Clover Honey • Neem oil • Methylsulfonylmethane (MSM) • Phytonadione (vitamin K) • Vitamin E Acetate • Retinol Palmitate (vitamin A) • Glyceryl Monostearate • Potassium Lauryl Lactylate • Harmonic Essence #5 • Gum Arabic • Guar Gum • Xanthan Gum • Potassium Sorbate • Orange essential oil • Lemon essential oil • Chamomile essential oil.

Repleniss (Répleniss) **-** InterPlexus
Each sachet contains: Proprietary Blend 55 billion organisms: Lactobacillus Acidophilus, Bifidobacterium Bifidus, L. Salivarius. Other Ingredients: Maltodextrin, Fructooligosaccharides (FOS).

Rescue Remedy **-** Nelson Bach
Active Ingredients: Rock Rose (helianthemum nummularium) 5X HPUS • Clematis (clematis vitalba) 5X HPUS • Impatiens (impatiens landulifera) 5X HPUS • Cherry Plum (prunus cerasifera) 5X HPUS • Star of Bethlehem (ornithogalum umbellatum) 5X HPUS.
See Editor's Note No. 50.

Resist **-** Pacific BioLogic
Astragalus root (Grade 1) • Ganoderma Fungus • Codonopsis root • Jujube fruit • Atractylodes (white) rhizome • Peony root (white) • Citrus peel (tangerine) • Cuscuta seeds • Dioscorea root • Schizandra fruit • Licorice root • Milletta root • Platycodon root • Ligustrum fruit • Glehnia root • Rehmannia root (prep.) • Ginger rhizome (fresh).

Resist 2 **-** Pacific BioLogic
Bitter Melon • St. John's Wort • Red Marine Algae • Echinacea Angustifolia • Tumeric rhizome • Licorice root (honey-baked) • Ligustrum root (Chinese) • Citrus peel (tangerine) • Viola (whole plant) • Prunella (selfheal spike) • Trichosanthis root • Knotweed rhizome (bushy) • Aucklandia root.

RespaClear **-** TriLight Herbs
Echinacea herb • Ginger • Whole Elderberries • Mullein.

Respa-Herb **-** Dial Herbs
Ma Huang • Mullein • Goldenseal • Colts Foot • Comfrey • Marshmallow • Lobelia • Cayenne.
See Editor's Note No. 30.

Some Brand Name Natural Products - What they Contain

www.NaturalDatabase.com contains MANY more listings than appear here.
Editor's Notes are located on pages 2155-2163.

Resphora - PhysioLogics
Each capsule contains: Tylophora (GPH: 0.1% tylophorine alkaloids) 30 mg • Piper Longum (GPH: 2% piperine) • Picrorhiza Kurroa (GPH: 4% kutkin) 50 mg.

Resphora + - PhysioLogics
Each capsule contains: Vitamin C (as ascorbic acid) 150 mg • Long Pepper fruit (piper longum, standardized to contain 1.5% piperine, 1.5 mg) 100 mg • Picrorhiza root (picrorhiza kurroa, standardized to contain 4% kutkin, 2 mg) 50 mg • Quercetin fruit (from dimorphandra mollis) 50 mg • Ginkgo Biloba leaf extract (standardized to contain 24% ginkgo flavone glycosides, 9.5 mg, 6% terpenes, 2.4 mg) • Tylophora leaf (tylophora asthmatica, standardized to contain 0.1% tylophorine alkaloids, 0.3 mg) 30 mg • Serratiopeptidase 7.5 mg. Other Ingredients: Gelatin, Vegetable Magnesium Stearate, Silica.

Respi-Oil - The Herbalist
Essential oils of Eucalyptus, Rosemary, Sage, Tea Tree & Nutmeg in a Sweet Almond oil base.

Respir-all - NOW Foods
Three tablets contain: Vitamin B5 (pantothenic acid) 100 mg • Vitamin B6 (pyridoxine HCL) 20 mg • Vitamin C (as magnesium ascorbate) 500 mg • Magnesium (as magnesium ascorbate) 40 mg • Zinc (as L-OptiZinc brand monomethionine) 10 mg • Quercetin 800 mg • Nettle root extract (urtica dioica, standardized 30 ppm scopoletin) 500 mg • Bromelain (2000 GDU) 500 mg • Licorice root 4:1 extract (glycyrrhiza glabra) 200 mg.

Respiratory Relief - Grandma's Herbs
Each capsule contains: Proprietary Blend 448 mg: Mullein leaf, Bayberry bark, Horehound leaf, Bladderpod herb, Heal All herb (prunella vulgaris), Elecampane root, Yerba Santa herb, Plantain herb, Nettle leaf, Coltsfoot powder, Cayenne pepper, Lungwort herb. Other Ingredients: Gelatin.

Respiratory Support Formula - PhysioLogics
Two capsules contain: Vitamin C (Ascorbic Acid) 130 mg • Ephedra root, stem (6% total Ephedrine Alkaloids, 12 mg) 200 mg • Citrus Bioflavonoids (lemon) 66 mg • Pleurisy root 45 mg • Mullein leaf 38 mg • Slippery Elm bark 38 mg • Licorice root 35 mg • Red Clover tops 35 mg • Ginkgo leaf (24% Ginkgo Flavonglycosides, 7.2 mg; 6% Terpene Lactones, 1.8 mg) 30 mg.
See Editor's Note No. 30.

Respi-Tea - The Herbalist
Wild Cherry bark • Slippery Elm bark • Coltsfoot leaf • Marshmallow root • Licorice root • Cinnamon bark • Yarrow blossom • Ginger root.

Respitonic - The Herbalist
Echinacea root • Golden Seal root • Osha root • Yerba Santa leaf • Horseradish root • Yarrow blossom • Cayenne pepper.

Res-Q 1250 - N3 Oceanic
Three capsules contain: EPA (Eicosapentaenoic Acid) 1200 mg • DHA (Docosahexaenoic Acid) 900 mg • Other Omega-3 150 mg.

Rest - Enzymes, Inc.
Two capsules contain: Calcium (100% as Calcium Citrate) 30 mg • Magnesium (aspartate) 60 mg • Proprietary Herbal Blend 520 mg: Valerian root extract, Passionflower herb extract • pHysioProtease 100 mg. Other Ingredients: Plant Cellulose, Water.

RestEZ - Melaleuca
Each capsule contains: Proprietary Blend 385 mg: Valerian root extract (0.8% valerenic acid) • Kava Kava extract (30% kavalactones) • Hops • natural Spearmint powder • Passion Flower extract (4% flavonoids). Inactive Ingredients: Cellulose, Gelatin.

Restful - BioDynamax
Two capsules contain: Kava Kava root extract 300 mg • Chamomile 100 mg • Passion flower 100 mg • Calcium 100 mg • Magnesium 50 mg.

Restorative Toner - Abra Therapeutics
Deionized Water • Extracts Blend: Elderflower, Calendula, Orange Blossom, Horsetail, Bulgarian Chamomile • Aloe Vera Gel, Sodium PCA, Almond Glycerides • Panthenol • Sea Kelp • Algae extract • Vegetable Glycerin • Sorbitol • Lecithin • Cucumber extract • Vitamin E • Vitamin A • Vitamin C • Chelated Trace Minerals • Essential Oils Blend: Geranium, Ylang Ylang, Clary Sage • Methyl/Propyl Paraben.

Restore-X - Cambridge Nutraceuticals
Each serving contains: L-Glutamine 10 g • N-Acetyl-Cysteine 600 mg • L-Arginine 140 mg • Vitamin A (mixed carotenoids) 5000 IU • Vitamin C 500 mg • Vitamin E 200 IU • Thiamin 6 mg • Riboflavin 6.8 mg • Niacin 80 mg • Vitamin B6 8 mg • Pantothenic Acid 40 mg • Magnesium 200 mg • Zinc 20 mg • Selenium 100 mcg • Copper 0.75 mg • Folate 400 mcg • Vitamin B12 50 mcg.

Restorex Tea Pill - Lanzhou Herbal Factory
Each tablet contains: Proprietary Blend 160 mg: Tangshen root, Atractylodis root, Lovage root, White Peony root, Di Huang root, Licorice root, Tang Kwei root.

RestPrep - HealthMinded
Two capsules contain: Vitamin B6 (as pyridoxine HCl) 12 mg • RestPrep Proprietary Blend 902 mg: Valerian root dried extract, Chamomile flower dried extract, Peppermint leaf, Hops flower, Passionflower leaf & stem, Scullcap herb, Melatonin. Other Ingredients: Gelatin, Stearic Acid, Magnesium Stearate.

Resveratone - Metabolic Response Modifiers
Each capsule contains: Polygonum cuspidatum (yielding 16 mg Resveratrol) 200 mg.

Resveratrol - Pure Encapsulations
Each vegetable capsule contains: Resveratrol (polygonum cuspidatum) extract 200 mg.

Resveratrol Synergy - Jarrow Formulas
Each tablet contains: Vitamin C (as ascorbic acid) 100 mg • Resveratrol (from 200 mg polygonum cuspidatum (tiger cane), 8% total resveratrol) 16 mg • Grapeskin extract (vitis vinifera, 95% polyphenols) 100 mg • Grapeseed extract (vitis vinifera, 95% polyphenols) 50 mg • Green Tea 5:1 extract (camellia sinensis, 45% polyphenolics) 200 mg. Other Ingredients: Cellulose, Stearic Acid, Magnesium Stearate, Silicon Dioxide, Modified Cellulose Gum, Modified Cellulose.

Retorol - Progressive Health Nutraceuticals
Vitamin B3 60 mg • Inositol 15 mg • Cassia Nomame 125 mg • Tumeric 50 mg • Gum Guggul 50 mg.

Revenge - Champion Nutrition
Each 29 g serving contains: Vitamin C 60 mg • Vitamin E 60 IU • Thiamine 5 mg • Riboflavin 3 mg • Vitamin B6 5 mg • Pantothenic Acid 10 mg • Magnesium 12 mg • Chromium 240 mcg • Potassium 160 mg. Tropical Mango Blast Ingredients: Metacarb VII (proprietary carbohydrate blend which contains Amylopectin Food Starch Modified, Glucose Polymer [Maltodextrin]) • Fructose • Peptol-7 (proprietary Protein-Amino Acid Blend which contains: Whey Protein Concentrate, L-Leucine, Glycine, L-Glutamine, Taurine, L-Isoleucine & L-Valine) • Lactate Blend (Sodium Potassium Lactate, Creatine Lactate, Glycerol Stearate, Magnesium Lactate, Glycerol Lactate) • Glucose (Dextrose) • Natural & Artificial Flavoring • Cellulose • Malic Acid • Trutina Dulcem (Natural Kiwi extract) • Phosphatidylcholine • D-Ribose • Vitamin E Acetate • Talc • Ginseng Root extract • Proteoglycan Support (proprietary blend which includes Glucosamine Hcl & Glucosamine Ascorbate) • Creatine Alpha-Ketoglutarate • Citric Acid • Potassium Phosphate • Guarana seed extract (standardized to 50% Caffeine) • Potassium Citrate • Ascorbic Acid • Quercetin • Willow Bark extract (standardized to 50% Salycin) • Sunett (Acesulfame-K) • Sodium Citrate • Omega-3 Fatty Acids (Fish oil) • Xanthan Gum • Feverfew extract • Vitamin B Blend (Vitamin B1, Vitamin B2, Vitamin B3, Vitamin B5, Vitamin B6, Pantethine) • Curcumin • N-Acetylcysteine • Periwinkle standardized extract • Coenzyme Q10 • Lipoic Acid • Chromium Polynicotinate • Annatto & Carmine (natural colors).

Some Brand Name Natural Products - What they Contain

www.NaturalDatabase.com contains MANY more listings than appear here.

Editor's Notes are located on pages 2155-2163.

BRAND NAMES

RevitaFem **-** The AIM Companies
Two capsules contain: Black Cohosh root standardized extract (2.5% triterpene glycosides) 40 mg • Dong Quai root standardized extract (1% ligustilide) 250 mg • Soy extract (standardized 40% isoflavones) 65 mg • Red Clover blossom standardized extract (8% isoflavones) 100 mg • Wild Yam root 100 mg • Panax Ginseng root standardized extract (6% ginsenosides) 100 mg • Burdock root 150 mg • Hesperidin complex 100 mg.

ReVitalize **-** Rx Vitamins
Three purecaps contain: Mixed Carotenoid complex (alpha, beta & gamma carotenes) 25000 IU • Vitamin C (ascorbic acid) 200 mg • Pantothenic Acid (calcium pantothenate) 100 mg • Calcium (amino acid chelate/complex) 50 mg • Magnesium (amino acid chelate/ complex) 50 mg • Vitamin B1 (thiamine) 50 mg • Vitamin B2 (riboflavin) 50 mg • Vitamin B3 (niacin) 50 mg • Vitamin B6 (pyridoxine HCl) 50 mg • Citrus Flavonoid complex (active flavonols, flavonones, flavones & naringen-44%) 50 mg • Choline (bitartrate) 50 mg • Inositol 50 mg • Potassium (glycero-phosphate) 25 mg • Zinc (amino acid chelate/complex) 15 mg • Manganese (amino acid chelate/complex) 5 mg • Iron (amino acid chelate/ complex) 4.5 mg • Copper (glycinate) 1 mg • Vanadium (as vanadyl sulfate) 1 mg • Vitamin D (calciferol) 400 IU • Vitamin E (d-alpha tocopherol) 200 IU • Folic Acid 400 mcg • Biotin 300 mcg • Iodine (kelp) 150 mcg • Vitamin B12 (cyanocobalamin) 100 mcg • Chromium (polynicotinate) 50 mcg • Selenium (amino acid complex) 50 mcg • Molybdenum (amino acid complex) 20 mcg • Korean Ginseng (Panax ginseng, standardized 5% ginsenosides) 50 mg • Chinese Green Tea extract (Camilla sinensis, standardized 40% polyphenols) 25 mg • Ginkgo Biloba (standardized 24% ginkgoflavoneglycosides, 6% terpene lactones) 10 mg • Bilberry (Vaccinium myrtillus, standardized 25% anthocyanosides) 5 mg • Mahonia Aquifolium (wild grape seed extract, standardized 95-100% leucoanthocyanins) 5 mg • Oleoresin Turmeric (Curcuma longa, standardized 90-95% curcuminoids) 5 mg • Milk Thistle (Silybum marianum, standardized 80% Silymarin) 75 mg • Parsley Leaves (Petroselinum crispum, naturally rich in apiin & luteolin-7-apiolglucoside) 75 mg • Juniper Berries (juniperus communis, naturally rich in glucuronic acid) 50 mg • Celery seed 4x (Aplum graveolens, naturally rich in limonene) 50 mg • Cayenne (Capsicum frutescens, naturally rich in capsaicin) 50 mg • Glucosamine Sulfate (aminomonosaccharide) 30 mg • Borage Seed Oil (Borago officinalis, standardized 25% gamma linolenic acid) 25 mg.

ReVitaMan **-** NorthStar Nutritionals
Each capsule contains: Maca root 67 mg • Muira Puama 167 mg • Catauba bark 33 mg • Ashwagandha powder 33 mg • Gotu Kola herb 14 mg • L-Arginine aspartate 67 mg • Thiamine 3 mg • Riboflavin (vitamin B2) 3 mg • Niacin 7 mg • Vitamin B6 8 mg • Folate 133 mcg • Vitamin B12 33 mg • Pantothenic Acid 8 mg.

Revitle **-** Progressive Health Nutraceuticals
Vitamin A 7500 IU • Vitamin C 250 mg • Vitamin E 45 IU • Selenium 100 mcg • Coenzyme Q10 2 mg • Omega 3 Fatty Acids 12.5 mg • Omega 6 Fatty Acids 12.5 mg • N-Acetyl L-Cysteine 50 mg • Alpha Lipoic Acid 25 mg • Ginkgo extract 10 mg • Hawthorne 25 mg • Siberian Ginseng 100 mg • Cordyceps Sinensis 25 mg • Bilberry 10 mg • Green Tea extract 100 mg • Grape seed extract 10 mg.

Revival Almond Amaretto **-** Physicians Laboratories
Eight fluid ounces contain: Certified Isoflavone 15 mg. Other Ingredients: Whole Roasted Soybeans, Natural and Artificial Flavors.

Revival Dark Roast **-** Physicians Laboratories
Eight fluid ounces Contain: Certified Isoflavone 15 mg. Other Ingredients: Whole Roasted Soybeans, Natural and Artificial Flavors.

Revival French Vanilla **-** Physicians Laboratories
Eight fluid ounces contain: Certified Isoflavone 15 mg. Other Ingredients: Whole Roasted Soybeans, Natural and Artificial Flavors.

Revival Hazelnut **-** Physicians Laboratories
Eight fluid ounces contain: Certified Isoflavone 15 mg. Other Ingredients: Whole Roasted Soybeans, Natural and Artificial Flavors.

Revival Hot Jalapeno & Cheddar Soynuts **-** Physicians Laboratories
Each 1/6 cup contains: Certified Isoflavone 10 mg. Other Ingredients: Soy Protein (whole roasted soybeans), Soybean Oil, Cheddar Cheese, Salt, Whey, Maltodextrin, Blue Cheese, Nonfat Milk, Citric Acid, Jalapeno Powder, Dextrose, Green Chile Pepper, Onion and Garlic Powder, Natural and Artificial Flavors, Artificial Color.

Revival Irish Cream **-** Physicians Laboratories
Eight fluid ounces contain: Certified Isoflavone 15 mg. Other Ingredients: Whole Roasted Soybeans, Natural and Artificial Flavors.

Revival Just Peachy Fructose **-** Physicians Laboratories
Each packet contains: Certified Isoflavone 160 mg. Other Ingredients: Soy Protein Isolate, Fructose, Sucrose, Natural and Artificial Flavor, Soy Lecithin, Calcium Phosphate, Maltodextrin, Potassium Chloride, Sodium Chloride, Xanthan Gum, Beta-carotene, Real Peach powder, Carboxymethylcellulose, Undegraded Carrageenan.

Revival Just Peachy Splenda **-** Physicians Laboratories
Each packet contains: Certified Isoflavone 160 mg. Other Ingredients: Soy Protein Isolate, Cocoa, Maltodextrin, Calcium Phosphate, Soy Lecithin, Salt, Potassium Chloride, Artificial Flavor, Carrageenan, Carboxymethylcellulose, Xanthan Gum, Sucralose.

Revival Just Peachy Unsweetened **-** Physicians Laboratories
Each packet contains: Certified Isoflavone 160 mg. Other Ingredients: Soy Protein Isolate, Natural and Artificial Flavor, Soy Lecithin, Calcium Phosphate, Maltodextrin, Potassium Chloride, Sodium Chloride, Xanthan Gum, Beta-Carotene, Real Peach Powder, Carboxymethylcellulose, Undegraded Carrageenan.

Revival Lightly Salted Soynuts **-** Physicians Laboratories
Each 1/6 cup contains: Certified Isoflavone 10 mg. Other Ingredients: Soy Protein (whole roasted soybeans), Soybean Oil, Salt.

Revival Low-Carb Apple Autumn Frost **-** Physicians Laboratories
Each bar contains: Certified Isoflavone 160 mg. Other Ingredients: Soy Protein Isolate, Rice Starch, Brown Rice Flour, Vegetable Protein, Whey Protein Isolate, Maltitol, Fractionated Palm Kernel Oil, Maltodextrin, Nonfat Yogurt Powder, Partially-Hydrogenated Palm oil, Calcium Caseinate, Soy Lecithin, Lactic Acid, Acesulfame K, Vanilla, Sulfite-Free Apples, Natural and Artificial Flavor, Glycerin, Corn Syrup Solids, Cinnamon, Potassium Sorbate, Citric Acid, Sucralose.

Revival Low-Carb Chocolate Raspberry Zing **-** Physicians Laboratories
Each Bar Contains: Certified Isoflavone 160 mg. Other Ingredients: Soy Protein Isolate, Rice Starch, Brown Rice Flour, Vegetable Protein, Whey Protein Isolate, Maltitol, Fractionated Palm Kernel Oil, Cocoa (processed with alkali), Partially-Hydrogenated Palm Oil, Soy Lecithin, Acesulfame K, Vanilla, Lactitol, Palm Kernel Oil, Polydextrose, Oat fiber, Dried Strawberries, Dried Raspberries, Natural and Artificial Flavors, Citric Acid, Vegetable Juice Coloring, Malic Acid, Glycerin, Corn Syrup Solids, Potassium Sorbate, Sucralose.

Revival Macaroni **-** Physicians Laboratories
Two Ounces Contain: Certified Isoflavone 15 mg. Ingredients: Soy Protein Isolate, Niacin, Iron (Ferrous Sulfate), Thiamin Mononitrate, Riboflavin, Folic Acid.

Revival Marshmallow Krunch **-** Physicians Laboratories
Each Bar Contains: Certified Isoflavone 160 mg. Ingredients: Corn syrup, Sugar, Corn starch, Water, Gelatin, Artificial Flavoring, Soy Protein Isolate, Rice flour, Malt, Salt, Glycerin, Sunflower oil, Soy Lecithin.

Revival Mocha **-** Physicians Laboratories
Eight Fluid Ounces Contain: Certified Isoflavone 15 mg. Ingredients: Whole Roasted Soybeans, Natural and Artificial Flavors.

Revival Original Roast - Physicians Laboratories
Eight Fluid Ounces Contain: Certified Isoflavone 15 mg. Ingredients: Whole Roasted Soybeans, Natural and Artificial Flavors.

Revival Peanut Butter Chocolate Pal - Physicians Laboratories
Each Bar Contains: Certified Isoflavone 160 mg. Ingredients: Corn syrup, Corn starch, Water, Gelatin, Artifical Flavoring, Soy Protein Isolate, Rice flour, Malt, Salt, Dry Roasted Peanuts, Glycerin, Cocoa processed with alkali, Chocolate Liquor, Dextrose, Gum Arabic, "High Oleic" Sunflower oil, Natural Flavors, Soy Lecithin.

Revival Peanut Butter Pal - Physicians Laboratories
Each Bar Contains: Certified Isoflavone 160 mg. Ingredients: Corn syrup, Sugar, Corn starch, Water, Gelatin, Soy Protein Isolate, Rice flour, Malt, Salt, Dry Roasted Peanuts, Glycerin, Sunflower oil, Natural and Artificial Flavors, Soy Lecithin.

Revival Penne - Physicians Laboratories
Two Ounces Contain: Certified Isoflavone 15 mg. Ingredients: Soy Protein Isolate, Niacin, Iron (Ferrous Sulfate), Thiamin Mononitrate, Riboflavin, Folic Acid.

Revival Plain Soy - Physicians Laboratories
Each Packet Contains: Certified Isoflavone 160 mg. Ingredients: Soy Protein Isolate, Soy Lecithin.

Revival Rotini - Physicians Laboratories
Two Ounces Contain: Certified Isoflavone 15 mg. Ingredients: Soy Protein Isolate, Niacin, Iron (Ferrous Sulfate), Thiamin Mononitrate, Riboflavin, Folic Acid.

Revival Southern Pecan - Physicians Laboratories
Eight Fluid Ounces Contain: Certified Isoflavone 15 mg. Ingredients: Whole Roasted Soybeans, Natural and Artificial Flavors.

Revival Strawberry Smile Fructose - Physicians Laboratories
Each Packet Contains: Certified Isoflavone 160 mg. Ingredients: Soy Protein Isolate, Fructose, Sucrose, Natural and Artificial Flavor, Soy Lecithin, Calcium Phosphate, Beet juice powder, Maltodextrin, Potassium Chloride, Sodium Chloride, Xanthan Gum, Real Strawberry powder, Carboxymethylcellulose, Carrageenan.

Revival Strawberry Smile Splenda - Physicians Laboratories
Each Packet Contains: Certified Isoflavone 160 mg. Ingredients: Soy Protein Isolate, Cocoa, Maltodextrin, Calcium Phosphate, Soy Lecithin, Salt, Potassium Chloride, Artificial Flavor, Carrageenan, Carboxymethylcellulose, Xanthan Gum, Sucralose.

Revival Strawberry Smile Unsweetened - Physicians Laboratories
Each Packet Contains: Certified Isoflavone 160 mg. Ingredients: Soy Protein Isolate, Natural and Artificial Flavor, Soy Lecithin, Calcium Phosphate, Beet juice powder, Maltodextrin, Potassium Chloride, Sodium Chloride, Xanthan Gum, Real Strawberry powder, Carboxymethylcellulose, Undegraded Carrageenan.

Revival Thin Spaghetti - Physicians Laboratories
Two Ounces Contain: Certified Isoflavone 15 mg. Ingredients: Soy Protein Isolate, Niacin, Iron (Ferrous Sulfate), Thiamin Mononitrate, Riboflavin, Folic Acid.

Revival Unsalted Soynuts - Physicians Laboratories
Each 1/6 Cup Contains: Isoflavones 10 mg: Soy Protein, Soybean Oil.

Revival Vanilla Pleasure Fructose - Physicians Laboratories
Each Packet Contains: Isoflavones 160 mg. Ingredients: Soy Protein Isolate, Fructose, Sucrose, Calcium Phosphate, Maltodextrin, Soy Lecithin, Salt, Potassium Chloride, Modified Corn Starch, Artificial Flavor, Carrageenan, Carboxymethylcellulose, Xanthan Gum.

Revival Vanilla Pleasure Splenda - Physicians Laboratories
Each Packet Contains: Certified Isoflavone 160 mg. Ingredients: Soy Protein Isolate, Cocoa, Maltodextrin, Calcium Phosphate, Soy Lecithin, Salt, Potassium Chloride, Artificial Flavor, Carrageenan, Carboxymethylcellulose, Xanthan Gum, Sucralose.

Revival Vanilla Pleasure Unsweetened - Physicians Laboratories
Each Packet Contains: Certified Isoflavone 160 mg. Ingredients: Soy Protein Isolate, Maltodextrin, Calcium Phosphate, Soy Lecithin, Salt, Potassium Chloride, Modified Corn Starch, Artificial Flavor, Carrageenan, Carboxymethylcellulose, Xanthan Gum.

Revival Yogurt-covered Soynuts - Physicians Laboratories
Each 1/6 Cup Contains: Certified Isoflavone 10 mg. Ingredients: Yogurt Coating (sugar, palm kernel oil, whey powder, yogurt powder, artificial color, lecithin), Soy Protein (whole roasted soybeans), Vanillin, Soybean Oil, Sucrose, Corn Syrup, Tapioca, Dextrin, Confectioner's Glaze.

RevivAll Classic PhytoSterols & Sterolins - Garden of Life, Inc.
Two capsules contain: Whole Food Vitality Blend 1424 mg: 100% pre-digested blend of Sweet Potato, Garbanzo beans, Soy beans, Red Lentils, Adzuki beans, Kidney beans, Brown Rice, Sesame seeds, Flax seeds, Sunflower seeds, Pumpkin seeds • Phytosterol Blend 76 mg: Beta-Sitosterol, Stigmasterol, Campesterol • HSO Probiotic Blend 1.6 billion CFU. Other Ingredients: Cellulose.

RevivAll Female Vitality Formula - Garden of Life, Inc.
Four capsules contain: Whole Food Vitality Blend 2000 mg: 100% pre-digested blend of Garbanzo beans, Red Lentils, Soy beans, Flax seeds, Sunflower seeds, Adzuki beans, Kidney beans, Brown Rice • Herbal Vitality Blend 720 mg: 100% pre-digested blend of Sweet Potato, Wild Yam, Dong Quai, Black Cohosh, Licorice, Clover, Horse Chestnut, Chasteberry • Red Clover standardized extract (containing 16% isoflavones) 200 mg • Phytosterol Blend 80 mg: Beta-Sitosterol, Stigmasterol, Campesterol • HSO Probiotic Blend 1.6 Billion CFU. Other Ingredients: Cellulose.

RevivAll Male Vitality Formula - Garden of Life, Inc.
Two capsules contain: Whole Food Vitality Blend 1092 mg: 100% pre-digested blend of Garbanzo beans, Red Lentils, Soy beans, Flax seeds, Sunflower seeds, Sesame seeds, Adzuki beans, Kidney beans, Brown rice • Herbal Vitality Blend 200 mg: 100% pre-digested blend of Sweet Potato, Ginger • Cemitin Swedish Flower Pollen extract 132 mg • Phytosterol Blend 76 mg: Beta-Sitosterol, Stigmasterol, Campesterol • HSO Probiotic blend 1.6 billion CFU. Other Ingredients: Cellulose.

Revivogen Bio-Cleansing Shampoo - Advanced Skin & Hair LLC
Deionized Water • Decyl Polyglucose • Cocoamphocarboxyglycinate • Cocamide MEA • Aloe Vera • Jojoba oil • Cocoyl Sarcosine • Dimethicone • Ethylene Glycol Stearate • Polyquatrenium-4 • Panthenol (vitamin B5) • Saw Palmetto extract • Niacin (vitamin B3) • Guar gum • Soy Protein • Pyridoxal Hydrochloride • Gamma Linolenic Acid • Linoleic Acid • Zinc Sulfate • Azaleic Acid • Menthol • Benzophnone-4 • Methyl Paraben.

Revivogen Scalp Therapy - Advanced Skin & Hair LLC
SD Alcohol-40 • Gamma Linolenic Acid • Alpha Linolenic Acid (GLA & ALA) • Linoleic Acid • Oleic Acid • Azelaic Acid • Saw Palmetto extract • Zinc Sulfate • Vitamin B6 • Ethyl Laurate • Phytol • Beta Sitosterol • Grape seed extract • Procyanidin Oligomers • Niacin (vitamin B3) • Tocopherol Acetate (vitamin E) • EDTA • Purified Water • Perfumes.

Rezoom - 4 Life
Each 1/2 oz. serving contains: Vitamin C (as calcium ascorbate, magnesium ascorbate) 6 mg • Thiamin (Vitamin B1) 168 mcg • Riboflavin (Vitamin B2) 189 mcg • Niacin 3.6 mg • Vitamin B6 (as pyridoxine HCl) 225 mcg • Folic Acid 50 mcg • Vitamin B12 (as cyanocobalamin) 0.05 mcg • Pantothenic Acid 0.4 mg • Zinc 50 mcg • Selenium (as selenomethionine) 1 mcg • Chromium (as chromium nicotinate) 2 mcg • Chloride (as sodium chloride) 1 mg • Sodium (as sodium chloride) 1 mg • Potassium (as potassium citrate) 3 mg • Yerba Mate (leaf) 266 mg • Aloe Vera 138 mg • Bio Essential Proprietary Blend 44 mg: Yerba Mate extract (leaf), Astragalus extract (root), English Hawthorn extract (leaf), Sarsaparilla extract (root),

Siberian Ginseng extract (root), Yarrow extract (flower), Echinacea Purpurea extract (root), Licorice extract (root), Charparral extract (root), Stillingia extract (root), Korean Ginseng extract (root) • Peppermint extract (leaf) 3 mg • Lime extract (blossom) 2 mg • Lemon Balm extract (peel) 2 mg • Boron 2 mcg. Other Ingredients: Water, Glycerin, High Fructose Corn Syrup, Alcohol, Potassium Sorbate, Sodium Benzoate, Phosphoric Acid, Malic Acid, Lactic Acid.

Rezyme - Nature's Secret
Vegetarian Enzyme that contains a proprietary blend of Amylase, Glucoamylase, Cellulase, Lipase, Lactase, Alpha Galactosidase, Bromelain, Papain, Betaine HCl, Gentian, Licorice, and Ginger root. Enzyme Rebuilder, which contains Bitters, Lecithin, L-Glutamine, and Piper longum fruit.

R-Form Lipoic Acid - Vital Nutrients
Each vegetarian capsule contains: "R" Isomer Lipoic Acid (D thioctic acid) 100 mg.

Rheumatex With S.O.D. Catalase - Life Extension
Each tablet contains: Superoxide Dismutase 4000 units • Catalase 8000 units • Glutathione Peroxidase 600 units (bovine liver base).

Rhinallergy - Boiron
Active Ingredients: Allium Cepa 5 CH 0.5 mg • Ambrosia Artemisiaefolia 5 CH 0.5 mg • Euphraisa Officinalis 5 CH 0.5 mg • Histaminum Muriaticum 9 CH 0.5 mg • Sabadilla 5 CH 0.5 mg • Solidago Virga Aurea 5 CH 0.5 mg. Inactive Ingredients: Lactose, Sucrose, Magnesium Stearate.
Available in France. See Editor's Note No. 1.

Rhino Acidophilus - Dial Herbs
Lactobacillus acidophilus • Bifidobacterium bifidum • Bifidobacterium infantis • FOS, in a base of rice powder & natural flavors • Vitamin C from Ester-C. Flavored & sweetened with all-natural raspberry fruit juice crystals, dextrose & fructose.

Rhino Actalin Bars - Nutrition Now
Soy Protein Isolate, Calcium Sodium Caseinate, Whey Protein Concentrate, Glucose, High Fructose Glucose Syrup, Fractionated Vegetable Oils, Turbinado Sugar, Non-Fat Dry Milk, Yogurt Solids, Vanilla, Lecithin, Raisins, Apple Paste, Natural Flavors, Apple Fiber, Graham Flour, and Cinnamon.

Rhino Actalin Dietary Supplement - Nutrition Now
Each tablet contains: Magnesium 20 mg • Inosine 50 mg • Phosphatidylserine 50 mg • Amino Acid Blend 50 mg.
See Editor's Note No. 21.

Rhino Chewy Vites - Dial Herbs
Vitamin A • Vitamin C • Vitamin D • Vitamin E • Vitamin B6 • Vitamin B12 • Calcium • Thiamin • Riboflavin • Folic Acid • Biotin • Pantothenic Acid • Iodine • Magnesium • Zinc • Choline • Inositol • Fruitrim: (Fruit juice, Natural grain dextrins) • Evaporated Cane juice (natural milled sugar) • Gelatin • Lactate • Gluconate • Ascorbic Acid • d-Alpha Tocopheryl Acetate • Citrate Palmitate • Betartrate • Citric Acid • Lactic Acid • Natural Flavors • Natural Colors added including Annatto, Turmeric, Carmine & Grape skin liquid • Beeswax.

Rhino Daily Pack - Nutrition Now
Two Rhino Vites contain: 100% natural daily multi-vitamin, two Rhino Calcium, one Rhino Ester-C (Vitamin C).

Rhino Echinacea - Dial Herbs
Two tablets contain: Echinacea 100 mg • Vitamin C 60 mg. Flavored & sweetened with all natural raspberry fruit juice crystals, dextrose & fructose.

Rhino Echinacea Pops Box - Dial Herbs
Each lollipop contains: Isomalt • Maltitol • Citric Acid • Ascorbic Acid 50 mg • Natural Flavor • Color from Beet liquid • Echinacea • Goldenseal • Phosphorus 6x • Drosera 6x • Kali Carbonicum 6x • Belladonna 6x • Rumex Crispus 6x • Hydrastis 6x.
See Editor's Note No. 1.

Rhino Ester-C - Dial Herbs
Vitamin C from Ester-C • Calcium. Flavored & sweetened with all-natural cherry flavorings, natural fruit flavors, fructose, dextrose & bilberry.

Rhino Support Pack - Nutrition Now
Each packet contains: Two Rhino Echinacea, two Rhino Acidophilus, one Rhino Ester-C (Vitamin C).

Rhizinate - PhytoPharmica
Two tablets contain: Deglycyrrizinated Licorice root 3:1 extract (DGL, glycyrrhiza glabra) 760 mg • Glycine 100 mg.

Rhizinate Chocolate-Mint flavor - PhytoPharmica
Two tablets contain: Licorice (Glycyrhiza glabra) root extract 4:1 (deglycyrrhizinated) 760 mg • Glycine (amino acid) in a base of fructose 100 mg. Flavored with Dutch Cocoa Powder, Creme Flavor, and Peppermint.

Rhodiola - Nature's Plus
Each capsule contains: Rhodiola root (rhodiola rosea, standardized 2.3% rosavin, 2.8% salidroside, 70% polyphenols, 5.4% beta-vicianosides, 1.4% rosin, 1.2% rosarin) 250 mg • Rhodiola powder 100 mg • Herbal Actives Base Powder 100 mcg: Green Tea extract, Grape seed extract, Red Wine extract, Elderberry extract, Broccoli extract, Spinach extract, Carrot extract, Tomato extract, Spirulina, Chlorella. Other Ingredients: Vegetable Cellulose, Microcrystalline Cellulose, Silica, Vegetable Glycerin, Purified Water.

Rhodiola - Vitamin World
Each capsule contains: Rhodiola Rosea root extract (rhodiola rosea L., standardized to contain 3% rosavins (4.5 mg), 0.8% salidrosides (1.2 mg)) 150 mg • Rhodiola Rosea (rhodiola rosea L.) 100 mg. Other Ingedients: Gelatin, Cellulose (plant origin), Vegetable Magnesium Stearate, Silica.

Rhodiola Extended Release 1000 mg - Nature's Plus
Each extended release tablet contains: Rhodiola root (rhodiola rosea, standardized 2.3% rosavin, 2.8% salidroside, 70% polyphenols, 5.4% beta-vicianosides, 1.4% rosin, 1.2% rosarin) 1000 mg • Active Whole Food Complex 100 mcg: Green Tea extract, Grape seed extract, Red Wine extract, Elderberry extract, Broccoli extract, Spinach extract, Carrot extract, Tomato extract, Spirulina, Chlorella. Other Ingredients: Di-calcium Phosphate, Stearic Acid, Hydroxypropyl Methylcellulose, Magnesium Stearate, Pharmaceutical Glaze, Silica.

Rhodiola Rosea - Pure Encapsulations
Each vegetable capsule contains: Rhodiola Rosea extract (standardized to 3% total rosavins and min. 1% salidrosides) 100 mg.

Rhodiola Rosea 3% - Vital Nutrients
Each capsule contains: Rhodiola Rosea extract (6 mg total rosavins as rosarin, rosavin, rosin) 200 mg.

Rhodiola Rosea 500 - Jarrow Formulas
Each capsule contains: Rhodiola root 30:1 extract (rhodiola rosea, 5% rosavins, including 3% minimum rosavin, from Russian root) 500 mg. Other Ingredients: Rice Powder, Magnesium Stearate, Silicon Dioxide.

Rhythm Right - J. R. Carlson Laboratories, Inc.
Two softgels contain: Vitamin E (as D-alpha tocopherol) 30 IU • Magnesium (as magnesium glycinate chelate) 200 mg • Potassium (as potassium chloride) 33 mg • Mixed Tocopherols 30 mg • Omega-3 Fish oil concentrate 300 mg • DHA (docosahexaenoic acid) 60 mg • EPA (eicosapentaenoic acid) 100 mg • Co-Q10 (coenzyme Q10) 20 mg • L-Arginine 50 mg • L-Carnitine 50 mg • L-Taurine 50 mg.

RiboCell brand - Nutratech
D-Ribose.
See Editor's Note No. 44.

Riboflavin - Pure Encapsulations
Each vegetable capsule contains: Riboflavin (vitamin B2) 400 mg • Vitamin C (as ascorbyl palmitate) 10 mg.

Riboflavin - PhytoPharmica
Each tablet contains: Riboflavin (vitamin B2) 400 mg.

Ribonucleic Acid (RNA) - Standard Process, Inc.
Each tablet contains: Calcium 15 mg • Ribonucleic Acid 185 mg. Other Ingredients: Magnesium Citrate, Cellulose, Arabic Gum.

Ribose - Jarrow Formulas
Each scoop contains: D-Ribose 2000 mg.

Ribose - Pure Encapsulations
Each supplied scoop contains: D-Ribose 2.2 g.

Ribose Rx-Energy - Nature's Plus
Each tablet contains: D-ribose 1100 mg • AMP (Adenosine-5'-monophosphoric acid) 1000 mcg. Other Ingredients: Di-calcium Phosphate, Microcrystalline Cellulose, Silica, Stearic Acid, Pharmaceutical Glaze.

Rice Bran Oil - Progressive Labs
Each tablespoon contains: Rice bran oil 14 g.

RiceMucille - NutraCea (formerly NutraStar)
Each 360 g canister contains: Stabailized Rice Bran and Germ.

Rich Moisture Cream - FreeLife International
Purified Water • Neroli Hydrolate (flower water) • Ahnfeltia Concinna seaweed • Willowherb • Olive Squalane • Cetyl Alcohol • Glyceryl Stearate • Jojoba oil (buxus chinensis) • Chrysanthellum Indicum extract • Vegetable Glycerin • Liposome: Sodium PCA, Phospholipids, Tocopheryl Acetate, Arginine, Lysine, Glycine, Proline • Ceramid 3 • Beta 1,3 Glucans • Sodium Hyaluronate • Saccharide Isomerate (moisture magnets) • Shea Butter • Vegetable Glycerin • BioEnhaced Grapefruit seed extract (BGSE) • Essential Bulgarian Rose oil • Essential Neroli oil (citrus aurantium) • Sodium Behenoyl Lactylate • Potassium Sorbate • Xanthan Gum.

Richardson Labs Arthred-G - Rexall - Sundown
Each rounded scoop contains: Arthred (enzymatically hydrolyzed collagen protein) 7 g • Glucosamine & Chondroitin Complex: Glucosamine HCl, Glucosamine Sulfate (potassium salt, sodium free), Chondroitin Sulfate.

Richardson Labs Chitosan-C with Biozan - Rexall - Sundown
Four caplets contain: BioZan 2500: Purified Chitosan, Betaine HCl, Oat Bran, Aloe, Beta Glucan • Chromium (picolinate) 200 mcg.

Richardson Labs Chroma Slim Biozan - Rexall - Sundown
Four caplets contain: BioZan 2500 mg: Purified Chitosan, Betaine HCl, Oat bran, Aloe, Beta Glucan 2500 mg • Chromium (picolinate) 250 mcg.

Richardson Labs Chroma Slim for Men - Rexall - Sundown
Four caplets contain: Trace Mineral Blend: Chromium Picolinate 400 mcg, Vanadium 120 mcg, Manganese Picolinate 2.5 mg • Proprietary Lipotropic Blend 3000 mg: Choline Bitartrate, L-Carnitine, Inositol, L-Methionine • Essential Nutrient & Amino Acid Blend 500 mg: Ferulic Acid Esters, Taurine, L-Lysine HCl, L-Glutamic Acid, Base, Glycine USP, Cernitin flower pollen extract 500 mg • Vitamin Blend: Pantothenic Acid 10 mg, Vitamin B6 5 mg • Thermogenic Herbal Blend 424 mg: Panax Ginseng powdered extract • Cayenne • Mustard seed powder • Cinnamon powder • Ginger root powdered extract • Uva Ursi • Standardized White Willow bark powder. In a base of Natural Peppermint, Saw Palmetto berries, Juniper berries, Spirulina.

Richardson Labs Chroma Slim Plus - Rexall - Sundown
Four caplets contain: Trace Mineral Blend: Chromium Picolinate 400 mcg, Vanadium 120 mcg, Manganese Picolinate 2.5 mg • Proprietary Lipotropic & Lipid Transport Blend 3000 mg: Choline Bitartrate, L-Carnitine, Inositol, L-Methionine • Essential Nutrient & Amino Acid Blend 500 mg: Ferulic Acid Esters, Taurine, L-Lysine HCl, L-Glutamic Acid, Base, Glycine USP, Cernitin flower pollen extract • Vitamin Blend: Potassium Chloride USP, Pantothenic Acid 10 mg, Vitamin B6 5 mg. Base: Peppermint and Bromelain.

Richardson Labs Chromium Picolinate - Rexall - Sundown
Each tablet contains: Chromium (Picolinate), derived from 3.2 mg of pure crystalline Chromium Picolinate.

Richardson Labs Pyruvate-C - Rexall - Sundown
Four caplets contain Pyruvate (Potassium Pyruvate, Calcium Pyruvate) 2 g • Chromium (Picolinate) 400 mcg.

Richardson Labs Ultra Chroma Slim Plan with Biotrol - Rexall - Sundown
Three caplets contain: Manganese (as manganese picolinate) 1.25 mg • Chromium (as chromium picolinate) 200 mcg • Blood Sugar Support blend 10.4 mg: Manganese Picolinate, Chromium Picolinate, Vanadium (as vanadyl sulfate) 60 mcg 10.4 mg • Lipotropic & Metabolic Support blend 1.1 grams: Choline Bitartrate, L-Carnitine Tartrate • Appetite Control & Neurotransmitter Support blend 1.6 g, Inulin, L-Phenylalanine, St. John's Wort extract leaves & flowers standardized to 0.3% hypercin, Capsicum fruit extract 10:1, Peppermint oil • Energy Support blend 252 mg: Siberian Ginseng root, Calcium Pyruvate. Other Ingredients: Cellulose, Modified Cellulose Gum, Stearic Acid, Silica, Hydroxypropyl Methylcellulose, Magnesium Stearate, Peppermint leaves.

Rich's MSM Eye and Ear Drops - Rich Distributing
Methylsulfonylmethane • Sterilized Activated Water.
See Editor's Note No. 10.

Rimostil - Novogen
Each tablet contains: Clovone Isoflavone Proprietary Blend 57 mg: Formononetin, Daidzein, Biochanin A, Genistein. Other Ingredients: Calcium Phosphate, Microcrystalline Cellulose, Soy Polysaccharide, Magnesium Sulfate, Titanium Dioxide.

Ripped Fuel - TwinLab
Ma Huang 20 mg • Guarana 200 mg • Chromium 200 mcg • L-Carnitine 100 mg.
See Editor's Note No. 21 and No. 30.

Ripped Fuel - MaHuang Free Formula - TwinLab
Each two capsules contain: Citrus Aurantium extract (standardized for 6% synephrine alkaloids) 325 mg • St. John's Wort extract (aerial parts, standardized for 0.3% hypericin) 300 mg • L-Phenylalanine 50 mg • Guarana seed extract (176 mg of caffeine) 800 mg. Other Ingredients: Thermogenic and Herbal Base Blend: Coleus Forskohlii (pashanabhedi) root extract, Green Tea extract, Citrus Bioflavonoids Complex, Ginger root, Cayenne, Yohimbe bark extract. Inactive Ingredients: Gelatin, Purified Water, MCT, Silica, Vegetable-based Stearic Acid, Magnesium Stearate.
See Editor's Note No. 40.

Ripped Fuel (Metabolic Enhancer) - TwinLab
Two capsules contain: Ma Huang extract (standardized for 6% Ephedrine) 334 mg • Guarana extract (standardized for 22% Caffeine) 910 mg • L-Carnitine 100 mg • Chromium (Chromium Picolinate) 200 mcg.

Ripped Fuel Extreme - TwinLab
Two capsules contain: Calcium (from calcium carbonate) 118 mg • Chromium (from chromium polynicotinate) 200 mcg • Proprietary Herbal Extract 125 mg: Baical Skullcap root, Black Catechu bark (standardized for 60% free-b-ring flavonoids and 10% flavans) • Cocoa seed extract (standardized for 10% theobromine as well as caffeine, tyramine and phenylethylamine) 315 mg • Green Tea extract (standardized for 45% epigallocatechin gallate and 6% caffeine) 315 mg • Caffeine (from caffeine anhydrous, green tea leaf extract and cocoa seed extract) 220 mg • L-Carnitine (from L-carnitine L-tartrate) 13 mg • Cayenne fruit extract 50 mg. Other Ingredients: Rice Flour, Gelatin, Purified Water, MCT, Magnesium Stearate, Silica.

Ripping Gel - Urban Biologics
Lecithin • Water (aqua) • Octyl Palmitate • Aminophylline • Fragrance • Vitamin E • Propylene Glycol • BHA • Propyl Gallate • Citric Acid • DMDM Hydantoin • Iodopropynyl Butylcarbamate • Caramel Color.

Some Brand Name Natural Products - What they Contain

www.NaturalDatabase.com contains MANY more listings than appear here.
Editor's Notes are located on pages 2155-2163.

Rise & Shine - Life Enhancement Products, Inc.
Each rounded tablespoon (14.5 g) contains: Vitamin A (as beta-carotene) 2500 IU • Vitamin C (as ascorbic acid and niacinamide ascorbate) 325 mg • Vitamin E (as D,L-alpha-tocopheryl acetate) 30 IU • Thiamine (vitamin B1 as thiamine hydrochloride) 1.5 mg • Riboflavin (vitamin B2) 3 mg • Niacin (vitamin B3 as niacinamide ascorbate) 75 mg • Vitamin B6 (as pyridoxine hydrochloride) 16 mg • Folic Acid 100 mcg • Vitamin B12 (cyanocobalamin) 20 mcg • Pantothenic Acid (vitamin B5 as calcium pantothenate) 18 mg • Zinc (as zinc gluconate) 3 mg • Copper (as copper gluconate) 420 mcg • Chromium (as chromium aspartate) 25 mcg • L-Phenylalanine 600 mg • Taurine 200 mg • Glycine 150 mg.

RiSolubles - NutraCea (formerly NutraStar)
Each 360 g canister contains: Stabilized Rice Bran and Germ.

Rite Life - 4 Life
Each 3 teaspoon serving contains: Vitamin C (as ascorbic acid) 200 mg • Sodium (from ionic rare earth minerals) 28 mg • Cranberry fruit 44 mg • English Hawthorn berry 1:6 dried extract (in 95% ethanol, 40 mg) 240 mg • Ginkgo Biloba 1:6 dried extract (in 95% ethanol, 40 mg) 240 mg • Licorice root 1:25 dried extrat (in water, 14 mg) 360 mg • Echinacea aerial parts 1:25 dried extract (echinacea purpurea, in water, 14 mg) 360 mg • Caffeine 13 mg • Korean Ginseng root 1:29 dried extract (in water, 12 mg) 360 mg • Guarana seed 1:29 dried extract (in water, 12 mg) 360 mg • Cat's Claw bark 1:63 dried extract (in water, 6 mg) 360 mg • Ionic Rare Earth Minerals 6 mg • Bilberry fruit 1:121 extract (in water, 3 mg) 360 mg • Grape Seed 1:309 dried extract (in water, 1 mg) 360 mg. Other Ingredients: High Fructose Corn Syrup, Water, Alcohol, Malic Acid, Potassium Sorbate, Citric Acid, Sodium Benzoate, Ionic Rare Earth Minerals: Tin, Titanium, Rubidium, Calcium, Zinc, Copper, Germanium, Potassium, Gallium, Iron, Cadmium, Boron, Silver, Cesium, Gold, Platinum, Cobalt, Silicon, Manganese, Chromium, Strontium, Iodine, Molybdenum, Antimony.

RiteStart Men - 4 Life
Each packet contains: Vitamin A (as 25% retinyl palmitate and 75% as beta carotene from Blakeslea trispora extract) 5,000 IU • Vitamin C (as calcium ascorbate, ascorbic acid, ascorbyl palmitate, erythorbic acid, magnesium ascorbate, dehydroascorbic acid, ascorbigen) 250 mg • Vitamin D (as cholecalciferol) 200 IU • Vitamin E (as D-alpha tocopheryl acetate) 108 IU • Vitamin K (phytonadione) 13 mcg • Thiamin (as thiamin mononitrate) 2 mg • Riboflavin 2 mg • Niacin (as niacinamide) 13 mg • Vitamin B6 (as pyrodoxine hydrochloride) 3 mg • Folate (as folic acid) 200 mcg • Vitamin B12 (as cyanocobalamin) 9 mcg • Biotin (D-biotin) 150 mcg • Pantothenic Acid (as D-calcium pantothenate) 13 mg • Calcium (as calcium carbonate, calcium amino acid chelate, calcium citrate) 163 mg • Iron (as iron amino acid chelate) 5 mg • Iodine (as potassium iodide) 38 mcg • Magnesium (as magnesium oxide, magnesium amino acid chelate) 50 mg • Zinc (as zinc amino acid chelate, monomethionine) 20 mg • Selenium (as I-selenomethionine) 100 mcg • Copper (as copper amino acid chelate) 0.5 mg • Manganese (as manganese amino acid chelate) 1 mg • Chromium (as chromium amino acid chelate) 120 mcg • Molybdenum (as molybdenum amino acid chelate) 20 mcg • Boron (as boron citrate) 1 mg • Vanadium (as bis glycinato oxovanadium) 10 mcg • Transfer Factor E-XF from Bovine Colostrum and Egg yolk 150 mg • Cordyvant Proprietary Polysaccharide Complex 440 mg: IP-6 (Inositol hexaphosphate), Soybean oil extract (phytosterols), Cordyceps sinensis (7% cordyceptic acids), Beta-Glucan from Baker's Yeast (saacharomyces cerevisiae), Beta-Glucan from Oat (avena sativa), Agaricus Blazeii extract, Mannans from aloe vera leaf, Olive Leaf extract (olea europaea), Maitake Mushroom (grifola frondosa whole plant), Shiitake Mushroom (lentinus edodes whole plant 5:1 extract). Alpha Linolenic Acid (ALA) from organic flax seed oil (linum usitatissimum seed)138 mg • Gamma Linolenic Acid (GLA) from borage seed oil (Borago officinalis seed) 35 mg • Eicosapentaenoic Acid (EPA) from Fish Oil 33 mg • Docosahexaenoic Acid (DHA) from Fish Oil 22 mg • Conjugated Linoleic Acid (CLA) from Safflower Oil (helianthus annuus seed) 122 mg • Proprietary OPC Blend (Oligomeric Proanthocyanidins) 50 mg: Grapeseed extract (vitis vinifera seed) with Oligomeric Proanthocyanidins, Pine bark extract (pinus maritima bark) with Oligomeric Proanthocyanidins. Proprietary Antioxidant Blend 68 mg: Lutein and Zeaxanthin (tagetes erecta petals), Bilberry (25% anthocyanidins), Coenzyme Q10, Alpha Lipoic Acid, Catechins (camellia sinensis leaf), Rutin. Men's Health Blend 116 mg: Soy Isoflavones including genistein and genistin (from soy extract), Quercitin, Sulforaphane from broccoli (brassica oleracea sprout), Curcumin from Turmeric (Curcuma longa root), Diindolyl Methane (DIM), Ipriflavone. Proprietary Blend 61 mg: Glucosamine Hydrochloride, Calcium D-Glucarate, N-Acetyl Cysteine, Ginkgo Biloba leaf (24% ginkgo flavone glycosides, 6% terpene lactones), Hyaluronic Acid, Tocotrienols (from palm oil).

RiteStart Women - 4 Life
Each packet contains: Vitamin A (as 25% retinyl palmitate and 75% as beta carotene from Blakeslea trispora extract) 5,000 IU • Vitamin C (as calcium ascorbate, ascorbic acid, ascorbyl palmitate, erythorbic acid, magnesium ascorbate, dehydroascorbic acid, ascorbigen) 250 mg • Vitamin D (as cholecalciferol) 200 IU • Vitamin E (as D-alpha tocopheryl acetate) 108 IU • Vitamin K (phytonadione) 13 mcg • Thiamin (as thiamin mononitrate) 2 mg • Riboflavin 2 mg • Niacin (as niacinamide) 13 mg • Vitamin B6 (as pyrodoxine hydrochloride) 3 mg • Folate (as folic acid) 400 mcg • Vitamin B12 (as cyanocobalamin) 9 mcg • Biotin (D-biotin) 150 mcg • Pantothenic Acid (as D-calcium pantothenate) 13 mg • Calcium (as calcium carbonate, calcium amino acid chelate, calcium citrate) 550 mg • Iron (as iron amino acid chelate) 9 mg • Iodine (as potassium iodide) 38 mcg • Magnesium (as magnesium oxide, magnesium amino acid chelate) 200 mg • Zinc (as zinc amino acid chelate, monomethionine) 13 mg • Selenium (as I-selenomethionine) 35 mcg • Copper (as copper amino acid chelate) 0.5 mg • Manganese (as manganese amino acid chelate) 1 mg • Chromium (as chromium amino acid chelate) 120 mcg • Molybdenum (as molybdenum amino acid chelate) 20 mcg • Boron (as boron citrate) 1 mg • Vanadium (as bis glycinato oxovanadium) 10 mcg • Transfer Factor E-XF from Bovine Colostrum and Egg yolk 150 mg • Cordyvant Proprietary Polysaccharide Complex 440 mg: IP-6 (Inositol hexaphosphate), Soybean oil extract (phytosterols), Cordyceps sinensis (7% cordyceptic acids), Beta-Glucan from Baker's Yeast (saacharomyces cerevisiae), Beta-Glucan from Oat (avena sativa), Agaricus Blazeii extract, Mannans from aloe vera leaf, Olive Leaf extract (olea europaea), Maitake Mushroom (grifola frondosa whole plant), Shiitake Mushroom (lentinus edodes whole plant 5:1 extract). Alpha Linolenic Acid (ALA) from organic flax seed oil (linum usitatissimum seed)138 mg • Gamma Linolenic Acid (GLA) from borage seed oil (Borago officinalis seed) 35 mg • Eicosapentaenoic Acid (EPA) from Fish Oil 33 mg • Docosahexaenoic Acid (DHA) from Fish Oil 22 mg • Conjugated Linoleic Acid (CLA) from Safflower Oil (helianthus annuus seed) 122 mg • Proprietary OPC Blend (Oligomeric Proanthocyanidins) 50 mg: Grapeseed extract (vitis vinifera seed) with Oligomeric Proanthocyanidins, Pine bark extract (pinus maritima bark) with Oligomeric Proanthocyanidins. Proprietary Antioxidant Blend 55 mg: Lutein and Zeaxanthin (tagetes erecta petals), Bilberry (25% anthocyanidins), Coenzyme Q10, Alpha Lipoic Acid, Catechins (camellia sinensis leaf), Rutin. Women's Health Blend 180 mg: Soy Isoflavones including genistein and genistin (from soy extract), Quercitin, Sulforaphane from broccoli (brassica oleracea sprout), Curcumin from Turmeric (Curcuma longa root), Diindolyl Methane (DIM), Ipriflavone. Proprietary Blend 61 mg: Glucosamine Hydrochloride, Calcium D-Glucarate, N-Acetyl Cysteine, Ginkgo Biloba leaf (24% ginkgo flavone glycosides, 6% terpene lactones), Hyaluronic Acid, Tocotrienols (from palm oil).

R-Lipoic Acid - Physician Formulas
Each capsule contains: R-Alpha Lipoic Acid 50 mg.

_RM-10_ - Garden of Life, Inc.
Two caplets contain: Proprietary Mushroom Blend 1455 mg: Cordyceps Sinensis, Ganoderma Lucidum (reishi), Grifola Frondosa (maitake), Agaricus Blazei, Lentinula Edodes (shiitake), Coriolus Versicolor, Hericium Erinaceus, Polyporus Umbellatus, Tremella Fuciformia, Poria Cocos • Uncaria Tomentosa 330 mg • Aloe Vera extract 15 mg. Other Ingredients: Cellulose, Stearates.

Some Brand Name Natural Products - What they Contain

www.NaturalDatabase.com contains MANY more listings than appear here.
Editor's Notes are located on pages 2155-2163.

RNA 125 & DNA 125 **-** GNC
Each tablet contains: RNA (Ribonucleic Acid) 125 mg • DNA (Deoxyribonucleic Acid) 125 mg. Other Ingredients: Dicalcium Phosphate, Cellulose, Food Glaze.

RNA Cream **-** Life Extension
RNA, PABA, NaPCA, Elastin, Collagen, Safflower oil, Apricot kernal oil, Coconut oil, Vitamin A, Vitamin D, Aloe gel, Squalene, Methylparaben, Propylparaben.

RNA/DNA **-** Puritan's Pride
Each tablet contains: RNA (Ribonucleic Acid) 100 mg • DNA (Deoxyribonucleic Acid) 100 mg. In a base containing 400 mg of Dried Debittered Brewer's Yeast.

Robert's Complex **-** Enzymatic Therapy
Each capsule contains: Niacinamide 5 m. Other Ingredients: American Cranesbill (Geranium maculatum) 100 mg • Cabbage extract (Braccica oleracea) 100 mg • Marshmallow extract 4:1 (Althaea officinalis) mucilage content 30-40%) 75 mg • Okra (Hibiscus esculentis) 75 mg • Slippery Elm (Ulma fulva) 75 mg • Duodenal Substance 75 mg • Echinacea root extract (Echinacea angustifolia) standardized to contain greater than 3.5% Echinacosides & 0.65% essential oils 25 mg • Goldenseal root extract (hydrastis canadensis, standardized to 5% total alkaloids including berberine, hydrastine, and canadine) 25 mg • Pancreatic Enzymes 25 mg. See Editor's Note No. 14.

Robert's Formula **-** PhytoPharmica
Two capsules contain: Niacinamide 10 mg • American Cranesbill (Geranium maculatum) root 200 mg • Cabbage (Brassica oleracea) leaf extract 4:1 200 mg • Marshmallow (althaea officinalis) root extract 4.25:1 150 mg •Okra (Abelmoschus esculentis) whole plant 150 mg • Slippery Elm (Ulma fulva) bark 150 mg •Duodenal substance 50 mg •Echinacea (Echinacea angustifolia) root extract (standardized to contain greater than 4% echinacosides) 50 mg • Goldenseal (Hydrastis canadensis) root and rhizome extract 4:1 (standardized to contain 5% total alkaloids including berberine, hydrastine, and canadine) 50 mg • Pancreatic enzymes 50 mg. See Editor's Note No. 21 and No. 53.

Rockstar Energy Cola **-** Rockstar, Inc.
Carbonated Water • High Fructose Corn Syrup • Glucose • Taurine 946 mg • Phosphoric Acid • Guarana seed extract 200 mg • Ascorbic Acid • Caffeine • L-Carnitine 25 mg • Inositol 25 mg • Milk Thistle extract 20 mg • Ginkgo Biloba leaf extract 15 mg • Niacinamide • Calcium Pantothenate • Eleutherococcus Senticosus 25 mg • Riboflavin • Pyridoxine Hydrochloride • Cyanocobalamin.

Rockstar Energy Drink **-** Rockstar, Inc.
Carbonated Water • High Fructose Corn Syrup • Dextrose • Citric Acid • Taurine 946 mg • Natural and Artificial Flavors • Guarana seed extract 200 mg • Ascorbic Acid • Caramel Color • Sodium Benzoate • Potassium Sorbate • Caffeine • Niacinamide • Inositol 25 mg • L-Carnitine 25 mg • Milk Thistle extract 20 mg • Ginkgo Biloba leaf extract 15 mg • Calcium Pantothenate • Siberian Ginseng root extract 25 mg • Cyanocobalamin • Riboflavin • Pyridoxine Hydrochloride.

Rodex B6 Forte **-** Pain & Stress Center
Each capsule contains: Pyridoxine HCl (B6) 150 mg • Cyanocobalamin (B12) 200 mcg • Folic Acid 800 mcg. Other Ingredients: Gelatin Capsule.

Rodex T.R B6 **-** Pain & Stress Center
Each capsule contains: Pyridoxine HCl (B) 150 mg. Other Ingredients: Gelatin Capsule.

Rogisen **-** Berkeley Premium Nutraceuticals
Each caplet contains: Vitamin A (100% as beta-carotene) 5000 IU • Vitamin C (as ascorbic acid) 250 mg • Vitamin E (as dl-alpha-tocopheryl acetate) 100 IU • Zinc (zinc citrate and as zinc oxide) 40 mg • Selenium (as selenium L-methionine complex) 200 mg • Copper (as cupric acid) 2 mg • Rogisen Proprietary Blend 307 mg: Red Wine Grape skin (37% total polyphenols), Orange Bioflavonoids (30%-40% total flavanones, flavonols, flavones), Ginkgo Biloba leaf standardized extract, European Bilberry standardized extract, L-Glutathione, Lutein / Zeaxanthin (active 5:1 ratio). Other Ingredients: Dicalcium Phosphate, Microcrystalline Cellulose, Croscarmellose Sodium, Stearic Acid, Silica, Magnesium Stearate, Film Coat Ingredients (hypromellose, hydroxypropyl cellulose, polyethylene glycol, propylene glycol, FD&C yellow #5 lake). See Editor's Note No. 61.

Rolaids - Extra Strength **-** Pfizer, Inc.
Each tablet contains: Calcium Carbonate (providing Calcium 271 mg) 675 mg • Magnesium Hydroxide (providing Magnesium 56 mg) 135 mg •Calcium Carbonate 675 mg •Magnesium Hydroxide 135 mg. Other Ingredients: Dextrose, Magnesium Stearate, Polyethylene Glycol, Pregelatinized Starch, Sucrose.

Roman Chamomile Pure Essential Oil **-** Nature's Sunshine
Chamaemelum Nobile oil.

Roniot Super **-** Hadas Natural Products
Each lozenge contains: Propolis standardized extract 125 mg • Echinacea Purpurea standardized extract 125 mg • Vitamin C 12.5 mg.

Root Food II **-** Life Enhancement Products, Inc.
Each capsule contains: Vitamin A (as beta-carotene) 1250 IU • Vitamin C (as ascorbic acid and niacinamide ascorbate) 375 mg • Vitamin D (as cholecalciferol) 50 mg • Vitamin E (as D,L-alpha-tocopheryl acetate) 25 mg • Thiamine (vitamin B1 as thiamine hydrochloride) 1.2 mg • Riboflavin (vitamin B2) 40 mg • Niacin (vitamin B3 as niacin and niacinamide ascorbate) 40 mg • Vitamin B6 (as pyridoxine hydrochloride) 1 mg • Folic Acid 100 mcg • Vitamin B12 (cyanocobalamin) 25 mcg • Biotin 250 mcg • Pantothenic Acid (vitamin B5 as calcium pantothenate) 20.7 mg • Calcium (as calcium pantothenate) 33 mg • Zinc (as zinc gluconate) 3.8 mg • Selenium (as sodium selenite) 6.25 mcg • Copper (as copper gluconate) 250 mcg • Manganese (as manganese gluconate) 250 mcg • Chromium (as chromium aspartate) 25 mcg • L-Cysteine Hydrochloride 175 mg • Taurine 63 mg • Inositol 25 mg.

Roplex **-** Medspan Laboratories
Each tablet contains: Proprietary Blend 600 mg: Scandenavian Flower Pollen, Saw Palmetto. Other Ingredients: Gelatin, Rice Flour, Dicalcium Phosphate, MCC, Stearic Acid, Crosscarmellose Sodium, Silica, Opedry 2 ns, Magnesium Stearate.

Rose-Hip C 1000 mg **-** J. R. Carlson Laboratories, Inc.
Each tablet contains: Vitamin C (as ascorbic acid) 100 mg • Rose Hips fruit powder (rosa L spp) 150 mg.

RosemarinX brand **-** Xymogen
Proprietary Rosemary extract.
See Editor's Note No. 44.

Rosemary **-** Nature's Way
Two capsules contain: Rosemary herb 800 mg. Other Ingredients: Gelatin, Magnesium Stearate.

RoseOx **-** Herbalife International of America, Inc.
Each tablet contains: Calcium (as calcium carbonate) 140 mg • Exclusive Herbal Blend 620 mg: Dried Rosemary leaf extract (RoseOx brand), Cruciferous Vegetable Concentrate: Broccoli, Cauliflower, Cabbage and Carrot extracts, Dried Turmeric root extract, Tomato concentrate, Sage leaf, Cloves flower. Other Ingredients: Corn Starch, Croscarmellose Sodium, Stearic Acid, Silicon Dioxide, Magnesium Stearate, Microcrystalline Cellulose, Sodium Carboxymethylcellulose, Dextrin, Dextrose, Soy Lecithin, Carnauba Wax, Sodium Citrate.

RoseOx **-** Natrol, Inc.
One capsule contains: Rosemary dried powdered extract leaf 250 mg. Other Ingredients: Rice powder, Magnesium Stearate, Gelatin.

Rosy Lucidity II **-** Life Enhancement Products, Inc.
Each capsule contains: Rhodiola Rosea (minimum 4% rosavins, 3% salidroside) 112.5 mg.

Some Brand Name Natural Products - What they Contain

www.NaturalDatabase.com contains MANY more listings than appear here.
Editor's Notes are located on pages 2155-2163.

BRAND NAMES

Rovicid **-** Berkeley Premium Nutraceuticals
Each tablet contains: Prostate Functional Blend 300 mg: Nettle leaf, Saw Palmetto berry extract, Pygeum bark, Pumpkin seed extract, Swedish Flower Pollen extract, Lycopene • Colon Health Blend 425 mg: Alfalfa leaf, Licorice root, Senna leaf, Ginger root, Psyllium husk, Oat Bran, Fennel seed, Anise seed • Sexual Response Blend 410 mg: Panax Ginseng root extract, Horny Goat Weed extract, L-Arginine HCl, Tribulus Terrestris fruit and root, Maca powder, Catuaba bark extract. Other Ingredients: Dicalcium Phosphate, Microcrystalline Cellulose, Croscarmellose Sodium, Stearic Acid, Magnesium Stearate, Silica, Pharmaceutical Glaze.
See Editor's Note No. 60.

Royal Bee Power **-** Nature's Plus
Two tablets contain: Bee Pollen 500 mg • Propolis from extract 500 mg Royal Jelly 50 mg. In a high energy natural base containing Gotu Kola, Ginseng & Fo-Ti.

Royal Brittany Evening Primrose Oil **-** American Health
Each softgel contains: Evening Primrose oil 500 mg: Cis-Linoleic Acid (LA) 350 mg, Gamma-Linolenic Acid (GLA) 350 mg. Other Ingredients: Gelatin, Glycerin.

Royal Jelly **-** DreamPharm
Each capsule contains: Royal Jelly (1.6% extract) 300 mg • Atractylodes Macrocephala 100 mg • Radix Dioscoreae Oppositae 100 mg.

Royal Silk Lotion (Royal Image Cosmetics) **-** InterPlexus
Aloe Barbadensis gel • Olive extract • Olive Squalane • Shea butter • Rose Hip oil • Olive oil • Coconut oil • Glycerin • Extracts Blend: Arnica, Comfrey, Ginkgo, Ginseng, Bioflavonoids • Hyaluronic Acid • Myrrh extract • Allantoin • Natural Gums • Natural Essences • Glucose Stearate • Tocopherol (vitamin E) • Retinyl Palmitate (vitamin A) • Cholecalciferol (vitamin D3) • Citric Acid.

Royaldophilus **-** Young Living Essential Oils
Each capsule contains: Plantain • Lemon Pectin • Magnesium Stearate • 250 Million Lactobacillus and Bifidus Cultures • Gelatin.

RTD 40 Advanced Mega Protein Shake **-** Nutripeak
Each can contains: Protein 40 g • Vitamin A (Retinyl Palmitate) 5000 IU • Vitamin C (Ascorbic Acid) 24 mg • Calcium Caseinate 24 mg • Iron (Ferrous Fumarate) 2.7 mg • Vitamin D (Cholecalciferol) 60 IU • Vitamin E (dl-Alpha Tocopheryl Acetate) 51 IU • Vitamin K (Phytonadione) 8 mcg • Thiamin Mononitrate 0.225 mg • Riboflavin 0.225 mg • Niacin (Niacinamide) 5 mg • Vitamin B6 (Pyridoxine Hydrochloride) 0.3 mg • Folic Acid 100 mcg • Vitamin B12 (Cyanocobalamin) 0.6 mcg • Biotin 45 mcg • Pantothenic Acid (Calcium D-Pantothenate) 1 mg • Phosphorus (Dipotassium Phosphorus and Potassium Triphosphate) 700 mg • Iodine (Potassium Iodide) 15 mcg • Magnesium Oxide 140 mg • Zinc Oxide 4.5 mg • Selenium (Sodium Selenate) 7 mcg • Copper (Cupric Sulfate) 0.2 mg • Manganese Sulfate 0.2 mg • Chromium Picolinate 12 mcg • Molybdenum (Sodium Molybdate) 15 mcg. Other Ingredients: Water; Metamyosyn V4 Protein Blend: Milk Protein Concentrate, Milk Protein Isolate, Calcium Sodium Casseinate, Hydrolyzed Wheat Protein (Gluten), Maltodextrin, High Fat Cocoa (processed with alkali); Sodium Phosphate; Sodium Citrate; Sodium Polyphosphate; Beta Carotene; Natural and Artificial Flavors; Microcrystalline Cellulose, Canola Oil, Soy Lecithin, Citric Acid, Sodium Carboxymethylcellulose, Salt, Carrageenan, Sucralose, Polysorbate 80, Dimethylpolysiloxane.

R-Throherb **-** Wild Rose
Each tablet contains: Devil's Claw root 175 mg • Red Clover blossom 75 mg • Yucca root 125 mg.

RU-21 **-** Spirit Sciences USA
Two tablets contain: Vitamin C 50 mg • Succinic Acid 200 mg • Fumaric Acid 75 mg • L-Glutamine 200 mg. Other Ingredients: Glucose (Dextrose).

Rubus-Ginger Tea **-** HerbaSway
Ginger • Green Tea • Blackberry • HerbaSwee (Cucurbitaceae fruit).

Rudofil **-** Berkeley Premium Nutraceuticals
Two caplets contain: Glucosamine HCl 1500 mg • Trans-Resveratrol 5 mg • COX-II Inhibitor Blend 675 mg: Feverfew leaf extract (0.2% parthenolide) 250 mg, Hops standardized extract 160 mg, Turmeric rhizome 40 mg. Other Ingredients: Dicalcium Phosphate, Microcrystalline Cellulose, Croscarmellose Sodium, Stearic Acid, Magnesium Stearate, Silica, Film Coat Ingredients (hypromellose, hydroxypropyl cellulose, polyethylene glycol with colors to be determined).

Rumalaya Cream **-** The Himalaya Drug Company
Karpoora oil (cinnamomum camphora) • Putiha oil (mentah arvensis) • Sarala oil (pinus roxburghii) • Thwak oil (cinnamomum zeylanicum syn. c.verum) • Tila Taila oil (sesamum indicum). Base: q.s. ad.

Rumalaya DS Tablets **-** The Himalaya Drug Company
Each tablet contains: Mahayograj Guggul 0.324 g • Shankh Bhasma (conch shell) 130 mg • Shilajeet (mineral pitch, purified) 32 mg • Latakasthuri (abelmoschus moshatus) 20 mg • Swarnamakshik Bhasma (chalcopyrites calx) 10 mg • Maharasnadi Quath 130 mg • Manjishtha (rubia cordifolia) 38 mg • Shigru (moringa pterygosperma) 32 mg • Gokshura (tribulus terrestris) 32 mg.

Rumalaya Forte Tablets **-** The Himalaya Drug Company
Each tablet contains: Shallaki (boswellia serrata) 240 mg • Guggulu Suddha (commiphora wightii) 200 mg • Rasna (alpinia galanga) 70 mg • Yashti-Madhu (glycyrrhiza glabra) 70 mg • Gokshura (tribulus terrestris) 60 mg • Guduchi (tinospora cordifolia) 60 mg.

Rumalaya Gel **-** The Himalaya Drug Company
Nirgundi (vitex negundo) 7.5 mg • Devadaru (cedrus deodara) 7.5 mg • Sunthi (zingiber officinale) 7.5 mg • Shallaki (boswellia serrata) 7.5 mg • Pudina (mentha arvensis) 60 mg • Tvak (cinnamomum zeylanicum) 30 mg • Sarala (pinus roxburghii) 55 mg • Gandhapura Taila (gaultheria fragrantissima) 55 mg • Base q.s. ad 770 mg.

Rumaplex **-** Standard Process, Inc.
Three capsules contain: Proprietary Blend 1075 mg: Nutritional Yeast, Bovine Bone, Magnesium Citrate, Dried Buckwheat leaf juice, Buckwheat seed, Veal Bone PMG extract, Dried Pea vine juice, Betaine Hydrochloride, Bovine Adrenal, Soy bean, Bovine Prostate Cytosol extract, Defatted Wheat germ, Oat flour, Carrot root, Veal Bone meal, Bovine Liver PMG extract, Bovine Spleen, Ovine Spleen, Bovine Liver, Licorice root, Dried Beet leaf juice, Peanut bran, Manganese Glycerophosphate, Enzymatically processed Tillandsia Usneoides, Beet root • Vitamin A 775 IU • Vitamin C 2.5 mg • Niacin 2.7 mg • Calcium 34 mg • Sodium 15 mg • Potassium 25 mg. Other Ingredients: Gelatin, Water, Colors.
See Editor's Note No. 14.

Runners' Shield **-** Source Naturals
Two tablets contain: Vitamin A (Beta Carotene 12,500 IU and Palmitate 5,000 IU) 17,500 IU • Vitamin C (Magnesium Ascorbate, Ascorbic Acid and Manganese Ascorbate) 500 mg • Fat-Soluble Vitamin C (from 186 mg of Ascorbyl Palmitate) 80 mg • Vitamin E (Natural d-alpha) 200 IU • Magnesium (Ascorbate) 30 mg • Zinc (OptiZinc Monomethionine) 15 mg • Manganese (Ascorbate) 5 mg • Copper (Sebacate) 750 mcg • Selenium (Selenomethionine) 100 mcg • Quercetin 200 mg • N-Acetyl-Cysteine 100 mg • Silymarin (Milk Thistle Seed Extract) 50 mg • Ginkgo Biloba extract 24% (50:1) 5 mg • Hawthorn Berry extract (4:1) 150 mg • Rosemary 150 mg • Schizandra 125 mg • Marshmallow root 85 mg • Astragalus 60 mg.

Russian Bear 5000 Weight Gainer **-** Vitol
Three Stage Carbohydrate Mix- (glucose polymers) Containing Complex • Medium Chain and Simple Carbohydrates • Pharmaceutical Grade Protein Blend: Non-Fat Milk Solids, Hydrolyzed Egg White (albumin) • Medium Chain Triglycerides • Vitamin, Mineral, Lipotropic Mixture (which includes Kreb's Cycle complexes) • Yohimbe bark • Eleutherococcus • Crystaline Fructose • Sika Deer Antler powder • Schizandra Chinensis • Inosine HXR • Colostrum • Boron • Chromium Picolinate • Natural Vanilla Flavor.

Some Brand Name Natural Products - What they Contain

www.NaturalDatabase.com contains MANY more listings than appear here.
Editor's Notes are located on pages 2155-2163.

Rutin 500 mg - GNC
Each tablet contains: Rutin 500 mg. Other Ingredients: Calcium Sulfate, Cellulose.

Rutin 500 mg - Nature's Plus
Each tablet contains: Rutin (from saphora japonica leaf) 500 mg. Other Ingredients: Microcrystalline Cellulose, Stearic Acid, Silica, Magnesium Stearate, Pharmaceutical Glaze.

Rutin-Quercetin - J. R. Carlson Laboratories, Inc.
Each tablet contains: Quercetin (from rutin) 250 mg • Rutin (from fava D. anta) 500 mg.

Rutozym - Wobenzym USA
Two tablets contain: Nattokinase (20,000 IU/gm) 25 mg • Bromelain (2450 GDU/gm) 90 mg • Papain N F (2400 USP units/mg) 100 mg • Rutin Bioflavonoid Copmlex 120 mg • White Willow Bark extract 100 mg. Other Ingredients: Plant Fiber, Povidone, Modified Cellulose Gum, Colloidal Silica, Titanium Dioxide Mineral, Vegetable Stearic Acid, pH Resistant Enteric Coating.

R-U-Ved Energy Tea - R-U Ved U.S.A.
Green Tea • Ginger • Ashwagandha • Bacopa Monnieri • Centella Asiatica • Cinnamon • Cardamom.

Rx for Life Cellular Essentials Pack (Bio-C) - Rexall - Sundown
Each tablet contains: Vitamin C (from ascorbyl palmitate, calcium ascorbate, magnesium ascorbate and ascorbic acid) 300 mg • Citrus Bioflavonoids 75 mg. Other Ingredients: Cellulose, Stearic Acid, Crospovidone, Croscarmellose Sodium, Silica, Magnesium Stearate.

Rx Fuel Bio-Designed Food Formula - TwinLab
Two servings contain: Branched Chain Amino Acids (L-Leucine, L-Isoleucine, L-Valine) • L-Glutamine 1000 mg • L-Carnitine 100 mg • Chromium (from Chromic Fuel Chromium Picolinate) 200 mcg.

Rx-Bone Ostivone - Nutritional Dynamics
Two tablets contain: Vitamin D 100 IU • Calcium 1000 mg • Ostivone 200 mg. Other Ingredients: Dicalcium Phosphate, Microcrystalline Cellulose, Silica, Stearic Acid, Pharmaceutical glaze.

S.O.D. - Lifewise
Each capsule contains: GliSODin brand complex 250 mg: SOD (superoxide dismutase), Gliadin.

S-4 (Sleep Enabler) - Oasis Wellness Network
Each capsule contains: Calcium (citrate, carbonate, phosphate) 61 mg • Magnesium (citrate) 11 mg • Niacin (niacinamide ascorbate) 25 mg • Valerian root extract 133 mg • Jujube roasted seed extract 133 mg • MaxCell Proprietary Blend 7 mg: Zisyphus Jujube, Aloe Vera gel, Piper Nigrum, Glycyrrhiza Glabra • Chamomile flower extract 20 mg • Kava Kava root stock extract 7 mg • Melatonin 0.2 mg. Other Ingredients: Cellulose, Magnesium Stearate, Silica.

Sabasol - Magistral Biotech
Each 1 tbsp serving contains: Proprietary Standardized Synergic Complex Blend 2900 mg: Saw Palmetto berry, Nettle root (urtica dioica), Asian Ginseng root, Ginkgo Biloba leaf, Suma root. Other Ingredients: Spring Water, Glycerine, Natural Flavours.

Saccharomyces Boulardii - Jarrow Formulas
Each tablet contains: Saccharomyces Boulardii (a subspecies of S. cerevisiae, 1.5 billion live cells at time of manufacture) 1.5 billion organisms • Bio-MOS brand MannanOligoSaccharide (derived from S. cerevisiae, souce of MOS) 200 mg. Other Ingredients: Maltodextrin, Magnesium Stearate, Ascorbic Acid, Gelatin.

Saccharomyces boulardii - Pure Encapsulations
Each vegetable capsule contains: Saccharomyces Boulardii (approximately 5 billion live cells per capsule) 250 mg.

SAF for Kids - Natrol, Inc.
Six capsules contain: Vitamin C (Ester-C brand) 60 mg • Calcium 100 mg • Vitamin B6 (pyridoxine HCl) 50 mg • Magnesium 50 mg • Additional Ingredients: GABA 800 mg • Glycine 800 mg • Passion flower extract 6:1 500 mg • L-Taurine 500 mg • Other Ingredients: Microcrystalline Cellulose, Magnesium Stearate, Gelatin.

SAF The Stress Formula - Natrol, Inc.
Four capsules contain: Vitamin C (Ester-C Brand) 100 mg • Thiamine (Vitamin B1) 3 mg • Riboflavin (Vitamin B2) 3.1 mg • Niacin (Niacinamide) 50 mg, • Vitamin B6 (Pyridoxine HCl) 4 mg • Magnesium 100 mg • GABA 650 mg • L-Tyrosine 650 mg • Siberian Ginseng 100 mg • Inositol 100 mg, Patent #4,973,467. Other Ingredients: Calcium Carbonate, Magnesium Stearate, Microcrystalline Cellulose, Gelatin.

Safeway Select Women's One Tablet Multivitamin - Safeway, Inc.
Each tablet contains: Vitamin A (50% as beta carotene) 5000 IU • Vitamin C 60 mg • Vitamin D 400 IU • Vitamin E 30 IU • Thiamin 1.5 mg • Riboflavin 1.7 mg • Niacin 20 mg • Vitamin B-6 2 mg • Folate 400 mcg • Vitamin B-12 6 mcg • Pantothenic Acid 10 mg • Calcium 450 mg • Iron 27 mg • Zinc 15 mg.

Sage - Motherlove Herbal Co.
Each 2 oz bottle contains: Sage. Base: Certified Kosher Alcohol, Glycerin.

Sage Leaf 285 mg - Vitamin World
Each capsule contains: Sage leaf (salvia officinails) 570 mg. Other Ingredients: Gelatin.

Sage Oil - NOW Foods
100% Pure Sage Oil (Salvia officinalis) USP.

Sage Tincture - American Health
100% Organic Sage (Salvia officinalis) tincture. Other Ingredients: R/O Water, 12-24% Alcohol.

Salad-Tabs - Wakunaga of America
Two tablets contain: Vitamin A (as palmitate & beta-carotene) 5000 IU • Vitamin C (as asorbic acid) 60 mg • Vitamin D (as cholecalciferol) 400 IU • Vitamin E (as d-alpha-tocopherol acid succinate) 30 IU • Thiamine (vitamin B1) 1.5 mg • Riboflavin (vitamin B2) 1.7 mg • Niacin 20 mg • Vitamin B6 (as pyridoxine hydrochloride) 2 mg • Folate (as folic acid) 400 mcg • Vitamin B12 (as cyanocobalamin) 6 mcg • Biotin 300 mcg • Pantothenic Acid (as calcium pantothenate) 10 mg • Iron (as ferrous fumarate) 18 mg • Iodine (as potassium iodide) 150 mcg • Zinc (as zinc oxide) 15 mg • Copper (as copper gluconate) 2 mg • Manganese (as manganese sulfate) 2 mg • Young Barley and Wheat Grass powder 600 mg • Chlorella 180 mg. Other Ingredients: Cellulose, Silica, Magnesium Stearate (vegetable source).

Salmix Pastilles - Functional Products
Each pastille contains: Ammonium Chloride 8 g • Succus Liquorice 12 g. Other Ingredients: Wheat Flour, Saccarose, Medical Coal, Glucose Syrup, Anise Oil, Shellac.

Salmon Oil - GNC
Each capsule contains: EPA (Eicosapentaenoic Acid) 180 mg • DHA (Docosahexaenoic Acid) 120 mg. Other Ingredients: Gelatin, Glycerin.

Salmon Oil - Puritan's Pride
Two softgels contain: EPA 240 mg • DHA 160 mg.

Salmon Oil 1000 mg - Jamieson
Each capsule contains: EPA (Eicosapentaenoic Acid) 180 mg • DHA (Docosahexaenoic Acid) 120 mg.

Salmon Oil and GLA - J. R. Carlson Laboratories, Inc.
Each softgel contains: Vitamin E (as D-alpha tocopherol) 10 IU • Omega-3 Fatty Acids (from fish oil) 260 mg • GLA (gamma linolenic acid) 40 mg • DHA (docosahexaenoic acid) 80 mg • EPA (eicosapenatenoic acid) 120 mg.

Salonpas - Hisamitsu Pharmaceutical Co., Inc.
Active Ingredients: Methyl Salicylate 132 mg • l-Menthol 120 mg • DL-Camphor 26 mg • Tocopherol Acetate 21 mg.

Some Brand Name Natural Products - What they Contain

www.NaturalDatabase.com contains MANY more listings than appear here.
Editor's Notes are located on pages 2155-2163.

Saloxicin - Xymogen
Each capsule contains: Salicin from 400 mg of White Willow bark (standardized to 30% salicin) 120 mg • Boswellic Acids from 320 mg of Boswellia Serrata (standardized to 65% boswellic acids) 280 mg • Berr-X brand Berry extract, standardized to 30% polyphenols 12 mg.

SaluGuard Tonic for Men - Flora Inc.
Each 20 mL serving contains: Proprietary aqueous extracts blend 662 mg: Bilberry fruit (vaccinium myrtillus) • Pumpkin seed (cucurbita pepo) • Ginseng root (Panax ginseng) • Nettle herb (urtica dioica) • Saw Palmetto fruit (serenoa serrulata) • Hawthorn berry (crataegus oxyacantha) • Artichoke leaf (cynara scolymus) • Dandelion herb (taraxacum officinale) • Ginkgo leaf (gingko biloba) • Grape Seed extract. Other Ingredients: Pear juice concentrate, Guava pulp, Orange juice concentrate, Mango concentrate, Passion Fruit juice, and Locust seed gum.

SaluGuard Tonic for Women - Flora Inc.
Each 20 mL contains: Proprietary aqueous extracts blend 518.27 mg: Bilberry fruit (vaccinium myrtillis), Ginseng root (Panax ginseng), Horse Chestnut leaves (hippocastani folium), Green Oat (avena sativa), Hawthorn berry (crataegus oxyacantha), Artichoke leaf (cynara scolymus), Ginkgo leaf (ginkgo biloba), Dandelion herb (taraxacum officinale), Horsetail herb (equisetum pratense), Black Cohosh root (cimicfuga racemosa), Red Clover blossom (trifolium pratense), Grape Seed extract (vitis vinifera). Other Ingredients: Pear Juice Concentrate, Guava Pulp, Orange Juice Concentrate, Mango Concentrate, Passion Fruit Juice, Locust Seed Gum.

Salusan Herbal Rest - Flora Inc.
St. John's Wort • Passion Flower • Valerian "& other calming herbs."

SAM 200 mg - Solgar
Each tablet contains: SAMe (as S-adenosyl-L-methionine) 200 mg. Other Ingredients: Vegetable Cellulose, Mannitol, Citric Acid, Sodium Starch, Glycinate, Triacetate, Croscarmellose Sodium, Vegetable Stearic Acid, Silica.

Sambu - Flora Inc.
Elderberry.

Sambucol Black Elder - Nature's Way
Each lozenge contains: Vitamin C (as ascorbic acid) 100 mg • Elderberry dried extract (berries) 130 mg. Other Ingredients: Sorbitol, Peppermint extract.

Sambucol Black Elderberry Extract - Nature's Way
Two teaspoons contain: Elderberry extract 3.8 g. Other Ingredients: Glucose Syrup, Raspberry Extract, Honey, Citric Acid, Natural Flavor.

Sambucol Black Elderberry Sugar Free Extract - Nature's Way
Two teaspoons contain: Sambucol patented Black Elderberry extract 3.8 g. Other Ingredients: Citric Acid, Raspberry Extract, Sorbitol, Water.

Sambucol for Kids - Nature's Way
Each 2 tsp serving contains: Proprietary Blend 1.93 g: Echinacea Angustifolia root, Echinacea Purpurea (stem, leaf, flower), Propolis, Sambucol patented Black Elderberry extract. Other Ingredients: Citric Acid, Glucose Syrup, Raspberry extract.

Sambucol Immune System - Nature's Way
Two teaspoons (10 mL) contain: Zinc 10 mg • Vitamin C 100 mg • Proprietary blend 4 g: Elderberry extract, Propolis, Echinacea Angustifolia root, Echinacea purpurea (stem, leaf, flower). Other Ingredients: Glucose syrup, Raspberry Extract, Honey, Citric Acid, Natural Flavors.

Sambucol Immune System Formula - Nature's Way
Two teaspoons contain: Proprietary Blend 4 g: Echinacea Angustifolia root, Echinacea Purpurea (stem, leaf, flower), Propolis, Sambucol patented Black Elderberry extract • Vitamin C 100 mg • Zinc Gluconate 10 mg. Other Ingredients: Citric Acid, Glucose Syrup, Honey, Raspberry Extract.

Sambucol Immune System Formula Lozenges - Nature's Way
Each lozenge contains: Proprietary Blend: Echinacea Purpurea (stem, leaf, flower), Sambucol patented Black Elderberry extract, Vitamin C, Zinc Gluconate. Other Ingredients: Peppermint Extract, Sorbitol.

Sambucol Lozenges - Nature's Way
Each lozenge contains: Sambucol patented Black Elderberry extract 130 mg • Vitamin C 100 mg. Other Ingredients: Peppermint Extract, Sorbitol.

Sambucol Original - Nature's Way
Each lozenge contains: Black Elder Tree extract (sambucus nigra).

Sambucol-D (Sugar Free) - Nature's Way
Each tablespoon contains: Elderberry juice (Black Elder tree, sambucus nigra 1). Other Ingredients: Liquid sorbitol, water, citric acid, natural flavor, & raspberry.

SambuGuard - Flora Inc.
Elder flower (sambucus nigra) • Elderberries (sambucus nigra) • Echinacea 22:1 concentrate • Vitamin C (ascorbic acid) • Acerola Cherry powder (malpighia punicifola) • Honey.

SAMe - NutraLife
Each tablet contains: S-adenosyl-methionine tosylate disulfate 200 mg.

SAMe - Olympian Labs
Each tablet contains: SAMe (S-adenosyl-L-methionine-tosylate-disulfate) 200 mg.

SAMe - Natrol, Inc.
Two tablets contain: S-Adenosyl-Methionine (SAMe) (as S-Adenosyl-Methionine Disulfate Ditosylate) 400 mg. Other Ingredients: Cellulose, Mannitol, Hydroxypropyl Methylcellulose Phthalate, Citric Acid, Sodium Starch Glycolate, Glyceryl Triacetate, Croscarmellose Sodium, Stearic Acid, Silica.

SAMe - Ortho Molecular Products
Each tablet contains: Vitamin C (as ascorbic acid USP) < 1 mg • Vitamin B6 (as pyridoxine HCl) 2 mg • Folic Acid 200 mcg • Vitamin B12 (as cyanocobalamin) 50 mcg • SAMe (as S-adenosyl-L-methionine disulfate tosylate) 200 mg. Other Ingredients: Cellulose, Citric Acid, Croscarmellose Sodium, Stearic Acid, Silica, Methacrylic Acid, Magnesium Stearate, Triethyl Citrate.

SAMe - Source Naturals
Two tablets contain: SAMe (S-Adenosyl-L-Methionine) from 800 mg of SAMe Disulfate Tosylate 400 mg.

SAM-e - DaVinci Laboratories
Each tablet contains: S-Adenosylmethionine Tosylate Disulfate (yields 200 mg S-adenosylmethionine) 400 mg. Other Ingredients: Cellulose, Mannitol, Hydroxypropylmethyl-Cellulose, Citric Acid, Sodium Starch Glycolate, Glyceryl Triacetate, Croscarmellose Sodium, Stearic Acid, Silica.

SAM-e - TwinLab
Two tablets contain: SAMe (S-adenosylmethionine tosylate) 400 mg. Other Ingredients: Cellulose, Mannitol, Hydroxypropyl Methylcellulose, Citric Acid, Sodium Starch, Glycolate, Glyceryl Triacetate, Croscarmellose Sodium, Stearic Acid.

SAM-e - The Vitamin Shoppe
Two tablets contain: S-Adenosyl-L-Methionine 400 mg. Other Ingredients: Colloidal Silica, Microcrystalline Cellulose, Sodium Starch Glycolate, Magnesium Stearate, Methacrylic Acid Copolymer, Polyethylene Glycol, Simethicone, Polysorbate 80, Sodium Hydroxide, Magnesium Silicate, Iron Oxide.

SAM-e - Quest
Each caplet contains: S-adenosyl-methionine tosylate (providing 50 mg S-adenosyl-methionine) 100 mg. Other Ingredients: Croscarmellose Sodium, Microcrystalline Cellulose, Calcium Phosphate, Vegetable Stearin, Magnesium Stearate.

BRAND NAMES

Some Brand Name Natural Products - What they Contain

www.NaturalDatabase.com contains MANY more listings than appear here.
Editor's Notes are located on pages 2155-2163.

Sam-e **-** Vitamin World
Two tablets contain: S-adenosylmethionine 400 mg. Other Ingredients: Cellulose (plant origin), Croscarmellose, Polymethacrylate, Silica, Magnesium Stearate, Triethyl Citrate, Vegetable Stearic Acid, Citric Acid, Ascorbic Acid, Riboflavin.

SAMe 100mg **-** GNC
Each tablet contains: S-Adenosyl-Methionine (SAMe) 100 mg. Other Ingredients: Microcrystalline Cellulose, Magnesium Stearate, Talc, Metacrylic Copolymer.

SAM-e 200 **-** Jarrow Formulas
Each tablet contains: S-Adenosyl Methionine (from 400 mg of SAM-e tosylate disulfate) 200 mg. Other Ingredients: Microcrystalline Cellulose, Methacrylate Copolymers, Glycerol Behenate, Magnesium Silicate, Triethyl Citrate, Magnesium Stearate, Mannitol, Titanium Dioxide, Yellow Ochre.

SAM-e 200 mg **-** Pro Health
Each tablet contains: SAM-e (S-adenosyl-L-methionine, from 400 mg disulphate tosylate) 200 mg. Other Ingredients: Cellulose, Mannitol, Hydroxypropyl Methylcellulose Phthalate, Citric Acid, Sodium Starch Glycolate, Glyceryl Triacetate, Croscarmellose Sodium, Magnesium Stearate, Silica.

SAM-e 400 mg **-** Pro Health
Each tablet contains: SAM-e (S-adenosyl-L-methionine, from 800 mg disulfate tosylate) 400 mg. Other Ingredients: Cellulose, Croscarmellose Sodium, Methacrylic Acid, Magnesium Stearate, Silica, Triethyl Citrate, Stearic Acid, Citric Acid, Asbcorbic Acid.

SAMe Extra Strength Super Size **-** Olympian Labs
Each tablet contains: SAMe (S-adenosyl-L-methionine-tosylate-disulfate) 400 mg.

SAMe Supersize **-** Olympian Labs
Each tablet contains: SAMe (s-adenosyl-l-methionine-tosylate-disulfate) 200 mg.

Samento 600 mg **-** NutraMedix
Each capsule contains: Cat's Claw bark (uncaria tomentosa, POA [pentacyclic oxindole alkaloids] 3 mg) 600 mg. Other Ingredients: Rice Bran Powder, Gelatin Capsule, Magnesium Stearate.

Samento Extract **-** NutraMedix
Five drops contain: Proprietary Blend 0.25 mL: Cat's Claw bark, Cat's Claw (TOA-free) extract, Mineral Water, Ethanol.

Samento Plus **-** NutraMedix
Each capsule contains: Cat's Claw bark (uncaria tomentosa [POA pentacyclic oxindole alkalodis 1.87 mg] 375 mg • Magnesium (From 150 mg of magnesium malate) 18.9 mg • Manganese (as manganese citrate) 30 mcg • Chromium (as chromium polynicotinate) 5 mcg • Malic Acid (from 150 mg magnesium malate) 103 mg • Protease 30,000 HUT • Cellulose 1600 CU. Other Ingredients: Bamboo Fiber, Hypromellose (vegetable capsule).

Sandal Turmeric (soap) **-** Auromere
Coconut oil • Palmyra oil • Rice Bran oil • Alkali • Water • Hydnocarpus oil (cactus) • Castor oil • Neem oil • Indian Beech oil • Mohwa oil (madhuca indica) • Sesame oil • Sandalwood oil • Neem bark • Dhub grass (cynodon dactylon) • Indian Gooseberry (amla) • Turmeric • Peepal (bodhi tree) • Licorice • Celastrus seed • Tulsi (holy basil) • Corallacarpus Epigaeus • Nutgrass • Zedoary • Indian Madder root • Costus • Mung bean • Fenugreek.

Sandalwood Essential Oil **-** Golden Glow Natural Health Products
Santalum Spicatum stem, wood and root essential oil.

Sandelios Beauty Caps **-** Health From The Sun
Each capsule contains: Wheat Germ oil 150 mg • Yeast 50 mg • Vitamin E (d-Alpha Tocopherol) 10 mg • Nicotinamide 10 mg • Vitamin B2 1 mg • Calcium D-Pantothenate 6.5 mg • Vitamin B1 1.2 mg • Vitamin B6 1 mg • Carotin 0.8 mg • D-Biotin 20 mcg • Vitamin B12 2 mcg.

Sandelios Garlic Caps **-** Health From The Sun
Each capsule contains: Garlic oil with Allicin 270 mg.

Sango Caps Coral Calcium **-** The Coral Connection
Two vegetable capsules contain: Coral Calcium Complex (75 trace minerals & elements) 1000 • Calcium (coral calcium/calcium carbonate) 250 mg • Magnesium (coral calcium/magnesium carbonate) 125 mg • Vitamin D (D3) 800 IU • Vitamin E 120 IU • Vitamin C (calcium ascorbate) 60 mg • Chromium (polynicotinate) 120 mcg • Zinc (monomethionine) 15 mg • Iodine (kelp) 15 mcg • Selenium 70 mcg • Copper 2 mg • Manganese 2 mg • Molybdenum 75 mcg • Rubidium (as amino acid chelate) 30 mcg • Vanadium (as amino acid chelate) 60 mcg • Boron (as amino acid chelate) 40 mcg • Silver (as silver nitrate) 10 mcg • Nickel (as amino acid chelate) 20 mcg • Betaine HCl 5 mg • Malic Acid 10 mg.

Sanhelios Circu Caps with Butcher's Broom **-** Health From The Sun
Each capsule contains: natural Rusci Aculeati (Butcher's Broom) extract 75 mg • Rosemary oil 2 mg.

Sanhelios Devil's Claw Caps **-** Health From The Sun
Each capsule contains: natural Devil's Claw extract 120 mg.

Sanhelios Garlic Forte **-** Health From The Sun
Each gelcap contains: Garlic oil, Maceration 2-3:1, 280 mg.

Sanhelios Kalm Caps **-** Health From The Sun
Each capsule contains: Valerian root extract 4:1 150 mg.

Sanhelios Onion Caps **-** Health From The Sun
Each capsule contains: natural etherial Onion oil from Allium Cepa Linne 1.5 mg.

Sanhelios Propolentum Capsules **-** Health From The Sun
Each capsule contains: Propolis 250 mg.

Sanhelios Propolentum Throat Lozenges **-** Health From The Sun
Each lozenge contains: Isomalt 1465 mg • Menthol Crystals 3 mg • Propolis powder 30 mg • Peppermint oil 2 mg.

Sanhelios Prosta Caps **-** Health From The Sun
Each capsule contains: Pumpkin seed oil with Cucurbitin 150 mg • Alpha-Tocopherolacetate equalling 40.8 IU • Vitamin E 30 mg.

Sanhelios Water Caps **-** Health From The Sun
Each capsule contains: natural Juniper berry oil 20 mg.

Satiet-ease **-** Pure Encapsulations
Two vegetable capsules contain: Relora brand Proprietary Blend 250 mg: Magnolia Officinalis bark extract, Phellodendron Amurense bark extract • Rhodiola Rosea root extract (standardized to contain 3% total rosavins and min. 1% salidrosides) 100 mg • L-Tyrosine (free-form) 800 mg • Vitamin C (as ascorbyl palmitate) 20 mg. Other Ingredients: Modified Food and Corn Starch, Silicon Dioxide.

Satietrol **-** PacificHealth Laboratories, Inc.
Each packet (18 g) contains: Casein from Whey Protein Isolate (enriched with glycomacropeptides) • Potato Fiber • Sunflower Oil • Corn Syrup Solids • Natural & Artificial Flavors • Konjac Flour • Maltodextrin • Guar Gum • Calcium Lactate • Sodium Caseinate • Soy Lecithin • Alfalfa Powder • Monoglycerides • Diglycerides • Dipotassium Phosphate • Sodium Silicoaluminate • Aspartame.

Saventaro **-** Enzymatic Therapy/PhytoPharmica
Each capsule contains: POA Cat's Claw root extract (uncaria tomentosa, pentacyclic chemotype, standardized to contain a minimum of 1.3% pentacyclic oxindole alkaloids) 20 mg. Other Ingredients: Cellulose, Calcium Carbonate, Gelatin, Magnesium Stearate, Silicon Dioxide, Titanium Dioxide Color.

Saw Palmetto **-** EcoNugenics
Each softgel contains: Saw Palmetto extract (85% fatty acids, esterols) 320 mg. Other Ingredients: Gelatin, Glycerin, Water.

Some Brand Name Natural Products - What they Contain

www.NaturalDatabase.com contains MANY more listings than appear here.
Editor's Notes are located on pages 2155-2163.

BRAND NAMES

Saw Palmetto - PhysioLogics
Each softgel contains: Saw Palmetto extract (standardized to 85-95% fatty acids, biologically active sterols, 136-152 mg) 160 mg. Other Ingredients: Pure Olive Oil, Gelatin, Glycerin.

Saw Palmetto - Celestial Seasonings
Two capsules contain: Vitamin E (as d-alpha tocopherol acetate) 90 IU • Zinc (as gluconate) 15 mg • Proprietary Blend: Saw Palmetto berries, Saw Palmetto extract, Stinging Nettle root extract 1230 mg.

Saw Palmetto - NSI - Nutraceutical Sciences Institute
Each two softgels contain: Saw Palmetto berry extract 160 mg • Pumpkin seed oil 160 mg.

Saw Palmetto - Benepure, Inc
Each capsule contains: Saw Palmetto berry extract (serenoa repens, yielding free fatty acids 80 mg) 320 mg. Other Ingredients: Rice Powder, Gelatin, Magnesium Stearate, Vegetable Cellulose.

Saw Palmetto - GNC
Two capsules contain: Saw Palmetto berry powder (Serenoa repens) 1000 mg. Other Ingredients: Gelatin, Cellulose.

Saw Palmetto - Puritan's Pride
Each softgel contains: Saw Palmetto extract berry (serenoa repens) 320 mg. Other Ingredients: Gelatin, Glycerin.

Saw Palmetto - Metabolic Response Modifiers
Each capsule contains: Saw Palmetto oil (Serenoa repens, containing 85-95% saponins) 160 mg.

Saw Palmetto - Natrol, Inc.
Each softgel contains: Saw Palmetto extract berries (serenoa repens) 160 mg. Other Ingredients: Olive Oil, Glycerin, Gelatin.

Saw Palmetto - Smart Basics
Each softgel contains: Saw Palmetto extract berry (Serenoa Repens)160 mg. Other Ingredients: Olive Oil, Gelatin, Glycerin.

Saw Palmetto - Gaia Herbs
Two capsules contain: Saw Palmetto supercritical CO2 extract (serenoa repens; 85% (320 mg) fatty acids) 375 mg. Other Ingredients: Lecithin, Vegetable Cellulose (capsule).

Saw Palmetto - Swanson Health Products
Each capsule contains: Saw Palmetto berries powder 540 mg.

Saw Palmetto - Pharmanex
Each softgel contains: Saw Palmetto berry 10:1 extract 160 mg. Other Ingredients: Olive Oil, Gelatin, Glycerin, Carob.

Saw Palmetto - Blessed Herbs
Saw Palmetto berry • Siberian Ginseng root • Jamaican Sarsaparilla root • Suma root • Astragalus root • Damiana • Grain alcohol & Distilled Water.

Saw Palmetto - Sundown
Two capsules contain: Saw Palmetto fruit 900 mg. Other Ingredients: Gelatin.

Saw Palmetto - Jarrow Formulas
Two softgels contain: Saw Palmetto extract 320 mg • Phytosterols (providing minimum 40 mg of beta-sitosterol) 100 mg • Pumpkin seed oil 320 mg • Gamma Tocopherol 4 mg. Other Ingredients: Gelatin, Glycerin, Water.

Saw Palmetto - Life Enhancement Products, Inc.
Each capsule contains: Saw Palmetto berries extract 640 mg.

Saw Palmetto - Leiner Health Products
Two softgels contain: Saw Palmetto extract (Serenoa repens) berry 160 mg. Other Ingredients: Soybean Oil, Gelatin, Glycerin, Caramel, Titanium Dioxide, Red 40, Blue 1.

Saw Palmetto 160 mg - Nature's Bounty
Two softgels contain: Saw Palmetto berry extract (serenoa repens, standardized to 85-95% fatty acids and active sterols) 160 mg. Other Ingredients: Pure Olive Oil, Gelatin, Glycerin.

Saw Palmetto 320 - Pure Encapsulations
Each softgel capsule contains: Saw Palmetto fruit extract 320 mg.

Saw Palmetto 320 mg Standardized Extract - Puritan's Pride
Each softgel contains: Saw Palmetto berry extract (serenoa repens, standardized to contain 85-95% fatty acids and sterols) 320 mg. Other Ingredients: Gelatin, Glycerin.

Saw Palmetto 450 mg Natural Whole Herb - Puritan's Pride
Each capsule contains: Saw Palmetto berry (serenoa repens) 450 mg. Other Ingredients: Gelatin.

Saw Palmetto Berry - Nature's Way
Each capsule contains: Saw Palmetto berry 585 mg. Other Ingredients: Gelatin, Magnesium Stearate, Silica.

Saw Palmetto Complex - Leiner Health Products
Each softgel contains: Zinc Gluconate 7.5 mg • Pumpkin Seed oil extract (Cucurbita pepeo) 40 mg • Saw Palmetto berry extract (serenoa repens) 160 mg. Other Ingredients: Gelatin, Glycerin, Vegetable Oil, Beeswax, Lecithin, Titanium Dioxide, Red 40, Yellow 6, Blue 1, Yellow 5.

Saw Palmetto Complex - PhytoPharmica
Two softgels contain: Pumpkin seed 2.5:1 extract (cucurbita pepeo) 80 mg • Pygeum bark extract (prunus africana, standardized to 12% total sterols, as beta sitosterol) 20 mg • Saw Palmetto berry extract (serenoa repens, standardized to 85-95% fatty acids, 0.2-0.4% total sterols, and 0.1-0.3% beta sitosterol) 160 mg • Uva-Ursi leaf extract (arctostaphylos uva-ursi, standardized to10% arbutin) 10 mg.

Saw Palmetto Complex - Enzymatic Therapy
Each capsule contains: Saw Palmetto Berry extract standardized to contain 85% to 95% fatty acids & sterols 80 mg • Pumpkin seed oil extract (Cucurbita pepo) 40 mg • Pygeum africanum extract standardized to contain 13% total sterols 10 mg • Bearberry extract (Uva Ursi) standardized to contain 10% Arbutin 5 mg.

Saw Palmetto Complex - Jamieson
Each capsule contains: Saw Palmetto Berry 200 mg • Pygeum Bark 7500 mg • Cranberry Fruit 250 mg • Pumpkin Seed Oil 100 mg.

Saw Palmetto Complex - Shaklee
Each capsule contains: Saw Palmetto extract (Serenoa repens berry, standardized to contain 85%-95% fatty acids and sterols) 160 mg • Beta Sitosterol (from soybean phytosterols) 15 mg. Other Ingredients: Pumpkin Seed Oil, Soybean Oil, Beeswax, Soy Lecithin, Ascorbyl Palmitate, Mixed Tocopherol Concentrate, Rosemary Extract, Gelatin, Glycerin, Water, Annatto, Caramel, Titanium Dioxide, Turmeric.

Saw Palmetto Extract - Pro Health
Each softgel contains: Saw Palmetto berry extract (serenoa repens fruit, standardized to contain between 85-95% fatty acids and biologically active sterol compounds) 160 mg. Other Ingredients: Extra Virgin Olive Oil, Gelatin, Glycerin, Water, Carob, Zinc Oxide.

Saw Palmetto Extract - Jamieson
Each capsule contains: Pumpkin seed oil (Curcubita pepo) 100 mg • Saw Palmetto berry 4:1 extract (Serenoa repens) 50 mg • Pygeum bark 150:1 extract (Pygeum africanum) 50 mg • Cranberry fruit 25:1 extract (Viccinum macrocarpon) 10 mg.

Saw Palmetto Extract - Ortho Molecular Products
Each capsule contains: Saw Palmetto fruit extract (standardized to contain 50% fatty acids) 320 mg. Other Ingredients: Magnesium Stearate, Microcrystalline Cellulose, Silicon Dioxide.

Saw Palmetto Formula - Quest
Each caplet contains: Saw Palmetto berry powder (Serenoa serrulate/ repens) 110 mg • Corn Silk powder (Zea mays) 110 mg • Pumpkin Seed powder 90 mg • Parsley leaf powder (Petroselinum crispum) 55 mg • Buchu leaf powder (Barosma betulina) 35 mg • Cayenne powder (Capsicum) 35 mg • Kelp powder (Fucus vesiculosis) 35 mg. Other Ingredients: Calcium Phosphate, Microcrystalline Cellulose, Vegetable Stearin, Croscarmellose Sodium, Magnesium Stearate.

Saw Palmetto Fruit - Aboca USA, Inc
Two capsules contain: Saw Palmetto fruit WPC (whole phytocomplex concentrate, serenoa repens, standardized to contain 14% total liposterolic extract, yielding 42 mg per capsule) 600 mg. Other Ingredients: Gelatin.

Saw Palmetto Male Toner - Traditional Medicinals
Hibiscus flower • Saw Palmetto berry • Nettle root • Uva Ursi leaf • Ginger rhizome • Saw Palmetto berry dry extract • Althea root • Rose Hip • natural Lemon flavor • Stevia leaf.

Saw Palmetto Plus - Pure Encapsulations
Each softgel capsule contains: Saw Palmetto extract (serenoa repens, standardized to contain 85% total fatty acids and 0.15% phytosterols) 160 mg • Pumpkin seed oil (cucurbita pepo) 320 mg • Pygeum Africanum extract (standardized to contain 13% total sterols) 20 mg • Nettle root 10:1 extract (urtica dioica L., standardized to contain 0.8% beta-sitosterol and 5% amino acids) 200 mg.

Saw Palmetto Plus - Atrium Biotechnologies
Each capsule contains: Saw Palmetto oil (50:1 extract) 160 mg • Olive oil 90 mg.

Saw Palmetto Plus - Nature's Bounty
Each softgel contains: Saw Palmetto Complex Blend 95 mg: Saw Palmetto berry extract (serenoa repens, standardized to contain 85-95% free fatty acids and sterols) 80 mg, Pygeum Africanum bark extract (standardized to contain 12% sterols) 10 mg, Bearberry leaf extract (arctostaphylos uva-ursi, standardized to contain 10% arbutin) 5 mg • Pumpkin Seed Oil extract (curcubita pepo) 40 mg. Other Ingredients: Soybean Oil, Gelatin, Glycerin, Lecithin, Silica, Caramel Color, Titanium Dioxide Color.

Saw Palmetto Prostate Health - DreamPharm
Each capsule contains: Saw Palmetto fruit 400 mg • Vaccaria Segetalis seeds 50 mg • Dianthus Superbus herb 50 mg • Pumpkin seeds 50 mg • Licorice 50 mg.

Saw Palmetto Pygeum Nettle Root - Vital Nutrients
Two capsules contain: Saw Palmetto CO2 extract 45% (equal to 320 mg of 85% fatty acids extract) 606 mg • Pygeum Africanum extract 4% (equal to 100 mg of 10% phytosterols extract) 250 mg • Nettle root 20:1 extract (source of plant phytosterols) 200 mg.

Saw Palmetto Standard - Sundown
Two softgels contain: Saw Palmetto fruit extract (standardized to 85%-95% fatty acids, 272 mg) 320 mg. Other Ingredients: Gelatin, Glycerin, Water, Titanium Dioxide, Yellow 6 Lake, Red 40 Lake, Blue 2 Lake.

Saw Palmetto Standardized Extract With Pumpkin Seed Oil and Zinc - NOW Foods
Each softgel contains: Zinc (as zinc gluconate) 30 mg • Saw Palmetto berry extract (serenoa repens, fruit) 160 mg • Pumpkin Seed Oil 1 g. Other Ingredients: Gelatin, Glycerine, Carob, Beeswax, Water.

Saw Palmetto Supreme - Gaia Herbs
Forty drops contain: Proprietary Blend 140 mg: Saw Palmetto berry (serenoa repens), Echinacea Supreme: Echinacea Angustifolia root, Echinacea Purpurea roots, flower head and seed, Fresh Stinging Nettle root (urtica dioica), Fresh Poplar bark and leaf (populus tremuloides), Pipsissewa herb (chimaphila umbellata), Fresh Thuja leaf (thuja occidentalis), 50-60% Pure Grain Alcohol USP.

Saw Palmetto with Lycopene - Health Smart Vitamins
Each soft gel contains: Saw Palmetto berry 320 mg • Lycopene (from tomato) 5 mg.

Saw Palmetto XTRA - Sundown
Two softgels contain: Vitamin E (as dl-alpha-tocopheryl acetate) 25 IU • Zinc (as zinc oxide) 7.5 mg • Saw Palmetto fruit extract (standardized to 85%-95% fatty acids, 272 mg) 320 mg • XTRA Premium Blend 59 mg: Vitamin E, Nettle root extract (10:1), Beta-Sitosterol, Zinc Oxide. Other Ingredients: Soybean oil, Soy Lecithin, Glycerin, Water, Titanium Dioxide (color), Yellow 6 Lake, Red 40 Lake, Blue 2 Lake.

Say Yes to Beans - Nature's Plus
Each Vegicap contains: Legumase (Saccharamyces cerevisae & Aspergillus enzyme complex) 125 mg • Licorice root (Glycyrrhiza glabra) standardized < 2% Glycyrrhizinic acid 75 mg • Ginger root (Zingiber officinale) standardized 5% gingerols 25 mg • Parsley seed (Petroselinum crispum) 20 mg.

SBR-Lipocream - Ferndale Laboratories, Inc.
30 grams contains: White Petrolaturn • Purified Water • Mineral Oil • Cetostearyl Alcohol • Ceteth-20 • Methyl Paraben • Citric Acid • Sodium Citrate.

ScalpBlock - Biotech Corp.
Octyl Methoxycinnamate • Octocylene • Oxybenzone • Octyl Dodecanol • Butyloctyl Salicylate • Cyclomethicone • C12-15 Alkyl Lactate • PVP/Hexadecene Copolymer • Tocopherol Acetate.

Schisandra - Pharmanex
Each capsule contains: Schisandra berry extract (Schisandra chinensis) (10:1) 200 mg. Other Ingredients: Rice Flour, Gelatin, Magnesium Stearate, Silicon Dioxide.

Schisandra Extract 30:1 - Vital Nutrients
Each capsule contains: Schisandra 30:1 extract 500 mg.

Schizandra Plus - Herbalife International of America, Inc.
Each tablet contains: Vitamin A (100% as beta-carotene) 2500 IU • Vitamin C (as ascorbic acid and ascorbyl palmitate) 40 mg • Vitamin E (as DL-alpha-tocopheryl acetate) 20 IU • Vitamin B6 (as pyridoxine hydrochloride) 10 mg • Pantothenic Acid (as D-calcium pantothenate) 5 mg • Calcium (as calcium sulfate) 79 mg • Selenium (as yeast) 50 mcg • Exclusive Blend 125 mg: Kelp, Cellulose, Ribonucleic Acid (yeast0, Deoxyribonucleic Acid (yeast), Superoxide Dismutase, Bee Pollen, Catalase, Citrus Bioflavonoids, Sea Bed Deposits • Schizandra fruit 90 mg • L-Cysteine 10 mg • L-Phenylalanine 10 mg. Other Ingredients: Micro-crystalline Cellulose, Stearic Acid, Silicon Dioxide, Cross-linked Sodium Carboxymethylcellulose, Food Grade Shellac, Hydroxypropyl Cellulose.

Schoomz - Cytotec Solutions, Inc.
Unknown.
See Editor's Note No. 49.

Scooter Rabbit - J. R. Carlson Laboratories, Inc.
Each tablet contains: Vitamin A (as palmitate) 5000 IU • Vitamin C (as calcium & sodium ascorbate) 120 mg • Vitamin D (D3) 400 IU • Vitamin E (as D-alpha tocopheryl succinate) 60 IU • Vitamin K 40 mcg • Thiamin (vitamin B1, as thiamin mononitrate) 1 mg • Riboflavin (vitamin B2) 1 mg • Niacin (vitamin B3, as niacinamide) 5 mg • Vitamin B6 (as pyridoxine hydrochloride) 2 mg • Folate (folic acid) 400 mcg • Vitamin B12 (cyanocobalamin) 6 mcg • Biotin 150 mcg • Calcium (as di-calcium phosphate) 50 mg • Iron (as iron glycinate chelate) 9 mg • Phosphorus (as di-calcium phosphate) 22 mg • Iodine (from potassium iodide) 75 mcg • Magnesium (as magnesium carbonate) 25 mg • Zinc (as zinc glycinate chelate) 7 mg • Selenium (as L-selenomethionine) 35 mcg • Copper (as copper gluconate) 1 mg • Manganese (as manganese sulfate) 1 mg • Chromium 60 mcg • Molybdenum 38 mcg • Potassium 2 mg • Pantothenic Acid (as D-calcium pantothenate) 10 mg • Lemon Bioflavonoids complex 10 mg.

Scooter Rabbit-C - J. R. Carlson Laboratories, Inc.
Each tablet contains: Vitamin C (as calcium ascorbate) 250 mg • Calcium (as calcium ascorbate) 25 mg.

Scudder's Alternative Supreme - Gaia Herbs
Forty drops contain: Proprietary Blend 50 mg: Corydalis tubers (dicentra canadensis), Fresh Black Alder bark (alnus serrulata), Mayapple root (podophyllum peltatum), Figwort flowering herb (scrophylaria nodos), Fresh Yellow Dock root (rumex crispus), 40-50% Pure Grain Alcohol USP, Spring Water.

Sea & Earth - The Vitamin Shoppe
Sea-life protein • Vitamin C • Zinc • Silica • Green Tea extract • Red Wine extract • Red Cabbage extract • Grape Juice extract • Pine Bark extract • Citrus Bioflavonoids • Carotene.

Some Brand Name Natural Products - What they Contain

www.NaturalDatabase.com contains MANY more listings than appear here.
Editor's Notes are located on pages 2155-2163.

BRAND NAMES

Sea Cal Oyster Shell Calcium - Nature's Life
Two tablets contain: Calcium (oyster shell) 500 mg • Vitamin D (vitamin D3, as cholecaciferol) 250 IU.

Sea Cucumber - Futurebiotics LLC
Sea Cucumber 500 mg.

Sea Mussel - Futurebiotics LLC
New Zealand Greenshell Mussel 500 mg.

Sea Nectar (Royal Image Cosmetics) - InterPlexus
Olive Squalane • Lavender • Olive oil • Olibanum • Tocopherol (vitamin E) • Seaweed extract • Rosemary • Retinyl Palmitate (vitamin A) • Cholecalciferol (vitamin D3).

Seacure - Proper Nutrition - PNI
Six capsules contain: Vitamin A 157 IU • Calcium 57 mg • Phosphorus 63 mg • Omega-3 32 mg. Ingredients: White Fish, Rosemary extract.

SeaHealth Plus - Zone Labs
Aloe Vera • Bladderwrack • Green Sea Lettuce • Irish Moss • Knotted Wrack • Popping Wrack • Purple Laver • Ribbon Kelp • Rockwrack • Sugar Wrack • Purified Water • Grape Seed extract • Wild Blueberry extract • Grape powder • Raspberry extract • Raspberry seed extract • Cranberry powder • Prune powder • Tart Cherry powder • Wild Bilberry extract • Strawberry powder • Dark Sweet Cherry • Honey • Citric Acid • Sodium Benzoate • Potassium Sorbate.

SeaSilver - SeaSilver, USA, Inc.
Each 32 ounce bottle contains: Matrix Aloe Vera leaf inner gel (barbadensis miller) • Sealogica Proprietary Blend: Ascophyllum Nodosum, Fucus Vesiculosus, Kelp, Fucus, Chondrus Crispus, Nori, Ulva Latuca • Pau d'Arco inner bark • Juice Concentrate Blend: White Grape, Cranberry, Concord Grape, Black Cherry.
See Editor's Note No. 34.

Seasonal Change - Progressive Health Nutraceuticals
Vitamin C 350 mg • Zinc 2 mg • Bromelain 100 mg • Spirulina 500 mg • Inositol 100 mg • Astragalus 140 mg • 1-3,1-6-Beta-Glucan 3 mg • Echinacea Purpurea 50 mg • Golden Seal 30 mg • Immune Enhancer AG 150 mg • Elderberry 70 mg.

Seasonal Defense - Nature's Sunshine
Each capsule contains: Proprietary Blend 470 mg: Andrographis Paniculata whole plant extract, Thyme leaf (thymus vulgaris), Bitter Orange fruit (fructus aurantia, synephrine 6% extract), Eleuthero root (eleutherococcus senticosus), Oregano leaf (origanum vulgare). Other Ingredients: Magnesium Stearate, Silicon Dioxide, Gelatin, Water.
See Editor's Note No. 40.

Seasonal Relief - Garden of Life, Inc.
Three caplets contain: Wild Oregano concentrate (6% volatile oils) 900 mg • Poten-Zyme Ginger juice 20:1 extract 180 mg • Olive leaf extract (20% oleuropin) 300 mg • Poten-Zyme Horseradish juice extract (20:1) 180 mg • Poten-Zyme Onion juice extract (20:1) 168 mg • Poten-Zyme Peppermint extract 168 mg • Poten-Zyme Yarrow extract 168 mg • Poten-Zyme Elder Flower extract 168 mg • Echinacea Angustifolia extract (24% echinacosides) 99 mg • Elderberry fruit extract (30% anthocyanins) 99 mg • Goldenseal extract (5% hydrastine) 99 mg • Poten-Zyme Garlic juice extract (20:1) 168 mg • Bayberry bark extract (70% myricetin) 24 mg • Lonicera Japonicum extract (40% polyphenols) 18 mg • Poten-Zyme Probiotic Blend 2.4 billion CFU. Other Ingredients: Cellulose, Acacia, Stearates.

Seatone Green Lipped Mussel Extract 350 mg - Peter Black
Each capsule contains: Green Lipped Mussel extract 350 mg. Other Ingredients: Gelatin.

Seatone Mussel Extract 230 mg - IT Pharmacy
Each capsule contains: Green Lipped Mussel extract 230 mg. Other Ingredients: Gelatin.

Seatone NZ Green-Lipped Mussel Extract 500 mg - McFarlane
Each capsule contains: Green Lipped Mussel extract 500 mg. Other Ingredients: Gelatin.

SeaVive - Proper Nutrition - PNI
Each capsule contains: Vitamin C (L-ascorbic acid) 50 mg • Omega-3 2.1 mg • White Fish (Seacure) 200 mg • Colostrum (casein- & lactose-free, bovine) 200 mg • Beta-1,3-D Glucan 50 mg. Other Ingredients: Gelatin.

Seaweed Virtue - Blessed Herbs
Kelp • Bladderwrack • Dulse & "Other Seaweeds as Available" • Grain alcohol & Distilled Water.

Secretagogue-One - MHP
Each packet contains: Anterior Pituitary Substance 25 mg • Glycoamino Acid-Glucose Complex 4200 mg • Novel polyose complex 2230 mg • Amino Acid Blend 500 mg • Broad Bean 10 mg.
See Editor's Note No. 31.

Seditol brand - Next Pharmaceuticals
Proprietary Magnolia Officinalis extract • Proprietary Ziziphus Spinosa extract.
See Editor's Note No. 44.

Sedivitax - Aboca USA, Inc
Two capsules contain: Passiflo 2-LMF Passionflower leaf multifraction freeze-dried extract (passiflora incarnata, standardized to 8% total flavonoids) 256 mg • Valerian root Whole Phytocomplex Concentrate (WPC) (valeriana officinalis, standardized to 0.25% total valerenic acids) 192 mg • Lemon Balm leaf WPC (melissa officinalis, standardized to 6.5% rosmarinic acid) 96 mg • California Poppy leaf/flower WPC (eschscholzia californica, standardized to 0.045% protopine) 89.6 mg. Other Ingredients: Gelatin (capsule), Essential Oils Of Lavender, Marjoram.

Sedivitax Drops - Aboca USA, Inc
Twenty-five drops contain: Passionflo 2-LMF Passionflower leaf multifraction freeze-dried extract (passiflora incarnata, standardized to 8% total flavonoids) 33.3 mg • Passionflower leaf extract (1:10 in organic grain alcohol 70% by volume, total flavonoids minimum 0.16%) 210.2 mg • Valerian root extract (1:10 in organic grain alcohol 70% by volume, total valerenic acids minimum 0.011%) 210.2 mg • Lemon Balm leaf extract (1:10 in organic grain alcohol 70% by volume, rosmarinic acid minimum 0.28%) 140.1 mg • California Poppy aerial part extract (1:10 in organic grain alcohol) 70% by volume, protopine minimum 0.0028% 140.1 mg. Other Ingredients: Essential Oil Of Lavender, Marjoram.

Sedivitax Herbal Tea - Aboca USA, Inc
Each bag contains: Passionflower leaf (passiflora incarnata) 0.36 g • Licorice root (glycyrrhiza glabra) 0.36 g • Chamomile flower (matricaria recutita) 0.27 g • Lemon Balm leaf (melissa officinalis) 0.27 g • Star Anise fruit (illicium verum) 0.18 g • Linden flower (tilia cordata) 0.18 g. Other Ingredients: Bitter Orange, Orange.

SEE - Quantum, Inc.
Three tablets contain: Bilberry extract 10 mg • Omega-3 Flax Meal 500 mg • Beta-Carotene (pro vitamin A) 25,000 IU • Vitamin A (palmitate) 5000 IU • Vitamin C 1000 mg • Natural Vitamin E (D-alpha succinate) 200 IU • Citrus Bioflavonoids 250 mg • Vitamin B2 (riboflavin) 40 mg • Rutin NF100 mg • Selenium (selenomethionine) 100 mcg • Pantothenic Acid (D-calcium pantothenate) 40 mg • Chromium 200 mcg • Zinc 25 mg • Lutein 5 mg.

SeLECT E-400 - Xymogen
Each softgel contains: Vitamin E (as D-alpha tocopherol) 400 IU • Selenium (as selenomethionine) 50 mcg. Other Ingredients: Gelatin, Glycerin, Beeswax, Lecithin.

Select Herbals Natural Whole Herb Aloe Vera 470 mg - Vitamin World
Each capsule contains: Aloe Vera leaf (aloe barbadensis) 470 mg. Other Ingredients: Gelatin, Silica, Vegetable Magnesium Stearate.

Some Brand Name Natural Products - What they Contain

www.NaturalDatabase.com contains MANY more listings than appear here.
Editor's Notes are located on pages 2155-2163.

Select Herbals Natural Whole Herb Astragalus 470 mg **-** Vitamin World
Each capsule cotnains: Astragalus root (astragalus membranaceus) 470 mg. Other Ingredients: Gelatin.

Select Herbals Natural Whole Herb Echinacea 400 mg **-** Vitamin World
Each capsule contains: Echinacea (echinacea purpurea, aerial) 400 mg. Other Ingredients: Gelatin.

Select Herbals Natural Whole Herb Saw Palmetto 450 mg **-** Vitamin World
Each capsule contains: Saw Palmetto berry (serenoa repens) 450 mg. Other Ingredients: Gelatin.

Select Herbals Natural Whole Herb Valerian Root 450 mg **-** Vitamin World
Each capsule contains: Valerian root (valeriana officinalis) 450 mg. Other Ingredients: Gelatin.

Selene-E **-** Schiff
Two softgels contain: Vitamin E (as D-alpha tocopherol and non-alpha tocopherols) 200 IU • Selenium (from selenium enriched yeast) 100 mcg • Lecithin 640 mg • Saccharomyces Cerevisiae (yeast, primary) 346 mg. Other Ingredients: Soybean Oil, Softgel (gelatin, glycerin, water), Yellow Beeswax.

Selenium **-** Pure Encapsulations
Each vegetable capsule contains: Selenium (selenomethionine) 200 mcg • Vitamin C (as ascorbyl palmitate) 2 mg.

Selenium **-** Golden Glow Natural Health Products
Each tablet contains: Selenomethionine 75 mcg: Selenium 25 mcg.

Selenium **-** Westcoast Naturals
Each tablet contains: Selenium (HVP chelate) 100 mcg.

Selenium **-** Source Naturals
Each tablet contains: Selenium (yeast free, from 40 mg of L-Selonomethionine) 200 mcg.

Selenium **-** Schiff
Each tablet contains: Selenium (as high selenium yeast) 200 mcg. Other Ingredients: Calcium Carbonate, Cellulose, Coating (dextrin, dextrose, soy lecithin, sodium carboxymethylcellulose, sodium citrate), Croscarmellose Sodium, Magnesium Stearate.

Selenium (as Selenomethionine) **-** EcoNugenics
Each capsule contains: Selenium (as selenomethionine) 200 mcg. Other Ingredients: Cellulose.

Selenium (citrate) **-** Pure Encapsulations
Each vegetable capsule contains: Selenium (citrate) 200 mcg.

Selenium 100 **-** GNC
Each tablet contains: Selenium (as selenium yeast) 100 mcg. Other Ingredients: Cellulose, Dicalcium Phosphate.

Selenium 100 mcg **-** Jamieson
Each tablet contains: Selenium (from Brewer's Yeast) 100 mcg.

Selenium 200 **-** Walgreens
Each tablet contains: Selenium (selenium yeast) 200 mcg. Other Ingredients: Dicalcium Phosphate, Microcrystalline Cellulose, Stearic Acid, Croscarmellose Sodium, Magnesium Stearate, Hydroxypropylmethyl Cellulose, Hydroxypropyl Cellulose, Polyethylene Glycol.

Selenium 200 **-** Leiner Health Products
Each tablet contains: Selenium (High Selenium yeast) 200 mcg. Other Ingredients: Calcium Carbonate, Maltodectrin, Cellulose, Croscarmellose Sodium, Tricalcium Phosphate, Crospovidone, Polyethylene Glycol 3350, Silicon Dioxide, Magnesium Stearate, Hydroxypropyl Methylcellulose, Hydroxypropyl Cellulose, Polysorbate 80.

Selenium 200 **-** GNC
Each tablet contains: Selenium (as selenomax selenium yeast) 200 mcg. Other Ingredients: Dicalcium Phosphate, Cellulose.

Selenium 200 mcg **-** Vital Nutrients
Each capsule contains: Selenium (50% sodium selenite, 50% selenomethionine) 200 mcg.

Selenium 200 mcg **-** Nature Made
Each tablet contains: Selenium (from selenium yeast) 200 mcg. Other Ingredients: Dibasic Calcium Phosphate, Cellulose, Stearic Acid, Silicon Dioxide, Hydroxypropyl Methylcellulose, Magnesium Stearate, Polyethylene Glycol, Carnauba Wax.
See Editor's Note No. 45.

Selenium 200 mcg **-** J. R. Carlson Laboratories, Inc.
Each tablet contains: Selenium (as L-selenomethionine) 200 mcg.

Selenium 200 mcg **-** Sunmark
Each tablet contains: Selenium 200 mcg. Other Ingredients: Dicalcium Phosphate, Microcrystalline Cellulose, Stearic Acid, Croscamellose Sodium, Magnesium Stearate, Hydroxypropylmethyl Cellulose, Hydroxypropyl Cellulose, Polyethylene Glycol.
See Editor's Note No. 45.

Selenium 200 mcg (L-Selenomethionine) **-** J. R. Carlson Laboratories, Inc.
Each capsule contains: Selenium (as L-selenomethionine) 200 mcg.

Selenium 50 **-** GNC
Each tablet contains: Selenium (as selenium yeast) 50 mcg. Other Ingredients: Cellulose, Dicalcium Phosphate.

Selenium 50 mcg **-** Jamieson
Each tablet contains: Selenium (from Brewer's Yeast) 50 mcg.

Selenium 50 mcg - Yeast Free **-** Jamieson
Each caplet contains: Selenium (Proteinate) 50 mcg • Beta-Carotene (Provitamin A) 5000 IU • Vitamin C (Ascorbic Acid) 60 mg • Vitamin E (Natural D-Alpha Tocopheryl Acetate) 10 IU.

Selenium Detoxification Formula - Smokers & Drinkers **-** Life Extension
Each 500 mcg tablet contains: Sodium Selenate 100 mcg • Selenomethionine (yeast free) 50 mcg • Seleno Di- Glutathione 50 mcg • Cysteine 100 mcg • Thiamide 100 mg • Nicotinic Acid 100 mg.

Selenium Forte **-** American Biologics
Each tablet contains: Selenium (as selenium proteinate, in an alfalfa base) 200 mcg. Other Ingredients: Dicalcium Phosphate, Cellulose, Magnesium Stearate.

Selenium Mineral Supplement **-** Eidon Inc.
Each 1 tbsp serving contains: Selenium (providing approx. 52 ppm selenium) 260 mcg. Other Ingredients: Purified Water.

Selenium Tablets **-** Leiner Health Products
Each tablet contains: Selenium Yeast 50 mcg. Other Ingredients: Brewer's Yeast, Dicalcium Phosphate, Cellulose, Stearic Acid, Croscarmellose Sodium, Silicon Dioxide.

Selenium Tablets 100 mcg **-** Solgar
Each tablet contains: Selenium (yeast) 100 mcg. Other Ingredients: Saccharomyces Cerevisiae.

Selenium Tablets 200 mcg **-** Solgar
Each tablet contains: Selenium (yeast) 200 mcg. Other Ingredients: Saccharomyces Cerevisiae, Vegetable Stearic Acid.

Selenium Tablets 50 mcg **-** Solgar
Each tablet contains: Selenium (yeast) 50 mcg. Other Ingredients: Saccharomyces Cerevisiae, Silica, Vegetable Stearic Acid.

SelenoExcell **-** BioGenesis Nutraceuticals
Each capsule contains: Selenium (from SelenoExcell brand selenium yeast) 200 mcg.

Selenomax **- Source Naturals**
Each tablet contains: Selenium (from 100 selenomax high selenium yeast) 100 mcg.

Selenomax brand **- Nutrition 21**
Selenium.
See Editor's Note No. 44.

Selenomax Selenium 200 Mcg **- Nature's Life**
Each tablet contains: Selenium (natural food yeast-based) (Nutrition 21 Selenomax) 200 mcg.

Selestro **- Metagenics**
Each tablet contains: Soybean concentrate 100 mg • Total Isoflavones (containing all forms of genistin, daidzin, glycitin) 40 mg • Black Cohosh root/rhizome extract (actaea racemosa, standardized to 2.5% triterpene glycosides as 27-deoxyactein) 80 mg.

Senaplex **- Standard Process, Inc.**
Two capsules contain: Proprietary Blend 950 mg: Nutritional Yeast, Choline Bitartrate, Tillandsia Usneoides, Bovine Liver PMG extract, Calcium Lactate, Betaine Hydrochloride, Defatted Wheat germ, Soy bean, Carrot root, Bovine Adrenal, Bovine Bone, Inositol, Soybean Lecithin, Ribonucleic Acid, Veal Bone meal, Bovine Kidney, Bovine Orchic extract, DL-Methionine, Bovine Spleen, Ovine Spleen, L-Lysine Mono-Hydrochloride, Dried Alfalfa juice, Glutamic Acid, Rice bran, Peanut bran • Vitamin A 390 IU • Vitamin D 135 IU • Riboflavin 0.1 mg • Niacin 4 mg • Vitamin B6 1.2 mg • Vitamin B12 0.6 mcg • Sodium 10 mg • Potassium 30 mg. Other Ingredients: Gelatin, Water, Colors, Cellulose.
See Editor's Note No. 14.

Senescegarl **- Olympian Labs**
Three capsules contain: Ginkgo Biloba leaf extract 120 mg • Garlic extract 600 mg • Coenzyme Q10 60 mg • Ascorbic Acid 300 mg • Grape Seed extract 90 mg • Vitamin B-6 (pyridoxine HCl) 30 mg • Zinc (gluconate) 15 mg • Copper (cupric oxide) 1800 mcg • Manganese (manganese sulfate) 1800 mcg.

Senior Moment **- Nutramax Laboratories, Inc.**
Each capsule contains: Cerebral Phospholipids 50 mg: Phosphatidylserine, Phosphatidylethanolamine, and Phosphatidylinositol • Docosahexaenoic acid 40mg. Other Ingredients: Sunflower Oil, Gelatin, Water, Ascorbyl Palmitate, Tocopherols, Titanium dioxide color, FD&C Red #3, Sodium Lauryl sulfate, FD&C Yellow #5, FD&C Blue #1.

Senior's One A Day Multi **- Golden Glow Natural Health Products**
Each tablet contains: Beta Carotene 2 mg • Retinyl Palmitate (vitamin A) 500 IU • Thiamine Nitrate (vitamin B1) 25 mg • Riboflavin (vitamin B2) 25 mg • Nicotinamide (vitamin B3) 30 mg • Calcium Pantothenate (vitamin B5) 25 mg • Pyridoxine Hydrochloride (vitamin B6) 25 mg • Cyanocobalamin (vitamin B12) 50 mcg • Ascorbic Acid (vitamin C, as calcium ascorbate) 160.3 mg • Cholecalciferol (vitamin D3 5 mcg) 200 IU • D-Alpha-Tocopheryl Acid Succinate 41.32 mg: Natural Vitamin E 50 IU • Biotin 50 mcg • Choline Bitartrate 25 mg • Folic Acid 99 mcg • Inositol 25 mg • Calcium (as citrate) 50 mg • Chromium (as picolinate) 25 mcg • Copper (as sulfate anhydrous) 128 mcg • Iodine (as potassium iodide) 157.8 mcg • Iron (as fumarate) 5 mg • Magnesium (as oxide) 50 mg • Manganese (as amino acid chelate) 1.5 mg • Selenium (as selenomethionine) 26 mcg • Zinc (as sulfate monohydrate) 15 mg • Ginkgo Biloba leaf extract 250 mg • Milk Thistle extract (silybum marianum) 200 mg • Brahmi extract (bacopa monnieri) 100 mg • Bilberry extract (vaccinium myrtillus) 100 mg • Cranberry extract (vaccinium macrocarpon) 100 mg • Grape seed extract (vitis vinifera) 100 mg • Horsetail extract (equisetum arvense) 50 mg • Pumpkin seed (cucurbita pepo) 50 mg • Citrus Bioflavonoid extract 50 mg • Fucus Vesiculosus extract (kelp) 20 mg: Iodine 1.6 mcg • Carica Papaya powder 10 mg • Natural Fish oil 6.5 mg • Glucosamine Sulfate (as potassium chloride complex) 100 mg • L-Glutamine 25 mg • Lecithin 25 mg • Taurine 25 mg. Other Ingredients: Lactose.

Senior-Vites Plus **- The Vitamin Shoppe**
Three tablets contain: Vitamin A Activity 20000 IU • Vitamin D 400 IU • Vitamin C 150 mg • Vitamin E 200 IU • Vitamin B1 35 mg • Vitamin B2 35 mg • Niacinamide 50 mg • Vitamin B6 35 mg • Vitamin B12 50 mcg • Pantothenic Acid 75 mg • Folic Acid 400 mcg • Biotin 300 mcg • PABA 35 mg • Inositol 100 mg • Choline 100 mg • Citrus Bioflavonoids 25 mg • Rutin 25 mg • Glutamine 100 mg • Taurine 100 mg • Glutamic Acid 50 mg • Pancreatin 25 mg • Ox Bile 10 mg • Calcium 100 mg • Magnesium 50 mg • Iron 18 mg • Zinc 15 mg • Manganese 6 mg • Potassium 45 mg • Iodine 225 mcg • Selenium 50 mcg • Chromium 25 mcg • Fo-Ti 50 mg • Gotu Kola 50 mg • Avena Sativa 25 mg • Siberian Ginseng 25 mg • Nettle extract 10 mg.
See Editor's Note No. 14.

Senna Leaves **- NOW Foods**
Each capsule contains: Senna leaves (Cassia Angustifolia) 470 mg. Other Ingredients: Gelatin (capsule), Magnesium Stearate.

Sentinel Multi Vitamin **- Health Center for Better Living**
Each tablet contains: Vitamin A (as retinyl acetate and beta-carotene) 5000 IU• Vitamin C (as ascorbic acid) 60 mg • Vitamin D (as cholecalciferol) 400 IU • Vitamin E (as dl-alpha-tocopheryl acetate) 30 IU • Vitamin K (as phytonadione) 25 mcg • Thiamin (as thiamin mononitrate) 1.5 mg • Riboflavin 1.7 mg • Niacin (as niacinamide) 20 mg • Vitamin B6 (as pyridoxine HCl) 2 mg • Folate (as folic acid) 400 mcg • Vitamin B12 (as cyancobalamin) 6 mcg • Biotin 30 mcg • Pantothenic acid (as D-calcium pantothenate) 10 mg • Calcium (as dicalcium phosphate) 162 mg • Iron (as ferrous fumarate) 18 mg • Phosphorus (as dicalcium phosphate) 125 mg • Iodine (as potassium iodide) 150 mcg • Magnesium (as magnesium oxide) 100 mg • Zinc (as zinc oxide) 15 mg • Selenium (as sodium selenate) 25 mcg • Copper (as cupric oxide) 2 mg • Manganese (as manganese sulfate) 2.5 mcg • Chromium (as chromium chloride) • Molybdenum (as sodium moybdate) 25 mcg • Chloride (as potassium choride) 36.3 mg Potassium (as potassium choride) 40 mg • Vanadium (as sodium metavandate) 10 mcg • Tin (as stannous chloride) 10 mcg • Silicon (as sodium metasilicate) 10 mcg • Nickel (nickelous sulfate) 5 mcg.

Septilin DS **- The Himalaya Drug Company**
Each tablet contains: Guggulu (balsamodendron mukul syn. commiphora wightii, purified) 0.324 g • Shankh Bhasma (conch shell calx/ash) 64 mg • Maharasnadi Quath 130 mg • Guduchi (tinospora cordifolia) 98 mg • Manjishtha (rubia cordifolia) 64 mg • Amalaki (emblica officinalis) 32 mg • Shigru (moringa pterygosperma) 32 mg • Yashti-Madhu (glycyrrhiza glabra) 12 mg.

Septilin Syrup **- The Himalaya Drug Company**
Each 1 tsp (5 mL) serving contains: Guggulu (balsamodendron mukul syn. commiphora wightii, purified) 80 mg • Maharasnadi Quath 30 mg • Manjishtha (rubia cordifolia) 15 mg • Guduchi (tinospora cordifolia) 14 mg • Trikatu 13 mg: Piper Nigrum, Piper Longum, Zingiber Officinale • Kushtah (saussurea lappa) 13 mg • Amalaki (emblica officinalis) 8 mg • Yashti-Madhu (glycyrrhiza glabra) 6 mg.

Seredrin **- Health Perception**
Each tablet contains: Ginkgo Biloba extract with Phytosome 120 mg (standardized to 9.6 mg ginkgo flavoneglycosides, 2.4 mg terpene lactones). Other Ingredients: Microcrystalline Cellulose, Croscarmellose, Magnesium Stearate, Hydroxypropylmethyl Cellulose.

Serenagen (formerly TCB 3) **- Metagenics**
Two tablets contain: 4:1 Proprietary Extract Blend 1000 mg: Rehmannia root (rehmannia glutinosa), Schisandra fruit (schisandra chinensis), Jujube fruit (zizyphus spinosa), Dong Quai root (angelica sinensis), Chinese Asparagus root (asparagus cochinchinensis), Ophiopogon root (ophiopogon japonicus), Scrophularia root (scrophularia ningpoensis), Asian Ginseng root (panax ginseng), Chinese Salvia root (salvia militiorrhiza), Poria fungus (wolfiporia cocos), Polygala root (polygala tenuifolia), Platycodon root (platycodon grandiflorum).

Some Brand Name Natural Products - What they Contain

www.NaturalDatabase.com contains MANY more listings than appear here.
Editor's Notes are located on pages 2155-2163.

SerenAid **-** Klaire Laboratories
Each capsule contains: Multi-Enzyme Complex (proprietary blend) 317 mg: L-Lysine, Peptidase FP, Papain, Protease, Protease, Lactase.

Serenitol **-** Truvae
Two capsules contain: Proprietary Blend 2092 mg: 5-Hydroxy Tryptophan, Blue Skullcap, Boswellia Serrata, Bromelain, Chondroitin, Chuchuhuasi, Curcuma Longa, DL-Phenylalanine, GABA, Gamma-Linolenic Acid, Ginseng, Melatonin, Passion Flower, Quercetin, Rosemary, Valerian 4:1 extract, White Willow bark. Other Ingredients: Di-Calcium Phosphate, Rice Powder, Gelatin.
See Editor's Note No. 15 and No. 16.

Serenity **-** Urban Nutrition Inc
Each capsule contains: Lithium Orotate 120 mg (provides elemental lithium 4.6 mg). Other Ingredients: Micro Vortex Enteric Coating.

Serenity capsules **-** Gaia Herbs
Three capsules contain: Skullcap herb extract (scutellaria lateriflora) 60 mg • Passionflower vine extract (passiflora incarnata) 60 mg • Kava Kava rhizome extract (piper methysticum) 60 mg • Chamomile flowers extract (matricaria recutita) 45 mg • Wild Oat milky seed extract (avena sativa) 27 mg • Hops Strobile extract (humulus lupulus) 24 mg • Mugwort herb extract (artemesia vulgaris) 15 mg • Peppermint leaf extract (mentha piperita) 9 mg. Other Ingredients: Vegetable Glycerin, Vegetable Cellulose.

Serenity with Kava Kava Root Elixir **-** Gaia Herbs
Sixty drops contain: Proprietary Extract Blend 400 mg: Passionflower (passiflora incarnata), Skullcap herb (scutellaria lateriflora), Kava Kava rhizome (piper methysticum), Chamomile flower (matricaria recutita), Hops strobile (humulus lupulus), Wild Oat seed (avena sativa), Mugwort herb (artemisia vulgaris), Peppermint leaf (mentha piperita), Hawthorn berry extract (crataegus spp.), Peppermint oil, Syrup of organic Mulberries and Apricots, Blend of Sea Vegetation, Vegetable Glycerin, 18-23% Pure Grain Alcohol, Spring Water.

Serenoa Repens **-** Progressive Labs
Each softgel contains: Saw Palmetto purified extract (95% free fatty acids) 160 mg • Olive oil 160 mg.

SerenPure brand **-** Soft Gel Technologies, Inc.
Saw Palmetto.
See Editor's Note No. 44.

Seren-X **-** Xymogen
Two capsules contain: 5:1 Herbal extract blend 1000 mg: Rehmannia root (rehmannia glutinosa), Schisandra fruit (schisandra chinensis), Jujube fruit (zizyphus spinosa), Biota seed (biota orientalis), Chinese Asparagus root (asparagus cochinensis), Ophiogon root (ophiogon japonicus) Scrophularia root (scrophularia ningpoensis), Dong Quai root (angelica sinensis), White Panax Ginseng root, Chinese Salvia root (salvia militorrhiza), Poria fungus (poria wolfiporia), Platycodon root (platycodon grandiflorum), Acorus rhizome (acorus gramineous).

Seriane **-** Dolisos
Each capsule contains: Milk Protein Hydrosylate (containing 1.5 mg of aeS1 casein decapeptide) 150 mg. Other Ingredients: Sodium Caseinate, Gelatin, Water, Titanium Dioxide, Glycerin.

Serious Mass **-** Optimum Nutrition
Two heaping scoops (334 g) contain: Creatine Monohydrate 1 g • L-Glutamine 500 mg • Glutamine Peptides 500 mg • Choline (bitartrate) 250 mg • Inositol 250 mg • PABA (para-aminobenzoic acid) 5 mg • Maltodextrin • Protein Blend: Whey Protein Concentrate, Calcium Caseinate, Egg Albumen, Sweet Dairy Whey • Cocoa • Natural and Artificial Flavor • Vitamin and Mineral Blend: DiPotassium Phosphate, Magnesium Aspartate, DiCalcium Phosphate, Calcium Citrate, Ascorbic Acid, Niacinamide, Zinc Citrate, Beta Carotene, D-Calcium Pantothenate, D-Alpha Tocopheryl Succinate, Selenomethionine, Copper Gluconate, Ferrous Fumarate, Pyridoxine Hydrochloride, Riboflavin, Chromium Polynicotinate, Folic Acid, Biotin, Molybdenum Amino Acid Chelate, Cholecalciferol, Potassium Iodide, Cyanocobalamin • Acesulfame Potassium • Medium Chain Triglycerides.

Seriphos **-** InterPlexus
Each capsule contains: Proprietary blend 1000 mg: Phosphoserine and Ethanolamine. Other Ingredients: Gelatin.

SeroCalm **-** Directly Young, LLC
Two caplets contain: Calcium (carbonate) 200 mg • Magnesium (oxide) 100 mg • Proprietary Blend 740 mg: L-Tyrosine, Wild Jujube seed extract, Griffonia Simplicifolia seed extract (5-HTP 50 mg), Stinging Nettle leaf extract (serotonin 50 mcg). Other Ingredients: Microcrystalline Cellulose, Croscarmellose Sodium, Stearic Acid, Hypromellose, Magnesium Stearate, Silica, Hydroxypropyl Cellulose.

SeroSlim **-** Directly Young, LLC
Two caplets contain: Thiamin (as thiamin hydrochloride) 1.5 mg • Riboflavin 1.7 mg • Niacin (as niacinamide) 20 mg • Vitamin B6 (as pyridoxine hydrochloride) 2 mg • Folate (as folic acid) 400 mcg • Vitamin B12 (as cyanocobalamin) 25 mcg • Biotin 300 mcg • Pantothenic Acid (as d-calcium pantothenate) 10 mg • Calcium (as dicalcium phosphate) 20 mg • Chromium (as chromium dinicotinate glycinate) 200 mcg • Proprietary Standardized Extract Blend 800 mg: Green Tea leaf (provides epigallocatechin gallate 90 mg, caffeine 50 mg), Cocoa bean (provides methylxanthines 50 mg), Griffonia Simplicifolia seed (provides 5-HTP 50 mg), Stinging Nettle leaf (provides serotonin 50 mcg). Other Ingredients: Microcrystalline Cellulose, Croscarmellose Sodium, Stearic Acid, Hypromellose, Magnesium Stearate, Silica, Hydroxypropyl Cellulose, Colorants.

SeroThin **-** Natural Balance
Two capsules contain: Vitamin B6 (pyridoxine HCl) 7.5 mg • Pantothenic Acid (D-calcium pantothenate) 200 mcg • DynaChrome brand Chromium (arginate/chelidamate) 200 mcg • L-Phenylalanine 100 mg • L-Tyrosine 100 mg • St. John's Wort flower extract (standardized to 0.3% hypericin) 50 mg • Rhodiola root extract 50 mg • 5-HTP (5-hydroxytryptophan, from griffonia simplicifolia seed extract) 15 mg • Citrus Aurantium fruit extract 20 mg. Other Ingredients: Gelatin, Cellulose, Magnesium Stearate.
See Editor's Note No. 40.

Serotone 5HTP 100 mg **-** Higher Nature
Each tablet contains: 5-HTP 100 mg • Vitamin B6 10 mg • Zinc (citrate) 5 mg • Biotin 0.05 mg • Folic Acid 100 mcg • Niacin (nicotinamide) 30 mg.

Serotone 5HTP 50 mg **-** Higher Nature
Each tablet contains: 5-HTP 50 mg • Vitamin B6 5 mg • Zinc (citrate) 2.5 mg • Biotin 0.025 mg • Folic Acid 50 mcg • Niacin (nicotinamide) 15 mg.

Serpina **-** The Himalaya Drug Company
Each tablet contains: Sarpagandha (rauwolfia serpentina) 4 mg.

Serraflazyme **-** Cardiovascular Research
Each tablet contains: Serrapeptase enzyme (serratio peptidase, enterically coated) 5 mg. Other Ingredients: Maltodextrin, Microcrystalline Cellulose, Stearic Acid, Silicon Dioxide.

Serrapeptase (Serraflazyme) **-** Olympia Nutrition
Silk worm enzyme.

Serrapeptase (Serratia Peptidase) **-** Davis Biotech Research Labs, Inc.
Each capsule contains: Serrapeptase (providing a minimum of 40,000 units) 450 mg. Other Ingredients: Vegetable Cellulose, Magnesium Stearate, Stearic Acid, Microcrystalline Cellulose.

Serum C **-** Nutraceutics Corp.
Active Ingredients: L-Ascorbic Acid • Maxogenol (botanical proanthoxidant complex). Inactive Ingredients: Ethoxydiglycol, Butylene Glycol, L-Tyrosine, Fruit & Citric Acid Complex, Phenoxyethanol, Purified Water, Methylparaben.

Sesa Hair Supplement **-** Rani-Pharma Inc.
Mukta Sukti 100 mg • Sudha Shilajeet 100 mg • Rohitak 60 mg • Sudh Bodar 50 mg • Rasayana 90 mg.

BRAND NAMES

Some Brand Name Natural Products - What they Contain

www.NaturalDatabase.com contains MANY more listings than appear here.
Editor's Notes are located on pages 2155-2163.

Sesame Herb - Herbalife International of America, Inc.
Tricalcium Phosphate • Calcium Carbonate • Black Sesame seed • Mung bean • Microcrystalline Cellulose • Corn Starch • Silicon Dioxide • Lecithin • Garlic Powder • Dextrin • Cider Vinegar • Chickweed herb powder • Ginger root powder • Couch grass powder • Echinacea extract • Black Walnut leaf powder • Fennelseed owder • Dandelion root • Parsley • Papaya fruit • Kelp powder • Dextrose • Sodium Citrate • Maltodextrin • Dicalcium Phosphate • Lactose. Product Available in Israel.

Sesame Seed Oil - Standard Process, Inc.
Each perle contains: Sesame seed oil 385 mg. Other Ingredients: Gelatin, Glycerin, Water, Carob.

Shake and Bake - The Herbalist
Oils of Sweet Almond, Aloe Vera, Safflower, St. John's Wort flower, Calendula flower, & Vitamin E • Extracts of St. John's Wort flower, Calendula flower & Chamomile flower • Essential oils of Sandalwood, Lite Musk, French Vanilla.

Shaman Botanicals SB Normal Stool Formula - P.S. Pharmaceuticals
Each tablet contains: Croton lechleri extract (sap) (standardized to contain 250 mg of SP-303). Other Ingredients: Microcrystalline Cellulose, Coating [Methacrylic Acid Copolymer, Magnesium Silicate, Triethyl Citrate], Glyceryl Monostearate, Sodium Starch Glycolate, Silicon Dioxide.

Shampoo Stuff - Blue Stuff, Inc.
Each 16 oz bottle contains: Whole leaf Aloe Vera concentrate • Purified Water • Tea-Lauryl Sulfate • Lauramide DEA • Pantothenol • Allantoin • Emu oil • Tea Tree oil • Sodium Hexametaphosphate • Methylparaben • Fragrance • Imidazolidinyl Urea • Retinol • Tocopherol • FD&C Blue No. 1 • FD&C Yellow No. 5.

Shape Up! Weight Management Supplement Intensifier for Apple or Pear Body Types - CSA Nutraceuticals, LLC
Each packet contains: Vitamin C 750 mg • CoQ10 100 mg • EPA (eicosapentaenoic acid) 300 mg • DHA (docosahexaenoic acid) 200 mg • CLA (conjugated linoleic acid) 2000 mg • Tyrosine 75 mg • L-Theanine 100 mg. Other Ingredients: Microcrystalline Cellulose, Maltodextrin, Gelatin, Tricalcium Phosphate, Magnesium Stearate, Silicon Dioxide, Corn Starch, Carboxymethylcellulose, Natural Color, Glycerin.

Shape Up! Apple Body Types Weight Management Supplement & Complete Multivitamin - CSA Nutraceuticals, LLC
Two packets contain: Vitamin A 5000 IU • Vitmain C 500 mg • Vitamin D 400 IU • Vitamin E 200 IU • Vitamin K 80 mcg • Thiamin (B1) 3 mg • Riboflavin (B2) 3.4 mg • Niacin (B3) 40 mg • Vitamin B6 4 mg • Folate, Folic Acid, Folacin 1 mcg • Vitamin B12 1 mcg • Biotin 600 mcg • Pantothenic Acid 20 mg • Calcium 500 mg • Iodine 75 mcg • Magnesium 400 mg • Zinc 30 mg •Selenium 140 mcg • Copper 2 mg • Manganese 2 mg • Chromium 400 mcg • Molybdenum 75 mcg • Vandium 10 mcg • Boron 1 mcg • Garcinia Cambogia fruit 3000 mg • Opuntia Cactus flesh (fics indica) 800 mg • Eleuthero root 100 mg • Kola Nut seed extract 300 mg • L-Carnitine (from L-carnitine tartrate) 100 mg • White Kidney Bean extract 500 mg • Gymnema Sylvestre leaves 300 mg. Other Ingredients: Glycerin, Microcrystalline Cellulose, Stearic Acid, Maltodextrin, Acacia, Corn Syrup Solids, Croscarmellose Sodium, Magnesium Stearate, Corn Starch, Hydroxypropyl Methylcellulose, Silicone Dioxide, Carnauba Wax, Sodium Starch Glyconate, Hydrolized Corn Syrup Solids, Lactose Monohydrate, Carrageenan, Propylene Glycol Alginate.

Shape Up! Complete Nutrition Bar, Chocolate Peanut Butter - CSA Nutraceuticals, LLC
Each bar contains: Syrup blend: Corn Syrup, Peanut Butter, Sugar, Hydrogenated Starch, High Fructose Corn Syrup, Salt, Lecithin, Natural Flavor, Carrageenan • Crisps: Soy Protein Isolate, Tapioca Starch, Soy Fiber, Oat Fiber, Rice Flour, Malt extract, Salt • Chocolate Flavored Coating: Lactitol, Fractionated Palm kernel oil, Chicory extract, Cocoa, Sucralose, Salt, Lecithin, Distilled Monoglycerides, Natural Flavor • Sodium Caseinate • Calcium Phosphate • Peanut Flour • Chicory • Partially Hydrolyzed Guar Gum • Acacia • Magnesium Oxide • Salt • Maltodextrin • Natural and Artificial Flavor • Ascorbic Acid (vitamin C) • Ferrous Fumarate • Biotin • Cholecalciferol (vitamin D) • Chromium Chloride • Copper Gluconate • Cyanocobalamin (vitamin B12) • D-Calcium Pantothenate • Dl-Alpha-Tocopheryl Acetate (vitamin E) • Folic Acid • Manganese Sulfate • Niacinamide (vitamin B3) • Phytonadione (vitamin K) • Potassium Iodide • Pyridoxine Hydrochloride (vitamin B6) • Retinyl Palmitate (vitamin A) • Riboflavin (vitamin B2) • Sodium Molybdate • Sodium Selenite • Thiamine Mononitrate (vitamin B1) • Zinc Oxide.

Shape Up! Complete Nutrition Bar, Chocolate Toffee Crunch - CSA Nutraceuticals, LLC
Each bar contains: Caramel Syrup: Corn Syrup, Hydrogenated Starch, High Fructose Corn Syrup, Sweetened Condensed Milk, Fractionated Palm Kernal Oil, Butter, Gelatin, Lecithin, Natural Flavor • Crisps: Soy Protein Isolate, Oat Fiber, Tapioca Starch, Rice Flour, Soy Fiber, Malt extract, Salt • Chocolate Flavored Coating: Lactitol, Fractionated Palm Kernal Oil, Chicory extract, Cocoa, Sucralose, Salt, Lecithin, Distilled Monoglycerides, Natural Flavor) • Sodium Caseinate • Partially Hydrolyzed Guar Gum • Calcium Phosphate • Peanut • Chicory • Magnesium Oxide • Maltodextrin • Ascorbic Acid (vitamin C) • Ferrous Fumarate • Biotin • Cholecalciferol (vitamin D) • Chromium Chloride • Copper Gluconate • Cyanocobalamin (vitamin B12) • D-Calcium Pantothenate • Dl-Alpha-Tocopheryl Acetate (vitamin E) • Folic Acid • Manganese Sulfate • Niacinamide (vitamin B3) • Phytonadione (vitamin K) • Potassium Iodide • Pyridoxine Hydrochloride (vitamin B6) • Retinyl Palmitate (vitamin A) • Riboflavin (vitamin B2) • Sodium Molybdate • Sodium Selenate • Thiamine Mononitrate (vitamin B1) • Zinc Oxide.

Shape Up! Complete Nutrition Bar, Fudge Brownie - CSA Nutraceuticals, LLC
Each bar contains: Fudge Syrup: Corn Syrup, Sugar, Hydrogenated Starch, High Fructose Corn Syrup, Fractionated Palm Kernal Oil, Glycerin, Sunflower Oil, Unsweetened Chocolate, Carrageenan, Natural Flavor • Crisps: Soy Protein Isolate, Tapioca Starch, Cocoa Powder, Calcium Carbonate, Oat Fiber, Rice Flour, Malt extract • Chocolate Flavored Coating: Lactitol, Fractionated Palm Kernal Oil, Chicory extract, Cocoa, Sucralose, Salt, Lecithin, Distilled Monoglycerides, Vanilla extract • Peanut • Sodium Caseinate • Partially Hydrolyzed Guar Gum • Calcium Phosphate • Chicory • Chicory extract • Magnesium Oxide • Maltodextrin • Ascorbic Acid (vitamin C) • Ferrous Fumarate • Biotin • Cholecalciferol (vitamin D) • Chromium Chloride • Copper Gluconate • Cyanocobalamin (vitamin B12) • D-Calcium Pantothenate • Dl-Alpha-Tocopheryl Acetate (vitamin E) • Folic Acid • Manganese Sulfate • Niacinamide (vitamin B3) • Phytonadione (vitamin K) • Potassium Iodide • Pyridoxine Hydrochloride (vitamin B6) • Retinyl Palmitate (vitamin A) • Riboflavin (vitamin B2) • Sodium Molybdate • Sodium Selenite • Thiamine Mononitrate (vitamin B1) • Zinc Oxide.

Shape Up! Complete Nutrition Bar, Oatmeal Raisin - CSA Nutraceuticals, LLC
Each bar contains: Syrup Blend: Raisin paste, Malitol syrup, Cocoa butter, High Fructose Corn syrup, Glycerin, Hydrogenated Starch, Molasses, Cinnamon, Caramel Color, Medium Chain Triglycerides, Lecithin • Protein Nuggets: Soy Protein Isolate, Tapioca Starch, Soy Fiber, Salt • Yogurt Coating: Lactitol, Fractionated Palm kernal oil, Nonfat Dry Milk, Chicory extract, Yogurt powder, Distilled Monoglycerides, Sucralose, Soy Lecithin, Vanilla, Salt • Rolled Oats/ Oat Crisps: Oat Fiber, Rice Flour, Malt extract • Calcium Caseinate • Soy Protein Isolate • Milk Protein Isolate • Natural, Artificial Flavor • Magnesium Oxide • Arabic Gum • Maltodextrin • Ascorbic Acid • Ferrous Fumarate • Biotin • Cholecalciferol • Chromium Chloride • Copper Gluconate • Cyanocobalamin • D-Calcium Pantothenate • Dl-Alpha-Tocopheryl Acetate • Folic Acid • Manganese Sulfate • Niacinamide • Phytonadione • Potassium Iodide • Pyridoxine Hydrochloride • Retinyl Palmitate • Riboflavin • Sodium Molybdate • Sodium Selenate • Thiamine Mononitrate • Tricalcium Phosphate • Zinc Oxide • Peanut (possible trace amounts).

Shape Up! Mix & Drink Nutrition Shake, Authentic Chocolate - CSA Nutraceuticals, LLC
Each packet (40 g) contains: Whey Protein Isolate • Nonfat Dry Milk • Alkalyzed Cocoa • Chicory extract • Acacia • Guar Gum • Oat Hull Fiber • Sunflower Oil • Maltodextrin • Cellulose Gel • Trimagnesium Phosphate • Disodium Phosphate • Tricalcium Phosphate • Salt • Carrageenan • Corn Bran • Medium Chain Triglycerides • Soy Lecithin • Cellulose Gum • Xanthan Gum • Sodium Caseinate • Ascorbic Acid • Sucralose • Selenium Yeast • Chromium Yeast • Molybdenum Yeast • D-Alpha-Tocopheryl Acetate • Manganese Gluconate • Copper Citrate • Niacinamide • Zinc Oxide • Electrolyte Iron • Calcium Pantothenate • Pyridoxine Hydrochloride • Vitamin A Palmitate • Riboflavin • Potassium Iodide • Folic Acid • Biotin • Phytonadione • Vitamin D (D3) • Vitamin B12.

Shape Up! Mix & Drink Nutrition Shake, Genuine Vanilla - CSA Nutraceuticals, LLC
Each packet (40 g) contains: Whey Protein Concentrate • Nonfat Dry Milk • Whey Protein Isolate • Chicory extract • Milk Protein Concentrate • Oat Hull Fiber • Acacia • Guar Gum • Sunflower Oil • Maltodextrin • Cellulose Gel • Trimagnesium Phosphate • Disodium Phosphate • Tricalcium Phosphate • Salt • Carrageenan • Corn Bran • Medium Chain Triglycerides • Soy Lecithin • Cellulose Gum • Xanthan Gum • Sodium Caseinate • Ascorbic Acid • Sucralose • Selenium Yeast • Chromium Yeast • Molybdenum Yeast • D-Alpha-Tocopheryl Acetate • Manganese Gluconate • Copper Citrate • Niacinamide • Zinc Oxide • Electrolyte Iron • Calcium Pantothenate • Pyridoxine Hydrochloride • Vitamin A Palmitate • Riboflavin • Potassium Iodide • Folic Acid • Biotin • Phytonadione • Vitamin D (D3) • Vitamin B12.

Shape Up! Pear Body Types Weight Management Supplement & Complete Multivitamin - CSA Nutraceuticals, LLC
Two packets contain: Vitamin A 5000 IU • Vitamin C 500 mg • Vitamin D 400 IU • Vitamin E 200 IU • Vitamin K 80 mcg • Thiamin (B1) 3 mg • Riboflavin (B2) 3.4 mg • Niacin (B3) 40 mg • Vitamin B6 40 mg • Folate, Folic Acid, Folacin 1 mcg • Vitamin B12 1 mcg • Biotin 600 mcg • Pantothenic Acid 20 mg • Calcium 500 mg • Iodine 75 mcg • Magnesium 400 mg • Zinc 30 mg • Selenium 140 mcg • Copper 2 mg • Manganese 2 mg • Chromium 200 mcg • Molybdenum 75 mcg • Boron 1 mcg • Garcinia Cambogia fruit 3000 mg • Opuntia Cactus flesh (fics indica) 800 mg • Eleuthero root 100 mg • Soybean extract 50 mg • Kola Nut seed extract 300 mg • L-Carnitine (from L-carnitine tartrate) 100 mg • Rhodiola Rosea root extract 200 mg • Green Tea leaves extract (camellia sinensis) 1000 mg • EGCG (epigallocatechin gallate, from green tea extract) 270 mg. Other Ingredients: Microcrystalline Cellulose, Stearic Acid, Maltodextrin, Croscarmellose Sodium, Acacia, Magnesium Stearate, Hydroxypropyl Methylcellulose, Corn Starch, Silicone Dioxide, Carnauba Wax, Sodium Starch Glycolate, Hydrogenated Cottonseed Oil, Glycerin, Corn Syrup Solids.

Shape4Life Type 1 - 4 Life
Each Red Packet contains: Aldimine EFX: Niacin 3 mg, Vitamin B6 4 mg, Folic Acid 700 mcg, Vitamin B12 12 mcg • Proprietary Blend 492 mg: Cocoa extract, Quercetin, L-Tyrosine, 5-Hydroxytryptophan, Bromelain, Schisandra Chinensis fruit • ChitoLite brand Proprietary Blend 340 mg: Chitosan, Ascorbic Acid, Erythorbic Acid, Aloe Vera • Carb BLX Type 1 Proprietary Blend 1470 mg: White Kidney Bean extract, Wheat Grass extract, Green Tea extract (polyphenols 90%, catechins 70%), Jaborandi extract, Arabinose.
Each Blue Packet contains: Aldimine EFX: Niacin 3 mg, Vitamin B6 4 mg, Folic Acid 700 mcg • Vitamin B12 12 mcg • Proprietary Blend 492 mg: Cocoa extract, Quercetin, L-Tyrosine, 5-Hydroxytryptophan, Bromelain, Schisandra Chinensis fruit • Catalyst Plus: Chromium (as glycinate nicotinate) 240 mcg • Proprietary Blend 820 mg: Gymnema Sylvestre powder, Gymnema Sylvestre extract, Momordica Charantia, Lagerstroemia Speciosa leaf extract, Vanadium (bis-glycinate oxo vanadium), Alpha-Lipoic Acid.

Shape4Life Type 2 - 4 Life
Each Red Packet contains: Aldimine EFX: Niacin 3 mg, Vitamin B6 4 mg, Folic Acid 700 mcg, Vitamin B12 12 mcg • Proprietary Blend 492 mg: Cocoa extract, Quercetin, L-Tyrosine, 5-Hydroxytryptophan, Bromelain, Schisandra Chinensis fruit • ChitoLite brand Proprietary Blend 680 mg: Chitosan, Ascorbic Acid, Erythorbic Acid, Aloe Vera • Carb BLX Type 2 Proprietary Blend 980 mg: Cassia Nomame extract, White Kidney Bean extract, Wheat Grass extract, Green Tea extract (polyphenols 90%, catechins 70%), Jaborandi extract, Arabinose.
Each Blue Packet contains: Aldimine EFX: Niacin 6 mg, Vitamin B6 8 mg, Folic Acid 1400 mcg, Vitamin B12 24 mcg • Proprietary Blend 984 mg: Cocoa extract, Quercetin, L-Tyrosine, 5-Hydroxytryptophan, Bromelain, Schisandra Chinensis fruit • Catalyst Plus: Chromium (as glycinate nicotinate) 120 mcg • Proprietary Blend 410 mg: Gymnema Sylvestre powder, Gymnema Sylvestre extract, Momordica Charantia, Lagerstroemia speciosa leaf extract, Vanadium (bis-glycinate oxo vanadium), Alpha-Lipoic Acid.

Shape-Fast EFX Type 1 - 4 Life
Each capsule contains: Niacin 3 mg • Vitamin B6 4 mg • Folic Acid 700 mcg • Vitamin B12 12 mcg • Proprietary Blend 492 mg: Cocoa extract, Quercetin, L-Tyrosine, 5-Hydroxytryptophan, Bromelain, Schisandra Chinensis fruit. Other Ingredients: Gelatin.

Shape-Fast EFX Type 2 - 4 Life
Each capsule contains: Niacin 2 mg • Vitamin B6 3 mg • Folic Acid 475 mcg • Vitamin B12 8 mcg • Proprietary Blend 377 mg: Cocoa extract, Quercetin, L-Tyrosine, Bromelain, Schisandra Chinensis • Cassia Nomame 43 mg • Cocoa 70 mg. Other Ingredients: Gelatin.

Shape-Fast Ultra - 4 Life
Each capsule contains: Niacin 10 mg • Vitamin B6 (pyridoxine hydrochloride) 61 mg • Vitamin B12 (cyanocobalamin) 20 mcg • Selenium (selenomethionine) 18 mcg • Chromium (glycinate-nicotinate) 25 mcg • Guarana (40% caffeine) 170 mg • ForsLean brand Coleus Forskohlii Extract (20% forskolin) 40 mg • Acetyl-L-Carnitine 100 mg • Alpha Lipoic Acid 25 mg • Proprietary Blend 247 mg: Transfer Factor E-XF, Cocoa - Almond extract, White Willow bark, Green Tea extract (90% epicatechin), Potassium, Cayenne, Panax Ginseng (24% ginsenosides), Ginkgo Biloba (24% glycosides, 6% terpines). Other Ingredients: Gelatin.

ShapeWorks Beverage Mix (peach mango flavor) - Herbalife International of America, Inc.
Hydrolyzed Gelatin • Whey Protein Concentrate • Citric Acid • Malic Acid • Natural and artificial flavors • Potassium Citrate • Soy Lecithin • Acesulfame Potassium • Beta Carotene color • Silicon Dioxide • Turmeric Oleoresin color • Red Beet powder color • Sucralose.

ShapeWorks Cell Activator - Herbalife International of America, Inc.
Each capsule contains: Magnesium (as potassium magnesium aspartate) 18 mg • Potassium (as potassium magnesium aspartate) 38 mg • Krebs Cycle powder 100 mg: Citric Acid, Fumaric Acid, Aspartic Acid, Glutamic Acid, Succinic Acid • Inositol 25 mg • Chlorella 20 mg • Shiitake whole mushroom 15 mg • L-Glutamine 10 mg • Dried Cordyceps extract (whole) 10 mg • Dried Rhodiola root extract 10 mg • Cayenne fruit powder 5 mg • Dried Reishie whole mushroom extract 5 mg • Dried Pine bark extract (Pycnogenol brand) 2.75 mg. Other Ingredients: Gelatin, Maltodextrin, Silicon Dioxide, Magnesium Stearate.

ShapeWorks Cell-U-Loss - Herbalife International of America, Inc.
Each tablet contains: Vitamin C (as ascorbic acid) 83 mg • Calcium (as calcium carbonate) 77 mg • Iron (as ferrous fumarate) 1 mg • Potassium (as potassium chloride) 99 mg • Herbal Blend 152 mg: Couch Grass root, Hydrangea root, Dried Short Buchu leaves extract, Dried Corn Silk extract, Dried Uva Ursi leaves extract • Kelp stems and leaves 33 mg. Other Ingredients: Stearic Acid, Apple Cider Vinegar, Soy Lecithin, Silicon Dioxide, Acacia, Sodium Carboxymethylcellulose, Dextrin, Dextrose, Sodium Citrate.

ShapeWorks Formula 1 (cookies n' cream flavor) - Herbalife International of America, Inc.
Fructose • Calcium Caseinate • Cookie crumbs (wheat flour, sugar, canola oil, cocoa powder, salt, sodium bicarbonate) • Isolated Soy Protein • Oat Fiber • Inulin • Powdered Cellulose • Natural and Artificial Banana flavor • Guar Gum • Casein • Sodium Caseinate • Rice Fiber • Canola oil • Soy Lecithin • Carrageenan • Natural and artificial Peach flavor • Potassium Chloride • Artifical Vanilla flavor • Medium Chain Triglycerides • Fructooligosaccharides • Magnesium Oxide • Silicon Dioxide • Licorice extract • Bacterially-Derived patented Proteases (from Aminogen) • Citrus Pectin • Psyllium husk • Ginger root • Ascorbic Acid • Vitamin E Acetate • Licorice root • Hawthorne berry • Gotu Kola • Dandelion root • Biotin • Parsley • Papaya • Ferrous Fumarate • FD&C Yellow No.5 • FD&C Yellow No.6 • Niacinamide • Sodium Selenite • Zinc Oxide • Copper Gluconate • Vitamin A Palmitate • Calcium Pantothenate • Papain • Bromelain • Pyridoxine Hydrochloride • Riboflavin • Thiamin Mononitrate • Cholecalciferol (vitamin D) • Cyanocobalamin • Folic Acid • Chromium Amino Acid Chelate • Chromium Aspartate • Honey powder • Sodium Molybdate • Chromium Nicotinate.

ShapeWorks Formula 1 (Dutch chocolate flavor) - Herbalife International of America, Inc.
Fructose • Calcium Caseinate • Dutch processed Cocoa • Nonfat Dry Milk • Isolated Soy Protein • Corn Bran Fiber • Powdered Cellulose • Natural and Artificial Vanilla flavor • Guar Gum • Casein • Sodium Caseinate • Rice Fiber • Canola oil • Soy Lecithin • Carrageenan • Potassium Chloride • Medium Chain Triglycerides • Fructooligosaccharides • Magnesium Oxide • Silicon Dioxide • Licorice extract • Bacterially-Derived patented Proteases (from Aminogen) • Citrus Pectin • Psyllium husk • Ginger root • Ascorbic Acid • Vitamin E Acetate • Licorice root • Hawthorne berry • Gotu Kola • Dandelion root • Biotin • Parsley • Papaya • Ferrous Fumarate • FD&C Yellow No.5 • FD&C Yellow No.6 • Niacinamide • Sodium Selenite • Zinc Oxide • Copper Gluconate • Vitamin A Palmitate • Calcium Pantothenate • Papain • Bromelain • Pyridoxine Hydrochloride • Riboflavin • Thiamin Mononitrate • Cholecalciferol (vitamin D) • Cyanocobalamin • Folic Acid • Chromium Amino Acid Chelate • Chromium Aspartate • Honey powder • Sodium Molybdate • Chromium Nicotinate.

ShapeWorks Formula 1 (French vanilla flavor) - Herbalife International of America, Inc.
Fructose • Calcium Caseinate • Nonfat Dry Milk • Isolated Soy Protein • Corn Bran Fiber • Powdered Cellulose • Artificial Vanilla flavor • Guar Gum • Casein • Sodium Caseinate • Rice Fiber • Canola oil • Soy Lecithin • Carrageenan • Natural Vanilla flavor • Potassium Chloride • Medium Chain Triglycerides • DL-Methionine • Fructooligosaccharides • Magnesium Oxide • Silicon Dioxide • Licorice extract • Bacterially-Derived patented Proteases (from Aminogen) • Citrus Pectin • Psyllium husk • Ginger root • Ascorbic Acid • Vitamin E Acetate • Licorice root • Hawthorne berry • Gotu Kola • Dandelion root • Biotin • Parsley • Papaya • Ferrous Fumarate • FD&C Yellow No.5 • FD&C Yellow No.6 • Niacinamide • Sodium Selenite • Zinc Oxide • Copper Gluconate • Vitamin A Palmitate • Calcium Pantothenate • Papain • Bromelain • Pyridoxine Hydrochloride • Riboflavin • Thiamin Mononitrate • Cholecalciferol (vitamin D) • Cyanocobalamin • Folic Acid • Chromium Amino Acid Chelate • Chromium Aspartate • Honey powder • Sodium Molybdate • Chromium Nicotinate.

ShapeWorks Formula 1 (tropical fruit flavor) - Herbalife International of America, Inc.
Fructose • Calcium Caseinate • Nonfat Dry Milk • Isolated Soy Protein • Corn Bran Fiber • Powdered Cellulose • Natural and Artificial Banana flavor • Guar Gum • Casein • Sodium Caseinate • Rice Fiber • Canola oil • Soy Lecithin • Carrageenan • Natural and artificial Peach flavor • Potassium Chloride • Artifical Vanilla flavor • Medium Chain Triglycerides • Fructooligosaccharides • Magnesium Oxide • Silicon Dioxide • Licorice extract • Bacterially-Derived patented Proteases (from Aminogen) • Citrus Pectin • Psyllium husk • Ginger root • Ascorbic Acid • Vitamin E Acetate • Licorice root • Hawthorne berry • Gotu Kola • Dandelion root • Biotin • Parsley • Papaya • Ferrous Fumarate • FD&C Yellow No.5 • FD&C Yellow No.6 • Niacinamide • Sodium Selenite • Zinc Oxide • Copper Gluconate • Vitamin A Palmitate • Calcium Pantothenate • Papain • Bromelain • Pyridoxine Hydrochloride • Riboflavin • Thiamin Mononitrate • Cholecalciferol (vitamin D) • Cyanocobalamin • Folic Acid • Chromium Amino Acid Chelate • Chromium Aspartate • Honey powder • Sodium Molybdate • Chromium Nicotinate.

ShapeWorks Formula 1 (wild berry flavor) - Herbalife International of America, Inc.
Fructose • Calcium Caseinate • Nonfat Dry Milk • Isolated Soy Protein • Corn Bran Fiber • Powdered Cellulose • Artificial Strawberry flavor • Guar Gum • Casein • Sodium Caseinate • Rice Fiber • Canola oil • Soy Lecithin • Carrageenan • Artificial Raspberry flavor • Potassium Chloride • Medium Chain Triglycerides • Fructooligosaccharides • Magnesium Oxide • Silicon Dioxide • Licorice extract • Bacterially-Derived patented Proteases (from Aminogen) • Citrus Pectin • Psyllium husk • Ginger root • Ascorbic Acid • Vitamin E Acetate • FD&C Red No. 40 • Licorice root • Hawthorne berry • Gotu Kola • Dandelion root • Biotin • FD&C Red No. 3 • FD&C Blue No.1 • FD&C Yellow No. 6 • Parsley • Papaya • Ferrous Fumarate • FD&C Yellow No.5 • FD&C Yellow No.6 • Niacinamide • Sodium Selenite • Zinc Oxide • Copper Gluconate • Vitamin A Palmitate • Calcium Pantothenate • Papain • Bromelain • Pyridoxine Hydrochloride • Riboflavin • Thiamin Mononitrate • Cholecalciferol (vitamin D) • Cyanocobalamin • Folic Acid • Chromium Amino Acid Chelate • Chromium Aspartate • Honey powder • Sodium Molybdate • Chromium Nicotinate.

ShapeWorks Formula 1 Strictly Kosher - Herbalife International of America, Inc.
Isolated Soy Protein • Fructose • Powdered Cellulose • Corn Bran Fiber • Guar Gum • Articifial French Vanilla flavor • Maltodextrin • Potassium Chloride • Dicalcium Phosphate • Canola Oil • Carrageenan • Soy Lecithin • Rice Fiber • DL-Methionine • Magnesium Oxide • Silicon Dioxide • Licorice extract • Natural Vanilla flavor • Citrus Pectin • Psyllium husk • Honey powder • Ascorbic Acid • Vitamin E Acetate • Biotin • Vitamin A Palmitate • Dandelion root • Parsley • Papaya • Ferrous Fumarate • Niacinamide • Zinc Oxide • Copper Gluconate • Calcium Pantothenate • Papain • Bromelain • Cholecalciferol (vitamin D) • Pyridoxine Hydrochloride • Riboflavin • Thiamin Mononitrate • Cyanocobalamin • Folic Acid.

ShapeWorks Formula 2 Multivitamin Complex - Herbalife International of America, Inc.
Each tablet contains: Vitamin A (50% as retinyl acetate and 50% as beta carotene) 1667 IU • Vitamin C (as ascorbic acid) 50 mg • Vitamin D (as cholecalciferol) 133 IU • Vitamin E (as dL-alpha tocopheryl acetate) 10 IU • Riboflavin 8.3 mg • Niacin (as nicainamide) 33.3 mg • Vitamin B6 (as pyridoxine hydrohcloride and pyridoxal-5-phosphate) 10 mg • Folate (as folic acid) 133 mcg • Vitamin B12 (as cyanocobalamin) 2 mcg • Biotin 100 mcg • Pantothenic Acid (as D-calcium pantothenate) 6.7 mg • Calcium (as calcium carbonate) 167 mg • Iron (as ferrous fumarate) 2 mg • Iodine (as potassium iodide) 50 mcg • Magnesium (as magnesium oxide) 66.7 mg • Zinc (as zinc gluconate) 5 mg • Selenium (as selenomethionine) 17 mcg • Copper (as copper gluconate) 0.5 mg • Manganese (as manganese gluconate) 1.7 mg • Chromium (as chromium GTF, polynicotinate and picolinate) 33 mcg • Potassium (as potassium gluconate and glycerophosphate) 30 mg • Vanadium (as vanadium amino acid chelate) 2 mcg • Herbal Blend 16 mg: Choline Bitartrate, Inositol, Bee Pollen, Broccoli, Cabbage, Carrot, Cauliflower, Citrus Bioflavonoids, Garlic, Liorice root, Limonene, Polyoids, Spinach, Vegetase. Other Ingredients: Stearic Acid, Silicon Dioxide, Croscarmellose Sodium, Acacia, Microcrystalline Cellulose, Magnesium Stearate, Betaine Hydrochloride, Dextrin, Para Amino Benzoic Acid, Dextrose, Soy Lecithin, Sodium Carboxymethylcellulose, Shellac, Ethyl Cellulose, Sodium Citrate.

ShapeWorks Formula 3 Personalized Protein Powder - Herbalife International of America, Inc.
Soy Protein Isolate • Whey Protein Concentrate • Natural Flavor • Silicon Dioxide.

ShapeWorks Garden 7 - Herbalife International of America, Inc.
Each packette contains: Vitamin A (as Betatene brand beta carotene and mixed carotenoids) 5028 IU • Vitamin C (as ascorbic acid) 195 mg • Calcium (as calcium phosphate) 550 mg • Riboflavin 2 mg • Phosphorus (as dicalcium phosphate) 130 mg • Magnesium 38 mg • Sodium 5 mg • Potassium 55 mg • Garlic powder 612 mg • Broccoli sprout extract 510 mg • Cranberry extract (20% organic acid) 500 mg • Carrot powder 400 mg • Olive oil 243 mg • Orange fruit Bioflavonoids 204 mg • Spinach powder 200 mg • Hesperidine (from orange fruit bioflavonoids) 100 mg • Pumpkin seed powder 100 mg • Quercetin 85 mg • Grape skin extract (20% polyphenols) 51 mg • Glucosinolates (from broccoli sprout extract) 20 mg • Alliin (from garlic powder) 14 mg • Lycopene 5 mg • Lutein 5 mg • Zeaxanthin 1 mg. Other Ingredients: Gelatin, Maltodextrin, Microcrystalline Cellulose, Croscarmellose Sodium, Methacrylic Acid Copolymer, Stearic Acid, Beeswax, Magnesium Stearate, Soy Lecithin, Silicon Dioxide, FD&C Yellow #6, Triethylcitrate, FD&C Yellow #5, Dextrose, FD&C Blue #2, Sodium Citrate.

ShapeWorks Herbal Concentrate - Herbalife International of America, Inc.
Camellia Sinensis (green tea and orange pekoe tea) • Fructose • Maltodextrin • Cadamom seed extract • Lemon peel extract • Natural Caffeine powder • Hibiscus flower powder • Malva Sylvestris extract.

ShapeWorks New & Improved Total Control - Herbalife International of America, Inc.
Each tablet contains: Calcium (as calcium carbonate) 50 mg • Herbal Blend 479 mg: Dried Green Tea leaves extract, Dried Ginger root extract, Dried Theobroma Cacao seeds extract, Dried Yerba Mate leaves extract, Astragalus root, Celery seeds, Fennel seeds, Hawthorne berry fruit, Licorice root, Marshmallow root, Parsley leaves, Suma root, Dried Cinnamon bark extract, Alfalfa leaves • Caffeine (80 mg from natural caffeine and 4 mg from herbal blend) 84 mg. Other Ingredients: Microcrystalline Cellulose, Maltodextrin, Corn Starch, Sodium Starch Glycolate, Silicon Dioxide, Sodium Carboxymethylcellulose, Magnesium Stearate, Hypromellose, Polyethylene Glycol.

ShapeWorks Protein Bar (chocolate coconut flavor) - Herbalife International of America, Inc.
Glycerin • Coconut pieces • Whey Protein Isolate • Hydrogenated Starch Hydolyzate • Soy Protein Isolate • Polydextrose • Casein • Modified Palm and Palm kernal oils • Milk Protein Concentrate • Maltitol • Oligofructose • Water • Calcium Caseinate • Natural Flavors • Cocoa powder processed with Alkali • Milk Mineral Concentrate • Soy Lecithin • Canola oil • Mono- and Diglycerides • Soybean oil • Dextrose • Magnesium Oxide • Potassium Lactate • Mixed Tocopherols • Potassium Sorbate • Ascorbic Acid • Copper Gluconate • Ferric Orthophosphate • DL-Alpha-Tocopheryl Acetate • Maltodextrin • Salt • Sucralose (non-nutritive sweetener) • Biotin • Niacinamide • Zinc Oxide • Beta-Carotene • Calcium Pantothenate • Vitamin A Palmitate • Phytonadione • Pyridoxine Hydrochloride • Manganese Sulphate • Riboflavin • Thiamine Mononitrate • Potassium Iodide • Cyanocobalamin • Chromium Chloride • Folic Acid • Sodium Molybdate • Sodium Selenite.

ShapeWorks Protein Bar (chocolate fudge flavor) - Herbalife International of America, Inc.
Casein • Glycerin • Hydrogenated Starch Hydrolysate • Modified Palm and Palm kernal oils • Oligofructose • Soy Protein Isolate • Whey Protein Isolate • Milk Protein Concentrate • Maltitol • Cocoa powder processed with Alkali • Polydextrose • Natural Flavors • Water • Soy Lecithin • Ground Almonds, Canola oil • Unsweetened Chocolate, Milk Mineral Concentrate, Cocoa Butter, Soybean oil, Dextrose, Mono- and Diglycerides, Potassium Lactate, Magnesium Oxide, Licorice Root Extract, Ascorbic Acid, Salt, Copper Gluconate, Ferric Orthophosphate, DL-Alpha-Tocopheryl Acetate, Maltodextrin, Biotin, Mixed Tocopherols, Sucralose (non-nutritive sweetener), Niacinamide, Zinc Oxide, Beta-Carotene, Calcium Pantothenate, Vitamin A Palmitate, Phytonadione, Pyridoxine Hydrochloride, Manganese Sulfate, Riboflavin, Thiamin Mononitrate, Potassium Iodide, Cyanocobalamin, Chromium Chloride, Folic Acid, Sodium Molybdate, Sodium Selenite.

ShapeWorks Protein Bar (lemon flavor) - Herbalife International of America, Inc.
Soy Protein Isolate • Calcium Caseinate • Modified Palm and Palm kernal oils • Whey Protein Isolate • Sugar • Glycerin • Polydextrose • Oligofructose • Hydrogenated Starch Hydrolysate • Water • Ground Almonds • Honey • Soy Lecithin • Canola oil • Skim Milk powder • Milk Mineral Concentrate • Natural Flavors • Soybean oil • Malic Acid • Potassium Lactate • Yoghurt solids • Citric Acid • Mono- and Diglycerides • Magnesium Oxide • Mixed Tocopherols • Potassium Sorbate • Ascorbic Acid • Copper Gluconate • Salt • Ferric Orthophosphate • DL-Alpha-Tocopheryl Acetate • Maltodextrin • Turmeric • Biotin • Sucralose (non-nutritive sweetener) • Niacinamide • Zinc Oxide • Beta-Carotene • Calcium Pantothenate • Vitamin A Palmitate • Phytonadione • Pyridoxine Hydrochloride • Manganese Sulphate • Riboflavin • Pyridoxine Hydrochloride • Manganese Sulphate • Riboflavin • Thiamine Mononitrate • Potassium Iodide • Cyanocobalamin • Chromium Chloride • Folic Acid • Sodium Molybdate • Sodium Selenite.

ShapeWorks Protein Bar (peanut butter flavor) - Herbalife International of America, Inc.
Maltitol syrup • Soy Protein Isolate • Peanut Flour • Peanut Butter (ground peanuts) • Hydrogenated Stach Hydrolysate • Modified Palm and Palm kernal oils • Glycerin • Whey Protein Isolate • Casein • Milk Protein Concentrate • Cocoa Powder processed with Alkali • Water • Soy Lecithin • Mono- and Diglycerides • Canola oil • Salt • Dextrose • Potassium Lactate • Mixed Tocohperols • Soybean oil • Magnesium Oxide • Citric Acid • Ascorbic Acid • Copper Gluconate • Ferric Orthophosphate • DL-Alpha-Tocopheryl Acetate • Maltodextrin • Biotin • Sucralose • Niacinamide • Zinc Oxide • Beta-Carotene • Calcium Pantothenate • Vitamin A Palmitate • Phytonadione • Pyridoxine Hydrochloride • Manganese Sulphate • Riboflavin • Thiamine Mononitrate • Potassium Iodide • Cyanocobalamin • Chromium Chloride • Folic Acid • Sodium Molybdate • Sodium Selenite.

ShapeWorks Roasted Soy Nuts - Herbalife International of America, Inc.
Roasted Soy nuts • Canola oil • Cardia Salt (sodium chloride, potassium chloride, magnesium sulfate, heptahydrate, L-lysine monohydrochloride, silicon dioxide).

ShapeWorks Soup Mix (creamy chicken flavor) - Herbalife International of America, Inc.
Total Milk Protein Concentrate • Soy Protein Isolate • Hydrolyzed Gelatin • Salt • Onion Powder • Hydrolyzed Corn Protein (contains thiamin hydrochloride, lactic acid) • Hydrolyzed Wheat Protein (contains autolyzed yeast extract, natural flavors). Other Ingredients: Potassium Bicarbonate • Natural and Artificial Flavors • Silicon Dioxide • Sodium Alginate • Xanthan Gum • Guar Gum • Spice Extractives • Green Onion Flakes.

Shark / Glucosamine Formula - Health Smart Vitamins
Three capsules contain: Protein 0.675 g • Calcium (from shark cartilage) 210 mg • Phosphorus (from shark cartilage) 135 mg • Potassium (from glucosamine sulfate) 98 mg • Shark Cartilage 1500 mg • Glucosamine Sulfate 750 mg.

Shark Cartilage - Swanson Health Products
Three capsules contain: Shark Cartilage 2.25 g.

Shark Cartilage - Leiner Health Products
Each capsule contains: Shark Cartilage 500 mg. Other Ingredients: Gelatin, Maltodextrin, Magnesium Stearate, Calcium Carbonate, Sodium Starch Glycolate.

Some Brand Name Natural Products - What they Contain

www.NaturalDatabase.com contains MANY more listings than appear here.
Editor's Notes are located on pages 2155-2163.

BRAND NAMES

Shark Cartilage - Olympian Labs
Each capsule contains: Shark Cartilage 750 mg.

Shark Cartilage - GNC
Each tablet contains: Shark Cartilage powder 750 mg. Other Ingredients: Cellulose, Povidone, Dicalcium Phosphate, Vegetable Acetoglycerides.

Shark Cartilage - Pure Encapsulations
Each vegetable capsule contains: Shark Cartilage concentrate 500 mg: Glycosaminoglycans 105 mg, Mucopolysaccharides, including chondroitin-4-sulfate and dermatan sulfate protein 135 mg • Vitamin C (as ascorbyl palmitate) 10 mg.

Shark Cartilage Plus - Life Extension
Each capsule contains: Shark Cartilage 800 mg • Devil's Claw 35 mg • Black Cohosh 20 mg • Goldenseal 15 mg • L-Histidine 20 mg.

Shark Energy Drink - Osotspa Co., Ltd.
Carbonated Water • Sucrose • Dextrose • Citric Acid • Choline Bitartrate • Natural Caffeine • Inositol • Caramel • Niacinamide • Taurine • Sodium Chloride • Pantothenyl Alcohol • Pyridoxine HCl • Guarana extract • Riboflavin-Phosphate Sodium • Thiamine Mononitrate.

Shark Oil - Futurebiotics LLC
Shark liver oil 460 mg.

Sharp Thinking - Goldshield Elite
Two caplets contain: Ginkgo Biloba leaf standardized extract (24% flavonglycosides, 6% terpene lactones) 120 mg • Huperzine A (from Huperzia serrata extract whole plant) 50 mcg • Green Tea leaf standardized extract (30% polyphenols, 20% methylxanthines) 500 mg • Panax Ginseng root standardized extract (4% ginsenosides) 200 mg • Brahmi leaf standardized extract (10% asiaticosides) 100 mg • Citrus aurantium fruit standardized extract (5-7% alkaloids) 50 mg. Other Ingredients: Dicalcium Phosphate, Vegetable Cellulose, Fractionated vegetable oil, Soy polysaccharides, Silica, and Vegetable resin glaze.
See Editor's Note No. 40.

Sheep Sorrel Burdock Supreme - Gaia Herbs
Forty drops contain: Proprietary Blend 70 mg: Fresh Sheep Sorrel (rumex acetosella), Fresh Burdock root (arctium lappa), Slippery Elm bark (ulmus rubra), Turkey Rhubarb root (rheum palmatum), Spring Water, 35-45% Pure Grain Alcohol USP.

Sheer Moisture Lotion - FreeLife International
Purified Water • Neroli Hydrolate (flower water) • Ahnfeltia Concinna seaweed • Willowherb • Olive Squalane • Vegetable Glycerin • Stearic Acid • Glyceryl Stearate • Chrysanthellum Indicum extract • Vegetable Glycerin • Liposomes: Sodium PCA, Soy Phospholipids, Tocopheryl Acetate, Arginine, Lysine, Glycine, Proline • Ceramide 3 • Beta 1,3 Glucans • Sodium Hyaluronate • Saccharide Isomerate (moisture magnets) • BioEnhanced Grapefruit seed extract (BGSE) • Vegetable Glycerin • Lonicera Japonica (Japanese honeysuckle) • Palmarose essential oil • Sweet Orange essential oil • Bulgarian rose essential oil • Sodium Behenoyl Lactylate • Potassium Sorbate • Xanthan Gum.

Shen Ling Bai Zhu San Plus - Secara
Organic Licorice root (gan cao) 630 mg • Asian Ginseng root 5:1 extract (ren shen) 243 mg • Atractylodes rhizome 5:1 extract (bai zhu) 204 mg • Chinese Yam rhizome 5:1 extract (shan yao) 204 mg • Poria sclerotium 5:1 extract (fu ling) 204 mg • Organic Cardamom seed 187 mg • Hyacinth bean 5:1 extract (bai bian dou) 153 mg • Dandelion leaf (3% vitexin (3 mg)) 113 mg • Job's Tears seed 5:1 extract (yi yi ren) 104 mg • Platycodon root 5:1 extract (jie geng) 104 mg • Sacred Lotus seed 5:1 extract (lian zi) 104 mg.

Shen Min - Puritan's Pride
Three tablets contain: Shen Min: He Shou Wu (Fo Ti) root powder 12:1 standardized extract: Chrysophanics and Resveratrol complex 1,775 mg • Bioperine brand Black Pepper extract (piper nigrum) 3.0 mg. Other Ingredients: Dicalcium Phosphate, Microcrystalline Cellulose, Croscarmellose Sodium, Stearic Acid, Magnesium Stearate, Pharmaceutical Glaze.

Shen Min - Biotech Corp.
Three tablets contain: Shen Min: a proprietary blend of 12:1 standardized He Shou Wu (Fo Ti) root extract and He Shou Wu root powder providing a synergistic complex of chrysophanics and resveratrol 1775 mg • Bioperine brand Black Pepper extract (piper nigrum) 3.0 mg. Other Ingredients: Dicalcium phosphate, Microcrystalline Cellulose, Croscarmellose Sodium, Stearic Acid, Magnesium Stearate, Pharmaceutical glaze.

Shen Min Activator with Progestoplex - Biotech Corp.
Purified Water • Jojoba oil • Herbal Blend Hair Complex: Henna extract, Horsetail extract, Nettle extract, Chamomile extract, Rosemary extract, Tormentil extract, Burdock extract, Honey extract, Golden Seal root extract • Lecithin • Peg-40 Stearate • Steareth-20 • Cholesterol • Trichopeptide (hydrolyzed keratin) • Lysine Carboxymethyl Cysteinate • Progestoplex Proprietary Blend: Progesterone, Copper Peptide • Retinyl Palmitate • Tocopheryl Acetate • He Shou Wu extract • Saw Palmetto extract • Nettle extract • Propyl Gallate • Biotin • Polysorbate 20 • Chamomile extract • Carbomer • Disodium EDTA • Aminomethyl Propanol • Phenoxyethanol • Methylparaben • Ethylparaben • Propylparaben • Butylparaben.

Shen Min DHT Blocker - Biotech Corp.
Each tablet contains: Zinc 10 mg • Selenium 100 mcg • He Shou Wu 100 mg • DHT Block Proprietary Blend 300 mg • Lycopene 2 mg • Isoflavones 20 mg. Other Ingredients: Dicalcium Phosphate, Microcrystalline Cellulose, Hypromellose, Stearic Acid, Vegetable Stearin, Magnesium Stearate, Silica, Calcium Silicate, Pharmaceutical Glaze.

Shen Min Hair Volumizing Serum - Biotech Corp.
Aqueous Extracts of Chamomile, Clary Sage, Rosemary, Rhatania root extract, Ginkgo extract • Liposomal Bio-Plex: Hydrolyzed Wheat Protein, Hydrolyzed Wheat Oligosaccharides, Panthenol, Sesame Oil, Lecithin, Retinyl Palmitate, Octyl Methoxycinnamate • Biotin • Carbomer • Henna extract • Methacryl Ethyl Betaine/Acrylates Copolymer • Sodium Hydroxide • Triethyl Citrate • Cyclomethicone • DMDM Hydantoin • Methylparaben • Propylparaben • Dimethicone Copolyol • Disodium EDTA • Fragrance.

Shen Min Hair, Skin & Nails - Biotech Corp.
Three tablets contain: Vitamin C (as ascorbic acid) 150 mg • Vitamin D (as cholecalciferol) 400 IU • Thiamin (as thiamine HCl) 10 mg • Riboflavin 10 mg • Vitamin B6 (as pyridoxine HCl) 25 mg • Folate (as folic acid) 400 mcg • Biotin 2000 mcg • Pantothenic Acid (D-calcium pantothenate) 500 mg • Iodine (from kelp) 150 mcg • Zinc (as zinc monomethionine) 5 mg • Selenium (as selenomethionine) 70 mcg • Shen Min (he shou wu standardized to 10% chrysophancis) 150 mg • Shen Min root powder (as he shou wu) 200 mg • Silica (from colloidals) 50 mg • Lecithin (from glycine max, providing 24% phosphatidyl choline and 14% phosphatidyl inositol) 200 mg • Collagen (spray dried) 300 mg • Isoflavones (from glycine max and peuraria lobata) 5 mg • Turmeric rhizome extract (curcuma longa, 92% curcuminoids minimum) 25 mg • Fatty Acids 25 mg • Bioperine brand Black Pepper extract (piper nigrum) 2.5 mg. Other Ingredients: Microcrystalline Cellulose, Croscarmellose Sodium, Stearic Acid, Magnesium Stearate, Pharmaceutical Glaze.

Shen Min Prostate Health Formula - Biotech Corp.
Two tablets contain: Zinc (as zinc citrate, zinc monomethionine) 7.5 mg • Selenium (as selenomethionine) 35 mcg • He Shou Wu root (polygonum multiflorum, 12:1 standardized extract, source of resveratrol and chrysophanics) 100 mg • Saw Palmetto berries (serenoa repens, standardized extract 85%-95% phytosterols) 160 mg • Pumpkin seed extract (curcubito pepo) 80 mg • Pygeum bark (pygeum africanum, 4:1 extract) 75 mg • Isoflavones (from pueraria lobata root standardized extract and soybeans) 10 mg • Tomato concentrate (200 ppm lycopene) 100 mg. Other Ingredients: Dicalcium Phosphate, Microcrystalline Cellulose, Croscarmellose Sodium, Stearic Acid, Magnesium Stearate, Pharmaceutical Glaze.

Shen Min Topical - Biotech Corp.
Purified Water • Glycerin (from vegetable) • Jojoba oil • Herbal Blend Complex: Henna, Horsetail, Rosemary, Tormentil, Burdock, Honey, Golden Seal • Lecithin • PEG-40 Stearate • Steareth 20 • Tilisina complex • Cholesterol • Trichopeptide • Hydrolyzed Soy Protein • Retinyl Palmitate • Tocopherol Acetate • He Shou Wu extract • Saw Palmetto extract • Nettle extract • Nicotinic Acid • Pantothenic Acid • Propyl Gallate • Biotin • Chamomile extract • Soap bark extract • Eucalyptus extract • Quaternium-51 • Carbomer • Polysorbate 20 • Phenoxyethanol • Methylparaben • Butylparaben • Ethylparaben • Propylparaben • Aminomethyl Propanol • Disodium EDTA.

Shiitake Mushroom - Pure Encapsulations
Each vegetable capsule contains: Shiitake mushroom extract (lentinus edodes, standardized to contain 6% polysaccharides) 500 mg.

Shiitake/Maitake Extract - Nature's Way
Each capsule contains: Maitake dried extract 100 mg • Oat grain 200 mg • Shiitake dried extract 100 mg. Other Ingredients: Gelatin, Magnesium stearate, Millet.

Ship-Assure - Nature's Plus
Two tablets contain: Ginger root (zingiber officinale, standardized 4% Volatile oils) 350 mg • Kava (piper methysticum, standardized 29-31% kavalactones) 50 mg • Chamomile flower (matricaria recutita) standardized 1% apigenin, 0.5% essential oil) 50 mg • Hops fruit (humulus lupulus, standardized 5.2% bitter acids, 4% flavonoids) 50 mg • Siberian Ginseng root (eleutherococcus senticosus, standardized 0.8% Eleutherosides) 50 mg • Passion Flower (passiflora incarnata, standardized 3.5-4% flavonoids, calculated as isovitexin) 50 mg • Wild Cherry (Prunus virginlana fruit) 50 mg.

SHN Skin-Hair-Nails - The Vitamin Shoppe
Three tablets contain: Vitamin A (beta carotene) 10,000 IU • Vitamin C 120 mg • Vitamin B1 10 mg • Vitamin B2 10 mg • Niacinamide 50 mg • Calcium 600 mg • Iron 6 mg • Vitamin D 200 IU • Vitamin E 30 IU • Vitamin B6 10 mg • Folic Acid 400 mcg • Vitamin B12 16 mcg • Phosphorus 300 mg • Iodine (kelp) 225 mcg • Magnesium 200 mg • Zinc 15 mg • Biotin 400 mcg • Pantothenic Acid 30 mg • Choline 150 mcg • Inositol 60 mg • PABA 50 mg • Selenium 25 mcg • Manganese 10 mg • RNA 60 mg • Bioflavonoids 50 mg • Rutin 25 mg • Betaine Hydrochloride 50 mg. In a base of L-Cysteine, Methionine, Gelatin, Papain, Oat Straw, Echinacea, Horse Tail, and Asparagus.

Shogun Imperial Green Tea - Green Foods Corp.
Each tablet contains: Green Tea 335 mg.

Short-Term Adrenal - Enzymes, Inc.
Each capsule contains: Vitamin C (100% from Acerola Cherries) 4 mg • Proprietary Herbal Blend 365 mg: Siberian Ginseng root extract, Chinese Thoroughwax root extract, Licorice root extract, Rice Bran • n-zimes Proprietary Blend 65 mg: Protease, CereCalase. Other Ingredients: Cellulose, Water.

Shot-O-B12 5000 mcg - Nature's Plus
Each vegetarian capsule contains: Vitamin B12 (as cyanocobalamin) 5000 mcg. Other Ingredients: Microcrystalline Cellulose, Vegetable Cellulose, Purified Water.

Shot-O-B12 5000 mcg - Sustained Release - Nature's Plus
Each extended-relase tablet contains: Vitamin B12 (as cyanocobalamin) 5000 mcg. Other Ingredients: Di-calcium Phosphate, Microcrystalline Cellulose, Stearic Acid, Hydroxypropyl Methylcellulose, Magnesium Stearate, Silica, Beet root (beta vulgaris), Pharmaceutical Glaze.

Shot-O-B12 5000 mcg Spray - Nature's Plus
Each spray contains: Vitamin E 3 IU • Vitamin B12 (as cyanocobalamin) 5000 mcg. Other Ingredients: Purified Water, Vegetable Glycerin, Purified Lecithin, Citrus seed Extract (citrus sinensis), Natural Cherry Flavor.

Si Wu Tang Plus - Secara
Dong Quai root 5:1 extract (dang gui) 513 mg • Rehmannia tuber 5:1 extract (shu di huang) 474 mg • Chinese Peony root 5:1 extract (bai shao) 450 mg • Organic Black Cohosh root 405 mg • Ligusticum Wallichii rhizome 5:1 extract (chuan xiong) 204 mg • Chastetree fruit 6:1 extract 204 mg.

Siberian Ginseng - Golden Glow Natural Health Products
Each capsule contains: Eleutherococcus Senticosus root (siberian ginseng) 1000 mg: Syringaresinol Diglucosides 400 mcg.

Siberian Ginseng - Olympian Labs
Each capsule contains: Siberian Ginseng 500 mg.

Siberian Ginseng - Quest
Each capsule contains: Siberian Ginseng 500 mg.

Siberian Ginseng - Gaia Herbs
Siberian Ginseng standardized for 0.8% eleutherosides B & E. Standardized Full Spectrum 200 mg of extract per capsule. Guaranteed Potency 100 mg of extract per capsule.

Siberian Ginseng - Pharmanex
Each capsule contains: Ginseng, Siberian root extract (Eleutherococcus senticosus Max)(10:1) 150 mg. Other Ingredients: Rice Flour, Gelatin, Magnesium Stearate, Silicon Dioxide.

Siberian Ginseng - Nature's Way
Three capsules contain: Siberian Ginseng root 1.23 g. Other Ingredients: Gelatin, Magnesium stearate.

Siberian Ginseng Extract - Ortho Molecular Products
Two capsules contain: Eleuthero root extract (siberian ginseng, standardized to contain 0.8% eleutherosides) 150 mg. Other Ingredients: Natural Vegetable Capsules, Magnesium Stearate, Microcrystalline Cellulose.

Siberian Ginseng Extract - PhytoPharmica
Each capsule contains: Siberian Ginseng (Eleutherococcus senticosus) root extract 10:1 (standardized to contain greater than 0.5% eleutheroside E) 200 mg.

Siberian Ginseng Rush - GNC
Each capsule contains: Siberian Ginseng root powder (Eleutherococcus) 500 mg • Guarana seed extract (Paullinia cupana) 95 mg. Other Ingredients: Gelatin, Calcium Carbonate, Cellulose.

Siberian Root 1000 mg, Concentrated - GNC
Each capsule contains: Siberian Root (eleutherococcus senticosus; from 28.5 mg siberian root extract 35:1) 1000 mg. Other Ingredients: Soybean Oil, Gelatin, Glycerin, Caramel Color, Titanium Dioxide (natural mineral whitener).

SierraSil Joint Formula - Sierra Mountain Minerals, Inc.
Each capsule contains: SierraSil blend 667 mg: Smectite, Calcium Sulfate, Silicon Dioxide, Feldspar, Potassium, Iron Sulfate, Kaolinite, and Zeolite minerals, each containing individual elements such as Calcium, Magnesium, Iron, Manganese, Copper, Zinc, Selenium, Chromium, Molybdenum, and Phosphorus. Other naturally occurring and trace elements: Strontium, Beryllium, Boron, Potassium and Sodium.

SierraSil Joint Formula powder - Sierra Mountain Minerals, Inc.
Each scoop contains: SierraSil blend 2 g: Smectite, Calcium Sulfate, Silicon Dioxide, Feldspar, Potassium, Iron Sulfate, Kaolinite, and Zeolite minerals, each containing individual elements such as Calcium, Magnesium, Iron, Manganese, Copper, Zinc, Selenium, Chromium, Molybdenum, and Phosphorus. Other naturally occurring and trace elements: Strontium, Beryllium, Boron, Potassium and Sodium.

SierraSil Joint Plus capsules - Sierra Mountain Minerals, Inc.
Each capsule contains: SierraSil blend 667 mg: Smectite, Calcium Sulfate, Silicon Dioxide, Feldspar, Potassium, Iron Sulfate, Kaolinite,

and Zeolite minerals, each containing individual elements such as Calcium, Magnesium, Iron, Manganese, Copper, Zinc, Selenium, Chromium, Molybdenum, and Phosphorus • Vincaria brand Cat's Claw bark extract (uncaria guianensis) 50 mg. Other naturally occurring and trace elements: Strontium, Beryllium, Boron, Potassium and Sodium.

SierraSil Osteo Formula - Sierra Mountain Minerals, Inc.
Six capsules contain: Vitamin D (D3, as cholecalciferol) 600 IU • Vitamin K (as phytonadione) 200 mcg • Calcium (as clacium malate and SierraSil) 250 mg • Magnesium (as magnesium citrate) 150 mg • Zinc (as OptiZinc brand zinc monomethionine) 12 mg • Proprietary Blend 2170 mg: Ipriflavone, Soy Isoflavones, SierraSil blend: Smectite, Calcium Sulfate, Silicon Dioxide, Feldspar, Potassium, Iron Sulfate, Kaolinite, and Zeolite minerals, each containing individual elements such as Calcium, Magnesium, Iron, Manganese, Copper, Zinc, Selenium, Chromium, Molybdenum, and Phosphorus. Other naturally occurring and trace elements: Strontium, Beryllium, Boron, Potassium and Sodium. Other Ingredients: Hydroxypropyl Methylcellulose.

Sil-150 - PhytoPharmica
Two sofgel capsules contain: Milk Thistle seed extract (silybum marianum, standardized to contain 80% silymarin (240 mg) calculated as silybin) 300 mg.

Silent Night Formula - Nature's Way
Four capsules contain: Proprietary Formula: Hops flower • Scullcap herb • Valerian root. Other Ingredients: Gelatin.

Silibinin Plus - Life Extension
Each capsule contains: Silibinin 266 mg • Silymarin 60 mg. Other Ingredients: Gelatin, Water.

Silica 10 mg - Jamieson
Each caplet contains: Standardized Silica from pure spring Horsetail herb 3080 mg (Equisetum arvense L 770 mg powdered extract 1:4) 10 mg. With natural occurring flavonoids, saponins and minerals.

Silica Complex - Puritan's Pride
Each tablet contains: Calcium (as calcium carbonate and calcium citrate) 200 mg • Magnesium (as magnesium oxide and magnesium citrate) 150 mg • Zinc (as zinc gluconate and zinc citrate) 15 mg • Boron (as Boron Citrate, Boron Glycinate, and Boron Aspartate) 1.5 mg • Betaine (as Betaine Hydrochloride) 38 mg • Horsetail extract (Euisetum arvense) arial (standardized to contain 7% Silica) 500 mg.

Silica Mineral Supplement - Eidon Inc.
Each 1 tbsp serving contains: Silica 375 mg. Other Ingredients: Purified Water.

Silica Plus - Global Health Trax
One quarter teaspoon contains: Global Health Trax Proprietary Blend 1240 mg: Silica, Ionic Trace Elements, Citric Acid, Gluconic Acid, Rice Vinegar, Hydrogen Sulfate, Purified Water, Amino Acid Blend, Enzyme Blend.

SiliCare - Holista
Each capsule contains Silicon (dioxide) derived from 410 mg 2.9% Spring Horsetail Equisetum arvense extract 5 mg.

Silk Essence Conditioner - FreeLife International
Water • Behentrimonium Methosulfate • Cetearyl Alcohol • Silt • Sorbitan Esters • Butyrospermum Parkii fruit (shea butter) • Simmondsia Chinensis seed oil (jojoba) • Limnanthes Alba seed oil (meadowfoam) • Chlorophyllin - Copper Complex • Panthenol • Sericin • Olibanum • Citrus Limonum peel oil (lemon) • Vanilla Planifolia fruit extract • Prunus Amygdalus Amara kernal oil (bitter almond) • Hydrolyzed Wheat Protein • Hydrolyzed Wheat Starch • Citric Acid • Sodium Hydroxymethylglycinate.

Silk Essence Shampoo - FreeLife International
Purified Water • Aloe Barbadensis gel • Sunflower • Sunflower seed • Quassia • Black Walnut leaves • Hibiscus flower • Horsetail • Elderflower • Henna • Nettle • Cranesbill • Burdock • Orange fruit • Vegetable Glycerin • Lauryl Glucoside • Decyl Glucoside • Sodium Isostearoyl Lactylate • Cellulose Gum • Cetyl Alcohol • DL Panthenol • Hydrolyzed Wheat Portein • Methylsulfonylmethane (MSM) • Chlorophyll • Clover Honey • Lotus Blossom essence • Potassium Sorbate • Citric Acid • Benzyl Alcohol • Phenoxyethanol • Essential Vanilla oil • Essential Frankincense oil • Essential Bitter Almond oil extracted from Apricot kernals • Essential Calophyllym oil • Essential Ylang Ylang oil • Essential Lemon oil • Vitamin E Acetate.

Silver Mineral Water - WaterOz
Each bottle contains: Colloidal Silver +/- 100 parts per million • Water.

Silybin Phytosome - PhytoPharmica
Each capsule contains: Silybin phytosome (milk thistle extract) bound to Phosphatidylcholine 120 mg.

Silymarin - Pure Encapsulations
Each vegetable capsule contains: Milk Thistle extract (silybum marianum, standardized to contain 80% silymarin) 250 mg.

Silymarin - Aspen Group, Inc.
Each capsule contains: Silymarin (Milk Thistle, standardized at 80%) 150 mg.

Silymarin 80 - Metagenics
Each tablet contains: Milk Thistle seed extract (silybum marianum, standardized to 80% silymarin) 70 mg.

Silymarin 80% - Jarrow Formulas
Each capsule contains: Milk Thistle seed 30:1 extract (silybum marianum, yielding 80% or 120 mg silymarin) 150 mg. Other Ingredients: Cellulose, Silicon Dioxide, Magnesium Stearate, Gelatin.

Silymarin Forte - Ortho Molecular Products
Each capsule contains: Milk Thistle extract (standardized to contain 80% silymarin) 200 mg. Other Ingredients: Natural Vegetable Capsules, Magnesium Stearate, Microcrystalline Cellulose.

Silymarin Plus - Futurebiotics LLC
Three tablets contain: Milk Thistle seed powder extract (standardized for 80% (420 mg) silymarin) 525 mg • Inositol 240 mg • Choline (as choline bitartrate) 240 mg • Dandelion root powder 300 mg • Alfalfa leaf powder extract 300 mg • Black Radish root powder 300 mg • Beet root powder 300 mg. Other Ingredients: Dicalcium phosphate, Magnesium stearate, Vegetable stearate, Silica, Cellulose.

Silymarin Plus - Source Naturals
Each tablet contains: Silymarin (from Milk Thistle Seed extract) 140 mg • Vitamin C 100 mg • Choline (Bitartrate) 50 mg • Inositol 50 mg • Vitamin E (d-alpha tocopheryl natural) 25 IU.

Simicort - Enzymatic Therapy
Active Ingredient: Salicylic Acid 1.8%. Other Ingredients: Purified Water, Organic Fatty Acid Complex (C11-C18), Glyceryl Stearate, Chamomile extract, 18-Beta-Glycyrrhetinic Acid from Licorice root extract, Allantoin 2.0% from Comfrey root extract, Dimethicone, Vitamin E antioxidant, & Hypoallergenic Fragrance.

Similasan Allergy Eye Relief - Similasan AG
Active Ingredients: Apis 6X • Euphrasia 6X • Sabadilla 6X. Inactive Ingredients: Borate Buffer, Sodium Nitrate, Silver Sulfate (as preservative), Purified Water.
See Editor's Note No. 1.

Similasan Computer Eyes - Similasan AG
Active Ingredients: Conium Maculatum 6X • Natrium Muriaticum 6X • Ruta Graveolens 6X • Senega Officinalis 6X. Inactive Ingredients: Borate Buffer, Sodium Nitrate, Silver Sulfate (as preservative), Purified Water.
See Editor's Note No. 1.

Similasan Dry Eye Relief - Similasan AG
Active Ingredients: Mercurius Sublimatus 6X • Belladonna 6X • Euphrasia 6X. Inactive Ingredients: Borate Buffer, Sodium Nitrate, Silver Sulfate (as preservative), Purified Water.
See Editor's Note No. 1.

Similasan Ear Wax Relief - Similasan AG
Active Ingredients: Causticum 12X • Graphites 15X • Lachesis 12X • Lycopodium 12X. Inactive Ingredients: Glycerin.
See Editor's Note No. 1.

Similasan Earache Relief - Similasan AG
Active Ingredients: Chamomilla 10X • Mercurius Solubilis 15X • Sulphur 12X. Inactive Ingredients: Glycerin.
See Editor's Note No. 1.

Similasan Hay Fever Relief - Similasan AG
Active Ingredients: Cardiospermum 6X • Galphimia Glauca 6X • Luffa Operculata 6X • Sabadilla 6X. Inactive Ingredients: Boric Acid, Sodium Nitrate, Silver Sulfate (as preservative), Purified Water.
See Editor's Note No. 1.

Similasan Pink Eye Relief - Similasan AG
Active Ingredients: Euphrasia 6X • Hepar Sulphurius 12X • Belladonna 6X. Inactive Ingredients: Borate Buffer, Sodium Nitrate, Silver Sulfate (as preservative), Purified Water.
See Editor's Note No. 1.

Similasan Sinus Relief - Similasan AG
Active Ingredients: Luffa Operculata 6X • Kali Bichromicum 6X • Sabadilla 6X. Inactive Ingredients: Boric Acid, Sodium Nitrate, Silver Sulfate (as preservative), Purified Water.
See Editor's Note No. 1.

Similasan Throat Relief - Similasan AG
Active Ingredients: Arnica Montana 6X • Calendula Officinalis 4X • Guaiacum 4X • Mercurius Sublimatus 12X • Thuja Occidentalis 6X. Inactive Ingredients: Alcohol, 23% v/v, Purified Water.
See Editor's Note No. 1.

Simple Cleanse - PhytoPharmica
Laxative Formula: Three tablets contain: Magnesium Hydroxide 2600 mg • Proprietary Mucilage Blend 650 mg: Slippery Elm bark (ulmus rubra), Marshmallow root 3.5:1 extract (althaea officinalis), Fenugreek seed 4:1 extract (trigonella foenum-graecum) • Proprietary Soothing Blend 150 mg: Peppermint leaf (mentha x piperita), Fennel seed (foeniculum vulgare), Ginger rhizome extract (zingiber officinale) • Other Ingredients: Cellulose, Modified Cellulose Gum, Modified Cellulose, Magnesium Stearate, Silicon Dioxide, Lecithin, Carnauba Wax.
Fiber Formula: Eight capsules contain: Proprietary Fiber Blend 3455 mg: Psyllium husk (plantago ovata), Oat bran (avena sativa), Guar Gum seed extract (cyamposis tetragonoloba), Pectin (from citrus fruit), Marshmallow root 3.5:1 extract. Other Ingredients: Cellulose, Gelatin, Magnesium Stearate, Silicon Dioxide.

Simply Creatine - PhytoPharmica
Each 1 1/2 tsp serving (5 g) contains: Creatine Monohydrate 5 g.

Sinatrol - Ortho Molecular Products
Three capsules contain: N-Acetyl-L-Cysteine USP 750 mg • Andrographis Paniculata leaf & stem extract (standardized to contain 20% andrographilides) 300 mg • Thyme aerial portion 5:1 extract 300 mg • Tumeric root extract (standardized to contain 95% curcumin) 300 mg • Eleuthero root extract (siberian ginseng, standardized to contain 0.8% eleutheroside) 250 mg • Bromelain (2400 GDU/g) 200 mg • Berberine sulfate 100 mg • Licorice root extract (standardized to contain 12% glycyrrhizin) 100 mg. Other Ingredients: Magnesium Stearate, Microcrystalline Cellulose.

SinEcch - Alpine Pharmaceuticals
Each capsule contains: Arnica Montana 12C 500 mg.
See Editor's Note No. 1.

Single Day - Schiff
Each tablet contains: Vitamin A (retinyl palmitate, 10% as beta carotene) 10,000 IU • Vitamin C (ascorbic acid) 250 mg • Vitamin D (cholecalciferol) 400 IU • Vitamin E (D-alpha tocopheryl succinate) 150 IU • Vitamin B1 (thiamin mononitrate) 75 mg • Vitamin B2 (riboflavin) 75 mg • Vitamin B3 (niacinamide) 75 mg • Vitamin B6 (pyridoxine hydrochloride) 75 mg • Folate (folic acid) 400 mcg • Vitamin B12 (cyanocobalamin) 75 mcg • Biotin 75 mcg • Pantothenic Acid (D-calcium pantothenate) 75 mg • Calcium (calcium amino acid chelate) 10 mg • Iron (iron amino acid chelate) 9 mg • Iodine (kelp) 150 mcg • Magnesium (amino acid chelate) 5 mg • Zinc (amino acid chelate) 5 mg • Selenium (selenomethionine) 50 mcg • Copper (amino acid chelate) 25 mcg • Manganese (amino acid chelate) 600 mcg • Chromium (polynicotinate) 25 mcg • Potassium (amino acid chelate) 5 mg • Choline Bitartrate 75 mg • Inositol 75 mg • PABA (para-aminobenzoic acid) 75 mg • Citrus Bioflavonoid Complex 25 mg • Rutin 25 mg • Hesperidin Complex 5 mg. Other Ingredients: Cellulose, Stearic Acid, Magnesium Stearate, Coating (pharmaceutical glaze, ethyl cellulose), Silicon Dioxide, Croscarmellose Sodium.

Single Day Sustained Release - Schiff
Each tablet contains: Vitamin A (as retinyl palmitate, 10% as beta carotene) 10,000 IU • Vitamin C (as ascorbic acid) 250 mg • Vitamin D (as cholecalciferol) 400 IU • Vitamin E (as d-alpha tocopheryl succinate) 150 IU • Vitamin B1 (as thiamin hydrochloride) 75 mg • Vitamin B2 (as riboflavin) 75 mg • Niacin 75 mg • Vitamin B6 (as pyridoxine hydrochloride) 75 mg • Folate (as folic acid) 400 mcg • Vitamin B12 (as cyanocobalamin) 75 mcg • Biotin 75 mcg • Pantothenic Acid (as d-calcium pantothenate) 75 mg • Calcium (as calcium amino acid chelate) 10 mg • Iron (as iron amino acid chelate) 9 mg • Iodine (from kelp) 150 mcg • Magnesium (as magnesium amino acid chelate) 5 mg • Zinc (as zinc amino acid chelate) 5 mg • Selenium (as selenomethionine) 50 mcg • Copper (as copper amino acid chelate) 25 mcg • Manganese (as manganese amino acid chelate) 600 mcg • Chromium (as chromium polynicotinate) 25 mcg • Potassium (as potassium amino acid chelate) 5 mg • Choline Bitartrate 75 mg • Inositol 75 mg • PABA (para aminobenzoic acid) 75 mg • Lemon Bioflavonoids 25 mg • Rutin 25 mg • Hesperidin Complex 5 mg. Other Ingredients: Stearic Acid, Methylcellulose, Silicon Dioxide, Magnesium Stearate, Coating (pharmaceutical glaze, ethylcellulose).

Single Herb Extract Bai Ji Li - Plum Flower Brand
Blackberry Lily Rhizome 5:1 extract powder (belamcanda chinensis; she gan) 100 g.

SinoFresh Antiseptic Nasal & Sinus Spray - SinoFresh Healthcare
Cetylpyridinium Chloride 0.05% • Dibasic Sodium Phosphate • Eucalyptus Oil • Monobasic Sodium Phosphate • Peppermint oil • Polysorbate 80 • Propylene Glycol • Purified Water • Sodium Chloride • Sorbitol solution • Spearmint oil • Wintergreen oil.

Sino-Lung Res-Q - Nutri-Quest Rx
Each tablet contains: Lung 35 mg • Thymus 35 mg • Spleen 35 mg • Vitamin C 75 mg • Beta Carotene 12600 IU • Lemon Bioflavonoids 125 mg • Rutin 20 mg • Hesperidin Complex 75 mg • N-Acetyl Cysteine 35 mg • Propolis 20 mg • Cranberry 36 mg • Echinacea 30 mg • Goldenseal 35 mg • Elderberry 10 mg • Scullcap 35 mg.
See Editor's Note No. 14.

SinuCheck - Enzymatic Therapy
Each capsule contains: Pseudoephedrine HCl (from ephedra sinensis) 30 mg • Scullcap 4:1 extract (scutellaria baicalensis) 100 mg • Chinese Thoroughwax extract (bupleurum falcatum) 100 mg • Chinese Peony 4:1 extract (paeonia lactiflora) 100 mg • Dong Quai 4:1 extract (angelica sinensis) 100 mg • Licorice root extract (glycyrrhiza glabra, standardized to 5% glycyrrhizic acid) 40 mg • Curcuma root extract (curcuma longa, standardized to 4% curcumin) 20 mg • Ginger root extract 6.5:1 (zingiber officinale) 20 mg.
See Editor's Note No. 30.

SinuClear - PhytoPharmica
Each capsule contains: Pseudoephedrine HCl 30 mg (from ephedra sinensis) • Scullcap extract (4:1, scutellaria baicalensis) 100 mg • Chinese Thoroughwax extract (bupleurum falcatum) 100 mg • Chinese Peony extract (4:1, paeonia lactiflora) 100 mg • Dong Quai extract (4:1, angelica sinensis) 100 mg • Licorice root extract (glycyrrhiza glabra, standardized to contain 5% glycyrrhizic acid) 40 mg • Curcuma root extract (curcuma longa, standardized to contain

BRAND NAMES

2.5% curcumin) 20 mg • Ginger root extract (6.5:1, zingiber officinale) 20 mg.
See Editor's Note No. 21 and No. 30.

SinuComp **- PhytoPharmica**
Each tablet contains: Cowslip flower (primula veris) 36 mg • Sour Dock aerial part (rumex acetosa) 36 mg • European Elder flower (sambucus nigra) 36 mg • European Vervain (verbena officinalis) 36 mg • Gentian root (gentiana lutea) 12 mg.

SinuFix **- NaturalCare**
Two capsules contain: Vitamin A (as mixed carotenes from dunaliella) 5000 IU • Vitamin C (as ascorbic acid) 250 mg • Vitamin B6 (as pyridoxine HCl) 30 mg • Vitamin B5 (as calcium pantothenate) 100 mg • Zinc (as zinc methionate) 15 mg • Bromelain (1600 MCU) 250 mg • Nettle leaf extract (urtica dioica, 4:1) 200 mg • Wild Mediterranean Oregano leaf extract (4:1) 150 mg • GoldenSeal root 150 mg • Quercetin Bioflavonoid 125 mg • N-Acetylcysteine (NAC) 100 mg • Garlic bulb powder (odor controlled) 100 mg • Echinacea Purpurea/Angustifolia root extract (4% phenols) 50 mg • Grapefruit seed extract 50 mg • Turmeric root extract (95% curcumin) 50 mg • Peppermint leaf extract (2% essential oil) 50 mg • Cryptoxanthin (from dunaliella) 12 mcg • Zeaxanthin (from dunaliella) 6 mcg. Other Ingredients: Gelatin, Purified Water, Glycerin, Titanium Dioxide.

SinuFix Mist **- NaturalCare**
Active Ingredients: Zinc Gluconate (zincum gluconicum) 2X, 6X • Euphorbium Officinarum 4X, 6X, 12X • Origanum Vulgare (oregano) 3X, 6X • Echinacea Angustifolia (cone flower) 3X, 6X, 12X • Hydrastis Candensis (golden seal) 3X, 6X, 12X • Argentum Metallicum (silver) 8X • Kali Sulphuricum (potassium sulfate) 3X, 6X, 12X • Allium Cepa (red onion) 6X • Ragweed (ambrosia artemisiaefolia) 6X • Calcium Sulfide (hepar sulphuris calcareum) 8X • Potassium Bichromate (kali dichromicum) 6X, 10X • Sanguinaria Canadensis (blood root) 6X • Lemna Minor (duckweed) 3X • Luffa Operculata (luffa fruit) 6X • Pulsatilla (windflower) 3X • Sabadilla (cevadilla seed) 6X • Silicea (silicon dioxide) 8X • Spigelia Anthelmia (pink root) 3X. Other Ingredients: Organically-Grown Aloe Vera Extract, Patented Process Colloidal Silver, Green Tea Extract, Water-Soluble Tea Tree Oil, D-Mannose (natural monosaccharide), Grapefruit Seed Extract 0.1%.
See Editor's Note No. 1.

SinuGuard **- Enzymatic Therapy**
Each tablet contains: Cowslip flower (Primula veris) 36 mg • Sour Dock (Rumex acetosa) 36 mg • Elder flower (Sambucus nigra) 36 mg • Verbena (Verbena officinalis) 36 mg • Gentian root (Gentiana lutea) 12 mg.

Sinuplex **- Metagenics**
Each tablet contains: Vitamin C (as ascorbic acid) 150 mg • Quercetin Dihydrate 200 mg • Nettle root 10:1 extract (urtica dioica) 100 mg • Bromelain (2400 GDU/g) 50 mg • N-Acetylcysteine 25 mg.

Sinupret **- Bionorica AG**
Each tablet contains: Gentian Root (gentian lutea) 9 mg • Elder Flower (sambucus nigra) 29 mg • European Vervain aerial parts (verbena) 29 mg • Primrose Flower (primula veris) 29 mg • Sorrel aerial parts (rumex acesota) 29 mg. Other Ingredients: Sucrose, Talc, Lactose Monohydrate, Calcium Carbonate, Potato Starch, Maize Starch, Maize Swell-Starch Flour, Colloidal Anhydrous Silica, Stearic Palmitic Acid, Titanium Dioxide, Glucose Syrup, Gelatin, Shellac, Magnesium Oxide, Sorbitol, Eudragit E 12.5, Montan Glycol Wax, Povidone, Castor Oil.
See Editor's Note No. 72.

Sinus **- Nelson Bach**
Active Ingredients: Hydrastis 6c HPUS • Kali bio 6c HPUS • Pulsatilla 6c HPUS • Thuja occ 6c HPUS. Inactive Ingredients: Lactose, Sucrose.
See Editor's Note No. 1.

Sinus Ease **- Nature's Life**
Three capsules contain: Bromelain 1200 mg • Quercetin 300 mg • Vitamin C (calcium ascorbic) 133 mg.

Sinus Essentials **- Swanson Health Products**
Three capsules contain: Ma Huang (8% ephedra) 252 mg • Fenugreek seed powder 100 mg • Slippery Elm bark 100 mg • Cayenne Pepper 100,000 HU 60 mg • Eucalyptus leaves powder 50 mg • Goldenseal root 50 mg • Aloe Vera leaf powder 25 mg.
See Editor's Note No. 30.

Sinus Remedy **- PhytoPharmica**
Two chewable tablets contain: Kalium bichromicum 5x • Silicea 5x • Mercurius sulphuratus ruber 4x • Kali sulphuricum 4x • Belladonna 3x • Calcarea carbonica 3x • Calcarea fluorica 3x • Hepar sulphuris calcareum 3x • Hydrastis canadensis 3x • Manganum sulphuricum 3x • Sabadilla 3x • Thuja 2x.
See Editor's Note No. 1 and No. 21.

Sinus Remedy (formerly HP 7) **- Metagenics**
Each drop contains: Euphrasia Officinalis 3X • Allium Cepa 3X • Kali Bichromicum 12X • Sticta Pulmonaria 30X • Arsenicum Album 30X • Ambrosia Artemisiaefolia 30X • Sabadilla 6X • Arundo Mauritanica 12X • Apis Mellifica 30X.
See Editor's Note No. 1.

Sinus Support EF **- Nature's Sunshine**
Two capsules contain: Proprietary Blend 886 mg: Capsicum fruit (capsicum annuum), Burdock root (arctium lappa), Goldenseal root (hydrastis canadensis), Parsley herb (petroselinum crispum), Horehound herb (marrubium vulgare), Althea root (althaea officinalis), Bitter Orange fruit (fructus aurantia, synephrine 6% extract), Yerba Santa herb (eriodictyon californicum). Other Ingredients: Gelatin, Water.
See Editor's Note No. 40.

SinusHealth **- Vita Pharmica - formerly Neopharmica**
Two tablets contain: Proprietary Blend 2500 mg: Baikal Skullcap root, Schizonepeta Tenuifolia, Angelica root, Cinnamon twig, Xanthium Strumarium, Astragalus root.

Sinustatin **- American Biologics**
Each drop contains: Arsen. Alb. 12X • Calc. Carb. 30X • Cinnabaris 12X • Kail Bichrom. 12X • Mercur. Sol. Hahnem 30X • Pulsatila 12X • Sepia 12X • Sulphur 30X. Other Ingredients: 20% Alcohol, Water.
See Editor's Note No. 1.

Sinutone **- The Herbalist**
Eyebright herb • Golden Seal root • Bayberry root bark • Osha root • Yarrow flower • Horseradish root • Cayenne pepper.

Sinu-X **- Olympian Labs**
Two capsules contain: Proteolytic Enzymes 150 mg • Spearmint 50 mg • Clove 10 mg • Sea Mussel 50 mg • Zinc Gluconate 20 mg • Echinacea 40 mg • Red Clover 20 mg • Goldenseal 30 mg • Citrus Aurantium 30 mg • Green Tea extract 20 mg.
See Editor's Note No. 40.

Sitol **- PharmaGen**
Each capsule contains: Serenoa repens extract (standardized) 320 mg.

Sitol PA **- PharmaGen**
Each capsule contains: Serenoa repens extract (standardized) 320 mg • Pygeum africanum extract (standardized) 100 mg.

Skeletal Strength **- Nature's Sunshine**
Two tablets contain: Vitamin A (beta-carotene) 250 IU • Vitamin C (ascorbic acid) 75 mg • Vitamin D 100 IU • Vitamin B6 (pyridoxine HCl) 2.5 mg • Vitamin B12 (cyanocobalamin) 15 mcg • Calcium (amino acid chelate, di-calcium phosphate, calcium citrate) 300 mg • Iron (ferrous gluconate) 1.5 mg • Phosphorus (di-calcium phosphate) 96 mg • Magnesium (amino acid chelate, magnesium oxide) 300 mg • Zinc (oxide) 7.5 mg • Copper (gluconate) 1 mg • Manganese (amino acid chelate) 0.5 mg • Potassium (citrate) 50 mg • Boron (amino acid chelate) 0.5 mg • Proprietary Blend 54 mg: Horsetail herb (equisetum arvense), Betaine HCl, Papaya fruit (carica papaya), Parsley herb (petroselinum crispum), Pineapple fruit (ananas comosus), Valerian root (valeriana officinalis), Licorice root concentrate (glycyrrhiza glabra). Other Ingredients: Cellulose, Stearic Acid.

Skin - Enzymes, Inc.
Each capsule contains: Proprietary Herbal Blend 315 mg: Safflower petals powder, Burdock root extract, Oregon Grape root extract, Dandelion root extract, Calendula flower extract, Black Currant seed extract, Grape seed extract • Proprietary Enzyme Blend 200 mg: Amylase, pHysioProtease, CereCalase, Lipase. Other Ingredients: Plant Cellulose, Water.

Skin & Joint Essentials Dietary Supplement - N.V. Perricone M.D. Cosmeceuticals
Each softgel contains: Vitamin E (as natural D-alpha tocopherol 6 mg) 7.5 IU • Evening Primrose oil (10% GLA) 166 mg • Borage seed oil (24% GLA) 166 mg • Black Currant seed oil (16% GLA) 166 mg • Flaxseed oil (cold pressed) 333 mg • Rosemary leaf extract 2.5 mg. Other Ingredients: Gelatin, Glycerin.

Skin & Nail Support - Gaia Herbs
Two capsules contain: Triphala Powder Extract Blend 200 mg: Emblica Officinalis, Terminalia Bellerica, Terminalia Chebula • Horsetail aerial parts (equisetum arvense) 150 mg • Alfalfa aerial parts (medicago sativa) 60 mg • Gotu Kola leaf and root (centella asiatica) 42 mg • Yellow Dock root (rumex crispus) 26 mg • Nettle leaf (urtica dioica) 22 mg • Burdock root (arctium lappa) 17 mg • Figwort aerial parts (scrophularia nodosa) 6 mg • Oregon Grape root (berberis aquifolium) 5 mg • Astaxanthan 4 mg. Other Ingredients: Vegetable Glycerin, Vegetable Cellulose (capsule).

Skin Answer - LaneLabs
Willow bark extract • Carbamide • Aloe Vera • Oil of Melaleuca • Menthol • Sandbrier extract (source of glycoalkaloid).
See Editor's Note No. 9 and No. 21.

Skin Clarity Supplement: - Abra Therapeutics
Vitamin A (50% from beta carotene) • Vitamin B1 (thiamine) • Vitamin B2 (riboflavin) • Vitamin B3 (niacin) • Vitamin B5 (pantothenic acid) • Vitamin B6 (pyridoxine HCl) • Biotin • Vitamin C (calcium ascorbate) • Vitamin E (succinate) • Magnesium Oxide • Zinc Ascorbate • Chromium Picolinate • Selenium (selenomethionine) • Methylsulfonylmethane (MSM) • L-Lysine HCl • L-Proline • Astragalus root • Burdock root • Dandelion root • Echinacea root • Horsetail (source of silica) • Yellow Dock root • Milk Thistle • Red Clover • Viola Tricolor • Calcium Sulfate • Cellulose • Vegetable Stearates.

Skin Clear - The Herbalist
Echinacea root • Yellow Dock root • Oregon Grape root • Burdock root • Red Clover blossom • Jamaican Sarsaparilla root.

Skin Eternal DMAE Serum - Source Naturals
Deionized water • Propylene Glycol • Polysorbate 80 • Glycerin • DMAE • Vitamin C - Ester (ascorbyl palmitate) • Polyethylene Glycol • MSM (methylsulfonylmethane) • Coconut fragrance • Alpha-Lipoic Acid • Kiwi fragrance • Simethicone • Aloe Vera • Methylparaben • Biotin • Vitamin A Palmitate • Vitamin D (D3) • Vitamin E • Calcium Pantothenate • Coenzyme Q10 • Chamomile flower extract.

Skin Eternal Hyaluronic Acid - Source Naturals
Two tablets contain: Protein 1 g • Calcium 140 mg • BioCell brand Collagen II 1 g, Type II Collagen 600 mg, Chondroitin Sulfate 200 mg, Hyaluronic Acid 100 mg. Other Ingredients: Dibasic Calcium Phosphate, Stearic Acid, Hydorxypropyl Cellulose, Modified Cellulose Gum, Peppermint Flavor, Colloidal Silicon Dioxide.

Skin Formula - HERBALmax
Astragalus root • Ledebouriellae root • Peppermint • Cnidium fruit • Vitex fruit • Tree Peony root bark • Rehmannia root.

Skin Nutrition Lotion - Abra Therapeutics
Purified Water • Aloe Vera • Coconut oil • Olive oil • Stearic Acid • Glycerin • Cetyl Stearate • Cetyl Alcohol • Alfalfa extract • Borage extract • Calendula extract • Lemon Balm extract • Marshmallow extract • Rosemary extract • Yarrow extract • Arnica extract • Comfrey extract • St. John's Wort extract • Sage extract • Vitamin E • Geranium oil • Chamomile oil • Palmarosa oil • Sodium PCA • TEA • Allantoin • Lecithin • Methylparaben • Propylparaben.

Skin Refining Scrub - Abra Therapeutics
Deionized Water • Vegetable Glycerin • Glyceryl Stearate • Jojoba Wax beads • Almond Glyceride • Stearyl Alcohol • Almond Meal • Oatmeal • Chamomile extract • Rosemary extract • Rosebud extract • Calendula extract • Horsetail extract • Lavender extract • Sea Kelp ash • Algae extract • Cucumber extract • Peppermint oil • Ylang Ylang oil • Allantoin • Methylparaben • Propylparaben.

Skin Relief Bar - All Terrain Company
Sodium Palmate • Sodium palm kernelate • Water • Glycerin • Malaleuca Alternifolia (tea tree) leaf oil • Melia Azadirachta leaf extract • Oat extract (water, butylene glycol, avena sativa kernel extract, major leaf extract) • Sodium Chloride • Plantain extract • Tetrasodium EDTA • Iron Oxides.

Skin Support for Women - Futurebiotics LLC
Two capsules contain: Vitamin A (5000 IU beta carotene, 5000 IU fish liver oil) 10000 IU • Vitamin C (ascorbic acid) 250 mg • Vitamin D (ergocalciferol) 200 IU • Vitamin E (d-alpha tocopherol succinate) 30 IU • Zinc (amino acid chelate) 30 mg • Selenium (amino acid chelate) 100 mcg • Boron (amino acid chelate) 3 mg • MSM (methylsulfonyl-methane) 500 mg • Collagen 500 mg • Glucosamine Sulfate 100 mg • Skin Support Herbal Base 200 mg: Citrus Bioflavonoids, Grape Seed extract, Horsetail leaf powder, Papain, Chamomile flower powder, Aloe Vera leaf powder. Other ingredients: Gelatin, Water.

Skin Tone Balancer - Jason
10% Complete Vitamin C Complex with Kojic Ester, beta Hydroxy Acids, and Barberry extract. Super Oxide Dismutase liposome.

Skin, Hair & Nails Formula - Puritan's Pride
Three tablets contain: Vitamin A (as Retinyl Palmitate) 5000 IU • Vitamin C (as Ascorbic Acid) 60 mg • Vitamin D (as Cholecalciferol) 100 IU • Vitamin E (as d-Alpha Tocopheryl Acetate) 15 IU • Thiamin (Vitamin B-1; as Thiamine Hydrochloride) 5 mg • Riboflavin (Vitamin B-2) 5 mg • Niacin (as Niacinamide) 25 mg • Vitamin B-6 (as Pyridoxine Hydrochloride) 5 mg • Folic Acid 200 mcg • Vitamin B-12 (as Cyanocobalamin) 8 mcg • Biotin (D-biotin) 200 mcg • Pantothenic Acid (as D-Calcium Pantothentate) 15 mg • Calcium (as Dicalcium Phosphate and Calcium Carbonate) 834 mg • Iron (as Ferrous Gluconate) 3 mg • Phosphorus (as Dicalcium Phosphate) 331 mg • Iodine (as Potassium Iodide) 112.5 mcg • Magnesium (as Magnesium Oxide) 100 mg • Zinc (as Zinc Gluconate) 7.5 mg • Selenium (as L-Selenomethionine) 12.5 mg • Manganese (as Manganese Gluconate) 5 mg • Para-Aminobenzoic Acid 25 mg • Choline Bitartrate 75 mg • Inositol 30 mg • RNA 30 mg • Citrus Bioflavonoid 25 mg • Rutin 12.5 mg • Betaine Hydrochloride 25 mg • Rose Hips 60 mg.

Skin, Hair and Nails - Aspen Group, Inc.
Three tablets contain: Vitamin A 5000 IU • Vitamin C 60 mg • Vitamin B1 5 mg • Riboflavin 5 mg • Niacinamide 25 mg • Calcium 300 mg • Iron 3 mg • Vitamin D 100 IU • Vitamin E 15 IU • Vitamin B6 5 mg • Folic Acid 200 mcg • Vitamin B12 8 mcg • Phosphorus 150 mg • Iodine 112.5 mg • Magnesium 100 mg • Zinc 7.5 mg • Biotin 200 mcg • Pantothenic Acid 15 mg • Choline 75 mg • Inositol 30 mg • PABA 25 mg • Selenium 12.5 mcg • Manganese 5 mg • RNA 30 mg • Bioflavonoids 25 mg • Rutin 12.5 mg • Betaine HCl 25 mg • Horsetail Silica 50 mg.

Skin, Hair, Nails - Natrol, Inc.
Two capsules contain: Vitamin A (as Vitamin A palmitate) 5000 mg • Vitamin C (ascorbic acid) 100 mg • Vitamin E (as d-alpha tocopherol succinate) 50 IU • Thiamine (Vitamin B1) (as Thiamine HCI) 10 mg • Riboflavin (Vitamin B2) 10 mg • Vitamin B6 (pyridoxine HCI) 20 mg • Vitamin B12 (as cobalamin) 50 mcg • Biotin 500 mcg • Zinc (as zinc oxide) 8 mg • Copper (as amino acid chelate) 2 mg • Manganese (as manganese carbonate) 2 mg • MSM (methyl sulfonyl methane) 250 mg • Trace Mineral Complex 100 mg • Cysteine (as L-cysteine hydrochloride) 75 mg • PABA (para amino benzoic acid) 50 mg • Burdock root 50 mg • Choline (as choline bitartrate) 25 mg • Inositol 25 mg • Silicon (as colloidal silicon) 20 mg • Glutathione (as L-glutathione reduced) 2 mg. Other Ingredients: Rice powder, Magnesium Stearate, Gelatin.

Skindulgence 30-Minute Non-Surgical Facelift Cleanser - Skindulgence
Purified Water • Aloe Vera Gel • Caprylic/Capric Triglyceride • Butylene Glycol • Triethanolamine • Glyceryl Stearate • PEG-100 Stearate • Laureth 4 • Neopentyl Glycol Dicaprylate/Dicaprate • Stearic Acid • C12-15 Alkyl Benzoate • Glyceryl Stearate • Jojoba oil • Cetyl Palmitate • Glycereth-26 • Carbomer • Cyclomethicone • Skindulgence Herbal Blend: Butylene Glycol, Water, Hops extract (humulus lupulus), Rosemary extract (rosemarinum officinalis), Horsetail extract (equistetum arvense), Pine Cone extract (pinus sylvestris), Lemon extract (citrus medica limonum), Borage extract (borago officinalis), Spirulina Maxima extract • Propylene Glycol • Ginkgo Biloba extract • Leucine • Valine • Tyrosine • Arginine • Lysine • Cysteine • Cetyl Alcohol • Stearyl Alcohol • Allantoin • Urea • Tocopheryl Acetate (vitamin E) • Retinol Palmitate (vitamin A) • Jojoba Esters • Polysorbate 20 • Ammonium Lauryl Sulfate • Tetrasodium EDTA • Diazolidinyl Urea • Methylparaben • Propylparaben • Fragrance.

Skindulgence 30-Minute Non-Surgical Facelift Mask - Skindulgence
Acacia Catechu • Purified Water • Aloe Vera Gel (from concentrate) • Corn Starch • Chondrus Crispus (carrageenan) • Polysorbate 20 • Skindulgence Herbal Blend: Butylene Glycol, Water, Hops extract (humulus lupus), Rosemary extract (rosemarinum officinalis), Horsetail extract (equisetum arvense), Pine Cone extract (pinus sylvestris), Lemon extract (citrus medica limonum), Borage extract (borago officinalis), Spirulina Maxima extract • Propylene Glycol • Ginkgo Biloba extract • Leucine • Valine • Tyrosine • Arginine • Lysine • Cysteine • TEA Lauryl Sulfate • Isoceceth-20 • Tetrasodium EDTA • Titanium Dioxide • Diazolidinyl Urea • Methylparaben • Fragrance.

Skindulgence 30-Minute Non-Surgical Facelift Moisturizer - Skindulgence
Purified Water • Aloe Vera Gel • Neopentyl Glycol Dicaprylate/ Dicaprate • Jojoba oil • Caprylic/Capric Triglyceride • Cetyl Alcohol • Butylene Glycol • Glyceryl Stearate • PEG-100 Stearate • Cetyl Palmitate • Laureth 4 • Skindulgence Herbal Blend: Butylene Glycol, Water, Hops extract (humulus lupus), Rosemary extract (rosmarinus officinalis), Horsetail extract (equisetum arvense), Pine Cone extract (pinus sylvestris), Lemon extract (citrus medica limonum), Borage extract (borago officinalis), Spirulina Maxima extract • Propylene Glycol • Comfrey extract (symphytum officinale) • Plantain extract (plantago ovata) • Hydrolyzed Wheat Protein • Glutamine • Proline • Leucine • Serine • Tocopheryl Acetate (vitamin E) • Retinyl Palmitate (vitamin A) • Sodium Hyaluronate • Panthenol • Allantoin • Glycereth-26 • Glycerin • Carbomer • Triethanolamine • Polysorbate 80 • Xanthan Gum • Tetrasodium EDTA • Ammonium Lauryl Sulfate • Diazolidinyl Urea • Methylparaben • Propylparaben • Fragrance.

Skinlogics Herbal Hydrating Mist - BeautiControl Inc.
Purified Water • Sodium Hyaluronate • Cucumber extract • Ivy extract • Arnica extract • Althea extract • Pellitory extract • Elder extract • Disodium EDTA • Diazolidinyl Urea • Phenoxyethanol • Methylparaben • Ethylparaben • Propylparaben • Butylparaben.

Skinny Mini - Nature's Plus
Two capsules contain: Vitamin B12 (as cyanocobalamin) 500 mcg • Chromium (as chromium polynicotinate, chloride) 120 mcg • Proprietary Skinny Mini Herbal Blend 620 mg: Guarana seed, Spirulina, Cacao fruit (theobroma cacao; metabromine), Green Tea leaf (camellia sinensis) • Rhodiola root (rhodiola rosea, with standardized rosavin, salidroside, polyphenols, beta-vicanosides, rosin and rosarin) 250 mg • CitriMax brand Garcinia Cambogia fruit extract (standardized 50% [-]hydroxycitrate) 100 mg • ForsLean brand Coleus Forskohlii extract (with standardized forskolin) 100 mg • Conjugated Linoleic Acid (CLA, standardized 1:1 c9-t11:t10-c12) 100 mg • Bioperine brand Piper Nigrum fruit extract (standardized to 95% 1-piperylpiperdine) 1 mg. Other Ingredients: Gelatin, Silica, Natural Color, Purified Water.

Skinny Mini Double Chocolate Fudge Crunch Shake - Nature's Plus
Each scoop (33 g) contains: Vitamin A 500 IU • Vitamin C 6 mg • Calcium • Iron 1.8 mg • Vitamin D 40 IU • Vitamin E 3 IU • Thiamin 0.15 mg • Riboflavin 0.17 mg • Niacin 2 mg • Vitamin B6 0.2 mg • Folic Acid 40 mcg • Vitamin B12 6 mcg • Biotin 30 mcg • Pantothenic Acid 1 mg • Iodine 3 mcg • Magnesium 40 mg • Zinc 1.5 mg • Selenium 7 mcg • Manganese 0.2 mg • ChromeMate brand Chromium 156 mcg • Molybdenum 7.5 mcg • Proprietary Skinny Mini Herbal Energy Blend 636 mg: Guarana seed, L-Phenylalanine, Aspartic Acid, Spirulina, Metabromine brand Cacao fruit (theobroma cacao), Green Tea leaf (camellia sinensis) • Rhodiola root (rhodiola rosea with standardized rosavin, salidroside, polyphenols, beta-vicianosides, rosin, rosarin) 250 mg • CitriMax brand Garcinia Cambogia fruit extract 100 mg • Conjugated Linoleic Acid (CLA) 100 mg • Bioperine brand Piper Nigrum fruit 1 mg. Other Ingredients: Vitasweet brand Proprietary Blend (maltitol, FOS, bromelain, papain), Skinny Mini Protein Blend (non-GMO isolated soy protein, soy crisps), Natural Flavors, Fructose, Xanthan Gum, Lecithin, Natural Color, Clarinol, Acacia Leaf Powder, Oat bran, ForsLean brand Coleus Forskohlii.

SkinZinc Cream - Selfworx
Active Ingredient: Salicylic Acid 2%. Inactive Ingredients: Water, Glyceryl Stearate SE, Propylene Glycol, Glycerin, Mineral oil, Stearic Acid, Ceteareth-20, Cetearyl Alcohol, DMDM Hydantoin, Methylparaben, Propylparaben, Melaleuca Alternifolia (tea tree) leaf oil, Tocopheryl Acetate, Medicago Sativa (alfalfa) extract, Arnica Montana flower extract, Sodium Hydroxide, Epilobium Angustifolium extract (willowherb).

SkinZinc Spray - Selfworx
Active Ingredient: Zinc Pyrithione 0.25%. Inactive Ingredients: Water, Glycerine, Propylene, Glycol, Epilobium Angustifolium Extract (Willowherb), Aloe Barbadensis leaf juice, Quarternarium 15.

Skullcap St. John's Wort Supreme - Gaia Herbs
Forty drops contain: Proprietary Blend 80 mg: Skullcap herb (scutellaria lateriflora), St. John's Wort flower buds (hypericum perforatum), Calendula flowers (calendula officinalis), German Chamomile flowers (matricaria recutita), California Poppy (eschscholzia californica), Fresh Wild Oats milky seed (avena sativa), Valerian root (valeriana officinalis), 45-55% Pure Grain Alcohol USP, Spring Water.

Sleep Aid - Nelson Bach
Active Ingredients: Kali brom 30c HPUS • Coffea cruda 30c HPUS • Passiflora 30c HPUS • Avena 30c HPUS • Alfalfa 30c HPUS • Valeriana 30c HPUS. Inactive Ingredients: Lactose, Sucrose.
See Editor's Note No. 1.

Sleep Ease - PhytoPharmica
Twenty drops contain: Secale cornutum 4x • Belladonna 3x • Avena sativa 1x • Passiflora incarnata 1x • Valeriana officinalis 1x. In a base of 40% USP alcohol by volume.
See Editor's Note No. 1 and No. 21.

Sleep Formula - Preventive Nutrition
One capsule contains: Kava Kava Root Extract (Piper methysticum; 55% Kavalactones) 90 mg • Griffonia Seed Extract (20% 5-Hydroxyl-L-Tryptophan) 50 mg • Melatonin (n-acetyl-5-Methoxytryptamine) 2 mg. Other Ingredients: Polyethylene Glycol, Gelatin, Glycerin, Chlorophyll, Titanium Dioxide.
See Editor's Note No. 16.

Sleep Link - Pain & Stress Center
Each capsule contains: Vitamin C (as Ester C brand calcium ascorbate and ascorbyl palmitate) 5 mg • Vitamin B6 (as pyridoxal 5' phosphate) 1 mg • Melatonin 500 mcg • L-Theanine (Suntheanine brand) 15 mg • L-5-HTP (5-hydroxytryptophan) 30 mg • Proprietary Blend 425 mg: GABA (gamma amino butyric acid), Passion Flower herb powder, Ashwagandha root 15:1 extract (withania somnifera), L-Glutamine. Other Ingredients: Gelatin Capsule.

BRAND NAMES

Sleep Miracle **-** Alternecare Health Products
Three sprays contain: Passion Flower extract (passiflora incarnata) 10 mg • Valerian root extract (valeriana officinalis) 10 mg • Stevia leaf extract • Melatonin 1 mg.
See Editor's Note No. 26.

Sleep Now **-** Herbalife International of America, Inc.
Each tablet contains: Calcium (as calcium carbonate) 144 mg • Exclusive Blend 300 mg: Dried Passionflower extract, Dried Valerian root extract, Dried Hops strobiles extract (humulus lupulus), Wild Lettuce leaves (latuca sativa), Cinnamon bark (cinnamomum aromaticum), Orange peel (citrus aurantium), Enlgish Lavender flower, Dried Amla fruit extract (phyllanthus emblica) • Melatonin 1 mg. Other Ingredients: Maltodextrin, Stearic Acid, Silicon Dioxide, Sodium Carboxymethylcellulose, Microcrystalline Cellulose, Dextrin, Dextrose Monohydrate, Soy Lecithin, Sodium Citrate, Hydroxypropyl Cellulose, Magnesium Stearate.

Sleep Secret **-** SleepSecret
Coffea Cruda 6X • Valeriana Officinalis 6X • Passiflora Incarnata 6X • Magnesia Phosphorica 7X • Medicago Sativa 6X • Avena Sativa 6X. Base: 40% Glycerin, 0.3% Citric Acid, 0.3% Ascorbic Acid, Purified Water, Vanilla Flavoring.
See Editor's Note No. 1.

Sleep Therapy Bath **-** Abra Therapeutics
Sodium Borate • Sodium Sulfate • Sodium Chloride • Sodium Sesquicarbonate • Olive oil • Mandarin oil • Neroli oil • Lavender oil • Mace • Vetiver oil • Tangerine oil • Peru Balsam oil • Artemisia leaf extract • Valerian root extract • Poppy extract • Chromium Oxide • Trace Mineral Salts.

Sleep-Assure **-** Nature's Plus
Each tablet contains: Rapid Release Layer: Melatonin (N-acetyl-5-methoxytryptamine) 1.5 mg • GABA (gamma aminobutyric acid) 10 mg • Pyridoxal-5-Phosphate (P5P) 10 mg. Sustained Release Layer: Melatonin (N-acetyl-5-methoxytryptamine) 1.5 mg • Herbal Blend 25 mg: Kava Kava root extract (piper methysticum, standardized 29-31% kavalactones), Passion Flower extract (passiflora incarnata. standardized 3.5-4% flavonoids calculated as isovitexin, Valerian root extract (valeriana officinalis, standardized 1% valerenic acid), Chamomile flower (matricaria recutita, standardized 1% Apigenin 0.5% essential oil).
See Editor's Note No. 16.

Sleep-N-Slim **-** EuroBotanicals, Inc.
L-Glutamine • L-Lysine HCl • Magnesium Citrate • L-Ornithine Glysine • L-Arginine • Collagen • Vitamin B6 (pyridoxine HCl) • L-Carnitine • Vitamin B3 (niacin) • Aloe Vera • Ascorbic Acid • Citric Acid • Sodium Benzoate • Potassium Sorbate • Carrageenan.

SleepRite **-** 4 Life
Each capsule contains: Vitamin B6 (as pyridoxine HCl) 15 mg • Melatonin 2.5 mg • 5-Hydroxytryptophan (Griffonia simplicitolia, seed) 30 mg • Proprietary Blend 215 mg: Valerian (0.8% valerinic acid, rood), Kava Kava extract (root), Scullcap (whole herb), Hops (aerial parts), Chamomile (aerial parts).

SleepTight **-** Life Enhancement Products, Inc.
Three capsules contain: Vitamin B6 (as pyridoxal-5-phosphate) 10 mg • Pantothenic Acid (vitamin B5) 100 mg • Choline (as choline bitartrate) 200 mg • Rhodiola Rosea extract 150 mg • 5-Hydroxytryptophan 100 mg • Melatonin 450 mcg.

Sleep-Tite **-** Wellness International Network, Ltd.
Two capsules contain: Herbal Blend (equivalent to 3330 mg of whole herbs) 790 mg: European Valerian root 4:1 extract, Celery seed 4:1 extract, Hops strobile 4:1 extract, Passion flower 4:1 extract, California Poppy 5:1 extract, Chamomile flower 5:1 extract, Chinese Fu Ling 5:1 extract (poria cocos), Kava Kava root 5:1 extract, Feverfew 5:1 extract, Skullcap. Other Ingredients: Dicalcium Phosphate, Micorcrystalline Cellulose, Croscarmellose Sodium, Stearic Acid, Silica, Magnesium Stearate, Sugar Coat (calcium sulfate, sucrose, kaolin, talc, gelatin, shellac, titanium dioxide, anise oil, beeswax, carnauba wax).

Sleepytime Extra **-** Celestial Seasonings
Two capsules contain: Calcium (as carbonate, citrate, and malate) 200 mg • Magnesium (as oxide) 100 mg • Proprietary Blend 800 mg: Valerian (root), Valerian (standardized extract), Kava Kava (root), Kava Kava (standardized extract). Other Ingredients: May contain one or more of the following: Dicalcium phosphate, gelatin, rice flour, stearic acid, spearmint extract, magnesium stearate, and silicon dioxide.

Slender Shaper **-** Pharmagel
E-L-A Complex.

Slender-Mist **-** KareMor International
Vitamin B6 • Pantothenic Acid • Chromium • Hydroxy-Citric Acid • L-Carnitine. Available in Arctic Mint, Berry Supreme, chocolate Fudge, and Tropical Delite.

Slim & Natural Shake (assorted flavors) **-** Nature's Plus
Each scoop (34 g) contains: Vitamin A 5000 IU • Vitamin C 60 mg • Calcium 200 mg • Iron 4.5 mg • Vitamin D 400 IU • Vitamin E 30 IU • Thiamin 1.5 mg • Riboflavin 1.7 mg • Niacin 20 mg • Vitamin B6 2 mg • Folic Acid 400 mcg • Vitamin B12 6 mcg • Biotin 300 mcg • Pantothenic Acid 10 mg • Iodine 150 mcg • Magnesium 80 mg • Zinc 15 mg • Selenium 20 mcg • Manganese 5 mg • Chromium 150 mcg • Molybdenum 20 mcg • Super CitriMax brand Garcinia Cambogia fruit extract 100 mg • Inositol 50 mg • Choline Bitartrate 21 mg. Other Ingredients: Non-GMO Isolated Soy Protein, Fructose, Microcrystalline Cellulose, Potassium Citrate, Guar Gum, Psyllium, Oat Bran, Apple Pectin, Bee Pollen, Bioflavonoids, Papaya, Bromelain. Vanilla flavor also contains: Natural Vanilla Flavor. Strawberry flavor also contains: Natural Strawberry Flavor, Beet Juice. Chocolate flavor also contains: Natural Dutch Cocoa.

Slim 7 **-** Swanson Health Products
Two tablets contain: Vitamin A (retinyl palmitate) 1667 IU • Vitamin C (as ascorbic acid) 20 mg • Vitamin E (as d-alpha tocopheryl succinate) 10 IU • Riboflavin (vitamin B-2) 0.6 mg • Niacin 6.6 mg • Vitamin B-6 (as pyridoxine HCl) 0.66 mg • Folic Acid 133.3 mcg • Vitamin B-12 (as cyanocobalamin) 2 mcg • Biotin 100 mcg • Iodine (from kelp) 50 mcg • Selenium (as selenomethionine) 16.6 mcg • Chromium (from Chromax chromium picolinate) 375 mcg • Chromium (from chromium polynicotinate) 375 mcg • CitriMax brand Garcinia Cambogia fruit extract 500 mg, (-) Hydroxycitric Acid 250 mg • Proprietary blend of 72 Trace Minerals 200 mg • L-Carnitine (as tartrate) 100 mg • Choline (as choline bitartrate) 67 mg • Green Tea extract (20% polyphenols) 50 mg • Kola Nut extract 50 mg • Capsicum 33.3 mg • Chitosan 33.3 mg • Ginger 33.3 mg • Inositol 33.3 mg • Spirulina 33.3 mg • Betaine HCl 8 mg.

Slim Down Apple Cider Vinegar **-** Jamieson
Each tablet contains: Apple Cider Vinegar Concentrate 500 mg.

Slim Down Bar **-** Jamieson
Each bar contains: Vitamin A 175 RE • Vitamin D 0.44 mcg • Vitamin C (Ascorbic Acid) 8.75 mg • Vitamin E (D-Alpha Acetate) 1.75 mg • Vitamin B1 245 mcg • Vitamin B2 315 mcg • Vitamin B6 315 mcg • Vitamin B12 0.525 mcg • Vitamin B3 1.5 NE • Vitamin B5 1.5 mg • Biotin 21 mcg • Calcium 306 mg • Phosphorus 175 mg • Iron 1.75 mg • Iodide 26.25 mcg • Magnesium 70 mg • Copper 0.26 mg • Zinc 2.45 mg • Manganese 0.79 mg • Selenium (Chelate) 7 mcg • Chromium (Chelate) 7 mcg • Molybdenum (Citrate) 14 mcg • Phaseolamin 2250 brand White Kidney bean extract 100 mg.

Slim Down Carb & Fat Burner **-** Jamieson
Each capsule contains: CitraMax HCA (hydroxycitric acid) 125 mg • Advantra Z Citrus Aurantium 125 mg • Kola Nut JKN-10 5 mg.
See Editor's Note No. 40.

Slim Down CLA 75 - Conjugated Linoleic Acid **-** Jamieson
Each capsule contains: Conjugated Linoleic Acid 1000 mg.

Slim Down GTF Chromium 200 mcg **-** Jamieson
Each tablet contains: Chromium (from brewer's yeast) 200 mcg.

Some Brand Name Natural Products - What they Contain

www.NaturalDatabase.com contains MANY more listings than appear here.

Editor's Notes are located on pages 2155-2163.

BRAND NAMES

Slim Down Natural Source Fibre **-** Jamieson
Each caplet contains: Dietary Fiber (derived from oat grains) 0.5 g.

Slim Essence **-** DreamPharm
Each capsule contains: Senna leaf 150 mg • Persimmon leaf 150 mg • Papaya leaf 100 mg • Orange peel 100 mg • Licorice root 50 mg • Chromium Picolinate 50 mcg.

Slim Form Diet Patch **-** Long Life Services, Inc.
Each 5x5 cm patch contains: Marine Algae • Mannitol • Chlorides • Potassium • Sodium • Magnesium • Amino Acids • Calcium • Glucose • Phosphates • Fucose. The glue contains: Natural Rubber, Natural Lanolin, Natural Parrafin (liquid), Zinc Oxide, Natural Resin.

Slim Smart **-** Health Center for Better Living
Chromium Picolinate 200 mcg; other herbs.

Slim Trim **-** Life Extension
L-Arginine 500 mg • L-Ornithine 250 mg.

Slimmer **-** Dr. Roopas Herbal Systems Pvt. Ltd
Each capsule contains: Propietary Formula 250 mg: Powder of Cassia Angustifolia, Cinnamomum Tamala, Garcinia Cambogia, Balsamodendron Mukul.

Slimming Formula **-** PhytoPharmica
Each tablet contains: Thyroidinum 8x • Antimonium crudum 3x • Calcarea acetica 2x • Fucus vesiculosus 2x.
See Editor's Note No. 1 and No. 21.

SlimPrep **-** HealthMinded
Three capsules contain: SlimPrep Proprietary Blend 2100 mg: CLA One brand Conjugated Linoleic Acid, Super CitriMax brand Garcinia Cambogia, Cayenne Pepper fruit extract (capsici fructus, 40,000 SHU), Ginger root (zingiber officinale), Bitter Orange peel extract (citrus aurantium, 6% synephrine, Advantra Z brand). Other Ingredients: Gelatin, Stearic Acid, Magnesium Stearate.
See Editor's Note No. 40.

SlimPro **-** HealthMinded
Four capsules contain: Vitamin C 100 mg • Vitamin B6 10 mg • Pantothenic Acid 12 mg • Magnesium 10 mg • Chromium 300 mcg • Garcinia Cambogia extract 200 mg • L-Tyrosine 200 mg • Cocoa extract 200 mg • L-Carnitine Fumarate 120 mg • Theobromine 100 mg • Dimethylaminoethanol (DMAE) 24 mg • SlimPro Proprietary Blend 200 mg: Green Tea extract (decaffeinated, 50% polyphenols), D/L Methionine, Ginger root extract, Quercetin, Bitter Orange extract, White Willow bark extract, Grape seed extract (95% OPC). Other Ingredients: Stearic Acid, Magnesium Stearate.
See Editor's Note No. 40.

SlimStyles with PGX (assorted flavors) **-** Natural Factors
Two scoops (57 g) contain: Protein 21 g • Vitamin A (as beta carotene) 2100 IU • Vitamin C (as ascorbic acid) 20 mg • Vitamin D (as ergocalciferol) 100 IU • Vitamin E (as D-alpha tocopheryl acetate) 6 IU • Thiamine (as thiamine hydrochloride) 0.75 mg • Riboflavin 0.8 mg • Niacin (as niacinamide) 12 mg • Vitamin B6 (as pyridoxine hydrochloride) 0.75 mg • Folic Acid 0.12 mg • Vitamin B12 (as cyanocobalamin) 0.5 mcg • Biotin 75 mcg • Pantothenic Acid (as calcium pantothenate) 2.5 mg • Calcium (as calcium citrate and dicalcium phospate) 400 mg • Iron (as ferrous fumarate) 2.5 g • Phosphorus (as dicalcium phosphate) 250 mg • Iodine (as potassium iodide) 40 mcg • Magnesium (as magnesium citrate) 120 mg • Zinc (as zinc citrate) 6 mg • Selenium (as selenium chelate) 20 mcg • Copper (as copper chelate) 0.5 mg • Manganese (as manganese citrate) 1 mg • Chromium (chelate) 20 mcg • Molybdenum (as molybdenum citrate) 25 mcg • Sodium 257 mg • Potassium 285 mg • Whey Protein 26.5 g • PGX Proprietary Blend 5 g: Konjac Mannan root (amorphophallus konjac, K. Koch), Sodium Alginate (laminaria digitata), Xanthan gum 5 g • Lecithin 4.7 g • Medium Chain Triglycerides 2.4 g • Stevia leaf powdered extract 125 mg.

SlimSure AM **-** Life Enhancement Products, Inc.
Two capsules contain: Vitamin B6 (as pyridoxine hydrochloride) 30 mg • Chromium (as chromium aspartate) 75 mcg • Tyrosine 500 mg • Caffeine 125 mg • Green Tea extract (55% EGCG) 100 mg • ForsLean brand Forskolin 50 mg • DHEA (dehydroepiandrosterone) 15 mg • 3,5-Diiodo-L-Thyronine (T2) 100 mcg. Other Ingredients: Gelatin.

SlimSure PM **-** Life Enhancement Products, Inc.
Two capsules contain: Vitamin B6 (pyridoxine hydrochloride) 30 mg • Chromium (chromium aspartate) 75 mcg • Green Tea extract (55% EGCG) 100 mg • 5-HTP (5-hydroxytryptophan) 75 mg • ForsLean brand Forskolin 50 mg • DHEA (dehydroepiandrosterone) 20 mg • 3,5-Diiodo-L-Thyronine (T2) 100 mcg. Other Ingredients: Gelatin.

SlimSure Thermogenic Booster **-** Life Enhancement Products, Inc.
Two capsules contain: Vitamin A (as beta-carotene) 2500 IU • Vitamin C (as ascorbic acid and niacinamide ascorbate) 160 mg • Vitamin E (as D,L-alpha-tocopheryl acetate) 60 mg • Thiamine (vitamin B1 as thiamine mononitrate) 4 mg • Riboflavin (vitamin B2) 8 mg • Niacin (vitamin B3 as niacinamide ascorbate) 20 mg • Vitamin B6 (as pyridoxine hydrochloride) 30 mg • Folic Acid 40 mcg • Vitamin B12 (cyanocobalamin) 300 mcg • Copper (as copper gluconate) 800 mcg • Magnesium (as magnesium hydroxide) 100 mg • Pantothenic Acid (vitamin B5 as calcium pantothenate) 40 mg • Zinc (as zinc gluconate) 6 mg • Chromium (as chromium aspartate) 50 mcg • 5-HTP (5-hydroxytryptophan) 100 mg • EGCG (epigallocatechin gallate, from green tea) 90 mg • Caffeine 50 mg.

Slim-Tech **-** Wild Rose
Each capsule contains: CitriMax brand Hydroxycitric Acid 275 mg 138 mg • Green Tea 1:4 extract 50 mg • Country Mallow leaf 75 mg • Feverfew leaf 25 mg • Cascara Sagrada bark 50 mg • Uva Ursi leaf 50 mg • Bladderwrack 25 mg.
See Editor's Note No. 39.

SlimTrax Forte **-** Pharmessen
Each tablet contains: Proprietary Blend 800 mg: Clove oil (eugenia caryophyllata, leaf), Cinnamon leaf oil (cinnamomum zeylonicum), Olive oil, Microcrystalline Cellulose, Hypromellose, Cab-o-sil, Talcum, Magnesium Stearate.

Slim-Trim **-** Life Extension
Each tablet contains: L-Arginine 500 mg • L-Ornithine 250 mg • Glutathione Peroxidase 600 mg.

Slippery Elm Bark Powder **-** Vital Nutrients
Each 1 rounded tsp serving contains: Slippery Elm bark powder (ulmus fulva) 2500 mg.

Slippery Elm Original Lozenges **-** Thayers Natural Pharmaceuticals
Each lozenge contains: Slippery Elm Bark 150 mg. Base: Corn Sweetener, Vegetable Stearate.

Slippery Elm Original Lozenges, Sugar-Free **-** Thayers Natural Pharmaceuticals
Each lozenge contains: Slippery Elm Bark 150 mg. Base: Sorbitol, Vegetable Stearate.

Slippery Elm Tangerine Lozenges with Rose Hips **-** Thayers Natural Pharmaceuticals
Each lozenge contains: Slippery Elm Bark 150 mg • Rose Hips 20 mg • Vitamin C 15 mg. Other Ingredients: Ascorbic Acid, Natural Tangerine Flavor, Corn Sweetener, Vegetable Stearate.

Slo-Niacin **-** Upsher-Smith Laboratories
Each tablet contains: Niacin 500 mg. Other Ingredients: Cellulose Polymer Derivative, Vegetable Stearine, Magnesium Stearate, Silicon Dioxide, Glyceryl Behenate, FD&C Red #40.

Slow Fe **-** Novartis
Each tablet contains: Dried Ferrous Sulfate USP (160 mg), USP (equivalent to 50 mg). Inactive Ingredients: Cetostearyl Alcohol, Hydroxypropyl Methylcellulose, Lactose, Magnesium Stearate, Polysorbate 80, Talc, Titanium Dioxide, Yellow Iron Oxide, FD&C Blue 32 Aluminum Lake.

Some Brand Name Natural Products - What they Contain

www.NaturalDatabase.com contains MANY more listings than appear here.
Editor's Notes are located on pages 2155-2163.

Slow-Mag - Roberts
Two tablets contain: Calcium (from calcium carbonate) 212 mg • Magnesium 128 mg & Chloride 373 mg (from magnesium chloride hexahydrate) • Cellulose Acetate Phthalate • Pregelatinized Starch • Povidone • Diethylphthalate • Talc • Titanium Dioxide • Magnesium Stearate & FD&C Blue No. 2 Lake.

Slumber - Nutrivention
Two tablets contain: Calcium (Amino Acid Chelate) 500 mg • Magnesium (Amino Acid Chelate) 500 mg • Inositol 200 mg • Niacinamide 20 mg • Biotin 100 mcg • Passion flower 200 mg • Blue Vervain 200 mg • Hops 100 mg • Valerian root (Star root) 100 mg • Wild Lettuce 100 mg.

Slumber EZ - Bios Biochemicals
Three capsules contain: Thiamin (as thiamin mononitrate) 30 mg • Riboflavin 30 mg • Niacin 30 mg • Vitamin B6 (as pyridoxal 5-phosphate) 15 mg • Magnesium (as magnesium chelate) 90 mg • Molybdenum (as molybdenum chelate) 300 mcg • Proprietary Blend 2160 mg: Glycine, L-Lysine HCl, L-Serine, GABA, Trimethylglycine, 5-HTP. Other Ingredients: Gelatin Capsule, Magnesium Stearate.

SlumberActin - Nature's Plus
Three capsules contain: Chamomile root (matricaria recutita, standardized to 1% Apigenin, 0.5% Essential oil) 200 mg • Valerian root (valeriana officinalis, standardized to 1% Valernic Acids) 100 mg • Passion Flower (passiflora incarnata, standardized to 3.5-4% Flavonoids) 75 mg • Hops (humulus lupulus, standardized to 5.2% Bitter Acids, 4% Flavonoids) 75 mg • Kava Kava root (piper methysticum, standardized to 29-31% kavalactones) 50 mg • English Hawthorne berry (crataegus laevigata, standardized to 3.2% Vitexin) 50 mg • Magnesium (amino acid chelate) 50 mg • Calcium (amino acid chelate) 25 mg.

Smart ALEC - Life Enhancement Products, Inc.
Each 2 rounded tsp serving contains: Vitamin C (from ascorbic acid) 500 mg • Niacin (vitamin B3 from niacin) 50 mg • Magnesium (from magnesium aspartate) 200 mg • Copper (from copper gluconate) 500 mcg • Chromium (chromium aspartate) 30 mcg • Potassium (from potassium aspartate) 99 mg • Acetyl L-Carnitine 500 mg • Glycine 200 mg. Other Ingredients: Fructose, Malic Acid, Citric Acid, Natural Flavors, Silicon Dioxide, Carmine.

Smart Coffee w/ Ginkgo Biloba - Nature's Plus
Each 3 g serving contains: Instant herbal coffee blend: naturally decaffeinated Brazilian coffee (coffea) • Ginkgo Biloba (standardized 24% ginkgo flavone-glycosides, 6% terpene lactones) • Rosemary (Rosmarinus officinalis) • Fo-Ti (Polygonum multiflorum) • Mahonia Aquifolium (wild grape, standardized 95-100% leucoanthocyanidins) • Chinese Apricot (Prunus armeniaca).

Smart Longevity - E'OLA
Ten drops contain: Vitamin C (as ascorbic acid) 16 mg • Vitamin E (as dl-alpha tocopheryl acetate) 7 IU • Proprietary Blend 324 mg: Choline Bitartrate, Dimethylaminoethanol Bitartrate, Siberian Ginseng (root), Schizandra (berry), Ginkgo Biloba (leaf). Other Ingredients: Water, Hydrochloric Acid, Sodium Benzoic Acid.

Smart Pill - Only Natural, Inc.
Two tablets contain: Ginkgo Biloba leaf extract 10:1 250 mg • Gotu Kola 250 mg • Ginseng 100 mg • Capsicum 50 mg • L-Phenylalanine 200 mg • L-Glutamine 500 mg • L-Tyrosine 200 mg • GABA 300 mg • Vitamin B1 50 mg • Vitamin B3 50 mg • Vitamin B5 100 mg • Vitamin B6 50 mg • Vitamin B12 500 mcg • Folic Acid 200 mcg • Inositol 100 mg • Phosphatidylcholine 500 mg • RNA 100 mg • TMG 50 mg.

Smart Vitamins - Jamieson
Each capsule contains: Choline Bitartrate • Molasses cone • L-Glutamine • Brewers Yeast (a natural source of the B complex vitamin family) • Acerola (a natural source of Vitamin C) • Taurine • Kola Nut • Korean Ginseng • Vegetable Magnesium Stearate • Wheat Germ Powder • Silica • Chromium Yeast • Turnera (Damiana aphrodesiaca) • Capsicum (Cayenne) • Ginkgo Biloba • Fo-Ti (polygonum multiflorum).

Smart Vitamins Phosphatidyl - Jamieson
Each capsule contains: Phosphatidyl Serine 10 mg • Phosphatidyl Choline (Derived from Pure Soy Lechtin) 9 mg • Omega 3 DHA (Derived from North Atlantic Fresh Fish Oil) 3 mg.

Smilax Damiana Supreme - Gaia Herbs
Forty drops contain: Proprietary Blend 300 mg: Sarsaparilla root solid extract and liquid extract (smilax officinalis), Damiana herb (turnera diffusa), American Ginseng (panax quinquefolium), Ashwagandha (withania somnifera), Shatavari (asparagus racemosa), Fresh Wild Oat (avena sativa), Licorice root (glycyrrhiza glabra), Hawthorn berry solid extract (crataegus oxycantha), Prickly Ash bark (xanthoxylum clava-herculis), 40-50% Pure Grain Alcohol USP, Spring Water.

Smoke Away Formula 1 - The Council On Natural Health
Six tablets contain: Vitamin C (as ascorbic acid) 316 mg • Iron (as ferrous fumarate) 2.4 mg • Iodine (from kelp) 192 mcg • Sodium (as sodium chloride) 25 mg • Proprietary Blend 4000 mg: Alfalfa leaf, Licorice root, Siberian Ginseng root, Cayenne pepper (40,000 scoville heat units), Dandelion root, Echinacea Purpurea (aerial parts), Ginger root, Peppermint leaf, Sarsaparilla root, Buckthorn bark, Burdock root, Hyssop (aerial parts), Lobelia leaf, Passionflower (plant, flower), Cascara Sagrada bark, Oregon Grape root, Barley Grass, Bayberry bark, Golden Seal (aerial parts), Lemon Verbena leaf, Ox bile extract, Safflower seed oil, Elderberry fruit 10:1 extract, Bioperine standardized Black Pepper extract (96-97% piperine). Other Ingredients: Dicalcium Phosphate, Microcrystalline Cellulose, Croscarmellose Sodium, Stearic Acid, Silica, Magnesium Stearate. See Editor's Note No. 14.

Smoke Away Formula 2 - The Council On Natural Health
Two tablets contain: Vitamin C (as ascorbic acid) 250 mg • Vitamin E (as dl-alpha-tocopheryl acetate) 30 IU • Pantothenic Acid (as D-calcium pantothenate) 10 mg • Selenium (as sodium selenite) 50 mcg • Long Health Blend 250 mg: Red Clover flower, Gotu Kola leaf, Burdock root • L-Glutamine 100 mg • MSM (methylsulfonylmethane) 100 mg • Korean Ginseng root (4% ginsenosides) 100 mg • Milk Thistle seed 100 mg • N-Acetyl-L-Cysteine 50 mg • Smoke Away Blend 100 mg: Rosemary (aerial parts), Thyme leaf, Black Cumin seed • Wild Jujube seed extract 50 mg • 5-HTP 50 mg • Lemon Verbena leaf 25 mg • Quercetin Dihydrate 25 mg. Other Ingredients: Dicalcium Phosphate, Microcrystalline Cellulose, Croscarmellose Sodium, Stearic Acid, Calcium Silicate, Silica, Magnesium Stearate.

Smoke Free - Boericke & Tafel
Each tablet contains: Caladium Seguinum 6X • Daphne Indica 6X • Graphite 12X • Valeriana Officinalis 6X • Lactose (HPU S). See Editor's Note No. 1.

SmokeAway Natural Homeopathic Medicine - The Council On Natural Health
Three pellets contain: Tabacum (tobacco) 5C-7C-9C • Lobelia Inflata (Indian tobacco) 5C • Cadmium Sulphuricum (cadmium sulphate) 5C • Nux Vomica (poison nut) 5C • Antimonium Crudum (antimony sulphide) 5C • Caladium Seguinum (American arum) 5C. See Editor's Note No. 1.

Smoke-Less - The Herbalist
Lobelia leaf • Milk Thistle seed • Oat seed • Siberian Ginseng root • Licorice root.

Smooth Food 2 - New Chapter, Inc.
Three capsules contain: Okra fruit 201 mg • Slippery Elm bark 201 mg • Psyllium husk 159 mg • Licorice root 159 mg • Ginger (rhizome) 159 mg • Marshmallow root 120 mg • Wheat Grass 21 mg • Bio Flora (100 million probiotic live cells per teaspoon) 21 mg • Chlorella regularis 6 mg • Cayenne fruit 3 mg. Other Ingredients: Vegetable cellulose.

Smooth Move - Traditional Medicinals
Sennosides A & B: 20 mg per cup as they naturally occur in Senna leaf (Casala angustifolia) present in the blend. Other Herbal Ingredients: Licorice root, Fennel seed, Orange peel, Cinnamon bark, Coriander seed, Ginger rhizome, Natural Orange Flavor.

Some Brand Name Natural Products - What they Contain

www.NaturalDatabase.com contains MANY more listings than appear here.
Editor's Notes are located on pages 2155-2163.

BRAND NAMES

Snack Defense **-** Herbalife International of America, Inc.
Each tablet contains: Calcium (carbonate) 130 mg • Chromium (polynicotinate) 75 mcg • Dried Garcinia Cambogia fruit extract 400 mcg • Dried Gymnema Sylvestre leaves extract 100 mg. Other Ingredients: Microcrystalline Cellulose, Stearic Acid, Hypromellose, Acacia, Croscarmellose Sodium, Shellac, Silicon Dioxide, Magnesium Stearate, Titanium Dioxide, Triethyl Citrate, Riboflavin. This product was formerly known as Thermojetics.

SneezEze **-** EuroPharma, Inc.
Active Ingredient: Kali Bichromicum (potassium bichromate) 3x. Inactive Ingredient: Cellulose.
See Editor's Note No. 1.

Snooze **-** Pacific BioLogic
Valerian root • Dragon Bone (fossilized) • Oyster Shell (untreated) • Mimosa Tree flower • Chamomile • Gotu Kola • Hops • Polygala root • Jujube seed (sour) • Passion flower • Scullcap • Melatonin 1.5 mg.
See Editor's Note No. 26.

Snooze-EZ **-** TriLight Herbs
Skullcap • German Chamomile • Passion Flower • Valerian • Oatstraw • Linden flower.

Snoreless **-** Nutrition for Life International
Three sprays (approx. 3 mL) contains: Vitamin C 4.5 mg • Vitamin E 7.5 mg • Vitamin B6 3 mg • Olive Oil 210 mg • Sunflower Oil 90 mg • Peppermint Oil 60 mg • Almond Oil 37.5 mg • Sesame Oil 30 mg. Other Ingredients: Purified Water, Glycerine.

SnoreMD **-** Long Life, Inc.
Each caplet contains: Calcium (as dicalcium phosphate) 105 mg • Phosphorus (as dicalcium phosphate) • Proprietary Blend 415 mg: Protease, Amylase, Lipase, Cellulase, Acerola fruit concentarate, Cayenne fruit, Fenugreek seed, Echinacea, Red Clover (aerial part), Yarrow flowers, Eucalyptus leaf, Elderberry flower/fruit. Other Ingredients: Croscarmellose Sodium, Magnesium Stearate, Microcrystalline Cellulose, Polyvinylpyrrolidone, Silica.

Snorenz **-** MedGen, Inc.
Peppermint Oil • Sunflower Oil • Sesame Oil • Olive Oil • Almond Oil.

SnoreStop **-** The Green Pharmacy
Each tablet contains: Nux vomica 4X • Nux vomica 6X • Belladonna 6X • Ephedra vulgaris 6X • Hydrastis canadensis 6X • Kali bichromicum 6X • Teucrium marum 6X • Histaminum hydrochloricum 12X.
See Editor's Note No. 1.

Snuffadelic **-** Cytotec Solutions, Inc.
Unknown.
See Editor's Note No. 49.

SoBe Adrenaline Rush **-** SoBe Beverage Co.
Filtered Water • High Fructose Corn Syrup • Citric Acid • Taurine 1000 mg • D-Ribose 500 mg • L-Carnitine 250 mg • Natural Flavor • Inositol 100 mg • Sodium Citrate • Ascorbic Acid • Caffeine • Monopotassium Phosphate • Salt • Gum Arabic • Ester Gum • Siberian Ginseng root extract 50 mg • Pyridoxine Hydrochloride • Guarana seed extract 50 mg • Caramel Color • Beta-Carotene • Folic Acid • Cyanocobalamin.

Sob'r-k Detoxifier HangoverStopper **-** Life Style Marketing, Inc.
Two capsules contain: Carbon 600 mg.

S-O-D **-** Nature's Sunshine
Each capsule contains: GliSODin brand complex 150 mg: SOD (superoxide dismutase), Gliadin. Other Ingredients: Cellulose (plant fiber), Magnesium Stearate, Silicon Dioxide, Gelatin, Water.

Soft Gelatin Multiple **-** Nature's Life
Two capsules contain: Beta Carotene 15,000 IU • Vitamin A (fish liver oil) 10,000 IU • Vitamin D (D3, as cholecalciferol) 400 IU • Vitamin E (D-alpha tocopherol) 400 IU • Vitamin C 300 mg • Rose Hips 20 mg • Folic Acid 400 mcg • Vitamin B1 (Thiamine Mononitrate) 50 mg • Vitamin B2 (Riboflavin) 50 mg • Niacinamide 50 mg • Vitamin B6 (Pyridoxine HCl) 50 mg • Vitamin B12 (Cyanocobalamin) 100 mcg • Biotin (d-Biotin) 300 mcg • Pantothenic Acid (d-Calcium Pantothenate) 50 mg • Choline (Bitartrate) 25 mg • Inositol 25 mg • PABA (Para Aminobenzoic Acid) 25 mg • Boron (Calcium Boron Gluconate) 25 mcg • Calcium (Carbonate, Citrate, Aspartate) 200 mg • Chromium (Nutrition 21 Picolinate) 25 mcg • Copper (Gluconate) 2 mg • Iodine (Potassium Iodide) 150 mcg • Iron (Peptonate) 10 mg • Magnesium (Magnesium Oxide) 100 mg • Manganese (Amino Acid Chelate) 15 mg • Molybdenum (Free-Form Amino Acid Chelate) 25 mcg • Potassium (Phosphate & Iodide) 15 mg • Selenium (l-Selenomethionine, yeast-free) 15 mcg • Silicon Dioxide 20 mg • Vanadium (Vanadyl Sulfate) 25 mcg • Zinc (Citrate, Gluconate, Picolinate) 15 mg • Essential Fatty Acids (Safflower oil) 540 mg.

Soft Tissue **-** Enzymes, Inc.
Each capsule contains: Vitamin C (100% from Acerola Cherries) 17 mg • Proprietary Herbal Blend 215 mg: Bladderwrack kelp extract, Quercetin, Tumeric root extract, Cramp bark extract, Corydalis root extract, Grape seed extract • Proprietary Enzyme Blend 227 mg: pHsyioProtease, Peptidase, Bromelain. Other Ingredients: Plant Cellulose, Water.

Solae brand **-** DuPont
Isolated Soy Protein.
See Editor's Note No. 44.

Solar Water **-** Cytotec Solutions, Inc.
Unknown.
See Editor's Note No. 49.

Solaray Bilberry **-** Nutraceutical Corp.
Each capsule contains: Bilberry berry extract 60 mg. Other Ingredients: Cellulose, Gelatin, Magnesium Stearate.

Solaray Continence with Flowtrol **-** Nutraceutical Corp.
Each two capsules contain: Butterbur root extract (Petasites hybridus) (Guaranteed to contain 15 mg sesquiterpenes) 100 mg • Flowtrol Proriteary Blend 870 mg: Cranberry berry extract (Vaccinium macrocarpon as CranActin Cranberry AF Extract), Morinda root extract 5:1, Psoralea fruit extract 5:1, Raspberry fruit extract 5:1 (Rubus chingii), Alpinia oxyphylla fruit and seed extract 5:1, Lobelia (aerial). Inactive Ingredients: Gelatin (capsule), Cellulose, Maltodextrin, Magnesium Stearate, Silica, Magnesium Hydroxide.

Solaray Cordyceps 520 mg **-** Nutraceutical Corp.
Each capsule contains: Cordyceps 520 mg. Inactive Ingredients: Gelatin, Cellulose, & Magnesium stearate.

Solaray DopaBean 333 mg **-** Nutraceutical Corp.
Each capsule contains: Velvet Bean seed extract (Mucuna pruriens) 333 mg • Catecholamines 66 mg • L-dopa 50 mg. Inactive Ingredients: Gelatin (capsule), Rice Flour, Maltodextrin, Magnesium Stearate, Silica, Alpha Galactosidase.

Solaray GP Cordyceps **-** Nutraceutical Corp.
Each two capsules contain: Cordyceps (Cordyceps sinensis) 520 mg. Inactive Ingredients: Gelatin, Cellulose, Magnesium.

Solaray Indole-3-Carbinol **-** Nutraceutical Corp.
Each capsule contains: Vitamin C (as ascorbic acid) 200 mg • Broccoli 50 mg • Brussel Sprouts 50 mg • Cabbage 50 mg • Cauliflower 50 mg • Kale 50 mg • Indole-3-Carbinol (I3C) 25 mg. Inactive Ingredients: Gelatin (capsule), Magnesium Stearate.

Solaray Iron 50 mg **-** Nutraceutical Corp.
Each capsule contains: Iron (Iron Amino Acid Chelate) 50 mg. Other Ingredients: Herb Base: Parsley leaf, Yellow Dock root, Gelatin, Whole Rice Concentrate (including bran, germ, and polishings), Magnesium Stearate.

Solaray Pure CoQ-10 **-** Nutraceutical Corp.
Each capsule contains: Coenzyme Q-10 30 mg. Inactive Ingredients: Cellulose, Gelatin (capsule).

Solaray Pure CoQ10-30 - Nutraceutical Corp.
Each capsule contains: Coenzyme Q-10 30 mg. Inactive Ingredients: Cellulose, Gelatin.

Solaray Pygeum and Saw Palmetto - Nutraceutical Corp.
Each six capsules contain: Vitamin B-6 (as pyridoxine HCl) 20 mg • Zinc (as optizinc) 15 mg • Cranberry extract 800 mg • Saw Palmetto berry oil 320 mg • Pygeum bark extract 100 mg. Inactive Ingredients: Gelatin, Cellulose, Pumpkin Seed, L-Glycerine, Glutamic Acid, L-Alanine, Magnesium Stearate.

Solaray Spectro 3 - Nutraceutical Corp.
Three tablets contain: Vitamin A (from Retinyl Palmitate, and 60% as natural Beta Carotene) 25,000 IU • Vitamin C (ascorbic acid, rose hips, acerola cherry) 1000 mg • Vitamin D (as Cholecalciferol D-3) 400 IU • Vitamin E (as natural d-Alpha Tocopheryl Succinate, D-Alpha Tocopheryl Acetate) 400 IU • Vitamin K 50 mcg • Thiamin (as Thiamine Mononitrate) (Vitamin B1) 25 mg • Riboflavin (Vitamin B2) 25 mg • Niacin (as Niacinamide) 125 mg • Vitamin B6 (as Pyridoxine HCl) 50 mg • Folic Acid 400 mcg • Vitamin B12 (as Cyanocobalamin) 100 mcg • Biotin 300 mcg • Pantothenic Acid (as d-Calcium Pantothenate) 125 mg • Calcium (as Calcium Carbonate, Calcium Amino Acid Chelate) 500 mg • Iron (as Iron Fumarate, Iron Amino Acid Chelate) 18 mg • Phosphorous (as Potassium Phosphate) 23 mg • Iodine (from Kelp) 225 mcg • Magnesium (Magnesium Oxide, Magnesium Amino Acid Chelate) 250 mg • Zinc (as Zinc Citrate, Zinc Picolinate, Zinc Amino Acid Chelate) 15 mg • Selenium (as yeast free I-Selenomethionine) 100 mcg • Copper (as Copper Amino Acid Chelate) 0.5 mg • Potassium (as Potassium Phosphate, Potassium Chloride) 88 mg • Choline Bitartrate 50 mg • Inositol 50 mg • PABA (Para-Aminobenzoic Acid) 30 mg • Lecithin 50 mg • Bioflavonoid concentrate (from Citrus) 150 mg • Rutin concentrate 50 mg • Hesperidin concentrate 50 mg • Pectin 25 mg • Boron (as Tetra-Boron: Boron Citrate, Boron Glycinate, Boron Aspartate, Boron Lysinate) 1.5 mg • Spirulina (Spirulina platensis) 50 mg • Alfalfa juice (aerial) 125 mg • Carrot and Yam concentrate 100 mg • Barley Grass juice concentrate 75 mg • Rosemary leaf extract 25 mg • Aloe Vera gel concentrate 200x (equivalent to 400 mg) 2 mg • Parsley leaf 50 mg • Pancreatin 4x (equivalent to 120 mg) 30 mg • Diatase 20 mg • Papain (from Papaya) 50 mg • Ox Bile extract 20 mg • Glutamic Acid HCl 50 mg • Propolis 2x (equivalent to 50 mg) 25 mg • Royal Jelly 3.5x (equivalent to 14 mg) 4 mg • Bee Pollen. Inactive Ingredients: Cellulose, Stearic Acid, Silica, Siberian Ginseng root, Calcium Phosphate, Whole Rice concentrate, Alfalfa herb, Montmorillonite Clay, Maltodextrin, Natural Flavors.
See Editor's Note No. 14.

Solaray ViraMax - Nutraceutical Corp.
Each two capsules contain: Catuaba 500 mg • Yohimbe bark extract (supplying 10 mg of yohimbine) 500 mg • Muira Puama root 250 mg • Peruvian Maca root extract (4:1) 100 mg.

Solidax ADX - Priority One Health & Nutrition
Each capsule contains: Synephrine 15 mg • Calcium Pyruvate 150 mg • Chromium Picolinate 500 mcg. Other Ingredients: Magnesium Stearate, Gelatin.
See Editor's Note No. 40.

Sollievo - Aboca USA, Inc
Each tablet contains: Senna leaf powder (cassia angustifolia, standardized to 2.5% sennosides) 122 mg • Cape Aloe juice (aloe ferox, standardized to 18% aloin A+B) 91.7 mg • Certified Organic Dandelion root powder (taraxacum officinale) 91 mg • Chicory root powder (cichorium intybus) 32 mg • Fennel fruit powder (foeniculum vulgare) 27 mg • Caraway fruit powder (carum carvi) 23 mg • Boldo leaf powder (peumus boldus) 7 mg • Cumin fruit powder (cuminum cyminum) 6 mg. Other Ingredients: Essential Oil of Fennel.

Sollievo Herbal Tea - Aboca USA, Inc
Each bag contains: Senna fruit (cassia angustifolia) 0.660 g • Licorice root (glycyrrhiza glabra) 0.550 g • Senna leaf (cassia angustifolia) 0.440 g • Fennel fruit (foeniculum vulgare) 0.132 g • Caraway fruit (carum carvi) 0.330 g • Lemon Balm fruit (melissa officinalis) 0.044 g • High Mallow flower and leaf (malva sylvestris) 0.044 g.

Solo Day Multi Vitamin - GNC
Each tablet contains: Vitamin A (29% as beta-carotene, 80% as acetate) 5000 IU • Vitamin C (as ascorbic acid) 60 mg • Vitamin D (as ergocalciferol) 400 IU • Vitamin E (as d-alpha tocopheryl acetate) 30 IU • Vitamin K (as phytonadione) 25 mcg • Thiamin (as thiamin mononitrate) 1.5 mg • Riboflavin 1.7 mg • Niacin (as niacinamide) 20 mg • Vitamin B6 (as pyridoxine hydrochloride) 2 mg • Folate, Folic Acid, Folacin 400 mcg • Vitamin B12 (as cyanocobalamin) 6 mcg • Biotin 30 mcg • Pantothenic Acid (calcium D-pantothenate) 10 mg • Calcium (as dicalcium phosphate and calcium carbonate) 162 mg • Iron (as ferrous fumarate) 18 mg • Phosphorus (as dicalcium phosphate) 109 mg • Iodine (as potassium iodide) 150 mcg • Magnesium (as magnesium oxide) 100 mg • Zinc (as zinc oxide) 15 mg • Selenium (as sodium selenate) 20 mcg • Copper (as cupric oxide) 2 mg • Manganese (as manganese sulfate) 2 mg • Chromium (as chromium chloride) 120 mcg • Molybdenum (as sodium molybdate) 75 mcg • Chloride (as potassium chloride) 72 mg • Potassium (as potassium chloride) 80 mg • Nickel (as nickel sulfate) 5 mcg • Tin (as stannous chloride) 10 mcg • Vanadium (as sodium meta vanadate) 10 mcg • Boron (as sodium borate) 150 mcg • Silica (as silicon dioxide) 2 mg • Lycopene 300 mcg. Other Ingredients: Cellulose, Vegetable Acetoglycerides, Artificial Color (FD&C Yellow #6), Titanium Dioxide.

Solovites - Puritan's Pride
Each tablet contains: Vitamin A 10,000 IU • Vitamin C 200 mg • Vitamin D 400 IU • Vitamin E 30 IU • Thiamin 30 mg • Riboflavin 30 mg • Niacin 30 mg • Vitamin B-6 30 mg • Folic Acid 400 mcg • Vitamin B-12 30 mcg • Biotin 30 mcg • Pantothenic Acid 30 mg • Calcium 60 mg • Iron 18 mg • Phosphorus 30 mg • Iodine 150 mcg • Magnesium 30 mg • Zinc 30 mg • Selenium 25 mcg • Copper 0.5 mg • Manganese 0.6 mg • Chromium 25 mcg • Molybdenum 25 mcg • Potassium 11 mg • PABA (Para-Aminobenzoic Acid) 30 mg • Choline Bitartrate 30 mg • Inositol 30 mcg • Citrus Bioflavonoid complex 25 mg • Betaine Hydrochloride 25 mg. In a base of Alfalfa, Parsley, Oyster Shell, Watercress, Kelp, and Lecithin.

Soluble Enzyme Caps - Atrium Biotechnologies
Each capsule contains: Papayotin 110 mg • Pancreatin (Bovine) 90 mg • Calf Thymus (Bovine) 50 mg • Bromelain 50 mg • Lipase 10 mg • Chymotrypsin 15 mg. Lemon flavor.
See Editor's Note No. 14.

Solu-Min - Aspen Group, Inc.
Calcium • Phosphorus • Magnesium • Potassium • Sulfur • Iron • Iodine • Copper • Cobalt • Zinc • Chromium • Manganese • Molybdenum • Selenium • Aluminum • Antimony • Barium • Bismuth • Cadmium • Sodium • Cesium • Carbon • Lithium • Nickel • Platinum • Rubidium • Silver • Strontium • Silicon • Tungsten • Tin • Titanium • Tantalum • Thorium • Vanadium • Zirconium • Yttrium. Plus up to 30 other randomly occurring trace minerals in natural combinations.

SomaLife gHP - SomaLife International Inc.
Six capsules contain: Proprietary Blend 5352 mg: L-Lysine, L-Arginine, L-Ornithine, L-Glutamine, Glycine, Leucine, Iso-Leucine, Valine. Other Ingredients: MCC, Magnesium Stearate.

SomaLife IQ150 - SomaLife International Inc.
Three capsules contain: Proprietary Blend 465 mg: Turmeric powder • Green Tea extract • Phosphatidyl Serine • Phosphatidyl Choline • Spanish Sage extract PE 5% Cineole (salvia lavandulifolia L.) • Ginkgo Biloba extract, 24%-6%. Other Ingredients: Brown Rice Flour, Magnesium Stearate, Silicon Oxide.

SomaLife Super X - SomaLife International Inc.
Each capsule contains: Proprietary Blend 680 mg: L-Carnitine • Broccoli powder extract (flavonones) • NAC (N-acetyl cysteine) • Grapeseed extract (proanthocyanidins) • ALA (alpha lipoic acid) • Coenzyme Q-10 • Bilberry fruit extract • Glutathione • Lycopene extract.

Some Brand Name Natural Products - What they Contain

www.NaturalDatabase.com contains MANY more listings than appear here.
Editor's Notes are located on pages 2155-2163.

BRAND NAMES

SomaSlim **-** SomaLife International Inc.
Two capsules contain: Proprietary Blend 400 mg: L-Carnitine, L-Carnosine, Amino Peptide Complex, 5 HTP, Chromium Picolinate. Other Ingredients: Magnesium Stearate, Rice Flour, Silicon Dioxide.

Soma-Slim **-** Soma-Slim.com
Two capsules contain: Pantothenic Acid 12 mg • Magnesium 10 mg • Proprietary Blend 1415 mg: Bitter Orange (synephrine), Tyrosine, Acetyl L-Tyrosine, Green Tea extract (50% polyphenols), Cocoa extract Yerba Mate (20% caffeine), Vitamin C 100 mg, Vitamin B6 10 mg, DL-methionine, Ginger root, Quercetin.
See Editor's Note No. 40.

SomaSlim C **-** SomaLife International Inc.
Two capsules contain: Phaseolus Vulgaris extract (white kidney bean) 300 mg • Amino Peptide Complex (whey protein isolate) 125 mg • 5 HTP (hydroxytryptophan) 50 mg • L-Carnosine 25 mg • Chromium Polynicotinate 25 mcg. Other Ingredients: Magnesium Stearate 5 mg, Silicon Dioxide 3 mg.

SomaTrim **-** SomaLife International Inc.
Two capsules contain: Proprietary Blend 572.5 mg: Calcium Pyruvate • Garcinia Cambogia • Amino Peptide Complex • Siberian Ginseng • Citrus Aurantium extract • Coleus Forskohlii 10% extract • Green Tea extract • Alpha Lipoic Acid (ALA). Other Ingredients: MCC, Magnesium Stearate, White or Brown Rice Flour, Silicon Dioxide.
See Editor's Note No. 40.

SomaVit Plus **-** SomaLife International Inc.
Two tablets contain: Beta-Carotene (pro-vitamin A) 15,000 IU • Vitamin C (ascorbic acid) 500 mg • Vitamin D (D3, cholecalciferol) 100 IU • Vitamin E (D-alpha tocopheryl acid succinate) 200 IU • Vitamin B1 (thiamine hydrochloride) 25 mg • Vitamin B2 (riboflavin) 25 mg • Niacinamide 25 mg • Vitamin B6 (pyridoxine hydrochloride) 25 mg • Folic Acid 400 mcg • Vitamin B12 (cyanocobalamin) 25 mcg • Pantothenic Acid (D-calcium pantothenate) 200 mg • Zinc (HVP chelate) 25 mg • Selenium (HVP chelate) 50 mcg • Copper (HVP chelate) 1 mg • Manganese (HVP chelate) 2 mg • Chromium (HVP chelate) 100 mcg.

Somnolin **-** Metagenics
Each tablet contains: L-5 Hydroxytryptophan (L-5-HTP from griffonia simplicifolia) 100 mg • Theanine 100 mg • Vitamin B6 20 mg • Vitamin B12 (as methylcobalamin) 250 mcg • L-5-Methyl Tetrahydrofolate 200 mcg.

SootheX Joint and Muscle Pain Relief Cream **-** Advocare International
Active Ingredient: Trolamine Salicylate 10%. Inactive Ingredients: Alkoxylated Diester, Caprylic/Capric Triglyceride, Cyclomethicone, Dimethicone, Ginger Extract, Glycerin, Glyceryl Stearate, Imidazolidinyl Urea, Isopropyl Myristate, Methylparaben, PEG-100 Stearate, Phenoxyethanol, Propylparaben, Purified Water, Stearyl Alcohol, Vanillyl Butyl Ether.

Sore Throat Lozenge **-** Jamieson
Each lozenge contains: Slippery Elm bark 50 mg • White Horehound leaves 50 mg • Parsley root 20 mg • Thyme leaves 10 mg • Menthol 5 mg. Other Ingredients: Camphor 50 mcg, Acerola Cherry 40 mg, Sugar, Glucose, Honey, Anise Oil, and natural flavors.

Sore Throat Remedy (formerly HP 8) **-** Metagenics
Each tablet contains: Belladonna 30X • Phytolacca Decandra 3X • Ferrum Phosphoricum 3X • Asclepias Tuberosa 3X • Mercurius Corrosivus 6X • Kali Muriaticum 3X.
See Editor's Note No. 1.

Sound Sleep **-** Gaia Herbs
Three capsules contain: Valerian root (valeriana off.) 150 mg • GABA (gamma aminobutyric acid) 106 mg • L-Glycine 106 mg • Kava Kava root and rhizome (piper methysticum) 26 mg • Passionflower vine (passiflora incarnata) 18 mg • California Poppy (escholzia californica) 16 mg • Skullcap herb (scutellaria lateriflora) 12 mg • Hops strobile (humulus lupulus) 12 mg. Other Ingredients: Vegetable Glycerin, Vegetable Cellulose (capsule).

Source of Life Adult's Chewable **-** Nature's Plus
Two wafers contain: Vitamin A (as beta carotene) 5000 IU • Vitamin C (as ascorbic acid) 300 mg • Vitamin D (as ergocalciferol) 400 IU • Vitamin E (as D-alpha tocopheryl succinate) 100 IU • Vitamin B1 (as thiamine HCl) 25 mg • Riboflavin (vitamin B2) 25 mg • Niacin (as niacinamide) 25 mg • Vitamin B6 (as pyridoxine HCl) 25 mg • Folate (as folic acid) 400 mcg • Biotin 100 mcg • Vitamin B12 (as cyanocobalamin) 50 mcg • Pantothenic Acid (as calcium pantothenate) 25 mg • Calcium (as aminoate complex) 100 mg • Iron (as aminoate complex) 4.5 mg • Iodine (from kelp) 150 mcg • Magnesium (as aminoate complex) 50 mg • Zinc (as aminoate complex) 10 mg • Copper (as aminoate complex) 1 mg • Manganese (as aminoate complex) 5 mg • Chromium (as aminoate complex) 25 mcg • Potassium (as aminoate complex) 5 mg • Nutrient Base 350 mg: Spirulina, Bee Pollen, Ginseng root (panax ginseng), Octacosanol • Enzyme Complex 50 mg: Bromelain (from pineapple fruit), Papain (from papaya fruit), Betaine HCl (from beet molasses), Apple Pectin, Amylase, Lipase • Lipid Complex 25 mg: Black Currant seed oil, Sunflower oil • Inositol 25 mg • Bioflavonoid Complex 20 mg: Flavonols, Flavonones, Flavones, Naringen, Hesperidin, Eriocitrin, Quercetin, Rutin • Choline (as bitartrate) 15 mg • PABA (para-aminobenzoic acid) 5 mg • Plant Pigment Complex 4 mg: Chlorophyll (from spirulina), Carotenoids. Other Ingredients: Fructose, Guar Gum, Natural Apple Flavor, Stearic Acid, Magnesium Stearate, Silica, Cinnamon, Natural Vanilla Flavor, Microcrystalline Cellulose, Astragalus Root, Ligustrum Berry, Schisandra, Young Barley Leaf, Echinacea Angustifolia Root, Irish Moss (chondrus crispus), Thyme Leaf, Rice Bran.

Source of Life Animal Parade Calcium **-** Nature's Plus
Two chewable tablets contain: Calcium (as amino acid chelate/complex) 250 mg • Magnesium (as aminoate complex) 50 mg. Other Ingredients: Fructose, Natural Vanilla, Spinach leaf extract (spinacia oleracea), Broccoli floret extract (brassica oleracea), Fig Concentrate (ficus carica), Date Concentrate (phoenix dactylifera), Stearic Acid, Magnesium Stearate.

Source of Life Cal/Mag 500/250 mg **-** Nature's Plus
Two tablets contain: Calcium (whole brown rice amino acid complex) 500 mg • Magnesium (whole brown rice amino acid complex) 250 mg • Proprietary Blend 200 mg: Fig, Date, Hazelnut, Sesame seed, Sunflower seed, Broccoli, Spinach. Other Ingredients: Stearic Acid, Microcrystalline Cellulose, Silica, Magnesium Stearate, Pharmaceutical Glaze.

Source of Life Caps **-** Nature's Plus
Nine capsules contain: Vitamin A (as beta carotene) 10,000 IU • Vitamin C (as ascorbic acid) 1000 mg • Vitamin D (as ergocalciferol) 400 IU • Vitamin E (as D-alpha tocopheryl succinate) 200 IU • Thiamin (vitamin B1, as thiamine hydrochloride) 25 mg • Riboflavin 25 mg • Niacin (as niacinamide) 40 mg • Vitamin B6 (as pyridoxine HCl) 25 mg • Folate (as folic acid) 400 mcg • Vitamin B12 (as cyanocobalamin) 200 mcg • Biotin 100 mcg • Pantothenic Acid (as calcium pantothenate) 60 mg • Calcium (as aminoate complex) 200 mg • Iron (as aminoate complex, ascorbate) 18 mg • Iodine (from kelp) 150 mcg • Magnesium (as aminoate complex) 100 mg • Zinc (as aminoate complex, picolinate) 15 mg • Selenium (as aminoate complex) 25 mcg • Copper (as aminoate complex) 0.5 mg • Manganese (as aminoate complex) 4 mg • Chromium (as aminoate complex) 20 mcg • Potassium (as aminoate complex) 50 mg • Spirulina 1000 mg • Bee Pollen 100 mg • Sunflower oil 70 mg: Linoleic Acid 54.1 mg, Oleic Acid 9.3 mg, Palmitic Acid 4.4 mg, Stearic Acid 2.2 mg • Citrus Bioflavonoids (from citrus limon exocarp, active flavonols, flavonones, flavones, naringen 26 mg) 60 mg • Black Currant seed oil 50 mg • Korean Ginseng root 50 mg • Bromelain (from pineapple fruit) 40 mg • Choline (as bitartrate) 30 mg • Inositol 30 mg • Quercetin (from saphora japonica leaf) 30 mg • Papain (from papaya fruit) 30 mg • Rutin (from saphora japonica leaf) 25 mg • Betaine HCl (from beet molasses) 25 mg • RNA (ribonucleic acid) 21 mg • Apple Pectin 20 mg • PABA (para-aminobenzoic acid) 15 mg • Hesperidin (from citrus limon exocarp) 10 mg • Chlorophyll (from spirulina) 7.5 mg • DNA (deoxyribonucleic acid) 6 mg • Amylase (from brown rice

fermentation) 5 mg • Lipase (from brown rice fermentation) 5 mg • Carotenoids 4 mg • Eriocitrin (from citrus limon exocarp) 3 mg • Octacosanol 200 mcg. Other Ingredients: Microcrystalline Cellulose, Silica, Magnesium Stearate, Schisandra Fruit, Astragalus Root, Young Barley Leaf, Echinacea Angustifolia Root, Irish Moss (chondrus crispus), Thyme Leaf, Ligustrum Berry, Gelatin, Rice Bran, Purified Water, Mineral Aminoates, Whole Brown Rice Chelates.

Source of Life Liquid - Nature's Plus
Each 2 tbsp serving contains: Vitamin A (as palmitate, beta carotene) 10,000 IU • Vitamin C (as ascorbic acid) 500 mg • Vitamin D (as ergocalciferol) 400 IU • Vitamin E (as D-alpha tocopherol acetate) 200 IU • Thiamine (vitamin B1, as thiamine mononitrate) 25 mg • Riboflavin (vitamin B2) 25 mg • Niacin (as niacinamide) 40 mg • Vitamin B6 (as pyridoxine HCl) 25 mg • Folate (as folic acid) 400 mcg • Vitamin B12 (as cyanocobalamin) 200 mcg • Biotin 100 mcg • Pantothenic Acid (as calcium pantothenate) 60 mg • Calcium (as citrate) 50 mg • Iron (as gluconate) 4.5 mg • Iodine (potassium iodide) 150 mcg • Magnesium (as citrate) 25 mg • Zinc (as gluconate) 7.5 mg • Selenium (as amino acid complex) 25 mcg • Copper (as chlorophyllin) 1.5 mg • Manganese (as gluconate) 4 mg • Chromium (as polynicotinate) 20 mcg • Potassium (as citrate) 50 mg • Source-70 brand Whole Food Complex 500 mg: Prehistoric Trace Element Concentrate, Spirulina (natural source of chlorophyll, ribonucleic acid, deoxyribonucleic acid, carotenoids), Alfalfa leaf juice (natural source of plant sitosterols), Barley grass juice (natural source of 2"-O-glycosyl isovitexin) • Bee Pollen (naturally providing vitamins, minerals and enzymes) 100 mg • Citrus Bioflavonoids (from citrus limon exocarp, containing active flavonols, flavonones, flavones, and naringen) 100 mg • Korean Ginseng root 50 mg • Inositol 30 mg • PABA (para-aminobenzoic acid) 15 mg • Choline (as bitartrate) 13 mg • Chlorophyll (from spirulina and copper chlorophyllin) 4 mg. Other Ingredients: Purified Water, Crystalline Fructose, Natural Flavors, Citric Acid, Xanthan Gum, Malic Acid, Potassium Benzoate, Potassium Sorbate, Flax Seed, Astragalus Root, Ligustrum Berry, Schisandra Fruit, Young Barley Leaf, Echinacea Angustifolia Root, Irish Moss (chondrus crispus), Thyme Leaf, Rice Bran.

Source of Life Men - Nature's Plus
Two tablets contain: Vitamin A (as beta carotene) 10,000 IU • Vitamin C (as ascorbic acid) 500 mg • Vitamin D (as ergocalciferol) 100 IU • Vitamin E (as D-alpha tocopheryl succinate) 200 IU • Vitamin K (as phytonadione) 150 mcg • Thiamin (vitamin B1, as thiamine HCl) 75 mg • Riboflavin (vitamin B2) 75 mg • Niacin (as niacinamide) 75 mg • Vitamin B6 (as pyridoxine HCl) 75 mg • Folate (as folic acid) 400 mcg • Vitamin B12 (as cyanocobalamin) 200 mcg • Biotin 300 mcg • Pantothenic Acid (as calcium pantothenate) 60 mg • Calcium (as aminoate complex) 250 mg • Iodine (from kelp) 150 mcg • Magnesium (as aminoate complex) 125 mg • Zinc (as monomethionine) 30 mg • Selenium (as aminoate complex) 100 mcg • Copper (as aminoate complex) 1 mg • Manganese (as aminoate complex) 2 mg • Chromium (as polynicotinate) 20 mcg • Molybdenum (as aminoate complex) 50 mcg • Spirulina 250 mg • Saw Palmetto berry (serenoa repens, standardized to 45% free fatty acids) 60 mg • Bee Pollen 50 mg • Bromelain (24 gelatin digesting units) 40 mg • Choline (as bitartrate) 30 mg • Inositol 30 mg • Citrus Bioflavonoids (from citrus limon exocarp) 25 mg • Herbal Antioxidant Complex 15 mg: Turmeric rhizome (curcuma longa, standardized to 95% curcumin), Bilberry extract (vaccinium myrtillus, standardized to 25% anthocyanosides), Green Tea leaf (camellia sinensis, decaffeinated, standardized to 50% polyphenols) • Rhodiola Rosea root 10 mg • Alpha Lipoic Acid 10 mg • Pumpkin seed (cucurbita maxima) 10 mg • L-Glycine (free form amino acid) 10 mg • L-Alanine (free form amino acid) 10 mg • L-Glutamine (free form amino acid) 10 mg • Amylase 5 mg • Lipase 5 mg • DairyMate brand Lactase 5 mg • Protease 5 mg • Lutein from Marigold flower extract 2 mg • Lycopene (from tomato) 1 mg. Other Ingredients: Microcrystalline Cellulose, Stearic Acid, Magnesium Stearate, Silica, Astragalus Root, Young Barley Leaf, Irish Moss (chondrus crispus), Thyme Leaf, Ligustrum Berry, Schisandra Fruit, Rice Bran, Pharmaceutical Glaze, Mineral Aminoates, Whole Brown Rice Chelates.

Source of Life Oxygenic - Nature's Plus
Three tablets contain: Mixed Wild Berry extract 300 mg: European Red Wine Grape, Bilberry, Blackberry, Black Raspberry, & Red Raspberry (standardized 20% Polyphenols, 4% Anthocyanosides) • Chinese Green Tea extract (standardized 20% Polyphenols) 300 mg • Horseradish concentrate 250 mg • Vitamin C fortified with Rose Hips, Mango, Guava & West Indian Cherry 100 mg • Beta Carotene (Dunaliella salina, Carrot) 2500 IU • Wild Grape seed extract standardized 95-100% Leucoanthocyanins 10 mg • Pycnogenol (Pine bark extract) standardized 85-95% Proanthocyanidins 5 mg. In a whole food base of Broccoli, Spinach, Cauliflower & Beet Greens.

Source of Life Power Teen - Nature's Plus
Two tablets contain: Vitamin A (67% as beta carotene, 33% as palmitate) 15,000 IU • Vitamin C (as ascorbic acid) 100 mg • Vitamin D (as ergocalciferol) 100 IU • Vitamin E (as D-alpha tocopheryl succinate) 100 IU • Thiamin (vitamin B1, as thiamine mononitrate) 50 mg • Riboflavin (vitamin B2) 50 mg • Niacin (as niacinamide) 50 mg • Vitamin B6 (as pyridoxine hydrochloride) 50 mg • Folate (as folic acid) 400 mcg • Vitamin B12 (as cyanocobalamin) 2 mcg • Biotin 75 mcg • Pantothenic Acid (as calcium pantothenate) 7 mg • Calcium (as amino acid chelate/complex) 250 mg • Iron (as amino acid chelate) 4.5 mg • Magnesium (as amino acid chelate/complex) 250 mg • Zinc (as amino acid chelate, gluconate) 20 mg • Selenium (as selenomethionine) 75 mcg • Copper (as amino acid chelate) 1 mg • Manganese (amino acid chelate) 2 mg • Chromium (polynicotinate) 50 mcg • Molybdenum (as sodium molybdate) 50 mcg • Potassium (amino acid complex) 20 mg • PhytoGreen blend 100 mg: Broccoli, Spinach, Carrot, Spirulina, Chlorella, Evening Primrose, Black Currant seed • Bioperine brand Black Pepper extract (piper nigrum fruit, standardized to 95% 1-piperoylpiperidine) 2.5 mg. Other Ingredients: Microcrystalline Cellulose, Di-Calcium Phosphate, Stearic Acid, Magnesium Stearate, Silica, Pharmaceutical Glaze.

Source of Life Prenatal - Nature's Plus
Two tablets contain: Vitamin A (as beta carotene) 10,000 IU • Vitamin C (as ascorbic acid) 150 mg • Vitamin D (as ergocalciferol) 100 IU • Vitamin E (as D-alpha tocopheryl succinate) 100 IU • Thiamin (vitamin B1, as thiamine HCl) 10 mg • Riboflavin (vitamin B2) 10 mg • Niacin (as niacinamide) 40 mg • Vitamin B6 (as pyridoxine HCl) 5 mg • Folate (as folic acid) 800 mcg • Vitamin B12 (as cyanocobalamin) 40 mcg • Biotin 800 mcg • Pantothenic Acid (as calcium pantothenate) 25 mg • Calcium (as amino acid chelate/complex) 400 mg • Iron (as amino acid chelate/complex) 18 mg • Phosphorus (as amino acid complex) 200 mg • Iodine (from kelp) 150 mcg • Magnesium (as amino acid chelate/complex) 200 mg • Zinc (as amino acid chelate/complex) 15 mg • Manganese (as amino acid chelate/complex) 6 mg • Potassium (as amino acid complex) 10 mg • Bromelain 50 mg • Papain 50 mg • Choline (as bitartrate) 5 mg • Inositol 5 mg • PABA (para-aminobenzoic acid) 5 mg • Probiotic Blend 100 million cells: Lactobacillus Acidophilus, Bifidobacterium Bifidum, Bifidobacterium Longum. Other Ingredients: Di-Calcium Phosphate, Stearic Acid, Magnesium Stearate, Silica, Brown Rice, Banana, Apricot, Apple, Alfalfa, Barley Leaves, Broccoli, Beet Juice, Collard Greens, Parsnips, Green Zucchini, Turnip Greens, Peach, Kale, Tomato, Spinach, Pharmaceutical Glaze.

Source of Life Vibra-Gest - Nature's Plus
Each vegicap contains: Brown rice fermentation: Amylase, 30000 units/gram 50 mg • Lactase, 1000 units/gram 50 mg • Lipase, 5000 units/gram 50 mg • Cellulase, 5000 units/gram 30 mg • Protease, 100000 units/gram 20 mg • Oxidase, 5000 units/gram 10 mg • Barley malt: Diastase, 1000 units/gram 10 mg • Maltase, 1000 units/gram 10 mg • Sweet potato: Phosphatase, 4000 units/gram 5 mg • Pineapple: Bromelain, 600 GDU/gram 35 mg • Papaya: Papain, 2 million units/gram 30 mg • Carrot powder: Lactobacillus acidophilus 4 billion viable cells/gram 100 mg • Natural cultures: Bifidobacterium longum 1 billion viable cells/gram 50 mg • Lactobacillus bulgaricus 1 billion viable cells/gram 50 mg.

Source of Life Vibran-C - Nature's Plus
Each tablet contains: Vitamin C 600 mg • Bioflavonoid Complex 60 mg: Ginkgo Biloba leaf, Saphora Japonica leaf, • West Indian Cherry

(malpighia glabra fruit) 40 mg • Amla fruit (emblica officinalis) 40 mg • Mammophen fruit (terminalia pentralis fruit) 40 mg • Rose Hips (rosa canina) 40 mg • Mango fruit(mangifera indica) 40 mg • Guava fruit (psidium guajava) 40 mg • Camu-Camu fruit (myrciaria dubia) 40 mg. Other Ingredients: Microcrystalline Cellulose, Stearic Acid, Magnesium Stearate, Silica, Pharmaceutical Glaze.

Source of Life Women **-** Nature's Plus
Two tablets contain: Vitamin A (as beta carotene) 10,000 IU • Vitamin C (as ascorbic acid) 500 mg • Vitamin D (as ergocalciferol) 100 IU • Vitamin E (as D-alpha tocopheryl succinate) 100 IU • Vitamin K (as phytonadione) 150 mcg • Thiamin (vitamin B1, as thiamine HCl) 50 mg • Riboflavin (vitamin B2) 50 mg • Niacin (as niacinamide) 50 mg • Vitamin B6 (as pyridoxine HCl) 50 mg • Folate (as folic acid) 800 mcg • Vitamin B12 (as cyanocobalamin) 200 mcg • Biotin 300 mcg • Pantothenic Acid (as calcium pantothenate) 60 mg • Calcium (as aminoate complex) 500 mg • Iron (as aminoate complex) 18 mg • Iodine (from kelp) 150 mcg • Magnesium (as aminoate complex) 250 mg • Zinc (as monomethionine) 15 mg • Selenium (as aminoate complex) 100 mcg • Copper (as aminoate complex) 1 mg • Manganese (as aminoate complex) 2 mg • Chromium (as polynicotinate) 120 mcg • Molybdenum (as aminoate complex) 50 mcg • Spirulina 250 mg • Ostivone brand Ipriflavone 50 mg • Bee Pollen 50 mg • Bromelain 40 mg • Novasoy brand Soy extract (standardized to 40% isoflavones) 40 mg • Fem-Effect Complex 40 mg: Chasteberry fruit (vitex agnus-castus, standardized to 0.5% agnuside, 0.6% aucubin), Damiana (whole herb), Dong Quai root (angelica sinensis), Black Cohosh root and rhizome (cimicifuga racemosa, standardized to 2.5% triterpene glycosides) • Choline (as bitartrate) 30 mg • Inositol 30 mg • Citrus Bioflavonoids (from citrus limon exocarp) 25 mg • Herbal Antioxidant Complex 15 mg: Turmeric rhizome (curcuma longa, standardized to 95% curcumin), Bilberry extract (vaccinium myrtillus, standardized to 25% anthocyanosides), Green Tea leaf (camellia sinensis, decaffeinated, standardized to 50% polyphenols) • Lipase 10 mg • Amylase 5 mg • DairyMate brand Lactase 5 mg • Protease 5 mg • Lutein from Marigold flower extract 2 mg • Boron (as citrate) 1 mg. Other Ingredients: Microcrystalline Cellulose, Stearic Acid, Magnesium Stearate, Silica, Astragalus Root, Young Barley Leaf, Irish Moss (chondrus crispus), Thyme Leaf, Ligustrum Berry, Schisandra Fruit, Rice Bran, Pharmaceutical Glaze, Mineral Aminoates, Whole Brown Rice Chelates.

Soy Almond Crunch StandardBar **-** Standard Process, Inc.
Brown Rice Syrup • Pure Wildflower Honey • Soy Protein • Almond Butter • Soy Nuggets • Textured Soy Protein • Rolled Oats • Dry Soy Milk • Glycerin • Sesame seed • Soybean Lecithin • Flaxseed oil • Natural Almond flavor • Soybean powder • Magnesium Lactate • Extra Virgin Olive oil • Natural Licorice extract • Pyridoxine Hydrochloride.

Soy Bean Lecithin **-** Standard Process, Inc.
Each perle contains: Soy Bean Lecithin 240 mg. Other Ingredients: Soybean Oil, Gelatin, Glycerin, Water, Carob.

Soy Defense **-** Goldshield Elite
Two caplets contain: Vitamin E (as D-Alpha-Tocopheryl Succinate and Dl-Alpha-Tocopheryl Acetate) 200 IU • Mixed Soy phytosterols 50 mg • Tri-source isoflavone concentrate 1333 mg: Soy Germ, Red Clover flower, and Kudzu root • Soy polysaccharides 150 mg. Other Ingredients: Dicalcium Phosphate, Vegetable Cellulose, Fractionated vegetable oil, Silica, Calcium Sulfate.

Soy Essentials **-** Health From The Sun
Four tablets contain: Genistein (Aglycone) 2.88 mg • Daidzein (Aglycone) 2.20 mg • Beta Glucans 7.87 mg. Ingredients: Certified GMO-Free Fermented Soymeal (Soynatto), Microcrystalline Cellulose, Stearic Acid, HPC (cellulose), Croscarmellose Sodium, Magnesium Stearate, Silicon Dioxide, Pharmaceutical Glaze.

Soy Extract **-** Enzymatic Therapy/PhytoPharmica
Each softgel contains: Soybean extract (glycine max, 15% isoflavones) 100 mg. Other Ingredients: Soybean Oil, Gelatin, Glycerin, Beeswax, Lecithin.

Soy Force Rx **-** Biotech Corp.
Two tablets contain: Soy Isoflavones 80 mg • Soy Protein Concentrate 500 mg • OPTiSOY Blend 300 mg.

Soy Isoflavone **-** Natrol, Inc.
Each capsule contains: Soy Isoflavone extract 100 mg containing: Isoflavones (10%) 10 mg • Daidzin & Daidzein (2%) 2 mg • Genistin & Genistein (9%) 9 mg • Glycitin & Glycitein (0.1%) 0.1 mg. Other Ingredients: Rice powder, Magnesium Stearate, Gelatin.

Soy Isoflavone **-** Jamieson
Each capsule contains: Isoflavone Concentrate derived from 125 mg of pure Soy 50 mg.

Soy Isoflavones **-** Olympian Labs
Each capsule contains: Soy Isoflavone dried extract 100 mg.

Soy Isoflavones **-** Pure Encapsulations
Each vegetable capsule contains: Full-spectrum Soy Isoflavone concentrate 850 mg: Genistin 3.61 mg, Genistein 0.14 mg, Glycitin 7.35 mg, Glycitein 0.714 mg, Daidzin 12.15 mg, Daidzein 0.391 mg, Total Isoflavones 25 mg.

Soy Isoflavones 40 **-** Pure Encapsulations
Each vegetable capsule contains: Soy Isoflavone extract (standardized to contain 40% total isoflavones) 100 mg: Genistin/Genistein 24-28 mg, Daidzin/Daidzein 10-14 mg, Glycitin/Glycitein 1.2-2.4 mg.

Soy Isoflavones 50 mg **-** Vital Nutrients
Each capsule contains: Soy Isoflavones (from soy isoflavone extract 40% 125 mg) 50 mg.

Soy Isoflavones Concentrate Caplet **-** Leiner Health Products
Each caplet contains: Isoflavones - Soy extract 50 mg • Lecithin 15 mg. Other Ingredients: Dicalcium Phosphate, Cellulose, Stearic Acid, Silicon Dioxide, Croscarmellose Sodium, Magnesium Stearate, Dextrin, Dextrose, Sodium Carboxymethylcellulose, Sodium Citrate.

Soy Isoflavones, 50mg **-** Nature Made
Each capsule contains: Soy bean extract 125 mg: Soy Isoflavones 50 mg.

Soy Lecithin Granules **-** GNC
Each tablespoon contains: Soy Lecithin Granules containing: Phosphatidyl Choline 1725 mg • Choline 250 mg.

Soy Lecithin Granules Apple Cinnamon Flavor **-** GNC
Each Tablespoon contains: Phosphorous 165 mg • Phosphatidyl Choline 1350 mg • Choline 200 mg. Ingredients: Soy Lecithin granules, Dried Apple juice, Dried Apples, Spices.

Soy Miracle Ultimate Antioxidant **-** FreeLife International
Two caplets contain: ProVitamin A (beta, alpha carotenes) 15,000 IU • Vitamin E (natural d-alpha tocopheryl succinate) 400 IU • Vitamin C (calcium ascorbate) 500 mg • Selenium (l-selenomethionine) 50 mcg • N-Acetyl Cysteine 50 mg • Ultra Soy Complex III 200 mg: standardized Soy kernel concentrate (source of daidzein, saponins), Soybean sprouts concentrate (source of antioxidant enzymes), Pine bark extract, Japanese Grape Seed extract, Glutathione, Red Cabbage, Green Tea, Carrots, Broccoli, Celery, Brussels sprouts, Kale, Cauliflower, Green Onion, Yam • Alfalfa Juice concentrate (medicago sativa) 200 mg • Bilberry extract (vaccinium myrtillis) 25 mg • Citrus Bioflavonoids (citrus limon) 100 mg • Grape Skin extract 50 mg • Ginger (zingiber officinale) 100 mg • Quercetin (sophora japonica) 25 mg • Rutin (sophora japonica) 50 mg • Turmeric (source of curcurmin) 50 mg.

Soy Miracle Ultimate Body Toner **-** FreeLife International
Two caplets contain: Vitamin B3 (niacinamide) 20 mg • Vitamin B6 (pyridoxine HCl, pyridoxal-5-phosphate) 10 mg • Chromium (yeast-free GTF, picolinate) 200 mcg • Choline Bitartrate 100 mg • Inositol 100 mg • L-Carnitine 50 mg • Methionine 50 mg • Taurine 50 mg • High-Esterase Plant Lipase Enzyme 1500 AP Units • Betaine HCl 100 mg • Panax Ginseng standardized extract (4% ginsenosides) 100 mg • Grapefruit extract (glycinated) 200 mg • Ultra Soy Complex

350 mg: Lecithin, Soy bran, Linoleic Acid, Phosphatidylcholine, Phytosterols (beta sitosterol, campesterol, stigmasterol, fucosterol), Cephalin, Inositol Phosphatides, Phosphatidylserine, Linolenic Acid • Active Herbal Blend 250 mg: Gotu Kola, Uva Ursi, Buchu, Apple Cider Vinegar, Spirulina, Peppermint, Cinnamon, Ginger, Licorice, Cayenne, Chinese Mustard, Spearmint Oil.

Soy Miracle Ultimate Shake - FreeLife International
Each level scoop contains: Ultra Soy Complex I: IPP SUPRO brand Soy protein isolate, Soy fiber, Soy Lecithin, Tofu powder, Soy flour, Tamari Soy powder, Miso powder, Cholestatin brand mixed Soy Phytosterols • Crystalline Fructose, Natural Flavors, Dahlulin brand dry Dahlia Inulin juice Complex • Gum Acacia • Xanthan Gum • Oat Fiber • Calcium Phosphate • Magnesium Oxide • Cellulose Gum • Guar Gum • Potassium Chloride • Eleuthero root • Ascorbic Acid • Inositol • Choline Bitartrate • Blue-Green Micro-Algae • L-Carnitine • Vitamin E Acetate • Spanish Bee Pollen • Apple Pectin • Citrus Bioflavonoid • Niacinamide • Zinc Oxide • Invertase (plant enzyme) • D-Calcium Pantothenate • Vitamin A Palmitate • Manganese Sulfate • Sucralose (non-nutritive sweetener) • Pyridoxine Hydrochloride • Riboflavin • Thiamine Hydrochloride • Bromelain • Papain • Folic Acid • Biotin • Vitamin D (D3) • Potassium Iodide • Chromium Picolinate • Selenomethionine • Sodium Molybdate • Cyanocobalamin. Chocolate Royale flavor also contains Dutch Cocoa powder (for flavoring).

Soy Preventive - GNC
Two capsules contain: Vitamin A (100% as Acetate) 5000 IU • Vitamin C (as Ascorbic Acid) 200 mg • Vitamin E (as d-alpha Tocopheryl Succinate) 100 IU • Selenium (as Selenium Yeast) 100 mcg • Soy Isoflavone Concentrate (34% Isoflavones = 8.5 mg) 25 mg. Other Ingredients: Cellulose, Calcium Carbonate, Gelatin.

Soy Protein Chocolate - GNC
One scoop (32g) contains: Isolated Soy Protein • Fructose • Maltodextrin • Cocoa • Natural Flavor • Salt.

Soy Protein Vanilla - GNC
One scoop (32g) contains: Isolated Soy Protein • Fructose • Maltodextrin • Natural Flavor • Salt.

Soy Special - Aspen Group, Inc.
Each tablet contains: Soy isoflavones 50 mg.

Soy2O Lemon Green Tea - Leading Brands, Inc.
Filtered Water • Sugar • Pear juice from concentrate • Natural Flavors • Citric Acid • Beta Carotene • Soy Isoflavones • Green Tea solids • Caramel Color.

Soy2O Peach Mango - Leading Brands, Inc.
Filtered Water • Sugar • Pear juice from concentrate • Natural Flavors • Citric Acid • Beta-Carotene • Black Carrot juice concentrate • Soy Isoflavones.

Soy2O Strawberry Guava - Leading Brands, Inc.
Filtered Water • Sugar • Pear juice from concentrate • Natural Flavors • Citric Acid • Black Carrot juice concentrate • Purple Sweet Potato juice extract • Soy Isoflavones.

Soya Lecithin - Golden Glow Natural Health Products
Each capsule contains: Lecithin 1200 mg.

Soya Lecithin 1200 mg - Sundown
Each softgel contains: Soya Lecithin 1200 mg (phospholipids 550 mg). Other Ingredients: Gelatin, Glycerin, Water.

SoyaMax - USANA Health Sciences
Two scoops contain: Potensoy: Soy Protein Isolate, Isoflavine Concentrate • Natural Vanilla Flavor.

Soy-Based Baby Formula - Bright Beginnings
Corn Syrup Solids • Soy Protein Isolate • Sucrose • Palm Oil (palm olein) • High Oleic Safflower or Sunflower oil • Coconut oil • Soybean oil • L-Carnitine • L-Methionine • Soybean Lecithin • Taurine • Cupric Sulfate • Ferrous Sulfate • Magnesium Chloride • Manganese Sulfate • Potassium Bicarbaonte • Potassium Chloride • Potassium Citrate • Potassium Hydroxide • Potassium Iodide • Sodium Citrate • Sodium Selenite • Tribasic Calcium Phosphate • Zinc Sulfate • Ascorbic Acid • Beta-Carotene • Biotin • Calcium Pantothenate • Choline Chloride • Cyanocobalamin • Folic Acid • Inositol • Niacinamide • Pyridoxine Hydrochloride • Riboflavin • Thiamine Hydrochloride • Vitamin A Palmitate • Vitamin D (cholecalciferol) • Vitamin E (DL-alpha tocopheryl acetate) • Vitamin K (phytonadione).

Soy-Based Milk-Free Lactobacillus Acidophilus powder - Nature's Life
Each level tablespoon (6 g) contains: Unrefined Apple Juice, Maltodextrin NF, SUPRO brand Soy Protein, pure Crystalline Fructose, Lactobacillus Acidophilus (95%), L. Bulgaricus (3%) & Bifidobacteria Bifidus (2%).

Soygenol 100 - FreeLife International
Each tablet contains: Soygenol 100 (soy-phosphatide-bonded premium Grape Seed OPCs) 100 mg • Green Tea leaf standardized extract (30% polyphenols) 100 mg • Ultra Soy Delivery System (Soy polysaccharides and plant enzymes) 5000 Units. Other Ingredients: Calcium Hydrogen Phosphate, Cellulose, Cellulose Gum, Vegetable Stearic Acid, Silica, Vegetable Magnesium Stearate, Calcium Silicate, Vita-Coat (vegetable resin, alpha-lipoic acid).

SoySwee Tea - HerbaSway
Soy • Ginger • Panax Ginseng • Siberian Ginseng • Blackberry • HerbaSwee (Cucurbitaceae fruit).

SP Cleanse - Standard Process, Inc.
Seven capsules contain: Proprietary Blend 3080 mg: Juniper berry powder (juniperus communis), Red Clover flower powder (trifolium pratense), Collinsonia root powder, Apple Pectin, Burdock root powder (arctium lappa), Barley grass powder, Celandine powder (chelidonium majus), Spanish Black Radish root, Oregon Grape root powder (berberis aquifolium), Cayenne pepper powder (capsicum annuum), Fenugreek seed powder, Choline Bitartrate, Inositol, Fringe tree root (chionanthus virginicus), Fennel seed, Oat flour, Beet leaf juice powder, Beet root powder, Milk Thistle (silybum marianum, 80% silymarin), Wildcrafted Tillandsia powder, Carrot powder, Broccoli powder, Kale powder • Vitamin C 3 mg • Iron 1 mg • Sodium 10 mg. Other Ingredients: Cellulose, Water.

SP Complete - Standard Process, Inc.
Two rounded tablespoons contain: Proprietary Blend 25 g: Whey Protein powder, Flax meal powder, Brown Rice Protein powder, Calcium Citrate, Magnesium Citrate, Buckwheat juice powder, Brussels Sprouts (whole plant), Kale, Choline Bitartrate, Inositol, Barley grass, Alfalfa juice powder, Soybean Lecithin powder, Grape seed extract (Masqueliers OPC-85; 98% total phenolic compounds; 65% proanthocyanidins), Carrot powder, Red Wine extract (95% total phenols) • Calcium 200 mg • Iron 2 mg • Sodium 60 mg.

SP Green Food - Standard Process, Inc.
Two capsules contain: Proprietary Blend 500 mg: Brussels sprout powder (whole plant), Kale powder, Alfalfa sprout powder • Buckwheat juice powder 200 mg • Barley grass juice powder 100 mg. Other Ingredients: Cellulose, Water, Calcium Stearate.

SP-500 - PhytoPharmica
Each capsule contains: Spleen Polypeptides (a mixture of highly purified bovine-derived spleen polypeptides naturally present in the spleen, including tuftsin, splenopentin, splenin and leukokinin) 375 mg • Goldenseal root extract (Hydrastis canadensis) standardized to contain 5% total alkaloids including Berberine, Hydrastine, and Canadine 125 mg.
See Editor's Note No. 14 and No. 21.

Spanish Black Radish - Standard Process, Inc.
Each tablet contains: Vitamin C 4.6 mg • Spanish Black Radish 360 mg. Other Ingredients: Honey, Calcium Stearate.

BRAND NAMES

Some Brand Name Natural Products - What they Contain

www.NaturalDatabase.com contains MANY more listings than appear here.

Editor's Notes are located on pages 2155-2163.

BRAND NAMES

Spark Drink Mix (original & cherry flavor) **- Advocare International**
Each scoop (0.53 oz/15 g) contains: Vitamin A (as mixed carotenes and vitamin A palmitate) 2500 IU • Vitamin C (as ascorbic acid) 180 mg • Vitamin E (as D-alpha tocopheryl acetate) 30 IU • Thiamine (as HCl) 3 mg • Riboflavin 3.4 mg • Niacin (as niacin and niacinamide) 60 mg • Vitamin B6 (as pyridoxine HCl) 15 mg • Vitamin B12 (as cyanocobalamin) 45 mcg • Pantothenic Acid (as calcium pantothenate) 50 mg • Zinc (as monomethionine - OptiZinc brand) 3 mg • Copper (as glycinate) 200 mcg • Chromium (as polynicotinate - ChromeMate brand) 24 mcg • Sodium (as phosphate) 20 mg • L-Carnitine (as tartrate) 10 mg • Taurine 200 mg • Gamma-Aminobutyric Acid (GABA) 50 mg • Glycine 100 mg • L-Phenylalanine 500 mg • Ribonucleic Acid 2 mg • Coenzyme Q-10 100 mcg • Choline (as citrate and bitartrate) 500 mg • Caffeine 120 mg. Other Ingredients: Maltodextrin, Citric Acid, Natural Flavor, Artificial Flavor (original flavor only), Beet Root Powder (for color, cherry flavor only), Sucralose, Sodium Phosphate, Silicon Dioxide, Sodium Carboxymethylcellulose.

Speak Easy Throat Spray **- The Herbalist**
Yerba Mansa root • Echinacea root • Marshmallow root • Propolis • Myrrh Gum • Licorice root in a base of Vegetable Glycerine.

Special B-Complex 50 mg **- Nature's Life**
Each capsule contains: Vitamin C 50 mg • Vitamin B1 (thiamine HCl) 50 mg • Vitamin B2 (riboflavin) 50 mg • Niacinamide 50 mg • Vitamin B6 (pyridoxine HCl) 50 mg • Folic Acid 800 mcg • Vitamin B12 (cobalamin concentrate) 50 mcg • Biotin 50 mcg • Pantothenic Acid (D-calcium pantothenate) 50 mg • Choline (bitartrate) 50 mg • Inositol 50 mg • PABA (Para-Aminobenzioc Acid) 50 mg. In a natural base of Rice Bran, Alfalfa, Parsley, Watercress, Rose Hips, Acerola.

Special Delivery B-12 Plus **- Bee-Alive Inc.**
Each softgel contains: Vitamin B6 (as pyridoxine hydrochloride) 25 mg • Folate (as folic acid) 400 mcg • Vitamin B12 (as cyanocobalamin) 500 mcg • Royal Jelly 25 mg. Other Ingredients: Honey, Gelatin, Glycerin, Sucralose.

Special Two **- NOW Foods**
Two tablets contain: Vitamin A (Beta Carotene) (6 mg) 10000 IU • Vitamin B1 (Thiamine HCL) 50 mg • Vitamin B2 (Riboflavin) 50 mg • Vitamin B3 (Niacinamide) 50 mg • Vitamin B5 (Pantothenic Acid) 50 mg • Vitamin B6 (Pyridoxine HCL) 50 mg • Vitamin B12 (Cyanocobalamin) 100 mcg • Biotin 100 mcg • Folic Acid 400 mcg • Vitamin C (Calcium Ascorbate) 500 mg • Vitamin D (Calciferol) 200 IU • Vitamin E (d-Alpha Succinate) 200 IU • Vitamin K (from green foods) 70 mcg • Calcium (Ascorbate, Carbonate) 100 mg • Magnesium (Oxide, Amino Acid Chelate) 50 mg • Zinc (Amino Acid Chelate) 15 mg • Iron (Amino Acid Chelate) 10 mg • Copper (Amino Acid Chelate) 1 mg • Iodine (Kelp) 150 mcg • Potassium 50 mg • Manganese (Amino Acid Chelate) 5 mg • Selenium (Amino Acid Chelate) 50 mcg • Chromium (Yeast-free GTF) 100 mcg • Molybdenum (Amino Acid Chelate) 50 mcg • Boron (Amino Acid Chelate) 1 mg • Vanadium (Amino Acid Chelate) 50 mcg • Choline (Bitartrate) 50 mg • Inositol 50 mg • PABA 30 mg • Spirulina 250 mg • Chlorella (broken cell wall) 250 mg • Barley grass organic 250 mg • Alfalfa juice concentrate 100 mg • Octacosanol wheat-free 100 mcg • Siberian Ginseng 50 mg • Bioflavonoids (40%) 50 mg • Rutin 25 mg • Psyllium husk fiber 50 mg • Echinacea 50 mg • Apple Pectin 25 mg • Betaine Hydrochloride 25 mg • Glutamic Acid 25 mg • Papain (Papaya) 25 mg • Lipase 10 mg • Amylase 10 mg • Chlorophyll 9 mg • 17 Amino Acids 380 mg derived from Spirulina, Chlorella , Barley grass & Alfalfa juice concentrate. Natural base includes Alfalfa, Rose Hips, Di-Calcium Phosphate, Cellulose, Stearic Acid, natural vegetable protein coating.

Spectra Senior Multi **- DaVinci Laboratories**
Three caplets contain: Vitamin A (2000 IU as palmitate and 7500 IU as beta-carotene) 9500 IU • Vitamin C 300 mg • Vitamin D 200 IU • Vitamin E (as D-alpha tocopheryl succinate) 200 IU • Vitamin K 2.5 mcg • Thiamin 25 mg • Riboflavin 25 mg • Niacin (and as niacinamide) 25 mg • Vitamin B6 (pyridoxine HCl 90%, P-5-P 10%) 25 mg • Folic Acid 200 mcg • Vitamin B12 (methylcobalamin) 25 mcg • Biotin 150 mcg • Pantothenic Acid 25 mg • Calcium (as calcium citrate) 300 mg • Iodine (from kelp) 35 mcg • Magnesium 150 mg • Zinc 10 mg • Selenium 25 mcg • Copper 0.025 mg • Manganese 2.5 mg • Chromium 25 mg • Molybdenum 25 mcg • Potassium 25 mg • Boron 0.5 mg • Silicon (horsetail rush) 3 mg • Vanadium 10 mcg • Choline 50 mg • Inositol 25 mg • PABA (para-aminobenzoic acid) 25 mg • L-Cysteine (enteric coated) 25 mg • Glutamic Acid 25 mg • DL-Methionine (enteric coated) 25 mg • L-Aspartic Acid 50 mg • Phosphatidylserine 12.5 mg • Octacosanol 500 mcg • Lecithin 50 mg • Gamma Linolenic Acid 2.5 mg • Alpha Lipoic Acid 15 mg • Coenzyme Q10 5 mg • Lycopene 2.5 mg • Bioperine brand Black Pepper extract 2.5 mg • Ginkgo Biloba 5 mg • Lutein 1.5 mg • Bilberry 4:1 extract 20 mg • RNA (ribonucleic acid) 5 mg • Mixed Citrus Bioflavonoids 100 mg • Hesperidin 12.5 mg • Rutin 12.5 mg • Pectin 12.5 mg • Betaine Hydrochloride 15 mg • Bromelain 2 gm • Papain (enteric coated) 2 mg • Cellulase enzymes 2 mg • Enzopharm Plus Proprietary Blend 9 mg: Amylase, Protease, Lipase, Hemicellulase, Lactase. Other Ingredients: Magnesium Carbonate, Calcium Ascorbate, Calcium Pantothenate, Potassium Citrate, Cellulose, Zinc Gluconate, Manganese Gluconate, Stearic Acid, Silica, Amino Acid Chelates (boron, copper, molybdenum, selenium), Chromium Polynicotinate.

Spectrabiotic **- Cell Tech**
Two capsules contain: Vitamin C (from acerola & rosehips) 75 mg • Vitamin K 4 mcg • Proprietary Blend 559 mg: Lactobacillus Acidophilus, Bifidobacterium Bifidum, Lactobacillus Casei, Lactobacillus Bulgaricus, Lactobacillus Plantarum, Lactobacillus Salivarius, Streptococcus Faecium, Streptococcus Thermophilius, Blue-Green Algae (aphanizomenon flos-aquae) 100 mg, Jerusalem Artichoke root, Lipase, Amylase, Protease, Cellulase. Other Ingredients: Maltodextrin, Vegetarian Capsule (plant fiber, water).

SpectraSoy **- Metagenics**
Each tablet contains: Soybean concentrate 113 mg • Total Isoflavones (contains glucoside and aglycone forms of genistin, daidzin, and glycitin) 45 mg.

SpectraZyme **- Metagenics**
Two tablets contain: Protease I 20,000 PC • Protease II 200,000 USP • Protease IIII 40,000 HUT • Amylase 20,000 DU • Lipase 20000 LU • Cellulase 2000 CU • Peptidase 600 units • Maltase 600 DP • Lactase 400 LAC U • Invertase 400 SUMNER • Amla fruit (phyllanthus emblica) 40 mg.

Speed Peel Facial Gel **- Cellex-C International Inc.**
Some ingredients include: Ficin Enzyme • Melon extract • Micro-Cylinders of Silica from natural Bamboo extract • Jojoba oil • Peppermint.
See Editor's Note No. 17.

Speman **- The Himalaya Drug Company**
Each tablet contains: Salabmisri (orchis mascula) 130 mg • Kokilaksha (hygrophila auriculata syn. asteracantha longifolia) 64 mg • Vanya Kahu (lactuca scariola syn. l.serriola) 32 mg • Kapikachchhu (mucuna pruriens) 32 mg • Suvarnavang (mosaic gold, unsublimed tin formulation) 32 mg • Vriddadaru (argyreia speciosa syn. a.nervosa) 32 mg • Gokshura (tribulus terrestris) 64 mg • Jeevanti (leptadenia reticulata) 64 mg • Shaileyam (parmelia perlata) 32 mg.

SPES **- BotanicLab**
Each capsule contains: Proprietary Blend 300 mg: Pyrola (pyrola rotundifolia L), Agrimony (agrimonia pilosa Ledeb), Corydalis (corydalis yanhusuo W.T. Wang), Reishi (ganoderma lucidum Karst), Rubescens (rabdosia rubescens Hara), Stephania (stephania delavayi Diels), Stephania (stephania sinica Diels), Lycoris (lycoris radiata Herb), Partinia (partrinia heterophylla Bunga), Oriental Ginseng (panax ginseng C.A. Meyer), Pollen (pollen), Prickly Ash (zanthoxylum nitidum DC), Chinese Licorice (glycyrrhiza uralensis Fisch), Cervus (cervus nippon Temmiinck), Broomrape (Cistanche deserticola Y.C. Ma).
See Editor's Note No. 2.

Sphingolin-MS - Ecological Formulas
Each capsule contains: Myelin Sheath extract (from bovine spinal cord) 200 mg • Ascorbic Acid 30 mg. Other Ingredients: Microcrystalline Cellulose, Cellulose, Magnesium Stearate, Silicon Dioxide.
See Editor's Note No. 31.

Spine Trac C2 - Health Logics
Four capsules contain: BioCell Collagen II 2000 mg: Type II Collagen 1400 mg, Hyaluronic Acid 200 mg, Depolymerized Chondroitin Sulfate (from chicken collagen) 400 mg • Glucosamine Sulfate Potassium 750 mg • Proprietary Blend 80 mg: Green Tea extract, Ginger root extract.

SpiruLEANe - NAI - Natural Alternatives International
Each tablet contains: Proprietary blend 1,545 mg: Ma Huang herb extract (24 mg) • Guarana seed extract (24 mg) • Chromium chelavite (400 mcg) • Spirulina Pacifica • White Willow bark • Green Tea leaf extract • Uva Ursi leaf • Kola Nut seed extract • Bromelain (from pineapple) • Ginger root • Siberian Ginseng root • Ginkgo Biloba leaf extract • Cayenne Pepper • Gotu Kola leaf • Grapefruit seed extract • Royal Jelly • Lecithin.
See Editor's Note No. 30.

Spirulina - Earthrise Nutritionals, LLC.
Six tablets contain: Sodium 35 mg • Vitamin A (100% Beta Carotene) 4,000 IU • Calcium 7 mg • Iron 2 mg • Riboflavin 0.06 mg • Niacin 0.35 mg • Potassium 50 mg • Total Carb. 0.5 g • Protein 2 g • Magnesium 7 mg • Thiamin 0.03 mg • Vitamin B12 4.2 mcg • Vitamin K 17 mcg • Phycocyanin 330 mg • Chlorophyll 30 mg • Mixed Carotenoids 8 mg • Gamma Linolenic Acid 30 mg • Sulfolipids 30 mg • Polysaccharides 140 mg.

Spirulina - Quest
Each capsule contains: Spirulina 500 mg.

Spirulina - Golden Glow Natural Health Products
Spirulina powder • Calcium Phosphate • Hydrogenated Vegetable oil • Anti-Caking Agents (551 & 572) • Thickener (414).

Spirulina - Source Naturals
Six tablets contain: Vitamin A (Beta Carotene) 14,000 IU • Vitamin B1 (Thiamin) 100 mcg • Vitamin B2 (Riboflavin) 99 mcg • Niacin 620 mcg • Vitamin B12 (Cobalamin) 6.6 mg • Boron 30 mcg • Iron 3.2 mg • Magnesium 14 mg • Phosphorus 31 mg • Protein 1,800 mg • Phycocyanin 333 mg • Linoleic Acid 33 mg • Gamma-Linolenic Acid (GLA) 30 mg • Omega-3 Fatty Acids 87 mcg • Chlorophyll 23.7 mg • Total Carotenoids 16.2 mg • Superoxide Dismutase (SOD) 1.2 mg.

Spirulina - Jamieson
Each caplet contains: 100% Pure Spirulina Blue-Green Microalgae 500 mg.

Spirulina & Chlorella - Earthrise Nutritionals, LLC.
Eight tablets contain: Vitamin A 2900 IU • Vitamin C 30 mg • Vitamin E 0.5 IU Vitamin K 17 mcg • Thiamin 0.04 mg • Riboflavin 0.1 mg • Niacin 0.35 mg • Vitamin B6 0.05 mg • Vitamin B12 2 mcg • Calcium 6 mg • Iron 2 mg • Magnesium 8 mg • Sodium 20 mg Potassium 45 mg • Phycocyanin 176 mg • Polysaccharides 75 mg • Chlorophyll 60 mg • Gamma Linolenic Acid 16 mg • Sulfolipids 16 mg • Mixed Carotenoids 8 mg.

Spirulina Bio - Earthrise Nutritionals, LLC.
Six tablets contain: Sodium 35 mg • Vitamin A (100% Beta Carotene) 4,000 IU • Calcium 7 mg • Iron 2 mg • Riboflavin 0.06 mg • Niacin 0.35 mg • Potassium 50 mg • Total Carb. 0.5 g • Protein 2 g • Magnesium 7 mg • Thiamin 0.03 mg • Vitamin B12 4.2 mcg • Vitamin K 17 mcg • Phycocyanin 330 mg • Chlorophyll 30 mg • Mixed Carotenoids 8 mg • Gamma Linolenic Acid 30 mg • Sulfolipids 30 mg • Polysaccharides 140 mg.

Spirulina Bio Powder - Earthrise Nutritionals, LLC.
Three grams contain: Sodium 60 mg • Vitamin A (100% Beta Carotene) 8300 IU • Calcium 12 mg • Iron 3.3 mg • Riboflavin 0.1 mg • Niacin 0.6 mg • Potassium 80 mg • Total Carb. 0.8 g • Protein 3 g • Magnesium 11 mg • Thiamin 0.05 mg • Vitamin B12 7 mcg • Vitamin K 29 mcg • Phycocyanin 550 mg • Chlorophyll 50 mg • Mixed Carotenoids 17 mg • Gamma Linolenic Acid 50 mg • Sulfolipids 50 mg • Polysaccharides 230 mg.

Spirulina Blue Green Algae - Leiner Health Products
Each capsule contains: Spirulina Blue Green Algae (Spirulina pacifica) cell 250 mg. Other Ingredients: Maltodextrin, Gelatin, Cellulose, Magnesium Stearate, Croscarmellose Sodium.

Spirulina Gold - Earthrise Nutritionals, LLC.
Twelve tablets contain: Vitamin A (100% beta carotene) 5000 IU • Calcium 7 mg • Iron 2 mg • Riboflavin 0.306 mg • Niacin 0.35 mg • Zinc 3 mg • Potassium 50 mg • Vitamin C 1.2 mg • Magnesium 7 mg • Thiamin 0.03 mg • Vitamin B12 4.2 mcg • Vitamin K 17 mcg • Phycocyanin 330 mg • Chlorophyll 30 mg • Mixed Carotenoids 10 mg • Gamma Linolenic Acid 30 mg • Sulfolipids 50 mg • Polysaccharides 140 mg.

Spirulina Gold Powder - Earthrise Nutritionals, LLC.
Five grams contain: Vitamin A (100% Beta Carotene) 10,000 IU • Vitamin C 2 mg • Vitamin K 29 mcg • Thiamin 0.05mg • Riboflavin 0.1 mg • Niacin 0.6 mg • Vitamin B12 7 mcg • Calcium 12 mg • Iron 3.3 mg • Magnesium 11 mg • Zinc 5 mg • Sodium 80 mg • Potassium 80 mg • Phycocyanin 550 mg • Polysaccharides 230 mg • Sulfolipids 50 mg • Chlorophyll 60 mg • Gamma Linolenic Acid 50 mg • Mixed Carotenoids 18.5 mg.

Spirulina Multiple - Source Naturals
Two tablets contain: Spirulina Plankton (Spirulina platensis) 200 mg • Rose Hips 25 mg • Beta Carotene (Pro-Vitamin A) 10,000 IU • Vitamin B1 (Thiamin Mononitrate) 25 mg • Vitamin B2 (Riboflavin) 25 mg • Niacin 25 mg • Vitamin B6 (Pyridoxine HCl) 25 mg • Vitamin B12 (Cobalamin) 100 mcg • Folic Acid 100 mcg • Vitamin C (Ascorbic Acid) 250 mg • Vitamin D (as Vitamin D3) (Cholecalciferol) 400 IU • Vitamin E d-alpha tocopheryl 60 IU • Calcium (Carbonate) 99 mg • Iodine (from Kelp) 150 mcg • Iron (Fumarate) 18 mg • Magnesium (Oxide) 33 mg • Potassium (Chelate) 7.5 mg • Zinc (Citrate) 5 mg.

Spirulina Powder - Source Naturals
Each teaspoon contains: Vitamin A (Beta Carotene) 42,000 IU • Vitamin B1 (Thiamin) 300 mcg • Vitamin B2 (Riboflavin) 300 mcg • Niacin 2 mg • Vitamin B12 (Cobalamin) 20 mg • Boron 90 mcg • Iron 9.5 mg • Magnesium 43 mg • Phosphorus 93 mg • Protein 5,400 mg • Phycocyanin 1,000 mg • Linoleic Acid 99 mg • Gamma-Linolenic Acid (GLA) 90 mg • Omega-3 Fatty Acids 261 mcg • Chlorophyll 71 mg • Total Carotenoids 48.6 mg • Superoxide Dismutase (SOD) 3.6 mg.

Spirulina Powder - Earthrise Nutritionals, LLC.
Three grams contain: Sodium 60 mg • Vitamin A (100% Beta Carotene) 8,300 IU • Calcium 12 mg • Iron 3.3 mg • Riboflavin 0.1 mg • Niacin 0.6 mg • Potassium 80 mg • Magnesium 11 mg • Thiamin 0.05 mg • Vitamin B12 7 mcg • Vitamin K 29 mcg • Phycocyanin 550 mg • Chlorophyll 50 mg • Mixed Carotenoids 17 mg • Gamma Linolenic Acid 50 mg • Sulfolipids 50 mg • Polysaccharides 230 mg.

Spirulina- Vegi-Capsules - Earthrise Nutritionals, LLC.
Seven Vegi-Capsules Contain: Sodium 35 mg • Vitamin A (100% Beta Carotene) 4,000 IU • Calcium 7 mg • Iron 2 mg • Riboflavin 0.06 mg • Niacin 0.35 mg • Potassium 50 mg • Total Carb. 0.5 mg • Protein 2 g • Magnesium 7 mg • Thiamin 0.03 mg • Vitamin B12 4.2 mcg • Vitamin K 17 mcg • Phycocyanin 330 mg • Chlorophyll 30 mg • Mixed Carotenoids 8 mg • Gamma Linolenic Acid 30 mg • Sulfolipids 30 mg • Polysaccharides 140 mg.

Spirulina Vegi-Capsules - Earthrise Nutritionals, LLC.
Three grams contain: Vitamin A 4000 IU • Vitamin K 17 mcg • Thiamin 0.03 mg • Riboflavin 0.06 mg • Niacin 0.35 mg • Vitamin B12 4.2 mcg • Calcium 7 mg • Iron 2 mg • Magnesium 7 mg • Sodium 35 mg • Potassium 50 mg • Phycocyanin 330 mg • Polysaccharides 30 mg • Chlorophyll 30 mg • Gamma Linolenic Acid 30 mg • Mixed Carotenoids 8 mg.

Spirulina+Chlorella **-** Earthrise Nutritionals, LLC.
Eight tablets contain: Sodium 20 mg • Vitamin A (100% Beta Carotene) 2900 IU • Calcium 6 mg • Iron 2 mg • Vitamin E 0.51 IU • Riboflavin 0.1 mg • Niacin 0.35 mg • Protein 2 g • Total Carb. 0.5 g • Potassium 45 mg • Vitamin C 30 mg • Magnesium 8.0 mg • Thiamin 0.04 mg • Vitamin B6 0.05 mg • Vitamin B12 2 mcg • Vitamin K 17 mcg • Phycocyanin 176 mg • Chlorophyll 60 mg • Mixed Carotenoids 8 mg • Gamma Linolenic Acid 16 mg • Sulfolipids 16 mg • Polysaccharides 75 mg.

Spiru-Tein Bar (assorted flavors) **-** Nature's Plus
Each bar contains: Vitamin A 2500 IU • Vitamin C 30 mg • Calcium 300 mg • Iron 4.5 mg • Vitamin E 15 IU • Thiamin 0.75 mg • Riboflavin 0.85 mg • Niacin 10 mg • Vitamin B6 1 mg • Folic Acid 200 mcg • Vitamin B12 3 mcg • Biotin 150 mcg • Pantothenic Acid 5 mg • Phosphorus 20 mg • Iodine 75 mcg • Magnesium 60 mg • Zinc 7.5 mg • Selenium 10 mcg • Manganese 2.5 mg • Chromium 10 mcg • Molybdenum 10 mcg. Other Ingredients: High Fructose Complex (from fruit concentrates, corn and/or malt), Non-GMO Isolated Soy Protein, Peanut Butter, Oat Bran, Maltodextrin, Natural Vanilla Flavor, Honey, Vegetable Glycerin, Guar Gum, Choline Bitartrate, Psyllium, Spirulina, Inositol, Potassium Citrate, Apple Pectin, Bee Pollen, Chlorophyll, Papaya, Malt, Vegetable Oil, Carob, Lecithin. Original Carob-Coated flavor also contains: Natural Vanilla Flavor. Coating: Malt, Vegetable Oil, Carob, Lecithin. Strawberry Yogurt-Coated flavor also contains: Malic Acid. Coating: Vegetable Oil, Fructose, Nonfat Dry Milk, Maltodextrin, Nonfat Yogurt Powder, Natural Color, Soy Lecithin, Natural Flavor. Carob Chocolate flavor also contains: Lowfat Cocoa. Coating: Malt, Vegetable Oil, Carob, Lecithin. Banana Yogurt-Coated flavor also contains: Coating: Vegetable Oil, Fructose, Nonfat Dry Milk, Maltodextrin, Nonfat Yogurt Powder, Soy Lecithin, Natural Flavor. Double Fudge Crunch flavor also contains: Soy Puffs, Dutch Processed Cocoa, Unsweetened Chocolate. Coating: Malt, Vegetable Oil, Carob, Lecithin.

Spiru-Tein Junior (chocolate and strawberry flavors) **-** Nature's Plus
Each scoop (33 g) contains: Vitamin A 2500 IU • Vitamin C 30 mg • Calcium 500 mg • Iron 9 mg • Vitamin D 200 IU • Vitamin E 15 IU • Thiamin 0.75 mg • Riboflavin 0.85 mg • Niacin 10 mg • Vitamin B6 1 mg • Folic Acid 200 mcg • Vitamin B12 3 mcg • Biotin 150 mcg • Pantothenic Acid 5 mg • Phosphorus 500 mg • Iodine 75 mcg • Magnesium 200 mg • Zinc 7.5 mg • Selenium 10 mcg • Manganese 2.5 mg • Chromium 10 mcg • Molybdenum 10 mcg • Inositol 25 mg • Choline (bitartrate) 11 mg. Other Ingredients: Fructose, Non-GMO Isolated Soy Protein, Oat Bran, Apple Pectin, Natural Vanilla Flavor, Papaya, Bromelain. Chocolate flavor also contains: Dutch Cocoa. Strawberry flavor also contains: Strawberry Flavor, Beet Juice.

Spiru-Tein Plus Shake **-** Nature's Plus
Each scoop (34 g) contains: Vitamin A 5000 IU • Vitamin C 60 mg • Calcium 400 mg • Iron 4.5 mg • Vitamin D 400 IU • Vitamin E 30 IU • Thiamin 1.5 mg • Riboflavin 1.7 mg • Niacin 20 mg • Vitamin B6 2 mg • Folic Acid 400 mcg • Vitamin B12 6 mcg • Biotin 300 mcg • Pantothenic Acid 10 mg • Phosphorus 300 mg • Iodine 150 mcg • Magnesium 80 mg • Zinc 15 mg • Selenium 21 mcg • Manganese 5 mg • Chromium 20 mcg • Molybdenum 20 mcg • Enzyme Complex 150 mg: Amylase 50 mg, Protease 50 mg, Lipase 50 mg • Marine Algae Duplex (ulva rigida and ulva fasciata) 100 mg • Modified Citrus Pectin 100 mg • Inositol 50 mg • Phosphatidylserine Complex 50 mg: Phosphatidylserine (PS) 10 mg, Phosphatidylcholine (PC) 10 mg, Cephalin (phosphatidylethanolamine) 6 mg, Phosphoinositides 3 mg • English Hawthorne berry (crataegus laevigata, standardized to 3.2% vitexin) 50 mg • Lactospore brand microencapsulated culture of B. Coagulans (provides 150 million viable cells) 25 mg • Choline (as bitartrate) 21 mg • Ginkgo Biloba leaf (standardized to 24% ginkgo flavone-glycosides and 6% terpene lactones) 10 mg • Lutein (from marigold flower extract) 3 mg • Boron (citrate) 150 mcg • Zeaxanthin (from marigold flower extract) 132 mcg. Other Ingredients: Non-GMO Isolated Soy Protein, Fructose, Natural Vanilla Flavor, Modified Citrus Pectin, Guar Gum, Psyllium, Oat Bran, Microcrystalline Cellulose, Spirulina, Leci-PS, Apple Pectin, Bee Pollen, Papaya fruit, Chlorophyll.

Spiru-Tein Shake (chocolate and strawberry flavors) **-** Nature's Plus
Each scoop (34 g) contains: Vitamin A 5000 IU • Vitamin C 60 mg • Calcium 300 mg • Iron 4.5 mg • Vitamin D 400 IU • Vitamin E 30 IU • Thiamin 1.5 mg • Riboflavin 1.7 mg • Niacin 20 mg • Vitamin B6 2 mg • Folic Acid 400 mcg • Vitamin B12 6 mcg • Biotin 300 mcg • Pantothenic Acid 10 mg • Phosphorus 200 mg • Iodine 150 mcg • Magnesium 80 mg • Zinc 15 mg • Selenium 21 mcg • Manganese 5 mg • Chromium 18 mcg • Molybdenum 20 mcg • Inositol 50 mg • Choline (as bitartrate) 21 mg. Other Ingredients: Non-GMO Isolated Soy Protein, Fructose, Guar Gum, Psyllium, Natural Vanilla Flavor, Oat Bran, Microcrystalline Cellulose, Spirulina, Apple Pectin, Bee Pollen, Lecithin, Lemon Bioflavonoids, Papaya, Bromelain, Chlorophyll. Chocolate flavor also contains: Dutch Cocoa. Strawberry flavor also contains: Strawberry Seeds, Beet Juice Powder.

Spiru-Tein Simply Natural Shake **-** Nature's Plus
Each scoop (34 g) contains: Vitamin A 5000 IU • Vitamin C 60 mg • Calcium 300 mg • Iron 4.5 mg • Vitamin D 400 IU • Vitamin E 30 IU • Thiamin 1.5 mg • Riboflavin 1.7 mg • Niacin 20 mg • Vitamin B6 2 mg • Folic Acid 400 mcg • Vitamin B12 6 mcg • Biotin 300 mcg • Pantothenic Acid 10 mg • Phosphorus 200 mg • Iodine 150 mcg • Magnesium 80 mg • Zinc 15 mg • Selenium 21 mcg • Manganese 5 mg • Chromium 18 mcg • Molybdenum 20 mcg • Inositol 50 mg • Choline (as bitartrate) 21 mg. Other Ingredients: Non-GMO Isolated Soy Protein, Maltodextrin, Natural Vanilla Flavor, Guar Gum, Psyllium, Oat Bran, Microcrystalline Cellulose, Spirulina, Apple Pectin, Bee Pollen, Lecithin, Lemon Bioflavonoids, Papaya, Bromelain, Chlorophyll.

Spiru-Tein Wafers (assorted flavors) **-** Nature's Plus
Six wafers contain: Vitamin A 5000 IU • Vitamin C 60 mg • Calcium 600 mg • Iron 4.5 mg • Vitamin D 400 IU • Vitamin E 30 IU • Thiamin 1.5 mg • Riboflavin 1.7 mg • Niacin 20 mg • Vitamin B6 2 mg • Folic Acid 400 mcg • Vitamin B12 6 mcg • Biotin 300 mcg • Pantothenic Acid 10 mg • Phosphorus 300 mg • Iodine 150 mcg • Magnesium 80 mg • Zinc 15 mg • Selenium 21 mcg • Manganese 5 mg • Chromium 21 mcg • Molybdenum 21 mcg • Inositol 50 mg • Choline (bitartrate) 21 mg. Other Ingredients: Non-GMO Isolated Soy Protein, Calcium Caseinate, Milk Protein Concentrate, Psyllium Seed Husk, Fructose, Guar Gum, Magnesium Stearate, Spirulina, Bee Pollen, Apple Pectin, Oat Bran, Lecithin, Papaya, Bromelain, Lemon Bioflavonoids, Chlorophyll. Vanilla flavor also contains: Natural Vanilla Flavor. Chocolate flavor also contains: Cocoa. Strawberry flavor also contains: Natural Strawberry Flavor, Natural Vanilla Flavor. Banana flavor also contains: Natural Banana Flavor.

Spiru-Tein Whey Shake (assorted flavors) **-** Nature's Plus
Each scoop (32 g) contains: Vitamin A 5000 IU • Vitamin C 60 mg • Calcium 300 mg • Iron 4.5 mg • Vitamin D 400 IU • Vitamin E 30 IU • Thiamin 1.5 mg • Riboflavin 1.7 mg • Niacin 20 mg • Vitamin B6 2 mg • Folic Acid 400 mcg • Vitamin B12 6 mcg • Biotin 300 mcg • Pantothenic Acid 10 mg • Phosphorus 200 mg • Iodine 150 mcg • Magnesium 80 mg • Zinc 15 mg • Selenium 21 mcg • Manganese 5 mg • Chromium 18 mcg • Molybdenum 18.75 mcg • Inositol 50 mg • Choline (bitartrate) 21 mg. Other Ingredients: Micro-filtered Whey Protein Concentrate, Di-Calcium Phosphate, Xanthan Gum, Fructooligosaccharides (FOS), Guar Gum, Psyllium, Maltodextrin, Potassium Citrate, Oat Bran, Microcrystalline Cellulose, Spirulina, Apple Pectin, Bee Pollen, Lecithin, Lemon Bioflavonoids, Papaya, Bromelain, Chlorophyll. Chocolate flavor also contains: Cocoa, Chocolate Flavor, Fructose. Strawberry flavor also contains: Strawberry Seeds, Fruit Punch Flavor, Beet Juice, Fructose. Vanilla Flavor also contains Vanilla Flavor, Fructose. Vanilla for Low Carb Diets flavor also contains: Vanilla Flavor, Vitasweet brand Proprietary Blend of Maltitol, FOS, Bromelain, Papain.

SPL and PAN **-** Dial Herbs
Chamomile • Dandelion • Goldenseal • Parsley • Uva Ursi • Yellow Dock • Cayenne • Yarrow.

Some Brand Name Natural Products - What they Contain

www.NaturalDatabase.com contains MANY more listings than appear here.
Editor's Notes are located on pages 2155-2163.

Splash C with Aloe Lemon - Pharmanex
Crystalline Fructose • Guam Arabic • Natural Orange Flavors • Citric Acid • Potassium Citrate • Silicon Dioxide • Maltodextrin • Dicalcium Phosphate • Ascorbic Acid • Tricalcium Phosphate • Sodium Chloride • Oat Fiber • Soy Fiber • Powdered Cellulose • DL-Alpha Tocopheryl Acetate • Beta-Carotene • Aloe Vera concentrate • Folic Acid.

Splash C with Aloe Orange - Pharmanex
Crystalline Fructose • Guam Arabic • Natural Orange Flavors • Citric Acid • Potassium Citrate • Silicon Dioxide • Maltodextrin • Dicalcium Phosphate • Ascorbic Acid • Tricalcium Phosphate • Sodium Chloride • Oat Fiber • Soy Fiber • Powdered Cellulose • DL-Alpha Tocopheryl Aceate • Beta-Carotene • Aloe Vera concentrate • Folic Acid.

Spleen Glandular - American Biologics
Each tablet contains: Raw Spleen concentrate (bovine origin) 40 mg. Other Ingredients: Dicalcium Phosphate, Magnesium Stearate. See Editor's Note No. 14.

Spleen PMG - Standard Process, Inc.
Each tablet contains: Proprietary Blend 183 mg: Bovine Spleen PMG extract, Magnesium Citrate • Calcium 30 mg. Other Ingredients: Cellulose.

Spleen, Desiccated - Standard Process, Inc.
Each tablet contains: Proprietary Blend 350 mg: Bovine Spleen, Ovine Spleen. Other Ingredients: Honey, Arabic Gum. See Editor's Note No. 14.

Spontane-ES - Warner Laboratories
Each tablet contains: Proprietary Blend 325 mg: Epimedium (20% extract, leaves), Xanthoparmelia Scabrosa (lichen), Cnidium Monnier (fruit), Quebracho (8% extract, bark), Ginkgo Biloba (leaves), Mucuna Pruriens (seed), L-Arginine. Other Ingredients: Microcrystalline Cellulose, Magnesium Stearate, Sodium Starch, FD&C Blue #1 Aluminum Lake.

Sport - Mannatech
Two capsules contain: Chromium (as chromium picolinate) 200 mcg • Proprietary Blend Sterol Complex 800 mg: Bovine Testes extract 400 mg, Wild Yam (root; standardized for 25 mg phytosterols) 200 mg, Sarsaparilla (root) 200 mg • Boron (as boron citrate) 2 mg • Ambrotose Complex (patent pending) 5 mg: Arabinogalactan (larix decidua gum), Manapol Aloe Vera gel extract (inner leaf gel), Gum Ghatti, Gum Tragacanth. Other Ingredients: Gelatin, Brown Rice Flour, Silicon Dioxide, Magnesium Stearate.

Sport Fuel - TwinLab
Six capsules contain: Beta-Carotene (pro-Vitamin A) 25000 IU • Vitamin D (from natural form Vitamin D3) 400 IU • Vitamin C 1000 mg • Natural Vitamin E (Succinate) 800 IU • CoQ10 (Coenzyme Q10) 30 mg • L-Glutathione 100 mg • N-Acetyl Cysteine (NAC) 200 mg • Alpha Lipoic Acid 100 mcg • Vitamin B1 (Thiamine) 50 mg • Vitamin B2 (Riboflavin) 50 mg • Vitamin B6 (Pyridoxine) 50 mg • Vitamin B12 (Cobalamin) 100 mcg • Folic Acid 400 mcg • Niacinamide 150 mg • Pantothenic Acid 250 mg • Biotin 300 mcg • PABA (Para-Aminobenzoic Acid) 25 mg • Choline Bitartrate 100 mg • Inositol 100 mg • L-Carnitine (from Carni Fuel L-Carnitine Magnesium Citrate) 100 mg • Magnesium (from L-Carnitine Magnesium Citrate, Aspartate, Oxide, and Alpha-Ketoglutarate) 600 mg • Potassium (from Potassium Aspartate, Citrate, and Alpha-Ketoglutarate) 100 mg • Zinc (from Zinc Picolinate) 30 mg • Manganese (from Manganese Gluconate) 5 mg • Copper (from Copper Gluconate) 2 mg • Iron (from Ferrous Fumarate) 10 mg • Iodine (from Potassium Iodide) 150 mcg • Selenium (from Selenomethionine & Selenate 50/50 mixture) 200 mcg • Chromium (from Chromic Fuel Chromium Picolinate) 400 mcg • Molybdenum (from natural Molybdic Acid) 150 mcg.

Sport Fuel With Iron - TwinLab
Six capsules contain: Beta-Carotene (pro-Vitamin A) 25000 IU • Vitamin D (from natural form Vitamin D3) 400 IU • Vitamin C 1000 mg • Natural Vitamin E (Succinate) 800 IU • CoQ10 (Coenzyme Q10) 30 mg • L-Glutathione 100 mg • N-Acetyl Cysteine (NAC) 200 mg • Alpha Lipoic Acid 100 mcg • Vitamin B1 (Thiamine) 50 mg • Vitamin B2 (Riboflavin) 50 mg • Vitamin B6 (Pyridoxine) 50 mg • Vitamin B12 (Cobalamin) 100 mcg • Folic Acid 400 mcg • Niacinamide 150 mg • Pantothenic Acid 250 mg • Biotin 300 mcg • PABA (Para-Aminobenzoic Acid) 25 mg • Choline Bitartrate 100 mg • Inositol 100 mg • L-Carnitine (from Carni Fuel L-Carnitine Magnesium Citrate) 100 mg • Calcium (from Calcium Citrate, Carbonate) 25 mg • Magnesium (from L-Carnitine Magnesium Citrate, Aspartate, Oxide, and Alpha-Ketoglutarate) 600 mg • Potassium (from Potassium Aspartate, Citrate, and Alpha-Ketoglutarate) 100 mg • Zinc (from Zinc Picolinate) 30 mg • Manganese (from Manganese Gluconate) 5 mg • Copper (from Copper Gluconate) 2 mg • Iron (from Ferrous Fumarate) 10 mg • Iodine (from Potassium Iodide) 150 mcg • Selenium (from Selenomethionine & Selenate‹50/50 mixture) 200 mcg • Chromium (from Chromic Fuel Chromium Picolinate) 400 mcg • Molybdenum (from natural Molybdic Acid) 150 mcg.

Sport Fuel Without Iron - TwinLab
Six capsules contain: Beta-Carotene (pro-Vitamin A) 25000 IU • Vitamin D (from natural form Vitamin D3) 400 IU • Vitamin C 1000 mg • Natural Vitamin E (Succinate) 800 IU • CoQ10 (Coenzyme Q10) 30 mg • L-Glutathione 100 mg • N-Acetyl Cysteine (NAC) 200 mg • Alpha Lipoic Acid 100 mcg • Vitamin B1 (Thiamine) 50 mg • Vitamin B2 (Riboflavin) 50 mg • Vitamin B6 (Pyridoxine) 50 mg • Vitamin B12 (Cobalamin) 100 mcg • Folic Acid 400 mcg • Niacinamide 150 mg • Pantothenic Acid 250 mg • Biotin 300 mcg • PABA (Para-Aminobenzoic Acid) 25 mg • Choline Bitartrate 100 mg • Inositol 100 mg • L-Carnitine (from Carni Fuel L-Carnitine Magnesium Citrate) 100 mg • Calcium (from Calcium Citrate, Carbonate) 25 mg • Magnesium (from L-Carnitine Magnesium Citrate, Aspartate, Oxide, and Alpha-Ketoglutarate) 600 mg • Potassium (from Potassium Aspartate, Citrate, and Alpha-Ketoglutarate) 100 mg • Zinc (from Zinc Picolinate) 30 mg • Manganese (from Manganese Gluconate) 5 mg • Copper (from Copper Gluconate) 2 mg • Iodine (from Potassium Iodide) 150 mcg • Selenium (from Selenomethionine & Selenate‹50/50 mixture) 200 mcg • Chromium (from Chromic Fuel Chromium Picolinate) 400 mcg • Molybdenum (from natural Molybdic Acid) 150 mcg.

Sportalyte - Pharmanex
Twenty grams contain: Glucose • Fructose • Maltodextrin • Citric Acid • Natural Flavor • Sodium Chloride • Silicon Dioxide • Sodium Citrate • Magnesium Carbonate • Tricalcium Phosphate • Potassium Citrate • Magnesium Oxide • Ascorbic Acid • D-Alpha Tocopheryl Acetate • Potassium Chloride • Hydromins • Taurine • Fructooligosaccharides.

Sports One DIOL XS - Sports One
Each capsule contains: Nor-4-Androstenediol 100 mg • 4-Androstenediol 100 mg
See Editor's Note No. 54.

Spring Valley Children's Chewables Complete - Leiner Health Products
Each tablet contains: Vitamin A Acetate (as Acetate and Beta Carotene) 5000 IU • Vitamin C (Ascorbic Acid) 60 mg • Vitamin D (Ergocalciferol) 400 IU • Vitamin E (dl-Alpha Tocopheryl Acetate) 30 IU • Thiamin Mononitrate (Vitamin B1) 1.5 mg • Riboflavin (Vitamin B2) 1.7 mg • Niacin (Niacinamide) 20 mg • Vitamin B-6 (Pyridoxine Hydrochloride) 2 mg • Folic Acid 400 mcg • Vitamin B-12 (Cyanocobalamin) 6 mcg • Biotin (USP Method 2) 40 mcg • Pantothenic Acid (d-Calcium Pantothenate) 10 mg • Calcium 100 mg • Iron (Ferrous Fumarate) 18 mg • Phosphorus 100 mg • Iodine (Potassium Iodide) 150 mcg • Magnesium Oxide 20 mg • Zinc Oxide 15 mg • Copper (Cupric Oxide) 2 mg. Other Ingredients: Sorbitol, Dicalcium Phosphate, Magnesium Phosphate, Fructose, Stearic Acid, Mono- & Diglycerides, Xylitol, Gelatin, Sodium Ascorbate, Carrageenan, Aspartame, Citric Acid, Red 40 Lake, Yellow 6 Lake, Starch, Silicon Dioxide, Magnesium Stearate, Blue 2 Lake, Hydroxypropyl Methylcellulose, Resin, Hydroxypropyl Cellulose, Lactose, Polyvinyl Pyrrolidone.

Spring Valley Glucosamine Sulfate - Nature's Bounty
Each capsule contains: Potassium 107 mg • Glucosamine Sulfate (2KCl) 1000 mg. Other Ingredients: Gelatin, Glycerin, Hydroxethyl Methylcellulose, Silica, Vegetable Magnesium Stearate.

Spring Valley High Potency Iron - Weider Nutrition
Each tablet contains: Iron (from 134 mg ferrous sulfate, USP) 27 mg. Other Ingredients: Calcium Carbonate, Cellulose, Maltodextrin, Corn Starch, Croscarmellose Sodium, Dextrin, Silicon Dioxide, Hypromellose, Red 40 Lake, Talc, Polyethylene Glycol, Dextrose, Magnesium Stearate, Titanium Dioxide, Lecithin, Blue 2 Lake, Sodium Carboxymethylcellulose, Sodium Citrate.

Spring Valley Natural Calcium 600 - Weider Nutrition
Each tablet contains: Calcium (as calcium carbonate) 600 mg. Other Ingredients: Corn Starch, Maltodextrin, Acacia, Coating (titanium dioxide, dextrose, hdyroxypropyl methylcellulose, polyethylene glycol, sodium carboxymethylcellulose, mineral oil, sodium citrate, polysorbate 80, dextrin), Magnesium Stearate.

Spring Valley Natural Fish Oil Concentrate - Weider Nutrition
Each softgel contains: Natural Fish oil concentrate 100 mg: EPA (eicosapentaenoic acid) 180 mg, DHA (docosahexaenoic acid) 120 mg. Other Ingredients: Gelatin, Glycerin, D-Sorbitol, D-Alpha Tocpherol.

Spring Valley Vitamin C with Rose Hips - Leiner Health Products
Each tablet contains: Vitamin C 500 mg. Other Ingredients: Ascorbic Acid, Starch, Cellulose, Rose Hips, Stearic Acid, Silicon Croscarmellose Sodium.

Springs of Life Water Enhancer - Garden of Life, Inc.
Twelve drops contain: Springs of Life Proprietary Blend 489 mg: Purified Water, Seawater extract, Ionic Plant Based Mineral blend, Plant Amino Acid blend, Plant Enzyme blend, Water.

Springtime Horsetail 2000 - Golden Glow Natural Health Products
Each tablet contains: Horsetail extract (equisetum arvense) 2000 mg.

SS Cream - Cheil Jedang Corporation
Each gram of cream contains: Bufonis venenum 10 mg • Extract blend 100 mg: Angelicae gigantis radix, Cistanchis herba, Torilis semen, Ginseng radix alba, Zanthoxyli fructos • Extract blend 10 mg: Asiasari radix, Caryophylli flos, Cinnamomi cortex.
See Editor's Note No. 13.

ST (Stomach Tonic) - Wild Rose
Each tablet contains: Meadowsweet 150 mg • Gentian root 100 mg • Fennel seed 75 mg • Goldenseal root 75 mg • Lobelia leaf 75 mg • Fenugreek seed 75 mg.

St John's Wort 2700 - Golden Glow Natural Health Products
Each tablet contains: Hypericum Perforatum herb extract (St. John's wort): Hypericun 1.37 mg.

St. John's Complex - Body Wise International, Inc.
Each tablet contains: St. John's Wort extract (0.3% Hypericin) 300 mg • Chamomile flowers (Anthemis flores) 25 mg • Passion Flower (Passiflora incarnata) 25 mg.

St. John's Formula - Health Smart Vitamins
Each capsule contains: Vitamin B6 (as pyridoxine hydrochloride) 10 mg • Folate (folic acid) 200 mcg • Vitamin B12 (as cyanocobalamin) 50 mcg • Magnesium (as magnesium oxide) 100 mg • St. John's Wort aerial parts (0.3% hypercins, 0.9 mg) 300 mg • Kava Kava root (30% kavalactones, 22.5 mg) 75 mg • Ginkgo leaf (24% ginkgo flavonglycosides, 9.6 mg; 6% terpene lactone, 2.4 mg) 40 mg.

St. John's Good Mood - Traditional Medicinals
St. John's Wort herb & dry extract • Lemon Balm leaf (Melissa) • Oatstraw herb • Damiana herb • Lavender flower • Berganot herb • Sage leaf • Spearmint leaf • Lemongrass leaf • Licorice root • Rose petals • Stevia leaf.

St. John's Plus - Nutri-Quest Rx
Each tablet contains: St. John's Wort herb 400 mg • Pyridoxal-5-Phosphate 5 mg • Riboflavin (as Riboflavin-5-Phosphate) 5 mg • Folic Acid 100 mcg • Vitamin B1 10 mg • Vitamin B12 250 mcg • Ginkgo Biloba extract 5 mg • Damiana herb 25 mg • Ginkgo Biloba herb 30 mg • Blue Vervain 25 mg • Kava Kava herb 10 mg • Hyssop herb 15 mg • Siberian Ginseng 10 mg • Niacinamide 50 mg • Calcium Citrate 100 mg • Magnesium Citrate 100 mg.

St. John's Plus - Rx Vitamins
Each caplet provides: St. John's Wort flower (Hypericum perforatum, standardized 0.3-0.5 hypericin) 300 mg • Kava root (Piper methylsticum, standardized 29-31% kavalactones) 50 mg • Siberian ginseng root (Eleutherococcus senticosis, standardized 0.8% eleutherosides) 50 mg • Feverfew leaf (Tanacetum parthenium, standardized 0.7% parthenolide) 25 mg • L-Tyrosine (free form amino acid) 25 mg • Zinc (l-monomethionine) 10 mg • Vitamin B6 (pyridoxine HCl) 5 mg • Vitamin B12 (cyanocobalamin) 10 mcg.

St. John's Plus Kava Kava - Progressive Labs
Each capsule contains: Vitamin B6 (pyridoxine HCl) 25 mg • St. John's Wort 0.3% Hypericin 200 mg • Kava Kava 100 mg.

St. John's Solution - Quantum, Inc.
One softgel contains: St. John's Wort (Hypericum perforatum Standardized 0.3% hypericin) 300 mg.
See Editor's Note No. 21.

St. Johns Wort - Pro Health
Each capsule contains: St. John's Wort leaf 0.3% extract 250 mg. Other Ingredients: Rice Bran, Talc, Silicon Dioxide.

St. John's Wort - USANA Health Sciences
Each tablet contains: St. John's wort (standardized extract 0.3% hypericin derivatives by UV analysis) 300 mg. Other Ingredients: Dextrose, Ascorbyl Palmitate, Colloidal Silicon Dioxide, Dextrin (modified food starch), Lecithin, Sodium Citrate.

St. John's Wort - GNC
Each capsule contains: St. John's Wort Herb powder (Hypericum perforatum) 500 mg. Other Ingredients: Gelatin.

St. John's Wort - Benepure, Inc
Each capsule contains: St. John's Wort extract (hypericum perforatum, hypericin 1 mg) 333 mg. Other Ingredients: St. John's Wort Herb Powder, Gelatin, Silicon Dioxide, Vegetable Stearate.

St. John's Wort - Leiner Health Products
Each caplet contains: St. John's Wort extract (Hypericum perforatum) herb 330 mg. Other Ingredients: Cellulose, Dicalcium Phosphate, Croscarmellose Sodium, Stearic Acid, Hydroxypropyl Methycellulose, Magnesium Stearate, Silicon Dioxide, Hydroxypropyl Cellulose, Red 40 Lake, Blue 2 Lake, Pharmaceutical Glaze, Polyethylene Glycol 3350, Polysorbate 80, Titanium Dioxide.

St. John's Wort - E'OLA
Two capsules contain: Vitamin C 30 mg • Vitamin D 200 IU • Vitamin B6 20 mg • Folic Acid 200 mcg • Magnesium 40 mg • Chromium 60 mcg • St. John's Wort (3% hypericin) 340 mg • St. John's Wort Herb 100 mg.

St. John's Wort - Celestial Seasonings
Three capsules contain: Proprietary Blend, 1800 mg: St. John's Wort (leaf, stem, flower), St. John's Wort (standardized extract). Other Ingredients: Dicalcium Phosphate, Gelatin, Rice Flour, Stearic Acid, Magnesium Stearate, Silicon Dioxide.

St. John's Wort - Metabolic Response Modifiers
Each capsule contains: Hypericum Perforatum (0.3%) 450 mg.

St. John's Wort - Quest
Each caplet contains: St. John's Wort (Hypericum perfortum) (provided by 300 mg P.E. 1:5 standardized to contain 0.3% Hypercin) 1500 mg. Other Ingredients: Microcrystalline Cellulose, Calcium phosphate, Croscarmellose Sodium Dioxide, Vegetable Stearin, Magnesium Stearate.

St. John's Wort - Nature's Way
Two capsules contain: St. John's Wort stem, leaf, flower 600 mg • St. John's Wort (dried extract 0.3% Dianthrones measures as Hypericin) 300 mg. Other Ingredients: Gelatin, Magnesium Stearate, Millet.

St. John's Wort - Jamieson
Each tablet contains: Vitamin C 2.5 mg • St. John's Wort 4.4:1 extract (Hypericum perforatum L. Aerial parts of flower, stamen and leaf Containing 0.3% hypericin) 225 mg.

St. John's Wort - Gaia Herbs
Three capsules contain: St. John's Wort flower buds (hypericum perforatum, 0.5% hypericins) 540 mg. Other Ingrediens: Vegetable Glycerin, Vegetable Cellulose.

St. John's Wort - Swanson Health Products
Each capsule contains: St. John's Wort powder 375 mg.

St. John's Wort - Ortho Molecular Products
Each capsule contains: St. John's Wort flower extract (standardized to contain 0.3% hypericin and 3% hyperforin) 500 mg. Other Ingredients: Natural Vegetable Capsules, Magnesium Stearate, Silicon Dioxide, Microcrystalline Cellulose.

St. John's Wort - Pharmanex
Each capsule contains: St. John's Wort flower tops/leaves (Hypericum perforatum 5:1) 300 mg. Other Ingredients: Rice Flour, Gelatin, Magnesium Stearate, Silicon Dioxide.

St. John's Wort .3% - Jarrow Formulas
Each capsule contains: St. John's Wort 0.3% extract 300 mg. Other Ingredients: Rice Powder, Magnesium Stearate, Silicon Dioxide, Gelatin.

St. John's Wort + Ginseng Caplet - Leiner Health Products
Each caplet contains: Lecithin 15 mg • Licorice extract (Glycyrrhiza glabra) root 20 mg • Siberian Ginseng extract (Eleutheroxoxxus senticosus) root 50 mg • Siberian Ginseng powder (Eleutherococcus senticosus) root 15 mg • St. John's Wort extract (Hypericum perforatum) aerial parts 300 mg. Other Ingredients: Cellulose, Dicalcium Phosphate, Croscarmellose Sodium, Silicon Dioxide, Stearic Acid, Magnesium Stearate, Hydroxypropyl Methylcellulose, Dextrin.

St. John's Wort + Kava Kava - Leiner Health Products
Each caplet contains: Kava Kava extract (Piper methysticum) root 60 mg • St. John's Wort extract (Hypericum perforatum) aerial parts 300 mg. Other Ingredients: Cellulose, Dicalcium Phosphate, Croscarmellose Sodium, Silicon Dioxide, Stearic Acid, Magnesium Stearate, Dextrin, Dextrose, Lecithin, Sodium Carboxymethylcellulose, Sodium Citrate.

St. John's Wort 1000 mg - GNC
Each capsule contains: St. John's Wort Leaves/Flowers (hypericum perforatum; from 166.7 mg of St. John's Wort Herb Extract 6:1) 1000 mg. Other Ingredients: Soybean Oil, Gelatin, Glycerin, Caramel Color, Titanium Dioxide (natural mineral whitener).

St. John's Wort 1000 mg, Concentrated - GNC
Each capsule contains: St. John's Wort leaf/flower (hypericum perforatum; 166.7 mg St. John's Wort 6:1 extract. Other Ingredients: Soybean Oil, Gelatin, Glycerin, Caramel Color, Titanium Dioxide.

St. John's Wort 250 mg - Nature's Plus
Each capsule contains: St. John's Wort flower (hypericum perforatum, standardized 0.3-0.5% hypericin) 250 mg. Other Ingredients: Di-calcium Phosphate, Silica, Gelatin, Purified Water.

St. John's Wort 300 mg - Nature's Plus
Each capsule contains: St. John's Wort flower (hypericum perforatum, standardized 0.3-0.5% hypericin) 300 mg. Other Ingredients: Di-calcium Phosphate, Silica, Vegetable Cellulose, Purified Water.

St. John's Wort Blend - VitaStore
Each capsule contains: St. John's Wort (standardized for 0.3% Hypericin) • Kava Kava • Ginkgo Biloba.

St. John's Wort Complete - Futurebiotics LLC
Two capsules contain: Vitamin C (as ascorbic acid) 300 mg • Thiamin 25 mg • Riboflavin 25 mg • Niacin (as niacinamide) 25 mg • Vitamin B6 (as pyridoxine hydrochloride) 25 mg • Folic Acid 400 mcg • Vitamin B12 (as cyanocobalamin) 250 mcg • Biotin 300 mcg • Pantothenic Acid (as calcium pantothenate) 25 mg • St. John's Wort flower powder extract (standardized for 0.3% (0.8 mg) hypericin) 250 mg • Choline (as choline bitartrate) 25 mg • Inositol 25 mg • Para-Aminobenzoic Acid 25 mg • L-Tyrosine 50 mg • L-Phenylalanine 100 mg. Other Ingredients: Gelatin, Water.

St. John's Wort Extract - NSI - Nutraceutical Sciences Institute
Each capsule contains: St. John's Wort extract (standardized to 0.3% hypericin and 3% hyperforin) 450 mg.

St. John's Wort Extract - Enzymatic Therapy
Each capsule contains: St. John's Wort flower head extract (hypericum perforatum, standardized to contain a minimum of 0.3% hypericin, 3% hyperforin) 300 mg. Other Ingredients: Gelatin, Magnesium Stearate, Silicon Dioxide, Titanium Dioxide.

St. John's Wort Flowering Top - Aboca USA, Inc
Two capsules contain: St. John's Wort flowering top WPC (whole phytocomplex concentrate, hypericum perforatum, standardized to contain 0.16% total hypericin, yielding 0.4 mg per capsule) 500 mg. Other Ingredients: Gelatin.

St. John's Wort Forte with Kava - PhytoPharmica
Each capsule contains: St. John's Wort (Hypericum peroratum) flower head extract (standardized to contain a minimum of 0.3% hypericin and 4% hyperforin) 300 mg • Valerian (Valeriana officinalis) root extract (standardized to contain a minimum of 0.8% valerenic acids) 100 mg • Kava (Piper methysticum) root extract (standardized to contain 30% kavalactones) 100 mg.
See Editor's Note No. 21.

St. John's Wort Hypericum Perforatum 300 mg - Puritan's Pride
Each capsule contains: St. John's Wort extract (hypericum perforatum, aerial, standardized to contain 0.3% hypericin, 0.9 mg) 300 mg. Other Ingredients: Maltodextrin, Gelatin, Magnesium Silicate, Vegetable Magnesium Stearate, Silica.

St. John's Wort NutraSpray - Source Naturals
Each spray contains: St. John's Wort standardized extract (Hypericum perforatum) 2.7 mg.

St. John's Wort Oil - Blessed Herbs
St. John's Wort flowering tops • organic cold-pressed Olive oil.

St. John's Wort Organic Extract - Wild Rose
Each 1 mL serving contains: St. John's Wort (hypericum perforatum) liquid 1:1 extract 1000 mg • Grain Alcohol 40-50% • Distilled Water.

St. John's Wort Plus - Wild Rose
Each tablet contains: St. John's Wort flower extract 300 mg • Reishi mushroom 100 mg • Oatstraw herb 50 mg • Lavender flower 50 mg.

St. John's Wort Plus - Aspen Group, Inc.
Each capsule contains: St. John's Wort herb extract standardized to 0.3% Hypericin 300 mg • Kava Kava 100 mg • Vitamin B6 25 mg • Standardized extract St. John's Wort herb extract Hypericum Perforatum.

St. John's Wort Standard Extract, 300mg - Nature Made
Each capsule contains: St. John's Wort aerial part extract 300 mg: Hypericin (by UV) 0.9 mg.

St. John's Wort Supreme - Gaia Herbs
St. John's Wort and Kava Kava standardized for 0.5% hypericins and 55% kavalactones. Standardized Full Spectrum 150 mg of extract per capsule. Guaranteed Potency 75 mg of extract per capsule.

St. John's Wort With Folic Acid & B12 - Metagenics
Each tablet contains: Folate (as folic acid, L-5-methyl tetrahydrofolate, and 5-formyl tetrahydrofolate) 400 mcg • Vitamin B12 (as cyanocobalamin) 250 mcg • St. John's Wort bud and flowering top extract (hypericum perforatum, standardized to 0.3% hypericins and 3% hyperforin) 450 mg.

St. John's Wort-Go! - Wakunaga of America
Each caplet contains: St. John's Wort standardized extract (herb with flower) standardized to 0.3% Hypericin 600 mg. Other Ingredients: Cellulose, Magnesium Stearate (vegetable source), Silica.

St. John's Wort-IMT - Standard Process, Inc.
Each capsule contains: Proprietary Blend 159 mg: Calcium Lactate, St. John's wort leaf and flower powder, Magnesium Citrate, Alfalfa meal, Carrot root powder • Vitamin A 40 IU • Iodine 30 mcg • St. John's Wort extract (0.3% hypericin) 300 mg • Inositol 50 mg. Other Ingredients: Gelatin, Kelp Powder, Water, Colors, Carrot Oil.

St. John's Wort-Kava Kava - Futurebiotics LLC
St. John's Wort flower powder extract standardized for 0.3% (0.8 mg) hypericin 250 mg • Kava Kava root powder extract standardized for 30% (30 mg) kavalactones 100 mg. Other ingredients: Gelatin, Water.

Stabilium - Smart Basics
Each capsule contains: Predigested Garum Armoricum 105 mg • Virgin Sunflower Oil 83 mg •Soya Lecithin Oil 12 mg.

Stabilized Acidophilus Three Billion - NOW Foods
Each tablet contains: Lactobacillus Acidophilus 3 billion. Other Ingredients: Anhydrous Dicalcium Phosphate, Microcrystalline Cellulose, Silica, Modified Cellulose Gum, Magnesium Stearate.

Stacker 2 - NVE Pharmaceuticals
Each capsule contains: Proprietary Blend 270 mg: Ephedra extract (leaves/stems, 25 mg ephedrine group alkaloids), Kola Nut (seeds, <1 mg caffeine group alkaloids) White Willow bark • Caffeine (anhydrous) 200 mg • Tri-GuggLyptoid Complex 25 mg: Green Tea (leaves, < 1 mg caffeine group alkaloids), Guggulsterone (whole plant), Gymnema (leaves). Other Ingredients: Dextrose, Gelatin, Stearic Acid, Magnesium Stearate, Titanium Dioxide, FD&C Yellow #5, FD&C Yellow #6.
See Editor's Note No. 30.

Stacker 2 Ephedra Free - NVE Pharmaceuticals
Each capsule contains: Proprietary Blend 196 mg: Kola Nut (seeds, caffeine group alkaloids 3 mg), Citrus Aurantium (fruit, synephrine 2 mg), Cassia Mimosoides extract (leaves/stems/pods), White Willow bark • Caffeine (anhydrous) 200 mg • Tri-GuggLyptoid Complex 25 mg: Green Tea (leaves, <1 mg caffeine group alkaloids), Guggulsterone (whole plant), Gymnema (leaves). Other Ingredients: Dextrose, Gelatin, Stearic Acid, Magnesium Stearate, Titanium Dioxide, FD&C Yellow #5, FD&C Blue #1, FD&C Red #3, FD&C Yellow #6.
See Editor's Note No. 40.

Stacker 2 LITE - NVE Pharmaceuticals
Each capsule contains: Proprietary Blend 320 mg: Kola Nut (seeds, 4 mg caffeine group alkaloids), Ephedra extract (leaves/stems, 12.5 mg ephedrine group alkaloids), White Willow bark • Caffeine (anhydrous) 100 mg • Tri-GuggLyptoid Complex 25 mg: Green Tea (leaves, <1 mg caffeine group alkaloids), Guggulsterone (whole plant), Gymnema (leaves). Other Ingredients: Dextrose, Gelatin, Stearic Acid, Magnesium Stearate, Titanium Dioxide, FD&C Yellow #5, FD&C Red #3, FD&CRed #40, FD&C Yellow #6.
See Editor's Note No. 30.

Stacker 2 Stackerdrene Ephedra Free - NVE Pharmaceuticals
Each capsule contains: Magnesium (as magnesium gluconate) 25 mg • Vitamin B6 (as pyridoxine hydrochloride) 6.8 mg • Zinc (as zinc gluconate) 5 mg • Vitamin B12 (as cyanocobalamin) 50 mcg • Proprietary Blend 277 mg: Green Tea leaves extract (60%, polyphenols 120 mg), Grape seed extract (80% of proanthocyanidins), Cactus extract (12:1), Yerba Mate fruit, Guarana seed • Caffeine Anhydrous 150 mg. Other Ingredients: Gelatin, Dibasic Calcium Phosphate, Stearic Acid, Titanium Dioxide, FD&C Yellow 6, Magnesium Stearate, Dextrose.

Stacker 2 Thermo Infusion Ephedra Free Glucodrene - NVE Pharmaceuticals
Two capsules contain: Glucomannan (form amorphophallus konjac root) 1200 mg. Other Ingredients: Gelatin, Microcrystalline Cellulose, Stearic Acid, Magnesium Stearate, Titanium Dioxide, FD&C Yellow 5, FD&C Yellow 6.

Stacker 3 - NVE Pharmaceuticals
Each capsule contains: Proprietary Blend 250 mg: Ephedra extract (leaves/stems, 25 mg ephedrine group alkaloids), Kola Nut (seeds, <1 mg caffeine group alkaloids), White Willow bark, Grapefruit extract (fruit), Chitosan (shellfish) • Caffeine (anhydrous) 250 mg • Tri-GuggLyptoid Complex 25 mg: Green Tea (leaves, <1 mg caffeine group alkaloids), Guggulsterone (whole plant), Gymnema (leaves). Other Ingredients: Gelatin, Dibasic Calcium Phosphate, Dextrose, Stearic Acid, Magnesium Stearate, Titanium Dioxide, FD&C Red #3, FD&C Blue #1, FD&C Red #40.
See Editor's Note No. 30.

Stacker 3 with Chitosan Ephedra Free Formula - NVE Pharmaceuticals
Each capsule contains: Proprietary Blend 225 mg: Kola nut seed (caffeine group alkaloids 4 mg), Cactus extract (whole plant, 12:1), White Willow bark, Grapefruit fruit extract, Chitosan (shellfish) • Caffeine (anhydrous) 250 mg • Tri-Guarcinia3 Complex 25 mg: Green tea leaves (caffeine group alkaloids <1 mg), Guarana seeds, Garcinia fruit. Other Ingredients: Gelatin, Dextrose, Stearic Acid, Magnesium Stearate, Titanium Dioxide, FD&C Red 3, FD&C Blue 1, FD&C Red 40, FD&C Yellow 5.

Stamanex - Sterling-Grant Laboratories
Two tablets contain: Niacin 25 mg • Horny Goat Weed (epimedium grandiflorum) 500 mg • Icarin (whole herb) 50 mg • Maca root extract (4:1, lepidium meyenii) • German Tribulus Terrestris fruit extract 250 mg • 70% Furostanolic Saponins Fenusterols (7.5% protodioscin) 150 mg • Avena Sativa extract (10:1, oat straw) 150 mg • Eurycoma Lonifolia (long jack root) 125 mg • Ginko Biloba 75 mg.

Stamina - HerbaSway
Horny Goat Weed • Yohimbe • Dong Quai • Knotweed • Panax Ginseng • Licorice • Blackberry • HerbaSwee (Cucurbitaceae fruit).

Stamina 100 - Jamieson
Three caplets contain: Vitamin A (as Retinyl Acetate) 7500 IU • Vitamin C (as Ascorbic Acid) 125 mg • Vitamin D (as Cholecalciferol) 200 IU • Vitamin E (as Dl-Alpha Tocopheryl Acetate) 25 IU • Thiamin (as Thiamine Mononitrate) 12.5 mg • Riboflavin (Vitamin B2) 12.5 mg • Niacin (as Nicacinamide) 190 mg • Vitamin B6 (as Pyridoxine Hydrochloride) 12.5 mg • Folate (as Folic Acid) 200 mcg • Vitamin B12 (as Cyanocobalamin) 50 mcg • Pantothenic Acid (as Calcium D-Pantothenate) 30 mg • Calcium (as Calcium Carbonate) 600 mg • Iron (as Ferrous Fumarate) 10 mg • Iodine (as Potassium Iodide) 150 mcg • Magnesium (as Magnesium Oxide) 100 mg • Zinc (as Zinc Gluconate) 5 mg • Selenium (as Seleium Brown Rice Protein Chelate) 12.5 mcg • Manganese (as Manganese Gluconate) 3.5 mg • Chromium (as Chromium Brown Rice Protein Chelate) 10 mcg • Potassium 50 mg.

Stamina Beverage - Jamieson
Each bottle contains: Purified Water • Canadian Maple Syrup • Glucose • Natural Lemon and Orange Flavor (Tocopherols, Soybean Oil) • Canadian Ginseng root (Panax Quinquegolium) • Citric Acid • Sodium Benzoate • Xanthan Gum • Caramel (natural color) • Potassium Sorbate.

Standardized Cat's Claw Extract - Nature's Way
Each capsule contains: Cat's Claw bark 160 mg • Cat's Claw dried extract 175 mg. Other Ingredients: Gelatin, Millet.

Some Brand Name Natural Products - What they Contain

www.NaturalDatabase.com contains MANY more listings than appear here.

Editor's Notes are located on pages 2155-2163.

Standardized Chamomile Extract - Nature's Way
Each capsule contains: Chamomile flower 220 mg • Chamomile dried extract 125 mg.

Standardized Cider Vinegar with Apple Pectin - The Vitamin Shoppe
Each tablet has been standardized to provide 27 mg of acetic acid and 27 mg of apple pectin.

Standardized Feverfew Extract - Nature's Way
Each capsule contains: Feverfew leaves (standardized 0.7% Parthenolide) 370 mg.

Standardized Ginkgo Extract - Nature's Way
Each capsule contains: Ginkgo Biloba leaf extract; standardized to 24% Ginkgo flavone glycosides & 6% terpene lactones) 60 mg • Gotu Kola stem & leaf 400 mg. Other Ingredients: Gelatin & Millet.

Standardized Kava Extract - Nature's Way
Each softgel contains: Concentrated 10:1 Kava Extract (rhizome, standardized to 55% kavalactones) 128 mg.

Standardized Lutein & Bilberry - Swanson Health Products
Each softgel contains: Bilberry extract (25% anthocyanidins) 20 mg • FloraGLO brand Lutein extract (from marigold) 6 mg.

Standardized Milk Thistle - GNC
Each capsule contains: Milk Thistle Seed Extract (silybum marianum; 80% silymarin = 160 mg) 200 mg. Other Ingredients: Cellulose, Dicalcium Phosphate, Gelatin.

Standardized Saw Palmetto - GNC
Each capsule contains: Saw Palmetto berries extract (Serenoa repens; 85% Fatty Acids=136 mg; 0.2% Sterols=0.32 mg) 160 mg. Other Ingredients: Olive Oil, Gelatin, Glycerin, Caramel Color, Titanium Dioxide (natural mineral whitener).

Standardized Saw Palmetto & Pygeum - Nature's Way
Each softgel contains: Pygeum dried extract 100 mg • Saw Palmetto dried extract 320 mg • Vitamin B6 (as pyridoxine HCl) 10 mg. Other Ingredients: Carob Color, Gelatin, Glycerin, Lecithin, Soybean Oil, Water, Yellow Wax.

Standardized Saw Palmetto Extract - Nature's Way
Each softgel contains: Saw Palmetto extract (berry, standardized to 85-95% Fatty Acids) 160 mg.

Starch Away - PhytoPharmica
Each soft chew contains: Phase 2 brand White Kidney bean (phaseolus vulgaris) 500 mg.

Starch Block - E'OLA
Each tablet contains: Chromium (as chromium polynicotinate) 100 mcg • Proprietary Blend 300 mg: Kidney Bean extract (10:1), Vanadium (as vanadyl sulfate).

Starch Blocker - Whole Health Discount Center
Each vegicap contains: Phaseolamin Phase 2 Phaseolus vulgaris extract • Water extracted from non-GMO White Kidney Beans.

Starch Blocker 1000 - R.P.M. Worldwide
Each capsule contains: Legume Protein Concentrate (Phase 2 brand) 500 mg. Other Ingredients: Gelatin, Magnesium Stearate, Stearic Acid, Microcrystalline Cellulose.

Starch Buster - Metabolife International, Inc.
Two tablets contain: Kidney Bean extract (Phaseolus vulgaris) 1000 mg. Other Ingredients: Modified Cellulose, Dicalcium Phosphate, Gum Acacia, Sodium Bicarbonate, Stearic Acid, Citric Acid, Dextrin, Dextrose, Lecithin, Sodium Carboxymethylcellulose, Sodium Citrate.

StarPac Daily Complex - Starlight International
Each packette contains: Vitamin A (50% as beta carotene and 50% as Vitamin A palmitate) 12,000 IU • Vitamin C (as ascorbic acid) 800 mg • Calcium (as calcium carbonate) 1,000 mg • Vitamin D (as cholecalciferol) 400 IU • Vitamin E (as D-alpha-tocopheryl acetate) 400 IU • Thiamin (as thiamine hydrochloride) 1.5 mg • Riboflavin 1.7 mg • Niacin (as niacinamide) 20 mg • Vitamin B6 (as pyridoxine hydrochloride) 2 mg • Folate (as folic acid) 400 mcg • Vitamin B12 (as cyanocobalamin) 6 mcg • Biotin 300 mcg • Pantothenic Acid (as calcium pantothenate) 10 mg • Iodine (as postassium iodide) 150 mcg • Magnesium (as magnesium oxide) 400 mg • Zinc (as zinc oxide) 15 mg • Selenium (as sodium selenite) 70 mcg • Copper (as copper sulfate) 2 mg • Manganese (as manganese sulfate) 2 mg • Chromium (as chromium picolinatinate) 120 mcg • Molybdenum (as sodium molybdate) 75 mcg • Potassium (as potassium chloride) 50 mg • Omega-3 Fatty Acids (from fish oil) 270 mg • Inositol 50 mg • Omega 6 Fatty Acids (from flaxseed oil) 28 mg • Para-Aminobenzoic Acid 25 mg • Betaine Hydrochloride 20 mg • Bromellain 20 mg • Boron.

Start Plus - 4 Life
Each packet contains: Vitamin A (50% beta-carotene, 50% retinyl palmitate) 10,000 IU • Vitamin C (as calcium ascorbate) 455 mg • Vitamin D (as cholecalciferol) 400 IU • Vitamin E (as D-alpha tocopheryl) 300 IU • Thiamin (as thiamine mononitrate) 10 mg • Riboflavin 10 mg • Niacin (as niacinamide) 20 mg • Vitamin B6 (as pyridoxine hydrochloride) 10 mg • Folate (as folic acid) 400 mcg • Vitamin B12 (as cyanocobalamin) 30 mcg • Biotin 300 mcg • Pantothenic Acid (as calcium pantothenate) 50 mg • Calcium (as carbonate, amino acid chelate, di-calcium phosphate, ascorbate, citrate from Calcite Super Brand) 454 mg • Iron (as amino acid chelate) 9 mg • Iodine (as potassium iodine) 150 mcg • Magnesium (as amino acid chelate, magnesium oxide) 175 mg • Zinc (as amino acid chelate) 16 mg • Selenium (as amino acid chelate) 105 mcg • Copper (as amino acid chelate) 2 mg • Manganese (as manganese glycinate) 4 mg • Chromium (as chromium chelate) 200 mcg • Molybdenum (as amino acid chelate) 75 mcg • Potassium (as amino acid chelate) 10 mg • NDS Digestive Enzyme Blend 100 mg: Fungal Protease, Fungal Amylase, Fungal Lipase, Cellulase, Pectinase • MDA Proprietary Blend 89 mg: Arabinogalactan, Amylase, Docosahexaenoic Acid, Lipase, Protease, Rose Hips, Siberian Ginseng, Coenzyme Q10, Tumeric • OPC Blend 50 mg: Grape extract (seed, bark), Maritime Pine bark extract. Grape skin extract 39 mg • Citrus Bioflavonoids (orange, grapefruit, lemon, lime, tangerine) 10 mg • Cranberry extract 10 mg • Horsetail extract (silica) 10 mg • Alfalfa root 10 mg • Hops 10 mg • Dandelion flower 10 mg • Echinacea Purpurea root 10 mg • Green Tea leaf extract 5 mg • Acerola (from cherry fruit) 5 mg • Rutin 5 mg • Quercitin 5 mg • Apple (fruit) 5 mg • Milk Thistle seed 2 mg • Ginkgo leaf 2 mg • Boron (as amino acid chelate) 500 mcg • Silicon Dioxide 50 mcg • Vanadium 10 mg. Other Ingredients: Gelatin, Microcrystalline Cellulose, Magnesium Stearate, Silicon Dioxide, Acacia Gum.

Start Up - TriLight Herbs
Pennyroyal • Feverfew • Blue Cohosh • Black Cohosh • Beth root.

Starters' Traditional Chinese Ephedra Herbal Tea - Life Enhancement Products, Inc.
Each rounded tablespoon contains: Vitamin A (as beta-carotene) 1250 IU • Vitamin C (ascorbic acid) 200 mg • Vitamin E (as DL-alpha-tocopheryl acetate) 30 IU • Zinc (as zinc gluconate) 5 mg • Copper (as copper gluconate) 750 mcg • Chromium (as chromium aspartate) 75 mcg • Taurine 300 mg • Glycine 200 mg • Ma Huang powder, leaves and stems 20 mg.
See Editor's Note No. 30.

Starters' Traditional Chinese Ephedra Herbal Tea - Sugar Free - Life Enhancement Products, Inc.
Each level tablespoon contains: Vitamin A (as beta-carotene) 1250 IU • Vitamin C (ascorbic acid) 200 mg • Vitamin E (as D,L-alpha tocopheryl acetate) 30 IU • Chromium (as chromium aspartate) 75 mcg • Taurine 300 mg • Glycine 200 mg • Ma Huang powder, leaves, and stems 20 mg.
See Editor's Note No. 30.

Start-Ups - Global Health Trax
Six capsules contain: Chromium (as chromium polynicotinate) 50 mcg • Guggulipid 250 mcg • Rhodiola root 150 mg • Acetyl-L-Carnitine (from hydrochloride) 250 mg • Alpha Lipoic Acid 50 mg •

Coleus Forskohlii root 500 mg • Gotu Kola root 350 mg • Astragalus root 250 mg • White Willow bark 250 mg • Green Tea leaf 450 mg • Bitter Orange rind 500 mg • Fructo Oligo Saccharides (FOS) 100 mg • Hydroxycitric Acid (HCA) 1.25 g • Dimethylglycine 30 mg • Rhemannia leaves 250 mg • Lutein 50 mg. Other Ingredients: Methylcellulose, Gelatin.
See Editor's Note No. 40.

StayCalm **- Resource Wellness**
Each caplet contains: Vitamin C (Ascorbic Acid) 10 mg • Thiamin Mononitrate 0.25 mg • Vitamin B6 (Pyridoxine HCl) 0.33 mg • Vitamin B12 (Cyanocobalamin) 1 mcg • Calcium 190 mg • St. John's Wort extract aerial parts 300 mg • Valerian root extract (root) 50 mg. Other Ingredients: Dicalcium Phosphate, Microcrystalline Cellulose, Croscarmellose Sodium, Magnesium Stearate, Stearic Acid, Maltodextrin, Silicon Dioxide, Hydroxypropyl Methylcellulose, Hydroxypropyl Cellulose, Polyethylene Glycol.

Steady On **- Allergy Research Group**
Each scoop (20 g) contains: Vitamin A (as beta-carotene) 1680 IU • Vitamin C (as ascorbic acid) 440 mg • Vitamin D (D3) 130 IU • Vitamin E (as mixed tocopherols) 360 IU • Vitamin K 45 mcg • Thiamin (vitamin B1) 22 mg • Riboflavin (vitamin B2) 22 mg • Niacin (as inositol hexanicotinate) 180 mg • Vitamin B6 22 mg • Folic Acid 350 mcg • Vitamin B12 22 mcg • Biotin 130 mcg • Pantothenic Acid 110 mg • Calcium (as calcium citrate/gluconate) 310 mg • Magnesium (as magnesium glycinate/gluconate) 130 mg • Zinc (as zinc arginate) 13 mg • Selenium (as sodium selenite/ selenomethionine) 90 mcg • Copper (as copper glycinate) 0.9 mg • Chromium (as chromium picolinate) 180 mcg • Potassium (as potassium gluconate) 45 mg • Alpha-Carotene 7 mg • Dehydroepiandrosterone (DHEA) 7 mg • Coenzyme Q10 67 mg • Inositol 22 mg • Choline 22 mg • Para-Aminobenzoic Acid 22 mg • Lecithin (26% phosphatidylcholine) 1440 mg • L-Alanine 35 mg • L-Arginine 110 mg • L-Aspartic Acid 95 mg • L-Carnitine 110 mg • L-Cystine 11 mg • L-Glutamine 67 mg • Glycine 67 mg • L-Histidine 22 mg • L-Isoleucine 45 mg • L-Lysine 50 mg • L-Methionine 180 mg • L-Ornithine Hydrochloride 220 mg • L-Phenylalanine 45 mg • L-Proline 45 mg • L-Serine 42 mg • Taurine 670 mg • L-Threonine 45 mg • L-Tyrosine 440 mg • N-Acetyl-L-Cysteine 440 mg • Glutathione (reduced) 110 mg • Pancreatin 13 mg • Papain 22 mg • Bromelain 22 mg • Grape skin extract 220 mg • Garlic (1% allicin) 45 mg • Lutein 1.8 mg • Lycopene 1.3 mg • Eicosapentaenoic Acid (EPA) 160 mg • Docosahexaenoic Acid (DHA) 110 mg • Palmitic Acid 130 mg • Stearic Acid 40 mg • Flax Seed Oil 440 mg • Lipoic Acid 45 mg • Methylsulfonylmethane 45 mg. Other Ingredients: Oat Bran, Rice Bran, Psyllium Bran, Stevia, Apple Fiber, Flavoring.

Sterisome Tea Tree Oil **- Jamieson**
Contains: 100% Tea Tree Oil (Derived from Australian Melalleuca Alterniflora) 50 ml • Pure Vitamin E Oil (Dl-Alpha Tocopheryl Acetate) 10 IU/50 ml.

Sterols/Sterolins **- Natur-Leaf**
Two capsules contain: Proprietary Sterol/Sitosterolin Blend 640 mg: Wild African Potato root, Lupins sprouts, Fenugreek sprouts, Barley sprouts, Wheat sprouts, Soybean sprouts, African Sunflower sprouts • Enzyme/Mineral Blend 60 mg. Other Ingredients: Gelatin (capsule).

Stevia Powder **- Optimum Nutrition**
Each scoop contains: Stevia leaf extract (stevia rebaudiana, standardized to 90% steviosides) 70 mg. Other Ingredients: Maltodextrin, Silica.

Stimulin **- Naturally Vitamins**
Two tablets contain: Calcium (di-calcium phosphate) 100 mg • Magnesium (oxide) 100 mg • Citruline 1875 mg. Other Ingredients: Colloidal Silica, Magnesium Stearate, Cholesterol free stearic acid.

Stimuliv **- Jarrow Formulas**
Two tablets contain: Andrographis Paniculata 8% 200 mg • Phyllanthus 10:1 100 mg • Eclipta Alba 4% 100 mg • Picrorhiza Kurroa 6% 100 mg • Boerhaavia Diffusa 8:1 50 mg • Berbris Aristata 8% 25 mg • Neem leaf 10:1 50 mg • Solanum Nigrum 10:1 25 mg • Tephrosia Purpurea 9:1 25 mg • Ipomoea Turpethum 30% 50 mg. Other Ingredients: Gum Tragacanth, Talc, Silica.

StimuMax for Men **- Natrol, Inc.**
Proprietary Blend 2.02 g: Maca 4:1 root extract (Lepidium meyenii), Muira Puama 5:1 root extract (Ptychopetalum olacoides), Wild Oats 10:1 extract (Avena sativa), Guarana seed extract (Paullinia Cupana) (20% Caffeine), Korean ginseng root extract (Panax Ginseng), Ginkgo Biloba leaf extract, Epimedium 10% aerial extract (epimedium grandiflorum). Other Ingredients: Rice powder, Silica, Magnesium Stearate, Gelatin.

StimuMax for Women **- Natrol, Inc.**
Proprietary Blend 1.90 g: Maca 4:1 root extract (lepidium meyenii), Muira Puama 5:1 root extract, Wild Oats 10:1 extract (Avena sativa), Kava Kava root extract (piper methsyticum), Dong Quai standardized extract (Angelica sinensis), Damiana 4:1 leaf extract (Turnera diffusa), Korean Ginseng root extract (Panax). Other Ingredients: Rice Powder, Silica, Magnesium Stearate, Gelatin.

Sting Soothe **- Quantum**
Purified Water • Hybrid Safflower oil • Aloe Vera gel • Echinacea extract • Propylene Glycol • Glyceryl Stearate • Nettle extract • Rosemary oil • Cetyl Alcohol • Bud oil • Peppermint oil • Sage oil • Camphor • Citronella oil • Stearic Acid • Menthol • Tea Tree oil • Panthenol • Tea-Carbomer 940 • Coconut oil • Dimethicone • Tocopherol (vitamin E) • PEG 40 Castor oil.

Stinging Nettle Leaf **- Aboca USA, Inc**
Two capsules contain: Stinging Nettle leaf WPC (whole phytocomplex concentrate, urtica dioica, standardized to 1% caffeic acid derivatives, yielding 2.48 mg per capsule) 496 mg. Other Ingredients: Gelatin.

Stinging Nettle Leaf Extract **- PhytoPharmica**
Two capsules contain: Stinging Nettle leaf extract (urtica dioica, standardized to contain 1% silicic acid) 600 mg.

Stomach Calm **- Enzymes, Inc.**
Each capsule contains: n-zimes Proprietary Enzyme Blend 128 mg: Peptidase, Lipase, Amylase, Glucoamylase, Malt Diastase, Lactase, Invertase, alpha-Galactosidase, CereCalase Plus, Cellulase, Xylanase, Pectinase • Proprietary Herbal Blend 355 mg: Marshmallow root extract, Ginger root extract (5% gingerols) plus whole root, Deglycyrrhizinized Licorice root, Papaya leaf, Lavender flower, Rosemary. Other Ingredients: Cellulose, Rice Bran, Water, Lecithin.

Stomach Comfort **- Nature's Sunshine**
Two tablets contain: Calcium (carbonate) 550 mg • Proprietary Herbal Blend 330 mg: Alginic Acid from Brown Seaweed (phaeophyceae), Papaya (carica papaya), Guar Gum (cyamopsis tetragonolobus), Slippery Elm bark (ulmus fulva), Ginger rhizome (zingiber officinale), Licorice root (glycyrrhiza glabra). Other Ingredients: Xylitol, Caseinate Powder (calcium, sodium, lecithin), Fructose, Stearic Acid, Magnesium Stearate, Natural Flavors.

Stomach Plus **- Atrium Biotechnologies**
Each tablet contains: Raw Stomach concentrate Bovine 323 mg • Folic Acid 100 mcg • Vitamin B12 50 mcg • Glycine 32 mg.
See Editor's Note No. 14.

Stomach Soothing Complex **- Shaklee**
Three tablets contain: Peppermint Ginger Proprietary Blend 750 mg: Peppermint leaf powder (mentha piperita), Anise seed powder (pimpinella anisum), Fennel powder (foeniculum vulgare), Ginger root powder (zingiber offinale) • Peppermint Oil (mentha piperita) 15 mg. Other Ingredients: Cellulose, Fructose, Maltodextrin, Corn Syrup Solids, Microcrystalline Cellulose.

Stomach-Aid **- Futurebiotics LLC**
Two capsules contain: Calcium (carbonate) 200 mg • MSM (methyl-sulfonyl-methane) 300 mg • Ginger root powder 400 mg • Peppermint leaf powder 100 mg • Bromelain 100 mg • Pancreatin 4X (supplying 1600 USP units lipase, 10000 USP units amylase, 10000 USP units protease) 100 mg • Aloe Vera (leaf powder) 50 mg • Papain 50 mg •

BRAND NAMES

Stomach Aid Herbal Base 200 mg: Chamomile (flower powder), Catnip (leaf powder), Parsley (leaf powder), Fennel (seed powder). Other Ingredients: Gelatin, Cellulose, Magnesium stearate, Water. See Editor's Note No. 14.

StomachEase - Vita Pharmica - formerly Neopharmica
Each two tablets contain: Proprietary Concentrate 1500 mg: Corydalis Tuber, Astragalus root, San-Qi Ginseng root, Chekiang Fritillary bulb, Chinese Licorice root, Gambir leaf and stem, Brown's Lilly bulb, Bletilla Striata, Sepia Esculenta shell.

Stomagic - DreamPharm
Two capsules contain: Proprietary Blend: Magnolia Cortex, Citrus Sinensis Exocarpium, Atractylodes Rhizoma, Sclerotium Poria Cocos, Licorice Root, Cinnamomum Cortex, Ginger (zingiber rhizoma), Hawthorn (crataegus fruit), Cyperus Tubercles, Euphoria Longan Arill, Lycium Fruit, Shen Chu Preparation, Lindera Radix, Agastache Herb, Areca Seed, Astragalus Root, Birthwort Root, Cardamom Fruit, Amomum Kravanh (Cluster) Fruit, Coptis Root, Pinellia Root, Curcuma Zedoaria Rhizome, Paeonia Albiflora Radix, Brunoton, Acidophilus, Papaya Leaf.
See Editor's Note No. 46.

Stone Root-Corn Silk Virtue - Blessed Herbs
Stone root • Gravel root • Hydrangea root • Goldenrod • Corn Silk • Nettle • Grain alcohol & Distilled Water.

Stopsmoking Herbal Tea - Health King
Each bag contains: Proprietary Blend: Licorice, Peppermint, Green Tea, Jasmine flower.

Strawberry Drinkable Yogurt - Stonyfield Farm
Each 10 fl oz bottle contains: Active Live Cultures: S. Thermophilus • L. Bulgaricus • L. Acidophilus • Bifidus • L. Casei • L. Reuteri. Ingredients: Cultured Pasturized Low Fat Milk • Organic Sugar • Organic Nonfat Dry Milk • Inulin • Pectin • Beet Juice Concentrate • Organic Strawberry Juice from concentrate • Natural Flavors.

Strawberry-Apple Lactobacillus Acidophilus - Nature's Life
Two tablespoons (1 fl.oz or 29.6 ml) contain: Purified Water • Strawberry concentrate • Unfiltered Apple Juice • Pasteurized Honey • Soy Protein Isolate • Lactobacillus Acidophilus Culture.

ST-Res-Q - Nutri-Quest Rx
Each tablet contains: Adrenal 25 mg • Thymus 70 mg • Spleen 20 mg • Stomach 10 mg • Parotid 80 mg (All bovine source) • Vitamin C 175 mg • Vitamin B2 15 mg • Vitamin B6 10 mg • Niacinamide 15 mg • Pantothenic Acid (D-Calcium Pantothenate) 105 mg • Grape seed extract 1 mg • Lemon Bioflavonoids 225 mg • L-Tyrosine 175 mg • Magnesium Oxide 75 mg • Zinc Chelate 5 mg • Chromium Chelate 50 mcg • Potassium Chelate 10 mg • Chlorella 50 mg.
See Editor's Note No. 14.

Stress Action - Nature's Plus
Two tablets contain: Vitamin C as Mineral Ascorbate 1000 mg • Desiccated Beef Liver 500 mg • Pantothenic Acid (calcium pantothenate) 125 mg • Vitamin B1 (thiamine) 100 mg • Vitamin B2 (riboflavin) 100 mg•Vitamin B6 (pyridoxine HCl) 100 mg • Niacinamide 100 mg • Vitamin E 100 IU • Choline (bitartrate) 75 mg • Inositol 75 mg • PABA (para-aminobenzoic acid) 50 mg • Bee Pollen 50 mg • Korean Ginseng 50 mg • Calcium Ascorbate 50 mg • Zinc Ascorbate 25 mg • Magnesium Ascorbate 25 mg • L-Phenylalanine (free form) 20 mg • Iron (gluconate) 20 mg • Potassium (citrate) 15 mg • L-Cysteine (free form) 15 mg • L-Methionine (free form) 15 mg • Folic Acid 400 mcg • Vitamin B12 from Cobalamin 250 mcg • Biotin 100 mcg • Octacosanol 50 mcg • Chromium chelate 20 mcg • Selenium amino acid complex 10 mcg.
See Editor's Note No. 14.

Stress Away - Futurebiotics LLC
Two tablets contain: Vitamin C (ascorbic acid/ascorbyl palmitate) 250 mg • Vitamin A (beta carotene) 5000 IU • Vitamin B1 (thiamin) 25 mg • Vitamin B2 (riboflavin) 25 mg • Niacinamide 200 mg • Calcium (phosphate, aspartate) 100 mg • Vitamin B6 5 mg • Folic Acid 400 mcg • Vitamin B12 50 mcg • Iodine (kelp) 75 mg • Magnesium (oxide, amino acid chelate) 100 mg • Zinc (oxide, picolinate) 15 mg • Biotin 300 mcg • Pantothenic Acid 50 mg • Inositol 50 mg • Choline Bitartrate 100 mg • Manganese (amino acid chelate) 3 mg • Chromium (amino acid chelate, polynicotinate) 40 mcg • Para Amino Benzoic Acid (PABA) 50 mg • Valerian 200 mg • Chamomile 100 mg • Skullcap 50 mg • Passion flower 50 mg • Methionine 50 mg • Ribonucleic Acid (RNA) 50 mg.

Stress B & C with Iron - Arrowroot
Three prolonged-release capsules contain: Vitamin B1 75 mg • Vitamin B2 37 mg • Vitamin B6 45 mg • Vitamin B12 25 mcg • Folic Acid 400 mcg • Pantothenic Acid 75 mg • PABA 75 mg • Vitamin C 600 mg • Niacinamide 150 mg • Iron 45 mg • Biotin 300 mcg.

Stress B Complex - Nature Made
Each tablet contains: Vitamin C 500 mg • Vitamin E 30 IU • Thiamin 10 mg • Riboflavin 10 mg • Niacin 100 mg • Vitamin B6 5 mg • Folic Acid 400 mcg • Vitamin B12 12 mcg • Biotin 45 mcg • Pantothenic Acid 20 mg.
See Editor's Note No. 45.

Stress B with C - Nature's Life
Two capsules contain: Vitamin B1 (Thiamine Mononitrate) 50 mg • Vitamin B2 (riboflavin and Riboflavin 5'-Phosphate) 50 mg • Vitamin B6 (pyridoxine HCl & Pyridoxal 5'-Phosphate) 50 mg • Vitamin B12 (cobalamin) 250 mcg • Niacinamide 100 mg • Folic Acid 400 mcg • Pantothenic Acid (D-calcium pantothenate) 250 mg • Biotin (d-Biotin) 100 mcg • PABA (para aminobenzoic acid) 50 mg • Choline (bitartrate) 100 mg • Vitamin C 1000 mg.

Stress B-Complex plus Vitamin C - Optimum Nutrition
Two capsules contain: Vitamin C (as ascorbic acid) 1 g • Thiamin (as thiamin hydrochloride) 50 mg • Riboflavin 50 mg • Niacin (as niacinamide) 100 mg • Vitamin B6 (as pyridoxine hydrochloride) 50 mg • Folic Acid 400 mcg • Vitamin B12 (as cyanocobalamin) 250 mcg • Biotin 100 mcg • Pantothenic Acid (as d-calcium pantothenate) 250 mg • PABA (as para-aminobenzoic acid) 50 mg • Choline (as choline bitartrate) 40 mg • Inositol 100 mg. Other Ingredients: Gelatin, Magnesium Stearate, Silica.

Stress B-Complex with Vitamin C & Zinc - Nature Made
Each tablet contains: Vitamin C (from ascorbic acid) 500 mg • Vitamin E (from dL-alpha tocopheryl acetate) 30 IU • Thiamin (B1, from thiamine mononitrate) 10 mg • Riboflavin (B2) 10 mg • Niacin (B3) 100 mg • Vitamin B6 (from pyridoxine hydrochloride) 50 mg • Folate, Folic Acid, Folacin 400 mcg • Vitamin B12 (from cyanocobalamin) 12 mcg • Biotin 45 mcg • Pantothenic Acid (from D-calcium pantothenate) 20 mg • Zinc (from zinc sulfate) 23.9 mg • Copper (from copper oxide) 3 mg. Other Ingredients: Calcium Carbonate, Cellulose, Magnesium Stearate, Hydroxypropyl Methylcellulose, Stearic Acid, Polyethylene Glycol, Carnauba Wax.
See Editor's Note No. 45.

Stress B-Complex with Vitamin C and Iron - Nature Made
Each tablet contains: Vitamin C (from ascorbic acid) 500 mg • Vitamin E (from dL-alpha tocopheryl acetate) 30 IU • Thiamin (from thiamin mononitrate) 10 mg • Riboflavin 10 mg • Niacin (from niacinamide ascorbate) 100 mg • Vitamin B6 (from pyridoxine hydrochloride) 5 mg • Folic Acid 400 mcg • Vitamin B12 (from cyanocobalamin) 12 mcg • Biotin 45 mcg • Pantothenic Acid (from D-calcium pantothenate) 20 mg • Iron (from ferrous fumarate) 18 mg. Other Ingredients: Cellulose, Calcium Carbonate, Gelatin, Croscarmellose Sodium, Corn Starch, Magnesium Stearate, Hydroxypropyl Methylcellulose, Polyethylene Glycol.
See Editor's Note No. 45.

Stress Complex - Natrol, Inc.
Two tablets contain: Thiamin HCl 20 mg • Riboflavin 20 mg • Niacin (niacinamide) 20 mg • Vitamin B6 (pyridoxine HCl) 20 mg • Folic Acid 200 mcg • Vitamin B12 (cyanocobalamin) 20 mcg • Melatonin 3 mg • Valerian root 5:1 extract 300 mg. Other Ingredients: Cellulose, Stearic Acid, Cellulose, Magnesium Stearate, Silica, Hydroxypropyl Methylcellulose, Polyethylene Glycol, Hydroxypropyl Cellulose.
See Editor's Note No. 26.

Some Brand Name Natural Products - What they Contain

www.NaturalDatabase.com contains MANY more listings than appear here.

Editor's Notes are located on pages 2155-2163.

BRAND NAMES

Stress Essentials - PhytoPharmica
Each capsule contains: Vitamin C (Ascorbic Acid & Rose Hips) 100 mg • Calcium (as calcium carbonate and calcium citrate) 50 mg • Magnesium (Oxide) 30 mg • Potassium (Citrate) 25 mg • Pantothenic Acid (D-Calcium Pantothenate) 20 mg • Vitamin B6 (Pyridoxine HCL) 15 mg • Thiamine HCL (Vitamin B1) 12.5 mg • Riboflavin (Vitamin B2) 12.5 mg • Niacin 10 mg • Manganese (Chelate) 5 mg • Zinc (Chelate) 1.5 mg • Biotin 100 mcg • Folic Acid 75 mcg • Vitamin B12 (Cyanocobalamin) 25 mcg • Inositol 50 mg • Siberian Ginseng extract 5:1 (Eleutherococcus senticosus) 50 mg • Valerian extract (Valeriana officinalis; standardized to contain 0.2% to 0.8% valerenic acids) 50 mg • L-Tyrosine 50 mg • Skullcap extract 4:1 (Scutellaria baicalensis) 50 mg • Passion flower extract (Passiflora) 50 mg • Hops extract (Humulus lupulus) 50 mg • PABA (Para-Aminobenzoic Acid) 5 mg.

Stress Fighter - Puritan's Pride
Each tablet contains: Vitamin B1 20 mg • Vitamin B2 15 mg • Vitamin B6 10 mg • Vitamin B12 25 mcg • Folic Acid 400 mcg • Niacinamide 100 mg • Pantothenic Acid 25 mg • Vitamin C 600 mg • Vitamin E 45 IU. Plus valuable minerals such as Zinc, Iron, and Copper.

Stress Formula - 4 Life
Each capsule contains: Peppermint leaf 110 mg • English Chamomile flower 70 mg • Stress Proprietary Extract Blend 45 mg: Ginkgo Biloba leaf extract • Valerian root extract • English Chamomile flower extract • Lime blossom extract • Lemon Balm extract • Peppermint leaf extract • Passion Flower aerial parts extract • Ginkgo Biloba leaf 36 mg • Passion Flower (aerial parts) 35 mg • Linden flower 35 mg • Lemon Balm peel 35 mg • Valerian root 34 mg. Other Ingredients: Gelatin, Magnesium Stearate.

Stress Formula B-Complex - Walgreens
Each caplet contains: Vitamin C 500 mg • Vitamin E • Thiamin (vitamin B1) 10 mg • Riboflavin (vitamin B2) 10 mg • Niacin (vitamin B3) 100 mg • Vitamin B6 5 mg • Folic Acid 400 mcg • Vitamin B12 12 mcg • Biotin 45 mcg • Pantothenic Acid 20 mg. Other Ingredients: Calcium Carbonate, Cellulose, Starch, Gelatin, Hydroxypropyl Methylcellulose, Croscarmellose Sodium, Sodium Starch Glycoate, Maltodextirn, Silicon Dioxide, Polyethylene Glycol, Hydroxypropyl Cellulose, Magnesium Stearate, Pharmaceutical Glaze, Dicalcium Phosphate, Titanium Dioxide, Yellow No. 6 Lake, Polysorbate 80, Resin, Mannitol, Blue No. 2 Lake.

Stress Formula B-Complex with Iron - Walgreens
Each caplet contains: Vitamin C 500 mg • Vitamin E • Thiamin (vitamin B1) 10 mg • Riboflavin (vitamin B2) 10 mg • Niacin (vitamin B3) 100 mg • Vitamin B6 5 mg • Folic Acid 400 mcg • Vitamin B12 12 mcg • Biotin 45 mcg • Pantothenic Acid 20 mg • Iron 18 mg. Other Ingredients: Calcium Carbonate, Starch, Hydroxypropyl Methylcellulose, Gelatin, Cellulose, Croscarmellose Sodium, Sodium Starch Glycolate, Maltodextrin, Silicon Dioxide, Hydroxypropyl Cellulose, Polyethylene Glycol 3350, Magnesium Stearate, Yellow No. 6 Lake, Dicalcium Phosphate, Pharmaceutical Glaze, Crospovidone, Titanium Dioxide, Polysorbate 80, Resin, Red No. 40 Lake, Mannitol.

Stress Formula B-Complex with Zinc - Walgreens
Each caplet contains: Vitamin C 500 mg • Vitamin E • Thiamin (vitamin B1) 10 mg • Riboflavin (vitamin B2) 10 mg • Niacin (vitamin B3) 100 mg • Vitamin B6 5 mg • Folic Acid 400 mcg • Vitamin B12 12 mcg • Biotin 45 mcg • Pantothenic Acid 20 mg • Zinc 23.9 mg • Copper 3 mg. Other Ingredients: Calcium Carbonate, Starch, Hydroxypropyl Methylcellulose, Gelatin, Cellulose, Croscarmellose Sodium, Sodium Starch Glycolate, Maltodextrin, Silicon Dioxide, Hydroxypropyl Cellulose, Polyethylene Glycol 3350, Magnesium Stearate, Yellow No. 6 Lake, Dicalcium Phosphate, Pharmaceutical Glaze, Crospovidone, Titanium Dioxide, Polysorbate 80, Resin, Red No. 40 Lake, Mannitol.

Stress Formula Calcet Plus - Mission Pharmacal
Each tablet contains: Vitamin A 5000 IU • Vitamin C 500 mg • Vitamin D (as Vitamin D3) 400 IU • Vitamin E 30 IU • Vitamin B1 2.25 mg • Vitamin B2 2.55 mg • Vitamin B3 30 mg • Vitamin B6 3 mg • Folate 0.8 mg • Vitamin B12 9 mcg • Vitamin B5 15 mg • Calcium 160 mg • Iron 18 mg • Zinc 15 mg. Other Ingredients: Sugar, Povidone, Magnesium Stearate, Color, Croscarmellose Sodium, Food Glaze, Carnauba Wax, White Beeswax, Sodium Benzoate, Cyanocobalamin.

Stress Manager - The Council On Natural Health
Two tablets contain: Thiamin (as thiamin HCl) 5 mg • Riboflavin 5 mg • Niacin (as niacinamide) 20 mg • Vitamin B6 (as pyridoxine HCl) 5 mg • Folate (as folic acid) 400 mcg • Vitamin B12 (as cyanocobalamin) 25 mcg • Pantothenic Acid (as d-calcium pantothenate) 10 mg • Kava Kava root 200 mg • Rhodiola Rosea root extract (40% total polyphenols) 10 mg • 5-HTP (from griffonia simplicifolia seeds) 10 mg • Adaptogenic Herbal Blend 150 mg: Ashwagandha root, Astragalus root, Panax Ginseng root, Suma root. Other Ingredients: Dicalcium Phosphate, Microcrystalline Cellulose, Croscarmellose Sodium, Stearic Acid, Silica, Magnesium Stearate, Pharmaceutical Glaze.

Stress Plex - Nature's Plus
Two tablets contain: Vitamin C with Rose Hips 500 mg • Pantothenic Acid (Calcium pantothenate) 100 mg • Niacinamide 100 mg • Choline (Bitartrate) 100 mg • Inositol 100 mg • PABA (Para-aminobenzoic acid) 30 mg • Vitamin B1 (Thiamine) 10 mg • Vitamin B2 (Riboflavin) 10 mg • Vitamin B6 (Pyridoxine HCL) 10 mg •Folic Acid 100 mcg • Vitamin B12 (from Cobalamin) 25 mcg • Biotin 25 mcg. B-Complex vitamins in a fortified rice bran base.

Stress Plex - Jamieson
Each tablet contains: Vitamin B1 3 mg • Vitamin B2 2.5 mg • Niacinamide 12 mg • Vitamin B6 3 mg • Vitamin B12 10 mcg • Biotin 10 mcg • Pantothenic Acid 5 mg • Folic Acid 0.05 mg • Vitamin C 250 mg • Zinc 5 mg • Lipotropic Factors: Choline Bitrate 5 mg, Inositol 5 mg.

Stress Plus - NOW Foods
Each tablet contains: Vitamin B1 (Thiamine) 30 mg • Vitamin B2 (Riboflavin) 30 mg • Vitamin B3 (Niacinamide) 150 mg • Vitamin B6 (Pyridoxine) 30 mg • Vitamin B12 50 mcg • Pantothenic Acid 150 mg • Vitamin C (Ascorbic Acid) 500 mg • Biotin 300 mcg • Folic Acid 400 mcg • Magnesium (Oxide) 100 mg • PABA 40 mg • Choline (Bitartrate) 150 mg • Inositol 150 mg • Valerian root (50 mg of 4:1 extract) 200 mg.

Stress Tab B - Nature's Life
Two tablets contain: Vitamin B1 (Thiamine HCl) 60 mg • Vitamin B2 (Riboflavin) 60 mg • Vitamin B6 (Pyridoxine HCl) 60 mg • Vitamin B12 (Cobalamin concentrate) 60 mcg • Vitamin C 600 mg • Niacin 30 mg • Niacinamide 30 mg • Folic Acid 600 mcg • Pantothenic Acid (d-Calcium Pantothenate) 600 mg • Biotin (D-Biotin) 600 mcg • Choline (Bitartrate) 60 mg • Inositol 60 mg • PABA (Para Aminobenzoic Acid) 60 mg.

Stress Therapy Bath - Abra Therapeutics
Sodium Borate • Sodium Sulfate • Sodium Chloride • Sodium Sesquicarbonate • Olive oil • Ylang Ylang oil • Lavender oil • Chamomile oil • Eucalyptus oil • Nutmeg oil • Peru Balsam oil • Valerian root extract • St. John's Wort flower extract • Hops flower extract • Chromium Oxide • Trace Mineral Salts.

Stressease - Jamieson
Each caplet contains: Vitamin B1 35 mg • Vitamin B2 35 mg • Niacinamide 50 mg • Vitamin B6 15 mg • Vitamin B12 30 mcg • Biotin 15 mcg • Vitamin C 500 mg • Vitamin E 30 IU • d-Pantothenic Acid 20 mg • Folic Acid 1 mg • Calcium (Carbonate) 150 mg • Magnesium 75 mg • Zinc 5 mg.

Stress-End - Enzymatic Therapy
Each capsule contains: Vitamin C (Ascorbic Acid/Rose Hips) 100 mg • Calcium (Oyster Shell) 50 mg • Magnesium (Oxide) 30 mg • Potassium (Citrate) 25 mg • Pantothenic Acid (D-Calcium Pantothenate) 20 mg • Vitamin B6 (Pyridoxine HCL) 15 mg • Thiamine HCL (Vitamin B1) 12.5 mg • Riboflavin (Vitamin B2) 12.5 mg • Niacin 10 mg • Manganese (Chelate) 5 mg • Zinc (Chelate)

1.5 mg • Biotin 100 mcg • Folic Acid 75 mcg • Vitamin B12 (Cyanocobalamin) 25 mcg • Other ingredients: Inositol 50 mg • Siberian Ginseng extract 5:1 (Eleutherococcus senticosus) 50 mg • Valerian extract (Valeriana officinalis) standardized to contain 0.2% to 0.8% Valerenic Acids 50 mg • L-Tyrosine 50 mg • Skullcap extract 4:1 (Scutellaria baicalensis) 50 mg • Passion flower extract (Passiflora) 50 mg • Hops extract (Humulus lupulus) 50 mg • PABA (Para-Aminobenzoic Acid) 5 mg.

Stresstabs - Inverness Medical Innovations, Inc.
Each tablet contains: Vitamin C 500 mg • Vitamin E 30 IU • Thiamin 10 mg • Riboflavin 10 mg • Niacinamide 100 mg • Vitamin B6 (as pyridoxine hydrochloride) 5 mg • Folic Acid 400 mcg • Vitamin B12 12 mcg • Biotin 45 mcg • Pantothenic Acid (as D-calcium pantothenate) 20 mg. Other Ingredients: Microcrystalline Cellulose, Starch, Calcium Carbonate Stearic Acid, Croscarmellose Sodium, Silicon Dioxide, Hydroxypropyl Methylcellulose, Titanium Dioxide, FD&C Yellow #6 Lake, Polyethylene Glycol, Polysorbate 80, FD&C Blue #2 Lake, Carnauba Wax.

Stresstabs + Zinc - Inverness Medical Innovations, Inc.
Each tablet contains: Vitamin C 500 mg • Vitamin E 30 IU • Thiamin 10 mg • Riboflavin 10 mg • Niacinamide 100 mg • Vitamin B6 5 mg • Folic Acid 400 mcg • Vitamin B12 12 mcg • Biotin 45 mcg • Pantothenic Acid 20 mg • Zinc 23.9 mg • Copper 3 mg. Ingredients: Ascorbic Acid • Calcium Carbonate • Cellulose • Niacinamide • dl-Alpha Tocopheryl Acetate (Vitamin E) • Starch • Zinc Oxide • d-Calcium Pantothenate • Hydroxypropyl Methylcellulose • Riboflavin (Vitamin B2) • Thiamine Mononitrate (Vitamin B1) • Dicalcium Phosphate • Pyridoxine Hydrochloride (Vitamin B6) • Silicon Dioxide • Triethyl Stearate • Stearic Acid • Magnesium Stearate • Cupric Oxide • Crospovidone • Providone • Mineral oil • Folic Acid • Titanium Dioxide • FD&C Yellow #6 Aluminum Lake • Biotin • Cyanocobalamin (Vitamin B12).

StriVectin-SD - Klein-Becker
Deionized Water • C12-15 Alkyl Benzoate • Sesame Oil • Caprylic/ Capric Triglyceride • Sweet Almond Oil • Cetearyl Olivate • Sorbitan Olivate • Striadil Complex: Phyllanthus Emblica fruit extract, Siegesbeckia Orietalis extract, Polyglyceryl Methyacrylate, Propylene Glycol, Palmitoyl Oligopeptide, Glucosamine HCl, Algae extract, Yeast extract, Urea, Butylene Glycol, Hydrocotyl extract, Coneflower extract, Hydrolyzed Wheat Protein, Hydrolyzed Wheat Starch, Imperata Cylindrica root extract, Bearberry extract, Licorice PTH • Glycerin • PPG-12/SMDI Copolymer • Glyceryl Stearate • PEG-100 Stearate • Cocoa Butter • Stearic Acid • Shea Butter • Tocopheryl Acetate • Mango Butter • Peppermint Oil • Methylparaben • Xanthan Gum • Propylparaben • Triethanolamine • Butylene Glycol • Disodium EDTA • Retinyl Palmitate • Tetrahexyldecyl Ascorbate.

Strixaderm MD - Pure Source
Deionized Water • C12-15 Alkyl Benzoate • Sesame oil • Caprylic / Capric / Triglycerides • Almond oil • Cetearyl Olivate • Sorbitan Olivate • Palmitoyl Pentapeptide • Phyllanthus Emblica fruit extract • Siegesbeckia Orietalis extract • Polyglyceryl Methacrylate • Propylene Glycol • Palmitoyl Oligopeptide • Glucosamine HCl • Algae extract • Stri Vera Blend: Aloe Vera, Yeast extract, Urea, Butylene Glycol, Hydrocotyl extract, Coneflower extract, Hydrolyzed Wheat Protein, Hydrolyzed Wheat Starch, Imperata Cylindrica root extract, Bearberry extract, Licorice extract • Glycerin • PPG-12/SMDI Copolymer • Glyceryl Stearate • PEG-100 Stearate • Cocoa Butter • Stearic Acid • Shea Butter • Tocopheryl Acetate • Mango Butter • Peppermint oil • Methylparaben • Xanthan gum • Propylparaben • Triethanolamine • DMDM Hydantoin • Iodopropynyl Butylcarbamate • Disodium EDTA • Retinyl Palmitate • Tetrahexyldecyl Ascorbate.

Strontium - Ortho Molecular Products
Two capsules contain: Strontium Citrate 1000 mg. Other Ingredients: Natural Vegetable Capsules, Magnesium Stearate, Microcrystalline Cellulose, Silicon Dioxide.

Strontium (citrate) - Vital Nutrients
Each vegetarian capsule contains: Strontium (citrate) 227 mg.

Stuart Prenatal Multivitamin/Multimineral Supplement - Integrity Pharmaceutical Corp.
Each tablet contains: Vitamin A Acetate (25% as Beta Carotene) 4000 IU • Vitamin C (Ascorbic Acid) 100 mg • Vitamin D (Cholecalciferol) 400 IU • Vitamin E (dl-Alpha Tocopheryl Acetate) 11 IU • Thiamin Mononitrate (Vitamin B1) 1.8 mg • Riboflavin (Vitamin B2) 1.7 mg • Niacin (Vitamin B3, Niacinamide) 18 mg • Vitamin B6 (Pyridoxine Hydrochloride) 2.6 mg • Folate (Folic Acid, Folacin) 0.8 mcg • Vitamin B12 (Cyanocobalamin) 4 mcg • Calcium Sulfate 200 mg • Iron (Ferrous Fumarate) 27 mg • Zinc Oxide 25 mg. Other Ingredients: Beta Carotene, Croscarmellose Sodium, Hydroxypropyl Methylcellulose, Microcrystalline Cellulose, Pregelatinized Starch, Red Iron Oxide, Titanium Dioxide.

Suan Zao Ren Tang Plus - Secara
Jujube seeds 5:1 extract (suan zao ren) 607 mg • Organic Licorice root (gan cao) 349 mg • Anemarrhena rhizome 5:1 extract (zhi mu) 242 mg • Poria sclerotium 5:1 extract (fu ling) 242 mg • Sichuan Lovage rhizome 5:1 extract (chuan xiong) 242 mg • Organic Skullcap herb 225 mg • Hawthorn leaf & flower (2.0% flavonoids (4 mg)) 180 mg • Passionflower herb (3.5% vitexin (5 mg)) 146 mg • Valerian oil 11 mg • Organic Lavender oil 6 mg.

Sub-Adrene - American Biologics
Each drop contains: Adrenal Cortex extract (from bovine source) 50 mcg. Other Ingredients: Natural Peppermint Flavoring, 5% Ethyl Alcohol, 1-Methionine.
See Editor's Note No. 14.

Sublingual B-12 Lozenge Tablets 2500 mcg - Puritan's Pride
Each lozenge contains: Vitamin B-12 2500 mcg.

Sublingual B-12 Lozenge Tablets 500 mcg - Puritan's Pride
Each lozenge contains: Vitamin B-12 500 mcg.

Sublingual B-12 Lozenge Tablets 5000 mcg - Puritan's Pride
Each lozenge contains: Vitamin B-12 5000 mcg.

Sublingual Vitamin B-12 - PhysioLogics
Each tablet contains: Vitamin B12 (as cyanocobalamin) 5000 mcg • Coenzyme B12 (as dibencozide) 100 mcg. Other Ingredients: Sorbitol, Vegetable Stearic Acid, Croscarmellose, Natural Cherry Flavor, Vegetable Magnesium Stearate.

Substrate Solutions Andro Heat - ErgoPharm/Proviant Technologies
Four capsules contain: Caffeine (naturally occuring in 2000 mg of kola nut herb) 200 mg • Ephedrine naturally occuring in 250 mg of Ma Huang herb 20 mg • 4-Androstenediol 100 mg.
See Editor's Note No. 30 and No. 54.

Substrate Solutions Andro Stack - ErgoPharm/Proviant Technologies
Each capsule contains: 4-Androstenediol 100 mg • 4-Androstenedione 100 mg.
See Editor's Note No. 54.

Substrate Solutions Di-Indolin - ErgoPharm/Proviant Technologies
Three tablets contain: Di-Indolin Proprietary Blend 300 mg: Diindolylmethane, Vitamin E (D-alpha tocopheryl succinate), Phosphatidylcholine. Other Ingredients: Calcium Carbonate, Cellulose, Starch, Magnesium Sterate, Tocophersolan, Silica.

Substrate Solutions Diol Stack - ErgoPharm/Proviant Technologies
Each tablet contains: Nor-4-Androstenediol 100 mg • 4-Androstenediol 100 mg.
See Editor's Note No. 54.

Substrate Solutions Nor Stack - ErgoPharm/Proviant Technologies
Each tablet contains: 19-Nor-4-Androstenediol 100 mg • 19-Nor-4-Androstenedione 100 mg.

Substrate Solutions Zinc Magnesium Aspartate **-** ErgoPharm/Proviant Technologies
Three capsules contain: Zinc (as L-OptiZinc & Aspartate) 30 mg • Magnesium (as Aspartate) 450 mg • Vitamin B6 (Pyridoxine Hydrochloride) 10.5 mg. Other Ingredients: Cellulose, Magnesium Stearate, Gelatin.

Sugar Balance capsules **-** Golden Glow Natural Health Products
Each capsule contains: Gymnema Sylvestre leaf extract 2000 mg • Vitis Vinifera seed extract (equivalent to 7.09 mg Procyanidins) 1000 mg • Pyridoxine Hydrochloride (vitamin B6) 15 mg • Ascorbic Acid (vitamin C) 200 mg • Magnesium Oxide 10 mg • D-Alpha-Tocopherol (natural vitamin E) 25 IU • Chromium Picolinate 50 mcg • Manganese (amino acid chelate) 5 mg • Zinc (gluconate) 5 mg • Rutin 25 mg.

Sugar Control **-** Nature's Plus
Each capsule contains: Chromium (as polynicotinate) 200 mcg • Rehmannia Glutinosa root 200 mg • L-Glutamine (as free form amino acid) 100 mg • L-Alanine (free form amino acid) 75 mg. Other Ingredients: Di-Calcium Phosphate, Microcrystalline Cellulose, Silica, Gelatin, Pharmaceutical Glaze.

Sugar Metabolism Formula **-** Pharmacist's Ultimate Health
Two tablets contain: Vitamin B1 (Thiamin) 20 mg • Vitamin B2 (as Riboflavin) 10 mg • Vitamin B5 (as Panthothic Acid) 60 mg • Vitamin B6 (as Pyridoxine HCl) 40 mg • Vitamin C (as Ascorbic Acid) 400 mg • Biotin (Vitamin H) 1 mg • Folate (as Folic Acid) 260 mcg • Chromium (as Picolinate) 133 mcg • Magnesium (as Oxide) 40 mg • Manganese (as Gluconate) 7 mg • Potassium (as Potassium Chloride) 40 mg • Selenium (as Chleate) 40 mcg • Zinc (as Oxide) 10 mg • Alpha Lipoic Acid 30 mg • Betaine HCl 60 mg • Citrus Bioflavonoids 200 mg • Black Radish powder 120 mg • Beet juice 120 mg • Inositol 80 mg • Blueberry powder 4:1 extract 100 mg • Choline (bitartrate) 60 mg • L-Methionine 60 mg • L-Taurine 120 mg.

Sugar Stopper **-** The Sports Nutrition Source, Inc.
Each capsule contains: Gymnena Sylvestre 300 mg • Chitosan shellfish 100 mg • Garcinia Cambogia 100 mg • Vitamin C 50 mg.

Sugar/Starch Digestion **-** Enzymes, Inc.
Each capsule contains: Proprietary Enzyme Blend 460 mg: Amylase, Protease, Invertase, Glucoamylase, Lipase, CereCalase, Malt Diastase, Lactase, alpha-Galactosidase, Cellulase, Peptidase. Other Ingredients: Plant Cellulose, Water.

SugarReg **-** Nature's Sunshine
Each capsule contains: Chromium (amino acid chelate) 200 mcg • Vanadium (amino acid chelate) 25 mcg • Proprietary Blend 476 mg: Nopal leaf (opuntia streptacantha), Fenugreek seed (trigonella foenum-graecum), Bitter Melon fruit (momordica charantia), Gymnema leaf extract (gymnema sylvestre), Banaba leaf (lagerstroemia speciosa corosolic acid 1%). Other Ingredients: Gelatin, Water.

Sulfur Mineral Supplement **-** Eidon Inc.
Each 1 tbsp serving contains: Sulfur (providing approx. 236 ppm sulfur) 1.2 mg. Other Ingredients: Purified Water.

Sul-Ray Acne Treatment Soap Bar **-** At Last Naturals, Inc.
Sulfur 5% • Aloe Vera • Trisodium HEDTA.

Summer Survivor **-** HOMS LLC
Soybean oil • Coconut oil • Glycerin • Lecithin • Water • Vanillin.

Summer Survivor Catnip! **-** HOMS LLC
Purified Water • Castor oil • Coconut oil • Mint oil • Citrus extract • Citric Acid • Catnip oil • Sodium Bicarbonate • Grapefruit seed extract • Inert Gas.

Summer Survivor Catnip-Emu **-** HOMS LLC
Purified Water • Castor oil • Coconut oil • Mint oil • Citrus extract • Citric Acid • Emu oil • Catnip oil • Sodium Bicarbonate • Grapefruit seed extract • Inert Gas.

Summer Survivor Outdoor Mist Body Oil **-** HOMS LLC
Purified Water • Geranium • Soybean oil • Coconut oil • Mint oil • Vanillin • Citric Acid • Sodium Bicarbonate • Germall Plus.

Sun Pollen **-** Futurebiotics LLC
Cracked Flower Pollen & Pollen Extract.

Sun Vitamines **-** The Fitzpatrick Group, Inc.
Two capsules contain: Polypodium Leucotomos 240 mg • Green Tea 50 mg • Beta-Carotene 10 mg.

Sundown Benefits Carbonyl Iron **-** Rexall - Sundown
Two tablets contain: Calcium 117 mg • Iron (as carbonyl iron) 50 mg. Other Ingredients: Dicalcium Phosphate, Maltodextrin, Corn Syrup Solids, Croscarmellose Sodium, Magnesium Stearate.

Sundown CoQ-10 75 Mg **-** Rexall - Sundown
Each softgel contains: Vitamin E (as D-alpha tocopherol) 5 IU • Coenzyme Q-10 75 mg. Other Ingredients: Soybean Oil, Gelatin, Glycerin, Water, Yellow Beeswax, Titanium Dioxide, Yellow 6 Lake, Red 40 Lake, Blue 1 Lake.

Sundown Echinacea **-** Rexall - Sundown
Each capsule contains: Echinacea Purpurea (aerial parts) 400 mg. Other Ingredients: Gelatin.

Sundown Zinc Gluconate 50 mg **-** Rexall - Sundown
Each tablet contains: Calcium 56 mg • Zinc (from zinc gluconate and zinc oxide) 50 mg. Other Ingredients: Dicalcium Phosphate, Microcrystalline Cellulose, Croscarmellose Sodium, Hydroxypropyl Methyl-Cellulose, Magnesium Stearate, Titanium Dioxide, PEG, Polysorbate 80.

Sunkist Vitamin C Citrus Complex **-** WN Pharmaceuticals, Ltd.
Each tablet contains: Vitamin C 250 mg. Other Ingredients: Fructose, Sorbitol, Sucrose, Sodium Ascorbate, Ascorbic Acid, Hydrogenated Soybean Oil, Maltodextrin, Magnesium Stearate, Corn Starch, Hydrogenated Castor oil, Silicon Dioxide, Lactose, Bioflavonoids.

SunSource Harmonex **-** Chattem, Inc.
Each caplet contains: Standardized St. John's Wort flower extract (0.3% hypericin) 450 mg • Standardized Siberian Ginseng root extract (0.8% eleutherosides) 90 mg. Other Ingredients: Microcrystalline Cellulose, Croscarmellose Sodium, Hydroxypropyl Methylcellulose, Sodium Carboxymethyl Cellulose, Magnesium Stearate, Dextrin, Dextrose, Mineral oil, Polyethylene Glycol, Caramel, Polysorbate 80, Propylene Glycol, Riboflavin, Silicon Dioxide, Sodium Citrate, Titanium Dioxide.

SunSource Melatonex **-** Chattem, Inc.
Each tablet contains: Vitamin B6 (as pyridoxine hydrochloride) 10 mg • Calcium 31 mg • Iron 1 mg Melatonin 3 mg. See Editor's Note No. 26.

SunSource New Phase **-** Chattem, Inc.
Each caplet contains: Proprietary Blend 410 mg: Soy Protein concentrate, standardized Kudzu extract root, standardized Red Clover extract leaf • standardized Chastetree extract berry 75 mg • standardized Black Cohosh extract root 40 mg.

SunSource Omnigest EZ **-** Chattem, Inc.
Each caplet contains: Plant-source Digestive Enzymes 230 mg: Acid Protease 340 APU, Amylase 3400 SKB, Cellulase 5400 C,-ASE, Glucoamylase 22 AG, Lactase 3000 FCC LacU, Lipase 2250 LU, Nautral Protease 11,000 HUT.

SunSource Propalmex Saw Palmetto **-** Chattem, Inc.
Each softgel contains: Zinc (as zinc gluconate) 75 mg •Saw Palmetto berry extract 160 mg •Pumpkin Seed Oil extract 40 mg •Lycopene (from Lyc-O-Mato tomato extract) 1.5 mg.

SunSource Rejuvex **-** Chattem, Inc.
Each caplet contains: Vitamin E (as DL-alpha tocopherol acetate) 30 IU • Thiamin HCl (vitamin B1) 2 mg • Riboflavin (vitamin B2) 2 mg • Niacin 10 mg • Vitamin B6 (as pyridoxine hydrochloride) 10 mg •

Pantothenic Acid (as D-calcium pantothenate) 10 mg • Magnesium (as magnesium oxide) 500 mg • Selenium (as sodium selenate) 25 mcg • Manganese (as manganese sulfate) 2 mg • Dong Quai root standardized extract 200 mg • Mammary gland powder 25 mg • Ovary gland powder 19 mg • Uterus gland powder 10 mg • Adrenal gland powder 10 mg • Pituitary gland powder 5 mg • Boron (chelated with citrate & aspartate) 3 mg. Other Ingredients: Microcrystalline Cellulose, Stearic Acid, Silicon Dioxide, Croscarmellose Sodium, Hydroxypropyl Methylcellulose, Magnesium Stearate, Polyethylene Glycol, Mineral oil, Shellac, Talc.
See Editor's Note No. 31.

SunSource Repose - Chattem, Inc.
One caplet contains: Vitamin C (calcium ascorbate) 100 mg • Vitamin B6 (pyridoxine HCl) 14 mg • Pantothenic Acid (D-calcium pantothenate) 17 mg • Magnesium (oxide) 70 mg • Standardized Kava root extract (30% kavalactones) 200 mg • Standardized Siberian Ginseng root extract (0.8% eleutherosides) 65 mg.

SunSpot ES - LaneLabs
Water • Aloe Vera • Propylene Glycol • Salicylic Acid • Urea • Carbomer 940 • Tea Tree Oil • Menthol • Glycoalkaloids extract • Imidazolidinylurea.
See Editor's Note No. 21.

Suntheanine brand - NutriScience Innovations, LLC
L-Theanine.
See Editor's Note No. 44.

SunVites With Lutein - Sundown
Each caplet contains: Vitamin A (20%/1000 IU as beta-carotene) 5000 IU • Vitamin C (as niacinamide ascorbate) 60 mg • Vitamin D (as cholecalciferol) 400 IU • Vitamin E (as dL-alpha tocopheryl acetate) 30 IU • Vitamin K (as phytonadione) 25 mcg • Thiamin (as thiamin mononitrate) 1.5 mg • Riboflavin (vitamin B2) 1.7 mg • Niacin (as niacinamide ascorbate) 20 mg • Vitamin B6 (as pyridoxine HCl) 2 mg • Folic Acid 400 mcg • Vitamin B12 (as cyanocobalamin) 6 mcg • Biotin 30 mcg • Pantothenic Acid (as calcium-D pantothenate) 10 mg • Calcium 170 mg • Iron (as ferrous fumarate) 18 mg • Phosphorus 109 mg • Iodine (as potassium iodide) 150 mcg • Magnesium (as magnesium oxide) 100 mg • Zinc (as zinc oxide) 15 mg • Selenium (as sodium selenate) 20 mcg • Copper (as cupric oxide) 2 mg • Manganese (as manganese sulfate) 2.5 mg • Chromium (chromium chloride) 120 mcg • Molybdenum (as sodium molybdate) 75 mcg • Chloride 36 mg • Potassium (as potassium chloride) 80 mg • Boron (as sodium borate and potassium borate) 150 mcg • Nickel (as nickel sulfate) 5 mcg • Silicon (as silica) 2 mg • Tin (as stannous chloride) 10 mcg • Vanadium (as sodium metavanadate) 10 mcg • Lutein 250 mcg. Other Ingredients: Microcrystalline Cellulose, Gelatin, Hydroxypropyl Methylcellulose, Croscarmellose Sodium, Triacetin, Titanium Dioxide (color), Magnesium Stearate, Corn Starch, Yellow 6 Lake, Retinyl Acetate, PEG.

Super 1000mg Cod Liver Oil - J. R. Carlson Laboratories, Inc.
Each softgel contains: Cod Liver Oil: Vitamin A 2000 IU, Vitamin D 250 IU • Vitamin E (as D-alpha tocopherol) 10 IU • Omega-3 Fatty Acids (from cod liver oil) 240 mg • ALA (alpha-linolenic acid) 20 mg • DPA (docosapentaenic acid) 10 mg • DHA (docosahexaenoic acid) 120 mg • EPA (eicosapentaenoic acid) 90 mg.

Super 2 Daily - J. R. Carlson Laboratories, Inc.
Two softgels contain: Vitamin A (as beta carotene) 10,000 IU • Vitamin C (as calcium ascorbate) 500 mg • Vitamin D (D3, from fish liver oil) 600 mg • VItamin E (as D-alpha tocopherol) 400 IU • Thiamin (vitamin B1, as thiamin hydrochloride) 25 mg • Riboflavin (vitamin B2) 25 mg • Niacin (vitamin B3, as niacinamide) 25 mg • Vitamin B6 (as pyridoxine hydrochloride) 25 mg • Folate (folic acid) 800 mcg • Vitamin B12 (cyanocobalamin) 100 mcg • Biotin 300 mcg • Pantothenic Acid (as di-calcium pantothenate) 25 mg • Calcium (as calcium ascorbate) 50 mg • Iodine (from kelp and potassium iodide) 150 mcg • Magnesium (as magnesium oxide) 100 mg • Zinc (as zinc gluconate) 15 mg • Selenium (from kelp) 200 mcg • Copper (as copper gluconate) 2 mg • Manganese (as manganese gluconate) 3 mg • Chromium (from kelp) 200 mcg • DHA (docosahexaenoic acid) 92 mg • EPA (eicosapentaenoic acid) 130 mg • Phosphatidyl Choline 50 mg • Phosphatidyl Ethanolamine 10 mg • Phosphatidyl Inositol 3 mg • Fish oil concentrate 770 mg • Lecithin 60 mg • Lemon Bioflavonoids complex 25 mg • Lutein 500 mcg.

Super All-Day Nutricom - Puritan's Pride
Each scoop contains: Vitamin A 10,000 IU • Vitamin C 1,000 mg • Vitamin D 500 IU • Vitamin E 400 IU • Vitamin K 5 mcg • Thiamin 25 mg • Riboflavin 25 mg • Niacin 100 mg • Vitamin B-6 25 mg • Biotin 25 mcg • Pantothenic Acid 100 mg • Calcium 500 mg • Iron 18 mg•Phosphorus 200 mg • Iodine 150 mcg • Magnesium 200 mg • Zinc 50 mg • Selenium 50 mcg • Copper 0.2 mg • Manganese 4 mg • Chromium 50 mcg • Molybdenum 50 mcg • Potassium 99 mg • Inositol 100 mg • Choline 100 mg • Para-Aminobenzoic Acid (PABA) 25 mg • Rutin 25 mg • Citrus Bioflavonoids 25 mg • Hesperidin complex 25 mg • Lecithin 350 mg. Typical Amino Acid content per 15 g serving: Alanine 235 mg, Arginine 285 mg, Aspartic Acid 518 mg, Cysteine 27 mg, Glutamic Acid 1,614 mg, Glycine 139 mg, Histidine 212 mg, Isoleucine 458 mg, Leucine 703 mg, Lysine 561 mg, Methionine 216 mg, Phenylalanine 377 mg, Proline 822 mg, Serine 469 mg, Threonine 300 mg, Tryptophan 93 mg, Tyrosine 407 mg, Valine 517 mg.

Super Aloe 250 - Ortho Molecular Products
Each capsule contains: Cape Aloe 250 mg. Other Ingredients: Natural Vegetable Capsules, Magnesium Stearate, Microcrystalline Cellulose.

Super Alor 450 - Ortho Molecular Products
Each capsule contains: Cape Aloe 450 mg.

Super Anti-OX - Nutri-Quest Rx
Each tablet contains: Grape seed extract 20 mg (92-95% Proanthocyanidins) • Zinc (as Ester-C 2 mg) 14 mg • Vitamin C 100 mg • Vitamin E (Succinate) 50 IU • L-Glutathione 2 mg • N-Acetyl Cysteine 5 mg • Magnesium Aspartate 5 mg • Manganese Chelate 1 mg • Selenium Chelate 50 mcg • Chromium Chelate 50 mcg • Milk Thistle 150 mg • Silymarin 5 mg.

Super Antioxidant - Health Center for Better Living
Vitamin C 500 mg • Vitamin E 300 IU.

Super Antioxidant Capsules - The Vitamin Shoppe
Two capsules contain: Vitamin A (beta carotene and mixed carotenoids) 10,000 IU • Vitamin E 200 IU • Vitamin C (Calcium ascorbate) 60 mg • Vitamin B1 25 mg • Vitamin B2 25 mg • Vitamin B3 25 mg • Vitamin B5 25 mg • Vitamin B6 25 mg • Vitamin B12 250 mcg • N-Acetyl Cysteine 50 mg • Glutathione 50 mg • Selenium 75 mcg • Zinc 15 mg • Green Tea Extract (30% Polyphenols) 25 mg • CoQ10 10 mg • Quercetin 25 mg • Alpha Lipoic Acid 10 mg • Garlic (odorless) 100 mg • Grape Seed Extract (minimum 85%-95% proanthocyanidins) 10 mg • Manganese (Gluconate/Citrate) 15 mg.

Super Anti-Oxidant Complex - Nature's Plus
Two extended-release tablets contain: Vitamin A (as beta carotene) 10,000 IU • Vitamin C (as ascorbic acid) 500 mg • Vitamin E (as D-alpha tocopheryl succinate) 200 IU • Selenium (as amino acid complex) 200 mcg • Chromium (as amino acid chelate) 200 mcg. Other Ingredients: Di-Calcium Phosphate, Microcrystalline Cellulose, Hydroxypropyl Methylcellulose, Stearic Acid, Silica, Rose Hips, Magnesium Stearate, Carrot, Broccoli, Spinach.

Super Antioxidant Formula - Puritan's Pride
Each softgel contains: Vitamin E 400 IU • Beta Carotene 25,000 IU • Vitamin C 500 mg • Selenium 50 mcg.

Super Antioxidant Formula - High Potency - Nature's Bounty
Each softgel contains: Vitamin A 25000 IU •Vitamin C (as Ascorbic Acid) 500 mg •Vitamin E (as d-Alpha Tocopherol) 400 IU •Selenium (as Selenium Yeast) 50 mcg. Other Ingredients: Gelatin, Glycerin, Soybean Oil, Soy Lecithin, Beeswax, St. John's Bread extract, Caramel Color.

BRAND NAMES

Some Brand Name Natural Products - What they Contain

www.NaturalDatabase.com contains MANY more listings than appear here.
Editor's Notes are located on pages 2155-2163.

BRAND NAMES

Super Antioxidants **-** NOW Foods
Two Vcaps contain: Green Tea extract (Camellia sinensis 40% Catechins) 200 mg • Milk Thistle extract (Silybum marianum 80% Silymarin) 100 mg • Curcumin extract (Curcuma longa min. 90% extract) 100 mg • Quercetin 100 mg • Bromelain from pineapple (2000 GDU) 100 mg • Cranberry powder extract 100 mg • Rosemary extract (Rosmarinus officinalis) 100 mg • Grape seed extract (95% Polyphenols) 30 mg • Ginkgo Biloba extract (24% Ginkgoflavoglycosides) 30 mg • Ginger root (Zingiber officinalis) 30 mg • Hawthorne berry extract (Crataegus oxyacantha 1.8% Vitexin-4"-Rhamnoside) 30 mg • Bilberry extract (Vaccimum myrtillus 25% Anthocyanidins) 20 mg.

Super Antioxidants with Folic Acid **-** Optimum Nutrition
Two capsules contain: Vitamin A (as CaroCare natural mixed carotenoids) 25,000 IU • Vitamin C 1000 mg • Vitamin E (as D-alpha tocopherol succinate) 400 IU • Folic Acid 400 mcg • Selenium 200 mcg • Alpha-Carotene 490 mcg • Zeaxanthin 94 mcg • Cryptoxanthin 114 mcg • Lutein 72 mcg. Other Ingredients: Gelatin, Microcrystalline Cellulose, Magnesium Stearate, Silica.

Super B + C **-** Golden Glow Natural Health Products
Each tablet contains: Thiamine Nitrate (vitamin B1) 50 mg • Riboflavin (vitamin B2) 25 mg • Nicotinamide (vitamin B3) 50 mg • Calcium Pantothenate (vitamin B5) 50 mg • Pyridoxine Hydrochloride (vitamin B6) 50 mg • Cyanocobalamin (vitamin B12) 50 mcg • Ascorbic Acid (vitamin C) 100 mg • Folic Acid 200 mcg • Biotin 50 mcg • Inositol 50 mcg • Choline Bitartrate 50 mcg.

Super B Caps **-** American Biologics
Two capsules contain: Vitamin B1 (thiamine HCl) 50 mg • Vitamin B2 (riboflavin) 50 mg • Vitamin B3 (niacinamide) 100 mg • Vitamin B5 (calcium pantothenate) 250 mg • Vitamin B6 (pyridoxine HCl) 100 mg • Pyridoxal-5-Phosphate 5 mg • PABA (para-amino-benzoic acid) 100 mg • Inositol (myo-inositol) 100 mg • Choline (bitartrate) 200 mg • Biotin 1000 mcg • Folic Acid 300 mcg • Vitamin B12 (cyanocobalamin) 500 mcg. Other Ingredients: Magnesium Stearate.

Super B Complex 100 **-** The Vitamin Shoppe
Each tablet contains: Vitamin B1 (Thiamin) 100 mg • Vitamin B2 (Riboflavin) 100 mg • Vitamin B6 (Pyridoxine HCl) 100 mg • Vitamin B12 (Cobalamin Concentrate) 100 mcg • Niacinamide 100 mg • Folic Acid 400 mcg • D-Biotin 100 mcg • Choline Bitartrate 100 mg • Inositol 100 mg • Pantothenic Acid (d-calcium pantothenate) 100 mg • PABA 100 mg. In a base of Alfalfa, Watercress, Parsley, Lecithin, and Rice Concentrate.

Super B Complex Vitamins plus Vitamin C **-** Nature's Bounty
Each caplet contains: Vitamin C (ascorbic acid) 150 mg • Thiamin (vitamin B1, as thiamin mononitrate) 100 mg • Riboflavin (vitamin B2) 20 mg • Niacin (niacinamide) 25 mg • Vitamin B6 (pyridoxine hydrochloride) 2 mg • Folic Acid 400 mcg • Vitamin B12 (cyanocobalamin) 15 mcg • Biotin 5 mcg • Pantothenic Acid (D-calcium pantothenate) 5.5 mg • Calcium (dicalcium phosphate) 29 mg • Brewer's Yeast 100 mg. Other Ingredients: Cellulose, Croscarmellose, Vegetable Stearic Acid, Stearic Acid, Silica, Vegetable Magnesium Stearate, Cellulose Coating.

Super B-50 **-** Nature's Plus
Each capsule contains: Thiamin (vitamin B1, as thiamine HCl) 50 mg • Riboflavin (vitamin B2) 50 mg • Niacin (as niacinamide) 50 mg • Vitamin B6 (as pyridoxine HCl) 50 mg • Folate (as folic acid) 100 mcg • Vitamin B12 (as cyanocobalamin) 50 mcg • Biotin 50 mcg • Pantothenic Acid (as calcium pantothenate) 50 mg • Inositol 50 mg • PABA (para-aminobenzoic acid) 30 mg • Choline (as bitartrate) 21 mg. Other Ingredients: Silica, Di-calcium Phosphate, Microcrystalline Cellulose, Rice Bran, Alfalfa, Watercress, Parsley, Vegetable Cellulose, Purified Water.

Super Balanced Neurotransmitter Complex (SBNC) **-** Pain & Stress Center
Each capsule contains: Vitamin B6 (as pyridoxal 5'phosphate) 25 mg • Proprietary Blend 750 mg: L-Glutamine, GABA (as gaba amino butyric acid), L-Taurine, L-Phenylalanine, Glycine, L-Arginine, L-Methionine, L-Valine, L-Lysine, L-Leucine, L-Alanine, L-Isoleucine, L-Histidine. Other Ingredients: Gelatin Capsule.

Super B-Complex **-** Walgreens
Each caplet contains: Vitamin C 300 mg • Thiamin (vitamin B1) 15 mg • Riboflavin (vitamin B2) 10 mg • Niacin 50 mg • Vitamin B6 5 mg • Vitamin B12 10 mg • Pantothenic Acid 20 mg. Other Ingredients: Calcium Carbonate, Dicalcium Phosphate, Maltodextrin, Hydroxypropyl Methylcellulose, Mineral Oil, Cellulose, Silicon Dioxide, Stearic Acid, Magnesium Stearate, FD&C Yellow No. 5 Aluminum Lake, Polysorbate 80, Polyethylene Glycol, FD&C Yellow No. 6 Aluminum Lake, Carnauba Wax, Crospovidone, Titanium Dioxide.

Super B-Complex **-** Nature Made
Each tablet contains: Vitamin C 150 mg • Thiamin 100 mg • Riboflavin 20 mg • Niacin 25 mg • Vitamin B6 2 mg • Vitamin B12 15 mcg • Biotin 5 mcg • Pantothenic Acid 5.5 mg • Dried Yeasts 100 mg. Other Ingredients: Dibasic Calcium Phosphate, Cellulose Gel, Croscarmellose Sodium, Corn Starch, Hydroxypropyl Methylcellulose, Magnesium Stearate, Polyethylene Glycol.
See Editor's Note No. 45.

Super Beta-Carotene **-** J. R. Carlson Laboratories, Inc.
Each softgel contains: Vitamin A (as beta carotene) 25,000 IU • Vitamin E (as D-alpha tocopherol) 1 IU.

Super Biotin 5000 mcg **-** Vitamin World
Each capsule contains: Biotin 5000 mcg. Other Ingredients: Gelatin, Rice Powder, Silica.

Super Blue Stuff **-** Blue Stuff, Inc.
Each jar, bottle, or roll-on contains: Whole leaf Aloe Vera concentrate • Purified Water • MSM • Arnica Extract • SD-Alcohol-40 • Emu Oil • Sorbitol • Menthol • Sodium Chondroitin Sulfate • Glucosamine HCl • Capsicum Oleoresin • Nettle Extract • Coriander Oil • Kava Kava Extract • Extracts of: Blue Bottle, Roman Chamomile, Marigold, Lime tree • Willow Bark Extract • Witch Hazel Extract • Carbomer-940 • Triethanolamine • Ascorbyl Palmitate • FD&C Blue No. 1.
See Editor's Note No. 15 and No. 17.

Super Booster **-** Life Extension
Each softgel contains: Gamma-Tocopherol 210 mg • Gamma-Tocotrienol 35.5 mg • Delta-Tocopherol 78.4 mg • Delta-Tocotrienol 9.3 mg • Alpha-Tocopherol 66.3 mg • Alpha-Tocotrienol 18.5 mg • Beta-Tocopherol 3.5 mg • Lycopene extract (from tomato extract) 10 mg • Lutein extract (from marigold extract) 2.2 mg • Ginkgo extract (28% ginkgo flavone glycosides/7% terpene lactones) 120 mg • Chlorophyllin 100 mg • Vitamin K (K1) 9 mg • Vitamin K (K2) 1 mg • Selenium 200 mcg • Sodium Selenate 50 mcg • Selenomethionine 50 mcg • Methyl-Selenocysteine 100 mcg • Folate (as folic acid) 800 mcg • Vitamin B12 (as cyanocobalamin) 500 mcg • Ascorbyl Palmitate 50 mg • Vitamin C (as calcium ascorbate, ascorbyl palmitate) 90 mg • Vitamin E (as d-alpha tocopherol) 98.8 IU • Calcium (as calcium ascorbate) 10 mg. Other Ingredients: Gelatin, Flaxseed Oil, Glycerine, Purified Water, Yellow Beeswax, Lecithin, Carob Color.

Super C Ascorbs **-** American Biologics
Each tablet contains: Vitamin C (as ascorbate) 1000 mg • Bioflavonoid complex (lemon) 100 mg • Calcium (as ascorbate) 53 mg • Magnesium (as ascorbate) 27 mg • Potassium (as citrate) 60 mg • Zinc (as ascorbate) 2.5 mg • Manganese 0.1 mg. Other Ingredients: Dicalcium Phosphate, Cellulose, Magnesium Stearate.

Super Cal Mag Plus **-** Shaklee
Ten tablets contain: Vitamin D (as cholecalciferol) 400 IU • Vitamin K (as phytonadione) 40 mcg • Calcium (as dicalcium phosphate, calcium carbonate and calcium citrate) 1200 mg • Phosphorus (as dicalcium phosphate) 700 mg • Magnesium (as magnesium oxide) 200 mg • Zinc (as zinc gluconate) 1.5 mg • Copper (as copper gluconate) 0.2 mg • Manganese (as manganese gluconate) 0.2 mg • Sodium 10 mg • Boron (as boron protein hydrolysate) 1 mg. Other Ingredients: Microcrystalline Cellulose, Croscarmellose Sodium.

Super Calcium 1200 with Vitamin D - Schiff
Two softgels contain: Vitamin D (as cholecalciferol) 400 IU • Calcium (as calcium carbonate) 1200 mg. Other Ingredients: Vegetable Oil, Gelatin, Glycerin, Lecithin, and Titanium Dioxide.

Super Calcium-Magnesium - Schiff
Three softgels contain: Vitamin D (as cholecalciferol) 400 IU • Calcium (as calcium carbonate) 1.2 g • Magnesium (as magnesium oxide) 400 mg • Boron (as boron glycinate) 3 mg. Other Ingredients: Soybean Oil, Gelatin, Glycerin, Water, Titanium Dioxide, Lecithin.

Super Cal-Mag - Nature's Life
Two tablets contain: Calcium (Chelated, Carbonate, Aspartate, Aminoate, Citrate Complex) 1000 mg • Magnesium (Chelated, Oxide, Aspartate, Aminoate, Citrate Complex) 500 mg.

Super Carb Blocker - Pro Health
Two tablets contain: White Kidney Bean 4:1 extract 250 mg • Garcinia Cambogia 50% extract 250 mg • Chromium (amino acid chelate) 100 mg. Other Ingredients: Dicalcium Phosphate, Cellulose, Stearic Acid, Silica, Magnesium, Stearate, Glaze.

Super Carnosine - Life Extension
Each capsule contains: Carnosine 500 mg • Benfotiamine 50 mg • Quercetin (water soluble) 50 mg. Other Ingredients: Magnesium Stearate, Dicalcium Phosphate, Gelatin, Water.

Super Cayenne - Swanson Health Products
Two capsules contain: Cayenne pepper (100,000 heating units) 450 mg • Ginger root powder 200 mg • Hawthorn berry powder 200 mg • Lecithin granules 50 mg.

Super C-Complex 500 - The Vitamin Shoppe
Each tablet contains: Vitamin C (with Rose Hips) 500 mg • Citrus Bioflavonoid Complex 100 mg • Hesperidin Complex 25 mg • Rutin 50 mg • Acerola 1 mg.

Super Chelated Multi-Mineral - Puritan's Pride
Three tablets contain: Calcium 750 mg • Phosphorus 300 mg • Magnesium 375 mg • Potassium 99 mg • Manganese 15 mg • Iron 15 mg • Zinc 15 mg • Copper 375 mcg • Iodine 225 mcg • Chromium 30 mcg • Selenium 38 mcg.

Super Chitosan - Genesis Nutrition
Two capsules contain: Chitosan 1 g.
See Editor's Note No. 37.

Super CitriMax - Vitamin World
Two capsules contain: Chromium (as ChromeMate brand chromium polynicotinate) 130 mcg • Gymnema leaf (gymnema sylvestre, standardized to contain 30 mg of gymnemic acid) 130 mg • (-) Hydroxycitric Acid (HCA, provided by 1500 mg of Super CitriMax Plus from garcinia cambogia rind) 900 mg. Other Ingredients: Gelatin, Silica, Magnesium Stearate.

Super CitriMax 750 mg - Natural Max
Two tablets contain: Super CitriMax brand Garcinia Cambogia (supplying 750 mg (60%) hydroxycitric acid-HCA) 1250 mg. Other Ingredients: Di-Calcium Phosphate, Cellulose, Stearic Acid, Magnesium Stearate.

Super CitriMax brand - InterHealth Nutraceuticals
Hydroxycitric Acid (HCA, extracted from garcinia cambogia fruit).
See Editor's Note No. 44.

Super CitriMax Clinical Strength brand - InterHealth Nutraceuticals
Hydroxycitric Acid (HCA, extracted from garcinia cambogia fruit).
See Editor's Note No. 44.

Super CitriMax Plus - Pure Encapsulations
Three vegetable capsules contain: Garcinia Cambogia extract (standardized to contain 60% (-)hydroxycitric acid) 1500 mg • Chromium (polynicotinate) 200 mcg • Gymnema Sylvestre extract (standardized to contain 75% gymnemic acids) 133 mg • Vitamin C (as ascorbyl palmitate) 30 mg.

Super CitriMax Plus - NOW Foods
Each capsule contains: Calcium (from CitriMax brand) 83 mg • Iodine (from kelp) 150 mcg • ChromeMate brand Chromium 100 mcg • Potassium 120 mg • Super CitriMax brand Garcinia Cambogia 750 mg • Panax Ginseng root 100 mg. Other Ingredients: Gelatin, Magnesium Stearate, Stearic Acid.

Super Citro Cee - Arrowroot
Each tablet contains: Vitamin C 500 mg • Rose Hips 500 mg • Lemon Bioflavonoids 500 mg • Rutin (from buckwheat) 50 mg.

Super Climax Cream - Media Dreamland Inc.
Organic Damiana leaf (folium terneraceae) • Organic Suma root (radix pfaffiae paniculatae) • Organic Motherwort (herba leonori) • Organic Wild Yam (rhizoma dioscorea villosae) • Organic Ginkgo Biloba • Organic Peppermint leaf (folium menthae piperitae).

Super Coenzyme Q-10 - Gary Null & Associates (GNA)
Each tablet contains: Coenzyme Q10 100 mg. Other Ingredients: Di-calcium Phosphate, Cellulose and Modified Cellulose, Stearic Acid, Magnesium Stearate, Silicon Dioxide, Pharmaceutical Glaze.

Super Complete capsules - Ultimate Nutrition
Nine capsules contain: Vitamin A 10000 IU • Vitamin D 400 IU • Vitamin E 400 IU • Vitamin B1 100 mg • Vitamin B2 100 mg • Vitamin B6 100 mg • Vitamin B12 100 mcg • Niacinamide 100 mg • Pantothenic Acid 100 mg • Folic Acid 400 mcg • Biotin 300 mcg • Choline 100 mg • Inositol 100 mg • PABA 100 mg • Vitamin C 1500 mg • Bioflavonoids 250 mg • Rutin 50 mg • Rose Hips powder 20 mg • Hesperidin 20 mg • Acerola Cherry 10 mg • Glutamic Acid HCL 100 mg • Betaine HCl 100 mg • Calcium 1000 mg • Magnesium 500 mg • Iodine 150 mcg • Potassium 95 mg • Iron 30 mg • Zinc 22.5 mg • Manganese 10 mg • Copper 3 mg • Boron 3 mg • Chromium 200 mcg • Selenium 50 mcg.

Super Concentrated Lecithin - Jamieson
Each capsule contains: Lecithin in a Super Concentrated form 400 mg. Derived from pure Soy. Standardized to Phosphatidylcholine 140 mg.

Super CoQ10 with Tocotrienols 100 mg - Life Extension
Each softgel contains: Coenzyme Q10 (Japanese pharmaceutical grade) 100 mg • Tocomin 30% (palm oil-derived tocotrienol complex) 45 mg • Rice Bran oil 350 mg • Vitamin E 5 IU. Other Ingredients: Gelatin, Glycerin, Water, Beeswax, Lecithin, Rosemary Extract.

Super CoQ10 with Tocotrienols 30 mg - Life Extension
Each softgel contains: Coenzyme Q10 (Japanese pharmaceutical grade) 30 mg • Tocomin 30% (palm oil-derived tocotrienol complex) 23 mg • Rice Bran oil 275 mg • Vitamin E 3 IU. Other Ingredients: Gelatin, Glycerin, Water, Beeswax, Lecithin, Rosemary Extract.

Super Cranberry Concentrate - Wellness for Women
Each softgel contains: Vitamin C USP (as ascorbic acid) 100 mg • Vitamin E (as dl-alpha tocopheryl acetate) 3 IU • Cranberry juice concentrate, 10:1 (equivalent to 800 mg) 80 mg.

Super Curcumin with Bioperine - Life Extension
Each tablet contains: Turmeric root powdered extract (curcuma longa, supplying curcumin 76.1% 685 mg) 900 mg • Demethoxycurcumin (15.7%) 142 mg • Bisdemethoxycurcumin (3.2%) 29 mg • Bioperine brand Black Pepper extract 5 mg. Other Ingredients: Magnesium Stearate, Gelatin, Water.

Super Daily Amino Blend - J. R. Carlson Laboratories, Inc.
Each level teaspoon contains: L-Ornithine (as L-ornithine monohydrochloride) 120 mg • L-Alanine 42 mg • L-Arginine 168 mg • L-Asparagine (monohydrate) 36 mg • L-Cysteine (N-acetyl) 200 mg • L-Cystine 99 mg • L-Glutamine 360 mg • L-Glycine 336 mg • L-Histidine (hydrochloride monohydrate) 60 mg • L-Lysine (as L-lysine monohydrochloride) 168 mg • L-Isoleucine 120 mg • L-Leucine 280 mg • L-Methionine 141 mg • L-Phenylalanine 159 mg • L-Proline 160 mg • L-Serine 42 mg • L-Taurine 99 mg • L-Threonine 111 mg • L-Tyrosine 99 mg • L-Valine 200 mg.

Super Daily Amino Blend capsules - J. R. Carlson Laboratories, Inc.
Each capsule contains: L-Ornithine (as L-ornithine monohydrochloride) 30 mg • L-Alanine 10 mg • L-Arginine 42 mg • L-Asparagine (monohydrate) 9 mg • L-Cysteine (N-Acetyl) 50 mg • L-Cystine 25 mg • L-Glutamine 90 mg • L-Glycine 84 mg • L-Histidine (hydrochloride monohydrate) 15 mg • L-Lysine (as L-lysine monohydrochloride) 42 mg • L-Isoleucine 30 mg • L-Leucine 70 mg • L-Methionine 35 mg • L-Phenylalanine 40 mg • L-Proline 40 mg • L-Serine 10 mg • L-Taurine 25 mg • L-Threonine 28 mg • L-Tyrosine 25 mg • L-Valine 50 mg.

Super Detox - 4 Life
Two capsules contain: Red Clover 450 mg • Milk Thistle extract (80% silymarin) 200 mg • Calcium d-Glucarate 130 mg • Sulforaphane (from broccoli, 25% DIM) 120 mg • Bupleurum 80 mg • N-Acetyl Cysteine 50 mg • Artichoke (leaf) 50 mg. Other Ingredient: Gelatin Capsule

Super DHA - J. R. Carlson Laboratories, Inc.
Each softgel contains: Vitamin E (as D-alpha tocopherol) 10 IU • DHA (docosahexaenoic acid) 500 mg • EPA (eicosapentaenoic acid) 100 mg • Fish oil concentrate 1000 mg.

Super Energy Oil - Puritan's Pride
Each softgel contains: Soybean oil 650 mg • Rice Bran oil 228 mg • Wheat Germ oil (cold pressed) 228 mg • Vitamin E (d-alpha tocopherol) 5 IU.

Super Energy Up - The Vitamin Shoppe
Each capsule contains: Standardized Panax Ginseng extract, Fo-Ti root, Sukday, Licorice, Lycii Berries, and Damiana leaves in a base of Royal Jelly, Bee Pollen, Vitamin B12, and Octacosanol.

Super Enzymes - NOW Foods
Each tablet contains: Betaine HCL (from beet molasses) 200 mg • Bromelain (2000 GDU from pineapple) 50 mg • Papain (140 MCU uncoated from papaya) 50 mg • Pancreatin 4x (equivalent to 800 mg) 200 mg supplying: Amylase (20000 USP Units) 100 mg, Protease [Chymotrypsin & Trypsin (20000 USP Units)] 100 mg, Lipase (3400 USP Units) 25 mg • Pepsin Enzymes NF 1:10000 50 mg • Cellulase 10 mg • Ox Bile extract 100 mg • Papaya Enzymes 45 mg • Pineapple Enzymes 45 mg.
See Editor's Note No. 14.

Super EPA DHA 500 mg - The Vitamin Shoppe
Each softgel contains: Vitamin E (as d-alpha tocopherol) 5 IU • EPA Eicosapentaenoic Acid (as marine fish oil) 300 mg • DHA Docosahexaenoic Acid (as marine fish oil) 200 mg.

Super Flex Joint Formula - Natural Balance
Each tablet contains: Vitamin C (as ascorbic acid) 40 mg • Manganese (as chelate) 6.7 mg • Glucosamine (as HCl/sulfate) 500 mg • MSM (methylsulfonylmethane) 333 mg • Boswellia Serrata Gum Resin (extract standardized to 65% total organic acids) 100 mg • Chondroitin Sulfate 50 mg • Ginger root 33 mg • Turmeric (curcumae longae standardized root extract) 15 mg • Polygonum Cuspidatum root (extract standardized to 50% trans-resveratrol) 5.4 mg. Other Ingredients: Microcrystalline Cellulose, Cellulose Gum, Magnesium Stearate, Stearic Acid, Silicon Dioxide.
See Editor's Note No. 15.

Super Food - Youngevity
Phosphorus • Sulfur • Chloride • Sodium • Vitamin A • Vitamin B1 • Vitamin B2 • Vitamin B3 • Vitamin B5 • Vitamin B6 • Vitamin B12 • Vitamin C • Vitamin D • Vitamin E • Vitamin K • Folic Acid • Biotin • Soy Protein • Soybean Oil • Soy Lecithin • Lactobacillus Acidophilus • FOS • Papaya • Protease • Bromelain • Amylase • Lipase • Cellulase • Soy • Rice • Barley • Oats • Prunes • Citrus • Alfalfa • Capsicum fruit • Chlorella • Garcinia fruit • Licorice.

Super Gainers Fuel - TwinLab
Each serving contains: Milk & Egg Proteins 100 g • High Levels of Complex Carbohydrates • Branched Chain Amino Acids (L-Leucine, L-Isoleucine & L-Valine) • L-Glutamine • L-Carnitine • Alpha-Ketoglutarate • Creatine Monohydrate • High Potencies of Vitamins & Minerals including Potassium 2000 mcg & Chromium 600 mcg • Fat 29 g [from Medium Chain Triglycerides (MCTs)]. MCTs are lipids composed of Medium Chain Fatty Acids.

Super Garlic - Pro Health
Each caplet contains: Garlic powder 600 mg • Allicin 3600 mcg • Thiosulfinates 4800 mcg • Alliin 4800 mcg • Gammaglutamyl Cysteines 12,000 mcg • Sulphur 3900 mcg. Other Ingredients: Microcrystalline Cellulose, Stearic Acid, Di-Calcium Phosphate, Magnesium Stearate, Silicon Dioxide, Silica.

Super Ginkgo (Ginkgo biloba) - Solgar
Each capsule contains: Ginkgo Biloba leaf 50:1 extract 60 mg • Raw Ginkgo Biloba leaf powder 30 mg. Other Ingredients: Vegetable Cellulose, Vegetable Magnesium Stearate, Water, Vegetable Glycerin.

Super Ginseng - Dial Herbs
Siberian Ginseng • Korean Ginseng • Brazilian Ginseng • Chinese Ginseng • American Ginseng.

Super GLA/DHA - Life Extension
Three softgels contain: Borage seed oil (borago officinalis) 2000 mg • GLA (gamma-linolenic acid) 460 mg • Marine Lipid concentrate 1000 mg • DHA (docosahexaenoic acid) 500 mg • EPA (eicosapentaenoic acid) 125 mg. Other Ingredients: Gelatin, Glycerin, Water, Carob Color, Rosemary Extract.

Super Glutamine 1000 mg (SG 1000) - Pain & Stress Center
Each scoop contains: Glutamine 1000 mg.

Super Gram II - Alacer
Each tablet contains: Vitamin C (as ascorbates) 1000 mg • Potassium (citrate, aspartate, ascorbate) 40 mg • Calcium (ascorbate) 35 mg • Magnesium (ascorbate, citrate) 35 mg • Zinc (ascorbate) • Manganese (ascorbate) 1 mg • Molybdenum (ascorbate) 50 mcg • Chromium (ascorbate, niacinate) 50 mcg • Quercetin 12.5 mg • 8 Bioflavonoids (from hesperidin: rose hips, acerola, pectin, orange, lemon, grapefruit, rutin) 100 mg. Other Ingredients: Acacia Gum, Magnesium Stearate, Vegetable Stearic Acid, Cellulose, Psyllium Husks, Parsley Seed, Silicon Dioxide, Chlorophyll, Titanium Dioxide, Polyentylene Glycol.

Super Gram III - Alacer
Each tablet contains: Vitamin C (as ascorbates) 1000 mg • Potassium (citrate, aspartate, ascorbate) 40 mg • Calcium (ascorbate) 35 mg • Magnesium (ascorbate, citrate) 35 mg • Zinc (ascorbate) • Manganese (ascorbate) 1 mg • Molybdenum (ascorbate) 50 mcg • Chromium (ascorbate, niacinate) 50 mcg • Quercetin 12.5 mg • 9 Mixed Bioflavonoids 12.5 mg • Vitamin B1 (thiamine HCl) 0.75 mg • Vitamin B2 (riboflavin) 0.85 mg • Vitamin B3 (as niacinates of potassium, calcium, magnesium, zinc, manganese, molybdenum, chromium) 10 mg • Vitamin B6 (pyridoxine HCl) 5 mg • Vitamin B12 (cyanocobalamin) 3 mcg • Vitamin E (tocopheryl acetate) 7.5 IU • Pantothenic Acid 5 mg • MSM (methylsulfonyl methane) 10 mg • D-Biotin 150 mcg • Folic Acid 200 mcg • Beta Carotene Complex (from S. salina) 2500 IU • Selenium (L-Selenomethionine) 50 mcg • Iodine (potassium iodide) 12.5 mcg. Other Ingredients: Acacia, Chlorophyllin, Ginkgo Biloba, Grapeseed Extract, Magnesium Stearate, Methyl- and Ethyl Cellulose, Methyl Nicotinate, Oregano Powder, Parsley Seed, Polyethylene Glycol, Potassium Aspartate, Potassium Citrate, Shellac, Silicon Dioxide, Vegetable Stearic Acid.

Super Greens - Jamieson
Each 8.5 g serving contains: Lecithin Powder 1220 mg • Concentrated Juice Blend 1710 mg: Alfalfa Leaf, Barley Grass, Buckwheat Seed, Kamut Seed, Red Beet Root, Wheat Grass • Spirulina Blue-Green Algae 1050 mg • Whole Brown Rice Hulls 549 mg • Stevia Root Extract 100 mg • Multi Algae Blend 427 mg: D. Salina Algae, Nori, Chlorella, Dulse, Kombu, Wakame • Sprouted Multi-Grains 427 mg: Barley Malt Seed, Mung Bean, Soybean, Wheat Berry • Dahlia Tuber and Chicory Root 225 mg • Beet Root Fiber 200 mg • Beta Glucans 200 mg • Soy Fiber 200 mg • Carrot Root Fiber 214 mg • Apple Pectin Fiber 214 mg • Bee Pollen 160 mg • Licorice Root 134 mg Acerola Fruit 134 mg • Astragalus Root 64 mg • Canary Island Brown Algae 50 mg • Sargassi Seaweed 50 mg

• Laminaria Seaweed 50 mg • Artichoke Leaf Extract 50 mg • Artichoke Leaf 50 mg • Dahlia Inulin Juice Complex 50 mg • Siberian Ginseng Root 47 mg • Royal Jelly 43 mg • Green Tea Leaf 33 mg • Milk Thistle Seed 32 mg • Jerusalem Artichoke Tuber 25 mg • Ginkgo Biloba Leaf 20 mg • Tomato Fruit 10 mg • Grape Seed Extract 10 mg • Papain Enzyme (from Papaya Fruit) 10 mg • Cellulase Enzyme 10 mg • Bilberry Fruit 11 mg • Natural Spearmint and Wintergreen Flavor.

Super Growth Enhancer - Optimum Nutrition
L-Arginine L-Ornithine Vitamin B6 20 mg • Vitamin C 200 mg.

Super Herbal V - MD Healthline
Two capsules contain: Yohimbe Bark 250 mg • Damiana Extract 50 mg • Bilberry Powder 100 mg • Gingko Biloba Extract (24%) 60 mg • Siberian Ginseng Extract 100 mg • Schisandra Extract 200 mg • Avena Sativa Extract 10:1 250 mg • Saw Palmetto (30%) 100 mg.

Super Immune - Oasis Wellness Network
Each tablet contains: Astragalus Membranaceus root extract 167 mg • Schisandra Chinensis fruit extract 100 mg • MaxCell Proprietary Blend 83 mg: Zisyphus Jujube, Aloe Vera gel, Glycyrrhiza Glabra, Piper Nigrum • L-Arginine (base) 67 mg • Reishi mushroom fruit extract (ganoderma lucidum) 50 mg. Other Ingredients: Stearic Acid, Cellulose, Calcium Sulfate, Magnesium Stearate, Silica.

Super Immunity - Susan Ambrosino's Herb Club, Inc.
Each capsule contains: Proprietary Blend 547 mg: Cat's Claw extract 3%, Goldenseal root extract 5%, Echinacea root extract 4%, Panax Ginseng extract 20%, Cat's Claw inner bark, Pau d'Arco, Astragalus root.

Super Immuno-Comp - Enzymatic Therapy
Two capsules contain: Vitamin A (Beta Carotene) non-toxic form of Vitamin A 5000 IU • Vitamin C (Ascorbic Acid/Rose Hips) 100 mg • Vitamin B6 (Pyridoxine HCl) 5 mg • Zinc (Picolinate) 3 mg • Other Ingredients: Astragalus extract (Astragalus membranaceus) 150 mg • Echinacea extract (Echinacea angustifolia) standardized to contain greater than 3.5% Echinacosides & 0.65% essential oils 150 mg • Goldenseal extract (Hydrastis canadensis) standardized to contain 5% total Alkaloids including: Berberine, Hydrastine & Canadine 150 mg • KS-2 (Peptidomannan Complex) Shiitake Mushroom, a purified extract of Lentinus Edodes 50 mg • Licorice root extract (Glycyrrhiza glabra) standardized to contain 5% Glycyrrhizic Acid 50 mg.

Super Immuno-Tone - PhytoPharmica
Two capsules contain: Vitamin A 5000 IU • Vitamin C 100 mg • Vitamin B6 5 mg • Zinc 3 mg • Astragalus extract 150 mg • Echinacea extract 150 mg • Goldenseal extract 150 mg • Shiitake Mushroom (KS-2) 50 mg • Licorice root extract 50 mg.

Super Joints - Baywood International
Three caplets contain: Methyl-sulfonyl-methane (LIGNISUL) 1500 mg • Glucosamine (HCl) 1200 mg • Boswellin extract 225 mg • Chondroitin Sulfate 200 mg • Manganese 25 mg • Proprietary Blend 300 mg: Bromelain, Peptizyme SP, Papain. Other Ingredients: Magnesium Stearate.
See Editor's Note No. 15.

Super K with K2 - Life Extension
Each softgel contains: Vitamin K (K1) 9 mg • Vitamin K (K2) 1 mg • Medium Chain Triglycerides (MCT oil) 215 mg • Ascorbyl Palmitate (antioxidant) 25 mg. Other Ingredients: Gelatin, Carob, Water.

Super KMH Chromium Liquid - Essential Nutrients Inc
Each fluid ounce contains: Potassium 585 mg • Magnesium 50 mg • Calcium 50 mg • Trace Minerals Blend: Aluminum, Antimony, Barium, Beryllium, Bismuth, Boron, Bromine, Cadmium, Calcium, Carbon, Cerium, Cesium, Chlorine, Chromium, Cobalt, Copper, Dysporosium, Erbium, Europium, Fluorine, Gadolinium, Gallium, Germanium, Hafnium, Homium, Hydrogen, Indium, Iodine, Iridium, Iron, Lanthanum, Lithium, Lutetium, Magnesium, Manganese, Molybdenum, Neodymium, Nickel, Niobium, Nitrogen, Oxygen, Palladium, Phosphorus, Potassium, Praseodymium, Rhenium, Thodium, Rubidium, Ruthenium, Samarium, Scandium, Selenium, Silicon, Silver, Sodium, Strontium, Sulfur, Tantalum, Terbium, Thallium, Thorium, Thulium, Tin, Titanium, Tungsten, Vanadium, Ytterbium, Yttrium, Zinc, Zirconium. Herb Blend: Thyme (thymus vulgaris), Senega Snakeroot (polygala senega), Saw Palmetto berries, Sarsaparilla (smilax officinalis), Passion Flower (passiflora incarnata), Licorice root (glycyrrhiza glabra), Horehound root (marrubium), Goldenseal (hydrastis canadensis), Ginseng (panax quinquefolius), Ginkgo (ginkgo biloba), Gentian root (gentiana lutea), Echinacea (echinacea augustifolia), Dandelion root (taraxacum officinalis), Chamomile (matricaria chamomilla), Celery seed (apium gloveclens), Angelica root (angelica archangelica), Alfalfa (medicago sativa).

Super Leci-Thins - Nature's Life
Three tablets contain: Lecithin (Soy) 1300 mg • Cider Vinegar 255 mg • Kelp 150 mg • Vitamin B6 (Pyridoxine HCl) 50 mg.

Super Liquid Absorbable Calcium - Puritan's Pride
Two softgels contain: Vitamin D (as Cholecalciferol) 100 IU • Calcium (as Calcium Carbonate) 1,000 mg.

Super Lysine Plus+ Cream - Quantum, Inc.
L-lysine • Lithium Carbonate 3X • Propolis extract • Calendula Flower extract • Echinacea Flower extract • Zinc Oxide • Goldenseal extract • Vitamin A • Vitamin D • Vitamin E • Cajeput Oil • Tea Tree Oil • Gum Benzoin Tincture. Prepared in a Beeswax and Olive Base.

Super Lysine Plus+ Tablets - Quantum, Inc.
Each three tablets contain: L-lysine 1500 mg • Vitamin C (ascorbic acid) 100 mg • Garlic (odorless) 200 mg • Echinacea extract (4:1 PE) 100 mg • Propolis 50 mg • Licorice extract (4:1 PE) 15 mg • Goldenseal root USP (Hydrastis) 15 mg.

Super Male Plex - The Vitamin Shoppe
Two tablets contain: Yohimbe extract 10 mg • Raw Testicular 250 mg • Damiana 250 mg • Ginseng (Korean/Siberian) 500 mg • Octacosanol 250 mcg • Vitamin E 250 IU • Histidine 200 mg • Sarsaparilla 100 mg • Saw Palmetto 100 mg • Raw Prostate 100 mg • Bee Pollen 100 mg • Zinc 100 mg • Oyster extract 50 mg • Cayenne 50 mg • Gotu Kola 50 mg • Selenium 50 mcg • Niacin 15 mg • Royal Jelly 5 mg.
See Editor's Note No. 14.

Super Male-Plex - Puritan's Pride
Two tablets contain: Raw Testicular 250 mg • Damiana 250 mg • Siberian Ginseng 250 mg • Korean Ginseng 250 mg • Octacosanol 250 mcg • Vitamin E 250 IU • Histidine 200 mg • Sarsaparilla 100 mg • Saw Palmetto 100 mg • Raw Prostate 100 mg • Bee Pollen 100 mg • Zinc 30 mg • Oyster extract 50 mg • Cayenne 50 mg • Gotu Kola 50 mg • Selenium 50 mcg • Niacin 15 mg • Royal Jelly 5 mg • Oatstraw 50 mg.
See Editor's Note No. 14.

Super Malic - Optimox
Six tablets contain: Magnesium (Hydroxide) 300 mg • Malic Acid 1200 mg.

Super Max 1600 Weight Gain - Aspen Group, Inc.
Each flavor (vanilla or chocolate) contains: Vitamin C 332 mg • Rose Hips 6.8 mg • Vitamin E 400 IU • Vitamin A 13,332 USP Units • Vitamin D 532 USP Units • Vitamin B1 20 mg • Vitamin B2 16 mg • Vitamin B6 68 mg • Vitamin B12 8 mcg • Niacin 56 mg • Choline 40 mg • Inositol 26.8 mg • Para Aminobenzoic Acid 1600 mg • Pantothenic 132 mg • Biotin 400 mcg • Folic Acid 532 mcg • Rutin 1700 mcg • Glutamic Acid 880 mg • Iodine 200 mcg • Calcium 1280 mg • Phosphorus 1200 mg • Potassium 10 mg • Iron 36 mg • Copper 2800 mg • Magnesium 13.2 mg • Manganese 3200 mg • Zinc 20 mg • Amino Acids: Arginine 7883 mg • Aspartic Acid 220 mg • Alanine 880 mg • Cystine 1100 mg • Glutamic Acid 880 mg • Glycine 1980 mg • Histidine 2332 mg • Isoleucine 7152 mg • Leucine 4840 mg • Lysine 5060 mg • Methionine 1100 mg • Phenylalanine 944 mg • Proline 328 mg • Serine 4840 mg • Threonine 3300 mg • Tyrosine 220 mg • Tryptophan 880 mg • Valine 4840 mg.

BRAND NAMES

Super Mega Vite II Multiple - Nature's Life
Each tablet contains: Beta Carotene (Vitamin A equivalent to 10,000 IU) 6 mg • Vitamin B1 (Thiamine HCl) 50 mg • Vitamin B2 (Riboflavin) 50 mg • Niacinamide 75 mg • Pantothenic Acid (Calcium Pantothenate) 75 mg • Vitamin B6 Pyridoxine HCl) 50 mg • Vitamin B12 (Cobalamin concentrate) 250 mcg • Folic Acid 400 mcg • Biotin (d-Biotin) 50 mcg • Choline (Bitartrate) 50 mg • Inositol 50mg • l-Methionine (free form) 25 mg • Vitamin E (d-Alpha Tocopherol plus mixed Tocopherols) 100 IU • Vitamin C 250 mg • Rutin 5 mg • Lemon Bioflavonoids Complex (TESTLAB 50%) 25 mg • Hesperidin Complex 5 mg • Calcium (Carbonate) 100 mg • Chromium (Chelate) 25 mcg • Copper (Chelate) 200 mcg • Iodine (Postassium Idodine) 100 mg • Iron (Chelate) 10 mg • Magnesium (Oxide) 40 mg • Manganese (Chelate) 7 mg • Phosporus (Potassium Phosphate) 45 mg • Potassium (Phosphate, Chloride, Iodide) 67 mg • Selenium (Nutrition 21) (l-Selenomethionine) 10 mcg • Silicon (Dioxide) 20 mg • Zinc (Chelate) 10 mg • Coenzyme Q-10 (Ubiquinone) 500 mcg • Betaine HCl 25 mg • Glutamic Acid HCL 25 mg. In a natural base of "72 Trace Minerals" from an ancient sedimentary sea bed, Chamomile, Rice Bran & Rose Hips.

Super Mega Vite Multiple - Nature's Life
Each tablet contains: Vitamin A (Fish Liver oil) 25000 IU • Vitamin D (as Vitamin D3, Cholecalciferol) 400 IU • Vitamin B1 (Thiamine HCl) 30 mg • Vitamin B2 (Riboflavin) 30 mg • Niacinamide 100 mg • Pantothenic Acid (d-Calcium Pantothenate) 100 mg • Vitamin B6 Pyridoxine HCl) 30 mg • Vitamin B12 (Cyanocobalamin) 250 mcg • Folic Acid 400 mcg • PABA (Para Aminobenzoic Acid) 60 mg • Biotin (d-Biotin) 50 mcg • Choline (Choline Bitartrate) 100 mg • Inositol 100 mg • Vitamin E (d-Alpha Tocopheryl Succinate) 100 IU • Vitamin C 250 mg • Lemon Bioflavonoids Complex (50% Total Flavanones) 25 mg • Rutin 25 mg • Hesperidin Complex (50% Total Flavanones) 5 mg • Calcium (Bone Meal) 82.5 mg • Chromium (Chelate) 25 mcg • Copper (Gluconate) 200 mcg • Iodine (Potassium Iodide) 100 mcg • Iron (Ferrous Fumarate) 10 mg • Magnesium (Oxide) 40 mg • Manganese (Gluconate) 7 mg • Phosphorus (Bone Meal) 37.5 mg • Potassium (Iodide) 10 mg • Selenium (Nutrition 21 L-Selenomethionine) 10 mcg • Zinc (Gluconate) 10 mg • Super Oxide Dismutase 30 IU • Betaine HCl 25 mg • Glutamic Acid HCl 25 mg • Methionine 50 mg. In a natural base of Lecithin, Alfalfa, Watercress, Parsley, Duodenal Substance, Rose Hips powder, Chamomile, Molasses, Kale, Cabbage, Goldenseal, Sarsaparilla, "72 Trace Minerals", Pepsin & Kelp.

Super Milk Thistle X - PhytoPharmica
Each capsule contains: Milk Thistle fruit extract (silybum marianum) bound to phosphatidylcholine 100 mg • Dandelion root 4:1 extract (taraxacum officinale) 10 mg • Artichoke leaf extract (cynara scolymus, standardized to contain 13%-18% caffeylquinic acids calculated as chlorogenic acid) 40 mg • Licorice root extract (glycyrrhiza glabra, standardized to 5% glycyrrhizic acid) 10 mg.

Super MiraForte with Maximum Strength Chrysin - Life Extension
Two capsules contain: Zinc (as zinc monomethionine) 7.5 mg • Chrysin 750 mg • Muira Puama (ptychopetalum olacoides) 425 mg • Maca root (lepidium meyenii) 160 mg • Nettle root (urtica dioica) powdered Methanolic extract 141 mg • Ginger root extract (zingiber officinale, rhizome) 25 mg • Piperine (from black pepper) 7.5 mg. Other Ingredients: Gelatin, Water.

Super Multi with Herbs - Leiner Health Products
Each tablet contains: Iron (Ferrous Fumarate) 9 mg • Magnesium (Magnesium Oxide) 100 mg • Calcium (Calcium Carbonate) 225 mg • Vitamin B12 (Cyanocobalamin) 12 mcg • Vitamin C (Ascorbic Acid) 120 mg • Vitamin E (dl-Tocopheryl Acetate) 60 IU • Chromium (Chromium Picolinate, Chromium Chloride) 120 mcg • Copper (Cupric Oxide) 2 mg • Folate (Folic Acid) 400 mcg • Iodine (Potassium Iodide) 150 mcg • Manganese (Manganese Sulfate) 2 mg • Molybdenum (Sodium Molybdate) 75 mcg • Niacin (Niacinamide) 20 mg • Pantothenic Acid (d-Calcium Pantothenate) 10 mg • Riboflavin (Vitamin B2) 1.7 mg • Selenium (Sodium Selenate) 70 mcg • Thiamin (Vitamin B1) 1.5 mg • Vitamin A (40% as Beta Carotene) 5000 IU • Vitamin B6 (Pyridoxine Hydrochloride) 2 mg • Vitamin D (Ergocalciferol) 400 IU • Vitamin K (Phytonadione) 80 mcg • Zinc (Zinc Oxide) 15 mg • Biotin (d-Biotin) 30 mcg • Boron (Boron Citrate) 150 mcg • Ginkgo Biloba (Ginkgo biloba) leaf 25 mg • Herbal Complex Blend 25 mg • Siberian Ginseng (Eleutherococcus senticosus) root 25 mg. Other Ingredients: Gelatin, Maltodextrin, Starch, Cellulose, Dicalcium Phosphate, Croscarmellose Sodium, Silicon Dioxide, Polyethylene Glycol 3350, Crospovidone, Tricalcium Phosphate, Hydroxypropyl Methylcellulose, Mannitol, Magnesium Stearate, Pharmaceutical Glaze, Hydroxypropyl Cellulose, Resin, Polysorbate 80.

Super Multi-Pak - Optimum Nutrition
Each pak (3 capsules/3 tablets) contains: Vitamin A (as fish liver oil) 10,000 IU • Vitamin C (as ascorbic acid) 1000 mg • Vitamin D (as fish liver oil) 400 IU • Vitamin E (as D-alpha tocopherol succinate) 400 IU • Thiamin (as thiamin hydrochloride) 75 mg • Riboflavin 75 mg • Niacin (as niacinamide) 75 mg • Vitamin B6 (as pyridoxine hydrochloride) 75 mg • Folic Acid 400 mcg • Vitamin B12 (as cyanocobalamin) 75 mcg • Biotin 300 mcg • Pantothenic Acid (as D-calcium pantothenate) 75 mg • Calcium (as calcium carbonate, citrate and dicalcium phosphate) 772 mg • Iron (as iron AA chelate) 9 mg • Phosphorus (as calcium phosphate) 203 mg • Iodine (as kelp) 75 mcg • Magnesium (as magnesium oxide) 250 mg • Zinc (as zinc AA chelate) 15 mg • Selenium (as selenium AA chelate) 56 mcg • Copper (as copper AA chelate) 2 mg • Manganese (as manganese AA chelate) 2 mg • Chromium (as chromium GTF) 96 mcg • Molybdenum (as molybdenum AA chelate) 60 mcg • Chloride (as potassium chloride) 44 mg • Potassium (as potassium chloride) 48.5 mg • Inositol 100 mg • Choline (as choline bitartrate) 100 mg • PABA (as para-aminobenzoic acid) 100 mcg • Lecithin 1200 mg • Citrus Bioflavonoids 100 mg • Rose Hips 10 mg • Betaine (as betaine hydrochloride) 50 mg. Other Ingredients: Microcrystalline Cellulose, Gelatin, Stearic Acid, Croscarmellose Sodium (disintegrant), Silica.

Super Multiple II - Pro Health
Two tablets contain: Vitamin A (as beta carotene) 10,000 IU • Vitamin C (from calcium ascorbate) 500 mg • Vitamin D (as calciferol) 200 IU • Vitamin E (as D-alpha tocopheryl acetate) 200 IU • Vitamin K (from green foods) 25 mcg • Thiamine (vitamin B1) 50 mg • Riboflavin (vitamin B2) 50 mg • Niacin (as niacinamide) 50 mg • Vitamin B6 (as pyridoxine HCl) 50 mg • Folate (folic acid) 400 mcg • Vitamin B12 (as cyanocobalamin) 100 mcg • Biotin 100 mcg • Pantothenic Acid 50 mg • Calcium (from calcium carbonate, ascorbate) 100 mg • Iron (from amino acid chelate) 10 mg • Iodine (from kelp) 150 mcg • Magnesium (from magnesium oxide and amino acid chelate) 50 mg • Zinc (from amino acid chelate) 15 mg • Selenium (from amino acid chelate) 50 mcg • Copper (from amino acid chelate) 1 mg • Manganese (from amino acid chelate) 5 mg • Chromium (from yeast free GTF) 100 mcg • Molybdenum (from amino acid chelate) 50 mcg • Potassium (from amino acid chelate) 50 mg • Boron (from amino acid chelate) 1 mg • Vanadium (from amino acid chelate) 50 mcg • Choline Bitartrate 50 mg • Inositol 50 mg • PABA 30 mg • Spirulina 250 mg • Chlorella (broken cell wall) 250 mg • Barley grass (organic) 250 mg • Alfalfa juice concentrate 100 mg • Octocosanol (wheat free) 100 mcg • Eleuthero 50 mg • Citrus Bioflavonoids (40% hesperidin) 50 mg • Rutin 25 mg • Psyllium husk fiber 50 mg • Echinacea 50 mg • Apple Pectin 25 mg • Betaine HCl 25 mg • Glutamic Acid 25 mg • Papain (from papaya) 25 mg • Lipase 10 mg • Amylase 10 mg • Chlorophyll 9 mg • Amino Acid Blend 380 mg. Other Ingredients: Alfalfa, Rose Hips, Dicalcium Phosphate, Cellulose, Stearic Acid, Croscarmellose, Sodium, Magnesium Stearate, Silica, Vegetable Protein.

Super Multiple without Iron - Pro Health
Two tablets contain: Vitamin A (as beta carotene) 25,000 IU • Vitamin C (from calcium ascorbate) 500 mg • Vitamin D (as ergocalciferol) 200 IU • Vitamin E (as tocopheryl) 200 IU • Vitamin K (from green foods) 70 mcg • Thiamine (vitamin B1) 50 mg • Riboflavin (vitamin B2) 50 mg • Niacin (as niacinamide) 50 mg • Vitamin B6 (as pyridoxine HCl) 50 mg • Folic Acid 800 mcg • Vitamin B12 (as cyanocobalamin) 200 mcg • Biotin 100 mcg • Pantothenic Acid (as calcium pantohtenate) 50 mg • Calcium (as

ascorbate, citrate, and carbonate) 100 mg • Iodine (from kelp) 150 mcg • Magnesium (as citrate oxide) 100 mg • Zinc (from zinc poicolinate) 15 mg • Selenium (as L-selenomethionine) 50 mcg • Copper (from amino acid chelate) 500 mcg • Manganese (from amino acid chelate) 5 mg • Chromium Picolinate 100 mcg • Molybdenum (from amino acid chelate) 50 mcg • Potassium (from potassium chloride) 25 mg • Boron (from amino acid chelate) 1 mg • Vanadium (from amino acid chelate) 50 mcg • Choline Bitartrate 50 mg • Inositol 50 mg • PABA 30 mg • Spirulina 250 mg • Chlorella (broken cell wall) 100 mg • Barley grass (organic) 250 mg • Wheat Grass (organic) 100 mg • Alfalfa juice concentrate 100 mg • Green Tea extract 50 mg • Trace Mineral Concentrate 100 mg • Panax Ginseng 100 mg • Citrus Bioflavonoids (37% hesperidin) 50 mg • Rutin 25 mg • Bromelain 50 mg • Papain (from papaya) 25 mg • Pepsin Enzymes 25 mg • Lipase 25 mg • Amylase 10 mg • Chlorophyll 8 mg • Amino Acid Blend 350 mg. Other Ingredients: Dicalcium Phosphate, Cellulose, Stearic Acid, Magnesium Stearate, Silica.

Super Nails - Puritan's Pride
Three tablets contain: Vitamin A (as Fish Liver Oil) 10,000 IU • Vitamin D (as Fish Liver Oil and Cholecalciferol) 400 IU • Riboflavin (Vitamin B2) 50 mg • Folic Acid 200 mcg • Vitamin B12 (as Cyanocobalamin) 100 mcg • Calcium (as Calcium Amino Acid Chelate and Dicalcium Phosphate) 730 mg • Iron (as Iron Amino Acid Chelate) 5 mg • Phosphorus (as Phosphorus Amino Acid Chelate and Dicalcium Phosphate) 372 mg • Magnesium (as Magnesium Amino Acid Chelate) 25 mg • Gelatin 260 mg • Horsetail (Equisetum arvense) stem 250 mg • L-Cysteine 100 mg • DL-Methionine 100 mg • Sulfur (as Potassium Sulfate and from amino acids) 25 mg • Oat Straw (Avena sativa) stem 25 mg • Rice Bran powder 12 mg.

Super Nutrients Jr - Ortho Molecular Products
Two tablets contain: Beta Carotene 4000 IU • Vitamin D (D3, fish liver oil) 100 IU • Vitamin E 50 IU • Vitamin C 250 mg • Thiamine HCl (B1) 10 mg • Riboflavin (B2) 10 mg • Pyridoxine HCl (B6) 10 mg • Niacin 5 mg • Niacinamide 5 mg • D-Calcium Pantothenate 10 mg • Pyridoxal 5-Phosphate 10 mg • Vitamin B12 25 mcg • Folic Acid 400 mcg • Biotin 30 mcg • Inositol 5 mg • Choline Bitartrate 5 mg • Calcium 100 mg • Iodine 75 mcg • Magnesium 100 mg • Potassium 25 mg • PABA 10 mcg • Vanadyl Sulfate 100 mcg • Boron (proteinate) 25 mcg • Molybdenum 1 mcg.

Super Nutrition Power - Mascot Enterprise
Deer Velvet • Shark Cartilage • Fish Oil (Salmon) • Royal Jelly • Oyster Extract • Orchic Substance • Siberian Ginseng extract 5:1 • Cinnamon • Garlic • Noni • Muira Puama • Guarana extract 4:1 • Smilax • Avena Sativa 10:1 • Damiana leaf extract 4:1 • Vitamin E • Vitamin C • Vitamin B6 • Boron (Citrate) • Zinc (Sulfate) • Niacinamide.
See Editor's Note No. 14.

Super Octacosanol - The Vitamin Shoppe
Each softgel contains: Octacosanol 3000 mcg • Wheat Germ Oil 235 mg • Lecithin 9 mg.

Super Odorless Garlic - NOW Foods
Each capsule contains: odorless Garlic extract 100:1 concentrate (equivalent to 5000 mg fresh Garlic) 50 mg • Hawthorne berry extract (standardized to contain 1.8% Vitexin-2"-Rhamnoside) 100 mg • Hawthorne berry powder 250 mg • Cayenne pepper (40,000 Heat units) 100 mg.

Super Omega 3 - Nutri-Quest Rx
Each capsule contains: Natural marine lipid concentrate 1 g • Omega-3 Fatty Acids 110 mg/1 g of Eicosapentaenoic Acid (EPA) • Omega-3 90 mg/1 g of Docosahexaenoic Acid (DHA).

Super Omega 3 EPA - Nature's Sunshine
Each capsule contains: Eicosapentaenoic Acid (EPA) 380 mg • Docosahexaenoic Acid (DHA) 190 mg. Other Ingredients: Natural Lemon Oil, Gelatin, Glycerin, Water.

Super Omega 3-9-6 - Wild Rose
Each capsule contains: Borage seed oil 400 mg • Organic Flax seed oil 400 mg • Deep Sea Cold Water Fish oil 400 mg • Alpha-Linolenic Acid (omega-3) 212 mg • Cis-Linoleic Acid (omega-6) 207 mg • Docosahexaenoic Acid (omega-3) 48 mg • Eicosapentaenoic Acid (omega-3) 72 mg • Gamma-Linolenic Acid (omega-6) 76 mg • Oleic Acid (omega-6) 173 mg.

Super Omega-3 Fish Oils - J. R. Carlson Laboratories, Inc.
Each capsule contains: Vitamin E (as D-alpha tocopherol) 10 IU • Other Omega-3 Fatty Acids 100 mg • Other Omega-3 Fatty Acids (from fish oil) 600 mg • DHA (docosahexaenoic acid) 200 mg • EPA (eicosapentaenoic acid) 300 mg.

Super Omega-3 Natural Fish Oil 1000 mg - Vitamin World
Each softgel contains: Fish Oil 1000 mg • EPA (eicosapentaenoic acid) 300 mg • DHA (docosahexaenoic acid) 200 mg. Other Ingredients: Gelatin, Glycerin.

Super One Daily - Arrowroot
Each tablet contains: Vitamin A 8000 IU • Vitamin D (D3) 400 IU • Vitamin E 100 IU • Vitamin C 250 mg • Vitamin B1 30 mg • Vitamin B2 30 mg • Niacinamide 100 mg • Vitamin B6 30 mg • Vitamin B12 250 mg • Folic Acid 400 mcg • Biotin 150 mcg • Pantothenic Acid 100 mg • Calcium 200 mg • Magnesium 100 mg • Iodine 150 mcg • Zinc 10 mg • Copper 2 mg • Manganese 7 mg • Selenium 50 mcg • Choline 117 mg • Inositol 250 mcg • PABA 30 mg • Rutin 25 mg • Lemon Bioflavonoids 25 mg • Hesperidin Complex 25 mg • Betaine HCl 25 mg • Glutamic Acid HCl 25 mg.

Super One-A-Day - Golden Glow Natural Health Products
Each capsule contains: Thiamine Nitrate (vitamin B1) 25 mg • Riboflavin (vitamin B2) 25 mg • Pyridoxine Hydrochloride (vitamin B6) 50 mg • Nicotinamide (vitamin B3) 50 mg • Ascorbic Acid (vitamin C) 100 mg • Calcium (as amino acid chelate) 10 mg • Cyanocobalamin (vitamin B12) 25 mcg • Calcium Pantothenate 50 mg: Pantothenic Acid (vitamin B5) 46 mg • Biotin 50 mcg • Folic Acid 400 mcg • D-Alpha-Tocopherol 67.1 mg: Natural Vitamin E 100 IU • Manganese (as amino acid chelate) 600 mcg • Zinc (as amino acid chelate) 8 mg • Citrus Bioflavonoid extract 25 mg • Hesperidin 25 mg • Rutin 25 mg • Beta Carotene 3 mg • Chromium (as chromium picolinate) 26.5 mcg • Cysteine Hydrochloride 36.3 mg • Inositol 25 mg • Potassium (as potassium gluconate) 2 mg • Selenium (as selenomethionine) 25 mcg • Kelp powder 10 mg: Iodine 30 mcg • Horsetail extract (equisetum arvense) 50 mg.

Super Orti Vite - Genestra - Seroyal
Each capsule contains: Vitamin A (palmitate) 1250 IU • Beta Carotene 2500 IU • Thiamin Hydrochloride (vitamin B1) 25 mg • Riboflavin (vitamin B2) 15 mg • Niacinamide (vitamin B3) 38 mg • Pantothenic Acid (d-calcium pantothenate) 25 mg • Pyridoxine Hydrochloride (vitamin B6) 15 mg • Pyridoxal 5-Phosphate 500 mcg • Cyanocobalamin (vitamin B12) 25 mcg • Folic Acid 100 mcg • Biotin 75 mcg • Vitamin C (ascorbic acid) 100 mg • Vitamin D (D3, cholecalciferol) 25 IU • Vitamin E (d-alpha tocopherol) 75 IU • Calcium (citrate) 50 mg • Chromium GTF (polynicotinate) 25 mcg • Iodine (potassium iodide) 56 mcg • Iron (aspartic acid chelate) 5 mg • Magnesium (aspartic acid chelate) 20 mg • Manganese (citrate) 5 mg • Potassium (citrate) 5 mg • Selenium (selenomethionine) 25 mcg • Zinc (citrate) 5 mg • Bromelain (pineapple) 5 mg • Choline (bitartrate) 10 mg • Coenzyme Q10 (ubiquinone) 1 mg • Inositol 10 mg • L-Cysteine 10 mg • Non-citrus Bioflavonoids 10 mg • Hesperidin 10 mg • Papain (papaya) 5 mg.

Super Phos 30 - Twenty First Century Products
Ninety drops contain: Phosphorus 360 mg • Inositol 51 mg • Choline Bitartrate 18 mg.

Super Phytonutrients with Pure Coral Calcium - Xtend-Life Nutraceuticals Inc.
Two level teaspoons contain: Coral Calcium 1500 mg • Green Phytonutrients 2750 mg • Red Phytonutrients 1750 mg.

Super Prostate Formula - Physician's Choice
Each tablet contains: Soy Phytosterol Complex 660 mg: Beta Sitosterol 300 mg, Campesterol 165 mg, Stigmasterol 138 mg, Brassicasterol 15 mg • Pygeum Africanum extract (standardized, providing 15 mg beta sitosterol) 120 mg • Saw Palmetto extract

BRAND NAMES

(standardized) 300 mg • L-Alanine 300 mg • L-Glycine 300 mg • L-Glutamic Acid 300 mg • Stinging Nettles 300 mg • Ginseng 150 mg • Pygeum Africanum powder 48 mg • Lycopene Complex (5% lycopene) 40 mg • Pumpkin seed 30 mg • Zinc 30 mg • PABA 30 mg • Vitamin B6 30 mg • Vitamin A 7500 IU • Vitamin E 30 IU • Bioperine brand Black Pepper extract (piper nigrum) 2 mg.

Super Q10 - Cell Tech
Two softgels contain: Vitamin A (beta-carotene) 4080 IU • Vitamin K 7 mcg • Proprietary Blend 1 g: Flax Seed oil, Blue-Green Algae (aphanizomenon flos-aquae) 170 mg, Coenzyme Q10 60 mg, Essential Oils (rosemary, fennel, ginger, cinnamon), Betatene Carotenoids (d. salina). Other Ingredients: Beeswax (encapsuling aid), Gelatin (gelatin, glycerin, water, carob, titanium dioxide).

Super Salve - The Herbalist
Oils of Sweet Almond, St. John's Wort flower, Plantain herb, Calendula flower, & Beeswax • Extracts of Poplar bud, Golden Seal root, Echinacea root, Plantain herb, Comfrey root, Marshmallow root, Yarrow flower.

Super SAM-e with Maximizers - Pro Health
Each tablet contains: Vitamin B6 (as pyridoxine HCl) 2 mg • Folic Acid 200 mcg • Vitamin B12 (as cyanocobalamin) 50 mcg • SAM-e (S-adenosyl-L-methionine, from 400 mg disulfate tosylate) 200 mg. Other Ingredients: Cellulose, Croscarmellose Sodium, Methacrylic Acid, Magnesium Stearate, Silica, Triethyl Citrate, Stearic Acid, Citric Acid, Ascorbic Acid.

Super Saw Palmetto - Enzymatic Therapy
Each softgel contains: Saw Palmetto berry extract 160 mg.

Super Seed Beyond Fiber - Garden of Life, Inc.
Two heaping tablespoons contain: Perfect Fiber Blend 18,360 mg: Flax seed meal, whole Chia seed • Poten-Zyme Whole Food Fiber Blend 1500 mg: Flax seeds, Sunflower seeds, Chia seeds, Sesame seeds, Pumpkin seeds, Adzuki beans, Millet, sprouted Quinoa, Garbanzo beans, Buckwheat, sprouted Amaranth, Red Lentils, Kidney beans • Organic Cinnamon 124 mg • Stevia 90% 16 mg • Poten-Zyme Probiotic Blend 1.6 Billion CFU.

Super Sel-E-Chrome - Alacer
Each tablet contains: Selenium (as L-selenomethionine) 50 mcg • Vitamin E (mixed tocopherols) 50 IU • Chromium (as ascorbate, aspartate, niacinate) 50 mcg • Vitamin A (Betatene brand carotenoid complex) 1000 IU • Ascorbyl Palmitate 25 mg • Vitamin C (as calcium-magnesium-zinc ascorbate) 125 mg • DL-Methionine 50 mg • Grape seed extract 5 mg • Quercetin bioflavonoid 10 mg.

Super Silica Complex - Futurebiotics LLC
One tablet contains: Calcium (as calcium carbonate, citrate) 200 mg • Magnesium (as magnesium oxide, citrate) 150 mg • Zinc (as zinc gluconate) 15 mg • Betaine hydrochloride 50 mg • Boron 1.5 mg • Horsetail leaf powder extract 275 mg. Other Ingredients: Dicalcium phosphate, Cellulose, Stearic acid, Magnesium stearate.

Super Snooze with Melatonin - Puritan's Pride
Each capsule contains: Valerian root 100 mg • Hops 75 mg • Scullcap 75 mg • Chamomile 75 mg • Passion Flower 50 mg • Calcium carbonate 100 mg • Magnesium oxide 50 mg • Inositol 50 mg • L-Taurine 50 mg • Melatonin 3 mg.
See Editor's Note No. 16.

Super Soy - Pro Health
Each Vcap contains: Soy Isoflavones extract providing minimum 20% Isoflavones including Genistein, Daidzein and Glycitein 300 mg. Other Ingredients: Rice Flour, Magnesium Stearate, Silica.

Super Sprouts & Algae - Cell Tech
Three tablets contain: Vitamin A (beta-carotene) 1845 IU • Vitamin D 24 IU • Vitamin K 8 mcg • Vitamin B12 0.4 mcg • Calcium 60 mg • Iron 0.5 mg • Phosphorus 60 mg • Proprietary Blend 2.4 g: Wheat sprouts, Blue-Green Algae (aphanizomenon flos-aquae) 180 mg, Red Beta Algae (d. salina). Other Ingredients: Dicalcium Phosphate, Glyceryl Monostearate, Croscarmellose Sodium, Silica Dioxide, Magnesium Stearate.

Super Strength Glucosamine Plus CSA - Optimum Nutrition
Two tablets contain: Glucosamine Sulfate (as glucosamine sulfate potassium) 1500 mg • Chondroitin Sulfate (as chondroitin sulfate A) 1200 mg. Other Ingredients: Pharmaceutical Glaze, Stearic Acid, Magnesium Stearate, Croscarmellose Sodium, Silica.

Super Stress Formula - The Vitamin Shoppe
Two capsules contain: Vitamin C 1000 mg • Vitamin B1 (Thiamin) 50 mg • Vitamin B2 (Riboflavin) 50 mg • Vitamin B6 (Pyridoxine HCl) 50 mg • Vitamin B12 400 mcg • Niacinamide 100 mg • Folic Acid 400 mcg • Pantothenic Acid 250 mg • Biotin 100 mcg • Choline Bitartrate 100 mg • Inositol 100 mg • PABA 50 mg.

Super Suppositories - The Herbalist
Tea Tree Oil • Herbal extracts of Usnea & Calendula in a base of Cocoa Butter & Purified Bees Wax.

Super Vanadyl Fuel - TwinLab
Four capsules contain: Vanadyl Sulfate (supplying elemental Vanadium IV 4.87 mg) 25 mg • BMOV (bis maltolato oxovanadium, supplying elemental vanadium IV 320 mcg) 2 mg • Chromium (from Chromic Fuel chromium picolinate and ChromeMate chromium nicotinate) 600 mcg • Natural Vitamin E 900 IU • Taurine 1000 mg • Selenium (sodium selenate) 150 mcg • Zinc (picolinate) 30 mg • Manganese (Gluconate) 5 mg • Magnesium (oxide and aspartate) 400 mg • Biotin 1000 mcg • Niacinamide 100 mg.

Super Vitamin B - Schiff
Each tablet contains: Vitamin B1 (as thiamin mononitrate) 30 mg • Vitamin B2 (as riboflavin) 35 mg • Niacin (as niacinamide) 50 mg • Vitamin B6 (as pyridoxine hydrochloride) 15 mg • Folate (as folic acid) 400 mcg • Vitamin B12 (as cyanocobalamin) 100 mcg • Biotin 300 mcg • Pantothenic Acid (as d-calcium pantothenate) 100 mg • Calcium (as dibasic calcium phosphate, d-calcium pantothenate) 37 mg • Choline Bitartrate 50 mg • Inositol 100 mcg • PABA (para-aminobenzoic acid) 50 mg • L-Methionine 25 mcg. Other Ingredients: Cellulose, Magnesium Stearate, Croscarmellose Sodium.

Super Vitamin E Creme - Aspen Group, Inc.
Each gram contains: Tocopheryl Acetate 25% • Panthenol 1% • Water • Glyceryl Stearate SE • Octyl Palmitate • Isoproyl Palmitate • Propylene Glycol • Cetearyl Alcohol • Cetyl Phosphate • Decyl Oleate • Aminomethyl Propanol • Carbomer • Allantoin • Diazolidinyl Urea • Methylparaben • Propylparaben.

Super Vita-Vim Level 3 Potency Multivitamin - Jamieson
Each caplet contains: Vitamin A 5000 IU • Beta Carotene 1500 IU • Vitamin C 200 mg • Vitamin D 400 IU • Vitamin E 60 IU • Vitamin B1 30 mg • Vitamin B2 30 mg • Vitamin B3 (No Flush Niacinamide) 50 mg • Vitamin B5 50 mg • Vitamin B6 50 mg • Vitamin B12 50 mg • Folic Acid 400 mcg • Biotin 30 mcg • Calcium 150 mg • Iron 4 mg • Copper 1 mg • Iodine 0.1 mg • Magnesium 75 mg • Zinc 10 mg • Potassium 25 mg • Manganese 1 mg • Chromium 10 mcg • Selenium 10 mcg • Vanadium 1 mcg • Molybdenum 1 mcg • Lutein 300 mcg • Lycopene 300 mcg • Citrus Bioflavonoids 2000 mcg • Ginseng (Canadian) 25 mg • Peppermint, Bromelain, Papain, Amylase, Lipase, Cellulose.

Super Vita-Vim with Beta Carotene - Jamieson
Each caplet contains: Vitamin A (as Tetinyl Acetate and 15% [1500] IU as Beta-Carotene) 10000 IU • Vitamin C (as Ascorbic Acid) 200 mg • Vitamin D (as Cholecalciferol) 400 IU • Vitamin E (as DL-Alpha Tocopheryl Acetate) 60 IU • Thiamin (as Thiamine Mononitrate) 30 mg • Riboflavin (Vitamin B2) 30 mg • Niacin (as Niacin and Nicacinamide) 60 mg • Vitamin B6 (as Pyridoxine Hydrochloride) 30 mg • Folate (as Folic Acid) 400 mcg • Vitamin B12 (as Cyanocobalamin) 60 mcg • Biotin 30 mg • Pantothenic Acid (as Calcium D-Pantothenate) 30 mg • Calcium (as Calcium Carbonate) 140 mg • Iron (as reduced Iron) 4 mg • Iodine (from kelp) 100 mcg • Magnesium (as Magnesium Oxide) 100 mg • Zinc (as Zinc Gluconate) 10 mg • Selenium (from yeast) 10 mcg • Copper (as Copper Gluconate) 1 mg • Chromium (as Chromium Rice Protein Chelate) 50 mcg • Potassium (as Potassium Gluconate) 30 mg • Choline Bitartrate 30 mg • Inositol 30 mg • Dl-Methionine 2.2 mg.

Some Brand Name Natural Products - What they Contain

www.NaturalDatabase.com contains MANY more listings than appear here.
Editor's Notes are located on pages 2155-2163.

Super VM - Puritan's Pride
Each tablet contains: Vitamin A (as Retinyl Palmitate) 10,000 IU • Vitamin C (as Ascorbic Acid and Rose Hips) 250 mg • Vitamin D (as Ergocalciferol) 400 IU • Vitamin E (as d-Alpha Tocopheryl Acetate) 150 IU • Thiamin (Vitamin B-1) 60.8 mg • Riboflavin (Vitamin B-2) 75 mg • Niacin (as Niacinamide) 75 mg • Vitamin B-6 (as Pyridoxine Hydrochloride) 61.5 mg • Folic Acid 400 mcg • Vitamin B-12 (as Cyanocobalamin) 75 mcg • Biotin (as D-Biotin) 75 mcg • Pantothenic Acid (as d-Calcium Pantothenate) 75 mg • Calcium (as Calcium Amino Acid Chelate) 50 mg • Iron (as Iron Amino Acid Chelate) 10 mg • Iodine (as Kelp) 150 mcg • Magnesium (as Magnesium Amino Acid Chelate) 25 mg • Zinc (as Zinc Amino Acid Chelate) 15 mg • Selenium (as Sodium Selenate) 10 mcg • Copper (as Cupric Amino Acid Chelate) 0.25 mg • Manganese (as Manganese Amino Acid Chelate) 6.1 mg • Potassium (as Potassium Amino Acid Chelate) 10 mg • PABA (Para-Aminobenzoic Acid) 75 mg • Choline Bitartrate 75 mg • Inositol 75 mg • Rutin 25 mg • Citrus Bioflavonoids 25 mg • Hesperidin 5 mg • Betaine Hydrochloride 25 mg • L-Glutamic Acid 25 mg • Proprietary Blend 3 mg: Alfalfa (leaf), Watercress (plant), Parsley (leaf).

Super Whey Fuel - TwinLab
Blend of Three key Whey Proteins: Micro-Filtered & Ion-Exchange Whey Protein Isolate, Modified Molecular Weight & Partially Pre-Digested Whey Protein, & Whey Protein Concentrate enriched with Glutamine, Taurine, Arginine, Leucine, Isoleucine, Valine, Carnitine & Carnosine.

Super Zinc-30 - Golden Glow Natural Health Products
Each tablet contains: Zinc Gluconate 234 mg: Zinc 30 mg • Magnesium Amino Acid Chelate 100 mg: Magnesium 20 mg • Manganese Amino Acid Chelate 25 mg: Manganese 2.5 mg • Pyridoxine Hydrochloride (vitamin B6) 15 mg • Beta Carotene 3 mg.

Super-1-Daily - J. R. Carlson Laboratories, Inc.
Each tablet contains: Vitamin A (as beta carotene) 10,000 IU • Vitamin C (as ascorbic acid) 250 mg • Vitamin D (D2, calciferol) 200 IU • Vitamin E (as D-alpha tocopheryl succinate) 200 IU • Vitamin K 40 mcg • Thiamin (vitamin B1, as thiamin hydrochloride) 25 mg • Riboflavin (vitamin B2) 25 mg • Niacin (vitamin B3, as niacinamide) 25 mg • Vitamin B6 (as pyridoxine hydrochloride) 25 mg • Folate (folic acid) 400 mcg • Vitamin B12 (cyanocobalamin) 100 mcg • Biotin 25 mcg • Pantothenic Acid (as di-calcium pantothenate) 25 mg • Calcium (as calcium citrate) 50 mg • Iron (as iron glycinate chelate) 9 mg • Iodine (from kelp & potassium iodide) 150 mcg • Magnesium (as magnesium oxide) 50 mg • Zinc (as zinc gluconate) 15 mg • Selenium (from kelp) 105 mcg • Copper (as copper gluconate) 1 mg • Manganese (as manganese gluconate) 3 mg • Chromium (from kelp) 120 mcg • Potassium (as potassium chloride) 45 mg • PABA (para-aminobenzoic acid) 25 mg • Lutein (FloraGlo brand, from marigolds) 500 mcg • Betaine (as betaine hydrochloride) 25 mg • Bioflavonoids 25 mg • Choline (as choline bitartrate) 25 mg • Inositol 25 mg • Lecithin 25 mg.

Super-75 - J. R. Carlson Laboratories, Inc.
Each tablet contains: Vitamin A (as beta carotene) 10,000 IU • Vitamin C (as calcium ascorbate) 250 mg • Vitamin D (D3, from fish liver oil) 400 IU • Vitamin D (as D-alpha tocopheryl succinate) 200 IU • Thiamin (vitamin B1, as thiamin mononitrate) 75 mg • Riboflavin (vitamin B2) 75 mg • Niacin (vitamin B3, as niacinamide) 75 mg • Vitamin B6 (as pyridoxine hydrochloride) 75 mg • Folate (folic acid) 400 mcg • Vitamin B12 (cyanocobalamin) 75 mcg • Biotin 75 mcg • Pantothenic Acid (as di-calcium pantothenate) 75 mg • Calcium (as calcium ascorbate and di-calcium pantothenate) 35 mg • Iron (as iron glycinate chelate) 9 mg • Iodine (from kelp and potassium iodide) 150 mcg • Magnesium (as magnesium oxide) 15 mg • Zinc (as zinc citrate) 10 mg • Selenium (from kelp) 25 mcg • Manganese (as manganese carbonate) 5 mg • Chromium (from kelp) 25 mcg • Potassium (as potassium citrate) 10 mg • PABA (para-aminobenzoic acid) 75 mg • Betaine (as betaine hydrochloride) 10 mg • Choline (as choline bitartrate) 75 mg • Inositol 75 mg • Lemon Bioflavonoids complex 25 mg.

Super-C-Complex - J. R. Carlson Laboratories, Inc.
Each tablet contains: Vitamin C (as ascorbic acid and from rose hips) 500 mg • Lemon Bioflavonoids complex 500 mg.

SuperCitriMax - NOW Foods
Each capsule contains: Calcium (from Citrimax) 90 mg • ChromeMate brand of Chromium (Chromium Polynicotinate) 100 mcg • Iodine (from Kelp) 150 mcg • CitriMax Garcinia cambogia extract 750 mg • Panax ginseng root powder 100 mg.

Superdrol - Anabolic Xtreme
Each capsule contains: Methasteron 10 mg.

Super-Eff - Standard Process, Inc.
Each capsule contains: Proprietary Blend 516 mg: Carbamide, Tillandsia Usneoides, Bovine Liver fat extract, Flaxseed oil extract, Mixed Tocopherols. Other Ingredients: Gelatin, Water, Calcium Stearate, Colors.

SuperGarlic 6000 - Metagenics
Each tablet contains: Raw Garlic concentrate (allium sativum, yields a minimum of 6000 mcg of allicin) 600 mg.

Super-Green Pro-96 Soy Protein - Nature's Life
Two scoops (28.35 g) contain: Full disclosure ingredients: SUPRO brand Soy Protein Isolate (including Lecithin) • Hawaiian Spirulina • natural Vanilla Flavor • Barley Grass • Psyllium seed husks • Apple Pectin • Oat Fiber • Chlorophyll • Lemon Bioflavonoids Complex • Bromelain • Papain • Kelp • Milk-free Lactobacillus acidophilus • Pyridoxine Hydrochloride (Vitamin B6).

Superior Amino 2222 Liquid - Optimum Nutrition
Each 4 tbsp (52 mL) serving contains: Proprietary Blend: Hydrolyzed Gelatin, Whey Protein Isolate • Crystalline Fructose • Natural and Artificial Flavors • FD&C Red #40 • Sodium Benzoate • Potassium Sorbate.

Superior Coral Calcium with Magnesium - NSI - Nutraceutical Sciences Institute
Two capsules contain: Calcium (from Coral calcium) 700 mg • Magnesium (from Coral calcium and Oxide) 350 mg • Marine Coral (from Okinawa, Japan) 2 g. Other Ingredients: Gelatin, Water, Magnesium Stearate.

Superior EFA Omega-3 - NSI - Nutraceutical Sciences Institute
Each softgel contains: Vitamin E (as miexed tocopherols) 3 IU • Fish Oil concentrate 500 mg containing DHA (Docosahexaenoic Acid) 250 mg, EPA (Eicosapentaenoic Acid) 100 mg, other Omega-3 (DPA & ALA) 50 mg.

Superior Fiber Blend - Waiora
Fiber Blend: Guar Gum, Oat Fiber, Carrot Fiber, Fibersol (digestive resistant maltodextrin) • Arabinogalactan • Sugar Cane Fiber and Citrus Pectin • Natural and Artificial Flavor • Orange Juice powder • Corn Syrup solids • Sterol Esters: Beta-Sitosterol 325 mg, Campesterol 160 mg, Stigmasterol 120 mg • Inulin 500 mg • Citric Acid • Malic Acid • Ascorbic Acid • Vitamin E Acetate • Sodium Caseinate • Sucralose • DiPotassium Phosphate • Beta Carotene.

Superior L-Arginine - NSI - Nutraceutical Sciences Institute
Each capsule contains: L-Arginine 750 mg.

Superior L-Carnitine Fumerate - NSI - Nutraceutical Sciences Institute
Each capsule contains: L-Carnitine (fumerate) 500 mg.

Superior L-Taurine - NSI - Nutraceutical Sciences Institute
Each capsule contains: L-Taurine 850 mg. Other Ingredients: Kosher Gelatin (capsule), Magnesium Stearate.

Superior Melatonin - NSI - Nutraceutical Sciences Institute
Each capsule contains: Melatonin 3 mg.

Superior One Plus - Swanson Health Products
Each tablet contains: Vitamin A (as beta-carotene) 25000 IU • Vitamin C USP (as ascorbic acid) 300 mg • Vitamin D (as cholecalciferol) 400 IU • Vitamin E USP (as d-alpha tocopheryl succinate) 15- IU • Thiamin USP (as thiamin HCl; vitamin B-1) 125 mg • Riboflavin (vitamin B-2) 125 mg • Niacinamide 125 mg • Vitamin B-6 USP (as pyridoxine HCl) 125 mg • Folic Acid USP 400 mcg • Vitamin B-12 USP (as cyanocobalamin) 125 mcg • Biotin 125 mcg • Pantothenic Acid USP (as d-calcium pantothenate) 125 mg • Calcium (from calcium carbonate) 75 mg • Iron USP (from ferrous fumarate) 18 mg • Iodine (from kelp) 225 mcg • Magnesium USP (from magnesium oxide) 40 mg • Zinc (from zinc gluconate) 20 mg • Selenium (from yeast) 100 mcg • Manganese USP (from manganese sulfate) 7 mg • Chromium (from yeast) 225 mcg • Inositol 125 mg • Choline (as choline bitartrate) 100 mg • Lemon Bioflavonoid Complex 50 mg • Betaine HCl 30 mg • PABA (para-aminobenzoic acid) 30 mg • Rutin 30 mg, Glutamic Acid HCl 25 mg, Hesperidin Complex 25 mg.

Superior Probiotic - NSI - Nutraceutical Sciences Institute
Each enteric coated capsule contains: Bacterial Cultures 50 mg: L. Acidophilus, L. Rhamnosus, S. Thermophilus, L. Bulgaricus.

Superior Selenium - NSI - Nutraceutical Sciences Institute
Each capsule contains: Selenium (as selenomethionine) 200 mcg.

Superior Smino 2222 Tabs - Optimum Nutrition
Each tablet contains: Whey Protein Concentrate • Soy Protein Isolate • Pharmaceutical Glaze • Stearic Acid • Croscarmellose Sodium • Silica • Hydrolyzed Whey Peptides • L-Carnitine Tartrate • L-Ornithine Hydrochloride.

Superlax - Grandma's Herbs
Each capsule contains: Proprietary Blend 0.476 g: Cascara Sagrada bark, Psyllium seeds, Senna herb, Turkey Rhubarb root, Aloe Vera leaf, Barberry root, Slippery Elm bark. Other Ingredients: Gelatin.

SuperNutrient - EnerGreens, Inc.
Six capsules contain: Beta Carotene 5000 IU • Vitamin D (D3, as cholicalciferol) 400 IU • Vitamin B1 (cocarboxylase) 11 mg • Vitamin B2 11 mg • Niacinamide 25 mg • Vitamin B5 100 mg • Vitamin B6 32 mg • Vitamin B12 100 mcg • Folic Acid 400 mcg • Biotin 300 mcg • Vitamin E (D-alpha tocopherol 400 IU • Vitamin C (from ester C) 600 mg • Quercetin 500 mg • Calcium (from citrate and ascorbate) 500 mg • Magnesium (from aspartate and ascorbate) 500 mg • TMG 150 mg • Selenium (as selenomethionine) 100 mcg • Manganese (from gluconate) 5 mg • Zinc (as gluconate) 15 mg • Copper (as gluconate and aspartate) 2 mg • Chromium (picolinate) 100 mcg • Potassium (chloride, gluconate and aspartate) 100 mg • Molybdenum (chelate) 130 mcg • Choline Bitartrate 125 mg • Phosphatidyl Choline 125 mg • Inositol 225 mg. Other Ingredients: Gelatin.

Supersalve - B2 Herbal Products
Calendula (calendula officinalis) • Eucalyptus (eucalyptus smithii) • Clove (eugenia caryophyllata) • Camphor (cinnamomum camphora) • Grapeseed oil (vitis vinifera) • Rosemary (rosmarinus officinalis) • Honey (mel) • St. John's Wort (hypericum perforatum).

Support - Ortho Molecular Products
Each capsule contains: Vitamin C (as ascorbic acid) 80 mg • Shepherds Purse aerial portion 125 mg • Panax Notoginseng Ginseng 100 mg • Dong Quai root extract (standardized to contain 1% ligustilide) 80 mg • Yarrow flowers 60 mg • Lady's Mantle aerial portion 60 mg • Organic Motherwort leaf 40 mg. Other Ingredients: Natural Vegetable Capsules, Magnesium Stearate, Microcrystalline Cellulose.

Supra Renal 220 - Atrium Biotechnologies
Each tablet contains: Raw Tissue concentrate from Bovine Sources (not extracts) 235 mg: Adrenal 220 mg, Pituitary 15 mg • Vitamin C 175 mg • Bioflavonoid Complex 45 mg • Pantothenic Acid 70 mg • Methionine 60 mg • Choline 60 mg • Vitamin B1 25 mg • Vitamin B2 25 mg • Vitamin B6 25 mg • Niacinamide 50 mg • Magnesium 100 mg • Folic Acid 400 mcg • RNA 25 mg.
See Editor's Note No. 31.

Supraene Creme - Atrium Biotechnologies
Two ounces contains: Squalene 30 mg • Triethanolamine 5 mg • Ceresin Wax 5 mg • Glucam F-20 4 mg • Amerchol L-101 2.5 mg • Solulan 16 2.5 mg • Steral 2.5 mg • Cetyl Alcohol 2.5 mg • Carbopol 934 0.5 mg • Methyl Paraben 10 mg • Propyl Paraben 0.05 mg.

Suprema C Powder - Gary Null & Associates (GNA)
One teaspoon contains: Vitamin C 2500 mg • Selenium 65 mcg • Bioflavonoids 150 mg.

Suprema C Tablets - Gary Null & Associates (GNA)
Each tablet contains Vitamin C 500 mg • Selenium 6 mcg • Bioflavonoids 10 mg.

Supreme Greens with MSM capsules - Dr. Alex Guerrero
Three capsules contain: Proprietary Blend 1925 mg: Alfalfa leaf (agrimonia eupatoria), Aloe leaf (aloe barbadensis), Barley grass (hordeum vulgare), Barley sprouts (hrodeum vulgare), Beet root (beta vulgaris), Bilberry leaf (vaccinium myrtillus), Broccoli stalk (brassica aleracea italica), Cabbage leaf (brassica aleracea), Carrot stalk (daucus carota), Celery seed (apium graveolens), Cornsilk silk (zea mays), Dandelion leaf (taraxacum officinale), Echinacea herb (echinacea purpurea), Garlic bulb (allium sativum), Ginger root (zingiber officinale), Goldenseal herb (hydrastis canadensis), Grapefruit pectin (citrus paradise), Kale leaf (brassica species), MSM, Okra pulp (abelmoschus esculentus), Parsley leaf (petroselinum sativum), Pau d'Arco bark (tabebuia heptaphylla), Peppermint leaf (mentha piperita), Raspberry berry (rubus idaeus), Rosemary leaf (rosmarinus officinalis), Sage leaf (salvia officinalis), Shavegrass herb (equisetum hyemal), Slippery Elm bark (almus rubra), Spearmint leaf (mentha spicaa), Spinach leaf (spinacea alaracea), Strawberry leaf (fragaria vesca), Watercress herb (nasturtium officinale), Wheatgrass herb (triticum vulgare), White Willow bark (salix alba), Wintergreen leaf (gaultheria procumbens). Other Ingredients: Rice Powder, Magnesium Stearate, Gelatin.

Supreme Greens with MSM powder - Dr. Alex Guerrero
Each 1 tsp (2 g) serving contains: Proprietary Blend 2000 mg: Alfalfa leaf (agrimonia eupatoria), Aloe leaf (aloe barbadensis), Barley grass (hordeum vulgare), Barley sprouts (hrodeum vulgare), Beet root (beta vulgaris), Bilberry leaf (vaccinium myrtillus), Broccoli stalk (brassica aleracea italica), Cabbage leaf (brassica aleracea), Carrot stalk (daucus carota), Celery seed (apium graveolens), Cornsilk silk (zea mays), Dandelion leaf (taraxacum officinale), Echinacea herb (echinacea purpurea), Garlic bulb (allium sativum), Ginger root (zingiber officinale), Goldenseal herb (hydrastis canadensis), Grapefruit pectin (citrus paradise), Kale leaf (brassica species), MSM, Okra pulp (abelmoschus esculentus), Parsley leaf (petroselinum sativum), Pau d'Arco bark (tabebuia heptaphylla), Peppermint leaf (mentha piperita), Raspberry berry (rubus idaeus), Rosemary leaf (rosmarinus officinalis), Sage leaf (salvia officinalis), Shavegrass herb (equisetum hyemal), Slippery Elm bark (almus rubra), Spearmint leaf (mentha spicaa), Spinach leaf (spinacea alaracea), Strawberry leaf (fragaria vesca), Watercress herb (nasturtium officinale), Wheatgrass herb (triticum vulgare), White Willow bark (salix alba), Wintergreen leaf (gaultheria procumbens).

Supreme Omega capsules - DaVinci Laboratories
Each capsule contains: Vitamin E (mixed tocopherols) 10 IU • Proprietary Blend 1200 mg: Borage oil, Fish oil, Flax seed oil (yielding alpha linolenic acid 169.6 mg, linoleic acid 156.6 mg, oleic acid 145 mg, gamma linolenic acid 60.8 mg, EPA 120 mg, DHA 80 mg). Other Ingredients: Gelatin, Glycerin.

Supreme Omega Liquid - DaVinci Laboratories
Each 1/2 tsp serving contains: Proprietary Blend 2300 mg: Borage seed oil, Fish oil, Flax seed oil. Other Ingredients: Rosemary, Mixed Tocopherols, Ascorbyl Palmitate, Citric acid, Natural Cherry Flavor.

Supreme Stress B Capsules - Arrowroot
Each capsule contains: Vitamin B1 100 mg • Vitamin B2 100 mg • Vitamin B6 100 mg • Vitamin B12 1000 mcg • PABA 100 mg • Niacinamide 200 mg • Choline 25 mg • Biotin 100 mcg • Inositol 25 mg • Folic Acid 400 mcg • Pantothenic Acid 200 mg.

Some Brand Name Natural Products - What they Contain

www.NaturalDatabase.com contains MANY more listings than appear here.
Editor's Notes are located on pages 2155-2163.

Sure Balance - Meta-Sure Health
Each two capsules contain: Manganese 2 mg • Vitamin B6 (as pyridoxine HCl) 10 mg • Niacinamide 20 mg • Vitamin C (as ascorbic acid) 60 mg • Folic Acid 400 mcg • Magnesium (as magnesium glycinate) 150 mg • SurePlex Proprietary Blend 300 mg: Red Clover extract (8% isoflavones), Chaste Berry (powder), White Willow bark (1% salicylates), Citrus Flavonoids, Turmeric (95% curcuminoids), L-Taurine • Boron 1 mg • Black Cohosh extract (2.5% triterpenes) 40 mg • Dong Quai (powder) 10 mg • Panax Ginseng (root) 50 mg • Soy Concentrate (40% isoflavones) 85 mg • St. John's Wort (3% hypericin) 75 mg • 5-HTP (griffonia seed) 3 mg.

Surf Buddies CONCENTRATE! - PhytoPharmica
Two capsules contain: DMAE (as dimethyalminoethanol bitartrate) 100 mg • L-Theanine 25 mg • N-Acetylcysteine (NAC) 25 mg • Phosphatidylserine (from purified soybean lecithin) 60 mg.

Surf Buddies Daily Multiple - PhytoPharmica
Two chewable tablets contain: Bilberry fruit 4:1 extract (vaccinium myrtillus) 2 mg • Biotin 150 mcg • Calcium (tricalcium phosphate) 100 mg • Chromium (picolinate) 60 mcg • Cranberry fruit 2:1 extract (vaccinium macrocarpon) 2 mg • European Elder berry 4:1 extract (sambucus nigra) 6 mg • Folic Acid 400 mcg • Iodine (potassium iodide) 150 mcg • Iron (ferrous fumarate) 5 mg • Magnesium (oxide) 10 mg • Manganese (citrate) 1 mg • Niacin (niacinamide) 5 mg • Pantothenic Acid (calcium D-pantothenate) 2.5 mg • Phosphorus (tricalcium phosphate) 50 mg • Riboflavin (vitamin B2) 1.7 mg • Selenium (L-selenomethionine) 20 mcg • Sour Cherry fruit 10:1 extract (prunus cerasus) 10 mg • Thiamin (vitamin B1) 1.5 mg • Vitamin A (retinyl acetate) 5000 IU • Vitamin B12 (cyanocobalamin) 6 mcg • Vitamin B6 (pyridoxine HCl) 1 mg • Vitamin C (ascorbic acid and calcium ascorbate) 120 mg • Vitamin D (cholecalciferol) 400 IU • Vitamin E (D-alpha tocopheryl acid succinate) 30 IU • Vitamin K (phytonadione) 40 mcg • Zinc (ascorbate) 5 mg.

Surf Buddies Immune Defense - PhytoPharmica
Each chewable tablet contains: European Elder berry 4:1 extract (sambucus nigra) 40 mg • Vitamin A (as beta carotene) 1000 IU • Vitamin B6 (as pyridoxine HCl) 2 mg • Vitamin C (ascorbic acid and as sodium ascorbate) 100 mg • Zinc (as zinc ascorbate) 2 mg.

Susan's Brain and Body - Susan Ambrosino's Herb Club, Inc.
Each capsule contains: Proprietary Blend 604 mg: Ginkgo 24/6 extract • Panax Ginseng 20% extract, Eleuthero 0.8% extract • Cat's Claw inner bark.

Suvaril - Berkeley Premium Nutraceuticals
Each caplet contains: Vitamin A (as retinyl palmitate) 2500 IU • Vitamin C (as ascorbic acid) 30 mg • Vitamin D (as cholecalciferol) 200 IU • Vitamin E (as DL-alpha-tocopheryl acetate) 15 IU • Thiamin (as thiamin HCl) 0.75 mg • Riboflavin 0.85 mg • Niacin (as niacinamide) 10 mg • Vitamin B6 (as pyridoxine HCl) 1 mg • Folate (as folic acid) 200 mcg • Vitamin B12 (as cyanocobalamin) 3 mcg • Biotin 150 mcg • Pantothenic Acid (as D-calcium pantothenate) 5 mg • Chromium (as chromium dinicotinate glycinate) 100 mcg • Vanadium (as vanadium chelate) 50 mcg • Suvaril Proprietary Blend 716 mg: Green Tea leaf extract (provides 50 mg caffeine and 90 mg epigallocatechin gallate), Panax Ginseng root extract (10% ginsenosides), Banaba leaf extract (lagerstroemia specioa, 1% corosolic acid), Vanadium (as vanadium chelate). Other Ingredients: Dicalcium Phospate, Microcrystalline Cellulose, Croscarmellose Sodium, Stearic Acid, Magnesium Stearate, Film Coat Ingredients (hypromellose, hydroxypropyl cellulose, polyethylene glycol with colors to be determined).

Swanson Ultra Celadrin - Swanson Health Products
Each softgel contains: Celadrin brand esterfied fatty acid carbons (EFAC) proprietary blend 350 mg: Cetyl Myristate, Cetylmyristoleate, Cetyl Oleate, Cetyl Palmitoleate, Cetyl Laurate • Soy oil 160 mg • Salmon oil 22 mg. Other Ingredients: Gelatin, Glycerin, Carob Color.

Swedish Bitters - Self Heal Natural Therapies, Ltd.
Aloe • Myrrh • Saffron • Senna leaf • Camphor • Rhubarb root • Zedoary • Manna • Theriaca Venezian • Carline root • Angelica root.

Sweet & Slender - Wisdom herbs
Each packet contains: Fructose • Luo Han Guo fruit extract.

Sweet Energy Formula - Bee-Alive Inc.
Each teaspoon contains: Royal Jelly (non-freeze dried) 1.06 g. Other Ingredients: Pure Honey.

Sweet Sixteen - Abundance Marketing
Special Marine Concentrate • Rice Protein Concentrate • Microcrystalline Cellulose • Iodine • Horsetail • Acerola extract in a base of Hydrolyzed Vegetable Protein • Vitamin A • Vitamin C • Vitamin D (D3) • Vitamin E • Zinc. Other Ingredients: Dicalcium Phosphate, Stearic Acid, Croscarmellose Sodium, Silica, Magnesium Stearate, Pharmaceutical Glaze.

SweetEase - Advocare International
Three capsules contain: L-Arabinose 500 mg • Gymnema leaf extract (gymnema sylvestre) 200 mg • Phaseolus Vulgaris seed extract (dry bean) 300 mg • Hibiscus flower extract (hibiscus sabdariffa) 500 mg • Green Tea leaf extract (camellia sinensis) 100 mg • Apple fruit extract (malus sylvestris) 20 mg • Lactobacillus Acidophilus 100 MM • Bifidobacterium Bifidus 100 MM. Other Ingredients: Silicon Dioxide, Magnesium Stearate, Gelatin.

Swiss Herbal - The Vitamin Shoppe
Each tablet contains: Senna (Cassia senna) leaves standardized to 3% sennosides 100 mg • Strawberry (Fragaria vesca) leaves 50 mg • Peach (Prunus persica) leaves 50 mg • Anise (Pimpinella anisum) fruit and seeds 50 mg • Cranberry (Vaccinium macrocarpon) fruit 50 mg • Calendula (Calendula officinalis) flower and leaves 25 mg.

Swiss Kriss Tabs - Swiss Kriss
Each tablet contains: Finely powdered sun-dried Senna leaves. Other Ingredients: Finely powdered Strawberry Leaf, Peach Leaf, Anise seed, Caraway seed, Hibiscus flowers, Calendula flowers.

Symbiotropin hGH - ASN - Advanced Sports Nutrition
Each two tablets contain: Anterior Pituitary Peptides Aminotrope-7 (a sequenced glycoamino acid complex) 4200 mg • Novel Polyose Complex (pharmaceutical mono, poly & oligo saccharides) 2230 mg. Base: L-Glutamine, L-Arginine, L-Pyroglutamate, GABA, L-Glycine, L-Lysine, L-Tyrosine, Vica Faba Major.

Sympathyl - Laboratoire Innotech International
Each tablet contains: Hawthorn flower (crataegus oxyacantha) 75 mg • California Poppy extract (eschscholzia californica) 20 mg • Elemental Magnesium (as 124.35 mg magnesium oxide) 75 mg. Product of France; not readily available in the U.S.

Symplex F - Standard Process, Inc.
Each tablet contains: Proprietary Blend 138 mg: Magnesium Citrate, Bovine Ovary extract, Bovine Adrenal extract, Bovine Pituitary extract, Bovine Thyroid extract (thyroxine removed). Other Ingredients: Calcium Lactate, Cellulose, Calcium Stearate.
See Editor's Note No. 31.

Symplex M - Standard Process, Inc.
Each tablet contains: Proprietary Blend 137 mg: Magnesium Citrate, Bovine Orchic extract, Bovine Adrenal extract, Bovine Pituitary extract, Bovine Thyroid extract (thyroxine removed). Other Ingredients: Calcium Lactate, Cellulose, Calcium Stearate.
See Editor's Note No. 14.

Sympt-X Plus - Cambridge Nutraceuticals
Each serving contains: Glutamine 10 g • Vitamin A (as mixed carotenoids) 6500 IU • Vitamin C 330 mg • Vitamin E 100 IU • Selenium 50 mcg. Available in 650 g jar and Single Dose Packets.

Synadrene - Metaphysics - Pro-Soma Enterprises
Each capsule contains: Citrus Aurantium (bitter orange Peel) 350 mg • Chromium Picolinate 400 mcg.
See Editor's Note No. 40.

SynBiotics-1 **-** NutraCea (formerly NutraStar)
Each capsule contains: Stabilized Rice Bran derivative 250 mg • Proprietary Probiotic Blend 250 mg (2.75 billion CFU when shipped): Bifidobacterium Longum, Lactobacillus Rhamnosus A, Lactobacillus Plantarum. Other Ingredients: Maltodextrin, Magnesium Stearate, Hydroxypropylmethyl Cellulose, Metacrylic Acid, Methyl Methacrylate Copolymer.

SynBiotics-2 **-** NutraCea (formerly NutraStar)
Each capsule contains: Stabilized Rice Bran derivative 250 mg • Proprietary Probiotic Blend 250 mg (3 billion CFU when shipped): Bifidobacterium Longum, Lactobacillus Rhamnosus A, Lactobacillus Plantarum. Other Ingredients: Maltodextrin, Magnesium Stearate, Hydroxypropylmethyl Cellulose, Metacrylic Acid, Methyl Methacyrlate Copolymer.

SynBiotics-3 **-** NutraCea (formerly NutraStar)
Each capsule contains: Stabilized Rice Bran derivative 250 mg • Proprietary Probiotic Blend 250 mg (4.5 billion CFU when shipped): Bifidobacterium Longum, Lactobacillus Rhamnosus A, Lactobacillus Plantarum. Other Ingredients: Maltodextrin, Magnesium Stearate, Hydroxypropylmethyl Cellulose, Metacrylic Acid, Methyl Methacrylate Copolymer.

Syndrome X **-** Wild Rose
Each tablet contains: FenuLife brand Fenugreek (trigonella foenum-graecum) 400 mg • Gymnema Sylvestre leaf 50 mg • Bitter Melon 5:1 extract (momordica charantia) 50 mg • Alpha-Lipoic Acid 5 mg.

SyneDrex **-** Metabolic Nutrition, Inc.
Four capsules contain: Advantra Z Citrus Aurantium (30%) 467 mg • Caffeine Anhydrous 700 mg • Green Tea extract (50%/35% polyphenols) 480 mg • Hydroxycitric Acid (garcinia cambogia 50%) 460 mg • Acetyl L-Carnitine 240 mg • L-Tyrosine 320 mg • Glucomannan 800 mg • Naringin 80 mg • Vitamin B6 14 mg • Vitamin B12 400 mcg • Chromium Polynicotinate 700 mcg • 5-HTP 4000 mcg • Simmondsin extract 4000 mcg.
See Editor's Note No. 40.

Synephrine 350 mg **-** GNC
Each capsule contains: Citrus Aurantium Fruit Extract 350 mg. Other Ingredients: Gelatin, Cellulose, Calcium Carbonate.
See Editor's Note No. 40.

Synergistic Iron **-** Quest
Each capsule contains: Iron (HVP Chelate) 25 mg • Copper (HVP Chelate) 2 mg • Molybdenum (HVP Chelate) 50 mcg • Vitamin C (Ascorbic Acid) 100 mg • Niacin 10 mg • Vitamin B1 (Thiamine HCl) 5 mg • Vitamin B6 (Pyridoxine HCl) 5 mg • Vitamin B2 (Riboflavin) 2 mg • Pantothenic Acid (d-Calcium Pantothenate) 10 mg • Folic Acid 0.2 mg • Vitamin B12 (Cobalamin) 20 mcg • Biotin 50 mcg. Other Ingredients: Magnesium Stearate (vegetable source), Microcrystalline Cellulose.

Synergistic Magnesium **-** Quest
Each tablet contains: Magnesium (HVP Chelate) 150 mg • Calcium (HVP Chelate) 30 mg • Phosphorus (HVP Complex) 15 mg • Vitamin B6 (Pyridoxine HCl) 20 mg. Other Ingredients: Croscarmellose Sodium, Magnesium Stearate (vegetable source), Microcrystalline Cellulose, Vegetable Stearin.

Synergistic Manganese **-** Quest
Each capsule contains: Manganese (HVP Chelate) 50 mg • Vitamin B1 (Thiamine HCl) 20 mg • Vitamin C 100 mg. Other Ingredients: Magnesium Stearate (vegetable source), Microcrystalline Cellulose.

Synergistic Multiple Mineral **-** Quest
Each tablet contains: Calcium (HVP Chelate) 100 mg • Magnesium (HVP Chelate) 100 mg • Potassium (HVP Chelate) 33 mg • Iron (HVP Chelate) 5 mg • Manganese (HVP Chelate) 5 mg • Zinc (HVP Chelate) 5 mg • Copper (HVP Chelate) 1 mg • Iodine (Potassium Iodide) 50 mcg • Molybdenum (HVP Chelate) 50 mcg • Chromium (HVP Chelate) 10 mcg • Selenium (HVP Complex) 10 mcg. Other Ingredients: Croscarmellose Sodium, Magnesium Stearate (vegetable source), Mircocrystalline Cellulose, Vegetable Stearin.

Synergistic Selenium **-** Quest
Each capsule contains: Selenium (chelate) 200 mcg • Vitamin E (D-alpha tocopheryl Acetate) 25 IU • Vitamin C 100 mg. Other Ingredients: Magnesium Stearate, Microcrystalline Cellulose.

Synergistic Zinc **-** Quest
Each tablet contains: Vitamin A (Palmitate) 5000 IU • Zinc (HVP Chelate) 20 mg • Copper (HVP Chelate) 1 mg. Other Ingredients: Calcium Phosphate, Croscarmellose Sodium, Magnesium Stearate (vegetable source), Microcrystalline Cellulose, Vegetable Stearin.

Synergy **-** NSI - Nutraceutical Sciences Institute
Each six capsules contain: Vitamin A (beta carotene, alpha carotene, lutein, zeaxanthin, cryptoaxanthin, and palmitate) 5000 IU • Vitamin C (calcium ascorbate) 500 mg • Vitamin D (D3, cholecalciferol) 700 IU • Vitamin E (D-alpha tocopherol succinate, gamma, delta, and beta) 500 IU • Thiamin 50 mg • Riboflavin (vitamin B2) 10 mg • Niacin (vitamin B3) 70 mg • Pyridoxine HCl (vitamin B6) 50 mg • Folic Acid (as folacin) 800 mcg • Vitamin B12 (methylcobalamin) 500 mcg • Biotin 1 mg • Pantothenic Acid (vitamin B5 as d-calcium pantothenate) 50 mg • Calcium from 2,430 mg citrate, malate, and Ester C) 500 mg • Zinc (as l-monomethoinine, OptiZinc) 15 mg • Selenium (selenomethionine) 200 mcg • Iodine (as kelp) 75 mcg • Magnesium (from 1,190 citrate) 200 mg • Manganese (as chelate, AAC) 2 mg • Chromium (as chromium picolinate, Chromates) 200 mcg • Molybdenum (as chelate, AAC) 75 mcg • Potassium (from 417 mg potassium citrate) 150 mg • Garlic (as aged, odorless, standardized 10,000 ppm allicin) 400 mg • Ginkgo Biloba (gonkoaceace, leaves, standardized 24% ginkgo flavon glycosides, 6% terpene lactones) 60 mg • CoEnzyme Q10 10 mg • Alpha Lipoic Acid 30 mg • Bioflavonoid (Citrus BioComplex Standardized to 50%) 50 mg • Bioflavonoid as Quercetin 50 mg • Grape seed extract 50 mg • Lutein extract (from 120 mg FloraGLO) 6 mg • Red Wine extract (standardized 30% polyphenols) 50 mg • Green Tea extract (standardized 98% polyphenols, 80% catechins, 45% EGCG) 50 mg • Plant Enzymes (amylase 2,000 SKB HUT, lipase 25 FIP, and lactase 250 ALU) 50 mg • Black Pepper extract (piper nigrum fruit extract, Bipoerine) 5 mg • Inositol 50 mg • Malic Acid (as calcium citrate malate) 367 mg • Copper (as chelate, AAC) 1 mg.

SynerPro Calcium-Magnesium **-** Nature's Sunshine
Two tablets contain: Vitamin D 100 IU • Calcium (amino acid chelate, di-calcium phosphate) 400 mg • Phosphorus (di-calcium phosphate) 250 mg • Magnesium (oxide) 200 mg • Zinc (oxide) 7.5 mg • Copper (gluconate) 1 mg • Boron (amino acid chelate) 0.5 mg • Proprietary Blend 100 mg: Broccoli flower (brassica oleracea), Carrot root (daucus carota), Red Beet root (beta vulgaris), Rosemary leaf (rosmarinus officinalis), Tomato fruit (solanum lycopersicum), Turmeric root (curcuma longa), Cabbage leaf (brassica oleracea), Chinese Cabbage leaf (brassica rapa), Citrus Bioflavonoids. Other Ingredients: Cellulose, Stearic Acid.

Synerpro Multiple Vitamins & Minerals **-** Nature's Sunshine
Each tablet contains: Vitamin A (beta-carotene) 2,500 IU • Vitamin C 30 mg • Vitamin D 200 IU • Vitamin E (D-alpha tocopherol) 15 IU • Thiamine (vitamin B1) 0.75 mg • Riboflavin (vitamin B2) 0.85 mg • Niacin (as nicotinic acid) 10 mg • Vitamin B6 (pyridoxine HCl) 1 mg • Folate (folic acid) 200 mcg • Vitamin B12 (cyanocobalamin) 3 mcg • Biotin 150 mcg • Pantothenic acid (D-calcium pantothenate) 5 mg • Calcium (D-calcium pantothenate and dicalcium phosphate) 125 mg • Iron (ferrous fumarate) 9 mg • Phosphorus (dicalcium phosphate) 90 mg • Iodine (potassium iodide) 75 mcg • Magnesium (magnesium oxide) 50 mg • Zinc (zinc oxide) 7.5 mg • Selenium (amino acid chelate) 25 mcg • Copper (copper gluconate) 1 mg • Manganese (amino acid chelate) 0.5 mg • Chromium (amino acid chelate) 50 mcg • Molybdenum (amino acid chelate) 38 mcg. Other Ingredients: Broccoli flowers (brassica oleracera), Turmeric root (curcuma longa), Red Beet root (beta vulgaris), Rosemary leaves (rosmarinus officinalis), Wild Carrot root (daucus carota), Tomato fruit (solanum lycopersicum), Chinese Cabbage leaves (brassica rapa), Cabbage leaves (brassica oleracea), Orange Bioflavonoids, Grapefruit Bioflavonoids, Hesperidin, Cellulose (plant fiber), Stearic Acid, Silicon Dioxide (powdered silica).

Some Brand Name Natural Products - What they Contain

www.NaturalDatabase.com contains MANY more listings than appear here.
Editor's Notes are located on pages 2155-2163.

SynoGlide II - Life Enhancement Products, Inc.
Two capsules contain: Molybdenum (as molybdenum gluconate) 100 mcg • N-Acetylglucosamine 187.5 mg • Glucosamine Sulfate 187.5 mg • Chondroitin 4,6-Sulfates 150 mg • Boswellin 300 mg • Curcumin 225 mg • Bromelain 160 mg • Papain 80 mg • Trypsin 50 mg • Pregnenolone 12.5 mg.

SynovoDerma - Allergy Research Group
Three softgels contain: Hyaluronic Acid powder 210 mg. Other Ingredients: Rice Bran Oil, Yellow Beeswax, Titanium Dioxide.

Synthovial 7 - Hyalogic LLC
Hyaluronic Acid 2.15 mg.
See Editor's Note No. 38.

System 343 - Advocare International
Fiber 10: Each pouch (0.7 oz / 20 g) contains: Vitamin A (as beta-carotene) 1000 IU • Vitamin C (as ascorbic acid) 30 mg • Sodium 10 mg • Fructose • Maltodextrin • Citric Acid • Natural Flavors • Artificial Flavors • Acesulfame Potassium • Papaya fruit powder • Prune powder • Rhubarb root extract • Black Walnut hull extract • Licorice root powder • Lactobacillus Acidophilus • Bifidobacterium Bifidum • Digestive Enzyme Complex: Lipase, Cellulase, Protease • Fiber Blend: Psyllium husk, Oats (oat fiber), Carboxymethylcellulose, Guar Gum, Citrus Pectin, Butternut Bark Powder.
Herbal Cleanse: Three caplets contain: Vitamin C (as ascorbic acid) 1200 mg • Thiamine (as HCI) 6 mg • Riboflavin 6.8 mg • Niacin/ Niacinamide 100 mg • Vitamin B6 (as pyridoxine HCI) 10 mg • Folic Acid 400 mcg • Vitamin B12 (as cyanocobalamin) 30 mcg • Biotin 300 mcg • Pantothenic Acid (as calcium pantothenate) 40 mg • OptiZinc Zinc (as monomethionine) 3 mg • Inositol 5 mg • Taurine 800 mg • System 343 Herbal Concentrate 1350 mg: Wheat Grass juice powder, Cranberry juice powder, Burdock root extract, Senna seed extract, Astragalus root extract, Echinacea Purpurea root extract, Milk Thistle leaf extract, Schisandra fruit extract, Beet root powder, Odorless Garlic bulb powder. Other Ingredients: Dicalcium Phosphate, Silicon Dioxide, Cellulose, Stearic Acid, Magnesium Stearate. ProBiotic Restore: Two capsules contain: Vitamin A (as palmitate) 2000 IU • Vitamin A (as beta-carotene) 2000 IU • OptiZinc Zinc (as monomethionine) 1 mg • Lactobacillus Acidophilus 1 billion • Bifidobacterium Bifidum 1 billion • Fructooligosaccharides 500 mg • Moomiyo 50 mg • Aloe Vera leaf extract 100 mg. Other Ingredients: Silicon Dioxide, Magnesium Stearate, Gelatin.

System D-Tox - Nutri-Quest Rx
Six capsules contain: Vitamin A Palmitate 2000 IU • Vitamin C 750 mg • Vitamin B1 20 mg • Niacin 25 mg • Vitamin B12 50 mcg • Folic Acid 300 mcg • Calcium Aspartate 75 mg • Magnesium Glycinate 200 mg • Magnesium Aspartate 100 mg • Chromium Picolinate 50 mcg • Zinc Picolinate 20 mg • N-Acetyl Cysteine 30 mg • L-Glutamine 200 mg • Silymarin extract 5 mg • Quercetin 25 mg • L-Taurine 50 mg • L-Ornithine 20 mg • L-Glutamic Acid 20 mg • L-Carnitine 20 mg • Choline 50 mg • Propolis 20 mg • Yellow Dock 25 mg • Beta Carotene 7500 IU • Vitamin E Succinate Natural 200 IU • Vitamin B2 20 mg • Pyridoxal 5 Phosphate 20 mg • Pantothenic Acid 50 mg • Biotin 200 mcg • Calcium Gluconate 75 mg • Magnesium Citrate 100 mg • Selenomethionine 150 mcg • Manganese Aspartate 5 mg • Molybdenum Citrate 50 mcg • Reduced Glutathione 20 mg • Milk Thistle 50 mg • Beet root 50 mg • Glucaronic Acid 5 mg • L-Glycine 50 mg • L-Methionine 50 mg • L-Arginine 20 mg • L-Tyrosine 20 mg • Inositol 50 mg • Curcumin 5 mg • Chlorophyll 10 mg • Asparagus 15 mg • Dandelion root 25 mg • Siberian Ginseng 30 mg • Broccoli 15 mg • Mullein 25 mg • Co-Enzyme Q-10 1 mg.

Syste-Max (SysteMax) - Goldshield Elite
One heaping teaspoonful (6.8 g) contains: Vitamin A 668 IU • Vitamin C 100 mg • Vitamin E 60 IU • Psyllium seed husk 4000 mg • Soy Germ flour (providing 15 mg of isoflavones) 500 mg • Chitosan 100 mg • Phytosterol complex 100 mg • Oat flour 100 mg.

Sytrinol - J. R. Carlson Laboratories, Inc.
Two softgels contain: Sytrinol Proprietary Blend 300 mg: Natural Citrus extract, Natural Palm fruit extract.

Sytrinol - Source Naturals
Each tablet contains: Calcium 35 mg • Sytrinol (proprietary blend of citrus polymethoxylated flavones and palm tocotrienols) 150 mg. Other Ingredients: Microcrystalline Cellulose, Dibasic Calcium Phosphate, Modified Cellulose Gum, Stearic Acid, Colloidal Dioxide.

Sytropin HGH - Speedwinds Nutrition Inc
Alpha GPC • GABA • Glycine • L-Arginine • L-Dopa bean extract • L-Glutamine • L-Isoleucine • L-Tyrosine • L-Valine • L-Lysine • Moomiyo extract • Ornithine Alpha Ketoglutarate. Inactive Ingredients: Deionized Water, Lecithin Phospholipids, Sodium Citrate, Potassium Sorbate, Maltodextrin, Paraben, Citric Acid.

T2 Pro-Thyroid Formula - BioTest Laboratories, LLC
Each cap contains: 3;5-diiodo-l-thyronine 50 mcg.

T-5W - Dial Herbs
Red Raspberry • Blue Cohosh • Bayberry • Squaw Vine • Blessed Thistle • Ginger • Motherwort • False Unicorn • Wild Yam • Lobelia • Cayenne.

T-ACN - Dial Herbs
Black Walnut • Burdock • Chaparral • Yellow Dock • Sassafras • Valerian.

Tadenan - European; Not available in the US.
Pygeum africanum extract standardized to contain 14% triterpenes and 0.5% n-docosanol usually in dosages of 100 - 200 mg.

T-AFT - Dial Herbs
Wild Lettuce • St. John's Wort • Valerian • Cayenne.

TAG - Metabolic Nutrition, Inc.
Each 2 tsp serving contains: Trans - Alanyl - Glutamine 10 g.

T-AIS - Dial Herbs
Rose Hips • Sage • Yarrow • Burdock • Echinacea • Goldenseal • Yellow Dock • Garlic • Nettle • Lemon Grass • White Oak bark • Black Cohosh • Fenugreek • Juniper berry • Oregon Grape • Plantain • Thyme.

T-AKE - Dial Herbs
Clove Oil • Oat Straw • Lobelia • Cayenne.

Take 10 Bars, Apple Cinnamon - Advocare International
Polydextrose • Dried Apples • Rolled Oats • Raisins • Maltitol Syrup • Figs • Rice Syrup • Oat Fiber • Corn Bran • Glycerin • High Fructose Corn Syrup • Soybean Oil • Natural Flavor • Spice • Arabinogalactan • Fructooligosaccharides • Guar Gum • Honey • Sunflower Oil • Sucralose • Soy Lecithin.

Take Control - Lipton
Water • Liquid Canola Oil • Vegetable Oil Sterol Esters • Liquid Sunflower Oil • Partially Hydrogenated Soybean Oil • Salt • Whey • Vegetable Mono- and Diglycerides • Potassium Sorbate • Lactic Acid • Calcium Disodium EDTA • Soy Lecithin • Artificial Flavor • Beta Carotene • Vitamin A (Palmitate).

Take Heart - Allergy Research Group
Each scoop (20 g) contains: Vitamin A (as beta-carotene) 2000 IU • Vitamin C (as ascorbic acid) 500 mg • Vitamin D (D3) 100 IU • Vitamin E (as D-alpha-tocopherol) 320 IU • Vitamin K 80 mcg • Thiamin (vitamin B1) 30 mg • Riboflavin (vitamin B2) 30 mg • Niacin 160 mg • Vitamin B6 16 mg • Folic Acid 320 mg • Vitamin B12 80 mcg • Biotin 240 mcg • Pantothenic Acid 100 mg • Calcium (as calcium citrate/gluconate) 280 mg • Magnesium (as magnesium glycinate/gluconate) 160 mg • Zinc (as zinc arginate) 12 mg • Selenium (as sodium selenite/selenomethionine) 80 mcg • Copper (as copper glycinate) 0.8 mg • Manganese (as manganese glycinate) 1 mg • Chromium (as chromium polynicotinate) 160 mcg • Molybdenum (as sodium molybdate) 40 mcg • Potassium (as potassium gluconate) 40 mg • Boron (as boron citrate) 0.4 mg • Vanadium (as vanadium pentoxide) 80 mcg • Alpha-Carotene 8 mg • Pregnenolone 6 mg • Dehydroepiandrosterone (DHEA) 6 mg • Coenzyme Q10 60 mg • Inositol 50 mg • Choline 50 mg • Para-Aminobenzoic Acid (PABA) 20 mg • Lecithin (26% phosphatidylcholine) 500 mg • L-Alanine

BRAND NAMES

30 mg • L-Arginine 480 mg • L-Aspartic Acid 85 mg • L-Carnitine 200 mg • L-Cystine 10 mg • L-Glutamine 600 mg • Glycine 30 mg • L-Histidine 20 mg • L-Isoleucine 35 mg • L-Leucine 60 mg • L-Lysine 45 mg • L-Methionine 160 mg • L-Ornithine 200 mg • L-Phenylalanine 38 mg • L-Proline 38 mg • L-Serine 38 mg • Taurine 500 mg • L-Threonine 28 mg • L-Tyrosine 220 mg • L-Valine 40 mg • N-Acetyl-L-Cysteine 200 mg • Glutathione 100 mg • Pancreatin 10 mg • Papain 16 mg • Bromelain 20 mg • Grape skin extract 200 mg • Hawthorn berry extract 200 mg • Garlic (1% allicin) 100 mg • Lutein 2 mg • Lycopene 0.4 mg • Tocotrienols 20 mg • Trimethylglycine 200 mg • Methylsulfonylmethane 80 mg • Eicosapentaenoic Acid (EPA) 145 mg • Docosahexaenoic Acid (DHA) 95 mg • Gamma-Linolenic Acid 90 mg • Linolenic Acid 220 mg • Oleic Acid 85 mg • Palmitic Acid 65 mg • Stearic Acid 25 mg • Flax Seed oil 400 mg • Lipoic Acid 30 mg. Other Ingredients: Oat Bran, Honey Powder, Rice Bran, Psyllium Bran, Apple Fiber, Lemon Flavor, Stevia.

Take Heart II without Hormones - Allergy Research Group
Each scoop (20 g) contains: Vitamin A (as beta-carotene) 2000 IU • Vitamin C (as ascorbic acid) 500 mg • Vitamin D (D3) 100 IU • Vitamin E (as D-alpha-tocopherol) 320 IU • Vitamin K 80 mcg • Thiamin (vitamin B1) 30 mg • Riboflavin (vitamin B2) 30 mg • Niacin 160 mg • Vitamin B6 16 mg • Folic Acid 320 mg • Vitamin B12 80 mcg • Biotin 240 mcg • Pantothenic Acid 100 mg • Calcium (citrate/gluconate) 280 mg • Magnesium (glycinate/gluconate) 160 mg • Zinc (as zinc arginate) 12 mg • Selenium (sodium selenite/ selenomethionine) 80 mcg • Copper (glycinate) 0.8 mg • Manganese (as manganese glycinate) 1 mg • Chromium (polynicotinate) 160 mcg • Molybdenum (as sodium molybdate) 40 mcg • Potassium (as potassium gluconate) 40 mg • Boron (citrate) 0.4 mg • Vanadium (as vanadium pentoxide) 80 mcg • Alpha-Carotene 8 mg • Coenzyme Q10 60 mg • Inositol 50 mg • Choline 50 mg • Para-Aminobenzoic Acid (PABA) 20 mg • Lecithin (26% phosphatidylcholine) 500 mg • L-Alanine 30 mg • L-Arginine 480 mg • L-Aspartic Acid 85 mg • L-Carnitine 200 mg • L-Cystine 10 mg • L-Glutamine 600 mg • Glycine 30 mg • L-Histidine 20 mg • L-Isoleucine 35 mg • L-Leucine 60 mg • L-Lysine 45 mg • L-Methionine 160 mg • L-Ornithine 200 mg • L-Phenylalanine 38 mg • L-Proline 38 mg • L-Serine 38 mg • Taurine 500 mg • L-Threonine 28 mg • L-Tyrosine 220 mg • L-Valine 40 mg • N-Acetyl-L-Cysteine 200 mg • Glutathione 100 mg • Pancreatin 10 mg • Papain 16 mg • Bromelain 20 mg • Grape skin extract 200 mg • Hawthorn berry extract 200 mg • Garlic (1% allicin) 100 mg • Lutein 2 mg • Lycopene 0.4 mg • Tocotrienols 20 mg • Trimethylglycine 200 mg • Methylsulfonylmethane 80 mg • Eicosapentaenoic Acid (EPA) 145 mg • Docosahexaenoic Acid (DHA) 95 mg • Gamma-Linolenic Acid 90 mg • Linolenic Acid 220 mg • Oleic Acid 85 mg • Palmitic Acid 65 mg • Stearic Acid 25 mg • Flax Seed oil 400 mg • Lipoic Acid 30 mg. Other Ingredients: Oat Bran, Honey Powder, Rice Bran, Psyllium Bran, Apple Fiber, Lemon Flavor, Stevia.

T-ALER - Dial Herbs
Bayberry • Echinacea • Yarrow • Wild Cherry • Cayenne • Goldenseal.

T-ANEM - Dial Herbs
Comfrey • Dandelion • Barberry • Parsley • Yellow Dock • Myrrh • Kelp.

Tang Kuei Plus - Herbalife International of America, Inc.
Each tablet contains: Calcium (as dicalcium phosphate) 40 mg • Tang Kuei root 200 mg • German Chamomile flower 200 mg. Other Ingredients: Starch, Stearic Acid, Hydrogenated Vegetable Oil, Silicon Dioxide, Magnesium Stearate, Dextrin, Sodium Dextrose Monohydrate, Carboxymethylcellulose, Soy Lecithin, Sodium Citrate.

Taraxatone - Cytodyne LLC
Six capsules contain: Vitamin B6 24 mg • Magnesium 8.4 mg • Dandelion leaf powder 1500 mg • Uva Ursi leaf extract 900 mg • Guarana extract 600 mg • Taurine 115 mg.

T-ARTH - Dial Herbs
Yucca • Alfalfa • Buckthorn • Burdock • Parsley • Slippery Elm • Yarrow • Cayenne.

Tarvil - SHS North America
Each 15 g packet contains: L-Leucine • L-Valine • L-Isoleucine • Sugar • Guar Gum • Artificial Color (beta carotene) • Soy Lecithin • Citric Acid • Artificial Flavor (pineapple) • Artificial Sweetener (Acesulfame K).

T-ASMA - Dial Herbs
Blood root • St. John's Wort • Mullein • Comfrey • Saw Palmetto • Wild Cherry bark • Goldenseal • Lobelia • Cayenne.

Taurine - Ortho Molecular Products
Each capsule contains: Taurine 500 mg. Other Ingredients: Natural Vegetable Capsules, Ascorbyl Palmitate, Microcrystalline Cellulose, Silicon Dioxide.

Taurine - J. R. Carlson Laboratories, Inc.
Each 1 tsp serving contains: Taurine 4000 mg.

Taurine 1000 - Pain & Stress Center
Each capsule contains: Vitamin C (ascorbyl palmitate) 10 mg • Taurine 1000 mg.

Taurine 1000 - Jarrow Formulas
Each capsule contains: Taurine 1000 mg. Other Ingredients: Magnesium Stearate, Gelatin.

Taurine 1000 mg - Pure Encapsulations
Each vegetable capsule contains: Taurine 1000 mg • Vitamin C (as ascorbyl palmitate) 10 mg.

Taurine 500 - GNC
Each tablet contains: Taurine 500 mg. Other Ingredients: Dicalcium Phosphate, Cellulose.

Taurine 500 mg - Pure Encapsulations
Each vegetable capsule contains: Taurine 500 mg • Vitamin C (as ascorbyl palmitate) 5 mg.

Taurine 500 mg - Solgar
Each capsule contains: Taurine 500 mg. Other Ingredients: Vegetable Cellulose, Microcrystalline Cellulose, Vegetable Stearic Acid, Water, Vegetable Glycerin.

Taurine 750 mg - Vital Nutrients
Each capsule contains: Taurine (free form) 750 mg.

Taurine Plus - American Biologics
Each 1 mL serving contains: Taurine 75 mg. Other Ingredients: Distilled Water.

Taurox SB 6X Enhanced - Allergy Research Group
Active Ingredients: Abies Nigra 6X (14%), 12X (1%), 30X (1%) • Aloe Socotrina 6X (14%), 12X (1%), 30X (1%) • Arnica Montana 6X (14%), 12X (1%), 30X (1%) • Cactus Grandiflora 6X (14%), 12X (1%), 30X (1%) • Lycopodium Clavatum 6X (14%), 12X (1%), 30X (1%) • Tauroxicum (carbobenzoxy beta-alanyl taurine or TAUROX SB) 6X (14%), 12X (1%), 30X (1%) • Calcarea Carbonica 8X (14%), 12X (1%), 30X (1%). Inactive Ingredients: 20% Ethanol, Water.
See Editor's Note No. 1.

Taurox SB 7X with Minerals - Allergy Research Group
Active Ingredients: Kalir Carbonicum 8X (13%), 12X (1%), 30X (1%) • Phosphoricum Acidum 8X (13%), 12X (1%), 30X (1%) • Selenium Metallicum 8X (13%), 12X (1%), 30X (1%) • Silicea 8X (13%), 12X (1%), 30X (1%) • Tauroxicum (carbobenzoxy beta-alanyl taurine or TAUROX SB) 7X (33&), 12X (1%), 30X (1%) • Zincum Metallicum 8X (13%), 12X (1%), 30X (1%). Inactive Ingredients: 20% Ethanol, Purified Water.
See Editor's Note No. 1.

Taurus Male Nutrient Complex - Starlight International
Each three tablets contain: Vitamin C (as calcium ascorbate and magnesium ascorbate) 180 mg • Vitamin E - Dry (as d alpha tocopheryl succinate) 75 IU • Vitamin B1 (as thiamine mononitrate) 30 mg • Vitamin B2 (riboflavin) 30 mg • Niacin 15 mg • Vitamin B6 (pyridoxine HCl) 30 mg • Folic Acid 150 mcg • Vitamin B12 (as cyanocobalamin) 30 mcg • Magnesium (as magnesium ascorbate)

18 mg • Potassium (as potassium glycerophosphate) 7.5 mg • Saw Palmetto berry extract, 4:1 (serenoa repens, fruit) 300 mg • Ashwagandha extract, 4:1 (Withania somnifera dunai, root) 300 mg • He Shou Wu extract, 4:1 (polygonum multiflorum thunb, root) 225 mg • Oriental Ginseng (panax ginseng, root) 150 mg • Kelp 30 mg • Spirulina 30 mg. Inactive Ingredients: Silicon Dioxide, Tricalcium Phosphate, Microcrystalline Cellulose, Hydroxypropylcellulose, Stearic Acid, Rice Flour, Dicalcium Phosphate, Croscarmellose Sodium, Magnesium Stearate, Dextrin , Dextrose, Lecithin, Sodium Citrate, Mono and Diglycerides.

T-BB **- Dial Herbs**
Buckthorn • Yellow Dock • Garlic • Cayenne • Dandelion • Poke root.

T-BC **- Dial Herbs**
White Oak bark • Comfrey • Black Walnut • Marshmallow root • Mullein • Gravel root • Wormwood • Lobelia • Scullcap • Glycerine.

T-BDW **- Dial Herbs**
Corn Silk • Plantain • St. John's Wort • Sanicle • Mullein • Sarsaparilla • Cubeb berries • Watermelon seeds • Cayenne.

T-BF **- Dial Herbs**
Oat Straw • Shavegrass • Comfrey • Slippery Elm • Burdock • Lobelia.

T-CAC **- Dial Herbs**
Buckthorn • Burdock • Chaparral • Dandelion • Cascara Sagrada • Licorice • Red Clover • Barberry.

T-CIRC **- Dial Herbs**
Witch Hazel • Garlic • Ginger • Cayenne.

T-CS **- Dial Herbs**
Bayberry • Myrrh • Echinacea • Goldenseal • Cayenne.

T-DI **- Dial Herbs**
Hyssop • Garlic • Hydrangea • Catnip • Peppermint • Cayenne.

T-DIA **- Dial Herbs**
Yarrow • Juniper berries • Huckleberry • Cayenne • Goldenseal.

T-DREA **- Dial Herbs**
Witch Hazel • Slippery Elm • Ginger • Shepherd's Purse • Raspberry.

T-DRY **- Dial Herbs**
Sage • Yarrow.

T-DTX **- Dial Herbs**
Echinacea • Yellow Dock • Garlic • Lobelia • Cayenne.

Tea Tree Oil **- Holista**
Tea Tree oil (Melaleuca alternifolia) 100% pure.

Tea4Life **- 4 Life**
Each teabag contains: Proprietary Blend 2 g: Senna leaf (cassia acutifolia), Stevia leaf (stevia rebaudiana), Cinnamon leaf (cinnamomum cassia), Buckthorn bark (rhamnus cathartica), Ginger root (zingiber officinale), Natural Apple flavor, Citri Sinensis peel (orange), Green Tea leaf (camellia sinensis), Bitter Orange fruit (citrus aurantium), Echinacea leaf (echinacea angustifolia), Rooibos leaf (aspalathus linearis), Astragalus root (astragalus membranaceus).
See Editor's Note No. 40.

Teavigo **- Pure Encapsulations**
Each vegetable capsule contains: Green Tea extract (standardized to 94% EGCG) 150 mg • Vitamin C (as ascorbyl palmitate) 10 mg.

T-EC **- Dial Herbs**
Eyebright • Bayberry • Passion flower • Goldenseal • Cayenne.

Teen Advantage Creatine Serum **- Muscle Marketing USA**
Each serving contains: Creatine Monohydrate • Glucosamine • Vitamin B12 • L-Glutamine • Sodium Pyruvate • Royal Jelly • Ginseng • Honey • Natural Glycerine • Natural Flavor • Water.

Teen Essentials **- Rexall - Sundown**
Two tablets contain: Vitamin A (from retinyl palmitate) 10000 IU • Vitamin C 400 mg • Vitamin D (as cholecalciferol) 400 IU • Vitamin E (as d-alpha-tocopheryl acid succinate and dl-alpha-tocopheryl acetate) 100 IU • Thiamin (as thiamin HCl) 50 mg • Riboflavin (Vitamin B2) 50 mg • Niacin (as niacinamide) 100 mg • Vitamin B-6 (from pyridoxine HCl) 50 mg • Folic Acid 400 mcg • Vitamin B-12 (as cyanocobalamin) 50 mcg • Biotin 150 mcg • Pantothenic Acid (from calcium d-pantothenate) 100 mg • Calcium 200 mg • Iron (from ferrous fumarate) 9 mg • Phosphorus 154 mg • Iodine (from potassium iodide) 75 mg • Magnesium (from magnesium oxide) 100 mg • Zinc (from zinc gluconate) 22 mg • Manganese (from manganese gluconate) 3 mg • Potassium (from potassium gluconate) 90 mg • Choline Bitartrate 100 mg • Para-Aminobenzoic Acid 30 mg • Inositol 10 mg. Other Ingredients: Dicalcium Phosphate, Cellulose, Stearic Acid, Croscarmellose Sodium, Silica, Magnesium Stearate, Hydroxypropyl Methylcellulose, PEG.

Teen Link **- Pain & Stress Center**
Each capsule contains: Vitamin C (as ascorbyl palmitate) 6 mg • Vitamin B6 (pyridoxine HCl) 5 mg • L-Tyrosine 175 mg • Gamma Amino Butyric Acid (GABA) 120 mg • L-Taurine 110 mg • L-Glutamine 100 mg • 5-Hydroxytryptophan (5-HTP) 25 mg. Other Ingredients: Gelatin Capsule.

Teething Gel **- Hyland's**
Calcarea phosphorica as Calcium phosphate 12X HPUS • Chamomilla as Chamomile 6X HPUS • Coffea cruda as Coffee 6X HPUS • Belladonna (Alkaloids 0.0000003%) 6X HPUS. In a base of Deionized Water, Vegetable Glycerin, Hydroxyethyl Cellulose, Methyl Paraben, Propyl Paraben.
See Editor's Note No. 1.

Teething Tablets **- Hyland's**
Each tablet contains: Calcarea phosphorica as Calcium Phosphate 3X HPUS • Chamomilla as Chamomile 3X HPUS • Coffea cruda as Coffee 3X HPUS • Belladonna as Alkaloids 0.0003% 3X HPUS. In a base of Lactose NF (Milk Sugar).
See Editor's Note No. 1.

Tegreen 97 **- Pharmanex**
Each 250 mg capsule contains a 15:1 extract of Green Tea extract that is standardized to contain a minimum of 97% pure polyphenols including >160 mg of catechins of which >100 mg is EGC.

Ten Mushroom Combination **- Smart Basics**
Each capsule contains: Cordyceps • Reishi • Maitake • Shiitake • Coriolus • Umbellatus Polyporus • Wood Ear • Tremella • Poria • Hericium.

T-ENDO **- Dial Herbs**
Chaparral • Pipsissewa • Licorice • Prickly Ash • Cramp bark • False Unicorn • Saw Palmetto • Red Clover.

Tenshin Essentials Elastase **- Taiko Healthcare, Inc.**
Each tablet contains: Elastase 20 mg. Other Ingredients: Dextran, Talc, Lactose Cellulose, Hydroxy Propyl Cellulose, Silicic Acid Anhydride, Magnesium Stearate, Titanium Dioxide, Methyl-Methacrylate Copolymer, Glycerol Fatty Acid Ester.

Tenshin Essentials Nattokin Plus **- Taiko Pharmaceutical Co., Ltd.**
Each tablet contains: Nattokin (bacillis subtilis) 7 mg • Oligosaccharide 100 mg • Enterocuccuss Faecium 21 mg. Other Ingredients: Vitamin B6, Vitamin B5, Vitamin B3, Vitamin B1, Vitamin C, Starch, Lactose, Glycerol Fatty Acid.

Tenshin Essentials Nattokin Plus Calcium **- Taiko Pharmaceutical Co., Ltd.**
Each tablet contains: Nattokin (bacillis subtilis) 7 mg • Oligosaccharide 100 mg • Calcium 100 mg. Other Ingredients: Vitamin B6, Vitamin B3, Vitamin B1, Vitamin B5, Vitamin C, Starch, Lactose, Glycerol Fatty Acid, Flavoring, Corn Starch.

Tenshin Essentials Nattokin Plus Iron - Taiko Pharmaceutical Co., Ltd.
Each tablet contains: Nattokin (bacillis subtilis) 7 mg • Oligosaccharide 100 mg • Iron 9.42 mg. Other Ingredients: Vitamin B6, Vitamin B3, Vitamin B1, Vitamin B5, Vitamin C, Starch, Lactose, Glycerol Fatty Acid.

Tenshin Essentials Nattokin Plus Vitamin C & E - Taiko Pharmaceutical Co., Ltd.
Each tablet contains: Nattokin (bacillis subtilis) 7 mg • Oligosaccharide 100 mg • Vitamin C 103 mg • Vitamin E 30 IU. Other Ingredients: Vitamin B6, Vitamin B3, Vitamin B1, Vitamin B5, Starch, Lactose, Glycerol Fatty Acid.

Tenshin Essentials Seirogan - Taiko Pharmaceutical Co., Ltd.
Three tablets contain: Creosote 67 mg • Geranium 75 mg • Phellodendron 75 mg. Other Ingredients: Talc, Calcium Carbonate, Carmellose Calcium.

tension & stress - Nelson Bach
Active Indredients: Kali Phos 6C HPUS • Arnica 6C HPUS. Other Ingredients: Lactose, Sucrose.
See Editor's Note No. 1.

Tension Tamer Extra - Celestial Seasonings
Two capsules contain: Vitamin B6 6 mg • Vitamin B12 (cyanocobalamin) 12 mcg • Magnesium (ascorbate and oxide) 60 mg • Proprietary Blend 1180 mg: Kava Kava root extract, Chamomile.

Tentex Forte - The Himalaya Drug Company
Each tablet contains: Latakasthuri (abelmoschus moshatus) 10 mg • Ashvagandha (withania somnifera) 65 mg • Vriddadaru (argyreia speciosa syn. a.nervosa) 32 mg • Kapikachchhu (mucuna pruriens) 32 mg • Trivang 32 mg: Lead (naga), Tin (vanga), Zinc (yasada) • Shilajeet (mineral pitch, purified) 32 mg • Kumkuma (crocus sativus) 16 mg • Shudha Kupilu (strychnos nux vomica, detoxified) 16 mg • Makardhwaj (sulphide of mercury) 16 mg • Salabmisri (orchis mascula) 16 mg • Akarakarabha (anacyclus pyrethrum) 16 mg • Bala (sida cordifolia) 16 mg • Shalmali (bombax ceiba) 16 mg • Maricha (piper nigrum) 5 mg.
See Editor's Note No. 39.

Tentex Royal - The Himalaya Drug Company
Each capsule contains: Kokilaksha (asteracantha longifolia) 145 mg • Vathada (prunus amygdalus) 126 mg • Sunishannaka (blepharis edulis) 115 mg • Kumkuma (crocus sativus) 14 mg • Gokshura (tribulus terrestris) 100 mg.

T-ER - Dial Herbs
Eyebright • Bayberry • Passion flower • Goldenseal • Cayenne • Mineral Water • Honey.

TerraSport Lotion SPF 15 - All Terrain Company
Active Ingredients: Zinc Oxide • Octyl Methoxycinnamate. Inactive Ingredients: Water, Aloe Vera Gel, Octyl Palmitate, Glycerin, Cetearyl Glucoside, Glyceryl Stearate, PEG-100 Stearate, Tricontanyl PVP, Beeswax, Magnesium Aluminum Silicate, Arginine, Rose Hip Seed Oil, Xanthan Gum, Arginine, Squalane, Glycereth-26, Tocopheryl Acetate (vitamin E acetate), Ascorbyl Palmitate (vitamin C palmitate), Retinyl Palmitate (vitamin A palmitate), Cholecalciferol (vitamin D3), Capryl Glycine, Methylparaben, Propylparaben.

TerraSport Lotion SPF 30+ - All Terrain Company
Active Ingredients: Zinc Oxide • Octyl Methoxycinnamate. Inactive Ingredients: Water, Aloe Vera Gel, Cetearyl Glucoside, Glyceryl Stearate, PEG-100 Stearate, Tricontanyl PVP, Starch, Magnesium Aluminum Silicate, Arginine, Rose Hip Seed Oil, Tocopheryl Acetate (vitamin E acetate), Ascorbyl Palmitate (vitamin C palmitate), Retinyl Palmitate (vitamin A palmitate), Cholecalciferol (vitamin D3), Capryl Glycine, Methylparaben, Propylparaben.

Testatropinol tablets - ASN - Advanced Sports Nutrition
Each 90 mg tablet contains: Testosterone, Growth Hormone (GH), Adrenalinum, Adrenocorticotropic Hormone (ACTH), Lutenizing Hormone (LH), Progesterone, Esterone.

Testomax - VitalMax Vitamins
Each tablet contains: Zinc (amino acid chelate) 15 mg • Vitamin B12 (as cyanocobalamin) 25 mcg • Tribulus Terrestris powder 250 mg • Saw Palmetto berry extract (25%) 250 mg • Yohimbe extract 250 mg • Damiana powder 100 mg • Korean Ginseng extract 80 mg • Ginkgo Biloba leaf 80 mg • Muira Puama powder 50 mg • Indole 3 Carbinol 50 mg • Chrysin powder 50 mg • 4-Androstenediol powder 5 mg • 19-Nor-4 Androstenedione powder 5 mg • 19-Nor-4 Androstenediol powder 5 mg. Other Ingredients: Stearic Acid, Terra Alba.
See Editor's Note No. 54.

Testostazine - MedLean
Each tablet contains: Proprietary Blend 1170 mg: Maca root (lepidium meyenii, standardized to 0.6% total glucosinolates), Yerba Mate extract (Ilex paraguariensis leaf, 4:1 extract), N-Acetyl-L-Tyrosine, Blueberry extract (Vaccinium corymbosum leaf, standardized to 25% total polyphenols), Elderberry extract (Sambucus nigra fruit, standardized to 15% total polyphenols, 5% total flavonoids), Pyridoxal-5-Phosphate. Other Ingredients: Rice Flour, Gelatin, Water, Silicon Dioxide.

Testosterone Booster - Life Extension
Each capsule contains: 4- Androstenedione 10 mg • 5-Androstenedione 10 mg • 5-Androstenediol 5 mg • 19-Nor-4-Androstenedione 5 mg • 19-Nor-5- Androstenedione 5 mg • Chrysin 50 mg • Velvet Deer Antler 50 mg.
See Editor's Note No. 47 and No. 54.

Testosterone Fuel Booster - TwinLab
Two capsules contain: Natural Testosterone Boosters DHEA (Dehydroepiandrosterone) (Pure Pharmaceutical Grade) 50 mg • Zinc (from Zinc Picolinate) 50 mg • Natural LH Boosters Acetyl-L-Carnitine 500 mg • Tribulus Terrestris extract 150 mg • Natural Aromatase Inhibitor (anti-estrogen) • Novasoy Purified Soy extract (providing 40% isoflavones)(providing isoflavones 80 mg including: Genistein39 mg, Daidzein 34 mg & Glycitein 7 mg) 200 mg • Natural DHT Inhibitors • Saw Palmetto (Serenoa repens) extract 120 mg • Phytosterol Complex (130 mg of Beta-Sitosterol) 250 mg.

Testralin - Metagenics
Three tablets contain: Vitamin A (50% as Betatene brand mixed carotenoids and 50% as retinyl palmitate) 2500 IU • Vitamin D (as cholecaliferol) 200 IU • Vitamin E (as D-alpha tocopheryl acetate) 200 Iu • Vitami K 40 mcg • Vitamin B6 (as pyridoxine hydrochloride) 50 mg • ActiFolate brand Folate (as Metafolin brand L-5-methyl tetrahydrofolate, folic acid, and 5-formyl tetrahydrofolate) 800 mcg • Vitamin B12 (as methylcobalamin and cyanocobalamin) 30 mcg • Trimethylglycine 200 mg • Chrysin 90 mg • Isoflavones (from a proprietary blend of red clover flowering tops extract (trifolium pratense), and kudzu root extract (pueraria lobata) 100 mg • Turmeric rhizome extract (curcuma longa, standardized to 95% (200 mg) curcuminoids) 210 mg • Rosemary leaf extract (rosmarinus officinalis, contains 5.1%-7.6% (10.2 mg-15.2 mg) carnosic acid/carnosol) 200 mg • Resveratrol 2 mg.

Testron SX - Nutraceutics Corp.
Two caplets contain: Boron (chelate) 3 mg • Proprietary Blend TSX Synergistic 1650 mg: Proteusterone (dioscorea machro stachya), Smilex Aristolochiafolii (dried root), Orchic Substance (bovine), Tribulus Terrestris (dried root), Leucine (as l-leucine hydrochloride) • Testrasterone Complex 360 mg: Ptychopetalum olacoides (dried root, dried trunk), Avena sativa (dried leaf and stem), Pfaffia paniculata (dried root), Urtica dioica (dried flowering plant and root).
See Editor's Note No. 14.

TestronRX - Nutraceutics Corp.
Two caplets contain: Boron (chelate) 3 mg • TSX Synergisitc Blend 1650 mg: Dioscorea Macrostachya (proteusterone), Smilax Aristolochiaefolii (dried root), Orchic Substance (bovine), Tribulus Terrestris (dried root), Leucine (as l-leucine hydrochloride) • Testrasterone Complex 360 mg: Ptychopetalum Olacoides (dried root, trunk), Avena Sativa (dried leaf, stem), Pfaffia Paniculata (dried root), Urtica Dioica (dried flowering plant, root).
See Editor's Note No. 14.

Tetrazene KGM-90 - BioQuest Pharmaceuticals
Two capsules contain: Vitamin B6 2 mg • Biotin 200 mcg • Proprietary Blend 507 mg: KGM-90 Glucomannan, Glutamine, Olive leaf extract. Other Ingredients: Magnesium Stearate, Gelatin, Water.

tf Age Defying Effects Hydrating Cleanser - 4 Life
Water • Sodium Laureth Sulfate • Sodium Cocoyl Isethionate • PEG-8 • Sodium Methyl Cocoyl Taurate • Aloe Barbadensis leaf juice • PEG-7 Glyceryl Cocoate • Lauramide MEA • Disodium Laureth Sulfosuccinate • Cocamidopropyl Betaine • Transfer Factor XF • Phospho-lipids • Sodium PCA • Panthenol • Algae extract • Citrus Aurantium var. Dulcis oil • PEG-120 Methyl Glucose Dioleate • Glycol Stearate • Disodium EDTA • Citric Acid • Sodium Chloride • Phenoxyethanol • Methylparaben • Ethyl-Paraben • Propylparaben • Butylparaben • Isobutylparaben.

tf Age Defying Effects Protective Moisturizer - 4 Life
Active Ingredients: (SPF 15 UVA/UVB) Ethylhexyl Methoxycinamate • Zinc Oxide. Other Ingredients: Water • Octyldodecyl Neopentanoate • Aloe Barbadensis leaf juice • Dicaprylyl Maleate • Cyclomethicone • Transfer Factor XF • Glycerin • Polyglyceryl-4 Isostearate • Cetyl Dimethicone Copolyol • Hexyl Laurate • Squalane • Ubiquinone (CoQ10) • Hyaluronic Acid • Tocopherol • Algae Extract • Retinyl Palmitate • Cetyl Laurate • Phospholipids • Citrus Aurantium var. Dulcis oil • Hydrogenated Casein • Ceratonia Siliqua Gum • Dimethicone • Microcrystaline Wax • Hydrogenated Castor Oil • Sodium Chloride • Phenoxyethanol • Methylparaben • Ethylparaben • Propylparaben • Butylparaben • Isobutylparaben.

tf Age Defying Effects Purifying Cleanser - 4 Life
Water • C12-15 Alkyl Benzoate • Dicaprylyl Maleate • Methyl Gluceth-20 • Glyceryl Stearate • PEG-100 Stearate • Cetyl Alcohol • Transfer Factor XF • Epilobium Angustifolium extract • Aloe Barbadensis leaf juice • Sodium Hyaluronate • Hamamelis Virginiana distillate (Witch Hazel) • Sodium Lactate • Sodium PCA • Sorbital • Proline • Citrus Aurantium var. Dulcis oil • Carbomer • Triethanolamine • Polysorbate 20 • Disodium EDTA • Phenoxyethonol • Methylparaben • Ethylparaben • Propylparaben • Butylparaben • Isobutylparaben.

tf Age Defying Effects Renewing Serum - 4 Life
Cyclomethicone • Polysilicone-11 • Ethylhexyl Hydroxystearate • Ascorbic Acid • Transfer Factor XF • Ubiquinone (coQ10) • Hyaluronic Acid • Tocopherol • Phospholipids • Retinyl Palmitate • Bisabolol • Squalane • Citrus Aurantium var. Dulcis oil.

TF Immune Spray - 4 Life
Each spray contains: Transfer Factor XF (bovine colostrum) 25 mg.

TF Kids - 4 Life
Each tablet contains: Vitamin A (as 60% beta carotene, 40% retinyl palmitate) 2500 IU • Vitamin C (as ascorbic acid, sodium ascorbate) 50 mg • Vitamin D (as cholecalciferol) 200 IU • Vitamin E (as D-alpha tocopheryl succinate) 12.5 IU • Vitamin K (phytonadione) 15 mcg • Thiamin (as thiamin mononitrate) 0.5 mg • Riboflavin 0.6 mg • Niacin (as niacinamide) 7 mg • Vitamin B6 (as pyridoxine hydrochloride) 0.7 mg • Folic Acid 140 mcg • Vitamin B12 (as cyanocobalamin) 2 mcg • Biotin (D-biotin) 100 mcg • Pantothenic Acid (as D-calcium pantothenate) 3.5 mg • Calcium (as carbonate) 25 mg • Iron (as carbonyl iron) 3 mg • Iodine (as potassium iodide) 38 mcg • Magnesium (as magnesium oxide, magnesium amino acid chelate) 25 mg • Zinc (as zinc oxide, amino acid chelate) 5 mg • Selenium (as L-selenomethionine) 25 mcg • Copper (as cupric gluconate) 0.7 mg • Manganese (as amino acid chelate) 0.7 mg • Chromium (as nicotinate) 40 mcg • Transfer Factor XF concentrate with other natural components from Bovine Colostrum 150 mg • Stevia extract 230 mcg. Other Ingredients: Fructose, Sorbitol, Mannitol, Grape Extract, Stearic Acid, Natural Flavors, Carrageenan, Cellulose, Magnesium Stearate, Citric Acid.

T-FC1 - Dial Herbs
Red Raspberry • Black Cohosh • Lady Slipper • Blessed Thistle • Damiana.

T-FC2 - Dial Herbs
Black Cohosh • Licorice root • Sarsaparilla • Ginseng • Goldenseal.

T-FC3 - Dial Herbs
Black Cohosh • Wood Betony • Blessed Thistle • Chamomile • Fennel • Ginger • Cayenne.

T-FC4 - Dial Herbs
Wood Betony • Sarsaparilla • Valerian • Blessed Thistle • Dandelion • Garlic • Chamomile.

T-FLO - Dial Herbs
Sanicle • Marshmallow • Fennel • Blessed Thistle • Ginger.

T-FVR - Dial Herbs
Peppermint • Garlic • Valerian • Yarrow • Echinacea • Goldenseal • Cayenne • Lobelia.

T-GB - Dial Herbs
Dandelion • Oregon Grape • Rhubarb • Bayberry • Yellow Dock • Lobelia.

T-GS - Dial Herbs
Catnip • Peppermint • Fennel • Cayenne • Lobelia.

T-H - Dial Herbs
White Willow bark • Valerian • Scullcap • Wood Betony.

TH-1 Probiotics - Jarrow Formulas
Each 1 tsp serving contains: Organic Fermented Soy milk (fermented with L. plantarum R202 and L. casei R256) 4.83 g • Tyndallized bacteria 100 mg: Lactobacillus Casei R256 50 mg, Lactobacillus Plantarum R206 50 mg • Bifidobacterium Longum BB536 10 mg.

Thai-Go - Nature's Sunshine
Reconstituted Mangosteen fruit (garcinia mangostana) • Concord Grape fruit concentrate (vitis labrusca) • Red Grape fruit concentrate (vitis vinifera) • Blueberry fruit concentrate (vaccinium corymbosum) • Red Raspberry fruit concentrate (rubus idaeus) • Red Grape skin extract (vitis vinifera) • Wolfberry Lycium fruit extract (lycium barbarum) • Sea Buckthorn fruit extract (hippophae rhamnoides) • Red Grape seed extract (vitis vinifera) • Green Tea leaf extract (camellia sinensis) • Apple fruit extract (malus domestica).

T-HBP - Dial Herbs
Black Cohosh • Blue Cohosh • Wild Cherry bark.

T-HBRN - Dial Herbs
Sarsaparilla • Thyme • Valerian • Wood Betony • Peppermint • Catnip • White Willow bark.

The Antioxidant Formula - Rx Vitamins
Three capsules contain: Vitamin C 500 mg • Beta Carotene 25000 IU • Phytonutrient Blend (Broccoli, Spinach, Tomato) 150 mg • Citrus Bioflavonoid Complex 50 mg • Vitamin E 200 IU • Selenium 50 mcg • Zinc 15 mg • NAC (N-Acetyl-Cysteine) 15 mg • Bilberry 10 mg • L-Glutathione 10 mg • Grape seed extract 10 mg.

The Antioxidant Phyters - The Vitamin Shoppe
Each tablet contains: Green and Red Wine 100 mg • Licorice 100 mg • Pine bark and Grape seed 30 mg • Bilberry 50 mg • Ginkgo Biloba 50 mg • Marigold, Sunflowers 60 mg.

The AstaFactor - Mera Pharmaceuticals
Two softgels contain: Natural Astaxanthin (6 mg total carotenoids) 5 mg. Ingredients: Algal meal (Haematococcus pluvialis), Rice Bran Oil, Natural Gelatin, Beeswax, Natural Vitamin E, Vegetal Glycerin.

The B-Total Solution with Extra B12 - Dial Herbs
Vitamin C • Vitamin B2 • Vitamin B3 • Vitamin B6 • Vitamin B12 • Pantothenic Acid. In a base of Distilled Water, Glycerine, Sorbitol, Sodium Bicarbonate, Citric Acid, Fruit flavors & Sodium Benzoate.

The Fat Metabolizer - The Vitamin Shoppe
Three tablets contain: Elemental Choline (from Choline Bitartrate) 1000 mg • Inositol 100 mg • L-Methionine 500 mg • Taurine 500 mg • Vitamin B6 (Pyridoxine HCl) 30 mg • Betaine HCl 150 mg • Barberry Extract (Berberis vulgaris) 100 mg.

The Fruit Phyters - The Vitamin Shoppe
Two tablets contain: Tomato, Red Grapefruit, Apricot, Watermelon 100 mg • Walnut, Berries, Grape, Apple, Tea • Orange, Lemon, Lime, Grapefruit, Tangerine, Cherry, Tomato, Strawberry 400 mg • Apricot, Cantaloupe, Citrus Fruit 150 mg • Citrus Fruit 100 mg • Papaya, Kiwi, Pineapple 50 mg • Mango, Citrus Fruit 100 mg.

The Greatest Vitamin in the World - The Greatest Vitamin In The World, LLC
Each capsule contains: Opti-Blend Delivery and Digestive Blend 108,918 Active Units: Amylase, Protease I, Protease II, Peptidase, Lipase, Invertase, Cellulase, Lactase, Maltase, Hemi Seb • Stabilized Probiotic Blend 3.510 Billion CFU: DDS-1 Lactobacillus Acidophilus, Bifidobacterium Bifidum, Enterococcus Faecium, Lactobacillus Bulgaricus, Lactobacillus Plantarum, Lactobacillus Salivarius, Streptococus Thermophilus, Bifidobacterium Infantis, Bacillus Caogulans • Calcium (amino acid chelate, dicalcium malate) 1004 mg • Iodine (potassium iodide) 150 mcg • Magnesium (amino acid chelate, oxie, glycyl glutamine) 400 mg • Zinc (amino acid chelate) 15 mg • Iron (Ferrochel, amino acid chelate) 18 mg • Selenium (amino acid complex) 70 mcg • Manganese (amino acid chelate) 2 mg • Copper (amino acid chelate) 2 mg • Chromium (amino acid chelate) 170 mcg • Molybdenum (amino acid chelate) 80 mcg • Potassium (amino acid chelate) 65 mcg • Vitamin A (Betatene, 2.5% beta carotene) 5000 IU • Vitamin C (natural source ascorbic acid) 60 mg • Vitamin E (D-alpha tocopherols from seed oil, Covitol 1185) 30 IU • Biotin 306 mcg • Thiamin (vitamin B1) 1.5 mg • Riboflavin (vitamin B2) 1.7 mg • Niacin (vitamin B3) 20 mg • Pantothenic Acid (vitamin B5) 10 mg • Vitamin B6 2 mg • Folate (folic acid) 400 mcg • Vitamin B12 (cyanocobalamin) 6 mcg • Garlic (pure gar A2000 +A22) 90 mg • Colostrum (Colostrum Gold) 315 mg • Ipriflavone (Ostivone - TSI) 180 mg • Garcinia Cambogia (super citrimax GarcinCambog) 252 mg • Conjugated Linoleic Acid 54 mg • Ginkgo Biloba 45 mg • Lecithin (non GMO) 90 mg • Grape seed extract (95% standardized proanthocyanidins) 45 mg • Pine bark (95% polyphenols) 45 mg • Opti SOD Precursor Blend 405 mcg • Gymnema Sylvestre 135 mg • Milk Thistle 27 mg • Licorice root (declycerinated) 90 mg • Lutein 5.4 mg • Glucosamine Sulfate 2KCl 180 mg • Whole Food Blend 603 mg: Carrot, Wild Yam, Broccoli, Spinach, Tomato, Kale, Nutritional Yeast, Acerola Cherry, Black Currant, Wheat Germ.

The Green Phyters - The Vitamin Shoppe
Two tablets contain: Spirulina 200 mg • Chlorella 200 mg • Barley Juice 200 mg • Wheat Grass 200 mg • Alfalfa Leaf 200 mg • Chlorophyll 200 mg.

The New Grapefruit Diet with Apple Cider Vinegar - Applied Nutrition
Two capsules contain: Vitamin B6 (as pyridoxine HCl) 25 mg • Iodine (kelp) 150 mcg • Chromate Chromium Polynicotinate 200 mcg • Proprietary Blend 774 mg: Soy Lecithin, Grapefruit powder extract, Cider Vinegar powder, Bioperine brand Black Pepper extract. Other Ingredients: Gelatin, Silica, Magnesium Stearate.

The Ocular Formula - Rx Vitamins
Three capsules contain: Vitamin C (Ascorbate) 200 mg • Citrus Flavonoid Complex 100 mg • Vitamin E 100 IU • Zinc 30 mg • Glutathione 10 mg • Beta Carotene 9 mg • Vitamin A (Retinol) 5000 IU • Selenium 50 mcg • Lutein 6 mg • Zeaxanthin 260 mcg • Bilberry 100 mg • Grape seed 10 mg • Essential Cofactors: CoQ10 5 mg, Copper 3 mg.

The One-Minute Facial - Jason
Seven different Vitamin Cs • Alpha Lipoic Acid.

The Original Happy PMS - Zeller
Purified Water • Stearal Konium Chloride • D-Alpha Tocopherol (vitamin E) • Natural Glycerin • Avocado oil • Natural Progesterone • Aloe Vera oil • Rosemary extract • Vitamin A Palmitate • Carrot oil • Lemon Grass oil.

The Original Hollywood Celebrity Diet Body Slimming & Contouring Creme - Celebrity Products Direct, Inc.
Purified Water • Sesame Seed Oil • Polysorbate 60 • PEG-100 Stearate • Cetyl Alcohol • Caffeine • Dimethicone • Glyceryl Stearate • Phenoxyethanol • Hydro C • Hydroxylated Lecithin • Carbomer • Triethanolamine • Methylparaben • Fragrance • Butylparaben • Theobromine • Vitamin E Acetate • Ethylparaben • Propylparaben.

The Original Hollywood Celebrity Diet Fat Metabolizers - Celebrity Products Direct, Inc.
Each capsule contains: Cocoa extract powder 225 mg • Choline Bitartrate 100 mg • Guarana seed extract 36 mg • Methyl Acetyl Pyruvic Acid 24 mg • Dimethyl Sulfone (MSM) 12 mg • Kava root extract 6 mg • Zhi Shi immature Orange fruit (citri seu ponchi, immaturus) 6 mg • Fennel seed extract 6 mg • White Willow bark extract 18 mg • Proprietary Blend 18 mg: Ginger root powder, L-Aspartic Acid, Gotu Kola, Aloe Vera powder, Garlic, Beet extract powder, Hawthorn berry powder, Saw Palmetto berry powder, Ginseng root powder, Ginkgo Biloba powder, Bladderwrack, Sea Kelp powder. Other Ingredients: Magnesium Trisilicate, Magnesium Stearate, Natural Gelatin Capsules.
See Editor's Note No. 40.

The Original Hollywood Celebrity Diet QuickStart Citrus Juice - Celebrity Products Direct, Inc.
Purified Water • Juice Concentrate Blend: Pineapple, Plum, White Grape, Orange, Apple, Lemon • Potassium Citrate (potassium) • Ascorbic Acid (vitamin C) • D-Alpha-Tocopheryl Acetate (vitamin E) • Niacinamide (vitamin B3) • Calcium Pantothenate (vitamin B5) • Beta Carotene • Bilberry extract • Green Tea extract • Ginkgo Biloba extract • Grape Seed extract • Pyridoxine Hydrochloride (vitamin B6) • Riboflavin - 5' Phosphate (vitamin B2) • Thiamine Mononitrate (vitamin B1) • Folic Acid • Cholecalciferol (vitamin D3) • Biotin • Cyanocobalamin (vitamin B12).

The Original Hollywood Celebrity Diet Tea - Celebrity Products Direct, Inc.
Each bag (1.8 g) contains: Blackberry leaves • Cassia Angustifolia • Raphamus Sativa • Cassia Tora • Orange peel • Chicory root • Lemon Grass • Lemon peel • Hawthorn berry • Barley • Natural Lemon flavor • Natural Orange flavor.

The Prostate Formula - Real Health Laboratories
Three tablets contain: Vitamin D 200.0 IU • Saw Palmetto powder 320.0 mg • Pygeum powder 300.0 mg • Vitamin E 100.0 IU • Stinging Nettle powder 100.0 mg • Vitamin B6 50.00 mg • Pumpkin seed powder 100.0 mg • Zinc 15.0 mg • L-Lysine HCl 250.0 mg • L-Glutamic acid 250.0 mg • Glycine 250.0 mg. Other Ingredients: Dicalcium Phosphate, Hydroxyproplyl Methylcellulose, Microcrystalline Cellulose, Croscarmellose Sodium, Stearic Acid, Polyethylene Glycos, Silica, Titanium Dioxide, Magnesium Stearate, Peppermint oil, Polysorbate 80.

The Sinus Buster - SiCap Industries, LLC
Purified Water • Oleoresin Capsicum • Eucalyptus Oil • Rosemary extract • Vitamin C (as ascorbic acid) • Sea Salt.

The Total EFA - Health From The Sun
Three capsules contain: Vitamin E 30 IU • Alpha-Linolenic Acid (ALA)(Omega-3) 699 mg • Docosahexaenoic Acid (DHA) (Omega-3) 138 mg • Eicosapentaenoic Acid (EPA)(Omega-3) 216 mg • Gamma Linolenic Acid (GLA)(Omega-6) 288 mg • Lenoleic Acid (Omega-6) 620 mg • Oleic Acid (Omega-9) 520 mg. Ingredients: Certified Organic Flax seed oil, Borage seed oil, Fish oil, Gelatin, Glycerine, Water, Mixed Tocopherols.

The Ultimate Anti-Oxidant Formula - Natrol, Inc.
Two capsules contain: Vitamin A (Beta Carotene from d-Salina) 10000 IU • Vitamin E (d-alpha tocopheryl) 200 IU • Vitamin C (Ester-C Brand) 250 mg • Niacinamide 40 mg • Zinc (Krebs Cycle) 25 mg • Copper (Krebs Cycle) 2 mg • Selenium (Selenomethionine) 125 mcg • Flavonoids, Herbs, & other selected ingredients: Spirulina 300 mg GP Flavonoids Complex+ 200 mg, a 30% guaranteed potency extract of mixed flavonoids extracted from: Rose Hips, Turmeric,

Acerola berry, Bilberry, Hawthorne berry, Grape skin, Milk Thistle, & Citrus fruits • Calendula 50 mg • Artichoke extract 10 mg. Other Ingredients: Silicon Dioxide, Magnesium Stearate, Gelatin.

The Ultimate Calcium Formula - Roex
Six tablets contain: Calcium (Chelate, Citrate, Hydroxyapatite, Aspartate, Lactate) 1000 mg • Magnesium (Chelate, Oxide, Aspartate) 500 mg • Zinc (Gluconate , Citrate, Aspartate) 15 mg • Manganese 5 mg • Copper 2 mg • Vitamin D (Cholecalciferol) 400 IU • Boron 3 mg • Trace Minerals 25 mg • Silica 150 mg • Selenium 50 mcg • Chromium 50 mcg • Molybdenum 10 mcg.

The Ultimate Natural Facelift Chin & Neck Treatment - Healthy Revelations Inc.
Urea • Carbomer • Isopropyl Alcohol • Glyceryl Stearate • Water • Caprylic/Capric Triglyceride • Glycerin • Panthenol • Glucose • Stearic Acid • Horse Chestnut extract (aesculus hippocastanum) • Hydrocotyl extract (centella asiatica) • Green Tea extract (camellia sinensis) • Arnica extract (arnica montana) • Ivy extract (hedera helix) • Yarrow extract (achillea millefolium) • Bladderwrack extract (fucus vesiculosus) • Lactoyl Methylsilanol Elastinate • Methylsilanol Elastinate • Methylsilanol Mannuronate • Hydroiodide T.E.A. • Ginkgo Biloba extract • Polysorbate 60 • PEG-7 Glyceryl Cocoate • Stearyl Alcohol • Sorbitol • Polysorbate 80 • Cetyl Acetate • Acetylated Lanolin Alcohol • Magnesium Aluminum Silicate • Hops extract (humulus lupulus) • Menthol • Aloe extract (aloe barbadensis) • Methylparaben • Camphor • Hydrolyzed Elastin • Hydrolyzed Collagen • Glycosaminoglycans • Saccharide Isomerate • Glycoproteins • Dibutyl Lauroyl Glutamide • Horsetail extract (equisetum arvense) • Propylparaben • Eucalyptus extract (eucalyptus globules) • Adenosine Phosphate • Adenosine Triphosphate • Niacinamide • Placental Enzymes • PVM/MA Decadience Crosspolymer • BHT • Glyceryl Oleate • Ascorbyl Palmitate • Citric Acid • Propylene Glycol • Lecithin • Coenzyme Q10 • Tocopherol • Meadowfoam (limnanthes alba) seed oil • Copper Protein Complex • Rosemary extract (rosmarinus officinalis) • Peppermint extract (mentha piperita) • DMDM Hydantoin • Iodopropynyl Butylcarbamate • Tocopheryl Nicotinate • FD&C Red #40.

The Ultimate Weight Loss & Nutrition System - Nature's Secret
Three tablets contain: Vitamin B6 30 mg • Garcinia cambogia extract 600 mg • Pantothenic Acid 100 mg • Magnesium (aspartate) 25 mg • Chromium 300 mcg • Potassium (citrate) 128 mg • L-Carnitine 250 mg • Betaine HCl 100 mg • Lipotropic factors 800 mg • Choline, L-Methionine, Inositol, Lecithin, Triphala powder, Echinacea angustifolia, Cascara sagrada • Astragalus. Thermogenic support factors 757 mg: N-Acetyl Glucosamine, Uva Ursi leaf, Gotu Kola, Siberian Ginseng, L-Glutamine, Parsley leaf, Ginger root, Borage oil, Shave Grass herb, Piper longum, Licorice root. L-Phenylalanine, Corn Silk, Guggulipid, Pacific Kelp, L-Tyrosine, Atractylodes, Bladderwrack, Dulse, Chickweed herb, Dandelion root, Capsicum fruit, Lipase, Mustard seed, Protease, Cellulase.

The Vegi Phyters - The Vitamin Shoppe
Two tablets contain: Red, Yellow, and Dark vegetable, Carrots, Kale, Parsley, Spinach, Sweet Potatoes, Turnip Greens, Winter Squash, and Yams 300 mg • Cruciferous Vegetable 300 mg • Horseradish 100 mg • Chili Peppers 100 mg • Cabbage, Brussel Sprouts, Kale, Collard Greens, Broccoli, Mustard Greens 200 mg.

TheaMune - Life Enhancement Products, Inc.
Each capsule contains: L-Theanine 80 mg. Other Ingredients: Rice Flour.

Theanine 100 - Jarrow Formulas
Each capsule contains: Theanine 100 mg. Other Ingredients: Rice Powder, Magnesium Stearate, Silicon Dioxide, Gelatin.

Theanine Serene - Source Naturals
Two tablets contain: Magnesium (as magnesium chelate) 300 mg • GABA 500 mg • Taurine 500 mg • L-Theanine 200 mg • Valerian root extract 100 mg. Other Ingredients: Sorbitol, Stearic Acid, Modified Cellulose Gum.

Thera Zinc Lozenges-Menthol - Natrol, Inc.
One lozenge contains: Vitamin C (as Calcium Ascorbate) 50 mg • Zinc (as Zinc Gluconate) 7.5 mg • Echinacea angustifolia entire plant 10 mg • Bee Propolis 10 mg • Slippery Elm Bark 10 mg • Elderberry 10 mg • Bee Pollen 10 mg. Other Ingredients: Hydrogenated Starch, Hydrolysate, natural Menthol Eucalyptus flavor.

Thera-C 3 Grams Lemon - Natrol, Inc.
One single serving contains: Vitamin C (Ascorbic Acid) 250 mg • Acerola berry extract 20 mg • Echinacea (Purpurea extract 16:1) 12.5 mg • White Willow bark 100 mg • Slippery Elm bark 75 mg • Stevia powder 20 mg. Other Ingredients: Lemon Juice powder, Citric Acid, Menthol from Peppermint, Honey powder, Fructose, Calcium Carbonate.

Theragran Heart Right - Bristol-Myers Squibb Co.
Two caplets contain: Vitamin A (8% as Beta-carotene, 2% as Alpha-carotene, Lutein, Lypcopene, Zeaxanthin, Cryptoxanthin 10 mg) 5000 IU • Vitamin C 120 mg • Vitamin D 400 IU • Vitamin E 400 IU • Vitamin K 14 mcg • Thiamin (B1) 3 mg • Riboflavin (B2) 3.4 mg • Niacin (B3) 20 mg • Vitamin B6 16 mg • Folate, Folic Acid, Folacin 600 mcg • Vitamin B12 30 mcg • Biotin 30 mcg • Pantothenic acid 10 mg • Calcium 55 mg • Iron 4 mg • Iodine 150 mcg • Magnesium 150 mg • Zinc 15 mg • Selenium 70 mcg • Copper 1.5 mg • Manganese 2 mg • Chromium 50 mcg • Molybdenum 75 mcg • Proprietary Blend 10 mg: Beta Carotene, Alpha Carotene, Lutein, Lycopene, Zeaxanthin, Cryptoxanthin.

Theragran-M - Bristol-Myers Squibb Co.
Each caplet contains: Boron 150 mcg • Vitamin A (20% as beta carotene) 5000 IU • Vitamin C 90 mg • Nickel 5 mcg • Vitamin D 400 IU • Silicon 2 mg • Vitamin E 60 IU • Tin 10 mcg • Vanadium 10 mcg • Vitamin K 28 mcg • Thiamin (B1) 3 mg • Riboflavin (B2) 3.4 mg • Niacin (B3) 20 mg • Vitamin B6 6 mg • Folate, Folic Acid 400 mcg • Vitamin B12 12 mcg • Biotin 30 mcg • Pantothenic Acid 10 mg • Calcium 40 mg • Iron 9 mg • Phosphorus 31 mg • Iodine 105 mcg • Magnesium 100 mg • Zinc 15 mg • Selenium 70 mcg • Copper 2 mg • Manganese 2 mg • Chromium 50 mcg • Molybdenum 75 mg • Chloride 7.5 mg • Potassium 7.5 mg. Other Ingredients: Carnauba Wax, Crospovidone, FD&C Blue No. 2 Aluminum Lake, FD&C Red No. 40 Aluminum Lake, Flavor, Hydroxypropyl Methylcellulose, Lactose, Magnesium Stearate, Maltodextrin, Microcrystalline Cellulose, Polyethylene Glycol, Polysorbate 80, Povidone, Stearic ACid, Titanium Dioxide, Triacetin.

Theragran-M Advanced Formula - Bristol-Myers Squibb Co.
Each caplet contains: Vitamin A Acetate (20% as beta carotene) 5000 IU • Vitamin C (ascorbic acid) 90 mg • Vitamin D (D3) 400 IU • Vitamin E (dL-alpha tocopheryl) 60 IU • Vitamin K (phytonadione) 28 mcg • Thiamin Mononitrate (vitamin B1) 3 mg • Riboflavin (vitamin B2) 3.4 mg • Niacin (vitamin B3, niacinamide) 20 mg • Vitamin B6 (pyridoxine hydrochloride) 6 mg • Folate (folic acid, folacin) 400 mcg • Vitamin B12 (cyanocobalamin) 12 mcg • Biotin 30 mcg • Pantothenic Acid (calcium pantothenate) 10 mg • Calcium 40 mg • Iron (ferrous fumarate) 9 mg • Phosphorus (calcium phosphate) 31 mg • Iodine (potassium iodide) 150 mcg • Magnesium Oxide 100 mg • Zinc Oxide 15 mg • Selenium (sodium selenate) 70 mcg • Copper (cupric sulfate) 2 mg • Manganese Sulfate 2 mg • Chromium Chloride 50 mcg • Molybdenum (sodium molybdate) 75 mcg • Chloride 7.5 mg • Potassium Chloride 7.5 mg • Nickel Sulfate 5 mcg • Tin 10 mcg • Silicon 2 mg • Vanadium 10 mcg • Boron (sodium borate) 150 mcg. Other Ingredients: Beta Carotene, Carnauba Wax, Crospovidone, FD&C Blue No.2 Aluminum Lake, FD&C Red No. 40 Aluminum Lake, Flavor, Gelatin, Hydroxypropyl Cellulose, Hydroxypropyl Methylcellulose, Lactose, Magnesium Stearate, Maltodextrin, Microcrystaline Cellulose, Polyethylene Glycol, Polysorbate 80, Potassium Citrate, Povidone, Silica Gel, Stearic Acid, Titanium Dioxide, Triacetin.

Theramune Black Cumin Seed Oil Softgel Capsules - TNC International, Inc.
Each capsule contains: Black Cumin Seed oil (100% pure) 500 mg.

Some Brand Name Natural Products - What they Contain

www.NaturalDatabase.com contains MANY more listings than appear here.
Editor's Notes are located on pages 2155-2163.

Theramune Black Seed & Garlic - TNC International, Inc.
Each capsule contains: Proprietary Blend: Black Seed herb, High Potency Garlic.

Theramune Black Seed Oil - TNC International, Inc.
Each ounce contains: Black Seed oil (black cumin oil, 100% pure) Which Contains The Following Fatty Acid/Nutrient Blend: Myristic Acid (0.5%), Palmitic Acid (13.7%), Palmitoleic Acid (0.1%), Stearic Acid (2.6%), Oleic Acid (23.7%), Linoleic Acid (Omega-6, 57.9%), Linolenic Acid (Omega-3, 0.2%), Arachidic Acid (1.3%), Protein, Thiamin, Riboflavin, Pyridoxine, Niacin, Folacin, Calcium, Iron, Copper, Zinc, Phosphorus.

Theramune Black Seed Ultimate - TNC International, Inc.
Each capsule contains: Proprietary Blend: Black Seed, Odorless Garlic extract, Ginger, Cayenne.

Theramune Ginseng Powder - TNC International, Inc.
Each capsule contains: Proprietary Blend: Black Seed, Korean Ginseng, Siberian Ginseng, American Ginseng.

Theramune Gold - TNC International, Inc.
Each capsule contains: Proprietary Blend: Echinacea, Goldenseal, Black Seed.

Therapeutic Foot Rub - All Terrain Company
Tea Tree Oil extract • Eucalyptus extract • Calendula flower extract • Rosemary extract • Lavender extract. Base: Canola Oil, Caster Oil, Beeswax, Corn Starch.

Therapeutic-M - Sunmark
Each caplet contains: Vitamin A (20% as beta carotene) 5000 IU • Thiamin (vitamin B1) 3 mg • Riboflavin (vitamin B2) 3.4 mg • Vitamin B6 6 mg • Vitamin B12 12 mcg • Vitamin C 90 mg • Vitamin D 400 IU • Vitamin E 60 IU • Vitamin K 28 mcg • Niacin 20 mg • Folate 400 mcg • Iodine 150 mcg • Magnesium 100 mg • Zinc 15 mg • Selenium 70 mcg • Copper 2 mg • Manganese 2 mg • Chromium 50 mcg • Molybdenum 75 mcg • Chloride 7.5 mg • Potassium 7.5 mg • Biotin 30 mcg • Pantothenic Acid 10 mg • Calcium 40 mg • Iron 9 mg • Phosphorus 31 mg • Boron 150 mcg • Nickel 5 mcg • Silicon 2 mg • Vanadium 10 mcg • Tin 10 mcg. Other Ingredients: Microcrystalline Cellulose, Gelatin, Modified Cellulose Gum, Stearic Acid, Hydroxypropyl Methylcellulose, Crospovidone, Polyethylene Glycol, Propylene Glycol, Artificial Colors (FD&C red no. 40 lake, titanium dioxide, FD&C blue no. 2 lake), Starch, Hydroxypropyl Cellulose, Lactose, Magnesium Stearate, Beta Carotene, Acacia, Cottonseed Oil, Sodium Lauryl Sulfate, Gluten.
See Editor's Note No. 45.

TheraStress liquid - Nutriceutical Technologies
Eleuthero root • Schizandra berry • Green Tea extract • Rhodiola root • Garcinia Cambogia • Chinese Ginseng • Reishi mushroom • Stevia herb. Other Ingredients: Glycerin, Deionized Water, Natural Flavors.

Theravim-M - Puritan's Pride
Each tablet contains: Vitamin A (retinyl acetate and beta carotene) 5000 IU • Vitamin C (ascorbic acid) 90 mg • Vitamin D (cholecalciferol) 400 IU • Vitamin E (DL-alpha tocopheryl acetate) 30 IU • Thiamin (vitamin B1) 3 mg • Riboflavin (vitamin B2) 3.4 mg • Niacin (niacinamide) 20 mg • Vitamin B6 (pyridoxine hydrochloride) 3 mg • Folic Acid 400 mcg • Vitamin B12 (cyancobalamin) 9 mcg • Biotin (D-biotin) 30 mcg • Pantothenic Acid (D-calcium pantothenate) 10 mg • Calcium (dicalcium phosphate) 40 mg • Iron (ferrous fumarate) 27 mg • Phosphorus (dicalcium phosphate) 31 mg • Iodine (potassium iodide) 150 mcg • Magnesium (oxide) 100 mg • Zinc (oxide) 15 mg • Selenium (sodium selenate) 10 mcg • Copper (sulfate) 2 mg • Manganese (sulfate) 5 mg • Chromium (chloride) 15 mcg • Molybdenum (sodium molybdate) 15 mcg • Chloride (potassium chloride) 7.5 mg • Potassium 7.5 mg.

Thermadrene - SportPharma
Each capsule contains: Ephedra extract 300 mg (24 mg ephedrine) • Caffeine 80 mg • Guarana extract 150 mg (15 mg caffeine) • Willow Bark extract 75 mg • Cayenne 60 mg • Ginger root 40 mg.
See Editor's Note No. 30.

ThermaLean-RX - MedaBiotics
Three capsules contain: Metabromine brand Theobroma Cacao fruit extract (providing 6% theobromine, 20 mg) 300 mg • Advantra Z brand Citrus Aurantium (providing 10% total amines, 35 mg) 350 mg • Serotain brand 5-HTP (providing 18/5% 5-hydroxytryptophan, 36 mg) 200 mg • Thermazide Proprietary Blend 1069 mg: Caffeine, Coral Calcium, Green Tea leaf extract (camellia sinensis, providing 30% tea polyphenols, 20% tea catechins), Glucuronolactone, L-Carnitine L-Tartrate, Taurine. Other Ingredients: Gelatin, Cellulose, Magnesium Stearate.
See Editor's Note No. 40.

Thermic Blast - Human Development Technologies (HDT)
Four sprays contain: Caffeine 100 mg • Ephedra extract 8% aerial (ephedrine 8 mg) 100 mg • Stevia extract 80% leaf (steviosides 32 mg) 40 mg • White Willow bark 1% bark (Salicin 200 mcg) 20 mg • Green Tea extract 30% leaf (polyphenols 6 mg) 20 mg • Guarana extract 10% seed (caffeine 2 mg) 20 mg • Chromium Picolinate 400 mcg. Other Ingredients: Water, Propylene Glycol, Cherry, Vanilla Flavors, Polysorbate 20, Benzyl Alcohol, Hydrochloric Acid Lecithin.
See Editor's Note No. 30.

Thermo Cuts - Optimum Nutrition
Four capsules contain: Citrimax 2000 mg • MaHuang extract 334 mg • Guarana extract 910 mg • Willow bark extract 100 mg • L-Carnitine 100 mg • Chromium Picolinate 300 mcg.
See Editor's Note No. 30.

Thermo DynamX - EAS, Inc.
Three capsules contain: Green Tea Leaf (carnellia sinensis; total catechins 213 mg, epigallocatechin gallates (EGCG) 110) 610 mg • Mate (ilex paraguarensis) leaves and stems 500 mg • Caffeine (from mate, caffeine anhydrous, green tea) 200 mg • Octopamine HCl 200 mg • Synephrine (from citrus aurantium) 20 mg. Other Ingredients: Gelatin, Microcellulose, Magnesium Stearate, Silica.
See Editor's Note No. 40.

Thermo Trim - Swanson Health Products
Three capsules contain: Chromium (Chromax chromium picolinate) 200 mcg • Guarana extract (standardized to 22% caffeine) 909 mg • Citrin Garcinia Cambogia extract (50% hydroxycitrate acid) 500 mg • Ma Huang extract (standardized to 20 mg ephedra alkaloids) 334 mg • L-Carnitine (tartrate) 100 mg.
See Editor's Note No. 30.

Thermo Tropic - Nature's Plus
Two tablets contain: Vitamin B6 (as pyridoxine HCl) 50 mg • Chromium (as polynicotinate, picolinate) 100 mcg • Choline (as bitartrate) 500 mg • Inositol 250 mg • L-Methionine (free form amino acid) 150 mg • L-Carnitine (L-carnitine-L-tartrate) 100 mg • Phytosterol complex 100 mg: 51% Beta Sitosterol 51 mg, 18% Campesterol 18 mg, 20% Stigmasterol 20 mg) • Garcinia Cambogia standardized extract 100 mg • Eleuthero root (eleutherococcus senticosus) 75 mg • Gotu Kola (centella asiatica) 75 mg • Fo-Ti (polygonum multiflorum) 75 mg • Lipase (fat-digesting enzyme) 25 mg. Other Ingredients: Stearic Acid, Di-Calcium Phosphate, Microcrystalline Cellulose, Silica, Magnesium Stearate.

Thermo Tropic Shake (mixed berry flavor) - Nature's Plus
Each scoop (35 g) contains: Vitamin A 5000 IU • Vitamin C 60 mg • Calcium 300 mg • Iron 4.5 mg • Vitamin D 400 IU • Vitamin E 30 IU • Thiamin 1.5 mg • Riboflavin 1.7 mg • Niacin 20 mg • Vitamin B6 2 mg • Folic Acid 400 mcg • Vitamin B12 6 mcg • Biotin 300 mcg • Pantothenic Acid 10 mg • Magnesium 80 mg • Zinc 15 mg • Selenium 20 mcg • Manganese 5 mg • Chromium 20 mcg • Molybdenum 20 mcg • Citrus Bioflavonoid Complex 25 mg. Other Ingredients: Fructose, Non-GMO Isolated Soy Protein, Natural Raspberry Flavor, Natural Strawberry Flavor, Natural Vanilla Flavor, Natural Blueberry Flavor, Amylase, Bromelain, Eleuthero, Gotu Kola, Fo-ti, Potassium Glycero-Phosphate, Medium-Chain Triglycerides, Lipase, Guar Gum, Psyllium, L-Carnitine-L-Tartrate, Wild Berry Powder, Natural Blackberry Flavor.

Some Brand Name Natural Products - What they Contain

www.NaturalDatabase.com contains MANY more listings than appear here.

Editor's Notes are located on pages 2155-2163.

Thermo-Actives - Natrol, Inc.
Each capsule contains: Ginger root extract (5% gingerols) 150 mg • Sida cordifolia extract (0.8% ephedrine) 100 mg • Mucuna pruriens 5:1 extract 100 mg • Cayenne extract (90000 SHU) 50 mg • Mustard extract seed (50% saponins) 15 mg • Bioperine brand Black Pepper 4:1 extract 15 mg. Other Ingredients: Rice Powder, Silicon Dioxide, Magnesium Stearate, Gelatin.
See Editor's Note No. 39.

ThermoAMP - E'OLA
0.25 mL contains: Proprietary Blend 31 mg: Ephedra extract (ephedra sinesis), White Willow Bark extract (salix alba), Guarana seed (paullinia cupana) , Atractylodes extract (atractylodes macrocephala), Licorice root (glycyrrhiza uralensis), DMAE (dimethyl amino ethenol bitartrate), Vitamin B12 (dibencozide). Inactive Ingredients: Water, Glycerin, Sodium Benzoic Acid, Sorbic Acid.
See Editor's Note No. 30.

ThermoAMP Herbal Chews - E'OLA
Each chew (8.6 g) contains: Calcium 245 mg • Vitamin B12 20 mcg • Proprietary Blend 31 mg: Ephedra extract (branch, ephedra sinica), White Willow Bark extract (salix alba), Guarana extract (seed, paullinia cupana), Atractylodes extract (herb, atractylodes macrocephala), Licorice root (glcyrrhiza uralensis), DMAE (dimethy amino ethanol bitatrate, Vitamin B12 (dibencozide). Other Ingredients: Corn Syrup, Sweetened Condensed Whole Milk, Sugar, Chocolate, Partially Hydrogenated Soybean Oil, Mono & Diglycerides, Soy Lecithin, Natural & Artificial Flavors.
See Editor's Note No. 30.

Thermochrome ephedra free - Market America, Inc.
Two tablets contain: Vitamin C (as ascorbic acid) 100 mg • Vitamin B6 (as pyridoxine HCl) 10 mg • Pantothenic Acid (as dicalcium pantothenate) 12 mg • Magnesium (as magnesium oxide) 10 mg • Chromium (chromium dinicotinate glycinate and chromium picolinate) 150 mcg • Proprietary Thermobolic Complex 1415 mg: Guarana seed extract (supplying 100 mg caffeine), Citrus Aurantium extract (immature fruit), DL-Phenylalanine, Green Tea leaf standardized extract, Theobroma Cacao standardized extract, Yerba Mate leaf extract, DL-Methionine, Ginger root, Dimethylaminoethanol (DMAE) bitartrate, Grape seed extract, Cinnamon twig extract, Galangal rhizome extract. Other Ingredients: Dicalcium Phosphate, Microcrystalline Cellulose, Croscarmellose Sodium, Stearic Acid, Magnesium Stearate, Silica.
See Editor's Note No. 40.

ThermoDiet for Men - Futurebiotics LLC
Two tablets contain: Spirulina 100 mg • MaHuang (Standardized Extract) 200 mg • Mustard Seed Powder 100 mg • Vitamin C 100 mg • Potassium (Citrate) 99 mg • Magnesium (Aspartate) 50 mg • Chromium (Picolinate) 200 mcg • Kelp 150 mg • Chinese Licorice 250 mg • Smilax.
See Editor's Note No. 30.

ThermoDiet For Women - Futurebiotics LLC
Two tablets contain: Spirulina 100 mg • Ma Huang standardized extract 200 mg • Mustard Seed powder 100 mg • Vitamin C 100 mg • Potassium (citrate) 99 mg • Magnesium (aspartate) 50 mg • Chromium (picolinate) 200 mcg • Kelp 150 mg • Peony 250 mg • Foti 250 mg • Dong Quai 250 mg.
See Editor's Note No. 30.

Thermo-G - Advocare International
Each caplet contains: Vitamin A (as beta-carotene) 1000 IU • Niacin 20 mg • Magnesium (as phosphate) 25 mg • Potassium (as phosphate) 50 mg • Green Orange pericarp extract (citrus aurantium) 500 mg • Guarana seed extract (paullinia cupana) 200 mg • Green Tea leaf extract (camellia sinensis) 10 mg. Other Ingredients: Dicalcium Phosphate, Silicon Dioxide, Cellulose, Stearic Acid, Magnesium Stearate, Beet Root Powder (for color).
See Editor's Note No. 40.

Thermogenic Herbal Complex - Starlight International
Each capsule contains: Chromium (as chromium picolinate) 6 mcg • Ma Huang (ephedra sinica, total ephedrine alkaloids 22 mg) 275 mg • Cascara Sagrada bark (rhamnus purshiana) 35 mg • Bladderwrack plant (focus vesiculosus) 35 mg • Uva Ursi leaf extract (4:1, arctostaphylos uva ursi, leaf) 25 mg • Parsley leaf extract, 4:1 (petroselinum crispum) 10 mg • Calcium Gluconate 5 mg • Corn Silk flower pistils (zea mays) 7 mg • Goldenrod leaf (solidago odora) 6 mg • Fumitory Herb aerial parts (fumaria officinalis) 6 mg • Magnesium Gluconate 7 mg • English Hawthorn fruit (crategus laevigata) 5 mg • Licorice root (glycyrrhiza glabra, root) 5 mg • Marshmallow root (athea officinalis) 5 mg • Apple Pectin 5 mg. Other Ingredients: Magnesium Stearate, Silicon Dioxide, Dicalcium Phosphate, Calcium Sulfate.
See Editor's Note No. 30.

Thermogenics Original Formula - SilverSage
Each capsule contains: Ephedrine Alkaloids from 310 mg standardized Ma Huang plant extract 25 mg • Caffeine (16.8 mg from standardized bissy nut 140 mg) 50 mg • Acetylsalicylic Acid (aspirin) 110 mg • Proprietary Blend of Synergistic Ingredients 249 mg: Siberian Ginseng root, Schizonepeta Spica extract 5:1, Forsythia fruit extract 5:1, Green Tea leaf extract standardized for Polyphenols/ Catechins content, Cayenne fruit, Ginger root • Vitamin C 50 mg • Pantothenic Acid 25 mg • Zinc amino acid chelate 7 mg • Selenium Amino Acid Chelate 1 mcg • Manganese Amino Acid Chelate 2.5 mg.
See Editor's Note No. 30.

ThermoGenics Plus - SilverSage
Each capsule contains: Ephedrine standardized extract (whole ma huang) 14 mg • Caffeine standardized extrac (from bissy nut) • Acetylsalicylic Acid • In a base of Vitamin C, Siberian Ginseng, Green Tea extract (standardized to 50% polyphenols/catechins), Schizonepeta Spica extract (5:1), Forsythia fruit extract (5:1), White Willow bark, Cayenne, Pantothenic Acid, Ginger root, Zinc (amino acid chelate), Manganese (amino acid chelate), Selenium (amino acid chelate).
See Editor's Note No. 30.

Thermogenics Plus, Stimulant Free - SilverSage
Two capsules contain: Proprietary Phosphosterine Blend 1330 mg: Calcium Phosphate, Commiphora Phytosterol extract, Garcinia Cambogia (HCA 125 mg), L-Tyrosine, Dipotassium Phosphate, Sodium Phosphate, Disodium Phosphate, Phosphatidyl Choline, Scutellaria root, Bupleurum root, Epimedium herb. Other Ingredients: Rice Flour.

Thermogenics Quick Start - SilverSage
Each capsule contains: Ephedrine Alkaloids standardized extract from 250 mg Ma Huang plant 20 mg • Caffeine (26 mg from standardized bissy nut 106 mg) 200 mg • Acetylsalicylic Acid (aspirin) 324 mg • Proprietary Synergistic Blend 198 mg: Siberian Ginseng root, Schizonepeta Spica extract (5:1), Forsythia fruit extract (5:1), Cayenne fruit, Ginger root • Vitamin C 40 mg • Pantothenic Acid 23 mg • Zinc Amino Acid Chelate 14 mg • Selenium Amino Acid Chelate 167 mcg • Manganese Amino Acid Chelate 5 mg.
See Editor's Note No. 30.

Thermojetics Activated Fiber tablets - Herbalife International of America, Inc.
Each tablet contains: Dietary Fiber 450 mg: Oat Fiber, Citrus Fiber, Lemon Pectin (citrus limon), Microcrystalline Cellulose, Gum Arabic root (acacia senega) • Sodium Choleate (from ox-bile extract) 56 mg • • L-Carnitine 25 mg. Other Ingredients: Corn Starch, Stearic Acid, Calcium Carbonate, Hydroxypropyl Cellulose, Croscarmellose Sodium, Sodium Lauryl Sulfate.

Thermojetics Active Fiber - Herbalife International of America, Inc.
Arabinogalactan • Maltodextrin • Hydrolyzed Guar Gum • Oligofiber • Silicon Dioxide • Glycerine.

BRAND NAMES

Some Brand Name Natural Products - What they Contain

www.NaturalDatabase.com contains MANY more listings than appear here.
Editor's Notes are located on pages 2155-2163.

BRAND NAMES

Thermojetics Aminogen - Herbalife International of America, Inc.
Each tablet contains: Calcium (carbonate) 76 mg • Patented Protease (Aminogen brand) 250 mg. Other Ingredients: Microcrystalline Cellulose, Stearic Acid, Hydroxypropyl Cellulose, Maltodextrin, Corn Starch, Sodium Starch Glycolate, Sodium Carboxymethylcellulose, Soy Lecithin, Sodium Citrate, Carnauba Wax.

Thermojetics Beige - Herbalife International of America, Inc.
Each tablet contains: English Hawthorn berry fruit 80 mg • Alfalfa leaves 70 mg • Parsley leaves 60 mg • Marshmallow root 55 mg •Uva Ursi leaves 50 mg • Cornsilk 50 mg •Magnolia bark 30 mg • Fennel seed 25 mg • Astragalus root 20 mg • Pfaffia root 20 mg • Pau d'Arco bark 20 mg • European Goldenrod leaves 15 mg • Licorice root 15 mg. Other Ingredients: Microcrystaline Cellulose, Tapioca & Corn Starches, Stearic Acid, Cross-linked Sodium Carboxymethylcellulose, Sodium Starch Glyconate, Silicon Dioxide, Magnesium Stearate, Food Grade Shellac, Hydroxypropyl Methylcellulose, Titianium Dioxide, Caramel.

Thermojetics Green Ephedra Free - Herbalife International of America, Inc.
Each tablet contains: Proprietary Blend: Green Tea extract, Cocoa extract, dried Citrus Aurantium extract (fruit), dried Bitter Orange extract (peel), Yerba Mate. Other Ingredients: Maltodextrin, Corn Starch, Silicon Dioxide, Methylcellulose, Colors, Titanium Dioxide, Sodium Carboxymethyl Cellulose, Hydroxypropylmethyl Cellulose, Magnesium Stearate, Trimethyl Citrate, Black Pepper extract, Flavor. See Editor's Note No. 40.

Thermojetics Green Refresh - Herbalife International of America, Inc.
Each tablet contains: Balu • Yerba Mate extract • Bladderwrack • Meadowsweet • Garcinia Cambogia • Valerian root • Green Tea extract • Fumitory herb • Honeysuckle • FD&C Blue No. 1 Lake.

Thermojetics Herbal Concentrate - Herbalife International of America, Inc.
Each serving contains: Camellia sinensis (Green Tea & Orange Pekoe Tea) extract • Maltodextrin • Fructose • Malva Sylvestris extract • Cardamom extract • Hibiscus extract • Lemon Peel extract.

Thermojetics N-R-G Nature's Raw Guarana instant tea mix - Herbalife International of America, Inc.
Maltodextrin • Roasted Guarana seed extract • Orange Pekoe extract • Lemon peel extract • Citric Acid • Natural Caffeine powder.

Thermojetics N-R-G Nature's Raw Guarana tablets - Herbalife International of America, Inc.
Each tablet contains: Calcium (as calcium sulfate) 250 mg • Guarana seed 800 mg. Other Ingredients: Stearic Acid, Hydrogenated Cotton Seed Oil, Silicon Dioxide, Magnesium Stearate, Sodium Carboxymethylcellulose, Glycerine, Polyvinyl Pyrrolidone.

Thermojetics Original Green - Herbalife International of America, Inc.
Each tablet contains: Calcium (as calcium carbonate) 58 mg • Iodine (from bladderwrack) 30 mg • Chinese Ephedra leaf 140 mg • Yerba Mate leaf 115 mg • Dried MaHuang extract 70 mg • Bladderwrack 40 mg • Valerian root 40 mg • Fumaria Officinalis 30 mg • Dried Salix Purpurea bark extract 30 mg • Chondrus Crispus 5 mg. Other Ingredients: Stearic Acid, Tapioca Starch, Microcrystalline Cellulose, Papain, Cross-linked Sodium Carboxymethylcellulose, Silicon Dioxide, Sodium Starch Glyconate, Magnesium Stearate, Sodium Laurel Sulfate, Food Grade Shellac, Titanium Dioxide, Polyethylene Glycol, Riboflavin, FD&C Blue #1.
See Editor's Note No. 21 and No. 30.

Thermojetics Thermo-Bond - Herbalife International of America, Inc.
Each tablet contains: Dietary Fiber 273 mg: Cellulose, Apple, Acacia, Oat, Citrus. Other Ingredients: Sodium Choleate, Stearic Acid, Sodium Carboxymethylcellulose, Silicon Dioxide, Magnesium Stearate, Dextrin, Dextrose, Soy Lecithin, Sodium Citrate.

Thermojetics Yellow - Herbalife International of America, Inc.
Each tablet contains: Garcinia (Garcinia Cambogia extract) 400 mg • GTF Chromium (Chomium Polynicotinate) 400 mg.

Thermo-Lift (ThermoLift) - Goldshield Elite
Each caplet contains: Chromium (dinicotinate glycinate, picolinate, niacin bound chromium) 200 mcg • Vanadium 100 mcg • Ma Huang stem standardized extract (supplying ephedrine alkaloids 25 mg) 310 mg • Thermogenic Herbal Blend 325 mg: Guarana seed standardized extract (20%,supplying caffeine 43 mg), Citrus Peel standardized extract (citrus aurantium, 5-7% alkaloids), White Willow bark, Siberian Ginseng root, Astragalus root, Bee Pollen, Bladderwrack kelp, Ginger root, Gotu Kola leaf, Licorice root, Rehmannia root, Reishi mushroom . Other Ingredients: Dicalcium Phosphate, Cellulose, Vegetable Oil, Soy Polysaccharides, Silica. See Editor's Note No. 30 and No. 40.

Thermo-Lift II (ThermoLift II) - Goldshield Elite
Each caplet contains: Niacin 10 mg • Chromium (as Chromium dinicotinate glycinate, Chromium polynicotinate and chromium picolinate) 100 mcg • Vanadium (as Vanadyl sulfate) 50 mcg • Panax Ginseng root standardized extract (8% ginsenosides) 100 mg • Guarana seed standardized extract (20% Caffeine) 225 mg • Yerba Mate leaf standardized extract 100 mg • L-Tyrosine 100 mg • Thermogenic herbal blend 75 mg: Standardized Citrus Peel extract (5% phenethylamines) (Citrus aurantium), Cayenne pepper, Cinnamon bark standardized extract, Ginger root, and White Willow bark • Supporting Herbal Blend 50 mg: Astragalus root, Bladderwrack kelp, Licorice root, Siberian Ginseng root, and Arctic root (Rhodiola rosea) standardized extract. Other Ingredients: Dicalcium phosphate, Vegetable cellulose, Fractionated Vegetable oil, Soy polysaccharides, Silica, and Vegetable resin glaze.
See Editor's Note No. 40.

Thermonex Ephedra Free Capsules - BSN Inc.
Three capsules contain: L-Tyrosine 300 mg • Caffeine Anhydrous 250 mg • Citrus Aurantium 10% extract (providing synephrine 20 mg) • Naringin 50 mg • Evodiamine 40 mg • Diiodotyrosine 100 mcg • Iodotyrosine 100 mcg • Yerba Mate (25% extract standardized for xanthines) 200 mg • Octopamine HCl 200 mg • Green Tea extract (catachins 243 mg/EGCG 112 mg) 375 mg. Other Ingredients: Magnesium Stearate, Gelatin.
See Editor's Note No. 40.

Thermo-Rx - Weightlosscontrol
Each capsule contains: Proprietary Blend 565 mg: Sida Cordifolia leaf 25 mg, Ephedrine Alkaloids, Citrus Aurantium fruit 10 mg, Synephrine Alkaloids, Caffeine 80 mg, Coleus Forskohlii root, Cassia Nomame, Green Tea, 5-Hydroxytryptophan, 5-Methoxtrytamine.
See Editor's Note No. 39 and No. 40.

ThermoSculpt - For Youthful Health
Four softgels contain: Vitamin B5 (pantothenic acid) 60 mg • Zinc Oxide 40 mg • ChromeMate brand Chromium 400 mcg • Vanadyl Sulfate, 31.25% 200 mcg • Advantra Z brand Citrus Aurantium 1000 mg: Total Amins 7.5%-8.2%; Synephrine 6%, N-Methyl Tyramine 0.9%-1.6%, Tyramine 0.2%-0.4%, Hordenine 0.2%-0.4%, Octopamine 0.2%-0.4% • Glucosol (corosolic acid) 48 mg.
See Editor's Note No. 40.

ThermoSyn - PharmAssure
One tablet contains: Chromium (as chromium picolinate) 400 mcg • MaHuang extract (ephedra sinica; 6% ephedrine, 20mcg) 333 mg • Guarana Seed extract (paullinia cupana; 365 caffeine 90mg) 250 mg • Citrus Aurantium fruit extract (4% synephrine, 6mg) 150 mg • White Willow bark extract (salix alba; 15% salicin 15mg) 100 mg. Other Ingredients: Dicalcium Phosphate, Croscarmellose Sodium, Cellulose. See Editor's Note No. 30 and No 40.

THERMOthin - Slimming and Nutrition Consultancy
Each capsule contains: Citrus aurantium • Citrin (HCA) • Guarana • Caffeine • White Willow bark • Chromium • Liquorice extract • Cayenne extract • Siberian Ginseng • Vitamin B6 • Iodine • Betaine.
See Editor's Note No. 40.

Ther-Rx PrimaCare - KV Pharmaceutical Co.
Each white softgel capsule contains: AM Regimen: Omega-3 Fatty Acids 150 mg • Linoleic Acid 25 mg • Linolenic Acid 25 mg • Calcium (carbonate) 150 mg • Vitamin D (D3, as cholecalciferol) 170 IU • Vitamin E (DL-alpha-tocopheryl acetate) 30 IU.
Each pink film-coated tablet contains: PM Regimin: Calcium (carbonate) 250 mg • Vitamin K 90 mcg • Vitamin C (as Ester-C) 100 mg • Vitamin D (vitamin D3, cholecalciferol) 230 IU • Folic Acid USP 1 mg • Thiamine (mononitrate, USP) 3 mg • Riboflavin USP 3.4 mg • Niacin (as niacinamide USP) 20 mg • Pyridoxine (as pyridoxine HCl USP) 10 mg • Cyanocobalamin (vitamin B12) 12 mcg • Biotin 35 mcg • Pantothenic Acid 7 mg • Iron (ferrous fumarate) 30 mg • Zinc (oxide) 13 mg • Copper (as cupric oxide) 1.3 mg • Selenium 75 mcg • Chromium 45 mcg • Molybdenum 50 mcg.

T-HFV - Dial Herbs
Bayberry • Cayenne • Mullein • Lobelia.

Thiamin B1 25 mg - Jarrow Formulas
Each capsule contains: Thiamin (as hydrochloride) 25 mg. Other Ingredients: Cellulose, Magnesium Stearate, Gelatin.

ThiaMind - Source Naturals
Each tablet contains: Vitamin B1 (Thiamin Mononitrate) 500 mg • Magnesium (Citrate, Malate, Succinate and Oxide) 100 mg.

Thin II - E'OLA
Each 0.60 g (Approx. 12 drops) serving contains: Vitamin B12 (as Cyanocobalamin) 20 mcg • Chromium (as Chromium Chloride) 200 mcg • Proprietary Blend 271 mg: Green Tea Extract, Guarana Extract, Caffeine, Kola Nut Extract, Stevia Extract. Other Ingredients: Purified Water, Glycerin, Hydroxylated Lecithin, Benzyl Alcohol, Potassium Sorbate, Potassium Hydroxide.

Thin II Herbal Chews - E'OLA
Each 8.6 g chew contains: Calcium 245 • Vitamin B12 20 mcg • Chromium 200 mcg • Proprietary Blend 271 mg: Green Tea extract (Camellia sinensis, leaf), Guarana extract (Paullina cupana, seed), Caffeine, Kola Nut extract (Cola ocuminoto), Stevia extract (stevia reboudiana, leaf). Other Ingredients: Corn Syrup, Sweetened Condensed Whole Milk, Sugar, Chocolate, Partially Hydrogenated Soybean Oil, Mono & Diglycerides, Soy Lecithin, Natural & Artificial Flavors, Maltodextrin.

Thinfat - VPX Sports
Conjugated Linoleic Acid • Triglyceride • Natural Lemon Flavor.

Think Clear - Pro Health
Each capsule contains: Ginkgo Biloba leaf extract (24% flavone glycosides, 6% terpene lactones) 60 mg • Vinpocetine 15 mg • Huperzine A 50 mcg • DHA 100 mg. Other Ingredients: Rice Flour, Magnesium Stearate.

Think Sharp - Health Smart Vitamins
Three capsules contain: Vitamin C (ascorbic acid) 250 mg • Thiamin (as thiamin mononitrate) 10 mg • Riboflavin 10 mg • Niacin (as 50% niacinamide, 50% nicotinic acid) 20 mg • Vitamin B6 (as pyridoxine HCl) 10 mg • Folic Acid 400 mcg • Vitamin B12 (as cyanocobalamin) 100 mcg • Biotin 300 mcg • Pantothenic Acid (as calcium pantothenate) 10 mg • Dimethylaminoethanol (DMAE; as Dimethylaminoethanol bitartrate) 500 mg • L-Glutamine 250 mg • L-Pyroglutamic Acid 100 mg • Acetyl-L-carnitine (as Acetyl-L-carnitine HCl) 50 mg.

Think-02 - Traditional Medicinals
Contains: Peppermint leaf • Ginkgo leaf and Ginkgo dry leaf extract • Gotu Kola leaf • Sage leaf • Siberian Ginseng root • Lemon Balm leaf • Rosemary leaf • natural Lemon flavor • Stevia leaf.

Thinker's Edge - Pro Health
Four tablets contain: Vitamin C (as ascorbic acid & zinc manganese ascorbates) 150 mg • Thiamin (vitamin B1) 50 mg • Riboflavin (vitamin B2) 20 mg • Niacinamide 80 mg • Niacin 40 mg • Vitamin B6 (as pyridoxine HCl) 25 mg • Folate (as folic acid) 400 mcg • Vitamin B12 (as cyanocobalamin) 50 mcg • Biotin 50 mcg • Pantothenic Acid (as calcium D-pantothenate) 120 mg • Calcium (as calcium citrate) 74 mg • Iron 7 mg • Magnesium (as magnesium oxide & citrate) 120 mg • Zinc (as zinc ascorbate) 10 mg • Manganese (as manganese ascorbate) 5 mg • Potassium (as potassium citrate) 99 mg • L-Glutamine 500 mg • L-Pyroglutamic Acid 500 mg • Super A brand Lecithin Gum 350 mg • L-Tyrosine 275 mg • Siberian Ginseng root 225 mg • DMAE (as DMAE bitartrate) 160 mg • Gotu Kola herb 150 mg • L-Phenylalanine 125 mg • Choline (as choline bitartrate) 100 mg • Taurine 100 mg • Ginger root 80 mg • Schizandra fruit 80 mg • Cayenne fruit 60 mg • Inositol 30 mg • Ginkgo Biloba leaf 50:1 extract 20 mg. Other Ingredients: Modified Cellulose Gum, Colloidal Silicon Dioxide, Zinc Stearate, Sorbitol, Tragacanth Gum.

Thinking Cap - Life Enhancement Products, Inc.
Each capsule contains: Pantothenic Acid (Vitamin B5) 100 mg • Choline (from choline citrate) 200 mg • Huperzine A 50 mcg. Other Ingredients: Silicon Dioxide, Gelatin, Maltodextrin.

Thinology - Abundance Marketing
Each tablet contains: Chromium (as chromium chloride) 150 mcg • Thinologic Blend 385 mg: Cyperus aerial parts, Green Tea leaf, Appestat brand from Green Tea leaf, Cinnamon twig, Galangal rhizome • Cocoa bean, Rhodiola root.

Thinz Back-To-Nature - Alva-Amco Pharmacal Cos., Inc.
Each tablet contains: Phenylpropanolamine HCl 75 mg. Other Ingredients: Apple Powder, Brown Lake Color Blend, Dicalcium Phosphate, D&C Yellow #10, FD&C Yellow #6, Hydroxypropyl Methylcellulose, Magnesium Stearate, Mineral Oil, Oat Bran, Polyethylene Glycol, Titanium Dioxide, Wheat Bran.

Thinz-Span - Alva-Amco Pharmacal Cos., Inc.
Each capsule contains: Phenylpropanolamine HCl 75 mg.

Thinzyme - General Vitamin
Each tablet contains: Vitamin B6 (pyridoxine HCl) 4 mg • Calcium (carbonatre, aminoate) 108 mg • Choline Bitartrate 300 mg • DL-Methionine 300 mg • Lecithin (phosphatide-rich soy extract) 10 mg • L-Arginine (free form amino acid) 10 mg • L-Ornithine HCl (free form amino acid) 10 mg • L-Carnitine (L-tartrate) 10 mg • Green Orange (citrus aurantium exocarp extract, standardized 4% synephrine) 100 mg • Super Citrimax brand Garcinia Cambogia exocarp extract (standardized 60% hydroxycitrate) 100 mg • Siberian Ginseng (eleutherococcus senticosis root) 100 mg • Lipase 10 mg. Other Ingredients: Dicalcium Phosphate, Microcrystalline Cellulose, Stearic Acid, Pharmaceutical Glaze.
See Editor's Note No. 40.

ThioNAC - Jarrow Formulas
Each tablet contains: N-Acetyl-L-Cysteine (NAC) 500 mg • Alpha Lipoic Acid (thioctic acid) 100 mg. Other Ingredients: Cellulose, Calcium Phosphate, Stearic Acid, Magnesium Stearate, Silicon Dioxide.

Thisilyn - Nature's Way
Each capsule contains: Milk thistle extract (standardized for a flavanoid content of 140 mg silymarin [80%], which includes silybinin, silychristin, and 85 mg of lactose) 175 mg.

ThistleComp - PhytoPharmica
Each capsule contains: Artichoke leaves extract (Cynara scolymus) 250 mg • Curcuma root extract (Curcuma longa) 150 mg • Boldo extract (Peumus boldo) 100 mg • Milk Thistle extract (Silybum marianum) (56 mg) calculated as silybin 70 mg.
See Editor's Note No. 21.

ThistlePlex - Enzymatic Therapy
Each capsule contains: Artichoke leaves extract (Cynara scolymus) standardized to contain 3% Caffeylquinic Acids 250 mg • Curcuma root extract (Curcuma longa) standardized to contain 2.5% Curcumin) 150 mg • Boldo extract (Peumus boldo) standardized to contain 1.52% essential oils) 100 mg • Milk Thistle extract (Silybum marianum) standardized to contain 80% Silymarin (56 mg) calculated as Silybin 70 mg.

Some Brand Name Natural Products - What they Contain

www.NaturalDatabase.com contains MANY more listings than appear here.
Editor's Notes are located on pages 2155-2163.

BRAND NAMES

ThistleRex - PhytoPharmica
Two capsules contain: Artichoke leaf extract (cynara scolymus, standardized to contain 13%-18% caffeylquinic acids) 20 mg • Dandelion root 4:1 exctract (taraxacum officinale) 20 mg • Licorice root and rhizome extract (glycyrrhiza glabra, standardized to contain 5% glycyrrhizic acids) 20 mg • Milk Thistle fruit extract (silybum marianum, standardized to contain 80% silymarin (240 mg) calculated as silybin) 300 mg.

Thistlezyme - Olympian Labs
Two capsules contain: Milk Thistle extract (standardized to contain at least 80% Silymarin) 200 mg.

Thorene - Thorne Research Inc.
Each capsule contains: Tylophora asthmatica 30 mg • Boswellia serrata extract (60% Boswellin) 150 mg • Piper longa 100 mg • Hesperidin Methyl Chalcone 100 mg.

Three-In-One - Goldshield Elite
Each capsule contains: Vitamin C (as Calcium Ascorbate) 120 mg • Aloe Vera leaf gel 200:1 concentrate 200 mg • Mexican Yam root 4:1 (equivalent to 150 mg) 37.5 mg. Other Ingredients: Gelatin, Maltodextrin, Calcium Sulfate, Magnesium Stearate, and Silica.

ThreeLac - Global Health Trax
Each packet contains: Vitamin C 10 mg • Thiamin 0.4 mg • Riboflavin 0.4 mg • Vitamin B6 0.4 mg • Sodium 10 mg. Other Ingredients: Spore Forming Lactic Acid Bacteria (lactobacillus sporogenes), Lemon juice powder, Refined Yeast powder, Castor Oil, Spore Forming Bacteria (bacillus subtills), Lactic Acid Bacteria (streptococcus faecalis).

Throat Coat - Traditional Medicinals
Active Ingredient: Slippery Elm bark (ulmus rubra). Inactive Ingredients: Licorice Root, Wild Cherry Bark, Fennel Seed, Cinnamon Bark, Orange Peel, Althea Root.

Throat Spray - Botanical Laboratories
Capsicum 6X • Echinacea Angustifolia 1X • Eucalyptus 1X • Kava 1X • Lycopodium Clavatum 4X • Peppermint 6X • Phosphorus 6X • Phytolacca Decandra 3X • Wild Thyme 1X.
See Editor's Note No. 1.

T-HRT - Dial Herbs
Hawthorne • Lecithin • Tansy • Fenugreek • Garlic • Cayenne.

T-HS - Dial Herbs
Ginseng • Damiana • Gotu Kola • Sarsaparilla • Sassafras • Saw Palmetto.

Thyax - Progressive Health Nutraceuticals
Acetyl L-Tyrosine 600 mg • L-Tyrosine 250 mg • Magnesium (magnesium aspartate) 200 mg • Zinc (picolinate) 10 mg • Iodine 450 mcg • Manganese 10 mg • L-Aspartic Acid 200 mg • Potassium (potassium aspartate) 198 mg • Niacin/Niacinamide (50/50) 50 mg • Vitamin B1 (thiamine HCl) 30 mg • Vitamin B2 (riboflavin) 50 mg.

Thyme and Myrrh - Dial Herbs
Thyme • Myrrh.

Thymex - Standard Process, Inc.
Each tablet contains: Proprietary Blend 195 mg: Bovine Thymus extract (Cytosol), Magnesium citrate. Other Ingredients: Calcium Lactate, Cellulose, Calcium Stearate, Ascorbic Acid.
See Editor's Note No. 14.

Thymic-Synergy - Metagenics
Each tablet contains: Vitamin A (retinyl acetate and beta-carotene) 5500 IU • Vitamin C (as ascorbic acid) 300 mg • Citrus Bioflavonoid Complex (standardized to 45% bioflavonoids) 150 mg • Ray Thymus concentrate (bovine) 40 mg • Pantothenic Acid (as D-calcium pantothenate) 30 mg • Raw Spleen concentrate (bovine) 20 mg • Vitamin B6 (as pyridoxine hydrochloride) 15 mg • Raw Adrenal concentrate (bovine) 10 mg • Zinc (as zinc citrate) 2 mg • Copper (as copper citrate) 200 mcg • Selenium (as selenium aspartate) 25 mcg • Molybdenum (as molybdenum aspartate) 20 mcg.

Thymucin - PhytoPharmica
Two capsules contain: Enzymatic Polypeptide Fractions (Thymus fractions) 750 mg • Astragalus root extract (astragalus membranaceus, standardized to 0.5% minimum of the isoflavone 4' hydroxy 3' methoxy isoflavone 7-SUG [GHMIF]) 250 mg.

Thymuplex Capsules - Enzymatic Therapy
Four capsules contain: Vitamin A (as beta carotene) 25,000 IU • Vitamin C (ascorbic acid) 250 mg • Vitamin E (as d-alpha tocopheryl acid succinate) 200 IU • Zinc (as zinc krebs cycle chelates) 15 mg • Selenium (as l-selenomethionine) 25 mcg • Proprietary Thymus Polypeptide Fraction/Glandular Complex 935 mg: Thymus Polypeptide fractions, Spleen extract (freeze-dried), Thymus extract, Lymphatic extract (freeze-dried), Bromelain (1200 M.C.U./g), Trypsin, Papain • Echinacea Purpurea root 300 mg • Lysine (as L-lysine HCl) 250 mg • Blue Flag root (iris versicolor) 130 mg • Goldenseal root (hydrastis canadensis) 64 mg. Other Ingredients: Gelatin, Fennel Seed, Magnesium Stearate, Silicon Dioxide, Titanium Dioxide Color.
See Editor's Note No. 14.

Thymuplex Tablets - Enzymatic Therapy
Two tablets contain: Vitamin A (as beta carotene) 25,000 IU • Vitamin C (ascorbic acid) 250 mg • Vitamin E (as d-alpha tocopheryl acid succinate) 200 IU • Zinc (as zinc krebs cycle chelates) 15 mg • Selenium (as l-selenomethionine) 25 mcg • Proprietary Thymus Polypeptide Fraction/Glandular Complex 935 mg: Thymus Polypeptide fractions, Spleen extract (freeze-dried), Thymus extract, Lymphatic extract (freeze-dried), Bromelain (1200 M.C.U./g), Trypsin, Papain • Echinacea Purpurea root 300 mg • Lysine (as L-lysine HCl) 250 mg • Blue Flag root (iris versicolor) 130 mg • Goldenseal root (hydrastis canadensis) 64 mg. Other Ingredients: Cellulose, Modified Cellulose Gum, Fennel Seed, Modified Cellulose, Magnesium Stearate, Lecithin, Carnauba Wax, Peppermint Leaf.
See Editor's Note No. 14.

Thymuril Capsules - PhytoPharmica
Four capsules contain: Vitamin A (beta-carotene) 25,000 IU • Vitamin C (ascorbic acid) 250 mg • Vitamin E (D-alpha tocopheryl acetate) 200 IU • Zinc (Krebs chelate) 15 mg • Selenium (L-selenomethionine) chelate 25 mcg • Polypeptide Fractions Thymus Complex (predigested, concentrated soluble extract standardized for peptides and polypeptides with molecular weight less than 10,000 daltons) 935 mg • Echinacea root (echinacea purpurea) 300 mg • L-Lysine (HCl) 250 mg • Blue Flag extract (iris versicolor) 130 mg • Goldenseal root extract (hydrastis canadensis) 64 mg.
See Editor's Note No. 14.

Thymuril Tablets - PhytoPharmica
Two tablets contain: Blue flag root (iris versicolor) 130 mg • Echinacea Purpurea root 300 mg • Goldenseal root (hydrastis canadensis) 64 mg • Lysine (as L-lysine HCl) 250 mg • Proprietary Thymus Polypeptide/Glandular Complex 935 mg: Thymus Polypeptide fractions, Spleen extract (freeze-dried), Thymus extract, Lymphatic extract (freeze-dried), Bromelain (1200 MCU/g), Trypsin, Papain • Selenium (as L-selenomethionine) 25 mcg • Vitamin A (as beta carotene) 25,000 IU • Vitamin C (ascorbic acid) 250 mg • Vitamin E (as D-alpha tocopheryl acid succinate) 200 IU • Zinc (as zinc Krebs cycle chelates) 15 mg.
See Editor's Note No. 14.

Thymus Cream - Atrium Biotechnologies
Three fluid ounces contain: Extract of Thymus (Viobin) • Glycerin Hexadecenol • Sodium Laureth Sulfate • Stearic Acid • Methylparaben • Sodium Sulfate • Propylparaben • Natural Fragrance.
See Editor's Note No. 14.

Thymus Glandular - American Biologics
Each tablet contains: Raw Thymus concentrate (bovine origin) 150 mg. Other Ingredients: Dicalcium Phosphate, Magnesium Stearate.
See Editor's Note No. 14.

Thymus PMG **-** Standard Process, Inc.
Each tablet contains: Proprietary Blend 230 mg: Bovine Thymus PMG extract, Magnesium Citrate • Calcium 18 mg • Sodium 22 mg. Other Ingredients: Calcium Lactate, Cellulose, Calcium Stearate.
See Editor's Note No. 14.

T-HYPO **-** Dial Herbs
Licorice • Juniper berry • Wild Yam • Dandelion • Ginger.

Thyrene **-** Metabolic Nutrition, Inc.
Six capsules contain: Guggulsterone (10%) 900 mg • L-Tyrosine 810 mg • Di Potassium Phosphate 600 mg • Coleus Forskohlii (20%) 260 mg • Sodium Phosphate 240 mg • Di Sodium Phosphate 240 mg • Iodine (organic) 900 mcg.

Thyrin-ATC **-** Rand Research Laboratories, LLC
Two capsules contain: Triphosrin Proprietary Blend 1637 mg: Sodium (as mono & disodium phosphate) 39 mg, Potassium (as dipotassium phosphate) 67 mg, Vitamin A (1000 IU as beta-carotene) 1325 IU, Vitamin C 13 mg, Calcium (as calcium phosphate) 73 mg, Vitamin E (as natural D-alpha tocopherol) 33 IU, Vitamin B1 (thiamin) 1 mg, Vitamin B2 (riboflavin) 7 mg, Vitamin B6 1.3 mg, Folic Acid 400 mcg, Vitamin B12 (cyanocobalamin) 6 mcg, Biotin 30 mcg, Pantothenic Acid 6 mg, Phosphorus (as mono & disodium dipotassium & calcium phosphate) 119 mg, Magnesium (as amino acid chelate) 13 mg, Zinc (as amino acid chelate) 4 mg, Selenium (as amino acid chelate) 4 mg, Copper (as amino acid chelate) 10 mcg, Manganese (as amino acid chelate) 690 mcg, Molybdenum (as amino acid chelate) 10 mcg, Commiphora Mukul SE, Garcinia Cambogia SE (HCA 125 mg), L-Tyrosine, Phopshatidylcholine, Caffeine 100 mg, Kelp meal (0.15% iodine [15 mg]), Niacinamide, L-Cysteine, Black Pepper fruit SE, Horsetail stem grass, Gentian root, Nettles herb, Radish root extract.

Thyro Complex **-** Progressive Labs
Each capsule contains: Raw Thyroid concentrate (thyroxin free) 60 mg • Raw Adrenal concentrate 30 mg • Raw Pituitary concentrate 10 mg • Raw Spleen concentrate 10 mg • Kelp 300 mg.
See Editor's Note No. 31.

Thyro-Calm **-** Ortho Molecular Products
Three capsules contain: Proprietary Blend 1.4 g: Bugleweed herb powder (lycopus virginicus), Lemon Balm flower extract (melissa officinalis, standardized to contain 5% rosmarinic acid). Other Ingredients: Natural Vegetable Capsules, Magnesium Stearate, Microcrystalline Cellulose.

Thyro-Dyne **-** InterPlexus
Two capsules contian: Iodine (as potassium iodide) 220 mcg • L-Tyrosine 200 mg • L-Cysteine HCl 150 mg • Proprietary Blend 1200 mg: Ashwaganda, Guggul. Other Ingredients: Magnesium Stearate, Silicon Dioxide.

ThyroFuel **-** E'OLA
Two capsules contain: Proprietary Blend 810 mg: Kelp, Thyroid Extract, Gugulipid Commiphora Mukul Extract, Tyrosine, Gentian (root). Other Ingredients: Gelatin, Rice Flour.

Thyroid **-** American Biologics
Each tablet contains: Raw Thyroid concentrate (bovine) 130 mg. Other Ingredients: Dicalcium Phosphate, Magnesium Stearate.
See Editor's Note No. 14.

Thyroid & L-Tyrosine Complex **-** Enzymatic Therapy
Two capsules contain: Vitamin B12 (as cyanocobalamin) 100 mcg • Iodine (as potassium iodide) 200 mcg • Magnesium (as magnesium oxide) 200 mg • Zinc (as zinc gluconate) 6 mg • Copper (as copper gluconate) 300 mcg • Manganese (as manganese gluconate) 2.3 mg • Molybdenum (as sodium molybdate) 100 mcg • L-Tyrosine 248 mg • Multi-Glandular Complex 70 mg: Liver, Lung, Pancreas, Heart, Kidney, Spleen • Thyroid extract (thyroxin-free) 8 mg. Other Ingredients: Gelatin, Modified Cellulose Gum, Magnesium Stearate, Silicon Dioxide, Titanium Dioxide Color.
See Editor's Note No. 14.

Thyroid Complex **-** The Vitamin Shoppe
Each capsule contains: Thiamine (Vitamin B1) 10 mg • Riboflavin (Vitamin B2) 10 mg • Vitamin B6 (as pyridoxine HCl) 10 mg • Vitamin B12 (as cyanocobalamin) 25 mcg • Iodine (from kelp) 150 mcg • Magnesium (as magnesium oxide) 100 mg • Zinc (as zinc chelate) 3 mg • Selenium (as selenium chelate) 70 mcg • Copper (as copper chelate) 150 mcg • Manganese (as manganese chelate) 3 mg • Molybdenum (as molybdenum chelate) 150 mcg • L-Tyrosine 150 mg • Multi Gland Complex 35 mg: Bovine Liver, Lung, Pancreas, Heart, Kidney, Spleen, Brain.
See Editor's Note No. 14.

Thyroid Essentials **-** Swanson Health Products
Each capsule contains: Thiamin USP (as thiamin HCl; vitamin B-1) 25 mg • Riboflavin USP (vitamin B-2) 25 mg • Niacinamide 25 mg • Vitamin B6 (as pyridoxine HCl) 25 mg • Folic Acid 25 mcg • Vitamin B12 (as cyanocobalamin) 25 mcg • Pantothenic Acid (as d-calcium pantothenate) 25 mg • Iodine (from kelp) 100 mcg • Magnesium (from magnesium oxide) 25 mg • Zinc (from zinc oxide) 25 mg • Selenium (as L-selenomethionine) 50 mcg • Copper (from copper gluconate) 2 mg • L-Tyrosine 150 mg • Coleus Forskohlii (18% forskolin) 50 mg.

Thyroid Factors **-** Michael's Naturopathic Programs
Three capsules contain: Vitamin B6 (as pyridoxine) 75 mg • Iodine (from kelp) 450 mcg • Chromium (as chromium polynicotinate) 300 mcg • Manganese (amino acid chelate) 90 mg • Proprietary Blend 675 mg: Gentian root (gentiana lutea), Irish Moss (whole plant, chondrus crispus), Bladderwrack (whole plant, fucus vesiculosus), Tyrosine (as L-tyrosine). Other Ingredients: Cellulose, Dicalcium Phosphate, Maltodextrin, Magnesium Stearate, Stearic Acid.

Thyroid Support **-** Gaia Herbs
Two capsules contain: L-Tyrosine 300 mg • Schizandra berry (schizandra chinensis) 156 mg • Coleus root (coleus forskohlii) 154 mg • Kelp fronds (nereocystis luetkeana) 130 mg • Ashwagandha root (withania somnifera) 120 mg • Bladderwrack fronds (fucus vesiculosus) 56 mg. Other Ingredients: Vegetable Glycerin, Lecithin, Vegetable Cellulose.

Thyroid Support Formula **-** PhysioLogics
Each capsule contains: Riboflavin 20 mg • Niacin (as niacinamide) 20 mg • Vitamin B6 (as pyridoxine hydrochloride) 1 mg • Iodine (from kelp) 110 mcg • Zinc (as zinc gluconate) 5 mg • Copper (as copper glycinate) 300 mcg • Chromium (as chromium chelavite) 75 mcg • L-Tyrosine 300 mg • Coleus Forskohlii leaf (standardized to contain 20% forskholin, 10 mg) 50 mg. Other Ingredients: Gelatin, Rice Powder, Vegetable Magnesium Stearate, Silica.

Thyroid T-3 **-** Absolute Nutrition
Two capsules contain: Calcium Phosphate 250 mg • Guggul gum extract (gugglesterone 10%) 300 mg • L-Tyrosine 300 mg • Garcinia Cambogia 200 mg • Dipotassium Phosphate 150 mg • Sodium Phosphate 75 mg • Disodium Phosphate 75 mg • Phosphatidyl Choline 25 mg. Other Ingredients: Microcrystalline Cellulose, Magnesium Stearate, Gelatin.

Thyro-Mel **-** Extreme Labs
Each capsule contains: Thyro-Mel (17-betahydroxy-5alpha-3andros T-1-ene-3-ether) 1000 mcg.

ThyroPlex for Men **-** Life Enhancement Products, Inc.
Each capsule contains: Hypothalamus (bovine, freeze-dried) 200 mg • Adrenal (bovine, freeze-dried) 200 mg • Pituitary, anterior (bovine, freeze-dried) 150 mg • Bovine Testicle extract (freeze-dried) 50 mg • Thyroid, whole (bovine, freeze-dried) 15 mg.
See Editor's Note No. 31.

ThyroPlex for Women **-** Life Enhancement Products, Inc.
Each capsule contains: Hypothalamus (bovine, freeze-dried) 200 mg • Adrenal (bovine, freeze-dried) 200 mg • Pituitary, anterior (bovine, freeze-dried) 150 mg • Ovary (bovine, freeze-dried) 50 mg • Thyroid, whole (bovine, freeze-dried) 15 mg.
See Editor's Note No. 31.

BRAND NAMES

Thyrosine Complex - PhytoPharmica
Two capsules contain: Copper (as copper gluconate) 300 mcg • Iodine (as potassium iodide) 200 mcg • L-Tyrosine 248 mg • Magnesium (as magnesium oxide) 200 mg • Manganese (as manganese gluconate) 2.3 mg • Molybdenum (as sodium molybdate) 100 mcg • Multi-Glandular Copmlex 70 mg: Liver, Lung, Pancreas, Heart, Kidney, Spleen • Thyroid extract (thyroxin-free) 8 mg • Vitamin B12 (as cyanocobalamin) 100 mcg • Zinc (as zinc gluconate) 6 mg.
See Editor's Note No. 31.

Thyrosol - Metagenics
Each tablet contains: Vitamin A (as retinyl palmitate) 3000 IU • Vitamin D (as cholecalciferol) 400 IU • Vitamin E (as D-alpha tocopheryl succinate) 100 IU • Riboflavin 3 mg • Niacin (as niacinamide) 4.5 mg • Iodine (as potassium iodide) 76 mcg • Zinc (as zinc glycinate) 10 mg • Selenium (as selenomethionine) 150 mcg • Rosemary leaf extract (rosmarinus officinalis) 79 mg.

ThyroStart - SilverSage
Two capsules contain: Kelp meal 500 mg • Vitamin C 20 mg • Magnesium 20 mg • L-Tryosine 20 mg • Vitamin B3 20 mg • Vitamin B2 10 mg • Zinc 10 mg • Vitamin B5 10 mg • Horsetail grass 5 mg • Gentian root 5 mg • Blue Flag 5 mg • Nettle leaf herb 5 mg • Radish extract 4:1 5 mg • Parathyroid substance 5 mg • Thymus substance 2.5 mg • Adrenal substance 2.5 mg • Pancreas substance 2.5 mg • Vitamin B6 2 mg • Vitamin B1 1.5 mg • Manganese 1 mg • Copper 0.02 mg • Vitamin A 2000 IU • Beta Carotene 2000 IU • Vitamin E 50 IU • Biotin 50 mcg • Folic Acid 50 mcg • Vitamin B12 10 mcg • Selenium 10 mcg • Molybdenum 10 mcg.
See Editor's Note No. 14.

Thyrotain - Ortho Molecular Products
Each capsule contains: Iodine (from kelp, potassium) 150 mcg • L-Tyrosine USP 500 mg • Ashwagandha root extract (standardized to contain 15% withanolides) 100 mg • Bladderwrack leaf 50 mg. Other Ingredients: Natural Vegetable Capsules, Ascorbyl Palmitate, Microcrystalline Cellulose, Silicon Dioxide.

Thyrotril - Sterling-Grant Laboratories
Two capsules contain: Selenium (as selenomethionine) 200 mcg • L-Tyrosine 500 mg • Olive leaf extract 100 mg • Pure Synthetic E & Z Guggelsterones 40 mg • Atlantic Kelp 30 mg • Bioperine brand Black Pepper extract 5 mg. Other Ingredients: Gelatin, Cellulose, Magnesium Stearate.

Thyrovarin - Klein-Becker
Two capsules contain: Vitamin A 3000 IU • Vitamin C 20 mg • Vitamin E 50 IU • Vitamin B1 1.65 mg • Vitamin B2 10 mg • Vitamin B6 2 mg • Vitamin B9 50 mcg • Vitamin B12 10 mcg • Biotin 50 mcg • Pantothenic Acid 10 mg • Magnesium 20 mg • Zinc 10 mg • Selenium 10 mcg • Copper 20 mcg • Manganese 1 mg • Molybdenum 10 mg • Proprietary Blend 690 mg: Kelp meal (0.15% iodine), L-Tyrosine, Niacinamide, Radish root 4:1 extract, Nettles herb, Horsetail grass stem, Gentian root. Other Ingredients: Rice Flour.

Thytrophin PMG - Standard Process, Inc.
Each tablet contains: Proprietary Blend 109 mg: Magnesium Citrate, Bovine Thyroid PMG extract (thyroxine removed) • Calcium 30 mg. Other Ingredients: Cellulose.
See Editor's Note No. 14.

Tian Ma Gou Teng Yin Plus - Secara
Organic Motherwort herb 265 mg • Organic Nettle leaf 225 mg • Poria sclerotium 5:1 extract (fu ling) 191 mg • Uncaria Rhynchophylla stem (gou teng) 5:1 extract 191 mg • Cyathula root 5:1 extract (chuan niu xi) 183 mg • Loranthus twig & leaf 5:1 extract (sang ji sheng) 172 mg • Fo-Ti stem 5:1 extract (ye jiao teng) 152 mg • Baikal Skullcap root 5:1 extract (huang qin) 133 mg • Eucommia bark 5:1 extract (du zhong) 133 mg • Gardenia fruit 5:1 extract (zhi zi) 133 mg • Gastrodia rhizome 5:1 extract (tian ma) 133 mg • Calcium (as calcium carbonate) 113 mg • Magnesium (as magnesium oxide) 113 mg • Horsetail shoots (2.6% silica (3 mg)) 113 mg.

Tian Wang Bu Xin Dan Plus - Secara
Rehmannia tuber 5:1 extract (sheng di huang) 414 mg • Organic Codonopsis root (dang shen) 246 mg • California Poppy 4:1 extract 165 mg • Hawthorn leaf and flower 6:1 extract 165 mg • Chinese Asparagus root 5:1 extract (tian men dong) 144 mg • Dong Quai root 5:1 extract 144 mg • Jujube seed 5:1 extract 144 mg • Juniper berry 5:1 extract 144 mg • Ophiopogon tuber 5:1 extract (mai dong) 144 mg • Schisandra fruit 5:12 extract (wu wei zi) 144 mg • Scrophularia root & rhizome 5:1 extract (xuan shen) 144 mg • Chinese Sage root & rhizome 5:1 extract (dan shen) 63 mg • Platycodon root 5:1 extract (jie geng) 63 mg • Polygala rhizome 5:1 extract (yuan zhi) 63 mg • Poria sclerotium 5:1 (fu ling) 63 mg.

Tiao He Cleanse - Nature's Sunshine
Each packet (6 capsules) contains: Chinese Liver Balance (one capsule) 485 mg: Bupleurum root (bupleurum chinense), Peony root (without bark, paeonia officinalis), Typhonium rhizome (typhonium flagelliforme), Cassia Cinnamon twig (cinnamomum cassia), Dong Quai root (angelica polymorpha var. sinensis), Fushen Sclerotium (with root, poria cocos), Scute root (scutellaria baicalensis), Zhishi fruit (citrus aurantium), Atractylodes rhizome (atractylodes lancea), Ginseng root (panax ginseng), Ginger rhizome (zingiber officinale), Licorice root (glycyrrhiza uralensis). All Cell Detox (one capsule) 475 mg: Gentian root (gentiana lutea), Irish Moss plant (chondrus crispus), Cascara Sagrada bark (rhamnus purhsiana), Golden Seal rhizome (hydrastis canadensis), Fenugreek seed (trigonella foenum-graecum), Slippery Elm bark (ulmus fulva), Safflower flowers (carthamus tinctorius), Black Walnut hulls (juglans nigra), Myrrh gum (commiphora molmol), Yellow Dock root (rumex crispus), Parthenium root (parthenium integrifolium), Oregon Grape root and rhizome (berberis aquifolium), Dandelion root (taraxacum officinale), Uva Ursi leaves (arctostaphylos uva ursi), Chickweed leaves and flowering tops (stellaria media), Catnip aerial parts (nepeta cataria), Cyani flowers (centaurea cyanus). LBS II (one capsule) 425 mg: Cascara Sagrada bark (rhamnus purshiana), Buckthorn bark (rhamnus frangula), Licorice root (glycyrrhiza glabra), Capsicum fruit (capsicum annuum), Ginger rhizome (zingiber officinale), Oregon Grape root and rhizome (berberis aquifolium), Turkey Rhubarb root (rheum officinale), Couch Grass rhizome (agropyron repens), Red Clover flowers (trifolium pratense). One capsule contains: Psyllium hulls (plantago ovata) 465 mg. One capsule contains: Burdock root (arctium lappa) 360 mg. One capsule contains: Black Walnut hulls (juglans nigra) 500 mg. Other Ingredients: Magnesium Stearate, Silicon dioxide, Gelatin, Water.
See Editor's Note No. 40.

Tiger Vites - Body Wise International, Inc.
Two caplets contain: Beta Carotene (vitamin A 5000 IU) 3 mg • Vitamin D (D3, cholecalciferol) 200 IU • Vitamin E (D-alpha tocopherol acid succinate and mixed tocopherols) 30 IU • Vitamin C 60 mg • Folic Acid 400 mcg • Vitamin B1 1.5 mg • Vitamin B2 1. 7 mg • Vitamin B6 2 mg • Niacin (niacinamide) 20 mg • Vitamin B12 6 mcg • Pantothenic Acid (D-calcium pantothenate) 5 mg • Biotin 150 mcg • Choline (bitartrate) 10 mcg • Inositol 10 mcg • Calcium chelate) 50 mg • Magnesium 40 mg • Copper 1 mg • Zinc 7.5 mg • Molybdenum 37.5 mcg • Iodine (kelp) 75 mcg • Chromium 120 mcg • Selenium (L-selenomethionine) 17.5 mcg • Manganese 0.5 mg • Potassium 0.5 mg • Iron 1.8 mg • PhytoNutrient Garden & Orchard Blend 50 mg: Broccoli, Bussels Sprout, Cabbage, Carrot, Cauliflower, Kale, Onion, Tomato, Acidophilus, Apple, Pectin, Bromelain, Cellulase, Cranberry, Date, Grape Seed extract, Grape Skin extract, Orange, Peach • Pineapple 12.5 mg • Papaya 12.5 mg • Citrus Bioflavonoids 12.5 mg. Other Ingredients: Spirulina, Whole Brown Rice, Spinach, Beet Leaf, Cherry, Rose Hips, Mango.

Tight! - SAN Nutrition
Each capsule contains: Thermogenic Proprietary Blend 325 mg: Caffeine Anhydrous • Forslean brand Coleus Forskohlii • Synephrine • Sclareolide • Pure Guggulsterones E & Z • Yohimbine • Vinpocetine • Bioperine brand Black Pepper extract. Other Ingredients: Microcrystalline Cellulose, Gelatin, Red #3, Orange #4.
See Editor's Note No. 40.

Tigra Pill - Universal Products, Performance Industries
Each tablet contains: Hydrolyzed protein rich in Arginine • D-Alpha-Tocopherol • Aromatic plant extracts: Damiana Aphrodisiaca, Dioscorea Villosa, Panax Ginseng, Smilax Officinalis • Choline sulfate • Vitamin B3 • Vitamin B1 • Zinc sulfate • Grape Seed extract • Peppermint oil • Savory oil • Clove oil • Magnesium stearate • Carboxymethylcellulose • Magnesium silicate.

Time C - J. R. Carlson Laboratories, Inc.
Each capsule contains: Vitamin C (as ascorbic acid) 500 mg.

Time Fighters For Men - Goldshield Elite
Four caplets contain: Vitamin A (as Beta-Carotene and mixed carotenoids from D. salina algae) 25000 IU • Vitamin C (as Ascorbic Acid) 500 mg • Vitamin D (as Cholecalciferol) 400 IU •Vitamin E (as Dl-Alpha-Tocopheryl and D-Alpha Tocopheryl Succinate) 200 IU • Vitamin B1 (as Thiamin HCI) 50 mg • Vitamin B2 (as Riboflavin) 50 mg • Niacin (as Niacinamide) 125 mg • Vitamin B6 (as Pyridoxine HCI) 50 mg •Folate (as Folic Acid) 800 mcg •Vitamin B12 (as Cyanocobalamin) 500 mcg • Biotin 300 mcg • Pantothenic acid (as D-Calcium Pantothenate) 50 mg • Calcium (as Calcium Carbonate and Citrate) 400 mg • Iodine (as Potassium Iodide) 150 mcg • Magnesium (as Magnesium Oxide and Aspartate) 500 mg • Zinc (as Zinc Citrate and Picolinate) 50 mg • Selenium (as Selenomethionine) 200 mcg • Copper (as Copper Gluconate) 2 mg • Manganese (as Manganese Gluconate) 2 mg • Chromium (as Chromium Dinicotinate Glycinate) 200 mcg • Molybdenum (as Sodium Molybdate) 150 mcg • Potassium (as Potassium Citrate and Chloride) 10 mg • Life Enhancement Men's Herbal Blend 360 mg: Soybean phytosterol complex (120 mg Beta-Sitosterol), Saw Palmetto berry 4:1 extract, Panax Ginseng extract (4% ginsenosides) • Marigold flower concentrate (2% Lutein) 50 mg • Tomato fruit concentrate (2% Lycopene) 50 mg • Choline Bitartrate 25 mg • Inositol 25 mg • PABA 10 mg • Whole Food Phytonutrient Concentrates 500 mg: Parsley, Dunaliela salina algae, Kale, Spinach, Cantoloupe, Carrot, Papaya, Red Peppers, Tomato, Yellow Squash, Turmeric, Cranberry, Tangerine, Grapefruit, Lemon, Orange, Pineapple, Leek, Onion, Garlic, Raspberry, Green Tea, Alfalfa, Soybean, Cherry, Peach, Pear, Red Grape, Strawberry, Asparagus, Broccoli, Bruessels Sprout, Cabbage, Cauliflower, Mustard Greens. Other Ingredients: Microcrystaline Cellulose, Croscarmellose Sodium, Stearic Acid, Silica, Caramel color, Magnesium Stearate, Vanillin.

Time Fighters For Women With Iron - Goldshield Elite
Four caplets contain: Vitamin A (beta-carotene and mixed carotenoids from D. salina algae) 25000 IU • Vitamin C (ascorbic acid) 500 mg • Vitamin D (cholecalciferol) 800 IU • Vitamin E (DL-alpha-tocopheryl Acetate and D-alpha tocopheryl succinate) 200 IU • Thiamin (Thiamin HCl) 25 mg • Riboflavin 25 mg • Niacin (niacinamide) 100 mg • Vitamin B6 (pyridoxine HCl) 25 mg • Folate (folic acid) 800 mcg • Vitamin B12 (cyanocobalamin) 250 mcg • Biotin 300 mcg • Pantothenic Acid (D-calcium pantothenate) 50 mg • Calcium (carbonate and citrate) 500 mg • Iron (ferrous fumarate) 18 mg • Iodine (potassium iodide) 150 mcg • Magnesium (oxide and aspartate) 400 mg • Zinc (citrate and picolinate) 30 mg • Selenium (selenomethionine) 200 mcg • Copper (gluconate) 2 mg • Manganese (gluconate) 2 mg • Chromium (dinicotinate glycinate) 200 mcg • Molybdenum (sodium molybdate) 150 mcg • Potassium (citrate and chloride) 10 mg • Boron (citrate) 3 mg • Marigold flower concentrate (2% lutein) 50 mg • Tomato fruit concentrate (2% lycopene) 50 mg • Choline Bitartrate 25 mg • Inositol 25 mg • PABA 10 mg • Life Enhancement Women's Herbal Blend 200 mg : Panax Ginseng root extract, Black Cohosh root, Chaste Tree fruit • Whole Food Phytonutrient Concentrates 500 mg: Parsley, Dunaliela Salina Algae, Kale, Spinach, Cantaloupe, Carrot, Papaya, Tomato, Yellow Squash, Turmeric rhizome, Tangerine, Grapefruit, Lemon, Orange, Red Pepper, Alfalfa, Soybean, Cranberry, Green Tea, Raspberry, Cherry, Peach, Pear, Pineapple, Red Grape, Strawberry, Asparagus spear, Brussesl sprouts, Garlic, Leek, Onion, Broccoli, Cauliflower, Cabbage, Mustard Greens. Other Ingredients: Microcrystalline Cellulose, Croscarmellose Sodium, Stearic Acid, Silica, Magnesium Stearate, Vanillin.

Time Fighters For Women Without Iron - Goldshield Elite
Four caplets contain: Vitamin A (beta-carotene and mixed carotenoids from D. salina algae) 25000 IU • Vitamin C (ascorbic acid) 500 mg • Vitamin D (cholecalciferol) 800 IU • Vitamin E (DL-alpha-tocopheryl acetate and D-alpha tocopheryl succinate) 200 IU • Thiamin (HCl) 25 mg • Riboflavin 25 mg • Niacin (niacinamide) 100 mg • Vitamin B6 (pyridoxine HCl) 25 mg • Folate (folic acid) 800 mcg • Vitamin B12 (cyanocobalamin) 250 mcg • Biotin 300 mcg • Pantothenic Acid (D-calcium pantothenate) 50 mg • Calcium (carbonate and citrate) 500 mg • Iodine (potassium iodide) 150 mcg • Magnesium (oxide and aspartate) 400 mg • Zinc (citrate and picolinate) 30 mg • Selenium (selenomethionine) 200 mcg • Copper (gluconate) 2 mg • Manganese (gluconate) 2 mg • Chromium (dinicotinate glycinate) 200 mcg • Molybdenum (sodium molybdate) 150 mcg • Potassium (citrate and chloride) 10 mg • Boron (citrate) 3 mg • Marigold flower concentrate (2% lutein) 50 mg • Tomato fruit concentrate (2% lycopene) 50 mg • Choline Bitartrate 25 mg • Inositol 25 mg • PABA 10 mg • Life Enhancement Women's Herbal Blend 200 mg: Panax Ginseng root extract, Black Cohosh root, Chaste Tree fruit • Whole Food Phytonutrient Concentrates 500 mg: Parsley, Dunaliela Salina Algae, Kale, Spinach, Cantaloupe, Carrot, Papaya, Tomato, Yellow Squash, Turmeric, Tangerine, Grapefruit, Lemon, Orange, Red Pepper, Alfalfa, Soybean, Cranberry, Green Tea, Raspberry, Cherry, Peach, Pear, Pineapple, Red Grape, Strawberry, Asparagus, Brussel sprouts, Garlic, Leek, Onion, Broccoli, Cauliflower, Cabbage, Mustard Greens. Other Ingredients: Microcrystalline Cellulose, Croscarmellose Sodium, Stearic Acid, Silica, Magnesium Stearate, Vanillin.

Time Release Athletes Formula - Puritan's Pride
Two caplets contain: Vitamin A 10,000 IU • Vitamin C 300 mg • Vitamin D 800 IU • Vitamin E 100 IU • Thiamin (Vitamin B1) 22.25 mg • Riboflavin (Vitamin B2) 25 mg • Niacin 100 mg • Vitamin B6 20.5 mg • Folic Acid 400 mcg • Vitamin B12 100 mcg • Biotin 50 mcg • Pantothenic Acid 25 mg • Calcium 250 mg • Iron 25 mg • Iodine 225 mcg • Magnesium 20 mg • Zinc 50 mg • Selenium (as Yeast) 25 mcg • Copper 0.05 mg • Manganese 5 mg • Chromium 50 mcg • Chloride 240 mg • Sodium 100 mg • Potassium 99 mg • Choline 25 mg • Inositol 25 mg • Lecithin 100 mg • RNA - DNA 25 mg • PABA 25 mg • Bee Pollen 50 mg • Rose Hips 20 mg • Isoleucine 389 mcg • Leucine 610 mcg • Lysine 632 mcg • Methionine 122 mcg • Phenylalanine 337 mcg • Threonine 390 mcg • Valine 500 mcg.

Time Release B-100 Ultra B-Complex - Puritan's Pride
Each tablet contains: Thiamin (Vitamin B1; as thiamine mononitrate) 100 mg • Riboflavin (Vitamin B2) 100 mg • Niacin (as niacinamide) 100 mg • Vitamin B6 (as pyridoxine hydrochloride) 100 mg • Folic Acid 100 mcg • Vitamin B12 (as cyanocobalamin) 100 mcg • Biotin (as D-Biotin) 100 mcg • Pantothenic Acid (as D-Calcium Pantothenate) 100 mg • Proprietary Blend 100 mg: Choline Bitartrate, Inositol, PABA (Para-Aminobenzoic Acid), Alfalfa, Watercress, Parsley, Lecithin, and Rice Bran.

Time Release B-50 Vitamin B-Complex - Puritan's Pride
Each tablet contains: Thiamin (vitamin B1) 50 mg • Riboflavin (vitamin B2) 50 mg • Niacin (niacinamide) 50 mg • Vitamin B6 (pyridoxine hydrochloride) 50 mg • Folic Acid 100 mcg • Vitamin B12 (cyanocobalamin) 50 mcg • Biotin (D-biotin) 50 mcg • Pantothenic Acid (D-calcium pantothenate) 50 mg • Proprietary Blend 50 mg: Choline Bitartrate, Inositol, PABA (Para-Aminobenzoic Acid), Alfalfa, Watercress, Parsley, Lecithin, Rice Bran.

Time Release B-Complex + C - Puritan's Pride
Each tablet contains: Vitamin C (as Ascorbic Acid and Rose Hips) 200 mg • Thiamin (Vitamin B1; as Thiamine Mononitrate) 10 mg • Riboflavin (Vitamin B2) 10 mg • Niacin (as Niacinamide) 50 mg • Vitamin B6 (as Pyridoxine Hydrochloride) 5 mg • Vitamin B12 (as Cyanocobalamin) 10 mcg • Pantothenic Acid (as D-Calcium Pantothenate) 10 mg.

Time Release Mega Vita-Min - Puritan's Pride
Each tablet contains: Vitamin A (as retinyl palmitate) 8000 IU • Vitamin C (as ascorbic acid and rose hips) 250 mg • Vitamin D (as cholecalciferol) 400 IU • Vitamin E (as D-alpha tocopheryl acetate)

125 IU • Thiamin (vitamin B1, as thiamine mononitrate) 80 mg • Riboflavin (vitamin B2) 80 mg • Niacin (as niacinamide) 80 mg • Vitamin B6 (as pyridoxine hydrochloride) 80 mg • Folic Acid 400 mcg • Vitamin B12 (as cyanocobalamin) 80 mcg • Biotin (as D-biotin) 80 mcg • Pantothenic Acid (as D-calcium pantothenate) 80 mg • Calcium (as calcium carbonate) 8 mg • Iron (as ferrous gluconate) 2 mg • Iodine (as kelp) 150 mcg • Magnesium (as magnesium oxide) 6 mg • Zinc (as zinc gluconate) 1.4 mg • Selenium (as sodium selenite) 25 mcg • Copper (as copper gluconate) 0.07 mg • Manganese (as manganese gluconate) 0.12 mg • Chromium (as chromium picolinate) 25 mcg • Molybdenum (as sodium molybdate) 25 mcg • Potassium (as potassium gluconate) 1.6 mg • Boron (as sodium borate) 0.5 mg • Choline Bitartrate 80 mg • Inositol 80 mg • PABA (para-aminobenzoic acid) 80 mg • Rutin fruit (dimorphandra mollis) 30 mg • Citrus Bioflavonoids fruit (citrus sinensis) 25 mg • Hesperidin fruit (citrus spp.) 5 mg • Betaine Hydrochloride 25 mg • Coenzyme Q-10 500 mg • Deodorized Garlic bulb (allium sativum) 1 mg • Korean Ginseng root (Panax ginseng) 1 mg • Pycnogenol 500 mcg • Proprietary Blend 4 mg: Alfalfa leaf, Watercress, Parsley leaf, Rice Bran, Lecithin. Other Ingredients: Methylcellulose, Vegetable Stearic Acid, Silica, Mannitol, Vegetable Magnesium Stearate, Cellulose Coating, Starch.

Time Release Mega Vitamins for the Hair - Puritan's Pride
Three tablets contain: Vitamin A (as 100% Beta Carotene) 10,000 IU • Vitamin C (as Ascorbic Acid) 1,000 mg • Thiamin (Vitamin B1; as Thiamine Hydrochloride) 89 mg • Riboflavin (Vitamin B2) 100 mg • Niacin (as niacinamide) 100 mg • Vitamin B6 (as Pyridoxine Hydrochloride) 82 mg • Folic Acid 400 mcg • Vitamin B12 (as Cyanocobalamin) 100 mcg • Biotin 2,000 mcg • Zinc (as Zinc Amino Acid Chelate) 5 mg • Copper (Cupric Sulfate) 2 mg • Choline Bitartrate 500 mg • Inositol 500 mg • PABA (Para-Aminobenzoic Acid) 100 mg • L-Cysteine Hydrochloride 334 mg.

Time Release Stress B with 500 mg Vitamin C - Puritan's Pride
Each tablet contains: Vitamin C (as ascorbic acid) 500 mg • Vitamin B1 (as thiamine hydrochloride) 100 mg • Vitamin B2 (riboflavin) 100 mg • Niacin (as niacinamide) 100 mg • Vitamin B6 (as pyridoxine hydrochloride) 100 mg • Folic Acid 400 mcg • Vitamin B12 (as cyanocobalamin) 500 mcg • Biotin (as D-Biotin) 50 mcg • Pantothenic Acid (as d-calcium pantothenate) 100 mg • Choline Bitartrate 50 mg • Inositol 50 mg • PABA (para-aminobenzoic acid) 50 mg • Citrus Bioflavonoids 50 mg.

Time Release Ultra Man - Puritan's Pride
Two tablets contain: Vitamin A (acetate) 5,000 IU • Vitamin E (D-alpha tocopheryl acetate) 100 IU • Vitamin C (ascorbic acid) 300 mg • Selenium (selenite) 25 mcg • Citrus Bioflavonoids 25 mg • Superoxide Dismutase (SOD) 10 mcg • Pycnogenol 1 mcg • Biotin 300 mcg • Silica 20 mcg • Inositol 10 mg • L-Cysteine 100 mg • Yohimbe extract 50 mg • Korean Ginseng root 50 mg • Swiss Avena Sativa (Oat Straw) 50 mg • Damiana leaves 50 mg • Muira Puama 50 mg • Nettles leaves 30 mg • Oyster Extract 25 mg • Saw Palmetto berries 50 mg • Prostate glandular 50 mg • Pumpkin Seed 30 mg • Pygeum 25 mg • Golden Seal herb 25 mg • Zinc (oxide) 2 mg • Vitamin B1 (thiamine mononitrate) 30 mg • Vitamin B2 (riboflavin) 30 mg • Vitamin B3 (Niacin) 30 mg • Vitamin B6 (pyridoxine HCl) 30 mg • Vitamin B12 (cyanocobalamin) 30 mcg • Folic Acid 400 mcg • Pantothenic Acid (calcium D-pantothenate) 30 mg • Choline (bitartrate) 10 mg • PABA (Para Aminobenzoic Acid) 10 mg • Vitamin D (cholecalciferol) 200 IU • Calcium (dicalcium phosphate) 275 mg • Phosphorus (dicalcium phosphate) 210 mg • Iodine (potassium iodide) 150 mcg • Magnesium (oxide) 100 mg • Manganese (gluconate) 5 mg • Potassium (chloride) 30 mg • Chromium (picolinate) 50 mcg • Vitamin K (Phytonadione) 25 mcg. Base: Garlic, Oat Bran, Spirulina, Alfalfa, Parsley, Lecithin, Watercress, Smilax (sarsaparilla), and Cayenne.
See Editor's Note No. 14.

Time Released B Complex Vitamin plus Vitamin C - Nature's Bounty
Each tablet contains: Vitamin C (as ascorbic acid and rose hips) 300 mg • Thiamin (vitamin B1, as thiamin mononitrate) 18 mg • Riboflavin (vitamin B2) 10 mg • Niacin (as niacinamide) 50 mg • Vitamin B6 (as pyridoxine hydrochloride) 5 mg • Folic Acid 400 mcg • Vitamin B12 (as cyanocobalamin) 10 mcg • Biotin 50 mcg • Pantothenic Acid (as D-calcium pantothenate) 10 mg. Other Ingredients: Dicalcium Phosphate, Cellulose (plant origin), Cellulose, Vegetable Stearic Acid, Silica, Vegetable Magnesium Stearate.

Time-B - J. R. Carlson Laboratories, Inc.
Each tablet contains: Thiamin (vitamin B1) 50 mg • Riboflavin (vitamin B2) 50 mg • Niacin (vitamin B3, as niacinamide) 50 mg • Vitamin B6 (pyridoxine hydrochloride) 50 mg • Folate (folic acid) 400 mcg • Vitamin B12 (cyanocobalamin) 50 mcg • Biotin 50 mcg • Pantothenic Acid (di-calcium pantothenate) 100 mg.

Time-C-Bio 1000 mg - J. R. Carlson Laboratories, Inc.
Each tablet contains: Vitamin C (as ascorbic acid) 1000 mg • Lemon Bioflavonoids complex 100 mg.

Time-C-Bio 500 mg - J. R. Carlson Laboratories, Inc.
Each tablet contains: Vitamin C (as ascorbic acid) 500 mg • Lemon Bioflavonoids complex 50 mg.

Timed Release Vitamin C - GNC
Each table contains: Vitamin C (as Ascorbic Acid) 1000 mg • Citrus Bioflavonoids Complex 100 mg. Other Ingredients: Calcium Sulfate, Cellulose, Stearic Acid, Magnesium Stearate, Rose hips, Acerola powder, Hesperidin Complex, Rutin.

Timed Release Vitamin C 500 mg - Walgreens
Each caplet contains: Vitamin C (ascorbic acid) 500 mg. Other Ingredients: Hydroxypropyl Methylcellulose, Dicalcium Phosphate, Stearic Acid, Talc, Silicon Dioxide, Magnesium Stearate, Colloidal Silicon Dioxide, Carnauba Wax.

Timed Release Vitamin C with Rose Hips - GNC
Each tablet contains: Vitamin C (as Ascorbic Acid) 500 mg. Other Ingredients: Dicalcium Phosphate, Cellulose, Food Glaze, Rose hips.

T-ING - Dial Herbs
Valerian root • Chamomile • Lobelia • Arnica • Cayenne.

T-JAUN - Dial Herbs
Barberry • Chamomile • Dandelion • Horehound • St. John's Wort • Tansy • Wood Betony • Yellow Dock.

T-KB - Dial Herbs
Peach bark • Marshmallow • Buchu Leaves • Corn Silk • Echinacea.

T-LB - Dial Herbs
Barberry • Cascara Sagrada • Licorice root • Senna Leaves • Red Raspberry • Lobelia • Cayenne.

TLC - Thymic Longevity Compound - EcoNugenics
Each packet contains: Purified Thymic Protein 4 mcg. Other Ingredients: Maltodextrin.

T-LS - Dial Herbs
Prickly Ash • Sarsaparilla • Poke root • Stillingia • Red Clover • Burdock • Barberry • Peach bark • Licorice root • Chaparral • Echinacea • Cayenne.

T-MEM - Dial Herbs
Lady Slipper • Rosemary • Gotu Kola • Borage • Siberian Ginseng • Licorice • Lobelia.

TMG (trimethylglycine) - Pure Encapsulations
Each vegetable capsule contains: Trimethylglycine (anhydrous betaine) 700 mg • Vitamin C (as ascorbyl palmitate) 14 mg.

TMG 500 - Jarrow Formulas
Each tablet contains: Trimethylglycine (anhydrous betaine) 500 mg. Other Ingredients: Dicalcium Phosphate, Modified Cellulose Gum, Silicon Dioxide, Magnesium Stearate.

Some Brand Name Natural Products - What they Contain

www.NaturalDatabase.com contains MANY more listings than appear here.
Editor's Notes are located on pages 2155-2163.

TMG Crystals - Jarrow Formulas
Each scoop contains: Trimethylglycine (anhydrous betaine) 500 mg.

TMG Plus - Progressive Labs
Each tablet contains: Trimethylglycine (anhydrous) 500 mg • Vitamin B6 (pyridoxine HCl) 37.5 mg • Vitamin B6 (pyridoxine-5'-phosphate) 7.5 mg • Folate (folic acid) 450 mcg • Vitamin B12 375 mcg • Selenium (from seleno-L-methionine) 7.5 mcg.

T-MISS - Dial Herbs
Wild Yam • Ginger • Red Raspberry • Catnip • False Unicorn • Squaw vine.

T-MSLE - Dial Herbs
Cleavers • Pleurisy root • Saffron • Valerian root • Yarrow • Bistort • Catnip • Cayenne • Lobelia.

T-MUSCL - Dial Herbs
Sarsaparilla • Saw Palmetto • Strawberry.

T-NAUS - Dial Herbs
Catnip • Peppermint • Cinnamon • Ginger • Alfalfa • Lobelia.

T-NRV - Dial Herbs
Black Cohosh • Blue Cohosh • Blue Vervain • Scullcap • Lobelia.

T-NSU - Dial Herbs
Cranesbill • Goldenseal • Marshmallow • Poke root • Echinacea.

Toco-Life - Jarrow Formulas
Each softgel contains: Vitamin E (D-alpha tocopherol) 27 IU • Palm fruit distillate 150 mg: D-Gamma Tocotrienol 33 mg, D-Delta Tocotrienol 7.5 mg, D-Alpha Tocotrienol 18 mg, Other Tocotrienols 1.5 mg, Squalene 15 mg, Phytosterols 5.3 mg. Other Ingredients: Gelatin, Glycerin, Water.

Tocotrien-All - Natrol, Inc.
One softgel contains: Tocotrienol Complex 50 mg containing Alpha-tocopherols 30 IU • Gamma-tocotrienols 45 mg • Alpha-tocotrienols 4 mg • Delta-tocotrienols 1 mg. Other Ingredients: Gelatin, Nutriene.

Tocotrienol Antioxidant Complex - Source Naturals
Each softgel contains: Vitamin E (as natural d-alpha tocopherol) 100 IU • Total Tocotrienols (gamma tocotrienol 31 mg) 50 mg.

Tocotrienols - Ortho Molecular Products
Each soft gel capsule contains: Vitamin E (D-alpha tocopherol with mixed tocopherols and tocotrienols) 100 IU • Tocotrienols 50 mg. Other Ingredients: Gelatin, Glycerin, Oryza Oil, Nutriene Rice Tocotrienol, Purified Water.

Tocotrienols - Pure Encapsulations
Each softgel capsule contains: Nutriene brand Rice Bran oil (standardized to 30% tocotrienols/tocopherols) 200 mg: D-gamma-tocotrienol 9 mg, D-alpha-tocotrienol 6 mg, D-alpha-tocopherol 30 IU, D-gamma-tocopherol 5 mg,

Tocotrienols - J. R. Carlson Laboratories, Inc.
Each softgel contains: Vitamin E (as D-alpha tocopherol) 100 IU • Delta Tocotrienol 6 mg • Gamma Tocotrienol 24 mg.

Tocotrienols plus E-100 I.U. - The Vitamin Shoppe
Each softgel contains: Vitamin E (as d-alpha, d-gamma, d-beta, d-delta tocopherols) 100 IU • Tocotrienols (NuTriene) (as d-alpha, d-gamma, d-beta, d-delta tocopherols) 35 mg.

Tofupill - Se-Cure Pharmaceuticals/Ventiv Health
Each capsule contains: Tofu concentrate 322 mg • Flaxseed 108 mg. Other Ingredients: Cellulose Capsule Shell.

Tomato Lycopene Softgels - TwinLab
Each softgel contains: Lycopene (lycopene10, from Lyc-O-Mato natural tomato) 10 mg. Other Ingredients: Rice Bran Oil, Gelatin, Glycerin, Water, MCT, Yellow Beeswax, Silica.

Tomentosin Plus - Atrium Biotechnologies
Each capsule contains: Uncaris tomentosa 400 mg • Bromelain 100 mg • Salix alba 50 mg • Curcuma longa 40 mg.

Tonalin - Natrol, Inc.
Each softgel contains: Proprietary Blend 1000 mg: CLA (conjugated linoleic acid), Oleic Acid, Palmitic Acid, Stearic Acid, Linoleic Acid. Other Ingredients: Glycerin, Water, Caramel Powder.

Tonalin 1000 - Source Naturals
Three softgels contain: Conjugated Linoleic Acid 2.22 g. Other Ingredients: Gelatin (capsule), Glycerin, Purified Water, Caramel, Titanium Dioxide, Carob.

Tonalin brand - Cognis
CLA (conjugated linoleic acid).

Tonalin CLA 1000 Mg - Natrol, Inc.
One softgel contains: Tonalin supplies 60-70% Conjugated Linoleic Acid from Sunflower oil 1000 mg. Other Ingredients: Lecithin, Beeswax, Soybean oil, Gelatin.

Tonalin CLA 750 Mg - Natrol, Inc.
One softgel contains: Tonalin supplies 60-70% Conjugated Linoleic Acid from Sunflower oil 750 mg • Chromium (Picolinate) 75 mcg • ThermoActives Capsicum (200 SCU) 100 mcg • Ginger root 100 mg. Other Ingredients: Lecithin, Beeswax, Soybean oil, Gelatin.

Tonalin CLA for Men - Natrol, Inc.
One capsule contains: Chromium (as Chromium Picolinate) 50 mcg • Sunflower oil 75 mg • CLA • Conjugated Linoleic Acid 150 mg • Alpha Lipoic Acid 8 mg • Vanadyl Sulfate 2 mg • Siberian Ginseng extract root 50 mg • Leucine (as L-Leucine Hydrochloride) 50 mg • Arginine (as L-Arginine Hydrochloride) 50 mg • Isoleucine (as L-Isoleucine Hydrochloride) 12 mg • Valine (as L-Valine Hydrochloride) 25 mg. Other Ingredients: Silicon Dioxide, Magnesium Stearate, Gelatin.

Tonalin XS-CLA - NSI - Nutraceutical Sciences Institute
Each softgel contains: Sunflower seed oil 1 g.

Tone 'N' Trim - Optimum Nutrition
Citrimax • L-Carnitine • Chromium Picolinate.

Tongkat Ali - Higher Power
Two tablets contain: Suma (pfaffia paniculata) 100 mg • Tongkat Ali 60 mg. Other Ingredients: Dicalcium Phosphate, Microcrystalline Cellulose, Stearic Acid, Croscarmellose Sodium, Magnesium Stearate, Silicon Dioxide, Klucel Nutra D.

Tongkat Ali - Physician Formulas
Each capsule contains: Tongkat Ali powder (eurycoma longifolia jack) 400 mg. Other Ingredients: Gelatin (capsules), Magnesium Stearate, Rice Powder, Silicon Dioxide.

Tongkat Ali Male Libido Tonic - Source Naturals
Each tablet contains: Eurycoma Longifolia extract (tongkat ali LJ100) 80 mg. Other Ingredients: Microcrystalline Cellulose, Stearic Acid, Modified Cellulose Gum, Colloidal Silicon Dioxide.

Top CLAss - Life Enhancement Products, Inc.
Each capsule contains: Conjugated Linoleic Acid (from safflower seed) 1000 mg. Other Ingredients: Glycerin, Gelatin, Carob Extract Concentrate, Water, Titanium Dioxide, Tertiarybutylhydroquinone (TBHQ), Citric Acid.

Topicure cream - SMG Enterprises Inc.
Bentonite • Calamine • Citric Acid • Diazolidinyl Urea • Glycerin • Iodopropynol Butylcarbamate • Lanolin • Methyl Glucose Sesquistearate • PEG-20 Methyl Glucose Sesquistearate • Petrolatum • Thuja Occidentalis leaf oil • Zinc Oxide • Water.

Tot Tonic - The Herbalist
Echinacea root • Golden Seal root • Lemon Balm herb • Yarrow flower • Yerba Santa leaf.

Total Balance Unisex - Xtend-Life Nutraceuticals Inc.
Six tablets contain: Boron (as boron citrate) 2 mg • Calcium (as calcium citrate) 100 mg • Copper (as copper gluconate) 2 mg • Magnesium (as magnesium citrate) 70 mg • Manganese (as manganese citrate) 8 mg • Sulfur as MSM 215 mg • Potassium (as

potassium citrate) 20 mg • Zinc (as zinc citrate) 10 mg • Mineral Sea Salts Proprietary Blend: Chromium, Indium, Iodine, Lithium, Molybdenum, Rubudium, Selenium, Strontium, Tungsten • Standardized Active Enzyems and Co-Factors Blend 140 mg: Betaine HCl, IsolasePro, Lipase, Papain • ATP Precursor 6 mg • Beta Carotene (natural) 7500 IU • Biotin 500 mcg • Folic Acid 500 mcg • Hesperidin 80 mg • Inositol Hexaphosphate 35 mg • Lutein 5 mg • Naringin 40 mg • PABA (para-aminobenzoic acid) 50 mg • Phosphatidyl Choline 75 mg • Piperine 10 mg • Rutin 10 mg • Tocotrienols (Tocomax 20% brand) 10 mg • Vitamin B1 (thiamine) 10 mg • Vitamin B2 (riboflavin) 10 mg • Vitamin B3 (niacinamide) 24 mg • Vitamin B5 (D-pantothenate) 40 mg • Vitamin B6 (pyridoxine HCl) 10 mg • Vitamin B12 (cyanocobalamin) 50 mcg • Vitamin C (ascorbic acid) 50 mg • Vitamin D3 (cholecalciferol) 150 IU • Vitamin E (succinate) 100 IU • Zeaxanthin 2 mg • Acetyl-L-Carnitine 100 mg • Alpha Lipoic Acid 50 mg • DIM, 3,3 Diindolylmethane 50 mg • DMAE, Dimethyl Amino Ethanol Bitartrate 200 mg • DMG, Di Methyl Glycine 25 mg • L-Arginine HCl 40 mg • L-Carnosine 100 mg • L-Lysine 100 mg • L-Methionine 20 mg • L-Proline 100 mg • L-Taurine 50 mg • L-Tyrosine 200 mg • Myricetin 70 mg • N-ACetyl L-Cysteine 35 mg • Policosanol 10 mg • Quercetin 50 mg • Resveratrol 32 mg • Ribonucleic Acid (RNA) 50 mg • Immunity Sitmulating Blend 157 mg: Aloe Vera, Beta Glucan, Tea Polysaccharides • Bilberry extract 50 mg • Black Cumin extract 50 mg • Cranberry extract 60 mg • Ginger extract 100 mg • Ginkgo Biloba extract 50 mg • Gotu Kola extract 100 mg • Green Tea extract 100 mg • Hawthorne berry extract 100 mg • Mahonia Grape extract 100 mg • Myrrh extract (guggulipid) 50 mg • Olive leaf extract 50 mg • Red Clover extract 50 mg • Turmeric extract 680 mg.

Total E **- Jarrow Formulas**
Each softgel contains: D-Alpha- Tocopherol 65 mg • D-Beta-Tocopherol 8 mg • D-Gamma- Tocopherol 210 mg • D-Delta-Tocopherol 82 mg • D-Alpha- Tocotrienol 15 mg • D-Beta-Tocotrienol 0.6 mg • D-Gamma- Tocotrienol 28 mg • D-Delta-Tocotrienol 6.3 mg • Coenzyme Q10 30 mg. Other Ingredients: Olive Oil, Rosemary Oil, Ascorbyl Palmitate, Gelatin, Carob.

Total Energy **- Jamieson**
Each caplet contains: Bee Pollen and Royal Jelly (from Organically Monitored Hives) 175 mg • Rocky Mountain Wheat Grass 125 mg • Siberian Ginseng 100 mg • Kola Nut 100 mg.

Total Flora (Total Flora Support) **- Infinity2**
Two capsules contain: Vitamin C (from calcium ascorbate) 60 mg • Manganese (as manganese chelazome) 0.1 mg • Probiotic Blend 260 mg: Lactobacillus Acidophilus 1 billion CFU, Bifidobacterium Bifidum 400 million CFU, Lactobacillus Bulgaricus 200 million CFU, Lactobacillus Plantarum 200 million CFU, Lactobacillus Salivarius 200 million CFU, Streptococcus Thermophilus 200 million CFU, Lactobacillus Reuteri 40 million CFU, Lactobacillus Brevis 40 million CFU, Bifidobacterium Longum 40 million CFU, Bifidobacterium Infantis 40 million CFU, Lactobacillus Lactis 40 million CFU, Lactobacillus Rhamnosus 200 million CFU • Jerusalem Artichoke (tubers) 60 mg • CAeDS (Chelate Activated Enzyme Delivery System) 40 mg: Amylase, Lipase, Cellulase, Calcium Chelazome, Protease, Zinc Chelazome, Magnesium Chelazome, Manganese Chelazome • Magnesium Glycyl Glutamine (MGG, stabilized glutamine) 10 mg. Other Ingredients: Gelatin.

Total Greens **- Solar Green/Nutraceutical**
Four tablets contains: Barley Grass Juice powder (Hordeum vulgare) 600 mg • Wheat Grass (Triticum aestivum) 600 mg • Alfalfa leaf (medicago sativa) 600 mg. Other Ingredients: Cellulose, Stearic Acid, Silica and Magnesium Stearate, Chlorella Broken Cell Algae (chlorella pyrenoidosa), Spirulina (algae pratensis), Norwegian Kelp (fucus vesiculosis).

Total Kal Plus Vitamin K **- Golden Glow Natural Health Products**
Each tablet contains: Calcium 2100 mg • Magnesium 84 mg • Vitamin D (D3, as cholecalciferol 5 mcg) 200 IU • Vitamin K (phytomenadione) 40 mcg.

Total Lean **- GNC**
Two tablets contain: Total Lean Proprietary Herbal Blend 1350 mg: Guarana seed extract (paullinia cupana, caffeine = 180 mg), Black Tea leaves extract (camellia sinensis), Grape skin extract (vitis vinifera), Ginger root extract (zingiber officinale), Grape seed extract (vitis vinifera), Dill weed extract (anethum graveolens). Other Ingredients: Dextrose, Cellulose, Starch, Caramel Color, Titanium Dioxide (natural mineral whitener), Ethyl Vanillin.

Total Lean - Reduce **- GNC**
Palm oil • Oat oil • Water.
See Editor's Note No. 64.

Total Lean Afternoon **- GNC**
Two tablets contain: Phase 2 brand White Kidney bean extract 500 mg. Other Ingredients: Calcium Carbonate, Cellulose, Titanium Dioxide (natural mineral whitener), Vegetable Acetoglycerides.

Total Lean Evening **- GNC**
Each capsule contains: Psyllium seed husks (plantago ovato) 500 mg • Curcumin (curcuma longa) 23 mg • Chamomile flower extract (matricaria chamomile) 14 mg • Menthol 8 mg. Other Ingredients: Gelatin, Maltodextrin, Titanium Dioxide (natural mineral whitener), Artificial Colors (FD&C blue #1, FD&C red #3, FD&C Red #40).

Total Lean Morning **- GNC**
Two tablets contain: Total Lean Proprietary Herbal Blend 1350 mg: Guarana seed extract (paullinia cupana, caffeine = 180 mg), Black Tea leaves (camellia sinensis), Grape skin extract (vitis vinifera), Ginger root extract (zingiber officinale), Grape seed extract (vitis vinifera), Dill weed extract (antheum graveolens). Other Ingredients: Dextrose, Cellulose, Starch, Artificial Color (FD&C red #40).

Total Lean MRP (vanilla and chocolate flavors) **- GNC**
Carb Blend: Maltodextrin, Oat Bran, Cellulose Gum, Resistant Starch, Fructooligosaccharides, Xanthan Gum, Carrageenan • Milk Protein Concentrate • Nonfat dry Milk • Creamer: Partially hydrogenated Soybean oil, Maltodextrin, Sodium Caseinate, Dipotassium Phosphate, Polysorbate 60, Monoglycerides • Total Lean MRP brand Vitamin and Mineral Blend: DiMagnesium Phosphate, Calcium Carbonate, Tricalcium Phosphate, Sodium Phosphate, Sodium Ascorbate, Maltodextrin, Ferric Orthophosphate, DL-Alpha Tocopheryl Acetate, Niacinamide, Zinc Oxide, D-Calcium Pantothenate, Manganese Sulfate, Pyridoxine Hydrochloride, Curpic Oxide, Thiamin Hydrochloride, Vitamin A Acetate, Riboflavin, Chromium Chloride, Folic Acid, Biotin, Sodium Molybdate, Potassium Iodide, Sodium Selenite, Cyanocobalamin • Salt • Natural and Artificial Flavors • Sucralose • Acesulfame Potassium. Chocolate flavor also contains: Cocoa.

Total Lean-Control **- GNC**
Two tablets contain: Thiamin (vitamin B1, as thiamin mononitrate) 1.5 mg • Riboflavin (vitamin B2) 1.7 mg • Niacin 20 mg • Vitamin B6 (as pyridoxine hydrochloride) 2 mg • Chromium (as hydrolyzed protein chelate) 120 mcg • Proprietary Herbal Blend 1762 mg: Yerba Mate extract (ilex paraguariensis, provides 180 mg caffeine), Black Tea leaves extract (camellia sinensis, provides 180 mg caffeine), Green Tea leaves extract (camellia sinensis, provides 180 mg caffeine), Coffee bean extract (provides 180 mg caffeine), Grape seed extract (vitis vinifera), Chrysin, Ginger root extract (zingiber officinale), Dill weed extract (antheum graveolens). Other Ingredients: Dicalcium Phosphate, Cellulose, Polyethylene Glycol, Vegetable Acetoglycerides, Titanium Dioxide (natural mineral whitener), Caramel Color, Ethyl Vanillin.

Total Life Care Nutrition System for Men **- Rexall - Sundown**
Each packet contains: Vitamin A 5000 IU • Vitamin C (ascorbic acid) 210 mg • Vitamin D (cholecalciferol) 400 IU • Vitamin E (DL-alpha-tocopheryl acetate and D-alpha-tocopherol) 100 IU • Thiamin (mononitrate) 1.5 mg • Riboflavin (vitamin B2) 1.7 mg • Niacin (niacinamide) 20 mg • Vitamin B-6 (pyridoxine HCl) 11 mg • Folic Acid 1 mg • Vitamin B-12 (cyanocobalamin) 101 mcg • Pantothenic Acid (calcium D-pantothenate) 1 mg • Calcium 100 mg • Magnesium

(oxide) 200 mg • Zinc (as zinc oxide) 5 mg • Selenium (as selenium amino acid chelate) 200 mcg • Fish Oil (EPA [eicosapentaenoic acid] 180 mg, DHA [docosahexaenoic acid] 120 mg) • L-Arginine (L-arginine and L-arginine HCl) 800 mg • Saw Palmetto fruit 450 mg • Calcium D-Glucarate 400 mg •Grape seed extract (vitis vinifera) 60 mg • Nettle root 50 mg • Pygeum (pygeum africanum) 50 mg • Coenzyme Q-10 20 mg. Other Ingredients: Gelatin, Cellulose, Dicalcium Phosphate, Glycerin, White Rice Powder, Croscarmellose Sodium, Calcium Silicate, Water, Hydroxypropyl Methylcellulose, Magnesium Stearate, PEG, Red 40 lake, Retinyl Acetate, Yellow 6 lake, Titanium Dioxide, Polysorbate 80, Blue 2 lake, Beta-Carotene.

Total Life Care Nutrition System for Women - Rexall - Sundown
One packet contains: Vitamin A 5000 IU • Vitamin C (as ascorbic acid) 410 mg • Vitamin D (as cholecalciferol) 400 IU • Vitamin E (as dl-alpha-tocopheryl acetate and d-alpha-tocopherol) 100 IU • Thiamin (vitamin B1); (as thiamin mononitrate) 1.5 mg • Riboflavin (vitamin B2) 1.7 mg • Niacin (as niacinamide) 20 mg • Vitamin B-6 (as pyridoxine HCl) 11 mg • Folic Acid 1 mg • Vitamin B-12 (as cyanocobalamin) 101 mcg • Pantothenic Acid (as calcium d-pantothenate) 1 mg • Calcium 100 mg • Magnesium (as magnesium oxide) 200 mg • Selenium (as selenium amino acid chelate) 200 mcg • Fish Oil (Eicosapentaenoic Acid [EPA] 180 mg, Docosahexaenoic acid [DHA] 120 mg) 1000 mg • L-Arginine (L-arginine and L-arginine HCl) 800 mg • Calcium D-Glucarate 400 mg • Cranberry fruit juice concentrate 140 mg • Grape seed extract (vitis vinifera) 60 mg • Coenzyme Q-10 20 mg. Other Ingredients: Gelatin, Cellulose, Soybean oil, Glycerin, Dicalcium Phosphate, White Rice Powder, Partially Hydrogenated Soybean Oil, Water, Croscarmellose Sodium, Calcium Silicate, Hydrogenated Soybean Oil, Yellow Beeswax, Hydroxypropyl Methylcellulose, Soy Lecithin, Magnesium Stearate, PEG, Red 40 lake, Retinyl acetate, Silica, Yellow 6 lake, Titanium Dioxide, Polysorbate 80, Blue 2 lake, Beta-carotene.

Total Woman Formula - Youngevity
Damiana leaf (Turnera aphrodisiaca) • Dong Quai root (Angelica sinensis) • Saw Palmetto (Serenoa repens) • Fennel seed (Foeniculum vulgare) • Oat Bran (Avena sativa) • Vilcabamba Mineral Essence: Potassium, Calcium, Magnesium, Zinc, Chromium, Selenium, Iron, Copper, Molybdenum, Vanadium, Iodine, Cobalt, Manganese.

Total-Cal - Golden Glow Natural Health Products
Each tablet contains: Calcium Carbonate 1.5 g: Calcium 600 mg • Manganese Sulfate Monohydrate 15.2 mg: Manganese 5 mg • Magnesium Oxide 25 mg: Magnesium 15 mg • Ferrous Fumarate 5 mg: Iron 1.6 mg • Vitamin D (D3, cholecalciferol 2.5 mcg) 100 IU.

Touku Natural Herbal Rheumatic Pills - Lishih
Korean Red Ginseng • Bark of Eucommiae • Pseudo Ginseng • Olibanum • Common Myrrh Tree • Starjasmine stem • Radix Astragali • Rhizoma Gastrodiae • Radix Morindae • Clematis root • Rhizoma Ligustici • Angelica root • Radix Dipsaci • Codonoptis Sinensis • Rhizoma Atractylodis Alba • Radix Heraclei • Fructus Chaenomelis • Fructus Liquidambaris • Uncaria Sinensis • Bee Honey.
See Editor's Note No. 46.

Toxi-Cleanse - Metagenics
Three tablets contain: DL-Methionine 600 mg • Vitamin C (as ascorbic acid) 600 mg • Sodium Alginate 450 mg • Sodium (as sodium alginate) 38 mg • Bentonite powder 300 mg • Citrus Bioflavonoid Complex (standardized to 45% [45 mg] full spectrum bioflavonoids) 100 mg • Garlic, odorless (allium sativum) 60 mg • Apple Pectin powder (malus domestica) 300 mg.

Toxoid OTC's Toxoid First Aid - HealthWatchers System
Zinc (as Zincboracyl crystals) • Menthol • Denatured Ethyl Alcohol 60%.

Toxoid OTC's Toxoid Pain - HealthWatchers System
Zinc (as Zincboracyl crystals) • Menthol • Camphor • Fang Fang Extract • Dong Quai Extract • Ling Man Zhin • Qin Jiu Extract.

Toxoid OTC's Toxoid Relief - HealthWatchers System
Trace Minerals • Zinc (as Zincboracyl crystals) • Red Cabbage Extract • Aluminum Acetate.

Toxoid OTC's Toxoid Skin - HealthWatchers System
Salicylic Acid • Zinc (as Zincoracyl crystals) • Purified Water.

T-PARA - Dial Herbs
Wormwood • Black Walnut • Senna • Wild Carrot.

T-PEP - Dial Herbs
Gotu Kola • Kelp • Alfalfa • Dandelion • Brigham Tea • Hydrangea • Saffron • Parsley.

T-PERSP - Dial Herbs
Pennyroyal • Cayenne • Catnip • Ginger • Chamomile • Mustard.

T-PNF - Dial Herbs
Wild Lettuce • Valerian • Scullcap • Blue Vervain • Arnica • Lobelia • Cayenne.

T-PR - Dial Herbs
Strawberry • Sassafras • Sarsaparilla • Echinacea • Garlic.

Trace Minerals-B12 - Standard Process, Inc.
Each tablet contains: Proprietary Blend 173 mg: Kelp, Alfalfa, Magnesium Citrate, Dried Pea vine juice, Bovine Orchic extract, Bovine Bone, Dried Buckwheat leaf juice, Buckwheat seed, Defatted Wheat germ, Oat flour, Dicalcium Phosphate, Carrot root, Peanut bran • Vitamin B12 5 mcg • Iron 1.4 mg • Iodine 145 mcg • Zinc 2.7 mg • Copper 0.3 mg • Manganese 16 mg • Potassium 10 mg. Other Ingredients: Honey, Calcium Stearate.

Trace-Min Plus - Progressive Labs
Three capsules contain: Vitamin B6 (pyridoxine HCl) 50 mg • Vitamin D (cholecalciferol) 50 IU • Calcium (as calcium carbonate and calcium citrate) 300 mg • Magnesium (as magnesium oxide and magnesium gluconate) 150 mg • Zinc (as zinc gluconate) 15 mg • Manganese (as manganese gluconate) 10 mg • Potassium (as potassium gluconate) 99 mg • Glutamic Acid HCl 325 mg.

Tran-Q (formerly TCB 12) - Metagenics
Two tablets contain: 4:1 Proprietary Blend 1000 mg: Polygala root (polygala tenuifolia), Biota seed (biota orientalis), Platycodon root (platycodon grandiflorum), Rehmannia root (rehmannia glutinosa), Tangerine peel (citrus reticulata), Jujube fruit (zizyphus spinosa), Chinese Licorice root (glycyrrhiza uralensis), Job's Tears seed (coix lachryma-jobi), Poria fungus (poria cocos), Bai-Zhu Atractylodes rhizome (atractylodes macrocephala), Gardenia fruit (gardenia jasminoides).

Tranquility - Nature's Plus
Each tablet contains: Valerian root 200 mg • Magnesium amino acid chelate/complex 200 mg • Calcium Caseinate, amino acid chelate/ complex 100 mg • Chamomile 50 mg. In a base of milk protein concentrate (750 mg), containing 10 mg of naturally occuring L-Tryptophan.

Tranquility - Wellness International Network, Ltd.
Each capsule contains: Vitamin A (as vitamin A palmitate) 3750 IU • Vitamin C (as ascorbic acid) 30 mg • Vitamin D (as cholecalciferol) 100 IU • Vitamin E (as dL-alpha tocopheryl acetate) 30 IU • Thiamin (as thiamin HCl) 5 mg • Riboflavin 1.6 mg • Niacin (as niacinamide) 18 mg • Vitamin B6 (as pyridoxine HCl) 2 mg • Folic Acid 300 mcg • Vitamin B12 (as cyanocobalamin) 2 mcg • Biotin 30 mcg • Pantothenic Acid (as D-calcium pantothenate) 5 mg • Magnesium (as magnesium amino acid chelate) 2.5 mg • Proprietary Blend 315.2 mg: Glutamic Acid (as isolated soy protein), Choline Bitartrate, Inositol, Lecithin, Ribonucleic Acid (RNA), Valerian root 4:1 extract (valeriana officinalis), Aspartic Acid (as isolated soy protein), Leucine (as isolated soy protein), Arginine (as isolated soy protein), Lysine (as isolated soy protein), Phenylalanine (as isolated soy protein), Serine (as isolated soy protein), Proline (as isolated soy protein), Valine (as isolated soy protein), Isoleucine (as isolated soy protein), Alanine (as isolated soy protein), Glycine (as isolated soy protein), Threonine (as isolated soy protein), Tyrosine (as isolated soy

protein), Histidine, Methionine (as isolated soy protein), Adenosine Triphosphate, Cysteine (as isolated soy protein). Other Ingredients: Talc, Silicon Dioxide, Hydroxypropyl Cellulose.

Transculpt XR **-** MedaBiotics
Yerba Mate • Algisium C • Forskolin • Hydroxypropylethyl Cellulose • Propylene Glycol • Rosemary leaf extract • Laminaria Digitata extract • Triethanolamine • Citric Acid • Methylparaben • Propylparaben.

Transfer Factor capsules **-** 4 Life
Each capsule contains: Transfer Factor E-XF from Bovine Colostrum 300 mg. Other Ingredients: Gelatin.

Transfer Factor Cardio **-** 4 Life
Four capsules contain: Vitamin A (as beta carotene) 2500 IU • Vitamin C (as magnesium dehydroascorbate, ascorbyl palmitate and ascorbic acid) 200 mg • Vitamin E (as D-alpha tocopherol succinate) 100 IU • Niacin (as niacinamide) 20 mg • Vitamin B6 (as pyridoxine hydrochloride) 2 mg • Folate (as folic acid) 400 mcg • Vitamin B12 (as cyanocobalamin) 8 mcg • Magnesium (as magnesium: chloride, dehydroascorbate, arginate and lysinate) 180 mg • Zinc (as zinc arginate) 10 mg • Selenium (as selenomethionine) 50 mcg • Copper (as copper glycinate) 2 mg • Potassium (as potassium citrate) 50 mg • Cardio Targeted Transfer Factor (from egg yolk) 200 mg • Proprietary Blend 478 mg: Butcher's Broom root (22% sterolic heterosides), Ginkgo Biloba leaf (24% ginkgo flavone glycosides, 6% terpene lactones), Hawthorn flower and leaf (1.8% rutin), Garlic clove (deodorized), Coenzyme Q10, Red Yeast extract, Resveratrol (from polygonum cuspidatum), Ginger oil. Other Ingredients: Gelatin.

Transfer Factor Chewable **-** 4 Life
Each capsule contains: Transfer Factor XF from Bovine Colostrum 200 mg. Other Ingredients: Fructose, Maltose, Sorbitol, Natural Flavors, Stearic Acid, Malic Acid, Silica.

Transfer Factor Classic **-** 4 Life
Each capsule contains: Transfer Factor XF from Bovine Colostrum 200 mg. Other Ingredients: Gelatin.

Transfer Factor Essentials **-** Pro Health
Two capsules contain: Folic Acid 100 mcg • Vitamin B12 (cyanocobalamin) 4 mcg • Zinc (oxide) 5 mg • Selenium (amino acid chelate) 25 mcg • Transfer Factor Matrix Blend 330 mg: Chicken-derived Transfer Factors, Bovine Colostrum extract • Beta Glucan 200 mg • Larch Arabinogalactan 333 mg • TMG 375 mg • IP-6 200 mg • Astragalus (1:5 extract) 70 mg. Other Ingredients: Gelatin, Dicalcium Phosphate, Cellulose, Magnesium Stearate, Magnesium Trisilicae, Silica.

Transfer Factor GluCoach **-** 4 Life
Each capsule contains: Chromium 70 mcg • Targeted Transfer Factor from Bovine Colostrum and Egg yolk 50 mg • Pterocarpus Marsupium 200 mg • Fenugreek 50 mg • Momordica Charantia 35 mg • Gymnema Sylvestre 25 mg • Korean Ginseng 20 mg • Alpha Lipoic Acid 30 mg • Vanadium (bis-glycinate oxo vanadium) 150 mg. Other Ingredients: Gelatin.

Transfer Factor Plus **-** 4 Life
Each capsule contains: Transfer Factor E-XF from Bovine Colostrum and Egg yolk 150 mg • Proprietary blend 440 mg: IP-6 (inositol hexaphosphate), Soya bean extract, Cordyceps Sinensis (7% cordyceptic acids), Beta Glucan from Baker's Yeast (saccharomyces cerevisiae), Beta Glucan from Oat (avena sativa), Agaricus Blazeii extract, Mannans from Aloe Vera leaf, Maitake mushroom (grifola frondosa whole plant), Shiitake mushroom 5:1 extract (Lentinus edodes whole plant). Other Ingredients: Gelatin, Lemon Peel.

Transfer Factor ReCall **-** 4 Life
Three capsules contain: Magnesium (oxide) 168 mg • Targeted Transfer Factor from Eggs 100 mg • Proprietary Blend 672 mg: Vinpocetine, Huperzine A, Soy Lecithin (30% phosphatidylserine), Glycerophosphocholine, N-Acetyl Tyrosine, N-Acetyl Cysteine, Bacopa Monnieri extract, Lemon Balm extract, Ginkgo Biloba extract (24% ginkgo flavone glycosides, 6% terpene lactones).

Transfer Factor RenewAll **-** 4 Life
Deionized water • Transfer Factor XF from Bovine Colostrum • Aloe Barbadensis leaf juice • Lavender extract (lavendula angustifolia) • Chamomile Recutita extract (matricaria) • Rosemary oil (rosmarinus officinalis, leaf) • Algae extract • Yeast polysaccharides • Panthenol • Allantoin • Sodium PCA • PPG-2 Isoceteth-20 Acetate • Dimethicone Copolyol • Carbomer • Triethanolamine • Butylene Glycol • Polysorbate 20 • Eucalyptus oil (eucalyptus globules, leaf) • Disodium EDTA • Phenoxyethanol • Methylparaben • Propylparaben • Butylparaben • Ethyl-Paraben • Isobutylparaben.

Transfer Factor tablets **-** 4 Life
Each tablet contains: Transfer Factor E-XF from Bovine Colostrum and Egg yolk 200 mg. Other Ingredients: Fructose, Maltose, Sorbitol, Natural Flavors, Stearic Acid, Malic ACid, Silica.

Transfer Factor Toothpaste **-** 4 Life
Sorbitol • Deionized Water • Hydrated Silica • Glycerin • Calcium Carbonate • Sodium Lauroyl Sarcosinate • Sodium Bicarbonate • Xylitol • Flavors • Transfer Factor E-XF • Lactoferrin • Carboxymethylcellulose • Titanium Dioxide • Coenzyme Q-10 • Stevia • Sodium Benzoate.

Transitions Carbohydrate Absorption Inhibitor **-** Market America, Inc.
Each capsule contains: Magnesium (as magnesium citrate) 50 mg • Chromium (as chromium dinicotinate glycinate) 100 mcg • Wheat Amylase Inhibitor 10 mg • Banaba leaf extract (lagerstroemia speciosa) 16 mg • Vanadium (as vanadium BMOV) 50 mcg • Bitter Melon fruit extract 100 mg. Other Ingredients: Gelatin, Cellulose, Magnesium Stearate, Silica.

Transitions CLA Conjugated Linoleic Acid **-** Market America, Inc.
Four capsules contain: Chromium (from Chromax chromium picolinate) 120 mg • Tonalin CLA (100% pure safflower oil, 2730 mg active CLA) 3500 mg • Caffeine (from guarana seed extract) 200 mg. Other Ingredients: Gelatin, Glycerin, Soybean Oil, Soy Lecithin, Beeswax, Carmine Color, Natural Lemon Flavor.

Transitions Fat Conversion Inhibitor **-** Market America, Inc.
Two tablets contain: Chromium (as chromium dinicotinate glycinate) 67 mcg • Gymnema Sylvestre leaf extract (25% gymnemic acids) 133 mg • Garcinia Cambogia fruit (60% hydroxycitric acid) 1500 mg • Bioperine brand Black Pepper extract 2.6 mg. Other Ingredients: Dicalcium Phosphate, Microcrystalline Cellulose, Sodium Starch Glycolate, Stearic Acid, Magnesium Stearate, Silica.

Trauma Cream (Royal Image Cosmetics) **-** InterPlexus
Aloe Barbadensis gel • Olive extract • Olive Squalane • Shea Butter • Rose Hip oil • Olive oil • Coconut oil • Spikenard • Extracts blend: Arnica, Comfrey, Ginkgo, Ginseng, Bioflavonoids • Glycerin • Olibanum • Hyaluronic Acid • Natural Essences • Allantoin • Menthol • Tocopherol (vitamin E) • Retinyl Palmitate (vitamin A) • Cholecalciferol (vitamin D3) • Citric Acid.

Traumatic Injury Remedy (formerly HP 16) **-** Metagenics
Each drop contains: Arnica Montana 200X • Ruta Graveolens 30X • Hypericum Perforatum 12X • Magnesia Phosphorica 30X • Symphytum Officinale 3X • Bellis Perennis 12X.
See Editor's Note No. 1.

Traumeel Gel **-** Heel/BHI, Inc.
Each 100 g serving contains: Calendula Officinalis 1X • Hamamelis Virginiana 1X • Arnica Montana radix 3X • Aconitum Napellus 3X • Belladonna 3X • Bellis Perennis 1X • Chamomilla 1X • Echinacea Angustifolia 1X • Echinacea Purpurea 1X • Millefolium 1X • Hepar Sulphuris Calcareum 8X • Mercurius Solubilis 8X • Symphytum Officinale 4X • Hypericum Perforatum 6X. Inactive Ingredients: Purified Water, Ethanol, Carbopol 980, Sodium Hydroxide.
See Editor's Note No. 1.

BRAND NAMES

Traumeel Ointment - Heel/BHI, Inc.
Each 100 g serving contains: Calendula Officinalis 1X • Hamamelis Virginiana 1X • Arnica Montana radix 3X • Aconitum Napellus 3X • Belladonna 3X • Bellis Perennis 1X • Chamomilla 1X • Echinacea Angustifolia 1X • Echinacea Purpurea 1X • Millefolium 1X • Hepar Sulphuris Calcareum 8X • Mercurius Solubilis 8X • Symphytum Officinale 4X • Hypericum Perforatum 6X. Inactive Ingredients: Water, Paraffin, White Petrolatum, Ethanol, Cetylstearyl Alcohol. See Editor's Note No. 1.

Traumeel Oral Drops - Heel/BHI, Inc.
Each 100 mL contains: Arnica Montana, Radix 3X 10 mL • Aconitum Napellus 3X 5 mL • Chamomilla 3X 5 mL • Belladonna 4X 5 mL • Symphytum Officinlae 8X 5 mL • Bellis Perennis 2X 2 mL • Calendula Officinalis 2X 2mL • Echinacea Angustifolia 2X 2 mL • Echinacea Purpurea 2X 2mL • Hamamelis Virginiana 2X 2mL • Hypericum Perforatum 3X 2 mL • Millefolium 3X 2 mL • Hepar Suphuris Calcareum 8X 2 mL • Mercurius Solubilis 8X 2 mL • 35% Ethyl Alcohol.
See Editor's Note No. 1.

Traumeel Pure Ear Drops - Heel/BHI, Inc.
Each 0.45 mL vial contains: Arnica Montana radix 2X • Belladonna 2X • Calendula Officinalis 2X • Chamomilla 3X • Millefoium 3X • Hepar Sulphurs Calcareum 6X • Symphytum Officinale 6X • Aconitum Napellus 2X • Bellis Perennis 2X • Mercurius Solubilis 6X • Hypericum Perforatum 2X • Echinacea Angustioflia 2X • Echinacea Purpurea 2X • Hamamelis Virginiana 1X.
See Editor's Note No. 1.

Traumeel Tablets - Heel/BHI, Inc.
Each tablet contains: Belladonna 4X 75 mg • Arnica Montana, Radix 3X 40 mg • Aconitum Napellus 3X 30 mg • Chamomilla 3X 24 mg • Symphytum Officinale 8X 24 mg • Calendula Officinalis 2X 15 mg • Hamamelis Virginiana 2X 15 mg • Millefolium 3X 15 mg • Hepar Sulphuris Calcareum 8X 15 mg • Mercurius Solubilis 8X 15 mg • Hypericum Perforatum 3X 8 mg • Bellis Perennis 2X 6 mg • Echinacea Angustifolia 2X 6 mg • Echinacea Purpurea 2X 6 mg. Other Ingredients: Lactose Base.
See Editor's Note No. 1.

Trenabol-X - Higher Power
Each 4 mL serving contains: 1-(5-alpha)-Androsten-17-Beta-0L-3-One 100 mg • 4-Androstene-3,17-Diol 100 mg • 1,4-Androstadienedione 100 mg.

Tres Bien Bars, Crunchy Lemon Burst - Advocare International
Red Clover extract 250 mg • Green Tea extract 100 mg • Phosphatidylcholine 50 mg • Docosahexaenoic Acid (DHA) 30 mg • Soy Protein Isolate • High Maltose Corn Syrup • High Fructose Corn Syrup • Sugar • Fractionated Palm Kernel Oil • Toasted Rolled Oats • Rice Syrup • Toasted Soy Pieces • Lemon Juice from Concentrate • Nonfat Milk • Dextrose • Maltodextrin • Crisp Rice (rice flour, rice bran, rosemary extract) • Natural Flavor • Tapioca Starch • Nonfat Yogurt Powder (cultured whey, nonfat milk) • Soy Lecithin • Soybean Oil • Ascorbic Acid • Pectin • Citric Acid • Guar Gum • Vegetable Oil (algae oil containing DHA, ascorbyl palmitate and tocopherols) • Beta-Carotene • Salt • Titanium Dioxide • Alpha-Tocopherol Acetate • Honey • Sodium Citrate • Folic Acid • Annatto.

T-RHU - Dial Herbs
Buchu Leaves • Oregon Grape • Cayenne • Black Cohosh • Buckthorn • Burdock • Hydrangea • Lobelia • Nettle • Scullcap • Wild Yam • White Willow bark • Yellow Dock • Arnica.

Tri Iron - TriLight Herbs
Nettle leaf • Yellow Dock • Red Raspberry • Dandelion • Anise.

Tri-40 - Progressive Labs
Each capsule contains: Iodine (from kelp) 150 mcg • Thyroid concentrate 40 mg • Spleen concentrate 40 mg • Thymus concentrate 40 mg • Pacific Sea Kelp 100 mg.
See Editor's Note No. 14.

Tri-Amino Supplement - Puritan's Pride
Four tablets contain: L-Arginine Hydrochloride 1447 mg • L-Ornithine Hydrochloride 900 mg • L-Lysine HCl 1200 mg.

Triaton - Progressive Health Nutraceuticals
Black Cohosh 160 mg • Dong Quai 150 mg • Licorice root 150 mg • Chasteberry 100 mg • Isoflavone 65 mg.

Triax - Syntrax Innovations
Each capsule contains: Tiratricol 1 mg. Other ingredients: Barley flour, gelatin, titanium dioxide, red #40, blue #1.
See Editor's Note No. 66.

Tri-B Homocysteine Formula - J. R. Carlson Laboratories, Inc.
Each tablet contains: Vitamin B6 (as pyridoxine hydrochloride) 25 mg • Folate (folic acid) 800 mcg • Vitamin B12 (cyanocobalamin) 400 mcg.

TRIBEST - New Hope Health Products
Each capsule contains: Tribulus terrestris (containing Furostanol and Protodioscin) 750 mg.

Tribest - Metabolic Response Modifiers
Each capsule contains: Tribulus terrestris (containing Furostanol and Protodioscin) 750 mg.

Tribestan - Sopharma
Each tablet contains: Tribestan from Tribulus Terrestris herb.

Tribestrone II - ASN - Advanced Sports Nutrition
Each tablet contains: Tribulus Terrestris L. extract 450 mg • Ashwaganda extract 100 mg • Mucuna extract 100 mg • Bioperine brand Black Pepper standardized extract 1.5 mg.

Tribex - BioTest Laboratories, LLC
Four capsules contain: Tribex Full-Spectrum Active Extracts 2000 mg: Tribulus Terrestris, Avena Sativa. Other Ingredients: Gelatin, Cellulose, Magnesium Stearate, FD&C Blue #1, FD&C Red #3, FD&C Red #40, Titanium Dioxide.

Tribulus - The Vitamin Shoppe
Each capsule contains: Tribulus Terrestris (fruit, standardized to 20% saponins) 625 mg.

Tribulus 625 Caps - Optimum Nutrition
Each capsule contains: Proprietary Tribulus Blend 625 mg: Tribulus Terrestris fruit extract (standardized to 40% furastanol saponins), Tribulus Terrestris powdered aerial parts. Other Ingredients: Gelatin, Silica, Magnesium Stearate.

Tribulus Complex - Jarrow Formulas
Each tablet contains: Tribulus extract (tribulus terrestris, 45% saponins as furanosterols) 500 mg • Aswagandha leaf extract (withania somnifera, 8% withanolides) 100 mg • Andrographis extract (andrographis paniculata, 10% andrographolide) 100 mg • Rhodioa extract (rhodioa rosea, 5% rosavins, including 3% minimum Rosavin) 50 mg • Green Tea extract (camellia sinensis, 40% polyphenols) 50 mg. Other Ingredients: Cellulose, Modified Cellulose Gum, Stearic Acid, Silicon Dioxide, Magnesium Stearate, Modified Cellulose Gum.

Tribulus Desire - Life Enhancement Products, Inc.
Each capsule contains: Tribulus Terrestris leaf etract 250 mg • Dehydroepiandrosterone (DHEA) 8.33 mg.

Tribulus Fuel - TwinLab
Each capsule contains: Tribulus Terrestris extract (standardized for 20-29% steroidal saponins) 625 mg.

Tribulus Fuel Stack - TwinLab
Two capsules contain: Tribulus Terrestris extract 1250 mg • DHEA (dehydroepiandrosterone) 50 mg.

Tribulus Gold - Mass Quantities, Inc.
Each capsule contains: Tribulus extract (standardized 42%) 675 mg.

Tribulus Synergy Male Response Formula - Metagenics
Each tablet contains: Proprietary Herbal Extract Blend 500 mg: Tribulus fruit (tribulus terrestris, 7:1 extract, containing saponins), Ashwagandha root (withania somnifera, 5:1 extract, containing withanolides), Cowhage seed (mucuna pruriens, containing naturally occurring levodopa), Sativari root (asparagus racemosus, 4:1 extract, containing saponins).

Tri-EFA - Pure Encapsulations
Each softgel capsule contains: Flax seed oil 400 mg • Borage seed oil 400 mg • Fish oil (50% omega-3) 400 mg. These oils typically provide: Alpha Linolenic Acid (ALA) 220 mg, EPA 120 mg, DHA 80 mg, Linoleic Acid 180 mg, Gamma Linolenic Acid (GLA) 96 mg, Oleic Acid 152 mg, Vitamin E (D-alpha tocopherol) 5 IU. Other Ingredients: Gelatin, Glycerin.

Triflex Dietary Supplement - GNC
Three tablets contain: Glucosamine HCl 1500 mg •Chondroitin Sulfate, Sodium 1200 mg • MSM (Metyhlsulfonylmethane) 900 mg. Ohter Ingredients: Titanium Dioxide.
See Editor's Note No. 15.

Tri-Flex Soft Chewables Chocolate - GNC
Each chew contains: Glucosamine HCl 500 mg • Chondroitin Sulfate 400 mg • Methylsulfonylmethane (MSM) 25 mg. Ingredients: Corn syrup, Sweetened Condensed Skim Milk, Partially Hydrogenated Soybean oil, Glucosamine HCl, Chondroitin Sulfate, Whey Chocolate liquor, Mono & Diglycerides, Methylsulfonylmethane (MSM), Soy Lecithin, Artificial Flavor.
See Editor's Note No. 15.

Triglic-Oil - Aboca USA, Inc
Three capsules contain: Fish Oil 930 mg (eicosapentaenoic acid 190 mg, docosahexaenoic acid 480 mg) • Turmeric root extract in Flaxseed oil (1:10) 230 mg. Other Ingredients: Gelatin (capsule), Essential Oils Of Rosemary, Lemon.

Trilean - VitaStore
Guarana (Paullinia Cupana) • Glutamine • Fennel • Choline • Spirulina • Hawthorne • Inositol • Bladderwrack • Vitamin A • Vitamin C • Vitamin D • Vitamin E • Vitamin B1 • Vitamin B2 • Vitamin B6 • Vitamin B12 • Folic Acid • Niacin • d-Biotin • Pantothenic Acid • Potassium • Calcium.

Trim Advantage Meal Replacement Shake (chocolate) - Quixtar, Inc.
Lowfat Milk • Filtered Water • Nonfat Milk • Soy Protein Isolate • Natural Flavors • Cocoa • Cottonseed Fiber • High Oleic Safflower oil • Magnesium Phosphate • Xanthan gum • Acesulfame Potassium • Sucralose • Vanilla extract • Soy Lecithin • Carrageenan • Calcium Carbonate • Sodium Ascorbate (vitamin C) • Sea Salt • Ferrous Amino Acid • Zinc Amino Acid • Tocopherol Acetate (vitamin E) • Biotin • Vitamin A Palmitate • Niacinamide • Phytonadione (vitamin K) • Potassium Iodide • Calcium Pantothenate • Chromium Chloride • Copper Amino Acid • Cyanocobalamin (vitamin B12) • Sodium Molybdate • Sodium Selenite • Folic Acid • Cholecalciferol (vitamin D3) • Pyridoxine Hydrochloride (vitamin B6) • Riboflavin • Thiamin Monohydrate • Manganese Sulfate.

Trim Advantage Meal Replacement Shake (french vanilla) - Quixtar, Inc.
Lowfat Milk • Filtered Water • Soy Protein Isolate • Nonfat Milk • Natural Flavors • Cottonseed fiber • High Oleic Safflower oil • Magnesium Phosphate • Sucralose • Xanthan gum • Calcium Carbonate • Sea Salt • Soy Lecithin • Carrageenan • Acesulfame Potassium • Vanilla extract • Sodium Ascorbate (vitamin C) • Ferrous Amino Acid • Zinc Amino Acid • Tocopherol Acetate (vitamin E) • Biotin • Vitamin A Palmitate • Niacinamide • Phytonadione (vitamin K) • Potassium Iodide • D-Calcium Pantothenate • Chromium Chloride • Copper Amino Acid • Cyanocobalamin (vitamin B12) • Sodium Molybdate • Sodium Selenite • Folic Acid • Cholecalciferol (vitamin D3) • Pyridoxine Hydrochloride (vitamin B6) • Riboflavin • Thiamine Mononitrate • Beta Carotene (color) • Manganese Sulfate.

Trim Advantage Protein Bar (banana creme flavor) - Quixtar, Inc.
Protein Blend: Whey Protein Isolate, Soy Protein Isolate, Whey Protein Concentrate, Hydrolyzed Whey Isolate • Glycerin • Maltitol • Sunflower oil • Soy Nuggets: Soy Protein Isolate, Rice Flour, Malt, Salt • Gum Arabic • Calcium Phosphate • Natural Flavors (natural banana flavor, natural graham cracker flavor) • Salt • Soy Lecithin • Sucralose.

Trim Advantage Protein Bar (caramel vanilla flavor) - Quixtar, Inc.
Protein Blend: Whey Protein Isolate, Soy Protein Isolate, Whey Protein Concentrate, Hydrolyzed Whey Isolate • Glycerin • Maltitol • Sunflower oil • Soy Nuggets: Soy Protein Isolate, Rice Flour, Malt, Calcium Carbonate • Gum Arabic • Natural Caramel type flavor • Natural Vanilla flavor with other Natural Flavors • Calcium Phosphate • Salt • Soy Lecithin • Sucralose.

Trim Advantage Protein Bar (chocolate mint flavor) - Quixtar, Inc.
Protein Blend: Whey Protein Isolate, Soy Protein Isolate, Whey Protein Concentrate, Hydrolyzed Whey Isolate • Glycerin • Maltitol • Sunflower oil • Soy Nuggets: Soy Protein Isolate, Rice Flour, Malt • Cocoa • Natural Peppermint flavor and other Natural Flavors • Calcium Phosphate • Salt • Soy Lecithin • Sucralose.

Trim Advantage Protein Bar (fudgy brownie flavor) - Quixtar, Inc.
Protein Blend: Whey Protein Isolate, Soy Protein Isolate, Whey Protein Concentrate, Hydrolyzed Whey Isolate • Glycerin • Maltitol • Sunflower oil • Soy Nuggets: Soy Protein Isolate, Rice Flour, Malt, Salt • Cocoa • Almonds • Natural Flavor • Calcium Phosphate • Salt • Soy Lecithin • Sucralose.

Trim Advantage Protein Bar (roasted peanut flavor) - Quixtar, Inc.
Protein Blend: Whey Protein Isolate, Soy Protein Isolate, Whey Protein Concentrate, Hydrolyzed Whey Isolate • Glycerin • Maltitol • Sunflower oil • Peanut Butter: Peanuts, Cottonseed oil, Dextrose, Salt • Soy Nuggets: Soy Protein Isolate, Rice Flour, Malt, Salt • Granulated Peanuts • Peanut Flour • Calcium Phosphate • Salt • Soy Lecithin • Sucralose.

Trim Advantage Protein Bar (strawberry creme flavor) - Quixtar, Inc.
Protein Blend: Whey Protein Isolate, Soy Protein Isolate, Whey Protein Concentrate, Hydrolyzed Whey Isolate • Glycerin • Maltitol • Sunflower oil • Soy Nuggets: Soy Protein Isolate, Rice Flour, Malt, Salt • Gum Arabic • Natural Strawberry flavor and other Natural Flavor • Calcium Phosphate • Salt • Soy Lecithin • Sucralose.

Trim Fit with Advantra Z-Tonalin Kit - Quest
Six capsules contain: Advantra-ZT Citrus Aurantium (standardized to 4% synephrine) 1050 mg • Green Tea extract (camellia sinensis, P.E. 1:6) 1050 mg • Tonalin (source of conjugated linoleic acid) 900 mg • Kelp (fucus vesiculosus) 300 mg • St. John's Wort extract (hypericum perforatum) 150 mg • Trim-Zyme Enzyme Blend (P.E. 1:5, standardized to 0.3% hypericin) 150 mg: Protease, Lipase, Amylase, Cellulase • Lipoic Acid 30 mg. Other Ingredients: Silicon Dioxide, Magnesium Stearate (vegetable source), Gelatin, Natural Color.
See Editor's Note No. 40.

Trim Fit with Advantra Z-Tonalin Kit Phase 2 - Quest
Each tablet contains: White Kidney Bean extract 500 mg. Other Ingredients: Calcium Phosphate, Microcrystalline Cellulose, Vegetable Stearin, Croscarmellose Sodium, Ascorbic Acid, Magnesium Stearate (vegetable source), Silicone Dioxide, Methylcellulose Complex (cellcote coating).

Trim Lite - Health Smart Vitamins
Three capsules contain: Vitamin C (ascorbic acid) 250 mg • Vitamin E (d-alpha tocopheryl succinate) 150 IU • Vitamin B6 (pyridoxine HCl) 7 mg • Chromium (as chromium nicotinate) 150 mcg • Cola Nut (14% caffeine, 70 mg) 500 mg • Ma Huang root (6% total

ephedrine alkaloids, 6 mg) 100 mg • DL-Phenylalanine 75 mg • English Hawthorn leaf & flower (1.8% vitexin, 0.9 mg) 50 mg • L-Carnitine (as L-carnitine tartrate) 30 mg.
See Editor's Note No. 30.

Trim4Life Appetite Control Phase II - FreeLife International
Each caplet contains: Herbal Energy Standardized Extract Blend 450 mg: Green Tea leaf, Chinese White Ginseng root (panax ginseng), Siberian Eleuthero Ginseng root, Korean Red Ginseng root (panax ginseng), American Five-Leaf Ginseng root (panax quinquefolius), Brazilian Suma Ginseng root (pfaffia paniculata), Central American Osha Ginseng root (ligusticum wallichi), Tibetian Tienchi Ginseng root (panax notoginseng), Manchurian Yellow Ginseng root (caulophyllum thalictrodies), Indian Ashwagandha Ginseng root (withania somnifera), Japanese Ginseng root (panax japonicus), Couchgrass herb, Buchu leaf, Uva Ursi leaf, Juniper berry, Hydrangea root, Cornsilk • Appetite Control Standardized Extract Blend 250 mg: Griffonia seed (griffonia simplicifolia), L-Tyrosine (soy amino acid), standardized Citrus peel extract (citrus aurantium) • Potassium Citrate 50 mg • Vanadium (from glycinate chelate) 50 mcg. Other Ingredients: Calcium Dihydrogen Phosphate, Cellulose, Fractionated Vegetable Oil, Silica, Vita-coat.

Trim4Life Thermogenic Phase 1 - FreeLife International
Each caplet contains: Vitamin B6 (as pyridoxine hydrochloride) 10 mg • Chromium (dinicotinate glycinate) 150 mcg • Thermonutrient Standardized Extract Blend 175 mg: Cinnamon bark, Country Mallow leaf, Piperine extract of Black Pepper • Adrenal Support Standardized Extract Blend 50 mg: Licorice root, Ginger root, Astragalus root. Other Ingredients: Calcium Dihydrogen Phosphate, Cellulose, Fractionated Vegetable Oil, Silica, Vita-Coat.
See Editor's Note No. 39.

Trimax - Enzymatic Therapy
Each capsule contains: St. John's Wort extract (Hypericum perforatum) standardized to contain 0.15% Hypericins, verified by HPLC 500 mg • Valerian extract (Valeriana officinalis) standardized to contain a minimum of 0.8%, 15 mg • Passionflower extract (Passiflora) 15 mg.

Trimelle - Progressive Health Nutraceuticals
Taurine 600 mg • L-Tyrosine 500 mg • Magnesium 300 mg • Potassium 290 mg • Choline (bitartrate) 250 mg • Hawthorne berries 250 mg • Calcium 150 mg • CoQ10 150 mg • L-Carnitine 150 mg • Raw Heart concentrate 150 mg • Thyroid extract 150 mg • Inositol 150 mg • Bromelain 100 mg • Chondroitin Sulfate A 50 mg • Gentian 50 mg • Methionine 30 mg.

TrimFast (Trim Fast) - Preferred Price Plus
Each capsule contains: Natural Ephedra • White Willow bark • Chromium Polynicotinate.
See Editor's Note No. 30.

TrimLife - Trimlife, Inc.
Each tablet contains: Vitamin E (as D-alpha tocopheryl succinate) 10 IU • Chromium (picolinate) 25 mcg • Guarana seed extract 4:1 (contains 100 mg caffeine) 455 mg • L-Tyrosine 167 mg • Ma Huang standardized extract (8% total alkaloids, contains 10 mg ephedrine) 143 mg • Hydroxy Citric Acid 125 mg • Ginger root 100 mg • Acetyl-L-Carnitine 12.5 mg • Siberian Ginseng root 10 mg • Capsicum fruit (providing approximately 0.126% capsaicin) 1 mg. Other Ingredients: Cellulose, Maltodextrin, Stearic Acid, Croscamellose Sodium, Silicon Dioxide, Magnesium Stearate, Cellulose.
See Editor's Note No. 30.

TrimLife Advanced - Trimlife, Inc.
Green Tea extract (camellia sinensis) 100 mg • Maca Force (lepidium meyenii) 450 mg • Bitter Orange (herbal synephrine) 83.3 mg • Yerba Mate and Guarana (200 mg standardized methylxanthines or caffeine) 490 mg • Calcium Pyruvate 10 mg • Botanical Energy Complex 530 mg: Peptide GX, D-Ribose, Mucuna Pruriens (standardized 15% L-dopa), Tricopus Zylanicus, Ashwagandha, Piper Longum, Vishnukranthi, Eleutherococcus Senticosus, Ginkgo Biloba, Astragalus Membranaceus, Panax Ginseng, Schizandra Chinensis, Polygonum Multiflorum, Eucommiae Ulmoides, Polyconatum Sibirica, Gynostemma Pentaphylla, Sargassum Fusiforme, Ganoderma Lucidum, Ziziphus Jujuba, Lycium Barbarum, Momordica Grosvenori.

Trim-Plex - Nature's Plus
Three softgels contain: Lecithin (soya) 600 mg • Kelp 300 mg • Apple Cider Vinegar 240 mg • Vitamin B6 (pyridoxine HCl) 50 mg. In a natural blend of Vegetable (soy) oil & Chlorophyll.

TrimSolution Bar (chocolate flavor) - Starlight International
Each bar contains: Starlight Protein Blend: Calcium caseinate, Soy protein isolate, Soy flour, Whey Protein concentrate, nonfat Milk • Rice Syrup • High Fructose Corn Syrup • Confectionary Coating: Sucrose, Fractionated Palm Kernel Oil, Cocoa powder, Whey powder, nonfat Milk, Lecithin, natural Vanilla •Fiber Blend: Guar Gum, Arabic Gum, Soy fiber, Corn bran • Chocolate • Natural Flavors • Garcinia Cambogia • Magnesium carbonate • Glycerin • Phytonutrients: Carrot powder, Spinach powder, Cabbage powder, Tomato powder, Broccoli powder • Ascorbic Acid • DL Alpha Tocopherol Acetate • Vitamin A palmitate • Niacinamide • Omega 3 and 6 Fatty Acids • Zinc oxide • Ferrous Fumarate • Copper gluconate • D-Calcium pantothenate • Schisandra berry extract • Vitamin D3 • Pyridoxine HCl • Riboflavin • Thiamine mononitrate • Vitamin B12 • Canola Oil • Folate • Biotin • Potassium iodide.

TrimSolution Bar (peanut butter flavor) - Starlight International
Each bar contains: Starlight Protein Blend: Calcium caseinate, Soy protein isolate, Peanut Butter, Soy flour, Whey Protein concentrate, nonfat Milk, defatted Peanut flour • Rice Syrup •High Fructose Corn Syrup • Confectionary Coating: Sucrose, Fractionated Palm Kernel Oil, Cocoa powder, Whey powder, nonfat milk, Lecithin, natural Vanilla • Fiber Blend: Guar Gum, Arabic Gum, Soy fiber, Corn Bran , Oat Bran • Natural Flavors • Tricalcium Phosphate • Garcinia Cambogia • Magnesium carbonate • Glycerin • Phytonutrients: Carrot powder, Spinach powder, Cabbage powder, Tomato powder, Broccoli powder •Ascorbic Acid • dl Alpha Tocopherol Acetate •Vitamin A palmitate • Niacinamide • Omega 3 and 6 Fatty Acids • Zinc oxide • Ferrous Fumarate • Copper gluconate • D-Calcium Pantothenate • Schisandra Berry extract • Vitamin D3 • Pyridoxine Hydrochloride • Riboflavin • Thiamine mononitrate • Vitamin B12 •Canola Oil • Folate • Biotin • Potassium iodide.

TrimSpa - Nutramerica Corp.
Each capsule contains: Chromium (as chromium dinicotinate glycinate) 150 mcg • Vanadium (as vanadium amino acid chelate) 50 mcg • Glucomannan 400 mg • Green Tea leaf extract (60 mg caffeine) 120 mg • Coleus Forskohlii tuber extract (10% forskolin) 250 mg • Sodium Carboxymethylcellulose 100 mg. Other Ingredients: Gelatin, Magnesium Stearate, Silica.

TrimSpa Carb Blocker - Nutramerica Corp.
Two tablets contain: Chromium (as chelavate chromium dinicotinate glycinate) 200 mcg • Phase 2 brand White Kidney bean extract (phaseolus vulgaris) 1000 mg • Vanadium (as vanadium amino acid chelate) 100 mcg. Other Ingredients: Dicalcium Phosphate, Microcrystalline Cellulose, Croscarmellose Sodium, Stearic Acid, Magnesium Stearate, Silica, Pharmaceutical Glaze.
See Editor's Note No. 37.

TrimSpa Fat Blocker - Nutramerica Corp.
Each capsule contains: Vitamin C (as ascorbic acid) 60 mg • Liposan Ultra Chitosan (marine fiber concentrate) 500 mg. Other Ingredients: Calcium Sulfate, Gelatin, Cellulose, Magnesium Stearate, Silica.
See Editor's Note No. 37.

Trimspa X32 - Nutramerica Corp.
Two tablets contain: Chromium (as chromium dinicotinate glycinate) 150 mcg • Vanadium (as vanadium amino acid chelate) 30 mcg • Glucomannan 400 mg • Sodium Carboxymethylcellulose 100 mg • Citrus Naringinine 10 mg • Glucosamine HCl 100 mg • Cocoa extract (standardized for phenylalanine, tyramine, 10% theobromine) 325 mg • Green Tea extract (40%, standardized for epigallocatechin gallate,

polyphenols, 40% caffeine) 250 mg • Hoodia Gordonii cactus (above ground parts) 150 mg. Other Ingredients: Dicalcium Phosphate, Microcrystalline Cellulose, Croscarmellose Sodium, Stearic Acid, Magnesium Stearate.

Trinovin - Novogen
Each tablet contains: Natural Isoflavones from Red Clover 40 mg. Other Ingredients: Dicalcium phosphate, Microcrystalline cellulose, Hydroxypropyl methylcellulose, Magnesium stearate, Mixed tocopherols, Silica, Soy polysaccharide, & Natural caramel color.

Triomega Omega-3 Softgels - Pronova Biocare
Each softgel contains: Triomega concentrated Fish oil 800 mg providing: EPA (eicosapentaenoic acid), DHA (docosahexaenoic acid, 62.5% EPA:DHA ratio approximately 2:1 as ethyl esters) 500 mg, total Omega-3 Fatty Acids (71.25%) 570 mg. Other Ingredients: Gelatin, USP Water, Glycerin, Natural Vitamin E.

Trioxalon 500 - AST Sports Science
Each capsule contains: Tribulus Terrestris extract 500 mg.

Tri-Oxy - Hillestad
Two tablets contain: Sodium Caprylate 120 mg • Pau d'Arco bark 50 mg • Horseradish root 12.5 mg • Clover extract oil 800 mcg • Goldenseal root 50 mg • Buchu leaves 50 gm • Caprylic Acid 75 mg. Other Ingredients: Oyster Shell, Cellulose, Fibrosol, Silicon Dioxide, Magnesium Stearate.

Trip2Night - Cytotec Solutions, Inc.
Some ingredients include: Ma-huang • Guarana • 5-HTP • Bioperine brand Black Pepper extract • Indian Bromine • Cinnamon • Cola Nut • Niacin • Fo Ti.
See Editor's Note No. 17, No. 30 and No. 49.

Trip2night-EF - Cytotec Solutions, Inc.
Citrus Aurantium • Guarana • 5-HTP • Bioperine brand Black Pepper extract • Indian Bromine • Cinnamon • Cola Nut • Niacin • Fo Ti.
See Editor's Note No. 40 and no. 49.

Triphala - The Himalaya Drug Company
Each capsule contains: Proprietary Blend 250 mg: Emblica officinalis, Terminalia chebula, Terminalia bellirica.

TriPhetamine - Pharmalogic
Two caplets contain: Sida Cordifolia Extract (standardized to 6% ephedrine alkaloids) 235 mg • Ma Huang Extract (standardized to 6% ephedrine alkaloids) 100 mg • Caffeinated Green Tea Leaf Extract (standardized to 50% polyphenols; 35% catechins) 200 mg • Cola Nut Extract (seed; standardized to 20% caffeine) 250 mg • Guarana Extract (seed; standardized to 20% caffeine) 250 mg • Caffeine (from caffeine anhydrous) 100 mg • Proprietary Blend 295 mg: L-Tyrosine, DMAE (2-dimethylaminoethanol bitartrate), Hypothalamic Peptides, L-Alanine, Cinnamon Extract (standardized to 5% cinnamonosides). Other Ingredients: Calcium Carbonate, Microcrystalline Cellulose, Stearic Acid, Magnesium Stearate, Titanium Dioxide.
See Editor's Note No. 30 and No. 39.

Triphla - R-U Ved U.S.A.
Amla (Indian gooseberry) standardized extract • Harar standardized extract • Bahera standardized extract.

Triple B Super Vision - DreamPharm
Each tablet contains: Bilberry fruit (standardized to 20% anthocyanin) 80 mg • Blackberry fruit (standardized to 20% anthocyanin) 60 mg • Blueberry fruit 400 mg • Eyebright herb (euphrasia officinalis) 250 mg • Cassia Obtusifolia seeds 100 mg • Eriocaulon Buergerianum 50 mg • Lutein (5% powder containing zeaxanthin, from marigold flower) 3 mg • Beta-Carotene 600 mcg.

Triple Berry Complex - Herbalife International of America, Inc.
Each capsule contains: Cranberry fruit powder 500 mg • Dried Bilberry fruit 4:1 extract 50 mg • Blueberry fruit powder 50 mg. Other Ingredients: Gelatin, Water, Calcium Carbonate, Silicon Dioxide, Magnesium Stearate, Maltodextrin, Sodium Lauryl Sulfate.

Triple Cod Liver Oil - GNC
Each capsule contains: Vitamin A (as cod liver oil) 1250 IU • Vitamin D (as cod liver oil) 135 IU • Vitamin E (as fish body oil) I IU • EPA (Eicosapentaenoic Acid) 173 mg • DHA (Docosahexaenoic Acid) 120 mg. Other Ingredients: Gelatin, Glycerin.

Triple Defense - Olympian Labs
Two capsules contain: Soy Isoflavone dried extract 100 mg • D-Glucarate 400 mg • Lycopene extract (5% Standardized Yielding 30 mg of pure Lycopene) 600 mg • Citrus Bioflavonoids 40 mg.

Triple Delicious High Protein Bar - Strength Systems USA
Each bar contains: Protein Blend: Whey Protein Isolate, Hydrolyzed Whey Protein, Calcium Caseinate, Soy Protein Isolate, Whey Protein Concentrate, Milk Protein Concentrate • Maltitol • Water • Glycerine • Hydrolyzed Gelatin • Lactitol • Fractionated Palm Kernal Oil • Almonds • Roasted Soybeans • Non-Fat Milk • Natural and Artificial Flavor • Cocoa • Modified Soybean Oil • Unsweetened Chocolate • Salt • Monoglycerides • Cream • Butter • Soy Lecithin • Inulin • Sodium Phosphate • Carrageenan • Sucralose • Potassium Sorbate.

Triple Flex - Nature Made
Three tablets contain: Sodium 20 mg • Glucosamine Hydrochloride 1500 mg • Chondroitin Sulfate 1200 mg • MSM (methylsulfonylmethane) 375 mg. Other Ingredients: Cellulose Gel, Povidone, Croscarmellose Sodium, Hydroxypropyl Methylcellulose, Magnesium Stearate, Titanium Dioxide, Polyethylene Glycol, Triethyl Citrate, Polysorbate 80, Sodium Citrate.
See Editor's Note No. 15.

Triple G Super Health - DreamPharm
Two capsules contain: Garlic 300 mg • Ginger 200 mg • Grape Seed extract 100 mg.

Triple Ginseng Rush - GNC
Each capsule contains: Korean Ginseng root (panax ginseng) 200 mg • American Ginseng root extract (panax quinquefolium) 200 mg • Siberian Ginseng root extract (eleutherococcus senticosus) 200 mg • Guarana seed extract (paullinia cupana) 100 mg. Other Ingredients: Gelatin.

Triple Lecithin 1200 - GNC
Each capsule contains: Chromium (picolinate) 100 mcg • High Choline Soy Lecithin (supplying phosphatidyl choline 420 mg) 1200 mg. Other Ingredients: Gelatin, Caramel Color, Titanium Dioxide.

Triple Lecithin 1200 with Phosphatidyl Choline - GNC
Each capsule contains: High Choline Lecithin 1200 mg • Phosphatidyl Choline (as soy lecithin) 420 mg. Other Ingredients: Gelatin, Glycerin.

Triple Lecithin 400 - GNC
Each capsule contains: Vitamin E (as d-alpha tocopherol) 5 IU • High Choline Soy Lecithin (supplying phosphatidyl choline 140 mg) 400 mg. Other Ingredients: Gelatin, Glycerin, Rosemary oil (rosmariunus officinalis).

Triple Mag - Vital Nutrients
Each capsule contains: Magnesium Glycinate 25 mg • Magnesium Citrate 75 mg • Magnesium Oxide 150 mg.

Triple Omega 3-6-9 Flax, Fish and Borage Oils - Vitamin World
Each softgel contains: Vitamin E (D-alpha tocopherol) 15 IU • Flaxseed Oil 1200 mg • Borage seed oil 1200 mg • Fish Oil (50% omega-3) 1200 mg • Omega-6 Fatty Acids 828 mg • Omega-9 Fatty Acids (oleic acid) 456 mg. Other Ingredients: Gelatin, Glycerin.

Triple Relief - Nature's Sunshine
Two capsules contain: Nexrutine brand Phellodendron extract (phellodendron amurense) 250 mg • Boswellia (boswellia serrata, standardized to 25% total boswellic acid) 250 mg • Willow bark extract (salix sp., (standardized to 15% total salicins) 120 mg. Other Ingredients: Cellulose, Magnesium Stearate, Silicon Dioxide, Gelatin, Water.

BRAND NAMES

Some Brand Name Natural Products - What they Contain

www.NaturalDatabase.com contains MANY more listings than appear here.
Editor's Notes are located on pages 2155-2163.

Triple Stack **-** Crystal Springs
Each tablet contains: Tribulis 250 mg • DHEA 50 mg • Androstenedione 50 mg • Saw Palmetto 200mg • Pygeum 100 mg. See Editor's Note No. 47.

Triple Strength Glucosamine 750 mg Chondroitin 600 mg **-** Vitamin World
Two caplets contain: Sodium (as chondroitin sulfate) 70 mg • Glucosamine Hydrochloride 1500 mg • Chondroitin Sulfate 1200 mg. Other Ingredients: Crospovidone, Beet Juice, Cellulose, Vegetable Magnesium Stearate.
See Editor's Note No. 15.

Triple Whey Fuel **-** TwinLab
Blend of three key Whey Proteins: Micro-Filtered & Ion-Exchange Whey Protein Isolate (with ~57% Beta-Lactoglobulin, ~24% Alpha-Lactalbumin, ~12% Immunoglobulins, ~7% Minor Peptones & Lactoferrin) •modified molecular weight & partially predigested (hydrolyzed) Whey Protein (providing di-, tri-, oligo- & poly-peptides) • Whey Protein Concentrate enriched with Glutamine.

Triple-Chrome **-** Alacer
Each timed-release tablet contains: Trivalent Chromium 400 mcg: Chromium Ascorbate 134 mcg, Chromium Nicotinate 133 mcg, Chromium Aspartate 133 mcg • Manganese (as ascorbate) 2 mg • Vitamin C (as mineral ascorbates) 16 mg • Calcium 49 mg.

TripleFlex Triple Strength **-** Nature Made
Two caplets contain: Glucosamine Hydrochloride 1.5 g • Chondroitin Sulfate 1.2 g • Methylsulfonylmethane (MSM) 250 mg. Other Ingredients: Croscarmellose Sodium, Beet Powder, Silicon Dioxide, Hydroxypropyl Methylcellulose, Magnesium Stearate, Polyethylene Glycol.

Tropical Fruit Drinkable Yogurt **-** Stonyfield Farm
Each 10 fl oz bottle contains: Active Live Cultures: S. Thermophilus • L. Bulgaricus • L. Acidophilus • Bifidus • L. Casei • L. Reuteri. Ingredients: Cultured Pasturized Low Fat Milk • Organic Sugar • Organic Nonfat Dry Milk • Inulin • Pectin • Pumpkin Juice Concentrate • Carrot Juice Concentrate • Organic Banana Puree • Natural Flavors.

Tropical Noni **-** NutraMed
Morinda citrifolia.

Tropical Ola Loa **-** Ola Loa, LLC
Each packet contains: Vitamin C 1000 mg • Vitamin B1 1 mg • Vitamin B2 1 mg • Vitamin B3 10 mg • Vitamin B6 10 mg • Folic Acid 600 mcg • Vitamin B12 100 mcg • Pantothenic Acid 10 mg • Biotin 100 mcg • Vitamin D (D3) 200 IU • Vitamin E 30 IU • Vitamin K (K1) 20 mcg • Coenzyme Q10 25 mg • Vitamin A 1000 IU • Lipoic Acid 1 mg • Choline Bitartrate 10 mg • Potassium (bicarbonate) 200 mg • Sodium (bicarbonate) 27 mg • Calcium (carbonate, ascorbate) 29 mg • Magnesium (ascorbate) 25 mg • Zinc (picolinate) 1.5 mg • Manganese (picolinate) 1.5 mg • Copper (aspartate) 500 mcg • Molybdenum (trioxide) 75 mcg • Selenium (selenite) 50 mcg • Chromium (picolinate) 100 mcg • Potassium Iodide 50 mcg • Boron (citrate) 1 mg • N-Acetyl Cysteine (NAC) 50 mg • Arginine 100 mg • Lysine 100 mg • Glycine 1000 mg • TMG - Betaine 1000 mg • Glutamine 100 mg • Bromelain 10 mg • Pineapple Bioflavonoids 100 mg. Other Ingredients: Fructose, Citric Acid, Aspartic Acid, Tartaric Acid, Malic Acid, Grape Flavor, Pineapple Strawberry Flavor, Lemon Juice Flavor.

True CMO **-** Jarrow Formulas
Two capsules contain: Cetyl Myristoleate extract (fatty acid complex) 760 mg. Other Ingredients: White Rice Flour, Magnesium Stearate, Gelatin, Titanium Dioxide.

TrueBlue Coral Calcium **-** CFU Distribution Co.
Each capsule contains: Calcium (from coral) 230 mg • Magnesium (from coral & chelated minerals) 51 mg • Vitamin D 400 IU • Malic Acid (from apples) 10 mg • Betaine HCl 5 mg • Vitamin C (as ascorbic acid) 5 mg • 73 Minerals from Coral 370 mg.

Trym Tone 1200 **-** Futurebiotics LLC
Four tablets contain: L-Arginine HCl 2100 mg • L-Glycine 1800 mg • L-Lysine HCl 300 mg • Vitamin C 30 mg • Pyridoxine HCl 15 mg • Chromium (polynicotinate) 75 mcg.

T-SEPT **-** Dial Herbs
Bayberry • Goldenseal • Myrrh • Mineral Water.

T-SHK **-** Dial Herbs
Lobelia • Cayenne • Mineral Water.

T-SKT **-** Dial Herbs
Myrrh • White Poplar bark • Balsam.

T-SLC **-** Dial Herbs
Comfrey • Mullein • Peppermint • Chickweed • Lobelia • Cayenne.

T-SS **-** Dial Herbs
Damiana • Licorice • Ginseng • Passion flower • Cayenne.

T-THD **-** Dial Herbs
Kelp • Parsley • Irish Moss • Cayenne • Licorice • Dulse • Bayberry • Bugleweed.

T-ULC **-** Dial Herbs
Goldenseal • Cayenne • Myrrh • Ginger • Comfrey • Poke root • Yellow Dock.

Tulsi-Neem soap **-** Auromere
Coconut oil • Palmyra oil • Rice Bran oil • Alkali • Water • Neem oil • Hydnocarpus oil (cactus) • Castor oil • Tulsi (holy basil) • Rose petals • Zedoary • Turmeric • Fenugreek • Psoralea Corlifolia seed (babchi) • Peepal (bodhi tree) • Alangium Salviifolium • Costus • Indian Sarsaparilla • Shiva Neem (variety of neem) • Hibiscus.

Tum-Ease **-** The Herbalist
Catnip leaf • Fennel seed • Angelica root • Gentian root • Oregon Grape root • Ginger root.

Tumeric Extract **-** Nature's Way
Each capsule contains: Tumeric root 50 mg • Tumeric dried extract 450 mg. Other Ingredients: Cellulose, Gelatin, Silica.

TUMS Calcium for Life Bone Health Calcium Supplement **-** GlaxoSmithKline (GSK)
Each tablet contains: Calcium Carbonate 500 mg. Other Ingredients: Sucrose, Corn Starch, Talc, Mineral Oil, Natural and Artificial Flavors, Adipic Acid, Sodium Polyphosphate, Red 40 Lake, Yellow 6 Lake, Yellow 5 Lake, Blue 1 Lake.

TUMS E-X (assorted berries flavor) **-** GlaxoSmithKline (GSK)
Each tablet contains: Calcium Carbonate 750 mg. Other Ingredients: Sucrose, Corn Starch, Talc, Mineral Oil, Artificial Flavors, Sodium Polyphosphate, Red 40 Lake, Blue 1 Lake.

TUMS Lasting Effects (mint flavor) **-** GlaxoSmithKline (GSK)
Active Ingredients: Calcium Carbonate USP 500 mg. Other Ingredients: Acesulfame Potassium, Alginic Acid, Blue 1 Lake, Calcium Stearate, Corn Starch, Mannitol, Mineral Oil, Natural Flavor, Potassium Bicarbonate, Sodium Polyphosphate, Sucralose, Sucrose, Talc.

TUMS Lasting Effects (mixed fruit flavor) **-** GlaxoSmithKline (GSK)
Active Ingredients: Calcium Carbonate USP 500 mg. Other Ingredients: Acesulfame Potassium, Alginic Acid, Calcium Stearate, Corn Starch, Mannitol, Mineral Oil, Natural and Artificial Flavors, Potassium Bicarbonate, Red 40 Lake, Sodium Polyphosphate, Sucralose, Sucrose, Talc, Yellow 5 (tartazine) Lake, Yellow 6 Lake.

TUMS Smooth Dissolve **-** GlaxoSmithKline (GSK)
Two tablets contain: Calcium Carbonate 750 mg. Other Ingredients: Calcium Carbonate, Sorbitol, Microcrystalline Cellulose, Magnesium Stearate, Natural and Artificial Flavors, Corn Starch, Guar Gum, Maltodextrin, Adipic Acid, Yellow 6 Lake, Red 40 Lake, Blue 1 Lake.

Some Brand Name Natural Products - What they Contain

www.NaturalDatabase.com contains MANY more listings than appear here.
Editor's Notes are located on pages 2155-2163.

BRAND NAMES

TUMS Ultra - GlaxoSmithKline (GSK)
Each tablet contains: Calcium Carbonate USP grade 1000 mg. Other Ingredients: Sucrose, Starch, Talc, Mineral Oil, Natural & Artificial Flavor, Sodium Polyphosphate, Blue 1 Lake, Red 40 Lake, Adipic Acid, Yellow 6 Lake, FD&C Yellow 5 Lake.

Turbo Charge Energy Formula (Ephedra Free) - Natural Balance
Each tablet contains: Proprietary Blend 985 mg: Guarana seed extract (contains caffeine), Korean Ginseng root standardized extract, Eleuthero root, Gotu Kola extract (aerial portion), Passion Flower extract (aerial portion), Wood Betony (aerial portion). Other Ingredients: Microcrystalline Cellulose, Silicon Dioxide, Cellulose Gum, Stearic Acid, Magnesium Stearate.

TurboBLAST II - Life Enhancement Products, Inc.
Each 1 tbsp (9.6 g) contains: Vitamin A (as beta-carotene) 2760 IU • Vitamin C (as ascorbic acid and niacinamide ascorbate) 400 mg • Vitamin E (as D,L-alpha-tocopheryl acetate) 60 IU • Thiamine (vitamin B1 as thiamine hydrochloride) 1.9 mg • Riboflavin (vitamin B2) 3 mg • Niacin (vitamin B3 as niacinamide ascorbate) 75 mg • Vitamin B6 (as pyridoxine hydrochloride) 19.5 mg • Folic Acid 100 mcg • Vitamin B12 (cyanocobalamin) 20 mcg • Pantothenic Acid (vitamin B5 as calcium pantothenate) 20 mg • Zinc (as zinc gluconate) 2.15 mg • Copper (as copper gluconate) 3 mg • Chromium (as chromium aspartate) 25 mcg • L-Phenylalanine 650 mg • Citric Acid 250 mg • Malic Acid 250 mg • Taurine 200 mg • Glycine 150 mg • Grape-seed extract 125 mg • Fumaric Acid 100 mg • Caffeine 42 mg • Tea Polyphenols 63 mg • Maltol 25 mg.

TurboShake, Choc-o-Blast - Advocare International
AdvoKids Protein Complex: Calcium Sodium Caseinates, Soy Protein, L-Lysine Hydrochloride, Whey Protein Isolate, L-Glutamine • Fructose • Maltodextrin • Cocoa powder • Guar Gum • Medium Chain Triglycerides • Calcium Phosphate • Potassium Chloride • Rice Syrup Solids • Cellulose • Magnesium Oxide • Natural Flavors • Artificial Flavors • Apple powder • Taurine • Calcium Ascorbate • Choline Citrate • Sodium Chloride • Oatgrass powder • Carrot powder • Vitamin E Acetate • Sucralose • Gum Acacia • Silicon Dioxide • Bromelain • Papain • Biotin • Boron Citrate • Niacinamide • Inositol • Folic Acid • Zinc Oxide • Selenomethionine • Copper Gluconate • Calcium Pantothenate • Vitamin A Palmitate • Vitamin K • Cholecalciferol • Chromium Polynicotinate (ChromeMate brand) • Manganese Carbonate • Pyridoxine Hydrochloride • Lactobacillus Acidophilus • Bifidobacterium Bifidus • Riboflavin • Thiamine Hydrochloride • Cyanocobalamin • Sodium Molybdate • Potassium Iodide.

TurboTrim Plus - Trim International
Each tablet contains: MaHuang • Guarana • Chromium Picolinate • Chitosan • Gymnema Sylvestre • Garcinia Cambogia • Vitamin E • Magnesium Chelate • Zinc Chelate • Proprietary Blend: Bee Pollen, Ginseng root, Ginger root, Lecithin, Bovine complex, Damiana herb, Sarsaparilla root, Goldenseal herb, Nettle leaf, Gotu Kola herb, Spirulina, Royal Jelly. Other Ingredients: Di-Calcium Phosphate, Magnesium Stearate, Stearic Acid.
See Editor's Note No. 14 and No. 30.

Turmeric Catechu Supreme - Gaia Herbs
Forty drops contain: Proprietary Blend 220 mg: Turmeric root (curcuma longa), Black Catechu (catechu nigrum), Grindelia floral buds (grindelia robusta), Licorice root (glycyrrhiza glabra), Rose Hip solid extract (rosa rugosa), Chinese Skullcap root (scutellaria baicalensis), Ginkgo leaf (ginkgo biloba), African Devil's Claw root (harpagophytum procumbens), Yarrow flowers (achillea millefolium), Lobelia herb and seed (lobelia inflata), 50-60% Pure Grain Alcohol USP, Spring Water.

T-VV - Dial Herbs
Oat Straw • Buckthorn • Yarrow • Brigham Tea • Witch Hazel • St. John's Wort • Cayenne.

Twinlab B-1 Caps - TwinLab
Each capsule contains: Thiamin (from thiamin monoitrate) 100 mg.

Two Trees Slippery Elm Lozenges - Thayers Natural Pharmaceuticals
Each lozenge contains: Slippery Elm Bark 150 mg. Base: Maple Sugar, Vegetable Stearate.

T-WRT - Dial Herbs
Garlic • Celandine • Mullein • Buckthorn.

Ty-Glute - Atrium Biotechnologies
Each tablet contains: L-Glutamine 255 mg • L-Tyrosine 155 mg • Vitamin C 150 mg • Adrenal concentrate 45 mg.
See Editor's Note No. 14.

T-YI - Dial Herbs
Echinacea • Goldenseal • Bayberry • Myrrh • Plantain • Slippery Elm • Wild Carrot.

Type II Collagen - Jarrow Formulas
Two capsules contain: Bovine Trachea Cartilage 1480 mg: Type II Collagen 740 mg, Chondroitin Sulfate 4,6/A,B 470 mg, Other Mucopolysaccharides 190 mg. Other Ingredients: Water, Magnesium Stearate, Gelatin.
See Editor's Note No. 15.

Tyroplex - Higher Nature
Each tablet contains: Tyrosine 500 mg • Magnesium (ascorbate) 25 mg • Niacin (nicotinamide) 15 mg • Vitamin C 12.5 mg • Zinc (citrate) 2.5 mg • Vitamin B6 5 mg • Manganese (chelate) 1.25 mg • Iron (chelate) 1.25 mg • Copper (chelate) 0.25 mg • Folic Acid 60 mcg • Vitamin B12 5 mcg.

Tyrosine - Golden Glow Natural Health Products
Each tablet contains: Tyrosine 500 mg.

Tyrosine 850 - Pain & Stress Center
Each capsule contains: Vitamin C (ascorbyl palmitate) 8 mg • Tyrosine 850 mg. Other Ingredients: Gelatin Capsule.

Tyrosine and Alpha Lipoic Acid Complex - N.V. Perricone M.D. Cosmeceuticals
Each capsule contains: Biotin 200 mcg • Chromium (as ChromeMate brand chromium polynicotinate) 100 mcg • L-Tyrosine 250 mg • Sustained release Alpha-Lipoic Acid 100 mg. Other Ingredients: Hydroxypropyl Methylcellulose, Gelatin, Calcium Sulfate, Magnesium Stearate, Silica.

Tyrosine and B-Vitamins - Vital Nutrients
Each capsule contains: Tyrosine 400 mg • Thiamine HCl (vitamin B1) 6 mg • Riboflavin (vitamin B2) 5 mg • Hydroxocobalamin (pure vitamin B12) 50 mcg • Niacinamide 25 mg • Biotin 50 mcg • Pyridoxine HCl (vitamin B6) 6 mg • Folic Acid 50 mcg • Calcium Pantothenate (vitamin B5) 10 mg.

UC - II - PhysioLogics
Each capsule contains: Undenatured Type II Collagen (from UC-II undenatured type II collagen complex 40 mg) 10 mg. Other Ingredients: Potassium Chloride, Cellulose (plant origin).

Udo's Choice Beyond Greens - Flora Inc.
Each 1 tsp serving (8 g) contains: Udo's Choice perfected seed blend: Certified Organic Flax seed, Defatted Flax, Certified Organic Sunflower seed, Defatted Sunflower seed, Certified Organic Sesame seed, Defatted Sesame seed, Rice germ, Bran powder, Oat germ, Bran powder • Pines Barley Grass powder • Cracked Golden Flax seed • Pumpkin seed • Pines Alfalfa Grass powder • Rice bran • Dried Cane juice • Carrot • Soyforce Sprouted Soybeans • Tomato • Pines Oat Grass • Pines Rye Grass • Red Beet • Cinnamon • Peppermint • Ginger • Bilberry leaf • Spirulina • Bee pollen • Dulse • Chlorella • Broccoli • Parsley • Kelp • Hawthorne berry • Milk Thistle • Burdock root • Red Clover • Kale • Licorice root • Chrysanthemum • Yucca • Natural Almond flavor • Lemon Grass • Udo's Choice Digestive Enzyme blend: Protease, Lipase, Amylase, Cellulase, Maltase, Glucoamylase, Invertase, Pectinase, with Phytase, Lactase • Beet juice • American Ginseng • Ginkgo extract • Psyllium • Slippery Elm • Stevia leaf • Artichoke • Dandelion root • Dandelion leaf • Rosemary • Thyme • Sage • Standardized Grape seed extract.

Some Brand Name Natural Products - What they Contain

www.NaturalDatabase.com contains MANY more listings than appear here.
Editor's Notes are located on pages 2155-2163.

Udo's Choice Fast Food Blend - Flora Inc.
Certified Organic Flax • Sunflower & Sesame seeds • Pines Organic Cereal Grasses • Soyforce Powdered Sprouted Soybeans.

Udo's Choice Oil Blend - Flora Inc.
Flax oil • Sunflower oil • Sesame oil • Medium Chain Triglycerides • Evening Primrose oil (12.6 mg GLA per tablespoon) • Rice germ & Bran oil • Soy Lecithin • d-Alpha Tocopherol (natural Vitamin E) • Oat germ & Bran oil.

Udo's Choice Perfect Oil Blend - Flora Inc.
Flax oil • sesame seed oil • Sunflower oil & other unrefined oils • medium triglycerides • Lecithin & d-alpha tocopherol.

Udo's Choice Super 5 - Flora Inc.
Each tablet contains: 1 billion plus viable organisms of Lactobacillus acidophilus DDS-1 • B. bifidum • L. bulgaricus • S. thermophilus & L. salivarius in a base of: (Maltodextrin, Fructose & Ascorbic Acid).

Ulcinex - Metagenics
Two tablets contain: Proprietary Ultra-Concentrate 1500 mg: Corydalis Yanhusuo tuber (corydalis yanhusuo), Astragalus root (astragalus membranaceus), Tienchi Ginseng root (panax pseudoginseng), Zhejiang Fritillary bulb (fritillaria thunbergii), Chinese Licorice root (glycyrrhiza uralensis), Gambir leaf and stem (uncaria gambir), Brown's Lily bulb (lilium brownii), Bletilla root (bletilla striata), Cuttlefish shell (sepia esculenta).

Ultimate Aloe - Market America, Inc.
Whole Leaf Aloe Vera Linne gel • Purified Water • Ascorbic Acid • Sodium Benzoate • Potassium Sorbate • Citric Acid • Malic Acid • Caramel.

Ultimate Antioxidant - Arrowroot
Two tablets contain: Beta Carotene 30,000 IU • Vitamin C 600 mg • Vitamin E 400 IU • Selenium 70 mcg • Lemon Bioflavonoids 600 mg.

Ultimate Antioxidant II - Gary Null & Associates (GNA)
Three capsules contain: Citrus Bioflavonoid Complex 300 mg • Rutin 25 mg • Bilberry extract 25 mg • Red Wine Concentrate 25 mg • Grape Skin extract 200 mg • China Green Tea 200 mg • Beta Carotene 10000 IU • L-Glutathione 5 mg • L-Cysteine 200 mg • Vitamin C 500 mg • Vitamin E 200 IU • Selenium 10 mcg • Zinc Picolinate 25 mg • CoQ10 10 mg • NAC 25 mg • Alpha Lipoic Acid 100 mg • Ascorbyl Palmitate 100 mg • SOD 25 mg • Vitamin B6 10 mg • Copper Lysinate 2 mg • Taurine 50 mg • Quercetin 50 mg • Pycnogenol 5 mg • Licorice 25 mg • Broccoli 25 mg • Lutein 25 mg • Cabbage 25 mg • Carrot powder 25 mg • Milk Thistle 25 mg.

Ultimate Ascorbate C - Source Naturals
Vitamin C (from magnesium, potassium, calcium, zinc, & manganese ascorbates) 1000 mg • Calcium (as calcium ascorbate) 20 mg • Magnesium (as magnesium ascorbate) 32 mg • Zinc (as zinc ascorbate) 3 mg • Manganese (as manganese ascorbate) 1 mg • Potassium (as potassium ascorbate) 90 mg.

Ultimate Balance - Antioxidant Formula - Bioadvantex Pharma
Two caplets contain: N-Acetyl Cysteine (NAC) 700 mg • Alpha-Lipoic Acid 200 mg • Milk Thistle seed extract 200 mg

Ultimate Caps - Arrowroot
Each capsule contains: Vitamin A 7500 IU • Biotin 50 mcg • Beta Carotene 5000 IU • Folic Acid 200 mcg • Vitamin D (D3) 200 IU • Copper 1.5 mg • Vitamin E 50 IU • Glutamic Acid 10 mg • Vitamin C 125 mg • Iron 9 mg • Vitamin B1 50 mg • Lemon Bioflavonoid Complex 12.5 mg • Vitamin B2 50 mg • Manganese 1.5 mg • Niacinamide 50 mg • Magnesium 12.5 mg • Vitamin B6 50 mg • Zinc 15 mg • Vitamin B12 50 mcg • Calcium 25 mg • Pantothenic Acid 50 mg • Selenium 12.5 mcg • Chromium 12.5 mcg • Chlorophyll 1 mg • Potassium 5 mg • PABA 50 mg • Choline 50 mg • Inositol 50 mg • Rutin 12.5 mg • Betaine HCl 12.5 mg.

Ultimate Cleanse - Nature's Secret
Each tablet contains: Multi-Herb: Alfalfa Leaf • Fenugreek Seed • Ginger Root • Dandelion root • Fennel Seed • Yarrow Flower • Hawthorne Berries • Horsetail Herb • Licorice Root • Marshmallow Root • Peppermint Leaf • Red Clover Tops • Red Raspberry Leaf • Safflower Oil • Scullcap Herb • Burdock Root • Chickweed Herb • Mullein Leaf • Papaya Leaf • Black Cohosh Root • Cayenne Fruit • Irish Moss • Pacific Kelp • Slippery Elm Bark • Yellow Dock Root • Plantain Herb • Echinacea Angustifolia Extract • Ginkgo Biloba Leaf Extract • Milk Thistle Extract. Multi-Fiber: Cascara Sagrada Bark • Fennel Seed • Psyllium Seed • Ginger Root • Acacia Gum • Alfalfa Leaf • Apple Pectin • Apple Powder • Barley Rice Fiber • Beet Root • Glucomannan • Karaya Gum • Peppermint Leaf • Lemon Peel • Oat Bran • Red Raspberry Leaf • Slippery Elm Bark • Shattered Cell Wall Chlorella • Lactobacillus Acidophilus (dairy free) • Guar Gum.

Ultimate Ester-C - Source Naturals
Each two tablets contain: Vitamin C (as magnesium, calcium, potassium, zinc, & manganese ascorbates) 2000 mg • Vitamin D (as cholecalciferol) 85 IU • Calcium (as calcium ascorbate & carbonate) 100 mg • Magnesium (as magnesium ascorbate & oxide) 100 mg • Zinc (as zinc ascorbate) 25 mg • Copper (as copper sebacate) 500 mcg • Manganese (as manganese ascorbate) 5 mg • Potassium (as potassium ascorbate & citrate) 99 mg • Bioflavonoids 250 mg • Rutin 31 mg • Hesperidin 30 mg.

Ultimate Eye Formula - Purity Products
Three capsules contain: Vitamin C (magnesium ascorbate) 360 mg • Vitamin E 50 IU • Vitamin B-6 10 mg • Vitamin B-12 500 mcg • Alpha-Lipoic Acid 150 mg • L-Taurine 250 mg • Bilberry fruit extract 120 mg • Lutein 10 mg • Wolfberry fruit powder 25 mg • Pomegranate fruit 50 mg • IP6 (inositol hexaphosphate) 150 mg • Soy Isoflavones 200 mg • Gamma Oryzanol 100 mg.

Ultimate Fiber - Nature's Secret
Psyllium husks, Slippery Elm bark, Acidophilus powder, Fructooligosaccharides.

Ultimate Green - Nature's Secret
Each packet contain: Shattered Cell Wall Chlorella • Hawaiian Blue-Green Algae • Barley Grass • Wheat Grass • Alfalfa • Spinach.

Ultimate H.A. Formula - Purity Products
Three capsules contain: Hyaluronic Acid 150 mg • Chondroitin Sulfate 300 mg • BioCell Collagen II 1500 mg.
See Editor's Note No. 15.

Ultimate Iron - Enzymatic Therapy
Two softgels contain: Vitamin C (ascorbic acid) 120 mg • Folic Acid 400 mcg • Vitamin B12 (as cyanocobalamin) 200 mcg • Iron (as ferrous succinate) 50 mg • Liquid Liver Fractions (predigested soluble concentrate) 500 mg • Chlorophyll (fat-soluble) 10 mg. Other Ingredients: Soybean Oil, Gelatin, Glycerin, Beeswax, Lecithin.
See Editor's Note No. 14.

Ultimate Libido Formula for Women - MD Healthline
Two capsules contain: Niacin 40 mg • Yohimbe bark 500 mg • Dong Quai 150 mg • Sativari (asparagus racemosus) 150 mg • DHEA 10 mg.• Ashwagandha 100 mg • L-Tyrosine 100 mg • L-Histidine 66 mg • Tree Peony 4:1 extract 50 mg • Royal Jelly 50 mg • Wild Yam 10:1 extract 40 mg • Quebracho bark 20 mg • Ginger root 5:1 extract 20 mg • Sundew 20 mg • Guarana 20 mg • Damiana 20 mg.

Ultimate Men's Peak Performance - Swanson Health Products
Each tablet contains: Vitamin E (as d-alpha tocopheryl succinate) 50 IU • Niacin 25 mg • Zinc (from zinc amino acid chelate) 7.5 mg • Yohimbe extract (2% yohimbine alkaloids) 250 mg • Tribulus Terrestris extract (40% steroidal saponins) 125 mg • Avena Sativa wild oats (5:1 extract) 50 mg • Cayenne Pepper 50 mg • Damiana leaf powder 50 mg • Ginger root powder 50 mg • Ginkgo Biloba leaf powder 50 mg • Ginseng extract (5% ginsenosides) 50 mg • Guarana extract (12.5% alkaloids) 50 mg • Hawthorn berry powder 50 mg • L-Arginine HCl 50 mg • Oyster extract 50 mg • Saw Palmetto berry powder 50 mg • Rhodiola Rosea extract (1% rosevin) 25 mg.

Some Brand Name Natural Products - What they Contain

www.NaturalDatabase.com contains MANY more listings than appear here.
Editor's Notes are located on pages 2155-2163.

Ultimate Multi Plus - Nature's Secret
Contains over 90 vitamins, minerals, amino acids, antioxidants, herbs, superfoods, digestive enzymes and Herbalgest.

Ultimate Oil - Nature's Secret
Blend of oils that offer a mixture of the essential fatty acids, Omega 3 and Omega 6.

Ultimate One - Arrowroot
Each tablet contains: Vitamin A 8000 IU • Biotin 100 mcg • Beta Carotene 10,000 IU • Folic Acid 400 mcg • Vitamin D (D3) 400 IU • Copper 2 mg • Vitamin E 100 IU • Phosphorus 30 mg • Vitamin C 250 mg • Iron 18 mg • Vitamin B1 100 mg • Iodine 225 mcg • Vitamin B2 100 mg • Manganese 7 mg • Vitamin B3 100 mg • Magnesium 40 mg • Vitamin B6 100 mg • Zinc 15 mg • Vitamin B12 100 mcg • Calcium 50 mg • Pantothenic Acid 100 mg • Selenium 50 mcg • Chromium 25 mcg • Molybdenum 15 mcg • Potassium 10 mg • PABA 30 mg • Choline 100 mg • Inositol 100 mg • Rutin 25 mg • Betaine HCl 25 mg • Lemon Bioflavonoid Complex 50 mg • Hesperidin Complex 25 mg.

Ultimate One Iron Free - Arrowroot
Each tablet contains: Vitamin A 8000 IU • Biotin 100 mcg • Beta Carotene 10,000 IU • Folic Acid 400 mcg • Vitamin D (D3) 400 IU • Copper 2 mg • Vitamin E 100 IU • Phosphorus 30 mg • Vitamin C 250 mg • Vitamin B1 100 mg • Iodine 225 mcg • Vitamin B2 100 mg • Manganese 7 mg • Vitamin B3 100 mg • Magnesium 40 mg • Vitamin B6 100 mg • Zinc 15 mg • Vitamin B12 100 mcg • Calcium 50 mg • Pantothenic Acid 100 mg • Selenium 50 mcg • Chromium 25 mcg • Molybdenum 15 mcg • Potassium 10 mg • PABA 30 mg • Choline 47 mg • Rose Hips 5 mg • Inositol 100 mg • Rutin 25 mg • Bioflavonoid Complex (from lemon, rutin, hesperidin) 100 mg • Betaine HCl 25 mg • Glutamic Acid HCl 25 mg.

Ultimate Orange Powercaps - Next Nutrition
Three softgels contain: Magnesium 9.7 mg • L-Tyrosine 500 mg • Ma Huang whole plant 313 mg • Guarana seed 227 mg • Caffeine 200 mg • Proprietary Blend 100 mg: Sida Cordifolia root, Korean Ginseng root, Green Tea leaf, Coleus Forskohlii root, Orange Peel Bioflavonoids, Grapefruit extract, Cayenne Pepper. Other Ingredients: Soybean Oil, Gelatin, Glycerin Water, Titanium Dioxide, FD&C Yellow 6, FD&C Red 40.
See Editor's Note No. 30 and No. 39.

Ultimate Performance Max Protein Bar (vanilla almond flavor) - Rexall - Sundown
Each bar contains: Protein 18 g • Vitamin A (as retinyl palmitate) 2500 IU • Vitamin C 30 mg • Vitamin D (as cholecalciferol) 200 IU • Vitamin E (as dl-alpha-tocopheryl acetate) 15 IU • Thiamin (as thiamine HCl) 0.75 mg • Riboflavin (Vitamin B-2) 0.85 mg • Niacin (as niacinamide) 10 mg • Vitamin B-6 (as pyridoxine HCl) 1 mg • Folic Acid 200 mcg • Vitamin B-12 (as cyanocobalamin) 3 mcg • Biotin 150 mcg • Pantothenic Acid (as calcium d-pantothenate) 5 mg • Calcium 500 mg • Iron (as ferrous fumarate) 9 mg • Phosphorus 700 mg • Iodine (as potassium iodide) 75 mcg • Magnesium (as magnesium oxide) 200 mg • Zinc (as zinc oxide) 7.5 mg • Copper (as copper gluconate) 1 mg • Chromium (as chromium picolinate) 5 mcg • Sodium 110 mg. Other Ingredients: Brown Rice Syrup, Cocoa Coating (sugar, fractionated palm kernel oil, cocoa powder, whey powder, nonfat dry milk powder, soy lecithin, natural vanilla flavor), Whey Protein Isolate, High Fructose Corn Syrup, Whey Protein Concentrate, Crystaline Fructose, Almond Butter, Natural flavor, Oat Fiber, Dicalcium Phosphate, L-Glutamine, Taurine.

Ultimate Plenamins - Rexall - Sundown
Each tablet contains: Vitamin A (from retinyl acetate) 5000 IU • Vitamin C (as niacinamide ascorbate and ascorbic acid) 120 mg • Vitamin D (as cholecalciferol) 400 IU • Vitamin E (as dl-alpha-tocopheryl acetate and d-alpha-tocopheryl acid succinate) 30 IU • Vitamin K (as phytonadione) 25 mcg • Thiamin (as thiamin HCl) 3 mg • Riboflavin (vitamin B-2) 3.4 mg • Niacin (from niacinamide ascorbate) 20 mg • Vitamin B-6 (from pyridoxine HCl) 4 mg • Folic Acid 400 mcg • Vitamin B-12 (as cyanocobalamin) 25 mcg • Biotin 50 mcg • Pantothenic Acid (from d-calcium pantothenate) 10 mg • Calcium (from dicalcium phosphate and calcium carbonate) 200 mg • Iron (from ferrous fumarate) 18 mg • Phosphorus (as dicalcium phosphate) 125 mg • Iodine (from potassium iodide) 150 mcg • Magnesium (from magnesium oxide) 100 mg • Zinc (from zinc sulfate) 15 mg • Selenium (from sodium selenate) 25 mcg • Copper (from cupric oxide) 2 mg • Manganese (from manganese sulfate) 5 mg • Chromium (from chromium chloride) 15 mcg • Molybdenum (from sodium molybdate) 25 mcg • Potassium (from potassium chloride) 30 mg • Vanadium (from vanadium aspartate) 10 mcg • Silicon (from silicon dioxide) 10 mcg • Nickel (from nickel sulfate) 5 mcg • PABA (para-aminobenzoic acid) 1 mg • Choline Bitartrate 1 mg • Inositol 100 mcg • Bee Pollen 25 mg • Siberian Ginseng root 25 mg • Fish Oil (EPA [eicosapentaenoic acid] 18 mg, DHA [docosahexaenoic acid] 12 mg) 100 mg • Plenamin nutritional catalyst base: Rose Hips and seed extract, Kelp, Soy Lecithin, Soy protein isolate, Wheat Germ, Hesperidin, Rutin, Acerola fruit extract, Citrus Bioflavonoids 3.5 mg. Other Ingredients: Cellulose, Croscarmellose sodium, Hydroxypropyl methylcellulose, Magnesium stearate, PEG, Red 40 lake, Blue 2 lake, Titanium dioxide, Polysorbate 80, Beta-carotene.

Ultimate Prostate Formula - Purity Products
Three capsules contain: Vitamin E 60 IU • Vitamin B-6 50 mg • Zinc (zinc citrate) 15 mg • Selenium (selenomethionine) 50 mcg • Saw Palmetto extract 575 mg • Pygeum extract 310 mg • Nettle root extract 300 mg • Lycopene 7 mg • L-Alanine 400 mg • Glutamic Acid 400 mg • Glycine 400 mg • Quercetin 100 mg.

Ultimate Prostate Formula - Herbalife International of America, Inc.
Each soft gel contains: Vitamin E (DL-alpha-tocopheryl acetate) 25 IU • Selenium yeast 25 mcg • Saw Palmetto fruit lipid extract 180 mg • Pumpkin seed oil 100 mg • Lycopene 1 mg • Dried Black Pepper fruit extract 1 mg. Other Ingredients: Gelatin, Glycerin, Beeswax, Water, Soy Lecithin, Carob Extract, Titanium Dioxide.

Ultimate Prostate Support - NorthStar Nutritionals
Each two softgel capsules contain: Saw Palmetto berry extract (85-90% fatty acids) 160 mg • Pygeum Africanum 50 mg • Nettle root extract 150 mg • Lycopene 5 mg • Vitamin E (d-alpha tocopherol, natural) 100 mg • Selenium 5 mcg • Zinc Arginate 7.5 mg.

Ultimate Senior - Arrowroot
Two tablets contain: Vitamin A (70% from palmitate, 30% from natural beta carotene D. salina) 10,000 IU • Zinc (OptiZinc brand) 15 mg • Vitamin C (calcium ascorbate) 150 mg • Selenium (L-selenomethionine) 70 mcg • Vitamin D (D3 as cholecalciferol) 500 IU • Copper • (copper gluconate) 2 mg • Vitamin E (D-alpha tocopheryl succinate) 100 IU • Manganese (manganous gluconate) 1 mg • Thiamine (thiamin mononitrate) 15 mg • Chromium (chromium picolinate) 60 mcg • Riboflavin 15 mg • Molybdenum (chelate) 10 mcg • Niacin (niacinamide) 20 mg • Betaine HCl 25 mg • Vitamin B6 (as pyridoxine HCl) 15 mg • Lemon Bioflavonoids 50 mg • Folic Acid 400 mcg • Boron (chelate) 200 mcg • Vitamin B12 (cyanocobalamin) 30 mcg • Choline (choline bitartrate) 25 mg • Biotin 300 mcg • Enzyme blend 60 mg: Papain, Lipase, Bromelain • Pantothenic Acid (D-calcium carbonate) 15 mg • Glutamic Acid HCl 25 mg • Calcium (calcium carbonate) 150 mg • PABA (para-aminobenzoic acid) 25 mg • Iron (iron fumarate) 4 mg • Inositol 25 mg • Iodine (potassium iodide) 150 mcg • Silica (colloidal silica) 25 mg • Magnesium (oxide) 75 mg • Vanadium (chelate) 2 mcg.

Ultimate Sleep System - Rainbow Light
Two tablets contain: Valerian rhizome (standardized to 0.8% valernic acid) 160 mg • Kava Kava root (standardized to 30% kavalactones) 40 mg • Spirulina 100 mg • 4:1 Custom Herbal extracts: [Valerian rhizome, Hops strobiles, Kava Kava root, Orange oil, Passion flower herb, Valerian oil, Reishi fruiting body (providing 3200 mg herbal powder equivalent)] 800 mg. Nutritional Cofactors: N-Acetyl-L-Carnitine (NAC) 10 mg • Niacin/Niacinamide (Vitamin B3) 115 mg • Magnesium (Oxide, Pyroglutamate) 47.3 mg • Chromium (Polynicotinate) 30 mcg.

Ultimate Two - Arrowroot
Two tablets contain: Vitamin A 8000 IU • Biotin 100 mcg • Beta Carotene 10,000 IU • Folic Acid 400 mcg • Vitamin D (D3) 400 IU • Copper 2 mg • Vitamin E 150 IU • Phosphorus 30 mg • Vitamin C 250 mg • Iron 18 mg • Vitamin B1 100 mg • Iodine 225 mcg • Vitamin B2 100 mg • Manganese 7 mg • Vitamin B3 100 mg • Magnesium 40 mg • Vitamin B6 100 mg • Zinc 15 mg • Vitamin B12 100 mcg • Calcium 50 mg • Pantothenic Acid 100 mg • Selenium 50 mcg • Chromium 25 mcg • Molybdenum 15 mcg • Potassium 10 mg • PABA 30 mg • Choline 100 mg • Inositol 100 mg • Rutin 25 mg • Betaine HCl 25 mg • Lemon Bioflavonoid Complex 50 mg • Hesperidin Complex 25 mg.

Ultimate Vegetarian - Arrowroot
Each tablet contains: Vitamin A 8000 IU • Biotin 75 mcg • Beta Carotene 10,000 IU • Folic Acid 400 mcg • Vitamin D (D3) 400 IU • Copper 1 mg • Vitamin E 100 IU • Para-Aminobenzoic Acid 75 mg • Vitamin C 250 mg • Iron 10 mg • Vitamin B1 75 mg • Iodine 150 mcg • Vitamin B2 75 mg • Manganese 6.1 mg • Vitamin B3 75 mg • Magnesium 7.2 mg • Vitamin B6 75 mg • Zinc 15 mg • Vitamin B12 75 mcg • Calcium 50 mg • Pantothenic Acid 75 mg • Selenium 100 mcg • Chromium Picolinate 50 mcg • Molybdenum 15 mcg • Potassium 10 mg • Glutamic Acid 25 mg • Choline 75 mg • Inositol 75 mg • Rutin 25 mg • Betaine HCl 25 mg • Lemon Bioflavonoid Complex 25 mg • Hesperidin Complex 25 mg.

Ultimate Wild Yam - Swanson Health Products
Four tablets contain: Yam extract 12 mg • Avena sativa 2 mg • Camellia sinensis 2 mg • Crataegus oxyacantha 2 mg • Dioscorea Quat 2 mg • Extracts of Barbasco 2 mg • Lactase 2 mg • Licorice root 2 mg • Medicago sativa 2 mg • Prunus SPP 2 mg • Smilax Aristolochiifolia (Mexican sarsaparilla) 2 mg • Soy extracts 2 mg.

Ultimate Women's Intimate Performance - Swanson Health Products
Each tablet contains: Niacin 8.3 mg • Ginseng extract (6% ginsenosides) 100 mg • Avena Sativa oats (5:1 extract) 33.3 mg • Cayenne pepper 33.3 mg • Damiana leaf powder 33.3 mg • Dong Quai extract (1% ligustilides) 33.3 mg • Ginger root powder 33.3 mg • Guarana extract (12.5% alkaloids) 33.3 mg • L-Arginine HCl 33.3 mg • Licorice extract (12% glycyrrhizic acid) 33.3 mg • Muira Puama root 33.3 mg • Agnus Castus (chasteberry) extract (0.5% agnusides) 8.3 mg • Black Cohosh extract (2.5% triterpene glycosides) 8.3 mg • Ovary extract 8.3 mg.
See Editor's Note No. 14.

Ultimate Zinc-C Lozenges - NOW Foods
Each lozenge contains: Vitamin A (from Fish Liver oil) 1000 IU • Vitamin C (as Ascorbic Acid) 150 mg • Zinc (as Zinc Gluconate) 24 mg • Echinacea root powder 100 mg • Bee Propolis 100 mg • Slippery Elm bark powder (Ulmus fulva) 25 mg.

Ultra 30/20 Fish oil - Health From The Sun
Two capsules contain: Vitamin E 4 IU • Omega-3 Fatty Acids 1.2 g [EPA (600 mg) DHA (400 mg)]. Ingredients: All natural Fish Body oil concentrate, Gelatin, Glycerine, Mixed Tocopherols.

Ultra AB-C - American Biologics
Each heaping teaspoon (5 g) contains: Ascorbic Acid (vitamin C) 2400 mg • Magnesium (as carbonate, generating ascorbate chelate in solution) 190 mg • Calcium (as carbonate, generating ascorbate chelate in solution) 350 mg • Potassium (as bicarboante, generating ascorbate chelate in solution) 198 mg • Zinc (as OptiZinc brand monomethionine) 6 mg • Quercetin Bioflavnonoid 200 mg. Other Ingredients: Silicon Dioxide, Microcrystalline Cellulose.

Ultra ActiVin Capsules - Nature's Plus
Each capsule contains: ActiVin brand Vitis Vinifera seed, standardized to a minimum of 85% Proanthocyanidins 100 mg • Bioperine brand Black Pepper extract (piper nigrum) 2.5 mg. Other Ingredients: Silica, Bilberry extract, Blackberry Extract, Chinese Green Tea Extract (decaffeinated), Black Raspberry, Red Raspberry, Gelatin, Purified Water.

Ultra Antioxidant - Pro Health
Two capsules contain: Vitamin A (as beta carotene, retinyl palmitate) 5000 IU • Vitamin C (as ascorbic acid, Ester C brand calcium ascorbate) 1000 mg • Vitamin E (as natural D-alpha tocopheryl succinate) 400 IU • OptiZinc brand Zinc 10 mg • Selenium (as L-selenomethionine) 100 mcg • Alpha Lipoic Acid 100 mg • Green Tea extract (camellia var. sinensis leaf, 75% polyphenols) 50 mg • Grape seed extract (vitis vinifera inner core, 95% proanthocyanidins) 30 mg • Lutein extract (from marigold flowers, 5% lutein) 30 mg • Lycopene extract (from Lycobeads brand, 1% lycopene) 30 mg • N-Acetyl Cysteine 30 mg • Odorless Garlic bulb powder (allium sativa) 30 mg • Quercetin Dihydrate 30 mg • L-Glutathione 20 mg • Coenzyme Q10 10 mg. Other Ingredients: Gelatin, Water, Magnesium Stearate, Silicon Dioxide, Hydrolyzed Gelatin, Vegetable Oil, Oleoresin, Sucrose, Corn Starch, Ascorbyl Palmitate, Natural Tocopherol.

Ultra ATP+ - Pro Health
Three tablets contain: Malic Acid from Apple 600 mg • Magnesium (from 150 mg magnesium hydroxide) 62.5 mg. Other Ingredients: Dicalcium Phosphate, Microcrystalline Cellulose, Stearic Acid, Magnesium Stearate, Silicon Dioxide, Pharmaceutical Glaze.

Ultra B-Complex High Potency with Folic Acid - Pro Health
Each capsule contains: Thiamin (vitamin B1 as thiamine HCl) 100 mg • Riboflavin (vitamin B2) 100 mg • Niacin (vitamin B3 as niacinamide) 100 mg • Vitamin B6 (as pyridoxine HCl) 100 mg • Folate (as folic acid) 400 mcg • Vitamin B12 (as cyanocobalamin) 100 mcg • Biotin 100 mcg • Pantothenic Acid (as D-calcium pantothenate) 100 mg • Choline (as choline bitartrate) 47 mg • Inositol 100 mg • PABA (para-aminobenzoic acid) 100 mg. Other Ingredients: Gelatin, Water, Magnesium Stearate, Silicon Dioxide.

Ultra Beauty Formula - Leiner Health Products
Two tablets contain: Biotin 266 mcg • Folate 266 mcg • Vitamin E (Mixed Tocopherols) 20 IU • Zinc Gluconate 10 mg • Thiamin (Vitamin B1) 6.6 mg • Calcium Carbonate 400 mg • Riboflavin (Vitamin B2) 6.6 mg • Manganese Oxide 6.6 mg • Vitamin B6 6.6 mg • Magnesium Oxide 133 mg • Vitamin D 133 IU • Iron 4 mg • Selenium 16 mcg • Pantothenic Acid 20 mg • Phosphorus 200 mg • Vitamin B12 10 mcg • Niacin 33 mg • Vitamin A 6666 IU • Vitamin C (Ascorbic Acid) 80 mg • Iodine 150 mcg • Betaine 33 mg • Bioflavonoids 33 mg • Choline Bitartrate 100 mg • Inositol 40 mg • L-Cysteine 680 mcg • PABA 33 mg • Ribonucleic Acid 40 mg • Rutin 16 mg. Other Ingredients: Dicalcium Phosphate, Cellulose, Stearic Acid, Croscarmellose Sodium, Sodium Starch Glycolate. In a base containing: Asparagus, Echinacea, Horsetail, L-Methionine, Gelatin, Oat Straw, and Papain.

Ultra Bifidis - Metagenics
Each 1/2 tsp serving contains: Bifidobacterium Lactis (formerly known as B. infantis) 15 billion live organisms.

Ultra Bifidus DF (dairy free) - Metagenics
Each 1/2 tsp serving contains: Bifidobacterium Lactis (formerly known as B. infantis) 15 billion live organisms.

Ultra Bone Balance - Source Naturals
Four tablets contain: Vitamin C (as Calcium, Magnesium, Manganese Ascorbates) 52 mg • Vitamin D (as Cholecalciferol) 300 IU • Vitamin B6 (as Pyridoxine HCl) 20 mg • Folate (as Folic Acid) 200 mcg • Calcium (as Calcium Carbonate, Citrate, Ethanolamine Phosphate, Malate, Ascorbate) 1200 mg • Magnesium (as Magnesium Oxide, Citrate, Fumarate, Malate, Ascorbate) 600 mg • Zinc (as Zinc Chelate) 7.5 mg • Copper (as Copper Sebacate) 1 mg • Manganese (as Manganese Ascorbate) 6 mg • Ipriflavone (Ostivone) 600 mg • Genistein Rich Soy concentrate (Yielding 50 mg total isoflavones) 125 mg • Silica (from Horsetail silica extract) 10 mg • Boron (as Boron Chelate) 3 mg.

Ultra Bone-Up - Jarrow Formulas
Six tablets contain: Vitamin C (ascorbic acid) 200 mg • Vitamin D (D3, cholecalciferol) 600 IU • Vitamin K (K1, phylloquinone) 100 mcg • Folic Acid 200 mcg • Microcrystalline Hydroxyapatite (MCHA) 4762 mg: Calcium (elemental from MCHA) 1000 mg,

Phosphorus (from MCHA) 510 mg, Protein (from MCHA) 1514 mg • Magnesium (as oxide) 600 mg • Zinc (as monomethionate) 10 mg • Copper (from gluconate) 1 mg • Manganese (as citrate) 1 mg • Ipriflavone 600 mg • Glucosamine HCl 300 gm • MSM (methylsulfonylmethate) 100 mg • Boron (as sodium borate) 3 mg. Other Ingredients: Dicalcium Phosphate, Cellulose, Stearic Acid, Modified Cellulose Gum, Magnesium Stearate, Modified Cellulose, Silicon Dioxide.

Ultra Brain Power **-** American Biologics
Three capsules contain: Vitamin B6 (as pyridoxine hydrochloride) 20 mg • Folic Acid (as folate) 400 mcg • Vitamin B12 (cyanocobalamin) 250 mcg • PhosphatidylSerine (PS, as LECI-PS brand) 100 mg • Ginkgo Biloba phytosome extract 30 mg • Choline (as phosphatidylcholine, PC) 100 mg • PhosphatidylCholine (PC) 127 mg • PhosphatidylEthanolamine (PE) 82 mg • PhosphatidylInositol (PI) 36 mg • Taurine 500 mg • L-Glutamine 125 mg • L-Glycine 125 mg. Other Ingredients: Magnesium Stearate, Silicon Dioxide, Microcrystalline Cellulose.

Ultra Calcium Complex **-** Pro Health
Two tablets contain: Vitamin D (from fish oil) 100 IU • Calcium (from calcium citrate) 600 mg • Magnesium (from magnesium oxide, magnesium aspartate) 300 mg • Zinc (from amino acid chelate) 15 mg • Manganese (from amino acid chelate) 5 mg • Copper (from amino acid chelate) 1 mg. Other Ingredients: Cellulose, Stearic Acid, Magnesium Stearate, Silica.

Ultra Carb **-** Sterling-Grant Laboratories
Two tablets contain: Chromium (as chromium dinicotinate glycinate) 100 mcg • Phaseolamin Northern White Kidney Bean extract 700 mg • Green Tea leaf extract (50% catechins, 35% polyphenols) 200 mg. Other Ingredients: Gelatin, Dicalcium Phosphate, Magnesium Stearate, Silica.

Ultra Carbo Blocker 2000 **-** Tiffin International, Inc.
Each capsule contains: Chromium 100 mcg • Proprietary Blend 200 mg: Phaseolus Vulgaris, Gymnema Sylvestre. Other Ingredients: Gelatin, Sodium Lauryl Sulfate, Colloidal Silicon Dioxide, Purified Water.
See Editor's Note No. 37.

Ultra Carbo Blocker 3000 **-** PotentHerbs
Each capsule contains: Chromium (as chromium polynicotinate) 100 mcg • Proprietary Blend 450 mg: Phaseolus Vulgaris (Phase 2), Gymnema Sylvestre. Other Ingredients: Kosher Capsules, Silicon Dioxide.
See Editor's Note No. 37.

Ultra Carotenoid Complex **-** The Vitamin Shoppe
Each softgel contains: Phytofluene 0.026 mg • Lycopene (LYC-O-MATO) 5 mg • Lutein 5 mg • Beta-carotene (25000 IU Vitamin A) 15 mg • Alpha-carotene (833 IU Vitamin A) 1 mg • Zeaxanthin 0.24 mg • Phytoene 0.055 mg.

Ultra Cee 500 mg **-** Puritan's Pride
Each capsule contains: Vitamin C 500 mg.

Ultra Chondroitin 600 **-** Nature's Plus
Each protein coated tablet contains: Chondroitin Sulfate A - CSA (glucuronic, N-acetyl-D-galactosamine 4-Sulfate) 600 mg • Bioperine brand Black Pepper extract (95% 1-piperoylpiperdine) 2.5 mg.
See Editor's Note No. 15.

Ultra Chromatone Plus **-** Abundance Marketing
Niacin • Chromium Polynicotinate • Guarana extract • Cayenne Pepper • Quebracho extract • Siberian Ginseng • Yerba Mate extract • Ligustrum berry • Cinnamon bark • Astragalus root • Bladderwrack • Reishi Mushroom • Sargassum Algae • Rehmannia root • Lemon Verbena • Chamomile flower • Ginger root • Licorice root.

Ultra Chromium GTF **-** Source Naturals
Each tablet contains: Chromium GTF (100 mcg of ChromeMate Chromium Polynicotinate and 100 mcg of Chromium Picolinate) 200 mcg • Niacin (Polynicotinate) 9 mg.

Ultra Chromium Picolinate **-** The Vitamin Shoppe
Each capsule contains: Chromium Picolinate, a compound of yeast-free trivalent chromium and picolinic acid 500 mcg.

Ultra Chromium Picolinate 500 **-** Source Naturals
Each tablet contains: Trivalent Chromium (from Chromax brand of yeast-free chromium picolinate) 500 mcg.

Ultra Citro Cee **-** Arrowroot
Each tablet contains: Vitamin C 1000 mg • Bioflavonoids 400 mg.

Ultra CLA **-** Metagenics
Two softgels contain: Conjugated Linoleic Acid (CLA) 1000 mg • Rosemary leaf extract (as RoseOx brand, rosmarinus officinalis, standardized to 6% [2.4 mg] carnosic acid) 40 mg.

Ultra Colloidal Silver **-** Olympia Nutrition
Deionized Water • Silver (10 ppm).

Ultra Connexin **-** American Biologics
Four capsules contain: Glucosamine Sulfate 250 mg • N-Acetyl Glucosamine 450 mg • Chondroitin Sulfate 50 mg • Hawthorn standardized extract 400 mg • Proanthocyanidin Flavonoids (grape seed) 10 mg • L-Proline amino acid 100 mg • L-Lysine amino acid 100 mg • Vitamin B6 (pyridoxine, as hydrochloride) 12 mg • Vitamin C (ascorbic acid from beet) 350 mg • Vitamin E (as D-alpha tocopherol) 125 IU • Magnesium (as citrate) 100 mg • Calcium (as citrate) 25 mg • Zinc (as citrate) 12 mg • Copper (as gluconate) 1 mg • Silicon (as horsetail extract 4X) 20 mg • Manganese (as citrate) 5 mg • Boron (as citrate) 3 mg • Selenium (as sodium selenite, selenomethionine) 150 mcg • Molybdenum (as sodium molybdate) 500 mcg • Bromelain 600 GDU 25 mg. Other Ingredients: Magnesium Stearate, Silica, Cellulose.
See Editor's Note No. 15.

Ultra CoQ10 **-** Nature's Plus
Each softgel contains: Coenzyme Q10 (ubiquinone) 100 mg.

Ultra Cranberry 1000 **-** Nature's Plus
Each protein coated tablet contains: Cranberry concentrate 45X 1000 mg • Vitamin C corn free 100 mg. In a highly active herbal base of Juniper berries (Juniperus communis), Parsley (Petroselinum crispum), Uva Ursi (Arctostaphylos uva ursi) & Red Clover (Trifolium pratense).

Ultra DHA 50 **-** Health From The Sun
Two capsules contain: Vitamin E 4 IU • Omega-3 Fatty Acids 700 mg [DHA (425 mg) EPA (200 mg)]. Ingredients: All natural Fish Body oil concentrate, Gelatin, Glycerine, Mixed Tocopherols.

Ultra Diet Pep **-** Natural Balance
Each tablet contains: Potassium (as chloride) 50 mg • Vitamin B6 (as pyridoxine HCl) 10 mg • Vitamin B12 (as cyanocobalamin) 6 mcg • Pantothenic Acid (as d-calcium pantothenate) 25 mg • Iodine (from kelp) 80 mcg • DynaChrome Chromium (as arginate/chelidamate) 120 mcg • Proprietary Blend 750 mg: Green Tea leaf extract (contains caffeine), L-Tyrosine, Kelp leaf, Dandelion leaf, Ginger root, Passion flower aerial portion extract. Other Ingredients: Microcrystalline Cellulose, Modified Cellulose Gum, Silicon Dioxide, Stearic Acid, Magnesium Stearate.

Ultra Diet Pep 2000 **-** Natural Balance
Two capsules contain: Vitamin C (ascorbic acid) 30 mg • Vitamin B6 (pyridoxine HCl) 7.5 mg • Pantothenic Acid (d-calcium pantothenate) 25 mg • DynaChrome Chromium (arginate/chelidamate) 100 mcg • Citrin (garcinia cambogia fruit extract standardized to 50% HCA) 750 mg • Proprietary Blend 495 mg: Kola Nut seed extract (contains caffeine), Siberian Ginseng root, Guarana seed extract (contains caffeine), Wild Yam rhizome, Dandelion leaf, standardized Kelp (thallus), Passion flower aerial portion extract, Licorice root, Gotu Kola aerial portion extract • Choline Bitartrate 25 mg • Inositol 25 mg. Other Ingredients: Gelatin, Magnesium Stearate, Silicon Dioxide.

Ultra Diet-Phen - Source Naturals
Each two tablets contain: St. John's Wort (Hypericum perforatum) standardized extract 0.3 %, yielding 1.2 of Hypericin 400 mg • Bitter Orange peel standardized extract, yielding 24 mg of Synepherine 570 mg • Green Tea standardized extract, yieldng 40 mg of Polypheols and 10 mg of Caffeine 100 mg • L-Phenylalanine 500 mg • Cayenne fruit 150 mg • Piper nigrum seed 150 mg • Mustard Seed 150 mg • Ginger root 150 mg • Dandelion Leaf 100 mg • Dandelion Root 100 mg • Chromium (300 mcg ChromeMate Polynicotinate and 100 mcg Chromium Picolinate) 400 mcg.
See Editor's Note No. 40.

Ultra Diet-Phen Calm Mood Night Formula - Source Naturals
Each tablet contains: Vitamin C (zinc ascorbate) 54 mg • Vitamin B6 (pyridoxine HCl) 10 mg • Folate (folic acid) 100 mcg • Magnesium (taurinate) 5 mg • Zinc (ascorbate) 10 mg • St. John's Wort leaf/ flower extract (standardized to 0.3%, 1.5 mg hypericin) 500 mg • L-Glutamine 150 mg • GABA (gamma amino butyric acid) 50 mg • Valerian root extract (0.8%) 50 mg • Lemon Balm leaf 50 mg • L-Carnitine (l-carnitine l-tartrate) 25 mg • Taurine (magnesium taurinate) 22 mg. Other Ingredients: Dibasic Calcium Phosphate, Stearic Acid, Colloidal Silicon Dioxide, Modified Cellulose Gum, Magnesium Stearate.

Ultra Dophilus DF - Metagenics
Each 1/2 tsp serving contains: Lactobacillus Acidophilus NCFM strain 15 billion live organisms.

Ultra EPA - Pro Health
Two softgels contain: Vitamin E (as mixed alpha-tocopherol) 2 IU • Omega-3 Fatty Acids 1.2 g: Eicosapentaenoic Acid (EPA) 720 mg • Docosahexaenoic Acid (DHA) 480 mg. Other Ingredients: Fish Oil Concentrate, Gelatin, Glycerin, Water.

Ultra Flora IB - Metagenics
Each capsule contains: Lactobacillus Acidophilus NCFM strain 30 billion live organisms • Bifidobacterium Lactis BI-07 strain 30 billion live organisms.

Ultra Flora Plus - Metagenics
Each 1/4 tsp serving contains: Lactobacillus Acidophilus NCFM strain 7.5 billion live organisms • Bifidobacterium Lactis (formerly known as B. infantis) 7.5 billion live organisms) • Globulin Protein concentrate 560 mg.

Ultra Flora Plus Capsules - Metagenics
Each capsule contains: Lactobacillus Acidophilus NCFM strain 7.5 billion live organisms • Bifidobacterium Lactis (B. infantis) 7.5 billion live organisms • Globulin Protein concentrate 170 mg.

Ultra Flora Plus DF (dairy-free) - Metagenics
Each 1/4 tsp serving contains: Lactobacillus Acidophilus NCFM strain 7.5 billion live organisms • Bifidobacterium Lactis (formerly B. infantis) 7.5 billion live organisms). Other Ingredients: Fructooligosaccharides.

Ultra Flora Plus DF (dairy-free) Capsules - Metagenics
Each capsule contains: Lactobacillus Acidophilus NCFM strain 7.5 billion live organisms • Bifidobacterium Lactis (formerly known as B. infantis) 7.5 billion live organisms.

Ultra Fuel - TwinLab
Each 16 ounce serving contains: Carbohydrates 100 g • Carbohydrate & Energy Metabolizers • Chromium • B Vitamins • Vitamin C.

Ultra Garlite - Nature's Plus
Each tablet contains: Garlic clove (allium sativum) 1000 mg. Other Ingredients: Di-Calcium Phosphate, Microcrystalline Cellulose, Stearic Acid, Hydroxypropyl Methylcellulose, Magnesium Stearate, Silica, Pharmaceutical Glaze.

Ultra Ginkgo 100 - Nature's Plus
Each capsule contains: Ginkgo Biloba leaf 50:1 extract (standardized 24% ginkgo flavone-glycosides and 6% terpene lactones) 100 mg. Other Ingredients: Silica, Gelatin, Purified Water.

Ultra Ginseng 500 - Nature's Plus
Each capsule contains: Standardized Korean Ginseng root (panax ginseng C.A. Meyer, minimum 5% ginsenosides) 500 mg. Other Ingredients: Silica, Gelatin, Purified Water.

Ultra H-3 - Uni Key Health Systems, Inc.
Each tablet contains: Procaine HCl 100 mg • Ascorbic Acid 25 mg • Citric Acid 25 mg • Niacin 16 mg • Folic Acid 0.4 mg • Biotin 0.3 mg • Potassium 11 mg • Magnesium 4 mg • Proprietary Blend 25 mg: Ginkgo Biloba 25:1 standardized extract, Bilberry 25:1 standardized extract.

Ultra Hair - Nature's Plus
Two tablets contain: Vitamin C with Rose Hips 500 mg • Pantothenic Acid 500 mg • Inositol 500 mg • Choline (bitartrate) 210 mg • L-Cysteine free form amino acid 100 mg • Vitamin B6 (pyridoxine HCl) 100 mg • Vitamin B2 (riboflavin) 100 mg • PABA (para-aminobenzoic acid) 100 mg • Vitamin B1 (thiamine) 30 mg • Niacinamide 30 mg • Zinc (amino acid chelate) 5 mg • Vitamin A (beta carotene) 10000 IU • Biotin 2000 mcg • Folic Acid 400 mcg. Base: Safflower Oil, Rice Bran, Spirulina.

Ultra Harmony - Wise Women Essentials
Purified Water • Wild Yam extract • Chaste Tree berry (vitex) • Apricot kernal oil • Jojoba oil • Aloe Vera • Retinyl Palmitate (vitamin A) • Tocopheryl Acetate (vitamin E) • Calciforal (vitamin D).

Ultra Hepa Trope - American Biologics
Four capsules contain: Vitamin A (as retinyl palmitate) 5000 IU • Thiamine (vitamin B1) 25 mg • Riboflavin (vitamin B2) 25 mg • Niacin (vitamin B3) 15 mg • Niacinamide (vitamin B3) 10 mg • Pantothenic Acid (vitamin B5) 40 mg • Vitamin B6 (as pyridoxine hydrochloride) 15 mg • Vitamin B6 (as pyridoxal-5'-phosphate) 5 mg • Folic Acid (as folate) 300 mcg • Vitamin B12 (as cyanocobalamin) 500 mcg • Ascorbic Acid (vitamin C) 200 mg • Vitamin E (as dL-alpha tocopheryl acetate) 200 IU • Magnesium (as citrate) 25 mg • Selenium (as selenomethionine) 100 mcg • Zinc (as citrate) 10 mg • Copper (as glycinate) 0.5 mg • Molybdenum (as sodium molybdate) 100 mcg • Siliphos brand bioavailable Milk Thistle extract 240 mg • PhosphatidylCholine (PC, phospholipid) 400 mg • PhosphatidylEthanolamine / Inositol complex 62 mg • Dandelion root 12:1 concentrate 80 mg • Trimethylglycine / Betaine 100 mg • Glutathione ("reduced glutathione") 50 mg • NAC (N-acetylcysteine) 100 mg • Alpha-Lipoic Acid 50 mg • MethylSulfonylMethane (MSM) 100 mg • Glycine 100 mg • Taurine 200 mg • Glutamine 100 mg. Other Ingredients: Magnesium Stearate, Silicon Dioxide, Microcrystalline Cellulose.

Ultra High Carb - The Sports Nutrition Source, Inc.
Four level scoops contain: Biotin 300 mcg • Chromium 200 mcg • Vitamin B-1 1.5 mg • Vitamin B-2 1.7 mg • Vitamin B-3 20 mg • Vitamin B-6 2 mg • Pantothenic Acid 100 mg • Vitamin C 60 mg • Potassium (from soluble potassium phosphate) 99 mg • Magnesium (from magnesium succinate) 25 mg.

Ultra I Iron-Free sustained release tablets - Nature's Plus
Each tablet contains: Vitamin A (as beta carotene) 25000 IU • Vitamin C (as ascorbic acid) 100 mg • Vitamin D (as ergocalciferol) 1000 IU • Vitamin E (as D-alpha tocopheryl succinate) 100 IU • Thiamin (vitamin B1 as thiamine HCl) 100 mg • Riboflavin (vitamin B2) 100 mg • Niacin (as niacinamide) 100 mg • Vitamin B6 (as pyridoxine HCl) 100 mg • Folate (as folic acid) 400 mcg • Vitamin B12 (as cyanocobalamin) 100 mcg • Biotin 100 mcg • Pantothenic Acid (as calcium pantothenate) 100 mg • Calcium (as amino acid chelate complex) 40 mg • Iodine (from kelp) 150 mcg • Magnesium (as amino acid chelate/complex) 20 mg • Zinc (as amino acid chelate/ complex) 20 mg • Selenium (as amino acid complex) 10 mcg • Manganese (as amino acid chelate/complex) 6.1 mg • Chromium (as amino acid chelate) 15 mcg • Potassium (as amino acid complex) 15 mg • PABA (para-aminobenzoic acid) 100 mg • Inositol 100 mg • Choline (as bitartrate) 42 mg • Rutin (from saphora japonica leaf) 25 mg • Bioflavonoids (from citrus limon exocarp) 25 mg • Betaine HCl (from beet molasses) 25 mg • Hesperidin (from citrus limon exocarp) 5 mg. Other Ingredients: Hydroxypropyl Methylcellulose, Stearic

Acid, Di-Calcium Phosphate, Calcium Carbonate, Isolated Soy Protein, Rice Bran, Silica, Papaya, Watercress, Parsley, Alfalfa, Green Cabbage, Acerola Cherry, Wheat Germ Flour, Bromelain (from pineapple fruit), Rose Hips, Pharmaceutical Glaze.

Ultra I Sustained Release Tablets - Nature's Plus
Each sustained-release tablet contains: Vitamin A (as beta carotene) 25,000 IU • Vitamin C (as ascorbic acid) 100 mg • Vitamin D (as ergocalciferol) 1000 IU • Vitamin E (as D-alpha tocopheryl succinate) 100 IU • Thiamin (vitamin B1, as thiamine hydrochloride) 100 mg • Riboflavin (vitamin B2) 100 mg • Niacin (as niacinamide) 100 mg • Vitamin B6 (as pyridoxine HCl) 100 mg • Folate (as folic acid) 400 mcg • Vitamin B12 (as cyanocobalamin) 100 mcg • Biotin 100 mcg • Pantothenic Acid (as calcium pantothenate) 100 mg • Calcium (as amino acid chelate complex) 40 mg • Iron (as amino acid chelate/complex) 25 mg • Iodine (from kelp) 150 mcg • Magnesium (as amino acid chelate/complex) 20 mg • Zinc (as amino acid chelate/complex) 20 mg • Selenium (as amino acid complex) 10 mcg • Manganese (as amino acid chelate/complex) 6.1 mg • Chromium (as amino acid chelate) 15 mcg • Potassium (as amino acid complex) 15 mg • PABA (para-aminobenzoic acid) 100 mg • Inositol 100 mg • Choline (as bitartrate) 42 mg • Rutin (from saphora japonica leaf) 25 mg • Citrus Bioflavonoids (from citrus limon exocarp) 25 mg • Hesperidin (from citrus limon exocarp) 5 mg • Betaine HCl (from beet molasses) 25 mg. Other Ingredients: Hydroxypropyl Methylcellulose, Stearic Acid, Di-Calcium Phosphate, Calcium Carbonate, Isolated Soy Protein, Rice Bran, Silica, Papaya, Watercress, Parsley, Alfalfa, Green Cabbage, Acerola Cherry, Wheat Germ Flour, Bromelain (from pineapple fruit), Rose Hips.

Ultra II Light sustained release tablets - Nature's Plus
Each tablet contains: Vitamin A (as beta carotene) 10,000 IU • Vitamin C (as ascorbic acid) 100 mg • Vitamin D (as ergocalciferol) 400 IU • Vitamin E (as D-alpha tocopheryl succinate) 100 IU • Thiamin (vitamin B1, as thiamine HCl) 100 mg • Riboflavin (vitamin B2) 100 mg • Niacin (as niacinamide) 100 mg • Vitamin B6 (as pyridoxine HCl) 100 mg • Folate (as folic acid) 400 mcg • Vitamin B12 (as cyanocobalamin) 100 mcg • Biotin 100 mcg • Pantothenic Acid (as calcium pantothenate) 100 mg • Calcium (as amino acid chelate complex) 40 mg • Iron (as amino acid chelate/complex) 25 mg • Iodine (from kelp) 150 mcg • Magnesium (as amino acid chelate/complex) 20 mg • Zinc (as amino acid chelate/complex) 20 mg • Selenium (as amino acid complex) 10 mcg • Manganese (as amino acid chelate/complex) 6.1 mg • Chromium (as amino acid chelate) 15 mcg • Potassium (as amino acid complex) 15 mg • PABA (para-aminobenzoic acid) 100 mg • Inositol 100 mg • Choline (as bitartrate) 42 mg • Rutin (from saphora japonica leaf) 25 mg • Bioflavonoids (from citrus limon exocarp) 25 mg • Betaine HCl (from beet molasses) 25 mg • Hesperidin (from citrus limon exocarp) 5 mg. Other Ingredients: Di-Calcium Phosphate, Hydroxypropyl Methylcellulose, Stearic Acid, Isolated Soy Protein, Rice Bran, Rose Hips, Magnesium Stearate, Pacific Kelp, Chlorella, Date, Barley Grass, Spirulina, Black Currant Seed, Bee Pollen, Garlic, Oat Bran, Apple Pectin, Broccoli, Spinach, Carrot, Chinese Cabbage (brassica campestris), Brown Rice, Sunflower Oil, Fig, Beet Greens, Lecithin, Silica, Alfalfa, Green Cabbage, Acerola Cherry, Parsley, Wheat Germ Flour, Bromelain (from pineapple fruit), Papaya, Watercress.

Ultra II sustained release tablets - Nature's Plus
Each tablet contains: Vitamin A (as beta carotene) 25,000 IU • Vitamin C (as ascorbic acid) 100 mg • Vitamin D (as ergocalciferol) 1000 IU • Vitamin E (as D-alpha tocopheryl succinate) 100 IU • Thiamin (vitamin B1, as thiamine HCl) 100 mg • Riboflavin (vitamin B2) 100 mg • Niacin (as niacinamide) 100 mg • Vitamin B6 (as pyridoxine HCl) 100 mg • Folate (as folic acid) 400 mcg • Vitamin B12 (as cyanocobalamin) 100 mcg • Biotin 100 mcg • Pantothenic Acid (as calcium pantothenate) 100 mg • Calcium (as amino acid chelate complex) 40 mg • Iron (as amino acid chelate/complex) 25 mg • Iodine (from kelp) 150 mcg • Magnesium (as amino acid chelate/complex) 20 mg • Zinc (as amino acid chelate/complex) 20 mg • Selenium (as amino acid complex) 10 mcg • Manganese (as amino acid chelate/complex) 6.1 mg • Chromium (as amino acid chelate) 15 mcg • Potassium (as amino acid complex) 15 mg • PABA (para-aminobenzoic acid) 100 mg • Inositol 100 mg • Choline (as bitartrate) 42 mg • Rutin (from saphora japonica leaf) 25 mg • Bioflavonoids (from citrus limon exocarp) 25 mg • Betaine HCl (from beet molasses) 25 mg • Hesperidin (from citrus limon exocarp) 5 mg. Other Ingredients: Stearic Acid, Microcrystalline Cellulose, Hydroxypropyl Methylcellulose, Silica, Ioslated Soy Protein, Rice Bran, Rose Hips, Magnesium Stearate, Parsley, Alfalfa, Green Cabbage, Acerola Cherry, Pacific Kelp, Chlorella, Date (phoenix dactylifera fruit), Barley Brass, Spirulina, Black Currant Seed, Bee Pollen, Garlic, Oat Bran, Apple Pectin, Broccoli, Spinach, Carrot, Chinese Cabbage (brassica campestris leaf), Brown Rice, Sunflower Oil, Fig, Beet Greens, Lecithin, Wheat Germ Flour, Bromelain (from pineapple fruit), Papaya, Watercress, Pharmaceutical Glaze.

Ultra II tablets - Nature's Plus
Each tablet contains: Vitamin A (as beta carotene) 25,000 IU • Vitamin C (as ascorbic acid) 100 mg • Vitamin D (as ergocalciferol) 1000 IU • Vitamin E (as D-alpha tocopheryl succinate) 100 IU • Thiamin (vitamin B1, as thiamine HCl) 100 mg • Riboflavin (vitamin B2) 100 mg • Niacin (as niacinamide) 100 mg • Vitamin B6 (as pyridoxine HCl) 100 mg • Folate (as folic acid) 400 mcg • Vitamin B12 (as cyanocobalamin) 100 mcg • Biotin 100 mcg • Pantothenic Acid (as calcium pantothenate) 100 mg • Calcium (as amino acid chelate complex) 40 mg • Iron (as amino acid chelate/complex) 25 mg • Iodine (from kelp) 150 mcg • Magnesium (as amino acid chelate/complex) 20 mg • Zinc (as amino acid chelate/complex) 20 mg • Selenium (as amino acid complex) 10 mcg • Manganese (as amino acid chelate/complex) 6.1 mg • Chromium (as amino acid chelate) 15 mcg • Potassium (as amino acid complex) 15 mg • PABA (para-aminobenzoic acid) 100 mg • Inositol 100 mg • Choline (as bitartrate) 42 mg • Rutin (from saphora japonica leaf) 25 mg • Bioflavonoids (from citrus limon exocarp) 25 mg • Betaine HCl (from beet molasses) 25 mg • Hesperidin (from citrus limon exocarp) 5 mg. Other Ingredients: Microcrystalline Cellulose, Isolated Soy Protein, Stearic Acid, Magnesium Stearate, Rice Bran, Pacific Kelp, Chlorella, Date, Barley Grass, Spirulina, Black Currant Seed, Bee Pollen, Garlic, Oat Bran, Apple Pectin, Broccoli, Spinach, Carrot, Chinese Cabbage (brassica campestris), Brown Rice, Sunflower Oil, Fig, Beet Greens, Lecithin, Rose Hips, Silica, Papaya, Watercress, Parsley, Alfalfa, Green Cabbage, Acerola Cherry, Wheat Germ Flour Parsley Bromelain (from pineapple fruit), Pharmaceutical Glaze.

Ultra ImmunoGlycans - American Biologics
Six capsules contain: Ascorbic Acid (vitamin C) 150 mg • Coriolus Versicolor mycelial extract 1500 mg • Grifola Frondosa mycelial extract 750 mg • Cordyceps Sinensis mycelial extract 125 mg • Lentinula Edodes mycelial extract 125 mg • Ganoderma Lucidum mycelial extract 125 mg • Tremella Fuciformis mycelial extract 125 mg • Schizophyllum Commune mycelial extract 125 mg • Agaricus Blazei mycelial extract 125 mg • Arabinogalactan (D-galacto-L-arabinan) 1500 mg. Other Ingredients: Magnesium Stearate, Silicon Dioxide, Microcrystalline Cellulose.

Ultra InflamX - HealthDesigns International
Two scoops (52 g) contain: Vitamin A (as retinyl palmitate) 2500 IU • Vitamin A (as mixed carotenoids) 2500 IU • Vitamin D 100 IU • Vitamin C (as sodium ascorbate) 180 mg • Vitamin E (as D-alpha tocopheryl acetate) 100 IU • Thiamin (as thiamin hydrochloride) 2 mg • Riboflavin 2 mg • Niacin (as niacinamide and niacin) 35 mg • Pantothenic Acid (as D-calcium pantothenate) 5 mg • Vitamin B6 (as pyridoxal-5-phosphate) 5 mg • Vitamin B12 (as cyanocobalamin) 3 mcg • Biotin 150 mcg • Folate (as folic acid) 80 mcg • Sodium 100 mg • Potassium (as potassium phosphate) 400 mg • Calcium (as calcium citrate) 275 mg • Iron 1 mg • Phosphorus 200 mg • Magnesium (as magnesium citrate) 280 mg • Zinc (as zinc methionate) 10 mg • Copper (as copper gluconate) 1 mg • Manganese (as manganese gluconate) 2 mg • Molybdenum (as molybdenum amino acid chelate) 38 mcg • Chromium (as chromium polynicotinate) 60 mcg • Selenium (as selenomethionine) 75 mcg • N-Acetylcysteine 100 mg • L-Glutamine 750 mg • L-Threonine 34 mg • L-Lysine 770 mg • Citrulline 100 mg • Hesperidin 200 mg • D-Limonene 100 mg • Rutin 200 mg • Quercetin 200 mg • Sodium Sulfate 75 mg • Ginger root extract (zingiber officinale, standardized

to 5 mg total pungent compounds) 100 mg • Turmeric rhizome extract (curcuma longa, standardized to 200 mg total pungent compounds) 210 mg • Rosemary leaf extract (rosmarinus officinalis) 100 mg. Other Ingredients: Rice Protein Concentrate, Rice Syrup Solids, Rice Bran, Olive Oil, Medium-Chain Triglycerides, Natural Flavors, Xanthan Gum, Carrageenan Gum, Cellulose Gum.

Ultra Infla-Zyme Forte powder - American Biologics
Each 1 tsp serving contains: Pancreatin 4X N.F. 1600 mg • Bromelain 250 mg • Papain 240 mg • Trypsin 240 mg • Chymotrypsin 5 mg • Lipase 70 mg • Amylase 70 mg • Rutin (eucalyptus) 170 mg • Zinc (gluconate) 5 mg • Superoxide Dismutase 200 units • Catalase 100 units • L-Cysteine (HCl) 20 mg.

Ultra Infla-Zyme Forte tablets - American Biologics
Each tablet contains: Pancreatin 4X (NF, 20,000 USP units of amylase activity; 1600 USP units of lipase activity; 20,000 USP units of protease activity) 800 mg • Bromelain 125 mg • Papain 120 mg • Trypsin (30,000 USP units of trypsin activity) 120 mg • Chymotrypsin (2500 USP units of chymotrypsin activity) 2.5 mg • Lipase (35 N.F. units of lipase activity) 25 mg • Rutin (from eucalyptus) 85 mg • Zinc (as the gluconate) 2.6 mg • Superoxide Dismutase (SOD) 100 units • Catalase 50 IU • L-Cysteine (as the hydrochloride) 10 mg. Other Ingredients: Sodium Formate, Calcium Gluconate, Magnesium Stearate.

Ultra Inosine - Source Naturals
Two tablets contain: Vitamin C (Potassium and Sodium Ascorbates) 350 mg • Calcium (carbonate) 100 mg • Vitamin B6 (pyridoxine HCl) 10 mg • Magnesium (oxide, aspartate) 100 mg • Vitamin B5 (pantothenic acid) 50 mg • Potassium (citrate, ascorbate and aspartate) 99 mg • Sodium (ascorbate) 20 mg • Inosine 1000 mg • Aspartic Acid (Potassium and Magnesium Aspartates and L-Aspartic Acid) 200 mg • Branched Chain Amino Acids (BCAAs) (L-Leucine 100 mg, L-Isoleucine 30 mg, L-Valine 44 mg) 174 mg • L-Carnitine L-Tartrate 20 mg • L-Lysine (HCl) 60 mg • Glycine 60 mg • Bee Pollen 200 mg • Octacosanol 4000 mcg • Spirulina 70 mg • Siberian Ginseng 100 mg • Tienchi Ginseng 100 mg.

Ultra Isoflavone 100 - Nature's Plus
Two tablets contain: Isoplex brand Proprietary Blend 1500 mg: Soybean concentrate, Soy germ extract, Radix Puerariae root • Isoflavones 100 mg • Puerarin 79.28 mg • Daidzin 15.97 mg • Daidzein 7.35 mg • Glycitin 6.1 mg • Genistin 1.8 mg • Glycitein 270 mcg • Genistein 100 mcg. Other Ingredients: Di-calcium Phosphate, Microcrystalline Cellulose, Stearic Acid, Silica, Magnesium Stearate.

Ultra Joint Response - Source Naturals
Three tablets contain: Vitamin A 5000 IU • Vitamin C 250 mg • Niacinamide 50 mg • Vitamin B6 12.5 mg • Zinc 15 mg • Selenium 100 mcg • Copper 1 mg • Manganese 10 mg • Molybdenum 130 mcg • MSM 1125 mg • Glucosamine Sulfate 900 mg • Boswellia serrata extract 321 mg • Quercetin 150 mg • Horse Chestnut extract 100 mg • Turmeric root extract 50 mg • Stinging Nettle leaf extract 50 mg • Ashwagandha root extract 50 mg • N-Acetyl Cysteine 50 mg • Sea Cucumber 40 mg • Grape Seed extract 25 mg • Aloe Vera whole leaf concentrate 25 mg • Black Pepper fruit extract 1 mg.

Ultra KLB6 - Puritan's Pride
Three tablets contain: Lecithin 1200 mg • Vitamin B6 (Pyridoxine HCl) 50 mg • Kelp powder 100 mg • Cider Vinegar 240 mg.

Ultra Lean - Schiff
Two tablets contains: Garcinia cambogia extract (min. 50% HCA) 500 mg • Dandelion root 4:1 extract (taraxacum officinate) 100 mg • Horsetail standardized extract (10% silicic acid, 6.3% organic silica - from Springtime Equisetum arvense) 50 mg • Juniper Berries 4:1 extract (juniper communis) 50 mg • Cayenne (oleoresin capsium 6:1 extract) 25 mg • Betaine HCl 50 mg • Iodine (Norwegian kelp) 150 mcg • Potassium (glycerophosphate) 25 mg • Magnesium (glycinate) 40 mg • Chromium (picolinate) 200 mcg.

Ultra L-Glutathione (Reduced) 200 mg - American Biologics
Each capsule contains: L-Glutathione 200 mg.

Ultra Lipo-Plex - Nature's Plus
Two tablets contain: Choline Bitartrate equivalent to 1000 mg of choline 2381 mg • Inositol 1000 mg • L-Methionine free form amino acid 500 mg • Vitamin B6 (Pyridoxine HCL) 100 mg. In a natural herbal base containing Dandelion root, Fennel seed, Barberry bark, Parsley, Capsicum & Ginger.

Ultra Lycopene, Advanced Heart Health Capsules - Natrol, Inc.
Each capsule contains: Vitamin E (as d-alpha-tocopheryl acid succinate) 400 IU • Lycopene (from natural tomato powder) 4 mg. Other Ingredients: Rice Powder, Gelatin.

Ultra Max 46 - Puritan's Pride
Each tablet contains: Vitamin A (13% as beta-carotene) 7,500 IU • Vitamin D 400 IU • Vitamin K 10 mcg • Thiamine (Vitamin B-1) 50 mg • Riboflavin (Vitamin B-2) 50 mg • Niacin 50 mg • Vitamin B-6 50 mg • Folic Acid 400 mcg • Vitamin B-12 50 mcg • Biotin 300 mcg • Pantothenic Acid 50 mg • Calcium 106 mg • Iron 9 mg • Iodine 150 mcg • Magnesium 100 mg • Zinc 50 mg • Selenium 50 mcg • Copper 1 mg • Manganese 5 mg • Chromium 50 mcg • Sodium 5 mg • Potassium 50 mg • Choline Bitartrate 50 mg • PABA (para-aminobenzoic acid) 25 mg • Inositol 10 mg.

Ultra Mega - GNC
Two tablets contain: Vitamin A (50% as beta-carotene;50% as retinyl acetate) 10,000 IU • Vitamin C (as ascorbic acid) 200 mg • Vitamin D (as cholecalciferol) 400 IU • Vitamin E (as d-alpha tocopheryl acetate) 100 IU • Vitamin K (as phytonadione) 75 mcg • Thiamin B1 (as thiamin mononitrate) 80 mg • Riboflavin B2 80 mg • Niacin B3 (as niacin and niacinamide) 80 mg • Vitamin B6 (as pyridoxine hydrochloride) 80 mg • Folate (folic acid, folacin) 400 mcg • Vitamin B12 (as cyanocobalamin) 80 mcg • Biotin 80 mcg • Pantothenic Acid (as calcium d-pantothenate) 80 mg • Calcium (as calcium carbonate) 500 mg • Iron (as hydrolyzed protein chelate) 27 mg • Iodine (as kelp) 150 mcg • Magnesium (as magnesium oxide) 200 mg • Zinc (as zinc oxide) 15 mg • Selenium (as hydrolyzed protein chelate) 100 mcg • Copper (as hydrolyzed protein chelate) 2 mg • Manganese (as hydrolyzed protein chelate) 5 mg • Chromium (as hydrolyzed protein chelate) 100 mcg • Molybdenum (as hydrolyzed protein chelate) 50 mcg • Boron (as hydrolyzed protein chelate) 2 mcg • Dong Quai Root Powder (angelica sinensis) 50 mg • Bee Pollen Powder 25 mg • Citrus Bioflavonoids Complex 25 mg • Choline (as choline bitartrate) 10 mg • Cranberry Concentrate (vaccinium macrocarpon) 10 mg • Para-Aminobenzoic Acid 10 mg • Royal Jelly 5 mg • Silica (as hydrolyzed protein chelate) 2 mg • Boron (as hydrolyzed protein chelate) 2 mg • Red Raspberry Leaves (rubus idaeus) 2 mg • Lutein 500 mcg • Inositol 10 mcg. Other Ingredients: Cellulose, Rice Protein Chelate, Titanium Dioxide (natural mineral whitener), Vegetable Acetoglycerides, Rose Hips Powder (rosina canina), Acerola, Chlorophyll.

Ultra Mega Gold Without Iron Timed Release - GNC
Two tablets contain: Vitamin A (75% as Betatene Beta-Carotene; 25% as Acetate) 20,000 IU • Vitamin C (as Ascorbic Acid) 500 mg • Vitamin D (as Cholecalciferol) 400 IU • Vitamin E (as d-alpha Tocopheryl Succinate) 300 IU • Thiamin (as Thiamin Mononitrate) 100 mg • Riboflavin 100 mg • Niacin (as Niacinamide) 100 mg • Vitamin B6 (as Pyridoxine Hydrochloride) 100 mg • Folate, Folic Acid, Folacin 400 mcg • Vitamin B12 (as Cyanocobalamin) 150 mcg • Biotin 100 mcg • Pantothenic Acid (as Calcium d-Pantothenate) 100 mg • Calcium (as Calcium Carbonate) 50 mg • Iodine (as Kelp) 100 mcg • Magnesium (as Magnesium Oxide) 50 mg • Zinc (as Zinc Oxide) 15 mg • Selenium (as Selenium Yeast) 150 mcg • Copper (as Cupric Oxide) 2 mg • Maganese (as Manganese Gluconate) 10 mg • Chromium (as GTF Chromium Yeast) 100 mcg • Molybdenum (as Molybdenum Yeast) 150 mcg • Potassium (as Potassium Chloride) 10 mg • Boron (as Boron Gluconate) 1 mg • Chlorine Bitartrate 50 mg • Inositol 25 mg • Para-Aminobenzoid Acid (PABA) 50 mg • Trimethylglycine (TMG) 25 mg • Citrus Bioflavanoid Complex 25 mg • Rutin Powder 10 mg • Hesperidin Complex 5 mg • Quercetin Dihydrate 10 mg • Natural Carotenoid Complex 15 mg • N-Acetyl-L-Cysteine (NAC) 10.5 mg • Amylase 10 mg • Lipase 5 mg • Protease

__2 mg • Cellulase 5 mg • Lycopene 200 mcg • Alpha-lipoic Acid 4.5 mg • Green Tea Leaves (Camellia sinensis) 15 mg. Other Ingredients: Cellulose, Vegetable Actoglycerides, Titanium Dioxide, Chlorophyll.

Ultra Mega Vite Multiple **-** Nature's Life
Each tablet contains: Vitamin A (Fish Liver oil) 10000 IU • Vitamin D (as Vitamin D3) (Cholecalciferol) 400 IU • Vitamin E (d-Alpha Tocopherol) 200 IU • Vitamin B1 (Thiamine Mononitrate) 100 mg • Vitamin B2 100 mg • Vitamin B3 (Niacinamide) 100 mg • Vitamin B6 (Pyridoxine HCl • Pyridoxal 5'-Phosphate) 100 mg • Vitamin B12 (Cobalamin concentrate) 100 mg • Folic Acid 400 mcg • Biotin 300 mcg • Pantothenic Acid (d-Calcium Pantothenate) 100 mg • Inositol 10 mg • Choline (Bitartrate) 10 mg • PABA (Para Aminobenzoic Acid) 10 mg • Vitamin C 300 mg • Lemon Bioflavonoids (TESTLAB 50% Flavonoids) 50 mg • Rutin 25 mg • Hesperidin Complex (10% Flavonoids) 25 mg • Boron (Citrate) 25 mcg • Calcium (Carbonate, Citrate/Malate) 100 mg • Chromium (Amino-Nicotinate) 100 mcg • Copper (Gluconate, Citrate) 1 mg • Iodine (Potassium) 25 mcg • Iron (Fumerate, Peptonate) 10 mg • Magnesium (Oxide, Citrate) 60 mg • Manganese (Citrate, Gluconate) 5 mg • Molybdenum (Molybdate) 25 mcg • Potassium (Citrate) 15 mg • Selenium (Yeast) 50 mcg • Silicon (Dioxide) 10 mg • Vanadium (Sulfate) 25 mcg • Zinc (Citrate) 20 mg • Chlorophyll 5 mg • Betaine HCl 30 mg • Glutamic Acid HCl 30 mg • Nature's Life Greens 20 mg.

Ultra Mega without Iron **-** GNC
Two tablets contain: Vitamin A (50% as beta-carotene; 50% as retinyl acetate) 10,000 IU • Vitamin C (as ascorbic acid) 200 mg • Vitamin D (as cholecalciferol) 400 IU • Vitamin E (as d-alpha tocopheryl acetate) 100 IU • Vitamin K (as phytonadione) 75 mcg • Thiamin B1 (as thiamin mononitrate) 80 mg • Riboflavin B2 (vitamin B2) 80 mg • Niacin B3 (as niacin and niacinamide) 80 mg • Vitamin B6 (as pyridoxine hydrochloride) 80 mg • Folate (folic acid, folacin) 400 mcg • Vitamin B12 (as cyanocobalamin) 80 mcg • Biotin 80 mcg • Pantothenic Acid (as calcium d-pantothenate) 80 mg • Calcium (as calcium carbonate) 500 mg • Iodine (as kelp) 150 mcg • Magnesium (oxide) 200 mg • Zinc (oxide) 15 mg • Selenium (as hydrolyzed protein chelate) 100 mcg • Copper (as hydrolyzed protein chelate) 2 mg • Manganese (as hydrolyzed protein chelate) 5 mg • Chromium (as hydrolyzed protein chelate) 100 mcg • Molybdenum (as hydrolyzed protein chelate) 50 mcg • Boron (as hydrolyzed protein chelate) 2 mcg • Dong Quai Root Powder (angelica sinensis) 50 mg • Bee Pollen Powder 25 mg • Citrus Bioflavonoids Complex 25 mg • Choline (as choline bitartrate) 10 mg • Cranberry Concentrate (vaccinium macrocarpon) 10 mg • Para-Aminobenzoic Acid 10 mg • Royal Jelly 5 mg • Silica (as hydrolyzed protein chelate) 2 mg • Red Raspberry Leaves (rubus idaeus) 2 mg • Lutein 500 mcg • Inositol 10 mcg. Other Ingredients: Cellulose, Rice Protein Chelate, Titanium Dioxide (natural mineral whitener), Vegetable Acetoglycerides, Rose Hips Powder (rosina canino), Acerola, Chlorophyll.

Ultra Micro-Plex **-** American Biologics
Each gram (approx. 1/4 tsp) contains: Lactobacillus Acidophilus 2.5 billion • Bifidobacterium Bifidum 2.5 billion • Bifidobacterium Infantis 2.5 billion • Lactobacillus Rhamnosus 2.5 billion • Protease 4545 units • Amylase 1636 units • Lipase 1364 units • Lactase 909 units • Peptidase 3030 units • Colostrum (bovine) 60 mg • FOS 30 mg. Other Ingredients: Herbal Stabilizers.

Ultra Minerals for Life **-** American Biologics
Three capsules contain: Vitamin B12 (cyanocobalamin) 500 mcg • Calcium (as microcyrstalline hydroxyapatite, citrate, malate) 100 mg • Iodine (as potassium iodide) 100 mcg • Magnesium (as citrate-malate) 150 mg • Zinc (as citrate) 20 mg • Selenium (as selenomethionine) 150 mcg • Copper (as gluconate) 1.5 mg • Manganese (as citrate) 5 mg • Chromium (as picolinate) 200 mcg • Molybdenum (as sodium molybdate) 150 mcg • Potassium (as citrate) 99 mg • Sulfur (as taurine) 50 mg • Cobalt (as cyanocobalamin, vitamin B12) 22 mcg • Boron (as citrate) 3 mg • Silicon as Equisetum Arvense whole plant extract 3.5 mg • Taurine 200 mg • L-Glutamine 200 mg. Other Ingredients: Magnesium Stearate, Silicon Dioxide, Microcrystalline Cellulose.

Ultra MSM Forte **-** American Biologics
Three capsules contain: Molybdenum (sodium molybdate) 100 mcg • Ascorbic Acid (vitamin C) 300 mg • MethylSulfonylMethane (MSM) 1500 mg • Glucosamine 100 mg • N-A-G 75 mg • Chondroitin Sulfate 50 mg. Other Ingredients: Magnesium Stearate, Silicon Dioxide, Microcrystalline Cellulose.
See Editor's Note No. 15.

Ultra Multiple **-** Source Naturals
Six tablets contain: Vitamin A (palmitate 10,000 IU and beta carotene 3000 IU) 13000 IU • Vitamin B-1 (thiamin) 100 mg • Vitamin B-2 (riboflavin) 75 mg • Niacinamide 75 mg and Niacin 25 mg 100mg • Vitamin B-5 (calcium D-Pantothenate) 150 mg • Vitamin B-6 (pyridoxine HCl) 125 mg • Vitamin B-12 (cyanocobalamin) 300 mcg • Biotin 150 mcg • Folic acid 420 mcg • Vitamin C (calcium, magnesium and ascorbates) 500 mg • Vitamin D-3 (cholecalciferol) 402 IU • Vitamin E (natural D-alpha succinate) 200 IU • Magnesium (ascorbate, oxide, citrate) 125 mg • Potassium (citrate) 10 mg • Iron (fumarate) 12 mg • Calcium (ascorbate, carbonate, citrate) 125 mg • Zinc (citrate) 15 mg • Manganese (ascorbate) 6 mg • Chromium (ChromeMate polynicotinate) 50 mcg • Copper (sebacate) 250 mcg • Selenium (sodium selenite) 100 mcg • Iodine (from kelp) 225 mcg.

Ultra Multiplex Advance **-** American Biologics
Two capsules contain: Vitamin A (retinyl palmitate) 5000 IU • Mixed Carotenoids 1500 IU • Thiamine (vitamin B1) 25 mg • Riboflavin (vitamin B2) 25 mg • Niacinamide (vitamin B3) 50 mg • Pantothenate (vitamin B5) 50 mg • Vitamin B6 (pyridoxine HCl) 20 mg • Pyridoxal-5-Phosphate (B6) 5 mg • Vitamin B12 (cyanocobalamin) 500 mcg • Folic Acid 200 mcg • Biotin 50 mcg • Lipoic Acid 5 mg • Vitamin C (ascorbic acid) 125 mg • Vitamin D (D3, cholecalciferol) 100 IU • Vitamin E (D-alpha tocopherol acetate) 100 IU • Quercetin 10 mg • Bioflavnonoids from Grape seed 10 mg • Taurine 50 mg • Potassium (as citrate) 30 mg • Magnesium (as citrate) 50 mg • Calcium (as citrate, pantothenate) 12 mg • Zinc (as citrate) 10 mg • Copper (as gluconate) 0.75 mg • Silicon as Horsetail extract 4X 0.5 mg • Manganese (as citrate) 2.5 mg • Boron (as citrate) 1.5 mg • Selenium (as sodium selenite) 75 mcg • Chromium (as picolinate) 50 mcg • Molybdenum (as sodium molybdate) 75 mcg • Iodine (as potassium iodide) 50 mcg • Inositol (as myo-inositol, phosphatidylinositol) 12 mg • Phosphatidylcholine (PC, other phospholipids) 50 mg. Other Ingredients: Magnesium Stearate, Silica.

Ultra Nails **-** Nature's Plus
Two tablets contain: Calcium amino acid chelate/complex 500 mg • Gelatin 260 mg • Horsetail supplying natural silica 250 mg • Phosphorus amino acid complex 200 mg • L-Cysteine free form amino acid 100 mg • L-Methionine free form amino acid 100 mg • Vitamin B2 (Riboflavin) 50 mg • Sulphur from Sulphur containing amino acids 25 mg • Oat straw 25 mg • Magnesium amino acid chelate/complex 25 mg • Iron (Amino Acid Chelate) 5 mg • Vitamin A Fish Liver oil 10000 IU • Folic Acid 200 mcg • Vitamin B12 from Cobalamin 100 mcg • Vitamin D Fish Liver oil 400 IU. In a natural Rice Bran base.

Ultra NeuroRecovery **-** American Biologics
Three capsules contain: Vitamin B6 (as pyridoxine HCl) 50 mg • Vitamin B12 (activated, as methylcobalamin) 1000 mcg • Vitamin B12 (as cyanocobalamin) 1000 mcg • Folic Acid 900 mcg • Alpha Lipoic Acid (ALA) 300 mg • N-Acetyl-L-Cysteine (NAC) 100 mg • Glutathione, reduced (GSH) 25 mg • Inositol 200 mg • L-Glutamine 300 mg. Other Ingredients: Magnesium Stearate, Silica, Cellulose.

Ultra Omega Essentials **-** American Biologics
Two softgels contain: DHA (docosahexaenoic acid, omega-3) 110 mg • EPA (eicosapentaenoic acid, omega-3) 150 mg • ALA (alpha-linolenic acid, other omega-3) 140 mg • GLA (gamma-linolenic acid, omega-6) 40 mg • LA (linolenic acid, other omega-6) 120 mg • OA (oleic acid, omega-9) 105 mg • Vitamin E 60 IU.

Ultra Omega-3 Fish Oil **-** Health From The Sun
Two capsules contain: Omega-3 Fatty Acids 600 mg [EPA (360) DHA (240 mg)]. Ingredients: All natural Fish Body Oil, Gelatin, Glycerine, Water, Carob powder, Mixed Tocopherols (Vitamin E).

Ultra Osteo Synergy - American Biologics
Six capsules contain: Vitamin D (as D3, cholecalciferol) 400 IU • Vitamin K (as K1, phylloquinone) 800 mcg • Vitamin B6 (as pyridoxine hydrochloride) 20 mg • Vitamin B6 (as pyridoxal-5'-phosphate) 5 mg • Folic Acid (as folate) 400 mcg • Vitamin B12 (as cyanocobalamin) 1000 mcg • Calcium (as microcrystalline hydroxyapatite, citrate-malate) 600 mg • Magnesium (as citrate-malate) 150 mg • Zinc (as citrate) 15 mg • Selenium (as selenomethionine) 150 mcg • Copper (as gluconate) 1.5 mg • Manganese (as citrate) 5 mg • Molybdenum (as sodium molybdate) 150 mcg • Ipriflavone 400 mg • Silicon, as Horsetail (equisetum arvense) 3.5 mg • Boron (as citrate) 3 mg. Other Ingredients: Magnesium Stearate, Silicon Dioxide, Microcrystalline Cellulose.

Ultra Parex - Metagenics
Three tablets contain: Coptis root and rhizome extract (coptis chinensis, standardized to 20% [80 mg] berberine) 400 mg • Ginger root and rhizome extract (zingiber officinale, standardized to 5% [15 mg] total pungent compounds [gingerols and shagauols]) 300 mg • Sour Plum fruit 5:1 extract (prunus mume) 450 mg.

Ultra Potassium - Source Naturals
Each tablet contains: Potassium (citrate, malate, ketoglutarate, fumarate, succinate, asparate, glycinate, and ascorbate) 99 mg.

Ultra Potent-C 1000 - Metagenics
Each tablet contains: Ultra Potent-C brand Vitamin C 1000 mg • Niacin (ascorbate) 77 mg • L-Glutathione 5 mg • L-Cysteine 10 mg • L-Lysine Hydrochloride 36 mg • Citrus Bioflavonoid Complex (standardized to 45% full spectrum bioflavonoids) 35 mg • Tetrasodium Pyrophosphate 15 mg • Alpha-D-Ribofuranose 14 mg • Xylitol 10 mg.

Ultra Potent-C 500 - Metagenics
Each tablet contains: Ultra Potent-C brand Vitamin C 500 mg • Niacin (as niacinamide ascorbate) 39 mg • L-Glutathione 3 mg • L-Cysteine 5 mg • L-Lysine Hydrochloride 18 mg • Citrus Bioflavonoid Complex (standardized to 45% full spectrum bioflavonoids) 18 mg • Tetrasodium Pyrophosphate 8 mg • Alpha-D-Ribofuranose 7 mg • Xylitol 5 mg.

Ultra Potent-C brand - Metagenics
Ascorbic Acid • Ascorbyl Palmitate • Niacinamide Ascorbate • Calcium Ascorbate • Magnesium Ascorbate • Potassium Ascorbate • Sodium Ascorbate • Xylitol • Lysine Acetate • Tetrasodium Pyrophosphate • Ribose • Cysteine • Hesperidin.
See Editor's Note No. 44.

Ultra Potent-C Chewable - Metagenics
Each tablet contains: Ultra Potent-C brand Vitamin C 250 mg • Niacin (as niacinamide ascorbate) 20 mg • Glutathione 1 mg • L-Cysteine (as monochloride) 2 mg • L-Lysine Hydrochloride 12 mg • Xylitol 344 mg • Citrus Bioflavonoid Complex 8 mg • Tetrasodium Pyrophosphate 3 mg • Alpha-D-Ribofuranose 3 mg. Other Ingredients: Fructose, Sorbitol, Natural Flavors.

Ultra Potent-C Powder - Metagenics
Each 1 tsp serving contains: Ultra Potent-C brand Vitamin C 4350 mg • Niacin (as niacinamide ascorbate) 337 mg • Calcium (as calcium ascorbate) 205 mg • Magnesium (as magnesium ascorbate) 30 mg • Potassium (as potassium ascorbate) 26 mg • Sodium (as sodium ascorbate) 59 mg • L-Glutathione 21 mg • L-Cysteine 43 mg • L-Lysine (as L-lysine hydrochloride) 158 mg • Xylitol 766 mg • Citrus Bioflavonoid Complex (standardized to 45% full spectrum bioflavonoids) 152 mg • Tetrasodium Pyrophosphate 65 mg • Alpha-D-Ribofuranose 61 mg.

Ultra Power Nutrient - Goldshield Elite
One packet (6g) contains: Vitamin A (as Retinyl palmitate with Lemongrass and Beta Carotene) 5000 IU • Vitamin C (as buffered mineral ascorbates) 60 mg • Vitamin D (as Cholecalciferol) 400 IU • Thiamin (Vitamin B1 as Thiamine hydrochloride) 1.5 mg • Riboflavin (Vitamin B2) 1.7 mg • Vitamin B6 (as Pyridoxine hydrochloride) 2 mg • Folate (as Folic acid) 400 mcg • Vitamin B12 (as Cyanocobalamin) 6 mcg • Biotin 300 mcg • Pantothenic acid (Vitamin B5, calcium pantothenate) 10 mg • Calcium (as Calcium citrate ascorbate) 40 mg • Magnesium (as Magnesium citrate ascorbate) 20 mg • Sodium (as Sodium citrate ascorbate) 60 mg • Potassium (as Potassium citrate ascorbate) 200 mg • Sea minerals from Celtic marine algae 10 mg. Other Ingredients: Crystalline fructose, Maltodextrin, Natural citrus flavors.

Ultra Pregnenolone - Nature's Plus
Each capsule contains: Pregnenolone 50 mg • Bioperine brand Black Pepper extract (piper nigrum fruit, standardized to 95% 1-piperoylpiperidine) 2.5 mg. Other Ingredients: Silica, Gelatin, Purified Water.

Ultra Prenatal Complex - Nature's Plus
Two tablets contain: Vitamin A (beta carotene) 10,000 IU • Vitamin C (ascorbic acid) 150 mg • Vitamin D (ergocalciferol) 400 IU • Vitamin E (D-alpha tocopheryl acetate) 100 IU • Vitamin B1 (thiamine HCl) 15 mg • Vitamin B2 (riboflavin) 15 mg • Niacin (niacinamide) 40 mg • Vitamin B6 (pyridoxine HCl) 50 mg • Folate (folic acid) 800 mcg • Vitamin B12 (cyanocobalamin) 20 mcg • Biotin 600 mcg • Pantothenic Acid (calcium pantothenate) 25 mg • Calcium (amino acid chelate/complex) 600 mg • Iron (amino acid chelate/complex) 36 mg • Phosporous (amino acid complex) 200 mg • Iodine (kelp) 225 mcg • Magnesium (amino acid chelate/complex) 300 mg • Zinc (amino acid chelate/complex) 15 mg • Manganese 6 mg • Potassium (amino acid complex) 6 mg • Choline (bitartrate) 10 mg • Inositol 10 mg • PABA (para-aminobenzoic acid) 10 mg. Other Ingredients: Microcrystalline Cellulose, Stearic Acid, Silica, Rice Bran, Rose Hips (rosa canina fruit).

Ultra Prime Secretagogue HGH Enhancer - Market America, Inc.
Each scoop (17.7 g) contains: Folate (as folic acid) 150 mcg • Magnesium (as magnesium citrate) 150 mg • L-Arginine Aspartate 2.5 g • Glycine 4 g • L-Arginine 3 g • Proprietary Blend 3.3 g: L-Glutamine, Colostrum, L-Lysine (as L-lysine HCl), Taurine, RNA/DNA (from brewer's yeast). Other Ingredients: Citric Acid, Malic Acid, Natural Flavors, Beet juice powder, Silica, Glucose Polymers, Ascesulfame Potassium, Sucralose.

Ultra Primrose Oil - Pro Health
Each softgel contains: Evening Primrose oil (oenothera biennis seed) 1.3 g • Gamma Linolenic Acid (GLA) 135 mg • Cis-Linoleic Acid (omega-6) 935 mg • Cis-Oleic Acid (omega-9) 105 mg. Other Ingredients: Gelatin, Glycerin, Water.

Ultra Prostagen - Metagenics
Each tablet contains: Vitamin A (as retinyl palmitate) 2500 IU • Vitamin E (as D-alpha tocopheryl succinate) 5 IU • Glycine 100 mg • L-Alanine 100 mg • L-Glutamic Acid 100 mg • Raw Prostate Concentrate (bovine) 90 mg • Vitamin B6 (as pyridoxine hydrochloride) 10 mg • Zinc (as zinc glycinate) 5 mg • Flaxseed oil (linum usitatissmum) 3 mg • Saw Palmetto berry extract (serenoa repens, standardized to 45% fatty acids and sterols) 80 mg • White Korean Ginseng root powder (panax ginseng) 50 mg • Pumpkin seed powder (curcurbita pepo) 10 mg.
See Editor's Note No. 14.

Ultra Prosta-Metto - The Vitamin Shoppe
Each softgel contains: Vitamin E 50 IU • Vitamin B6 5 mg • Zinc 15 mg • Saw Palmetto berries 160 mg • Pumpkin seed 40 mg • Pygeum Africanum bark 10 mg • Nettle leaf 50 mg • Lycopene 2.5 mg.

Ultra Pure Fish Oil - Vital Nutrients
Each 1 tsp serving contains: EPA min. 2200 mg • DHA max. 750 mg • Other Omega 3 Fatty Acids 300 mg • Antioxidant Blend 25 mg: Rosemary extract, Natural Mixed Tocopherols. Other Ingredients: Natural Lemon Flavor.

Ultra Pure Fish Oil "RS" - Vital Nutrients
Each 1 tsp serving contains: EPA 900 mg • DHA 600 mg • Other Omega 3 Fatty Acids 350 mg • Antioxidant Blend 18 mg: Rosemary extract, Natural Mixed Tocopherols. Other Ingredients: Natural Lemon Flavor.

Ultra Pure Fish Oil & Coenzyme Q10 100 mg/tsp - Vital Nutrients
Each 1 tsp serving contains: EPA min. 2154 mg • DHA max. 734 mg • Other Omega 3 Fatty Acids 293 mg • Coenzyme Q10 100 mg • Antioxidant Blend 25 mg: Rosemary extract, Natural Mixed Tocopherols. Other Ingredients: Natural Lemon Flavor.

Ultra Pure Fish Oil & Coenzyme Q10 50 mg/tsp - Vital Nutrients
Each 1 tsp serving contains: EPA min. 2200 mg • DHA max. 750 mg • Other Omega 3 Fatty Acids 300 mg • Coenzyme Q10 50 mg • Antioxidant Blend 25 mg: Rosemary extract, Natural Mixed Tocopherols. Other Ingredients: Natural Lemon Flavor.

Ultra Pure Fish Oil 360 EPA/240 DHA - Vital Nutrients
Each softgel contains: Pure Fish Oil 1200 mg: EPA 360 mg, DHA 240 mg.

Ultra Quercetin - Flavonoid Complex - Jamieson
Each caplet contains: Quercetin Pure Flavonoid 165 mg • Nettle leaf 1:6 extract • Perilla fruit 1:37 extract 35 mg.

Ultra S - E'OLA
Each 1/2 tsp contains: Silver 25 mcg.

Ultra Saw Palmetto + Pygeum - Jarrow Formulas
Two softgels contain: Saw Palmetto berry extract (serenoa repens 85%-90% fatty acids and sterols) 300 mg • Pygeum Africanum bark extract (prunus african, 13% sterols) 100 mg • Phytosterols (providing minimum 40 mg of beta-sitosterol) 100 mg • Pumpkin seed oil 320 mg • Gamma Tocopherol 4 mg. Other Ingredients: Gelatin, Glycerin, Carob, Water.

Ultra Skin - Nature's Plus
Two tablets contain: Unsaturated Fatty Acids from natural Safflower oil 500 mg • Vitamin C with Rose Hips 200 mg • Vitamin B2 (Riboflavin) 200 mg • Vitamin B6 (Pyridoxine HCL) 200 mg • Vitamin E natural 200 IU • Niacinamide 150 mg • PABA (Para-Aminobenzoic Acid) 150 mg • Pantothenic Acid 150 mg • Vitamin B1 (Thiamine) 100 mg • Zinc amino acid chelate/complex 50 mg • Vitamin A (Beta Carotene) 25000 IU • Biotin 400 mcg • Folic Acid 100 mcg • Vitamin B12 (from Cobalamin) 100 mcg • Vitamin D (Calciferol) 1000 IU. In a natural base of rice bran & spirulina.

Ultra Slim Down - Jamieson
Carb & Fat Burner: Each capsule contains: CitraMax 50% HCA Hydroxycitric Acid (derived from fruit of garcinia cambogia) 125 mg • Advantra Z Citrus Aurantium (derived from fruit of bitter orange) 125 mg • Kola nut JKN-10 (P.E. 10%) 5 mg.
Calorie & Fat Eliminator: Each capsule contains: Natural soluble and insoluble Fibre Complex 343 mg: Derived from Chitosan of North Atlantic Shellfish, Mediterranean Nopal Cactus, and Organic Citrus Orange fruit fibre.
See Editor's Note No. 40.

Ultra Stress with Iron - Nature's Plus
Each tablet contains: Vitamin C with Rose Hips 500 mg • Pantothenic Acid 200 mg • Vitamin B1 (Thiamine) 125 mg • Vitamin B2 (Riboflavin) 125 mg • Vitamin B6 (Pyridoxine HCL) 125 mg • Niacinamide 125 mg • Inositol 75 mg • PABA (Para-aminobenzoic acid) 50 mg • Choline (Bitartrate) 32 mg • Iron amino acid chelate/complex 20 mg • Vitamin B12 from Cobalamin 500 mcg • Folic Acid 400 mcg • Biotin 125 mcg. B-Complex vitamins in a fortified rice bran base.

Ultra Sugar Control - Nature's Plus
Two tablets contain: Chromium (as polynicotinate) 500 mcg • Citrimax brand Garcinia Cambogia fruit (standardized to 50% (-) hydroxycitrate) 500 mg • Rehmannia Glutinosa root 400 mg • L-Glutamine (free form amino acid) 250 mg • L-Alanine (free form amino acid) 250 mg • Gymnema Sylvestre leaf (standardized to 75% gymnemic acids) 200 mg. Other Ingredients: Di-Calcium Phosphate, Microcrystalline Cellulose, Stearic Acid, Magnesium Stearate, Silica, Pharmaceutical Glaze.

Ultra True E - American Biologics
Each softgel contains: Vitamin E (D-alpha-tocopherol, from pure soy oil) 400 IU.

Ultra Vein-Gard - NaturalCare
Active Ingredients: Horse Chestnut (aesculus hippocastanum)3X, 6X, 3C • Witch Hazel (hamamelis virginica) 1X, 4X, 3C • Honeybee (apis mellifica) 3X, 6X, 12X, 30X • Wind Flower (pulsatilla) 3X, 6X, 30X • St. Mary's Thistle (carduus marianus) 3X, 6X • Club Moss (lycopodium clavatum) 6X, 30X • Vegetable Charcoal (carbo vegetabilis) 6X, 30X • Ergot (secale cornutum) 3X. Other Ingredients: Aloe Vera Gel, Horse Chestnut Seed Extract (at 20% Escin), Purified Water, Butcher's Broom Extract (at 10% Ruscogenin), Rutin, Gotu Kola Extract (at 10% triterpenoids), Vegetable Glycerin, Glyceryl Stearate (vegetable), Cetyl Alcohol, Cetearyl Alcohol, Caprylic/Capric Triglyceride (from coconut), Stearic Acid (from vegetable oil), Beeswax, Jojoba Oil, Vitamin C (ascorbyl palmitate), Vitamin E (d-alpha tocopherol), Vitamin A (retinyl palmitate), Quercetin, Methyl Glucoses (from fruit), Xanthan Gum, Grapefruit Seed Extract, Rosemary Extract, Neem Oil, Tea Tree Oil, Glycyrrhetinic Acid (from licorice root), St. John's Wort Oil, Lavender Oil.
See Editor's Note No. 1.

Ultra Virile-Actin - Nature's Plus
Two protein coated tablets contain: Vitamin E natural 200 IU • Korean Ginseng (panax ginseng root, standardized 15% Ginsenosides) 100 mg • Siberian Ginseng (eleutherococcus senticosus root, standardized 0.8% Eleutherosides) 100 mg • Bee Pollen, Spanish 75 mg • Saw Palmetto [(Serenoa repens berry) standardized 35%-45% free fatty acids] 60 mg • Brazilian Muirapuama (Phychopetalum olacoides root & rhizome) 50 mg • L-Histidine, pharmaceutical grade free form amino acid 50 mg • Zinc (Monomethionine) 50 mg • Cayenne [(Capsicum frutescens fruit) standardized 125000 STU/gram] 50 mg • L-Phenylalanine pharmaceutical grade free form amino acid 50 mg • St. John's Wort [(Hypericum perforatum flower) 0.3%-0.5% Hypericin] 50 mg • Royal Jelly 25 mg • L-Carnitine (L-Carnitine-L-Tartrate) 25 mg • Pacific Oyster extract [(Crassostreagis thunberg) naturally rich in trace elements & amino acids] 10 mg • Vitamin B6 (Pyridoxine HCL) 5 mg • Coenzyme Q10 (Ubiquinone) 2500 mcg.

Ultra Vita-Min - Puritan's Pride
Each tablet contains: Vitamin A (as retinyl palmitate and beta carotene) 10,000 IU • Vitamin C (as ascorbic acid) 150 mg • Vitamin D (as cholecalciferol) 400 IU • Vitamin E (as d-alpha tocopheryl succinate) 12.5 IU • Thiamin (Vitamin B-1; as thiamine hydrochloride) 25 mg • Riboflavin (Vitamin B-2) 25 mg • Niacin (as niacinamide) 50 mg • Vitamin B6 (pyridoxine hydrochloride) 15 mg • Folic Acid 400 mcg • Vitamin B12 (as cyanocobalamin) 50 mcg • Biotin 1 mcg • Pantothenic Acid (as d-calcium pantothenate) 12.5 mg • Calcium (as oyster shell and bone meal) 60 mg • Iron (as ferrous gluconate) 6.26 mg • Phosphorus (as bone meal) 24.3 mg • Iodine (as potassium iodide) 100 mcg • Magnesium (as magnesium gluconate) 0.42 mg • Zinc (as zinc gluconate) 0.72 mg • Selenium (as sodium selenate) 10 mcg • Copper (as cupric gluconate) 0.035 mg • Manganese (as manganese gluconate) 0.76 mg • Chromium (as chromium picolinate) 2.35 mg • Molybdenum (as sodium molybdate) 10 mcg • Potassium (as potassium gluconate) _0.5 mg • PABA 15 mg • Choline Bitartrate 25 mg • Inositol 25 mg • Boron (as sodium borate) 500 mcg • Betaine Hydrochloride 25 mg • Rose Hips powder 10 mg • Rutin 5 mg • Citrus Bioflavonoids complex 15 mg • Royal Jelly 5 mg • Bee Propolis powder 5 mg • Coenzyme Q10 30 mcg • Octacosanol 50 mcg • Deodorized Garlic powder 10 mg • Ginseng root 15 mg • RNA 2 mg • DNA 2 mg.

Ultra Zinc Lozenge - GNC
Two lozenges contain: Beta-Carotene 1.2 mg • Vitamin C (ascorbic acid) 200 mg •Zinc (zinc oxide) 20 mg • Copper (copper oxide) 1 mg • Bee Propolis extract 1:5 20 mg •Echinacea Purpurea powder 20 mg. Other Ingredients: Sorbital, Fructose, Stearic Acid, Magnesium Stearate, Citric Acid, Natural Flavors.

UltraAC **-** Great American Nutrition
Four capsules contain: Potassium (as potassium glycerophosphate) 112 mg • Chromium (as chromium picolinate) 200 mcg • Potassium Glycerophosphate 450 mg • DL-Phenylalanine 1000 mg • Zhi Shi fruit (Citrus aurantium (Bitter Orange peel) containing 10 mg synephrine from a 4% standardized extract) 250 mg • Kola Nut nut (Cola acuminata, containing 50 mg caffeine from a 10% standardized extract) 500 mg • Ginger root (Zingiber officinale) 100 mg. Other Ingredients: Rice powder, Magnesium Silicate, Magnesium Stearate. See Editor's Note No. 40.

UltraAP Activated Pyruvate **-** Great American Nutrition
Four capsules contain: Potassium (as potassium glycerophosphate) 125 mg • Potassium Glycerophosphate 500 mg • Caffeine (from caffeine citrate & kola nut) 150 mg • Zhi Shi fruit (citrus aurantium peel, synephrine from a 4% standardized extract 10 mg) 250 mg • Kola Nut (cola acuminata) 500 mg • Siberian Ginseng root (eleutherococcus senticosus) 200 mg • Quercetin 100 mg • Jing Jie leaf (schizonepeta divaricata, 5:1 extract) 10 mg • Fang Feng leaf (ledebouriella tenuifolia, 5:1 extract) 10 mg. Other Ingredients: Rice powder, Maltodextrin, Magnesium Silicate and Magnesium Stearate. See Editor's Note No. 40.

UltraBalance Protein **-** Metagenics
Each scoop (24 g) contains: Vitamin A (mixed carotenoids) 1750 IU • Vitamin D (as cholecalciferol) 80 IU • VItamin C (as ascorbic acid) 48 mg • Vitamin E (as D-alpha tocopheryl acetate) 13.5 IU • Thiamin (as thiamin hydrochloride) 675 mcg • Riboflavin 1.4 mg • Niacin (as niacinamide) 7 mg • Pantothenic Acid (as D-calcium pantothenate) 3.5 mg • Vitamin B6 (as pyridoxine hydrochloride) 3.4 mg • Vitamin B12 (as cyanocobalamin) 3.6 mcg • Biotin 135 mcg • Folate (as folic acid) 133 mcg • Sodium 90 mg • Potassium (as potassium citrate, chloride) 390 mg • Calcium (as calcium citrate, tricalcium phosphate) 150 mg • Iron (as iron amino acid chelate) 3.8 mg • Phosphorus 100 mg • Iodine 53 mcg • Magnesium (as magnesium glycinate) 130 mg • Zinc (as zinc amino acid chelate) 5.25 mg • Copper (as copper amino acid chelate) 1.6 mg • Manganese (as manganese amino acid chelate) 1.3 mg • Molybdenum (as molybdenum amino acid chelate) 50 mcg • Chromium (as ChromeMate brand GTF) 50 mcg • Selenium (as selenium amino acid chelate) 33 mcg. Other Ingredients: Hydrolyzed Lactalbumin, Rice Protein Concentrate, Olive Oil, Natural Flavors.

Ultra-Cal Night **-** Source Naturals
Four tablets contain: Calcium 600 mg • Magnesium (Oxide, Citrate, Fumarate, Malate, and Ascorbate) 600 mg • SoyLife Genistein Rich Soy Concentrate (Daidzein 13 mg, Glycitein 9 mg, Genistein 3 mg, total Isoflavones 25 mg) 830 mg • Vitamin C (Magnesium and Calcium Ascorbates, Ascorbic Acid and Manganese Ascorbate) 285 mg • Vitamin B6 (Pyridoxine HCl) 20 mg • Vitamin D (as Vitamin D3) (Cholecalciferol) 200 IU • Folic Acid 200 mcg • L-Lysine (HCl) 60 mg • Silica (Horsetail Silica Extract) 10 mg • Zinc (Chelate) 7.5 mg • Manganese (Ascorbate) 6 mg • Boron (Amino Acid Chelate) 3 mg • Copper (Sebacate) 1 mg.

Ultracare for Kids **-** Metagenics
Each scoop (35 g) contains: Vitamin A (as retinyl palmitate) 275 IU • Vitamin A (as mixed carotenoids) 200 IU • Vitamin D 130 IU • Vitamin C (as ascorbic acid) 10 mg • Vitamin E (as D-alpha tocopheryl acetate) 5 IU • Thiamin (as thiamin hydrochloride) 150 mcg • Riboflavin 170 mcg • Niacin (as niacinamide) 2.5 mg • Pantothenic Acid (as D-calcium pantothenate) 500 mcg • Vitamin B6 (as pyridoxine hydrochloride) 100 mcg • Vitamin B12 (as cyanocobalamin) 0.5 mcg • Biotin 6 mcg • Folate (as folic acid) 25 mcg • Potassium 350 mg • Calcium (as calcium citrate, phosphate) 250 mg • Iron (as ferrous fumarate) 500 mcg • Phosphorus 150 mg • Iodine (as potassium iodide) 15 mcg • Magnesium (as magnesium oxide) 20 mg • Molybdenum (as sodium molybdate) 40 mcg • Chromium (as chromium polynicotinate) 5 mcg • Selenium (as sodium selenite) 5 mcg • Chloride 225 mg • L-Threonine 6 mg • L-Lysine 6 mg • Taurine 10.6 mg • Inositol 18 mg • Choline 10 mg • Fructooligosaccharides 500 mg • Docosahexaenoic Acid (DHA) 100 mg. Other Ingredients: Rice Syrup Solids, Rice Protein Concentrate, Rice Flour, Olive Oil, Natural Flavors, Vegetable Oil from Algae.

UltraClear **-** Metagenics
Two scoops (44 g) contain: Vitamin A (as retinyl palmitate) 1000 IU • Vitamin A (as mixed carotenoids) 4000 IU • Vitamin D 80 IU • Vitamin C (Ester-C brand) 110 mg • Vitamin E (as D-alpha tocopheryl acetate) 80 IU • Thiamin (as thiamin hydrochloride) 2 mg • Riboflavin 2 mg • Niacin (as niacinamide) 7 mg • Pantothenic Acid (as D-calcium pantothenate) 3.5 mg • Vitamin B6 (as pyridoxine hydrochloride) 3.4 mg • Vitamin B12 (as cyanocobalamin) 3.6 mcg • Folate (as folic acid) 80 mcg • Biotin 135 mcg • Sodium 60 mg • Potassium (as phosphate, iodide) 420 mg • Calcium (as calcium citrate, phosphate) 75 mg • Iron (as ferrous fumarate) 3.6 mg • Phosphorus 200 mg • Iodine (as potassium iodide) 53 mcg • Magnesium (as magnesium citrate) 140 mg • Zinc (OptiZinc brand) 10 mg • Copper (as copper gluconate) 1 mg • Manganese (as manganese gluconate) 1.3 mg • Molybdenum (as amino acid chelate) 120 mcg • Chromium (ChromeMate GTF brand) 50 mcg • Selenium (as selenomethionine) 40 mcg • N-Acetylcysteine 35 mg • L-Glutathione 10 mg • L-Cysteine 30 mg • L-Threonine 35 mg • L-Lysine 35 mg. Other Ingredients: Rice Protein Concentrate, Rice Syrup Solids, Olive Oil, Medium-Chain Trigylcerides, Natural Flavors.

UltraClear MACRO **-** Metagenics
Two scoops (40 g) contain: Potassium (as potassium phosphate, chloride) 730 mg • Calcium 40 mg • Phosphorus 250 mg • Manganese 1 mg • Iron 1 mg • Magnesium (as magnesium citrate) 160 mg • L-Glycine 1.6 g • L-Glutamin 500 mg • L-Lysine 35 mg • L-Threonine 35 mg. Other Ingredients: Rice Protein Concentrate, Rice Syrup Solids, Sesame Seed Flour, Rice Bran, Beet Fiber, Medium-Chain Triglycerides, Olive Oil, Natural Flavors, Cellulose Gum, Silica.

UltraClear PLUS **-** Metagenics
Two scoops (44 g) contain: Vitamin A (as retinyl palmitate) 1000 IU • Vitamin A (mixed carotenoids) 4000 IU • Vitamin D 80 IU • Vitamin C (sodium asocrbate) 300 mg • Vitamin E (D-alpha tocopheryl acetate) 42 IU • Thiamin (hydrochloride) 2 mg • Riboflavin 2 mg • Niacin (niacinamide) 7 mg • Pantothenic Acid (D-calcium pantothenate) 36 mg • Vitamin B6 (pyridoxine HCl) 3.4 mg • Vitamin B12 (cyanocobalamin) 3.6 mcg • Folate (folic acid) 80 mcg • Biotin 135 mcg • Sodium 70 mg • Potassium (phosphate, iodide) 420 mg • Calcium (citrate, pohsphate) 200 mg • Phosphorus 200 mg • Iodin (as potassium iodide) 53 mcg • Magnesium (citrate) 200 mg • Zinc (citrate) 10 mg • Copper (as copper gluconate) 1 mg • Manganese (as manganese gluconate) 1.3 mg • Chromium (as chromium chloride) 50 mcg • Selenium (as selenomethionine) 40 mcg • N-Acetylcysteine 20 mg • L-Glutathione 10 mg • L-Cysteine 5 mg • Glycine 1.6 g • Taurine 100 mg • L-Lysine 35 mg • L-Threonine 35 mg • Sodium Sulfate 30 mg • Catechins from decaffeinated Green Tea extract 15 mg. Other Ingredients: Rice Protein Concentrate, Rice Syrup Solids, Olive Oil, Medium-Chain Triglycerides, Natural Flavors.

UltraClear SUSTAIN **-** Metagenics
Two scoops (60 g) contain: Vitamin A (as retinyl palmitate) 2500 IU • Vitamin A (as mixed carotenoids) 2500 IU • Vitamin D 100 IU • Ester-C brand Vitamin C 102 mg • Vitamin K 80 mcg • Vitamin E (as D-alpha tocopheryl acetate) 51 IU • Thiamin (as thiamin hydrochloride) 525 mcg • Riboflavin 595 mcg • Niacin (as niacinamide) 7 mg • Pantothenic Acid (as D-calcium pantothenate) 100 mg • Vitamin B6 (as pyridoxine hydrochloride) 0.7 mg • Vitamin B12 (as cyanocobalamin) 2.1 mcg • Biotin 105 mcg • Folate (as folic acid) 140 mcg • Sodium 20 mg • Potassium (as potassium phosphate, iodide) 300 mg • Calcium (as calcium citrate, phosphate) 275 mg • Iron (as ferrous fumarate) 3.6 mg • Phosphorus 175 mg • Magnesium (as magnesium citrate) 121 mg • Zinc (as zinc picolinate) 7.5 mg • Copper (as copper gluconate) 0.5 mg • Manganese (as manganese gluconate) 2 mg • Molybdenum (as amino acid chelate) 50 mcg • ChromeMate GTF brand Chromium 75 mcg • Selenium (as selenomethionine) 50 mcg • N-Acetylcysteine 5 mg • L-Glutathione 5 mg • L-Cysteine 5 mg • L-Glutamine 500 mg • L-Lysine 35 mg • L-Threonine 35 mg • Fructooligosaccharides 2 g • Inulin 1.4 g. Other Ingredients: Rice Protein Concentrate, Rice Syrup Solids, Rice Flour, Olive Oil, Medium-chain Triglycerides, Natural Flavors.

Ultra-Eyebright **-** Nutri-Quest Rx
Each tablet contains: Eyebright 100 mg • Bilberry extract 6 mg • Ginkgo Biloba 6 mg • Siberian Ginseng 15 mg • Gymnema sylvestre 100 mg • Tumeric 25 mg • Quercetin 10 mg • Lemon Bioflavonoids 40 mg • Bromelain 30 mg • Pancreatin 30 mg • Papain 30 mg • Trypsin 40 mg (Chymotrypsin 8 mg) • Pancreolipase 15 mg • Amylase-Diastase 15 mg • Ox Bile 30 mg • Betaine HCL 10 mg • Rutin 50 mg • L-Glutathione 2.5 mg • L-Taurine 15 mg • N-Acetyl Cysteine 10 mg • Selenium Chelate 10 mcg • Zinc Chelate 15 mg • Chromium Aspartate 1 mg • Parotid 1 mg • Beta Carotene 1000 IU • Vitamin C 75 mg • Vitamin D 200 IU • Vitamin E (Succinate) 20 IU • Vitamin B2 20 mg • Vitamin B6 10 mg • Folic Acid 50 mcg.
See Editor's Note No. 14.

UltraFlax **-** Aidan Products, LLC
Each capsule contains: Omega-3 667 mg • Omega-6 194 mg • Omega-9 218 mg • Flaxseed particulate (containing lignan) 285 mg. Other Ingredients: Gelatin, Carob.

UltraGlycemX **-** Metagenics
Two scoops (50 g) contain: Dietary Fiber 9g • Vitamin A (as retinyl palmitate) 2500 IU • Beta-Carotene (as mixed carotenoids) 2500 IU • Vitamin D 100 IU • Vitamin C (as Ultra Potent-C) 250 mg • Vitamin E (as d-alpha tocopheryl succinate) 200 IU • Thiamin (as thiamin hydrochloride) 1 mg • Riboflavin 1 mg • Niacin (as niacin, niacinamide, niacinamide ascorbate) 39 mg • Pantothenic Acid (as d-calcium pantothenate) 5 mg • Vitamin B6 (as pyridoxine hydrochloride) 1 mg • Vitamin B12 (as cyanocobalamin) 3 mcg • Biotin 5 mg • Folic Acid 200 mcg • Sodium 170 mg • Potassium 580 mg • Calcium (as calcium phosphate) 500 mg • Phosphorus 400 mg • Magnesium (as magnesium citrate) 200 mg • Zinc (as zinc glycinate) 15 mg • Copper (as copper lysinate) 1.5 mg • Manganese (as manganese glycinate) 1 mg • Molybdenum (as molybdenum amino acid chelate) 38 mcg • Chromium (as polynicotinate) 500 mcg • Selenium (as selenomethionine) 150 mcg • Soy Isoflavones 17 mg • Alpha-Lipoic Acid 200 mg • Inositol 100 mg • Vanadium (as vanadyl sulfate) 2.5 mg. Other Ingredients: Soy Protein Isolate (PharmaSoy), Corn Maltodextrin, Modified High Amylose Starch, Rice Polishings, Partially Hydrolyzed Guar Gum, Fructose, Natural Flavors, Locust Bean Gum, Lecithin.

UltraInflamX **-** Metagenics
Two scoops (52 g) contain: Vitamin A (as retinyl palmitate) 2500 IU • Vitamin A (as mixed carotenoids) 2500 IU • Vitamin D 100 IU • Vitamin C (as sodium ascorbate) 180 mg • Vitamin E (as D-alpha tocopheryl acetate) 100 IU • Thiamin (as thiamin hydrochloride) 2 mg • Riboflavin 2 mg • Niacin (as niacinamide and niacin) 35 mg • Pantothenic Acid (as D-calcium pantothenate) 5 mg • Vitamin B6 (as pyridoxal-5-phosphate) 5 mg • Vitamin B12 (as cyanocobalamin) 3 mcg • Bitoin 150 mcg • Folate (as folic acid) 80 mcg • Sodium 100 mg • Potassium (as potassium phosphate) 400 mg • Calcium (as calcium citrate) 275 mg • Iron 1 mg • Phosphorus 200 mg • Magnesium (as magnesium citrate) 280 mg • Zinc (as zinc methionate) 10 mg • Copper (as copper gluconate) 1 mg • Manganese (as manganese gluconate) 2 mg • Molybdenum (as molybdenum amino acid chelate) 38 mcg • Chromium (as chromium polynicotinate) 60 mcg • Selenium (as selenomethionine) 75 mg • N-Acetylcysteine 100 mg • L-Glutamine 750 mg • L-Threonine 34 mg • L-Lysine 770 mg • Citrulline 100 mg • Hesperidin 200 mg • D-Limonene 100 mg • Rutin 200 mg • Quercetin 200 mg • Sodium Sulfate 75 mg • Ginger root extract (zingiber officinale, standardized to 5% (5 mg) total pungent compounds) 100 mg • Turmeric rhizome extract (curcuma longa, standardized to 95% (200 mg) total pungent compounds) 210 mg • Rosemary leaf extract (rosmarinus officinalis) 100 mg. Other Ingredients: Rice Protein Concentrate, Rice Syrup Solids, Rice Bran, Olive Oil, Medium-Chain Triglycerides, Natural Flavors, Xanthan, Carrageenan, Cellulose Gum.

UltraLean **-** MK Supplements
Two capsules contain: Chitosan (from shellfish) 500 mg • Hydroxycitric Acid 300 mg • L-Carnitine 200 mg • Gymnema Sylvestre 100 mg • Chromium (polynicotinate) 200 mcg • Vanadium (aspartate) 200 mcg • Lipase 1500 LU.

Ultralec brand **-** ADM
Lecithin.
See Editor's Note No. 44.

Ultra-Mag **-** Source Naturals
Two tablets contain: Magnesium (citrate, taurinate, glycinate, malate and succinate) 400 mg • Vitamin B-6 (pyridoxine HCl) 50 mg.

UltraMeal (assorted flavors) **-** Metagenics
Two scoops (47 g) contain: Soy Isoflavones 17 mg • Vitamin A (as retinyl palmitate) 1750 IU • Vitamin D (as cholecalciferol) 200 IU • Vitamin C (as ascorbic acid) 60 mg • Vitamin E (as D-alpha tocopheryl acetate) 11 IU • Thiamin (as thiamin hydrochloride) 750 mcg • Riboflavin 850 mcg • Niacin (as niacinamide) 10 mg • Pantothenic Acid (as D-calcium pantothenate) 5 mg • Vitamin B6 (as pyridoxine hydrochloride) 25 mg • Vitamin B12 (as methylcobalamin and cyanocobalamin) 30 mcg • Biotin 150 mcg • Folate (as folic acid, L-5-methyl tetrahydrofolate, and 5-formyl tetrahydrofolate) 500 mcg • Vitamin K 40 mcg • Sodium 180 mg • Potassium 510 mg • Calcium (as calcium phosphate) 600 mg • Iron (as ferrous fumarate) 3 mg • Phosphorus 460 mg • Iodine (as potassium iodide) 75 mcg • Magnesium (as magnesium citrate) 150 mg • Zinc (as zinc citrate) 9 mg • Copper (as copper gluconate) 1 mg • Manganese (as manganese gluconate) 1 mg • Molybdenum (as molybdenum amino acid chelate) 75 mcg • Chromium (as chromium polynicotinate) 100 mcg • Selenium (as selenomethionine) 35 mcg. Other Ingredients: PharmaSoy brand Soy Protein Isolate, Fructose, Maltodextrin, Soy Fiber, Corn Bran, Natural Flavors, Lecithin, Olive Oil, Xanthan, Carrageenan, Cellulose Gum.

UltraMeal Bar (chocolate raspberry flavor) **-** Metagenics
Each bar contains: Vitamin A (retinyl palmitate) 1750 IU • Vitamin D (cholecalciferol) 200 IU • Vitamin C (ascorbic acid) 60 mg • Vitamin E (D-alpha tocopheryl acetate) 11 IU • Vitamin B1 (thiamin mononitrate) 1 mg • Vitamin B2 (riboflavin) 1 mg • Vitamin B3 (niacinamide) 10 mg • Pantothenic Acid (D-calcium pantothenate) 5 mg • Vitamin B6 (pyridoxine hydrochloride) 25 mg • Vitamin B12 (cyanocobalamin, methylcobalamin) 30 mcg • Biotin 150 mcg • Folate (folic acid) 400 mcg • Vitamin K 40 mcg • Sodium 220 mg • Potassium 170 mg • Calcium 600 mg • Iron 3 mg •Phosphorus 400 mg • Iodine (potassium iodide) 150 mcg • Magnesium (oxide) 150 mg • Zinc (arginate) 8 mg • Copper (gluconate) 1 mg • Manganese (sulfate) 1 mg • Molybdenum (glycinate) 50 mcg • Chromium (polynicotinate) 100 mcg • Selenium (selenomethionine) 35 mcg. Other Ingredients: Metagenics Soy Blend: Non-genetically engineered, identity-preserved Soy Protein Isolate, Soy Crisps (contains non-genetically engineered, identity-preserved soy protein isolate, tapioca starch and malt extract or salt), Toasted Soy pieces, Liquid Fructose, ActivCoat (contains fractionated palm kernel oil, fructose, alkalized cocoa, soy protein isolate, polydextrose, soy lecithin, and vanilla), Maltitol syrup, Hydrolyzed Collagen, Glycerine, Inulin (natural chicory root extract), Alkalized Cocoa powder, Natural Flavor, Maltodextrin, Extra Virgin Olive Oil, Malt Powder, Soy Lecithin.

UltraMeal Carb Conscious (vanilla) **-** Metagenics
Two scoops contain: PharmaSoy brand Soy Protein Isolate • Maltitol • Inulin • Glycine • Natural Flavors • Olive Oil • Lecithin • Xanthan • Carrageenan • Cellulose Gum providing Vitamin A (retinyl palmitate) 1750 IU • Vitamin D (cholecalciferol) 200 IU • Vitamin C (ascorbic acid) 60 mg • Vitamin E (D-alpha tocopheryl acetate) 11 IU • Thiamin (hydrochloride) 750 mcg • Riboflavin 850 mcg • Niacin (niacinamide) 10 gm • Pantothenic Acid (D-calcium pantothenate) 5 mg • Vitamin B6 (pyridoxine HCl) 25 mg • Vitamin B12 (methylcobalamin, cyanocobalamin) 15 mcg • Biotin 150 mcg • Folate (Metafolin brand, folic acid, ActiFolate brand L-5-methyl tetrahydrofolate, and 5-formyl tetrahydrofolate) 400 mcg • Vitamin K 40 mcg • Calcium (phosphate) 600 mg • Iron (ferrous fumarate) 3 mg • Phosphorus 460 mg • Iodine (potassium iodide) 75 mcg • Magnesium (citrate) 180 mg • Zinc (citrate) 8 mg • Copper (gluconate) 1 mg • Manganese (gluconate) 1 mg • Molybdenum (amino acid chelate) 75 mcg • Chromium (polynicotinate) 100 mcg • Selenium (selenomethionine) 35 mcg.

UltraMeal Plus (assorted flavors) - Metagenics
Two scoops (50 g) contain: Soy Isoflavones 17 mg • Vitamin A (as retinyl palmitate) 1750 IU • Vitamin D (as cholecalciferol) 200 IU • Vitamin C (as ascorbic acid) 60 mg • Vitamin E (as D-alpha tocopheryl acetate) 11 IU • Thiamin (as thiamin hydrochloride) 750 mcg • Riboflavin 850 mcg • Niacin (as niacinamide) 10 mg • Pantothenic Acid (as D-calcium pantothenate) 5 mg • Vitamin B6 (as pyridoxine hydrochloride) 25 mg • Vitamin B12 (as methylcobalamin & cyanocobalamin) 30 mcg • Biotin 150 mcg • Folate (as folic acid, L-5-methyl tetrahydrofolate and 5-formyl tetrahydrofolate) 500 mcg • Vitamin K 40 mcg • Calcium (as calcium phosphate) 600 mg • Iron (as ferrous fumarate) 3 mg • Phosphorus 460 mg • Iodine (as potassium iodide) 75 mcg • Magnesium (as magnesium citrate) 9 mg • Zinc (as zinc citrate) 9 mg • Copper (as copper gluconate) 1 mg • Manganese (as manganese gluconate) 1 mg • Molybdenum (as molybdenum amino acid chelate) 75 mcg • Chromium (as chromium polynicotinate) 100 mcg • Selenium (as selenomethionine) 35 mcg.

UltraMeal RICE - Metagenics
Two scoops (56 g) contain: Vitamin A (as retinyl palmitate) 1750 IU • Vitamin C (as ascorbic acid) 60 mg • Calcium (as dicalcium phosphate) 600 mg • Iron 3 mg • Vitamin D (as cholecalciferol) 200 IU • Vitamin E (as D-alpha tocopheryl acetate) 11 IU • Vitamin K 40 mcg • Thiamin (as thiamin hydrochloride) 0.75 mg • Riboflavin 0.85 mg • Niacin (as niacinamide) 10 mg • Vitamin B6 (as pyridoxine hydrochloride) 25 mg • Folate (as L-5-methyl tetrahydrofolate, 5-formyl tetrahydrofolate, folic acid) 500 mcg • Vitamin B12 (as methylcobalamin, cyanocobalamin) 30 mcg • Biotin 150 mcg • Pantothetic Acid (as D-calcium pantothenate) 5 mg • Phosphorus 600 mg • Iodine (as potassium iodide) 75 mcg • Magnesium (as magnesium citrate) 150 mg • Zinc (as zinc citrate) 7.5 mg • Selenium (as selenomethionine) 35 mcg • Copper (as copper gluconate) 1 mg • Manganese (as manganese gluconate) 2 mg • Chromium (as chromium polynicotinate) 100 mcg • Molybdenum (as molybdenum amino acid chelate) 75 mcg • Sodium 65 mg • Potassium (as potassium chloride) 450 mg • L-Lysine (as lysine hydrochloride) 35 mg • L-Threonine 35 mg. Other Ingredients: Rice Protein Concentrate, Fructose, Olive Oil, Dutch Processed Cocoa, Natural Flavors, Cellulose Gum, Silica.

UltraMeal WHEY - Metagenics
Two scoops (47 g) contain: Soy Isoflavones 17 mg • Vitamin A (as retinyl palmitate) 1750 IU • Vitamin D (as cholecalciferol) 200 IU • Vitamin C (as ascorbic acid) 60 mg • Vitamin E (as D-alpha tocopheryl acetate) 11 IU • Thiamin (as thiamin hydrochloride) 750 mcg • Riboflavin 850 mcg • Niacin (as niacinamide) 10 mg • Pantothenic Acid (as D-calcium pantothenate) 5 mg • Vitamin B6 (as pyridoxine hydrochloride) 25 mg • Vitamin B12 (as methylcobalamin and cyanocobalamin) 30 mcg • Biotin 150 mcg • Folate (as folic acid, L-5-methyl tetrahydrofolate, and 5-formyl tetrahydrofolate) 500 mcg • Vitamin K 40 mcg • Calcium (as calcium phosphate) 600 mg • Iron (as ferrous fumarate) 3 mg • Phosphorus 460 mg • Iodine (as potassium iodide) 75 mcg • Magnesium (as magnesium citrate) 160 mg • Zinc (as zinc citrate) 9 mg • Copper (as copper gluconate) 1 mg • Manganese (as manganese gluconate) 1 mg • Molybdenum (as molybdenum amino acid chelate) 75 mcg • Chromium (as chromium polynicotinate) 100 mcg • Selenium (as selenomethionine) 35 mcg. Other Ingredients: Whey Protein Isolate, Whey Protein Hydrosolate, Fructose, Rice Syrup Solids, Maltodextrin, Corn Bran, Natural Flavors, Cellulose, Olive Oil, Guar Gum, Xanthan Gum.

Ultramet (vanilla flavor) - Champion Nutrition
Each packet contains: Peptol-EX protein 42 grams including Ion-Exchange Whey Protein Isolate, Calcium Caseinate, Milk Protein Isolate, Potassium Caseinate, Egg Albumen, Whey Protein Concentrate, Sodium Caseinate, L-Glutamine, Taurine, Calcium Alpha-Ketoglutarate & L-Arginine.

Ultra-Mins - Nature's Plus
Two tablets contain: Calcium (as amino acid chelate/complex) 1000 mg • Iron (as amino acid chelate/complex) 27 mg • Phosphorus (as amino acid complex) 200 mg • Iodine (from kelp) 225 mcg • Magnesium (as amino acid chelate/complex) 500 mg • Zinc (as amino acid complex) 50 mg • Selenium (as amino acid complex) 50 mcg • Manganese (as amino acid chelate/complex) 10 mg • Chromium (as amino acid chelate) 100 mcg • Potassium (as amino acid complex) 99 mg. Other Ingredients: Stearic Acid, Magnesium Stearate, Isolated Soy Protein, Fig, Date, Hazelnut, Sesame Seed, Sunflower Seed, Broccoli, Spinach, Pacific Kelp, Spirulina, Black Currant Seed, Barley Grass, Pharmaceutical Glaze, Silica.

UltraNutrient - Pure Encapsulations
Six vegetable capsules contain: Mixed Carotenoids 25,000 IU: Beta Carotene 14,280 mcg, Alpha Carotene 450 mcg, Zeaxanthin 90 mcg, Cryptoxanthin 110 mcg, Lutein 70 mcg • Vitamin D (as D3) 400 IU • Vitamin E (D-alpha tocopherol succinate) 400 IU • Ascorbyl Palmitate (fat soluble vitamin C) 100 mg • Pantothenic Acid (calcium pantothenate) 400 mg • Niacinamide 100 mg • Thiamine HCl (vitamin B1) 100 mg • Inositol Hexaniacinate (no-flush niacin) 90 mg • Riboflavin (vitamin B2) 50 mg • Riboflavin 5' Phosphate (activated B2) 25 mg • Pyridoxine HCl (vitamin B6) 25 mg • Pyridoxal 5' Phosphate (activated B6) 25 mg • Methylcobalamin (vitamin B12) 1000 mcg • Folic Acid 800 mcg • Biotin 800 mcg • Calcium (citrate/malate) 300 mg • Magnesium (aspartate) 200 mg • Potassium (aspartate) 99 mg • Zinc (picolinate) 25 mg • Manganese (aspartate) 10 mg • Boron (glycinate) 2 mg • Copper (glycinate) 2 mg • Chromium (polynicotinate) 500 mcg • Selenium (selenomethionine) 200 mcg • Vanadium (aspartate) 200 mcg • Molybdenum (aspartate) 100 mcg • Alpha Lipoic Acid (thioctic acid) 100 mg • Hawthorn extract (crataegus oxyacantha, standardized to contain 2% vitexins) 100 mg • Ginger extract (zingiber officinale, standardized to contain 5% gingerols) 100 mg • Milk Thistle extract (silybum marianum, standardized to contain 80% silymarin) 100 mg • Turmeric extract (curcuma longa, standardized to contain 97% curcuminoids) 200 mg • Reduced Glutathione 50 mg • Coenzyme Q10 (ubiquinone) 50 mg.

Ultra-One tablets - Nature's Plus
Each tablet contains: Vitamin A (as beta carotene) 25000 IU • Vitamin C (as ascorbic acid) 100 mg • Vitamin D (as ergocalciferol) 1000 IU • Vitamin E (as D-alpha tocopheryl succinate) 100 IU • Thiamin (vitamin B1 as thiamine HCl) 100 mg • Riboflavin (vitamin B2) 100 mg • Niacin (as niacinamide) 100 gm • Vitamin B6 (as pyridoxine HCl) 100 mg • Folate (as folic acid) 400 mcg • Vitamin B12 (as cyanocobalamin) 100 mcg • Biotin 100 mcg • Pantothenic Acid (as calcium pantothenate) 100 mg • Calcium (as amino acid chelate/complex) 40 mg • Iron (as amino acid chelate/complex) 25 mg • Iodine (from kelp) 150 mcg • Magnesium (as amino acid chelate/complex) 20 mg • Zinc (as amino acid chelate/complex) 20 mg • Selenium (as amino acid complex) 10 mcg • Manganese (as amino acid chelate/complex) 6.1 mg • Chromium (as amino acid chelate) 15 mcg • Potassium (as amino acid complex) 15 mg • PABA (para-aminobenzoic acid) 100 mg • Inositol 100 mg • Choline (as bitartrate) 42 mg • Rutin (from saphora japonica leaf) 25 mg • Bioflavonoids (from citrus limon exocarp) 25 mg • Betaine HCl (from beet molasses) 25 mg • Hesperidin (from citrus limon exocarp) 5 mg. Other Ingredients: Microcrystalline Cellulose, Stearic Acid, Isolated Soy Protein, Rice Bran, Rose Hips, Magnesium Stearate, Parsley, Alfalfa, Green Cabbage, Acerola Cherry, Bromelain (from pineapple fruit), Wheat Germ Flour, Papaya, Watercress, Silica.

Ultra-Pro Training Pak - The Sports Nutrition Source, Inc.
One packet of eight tablets contains: Vitamin A 20,000 IU • Vitamin C 1000 mg • Vitamin D 200 IU • Vitamin E 400 IU • Thiamin (B1) 100 mg • Riboflavin (B2) 120 mg • Niacin 125 mg • Vitamin B-6 100 mg • Biotin 300 mcg • Pantothenic Acid 200 mg • Folic Acid 400 mcg • Vitamin B-12 200 mcg • Calcium 1000 mg • Iron 25 mg • Iodine 150 mcg • Magnesium 600 mg • Zinc 25 mg • Selenium 200 mcg • Copper 500 mcg • Manganese 15 mg • Chromium 100 mcg • Molybdenum 20 mcg • Potassium 99 mg • Rutin 100 mg • Bioflavonoids 100 mg • Gamma Oryzanol 40 mg • Inosine 10 mg • Coenzyme Q10 5 mg • Germanium 100 mcg • PABA 25 mcg • Choline 200 mg • Inositol 100 mg • Bromelain 25 mg • Papain 25 mg • Beta Sitosterol 20 mg • L-Carnitine 10 mg • Cayenne 20 mg • Gotu Kola 10 mg • Sarsaparilla 10 mg • Ginseng 10 mg • L-Leucine 78 mg • L-Isoleucine 48 mg • L-Valine 60 mg • L-Alanine 47 mg • L-Arginine 84 mg • L-Aspartic Acid 77 mg • L-Cystine 14 mg •

L-Glutamic Acid 193 mg • L-Glycine 50 mg • L-Histidine 15 mg • L-Lysine 47 mg • L-Methionine 50 mg • L-Ornithine 46 mg • L-Phenylalanine 58 mg • L-Proline 35 mg • L-Serine 47 mg • L-Taurine 50 mg • Threonine 35 mg • L-Tryptophan 13 mg • L-Tyrosine 53 mg.

Ultrasex **- Life Extension**
Three capsules contain: Yohimbe extract (4:1, equal to 1000 mg) 250 mg • Avena Sativa (wild oats) 200 mg • Siberian Ginseng 200 mg • Damiana 200 mg • Saw Palmetto 200 mg • Sarsaparilla 200 mg • Fo-Ti 100 mg • Ginkgo Biloba 50 mg • Yerba Mate 50 mg • Irish Moss 50 mg • White Yellow 50 mg • Cayenne 25 mg.

Ultra-Synergist E **- Pure Encapsulations**
Each softgel capsule contains: Natural Vitamin E (from mixed tocopherols) 1000 mg: D-alpha tocopherol 336 mg, D-beta tocopherol 25 mg, D-gamma tocopherol 400 mg, D-delta tocopherol 117 mg.

Ultra-Two softgels **- Nature's Plus**
Three softgels contain: Vitamin A (beta carotene) 25,000 IU • Vitamin C (ascorbic acid) 100 mg • Vitamin D (ergocalciferol) 200 IU • Vitamin E (D-alpha tocopheryl succinate) 100 IU • Thiamin (vitamin B1, as thiamine HCl) 100 mg • Riboflavin (vitamin B2) 100 mg • Niacin (niacinamide) 100 mg • Vitamin B6 (pyridoxine HCl) 100 mg • Folate (folic acid) 400 mcg • Vitamin B12 (as cyanocobalamin) 100 mcg • Biotin 100 mcg • Pantothenic Acid (as calcium pantothenate) 100 mg • Calcium (as amino acid chelate complex) 40 mg • Iron (as amino acid chelate/complex) 25 mg • Iodine (from kelp) 150 mcg • Magnesium (as amino acid chelate/complex) 20 mg • Zinc (as amino acid chelate/complex) 20 mg • Selenium (as amino acid complex) 10 mcg • Manganese (as amino acid chelate/complex) 6.1 mg • Chromium (as amino acid chelate) 15 mcg • Potassium (as amino acid complex) 15 mg • PABA (para-aminobenzoic acid) 100 mg • Inositol 100 mg • Choline (bitartrate) 42 mg • Rutin (from saphora japonica leaf) 25 mg • Bioflavonoids (citrus limon) 25 mg • Betaine HCl (from beet molasses) 25 mg • Boron (as citrate, glycinate, aspartate) 3 mg. Other Ingredients: Gelatin, Carob, Glycerin, Purified Water, Soy Oil, Rice Bran, Papaya Fruit, Watercress, Parsley Leaf, Pacific Kelp, Alfalfa Sprout, Green Cabbage Leaf, Rice Polishings, Acerola Cherry (malpighia glabra fruit), Wheat Germ Flour, Bromelain (from pineapple fruit), Chlorella, Date (phoenix dactylifera fruit), Barley Grass, Spirulina, Black Currant Seed, Bee Pollen, Rose Hips (rosa canina fruit), Garlic Bulb, Oat Leaf and Stem, Apple Pectin, Broccoli Floret, Spinach Leaf, Carrot Root, Chinese Cabbage (brassica campestris leaf), Brown Rice, Sunflower Oil, Fig (ficus carica fruit), Beet (beta vulgaris leaf), Lecithin.

Ultra-Zyme **- Nature's Plus**
Two tablets contain: Pancreatin 4X quadruple strength 325 mg, supplying: Amylase 32500 USP Units, Protease (Trypsin & Chymotrypsin) 32500 USP Units, Lipase (Pancreatic lipase) 2600 USP Units • Glutamic Acid HCL 200 mg • Acidophilus (Lactobacillus, Bulgaricus, Bifidus) 150 mg • Ox Bile 120 mg • Bromelain, 1:10, pineapple, 100 mg • Pepsin NF 1:15000 65 mg • Malt Diastase 65 mg • Cellulase • Hemicellulase • 5 mg • Lactase 5 mg. Base: Peppermint, Fennel seed, Ginger & Rosemary.
See Editor's Note No. 14.

Ultrim-fx **- Johnston-Keay Laboratories, Inc**
Two capsules contain: Vitamin B6 30 mg • Vitamin B12 • Folic Acid 250 mcg • Chromium (as chromium nicotinate) 70 mcg • L-Phenylalanine 100 mg • Adenosine Monophosphate 50 mg • Carboxymethylcellulose 500 mg • Tyrosine Hydroxylase 10 mg • Activated Charcoal 10 mg.

Umcka ColdCare Alcohol Free Drops **- Nature's Way**
Active Ingredient: Pelargonium sidoides 1x. Other Ingredients: Purified Water, Vegetable-Source Glycerin.
See Editor's Note No. 1.

Umcka ColdCare Cherry Syrup **- Nature's Way**
Active Ingredients: Pelargonium sidoides 1x. Other Ingredients: Aronia Juice, Citric Acid, Fructose, Natural Cherry Flavor, Purified Water, Vegetable-source Glycerin.
See Editor's Note No. 1.

Umcka ColdCare Menthol Syrup **- Nature's Way**
Active Ingredient: Pelargonium sidoides 1x. Other Ingredients: Alcohol (8.2%), Fructose, Spearmint Flavor, Purified Water, Vegetable-source Glycerin.
See Editor's Note No. 1.

Umcka ColdCare Original Drops **- Nature's Way**
Active Ingredient: Pelargonium sidoides 1x. Other Ingredients: Purified Water, Vegetable-Source Glycerin.
See Editor's Note No. 1.

Umph **- Frontsiders, LLC**
Each tablet contains: Vitamin B6 0.75 mg • Sodium 188 mg • Potassium 116 mg • Ginseng root (panax) 30 mg • Caffeine 99 mg. Other Ingredients: Citric Acid, Sorbitol, Polyethylene Glycol, Natural Flavors, Acesulfame Potassium.

Una De Gato-Go! Cat's Claw Extract **- Wakunaga of America**
Each capsule contains: Cat's Claw standardized extract (Una De Gato)(bark) 250 mg. Other Ingredients: Cellulose, Colloidal Silica, Magnesium Stearate (vegetable source).

UnDo **- Lindsey Duncan's Home Nutrition**
Blended Fiber Formula: Each tablet contains: Proprietary blend 495 mg: Fiber blend: [Apple pectin, Beet fiber, Barley fiber, Psyllium husk, Karaya Gum, Oat Bran] • Fennel seed • Buckthorn bark • Cascara Sagrada bark • Kava Kava root • Red Raspberry leaf • Ginger root • Capsicum Fruit. Blended Herb Formula: Each tablet contains: Proprietary blend 368 mg: Panax Ginseng root • Ginkgo Biloba leaf extract (50:1) • Garlic bulb • Milk Thistle extract (80% Silymarin) • Echinacea Angustifolia leaf extract (6:1) • Cat's Claw bark • Uva Ursi leaf • Alfalfa leaf • Hawthorn berries • Licorice root • Ginger root • Rosemary leaf • Oregon Grape root • Turmeric root • Dandelion leaf • Burdock root • Yellow Dock root • Mullein leaf • Fenugreek seed • Horsetail herb • Safflower flower • Butcher's Broom root • Red root • Capsicum fruit • Schizandra fruit.

Unique E **- A.C. Grace Company**
Mixed Tocopherols concentrate pure Vitamin E 700 mg, 400 IU high D-Gamma Tocopherol.

Univase **- Rocky Fork Formulas**
Each tablet contains: Pancreatin 4X (equivalend to 1250 mg) 313 mg • Papain 150 mg • Bromelain 150 mg • Trypsin 125 mg • Alpha-Chymotrypsin 3 mg • Superoxide Dismutase (SOD) 50 mcg • Catalase 200 units • L-Glutathione 10 mg • Lipase 50 mg • Amylase 50 mg • Rutin 100 mg • Lyophilized Calf Thymus 55 mg • Zinc (as gluconate) 1.4 mg.
This product was formerly known as Megazyme.
See Editor's Note No. 14.

Univase Forte **- Rocky Fork Formulas**
Each tablet contains: Pancreatin (4X, equivalent to 1250 mg) 313 mg • Papain 150 mg • Bromelain 150 mg • Trypsin 125 mg • Alpha-Chymotrypsin 45 mg • Super Oxide Dismutase (SOD) 50 mcg • Catalase 200 units • L-Glutathione 10 mg • Lipase 50 mg • Amylase 50 mg • Rutin 100 mg • Lyophilized Calf Thymus 55 mg • Zinc (as gluconate) 1.4 mg.
This product was formerly known as Megazyme Forte.
See Editor's Note No. 14.

Up Your Gas (Ma Huang Formula) **- National Health Products**
Each tablet contains: Proprietary Blend 1200 mg: Guarana seed (aullinia cupana) • Ma Huang herb (ephedra sinica, standardized 6% extract) 285 mg • Korean Ginseng root (panax ginseng) • Bee Pollen • Vitamin E (d-alpha-tocopheryl acetate) • Spirulina Blue-Green Algae (spirulina pratensis) • Gotu Kola (centella asiatica) • Inosine • Octacosanol • Pyridoxal-Alpha-Ketoglutarate • Wheat Grass (triticum aestivum) • Cayenne pepper (capsicum frutescens) • Lipoic Acid • Cytochrome C. In Calcium, Magnesium, Potassium Succinate Base.
See Editor's Note No. 21 and No. 30.

Some Brand Name Natural Products - What they Contain

www.NaturalDatabase.com contains MANY more listings than appear here.
Editor's Notes are located on pages 2155-2163.

Up Your Gas (No Ma Huang) **-** National Health Products
Each tablet contains: Niacin 15 mg • Guarana seed standardized extract (caffeine 90 mg) 450 mg • Kola nut standardized extract (caffeine 10 mg) 50 mg • Yerba Mate leaf 125 mg • Panax Ginseng root standardized ginseng (ginsenosides 8 mg) 100 mg • Herbal Base 65 mg: Gotu Kola leaf, Bee Pollen, Barley Grass, Spirulina, Wheat Grass • Krebs Cycle Chelates 65 mg: Calcium Carbonate, Magnesium Carbonate, Potassium Citrate • Activator Base 25 mg: Cayenne Pepper fruit, Octacosanol, Ginkgo Biloba leaf extract, Inosine, Lipoic Acid. Other Ingredients: Dicalcium Phosphate, Microcrystalline Cellulose, Croscarmellose Sodium, Stearic Acid, Magnesium Stearate, Silica, Pharmaceutical Glaze.

Upper Di-GST **-** Nutri-Quest Rx
Each tablet contains: L-Glutamine 50 mg • Okra 25 mg • Stomach 125 mg • Folic Acid 250 mcg • Vitamin A 1500 IU • Parotid 10 mg • Aloe Vera 5 mg • N-Acetyl Glucosamine 50 mg • Bromelain 25 mg • Duodenum 125 mg • Deglycerrized Licorice root 156 mg • Cabigen extract (Vitamin U) 20 mg • Slippery Elm 25 mg • Magnesium Chelate 75 mg.
See Editor's Note No. 14.

UpSwing **-** Life Enhancement Products, Inc.
Three capsules contain: Vitamin C (from niacinamide ascorbate) 75 mg • Niacin (from niacinamide ascorbate) 25 mg • Vitamin B6 (from pyridoxal 5-phosphate) 10 mg • Magnesium (from magnesium aspartate) 200 mg • Potassium (from potassium aspartate) 99 mg • L-Phenylalanine 200 mg • DHEA 30 mg • 5-HTP 25 mg • Hypericum (from St. John's wort extract, flower) 15 mg. Other Ingredients: Silicone Dioxide, Gelatin.

UpTime Herbal **-** Uptime Sports Nutrition
Three caplets contain: Vitamin A (beta-carotene) (10% DV) 501 IU • Vitamin C (150% DV) 90 mg • Thiamin (thiamin mononitrate) (100% DV) 1.5 mg • Riboflavin (100% DV) 1.71 mg • Niacin (niacinamide) (225% DV) 45 mg • Vitamin B6 (pyridoxine hydrochloride) (300% DV) 6 mg • Folate (folic acid) (98% DV) 390 mcg • Vitamin B12 (cyanocabalamin) (300% DV) 18 mcg • Pantothenic Acid (Calcium pantothenate) (300% DV) 30 mg • Chromium (aspartate) (250% DV) 300 mcg • Molybdenum (amino acid chelate) (300% DV) 225 mcg • Vanadium (vanadyl sulfate) 2.85 mcg • Herbal Powder Base 1014 mg: Green Tea leaf, Dong Quai, Schisandra berry, Kola Nut seed, Ashwaganda leaf, Organic Bee Pollen, Yerba Mate leaf, Siberian Ginseng root, Papain (from papaya), Long Pepper fruit, Jujube fruit, Gamma Oryzanol, Wild Yam root, White Ginseng root, Fo-ti root, Ligustrum fruit, Astragalus root, Ginger root.

UpTime Nutritional Fitness **-** Uptime Sports Nutrition
Three caplets contain: Vitamin C (as ascorbic acid) (1500% DV) 900 mg • Calcium (as Calcium carbonate) (70% DV) 700 mg • Chromium (as picolinate) (8% DV) 10 mcg • Uptime Power Base: Spirulina Blue Green Algae, Wheat Grass, Alfalfa leaf, Caffeine, Papaya fruit, Silica, Cayenne fruit, Siberian Ginseng extract, Echinacea herb, Ginkgo Biloba extract, Carnitine (tartrate), Coenzyme Q10, Chromium (picolinate) 750 mg.

Urban Air Defense **-** Source Naturals
Two tablets contain: Vitamin A (Beta Carotene 12500 IU and Palmitate 5000 IU) 17500 IU • Vitamin C (Magnesium Ascorbate, Vitamin C and Manganese Ascorbate) 500 mg • Fat-Soluble Vitamin C (from 186 mg of Ascorbyl Palmitate) 80 mg • Vitamin E (D-Alpha Tocopheryl)(Natural) 200 IU • Magnesium (Ascorbate) 30 mg • Zinc (OptiZinc Monomethionine) 15 mg • Manganese (Ascorbate) 5 mg • Copper (Sebacate) 750 mcg • Selenium (as L-Selenomethionine) 100 mcg • Quercetin 200 mg • N-Acetyl Cysteine 100 mg • Silymarin (Milk Thistle seed extract) 50 mg • Ginkgo Biloba extract 24% (50:1) 5 mg • Hawthorn berry 150 mg • Rosemary 150 mg • Schizandra 125 mg • Marshmallow root 85 mg • Astragalus 60 mg.

UriCare with Cranberry **-** TriLight Herbs
Dandelion • Marshmallow • Cornsilk • Cleavers herb • Cranberry.

Urinary & Kidney Care **-** Wellness for Women
Each capsule contains: Vitamin C (as ascorbic acid) 50 mg • Thiamin USP (as thiamin HCl; vitamin B-1) 12.5 mg • Riboflavin (vitamin B-2) 12.5 mg • Niacinamide 12.5 mg • Vitamin B-6 (as pyridoxine HCl) 12.5 mg • Folic Acid 100 mcg • Vitamin B-12 (as cyanocobalamin) 100 mcg • Biotin 12.5 mcg • Pantothenic Acid (as d-calcium pantothenate) 12.5 mg • Potassium (from potassium gluconate and potassium chloride) 99 mg • Cranberry extract (10:1 concentrate) 200 mg • Juniper berry powder 50 mg • Corn Silk 25 mg • Uva Ursi 25 mg • Choline (as choline bitartrate) 12.5 mg • Inositol 12.5 mg • PABA (para-aminobenzoic acid) 12.5 mg.

Urinary Formula **-** Nature's Way
Three capsules contain: Cleavers herb 180 mg • Corn Silk 150 mg • Cranberry concentrate fruit 600 mg • Dandelion leaf 180 mg • Goldenseal stem, leaf, flower 60 mg • Marshmallow root 180 mg. Other Ingredients: Gelatin, Magnesium Stearate, Millet.

Urinary Support **-** Gaia Herbs
Three capsules contain: Uva Ursi extract (arctostaphylos uva ursi) 370 mg • Pipsissewa leaf (chimaphila umbellata) 92 mg • Coptis rhizome (coptis chenensis) 50 mg • Echinacea (echinacea pupurea flowering top, echinacea pupurea root, echinacea angustifolia root, echinacea purpurea seed) 30 mg • Usnea lichen (usnea spp.) 14 mg. Other Ingredients: Vegetable Glycerin, Vegetable Cellulose (capsule).

Uriphron **-** PhytoPharmica
Two tablets contain: Birch leaf 5.5:1 extract (betula pendula) 218 mg • European Goldenrod aerial part 5.9:1 extract (solidago virgaurea) 272 mg • Java Tea leaf 6.2:1 extract (orthosiphon aristatus) 194 mg.

Uriplex **-** Enzymatic Therapy
Each tablet contains: Goldenrod extract 5.9:1 (Solidago virgaurea) 136 mg • Birch Leaf extract 5.5:1 (Betula pendula) 109 mg • Orthosiphon Leaf extract 6.2:1 (O. aristata) 97 mg.

UritraX **-** Xymogen
Each 1/2 tsp (0.9 g) serving contains: D-Mannose 0.9 g.

Usanimals **-** USANA Health Sciences
One tablet contains: Vitamin A (as Beta Carotene) 2500 IU • Vitamin C (as Ascorbic Acid and Calcium Ascorbate) 100 mg • Vitamin D (as Cholecalciferol) 150 IU • Vitamin E (as D-Alpha Tocopheryl Succinate 36 IU • Vitamin K (as Phylloquinone) 10 mcg • Thiamine (as Thiamine Mononitrate) 0.75 mg • Riboflavin 1 mg • Niacin (as Niacinamide) 10 mg • Vitamin B6 (as Pyridoxine Hydrochloride) 1.25 mg • Folate (as Folic Acid) 200 mcg • Vitamin B12 (as Cyanocobalamin) 3 mcg • Biotin 15 mcg • Pantothenic Acid (as D-Calcium Pantothenate) 2.5 mg • Calcium (as Carbonate and Ascorbate) 75 mg • Iodine (as Sodium Iodide) 37.5 mcg • Magnesium (as Oxide and Amino Acid Chelate) 25 mg • Zinc (as Citrate) 2.5 mg • Selenium (as Amino Acid Complex) 10 mcg • Manganese (as Amino Acid Chelate) 0.5 mg • Chromium (as Amino Acid Chelate) 10 mcg • Molybdenum (as Amino Acid Chelate) 12.5 mcg • Hesperidin (Citrus SPP. L.) Fruit 4 mg. Other Ingredients: Xylitol, Natural Flavor Blend, Vegetable-Derived Stearic Acid, Ascorbyl Palmitate, Collodial Silicon Dioxide.

USF Ointment **-** Standard Process, Inc.
Lard • Lanolin • Linseed oil • Soybean Lecithin • Beeswax • Bovine Orchic extract • Fragrance.

Usnea Uva Ursi Supreme **-** Gaia Herbs
Forty drops contain: Proprietary Blend 90 mg: Usnea lichen extract (usnea spp.), Uva Ursi leaf extract (arctostaphylos uva ursi), Pipsissewa herb extract (chimaphila umbellata), Echinacea Supreme (echinacea angustifolia root, echinacea purpurea root, flower head and seed) • 40-50% Pure Grain Alcohol USP • Spring Water.

Usnea-Propolis Virtue **-** Blessed Herbs
Usnea lichen • Pau d'Arco bark • Echinacea Angustifolia root • Propolis • Goldenseal root • Myrrh Gum • Grain Alcohol, Water.

U-Tract **-** Progressive Labs
Each level tsp contains: Pure Mannoplex D-Alpha-Mannose 1.9 g.

Some Brand Name Natural Products - What they Contain

www.NaturalDatabase.com contains MANY more listings than appear here.
Editor's Notes are located on pages 2155-2163.

Utrophin PMG - Standard Process, Inc.
Each tablet contains: Proprietary Blend 192 mg: Bovine Uterus PMG extract, Magnesium Citrate. Other Ingredients: Calcium Lactate, Cellulose, Calcium stearate.
See Editor's Note No. 14.

Uva Ursi - Ortho Molecular Products
Each capsule contains: Uva Ursi leaf extract (standardized to contain 20% arbutin) 250 mg. Other Ingredients: Natural Vegetable Capsules, Magnesium Stearate, Microcrystalline Cellulose.

Uva Ursi Formula - Quest
Each caplet contains: Uva Ursi leaf powder (Arctostaphylos uva-ursi) 85 mg • Dandelion root powder (Taraxacum officinale) 60 mg • Gentian root powder (Gentiana lutea) 55 mg • Huckleberry leaf powder (Vaccinium Myrtillus) 55 mg • Parsley leaf powder (Petroselinum crispum) 45 mg • Buchu leaf powder (Barosma betulina) 35 mg • Kelp powder (Fucus vesiculosis) 35 mg • Raspberry leaf powder (Rubus idaeus) 35 mg • Saw Palmetto berry powder (Serenoa serrulata/repens) 35 mg • Bladderwrack powder (Fuccus vesiculosis) 20 mg. Other Ingredients: Calcium Phosphate, Microcrystalline Cellulose, Vegetable Stearin, Croscarmellose Sodium, Magnesium Stearate.

U-Viva Vitamin E (Chewable) - Uviva
Each tablet contains: Vitamin E (d-alpha tocopheryl succinate) 400 IU. Other Ingredients: Sucrose, Wheat Starch, Talc Purified, Kaolin, CL 75470, Gelatin.

V12 (V-12) - SAN Nutrition
Each 9.5 g serving contains: TriCreatine Malate 3 g • Betaine-Glycocyamine 1.5 g • NitroArginine (arginine alpha-ketoglutarate) 1 g • NAG (N-acetyl-L-glutamine) 1 g • Micronized Taurine 1 g. Other Ingredients: Citric Acid, Natural Flavors, Acesulfame K, Aspartame, Orange Extract Powder, Calcium Silicate.

V2G - EAS, Inc.
Each capsule contains: Vanadyl Sulfate 7.5 mg • Taurine 800 mg • Selenium (Sodium Selenate) 33 mcg.

Vaginitis - Hyland's
Two tablets contain: Natrum Muriaticum 12X • Candida Albicans 30X • Kreosotum 12X • Carbolicum Acidum 12X. Base: Lactose.
See Editor's Note No. 1.

Vag-Mend - The Herbalist
Golden Seal root • Thuja leaf • Usnea lichen • Bayberry root bark • Echinacea root • Red Raspberry leaf.

Valaxin - Nutraceutics Corp.
Each caplet contains: Niacinamide 10 mg • Magnesium (as magnesium oxide) 10 mg • Suanzaorentang Extract (dried root) 400 mg • Valeriana Officinalis Extract (dried root) 400 mg • Passiflora Incarnata Extract (aerial parts) 25 mg • Proprietary Blend 150 mg: Bupleurum Chinensis (root), L-Glycine, Gaba (as gamma aminobutyric acid). Other Ingredients: Magnesium Stearate, DiCalcium Phosphate, Microcrystalline Cellulose, FD&C Lake Blue #1, Yellow #6.

Valer-A-Somn - PhytoPharmica
Each capsule contains: Valerian extract (Valeriana officinalis) - (standardized to contain 0.2%-0.8% valerenic acids) 150 mg.
See Editor's Note No. 21.

Valerian - Pure Encapsulations
Each vegetable capsule contains: Valerian root extract (valeriana officinalis, standardized to contain 0.8% valerenic acids) 250 mg • Vitamin C (as ascorbyl palmitate) 5 mg.

Valerian - Pharmanex
Each capsule contains: Valerian root extract (6:1) (Valerian officinalis) 350 mg. Other Ingredients: Gelatin, Rice Flour, Magnesium Stearate, Silicon Dioxide.

Valerian - Leiner Health Products
Two caplets contain: Valerian extract (Valeriana officinalis) root 200 mg. Other Ingredients: Calcium Carbonate, Cellulose, Maltodextrin, Hydroxypropyl Methylcellulose, Silicon Dioxide, Polyethylene Glycol 3350, Croscarmellose Sodium, Hydroxypropyl Cellulose, Pharmaceutical Glaze, Crospovidone, Magnesium Stearate, Blue 1 Lake, Polysorbate 80, Titanium Dioxide, Sodium Citrate.

Valerian - Jamieson
Each capsule contains: Valerian Root 400 mg.

Valerian 2000 - Golden Glow Natural Health Products
Each capsule contains: Valerian root extract (valeriana officinalis) 2000 mg.

Valerian 400 - Enzymatic Therapy
Two capsules contain: Valerian root extract (valeriana officinalis, standardized to 0.8% valerenic acids) 800 mg. Other Ingredients: Gelatin, Magnesium Stearate, Silicon Dioxide, Titanium Dioxide.

Valerian Extract - Vital Nutrients
Each capsule contains: Valeriana Officinalis root extract (standardized to 0.8% valerenic acids) 250 mg.

Valerian Extract - Nature's Way
Two capsules contain: Calcium 30 mg • Valerian (dried extract) 220 mg • Valerian root 800 mg. Other Ingredients: Gelatin.

Valerian Nighttime - Nature's Way
Each tablet contains: Lemon Balm dried extract 80 mg • Valerian Nighttime (dried valerian extract) 160 mg.

Valerian Plus - PhysioLogics
Each capsule contains: Valerian (0.8% Valerenic Acids, 1.52 mg) 190 mg • Chamomile 90 mg • Peppermint 90 mg • Propolis 45 mg • Passion flower 45 mg • American Ginseng 40 mg.

Valerian Poppy Supreme - Gaia Herbs
Forty drops contain: Proprietary Blend 90 mg: Valerian root (valeriana officinalis), Fresh Skullcap herb (scutellaria lateriflora), California Poppy herb (eschscholzia californía), Kava Kava rhizome and root (piper methysticum), Passionflower vine (passiflora incarnata), German Chamomile flowers (matricaria recutita), Mugwort herb (artemisia vulgaris), 50-60% Pure Grain Alcohol USP.

Valerian Root - Gaia Herbs
Two capsules contain: Valerian root (valeriana off.; 0.9% (1.8 mg) valerenic acid) 50 mg. Other Ingredients: Vegetable Glycerin, Vegetable Cellulose (capsule).

Valerian Root - Aboca USA, Inc
Two capsules contain: Valerian root WPC (whole phytocomplex concentrate, valeriana officinalis, standardized to 0.24% total valerenic acids, yielding 0.6 mg per capsule) 496 mg. Other Ingredients: Gelatin.

Valerian Root - Olympian Labs
Each capsule contains: Valerian root 500 mg.

Valerian Root 450 mg - Puritan's Pride
Each capsule contains: Valerian root (valeriana officinalis) 450 mg. Other Ingredients: Gelatin.

Valerian Root Concentrated Herb 1000 mg - Puritan's Pride
Each softgel contains: Valerian root (valeriana officinalis, from 250 mg of 4:1 extract) 1000 mg. Other Ingredients: Soybean Oil, Gelatin, Glycerin, Beeswax / Soybean Oil Mixture, Lecithin, Caramel Color, Titanium Dioxide Color.

Valerian Root Extract, 100mg - Nature Made
Two softgels contain: Valerian root extract 200 mg: Valerenic Acid 1.6 mg.

Valerian with Lemon Balm - Pro Health
Two tablets contain: Valerian root 320 mg • Lemon Balm 160 mg. Other Ingredients: Cellulose, Stearic Acid, Magnesium Stearate, Silicon Dioxide, Croscarmellose Sodium, Titanium Dioxide, HPMC.

Valerian-400 - PhytoPharmica
Two capsules contain: Valerian (Valeriana officinalis) root extract (standardized to a minimum of 0.8% valerenic acids) 800 mg. See Editor's Note No. 21.

Valerianets - At Last Naturals, Inc.
Three tablets contain: Vitamin B1 (thiamine HCl) 0.9 mg • Vitamin B2 9riboflavin) 0.3 mg • Niacin 1.4 mg • Vitamin B5 39 mcg • Folic Acid 15 mcg • Biotin 3 mcg • Pantothenic Acid 0.1 mg • Valerian root extract 150 mg • Inositol 6.7 mg • Choline 5.7 mg • PABA 57 mcg.

Valerian-Primrose Virtue - Blessed Herbs
Valerian root • Primrose flower & leaf • California Poppy flower & leaf • Hops strobile • Wild Lettuce • Passion flower • Scullcap • Grain alcohol & Distilled Water.

Val-Tran - Atrium Biotechnologies
Each tablet contains: Valerian (standardized extract) 100 mg • Vitamin B6 5 mg • Magnesium Gluconate 50 mg • Magnesium Oxide 50 mg. In a base containing Chamomile, Anise & Peppermint.

Vanadyl Factors - Jarrow Formulas
Each capsule contains: Vanadyl Sulfate 7.5 mg • Taurine 800 mg • L-Arginine 100 mg. Other Ingredients: Rice Powder, Magnesium Stearate, Silicon Dioxide, Gelatin.

Vanadyl Factors - Olympia Nutrition
Vanadyl Sulfate + 800 mg Taurine.

Vanadyl pH - SportPharma
Each capsule contains: Vanadyl Sulfate 7.5 mg.

Vanadyl Plus with Chromium - Olympian Labs
Each capsule contains: Chromium Picolinate 200 mcg • Vanadyl Sulfate 10 mg • Niacin 20 mg.

Vanadyl Sulfate - Ultimate Nutrition
Each tablet contains: Vanadyl Sulfate 10 mg.

Vanadyl Sulfate - Life Extension
Each capsule contains: Vanadyl Sulfate 10 mg • Choline Complex 25 mg.

Vanadyl Sulfate with Niacin - Olympian Labs
Each capsule contains: Vanadyl Sulfate 20 mg • Niacin 25 mg.

Vancol (Cholesterol Lowering Plan) - Omnicron International
Two chewable tablets contain: Beta Sitosterol 10 mg • Psyllium 200 mg • Chromium from Picolinate 50 mcg with natural Quinone Antioxidants. In a base of Calcium Carbonate & Magnesium Stearate.

Vanilla PerfectRx - Nature's Best
Chocolate flavor contains: Perfect Unique Protein Blend: Milk Protein Isolate, Calcium Caseinate, Whey Protein Concentrates, Egg Albumin • Maltodextrin • Potassium Chloride • Potassium Citrate • Sodium Chloride • Sodium Citrate • Dipotassium Phosphate • Natural & Artificial Flavors • Aspartame • Magnesium Oxide • Choline Bitartrate • Cellulose • Ascorbic Acid • D-Alpha-Tocopheryl Acetate • Ferrous Fumarate • Niacin • Biotin • Xanthan gum • Vitamin A Palmitate • Zinc • Oxide • D-Calcium Pantothenate • Vitamin K • Manganese Sulfate • Beta-Carotene • Copper Sulfate • Pyridoxine HCl • Riboflavin • Thiamine HCl • L-Glutamine • Chromium Picolinate • Cobalamin Concentrate (vitamin B12) • Vitamin D (D3) • Folic Acid • Sodium Molybdate • Potassium Iodide • Sodium Selenite.

Vanilla Phosphagain 2 - EAS, Inc.
Each 59 gram serving contains: Potassium 730 mg • Chromium 50 mcg • Selenium 30 mcg • Manganese 1 mg • Vitamin K 40 mcg • Molybdenum 60 mcg • Choline 80 mg. Ingredients: Nitrogenin 2 proprietary Protein/Nitrogen reinforcing matrix [Milk Protein Isolate, Calcium Caseinate, L-Glutamine, Taurine, Calcium Alpha-Ketoglutarate (AKG) & Egg Albumin] • Phosphagen (HPCE Pure Creatine Monohydrate) • Maltodextrin, Dextrose • Vitamin & Mineral Blend: Potassium Phosphate, Potassium Citrate, Salt, Magnesium Oxide, Choline Bitartrate, Disodium Phosphate, Beta-Carotene, Ascorbic Acid, Dl-Alpha Tocopheryl Acetate, Ferrous Fumarate, Niacin, Zinc Oxide, D-Calcium Pantothenate, Copper Sulfate,Vitamin A Palmitate, Manganese Sulfate, Chromium Citrate, Pyridoxine Hydrochloride, Riboflavin, Thiamine Hydrochloride, Sodium Molybdate, Vitamin D (as Vitamin D3), Folic Acid, Biotin, Potassium Iodide, Sodium Selenate, Vitamin K, & Cyanocobalamin • Corn Syrup Solids • Partially Hydrogenated Canola oil • Xanthan Gum • Natural & Artificial Flavors • Sodium RNA • Soy Lecithin • Aspartame • Carrageenan • Phenylalanine.

VariCare - Enzymatic Therapy
Each tablet contains: Butcher's Broom extract (Ruscus aculeatus) standardized to contain 9 - 11% Saponins calculated as Ruscogenin 150 mg • Horse Chestnut extract (Aesculus hippocastanum) standardized to contain 20 - 22% Saponins calculated as Escin 125 mg • Gotu Kola Phytosome (Centella asiatica) standardized to contain 30 - 35% Centella Triterpenes 15 mg.

Varicosin - PhytoPharmica
Two tablets contain: Butcher's Broom root and rhizome extract (ruscus aculeatus, standardized to contain 9-11% saponins calculated as ruscogenins) 300 mg • Gotu Kola leaf phytosome (centella asiatica, one part gotu kola extract, standardized to contain 90% centella triterpenes, bound to two parts phosphatidylcholine) 30 mg • Horse Chestnut seed extract (aesculus hippocastanum, standardized to contain 20% triterpene glycosides calculated as escin) 250 mg.

Vascular Complete - Rexall - Sundown
Each tablet contains: Vitamin C 33.3 mg • Calcium 260 mg • Sodium 10 mg • Chondroitin Sulfate 66.7 mg • Alpha-Ketoglutaric Acid (from calcium alpha-ketoglutarate) 33.3 mg • Citric Acid 33.3 mg • L-Arginine (from L-arginine HCl) 33.3 mg • L-Lysine (from L-lysine HCl) 33.3 mg • L-Proline 33.3 mg • L-Ornithine (from L-ornithine HCl) 16.7 mg • Choline (from choline bitartrate) 16.7 mg • Silica 7 mg • Vascular Complete base blend: Rose Hips and seeds extract (Rosa canina), Citrus Bioflavonoids, rutin, Hesperidin, Acerola Fruit extract (malpighia punicifolia) 7 mg. Other Ingredients: Calcium Carbonate, Cellulose, Croscarmellose Sodium, Hydroxypropyl Methylcellulose, Talc, Magnesium Stearate, Riboflavin (colorant), Titanium Dioxide, Calcium Sulfate, Polysaccharides.

Vascular Maintenance - Enzymes, Inc.
Each capsule contains: Vitamin E (100% from d-Alpha Tocopheryl Acid Succinate) 20 IU • Proprietary Herbal Blend 350 mg: Garlic bulb extract, Guggulipids extract, Lecithin (Soy Phospholipids), Turmeric root extract, Flaxseed oil powder, Globe Artichoke leaf extract • Proprietary Enzyme Blend 150 mg: Lipase, pHysioProtease. Other Ingredients: Plant Cellulose, Water.

Vascular Support Formula - The Vitamin Factory
Each tablet contains: Vitamin C (Ascorbic Acid) 500 mg • Pycnogenol (Maritime Pine bark extract) 100 mg.

Vasculin - Standard Process, Inc.
Two tablets contain: Proprietary Blend 638 mg: Bovine Heart PMG extract, Nutritional Yeast, Veal Bone PMG extract, Rice bran, Bovine Liver, Oat flour, Porcine Duodenum, Inositol, Dried Pea vine juice, Bovine Adrenal Cytosol extract, Dried Beet root juice, Ribonucleic Acid, Defatted Wheat germ, Choline Bitartrate, Dried Alfalfa juice, Dried Buckwheat leaf juice, Buckwheat seed, Mushroom, Alfalfa flour, Bovine Spleen, Ovine Spleen, Soybean Lecithin • Vitamin C 3.8 mg • Vitamin E 1.1 IU • Thiamine 0.3 mg • Niacin 10.9 mg • Vitamin B6 0.6 mg • Vitamin B12 0.3 mcg • Calcium 19.4 mg • Sodium 10 mg • Potassium 10 mg. Other Ingredients: Honey, Gelatin, Cellulose.

Vascuzyme - Ortho Molecular Products
Each tablet contains: Pancreatin 6X 200 mg • Papain 100 mg • Bromelain 75 mg • Rutin 60 mg • Thymus 35 mg • Trypsin 35 mg • Amylase 15 mg • Lipase 15 mg • Lysozyme 10 mg • Cellulase 2 mg • Alpha Chymotrypsin 1 mg. Other Ingredients: Dicalcium Phosphate, Magnesium Stearate, Sorbitol, Pharmaceutical Glaze.

Some Brand Name Natural Products - What they Contain

www.NaturalDatabase.com contains MANY more listings than appear here.
Editor's Notes are located on pages 2155-2163.

Vasko - Ayurvedanta
Triphala: Indian Gooseberry (amla), Terminalia Chebula, Terminalia Bellerika • Tinospora Cordifolia • Kummifora Mugul • Terminalia Arjuna • Curcuma Longa • Bohrevia Diffusa • Cyperus Rotundum • Nimba • Picrorhiza Kurroa (katki) • Trikadu: Dry Ginger, Piper Longum, Piper Nigrum.

VasoRect - Real Health Laboratories
Each capsule contains: L-Arginine 625 mg • Calcium 12.5 mg.

Vasotensin - Metagenics
Four tablets contain: Bonito peptides (sarda orientalis) 2 g.

Vazoplex - Gerovicap
Propylene Glycol • Deionized Water • Hydroxyethyl Cellulose • Wild Yam extract • Nicotinate • DHEA • Menthol • L-Arginine • Methylparaben.

Veg E-Gems - J. R. Carlson Laboratories, Inc.
Each softgel contains: Vitamin E (as D-alpha tocopheryl acetate) 400 IU.

Vege Fuel - TwinLab
Pure Isolated Soy (All-Vegetable) Protein 100%.

Vege Fuel (Aspartame Free) - TwinLab
Pure Isolated Soy (All-Vegetable) Protein 100%.

Veg-Easy - Progressive Labs
Two tablets contain: Blend 1400 mg: Broccoli powder • Spirulina • Wheat Grass • Alfalfa powder • Spinach powder • Cabbage powder • Green Tea • Carrot • Barley grass • Parsley • Beet root powder • Kale • Oat fiber medium • Brussels Sprouts • Lipase • Amylase • Protease • Cellulase • Powdered Cellulose • Beet leaf powder • Barley fiber • Oat bran • Lactobacillus Acidophilus • Glucomannan & Calcium Gluconate.

Veg-Enzyme - Atrium Biotechnologies
Each capsule contains: Protease Enzymes 150 mg • Amylase Enzymes 140 mg • Lipase Enzymes 25 mg • Cellulase Enzymes 10 mg.

VegeSil - Flora Inc.
Silica extract • Spring Horsetail.

Vegetarian Children's Chewable - Nature's Plus
Each tablet contains: Vitamin A (beta carotene) 5000 IU • Vitamin C (with rose hips) 90 mg • Vitamin D (calciferol) 400 IU • Vitamin E (natural) 30 IU • Vitamin B1 (as thiamin HCl) 10 mg • Vitamin B2 (as riboflavin) 10 mg • Niacin (as niacinamide) 20 mg • Vitamin B6 (pyridoxine HCl) 10 mg • Folate (as folic acid) 15 mcg • Vitamin B12 (as cyanocobalamin) 15 mcg • Biotin 50 mcg • Pantothenic Acid 10 mg • Calcium (gluconate) 15 mg • Iron (gluconate) 10 mg • Iodine (kelp) 0.1 mg • Magnesium (gluconate) 0.25 mg • Zinc (gluconate) 0.25 mg • Manganese (gluconate) 50 mcg • Potassium (gluconate) 1 mg • Choline (as bitartrate) 15 mcg • Inositol 15 mcg • PABA (para-aminobenzoic acid) 0.6 mg.

Vegetarian Digestive Enzymes - NSI - Nutraceutical Sciences Institute
Each capsule contains: Protease 82,000 HUT • Amylase 8,000 SKB • Lipase 90 FIP • Cellulase 600 CU • Malt Diastase 215 DP • Invertase 525 SUMNER • Lactase 1,000 ALU • Pectinase 55 ENDO-PG • Alpha Galactosidase 300 GAL.

Vegetarian Enzyme Complex - Futurebiotics LLC
Protease 6500 HUT • Amylase 2000 DU • Cellulase 20 CU • Lipase 14.5 LU • Papaya enzyme (papain) 50 mg • Lactase 100 LacU • Alfalfa powder 50 mg • Pineapple enzyme (bromelain) 50 mg • Betaine HCl 3 mg.

Vegetarian Enzyme Complex 50 Plus - Futurebiotics LLC
Protease 8000 HUT • Amylase 4000 DU • Cellulase 100 CU • Lipase 40 LU • Invertase 0.2 IAU • Lactase 240 LacU • Papain 10 mg • Maltase 15 AGU • Gentian root 100 mg • Bromelain 10 mg • Fennel seed 50 mg.

Vegetarian Glucosamine & MSM - NOW Foods
Two Vcaps contain: Regenasure Glucosamine HCl (vegetarian source) 1 g • Lignisul MSM (methylsulfonylmethane) 1g. Other Ingredients: Cellulose (capsule), Magnesium Stearate (vegetable source), Stearic Acid (vegetable source), Silica.
See Editor's Note No. 43.

Vegetarian Mega Minerals - Nature's Life
Two tablets contain: Boron (Citrate) 1 mg • Calcium (carbonate, citrate/malate) 1000 mg • Chromium (picolinate, polynicotinate) 200 mcg • Copper (glyconate, citrate) 1 mg • Iodine (kelp) 25 mcg • Iron (fumarate, peptonate) 15 mg • Magnesium (oxide, citrate) 500 mg • Manganese (citrate) 10 mg • Molybdenum (sodium molybdate) 20 mcg • Potassium (citrate) 99 mg • Selenium (L-selenomethionine) 100 mcg • Silicon Dioxide 20 mg • Vanadium (vanadyl sulfate) 20 mcg • Zinc (picolinate, citrate) 15 mg • Betaine HCl 100 mg • Glutamic Acid HCl 100 mg.

Vegetarian Super Multi - Futurebiotics LLC
Three tablets contain: Vitamin C 500 mg • Beta Carotene 15,000 IU • Vitamin B1 (thiamin) 20 mg • Vitamin B2 (riboflavin) 20 mg • Niacinamide 75 mg • Vitamin D 200 IU • Vitamin E (natural succinate) 100 IU • Vitamin B6 20 mg • Folic Acid 400 mcg • Vitamin B12 100 mcg • Biotin 300 mcg • Pantothenic Acid 50 mg • Inositol 50 mg. Minerals: Calcium: (carbonate, phosphate, ascorbate) 200 mg • Iron (gluconate) 8 mg • Phosphorus 100 mg • Iodine (kelp) 150 mcg • Magnesium: (oxide, ascorbate, amino acid chelate) 25 mcg • Zinc (gluconate, oxide) 25 mg • Copper (gluconate) 1 mg • Selenium (amino acid chelate) 200 mcg • Chromium (amino acid chelate) 200 mcg • Manganese (proteinate) 5 mg • Molybdenum (amino acid chelate) 25 mcg. Other Ingredients: Choline 150 mg • Para Amino Benzoic Acid (PABA) 75 mg • Bioflavonoid complex 100 mg • Sodium Phosphate 1 mg • Methionine 75 mg • Betaine HCl 75 mg • Bromelain 75 mg • RNA/DNA (chlorella) 50 mg • Chlorella 400 mg. Other Ingredients: Sea Vegetable, Ginkgo Biloba, Milk Thistle, Goldenseal, Dandelion, Burdock root, Alfalfa & Horsetail 500 mg.

Veggie Carotenoids - NOW Foods
Two VCaps contain: natural Beta-Carotene (D. salina) 12 mg/ 20000 IU • Alpha Carotene (D. salina) 400 mcg containing additional Carotenoids from D. salina algae: Xeaxanthin, Cryptoxanthin, Lycopene & Lutein • Lutein Floraglo Marigolds 3 mg • Lycopene natural source 3 mg • Broccoli concentrate (250 mcg Sulforaphane) 250 mg • Spinach concentrate (75 mcg Lutein) 100 mg • Tomato concentrate (140 mcg Lycopene) 100 mg • Kale powder 50 mg • Cabbage powder 50 mg • Brussels Sprouts powder 50 mg.

Veggie Magma - Green Foods Corp.
Each 5.3 oz jar contains: Proprietary Blend 150 g: Powdered Barley Grass juice, Maltodextrin, Alfalfa juice, Carrot juice, Tomato juice, Celery juice, dried Spinach, Cilantro juice, Broccoli juice, Broccoli Sprout juice, dried Green Pepper, Cucumber juice, dried Kale, Red Beet juice, Shiitake extract, Ginger root extract, dried Garlic, Aloe Vera.

Veggies4Life - Swanson Health Products
Two tablets contain: Alfalfa leaf powder 100 mg • Beet powder 100 mg • Broccoli powder 100 mg • Carrot powder 100 mg • Odor-Controlled Garlic bulb (PureGar® 10,000 ppm allicin potential) 100 mg • Parsley powder 100 mg • Spinach powder 100 mg • Tomato powder 100 mg • Barley Grass powder 50 mg • Cabbage powder 50 mg • Celery Seed powder 50 mg • Kale powder 50 mg • Kelp powder 50 mg • Wheat Grass powder 50 mg • Oregano powder 40 mg.

Vegie-Tabs One - Dial Herbs
Parsley • Garlic • Black Walnut hulls • Red Beet • Kelp • Dulse • Wheat bran • Wheat germ • Oat straw • Honey • Spinach • Cabbage • Carrots • Squash • Onion • Broccoli • Yellow Dock • Chickweed • Echinacea • Ginger • Cloves • Alfalfa • Alfalfa seeds • Papaya seeds • Rice Bran Capsicum • Sweet Potato.

Vegie-Tabs Two - Dial Herbs
Parsley • Hawthorne • Black Walnut hulls • Red Beet • Kelp • Dulse • Millet • Oat Straw • Honey • Spinach • Cabbage • Carrots • Squash • Onion • Broccoli • Yellow Dock • Chickweed • Echinacea • Alfalfa • Alfalfa seed • Papaya seed • Rice Bran • Capsicum • Ginger • Clove.

Vegiplex - HealthWatchers System
Brocolli • Kale • Sprouts • Spinach • Radish • Carrot • Beet • Tomato • Celery • Onion • Leek • Cauliflower • Brussel Sprouts.

Vegzyme - Progressive Labs
Each 500 mg capsule contains: Protease 10000 NP Units • Lipase 3600 NL Units • Amylase 4000 NA Units • Cellulase 30 NC Units • Papaya leaf powder 25 mg. Other Ingredients: Plant fiber. Cultures of Aspergillus Oryzae & Niger & Papaya. Naturally occurring Invertase, Maltase, Beta-Amylase, Hemicellulase, Phosphatase, Peroxidase, Catalase & Hydrolase are also present.

Vein Formula - Pharmanex
Each tablet contains: Vitamin C (as Calcium Ascorbate) 60 mg • Grape Seed Extract (as Masquelier's Original OPC's) 75 mg. Other Ingredients: Gelatin, Maltodextrin, Microcrystalline Cellulose, Magnesium stearate, Silicon dioxide.

Vein Guard Horse Chestnut Standardized - Sundown
Each capsule contains: Horse Chestnut seed extract (standardized to 18% escin, 54 mg) 300 mg. Other Ingredients: Maltodextrin, Gelatin, Magnesium Stearate.

Vein Support Formula - Baywood International
Each tablet contains: Proprietary Flavonoid Blend: Diosmin • Hesperidin 500 mg. Other Ingredients: Microcrystalline Cellulose, Maize Starch, Opadry II Orange, Povidone.

VeinAway Capsules - Quantum
Each capsule contains: Horse Chestnut seed extract (standardized to 18% escin) 300 mg • Grape seed 5:1 extract 20 mg • Bromelain 100 mg. Other Ingredients: Rice Flour, Calcium Stearate, Magnesium Silicate.

Veinaway Cream - Quantum
Purified Water • Caprylic/Capric Triglyceride • PEG-40 & PEG-100 Stearate • Cetyl, Stearyl & Benzyl Alcohol • Cyclomethicone • Sorbitan Oleate • Hydroxylated Lecithin • Horse Chestnut extract 2% • Myristyl Myristate • Dimethicone • Allantoin • Sodium Metabisulfite • Natural Vanilla Frangrance • Xanthan Gum • Vitamin K (mendaione, vitamin K3) 0.20% • Cholesterol • Aloe Vera extract • Linoleic Acid • Retinyl Palmitate • Alpha Tocopherol • Alpha-Bisabolol • Magnesium Ascorbyl Phosphate.

VeinFlow - Life Enhancement Products, Inc.
Each capsule contains: Centella Asiatica, purified triterpenes 15 mg.

Vein-Gard - NaturalCare
Active Ingredients: Horse Chestnut (aesculus hippocastanum)3X, 6X, 3C • Witch Hazel (hamamelis virginica) 1X, 4X, 3C • Honeybee (apis mellifica) 3X, 6X, 12X, 30X • Wind Flower (pulsatilla) 3X, 6X, 30X • St. Mary's Thistle (carduus marianus) 3X, 6X • Club Moss (lycopodium clavatum) 6X, 30X • Vegetable Charcoal (carbo vegetabilis) 6X, 30X • Ergot (secale cornutum) 3X. Other Ingredients: Bromelain (1500 mcu), Vitamin C, Rutin, Horse Chestnut Seed Extract (at 20% escin), Butcher's Broom (at 9-11% ruscogenin), Ginger, Cayenne, Lecithin, Gotu Kola Extract (8-10% triterpenoids), Quercetin, Grape seed extract (95% proanthocyanidins).
See Editor's Note No. 1.

Veinicin - Gero Vita International
Each capsule contains: Diosmin Complex (92% diosmin) 450 mg • Hesperidin Complex (98% bioflavonoids). Other Ingredients: Gelatin, Silicon Dioxide, Magnesium Stearate.

Veinish - WellQuest International, Inc.
Sesame Oil • Emulsifying Wax • Stearic Acid • Marine Algae • Propylene Glycol • Cetyl Alcohol • Canola Oil • Calendula Oil • Marigold Extract • Chickweed Extract • Lecithin • Essence of Lemon.

VeinoTonic II - Life Enhancement Products, Inc.
Two capsules contain: Troxerutin 300 mg • Diosmin 300 mg • Horse Chestnut seed extract 166 mg • Centella Asiatica, purified triterpenes 20 mg • Hesperidin 33 mg.

VeinPro (horse chestnut extract) - Pure Encapsulations
each vegetable capsule contains: Horse Chestnut extract (aesculus hippocastanum, standardized to contain 20-22% triterpene saponins as escin) 300 mg • Vitamin C (as ascorbyl palmitate) 4 mg.

VeinTain - Resource Wellness
Each caplet contains: Vitamin A 250 IU • Vitamin C 30 mg • Calcium 175 mg • Grape Seed extract 25 mg • Horse Chestnut extract 250 mg. Other Ingredients: Dicalcium Phosphate, Microcrystalline Cellulose, Croscarmellose Sodium, Stearic Acid, Magnesium Stearate, Silicon Dioxide, Hydroxypropyl Methylcellulose, Hydroxypropyl Cellulose, Polyethylene Glycol.

VelvaMax - Gold Mountain Trading
Ginseng (Panax Ginseng) • Reishi (Ganoderma lucidum) • Tienchi (Radix Pseudoginseng) • Astragalus (Astragalus membranaceus) • Licorice (Radix glycyrrhizae uralensis).

Vemma Minerals - Vemma
Each 2 tbsp serving contains: Proprietary Mineral Blend 956 mg: Carbon (organic), Calcium, Sodium, Sulfur, Magnesium, Chloride, Bromide, Flouride, Iodine, Potassium, Niobium, Aluminum, Iron, Phosphorus, Silica, Magnanese, Boron, Strontium, Titanium, Tungsten, Copper, Zinc, Tin, Zirconium, Molybdenum, Vanadium, Chromium, Selenium, Nickel, Cobalt, Lithium, Gallium, Barium, Yttrium, Neodymium, Hafnium, Cadmium, Thorium, Antimony, Cerium, Tellurium, Beryllium, Samarium, Dysprosium, Erbium, Bismuth, Gadolinium, Cesium, Lathanum, Praseodymium, Europium, Lutetium, Terbium, Holmium, Thallium, Thulium, Tantalum, Germanium, Gold, Platinum, Rhodium, Rubidium, Ruthenium, Scandium, Silver, Indium. Other Ingredients: Purified Water, Fructose, Plant Mineral Extract, Natural Kiwi Flavor, Natural Strawberry Flavor, Citric Acid, Xanthan Gum, Carmine Color.

Vemma Vitamins - Vemma
Each 2 tbsp serving contains: Vitamin A (100% as beta carotene) 5000 IU • Vitamin C (as ascorbic acid) 300 mg • Vitamin D (as cholecalciferol) 400 IU • Vitamin E (as D-alpha-tocopherol acetate) 60 IU • Thiamin (as thiamine hydrochloride) 1.5 mg • Riboflavin (as riboflavin USP) 1.7 mg • Niacin (as niacinamide) 20 mg • Vitamin B6 (as pyridoxine hydrochloride) 5 mg • Folate (as folic acid) 800 mcg • Vitamin B12 (as cyanocobalamin) 15 mcg • Biotin as D-biotin) 300 mcg • Pantothenic Acid (as calcium D-pantothenate) 10 mg • Selenium (as amino acid chelate) 140 mcg • Proprietary Blend 25.2 g: Reconstituted Mangosteen juice (garcinia mangostana L. whole fruit and pericarp), Aloe Vera leaf gel (aloe barbadensis miller), Green Tea leaf (camellia sinensis). Other Ingredients: Fructose, Natural Flavors, Potassium Sorbate, Sodium Benzoate, Malic Acid, Xanthan Gum.

VenaFit - Biotech Corp.
Two tablets contain: Horse Chestnut standardized extract (18%-22% aescin, aesculin free) 280 mg • Niacin (as nicotinic acid) 20 mg • Ginkgo leaf powder 250 mg • Garlic (5:1 standardized extract) 100 mg • Hawthorne berries standardized extract 100 mg • Ginger root powder 100 mg • Citrus Bioflavonoids 100 mg.

Venaplex - Metagenics
Each tablet contains: Rutin 500 mg • Horse Chestnut seed extract (aesculus hippocastanum, standardized to 20% aescins) 250 mg • Arjuna bark 8:1 extract (terminalia arjuna) 38 mg • Forskohlii root extract (coleus forskohlii) 38 mg • Pushkaramula root extract (inula racemosa, standardized to 2.5% alantolactones) 25 mg • Guggul resin 5:1 extract (commiphora mukul, standardized to 2.5% guggulsterones) 25 mg.

Venapro - Ultra Herbal, LLC
Each caplet contains: Vitamin E (D-alpha tocopheryl succinate) 100 IU • Zinc (oxide) 5 mg • L-Arginine HCl 100 mg • Horse Chestnut (equisetum arvense, standardized to 20% naturally

BRAND NAMES

occurring silica) 100 mg • Oat straw (avena sativa) • Plantain (musa pardisiaca) 75 mg • Cascara Sagrada root (rhamnus purshiana) 60 mg • Bilberry fruit (vaccinium myrtillus) 50 mg • Butcher's Broom herb (ruscus aculeatus) 40 mg • Mullein leaf (verbascum densiflorum) 25 mg • Cayenne (capsicum sp.) 15 mg • Red Sage leaf (salvia miltiorrhiza) 15 mg. Other Ingredients: Gelatin, Rice Flour, Magnesium Stearate, Silicon Dioxide, Maltodextrin, Water.

Venastat - PanGeo Health Brands, Inc.
Each Supro Cap contains: Horse Chestnut seed extract as Triterpene glycosides calculated as Escin (16%) 300 mg. Other Ingredients: Dextrin, Gelatin, Copolyvidone, Talc, Polymethacrylic Acid Derivatives, Titanium Dioxide, Dibutyl Phthalate, Iron Oxide.

Venex - Johnston-Keay Laboratories, Inc
Each tablet contains: VASX Proprietary Blend 500 mg: Cassia tree, Dodder seeds, Epimedium, Wolfberry, Saling, Cistanche, Magnolia vine fruit, Red Raspberry, Narrow Leaved Polygala, Rehmannia root, Eucommia bark, Hindo Lotus seed, Bidemate bark, Milk Vetch seed, Cherokee Rose, Arborvitae seed, American Ginseng, Gingko Biloba. Other Ingredients: Microcrystalline Cellulose, Stearic Acid, Silicon Dioxide, Magnesium Stearate, Pharmaceutical Coating.

Venix - Pharmanex
Two capsules contain: Triacin, a proprietary blend of 1325 mg: Cs-4 Mushroom Mycelia Cordyceps Sinensis, L-Arginine HCl, Ginkgo Biloba leaf extract (50:1). Other Ingredients: Gelatin, Magnesium Stearate, Silicon Dioxide.

VenoBalance - Pure Encapsulations
Two vegetable capsules contain: Dandelion leaf 4:1 extract (taraxacum officinale) 250 mg • Parsley root 4:1 extract (petroselinum crispum) 250 mg • Cornsilk 4:1 extract (zea mays) extract 250 mg • Butcher's Broom root extract (ruscus aculeatus, standardized to contain 10% ruscogenins) 100 mg • Rutin 20 mg • Vitamin C (as ascorbyl palmitate) 20 mg.

Ventilean - PharmaGenX
Two LipoGels contain: Guarana 750 mg • Zhi Shi (95% synephrine) 20 mg • Vinpocetine • Yohimbe 5.3 mg • Vitamin B1 1.4 mg • Vitamin B2 1.3 mg • Vitamin B6 1.3 mg • Vitamin B12 24 mcg. Other Ingredients: Water, Glycerin, Propylene Glycol, Emulsifiers, Phospholipids, Licorice Flavor, Peppermint Oil, Medium Chain Triglycerides, Sucralose, Aspartame, Cinnamon Oil, Potassium Sorbate, Sodium Benzoate, Phosphoric Acid, Natural and Artificial Colors, Kelp, Sodium Citrate, Sodium Phosphate, Mono Potassium Phosphate, Collagen.
See Editor's Note No. 40.

Vermex - American Biologics
Each drop contains: Cina 4X • Tanacet Vulg. 1X • Astemsia Vulg. 1X • Filix 2X • Mercur. Subl. Corr 8X • Graphites 30X. Other Ingredients: 30% Alcohol, Distilled Water.
See Editor's Note No. 1.

Veromax for Men - Veromax International
Each tablet contains: Jujube Dates (Zizyphi fructus) fruit 100 mg • Proprietary Amino Blend: L-Arginine, L-Alanine, Glutamic Acid, Lysine (L-Lysine hydrochloride) 213 mg • Proprietary Herbal Blend: Korean Ginseng root powder, Ginkgo Biloba leaf powder, Saw Palmetto berry powder 238 mg. Other Ingredients: Calcium Carbonate, Cellulose, Croscarmellose Sodium, Stearic Acid, Silica, Magnesium Stearate, Hydroxypropyl Methylcellulose.

Veromax Sexual Performance Enhancer for Women - Nx Nutraceuticals
Each tablet contains: Jujube Dates fruit (zizyphi fructus) 100 mg • Proprietary Amino Potency Power Blend 175 mg: Arginine (as l-arginine hydrochloride), Alanine, Glutamic Acid, Lysine (as l-lysine hydrochloride) • Proprietary Veromax Herbal Blend 177.5 mg: Siberian Ginseng root powder, Ginkgo Biloba leaf powder, Isoflavones (from kudzo root extract). Other Ingredients: Calcium Carbonate, Microcrystalline Cellulose, Croscarmellose Sodium, Stearic Acid, Silica, Magnesium Stearate, Hydroxypropyl Methylcellulose.

Vertigoheel - Heel/BHI, Inc.
Each 50 mL contains: Cocculus (Indian berries) 4X 35 ml • Conium (Spotted Hemlock) 3x • Ambra (Amber) 6X • Petroleum (Mineral Oil) 8X 5 mg. Contains 35 Vol.% alcohol.
See Editor's Note No. 1.

Vertigoheel Tablets - Heel/BHI, Inc.
Each tablet contains: Cocculus (Indian berries) 4X 210 mg • Conium (Spotted Hemlock) 3X • Ambra (Amber) 6X • Petroleum (Mineral Oil) 8X ana 30 mg.
See Editor's Note No. 1.

VesPro GHS - Pro Health
Three tablets contain: NGH Protein/Peptide Complex 1500 mg: Naturally occurring Peptides, Amino Acids, Valine, Leucine, Isoleucine Ornithine, Glutamine, Arginine, Glycine • GH Support Herbal Blend 600 mg: Shilajit (mineral pitch) extract, Licorice, Tribulus extract, Chinese Licorice extract, Schizandra extract • Nutraceutic Matrix 450 mg: Colostrum, GABA, Mucuna Pruriens, Alpha-glycerylphosphorylcholine (alpha GPC) • Calcium Phosphate 71 mg. Other Ingredients: Cellulose, Vegetable Fatty Acids.

Vessel Care - Metagenics
Each tablet contains: Riboflavin 5 mg • Vitamin B6 (as pyridoxine hydrochloride) 25 mg • Folate (as folic acid, L-5-methyl tetrahydrofolate, 5-formyl tetrahydrofolate) 800 mcg • Vitamin B12 (as cyanocobalamin) 500 mcg • Zinc (as zinc glycinate) 5 mg • Trimethylglycine (as betaine hydrochloride) 500 mg • Choline (as choline bitartrate) 100 mg • Intrinsic Factor 20 mg.

Vessel Max - Ortho Molecular Products
Three capsules contain: Troxerutin 600 mg • Horsechestnut seed extract (standardized to contain 20% aescin) 500 mg • Butcher's Broom (standardized to contain 9-11% ruscogenins) 200 mg • Gotu Kola leaf extract (standardized to contain 10% asiaticoside) 200 mg • Centella Asiatica purified triterpenes 60 mg. Other Ingredients: Natural Vegetable Capsules, Ascorbyl Palmitate, Magnesium Stearate, Microcrystalline Cellulose, Silicon Dioxide.

V-Gel - The Himalaya Drug Company
Each 1 gm serving contains: Triphala 4 mg: Emblica Officinalis, Terminalia Chebula, Terminalia Bellirica • Satapatri (rosa damascena) 3.6 mg • Ela (elattaria cardamomum) 3.6 mg • Punarnava (boerhaavia diffusa) 3.6 mg • Shaileyam (parmelia perlata) 2 mg • Nirgundi (vitex negundo) 1.6 mg • Haridra (curcuma longa) 1.6 mg.

VHandC Tabs - Dial Herbs
Vinegar • Honey • Cayenne.

Viactiv Soft Calcium Chews - Mead Johnson Nutritionals
Each chew contains: Calcium (as calcium carbonate) 500 mg • Vitamin D 100 IU • Vitamin K 40 mcg • Potassium 15 mg • Phosphorus 8 mg • Lactose 0.5 mg • Caffeine 1.14 mg. Other Ingredients: Corn syrup, calcium carbonate, sugar, chocolate, nonfat milk, cocoa butter, salt, soy lecithin, glyceryl monostearate, artificial flavor, carrageenan, & sodium phosphate.

Viacyn - Live Well Nutrition, LLC
Two capsules contain: Zinc 50 mg • L-Arginine 250 mg • Catuaba 100 mg • Oatstraw 150 mg • Nettle leaf 75 mg • Tribulus 50 mg • Cayenne 50 mg • Astragalus 25 mg • Sarsaparilla 25 mg • Boron 2 mg • Pumpkin seed 20 mg • Licorice root 20 mg • Siberian Ginseng 125 mg • Orchic Substance. Other Ingredients: Magnesium Stearate, Gelatin, Water, Epimedium Sagittatum (horny goat weed extract, 20:1), Maca, Oyster Meat, Muira Puama.
See Editor's Note No. 14.

Viastat - Optimal Therapeutics
Two capsules contain: Niacin 25 mg • Horny Goat Weed (10% icarin) 250 mg • Di-Arginine Malate 250 mg • Avena Sativa 10:1 extract (oat straw) 250 mg • Maca 4:1 extract 160 mg • Eurycoma Longifolia 125 mg • Damiana leaf 4:1 extract 120 mg • Tribulus Terrestris (70% saponins) 100 mg • Ginkgo Biloba 50 mg • Cnidium Monnier extract (35% ostole) 25 mg • Bioperine brand Piperine extract 3 mg. Other Ingredients: Gelatin, Cellulose, Magnesium Stearate.

Some Brand Name Natural Products - What they Contain

www.NaturalDatabase.com contains MANY more listings than appear here.
Editor's Notes are located on pages 2155-2163.

ViaViente - ViaViente
Two tablespoons (25 ml) contain: Proprietary PhytoNectar Blend 13,500 mg: Grape PhytoNectar, Whole leaf Aloe Vera PhytoNectar (aloe barbadensis), Apple PhytoNectar (malva pumila), Morinda Citrifolia PhytoNectar, Chinese Scullcap PhytoNectar (scutellaria biacalensis), Blueberry PhytoNectar (vaccinium spp.), Prune PhytoNectar (prunus domestica), Cranberry PhytoNectar (vaccinium macrocarpon), Elderberry PhytoNectar (sambucus cerulea), Bilberry PhytoNectar (vaccinium myrtillus), Gentian PhytoNectar (gentiana lutea) • Proprietary Vilcabamba Mineral Essence Blend 150 mg: Potassium, Calcium, Magnesium, Zinc, Chromium, Selenium, Iron, Copper, Molybdenum, Vanadium, Iodine, Cobalt, Manganese. Other Ingredients: Vilcabamba Mineral Water, Citric Acid, Natural Flavors, Sodium Benzoate (0.1%), Potassium Sorbate (0.1%).

ViaVita - DreamPharm
Two tablets contain: Proprietary Blend: Lecithin (soya), Calcium (carbonate), Citric Acid, Iron (ferrous fumarate), Vitamin B12.

Vibrant Celcaps - Vibrant Health
Three celcaps contain: Celadrin Proprietary Blend 1050 mg: Cetyl Myristate, Cetyl Myristoleate, Cetyl Esters. Other Ingredients: Soy Lecithin, Fish Oil.

Vibrant Creme with Celadrin - Vibrant Health
Menthol • Benzyl Alcohol • Butylparaben • Carbomer • Proprietary Cetyl Ester Blend (Celadrin): Cetyl Myristate, Cetyl Oleate • Cetyl Palmitoleate • Cetyl Laurate • Cetyl Myristoleate • Ethylparaben • Glycerin • Glyceryl Stearate • Isobutylparaben • Lecithin • Methylparaben • Olea Europaea fruit oil (olive) • PEG 100 Stearate • Peppermint oil • Phenoxyethanol • Potassium Hydroxide • Propylparaben • Tocopheryl Acetate • Water.

Viburcol monodose vials - Heel/BHI, Inc.
Each 1 mL vial contains: Calcarea Carbonica 8X • Pulsatilla 6X • Chamomilla 4X • Plantago Major 4X • Dulcamara 6X • Belladonna 6X. Base: Isotonic Saline Solution.
See Editor's Note No. 1.

Viburcol suppositories - Heel/BHI, Inc.
Each suppository contains: Calcarea Carbonica 8X • Pulsatilla 2X • Chamomilla 1X • Belladonna 2X • Plantago Major 3X • Dulcamara 4X.
See Editor's Note No. 1.

Vicco Toothpaste (Royal Image Cosmetics) - InterPlexus
Fine Chalk • Water • Sorbitol • Sodium Lauryl Sulphate • Gum Tragacanth • Indian Licorice root • Currant • Common Jujube • Rose Apple • Barleria Prionitis • Asian Holly Oak • Persian Walnut • Prickly Ash • Indian Almond • Beeda nut • Bishop's Weed • Sarsaparilla • Catechu • Sappan wood • Medlar • Cinnamon • Gum Arabic • Bengal Madder • Mayweed • Flavour • Sodium Saccharin • Methyl Hydroxy Benzoate Sodium.

Viga - Health Nutrition (RMA Labs)
Each tablet contains: Yohimbe extract 40 mg • Muira Puama 10 mg • Tribulus Terrestris 40 mg • Ginseng 40 mg • Saw Palmetto 40 mg • Oat straw 10 mg • DHEA 10 mg • Androstenedione 10 mg.
See Editor's Note No. 47.

Viga for Women - Health Nutrition (RMA Labs)
Muira Puama • Ginseng • Maca • Wild Yam • Damiana • L-Arginine • Dong Quai • Guarana • Horny Goat Weed • Macuna Prurions extract.

Vigorelle - Leading Edge Herbals
Organic Damiana leaf (folium turneraceae) • Organic Suma root (radix pfaffiae paniculatae) • Organic Motherwort (herba leonori) • Organic Wild Yam (rhizoma dioscorea villosae) • Organic Ginkgo Biloba • Organic Peppermint leaf (folium menthae piperitae).

Vigorex Femme - New Hope Health Products
Each tablet contains: Sabal Serrulata (saw palmetto) • Avena Sativa.

Vigorex forte - Doc Johnson Enterprises
Active Ingredient: Avena sativa 1X. Base: Lactose.
See Editor's Note No. 1.

Vigorex Forte - New Hope Health Products
Each capsule contains: Avena Sativa extract 300 mg.

Vigrex - Puritan's Pride
Each tablet contains: Yohimbe 500 mg • Tribulus Terrestris 225 mg • Maca root 200 mg • Muira Puama root 200 mg • Panax Ginseng 150 mg • Ginger extract 100 mg • Citrus Aurantium extract 50 mg • Fructooligosaccharides (FOS) 50 mg • Saw Palmetto (standardized for 30% fatty acids) 15 mg. Other Ingredients: Dicalcium Phosphate, Cellulose, Magnesium Stearate, Silica, Stearic Acid.
See Editor's Note No. 40.

VigroMax - AIE Pharmaceuticals
L-Arginine • Passion Flower • Pregnenolone • DHEA • Zinc • Wild Oat • Semen Cuscutae • Niacin • Saw Palmetto.

VigRx - Albion Medical
Each capsule contains: Epimedium Sagittatum extract 330 mg • Cuscuta seed 100 mg • Ginkgo Biloba 100 mg • Korean Red Ginseng (panax ginseng) 100 mg • Saw Palmetto (fructus serenoae) 100 mg • Muira Puama extract (4:1) 50 mg. Other Ingredients: MCC, Magnesium Stearate, D-Calcium Phosphate, Croscarmellose Sodium, PVP K90, Silicon Dioxide.

Vimax Pills - PillsExpert.com
Two capsules contain: Vitamin E (as natural d-alpha tocopheryl) 20 IU • Inosine 50 mg • Proprietary Blend 938 mg: Yohimbe bark 4:1, Muira Puama balsam, Deer Antler Velvet, Ginkgo leaf, Damiana leaf, Cayenne fruit, Oats (entire plant), Panax Ginseng root, Tribulus fruit. Other Ingredients: Cellulose, Vegetable Stearate, Silica.

Vinarol - Johnston-Keay Laboratories, Inc
Each tablet contains: VASX Proprietary Blend 500 mg: Cassia tree, Dodder seed, Epimedium, Wolfberry, Saling, Cistanche, Magnolia vine fruit, Red Raspberry, Narrow-leaved Polygala, Rehmannia root, Eucommia bark, Hindo Lotus seed, Bidemate bark, Milk Vetch seed, Cherokee Rose, Arborvitae seed, American Ginseng, Gingko Biloba. Other Ingredients: Microcrystalline Cellulose, Stearic Acid, Silicon Dioxide, Magnesium Stearate, Pharmaceutical Coating.
See Editor's Note No. 25.

VincaClear - Life Enhancement Products, Inc.
Each capsule contains: Vitamin C (as calcium ascorbate) 200 mg • Calcium (as calcium ascorbate) 26 mg • L-Arginine (as L-arginine hydrochloride) 375 mg • Vinpocetine 10 mg.

VincaHear - Life Enhancement Products, Inc.
Each capsule contains: Vitamin D (D3, as cholicalciferol) 25 IU • Niacin (vitamin B3) 6 mg • Calcium (as calcium citrate) 50 mg • Magnesium (as magnesium aspartate) 42 mg • Zinc (as zinc gluconate) • 3 mg • Quercetin 25 mg • Ginkgo Biloba leaf extract 15 mg • Vinpocetine 5 mg. Other Ingredients: Gelatin.

VincaHear Plus - Life Enhancement Products, Inc.
Each capsule contains: Vitamin D (D3, as cholicalciferol) 25 IU • Niacin (vitamin B3) 6 mg • Calcium (as calcium citrate) 38 mg • Magnesium (as magnesium aspartate) 42 mg • Zinc (as zinc gluconate) 3 mg • Alpha Lipoic Acid 100 mg • Quercetin 25 mg • Ginkgo Biloba leaf extract 15 mg • Vinpocetine 5 mg.
Other Ingredients: Gelatin.

Vincamine - Source Naturals
Each tablet contains: Vincamine 30 mg.

VincaSee - Life Enhancement Products, Inc.
Each capsule contains: Vitamin A (from beta carotene) 2000 IU • Vitamin C (from calcium ascorbate) 187.5 mg • Vitamin E (from dL-alpha tocopheryl acetate) 50 IU • Riboflavin (vitamin B2) 6.25 mg • Calcium (from calcium ascorbate) 25 mg • Zinc (from zinc gluconate) 3 mg • Selenium (from sodium selenite) 12.5 mcg • Chromium (from chromium aspartate) 25 mcg • Taurine 50 mg • L-Cysteine Hydrochloride 25 mg • Hesperidin 25 mg • Ginkgo Biloba 60 mg • Vinpocetine 5 mg • Lutein 3.75 mg • Bilberry fruit extract 1.25 mg • Quercetin 1.25 mg • Zeaxanthin 750 mcg. Other Ingredients: Gelatin, Silicon Dioxide.

Vincazine **-** Smart Basics
Each capsule contains: Vinpocetine 10 mg • (-) Huperzine A 50 mcg.

Vine Essence **-** Capital United (Beijing) Medical Manufacturer Co
Active ingredients: Geranium herb (geranium eriostemon), Erycibe stem (erycibe obtusifolia Benth, ding-gong-teng), Chinese Angelica Tree herb (aralia chinensis L.), Futokadsura stem(piper futokadsura Sieb. Et Zucc., hai-feng-teng), Oriental Ren-Shen, Pipefish, Ilicis (ilex pubescens hook et arn), Kadsura root (kadsura cocchinea [Lem] A.C.), Epimedium (epimedium sagittatum [Sieb. et Zucc.] maxim, yin-yang-huo), Dong-Quai root, Homalomeana rhizome (homalomeana sagittaefolia Jungh., qian-nian-jian), Chinese Licorice root (gan-cao), Sichuan Lovage rhizome (chuan-xiong), Morinda (ba-ji-tian), Ligusticum rhizome (gao-ben), Gastrodia rhizome (tian-ma), Sichuan Teasel root (xu-duan), Fo-Ti root (he-shou-wu).
See Editor's Note No. 17.

Vinpocetine **-** PhysioLogics
Each softgel contains: Vinpocetine 10 mg. Other Ingredients: Lecithin, Soybean Oil, Gelatin, Beeswax / Soybean Oil Mixture, Glycerin, Titanium Dioxide Color.

Vinpocetine **-** Pro Health
Each tablet contains: Vinpocetine 5 mg. Other Ingredients: Dicalcium Phosphate, Microcrystalline Cellulose, Stearic Acid, Magnesium Stearate, Pharmaceutical Glaze.

Vinpocetine **-** Source Naturals
Each tablet contains: Vinpocetine 10 mg. Other Ingredients: Microcrystalline Cellulose, Stearic Acid, Magnesium.

Vinpocetine **-** Life Enhancement Products, Inc.
Each capsule contains: Vinpocetine 10 mg.

Vinpocetine **-** Jarrow Formulas
Each capsule contains: Vinpocetine 5 mg. Other Ingredients: Cellulose, Magnesium Stearate, Gelatin.

Vinpocetine **-** Amerifit Nutrition
Each tablet contains: Vinpocetine 5 mg • Green Tea standardized extract 200 mg. Other Ingredients: Dicalcium Phosphate, Croscarmellose Sodium, Microcrystalline Cellulose, Magnesium Stearate, Silica, Stearic Acid, Pharmaceutical Glaze.
See Editor's Note No. 21.

Vinpocetine 20 mg **-** Pure Encapsulations
Each vegetable capsule contains: Vinpocetine 20 mg.

Vinpo-Zine **-** Smart Nutrition
Each capsule contains: Vinpocetine 10 mg • Huperzine A 50 mcg.

Viper **-** Puritan's Pride
Each capsule contains: Kola Nut 175 mg • Oatstraw 150 mg • Nettle 100 mg • Yohimbe 2% extract 50 mg • Siberian Ginseng 50 mg • Horny Goat Weed 20 mg • Catuaba 10 mg • Muira Puama 10 mg • Korean Ginseng 10 mg • Turnera Aphrodisiaca 10 mg • Saw Palmetto 10 mg.

Viracid **-** Ortho Molecular Products
Each capsule contains: Vitamin A (as palmitate, Betatene brand natural mixed carotenoids) 15,000 IU • Vitamin C (as ascorbic acid USP, acerola fruit extract) 300 mg • Vitamin B12 (as methylcobalamin) s.5 mcg • Pantothenic Acid (as D-calcium pantothenate) 10 mg • Zinc (as Chelazome brand amino acid chelate) 4 mg • L-Lysine USP 100 mg • Echinacea Purpurea aerial portion 16:1 extract 50 mg • Pau d'Arco inner bark 5:1 extract 50 mg • Thumus (bovine) 50 mg • Acerola fruit extract (standardized to contain 17% vitamin C) 25 mg • Lung (bovine) 25 mg • Lymph (bovine) 25 mg • Spleen (bovine) 25 mg. Other Ingredients: Natural Vegetable Capsules, Magnesium Stearate, Microcrystalline Cellulose.

ViraCon **-** Vital Nutrients
Two capsules contain: Sambucus Nigra fruit 50:1 extract (elderberry) 125 mg • Scutellaria Baicalensis 8:1 extract 125 mg • Propolis 100 mg • Astragalus root 15:1 extract 100 mg • Isatis root 15:1 extract 100 mg • Coptis Chinensis 10:1 extract 50 mg • Hypericum Perforatum 0.3% extract 50 mg • Glycyrrhiza Glabra root extract (licorice) 50 mg • Zinc (citrate) 5 mg.

ViraPlex **-** Enzymatic Therapy
Each tablet contains: Vitamin A (Fish Liver oil) 10000 IU • Vitamin D (Fish Liver oil) 35 IU • Vitamin C (Ascorbic Acid/Rose Hips) 200 mg • Calcium (Lactate) 41 mg • Pantothenic Acid (D-Calcium Pantothenate) 25 mg • Zinc (Gluconate) 10.5 mg • Magnesium (Citrate) 6.7 mg • Vitamin B12 (Cyanocobalamin) 2.5 mcg • Other ingredients: RNA Powder 60 mg • Alfalfa juice powder 50 mg • Lemon Bioflavonoids 30 mg • Spleen extract 30 mg • Thymus extract 25 mg • Trace Mineral concentrate (Kelp) 25 mg • Unsaturated Free Fatty Acids 15 mg • Lung extract 10 mg. In a base of Chlorophyll, Lymph, & Fermentation extract.
See Editor's Note No. 14.

Viraplex EB with Elderberry **-** Enzymatic Therapy
Each tablet contains: Vitamin A (as acetate) 10,000 IU • Vitamin C (ascorbic acid) 200 mg • Vitamin D (as cholecalciferol) 35 IU • Vitamin B12 (as cyanocobalamin) 50 mcg • Pantothenic Acid (as calcium d-pantothenate) 25 mg • Calcium (as calcium lactate) 41 mg • Magnesium (as magnesium citrate) 6.7 mg • Zinc (as zinc gluconate) 10.5 mg • European Elderberry extract (sambucus nigra, 4:1) 100 mg • Alfalfa aerial part extract (medicago sativa, 10:1) 50 mg • Astragalus root extract (astragalus membranaceus, standardized to contain a minimum of 0.5% 4-hydroxy-3#-methoxyisoflavone-7-glucoside) 50 mg • Mixed Bioflavonoids 50% (from citrus fruits) 30 mg • Proprietary Trace Mineral Blend 24 mg: Selenium (as selenium yeast), Silicon (as magnesium trisilicate), Boron (as sodium borate), Nickel (as nickel chelate). Other Ingredients: Cellulose, Modified Cellulose, Magnesium Stearate, Carnauba Wax, Lecithin.

Virile 1 **-** Biotech Corp.
Two tablets contain: Yohimbine bark 5.4 mg • Shen Min 4:1 extract 100 mg • DHEA (dehydroepiandrosterone) 12.5 mg • Pregnenolone (pharmaceutical grade) 2.5 mg • Virile 1 Formula Proprietary Herb Blend 635 mg: Saw Palmetto berry 4:1 extract, Licorice root 4:1 extract, Muira Puama 4:1 extract, Fennel seed, Damiana leaf, Avena Sativa straw extract, Pygeum bark, Nettle.

Virile V for Him **-** USA Pharmacal Sales
Two tablets contain: Niacin 10 mg •Yohimbe 250 mg •Avena Sativa 150 mg •Androstenedione 100 mg •Saw Palmetto 100 mg •Guarana 300 mg •Taurine 200 mg •Siberian Ginseng 30 mg •Panax Ginseng 30 mg •Tribulus Terrestris 50 mg •Rhodiola Roseo 10 mg •Wild Yam 250 mg •Maca 100 mg •Arginine 100 mg.
See Editor's Note No. 47.

Viriligen **-** Xymogen
Each softgel contains: Horny Goat Weed (20% icarin) 75 mg • Yohimbe (10% yohimbine) 37.5 mg • Tribulus (45% saponins) 125 mg • Yanhusuo (25% corydaline) 12.5 mg.

Virility Elixir **-** Gaia Herbs
Sixty drops contain: Proprietary Extract Blend 600 mg: Siberian Ginseng solid extract (eleutherococcus senticosus), Wild Sarsaparilla root (smilax officinalis), Fresh Saw Palmetto berries (serenoa repens), Muira Puama root (ptychopetalum olacoides), Damiana herb (turnera diffusa), Fresh Wild Oats milky seed (avena sativa), Prickly Ash bark (xanthoxylum clava-herculis), Rose Hips solid extract (rosa canina), Hawthorn berry solid extract (crataegus spp.), Blend of Sea Vegetation, Vegetable Glycerin, 18-25% Pure Grain Alcohol USP, Spring Water.

Virility EX (International Formula) **-** Ultra Herbal, LLC
Two tablets contain: Niacin 50 mg • Zinc (as zinc oxide) 26 mg • Maca tuber 333 mg • Catuaba bark 83 mg • Muira Puama bark 83 mg • L-Arginine HCl 67 mg • Heart-Leaf Sida (entire plant) 80 mg • Barrenwort (aerial parts) 73 mg • Tribulus herb 67 mg • Cola seed 50 mg • Oat straw 50 mg • Stinging Nettle leaf 50 mg • Pumpkin seed 50 mg • Ginger root 40 mg • Cayenne (25,000 HU) 40 mg • American Ginseng root 33 mg • Eleuthero root 33 mg • Asian Ginseng root 33 mg • Sarsaparilla root 33 mg • Orchic Substance (bovine) 20 mg •

Boron Citrate 7 mg. Other Ingredients: Cellulose, Gum Arabic (acacia), Vegetable Stearic Acid, Modified Cellulose, Silicon Dioxide, Magnesium Stearate, FD&C Blue #2, FD&C Indigo Carmine Lake. See Editor's Note No. 14 and No. 39.

Virility EX (US Formula) - Ultra Herbal, LLC
Two tablets contain: Yohimbe bark (pausinystalia johimbe, standardized to 8% yohimbe group alkaloids) 250 mg • Maca root (lypedium meyenii) 240 mg • Tribulus fruit (tribulus terrestris) 200 mg • Horny Goat Weed (epimedium sagittatum) 160 mg • Elk Velvet Antler 100 mg • Eleuthero (eleutherococcus senticosus) 100 mg • Tongkat Ali root (eurycoma longifolia) 10 mg • Catuaba (erythroxylum catuaba) 20 mg • Muira Puama bark (ptychopetalum olacoides) 20 mg • Oat straw (avena sativa) 20 mg • Damiana leaf (turnera diffusa) 20 mg • Sarsaparilla root (smilax sp.) 20 mg. Other Ingredients: Calcium Carbonate, Dibasic Calcium Phosphate, Tribasic Calcium Phosphate, Microcrystalline Cellulose, Croscarmellose Sodium, Stearic Acid, Magnesium Stearate, Silicon Dioxide, Modified Cellulose, Maltodextrin, Hydroxypropyl Methylcellulose, Hydroxypropyl Cellulose, Water.

Virility Pills VP-RX - EyeFive, Inc.
Two capsules contain: Vitamin E (as d-alpha tocopheryl acetate) 20 IU • Soy Protein concentrate 550 mg • Damiana leaf 200 mg • Muira Puama herb (ptychopetalum olacoides) 200 mg • Ginkgo Biloba leaf 120 mg • Panax Ginseng root 120 mg • Tribulus Terrestris herb extract 120 mg • Yohimbe bark extract 4:1 120 mg • Inosine 50 mg • Oat Straw 32 mg • Cayenne fruit 20 mg • Velvet Deer Antler 6 mg. Other Ingredients: Gelatin, Microcrystalline Cellulose, Magnesium Stearate, Silicon Dioxide.

Virility Support Formula - The Vitamin Factory
Each tablet contains: Niacin 10 mg • L-Arginine 250 mg • Muirapuama root & bark extract 10:1 100 mg • Yohimbe bark extract (min 1% Yohimbe) 100 mg • Quebracho Branco bark extract (Aspidosperma • min. 6% Quebrachine) 25 mg • Catuaba bark extract 4:1 50 mg • Pycnogenol (Maritime Pine bark extract) 10 mg.

VirilityPrep - HealthMinded
Two capsules contain: VirilityPrep Proprietary Blend 1080 mg: Asian Ginseng root, Ginkgo Biloba leaf dried extract, Hawthorn berry, Saw Palmetto berry, Chinese Dodder seed dried extract, Muira Puama root dried extract, Catuaba bark dried extract, Epimedium aerial parts dried extract. Other Ingredients: Gelatin, Stearic Acid, Magnesium Stearate.

Virility-V - Aspen Group, Inc.
Two tablets contain: Yohimbe extract 2% 500 mg • Avena Sativa extract 10.1 150 mg • Androstenedione 90 mg • Saw Palmetto extract 4.1 100 mg • Guarana extract 22% 300 mg • Taurine 200 mg • Siberian Ginseng extract 35.1 30 mg • Tribulus Terrestris extract 40% 50 mg. Other ingredients: Dicalcium Phosphate, Microcrystaline Cellulose, Magnesium Stearte, Stearic Acid. See Editor's Note No. 47.

Virility-V Female - Aspen Group, Inc.
Three tablets contain: Vitamin D (cholecalciferol) 21 IU • Niacin (niacinamide) 20 mg • Vitamin B6 (pyridoxine hydrochloride) 2.4 mg • Folic Acid (folacin) 6.4 mg • Vitamin B12 (cyanocobalamin) 6 mg. Other Ingredients: Avena Sativa (10:1) 150 mg, Kava Kava (30%) 10 mg, Muira Puama (4:1) 20 mg, St. John's Wort (0.3%) 250 mg, Siberian Ginseng (35:1) 30 mg, Gingko Biloba (24%) 40 mg, Cordyceps 100 mg, Damiana 20 mg, L-Taurine 200 mg.

Virilogarl - Olympian Labs
Three capsules contain: Ginkgo Biloba leaf extract 120 mg • Garlic extract 600 mg • L-Arginine 390 mg • Bilberry extract 150 mg • Grape Seed extract 75 mg • Green Tea leaf extract 225 mg.

Virx - Nutri-Quest Rx
Each tablet contains: Olive leaf 100 mg • L-Lysine 100 mg • Vitamin C 25 mg • Zinc Chelate 10 mg • Elderberry extract 100 mg • Selenium Chelate 50 mcg • Olive leaf extract 5 mg • Vitamin A 3333.33 IU • Echinacea 100 mg • Goldenseal 50 mg • Astragalus 100 mg • natural Beta Carotene 3333.33 IU.

Vision Answer for Women - Doctor's Preferred, Inc.
Two softgels contain: Vitamin A (beta carotene) 250 IU • Vitamin C (ascorbic acid) 250 mg • Zinc (chelate) 10 mg • Selenium (chelate) 50 mcg • Copper (gluconate) 1000 mcg • Rutin (from pod) 250 mg • Vegetable Blend 134 mg: Green Tea extract, Pine bark extract, Broccoli, Tomato, Carrot, Spinach, Kale, Brussels Sprouts • Grape seed extract 50 mg • Lutein (from marigold) 15 mg • Lycopene (from tomato) 4 mg • Polygonum Cuspidatum root extract 4 mg • Astaxanthin (from algae) 3 mg • Zeaxanthin (from marigold) 3 mg.

Vision Complete - Rexall - Sundown
Two capsules contain: Vitamin A (100% as beta-carotene) 5000 IU • Vitamin C (as ascorbic acid, ascorbyl palmitate) 60 mg • Vitamin E (as dl-alpha-tocopheryl acetate and d-alpha-tocopheryl succinate) 30 IU • Riboflavin (Vitamin B2) 3.4 mg • Vitamin B-6 (as pyridoxine HCl) 2 mg • Lutein (from marigold flower extract) 5 mg • Bilberry leaf 10 mg • Piperine (black pepper extract) 4.75 mg • Alpha-Lipoic Acid 10 mg • Glutathione 5 mg • Spinach leaf 20 mg. Other Ingredients: Maltodextrin, Gelatin, Water, Magnesium Stearate.

Vision Enhancement - Gaia Herbs
Two capsules contain: Bilberry berry (vaccinium myrtillus) 50 mg • Grape seed (vitis vinifera) 20 mg • Lutein 10 mg • Astaxanthan 2 mg. Other Ingredients: Vegetable Glycerin, Lecithin, Vegetable Cellulose.

Vision Essentials - Enzymatic Therapy
Each capsule contains: Vitamin A (Beta Carotene) non-toxic form of Vitamin A 5000 IU • Vitamin C (Ascorbic Acid) 100 mg • Riboflavin (Vitamin B2) 5 mg • Other Ingredients: Bilberry extract (Vaccinium myrtillus Fructus) standardized to contain 25% Anthocyanosides (20 mg per capsule) calculated as Anthocyanidins 80 mg.

Vision Formula - Nature's Way
Two capsules contain: Bilberry fruit (dried extract 25% Anthocyanins) 50 mg • Biotin (Biotin Triurate) 40 mcg • Cayenne pepper fruit 100 mg • Citrus Bioflavonoids 150 mg • Copper (Amino Acid Chelate) 1 mg • Lutein 6 mg • Niacin (Vitamin B3) 20 mg • Riboflavin (Vitamin B2) 8 mg • Siberian Ginseng root 50 mg • Taurine 150 mg • Tru-OPCs (dried Grape seed extract) 20 mg • Vitamin A (Retinol Palmitate) 2000 IU • Vitamin E (d-Alpha Tocopheryl) 80 IU • Zinc (Amino Acid Chelate) 16 mg. Other Ingredients: Gelatin, Magnesium Stearate, Millet.

Vision Nutrients - Puritan's Pride
Each tablet contains: Pro-Vitamin A (beta carotene) 5,000 IU • Vitamin E (dl-alpha Tocopheryl) 30 IU • Vitamin C (ascorbic acid) 60 mg • Zinc (oxide) 40 mg • Copper (oxide) 2 mg • Selenium 40 mcg.

Vision Spray - Natural Ophthalmics
Three sprays contain: Vitamin A (beta carotene) 500 IU • Vitamin B3 (niacin) 5 mg • Vitamin C (Ester-C) 15 mg • Vitamin E 4 IU • Zinc 5 mg • Lutein (FloraGLO) 10 mg • Zeaxanthin 0.1 mg • Vinpocetine 1 mg • Bilberry extract 5 mg • Eyebright 2 mg • Glutathione 2 mg • Ginkgo Biloba 1 mg • MSM 5 mg • L-Taurine 5 mg • L-Glycine 5 mg • Rutin 5 mg • Quercetin 5 mg. Other Ingredients: Purified Water, Vegetable Glycerin, Aloe Vera, Trace Minerals, Grapefruit Seed extract, Potassium Sorbate, Stevia, Flavorings.

Visionace - Vitabiotics
Each tablet contains: Vitamin A (1000 IU) 300 mcg • Vitamin D (100 IU) 2.5 mcg • Vitamin E (natural source) 60 mg • Vitamin C 150 mg • Vitamin B1 (thiamin) 12 mg • Vitamin B2 (riboflavin) 4.8 mg • Vitamin B3 (niacin) 18 mg • Vitamin B6 (pyridoxine HCl) 10 mg • Folacin (as folic acid) 400 mcg • Vitamin B12 9 mcg • Pantothenic Acid 20 mg • Iron 6 mg • Magnesium 50 mg • Zinc 15 mg • Iodine 100 mcg • Copper 1 mg • Manganese 4 mg • Selenium 150 mcg • Chromium 50 mcg • Natural Mixed Carotenoids 3 mg • Citrus Bioflavonoids 15 mg • Bilberry extract 60 mg • Lutein Esters 4 mg.

Visionex - USANA Health Sciences
Two tablets contain: Vitamin C (as Calcium, Potassium, Magnesium, Zinc Ascorbates) 500 mg • Zinc (as Citrate) 20 mg • Lutein 10 mg • Zeaxanthin 2000 mg • Bilberry Extract (Vaccinium Myrtillus L.) Fruit 50 mg. Other Ingredients: Microcrystalline Cellulose, Croscarmellose Sodium, Ascorbyl Palmitate, Dextrin, Dextrose.

VisionPrep **-** HealthMinded
Two capsules contain: Vitamin A (50% as beta-carotene, 50% as acetate) 5000 IU • Vitamin C (as ascorbic acid) 500 mg • Vitamin E (as D-alpha tocopheryl acetate) 400 IU • Riboflavin (vitamin B2) 5 mg • Zinc (as zinc gluconate) 15 mg • Selenium (as sodium selenate) 70 mcg • Copper (as copper gluconate) 2 mg • VisionPrep Proprietary Blend 224 mg: Bilberry extract (25% anthocyanosides = 40 mg), Quercetin, Green Tea leaf extract (camellia sinensis), Lutein, Zeaxanthin, Lycopene. Other Ingredients: Gelatin, Stearic Acid, Magnesium Stearate.

VisionPro **-** HealthMinded
Four capsules contain: Vitamin A 20,000 IU • Vitamin C 200 mg • Vitamin E 440 IU • Calcium 117 mg • Zinc 60 mg • Selenium 20 mcg • Copper 8 mg • Chromium 200 mcg • VisionPro Proprietary Blend 782.5 mg: Citrus Bioflavonoids, L-Taurine, Quercetin, Rutin, Eyebright, N-Acetyl-Cysteine, Bilberry fruit extract, L-Glutathione, Lutein complex, Astaxanthin, Zeaxanthin. Other Ingredients: Stearic Acid, Magnesium Stearate.

Visioplex **-** Progressive Labs
Each capsule contains: Vitamin A (acetate) 937 IU • Vitamin A (beta carotene) 3125 IU • Vitamin C 62.5 mg • Calcium (as calcium citrate) 12.5 mg • Vitamin E (dl-alpha tocopherol) 50 IU • Thiamin (vitamin B1) 2.5 mg • Riboflavin (vitamin B2) 3.1 mg • Niacin 1.25 mg • Niacinamide 6.25 mg • Vitamin B6 (pyridoxine HCl) 3.75 mg • Folate (folic acid) 100 mcg • Vitamin B12 6.25 mcg • Pantothenic Acid 12.5 mg • Magnesium (citrate) 31.25 mg • Zinc (picolinate) 6.25 mg • Selenium (selenomethionine) 25 mcg • Copper (amino acid chelate) 0.375 mg • Raw Eye concentrate 8.75 mg • Eyebright (Euphrasia officinalis) 18.75 mg • Bilberry powder (vaccinium myrtillis) 5 mg • Ginkgo extract (Ginkgo biloba) 7.5 mg • N-Acetyl-Cysteine (NAC) 31.25 • Quercetin 37.5 mg • Taurine 62.5 mg • L-Methionine 25 mg • Glutamic Acid 6.25 mg • Glycine 6.25 mg. See Editor's Note No. 14.

Visual Eyes **-** Source Naturals
Four tablets contain: Vitamin A (Beta Carotene) 25000 IU • Vitamin A (Palmitate) 7500 IU • Vitamin B2 50 mg • Inositol Hexanicotinate 100 mg • Vitamin C (Magnesium Ascorbate) 1500 mg • Vitamin E (D-Alpha Tocopheryl Succinate) 400 IU • Chromium (ChromeMate Polynicotinate 125 mcg and Chromium Picolinate 125 mcg) 250 mcg • Copper (Sebacate) 1 mg • Magnesium (Ascorbate, Taurinate) 164 mg • Selenium (L-Selenomethionine) 200 mcg • Zinc (Monomethionine) 30 mg • Bilberry extract (Yielding 37 mg of Anthocyanosides)100 mg • Lutein 10 mg • Alpha-Lipoic Acid 25 mg • Ginkgo Biloba 24% (50:1 Extract) 45 mg • Grape Seed extract (Proanthodyn with a Proanthocyanidolic Value of 95) 45 mg • Quercetin 320 mg • N-Acetyl Cysteine 400 mg • Taurine (Magnesium Taurinate) 500 mg • Inositol (Hexanicotinate) 10 mg.

Vita C **-** Shaklee
Each tablet contains: Vitamin C (as Ascorbic acid) 500 mg • Sodium 5 mg. Other Ingredients: Bioflavonoid Complex (Lemon, Orange, Grapefruit, and Hesperidin Complex), Rose Hips, Dicalcium Phosphate, Alginic Acid, Carnauba Wax, Carrageenan, Pectin, Acacia Gum, Guar Gum, Locust Bean Gum, Agar-Agar, Grapefruit Oil.

Vita E **-** Shaklee
Each tablet contains: Vitamin E (as D-alpha tocopheryl acid succinate) 400 IU • Selenium (as Selenium yeast) 10 mcg. Other Ingredients: Dicalcium Phosphate, Silicon Dioxide, Modified Food Starch, Mixed Tocopherol Concentrate, Wheat Germ Flour, Natural Beet Powder.

Vita E Complex **-** Shaklee
Two capsules contain: Vitamin E (as D-alpha Tocopherol concentrate and mixed Tocopherols concentrate) 800 IU • Selenium (as Selenium protein hydrolysate) 130 mcg • Grapeseed extract (Vitis vinifera) seed/skin 76 mg. Other Ingredients: Soybean Oil, Beeswax, Soy Lecithin, Gelatin, Glycerin, Water, Annatto, Caramel.

Vita Fuel With Iron **-** TwinLab
Nine capsules contain: Beta-Carotene (pro-Vitamin A) 25000 IU • Vitamin D (from natural form Vitamin D3) 400 IU • Vitamin C 2000 mg • Natural Vitamin E (Succinate) 800 IU • CoQ10 (Coenzyme Q10) 30 mg • L-Glutathione 100 mg • N-Acetyl Cysteine (NAC) 200 mg • Alpha-Lipoic Acid 100 mcg • Vitamin B1 (Thiamine) 50 mg • Vitamin B2 (Riboflavin) 50 mg • Vitamin B6 (Pyridoxine) 50 mg • Vitamin B12 (Cobalamin) 100 mcg • Niacinamide 75 mg • Pantothenic Acid 100 mg • Folic Acid 800 mcg • Biotin 600 mcg • PABA 10 mg • Choline Bitartrate 100 mg • Inositol 100 mg • L-Carnitine (from Carni Fuel L-Carnitine Magnesium Citrate) 100 mg • Creatine (Monohydrate) 1000 mg • Calcium (from Calcium Citrate & Carbonate) 500 mg • Magnesium (from L-Carnitine Magnesium Citrate, Aspartate, Alpha-Ketoglutarate & Oxide) 500 mg • Potassium (from Potassium Alpha-Ketoglutarate, Citrate & Aspartate) 500 mg • Zinc (from Zinc Picolinate) 50 mg • Manganese (from Manganese Gluconate) 10 mg • Iron (from Ferrous Fumarate) 10 mg • Copper (from Copper Gluconate) 2 mg • Iodine (from Potassium Iodide) 150 mcg • Selenium (from Selenomethionine & Selenate<50/50 mixture) 200 mcg • Chromium (from Chromic Fuel patented Chromium Picolinate) 400 mcg • Molybdenum 150 mcg.

Vita Fuel Without Iron **-** TwinLab
Nine capsules contain: Beta-Carotene (pro-Vitamin A) 25000 IU • Vitamin D (from natural form Vitamin D3) 400 IU • Vitamin C 2000 mg • Natural Vitamin E (Succinate) 800 IU • CoQ10 (Coenzyme Q10) 30 mg • L-Glutathione 100 mg • N-Acetyl Cysteine (NAC) 200 mg • Alpha-Lipoic Acid 100 mcg • Vitamin B1 (Thiamine) 50 mg • Vitamin B2 (Riboflavin) 50 mg • Vitamin B6 (Pyridoxine) 50 mg • Vitamin B12 (Cobalamin) 100 mcg • Niacinamide 75 mg • Pantothenic Acid 100 mg • Folic Acid 800 mcg • Biotin 600 mcg • PABA 10 mg • Choline Bitartrate 100 mg • Inositol 100 mg • L-Carnitine (from Carni Fuel L-Carnitine Magnesium Citrate) 100 mg • Creatine (Monohydrate) 1000 mg • Calcium (from Calcium Citrate & Carbonate) 500 mg • Magnesium (from L-Carnitine Magnesium Citrate, Aspartate, Alpha-Ketoglutarate & Oxide) 500 mg • Potassium (from Potassium Alpha-Ketoglutarate, Citrate & Aspartate) 500 mg • Zinc (from Zinc Picolinate) 50 mg • Manganese (from Manganese Gluconate) 10 mg • Copper (from Copper Gluconate) 2 mg • Iodine (from Potassium Iodide) 150 mcg • Selenium (from Selenomethionine & Selenate 50/50 mixture) 200 mcg • Chromium (from Chromic Fuel patented Chromium Picolinate) 400 mcg • Molybdenum (from natural Molybdic Acid) 150 mcg.

Vita Lea for Children Fruit **-** Shaklee
Two tablets contain: Vitamin A (as Vitamin A acetate) 2500 IU • Vitamin C (as Ascorbic acid) 60 mg • Vitamin D (as Choloecalciferol) 400 IU • Vitamin E (as D-alpha tocopheryl acetate) 30 IU • Vitamin K (as Phytonadione) 10 mcg • Thiamin (as Thiamin mononitrate) 1.5 mg • Riboflavin 1.7 mg • Niacin (as Niacinamide) 20 mg • Vitamin B6 (as Pyridoxine hydrochloride) 2 mg • Folate (as Folic acid) 400 mcg • Vitamin B12 (as Cyanocobalamin) 6 mcg • Biotin (as D-biotin) 300 mcg • Pantothenic acid (as D-calcium pantothenate) 10 mg • Calcium (as Dicalcium iphosphate) 200 mg • Iron (as Ferrous fumerate) 10 mg • Phosphorus (as Dicalcium phosphate) 160 mg • Iodine (as Potassium iodide) 90 mcg • Magnesium (as Magnesium oxide) 80 mg • Zinc (as Zinc gluconate) 10 mg • Selenium (as trace mineral Protein hydrolysate) 20 mcg • Copper (as Copper oxide) 1 mg • Manganese (as Manganese gluconate) 1.5 mg • Chromium (as trace mineral Protein hydrolysate) 50 mcg • Molybdenum 50 mcg. Other Ingredients: Sorbitol, Fructose, Natural Flavors, Vegetable Juice Extracts (Beet, Carrot, Cabbage) and Annatto, Acacia Gum, Citric Acid, Inositol, Choline Bitartrate, Mixed Tocopherols, Rice Bran Powder, Rose Hips Powder, Alfalfa Powder, Acerola Extract, Grapefruit Bioflavonoid, Hesperidin Complex, Lemon Bioflavonoid, Orange Bioflavonoid, Sea Kelp Powder.

Vita Lea Iron Formula **-** Shaklee
Two tablets contain: Vitamin A (as Vitamin A acetate) 5000 IU • Vitamin C (as Ascorbic acid) 120 mg • Vitamin D (as Cholecalciferol) 400 IU • Vitamin E (as D-alpha tocopheryl acid succinate) 60 IU • Vitamin K (as Phytonadione) 80 mcg • Thiamin (as Thiamin mononitrate) 1.5 mg • Riboflavin 1.7 mg • Niacin (as

Niacinamide) 20 mg • Vitamin B6 (as Pyridoxine hydrochloride) 2 mg • Folate (as Folic acid) 400 mcg • Vitamin B12 (as Cyanocobalamin) 6 mcg • Biotin (as D-biotin) 300 mcg • Pantothenic acid (as D-calcium pantothenate) 10 mg • Calcium (as Dicalcium phosphate) 450 mg • Iron (as Ferrous fumarate) 18 mg • Phosphorus (as Dicalcium phosphate) 350 mg • Iodine (as Potassium iodide and sea kelp) 150 mcg • Magnesium (as Magnesium oxide) 200 mg • Zinc (as Zinc gluconate) 15 mg • Selenium (as trace mineral Protein hydrolysate) 70 mcg • Copper (as Copper gluconate) 2 mg • Manganese (as Manganese gluconate) 3.5 mg • Chromium (as trace mineral Protein hydrolysate) 130 mcg • Molybdenum (as trace mineral Protein hydrolysate) 130 mcg • Sodium 5 mg • Nickel (as trace mineral Protein hydrolysate) 15 mcg • Tin (as trace mineral Protein hydrolysate) 10 mcg • Vanadium (as trace mineral Protein hydrolysate) 2 mcg • Boron (as trace mineral Protein hydrolysate) 1 mg • Silicon (as Silicon dioxide) 2 mg. Other Ingredients: Microcrystalline Cellulose, Hydroxypropyl Methylcellulose, Croscarmellose Sodium, Spirulina, Inositol, Choline Bitartrate, Alfalfa Powder, Grapefruit Bioflavonoid, Hesperidin Complex, Lemon Bioflavonoid, Mixed Tocopherols, Orange Bioflavonoid, Rice Bran Powder, Rose Hips Powder, Acerola Extract, Hydroxylated Soy Lecithin, Carnauba Wax.

Vita Lea No Iron Formula - Shaklee
Two tablets contain: Vitamin A (as Vitamin A acetate) 5000 IU • Vitamin C (as Ascorbic acid) 120 mg • Vitamin D (as Cholecalciferol) 400 IU • Vitamin E (as D-alpha tocopheryl acid succinate) 60 IU • Vitamin K (as Phytonadione) 80 mcg • Thiamin (as Thiamin mononitrate) 1.5 mg • Riboflavin 1.7 mg • Niacin (as Niacinamide) 20 mg • Vitamin B6 (as Pyridoxine hydrochloride) 2 mg • Folate (as Folic acid) 400 mcg • Vitamin B12 (as Cyanocobalamin) 6 mcg • Biotin (as D-biotin) 300 mcg • Pantothenic Acid (as D-calcium pantothenate) 10 mg • Calcium (as Dicalcium phosphate) 450 mg • Phosphorus (as Dicalcium phosphate) 350 mg • Iodine (as Potassium iodide and sea kelp) 150 mcg • Magnesium (as Magnesium oxide) 200 mg • Zinc (as Zinc gluconate) 15 mg • Selenium (as Trace mineral protein hydrolysate) 70 mcg • Copper (as Copper gluconate) 2 mg • Manganese (as Manganese gluconate) 3.5 mg • Chromium (as Trace mineral protein hydrolysate) 130 mcg • Molybdenum (as Trace mineral protein hydrolysate) 160 mcg • Sodium 5 mg • Nickel (as Trace mineral protein hydrolysate) 15 mcg • Tin (as Trace mineral protein hydrolysate) 10 mcg • Vanadium (as Trace mineral protein hydrolysate) 2 mcg • Boron (as Trace mineral protein hydrolysate) 1 mg • Silicon (as Silicon dioxide) 2 mg. Other Ingredients: Microcrystalline Cellulose, Hydroxypropyl Methylcellulose, Croscarmellose Sodium, Spirulina, Inositol, Choline Bitartrate, Alfalfa Powder, Grapefruit Bioflavonoid, Hesperidin Complex, Lemon Bioflavonoid, Mixed Tocopherols, Orange Bioflavonoid, Rice Bran Powder, Rose Hips Powder, Acerola Extract, Hydroxylated Soy Lecithin, Carnauba Wax.

Vita Male - Nutri-Quest Rx
Each tablet contains: Yohimbe bark 250 mg • Damiana 40 mg • Gotu Kola 25 mg • Hawthorne berries 25 mg • Beet root.

Vita-Bears - Melaleuca
Four tablets contain: Vitamin A (as beta-carotene) 5000 IU • Vitamin C 80 mg • Vitamin D 400 IU • Vitamin E 30 IU • Vitamin B1 (thiamine) 2 mg • Vitamin B2 (riboflavin) 2 mg • Niacinamide 20 mg • Vitamin B6 (pyridoxine) 2 mg • Folic Acid 400 mcg • Vitamin B12 (cyanocobalamin) 6 mcg • Biotin 40 mcg • Pantothenic Acid 10 mg • Calcium 10 mg • Iron 18 mg • Phosphorous 40 mg • Iodine 150 mcg • Magnesium 20 mg • Zinc 16 mg • Copper 2 mg • Chromium 10 mcg.

VitaCardia - PhysioLogics
Three capsules contain: Vitamin B6 (as pyridoxine HCl) 10 mg • Folic Acid 810 mcg • Vitamin B12 (as cyanocobalamin) 510 mcg • Magnesium (as magnesium glycinate) 50 mg • Potassium (as potassium chloride) 95 mg • Hawthorn fruit extract (crataegus oxyacantha, standardized to contain 1.8% vitexin, 10.8 mg) 600 mg • Cordyceps (standardized to contain 7% cordyceptic acid, 28 mg) 400 mg • Taurine 200 mg. Other Ingredients: Gelatin, Silica, Vegetable Magnesium Stearate.

Vitacor Plus - Matthias Rath, Inc.
Each tablet contains: Ascorbic Acid 230 mg • Ascorbyl Palmitate 170 mg • Calcium Ascorbate 100 mg • Magnesium Ascorbate 100 mg • Vitamin E (d-Alpha-Tocopherol) 130 IU • Vitamin A (Beta-Carotene) 1665 IU • Vitamin B1 (Thiamine) 7 mg • Vitamin B2 (Riboflavin) 7 mg • Niacin 10 mg • Niacinamide 35 mg • Pantothenic Acid (d-Calcium Pantothenate) 40 mg • Vitamin B6 (Pyridoxal Phosphate) 10 mg • Vitamin B12 (Cyanocobalamin) 20 mcg • Vitamin D (as Vitamin D3) (Cholecalciferol) 130 IU • Folic Acid 90 mcg • Biotin 65 mcg • L-Proline 110 mg • L-Lysine 110 mg • L-Carnitine 35 mg • L-Arginine 40 mg • L-Cysteine 35 mg • Calcium (Glycinate, Ascorbate) 35 mg • Magnesium (Glycinate, Ascorbate) 40 mg • Potassium (Chelate) 20 mg • Zinc (Glycinate) 7 mg • Manganese (Chelate) 1.3 mg • Copper (Glycinate) 330 mcg • Selenium (L-Seleno Methionine) 20 mcg • Chromium (Glycinate) 10 mcg • Molybdenum (Glycinate) 4 mcg • Inositol 35 mg • Coenzyme Q10 7 mg • Phosphorous (Dicalcium Phosphate) 15 mg • Pycnogenol 7 mg • Citrus Bioflavonoids 100 mg • Vitamin E (Beta, Gamma & Delta Tocopherols) 22 mg • Carotenoids (Alpha-Carotene, Lutein, Zeaxanthin, & Cryptoxanthin) 50 mcg.

VitAdvance Immune Advance Formula - Avon
Each tablet contains: Vitamin A (as beta-carotene) 3333 IU • Vitamin C (as ascorbic acid) 200 mg • Vitamin E (as d-alpha tocopheryl acetate) 200 IU • Vitamin B6 (as pyridoxine HCl) 6 mg • Zinc (as zinc gluconate) • Astragalus root extract (astragalus membranaceus, standardized to 0.4% 7-glyco-4'-hydroxy-3'-methyoxyisoflavone) 50 mg • Green Tea leaf extract (camellia sinensis, standardized to 50% polyphenols) 50 mg. Other Ingredients: Microcrystalline Cellulose, Croscarmellose Sodium, Silicon Dioxide, Hydroxypropyl Methylcellulose, Stearic Acid, Titanium Dioxide, Magnesium Stearate, Polyethylene Glycol, Caramel, Riboflavin.

VitAdvance Joint Formula - Avon
Each tablet contains: Vitamin C (as ascorbic acid) 30 mg • Manganese (as manganese gluconate) 1.5 mg • Glucosamine Sulfate powder (includes potassium chloride 125 mg) 500 mg • Devil's Claw (harpagophytum procumbens) root extract (standardized to 2% harpagosides) 150 mg. Other Ingredients: Microcrystalline Cellulose, Croscarmellose Sodium, Stearic Acid, Magnesium Stearate, Hydroxypropyl Methylcellulose, Polyethylene Glycol, Carnauba Wax.

VitAdvance Menopause Support - Avon
Each tablet contains: Calcium (as dicalcium phosphate) 61 mg • Chaste Tree berry fruit (vitex angus-castus, standardized to 0.5% angusides) 50 mg • Black Cohosh roots extract (cimicifuga racemosa, standardized to 2.5% triterpene glycosides) 40 mg • Soy Isoflavones 22.5 mg • Boron (as sodium borate) 1.5 mg. Other Ingredients: Microcrystalline Cellulose, Stearic Acid, Magnesium Stearate, Silicon Dioxide, Hydroxypropyl Methylcellulose, Polyethylene Glycol, Carnauba Wax.

VitAdvance Men's Complete Multivitamin - Avon
Each tablet contains: Vitamin A (as retinyl acetate and 20% (1000 IU) as beta-carotene) 5000 IU • Vitamin C (as ascotbic acid) 90 mg • Vitamin D (as cholecalciferol) 400 IU • Vitamin E (as d-alpha tocopheryl acetate) 45 IU • Vitamin K (as phytonadione) 80 mcg • Thiamin (a thiamin mononitrate) 2.25 mcg • Niacin (as niacinamide) 20 mg • Vitamin B6 (as pyridoxine hydrochloride) 3 mg • Folate (as folic acid) 400 mcg • Vitamin B12 (as cyanocobalamin) 12 mcg • Biotin 60 mcg • Pantothenic Acid (as calcium d-pantothenate) 10 mg • Calcium (as dicalcium phosphate) 100 mg • Iron (as ferrous gluconate) 18 mg • Phosphorous (as dicalcium phosphate) 78 mg • Iodine (as potassium iodide) 150 mcg • Magnesium (as magnesium oxide) 100 mg • Zinc (as zinc gluconate) 15 mg • Selenium (as selenium-brown rice protein chelate) 70 mcg • Copper (as copper gluconate) 2 mg • Manganese (as manganese gluconate) 2 mg • Chromium (as chromium-brown rice protein chelate) 120 mcg • Molybdenum (as molybdenum citrate) 75 mcg • Chloride (as potassium chloride) 72 mg • Potassium (as potassium chloride) 82 mg • Silicon (as silicon dioxide) 2 mg • Lycopene 400 mcg • Lutein 250 mcg • Boron (as sodium borate) 150 mcg • Vanadium (as vanadium citrate) 10 mcg • Tin (as stannous chloride) 10 mcg • Nickel (as

nickel sulphate) 5 mcg. Inactive Ingredients: Microcrystalline Celluslose, Croscarmellose Sodium, Stearic Acid, Magnesium Stearate, Hydroxypropyl Methylcellulose, Titanium Dioxide, Hydroxypropyl Cellulose, Polyethylene Glycol, Caramel, Polysorbate 80, Carnauba Wax, Acetylated Monoglycerides, Xanthan Gum.

VitAdvance Menstrual Comfort I - Avon
Each tablet contains: Vitamin B6 (pyridoxine HCl) 50 mg • Magnesium (oxide) 250 mg • Calcium (dicalcium phosphate) 85 mg • Chaste Tree berry standardized extract (vitex angus-castus, 0.5% angusides) 30 mg. Other Ingredients: Microcrystalline Cellulose, Stearic Acid, Magnesium Stearate, Silicon Dioxide, Hydroxypropyl Methylcellulose, Polyethylene Glycol, Carnauba Wax.

VitAdvance Menstrual Comfort II - Avon
Each softgel contains: Vitamin E (D-alpha tocopheryl acetate) 10 IU • Evening Primrose Oil (oenothera biennis) 500 mg • Fatty Acid Profile: Linoleic Acid (omega 6) 350 mg • Oleic Acid (omega 9) 55 mg • Gamma Linolenic Acid (omega 6) 50 mg • Palmitic Acid 30 mg • Linolenic Acid (omega 3) 12 mg. Other Ingredients: Soybean Oil, Gelatin, Glycerin, Stearic Acid.

VitAdvance Multi-Kids Complete - Avon
Each tablet contains: Vitamin A (retinyl acetate and beta-carotene) 5000 IU • Vitamin C (ascorbic acid) 60 mg • Vitamin D (cholecalciferol) 400 IU • Vitamin E (D-alpha tocopheryl acetate) 30 IU • Vitamin K (phytonadione) 80 mcg • Thiamin (mononitrate) 1.5 mg • Riboflavin (vitamin B2) 1.7 mg • Niacin (niacinamide) 20 mg • Vitamin B6 (pyridoxine HCl) 2 mg • Folate (folic acid) 400 mcg • Vitamin B12 (cyanocobalamin) 6 mcg • Biotin 50 mcg • Pantothenic Acid (calcium d-pantothenate) 10 mg • Calcium (carbonate) 100 mg • Iron (ferrous fumarate) 10 mg • Iodine (potassium iodide) 150 mcg • Magnesium (oxide) 20 mg • Zinc (citrate) 15 mg • Copper (cupric acid) 2 mg • Manganese (citrate) 2 mg. Inactive Ingredients: Sorbitol, Fructose, Natural Flavor, Microcrystalline Cellulose, Stearic Acid, Magnesium Stearate, Silicon Dioxide, Carmine (natural colorant), Sucralose.

VitAdvance Restful Sleep - Avon
Each tablet contains: Valerian root extract (valeriana officinalis, standardized to 0.8% valerenic acid) 250 mg • Passionflower herb extract (passiflora incarnata, standardized to 4% vitexin) 150 mg. Other Ingredients: Mircrocrystalline Cellulose, Croscarmellose Sodium, Hydroxypropyl Methylcellulose, Stearic Acid, Silicon Dioxide, Titanium Dioxide, Polyethylene Glycol, Magnesium Stearate, Caramel, Peppermint Oil, Riboflavin.

Vita-E - Shaklee
Each tablet contains: Vitamin E (as D-alpha tocopheryl acid succinate) 400 IU • Selenium (as selenium yeast) 10 mcg. Other Ingredients: Dicalcium Phosphate, Silicon Dioxide, Modified Food Starch, Wheat Germ Flour, Natural Beet Powder.

VitaGreen - Young Living Essential Oils
Each capsule contains: Bee Pollen • Barley Juice Concentrate • Spirulina • Choline Bitartrate • Ginseng • Alfalfa Juice Concentrate • Pacific Kelp • L-Arginine • L-Cysteine • L-Tyrosine • Lemon Oil • Lemongrass Oil • Melissa Oil • Rosemary Oil • Gelatin.

Vital - Hillestad
Each tablet contains: Vitamin A (60% as beta carotene) 3750 IU • Vitamin C (ascorbic acid, rose hips) 150 mg • Vitamin D (D3, fish oil) 500 IU • Vitamin E (D-alpha tocopheryl succinate) 150 IU • Niacin (molasses culture, niacinamide) 37.5 mg • Magnesium (oxide) 55 mg • Zinc (gluconate) 3.75 mg • Selenium (kelp) 37.5 mcg • Manganese (amino acid chelate) 0.5 mg • Chromium (chromium nicotinate) 37.5 mcg • Co-Enzyme Q-10 25 mg • PABA (para amino benzoic acid) 37.5 mg • Choline (bitartrate) 25 mg • Inositol 25 mg • SOD (super oxide dismutase) 37.5 mg • Hesperidin Complex 20 mg • Citrus Bioflavonoids 20 mg • Bee Pollen 20 mg • Herbal Blend: Fennel, Goldenseal, Black Cohosh, Dandelion, Pau d'Arco, Comfrey, Flax seed, Psyllium seed, Chickweed, Garlic (odorless), Ginseng (American), Echinacea, Cellulose, Oyster shell, Magnesium Stearate, Silicon Dioxide, Food Glaze, Gum Arabic, L-Carnitine.

Vital #1 - J. R. Carlson Laboratories, Inc.
Each tablet contains: Whole Bovine Adrenal concentrate 100 mg.

Vital #27 (Thymus) - J. R. Carlson Laboratories, Inc.
Each tablet contains: Whole Bovine Thymus concentrate 200 mg.

Vital Adrenal - Vital Nutrients
Each dropper contains: Eleuthero (siberian ginseng) • Licorice • Gum Guggal • Gotu Kola • Ginger root • Dandelion • Cayenne • Fenugreek • Hawthorn • Red Clover.

Vital Brain - Vital Nutrients
Each dropper contains: Gotu Kola • Skullcap • Passionflower • Gum Guggal • Valerian • Hawthorn • Horsetail • Cayenne • Elecampane • Milk Thistle • Eleuthero (siberian ginseng) • Licorice • Fo-Ti root.

Vital D-Tox/Lymph - Vital Nutrients
Each dropper contains: Burdock • Oregon Grape • Red Clover • Buckthorn • Garlic • Ginger • Clove • Echinacea • Cayenne • Skullcap • Licorice • Slippery Elm • Fo-Ti root • Milk Thistle.

Vital Enzymes - Pro Health
Each tablet contains: Betaine (as betaine HCl from beets & molasses) 200 mg • Pancreatin 200 mg: Amylase 20,000 USP units, Protease 20,000 USP units, Lipase 3400 USP units • Papain (70 MCU from papaya) 50 mg • Cellulase (10 FCC units) 10 mg • Ox Bile extract 100 mg • Pepsin Enzymes (NF 1:10,000) 50 mg • Bromelain (2400 GDU from pineapple) 50 mg • Papaya powder 45 mg • Bromelain 10:1 (80 GDU) 45 mg. Other Ingredients: Calcium Carbonate, Cellulose, Stearic Acid, Magnesium Stearate.

Vital Female - Vital Nutrients
Each dropper contains: Partridge berry • Cramp Bark • Wild Yam • Dandelion • Damiana • Gum Guggal • Blessed Thistle • Red Raspberry leaf • Licorice • Ginger • Shepherd's Purse • Hawthorn • Red Clover • Fo-Ti root.

Vital Green - Futurebiotics LLC
Ten tablets contain: Alfalfa leaf juice powder concentrate 1350 mg • Barley grass juice powder concentrate 100 mg • Wheat Grass juice powder concentrate 250 mg • Spirulina powder 150 mg • Chlorella powder (broken cell) 150 mg. Other Ingredients: Dicalcium phosphate, Cellulose, Magnesium stearate, Vegetable stearate, Silica.

Vital Heart/Lung - Vital Nutrients
Each dropper contains: Hawthorn • Mullein • Red Clover • Eleuthero (siberian ginseng) • Garlic • Ginger • Gum Guggal • Burdock • Wild Cherry bark • Slippery Elm • Skullcap • Licorice • Oregon Grape • Dandelion • Fenugreek • Cramp Bark • Elecampane.

Vital Immune - Vital Nutrients
Each dropper contains: Para Cress • Pau d'Arco • Red Clover • Astragalus • Echinacea • Garlic • Elecampane • Licorice • Ginger • Turmeric • Buckthorn.

Vital K + Ginseng Capsules - Futurebiotics LLC
Potassium • Calcium • Magnesium • 16 Herbal extracts Plus the Triple Ginseng Action of Korean, Siberian & American Ginseng.

Vital K + Ginseng Extra - Futurebiotics LLC
Siberian, Korean, & American Ginseng • "16 Invigorating Herbal extracts" • Potassium • Calcium & Iron found in the Original Vital K.

Vital K Original with Magnesium - Futurebiotics LLC
Potassium • Magnesium • Calcium • Iron, "17 Herbal extracts" including Ginseng, Astragalus, Schizandra, Dong Quai.

Vital Kidney/Bladder - Vital Nutrients
Each dropper contains: Nettles • Uva Ursi • Fo-Ti root • Red Clover • Dandelion leaf • Burdock • Slippery Elm • Echinacea • Skullcap • Parsley • Licorice • Oregon Grape • Hawthorn.

Vital Liver/Digest - Vital Nutrients
Each dropper contains: Oregon Grape • Fenugreek • Turmeric • Red Clover • Bupleurum • Eleuthero (siberian ginseng) • Fo-Ti root • Pau D'Arco • Hawthorn • Milk Thistle • Licorice • Wild Yam • Buckthorn • Ginger • Dandelion.

Vital Male - Vital Nutrients
Each dropper contains: Saw Palmetto • Muira Puama • Eleuthero (siberian ginseng) • Turmeric • Parsley • Fo-Ti root • Hawthorn • Damiana • Gum Guggal • Cayenne • Juniper berry • Licorice • Elecampane • Sarsaparilla.

Vital Memory - TwinLab
Each tablet contains: Vitamin C (ascorbic acid) 50 mg • Vitamin E (D-alpha tocopheryl acid succinate) 33.34 IU • Folic Acid 133.34 mcg • Vitamin B12 (cyanocobalamin) 16.67 mcg • Calcium (phosphate, carbonate, silicate) 336 mg • Phosphorus (calcium phosphate) 192 mg • Phosphatidylserine 100 mg • Acetyl L-Carnitine Hydrochloride 50 mg • Alpha Lipoic Acid 16.67 mg. Other Ingredients: Cellulose, Croscarmellose Sodium, Maltodextrin, Vegetable Stearate, Magnesium Stearate, Silica.

Vital Multiple - Vital Nutrients
Each dropper contains: Bladderwrack • Parsley • Dandelion • Burdock • Ginger • Slippery Elm • Fo-Ti root.

Vital PSP+ - Healthywize
Each 50 g scoop contains: Proprietary Blend 5000 mg: Alpha-Glycan Polysaccharidepeptides of Rice Flour, Natural Spirulina.

Vital Thyroid - Vital Nutrients
Each dropper contains: Gum Guggal • Wild Yam • Dandelion • Hawthorn • Saw Palmetto • Eleuthero (siberian ginseng) • Cayenne • Ginger • Licorice • Turmeric • Gotu Kola.

Vital Vein - Puritan's Pride
Three capsules contain: Vitamin A 10,000 IU • Vitamin C 250 mg • Vitamin E 100 IU • Magnesium 100 mg • Zinc 3 mg • Selenium 0.42 mcg • Grape Seed extract 15 mg • Gotu Kola herb (centella asiatica) 800 mg • Lecithin 200 mg • Butchers' Broom herb (Ruscus aculeatus) 400 mg • Rutin 125 mg • Spirulina 100 mg • White Oak Bark (Quercus alba) 75 mg • Ginkgo Biloba leaf (Ginkgo biloba) 100 mg • Kelp 100 mg • Bromelain 50 mg • Ginger root (Zingiber officinate) 50 mg • Hawthorn berry (Crataegus laevigata) 50 mg.

Vital-Greens Rx - Alternecare Health Products
Each 1 tbsp serving contains: Soy Lecithin (99% oil free) 2000 mg • Spirulina powder 1000 mg • Apple Pectin 670 mg • Apple fiber 670 mg • Barley grass leaf juice powder 430 mg • Alfalfa juice powder 430 mg • Wheat Grass juice powder 430 mg • Brown Rice Bran 400 mg • Wheat sprout powder 300 mg • Barley malt 300 mg • Chlorella 250 mg • Beet root juice 250 mg • Nova Scotia Dulse leaf 250 mg • Bee Pollen 200 mg • Probiotic Culture (2.5 billion) 135 mg • Acerola berry 100 mg • Siberian Ginseng root 80 mg • Echinacea Angustifolia herb 80 mg • Astragalus root 80 mg • Bilberry extract 60 mg • Royal Jelly 3.3x Concentrate 60 mg • Suma root powder 60 mg • Silymarin 83.5% (as milk thistle seed) • Licorice root powder 50 mg • Ginkgo Biloba leaf (24% extract) 30 mg • Licorice root 4:1 extract 20 mg • Grape seed extract 10 mg • Green Tea catechins 10 mg.

Vita-Licious Vitamin Chews - Bronson Laboratories
Each chew contains: Vitamin C 500 mg.

Vitaline Chewable CoQ10 (100 mg, maple nut/orange creme/chocolate) - PhytoPharmica
Each chewable tablet contains: Coenzyme Q10 (coq10, ubiquinone 10) 100 mg • Vitamin E (as D-alpha tocopheryl acetate) 300 IU.

Vitaline Chewable CoQ10 (200 mg, maple nut) - PhytoPharmica
Each chewable tablet contains: Coenzyme Q10 (coq10, ubiquinone 10) 200 mg • Vitamin E (as dL-alpha tocopheryl aceate, D-alpha tocopheryl acetate, and mixed tocopherols) 400 IU.

Vitaline CoQ10 100 mg (chocolate flavor) - PhytoPharmica
Each chewable wafer contains: Vitamin E 300 IU • Coenzyme Q10 100 mg.

Vitaline CoQ10 100 mg (maple nut flavor) - PhytoPharmica
Each chewable wafer contains: Vitamin E (as dl-alpha tocopheryl acetate, d-alpha tocopheryl acetate, and mixed tocopherols) 300 IU • Coenzyme Q10 (CoQ10; Ubiquinone) certified by Assay 100 mg.

Vitaline CoQ10 200 mg (chocolate flavor) - PhytoPharmica
Each chewable wafer contains: Vitamin E (as dl-alpha tocopheryl acetate, d-alpha tocopheryl acetate, and mixed tocopherols) 400 IU • Coenzyme Q10 (CoQ10; Ubiquinone) certified by Assay 200 mg.

Vitaline CoQ10 200 mg (maple nut flavor) - PhytoPharmica
Each chewable wafer contains: Vitamin E (as dl-alpha tocopheryl acetate, d-alpha tocopheryl acetate, and mixed tocopherols) 400 IU • Coenzyme Q10 (CoQ10; Ubiquinone) certified by Assay 200 mg.

Vitaline CoQ10 60 mg (chocolate flavor) - PhytoPharmica
Each chewable wafer contains: Vitamin E (as dl-alpha tocopheryl acetate, d-alpha tocopheryl acetate, and mixed tocopherols) 180 IU • Coenzyme Q10 (CoQ10; Ubiquinone) certified by Assay 60 mg.

Vitaline CoQ10 60 mg (maple nut flavor) - PhytoPharmica
Each chewable wafer contains: Vitamin E (as dl-alpha tocopheryl acetate, d-alpha tocopheryl acetate, and mixed tocopherols) 180 IU • Coenzyme Q10 (CoQ10; Ubiquinone) certified by Assay 60 mg.

Vitaline CoQ10, Creatine, and Acetyl-L-Carnitine - PhytoPharmica
Each scoop contains: Acetyl-L-Carnitine HCl 2.5 g • Creatine (pyruvate) 5 g • Natural Coenzyme Q10 (trans-coq10, ubiquinone 10 1.2 g • Vitamin E (as DL-alpha tocopheryl acetate) 1200 IU.

Vitaline Formulas 3 mg Biotin Forte - Integrative Therapeutics
Each tablet contains: Vitamin C (ascorbic acid) 200 mg • Thiamin (mononitrate) 10 mg • Riboflavin 10 mg • Niacin (niacinamide) 40 mg • Vitamin B6 (pyridoxine HCl) 25 mg • Folic Acid 800 mcg • Vitamin B12 (cyanocobalamin) 10 mcg • Biotin 3 mg • Pantothenic Acid (calcium pantothenate) 10 mg • Zinc (acetate) 30 mg. Other Ingredients: Microcrystalline Cellulose, Cellulose, Sodium Starch Glycolate, Silicon Dioxide, Vegetable Stearine, Calcium Stearate, Hydroxypropyl Methylcellulose, Titanium Dioxide.

Vitaline Formulas Coenzyme Q10 100 mg with Vitamin E - Integrative Therapeutics
Each wafer contains: Vitamin E (as dl-alpha tocopheryl acetate, d-alpha tocopheryl acetate, mixed tocopherols) 300 IU • Coenzyme Q10 (ubiquinone) 100 mg. Other Ingredients: Fructose, Dextrates, Silicone Dioxide, Vanilla Flavor, Maple Nut Flavor, Licorice Extract, Vegetable Fatty Acids, Magnesium Sulfate.

Vitaline Formulas Coenzyme Q10 200 mg - Integrative Therapeutics
Each tablet contains: Coenzyme Q10 (ubiquinone) 200 mg. Other Ingredients: Vegetable Fatty Acids, Silicon Dioxide, Magnesium Sulfate, Microcrystalline Cellulose, Stearic Acid, Croscarmellose Sodium, Magnesium Stearate.

Vitaline Formulas Coenzyme Q10 200 mg with Vitamin E - Integrative Therapeutics
Each wafer contains: Vitamin E (from dl-alpha tocopheryl acetate, d-alpha tocopheryl acetate, and mixed tocopherols) 400 IU • Coenzyme Q10 (ubiquinone) 200 mg. Other Ingredients: Fructose, Dextrates, Silicon Dioxide, Calcium Silicate, Magnesium Stearate, Natural Vanilla flavor, Maple Nut Flavor, Licorice Root Extract, Vegetable Fatty Acids, Magnesium Sulfate.

Vitaline Formulas Coenzyme Q10 60 mg - Integrative Therapeutics
Each tablet contains: Coenzyme Q10 60 mg. Other Ingredients: Vegetable Fatty Acids, Silicon Dioxide, Magnesium Sulfate, Microcrystalline Cellulose, Stearic Acid, Magnesium Stearate.

Vitaline L-Carnitine - PhytoPharmica
Each caplet contains: L-Carnitine 500 mg.

Vitality Rx - Athletic Technologies Inc.
Two capsules contain: L-Arginine 200 mg • L-Ornithine 150 mg • L-Lysine 50 mg • L-Glutamine 150 mg • Colostrum 100 mg • Anterior Pituitary 50 mg • Ornithine AKG 50 mg • L-Glycine 50 mg. See Editor's Note No. 31.

Some Brand Name Natural Products - What they Contain

www.NaturalDatabase.com contains MANY more listings than appear here.
Editor's Notes are located on pages 2155-2163.

BRAND NAMES

Vitaliza **- HerbaSway**
Horny Goat Weed • Dong Quai • He Sho Wu • Panax Ginseng • Knotweed • Schisandra • Blackberry • HerbaSwee (Cucurbitaceae fruit).

Vitalize Shampoo **- Biotech Corp.**
Purified Water • Saponified Oils of Coconut Oil and Olive Oil • Vegetable Glycerin • Methylsulfonylmethane (MSM) • Aloe Vera gel • Jojoba oil • PEG-150 Distearate (from plant) • Hydrolyzed Wheat Protein • Natural Essential Oils • Avena Sativa (oat) extract • Citric Acid • Rosemary Oil.

Vitalizer VitaSerum **- Abra Therapeutics**
Cranberry juice • Vitamin C (as acerola L-ascorbic acid) • Glycosaminoglycans • Hyaluronic Acid • Zinc Sulfate • Vegetable Glycerine • ABRA3 PhytoSerum Complex: Red Grape seed extract, Green Tea extract, Horsetail extract, Elder flower extract • Citrus Bioflavonoids • Sweet Orange oil • Lavender oil • Rose Geranium oil • Methylparaben • Propylparaben.

Vitalux AREDS **- Novartis**
Each tablet contains: Beta Carotene (provitamin A) 12,500 IU • Vitamin C (ascorbic acid) 250 mg • Vitamin E (d-alpha tocopheryl acetate) 200 IU • Zinc (zinc gluconate) 40 mg • Copper (HVP chelate) 1 mg • Lutein (supplying 132 mg of Zeaxanthin).

Vitalux with Lutein **- Novartis**
Each tablet contains: Beta-Carotene (provitamin A) 10,000 IU • Vitamin C (ascorbic acid) 300 mg • Vitamin E (acetate) 100 IU • Vitamin B2 (riboflavin) 20 mg • Selenium (HVP chelate) 50 mcg • Zinc (gluconate) 40 mg • Copper (HVP chelate) 2 mg • Lutein 4 mg (supplying 176 mcg of Zeaxanthin) 4 mg. Other Ingredients: Cellulose, Calcium Silicate, Hydroxypropyl Methylcellulose, Stearic Acid, Magnesium Stearate, Silicon Dioxide, Titanium Dioxide, Hydroxypropyl Cellulose, Polyethylene Glycol, Caramel Color, Polysorbate 80, Vegetable Wax, Ethyl Vanillin, Diacetylated Monoglycerides, Xanthan Gum.

Vitalzym **- World Nutrition**
Three capsules contain: Proprietary Enzyme Blend 1500 mg: Protease, Serrapeptase, Papain, Bromelain, Amylase, Lipase, Rutin, Amla. Other Ingredients: Cellulose, Maltodextrin, Silicon Dioxide, Magnesium Stearate, Titanium Dioxide, Chlorophyllin.

Vita-Min **- Puritan's Pride**
Six tablets contain: Vitamin A (as Retinyl Acetate and Beta Carotene) 7,650 IU •Vitamin D (as Cholecalciferol) 200 IU • Vitamin C (as Ascorbic Acid) 200 mg • Vitamin E (as d-Alpha Tocopheryl Acid Succinate) 10 IU • Thiamin (Vitamin B-1; as Thiamine Hydrochloride) 6 mg • Riboflavin (Vitamin B-2) 12 mg • Niacin 3 mg • Vitamin B-6 (as Pyridoxine Hydrochloride) 2 mg • Folic Acid 400 mcg • Vitamin B-12 (as Cyanocobalamin) 5 mcg • Biotin (as D-Biotin) 5 mcg • Pantothenic Acid (as D-Calcium Pantothenate) 0.12 mg • Calcium (as Dicalcium Phosphate) 800 mg • Iron (as Ferrous Gluconate) 14 mg • Phosphorus (as Dicalcium Phosphate) 600 mg • Iodine (as Potassium Iodide) 100 mcg • Magnesium (as Magnesium Oxide) 50 mg • Zinc (as Zinc Sulfate) 0.022 mg • Selenium (as Sodium Selenate) 70 mcg • Copper (as Copper Sulfate) 0.022 mg • Manganese (as Manganese Sulfate) 0.0042 mg • Potassium (as Potassium Chloride and Potassium Iodide) 0.0574 mg • Silicon (as Silicon Dioxide) 0.097 mcg • Boron (as Sodium Borate Decahydrate) 300 mcg • PABA (Para-Aminobenzoic Acid) 37.5 mg • Choline Bitartrate 5.25 mg • Inositol 10 mg • Alfalfa 40 mg • L-Lysine 10 mg • Methionine 1.25 mg • Leucine 4.5 mg • Cysteine 1.25 mg • Isoleucine 4.5 mg • Phenylalanine 2.6 mg • Arginine 1.93 mg • Histidine 1.09 mg • Threonine 2.08 mg • Valine 3.16 mg • Wheat Germ powder 60 mg • Papain 20 mg • Chlorophyll 10 mg • Citrus Bioflavonoid 30 mg • Wheat Germ oil 20 mg • Peppermint leaves 20 mg • Ginkgo Biloba leaf 30 mg • Coenzyme Q-10 30 mcg • Ginseng 12 mg • Deodorized Garlic 12 mg • Echinacea Purpurea 24 mg • Spirulina 12 mg • Chlorella 12 mg • Klamath Lake Blue Green Algae 12 mg • Grapeseed extract complex 200 mcg. In a natural base of Watercress, Parsley, Kelp, and Lecithin.

Vitamin & Aloe Mosturizing Creme **- Aspen Group, Inc.**
Each gram contains: Tocopheryl Acetate 1% • Panthenol 1% • Water • Hydrogenated Polyisobutane • Octyl Methoxycinnamate • Mineral Oil • Ceteraryl Alcohol • Cetyl Phosphate • Dimethicone • Aloe Vera Gel • Aminomethyl Propanol • Fragrance • Carbomer • Propylene Glycol • Diazolidinyl Urea • Methylparaben • Propylparaben.

Vitamin A **- Puritan's Pride**
Each softgel contains: Vitamin A (as derived from fish liver oils) 10,000 IU.

Vitamin A **- GNC**
Each capsule contains: Vitamin A (as Fish Liver Oil) 10,000 IU. Other Ingredients: Soybean oil, Gelatin, Glycerin.

Vitamin A **- Nature's Bounty**
Each softgel contains: Vitamin A (from Fish Liver Oils) 10000 IU. Other Ingredients: Soybean Oil, Gelatin, Glycerin.

Vitamin A **- Nature's Way**
Each softgel contains: Vitamin A (cod liver oil) 10,000 IU. Other Ingredients: Gelatin, Glycerin, Soybean Oil, Water.

Vitamin A **- Jamieson**
Each capsule contains: Vitamin A (from Halibut liver oil) 10000 IU.

Vitamin A **- Golden Glow Natural Health Products**
Each softgel contains: Retinyl Palmitate (vitamin A) 2500 IU. Other Ingredients: Peanut Oil.

Vitamin A **- Pure Encapsulations**
Each softgel capsule contains: Vitamin A (from fish oil) 25,000 IU.

Vitamin A - In Water Soluble Base **- Nature's Bounty**
Each softgel contains: Vitamin A (as Retinyl Palmitate) 10000 IU. Other Ingredients: Polysorbate 80, Gelatin, Glycerin, Propylene Glycol.

Vitamin A & D **- Nature's Sunshine**
Each capsule contains: Vitamin A (from fish oil) 10,000 IU • Vitamin D (from fish oil) 400 IU. Other Ingredients: Gelatin, Water.

Vitamin A & D **- Nature's Bounty**
Each tablet contains: Vitamin A (as retinyl palmitate) 10,000 IU • Vitamin D (as cholecalciferol) 400 IU. Other Ingredients: Dicalcium Phosphate, Cellulose, Calcium Sulfate, Vegetable Stearic Acid, Cellulose Coating, Vegetable Magnesium Stearate, Silica.

Vitamin A & D **- GNC**
Each capsule contains: Vitamin A (as fish liver oil) 5000 IU •Vitamin D (as fish liver oil) 400 IU. Other Ingredients: Soybean Oil, Gelatin, Glycerin.

Vitamin A & D **- Health Smart Vitamins**
Each softgel contains: Vitamin A (from cod liver oil) 10,000 IU • Vitamin D (from cod liver oil) 400 IU.

Vitamin A & D **- Jamieson**
Each capsule contains: Vitamin A (Retinol) 5000 IU • Vitamin D 400 IU.

Vitamin A & D **- Source Naturals**
Each tablet contains: vitamin A (as palmitate) 10,000 IU • Vitamin D (as cholecalciferol) 400 IU.

Vitamin A & D 10,000/400 IU **- Arrowroot**
Each gelcap contains: Vitamin A 10,000 IU • Vitamin D 400 IU.

Vitamin A & D Fortified **- Jamieson**
Each capsule contains: Vitamin A 10,000 IU • Vitamin D 400 IU.

Vitamin A (from fish oil) 10,000 IU **- Vital Nutrients**
Each softgel contains: Vitamin A (from fish liver oil) 10,000 IU.

Vitamin A (from fish oil) 25,000 IU **- Vital Nutrients**
Each softgel contains: Vitamin A (from fish liver oil) 25,000 IU.

Vitamin A 10,000 IU - Jamieson
Each capsule contains: Vitamin A Retinol (Derived from fresh, pure fish liver oil) 10,000 IU.

Vitamin A 10,000 IU - GNC
Each capsule contains: Vitamin A (as fish liver oil) 10,000 IU. Other Ingredients: Soybean Oil, Gelatin, Glycerin.

Vitamin A 10,000 IU - Nature Made
Each softgel contains: Vitamin A (from fish liver oil) 10,000 IU. Other Ingredients: Soybean Oil, Gelatin, Glycerin, Water. See Editor's Note No. 45.

Vitamin A 10,000 IU - Arrowroot
Each gelcap contains: Vitamin A 10,000 IU.

Vitamin A 8000 IU - Nature Made
Each softgel contains: Vitamin A (from fish liver oil) 8000 IU. Other Ingredients: Soybean Oil, Gelatin, Glycerin, Water. See Editor's Note No. 45.

Vitamin A 8000 IU - Nature's Valley
Each softgel contains: Vitamin A (as fish liver oil) 8000 IU. Other Ingredients: Vegetable Oil, Gelatin, Glycerin. See Editor's Note No. 45.

Vitamin A Cream - Life Extension
Vitamin A, De-Ionized Water, Aloe, Emollients, Cetearyl Alcohol, Methyl Glucose, Sesquisterate, Mink oil, Vitamin D oil (vitamin D2), Vitamin E oil, BHT, BHA, Tea, Sesame oil, Lanolin.

Vitamin A Emulsified 25,000 IU - J. R. Carlson Laboratories, Inc.
Each softgel contains: Vitamin A (from fish liver oil) 25,000 IU.

Vitamin A Micellized with Beta-Carotene - American Biologics
Each drop contains: Micellized Vitamin A (as vitamin A palmitate) 5000 IU. Other Ingredients: Water, Castor Bean Oil (ethoxyiated), Glycerin, Citric Acid, Potassium Sorbate, Potassium Benzoate.

Vitamin A Natural 10,000 IU - J. R. Carlson Laboratories, Inc.
Each softgel contains: Vitamin A (from fish liver oil) 10,000 IU.

Vitamin A Natural 25,000 IU - J. R. Carlson Laboratories, Inc.
Each softgel contains: Vitamin A (from fish liver oil) 25,000 IU.

Vitamin A Palmitate - Source Naturals
Each tablet contains: Vitamin A (as palmitate) 10,000 IU.

Vitamin A Palmitate 15,000 IU - J. R. Carlson Laboratories, Inc.
Each softgel contains: Vitamin A (as retinyl palmitate) 15,000 IU.

Vitamin A Palmitate 15,000 IU - J. R. Carlson Laboratories, Inc.
Each softgel contains: Vitamin A (as retinyl palmitate) 15,000 IU.

Vitamin A Retinol - Anti-Aging Moisturizer - Jamieson
Contains: Vitamin A Retinol (Retinyl Palmitate) • SPF Active Ingredients • Aloe Vera Extract • Bee Pollen Extract • Chamomile Extract • Comfrey Extract • Watercress Extract.

Vitamin A Retinol - Night Treatment Moisturizer - Jamieson
Vitamin A Retinol (Retinyl Palmitate) • Tocopheryl Acetate • Aloe Vera Extract • Fennel Extract • Hops Extract • Chamomile Extract • Balm Mint Extract • Mistletoe Extract • Bee Pollen Extract • Jojoba Oil • Wheat Germ Oil • Fructose • Glucose • Sucrose.

Vitamin A Retinyl Palmitate Wrinkle Treatment - Derma E
Vitamin A 10000 IU/100 gm • Vitamin E • Vitamin D • Allantoin.

Vitamin A Solubilized 10,000 IU - J. R. Carlson Laboratories, Inc.
Each softgel contains: Vitamin A (as palmitate) 10,000 IU.

Vitamin A Tablets 15,000 IU - Arrowroot
Each tablet contains: Vitamin A 15,000 IU.

Vitamin and Mineral Supplement - Alotek Supplement Company
Two tablets contain: Vitamin E (D-alpha-tocopherol) 133 IU • Vitamin A 3333 IU • Beta Carotene 3333 IU • Vitamin D 267 IU • Vitamin C 267 mg • Folic Acid 267 mcg • Thiamine 1 mg • Riboflavin 1.1 mg • Niacin 13.3 mg • Vitamin B6 1.3 mg • Vitamin B12 4 mcg • Biotin 200 mcg • Pantothenic Acid 6.7 mg • Calcium Citrate 400 mg • Phosphorus 300 mg • Iodine (kelp) 100 mcg • Magnesium Carbonate 133 mg • Copper (as gluconate) 1.3 mg • Zinc (as gluconate) 10 mg • Vitamin K 67 mcg • Selenium 50 mcg • Manganese Gluconate 3.3 mg • Chromium (as aspartate) 133 mcg • Molybdenum 100 mcg • Nickel 10 mcg • Tin 10 mcg • Vanadium 3.3 mg • Boron (as citrate) 1.3 mg • Potassium Gluconate 67 mg • Grape seed extract 6.7 mg • CoQ10 6.7 mg. Other Ingredients: Magnesium Stearate, Stearic Acid.

Vitamin B 100 Complex - Jamieson
Each caplet contains: Thiamin (mononitrate) 100 mg • Riboflavin (vitamin B2) 100 mg • Niacin (niacinamide) 100 mg • Vitamin B6 (pyridoxine hydrochloride) 100 mg • Folate (folic acid) 400 mcg • vitamin B12 (cyanocobalamin) 100 mcg • Biotin 100 mcg • Pantothenic Acid (calcium D-pantothenate) 100 mg • Calcium 555 mg • Choline Bitartrate 100 mg • Inositol 100 mg.

Vitamin B Complete - AIE Pharmaceuticals
Thiamin • Riboflavin • Niacin • Vitamin B6 • Folic Acid • Vitamin B12 • Biotin • Pantothenic Acid • Inositol • Choline • Para-Aminobenzoic Acid.

Vitamin B Complex - Westcoast Naturals
Each caplet contains: Vitamin B1 (thiamine hydrochloride) 50 mg • Vitamin B2 (riboflavin) 50 mg • Vitamin B3 (niacinamide) 100 mg • Vitamin B5 (pantothenic acid-calcium pantothenate) 100 mg • Vitamin B6 (pyridoxine hydrochloride) 50 mg • Vitamin B12 (cyanocobalamin) 100 mcg • Biotin 50 mcg • Folic Acid 1 mg • Choline (bitartrate) 100 mg • Inositol 100 mg.

Vitamin B Complex - NSI - Nutraceutical Sciences Institute
Each capsule contains: Thiamine HCl (B1) 250 mg • Riboflavin (B2) 10 mg • Niacinamide (B3) 100 mg • Pantothenic Acid (B6) 100 mg • Methylcobalamin (B12) 500 mcg • Folic Acid 800 mcg • Biotin 500 mcg • Vitamin C (magnesium acorbate, Ester C) 100 mg.

Vitamin B Complex - PhysioLogics
Each capsule contains: Thiamin (vitamin B1, as thiamin mononitrate) 100 mg • Riboflavin (vitamin B2) 100 mg • Niacin (as niacinamide) 100 mg • Vitamin B6 (as pyrdioxine hydrochloride) 100 mg • Folic Acid 400 mcg • Vitamin B12 (as cyanocobalamin) 100 mcg • Biotin 100 mcg • Pantothenic Acid (as d-calcium pantothenate) 100 mg • Choline Bitartrate 100 mg • PABA (para-aminobenzoic acid) 100 mg • Inositol 100 mg • Proprietary Blend 7.5 mg: Alfalfa, Watercress, Parsley, Lecithin, Rice Bran. Other Ingredients: Gelatin, Vegetable Magnesium Stearate, Silica.

Vitamin B Complex With C - Nature's Valley
Each caplet contains: Vitamin C 300 mg • Thiamine (vitamin B1) 15 mg • Riboflavin (vitamin B2) 10.2 mg • Niacin 50 mg • Vitamin B6 5 mg • Folic Acid 400 mcg • Vitamin B12 6 mcg • Pantothenic Acid 10 mg. Other Ingredients: Dextrose, Cellulose, D-Calcium Pantothenate, Croscarmellose Sodium, Hydroxpropyl Methycellulose, Starch Oligosaccharides, Stearic Acid, Starch, Dextrin, Magnesium Stearate, Silicon Dioxide, Resin, Lecithin, Sodium Carboxymethylcellulose, Sodium Citrate. See Editor's Note No. 45.

Vitamin B1 - Source Naturals
Each tablet contains: Thiamin (vitamin B1) 100 mg.

Vitamin B-1 - J. R. Carlson Laboratories, Inc.
Each tablet contains: Thiamin (vitamin B1) 100 mg.

Vitamin B-1 **-** Nature's Bounty
Each tablet contains: Thiamin (as Thiamine Hydrochloride) 100 mg. Other Ingredients: Dicalcium Phosphate, Cellulose, Vegetable Stearic Acid, Silica, Vegetable Magnesium Stearate.

Vitamin B1 (Thiamin) 100 mg **-** Solgar
Each vegetable capsule contains: Thiamin (as thiamin HCl, vitamin B1) 100 mg. Other Ingredients: Vegetable Cellulose, Microcrystalline Cellulose, Silica, Vegetable Magnesium Stearate, Water.

Vitamin B1 (Thiamin) 50 mg **-** Solgar
Each tablet contains: Thiamin (as thiamin HCl, vitamin B1) 50 mg • Calcium (as dicalcium phosphate) 85 mg. Other Ingredients: Dicalcium Phosphate, Vegetable Cellulose, Vegetable Stearic Acid.

Vitamin B1 (Thiamin) 500 mg **-** Solgar
Each tablet contains: Thiamin (HCl, vitamin B1) 500 mg • Calcium (dicalcium phosphate) 75 mg. Other Ingredients: Dicalcium Phosphate, Microcrystalline Cellulose, Vegetable Cellulose, Silica, Vegetable Stearic Acid, Magnesium Stearate.

Vitamin B1 (Thiamine) **-** Gold Mountain Trading
Each tablet contains: Thiamine Nitrate (vitamin B1) 100 mg.

Vitamin B1 100 mg **-** Nature Made
Each tablet contains: Thiamin (B1, from thiamine hydrochloride) 100 mg. Other Ingredients: Dibasic Calcium Phosphate, Cellulose, Magnesium Stearate, Silicon Dioxide.
See Editor's Note No. 45.

Vitamin B1 100 mg **-** Nature's Valley
Each tablet contains: Vitamin B1 100 mg. Other Ingredients: Dicalcium Phosphate, Cellulose, Stearic Acid, Croscarmellose Sodium, Vegetable Oil, Magnesium Stearate, Silicon Dioxide.
See Editor's Note No. 45.

Vitamin B1 100 mg **-** Jamieson
Each tablet contains: Vitamin B1 (Thiamine Mononitrate) 100 mg.

Vitamin B1 100 mg **-** Solgar
Each tablet contains: Thiamin (as thiamin HCl, vitamin B1) 100 mg • Calcium (as dicalcium phosphate) 85 mg. Other Ingredients: Microcrystalline Cellulose, Silica, Vegetable Cellulose, Vegetable Stearic Acid, Vegetable Magnesium Stearate.

Vitamin B1 100 mg Tablets **-** Nature's Plus
Each tablet contains: Thiamin (vitamin B1, as thiamine hydrochloride) 100 mg. Other Ingredients: Di-calcium Phosphate, Microcrystalline Cellulose, Stearic Acid, Magnesium Stearate, Rice Bran, Pharmaceutical Glaze, Silica.

Vitamin B1 300 mg Sustained Release tablets **-** Nature's Plus
Each extended-release tablet contains: Thiamin (vitamin B1, as thiamine hydrochloride) 300 mg. Other Ingredients: Microcrystalline Cellulose, Microcrystalline Cellulose, Hydroxypropyl Methylcellulose, Rice Bran, Di-calcium Phosphate, Stearic Acid, Magnesium Stearate, Pharmaceutical Glaze, Silica.

Vitamin B1 50 mg **-** Solgar
Each tablet contains: Thiamin (as thiamin HCl, vitamin B1) 50 mg • Calcium (as dicalcium phosphate) 85 mg. Other Ingredients: Dicalcium Phosphate, Vegetable Cellulose, Vegetable Stearic Acid.

Vitamin B12 **-** Source Naturals
Each tablet contains: Vitamin B12 2 mg.

Vitamin B12 **-** Jamieson
Each tablet contains: Vitamin B12 (as Cyanocobalamin) 1200 mcg • Calcium 80 mg.

Vitamin B12 **-** AIE Pharmaceuticals
Each tablet contains: Vitamin B12 (as cyanocobalamin) 1000 mcg.

Vitamin B-12 **-** GNC
Each tablet contains: Vitamin B12 (as cyanocobalamin) 1000 mcg. Other Ingredients: Dicalcium Phosphate, Cellulose, Vegetable Stearate, Food Glaze, Whole Brown Rice powder (oryza sativa).

Vitamin B-12 **-** Nature's Bounty
Each tablet contains: Vitamin B-12 (as Cyanocobalamin) 100 mcg. Other Ingredients: Dicalcium Phosphate, Cellulose, Vegetable Stearic Acid, Mannitol, Silica, Vegetable Magnesium Stearate.

Vitamin B-12 **-** Leiner Health Products
Each tablet contains: Vitamin B12 (Cyanocobalamin) 100 mcg. Other Ingredients: Lactose, Starch, Dicalcium Phosphate, Magnesium Stearate, Red 40 Lake.

Vitamin B-12 **-** Vital Nutrients
Each capsule contains: Vitamin B12 (as hydroxocobalamin powder) 1000 mcg.

Vitamin B-12 **-** GNC
Each tablet contains: Vitamin B12 (as Cyanocobalamin) 500 mcg. Other Ingredients: Dextrose, Stearic Acid, Magnesium Stearate, Whole Brown rice powder.

Vitamin B12 (Cyanocobalamin) **-** Golden Glow Natural Health Products
Each tablet contains: Cyanocobalamin (vitamin B12) 1000 mcg.

Vitamin B12 (Sublingual) **-** Westcoast Naturals
Each sublingual tablet contains: Vitamin B12 (cyanocobalamin) 1000 mcg. Base: Natural Cherry Juice Powder, Stearic Acid.

Vitamin B12 100 mcg **-** Sunmark
Each tablet contains: Vitamin B12 100 mcg. Other Ingredients: Dicalcium Phosphate, Microcrystalline Cellulose, Stearic Acid, Croscarmellose Sodium, Crospovidone, Magnesium Stearate.
See Editor's Note No. 45.

Vitamin B12 100 mcg **-** Solgar
Each tablet contains: Vitamin B12 (as cobalamin) 100 mcg • Calcium (as dicalcium phosphate) 40 mg. Other Ingredients: Dicalcium Phosphate, Microcrystalline Cellulose, Vegetable Cellulose, Vegetable Stearic Acid, Silica, Vegetable Magnesium Stearate.

Vitamin B12 100 mcg **-** Jamieson
Each tablet contains: Vitamin B12 (Cyanocobalamin) 100 mcg.

Vitamin B-12 1000 **-** GNC
Each tablet contains: Vitamin B12 (as cyanocobalamin) 1000 mcg. Other Ingredients: Dicalcium Phosphate, Cellulose, Whole Brown Rice powder (oryza sativa).

Vitamin B12 1000 mcg Chewable **-** Solgar
Each nugget contains: Vitamin B12 (as cobalamin) 1000 mcg. Other Ingredients: Mannitol, Vegetable Magnesium Stearate, Vegetable Stearic Acid, Natural Cherry Flavor.

Vitamin B12 1000 mcg Tablets **-** Nature's Plus
Each tablet contains: Vitamin B12 (as cyanocobalamin) 1000 mcg. Other Ingredients: Microcrystalline Cellulose, Di-calcium Phosphate, Stearic Acid, Magnesium Stearate, Beet Juice, Pharmaceutical Glaze, Silica.

Vitamin B12 1200 mcg Timed Release **-** Jamieson
Each tablet contains: Vitamin B12 (Cyanocobalamin) 1200 mcg.

Vitamin B-12 1500 **-** GNC
Each capsule contains: Vitamin B12 (as cyanocobalamin) 1500 mcg. Other Ingredients: Dicalcium Phosphate, Cellulose, Calcium Carbonate, Gelatin.

Vitamin B12 2000 mcg Sustained Release tablets **-** Nature's Plus
Each extended-release tablet contains: Vitamin B12 (as cyanocobalamin) 2000 mcg. Other Ingredients: Di-calcium Phosphate, Microcrystalline Cellulose, Stearic Acid, Hydroxypropyl Methylcellulose, Magnesium Stearate, Beet Juice Powder, Silica, Pharmaceutical Glaze.

Vitamin B12 25 mcg **-** Jamieson
Each tablet contains: Vitamin B12 (Cyanocobalamin) 25 mcg.

Vitamin B12 250 mcg - Jamieson
Each tablet contains: Vitamin B12 (Cyanocobalamin) 250 mcg.

Vitamin B12 250 mcg - Nature Made
Each tablet contains: Vitamin B12 (from cyanocobalamin) 250 mcg. Other Ingredients: Dibasic Calcium Phosphate, Cellulose, Stearic Acid, Croscarmellose Sodium, Magnesium Stearate.
See Editor's Note No. 45.

Vitamin B12 250 mcg - Solgar
Each tablet contains: Vitamin B12 (as cobalamin) 250 mcg • Calcium (as dicalcium phosphate) 50 mg. Other Ingredients: Dicalcium Phosphate, Microcrystalline Cellulose, Vegetable Stearic Acid, Vegetable Cellulose, Silica, Vegetable Magnesium Stearate.

Vitamin B12 50 mcg - Jamieson
Each tablet contains: Vitamin B12 (Cyanocobalamin) 50 mcg.

Vitamin B12 50 mcg - Walgreens
Each tablet contains: Vitamin B12 (cyanocobalamin) 50 mcg. Other Ingredients: Dicalcium Phosphate, Microcrystalline Cellulose, Stearic Acid, Modified Cellulose Gum, Magnesium Stearate.

Vitamin B-12 500 - GNC
Each tablet contains: Vitamin B12 (as cyanocobalamin) 500 mcg. Ingredients: Cyanocobalamin, Dextrose, Dicalcium Phosphate, Whole Brown Rice powder (oryza sativa).

Vitamin B12 500 mcg - Nature's Valley
Each tablet contains: Vitamin B12 (cyanocobalamin) 500 mcg. Other Ingredients: Lactose, Dicalcium Phosphate, Starch, Magnesium Sterate, Red 40 Lake.
See Editor's Note No. 45.

Vitamin B12 500 mcg - Sunmark
Each tablet contains: Vitamin B12 500 mcg. Other Ingredients: Dicalcium Phosphate, Microcrystalline Cellulose, Stearic Acid, Croscamellose Sodium, Crospovidone, Magnesium Stearate, Silicon Dioxide.
See Editor's Note No. 45.

Vitamin B12 500 mcg - Nature Made
Each tablet contains: Vitamin B12 (from cyanocobalamin) 500 mcg. Other Ingredients: Dibasic Calcium Phosphate, Cellulose Gel, Stearic Acid, Croscarmellose Sodium, Magnesium Stearate.
See Editor's Note No. 45.

Vitamin B-12 500 mcg - Puritan's Pride
Each tablet contains: Ener-B Vitamin B12 (as cyanocobalamin) 500 mcg. Other Ingredients: Dicalcium Phosphate, Cellulose (plant origin), Croscarmellose, Vegetable Stearic Acid, Silica, Vegetable Magnesium Stearate.

Vitamin B12 500 mcg Tablets - Nature's Plus
Each tablet contains: Vitamin B12 (as cyanocobalamin) 500 mcg. Other Ingredients: Microcrystalline Cellulose, Di-calcium Phosphate, Stearic Acid, Magnesium Stearate, Beet Juice, Pharmaceutical Glaze, Silica.

Vitamin B12 500 mcg Tablets - Solgar
Each tablet contains: Vitamin B12 (as cobalamin) 500 mcg • Calcium (as dicalcium phosphate) 130 mg. Other Ingredients: Dicalcium Phosphate, Microcrystalline Cellulose, Silica, Vegetable Stearic Acid, Vegetable Cellulose.

Vitamin B12 500 mcg Vegetable Capsules - Solgar
Each vegetable capsule contains: Vitamin B12 (as cobalamin) 500 mcg. Other Ingredients: Microcrystalline Cellulose, Vegetable Cellulose, Vegetable Magnesium Stearate, Silica, Water.

Vitamin B12 Timed Release 1000 mcg - Nature Made
Each tablet contains: Vitamin B12 (cyanocobalamin) 1000 mg. Other Ingredients: Dibasic Calcium Phosphate, Cellulose Gel, Stearic Acid, Magnesium Stearate.

Vitamin B125 - Source Naturals
Each tablet contains: Thiamin (vitamin B1) 125 mg • Riboflavin (as vitamin B2) 125 mg • Niacinamide 100 mg • Niacin 25 mg • Vitamin B6 (as pyridoxine HCl) 125 mg • Folate (as folic acid) 400 mcg • Vitamin B12 (as cyanocobalamin) 125 mcg • Biotin 125 mcg • Pantothenic Acid (as calcium d-pantotehnate) 125 mcg • Choline (as choline bitartrate) 125 mcg • Inositol 125 mcg • PABA (para-aminobenzoic acid) 125 mcg.

Vitamin B2 - Source Naturals
Each tablet contains: Riboflavin (vitamin B2) 100 mg.

Vitamin B-2 - J. R. Carlson Laboratories, Inc.
Each tablet contains: Riboflavin (vitamin B2) 100 mg.

Vitamin B-2 - Nature's Bounty
Each tablet contains: Riboflavin 100 mg. Other Ingredients: Dicalcium Phosphate, Cellulose, Vegetable Stearic Acid, Guar Gum, Croscarmellose, Silica.

Vitamin B2 (Riboflavin) - Golden Glow Natural Health Products
Each tablet contains: Riboflavin (vitamin B2) 100 mg.

Vitamin B2 (Riboflavin) 100 mg Tablets - Solgar
Each tablet contains: Riboflavin (vitamin B2) 100 mg • Calcium (as dicalcium phosphate) 40 mg. Other Ingredients: Dicalcium Phosphate, Microcrystalline Cellulose, Vegetable Cellulose, Silica, Vegetable Magnesium Stearate, Vegetable Stearic Acid.

Vitamin B2 (Riboflavin) 100 mg Vegetable Capsules - Solgar
Each vegetable capsule contians: Riboflavin (vitamin B2) 100 mg. Other Ingredients: Microcrystalline Cellulose, Vegetable Cellulose, Vegetable Magnesium Stearate, Water.

Vitamin B2 (Riboflavin) 50 mg - Solgar
Each tablet contains: Riboflavin (vitamin B2) 50 mg • Calcium (as dicalcium phosphate) 100 mg. Other Ingredients: Dicalcium Phosphate, Vegetable Stearic Acid, Silica, Vegetable Cellulose, Vegetable Magnesium Stearate.

Vitamin B2 100 mg - Jamieson
Each tablet contains: Vitamin B2 (Riboflavin) 100 mg.

Vitamin B2 100 mg Tablets - Nature's Plus
Each tablet contains: Riboflavin (vitamin B2) 100 mg. Other Ingredients: Microcrystalline Cellulose, Stearic Acid, Rice Bran, Magnesium Stearate, Pharmaceutical Glaze, Silica.

Vitamin B2 250 mg Sustained Release Tablets - Nature's Plus
Each extended-release tablet contains: Riboflavin (vitamin B2) 250 mg. Other Ingredients: Microcrystalline Cellulose, Microcrystalline Cellulose, Hydroxypropyl Methylcellulose, Di-calcium Phosphate, Stearic Acid, Rice Bran, Magnesium Stearate, Silica.

Vitamin B-2 50 - GNC
Each tablet contains: Riboflavin (as vitamin B-2) 50 mg. Other Ingredients: Dicalcium Phosphate, Cellulose, Vegetable Acetoglycerides, Whole Brown Rice powder (oryza sativa).

Vitamin B3 (Niacinamide) - Golden Glow Natural Health Products
Each tablet contains: Niacinamide (vitamin B3) 500 mg.

Vitamin B50 Complex - Source Naturals
Each tablet contains: Thiamin (vitamin B1) 50 mg • Riboflavin (vitamin B2) 50 mg • Niacinamide 50 mg • Vitamin B6 (as pyridoxine HCl) 50 mg • Folate (as folic acid) 100 mcg • Vitamin B12 (as cyanocobalamin) 50 mcg • Biotin 50 mcg • Pantothenic Acid (as calcium d-pantothenate) 100 mg • Choline (as bitartrate) 50 mg • Inositol 50 mg • PABA (as para amino benzoic Acid) 30 mg.

Vitamin B-50 Complex - GNC
Each tablet contains: Thiamin (as Thiamin Mononitrate) 50 mg • Riboflavin 50 mg • Niacin (as Niacinamide) 50 mg • Vitamin B6 (as Pyridoxine Hydrochloride) 50 mg • Folate, Folic Acid, Folacin

BRAND NAMES

400 mg • Vitamin B12 (as Cyanocobalamin) 50 mcg •Biotin 50 mcg • Pantothenic Acid (as Calcium d-Pantothenate) 50 mg • Choline Bitartrate 50 mg • Inositol 50 mcg • Para-aminobenzoic acid (PABA) 50 mcg. Other Ingredients: Dicalcium Phosphate, Cellulose, Magnesium Stearate, Yeast, Alfalfa, Watercress, Parsley, Lecithin, Rice Bran, Vegetable Acetoglycerides.

Vitamin B6 - Ortho Molecular Products
Each capsule contains: Vitamin B6 (as pyridoxine HCl USP) 250 mg. Other Ingredients: Natural Vegetable Capsules, Ascorbyl Palmitate, Magnesium Stearate, Microcrystalline Cellulose, Silicon Dioxide.

Vitamin B6 - Jamieson
Each tablet contains: Vitamin B6 (pyridoxine HCl) 100 mg.

Vitamin B-6 - Nature's Bounty
Each tablet contains: Vitamin B-6 (Pyridoxine Hydrochloride) 50 mg. Other Ingredients: Dicalcium Phosphate, Cellulose, Vegetable Stearic Acid, Croscarmellose, Vegetable Magnesium Stearate, Silica.

Vitamin B-6 - PhysioLogics
Each tablet contains: Vitamin B6 (as pyridoxine hydrochloride) 100 mg. Other Ingredients: Cellulose (plant origin), Dicalcium Phosphate, Vegetable Stearic Acid, Croscarmllose, Cellulose Coating, Silica, Vegetable Magnesium Stearate.

Vitamin B-6 - Leiner Health Products
Each tablet contains: Vitamin B6 (Pyridoxine Hydrochloride) 100 mg. Other Ingredients: Dicalcium Phosphate, Cellulose, Starch, Croscarmellose Sodium, Polyethylene Glycol 3350, Silicon Dioxide, Magnesium Stearate.

Vitamin B-6 - GNC
Each tablet contains: Vitamin B6 (as Pyridoxine Hydrochloride) 50 mg. Other Ingredients: Dextrose, Stearic Acid, Magnesium Stearate, Cellulose, Whole Brown Rice powder.

Vitamin B6 (Pyridoxine Hydrochloride) - Golden Glow Natural Health Products
Each tablet contains: Pyridoxine (vitamin B6) 200 mg (from pyridoxine hydrochloride 243 mg).

Vitamin B-6 100 - GNC
Each tablet contains: Vitamin B6 (as Pyridoxine hydrochloride) 100 mg. Other Ingredients: Dicalcium Phosphate, Whole Brown Rice powder (oryza sativa).

Vitamin B6 100 mg - Vital Nutrients
Each capsule contains: Vitamin B6 (from 122 mg pyridoxine HCl) 100 mg.

Vitamin B6 100 mg - Jamieson
Each tablet contains: Vitamin B6 (pyridoxine HCl) 100 mg.

Vitamin B6 100 mg - Nature Made
Each tablet contains: Vitamin B6 (from pyridoxine hydrochloride) 100 mg. Other Ingredients: Dibasic Calcium Phosphate, Cellulose Gel, Croscarmellose Sodium, Stearic Acid, Magnesium Stearate. See Editor's Note No. 45.

Vitamin B6 100 mg - Source Naturals
Each tablet contains: Vitamin B6 (as pyridoxine HCl) 100 mg.

Vitamin B6 100 mg - Westcoast Naturals
Each capsule contains: Vitamin B6 (pyridoxine HCl USP) 100 mg.

Vitamin B6 100 mg - Nature's Valley
Each tablet contains: Vitamin B6 (pyridoxine hydrochloride) 100 mg. Other Ingredients: Cellulose, Dicalcium Phosphate, Starch, Croscarmellose Sodium, Polyethylene Glycol, Silicon Dioxide, Magnesium Stearate.
See Editor's Note No. 45.

Vitamin B6 100 mg Capsules - Nature's Plus
Each capsule contains: Vitamin B6 (as pyridoxine HCl) 100 mg. Other Ingredients: Microcrystalline Cellulose, Silica, Rice Bran, Gelatin, Purified Water.

Vitamin B6 100 mg Tablets - Nature's Plus
Each tablet contains: Vitamin B6 (as pyridoxine HCl) 100 mg. Other Ingredients: Di-calcium Phosphate, Microcrystalline Cellulose, Stearic Acid, Rice Bran, Magnesium Stearate, Pharmaceutical Glaze, Silica.

Vitamin B6 100 mg Tablets - Solgar
Each tablet contains: Vitamin B6 (as pyridoxine HCl) 100 mg • Calcium (as dicalcium phosphate) 55 mg. Other Ingredients: Dicalcium Phosphate, Microcrystalline Cellulose, Vegetable Cellulose, Vegetable Stearic Acid, Vegetable Magnesium Stearate.

Vitamin B6 100 mg Vegetable Capsules - Solgar
Each vegetable capsule contains: Vitamin B6 (as pyridoxine HCl) 100 mg. Other Ingredients: Vegetable Cellulose, Vegetable Magnesium Stearate, Vegetable Stearic Acid, Silica, Microcrystalline Cellulose, Water.

Vitamin B-6 200 - GNC
Each tablet contains: Vitamin B6 (as pyridoxine hydrochloride) 200 mg. Other Ingredients: Dicalcium Phosphate, Cellulose, Whole Brown Rice powder (oryza sativa).

Vitamin B6 25 mg - Jamieson
Each tablet contains: Vitamin B6 (Pyridoxine Hydrochloride) 25 mg.

Vitamin B6 25 mg - Solgar
Each tablet contains: Vitamin B6 (as pyridoxine HCl) 25 mg • Calcium (as dicalcium phosphate) 40 mg. Other Ingredients: Dicalcium Phosphate, Microcrystalline Cellulose, Vegetable Cellulose, Vegetable Stearic Acid.

Vitamin B6 250 mg - Vital Nutrients
Each capsule contains: Vitamin B6 (from 305 mg pyridoxine HCl) 250 mg.

Vitamin B6 250 mg - Jamieson
Each tablet contains: Vitamin B6 (pyridoxine hydrochloride) 250 mg.

Vitamin B6 250 mg - Solgar
Each vegetable capsule contains: Vitamin B6 (as pyridoxine HCl) 250 mg. Other Ingredients: Vegetable Cellulose, Microcrystalline Cellulose, Vegetable Magnesium Stearate, Water.

Vitamin B-6 250 mg - J. R. Carlson Laboratories, Inc.
Each tablet contains: Vitamin B6 (pyridoxine hydrochloride) 250 mg.

Vitamin B-6 50 - GNC
Each tablet contains: Vitamin B6 (as pyridoxine hydrochloride) 50 mg. Other Ingredients: Dextrose, Whole Brown Rice powder (oryza sativa).

Vitamin B6 50 mg - Nature's Sunshine
Each tablet contains: Vitamin B6 (pyridoxine HCl) 50 mg • Calcium (di-calcium phosphate) 65 mg • Phosphorus (di-calcium phosphate) 50 mg. Other Ingredients: Cellulose, Wheat Germ Flour, Stearic Acid, Magnesium Stearate.

Vitamin B6 50 mg - Solgar
Each tablet contains: Vitamin B6 (as pyridoxine HCl) 50 mg • Calcium (as dicalcium phosphate) 50 mg. Other Ingredients: Dicalcium Phosphate, Microcrystalline Cellulose, Vegetable Stearic Acid, Vegetable Magnesium Stearate, Vegetable Cellulose.

Vitamin B6 50 mg - Jamieson
Each tablet contains: Vitamin B6 (Pyridoxine Hydrochloride) 50 mg.

Vitamin B6 50 mg - Nature Made
Each tablet contains: Vitamin B6 (from pyridoxine HCl) 50 mg. Other Ingredients: Dibasic Calcium Phosphate, Cellulose, Croscarmellose Sodium, Magnesium Stearate.
See Editor's Note No. 45.

Vitamin B6 50 mg - Source Naturals
Each tablet contains: Vitamin B6 (as pyridoxine HCl) 50 mg.

Some Brand Name Natural Products - What they Contain

www.NaturalDatabase.com contains MANY more listings than appear here.
Editor's Notes are located on pages 2155-2163.

Vitamin B-6 50 mg - J. R. Carlson Laboratories, Inc.
Each tablet contains: Vitamin B6 (pyridoxine hydrochloride) 50 mg.

Vitamin B6 500 mg - Solgar
Each capsule contains: Vitamin B6 (as pyridoxine HCl) 500 mg. Other Ingredients: Vegetable Cellulose, Vegetable Magnesium Stearate, Water, Vegetable Glycerin.

Vitamin B6 500 mg Sustained Release tablets - Nature's Plus
Each extended-release tablet contains: Vitamin B6 (as pyridoxine HCl) 500 mg. Other Ingredients: Hydroxypropyl Methylcellulose, Stearic Acid, Rice Bran, Magnesium Stearate, Di-calcium Phosphate, Silica, Pharmaceutical Glaze.

Vitamin B6 500 mg Time Release - Source Naturals
Each tablet contains: Vitamin B6 (pyridoxine HCl) 500 mg • Calcium 27 mg.

Vitamin B-6 Liquid - J. R. Carlson Laboratories, Inc.
Each 1 tsp serving contains: Vitamin B6 (as pyridoxine hydrochloride) 200 mg.

Vitamin B-Complex - PhysioLogics
Each capsule contains: Thiamine (mononitrate) 50 mg • Riboflavin 50 mg • Niacin 55 mg • Pantothenic Acid (calcium pantothenate) 100 mg • Vitamin B6 (pyridoxine HCl) 50 mg • Vitamin B12 (cyanocobalamin) 50 mcg • Folic Acid 400 mcg • Biotin 300 mcg • Inositol 50 mg • Choline (bitartrate) 50 mg • PABA 50 mg.

Vitamin C - Jarrow Formulas
Each 1/4 tsp contains: Vitamin C (USP grade) 1000 mg.

Vitamin C - Leiner Health Products
Each tablet contains: Vitamin C (Ascorbic Acid) 250 mg. Other Ingredients: Calcium Carbonate, Maltodextrin, Cellulose, Starch, Silicon Dioxide, Stearic Acid, Magnesium Stearate, Sodium Starch Glycolate, Croscarmellose Sodium.

Vitamin C - CVS Pharmacy
Each tablet contains: Vitamin C 500 mg. Other Ingredients: Ascorbic Acid, Starch, Cellulose, Stearic Acid, Croscarmellose Sodium, Lactose, Magnesium Stearate, Silicon Dioxide.

Vitamin C - NSI - Nutraceutical Sciences Institute
Each capsule contains: Vitamin C (ascorbic acid) 1000 mg.

Vitamin C - Optimum Nutrition
Each capsule contains: Vitamin C (as ascorbic acid) 500 mg. Other Ingredients: Microcrystalline Cellulose, Gelatin, Magnesium Stearate.

Vitamin C - GNC
Each tablet contains: Vitamin E (as dl-alpha Tocopheryl Acetate) 1000 IU • Vitamin C (as Ascorbic Acid) 500 mg. Other Ingredients: Cellulose, Magnesium Stearate, Stearic Acid.

Vitamin C - 1000 - Nature's Bounty
Each tablet contains: Vitamin C (as ascorbic acid) 1000 mg. Other Ingredients: Cellulose Plant Origin, Vegetable Magnesium Stearate, Vegetable Stearic Acid, Silica.

Vitamin C - Ascorbic Acid Crystals - Source Naturals
Each 1/4 tsp contains: Vitamin C (as ascorbic acid) 1.065 g.

Vitamin C & Zinc Lozenges - Puritan's Pride
Each lozenge contains: Vitamin C (as Ascorbic Acid and Rose Hips) 300 mg • Zinc (as Zinc Citrate) 7 mg • Natural Food Base 15 mg: Rutin, Hesperidin, Acerola, Citrus Bioflavonoids, Black Currant.

Vitamin C (Chewable Grape) - Westcoast Naturals
Each tablet contains: Vitamin C 500 mg. Other Ingredients: Rose Hips, Natural Grape Flavor, Fructose.

Vitamin C (Chewable Orange) - Westcoast Naturals
Each tablet contains: Vitamin C (from sodium ascorbate and ascorbic acid) 500 mg • Rosehips 4:1 extract 50 mg • Hesperidin Complex 10 mg • Lemon Bioflavonoids 4:1 extract 10 mg • Rutin Powder 2.5 mg.

Vitamin C + Echinacea - Leiner Health Products
Each tablet contains: Vitamin C (Ascorbic Acid) 500 mg • Echinacea (Echinacea angustifolia) herb 35 mg • Echinacea (Echinacea angustifolia) root 15 mg • Echinacea (Echinacea purpurea) herb 50 mg. Other Ingredients: Cellulose, Hydroxypropyl Methylcellulose, Croscarmellose Sodium, Magnesium Stearate, Silicon Dioxide, Lemon Bioflavonoids, Rose Hips, Acerola, Hesperidin, Orange Peel, Quercetin, Rutin, Polyethylene Glycol 3350.

Vitamin C 1000 - Olympian Labs
Each capsule contains: Vitamin C 1000 mg •Rose Hips 50 mg •Citrus Bioflavonoids 100 mg.

Vitamin C 1000 - PhysioLogics
Each tablet contains: Vitamin C (ascorbic acid) 1000 mg • Bioflavonoids lemon 30 mg.

Vitamin C 1000 mg - Nature's Valley
Each tablet contains: Vitamin C (ascorbic acid) 1000 mg. Other Ingredients: Cellulose, Hydroxypropyl Methylcellulose, Croscarmellose Sodium, Talc, Hydrogenated Vegetable Oil, Crospovidone, Silicon Dioxide, Magnesium Stearate, Hydroxypropyl Cellulose, Polysorbate 80, Polyethylene Glycol 3350.
See Editor's Note No. 45.

Vitamin C 1000 mg - Walgreens
Each caplet contains: Vitamin C (ascorbic acid) 1000 mg. Other Ingredients: Microcrystalline Cellulose, Croscarmellose Sodium, Powdered Cellulose, Stearic Acid, Colloidal Silicon Dioxide, Magnesium Stearate.

Vitamin C 1000 mg - Jamieson
Each caplet contains: Vitamin C (Ascorbic Acid) 1000 mg.

Vitamin C 1000 mg - Nature Made
Each tablet contains: Vitamin C (from ascorbic acid) 1000 mg. Other Ingredients: Corn Starch, Cellulose, Magnesium Stearate, Stearic Acid, Silica Gel.
See Editor's Note No. 45.

Vitamin C 1000 mg - Nature Made
Each tablet contains: Vitamin C 1000 mg.
See Editor's Note No. 45.

Vitamin C 1000 mg - Arrowroot
Each tablet contains: Vitamin C 1000 mg.

Vitamin C 1000 mg - Timed Release - Jamieson
Each caplet contains: Vitamin C (Ascorbic Acid) 1000 mg.

Vitamin C 1000 mg Capsules with Bioflavonoids - Puritan's Pride
Each capsule contains: Vitamin C 1000 mg • Bioflavonoids 30 mg.

Vitamin C 1000 mg Time Release - Nature's Sunshine
Each time-release tablet contains: Vitamin C (ascorbic acid) 1000 mg • Proprietary Blend 25 mg: Rose Hips fruit (rosa canina), Acerola fruit (malpighia glabra), Rutin, Hesperidin, Lemon Bioflavonoid. Other Ingredients: Cellulose, Stearic Acid, Magnesium Stearate, Silicon Dioxide, Di-Calcium Phosphate.

Vitamin C 1000 mg Timed Release - Jamieson
Each caplet contains: Vitamin C (as ascorbic acid) 1000. Other Ingredients: Rutin, Hesperidin, Lemon Bioflavonoids, Acerola, Rosehips.

Vitamin C 1000 mg Veg Caps - Vital Nutrients
Each vegetarian capsule contains: Vitamin C (ascorbic acid) 1000 mg.

Vitamin C 1000 mg With Rose Hips - Nature's Valley
Each tablet contains: Vitamin C 1000 mg. Other Ingredients: Starch, Cellulose, Dicalcium Phosphate, Hydroxypropyl Methylcellulose, Rose Hips, Stearic Acid, Crospovidone, Hydroxypropyl Cellulose, Magnesium Stearate, Silicon Dioxide, Croscarmellose Sodium, Sodium Starch Glycolate, Polysorbate 80, Polyethylene Glycol.
See Editor's Note No. 45.

Some Brand Name Natural Products - What they Contain

www.NaturalDatabase.com contains MANY more listings than appear here.
Editor's Notes are located on pages 2155-2163.

BRAND NAMES

Vitamin C 1000 mg with Rose Hips - GNC
Each tablet contains: Vitamin C 1000 mg. Other Ingredients: Rose Hips powder, Cellulose, Magnesium Stearate, Dicalcium Phosphate, Food Glaze, Stearic Acid, Silica.

Vitamin C 1000 mg with Rose Hips capsules - Arrowroot
Each capsule contains: Vitamin C (from rose hips) 1000 mg.

Vitamin C 1000 mg with Rose Hips tablets - Arrowroot
Each tablet contains: Vitamin C (from rose hips) 1000 mg.

Vitamin C 1000 mg with Rose Hips Timed Release - Nature Made
Each tablet contains: Vitamin C (from rose hips) 1000 mg.
Other Ingredients: Hydroxypropyl Methylcellulose, Corn Starch, Stearic Acid, Magnesium Stearate, Polyethylene Glycol, Riboflavin, Carnauba Wax.
See Editor's Note No. 45.

Vitamin C 1000 with Bioflavonoids and Rose Hips - GNC
Each tablet contains: Vitamin C (ascorbic acid) 1000 mg. Other Ingredients: Cellulose, Calcium Sulfate, Rose Hips powder.

Vitamin C 1000 with Rose Hips - Nature's Way
Each capsule contains: Vitamin C 1000 mg. Other Ingredients: Cellulose, Gelatin, Magnesium Stearate, Rose Hips.

Vitamin C 1000mg - Vital Nutrients
Each capsule contains: Vitamin C (ascorbic acid) 1000 mg.

Vitamin C 1500 mg Tablets with Rose Hips - Puritan's Pride
Each tablet contains: Vitamin C with Rose Hips 1500 mg.

Vitamin C 1500 mg with Rose Hips - Arrowroot
Each tablet contains: Vitamin C (from rose hips) 1500 mg.

Vitamin C 1500 mg with Rose Hips - Nature Made
Each tablet contains: Vitamin C 1500 mg.
See Editor's Note No. 45.

Vitamin C 200 mg - The Vitamin Shoppe
Each tablet contains: Vitamin C 200 mg • Citrus Bioflavonoid Complex 20 mg.

Vitamin C 2000 mg with Rose Hips - GNC
Each tablet contains: Vitamin C (as ascorbic acid) 2000 mg.
Other Ingredients: Cellulose, Rose Hips (rosina canina).

Vitamin C 250 mg - Walgreens
Each tablet contains: Vitamin C (ascorbic acid) 250 mg.
Other Ingredients: Microcrystalline Cellulose, Croscarmellose Sodium, Stearic Acid, Powdered Cellulose, Colloidal Silicon Dioxide, Magnesium Stearate.

Vitamin C 250 mg - Nature Made
Each tablet contains: Vitamin C 250 mg.
See Editor's Note No. 45.

Vitamin C 250 mg - Sunmark
Each tablet contains: Vitamin C 250 mg. Other Ingredients: Dicalcium Phosphate, Microcrystalline Cellulose, Crospovidone, Stearic Acid, Magnesium Stearate, Silicon Dioxide.
See Editor's Note No. 45.

Vitamin C 500 mg - GNC
Each tablet contains: Vitamin C 500 mg. Other Ingredients: Cellulose.

Vitamin C 500 mg - Nature Made
Each tablet contains: Vitamin C 500 mg.
See Editor's Note No. 45.

Vitamin C 500 mg - Walgreens
Each tablet contains: Vitamin C 500 mg.

Vitamin C 500 mg - Jamieson
Each tablet contains: Vitamin C (ascorbic acid, sodium ascorbate) 500 mg • Sodium (sodium ascorbate) 35 mg. Available in Chewable Orange, Grape Juice-Chewable, and Chewable Tropical Fruit flavors.

Vitamin C 500 mg - Sunmark
Each caplet contains: Vitamin C 500 mg. Other Ingredients: Cellulose, Crospovidone, Microcrystalline Cellulose, Magnesium Stearate, Stearic Acid, Silicon Dioxide, Hydroxypropyl Methylcellulose, Hydryoxypropyl Cellulose, Polyethylene Glycol.
See Editor's Note No. 45.

Vitamin C 500 mg - Arrowroot
Each tablet contains: Vitamin C 500 mg.

Vitamin C 500 mg - Nature's Valley
Each tablet contains: Vitamin C (ascorbic acid) 500 mg.
Other Ingredients: Starch, Cellulose, Crospovidone, Magnesium Stearate, Hydroxypropyl Cellulose, Stearic Acid, Silicon Dioxide, Croscarmellose Sodium.
See Editor's Note No. 45.

Vitamin C 500 mg (citrus juice flavor) - Jamieson
Each tablet contains: Vitamin C (ascorbic acid and sodium ascorbate) 500 mg.

Vitamin C 500 mg (grape juice flavor) - Jamieson
Each tablet contains: Vitamin C (ascorbic acid and sodium ascorbate) 500 mg.

Vitamin C 500 mg (tangy orange flavor) - Jamieson
Each tablet contains: Vitamin C 500 mg.

Vitamin C 500 mg (tropical fruit flavor) - Jamieson
Each tablet contains: Vitamin C (ascorbic acid and sodium ascorbate) 500 mg.

Vitamin C 500 mg + Echinacea - Walgreens
Each caplet contains: Vitamin C (ascorbic acid, rose hips, hesperidine complex, citric bioflavonoid complex acerola, lemon bioflavonoid complex, rutin, quercetin, sweet orange peels) 500 mg • Echinacea aerial parts (echinacea purpurea, echinacea angustifolia) 50 mg.
Other Ingredients: Microcrystalline Cellulose, Croscarmellose Sodium, Stearic Acid, Magnesium Stearate, Silicon Dioxide, Hydroxypropyl Methylcellulose, Carnauba Wax.

Vitamin C 500 mg Tablets with Rose Hips - Puritan's Pride
Each tablet contains: Vitamin C with Rose Hips 500 mg.

Vitamin C 500 mg Timed Release caplets - Jamieson
Each caplet contains: Vitamin C 500 mg.

Vitamin C 500 mg Timed Release capsules - Jamieson
Each capsule contains: Vitamin C (ascorbic acid) 500 mg.

Vitamin C 500 mg with Rose Hips - Nature Made
Each tablet contains: Vitamin C 500 mg.
See Editor's Note No. 45.

Vitamin C 500 mg with Rose Hips - Nature's Valley
Each tablet contains: Vitamin C 500 mg. Other Ingredients: Starch, Cellulose, Hydroxypropyl Methylcellulose, Crospovidone, Stearic Acid, Rose Hips, Magnesium Stearate, Silicon Dioxide, Hydroxypropyl Cellulose, Croscarmellose Sodium.
See Editor's Note No. 45.

Vitamin C 500 mg with Rose Hips - Arrowroot
Each tablet contains: Vitamin C (from rose hips) 500 mg.

Vitamin C 500 mg with Rose Hips - Nature Made
Each tablet contains: Vitamin C (from ascorbic acid, rose hips) 500 mg. Other Ingredients: Corn Starch, Cellulose Gel, Croscarmellose Sodium, Stearic Acid, Silicon Dioxide, Magnesium Stearate.
See Editor's Note No. 45.

Vitamin C 500 mg with Rose Hips Timed Release - GNC
Each capsule contains: Vitamin C (as ascorbic acid) 500 mg.
Other Ingredients: Sucrose, Starch, Gelatin, Food Glaze, Rose Hips powder (rosina canina).

Vitamin C 500 with Bioflavonoids - Nature's Way
Two capsules contain: Citrus Bioflavonoids 600 mg • Vitamin C (ascorbic acid) 1000 mg.

Some Brand Name Natural Products - What they Contain

www.NaturalDatabase.com contains MANY more listings than appear here.
Editor's Notes are located on pages 2155-2163.

Vitamin C 500 with Rose Hips - Windmill Health Products
Each tablet contains: Vitamin C 500 mg •Ascorbic Acid 500 mg • Rose Hips 30 mg.

Vitamin C 500 with Rose Hips - GNC
Each tablet contains: Vitamin C (as ascorbic acid) 500 mg. Other Ingredients: Dicalcium Phosphate, Cellulose, Rose Hips powder (rosina canina), Food Glaze.

Vitamin C Ascorbates - Nature's Sunshine
Each 1 slightly rounded tsp (4.5 g) serving contains: Vitamin C (calcium ascorbate, potassium ascorbate, magnesium ascorbate) 2000 mg. Other Ingredients: Maltodextrin, Acerola Fruit Extract (malpighia glabra), Xanthan Gum, Natural Orange Flavor, Rutin, Hesperidin, Beta Carotene.

Vitamin C Chewable - Leiner Health Products
Each tablet contains: Vitamin C (ascorbic acid) 500 mg • Sodium 40 mg. Other Ingredients: Sucrose, Sodium Ascorbate, Stearic Acid, Starch, Natural Flavor, Magnesium Stearate, Silicon Dioxide, Sorbitol, Yellow 6 Lake, Lactose, Ethylmaltol.

Vitamin C Crystals - Puritan's Pride
Each teaspoon contains: Vitamin C 5000 mg.

Vitamin C Crystals - J. R. Carlson Laboratories, Inc.
Each 1 tsp serving contains: Vitamin C (as ascorbic acid) 4000 mg.

Vitamin C Crystals Buffered - GNC
1/2 Teaspoon contains: Vitamin C (as calcium ascorbate) 2000 mg • Calcium (as calcium ascorbate) 230 mg. Other Ingredients: Calcium Ascorbate.

Vitamin C Crystals with Rose Hips - GNC
1/2 Teaspoon contains: Vitamin C (as ascorbic acid) 2000 mg. Other Ingredients: Rose Hips powder.

Vitamin C Ester Eye Area Therapy - N.V. Perricone M.D. Cosmeceuticals
Cyclomethicone • Tetrahexyldecyl Ascorbate • Squalane • Tocopheryl Acetate • Tocotrienols • Bisabolol • Ascorbyl Palmitate • DMAE (dimethyl MEA).

Vitamin C Moisturizing Lotion - Jamieson
Maleated Soybean Oil • Propylene Glycol • Glycerin • Panthenol • Aloe Barbadenis Gel • SPF Active Ingredients: Octocrylene 7%, Octyl Methoxycinnamate 7%, Oxybenzone 3%.

Vitamin C Plex - Olympian Labs
Each capsule contains: Vitamin C (calcium ascorbate) 500 mg • Calcium (ascorbate) 55 mg • Citrus Bioflavonoid Complex 50 mg • Hesperidin 25 mg • Rutin 20 mg • Ascorbyl Palmitate 10 mg.

Vitamin C Skin Supplement Cream - Orjene
Antioxidants • Vitamin C • Ginkgo Biloba • Germanium • Chamomile.

Vitamin C Solution - Dial Herbs
Vitamin C • Vitamin B3 • Citrus bioflavonoids extract. In a base of Distilled Water, Fructose, Sorbitol, Vegetable Glycerine (kosher), Fruit flavors, Sodium Benzoate & Caramel color.

Vitamin C Timed Release with Rose Hips - Pro Health
Each tablet contains: Vitamin C (as ascorbic acid) 1000 mg • Rose Hips powder (rosae pseudofructus seed) 25 mg. Other Ingredients: Cellulose, Stearic Acid, Magnesium Stearate, Dicalcium Phosphate.

Vitamin C Ultra - FreeLife International
Each caplet contains: Vitamin C (as ascorbates of calcium, magnesium, potassium and zinc) 500 mg • Calcium (from calcium ascorbate) 50 mg • Magnesium (from magnesium ascorbate) 25 mg • Zinc (from zinc ascorbate) 2.5 mg • Potassium (from potassium ascorbate) 5 mg • Proprietary Citri-C brand Complex 875 mg: Ascorbates and Citrates of Calcium, Magnesium, Potassium and Zinc, Sodium Isoascorbate, Citrus Glycosyl Flavones (cirantin, isosakuranetin-7-beta-rutinoside, narirutin, eriocitrin, nobiletin, tangeretin, heptamethoxyflavone), Natural Orange essence. Other Ingredients: Cellulose, Cellulose Gum, Vegetable Stearic Acid, Silica, Vegetable Magnesium Stearate, Vita-Coat (vegetable resin, alpha-lipoic acid).

Vitamin C with Bioflavonoids 500 mg - Vital Nutrients
Each capsule contains: Vitamin C (ascorbic acid) 500 mg • Citrus Bioflavonoid Complex 250 mg: Hesperidin 41.4%; Naringin, Naringenin, 7-B Rutinoside 17.4%; Flavonols, Flavones and Phenolics 1.2%.

Vitamin C with Citrus Bioflavonoids & Rose Hips - Optimum Nutrition
Two capsules contain: Vitamin C (as ascorbic acid) 1000 mg • Proprietary Citrus Blend 751 mg: Citrus Bioflavonoids, Rose Hips. Other Ingredients: Gelatin, Magnesium Stearate.

Vitamin C with Echinacea - Holista
Each tablet contains: Vitamin C 500 mg • Echinacea 100 mg.

Vitamin C with Natural Rosehips - Westcoast Naturals
Each capsule contains: Vitamin C 500 mg • Rosehips 50 mg.

Vitamin C with Rose Hips and Echinacea - PhysioLogics
Each tablet contains: Vitamin C (as ascorbic acid, rose hips (rosa canina) 500 mg • Echinacea aerial parts, root (echinacea purpurea, echinacea angustifolia) 100 mg. Other Ingredients: Dicalcium Phosphate, Cellulose, Vegetable Stearic Acid, Croscarmellose, Silica, Vegetable Magnesium Stearate, Cellulose Coating.

Vitamin C, 500 mg (special) - Nature's Life
Vitamin C (Ascorbic Acid), 500 mg. In a natural base of Rose Hips Powder. Excipients: Cellulose, Magnesium stearate and Micro-Cellulose coating.

Vitamin C, Hesperidin & Mineral Powder - Wonder Foods
Two grams of powder contain: Ascorbic Acid 800 mg • Calcium Ascorbate 200 mg • Hesperidin 190 mg • Calcium Phosphate 100 mg • Magnesium Phosphate 190 mg • Zinc Sulfate Monohydrate 2.9 mg.

Vitamin D - Puritan's Pride
Each tablet contains: Vitamin D 400 IU.

Vitamin D - Ortho Molecular Products
Each capsule contains: Vitamin D 1000 IU.

Vitamin D - GNC
Each tablet contains: Vitamin D (as Ergocalciferol) 400 IU. Other Ingredients: Dicalcium Phosphate, Cellulose.

Vitamin D (Cholecalciferol) 1000 - Solgar
Each softgel contains: Vitamin A (naturally occurring from fish liver oil) 3000 IU • Vitamin D (as cholecalciferol, naturally occurring from fish liver oil) 1000 IU. Other Ingredients: Safflower Oil, Gelatin, Glycerin, Water.

Vitamin D (Cholecalciferol) 400 IU - Solgar
Each softgel contains: Vitamin A (naturally occurring from fish liver oil) 1000 IU • Vitamin D (as cholecalciferol naturally occurring from fish liver oil) 400 IU. Other Ingredients: Safflower Oil, Gelatin, Glycerin, Water.

Vitamin D 1000 IU - Jamieson
Each tablet contains: Vitamin D 1000 IU.

Vitamin D 1000 IU - Jamieson
Each tablet contains: Vitamin D (as Cholecaliciferol) 1000 IU • Calcium (as Dicalcium Phosphate) 20 mg • Peanut oil.

Vitamin D 1000 IU - J. R. Carlson Laboratories, Inc.
Each softgel contains: Vitamin A (from fish liver oil) 1600 IU • VItamin D (D3, from fish liver oil) 1000 IU.

Vitamin D 2000 IU - J. R. Carlson Laboratories, Inc.
Each softgel contains: Vitamin D (D3, cholecalciferol) 2000 IU.

Vitamin D 400 - GNC
Each tablet contains: Vitamin D (as ergocalciferol) 400 IU. Other Ingredients: Dicalcium Phosphate, Cellulose.

Some Brand Name Natural Products - What they Contain

www.NaturalDatabase.com contains MANY more listings than appear here.
Editor's Notes are located on pages 2155-2163.

BRAND NAMES

Vitamin D 400 IU - Jamieson
Each tablet contains: Vitamin D (as Vitamin D3) 400 IU.

Vitamin D 400 IU - J. R. Carlson Laboratories, Inc.
Each softgel contains: Vitamin A (from fish liver oil) 1000 IU • Vitamin D (D3, from fish liver oil) 400 IU.

Vitamin D 400IU - Vital Nutrients
Each capsule contains: Vitamin D (D3 as cholecalciferol from lanolin) 400 IU.

Vitamin D3 - Pure Encapsulations
Each vegetable capsule contains: Vitamin D (as D3) 400 IU.

Vitamin D3 1000 IU - Pure Encapsulations
Each vegetable capsule contains: Vitamin D (as D3) 1000 IU.

Vitamin D3 2000IU - Vital Nutrients
Each vegetarian capsule contains: Vitamin D (D3 as cholecalciferol from lanolin) 2000 IU.

Vitamin D3 400 IU - Jarrow Formulas
Each softgel contains: Vitamin D (D3, cholecalciferol) 400 IU. Other Ingredients: Soybean Oil, Gelatin, Glycerin, Water.

Vitamin D3 5000 IU - Pure Encapsulations
Each vegetable capsule contains: Vitamin D (as D3) 5000 IU.

Vitamin E - Health Smart Vitamins
Each softgel contains: Vitamin E (as 50% d-alpha tocopherol, 50% dl-alpha tocopheryl acetate) 1,000 IU.

Vitamin E - Nature's Way
Each softgel contains: Vitamin E (d-alpha tocopheryl) 400 IU. Other Ingredients: Gelatin.

Vitamin E - Pain & Stress Center
Each capsule contains: Vitamin E (as D-alpha tocopherol) 400 IU. Other Ingredients: Soybean Oil, Glycerin, Purified Water, Gelatin.

Vitamin E - Vitamins.com
Each softgel contains: Vitamin E Complex 400 IU. Other Ingredients: Glycerin, Gelatin.

Vitamin E - Pure Encapsulations
Each softgel capsule contains: Natural Vitamin E (mixed tocopherols): D-alpha tocopherol 268 mg, Other Tocopherols 67 mg. Other ingredients: Soybean Oil.

Vitamin E - Olympian Labs
Each capsule contains: Vitamin E (d-alpha tocopherol) 400 IU. In a base of Soybean Oil or Safflower Oil.

Vitamin E - A&D Cream - Atrium Biotechnologies
Three ounces contain: Vitamin E 1500 IU • Vitamin A 750 IU • Vitamin D 300 IU. In a Silicone Cream Base: Stearic Acid, Glycerol, Cetyl Alcohol, Beeswax, Apricot Kernel oil, Triethanolamine, Borax, Allantoin, Methyl Parasept.

Vitamin E & Selenium - Swanson Health Products
Each softgel contains: Vitamin E (as D-alpha tocopherol) 400 IU • Selenium (as selenomethionine) 50 mcg.

Vitamin E (Natural Source) - Westcoast Naturals
Each softgel contains: Vitamin E (from D-alpha tocopherol) 400 IU.

Vitamin E 100 IU - Jamieson
Each capsule contains: Natural Source Vitamin E (D-Alpha Tocopheryl Acetate from Purified Soy Oil) 100 IU.

Vitamin E 1000 I.U. - Walgreens
Each softgel contains: Vitamin E (dL-alpha tocopheryl acetate) 1000 IU. Other Ingredients: USP Water, Glycerin.

Vitamin E 1000 IU - Sunmark
Each softgel contains: Vitamin E 1000 IU. Other Ingredients: Gelatin, Glycerin, Soybean Oil, Purified Water.
See Editor's Note No. 45.

Vitamin E 1000 IU - GNC
Each capsule contains: Vitamin E (as D-alpha tocopheryl acetate) 1000 IU. Other Ingredients: Gelatin, Glycerin.

Vitamin E 1000 IU - Nature's Valley
Each softgel contains: Vitamin E (from DL-alpha tocopheryl acetate) 1000 IU. Other Ingredients: Gelatin, Glycerin, Vegetable Oil.
See Editor's Note No. 45.

Vitamin E 1000 IU - GNC
Each capsule contains: Vitamin E (as DL-alpha tocopheryl acetate) 1000 IU. Other Ingredients: Gelatin, Glycerin.

Vitamin E 1000 IU Blended - Sunmark
Each softgel contains: Vitamin E (DL-alpha tocopheryl acetate, D-alpha tocopherol) 1000 IU. Other Ingredients: Gelatin, Glycerin, Soybean Oil.
See Editor's Note No. 45.

Vitamin E 200 I.U. - Walgreens
Each softgel contains: Vitamin E (DL-alpha tocopheryl acetate) 200 IU. Other Ingredients: USP Water, Glycerin.

Vitamin E 200 IU - Leiner Health Products
Each softgel contains: Vitamin E (DL-alpha tocopheryl acetate) 200 IU. Other Ingredients: Gelatin, Glycerin, Vegetable Oil.

Vitamin E 200 IU - Jamieson
Each capsule contains: Natural Source Vitamin E (D-alpha tocopheryl acetate from purified soy oil) 200 IU.

Vitamin E 200 IU - GNC
Each capsule contains: Vitamin E (as DL-alpha tocopheryl acetate) 200 IU. Other Ingredients: Gelatin, Glycerin.

Vitamin E 200 IU - Sunmark
Each softgel contains: Vitamin E 200 IU.
See Editor's Note No. 45.

Vitamin E 200 IU - Chewable - Jamieson
Each tablet contains: Vitamin E 200 IU.

Vitamin E 200 IU with Selenium - Jamieson
Each caplet contains: Natural Source Vitamin E (D-alpha tocopheryl acetate) 200 IU • Selenium (from yeast) 2 mcg.

Vitamin E 2000 IU Moisture Cream - Jamieson
4% Antioxidant Vitamin E • Chamomile.

Vitamin E 30,000 IU Moisture Cream - Jamieson
27% Antioxidant Vitamin E (Tocopheyrl Acetate) with Swiss Alpine Herbs: Fennel, Hops, Chamomile, Balm Mint, Mistletoe.

Vitamin E 400 I.U. - Walgreens
Each softgel contains: Vitamin E (dL-alpha tocopheryl acetate) 400 IU. Other Ingredients: Gelatin, Polysorbate 80, USP Water, Glycerin, Mono- and Diglycerides.

Vitamin E 400 IU - American Biologics
Each tablet contains: Vitamin E (D-alpha-tocopherol) 400 IU. Other Ingredients: Cellulose, Magnesium Stearate.

Vitamin E 400 IU - Nature's Valley
Each softgel contains: Vitamin E 400 IU. Other Ingredients: Gelatin, Soybean Oil, Glycerin.
See Editor's Note No. 45.

Vitamin E 400 IU - PhytoPharmica
Each softgel capsule contains: Mixed Tocopherols (gamma, delta, alpha, and beta) 50 mg • Vitamin E (as D-alpha tocopherol) 400 IU.

Vitamin E 400 IU - Jamieson
Each capsule contains: Vitamin E 400 IU.

Vitamin E 400 IU - Sunmark
Each softgel contains: Vitamin E 400 IU. Other Ingredients: Gelatin, Glycerin, Soybean Oil, Purified Water.
See Editor's Note No. 45.

Vitamin E 400 IU (Natural Source) - Jamieson
Each capsule contains: Natural Source Vitamin E (D-alpha tocopheryl acetate from purified soy oil) 400 IU.

Vitamin E 400 IU Blended - Sunmark
Each softgel contains: Vitamin E (as dL-alpha tocopheryl acetate and D-alpha tocopherol) 400 IU. Other Ingredients: Gelatin, Glycerin, Soybean Oil.
See Editor's Note No. 45.

Vitamin E 400 IU softgels - GNC
Each capsule contains: Vitamin E (as dL-alpha tocopheryl acetate). Other Ingredients: Gelatin, Glycerin.

Vitamin E 400 IU Water Dispersible - Sunmark
Each softgel contains: Vitamin E 400 IU. Other Ingredients: Gelatin, Glycerin, Polysorbate 80, Purified Water.
See Editor's Note No. 45.

Vitamin E 400 IU, Blended - GNC
Each capsule contains: Vitamin E (as dL-alpha tocopheryl acetate and D-alpha tocopherol) 400 IU. Other Ingredients: Gelatin, Glycerin.

Vitamin E 400 IU, dl-alpha Form - GNC
Each capsule contains: Vitamin E (as dL-alpha tocopheryl acetate) 400 IU. Other Ingredients: Gelatin, Glycerin.

Vitamin E 400 IU, Naturally Blended - GNC
Each capsule contains: Vitamin E (as dL-alpha tocopheryl acetate and D-alpha tocopherol) 400 IU. Other Ingredients: Gelatin, Glycerin.

Vitamin E 400IU 294mg - Nature's Sunshine
Each capsule contains: Vitamin E (D-alpha tocopherol) 294 mg.

Vitamin E 800 I.U. - Leiner Health Products
Each softgel contains: Vitamin E (DL-alpha tocopheryl acetate) 800 IU. Other Ingredients: Gelatin, Glycerin.

Vitamin E 800 IU - Jamieson
Each capsule contains: Vitamin E (D-alpha tocopheryl acetate) 800 IU.

Vitamin E Complex - Optimum Nutrition
Each softgel contains: Vitamin E (as D-alpha tocopherol plus D-beta, D-gamma, D-delta tocopherols) 400 IU. Other Ingredients: Gelatin, Soy Oil.

Vitamin E Complex 1000 IU - Schiff
Each softgel contains: Vitamin E 100 IU. Other Ingredients: Soybean Oil, Gelatin, Glycerin, Purified Water.

Vitamin E Complex 200 IU - Schiff
Each softgel contains: Vitamin E 200 IU. Other Ingredients: Soybean Oil, Gelatin, Glycerin, Purified Water.

Vitamin E Complex 400 IU - Schiff
Each softgel contains: Vitamin E 400 IU. Other Ingredients: Soybean Oil, Gelatin, Glycerin, Purified Water.

Vitamin E Essential Skin Cream - Orjene
Vitamin E 6000 IU • Vitamin A 20,000 USP units • Vitamin D 5000 USP units.

Vitamin E Microtargeted Moisture Oil - Jamieson
Each capsule contains: Grape Seed Oil • Sesame Seed Oil • Coconut Oil • Squalane • Phytosterol • Glycolipids • Tocopheryl Acetate • Chamomile Oil • Tocopheryl Linoleate.

Vitamin E Natural 100 IU - Nature Made
Each softgel contains: Vitamin E 100 IU. Other Ingredients: Soybean Oil, Gelatin, Glycerin, Water, Polysorbate 80.
See Editor's Note No. 45.

Vitamin E Natural 1000 IU - Nature Made
Each softgel contains: Vitamin E 1000 IU. Other Ingredients: Soybean Oil, Gelatin, Glycerin, Water.
See Editor's Note No. 45.

Vitamin E Natural 200 IU - Nature Made
Each softgel contains: Vitamin E (DL-alpha tocopherol acetate) 200 IU. Other Ingredients: Gelatin, Glycerin, water.
See Editor's Note No. 45.

Vitamin E Natural 400 IU - Nature Made
Each softgel contains: Vitamin E (from dL-alpha tocopheryl acetate) 400 IU. Other Ingredients: Gelatin, Glcyerin, Polysorbate 80, Water.
See Editor's Note No. 45.

Vitamin E Natural 800 IU - Nature Made
Each softgel contains: Vitamin E 800 IU. Other Ingredients: Soybean Oil, Gelatin, Glycerin, Water.
See Editor's Note No. 45.

Vitamin E Oil - Orjene
6000 IU of Vitamin E and Vitamin A and Vitamin D.

Vitamin E Oil 20,000 IU - Nature's Valley
Soybean Oil • Vitamin E (dL-alpha tocopheryl acetate).
See Editor's Note No. 45.

Vitamin E Oil 28,000 IU - Jamieson
Contains: 100% Vitamin E (Tocopheryl Acetate) 28,000 IU.

Vitamin E Soothing Ointment - Jamieson
Contains: Petrolatum • Mineral Oil • Vitamin E.

Vitamin E Succinate 400 IU - Life Extension Foundation
Each capsule contains: Vitamin E (as d-alpha-tocopheryl succinate) 400 IU. Other Ingredients: Magnesium Stearate, Rice Flour, Gelatin, Water.

Vitamin E Synthetic 1000 IU - Nature Made
Each softgel contains: Vitamin E (from dL-alpha tocopheryl acetate) 1000 IU. Other Ingredients: Gelatin, Glycerin, Water.
See Editor's Note No. 45.

Vitamin E Synthetic 200 IU - Nature Made
Each softgel contains: Vitamin E (from dL-alpha tocopheryl acetate) 200 IU. Other Ingredients: Gelatin, Glycerin, Water.
See Editor's Note No. 45.

Vitamin E Synthetic 400 IU - Nature Made
Each softgel contains: Vitamin E (from dL-alpha tocopheryl acetate) 400 IU. Other Ingredients: Gelatin, Glycerin, Water.
See Editor's Note No. 45.

Vitamin E Water Dispersible - Leiner Health Products
Each softgel contains: Vitamin E (dl-Alpha Tocopheryl Acetate) 400 IU. Other Ingredients: Gelatin, Polysorbate 80, Glycerin, Soybean Oil.

Vitamin E Water Soluble 400 IU - Nature's Valley
Each softgel contains: Vitamin E 400 IU. Other Ingredients: Gelatin, Polysorbate 80, Glycerin, Vegetable oil.
See Editor's Note No. 45.

Vitamin E with Mixed Tocopherols 1000 IU - Pro Health
Each softgel contains: Vitamin E (as D-alpha-tocopherol plus D-beta, D-delta, and D-gamma tocopherols) 1000 IU. Other Ingredients: Gelatin, Glycerin, Vegetable Oil Concentrate.

Vitamin E with Mixed Tocopherols 400 IU - Pro Health
Each softgel contains: Vitamin E (as unesterified D-alpha tocopherol plus D-beta, D-delta, and D-gamma tocopherols) 400 IU. Other Ingredients: Vegetable Oil Concentrate, Gelatin, Glycerin, Water.

Vitamin E with Tocotrienols - PhysioLogics
Each softgel contains: Vitamin E (as d-alpha tocopherol) 400 IU • Tocotrienols 35 mg. Other Ingredients: Gelatin, Glycerin.

Vitamin for the Hair - Puritan's Pride
Each tablet contains: Calcium Pantothenate 100 mg • Choline Bitartrate 125 mg • Inositol 50 mg • Niacin (nicotinic acid) 35 mg • Para-Aminobenzoic Acid 30 mg • Folic Acid 0.4 mg • Cobalamin (vitamin B12) 6 mcg • Iron (ferrous sulfate) 18 mg • Copper (gluconate) 2 mg • Iodine (kelp) 0.15 mg • Manganese (gluconate) 5 mg • Protein (from soy protein) 100 mg • Zinc (gluconate) 15 mg.

BRAND NAMES

Some Brand Name Natural Products - What they Contain

www.NaturalDatabase.com contains MANY more listings than appear here.
Editor's Notes are located on pages 2155-2163.

BRAND NAMES

Vitamin Foundation Creme - Aspen Group, Inc.
Each gram contains: Tocopheryl Acetate • Panthenol • Water • Octyldodecyl Neopetanoate • Octyl Methoxycinnmate • Cetearyl Alcohol • Cetyl Phosphate • Dimethicone • Beeswax • Carbomer • Aminomethyl Propanol • Propylene Glycol • Diazolidinyl Urea • Methylparaben • Propylparaben.

Vitamin K 100 mcg - GNC
Each tablet contains: Vitamin K (as phytonadione) 100 mcg. Other Ingredients: Dicalcium Phosphate, Cellulose.

Vitamin O - R-Garden Internationale
Stabilized Oxygen in a solution of distilled water, Sodium Chloride, and trace minerals.

Vita-Mind - Market America, Inc.
Two tablets contain: Vitamin C (L-ascorbate) 300 mg • Folic Acid 600 mcg • Vitamin B12 300 mcg • Potassium (chloride) 300 mg • Lecithin (phosphatidyl choline) 200 mg • Choline Bitartrate 150 mg • L-Phenylalanine 150 mg • L-Glutamine 45 mg • Coenzyme Q10 10 mg • Ginkgo Biloba 30 mg • Gotu Kola 30 mg • Korean Ginseng (Panax ginseng) 15 mg • Siberian Ginseng (Eleutherococcus senticosus) 15 mg. Other Ingredients: Microcrystalline Cellulose, Steraic Acid, Magnesium Stearate, Silicon Dioxide, Croscarmellose Sodium, Dicalcium Phosphate.

Vitamins A & D 10,000 IU + 400 IU - J. R. Carlson Laboratories, Inc.
Each softgel contains: Vitamin A (from fish liver oil) 10,000 IU • Vitamin D (D3, from fish liver oil) 1000 IU.

Vitamins A & D 25,000 IU + 1000 IU - J. R. Carlson Laboratories, Inc.
Each softgel contains: Vitamin A (from fish liver oil) 25,000 IU • Vitamin D (D3, from fish liver oil) 1000 IU.

Vitargo CGL - Nutrex, Inc.
Two level scoops contain: Magnesium 50 mg • Phosphorus 200 mg • Potassium 150 mg • Creatine Monohydrate 10 g • Vitargo (sugar free high molecular weight (500.000-700.000) carbohydrate from Swedish waxy maize starch) 60 mg. Other Ingredients: Natural and Artificial Flavors, Citric Acid, Osmosis Balancing Electrolytes (dipotassium phosphate, disodium phosphate, dimagnesium phosphate), Silicon Dioxide, Sucralose, FD&C Red 40.

Vitasana - Boehringer Ingelheim
Two gelcaps contain: Vitamin A (beta carotene) 4000 IU • Vitamin C (ascorbic acid) 120 mg • Vitamin D (cholecalciferol) 400 IU • Vitamin E (DL-alpha tocopheryl acetate) 30 IU • Vitamin B1 (thiamine mononitrate) 2.4 mg • Vitamin B2 (riboflavin) 3.4 mg • Vitamin B3 (niacinamide) 30 mg • Vitamin B6 (pyridoxine HCl) 4 mg • Folic Acid 400 mcg • Vitamin B12 (cobalamin) 2 mcg • Calcium (phosphate) 200 mg • Iron (ferrous sulfate) 18 mg • Phosphorus (calcium phosphate) 160 mg • Magnesium (oxide) 20 mg • Zinc (sulfate) 2 mg • Copper (sulfate) 2 mg • Manganese (sulfate) 2 mg • G115 Ginseng extract (from panax ginseng) 80 mg.

Vitase Digestion Formula - Enzymatic Therapy
Two capsules contain: Pure Plant Enzymes Blend 352 mg: Amylase (USP XXI [pH6.8]) 33,000 USP (FCC IV [pH4.8]) 14,300 DU, Protease I,II,III,IV (USP XXIII [pH7.5]) 29,150 USP (FCC IV [pH7.0]) 46,500 PC.. (FCC IV [pH5.7]) 36,150 HUT, Lactase I,II (FCC III [pH4.5]) 840 LacU, Cellulase I (FCC IV[pH4.5]) 142 CU, Lipase II (FCC III [pH6.5]) 215 LU, Maltase (malt diatase) (FCC IV[pH4.6]) 19,650 DP, Sucrase (invertase) (FCC IV[pH4.6]) 240 INVU.

Vita-Smart High Potency Vitamins and Minerals - K-mart
Each tablet contains: Vitamin A 8000 IU • Vitamin C 120 mg • Vitamin D 400 IU • Vitamin E 30 IU • Thiamin 5 mg • Riboflavin 5 mg • Niacin 30 mg • Vitamin B-6 5 mg • Folic Acid 400 mcg • Vitamin B-12 10 mcg • Biotin 10 mcg • Pantothenic Acid 10 mg • Calcium 100 mg • Iron 18 mg • Phosphorous 78 mg • Iodine 150 mcg • Magnesium 100 mg • Zinc 15 mg • Copper 2 mg • Chloride 15 mg • Potassium 15 mg.

Vitastic Body Revitalizer - Alacer
Purified Water • Ethanol • Aloe Vera • Cellulose • Propylene Glycol • Vitamin C • Vitamin B2 (riboflavin) • Vitamin B3 (niacin complex) • Vitamin B6 (pyridoxine) • Vitamin B12 (cyanocobalamin) • Vitamin E (D-alpha tocopherol) • Panthenol • PABA • Folic Acid • Zinc Gluconate • Magnesium Citrate • Manganese Gluconate • Chromium Picolinate • MSM (methylsulfonyl methane) • Polysorbate 80 • Selenium (sodium selenite) • Glycerine • Paraben • Peppermint Oil • Mineral Complexes of Magnesium, Potassium, Sodium • Lavender • Over 200 Trace Elements from Flower Pollen extract.

Vitastic Facial Mist - Alacer
Purified Water • Ethanol • Aloe Vera • Cellulose • Propylene Glycol • Vitamin C • Vitamin B12 (cyanocobalamin) • Vitamin B6 (pyridoxine) • Vitamin B2 (riboflavin) • Vitamin B3 (niacin complex) • Panthenol • MSM (methylsulfonyl methane) • Vitamin E • PABA • Folic Acid • Zinc Gluconate • Magnesium Citrate • Manganese Gluconate • Selenium (sodium selenite) • Methionine • Polysorbate 80 • Glycerine • Chromium Picolinate • Paraben • Peppermint Oil • Mineral Complexes of Magnesium, Potassium, Sodium • Lavender • Over 200 Trace Elements from Flower Pollen extract.

Vitastic Foot Revitalizer - Alacer
Purified Water • Ethanol • Aloe Vera • Cellulose • Propylene Glycol • Vitamin C • Vitamin B2 (riboflavin) • Vitamin B3 (niacin complex) • Polysorbate 80 • Vitamin B6 (pyridoxine) • Vitamin B12 (cyanocobalamin) • Vitamin E (D-alpha tocopherol) • Panthenol • PABA • Folic Acid • Zinc Gluconate • Magnesium Citrate • Manganese Gluconate • Chromium Picolinate • MSM (methylsulfonyl methane) • Selenium (sodium selenite) • Glycerine • Paraben • Peppermint Oil • Mineral Complexes of Magnesium, Potassium, Sodium • Lavender • Over 200 Trace Elements from Flower Pollen extract.

Vitastic Miracle Mist - Alacer
Purified Water • Magnesium • Manganese • Chelated Potassium • Chelated Chromium • Chelated Calcium • Chelated Zinc • Aloe Vera • Propylene Glycol • Vitamin B2 (riboflavin) • Vitamin B3 (niacin complex) • Vitamin B6 (pyridoxine) • MSM (methylsulfonyl methane) • Peppermint oil • Lavender.

Vitastic Muscle Pow'r Gel - Alacer
Purified Water • Ethanol • Aloe Vera • Lanolin • Propylene Glycol • Cellulose • Glycerin • Magnesium Citrate • Chelated Zinc • Chelated Manganese • MSM (methylsulfonyl methane) • Panthenol • Vitamin B1 (thiamine) • Vitamin B2 (riboflavin) • Vitamin B3 (niacin complex) • Vitamin B6 (pyridoxine) • Vitamin B12 (cyanocobalamin) • Vitamin E (D-alpha tocopherol) • Folic Acid • Selenium (sodium selenate) • Chromium Picolinate • Peppermint oil • Polysorbate 80 • Methylparaben • Propylparaben • PABA • Ginkgo Biloba • Methionine • Lavender • Over 200 Trace Elements from Flower Pollen extract.

Vitastic Soothing Shave - Alacer
Purified Water • Ethanol • Aloe Vera • Cellulose • Propylene Glycol • Vitamin C • Vitamin B2 (riboflavin) • Vitamin B3 (niacin complex) • Vitamin B6 (pyridoxine) • Vitamin B12 (cyanocobalamin) • Vitamin E (D-alpha tocopherol) • Panthenol • PABA • Folic Acid • Zinc (gluconate) • Magnesium Citrate • Manganese (gluconate) • Chromium (picolinate) • MSM (methylsulfonyl methane) • Polysorbate 80 • Lavender • Selenium • Glycerin • Paraben • Peppermint oil • Mineral Complexes of Magnesium, Potassium and Sodium • 200 Trace Elements from Flower Pollen extract.

Vitastic Spray Alive - Alacer
Purified Water • Glycerin • Ethanol • Aloe Vera • Propylene Glycol • Vitamin E • Vitamin B1 (thiamin) • Vitamin B2 (riboflavin) • Vitamin B3 (niacin complex) • Vitamin B6 (pyridoxine) • Vitamin B12 (cyanocobalamin) • PABA • Folic Acid • Selenium (sodium selenite) • MSM (methylsulfonyl methane) • D-Panthenol • Chelated Zinc • Chelated Manganese • D-Biotin • Chromium Picolinate • Melatonin • Peppermint oil • Ginkgo Biloba • Magnesium Citrate • Methionine • 200 Trace Elements from Flower Pollen extract.
See Editor's Note No. 26.

Vitastic Throat Power - Alacer
Distilled Water • Vitamin C • Propylene Glycol • Aloe Vera • Vitamin B2 (riboflavin) • Vitamin B6 (pyridoxine) • Niacin Complex • Parsley seed oil • MSM (methylsulfonyl methane) • Peppermint oil • Magnesium Niacinate • Tea Tree oil • Eucalyptus oil • Lime oil • Echinacea extract • White Willow bark extract • 200 trace elements from Flower Pollen extract.

Vita-Vim - Jamieson
Each caplet contains: Vitamin A (retinyl acetate) 10000 IU • Vitamin C (as Ascorbic Acid) 150 mg • Vitamin D (as Cholecalciferol) 400 IU • Vitamin E (as Dl-Alpha Tocopheryl Acetate) 15 IU • Thiamin (as Thiamine Mononitrate) 4.5 mg • Riboflavin (Vitamin B2) 7.5 mg • Niacin (as Niacin and Nicacinamide) 65 mg • Vitamin B6 (as Pyridoxine Hydrochloride) 3 mg • Folate (as Folic Acid) 400 mcg • Vitamin B12 (as Cyanocobalamin) 14 mcg • Biotin 10 mcg • Pantothenic Acid (as Calcium D-Pantothenate) 15 mg • Calcium (as Calcium Carbonate) 130 mg • Iron (as reduced Iron) 4 mg • Iodine (as from Kelp) 100 mcg • Magnesium (as Magnesium Oxide) 100 mg • Zinc (as Zinc Gluconate) 10 mg • Selenium (from yeast) 15 mcg • Copper (as Copper Gluconate) 1 mg • Choline Bitartrate 20 mg • Inositol 20 mg • Dl-Methionine 2.2 mg.

Vita-Vitamin - Olympian Labs
Two tablets contain: Vitamin A (palmitate) 5000 IU • Vitamin B-1 (thiamine HCl) 50 mg • Vitamin B-2 (riboflavin) 80 mg • Vitamin B-3 (inositol hexanicotinate) 80 mg • Vitamin B-5 (calcium pantothenate) 80 mg • Vitamin B-6 (pyridoxine HCl) 80 mg • Vitamin B-9 (folic acid) 400 mcg • Vitamin B-12 (cyanocobalamin) 60 mcg • Vitamin C (ascorbic acid) 300 mg • Vitamin D (cholecalciferol) 400 IU • Vitamin E (d-alpha-tocopherol acetate) 100 IU • Alpha Lipoic Acid 10 mg • Betaine HCl 30 mg • Boron 100 mcg • Calcium (citrate and phosphate) 120 mg • Choline Bitartrate 50 mg • Chromium 120 mcg • Citrus Bioflavonoid Complex 30 mg • Coenzyme Q10 10 mg • d-Biotin 300 mcg • Grape Skin extract 50 mg • Hesperidin 5 mg • Inositol 50 mg • Iodine (Kelp) 150 mcg • Lutein/Zeaxanthin 3 mg • Lycopene (100 mg Yielding 5 mg Pure Lycopene) 5 mg • Magnesium (Citrate and Magnesium Oxide) 40 mg • Manganese (Amino Acid Chelate) 2 mg • Molybdenum (Amino Acid Chelate) 75 mcg • PABA 50 mg • Potassium (Amino Acid Chelate) 7 mg • Rutin 30 mg • Selenium (L-Selenomethionine) 50 mcg • Vanadium (Amino Acid Chelate) 5 mcg • Zinc (Amino Acid Chelate) 20 mg. In a Proprietary Base: Barley Grass, Echinacea purpurea, Goldenseal root, Lecithin, Parsley, Pau d' Arco, Rice Bran, and Watercress.

Vitera-XT - Asia MedLabs, Inc.
Each capsule contains: Proprietary Blend 250 mg: Ephedra 4.22% (17 mg of plant derived ephedrines), Aimisu grass, 2,3,5,6-Tetramethyl Pyrazine (TMP). Other Ingredients: Gelatin Capsule, Cellulose.
See Editor's Note No. 30.

Vitex - Pharmanex
Each capsule contains: Vitex fruit 20:1 extract 175 mg.
Other Ingredients: Rice flour, Gelatin.

Vitex - Puritan's Pride
Each capsule contains: Vitex (Chastetree fruit powder: Vitex agnus-castus) 400 mg.

Vitex - Ortho Molecular Products
Each capsule contains: Chaste berry 10:1 extract 20 mg.
Other Ingredients: Natural Vegetable Capsules, Magnesium Stearate, Microcrystalline Cellulose.

Vitex Alfalfa - Gaia Herbs
Thirty drops contain: Proprietary Blend 240 mg: Chaste Tree berry (vitex agnus-castus), Alfalfa leaf solid extract (medicago sativa), Fresh Night Blooming Cereus stems (cactus grandiflorus), Fresh St. John's Wort flower buds (hypericum perforatum), Fresh Sage leaf (salvia officinalis), Wild Oats milky seed (avena sativa), Fresh Motherwort flowering tops (leonurus cardiaca), Essential oil of Lavender, Spring Water, 40-50% Pure Grain Alcohol USP.

Vitex Chaste Berry - Jamieson
Each capsule contains: Vitex Chaste Berry Formula VH1 (Vitex Agnuscastus, 200 mg powdered extract 1:20) 4000 mg. Derived only from the fruit of the Chaste Berry.

Vitex Elixir - Gaia Herbs
Thirty drops contain: Proprietary Blend 220 mg: Chaste Tree berry (vitex agnus-castus), Partridgeberry (mitchella repens), Black Haw root and tree bark (viburnum prunifolium), Red Raspberry leaf (rubus idaeus), Butterbur root (petasites frigida), Mugwort leaf (artemesia vulgaris), Dandelion root and leaf (taraxacum officinalis), Usnea lichen (usnea barbate), Prickly Ash bark (xanthoxylum clava-herculis), Rose Hip solid extract (rosa canina), Syrup of sweet Grapes and Mulberries, Blend of Sea Vegetation, Vegetable Glycerin, 18-25% Pure Grain Alcohol USP, Spring Water.

Vitex Extract - PhytoPharmica
Each capsule contains: Chaste Tree berry extract (vitex agnus-castus, standardized to contain a minimum of 0.5% agnuside) 225 mg.

Vitex/Chaste Tree - PhysioLogics
Two capsules contain: Vitex (agnus castus, chaste tree fruit powder) 800 mg. Other Ingredients: Gelatin, Calcium Sulfate, Cellulose (plant origin), Vegetable Magnesium Stearate, Silica.

Vit-Min 100+ - NOW Foods
Each tablet contains: Vitamin A (6 mg Beta-Carotene) 10000 IU • Vitamin A (Acetate) 10000 IU • Vitamin B1 (Thiamine HCL) 100 mg • Vitamin B2 (Riboflavin) 100 mg • Vitamin B3 (Niacinamide) 100 mg • Vitamin B5 (Pantothenic Acid) 100 mg • Vitamin B6 (Pyridoxine HCL) 100 mg • Vitamin B12 (Cyanocobalamin) 100 mcg • Biotin 100 mcg • Folic Acid 400 mcg • Vitamin C (Calcium Ascorbate) 250 mg • Vitamin D (Calciferol) 400 IU • Vitamin E (d-Alpha Tocopheryl Succinate) 150 IU • Calcium (Ascorbate, Carbonate) 50 mg • Magnesium (Oxide • Amino Acid Chelate) 30 mg • Zinc (Amino Acid Chelate) 15 mg • Copper (Amino Acid Chelate) 500 mcg • Iodine (Kelp) 150 mcg • Iron (Amino Acid Chelate) 10 mg • Potassium 10 mg • Manganese (Amino Acid Chelate) 5 mg • Selenium (Amino Acid Chelate) 25 mcg • Chromium (Yeast-free GTF) 100 mcg • Molybdenum (Amino Acid Chelate) 50 mcg • Boron (Amino Acid Chelate) 500 mcg • Vanadium (Amino Acid Chelate) 50 mcg • Choline (Bitartrate) 100 mg • Inositol 100 mg • PABA 50 mg • Rutin 25 mg • Betaine (HCL) 25 mg • Glutamic Acid 25 mg • Spirulina 50 mg • Barley grass organic 50 mg • Citrus Bioflavonoids (40% Hesperidin) 25 mg • Psyllium husk fiber 25 mg. This timed release multiple is formulated in a base of 72 Trace Minerals, Dicalcium Phosphate, Cellulose, Stearic Acid, Silica & natural vegetable protein coating.

Vit-Min 75+ - NOW Foods
Each tablet contains: Vitamin A (natural Fish Liver oil) 10000 IU • Beta-Carotene (6 mg) 10000 IU • Vitamin B1 (Thiamine HCL) 75 mg • Vitamin B2 (Riboflavin) 75 mg • Vitamin B3 (Niacinamide) 75 mg • Vitamin B5 (Pantothenic Acid) 75 mg • Vitamin B6 (Pyridoxine HCL) 75 mg • Vitamin B12 (Cyanocobalamin) 100 mcg • Biotin 100 mcg • Folic Acid 400 mcg • Vitamin C (Ascorbic Acid) 250 mg • Vitamin D (natural Fish Liver oil) 400 IU • Vitamin E (100% d-Alpha) 150 IU • Calcium (Amino Acid Chelate, Oystershell) 100 mg • Magnesium (Oxide, Amino Acid Chelate) 60 mg • Zinc (Amino Acid Chelate) 15 mg • Copper (Amino Acid Chelate) 1 mg • Iodine (Kelp) 150 mcg • Iron (Amino Acid Chelate) 10 mg • Choline (Bitartrate) 100 mg • Inositol 75 mg • PABA 30 mg • Rutin 25 mg • Citrus Bioflavonoids (40%) 100 mg • Betaine (HCL) 25 mg • Glutamic Acid 25 mg • Potassium (Amino Acid Chelate) 10 mg • Manganese (Amino Acid Chelate) 5 mg • Selenium (Amino Acid Chelate) 25 mcg • Chromium (Yeast-free GTF) 50 mcg • Boron (Amino Acid Chelate) 500 mcg • Molybdenum (Amino Acid Chelate) 50 mcg • Nucleic Acid 50 mg. In a natural base containing Alfalfa, Parsley, Rice polishings, Lecithin & Rose Hips, Dicalcium Phosphate, Cellulose, Stearic Acid & Silica.

Some Brand Name Natural Products - What they Contain

www.NaturalDatabase.com contains MANY more listings than appear here.
Editor's Notes are located on pages 2155-2163.

BRAND NAMES

Vitox - Pharmanex
Two capsules contain: Vitamin A (Vitamin A Palmitate) 3750 IU • Beta-Carotene (Beta-Carotene, Spirulina Pacifica) 6250 IU • Vitamin C (Calcium Ascorbate Complex-Ester-C, Acorbyl Palmitate) 250 mg • Vitamin D (as Vitamin D3, Cholecalciferol) 200 IU • Vitamin E (d-Alpha Tocopheryl Succinate, Beta, Gamma, Delta Tocopherols) 150 IU • Vitamin K (Phylloquinone) 35 mcg • Thiamin (Thiamine Mononitrate) 1.5 mg • Riboflavin (Riboflavin, Riboflavin-5-Phosphate) 1.7 mg • Niacin (Niacinamide Ascorbate) 20 mg • Vitamin B6 (Pyridoxine Hydrochloride, Pyridoxal-5-Phosphate) 2 mg • Folate (Folic Acid) 200 mcg • Vitamin B12 (Cyanocobalamin, Dibencozide) 6 mg • Biotin (Biotin) 150 mcg • Pantothenic Acid (d-Calcium Pantothenate) 25 mg • Calcium (Calcium Carbonate, Calcium Citrate, Calcium Chelate) 250 mg • Iron (Iron Chelate) 3 mg • Magnesium (Magnesium Oxide, Magnesium Citrate, Magnesium Chelate) 100 mg • Zinc (Zinc Chelate) 7.5 mg • Selenium (L-Selenomethionine) 50 mcg • Copper (Copper Chelate) 2.5 mg • Manganese (Manganese Chelate) 2.5 mg • Chromium (Chromium Chelate, Chromium Picolinate) 50 mcg • Boron (Boron) 0.5 mg • Glutathione 0.5 mg • Leucoanthocyanin (Grape Seed extract) 0.5 mg.

Vitrin - Nutraceutics Corp.
Two caplets contain: Vitamin A (20% as b-carotene) 5000 IU • Vitamin C 60 mg • Vitamin D 400 IU • Vitamin E 30 IU • Vitamin K 50 mcg • Vitamin B1 (thiamine) 1.5 mg • Vitamin B2 (riboflavin) 1.7 mg • Niacinamide 20 mg • Vitamin B6 (pyridoxine) 2 mg • Vitamin B12 6 mcg • Folic Acid 400 mcg • Pantothenic Acid 10 mg • Calcium 170 mg • Phosphorus 114 mg • Magnesium 100 mg • Zinc 15 mg • Iodine 150 mcg • Manganese 2 mg • Copper 2 mg • Potassium 80 mg • Chloride 72 mg • Selenium 20 mcg • Chromium 120 mcg • Molybdenum 75 mcg • Boron 150 mcg • Nickel 5 mcg • Silicon 2 mg • Tin 10 mcg • Vanadium 10 mcg • Lutein 250 mcg • Proprietary Blend HiORAC 600 mg: Grape Seed Extract, Dried Apple Juice Concentrate, Dried Orange Juice Concentrate, Dried Pineapple Juice Concentrate, Dried Peach Juice Concentrate, Dried Broccoli Concentrate, Dried Cauliflower Concentrate, Dried Spinach Concentrate, Dried Carrot Concentrate. Other Ingredients: Microcrystalline Cellulose, Gelatin, Crospovidone, Hydroxypropyl Methylcellulose, Starch, Lactose, Sodium Benzoate.

Vitrix - Nutrex, Inc.
Six liqui-caps contain: Liquid German Tribulus Terrestris (total saponins 80%, protodioscin 20%) 1000 mg • NTS-5 Liquid Proprietary Phyto-Nutrient Blend 500 mg: Vitex Agnus Castus, Avena Sativa, Epimedium, Eurycomo Longfolia Jack. Other Ingredients: Sesame Oil, Gelatin.

Viva Cell Plus - E'OLA
Three capsules contain: Proprietary Blend 2125 mg: Arabinogalactan (larix occidentalis), Bladderwrack, Pau D'Arco, Cat's Claw (Uncaria Tomentosa), Astragalus, Thymus Gland Extract. Other Ingredients: Rice Flour, Maltodexrin, Magnesium Stearate, Gelatin.

Vivace - Veromax International
Each tablet contains: Siberian Ginseng root 100 mg • Ginkgo Biloba leaf 37.5 mg • Jujube Dates (Zizyphi fructus) 100 mg • Isoflavones 40 mg • Proprietary Blend 175 mg: Glutamic acid, L-lysine HCL, L-Alanine. Other Ingredients: Dicalcium Phosphate, Microcrystalline Cellulose, Croscarmellose Sodium, Stearic Acid, Magnesium Stearate, Silicon Dioxide.

Vivarin - GlaxoSmithKline (GSK)
Each tablet contains: Caffeine 200 mg. Other Ingredients: Carnauba Wax, Colloidal Silicon Dioxide, FD&C Yellow #10 Lake, Dextrose, FD&C Yellow #6 Lake, Hydroxypropyl Methylcellulose, Magnesium Stearate, Microcrystalline Cellulose, Polyethylene Glycol, Polysorbate 80, Starch, Titanium Dioxide.

Vivaxl - Nutraceutics Corp.
Each packet contains: Thiamine (as HCl) 13 mg • Riboflavin (as 5-phosphate) 15 mg • Niacin 50 mg • Pyridoxine (as HCl) 40 mg • Vitamin B12 (cyanocobalamin) 300 mcg • Biotin 150 mcg • Pantothenic Acid (calcium pantothenate) 21 mg • Folic Acid 400 mcg • L-Arginine HCl 2800 mg • DL-Phenylalanine 400 mg • D-Phenylalanine 500 mcg • DMAE (2-dimethylaminoethanol bitartrate) 200 mg • GNS2 Ginseng extract (panax ginseng, standardized to 20% ginsenosides) 200 mg • Kola nut (cola acumenata) 175 mg • Inositol 100 mg • Trimethyl Glycine 100 mg • L-Taurine 50 mg • L-Citruline 50 mg • Sodium (carbonates) 98 mg. Other Ingredients: Dextrose, Citric Acid, Sodium Bicarbonate, Natural/Artificial Flavors, Sodium Carbonate, Sucralose.

VIVEX Beet Root Adjuvant - Functional Products
Each capsule contains: Beet Root Powder 435 mg • Celljuvant 4.35 mg. Other Ingredients:Gelatin, Magnesium Stearate.

VIVEX Brain Adjuvant - Functional Products
Each capsule contains: Siberian Ginseng Root Extract, Standardized to 0.8% 200 mg • Ginkgo Biloba Extract Standardized to 24% Flavon 50 mg. Other Ingredients: Gelatin, Eleutherococcus Senticosus Radix, Magnesium Stearate.

VIVEX Digestion Adjuvant - Functional Products
Each capsule contains: Pancreatin 6x 30 mg • Bromelain (600 GDU) 65 mg • Papain (100) 60 mg • Papaya Leaves 30 mg • Pepsin (1:3000) 60 mg • Betain HCl 55 mg • Bile Salt 30 mg. Other Ingredients: Gelatin, Magnesium Stearate.

VIVEX Heart Adjuvant - Functional Products
Three capsules contain: Hawthorn Extract 1.8% Vitexin 1100 mg. Other Ingredients: Gelatin, Crataegi Fructus Pulvis.

VIVEX Immune Adjuvant - Functional Products
Each capsule contains: Vitamin C 235 mg • Echinacea Angustifolia Extract, 4% Echinacosides 100 mg • Astragalus Extract 70% Polysaccharides 100 mg • Siberian Ginseng Extract, 0.8% Eleutherosides 50 mg. Other Ingredients: Gelatin.

VIVEX Joint Adjuvant - Functional Products
Two capsules contain: Devil's Claw Root Extract (2% Harpagoside) 850 mg. Other Ingredients: Gelatin, Magnesium Stearate, Harpagophytum Procumbensens.

VIVEX Laxative Adjuvant - Functional Products
Each capsule contains: Senna Pods 89 mg • Aloe Juice 78.5 mg • Buckthorn Bark 59.5 mg • Caraway Seed 33.5 mg • Rhubarb Root 26 mg • Fennel Seed 26 mg • Cascara Bark 14 mg. Other Ingredients: Gelatin, Magnesium Stearate.

VIVEX Migra-Feverfew Adjuvant - Functional Products
Two capsules contain: Feverfew Extract 66.66 mg. Other Ingredients: Chrysanthenum Partenium Herb, Gelatin, Magnesium Stearate.

VIVEX Mood Adjustment - Functional Products
Each capsule contains: St. John's Wort, 0.3% Hypericin 300 mg • Kava Kava Extract, 30% Kavapyrones. Other Ingredients: Gelatin, Kava Kava Radix, Fumed Silica, Magnesium Stearate.

VIVEX Nerve Adjuvant - Functional Products
Each capsule contains: Valerian Root 243 mg • Lemon Balm Herb 41 mg • Hops 81 mg • St. John's Wort Tops 81 mg • Chamomile 81 mg • Celljuvant 5.2 mg. Other Ingredients: Gelatin, Kava Kava Radix, Fumed Silica, Magnesium Stearate.

VIVEX Prostate Adjuvant - Functional Products
Each capsule contains: Saw Palmetto Extract, 905 Fatty Acids and Sterols 220 mg • Nettle Root Extract, 0.85% Belasitosterols 100 mg • Pumpkin seed oil, 90% Fatty Acids and Sterols 50 mg. Other Ingredients: Gelatin, Vegetable Oil, Glycerin (Kosher), Caramel, Soybean, Lecithin, Yellow Bees Wax, Water.

VIVEX Stomach Adjuvant - Functional Products
Each capsule contains: Yarrow Herb 61 mg • Chamomile Flower 61 mg • Peppermint Leaves 61 mg • Caraway Seed 61 mg • Ginger Root 61 mg • Thyme Leaves 61 mg • Licorice Root 61 mg. Other Ingredients: Gelatin, Magnesium Stearate.

VIVEX Vein & Artery Adjuvant - Functional Products
Each capsule contains: Vitamin E 50 IU • Garlic Powder 970 mg • Celljuvant 9.7 mg. Other Ingredients: Gelatin, Cellulose, Magnesium Stearate.

VIVEX Vitamin Mineral Complex **-** Functional Products
Three capsules contain: Vitamin A 3000 IU • Vitamin C 250 mg • Vitamin E 22 IU • Vitamin B1 10 mg • Vitamin B2 10 mg • Niacinamide 100 mg • Vitamin B6 5 mg • Vitamin B12 0.005 mg • Calcium 80 mg • Iron 17 mg • Magnesium 15 mg • Manganese 0.6 mg • Molybdenum 0.2 mg. Ingredients: Soybean Oil, Gelatin, Ascorbic Acid, Calcium Carbonate, Glycerin (Kosher), Niacinamide, Water, Soybean Lecithin, Ferrous Sulfate, Magnesium Oxide, Bees Wax, d-Alpha Tocopherol, Thiamine HCl, Vitamin A Palmitate, Manganese Gluconate, Molybdenum Glycinate, Cyanocobalamin 1%.

VIVEX Women's Adjuvant **-** Functional Products
Each capsule contain: Vitamin E 42.19 mg • Black Cohosh Root Extract, 2.5% Triterpene Glycosides 500 mg. Other Intredients: Gelatin, Magnesium Stearate.

Volkov's V16 **-** Advocare International
Each wafer contains: Vitamin A (as acetate and beta-carotene) 2000 IU • Vitamin C (as ascorbic acid) 75 mg • Vitamin D (as cholecalciferol) 200 IU • Vitamin E (as acetate) 10 IU • Vitamin K (as phylloquinone) 60 mcg • Thiamine (as mononitrate) 2 mg • Riboflavin 2 mg • Niacin (as niacinamide) 20 mg • Vitamin B6 (as pyridoxine HCl) 2 mg • Folic Acid 200 mcg • Vitamin B12 (as cyanocobalamin) 5 mcg • Biotin 60 mcg • Pantothenic Acid (as calcium pantothenate) 10 mg • Sodium (as bicarbonate) 95 mg • Golden Root extract (rhodiola rosea) 30 mg • Leuzea root extract (rhaponticum carthamoides) 20 mg • Wild Schisandra fruit extract (schisandra chinensis) 10 mg. Other Ingredients: Citric Acid, Dextrose, Potassium Bicarbonate, Silica, Modified Cellulose, Polysorbate, Stearic Acid, Sucralose, Natural Flavor, Magnesium Stearate.

Volumex **-** Mass Quantities, Inc.
Each rounded teaspoon contains: Creatine Monohydrate 5 grams.

VP2 **-** AST Sports Science
Each serving contains: 100% Hydrolyzed "Oligopeptide" Isolated Whey Protein Fractions consisting of precision engineered Whey Protein Isolate Fractions: Beta-Lactoglobulin, Alpha-Lacalbumin, Immunoglobulin, Proteose-Peptone, Glycomacropeptides (GMP), Bovine Serum Albumin, Lactoferrin, Lactoperoxidase. Lysozyme, Relaxin, Lactollin, Beta-Microglobulin • Natural & Artificial Flavors • Aspartame.

V-Pro **-** HealthMinded
Two capsules contain: V-Pro Proprietary Blend 1080 mg: Korean Red Ginseng, Saw Palmetto berry powder, Hawthorn berry, Ginkgo Biloba, Muira Puama powder extract (5:1), Catuaba bark extract (4:1), Cuscuta seed (4:1), Epimedium extract (20:1). Other Ingredients: Stearic Acid, Magnesium Stearate.

VPS Coriolus versicolor **-** JHS Natural Products
Each capsule contains: Coriolus extract 625 mg.

VS-10 Vanadyl Sulfate **-** Optimum Nutrition
Each tablet contains: Vanadyl Sulfate 10 mg.

VS-C Capsules **-** Nature's Sunshine
Four capsules contain: Proprietary Blend 1600 mg: Dandelion entire plant (taraxacum officinale), Purslane tops (portulaca oleracea), Indigo leaf and root (indigofera tinctoria), Thlaspi whole plant (thlaspi arvense), Bupleurum root (bupleurum chinense), Typhonium rhizome (typhonium flagelliforme), Scute root (scutellaria baicalensis), Cinnamon twig (cinnamomum cassia), Licorice root (glycyrrhiza uralensis), Panax Ginseng root. Other Ingredients: Gelatin, Water.

VS-C Liquid **-** Nature's Sunshine
Dandelion root (taraxacum officinale) • Purslane tops (portulaca oleracea) • Indigo leaf and root (indigofera tinctoria) • Thlaspi whole plant (thlaspi arvense) • Bupleurum root (burpleurum chinense) • Scute root (scutellaria baicalensis) • Typhonium rhizome (typhonium flagelliforme) • Panax Ginseng root • Cinnamon twig (cinnamomum cassia) • Licorice root (glycyrrhiza glabra). Base: 80% Glycerin, 20% Water.

VSL #3 **-** Questcor Pharmaceuticals
Each packet contains: Yougurt bacteria 450 billion.

VyoPro **-** AST Sports Science
Each serving contains: Fat-Free Whey Protein (L-Glutamine & B Vitamins) 18 g • 100% cool processed, (partially digested) "amino-specific" controlled Chymotrypsin/ Trypsin Hydrolyzed CCTH (Tryptic Hydrolysate) Oligopeptide Whey Protein from "Micro Filtered" & "Stirred-Bed Reactor" Ion-Exchange Whey Protein providing the highest percentage of Oligopeptides along with Di-, Tri-, & Poly-Peptides (multi-spectrum short & long amino acid chains) with specifically tailored & precision engineered molecular weight profiles [isolate fractions 53% Beta-Lactalbumin (molecular weight - MW 18,400 - 36,800D), 24% Alpha-Lactalbumin (MW 14,200) 17% Immunoglobulin (MW 16,000-160,000D) 6% Minor Peptones {lactoferrin, lactoperoxidase, lysozyme, relaxin, lactollin, & Beta-microglobulin (MW 4,000 - 40,000D)}] • Dual Stage Glutamine Composite, consisting of low molecular weight Whey Glutamine Peptides (MW 500 - 10,000) & Microencapsulated Pure Crystalline L-Glutamine • Protein Absorption Enhancing Matrix (Cyanocobalamin, Pyridoxine HCL, Thiamin, Riboflavin, & Calcium Pantothenate) •Natural Flavors • Aspartame.

Walgreens Multiple Vitamins **-** Walgreens
Each tablet contains: Vitamin A 5000 IU • Vitamin C 60 mg • Vitamin D 400 IU • Vitamin E 30 IU • Thiamin 1.5 mg • Riboflavin 1.7 mg • Niacin 20 mg • Vitamin B-6 2 mg • Folic Acid 400 mcg • Vitamin B-12 6 mcg • Pantothenic Acid 10 mg • Iron 18 mg.

Wal-Mart Equate Ultra Dairy Digest **-** Perrigo
Each caplet contains: Lactase 9000 FCC Units. Inactive Ingredients: Dextrates, Microcrystalline Cellulose, Dextrose, Sodium Citrate, Calcium Carbomethylcellulose, Magnesium Stearate, Silicon Dioxide.

Warm Cream **-** Strategic Science & Technology
Water • Choline chloride • L-Arginine • Sodium chloride • Mineral oil • Glyceryl stearate SE • Squalane • Cetyl alcohol • Magnesium chloride • Propylene glycol stearate SE • Wheat germ oil • Glyceryl stearate • Isopropyl myristate • Stearyl stearate • Polysorbate-60 • Propylene gylcol • Oleic acid • Tocopherol acetate • Collagen • Sorbitan stearate • Vitamin A • Vitamin D • Triethanolamine • O capsic • Methylparaben • Aloe vera extract • Imidazolidinyl urea • Propylparaben • BHA.

Water Balance **-** Nutrivention
Three tablets contain: Vitamin B6 (Pyridoxine) 150 mg • Potassium (Amino Acid Complex) 149 mg • Corn Silk (Stigmata maidis) 900 mg • Buchu (Barosma betulina) 600 mg • Elder flowers (Sambuccua canadensis nigra) 300 mg • Hydrangea (Hydrangea arborescens) 300 mg • Uva Ursi (Arctostaphylos uva ursi) 300 mg • Parsley (Petroselinum sativum) 150 mg • Samphire (Crithmum maritimum) 150 mg • Watermelon seed (Citrullus vulgaris) 150 mg.

Water Garden Pycnogenol Skin Lotion **-** Quantum, Inc.
Purified Water • Aloe Vera gel • Propylene Glycol • Hybrid Safflower Oil • Glyceryl Stearate • Stearic Acid • Octyl Palmitate • Sorbitol • Cetyl Alcohol • Tocopherol Acetate (vitamin E) • Panthenol • Allantoin • Sodium PCA • Jojoba Oil • Shea Butter • Kelp extract • Chamomile extract • Calendula extract • Lecithin • Tocopherol • Dimethicone • Triethanolamine • Methylparaben • Propylparaben • Vitamin A • Vitamin D (D3) • Diazolidinyl Urea • Pycnogenol • Super Oxide Dismutase.

Water Garden Pycnogenol Wrinkle Therapy Cream **-** Quantum, Inc.
Deionized Water • Aloe Vera gel • Dioctyl Dodecyl Dodecane Dioate • Propylene Glycol • Dimethicone • Toccopheryl Acetate • Stearic Acid • Emulsifying Wax • Cetyl Alcohol • Jojoba Oil • Pycnogenol • Lecithin • Panthenol • Allantoin • Extracts of Ginkgo Biloba • Echinacea • Chamomile • Super Oxide Dismutase SOD • Lipoderm • Glyceryl Stearate • Xanthan Gum • Triethanolamine • Methylparaben • Propylparaben • Diazolidinyl Urea • Tocopherol (Vitamin E).

Some Brand Name Natural Products - What they Contain

www.NaturalDatabase.com contains MANY more listings than appear here.
Editor's Notes are located on pages 2155-2163.

Water Garden Pycnogenol+ - Quantum, Inc.
Each tablet contains: Pycnogenol Atlantic Pine Bark extract (Pinus maritma) 30 mg • Grape Seed extract standardized 85% proanthocyanidins (Vinus vinifera) 20 mg.

Water Pill - Puritan's Pride
Two tablets contain: Potassium (as Potassium Gluconate) 40 mg • Buchu (Barosma betulina) leaf (25 mg of Buchu leaves 4:1 extract) 100 mg • Uva Ursi (Arctostaphylos uva-ursi) leaf (33.4 mg of Uva Ursi 3:1 extract) 100 mg • Juniper (Juniperus communis) berry 20 mg • Parsley (Petroselinum crispum) leaf 100 mg.

Water Pill - Natrol, Inc.
Two tablets contain: Vitamin B6 (as Pyridoxine HCl) 150 mg • Potassium (as Potassium Gluconate) 99 mg • Buchu extract leaf 4:1 100 mg • Parsley extract leaf 4:1 100 mg • Uva Ursi extract leaf 4:1 100 mg • Juniper extract berry 4:1 20 mg. Other Ingredients: Calcium Carbonate, Mono & Di-Glycerides, Stearic Acid, Croscarmellose Sodium, Silicon Dioxide, Magnesium Stearate.

Watershed - Absolute Nutrition
Two tablets contain: Potassium (from potassium gluconate) 200 mg • Proprietary Botanical Blend 200 mg: Cornsilk stylus, Couchgrass rhizome, Rose Hips 4:1 extract, Elecampane root, Goldenrod herb (aerial parts), Celery seed 4:1 extract, Dandelion root standardized 5:1 extract (20% taraxasterol) • Uva Ursi 4:1 extract 250 mg • Parsley 4:1 extract 250 mg. Other Ingredients: Dicalcium Phosphate, Microcrystalline Cellulose, Croscarmellose Sodium, Stearic Acid, Silica, Magnesium Stearate, Pharmaceutical Glaze.

Wei An Le capsules - Eu Yan Sang
Fructus Amomi • Cortex Cinnamomi • Rhizoma Zingibers • Rhizoma Atractylodis • Radix Paeoniae Alba • Flos Carthami • Rhizoma Corydalis • Fructus Aurantii • Oryza Sativa L • Fructus Evodiae • Radix Astragali.

Weight Gain - Vidafit
Each serving contains: Folate 300 mcg • Niacin 16 mg • Pantothenic Acid 5 mg • Riboflavin 1.3 mg • Thiamine 1.2 mg • Vitamin A 3300 IU • Vitamin B12 2.4 mcg • Vitamin B6 1.3 mg • Vitamin C 75 mg • Vitamin D 200 IU • Vitamin E 10 IU • Calcium 500 mg • Chromium 50 mcg • Copper 1 mg • Iodine 150 mcg • Magnesium 420 mg • Phosphorus 500 mg • Potassium 100 mg • Zinc 15 mg • Complex Carbohydrates 13 grams • Soy Protein 7 grams • Whey Protein 13 g.

Weight Gain Plus Appetite Increaser - VitaSalveo
Two capsules contain: Vitamin A Acetate 5000 IU • Ascorbic Acid 30 mg • Vitamin D (D3) 200 IU • Vitamin E 15 IU • Thiamine HCl 2.4 mg • Riboflavin 2.6 mg • Niacinamide 10 mg • Pyridoxine HCl 2.6 mg • Folic Acid 300 mcg • Vitamin B12 6 mcg • D-Calcium 10 mg • Iodine 150 mcg • Phosphorus Proteinate 10 mg • Magnesium Oxide powder 80 mg • Zinc Citrate powder 15 mg • Chromium Chloride 50 mcg • Potassium Chelate 10 mg • Whey Protein 200 mg • Soy Protein (isolated) 150 mg.

Weight Wellness - NorthStar Nutritionals
Each capsule contains: Rhodiola Rosea extract 100 mg • Rhododendron Caucasicum extract 50 mg • Blueberry extract 100 mg • Kelp extract 200 mg.

Weightless Cinnamon-Spice - Traditional Medicinals
Cinnamon bark • Fennel seed • Chicory root • Uva Ursi leaf • Flax seed • Cleavers herb • Licorice root • Red Clover top • Clove stem • Star Anise seed • Hibiscus flower • Buchu leaf • Natural Flavors.

Weightless Cranberry - Traditional Medicinals
Contains: Hibiscus flower • Roasted Chicory root • Fennel seed • Red Clover top • Uva Ursi leaf • Parsley leaf • Cleavers herb • Cranberry • Other natural flavors.

Weightless Tea - Traditional Medicinals
Fennel seed • Hibiscus flower • Lemongrass leaf • Uva Ursi leaf • Lemon Verbena leaf • Flax seed • Spearmint leaf • Cleavers herb • Red Clover top • Parsley leaf • Buchu leaf • Natural flavors.

Welah Mide - Shawnee Moon
Buchu leaf • Red Clover • Saw Palmetto • Uva Ursi.

WellBetX PGX capsules - Natural Factors
Two capsules contain: Calcium 6 mg • PGX Proprietary Blend 1000 mg: Konjac root extract (amorphophallus konjac, K. Koch), Sodium Alginate, Xanthan gum • Mulberry leaf powdered extract (morus alba) 50 mg. Other Ingredients: Gelatin Capsule (gelatin, purified water), Rice Powder, Magnesium Stearate.

WellBetX with PGX powder (chocolate and French vanilla flavors) - Natural Factors
Two scoops (61 g) contain: Potassium Citrate 225 mg • Vitamin A (beta carotene) 6300 IU • Vitamin C (ascorbic acid) 20 mg • Calcium (citrate and dicalcium phosphate) 400 mg • Iron (ferrous fumarate) 2.5 mg • Vitamin D (ergocalciferol) 100 IU • Vitamin E (D-alpha tocopheryl acetate) 6 IU • Thiamin (hydrochloride) 0.75 mg • Riboflavin 0.8 mg • Niacin (niacinamide) 12 mg • Vitamin B6 (pyridoxine hydrochloride) 0.75 mg • Folacin 0.11 mg • Vitamin B12 (cyanocobalamin) 0.5 mcg • Biotin 75 mcg • Pantothenic Acid (calcium pantothenate) 2.5 mg • Phosphorus (dicalcium phosphate) 2.5 mg • Iodine (potassium iodide) 40 mcg • Magnesium (citrate) 120 mg • Zinc (citrate) 6 mg • Selenium (chelate) 20 mcg • Copper (chelate) 0.5 mg • Manganese (citrate) 1 mg • Chromium (chelate) 20 mcg • Molybdenum (citrate) 25 mcg • Whey Protein 28 g • PGX Proprietary Blend 5 g: Konjac root extract (amorphophallus konjac, K. Koch), Sodium Alginate extract powder (laminaria digitata), Xanthan gum • Lecithin 4 g • Medium Chain Triglycerides 0.9 g • Stevia leaf powdered extract 100 mg • Bilberry fruit extract (vaccinium myrtillus, 25% anthocyanidins) 25 mg • Taurine 25 mg • Lutein 4 mg.

Wellman Fizz - Vitabiotics
Each tablet contains: Vitamin C 30 mg • Vitamin B1 (thiamin) 12 mg • Vitamin B2 (riboflavin) 5 mg • Vitamin B3 (niacin) 27 mg • Vitamin B6 (pyridoxine HCl) 10 mg • Folic Acid 400 mcg • Vitamin B12 (cyanocobalamin) 30 mcg • Biotin 50 mcg • Pantothenic Acid 6 mg • Iron 5 mg • Magnesium 50 mg • Zinc 5 mg • Selenium 30 mcg • L-Tyrosine 20 mg • Siberian Ginseng extract 150 mg • Co-Enzyme Q10 5 mg • L-Carnitine 75 mg.

Wellman Tablets - Vitabiotics
Each tablet contains: Vitamin A 750 mcg • Vitamin D 5 mcg • Vitamin E 20 mg • Vitamin C 60 mg • Vitamin B1 (thiamin) 12 mg • Vitamin B2 (riboflavin) 5 mg • Vitamin B3 (niacin) 20 mg • Vitamin B6 (pyridoxine HCl) 9 mg • Folic Acid 500 mcg • Vitamin B12 (cyanocobalamin) 9 mcg • Biotin 0.05 mg • Pantothenic Acid 10 mg • Iron 6 mg • Magnesium 50 mg • Zinc 15 mg • Iodine 150 mcg • Manganese 3 mg • Copper 1.5 mg • Chromium 50 mcg • Selenium 150 mcg • Silicon 10 mg • Arginine 20 mg • Methionine 20 mg • Betacarotene 2 mg • PABA (para-aminobenzoic acid) 20 mg • Ginseng 20 mg • Bioflavonoids 10 mg • Co-Enzyme Q10 2 mg • L-Carnitine 30 mg.

Wellness C-1000 - Source Naturals
Each tablet contains: Vitamin C (as ascorbic acid, potassium, magnesium and calcium ascorbates, ascorbyl palmitate, zinc and manganese ascorbates) 1000 mg • Bioflavonoids 100 mg • Ascorbyl Palmitate 60 mg • Rose Hips fruit 25 mg • Rutin 25 mg • Quercetin 25 mg • Grape seed extract (Proanthodyn, with a proanthocyanidolic value of 95) 15 mg • Alpha-Lipoic Acid 10 mg.

Wellness Cell Response - Source Naturals
Each capsule contains: Polyvalent Transfer Factor (as colostral fraction with minimum 20 potency units) 5 mg.

Wellness Cold and Flu - Source Naturals
Each tablet contains: Echinacea angustifolia 3X • Allium cepa (red onion) 4X • Bryonia alba (white bryony) 4X • Eupatorium perfoliatum (boneset) 4X • Gelsemium sempervirens (yellow jasmine) 4X • Sanguinaria canadensis (blood root) 4X • Kali bichromicum (potassium dichromate) 6X • Phosphorus 6X • Aconitum napellus (monkshood) 12X • Influenzinum 12X.
See Editor's Note No. 1.

BRAND NAMES

Some Brand Name Natural Products - What they Contain

www.NaturalDatabase.com contains MANY more listings than appear here.
Editor's Notes are located on pages 2155-2163.

Wellness Colloidal Silver Liquid - Source Naturals
Each two tablespoons contain: Silver 30 ppm.

Wellness Colloidal Silver Nasal Spray - Source Naturals
Each spray contains: Silver 30 ppm.

Wellness Colloidal Silver Throat Spray - Source Naturals
Each spray contains: Silver 30 ppm.

Wellness Earache - Source Naturals
Each tablet contains: Capsicum annuum (Cayenne Pepper) 6X • Silicea (Silica) 6X • Verbascum thapsus (Mullein) 6X • Ferrum phosphoricum (Ferrosoferric Phosphate) 12X • Kali muriaticum (Potassium Chloride) 12X • Aconitum napellus (Aconite) 30X • Belladonna (Nightshade) 30X • Calcarea carbonica (Calcium Carbonate) 30X • Pulsatilla (Wind Flower) 30X.
See Editor's Note No. 1.

Wellness Elderberry Extract Liquid - Source Naturals
Each 1 tsp contains: Elderberry & flower extract 2 mL.

Wellness Elderberry Extract Tablets - Source Naturals
Each three tablets contain: Elder berry and flower (standardized extract yielding 81 mg bioflavonoids and anthocyanins) 1020 mg • Elderberries and flowers 480 mg.

Wellness Essentials - Metagenics
Two packets (one AM packet and one PM packet) contain: Multigenics Intensive Care Formula without Iron (five tablets): Vitamin A (beta carotene) 9375 IU • Vitamin A (retinyl acetate) 3125 IU • Vitamin C (ascorbic acid) 750 mg • Vitamin D (cholecalciferol) 250 IU • Vitamin E (D-alpha tocopheryl succinate) 62 IU • Thiamin (mononitrate) 18 mg • Riboflavin 21 mg • Niacin (niacinamide, niacin) 262 mg • Vitamin B6 (pyridoxine HCl) 25 mg • Folate (as folic acid, L-5-methyl tetrahydrofolate, 5-formyl tetrahydrofolate) 500 mcg • Vitamin B12 (as cyanocobalamin) 125 mcg • Biotin 125 mcg • Pantothenic Acid (as D-calcium pantothenate) 125 mg • Calcium (as calcium citrate, MCHC, calcium glycinate) 312 mg • Phosphorus (as MCHC) 68 mg • Iodine (as potassium iodide) 95 mg • Magnesium (as magnesium bis-glycinate, citrate) 156 mg • Zinc (as zinc glycinate, histidinate) 12 mg • Selenium (as selenium aspartate) 125 mcg • Copper (as copper lysinate) 1.25 mg • Manganese (as manganese glycinate) 625 mcg • Chromium (as chromium dinicotinate glycinate) 125 mcg • Molybdenum (as molybdenum aspartate) 65 mcg • Potassium (as potassium aspartate) 61 mg • Betaine Hydrochloride 109 mg • Choline (as choline bitartrate) 78 mg • Inositol 75 mg • Citrus Bioflavonoid Complex 65 mg • Para-Aminobenzoic Acid (PABA) 31 mg • Vanadium (as vanadyl sulfate) 25 mcg • Quercetin Dihydrate 15 mg • Alpha-Carotene 121 mcg • Cryptoxanthin 34 mg • Zeaxanthin 16 mcg • Lutein 16 mcg. AdvaClear blend (two capsules): Vitamin A (33% as retinyl palmitate and 67% as beta-carotene) 2500 IU • Vitamin C (as magnesium ascorbate) 33 mg • Vitamin D (as cholecalciferol) 33 IU • Vitamin E (as D-alpha tocopheryl acetate and mixed tocopherols) 66 IU • Thiamin (as thiamin hydrochloride) 10 mg • Riboflavin 5 mg • Niacin (as niacinamide, niacin) 23 mg • Vitamin B6 (as pyridoxine hydrochloride) 17 mg • Folate (L-5-methyl tetrahydrofolate, 5-formyl tetrahydrofolate) 267 mg • Vitamin B12 (as cyanocobalamin) 33 mcg • Biotin 66 mcg • Pantothenic Acid (as D-calcium pantothenate) 33 mg • Magnesium (as magnesium ascorbate) 19 mg • Zinc (as zinc citrate) 6.5 mg • Selenium (as selenomethionine) 50 mcg • Copper (as copper citrate) 0.65 mg • Manganese (as manganese citrate) 1.65 mg • Molybdenum (as molybdenum amino acid chelate) 66 mcg • Choline (as choline bitartrate) 66 mg • N-Acetylcysteine 66 mg • Sodium Sulfate 100 mg • Taurine 117 mg • Silymarin (as silybin, silychristin, silydianin, from milk thistle seed extract, silybum marianum) 50 mg • Catechins 34 mg • Epigallocatechin Gallate (EGCG, from decaffeinated green tea leaf, camellia sinensis) 22 mg • Artichoke leaf extract (cynara scolymus, containing cynarin and chlorogenic acid) 166 mg • Watercress whole plant 4:1 extract (nasturtium officinale) 134 mg • Ellagic Acid (from pomegranate rind extract, punica granatum) 33 mg. EPA-DHA Complex (two softgels): Natural Marine Lipid Concentrate 2 g • EPA (eicosapentaenoic acid) 360 mg • DHA (docosahexaenoic acid) 240 mg.

Wellness Essentials for Men - Metagenics
Two packets (one AM packet and one PM packet) contain: Tribulus Synergy blend (two tablets) 2000 mg: Tribulus fruit 7:1 extract (tribulus terrestris, containing saponins) • Ashwagandha root 5:1 extract (withania somnifera, containing withanolides) • Cowhage seed extract (mucuna pruriens, containing naturally occuring levadopa) • Shatavari root 4:1 extract (asparagus racemosus, containing saponins). EPA-DHA Lemon Softgels (two softgels): Natural Marine Lipid Concentrate 2.5 g • EPA (eicosapentaenoic acid) 720 mg • DHA (docosahexaenoic acid) 560 mg. Multigenics Intensive Care without Iron (two tablets): Vitamin A (as beta-carotene) 3750 IU • Vitamin A (as retinyl acetate) 1250 IU • Vitamin C (as ascorbic acid) 300 mg • Vitamin D (as cholecalciferol) 100 IU • Vitamin E (as D-alpha tocopheryl succinate) 25 IU • Thiamin (as thiamin mononitrate) 7.5 mg • Riboflavin 8.5 mg • Niacin (as niacinamide, niacin) 105 mg • Vitamin B6 (as pyridoxine hydrochloride) 10 mg • Folate (as folic acid, L-5-methyl tetrahydrofolate, 5-formyl tetrahydrofolate) 200 mcg • Vitamin B12 (as cyanocobalamin) 50 mcg • Biotin 50 mcg • Pantothenic Acid (as D-calcium pantothenate) 50 mg • Calcium (as citrate, MCHC, glycinate) 125 mg • Phosphorus (as MCHC) 28 mg • Iodine (as potassium iodide) 38 mcg • Magnesium (as magnesium bis-glycinate, magnesium citrate) 62 mg • Zinc (as zinc glycinate, zinc histidinate) 5 mg • Selenium (as selenium aspartate) 50 mcg • Copper (as copper lysinate) 0.5 mg • Manganese (manganese glycinate) 0.25 mg • Chromium (as chromium dinicotinate glycinate) 50 mcg • Molybdenum (as molybdenum aspartate) 25 mcg • Potassium (as potassium aspartate) 24 mg • Betaine Hydrochloride 43 mg • Choline (as choline bitartrate) 31 mg • Inositol 30 mg • L-Glutamine 25 mg • Citrus Bioflavonoid Complex 25 mg • Para-Aminobenzoic Acid (PABA) 12 mg • Vanadium (as vanadyl sulfate) 9 mcg • Quercetin Dihydrate 6 mg • Alpha-Carotene 48 mcg • Cryptoxanthin 13 mcg • Zeaxanthin 6 mcg • Lutein 6 mcg. Zinc A.G. blend (one tablet): Zinc (as zinc arginate, glycinate) 20 mg.

Wellness Essentials for Women - Metagenics
Two packets (one AM packet and one PM packet) contain: Multigenics Intensive Care Formula (four tablets): Vitamin A (as beta carotene) 7500 IU • Vitamin A (retinyl acetate) 2500 IU • Vitamin C (as ascorbic acid) 600 mg • Vitamin D (as cholecalciferol) 200 IU • Vitamin E (as D-alpha tocopheryl succinate) 50 IU • Thiamin (as thiamin mononitrate) 15 mg • Riboflavin 17 mg • Niacin (as niacinamide, niacin) 210 mg • Vitamin B6 (as pyridoxine hydrochloride) 20 mg • Folate (as folic acid, L-5-methyl tetrahydrofolate, 5-formyl tetrahydrofolate) 400 mcg • Vitamin B12 (as cyanocobalamin) 100 mcg • Biotin 100 mcg • Pantothenic Acid (as D-calcium pantothenate) 100 mg • Calcium (as calcium citrate, MCHC, calcium glycinate) 250 mg • Iron (as iron glycinate) 5 mg • Phosphorus (as MCHC) 57 mg • Iodine (as potassium iodide) 76 mcg • Magnesium (as magnesium bis-gylcinate, citrate) 125 mg • Zinc (as zinc glycinate, histidinate) 10 mg • Selenium (as selenium aspartate) 100 mcg • Copper (as copper lysinate) 1 mg • Manganese (as manganese glycinate) 500 mcg • Chromium (as chromium dinicotinate glycinate) 100 mcg • Molybdenum (as molybdenum aspartate) 50 mcg • Potassium (as potassium aspartate) 49 mg • Betaine Hydrochloride 87 mg • Choline (as choline bitartrate) 62 mg • Inositol 60 mg • L-Glutamine 50 mg • Citrus Bioflavonoid Complex 50 mg • Para-Aminobenzoic Acid (PABA) 25 mg • Vanadium (as vanadyl sulfate) 19 mcg • Quercetin Dihydrate 12 mg • Alpha-Carotene 97 mcg • Cryptoxanthin 27 mcg • Zeaxanthin 13 mcg • Lutein 13 mcg. E Complex-1:1 blend (one softgel): Vitamin E (as D-alpha tocopherol) 200 IU • Gamma-Tocopherol 135 mg • Delta-Tocopherol 49 mg • Beta-Tocopherol 3 mg. EPA-DHA Extra Strength blend (two softgels): Natural Marine Lipid Concentrate 2 g • EPA (eicosapentaenoic acid) 600 mg • DHA (docosahexaenoic acid) 400 mg • Vitamin E (as D-alpha-tocopherol and mixed tocopherols) 20 IU. Cal Apatite with Magnesium blend (two tablets): Microcrystalline Hydroxyapatite Concentrate (MCHC) 1000 mg • Calcium (as MCHC and dicalcium phosphate) 400 mg • Phosphorus (as MCHC and dicalcium phosphate) 252 mg • Magnesium (as magnesium citrate, aspartate, and magnesium bis-glycinate) 200 mg.

Wellness Essentials JOINT FOCUS - Metagenics
Two packets (one AM packet and one PM packet) contain: Kaprex blend 880 mg (two tablets): Luduxin brand Iso-Alpha Acids from Hops extract (humulus lupulus), Magnesium Salt • Oleanolic Acid from Olive leaf extract (olea europaea) • Rosemary leaf extract (rosmarinus officinalis). Glucosamine Sulfate blend (three tablets): Glucosamine Sulfate 1500 mg • Vitamin C 90 mg. EPA-DHA Extra Strength (two softgels): Natural Marine Lipid Concentrate 2 g • EPA (eicosapentaenoic acid) 600 mg • DHA (docosahexaenoic acid) 400 mg • Vitamin E (mixed tocopherols) 10 IU.

Wellness Formula - Source Naturals
Three tablets contain: Vitamin A (Palmitate 4000 IU, Beta Carotene 1000 IU) 5000 IU • Vitamin C (Ascorbic Acid, and Zinc, Calcium, and Magnesium Ascorbates) 1075 mg • Calcium (Ascorbate) 7.5 mg • Copper (Sebacate) 300 mcg • Magnesium (Ascorbate) 3.8 mg • Selenium (Sodium Selenite) 25 mcg • Zinc (Ascorbate) 23 mg • Propolis 324 mg • Propolis extract 126 mg • Garlic clove 360 mg • Boneset leaf 328 mg • Polygonum Odoratum 200 mg • Echinacea root 196 mg • Echinacea extract 164 mg • Isatis (root and leaf) 159 mg • Horehound stems 150 mg • Bioflavonoids 120 mg • Astragalus root 90 mg • Angelica Archangelica root 87 mg • Mullein leaf 80 mg • Goldenseal root 75 mg • Siberian Ginseng root 66 mg • Hawthorn berry 55 mg • Oregon Grape root 55 mg • Siberian Ginseng extract 54 mg • Pau d'Arco extract 36 mg • Cayenne fruit 30 mg.

Wellness GarliCell - Source Naturals
Each tablet contains: Garlic clove 650 mg.

Wellness Herbal Resistance - Alcohol Free - Source Naturals
Each 1/2 tsp contains: Proprietary Extract 1.7 mL: Echinacea (E. purpurea & E. angustifolia standardized extract), Goldenseal root, Yin Chiao formula (lonicera, forsythia, mint, prepared sojae, licorice, schizonepeta phragmitis, platycodon, arctium, lophatherum), Ginger root, Boneset leaf & stem, Siberian Ginseng root, Elderberry flowers, Isatis leaf & root, Horehound aerial parts, Bayberry bark.

Wellness Herbal Resistance Liquid - Source Naturals
Each 1/2 tsp contains: Proprietary Extract 2.5 mL: Echinacea (E. purpurea & E. angustifolia standardized extract), Goldenseal root, Yin Chiao formula (lonicera, forsythia, mint, prepared sojae, licorice, schizonepeta phragmitis, platycodon, arctium, lophatherum), Ginger root, Boneset leaf & stem, Siberian Ginseng root, Elderberry flowers, Isatis leaf & root, Horehound aerial parts, Bayberry bark.

Wellness Larchtree Extract - Source Naturals
Two tablets contain: Larch Tree extract (Larix occidentalis, standardized to 85% arabinogalactans yielding 1.7 grams of arabinogalactans) 2 g • Calcium 91 mg.

Wellness Multiple - Source Naturals
Four tablets contain: Vitamin A (as palmitate 15,000 IU & beta carotene 10,000 IU) 25,000 IU • Vitamin C (as magnesium ascorbate, ascorbic acid, calcium, potassium, zinc & manganese ascorbates) 1000 mg • Vitamin E (as natural d-alpha tocopheryl) 400 IU • Thiamin (vitamin B1) 50 mg • Riboflavin (vitamin B-2) 50 mg • Niacinamide 50 mg • Niacin 25 mg • Vitamin B6 (as pyridoxine HCl) 50 mg • Folate (as folic acid) 400 mcg • Vitamin B12 (as cyanocobalamin) 100 mcg • Biotin 100 mcg • Pantothenic Acid (as calcium d-pantothenate) 50 mg • Calcium (as calcium ascorbate) 25 mg • Magnesium (as magnesium ascorbate) 25 mg • Zinc (as zinc ascorbate) 15 mg • Selenium (as l-selenomethionine [Selenomax] & sodium selenite) 200 mcg • Copper (as copper sebacate) 2 mg • Manganese (as manganese ascorbate) 3 mg • Chromium (as chromium polynicotinate [ChromeMate] & picolinate) 200 mcg • Molybdenum (as molybdenum chelate) 200 mcg • Potassium (as potassium ascorbate) 25 mg • N-Acetyl Cysteine 400 mg • Quercetin 200 mg • whole leaf Aloe Vera concentrate (200:1) 100 mg • Turmeric root extract 100 mg • Milk Thistle seed extract yielding 50 mg silymarin) 60 mg • Choline (as choline bitartrate) 50 mg • Grape seed extract (Proanthodyn, with a proanthocyanidolic value of 95) 50 mg • Inositol 50 mg • Coenzyme Q10 (ubiquinone) 30 mg • Alpha-Lipoic Acid 30 mg • Green Tea leaf extract 20 mg. Proprietary Blend 1310 mg: Cat's Claw bark, Elderberry flowers, St. John's Wort leaf & flower extract, Reishi Mycelia, Astragalus root, Schizandra fruit, Garlic clove, Maitake Mycelia, Shiitake Mycelia, Elderberry extract, Siberian Ginseng root extract, Atractylodes rhizome.

Wellness Olive Leaf - Source Naturals
Two tablets contain: Olive leaf (standardized extract of olea europaea yielding 75 mg of Oleuropein) 1000 mg.

Wellness Plus Capsules - Vista Vitamins
Each packet contains: Vitamin A (as retinyl palmitate) 5000 IU • Vitamin A (as alpha and beta carotene) 2500 IU • Vitamin C (as ascorbic acid) 120 mg • Vitamin D (as cholecalciferol) 400 IU • Vitamin E (as d-alpha tocopheryl acetate) 50 IU • Vitamin K (as phylloquinone) 60 mcg • Thiamin (as thiamin hydrochloride) 12 mg • Riboflavin 13 mg • Niacin (as niacinamide) 16 mg • Vitamin B6 (as pyridoxine hydrochloride) 14 mg • Folic Acid 400 mcg • Vitamin B12 (as methylcobalamin) 120 mcg • Biotin 150 mcg • Pantothenic Acid (as d-calcium pantothenate) 10 mg • Calcium (as calcium amino acid chelate) 150 mg • Iron (as ferrochel ferrous bis-glycine) 4 mg • Iodine (as potassium iodide) 75 mcg • Magnesium (as magnesium amino acid chelate) 100 mg • Zinc (as chelazome amino acid chelate) 11 mg • Selenium (as selenium amino acid complex) 70 mcg • Copper (as chelazome amino acid chelate) 0.45 mg • Manganese (as chelazome amino acid chelate) 1.15 mg • Chromium (as chelavite amino acid chelate) 75 mcg • Molybdenum (as molybdenum amino acid chelate) 22.5 mcg • Potassium (as potassium chloride) 49.5 mg • Boron (as boron amino acid complex) 0.75 mg • Larix occidentalis (arabinogalatans) 250 mg • Lactobacillus sporogenes 5 million. Other Ingredients: Gelatin, Cellulose, Stearic Acid, Silicon Dioxide, Magnesium Stearate, Titanium Dioxide.

Wellness Source - HealthWatchers System
Vitamin A • Vitamin D • Vitamin E • Vitamin C • Vitamin B6 • Vitamin B2 • Vitamin B1 • Vitamin B12 • Vitamin U • Bioflavonoids • Choline Bitartrate • Niacin-Niacinamide • Pantothenic Acid • Inositol • Rutin • Papain • PABA • Lecithin • Quercetin • RNA • Hesperidin • DNA • CoQ10 • Folic Acid • Octacosanol • Biotin • Magnesium • Calcium • Zinc • Boron • Potassium • Manganese • Copper • Iodine (Kelp) • Selenium • Chromium.

Wellness Source Booster - HealthWatchers System
Beta Carotene • Vitamin E • Vitamin C • Calcium • Magnesium • Choline • Potassium • Silica • Niacinamide.

Wellness Zinc Lozenges - Source Naturals
Each lozenge contains: Zinc (as zinc gluconate, ascorbate, & chelate) 23 mg • Vitamin C (as zinc ascorbate) 30 mg.

Wellness Zinc Throat Spray - Source Naturals
Each two oz serving contains: Vitamin C 11 mg • Zinc (gluconate) 23 mg • Echinacea extract 40 mg • Elderberry extract 34 mg.

Wellwoman Capsules - Vitabiotics
Each capsule contains: Starflower Oil 100 mg • Evening Primrose Oil 100 mg • Vitamin D (200 IU) 5 mcg • Vitamin E (natural source) 30 mg • Vitamin C 60 mg • Vitamin B1 (thiamin) 10 mg • Vitamin B2 (riboflavin) 5 mg • Vitamin B3 (niacin) 36 mg • Vitamin B6 (pyridoxine HCl) 20 mg • Folic Acid 400 mcg • Vitamin B12 (cyanocobalamin) 20 mcg • Biotin 50 mcg • Pantothenic Acid 6 mg • Vitamin K 90 mcg • Natural Mixed Carotenoids 2 mg • Iron 12 mg • Magnesium 100 mg • Zinc 12 mg • Manganese 2.5 mg • Copper 1.5 mg • Selenium 100 mcg • Chromium 50 mcg • PABA (para-aminobenzoic acid) 30 mg • Citrus Bioflavonoids 10 mg.

Wellwoman Fizz - Vitabiotics
Each tablet contains: Vitamin C 30 mg • Vitamin B1 (thiamin) 10 mg • Vitamin B2 (riboflavin) 5 mg • Vitamin B3 (niacin) 27 mg • Vitamin B6 (pyridoxine HCl) 10 mg • Folic Acid 400 mcg • Vitamin B12 (cyanocobalamin) 40 mcg • Biotin 100 mcg • Pantothenic Acid 6 mg • Iron 8 mg • Magnesium 50 mg • Zinc 5 mg • L-Carnitine 100 mg • Gotu Kola extract 40 mg • Guarana extract 150 mcg.

Wellzymes Blood Sugar Balance - Enzymes, Inc.
Two capsules contain: Vitamin E (from d-Alpha Tocopheryl Acid Succinate) 40 IU • Chromium (from Chromium GTF Polynicolinate)

100 mcg • n-zimes Proprietary Enzyme Blend 20 mg: Lipase, CereCalase Plus • Proprietary Herbal Blend 330 mg: Gymnema leaf extract (standardized to contain 25% gymnemic acid), Fenugreek seed extract (equivalent to 400 mg raw herb), Rice Bran, Quercetin. Other Ingredients: Plant Cellulose, Water.

Wellzymes Colon Health **-** Enzymes, Inc.
Each capsule contains: Proprietary Blend 225 mg: Lactobacillus Acidophilus, Lactobacillus Plantarum, Bifidobacterium Bifidum, Lactobacillus Casei, Lactobacillus Salivarius. Other Ingredients: Plant Cellulose, Water.

Wellzymes Digestive Health **-** Enzymes, Inc.
Each capsule contains: n-zimes Proprietary Enzyme Blend 215 mg: Protease Blend (alkaline, neutral and acid proteases plus peptidase), Lipase, Amylase, Glucoamylase, Malt Diastase, Invertase, Lactase, alpha-Galactosidase, Cellulase, CereCalase Plus, Xylanase, Pectinase. Other Ingredients: Plant Cellulose, Water.

Wellzymes Gastric Ease **-** Enzymes, Inc.
Each capsule contains: n-zimes Proprietary Enzyme Blend 73 mg: Catalase, Peptidase, Lipase, Amylase, Glucoamylase, Malt Diastase, Invertase, Lactase, alpha-Galactosidase, Cellulase, CereCalase Plus, Xylanase, Pectinase • Proprietary Herbal Blend 145 mg: Marshmallow root, Marshmallow root extract (equivalent to 200 mg of raw herb), Aloe Vera gel extract (equivalent to 2000 mg of raw gel). Other Ingredients: Plant Cellulose, Water.

Wellzymes Immune Health **-** Enzymes, Inc.
Two capsules contain: n-zimes Proprietary Enzyme Blend 82 mg: pHysioProtease (236,800 pHysio-U), CereCalase Plus • Proprietary Herbal Blend 360 mg: Astragalus root extract (equivalent to 640 mg raw herb), Reishi Mushroom extract (equivalent to 160 mg raw herb), Cat's Claw herb extract (standardized to contain 1% oxindole alkaloids), Burdock root extract (equivalent to 160 mg raw herb). Other Ingredients: Plant Cellulose, Water.

Wellzymes Joint Health **-** Enzymes, Inc.
Two capsules contain: Zinc (citrate) 14 mg • Copper (citrate) 1 mg • Manganese (citrate) 8 mg • Boron (citrate) 0.4 mg • n-zimes Proprietary Enzyme Blend 108 mg: pHysioProtease (236,800 pHysio-U), Bromelain, CereCalase Plus • Proprietary Herbal Blend 235 mg: Boswellia resin extract (standardized to contain 60% boswellic acid), Horsetail herb extract (equivalent to 200 mg raw herb), Rice Bran, Turmeric root extract (standardized to 95% curcumin), White Willow bark extract (standardized to contain 12% salicin). Other Ingredients: Plant Cellulose, Water.

Wellzymes Lung Health **-** Enzymes, Inc.
Two capsules contain: n-zimes Proprietary Enzyme Blend 84 mg: pHysioProtease (213,120 pHysio-U), Amylase, CereCalse Plus • Proprietary Herbal Blend 350 mg: Thyme herb extract (equivalent to 520 mg raw herb), Mullein leaf extract (equivalent to 400 mg raw herb), Great Plantain leaf extract (equivalent to 160 mg raw herb), Acerola Cherries extract (standardized to contain 17% Vitamin C), Quercetin, Rice Bran. Other Ingredients: Plant Cellulose, Water.

Wellzymes Male Vigor **-** Enzymes, Inc.
Two capsules contain: Vitamin E (from d-Alpha Tocopheryl Acid Succinate) 40 IU • Zinc (from Zinc Citrate) 14 mg • n-zimes Proprietary Enzyme Blend 32 mg: pHysioProtease, CereCalase Plus • Proprietary Herbal Blend 320 mg: Panax Ginseng root extract (standardized to contain 8% ginsenosides), Damiana leaf extract (equivalent to 400 mg raw herb), Yohimbe bark extract (standardized to contain 3% yohimbine), Ginkgo Biloba leaf extract (standardized to contain 24% flavonoid glycosides), Rice Bran. Other Ingredients: Plant Cellulose, Water.

Wellzymes Mature Woman **-** Enzymes, Inc.
Two capsules contain: Vitamin E (from d-Alpha Tocopheryl Acid Succinate) 20 IU • n-zimes Proprietary Enzyme Blend 36 mg: pHysioProtease (94,720 pHysio-U), CereCalase Plus • Proprietary Herbal Blend 386 mg: Black Cohosh root extract (standardized to contain 2.5% triterpene glycosides), Deglycyrrhizinized Licorice root extract (equivalent to 400 mg of raw herb), St. John's Wort herb extract (standarized to contain 0.3% hypericin), Rice Bran, Soy Isoflavone extract (standardized to contain 23% genistein & 18% daidzein). Other Ingredients: Plant Cellulose, Water.

Wellzymes Mental Focus **-** Enzymes, Inc.
Two capsules contain: n-zimes Proprietary Enzyme Blend 34 mg: pHysioProtease (82,880 pHysio-U), CereCalase Plus • Proprietary Herbal Blend 400 mg: Ginkgo Biloba leaf extract (standardized to contain 24% ginkgolides), Gotu Kola herb extract (standardized to contain 10% asiaticosides), Panax Ginseng root extract (standardized to contain 8% ginsenosides), Rice Bran, Water Hyssop herb extract (standardized to contain 20% bacosides). Other Ingredients: Plant Cellulose, Water.

Wellzymes Migra-Min **-** Enzymes, Inc.
Two capsules contain: n-zimes Proprietary Enzyme Blend 58 mg: pHysio-Protease (142,080 pHysio-U), CereCalase Plus • Proprietary Herbal Blend 390 mg: Feverfew leaf, Feverfew leaf extract (standardized to contain 0.6% parthenolides), Rosemary leaf extract (equivalent to 320 mg raw herb), Passionflower herb extract (equivalent to 160 mg raw herb), Rice Bran. Other Ingredients: Plant Cellulose, Water.

Wellzymes Mood Enhance **-** Enzymes, Inc.
Each capsule contains: n-zimes Proprietary Enzyme Blend 15 mg: pHysioProtease (41,440 pHysio-U), CereCalase Plus • Proprietary Herbal Blend 205 mg: St. John's Wort herb extract (standardized to contain 0.3% hypericin), Ginkgo Biloba leaf extract (standardized to contain 24% ginkgolides), Oat Straw extract (equivalent to 200 mg raw herb), Rice Bran. Other Ingredients: Plant Cellulose, Water.

Wellzymes Nasal Clear **-** Enzymes, Inc.
Three capsules contain: Zinc (from Zinc Citrate) 9 mg • n-zimes Proprietary Enzyme Blend 126 mg: pHysioProtease (257,520 pHysio-U), Peptidase, Amylase, CereCalase Plus • Proprietary Herbal Blend 510 mg: Elder flower ext. (equivalent to 600 mg raw herb), Echinacea Purpurea Angustifolia root ext. (equivalent to 600 mg raw herb), Acerola Cherries ext. (standardized to contain 17% vitamin C), Quercetin, Eyebright herb ext. (equivalent to 180 mg raw herb), Goldenseal root ext. (standardized to contain 5% total alkaloids), Rice Bran. Other Ingredients: Plant Cellulose, Water.

Wellzymes PMS Comfort **-** Enzymes, Inc.
Two capsules contain: Vitamin E (from d-Alpha Tocopheryl Succinate) 20 IU • n-zimes Proprietary Enzyme Blend 34 mg: pHysioProtease (94,720 pHysio-U), CereCalase Plus • Proprietary Herbal Blend 390 mg: Chasteberry extract (equivalent to 480 mg raw herb), Dong Quai root extract (equivalent to 480 mg raw herb), Cramp Bark extract (equivalent to 360 mg raw herb), Parsley leaf extract (equivalent to 200 mg raw herb), Rice Bran. Other Ingredients: Plant Cellulose, Water.

Wellzymes Skin, Hair and Nails **-** Enzymes, Inc.
Three capsules contain: Vitamin A (as Beta Carotene from Dunaliella Algae) 10,500 IU • Zinc (from Zinc Citrate) 15 mg • n-zimes Proprietary Enzyme Blend 75 mg: pHysioProtease (177,600 pHysio-U), CereCalase Plus • Proprietary Herbal Blend 450 mg: Calendula flower extract (standardized to contain 3% lutein), Bladderwrack Kelp extract (equivalent to 450 mg raw herb), Horsetail herb extract (equivalent to 300 mg raw herb), Oregon Grape root extract (equivalent to 240 mg raw herb), Safflower petals, Fo Ti root extract (equivalent to 150 mg raw herb), Rice Bran, Grape seed extract (standardized to contain 95% proanthocyanidins). Other Ingredients: Plant Cellulose, Water.

Wellzymes Sleep Enhance **-** Enzymes, Inc.
Two capsules contain: n-zimes Proprietary Enzyme Blend 34 mg: pHysioProtease (94,720 pHysio-U), CereCalase Plus • Proprietary Herbal Blend 410 mg: Valerian root extract (equivalent to 800 mg raw herb), Passionflower herb extract (equivalent to 480 mg raw herb), Wild Lettuce leaf extract (equivalent to 160 mg raw herb), Oat Straw extract (equivalent to 300 mg raw herb), Rice Bran. Other Ingredients: Plant Cellulose, Water.

Some Brand Name Natural Products - What they Contain

www.NaturalDatabase.com contains MANY more listings than appear here.
Editor's Notes are located on pages 2155-2163.

Wheat Germ Oil - Standard Process, Inc.
Each perle contains: Wheat Germ oil 385 mg. Other Ingredients: Gelatin, Glycerin, Water, Carob.

Wheat Germ Oil 1000 mg - GNC
Each capsule contains: Wheat Germ oil 1 g. Other Ingredients: Gelatin, Glycerin.

Wheat Germ Oil Fortified - Standard Process, Inc.
Each perle contains: Vitamin E 50 IU • Wheat Germ oil 245 mg. Other Ingredients: Gelatin, Soybean Oil, Glycerin, Water, Carob.

Wheat Grass - Pines International
Seven tablets (or 1 tsp of powder) contain: Protein 860 mg • Chlorophyll 18.5 mg • Biotin 4 mcg • Choline 5 mg • Lutein 1 mg • Lycopene 29 mcg • Vitamin A (beta-carotene) 1668 IU • Vitamin B-1 (thiamine) 11 mcg • Vitamin B-2 (riboflavin) 260 mcg • Vitamin B-3 252 mcg • Vitamin B-5 (pantothenic acid) 36 mcg • Vitamin B-6 (pyridoxine) 39 mcg • Vitamin B-8 (folic acid) 21 mcg • Vitamin B-12 0.05 mcg • Vitamin C 7.5 mg • Vitamin E 320 mcg • Vitamin K 35 mcg • Zeaxanthin 279 mcg • Calcium 15 mg • Cobalt 1.7 mcg • Copper 17 mcg • Iodine 8 mcg • Iron 870 mcg • Magnesium 3.9 mcg • Manganese 240 mcg • Phosphorus 14 mg • Potassium 137 mg • Selenium 3.5 mcg • Sodium 1 mg • Sulfur 10.5 mg • Zinc 62 mcg • Alanine 69 mg • Arginine 66 mg • Aspartic Acid 50 mg • Cystine 11 mg • Glutamic Acid 76 mg • Glycine 49 mg • Histidine 18 mg • Isoleucine 35 mg • Leucine 72 mg • Lysine 38 mg • Methionine 18 mg • Phenylalanine 36 mg • Proline 46 mg • Serine 31 mg • Valine 48 mg • Threonine 42 mg • Tryptophan 6 mg • Tyrosine 33 mg.

Whey MRP - Optimum Nutrition
Each packet (76 g) contains: Protein Blend: Whey Protein Concentrate, Whey Protein Isolate, Hydrolyzed Whey Peptides • Maltodextrin • Gum Blend: Cellulose Gum, Xanthan Gum, Carrageenan • Vitamin/Mineral Blend: DiMagnesium Phosphate, Calcium Carbonate, Tricalcium Phosphate, Ascorbic Acid, Ferric Orthophosphate, D-Alpha Tocopheryl Acetate, Boron Proteinate, Maltodextrin, Niacinamide, Zinc Oxide, Manganese Sulfate, D-Calcium Pantothenate, Molybdenum AA Chelate, Selenomethionine, Pyridoxine Hydrochloride, Riboflavin, Beta Carotene, Folic Acid, Biotin, Potassium Iodide, Cyanocobalamin • Brown Rice Syrup Solids • Natural & Artificial Flavor • Salt • Sucralose • Acesulfame Potassium • Aminogen • Carbogen • Lactase.

Whey Protein - The Sports Nutrition Source, Inc.
Each scoop contains: Potassium 75 mg • Protein 16 g.

Whey Protein - Jarrow Formulas
100% Ultrafiltered Whey Protein (comprising major isolate fractions: 51% beta lactoglobulin, 20% alpha-lactalbumin, 10% immunoglobulin, 10% albumin, 7% minor fractions, betamicroglobulin, lactoferrin, relaxin).

Whey Protein (chocolate) - Jarrow Formulas
100% Ultrafiltered Whey Protein (comprising major isolate fractions: 51% beta lactoglobulin, 20% alpha-lactalbumin, 10% albumin, 10% immunoglobulin, 7% minor fractions, betamicroglobulin, lactoferrin, relaxin) • Fructose • Natural Chocolate flavor • Natural Cocoa powder • Lo Han • Vanilla flavor • Guar Gum • Lecithin.

Whey Protein (vanilla) - Jarrow Formulas
100% Ultrafiltered Whey Protein (comprising major isolate fractions: 51% beta lactoglobulin, 20% alpha-lactalbumin, 10% albumin, 10% immunoglobulin, 7% minor fractions, betamicroglobulin, lactoferrin, relaxin) • Fructose • Vanilla flavor • Lo Han • Guar Gum • Lecithin.

Whey To Go (chocolate flavor) - Solgar
Whey Protein Concentrate: 8.3 g B-Lactoglobulin, 4.8 g A-Lactalbumin, 2 g Glycomacropeptides, 0.85 g Immunoglobulin, 0.51 g Bovine Serum Albumin, 0.34 g Residual Caseins, 0.20 g Protease Peptides, Lactoferrin • Dutch Cocoa • Hydrolyzed Whey Protein Concentrate: Dipeptides, Tripeptides, Oligopeptides, Polypeptides • Crystalline Fructose • Natural Chocolate and Vanilla Bean Flavors • Vegetable gum • Free-Form L-Glutamine • Free-Form BCAA's: Leucine, Valine, Isoleucine • Medium Chain Triglycerides.

Whey To Go (honey nut flavor) - Solgar
Whey Protein Concentrate: 8.3 g B-Lactoglobulin, 4.8 g A-Lactalbumin, 2 g Glycomacropeptides, 0.85 g Immunoglobulin, 0.51 g Bovine Serum Albumin, 0.34 g Residual Caseins, 0.20 g Protease Peptides, Lactoferrin • Hydrolyzed Whey Protein Concentrate: Dipeptides, Tripeptides, Oligopeptides, Polypeptides • Crystalline Fructose • Natural Honey Nut flavor • Vegetable gum • Dried Honey • Free-Form L-Glutamine • Free-Form BCAA's: Leucine, Valine, Isoleucine • Medium Chain Triglycerides.

Whey To Go (mixed berry flavor) - Solgar
Whey Protein Concentrate: 8.3 g B-Lactoglobulin, 4.8 g A-Lactalbumin, 2 g Glycomacropeptides, 0.85 g Immunoglobulin, 0.51 g Bovine Serum Albumin, 0.34 g Residual Caseins, 0.20 g Protease Peptides, Lactoferrin • Hydrolyzed Whey Protein Concentrate: Dipeptides, Tripeptides, Oligopeptides, Polypeptides • Crystalline Fructose • Natural Mixed Berry flavor • Vegetable gum • Free-Form L-Glutamine • Free-Form BCAA's: Leucine, Valine, Isoleucine • Medium Chain Triglycerides.

Whey To Go (vanilla bean flavor) - Solgar
Micro-Filtered Whey Protein Isolate • Micro-Filtered Ion-Exchanged Whey Protein Concentrate • Natural Vanilla Bean Flavor • Hydrolyzed Whey Protein Concentrate: Dipeptides, Tripeptides, Oligopeptides, and Polypeptides • Free-Form BCAA's: Leucine, Valine, Isoleucine • Free-Form L-Glutamine.

WheyFit 2000 - Young Living Essential Oils
Each scoop contains: Whey Protein • Egg Whites • Soy Protein • Lecithin • Fructooligosaccharides (FOS) • Stevia • Blueberry Powder • Strawberry Powder • Blueberry Flavor (liquid) • Natural Flavors • Vanilla Extract • Zinc Citrate • Sodium Selenate • Magnesium Citrate • Citric Acid • Lemon Oil • Enzyme Complex Blend: Amylase, Cellulase, Lactase, Lipase, Natural Protease.

White Stuff - Blue Stuff, Inc.
Each 1 oz jar contains: Whole leaf Aloe Vera concentrate • Squalene • Petroleum • Glycerin • Ceresin • Cetyl Dimethicone • Copolyol • Octyl Palmitate • Emu oil • Phenylephrine HCL • Alpha Bisabolol • Grapefruit Seed extract • Fragrance.

White Willow Bark Extract - Nature's Way
Each capsule contains: White Willow Bark 250 mg • White Willow Bark, dried extract 200 mg. Other Ingredients: Gelatin.

Whole Body - American Biologics
Three tablets contain: Calcium 450 mg • Proprietary Blend 2043 mg: Burdock root, Barberry bark, Peppermint leaf, Sarsaparilla, Chickweed, Yarrow, Fenugreek, Mullein herb, Bupleurum, Dandelion root, Ginger root, Irish Moss, Licorice root, Milk Thistle, Yellow Dock, Safflower herb, Echinacea, Peach leaves, Slippery Elm, Capsicum, Gentian. Other Ingredients: Calcium Carbonate, Silicon Dioxide, Stearic Acid.

Whole Body Cleanse - PhytoPharmica
Whole Body Cleanse Laxative Formula: Three tablets contain: Magnesium Hydroxide 2600 mg • Proprietary Mucilage Blend 650 mg: Slippery Elm bark (ulmus rubra), Marshmallow root 3.5:1 extract (althaea officinalis), Fenugreek seed 4:1 extract (trigonella foenum-graecum) • Burdock root 3:1 extract (arctium lappa) 300 mg • Proprietary Soothing Blend 150 mg: Peppermint leaf (mentha x piperita), Fennel seed (foeniculum vulgare), Ginger rhizome extract (zingiber officinale) • Red Clover blossom 4:1 extract (trifolium pratense) 100 mg. Other Ingredients: Cellulose, Modified Cellulose Gum, Modified Cellulose, Magnesium Stearate, Silicon Dioxide, Lecithin, Carnauba Wax.
Fiber Formula: Eight capsules contain: Proprietary Fiber Blend 3455 mg: Psyllium husk (plantago ovata), Oat bran (avena sativa), Guar Gum seed extract (cyamposis tetragonoloba), Pectin (from citrus fruit), Marshmallow root 3.5:1 extract (althaea officinalis). Other Ingredients: Cellulose, Gelatin, Magnesium Stearate, Silicon Dioxide.
Super Milk Thistle: Each softgel contains: Milk Thistle fruit phytosome (silybum marianum, one part milk thistle extract, standardized to contain 80% silymarin, bound to two parts

phosphatidylcholine) 100 mg • Artichoke leaf extract (cynara scolymus, standardized to contaon 13-18% caffeylquinic acids calculated as chlorogenic acid) 40 mg • Dandelion root 4:1 extract (taraxacum officinale) 10 mg • Licorice root and rhizome extract (glycyrrhiza glabra, standardized to contain 5% glycyrrhizic acid) 10 mg. Other Ingredients: Soybean Oil, Gelatin, Glycerin, Beeswax, Lecithin.

Whole Heart Multivitamin - PhytoPharmica
Two tablets contain: Alpha Lipoic Acid 100 mg • Biooin 300 mcg • Calcium (as calcium carbonate and calcium citrate) 200 mg • Choline Bitartrate 138 mg • Chromium (as chromium picolinate) 100 mcg • Copper (as copper gluconate) 1 mg • Folic Acid 450 mcg • Iodine (as potassium iodide) 150 mcg • Lutein (from calendula officinalis) 750 mcg • Lycopene 3 mg • Magnesium (as magnesium aspartate and magnesium oxide) 125 mg • Manganese (as manganese citrate) 1 mg • Molybdenum (as sodium molybdate) 38 mcg • Niacin (as niacinamide and niacin) 60 mg • Pantothenic Acid (as calcium D-pantothenate) 50 mg • Riboflavin (vitamin B2) 30 mg • Selenium (as L-selenomethionine) 100 mcg • Sodium 5 mg • Thiamin (as thiamin HCl, vitamin B1) 30 mg • Vanadium (as vanadyl sulfate) 50 mcg • Vitamin A (75% as beta carotene and as retinyl acetate) 5000 IU • Vitamin B12 (as cyanocobalamin) 500 mcg • Vitamin B6 (as pyridoxine HCl) 30 mg • Vitamin C (ascorbic acid) 250 mg • Vitamin D (as cholecalciferol) 200 IU • Vitamine E (as D-alpha tocopheryl acid succinate) 200 IU • Zeaxanthin (from calendula officinalis) 33 mcg • Zinc (as zinc gluconate) 15 mg.
This product was formerly known as Clinical Nutrients for Heart Health.

Wild BlueBerry IQ - Flavonoid Sciences
Each softgel contains: Wild Blueberries: Anthocyanins 40 mg, Flavones 10 mg. Other Ingredients: Olive Oil, Gelatin, Glycerin, Purified Water, Beeswax.

Wild Brazilian SUMA-750 - Nature's Plus
Each capsule contains: Wild Brazilian SUMA (Pfaffia paniculata [Martius] Kuntze) 750 mg. Naturally rich in the 6 Saponins, Pfaffosides A,B,C,D,E & F - average 6%; 100% pure.

Wild Cherry Syrup - Dial Herbs
Wild Cherry bark • Cubeb berry • Mullein • Skunk Cabbage • Lobelia • Honey • Clove.

Wild Cherry Virtue - Blessed Herbs
Wild Cherry bark • Plantain leaf • Mullein leaf • Mullein flower • Licorice root • Black Cherry concentrate.

Wild Cherry-Slippery Elm Bark Formula - Quest
Each caplet contains: Wild Cherry bark powder (Prunus serotina) 60 mg • Slippery Elm bark powder (Ulmus fulva) 60 mg • Pleurisy Root powder (Asclepias tuberosa) 60 mg • Chickweed powder (Stellaria media) 40 mg • Horehound powder (Marrubium vulgare) 40 mg • Kelp powder (Fucus vesiculosus) 40 mg • Licorice root powder (Glycyrrhiza glabra) 40 mg • Mullein leaf powder (Verbascum thapsus) 40 mg • Cayenne powder (Capsicum minimum) 35 mg • Saw Palmetto berry powder (Serenoa serrulata) 15 mg. Other Ingredients: Calcium Phosphate, Microcrystalline Cellulose, Vegetable Stearin, Croscarmellose Sodium, Magnesium Stearate (vegetable source).

Wild Rose Nerve Formula - Dial Herbs
Valerian root • Mistletoe • Scullcap • Hops • Lady Slipper • Passion flower.

Wild Vites - Nature's Life
Each tablet contains: Vitamin A (Acetate) 5000 IU • Vitamin D3 (Cholecalciferol) 400 IU • Vitamin E (d-Alpha Tocopheryl acetate) 30 IU • Vitamin C (Ascorbic Acid) 60 mg • Vitamin B1 (Thiamine Monoitrate) 1.5 mg • Vitamin B2 (Riboflavin) 1.7 mg • Vitamin B3 (Niacinamide) 20 mg • Vitamin B5 (Pantothenic Acid) 10 mg • Vitamin B6 Pyridoxine HCl) 2 mg • Vitamin B12 (Cobalamin) 6 mcg • Folic Acid 400 mcg • Biotin 300 mg. In a natural base of low-Glycemic pure Crystalline Fructose & Sorbitol.

Wild Yam - Alvin Last
Wild Yam extract • Aloe Vera gel • Soybean Oil • Stearic Acid • Cetyl Alcohol • Triethanolamine • Tocopheryl Acetate • Glycerin • Methylparaben • Propylparaben.

Wild Yam & Progesterone+ - Wise Women Essentials
Wild Yam extract • Natural Progesterone USP (origin from wild yam) • Chaste Tree (vitex) • Liposome-Water / Soy Lecithin • Jojoba oil • Squalane (from olives) • Allantoin • Retinyl Palmitate • Ascorbyl Palmitate • Tocopheryl Acetate (liposomes of vitmains A, C and E) • Dong Quai extract • Licorice extract • Black Cohosh extract • Grapefruit seed extract • Ascorbic Acid.

Wild Yam Cream - Youngevity
Wild Yam root extract (Dioscorea villosa) • Aloe Vera gel • Natural Emollients and Moisturizers • Avocado oil • Oat oil • Key Lime fragrance • Chamomile (Matricaria chamomilla) • Burdock root (Arctium lappa) • Black Cohosh (Cimicifuga racemosa) • Siberian Ginseng (Eleutherococcus senticosus) • D-Alpha Tocopherol Acetate • Methylparaben • Propylparaben.

Wild Yam Extract - PhytoPharmica
Two capsules contain: Wild (Mexican) Yam (Dioscorea villosa) root extract 10:1 (standardized to contain 10% diosgenin) 480 mg • Adrenal extract (freeze-dried) 200 mg • Beta-sitosterol 42 mg.

Wild Yam Root - Nature's Bounty
Two capsules contain: Wild Yam root (Dioscorea Villosa) 810 mg. Other Ingredients: Cellulose, Gelatin, Vegetable Magnesium Stearate, Silica.

Wild Yam/Dong Quai Formula - PhysioLogics
Each capsule contains: Dong Quai root extract (angelica sinensis, standardized to contain 1% lingustilides, 2 mg) 200 mg • Wild Yam root extract (dioscorea villosa, standardized to contain 6% saponins, 12 mg) 200 mg • Soybean seed extract (glycine max, standardized to contain 5% isoflavones, 5 mg) 100 mg. Other Ingredients: Gelatin, Rice Powder, Vegetable Magnesium Stearate, Silica.

Wild Yam-False Unicorn Virtue - Blessed Herbs
False Unicorn root • Black Haw bark • Wild Yam root • Lobelia • Grain alcohol & Distilled Water.

Winter Wellness - NOW Foods
Two tablets contain: Vitamin A 5000 IU • Vitamin C 500 mg • Potassium 20 mg • Zinc 15 mg • Bee Propolis 200 mg • Deodorized Garlic Extract 200 mg • Ginger root 200 mg • Oregon Grape root 150 mg • Peptizyme 125 mg • Echinacea angustifolia root extract 100 mg • Elderberry extract 100 mg • Olive leaf extract 100 mg • Quercetin 100 mg • Shitake mushroom extract 100 mg • Reishi mushroom 100 mg • American Ginseng root 100 mg • Licorice root extract 100 mg • Goldenseal root 75 mg • Cayenne pepper 50 mg.

Wobenzym N (Wobenzym-N) - Mucos Pharma GMBH & Co
Each tablet contains: Pancreatin 100 mg • Trypsin 24 mg • Papain 60 mg • Chymotrypsin 1 mg • Bromelain 45 mg • Rutoside 50 mg. See Editor's Note No. 18.

Woman's Choice - Herbalife International of America, Inc.
Each tablet contains: Calcium (as dicalcium phosphate) 124 mg • Dried Soy bean extract (38% isoflavones) 83 mg • Dried Red Clover aerial parts extract (1% biochanins) 50 mg • Dried Kudzu root extract (40% isoflavones) 30 mg • Bio-Absorption Complex-5 23 mg: Soy Lecithin, Vitamin C (as ascorbyl palmitate), Plant Cellulose Enzyme, Cinnamon bark powder, Dried Black Pepper fruit extract (Bioperine brand, NLT 95% piperine) • Dried Black Cohosh root extract (8% triterpene glycosides) 10 mg. Other Ingredients: Microcrystalline Cellulose, Stearic Acid, Silicon Dioxide, Hydroxypropyl Methylcellulose, Magnesium Stearate, Hydroxypropyl Cellulose, Polysorbate, Polyethylene Glycol.

Woman's Choice - PhytoPharmica
Three capsules contain: Vitamin A (Beta Carotene) - (Non-toxic form of Vitamin A) 16665 IU • Vitamin E (D-Alpha Tocopherol Succinate) 200 IU • Vitamin C (Ascorbic Acid) 200 mg • Magnesium

L-Aspartate 150 mg • Pantothenic Acid (D-Calcium Pantothenate) 100 mg • Thiamine HCL (Vitamin B1) 50 mg • Riboflavin (Vitamin B2) 50 mg • Calcium Citrate 50 mg • Iron (Ferrous Succinate) 18 mg • Zinc (Gluconate) 15 mg • Chromium (Polynicotinate) 250 mcg • Folic Acid 100 mcg • Vitamin B12 (Cyanocobalamin) 50 mcg • Selenium (L-Selenomethionine) 50 mcg • Dong Quai extract 4:1 (Angelica sinensis) 75 mg • Licorice root extract (Glycyrrhiza glabra) 60 mg • Milk Thistle extract 50 mg (Silybum marianum) • Black Cohosh extract 4:1 (Cimicifuga racemosa) 30 mg • Chaste Tree berry extract (Vitex agnus-castus) 20 mg • Pyridoxal-5'-Phosphate 10 mg.

Women Over 40 DailyFoods **-** MegaFood
Six tablets contain: Vitamin A 5000 IU • Vitamin C 200 mg • Vitamin D (D3) 200 IU • Vitamin E 200 IU • Vitamin K (K1) 65 mcg • Thiamine (B1) 5 mg • Riboflavin (B2) 5 mg • Niacinamide 25 mg • Vitamin B6 15 mg • Folic Acid 400 mcg • Vitamin B12 50 mcg • Biotin 300 mcg • Pantothenic Acid 20 mg • Calcium 100 mg • Iron 9 mg • Phopshorous 1 mg • Iodine 100 mcg • Magnesium 75 mg • Zinc 15 mg • Selenium 50 mcg • Copper 500 mcg • Manganese 2.5 mg • Chromium (GTF) 50 mcg • Molybdenum 25 mcg • Beta Carotene 5000 IU • Bioflavonoids 95 mg • Choline 25 mg • Inositol 20 mg • Potassium 10 mg • Boron 3 mg • Silicon 1 mg • Vanadium 10 mcg • Alfalfa 100 mg • Hydrilla Verticillata 50:1 100 mg • Sea Vegetable Blend Laminaria 100 mg • Evening Primrose oil 100 mg • Barley grass & juice concentrate 50 mg • Chaste tree berry (vitex) 5:1 125 mg • Shatavari root 50 mg • Eleuthero root 5:1 50 mg • Wild Yam root 10:1 50 mg • Schizandra berry 4:1 45 mg • Gotu Kola leaf 5:1 35 mg • Red Clover blossom 5:1 35 mg • Motherwort 7:1 25 mg • Turmeric root 10:1 25 mg • Bilberry fruit (25% anthocyanidins) 20 mg • Ginkgo leaf 8:1 20 mg • Licorice root 4:1 20 mg • Fo-Ti root 5:1 20 mg • Nettle leaf 4:1 20 mg • Damiana leaf 4:1 20 mg • Saw Palmetto berry (20-25% fatty acids) 20 mg • Hawthorn berry 4:1 15 mg • Dandelion leaf 4:1 10 mg • Dandelion root 4:1 10 mg • Hawthorn leaf 10 mg • Spring Horsetail leaf 5:1 10 mg • Wild Green Oats seed 4:1 10 mg • Sage leaf 4:1 5 mg • Fermented super Soy 250 mg • Alfalfa 4:1 50 mg • Kudzu root 10:1 25 mg • Blueberry fruit 6:1 20 mg • Cranberry fruit 25:1 10 mg • Reishi mushroom mycelia 7:1 10 mg • Shiitake mushroom 4:1 10 mg • Cordyceps mycelia 4:1 10 mg • Grape seed extract with 500 ppm Resveratrol 5:1 10 mg • Tangerine peel 7 mg • Lecithin 50 mg • Ginger root 5:1 20 mg • Cumin seed 3 mg • Black Pepper fruit 3 mg • Dendrobium Orchid herb 20 mg • Lavender flowers 4:1 7 mg • Hibiscus flower 5 mg • Rose petals 3 mg • Elder flower 4:1 3 mg • Jasmine flower 3 mg. Other Ingredients: Vegetable Lubricant, Guar Gum, Silica.

Women's Arginmax **-** GNC
Six tablets contain: Vitamin A (as retinyl palmitate) 5000 IU •Vitamin C (as ascorbic acid) 60 mg •Vitamin E (as d-alpha tocopherol succinate) 30 IU •Thiamin (as thiamin mononitrate) 1.5 mg •Riboflavin (B2) 1.7 mg •Niacin (as niacinamide) 20 mg •Vitamin B-6 (pyridoxine hydrochloride) 2 mg •Folic Acid 400 mcg • Vitamin B-12 (cyanocobalamin) 6 mcg • Biotin 300 mcg •Pantothenic Acid (as calcium d-pantothenate) 10 mg •Calcium (as calcium carbonate) 500 mg •Iron (as ferrous gluconate) 9 mg • Zinc (as zinc gluconate) 7.5 mg •L-Arginine 2500 mg •Korean Ginseng extract aerial parts and roots 100 mg • Ginkgo Biloba extract leaf 50 mg •Damiana leaf 50 mg.Other Ingredients: Microcrystalline Cellulose, Hydroxypropyl Methylcellulose, Pharmaceutical Glaze, Silica, Titanium Dioxide, Magnesium Stearate, PEG, Polysorbate 80.

Women's Cycle Multivitamins **-** Leiner Health Products
Each caplet contains: Iron (Ferrous Fumarate) 15 mg • Vitamin K (Phytonadione) 65 mcg • Folate (Folic Acid) 300 mcg • Biotin 200 mcg• Molybdenum (Sodium Molybdate) 38 mcg • Niacin (Niacinamide) 8.5 mg • Calcium 160 mg • Vitamin B6 (Pyridoxine Hydrochloride) 3 mg • Vitamin E (dl-Alpha Tocopheryl Acetate) 45 IU • Riboflavin (Vitamin B2) 2.5 mg • Selenium 100 mcg • Thiamin Mononitrate (Vitamin B1) 2 mg •Magnesium Oxide 50 mg •Phosphorus 124 mg •Chromium Chloride 120 mcg • Copper (Cupric Oxide) 2 mg • Iodine 10 mcg • Manganese Sulfate 2 mg •Pantothenic Acid (d-Calcium Pantothenate) 10 mg • Vitamin A Acetate 5000 IU • Vitamin B12 (Cyanocobalamin - USP Method 2) 6 mcg • Vitamin C (Ascorbic Acid) 60 mg •Vitamin D (Ergocalciferol) 400 IU • Zinc Oxide 15 mg • Borage Oil complex (Borage officinalis) seed (Standardized to 10% GLA) 25 mg • Chloride 18 mg • Isoflavones from Soy extract 5 mg • Kelp (Macrocystis pyrifera) frond 5 mg • Lecithin powder (Glycine max) bean 20 mg • Nickel (Nickelous Sulfate) 5 mcg • Potassium Chloride 20 mg • Silicon Dioxide 2 mg • Tin (Stannous Chloride) 10 mcg • Trace Mineral complex 5 mg • Vanadium (Sodium Metavanadate) 10 mcg. Other Ingredients: Dicalcium Phosphate, Cellulose, Gelatin, Stearic Acid, Croscarmellose Sodium, Hydroxypropyl Methylcellulose, Titanium Dioxide, Red Raspberry Powder, Dextrin, Maltodextrin, Mannitol, Hydroxypropyl Cellulose, Polyethylene Glycol, Kelp Powder, Trace Mineral Complex, Starch, Polysorbate 80, Blue 1 Lake, Red 40 Lake, Dextrose.

Women's DailyFoods **-** MegaFood
Three tablets contain: Vitamin A 5000 IU • Vitamin C 150 mg • Vitamin D (D3) 200 IU • Vitamin E 100 IU • Vitamin K (K1) 40 mcg • Thiamine (B1) 11 mg • Riboflavin (B2) 9 mg • Niacinamide 30 mg • Vitamin B6 11 mg • Folic Acid 800 mcg • Vitamin B12 25 mcg • Biotin 300 mcg • Pantothenic Acid 23 mg • Calcium 25 mg • Iron 18 mg • Iodine 150 mcg • Magnesium 25 mg • Zinc 10 mg • Selenium 100 mcg • Copper 100 mcg • Manganese 2 mg • Chromium (GTF) 100 mcg • Molybdenum 25 mcg • Beta Carotene 5000 IU • Bioflavonoids (from FoodState brand vitamin C) 63 mg • Choline 30 mg • Inositol 15 mg • Potassium 10 mg • PABA 3 mg • Boron 1 mg • Vanadium 10 mcg • Hydrilla Verticillata 50:1 250 mg • Alfalfa 100 mg • Chastetree berry (vitex) 5:1 50 gm • Red Raspberry leaf 4;1 20 mg • Nettle leaf 4:1 20 mg • Wild Green Oats seed 4:1 15 mg • Eleuthero root 5:1 15 mg • Licorice root 4:1 15 mg • Spring Horsetail leaf 5:1 10 mg • Rosemary leaf 4:1 10 mg • Ginger root 5:1 10 mg • Yellowdock root 4:1 10 mg • Dandelion leaf 4:1 5 mg • Dandelion root 4:1 5 mg. Other Ingredients: Vegetable Lubricant, Food Glaze.

Women's Exclusive Formula **-** Puritan's Pride
Two tablets contain: Vitamin A 5,000 IU • Vitamin C 60 mg • Vitamin D 400 IU • Vitamin E (as d-Alpha Tocopheryl Acetate) 30 IU • Thiamin (Vitamin B-1) 26.7 mg • Riboflavin (Vitamin B-2) 30 mg • Niacin 30 mg • Vitamin B-6 24.6 mg • Folic Acid 400 mcg • Vitamin B-12 100 mcg • Biotin 30 mcg • Pantothenic Acid 30 mg • Calcium 500 mg • Iron 15 mg • Phosphorus 30 mg • Iodine 150 mcg • Magnesium 250 mg • Zinc 15 mg • Selenium 25 mcg • Copper 0.5 mg • Manganese 5 mg • Chromium 25 mcg • Molybdenum 25 mcg • Potassium 11.5 mg • Inositol 30 mg • Choline Bitartrate 30 mg • PABA (Para-Aminobenzoic Acid) 30 mg • Citrus Bioflavonoids 25 mg • Betaine Hydrochloride 25 mg • L-Cysteine 50 mg • Dong Quai 50 mg • Rose Hips 6 mg.

Women's Formula 1 **-** Rexall - Sundown
Two tablets contain: Vitamin C 67 mg • Vitamin D (cholecalciferol) 67 IU • Vitamin B-6 (pyridoxine HCl) 3.3 mg • Folic Acid 100 mcg • Vitamin B-12 (cyanocobalamin) 3.3 mcg • Calcium (carbonate, citrate and gluconate) 333 mg • Iron (carbonyl iron) 3 mg • Magnesium (gluconate and oxide) 133 mg • Zinc (gluconate) 3.3 mg • Selenium (sodium selenate) 16.7 mcg • Copper (gluconate) 0.17 mg • Manganese (sulfate) 5 mg • Molybdenum (sodium molybdate) 16.7 mcg • Potassium (chloride) 35 mg • Boron (potassium borate and sodium borate) 16.7 mcg • Silica 7 mg • Phytonutrient Vegetable Blend (Broccoli, Carrot, Spinach, Tomato) 40 mg. Other Ingredients: Cellulose, Croscarmellose Sodium, Hydroxypropyl Methylcellulose, Magnesium Stearate, PEG.

Women's Formula 2 **-** Rexall - Sundown
Two tablets contain: Vitamin C 33 mg • Vitamin D (as cholecalciferol) 67 IU • Vitamin K (as phytonadione) 3.3 mcg • Vitamin B-6 (as pyridoxine HCl) 3.3 mg • Folic Acid 33.3 mcg • Vitamin B-12 (as cyanocobalamin) 6.7 mcg • Calcium (as calcium carbonate, calcium citrate and calciulm gluconate) 400 mg • Iodine (as potassium iodide) 16.7 mcg • Magnesium (as magnesium gluconate and magnesium oxide) 150 mg • Zinc (as zinc gluconate) 1.7 mg • Selenium (as sodium selenate) 16.7 mcg • Copper (as copper gluconate) 0.1 mg • Manganese (as manganese sulfate) 5 mg • Molybdenum (as sodium molybdate) 16.7 mcg • Potassium (as potassium chloride) 35 mg • Boron (as potassium borate and sodium

borate) 16.7 mcg • Betaine (as betaine HCl) 33.3 mg • Silica 6.9 mg • Phytonutrient Vegetable Blend (Broccoli, Carrot, Spinach,Tomato) 40 mg. Other Ingredients: Cellulose, Croscarmellose Sodium, Magnesium Stearate, Hydroxypropyl Methylcellulose, PEG.

Women's Formula Plus - Rexall - Sundown
Two caplets contain: Calcium 518 mg • Calcium D-Glucarate 400 mg • Women's Nutritional Blend: Flaxseed, Citrus Bioflavonoids, Red Clover (flower head), Soybean (standardized to 3.5% Isoflavones) 176 mg. Other Ingredients: Calcium Carbonate, Cellulose, Croscarmellose Sodium, Stearic Acid, Magnesium Stearate.

Women's Harmony - FreeLife International
Each caplet contains: Vitamin B6 (as pyridoxine HCl) 10 mg • Folate (as folic acid) 400 mcg • Vitamin B12 (as cyanocobalamin) 100 mcg • Calcium (as hydroxyapatite and purified calcite) 150 mg • Boron (as boron chelate) 3 mg • Isoflavones from Kudzu root (pueraria lobata), Non-GMO Soybeans, and Red Clover blossoms 80 mg • Trans-Resveratrol 2 mg • Wild Jujube seed extract 150 mg • Black Cohosh root standardized extract 40 mg • Other Ingredients: Cellulose Gum, Fractionated Vegetable Oil, Silica, Vita-Coat.

Women's Hormonal Health - EnerGreens, Inc.
Each capsule contains: Beta Sitosterol 50 mg • IP-6 (inositol hexaphosphate) 50 mg • Magnesium Aspartate 50 mg • Vitamin B6 12.5 mg • Folic Acid 50 mcg • Quercetin 50 mg • Iodine 400 mcg • Proprietary Blend 195 mg: Chaste Tree berry 4:1 extract, Silymarin standardized extract, Dong Quai, Motherwort, Black Cohosh, Wild Yam, Licorice root, Dandelion root, Ginger root, Primrose oil powder. Other Ingredients: Gelatin.

Women's Liberty - Traditional Medicinals
Licorice root • Orange peel • Wild Yam root • Ginger rhizome • Cinnamon bark • Dong Quai root • Clove stem • Fo Ti root • Angelica root.

Women's Libido - Gaia Herbs
Two capsules contain: Suma root (pfaffia paniculata) 50 mg • Catuaba bark (juniperus brasiliensis) 50 mg • Chuchuhasi bark (maytenus krukovit) 30 mg • Damiana leaf (turnera diffusa) 26 mg • Sarsaparilla rhizome (smilax ornata) 26 mg • Horny Goat Weed (epimedium grandiflorum) 26 mg • Wild Oats milky seed (avena sativa) 16 mg • Helonias root (chamaelirium luteum) 16 mg • Ginger rhizome, supercritical CO2 extract 8 mg. Other Ingredients: Vegetable Glycerin, Vegetable Cellulose (capsule).

Women's Longevity Integrative Breast Care - EcoNugenics
Two capsules contain: Vitamin A (as betacarotene) 5000 IU • Vitamin C (as magnesium and calcium ascorbate) 75 mg • Vitamin E (as alpha tocopherol) 50 IU • Zinc (as orotate, picolinate) 15 mg • Selenium (as selenomethionine) 75 mcg • Women's Longevity Breast Health Blend 370 mg: Turmeric rhizome extract, Garlic bulb, Red Clover leaf and flower, Milk Thistle seed extract, Snake Grass herb (oldenlandia difusae), Heal-All spikelets, Scutellae Barbatae herb, Green Tea leaf, Reishi (ganoderma lucidum), Rehmannia root, Job's Tears seed, Astragalus root, Cat's Claw bark, Umbellatus (polyprous umbellatus), Peah seed, Dong Quai root, White Peony root, Atractylodes root, Poria Cocos, Sichuan Lovage root, Licorice root extract, Cinnamon bark, Oriental Ginseng root • Calcium D-Glucarate 150 mg • Bovine Cartilage 100 mg • Alpha-Lipoic Acid 75 mg • Indole-3-Carbinol 50 mg • PectaSol brand Modified Citrus Pectin 50 mg • Quercetin 50 mg • Thymus gland extract 50 mg • L-Glutathione 25 mg • Lactobacillus Acidophilus 20 mg • Co-Enzyme Q-10 10 mg • Grape seed extract 10 mg • Beta 1,3 Glucans (from purified yeast) 8 mg. Other Ingredients: Gelatin, Dicalcium Phosphate, Cellulose, Silica, Vegetable Stearate. See Editor's Note No. 14.

Women's Longevity Rhythms - EcoNugenics
Five capsules contain: Vitamin A (as beta carotene) 5000 IU • Vitamin C (as ascorbic acid) 200 mg • Vitamin D 50 IU • Vitamin E (as d-alpha tocopherol) 150 IU • Vitamin B1 (as thiamine hydrochloride) 40 mg • Vitamin B2 (as riboflavin-5-phosphate) 40 mg • Vitamin B3 (as niacinamide) 125 mg • Vitamin B6 (as pyridoxine hydrochloride) 40 mg • Folic Acid 400 mcg • Vitamin B12 (as cyanocobalamin) 50 mcg • Biotin 200 mcg • Vitamin B5 (as calcium pantothenate) 40 mg • Calcium (as citrate, carbonate, aspartate) 300 mg • Iodine (from kelp) 17.5 mcg • Magnesium (as oxide, citrate, aspartate) 160 mcg • Zinc (as citrate) 15 mg • Selenium (as selenomethionine) 70 mcg • Copper (as sebacate) 1 mg • Manganese (as sulfate) 2 mg • EcoGen Soy Isoflavone concentrate 400 mg • Women's Longevity Blend 350 mg: Dried extracts of Burdock root, Eleuthero root, Blue Cohosh root, Horsetail herb, Alfalfa leaf, Green Tea leaf, Uva Ursi leaf, Thymus Gland extract, Chaste Tree berry (vitex), Cranberry fruit • Chinese Herbal Extract Blend 310 mg: Dong Quai root, White Peony root, Sichuan Lovage root, Poria Cocos, Rehmannia root, Ginseng root, Atractylodes root, Ginger root, Jujube fruit • Royal Jelly 250 mg • MycoCeutics 10 Mushroom Proprietary Blend 100 mg: Reishi (ganoderma lucidum), Poria cocos, Cordyceps (cordyceps sinensis), Tremella Fuciformis, Umbellatus (polyporus umbellatus), Coriolus (coriolus versicolor), Maitake (grifola frondosa), Shitake (lentinula edodes), Wood Ear (auricularia auricula), Hericium Erinaceus • Inositol 50 mg • Choline (as bitartrate) 40 mg • Para-Aminobenzoic Acid (PABA) 40 mg • Citrus Bioflavonoid complex 20 mg • Taurine 10 mg • Beta-1,3-Glucan (from purified yeast, baker's yeast) 5 mg • Boron (as boric acid) 1 mg. Other Ingredients: Gelatin, Cellulose, Silica, Magnesium Stearate.
See Editor's Note No. 14.

Women's Longevity Rhythms Gold - EcoNugenics
Six capsules contain: Vitamin A (beta-carotene) 5000 IU • Vitamin C (ascorbic acid, corn-free) 200 mg • Vitamin D (ergocalciferol, from fish oil) 100 IU • Vitamin D (D3, cholecalciferol, from fish oil) 50 IU • Vitamin E (d-alpha tocopherol natural) 175 IU • Vitamin B1 (thiamine hydrochloride) 50 mg • Vitamin B2 (riboflavin 5-phosphate) 50 mg • Vitamin B3 (niacinamide) 150 mg • Vitamin B6 (pyridoxine hydrochloride) 50 mg • Folic Acid 0.5 mg • Vitamin B12 (cyanocobalamin) 100 mcg • Biotin 200 mcg • Vitamin B5 (calcium pantothenate) 50 mg • Calcium (as carbonate, citrate, hydroxyapatite, aspartate) 500 mg • Iodine (as kelp) 17.5 mcg • Magnesium (as oxide, citrate, aspartate) 200 mg • Zinc (as citrate) 15 mg • Selenium (as selenomethionine) 80 mcg • Copper (as sebacate) 1.5 mg • Manganese (as sulfate) 4 mg • Chromium (as picolinate, non-yeast) 120 mcg • Chinese Herbal Blend 535 mg: Dried Extracts of Dong Quai, White Peony root, Chinese Yam, Chinese Licorice root, Chinese Hawthorne fruit, Chinese Motherwort herb • Women's Longevity Blend 642 mg: Dried Extracts of Wild Oats, Korean Ginseng root, Black Cohosh root, Burdock root, Chaste Tree berry (vitex), Damiana herb, Ginkgo Biloba leaf (24%), Horsetail herb, Uva Ursi herb • EcoGen Soy Isoflavone concentrate 400 mg • Royal Jelly (freeze dried) 300 mg • MycoCeutics 10 Mushroom Proprietary Blend 300 mg: Reishi (ganoderma lucidum), Poria Cocos, Cordyceps (cordyceps sinensis), Tremella Fuciformis, Umbellatus (polyporus umbellatus), Coriolus (coriolus versicolor), Maitake (grifola frondosa), Shitake (lentinula edodes), Wood Ear (auricularia auricula), Hericium Erinaceus • Inositol 50 mg • Choline (as bitartrate) 50 mg • PABA (para-amino-benzoic acid) 50 mg • N-Acetyl Cysteine 50 mg • Saw Palmetto berry extract 50 mg • Glucosamine Sulfate 50 mg • Hesperidin complex 50 mg • Taurine 50 mg • Beta-1,3-Glucan (from purified yeast) 6 mg • Co-Enzyme Q-10 5 mg • Boron (as boric acid) 2 mg. Other Ingredients: Gelatin, Cellulose, Silica, Magnesium Stearate.

Women's Mood-Enhancer - HerbaSway
St. John's Wort • Dong Quai • Rehmannia • Schisandra • Coptis • Ginkgo biloba • Cassia tora • Astragalus • Blackberry • HerbaSwee (cucurbitaceae fruit).

Women's Multi - Jarrow Formulas
Six tablets contain: Vitamin A (as palmitate) 2500 IU • Beta-Carotene (from dunaliella salina) 5000 IU • Vitamin C (from calcium ascorbate) 40 mg • Vitamin D (D2, ergocalciferol) 400 IU • Vitamin E (alpha tocopheryl succinate) 200 IU • Vitamin K (phylloquinone) 25 mcg • Vitamin B1 (thiamin mononitrate) 10 mg • Vitamin B2 (riboflavin) 10 mg • Vitamin B3 (niacin) 10 mg • Niacinamide 50 mg • Vitamin B6 (as pyridoxine HCl) 15 mg • Folic Acid 400 mcg • Vitamin B12 (as methylcobalamin) 20 mcg • Biotin 300 mcg •

Pantothenic Acid (as D-calcium pantothenate) 25 mg • Calcium (from calcium citrate/ascorbate) 540 mg • Iron (as ferrous gluconate) 15 mg • Iodine (as potassium iodide) 153 mcg • Magnesium (as magnesium citrate) 253 mg • Zinc (as zinc monomethionate) 15 mg • Selenium (as L-selenomethionine/sodium selenate 50/50) 100 mcg • Copper (as copper gluconate) 1 mg • Manganese (as manganese citrate) 2 mg • Chromium (fermentation by saccharomyces boulardii) 200 mcg • Molybdenum (as sodium molybdate) 75 mcg • Potassium (as potassium chloride) 99 mg • Choline (as choline bitartrate) 110 mg • Inositol 100 mg • Boron (as sodium borate) 1 mg • Bilberry extract (vaccinium myrtillus, 25% flavonoids) 20 mg • Grape seed extract (vitis vinifera, 95% polyphenols) 25 mg • Lutein (from calendula officinalis) 3 mg • Citrus Bioflavonoids complex 50 mg • Cranberry (vaccinium macrocarpon, juice infused cranberry fiber) 100 mg • Shatabari (asparagus racemosus) 200 mg. Other Ingredients: Calcium Carbonate, Micorcrystalline Cellulose, Modified Cellulose Gum, Magnesium Stearate, Silicon Dioxide.

Women's Nutra-Pack - Nature's Plus
Each pack contains: Vitamin A (beta carotene) 10,000 IU • Vitamin C (ascorbic acid) 800 mg • Vitamin D (ergocalciferol) 400 IU • Vitamin E (D-alpha tocopheryl acetate, succinate) 300 IU • Thiamin (vitamin B1, as thiamine HCl) 25 mg • Riboflavin (vitamin B2) 25 mg • Niacin (niacinamide) 100 mg • Vitamin B6 (pyridoxine HCl) 25 mg • Folate (folic acid) 100 mcg • Vitamin B12 (cyanocobalamin) 250 mcg • Biotin 20 mcg • Pantothenic Acid (calcium pantothenate) 50 mg • Calcium (amino acid chelate/complex) 776 mg • Iron (amino acid chelate/complex) 39 mg • Phosphorus (amino acid complex) 114 mg • Iodine (from kelp) 113 mcg • Magnesium (amino acid chelate/complex) 257 mg • Zinc (amino acid chelate/complex) 25 mg • Selenium (amino acid complex) 25 mcg • Manganese (amino acid chelate/complex) 11.1 mg • Copper (amino acid chelate) 0.28 mg • Chromium (amino acid chelate) 50 mcg • Potassium (amino acid complex) 50 mg • Pancreatin 4X 129 mg • Ox Bile Extract 129 mg • Citrus Bioflavonoids (from citrus spp. exocarp) 125 mg • Rutin (from saphora japonica leaf) 75 mg • L-Glutamic Acid HCl 60 mg • Malt Diastase 60 mg • Inositol 50 mg • Hesperidin (from citrus limon exocarp) 30 mg • Pepsin 1:15,000 (equivalent to pepsin NF 150 mg) 30 mg • Papain (from papaya) 30 mg • Betaine HCl (from beet molasses) 25 mg • PABA (para-aminobenzoic acid) 25 mg • Lecithin (from soy) 25 mg • Choline (as bitartrate) 21 mg • Methylcellulose 15 mg. Other Ingredients: Di-calcium Phosphate, Microcrystalline Cellulose, Stearic Acid, Hydroxypropyl Methylcellulose, Rose Hips (rosa canina fruit), Magnesium Stearate, Silica, Isolated Soy Protein, Watercress, Horsetail Root, Rice Bran, Papaya, Parsley, Alfalfa, Green Cabbage, Acerola Cherry, Wheat Germ Flour, Fig, Date, Hazelnut, Sesame Seed, Sunflower Seed, Broccoli, Pacific Kelp, Spirulina, Black Currant Seed, Barley Grass, Pharmaceutical Glaze, Gelatin, Glycerin, Purified Water.

Women's Nutritional System - Rainbow Light
Six tablets contain: Beta Carotene 10000 IU • Vitamin D 400 IU • Vitamin E natural 120 IU • Vitamin K 30 mcg • Thiamin (Vitamin B1) 36 mg • Riboflavin (Vitamin B2) 41 mg • Niacinamide 80 mg • Pantothenic Acid 80 mg • Pyridoxine (Vitamin B6) 48 mg • Folic Acid 800 mcg • Biotin (d-Biotin) 300 mcg • Cyanocobalamin (Vitamin B12) 144 mcg • Vitamin C 500 mg • Calcium (Amino Acid Chelate, Citrate) 200 mg • Magnesium (Amino Acid Chelate, Ascorbate, Oxide) 400 mg • Potassium (Aspartate, Chloride) 99 mg • Manganese (Amino Acid Chelate) 2.5 mg • Iron (Amino Chelate) 22.5 mg • Zinc (Picolinate) 15 mg • Copper (Amino Acid Chelate) 1 mg • GTF Chromium (Polynicotinate) 30 mcg • Selenium (l-Selenomethionine) 40 mcg • Iodine (Kelp) 150 mcg • Molybdenum (Aspartate) 50 mcg • Choline (Bitartrate) 40 mg • Inositol 40 mg • PABA (Para Aminobenzioc Acid) 30 mg • Octacosanol (Spinach) 300 mcg • Black Currant (seed) 30 mg • Bioflavonoids 250 mg • Rutin 20 mg • L-Tyrosine 20 mg • Hesperidin Complex 15 mg • Protease 3600 HUT • Amylase 282 DU • Lipase 3 LU • Cellulase 3.2 CU. Superfood & Herbal Ingredients: Bee Pollen • Spirulina • Lemon juice powder • Wheatgrass • Dong Quai • Barley Grass • Echinacea agustifolia • Reishi (Ling Chi) • Rosemary oil • Blue Cohosh 4:1) 530 mg. Custom Herbal extracts: Vitex • Red Raspberry • Mulberry • Fo-Ti • Bladderwrack • Tumeric • Peony Cistanche • Cynomorium 270 mg.

Women's Prime Multi - Swanson Health Products
Each tablet contains: Vitamin A (as beta-carotene) 3000 IU • Vitamin C (as ascorbic acid) 100 mg • Vitamin D (as cholecalciferol) 60 IU • Vitamin E (as d-alpha tocopheryl succinate) 60 IU • Thiamin USP (as thiamin HCl; Vitamin B-1) 5 mg • Riboflavin USP (Vitamin B-2) 5 mg • Niacin (as niacinamide) 5 mg • Vitamin B-6 (as pyridoxine HCl) 5 mg • Folic Acid 200 mcg • Vitamin B-12 (as cyanocobalamin) 50 mcg • Biotin 5 mcg • Pantothenic Acid (as d-calcium pantothenate) 5 mg • Calcium (50 mg from calcium citrate, 12 mg from calcium glucarate, 4 mg from calcium phytate) 66 mg • Iron (from Albion amino acid chelate) 5 mg • Iodine (from kelp) 50 mcg • Magnesium (from magnesium oxide) 30 mg • Zinc (from Albion® amino acid chelate) 7.5 mg • Selenium (from Albion amino acid chelate) 100 mcg • Manganese (from Albion® amino acid chelate) 2 mg • Chromium (from Albion amino acid chelate) 25 mcg • Dong Quai powder 50 mg • Green Tea powder 50 mg • Soy powder 50 mg • IP-6 (inositol hexaphosphate)-(from calcium phytate) 25 mg • Korean Ginseng powder (5% ginsenosides) 15 mg • Black Cohosh (2.5% triterpenoids) 10 mg • Choline (as choline bitartrate) 10 mg • GLA (gamma-linolenic acid from borage) 10 mg • Inositol 10 mg • Bilberry powder (25% anthocyanidins) 5 mg • Ginkgo Biloba leaf extract (24% flavon glycosides, 6% terpene lactones) 5 mg • PABA (para-aminobenzoic acid) 5 mg • Rutin (from buckwheat) 5 mg • Coenzyme Q10 2 mg • Boron 1 mg.

Women's Stress System - Rainbow Light
Two tablets contain: Vitamin A (Beta Carotene) 250 IU • Vitamin E (d-Alpa Tocopheryl Acetate) 30 IU • Vitamin C (Ascorbic Acid) 120 mg • Magnesium (Citrate) 60 mg • Potassium (Chloride) 40 mg • Niacin-Niacinamide (Vitamin B3) 40 mg • Pantothenic Acid (Vitamin B5) 20 mg • Pyridoxine (Vitamin B6) 10 mg • Zinc (Glycinate) 8 mg • Riboflavin (Vitamin B2) 3 mg • Thiamin (Vitamin B1) 3 mcg • Copper (Glycinate) 750 mcg • Folic Acid 400 mcg • Biotin 300 mcg • Cyanocobalamin (Vitamin B12) 12 mcg • Soy extract 150 mg • Hawaiian Spirulina 70 mg • standardized to 1.5% Isoflavonoids Citrus Bioflavonoids 50 mg • Wheat Grass 80 mg • 4:1 Custom Herbal extracts containing 302 mg: [Siberian Ginseng (Eleuthero root), St. John's Wort herb, Kava root, Codonopsis root, Vitex berry, Lavender oil]. Other Nutritional Ingredients: L-Glutamine 50 mg, L-Taurine 20 mg, Alpha-Lipoic Acid 25 mg, L-Methionine 15 mg, L-Tyrosine 25 mg.

Women's Support Formula - PhysioLogics
Each capsule contains: Vitamin E (as d-alpha tocopheryl acetate) 5 0 IU • Vitamin B6 (as pyridoxine HCl) 25 mg • Folic Acid 200 mcg • Magnesium (as magnesium oxide) 100 mg • Zinc (as zinc amino acid chelate) 3.75 mg • Copper (as copper amino acid chelate) 0.5 mg • Black Cohosh root (cimicifuga racemosa) 100 mg • Chastetree fruit (vitex agnus-castus, standardized to contain 5% flavonoids, 5 mg) 100 mg • Dong Quai root (angelica sinensis, standardized to contain 1% ligustilides) 100 mg • Soy Isoflavones 50 mg • Kava Kava root (piper methysticum, standardized to conatin 30% kavalactones, 7.5 mg) 25 mg. Other Ingredients: Rice Powder, Gelatin, Vegetable Magnesium Stearate, Silica.

WOW - Life Enhancement Products, Inc.
Each 1 rounded tsp serving contains: Vitamin A (as beta-carotene) 2500 IU • Vitamin C (as ascorbic acid and niacinamide ascorbate) 325 mg • Vitamin E (as DL-alpha-tocopheryl acetate) 30 IU • Thiamine (vitamin B1, as thiamine hydrochloride) 1.5 mg • Riboflavin (vitamin B2) 3 mg • Niacin (vitamin B3, as niacinamide ascorbate) 75 mg • Vitamin B6 (as pyridoxine hydrochloride) 16 mg • Folic Acid 100 mcg • Vitamin B12 (as cyanocobalamin) 20 mcg • Pantothenic Acid (vitamin B5, as calcium pantothenate) 18 mg • Zinc (as zinc gluconate) 3 mg • Copper (as copper gluconate) 420 mcg • Chromium (as chromium aspartate) 25 mcg • L-Phenylalanine 600 mg • Taurine 200 mg • Glycine 150 mg • Caffeine 80 mg • Polyphenols (from green tea) 50 mg.

X-Action Gel - Nature's Sunshine
Water • Glycerin • Butylene Glycol • Pentylene Glycol • Cellulose Gum • Carbomer • Methylparaben • Menthol • Arginine PCA • Sodium Hydroxide • Dipotassium Glycyrrhizinate • Red Clover

flower extract (trifolium pratense) • Panax Ginseng root extract • Dulse plant extract (palmaria palmata) • Propylparaben • Green Tea extract (camellia oleifera) • Black Cohosh root extract (cimicifuga racemosa) • Saw Palmetto fruit extract (serenoa serrulata) • Red Raspberry fruit extract (rubus idaeus) • Dong Quai root extract (angelica polymorpha sinensis).

X-Action Men's Formula - Nature's Sunshine
Each capsule contains: Proprietary Blend 452 mg: L-Arginine, Horny Goat Weed (epimedium sagittatum), Damiana leaf (turnera diffusa), Oat straw (avena sativa), Muira Puama (ptychopetalum olacoides), Saw Palmetto berry, Yohimbe bark (pausinystalia yohimbe), DHEA. Other Ingredients: Cellulose, Magnesium Stearate, Gelatin, Water.

XanGo Juice - XanGo Corp
Garcinia Mangostana (reconstituted juice from whole fruit) • Apple juice concentrate • Pear juice concentrate • Grape juice concentrate • Pear puree • Blueberry juice concentrate • Raspberry juice concentrate • Strawberry juice concentrate • Cranberry juice concentrate • Cherry juice concentrate • Citric Acid • Natural Flavor • Pectin • Xanthan Gum • Sodium Benzoate • Potassium Sorbate.

Xantrex ThermoGenics Plus Rapid Weight Loss for Men - SilverSage
Two capsules contain: Niacin 50 mg • Proprietary Xantrex Blend 1243.5 mg: Yerba Mate bark standardized extract (SE), Caffeine, Guarana seed SE, Damiana leaf/stem SE, Schizonepeta Spica SE, Green Tea leaf SE, Piper Nigrum fruit SE, Tibetan Ginseng root SE, Panax Ginseng root SE, Maca herb SE, Cocoa bean SE, Tribulus Terrestris root SE, Kola Nut SE, Thea Sinensis leaf complex, NADH. Other Ingredients: Rice Flour.

Xantrex ThermoGenics Plus Rapid Weight Loss for Women - SilverSage
Two capsules contain: Niacin 50 mg • Proprietary Xantrex Blend 1243.5 mg: Yerba Mate bark standardized extract (SE), Caffeine, Guarana seed SE, Damiana leaf/stem SE, Schizonepeta spica SE, Green Tea leaf SE, Piper Nigrum fruit SE, Tibetan Ginseng root SE, Panax Ginseng root SE, Vitex Agnus Castus fruit SE, Hawthorne berry SE, Sodium Bicarbonate, Kola nut SE, Thea Sinensis leaf complex, NADH. Other Ingredients: Rice Flour.

Xcel Patch - Unknown
L-Arginine • Nettle leaf • Cayenne • Muira Puama • Orchic substance • Oyster meat • Tribulus • Zinc • Sarsaparilla • Astragalus • Licorice root • Pumpkin seed • Boron • Pygeum • Maca • Horny Goat Weed • Oat straw • Catuaba.

Xcellent C - Xymogen
Each capsule contains: Vitamin C 750 mg • Bioperine brand Black Pepper extract 7.5 mg.

Xcellent E HG-400 - Xymogen
Each softgel contains: Natural Vitamin E (from mixed tocopherols) 400 mg: D-Alpha-Tocopherol 134 mg (200 IU) • D-Beta-Tocopherol 12 mg • D-Gamma-Tocopherol 200 mg • D-Delta-Tocopherol 54 mg • Tocotrienols 2 mg. Other Ingredients: Gelatin, Glycerin, Soybean Oil.

Xenadrine EFX - Cytodyne LLC
Two capsules contain: Vitamin C 100 mg • Vitamin B6 10 mg • Pantothenic Acid 12 mg • Magnesium 10 mg • Proprietary Thermodyne Complex 1415 mg: Tyroplex proprietary blend of L-Tyrosine and Acetyl L-Tyrosine, Green Tea extract (standardized for EGCG and caffeine), Seropro propreitary Cocoa extract (standardized for phenylethylamine, tyramine and theobromine), Yerba Mate (standardized for caffeine), DL-Methionine, Ginger root (standardized for gingerols), Isotherm proprietary blend of Quercetin and Fisetin, Bitter Orange (standardized for synephrine), DMAE (2-diemthylaminoethanol), Grape Seed extract.
See Editor's Note No. 40.

Xenadrine NRG - Cytodyne LLC
Two tablets contain: Vitamin B12 188 mcg • Norambrolide 37.5 mg • Proprietary Thermoxanthin Blend 454 mg: L-Tyrosine, L-Theanine, Yerba Mate leaf, Guarana seed, Cocoa seed, Green Tea leaf, Green Coffee bean extract, infused with natural Caffeine. Other Ingredients: Calcium Phosphate, Cellulose, Sorbitol, Gamma Cyclodextrin, Cephalins, Xanthan, Inulin, Magnesium Stearate.

Xenadrine RFA-1 - Cytodyne LLC
Two capsules contain: Citrus Aurantium peel (bitter orange, standardized for 4% synephrine) 125 mg • Ma Huang (standardized for 6% ephedrine) 335 mg • Guarana extract (standardized for 22% caffeine) 910 mg • White Willow bark extract (standardized for 15% salicin) 105 mg • Acetyl L-Carnitine 100 mg • L-Tyrosine 80 mg • Ginger root 50 mg • Vitamin B5 (pantothenic acid) 40 mg.
See Editor's Note No. 30 and No. 40.

Xiao Chai Hu Tang Plus - Secara
Bupleurum root 5:1 extract (chai hu) 360 mg • Pinellia Ternata rhizome 5:1 extract (ban xia) 360 mg • Organic Licorice root (gan cao) 353 mg • Jujube fruit 5:1 extract (da zao) 299 mg • Asian Ginseng root 5:1 extract (ren shen) 270 mg • Chinese Skullcap root 5:1 extract (huang qin) 270 mg • Ginger rhizome 5:1 extract (sheng jiang) 270 mg • Cinchona bark extract 68 mg.

Xiao Yao San Plus - Secara
Organic Licorice root (gan cao) 450 mg • Artichoke leaf extract (2% cynarin, 7 mg) 333 mg • Bupleurum rhizome 5:1 extract (chai hu) 279 mg • Dong Quai root 5:1 extract (dang gui) 279 mg • Atractylodes root 5:1 extract (bai zhu) 240 mg • Chinese Peony root 5:1 extract (bai shao) 240 mg • Poria sclerotium 5:1 extract (fu ling) 222 mg • Organic Peppermint leaf 189 mg • Organic Peppermint oil 18 mg.

Xo3 Hangover Prevention - DietBlends, Inc.
Each twin-pack (8 g) contains: Vitamin C 240 mg • Vitamin B Complex 44 mg • Calcium 24 mg • Zinc 7.8 mg • Magnesium Blend 7 mg • Chromium Blend 66 mcg • Amino Acids • Caffeine 25 mg • Trace Minerals • Tartaric Acid • Sodium Bicarbonate • Potassium Chloride • FD&C Colors • Natural Flavors.

Xomatropin hGH Spray - ASN - Advanced Sports Nutrition
Each two part formula contains: Part One: Secreatagoges • GH & IGF-1 Peptides. Part Two: Anti-Soatosatin called Revosatin (a power suppressor of an antagonistic hormone called somatosatin responsible for what is called the negative feedback loop for GH).

XS Energy Drink (assorted flavors) - XS Energy, LLC / QUIXTAR
Carbonated Water • L-Taurine • L-Glutamine • Citric Acid • Eleutherococcus Senticosus • Panax Ginseng • Panax Quinquefolium • Schisandra • Astragalus • Reishi • Acesulfame Potassium • Caffeine • Potassium Sorbate • Sucralose • Niacin • Pyridoxine HCl • Cyanocobalamin • Pantothenic Acid. Cherry Blast flavor also contains: Sodium Benzoate, Natural Flavors. Electric Lemon Blast flavor also contains: Lemon juice concentrate. Tropical Blast flavor also contains: Natural Flavors, Yellow 6. Tea Berry Typhoon flavor also contains: Green Tea extract, Black Tea extract, Natural Flavors. Citrus Blast flavor also contains: Echinacea Purpurea, Natural Flavors, Yellow 5. Cranberry-Grape flavor also contains: Cranberry juice concentrate, Echinacea Purpurea, Natural Flavors, Red 40.

XS Energy Drink caffeine free (tropical blast flavor) - XS Energy, LLC / QUIXTAR
Carbonated Water • L-Taurine • L-Glutamine • Citric Acid • Acesulfame Potassium • Sodium Benzoate • Potassium Sorbate • Sucralose • Niacin • Pyridoxine HCl • Cyanocobalamin • Pantothenic Acid • Folic Acid • Yellow 6.

XTEND-LIFE Prostate - Xtend-Life Nutraceuticals Inc.
Each capsule contains: Saw Palmetto extract 160 mg • Pygeum extract 50 mg • Pumpkin Seed extract 40 mg.

XTEND-LIFE Total Balance - Xtend-Life Nutraceuticals Inc.
Each tablet contains: Amino Acid Blend: L-Arginine, Aspartic Acid, L-Glutamic Acid, L-Lysine, Glycine, Tryptophan, L-Phenylalanine, L-Serine, L-Methionine, L-Leucine, L-Isoleucine, L-Alanine, L-Proline, L-Threonine, L-Histidine 200 mg • N-Acetyl L-Tyrosine 20 mg • L-Carnitine 20 mg • L-Glutathione 20 mg • N-Acetyl

Cysteine 20 mg • L-Taurine 20 mg • Bromelain 2000 GUI 10 mg • Lipase 10 mg • Catalase 10 mg • Betaine HCl 10 mg • Citrus Bioflavonoids 30 mg • Hesperidin 10 mg • Quercetin 10 mg • Trimethylglycine 15 mg • Inositol 20 mg • N-Acetyl Glucosamine 20 mg • Chondroitin Sulfate 20 mg • MSM (Methyl Sulfonyl Methane) 20 mg • DMAE (Bitartrate) 20 mg • Lutein 2 mg •Lycopene 2 mg • Alpha-Lipoic Acid 10 mg • Rutin 10 mg • Phosphatidyl Choline 25 mg • Choline (Bitartrate) 25 mg • Octacosanol 5 mg • 1,3-Beta Glucan 10 mg • Hawthorne berry extract 25 mg • Grape Seed extract 25 mg • Ginkgo Biloba 40 mg • Bilberry extract 20 mg • Whole Leaf Aloe Vera extract 20 mg • Turmeric extract 20 mg • Green Tea extract 60 mg • Silymarin (Milk Thistle Seed extract) 20 mg • Ginger root extract 25 mg • Barley Grass Juice powder 80 mg • Artichoke powder 50 mg • Green Oat Juice powder 50 mg • Beet Juice powder 50 mg • Vitamin A (Beta Carotene) 2500 IU • Vitamin A (Palmitate) 1000 IU • Vitamin B-1 (Thiamin Nitrate) 2 mg • Vitamin B-2 (Riboflavin) 2 mg • Vitamin B-3 (Niacinamide) 12 mg • Vitamin B-5 (d-Pantothenate) 12 mg • Vitamin B-6 (Pyridoxine HCl) 6 mg • Vitamin B-12 (Cyanocobalamin) 24 mcg • Biotin 100 mcg •Folic Acid 200 mcg • Vitamin C 20 mg • Vitamin D (Cholecalciferol) 100 IU • Vitamin E (d-Alpha Tocopheryl) 25 mg • Vitamin K (Phytonadione) 20 mcg • PABA 10 mg • Boron (Chelate) 1 mg • Calcium (Citrate) 50 mg • Chromium (Polynicotinate) 120 mcg • Copper (Gluconate) 150 mcg • Iodine (from Kelp) 50 mcg • Magnesium (Aspartate) 50 mg • Manganese (Chelate) 1.5 mg • Molybdenum 75 mcg • Potassium (Aspartate) 20 mg • Selenium 70 mcg • Vanadium 25 mcg • Zinc (Gluconate) 10 mg. Other Ingredients: Cellulose Powder, Hydroxypropylcellulose, Magnesium Stearate, Silicon Dioxide.
See Editor's Note No. 15.

BRAND NAMES

Xtra Advantage Creatine Serum **-** Muscle Marketing USA
Each 5 mL serving contains: Creatine Monohydrate • Glucosamine • L-Glutamine • L-Taurine • L-Carnitine • Magnesium • Zinc • Calcium • Vitamin B12 • Royal Jelly • Ginseng • Honey • Natural Glycerine • Natural Flavor • Distilled Water.

Xtra Fuel **-** TwinLab
Three capsules contain: Guarana extract (22% caffeine) 910 mg • Citrus Aurantium extract (bitter orange, standardized to 4% synephrine) 325 mg • L-Tyrosine 500 mg • Vitamin C 250 mg • Vitamin B6 10 mg • Ginkgo Biloba extract (standardized to 24% flavonoid glycoside) 60 mg • DMAE (2-dimethylaminoethanol) 100 mg • Vitamin B5 (pantothenic acid) 100 mg.
See Editor's Note No. 40.

Xtra Strength 5 HTP **-** Pro Health
Each capsule contains: 5HTP (5-hydroxy-l-tryptophan, from griffonia seed) 200 mg. Other Ingredients: Gelatin, Rice Flour, Magnesium Trisilicate, Magnesium Stearate.

Xtra Strength Glucosamine Chondroitin **-** Pro Health
Two tablets contain: Glucosamine Sulfate (as glucosamine sulfate 2KCI) 1500 mg • Chondroitin Sulfate 1200 mg. Other Ingredients: Stearic Acid, Microcrystalline Cellulose, Magnesium Stearate, Croscarmellose Sodium, Pharmaceutical Glaze.
See Editor's Note No. 15.

Xtra-Cal **-** Herbalife International of America, Inc.
Each tablet contains: Vitamin C (as ascorbic acid) 20 mg • Vitamin D (as ergocalciferol) 30 IU • Vitamin E (as dL-alpha tocopheryl acetate) 10 IU • Calcium (as calcium carbonate and citrate) 334 mg • Magnesium (as magnesium oxide and citrate) 134 mg • Zinc (as zinc gluconate) 1.7 mg • Copper (as copper amino acid chelate) 0.167 mg • Manganese (as manganese amino acid chelate) 0.7 mg • Exclusive Blend 30 mg: Horsetail herb stem, Glutamic Acid Hydrochloride, Kelp leaves, Licorice root, Spirulina algae. Other Ingredients: Microcrystalline Cellulose, Croscarmellose Sodium, Silicon Dioxide, Magnesium Stearate, Betaine Hydrochloride, Vegetable Oil, Stearic Acid, Dextrin, Dextrose, Lecithin, Sodium Carboxymethylcellulose, Sodium Citrate.

Xtra-Mineral **-** The Herbalist
Yellow Dock root • Red Raspberry leaf • Nettles leaf • Dandelion root.

Xtreme Cut with Super CitriMax **-** Vitamin World
Two capsules contain: Chromium (as chromium polynicotinate) 120 mcg • (-) Hydroxycitric Acid (HCA, provided by 1500 mg of Super CitriMax Plus brand from garcinia cambogia rind) 825 mg • Guarana bark extract (paullinia cupana, standardized to contain 36% caffeine) 430 mg • Kola Nut seed extract (cola acuminata, standardized to contain 10% caffeine) 320 mg • Gymnema leaf (gymnema sylvestre, standardized to contain 25% gymnemic acid) 120 mg • Black Tea leaf extract (camellia sinensis, stnadardized to contain 60% polyphenols and 15% EGCG) 100 mg • Green Tea leaf extract (camellia sinensis, standardized to contain 90% polyphenols, 45% EGCG and 70% catechins) 100 mg • Caffeine (from guarana, kola nut and tea extracts) 200 mg • Alpha Lipoic Acid 30 mg • L-Carnitine (as carnitine fumarate) 20 mg. Other Ingredients: Gelatin, Vegetable Magnesium Stearate, Silica.

Xtreme Trim **-** Puritan's Pride
Two capsules contain: Pantothenic Acid (D-calcium pantothenate) 10 mg • Citrus Aurantium extract (4% synephrine) 125 mg • Ma Huang extract (ephedra sinica, 6% ephedrine) 335 mg • Guarana extract (paullinia cupana, standardized for 22% caffeine) 910 mg • White Willow extract (salix alba, standardized for 15% silicin) 105 mg • Acetyl-L-Carnitine Hydrochloride 50 mg • L-Tyrosine 40 mg • Ginger root (zingiber officinale) 25 mg.
See Editor's Note No. 30 and No. 40.

Xtreme Trim Ephedra Free **-** Puritan's Pride
Two capsules contain: Vitamin C (ascorbic acid) 100 mg • Vitamin B6 (pyridoxine HCl) 10 mg • Pantothenic Acid (D-calcium pantothenate) 12 mg • Magnesium (oxide) 10 mg • Xtreme Trim Thermo Complex 1415 mg: Yerba Mate leaf extract (standardized for methylxanthines), Green Tea leaf extract (camellia sinensis, standardized for epigallocatechin gallate, caffeine, polyphenols), Metabromine Cocoa extract (standardized for theobromine, caffeine), Bitter Orange fruit extract (citrus aurantium, standardized for synephrine, n-methyltyramine, hordenine, octopamine, tyramine), Tyrosine Complex (l-tyrosine, acetyl l-tyrosine), L-Methionine, Ginger root extract (zingiber officinale), Grape seed extract, Flavone complex (proprietary blend of 3, 3', 4', 5-7-pentahydroxyflavone, 3, 3', 4', 7 tetrahydroxyflavone), DMAE (dimethylaminoethanol). Other Ingredients: Gelatin, Vegetable Magnesium Stearate, Silica.
See Editor's Note No. 40.

Xtreme Trim Phase 2 White Kidney Bean Extract **-** Vitamin World
Each tablet contains: Calcium (as dicalcium phosphate) 182 mg • Phase 2 Brand Phaseolus Vulgaris (from white kidney bean extract) 1000 mg. Other Ingredients: Cellulose (plant origin), Croscarmellose, Vegetable Stearic Acid, Silica, Cellulose Coating, Vegetable Magnesium Stearate.

Xzite Female Sexual Enhancement **-** BJH Laboratories
Each capsule contains: Proprietary Xzite Blend 500 mg: Ligusticom Wallichi 166 mg, Acanthopanax 166 mg, Chrysanthemum 168 mg. Other Ingredients: Rice Protein, Magnesium Stearate, Gelatin.

Yaeyama Chlorella + Barley **-** Jarrow Formulas
Ten tablets contain: Vitamin A (as beta-carotene) 1865 IU • Vitamin C 7 mg • Calcium 30 mg • Iron 4.5 mg • Magnesium 32 mg • Potassium 105 mg • Yaeyama Chlorella 2.5 g: Chlorella Growth Factor (CGF) 475 mg • Barley 2.5 g. Other Ingredients: Calcium Phosphate, Cellulose, Modified Cellulose Gum, Stearic Acid, Magnesium Stearate, Silicon Dioxide.

Yaeyama Chlorella capsules **-** Jarrow Formulas
Five capsules contain: Vitamin A (as beta carotene)804 IU • Vitamin C 2 mg • Thiamin (B1) 30 mcg • Riboflavin 100 mcg • Niacin (B3) 0.5 mg • Vitamin B6 50 mcg • Vitamin B12 0.3 mcg • Magnesium 7 mg • Manganese 0.12 mg • Iron 2 mg • Potassium 30 mg • Yaeyama Chlorella 2 g: Chlorophyll 86 mg, Chlorella Growth Factor 380 mg. Other Ingredients: Rice Powder, Magnesium Stearate, Silicon Dioxide, Gelatin.

Some Brand Name Natural Products - What they Contain

www.NaturalDatabase.com contains MANY more listings than appear here.
Editor's Notes are located on pages 2155-2163.

Yaeyama Chlorella tablets - Jarrow Formulas
Five tablets contain: Vitamin A (as beta carotene) 402 IU • Riboflavin 0.05 mg • Vitamin B12 0.2 mc g • Manganese 60 mcg • Iron 1 mg • Yaeyama Chlorella (chlorella vulgaris) 1 g: Chlorophyll 35 mg, Chlorella Growth Factor 212 mg. Other Ingredients: Calcium Phosphate, Modified Cellulose Gum, Cellulose, Stearic Acid, Modified Cellulose, Magnesium Stearate, Silicon Dioxide.

Yaeyama Chlorophyll liquid - Jarrow Formulas
Each 1 tsp (5 g) serving conatins: Vitamin A (as beta carotene) 2010 IU • Vitamin C 5 mg • Thiamin (B1) 80 mcg • Riboflavin 0.3 mcg • Niacin (B3) 1.3 mg • Vitamin B6 130 mcg • Vitamin B12 0.7 mcg • Magnesium 17 mg • Manganese 0.3 mg • Iron 4 mg • Potassium 69 mg • Yaeyama Chlorella 5 g: Chlorophyll 215 mg, Chlorella Growth Factor 950 mg.

Yam Extract Plus 30 - Aspen Group, Inc.
Each capsule contains: Mexican Yam extract 500 mg • Adrenal substance (freeze dried) 200 mg.
See Editor's Note No. 14.

Yam Extract Plus 30 - Atrium Biotechnologies
Each capsule contains: Mexican Yam extract 500 mg • Adrenal Substance (freeze dried) 200 mg.
See Editor's Note No. 14.

Yamoa Powder - Yamoapowder.com
Each capsule contains: Funtumia Elastica Gum Tree powdered bark 500 mg. Other Ingredients: Magnesium Stearate 10 mg.

Yarrow-Pipsissewa Virtue - Blessed Herbs
Echinacea Angustifolia root • Yarrow flower • Pipsissewa • Oregon Grape root • Corn Silk • Kava Kava root • Hydrangea root • Grain alcohol & Distilled Water.

Yeast Fighters - TwinLab
Five hard gelatin capsules contain: High Potency Freeze Dried Lactobacillus Acidophilus (milk free, supplying 2.5 billion viable cells) 1000 mg • Concentrated Odorless Garlic extract powder (equivalent to 1500 mg of fresh garlic) 100 mg • Natural Caprylic Acid 100 mg • Biotin 900 mcg • Fiber Blend 3000 mg: Psyllium seed husks, Guar Gum, Apple Pectin. Base: Pau d'Arco, Onion, Black Walnut, Echinacea, Golden Seal root.

Yeast Formula - PhytoPharmica
Two softgel capsules contain: Goldenseal root and rhizome extract (hydrastis canadensis, standardized to contain 5% total alkaloids including berberine, hydrastine and canadine) 100 mg • Oregano oil of aerial part extract (origanum vulgare) 0.2 mL • Peppermint oil of leaf extract (mentha x piperita) 0.2 mL • Thyme oil of leaf and stem extract (thymus vulgaris) 0.1 mL.
This product was formerly known as Candimyacin.

Yeast Raiders - Puritan's Pride
Five capsules contain: Vitamin C 60 mg • Biotin 900 mcg • Zinc 10 mg • Selenium 50 mcg • Freeze Dried Lactobacillus Acidophilus 1,000 mg • Concentrated Odorless Garlic extract (equivalent to 1,500 mg of fresh Garlic) 100 mg • Natural Caprylic Acid 100 mg • Fiber Blend: Psyllium seed husks (Plantago ovata), Guar Gum, Apple Pectin 3,000 mg • Barberry (Berberis vulgaris) root 100 mg • Ginger (Zingiber officinale) root 10 mg • Thyme (Thymus vulgaris) herb 10 mg • Cinnamon bark (cinnamomum verum) 10 mg • Proprietary Blend 50 mg: Pau D'Arco, Onion powder, Black Walnut, Echinacea, Goldenseal root.

Yeast Rx - Pro Health
Each level scoop (1 g) contains: Egg powder 1000 mg.

Yellow Dock - Nature's Way
Two capsules contain: Yellow Dock root 1 g. Other Ingredients: Gelatin.

Yellow Swarm - NVE Pharmaceuticals
Each capsule contains: Proprietary Blend 261 mg: Ephedra extract (leaf, stem, 25 mg ephedrine group alkaloids), Capsicum Annum (whole pepper), Kola Nut (<1 mg caffeine group alkaloids), Ginseng (root) • Caffeine (anhydrous) 300 mg • Other Ingredients: Gelatin, Dextrose, Stearic Acid, Magnesium Stearate, Titanium Dioxide, FD&C Red #40, FD&C Blue #1, FD&C Yellow #5, FD&C Yellow #6.
See Editor's Note No. 30.

Yerba Manza-Eyebright Virtue - Blessed Herbs
Yerba Manza root • Yerba Santa leaf • Usnea lichen • Osha root • Eyebright • Propolis • Goldenseal root • Myrrh Gum • Licorice root • Grain alcohol & Distilled Water.

Yerba Santa-Echinacea Virtue - Blessed Herbs
Yerba Santa leaf • Osha root • Usnea lichen • Lomatium root • Pau d'Arco bark • Echinacea Angustifolia root • Goldenseal root • Myrrh Gum • Shitake mycelium • Propolis • Licorice root • Grain alcohol & Distilled Water.

Y-Factors - Advocare International
Three capsules contain: Niacin 25 mg • Zinc (as monomethionine OptiZinc) 7.5 mg • Proprietary Blend a-MPC 1130 mg: Yohimbe extract (bark - pausinystalia yohimbe), Saw Palmetto extract (berry - serenoa repens), Pygeum extract (bark - pygeum africanum) • Ginkgo extract (leaf - ginkgo biloba) 120 mg • Cranberry extract (fruit - vaccinium macrocarpon) 100 mg • Swedish Flower pollen extract (cernitin - secale cereal) 100 mg • American Ginseng extract (root - panax quinquefolius) 15 mg. Other Ingredients: Cellulose, Silicon Dioxide, Magnesium Stearate, Gelatin.

Yigan Jiedu capsules (Liver Formula) - Hubei Yichang Minkang factory
Each capsule contains: Proprietary Blend 350 mg: Phellodendron stem bark, Chinese Skullcap root, Indian Goldthread rhizome, Poria sclerotium, Bupleurum root, Magnolia stem, Chinese Amomum fruit, Fragrant Angelica root.

Yin Qiao San Plus - Secara
Three tablets contain: Forsythia fruit (lian qiao, 5:1 extract) 255 mg • Japanese Honeysuckle flower (jin yin hua, 5:1 extract) 255 mg • Phragmites root/rhizome (lu gen, 5:1 extract) 237 mg • Organic Peppermint leaf 234 mg • Organic Licorice root (gan cao) 228 mg • Lophatherum stem/leaf (dan zhu ye, 5:1 extract) 183 mg • Organic Thyme herb 180 mg • Organic Goldenseal root/rhizome 156 mg • American Elder fruit (10:1 extract) 147 mg • Platycodon root (jie geng), 5:1 extract) 129 mg • Soy Bean (dan dou chi, 5:1 extract) 111 mg • Burdock seed (niu bang zi, 5:1 extract) 54 mg • Yarrow tops 54 mg • Organic Peppermint Oil 21 mg • Thyme Oil 6 mg.

Yin-Yang Athletic Tone - Flora Inc.
Chinese Red Ginseng • American Ginseng • Astragalus • Reishi Mushroom • Schisandra • Panax Notoginseng • He Shou Wu • Codonopsis • Lycii berries • Licorice • Rehmania • Du Zhong • Prince Ginseng • Dodder Seed • Asparagus root.

Yin-Yang Beautiful Lady - Flora Inc.
Peony • Schisandra • Lycii berries • Licorice • He Shou Wu • Asparagus root • Noto Ginseng • Dang Gui • Codonopsis • Atractylodes • Poria.

Yin-Yang Crystal Clear Vision - Flora Inc.
Rehmania • Dodder Seed • Lycii berries • Chrysanthemum • He Shou Wu • Poria • Ligusticum • Acorus • Plantago Seeds.

Yin-Yang Golden Passage - Flora Inc.
Curculigo • Epimedii • Morinda root • Dang Gui • Phellodendron bark • Anemarrhena • Schisandra • Lycii berries • He Shou Wu • Licorice.

Yin-Yang Premenstrual Harmony - Flora Inc.
Bupleurum • Dang Gui • Peony • Poria • Atractylodes • Ginger • Licorice • Peppermint • Peony root bark • Cyperus berries • Ligusticum • Citrus Peel.

Yin-Yang Secret of Longevity - Flora Inc.
Chinese Red Ginseng • Astragalus • Noto Ginseng • Reishi Mushroom • Dang gui • Lycii berries • Asparagus root • Licorice • Poria • Prince Ginseng • Rehmania • Ligustrum Fruit • Schisandra • He Shou Wu.

BRAND NAMES

Yin-Yang Tranquil Spirit - Flora Inc.
Zizyphus Jujube seed • Poria • Biota Seed • Anemarrhena • Licorice • Schisandra • Dang Gui.

YoHIMbe - HVL, Inc
Two capsules contain: Yohimbe 4:1 extract 500 mg • Cellulose • Gelatin • Silica and Magnesium Stearate.

Yohimbe 1111 Caps - Optimum Nutrition
Each capsule contains: Yohimbe extract (2% yohimbine) 1111 mg. Other Ingredients: Gelatin, Magnesium Stearate.

Yohimbe B-12 - Puritan's Pride
Each 1 ml serving contains: Yohimbe extract (pausinystalia yohimbe) bark 1000 mg • Co-Enzyme B-12 (dibencozide) 5,000 mcg.

Yohimbe Fuel - TwinLab
Yohimbine (the active component in Yohimbe bark) 8 mg.

Young Again - Aspen Group, Inc.
Four tablets contain: Vitamin A Palmitate 500,000 IU/GR 8000 IU • Niacinamide 80 mg • Vitamin B6 20 mg • Vitamin C (magnesium ascorbate) 400 mg • Vitamin E (succinate) 100 IU • N-Acetyl Glucosamine 160 mg • L-Proline 360 mg • L-Lysine 320 mg • Glucosamine Sulfate 560 mg • Chondroitin Sulfate 160 mg • N-Acetyl Cysteine 120 mg • Quercetin 80 mg • Grape seed extract 30 mg • Zinc (gluconate) 12 mg • Manganese Ascorbate 12 mg • Copper (gluconate) 0.5 mg • Selenomethionine 80 mcg.
See Editor's Note No. 15.

YourLife B-100 Complex - Leiner Health Products
Each tablet contains: Biotin 100 mcg • Folic Acid (folate) 400 mcg • Niacin (vitamin B3) 100 mg • Pantothenic Acid (vitamin B5) 100 mg • Riboflavin (vitamin B2) 100 mg • Thiamin (vitamin B1) 100 mg • Vitamin B12 100 mcg • Vitamin B6 100 mg. Other Ingredients: Calcium Carbonate, D-Calcium Pantothenate, Cellulose, Maltodextrin, Croscarmellose Sodium, Silicon Dioxide, Polyethylene Glycol 3350, Dicalcium Phosphate, Crospovidone.
See Editor's Note No. 45.

YourLife B-50 Complex - Leiner Health Products
Each tablet contains: Biotin 50 mcg • Folic Acid (folate) 100 mcg • Niacin (vitamin B3) 50 mg • Pantothenic Acid (vitamin B5) 50 mg • Riboflavin (vitamin B2) 50 mg • Thiamin (vitamin B1) 50 mg • Vitamin B12 50 mcg • Vitamin B6 50 mg. Other Ingredients: Calcium Carbonate, Cellulose, D-Calcium Pantothenate, Maltodextrin, Croscarmellose Sodium, Sodium Starch Glycolate, Silicon Dioxide, Polyethylene Glycol 3350, Tricalcium Phosphate.
See Editor's Note No. 45.

YourLife B-Complex Supplement - Leiner Health Products
Each tablet contains: Biotin 10 mcg • Folic Acid (folate) 100 mcg • Niacin (vitamin B3) 10 mg • Pantothenic Acid (vitamin B5) 10 mg • Riboflavin (vitamin B2) 10 mg • Thiamin (vitamin B1) 10 mg • Vitamin B12 10 mcg • Vitamin B6 10 mg. Other Ingredients: Maltodextrin, Hydroxypropyl Methylcellulose, Cellulose, Starch, Para-Aminobenzoic Acid, Croscarmellose Sodium, Sodium Starch Glycolate, Silicon Dioxide, Hydroxypropyl Cellulose, Red 40 Lake, Polyethylene Glycol 3350, Magnesium Stearate, Resin, Dicalcium Phosphate, Polysorbate 80, Titanium Dioxide, Povidone.
See Editor's Note No. 45.

YourLife Beta Carotene 25,000 IU - Leiner Health Products
Each softgel contains: Vitamin A from Beta Carotene 25,000 IU. Other Ingredients: Soybean Oil, Gelatin, Glycerin, Vegetable Oil (partially hydrogenated cottonseed and soybean oils), Yellow Beeswax, Carrot Oil.
See Editor's Note No. 45.

YourLife Calcium 600 mg - Leiner Health Products
Each tablet contains: Calcium (carbonate) 600 mg. Other Ingredients: Maltodextrin, Soy Polysaccharide, Cellulose, Croscarmellose Sodium, Gum Arabic, Mineral Oil, Talc, Starch, Polyethylene Glycol 3350, Hydroxypropyl Methylcellulose, Magnesium Stearate, Hydroxypropyl Cellulose, Polysorbate 80, Crospovidone, Stearic Acid.
See Editor's Note No. 45.

YourLife Calcium 600 mg Plus D - Leiner Health Products
Each tablet contains: Calcium (as calcium carbonate) 600 mg • Vitamin D (cholecalciferol) 200 IU. Other Ingredients: Maltodextrin, Hydroxypropyl Methylcellulose, Talc, Croscarmellose Sodium, Acacia, Hydroxypropyl Cellulose, Titanium Dioxide, Silicon Dioxide, Starch, Magnesium Stearate, Polysorbate 80, Polyethylene Glycol 3350, Sodium Citrate, Yellow 6 Lake.
See Editor's Note No. 45.

YourLife Calcium Plus Vitamin D & Minerals - Leiner Health Products
Each tablet contains: Calcium 600 mg • Copper 1 mg • Magnesium 40 mg • Manganese 1.8 mg • Vitamin D 200 IU • Zinc 7.5 mg • Boron 250 mcg. Other Ingredients: Maltodextrin, Hydroxypropyl Methylcellulose, Titanium Dioxide, Magnesium Stearate, Red 40 Lake, Yellow 6 Lake, Blue 1 Lake, Cellulose, Talc, Starch, Mineral Oil, Croscarmellose Sodium, Hydroxypropyl Cellulose, Silicon Dioxide, Polyethylene Glycol 8000, Polysorbate 80, Sodium Lauryl Sulfate, Polyethylene Glycol 3350, Crospovidone, Gelatin, Stearic Acid.
See Editor's Note No. 45.

YourLife Calcium, Magnesium & Zinc - Leiner Health Products
Each tablet contains: Calcium (as calcium carbonate) 333 mg • Magnesium (as magnesium oxide) 133 mg • Zinc (as zinc sulfate) 5 mg. Other Ingredients: Maltodextrin, Cellulose, Croscarmellose Sodium, Talc, Hydroxypropyl Methylcellulose, Acacia, Soy Polysaccharide, Mineral Oil, Silicon Dioxide, Starch, Magnesium Stearate, Stearic Acid, Citric Acid, Sodium Starch Glycolate, Polyethylene Glycol, Hydroxypropyl Cellulose, Polysorbate 80, Crospovidone.
See Editor's Note No. 45.

YourLife Central-Vite - Leiner Health Products
Each tablet contains: Vitamin A 5000 IU • Iodine 150 mcg • Vitamin C 60 mg • Magnesium 100 mg • Vitamin D 400 IU • Zinc 15 mg • Vitamin E 30 IU • Selenium 20 mcg • Vitamin K 25 mcg • Copper 2 mg • Thiamin (vitamin B1) 1.5 mg • Manganese 2 mg • Riboflavin (vitamin B2) 1.7 mg • Chromium 120 mcg • Niacin 20 mg • Molybdenum 75 mcg • Vitamin B6 2 mg • Chloride 72 mg • Folic Acid 400 mcg • Potassium 80 mg • Vitamin B12 6 mcg • Nickel 5 mcg • Biotin 30 mcg • Tin 10 mcg • Pantothenic Acid 10 mg • Silicon 2 mg • Calcium 162 mg • Vanadium 10 mcg • Iron 18 mg • Lutein 250 mcg • Phosphorus 109 mg • Boron 150 mcg.
See Editor's Note No. 45.

YourLife Chewable Calcium Plus D - Leiner Health Products
Each tablet contains: Calcium (as calcium carbonate) 300 mg • Vitamin D (as ergocalciferol) 100 IU. Other Ingredients: Sorbitol, Stearic Acid, Cocoa, Magnesium Stearate, Maltodextrin, Silicon Dioxide, Natural Vanilla, Maltol, Gelatin.
See Editor's Note No. 45.

YourLife Chewable Vitamin C 500 mg - Leiner Health Products
Each tablet contains: Vitamin C 500 mg. Other Ingredients: Sucrose, Sodium Ascorbate, Stearic Acid, Starch, Natural Flavor, Magnesium Stearate, Silicon Dioxide, Sorbitol, Yellow 6 Lake, Lactose, Ethylmaltol.
See Editor's Note No. 45.

YourLife Chewable Vitamin C 500 mg With Acerola - Leiner Health Products
Each wafer contains: Vitamin C 500 mg. Other Ingredients: Sugar, Stearic Acid, Cellulose, Silicon Dioxide, Artificial Flavor, Acerola, Magnesium Stearate, Starch, Rose Hips, Lemon Bioflavonoids Complex, Hesperidin Complex, Buckwheat, Caramel, Rutin, Green Pepper Extract, Black Currant Extract.
See Editor's Note No. 45.

YourLife Chromium Picolinate 200 mcg - Leiner Health Products
Each tablet contains: Chromium (as chromium picolinate) 200 mcg. Other Ingredients: Calcium Carbonate, Maltodextrin, Cellulose, Croscarmellose Sodium, Talc, Tricalcium Phosphate, Crospovidone, Polyethylene Glycol 3350, Silicon Dioxide, Magnesium Stearate.
See Editor's Note No. 45.

YourLife Chromium Picolinate 400 mcg - Leiner Health Products
Each tablet contains: Chromium (as chromium picolinate) 400 mcg. Other Ingredients: Calcium Carbonate, Maltodextrin, Cellulose, Croscarmellose Sodium, Talc, Tricalcium Phosphate, Polyethylene Glycol, Crospovidone, Silicon Dioxide, Magnesium Stearate, Hydroxypropyl Methylcellulose, Hydroxypropyl Cellulose, Polysorbate 80.
See Editor's Note No. 45.

YourLife Cod Liver Oil - Leiner Health Products
Each softgel contains: Vitamin A 1250 IU • Vitamin D 135 IU. Other Ingredients: Gelatin, Glycerin, Water.
See Editor's Note No. 45.

YourLife Coenzyme Q10 - Leiner Health Products
Each softgel contains: Coenzyme Q10 30 mg. Other Ingredients: Hydrogenated Vegetable Oil, Refined Soybean Oil, Gelatin, Glycerin, Lecithin, Titanium Dioxide, Red 40 Lake, d-Alpha Tocopherol, Yellow 6 Lake, Blue 1 Lake.

YourLife Daily Pak Essential - Leiner Health Products
Each packet contains: Biotin 60 mcg • Calcium 498 mg • Chloride 72 mg • Chromium 200 mcg • Copper 2.5 mg • Folic Acid (folate) 400 mcg • Iodine 150 mcg • Iron 8 mg • Magnesium 233 mg • Manganese 7.5 mg • Molybdenum 208 mcg • Niacin (vitamin B3) 40 mg • Pantothenic Acid (vitamin B5) 10 mg • Phosphorus 130 mg • Potassium 80 mg • Riboflavin (vitamin B2) 5.1 mg • Selenium 200 mcg • Thiamin (vitamin B1) 4.5 mg • Vitamin A 7500 IU • Vitamin B12 18 mcg • Vitamin B6 6 mg • Vitamin C 620 mg • Vitamin D 400 IU • Vitamin E 460 IU • Vitamin K 80 mcg • Boron 200 mcg • Citrus Bioflavonoids complex 10 mg • Ginkgo Biloba leaf 25 mg • Grape Seed extract (vitis vinefera) 1 mg • Hesperidin complex 5 mg • Kelp frond powder (macrocystis pyrifera) 5 mg • Lecithin 10 mg • Mixed Carotenoids complex 10 mg • Nickel 6.5 mcg • Siberian Ginseng root powder (eleutherococcus senticosus) 25 mg • Silicon 2 mg • Tin 13 mcg • Tocotrienol complex 5 mg • Trace Mineral complex 10 mg • Vanadium 13 mcg. Other Ingredients: Calcium Carbonate, Glucosamine Sulfate, Glucosamine Hydrochloride, Cellulose, Methylcellulose, Maltodextrin, Silicon Dioxide, Hydroxypropyl Methylcellulose, Polyethylene Glycol 3350, Propylene Glycol, Starch, Crospovidone, Croscarmellose Sodium, Acacia.

YourLife Daily Pak Maximum - Leiner Health Products
Each packet contains: Zinc 12.5 mg • Biotin 25 mg • Copper 1.5 mg • Iodine 112.5 mg • Manganese 1.5 mg • Vitamin D 200 IU • Vitamin B12 25 mg • Chromium 425 mcg • Vitamin E (dl-alpha tocopheryl acetate) 900 IU • Pantothenic Acid 25 mg • Iron 4.1 mg • Vitamin C (ascorbic acid) 1200 mg •Selenium 12.5 mcg • Thiamin (vitamin B1) 25 mg • Riboflavin (vitamin B2) 25 mg • Calcium Carbonate 130 mg • Vitamin B6 25 mg • Niacin 25 mg • Magnesium 54.55 mg • Folate 400 mg • Vitamin A 5000 IU • Molybdenum 7.5 mcg • Phosphorus 100 mg • Ginseng 250 mg • Inositol 5 mg • PABA 2.5 mg. Other Ingredients: Dicalcium Phosphate, Gelatin, Glycerin, Cellulose, Hydroxypropyl Methylcellulose, Hydrogenated Vegetable Oil, Stearic Acid, Magnesium Oxide, Starch, Silicon Dioxide, Maltodextrin.

YourLife Daily Pak Men's 50+ - Leiner Health Products
Each packet contains: Biotin 60 mcg • Calcium 533 mg • Chloride 90 mg • Chromium 200 mcg • Folate (folic acid) 400 mcg • Iodine 150 mcg • Magnesium 267 mg • Manganese 7.5 mg • Molybdenum 200 mcg • Niacin (vitamin B3) 40 mg • Pantothenic Acid (vitamin B5) 10 mg • Phosphorus 130 mg • Potassium 100 mg • Riboflavin (vitamin B2) 5.1 mg • Selenium 200 mcg • Thiamin (vitamin B1) 4.5 mg • Vitamin A 7500 IU • Vitamin B12 30 mcg • Vitamin B6 6 mg • Vitamin C 120 mg • Vitamin D 400 IU • Vitamin E 460 IU • Vitamin K 10 mcg • Zinc 15 mg • Bilberry 25 mg • Bilberry berry extract (vaccinium myrtillus) 500 mcg • Boron 1 mg • Citrus Bioflavonoids complex 5 mg • DHA (docosahexaenoic acid) 500 mcg • Grape Seed extract (vitis vinifera) 1 mg • Hesperidin 10 mg • Korean Ginseng root extract (panax ginseng) 100 mg • Lecithin 5 mg • Lutein 500 mcg • Mixed Carotenoids complex 1 mg • Nickel 6.5 mg • Saw Palmetto berry extract (serenoa repens) 160 mg • Siberian Ginseng root powder (eleutherococcus senticosus) 25 mg • Silicon 2 mg • Tin 13 mcg • Tocotrienol complex 1 mg • Trace Mineral complex 1 mg • Vanadium 13 mcg. Other Ingredients: Gelatin, Cellulose, Maltodextrin, Olive Oil, Glycerin, Croscarmellose Sodium, Hypromellose, Silicon Dioxide, Talc, Crospovidone, Magnesium Stearate, Acacia, Mineral Oil, Corn Starch, Soy Polysaccharide, Polyethylene Glycol, Dextrose, Methylcellulose, Dextrin, Lecithin, Hydroxypropyl Cellulose, Caramel, Pharmaceutical Glaze, Sodium Carboxymethylcellulose, Polysorbate 80, Yellow 6 Lake, Kelp, Stearic Acid, Red 40 Lake, Sodium Lauryl Sulfate, Blue 1 Lake, Carnauba Wax.

YourLife Daily Pak Women's - Leiner Health Products
Each packet contains: Vitamin A (Acetate) 2500 IU • Vitamin A (Beta Carotene) 5000 IU • Vitamin C (Ascorbic Acid) 120 mg • Vitamin D (Ergocalciferol) 200 IU • Vitamin E (dl-Alpha Tocopheryl Acetate) 230 IU • Vitamin K (Phytonadione) 10 mcg • Vitamin B1 (Thiamine Mononitrate) 2 mg • Vitamin B2 (Riboflavin) 3 mg • Niacin (Niacinamide) 20 mg • Vitamin B6 (Pyridoxine HCl) 2 mg • Folate (Folic Acid) 400 mcg • Vitamin B12 (Cyanocobalamin) 3 mcg • Biotin (d-Biotin) 30 mcg • Pantothenic Acid (d-Calcium Pantothenate) 10 mg • Calcium (Oyster Shell, Calcium Carbonate, Calcium Phosphate) 725 mg • Iron (Ferrous Fumarate) 4 mg • Phosphorus (Calcium Phosphate) 50 mg • Iodine (Potassium Iodide) 100 mcg • Magnesium (Magnesium Oxide) 100 mg • Zinc (Zinc Oxide) 20 mg • Selenium (Selenium Amino Acid Chelate) 30 mcg • Copper (Copper Oxide) 3 mg • Manganese (Manganese Sulfate) 4 mg • Chromium (Chromium Amino Acid Chelate) 20 mcg • Molybdenum (Molybdenum Amino Acid Chelate) 25 mcg • Chloride (Potassium Chloride) 36 mg • Evening Primrose oil (Evening Primrose Seed) 500 mg. 7 day iron strip contains: Iron (Ferrous Sulfate) 18 mg. Contains colors: Titanium Dioxide, Yellow 6 Lake, Red 40 Lake, Blue 2 Lake.

YourLife Daily Pak Women's 50+ - Leiner Health Products
Each packet contains: Biotin 30 mcg • Calcium 1362 mg • Chloride 36.3 mg • Chromium 25 mcg • Copper 2 mg • Folic Acid (folate) 400 mcg • Iodine 150 mcg • Magnesium 100 mg • Manganese 2.5 mg • Molybdenum 25 mcg • Niacin (vitamin B3) 20 mg • Pantothenic Acid (vitamin B5) 10 mg • Phosphorus 109 mg • Potassium 40 mg • Riboflavin (vitamin B2) 1.7 mg • Selenium 20 mcg • Thiamin (vitamin B1) 1.5 mg • Vitamin A 5000 IU • Vitamin B12 6 mcg • Vitamin B6 2 mg • Vitamin C 560 mg • Vitamin D 400 IU • Vitamin E 430 IU • Vitamin K 25 mcg • Zinc 15 mg • Boron 150 mcg • Deoiled Lecithin bean (glycine max) 25 mg • Devil's Claw root extract (harpogophytum procumbens) 40 mg • Glucosamine Sulfate 500 mg • MSM (methylsulfonylmethane) 200 mg • Nickel 5 mcg • Silicon 2 mg • Vanadium 10 mcg. Other Ingredients: Cellulose, Gelatin, Maltodextrin, Glycerin, Soybean Oil, Croscarmellose Sodium, Silicon Dioxide, Hydroxypropyl Methylcellulose, Talc, Yellow Wax, Magnesium Stearate, Stearic Acid, Glycolate, Dextrin, Crospovidone, Hydroxypropyl Cellulose, Polythylene Glycol 3350, Mannitol, Dextrose, Red 40 • Polysorbate 80, Sodium Carboxymethylcellulose, Resin, Blue 1.

YourLife Energy B-Complex - Leiner Health Products
Each tablet contains: Biotin 10 mcg • Folic Acid (folate) 100 mcg • Niacin (vitamin B3) 10 mg • Pantothenic Acid (vitamin B5) 10 mg • Riboflavin (vitamin B2) 10 mg • Thiamin (vitamin B1) 10 mg • Vitamin B12 10 mcg • Vitamin B6 10 mg. Other Ingredients: Calcium Carbonate, Maltodextrin, Hydroxypropyl Methylcellulose, Cellulose, Starch, Para-Aminobenzoic Acid, Croscarmellose Sodium, Sodium Starch Glycolate, Silicon Dioxide, Hydroxypropyl Cellulose, Red 40 Lake, Polyethylene Glycol 3350, Magnesium Stearate, Resin, Polysorbate 80, Titanium Dioxide, Povidone, Pharmaceutical Glaze.

YourLife Energy Daily Pak **-** Leiner Health Products
Each packet contains: Biotin 100 mcg • Folic Acid (folate) 400 mcg • Niacin (vitamin B3) 100 mg • Pantothenic Acid (vitamin B5) 100 mg • Riboflavin (vitamin B2) 100 mg • Thiamin (vitamin B1) 100 mg • Vitamin B12 100 mcg • Vitamin B6 100 mg • American Ginseng root extract (panax quinquefolium) 70 mg • Chinese Panax Ginseng root extract (panax ginseng) 260 mg • Damiana leaf (turmera diffusa) 2 mg • Fo-Ti root (polygonum multiflorum) 2 mg • Gotu Kola whole plant (centella asiatica) 78 mg • Green Tea leaf extract (camellia sinensis, 50% catechins) 2 mg • Jamaican Ginger root (zingiber officinalis) 2 mg • Korean Ginseng root extract (panax ginseng) 70 mg • Yerba Mate leaf extract (ilex paraguariensis) 575 mg. Other Ingredients: Calcium Carbonate, Cellulose, Maltodextrin, Dicalcium Phosphate, Croscarmellose Sodium, Polyethylene Glycol, Magnesium Stearate, Silicon Dioxide, Hydroxypropyl Cellulose, Hypromellose, Crospovidone, Tricalcium Phosphate, Dextrin, Corn Starch, Wheat Bran, Lecithin, Alfalfa Powder, Brewer's Yeast, Para-Aminobenzoic Acid, Parsley Powder, Watercress, Dextrose, Sodium Carboxymethylcellulose, Polysorbate 80, Sodium Citrate.

YourLife Energy Natural Balance B-100 Complex **-** Leiner Health Products
Each tablet contains: Biotin 100 mcg • Folic Acid (folate) 400 mcg • Niacin (vitamin B3) 100 mg • Pantothenic Acid (vitmain B5) 100 mg • Riboflavin (vitamin B2) 100 mg • Thiamin (vitamin B1) 100 mg • Vitamin B12 100 mcg • Vitamin B6 100 mg. Other Ingredients: Calcium Carbonate, Cellulose, Maltodextrin, Croscarmellose Sodium, Silicon Dioxide, Polyethylene Glycol 3350, Dicalcium Phosphate, Crospovidone, Tricalcium Phosphate.

YourLife Energy Natural Balance B-50 Complex **-** Leiner Health Products
Each tablet contains: Biotin 50 mcg • Folic Acid (folate) 100 mcg • Niacin (vitamin B3) 50 mg • Pantothenic Acid (vitamin B5) 50 mg • Riboflavin (vitamin B2) 50 mg • Thiamin (vitamin B1) 50 mg • Vitamin B12 50 mcg • Vitamin B6 50 mg. Other Ingredients: Calcium Carbonate, Cellulose, Maltodextrin, Croscarmellose Sodium, Sodium Starch Glycolate, Silicon Dioxide, Polyethylene Glycol 3350, Tricalcium Phosphate.

YourLife Ester C with Bioflavonoids **-** Leiner Health Products
Each tablet contains: Vitamin C (Ester-C brand calcium ascorbate) 500 mg • Citrus Bioflavonoids Complex 200 mg. Other Ingredients: Calcium Carbonate, Cellulose, Croscarmellose Sodium, Crospovidone, Silicon Dioxide, Maltodextrin, Polyethylene Glycol 3350, Talc, Magnesium Stearate, Hydroxypropyl Methylcellulose, Hydroxypropyl Cellulose, Polysorbate 80.
See Editor's Note No. 45.

YourLife Folic Acid 800 mcg **-** Leiner Health Products
Each tablet contains: Folic Acid 800 mcg. Other Ingredients: Dicalcium Phosphate, Cellulose, Croscarmellose Sodium, Stearic Acid, Corn Starch, Magnesium Stearate, Silicon Dioxide.
See Editor's Note No. 45.

YourLife High Potency Iron from Ferrous Sulfate **-** Leiner Health Products
Each tablet contains: Iron (ferrous sulfate) 27 mg. Other Ingredients: Calcium Carbonate, Starch, Maltodextrin, Cellulose, Croscarmellose Sodium, Tricalcium Phosphate, Hydroxypropyl Methylcellulose, Polyethylene Glycol 3350, Silicon Dioxide, Talc, Magnesium Stearate, Hydroxypropyl Cellulose, Red 40 Lake, Polysorbate 80, Titanium Dioxide, Povidone.
See Editor's Note No. 45.

YourLife High Potency Multivitamin & Mineral **-** Leiner Health Products
Each tablet contains: Biotin 10 mcg • Calcium 162 mg • Copper 2 mg • Folic Acid (folate) 400 mcg • Iodine 150 mcg • Iron 27 mg • Magnesium 100 mg • Niacin (vitamin B3) 20 mg • Pantothenic Acid (vitamin B5) 10 mg • Phosphorus 40 mg • Riboflavin (vitamin B2) 10 mg • Selenium 10 mcg • Thiamin (vitamin B1) 10 mg • Vitamin A 7500 IU • Vitamin B12 12 mcg • Vitamin B6 3 mg • Vitamin C 100 mg • Vitamin D 400 IU • Vitamin E 30 IU • Zinc 15 mg. Other Ingredients: Cellulose, Gelatin, Starch, Maltodextrin, Croscarmellose Sodium, Sodium Starch Glycolate, Kelp, Silicon Dioxide.
See Editor's Note No. 45.

YourLife Immune System Natural Vitamin A **-** Leiner Health Products
Each softgel contains: Vitamin A 8000 IU. Other Ingredients: Vegetable Oil, Gelatin, Glycerin, Fish Liver Oil.

YourLife Immune System Natural Vitamin A & D **-** Leiner Health Products
Each softgel contains: Vitamin A (from cod liver oil) 1250 IU • Vitamin D 135 IU. Other Ingredients: Gelatin, Glycerin, Water.

YourLife Lutein Formula **-** Leiner Health Products
Each tablet contains: Selenium 40 mcg • Vitamin A 2500 IU • Vitamin C 30 mg • Bilberry 30 mg • Lutein/Zeaxanthin Complex: Lutein 8 mg • Zeaxanthin 640 mcg. Other Ingredients: Calcium Carbonate, Spinach, Gelatin, Glycerol, Starch, Cellulose, Maltodextrin, Hydroxypropyl Methylcellulose, Croscarmellose Sodium, Crospovidone, Silicon Dioxide, Ascorbyl Palmitate, Dicalcium Phosphate, Polyethylene Glycol 3350, Tocopherols, Hydroxypropyl Cellulose, Magnesium Stearate, Riboflavin, Blue 1 Lake, Titanium Dioxide, Polysorbate 80.
See Editor's Note No. 45.

YourLife Magnesium 250 mg **-** Leiner Health Products
Each tablet contains: Magnesium (oxide) 250 mg. Other Ingredients: Cellulose, Talc, Silicon Dioxide, Croscarmellose Sodium, Polyethylene Glycol, Kelp, Magnesium Stearate.
See Editor's Note No. 45.

YourLife Natural High Potency Iron **-** Leiner Health Products
Each softgel contains: Iron (ferrous fumarate) 27 mg. Other Ingredients: Vegetable Oil, Gelatin, Vegetable Shortening, Glycerin, Blackstrap Molasses, Yellow Beeswax, Hydrogenated Soybean Oil, Lecithin, Polysorbate 80, Caramel Color, Titanium Dioxide.
See Editor's Note No. 45.

YourLife Niacin 100 mg **-** Leiner Health Products
Each tablet contains: Niacin (vitamin B3) 100 mg. Other Ingredients: Lactose, Starch, Stearic Acid, Silicon Dioxide, Magnesium Stearate.
See Editor's Note No. 45.

YourLife One Daily **-** Leiner Health Products
Each tablet contains: Folic Acid (folate) 400 mcg • Niacin (vitamin B3) 20 mg • Pantothenic Acid (vitamin B5) 10 mg • Riboflavin (vitamin B2) 1.7 mg • Thiamin (vitamin B1) 1.5 mg • Vitamin A 5000 IU • Vitamin B12 6 mcg • Vitamin B6 2 mg • Vitamin C 60 mg • Vitamin D 400 IU • Vitamin E 30 IU. Other Ingredients: Calcium Carbonate, Gelatin, D-Calcium Pantothenate, Maltodextrin, Hydroxypropyl Methylcellulose, Starch, Cellulose, Croscarmellose Sodium, Sodium Starch Glycolate, Silicon Dioxide, Hydroxypropyl Cellulose, Red 40 Lake, Magnesium Stearate, Polysorbate 80, Titanium Dioxide, Povidone, Beta Carotene, Ergocalciferol.
See Editor's Note No. 45.

YourLife One Daily 50 + **-** Leiner Health Products
Each tablet contains: Biotin 30 mcg • Calcium 120 mg • Chloride 34 mg • Chromium 180 mcg • Copper 2 mg • Iodine 150 mcg • Magnesium 100 mg • Manganese 4 mg • Molybdenum 93.75 mcg • Potassium 37.5 mg • Selenium 105 mcg • Vitamin A 5000 IU • Vitamin B12 30 mcg • Vitamin B6 6 mg • Vitamin C 120 mg • Vitamin D 400 IU • Vitamin E 60 IU • Vitamin K 20 mcg • Zinc 22.5 mg. Other Ingredients: Niacinamide Ascorbate, Starch, Cellulose, Maltodextrin, Hydroxypropyl Methylcellulose, Croscarmellose Sodium, Gelatin, Titanium Dioxide, Silicon Dioxide, Crospovidone, Magnesium Stearate, Thiamine Mononitrate, Hydroxypropyl Cellulose, Riboflavin, Resin, Mannitol, Yellow 6 Lake, Blue 2 Lake, Beta Carotene, Folic Acid, Sodium Molybdate, Sodium Selenate.
See Editor's Note No. 45.

YourLife One Daily Men's Formula - Leiner Health Products
Each tablet contains: Chloride 34 mg • Chromium 150 mcg • Copper 2 mg • Iodine 150 mcg • Magnesium 100 mg • Manganese 3.5 mg • Molybdenum 75 mcg • Potassium 37.5 mg • Selenium 87.5 mcg • Vitamin A 5000 IU • Vitamin B12 9 mcg • Vitamin B6 3 mg • Vitamin C 90 mg • Vitamin D 400 IU • Vitamin E 45 IU • Zinc 15 mg. Other Ingredients: Niacinamide Ascorbate, Starch, Cellulose, Gelatin, Croscarmellose Sodium, Hydroxypropyl Methylcellulose, Crospovidone, Hydroxypropyl Cellulose, Silicon Dioxide, Pharmaceutical Glaze, Polyethylene Glycol 3350, Magnesium Stearate, Yellow 6 Lake, Riboflavin, Thiamine Mononitrate, Titanium Dioxide, Resin, Beta Carotene, Folic Acid, Sodium Molybdate, Polysorbate 80.
See Editor's Note No. 45.

YourLife One Daily Plus Minerals - Leiner Health Products
Each tablet contains: Biotin 30 mcg • Calcium 130 mg • Chloride 34 mg • Chromium 10 mcg • Copper 2 mg • Folic Acid (folate) 400 mcg • Iodine 150 mcg • Iron 18 mg • Magnesium 100 mg • Manganese 2.5 mg • Molybdenum 10 mcg • Niacin (vitamin B3) 20 mg • Pantothenic Acid (vitamin B5) 10 mg • Phosphorus 100 mg • Potassium 37.5 mg • Riboflavin (vitamin B2) 1.7 mg • Selenium 10 mcg • Thiamin (vitamin B1) 1.5 mg • Vitamin A 5000 IU • Vitamin B12 6 mcg • Vitamin B6 2 mg • Vitamin C 60 mg • Vitamin D 400 IU • Vitamin E 30 IU • Zinc 15 mg. Other Ingredients: Gelatin, Pregelatinized Starch, Cellulose, Sodium Starch Glycolate, Hydroxypropyl Methylcellulose, Croscarmellose Sodium, Silicon Dioxide, Tricalcium Phosphate, Red 40 Lake, Polyethylene Glycol 3350, Hydroxypropyl Cellulose, Pharmaceutical Glaze, Magnesium Stearate, Crospovidone, Polysorbate 80, Titanium Dioxide, Resin, Povidone, Molybdenum Yeast, Ergocalciferol.
See Editor's Note No. 45.

YourLife One Daily Women's Formula - Leiner Health Products
Each tablet contains: Calcium 450 mg • Iron 27 mg • Vitamin A 5000 IU • Vitamin B12 6 mcg • Vitamin B6 2 mg • Vitamin C 60 mg • Vitamin D 400 IU • Vitamin E 30 IU • Zinc 15 mg. Other Ingredients: Maltodextrin, Gelatin, Hydroxypropyl Methylcellulose, Croscarmellose Sodium, Sodium Starch Glycolate, Niacinamide, Silicon Dioxide, Propylene Glycol, Titanium Dioxide, Hydroxypropyl Cellulose, Polyethylene Glycol 3350, Pharmaceutical Glaze, Starch, Magnesium Stearate, Yellow 5 Lake, Yellow 6 Lake, Polysorbate 80, Beta Carotene, Riboflavin, Povidone, Resin, Folic Acid.
See Editor's Note No. 45.

YourLife Oyster Shell Calcium 250 mg With D - Leiner Health Products
Each tablet contains: Calcium (oyster shell) 250 mg • Vitamin D (ergocalciferol) 125 IU. Other Ingredients: Maltodextrin, Acacia, Cellulose, Mineral Oil, Croscarmellose Sodium, Tricalcium Phosphate, Soy Fiber, Magnesium Stearate, Crospovidone, Stearic Acid.
See Editor's Note No. 45.

YourLife Oyster Shell Calcium 500 mg - Leiner Health Products
Each tablet contains: Calcium (oyster shell) 500 mg. Other Ingredients: Maltodextrin, Acacia Gum, Croscarmellose Sodium, Tricalcium Phosphate, Magnesium Stearate.
See Editor's Note No. 45.

YourLife Oyster Shell Calcium 500 mg With D - Leiner Health Products
Each tablet contains: Calcium (oyster shell) 500 mg • Vitamin D (as ergocalciferol) 200 IU. Other Ingredients: Maltodextrin, Croscarmellose Sodium, Cellulose, Mineral Oil, Gelatin, Magnesium Stearate.
See Editor's Note No. 45.

YourLife Potassium Gluconate 550 mg - Leiner Health Products
Each tablet contains: Potassium (from potassium gluconate) 90 mg. Other Ingredients: Cellulose, Croscarmellose Sodium, Starch, Silicon Dioxide, Stearic Acid, Magnesium Stearate.
See Editor's Note No. 45.

YourLife Prenatal Tablets - Leiner Health Products
Each tablet contains: Calcium 200 mg • Iron 27 mg • Vitamin A 4000 IU • Vitamin B12 4 mcg • Vitamin B6 2.6 mg • Vitamin C 100 mg • Vitamin D 400 IU • Vitamin E 11 IU • Zinc 25 mg. Other Ingredients: Cellulose, Maltodextrin, Starch, Hydroxypropyl Methylcellulose, Croscarmellose Sodium, Sodium Starch Glycolate, Gelatin, Silicon Dioxide, Tricalcium Phosphate, Polyethylene Glycol 3350, Hydroxypropyl Cellulose, Titanium Dioxide, Magnesium Stearate, Pharmaceutical Glaze, Thiamine Mononitrate, Polysorbate 80, Riboflavin, Lactose, Folic Acid, Yellow 6 Lake, Red 40 Lake, Blue 1 Lake, Beta Carotene, Resin.
See Editor's Note No. 45.

YourLife Selenium 200 mcg - Leiner Health Products
Each tablet contains: Selenium (as Selenoexcell brand selenium yeast) 200 mcg. Other Ingredients: Calcium Carbonate, Maltodextrin, Cellulose, Croscarmellose Sodium, Tricalcium Phosphate, Crospovidone, Polyethylene Glycol 3350, Silicon Dioxide, Magnesium Stearate, Hydroxypropyl Methylcellulose, Hydroxypropyl Cellulose, Polysorbate 80.
See Editor's Note No. 45.

YourLife Vitamin A 8000 IU - Leiner Health Products
Each softgel contains: Vitamin A 8000 IU. Other Ingredients: Vegetable Oil, Gelatin, Glycerin, Fish Liver Oil.
See Editor's Note No. 45.

YourLife Vitamin B-12 100 mcg - Leiner Health Products
Each tablet contains: Vitamin B12 100 mcg. Other Ingredients: Lactose, Starch, Dicalcium Phosphate, Magnesium Stearate, Red 40 Lake.
See Editor's Note No. 45.

YourLife Vitamin B-6 - Leiner Health Products
Each tablet contains: Vitamin B6 100 mg. Other Ingredients: Dicalcium Phosphate, Cellulose, Starch, Croscarmellose Sodium, Polyethylene Glycol 3350, Silicon Dioxide, Magnesium Stearate.
See Editor's Note No. 45.

YourLife Vitamin C 1000 mg - Leiner Health Products
Each tablet contains: Vitamin C 1000 mg. Other Ingredients: Starch, Cellulose, Crospovidone, Magnesium Stearate, Silicon Dioxide, Stearic Acid.
See Editor's Note No. 45.

YourLife Vitamin C 1000 mg with Rose Hips - Leiner Health Products
Each tablet contains: Vitamin C 1000 mg. Other Ingredients: Starch, Cellulose, Dicalcium Phosphate, Rose Hips, Stearic Acid, Hydroxypropyl Methylcellulose, Magnesium Stearate, Silicon Dioxide, Croscarmellose Sodium, Sodium Starch Glycolate.
See Editor's Note No. 45.

YourLife Vitamin C 250 mg - Leiner Health Products
Each tablet contains: Vitamin C 250 mg. Other Ingredients: Calcium Carbonate, Maltodextrin, Cellulose, Starch, Silicon Dioxide, Stearic Acid, Magnesium Stearate, Sodium Starch Glycolate, Croscarmellose Sodium.
See Editor's Note No. 45.

YourLife Vitamin C 500 mg - Leiner Health Products
Each tablet contains: Vitamin C 500 mg. Other Ingredients: Starch, Crospovidone, Cellulose, Magnesium Stearate, Stearic Acid, Croscarmellose Sodium, Silicon Dioxide, Lactose.
See Editor's Note No. 45.

BRAND NAMES

YourLife Vitamin C 500 mg with Rose Hips - Leiner Health Products
Each tablet contains: Vitamin C 500 mg. Other Ingredients: Starch, Cellulose, Rose Hips, Stearic Acid, Silicon Dioxide, Magnesium Stearate, Croscarmellose Sodium.
See Editor's Note No. 45.

YourLife Vitamin D 400 IU - Leiner Health Products
Each tablet contains: Vitamin D 400 IU. Other Ingredients: Dicalcium Phosphate, Cellulose, Corn Starch, Croscarmellose Sodium, Silicon Dioxide, Magnesium Stearate, Stearic Acid, Dextrin, Dextrose, Lecithin, Sodium Carboxymethylcellulose, Sodium Citrate.
See Editor's Note No. 45.

YourLife Vitamin E 1000 IU - Leiner Health Products
Each softgel contains: Vitamin E 1000 IU. Other Ingredients: Gelatin, Glycerin, Vegetable Oil.
See Editor's Note No. 45.

YourLife Vitamin E 200 IU - Leiner Health Products
Each softgel contains: Vitamin E 200 IU. Other Ingredients: Gelatin, Glycerin, Vegetable Oil.
See Editor's Note No. 45.

YourLife Vitamin E 400 IU - Leiner Health Products
Each softgel contains: Vitamin E 400 IU. Other Ingredients: Gelatin, Glycerin, Vegetable Oil.
See Editor's Note No. 45.

YourLife Vitamin E 400 IU Water Dispersible - Leiner Health Products
Each softgel contains: Vitamin E 400 IU. Other Ingredients: Gelatin, Polysorbate 80, Glycerin, Soybean Oil.
See Editor's Note No. 45.

YourLife Vitamin E 400 IU with C 500 mg - Leiner Health Products
Each softgel contains: Vitamin C 500 mg • Vitamin E 400 IU. Other Ingredients: Gelatin, Glycerin, Soybean Oil, Yellow Beeswax, Vegetable Shortening (soybean and cottonseed oil), Lecithin, Red 40, Titanium Dioxide, Red 3, Blue 1.
See Editor's Note No. 45.

YourLife Vitamin E 800 IU - Leiner Health Products
Each softgel contains: Vitamin E 800 IU. Other Ingredients: Gelatin, Glycerin.
See Editor's Note No. 45.

YourLife Zinc Gluconate 50 mg - Leiner Health Products
Each tablet contains: Zinc (as zinc gluconate) 50 mg. Other Ingredients: Starch, Croscarmellose Sodium, Sodium Starch Glycolate, Magnesium Stearate.
See Editor's Note No. 45.

Youth Flex - Nature's Youth
Two capsules contain: Vitamin C (as Ester C brand calcium ascorbate) 40 mg • Zinc (as zinc monomethionine) 10 mg • Copper (as copper gluconate) 0.83 mg • Manganese (as manganese gluconate) 10 mg • Glucosamine Sulfate 2KCl 500 mg • Cetyl Myristoleate complex 200 mg • IsoOxygene brand Hops strobile extract 500 mg • Boron (as boron chelate) 67 mcg • Boswellia Serrata gum extract 50 mg. Other Ingredients: Gelatin, Calcium Sulfate, Magnesium Stearate, Silica.

Youth-Assure - Nature's Plus
Two tablets contain: Rapid Release Layer: Melatonin (N-Acetyl-5-Methoxytryptamine) 3 mg. Sustained Release Layer: Pregnenolone 50 mg • DHEA pharmaceutical grade Dehydroepiandrosterone 25 mg • LECI-PS 25 mg: Phosphatidylserine (PS) 5 mg, Phosphatidylcholine (PC) 5 mg, Phosphoinositides 1.5 mg, Cephalin (phosphatidylethanolamine) 3 mg.
See Editor's Note No. 16.

YouthPrep - HealthMinded
Four capsules contain: YouthPrep Proprietary Blend 2715 mg: Amino Acid Peptide Complex (from wheat gluten), Colostrum (bovine source), Tribulus herb dried extract, Citrus Bioflavonoids complex (from grapefruit), Chrysin (as dihydroxy flavone), Phosphatidyl Serine (from soy lecithin), Phosphatidyl Choline (from soy lecithin). Other Ingredients: Gelatin, Stearic Acid, Magnesium Stearate.
See Editor's Note No. 14.

YouthPrep15 - HealthMinded
Four capsules contain: Anterior Pituitary 80 mg • Hypothalamus 20 mg • Amino Acid Blend (essential amino acids) 1200 mg • Phytosterol Complex 40 mg: Beta Sitosterol, Campesterol, Stigmasterol • Soy Phosphatide Complex 80 mg: Phosphatidylserine, Phosphatidylcholine, Phosphatidylehtanolamine, Phosphatidylinositol • Panax Ginseng 80 mg. Other Ingredients: Gelatin, Stearic Acid, Magnesium Stearate.
See Editor's Note No. 31.

YST-RES-Q - Nutri-Quest Rx
Two tablets contain: Lacto Bacillus 1 million IU • Caprylic Acid 50 mg • Grapefruit seed extract 100 mg • Garlic 25 mg • Berberis aquifolium 100 mg • Aloe Vera 25 mg • Undecenoic Acid 50 mg.

Yu Ping Feng San Plus - Secara
Astragalus root 5:1 extract (huang qi) 736 mg • Atractylodes rhizome 5:1 extract (bai zhu) 614 mg • Siler root 5:1 extract (fang feng) 450 mg • Organic Echinacea root 225 mg • Shiitake fruit body (20% polysaccharides, 45 mg) 225 mg.

Yu Xiao San 8805 - Chong's Health Care Enterprise, Inc.
Two tablets contain: Euonymus 374 mg • Lycium bark 544 mg • Burdock 238 mg • Platycodon root 238 mg • Lichi seed 204 mg • Turmeric 68 mg • American Ginseng 34 mg.

Yucca Burdock Supreme - Gaia Herbs
Thirty drops contain: Proprietary Blend 50 mg: Yucca root, Echinacea Supreme (echinacea angustifolia root, echinacea purpurea root, flower head and stem), Burdock root and seed (arctium lappa), Poke root (phytolacca americana), Dried Celery seed (apium graveolens), Dried Bladderwrack fronds (fucus vesiculosus), Pipsissewa herb (chimaphila umbellata), Spring Water, 45-55% Pure Grain Alcohol.

Yucca extract 4:1 - Jarrow Formulas
Each capsule contains: Yucca juice 4:1 extract (yucca schidigera) 500 mg. Other Ingredients: Magnesium Stearate, Gelatin.

Yucca-AR Formula - Nature's Way
Two capsules contain: Proprietary Formula: Black Cohosh root • Black Walnut hulls • Brigham Tea herb • Burdock root • Cayenne pepper fruit • Hydrangea root • Rosemary herb • Sarsaparilla root • Valerian root • Wild Lettuce leaf • Wild Yam root • Yucca stalk. Other Ingredients: Gelatin.

Yunnan Paiyao - Yunnan Paiyao Group
Active Ingredients: San-Qi Ginseng root, Herb of Clarke, Chinese Yam root, Wild Yam root, Geranium, Lesser Galangal herb, Ox Gallbladder. Inactive Ingredients: Gelatin, Water, FD&C Red No. 40.

Z 23 - Hillestad
Two tablets contain: Vitamin A (100% as beta carotene) 15,000 IU • Vitamin C (as ascorbic acid) 200 mg • Vitamin E (as D-atocopheryl succinate) 120 IU • Vitamin B6 (as pyridoxine HCl) 100 mg • Magnesium (as magnesium oxide) 100 mg • Zinc (as zinc oxide and zinc gluconate) 150 mg • Bee Pollen 200 mg • L-Lysine 100 mg • Saw Palmetto fruit 200 mg • American Ginseng root 100 mg • Glycine 100 mg • Parsley root 50 mg • Chamomile flower 50 mg • Prostate gland 50 mg • Gotu Kola leaf 50 mg • Juniper berry 50 mg • Milkweed seed 50 mg • Uva Ursi leaf 50 mg • Yucca root 50 mg • Echinacea root 50 mg • Gravel root 50 mg • Hydrangea root 50 mg • Buchu leaf extract 50 mg • Pygeum bark 50 mg. Other Ingredients: Cellulose, Glyceryl Stearate, Gum Arabic, Silica, Magnesium Stearate, Oyster Shell, Sorbitol, Chlorophyll.
See Editor's Note No. 14.

Zaizao - Balanceuticals
Each capsule contains: Proprietary Blend 500 mg: Herba Hedyotis Diffusae, Radix Sophorae Tonkinenisis, Radix Astragali Seu Hedysari, Aloe, Garlic, Fructus Chebulae, Fructus Chaenomelis, Radix Ginseng.

Zalestra - Optimal Therapeutics
Two capsules contain: Green Tea leaf extract (camellia sinensis, 80% catechins, 60% EGCG) 200 mg • Guggul extract (2.5% E + G guggulsterones) 200 mg • Octopalean brand Octopamine HCl 100 mg • Maca root powder (lepidium meyenii) 80 mg • Jojoba meal extract (60% simmondsin) 40 mg • Indole-3-Carbinol 30 mg • Borage oil powder (borago officinalis) 25 mg • Mega Soy extract 20 mg • Manganese 10 mg • Black Cohosh (2.5% triterpene) 10 mg • DHEA (dehydroepiandrosterone) 7.5 mg • Vitex fruit extract (5% vitexicarpin) 5 mg • Bioperine brand Black Pepper extract 2 mg. Other Ingredients: Gelatin, Cellulose, Magnesium Stearate.

Zallnex Male Formula - Nutranex
Two capsules contain: Vitamin B6 (pyridoxine HCl) 3 mg • Magnesium (magnesium aspartate) 8.5 mg • Zinc (zinc aspartate) 1.6 mg • Zallouh root (Ferula harmonis L.) 250 mg • Muira Puama bark (pxchopetalum olecosides) 250 mg • Arginine HCl 200 mg • Tribulis terrestris L. fruit 100 mg. Other Ingredients: Gelatin, Rice Flour.

Zamoreve Female Formula - Nutranex
Two capsules contain: Vitamin B6 (pyridoxine HCl) 3 mg • Magnesium (magnesium aspartate) 8.5 mg • Zinc (zinc aspartate) 1.6 mg • Zallouh root (ferula harmonis L) 200 mg • Tribulis terrestris L. fruit 100 mg • Avena sativa L. fruit 100 mg • Nettle root 100 mg. Other Ingredients: Gelatin, Rice Flour.

Zand Quietussin - Botanical Laboratories
Each 1 tsp serving contains: Chinese Fritillaria bulb • Loquat leaf • Mullein leaf • Platycodon Grandiflorum root • Schisandra fruit • Pinellia rhizome • Peucedanum root • Marshmallow root • Trichosanthes root • Licorice root • Horehound herb • Fritillaria Cirrhosa bulb • Scullcap herb • Coptis rhizome.

Zantrex-3 - Zoller Laboratories
Two capsules contain: Niacin (vitamin B3) 50 mg • Zantrex-3 Proprietary Blend 1312 mg: Yerba Mate bark standardized extract (SE), Caffeine, Guarana seed SE, Damiana leaf/stem SE, Schizonepeta Spica SE, Green Tea leaf SE, Piper Nigrum fruit SE, Tibetan Ginseng root SE, Panax Ginseng root SE, Maca root SE, Cocoa Nut SE, Kola Nut SE, Thea Sinensis leaf complex. Other Ingredients: Rice Flour.

ZeaVision - ZeaVision, LLC
Each capsule contains: Zeaxanthin 10 mg. Inactive Ingredients: Gelatin, Sodium Laurel Sulfate, Cellulose, Vegetable Stearate, Sucrose, Corn Starch, Sodium Ascorbate, Ascorbyl Palmitate, dl-Alpha-Tocopherol, Titanium Dioxide, Colors.

Zeel ointment - Heel/BHI, Inc.
Each 100 g serving contains: Silicea 6X • Symphytum Officinale 8X • Arnica Montana radix 2X • Rhus Toxicodendron 2X • Sulphur 6X • Sanguinaria Canadensis 2X • Dulcamara 2X • Coenzyme A 6X • Alpha-Lipoicum Acidum 6X • Nadidum 6X • Natrum Oxalaceticum 6X • Cartilago Suis 2X • Embryo Totalis Suis 2X • Funiculus Umbilicalis Suis 2X • Placenta Suis 2X.
See Editor's Note No. 1.

Zeel Tablets - Heel/BHI, Inc.
Each tablet contains: Silicea 6X 3 mg • Arnica Montana, Radix 1X 0.6 mg • Rhus Toxicodendron 1X 0.54 mg • Sulphur 6X 0.54 mg • Sanguinaria Canadensis 3X 0.45 mg • Cartilago Suis 4X 0.3 mg • Embryo Totalis Suis 4X 0.3 mg • Funiculus Umbilicalis Suis 4X 0.3 mg • Placenta Suis 4X 0.3 mg • Dulcamara 2X 0.15 mg • Symphytum Officinale 8X 0.15 mg • Coenzyme A 6X 0.03 mg • Lipoicum Acidum 6X 0.03 mg • Nadidum 6X 0.03 mg • Natrum Oxalaceticum 6X 0.03 mg. Other Ingredients: Lactose Base.
See Editor's Note No. 1.

Zenibolin - Syntrax Innovations
Each .25 mL contains: 19-Nor (5) Androstenediol • Isotonic Saline • Carboxymethylcellulose • Benzyl Alcohol.
See Editor's Note No. 54.

Zero Gravity Weight Management Formula - Garden of Life, Inc.
Three caplets contain: Poten-Zyme Organic Grapefruit extract 1320 mg • Sea Vegetable Blend (45% fucoidans) 600 mg: Ecklonia, Ascophyllum Nodosum, Laminaria Japonica, Macrocystis, Alaria • Rhododendron Caucasicum extract (40% polyphenols) 450 mg • Rhodiola Rosea extract (3% rosavin) 300 mg • Blueberry leaf extract (20% chlorogenic acid) 150 mg • Magnolia extract (60% magnolol) 30 mg • Poten-Zyme Probiotic blend 2.4 Billion CFU. Other Ingredients: Cellulose, Silicon Dioxide, Stearates.

Zestra Feminine Arousal Fluid - QualiLife Pharmaceuticals
Borage Seed Oil • Evening Primrose Oil • Angelica Extract • Coleus Extract • Vitamin C • Vitamin E • Natural Fragrances.
See Editor's Note No. 29.

Zesty Onion & Garlic Soynuts - Physicians Laboratories
Each 1/6 Cup Contains: Certified Isoflavone 10 mg. Ingredients: Soy Protein (whole roasted soybeans), Soybean Oil, Dehydrated Onion and Garlic, Salt, Dextrose, Corn Starch, Parsley, Natural Flavor.

Zhi Bai Di Huang Wan Plus - Secara
Rehmannia cured root tuber 5:1 extract (shu di huang) 487 mg • Asiatic Dogwood fruit 5:1 extract (shan zhu yu) 243 mg • Chinese Yam rhizome 5:1 extract (shan yao) 243 mg • Organic American Ginseng root 225 mg • Asian Water Plantain rhizome 5:1 extract (ze xie) 218 mg • Poria sclerotium 5:1 extract (fu ling) 218 mg • Ginkgo leaf (24% flavone glycosides, 43 mg) 178 mg • Anemarrhena rhizome 5:1 extract (zhi mu) 146 mg • Tree Peony root bark 5:1 extract (mu dan pi) 146 mg • Phellodendron bark 5:1 extract (huang bai) 146 mg.

Zicam Cold Remedy Nasal Spray - Zicam, LLC
Active Ingredients: Zinc (zincum gluconium) 2X. Inactive Ingredients: Benzalkonium Chloride, Glycerine, Purified Water, Hydroxyethylcellulose, Sodium Chloride, Sodium Hydroxide.
See Editor's Note No. 1.

Zicam Nasal Moisturizer - Zicam, LLC
Purified Water • Sodium Phosphate • Hydroxyethylcellulose • Disodium Phosphate • Glycerin • Alkoxylated Diester • Aloe Barbadensis gel • Hydrolyzed Algin • Chlorella Vulgaris extract • Sea Water • Benzalkonium Chloride • Benzyl Alcohol • Disodium EDTA • Hydroxylated Lecithin • Tocopherol • Polysorbate 80.

Zicam Seasonal Allergy Relief - Zicam, LLC
Active Ingredients: Luffa Operculata 4X, 12X, 30X • Galphimia Glauca 12X, 30X • Histaminum Hydrochloricum 12X, 30X, 200X • Sulphur 12X, 30X, 200X. Inactive Ingredients: Benzalkonium Chloride, Benzyl Alcohol, Edetate Disodium, Glycerine, Hydroxyethylcellulose, Potassium Chloride, Potassium Phosphate, Purified Water, Sodium Chloride, Sodium Phosphate.
See Editor's Note No. 1.

Zinaxin - FreeLife International
Each softgel contains: Patented Ginger extract EV.EXT 33 (Zingiber officinale) root 255 mg. Other Ingredients: Soybean oil, Silicon Dioxide, Lecithin, Gelatine, Glycerin, Sorbitol, Water, Natural Chlorophyll Complex, Titanium Dioxide (natural mineral color).

Zinaxin (HMP-33) - Eurovita A/S, Denmark
Each capsule contains: Zingiber Officinale Roscoe Extract (HMP-33 Extract) 255 mg.

Zinaxin Rapid - Eurovita A/S, Denmark
Each capsule contains: Ginger Extract EV.EXT 77 (255 mg is equivalent to approximately 3000 mg of dried ginger rhizome and 1500 mg of dried galanga rhizome) • Sunflower Seed Oil • Gelatin • Glycerol • Beeswax Yellow • Lecithin • Titanium Dioxide • Copper Chlorophyllins.

Zinc **-** Benepure, Inc
Each capsule contains: Vitamin C (ascorbic acid) 100 mg • Zinc (as zinc picolinate) 15 mg. Other Ingredients: Gelatin, Calcium Carbonate, Cellulose, Silica, Vegetable Stearate.

Zinc **-** Source Naturals
Each tablet contains: Zinc (from 500 mg of zinc amino acid chelate) 50 mg • Copper (from 3.57 mg of copper sebacate) 500 mcg.

Zinc **-** EcoNugenics
Each capsule contains: Zinc (as methionine, orotate, picolinate) 30 mg. Other Ingredients: Dicalcium Phosphate, Gelatin, Cellulose, Magnesium Stearate, Silica.

Zinc (citrate) **-** Pure Encapsulations
Each vegetable capsule contains: Zinc (citrate) 30 mg • Vitamin C (as ascorbyl palmitate) 4 mg.

Zinc + C **-** Golden Glow Natural Health Products
Each tablet contains: Zinc (from gluconate) 6.5 mg • Vitamin C (from ascorbic acid 150 mg and sodium ascorbate 112.5 mg) 250 mg. Other Ingredients: Glucose, Sucrose.

Zinc 10 mg **-** Jamieson
Each tablet contains: Elemental Zinc 10 mg.

Zinc 10 mg - Chelated **-** Jamieson
Each tablet contains: Elemental Zinc 10 mg. Chelated (microbound) to Amino Acid from organic Soy to aid in Zinc assimilation.

Zinc 100 mg **-** GNC
Each tablet contains: Zinc (as zinc gluconate) 100 mg. Other Ingredients: Cellulose.

Zinc 15 **-** Pure Encapsulations
Each vegetable capsule contains: Zinc (picolinate) 15 mg.

Zinc 15 mg **-** J. R. Carlson Laboratories, Inc.
Each tablet contains: Zinc (as zinc gluconate) 15 mg.

Zinc 25 mg **-** Nature's Sunshine
Each tablet contains: Calcium (di-calcium phosphate) 45 mg • Phosphorus (di-calcium phosphate) 35 mg • Zinc (zinc gluconate) 25 mg • Proprietary Blend 130 mg: Kelp plant (ascophyllum nodosum and laminaria digitata), Thyme herb (thymus vulgaris), Alfalfa herb (medicago sativa). Other Ingredients: Cellulose, Magnesium Stearate.

Zinc 25 mg **-** Jamieson
Each tablet contains: Elemental Zinc (gluconate) 25 mg.

Zinc 30 **-** Pure Encapsulations
Each vegetable capsule contains: Zinc (picolinate) 30 mg • Vitamin C (as ascorbyl palmitate) 4 mg.

Zinc 30 mg **-** Nature Made
Each tablet contains: Zinc (from zinc gluconate) 30 mg.
Other Ingredients: Dibasic Calcium Phosphate, Magnesium Stearate, Croscarmellose Sodium.
See Editor's Note No. 45.

Zinc 30mg **-** Vital Nutrients
Each capsule contains: Zinc (citrate) 30 mg.

Zinc 50 mg **-** Nature Made
Each tablet contains: Zinc 50 mg.
See Editor's Note No. 45.

Zinc 50 mg **-** GNC
Each tablet contains: Zinc (as zinc gluconate) 50 mg.
Other Ingredients: Cellulose.

Zinc 50 mg **-** Jamieson
Each tablet contains: Elemental Zinc (gluconate) 50 mg.

Zinc 50 mg **-** J. R. Carlson Laboratories, Inc.
Each tablet contains: Zinc (as zinc gluconate) 50 mg.

Zinc 50 mg **-** Sunmark
Each tablet contains: Zinc 50 mg. Other Ingredients: Microcrystalline Cellulose, Dicalcium Phosphate, Croscamellose Sodium, Stearic Acid, Magnesium Stearate.
See Editor's Note No. 45.

Zinc 50 mg - Timed Release **-** Jamieson
Each tablet contains: Zinc (organic gluconate) 50 mg. Prepared in a special time-diffused micro-encapsulation allowing for a gradual release of Zinc over six to eight hours.

Zinc 60 mg **-** Nature Made
Each tablet contains: Zinc (from zinc gluconate) 60 mg.
Other Ingredients: Dibasic Calcium Phosphate, Cellulose Gel, Stearic Acid, Magnesium Stearate, Croscarmellose Sodium.
See Editor's Note No. 45.

Zinc A.G. **-** Metagenics
Each tablet contains: Zinc (as zinc arginate, glycinate) 20 mg.

Zinc Ascorbs **-** Alacer
Each tablet contains: Vitamin C (zinc ascorbate) 90 mg • Zinc (zinc ascorbate) 10 mg • Vitamin B6 (pyridoxine HCl) 5 mg • Bioflavonoids 50 mg. Base: Cellulose, Bioflavonoids.

Zinc Balance **-** Jarrow Formulas
Each capsule contains: Zinc (OptiZinc brand monomethionine) 15 mg • Copper (gluconate) 1 mg. Other Ingredients: Cellulose, Magnesium Stearate, Gelatin.

Zinc Boost **-** Golden Glow Natural Health Products
Each tablet contains: Zinc Amino Acid Chelate 220 mg: Zinc 22 mg.

Zinc Chelate **-** Pro Health
Each tablet contains: Zinc (amino chelate) 50 mg • Copper (sebacate) 500 mcg. Other Ingredients: Dibasic Calcium Phosphate, Stearic Acid, Sorbitol, Modified Cellulose Gum, Vegetable Fiber, Colloidal Silicon Dioxide, Magnesium Stearate.

Zinc Chewable **-** Aspen Group, Inc.
Each tablet contains: Amino Acid Chelated Minerals as Zinc 29 mg • Raw Tissue concentrates (bovine source) from: Spleen 29 mg, Brain 8 mg, Liver 5 mg, Heart 4 mg, Kidney 4 mg, Thymus 2 mg, Adrenal 2 mg, Pituitary 1 mg, Duodenum 1 mg.
See Editor's Note No. 31.

Zinc Citrate **-** Quest
Each tablet contains: Zinc (Citrate) 50 mg. Other Ingredients: Croscarmellose Sodium, Calcium Phosphate, Magnesium Stearate, Microcrystalline Cellulose, Silicon Dioxide, Vegetable Stearin.

Zinc Citrate + **-** American Biologics
Each capsule contains: Zinc (as citrate) 50 mg • Copper (as citrate) 1.5 mg. Other Ingredients: Cellulose, Magnesium Stearate.

Zinc Drink **-** Metagenics
Each 1 tsp serving contains: Zinc (sulfate) 15 mg.

Zinc Ease **-** J. R. Carlson Laboratories, Inc.
Each tablet contains: Zinc (citrate) 10 mg.

Zinc for Acne **-** Puritan's Pride
Two tablets contain: Vitamin A (retinyl palmitate) 1,000 IU • Vitamin C (with rose hips) 150 mg • Vitamin E (DL-alpha tocopheryl acetate) 50 IU • Vitamin B6 20 mg • Zinc (gluconate) 50 mg.

Zinc Liver Chelate **-** Standard Process, Inc.
Each tablet contains: Proprietary Blend 296 mg: Bovine Liver, Carrot root, Beet root, Dried Beet root juice, Oat flour • Zinc 10 mg. Other Ingredients: Honey, Arabic Gum, Calcium Stearate.

Zinc Lozenge **-** Benepure, Inc
Each lozenge contains: Zinc (gluconate and citrate) 23 mg. Other Ingredients: Fructose, Sorbitol, Microcrystalline Cellulose, Honey Powder, Stearic Acid, Citric Acid, Natural and Artifical Flavors, Magnesium Stearate, Silica.

Zinc Lozenge - Nutri-Quest Rx
Each lozenge contains: Zinc Gluconate 75 mg.

Zinc Lozenge - Nature's Way
Each lozenge contains: Echinacea Purpurea (stem, leaf, flower) 20 mg • Stevia dried extract 3 mg • Vitamin C (ascorbic acid) 100 mg • Zinc Citrate 23 mg. Other Ingredients: French Vanilla flavor, Fructose, Magnesium stearate, Mannitol, Sodium, Sorbitol, Wild Berry flavor.

Zinc Lozenges - Nature's Plus
Each lozenge contains: Zinc (as aspartate) 15 mg. Other Ingredients: Fructose, Natural Flavors, Stearic Acid, Carob, Magnesium Stearate, Silica.

Zinc Lozenges - Jamieson
Each lozenge contains: Vitamin C (as Ascorbic Acid) 50 mg • Zinc (as Zinc Gluconate) 5 mg. Other Ingredients: Eucalyptus, Anise Oil, Menthol, Camphor, Lemon.

Zinc Lozenges - Futurebiotics LLC
One lozenge contains: Vitamin C (from ascorbic acid) 60 mg • Zinc (as zinc citrate) 15 mg • Herbal Lozenge Blend, 8 mg: Echinacea leaf powder 4:1 extract, Goldenseal root powder 4:1 extract, Elderberry flower powder, Bee Propolis powder, Peppermint leaf powder, Kava Kava root powder. Other Ingredients: Orange crystals, Orange flavor, Magnesium stearate, Stearic acid, Mannitol, Fructose, Cane sugar.

Zinc Lozenges - Nature's Life
Each lozenge contains: Zinc (Gluconate) 10 mg • Vitamin C 100 mg • Beta Carotene (equivalent to 500 IU Vitamin A) 300 mcg • Purple Cone Flower root (Echinacea purpurea) 25 mg. In a natural base of low-Glycemic, pure Crystalline Fructose, pasteurized Honey powder, Hydrogenated Vegetable oil, natural Peppermint flavor, Eucalyptus leaf (Eucalyptus globulus) Licorice root (Glycyrrhiza glabra), Goldenseal root (Hydrastis canadensis), Slippery Elm bark (Ulmus ruba), & Fenugreek seed (Trigonella foenum-graecum).

Zinc Lozenges - Oringinal Formula - Jamieson
Each lozenge contains: Zinc Gluconate 35 mg.

Zinc Lozenges - Vitamin C, Anise, Menthol, Camphor, Eucalyptus - Jamieson
Each lozenge contains: Vitamin C (as Ascorbic Acid) 50 mg • Zinc (as Zinc Gluconate) 5 mg • In a base of Eucalyptus, Anise Oil, Menthol, Camphor, Lemon.

Zinc Lozenges Cherry with Vitamin C and B-6 - Leiner Health Products
Each lozenge contains: Vitamin B6 (Pyridoxine Hydrochloride) 5 mg • Vitamin C 60 mg • Zinc 15 mg • Other Ingredients: Sugar, Zinc Aspartate, Stearic Acid, Sodium Ascorbate, Maltodextrin, Ascorbic Acid, Mono- and Diglycerides, Magnesium Stearate, Silicon Dioxide, Aspartame, Red 40 Lake, Artificial Cherry Flavor, Starch. Phenylketonurics: Contains Phenylalanine.

Zinc Lozenges Plus - The Vitamin Shoppe
Each lozenge contains: Zinc 24 mg • Echinacea 100 mg • Vitamin C 150 mg • Propolis 100 mg • Vitamin A 1000 IU • Slippery Elm 25 mg. In a base of Golden Seal, Acerola, Fructose Cellulose, with Vanilla and Orange flavor.

Zinc Lozenges with Echinacea and Vitamin C - Jamieson
Each lozenge contains: Elemental Zinc (from Zinc Citrate) 5 mg • Vitamin C (Ascorbic Acid) 50 mg • Echinacea (Derived from 12.5 mg root extract, 1:4 of Echinanea Purpurea) 50 mg • Sorbitol • Fructose • Wild Cherry Flavor.

Zinc Lozenges with Vitamin C - GNC
Two lozenges contain: Sodium 10 mg • Vitamin C 120 mg (as Ascorbic Acid and Sodium Ascorbate) • Zinc (as Zinc Oxide, Zinc Gluconate). Ingredients: Sorbitol, Lactitol, Cellulose, Natural Flavors, Peppermint oil, Eucalyptus oil, Anise oil, Sucralose, Camphor.

Zinc Lozenges with Vitamin C - Jamieson
Each lozenge contains: Elemental Zinc (from Zinc Citrate) 5 mg • Vitamin C (Ascorbic Acid) 50 mg • Echinacea Root (Echinacea Purpurea) 50 mg • Sorbitol • Fructose.

Zinc Mineral Supplement - Eidon Inc.
Each 1 tbsp serving contains: Zinc 3 mg. Other Ingredients: Purified Water.

Zinc Picolinate 30 mg - GNC
Each tablet contains: Zinc (picolinate) 30 mg • Copper (as copper gluconate) 2 mg. Other Ingredients: Dicalcium Phosphate, Cellulose.

Zinc Plex - PhysioLogics
Each capsule contains: Zinc (50% as zinc arginine amino acid chelate, 25% as zinc histidinate amino acid chelate, 25% as zinc glycinate) 30 mg • Copper (53% as copper amino acid chelate, 47% as copper lysine amino acid chelate) 2 mg. Other Ingredients: Rice Powder, Gelatin, Silica, Vegetable Magnesium Stearate.

Zinc Plus - Olympian Labs
Each capsule contains: Zinc Chelate 30 mg. In a base of Pumpkin Seeds, Kelp, and Dulse.

Zinc Tally - Metagenics
Each 2 tsp serving contains: Zinc (as zinc sulfate, in a base of distilled water) 2.2 mg.

Zinc Test - Standard Process, Inc.
Each 2 tsp serving contains: Zinc 2.5 mg. Other Ingredients: Deionized Water.

ZincEchinacea Drops - Quantum, Inc.
Each drop contains: Vitamin A acetate 500 IU • Elemental Zinc (Zinc acetate) 14 mg • Echinacea purpurea extract (4:1) 20 mg • Slippery Elm bark (Ulmus fulva) 20 mg • Bee Propolis extract powder (5:1) 5 mg • Goldenseal 2 mg. Other Ingredients: Sugar, Corn Syrup, Natural and Artificial Flavors.

ZincEchinacea Lozenges - Quantum, Inc.
Each lozenge contains: Zinc acetate 14 mg • Vitamin A acetate 500 IU • Slippery Elm bark (Ulmus fulva) 20 mg • Echinacea (4:1) 20 mg • Propolis 5 mg. In a base of Goldenseal, Sugar, Dextrose, Fructose.

ZincEchinacea Pops - Quantum, Inc.
Each pop contains: Vitamin A acetate 167 IU • Elemental Zinc (Zinc acetate) 5 mg • Echinacea purpurea extract (4:1) 7 mg • Slippery Elm bark 7 mg • Bee Propolis extract powder (5:1) 2 mg • Goldenseal 1 mg. Other Ingredients: Sugar, Corn Syrup, Natural Flavor.

Zincosamine - FreeLife International
Each softgel contains: EV.EXT 77 Extract 170 mg: Ginger extract with Zingiber officinale and Alpinia rhizome • Glucosamine Sulfate Potassium 350 mg. Other Ingredients: Gelatin, Coconut Oil, Glycerin, Silica, Sorbitol, Wax, Palm Kernel Oil, Caramel Color.

Zing! - Health Center for Better Living
Each capsule contains: Siberian Ginseng Root 106 mg • Ginkgo Biloba Leaf 79 mg • Gota Kola Herb 79 mg • Kola Nut 79 mg • Bee Pollen 53 mg • Foti Root 26 mg • Rehmannia Root 26 mg • Spirulina 26 mg.

Zingiforce - New Chapter, Inc.
One softgel contains: Ginger (rhizome), certified organic, supercritical extract (minimum 20% pungent compounds- 20 mg, 4% zingiberene- 4 mg) 100 mg • Rosemary leaf & essential oil, supercritical extract (23% total phenolic antioxidants [TPA] - 1.15 mg) 5 mg. Other Ingredients: Olive Oil - certified organic, Yellow Beeswax, Gelatin, Vegetable Glycerin, Purified Water, Carob.

Zinlori 75 - Metagenics
Each tablet contains: Zinc Carnosine 75 mg.

Zinopin - DKSH North America, Inc.
Each capsule contains: Pycnogenol (French maritime pine bark extract) 100 mg • Ginger root extract (standardized) 150 mg. Other Ingredients: Vcap (cellulosic raw materials).

Some Brand Name Natural Products - What they Contain

www.NaturalDatabase.com contains MANY more listings than appear here.
Editor's Notes are located on pages 2155-2163.

BRAND NAMES

ZMA - SNAC Systems, Inc.
Each capsule contains: Zinc (Monomethionine/Asparate) 10 mg • Magnesium (Aspartate) 150 mg • Vitamin B6 3.5 mg.

ZMA - Pro Health
Three capsules contain: Vitamin B6 (as pyridoxine HCl) 15 mg • Magnesium (as magnesium aspartate) 450 mg • Zinc 30 mg. Other Ingredients: Gelatin, Magnesium Stearate.

ZMA for Men - Optimum Nutrition
Three capsules contain: Zinc (monomethionine and aspartate) 30 mg • Magnesium (aspartate) 450 mg • Vitamin B6 (pyridoxine HCl) 10.5 mg. Other Ingredients: Rice Powder, Gelatin, Magnesium Stearate.

ZMA for Women - Optimum Nutrition
Two capsules contain: Zinc (monomethionine and aspartate) 30 mg • Magnesium (aspartate) 450 mg • Vitamin B6 (pyridoxine HCl) 10.5 mg. Other Ingredients: Rice Powder, Gelatin, Magnesium Stearate.

ZMA Pro - VitaCube Systems (V3S)
Each tablet contains: Vitamin B6 (as ZMA) 6 mg • Magnesium (as ZMA) 255 mg • Zinc (as ZMA) 17 mg • VitaCube Activating Proprietary Blend 50 mg: Orange fruit Bioflavonoid Complex, Grapefruit Bioflavonoid Complex, Alfalfa leaf, Ginkgo Biloba leaf, Spirulina algae, Cayenne, Apple Pectin, Odorles Garlic, 7-Isopropoxy Isoflavone, L-Glutathione, Lemon fruit Bioflavonoid, Glycerophosphate, Dimethylglycine, Potassium Glycerophosphate, Rutin, Bromelain, Lutein 5% • Epimedium Sagittatum (horny goat weed) 25 mg • Potassium Glycerophosphate 100 mg • Capsicum fruit (cayenne pepper) 5 mg. Other Ingredients: Cellulose, Stearic Acid, Croscarmellose Sodium, Silicon Dioxide, Magnesium Stearate, Light Green Cellulose Film Coat containing Titanium Dioxide.

ZMA Rx-Strength - Nature's Plus
Three capsules contain: Vitamin B6 (pyridoxine HCl) 0.5 mg • Magnesium (aspartate) 450 mg • Zinc (aspartate/monomethionine) 30 mg • ZMA brand Proprietary Anabolic Support Factor 2424 mg. Other Ingredients: Magnesium Stearate, Gelatin, Purified Water.

Z-Mass PM - Cytodyne LLC
Four capsules contain: Vitamin B6 11 mg • Magnesium 450 mg • Zinc 30 mg • Potassium 10 mg • Proprietary Anabolic Herbal Blend 706 mg: Mucuna Pruriens seeds (standardized for L-dopa), Polypodium Vulgare / Suma (root, standardized for 20-hydroxyecdysone).

ZonePerfect Fish Oil Capsules - ZonePerfect
Each capsule contains: Molecularly Distilled Fish oil • Natural Vitamin E 20 IU • EPA 160 mg • DHA 107 mg.

Zostrix - Rodlen Laboratories, Inc.
Active Ingredients: Capsaicin (0.025%). Inactive Ingredients: Benzyl Alcohol, Cetyl Alcohol, Glyceryl Monostearate, Isopropyl Myristate, PEG-100 Stearate, Purified Water, Sorbitol Solution, White Petrolatum.

Zotrin (Zotril) for Men - Klein-Becker
Two capsules contain: Zotril brand Proprietary Blend 847.8 mg: Yerba Mate bark (standardized proprietary extract), Guarana seed (standardized proprietary extract), Damiana leaf, stem (standardized proprietary extract), Calcium Phosphate, Microcrystalline Cellulose, Magnesium Stearate, L-Tyrosine, Trimethylglycine • Proprietary Blend for Men 128 mg: Schizonepeta Spica SE, Yucca plant, Passion Flower, Panax Ginseng root SE, Maca root SE, St. John's Wort SE, L-Leucine, L-Glutamine, NADH.

Zotrin (Zotril) for Women - Klein-Becker
Two capsules contain: Proprietary Blend 847.8 mg: Yerba Mate bark (standardized proprietary extract), Guarana seed (standardized proprietary extract), Damiana leaf/stem (standardized proprietary extract), Calcium Phosphate, Microcrystallene Cellulose, Magnesium Stearate, Barberry root/bark SE, L-Tyrosine, Trimethylglycine • Proprietary Blend 158 mg: Rosemary leaf/twig SE, Forsythia fruit, Sage leaf, Black Cohosh root SE, Chasteberry fruit SE, Shisandra herb, Chlorella, St. John's Wort herb. Other Ingredients: Rice Flour.

Zotrin Women's Formula - AlphaGen Biotech
Two capsules contain: Zotril brand Proprietary Blend 847 mg: Yerba Mate bark (standardized proprietary extract), Guarana seed (standardized proprietary extract), Damiana leaf & stem (standardized proprietary extract), Calcium Phosphate, Microcrystalline Cellulose, Magnesium Stearate, Ginger root, Trimethylglycine • Proprietary Blend for Women 144 mg: Rosemary leaf SE, Forsythia, Sage, Chasteberry SE, Schisandra, Chlorella.

Z-Plex - PharmAssure
Each softgel contains: Kava Kava Root Extract (piper methysticum; 55% kavalactones) 100 mg • Griffonia seed extract (griffonia simplicifolia; 20% 5-hydroxy-L-tryptophan) 50 mg • Melatonin (N-acetyl-5-methoxytryptamine) 2 mg. Other ingredients: Polyethylene Glycol, Gelatin, Glycerin, Chlorophyll, Titanium Dioxide.
See Editor's Note No. 16.

Zyflamend - New Chapter, Inc.
Two softgels contain: Rosemary leaf (100 mg supercritical extract and 50 mg extract, 23% total phenolic antioxidants (TPA)-34.5 mg) 150 mg • Turmeric rhizome (10 mg supercritical extract, 45% turmerones-4.5 mg and 100 mg ethanolic extract (7% curcuminoids-7 mg)) 100 mg • Ginger rhizome (54 mg supercritical extract (30% pungent compounds-16.2 mg, 8% zingiberene-4.3 mg) and 46 mg PSE extract (3% pungent compounds-1.4 mg)) 100 mg • Holy Basil leaf extract (2% ursolic acid-2 mg) 100 mg • Green Tea leaf extract (45% polyphenols-45 mg) 100 mg • Hu Zhang root and rhizome extract (polygonum cuspidatum, 8% resveratrol-6.4 mg) 80 mg • Chinese Goldthread root extract (6% berberine-2.4 mg) 40 mg • Barberry root extract (6% berberine-2.4 mg) 40 mg • Oregano leaf supercritical extract (0.8% TPA-0.32 mg) 40 mg • Scutellaria Baicalensis root extract 5:1 20 mg. Other Ingredients: Olive Oil (certified organic), Yellow Beeswax, Gelatin, Vegetable Glycerin, Purified Water, Carob.

Zyflamend PM - New Chapter, Inc.
Two softgels contain: Holy Basil leaf, extract (2% ursolic acid- mg) 150 mg • Melissa leaf, extract (1% essential oil- 0.85 mg) (including neral and geranial) 85 mg • Tumeric (rhizome) extract (7% curcumin-7 mg) 100 mg • Scutellaria baicalensis root, extract 5:1 100 mg • Ginger (rhizome) certified organic (post-ethanolic extract) (3% pungent compunds- 1.5 mg) 50 mg • Ginger, SBSC (rhizome), certified organic (minimum 20% pungent compounds 5 mg, 4% zingiberene-1 mg) 25 mg • Chamomile flower, extract (25% alpha-bisabolol- 12.5 mg) 50 mg • Hops (strobiles) ethanolic extract (1.5% xanthohumol- 0.37 mg) 25 mg • Chamomile flower, extract (3% apigeninglycosides- 0.75 mg) 25 mg • Mexican Valerian and Valerian root, extract 30:1 20 mg. Other Ingredients: Olive oil - certified organic, Yellow Beeswax.

Zygest - PhysioLogics
Two capsules contain: Zygest Blend 104 mg: Bromelain (from pineapple) 120 GDU, Papain (from papaya fruit) 600,000 FCCPU, Protease 3.0 (from aspergillus oryzae) 10 SAPU, Amylase (from aspergillus oryzae) 400 DU, Lipase (from aspergillus niger 60 FCCLU, Protease 4.5 (from aspergillus oryzae) 400 HUT, Lactase (from aspergillus oryzae) 20 ALU, Cellulase (from trichoderma longbrachiatum) 10 CU, Hemicellulase (from aspergillus niger) 10 HCU. Other Ingredients: Rice Powder, Gelatin, Vegetable Magnesium Stearate, Silica.

Zyladex Plus - Medlabs
Each tablet contains: Proprietary Blend 717 mg: Desert Tea, Guarana extract, Hawthorne berry, Citrin, Choline, White Willow bark, Borage seed, Wild Yam, Couch Grass, Hydrangea, Corn Silk, Bucchu, Alisma, Inositol, L-Methionine, L-Carnitine, Chromium picolinate, L-Tyrosine, Vitamin B12, Whey, Croscarmellos, Silica, Steric Acid, Magnesium stearate.

Zylodrine XP - Unknown
Each tablet contains: Chromium Picolinate 50 mcg • Betaine 25 mg • Choline complex 25 mg • Korean Ginseng 100 mg • Metabolism Booster Complex 50 mg: L-Phenylalanine 25 mg, L-Tyrosine 25 mg • Cascara Sagrada 25 mg.

Zymatein - Metabolic Nutrition, Inc.
Each scoop (30 g) contains: Whey Protein Concentrate • Vitamin Mineral Matrix • Cocoa • Natural Flavors • Nutrient Stabilizers • Sucralose • Sodium Chloride • Digestive Enzyme Complex: Amylase, Cellulase, Lactase, Lipase, Protease.

Zymax - HealthWatchers System
Pancreatin • Papain • Rutin • Bromelain • Pancrelipase • Peppermint • Trypsin • Lipase • Amylase • Lysozyme • Cellulase • Chymotrypsin. See Editor's Note No. 14.

ZymaX A.M. Formula - Denman Scientific Research
Two tablets contain: Vitamin E 6 IU • Magnesium (chelate) 75 mg • Zinc (chelate) 5 mg • Chromium (picolinate) 75 mcg • Proprietary Blend 175 mcg: Evening Primrose Oil (contains gamma linolenic acid), Borage seed oil, Bladderwrack extract (dried fucus vesiculosus), Grape Seed extract, Bioflavonoids, Soya Lecithin, Fatty Acids, Dried Sweet Red Clover extract (mellotus officinalis, tri foliumratense, 50 mg methylxanthines) • Proprietary Blend 100 mg: Bee Pollen, Ginseng root, Ginger root, Lecithin, Bovine complex, Damiana leaf, Sarsaparilla root, Golden Seal aerial part, Nettles leaf, Gotu Kola aerial part, Spirulina Algae, Royal Jelly • Proprietary Blend 500 mg: Ma Huang extract (15 mg ephedrine), Guarana extract (50 mg caffeine), White Willow bark extract (3 mg salicin).
See Editor's Note No. 14 and No. 30.

ZymaX Accelerator Formula - Denman Scientific Research
Each capsule contains: Garcinia cambogia 500 mg. Inactive Ingredients: Calcium Carbonate, Calcium Phosphate, Cellulose, Gelatin, Stearic Acid, Croscarmellose, and Magnesium Stearate.

ZymaX P.M. Formula - Denman Scientific Research
Each tablet contains: Proprietary Blend 400 mg: Evening Primrose oil, Borage seed oil, Bladderwrack extract, Fucus Vesiculosus extract, Grape Seed extract, Bioflavonoids, Soya Lecithin, Fatty Acids, dried sweet Red Clover extract, Griffonia simplicifolia (20 mg 5-HTP).

Zymex capsules - Standard Process, Inc.
Two capsules contain: Proprietary Blend 1113 mg: Defatted Wheat germ, Lactose, Enzymatically Processed Tillandsia Usneoides, Beet root. Other Ingredients: Gelatin, Water, Calcium Stearate, Colors.

Zymex II - Standard Process, Inc.
Two capsules contain: Proprietary Blend 884 mg: Defatted Almond, Fig fruit, Papain, Bromelain, Amylase, Lipase, Cellulose • Ficin 20 mg. Other Ingredients: Gelatin, Water, Colors.

Zymex wafers - Standard Process, Inc.
Two wafers contain: Proprietary Blend 1680 mg: Defatted Wheat germ, Lactose, Date fruit, Whey, Tillandsia Usneoides, Beet root. Other Ingredients: Honey, Calcium Lactate, Calcium Stearate.

Zymitol - Generation+
Three vegetable capsules contain: Proprietary Blend 2265 mg: Serrapeptase 45 mg, MSM, Protease, Bromelain, Papain, Amylase, Lipase, Alpha Lipoic Acid, Magnesium Citrate, Rutin.

Zypan - Standard Process, Inc.
Each two tablets contain: Proprietary Blend 700 mg: Betaine hydrochloride, Pancreas extract (Cytosol), Pancreatin (3X), Fatty Acid, Pepsin (1:10,000), Ammonium chloride, Bovine Spleen, Ovine Spleen. Other Ingredients: Cellulose, Lactose, Calcium stearate.
See Editor's Note No. 14.

Zyroxin - Optimal Therapeutics
Three capsules contain: Thiamin (B1) 20 mg • Niacin (B3) 20 mg • Pantothenic Acid 20 mg • Vitamin B6 (6 mg • Vitamin B12 (500 mcg) • L-Tyrosine 500 mg • Green Tea leaf extract (camellia sinensis, 80% catechins, 60% EGCG) 225 mg • Caffeine 200 mg • Rhodiola Rosea 150 mg • Octopalean brand Octopamine HCl 150 mg • Hoodia Gordonii 125 mg • Colues Forskohlii (10% forskohlin) 100 mg • Yerba Mate 60 mg • 5 HTP (5-hydroxytryptophan) 5 mg • Evodiamine 25 mg • Vinpocetine 20 mg • Pure Synthetic E+Z Guggulsterones 10 mg • Bioperine brand Black Pepper extract 3 mg. Other Ingredients: Gelatin, Cellulose, Magnesium Stearate.

Zzz (Lipospray) - Advocare International
Each full spray contains: Vitamin E (as dL-alpha tocopheryl acetate) 1.5 IU • Vitamin B6 (as pyridoxine HCl) 35 mg • Zinc (as gluconate) 500 mcg • Valerian root extract (valeriana officinalis) 20 mg • Griffonia seed extract (griffonia simplicifolia) 20 mg • Melatonin 1.5 mg. Other Ingredients: Purified Water, Propylene Glycol, Natural Flavors, Polysorbate 80, Hydroxylated Lecithin, Sucralose, Potassium Sorbate, Modified Pectin.
See Editor's Note No. 26.

Zzz capsules - Advocare International
Each capsule contains: Vitamin B6 (as pyridoxine HCl) 30 mg • Zinc (as OptiZinc brand monomethionine) 1 mg • Hops flower extract (humulus lupulus) 25 mg • Passionflower herb/flower extract (passiflora incarnata) 75 mg • White Willow bark extract (salix alba) 50 mg • Valerian root extract (valeriana officinalis) 100 mg • Chamomile flower extract (matricaria chamomilla) 50 mg • Melatonin 2 mg. Other Ingredients: Silicon Dioxide, Magnesium Stearate, Gelatin.
See Editor's Note No. 26.

Editor's Note No. 1
This is a homeopathic preparation. Homeopathy is a system of medicine established in the 19th century by a German physician named Samuel Hahnemann. Its basic principles are that "like treats like" and "potentiation through dilution." For example, in homeopathy, diarrhea would be treated with an extreme dilution of a substance that normally causes diarrhea when taken in high doses. Practitioners of homeopathy believe that more dilute preparations are more potent. Many homeopathic preparations are so diluted that they contain little or no active ingredient. Therefore, most homeopathic products are not expected to have any pharmacological effects, drug interactions, or other harmful effects. Any beneficial effects are controversial and cannot be explained by current scientific methods.
Dilutions of 1 to 10 are designated by an "X." So a 1X dilution = 1:10, 3X=1:1000; 6X=1:1,000,000. Dilutions of 1 to 100 are designated by a "C." So a 1C dilution = 1:100; 3C = 1:1,000,000. Dilutions of 24X or 12C or more contain zero molecules of the original active ingredient.
Homeopathic products are permitted for sale in the US due to legislation passed in 1938 sponsored by a homeopathic physician who was also a Senator. The law still requires that the FDA allow the sale of products listed in the Homeopathic Pharmacopeia of the United States. However, homeopathic preparations are not held to the same safety and effectiveness standards as conventional medicines.

Editor's Note No. 2
Product Recall: On January 28, 2002, this product was voluntarily withdrawn from the market. Lab testing by the California Department of Health Services discovered amounts of the prescription drug alprazolam (Xanax) in a sample of the product (8010). Advise patients using this product to discontinue taking it. Patients can return this product to BotanicLab for a refund.

Editor's Note No. 3
Product Recall: On February 15, 2002, Health Canada required the withdrawal of this product from the market. Lab testing discovered amounts of a drug similar to sildenafil (Viagra) in a sample of the product (7093). Advise patients using this product to discontinue taking it.

Editor's Note No. 4
The potential risk of transmission of bovine spongiform encephalopathy (BSE, mad cow disease) is raising patients' concerns about products containing chondroitin. Chondroitin is produced from bovine trachea. Although bovine trachea tissue does not seem to carry a high risk of BSE disease infectivity, in some cases manufacturing methods might lead to with other diseased animal tissues. So far there are no reports of BSE, or other disease transmission to humans from dietary supplements containing animal materials and the risk of potential disease transmission is thought to be low. The manufacturer of this product reports taking extensive steps to ensure that their chondroitin is not contaminated

Editor's Note No. 5
Herbal Ecstacy is no longer being produced under an agreement with the FDA. Global World Media now produces Organic Ecstacy which they claim to be ephedra free. The ingredients of Organic Ecstacy are currently unknown.

Editor's Note No. 6
In April 2000, the Federal Trade Commission filed a complaint against manufacturers of natural or herbal cigarettes for making claims that these products were safer than conventional cigarettes. The labeling on these products is now required to state "Herbal cigarettes are dangerous to your health. They produce tar and carbon monoxide." If they use the term "No additives" they must also state "No additives in our tobacco does NOT mean a safer cigarette."

Editor's Note No. 7
Product Recall: On February 8, 2002, this product was voluntarily withdrawn from the market. Lab testing by the California Department of Health Services discovered amounts of the prescription drug warfarin (Coumadin) in a sample of the product (8010). Advise patients using this product to discontinue taking it. On June 1, 2002, BotanicLab closed operations, following product recalls. The future availability of PC-SPES is unknown (8136).
PC-SPES is a combination product containing eight Chinese herbs that has been available commercially since 1996. It is used therapeutically for prostate cancer. "PC" stands for prostate cancer and "spes" is Latin for hope (5548). So far, studies look promising. Preliminary clinical evidence from several small uncontrolled studies and anecdotal reports show that PC-SPES can benefit patients with both hormone-sensitive and hormone-insensitive or refractory prostate cancers. In both groups of patients, PC-SPES can significantly decrease serum prostate-specific antigen (PSA) levels (5122,5548,6284,6286,6483,7785,7786,11764,11765). In patients with hormone-sensitive prostate cancer, PC-SPES can decrease PSA levels by at least 50% in 78-100% of patients (3577,5548,6483,6484,11764,11765). In 56-80% of patients PSA levels become undetectable after approximately 6 months (3577,6484). PC-SPES also seems to significantly decrease PSA in patients with hormone-insensitive prostate cancer. PSA levels decrease more than 50% in about 50-90% of patients

BRAND NAMES

after 6 months of treatment (3577,6286,6483,6484,7786,11764,11765). This effect rapidly reverses when PC-SPES is discontinued; PSA levels may rise dramatically within 2 to 6 weeks; increases up to 1300% can occur in some patients (5548,8137). PC-SPES also seems to cause clinically significant reductions in serum testosterone (5548,6484), improve quality of life, and reduce pain and analgesic use (6286) in patients with prostate cancer.
There is also some evidence that PC-SPES in combination with conventional hormonal therapy for 5 months can improve quality of life, reduce PSA levels, and reduce pain in patients with metastatic prostate cancer (6286). Although PC-SPES does not contain estrogen, the licorice and Panax-pseudoginseng constituents have estrogenic activity. The saw palmetto constituent also inhibits 5-alpha reductase, an enzyme involved in conversion of testosterone to the more biologically active dihydrotestosterone (5548).
Laboratory studies on prostate cancer cell lines show PC-SPES might decrease tumor cell proliferation and might induce apoptosis in both hormone sensitive and insensitive cancer cells, indicating that its estrogenic effects are not the sole mechanism of action (6284,6285,6483,7784). However, PC-SPES seems to reduce tumor cell proliferation more in hormone sensitive prostate cancer (6483). Some retrospective research suggests that PC-SPES might be more effective against androgen-independent prostate cancer in older men and in men with a longer duration of initial antiandrogen therapy (7785). Laboratory studies also suggest that PC-SPES might protect prostate cells from cancer. Licorice seems to have antimutagenic activity (7783). Reduction in pain by PC-SPES could result from the antitumor effect or from some of its components with reported anti-inflammatory and analgesic properties: licorice, reishi mushroom, chrysanthemum, and Panax-pseudoginseng (7784).
The composition of PC-SPES has been inconsistent. Various lots of PC-SPES contain differing amounts of phytoestrogens, licochalcone A (a constituent of licorice), and baicalin (a constituent of Baikal scullcap). PC-SPES may also contain diethylstilbestrol, indomethacin, and warfarin (11763).
Although PC-SPES is generally well-tolerated, some side effects are relatively common. Most side effects can be attributed to the estrogenic effects of PC-SPES, similar to those of diethylstilbestrol (DES) (7784,7785). One of the most common side effects is nipple and breast tenderness and breast enlargement. This seems to occur in up to 90% of patients (3577,6483). Other frequently reported side effects include leg cramps, indigestion, nausea, diarrhea, decreased libido, erectile dysfunction, and hot flashes. Other side effects that might occur are reduction in overall body hair, pitting edema, significant drop in lipoprotein a, hypertriglyceridemia, and venous and pulmonary thrombosis (5122,5548,6287,6483,6484,7785,11764,11765). There is a lot of concern about the potential for thrombosis formation in patients taking PC-SPES. So far, it seems to occur in about 2-4% of patients (3577,6483). Pulmonary embolus has been reported, leading some practitioners to suggest prophylactic anticoagulation (7785,7787). Since PC-SPES has estrogenic effects, there is also some concern that it might interfere with conventional hormone therapies for prostate cancer if used concurrently. In vitro evidence suggests combination therapy of PC-SPES and paclitaxel decreases the effectiveness of paclitaxel therapy alone, in both androgen-independent and androgen-sensitive prostate carcinoma situations (11482). Because of these risks patients should avoid using PC-SPES without the supervision of a healthcare provider. Tell patients not to attempt to self-treat prostate cancer with PC-SPES.
Although PC-SPES might be helpful for some patients, it should only be used in conjunction with a comprehensive treatment plan developed between the patient and oncologist. Clinical trials have used 6-9 capsules daily. Each capsule contains 320 mg of the herbal combination. In some studies patients started with one capsule three times daily during the first week and 2 capsules three times daily during the second week. Then, if this dose was tolerated, it was increased to 3 capsules three times daily. PC-SPES should be taken on an empty stomach and should not be administered concurrently with antacids or other medicines (3577).
Depending on the dose required, cost is estimated to range from $162-$486/month (5233).

Editor's Note No. 8
The FDA has recently declared this product as adulterated and misbranded. It is adulterated because it is promoted for use during the last 6 weeks of pregnancy, but contains ingredients that should not be used during any stage of pregnancy. These include black cohosh, blessed thistle, false unicorn root, and pennyroyal. It also contains raspberry leaf which should be avoided during pregnancy unless used under the guidance of a health professional. It is misbranded because its labeling does not state that it should not be used by pregnant women.

Editor's Note No. 9
This product is considered by the FDA to be an unapproved drug due to promotion of the product for the treatment of cancer and other diseases. The manufacturer has been barred from selling these products without first gaining FDA approval as a new drug (12069). The FDA first cited this manufacturer for marketing an unapproved drug in 1999 (387). In June 2000, the manufacturer of this product also settled

Federal Trade Commission charges of making unsubstantiated claims for a one million dollar judgement (6999).

Editor's Note No. 10
The manufacturer has voluntarily recalled this product after FDA laboratories found contamination problems. It might be contaminated with yeast and Pseudomonas fluorescens. Use of this contaminated product might result in severe eye injury and loss of sight. This product should not be used. People who have used this product should contact their physician or other health care professional.

Editor's Note No. 11
There are serious concerns about the safety of this product. LipoKinetix is marketed for weight loss. However, there is no reliable evidence it works. From July to December 2000 there have been at least seven cases of acute hepatotoxicity in patients taking LipoKinetix. Symptoms including nausea, weakness and fatigue, abdominal pain, and yellowing of the skin usually develop from 2 weeks to 3 months after starting LipoKinetix. Symptoms resolve when it is discontinued (7091). Tell patients not to use this product.

Editor's Note No. 12
The manufacturer refuses to disclose the ingredients of this product. Anecdotal evidence suggests that this product may have induced a seizure in one patient. Patients should be strongly encouraged to avoid using this product until more is known about its contents and safety.

Editor's Note No. 13
There is some evidence that SS Cream can be helpful for premature ejaculation. Applying SS Cream to the glans penis one hour prior to intercourse and washing off immediately before intercourse seems to significantly delay ejaculation compared to placebo. A single application of SS Cream seems to be safe. However, the safety of SS Cream with repeated application is not known. SS Cream seems to be well tolerated, but can sometimes cause sporadic erectile dysfunction, excessively delayed ejaculation, mild pain, and local irritation and burning.

Editor's Note No. 14
There is some concern about the safety of this product because it contains glandular or organ material derived from animals. The concern is that animal materials might be obtained from diseased animals, including those harboring bovine spongiform encephalopathy (BSE, mad cow disease). There are no reports of BSE or other disease transmission to humans from dietary supplements containing glandular or organ material and the risk of potential disease transmission is thought to be low. However, until more is known about the safety of these products, tell patients to avoid this and other supplements containing glandular or organ materials.

Editor's Note No. 15
The potential risk of transmission of bovine spongiform encephalopathy (BSE, mad cow disease) is raising patients' concerns about products containing chondroitin. Chondroitin is produced from bovine trachea. Although bovine trachea tissue does not seem to carry a high risk of BSE disease infectivity, in some cases manufacturing methods might lead to contamination with other diseased animal tissues. So far there are no reports of BSE or other disease transmission to humans from dietary supplements containing animal materials and the risk of potential disease transmission is thought to be low. However, until more is known about the quality of manufacturing practices, tell patients to avoid this product.

Editor's Note No. 16
The potential risk of transmission of bovine spongiform encephalopathy (BSE, mad cow disease) is raising patients' concerns about products containing melatonin. Melatonin is a hormone sometimes harvested from the pineal gland of animals. However, some melatonin products are made synthetically and are free of this potential risk. The manufacturer of this product has not disclosed its source of melatonin. Until more is known, tell patients to avoid this product.

Editor's Note No. 17
The manufacturer of this product refuses to disclose specific details about the ingredients. Because the exact amounts of ingredients are unknown, tell patients to avoid this product.

Editor's Note No. 18
Wobenzym N is promoted for reducing inflammation and edema, and speeding recovery from certain injuries. Often it is used by individuals with arthritis and by athletes, including some professional and Olympic athletes. Enzymes in this product are thought to activate macrophages that attack inflammation-causing circulating immune complexes. Rutoside, an additional ingredient, acts as an antioxidant. To date there is no convincing clinical evidence that Wobenzym is effective for these uses. Because these enzymes do not affect prostaglandin synthesis, Wobenzym N is also promoted to be free of many of the side effects associated with non-steroidal anti-inflammatory drugs (NSAIDS). Adverse reactions reported after oral administration include loose stools, increased gas, and skin reactions. Wobenzym N contains enzymes with fibrinolytic activity and might affect coagulation. It should be used

cautiously by people on anticoagulant medications such as aspirin, clopidogrel (Plavix), dalteparin (Fragmin), enoxaparin (Lovenox), heparin, ticlopidine (Ticlid), warfarin (Coumadin), and others (6060).

Editor's Note No. 19
This product is utilized at the Mexican cancer clinic American Metabolic Institute and promoted by Geronimo Rubio, MD, the clinic's medical director. However, the clinic does not disclose the ingredients of this preparation. Tell patients to avoid this and other products that do not disclose ingredients.

Editor's Note No. 20
This product was recently reformulated. Many of the ingredients increased in strength. For example, amounts of procaine, thiamine, riboflavin, pyridoxine, niacin, and chromium doubled.

Editor's Note No. 21
This product has been discontinued by the manufacturer.

Editor's Note No. 22
This product has been discontinued by the manufacturer. See Leptoprin-SF.

Editor's Note No. 23
Lab testing has discovered amounts of the drug tadalafil (Cialis) in a sample of the product (9605). This drug is a prescription product in many conutries and is similar to sildenafil (Viagra). Advise patients using this product to discontinue taking it.

Editor's Note No. 24
Poly-MVA is a combination of minerals, vitamins, and amino acids (hence, the acronym "MVA") that was patented in 1995. It's promoted as a "metalo-vitamin"...as a cancer preventative and as a nontoxic alternative to chemotherapy for treating cancer. There is no reliable clinical research or preclinical research about Poly-MVA...no credible evidence to support anecdotal claims of tumor regression, pain reduction, and prolonged survival in patients with various kinds of cancer. There is no reliable information about potential risks or adverse reactions.
The ingredients of Poly-MVA are a "proprietary blend." Under dietary supplement regulations, the manufacturer is not required to include specific amounts of any ingredient on the product label. Poly-MVA is available as a reddish brown liquid that is mixed with juice or water. Poly-MVA is very expensive...$165 for a 4-ounce bottle, which is less than a one-week supply.

Editor's Note No. 25
Product Recall: On April 4, 2003, this product was voluntarily withdrawn from the market. Lab testing found that it contained the prescription drug sildenafil (Viagra). Advise patients using this product to discontinue taking it.

Editor's Note No. 26
The potential risk of transmission of bovine spongiform encephalopathy (BSE, mad cow disease) is raising patients concerns about products containing melatonin. Melatonin is a hormone sometimes harvested from the pineal gland of animals. However, the melatonin contained in this product is produced synthetically and is free of this potential risk.

Editor's Note No. 27
This product is not available in the U.S.

Editor's Note No. 28
This product may contain excessive levels of lead. An analysis shows it can contain as much as 2.5 mcg of lead per gram of calcium (9598). Advise patients not to use this product.

Editor's Note No. 29
Using Zestra topically might improve symptoms of female sexual arousal disorder. A small clinical study suggests massaging 0.5 to 1 ml into the external female genitalia, clitoris, labia, and vaginal opening for 3 to 5 minutes prior to intercourse may improve sexual pleasure (11968). More evidence is needed to rate Zestra for this use. Topically, Zestra appears to be safe for short term use (11968,11969). Zestra can cause mild genital burning sensations that last 5 to 30 minutes (11968).

Editor's Note No. 30
This product contains ephedra, also commonly known as ma huang. On April 14, 2004, the FDA issued its final ruling, stating that it will ban ephedra-containing products in the U.S. This is due to numerous reports that link ephedra use to severe adverse reactions including heart attack, stroke, hypertension, seizure, and others (10055). Advise patients not to use this or other products containing ephedra.

Editor's Note No. 31
There is concern about the safety of this product because it contains glandular or organ material derived from animals. The concern is that animal materials might be obtained from diseased animals, including those harboring bovine spongiform encephalopathy (BSE, mad cow disease). There are no reports of BSE or other disease transmission to humans from dietary supplements containing glandular or organ material and the risk of potential disease transmission is thought to be low. However, as of July 1, 2004, the FDA has banned all dietary supplements containing brain or spinal cord

material from cows over 30 months of age (4953). This product appears to contain brain materials. Tell patients to avoid this and other supplements containing glandular or organ materials.

Editor's Note No. 32
Immunace (Immunance) is a high-dose combination micronutrient product containing vitamins, minerals, and the amino acid cystine. In the recommended daily dose of 2 tablets, some of the ingredients exceed the recommended dietary allowance (RDA) set for healthy people. Some clinical research suggests that this supplement might improve survival of HIV-infected patients with CD4 cell counts below 200 million cells per liter. The mechanism of action is unknown, but seems to be independent of change in CD4 cell count (11348). Immunace (Immunance) is not available in the US, but can be ordered from the UK via the Internet. Tell patients not to attempt to self-treat with Immunace (Immunance). Although Immunace (Immunance) might be helpful for some patients, it should only be used in conjunction with a comprehensive treatment plan developed between the patient and health care provider. Although tablets were used in the study, Immunace (Immunance) is only available in capsule form.

Editor's Note No. 33
In August 2004 the manufacturer of this product was warned by the US Food and Drug Administration (FDA) for making unsubstantiated claims about the benefits of this product. The FDA indicates that claims made in promotional materials such as "controls appetite", "burn calories more efficiently", "controls cortisol levels within a healthy range" and several other claims are false and misleading and therefore the product is misbranded (12141).

Editor's Note No. 34
In March 2004, the US Food and Drug Administration ordered the manufacturer and distributors of SeaSilver to discontinue marketing it and to recall existing product. This is due to their unsubstantiated claims that SeaSilver can treat over 650 diseases including cancer, AIDS, diabetes, heart disease, hepatitis, and many others. Due to these claims this product is considered by the FDA to be a misbranded drug (6814).

Editor's Note No. 35
Juice Plus+ Garden Blend is a commercially available mixed vegetable supplement made from dehydrated juice concentrates. It is used with Juice Plus+ Orchard Blend, a mixed fruit supplement made from dehydrated juice concentrates, to reduce coronary heart disease (CHD) risk. Preliminary clinical evidence from several small studies suggests Juice Plus+ may have pharmacologic activity that could reduce CHD risk (11374,11375,11376,11377). It may lower plasma homocysteine levels, raise plasma antioxidant vitamin and folate levels, and raise serum nitrate and nitrite levels (11374,11375). Juice Plus+ may also improve flow-mediated vasoactivity and reduce oxidative changes in DNA (11376,11377). But there's no reliable evidence showing Juice Plus+ decreases risk of death or cardiovascular events such as stroke or myocardial infarction. Preliminary clinical research trials have used two capsules Juice Plus+ Garden Blend and two capsules Juice Plus+ Orchard Blend divided twice daily (11374,11375,11376,11377).

Editor's Note No. 36
Juice Plus+ Orchard Blend is a commercially available mixed fruit supplement made from dehydrated juice concentrates. It is used with Juice Plus+ Garden Blend, a mixed vegetable supplement made from dehydrated juice concentrates, to reduce coronary heart disease (CHD) risk. Preliminary clinical evidence from several small studies suggests Juice Plus+ may have pharmacologic activity that could reduce CHD risk (11374,11375,11376,11377). It may lower plasma homocysteine levels, raise plasma antioxidant vitamin and folate levels, and raise serum nitrate and nitrite levels (11374,11375). Juice Plus+ may also improve flow-mediated vasoactivity and reduce oxidative changes in DNA (11376,11377). But there's no reliable evidence showing Juice Plus+ decreases risk of death or cardiovascular events such as stroke or myocardial infarction. Preliminary clinical research trials have used two capsules Juice Plus+ Garden Blend and two capsules Juice Plus+ Orchard Blend divided twice daily (11374,11375,11376,11377).

Editor's Note No. 37
On April 1, 2004, the FDA warned the distributor of this product to stop making false and misleading claims about this product's use for weight loss. This and other similar products sometimes claim to block starch, carbohydrates, and calories to help users lose weight without making any lifestyle changes such as calorie restriction or exercise. The FDA indicates that these claims are not supported by reliable scientific evidence (12005).

Editor's Note No. 38
On May 5, 2004, the FDA warned the company that produces this product to stop making false and misleading claims about this product's use. The labeling for this product stated that it provides "cushioning" and "lubrication" for the joints and that it alleviates pain from arthritis and fibromyalgia. The FDA indicates that these claims are not supported by reliable scientific evidence (12029).

Editor's Note No. 39
This product contains country mallow, which is a source of ephedrine. On April 14, 2004, the FDA issued its final ruling, stating that it will ban ephedrine-containing products such as country mallow and ephedra in the U.S. This is due to numerous reports that link the ephedrine-containing product ephedra to severe adverse reactions including heart attack, stroke, hypertension, seizure, and others (10055). Advise patients not to use this or other products containing ephedrine.

Editor's Note No. 40
This product contains the ingredient synephrine. Synephrine is a stimulant similar to ephedrine, which is contained in the herb ephedra (ma huang). Ephedra products were removed from the U.S. market due to safety concerns. Ephedra is linked to stroke, heart attack, seizure, and other serious side effects.
Many manufacturers have now substituted synephrine in products that used to contain ephedra. These products are typically promoted for weight loss. Many of these products are now labeled as ephedra-free or ma huang-free, but they often still contain the stimulant synephrine. These synephrine-containing products likely have the same risks as the ephedra-containing products. Synephrine is a constituent of the bitter orange (Citrus aurantium). Products that list bitter orange or Citrus aurantium on the label also likely contain synephrine. Advise patients about the potential risks associated with this and other synephrine-containing products.

Editor's Note No. 41
The manufacturer refuses to disclose the ingredients of this product. Because the ingredients are unknown, tell patients to avoid this product.

Editor's Note No. 42
There is preliminary clinical evidence that drinking 250 mL or 1 can of Red Bull Energy Drink might improve anaerobic exercise endurance by 24% and aerobic exercise endurance by 9% in patients on cycle ergometers. Red Bull Energy Drink might also improve subjective mental performance in the areas of concentration, immediate memory recall, and reaction time (11470).

Editor's Note No. 43
This formulation of glucosamine is corn-derived. Most glucosamine products are animal-derived, from the shell of crustaceans. This product may be a safer alternative for people with a shellfish allergy. However, clinical studies have only evaluated glucosamine products derived from shellfish.

Editor's Note No. 44
This is a "branded ingredient." This means that it is an ingredient used in other companies' products. For example, this product might be just one ingredient used in another companys product that contains multiple ingredients. These branded ingredients usually are not available for sale as stand alone products for consumers.

Editor's Note No. 45
This product has been certified by the United States Pharmacopeia (USP) Dietary Supplement Verification Program. This certification ensures that this product contains the ingredients listed on the label and meets USP standards for purity and good manufacturing practices. This certification does not ensure safety or effectiveness. For information about safety, effectiveness, side effects, interactions and other clinical information, click the links for the individual ingredients to review the detailed ingredient monographs.
For more information about the USP certification program, click here: www.usp.org/USPVerified/

Editor's Note No. 46
This product contains aristolochic acid. The FDA considers all products containing aristolochic acid to be unsafe and adulterated (6118). The FDA intends to automatically detain, without physical examination, any product which contains plants known or suspected to contain aristolochic acid, or which might be adulterated with plants known to contain aristolochic acid. Each detained product will be released only after the responsible party provides direct analytical evidence that it is free of aristolochic acid (6118). Aristolochia is also banned in Germany, Austria, France, Great Britain, Belgium, and Japan (367).
Health Canada, the Canadian health authority, removed five aristolochia-containing Chinese herbal medicine products from sale. The products include Touku Natural Herbal Rheumatic Pills, two brands of Tri-Snakegall & Fritillary Powder, Tracheitis Pills, and Gastropathy Capsules (367).

Editor's Note No. 47
This product contains the ingredient androstenedione. In March 2004, the U.S. Food and Drug Administration told manufacturers of products containing this ingredient to immediately stop distribution. The FDA considers these dietary supplements to be adulterated drugs due the lack of historical data regarding dietary use that establishes a reasonable expectation of safety. There are concerns that these products are unsafe. Androstenedione might have potent androgenic effects and lead to serious side effects including impotence, liver problems, and increased cancer risk (12001).
In January 2005 legislation went into affect in the United States called the Anabolic Steroid Control Act of 2004. This reclassifies androstenedione from a dietary

supplement to an anabolic steroid, which is a schedule III controlled substance (8639).

Editor's Note No. 48
The potential risk of transmission of bovine spongiform encephalopathy (BSE, mad cow disease) is raising patients' concerns about products containing chondroitin. Chondroitin is sometimes produced from bovine trachea. However, the chondroitin in this product is not from a bovine source, so this product is free of this potential risk.

Editor's Note No. 49
This product is marketed as a street drug alternative and is claimed to produce a safe legal high. This and other products marketed by Cytotec Solutions have been found to contain high levels of over-the-counter drugs such as diphenhydramine, dextromethorphan, or ephedrine. In some cases, the controlled substances gamma-butyrolactone (GBL) and gamma-hydroxybutyrate (GHB) have been found in these products. The FDA considers these products to be illegal unapproved drugs (12007). Advise patients against using this or other products marketed by Cytotec Solutions.

Editor's Note No. 50
This product is a Bach flower remedy. Bach (pronounced Batch) flower remedies were developed by Dr. Edward Bach in the 1930's. Dr. Bach believed that illnesses are "manifestations of flaws" in one's personality. He believed that a person's own nature, character, and feelings play a key role in the development of diseases. Therefore, Bach flower remedies are often promoted to help mental and emotional problems, rather than to directly treat physical ailments.
Bach flower remedies are produced from a "mother tincture" by adding only a few drops of extract to distilled water, which are then preserved with brandy. Many people often refer to Bach flower remedies as homeopathic products because they are diluted like homeopathic remedies. In fact, Dr. Bach developed the first 7 of his 38 remedies while working at the London Homeopathic Hospital.
Bach flower remedies are often so dilute that they contain little or no detectable amounts of active ingredients. Therefore, just as with homeopathic preparations, Bach flower remedies are not expected to have any beneficial pharmacological effects, or any drug interactions, or side effects.

Editor's Note No. 51
This product has been discontinued by the manufacturer. See Leptoprin.

Editor's Note No. 52
This product has been discontinued by the manufacturer. This product is marketed as "Sinupret" in Germany.

Editor's Note No. 53
There is some concern about the safety of this product because it contains glandular or organ material derived from animals.

Editor's Note No. 54
This product contains androstenediol. In January 2005 legislation went into affect in the United States called the Anabolic Steroid Control Act of 2004. This reclassifies androstenediol from a dietary supplement to an anabolic steroid, which is a schedule III controlled substance (8639).

Editor's Note No. 55
In November 2004, this product was removed from the market in the US. This product was shown to contain aristolochic acid which is a potent carcinogen and can cause kidney failure. Advise patients using this product to discontinue using it.

Editor's Note No. 56
Do not confuse this product with the Menofem product by Pharmaton that has been used in clinical research. Menofem by Pharmaton contains black cohosh extract 20 mg per capsule. This product is not available in the US or Canada.

Editor's Note No. 57
In May 2004, the US Food and Drug Administration issued a warning letter to the manufacturer of this product due to marketing materials that claim it is a cure for cancer. Marketing materials claim that it treats cancer and that it "reverts cancer cells back to normal cells" as well as other unsubstantiated claims. Based on these materials, the product is misbranded and is being promoted as an unapproved drug. Other materials falsly imply that it is an FDA-approved product (12224). Advise patients that there is no proof that this product can treat or cure cancer.

Editor's Note No. 58
In November 2004, this product was removed from the market by the U.S. Food and Drug Administration. It has been found to contain prescription strength quantities of the drug sildenafil (Viagra). Advise patients using this product to discontinue taking it.

Editor's Note No. 59
In October 2004, the manufacturer of this product was cited by the U.S Food and Drug Administration for making false and misleading claims. Content analysis of this product indicates that the product does not contain

BRAND NAMES

the amount of ingredients listed on the label and therefore the product is misbranded (12223).

Editor's Note No. 60
In October 2004, the manufacturer of this product was cited by the U.S Food and Drug Administration for making false and misleading claims. Marketing and promotional materials claim that this product lowers cholesterol, reduces the risk of heart disease and prevents heart disease. However, this product is not generally recognized as safe and effective for these indications. Content analysis of this product also indicates that the product does not contain the amount of ingredients listed on the label and therefore the product is misbranded (12223).
Advise patients that there is no reliable evidence that this product is safe and effective for treating high cholesterol or preventing heart disease.

Editor's Note No. 61
In October 2004, the manufacturer of this product was cited by the U.S Food and Drug Administration for making false and misleading claims. Marketing and promotional materials claim that this product treats macular degeneration and "may be your best defense against AMD." However, this product is not generally recognized as safe and effective for these indications (12223).
Advise patients that there is no reliable evidence that this product is safe and effective for treating macular degeneration.

Editor's Note No. 62
Manufacturers of this product have been warned by the Food and Drug Administration (FDA) for making misleading claims. The product website suggests that the product increases lean muscle mass and decreases fat. The FDA considers these claims to be misleading and not supported by scientific evidence (13062).

Editor's Note No. 63
On June 7, 2005, Health Canada warned consumers against using this product. The Health Canada warning indicates that the manufacturer of this product makes unsubstantiated health claims by suggesting that this product can cure or help prevent diabetes, cancer, arthritis, multiple sclerosis, and heart disease. This product has also been linked to reports of hyperthyroidism, allergic reactions, and potential interactions with drugs (13097). Advise patients against using this product.

Editor's Note No. 64
Preliminary evidence suggests that the ingredients in this product, palm oil and oat oil (Olibra), might help reduce calorie intake. In several small-scale studies, people who consumed a yogurt product containing 2-6 grams of Olibra 4 hours before eating a meal, consumed fewer calories at mealtime compared to those who consumed yogurt that did not contain Olibra, but which contained an equal quantity of fat and other nutrients (13078,13090). It is thought that Olibra increases fat-specific satiety. More evidence is needed to determine if this product has any effect on long-term calorie intake or weight loss.

Editor's Note No. 65
The manufacturer of this product has been permanently banned from marketing any supplements used for weight loss. This stems from charges filed by the US Federeal Trade Commission (FTC) that Enforma made repeated unsubstantiated and false claims about its weight loss products (13005).

Editor's Note No. 66
The FDA has determined that this product is not a dietary supplement but an unapproved new drug containing a potent thyroid hormone, which may cause serious health consequences. The State of Missouri embargoed the product at its distributor (Syntrax) and the Utah-based manufacturer (Pharmatech) has agreed to stop distributing any product containing the ingredient TRIAC. The FDA has issued recalls for other tiratricol-containing products, including Tricana Metabolic Hormone Analogue, Tria-Cutz Thyroid Stimulator Dietary Supplement Capsules, and Sci-Fi-Tri-Cuts Dietary Supplement Capsules (6675).

Editor's Note No. 67
This product contains ephedra, also commonly known as ma huang. On April 14, 2004, the FDA issued its final ruling, stating that it will ban ephedra-containing products in the U.S. This is due to numerous reports that link ephedra use to severe adverse reactions including heart attack, stroke, hypertension, seizure, and others (10055). A report specific to Metabolife 356 indicates that a single dose can significantly prolong the QT interval and P wave duration. Both are risk factors for the development of arrhythmias. In addition, systolic blood pressure may also increase after one dose (11355). Advise patients not to use this or other products containing ephedra.

Editor's Note No. 68
This product has been linked to two cases of hepatotoxicity (13037). In both cases symptoms resolved when the product was discontinued. It is not known which ingredient(s) might be responsible for this side effect. But there is a previous report of acute hepatitis in a patient who took the ingredient chromium polynicotinate, which is also contained in this product.

Advise patients with liver disease to avoid taking this or other products containing chromium polynicotinate.

Editor's Note No. 69
This product is also known as STW 5. It is typically used for dyspepsia, nausea, gastroesophageal reflux disease (GERD), irritable bowel syndrome (IBS) and other gastrointestinal conditions. This specific combination has been evaluated in several clinical studies of functional dyspepsia (7049,12724,13089). An analysis of these studies suggests that taking 1 mL orally three times daily over a period of 4-weeks significantly reduces severity of acid reflux, epigastric pain, cramping, nausea and vomiting compared to placebo (13089). Iberogast seems to be well-tolerated by most patients. The incidence of side effects appears to be similar to placebo (13089).

Editor's Note No. 70
This product is marketed for erectile dysfunction. In November 2004, this product was voluntarily removed from the market in North America because it might contain quantities of the prescription drug tadalafil (Cialis) (12225). Advise patients who use this product to discontinue taking it.

Editor's Note No. 71
This product is promoted for diabetes. It is also known as Liqiang Xiao Ke Ling. On July 1, 2005, the FDA warned that this product is adulterated with unspecified amounts of the prescription diabetes drug glyburide (13130). People taking this product could be at risk for hypoglycemia, especially if they are already taking other diabetes drugs. Advise patients not to use this product.

Editor's Note No. 72
This product was marketed in the US as "Quanterra Sinus Defense" before being discontinued by its manufacturer, Warner-Lambert Company.

Editor's Note No. 73
We have published the following in *Pharmacist's Letter* and *Prscriber's Letter*:

People are asking about *Limbrel* (flavocoxid) for osteoarthritis.

The name, flavocoxid, sounds like a COX-2 inhibitor.

The product labeling looks like an Rx drug package insert... complete with chemical structure and NDC number.

But *Limbrel* is NOT an Rx drug...NOT an OTC drug...and NOT a dietary supplement.

The manufacturer is marketing it in the little-known category of "medical food."

Medical foods are supposed to meet unique nutritional needs due to a specific disease that can't be met by ordinary foods.

Some examples are *Phenyl-Free-1* for babies with phenylketonuria... *Pro-Phree* for celiac disease...and *Ketonex-1* for maple syrup disease.

Ensure and many other enteral formulas aren't medical foods... because they're supplements to a normal diet, for the general population.

"Medical foods" have a marketing advantage over "dietary supplements." Medical foods CAN claim to treat a medical condition such as arthritis. Supplements can only make structure and function claims such as "maintain healthy joints."

Limbrel contains a combination of plant extracts called flavonoids.

There's no proof it's effective for osteoarthritis...and it costs over $90 a month. Don't recommend it.

Therapeutic Efficacy

For more information on any of the natural medicines identified in this list, review the listing for that monograph in the database. Just because a product has a positive effectiveness rating does not mean it is appropriate for all patients. In some cases natural medicines that are rated effective might be unsafe for certain patients due to contraindications, drug interactions, or other reasons.

Abortion
Possibly Ineffective
Rosemary
ACE inhibitor-associated cough
Possibly Effective
Iron
Acetaminophen poisoning
Effective
N-Acetyl Cysteine
Possibly Effective
Methionine
Acne
Possibly Effective
Alpha Hydroxy Acids
Bovine Cartilage
Saccharomyces Boulardii
Tea Tree Oil
Zinc
Acrodermatitis enteropathica
Possibly Effective
Zinc
Acute bronchitis
Possibly Ineffective
Vitamin C
Acute Myocardial infarction (MI)
[see also Myocardial infarction (MI)]
Possibly Effective
Magnesium
Acute respiratory distress syndrome (ARDS)
[see also Respiratory distress syndrome (ARDS)]
Possibly Effective
Borage
Adjustment disorder with anxious mood
Possibly Effective
Passionflower
Adrenal insufficiency
Possibly Effective
DHEA
Adrenoleukodystrophy and Adrenomyeloneuropathy
Likely Ineffective
Lorenzo's Oil
Age-related cognitive impairment
Possibly Effective
Acetyl-L-Carnitine
Citicoline
Phosphatidylserine

Age-related macular degeneration (AMD)
Possibly Effective
Beta-Carotene
DHA
Lutein
Vitamin C
Vitamin E
Zinc
Possibly Ineffective
EPA
Age-related maculopathy
Possibly Effective
Fish Oil
Age-related memory impairment
Possibly Effective
Ginkgo
Likely Ineffective
Choline
Age-related testosterone deficiency
Possibly Effective
Acetyl-L-Carnitine
Propionyl-L-Carnitine
Aging skin
Possibly Effective
DHEA
Pyruvate
AIDS diarrhea-wasting syndrome
Possibly Ineffective
Zinc
AIDS
(see HIV/AIDS)
AIDS-related diarrhea
(see also HIV/AIDS-related diarrhea)
Possibly Effective
Sangre de Grado
AIDS-related myelopathy
Possibly Effective
SAMe
AIDS-related wasting
(see also HIV/AIDS-related wasting)
Possibly Effective
HMB
L-Arginine
Possibly Ineffective
Medium Chain Triglycerides
Albuminuria
Possibly Effective
Vitamin C
Alcoholism
Possibly Effective
GHB
Alcohol-related liver disease
(see also Cirrhosis and Liver disease)
Possibly Ineffective
Alpha-Lipoic Acid

Allergic rhinitis (hayfever)
Possibly Effective
Butterbur
Thymus Extract
Possibly Ineffective
EPA
Grape
Alopecia areata
Possibly Effective
Cedarwood Oil
Lavender
Rosemary
Possibly Ineffective
Zinc
Altitude sickness
Possibly Ineffective
Ginkgo
Alzheimer's disease
(see also Dementia)
Possibly Effective
Acetyl-L-Carnitine
Idebenone
Lemon Balm
Niacin and Niacinamide
Phosphatidylserine
Sage
Vitamin E
Possibly Ineffective
Beta-Carotene
Choline
DHEA
Inositol
Vitamin C
Likely Ineffective
Deanol
Lecithin
N-Acetyl Cysteine
Amenorrhea
Likely Effective
Progesterone
Amyloidosis
Possibly Effective
DMSO
Amyotrophic lateral sclerosis (ALS, Lou Gehrig's disease)
Possibly Ineffective
Creatine
N-Acetyl Cysteine
Threonine
Transfer Factor
Likely Ineffective
Branched-Chain Amino Acids
Anal fissures
Possibly Effective
Bovine Cartilage
Anal pruritus
Possibly Effective
Bovine Cartilage

Therapeutic Efficacy

For additional data, refer to the database.

Anemia
(see also Hereditary sideroblastic anemia, Iron deficiency anemia, and Pernicious anemia)
Possibly Effective
Vitamin E
Possibly Ineffective
Histidine
Vitamin A

Anemia of chronic disease
Effective
Iron

Angina
Possibly Effective
L-Arginine
L-Carnitine
N-Acetyl Cysteine
Propionyl-L-Carnitine
Terminalia
Possibly Ineffective
Vitamin E

Angioplasty
Possibly Effective
Fish Oil

Anorexia
Possibly Effective
Branched-Chain Amino Acids

Anorexia nervosa
Possibly Effective
Zinc

Antibiotic-associated diarrhea
Possibly Effective
Lactobacillus
Saccharomyces Boulardii
Yogurt

Antibiotic-induced gastrointestinal adverse effects
Possibly Effective
Bifidobacteria

Antidepressant-induced sexual dysfunction
Possibly Ineffective
Ginkgo

Antiphospholipid syndrome-associated miscarriage
Possibly Effective
Fish Oil

Anxiety
Likely Effective
Kava
Possibly Effective
Valerian

Ariboflavinosis
Effective
Riboflavin

Arrhythmias
(see also Cardiac glycoside-induced arrhythmias)
Possibly Effective
Magnesium

Asthma
(see also Exercise-induced Asthma)
Possibly Effective
Caffeine
Choline
Fish Oil
Forskolin
Lycopene
Magnesium
Pycnogenol
Thymus Extract
Possibly Ineffective
EPA
Picrorhiza
Yogurt

Atelectasis
Effective
N-Acetyl Cysteine

Atherosclerosis
Possibly Effective
Alpha-Linolenic Acid
Black Tea
Fish Oil
Garlic
Niacin and Niacinamide
Possibly Ineffective
Vitamin C
Vitamin E

Athletic conditioning
Possibly Ineffective
Androstenediol
Boron
Chromium
Chrysin
Likely Ineffective
Androstenedione
Creatine

Athletic performance
Possibly Effective
Caffeine
Creatine
Deanol
Pycnogenol
Possibly Ineffective
Bee Pollen
Branched-Chain Amino Acids
Choline
Cordyceps
Ginseng, Panax
Ginseng, Siberian
Glutamine
L-Tryptophan
Magnesium
Ornithine
Ornithine Ketoglutarate
Pangamic Acid
Puncture Vine
Likely Ineffective
Coca
Coenzyme Q-10
Glycerol
Inosine
L-Carnitine
Phosphate Salts

Atopic dermatitis (eczema)
Possibly Effective
Bifidobacteria
Lactobacillus
Rice Bran
Possibly Ineffective
Borage
Evening Primrose Oil
Zinc

Atopic disease
Possibly Effective
Lactobacillus
Whey Protein

Atrial fibrillation
Likely Effective
Digitalis

Atrophic acne scars
Possibly Effective
Alpha Hydroxy Acids

Attention deficit disorder (ADD)
Possibly Ineffective
Tyrosine

Attention deficit-hyperactivity disorder (ADHD)
Possibly Effective
Lithium
Zinc
Possibly Ineffective
Caffeine
DHA
Evening Primrose Oil
Phenylalanine
Pycnogenol
Tyrosine
Vitamin C

Autism
Possibly Ineffective
Dimethylglycine
Inositol
Pyridoxine
Secretin

Back pain
Possibly Effective
Devil's Claw
Willow Bark

Bacterial vaginosis
Possibly Effective
Yogurt

Barium enema-related colonic spasm
Possibly Effective
Peppermint

Bee sting allergy
Likely Effective
Bee Venom

Benign breast disease
Likely Ineffective
Vitamin E

CHARTS

Therapeutic Efficacy

For additional data, refer to the database.

Benign prostatic hyperplasia (BPH)
Likely Effective
Beta-Sitosterol
Pygeum
Saw Palmetto
Possibly Effective
African Wild Potato
Pumpkin
Rye Grass
Possibly Ineffective
Stinging Nettle

Benzodiazepine withdrawal
Possibly Effective
Kava
Melatonin
Possibly Ineffective
Progesterone

Beta blocker-induced dyslipidemia
Possibly Effective
Chromium

Beta-thalassemia
Possibly Effective
Vitamin E

Biliary stones
Possibly Effective
DMSO

Biotin deficiency
Likely Effective
Biotin

Bipolar disorder
Effective
Lithium
Possibly Effective
Fish Oil

Bladder cancer
Possibly Effective
Green Tea
Vitamin E
Possibly Ineffective
Lycopene
Tomato

Bone substitute
Likely Effective
Coral

Breast cancer
Possibly Effective
Beta-Carotene
Folic Acid
Green Tea
Lentinan
Olive
Soy
Vitamin A
Possibly Ineffective
Black Tea
Coffee
Garlic
Likely Ineffective
Vitamin E

Breast cancer-related hot flashes
Possibly Ineffective
Black Cohosh
Vitamin E

Breast engorgement
Possibly Effective
Cabbage

Breast pain
(see Mastalgia)

Brittle nails
Possibly Effective
Biotin

Bronchial diagnostic studies
Effective
N-Acetyl Cysteine

Bronchitis
(see also Acute bronchitis and Chronic obstructive bronchitis)
Possibly Effective
N-Acetyl Cysteine

Bronchopulmonary disorders
Effective
N-Acetyl Cysteine

Bronchopulmonary dysplasia
Possibly Effective
Superoxide Dismutase
Possibly Ineffective
Vitamin E

Bruxism
Possibly Ineffective
L-Tryptophan

Burns
Possibly Effective
Chymotrypsin
Honey
Ornithine Ketoglutarate
Zinc
Possibly Ineffective
RNA and DNA
Tannic Acid

Cachexia
Possibly Effective
Adenosine
Fish Oil
Medium Chain Triglycerides

Cancer
(see also various types of Cancer)
Possibly Effective
Beta Glucans
Coriolus Mushroom
Fish Oil
Vitamin C
Possibly Ineffective
Beer
Likely Ineffective
Beta-Carotene
DMSO
European Mistletoe
Shark Cartilage
Ineffective
Apricot

Cancer-associated neuropathic pain
Possibly Effective
Magnesium

Cardiac arrest
Possibly Ineffective
Magnesium

Cardiac autonomic neuropathy
Possibly Ineffective
Alpha-Lipoic Acid

Cardiac glycoside-induced ventricular arrhythmias
(see also arrhythmias)
Likely Effective
EDTA

Cardiovascular disease
Likely Effective
Beer
Fish Oil
Oats
Wine
Possibly Effective
Alpha-Linolenic Acid
Niacin and Niacinamide
Olive
Tomato
Possibly Ineffective
Lycopene
Selenium
Possibly Ineffective
Soy
Likely Ineffective
Beta-Carotene
Vitamin E

Carpal tunnel syndrome
Possibly Ineffective
Pyridoxine

Cataracts
Effective
Chymotrypsin
Likely Effective
Hyaluronic Acid
Possibly Effective
Fish Oil
Lutein
Niacin and Niacinamide
Riboflavin
Thiamine
Tomato
Vitamin A
Possibly Ineffective
Beta-Carotene
Zinc

Cerebellar ataxia
Possibly Ineffective
Choline

Cerebral palsy
Possibly Ineffective
Magnesium

Cerebrovascular disease
Possibly Effective
Citicoline
Mesoglycan

Cervical dysplasia
Possibly Effective
Green Tea
Indole-3-Carbinol

Chemotherapy extravasation
Possibly Effective
Vitamin E

CHARTS

Therapeutic Efficacy

For additional data, refer to the database.

Chemotherapy toxicity
Possibly Effective
Glutathione

Chemotherapy-induced gastrointestinal (GI) adverse effects
Possibly Ineffective
Vitamin A

Chemotherapy-induced nausea and vomiting
Possibly Effective
Ginger

Cholera
Possibly Effective
Niacin and Niacinamide

Chronic cerebral ischemia
Possibly Effective
Acetyl-L-Carnitine

Chronic fatigue syndrome (CFS)
Possibly Effective
Magnesium
Possibly Ineffective
Folic Acid
Melatonin
Transfer Factor

Chronic ischemic heart disease
Possibly Effective
Propionyl-L-Carnitine

Chronic obstructive bronchitis
(see also Bronchitis)
Possibly Effective
English Ivy

Chronic obstructive pulmonary disease (COPD)
Possibly Effective
Beta-Carotene
Magnesium
N-Acetyl Cysteine

Chronic pouchitis
Possibly Effective
Bifidobacteria
Lactobacillus

Chronic venous insufficiency
Likely Effective
Horse Chestnut
Possibly Effective
Butcher's Broom
Grape
Pycnogenol
Sweet Clover

Circadian rhythm sleep disorders
Likely Effective
Melatonin
Possibly Ineffective
Vitamin B12

Cirrhosis
(see also Alcohol-related liver disease and Liver disease)
Possibly Ineffective
Fish Oil

Cisplatin-induced neurotoxicity
Possibly Effective
Vitamin E

Claudication
Possibly Ineffective
Fish Oil

Clostridium difficile diarrhea
Possibly Effective
Lactobacillus
Saccharomyces Boulardii

Cluster headache
(see also Headache)
Possibly Effective
Magnesium
Melatonin

Coenzyme Q-10 deficiency
Likely Effective
Coenzyme Q-10

Cognitive function
Possibly Effective
Beer
Brahmi
Ginkgo
Ginseng, Panax
Huperzine A
Iron
Wine
Possibly Ineffective
DHEA

Cognitive impairment
Possibly Effective
Acetyl-L-Carnitine

Cold sores
(see Herpes labialis)

Colorectal adenoma
Possibly Ineffective
Blond Psyllium

Colorectal cancer
Possibly Effective
Calcium
Coffee
Folic Acid
Garlic
Lutein
Olive
Possibly Ineffective
Barley
Green Tea
Hydrazine Sulfate
Lycopene
Oats
Rice Bran
Vitamin E
Wheat Bran

Colostomy odor
Possibly Ineffective
Chlorophyll

Common cold
Possibly Effective
Andrographis
Echinacea
Vitamin C
Zinc

Concentration, coordination, and endurance
Possibly Effective
Schisandra

Condylomata acuminata
(see Genital warts)

Congestive heart failure (CHF)
Likely Effective
Digitalis
Possibly Effective
Coenzyme Q-10
Creatine
Hawthorn
L-Arginine
L-Carnitine
Propionyl-L-Carnitine
Taurine
Terminalia
Possibly Ineffective
Vitamin E

Constipation
Effective
Agar
Black Psyllium
Blond Psyllium
Magnesium
Likely Effective
Cascara
European Buckthorn
Flaxseed
Glycerol
Olive
Senna
Possibly Effective
Alder Buckthorn
Aloe
Castor
Guar Gum
Inulin
Karaya Gum
Sweet Almond
Wheat Bran
Xanthan Gum

Contraception
Possibly Effective
Castor
Gossypol

Contrast agent-induced nephropathy
Possibly Effective
N-Acetyl Cysteine

Contrast-mediated nephropathy
Possibly Effective
Vitamin C

Copper deficiency
Likely Effective
Copper

Corneal calcium deposits
Possibly Effective
EDTA

Coronary artery bypass
Possibly Effective
Fish Oil

Coronary artery disease
Possibly Effective
DHA
EPA
Magnesium
Ribose

CHARTS

Therapeutic Efficacy

For additional data, refer to the database.

Coronary artery disease (cont.)
Possibly Ineffective
Folic Acid

Coronary heart disease
Possibly Effective
English Walnut
Likely Ineffective
L-Arginine
EDTA

Corticosteroid-induced osteoporosis
Likely Effective
Calcium
Vitamin D

Cough
Effective
Camphor

Critical illness (trauma)
Possibly Effective
Glutamine

Crohn's disease
Possibly Effective
Saccharomyces Boulardii
Possibly Ineffective
Glutamine

Cutaneous sporotrichosis
Effective
Iodine

Cyclosporine-induced hypertension
Possibly Effective
Fish Oil

Cyclosporine-induced nephrotoxicity
Possibly Effective
Fish Oil

Cystic fibrosis
Effective
N-Acetyl Cysteine
Possibly Ineffective
EPA

Cystinuria
Possibly Ineffective
Glutamine

Deep vein thrombosis (DVT)
Possibly Ineffective
Mesoglycan

Delayed sleep phase syndrome (DSPS)
Possibly Effective
Melatonin

Dementia
(see also Alzheimer's disease)
Possibly Effective
Ginkgo
Huperzine A
Vinpocetine
Vitamin E
Possibly Ineffective
NADH
Likely Ineffective
Lecithin

Dental caries
Effective
Fluoride
Likely Effective
Xylitol

Dental hypersensitivity
Effective
Strontium

Depression
Likely Effective
Lithium
SAMe
St. John's Wort
Possibly Effective
5-HTP
EPA
Fish Oil
Folic Acid
Saffron
Possibly Ineffective
DHA
Inositol
Tyrosine
Likely Ineffective
Melatonin

Dermatitis
Likely Effective
Lecithin
Possibly Ineffective
German Chamomile

Diabetes
Possibly Effective
Alpha-Lipoic Acid
Beer
Blond Psyllium
Cassia Cinnamon
Chromium
Coffee
Ginseng, American
Ginseng, Panax
Glucomannan
Guar Gum
Magnesium
Niacin and Niacinamide
Oats
Prickly Pear Cactus
Soy
Vitamin D
Wine
Xanthan Gum
Possibly Ineffective
Cranberry
DHA
EPA
Garlic
Jambolan
Wheat Bran
Likely Ineffective
Fish Oil

Diabetic foot ulcers
Possibly Effective
Iodine

Diabetic nephropathy
Possibly Effective
Cod Liver Oil
Fish Oil
Soy

Diabetic neuropathy
Possibly Effective
Acetyl-L-Carnitine
Gamma Linolenic Acid
Likely Ineffective
Inositol

Diabetic retinopathy
(see also Retinopathy)
Possibly Effective
Ginkgo

Diaper rash
Possibly Ineffective
Tannic Acid

Diarrhea
(see also AIDS-related diarrhea, Antibiotic-associated diarrhea, and HIV-related diarrhea)
Likely Effective
Zinc
Possibly Effective
Blond Psyllium
Guar Gum
Lactobacillus
Saccharomyces Boulardii
Soy
Yogurt
Possibly Ineffective
Glutamine

Digestive disorders
Likely Ineffective
Pancreatin

Digestive tract cancers
Possibly Ineffective
Coffee

Doxorubicin-induced cardiac toxicity
Possibly Ineffective
N-Acetyl Cysteine

Dry eyes
Possibly Effective
Chondroitin Sulfate

Dry mouth
Possibly Effective
Betaine Anhydrous

Dry skin
Likely Effective
Alpha Hydroxy Acids
Lecithin

Duchenne muscular dystrophy
Possibly Ineffective
Vitamin E

Dyslexia
Possibly Effective
Fish Oil

Dyslipidemia
Possibly Effective
Fish Oil
Gamma Oryzanol

Dysmenorrhea
Possibly Effective
Fish Oil

Therapeutic Efficacy

For additional data, refer to the database.

Dyspepsia
Effective
Calcium
Possibly Effective
Angelica
Artichoke
Caraway
Clown's Mustard Plant
German Chamomile
Greater Celandine
Lemon Balm
Licorice
Milk Thistle
Peppermint
Turmeric

Dyspraxia
Possibly Effective
Fish Oil
Vitamin E

Earwax
Possibly Ineffective
Olive

Eclampsia
Likely Effective
Magnesium

Eczema
(see Atopic dermatitis)

Elevated lead concentrations
Possibly Ineffective
Calcium

Endometrial cancer
Possibly Effective
Fish Oil

Endometrial hyperplasia
Possibly Effective
Progesterone

End-stage renal disease (ESRD)
Effective
L-Carnitine
Likely Effective
Folic Acid
Possibly Effective
N-Acetyl Cysteine
Possibly Ineffective
Blond Psyllium

Enhancing infant development
Possibly Ineffective
Omega-6 Fatty Acids

Epilepsy
Possibly Effective
N-Acetyl Cysteine
Possibly Ineffective
Dimethylglycine

Erectile dysfunction (ED)
Possibly Effective
DHEA
Ginseng, Panax
L-Arginine
Melanotan-II
Propionyl-L-Carnitine
Yohimbe

Erythema
Possibly Effective
Vitamin C

Erythropoietic protoporphyria (EPP)
Effective
Beta-Carotene
Possibly Effective
Canthaxanthin

Esophageal cancer
Possibly Ineffective
Green Tea

Exercise-induced asthma
(see also Asthma)
Possibly Effective
Beta-Carotene

Exercise-induced muscle soreness
Possibly Ineffective
Soy

Exercise-induced respiratory infections
Possibly Effective
Vitamin C

Extrapyramidal disorders
Likely Ineffective
Lecithin

Extravasation
Possibly Effective
DMSO

Eye surgery
Likely Effective
Chondroitin Sulfate

Fall prevention
Likely Effective
Vitamin D

Familial hypercholesterolemia
Possibly Effective
Sitostanol
Possibly Ineffective
Garlic

Familial hypophosphatemia
Effective
Vitamin D

Fanconi syndrome
Effective
Vitamin D

Fetal and early infant mortality
Possibly Ineffective
Vitamin A

Fetal bone mineralization
Likely Effective
Calcium

Fibrocystic breast disease
Possibly Effective
Iodine

Fibromyalgia
Possibly Effective
5-HTP
Capsicum
GHB
SAMe

Fibrosing alveolitis
Possibly Effective
N-Acetyl Cysteine

Fluorosis
Possibly Effective
Calcium

Folate deficiency
Effective
Folic Acid

Food allergies
Possibly Effective
Thymus Extract

Fractures
Possibly Effective
Chymotrypsin

Fragile-X syndrome
Likely Ineffective
Folic Acid

Galactosemia
Possibly Effective
Soy

Gallbladder disease
Possibly Effective
Caffeine
Coffee
Vitamin C
Possibly Ineffective
Lecithin
Likely Ineffective
Beta-Sitosterol

Gastric cancer
Possibly Effective
Barley
Garlic
Green Tea
Lentinan
Oats
Rice Bran
Wheat Bran

Gastroesophageal reflux disease (GERD)
Effective
Magnesium

Gastrointestinal cancer
Possibly Ineffective
Black Tea

Generalized anxiety disorder (GAD)
Possibly Effective
Passionflower

Genital warts (condylomata acuminata)
Likely Effective
Podophyllum

Gingivitis
Possibly Effective
Zinc
Possibly Ineffective
Fish Oil

Glaucoma
Possibly Effective
Ginkgo
Marijuana

Glomerulosclerosis
Possibly Effective
Vitamin E

Glucose-6-phosphate dehydrogenase (G6PD) deficiency
Possibly Effective
Vitamin E

Therapeutic Efficacy

For additional data, refer to the database.

Granuloma annulare
Possibly Effective
Vitamin E

Gyrate atrophy of the choroid and retina
Possibly Effective
Creatine

Hangover
Possibly Effective
Prickly Pear Cactus
Possibly Ineffective
Artichoke

Hayfever
(see Allergic rhinitis)

Head and neck cancer
Possibly Ineffective
Vitamin E
Likely Ineffective
N-Acetyl Cysteine
Vitamin A

Headache
(see also Cluster headache, Migraine headache, Postoperative headache, and Tension headache)
Effective
Caffeine

Hearing loss
Possibly Effective
Magnesium

Heart failure
Possibly Effective
Beer
Wine

Heart transplant
Possibly Effective
Fish Oil

Helicobacter pylori (H. pylori)
Possibly Effective
Beer
Bifidobacteria
Lactobacillus
Saccharomyces Boulardii
Wine
Yogurt
Vitamin C
Possibly Ineffective
Fish Oil
Garlic

Hemodialysis grafts
Possibly Effective
Fish Oil

Hemolytic anemia
Possibly Ineffective
Vitamin E

Hemorrhagic disease
Effective
Vitamin K

Hemorrhoids
Possibly Effective
Blond Psyllium
Bovine Cartilage
Diosmin
Hesperidin
Wheat Bran
Witch Hazel

Hepatic encephalopathy
Possibly Effective
Branched-Chain Amino Acids
Likely Ineffective
Ornithine Ketoglutarate

Hepatic steatosis
Likely Effective
Choline
Possibly Effective
Lecithin

Hepatitis
Possibly Effective
Schisandra
Taurine

Hepatitis A
Possibly Ineffective
Phosphatidylcholine

Hepatitis B
Possibly Ineffective
Chanca Piedra

Hepatitis C
Possibly Effective
Phosphatidylcholine
Possibly Ineffective
St. John's Wort

Hereditary lactase deficiency
Possibly Effective
Soy

Hereditary sideroblastic anemia
Effective
Pyridoxine

Herpes labialis (cold sores)
Possibly Effective
Lemon Balm
Lysine
Rhubarb
Sage
Possibly Ineffective
Tannic Acid
Tea Tree Oil

Herpes simplex virus (HSV)
Possibly Effective
Sangre de Grado
Zinc
Possibly Ineffective
Echinacea

Herpes simplex virus type 2 (HSV-2)
Possibly Effective
Ginseng, Siberian
Propolis

Herpes zoster (shingles)
Possibly Effective
DMSO
Papain
Transfer Factor

HIV
(see HIV/AIDS)

HIV transmission
Possibly Effective
Vitamin C
Possibly Ineffective
Vitamin A

HIV/AIDS
Possibly Effective
Beta Glucans
Coenzyme Q-10
Lentinan
Red Yeast
Possibly Ineffective
St. John's Wort

HIV/AIDS-related wasting
(see also AIDS-related wasting)
Possibly Effective
Glutamine

HIV/AIDS-related weight loss
Possibly Effective
Marijuana
Whey Protein

HIV-associated peripheral neuropathy
Possibly Ineffective
Capsicum

HIV-related dementia
Possibly Ineffective
Alpha-Lipoic Acid

HIV-related diarrhea
Possibly Effective
Saccharomyces Boulardii
Vitamin A

Homocystinuria
Effective
Betaine Anhydrous

Hormone replacement therapy (HRT)
Likely Effective
Progesterone

Hot flashes
(see Menopausal symptoms)

Huntington's disease
Possibly Effective
Coenzyme Q-10
Vitamin E

Hypercalcemia
Likely Effective
EDTA
Phosphate Salts

Hypercalciuria
Possibly Effective
Potassium
Rice Bran

Hypercholesterolemia
(see also Familial hypercholesterolemia)
Likely Effective
Beta-Sitosterol
Flaxseed
Oats
Red Yeast
Sitostanol
Possibly Effective
Alfalfa
Avocado

CHARTS

Hypercholesterolemia (cont.)
Possibly Effective (cont.)
Barley
Beta Glucans
Black Psyllium
Calcium
English Walnut
Guar Gum
Jiaogulan
Macadamia Nut
Magnesium
Olive
Pectin
Policosanol
Rice Bran
Safflower
Soybean Oil
Sweet Orange
Possibly Ineffective
Acacia
Amaranth
Cod Liver Oil
Guggul
Inulin
Lecithin
Red Clover
Hyperhomocysteinemia
Likely Effective
Folic Acid
Pyridoxine
Vitamin B12
Possibly Effective
N-Acetyl Cysteine
Hyperkalemia
Effective
Calcium
Hyperkinetic cerebral dysfunction syndrome
Possibly Effective
Pyridoxine
Hyperlipidemia
Effective
Niacin and Niacinamide
Likely Effective
Blond Psyllium
Soy
Possibly Effective
Artichoke
Garlic
Green Tea
Inositol Nicotinate
Yogurt
Likely Ineffective
Kefir
Hyperlipoproteinemia
Possibly Effective
Pantethine
Hyperparathyroidism
Likely Effective
Calcium
Hyperparathyroidism-related bone loss
Possibly Effective
Vitamin D

Hypertension
Possibly Effective
Alpha-Linolenic Acid
Blond Psyllium
Calcium
Cod Liver Oil
Coenzyme Q-10
Fish Oil
Garlic
Green Tea
Magnesium
Olive
Oolong Tea
Potassium
Pycnogenol
Soy
Stevia
Sweet Orange
Vitamin C
Wheat Bran
Possibly Ineffective
Oats
Vitamin E
Hyperthyroidism
Possibly Effective
L-Carnitine
Hypertriglyceridemia
Effective
Fish Oil
Likely Effective
Cod Liver Oil
Possibly Effective
Inulin
Mesoglycan
Hypocalcemia
Effective
Calcium
Hypogeusia
Possibly Effective
Zinc
Hypoglycemia
Possibly Effective
Chromium
Hypokalemia
Effective
Potassium
Hypomagnesemia
Effective
Magnesium
Hypoparathyroidism
Effective
Vitamin D
Hypophosphatemia
Effective
Phosphate Salts
Hypoprothrombinemia
Effective
Vitamin K
Hypotension
Possibly Effective
Black Tea
Caffeine
Coffee
Green Tea

Hypothyroidism
Possibly Effective
Tiratricol
Idiopathic congestive cardiomyopathy
Possibly Effective
Forskolin
Ifosfamide (Ifex) toxicity
Possibly Effective
N-Acetyl Cysteine
IgA nephropathy
Possibly Effective
Fish Oil
Imerslund-Grasbeck disease
Effective
Vitamin B12
Imparied glucose tolerance (Prediabetes)
Possibly Ineffective
Chromium
Infectious diarrhea
Possibly Effective
Colostrum
Infertility
Likely Effective
Progesterone
Possibly Effective
Acetyl-L-Carnitine
L-Carnitine
Vitamin E
Inflammatory bladder disease
Possibly Effective
DMSO
Inflammatory bowel disease (IBD)
Possibly Ineffective
Zinc
Influenza
Possibly Effective
Elderberry
N-Acetyl Cysteine
Possibly Ineffective
Zinc
Insomnia
Possibly Effective
Melatonin
Valerian
Interferon-related retinopathy
Possibly Ineffective
Vitamin C
Intermittent claudication
Possibly Effective
Ginkgo
Policosanol
Propionyl-L-Carnitine
Possibly Ineffective
Vitamin E
Interstitial cystitis
Effective
DMSO
Possibly Effective
L-Arginine
Superoxide Dismutase
Intestinal bacterial overgrowth
Possibly Ineffective
Lactobacillus

Therapeutic Efficacy

For additional data, refer to the database.

Intestinal parasitic infection
Possibly Effective
Oregano
Intracranial hemorrhage
Possibly Effective
Vitamin E
Intracranial pressure
Possibly Effective
DMSO
Intrahepatic cholestasis
Possibly Effective
SAMe
Intrauterine growth
Possibly Ineffective
EPA
Intraventricular hemorrhage
Possibly Effective
Vitamin E
Iron absorption
Likely Effective
Vitamin C
Iron deficiency anemia
Effective
Iron
Irradiated skin
Possibly Ineffective
Pantothenic Acid
Irritable bowel syndrome (IBS)
Possibly Effective
Bifidobacteria
Blond Psyllium
Guar Gum
Wheat Bran
Possibly Ineffective
Brahmi
Ischemic reperfusion injury
Possibly Effective
Alpha-Ketoglutarate
Coenzyme Q-10
Ischemic stroke
(see also Stroke)
Possibly Effective
Calcium
Citicoline
Isolated systolic hypertension
Possibly Effective
Coenzyme Q-10
Jet lag
Possibly Effective
Melatonin
Kidney disease
Possibly Effective
Soy
Kidney failure
(see Renal failure)
Kidney stones (nephrolithiasis)
Possibly Effective
Black Tea
IP-6
Magnesium
Phosphate Salts
Pyridoxine

Labor facilitation
(see Parturition)
Possibly Ineffective
Raspberry Leaf
Lactose intolerance
Likely Effective
Lactase
Possibly Effective
Yogurt
Possibly Ineffective
Lactobacillus
L-carnitine deficiency
Effective
L-Carnitine
Lead toxicity
Effective
EDTA
Possibly Effective
Vitamin C
Leg ulcers
Possibly Effective
Glycine
Leprosy
Possibly Effective
Zinc
Lice
Effective
Pyrethrum
Possibly Effective
Quassia
Lithium-induced side effects
Possibly Effective
Inositol
Liver disease
Possibly Effective
SAMe
Lometrexol toxicity
Possibly Ineffective
Folic Acid
Low birth weight
Possibly Effective
L-Carnitine
Lung cancer
Possibly Effective
Lycopene
Pyridoxine
Possibly Ineffective
Garlic
Selenium
Transfer Factor
Likely Ineffective
Beta-Carotene
Hydrazine Sulfate
N-Acetyl Cysteine
Vitamin E
Lymphedema
Possibly Ineffective
Diosmin
Hesperidin
Malaria
Possibly Effective
Vitamin A
Possibly Ineffective
Zinc

Malignant melanoma
(see also Skin cancer)
Possibly Ineffective
Transfer Factor
Malnourishment-related diarrhea
Possibly Ineffective
Yogurt
Mandibular alveolitis
Possibly Effective
Bovine Cartilage
Manganese deficiency
Effective
Manganese
Mania
Possibly Effective
Branched-Chain Amino Acids
Mastalgia
Possibly Effective
Evening Primrose Oil
Possibly Ineffective
Fish Oil
Mastodynia
Possibly Effective
Progesterone
McArdle's disease
Possibly Effective
Creatine
Likely Ineffective
Ribose
Measles
Possibly Effective
Vitamin A
Melasma
Possibly Effective
Alpha Hydroxy Acids
Menopausal anxiety
Possibly Effective
Kava
Menopausal symptoms
Possibly Effective
Black Cohosh
DHEA
Flaxseed
Progesterone
Soy
Possibly Ineffective
Dong Quai
Evening Primrose Oil
Ginseng, Panax
Red Clover
Wild Yam
Mental alertness
Likely Effective
Black Tea
Caffeine
Coffee
Green Tea
Oolong Tea
Metabolic disorders
Effective
Thiamine
Methotrexate toxicity
Likely Effective
Folic Acid

CHARTS

Therapeutic Efficacy

For additional data, refer to the database.

Migraine headache
Effective
Caffeine
Possibly Effective
Butterbur
Coenzyme Q-10
Feverfew
Magnesium
Riboflavin
Possibly Ineffective
Fish Oil

Minor bleeding
Possibly Effective
Witch Hazel

Mitochondrial encephalomyopathies
Likely Effective
Coenzyme Q-10

Mitral valve prolapse
Possibly Effective
Magnesium

Morning sickness
Possibly Effective
Ginger

Mosquito repellent
Likely Effective
Lemon Eucalyptus
Soybean Oil
Possibly Effective
Citronella Oil

Motion sickness
Possibly Ineffective
Ginger

Multiple sclerosis (MS)
Possibly Effective
Marijuana
Vitamin D

Multisystem organ failure
Likely Ineffective
N-Acetyl Cysteine

Muscle breakdown
Possibly Effective
Branched-Chain Amino Acids

Muscle catabolism
Possibly Effective
Alpha-Ketoglutarate

Muscle cramps
Possibly Effective
Zinc

Muscle strength
Possibly Ineffective
Vitamin D

Muscular dystrophy
(see also Myotonic dystrophy)
Possibly Effective
Coenzyme Q-10
Creatine

Myalgia
(see also Pain)
Possibly Ineffective
Bromelain
Fish Oil

Myasthenia gravis
Possibly Effective
Huperzine A

Myoadenylate deaminase deficiency (MAD)
Possibly Effective
Ribose

Myocardial infarction (MI)
[see also Acute myocardial infarction (MI)]
Possibly Effective
Black Tea
Coenzyme Q-10
L-Carnitine
Likely Ineffective
Superoxide Dismutase

Myocarditis
Possibly Effective
L-Carnitine

Myofascial pain
Possibly Ineffective
L-Tryptophan

Myotonic dystrophy
(See also Muscular dystrophy)
Possibly Ineffective
Vitamin E

Narcolepsy
Possibly Effective
GHB

Necrotizing enterocolitis (NEC)
Possibly Effective
Bifidobacteria
L-Arginine

Neonatal apnea
Possibly Effective
Caffeine

Nephrolithiasis
(see Kidney stones)

Neural tube birth defects
Likely Effective
Folic Acid
Possibly Effective
Choline

Niacin deficiency
Effective
Niacin and Niacinamide

Nicotine withdrawal
Possibly Effective
Melatonin

Night vision
Possibly Ineffective
Bilberry

Nitrate tolerance
Possibly Effective
L-Arginine
Vitamin C
Vitamin E
Likely Ineffective
N-Acetyl Cysteine

Nodulocystic acne
Possibly Effective
Guggul

Obesity
Possibly Effective
Conjugated Linoleic Acid
Diacylglycerol
Ephedra
Fish Oil
Possibly Ineffective
Garcinia
Inulin

Obsessive-compulsive disorder (OCD)
Possibly Effective
Inositol

Ocular stress
Possibly Effective
Grape

Onychomycosis
Possibly Effective
Tea Tree Oil

Opiate withdrawal
Possibly Effective
GHB
Passionflower

Oral leukoplakia
Possibly Effective
Beta-Carotene
Blue-Green Algae
Green Tea

Oral mucosal lesions
Possibly Ineffective
Vitamin E

Oral mucositis
Likely Effective
Hyaluronic Acid
Possibly Effective
German Chamomile
Glutamine
Iodine
Kaolin

Orlistat (*Xenical*) side effects
Possibly Effective
Blond Psyllium

Osteoarthritis
Likely Effective
Chondroitin Sulfate
Glucosamine Sulfate
SAMe
Possibly Effective
Avocado
Beta-Carotene
Bovine Cartilage
Bromelain
Camphor
Cat's Claw
Cetylated Fatty Acids
Devil's Claw
DMSO
Glucosamine Hydrochloride
Hyaluronic Acid
Niacin And Niacinamide
Rutin
Soybean Oil
Superoxide Dismutase
Trypsin
Vitamin C

Osteoarthritis (cont.)
Possibly Ineffective
Bee Venom
Cod Liver Oil
Vitamin E
Osteogenesis imperfecta
Possibly Effective
Vitamin D
Osteomalacia
Effective
Vitamin D
Osteoporosis
(see also Corticosteroid-induced osteoporosis)
Likely Effective
Calcium
Ipriflavone
Vitamin D
Possibly Effective
DHEA
Evening Primrose Oil
Fish Oil
Fluoride
Magnesium
Manganese
Silicon
Soy
Strontium
Possibly Ineffective
Progesterone
Otitis media
Possibly Effective
Xylitol
Possibly Ineffective
Olive
Ovarian cancer
Possibly Effective
Beta-Carotene
Green Tea
Lycopene
Possibly Ineffective
Black Tea
Paget's disease
Possibly Effective
Ipriflavone
Pain
(see also Myalgia)
Effective
Camphor
Procaine
Likely Effective
Capsicum
Possibly Ineffective
Phenylalanine
Painful bony metastases
Effective
Strontium
Pancreatic cancer
Possibly Effective
Folic Acid
Possibly Ineffective
Green Tea
Vitamin E
Pancreatic insufficiency
Effective
Lipase
Pancreatin
Pancreatitis
Possibly Effective
Chlorophyll
Panic disorder
Possibly Effective
Inositol
Pantothenic acid deficiency
Effective
Pantothenic Acid
Parkinson's disease
Possibly Effective
Black Tea
Caffeine
Coenzyme Q-10
Coffee
Green Tea
Vitamin E
Paroxysmal supraventricular tachycardia
Effective
Adenosine
Parturition
(see also Labor facilitation)
Possibly Effective
Castor
Possibly Ineffective
Laminaria
Pellagra
Effective
Niacin and Niacinamide
Peptic ulcers
Possibly Effective
Zinc
Periodontal disease
Likely Ineffective
Coenzyme Q-10
Periodontitis
Possibly Effective
Chitosan
Peripheral arterial disease
Possibly Effective
L-Arginine
Mesoglycan
Vitamin C
Possibly Ineffective
Garlic
Peripheral neuropathy
Possibly Effective
Alpha-Lipoic Acid
Peripheral vascular disease
Possibly Effective
Inositol Nicotinate
Peritoneal dialysis
Possibly Ineffective
Phosphatidylcholine
Pernicious anemia
Effective
Vitamin B12
Pervasive developmental disorder
Likely Ineffective
Secretin
Peyronie's disease
Possibly Effective
Acetyl-L-Carnitine
Propionyl-L-Carnitine
Pharyngitis
Possibly Effective
Papain
Pharyngotonsillitis
Possibly Effective
Andrographis
Phenylketonuria (PKU)
Effective
Tyrosine
Phenytoin-induced gingival hyperplasia
Possibly Effective
Folic Acid
Photoreactive keratectomy
Possibly Effective
Vitamin A
Vitamin E
Pituitary resistance to thyroid hormone (PRTH)
Likely Effective
Tiratricol
Plastic surgery
Possibly Effective
Chitosan
Pneumonia
Possibly Effective
Zinc
Likely Ineffective
Vitamin A
Poison oak and poison ivy dermatitis
Possibly Effective
Bovine Cartilage
Poisoning
Likely Effective
Activated Charcoal
Possibly Effective
Ipecac
Polycystic ovary syndrome
Possibly Effective
Inositol
Polyneuropathy
Possibly Ineffective
St. John's Wort
Postdural puncture headache
Possibly Effective
Caffeine
Postherpetic neuralgia
Possibly Effective
DMSO
Post-hysterectomy pain
Possibly Effective
Magnesium
Postoperative headache
Effective
Caffeine

CHARTS

Postoperative infection
Possibly Effective
Beta Glucans

Postoperative nausea
Possibly Effective
Peppermint

Postoperative nausea and vomiting
Possibly Effective
Ginger

Postoperative swelling
Possibly Effective
Serrapeptase

Post-partum complications
Possibly Effective
Beta-Carotene
Vitamin A

Post-surgery recovery
Possibly Effective
L-Arginine

Pre-eclampsia
Likely Effective
Magnesium
Possibly Effective
Vitamin C
Vitamin E
Possibly Ineffective
L-Arginine

Pregnancy-induced hypertension
Possibly Ineffective
EPA

Pregnancy-induced leg cramps
Possibly Effective
Magnesium

Pregnancy-induced nausea and vomiting
Possibly Effective
Pyridoxine

Pregnancy-related complications
Possibly Effective
Beta-Carotene
Calcium
Vitamin A

Pregnancy-related gingivitis
Possibly Effective
Folic Acid

Pregnancy-related iron deficiency
Possibly Ineffective
Zinc

Premature ejaculation
Possibly Effective
Angelica
Cinnamon Bark
Clove
Dong Quai
Ginseng, Panax

Premenstrual dysphoric disorder (PMDD)
Possibly Effective
Chasteberry
L-Tryptophan

Premenstrual syndrome (PMS)
Likely Effective
Calcium
Possibly Effective
Brewer's Yeast
Chasteberry
Ginkgo
Magnesium
Pyridoxine
Vitamin E
Possibly Ineffective
Evening Primrose Oil
Progesterone

Preoperative anxiety and sedation
Possibly Effective
Melatonin

Preterm labor
Possibly Effective
Magnesium

Prickly heat
Possibly Ineffective
Tannic Acid

Prostate cancer
Possibly Effective
Fish Oil
Garlic
Lentinan
Lycopene
Melatonin
Selenium
Strontium
Tomato
Possibly Ineffective
Beta-Carotene
Shiitake Mushroom

Prostatitis
Possibly Effective
Quercetin

Prurigo nodularis
Possibly Effective
Capsicum

Pruritus (itching)
(see also Anal pruritus)
Effective
Camphor

Psoriasis
Effective
Vitamin D
Possibly Effective
Aloe
Bovine Cartilage
DHA
EPA
Fish Oil
Possibly Ineffective
Zinc

Psoriatic arthritis
Possibly Ineffective
Zinc

Pyridoxine deficiency
Effective
Pyridoxine

Pyridoxine-dependent seizures
Effective
Pyridoxine

Quality of life
Possibly Ineffective
Ginseng, Panax

Radiation
Effective
Iodine

Radiation dermatitis
Possibly Ineffective
Vitamin C

Radiation-induced fibrosis
Possibly Effective
Vitamin E

Raynaud's syndrome
Possibly Effective
Fish Oil
Ginkgo

Reflex sympathetic dystrophy (RSD)
Possibly Effective
Vitamin C

Renal failure
Effective
Calcium
Possibly Effective
Chitosan

Renal osteodystrophy
Effective
Vitamin D
Possibly Effective
Ipriflavone

Renal transplant
Possibly Effective
L-Arginine

Renal transplant-related bone loss
Possibly Ineffective
Vitamin D

Respiratory congestion
Effective
Iodine

Respiratory distress syndrome
Possibly Effective
Inositol

Respiratory infections
Possibly Effective
Lactobacillus
Thymus Extract
Possibly Ineffective
Vitamin E

Retinitis pigmentosa
Possibly Ineffective
Vitamin E

Retinopathy
(see also Diabetic retinopathy)
Possibly Effective
Bilberry
Pycnogenol

Retrolental fibroplasia
Possibly Effective
Vitamin E

CHARTS

Therapeutic Efficacy

For additional data, refer to the database.

Rheumatoid arthritis (RA)
Possibly Effective
Borage
Bovine Cartilage
Cat's Claw
DMSO
Fish Oil
Olive
Superoxide Dismutase
Thunder God Vine
Vitamin D
Vitamin E
Possibly Ineffective
Creatine
Feverfew
Flaxseed Oil
Histidine
New Zealand Green-Lipped Mussel
Selenium
Zinc

Rickets
Effective
Vitamin D

Rotating shift work
Possibly Ineffective
Melatonin

Rotaviral diarrhea
Likely Effective
Lactobacillus
Possibly Effective
Bifidobacteria

Scabies
Ineffective
Pyrethrum

Scarring
Possibly Ineffective
Vitamin E

Schistosomiasis
Possibly Effective
Gotu Kola

Schizophrenia
Possibly Effective
DHEA
Glycine
Lithium
Possibly Ineffective
EPA
Inositol
Likely Ineffective
Choline

Scleroderma
Possibly Ineffective
DMSO
EDTA
Gamma Linolenic Acid
PABA

Scurvy
Possibly Effective
Acerola

Seasonal affective disorder (SAD)
Possibly Ineffective
Ginkgo

Seborrheic dermatitis
Possibly Ineffective
Biotin

Seizures
Possibly Effective
Medium Chain Triglycerides

Sexual arousal
Possibly Ineffective
DHEA

Sexual desire
Possibly Effective
Maca

Sexual dysfunction
Possibly Effective
Yohimbe

Shingles
(see also Herpes zoster)

Sickle cell disease
Possibly Effective
Zinc

Sinusitis
Possibly Effective
Cowslip
Elderflower
Gentian
Sorrel
Verbena

Sjogren's syndrome
Possibly Effective
Xanthan Gum

Skin cancer
(see also Malignant melanoma)
Possibly Ineffective
Selenium

Skin flap ischemia
Possibly Effective
DMSO

Skin infection
Effective
Iodine

Skin irritation
Possibly Effective
Sweet Almond
Witch Hazel

Sleep
Possibly Effective
Lemon Balm

Sleep deprivation
Possibly Effective
Tyrosine

Sleep-wake cycle disturbances
Likely Effective
Melatonin

Smoking cessation
Possibly Effective
L-Tryptophan
Likely Ineffective
Lobelia

Solid tumors
Possibly Effective
Melatonin

Somatization disorder
Possibly Effective
St. John's Wort

Sore throat
Possibly Effective
Slippery Elm

Spinal spasticity
Possibly Effective
Threonine

Stroke
(see also Ischemic stroke)
Possibly Effective
Fish Oil
Glycine
Magnesium
Potassium
Soy
Possibly Ineffective
Beta-Carotene
Folic Acid
Mesoglycan
Pyridoxine
Vitamin B12
Vitamin C
Likely Ineffective
Glycerol

Sulcoplasty
Possibly Effective
Propolis

Sunburn
Effective
PABA
Possibly Effective
Beta-Carotene
Melatonin
Vitamin C
Vitamin E

Surgery
Possibly Effective
EPA
Glutamine

Surgical recovery
Possibly Effective
RNA and DNA

Systemic lupus erythematosus (SLE)
Possibly Effective
DHEA

Systemic lupus erythematosus (SLE) nephritis
Possibly Effective
Flaxseed

Tanning skin
Possibly Effective
Melanotan-II

Tardive dyskinesia
Possibly Effective
Branched-Chain Amino Acids
Melatonin
Pyridoxine
Vitamin E
Possibly Ineffective
Phosphatidylcholine
Likely Ineffective
Deanol

Therapeutic Efficacy

For additional data, refer to the database.

Temporomandibular joint (TMJ) arthritis
Possibly Effective
Glucosamine Sulfate

Tension headache
Possibly Effective
Peppermint
Possibly Ineffective
5-HTP

Thiamine deficiency
Effective
Thiamine

Thrombocytopenia
Possibly Effective
Melatonin

Thyroid cancer
Possibly Effective
Tiratricol

Thyroid conditions
Effective
Iodine

Tick bites
Possibly Effective
Garlic

Tick repellent
Possibly Effective
Lemon Eucalyptus

Tinea corporis
Possibly Effective
Bitter Orange
Garlic

Tinea cruris
Possibly Effective
Bitter Orange
Garlic

Tinea pedis (athlete's foot)
Possibly Effective
Bitter Orange
Garlic
Tea Tree Oil

Tinnitus
Possibly Ineffective
Ginkgo
Zinc

Tooth retention
Possibly Effective
Calcium

Torsade de pointes
Likely Effective
Magnesium

Tracheostomy care
Effective
N-Acetyl Cysteine

Traveler's diarrhea
Possibly Effective
Bifidobacteria
Saccharomyces Boulardii
Sangre de Grado
Lactobacillus
Possibly Ineffective
Fructo-Oligosaccharides

Tuberculosis
Possibly Ineffective
Beta-Sitosterol

Tyrosinemia
Likely Effective
Vitamin C

Ulcerative colitis
Possibly Effective
Blond Psyllium

Urinary odor
Possibly Effective
Cranberry
Possibly Ineffective
Chlorophyllin

Urinary tract infections (UTIs)
Possibly Effective
Cranberry

Urine drug tests
Possibly Ineffective
Goldenseal

Uveitis
Possibly Effective
Vitamin E

Vaginal candidiasis
Possibly Effective
Echinacea
Yogurt

Valproic acid-induced toxicities
Possibly Effective
L-Carnitine

Vascular dementia
Possibly Ineffective
Vitamin C

Vasospastic angina
(see also Angina)
Possibly Effective
Magnesium

Venous insufficiency
Possibly Effective
Gotu Kola
Mesoglycan

Venous leg ulcers
Possibly Effective
Zinc

Venous stasis ulcers
Possibly Effective
Adenosine
Diosmin
Hesperidin
Mesoglycan

Vertigo
Possibly Effective
Ginger
Ginkgo

Vitamin A deficiency
Effective
Vitamin A
Possibly Effective
Zinc

Vitamin B12 deficiency
Effective
Vitamin B12

Vitamin C deficiency
Effective
Vitamin C

Vitamin E deficiency
Effective
Vitamin E

Vitiligo
Possibly Effective
Folic Acid
Phenylalanine
Picrorhiza

Vulval lichen sclerosis
Possibly Ineffective
Progesterone

Vulvovaginitis
Possibly Ineffective
Lactobacillus

Warfarin anticoagulation
Effective
Vitamin K

Water purification
Effective
Iodine

Weight loss
Possibly Effective
Caffeine
Calcium
Pyruvate
Possibly Ineffective
Blue-Green Algae
Chitosan
Glycerol
Guar Gum
Likely Ineffective
Tiratricol

Wilson's disease
Effective
Zinc

Wisdom tooth extraction
Possibly Ineffective
Arnica

Wound healing
Possibly Effective
Magnesium
Trypsin

Wrinkled skin
Likely Effective
Alpha Hydroxy Acids
Possibly Effective
Vitamin C

Zinc deficiency
Effective
Zinc

Potential Interactions Between Drugs and Natural Medicines

For details on possible interactions between drugs and natural medicines, see the listing for the specific natural medicine in the body of this database. This chart does not contain all theoretical or unknown interactions.

Drug	Natural Medicine
5-HT1 AGONISTS ("Triptans") Some drugs in this category include: Eletriptan (*Relpax*) • Naratriptan (*Amerge*) • Rizatriptan (*Maxalt*) • Sumatriptan (*Imitrex*) • Zolmitriptan (*Zomig*)	St. John's Wort
ACARBOSE (*Precose*, *Prandase*)	Pancreatin
ACE INHIBITORS (ACEIs) Some drugs in this category include: Captopril (*Capoten*) • Enalapril (*Vasotec*) • Lisinopril (*Prinivil*, *Zestril*) • Fosinopril (*Monopril*) • Moexipril (*Univasc*) • Perindopril (*Aceon*) • Quinapril (*Accupril*) • Ramipril (*Altace*) • Spirapril (*Renormax*) • Trandolapril (*Mavik*)	Capsicum • Iodine • Laminaria • Lithium • Morinda • Pomegranate • Potassium
ACENOCOUMAROL (*Sintrom*)	Acetyl-L-Carnitine • L-Carnitine • Propionyl-L-Carnitine
ACETAMINOPHEN (*Tylenol*, others)	Ambrette • Cabbage • Glucosamine Sulfate • Hibiscus • Vitamin C
ACETYLCHOLINESTERASE (AChE) INHIBITORS Some drugs in this category include: Donepezil (*Aricept*) • Galantamine (*Reminyl*) • Rivastigmine (*Exelon*) • Tacrine (*Cognex*)	Chinese Club Moss • Huperzine A
ACTIVATED CHARCOAL	Ipecac • N-Acetyl Cysteine
ADENOSINE (*Adenocard*)	Black Tea • Caffeine • Cocoa • Coffee • Cola Nut • Green Tea • Guarana • Mate • Oolong Tea
ALCOHOL (Ethanol)	Activated Charcoal • Baikal Skullcap • Black Tea • Butanediol • Caffeine • Calcium D-Glucarate • Coca • Coffee • Cola Nut • GBL • GHB • Ginseng, Siberian • Green Tea • Guarana • Hops • Indian Snakeroot • Magnolia • Mate • Oolong Tea • Red Yeast • Ribose • Tansy • Valerian
ALENDRONATE (*Fosamax*)	Coffee • Whey Protein
ALPHA-ADRENERGIC AGONISTS Some drugs in this category include: Pseudoephedrine (*Sudafed*, others) • Phenylephrine • Phenylpropanolamine	Butcher's Broom
ALPHA-ADRENERGIC ANTAGONISTS Some drugs in this category include: Phenoxybenzamine (*Dibenzyline*) • Phentolamine (*Regitine*) • Tamsulosin (*Flomax*) • Terazosin (*Hytrin*) • Prazosin (*Minipress*) • Doxazosin (*Cardura*)	Butcher's Broom
ALPRAZOLAM (*Xanax*)	Kava • St. John's Wort • Valerian
ALUMINUM	Cherokee Rosehip • Rose Hip • Vitamin C • Vitamin D
AMILORIDE (*Midamor*)	Zinc
AMINOGLYCOSIDES Some drugs in this category include: Gentamicin (*Garamycin*) • Amikacin (*Amikin*) • Tobramycin (*Tobrex*)	Magnesium
AMINOLEVULINIC ACID	St. John's Wort
AMINOSALICYLIC ACID (*Paser*, *Teebacin*, *Tubasal*)	Procaine
AMIODARONE (*Cordarone*)	Iodine • Pyridoxine
AMITRIPTYLINE (*Elavil*)	St. John's Wort
AMOXICILLIN (*Amoxil*, *Trimox*)	Acacia
AMPHETAMINES	Butanediol • Cola Nut • GBL • GHB • Green Tea • Guarana • Mate • Oolong Tea
ANASTROZOLE (*Arimidex*)	DHEA
ANESTHESIA Some drugs in this category include: Thiopental Sodium (*Pentothal*) • Methohexital Sodium (*Brevital*) • Etomidate (*Amidate*) • Ketamine (*Ketalar*) • Propofol (*Diprivan*) • Nitrous Oxide • Enflurane (*Ethrane*) • Halothane (*Fluothane*) • Methoxyflurane (*Penthrane*) • Sevoflurane (*Ultane*) • Isoflurane (*Forane*) • Desflurane (*Suprane*)	Borage • Cowhage • Evening Primrose Oil • Fever Bark

CHARTS

Potential Interactions: Drug/Natural Medicine

For additional data, refer to the database.

Drug	Natural Medicine
ANGIOTENSIN RECEPTOR BLOCKERS (ARBs) Some drugs in this category include: Candesartan (*Atacand*) • Eprosartan (*Teveten*) • Irbesartan (*Avapro*) • Losartan (*Cozaar*) • Telmisartan (*Micardis*) • Valsartan (*Diovan*)	Iodine • Morinda • Potassium
ANTACIDS Some drugs in this category include: Aluminum Hydroxide (*Amphojel*, others) • Calcium Carbonate (*Tums*, others) • Aluminum and Magnesium Hydroxide (*Maalox*, *Mylanta*)	Aletris • Alpinia • Angelica • Black Mustard • Blessed Thistle • Calamus • Cinchona • Colombo • Cubebs • Dandelion • Devil's Claw • Gentian • Goldenseal • Goldthread • Northern Prickly Ash • Peppermint • Phosphate Salts • Quassia • Southern Prickly Ash • Yarrow
ANTIBIOTICS (see also individual listings) Some drugs in this category include: Fluoroquinolones: Ciprofloxacin (*Cipro*) • Levofloxacin (*Levaquin*) • Norfloxacin (*Noroxin*) • Ofloxacin (*Floxin*) • Enoxacin (*Penetrex*) • Lomefloxacin (*Maxaquin*) • Trovafloxacin; Alatrofloxacin (*Trovan*) Penicillins: Penicillin (*Bicillin*, *Veetids*) • Nafcillin (*Unipen*) • Oxacillin (*Bactocill*) • Dicloxacillin (*Dynapen*) • Cloxacillin (*Cloxapen*) • Ampicillin (*Principen*) • Amoxicillin (*Amoxil*) • Amoxicillin;Potassium Clavulanate (*Augmentin*) • Ticarcillin (*Ticar*) • Ticarcillin;Clavulanate (*Timentin*) • Mezlocillin (*Mezlin*) • Piperacillin (*Pipracil*) • Piperacillin;Tazobactam (*Zosyn*) • Carbenicillin (*Geocillin*) Macrolides: Clarithromycin (*Biaxin*) • Azithromycin (*Zithromax*) • Dirithromycin (*Dynabac*) • Erythromycin Base (*E-Mycin*, *Ery-Tab*) • Erythromycin Ethylsuccinate (*E.E.S.*) Vancomycin (*Vancocin*) Clindamycin (*Cleocin*) Aminoglycosides: Tobramycin (*Nebcin*) • Amikacin (*Amikin*) • Kanamycin (*Kantrex*) • Gentamicin (*Garamycin*) Metronidazole (*Flagyl*) Sulfadiazine • Sulfisoxazole • Sulfamethoxazole (*Gantanol*) • Sulfamethoxazole;Trimethoprim (*Bactrim*) Nitrofurantoin (*Macrodantin*) Tetracycline (*Sumycin*) • Doxycycline (*Vibramycin*) • Minocycline (*Minocin*) Cefpodoxime (*Vantin*) • Cefaclor (*Ceclor*) • Cephalexin (*Keflex*) • Cefadroxil (*Duricef*) • Cephradine (*Velosef*) • Loracarbef (*Lorabid*) • Cefprozil (*Cefzil*) • Cefitbuten (*Cedax*) • Cefdinir (*Omnicef*) • Cephapirin (*Cefadyl*) • Cefazolin (*Ancef*) • Cefoxitin (*Mefoxin*) • Cefuroxime (*Ceftin*) • Cefonicid (*Monocid*) • Ceftriaxone (*Rocephin*) • Cefixime (*Suprax*) • Cefoperazone (*Cefobid*) • Cefotaxime (*Claforan*) • Cefotetan (*Cefotan*) • Ceftazidime (*Fortaz*) • Cefamandole (*Mandol*) • Imipenem;Cilastatin (*Primaxin*) • Aztreonam (*Azactam*)	Bifidobacteria • Lactobacillus • Soy
ANTICHOLINERGIC DRUGS Some drugs in this category include: Amitriptyline (*Elavil*) • Diphenhydramine (*Benadryl*) • Cyproheptadine (*Periactin*) • Amantadine (*Symmetrel*) • Atropine;Belladonna;Scopolamine (*Donnatal*) • Clozapine (*Clozaril*) • Prochlorperazine (*Compazine*)	Angel's Trumpet • Areca • Belladonna • Calabar Bean • Chinese Club Moss • Deanol • European Mandrake • Henbane • Huperzine A • Iboga • Jimson Weed • Riboflavin • Scopolia

CHARTS

Potential Interactions: Drug/Natural Medicine

For additional data, refer to the database.

Drug	Natural Medicine
ANTICOAGULANT / ANTIPLATELET DRUGS Some drugs in this category include: Ardeparin (*Normiflo*) • Dalteparin (*Fragmin*) • Danaparoid (*Orgaran*) • Enoxaparin (*Lovenox*) Heparin Antithrombin III (*Thrombate III*) Lepirudin (*Refludan*) Warfarin (*Coumadin*) • Dicumarol • Clopidogrel (*Plavix*) • Cilostazol (*Pletal*) • Dipyridamole (*Persantine*) • Ticlopidine (*Ticlid*) • Tirofiban (*Aggrastat*) • Eptifibatide (*Integrilin*) • Abciximab (*ReoPro*) • Anagrelide (*Agrylin*)	Allspice • Andrographis • Angelica • Arnica • Asafoetida • Bishop's Weed • Black Tea • Bladderwrack • Bogbean • Boldo • Borage • Bromelain • Buchu • Burdock • Caffeine • Capsicum • Carrageenan • Cinchona • Clove • Cod Liver Oil • Coffee • Coltsfoot • Danshen • Deertongue • DHA • Dong Quai • EPA • Epimedium • Evening Primrose Oil • Fenugreek • Feverfew • Fish Oil • Flaxseed • Flaxseed Oil • Forskolin • Forsythia • Gamma Linolenic Acid • Garlic • Ginger • Ginseng, Panax • Ginseng, Siberian • Green Tea • Guarana • Guggul • Holy Basil • Honeysuckle • Horse Chestnut • Inositol Nicotinate • IP-6 • Jiaogulan • Kudzu • Mate • Melatonin • Mesoglycan • Nattokinase • Onion • Oolong Tea • Pantethine • Pau D'arco • Policosanol • Red Clover • Reishi Mushroom • Resveratrol • Safflower • Saw Palmetto • Sea Buckthorn • Sweet Clover • Sweet Vernal Grass • Tiratricol • Turmeric • Vanadium • Vinpocetine • Vitamin E • Willow Bark • Yarrow
ANTICONVULSANTS Some drugs in this category include: Carbamazepine (*Tegretol*) • Clonazepam (*Klonopin*) • Ethosuximide (*Zarontin*) • Gabapentin (*Neurontin*) • Lamotrigine (*Lamictal*) • Levetiracetam (*Keppra*) • Methsuximide (*Celontin*) • Oxcarbazepine (*Trileptal*) • Tiagabine (*Gabitril*) • Topiramate (*Topamax*) • Valproic Acid (*Depakote*) • Zonisamide (*Zonegran*)	Butanediol • Cedar Leaf • Cedar Leaf Oil • Ephedra • GBL • GHB • Ginkgo • Glutamine • Lithium • Sage • Wormwood
ANTIDEPRESSANTS Some drugs in this category include: Bupropion (*Wellbutrin*) Nefazodone (*Serzone*) Tetracyclics: Maprotiline (*Ludiomil*) • Mirtazapine (*Remeron*) Trazodone (*Desyrel*) Monoamine Oxidase Inhibitors: Phenelzine (*Nardil*) • Tranylcypromine (*Parnate*) • Isocarboxazid (*Marplan*) Selective Serotonin Reuptake Inhibitors: Citalopram (*Celexa*) • Fluoxetine (*Prozac*) • Fluvoxamine (*Luvox*) • Paroxetine (*Paxil*) • Sertraline (*Zoloft*) • Venlafaxine (*Effexor*) Tricyclics: Amitriptyline (*Elavil*) • Clomipramine (*Anafranil*) • Amoxapine (*Asendin*) • Desipramine (*Norpramin*) • Doxepin (*Sinequan*) • Imipramine (*Tofranil*) • Nortriptyline (*Pamelor*)	5-HTP • Ergot • Hawaiian Baby Woodrose • Lithium • L-Tryptophan • SAMe • St. John's Wort
ANTIDIABETES DRUGS Some drugs in this category include: Insulins: (*Humulin*, *Novolin*, *Lantus*, *Humalog*, *Novolog*) Biguanides: Metformin (*Glucophage*) Meglitinides: Repaglinide (*Prandin*) • Nateglinide (*Starlix*) Alpha-Glucosidase Inhibitors: Acarbose (*Precose*) • Miglitol (*Glyset*) Sulfonylureas: Chlorpropamide (*Diabinese*) • Glimepiride (*Amaryl*) • Glipizide (*Glucotrol*) • Glyburide (*DiaBeta*, *Glynase*, *Micronase*) • Tolbutamide (*Orinase*) Thiazolidinediones: Pioglitazone (*Actos*) • Rosiglitazone (*Avandia*)	Agrimony • Aloe • Alpha-Lipoic Acid • Annatto • Baikal Skullcap • Banaba • Barley • Bean Pod • Bilberry • Bitter Melon • Black Mulberry • Black Psyllium • Black Tea • Blond Psyllium • Blue Cohosh • Blueberry • Branched-Chain Amino Acids • Bugleweed • Caffeine • Capers • Caraway • Cassia Auriculata • Cassia Cinnamon • Chanca Piedra • Chinese Cucumber • Cinnamon Bark • Cocoa • Coffee • Cola Nut • Corn Silk • Country Mallow • Cowhage • Cumin • Damiana • Devil's Claw • Ephedra • Eucalyptus • Fenugreek • Fig • Flaxseed • Fo-Ti • Ginger • Ginseng, American • Ginseng, Panax • Ginseng, Siberian • Glucomannan • Glucosamine Hydrochloride • Glucosamine Sulfate • Goat's Rue • Green Tea • Guar Gum • Guarana • Gymnema • Horse Chestnut • Hydrazine Sulfate • Inositol Nicotinate • Ivy Gourd • Juniper • Kudzu • Lycium • Madagascar Periwinkle • Maitake Mushroom • Marshmallow • Mate • Melatonin • Myrrh • N-Acetyl Glucosamine • Neem • Niacin and Niacinamide • Olive • Onion • Oolong Tea • Puncture Vine • Ribose • Sage • Solomon's Seal • Spinach • Stevia • Stinging Nettle • Tiratricol • Vanadium • Xanthan Gum

CHARTS

Potential Interactions: Drug/Natural Medicine

For additional data, refer to the database.

Drug	Natural Medicine
ANTIFUNGALS Some drugs in this category include: Ciclopirox (*Loprox*) • Griseofulvin (*Grisactin, Gris-PEG*) • Terbinafine (*Lamisil*) • Clotrimazole (*Lotrimin, Mycelex*) • Fluconazole (*Diflucan*) • Itraconazole (*Sporanox*) • Ketoconazole (*Nizoral*) • Miconazole (*Desenex, Monistat*) • Terconazole (*Terazol*) • Amphotericin B (*Amphotec*) • Nystatin (*Mycostatin*)	Brewer's Yeast • Saccharomyces Boulardii
ANTIGOUT DRUGS Some drugs in this category include: Allopurinol (*Zyloprim*) • Probenecid (*Benemid*) • Colchicine	Adenosine
ANTIHYPERTENSIVE DRUGS Some drugs in this category include: Beta-Adrenergic Blockers: Atenolol (*Tenormin*) • Labetalol (*Normodyne*) • Metoprolol (*Lopressor*) • Nadolol (*Corgard*) • Propranolol (*Inderal*) Calcium Channel Blockers: Amlodipine (*Norvasc*) • Diltiazem (*Cardizem*) • Felodipine (*Plendil*) • Nifedipine (*Adalat, Procardia*) • Verapamil (*Calan*) Antiadrenergic Agents: Reserpine • Methyldopa (*Aldomet*) • Clonidine (*Catapres*) • Guanfacine (*Tenex*) • Guanabenz (*Wytensin*) Alpha-1 Adrenergic Blockers: Doxazosin (*Cardura*) • Prazosin (*Minipress*) • Terazosin (*Hytrin*) Angiotensin II Receptor Antagonists: Irbesartan (*Avapro*) • Losartan (*Cozaar*) • Valsartan (*Diovan*) Angiotensin-Converting Enzyme Inhibitors: Benazepril (*Lotensin*) • Captopril (*Capoten*) • Enalapril (*Vasotec*) • Fosinopril (*Monopril*) • Lisinopril (*Prinivil*) • Quinapril (*Accupril*) • Ramipril (*Altace*)	Andrographis • Asafoetida • Betony • Blue Cohosh • Carrageenan • Casein Peptides • Cat's Claw • Cod Liver Oil • Coenzyme Q-10 • Coltsfoot • Corn Silk • Devil's Claw • DHA • EPA • Epimedium • European Mistletoe • Fish Oil • Goldenseal • L-Arginine • Licorice • Lycium • Olive • Periwinkle • Pomegranate • Reishi Mushroom • Stevia • Stinging Nettle • Theanine • Verbena • Wild Carrot • Yohimbe
ANTIMITOTIC CHEMOTHERAPY Some drugs in this category include: Etoposide (*VePesid*) • Teniposide (*Vumon*) • Vinblastine (*Velban*) • Vincristine (*Oncovin*) • Vinorelbine (*Navelbine*)	Glucosamine Hydrochloride • Glucosamine Sulfate
ANTIPSYCHOTIC DRUGS Some drugs in this category include: Benzisoxazoles: Risperidone (*Risperdal*) Dibenzapines: Clozapine (*Clozaril*) • Loxapine (*Loxitane*) • Olanzapine (*Zyprexa*) • Quetiapine (*Seroquel*) • Ziprasidone (*Geodon*) Thioanthenes: Thiothixene (*Navane*) Phenylbutylpiperadines: Haloperidol (*Haldol*) Phenothiazines: Chlorpromazine (*Thorazine*) • Fluphenazine (*Prolixin*) • Mesoridazine (*Serentil*) • Perphenazine (*Trilafon*) • Thioridazine (*Mellaril*) • Trifluoperazine (*Stelazine*)	Butanediol • Chasteberry • Cowhage • GBL • GHB • Ginseng, American • Indian Snakeroot • Phenylalanine
ANTITHYROID DRUGS Some drugs in this category include: Methimazole (*Tapazole*) • Potassium Iodide (*SSKI, Pima*) • Propylthiouracil; PTU	Bladderwrack • Iodine
AROMATASE INHIBITORS Some drugs in this category include: Anastrozole (*Arimidex*) • Exemestane (*Aromasin*) • Letrozole (*Femara*)	Chrysin
ARTEMETHER (*Artenam, Paluther*)	Grapefruit
ASPIRIN	Beer • Cherokee Rosehip • Kudzu • Meadowsweet • Onion • Parsley • Ribose • Rose Hip • Tamarind • Vitamin C • Willow Bark • Wine • Wintergreen
BARBITURATES Some drugs in this category include: Pentobarbital (*Nembutal*) • Phenobarbital • Primidone (*Mysoline*) • Secobarbital (*Seconal*)	Beer • Cedarwood • Indian Snakeroot • Lavender • Magnolia • Marijuana • Passionflower • St. John's Wort • Wine • Yarrow

CHARTS

Potential Interactions: Drug/Natural Medicine

For additional data, refer to the database.

Drug	Natural Medicine
BENZODIAZEPINES Some drugs in this category include: Alprazolam (*Xanax*) • Lorazepam (*Ativan*) • Clonazepam (*Klonopin*) • Clorazepate (*Tranxene*) • Chlordiazepoxide (*Librium*) • Diazepam (*Valium*) • Estazolam (*Prosom*) • Flurazepam (*Dalmane*) • Midazolam (*Versed*) • Oxazepam (*Serax*) • Quazepam (*Doral*) • Triazolam (*Halcion*) • Temazepam (*Restoril*)	Ashwagandha • Baikal Skullcap • Beer • Butanediol (BD) • California Poppy • GBL • GHB • German Chamomile • Grapefruit • L-Tryptophan • Magnolia • Melatonin • Valerian • Wine
BETA-ADRENERGIC AGONISTS Some drugs in this category include: Albuterol (*Ventolin*) • Metaproterenol (*Alupent*) • Terbutaline (*Brethine*) • Isoproterenol (*Isuprel*)	Cocoa
BETA-BLOCKERS Some drugs in this category include: Atenolol (*Tenormin*) • Metoprolol (*Lopressor, Toprol XL*) • Nadolol (*Corgard*) • Propranolol (*Inderal*)	Hawthorn
BISPHOSPHONATES Some drugs in this category include: Alendronate (*Fosamax*) • Etidronate (*Didronel*) • Pamidronate (*Aredia*) • Risedronate (*Actonel*) • Tiludronate (*Skelid*)	Calcium • Dolomite • Iron • Magnesium
BUSPIRONE (*BuSpar*)	Ginkgo • Grapefruit
CAFFEINE (*NoDoz, Stay Alert, Vivarin*)	Creatine • Ginseng, Panax • Grapefruit • Melatonin
CALCIPOTRIENE (*Dovonex*)	Calcium • Vitamin D
CALCIUM CHANNEL BLOCKERS Some drugs in this category include: Amlodipine (*Norvasc*) • Diltiazem (*Cardizem*) • Felodipine (*Plendil*) • Isradipine (*DynaCirc*) • Nicardipine (*Cardene*) • Nifedipine (*Procardia, Adalat*) • Nisoldipine (*Sular*) • Verapamil (*Calan*)	Calcium • Forskolin • Ginger • Grapefruit • Hawthorn • Lithium • Magnesium • Pangamic Acid • Stevia
CALCIUM SUPPLEMENTS (*Citracal, Caltrate, Os-Cal, Titrilac*)	Lily-of-the-Valley • Lysine • Oleander • Pheasant's Eye • Squill • Strophanthus • Wallflower
CARBAMAZEPINE (*Tegretol*)	Adenosine • Black Psyllium • Blond Psyllium • Cassia Auriculata • Cinchona • Grapefruit
CARBIDOPA (*Lodosyn*)	5-HTP
CARVEDILOL (*Coreg*)	Grapefruit
CEFAMANDOLE (*Mandol*)	Beer • Wine
CEFOPERAZONE (*Cefobid*)	Beer • Wine
CELIPROLOL (*Celicard*)	Sweet Orange
CHEMOTHERAPY Some drugs in this category include: Alkyl Sulfonates: Busulfan (*Myleran*) Triazines: Dacarbazine (*DTIC-Dome*) Nitrogen Mustards: Chlorambucil (*Leukeran*) • Cyclophosphamide (*Cytoxan*) • Ifosfamide (*Ifex*) • Melphalan (*Alkeran*) Nitrosoureas: Carmustine, BCNU (*Gliadel*) • Lomustine (*CeeNu*) • Streptozocin (*Zanosar*) Platinum Coordination Complex: Carboplatin (*Paraplatin*) • Cisplatin (*Platinol-AQ*) Antimetabolites: Hydroxyurea (*Hydrea*) Folic Acid Analogs: Methotrexate (*Rheumatrex*) Pyrimidine Analogs: Cytarabine ARA-C (*Cytosar-U*) • Fluorouracil, 5-FU (*Efudex*) • Gemcitabine (*Gemzar*) Purine Analogs: Cladribine (*Leustatin*) • Fludarabine (*Fludara*) • Mercaptopurine (*Purinethol*) • Pentostatin (*Nipent*) • Thioguanine Vinca Alkaloids: Vinblastine (*Velban*) • Vincristine (*Oncovin*) Taxoids: Paclitaxel (*Taxol*) • Docetaxel (*Taxotere*) Anthracyclines: Daunorubicin (*DaunoXome*) • Doxorubicin (*Adriamycin*) • Idarubicin (*Idamycin*) • Valrubicin (*Valstar*)	Alpha-Lipoic Acid • Coenzyme Q-10 • Glutamine • N-Acetyl Glucosamine • Vitamin C • Vitamin E
CHLORAL HYDRATE (*Aquachloral*)	Clary Sage • Lavender

CHARTS

Potential Interactions: Drug/Natural Medicine

For additional data, refer to the database.

Drug	Natural Medicine
CHLORAMPHENICOL (*Chloromycetin*)	Dibencozide • Iron • Vitamin B12
CHLORPROPAMIDE (*Diabinese*)	Beer • Prickly Pear Cactus • Solomon's Seal • Wine
CHLORZOXAZONE (*Parafon Forte, Paraflex*)	Watercress
CHOLESTYRAMINE (*Questran*)	Phosphate Salts • Tiratricol
CHOLINE MAGNESIUM TRISALICYLATE (*Trilisate*)	Cherokee Rosehip • Meadowsweet • Ribose • Rose Hip • Vitamin C • Willow Bark
CHOLINERGIC DRUGS Some drugs in this category include: Bethanechol (*Urecholine*) • Echothiophate (*Phospholine Iodide*) • Neostigmine (*Prostigmin*) • Physostigmine (*Antilirium*) • Pyridostigmine (*Mestinon*) • Succinylcholine (*Anectine*)	Areca • Chinese Club Moss • Huperzine A • Iboga
CIMETIDINE (*Tagamet*)	Black Tea • Caffeine • Cocoa • Coffee • Cola Nut • Green Tea • Guarana • Mate • Oolong Tea • Vitamin D
CIPROFLOXACIN (*Cipro*)	Fennel • Yogurt
CISAPRIDE (*Propulsid*)	Beer • Grapefruit • Wine
CISPLATIN (*Platinol-AQ*)	Black Cohosh • Zinc
CLINDAMYCIN (*Cleocin*)	Kaolin
CLOMIPRAMINE (*Anafranil*)	Grapefruit
CLONIDINE (*Catapres*)	Yohimbe
CLOPIDOGREL (*Plavix*)	St. John's Wort
CLOZAPINE (*Clozaril*)	Black Tea • Caffeine • Cocoa • Coffee • Cola Nut • Glycine • Green Tea • Guarana • Hawaiian Baby Woodrose • Mate • Oolong Tea
CNS DEPRESSANTS Some drugs in this category include: Secobarbital (*Seconal*) • Pentobarbital (*Nembutal*) • Clonazepam (*Klonopin*) • Diazepam (*Valium*) • Midazolam (*Versed*) • Zolpidem (*Ambien*) • Zaleplon (*Sonata*) • Hydroxyzine (*Atarax*) • Temazepam (*Restoril*) • Flurazepam (*Dalmane*) • Triazolam (*Halcion*) • Lorazepam (*Ativan*) • Estazolam (*Prosom*) • Secobarbital (*Seconal*) • Phenobarbital (*Luminal*)	Ashwagandha • Baikal Skullcap • Beer • Bitter Almond • Butanediol • Calamus • Calendula • California Poppy • Catnip • Celery • Cowslip • Elecampane • GBL • GHB • German Chamomile • Ginseng, Siberian • Goldenseal • Gotu Kola • Hops • Hydrazine Sulfate • Jamaican Dogwood • Kava • Lavender • L-Tryptophan • Lemon Balm • Magnolia • Marijuana • Marsh Tea • Melatonin • Motherwort • Passionflower • Sage • Sassafras • Shepherd's Purse • Stinging Nettle • Sweet Bay • Valerian • Wild Lettuce • Wine • Yerba Mansa
COCAINE	Capsicum • Cola Nut • Green Tea • Guarana • Mate • Oolong Tea
COLCHICINE	Autumn Crocus
COLESTIPOL (*Colestid*)	Phosphate Salts
CONTRACEPTIVE DRUGS Some drugs in this category include: Ethinyl Estradiol and Levonorgestrel (*Alesse, Levlen, Triphasil*, others) • Ethinyl Estradiol and Norethindrone (*Brevicon, Demulen, Loestrin, Ortho Novum*, others)	Alfalfa • Anise • Black Tea • Caffeine • Chasteberry • Cocoa • Coffee • Cola Nut • Fennel • Fish Oil • Garlic • Green Tea • Guarana • Guggul • Kudzu • Mate • Melatonin • Oolong Tea • Red Clover • Saw Palmetto • St. John's Wort
CORTICOSTEROIDS Some drugs in this category include: Beclomethasone (*Beclovent, Celestone*) • Betamethasone (*Valisone*) • Budesonide (*Rhinocort*) • Cortisone (*Cortone*) • Dexamethasone (*Adrenocot, Decadron*) • Fludrocortisone (*Florinef*) • Flunisolide (*Aerobid*) • Fluocinonide (*Lidex*) • Fluticasone (*Flovent*) • Hydrocortisone (*Cortef*) • Methylprednisolone (*Medrol*) • Prednisolone (*Econopred, Orapred*) • Prednisone (*Orasone, Deltasone*) • Triamcinolone (*Kenalog*)	Alder Buckthorn • Branched-Chain Amino Acids • Butternut • Cascara • Castor • Cesium • Corn Silk • DHEA • Gamboge • Horsetail • Licorice • Lily-of-the-Valley • Pheasant's Eye • Rhubarb • Squill • Strophanthus • Wallflower
CORTISONE (*Cortisone Acetate*)	PABA
CYCLOPHOSPHAMIDE (*Cytoxan*)	Astragalus • Cordyceps
CYCLOSPORINE (*Neoral, Sandimmune*)	Garlic • Grapefruit • Peppermint • Red Yeast • St. John's Wort • Vitamin E • Wine

CHARTS

Potential Interactions: Drug/Natural Medicine

For additional data, refer to the database.

Drug	Natural Medicine
CYPROHEPTADINE (*Periactin*)	Hawaiian Baby Woodrose
CYTOCHROME P450 1A1 (CYP1A1) SUBSTRATES Some drugs in this category include: Chlorzoxazone • Theophylline • Bufuralol	Nutmeg and Mace
CYTOCHROME P450 1A2 (CYP1A2) SUBSTRATES Some drugs in this category include: Clozapine (*Clozaril*) • Cyclobenzaprine (*Flexeril*) • Fluvoxamine (*Luvox*) • Haloperidol (*Haldol*) • Imipramine (*Tofranil*) • Mexiletine (*Mexitil*) • Olanzapine (*Zyprexa*) • Pentazocine (*Talwin*) • Propranolol (*Inderal*) • Tacrine (*Cognex*) • Theophylline • Zileuton (*Zyflo*) • Zolmitriptan (*Zomig*)	Cabbage • Chrysin • Diindolylmethane • Eucalyptus • Feverfew • Fo-Ti • Ginkgo • Ginseng, Siberian • Grape • Grapefruit • Indole-3-Carbinol • Ipriflavone • Kava • Methoxylated Flavones • Nutmeg and Mace • Peppermint • Red Clover • St. John's Wort • Sulforaphane
CYTOCHROME P450 2B1 (CYP2B1) SUBSTRATES	Nutmeg and Mace
CYTOCHROME P450 2B2 (CYP2B2) SUBSTRATES	Nutmeg and Mace
CYTOCHROME P450 2B6 (CYP2B6) SUBSTRATES Some drugs in this category include: Ketamine (*Ketalar*) • Phenobarbital (*Luminal*) • Orphenadrine (*Norflex*) • Secobarbital (*Seconal*) • Dexamethasone (*Decadron*)	Licorice
CYTOCHROME P450 2C19 (CYP2C19) INDUCERS	Limonene
CYTOCHROME P450 2C19 (CYP2C19) INHIBITORS	Limonene
CYTOCHROME P450 2C19 (CYP2C19) SUBSTRATES Some drugs in this category include: Amitriptyline (*Elavil*) • Clomipramine (*Anafranil*) • Cyclophosphamide (*Cytoxan*) • Diazepam (*Valium*) • Lanzoprazole (*Prevacid*) • Omeprazole (*Prilosec*) • Lansoprazole (*Protonix*) • Phenytoin (*Dilantin*) • Phenobarbital (*Luminal*)	Devil's Claw • Eucalyptus • Feverfew • Fo-Ti • Ginkgo • Grapefruit • Kava • Peppermint • Red Clover
CYTOCHROME P450 2C9 (CYP2C9) INDUCERS	Limonene
CYTOCHROME P450 2C9 (CYP2C9) INHIBITORS	Limonene
CYTOCHROME P450 2C9 (CYP2C9) SUBSTRATES Some drugs in this category include: Celecoxib (*Celebrex*) • Diclofenac (*Voltaren*) • Fluvastatin (*Lescol*) • Glipizide (*Glucotrol*) • Ibuprofen (*Advil, Motrin*) • Irbesartan (*Avapro*) • Losartan (*Cozaar*) • Phenytoin (*Dilantin*) • Piroxicam (*Feldene*) • Tamoxifen (*Nolvadex*) • Tolbutamide (*Tolinase*) • Torsemide (*Demadex*) • Warfarin (*Coumadin*)	Cranberry • Devil's Claw • Eucalyptus • Feverfew • Fo-Ti • Ginkgo • Ginseng, Siberian • Grapefruit • Ipriflavone • Kava • Limonene • Lycium • Milk Thistle • Peppermint • Red Clover • St. John's Wort
CYTOCHROME P450 2D6 (CYP2D6) SUBSTRATES Some drugs in this category include: Amitriptyline (*Elavil*) • Codeine • Desipramine (*Norpramin*) • Flecainide (*Tambocor*) • Haloperidol (*Haldol*) • Imipramine (*Tofranil*) • Metoprolol (*Lopressor*, *Toprol XL*) • Ondansetron (*Zofran*) • Paroxetine (*Paxil*) • Risperidone (*Risperdal*) • Tramadol (*Ultram*) • Venlafaxine (*Effexor*)	Ginkgo • Ginseng, Panax • Ginseng, Siberian • Kava
CYTOCHROME P450 3A4 (CYP3A4) INDUCERS Some drugs in this category include: Aminoglutethimide (*Cytadren*) • Aprepitant (*Emend*) • Carbamazepine (*Tegretol*) • Dexamethasone (*Dexone, Hexadrol*) • Efavirenz (*Sustiva*) • Ethosuximide (*Zarontin*) • Glucocorticoids • Glutethimide (*Doriden*) • Griseofulvin (*Fulvicin, Grisactin*) • Modafinil (*Provigil*) • Nafcillin (*Nallpen, Unipen*) • Nevirapine (*Viramune*) • Oxcarbazepine (*Trileptal*) • Phenobarbital (*Luminal*) • Phenytoin (*Dilantin, Phenytek*) • Primidone (*Mysoline*) • Rifabutin (*Mycobutin*) • Rifampin (*Rifadin, Rimactane*) • Rifapentine (*Priftin*)	Alkanna • Alpine Ragwort • Borage • Butterbur • Coltsfoot • Comfrey • Dusty Miller • Golden Ragwort • Gravel Root • Groundsel • Hemp Agrimony • Hound's Tongue • Tansy Ragwort
CYTOCHROME P450 3A4 (CYP3A4) INHIBITORS Some drugs in this category include: Clarithromycin (*Biaxin*) • Erythromycin • Itraconazole • Ketoconazole • Cimetidine • Nefazodone (*Serzone*) • Indinavir (*Crixivan*) • Nelfinavir (*Viracept*) • Saquinavir (*Invirase*)	Ergot • Red Yeast
CYTOCHROME P450 3A4 (CYP3A4) SUBSTRATES Some drugs in this category include: Alprazolam (*Xanax*) • Amlodipine (*Norvasc*) • Clarithromycin (*Biaxin*) • Cyclosporine (*Sandimmune*) • Erythromycin • Lovastatin (*Mevacor*) • Ketoconazole (*Nizoral*) • Itraconazole (*Sporanox*) • Fexofenadine (*Allegra*) • Triazolam (*Halcion*) • Verapamil (*Calan, Isoptin*)	American Elder • Bishop's Weed • Bitter Orange • Cat's Claw • Devil's Claw • DHEA • Echinacea • Eucalyptus • Feverfew • Fo-Ti • Garlic • German Chamomile • Ginkgo • Ginseng, Siberian • Goldenseal • Grapefruit • Guggul • Kava • Licorice • Lime • Milk Thistle • Peppermint • Red Clover • Resveratrol • St. John's Wort • Valerian • Wild Cherry
DAPSONE (*Avlosulfon*)	PABA

Potential Interactions: Drug/Natural Medicine

For additional data, refer to the database.

Drug	Natural Medicine
DEXAMETHASONE (*Decadron*)	Country Mallow • Ephedra
DEXTROMETHORPHAN (*Robitussin DM*, and others)	5-HTP • Bitter Orange • Ergot • Grapefruit • Hawaiian Baby Woodrose • Lithium • L-Tryptophan • SAMe • St. John's Wort
DIAZOXIDE (*Hyperstat*, *Proglycem*)	Branched-Chain Amino Acids
DIGOXIN (*Lanoxin*)	Alder Buckthorn • Aloe • Apple Cider Vinegar • Black Hellebore • Black Psyllium • Black Root • Blond Psyllium • Blue Flag • Butternut • Calcium • Calotropis • Canadian Hemp • Cascara • Castor • Cereus • Colocynth • Danshen • Digitalis • European Buckthorn • Fo-Ti • Gamboge • Ginseng, Siberian • Gossypol • Greater Bindweed • Guar Gum • Hawthorn • Hedge Mustard • Horsetail • Indian Snakeroot • Jalap • Kaolin • Khella • Laminaria • Licorice • Lily-of-the-Valley • Manna • Mexican Scammony Root • Oleander • Pangamic Acid • Pectin • Pheasant's Eye • Pleurisy Root • Procaine • Quassia • Rhubarb • Sarsaparilla • Senna • Squill • St. John's Wort • Strophanthus • Swamp Milkweed • Uzara • Vitamin D • Wahoo • Wallflower • Wheat Bran • Yellow Dock
DILTIAZEM (*Cardizem*)	Calcium • Guggul • Vitamin D
DIPYRIDAMOLE (*Persantine*)	Adenosine • Black Tea • Caffeine • Cocoa • Coffee • Cola Nut • Green Tea • Guarana • Mate • Oolong Tea
DISULFIRAM (*Antabuse*)	Beer • Black Tea • Caffeine • Cocoa • Coffee • Cola Nut • Green Tea • Guarana • Kombucha Tea • Marijuana • Mate • Oolong Tea • Wine
DIURETIC DRUGS Some drugs in this category include: Thiazides: Indapamide (*Lozol*) • Chlorothiazide (*Diuril*) • Hydrochlorothiazide (*Esidrix*, *Hydrodiuril*, others) • Chlorthalidone (*Hygroton*) • Metolazone (*Zaroxolyn*) Loop Diuretics: Bumetanide (*Bumex*) • Ethacrynic Acid (*Edecrin*) • Furosemide (*Lasix*) • Torsemide (*Demadex*)	Alder Buckthorn • Aloe • Apple Cider Vinegar • Birch • Black Hellebore • Black Root • Blue Flag • Butternut • Calotropis • Canadian Hemp • Cascara • Castor • Cesium • Colocynth • Corn Silk • Cowslip • Digitalis • EDTA • European Buckthorn • Figwort • Fo-Ti • Gamboge • Goldenrod • Gossypol • Greater Bindweed • Hedge Mustard • Horsetail • Indian Snakeroot • Jalap • Juniper • Licorice • Lily-of-the-Valley • Lovage • Manna • Mexican Scammony Root • Oleander • Parsley • Pheasant's Eye • Pleurisy Root • Quassia • Rhubarb • Senna • Squill • Stone Root • Strophanthus • Swamp Milkweed • Uzara • Wahoo • Wallflower • Yellow Dock
DOPAMINE AGONISTS Some drugs in this category include: Bromocriptine (*Parlodel*) • Carbidopa (*Lodosyn*) • Carbidopa;Levodopa (*Sinemet*) • Pergolide (*Permax*) • Pramipexole (*Mirapex*) • Ropinirole (*Requip*)	Black Horehound • Chasteberry
EPHEDRINE (*Pretz-D*)	Black Tea • Caffeine • Coffee • Cola Nut • Green Tea • Guarana • Indian Snakeroot • Mate • Oolong Tea
ERGOT DERIVATIVES Some drugs in this category include: Bromocriptine (*Parlodel*) • Caffeine;Ergotamine (*Cafergot*) • Dihydroergotamine (*D.H.E.*) • Ergotamine (*Ergostat*) • Methylergonovine (*Methergine*) • Methysergide (*Sansert*)	Country Mallow • Ephedra • Ergot
ERGOTAMINE (*Ergomar*)	Cocoa
ERYTHROMYCIN (*E.E.S.*, *E-Mycin*, *PCE*)	Beer • Grapefruit • Wine
ESTRADIOL (*Alora*, *Climara*, and others)	Vitamin C
ESTROGENS (*Estrace*, *Estratest*, *Ogen*, *Premarin*)	Acerola • Alfalfa • Androstenediol • Androstenedione • Anise • Black Tea • Boron • Caffeine • Calcium • Chasteberry • Cherokee Rosehip • Cocoa • Coffee • Cola Nut • Dolomite • Fennel • Grapefruit • Green Tea • Guarana • Guggul • Hu Zhang • Kudzu • Licorice • Mate • Milk Thistle • Oolong Tea • Pleurisy Root • Pregnenolone • Progesterone • Red Clover • Rose Hip • Saw Palmetto • Soy • Vitamin C • Wild Carrot
ETHACRYNIC ACID (*Edecrin*)	Licorice
ETHINYL ESTRADIOL	Blond Psyllium • Guar Gum

CHARTS

Potential Interactions: Drug/Natural Medicine

For additional data, refer to the database.

Drug	Natural Medicine
ETOPOSIDE (*VePesid*)	Grapefruit
EXEMESTANE (*Aromasin*)	DHEA
EZETIMIBE (*Zetia*)	Beta-Sitosterol
FELODIPINE (*Plendil*)	Bitter Orange • Wine
FENFLURAMINE (*Pondimin*)	St. John's Wort
FEXOFENADINE (*Allegra*)	Apple • Grapefruit • St. John's Wort • Sweet Orange
FLUCONAZOLE (*Diflucan*)	Black Tea • Caffeine • Cocoa • Coffee • Cola Nut • Green Tea • Guarana • Mate • Oolong Tea
FLUMAZENIL (*Romazicon*)	Melatonin
FLUOXETINE (*Prozac*)	Ginkgo • Marijuana
FLUPHENAZINE (*Prolixin*)	Acerola • Cherokee Rosehip • Rose Hip • Vitamin C
FLUVOXAMINE (*Luvox*)	Black Tea • Caffeine • Coffee • Cola Nut • Green Tea • Guarana • Mate • Melatonin • Oolong Tea
FOSPHENYTOIN (*Cerebyx*)	Folic Acid
FULVESTRANT (*Faslodex*)	DHEA
FUROSEMIDE (*Lasix*)	Germanium • Ginseng, Panax • Licorice
GEMFIBROZIL (*Lopid*)	Red Yeast
GLUCURONIDATED DRUGS Some drugs in this category include: Acetaminophen (*Tylenol*) • Estrogens (*Estrace*, *Premarin*, others) and Oral Contraceptives • Entacapone (*Comtan*) • Irinotecan (*Camptosar*) • Atorvastatin (*Lipitor*) • Diazepam (*Valium*) • Digoxin • Lamotrigine (*Lamictal*) • Lorazepam (*Ativan*) • Lovastatin (*Mevacor*) • Meprobamate • Morphine • Oxazepam (*Serax*)	Cabbage • Calcium D-Glucarate • Chrysin • Milk Thistle
GRISEOFULVIN (*Fulvicin*)	Beer • Wine
GUANABENZ (*Wytensin*)	Yohimbe
GUANETHIDINE (*Ismelin*)	Cowhage
H2-BLOCKERS Some drugs in this category include: Famotidine (*Pepcid*) • Ranitidine (*Zantac*) • Nixatidine (*Axid*) • Cimetidine (*Tagamet*)	Aletris • Alpinia • Angelica • Beer • Black Mustard • Blessed Thistle • Calamus • Cinchona • Colombo • Cubebs • Dandelion • Devil's Claw • Gentian • Goldenseal • Goldthread • Northern Prickly Ash • Peppermint • Quassia • Southern Prickly Ash • Wine • Yarrow
HALOPERIDOL (*Haldol*)	Butanediol • GBL • GHB • Scotch Broom
HEPARIN	Vitamin D
HEPATOTOXIC DRUGS Some drugs in this category include: Amphotericin B (*Fungizone*) • Azathioprine (*Imuran*) • Carbamazepine (*Tegretol*) • Disulfiram (*Antabuse*) • Felbamate (*Felbatol*) • Flutamide (*Eulexin*) • Hydroxychloroquine (*Plaquenil*) • Indinavir (*Crixivan*) • Interferon (*Roferon, Intron, Wellferon*) • Itraconazole (*Sporanox*) • Leflunomide (*Arava*) • Methotrexate (*Rheumatrex*) • Procainamide (*Procan*) • Rosiglitazone (*Avandia*) • Stavudine, d4T (*Zerit*) • Tacrine (*Cognex*) • Terbinafine (*Lamisil*) • Ticlopidine (*Ticlid*) • Tolcapone (*Tasmar*) • Zalcitabine, ddC (*Hivid*)	Beer • Bishop's Weed • Black Cohosh • Chaparral • Comfrey • Kava • Khella • Sweet Clover • Vitamin A • Wine
HEXOBARBITAL	Greek Sage
HEXOBARBITONE	Clary Sage
HMG-COA REDUCTASE INHIBITORS ("Statins") Some drugs in this category include: Atorvastatin (*Lipitor*) • Fluvastatin (*Lescol*) • Lovastatin (*Mevacor*) • Pravastatin (*Pravachol*) • Simvastatin (*Zocor*)	Beta-Carotene • Grapefruit • Inositol Nicotinate • Niacin and Niacinamide • Red Yeast • Selenium • Vitamin C • Vitamin E
IBUPROFEN (*Advil, Motrin,* and others)	Tamarind
IMATINIB (*Gleevec*)	St. John's Wort

Potential Interactions: Drug/Natural Medicine

For additional data, refer to the database.

Drug	Natural Medicine
IMMUNOSUPPRESSANTS Some drugs in this category include: Azathioprine (*Imuran*) • Basiliximab (*Simulect*) • Cyclosporine (*Neoral, Sandimmune*) • Daclizumab (*Zenapax*) • Muromonab-CD3 (*OKT3*) • Mycophenolate (*CellCept*) • Prednisone (*Orasone, Deltasone*) • Sirolimus (*Rapamune*) • Tacrolimus (*FK506, Prograf*)	Andrographis • Ashwagandha • Astragalus • Beta Glucans • Cat's Claw • Echinacea • Elderberry • European Mistletoe • Ginseng, Panax • Ipriflavone • Jiaogulan • Kefir • Lactobacillus • Larch Arabinogalactan • Melatonin • Neem • Picrorhiza • Pycnogenol • Thunder God Vine • Thymus Extract • Yogurt
INDINAVIR (*Crixivan*)	Bitter Orange • Milk Thistle
INJECTABLE DRUGS	DMSO (Dimethylsulfoxide)
INSULIN	Apple Cider Vinegar • Burdock • Chromium • DHEA • EDTA • Fig • Ginkgo • Ginseng, Panax • Gymnema • Ribose • Solomon's Seal
IRINOTECAN (*Camptosar*)	St. John's Wort
ISONIAZID (INH)	Hydrazine Sulfate
ITRACONAZOLE (*Sporanox*)	Grapefruit
IVERMECTIN (*Stromectol*)	Sweet Orange
KANAMYCIN (*Kanatrex*)	Calcium D-Glucarate
LACTULOSE	Glutamine
LETROZOLE (*Femara*)	DHEA
LEVODOPA	Branched-Chain Amino Acids • Indian Snakeroot • Iron • Kava • Phenylalanine • Pyridoxine • SAMe • Tyrosine • Whey Protein
LEVODOPA/CARBIDOPA (*Sinemet*)	Octacosanol
LEVOTHYROXINE (*Levothroid, Levoxyl, Synthroid*, and others)	Calcium • Celery • Colloidal Silver • Dolomite • Horseradish • Iron • Red Yeast
LITHIUM (*Eskalith, Lithobid*)	Black Psyllium • Black Tea • Blond Psyllium • Caffeine • Cocoa • Coffee • Cola Nut • Dandelion • Green Tea • Guarana • Iodine • Mate • Oolong Tea
LOOP DIURETICS Some drugs in this category include: Bumetanide (*Bumex*) • Ethacrynic Acid (*Edecrin*) • Furosemide (*Lasix*)	Lithium
LOSARTAN (*Cozaar*)	Grapefruit
LOVASTATIN (*Mevacor*)	Pectin
LOW MOLECULAR WEIGHT HEPARINS (LMWHs)	Vitamin D
MACROLIDE ANTIBIOTICS Some drugs in this category include: Azithromycin (*Zithromax*) • Clarithromycin (*Biaxin*) • Dirithromycin (*Dynabec*) • Erythromycin (*E.E.S., E-Mycin, Ery-Tab*)	Black Hellebore • Digitalis • Hedge Mustard • Lily-of-the-Valley • Oleander • Swamp Milkweed • Uzara • Wahoo
MEPERIDINE (*Demerol*)	5-HTP • Ergot • Hawaiian Baby Woodrose • Lithium • L-Tryptophan • SAMe • St. John's Wort
METFORMIN (*Glucophage*)	Beer • Guar Gum • Quillaia • Raspberry Leaf • Water Avens • Wine
METHOTREXATE (*MTX, Rheumatrex*)	Folic Acid • Kudzu
METHYLDOPA (*Aldomet*)	Cowhage • Iron • Lithium
METHYLPREDNISOLONE (*Adlone, A-Methapred, depMedalone, Depoject, Medrol, Solu-Medrol*)	Grapefruit
METHYLXANTHINES Some drugs in this category include: Caffeine (*NoDoz, Vivarin*) • Theophylline (*Slo-Bid, Theo-Dur, Theolair*)	Adenosine • Country Mallow • Ephedra • Lithium
METOCLOPRAMIDE (*Reglan*)	Chasteberry
METRONIDAZOLE (*Flagyl*)	Beer • Wine
MEXILETINE (*Mexitil*)	Black Tea • Caffeine • Cocoa • Coffee • Cola Nut • Green Tea • Guarana • Mate • Oolong Tea
MIDAZOLAM (*Versed*)	Bitter Orange • Echinacea

Potential Interactions: Drug/Natural Medicine

For additional data, refer to the database.

Drug	Natural Medicine
MONOAMINE OXIDASE INHIBITORS (MAOIs) Some drugs in this category include: Phenelzine (*Nardil*) • Tranylcypromine (*Parnate*)	5-HTP • Anise • Bitter Orange • Black Tea • Brewer's Yeast • Caffeine • Calamus • Cereus • Cocoa • Coffee • Cola Nut • Country Mallow • Cowhage • Ephedra • Ergot • Ginseng, American • Ginseng, Panax • Green Tea • Guarana • Hawaiian Baby Woodrose • Hydrazine Sulfate • Indian Snakeroot • Lithium • L-Tryptophan • Mate • Oolong Tea • Phenylalanine • SAMe • Scotch Broom • St. John's Wort • Wine • Yohimbe
MORPHINE (*Kadian, MS Contin, MSIR, Oramorph, Roxanol*)	Oats
MYCOPHENOLATE MOFETIL (*CellCept*)	Iron
NALOXONE (*Narcan*)	Butanediol • Fever Bark • GBL • GHB • Yohimbe
NARCOTIC DRUGS Some drugs in this category include: Acetaminophen;Oxycodone (*Percocet*) • Acetaminophen;Propoxyphene (*Darvocet*) • Aspirin;Oxycodone (*Percodan*) • Fentanyl (*Duragesic*) • Hydromorphone (*Dilaudid*) • Meperidine (*Demerol*) • Methadone (*Methadose, Dolophine*) • Morphine (*MS Contin, Roxanol*) • Oxycodone (*OxyContin*) • Propoxyphene (*Darvon*) • Sufentanil (*Sufenta*)	Beer • Butanediol • GBL • GHB • Meadowsweet • St. John's Wort • Sweet Bay • Wine
NEFAZODONE (*Serzone*)	St. John's Wort
NEPHROTOXIC DRUGS Some drugs in this category include: Carbamazepine (*Tegretol*) • Diclofenac (*Voltaren*) • Diflunisal (*Dolobid*) • Ganciclovir (*Cytovene*) • Gatifloxacin (*Tequin*) • Interferon • Meloxicam (*Mobic*) • Spironolactone (*Aldactone*) • Tacrolimus (*Prograf*) • Valacyclovir (*Valtrex*) • Amphotericin B (*Fungizone*) • Cisplatin (*Platinol*) • Cyclosporine (*Neoral*) • Enalapril (*Vasotec*) • Nafcillin (*Unipen*) • Tobramycin (*Nebcin*)	Creatine
NIACIN (*Niacor, Niaspan, Nicobid, Slo-Niacin*)	Beta-Carotene • Red Yeast • Selenium • Vitamin C • Vitamin E
NICARDIPINE (*Cardene*)	Vitamin C
NICOTINE (*Habitrol, Nicoderm, Nicorette, Nicotrol, Prestep*)	Blue Cohosh • Cola Nut • Green Tea • Guarana • Mate • Oolong Tea
NIFEDIPINE (*Adalat, Procardia*)	Coca • Melatonin • Vitamin C
NITRATES Some drugs in this category include: Isosorbide Dinitrate (*Isordil*) • Isosorbide Mononitrate (*Imdur*) • Nitroglycerin (*Nitrostat*)	Forskolin • Hawthorn • L-Arginine
NITROGLYCERIN (*Minitran, Nitrek, Nitrostat*)	N-Acetyl Cysteine
NMDA ANTAGONISTS (*Namenda*)	Threonine
NON-NUCLEOSIDE REVERSE TRANSCRIPTASE INHIBITORS (NNRTIs) Some drugs in this category include: Nevirapine (*Viramune*) • Delavirdine (*Rescriptor*) • Efavirenz (*Sustiva*)	Garlic • St. John's Wort
NONSTEROIDAL ANTI-INFLAMMATORY DRUGS (NSAIDs) Some drugs in this category include: Diclofenac (*Voltaren*) • Etodolac (*Lodine*) • Flurbiprofen (*Ansaid*) • Ibuprofen (*Motrin*) • Indomethacin (*Indocin*) • Ketoprofen (*Orudis*) • Ketorolac (*Toradol*) • Meclofenamate; Mefenamic Acid (*Ponstel*) • Nabumetone (*Relafen*) • Naproxen (*Naprosyn*) • Oxaprozine (*Daypro*) • Piroxicam (*Feldene*) • Sulindac (*Clinoril*)	Beer • Borage • Chromium • Gossypol • Lithium • Wine
NORTRIPTYLINE (*Pamelor, Aventyl*)	St. John's Wort

CHARTS

Potential Interactions: Drug/Natural Medicine

For additional data, refer to the database.

Drug	Natural Medicine
OMEPRAZOLE (*Prilosec*)	Ginkgo
ORAL DRUGS	Activated Charcoal • Agar • Alder Buckthorn • Algin • Aloe • American Chestnut • Barley • Bistort • Black Walnut • Butternut • Carrageenan • Cascara • Castor • Coffee Charcoal • DMSO • European Buckthorn • European Chestnut • European Mandrake • Flaxseed • Glucomannan • Iceland Moss • Jalap • Karaya Gum • Larch Arabinogalactan • Marshmallow • Mexican Scammony Root • Mormon Tea • Pinus Bark • Pomegranate • Quillaia • Quince • Raspberry Leaf • Rhatany • Rhubarb • Rice Bran • Slippery Elm • Sorrel • Tannic Acid • Tragacanth • Water Avens
OXAZEPAM (*Serax*)	Cabbage
PAROXETINE (*Paxil*)	St. John's Wort
PENICILLAMINE (*Cuprimine*)	Colloidal Silver • Copper • Iron • Zinc
PENICILLIN (*Penicillin VK, Pen VK, Veetids*)	Guar Gum
PENTAZOCINE (*Talwin*)	5-HTP • Ergot • Hawaiian Baby Woodrose • Lithium • L-Tryptophan • SAMe • St. John's Wort
PENTOBARBITAL (*Nembutal*)	Holy Basil
P-GLYCOPROTEIN SUBSTRATES Some drugs in this category include: Etoposide (*VePesid*) • Paclitaxel (*Taxol*) • Vinblastine (*Velban*) • Vincristine (*Oncovin*) • Ketoconazole • Itraconazole • Amprenavir (*Agenerase*) • Indinavir (*Crixivan*) • Nelfinavir (*Viracept*) • Squinavir (*Fortovase, Invirase*) • Cimetidine • Ranitidine • Diltiazem • Verapamil • Corticosteroids • Erythromycin • Fexofenadine (*Allegra*) • Cyclosporine • Loperamide (*Imodium*) • Quinidine	St. John's Wort
PHENACETIN	Grape
PHENOBARBITAL (*Luminal*)	Cinchona • Folic Acid • Nutmeg and Mace • Pyridoxine • Riboflavin • St. John's Wort
PENTOBARBITONE	Holy Basil
PHENOTHIAZINES Some drugs in this category include: Thioridazine (*Mellaril*) • Mesoridazine (*Serentil*) • Trifluoperazine (*Stelazine*) • Chlorpromazine (*Thorazine*) • Fluphenazine (*Prolixin*)	Black Tea • Coffee • Evening Primrose Oil • Fever Bark • Gamma Linolenic Acid • Lithium • L-Tryptophan • Yohimbe
PHENPROCOUMON	Ginger • St. John's Wort
PHENYLPROPANOLAMINE (*Propagest, Rhindecon*)	Black Tea • Caffeine • Cocoa • Coffee • Cola Nut • Green Tea • Guarana • Mate • Oolong Tea
PHENYTOIN (*Dilantin*)	Beer • Black Pepper and White Pepper • Folic Acid • Indian Long Pepper • Peony • Pyridoxine • St. John's Wort • Wine
PHOSPHODIETERASE-5 INHIBITORS Some drugs in this category include: Sildenafil (*Viagra*) • Tadalafil (*Cialis*) • Vardenafil (*Levitra*)	Hawthorn
PHOTOSENSITIZING DRUGS Some drugs in this category include: Acyclovir (*Zovirax*) • Amitriptyline (*Elavil*) • Azithromycin (*Zithromax*) • Captopril (*Capoten*) • Carbamazepine (*Tegretol*) • Chloroquine (*Aralen*) • Chlorthiazide (*Diuril*) • Chlorpromazine (*Thorazine*) • Ciprofloxacin (*Cipro*) • Dantrolene (*Dantrium*) • Dapsone • Divalproex (*Depakote*) • Oral Contraceptives • Felbamate (*Felbatol*) • Fluorouracil (*Efudex, Carac*) • Flutamide (*Eulexin*) • Furosemide (*Lasix*) • Glipizide (*Glucotrol*) • Glyburide (*Micronase*) • Hydroxychloroquine (*Plaquenil*) • Isotretinoin (*Accutane*) • Methoxsalen (*Oxsoralen*) • Minocycline (*Minocin*) • Phenobarbital • Promethazine (*Phenergan*) • Quinidine (*Quinidex*) • Sulfamethoxazole;Trimethoprim (*Bactrim, Septra*) • Tacrolimus (*Prograf*) • Tolbutamide (*Orinase*) • Trazodone (*Desyrel*) • Tretinoin (*Retin-A*) • Valproic Acid (*Depakene*)	Alfalfa • Angelica • Arrach • Bergamot Oil • Bishop's Weed • Celery • Chenopodium Oil • Chlorophyll • Khella • Lime • Masterwort • Rue • St. John's Wort • Wild Carrot
POTASSIUM SUPPLEMENTS	Laminaria

CHARTS

Potential Interactions: Drug/Natural Medicine

For additional data, refer to the database.

Drug	Natural Medicine
POTASSIUM-SPARING DIURETICS Some of the drugs in this category include: Amiloride (*Midamor*) • Triamterene (*Dyrenium*) • Spironolactone (*Aldacton*)	Dandelion • Dolomite • Iodine • Laminaria • Magnesium • Morinda • Potassium • Zinc
PRAVASTATIN (*Pravachol*)	Beta-Sitosterol
PRAZIQUANTEL (*Biltricide*)	Grapefruit
PREDNISOLONE (*Pediapred*)	Cordyceps
PRIMIDONE (*Mysoline*)	Folic Acid
PROBENECID (*Benemid*)	Riboflavin
PROCYCLIDINE (*Kemadrin*)	Areca
PROGESTIN	Pregnenolone
PROPRANOLOL (*Inderal*)	Black Pepper and White Pepper • Guggul • Indian Long Pepper • Indian Snakeroot • Ribose
PROTEASE INHIBITORS (PIs) Some drugs in this category include: Indinavir (*Crixivan*) • Nelfinavir (*Viracept*) • Squinavir (*Invirase*)	St. John's Wort • Vitamin C
PROTON PUMP INHIBITORS (PPIs) Some drugs in this category include: Esomeprazole (*Nexium*) • Lansoprazole (*Prevacid*) • Omeprazole (*Prilosec*) • Pantoprazole (*Protonix*) • Rabeprazole (*Aciphex*)	Aletris • Alpinia • Angelica • Black Mustard • Blessed Thistle • Calamus • Cinchona • Colombo • Cubebs • Dandelion • Devil's Claw • Gentian • Ginger • Goldenseal • Goldthread • Northern Prickly Ash • Peppermint • Quassia • Southern Prickly Ash • Yarrow
PSYLLIUM	Riboflavin
PYRIMETHAMINE (*Daraprim*)	Folic Acid
QT INTERVAL-PROLONGING DRUGS Some drugs in this category include: • Amitriptyline • Clarithromycin (*Biaxin*) • Erythromycin • Quinidine • Sotalol (*Betapace*) • Thioridazine • Indapamide (*Lozol*) • Risperidone (*Risperdal*) • Moxifloxacin (*Avelox*) • Ziprasidone (*Geodon*)	Bitter Orange • Country Mallow • Ephedra
QUINIDINE (*Quinidex*)	Cinchona • Grapefruit • Kaolin • Pheasant's Eye • Scopolia • Scotch Broom • Squill • Strophanthus • Wallflower
QUININE	Black Hellebore • Cinchona • Digitalis • Hedge Mustard • Lily-of-the-Valley • Oleander • Strophanthus • Swamp Milkweed • Uzara • Wahoo • Wallflower
QUINOLONE ANTIBIOTICS Some drugs in this category include: Ciprofloxacin (*Cipro*) • Gatifloxacin (*Tequin*) • Levofloxacin (*Levaquin*) • Moxifloxacin (*Avelox*) • Norfloxacin (*Noroxin*) • Ofloxacin (*Floxin*) • Trovafloxacin (*Trovan*)	Black Tea • Caffeine • Calcium • Cocoa • Coffee • Cola Nut • Colloidal Silver • Dolomite • Green Tea • Guarana • Iron • Magnesium • Manganese • Mate • Oolong Tea • Quercetin • Whey Protein • Zinc
RESERPINE	St. John's Wort
RETINOIDS Some drugs in this category include: Adapelene (*Differin*) • Isotretinoin (*Isotrex*) • Tretinon (*Retin-A, Retinova*)	Vitamin A
RILUZOLE (*Rilutek*)	Black Tea • Caffeine • Coffee • Cola Nut • Green Tea • Guarana • Mate • Oolong Tea
RISPERIDONE (*Risperdal*)	Hawaiian Baby Woodrose
RITONAVIR (*Norvir*)	Butanediol • GBL • GHB
SALSALATE (*Disalcid*)	Meadowsweet • Ribose • Rose Hip • Vitamin C • Willow Bark
SAQUINAVIR (*Fortovase, Invirase*)	Butanediol • GBL • GHB • Garlic • Grapefruit
SCOPOLAMINE (*Transderm Scop*)	Alpha-GPC • Grapefruit

Potential Interactions: Drug/Natural Medicine

For additional data, refer to the database.

Drug	Natural Medicine
SEIZURE THRESHOLD LOWERING DRUGS Some of the drugs in this category include: Anesthetics (*Propofol*, others) • Antiarrhythmics (*Mexiletine*) • Antibiotics (*Amphotericin, Penicillin, Cephalosporins, Imipenem*) • Antidepressants (*Bupropion*, others) • Antihistamines (*Cyproheptadine*, others) • Immunosuppressants (*Cyclosporin*) • Narcotics (*Fentanyl*, others) • Stimulants (*Methylphenidate*, others) • Theophylline	Ginkgo
SERTRALINE (*Zoloft*)	St. John's Wort
SEVOFLURANE (*Ultane*)	Aloe
SILDENAFIL (*Viagra*)	Grapefruit • L-Arginine
SIMVASTATIN (*Zocor*)	St. John's Wort
SKELETAL MUSCLE RELAXANTS Some drugs in this category include: Baclofen (*Lioresal*) • Botulinum Toxin Type A (*Botox*) • Chlorzaoxazone (*Parafon Forte*) • Cyclobenzaprine (*Flexeril*) • Dantrolene (*Dantrium*) • Metaxalone (*Skelaxin*) • Orphenadrine (*Norflex*)	Butanediol • GBL • GHB • Lithium • Magnesium • Procaine
SOTALOL (*Betapace*)	Calcium • Dolomite
STIMULANT DRUGS Some drugs in this category include: Pemoline (*Cylert*) • Methylphenidate (*Ritalin*) • Fenfluramine (*Pondimin*) • Dextroamphetamine (*Dexedrine*) • Dexfenfluramine (*Redux*) • Caffeine (*NoDoz*) • Pseudoephedrine	Bitter Orange • Black Tea • Caffeine • Coffee • Country Mallow • Ephedra • Ergot • Fever Bark • Ginseng, American • Ginseng, Panax • Indian Snakeroot • Peyote • Theanine • Tiratricol • Yohimbe
STIMULANT LAXATIVES Some drugs in this category include: Senna (*Senokot*) • Bisacodyl (*Dulcolax*)	Alder Buckthorn • Aloe • Black Hellebore • Butternut • Calotropis • Cascara • Castor • Digitalis • Fo-Ti • Gamboge • Gossypol • Hedge Mustard • Jalap • Lily-of-the-Valley • Mexican Scammony Root • Oleander • Pheasant's Eye • Rhubarb • Squill • Strophanthus • Swamp Milkweed • Uzara • Wahoo • Wallflower
SUCCINYLCHOLINE	Procaine
SULFONAMIDE ANTIBIOTICS Some drugs in this category include: Sulfamethoxazole; Trimethoprim (*Bactrim*) • Sulfacetamide (*Sodium Sulamyd*) • Sulfisoxazole (*Gantrisin*)	Beer • PABA • Procaine • Wine
SYRUP OF IPECAC	Activated Charcoal
TACROLIMUS (*Prograf, Protopic*)	St. John's Wort
TAMOXIFEN (*Nolvadex*)	Anise • DHEA • Fennel • Guggul • Kudzu • Red Clover • Soy
TERBINAFINE (*Lamisil*)	Black Tea • Caffeine • Coffee • Cola Nut • Green Tea • Guarana • Mate • Oolong Tea
TERFENADINE (*Seldane*)	Grapefruit
TESTOSTERONE	Androstenediol • Pregnenolone
TETRACYCLINES Demeclocycline (*Declomycin*) • Doxycycline (*Vibramycin*) • Minocycline (*Minocin*) • Tetracyline (*Achromycin, Sumycin*) •	Black Hellebore • Bromelain • Calcium • Colloidal Silver • Digitalis • Dolomite • Hedge Mustard • Iron • Lily-of-the-Valley • Magnesium • Manganese • Oleander • Pectin • Swamp Milkweed • Uzara • Vitamin A • Wahoo • Whey Protein • Yogurt • Zinc
THEOPHYLLINE (*Theo-Dur*)	Black Pepper and White Pepper • Black Tea • Caffeine • Capsicum • Cocoa • Coffee • Cola Nut • Gossypol • Grapefruit • Green Tea • Guarana • Indian Long Pepper • Ipriflavone • Marijuana • Mate • Oolong Tea • St. John's Wort
THIAZIDE DIURETICS Some drugs in this category include: Chlorothiazide (*Diuril*) • Metolazone (*Zaroxolyn*)	Calcium • Dolomite • Lithium • Pangamic Acid • Vitamin D • Zinc
THROMBOLYTIC DRUGS (*tPA, Alteplase*)	Mesoglycan • Potato
THYROID HORMONE Some drugs in this category include: Levothyroxine (*Synthroid, Levothroid, Levoxyl*)	Ashwagandha • Branched-Chain Amino Acids • Bugleweed • Guggul • Laminaria • Shepherd's Purse • Tiratricol • Tyrosine

Potential Interactions: Drug/Natural Medicine

For additional data, refer to the database.

Drug	Natural Medicine
TOLBUTAMIDE (*Orinase*)	Beer • Wine
TOPICAL DRUGS	DMSO
TRAMADOL (*Ultram*)	5-HTP • Ergot • Hawaiian Baby Woodrose • Lithium • L-Tryptophan • SAMe • St. John's Wort
TRANSDERMAL NICOTINE (*Nicoderm*, *Nicotrol*)	Inositol Nicotinate • Niacin and Niacinamide
TRAZODONE (*Desyrel*)	Ginkgo
TRIAZOLAM (*Halcion*)	DHEA
TRICYCLIC ANTIDEPRESSANTS (TCAs) Some drugs in this category include: Amitriptyline (*Elavil*) • Clomipramine (*Anafranil*) • Desipramine (*Norpramin*) • Doxepin (*Sinequan*) • Imipramine (*Tofranil*) • Nortriptyline (*Pamelor*) • Protriptyline (*Vivactil*)	Black Tea • Coffee • Cowhage • Indian Snakeroot • Riboflavin • Scopolia • Yohimbe
TRIMETHOPRIM (*Proloprim*)	Kaolin
VERAPAMIL (*Calan*, *Covera*, *Isoptin*, *Verelan*)	Black Tea • Caffeine • Calcium • Cocoa • Coffee • Cola Nut • Green Tea • Guarana • Mate • Melatonin • Oolong Tea • Vitamin D
WARFARIN (*Coumadin*)	Acerola • Acetyl-L-Carnitine • Alfalfa • Avocado • Beer • Blond Psyllium • Boldo • Cabbage • Cherokee Rosehip • Chlorella • Chondroitin Sulfate • Coenzyme Q-10 • Corn Silk • Cranberry • Danshen • Devil's Claw • Dong Quai • EDTA • Fenugreek • Garlic • Ginger • Ginkgo • Ginseng, American • Ginseng, Panax • Glucosamine Hydrochloride • Glucosamine Sulfate • Grape • Grapefruit • Great Plantain • Green Tea • L-Carnitine • Lycium • N-Acetyl Glucosamine • Papaya • Parsley • Propionyl-L-Carnitine • Rose Hip • Smartweed • Soy • Spinach • St. John's Wort • Stinging Nettle • Vinpocetine • Vitamin A • Vitamin C • Vitamin E • Vitamin K • Watercress • Wine • Wintergreen
ZIDOVUDINE (AZT, *Retrovir*)	Acetyl-L-Carnitine • L-Carnitine • Propionyl-L-Carnitine

Potential Interactions Between Natural Medicines and Drugs

For details on possible interactions between natural medicines and drugs, see the listing for the specific natural medicine in the body of this database. This chart does not contain all theoretical or unknown interactions.

Natural Medicine	Drug
5-HTP	Antidepressant Drugs • Carbidopa (*Lodosyn*) • Dextromethorphan (*Robitussin DM*, others) • Meperidine (*Demerol*) • Monoamine Oxidase Inhibitors (MAOIs) • Pentazocine (*Talwin*) • Tramadol (*Ultram*)
Acacia	Amoxicillin (*Amoxil*, *Trimox*)
Acerola	Estrogens • Fluphenazine (*Prolixin*) • Warfarin (*Coumadin*)
Acetyl-L-Carnitine	Acenocoumarol (*Sintrom*) • Warfarin (*Coumadin*) • Zidovudine (AZT, *Retrovir*)
Activated Charcoal	Alcohol (Ethanol) • Oral Drugs • Syrup of Ipecac
Adenosine	Antigout Drugs • Carbamazepine (*Tegretol*) • Dipyridamole (*Persantine*) • Methylxanthines
Agar	Oral Drugs
Agrimony	Antidiabetes Drugs
Alder Buckthorn	Corticosteroids • Digoxin (*Lanoxin*) • Diuretic Drugs • Oral Drugs • Stimulant Laxatives
Aletris	Antacids • H2-Blockers • Proton Pump Inhibitors (PPIs)
Alfalfa	Contraceptive Drugs • Estrogens • Photosensitizing Drugs • Warfarin (*Coumadin*)
Algin	Oral Drugs
Alkanna	Cytochrome P450 3A4 (CYP3A4) Inducers
Allspice	Anticoagulant/Antiplatelet Drugs
Aloe	Antidiabetes Drugs • Digoxin (*Lanoxin*) • Diuretic Drugs • Oral Drugs • Sevoflurane (*Ultane*) • Stimulant Laxatives
Alpha-GPC	Scopolamine
Alpha-Lipoic Acid	Antidiabetes Drugs • Chemotherapy
Alpine Ragwort	Cytochrome P450 3A4 (CYP3A4) Inducers
Alpinia	Antacids • H2-Blockers • Proton Pump Inhibitors (PPIs)
Ambrette	Acetaminophen (*Tylenol*, others)
American Chestnut	Oral Drugs
American Elder	Cytochrome P450 3A4 (CYP3A4) Substrates
Andrographis	Anticoagulant/Antiplatelet Drugs • Antihypertensive Drugs • Immunosuppressants
Androstenediol	Estrogens • Testosterone
Androstenedione	Estrogens
Angelica	Antacids • Anticoagulant/Antiplatelet Drugs • H2-Blockers • Photosensitizing Drugs • Proton Pump Inhibitors (PPIs)
Angel's Trumpet	Anticholinergic Drugs
Anise	Contraceptive Drugs • Estrogens • Monoamine Oxidase Inhibitors (MAOIs) • Tamoxifen (*Nolvadex*)
Annatto	Antidiabetes Drugs
Apple	Fexofenadine (*Allegra*)
Apple Cider Vinegar	Digoxin (*Lanoxin*) • Diuretic Drugs • Insulin
Areca	Anticholinergic Drugs • Cholinergic Drugs • Procyclidine (*Kemadrin*)
Arnica	Anticoagulant/Antiplatelet Drugs
Arrach	Photosensitizing Drugs
Asafoetida	Anticoagulant/Antiplatelet Drugs • Antihypertensive Drugs
Ashwagandha	Benzodiazepines • CNS Depressants • Immunosuppressants • Thyroid Hormone
Astragalus	Cyclophosphamide (*Cytoxan*) • Immunosuppressants

CHARTS

Potential Interactions: Natural Medicine/Drug

For additional data, refer to the database.

Natural Medicine	Drug
Autumn Crocus	Colchicine
Avocado	Warfarin (*Coumadin*)
Baikal Skullcap	Alcohol (Ethanol) • Antidiabetes Drugs • Benzodiazepines • CNS Depressants
Banaba	Antidiabetes Drugs
Barley	Antidiabetes Drugs • Oral Drugs
Bean Pod	Antidiabetes Drugs
Beer	Aspirin • Barbiturates • Benzodiazepines • Cefamandole (*Mandol*) • Cefoperazone (*Cefobid*) • Chlorpropamide (*Diabinese*) • Cisapride (*Propulsid*) • CNS Depressants • Disulfiram (*Antabuse*) • Erythromycin (*E.E.S.*, *E-Mycin*, *PCD*) • Griseofulvin (*Fulvicin*) • H2-Blockers • Hepatotoxic Drugs • Metformin (*Glucophage*) • Metronidazole (*Flagyl*) • Narcotic Drugs • Nonsteroidal Anti-Inflammatory Drugs (NSAIDs) • Phenytoin (*Dilantin*) • Sulfonamide Antibiotics • Tolbutamide (*Orinase*) • Warfarin (*Coumadin*)
Belladonna	Anticholinergic Drugs
Bergamot Oil	Photosensitizing Drugs
Beta Glucans	Immunosuppressants
Beta-Carotene	HMG-CoA Reductase Inhibitors ("Statins") • Niacin
Beta-Sitosterol	Ezetimibe (*Zetia*) • Pravastatin (*Pravachol*)
Betony	Antihypertensive Drugs
Bifidobacteria	Antibiotic Drugs
Bilberry	Antidiabetes Drugs
Birch	Diuretic Drugs
Bishop's Weed	Anticoagulant/Antiplatelet Drugs • Cytochrome P450 3A4 (CYP3A4) Substrates • Hepatotoxic Drugs • Photosensitizing Drugs
Bistort	Oral Drugs
Bitter Almond	CNS Depressants
Bitter Melon	Antidiabetes Drugs
Bitter Orange	Cytochrome P450 3A4 (CYP3A4) Substrates • Dextromethorphan (*Robitussin DM*, and others) • Felodipine (*Plendil*) • Indinavir (*Crixivan*) • Midazolam (*Versed*) • Monoamine Oxidase Inhibitors (MAOIs) • QT Interval-Prolonging Drugs • Stimulant Drugs
Black Cohosh	Cisplatin (*Platinol-AQ*) • Hepatotoxic Drugs
Black Hellebore	Digoxin (*Lanoxin*) • Diuretic Drugs • Macrolide Antibiotics • Quinine • Stimulant Laxatives • Tetracycline Antibiotics
Black Horehound	Dopamine Agonists
Black Mulberry	Antidiabetes Drugs
Black Mustard	Antacids • H2-Blockers • Proton Pump Inhibitors (PPIs)
Black Pepper and White Pepper	Phenytoin (*Dilantin*) • Propranolol (*Inderal*) • Theophylline (*Theo-Dur*)
Black Psyllium	Antidiabetes Drugs • Carbamazepine (*Tegretol*) • Digoxin (*Lanoxin*) • Lithium (*Eskalith*, *Lithobid*)
Black Root	Digoxin (Lanoxin) • Diuretic Drugs

Potential Interactions: Natural Medicine/Drug

For additional data, refer to the database.

Natural Medicine	Drug
Black Tea	Adenosine (*Adenocard*) • Alcohol (Ethanol) • Anticoagulant/Antiplatelet Drugs • Antidiabetes Drugs • Cimetidine (*Tagamet*) • Clozapine (*Clozaril*) • Contraceptive Drugs • Dipyridamole (*Persantine*) • Disulfiram (*Antabuse*) • Ephedrine (*Pretz-D*) • Estrogens • Fluconazole (*Diflucan*) • Fluvoxamine (*Luvox*) • Lithium (*Eskalith, Lithobid*) • Mexiletine (*Mexitil*) • Monoamine Oxidase Inhibitors (MAOIs) • Phenothiazines • Phenylpropanolamine (*Propagest, Rhindicon*) • Quinolone Antibiotics • Riluzole (*Rilutek*) • Stimulant Drugs • Terbinafine (*Lamisil*) • Theophylline (*Theo-Dur*) • Tricyclic Antidepressants (TCAs) • Verapamil (*Calan, Covera, Isoptin, Verelan*)
Black Walnut	Oral Drugs
Bladderwrack	Anticoagulant/Antiplatelet Drugs • Antithyroid Drugs
Blessed Thistle	Antacids • H2-Blockers • Proton Pump Inhibitors (PPIs)
Blond Psyllium	Antidiabetes Drugs • Carbamazepine (*Tegretol*) • Digoxin (*Lanoxin*) • Lithium (*Eskalith, Lithobid*) • Ethinyl Estradiol • Warfarin (*Coumadin*)
Blue Cohosh	Antidiabetes Drugs • Antihypertensive Drugs • Nicotine (*Habitrol, Nicoderm, Nicorette, Prestep*)
Blue Flag	Digoxin (*Lanoxin*) • Diuretic Drugs
Blueberry	Antidiabetes Drugs
Bogbean	Anticoagulant/Antiplatelet Drugs
Boldo	Anticoagulant/Antiplatelet Drugs • Warfarin (*Coumadin*)
Borage	Anesthesia • Anticoagulant/Antiplatelet Drugs • Cytochrome P450 3A4 (CYP3A4) Inducers • Nonsteroidal Anti-Inflammatory Drugs (NSAIDs)
Boron	Estrogens
Branched-Chain Amino Acids	Antidiabetes Drugs • Corticosteroids • Diazoxide (*Hyperstat, Proglycem*) • Levodopa • Thyroid Hormone (*Cytomel, Triostat*)
Brewer's Yeast	Antifungals • Monoamine Oxidase Inhibitors (MAOIs)
Bromelain	Anticoagulant/Antiplatelet Drugs • Tetracycline Antibiotics
Buchu	Anticoagulant/Antiplatelet Drugs
Bugleweed	Antidiabetes Drugs • Thyroid Hormone
Burdock	Anticoagulant/Antiplatelet Drugs
Butanediol (BD)	Alcohol (Ethanol) • Amphetamines • Anticonvulsants • Antipsychotic Drugs • Benzodiazepines • CNS Depressants • Haloperidol (*Haldol*) • Naloxone (*Narcan*) • Narcotic Drugs • Ritonavir (*Norvir*) • Saquinavir (*Fortovase, Invirase*) • Skeletal Muscle Relaxants
Butcher's Broom	Alpha-Adrenergic Agonists • Alpha-Adrenergic Antagonists
Butterbur	Cytochrome P450 3A4 (CYP3A4) Inducers
Butternut	Corticosteroids • Digoxin (*Lanoxin*) • Diuretic Drugs • Oral Drugs • Stimulant Laxatives
Cabbage	Acetaminophen (*Tylenol*, others) • Cytochrome P450 1A2 (CYP1A2) Substrates • Glucuronidated Drugs • Oxazepam (*Serax*) • Warfarin (*Coumadin*)
Caffeine	Adenosine (*Adenocard*) • Alcohol (Ethanol) • Anticoagulant/Antiplatelet Drugs • Antidiabetes Drugs • Cimetidine (*Tagamet*) • Clozapine (*Clozaril*) • Contraceptive Drugs • Dipyridamole (*Persantine*) • Disulfiram (*Antabuse*) • Ephedrine (*Pretz-D*) • Estrogens • Fluconazole (*Diflucan*) • Fluvoxamine (*Luvox*) • Lithium (*Eskalith, Lithobid*) • Mexiletine (*Mexitil*) • Monoamine Oxidase Inhibitors (MAOIs) • Phenylpropanolamine (*Propagest, Rhindicon*) • Quinolone Antibiotics • Riluzole (*Rilutek*) • Stimulant Drugs • Terbinafine (*Lamisil*) • Theophylline (*Theo-Dur*) • Verapamil (*Calan, Covera, Isoptin, Verelan*)
Calabar Bean	Anticholinergic Drugs
Calamus	Antacids • CNS Depressants • H2-Blockers • Monoamine Oxidase Inhibitors (MAOIs) • Proton Pump Inhibitors (PPIs)

Potential Interactions: Natural Medicine/Drug

For additional data, refer to the database.

Natural Medicine	Drug
Calcium	Bisphosphonates • Calcipotriene (*Dovonex*) • Calcium Channel Blockers • Digoxin (*Lanoxin*) • Diltiazem (*Cardizem, Dilacor, Tiazac*) • Estrogens • Levothyroxine (*Synthroid, Levothroid, Levoxyl*, and others) • Quinolone Antibiotics • Sotalol (*Betapace*) • Tetracycline Antibiotics • Thiazide Diuretics • Verapamil (*Calan, Covera, Isoptin, Verelan*)
Calcium D-Glucarate	Alcohol (Ethanol) • Glucuronidated Drugs • Kanamycin (*Kanatrex*)
Calendula	CNS Depressants
California Poppy	Benzodiazepines • CNS Depressants
Calotropis	Digoxin (*Lanoxin*) • Diuretic Drugs • Stimulant Laxatives
Canadian Hemp	Digoxin (*Lanoxin*) • Diuretic Drugs
Capers	Antidiabetes Drugs
Capsicum	ACE Inhibitors (ACEIs) • Antacids • Anticoagulant/Antiplatelet Drugs • Cocaine • Theophylline (*Theo-Dur*)
Caraway	Antidiabetes Drugs
Carrageenan	Anticoagulant/Antiplatelet Drugs • Antihypertensive Drugs • Oral Drugs
Cascara	Corticosteroids • Digoxin (*Lanoxin*) • Diuretic Drugs • Oral Drugs • Stimulant Laxatives
Casein Peptides	Antihypertensive Drugs
Cassia Auriculata	Antidiabetes Drugs • Carbamazepine (*Tegretol*)
Cassia Cinnamon	Antidiabetes Drugs
Castor	Corticosteroids • Digoxin (*Lanoxin*) • Diuretic Drugs • Oral Drugs • Stimulant Laxatives
Catnip	CNS Depressants
Cat's Claw	Antihypertensive Drugs • Cytochrome P450 3A4 (CYP3A4) Substrates • Immunosuppressants
Cedar Leaf	Anticonvulsants
Cedar Leaf Oil	Anticonvulsants
Cedarwood	Barbiturates
Celery	CNS Depressants • Levothyroxine (*Synthroid, Levothroid, Levoxyl*, and others) • Photosensitizing Drugs
Cereus	Digoxin (*Lanoxin*) • Monoamine Oxidase Inhibitors (MAOIs)
Cesium	Corticosteroids • Diuretic Drugs
Chanca Piedra	Antidiabetes Drugs
Chaparral	Hepatotoxic Drugs
Chasteberry	Antipsychotic Drugs • Contraceptive Drugs • Dopamine Agonists • Estrogens • Metoclopramide (*Reglan*)
Chenopodium Oil	Photosensitizing Drugs
Cherokee Rosehip	Aluminum • Aspirin • Choline Magnesium Trisalicylate (*Trilisate*) • Estrogens • Fluphenazine (*Prolixin*) • Warfarin (*Coumadin*)
Chinese Club Moss	Acetylcholinesterase (AChE) Inhibitors • Anticholinergic Drugs • Cholinergic Drugs
Chinese Cucumber	Antidiabetes Drugs
Chlorella	Warfarin (*Coumadin*)
Chlorophyll	Photosensitizing Drugs
Chondroitin Sulfate	Warfarin (*Coumadin*)
Chromium	Insulin • Nonsteroidal Anti-Inflammatory Drugs (NSAIDs)
Chrysin	Aromatase Inhibitors • Cytochrome P450 1A2 (CYP1A2) Substrates • Glucuronidated Drugs

Potential Interactions: Natural Medicine/Drug

For additional data, refer to the database.

Natural Medicine	Drug
Cinchona	Antacids • Anticoagulant/Antiplatelet Drugs • Carbamazepine (*Tegretol*) • H2 Blockers • Phenobarbital (*Luminal*) • Proton Pump Inhibitors (PPIs) • Quinidine (*Quinidex*) • Quinine
Cinnamon Bark	Antidiabetes Drugs
Clary Sage	Chloral Hydrate • Hexobarbitone
Clove	Anticoagulant/Antiplatelet Drugs
Coca	Alcohol (Ethanol) • Nifedipine (*Adalat*, *Procardia*)
Cocoa	Adenosine (*Adenocard*) • Antidiabetes Drugs • Beta-Adrenergic Agonists • Cimetidine (*Tagamet*) • Clozapine (*Clozaril*) • Contraceptive Drugs • Dipyridamole (*Persantine*) • Disulfiram (*Antabuse*) • Ergotamine (*Ergomar*) • Estrogens • Fluconazole (*Diflucan*) • Lithium (*Eskalith, Lithobid*) • Mexiletine (*Mexitil*) • Monoamine Oxidase Inhibitors (MAOIs) • Phenylpropanolamine (*Propagest*, *Rhindicon*) • Quinolone Antibiotics • Theophylline (*Theo-Dur*) • Verapamil (*Calan*, *Covera*, *Isoptin*, *Verelan*)
Cod Liver Oil	Anticoagulant/Antiplatelet Drugs • Antihypertensive Drugs
Coenzyme Q-10	Antihypertensive Drugs • Chemotherapy • Warfarin (*Coumadin*)
Coffee	Adenosine (*Adenocard*) • Alcohol (Ethanol) • Alendronate (*Fosamax*) • Anticoagulant/ Antiplatelet Drugs • Antidiabetes Drugs • Cimetidine (*Tagamet*) • Clozapine (*Clozaril*) • Contraceptive Drugs • Dipyridamole (*Persantine*) • Disulfiram (*Antabuse*) • Ephedrine (*Pretz-D*) • Estrogens • Fluconazole (*Diflucan*) • Fluvoxamine (*Luvox*) • Lithium (*Eskalith, Lithobid*) • Mexiletine (*Mexitil*) • Monoamine Oxidase Inhibitors (MAOIs) • Phenothiazines • Phenylpropanolamine • Quinolone Antibiotics • Riluzole (*Rilutek*) • Stimulant Drugs • Terbinafine (*Lamisil*) • Theophylline (*Theo-Dur*) • Tricyclic Antidepressants (TCAs) • Verapamil (*Calan*, *Covera*, *Isoptin*, *Verelan*)
Coffee Charcoal	Oral Drugs
Cola Nut	Adenosine (*Adenocard*) • Alcohol (*Ethanol*) • Amphetamines • Antidiabetes Drugs • Cimetidine (*Tagamet*) • Clozapine (*Clozaril*) • Cocaine • Contraceptive Drugs • Dipyridamole (*Persantine*) • Disulfiram (*Antabuse*) • Ephedrine (*Pretz-D*) • Estrogens • Fluconazole (*Diflucan*) • Fluvoxamine (*Luvox*) • Lithium (*Eskalith, Lithobid*) • Mexiletine (*Mexitil*) • Monoamine Oxidase Inhibitors (MAOIs) • Nicotine • Phenylpropanolamine • Quinolone Antibiotics • Riluzole (*Rilutek*) • Terbinafine (*Lamisil*) • Theophylline (*Theo-Dur*) • Verapamil (*Calan*, *Covera*, *Isoptin*, *Verelan*)
Colloidal Silver	Levothyroxine (*Synthroid, Levothroid, Levoxyl*) • Penicillamine (*Curpimine*) • Quinolone Antibiotics • Tetracycline Antibiotics
Colocynth	Digoxin (*Lanoxin*) • Diuretic Drugs
Colombo	Antacids • H2-Blockers • Proton Pump Inhibitors (PPIs)
Coltsfoot	Anticoagulant/Antiplatelet Drugs • Antihypertensive Drugs • Cytochrome P450 3A4 (CYP3A4) Inducers
Comfrey	Cytochrome P450 3A4 (CYP3A4) Inducers • Hepatotoxic Drugs
Copper	Penicillamine (*Curpimine*)
Cordyceps	Cyclophosphamide (*Cytoxcin, Neosar*) • Prednisolone (*Pediapred*)
Corn Silk	Antidiabetes Drugs • Antihypertensive Drugs • Corticosteroids • Diuretic Drugs • Warfarin (*Coumadin*)
Country Mallow	Antidiabetes Drugs • Dexamethasone (*Decadron*) • Ergot Derivatives • Methylxanthines • Monoamine Oxidase Inhibitors (MAOIs) • QT Interval-Prolonging Drugs • Stimulant Drugs
Cowhage	Anesthesia • Antidiabetes Drugs • Antipsychotic Drugs • Guanethidine (*Ismelin*) • Methyldopa (*Aldomet*) • Monoamine Oxidase Inhibitors (MAOIs) • Tricyclic Antidepressants (TCAs)
Cowslip	CNS Depressants • Diuretic Drugs
Cranberry	Cytochrome P450 2C9 (CYP2C9) Substrates • Warfarin (*Coumadin*)
Creatine	Nephrotoxic Drugs
Cubebs	Antacids • H2-Blockers • Proton Pump Inhibitors (PPIs)

CHARTS

Potential Interactions: Natural Medicine/Drug

For additional data, refer to the database.

Natural Medicine	Drug
Cumin	Antidiabetes Drugs
Damiana	Antidiabetes Drugs
Dandelion	Antacids • H2-Blockers • Lithium (*Eskalith, Lithobid*) • Potassium-Sparing Diuretics • Proton Pump Inhibitors (PPIs)
Danshen	Anticoagulant/Antiplatelet Drugs • Digoxin (*Lanoxin*) • Warfarin (*Coumadin*)
Deanol	Anticholinergic Drugs
Deertongue	Anticoagulant/Antiplatelet Drugs
Devil's Claw	Antacids • Antidiabetes Drugs • Antihypertensive Drugs • Cytochrome P450 2C19 (CYP2C19) Substrates • Cytochrome P450 2C9 (CYP2C9) Substrates • Cytochrome P450 3A4 (CYP3A4) Substrates • H2 Blockers • Proton Pump Inhibitors (PPIs) • Warfarin (*Coumadin*)
DHA (Docosahexaenoic Acid)	Anticoagulant/Antiplatelet Drugs • Antihypertensive Drugs
DHEA	Anastrozole (*Arimidex*) • Corticosteroids • Cytochrome P450 3A4 (CYP3A4) Substrates • Exemestane (*Aromasin*) • Fulvestrant (*Faslodex*) • Insulin • Letrozole (*Femara*) • Tamoxifen (*Nolvadex*) • Triazolam (*Halcion*)
Dibencozide	Chloramphenicol (*Chloromycetin*)
Digitalis	Digoxin (*Lanoxin*) • Diuretic Drugs • Macrolide Antibiotics • Quinine • Stimulant Laxatives • Tetracycline Antibiotics
Diindolylmethane	Cytochrome P450 1A2 (CYP1A2) Substrates
DMSO (Dimethylsulfoxide)	Injectable Drugs • Oral Drugs • Topical Drugs
Dolomite	Bisphosphonates • Estrogens • Levothyroxine (*Synthroid*, *Levothroid*, *Levoxyl*, and others) • Potassium-Sparing Diuretics • Quinolone Antibiotics • Sotalol (*Betapace*) • Tetracycline Antibiotics • Thiazide Diuretics
Dong Quai	Anticoagulant/Antiplatelet Drugs • Warfarin (*Coumadin*)
Dusty Miller	Cytochrome P450 3A4 (CYP3A4) Inducers
Echinacea	Cytochrome P450 3A4 (CYP3A4) Substrates • Immunosuppressants • Midazolam (*Versed*)
EDTA	Diuretic Drugs • Insulin • Warfarin (*Coumadin*)
Elderberry	Immunosuppressants
Elecampane	CNS Depressants
EPA (Eicosapentaenoic Acid)	Anticoagulant/Antiplatelet Drugs • Antihypertensive Drugs
Ephedra	Anticonvulsants • Antidiabetes Drugs • Dexamethasone (*Decadron*) • Ergot Derivatives • Methylxanthines • Monoamine Oxidase Inhibitors (MAOIs) • QT Interval-Prolonging Drugs • Stimulant Drugs
Epimedium	Anticoagulant/Antiplatelet Drugs • Antihypertensive Drugs
Ergot	Antidepressant Drugs • Cytochrome P450 3A4 (CYP3A4) Inhibitors • Dextromethorphan (*Robitussin DM*, and others) • Ergot Derivatives • Meperidine (*Demerol*) • Monoamine Oxidase Inhibitors (MAOIs) • Pentazocine (*Talwin*) • Stimulant Drugs • Tramadol (*Ultram*)
Eucalyptus	Antidiabetes Drugs • Cytochrome P450 1A2 (CYP1A2) Substrates • Cytochrome P450 2C19 (CYP2C19) Substrates • Cytochrome P450 2C9 (CYP2C9) Substrates • Cytochrome P450 3A4 (CYP3A4) Substrates
European Buckthorn	Digoxin (*Lanoxin*) • Diuretic Drugs • Oral Drugs
European Chestnut	Oral Drugs
European Mandrake	Anticholinergic Drugs • Oral Drugs
European Mistletoe	Antihypertensive Drugs • Immunosuppressants
Evening Primrose Oil	Anesthesia • Anticoagulant/Antiplatelet Drugs • Phenothiazines
Fennel	Ciprofloxacin (*Cipro*) • Contraceptive Drugs • Estrogens • Tamoxifen (*Nolvadex*)

CHARTS

Potential Interactions: Natural Medicine/Drug

For additional data, refer to the database.

Natural Medicine	Drug
Fenugreek	Anticoagulant/Antiplatelet Drugs • Antidiabetes Drugs • Warfarin (*Coumadin*)
Fever Bark	Anesthesia • Naloxone (*Narcan*) • Phenothiazines • Stimulant Drugs
Feverfew	Anticoagulant/Antiplatelet Drugs • Cytochrome P450 1A2 (CYP1A2) Substrates • Cytochrome P450 2C19 (CYP2C19) Substrates • Cytochrome P450 2C9 (CYP2C9) Substrates • Cytochrome P450 3A4 (CYP3A4) Substrates
Fig	Antidiabetes Drugs • Insulin
Figwort	Diuretic Drugs
Fish Oil	Anticoagulant/Antiplatelet Drugs • Antihypertensive Drugs • Contraceptive Drugs
Flaxseed	Anticoagulant/Antiplatelet Drugs • Antidiabetes Drugs • Oral Drugs
Flaxseed Oil	Anticoagulant/Antiplatelet Drugs
Folic Acid	Fosphenytoin (*Cerebyx*) • Methotrexate (*MTX*, *Rheumatrex*) • Phenobarbital (*Luminal*) • Phenytoin (*Dilantin*) • Primidone (*Mysoline*) • Pyrimethamine (*Daraprim*)
Forskolin	Anticoagulant/Antiplatelet Drugs • Calcium Channel Blockers • Nitrates
Forsythia	Anticoagulant/Antiplatelet Drugs
Fo-Ti	Antidiabetes Drugs • Cytochrome P450 1A2 (CYP1A2) Substrates • Cytochrome P450 2C19 (CYP2C19) Substrates • Cytochrome P450 2C9 (CYP2C9) Substrates • Cytochrome P450 3A4 (CYP3A4) Substrates • Digoxin (*Lanoxin*) • Diuretic Drugs • Stimulant Laxatives
Gamboge	Corticosteroids • Digoxin (*Lanoxin*) • Diuretic Drugs • Stimulant Laxatives
Gamma Butyrolactone (GBL)	Alcohol (Ethanol) • Amphetamines • Anticonvulsants • Antipsychotic Drugs • Benzodiazepines • CNS Depressants • Haloperidol (*Haldol*) • Naloxone (*Narcan*) • Narcotic Drugs • Ritonavir (*Norvir*) • Saquinavir (*Fortovase*, *Invirase*) • Skeletal Muscle Relaxants
Gamma Linolenic Acid	Anticoagulant/Antiplatelet Drugs • Phenothiazines
Gamma-Hydroxybutyrate (GHB)	Alcohol (Ethanol) • Amphetamines • Anticonvulsants • Antipsychotic Drugs • Benzodiazepines • CNS Depressants • Haloperidol (*Haldol*) • Naloxone (*Narcan*) • Narcotic Drugs • Ritonavir (*Norvir*) • Saquinavir (*Fortovase*, *Invirase*) • Skeletal Muscle Relaxants
Garlic	Anticoagulant/Antiplatelet Drugs • Contraceptive Drugs • Cyclosporine (*Neoral*, *Sandimmune*) • Cytochrome P450 3A4 (CYP3A4) Substrates • Non-Nucleoside Reverse Transcriptase Inhibitors (NNRTIs) • Saquinavir (*Fortovase*, *Invirase*) • Warfarin (*Coumadin*)
Gentian	Antacids • H2-Blockers • Proton Pump Inhibitors (PPIs)
German Chamomile	Benzodiazepines • CNS Depressants • Cytochrome P450 3A4 (CYP3A4) Substrates
Germanium	Furosemide (*Lasix*)
Ginger	Anticoagulant/Antiplatelet Drugs • Antidiabetes Drugs • Calcium Channel Blockers • Phenprocoumon • Warfarin (*Coumadin*)
Ginkgo	Anticoagulant/Antiplatelet Drugs • Anticonvulsants • Buspirone (*BuSpar*) • Cytochrome P450 1A2 (CYP1A2) Substrates • Cytochrome P450 2C19 (CYP2C19) Substrates • Cytochrome P450 2C9 (CYP2C9) Substrates • Cytochrome P450 2D6 (CYP2D6) Substrates • Cytochrome P450 3A4 (CYP3A4) Substrates • Fluoxetine (*Prozac*) • Insulin • Omeprazole (*Prilosec*) • Seizure Threshold Lowering Drugs • Trazodone (*Desyrel*) • Warfarin (*Coumadin*)
Ginseng, American	Antidiabetes Drugs • Antipsychotic Drugs • Monoamine Oxidase Inhibitors (MAOIs) • Stimulant Drugs • Warfarin (*Coumadin*)
Ginseng, Panax	Alcohol (Ethanol) • Anticoagulant/Antiplatelet Drugs • Antidiabetes Drugs • Caffeine (*No-Doz, Stay Alert, Vivarin*) • Cytochrome P450 2D6 (CYP2D6) Substrates • Furosemide (*Lasix*) • Immunosuppressants • Insulin • Monoamine Oxidase Inhibitors (MAOIs) • Stimulant Drugs • Warfarin (*Coumadin*)

Potential Interactions: Natural Medicine/Drug

For additional data, refer to the database.

Natural Medicine	Drug
Ginseng, Siberian	Alcohol (Ethanol) • Anticoagulant/Antiplatelet Drugs • Antidiabetes Drugs • CNS Depressants • Cytochrome P450 1A2 (CYP1A2) Substrates • Cytochrome P450 2C9 (CYP2C9) Substrates • Cytochrome P450 2D6 (CYP2D6) Substrates • Cytochrome P450 3A4 (CYP3A4) Substrates • Digoxin (*Lanoxin*)
Glucomannan	Antidiabetes Drugs • Oral Drugs
Glucosamine Hydrochloride	Antidiabetes Drugs • Antimitotic Chemotherapy • Warfarin (*Coumadin*)
Glucosamine Sulfate	Acetaminophen (*Tylenol*, others) • Antidiabetes Drugs • Antimitotic Chemotherapy • Warfarin (*Coumadin*)
Glutamine	Anticonvulsants • Chemotherapy • Lactulose
Glycine	Clozapine (*Clozaril*)
Goat's Rue	Antidiabetes Drugs
Golden Ragwort	Cytochrome P450 3A4 (CYP3A4) Inducers
Goldenrod	Diuretic Drugs
Goldenseal	Antacids • Antihypertensive Drugs • CNS Depressants • Cytochrome P450 3A4 (CYP3A4) Substrates • H2-Blockers • Proton Pump Inhibitors (PPIs)
Goldthread	Antacids • H2-Blockers • Proton Pump Inhibitors (PPIs)
Gossypol	Digoxin (*Lanoxin*) • Diuretic Drugs • Nonsteroidal Anti-Inflammatory Drugs (NSAIDs) • Stimulant Laxatives • Theophylline (*Theo-Dur*)
Gotu Kola	CNS Depressants
Grape	Cytochrome P450 1A2 (CYP1A2) Substrates • Phenacetin • Warfarin (*Coumadin*)
Grapefruit	Artemether (*Artenam, Paluther*) • Benzodiazepines • Buspirone (*BuSpar*) • Caffeine (*NoDoz, Stay Alert, Vivarin*) • Calcium Channel Blockers • Carbamazepine (*Tegretol*) • Carvedilol (*Coreg*) • Cisapride (*Propulsid*) • Clomipramine (*Anafranil*) • Cyclosporine (*Neoral, Sandimmune*) • Cytochrome P450 1A2 (CYP1A2) Substrates • Cytochrome P450 2C19 (CYP2C19) Substrates • Cytochrome P450 2C9 (CYP2C9) Substrates • Cytochrome P450 3A4 (CYP3A4) Substrates • Dextromethorphan (*Robitussin DM*, and others) • Erythromycin (*E.E.S., E-Mycin, PCE*) • Estrogens • Etoposide (*VePesid*) • Fexofenadine (*Allegra*) • HMG-CoA Reductase Inhibitors ("Statins") • Itraconazole (*Sporanox*) • Losartan (*Cozaar*) • Methylprednisolone (*Aldone, A-Methapred, depMedalone, Depoject, Medrol, Solu-Medrol*) • Praziquantel (*Biltricide*) • Quinidine (*Quinidex*) • Saquinavir (*Fortovase, Invirase*) • Scopolamine (*Transderm Scope*) • Sildenafil (*Viagra*) • Terfenadine (*Seldane*) • Theophylline (*Theo-Dur*) • Warfarin (*Coumadin*)
Gravel Root	Cytochrome P450 3A4 (CYP3A4) Inducers
Great Plantain	Warfarin (*Coumadin*)
Greater Bindweed	Digoxin (*Lanoxin*) • Diuretic Drugs
Greek Sage	Hexobarbital
Green Tea	Adenosine (*Adenocard*) • Alcohol (Ethanol) • Amphetamines • Anticoagulant/Antiplatelet Drugs • Antidiabetes Drugs • Cimetidine (*Tagamet*) • Clozapine (*Clozaril*) • Cocaine • Contraceptive Drugs • Dipyridamole (*Persantine*) • Disulfiram (*Antabuse*) • Ephedrine (*Pretz-D*) • Estrogens • Fluconazole (*Diflucan*) • Fluvoxamine (*Luvox*) • Lithium (*Eskalith, Lithobid*) • Mexiletine (*Mexitil*) • Monoamine Oxidase Inhibitors (MAOIs) • Nicotine (*Habitrol, Nicoderm, Nicorette, Prestep*) • Phenylpropanolamine (*Propagest, Rhindicon*) • Quinolone Antibiotics • Riluzole (*Rilutek*) • Terbinafine (*Lamisil*) • Theophylline (*Theo-Dur*) • Verapamil (*Calan, Covera, Isoptin, Verelan*) • Warfarin (*Coumadin*)
Groundsel	Cytochrome P450 3A4 (CYP3A4) Inducers
Guar Gum	Antidiabetes Drugs • Digoxin (*Lanoxin*) • Ethinyl Estradiol • Metformin (*Glucophage*) • Penicillin (*Penicillin VK, Pen VK, Veetids*)

Potential Interactions: Natural Medicine/Drug

For additional data, refer to the database.

Natural Medicine	Drug
Guarana	Adenosine (*Adenocard*) • Alcohol (Ethanol) • Amphetamines • Anticoagulant/ Antiplatelet Drugs • Antidiabetes Drugs • Cimetidine (*Tagamet*) • Clozapine (*Clozaril*) • Cocaine • Contraceptive Drugs • Dipyridamole (*Persantine*) • Disulfiram (*Antabuse*) • Ephedrine (*Pretz-D*) • Estrogens • Fluconazole (*Diflucan*) • Fluvoxamine (*Luvox*) • Lithium (*Eskalith, Lithobid*) • Mexiletine (*Mexitil*) • Monoamine Oxidase Inhibitors (MAOIs) • Nicotine (*Habitrol, Nicoderm, Nicorette, Prestep*) • Phenylpropanolamine (*Propagest, Rhindicon*) • Quinolone Antibiotics • Riluzole (*Rilutek*) • Terbinafine (*Lamisil*) • Theophylline (*Theo-Dur*) • Verapamil (*Calan, Covera, Isoptin, Verelan*)
Guggul	Anticoagulant/Antiplatelet Drugs • Contraceptive Drugs • Cytochrome P450 3A4 (CYP3A4) Substrates • Diltiazem (*Cardizem, Dilacor, Tiazac*) • Estrogens • Propranolol (*Inderal*) • Tamoxifen (*Nolvadex*) • Thyroid Hormone
Gymnema	Antidiabetes Drugs • Insulin
Hawaiian Baby Woodrose	Antidepressant Drugs • Clozapine (*Clozaril*) • Cyproheptadine (*Periactin*) • Dextromethorphan (*Robitussin DM*, and others) • Meperidine (*Demerol*) • Monoamine Oxidase Inhibitors (MAOIs) • Pentazocine (*Talwin*) • Risperidone (*Risperdal*) • Tramadol (*Ultram*)
Hawthorn	Beta-Blockers • Calcium Channel Blockers • Digoxin (*Lanoxin*) • Nitrates • Phosphodieterase-5 Inhibitors
Hedge Mustard	Digoxin (*Lanoxin*) • Diuretic Drugs • Macrolide Antibiotics • Quinine • Stimulant Laxatives • Tetracycline Antibiotics
Hemp Agrimony	Cytochrome P450 3A4 (CYP3A4) Inducers
Henbane	Anticholinergic Drugs
Hibiscus	Acetaminophen (*Tylenol*, others)
Holy Basil	Anticoagulant/Antiplatelet Drugs • Pentobarbitone
Honeysuckle	Anticoagulant/Antiplatelet Drugs
Hops	Alcohol (Ethanol) • CNS Depressants
Horse Chestnut	Anticoagulant/Antiplatelet Drugs • Antidiabetes Drugs
Horseradish	Levothyroxine (*Synthroid*, *Levothroid*, *Levoxyl*, others)
Horsetail	Corticosteroids • Digoxin (*Lanoxin*) • Diuretic Drugs
Hound's Tongue	Cytochrome P450 3A4 (CYP3A4) Inducers
Hu Zhang	Estrogens
Huperzine A	Acetylcholinesterase (AChE) Inhibitors • Anticholinergic Drugs • Cholinergic Drugs
Hydrazine Sulfate	Antidiabetes Drugs • CNS Depressants • Isoniazid (INH) • Monoamine Oxidase Inhibitors (MAOIs)
Iboga	Anticholinergic Drugs • Cholinergic Drugs
Iceland Moss	Oral Drugs
Indian Long Pepper	Phenytoin (*Dilantin*) • Propranolol (*Inderal*) • Theophylline (*Theo-Dur*)
Indian Snakeroot	Alcohol (Ethanol) • Antipsychotic Drugs • Barbiturates • Digoxin (*Lanoxin*) • Diuretic Drugs • Ephedrine (*Pretz-D*) • Levodopa • Monoamine Oxidase Inhibitors (MAOIs) • Propranolol (*Inderal*) • Stimulant Drugs • Tricyclic Antidepressants (TCAs)
Indole-3-Carbinol	Cytochrome P450 1A2 (CYP1A2) Substrates
Inositol Nicotinate	Anticoagulant/Antiplatelet Drugs • Antidiabetes Drugs • HMG-CoA Reductase Inhibitors ("Statins") • Nicotine (*Nicoderm, Nicotrol*)
Iodine	ACE Inhibitors (ACEIs) • Amiodarone (*Cordarone*) • Angiotensin Receptor Blockers (ARBs) • Antithyroid Drugs • Lithium (*Eskalith, Lithobid*) • Potassium-Sparing Diuretics
IP-6	Anticoagulant/Antiplatelet Drugs
Ipecac	Activated Charcoal
Ipriflavone	Cytochrome P450 1A2 (CYP1A2) Substrates • Cytochrome P450 2C9 (CYP2C9) Substrates • Immunosuppressants • Theophylline

CHARTS

Potential Interactions: Natural Medicine/Drug

For additional data, refer to the database.

Natural Medicine	Drug
Iron	Bisphosphonates • Chloramphenicol • Levodopa • Levothyroxine (*Levothroid*, *Levoxyl*, *Synthroid*, and others) • Methyldopa (*Aldomet*) • Mycophenolate Mofetil (*CellCept*) • Penicillamine • Quinolone Antibiotics • Tetracycline Antibiotics
Ivy Gourd	Antidiabetes Drugs
Jalap	Digoxin (*Lanoxin*) • Diuretic Drugs • Oral Drugs • Stimulant Laxatives
Jamaican Dogwood	CNS Depressants
Jiaogulan	Anticoagulant/Antiplatelet Drugs • Immunosuppressants
Jimson Weed	Anticholinergic Drugs
Juniper	Antidiabetes Drugs • Diuretic Drugs
Kaolin	Clindamycin (*Cleocin*) • Digoxin (*Lanoxin*) • Quinidine (*Quinidex*) • Trimethoprim (*Proloprim*)
Karaya Gum	Oral Drugs
Kava	Alprazolam (*Xanax*) • CNS Depressants • Cytochrome P450 1A2 (CYP1A2) Substrates • Cytochrome P450 2C19 (CYP2C19) Substrates • Cytochrome P450 2C9 (CYP2C9) Substrates • Cytochrome P450 2D6 (CYP2D6) Substrates • Cytochrome P450 3A4 (CYP3A4) Substrates • Hepatotoxic Drugs • Levodopa
Kefir	Immunosuppressants
Khella	Digoxin (*Lanoxin*) • Hepatotoxic Drugs • Photosensitizing Drugs
Kombucha Tea	Disulfiram (*Antabuse*)
Kudzu	Anticoagulant/Antiplatelet Drugs • Antidiabetes Drugs • Contraceptive Drugs • Estrogens • Methotrexate (*Rheumatrex*) • Tamoxifen (*Nolvadex*)
Lactobacillus	Antibiotic Drugs • Immunosuppressants
Laminaria	ACE Inhibitors (ACEIs) • Digoxin (*Lanoxin*) • Potassium-Sparing Diuretics • Thyroid Hormone
Larch Arabinogalactan	Immunosuppressants • Oral Drugs
L-Arginine	Antihypertensive Drugs • Nitrates • Sildenafil (*Viagra*)
Lavender	Barbiturates • Chloral Hydrate • CNS Depressants
L-Carnitine	Acenocoumarol (*Sintrom*) • Warfarin (*Coumadin*) • Zidovudine (AZT, *Retrovir*)
Lemon Balm	CNS Depressants
Licorice	Antihypertensive Drugs • Corticosteroids • Cytochrome P450 2B6 (CYP2B6) Substrates • Cytochrome P450 3A4 (CYP3A4) Substrates • Digoxin (*Lanoxin*) • Diuretic Drugs • Estrogens • Ethacrynic Acid (*Edecrin*) • Furosemide (*Lasix*)
Lily-of-the-Valley	Calcium Supplements • Corticosteroids • Digoxin (*Lanoxin*) • Diuretic Drugs • Macrolide Antibiotics • Quinine • Stimulant Laxatives • Tetracycline Antibiotics
Lime	Cytochrome P450 3A4 (CYP3A4) Substrates • Photosensitizing Drugs
Limonene	Cytochrome P450 2C19 (CYP2C19) Inducers • Cytochrome P450 2C19 (CYP2C19) Inhibitors • Cytochrome P450 2C9 (CYP2C9) Inducers • Cytochrome P450 2C9 (CYP2C9) Inhibitors • Cytochrome P450 2C9 (CYP2C9) Substrates
Lithium	ACE Inhibitors (ACEIs) • Anticonvulsants • Antidepressant Drugs • Calcium Channel Blockers • Dextromethorphan (*Robitussin DM*, others) • Loop Diuretics • Meperidine (*Demerol*) • Methyldopa (*Aldomet*) • Methylxanthines • Monoamine Oxidase Inhibitors (MAOIs) • Nonsteroidal Anti-Inflammatory Drugs (NSAIDs) • Pentazocine (*Talwin*) • Phenothiazines • Skeletal Muscle Relaxants • Thiazide Diuretics • Tramadol (*Ultram*)
Lovage	Diuretic Drugs
L-Tryptophan	Antidepressant Drugs • Benzodiazepines • CNS Depressants • Dextromethorphan (*Robitussin DM*, others) • Meperidine (*Demerol*) • Monoamine Oxidase Inhibitors (MAOIs) • Pentazocine (*Talwin*) • Phenothiazines • Tramadol (*Ultram*)
Lycium	Antidiabetes Drugs • Antihypertensive Drugs • Cytochrome P450 2C9 (CYP2C9) Substrates • Warfarin (*Coumadin*)

CHARTS

Potential Interactions: Natural Medicine/Drug For additional data, refer to the database.

Natural Medicine	Drug
Lysine	Calcium Supplements
Madagascar Periwinkle	Antidiabetes Drugs
Magnesium	Aminoglycoside Antibiotics • Bisphosphonates • Calcium Channel Blockers • Potassium-Sparing Diuretics • Quinolone Antibiotics • Skeletal Muscle Relaxants • Tetracycline Antibiotics
Magnolia	Alcohol (Ethanol) • Barbiturates • Benzodiazepines • CNS Depressants
Maitake Mushroom	Antidiabetes Drugs
Manganese	Quinolone Antibiotics • Tetracycline Antibiotics
Manna	Digoxin (*Lanoxin*) • Diuretic Drugs
Marijuana	Barbiturates • CNS Depressants • Disulfiram (*Antabuse*) • Fluoxetine (*Prozac*) • Theophylline (*Theo-Dur*, *Slo-Bid*)
Marsh Tea	CNS Depressants
Marshmallow	Antidiabetes Drugs • Oral Drugs
Masterwort	Photosensitizing Drugs
Mate	Adenosine (*Adenocard*) • Alcohol (Ethanol) • Amphetamines • Anticoagulant/ Antiplatelet Drugs • Antidiabetes Drugs • Cimetidine (*Tagamet*) • Clozapine (*Clozaril*) • Cocaine • Contraceptive Drugs • Dipyridamole (*Persantine*) • Disulfiram (*Antabuse*) • Ephedrine (*Pretz-D*) • Estrogens • Fluconazole (*Diflucan*) • Fluvoxamine (*Luvox*) • Lithium (*Eskalith*) • Mexiletine (*Mexitil*) • Monoamine Oxidase Inhibitors (MAOIs) • Nicotine (*Habitrol, Nicoderm, Nicorette, Prestep*) • Phenylpropanolamine (*Propagest, Rhindicon*) • Quinolone Antibiotics • Riluzole (*Rilutek*) • Terbinafine (*Lamisil*) • Theophylline (*Theo-Dur*) • Verapamil (*Calan*, *Covera*, *Isoptin*, *Verelan*)
Meadowsweet	Aspirin • Choline Magnesium Trisalicylate (*Trilisate*) • Narcotic Drugs • Salsalate (*Disalcid*)
Melatonin	Anticoagulant/Antiplatelet Drugs • Antidiabetes Drugs • Benzodiazepines • Caffeine (*NoDoz, Stay Alert, Vivarin*) • CNS Depressants • Contraceptive Drugs • Flumazenil (*Romazicon*) • Fluvoxamine (*Luvox*) • Immunosuppressants • Nifedipine GITS (*Procardia* XL) • Verapamil (*Calan*, *Covera*, *Isoptin*, *Verelan*)
Mesoglycan	Anticoagulant/Antiplatelet Drugs • Thrombolytic Drugs
Methoxylated Flavones	Cytochrome P450 1A2 (CYP1A2) Substrates
Mexican Scammony Root	Digoxin (*Lanoxin*) • Diuretic Drugs • Oral Drugs • Stimulant Laxatives
Milk Thistle	Cytochrome P450 2C9 (CYP2C9) Substrates • Cytochrome P450 3A4 (CYP3A4) Substrates • Estrogens • Glucuronidated Drugs • Indinavir (*Crixivan*)
Morinda	ACE Inhibitors (ACEIs) • Angiotensin Receptor Blockers (ARBs) • Potassium-Sparing Diuretics
Mormon Tea	Oral Drugs
Motherwort	CNS Depressants
Myrrh	Antidiabetes Drugs
N-Acetyl Cysteine	Activated Charcoal • Nitroglycerin (*Minitran, Nitrek, Nitrostat*)
N-Acetyl Glucosamine	Antidiabetes Drugs • Chemotherapy • Warfarin (*Coumadin*)
Nattokinase	Anticoagulant/Antiplatelet Drugs
Neem	Antidiabetes Drugs • Immunosuppressants
Niacin and Niacinamide (Vitamin B3)	Antidiabetes Drugs • HMG-CoA Reductase Inhibitors ("Statins") • Nicotine (*Nicoderm, Nicotrol*)
Northern Prickly Ash	Antacids • H2-Blockers • Proton Pump Inhibitors (PPIs)
Nutmeg and Mace	Cytochrome P450 1A1 (CYP1A1) Substrates • Cytochrome P450 1A2 (CYP1A2) Substrates • Cytochrome P450 2B1 (CYP2B1) Substrates • Cytochrome P450 2B2 (CYP2B2) Substrates • Phenobarbital (*Luminal*)
Oats	Morphine (*Kadian, MS Contin, MSIR, Oramorph, Roxanol*)

CHARTS

Potential Interactions: Natural Medicine/Drug

For additional data, refer to the database.

Natural Medicine	Drug
Octacosanol	Levodopa/Carbidopa (*Sinemet*)
Oleander	Calcium Supplements • Digoxin (*Lanoxin*) • Diuretic Drugs • Macrolide Antibiotics • Quinine • Stimulant Laxatives • Tetracycline Antibiotics
Olive	Antidiabetes Drugs • Antihypertensive Drugs
Onion	Anticoagulant/Antiplatelet Drugs • Antidiabetes Drugs • Aspirin
Oolong Tea	Adenosine (*Adenocard*) • Alcohol (Ethanol) • Amphetamines • Anticoagulant/ Antiplatelet Drugs • Antidiabetes Drugs • Cimetidine (*Tagamet*) • Clozapine (*Clozaril*) • Cocaine • Contraceptive Drugs • Dipyridamole (*Persantine*) • Disulfiram (*Antabuse*) • Ephedrine (*Pretz-D*) • Estrogens • Fluconazole (*Diflucan*) • Fluvoxamine (*Luvox*) • Lithium (*Eskalith, Lithobid*) • Mexiletine (*Mexitil*) • Monoamine Oxidase Inhibitors (MAOIs) • Nicotine (*Habitrol, Nicoderm, Nicorette, Prestep*) • Phenylpropanolamine (*Propagest, Rhindicon*) • Quinolone Antibiotics • Riluzole (*Rilutek*) • Terbinafine (*Lamisil*) • Theophylline (*Theo-Dur*) • Verapamil (*Calan, Covera, Isoptin, Verelan*)
Pancreatin	Acarbose (*Precose, Prandase*)
Pangamic Acid	Calcium Channel Blockers • Digoxin (*Lanoxin*) • Thiazide Diuretics
Pantethine	Anticoagulant/Antiplatelet Drugs
Papaya	Warfarin (*Coumadin*)
Para-Aminobenzoic Acid (PABA)	Cortisone (*Cortisone Acetate*) • Dapsone (*Avlosulfon*) • Sulfonamide Antibiotics
Parsley	Aspirin • Diuretic Drugs • Warfarin (*Coumadin*)
Passionflower	Barbiturates • CNS Depressants
Pau d'Arco	Anticoagulant/Antiplatelet Drugs
Pectin	Digoxin (*Lanoxin*) • Lovastatin (*Mevacor*) • Tetracycline Antibiotics
Peony	Phenytoin (*Dilantin*)
Peppermint Oil	Antacids • Cyclosporine (*Neoral, Sandimmune*) • Cytochrome P450 1A2 (CYP1A2) Substrates • Cytochrome P450 2C19 (CYP2C19) Substrates • Cytochrome P450 2C9 (CYP2C9) Substrates • Cytochrome P450 3A4 (CYP3A4) Substrates • H2 Blockers • Proton Pump Inhibitors (PPIs)
Periwinkle	Antihypertensive Drugs
Peyote	Stimulant Drugs
Pheasant's Eye	Calcium Supplements • Corticosteroids • Digoxin (*Lanoxin*) • Diuretic Drugs • Quinidine (*Quinidex*) • Stimulant Laxatives
Phenylalanine	Antipsychotic Drugs • Levodopa • Monoamine Oxidase Inihbitors (MAOIs)
Phosphate Salts	Antacids • Cholestyramine (*Questran*) • Colestipol (*Colestid*)
Picrorhiza	Immunosuppressants
Pinus Bark	Oral Drugs
Pleurisy Root	Digoxin (*Lanoxin*) • Diuretic Drugs • Estrogens
Policosanol	Anticoagulant/Antiplatelet Drugs
Pomegranate	ACE Inhibitors (ACEIs) • Antihypertensive Drugs • Oral Drugs
Potassium	ACE Inhibitors (ACEIs) • Angiotensin Receptor Blockers (ARBs) • Potassium-Sparing Diuretics
Potato	Thrombolytic Drugs
Pregnenolone	Estrogens • Progestin • Testosterone
Prickly Pear Cactus	Chlorpropamide (*Diabinese*)
Procaine	Aminosalicylic Acid (*Paser, Teebacin, Tubasal*) • Digoxin (*Lanoxin*) • Skeletal Muscle Relaxants • Succinylcholine • Sulfonamide Antibiotics
Progesterone	Estrogens
Propionyl-L-Carnitine	Acenocoumarol (*Sintrom*) • Warfarin (*Coumadin*) • Zidovudine (AZT, *Retrovir*)

Potential Interactions: Natural Medicine/Drug For additional data, refer to the database.	
Natural Medicine	**Drug**
Puncture Vine	Antidiabetes Drugs
Pycnogenol	Immunosuppressants
Pyridoxine (Vitamin B6)	Amiodarone (*Cordarone*) • Levodopa • Phenobarbital (*Luminal*) • Phenytoin (*Dilantin*)
Quassia	Antacids • Digoxin (*Lanoxin*) • Diuretic Drugs • H2-Blockers • Proton Pump Inhibitors (PPIs)
Quercetin	Quinolone Antibiotics
Quillaia	Metformin (*Glucophage*) • Oral Drugs
Quince	Oral Drugs
Raspberry Leaf	Metformin (*Glucophage*) • Oral Drugs
Red Clover	Anticoagulant/Antiplatelet Drugs • Contraceptive Drugs • Cytochrome P450 1A2 (CYP1A2) Substrates • Cytochrome P450 2C19 (CYP2C19) Substrates • Cytochrome P450 2C9 (CYP2C9) Substrates • Cytochrome P450 3A4 (CYP3A4) Substrates • Estrogens • Tamoxifen (*Nolvadex*)
Red Yeast	Alcohol (Ethanol) • Cyclosporine (*Neoral*, *Sandimmune*) • Cytochrome P450 3A4 (CYP3A4) Inhibitors • Gemfibrozil (*Lopid*) • HMG-CoA Reductase Inhibitors ("Statins") • Levothyroxine (*Synthroid*, *Levothroid*, *Levoxyl*, and others) • Niacin (*Niacor, Niaspan, Nicobid, Slo-Niacin*)
Reishi Mushroom	Anticoagulant/Antiplatelet Drugs • Antihypertensive Drugs
Resveratrol	Anticoagulant/Antiplatelet Drugs • Cytochrome P450 3A4 (CYP3A4) Substrates
Rhatany	Oral Drugs
Rhubarb	Corticosteroids • Digoxin (*Lanoxin*) • Diuretic Drugs • Oral Drugs • Stimulant Laxatives
Riboflavin (Vitamin B2)	Anticholinergic Drugs • Phenobarbital (*Luminal*) • Probenecid (*Benemid*) • Psyllium • Tricyclic Antidepressants
Ribose	Alcohol (Ethanol) • Antidiabetes Drugs • Aspirin • Choline Magnesium Trisalicylate (*Trilisate*) • Insulin • Propranolol (*Inderal*) • Salsalate (*Disalcid*)
Rice Bran	Oral Drugs
Rose Hip	Aluminum • Aspirin • Choline Magnesium Trisalicylate (*Trilisate*) • Estrogens • Fluphenazine (*Prolixin*) • Salsalate (*Disalcid*) • Warfarin (*Coumadin*)
Rue	Photosensitizing Drugs
Saccharomyces Boulardii	Antifungals
Safflower	Anticoagulant/Antiplatelet Drugs
Sage	Anticonvulsants • Antidiabetes Drugs • CNS Depressants
SAMe	Antidepressant Drugs • Dextromethorphan (*Robitussin DM*, and others) • Levodopa • Meperidine (*Demerol*) • Monoamine Oxidase Inhibitors (MAOIs) • Pentazocine (*Talwin*) • Tramadol (*Ultram*)
Sarsaparilla	Digoxin (*Lanoxin*)
Sassafras	CNS Depressants
Saw Palmetto	Anticoagulant/Antiplatelet Drugs • Contraceptive Drugs • Estrogens
Scopolia	Anticholinergic Drugs • Quinidine (*Quinidex*) • Tricyclic Antidepressants (TCAs)
Scotch Broom	Haloperidol (*Haldol*) • Monoamine Oxidase Inhibitors (MAOIs) • Quinidine
Sea Buckthorn	Anticoagulant/Antiplatelet Drugs
Selenium	HMG-CoA Reductase Inhibitors ("Statins")
Senna	Digoxin (*Lanoxin*) • Diuretic Drugs
Shepherd's Purse	CNS Depressants • Thyroid Hormone
Slippery Elm	Oral Drugs
Smartweed	Warfarin (*Coumadin*)

CHARTS

Potential Interactions: Natural Medicine/Drug For additional data, refer to the database.

Natural Medicine	Drug
Solomon's Seal	Antidiabetes Drugs • Chlorpropamide (*Diabinese*) • Insulin
Sorrel	Oral Drugs
Southern Prickly Ash	Antacids • H2-Blockers • Proton Pump Inhibitors (PPIs)
Soy	Antibiotic Drugs • Estrogens • Tamoxifen (*Nolvadex*) • Warfarin (*Coumadin*)
Spinach	Antidiabetes Drugs • Warfarin (*Coumadin*)
Squill	Calcium Supplements • Corticosteroids • Digoxin (*Lanoxin*) • Diuretic Drugs • Quinidine (*Quinidex*) • Stimulant Laxatives
St. John's Wort	5-HT1 Agonists (Triptans) • Alprazolam (*Xanax*) • Aminolevulinic Acid • Amitriptyline (*Elavil*) • Antidepressant Drugs • Barbiturates • Clopidogrel (*Plavix*) • Contraceptive Drugs • Cyclosporine (*Neoral*, *Sandimmune*) • Cytochrome P450 1A2 (CYP1A2) Substrates • Cytochrome P450 2C9 (CYP2C9) Substrates • Cytochrome P450 3A4 (CYP3A4) Substrates • Dextromethorphan (*Robitussin DM*, and others) • Digoxin (*Lanoxin*) • Fenfluramine (*Pondimin*) • Fexofenadine (*Allegra*) • Imatinib (*Gleevec*) • Irinotecan (*Camptosar*) • Meperidine (*Demerol*) • Monoamine Oxidase Inhibitors (MAOIs) • Narcotic Drugs • Nefazodone (*Serzone*) • Non-Nucleoside Reverse Transcriptase Inhibitors (NNRTIs) • Nortriptyline (*Pamelor*) • P-Glycoprotein Substrates • Pentazocine (*Talwin*) • Paroxetine (*Paxil*) • Phenobarbital (*Luminal*) • Phenprocoumon • Phenytoin (*Dilantin*) • Photosensitizing Drugs • Protease Inhibitors (PIs) • Reserpine • Sertraline (*Zoloft*) • Simvastatin (*Zocor*) • Tacrolimus (*Prograf*, *Protopic*) • Theophylline (*Theo-Dur*) • Tramadol (*Ultram*) • Warfarin (*Coumadin*)
Stevia	Antidiabetes Drugs • Antihypertensive Drugs • Calcium Channel Blockers
Stinging Nettle	Antidiabetes Drugs • Antihypertensive Drugs • CNS Depressants • Warfarin (*Coumadin*)
Stone Root	Diuretic Drugs
Strophanthus	Calcium Supplements • Corticosteroids • Digoxin (*Lanoxin*) • Diuretic Drugs • Quinidine (*Quinidex*) • Quinine • Stimulant Laxatives
Sulforaphane	Cytochrome P450 1A2 (CYP1A2) Substrates
Swamp Milkweed	Digoxin (*Lanoxin*) • Diuretic Drugs • Macrolide Antibiotics • Quinine • Stimulant Laxatives • Tetracycline Antibiotics
Sweet Bay	CNS Depressants • Narcotic Drugs
Sweet Clover	Anticoagulant/Antiplatelet Drugs • Hepatotoxic Drugs
Sweet Orange	Celiprolol (*Celicard*) • Fexofenadine (*Allegra*) • Ivermectin (*Stromectol*)
Sweet Vernal Grass	Anticoagulant/Antiplatelet Drugs
Tamarind	Aspirin • Ibuprofen (*Advil*, *Motrin*, and others)
Tannic Acid	Oral Drugs
Tansy	Alcohol (Ethanol)
Tansy Ragwort	Cytochrome P450 3A4 (CYP3A4) Inducers
Theanine	Antihypertensive Drugs • Stimulant Drugs
Threonine	NMDA Antagonists
Thunder God Vine	Immunosuppressants
Thymus Extract	Immunosuppressants
Tiratricol	Anticoagulant/Antiplatelet Drugs • Antidiabetes Drugs • Cholestyramine (*Questran*) • Stimulant Drugs • Thyroid Hormone
Tragacanth	Oral Drugs
Turmeric	Anticoagulant/Antiplatelet Drugs
Tyrosine	Levodopa
Uzara	Digoxin (*Lanoxin*) • Diuretic Drugs • Macrolide Antibiotics • Quinine • Stimulant Laxatives • Tetracycline Antibiotics

CHARTS

Potential Interactions: Natural Medicine/Drug

For additional data, refer to the database.

Natural Medicine	Drug
Valerian	Alcohol (Ethanol) • Alprazolam (*Xanax*) • Benzodiazepines • CNS Depressants • Cytochrome P450 3A4 (CYP3A4) Substrates
Vanadium	Anticoagulant/Antiplatelet Drugs • Antidiabetes Drugs
Verbena	Antihypertensive Drugs
Vinpocetine	Anticoagulant/Antiplatelet Drugs • Warfarin (*Coumadin*)
Vitamin A	Hepatotoxic Drugs • Retinoids • Tetracycline Antibiotics • Warfarin (*Coumadin*)
Vitamin B12	Chloramphenicol
Vitamin C (Ascorbic Acid)	Acetaminophen (*Tylenol*, others) • Aluminum • Aspirin • Chemotherapy • Choline Magnesium Trisalicylate (*Trilisate*) • Estrogens • Fluphenazine (*Prolixin*) • HMG-CoA Reductase Inhibitors ("Statins") • Niacin (*Niacor, Niaspan, Nicobid, Slo-Niacin*) • Nicardipine (*Cardene*) • Nifedipine (*Adalat*, Procardia) • Protease Inhibitors (PIs) • Salsalate (*Disalcid*) • Warfarin (*Coumadin*)
Vitamin D	Aluminum • Calcipotriene (*Dovonex*) • Cimetidine (*Tagamet*) • Digoxin (*Lanoxin*) • Diltiazem (*Cardizem*, *Dilacor*, *Tiazac*) • Heparin • Low Molecular Weight Heparins (LMWHs) • Thiazide Diuretics • Verapamil (*Calan*, *Covera*, *Isoptin*, *Verelan*)
Vitamin E	Anticoagulant/Antiplatelet Drugs • Chemotherapy • Cyclosporine (*Neoral, Sandimmune*) • HMG-CoA Reductase Inhibitors ("Statins") • Niacin (*Niacor, Niaspan, Nicobid, Slo-Niacin*) • Warfarin (*Coumadin*)
Vitamin K	Warfarin (*Coumadin*)
Wahoo	Digoxin (*Lanoxin*) • Diuretic Drugs • Macrolide Antibiotics • Quinine • Stimulant Laxatives • Tetracycline Antibiotics
Wallflower	Calcium Supplements • Corticosteroids • Digoxin (*Lanoxin*) • Diuretic Drugs • Quinidine (*Quinidex*) • Quinine • Stimulant Laxatives
Water Avens	Metformin (*Glucophage*) • Oral Drugs
Watercress	Chlorzoxazone (*Parafon Forte*, *Paraflex*) • Warfarin (*Coumadin*)
Wheat Bran	Digoxin (*Lanoxin*)
Whey Protein	Alendronate (*Fosamax*) • Levodopa • Quinolone Antibiotics • Tetracycline Antibiotics
Wild Carrot	Antihypertensive Drugs • Estrogens • Photosensitizing Drugs
Wild Cherry	Cytochrome P450 3A4 (CYP3A4) Substrates
Wild Lettuce	CNS Depressants
Willow Bark	Anticoagulant/Antiplatelet Drugs • Aspirin • Choline Magnesium Trisalicylate (*Trilisate*) • Salsalate (*Disalcid*)
Wine	Aspirin • Barbiturates • Benzodiazepines • Cefamandole (*Mandol*) • Cefoperazone (*Cefobid*) • Chlorpropamide (*Diabinese*) • Cisapride (*Propulsid*) • CNS Depressants • Cyclosporine (*Neoral*, *Sandimmune*) • Disulfiram (*Antabuse*) • Erythromycin (*E.E.S., E-Mycin, PCE*) • Felodipine (*Plendil*) • Griseofulvin (*Fulvicin*) • H2-Blockers • Hepatotoxic Drugs • Metformin (*Glucophage*) • Metronidazole (*Flagyl*) • Monoamine Oxidase Inhibitors (MAOIs) • Narcotic Drugs • Nonsteroidal Anti-Inflammatory Drugs (NSAIDs) • Phenytoin (*Dilantin*) • Sulfonamide Antibiotics • Tolbutamide (*Orinase*) • Warfarin (*Coumadin*)
Wintergreen	Aspirin • Warfarin (*Coumadin*)
Wormwood	Anticonvulsants
Xanthan Gum	Antidiabetes Drugs
Yarrow	Antacids • Anticoagulant/Antiplatelet Drugs • Barbiturates • H2-Blockers • Proton Pump Inhibitors (PPIs)
Yellow Dock	Digoxin (*Lanoxin*) • Diuretic Drugs
Yerba Mansa	CNS Depressants

Potential Interactions: Natural Medicine/Drug	For additional data, refer to the database.
Natural Medicine	**Drug**
Yogurt	Ciprofloxacin (*Cipro*) • Immunosuppressants • Tetracycline Antibiotics
Yohimbe	Antihypertensive Drugs • Clonidine (*Catapres*) • Guanabenz (*Wytensin*) • Monoamine Oxidase Inhibitors (MAOIs) • Naloxone (*Narcan*) • Phenothiazines • Stimulant Drugs • Tricyclic Antidepressants (TCAs)
Zinc	Amiloride (*Midamor*) • Cisplatin (*Platinol-AQ*) • Penicillamine (*Curpimine*)• Potassium-Sparing Diuretics • Quinolone Antibiotics • Tetracycline Antibiotics • Thiazide Diuretics

CHARTS

Drug Influences on Nutrient Levels and Depletion

Some medications can affect the levels of certain nutrients in the body. There is considerable interest in using nutritional supplements to counteract these possible drug-induced "nutrient depletions." The chart below shows the current scientific understanding of these relationships, and suggested actions.

DRUGS (Includes some representative U.S. and Canadian Brand Names.	NUTRIENT DEPLETED	POSSIBLE MECHANISM	COMMENTS & REFERENCES
ANALGESICS/ANTI-INFLAMMATORIES			
Acetaminophen (*Tylenol*)	Glutathione	Acetaminophen depletes endogenous glutathione.	It's not known if glutathione supplements would be beneficial.[5394]
Aspirin, other salicylates	Folic Acid	Decreases protein binding and serum levels.	Folic acid appears to be redistributed rather than lost from the body. Red blood cell folate levels are normal. Supplements are not needed.[2677,9351,9360]
	Iron	Mucosal damage and GI bleeding, even if asymptomatic, can cause chronic blood loss.	Monitor for signs and symptoms of anemia. Encourage intake of iron-fortified foods since supplements may exacerbate GI irritation.[8888,9515,9576-7]
	Vitamin C	Increases urinary excretion.	Deficiency of vitamin C is unlikely. Only consider supplementation with long-term therapy and symptoms of deficiency.[10590-2,11526-7]
Nonsteroidal Anti-Inflammatory Drugs (NSAIDS): Diclofenac (*Voltaren*), Etodolac (*Lodine*), Fenoprofen (*Nalfon*), Flurbiprofen (*Ansaid*), Ibuprofen (*Advil*, *Motrin*, etc), Indomethacin (*Indocin*), Ketoprofen (*Orudis*, *Oruvail*), Ketorolac (*Toradol*), Meclofenamate, Mefenamic Acid (*Ponstel*), Meloxicam (*Mobic*), Nabumetone (*Relafen*), Naproxen (*Anaprox*, *Naprosyn*, *Naprelan*), Oxaprozin (*Daypro*), Piroxicam (*Feldene*), Sulindac (*Clinoril*), Tolmetin (*Tolectin*)	Iron	Mucosal damage and GI bleeding, even if asymptomatic, can cause chronic blood loss.	Monitor for signs and symptoms of anemia. Encourage intake of iron-rich foods since supplements may exacerbate GI irritation.[8888,9515,9576-7]
ANTI-INFECTIVES			
ANTIBIOTICS			
Antibiotics - General: Cephalosporins, Fluoroquinolones, Isoniazid, Macrolides, Penicillins, Sulfonamides, Tetracyclines, Trimethoprim/Sulfamethoxazole	Dibencozide Niacin and Niacinamide Pantothenic Acid (B5) Pyridoxine (B6) Riboflavin (B2) Thiamine (B1) Vitamin B12 Vitamin K	Destruction of normal intestinal microflora may lead to decreased production of various B vitamins and vitamin K. Some cephalosporins interfere directly with vitamin K-dependent clotting factor production.	The intestinal microflora is reduced by antibiotics. However, the B vitamins are mainly obtained from the diet, and any changes in their production by intestinal bacteria is unlikely to be clinically significant.[4434-43,6243,9502,9530] Reduction in vitamin K-dependent clotting factor production may be significant in people with other risk factors for low vitamin K levels. Monitor these patients closely.[4437,4439,7135,9502,11513-6]

CHARTS

Drug Influences on Nutrient Levels and Depletion

Some medications can affect the levels of certain nutrients in the body. There is considerable interest in using nutritional supplements to counteract these possible drug-induced "nutrient depletions." The chart below shows the current scientific understanding of these relationships, and suggested actions.

DRUGS (Includes some representative U.S. and Canadian Brand Names.)	NUTRIENT DEPLETED	POSSIBLE MECHANISM	COMMENTS & REFERENCES
ANTI-INFECTIVES (CONT.)			
ANTIBIOTICS (CONT.)			
Antibiotics - General: Cephalosporins, Fluoroquinolones, Isoniazid, Macrolides, Penicillins, Sulfonamides, Tetracyclines, Trimethoprim/Sulfamethoxazole (Continued from previous page.)	Folic Acid	Disruption of normal intestinal microflora decreases enterohepatic circulation and reabsorption of folic acid, and may reduce synthesis. Trimethoprim inhibits conversion of folic acid to its active form.	Folic acid synthesized by intestinal microflora probably doesn't contribute significantly to overall folate status, and supplements aren't necessary with normal courses of antibiotics.[2677,4436-7,6243] Prolonged courses of high-dose trimethoprim rarely cause megaloblastic anemia, and folic acid supplements have been used to prevent this. However, some evidence suggests folic acid supplements can reduce the efficacy of trimethoprim. Avoid supplements unless recommended by a physician.[2677,4468,4531,9382-7,9398-9]
Aminoglycosides: Amikacin (*Amikin*) Gentamicin (*Garamycin*) Kanamycin (*Kantrex*) Netilmicin (*Netromycin*) Streptomycin Tobramycin (*Nebcin*)	Magnesium Potassium	Increased urinary excretion, associated with drug-induced renal damage.	Monitor patients for electrolyte disturbances and declining renal funciton. Give intravenous electrolyte replacement if necessary.[9519]
Fluoroquinolones: Ciprofloxacin (*Cipro*), Enoxacin (*Penetrex*), Gatifloxacin (*Tequin*), Levofloxacin (*Levaquin*), Lomefloxacin (*Maxaquin*), Moxifloxacin (*Avelox*), Norfloxacin (*Noroxin*), Ofloxacin (*Floxin*), Sparfloxacin (*Zagam*), Trovafloxacin (*Trovan*)	Calcium Iron Magnesium Zinc	Formation of insoluble complexes (prevents absorption of both nutrient and fluoroquinolone).	Significant effects on levels of these nutrients are unlikely when fluoroquinolones are taken at least 2 hours before, or 4-6 hours after calcium/iron/magnesium/zinc-containing foods or supplements.[828,2682,3046,4412,4531]
Cefditoren Pivoxil (*Spectracef*)	L-Carnitine Acetyl-L-Carnitine Propionyl-L-Carnitine	Chronic use of cefditoren can induce carnitine deficiency.	Long-term use of cefditoren might require supplementation, but short-term use does not seem to have a clinically significant effect on carnitine levels.[12759]
Neomycin (*Mycifradin*)	Beta-Carotene Dibencozide Vitamin A Vitamin B12	Reduced absorption.	Not clinically significant with short-term use of neomycin.[3046,5916,8434,10565-6]
Pivampicillin (*Pondocillin*)	L-Carnitine Acetyl-L-Carnitine Propionyl-L-Carnitine	Chronic use of pivampicillin can induce carnitine deficiency.	Long-term use of pivampicillin might require supplementation, but short-term use does not seem to have a clinically significant effect on carnitine levels.[12759]

Drug Influences on Nutrient Levels and Depletion

Some medications can affect the levels of certain nutrients in the body. There is considerable interest in using nutritional supplements to counteract these possible drug-induced "nutrient depletions." The chart below shows the current scientific understanding of these relationships, and suggested actions.

DRUGS (Includes some representative U.S. and Canadian Brand Names.)	NUTRIENT DEPLETED	POSSIBLE MECHANISM	COMMENTS & REFERENCES
ANTI-INFECTIVES (CONT.)			
ANTIBIOTICS (CONT.)			
Penicillins (sodium-containing): Carbenicillin (*Geocillin*), Mezlocillin (*Mezlin*), Penicillin G sodium (*Pfizerpen*), Piperacillin (*Pipracil*), Ticarcillin (*Ticar*)	Potassium	Large sodium load is presented to the kidneys, resulting in sodium reabsorption and potassium excretion.	Monitor potassium levels, and give supplements or switch to a different antibiotic if necessary.[9519]
Tetracyclines: Tetracycline (*Achromycin V, Panmycin, Robitet, Robicaps, Sumycin, Teline, Tetracap, Tetracyn, Tetralan*), Demeclocycline (*Declomycin*), Doxycycline (*Bio-Tab, Doryx, Doxy Caps, Doxychel, Doxychel Hyclate, Monodox, Periostat, Vibra-Tabs, Vibramycin*), Minocycline (*Dynacin, Vectrin*), Oxytetracycline (*Terramycin, Uri-Tet*)	Calcium Iron Magnesium Zinc	Formation of insoluble complexes prevents absorption of both nutrient and tetracycline. Doxycycline does not reduce zinc absorption.	Significant effects on levels of these nutrients are unlikely when tetracyclines are taken at least 2 hours before, or 4-6 hours after calcium/iron/magnesium/zinc-containing foods or supplements.[4412,4531,4549-50,4945]
	Potassium	Increased renal excretion associated with nephropathy.	Due to a toxic degradation product in outdated tetracyclines. Avoid outdated drugs.[4425]
ANTIFUNGALS			
Amphotericin B (*Abelcet, AmBisome, Amphocin, Amphotec, Fungizone*)	Magnesium Potassium	Increased urinary excretion, associated with drug-induced renal damage.	Monitor patients for electrolyte disturbances and declining renal function. Give intravenous electrolyte replacement if necessary.[9519]
Fluconazole (*Diflucan*)	Potassium	Increased urinary excretion, associated with drug-induced renal damage.	Monitor potassium levels and renal function in people on prolonged fluconazole therapy, and in those with other risk factors for hypokalemia.[9519]
ANTIMALARIALS			
Pyrimethamine (*Daraprim*)	Folic Acid	Folate antagonism. Binds to dihydrofolate reductase, preventing conversion of folic acid to its active form.	At lower pyrimethamine doses, the need for supplementation has not been adequately studied. Advise patients to maintain good dietary folate intake. People receiving larger pyrimethamine doses (those required to treat toxoplasmosis), should receive folinic acid (leucovorin) to prevent megaloblastic anemia. Avoid folic acid (antagonizes therapeutic effects of pyrimethamine).[4425,4532,9380]
Quinacrine	Riboflavin (B2)	Can interfere with conversion to the active form flavin adenine dinubleotide (FAD).	May cause riboflavin deficiency. Clinical significance is not known.[505,10521-2]

CHARTS

Drug Influences on Nutrient Levels and Depletion

Some medications can affect the levels of certain nutrients in the body. There is considerable interest in using nutritional supplements to counteract these possible drug-induced "nutrient depletions." The chart below shows the current scientific understanding of these relationships, and suggested actions.

DRUGS (Includes some representative U.S. and Canadian Brand Names.	NUTRIENT DEPLETED	POSSIBLE MECHANISM	COMMENTS & REFERENCES
ANTI-INFECTIVES (CONT.)			
ANTIPROTAZOALS			
Pentamidine (*NebuPent, Pentacarinat, Pentam 300*)	Folic Acid	Weak folate antagonist, preventing conversion of folic acid to its active form.	Rare cases of megaloblastic anemia, but only with prolonged parenteral therapy. Folic acid supplements are usually not necessary.[9378]
	Magnesium	Increased urinary excretion, associated with drug-induced renal damage.	Monitor serum magnesium levels and give oral or intravenous supplements as needed.[8872,9618-9]
ANTIRETROVIRALS			
Zidovudine (AZT, *Combivir, Retrovir*)	Copper Dibencozide Vitamin B12	Some HIV patients taking zidovudine have subnormal copper and vitamin B12 levels. Mechanism unknown.	Preliminary evidence suggests lower copper levels are not harmful and supplements shouldn't be used.[4986,8970] Preliminary data suggests vitamin B12 supplements aren't helpful.[10531-3]
ANTITUBERCULOSIS AGENTS			
Aminosalicylic Acid (Para-aminosalicylic Acid, *Paser*)	Folic Acid	Inhibits absorption in the gastrointestinal tract.	May worsen the folic acid deficiency associated with tuberculosis. Recommend supplements if diet is folate-deficient.[4459,8441,9363,9388,9395-7]
	Iron	Reduced gastrointestinal absorption.	Monitor for signs and symptoms of iron deficiency and give supplements if needed.[9574]
	Dibencozide Vitamin B12	Reduced gastrointestinal absorption.	Monitor vitamin B12 levels if treatment lasts more than one month.[4558,9395,9397,9574]
Cycloserine (*Seromycin*)	Folic Acid	Possibly reduces absorption or increases metabolism.	Rare cases of megaloblastic anemia reported, but usually with other factors contributing to folate deficiency. Recommend supplements only if dietary intake is deficient.[4531,4536,9363]
Ethambutol (*Myambutol*)	Copper	Ethambutol and its metabolite chelate copper in the gastrointestinal tract and decrease copper absorption.	It is not known if copper supplementation is beneficial.[4535,8971]
Isoniazid (INH, *Laniazid*)	Pyridoxine (B6)	Interferes with pyridoxine metabolism.	Patients receiving > 10 mg/kg/day of INH should be supplemented with 50 - 100 mg of pyridoxine per day.[4481-2]
	Niacin and Niacinamide	Isoniazid inhibits the conversion of tryptophan to niacin.	Might induce pellagra, particularly in poorly nourished patients.[4865-6]

CHARTS

Drug Influences on Nutrient Levels and Depletion

Some medications can affect the levels of certain nutrients in the body. There is considerable interest in using nutritional supplements to counteract these possible drug-induced "nutrient depletions." The chart below shows the current scientific understanding of these relationships, and suggested actions.

DRUGS (Includes some representative U.S. and Canadian Brand Names.	NUTRIENT DEPLETED	POSSIBLE MECHANISM	COMMENTS & REFERENCES
ANTI-INFECTIVES (CONT.)			
ANTITUBERCULOSIS AGENTS (CONT.)			
Rifampin (*Rifadin, Rimactane, Rofact)*	Vitamin D	Increased vitamin D metabolism.	There is no consensus that vitamin D supplementation is always required. Give supplements of vitamin D only if clinical judgment warrants it.[11561-5]
	Vitamin K	Possibly decreased gastrointestinal absorption, destruction of vitamin K-producing bacteria, and interference with regeneration of vitamin K from inactive metabolite.	Consider supplements in people with other risk factors for vitamin K deficiency.[11517-8]
ANTIVIRALS			
Foscarnet (*Foscavir*)	Magnesium	Chelation and increased excretion.	Monitor magnesium levels and give supplements as necessary.[8869,9617]
ANTI-CANCER DRUGS			
Aldesleukin (Interleukin-2, IL-2, *Proleukin*)	Magnesium	Intracellular shift of magnesium.	Supplements usually not needed - serum magnesium levels normalize after course complete.[8874]
Amifostine (*Ethyol*)	Magnesium	Increased urinary excretion.	This is usually only a transient effect, with levels returning to baseline in 24 hours.[9625]
Busulfan	Vitamin E	High doses of chemotherapy seems to reduce levels of vitamin E.	The clinical significance is unknown. It's not known if supplementation with vitamin E is beneficial.[98,10366,11588,11589]
Cisplatin (*Platinol-AQ*), Carboplatin (*Paraplatin*)	Magnesium	Increased urinary excretion probably associated with drug-induced renal damage.	Hypomagnesemia worsens with repeated courses of treatment, and is more severe with cisplatin. Monitor magnesium levels and give supplements as necessary.[9626]
	Vitamin E	High doses of chemotherapy seems to reduce levels of vitamin E.	The clinical significance is unknown. It's not known if supplementation with vitamin E is beneficial.[98,10366,11588,11589]
Cyclophosphamide (*Cytoxan, Neosar*)	Vitamin E	High doses of chemotherapy seems to reduce levels of vitamin E.	The clinical significance is unknown. It's not known if supplementation with vitamin E is beneficial.[98,10366,11588,11589]
Cytosine Arabinoside (*Cytosar-U*)	Vitamin E	High doses of chemotherapy seems to reduce levels of vitamin E.	The clinical significance is unknown. It's not known if supplementation with vitamin E is beneficial.[98,10366,11588,11589]
Doxorubicin (*Adriamycin, Rubex, Doxil*)	Riboflavin (B2)	Formation of inactive complexes, interference with binding and conversion to active form, increased renal excretion.	This might contribute to doxorubicin toxicity, but it isn't known if riboflavin supplements are helpful.[9533,10528-30]
	Vitamin E	High doses of chemotherapy seems to reduce levels of vitamin E.	The clinical significance is unknown. It's not known if supplementation with vitamin E is beneficial.[98,10366,11588,11589]

CHARTS

Drug Influences on Nutrient Levels and Depletion

Some medications can affect the levels of certain nutrients in the body. There is considerable interest in using nutritional supplements to counteract these possible drug-induced "nutrient depletions." The chart below shows the current scientific understanding of these relationships, and suggested actions.

DRUGS (Includes some representative U.S. and Canadian Brand Names.)	NUTRIENT DEPLETED	POSSIBLE MECHANISM	COMMENTS & REFERENCES
ANTI-CANCER DRUGS (CONT.)			
Etoposide (*Etopophos, VePesid, Toposar*)	Vitamin E	High doses of chemotherapy seems to reduce levels of vitamin E.	The clinical significance is unknown. It's not known if supplementation with vitamin E is beneficial.[98,10366,11588,11589]
Fluorouracil (5-FU, *Adrucil*)	Thiamine (B1)	Interference with activation, increased breakdown.	There isn't sufficient data to recommend routine use of supplements.[10522-4]
	Vitamin E	High doses of chemotherapy seems to reduce levels of vitamin E.	The clinical significance is unknown. It's not known if supplementation with vitamin E is beneficial.[98,10366,11588,11589]
Methotrexate (*Rheumatrex*)	Vitamin E	High doses of chemotherapy seems to reduce levels of vitamin E.	The clinical significance is unknown. It's not known if supplementation with vitamin E is beneficial.[98,10366,11588,11589]
Thiotepa (*Thioplex*)	Vitamin E	High doses of chemotherapy seems to reduce levels of vitamin E.	The clinical significance is unknown. It's not known if supplementation with vitamin E is beneficial.[98,10366,11588,11589]
ANTI-DIABETES AGENTS			
Metformin (*Glucophage*)	Dibencozide Folic Acid Vitamin B12	Causes malabsorption of dietary vitamin B12 and possibly folic acid.	The *Glucophage* package insert recommends obtaining hematological parameters annually and obtaining B12 levels at 2-3 year intervals in patients at increased risk for B12 deficiency. Symptomatic folic acid deficiency is unlikely.[9366-8] Give supplements only if clinical judgment warrants it.[32,4490-1,7839,7841,8834,9520-3]
	Thiamine (B1)	Might reduce thiamine activity.	Theoretically, reducing thiamine activity could result in more pyruvate entering the Kreb's cycle and being converted to lactic acid. This might be associated with metformin-related lactic acidosis. But this has not be substantiated.[9536,11466]
ANTIGOUT/ANTIRHEUMATIC			
Colchicine	Beta-Carotene	Reduced absorption	Colchicine 1-2 mg/day doesn't affect beta-carotene serum levels, but higher doses may. Give supplements only if clinical judgement warrants it.[4543,5921]
	Dibencozide Vitamin B12	Decreases intestinal absorption of vitamin B12.	There is limited evidence that people on colchicine may have reduced levels of vitamin B12. Give supplements only if clinical judgment warrants it.[4543-5,5921]

CHARTS

Drug Influences on Nutrient Levels and Depletion

Some medications can affect the levels of certain nutrients in the body. There is considerable interest in using nutritional supplements to counteract these possible drug-induced "nutrient depletions." The chart below shows the current scientific understanding of these relationships, and suggested actions.

DRUGS (Includes some representative U.S. and Canadian Brand Names.	NUTRIENT DEPLETED	POSSIBLE MECHANISM	COMMENTS & REFERENCES
ANTIGOUT/ANTIRHEUMATIC (CONT.)			
Methotrexate (*Rheumatrex*)	Folic Acid	Folate antagonism. Binds to dihydrofolate reductase, preventing conversion of folic acid to its active form.	In people taking long-term, low-dose methotrexate for rheumatoid arthritis or psoriasis, reduced folate levels increase the risk of side effects. Recommend folic acid 1 mg/day, especially in people with a low dietary folate intake or who are experiencing side effects. This doesn't reduce the efficacy of methotrexate in these conditions.[768,2162,4492-4,4546,9369,9418-20] People taking methotrexate for cancer should avoid folic acid supplements unless recommended by their oncologist, since they may interfere with the anticancer effects.[9420]
Penicillamine (*Cuprimine, Depen*)	Copper Iron Magnesium Pyridoxine (B6) Zinc	Pyridoxine - inactivates pyridoxal-5'-phosphate, increasing pyridoxine requirements. Copper, Iron, Magnesium, Zinc - Forms chelation complexes in the GI tract. Decreases absorption of these elements.	Magnesium, pyridoxine, zinc - The need for supplementation has not been adequately studied. Give supplements of these nutrients only if clinical judgment warrants it.[4453,4531,4534,9630] Copper, Iron - Separate copper or iron and penicillamine administration by at least 2 hours.[4453,4531,4535,9630]
CARDIOVASCULAR			
ANTIHYPERTENSIVES			
Hydralazine (*Apresoline*)	Pyridoxine (B6)	Inactivates pyridoxal-5'-phosphate, increasing pyridoxine requirements.	The need for supplementation has not bee adequately studied. Give supplements of pyridoxine only if clinical judgment warrants it.[4453,4531,4533]
Captopril (*Capoten*)	Zinc	Captopril increases urinary elimination of zinc.	Clinical significance is unknown.[25,26,6543]
CARDIAC GLYCOSIDES			
Digoxin (*Lanoxicaps, Lanoxin*)	Magnesium	Limits reabsorption of magnesium in the renal tubule, leading to magnesium excretion.	Low magnesium levels can increase the risk of arrhythmias. Hypomagnesemia more likely with concurrent diuretic use. Monitor magnesium levels as clinical judgment warrants and give supplements if necessary.[4556,9613,9631]
CHOLESTEROL-REDUCING DRUGS			
HMG CoA Reductase Inhibitors ("Statins"): Atorvastatin (*Lipitor*) Fluvastatin (*Lescol*) Lovastatin (*Mevacor*) Pravastatin (*Pravachol*) Simvastatin (*Zocor*)	Coenzyme Q10	HMG CoA reductase inhibitors block synthesis of mevalonic acid, which is a precursor of coenzyme Q10. Therefore, production of coenzyme Q10 is decreased.	Serum levels of coenzyme Q-10 are reduced but muscle levels are not affected. Therefore, this is probably not clinically significant.[3367,3370,4404-10,8915,12099]

Drug Influences on Nutrient Levels and Depletion

Some medications can affect the levels of certain nutrients in the body. There is considerable interest in using nutritional supplements to counteract these possible drug-induced "nutrient depletions." The chart below shows the current scientific understanding of these relationships, and suggested actions.

DRUGS (Includes some representative U.S. and Canadian Brand Names.	NUTRIENT DEPLETED	POSSIBLE MECHANISM	COMMENTS & REFERENCES
CARDIOVASCULAR (CONT.)			
CHOLESTEROL-REDUCING DRUGS (CONT.)			
Cholestyramine (*LoCHOLEST, Prevalite, Questran*)	Beta-Carotene Folic Acid Dibencozide Iron Niacin and Niacinamide Vitamins A, B12, D, E, K	All nutrients – Reduces gastrointestinal absorption.	Cholestyramine binds with some of these nutrients but there isn't clinical proof that supplements are necessary. Supplementation may be valuable in some patients. Separate dosing times of cholestyramine and supplements as much as possible.[2672,4455-8, 4460-1,9566,10542-3,10566-7,10566-9,11519]
	Calcium		Taking over 32 g-day of cholesyramine or >2 years could result in vitamin D and calcium deficiency and related complications. Supplemental vitamin D and calcium may be necessary.[4458,5655,5809,5838]
	Magnesium	Reduces absorption and increases urinary magnesium excretion.	Magnesium deficiency has not been reported. Supplements aren't likely to be needed.[9566,9627]
Colestipol (*Colestid*)	Beta-Carotene Dibencozide Folic Acid Iron Niacin and Niacinamide Vitamins A, B12, D, E, K	All nutrients – Reduces gastrointestinal absorption.	It is possible that supplementation with folic acid and vitamin D may be appropriate. In some cases it may be appropriate to supplement all nutrients depleted by colestipol.[4457,4460-1,9566]
Gemfibrozil (*Lopid*)	Vitamin E	Gemfibrozil can decrease vitamin E serum levels.	The clinical significance is unknown.[4096,11548,11587]
DIURETICS			
Loop Diuretics: Bumetanide (*Bumex, Burinex),* Ethacrynic acid (*Edecrin*), Furosemide (*Lasix*), Torsemide (*Demadex*)	Calcium Folic Acid Magnesium Potassium Sodium Thiamine (B1) Zinc	Increased urinary excretion.	Electrolyte disturbances more likely with higher doses. Hypokalemia and hypomagnesemia occur most commonly. May need to use potassium and/or magnesium supplements, or add a potassium-sparing diuretic (which will also spare magnesium).[4412,9613-4,9622] Thiamine deficiency may occur in elderly people with poor dietary intake who are on high doses of diuretics (e.g. > 80 mg furosemide/day) for several months. Thiamine deficiency may worsen heart failure. Supplement of 200mg/day has improved cardiac function in some thiamine-deficient people on diuretics, but there isn't enough data to recommend routine use.[1283-6,10507-9] The need for folic acid supplementation has not been adequately studied.[1898]

CHARTS

Drug Influences on Nutrient Levels and Depletion

Some medications can affect the levels of certain nutrients in the body. There is considerable interest in using nutritional supplements to counteract these possible drug-induced "nutrient depletions." The chart below shows the current scientific understanding of these relationships, and suggested actions.

DRUGS (Includes some representative U.S. and Canadian Brand Names.	NUTRIENT DEPLETED	POSSIBLE MECHANISM	COMMENTS & REFERENCES
CARDIOVASCULAR (CONT.)			
DIURETICS (CONT.)			
Loop Diuretics (Cont.): Bumetanide (*Bumex*, *Burinex*), Ethacrynic acid (*Edecrin*), Furosemide (*Lasix*), Torsemide (*Demadex*)	Vitamin C	In people with chronic renal failure, a 20 mg intravenous dose of furosemide increases urinary losses of vitamin C, probably due to increased water excretion.	Significant vitamin C depletion hasn't been reported with chronic oral use of furosemide or other diuretics.[9525]
Thiazide and Thiazide Derivatives: Bendroflumethiazide (*Naturetin*), Benzthiazide (*Exna*), Chlorothiazide (*Diuril*), Chlorthalidone (*Hygroton, Thalitone*), Hydrochlorothiazide (*Esidrix, Hydrodiuril, Oretic*), Hydroflumethiazide (*Diucardin, Saluron*), Indapamide (*Lozide, Lozol*), Methyclothiazide (*Aquatensen, Enduron*), Metolazone (*Mykrox, Zaroxolyn*), Polythiazide (*Renese*), Quinethazone (*Hydromox*), Trichlormethiazide (*Diurese, Metahydrin, Naqua*)	Folic Acid Magnesium Potassium Sodium Thiamine (B1) Zinc	Increased urinary excretion.	Electrolyte disturbances are more likely with higher doses. Hypokalemia and hypomagnesemia occur most commonly. May need to use potassium and/or magnesium supplements, or add a potassium sparing diuretic (which will also spare magnesium).[4412,9613-4,9622] The need for folic acid supplementation has not been adequately studied.[1898] Thiamine deficiency may occur in elderly people with poor dietary intake who are on high doses of diuretics for several months. Thiamine deficiency may worsen heart failure. Supplement of 200 mg/day has improved cardiac function in some thiamine-deficient people on diuretics, but there isn't enough data to recommend routine use.[1283-6,10506-9]
Triamterene (*Dyrenium*)	Folic Acid	Reduces absorption of folic acid and prevents its conversion to the active form	The need for supplementation has not been adequately studied. Give supplements of this vitamin only if dietary intake is inadequate.[4425,4536-7,9375]
CENTRAL NERVOUS SYSTEM			
ANTICONVULSANTS			
Carbamazepine (*Atretol, Epitol, Tegretol*)	Biotin	Carbamazepine seems to increase the break down of biotin and decrease biotin levels.	The clinical significance of this is not known. It is not known if taking biotin supplements is necessary.[172,175,176]
	L-Carnitine Acetyl-L-Carnitine Propionyl-L-Carnitine	Carbamazepine lowers serum carnitine levels possibly by increasing metabolism or decreasing synthesis.	It is not known if carnitine supplementation is necessary.[1911,12758]
	Folic Acid	Two mechanisms have been proposed: Induction of hepatic microsomal enzymes leading to increased folic acid metabolism and decreased intestinal absorption.	Megaloblastic anemia due to folic acid deficiency hasn't been reported with carbamazepine. Low folic acid levels might contribute to mental changes in some people on carbamazepine, but folic acid supplements may worsen seizure control. Advise patients to consult their physician before starting folic acid supplements.[4426-9,9359]

CHARTS

Drug Influences on Nutrient Levels and Depletion

Some medications can affect the levels of certain nutrients in the body. There is considerable interest in using nutritional supplements to counteract these possible drug-induced "nutrient depletions." The chart below shows the current scientific understanding of these relationships, and suggested actions.

DRUGS (Includes some representative U.S. and Canadian Brand Names.)	NUTRIENT DEPLETED	POSSIBLE MECHANISM	COMMENTS & REFERENCES
CENTRAL NERVOUS SYSTEM (CONT.)			
ANTICONVULSANTS (CONT.)			
Carbamazepine (*Atretol, Epitol, Tegretol*) (Cont.)	Vitamin D Calcium	Increases the rate of vitamin D metabolism leading to decreased levels of various forms of vitamin D. Decreased vitamin D levels reduce calcium absorption.	Hypocalcemia and osteomalacia have occurred with long-term anticonvulsant therapy. Advise patients taking carbamazepine for 6 months or longer to have their vitamin D and calcium levels checked, and that they may need supplements.[2675,10578]
	Vitamin K	Induction of liver enzymes may increase vitamin K metabolism, producing a significant decrease in vitamin K levels in neonates, who haven't built up stores of the vitamin.	Increases risk of neonatal intracranial hemorrhage. Women who need to take carbamazepine during pregnancy should take vitamin K, 10-20 mg/day, during the last month of pregnancy. The baby should receive vitamin K immediately after delivery.[11521-5,10582,11533-4]
	Vitamin E	Children taking carbamazepine seem to have lower vitamin E levels compared to children not receiving carbamazepine.	The clinical significance is unknown. It's not known if supplementation with vitamin E is beneficial.[11574-8]
Phenytoin (*Dilantin*), Fosphenytoin (*Cerebyx*)	Biotin	Phenytoin seems to increase break down of biotin and decrease biotin levels.	The clinical significance of this is not known. It is not known if taking biotin supplements is necessary.[172,175,176]
	Folic Acid	Reduced absorption, increased metabolism, and increased demand for folate as a coenzyme for induced hepatic enzymes.	Folic acid supplements may reduce phenytoin side effects, but can also reduce phenytoin serum levels and may independently worsen seizure control. Advise patients to consult a physician before starting folic acid supplements.[4427,4471,4477,4536,9354-9]
	L-carnitine Acetyl-L-Carnitine Propionyl-L-Carnitine	Phenytoin lowers serum carnitine levels possibly by increasing metabolism or decreasing synthesis.	It is not known if carnitine supplementation is necessary.[1911,12758]
	Thiamine (B1)	Mechanism unknown.	Thiamine deficiency might contribute to neurologic side effects, but there's insufficient evidence to recommend supplements.[10510-2]
	Dibencozide Vitamin B12	Reduces absorption of vitamin B12.	This may contribute to the megaloblastic anemia, primarily caused by folate deficiency. Encourage patients to maintain adequate dietary vitamin B12 intake. Monitor vitamin B12 and folate if symptoms of anemia develop.[7843,10502-5]
	Vitamin D Calcium	Increases the rate of vitamin D metabolism leading to decreased levels of various forms of vitamin D. Phenytoin may also increase the renal excretion of polar vitamin D metabolites. Decreased vitamin D levels reduce calcium absorption.	Hypocalcemia and osteomalacia have occurred with long-term anticonvulsant therapy. Advise patients taking phenytoin for 6 months or longer that they should have their vitamin D and calcium levels checked, and that they may need supplements.[2675,4430-1,4475,10578]

CHARTS

Drug Influences on Nutrient Levels and Depletion

Some medications can affect the levels of certain nutrients in the body. There is considerable interest in using nutritional supplements to counteract these possible drug-induced "nutrient depletions." The chart below shows the current scientific understanding of these relationships, and suggested actions.

DRUGS (Includes some representative U.S. and Canadian Brand Names.	NUTRIENT DEPLETED	POSSIBLE MECHANISM	COMMENTS & REFERENCES
CENTRAL NERVOUS SYSTEM (CONT.)			
ANTICONVULSANTS (CONT.)			
Phenytoin (*Dilantin*), Fosphenytoin (*Cerebyx*) (Cont.)	Vitamin E	Children taking phenytoin seem to have lower vitamin E levels compared to children not receiving phenytoin.	The clinical significance is unknown. It's not known if supplementation with vitamin E is beneficial.[11574-8]
	Vitamin K	Induction of liver enzymes may increase vitamin K metabolism, producing a significant decrease in vitamin K levels in neonates who haven't built up stores of the vitamin.	Increased risk of neonatal intracranial hemorrhage. Women who need to take these anticonvulsants during pregnancy should take vitamin K, 10-20 mg/day, during the last month of pregnancy. The baby should receive vitamin K immediately after delivery.[11521-5,10582,11533-4]
Phenobarbital (*Luminal, Solfoton*) Primidone (*Mysoline*)	Biotin	Might increase the break down of biotin and decrease biotin levels.	The clinical significance of this is not known. It is not known if taking biotin supplements is necessary.[172,175,176]
	Folic Acid	Reduced absorption, increased metabolism, and increased demand for folate as a coenzyme for induced hepatic enzymes.	Reduced folic acid levels due to treatment with phenobarbital or primidone occasionally lead to megaloblastic anemia, and may contribute to neurological side effects and mental changes. However, folic acid supplements can worsen seizure control. Advise patients to consult a physician before starting folic acid supplements.[4427,4530,4536,9333,9354-9]
	Dibecozide Vitamin B12	Reduced absorption	Encourage patients to maintain adequate dietary vitamin B12 intake. Monitor vitamin B12 status if symptoms of anemia develop.[7843, 10502-5]
	L-Carnitine Acetyl-L-Carnitine Propionyl-L-Carnitine	Phenobarbital lowers serum carnitine levels possibly by increasing metabolism or decreasing synthesis.	It is not known if carnitine supplementation is necessary.[1911,12758]
	Vitamin E	Children taking phenobarbital seem to have lower vitamin E levels compared to children not receiving phenobarbital.	The clinical significance is unknown. It's not known if supplementation with vitamin E is beneficial.[11574-8]
	Vitamin D Calcium	Increases the rate of vitamin D metabolism leading to decreased levels of various forms of vitamin D. Decreased vitamin D levels reduce calcium absorption.	Hypocalcemia and osteomalacia have occurred with long-term anticonvulsant therapy. Advise patients taking phenobarbital or primidone for 6 months or longer that they should have their vitamin D and calcium levels checked, and that they may need supplements.[2675]

Drug Influences on Nutrient Levels and Depletion

Some medications can affect the levels of certain nutrients in the body. There is considerable interest in using nutritional supplements to counteract these possible drug-induced "nutrient depletions." The chart below shows the current scientific understanding of these relationships, and suggested actions.

DRUGS (Includes some representative U.S. and Canadian Brand Names.)	NUTRIENT DEPLETED	POSSIBLE MECHANISM	COMMENTS & REFERENCES
CENTRAL NERVOUS SYSTEM (CONT.)			
ANTICONVULSANTS (CONT.)			
Phenobarbital (*Luminal, Solfoton*) Primidone (*Mysoline*) (Cont.)	Vitamin K	Induction of liver enzymes may increase vitamin K metabolism, producing a significant decrease in vitamin K levels in neonates, who haven't built up stores of the vitamin.	Increased risk of neonatal intracranial hemorrhage. Women who need to take these anticonvulsants during pregnancy should take vitamin K, 10-20 mg/day, during the last month of pregnancy. The baby should receive vitamin K immediately after delivery.[11521-5,10582,1533-4]
Valproic Acid (*Depakene, Depakote*)	Folic Acid	Reduced levels occur occasionally but mechanism is unclear.	Symptomatic folic acid deficiency has not been reported. Avoid supplements since they may worsen seizure control.[4427-8,9355-6,9359]
	L-Carnitine Acetyl-L-Carnitine Propionyl-L-Carnitine	Valproic acid lowers serum carnitine levels possibly by increasing metabolism or decreasing synthesis.	Valproic acid supplement may not be necessary in patients who have adequate nutrition intake.[1911,4528-9,5798,9612,12758]
DOPAMINE AGONISTS			
Levodopa (*L-DOPA, Larodopa, Dopar*)	Potassium	Increased urinary potassium losses occur in some people treated with levodopa. The mechanism isn't clear, but the effect doesn't occur when a peripheral decarboxylase inhibitor, such as carbidopa, is used with levodopa (as in *Sinemet*).	This interaction is unlikely to be significant since most patient get levodopa in combination with carbidopa.[7201]
PHENOTHIAZINES			
Chlorpromazine (*Thorazine*)	Riboflavin (B2)	Interference with conversion to active form of vitamin; increased renal excretion.	These effects occur in animals, but there isn't enough data in humans to recommend supplements.[10515,10518-21]
GASTROINTESTINALS			
ANTACIDS			
Aluminum Salts (*Amphojel, Alternajel, Basaljel,* etc), Magnesium Salts (*Mag-Ox, Milk of Magnesia,* etc), Aluminum Salt/Magnesium Salt mixtures (*Maalox,* etc)	Calcium Phosphate Salts	Aluminum salts bind phosphate in the gastrointestinal tract. This reduces phosphate levels, which induces movement of calcium from bones into the blood, increasing urinary calcium excretion. High serum magnesium levels can increase urinary calcium excretion.	Prolonged administration of large doses of antacids may lead to hypocalcemia and/or hypophosphatemia. Avoid prolonged administration of large doses.[2730-1,3371,4400,4623,5979]
	Chromium	Antacids may reduce chromium absorption from the gastrointestinal tract	Unlikely to be clinically significant.[7135]
	Folic Acid	Increased intestinal pH produced by antacids may reduce folic acid absorption.	Long-term use of large doses of antacids can cause folate depletion if dietary intake is very low. Most people don't need supplements.[2677,8441]

CHARTS

Drug Influences on Nutrient Levels and Depletion

Some medications can affect the levels of certain nutrients in the body. There is considerable interest in using nutritional supplements to counteract these possible drug-induced "nutrient depletions." The chart below shows the current scientific understanding of these relationships, and suggested actions.

DRUGS (Includes some representative U.S. and Canadian Brand Names.)	NUTRIENT DEPLETED	POSSIBLE MECHANISM	COMMENTS & REFERENCES
GASTROINTESTINALS (cont.)			
ANTACIDS (CONT.)			
Aluminum Salts (Cont.)	Iron	Increased gastric pH reduces iron solubility and absorption.	Separate dosing times as much as possible. Monitor for adequate response to iron.[3046,3072,4539]
GI ANTI-INFLAMMATORIES			
Sulfasalazine (*Azulfidine, Salazopyrin*)	Folic Acid	Interferes with breakdown of dietary folate to its active form. Can also cause hemolysis, which increases folate requirements for red blood cell formation.	Decreased folate levels may lead to megaloblastic anemia, hyperhomocysteinemia, and an increased risk of colon cancer. Recommend that patients increase their dietary folate intake if possible, or take a supplement, especially if they have other factors contributing to folate deficiency.[2677,4515-7,4536,4560,9353,9376-7,9379]
HISTAMINE-2 BLOCKERS			
H2 Blockers: Cimetidine (*Tagamet*), Famotidine (*Pepcid*), Nizatidine (*Axid*), Ranitidine (*Zantac*)	Calcium	Absorption of some calcium supplements, especially the carbonate salt, is decreased by increased gastric pH.	There isn't any evidence of a clinically significant effect on calcium levels.[2738,4330-1,5060]
	Chromium Folic Acid	Chromium and folic acid absorption from the gastrointestinal tract may be decreased by increased pH.	The clinical significance of the effect on chromium absorption isn't known.[7135] A significant effect on folic acid levels is unlikely unless dietary intake is very low.[4483,8441]
	Dibencozide Iron Vitamin B12	May decrease iron and vitamin B12 absorption from the gastrointestinal tract.	The need for iron and vitamin B12 supplementation hasn't been adequately studied. Depletion may be significant in people with inadequate dietary intake, poor stores of iron and B12, or continuous intake of H2 blockers for more than 2 years. Monitor for anemia and give supplements if clinical judgement warrants it.[4483,4539,4540-1,8876,9513-4,9528,9578]
LAXATIVES			
Mineral Oil	Beta-Carotene Calcium Vitamins A, D, E, K	Decreases gastrointestinal absorption.	May be avoided by limiting duration of use to less than 4 months.[4454,4495-6]
Sodium Phosphates (*Fleet Phospho-Soda*)	Magnesium Potassium	Increased loss of electrolytes from gastrointestinal tract.	High doses (such as those used for preoperative bowel cleansing) can cause severe electrolyte disturbances. Avoid high doses and monitor electrolyte levels in the elderly and others with risk factors for hypomagnesemia or hypokalemia.[8877,9531,9615-6]

CHARTS

Drug Influences on Nutrient Levels and Depletion

Some medications can affect the levels of certain nutrients in the body. There is considerable interest in using nutritional supplements to counteract these possible drug-induced "nutrient depletions." The chart below shows the current scientific understanding of these relationships, and suggested actions.

DRUGS (Includes some representative U.S. and Canadian Brand Names.	NUTRIENT DEPLETED	POSSIBLE MECHANISM	COMMENTS & REFERENCES
GASTROINTESTINALS (cont.)			
LAXATIVES (CONT.)			
Stimulant Laxatives: Senna (*Senexon, Senolax, Senokot, Senna-Gen, Senokotxtra, Black-Draught, Gentlax, Dr. Caldwell Senna, Fletcher's Castoria, Dosalax*), Bisacodyl Tablets (*Bisacodyl, Uniserts, Bisco-Lax, Correctol, Dulcagen, Dulcolax, Feen-a-mint, Fleet Laxative*)	Calcium Potassium Sodium Vitamin D	Calcium and Vitamin D - Decreases gastrointestinal absorption. Sodium and Potassium – Increases gastrointestinal losses.	Excessive use of stimulant laxatives may result in depletion of these elements and vitamin D. Limit to short-term use of recommended doses.[506,11530] Hypokalemia has been reported in patients undergoing short-term bowel-cleansing regimens. Use caution in patients who may be predisposed to hypokalemia (i.e. aggressive diuretic therapy). Give supplements of potassium if clinical judgment warrants it.[4411-2]
PANCREATIC ENZYMES			
Pancreatin (*Donnazyme, Pancrezyme*) Pancrelipase (*Cotazym, Creon, Pancrease, Ultrase, Viokase*)	Folic Acid Iron	Forms complexes with folic acid/iron in the gastrointestinal tract, reducing absorption.	Supplements may be needed with prolonged pancreatic enzyme therapy.[9374,9575,9585]
PROTON PUMP INHIBITORS			
Proton Pump Inhibitors: Lansoprazole (*Prevacid*), Omeprazole (*Losec, Prilosec*), Rabeprazole (*Aciphex*), Pantoprazole (*Pantoloc, Protonix*)	Beta-Carotene Calcium Chromium Dibencozide Folic Acid Iron Vitamin B12	May decrease beta carotene, calcium, chromium, folic acid, iron and vitamin B12 absorption from the gastrointestinal tract, due to increased pH.	There isn't any evidence of a clinically significant effect on calcium levels.[2738,5060] A significant effect on folic acid levels is unlikely unless dietary intake is very low.[4483,8441] The clinical significance of the effect on beta-carotene, chromium, iron, and vitamin B12 absorption isn't known. Give supplements of these vitamins and minerals only if clinical judgement warrants it.[31,4483-6,4539,8441,9513,9528,9578]
	Vitamin C	Preliminary data suggests omeprazole reduces vitamin C levels, possibly due to increased destruction of vitamin C at higher gastric pH levels.	It isn't known if this is clinically significant.[10572]
HORMONES			
Corticosteroids [Glucocorticoids]: **Short-acting** Cortisone (*Cortone*), Hydrocortisone [Cortisol] (*Cortef, Hydrocortone*) **Intermediate-acting** Prednisone (*Deltasone, Meticorten, Orasone, Panasol-S*), Prednisolone (*Delta-Cortef, Prelone, Pediapred*), Triamcinolone (*Aristocort, Atolone, Kenacort*), Methylprednisolone (*Medrol*) **Long-acting** Dexamethasone (*Decadron, Dexameth, Dexone*), Betamethasone (*Celestone*)	Calcium (Indirectly – Vitamin D)	Calcium – Increases renal calcium excretion and decreases intestinal calcium absorption. Vitamin D - Depletion of calcium by steroids creates a greater need for vitamin D, which is necessary for appropriate GI absorption of calcium.	Steroid-induced osteoporosis, and the associated increase in fracture risk, are well-recognized consequences of long-term administration of corticosteroids, in doses equivalent to prednisone 7.5 mg/day or higher. Recommend patients maintain a calcium intake of 1500 mg/day. Monitor serum calcium levels regularly. Vitamin D supplements may also be needed.[1832,4462-7]

CHARTS

Drug Influences on Nutrient Levels and Depletion

Some medications can affect the levels of certain nutrients in the body. There is considerable interest in using nutritional supplements to counteract these possible drug-induced "nutrient depletions." The chart below shows the current scientific understanding of these relationships, and suggested actions.

DRUGS (Includes some representative U.S. and Canadian Brand Names.	NUTRIENT DEPLETED	POSSIBLE MECHANISM	COMMENTS & REFERENCES
HORMONES (CONT.)			
Corticosteroids [Glucocorticoids] (Cont.)	Chromium	Increases renal excretion of chromium, possibly leading to chromium deficiency, which may contribute to corticosteroid-induced hyperglycemia.	The need for chromium supplementation has not been adequately studied. Give supplements only if clinical judgment warrants it.[5039]
	Dolomite	Corticosteroids can decrease calcium absorption from dolomite and increase calcium elimination.	Calcium supplements might be necessary with long-term use of corticosteroids.[15]
	Folic Acid	Patients with multiple sclerosis treated with methylprednisolone seem to have decreased levels of serum folate.	The clinical significance of this is not known. It's not known if supplementation is beneficial.[9362]
	Magnesium	Drug-induced bone loss releases magnesium from bone and increases urinary excretion.	Serum magnesium levels are usually not affected and no supplements are needed.[9507-9,9628-9]
	Potassium	Corticosteroids cause sodium retention, resulting in compensatory renal potassium excretion.	Hypokalemia is dose-dependent and more common with steroids having high mineralocorticoid activity (hydrocortisone, cortisone, fludrocortisone, prednisone, prednisolone). Monitor potassium levels with chronic therapy. If necessary, give supplements, or switch to a steroid with no mineralocorticoid activity (betamethasone, dexamethasone, methylprednisolone, triamcinolone).[4425]
	Strontium	Might increase urinary excretion of strontium.	Dose adjustments for strontium might be necessary.[11405]
Estrogens: (*Alora, Cenestin, Climara, Estinyl, Estrace, Estraderm, Estratab, FemPatch, Menest, Ogen, Premarin, Premphase, Prempro, Vivelle*) Estrogen-containing Oral Contraceptives	Folic Acid	Folic Acid - Possibly reduced absorption, increased excretion, increased protein binding and induction of liver enzymes which use folate.	Folic acid supplements should be considered only in people with a very low dietary intake, or with other conditions which contribute to folate deficiency.[4459,4498,7843-4,9532,9371-3]
	Strontium	Might decrease urinary excretion of strontium.	Dose adjustments for strontium might be necessary.[11405]
	Magnesium	Magnesium – Shift from plasma to other tissues.	Monitor magnesium levels in people with other risk factors for hypomagnesemia.[9621,9638-40]
	Pyridoxine (B6)	Pyridoxine – Interference with metabolism.	Although there is much talk about giving pyridoxine supplements to people on estrogens, the need for this hasn't been proven.[4459,4498,4547]
	Riboflavin (B2)	Riboflavin - possibly reduced absorption or interference with conversion to active form.	Riboflavin supplements aren't necessary unless dietary intake is inadequate.[4548,9373,9505,10523-7,10536]
	Vitamin A	Vitamin A - Estrogens stimulate production of retinol binding protein, increasing amount of vitamin removed from liver storage and carried in blood.	Vitamin A supplements might help maintain liver stores, but the need for this hasn't been proven.[9373,9505,10523,10548]

Drug Influences on Nutrient Levels and Depletion

Some medications can affect the levels of certain nutrients in the body. There is considerable interest in using nutritional supplements to counteract these possible drug-induced "nutrient depletions." The chart below shows the current scientific understanding of these relationships, and suggested actions.

DRUGS (Includes some representative U.S. and Canadian Brand Names.	NUTRIENT DEPLETED	POSSIBLE MECHANISM	COMMENTS & REFERENCES
HORMONES (CONT.)			
Estrogens (Cont.)	Dibencozide Vitamin B12	Vitamin B12 - Reduced protein binding, leading to increased tissue uptake.	Vitamin B12 supplements aren't necessary.[4498,4547,7843,9371-3,9505,10123]
	Vitamin C	Vitamin C - Rossibly increased elimination.	Data are limited, but vitamin C supplements probably aren't necessary.[10548,10583,10585-7,11528,11161]
	Thiamine (B1)	Some studies have reported a small reduction in activity of the thiamine-dependent enzyme erythrocyte transketolase in women taking oral contraceptives, suggesting mild thiamine deficiency.	Routine use of thiamine supplements with oral contraceptives is not necessary.[10548,10555]
Androgens	Strontium	Might decrease urinary excretion of strontium.	Dose adjustments for strontium might be necessary.[11405]
Levothyroxine	Calcium	Increased bone turnover may lead to increased urinary calcium losses.	Calcium loss is unlikely to be clinically significant with doses of thyroid hormones used to treat hypothyroidism. Check thyroid function tests to ensure patients are not receiving excessive thyroid hormone doses, which may increase calcium losses.[27-9,2684-5,2695,2697-8,2721]
RESPIRATORY			
Beta-2-Agonists: Albuterol (salbutamol, *Proventil*, *Ventolin*), Bitolterol (*Tornalate*), Isoetharine, Levalbuterol (*Xopenex*), Metaproterenol (*Alupent*), Pirbuterol (*Maxair*), Salmeterol (*Serevent*), Terbutaline (*Brethine*)	Magnesium Potassium	Intracellular shift of magnesium and potassium.	May contribute to arrhythmias, especially at high doses and in people with other risk factors. Monitor electrolyte levels during acute use of high doses (e.g. in preterm labor or acute asthma attacks), and in people with other risk factors. With chronic use of beta-2-agonists, electrolyte levels may return to baseline.[2644,6203,6205,6209-10,6217,7001,8880-6,8889-91,9507,9517,9534,9599,9641]
Methylxanthines	Potassium	Possibly increased intracellular uptake.	Risk for hypokalemia is dose-dependent. Monitor potassium levels in people on high doses or with other risk factors.[9534,9537-9]
Theophylline (*Slobid, Theo-24, Theo-Dur, Theolair*)	Pyridoxine (B6)	Interferes with pyridoxine metabolism.	Studies of the use of pyridoxine supplements with theophylline have given conflicting results. Give supplements of this vitamin only if clinical judgment warrants it.[4522,7064-6,9480,9503]
MICELLANEOUS			
Alcohol (Ethanol)	Glutathione	Alcohol depletes endogenous glutathione.	It's not known if glutathione supplements would be beneficial.[5394]
Cobalt Irradiation	Dibencozide Vitamin B12	Decreases absorption of vitamin B12 and dibencozide.	Monitor serum vitamin B12.[15]
Cyclosporine (*Neoral, Sandimmune*)	Magnesium	Increased urinary excretion probably associated with drug-induced renal damage.	Monitor serum magnesium levels.[9117,9632-3]

CHARTS

Drug Influences on Nutrient Levels and Depletion

Some medications can affect the levels of certain nutrients in the body. There is considerable interest in using nutritional supplements to counteract these possible drug-induced "nutrient depletions." The chart below shows the current scientific understanding of these relationships, and suggested actions.

DRUGS (Includes some representative U.S. and Canadian Brand Names.	NUTRIENT DEPLETED	POSSIBLE MECHANISM	COMMENTS & REFERENCES
MICELLANEOUS (CONT.)			
Deferoxamine (*Desferal*)	Zinc	Deferozamine increases urinary zinc elimination.	It is not known if zinc supplementation is necessary.[6597-8]
Nitrous oxide (N_2O)	Dibencozide Vitamin B12	Inactivates the cobalamin form of vitamin B12.	Deficiency symptoms may occur after a single dose of nitrous oxide in people with pre-existing, subclinical deficiency. Check B12 levels before using N_2O anesthesia in people with risk factors for vitamin B12 deficiency.[9527,9532]
Orlistat (*Xenical*)	Beta-Carotene	Decreased absorption of beta-carotene supplements by 30%.	Recommend people on orlistat also take a multivitamin supplement. Separate administration of orlistat and beta-carotene, vitamin A, vitamin D, vitamin E, and vitamin K supplements by 2 hours to avoid this interaction.[1727,1730,6001,9595,10570-1]
	Vitamin E	Decreased absorption of vitamin E supplements by 60%.	
	Vitamin A Vitamin D Vitamin K	Possibly decreases the absorption from the gastrointestinal tract.	
Sunscreens	Vitamin D	Frequent and extensive application of sunscreens can reduce vitamin D synthesis in the skin and plasma levels.	Sunscreens are not likely to cause clinically significant vitamin D deficiency in most people.[6855,11507,11508,11509]
Tacrolimus (FK506, *Prograf*)	Magnesium	Reduced renal tubular reabsorption leads to increased excretion of magnesium.	Hypomagnesemia occurs in a significant proportion of patients. Monitor levels and give supplements as necessary.[8900,9620]

Footnote: Oral L-carnitine supplementation is strongly suggested for the following groups: patients with certain secondary carnitine deficiency syndromes; symptomatic VPA-associated hyperammonemia; multiple risk factors for VPA-associated hepatotoxicity; infants and young children taking VPA. An oral L-carnitine dosage of 100 mg/kg/day, up to a maximum of 2 g/day has been recommended.

INDEX

INDEX

INDEX

INDEX

INDEX

INDEX

INDEX

INDEX

INDEX

INDEX

INDEX

INDEX

INDEX

INDEX

INDEX

INDEX

INDEX

INDEX

INDEX

INDEX

INDEX

INDEX

INDEX

INDEX

INDEX

INDEX

INDEX

INDEX

INDEX

INDEX

INDEX

INDEX

INDEX

INDEX

INDEX

INDEX

INDEX

INDEX

INDEX

INDEX

INDEX

INDEX

INDEX

INDEX

INDEX

INDEX

INDEX

INDEX

INDEX

INDEX

Call, fax, or email your comments. Thanks!

"Tell the Editors..."

This *Database* is constantly evolving. We invite your help in keeping this database current and clinically relevant. Please alert the editors if you spot a statement that needs to be changed, or a place where information needs to be added. You can use this form, or a copy of it, to communicate directly with the editors. Feel free to mail, email, or fax. We appreciate your help!

1. What part of the *Database* are you commenting about?

Section ______________________

Paragraph ______________________

2. What this area says currently:

____

____

3. What should be changed:

Please be specific about the exact wording you're proposing. Use additional pages if needed.

____

____

4. Which words should be eliminated:

____

____

5. Which words should be added:

____

____

6. What reference citations support this change? Please give us specific reference citations. We base entries into this *Database* on reliable studies published in peer-reviewed professional literature. Please give enough information for us to find the reference.

____

____

7. How can we contact you?

Name ______________________

Address ______________________

Phone ______________________ Email ______________________

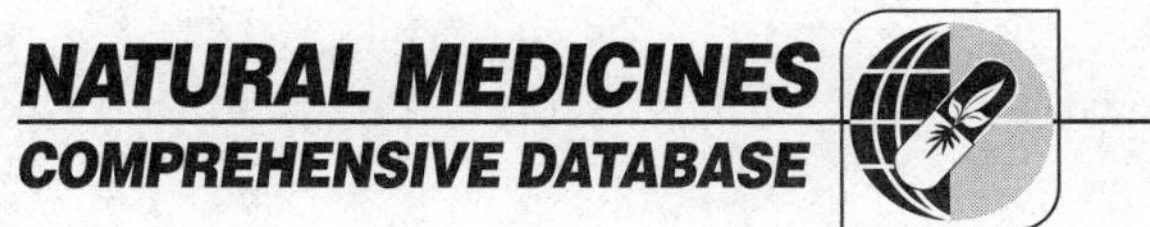

For your convenience, fax to (209) 472-2249.
Call (209) 472-2244 • mail@naturaldatabase.com
Visit us online at www.naturaldatabase.com
3120 W. March Lane, PO Box 8190, Stockton, CA 95208

Call, fax, or email your comments. Thanks!

"Tell the Editors..."

This *Database* is constantly evolving. We invite your help in keeping this database current and clinically relevant. Please alert the editors if you spot a statement that needs to be changed, or a place where information needs to be added. You can use this form, or a copy of it, to communicate directly with the editors. Feel free to mail, email, or fax. We appreciate your help!

1. What part of the *Database* are you commenting about?

Section ________________________

Paragraph ________________________

2. What this area says currently:

3. What should be changed:

Please be specific about the exact wording you're proposing. Use additional pages if needed.

4. Which words should be eliminated:

5. Which words should be added:

6. What reference citations support this change? Please give us specific reference citations. We base entries into this *Database* on reliable studies published in peer-reviewed professional literature. Please give enough information for us to find the reference.

7. How can we contact you?

Name ________________________

Address ________________________

Phone ____________ Email ____________

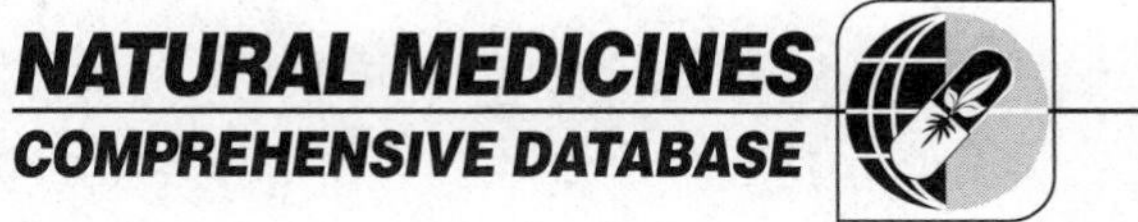

For your convenience, fax to (209) 472-2249.

Call (209) 472-2244 • mail@naturaldatabase.com

Visit us online at www.naturaldatabase.com

3120 W. March Lane, PO Box 8190, Stockton, CA 95208

Call, fax, or email your comments. Thanks!

"Tell the Editors..."

This *Database* is constantly evolving. We invite your help in keeping this database current and clinically relevant. Please alert the editors if you spot a statement that needs to be changed, or a place where information needs to be added. You can use this form, or a copy of it, to communicate directly with the editors. Feel free to mail, email, or fax. We appreciate your help!

1. What part of the *Database* are you commenting about?

Section ______________________________

Paragraph ______________________________

2. What this area says currently:

____

____

3. What should be changed:

Please be specific about the exact wording you're proposing. Use additional pages if needed.

____

____

4. Which words should be eliminated:

____

____

5. Which words should be added:

____

____

6. What reference citations support this change? Please give us specific reference citations. We base entries into this *Database* on reliable studies published in peer-reviewed professional literature. Please give enough information for us to find the reference.

____

____

7. How can we contact you?

Name ______________________________

Address ______________________________

Phone ______________ Email ______________

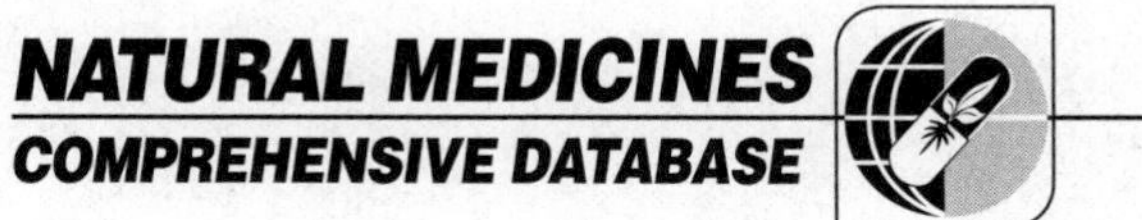

For your convenience, fax to (209)472-2249.
Call (209)472-2244 • mail@naturaldatabase.com
Visit us online at www.naturaldatabase.com
3120 W. March Lane, PO Box 8190, Stockton, CA 95208

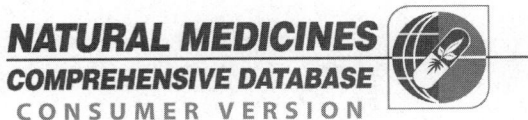

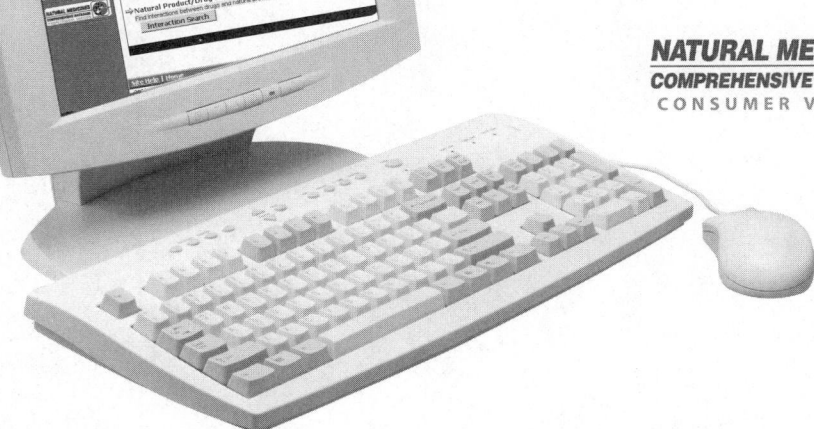

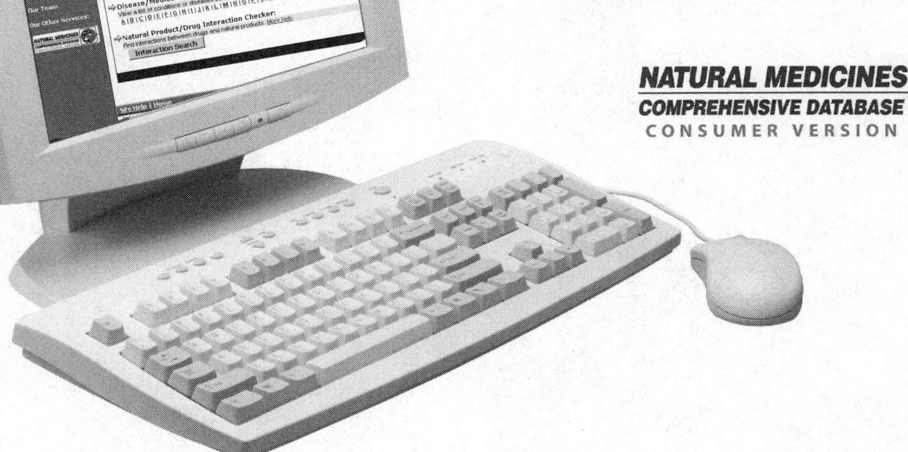

NATURAL MEDICINES
COMPREHENSIVE DATABASE
CONSUMER VERSION
Search
Product Search:
Browse the List of Products:
Natural Product Effectiveness Checker:
Disease/Medical Conditions Search:
Natural Product/Drug Interaction Checker:
Interaction Search

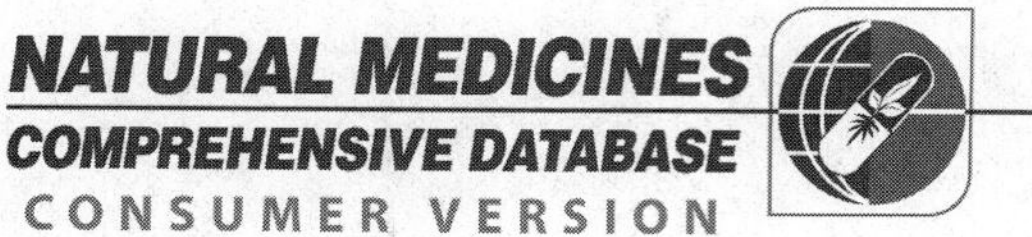

NATURAL MEDICINES
COMPREHENSIVE DATABASE
CONSUMER VERSION

Order Additional Copies

☐ **Yes, START MY NEW SUBSCRIPTION.** ***BONUS: Online CE FREE with Web Access.***

- ☐ Book . . . . $92 ($131 CAN)
- ☐ Online Version: 1 year Web access to www.naturaldatabase.com (single-user price) $92 ($131 CAN)
- ☐ **NEW** PDA Version with full featured searches & updates available daily . . . . $92 ($131 CAN)
- ☐ Online + PDA Version - 1 year single-user access . . . .$132 ($171 CAN)

☐ **Yes, EXTEND MY EXISTING SUBSCRIPTION.** ***BONUS: Online CE FREE with Web Access.***

- ☐ Send me a new edition of the Book when it's published . . . . $92 ($131 CAN)
- ☐ Online Version: 1 year Web access to www.naturaldatabase.com (single-user price) $92 ($131 CAN)
- ☐ **NEW** PDA Version with full featured searches & updates available daily . . . . $92 ($131 CAN)
- ☐ Online + PDA Version - 1 year single-user access . . . .$132 ($171 CAN)

For the book only, please add:

In California, add 8% sales tax . . . . $ ________

Shipping in U.S and Canada.. . . . . FREE

Shipping outside of North America. . . . . $24 US

TOTAL . . . .$ ________

Website users will have an opportunity to agree to the license agreement on the website, or get a full refund.

Name ____________________ Degree ________ Member # (optional) ____________

Address ____

City ____________________ State/Province ________ Zip/Postal Code ________

Email ____________________ Phone ____________________

☐ Payment enclosed (please make check payable to *Natural Database*).

☐ Charge my VISA, MasterCard, American Express, or Discover Card.

Card No. ____________________ Exp. Date ____________

☐ Bill my business or institution with this Purchase Order # ____________________

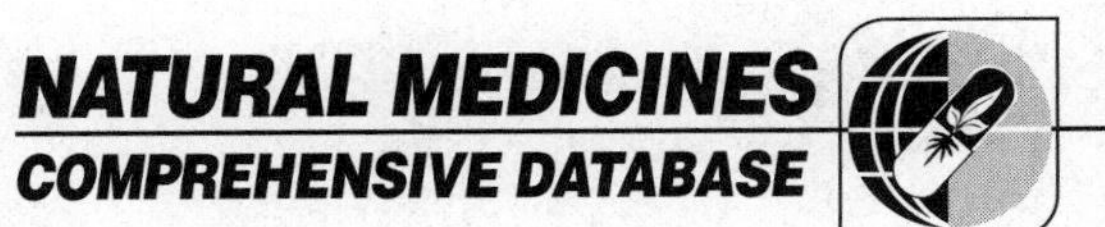

For fastest ordering, call (209)472-2244.
Fax (209)472-2249 • mail@naturaldatabase.com
Visit us online at www.naturaldatabase.com
3120 W. March Lane, PO Box 8190, Stockton, CA 95208

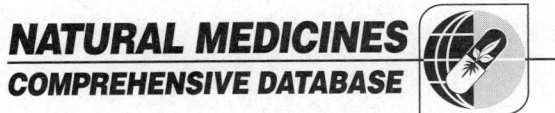

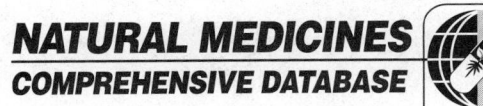

Sign-up today for the most current information online!

Want Web Access too?

This book version of the *Natural Medicines Comprehensive Database* was current the day it was printed.

But a large amount of new information comes in every day. So, our website is **updated daily** to give you the latest info.

The website gives you everything in this book plus lots more. We constantly add brand name products and the latest research on natural medicines.

Use NaturalDatabase.com to search:

- Interactions, uses, and side effects
- Brand names and ingredients
- Diseases or medical conditions

Or narrow your search further with the *Natural Product Effectiveness Checker, Natural Product/Drug Interaction Checker, Disease/Medical Conditions Checker,* and *Brand Product Finder.*

For each monograph, click to see all the references used. Then click on any of the thousands of reference citations and read the original journal abstract. You can also post questions and comments and interact with the editors and other health professionals around the world.

You can also get the latest news emailed to you with *eUPDATE* and *eCE*. With Web Access you get FREE continuing education credits accredited for pharmacists, MDs, DOs, PAs, NPs, and RDs.

At NaturalDatabase.com you can click and print a Patient Education Handout for any product anytime.

If you are part of an organization, you can also arrange to have your name and logo included on these Patient Handouts.

Sign up today to get these great features for yourself or for everyone in your organization.

YES, please send me my single-user access code so I can use www.naturaldatabase.com

Name ______________________________

Address ______________________________

City ______________________ State/Province ________ Zip/Postal Code ____________

Email ______________________ Phone ______________________

If you are currently a subscriber, please write your member number: ______________________

☐ Payment enclosed for $92 ($131CAN) per year (payable to *Natural Database*).

☐ Please charge my VISA, MasterCard, American Express, or Discover Card.

Card No. ______________________ Exp. Date ____________

☐ Bill my business or institution with this Purchase Order #

☐ **Contact me to arrange a multi-user license for my whole organization.**

Website users will have an opportunity to agree to the license agreement on the website, or get a full refund.

NATURAL MEDICINES
COMPREHENSIVE DATABASE

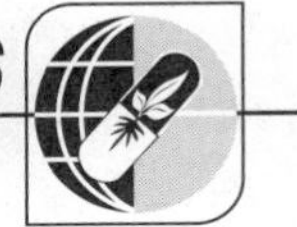

For fastest ordering, call (209) 472-2244.
Fax (209) 472-2249 • mail@naturaldatabase.com
Visit us online at www.naturaldatabase.com
3120 W. March Lane, PO Box 8190, Stockton, CA 95208

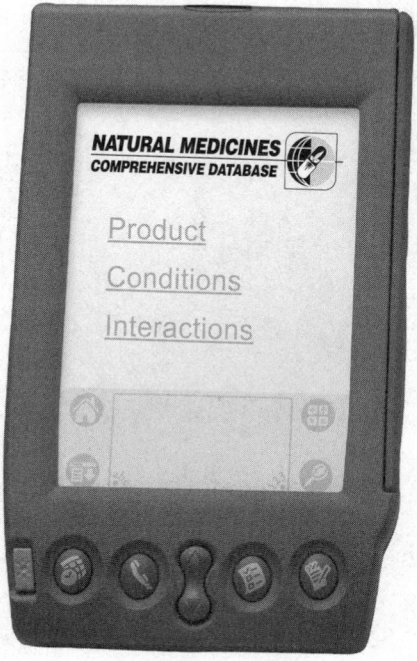

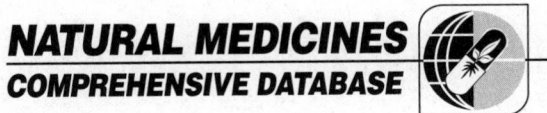

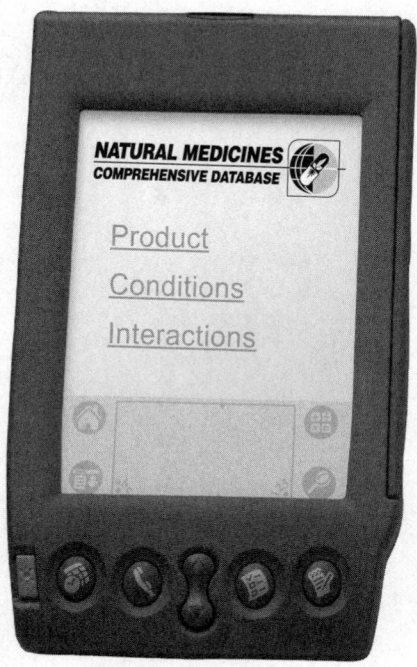

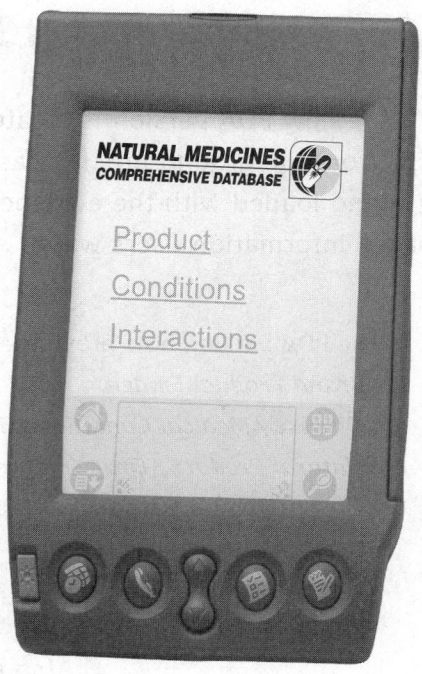

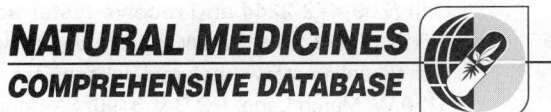

New PDA Version Lets You
the Whole Database with Y
Wherever You Go

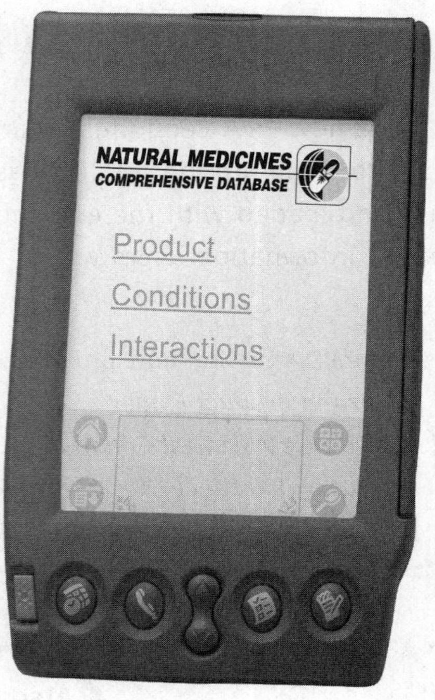

For Palm & Pocket PC

The new PDA version is created from the ground up...it's easy to use and loaded with the evidence-based information users want.

The PDA version now provides:

- *Brand Product Finder*
- *Disease / Medical Conditions Checker*
- *Natural Product / Drug Interaction Checker*
- Full Safety and Effectiveness Ratings
- New Updates available DAILY

Also purchase with Web Access and save even more!

✔ YES! I want to purchase the PDA version.

☐ PDA version for your Palm or Pocket PC*. . . . . $92 per year ($131CAN)

☐ **SAVE with the combo!** Buy PDA version + 1-year web access (single-user price). $132 ($171CAN)

Name ____________ Degree ______ Member # (optional) ____________

Address ____________

City ____________ State/Province ________ Zip/Postal Code ________

Email ____________ Phone ____________

☐ Payment enclosed (please make check payable to *Natural Database*).

☐ Charge my VISA, MasterCard, American Express, or Discover Card.
Card No. ____________ Exp. Date ________

☐ Bill my business or institution with this Purchase Order # ____________

PDA version for Palm and Pocket PC requires 8 MB or 11.5 MB

Website users will have an opportunity to agree to the license agreement on the website, or get a full refund.

NATURAL MEDICINES
COMPREHENSIVE DATABASE

Call (209) 472-2244 and receive faster access.
Fax (209) 472-2249 • mail@naturaldatabase.com
Visit us online at www.naturaldatabase.com
3120 W. March Lane, PO Box 8190, Stockton, CA 95208